ORTHOPAEDICS

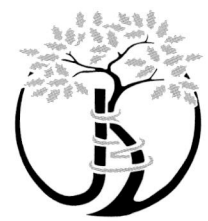

ORTHOPAEDICS

Robert H. Fitzgerald, Jr, M.D.
Bell Medical Center
Ishpeming, Michigan

Herbert Kaufer, M.D.
Professor and Chairman Emeritus
of Orthopaedic Surgery
University of Kentucky
Chandler Medical Center
Lexington, Kentucky
Visiting Professor of Orthopaedic
Surgery
University of Michigan
Ann Arbor, Michigan

Arthur L. Malkani, M.D.
Associate Professor and Chief,
Adult Reconstruction
Department of Orthopaedic Surgery
University of Louisville
Louisville, Kentucky

SECTION EDITORS

Christoper T. Born, M.D.
DeLong and Born Orthopaedics
Haddonfield, New Jersey

William G. DeLong, Jr, M.D.
DeLong and Born Orthopaedics
Haddonfield, New Jersey

James C. Drennan, M.D.
Carrie Tingley Hospital
Albuquerque, New Mexico

Steven R. Garfin, M.D.
Department of Orthopaedics
UCSD Medical Center
San Diego, California

Victor M. Goldberg, M.D.
Charles H. Herndon Professor and
Chairman
Department of Orthopaedics
Case Western Reserve University
University Hospital of Cleveland
Cleveland, Ohio

Walter B. Greene, M.D.
Department of Orthopaedic Surgery
University of Missouri Hospital
Columbia, Missouri

Kenneth J. Guidera, M.D.
Shriner's Hospital for Children–
Tampa
Tampa, Florida

Arlen D. Hanssen, M.D.
Mayo Clinic
Rochester, Minnesota

Darren L. Johnson, M.D.
Chief, Section of Sports Medicine
University of Kentucky
Kentucky Clinic
Lexington, Kentucky

Brian Johnstone, M.D.
Case Western Reserve University
Cleveland, Ohio

Courtland G. Lewis, M.D.
Department of Orthopaedic Surgery
University of Connecticut School of
Medicine
Farmington, Connecticut

Harry E. Rubash, M.D.
Department of Orthopaedics
Massachusetts General Hospital
Boston, Massachusetts

Charles L. Saltzman, M.D.
Department of Orthopaedics
University of Iowa Hospitals &
Clinics
Iowa City, Iowa

Raj K. Sinha, M.D., Ph.D.
Division of Adult Reconstructive
Surgery
University of Pittsburgh Medical
Center
Pittsburgh, Pennsylvania

Dempsey S. Springfield, M.D.
Department of Orthopaedics
Mount Sinai Hospital
New York, New York

Peter J. Stern, M.D.
Hand Surgery Specialists, Inc.
Cincinnati, Ohio

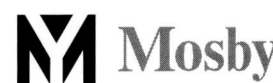 **Mosby**

An Imprint of Elsevier Science
St. Louis   London   Philadelphia   Sydney   Toronto

MOSBY, INC.
An Imprint of Elsevier Science

11830 Westline Industrial Drive
St. Louis, Missouri 63146

Library of Congress Cataloging-in-Publication Data

Orthopaedics / [edited by] Robert Fitzgerald, Herbert Kaufer, Arthur L. Malkani.—1st ed.

p.; cm.

ISBN 0-323-01318-X

1. Orthopedics. 2. Musculoskeletal system—Diseases. I. Fitzgerald, Robert H. (Robert Hannon), 1942– II. Kaufer, Herbert. III. Malkani, Arthur L.
[DNLM: 1. Orthopedics. WE 168 O76276 2002]

RD731.O7782 2002

616.7—dc21

00-056257

NOTICE

Medicine is an ever-changing field. Standard safety precautions must be followed, but as new research and clinical experience broaden our knowledge, changes in treatment and drug therapy may become necessary or appropriate. Readers are advised to check the most current product information provided by the manufacturer of each drug to be administered to verify the recommended dose, the method and duration of administration, and contraindications. It is the responsibility of the treating physician, relying on experience and knowledge of the patient, to determine dosages and the best treatment for each individual patient. Neither the publisher nor the editor assumes any liability for any injury and/or damage to persons or property arising from this publication.

THE PUBLISHER

Acquisitions Editor: Richard Lampert
Production Manager: Frank Polizzano
Illustration Specialist: Lisa Lambert

ORTHOPAEDICS   ISBN 0-323-01318-X

Printed in the United States of America

Last digit is the print number   9   8   7   6   5   4   3   2   1

CONTRIBUTORS

Nicholas A. Abidi, M.D.
Attending Physician, Orthopaedic Surgery of Santa
Cruz, Dominican Hospital, Santa Cruz, CA; Formerly,
Assistant Professor of Orthopaedic Surgery, Thomas
Jefferson University Medical College; Former Director,
Orthopaedic Foot and Ankle Surgery, Rothman Institute
at Jefferson, Philadelphia, PA
**ANKLE ARTHRITIS DIAGNOSIS AND
MANAGEMENT**

Brian D. Adams, M.D.
Professor of Orthopaedic Surgery, University of Iowa,
Iowa City, IA
ULNAR NERVE COMPRESSION

Christopher J. Aiken
Staff Orthotist, Hanger Prosthetics and Orthotics, New
London, CT
**LOWER EXTREMITY ORTHOTICS AND
PROSTHETICS**

Michael D. Aiona, M.D.
Assistant Chief of Staff, Shriners Hospitals for Children,
Portland, OR
**GUIDELINES FOR MANAGING LOWER EXTREMITY
PROBLEMS IN CEREBRAL PALSY**

Todd J. Albert, M.D.
Associate Professor & Vice Chairman, Dept. of
Orthopaedic Surgery, Thomas Jefferson University
Medical College; Attending Surgeon, Rothman Institute,
Philadelphia, PA 19107
**CERVICAL SPINE TRAUMA; THORACOLUMBAR
SPINE INJURIES; LOW BACK PAIN AND SCIATICA**

Benjamin A. Alman, M.D.
Associate Professor and Scientist, Division of
Orthopaedics and Program in Developmental Biology,
University of Toronto; Surgeon, Hospital for Sick
Children, Toronto, Ontario, Canada
GENETICS I

John Amory, M.D.
Assistant Professor of Medicine, University of
Washington; Medical Director, Pre-Op Clinic, Veterans
Affairs—Puget Sound Health Care System, Seattle, WA
**ANESTHETIC AND PERIOPERATIVE MANAGEMENT
OF THE GERIATRIC PATIENT**

Glenn M. Amundson, M.D.
Heartland Hand and Spine Orthopaedic Center P.A.
Shawnee Mission, KS
ADULT SCOLIOSIS

Howard S. An, M.D.
Rush-Presbyterian St. Luke's Medical Center, Chicago, IL
LUMBAR SPONDYLOLISTHESIS

Devry C. Anderson
Thomas Jefferson University Medical College,
Philadelphia, PA
CERVICAL SPINE TRAUMA

Jeff Anglen, M.D.
Associate Professor of Orthopaedics; Chief,
Orthopaedic Trauma Service, University of Missouri,
Columbia, MO
CALCANEUS AND TALUS

Thomas D. Armsey, M.D.
Assistant Professor, Depts. of Family Practice
and Orthopaedics, University of Kentucky,
Lexington, KY
**MEDICAL ASPECTS OF SPORTS: EPIDEMIOLOGY
OF INJURIES, PREPARTICIPATION PHYSICAL
EXAMINATION, AND DRUGS IN SPORTS**

Peter F. Armstrong, M.D.
Director of Medical Affairs, Shriners Hospitals for
Children, Tampa, FL
PRINCIPLES OF PEDIATRIC FRACTURES

Michael S. Aronow, M.D.
Dept. of Orthopaedic Surgery, University of Connecticut
Health Center, Farmington, CT
FRACTURES OF THE FOREFOOT AND MIDFOOT

James Aronson, M.D.
Professor, Dept. of Orthopaedics, University of
Arkansas for Medical Sciences; Chief of Pediatric
Orthopaedics, Arkansas Children's Hospital, Little
Rock, AR
HEMATOPOIETIC CONDITIONS

Marc A. Asher, M.D.
Professor, Dept. of Orthopaedic Surgery, University of
Kansas Medical Center, Kansas City, KS
ADULT SCOLIOSIS

Champ L. Baker, Jr, M.D.
Clinical Assistant Professor, Dept. of Orthopaedic
Surgery, Tulane University School of Medicine, New
Orleans, LA; The Hughston Clinic, Columbus, GA
**THE ARTHROSCOPIC MANAGEMENT OF ANKLE
INJURIES IN ATHLETES**

John V. Banta, M.D.
Director, Newington Dept. of Orthopaedics, Connecticut
Children's Medical Center; Professor of Orthopaedic
Surgery, University of Connecticut School of Medicine;
Surgeon-in-Chief, Connecticut Children's Medical
Center, Hartford, CT
MYELOMENINGOCELE

M. Janet Barger-Lux, M.S.
Senior Research Associate in Medicine, Creighton University School of Medicine, Omaha, NE
OSTEOPOROSIS: ETIOLOGY, DIAGNOSIS, AND TREATMENT

Roland Baron, D.D.S
Professor, Depts. of Orthopaedics and Cell Biology, Yale University School of Medicine, New Haven, CT
BONE: STRUCTURE, FUNCTION, GROWTH, AND REMODELING

Robert L. Bass, M.D.
Assistant Professor, Chief, Hand/Upper Extremity Service, Dept. of Orthopaedic Surgery, University of Texas Southwestern Medical Center, Dallas, TX
NAIL BED AND FINGERTIP INJURIES

Judith F. Baumhauer, M.D.
Associate Professor of Orthopaedics, Dept. of Orthopaedics, University of Rochester School of Medicine, Rochester, NY
THE RHEUMATOID FOOT AND ANKLE

Michael T. Bayliss, Ph.D.
Professor of Connective Tissue Biochemistry, The Royal Veterinary College, London, England
ARTICULAR CARTILAGE: STRUCTURE, FUNCTION, AND PHYSIOLOGY

Douglas Beaman, M.D.
Clinical Assistant Professor, Oregon Health Sciences University, Portland, OR
MIDFOOT ARTHRITIS

James H. Beaty, M.D.
Professor, University of Tennessee Campbell Clinic, Dept. of Orthopaedic Surgery; Chief, Pediatric Orthopaedics, Le Bonheur Children's Hospital, Memphis, TN
CONGENITAL DEFORMITIES OF THE KNEE

Gordon R. Bell, M.D.
Head, Section of Spinal Surgery; Vice Chairman, Dept. of Orthopaedic Surgery, Cleveland Clinic Foundation, Cleveland, OH
MECHANISMS OF DISK AND MUSCULOSKELETAL BACK PAIN

Frederick S. Bennett, M.D.
UCSF School of Medicine, Santa Rosa, CA
FRACTURES OF THE DISTAL FEMUR

R. M. Bernstein, M.D.
Assistant Clinical Professor, UCLA School of Medicine; Assistant Chief of Staff, Shriners Hospitals for Children, Los Angeles, CA
FAILURE OF FORMATION OF THE LIMBS; ARTHROGRYPOSIS

Allen T. Bishop, M.D.
Professor of Orthopaedic Surgery, Mayo Medical School; Chair, Division of Hand Surgery, Dept. of Orthopaedic Surgery, The Mayo Clinic, Rochester, MN
NECROTIZING FASCIITIS AND SOFT-TISSUE INFECTIONS

Laura C. Blakemore, M.D.
Assistant Professor, Dept. of Orthopaedics, Division of Pediatric Orthopaedics, University of Michigan Medical Center, Ann Arbor, MI
KYPHOSIS

Oren G. Blam, M.D.
Spine Fellow, Dept. of Orthopaedic Surgery, Thomas Jefferson University Hospital, Philadelphia, PA
CERVICAL SPINE TRAUMA

David L. Boardman, M.D.
Orthopaedic Surgeon, Kaiser Sunnyside Medical Center, Clackamas, OR
ARTHRITIS OF THE HIP

Vladimir Bobic, M.D.
The Grosvenor Nuffield Hospital, Chester, England
ARTICULAR CARTILAGE INJURIES OF THE KNEE

Delmas J. Bolin, M.D.
Assistant Director, Primary Care Sports Medicine Fellowship, University of Pittsburgh Medical Center, St. Margaret Hospital; Clinical Instructor, Dept. of Family Medicine, Pittsburgh, PA
OVERUSE INJURIES

Frédérique Bonnet
Physiotherapist, Pediatric Orthopaedic Dept., Institut St. Pierre, Palavas, France
CLUBFOOT

Peter S. Borden, M.D.
Section of Sports Medicine, Kentucky Clinic, Lexington, KY
ARTICULAR CARTILAGE INJURIES OF THE KNEE

Christopher T. Born, M.D.
Attending Orthopaedic Surgeon, Hospital of the University of Pennsylvania, University of Pennsylvania School of Medicine; Associate Director of Orthopaedic Trauma, University of Pennsylvania Health System; Associate Professor of Orthopaedic Surgery; Co-Director of Orthopaedic Trauma, University of Pennsylvania Health System, Philadelphia, PA
PRIORITIZATION AND MANAGEMENT OF THE POLYTRAUMA PATIENT; ACETABULAR FRACTURES

Michael Bothwell, P.A.–C.
Plancher Hand and Sports Medicine, Stamford, CT
BENIGN BONE AND SOFT-TISSUE TUMORS OF THE HAND AND WRIST

Declan J. M. Bowler, M.Med.Sci.
Dept. of Orthopaedics, James Connolly Memorial Hospital, Dublin, Ireland
INFECTED FRACTURES AND NONUNIONS

Jeff Brand, Jr, M.D.
Alexandria Orthopaedics Associates, Alexandria, MN
TECHNIQUES IN KNEE LIGAMENT SURGERY

Eric A. Brandser, M.D.
Associate Professor, Dept. of Radiology, University of Iowa College of Medicine, Iowa City, IA
MUSCULOSKELETAL HELICAL COMPUTED TOMOGRAPHY

Brad E. Brautigan, M.D.
Orthopaedic Surgeon, Orthopaedic Associates, Zanesville, OH
SHOULDER INSTABILITY AND LABRAL INJURIES: SURGICAL INDICATIONS AND TECHNIQUES

Thomas Breen, M.D.
Associate Professor of Orthopaedics, Dept. of Orthopaedics, University of Massachusetts School of Medicine, Worcester, MA
RADIAL NERVE COMPRESSION SYNDROMES

Patrick J. Brogle, M.D.

Hospital of the University of Pennsylvania, Dept. of Orthopaedic Surgery; St. Luke's Hospital, Dept. of Orthopaedic Trauma, Philadelphia, PA
ACETABULAR FRACTURES

W. David Bruce, M.D.

Associate Professor, Dept. of Pediatric Orthopaedics, University of Tennessee at Chattanooga; Physician, Chattanooga Bone and Joint Surgeons, Chattanooga, TN
THE ARTHROSCOPIC MANAGEMENT OF ANKLE INJURIES IN ATHLETES

James D. Bruckner, M.D.

Department of Orthopaedics, University of Washington, Seattle, WA
SURGICAL MANAGEMENT OF THE SPINE

David N. M. Caborn, M.D.

Associate Professor, University of Kentucky Sports Medicine, Lexington, KY
SHOULDER INSTABILITY AND LABRAL INJURIES: SURGICAL INDICATIONS AND TECHNIQUES

Domenico A. Campanacci, M.D.

Consultant, Dept. of Orthopaedic Oncology, Centro Traumatologico Ortopedico, Florence, Italy
MANAGEMENT AND SURGERY

S. Terry Canale, M.D.

Professor, Dept. of Orthopaedic Surgery, University of Tennessee Campbell Clinic; Chief of Staff, Campbell Clinic; Staff Member, Baptist Memorial Hospital, Le Bonheur Children's Hospital, Memphis, TN
CONGENITAL DEFORMITIES OF THE KNEE

Rodolfo Capanna, M.D.

Chairman, Dept. of Orthopaedic Oncology, Centro Traumatologico Ortopedico, Florence, Italy
MANAGEMENT AND SURGERY

Timothy P. Carey, M.D.

London, Ontario, Canada
INFLAMMATORY ARTHRITIDES: JUVENILE RHEUMATOID ARTHRITIS, SERONEGATIVE SPONDYLOARTHROPATHIES, TRANSIENT SYNOVITIS, HEMOPHILIC ARTHROPATHY

Michell G. Carlson, M.D.

Hospital for Special Surgery, New York, NY

Jack Choueka, M.D.

Director of Hand and Upper Extremity Surgery, Maimonides Medical Center, Brooklyn, NY; Attending Physician, Hospital for Joint Diseases, New York, NY
TENDON TRANSFERS IN THE UPPER EXTREMITY

George Cierny III, M.D.

Clinical Professor, Dept. of Orthopaedics, Emory University School of Medicine, Atlanta, GA
ADULT OSTEOMYELITIS AND SEPTIC ARTHRITIS

Henry D. Clarke, M.D.

Attending Orthopaedic Surgeon, Beth Israel Medical Center; Director, Insall Scott Kelly Institute for Orthopaedics and Sports Medicine, New York, NY
INFECTED TOTAL KNEE ARTHROPLASTY

Dennis R. Clohisy, M.D.

Professor, Dept. of Orthopaedic Surgery, University of Minnesota Medical School; Attending Physician, Fairview University Hospital, Minneapolis, MN
METASTATIC SKELETAL DISEASE

Ilan Cohen, M.D.

Hertzlia, Israel
NERVE PROBLEMS OF THE FOOT AND ANKLE

Evan Collins, M.D.

Assistant Professor, Dept. of Orthopaedic Surgery, Baylor College of Medicine, Houston, TX
COMPLEX REGIONAL PAIN SYNDROME IN THE UPPER EXTREMITY

Daniel R. Cooperman, M.D.

Associate Professor, Dept. of Orthopaedic Surgery, Case Western Reserve University; Rainbow Babies and Children's Hospital, Cleveland, OH
LEGG-CALVÉ-PERTHES

Karl B. Coyner, M.D.

Dept. of Radiology, Hartford Hospital, Hartford, CT
GENERAL ORTHOPAEDIC RADIOLOGY: RADIOGRAPHY, ARTHROGRAPHY, TOMOGRAPHY, MYELOGRAPHY, AND DISKOGRAPHY

Lawrence S. Crossett, M.D.

Dept. of Orthopaedic Surgery, University of Pittsburgh Medical Center, Pittsburgh, PA
KNEE ARTHROPLASTY

Randall W. Culp, M.D.

Associate Professor of Orthopaedics, Hand, and Microsurgery, Philadelphia Hand Center, Thomas Jefferson University, Philadelphia, PA
NONUNION OF THE SCAPHOID

Brian L. Davison, M.D.

Associate Director of Orthopaedic Trauma, Grant Medical Center, Columbus, OH
FEMORAL SHAFT FRACTURES

Mark B. Dekutoski, M.D.

Dept. of Orthopaedics, Mayo Clinic Foundation, Rochester, MN
SPINAL INFECTIONS

Jonathan T. Deland, M.D.

Associate Professor of Orthopaedic Surgery, Cornell University Medical College; Attending Orthopaedic Surgeon, Hospital for Special Surgery, New York, NY
ACQUIRED ADULT FLATFOOT DEFORMITY

William G. DeLong, Jr, M.D.

DeLong and Born Orthopaedics, Haddonfield, NJ
ACETABULAR FRACTURES

Vincent J. Devlin, M.D.

Dept. of Orthopaedic Surgery, Loma Linda University Medical Center, Loma Linda, CA; Orthopaedic Spine Surgeon, Southern California Permanente Medical Group, Kaiser Fontana Medical Center, Fontana, CA
IDIOPATHIC SCOLIOSIS

Edward Diao, M.D.

Associate Professor of Orthopaedic Surgery; Chief, Division of Hand, Upper Extremity and Microvascular Surgery; Director, UCSF Combined Hand Fellowship; Director, Hand Vascular Laboratory; Attending Surgeon, UCSF Hospital, San Francisco General Hospital, San Francisco Veterans Administration Hospital, San Francisco, CA
ARTHRODESIS

Alain Diméglio, M.D.

Orthopaedics and Trauma, Hopital Lapevronie, Montpellier, France
CLUBFOOT

Brian G. Donley, M.D.

Staff Physician, Cleveland Clinic Foundation, Cleveland, OH
DISORDERS OF THE FIRST RAY

John Dormans, M.D.

Chief of Orthopaedic Surgery, Children's Hospital of Philadelphia; Professor of Orthopaedic Surgery, University of Pennsylvania School of Medicine, Philadelphia, PA
SPINE AND PELVIS

James C. Drennan, M.D.

Carrie Tingley Hospital, Albuquerque, NM

Jayesh Dudhia, Ph.D.

Senior Research Fellow, Royal Veterinary College, London, England
ARTICULAR CARTILAGE: STRUCTURE, FUNCTION, AND PHYSIOLOGY

Clive P. Duncan

Professor and Chairman, Dept. of Orthopaedics, University of British Columbia; Head, Dept. of Orthopaedics, Vancouver Hospital and Health Sciences Center, Vancouver, British Columbia, Canada
REVISION THA: ACETABULUM

Mark E. Easley, M.D.

Duke University Medical Center, Durham, NC
NERVE PROBLEMS OF THE FOOT AND ANKLE

Thomas A. Einhorn, M.D.

Professor and Chairman, Dept. of Orthopaedic Surgery, Boston University School of Medicine; Chief of Orthopaedic Surgery, Boston Medical Center, Boston, MA
CALCIUM HOMEOSTASIS

Tomas Epeldegui, M.D.

Honorary Professor, Universidad Autonoma Madrid, Spain; Head, Pediatric Orthopaedic Division, Hospital Niño Jesus, Madrid, Spain
TARSAL COALITION

John L. Esterhai, M.D.

Dept. of Orthopaedic Surgery, University of Pennsylvania Medical Center, Philadelphia, PA
COMPLICATIONS OF FRACTURES: CHRONIC

Stephen J. Eustace

Senior Lecturer, Radiology, University College; Director of Radiology, Coppagh National Orthopaedic Hospital, Dublin, Ireland
MAGNETIC RESONANCE IMAGING

J. David Evanich, M.D.

Clinical Instructor, University of Utah Dept. of Orthopaedics, Salt Lake City, UT; Orthopaedic Surgeon, Raleigh Orthopaedic Clinic, Raleigh, NC
FOREARM FRACTURES

Peter J. Evans, M.D.

Hand and Upper Extremity Surgery, Dept. of Orthopaedic Surgery, Cleveland Clinic Foundation, Cleveland, OH
GENERAL ASPECTS OF MICROVASCULAR TISSUE REPLANTATION

Trent H. Evans, Ph.D.

Clinical Psychologist, Pride Research Foundation, Dallas, TX
CHRONIC LOW BACK PAIN

Marybeth Ezaki, M.D.

Associate Professor of Orthopaedics, University of Texas Southwestern; Director of Hand Surgery, Texas Scottish Rite Hospital for Children, Dallas, TX
THUMB (INCLUDING FLEXED, DUPLICATED, AND HYPOPLASTIC)

Joseph M. Failla, M.D.

Dept. of Orthopaedic Surgery, Henry Ford Health System, Detroit, MI
MEDIAN NERVE COMPRESSION

Gregory C. Fanelli, M.D.

Chief, Arthroscopic Surgery and Orthopaedic Sports Medicine, Dept. of Orthopaedic Surgery, Geisinger Clinic Medical Center, Danville, PA
KNEE LIGAMENT INJURIES: EPIDEMIOLOGY, MECHANISM, DIAGNOSIS, AND NATURAL HISTORY

Alexander Fedenko, M.D.

Chief of Anatomic Pathology, University of Southern California Keck School of Medicine, Los Angeles, CA
BENIGN SOFT-TISSUE TUMORS

Chris Fellner

Orthotist, University of Iowa Hospitals, Iowa City, IA
ORTHOTIC MANAGEMENT OF FOOT AND ANKLE PROBLEMS

J. Dominic Femino, M.D.

Orthopaedic Surgeon, Children's Hospital of Los Angeles; Assistant Professor of Clinical Orthopaedic Surgery, University of Southern California Keck School of Medicine, Los Angeles, CA
SURGICAL MANAGEMENT OF THE SPINE

C. Fennell, M.D.

Clinical Associate Professor of Surgery, University of North Dakota; Chief, Orthopaedic Service, Altru Hospital, Grand Forks, ND
BONE GRAFT AND BONE SUBSTITUTES

Jeffrey S. Fischgrund, M.D.

Attending Spine Surgeon, Weissman, Gitlin, Herkowitz Orthopedic Surgery, Southfield, MI
CERVICAL DISK DISEASE

John R. Fisk, M.D.

Professor, Division of Orthopaedics and Rehabilitation, Southern Illinois University School of Medicine—Surgery, Springfield, IL
ANTERIOR HORN CELL DISEASES

Robert H. Fitzgerald, Jr, M.D.

Bell Medical Center, Ishpeming, Michigan
ADULT OSTEOMYELITIS AND SEPTIC ARTHRITIS

Timothy C. Fitzgibbons, M.D.

Assistant Clinical Professor Orthopaedic Surgery, Clinical
Instructor, Dept. of Orthopaedics, Creighton University School of
Medicine, University of Nebraska Medical Center, Omaha, NE
TENDINOPATHIES OF THE FOOT AND ANKLE

John M. Flynn, M.D.

Assistant Orthopaedic Surgeon, Children's Hospital of
Philadelphia; Assistant Professor of Orthopaedic Surgery,
University of Pennsylvania School of Medicine, Philadelphia, PA
SPINE AND PELVIS

Guy Foucher, M.D.

Strasbourg, France
POST-TRAUMATIC THUMB RECONSTRUCTION

Deborah Anne Frassica, M.D.

Assistant Professor of Radiation Oncology, Johns Hopkins
University, Baltimore, MD
LOWER EXTREMITY METASTASES

Frank J. Frassica, M.D.

Chairman and Professor of Orthopaedic Surgery, Johns Hopkins
University, Baltimore, MD
LOWER EXTREMITY METASTASES

Bruce French, M.D.

Assistant Professor of Orthopaedics, University of Massachusetts
Medical School, Dept. of Orthopaedics and Physical
Rehabilitation, Worcester, MA
DISTAL TIBIA FRACTURES

Freddie H. Fu, M.D.

Chairman, Dept. of Orthopaedic Surgery, University of Pittsburgh
Medical Center Health System, Pittsburgh, PA
SHOULDER INJURIES IN ATHLETES

Keith R. Gabriel, M.D.

Clinical Associate Professor, Dept. of Orthopaedic Surgery,
University of Minnesota School of Medicine; Assistant Chief of
Staff, Shriners Hospitals for Children—Twin Cities, Minneapolis,
MN
GENETICS II: GENETIC SYNDROMES WITH ORTHOPAEDIC
MANIFESTATIONS

Timothy M. Ganey, Ph.D.

Director of Orthopaedic Research, Atlanta, GA
EMBRYOLOGY AND ANATOMY

Donald S. Garbuz, M.D.

Assistant Professor, Dept. of Orthopaedics, University of British
Columbia; Vancouver Hospital and Health Sciences Center,
Vancouver, British Columbia, Canada
REVISION THA: ACETABULUM

Peter J. Gard, MBBS FRACS

Joint Replacement Surgeon, Melbourne, Australia
ARTHRITIS OF THE KNEE

Steven R. Garfin, M.D.

Dept. of Orthopaedics, University of California at San Diego
Medical Center, San Diego, CA
SPINE FUSION: BIOLOGICAL AND MECHANICAL
CONSIDERATIONS

William E. Garrett, Jr, M.D.

Professor and Chair, Dept. of Orthopaedics, University of North
Carolina, Chapel Hill, NC
MUSCLE, TENDON, AND LIGAMENT: STRUCTURE,
FUNCTION, AND PHYSIOLOGY; INJURIES TO THE MUSCLE-
TENDON UNIT

Kevin L. Garvin, M.D.

Professor, Dept. of Orthopaedic Surgery and Rehabilitation,
University of Nebraska Medical Center, Omaha, NE
INFECTED TOTAL HIP ARTHROPLASTY

Robert J. Gatchel, Ph.D.

Professor of Psychiatry, University of Texas Southwestern
Medical Center at Dallas; Program Director, Eugene McDermott
Center for Pain Management, Dallas, TX
CHRONIC LOW BACK PAIN

William B. Geissler, M.D.

Associate Professor, Division of Hand and Upper Extremity,
Dept. of Orthopaedic Surgery, University of Mississippi Medical
Center, Jackson, MS
METACARPAL AND PHALANGEAL NONUNIONS

Harris Gellman, M.D.

Professor and Co-Director, Division of Hand and Upper
Extremity Surgery, Dept. of Orthopaedic Surgery, University of
Miami, Miami, FL
COMPLEX REGIONAL PAIN SYNDROME IN THE UPPER
EXTREMITY

Michell Gerwin
KIENBÖCK'S DISEASE

Thomas J. Gill, M.D.

Instructor in Orthopaedic Surgery, Harvard Medical School;
Assistant Orthopaedic Surgeon, Dept. of Orthopaedic Surgery,
Division of Sports Medicine, Massachusetts General Hospital,
Boston, MA
OSTEOTOMIES ABOUT THE KNEE

William J. Glucksman, M.D.

Section Chief, Musculoskeletal Radiology, Jefferson X-Ray
Group, Hartford Hospital, Hartford, CT
GENERAL ORTHOPAEDIC RADIOLOGY: RADIOGRAPHY,
ARTHROGRAPHY, TOMOGRAPHY, MYELOGRAPHY, AND
DISKOGRAPHY

Robert J. Goitz, M.D.

Assistant Professor, Dept. of Orthopaedic Surgery, University of
Pittsburgh Medical Center, Pittsburgh, PA
REGIONAL FLAPS

Michael J. Goldberg, M.D.

Professor and Chairman, Dept. of Orthopaedics, Tufts University
School of Medicine; Orthopaedist-in-Chief, New England Medical
Center, Boston, MA
GENETICS I

Victor M. Goldberg, M.D.
Charles H. Herndon Professor and Chairman, Dept. of Orthopaedics, Case Western Reserve University, University Hospitals of Cleveland, Cleveland, OH

Stuart B. Goodman, M.D.
Professor of Orthopaedic Surgery, Stanford University Medical Center; Attending Orthopaedic Surgeon, Stanford University Medical Center, Lucile Packard Children's Hospital, Palo Alto Veterans Administration Hospital, Stanford, CA
PARTICULATE DISEASE

John T. Gorczyca, M.D.
Associate Professor, University of Rochester Medical Center; Chief, Division of Musculoskeletal Trauma, Strong Memorial Hospital, Rochester, NY
TRAUMATIC KNEE INJURIES

James A. Goulet, M.D.
Professor of Orthopaedic Surgery, University of Michigan Medical School; Director of Orthopaedic Trauma Service, Ann Arbor, MI
PELVIS AND SACRUM

Thomas J. Graham, M.D.
Chief, The Curtis National Hand Center, Union Memorial Hospital, Baltimore, MD
DUPUYTREN'S CONTRACTURE

Linda Granowetter, M.D.
Associate Professor of Clinical Pediatrics, Columbia University College of Physicians and Surgeons; Director of Clinical Services, Hope and Heroes Division of Pediatric Oncology, Children's Hospital of New York, Columbia Presbyterian Medical Center, New York, NY
CHEMOTHERAPY

Walter B. Greene, M.D.
Dept. of Orthopaedic Surgery, University of Missouri Hospital, Columbia, MO
NEUROFIBROMATOSIS TYPE I

Edward M. Greenfield, Ph.D.
Associate Professor of Orthopaedics, Case Western Reserve University, Cleveland, OH
CALCIUM HOMEOSTASIS

Rupinder Grewal, M.D.
Fellow, Christine M. Kleinert Institute for Hand and Microsurgery, Inc., University of Louisville, Louisville, KY
WRIST FRACTURES

Yram J. Groff, M.D.
Fellow in Sports Medicine, University of Pittsburgh Medical Center, Pittsburgh, PA
KNEE ARTHROPLASTY

Dennis P. Grogan, M.D.
Clinical Professor, University of South Florida College of Medicine; Chief of Staff, Shriners Hospital for Children, Tampa, FL
METABOLIC CONDITIONS

Gary S. Gruen, M.D.
Associate Professor and Vice-Chairman, Dept. of Orthopaedic Surgery; Chief, Orthopaedic Trauma, University of Pittsburgh Medical Center, Pittsburgh, PA
PRINCIPLES OF OPERATIVE FRACTURE STABILIZATION AND FIXATION

Kenneth J. Guidera, M.D.
Shriners Hospital for Children, Tampa, FL

Lawrence L. Haber, M.D.
Assistant Professor of Orthopaedic Surgery, Case Western Reserve University, Cleveland, OH; Director, Pediatric Orthopaedics, Tod Children's Hospital, Youngstown, OH
UPPER EXTREMITY

Fares S. Haddad, M.Ch.(Orth.)
Honorary Senior Lecturer, Institute of Orthopaedics, Roth National Orthopaedic Hospital; Consultant Orthopaedic Surgeon, University College London Hospitals, London, England
REVISION THA: ACETABULUM

Douglas P. Hanel, M.D.
Associate Professor, Orthopaedic Surgery, University of Washington; Harborview Medical Center; Children's Hospital and Regional Medical Center, Seattle, WA
DISTANT FLAPS: PEDICLE AND FREE

Arlen D. Hanssen, M.D.
Professor of Orthopaedic Surgery, Mayo Medical School; Consultant in Orthopaedic Surgery, Mayo Clinic, Rochester, MN
INFECTED TOTAL KNEE ARTHROPLASTY

James A. Harder, M.D.
Division of Pediatric Surgery, Alberta Children's Hospital, Calgary, Alberta, Canada
CONGENITAL ABSENCE OF THE FIBULAE

Carl T. Hasselman, M.D.
Instructor, Orthopaedic Surgery, University of Pittsburgh, Pittsburgh, PA
PRINCIPLES OF OPERATIVE FRACTURE STABILIZATION AND FIXATION

David Hatfield, M.D.
Resident Physician, Division of Orthopaedics and Rehabilitation, Southern Illinois University School of Medicine, Springfield, IL
ANTERIOR HORN CELL DISEASES

Justin P. Hawes, M.D.
Dept. of Orthopaedic Surgery, University of Pennsylvania, Philadelphia, PA
TIBIAL SHAFT FRACTURES

Roman A. Hayda, M.D.
Chief, Orthopaedic Trauma, Brooke Army Medical Center, Fort Sam Houston, TX
ELBOW

Amira A. Helal, M.D.
Assistant Professor, University of South Florida, Dept. of Pediatrics; Staff Pediatrician, Shriners Hospitals for Children, Tampa, FL
LIMB LENGTH DISCREPANCY

Jill A. Helms, D.D.S.
University of California San Francisco, San Francisco, CA
EMBRYOLOGY OF BONE

M. Bradford Henley, M.D.
Associate Professor, Dept. of Orthopaedic Surgery and Sports Medicine, University of Washington School of Medicine, Seattle, WA
FRACTURES OF THE HUMERAL SHAFT

Stephen A. Herbst, M.D.
University of Iowa Hospitals and Clinics, Iowa City, IA
MIDFOOT ARTHRITIS

Harry N. Herkowitz, M.D.
Weissman, Gitlin, Herkowitz Orthopaedic Surgery, Southfield, MI
CERVICAL DISK DISEASE

James H. Herndon, M.D.
Chairman and Professor of Orthopaedic Surgery, Harvard Medical School, Boston, MA
ARTHRITIS OF THE ELBOW

M. Mark Hoffer, M.D.
Professor and Chair Emeritus, Orthopaedic Surgery, University of California at Irvine; Lowman Professor, Orthopaedic Hospital, Los Angeles, CA
UPPER EXTREMITY (ACQUIRED ERB'S)

Scott A. Hoffinger, M.D.
Assistant Clinical Professor, Dept. of Orthopaedics, University of California at San Francisco School of Medicine; Chief, Pediatric Orthopaedics, Children's Hospital Oakland, Oakland, CA
SLIPPED CAPITAL FEMORAL EPIPHYSIS; KNEE DISORDERS IN ADOLESCENCE

Daniel S. Horwitz, M.D.
Professor; Director, Orthopaedic Trauma, University of Utah, Salt Lake City, UT
HIP

Robert G. Hosey, M.D.
Assistant Professor, Dept. of Family Medicine, University of Kentucky, Lexington, KY
MEDICAL ASPECTS OF SPORTS: EPIDEMIOLOGY OF INJURIES, PREPARTICIPATION PHYSICAL EXAMINATION, AND DRUGS IN SPORTS

John D. Hsu, M.D.
Clinical Professor, Dept. of Orthopaedics, University of Southern California Keck School of Medicine, Los Aangeles, CA; Chief of Orthopaedics; Chair, Dept. of Surgery, Rancho Los Amigos National Rehabilitation Center, Downey, CA
ACQUIRED CEREBROSPASTIC DISORDER: STROKE, BRAIN INJURY

Serena S. Hu, M.D.
Dept. of Orthopaedic Surgery, University of California at San Francisco, San Francisco, CA
COMPLICATIONS OF SPINAL SURGERY

Robert F. Hube, M.D.
Professor of Orthopaedic Surgery, Martin Luther University Orthopaedic Clinic, Halle, Germany
MANAGEMENT OF COMPLICATIONS AFTER JOINT ARTHROPLASTY

Laurie O. Hughes, M.D.
Assistant Professor of Othopaedic Surgery, University of Arkansas for Medical Sciences; Staff Orthopaedic Surgeon, Arkansas Children's Hospital, Little Rock, AR
HEMATOPOIETIC CONDITIONS

Thomas R. Hunt, M.D.
The Cleveland Clinic, Cleveland, OH
OVERVIEW OF ARTHRITIS; DUPUYTREN'S CONTRACTURE

Michael H. Huo, M.D.
Dept. of Orthopaedic Surgery, Baylor College of Medicine, Houston, TX
OVERVIEW OF ARTHRITIS

Mary E. Hurley, M.D.
Clinical Professor of Pediatric Orthopaedics, Loma Linda University, Loma Linda, CA; Pediatric Orthopaedic Surgeon, Kaiser Permanente Dept. of Orthopaedics, Fontana, CA
IDIOPATHIC SCOLIOSIS

Dawn Marie Ickes, M.P.T.
Physical Therapist, Child Amputee Prosthetics Project, Shriners Hospital for Children, Los Angeles, CA
ACQUIRED AMPUTATIONS IN CHILDREN

Takaaki Ikata, M.D.
University of Tokushima, Tokushima, Japan
ELBOW INJURIES IN THE THROWING ATHLETE, INCLUDING INSTABILITY AND OSTEOCHONDRAL/CHONDRAL LESIONS

Omer A. Ilahi
Orthopaedic Surgery, University of Kansas School of Medicine, Kansas City, KS
OVERVIEW OF ARTHRITIS

Mary Lloyd Ireland, M.D.
Team Physician, Eastern Kentucky University, Richmond, KY; Orthopaedic Consultant, Georgetown College, Georgetown, KY; Medical Director, Women's United Soccer Association; Consultant, Orthopaedic Surgery, Shriners Hospital, Lexington, KY
SPECIAL CONCERNS OF THE FEMALE ATHLETE

Larissa B. Isterabadi, M.S.
University of Southern California Keck School of Medicine, Los Angeles, CA
BENIGN SOFT-TISSUE TUMORS

Jon A. Jacobson, M.D.
Clinical Assistant Professor of Radiology, Dept. of Radiology, University of Michigan Medical Center, Ann Arbor, MI
MUSCULOSKELETAL SONOGRAPHY

Peter J. L. Jebson, M.D.
Assistant Professor, Orthopaedic Surgery, University of Michigan Medical Center, Ann Arbor, MI
PERIPHERAL NERVE INJURIES

Louis G. Jenis, M.D.
New England Baptist Hospital, Clinical Instructor Orthopaedic Surgery, Tufts University School of Medicine, Boston, MA
LUMBAR SPONDYLOLISTHESIS

Darren L. Johnson, M.D.

Associate Professor and Chief, Section of Sports Medicine, University of Kentucky, Lexington, KY
TECHNIQUES IN KNEE LIGAMENT SURGERY; ARTICULAR CARTILAGE INJURIES OF THE KNEE

Brian Johnstone, M.D.

Chief, Orthopaedic Laboratories, Case Western Reserve University, Cleveland, OH

Subir Jossan, M.D.

Georgetown University Medical Center, Washington, D.C.
WRIST INSTABILITY

Alexander Kalenak, M.D.

Professor of Orthopaedic Surgery (Ret.), College of Medicine, Pennsylvania State University; Associate Orthopaedic Surgeon, Orthopaedic Institute of Pennsylvania, Camp Hill, PA; Attending Orthopaedic Surgeon, Harrisburg Hospital, Harrisburg, PA
ANTERIOR KNEE PAIN AND PATELLOFEMORAL JOINT INSTABILITY

Madhav Karunakar, M.D.

Assistant Professor of Orthopaedic Surgery, University of Michigan Medical Center; University of Michigan Hospitals, Ann Arbor, MI
PELVIS AND SACRUM

Shinji Kashiwagucgi, M.D.

Division of Sports Medicine, University of Tokushima, Kuramoto-Cho, Tokushima, Japan
ELBOW INJURIES IN THE THROWING ATHLETE, INCLUDING INSTABILITY AND OSTEOCHONDRAL/ CHONDRAL LESIONS

Mary Ann Keenan, M.D.

Professor of Orthopaedic Surgery, Thomas Jefferson University School of Medicine; Director, Neuro-Orthopaedics Program, Albert Einstein Medical Center, Philadelphia, PA
PRINCIPLES OF NEURO-ORTHOPAEDIC REHABILITATION

Michael A. Kelly, M.D.

Assistant Clinical Professor of Orthopaedic Surgery, Albert Einstein College of Medicine, Bronx, NY; Director, Insall Scott Kelly Institute for Orthopaedic and Sports Medicine, Beth Israel Medical Center—Singer Division, New York, NY
OSTEOTOMIES ABOUT THE KNEE

Peter Keogh, M.D.

Consultant Orthopaedic Surgeon, Dept. of Orthopaedics, James Connolly Memorial Hospital, Dublin, Ireland
INFECTED FRACTURES AND NONUNIONS

Safdar N. Khan, M.D.

Research Associate, Spinal Surgical Service and Spine Care Institute, The Hospital for Special Surgery, New York, NY
MUSCULOSKELETAL TUMORS, PAGET'S DISEASE, AND FIBROUS DYSPLASIA

Navin Kilambi

Staff Physician, Naval Medical Center, San Diego, CA
SPINE FUSION: BIOLOGICAL AND MECHANICAL CONSIDERATIONS

Harry K. W. Kim, M.D.

Pediatric Orthopaedic Surgeon, Section Chief—Tissue Repair, Shriners Hospital for Children, Tampa, FL
METABOLIC CONDITIONS

John A. King, M.D.

Staff Orthopaedic Hand Surgeon, Lakelands Orthopaedic Clinic, Self Memorial Hospital, Greenwood, SC
ARTHRITIS OF THE ELBOW

John S. Kirchner, M.D.

Assistant Professor, University of Pittsburgh; Dept. of Orthopaedic Surgery, Division of Foot and Ankle Surgery, University of Pittsburgh Medical Center—Presbyterian, Pittsburgh, PA
NEUROPATHIC ARTHROPATHIES

Peter Kirkbride

Honorary Lecturer, Dept. of Clinical Oncology, University of Sheffield; Consultant Clinical Oncologist, Weston Park Hospital, Sheffield, England
NONSURGICAL MANAGEMENT OF BONE METASTASES

Donald T. Kirkendall, Ph.D.

Clinical Assistant Professor, Dept. of Orthopaedics, University of North Carolina, Chapel Hill, NC
MUSCLE, TENDON, AND LIGAMENT: STRUCTURE, FUNCTION, AND PHYSIOLOGY; INJURIES TO THE MUSCLE-TENDON UNIT

Michael J. Klein, M.D.

Department of Pathology, Mount Sinai Medical Center, New York, NY
PATHOPHYSIOLOGY OF BONE TUMORS

Steven E. Koop, M.D.

Gillette Children's Hospital, St. Paul, MN
CEREBRAL PALSY: OVERVIEW AND MANAGEMENT OF SPINAL DEFORMITIES

Stephen Kottmeier, M.D.

Assistant Professor, Dept. of Orthopaedics, State University of New York at Stony Brook, Stony Brook, NY
SHOULDER GIRDLE AND PROXIMAL HUMERAL FRACTURES

Scott H. Kozin, M.D.

Associate Professor, Dept. of Orthopaedic Surgery, Temple University; Pediatric Hand and Upper Extremity Surgeon, Shriners Hospital for Children, Philadelphia, PA
RADIAL CLUBHAND

P. John Kumar, M.D.

Assistant Clinical Professor, Dept. of Orthopaedic Surgery, University of Southern California, Los Angeles, CA; Associate Physician, Southern California Permanente Group, Bellflower, CA
OSTEOARTHRITIS

Patrick W. Kwok, M.D.

Resident, Dept. of Orthopaedic Surgery, University of Connecticut School of Medicine, Farmington, CT
ORTHOPAEDIC BIOMATERIALS

Hubert Labelle, M.D.

Professor of Surgery, University of Montreal; Pediatric Orthopaedic Surgeon, Sainte-Justine Mother-Child University Center, Montreal, Quebec, Canada
FRIEDREICH'S ATAXIA AND RETT'S SYNDROME

Stephen H. Lacey, M.D.

Dept. of Orthopaedic Surgery, Case Western Reserve University, Cleveland, OH
TENDINITIS OF THE HAND AND WRIST

A. Ladd, M.D.

Associate Professor, Stanford University, Dept. of Orthopaedics; Chief, Lucile Salter Packard Children's Hospital, Hand and Upper Extremity Clinic, Palo Alto, CA
BONE GRAFT AND BONE SUBSTITUTES

Naomi Laird, P.A.–C.

Dept. of Orthopaedic Surgery, University of Iowa Hospitals, Iowa City, IA
THE DIABETIC FOOT

Joseph M. Lane

Professor of Orthopaedic Surgery, Assistant Dean, Medical Students, Weill Medical College of Cornell University; Chief, Metabolic Bone Disease Service, The Hospital for Special Surgery, New York, NY
MUSCULOSKELETAL TUMORS, PAGET'S DISEASE, AND FIBROUS DYSPLASIA

Ian D. Learmonth, M.D.

Professor and Head, Dept. of Orthopaedic Surgery, University of Bristol; Consultant Orthopaedic Surgeon, Bristol Royal Infirmary, Bristol, England
CLINICAL HISTORY AND PHYSICAL EXAMINATION

Henry T. Leis, M.D.

Wilford Hall Medical Center, Dept. of Orthopaedic Surgery, Lackland AFB, TX
DIAGNOSIS OF SHOULDER INSTABILITY AND LABRUM INJURIES

Fraser J. Leversedge, M.D.

Resident, Dept. of Orthopaedic Surgery, Emory University School of Medicine, Atlanta, GA
FLEXOR TENDON INJURIES

Gerald Levy, M.D.

Assistant Clinical Professor, College of Medicine, University of California at Irvine, Irvine, CA; Staff Physician, Southern California Permanente Medical Group, Bellflower, CA
OSTEOARTHRITIS

Courtland G. Lewis, M.D.

Clinical Professor, Dept. of Orthopaedic Surgery, University of Connecticut School of Medicine, Farmington, CT
ORTHOPAEDIC BIOMATERIALS

Jay R. Lieberman, M.D.

Associate Professor of Orthopaedic Surgery, University of California at Los Angeles School of Medicine, Los Angeles, CA
ARTHRITIS OF THE HIP

Steven A. Lietman, M.D.

Assistant Professor of Orthopaedics, Johns Hopkins University, Baltimore, MD
LOWER EXTREMITY METASTASES

Robert S. Lin

LOWER EXTREMITY ORTHOTICS AND PROSTHETICS

Sheldon S. Lin, M.D.

Assistant Professor of Orthopaedic Surgery, University of Medicine and Dentistry of New Jersey; Director, Foot and Ankle Division, Dept. of Orthopaedics, UMDNJ Hospital, Newark, NJ
ANKLE ARTHRITIS DIAGNOSIS AND MANAGEMENT

Margaret Lobo

Weill Medical College of Cornell University, New York, NY
MUSCULOSKELETAL TUMORS, PAGET'S DISEASE, AND FIBROUS DYSPLASIA

Aldo Vincent Londino, M.D.

Associate Professor of Medicine and Pediatrics, University of Pittsburgh School of Medicine; Chief, Division of Pediatric Rheumatology, Childrens Hospital of Pittsburgh, Pittsburgh, PA
INFLAMMATORY ARTHRITIS

Gary E. Loyd, M.D.

Associate Professor, Vice-Chair, Dept. of Anesthesiology, University of Louisville, Louisville, KY
ANESTHESIA AND PAIN MANAGEMENT

John D. Lubahn, M.D.

Chairman, Dept. of Orthopaedics, Residency Program Director—Orthopaedics, Hamot Medical Center; Instructor, Shriners Hospital for Children, St. Vincent Health Center, and Hamot Medical Center, Erie, PA
SYNDACTYLY

John P. Lubicky, M.D.

Professor of Orthopaedic Surgery, Rush Medical College; Chief of Staff, Shriners Hospital for Children, Chicago, IL
PEDIATRIC SPINAL CORD INJURY: LONG-TERM MANAGEMENT

James V. Luck, Jr, M.D.

Dept. of Orthopaedic Surgery, University of California at Los Angeles Orthopaedic Hospital, Los Angeles, CA
ORTHOPAEDIC SURGERY IN THE IMMUNOCOMPROMISED HOST

William B. Macaulay, M.D.

Assistant Professor of Orthopaedic Surgery, Columbia University; Adjunct Professor of Biochemistry, Rockefeller University; Attending Surgeon, New York Presbyterian Hospital of Columbia University, New York, NY
PRIMARY TOTAL HIP ARTHROPLASTY

Scott D. Mair, M.D.

Assistant Professor, University of Kentucky Sports Medicine, Lexington, KY
SHOULDER INSTABILITY AND LABRAL INJURIES: SURGICAL INDICATIONS AND TECHNIQUES; ARTICULAR CARTILAGE INJURIES OF THE KNEE

David R. Maish, M.D.

Resident, Orthopaedic Surgery, Geisinger Medical Center, Danville, PA
KNEE LIGAMENT INJURIES: EPIDEMIOLOGY, MECHANISM, DIAGNOSIS, AND NATURAL HISTORY

Arthur L. Malkani, M.D.

Associate Professor and Chief, Adult Reconstruction, Dept. of Orthopaedic Surgery, University of Louisville, Louisville, KY
REVISION TOTAL HIP ARTHROPLASTY: THE FEMORAL SIDE

Bert R. Mandelbaum, M.D.

Fellowship Co-Director, Orthopedics and Sports Medicine Group; Team Physician, U.S. Men's National Team; St. John's Health Center, Santa Monica, CA
PAINFUL ELBOW ENTHESOPATHY, ENTRAPMENT, AND NEUROPATHY

Marco Manfrini, M.D.

Orthopaedic Surgeon, Dept. of Musculoskeletal Oncology, Instituti Ortopedici Rizzoli, Bologna, Italy
MALIGNANT BONE TUMORS

Stephen G. Manifold, M.D.

Fellow, Insall Scott Kelly Institute for Orthopaedics and Sports Medicine, Beth Israel Medical Center—Singer Division, New York, NY
OSTEOTOMIES ABOUT THE KNEE

F. W. Marsden, M.D.

Professor Emeritus, Orthopaedic Surgery, University of Queensland, Australia; Consultant Orthopaedic Surgeon, Royal Prince Alfred Hospital, The New Children's Hospital, Sydney, Australia
MANAGEMENT/SURGERY

Bassam A. Masri, M.D.

Associate Professor and Head, Division of Reconstructive Orthopaedics, University of British Columbia; Head, Division of Reconstructive Orthopaedics, Vancouver Hospital and Health Sciences Center, Vancouver, British Columbia, Canada
REVISION THA: ACETABULUM

Daniel P. Mass, M.D.

Professor of Clinical Surgery, University of Chicago; University of Chicago Hospitals, Chicago, IL
TENDON TRANSFERS IN THE UPPER EXTREMITY

Tom G. Mayer, M.D.

Dept. of Orthopaedic Surgery, University of Texas Southwestern Medical Center at Dallas; Medical Director, Dallas, TX
CHRONIC LOW BACK PAIN

Wren V. McCallister, M.D.

Resident in Orthopaedic Surgery, University of Washington Medical Center, University of Washington Dept. of Orthopaedics and Sports Medicine, Seattle, WA
NERVE PHYSIOLOGY AND REPAIRS

Geoffrey M. McCullen, M.D.

Neurological and Spinal Surgery, Lincoln, NE
SPINAL BIOMECHANICS; SPINE FUSION: BIOLOGICAL AND MECHANICAL CONSIDERATIONS

Marion McGregor, M.S.

Associate Professor, Texas Chiropractic College, Pasadena, TX
WHIPLASH

Robert F. McLain, M.D.

Associate Professor, Dept. of Orthopaedic Surgery, Ohio State University School of Medicine, Columbus, OH; Director, Spine Research, Spine Research Laboratory, Dept. of Orthopaedic Surgery, The Cleveland Clinic Foundation, Cleveland, OH
MECHANISMS OF DISK AND MUSCULOSKELETAL BACK PAIN

Scott T. McMullen, M.D.

Clinical Adjunct Assistant Professor, University of Nebraska Medical Center, Omaha, NE
TENDINOPATHIES OF THE FOOT AND ANKLE

Lawrence R. Menendez, M.D.

Professor of Orthopaedic Oncology, University of Southern California Keck School of Medicine, Los Angeles, CA
BENIGN SOFT-TISSUE TUMORS

Theodore Miclau, M.D.

Assistant Professor, Dept. of Orthopaedic Surgery, University of California at San Francisco, San Francisco, CA
EMBRYOLOGY OF BONE

Mark D. Miller, M.D.

Associate Professor of Orthopaedic Surgery, University of Virginia, Charlottesville, VA
DIAGNOSIS OF SHOULDER INSTABILITY AND LABRUM INJURIES

Srdjan Mirkovic, M.D.

Assistant Professor, Chicago, IL
THORACIC DISK HERNIATIONS

M. Ramin Modabber, M.D.

Orthopaedic Surgeon, St. John's Health Center, Santa Monica, CA
PAINFUL ELBOW ENTHESOPATHY, ENTRAPMENT, AND NEUROPATHY

Rodrigo Moreno, M.D.

Fellow, Christine M. Kleinert Institute for Hand and Microsurgery, Inc., University of Louisville, Louisville, KY
WRIST FRACTURES

Errol Mortimer, M.D.

Assistant Professor, Dept. of Orthopaedics, University of Massachusetts Memorial Health Care, Worcester, MA
LEG DEFORMITIES

Vincent S. Mosca, M.D.

Associate Professor, Chief of Pediatric Orthopaedists, University of Washington School of Medicine; Director, Dept. of Orthopaedics, Children's Hospital and Regional Medical Center, Seattle, WA
FLEXIBLE FLATFOOT, METATARSUS ADDUCTUS, SKEWFOOT

Marek Napiontek, M.D.

Associate Professor, Karol Marcinkowski University of Medical Sciences; Vice-Chief of Department, Samodzielny Publiczny Szpital, Poznan, Poland
VERTICAL TALUS

Robert S. Negrin, M.D.

Associate Professor of Medicine, Stanford University, Stanford, CA

Mary Lynn Newport, M.D.

Associate Professor, Dept. of Orthopaedic Surgery, University of Connecticut School of Medicine, Farmington, CT
EXTENSOR TENDON INJURIES

Michael F. Nolan, Ph.D.

Professor of Anatomy and Neurology, Dept. of Anatomy, University of South Florida College of Medicine, Tampa, FL
THERAPEUTIC MODALITY: REHABILITATION OF THE INJURED ATHLETE

Sean Nork, M.D.

Assistant Professor, Dept. of Orthopaedic Surgery and Sports Medicine, University of Washington School of Medicine, Seattle, WA
FRACTURES OF THE HUMERAL SHAFT

Markku T. Nousiainen

COMPLICATIONS OF FRACTURES: ACUTE

John Nyland, Ed.D.

Associate Professor, School of Physical Therapy, University of South Florida College of Medicine, Tampa, FL
THERAPEUTIC MODALITY: REHABILITATION OF THE INJURED ATHLETE

Mary I. O'Connor, M.D.

Assistant Professor of Orthopaedics, Mayo Medical Center, Mayo Graduate School of Medicine, Rochester, MN; Consultant, Mayo Clinic, Jacksonville, FL
SURGICAL MANAGEMENT OF METASTATIC DISEASE OF THE PELVIS

John A. Ogden, M.D.

Clinical Professor of Orthopaedics, Emory Hospital; Director of Orthopaedics, Atlanta Medical Hospital, Atlanta, GA
EMBRYOLOGY AND ANATOMY

James A. O'Leary, M.D.

Clinical Fellow in Sports Medicine, Knee and Shoulder Surgery, University of Pittsburgh Medical Center, Pittsburgh, PA
SHOULDER INJURIES IN ATHLETES

George E. Omer, Jr, M.D.

Professor and Chairman Emeritus, Dept. of Orthopaedics and Rehabilitation, University of New Mexico; Consultant Hand Surgeon, Carrie Tingley Children's Hospital, Albuquerque, NM
THE CONGENITAL HAND

William L. Oppenheim, M.D.

Professor, Pediatric Orthopaedics, University of California at Los Angeles School of Medicine; Consultant, Shriners Hospital for Children, Los Angeles, CA
ARTHROGRYPOSIS

Nathaniel Ordway, M.S.P.E.

Assistant Professor, Dept. of Orthopaedic Surgery, State University of New York Upstate Medical University, Syracuse, NY
SPINAL BIOMECHANICS

Douglas R. Osmon, M.D.

Assistant Professor of Medicine, Mayo Clinic, Rochester, MN
DIAGNOSIS AND MANAGEMENT OF MUSCULOSKELETAL INFECTION

Robert F. Ostrum, M.D.

Clinical Associate Professor of Orthopaedic Surgery, Ohio State University; Associate Director of Orthopaedic Trauma, Grant Medical Center, Columbus, OH
FEMORAL SHAFT FRACTURES

T. Otsuka, M.D.

Associate Professor, Nagoya CIty University Medical School, Nagoya, Japan
BONE GRAFT AND BONE SUBSTITUTES

Susan M. Ott, D.O.

Orthopaedic Surgeon, Guthrie Clinic, Sayre, PA
SPECIAL CONCERNS OF THE FEMALE ATHLETE

Sylvia Õunpuu, MSc

Center for Motion Analysis, Connecticut Children's Medical Center, Hartford, CT
GAIT ANALYSIS IN ORTHOPAEDICS

M. Hakan Öszoy, M.D.

Assistant Professor, Kocatepe University Medical School, Afyon, Turkey
MENISCAL INJURY

Christopher J. Palestro, M.D.

Professor of Nuclear Medicine and Radiology, Albert Einstein College of Medicine, Bronx, NY; Director of Nuclear Medicine, Long Island Jewish Medical Center, New Hyde Park, NY
NUCLEAR MEDICINE

Arthur Pappas, M.D.

Professor, University of Massachusetts Medical School; Chair, Dept. of Orthopaedics, University of Massachusetts Memorial Health Care, Worcester, MA
LEG DEFORMITIES

Theodore W. Parsons III, M.D.

Clinical Associate Professor of Orthopaedics, University of Texas at San Antonio Health Sciences Center; Assistant Professor of Surgery, Uniformed Services University of Health Sciences, Bethesda, MD; Chairman and Program Director, Dept. of Orthopaedics, Wilford Hall Medical Center, San Antonio, TX
BENIGN BONE TUMORS

Terrance D. Peabody, M.D.

Assistant Professor, Dept. of Surgery, University of Chicago, Chicago, IL
CLINICAL PRESENTATION AND RECOMMENDED EVALUATION OF A PATIENT WITH A SUSPECTED BONE TUMOR

Matthew D. Pepe, M.D.

Fellow, Dept. of Orthopaedic Surgery, University of Pittsburgh School of Medicine, Pittsburgh, PA
COMPLICATIONS OF FRACTURES: CHRONIC

David Pienkowski, Ph.D.

Associate Professor, University of Kentucky, Lexington, KY
BASIC CONCEPTS OF BIOMECHANICS

Miguel A. Pirela-Cruz, M.D.

Clinical Assistant Professor, Dept. of Orthopaedics, University of New Mexico, Albuquerque, NM; Clinical Assistant Professor, Texas Tech University, EL Paso, TX; Director of Orthopaedics, Memorial Medical Center, Las Cruces, NM
THE CONGENITAL HAND

Peter D. Pizzutillo, M.D.

Professor of Orthopaedic Surgery and Pediatrics, Hahnemann School of Medicine; Director, Section of Orthopaedic Surgery, St. Christopher's Hospital for Children, Philadelphia, PA
CERVICAL: KLIPPEL-FEIL, TORTICOLLIS

Rick Placide, M.D.

Resident, Hospital of the University of Pennsylvania, Philadelphia, PA
GLENOHUMERAL ARTHRITIS

Anton Y. Plakseychuk, M.D.

Dept. of Orthopaedic Surgery, University of Pittsburgh Medical Center, Pittsburgh, PA
KNEE ARTHROPLASTY

Kevin D. Plancher, M.D.

Plancher Hand and Sports Medicine, Stamford, CT
BENIGN BONE AND SOFT-TISSUE TUMORS OF THE HAND AND WRIST

David A. Porter, M.D.

Co-Director, Research Education, Methodist Sports Medicine Complex; Foot and Ankle Consultant, Indianapolis Colts, Purdue University, Indiana University, Indianapolis, IN
LIGAMENT INJURIES OF THE FOOT AND ANKLE

Gerard Powell, M.D.

Orthopaedic Surgeon, Dept. of Orthopaedics, St. Vincent's Hospital, Fitzroy, Australia
BIOPSY

David C. Preston, M.D.

Associate Professor of Neurology, Case Western Reserve University; Director, Neuromuscular Service, University Hospitals of Cleveland, Cleveland, OH
PERIPHERAL NERVE STRUCTURE: FUNCTION AND PHYSIOLOGY

Kevin J. Pugh, M.D.

Director, Division of Trauma, Dept. of Orthopaedics, Ohio State University, Columbus, OH
FRACTURES AND SOFT-TISSUE INJURIES ABOUT THE ANKLE

George T. Rab, M.D.

Professor and Chair of Orthopaedic Surgery, University of California at Davis; Ben Ali Shriners Chair in Pediatric Orthopaedics, Shriners Hospital for Children Northern California, Sacramento, CA
DIAGNOSIS AND TREATMENT IN THE AMBULATORY CHILD WITH DEVELOPMENTAL DYSPLASIA OF THE HIP

Ellen M. Raney, M.D.

Associate Clinical Professor, University of Hawaii John A. Burns School of Medicine; Assistant Chief of Staff, Shriners Hospital for Children, Honolulu, HI
LIMB LENGTH DISCREPANCY

Robert R. Recker, M.D.

Professor of Medicine, Director, Creighton University Osteoporosis Research Center, Chief, Section of Endocrinology, Creighton University School of Medicine; Senior Staff, St. Joseph Hospital; Attending Physician, Omaha Veterans Administration Hospital, Omaha, NE
OSTEOPOROSIS: ETIOLOGY, DIAGNOSIS, AND TREATMENT

Thomas S. Renshaw, M.D.

Professor of Orthopaedic Surgery, Yale University, New Haven, CT
SCOLIOSIS: CONGENITAL AND NEUROMUSCULAR

Sylvia Resch, M.D.

Head of Dept. of Orthopaedics, Blekinge Hospital, Karlshamn, Sweden
PROBLEMS OF THE LESSER TOES

E. Greer Richardson, M.D.

Professor, Dept. of Orthopaedic Surgery, University of Tennessee Campbell Clinic, Memphis, TN
DISORDERS OF THE FIRST RAY

Lars Richardson, M.D.

Resident, Dept. of Orthopaedic Surgery, Harvard Medical School, Boston, MA
OSTEOTOMIES ABOUT THE KNEE

John M. Roberts, M.D.

Professor of Orthopaedic Surgery Emeritus, Boston University School of Medicine, Boston, MA; Emeritus Chief of Staff, Shriners Hospital for Children, Springfield, MA
DEVELOPMENTAL DYSPLASIA OF THE HIP: DIAGNOSIS AND TREATMENT OF THE NON-AMBULATOR

Mark W. Rodosky, M.D.

Assistant Professor and Chief of Shoulder Service, University of Pittsburgh Medical Center, Pittsburgh, PA
SHOULDER INJURIES IN ATHLETES

G. Alec Rooke, M.D.

Associate Professor of Anesthesiology, University of Washington School of Medicine; Staff Anesthesiologist, Veterans Affairs Puget Sound Health Care System, Seattle, WA
ANESTHETIC AND PERIOPERATIVE MANAGEMENT OF THE GERIATRIC PATIENT

Harry E. Rubash, M.D.

Dept. of Orthopaedics, Massachusetts General Hospital, Boston, MA

David S. Ruch, M.D.

Associate Professor, Co-Director, Hand Surgery Fellowship, Wake Forest University Baptist Medical Center, Winston-Salem, NC
GENERAL ASPECTS OF MICROVASCULAR TISSUE REPLANTATION

Charles L. Saltzman, M.D.

Associate Professor, Dept. of Orthopaedic Surgery, Dept. of Biomedical Engineering, University of Iowa College of Medicine, Iowa City, IA
THE DIABETIC FOOT; MIDFOOT ARTHRITIS

Rajit Saluja, M.D.

Milwaukee, WI
OSTEOTOMY/ARTHRODESIS/RESECTION

Eduardo A. Salvati, M.D.

Director of Hip Service, Attending Surgeon, Hospital for Special Surgery, New York, NY
PRIMARY TOTAL HIP ARTHROPLASTY

Steven P. Sampson, M.D.

Dept. of Orthopaedics, University Medical Center at Stony Brook, Stony Brook, NY
HAND FRACTURES

Paul E. Savas, M.D.

Spine Fellow, Rothman Institute, Thomas Jefferson University Medical College, Philadelphia, PA
THORACOLUMBAR SPINE INJURIES

Mark T. Scarborough, M.D.

Associate Professor of Orthopaedic Surgery, Dept. of Orthopaedic Surgery and Rehabilitation, University of Florida, Gainesville, FL
BIOPSY

N. Schachar, M.D.

Professor of Surgery, Division of Orthopaedic Surgery, University of Calgary; Foothills Hospital, Calgary, Alberta, Canada
BONE GRAFT AND BONE SUBSTITUTES

Jonathan L. Schaffer, M.D.

Managing Director, e-Cleveland Clinic, Information Technology Division; Staff, Adult Reconstruction Section, Department of Orthopaedic Surgery; Assistant Director, Orthopaedic Clinical Research Center, The Cleveland Clinic, Cleveland, Ohio
ARTHRITIS OF THE KNEE

Luis R. Scheker, M.D.

Assistant Clinical Professor, Division of Plastic and Reconstructive Surgery, University of Louisville School of Medicine; Statt, Kleinert, Kutz, and Associates, Hand Care Center, Louisville, KY
WRIST FRACTURES

E. H. Schemitsch, M.D.

St. Michael's Hospital, University of Toronto, Toronto, Ontario, Canada
COMPLICATIONS OF FRACTURES: ACUTE

Ulrich Schietsch, Ph.D.

Professor of Orthopaedic Surgery, Martin Luther University Orthopaedic Clinic, Halle, Germany
MANAGEMENT OF COMPLICATIONS AFTER JOINT ARTHROPLASTY

Gregory J. Schmeling, M.D.

Associate Professor, Director, Division of Orthopaedic Trauma, Dept. of Orthopaedics, MCW Clinics, Milwaukee, WI
FOREARM FRACTURES

Stephen Schnall, M.D.

Associate Professor of Clinical Orthopaedics, Keck School of Medicine, University of Southern California; Chief of Hand Surgery, Director USC/Joseph Boyes Hand Fellowship, Los Angeles, CA
HAND INFECTIONS; NECROTIZING FASCIITIS AND SOFT-TISSUE INFECTIONS

Richard A. Schneider

Assistant Adjunct Professor, Dept. of Orthopaedic Surgery, University of California at San Francisco, San Francisco, CA
EMBRYOLOGY OF BONE

Perry L. Schoenecker, M.D.

Professor, University of Washington School of Medicine; Chief of Staff, Shriners Hospital for Children, St. Louis Children's Hospital, St. Louis, MO
COMPLICATIONS IN THE TREATMENT OF HIP DYSPLASIA

Lew C. Schon, M.D.

Dept. of Orthopaedic Surgery, Union Memorial Hospital, Baltimore, MD
NERVE PROBLEMS OF THE FOOT AND ANKLE

C. William Schwab, M.D.

Professor of Surgery, University of Pennsylvania; Chief, Division of Traumatology and Surgical Critical Care, Hospital of the University of Pennsylvania, Philadelphia, PA
PRIORITIZATION AND MANAGEMENT OF THE POLYTRAUMA PATIENT

Giles R. Scuderi, M.D.

Assistant Clinical Professor of Orthopaedic Surgery, Albert Einstein College of Medicine; Associate Chief, Adult Knee Reconstruction, Dept. of Orthopaedics, Beth Israel Medical Center, New York, NY
INFECTED TOTAL KNEE ARTHROPLASTY

John G. Seiler III, M.D.

Georgia Hand and Microsurgery, Atlanta, GA
FLEXOR TENDON INJURIES

Yoshio Setoguchi, M.D.

Emeritus Clinical Professor of Pediatrics, University of California at Los Angeles School of Medicine; Medical Director, Child Amputee Prosthetics Project, Shriners Hospital for Children, Los Angeles, CA
ACQUIRED AMPUTATIONS IN CHILDREN

William J. Shaughnessy, M.D.

Assistant Professor of Orthopaedic Surgery, Mayo Medical School; Chair, Division of Pediatric Orthopaedic Surgery, Mayo Clinic, Rochester, MN
PEDIATRIC OSTEOMYELITIS AND SEPTIC ARTHRITIS

Donald G. Shurr, C.P.O.

Adjunct Lecturer, University of Iowa Physical Therapy Education; Director of Orthotic and Prosthetic Services, American Prosthetics and Orthotics, Inc., University of Iowa Hospitals and Clinics, Iowa City, IA
ORTHOTIC MANAGEMENT OF FOOT AND ANKLE PROBLEMS

Natalie Sims, Ph.D.

St. Vincent's Institute of Medical Research, Fitzroy, Australia
BONE: STRUCTURE, FUNCTION, GROWTH, AND REMODELING

Divya Singh, M.D.

Chief Resident, Dept. of Orthopaedics, University of Massachusetts School of Medicine, Worcester, MA
RADIAL NERVE COMPRESSION SYNDROMES

Kush Singh

Thomas Jefferson University Medical College, Philadelphia, PA
LOW BACK PAIN AND SCIATICA

Raj K. Sinha, M.D.

Division of Adult Reconstructive Surgery, University of Pittsburgh Medical Center, Pittsburgh, PA
REVISION TOTAL KNEE ARTHROPLASTY

Mark Slovenkai, M.D.

Lahey Clinic, Burlington, MA
THE DIABETIC FOOT

Brian G. Smith, M.D.

Associate Professor, Dept. of Orthopaedics, University of Connecticut Health Center, Farmington, CT; Staff Orthopaedic Surgeon, Connecticut Children's Medical Center, Hartford, CT
HEREDITARY SENSORY MOTOR NEUROPATHIES

Daniel Solomon, M.D., MPH

Instructor in Medicine, Division of Rheumatology and Division of Pharmacoepidemiology and Pharmaeconomics, Harvard Medical School; Associate Physician, Division of Rheumatology, Brigham and Women's Hospital, Boston, MA
ARTHRITIS OF THE KNEE

Dean G. Sotereanos, M.D.

Chief, Division of Hand and Upper Extremity Surgery, Dept. of Orthopaedic Surgery, University of Pittsburgh Medical Center, Pittsburgh, PA
GAMEKEEPER'S THUMB

Nicholas G. Sotereanos, M.D.

Assistant Professor of Orthopaedic Surgery, Hahnemann University, Philadelphia, PA; Director, Division of Adult Reconstruction, Allegheny General Hospital, Pittsburgh, PA
MANAGEMENT OF COMPLICATIONS AFTER JOINT ARTHROPLASTY

Dempsey S. Springfield, M.D.

Professor and Chairman, Dept. of Orthopaedics, Mount Sinai Hospital, New York, NY
IRRADIATION FOR MUSCULOSKELETAL TUMORS

David R. Steinberg, M.D.

Assistant Professor, Dept. of Orthopaedic Surgery, University of Pennsylvania; Director of Hand Fellowship, Penn Orthopaedic Institute, University of Pennsylvania Health System, Philadelphia, PA
OSTEOARTHRITIS OF THE HAND

Heidi M. Stephens, M.D.

Associate Professor of Orthopaedic Surgery, University of South Florida, Tampa, FL
BUNIONS

Peter J. Stern, M.D.

Hand Surgery Specialists, Inc, Cincinnati, OH

David A. Stone, M.D.

Assistant Professor, Dept. of Orthopaedic Surgery and Family Medicine, University of Pittsburgh; Director, Primary Care Sports Medicine Fellowship, University of Pittsburgh Medical Center— St. Margaret Hospital, Pittsburgh, PA
OVERUSE INJURIES

William B. Strecker, M.D.

Orthopaedic Associates, St. Louis, MO
CEREBRAL PALSY: UPPER EXTREMITY

Peter F. Sturm, M.D.

Clinical Associate Professor of Orthopaedic Surgery, George Washington University School of Medicine, Washington, D.C.; Clinical Associate Professor of Pediatrics, University of Virginia School of Medicine, Charlottesville, VA; Pediatric Orthopaedic and Scoliosis Associates, Annandale, VA
LOWER EXTREMITY

Nobuhiko Sugano, M.D.

Assistant Professor, Dept. of Orthopaedics, Osaka University Medical School, Osaka, Japan
OSTEONECROSIS

Raymond J. Sullivan, M.D.

Clinical Assistant Professor, University of Connecticut Health Center, Farmington, CT
FRACTURES OF THE FOREFOOT AND MIDFOOT

Il Hoon Sung, M.D.

The Hospital for Special Surgery, New York, NY
ACQUIRED ADULT FLATFOOT DEFORMITY

Michael D. Sussman, M.D.

Clinical Professor of Orthopaedic Surgery, Oregon Health Science University; Staff Orthopaedic Surgeon, Former Chief of Staff, Shriners Hospital for Children, Portland, OR
MUSCULAR DYSTROPHY

Emin Taskiran, M.D.

Orthopaedic and Trauma Subdivision of Sports, Trauma Arthroscopy and Knee Surgery, Izmir, Turkey
MENISCAL INJURY

H. Thomas Temple, M.D.

Professor of Orthopaedics and Pathology, Chief, Orthopaedic Oncology Division, University of Miami School of Medicine, Miami, FL
MALIGNANT SOFT-TISSUE TUMORS; METASTATIC DISEASE OF THE UPPER EXTREMITY

Andrew L. Terrono, M.D.

Associate Clinical Professor, Tufts University School of Medicine; Hand Surgeon, New England Baptist Bone and Joint Institute, Boston, MA
RHEUMATOID ARTHRITIC HAND

George H. Thompson, M.D.

Professor of Orthopaedic Surgery and Radiatrics, Case Western Reserve University; Director, Pediatric Orthopaedics, Rainbow Babies and Children's Hospital, Cleveland, OH
UPPER EXTREMITY; KYPHOSIS

Matthew M. Tomaino, M.D.

Associate Professor, Department of Orthopaedic Surgery, University of Pittsburgh Medical Center, Pittsburgh, PA
ARTHRITIS OF THE ELBOW; REGIONAL FLAPS

Maria B. Tomas, M.D.

Assistant Professor of Nuclear Medicine, Albert Einstein College of Medicine, Bronx, NY; Attending Physician, Division of Nuclear Medicine, Long Island Jewish Medical Center, New Hyde Park, NY
NUCLEAR MEDICINE

Paul Tornetta, III, M.D.

Associate Professor and Vice-Chairman, Boston University School of Medicine, Boston, MA
DISTAL TIBIA FRACTURES

John J. Triano, Ph.D.

Adjunct Faculty, University of Texas Southwestern Medical School, University of Texas Arlington Joint Biomedical Engineering Program; Co-Director, Conservative Care; Director, Chiropractic Division, Texas Back Institute, Plano, TX
WHIPLASH

Todd J. Troshynski, M.D.

Associate Director Operating Room, Children's Hospital of Wisconsin, Assistant Professor of Anesthesiology, Medical College at Wisconsin, Milwaukee, WI
ANESTHESIA FOR PEDIATRIC PATIENTS UNDERGOING ORTHOPAEDIC PROCEDURES

Thomas E. Trumble, M.D.

Professor and Chief, Hand and Microvascular Surgery Service, Dept. of Orthopaedics and Sports Medicine, University of Washington Medical Center, Seattle, WA
NERVE PHYSIOLOGY AND REPAIRS

Kentaro Tsueda, M.D.

Professor of Anesthesiology, University of Louisville School of Medicine, Louisville, KY
ANESTHESIA AND PAIN MANAGEMENT

Joshua A. Urban, M.D.

Resident, Dept. of Orthopaedic Surgery and Rehabilitation, University of Nebraska Medical Center, Omaha, NE
INFECTED TOTAL HIP ARTHROPLASTY

Marc W. Urquhart, M.D.

The Hospital for Special Surgery, New York, NY
SHOULDER INJURIES IN ATHLETES

Alexander R. Vaccaro, M.D.

Professor, Co-Chief of Spine Surgery, Dept. of Orthopaedic Surgery, Thomas Jefferson University Hospital; Co-Director, Regional Spinal Cord Injury Center of the Delaware Valley, Philadelphia, PA
CERVICAL SPINE TRAUMA; THORACOLUMBAR SPINE INJURIES; SPINAL STENOSIS

Sokratis E. Varitimidis, M.D.

Attending Hand Surgeon, University of Larissa, Larissa, Greece
MANAGEMENT OF COMPLICATIONS AFTER JOINT ARTHROPLASTY; GAMEKEEPER'S THUMB

Scott Waller, M.D.

Howard Beach, NY
HAND INFECTIONS

William G. Ward, Sr, M.D.

Professor of Orthopaedic Surgery, Wake Forest University School of Medicine; Director, Orthopaedic Oncology, Baptist Medical Center, Winston-Salem, NC
PRESENTATION AND EVALUATION

William C. Warner, Jr, M.D.

Associate Professor, Dept. of Orthopaedic Surgery, University of Tennessee; Staff, Campbell Clinic and Baptist Memorial Hospital; Chief, Mississippi Crippled Children's Service, Memphis, TN
CONGENITAL DEFORMITIES OF THE KNEE

Mary Chester M. Wasko, M.D.

Assistant Professor of Medicine, University of Pittsburgh School of Medicine, Pittsburgh, PA
CRYSTALLINE ARTHROPATHIES

Peter M. Waters, M.D.

Associate Professor, Dept. of Orthopaedic Surgery, Harvard Medical Center; Clinical Director, Hand and Upper Extremity Program, Children's Hospital, Boston, MA
BRACHIAL PLEXUS INJURIES

H. G. Watts, M.D.

Shriners Hospital
FAILURE OF FORMATION OF THE LIMBS

Steven Weisman, M.D.

Anesthesiology, New Haven, CT
ANESTHESIA FOR PEDIATRIC PATIENTS UNDERGOING ORTHOPAEDIC PROCEDURES

Neil J. Wells, M.D.

Division of Plastic Surgery, St. Paul's Hospital, University of British Columbia, Vancouver, British Columbia, Canada
DISTANT FLAPS: PEDICLE AND FREE

A. Paige Whittle, M.D.

Dept. of Orthopaedics, Regional Medical Center, Memphis, TN
TIBIAL SHAFT FRACTURES

Gerald R. Williams, Jr, M.D.

Associate Professor of Orthopaedic Surgery, University of Pennsylvania; Chief of Shoulder and Elbow Service, Hospital of the University of Pennsylvania, Philadelphia, PA
GLENOHUMERAL ARTHRITIS

Scott W. Wolfe, M.D.

Professor of Orthopaedics, Weill-Cornell Medical College; Attending Orthopaedic Surgeon, The Hospital for Special Surgery, New York, NY
WRIST INSTABILITY

Timothy M. Wright, M.D.

Associate Professor of Medicine, Associate Professor of Molecular Genetics and Biochemistry; Chief, Division of Rheumatology and Clinical Immunology, University of Pittsburgh School of Medicine; Director, University of Pittsburgh Arthritis Institute, Pittsburgh, PA
INFLAMMATORY ARTHRITIS; CRYSTALLINE ARTHROPATHIES

Hansen A. Yuan, M.D.

Professor of Orthopaedic and Neurological Surgery, State University of New York, Syracuse, NY
SPINAL BIOMECHANICS

S. Tim Yoon

COMPLICATIONS OF SPINAL SURGERY

Colby Young

ORTHOPAEDIC SURGERY IN THE IMMUNOCOMPROMISED HOST

Jack E. Zigler, M.D.

Texas Back Institute, Plano, TX
WHIPLASH

Dan A. Zlotolow, M.D.

Clinical Research Fellow, The Rothman Institute, Philadelphia, PA
SPINAL STENOSIS

PREFACE

Orthopaedics was envisioned and developed to provide concise, systematic coverage of the essential principles of orthopaedics, including the relevant scientific information on which those principles are based. While scientific literature remains the foundation of knowledge of the musculoskeletal system, its prodigious nature in an ever-expanding number of specialty journals precludes assimilation of all of the information. The editors sought to develop a single source of authoritative information reflecting knowledge synthesized from the literature and clinical experience, with integration of pertinent basic research investigations and clinical outcomes.

Orthopaedics was not intended to compete with multivolume reference works nor with monographs on circumscribed topics. Rather, it represents core orthopaedic knowledge that will provide the reader with information and concepts pertinent to the essential principles that guide modern orthopaedic practice.

One of the main goals of this textbook is to integrate current discussion of the clinical aspects of musculoskeletal disorders with rapidly evolving scientific information that is altering knowledge of diseases and their treatments. Another, closely related goal is to provide information that will facilitate preparation for the American Board of Orthopaedic Surgery Certification Examination, for the Recertification Examination, for the American Academy of Orthopaedic Surgeons In-Training Examination, and for other certifying examinations throughout the world.

Diseases of the musculoskeletal system are increasing with an aging world population and are highly prevalent throughout the world. As a result, a wide range of individuals have a keen interest in the principles of musculoskeletal medicine and surgery who we hope will find *Orthopaedics* useful. We believe this book will have value to orthopaedic surgeons at all stages of their professional lives. Beginning residents can read through this book for an overview of their new specialty; trainees or clinicians preparing for certification or recertification examinations can read portions of this book as a broad review; and practicing clinicians can use this book as a convenient shelf reference. We also believe that other physicians, including rheumatologists, physiatrists, and a wide range of primary care physicians, will find this book advantageous both for treating patients and deciding which patients require referral for musculoskeletal care. In addition, the many other health professionals who care for patients with musculoskeletal disorders should find this book to be an accessible, authoritative, and reliable guide to the foremost, up-to-date medical and surgical thinking.

In order to avoid the lengthy tracts of dense text so often encountered in modern multivolume orthopaedic reference works, *Orthopaedics* has a unique user-friendly format with a high degree of consistency in style and presentation designed to impart knowledge without unnecessary minutiae. Each chapter opens with a Summary Box featuring several concise statements that highlight the key principles detailed in the chapter. These summaries not only provide a preview of the chapter but also serve as a rapid-recall trigger for readers who have studied the chapter. Each chapter is then developed in a consistent manner. Rather than an exhaustive list of references, each chapter contains highly selected and relevant references.

Chapters devoted to various diseases of the musculoskeletal system begin with a concise definition of the disease followed by a discussion of its history, epidemiology, pathophysiology, clinical findings, differential diagnosis, and mangement. *Orthopaedics* was not envisioned to be a treatise on surgical technique; pearls of surgical wisdom are provided in operative pictures, artwork, and text. Applications of new devices and techniques are emphasized with diagrams and operative photographs. Each of the chapters that focuses on diagnostic and therapeutic interventions discusses the various options for achieving a desired goal and clearly identifies the pros and cons, priorities, and controversies of each option. Chapters concerned with basic science of the musculoskeletal system contain a brief historical review of the development of the scientific issues and clearly identify the clinical or practical relevance of each biological or engineering issue that is discussed. This approach will appeal to the reader who desires an in-depth understanding of the disease and also allows for easy retrieval of specific information on the subject.

In *Orthopaedics* there is a strong emphasis on illustrations, with the belief that visual images facilitate rapid learning with long-term retention. Medical and surgical treatments have been summarized with tables and graphs to present easily digested comparisons. Artists working with the contributors in a consistent style and format created hundreds of new drawings. In addition to these drawings, each of the chapters includes clinical photographs and high-quality reproductions of pathological specimens, radiographs, and other clinical imaging techniques.

The editors wish to thank all whose efforts have been responsible for the development of this readable and informative textbook. The contributing authors were carefully selected to provide information that is accurate, up-to-date, and easy to understand. We are grateful to them for their effort, their knowledge, and their skill. We are particularly grateful to the section editors who shared our enthusiasm and played a critical role in the development of their sec-

tions, choice of authors, and editing. Geoff Greenwood should be commended for his efforts with the initial impetus for the development of *Orthopaedics,* and Richard Lampert has been a stalwart through the various difficulties we have encountered.

Robert H. Fitzgerald, Jr, M.D.
Herbert Kaufer, M.D.
Arthur L. Malkani, M.D.

CONTENTS

SECTION 4   ORTHOPAEDIC SPORTS MEDICINE
DARREN L. JOHNSON

SECTION 5   INFECTION
ARLEN D. HANSSEN

SECTION 6 ARTHRITIDES ARTHROPATHIES

RAJ SINHA, HARRY RUBASH

UPPER EXTREMITY RECOUNT

THE HIP

COMPLICATIONS

SECTION 7 MUSCULOSKELETAL TUMORS

DEMPSEY S. SPRINGFIELD

BONE TUMORS

SOFT-TISSUE TUMORS

SECTION 8   SPINE
STEVEN R. GARFIN

SECTION 9   PEDIATRIC ORTHOPAEDICS
JAMES C. DRENNAN, KENNETH GUIDERA

GENERAL ORTHOPAEDICS

COURTLAND G. LEWIS

CLINICAL HISTORY AND PHYSICAL EXAMINATION

Ian D. Learmonth

Summary
- The musculoskeletal system provides locomotor function.
- Disorders of the musculoskeletal system are associated with pain and loss of function.
- A good history qualitatively and quantitatively characterizes the pain and quantifies the disability based on the functional requirements peculiar to each individual patient.
- A structured routine of clinical history and examination usually elicits the clinical symptoms and signs that will confirm the diagnosis.

Orthopaedic surgeons deal with injuries, diseases, and disorders of the musculoskeletal system. Patients are unaware of the autonomic control of many of the systems of the body; for example, they are unaware of an increased production of insulin after a glucose-rich meal, or of the liver's response to a cholesterol challenge. The function of the musculoskeletal system, however, is most often recruited by a conscious act of volition. A failure to provide the desired function is therefore usually readily apparent.

A PHILOSOPHY OF ORTHOPAEDIC DIAGNOSIS

I do not believe that the orthopaedic clinical examination should be based on the symptoms and signs traditionally associated with pathogenetic groupings of disease entities—inflammatory, infective, vascular, neoplastic, degenerative. These should rather be unbundled and applied to problem solving in specific clinical areas—the painful knee, the painful shoulder, and so on. A careful history will often provide sufficient information for a provisional diagnosis, which can usually be affirmed by methodical clinical examination. Special investigations are then only required to confirm the diagnosis.

In orthopaedic surgery, it is often easy to make the diagnosis; it is the choice of management that provides the greatest challenge. In deciding on the optimal treatment, it is essential to attempt to assess the pain and to quantify the associated disability. Disability will to some extent be determined by deformity, rate of progression, and so on. However, it will mainly depend on the degree to which the patient's social, domestic, recreational, and professional activities are restricted. Although expectations will clearly differ enormously from patient to patient, one needs to define to what degree quality of life is compromised. This will be very patient-specific. Only when armed with this information can the surgeon make a rational decision about management (Fig. 1).

HISTORY

The history should consist of the following points.

Presenting Complaint. What was the patient's main complaint that persuaded him or her to visit the doctor? How long has it been present? Is it deteriorating, and if so, how rapidly?

Personal History and Background. It is important to establish the patient's age, social circumstances (e.g., family, type of abode), work environment, recreational pursuits, and general psychological condition. This allows the orthopaedic surgeon to establish a patient profile. Souter[1] has emphasized the importance of "picking a winner" when choosing the first operation in a program of reconstructive surgery in a patient with rheumatoid arthritis. A successful procedure establishes patient trust, and the more complex surgery can then be contemplated "together" with more confidence. It is only when the patient's expectations and attitude have been identified that it becomes possible to "pick a winner" in patient terms (Table 1).

Family History. A pertinent family history should be sought only when the presenting complaint has been defined. The interrogation should include any history of a similar complaint in any member of the family.

Some orthopaedic conditions are autosomal dominant (e.g., Ehlers-Danlos and Marfan's syndromes) whereas others are autosomal recessive (e.g., diastrophic dysplasia). However, the majority of orthopaedic conditions that have any genetic association are characterized by a familial predisposition, such as osteoarthritis, rheumatoid arthritis, and gout.

Past Medical History. Musculoskeletal symptoms in the adult are often a late expression of treated or untreated orthopaedic disorders. It is therefore important to try to establish whether the patient had any musculoskeletal disorder as a child. As much detail as possible should be gleaned about any previous orthopaedic surgery. In some cases, this may merely assist with the diagnosis (e.g., degeneration secondary to a dysplastic hip), whereas in other cases it may have management implications (e.g., ankylosis and scarring from drainage of previous septic arthritis).

Trauma of bones, joints, and soft tissues often predisposes to degenerative conditions of the musculoskeletal system. A detailed history of all severe trauma should therefore be obtained. It must be recognized that all children suffer intermittent episodes of minor trauma, but these will invariably be implicated in the etiology of many nontraumatic childhood conditions (e.g., Perthes' disease, slipped capital femoral epiphysis).

In arthritis, any history of the involvement of other joints should be sought. This may suggest a polyarticular inflammatory arthropathy. Do these patients fit the American Rheumatism Association criteria for rheumatoid arthritis? Similarly, arthritic patients should be specifically questioned

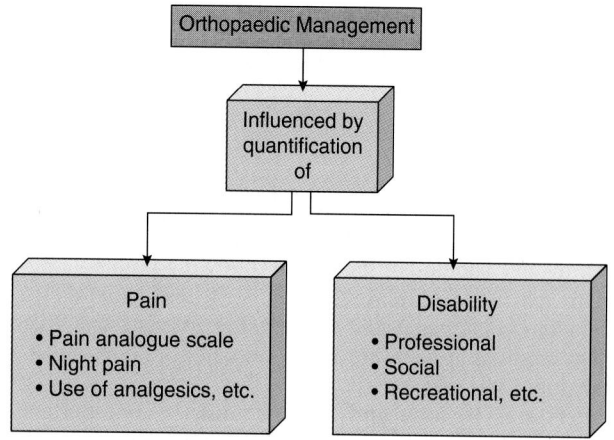

Fig. 1. Orthopaedic management.

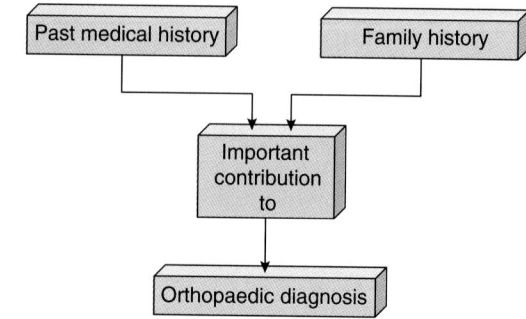

Fig. 2. Orthopaedic diagnosis.

regarding the stigmata of reactive arthritis—psoriasis, regional ileitis, urethritis, and so on.

Examination and special investigations may suggest diagnoses that invite more specific details of the medical history. Thus a suspected diagnosis of osteosarcoma in the middle-aged patient demands further questioning regarding a history of previous radiotherapy. An overview of other systems should always be included in the past medical history. This may contribute to the diagnosis and should expose any conditions from which the patient suffers that might adversely affect proposed surgery and anesthesia. Risk factors should be identified, such as diabetes mellitus or steroid therapy (Fig. 2).

The prevalence rate of familial predisposition in inflammatory arthropathies, and the association of mechanical derangement and osteoarthritis, makes the past medical history particularly relevant in making an orthopaedic diagnosis.

PREDISPOSING FACTORS

In cases in which predisposing factors are associated with specific diagnoses, the surgeon should expose the relevant history. Thus a patient with suspected osteonecrosis of the

hip should be carefully questioned regarding exposure to a dysbaric environment, abuse of alcohol, steroid therapy, and so on. Likewise, a patient with a suspected infective lesion of the spine should be asked about previous exposure to tuberculosis and brucellosis.

Overuse injuries occur in athletes and dancers, or indeed in anyone after excessive activity without adequate training. The three main causes of overuse trauma are friction, stress, and ischemia.

Excessive friction of a tendon or bursa during joint movement may provoke an inflammatory reaction (e.g., iliotibial band syndrome). Repeated stress may result in an incomplete fracture of bone (e.g., March fracture of the second or third metatarsal). Ischemia usually occurs in muscles that are tightly contained within fascial compartments. Overuse causes relative ischemia, swelling, and, occasionally, a recurring low-grade compartment syndrome.

Table 2 lists some of the better known clinical overuse syndromes.

SYMPTOMS

PAIN

Pain is probably the most common presenting symptom in orthopaedic conditions (Table 3). It is traditional to discuss the pain's location, duration, progression, nature (e.g., stabbing, burning), intensity, and presence of radiation. It is important to elicit this history; however, this should not be undertaken by rote. The specific characterization of the pain is often diagnostic. Thus a sharp shooting pain in the back (often with radiation) is usually radicular, whereas a chronic ache aggravated by activity is caused by degenerative changes, and a constant boring pain is usually infective or neoplastic.

TABLE 1. ELEMENTS OF THE ORTHOPAEDIC PATIENT'S HISTORY

Main complaint
Pain
Disability

Other complaints
Musculoskeletal
Nonorthopaedic

Personal history and social background
Determine sociodomestic and work environment

Past medical history
Musculoskeletal
Other

Family history
Musculoskeletal
Other

TABLE 2. OVERUSE SYNDROMES

Tennis elbow (lateral epicondylitis)
Golfer's elbow (medial epicondylitis)
Trochanteric bursitis
Patellar tendinitis (jumper's knee)
Iliotibial band syndrome
Achilles tendinitis
Calcaneal bursitis
Shin splints
Stress fractures (tibia and metatarsals)

TABLE 3. PRESENTING SYMPTOMS IN ORTHOPAEDIC CONDITIONS

Pain
Stiffness
Swelling
Deformity
Altered sensation
Limp
Loss of function

Groin pain is typically hip pain. As a rule of thumb, pain anterior to a midline coronal plane usually arises from the hip whereas pain posterior to this line is most often attributable to the spine (Fig. 3).

It is often useful to ask a patient to point to the site of pain. Thus pain in the neck/shoulder interval is usually caused by cervical spondylosis, whereas the patient will point with one finger to the source of acromioclavicular joint pain. The shoulder is clasped for glenohumeral pain

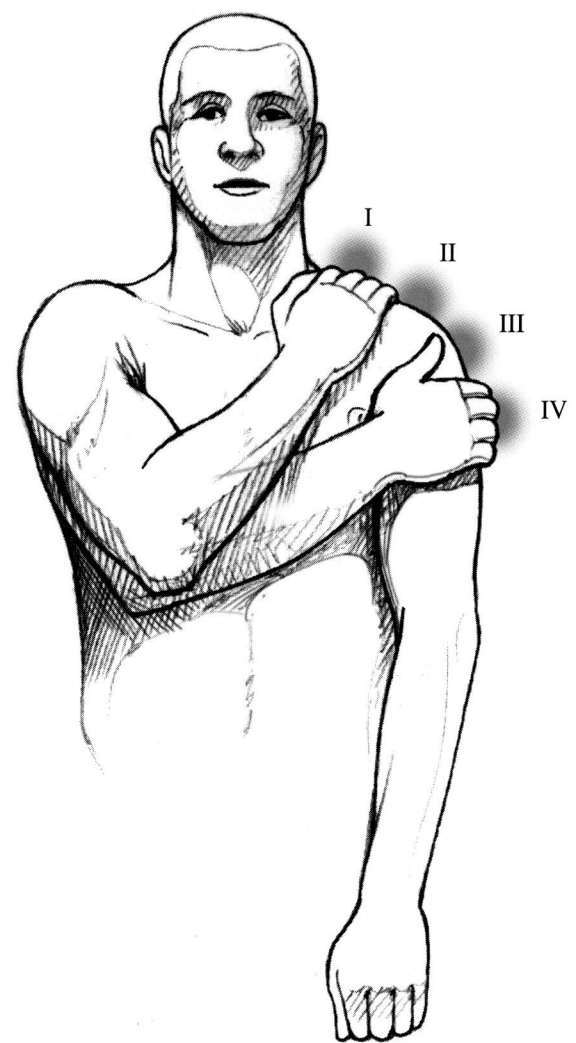

Fig. 4. **Pain.** The patient's localization of pain is often diagnostic around the shoulder: I. cervical spondylosis; II. arthritis of the acromioclavicular joint; III. glenohumeral arthritis; IV. rotator cuff syndrome.

and a hand over the badge area indicates a rotator cuff problem (Fig. 4).

If the pain has been present for a long time, the condition is likely to be chronic and degenerative. The severity and rate of deterioration will certainly influence decisions regarding management. It is often useful to use a pain analogue scale in an attempt to quantify pain (Fig. 5).

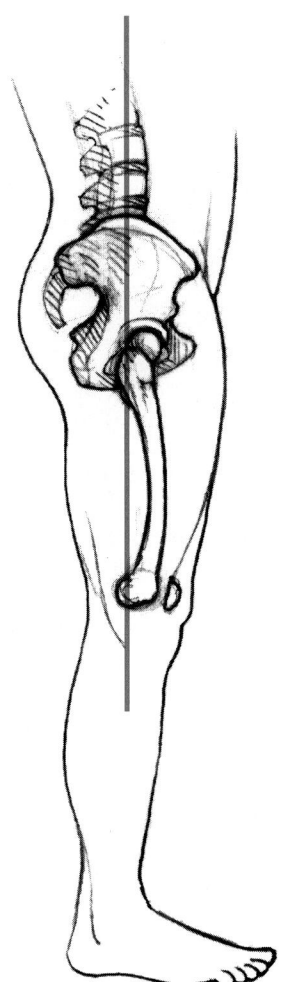

Fig. 3. **Pain.** Pain anterior to the midcoronal plane generally arises from the hip, whereas pain posterior to this line is usually attributable to the spine.

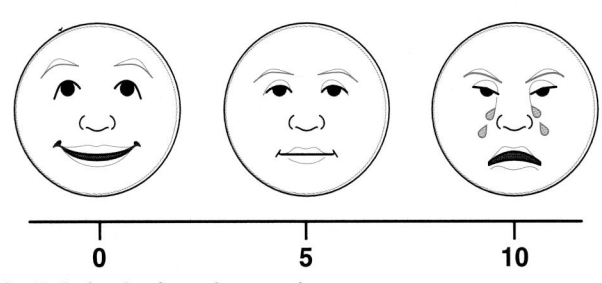

Fig. 5. **A visual pain analogue scale.**

TABLE 4. GRADING OF PAIN	
Grade	Criteria
1	No pain
2	Mild, can be ignored
3	Moderate, requires analgesics
4	Severe, intrusive despite an analgesic
5	Very severe; inhibits virtually all activities

Although pain is subjective, its intrusiveness and the need for an analgesic have been recruited in an attempt to classify its severity (Table 4).

Patients should also be carefully questioned regarding their analgesic regimen. This can be used to monitor pain in much the same way as the patient-controlled analgesia method is used in the postoperative period. Some patients are stoic and will deny significant pain despite taking a substantial regular dose of analgesia. Alternatively, an impressionable person who has witnessed a loved one die with excruciating pain may grossly exaggerate his or her own pain as a result of anxiety bordering on neurosis.

When considering the identified site of the pain, it should be remembered that it could be referred. Pain referred into the upper and lower limbs is commonly referred from the cervical or lumbar region. Osteonecrosis of the hip may present exclusively with pain in the knee. Referred pain may originate from very different areas. For example, avascular necrosis and an obturator hernia can both present with pain in the knee. This is not the result of shared sensory pathways but reflects the inability of the cerebral cortex to distinguish between sensory messages from embryologically related sites (Fig. 6).

I am aware of at least three patients with osteonecrosis of the femoral head who underwent arthroscopies of the knee because the possibility of referred pain was not considered in their symptomatic presentation.

STIFFNESS

Stiffness may represent a subjective impression or may denote an absolute reduction in movement. Stiffness is commonly encountered with soft tissue scarring, periarticular fibrosis, or intra-articular adhesions. This is nonspecific; however, establishing when the stiffness is at its worst may provide a valuable clue to the diagnosis. Thus osteoarthritic joints are painful on rising after an interval of rest following a period of vigorous physical activity. Prolonged morning stiffness characterizes the inflammatory arthropathies. For example, a young man in his 20s who complains of recurring severe stiffness (and pain) in his back on rising in the morning should be regarded as having ankylosing spondylitis until it is proved otherwise. Stiffness will of course also contribute to loss of function.

SWELLING

The patient may be aware of a swelling. Is this hard or soft and does it fluctuate? Is it progressive? If the knee has swollen following trauma, it is important to distinguish

between early swelling (within an hour) and late swelling (within 12 to 24 hours). The former is probably hemarthrosis consequent on disruption of intracapsular soft tissue, whereas the latter is likely to be an effusion (possibly a meniscal tear).

INSTABILITY

Instability may be the presenting symptom of the patient. It is then necessary to obtain a detailed account of the mechanism of injury and to establish the movements or positions that give rise to the feeling of instability. Structurally, the instability may be the result of ligamentous disruption, or it may be spurious to avoid pain because soft tissue is trapped in the joint. The latter case will then often be associated with locking. This may be the presenting feature of a bucket handle tear of the meniscus. Muscle weakness may also lead to a feeling of instability.

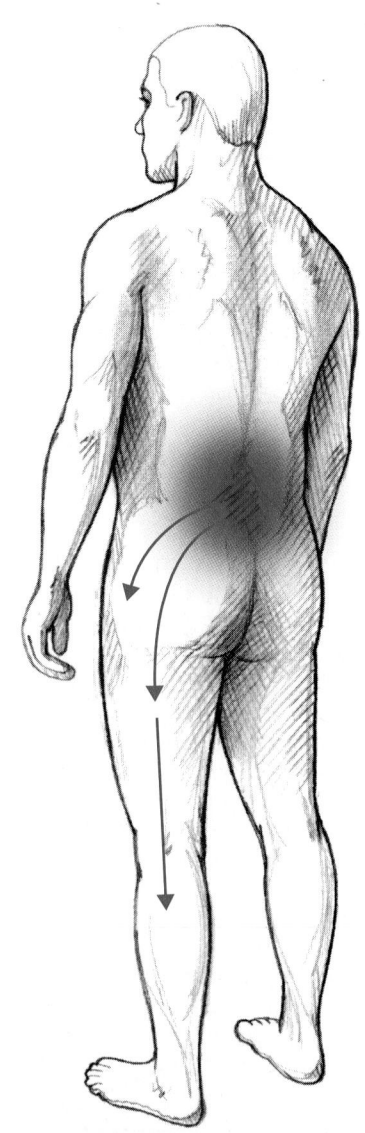

Fig. 6. Referred pain. A disorder in the lower back can produce nonradicular pain that radiates down the leg.

DEFORMITY

Deformity may on occasion be the presenting complaint, although it is more frequently associated with pain and stiffness. The patient may report the recent development of bowlegs or knock-knees. It is important to establish whether the deformity is progressing and, if so, how rapidly.

Deformities of the feet may prevent the patient from purchasing "off the shelf" shoes, and this could be the presenting complaint.

LIMP

A limp may be caused by involvement of the joint, dysfunctional muscle, deformity (short limb), and so on. How long has the limp been present and is it getting worse? Does the patient use walking aids and if so for how long? The presence of a limp seems to be particularly discomfiting to women and often constitutes one of their main concerns.

ALTERED SENSATION

Patients may complain of altered sensation, which is usually the result of neurological involvement. An attempt should be made to elicit a history of associated conditions (e.g., diabetic neuropathy, radiculopathy, laceration). Once again, the pattern of progression must be established. Specific inquiries should also be made about associated weakness.

LOSS OF FUNCTION

It is relatively easy to establish the effect of musculoskeletal dysfunction in a particular joint. Thus there may be a quantifiable loss of flexion or extension at the elbow. Many daily activities are recruited to assess integrated musculoskeletal function and to quantify disability. When assessing function at the hip, for example, patients are asked about their ability to cut their toenails, negotiate stairs, or get in and out of a car or how far they can walk. It is critically important to establish the extent to which the pain, deformity, and loss of movement are compromising the functions of the patient on a day-to-day basis. This must be assessed against the patient's social, professional, domestic, and recreational demands.

When loss of function is judged in these terms, it is highly individualized and linked with patient expectations. A painter with a family of four cannot confine himself to painting baseboards until the frozen shoulder in his dominant upper limb has resolved. He may demand aggressive treatment. A similar condition, however, in the nondominant shoulder of an inactive retiree may be of little inconvenience and require no treatment. Equally, moderate osteoarthritis of the hip might present an unacceptable disability to a middle-aged executive who finds it impossible to negotiate the corridor of an air terminal or board an aircraft. The same hip might constitute little or no disability in a septuagenarian who is a bridge fanatic and who never ventures much beyond the confines of the living room. It is therefore necessary to try to quantify the loss of function and disability based on realistic expectations and requirements identified by the patient. Only then can a rational decision be made regarding appropriate management.

EXAMINATION

Clinical examination is the second basis on which to form a diagnosis. A good history allows the formulation of a provisional diagnosis; a good clinical examination usually establishes the diagnosis, and special investigations are recruited for detailed confirmation. **It is bad practice to use the availability of sophisticated imaging techniques as a surrogate for a thorough clinical examination.**

This chapter can deal only with the generalities of examination of the musculoskeletal system. Specific clinical signs and tests will be detailed and dealt with on a regional basis later in the book.

It is essential that a structured routine be followed during the course of the examination. Only by always proceeding in a systematic way is it possible to avoid missing important clinical signs. The patient should always be suitably undressed to expose the involved area. If a limb is involved, the contralateral side should be exposed for comparison. It is usually wise to avoid immediately targeting the affected area, and to examine the uninvolved side first. This helps the examining physician to gain the confidence of the patient.

Simplicity remains the key to a systematic approach. First look (inspect), then feel (palpate), and then move.[2] This routine must embrace flexibility to cater for specific clinical situations. It may, for example, be necessary to move a swollen joint to be able to feel the joint margins.

INSPECTION

The patient should be carefully observed from the moment he or she sets foot in the consulting rooms. Observe the patient's general appearance, posture, and gait. Are the movements smooth and coordinated? Note any difficulty the patient has in getting in or out of a chair and on and off the examination couch and in undressing and dressing. Does the patient use trick movements to perform simple tasks?

Gait

Look at the symmetry of the gait and for any evidence of a limp. Pain from any source in a weightbearing lower limb will produce an *antalgic gait*. There is an altered gait cadence, and during the gait cycle the patient will spend less time on one foot than the other. With a *short-limb limp* the ipsilateral shoulder dips with weightbearing on the affected side. A *Trendelenburg gait* is characterized by the whole trunk swaying across the affected limb on weightbearing. Although the Trendelenburg gait is normally attributable to dysfunctional abductors, it should be remembered that it can accompany an antalgic gait with a painful hip where it represents an attempt to reduce the load across the hip joint. The functional integrity of the abductors can be assessed by the Trendelenburg test (Fig. 7). This can be performed in a variety of different ways, but it is important that the knee be flexed with the hip extended so that iliopsoas does not contribute to stabilization of the pelvis.

A stiff hip or a stiff knee will lead to an asymmetrical gait. An inability to heelstrike may be due to a fixed equinus deformity, foot drop, or a painful heel. Foot drop is obvious during the swing phase of gait, as the patient adopts a high-stepping gait and "flaps" the foot upward to

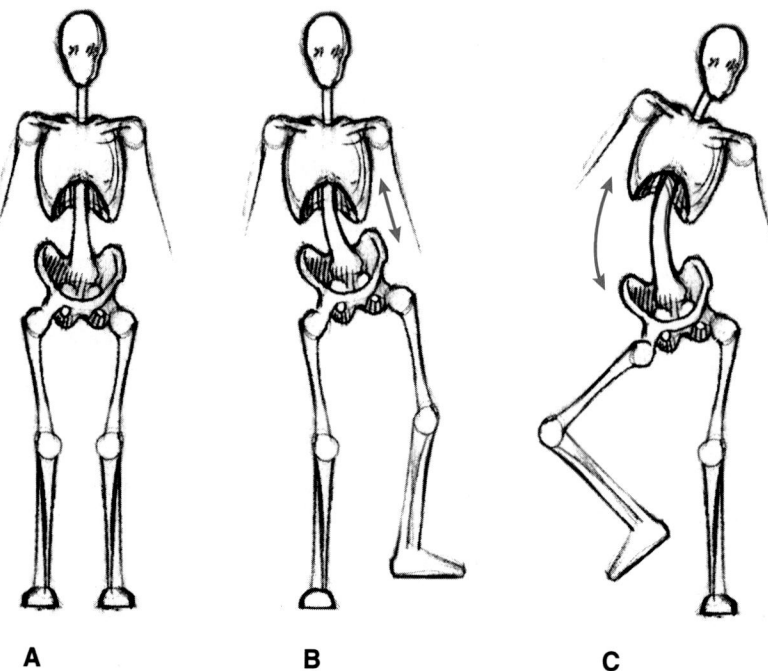

A B C

Fig. 7. Trendelenburg's sign. *A*, Standing on two legs. *B*, Standing on the right leg with normal abductor muscles. *C*, Standing on the left leg with dysfunctional abductors: pelvis drops to the opposite side, and the trunk swings over to the involved side to maintain balance.

obtain a plantigrade foot. When bilateral, it may be due to loss of position sense.

Deformities of the knee, foot, and ankle are often obvious as the patient walks. A flexion deformity of the hip may declare itself with a shortened stride length, whereas an adduction deformity may present with a short-limb gait.

Skin

The skin should be inspected for scars (surgical and traumatic), discoloration, and asymmetrical creases. The latter may denote contractures or, for example, scoliosis. A patch of hair at the base of the spine may identify the spinal dysraphism as the cause of a child's clubfoot, whereas café au lait spots signify the presence of neurofibromatosis. A patch of psoriasis or pitting of the nails may explain the presence of psoriatic arthritis.

The description by patients of little hard knobs, about the size of a pea, frequently seen on the fingers, and unsightly rather than inconvenient indicates Heberden's nodes,[3] the presence of which is highly suggestive of a primary polyarticular osteoarthritis with a familial predisposition.

Look for varicose veins or any other evidence of venous insufficiency.

Deformity

Deformity is defined by the Oxford English Dictionary as "bodily misshapenness or malformation." Thus any abnormality of shape or position may produce a deformity. It is important to try to ascertain whether the deformity is in the soft tissues, the bones, or the joints.

The *soft tissues* may be deformed by swelling, by scarring (i.e., consequent to ischemic necrosis of the muscles), by overgrowth, or, most commonly, by wasting. It is important to look for any asymmetry of muscle bulk, which denotes muscle atrophy.

Bones may be short, thickened, or bent. Thickening may occur following fracture healing or with chronic infective conditions. "Soft" bone (i.e., rickets in children, Paget's disease in adults) may bend, and malunited fractures may also produce obvious deformities. Tumors of any description may give rise to swelling (Table 5). *Joints* may be malaligned, or they may be held in an abnormal position because they lack full movement. Specific terms are used to denote specific deformities. Thus *varus* denotes a deformity in which the convexity of the malalignment is directed away from the midline, and *valgus* denotes a deformity that is directed toward the midline (Fig. 8). A kyphotic deformity of the spine is an excessive curvature of the spine, which is convex posteriorly, whereas a lordotic deformity is the reverse. Any curvature of the spine in a coronal plane represents a scoliosis. This is either fixed (or structural) and cannot be corrected by any movement or posture, or mobile (postural), where the curvature corrects on sitting or on lateral bending.

A fixed deformity of a joint occurs when it cannot be returned to its normal position. There are basically three causes of joint deformity:

1. Contracture of the juxtaposed soft tissue, which pulls the joint into an abnormal position. This occurs as a

TABLE 5. CAUSES OF DEFORMED BONES	
1	Malunited fracture
2	Growth plate injury
3	Metabolic bone disease (rickets, osteomalacia)
4	Congenital disorders (pseudarthrosis)
5	Paget's disease
6	Multiple exostosis

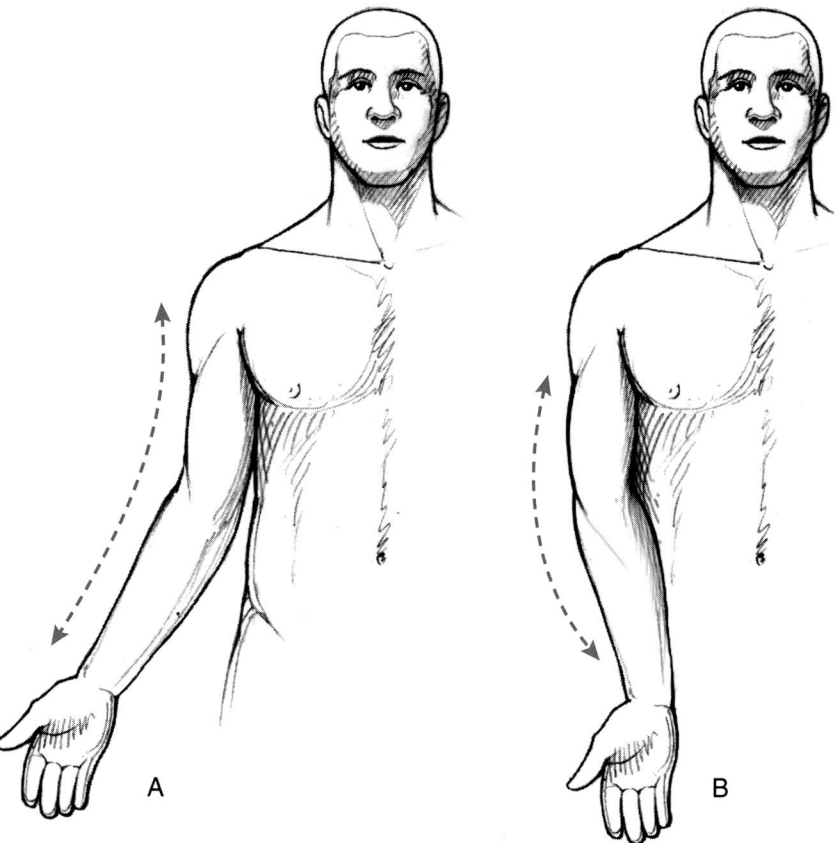

Fig. 8. Cubitus valgus and varus. *A*, Cubitus valgus: the convexity of the deformity is directed towards the midline. *B*, Cubitus varus: the convexity is directed away from the midline.

result of scarring, either of the skin (burns) or of the underlying muscles (ischemic necrosis).

2. Muscle imbalance. This may occur as a result of neuromuscular disorder or following tendon rupture.

3. Chronic arthritis, which results in periarticular fibrosis and joint destruction.

PALPATION

The soft tissues should not merely be kneaded haphazardly in the hope that thus abused they will yield their secret. They should be systematically palpated using the same routine each time. This routine should be based on a knowledge and understanding of the subjacent anatomy.

Feel the skin. Is it sweaty, dry, cold, or warm? Any mass should be carefully palpated to ascertain its consistency (hard or soft), attachment to underlying tissues (mobile or fixed), and whether it is well delineated or not. If the mass is tender, it may be infective or inflammatory. If it is soft, look for fluctuance. Remember that a lump near a joint is likely to be a tumor, and benign tumors frequently feel hard whereas malignant tumors often feel slightly soft with increased vascularity (prominent vessels may be visible on the overlying skin).

The exact site of tenderness should be carefully located while observing the patient's reactions. Precise localization of the tenderness will often provide the diagnosis. The knee perhaps provides a useful example of the benefit of systematic palpation looking for regional tenderness. Starting over the tibial tubercle (Osgood-Schlatter, infrapatellar tendinitis), one moves medially to the proximomedial flare of the tibia (pes anserinus bursitis) and up to the medial joint line. The substance and attachments of the medial collateral are palpated, as is the full extent of the joint line (e.g., for meniscal injury, arthritis). The presence of bony thickening at the joint margin is suggestive of osteophyte formation, whereas soft tissue swelling is probably synovitis. The suprapatellar pouch is then palpated, followed by the substance and proximal and distal attachment of the lateral collateral ligament. Finally, the iliotibial tract and Gerdy's tubercle (for iliotibial band syndrome) are explored (Fig. 9).

Transverse and longitudinal patellofemoral compressions are assessed for pain, and the reciprocal medial and lateral patellofemoral articulations are palpated for tenderness.

Muscles should be palpated for both tenderness and spasm. Spasm of the paraspinal muscles is often indicative of a back injury or a disk lesion and is often associated with an uncompensated scoliosis. A similar routine should be established for each joint and systematically followed.

It is also important to establish whether there is excess fluid in the joint (effusion). At the knee, clinical examination allows the effusion to be categorized as mild, moderate, or severe. The wipe or blow-out test, in which the fluid is wiped away from the medial parapatellar gutter before being milked back into it, will identify a collection of fluid of 10 to 20 mL. A patellar tap (balloting the patella on the underlying femur) indicates an effusion of 20 to 100 mL, while the hydrodynamic resistance of a larger

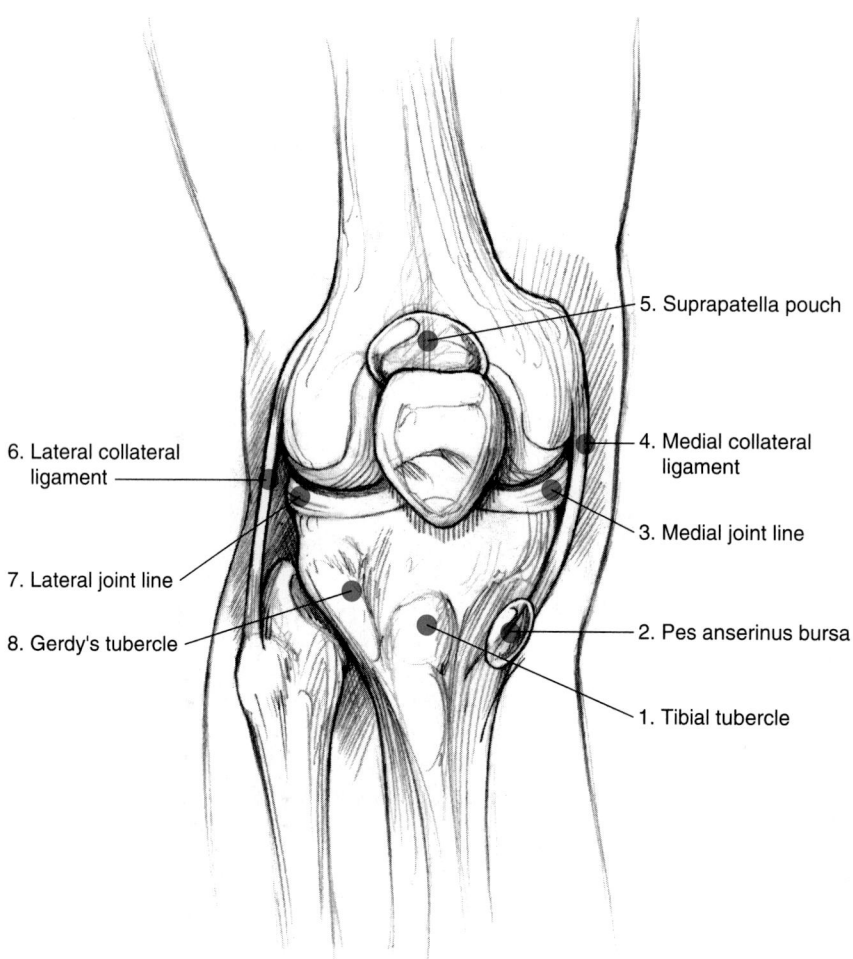

5. Suprapatella pouch

6. Lateral collateral ligament

7. Lateral joint line

8. Gerdy's tubercle

4. Medial collateral ligament

3. Medial joint line

2. Pes anserinus bursa

1. Tibial tubercle

Fig. 9. Systematic palpation of the tibiofemoral joint. 1. Tibial tubercle; 2. Pes anserinus bursa; 3. Medial joint line (tenderness/osteophytes, soft-tissue swelling); 4. Medial collateral ligament; 5. Suprapatella pouch; 6. Lateral collateral ligament; 7. Lateral joint line; 8. Gerdy's tubercle.

effusion resists balloting but permits cross-fluctuation (>100 mL).

MOVEMENT

It is the pain-free movement of stable joints that provides the integrated function of the musculoskeletal system.

Movements can be tested actively and passively. Any discrepancy between active and passive movement is probably attributable to pain or abnormal neuromuscular function (i.e., tendon rupture or muscle weakness). If any such dysfunction is suspected, it is important to test the full range of active movements and muscle strength. Function can be impaired by an intact but mechanically disadvantaged musculotendinous unit. Thus it is important to distinguish between a "dropped finger" due to a ruptured extensor tendon, and an inability to extend the metacarpophalangeal joint because of subluxation of the extensor tendon between the metacarpal heads. In the latter instance, the patient will be able to hold the passively extended finger in extension, as in this position the extensor tendon is restored to its functional position over the dorsum of the metacarpophalangeal joint (Fig. 10).

When testing the range of movement, it is important to ascertain the contribution of adjacent joints and muscles to limiting or concealing loss of movement or fixed deformities. Thus a tight gastrocnemius may limit dorsiflexion at the ankle. However, flexing the knee relaxes the muscle, with a resultant increase in the range of dorsiflexion. Equally, loss of abduction at the hip may be masked by compensatory movement of the pelvis. Pelvic bony landmarks should therefore be carefully monitored when testing for movements at the hip. A flexion deformity at the hip may be masked by excessive lumbar lordosis. Thomas' test flattens the lumbar lordosis and exposes the loss of extension (Fig. 11).

The range of movement should be recorded with the anatomic position as the neutral position. Excessive movement (i.e., hyperextension) should also be recorded. If it is present, it is important to note whether it is localized or generalized (indicating collagen abnormality).

When moving the joint one should feel for crepitus. This can be coarse and pain-free (of no significance) or a painful grating sensation. The latter is often indicative of bone-on-bone articulation. Fine crepitus felt over tenosynovial sheaths during movement of the adjacent joints usually denotes a tenosynovitis. This is often associated with a soft tissue swelling or a feeling of fullness.

Active movements load joints and may be of use in localizing the site of the symptomatic pathology. Degenerative changes in the spine and hip often coexist. If the hip is the source of pain, unilateral active straight leg raising

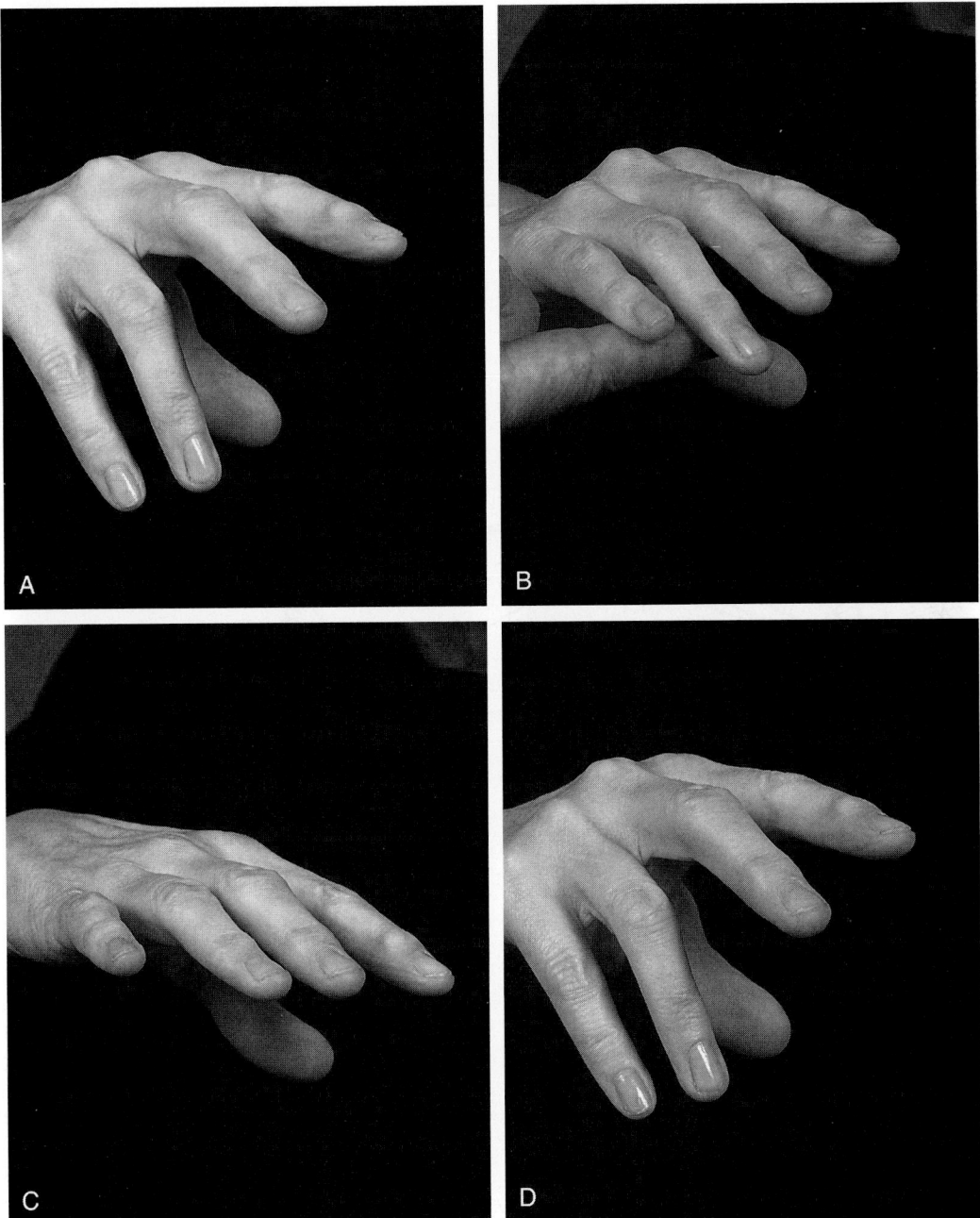

Fig. 10. MCP extensor lag. *A,* "Dropped" fingers. *B,* The fingers are passively extended. *C,* If the extensor tendons were subluxed, full extension restores them to their functional position on the dorsum of the metacarpophalangeal joint, and they are able to hold the finger extended. *D,* If the extensor tendons are ruptured, they "drop" again as soon as the support is removed.

loads the hip and will usually provoke pain in the groin. However, if the lower lumbar spine is the cause of the symptoms, bilateral active straight leg raising will place strain on the lumbosacral junction and cause pain in the lower back.

Symptoms may be provoked by derangement of intra-articular structures. Specific tests are designed to diagnose the pathology. Thus numerous rotation tests have been designed to trap abnormally mobile or torn fragments of menisci between two joint surfaces, thus causing either pain or a palpable clicking. The three most widely used

tests are the McMurray, the Apley, and the Steinmann tests.

If a joint is stiff, it is useful to discriminate between the loss of all movements, a reduction of all movements, and a limitation of only certain movements. Abolition of all movement is an indication of a fibrous or bony ankylosis. Reduced movement in all directions is indicative of a mechanical block, as in loss of full extension at the knee as a result of a torn meniscus. Loss of certain movements at the shoulder have persuaded rheumatologists to distinguish between a capsular and glenohumeral joint pattern.

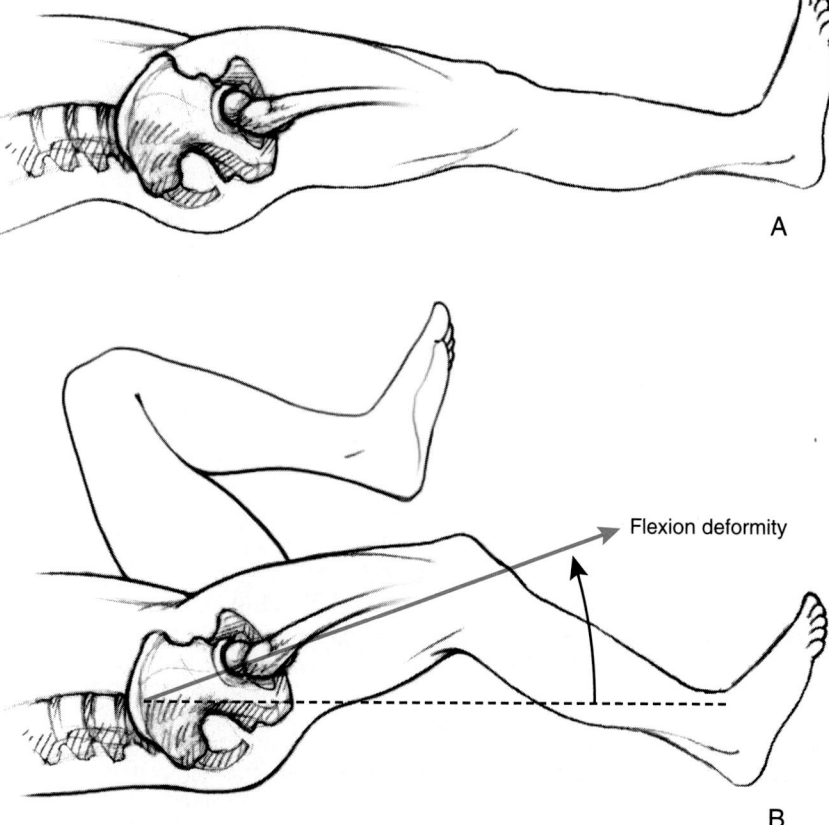

Flexion deformity

Fig. 11. Thomas' test. *A,* Flexion deformity. *B,* Fully flexing the contralateral hip flattens the lumbar lordosis and exposes the flexion deformity in the involved hip.

It is then necessary to examine the joint for abnormal out of plane movements. If present, these should always be compared with the contralateral side. Universal laxity is a sign of a connective tissue disorder. Abnormal movement in one joint suggests previous trauma with disruption of ligaments or loss of bone support. Poor muscle tone and control can also contribute to this type of instability. Specific tests are required to assess the integrity of the specific periarticular soft tissues that may have been damaged (Tables 6 and 7).

These issues will be considered in more detail in the chapters dealing with specific anatomical regions. It should be noted, however, that the clinical examination of laxity is highly subjective. Classifications (mild, moderate, severe) are therefore subject to different interpretations. It is preferable, if possible, to describe laxity as the estimated displacement at the joint margin (in millimeters).

If the joint is painful, it may be necessary to carry out an examination with the patient under anesthesia to assess structural integrity. The installation of local anesthetic may also be of assistance in assessing functional integrity. A

TABLE 6. LIGAMENT TESTS: THE KNEE		
Ligaments	**Test**	**Pathological Finding**
Cruciate ligaments Anterior (ACL) Posterior (PCL)	Anterior drawer	ACL rupture (± torn or lax posteromedial structures)
	Posterior drawer	PCL rupture
	Lachman's	ACL/PCL rupture
	Posterior sag	PCL rupture
	Pivot shift	ACL rupture
Collateral ligaments	Valgus stress in full extension	Medial collateral and secondary stabilizers ruptured
	Valgus stress in 30-degree flexion	Isolated rupture of medial collateral
	Varus stress	Lateral collateral rupture

TABLE 7. INSTABILITY TESTS: THE SHOULDER*	
Area of Instability	**Test**
Anterior	Anterior apprehension (arm placed in abduction and external rotation behind the coronal plane)
Posterior	Posterior apprehension (flexion and internal rotation)
Multidirectional	Anterior drawer Posterior drawer Sulcus sign (inferior laxity)

* These tests are best performed with the patient lying down.

patient may be reluctant to abduct his arm following an injury of the rotator cuff, making it is difficult to distinguish between discontinuity of the supraspinatus and reflex pain-mediated inhibition. However, if he is still unable to abduct the arm following abolition of the pain with local anesthetic, this finding is highly suggestive of a complete tear of the supraspinatus tendon.

NEUROLOGICAL EXAMINATION

It is probable that an orthopaedic surgeon will recruit the assistance of a neurologist for any complex neuromuscular problem. However, a thorough neuromuscular assessment is central to a complete examination of the musculoskeletal system. It is essential to be able to identify long tract signs (upper motor neuron lesion), diagnose nerve root and peripheral nerve lesions, and recognize progressive muscular dystrophy. Although some neurological lesions are characteristic, attempted movement often best defines the type and extent of the motor disorders. Upper motor neuron lesions result in undamped reflex contraction and spastic paralysis, whereas damage to the peripheral nerves (or anterior horn cells) causes flaccid paralysis.

UPPER MOTOR NEURON LESION

Any central lesion of the spinal cord can give rise to positive long tract signs. Many of these will fall within the domain of the neurosurgeon. However, the spinal cord can be damaged by trauma to the spine, and involvement of the upper cervical spine is exceedingly common in rheumatoid arthritis and is not infrequently associated with positive long tract signs. These signs include a somewhat ataxic gait, an upgoing plantar reflex (positive Babinski's sign), ankle clonus (sharp dorsiflexion causes repetitive clonic movement of the foot), increased muscle tone (not to be confused with the lead-pipe rigidity of Parkinson's disease), and brisk reflexes. Polyarticular involvement and peripheral neuropathies can make neurological examination particularly difficult in patients with rheumatoid arthritis.

NEUROMUSCULAR AND MUSCULAR DYSTROPHIES

There are a number of conditions in which progressive neuromuscular degeneration produces progressive paresis. There is no loss of sensation. It is important to test each muscle action, and to quantify the strength of the muscles involved. Muscle strength has been classified on a scale of 0 to 5. It has been customary for some time now to use the Medical Research Council scale for recording muscle power:

0   no contraction
1   flicker or trace of contraction
2   active movement with gravity eliminated
3   active movement against gravity
4   active movement against gravity and resistance
5   normal power

Subdividing grade 4 may be helpful: 4−, 4, and 4+ can be used to indicate movement against slight, moderate, and strong resistance, respectively.

Table 8 gives examples of common neuropathies and muscular dystrophies. Weakness of syndromically deter-

TABLE 8. COMMON NEUROPATHIES AND MUSCULAR DYSTROPHIES	
Neuropathies	**Muscular Dystrophies**
Hereditary 　Peroneal muscle atrophy (Charcot-Marie-Tooth disease) 　Friedrich's ataxia 　Hereditary sensory neuropathy Acquired 　Diabetic neuropathy 　Herpes zoster 　Neuralgic amyotrophy 　Leprosy (still common in Africa and Asia)	Duchenne muscular dystrophy Limb girdle dystrophy Fascioscapulohumeral dystrophy

mined groups of muscles often gives rise to characteristic deformities. The high arch, varus heel, and wasted calf are, for example, typical of peroneal muscular dystrophy.

It is only by retaining the awareness of the possibility that an early diagnosis of these conditions can be made by a careful and thorough examination.

NERVE ROOT LESIONS

Nerve root lesions can usually be identified by the sensory deficit in the specific dermatome and motor weakness in the relevant myotome. The deep tendon reflex (elicited by rapidly stretching the tendon near its insertion) controlled by the involved nerve root is suppressed or absent. Thus a depressed biceps jerk would be suggestive of pressure on the fifth or sixth cervical nerve, whereas an absent knee jerk is associated with a L3-4 lesion.

It is important for the orthopaedic surgeon to know which nerve roots innervate the different muscle groups.

Sensory testing should include light touch, pain, two-point discrimination, and position sense. Position sense (together with vibration sense and stereognosis, the ability to recognize shape and texture) is used to test deep sensibility. The pathways for deep sensibility run in the posterior columns of the spinal cord, and disturbances are therefore found with spinal cord lesions and peripheral neuropathies. It is well recognized that the area of skin supplied by a nerve root or a peripheral nerve will vary from patient to patient. However, it is essential to be familiar with the common dermatomes and with common sensory distribution of peripheral nerves (Fig. 12).

It should be recognized that sensibility to touch and to pinprick may be increased (hyperesthesia, occurs in irritative nerve lesions), decreased (hypoesthesia), or absent (anesthesia).

PERIPHERAL NERVE INJURY

Peripheral nerves may be involved in neuropathies (e.g., diabetic, vasculitic), entrapment syndromes, and direct trauma. Carpal tunnel syndrome is the most common entrapment syndrome. It is characterized both by symptomatic presentation (night pain, pain in the median distribution of the hand) and by altered sensation in the radial 3½ digits. There may be wasting of the thenar mus-

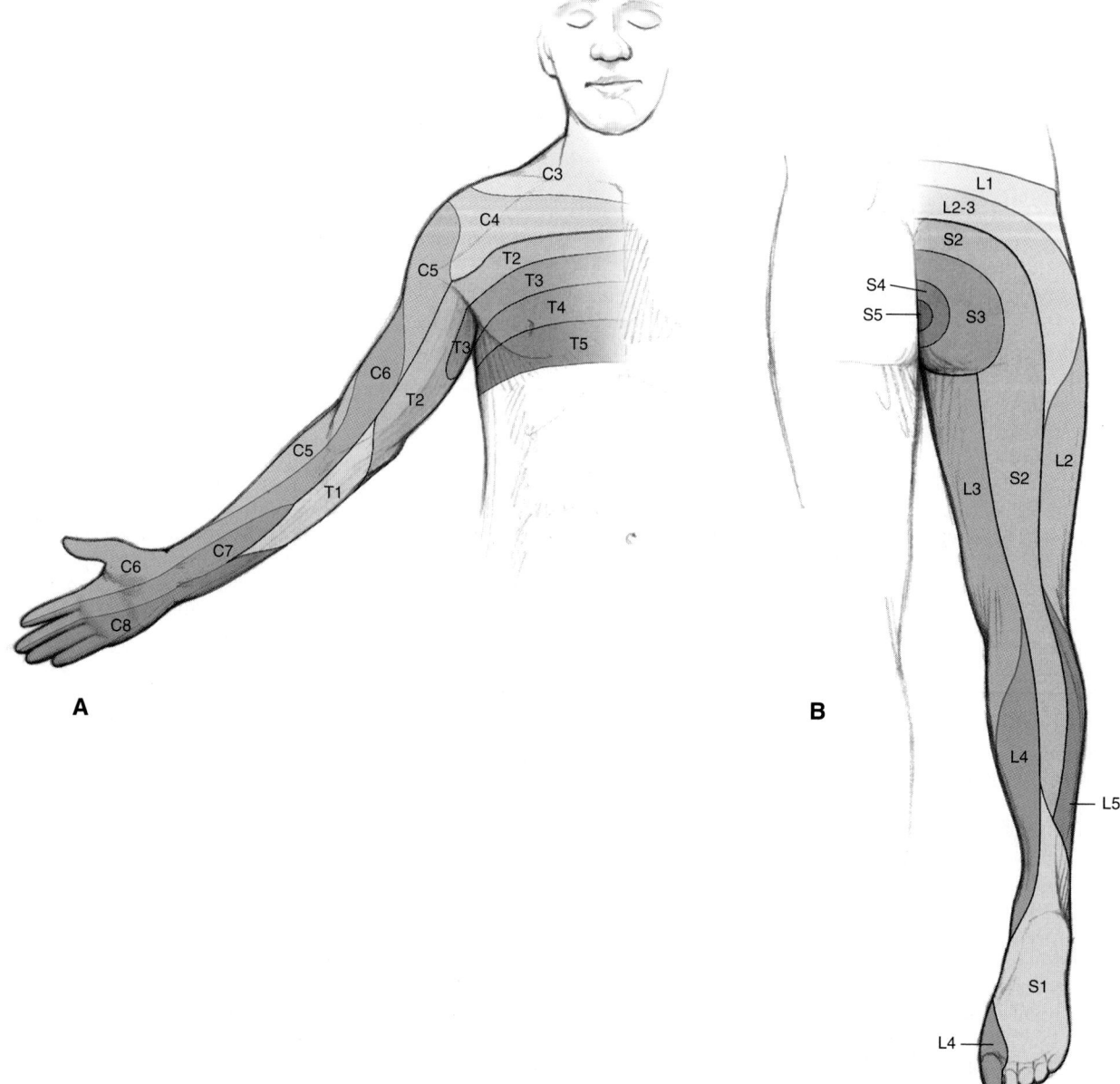

Fig. 12. Approximate distribution of dermatomes. *A,* The anterior aspect of the upper limb. *B,* The posterior aspect of the lower limb.

cles and weakness of the abductor pollicis brevis. Certain tests may provoke the symptoms (e.g., Tinel, Madonna, Phalen).

Other entrapment syndromes occur at the elbow (median, ulnar, and posterior interosseous nerves) and at the ankle (tibialis posterior nerve). The symptoms and motor and sensory signs generally provide the diagnosis.

Peripheral nerves may be damaged by laceration or at the time of fractures. Look for any scars. Some nerve injuries produce postures that are diagnostic—the ulnar claw hand, the simian hand of a distal median and ulnar nerve lesion, wristdrop following a radial nerve palsy, and so on. Inspection may reveal trophic changes, ulcers that

refuse to heal, or scars of old burns, all signifying a loss of sensibility. The skin is often smooth and hairless, and there may be trophic changes of the fingertips and nails.

Localized and asymmetrical muscle wasting suggests dysfunction of a specific motor nerve. The paralysis is flaccid. In testing for muscle action, it is important to palpate for muscle contraction.

CONCLUSION

The preceding is a brief overview of examination of the neuromuscular system. It remains important, however, that when appropriate the orthopaedic surgeon can summon the clinical skills to expose early neuromuscular abnormalities, as these often represent the precursors of important and potentially disabling disorders.

I believe that a detailed history and clinical examination establishes a rapport with the patient and represents the first move toward securing the patient's confidence. A good doctor/patient relationship remains the cornerstone of successful clinical practice. It has been our neglect of these basic tenets—which have been superseded by a reliance on sophisticated imaging technologies—that has driven so many patients to seek help from nonmedical practitioners. Let us return to the basics, use technology appropriately, and preserve our status as clinicians and surgeons, not merely technicians.

REFERENCES

1. Souter WA: Planning treatment of the rheumatoid hand. The Hand, vol 2. 1979; 3:16.
2. Apley AG, Solomon L: Apley's System of Orthopaedics and Fractures, 7th ed. Oxford, Butterworth-Heinemann, 1993, p 8.
3. Heberden W: Commentaries on the History and Cure of Diseases. Classics of Medicine Library, Division of Gryphon Editions Ltd, Alabama, 1982, p 148.
4. Arnett FC, Edworthy SM, Block DA: The American Rheumatism Association 1987 revised criteria for the classification of rheumatoid arthritis. Arth Rheum 1988; 31:315.

section 1 chapter 2

ANESTHESIA FOR PEDIATRIC PATIENTS UNDERGOING ORTHOPAEDIC PROCEDURES

Todd J. Troshynski and Steven J. Weisman

Summary
- The need for an anesthetic as part of a procedure to correct a pediatric musculoskeletal problem is common.
- Frequent upper respiratory tract infections are a frequent issue in the pediatric patient.
- The increasing frequency of asthma is a special challenge for administering a child's anesthetics.
- Children who need an orthopaedic operation are especially likely to have a latex allergy, which often leads to anaphylaxis.
- The younger the child, the more likely is a serious anesthetic complication (cardiac arrest or death).
- Regional anesthesia is much less useful in children than in adults.

Many children undergo some type of orthopaedic surgical procedure prior to maturity. These procedures make up a significant and sometimes large percentage of cases performed in most children's hospitals and in other hospitals where children are treated. The majority of these children are healthy, but many of them have coinciding medical illnesses or conditions. These illnesses or conditions may range from a simple upper respiratory tract infection to the most complex congenital heart disease.

The purpose of this chapter is to provide a general approach to providing perioperative medical care and anesthesia applicable to all children undergoing orthopaedic surgical procedures. Also, in this chapter we consider the impact of a number of illnesses and conditions that are likely to occur in pediatric patients and provide approaches to the care of children with these conditions. We discuss some special situations and topics applicable to the perioperative care of children undergoing orthopaedic procedures.

PREOPERATIVE EVALUATION

HISTORY AND PHYSICAL

Every child scheduled for surgery should have a basic history and physical examination, even though many are otherwise healthy. This should include a medical history and review of systems as well as a physical examination concentrating on evaluation of the airway, cardiac, and respiratory systems. The preoperative evaluation must take into consideration the child's physical as well as psychological health and developmental well-being, because all of these aspects may affect the postoperative course.

The evaluation should begin with a perinatal history. Premature birth is a frequent cause of morbidity in children. As improved methods of ventilation and the use of exogenous surfactant have become widespread, increasing numbers of survivors of premature birth return into the health care system for further care. These children may have suffered morbidity to any organ system as a consequence of their prematurity. Central nervous system abnormalities may include cerebral palsy, seizure disorders, hydrocephalus, and apnea of prematurity. They may have lung disease resulting in bronchopulmonary dysplasia (chronic lung disease occurring in premature infants secondary to exogenous surfactant deficiency and mechanical ventilation). They may have cardiac disease secondary to their lung disease or as a result of congenital heart disease. Children with a history of premature birth also have a higher incidence of hypertension than their full-term counterparts. They have a higher incidence of gastroesophageal reflux and other gastrointestinal abnormalities as well.

The medical history should include questions about medical illnesses, surgical history, medications, allergies, and previous anesthetics. Particular attention should be paid to cardiac and respiratory illnesses. Any history of congenital heart disease should be noted in detail, including the original diagnosis, any procedures the child has undergone to correct or palliate the defect, and information regarding cardiac function as well as data from cardiac catheterizations or echocardiograms. Many children with congenital heart disease will, as a result of shunting of blood, have lower blood oxygen saturation than their normal counterparts. Therefore, children with congenital heart disease should have their usual oxygen saturation recorded while breathing room air and while at rest at their preanesthetic visit. Patients with complex lesions or serious cardiac illness should have their anesthesia care provided by anesthesiologists experienced in the care of these patients. It is often helpful to consult with the child's cardiologist before surgery to help further delineate cardiac function and reserve.

A thorough history of anesthetics and surgical procedures should be included in the preoperative evaluation. Any history of difficulty in managing the airway is essential to note in detail. This includes difficulty with the mask airway as well as difficulty with intubation. If a difficult intubation has occurred in a previous anesthetic at the same institution, the prior records should be studied in detail so that techniques that failed previously are not repeated. If the parents indicate that there was difficulty with airway management at a different hospital, attempts should be made to obtain a copy of the anesthetic record via fax. In either case, it may be helpful to discuss with the anesthesiologist of record for the previous case the details of the difficult airway management. A history of unexpected severe bleeding should also be noted and a coagulation study work-up performed and a hematologist consulted, if necessary for history of postoperative nausea and vomiting. Antiemetics can be given prophylactically. Of course, any family history of malignant hyperthermia or the presence of atypical pseudocholinesterase should be sought.

ASTHMA/UPPER RESPIRATORY TRACT ILLNESS

Important respiratory illnesses occurring in children include asthma and upper respiratory tract viral infections (URTIs). Cystic fibrosis is a less common but more severe illness. Asthma is a disease that is relatively common in children and has become more prevalent in the past 10 years. Preoperative evaluation for a child with asthma should include an assessment of the severity of the illness. For example, the number of hospitalizations and the level of care required for these admissions can provide information about the severity of the asthma. It is also important to note the medications used for treatment and their frequency of use. The most common medication used by asthmatics is inhaled β-agonists, such as albuterol. Any recent or chronic use of corticosteroids should be noted, because "stress" doses may be required during surgery. Children with a history of asthma and a current URTI should probably not be anesthetized for elective surgery because they are at increased risk for bronchospasm and other respiratory complications.

The presence of URTI in a child about to undergo an anesthetic and surgical procedure sometimes results in controversy regarding whether or not the case should be canceled. Clearly, there are risks associated with providing an anesthetic for these children. The risks of laryngospasm, bronchospasm, postoperative croup (primarily in younger children), atelectasis, pneumonia, and postoperative oxygen requirement are increased for a child with a URTI. However, some children have such frequent URTIs that there are only infrequent times during which some URTI symptoms are not present. Young children average about six to nine URTIs per year. If they attend day care or live with parents who smoke, the incidence may even be higher. Any URTI may also be accompanied by lower respiratory tract involvement, although this might not be clinically obvious. Lower airway edema and increased secretions may contribute to bronchospasm, cough, and atelectasis. Signs of lower respiratory tract involvement include productive cough, bronchospastic or brassy cough, wheezing, rales, and rhonchi. What appears to be the onset of a URTI may actually be the prodromal stage of a more serious systemic viral or bacterial infection. Fever, lethargy, decreased activity level, and decreased appetite are all early signs of systemic illness, as is purulent nasal discharge. For purely elective procedures, any sign of lower respiratory involvement (productive or bronchospastic cough, wheezes, rales, or rhonchi) or onset of systemic illness should result in cancellation of the case.

Lower respiratory involvement may not clear for 6 to 8 weeks once symptoms are resolved. However, the children can generally be rescheduled in 3 to 4 weeks. Children with uncomplicated URTI (no lower respiratory tract symptoms) are seldom turned away when they present for elective procedures. Some anesthesiologists would avoid, when possible, intubation of the trachea in these children, opting instead for either a mask anesthetic or the use of a laryngeal mask airway as appropriate.

CYSTIC FIBROSIS

Children with cystic fibrosis present some special problems for the anesthesiologist. Cystic fibrosis, transmitted by an autosomal-recessive gene, occurs in about 1 in 2000 live births among Caucasians. This disorder is characterized by obstruction of exocrine glands and abnormal secretion of mucus and electrolytes. This primarily affects the lungs, gastrointestinal tract, and pancreas. Information quantifying the child's pulmonary function is important to establish a baseline and to determine the child's suitability for surgery. Recent pulmonary function testing is ideal. If these data are not available, evaluation of several other clinical data points, such as room air oxygen saturation (compared with baseline), activity level, and physical examination may have to substitute. Consultation with the child's physician (pediatrician or pulmonologist) is necessary both to determine where the child is compared with baseline and to arrange for assistance in postoperative management. There is no specific anesthetic technique recommended for the care of cystic fibrosis patients. Any technique that allows the patient to return as quickly as possible to preoperative respiratory function is preferred.

ALLERGY

Allergies to specific medications must be identified and those medications avoided. If possible, specific information about the exact nature of any allergic reaction must be obtained. Of course, once a medication allergy is identified, it is relatively simple to avoid the allergic reaction by avoiding the medication. Latex allergy occurs as a result of exposure to latex-containing products and a hypersensitivity response to repeated exposures. The reaction may range from mild skin erythema to a full-blown anaphylactic reaction with severe bronchospasm and cardiovascular collapse. Patients at risk for the development of latex allergy include all children with neural tube defects and children with congenital urologic abnormalities, who require frequent or chronic bladder catheterization. Exposure to latex should be avoided in these at-risk patients. Patients who have had full-blown anaphylactic reactions to latex should probably be premedicated with histamine (H_1 and H_2) blockers and corticosteroids before proceeding to the operating room, although this has become somewhat controversial. Obviously, exposure to latex, especially powdered latex gloves, should be strictly avoided for patients at risk for latex allergy, especially those who have had a documented reaction to latex. We usually attempt to schedule these patients as the first case of the day when possible to avoid any latex exposure from previous cases in the same room.

PREOPERATIVE EVALUATION FOR PAIN MANAGEMENT

An additional consideration during the preoperative evaluation is some discussion with the patient and family regarding plans for postoperative pain management. If the use of patient-controlled analgesia (PCA) is being considered, the patient should receive preoperative instruction in how to use the PCA pump, so that this information does not have to be processed by the patient in the initial postanesthetic time period. Also any discussion about the use of any regional anesthetic techniques should be discussed with the family at this time.

RISK OF ANESTHESIA

Parents will often ask about the risk of anesthesia during the preoperative surgical visit. Discussion of the specifics of anesthetic risk is probably best left to the anesthesiologist. It is unwise to quote outdated data gathered before the current era of monitoring in anesthesia. The American Society of Anesthesiologists (ASA) Closed Claims Project showed a clear decrease in respiratory system damaging events, brain damage, and death when comparing claims from 1975 and 1978 with those submitted after 1990. This coincides with changes in the ASA Standards for Basic Anesthetic Monitoring[1] that included the addition of pulse oximetry (January 1, 1990) and capnometry (January 1, 1991).

As in adults, the age of the patient is a consideration affecting perioperative risk. However, the youngest patients are at greatest risk; children younger than 1 year are at the highest risk. The Pediatric Perioperative Cardiac Arrest (POCA) registry, started in 1994 and continuing through the present date, has also followed this trend.[2] In fact, POCA data indicate that the cardiac arrest incidence and death rate can be further delineated by age and indicate that those children younger than 1 month have the highest incidence of cardiac arrest, the highest mortality per cardiac arrest, and the highest rate of mortality per anesthetic. POCA data also conflict with the Closed Claims study in cause of death. In the Closed Claims data, the cause of arrest was respiratory 43% of the time, whereas in the POCA data respiratory events accounted for only 9% of arrests. Once again, the decreased fraction of respiratory cause for cardiac arrest is probably a function of changes in monitoring practice.

So what is the "risk of death" for a child undergoing an anesthetic? This is difficult to ascertain. The POCA data indicate a cardiac arrest rate of 2.8 per 10,000 anesthetics. This is the incidence of cardiac arrest, not the incidence of death. Also, the incidence of cardiac arrest was much less in ASA I–II patients older than 1 year compared with ASA III–V patients younger than 1 year. In addition, the incidence of death, when cardiac arrest occurs, is much higher at age less than 1 month than in children 1 to 5 months of age and much less in children older than 1 year. Accurate numbers for perioperative mortality and morbidity in children are then quite difficult to estimate. For previously healthy children, the risk of an adverse event is probably about 1:200,000 anesthetics.[3]

LABORATORY STUDIES

With few exceptions, children undergoing procedures with little risk of blood loss have no need for preoperative laboratory studies. One possible exception is that all young women who have begun menstruating should have a urine or blood pregnancy test. Routine urinalysis is neither helpful nor cost effective. A routine complete blood count (CBC) is also not helpful. Laboratory studies should be tailored to the medical condition of the patient and the nature of the procedure. For example, a healthy patient scheduled for a femoral or pelvic osteotomy should probably have a preoperative hematocrit level check to serve as a baseline in case of greater than expected bleeding, but no other studies are needed. Patients with a history of anemia should have a baseline hematocrit. Patients with renal failure should have electrolyte, blood urea nitrogen, and creatinine measurement and a CBC. Routine coagulation studies are not needed unless there is a history of bleeding problems. An example of this is the scoliosis patients undergoing spine fusion who should have a CBC, coagulation studies, and a crossmatch, so that crossmatched blood will be available in the likely event of significant blood loss. In the past, many anesthesiologists used unproven guidelines requiring hematocrit levels of 30% or more for children before anesthesia and surgery. Fortunately, these guidelines are no longer followed, and the need for blood during surgery is quite rare in children. Certainly, complicated procedures such as open heart surgery or spine fusions have specific reasons for the frequent need for blood products, but even these children are now routinely taken to surgery with hematocrits below 30%. In children who weight 40 kg or more, it is also possible to collect blood preoperatively for autologous blood transfusion. The "directed donation" of blood by family members is another method of blood procurement aimed at reducing, at least theoretically, the risk of transmission of viral disease.

FASTING GUIDELINES

In the past, all patients were placed on orders of "nothing by mouth (NPO) after midnight" regardless of age. Out of concern for the comfort of younger patients and in an effort to avoid hypoglycemia or hypotension resulting from hypovolemia in infants, many clinicians advocated lesser NPO times, at least for infants and younger children. In fact, in a 1990 editorial, Charles Coté recommended investigation of the practice of preoperative fasting. Many institutions have since developed more liberal fasting guidelines.[4] However, because different institutions have responded to this in different ways, we find that there is little uniformity among institutions regarding fasting guidelines for children.[5] In most institutions, ingestion of clear fluids 2 to 4 hours preoperatively is acceptable. Hospital policies regarding time intervals between consumption of breast milk, formula, and solid foods and surgery vary among institutions, although no institutions allow solid foods less than 6 hours before surgery. In 1999, the ASA published practice guidelines[6] that are summarized in Table 1. The Medical College of Wisconsin uses guidelines that are similar but slightly more conservative.

PREOPERATIVE MEDICATIONS

Children undergoing anesthesia and surgery understandably are anxious before coming to the operating room. Currently, many, but not all, institutions provide anxiolytic preoperative medication for all children older than about 8 months who present for surgery. The most commonly used preoperative medication used for children is midazolam.[7] Typically, 0.5 mg/kg is given, up to a maximum dose of

10 to 15 mg 20 to 30 minutes before surgery. Sometimes teenagers respond better to oral diazepam, 5 to 10 mg given about 1 hour before coming to the operating room. Another choice for preoperative medication is oral ketamine (5 to 10 mg/kg).

Other institutions make use of "parent-present inductions," in which one parent is present while the child undergoes induction of anesthesia, usually via inhalation technique. This is done in induction rooms, if they are available, or in the operating room if they are not. Parent-present inductions are still considered controversial. Although it seems that the presence of a parent would attenuate anxiety, a 2000 study by Kain et al showed no difference in anxiety between midazolam premedication alone and midazolam plus parent-present induction.[8] Still, in carefully selected cases, having a parent present may be helpful for the child undergoing induction of anesthesia.

INDUCTION OF ANESTHESIA

In children, the technique chosen for induction of anesthesia depends on the child's age, NPO status, medical condition, and preference. In younger children, the most common technique used is inhalation induction. This is usually accomplished with either halothane or sevoflurane along with a mixture of nitrous oxide and oxygen. The child breathes this mixture at increasing concentrations until sleep is induced. At that point, an intravenous cannula is placed. If intubation of the trachea is planned, a neuromuscular blocking drug may be given. One advantage of this induction technique is that the patient does not have to tolerate intravenous placement while awake. The major disadvantage is that there is a significant period of time during which airway reflexes are obtunded, but the airway is not protected. Clearly, inhalation induction is not an option in patients with a full stomach.

Patients presenting with orthopaedic emergencies are most often considered to have "full stomachs." Either the NPO time is not sufficient or the patient is considered to have increased gastric acid secretion and delayed gastric emptying because of stress associated with the injury. Although the length of NPO time required before a patient is considered not to be at risk for aspiration is controversial, most clinicians accept that a patient should have been NPO for at least 6 to 8 hours before anesthesia and surgery. In emergency cases, in which patients may not be NPO for the recommended length of time or the patient may have a full stomach, a rapid-sequence induction should be used. Classically, this is accomplished with a hypnotic drug such as sodium thiopental, propofol, or etomidate along with the depolarizing neuromuscular blocking agent succinylcholine. Because of the rare occurrence of malignant hyperthermia or bradycardia with succinylcholine, it is now indicated only for emergency management of the airway or for rapid management of the airway when risk of aspiration is considered to be high. In young children, atropine should be administered before using drugs including the newer agents, rocuronium and rapacuronium.

Of course, for older pediatric patients, an intravenous induction may be the best choice. This can be accomplished using any induction drug (e.g., thiopental, propofol,

TABLE 1. AMERICAN SOCIETY OF ANESTHESIOLOGISTS GUIDELINES FOR FASTING BEFORE SURGERY	
Ingested Material	**Minimum Fasting Period (Hours)**
Clear liquids	2
Breast milk	4
Infant formula	6
Nonbreast milk	6
Light meal	6

etomidate, midazolam, ketamine) and any neuromuscular blocking drug. With an intravenous catheter already in place, most anesthesiologists would choose an intravenous induction. When an intravenous induction is preferred but no catheter is in place, starting the intravenous administration can be made more tolerable by applying a combination of lidocaine and prilocaine (EMLA) cream or using iontophoretic lidocaine at potential intravenous sites. Also, the inhalation of nitrous oxide mixed with oxygen can help to facilitate intravenous placement.

MAINTENANCE OF ANESTHESIA

Techniques and medications for maintenance of anesthesia are based on the type and length of the procedure and on the patient's medical condition. Most children do well with the use of volatile anesthetic agents. Alternatively, primarily intravenous-based anesthetics can be very useful. In the case of spine fusion surgery, an anesthetic technique that is primarily opioid based, typically with remifentanil, fentanyl, or sufentanil, provides excellent hemodynamic stability. In addition, an opioid-based technique is a good choice when the depth of anesthesia must be adjusted rapidly, as when a "wake-up" test is required.

Patients with poor cardiac reserve as a result of complex congenital heart disease or cardiomyopathy also benefit from the hemodynamic stability that is characteristic of a primarily opioid anesthetic technique. Remifentanil is particularly useful for these patients and has the advantage of a very short duration of action, providing precise hemodynamic control.

The use of primary regional anesthetic techniques has become quite common in adult orthopaedic surgery. Procedures such as fixation of hip fractures performed with a spinal anesthetic, replacement of a knee or hip with an indwelling epidural catheter, or a carpal tunnel release under Bier block anesthesia are performed frequently. Unfortunately, most children are developmentally unable to cooperate for such "awake" anesthetics. In addition, there is no evidence that there is any safety advantage of pure regional anesthesia in children over general or combined general/regional techniques. Therefore, the use of regional techniques is mainly directed at improving postoperative pain management. The range of possible techniques is from simple combinations of peripheral nerve blocks to neuraxial techniques. It is possible to perform brachial plexus blocks for upper extremity procedures using long-acting local anesthetics, such as bupivacaine. These techniques can provide excellent pain relief for as long as 24 hours. Femoral nerve blocks or combinations of nerve blocks (three-in-one block or fascia iliaca compartment block) can be used to provide postoperative pain control for procedures involving the femur or the knee. Epidural analgesia can also be used for pain relief for lower extremity procedures using either catheter techniques, when several days of analgesia are anticipated, or "single-shot" techniques. Epidural analgesia can be provided with low concentrations of local anesthetics combined with an opioid analgesic (usually morphine or hydromorphone) so that the amount of motor block is minimized.

MONITORING

Appropriate monitoring for pediatric patients begins with the use of a precordial stethoscope. This simple device allows direct assessment of both heart tones and breath sounds. When a precordial stethoscope cannot be used, such as in the prone position, an esophageal stethoscope can substitute. Electrocardiographic monitoring, pulse oximetry, capnometry, temperature monitoring, blood pressure monitoring at least every 5 minutes, and monitoring of inspired oxygen concentration are all part of the ASA standards for monitoring and should be used in every case.

When considerable blood loss is anticipated, an arterial catheter should be placed for continuous hemodynamic monitoring as well as the ability to easily sample blood for laboratory evaluation. Central venous catheters are rarely indicated. Patients with congenital heart disease or with cardiomyopathy may benefit from monitoring central venous pressure. Also, a central venous catheter may be required if peripheral access is difficult.

PAIN MANAGEMENT

Consideration of postoperative pain management is a part of any anesthetic plan. It is essential to provide regularly scheduled analgesic administration and not utilize as-needed dosing. It is also essential to avoid painful techniques for delivery of analgesia in children. In fact, young children will decline painful intramuscular injections, even though they have severe pain. Therefore, postoperative analgesia should be administered intravenously, orally, or by some other regulated regional technique. A very popular method for providing postoperative pain control for orthopaedic patients is patient-controlled analgesia (PCA), which has the advantage of providing the patient with a potent analgesic (usually morphine, hydromorphone, or fentanyl) and in a way that they can use with some degree of self-regulation. Clearly, this is an advantage compared with methods in which patients have to wait for an individual dose to be administered by nursing staff. Most patients report good pain control with this method. Effective use of PCA is limited by the developmental stage of the patient. As a general rule of thumb, patients must have the cognitive capabilities of a normal 7- to 8-year-old to use PCA effectively. In some circumstances, responsibility for drug administration can be delegated to a nurse or parent.

As mentioned, regional anesthetic techniques may be extremely useful in providing for pain control in the postoperative period. Epidural analgesia can be provided for many extensive orthopaedic procedures, including clubfoot repair, femoral or tibial osteotomy, and even spine fusion procedures. Although theoretical concerns may exist regarding difficulty with evaluating peripheral nerve function while using epidural analgesia, the fact is that, by using low concentrations of local anesthetics along with epidural opioids, one can avoid dense motor blockade. Also, epidural opioids can be used alone with no resultant motor block. Epidural analgesia can be provided as a continuous infusion or with a "patient-controlled" option.

REFERENCES

1. Cheny FW: The ASA closed claims project: Lessons learned. In Annual Refresher Course Lectures. City, American Society of Anesthesiologists, 1995, p 422.
2. Morray JP: Pediatric arrest stats kept in National Registry. APSF Newsletter 1998.
3. Eichorn JH: Effect of monitoring standards on anesthesia outcome. Int Anesthesiol Clin 1993; 31:181.
4. Coté CJ: NPO after midnight for children— A reappraisal. Anesthesiology 1990; 72:589.
5. Ferrari LR, Rooney FM, Rockoff MA: Preoperative fasting practices in pediatrics. Anesthesiology 1999; 90:978.
6. American Society of Anesthesiologists: A Report by the American Society of Anesthesiologists Task Force on Preoperative Fasting. Anesthesiology 1999; 90:896.
7. Feld LH, Negus JB, White PF: Oral midazolam preanesthetic medication in pediatric outpatients. Anesthesiology 1990; 73:831.
8. Kain ZN, Mayes LC, Wang SM, et al: Parental presence and a sedative premedicant for children undergoing surgery. Anesthesiology 2000; 92:939.

section 1

chapter 3

ANESTHETIC AND PERIOPERATIVE MANAGEMENT OF THE GERIATRIC PATIENT

G. Alec Rooke and John Amory

Summary
- Patients older than 65 years of age undergo orthopaedic surgery twice as often as those younger than 65 years of age.
- Twenty percent of elderly patients will have at least one complication postoperatively.
- Although age and comorbidity both contribute to complications, the combination results in a dramatic increase in the rate of complications.

"My diseases are an asthma and a dropsy and, what is less curable, seventy-five."

Samuel Johnson

AGE AND PERIOPERATIVE RISK

Adults older than 65 years of age undergo orthopaedic surgery at twice the rate of those younger than 65 years, are more likely to have comorbid illness, and account for a disproportionate number of postoperative deaths. The good news, however, is that surgical mortality rates have fallen dramatically over the last 40 years for all ages, and some evidence suggests that elderly patients who survive surgery outlive their counterparts.[1] Nevertheless, almost 20% of elderly patients will have at least one complication postoperatively and upward of 3% of elderly patients will die within 30 days of surgery.[2] These data suggest, particularly for orthopaedic surgery, that mortality invariably involves organ systems not subjected to surgery. The aging process decreases organ physiological reserve, as will be discussed shortly. Age-related disease is also important, as it further compromises organ function. In fact, the interaction of age-related disease and physiological aging may contribute more to perioperative complications than either factor by itself. If one examines healthy adults, age is associated with only a small increase in the perioperative complication rate (Fig. 1).[3] The presence of chronic disease increases risk at any age, but the combination of old age and chronic disease results in very high complication rates.

This observation suggests that the decrease in physiological reserve by normal aging primarily contributes to risk when superimposed on medical illness.

THE MEDICAL CONSULT

Given the influence of aging and disease on outcome, the preoperative medical consult may provide the best mecha-

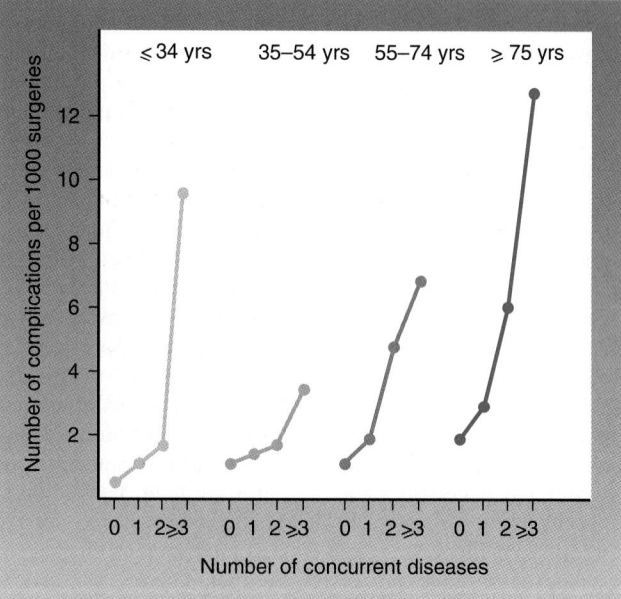

Fig. 1. The interaction of age and concurrent disease is demonstrated in this figure. This figure shows 268 major complications that occurred during or within 24 hours of 198,103 surgeries. Data are stratified by patient age bracket and by the number of chronic illnesses present at the time of surgery. When zero or one illness was present, age had only a modest effect on complication rate, but at two or more illnesses the complication rate became heavily dependent on age. (Modified from Tiret L, Desmonts JM, Hatton F, et al: Complications associated with anaesthesia—a prospective survey in France. Can Anaesth Soc J 1986; 33:336.)

CLINICAL RELEVANCE

- Preoperative medical consultations may provide the best mechanism to decrease morbidity if problems are identified *and* managed.
- Communication among orthopaedist, anesthesiologist, and internist is paramount in treating the ill elderly patient.
- Physiological response to anesthesia changes dramatically with age.
- Postoperative analysis is important and requires close monitoring to prevent complications.

nism to reduce perioperative risk. Unfortunately, this opportunity is frequently lost because of a poor understanding of the goals of the medical consult by all parties involved. Sometimes it seems as if the only purpose is to "keep anesthesia from cancelling the case." The goal of preoperative care is to bring the patient to surgery in the most optimal condition possible, regardless of which service performs the preparation.

There are five components to complete perioperative medical care (Table 1). A medical consult becomes necessary only when the orthopaedist or the anesthesiologist desires assistance with one or more of the components. If scheduling permits, an anesthesiologist should see the patient well in advance of surgery, as this meeting provides an opportunity for the anesthesiologist to add to the list of issues to be addressed by the medical consult. After our medical center instituted an anesthesiology preoperative clinic that includes both anesthesiologists and a general internist, the number of consult requests to the cardiology section decreased by more than 80%. When a consult is requested, the consultant should receive explicit instructions regarding both the components of Table 1 and the illnesses for which help is requested. Specific requests allow the consultant to concentrate on the areas of need and not waste time on extraneous issues or be left with nothing better to write than "Patient with stable angina. Cleared for surgery. Thank you for this interesting consult."

The first component is a good history and physical examination with emphasis on historical highlights and the current status of each problem. The next issue is to decide whether further evaluation is needed. If so, the timing of these tests sometimes becomes an issue. If surgery is impending, the temptation will be to postpone the test until after surgery. An argument can be made for performing the tests before surgery, even if this postpones surgery, if the information obtained would influence perioperative care or provide significant information about the medical status of

TABLE 1. COMPONENTS OF THE PREOPERATIVE MEDICAL EVALUATION

1. History and physical examination with problem-oriented assessment
2. Further evaluation as needed
3. Risk stratification
4. Optimization of medical status prior to surgery
5. Perioperative management of medical illness

the patient. Clinical judgment is necessary to balance the disadvantages of delaying surgery against the benefits of the additional information. The best solution to this awkward situation is to prevent its occurrence, and the ability to send the patient to a preoperative clinic in advance of surgery can markedly reduce cancellations.

The third component of the medical consult is risk stratification. This process includes the decision as to whether the benefits of surgery warrant the risks. A good example of risk stratification plus recommendations for evaluation is the American College of Cardiology/American Heart Association guidelines for cardiac disease discussed later in the chapter. Occasionally a patient will be found whose risk is high enough to question the benefits of surgery. Whenever any one of the caregivers, be it surgeon, internist, or anesthesiologist, raises this concern, the best solution is for all three parties to share their individual evaluations and assessments and come to a consensus. It is not uncommon for one of the three parties to over- or underestimate the concerns of either or both of the other two parties. For example, it is quite common for internists to have a poor understanding of the stress of a particular surgery. In this regard, anesthesiologists are pretty good at anticipating the stress of a particular surgery after working with a surgeon for a while, but they can be misdirected if the surgeon plans something unusual that is not reflected in how the case is booked. Ideally such sharing of information would occur for all patients, but on a practical basis the three-way conversation may be needed only for the most difficult patient. Once a consensus is reached, the medical opinion needs to be shared with the patient. Ultimately, it is the patient's decision, and only the patient can determine what constitutes acceptable risk.

Unfortunately, medical consults often seem to end after the risk has been assessed, especially if the perceived risk is low. This endpoint constitutes the proverbial "clearing" of the patient for surgery, and as such represents a failure to proceed to the most important part of the consult: optimization of the patient's medical status. No one argues the importance of improving the condition of a serious medical problem, but why not at least consider trying to make the "low risk" patient even better? If we believe that improved medical status reduces risk, then we should endeavor to have every patient present to surgery in the most optimal condition. One provocative study took 148 elderly patients scheduled for major surgery, all of whom had been "cleared" by an internist.[4] Shortly before surgery the patients underwent an extensive physiological evaluation, including the gathering of pulmonary artery catheter data. Patients with no abnormalities (13.5%) had no further intervention and underwent surgery without mortality. Patients with minor baseline abnormalities, patients with major abnormalities that improved to normal, and patients with minor abnormalities after treatment constituted the bulk of the patients (63.5%). This group underwent surgery with a 8.5% mortality rate. Of the patients with major abnormalities who failed to improve with therapy (23%), those who had their surgery canceled or for whom a minor surgery was substituted all survived. There were, however, eight patients with major physiological abnormalities who did not improve with treatment and who, nevertheless, underwent major surgery. All eight died.

The last component of the medical consult involves the intraoperative and postoperative management of medical illnesses, many of which become exacerbated by surgical stress. Management is often best left to physicians who treat such illnesses as a matter of routine. This approach is especially important if the patient has an unusual disease, in which case the consultant can also help educate both the surgeon and the anesthesiologist. For unusual illnesses, or diseases that are particularly difficult to manage, the orthopaedist, anesthesiologist, and internist should discuss medical management before surgery. Postoperatively, the orthopaedist may choose to have the consultant manage some or all of the patient's medical illnesses.

A final comment about the medical consult is in order. Sometimes consultants are inclined to make recommendations about invasive monitoring, anesthetic management, and the intraoperative management of medical illnesses. Anesthetic management should be left to the anesthesiologist, however, and it is in the best interest of the patient for the orthopaedist to not let the consultant dictate the anesthetic plan. It is a mistake for the consultant or orthopaedist to put the recommendation in writing. First of all, there may be considerations of which the consultant or orthopaedist is unaware. Second, regional anesthetics may fail, and a general anesthetic may have to be instituted. Third, division of opinion in the medical record is a bad idea from a medicolegal point of view. If the consultant or orthopaedist is concerned about issues that involve intraoperative care, an anesthesiologist needs to be involved in the decision-making process. Two- and three-way discussions with consensus prior to note writing will go a long way to preserving a collegial and friendly atmosphere among the specialties and will ultimately result in optimal patient care.

PERIOPERATIVE MANAGEMENT OF MEDICAL ILLNESS

A comprehensive review of medical disease is beyond the scope of a single chapter. Nevertheless, it is worth reviewing a few aspects of selected medical problems that are common to the elderly.

CARDIAC RISK STRATIFICATION

Cardiac risk stratification identifies patients at increased risk for major cardiac complications such as myocardial infarction, ventricular dysrhythmias, and cardiac death. Risk stratification allows for better informed consent and preoperative planning. Until recently, cardiac risk stratification has been accomplished by the use of clinical risk indices, which compute scores based on the presence or absence of certain clinical, electrocardiographic, and laboratory parameters. Models of this type have been validated as predictors of cardiac risk in several populations, although they share a flaw in their inability to predict postoperative events in the large numbers of patients with low scores.[5]

Recent guidelines for perioperative cardiovascular evaluation for noncardiac surgery were published jointly by the American Heart Association and the American College of Cardiology.[6] These guidelines divide patients into two groups: those who can proceed directly to surgery and those who may require further cardiac testing. These guidelines are based on a stepwise bayesian approach that incorporates clinical markers of cardiac disease, prior cardiac evaluation, surgery-specific risk, and a patient's functional capacity.

The algorithmic representation of these guidelines, modified slightly for orthopaedic surgery, is reproduced in Figure 2.

Most major orthopaedic procedures are classified as intermediate surgical risk (cardiac risk 1% to 5%). Superficial procedures such as carpal tunnel repair are considered low risk and rarely require cardiac testing unless a patient has a "high risk" clinical predictor (Fig. 2). Functional status is best ascertained by direct testing in the clinic. As a rule of thumb, a patient who can climb one flight of stairs without stopping has a functional capacity of greater than 4 METs (metabolic equivalents). With clinical predictors of cardiac risk and functional status, the clinician can make the decision about the need for further cardiac testing prior to surgery. This approach is somewhat conservative, reflecting both the power of functional capacity to predict successful outcomes[7] and evidence that preoperative angiography and revascularization are appropriate for a very small number of patients who mostly meet criteria for revascularization independent of their need for surgery.[8]

The patient with an implanted pacemaker or cardioverter/defibrillator should be thoroughly evaluated prior to surgery. Pacemaker function should ideally be checked within a month of an operation, and arrangements for deactivating an implantable defibrillator should be made, as electrocautery devices may trigger unnecessary discharges.[9]

NONCARDIAC RISK STRATIFICATION

Postoperative pulmonary complications account for 40% of all complications and up to 20% of postoperative deaths. Risk factors for pulmonary complications include resting hypoxemia or hypercarbia, obesity, dyspnea, smoking, and pulmonary or upper abdominal surgery.[10] Pulmonary function testing is often performed preoperatively and can be helpful as a baseline for later comparison, but its ability to stratify patients undergoing surgery other than lung resection is poor.[11] Smoking cessation can reduce the rate of pulmonary complications if undertaken more than 8 weeks prior to an operation, but the improvement is small unless many months transpire to permit maximal pulmonary mucosal recovery.

Renal disease itself is an uncommon cause of perioperative mortality; however, it is a frequent cause of morbidity, especially in an elderly population. Most perioperative renal dysfunction results from acute tubular necrosis due to hypovolemia or nephrotoxic drugs.

Cirrhosis of the liver, if severe, carries a markedly increased perioperative mortality. In patients with Child's stage A or B cirrhosis, operative mortality is usually less than 10%. Child's class C disease, however, is associated with upwards of 50% mortality.[12]

HIP FRACTURES

Approximately 250,000 hip fractures occur annually in the United States and are associated with appreciable morbidity and mortality. In a Medicare population, the mortality rate was 7% at 1 month and 13% at 3 months.[13] In addition to routine concerns, these patients are at increased risk of

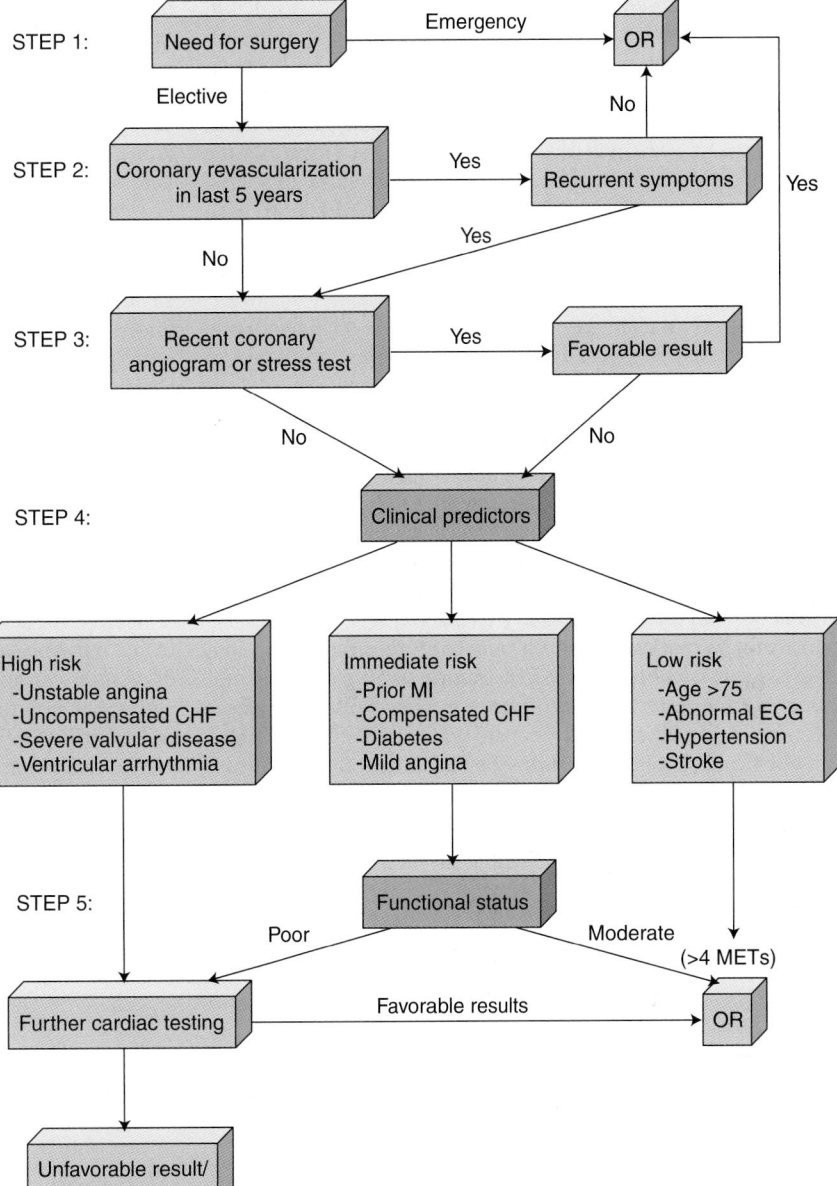

Fig. 2. American Heart Association/American College of Cardiology guidelines. Guidelines for the preoperative evaluation and management of patients undergoing noncardiac surgery as modified for orthopaedic surgeries. The algorithm first examines whether the patient has had coronary testing and, if so, the current symptomatology. Patients without clear evidence of absent disease are then categorized by their clinical predictor profile and functional status to determine if further evaluation is necessary. (Modified from ACC/AHA Guidelines for perioperative cardiovascular examination for non-cardiac surgery. Circulation 1996; 93:1278.)

postoperative delirium, subsequent falls, and malnutrition. Many authors feel that surgical repair should be undertaken in 24 to 48 hours of the injury, but this is not an absolute, and a medically unstable patient should be aggressively medically managed prior to surgery with particular attention to hypovolemia and the hematocrit level.

There are several other points that must be made about these patients:

- All patients should receive prophylactic antibiotics and the dose should be given 0 to 2 hours prior to surgery.
- All patients should receive thromboembolic prophylaxis unless contraindicated.
- Indwelling Foley catheters should be removed within 24 hours.
- Sedative-hypnotics and drugs with anticholinergic effects should be avoided.

- Electrolyte levels should be maintained within normal ranges.
- Exercise and balance training should be undertaken.
- Early mobilization can be done safely in the appropriate circumstances.

MANAGEMENT OF CARDIAC DISEASE IN THE PERIOPERATIVE PERIOD

No anesthetic agent or technique has been associated with clear-cut reductions in cardiac morbidity or mortality rates.[14] Furthermore, until recently, there was no cardiac medication proven to prevent perioperative myocardial ischemia. The prophylactic administration of medications such as nitrates, calcium-channel blockers, and digitalis has not been shown to be beneficial. However, recently a trial of atenolol administered for 7 days beginning the day of surgery showed statistically significant reductions in death, heart failure, angina, and the need for revascularization at 6 and 12 months postoperatively.[15] Contraindications to perioperative β-blockade include evidence of current congestive heart failure (e.g., rales, jugular venous distention), bronchospasm on physical examination, or third-degree heart block on the electrocardiogram. Given the low cost and substantial benefit of this intervention, perioperative β-blockade should be strongly considered in any patient with known coronary disease or substantial risk factors for coronary disease.

Severe valvular heart disease, especially critical aortic stenosis, poses a significant risk to a patient undergoing surgery. Mortality rates for critical aortic stenosis are upward of 13% and should prompt consideration of valve repair prior to elective surgery. Less critical degrees of stenosis can be managed with close hemodynamic monitoring and maintenance of sinus rhythm, as these patients tolerate hypovolemia and atrial fibrillation poorly.

MANAGEMENT OF NONCARDIAC DISEASE IN THE PERIOPERATIVE PERIOD

Most elderly patients with chronic lung disease have some degree of reversible airway constriction even if they do not have overt asthma. Bronchodilator therapy with inhaled β-agonists and anticholinergics are safe and effective and should be used liberally, with special attention to administering them shortly before induction of anesthesia. A brief course of corticosteroids should be considered for patients with recent worsening of their breathing. Any significant subjective worsening warrants delay of elective surgery until improvement to baseline is achieved.

Pneumonia is the most common postoperative complication, occurring in upwards of 6% of surgical patients postoperatively. Patients are subject to typical causative organisms as well as being at risk of aspiration pneumonitis due to anesthesia, sedation, decreased mucociliary clearance of the lung, and decreased gag and cough reflexes. The antibiotic treatment of postoperative pneumonia should be based on the most likely organism until culture provides identification. In complicated or severe pneumonia, medical consultation is highly advisable.

Malnutrition is associated with increased surgical morbidity and mortality rates; however, interventions that improve nutritional status rarely have dramatic beneficial effects. Nevertheless, there is some improvement from measures such as protein supplementation and nocturnal nasogastric feedings. Such interventions should be reserved for the patients with severe malnutrition who may benefit the most.[16] A serum albumin level of less than 2.5 g/dL and physical examination should help identify patients at risk. Even if improvement cannot be achieved prior to surgery, treatment can begin promptly, thereby minimizing the adverse consequences of postoperative negative nitrogen balance imposed on an already nutritionally compromised patient.

PERIOPERATIVE CHANGES IN CHRONIC MEDICATIONS

Most chronic medications can and should be continued during the perioperative period. Notable exceptions include aspirin (hold for 7 days before surgery), nonsteroidal anti-inflammatory drugs (3 days' abstinence) and of course, Coumadin (see later discussion). Diabetic medications (metformin, sulfonylureas, insulin) should be held as of the day of surgery. Ticlopidine, dipyridamole, pentoxifylline, and clopidogrel should probably be held for 7 days before surgery. In the majority of diabetic patients, oral agents can be safely restarted when the patient resumes eating. Metformin should not be resumed until at least 48 hours after the surgery and after kidney function has been reevaluated. Insulin will often need to be given during surgery, especially with type I diabetic patients or otherwise brittle diabetic patients. The patient on chronic corticosteroid therapy should be managed with "stress-dose steroids" for any major operation. The most frequently used dose is 100 mg of hydrocortisone 30 minutes prior to surgery and every 8 hours for three doses. This can be rapidly tapered over the next 2 days, after which the patient can resume preoperative corticosteroid dosing.

The management of anticoagulation for patients on long-term anticoagulants in the perioperative period was recently reviewed.[17] The approach is to balance the risk of bleeding from intravenous heparin with the benefits provided by prevention of thromboembolic disease afforded by anticoagulation. For most indications, including atrial fibrillation, recurrent thromboembolic disease and even the presence of mechanical heart valves, Coumadin can be held for four doses prior to surgery without the need for intravenous heparin. The exceptions to this approach are those patients with recent (within 3 months) thromboembolic events such as pulmonary emboli, deep venous thrombosis, or arterial embolism. In these patients, the benefits of intravenous heparin in the prevention of further thromboembolic events may outweigh the risks.

PROPHYLAXIS OF WOUND INFECTIONS

Prophylactic antibiotics are used in most surgeries. They are most effective when administered prior to surgery, and their efficacy decreases if given too early or too late. In most orthopaedic patients, cefazolin is a good choice. Vancomycin should be reserved for the patient with documented allergies to cephalosporins.

THROMBOEMBOLIC PROPHYLAXIS

Without prophylaxis, deep vein thrombosis would occur in upwards of 50% of patients undergoing total joint replacement or hip fracture repair. Several recent trials have demonstrated the relative superiority and ease of administration of low-molecular weight heparins, such as enoxaparin, to *fixed-dose* heparin and Coumadin, although *adjusted-dose* heparin and Coumadin remain reasonable alternatives.[18] The recommended doses are 30 mg SQ of enoxaparin twice daily starting 12 hours after surgery or 40 mg SQ once daily starting 10 to 12 hours before surgery (see also Anticoagulation and Neuraxial Block).

INTRAOPERATIVE CONSIDERATIONS

Aging alters virtually every organ system of the body. These changes influence the response to anesthesia, invaria-

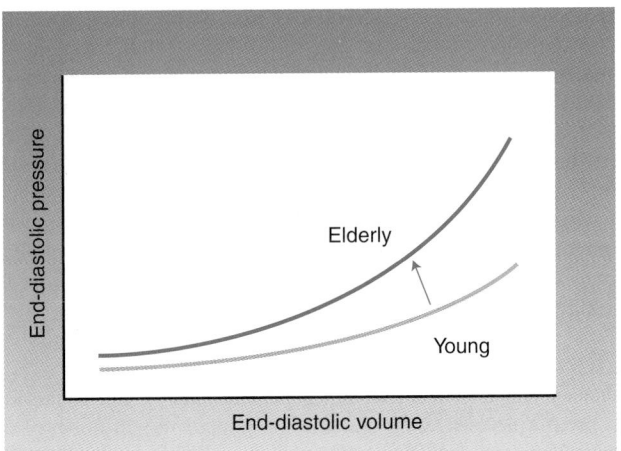

Fig. 3. Schematized illustration of the change in the passive end-diastolic volume/end-diastolic pressure relationship with age. Due to myocyte death without replacement, connective tissue changes and the increase in systolic pressure, the left ventricle becomes more stiff with age. This change requires end-diastolic pressure to be higher than in a young adult to achieve the same end-diastolic volume. (Modified from Rooke GA, Robinson BJ: Cardiovascular and autonomic aging. In Dauchot PJ, Cascorbi H [eds]: Management of the Elderly Surgical Patient. Problems in Anesthesia, vol 9, no 4. Philadelphia, Lippincott-Raven, 1997, pp 482–497.)

bly in a negative way. The physiology of aging is reviewed briefly along with comments on how anesthetic and postoperative management can be complicated by the changes.

CARDIOVASCULAR SYSTEM

The key changes to the cardiovascular system are a decreased response to β-receptor stimulation and connective tissue stiffening of the arteries, veins, and myocardium.[19] What does not change in the healthy elderly patient is the strength of the cardiac muscle, that is, the ability of the ventricles to eject blood against pressure in the aorta or pulmonary artery. The decreased response to β-receptor stimulation translates into a lesser increase in heart rate and contractility whenever exogenous catecholamines are administered or the sympathetic nervous system is activated by the baroreflex, exercise, or pain. Arterial stiffening alters the arterial waveform and places a strain on the left ventricle at the end of ejection due to late systolic hypertension. This strain causes hypertrophy that leads to a slowed contraction and a slowed ventricular relaxation. When the ventricle relaxes slowly, the early phase of diastolic filling diminishes and the ventricle must depend more on the atrial pressure to push blood into the ventricle. In extreme cases, the atrial pressure may increase to high levels and cause symptoms of heart failure. This phenomenon, termed *diastolic dysfunction*, can occur even in the absence of impaired contractility (systolic dysfunction). In fact, diastolic dysfunction with normal or nearly normal systolic function accounts for half the cases of heart failure in patients older than 75 years of age.

The limited response to β-receptor activation increases the dependence on the Frank-Starling (length-tension) relationship for cardiac muscle. The elderly heart must remain more "full" than its younger counterpart. Keeping the heart full, however, requires increased atrial pressures because of impaired ventricular relaxation and increased stiffness due to hypertrophy and connective tissue changes (Fig. 3).[20] To maintain an adequate atrial pressure, central blood volume must be preserved. The systemic veins are responsible for buffering changes in blood volume and shifts in the distribution of blood throughout the body. Unfortunately, connective tissue changes stiffen the veins, too, and make it more difficult to maintain a constant blood volume to the heart. Hypovolemia is particularly poorly tolerated, as demonstrated in Figure 4.[21]

Changes in blood volume and variable fluid resuscitation are common during major orthopaedic surgery. In addition, during general anesthesia sympathetic nervous system activity can increase or decrease depending on the balance between the surgical stimulation and the depth of anesthesia. Changes in sympathetic tone cause changes in vascular resistance, heart rate, and venoconstriction. Increased sympathetic tone leads to hypertension by increased vascular resistance and increased cardiac output by raising heart rate and contractility and shifting blood from the periphery to the heart. If sympathetic tone decreases, the reverse occurs and blood pressure decreases, often precipitously. The elderly generally exhibit greater changes in sympathetic tone than young people, and the consequences of the changes in vascular filling and blood distribution are more dramatic

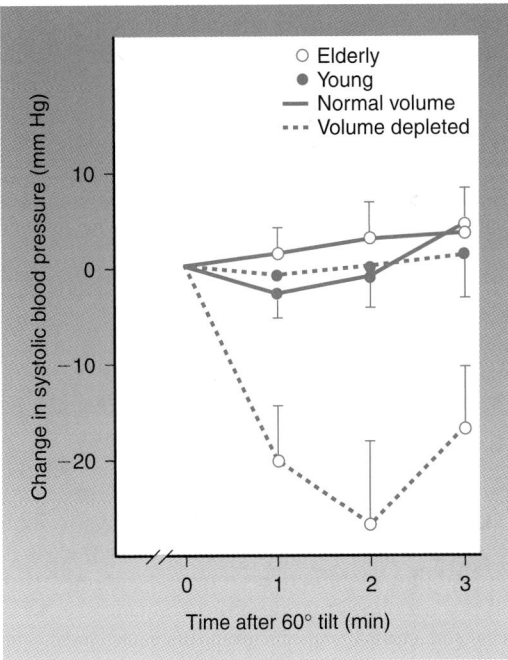

Fig. 4. Demonstration of the sensitivity of healthy elderly to volume depletion. When subjected to a tilt test in a state of normal hydration, both young and old adults exhibited tight blood pressure stability. After 2 days of restricted fluid intake and diuretic induced salt loss, the young adults still demonstrated good blood pressure control. In contrast, the elderly subjects suffered significant decreases in systolic blood pressure to levels associated with postural hypotension. (Modified from Shannon RP, Wei JY, Rosa RM, et al: The effect of age and sodium depletion on cardiovascular response to orthostasis. Hypertension 1986; 8:438.)

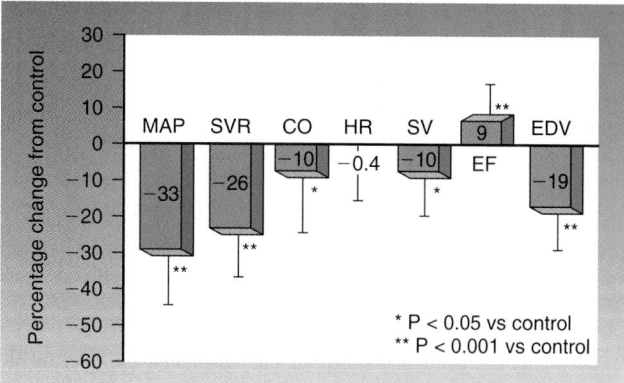

Fig. 5. Spinal anesthesia produces major hemodynamic changes in elderly men with a history of cardiac disease. MAP = mean arterial pressure, SVR = systemic vascular resistance, CO = cardiac output, HR = heart rate, SV = stroke volume, EF = left ventricular ejection fraction, EDV = left ventricular end-diastolic volume. Levels of spinal blockade high enough to cause total or near total sympathectomy produced major decreases in blood pressure, primarily from a decrease in SVR and not so much from decreases in CO. Blood distribution shifted from the heart (EDV) to the legs and abdomen (data not shown), but the expected decrease in SV was lessened by the increase in the EF. (Modified from Rooke GA, Freund PR, Jacobson AF: Hemodynamic response and change in organ blood volume during spinal anesthesia in elderly men with cardiac disease. Anesth Analg 1997; 85:99.)

than in young adults. Stability of blood pressure is difficult to achieve during general anesthesia, and the elderly therefore demonstrate more hypotension and greater blood pressure lability during anesthesia than do young adults.[22, 23] During general anesthesia, one approach to this problem is to use large amounts of opioid and less gas anesthetic. This permits a high depth of anesthesia to be present at all times that will block the periods of high surgical stimulation, yet not depress the blood pressure as much as a pure gas anesthetic would during periods of low surgical stimulation. Sometimes a high depth of anesthesia is deliberately applied, and fluid, α-agonists such as phenylephrine, or mixed agents such as ephedrine, dopamine, or epinephrine are used to support blood pressure. During spinal anesthesia, much or even all of the sympathetic tone is eliminated (Fig. 5).[24] The ensuing hypotension often requires therapy, but the blood pressure is less labile because sympathetic tone cannot change very much. Once the blood pressure has been stabilized after the onset of the spinal anesthetic, subsequent hypotension is usually due to hypovolemia and can be easily recognized and treated. Nevertheless, the inherent instability of blood pressure and volume status during surgery accounts for the more frequent use of arterial catheters and central venous or pulmonary artery monitoring in the elderly.

RESPIRATORY SYSTEM

Unlike the cardiovascular system, in which connective tissue stiffening occurs, the lungs lose elastin and actually become more compliant with age (Fig. 6).[25] The loss of "springiness" has a deleterious effect on the small airways that are dependent on the pull of the surrounding tissue to hold them open. At any given stretch of the surrounding

tissue, the pull on the airways is less, so the lungs must be more inflated to achieve the minimum stretch to keep the small airways from collapsing. General anesthesia is associated with a decrease in end-expiratory lung volume and a decrease in pull on the airways. This problem is handled by the use of controlled ventilation with large tidal volumes so that all the airways become open during at least a portion of the respiratory cycle. Postoperatively, supplemental oxygen is commonly required to maintain arterial oxygenation. Even after leaving the recovery room, hypoxia is a common problem in the elderly.

URINARY SYSTEM

One of the best-known aging phenomena is the reduction in creatinine clearance and the associated reduction in renal drug elimination. Less well appreciated is a decrease in the ability to retain salt and urine when hypovolemic and a decreased ability to eliminate free water. Central nervous system changes contribute to elderly people's diminished fluid homeostasis through a decreased sensation of thirst. Coupled with the fact that the elderly are often taking diuretics, it is not surprising that they are prone to hypovolemia. Volume resuscitation becomes an important aspect of preoperative preparation, especially after a fracture that can lead to internal bleeding as well as decreased mobility with poor oral intake.

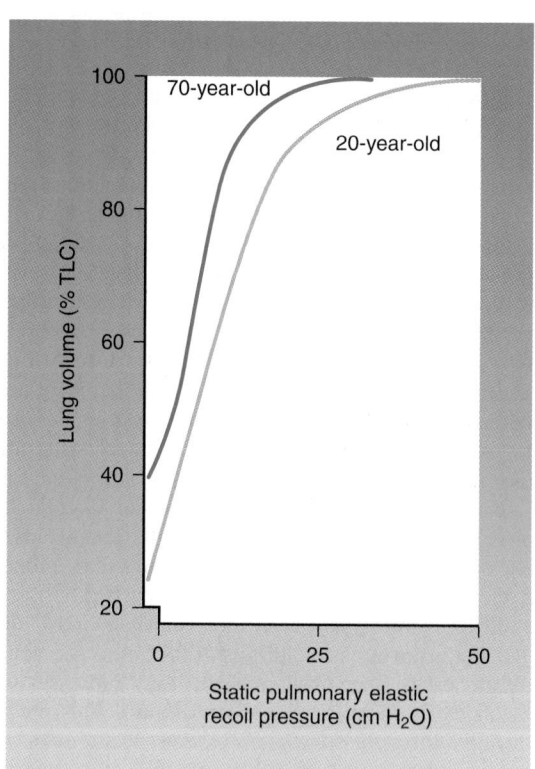

Fig. 6. Aging increases pulmonary compliance. Improved ease of inflation with age is actually deleterious because the tethering of small airways decreases. If the lungs do not remain adequately inflated, the small airways collapse and cause atelectasis, shunt, and hypoxia. (Reprinted from Wahba WM: Influence of aging on lung function: Clinical significance of changes from age 20. Anesth Analg 1983: 62:764.)

TEMPERATURE REGULATION

With age comes a gradual reduction in metabolic rate and therefore less heat production. There is also a decrease in the ability to vasoconstrict that compromises heat retention. For these reasons, elderly patients are particularly prone to hypothermia during surgery. All patients are challenged in the operating room by a cold environment. Isoflurane, sevoflurane, and spinal anesthesia vasodilate the skin, further compromising heat conservation. All gas and some intravenous anesthetics have central nervous system effects that further impair temperature regulation by lowering the body temperature necessary to trigger vasoconstriction and shivering. Hypothermia has serious adverse consequences, including a fourfold increased risk of morbid cardiac events and a threefold increase in wound infections (in a study of abdominal surgery).[26, 27] The use of warming devices such as forced-air blankets represent a significant advancement, but care must still be taken with respect to a cold operating room, evaporative heat loss from the preparation, and cold irrigating solutions.

ANESTHETIC AGENT ADMINISTRATION

Elderly patients require lower levels of gas anesthetic to achieve the same depth of anesthesia. The residual effects of gas anesthetics take longer to wear off as well. Almost every intravenous anesthetic drug can also be expected to have a greater effect on the elderly, but often for different reasons. The initial effects of most anesthetic intravenous drugs dissipate not by metabolism, but by shifting the drug into fat and therefore out of the central nervous system. The therapeutic goal (e.g., unconsciousness, analgesia) is only achieved during the time that the drug is moving from blood to fat (redistribution phase). Ultimately the drug is released by the fat and metabolized by the liver or kidneys (elimination phase), but the blood levels during this elimination phase are usually low and subtherapeutic for surgery. The sedative-hypnotic agent propofol is probably the best example of a drug that exhibits minimal residual effects once the drug has redistributed into fat. Most drugs, though, generate a residual blood level after redistribution that is associated with some degree of central nervous system effect. Sodium pentothal can be expected to provide some residual grogginess, for example, especially if repetitive doses are given. Sometimes this is useful; for example with fentanyl, high levels are desired during surgery, but a modest level after surgery aids postoperative analgesia. If too much is given, however, the residual levels are too high. In the case of fentanyl, prolonged time to awakening or respiratory depression may result. Excessive residual drug levels are especially problematic in the elderly because the elimination half-life is commonly two to four times longer than in young adults. Furthermore, the brain is more sensitive to some drugs in the elderly. Anesthetic drugs are therefore administered more carefully to the elderly. Bolus administration of drugs must be reduced in amount, and more time allowed for their peak effect (slower circulation). Drug selection favors the use of drugs with relatively low residual levels after redistribution and short metabolic half-lives. The goal at any age is to have an awake, responsive patient who is pain free at the con-

clusion of surgery. Unfortunately, these goals are hardest to achieve in the elderly, the very group who would benefit the most from their achievement.

GENERAL VERSUS REGIONAL ANESTHESIA

As mentioned previously, spinal or epidural anesthesia may provide more stable hemodynamics than a general anesthetic. Extremity blocks produce even less perturbations. Nerve blocks can be performed with either short- or long-acting local anesthetics, and therefore provide the choice of relatively quick recovery or 12 to 24 hours of postoperative analgesia. Spinal or epidural anesthesia has been shown to decrease intraoperative blood loss during total hip arthroplasty when compared with general anesthesia.[28] Many, but not all, anesthesiologists prefer to use regional techniques over general anesthesia whenever possible, not only because of the simplicity, but out of the belief that regional anesthesia is safer. Yet there is little published evidence to support greater safety of regional anesthesia. This observation is not surprising, however, as good evidence would require a randomized study of enormous size. Thus one is left with the bias and preference of the anesthesiologist taking care of the patient. Even if all parties agree that regional anesthesia is best for the patient, it would be a mistake to assume that since a regional anesthetic is to be used, the patient's status can be worse than what one would tolerate for a general anesthetic. First of all, the major stress to the patient may not be the anesthetic, but rather the surgery. Second, regional anesthesia may not be safer. Lastly, the regional anesthetic may fail and a general anesthetic would have to be administered anyway. Therefore it is imperative that all patients present for surgery prepared for all eventualities.

ANTICOAGULATION AND NEURAXIAL BLOCK

One major concern with the use of regional anesthesia, especially spinal and epidural anesthesia (neuraxial block), is the issue of thromboembolic prophylaxis with heparin or warfarin. The actual incidence of epidural hematoma in anticoagulated patients who receive a needle placed in their back is unknown and undoubtedly low, but it clearly can occur.[29] Epidural hematoma formation usually presents with pain and paralysis. Unfortunately, even prompt surgical decompression is unlikely to prevent permanent neurological damage. Anticoagulation that is instituted a minimum of 1 hour after spinal block or epidural catheter placement appears to be safe, but removal of an epidural catheter may be as risky as catheter placement and therefore the catheter should be removed only when coagulation is normal. Clearly these caveats require coordination between the surgical service and anesthesia. Anticoagulation with warfarin or a heparin infusion would have to be postponed until at least 1 hour after a spinal block or epidural catheter removal. Anticoagulation with twice daily subcutaneous heparin requires careful coordination. The worst time for spinal or epidural placement or removal is approximately 2 hours after subcutaneous heparin when the blood levels peak and a substantial percentage of patients will actually have therapeutic partial thromboplastin time values. The best solution is to hold a dose of twice-daily heparin and then place or remove the needle or catheter 1 to 4 hours before the next dose of heparin (i.e., 20 to 23 hours after the last dose). Waiting more than 12 hours after heparin may be particularly important if low molecular weight heparin is employed. Fortunately, once-a-day dosing for low molecular weight heparin appears to be effective. The message is that both the anesthesiologist and the surgeon need to decide how anticoagulation will proceed before the patient arrives for surgery, to avoid confusion and disagreements later.

POSTOPERATIVE CONSIDERATIONS

Both the internist and the anesthesiologist may be able to provide significant contributions to the postoperative care of the patient. Specifically, medical illnesses may be best managed by the internist, and the anesthesiologist may be able to provide assistance with postoperative analgesia. It is beyond the scope of this chapter to cover the management of medical illnesses, but the issues of postoperative delirium and postoperative analgesia are particularly relevant to the care of the elderly patient and will be discussed.

POSTOPERATIVE DELIRIUM

The effects of aging on the nervous system, particularly the brain, are complex and poorly understood. Nerve conduction slows and cognitive skills decline in some areas, but not all. The area of greatest concern in the perioperative period is postoperative delirium. The new onset of confusion, decreased alertness, and misperception of the surrounding environment characterizes delirium. Agitation often accompanies delirium in young adults, but the elderly more commonly demonstrate withdrawal from their environment, making recognition of the delirium more difficult. Delirium is a common occurrence in the hospitalized elderly regardless of whether surgery has been performed, but delirium is especially common after major orthopaedic surgery, with an incidence as high as 60% after hip surgery or knee replacement. Why orthopaedic surgery should represent an especially high risk is not clear, although fat embolism is a logical concern. The list of contributing factors for delirium is so long as to bring into question our understanding of the affliction. Certainly almost any drug can contribute, including anesthetic agents as well as any of the chronic medications typically taken by the elderly. Drugs with anticholinergic effects are perhaps the most commonly cited offending agents. Poor baseline mental function, electrolyte imbalance, an unfamiliar environment, sleep deprivation, sensory deprivation (loss of hearing aids, eyeglasses), alcohol withdrawal, and infection are other factors. Despite the tendency to attribute delirium to "anesthesia," it is unlikely that anesthetic agents are any more or less likely to cause delirium than any other class of drug. In fact, the use of regional anesthesia does not appear to be protective over general anesthesia. Delirium is usually transient, but merely its occurrence is associated with prolonged hospitalization, increased hospital costs, and an increased likelihood of requiring extended care after discharge, such as a nursing home.[30] There is also the issue of those patients who never seem to recover from the stress of the surgery and hospitalization. Documentation of the fact that "grandma has never been the same since" is largely anecdotal, but a recent study did demonstrate that 10% of elderly patients continue to exhibit significant cognitive dysfunction 3 months after major surgery.[31] If delirium is detected, attempts should be made to rule out correctable problems such as hypotension, hypoxia, electrolyte imbalance, infection, cardiac failure, or other illnesses. Sleep and sensory deprivation are likely very important; even simple things such as items from home may help keep the patient oriented. An attempt should be made to review current medications to see if changes or deletions can be made. If agitation is a problem, haloperidol in small doses may be useful.

POSTOPERATIVE ANALGESIA

Patient-controlled analgesia, typically with morphine, is a simple and effective means of controlling pain after most orthopaedic procedures. The use of meperidine is absolutely contraindicated in the elderly. Overdose with patient-controlled analgesia is rare in the absence of other individuals pushing the button for the patient.

On occasion, epidural analgesia with continuous infusion of local anesthetic, morphine, or both will prove useful after major orthopaedic surgery.[32] Likely candidates include patients for whom other methods would fail or are impractical, patients at high risk for medical complications, and patients in whom epidural local anesthetic infusion is used to decrease postoperative bleeding or as an adjunct for deep vein thrombosis prophylaxis. Epidural analgesia is time intensive, and there are significant risks, including epidural hematoma, hypotension, and inadvertent injection of some other medication through the epidural catheter. Medical benefits in high-risk patients include decreased myocardial infarction and cardiac death, decreased pneumonia, and shorter intensive care unit length of stay.[32] If epidural analgesia is employed, it must be remembered that it is impossible to achieve analgesia without also causing some degree of sympathetic nervous system blockade. Mild to moderate hypotension may result, but the lumbar epidural catheters used for lower extremity surgery are less likely to cause hypotension than are the thoracic catheters employed for thoracic and upper abdominal surgery.

CONCLUSION

The aging process decreases organ reserve and accentuates the adverse effects of disease, thereby increasing the risk of perioperative complications and death. The goal of preoperative assessment and improvement in medical status is to prepare the patient both mentally and physically for surgery. Good anesthetic care should not only provide an uneventful visit to the operating room, but also lay the groundwork for a successful postoperative course. Continued follow-up and assistance in the management of medical illness by the internist should smooth the recovery process as well. Therapeutic choices made by the orthopaedist, anesthesiologist, and internist will have an impact on the others' plans; therefore, timely communication among the services is essential for coordinated, optimal care.

REFERENCES

1. Thomas DR, Ritchie CS: Preoperative assessment of older patients. J Am Geriatr Soc 1995; 43(7):811.
2. Khuri SF, Daley J, Henderson W, et al: The National Veterans Administration Surgical Risk Study: Risk adjustment for the comparative assessment of the quality of surgical care. J Am Coll Surg 1995; 180: 519.
3. Tiret L, Desmonts JM, Hatton F, et al: Complications associated with anaesthesia: A prospective survey in France. Can Anesth Soc J 1986; 33:336.
4. Del Guercio LRM, Cohn JD: Monitoring operative risk in the elderly. JAMA 1980; 243:1350.
5. Palde VA, Detsky AS: Perioperative assessment and management of risk from coronary artery disease. Ann Intern Med 1997; 127:313.
6. ACC/AHA: Guidelines for perioperative cardiovascular examination for non-cardiac surgery. Circulation 1996; 93:1278.
7. Browner WS, Li J, Mangano ET: In-hospital and long-term mortality in male veterans following noncardiac surgery: The Study of Perioperative Ischemia Research Group. JAMA 1992; 268:228.
8. Huber KC, Evans MA, Bresnahan JF, et al: Outcome of noncardiac operation in patients with severe coronary artery disease successfully treated preoperatively with coronary angioplasty. Mayo Clin Proc 1992; 67:15.
9. Pinski SL, Trohman RG: Implantable cardioverter-defibrillators: Implications for the nonelectrophysiologist. Ann Intern Med 1995; 122:770.
10. Mohr DN, Jett JR: Pre-operative evaluation of pulmonary risk factors. J Gen Intern Med 1988; 3:277.
11. Jackson CJ: Preoperative pulmonary evaluation. Arch Intern Med. 1988; 148:2120.
12. Friedman LS, Maddrey WL: Surgery in the patient with liver disease. Med Clin North Am 1987; 71:453.
13. Lu-Yao GL, Baron JA, Barrett JA, et al: Treatment and survival among elderly Americans with hip fracture: A population-based study. Am J Pub Health 1994; 84:1287.
14. Christopherson R, Beattie C, Frank SM, et al: Perioperative morbidity in patients randomized to epidural or general anesthesia for lower extremity vascular surgery. Perioperative Ischemia Randomized Anesthesia Trial Study Group. Anesthesiology 1993; 79:422.
15. Mangano DT, Layug EL, Wallace A, et al: Effects of atenolol on mortality and cardiovascular morbidity after noncardiac surgery. The Multicenter Study of Perioperative Ischemia Research Group. N Engl J Med. 1996; 335:1713.
16. Morrison RS, Chassin MR, Siu AL: The medical consultant's role in caring for patients with hip fracture. Ann Intern Med 1998; 128:1010.
17. Kearon C, Hirsh J: Management of anticoagulation before and after elective surgery. N Engl J Med 1997; 336:1506.
18. Imperiale RF, Speroff T: A meta-analysis of methods to prevent venous thromboembolism following total hip replacement. JAMA 1994; 271:1780.
19. Folkow B, Svanborg A: Physiology of cardiovascular aging. Physiol Rev 1993; 73: 725.
20. Rooke GA, Robinson BJ: Cardiovascular and autonomic aging. In Dauchot PJ, Cascorbi H (eds): Management of the Elderly Surgical Patient: Problems in Anesthesia, vol 9, no. 4. Philadelphia, Lippincott-Raven, 1997, p 482.
21. Shannon RP, Wei JY, Rosa RM, et al: The effect of age and sodium depletion on cardiovascular response to orthostasis. Hypertension 1986; 8:438.
22. Carpenter RL, Caplan RA, Brown DL, et al: Incidence and risk factors for side effects of spinal anesthesia. Anesthesiology 1992; 76:906.
23. Forrest JB, Rehder K, Cahalan MK: Multicenter study of general anesthesia: III. Predictors of severe perioperative adverse outcomes. Anesthesiology 1992; 76:3.
24. Rooke GA, Freund PR, Jacobson AF: Hemodynamic response and change in organ blood volume during spinal anesthesia in elderly men with cardiac disease. Anesth Analg 1997; 85:99.
25. Wahba WM: Influence of aging on lung function; Clinical significance of changes from age 20. Anesth Analg 1983; 62:764.
26. Frank SM, Fleisher LA, Breslow MJ, et al: Perioperative maintenance of normothermia reduces the incidence of morbid cardiac events. JAMA 1997; 277:1127.
27. Kurz A, Sessler DI, Lenhardt R: Perioperative normothermia to reduce the incidence of surgical-wound infection and shorten hospitalization. N Engl J Med 1996; 334:1209.
28. Rose SH: A comparison of regional and general anesthesia. In Wedel DJ (ed): Orthopedic Anesthesia. New York, Churchill Livingstone, 1993, p 69.
29. Vandermeulen EP, Van Aken H, Vermylen J: Anticoagulants and spinal-epidural anesthesia. Anesth Analg 1994; 79:1165.
30. Marcantonio ER, Goldman L, Mangione CM, et al: A clinical prediction rule for delirium after elective noncardiac surgery. JAMA 1994; 271:134.
31. Moller JT, Cluitmans P, Rasmussen LS, et al: Long-term postoperative cognitive dysfunction in the elderly: ISPOCD1 study. Lancet 1998; 351:857.
32. Liu S, Carpenter RL, Neal JM: Epidural anesthesia and analgesia-their role in postoperative outcome. Anesthesiology 1995; 85:1474.

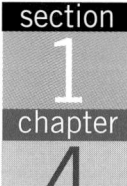

ANESTHESIA AND PAIN MANAGEMENT

Kentaro Tsueda and Gary E. Loyd

Summary

- Regional anesthesia also provides analgesia in the immediate postoperative period.
- Neuraxial (spinal and epidural) anesthesia substantially reduces perioperative blood loss.
- Neuraxial anesthesia decreases the incidence of deep vein thrombosis associated with total hip and knee arthroplasty.
- Neuraxial analgesia with opiates and/or local anesthetics via indwelling catheters provides antinociception in the postoperative period.
- Recommendations by the American Society of Regional Anesthesia should be closely followed when neuraxial analgesia is implemented in patients on anticoagulant regimens.

Orthopaedic surgical procedures can be performed under general anesthesia. Regional anesthesia, however, offers certain advantages, including continuous analgesia in the postoperative period, possibly facilitating early ambulation and joint mobilization. Neuraxial (spinal and epidural) anesthesia reduces blood loss and probably decreases the incidence of deep vein thrombosis. Procedures to the extremities, those involving the lower extremity and the pelvic structure, are particularly amenable to and are frequently performed under regional anesthesia with light sedation or combined regional/general techniques.

PREOPERATIVE ASSESSMENT

Coexisting diseases affect anesthetic management and may require preoperative treatment, depending on the severity of the disease. For example, in hypertensive patients, blood pressure fluctuates widely during surgery. Light anesthesia may lead to exaggerated hypertensive responses, and induction of general or neuraxial anesthesia may result in a marked decrease in blood pressure. In another scenario, delay of major elective procedures may be considered in high-risk patients with a recent myocardial infarction (less than 6 months' preoperative) to reduce the likelihood of reinfarction.[1] The extent of coronary disease should be evaluated before elective surgery in patients with unstable angina, and blood pressure and heart rate need to be controlled to within optimal ranges in the perioperative period. Orthopaedic trauma patients having emergency surgery must be considered to have "a full stomach" as the result of delayed gastric emptying because of stress reaction to the trauma as well as use of opiates. Concomitant injuries to organs other than bone may result in substantial blood loss, requiring more extensive preparation and monitoring.

Patients with arthritis (e.g., rheumatoid arthritis and an-kylosing spondylitis) may present specific technical difficulties related to the arthritis in the management of airway and cervical instability. In rheumatoid arthritis, atlantoaxial instability and subluxation may result from the erosion of ligaments and attenuation of supporting structures.[2] Flexion of the neck may result in quadriplegia or sudden death secondary to compression of the cord and/or the vertebral artery. Orotracheal intubation is difficult or may be impossible in these patients because of limited extension and instability of the cervical spine as well as ankylosed temporomandibular and laryngeal joints.

Ankylosing spondylitis is an inflammatory disease largely involving the axial skeleton. Ossification of ligaments and syndesmophyte formation lead to ankylosis of the spine and the afflicted joints. Awake nasotracheal intubation under topical anesthesia with the use of fiberoptic bronchoscopy is frequently required in these patients.

CHOICE OF ANESTHETIC TECHNIQUE

General endotracheal anesthesia provides total control of airway and respiration, amnesia, analgesia, and muscle relaxation. General anesthesia may be preferred for major orthopaedic surgery in which patients are positioned other than supine, undergo lengthy procedures, and lose a substantial amount of blood. Although orthopaedic procedures to the extremities can all be performed satisfactorily under regional anesthesia, general endotracheal anesthesia may be indicated for surgery in the vicinity of the face and neck, particularly in patients in whom maintenance of patent airway is expected to be difficult. Combined general/regional technique is frequently employed for surgery of the shoulder and the upper arm as well as for surgery of the hip or knee joint in order to alleviate apprehension and discomfort from remaining in the same position for a prolonged period.

NEURAXIAL BLOCK AND BLOOD LOSS

Several studies have reported that blood loss under neuraxial anesthesia is significantly less than that under general anesthesia during total hip arthroplasty (Table 1).[3–8] The reduction in blood loss in these reports ranged from 25% to 50%. In one report, continuation of epidural analgesia after operation also resulted in a significant reduction (approximately 30%) in postoperative blood loss.[7] The mechanism for blood loss reduction has not been elucidated. Reduction in mean arterial pressure and decrease in local venous pressure induced by sympathetic blockade have been suggested to be among the contributing factors.

Major spine surgery, revision of joint replacements, and major tumor resections are often associated with substantial blood loss. A variety of techniques (predonation of autolo-

TABLE 1. EFFECT OF ANESTHETIC TECHNIQUE AND METHOD OF POSTOPERATIVE ANALGESIA ON PERIOPERATIVE BLOOD LOSS (MEAN ± SD AND MEDIAN WITH RANGE IN PARENTHESIS) DURING AND AFTER TOTAL HIP ARTHROPLASTY

| Study | Anesthesia | Pain Relief | n | Blood Loss | |
				During Operation	After Operation
Keith[3]	Halothane	Parenteral	9	648 ± 58[a]	338 ± 61
	Neurolept	Parenteral	8	744 ± 99	424 ± 98
	Epidural	Parenteral	10	341 ± 59	393 ± 96
Thorburn[4]	General	Not specified	47	848 ± 61[b]	656 ± 38
	Spinal	Not specified	38	420 ± 41	582 ± 39
Modig[5]	General	Parenteral	15	757 ± 426[c]	
	Epidural	Epidural	15	100 ± 316	
Modig[6]	General	Parenteral	16	1616 ± 313[a]	
	Epidural	Epidural	14	1100 ± 316	
Modig[7]	General	Parenteral	30	1548 ± 410[c]	427 ± 175[c]
	Epidural	Epidural	30	1158 ± 446	294 ± 64
Wille-Jorgensen[8]	General	Parenteral	65	899 (0–1800)[a]	450 (0–880)
	Epidural/spinal	Parenteral	33	450 (0–3600)	510 (0–5000)

[a] P < .01.
[b] P < .05.
[c] P < .001.

gous blood, preoperative erythropoietin in patients who are anemic or refuse transfusion, neuraxial anesthesia, intraoperative hemodilution and maintenance of normothermia, induced hypotension, use of cell-saver, and lowering the transfusion trigger) have been successfully employed to minimize allogeneic transfusion.

NEURAXIAL BLOCK AND DEEP VEIN THROMBOSIS

Deep vein thrombosis and pulmonary embolus are major postoperative morbidities associated with orthopaedic procedures of the lower extremities. The prevalence of deep vein thrombosis following total hip and knee arthroplasty is 50% and 60%, respectively, in patients not administered prophylactic measures.[9] Various prophylactic regimens (e.g., adjusted-dose heparin, low molecular weight heparin [LMWH], low-intensity warfarin, intermittent pneumatic compression, or graded compression elastic stockings) have been reported to reduce the prevalence to 15% to 30% following hip or to 40% to 50% following knee arthroplasty.[9]

Several reports show that the incidence of deep vein thrombosis following hip[4–6, 8, 10] or knee arthroplasty[11–13] is substantially lower in patients who received neuraxial anesthesia than in those who received general anesthesia (Table 2). Proposed mechanisms for the lower incidence of deep vein thrombosis under neuraxial anesthesia include rheological alterations resulting in hyperkinetic lower extremity blood flow, increased lower extremity blood flow secondary to epinephrine added to local anesthetic, alteration induced by neuraxial blockade in coagulation and fibrinolytic responses to surgery, absence of positive pressure ventilation, and effects of local anesthetics (e.g., decreased platelet aggregation). Early ambulation as the result of epidural

analgesia extended into the postoperative period may also have played a role in the reduction of the incidence in some of these reports.

REGIONAL ANESTHESIA FOR THE UPPER EXTREMITY

The shoulder is innervated mostly by the C5 and C6 dermatomes. Interscalene or supraclavicular brachial plexus block provides good surgical anesthesia for surgery to the shoulder and the proximal humerus (Fig. 1A). Interscalene block is associated with a 100% prevalence of ipsilateral phrenic nerve paralysis. In the presence of abnormal processes in the contralateral lung (e.g., pneumonitis, atelectasis) or chest cage (flail chest, hemothorax, pneumothorax), arterial oxygenation must be monitored closely following the block. Supraclavicular and infraclavicular approaches (see Fig. 1A and 1B) provide reliable anesthesia for procedures to the distal humerus, elbow, and forearm. The axillary approach (see Fig. 1B), although devoid of the risk of pneumothorax that is associated with interscalene, supraclavicular, and infraclavicular approaches, may require a supplemental block of intercostobrachialis (T1-2) for procedures to the distal humerus and elbow. Axillary block provides excellent anesthesia for surgery of the forearm and hand. The interscalene approach produces incomplete (or delayed) block of the ulnar nerve (C7, C8, T1) and is not used for surgery of the forearm and hand.

Minor procedures of the hand, when a tourniquet is not used, may be performed under local infiltration or peripheral nerve block at the elbow, wrist, phalanx, or digit. An intravenous regional (Bier) block with a double tourniquet provides adequate anesthesia of the elbow and the structures distal to the elbow. The maximal duration (imposed by tourniquet-induced ischemia), however, is limited to 2

TABLE 2. EFFECT OF ANESTHETIC TECHNIQUE ON PREVALENCE OF VENOUS THROMBOEMBOLISM (%) FOLLOWING TOTAL HIP OR KNEE ARTHROPLASTY

Study	Procedure	Anesthesia	n	Deep Vein Thrombosis (%)	Pulmonary Embolism (%)
Thorburn[4]	Total hip	General	47	25 (53)[a]	
		Epidural	38	11 (29)	
Modig[5]	Total hip	General	15	11 (73)[a]	7 (47)
		Epidural	15	5 (33)	2 (13)
Modig[6]	Total hip	General	30	23 (77)[b]	10 (33)[a]
		Epidural	30	12 (40)	3 (10)
Davis[10]	Total hip	General	71	19 (27)[a]	
		Spinal	69	9 (13)	
Wille-Jorgensen[8]	Total hip	General	65	20 (31)[a]	6 (9)
		Epidural	33	3 (9)	1 (3)
Nielsen[11]	Total knee	General	18	10 (63)[a]	
		Epidural	18	2 (15)	
Sharrock[12]	Total knee	General	264	169 (64)[c]	
		Epidural	227	109 (48)	
Williams-Russo[13]	Total knee	General	81	39 (48)	7 (9)
		Epidural	97	39 (40)	12 (12)

[a] $P < .05$.
[b] $P < .01$.
[c] $P < .001$.

hours; anesthesia is terminated rapidly on release of the tourniquet, and there is a potential risk of local anesthetic toxicity when the tourniquet is released. A Bier block may not provide satisfactory anesthesia for obese patients.

The use of an indwelling brachial plexus catheter provides long-term postoperative analgesia of the upper extremity. Infusion of low-dose anesthetic solution (e.g., 0.125% or 0.25% bupivacaine) prevents vasospasm after

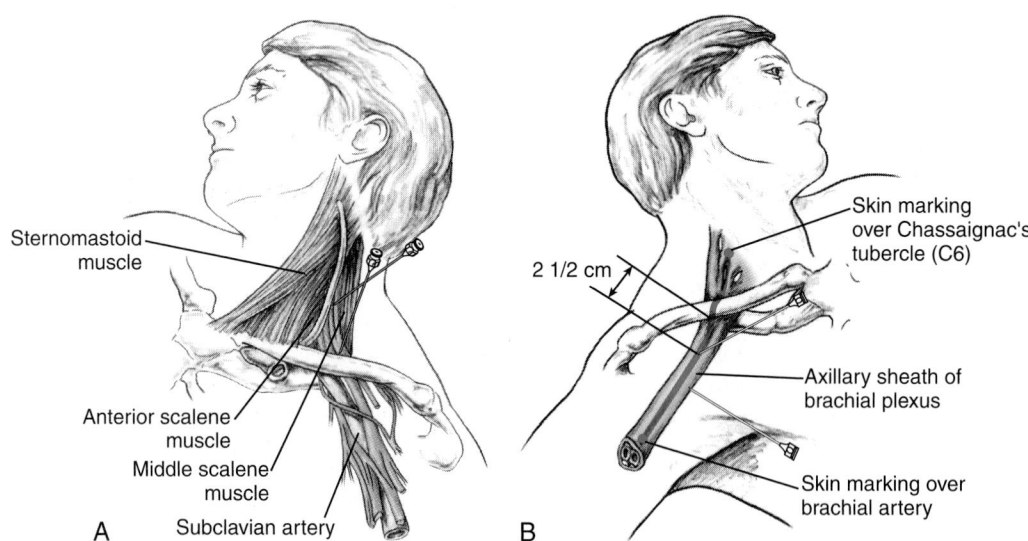

Fig. 1. Brachial plexus block. *A,* Interscalene and supraclavicular approaches. The patient lies supine without a pillow, arms at the side, and head turned slightly to the opposite side, with the shoulder depressed. For interscalene block, the needle is inserted in the interscalene groove at the cricoid level and advanced toward the C6 transverse process. For supraclavicular approach, the needle is inserted perpendicular to the plane of the skin at the posterior border of the sternocleidomastoid muscle and advanced to the first rib just posterior to the subclavian or innominate artery (a paresthesia or nerve stimulator is required). *B,* Infraclavicular and axillary approaches. For infraclavicular block, the patient lies supine with the head turned to the opposite side. The arm is abducted to 90 degrees and supinated. The needle is inserted 2.5 cm below the midclavicular point and directed toward the brachial artery using a nerve stimulator. For axillary block the patient lies in a supine position with the head turned away from the side to be blocked. The arm is abducted to approximately 90 degrees, and the forearm is flexed to 90 degrees and externally rotated. The needle is inserted perpendicular to the plane of the skin and directed as high into the axilla as the axillary artery can be palpated and advanced toward and through the artery (the vascular approach). A local anesthetic is injected behind and in front of the artery. Alternately, the needle is advanced lateral or medial to the artery until paresthesia is obtained. (From Bridenbaugh LD: The upper extremity: Somatic blockade. In Cousins MJ, Bridenbaugh PO [eds]: Neural Blockade in Clinical Anesthesia and Management of Pain, 2nd ed. Philadelphia, JB Lippincott, 1998, p 378.)

vascular repair or limb replantation. Continued analgesia in the postoperative period permits early mobilization of shoulder and elbow joints. The catheter may be used for several days without adverse effects.

REGIONAL ANESTHESIA FOR THE LOWER EXTREMITY

Orthopaedic procedures to the hip and the pelvic bones may be performed under general, regional, or combined general and regional anesthesia. For prolonged and complex orthopaedic procedures, however, general anesthesia or the combined technique may be preferred to regional techniques. Less extensive procedures to the lower extremity may be performed under neuraxial or regional nerve blocks with sedation or concurrently with general anesthesia.

The perivascular technique of femoral nerve block anesthetizes the lateral femoral cutaneous nerve, the obturator nerve, and the femoral nerve. Arthroscopic procedures to the knee may be performed with the perivascular femoral block (Fig. 2) and intra-articular local anesthetic. More extensive procedures may be performed with the neuraxial block or block of the femoral and sciatic nerves (Fig. 3). Femoral nerve block provides satisfactory

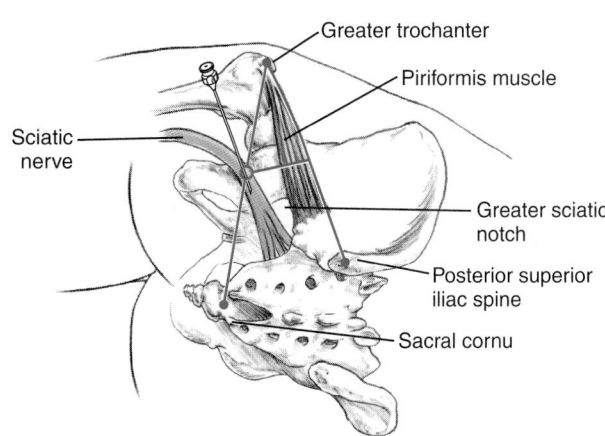

Fig. 3. Sciatic nerve block. The patient lies on the side opposite the one to be blocked and is rolled forward onto the flexed knee with the heel in opposition to the knee of the outstretched dependent leg. The needle is advanced perpendicular to the skin 3 cm below the midpoint between the greater trochanter and the posterior iliac spine until a paresthesia is obtained. Alternately, use a nerve stimulator. (From Bridenbaugh PO: The lower extremity: Somatic blockade. In Cousins MJ, Bridenbaugh PO [eds]: Neural Blockade in Clinical Anesthesia and Management of Pain, 2nd ed. Philadelphia, JB Lippincott, 1998, p 417.)

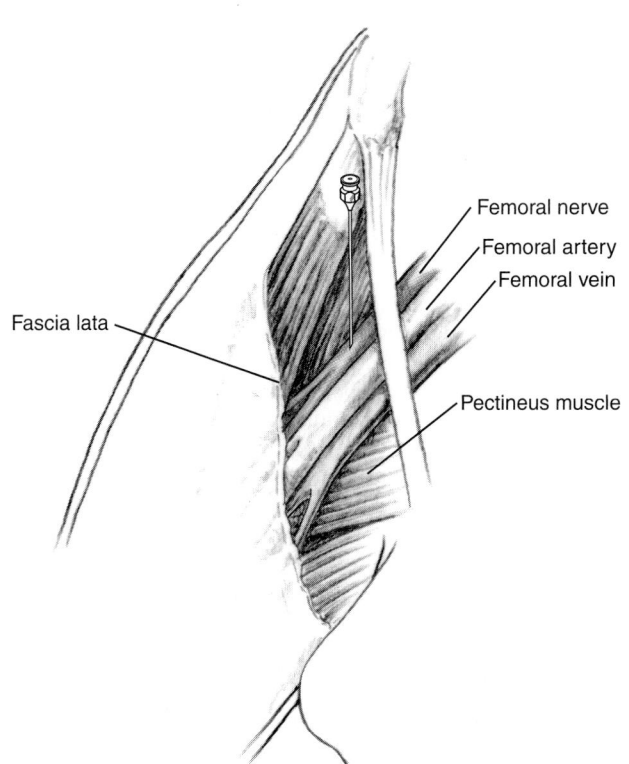

Fig. 2. Femoral nerve block. The needle is inserted and advanced lateral to the femoral artery where it emerges distal to the inguinal ligament until a paresthesia is elicited. Alternately, a nerve stimulator must be used. (From Bridenbaugh PO: The lower extremity: Somatic blockade. In Cousins MJ, Bridenbaugh PO [eds]: Neural Blockade in Clinical Anesthesia and Management of Pain, 2nd ed. Philadelphia, JB Lippincott, 1998, p 417.)

postoperative analgesia following surgery to the hip, femur, and knee.

Surgery to the ankle may be performed under a neuraxial block. With an epidural block, the onset of adequate analgesia may be delayed up to 30 min until L5 and S1 nerve roots are anesthetized. Spinal or caudal anesthesia may be a preferable technique. Deep structures of the ankle are innervated by the sciatic nerve. Sciatic block alone produces anesthesia that is adequate for closed reduction of an ankle fracture. Tibial, femoral, and saphenous nerve blocks provide anesthesia for ankle surgery if tourniquets are not used. Ankle or midtarsal blocks produce adequate anesthesia for surgery to the forefoot as does the block of sciatic and femoral nerve at proximal sites.

POSTOPERATIVE PAIN MANAGEMENT

Orthopaedic procedures to the shoulder, humerus, hip, and knee are associated with significant pain after operation, particularly procedures to the knee when continuous passive motion devices are used. Intensity of pain depends on the location and extent of surgery as well as the presence of chronic pain and use of analgesics before operation. Following general anesthesia, postoperative pain is typically managed by systemic analgesics such as oral opiates, intravenous or intramuscular opiates, or intravenous patient-controlled analgesia (PCA) with opiates. Regional anesthesia with long-acting local anesthetics (e.g., bupivacaine or ropivacaine) provides up to 24 hours of analgesia, obviating the need for parenteral narcotics in minor procedures. Intra-articular injections of local anesthetic and opiate may facilitate early discharge after ambulatory arthroscopic surgery.

Epidural PCA with a combination of low concentrations

of opiate (e.g., 2–5 μg/mL) and local anesthetic (e.g., 0.05% to 0.1% bupivacaine) provide excellent analgesia following pelvic and lower extremity surgery. The infusion rate (3–10 mL/h) must be adjusted frequently according to the change in pain intensity and the cumulative doses of the drugs. Level of anesthesia and motor function, as well as symptoms of sympathetic nervous dysfunction, must be closely monitored during epidural or intrathecal infusion of local anesthetics in the postoperative period.

Epidural PCA with a hydrophilic opiate (e.g., morphine) or a lipophilic opiate (e.g., fentanyl or meperidine) provide satisfactory analgesia without impairment of sensory, motor, or sympathetic function. Nausea and pruritus are fairly common side effects that are both amenable to μ-receptor antagonists. Respiratory depression and/or deep sedation require immediate treatment with a μ-receptor antagonist. Rapid egress from the epidural space of lipophilic epidural opiates into the systemic circulation increases plasma concentration of these opiates toward analgesic levels. Patients having epidural PCA fentanyl tend to be drowsy and dysphoric.

EPIDURAL ANALGESIA AND ANTICOAGULATION

The incidence of spinal hematoma resulting from neuraxial anesthesia has been estimated to be less than 1:150,000 for spinal anesthesia and less than 1:220,000 for epidural procedures.[14] Currently, in the United States, oral anticoagulants and LMWH are frequently used in patients having major orthopaedic procedures. Epidural catheter insertion or removal concurrent with anticoagulant therapy is ex-

---

TABLE 4. RECOMMENDATIONS OF 1998 ASRA CONSENSUS CONFERENCE ON STANDARD (UNFRACTIONATED) HEPARIN AND NEURAXIAL BLOCK

1. There is no contraindication to the use of neuraxial techniques during minidose prophylaxis.
2. Combining neuraxial techniques with intraoperative anticoagulation with heparin during vascular surgery may be acceptable with the following precautions:
   a. Avoid the technique in patients with other coagulopathies.
   b. Heparin administration should be delayed for 1 hour after needle placement.
   c. Remove the catheter 1 hour before subsequent heparin administration or 2 to 4 hours after the last heparin dose.
   d. Monitor the patient postoperatively to provide early detection of motor blockade, and consider use of minimal concentration of local anesthetics to enhance the early detection of a spinal hematoma.
   e. No data support mandatory cancellation of surgery when neuraxial needle placement is difficult or bloody. If a decision is made to proceed, full discussion with the surgeon and close monitoring are warranted.
3. Sufficient data and experience are not available to determine if the risk of neuraxial hematoma is increased when combining neuraxial techniques with full anticoagulation of cardiac surgery.
4. Neuraxial blocks should be avoided during prolonged therapeutic anticoagulation because it appears to increase risk of spinal hematoma, especially if combined with other anticoagulants or thrombolytics. But if anticoagulation therapy is begun with an epidural catheter already in place, delay of catheter removal for 2 to 4 hours following therapy discontinuation and evaluation of coagulation status is recommended.
5. Concurrent use of medications that affect other components of the clotting mechanisms (e.g., aspirin, nonsteroidal anti-inflammatory drugs, LMWH, and oral anticoagulants) may increase the risk of bleeding in patients receiving standard heparin.

From Liu SS, Mulroy MF: Neuraxial anesthesia and analgesia in the presence of standard heparin. Reg Anesth Pain Block 23:157, 1998.

TABLE 3. RECOMMENDATIONS OF 1998 ASRA CONSENSUS CONFERENCE ON ORAL ANTICOAGULANTS AND NEURAXIAL BLOCK

1. The prothrombin time (PT) and international normalized ratio (INR) must be assessed before neuraxial block in patients on chronic anticoagulant therapy, and interactions with concurrent medications that affect other components of clotting mechanisms without influencing the PT and INR (e.g., aspirin and nonsteroidal anti-inflammatory drugs) should be taken into consideration.
2. The PT and INR should be measured before neuraxial block if the initial preoperative dose of warfarin was given more than 24 hours earlier or if the second dose has already been given.
3. The PT and INR should be monitored daily in those patients receiving low-dose warfarin therapy (daily dose of approximately 5 mg) during epidural analgesia and should be checked before catheter removal if the initial dose of warfarin is 36 or more hours before.
4. Sensory and motor function should be tested routinely during epidural analgesia in patients receiving warfarin therapy. The testing should be continued for at least 24 hours and longer if the INR is greater than 1.5 at the time of catheter removal.
5. If an INR is 3.0 or greater, warfarin dose should be withheld or reduced in the patient with an indwelling epidural catheter. In patients with therapeutic levels of anticoagulation, clinical judgment must be exercised in making decisions regarding removal or maintenance of the catheters.

From Enneking KF, Benzon HT: Oral anticoagulants and regional anesthesia: A perspective. Reg Anesth Pain Block 23:140, 1998.

---

pected to increase the risk of spinal hematoma. The incidence of spinal hematoma secondary to neuraxial block and anticoagulation is not known. Only a few anecdotal cases of hematoma have been reported in association with both low-dose oral anticoagulants and unfractionated heparin, suggesting the relative safety of these drugs. Only one case of spinal hematoma was reported in Europe out of more than 1 million patients who received LMWH (enoxaparin)[15]; in the United States, six cases of spinal hematoma associated with neuraxial anesthesia and enoxaparin thromboprophylaxis were reported to the manufacturer within 18 months of its introduction in 1993.[16] The recommendations developed by a 1998 consensus conference of the American Society of Regional Anesthesia (ASRA) on neuraxial block and oral anticoagulants, antiplatelet drugs, fibrinolytic and thrombolytic drugs, standard heparin, and LMWH should be consulted when an epidural catheter is inserted or removed in patients on anticoagulant regimens (Tables 3–5).[17–19] Prothrombin time (international normalized ratio) must be closely monitored for patients on perioperative warfarin. Timely communication between surgeons and anesthesiologists is essential for a successful outcome of epidural PCA.

TABLE 5. RECOMMENDATIONS OF 1998 ASRA CONSENSUS CONFERENCE ON LMWH AND NEURAXIAL BLOCK

1. Antiplatelets or oral anticoagulants may increase the risk of spinal hematoma in patients receiving LMWH.
2. Initiation of LMWH therapy should be delayed for 24 hours postoperatively if needle and catheter placement was traumatic. In this event, increased risk of spinal hematoma should be discussed with the surgeon.
3. In patients on LMWH therapy preoperatively, single-dose spinal anesthetic may be the safest neuraxial technique, and needle placement should occur at least 10 to 12 hours after the last LMWH dose; patients receiving higher doses of LMWH (e.g., enoxaparin, 1 mg/kg, twice a day) may require longer delays (e.g., 24 hours).
4. Patients placed on LMWH thromboprophylaxis after operation may safely undergo single-dose and continuous catheter techniques. If a continuous technique is selected, the epidural catheter may be left indwelling overnight and removed the following day, with the first dose of LMWH administered 2 hours after catheter removal.
5. The decision to implement LMWH thromboprophylaxis in the presence of an indwelling catheter must be made with care. Extreme vigilance of the patient's neurological status is warranted. An opioid or dilute local anesthetic solution is recommended in these patients in order to allow frequent monitoring of neurological function. If epidural analgesia is expected to continue for more than 24 hours, LMWH administration may be delayed, or an alternate method used, based on the risk profile of the patient. The decision should be made preoperatively to allow optimal management of both postoperative analgesia and thromboprophylaxis.
6. Catheter removal should be delayed for at least 10 to 12 hours after a dose of LMWH. A normalization of the coagulation status may be achieved if the evening dose of LMWH is withheld and the catheter is removed the following morning (24 hours after the last dose). Subsequent dosing should not occur for at least 2 hours after catheter removal.

From Horlocker TT, Wedel DJ: Neuraxial block and low molecular weight heparin: Balancing perioperative analgesia and thromboprophylaxis. Reg Anesth Pain Block 23:164, 1998.

LIMITATIONS OF NEURAXIAL ANALGESIA

Epidural infusion of local anesthetic or continuous nerve blocks of the lower extremities may be contraindicated in patients at risk of developing a compartment syndrome. Patients with fractures of the tibia and fibula are particularly vulnerable to this syndrome. These blocks may obscure early symptoms and signs of compartment syndrome (e.g., severe pain, numbness, or weakness of muscle) and thus may delay the treatment that is urgently needed. These techniques may best be avoided in such a setting.

Peroneal nerve palsy is the most frequent mononeuropathy in the lower extremity caused by mechanical irritation, traction, crushing injuries, and laceration. The prevalence ranges from 0.3% to 10% following total knee arthroplasty, and that after proximal tibial osteotomy is approximately 10%. Epidural opioid may be used, but patients should be monitored closely and lengthy postoperative anesthesia avoided.

COMPLEX REGIONAL PAIN SYNDROME

The syndromes previously described as "reflex sympathetic dystrophy" and "causalgia" are now classified as complex regional pain syndromes (CRPS) type I and, when associated with a nerve injury, type II, which may lead to severe pain and crippling disability following relatively minor injuries.[20] CRPS usually follows an initiating noxious event. Spontaneous pain and/or allodynia-hyperalgesia is present beyond the area of peripheral nerve distribution and is disproportionate in intensity to the inciting event. There is typically evidence of edema and abnormality in skin blood flow and sudomotor activity in the region of pain. Trophic changes may develop in the skin, muscles, tendons, and joints. Impairment of motor function (e.g., weakness, tremor, and dystonia) may occur. CRPS is usually limited to the limbs but may also develop in central nervous system lesions, visceral diseases (e.g., involvement of coeliac plexus), soft-tissue lesions, and amputation syndromes such as after mastectomy. Most frequently involved in the type II CRPS are the median, sciatic, tibial, and ulnar nerves.

Following nerve damage, a subset of C-polymodal nociceptors becomes highly sensitive to sympathetic stimulation. In CRPS, norepinephrine released from sympathetic postganglionic neurons releases prostaglandins that may stimulate the nociceptor. Exacerbation of hyperalgesia (produced in rats following sciatic nerve injury) by peripheral norepinephrine injection is eliminated by peripheral injection of indomethacin. The α_2-adrenergic blocker, yohimbine, relieves the hyperalgesia, whereas the α_1-adrenergic blocker, prazosin, does not, indicating that the α_2-adrenergic receptor is involved in the hyperalgesia. In the central nervous system, prolonged activation of C-polymodal receptors results in the N-methyl-D-aspartate receptor–mediated sensitization of wide-dynamic range neurons in the dorsal horn of the spinal cord. Sensitized wide-dynamic range neurons respond to low-threshold A-mechanoreceptors that are activated by light touch, perceiving the activity as pain. In sympathetically maintained pain, A-mechanoreceptor activity is maintained by sympathetic efferent activity in the absence of cutaneous stimulation. After nerve injury, noradrenergic perivascular axons have been shown to sprout into the dorsal root ganglion and form basket-like structures around large-diameter sensory neurons.

The incidence of CRPS is a controversial issue. CRPS has been well recognized in France and Italy but has been considered rare in the United States and United Kingdom. Retrospective studies have reported a prevalence of 1% to 2% in the latter. However, a prospective study in 274 patients with Colles' fracture reported a 28% prevalence of CRPS (defined by the presence of bony tenderness of the hand, pain, vasomotor symptoms, swelling, and stiffness) 2 weeks following removal of the cast, suggesting that CRPS may be far more common than previously recognized.[21] Pain, tenderness, vasomotor instability, or edema were present 1 year later in 12% to 29% of the patients with CRPS. The hand was still stiff in 65% of the patients with CRPS. Early recognition and treatment are associated with a successful amelioration of CRPS. Management of CRPS must include prompt and appropriate treatment of the precipitating injury to minimize nociceptive stimulation from traumatized tissue, inflammation, and/or infection.

REFERENCES

1. Rao TL, Jacobs KH, El-Etr AA: Reinfarction following anesthesia in patients with myocardial infarction. Anesthesiology 59: 499, 1983.
2. MacArthur A, Kleiman S: Rheumatoid cervical joint disease: A challenge to anaesthetists. Can J Anaesth 40:154, 1993.
3. Keith I: Anaesthesia and blood loss in total hip replacement. Anaesthesia 32:444, 1977.
4. Thorburn J, Louden JR, Vallance R: Spinal and general anaesthesia in total hip replacement: Frequency of deep vein thrombosis. Br J Anaesth 52:1117, 1980.
5. Modig J, Hjelmstedt Å, Sahlstedt B, et al: Comparative influences of epidural and general anesthesia on deep venous thrombosis and pulmonary embolism after total hip replacement. Acta Chir Scand 147: 125, 1981.
6. Modig J, Borg T, Karlström G, et al: Thromboembolism after total hip replacement: Role of epidural and general anesthesia. Anesth Analg 62:174, 1983.
7. Modig J, Borg R, Bagge L, et al: Role of extradural and general anesthesia in fibrinolysis and coagulation after total hip replacement. Br J Anaesth 55:625, 1983.
8. Wille-Jorgensen P, Christensen SW, Bjerg-Nielsen A, et al: Prevention of thromboembolism following elective hip surgery. Clin Orthop Rel Res 247:163, 1989.
9. Clagett GP, Anderson FA Jr, Heit J, et al: Prevention of venous thromboembolism. Chest 108:312S, 1995.
10. Davis FM, Laurenson VG, Gillespie WJ, et al: Deep vein thrombosis after total hip replacement: A comparison between spinal and general anaesthesia. J Bone Joint Surg Br 71:181, 1989.
11. Nielsen PT, Jorgensen LN, Albrecht-Beste E, et al: Lower thrombosis risk with epidural blockade in knee arthroplasty. Acta Orthop Scand 61:29, 1990.
12. Sharrock NE, Haas SB, Hargett MJ, et al: Effects of epidural anesthesia on the incidence of deep vein thrombosis after total knee arthroplasty. J Bone Joint Surg Am 73:502, 1991.
13. Williams-Russo P, Sharrock NE, Haas SB: Randomized trial of epidural versus general anesthesia: Outcomes after primary total knee replacement. Clin Orthop Rel Res 331:199, 1996.
14. Tryba M: Epidural regional anesthesia and low molecular heparin: Pro Anasthesiol Intensivmed Notfallmed Schmerzther 28: 179, 1993.
15. Bergqvist D, Lindblad B, Matzsch T: Low molecular weight heparin for thromboprophylaxis and epidural/spinal anaesthesia: Is there a risk? Acta Anaesthesiol Scand 36: 605, 1992.
16. Hynson JM, Katz JA, Bueff HU: Epidural hematoma associated with enoxaparin. Anesth Analg 82:1072, 1996.
17. Enneking KF, Benzon HT: Oral anticoagulants and regional anesthesia: A perspective. Reg Anesth Pain Block 23:140, 1998.
18. Liu SS, Mulroy MF: Neuraxial anesthesia and analgesia in the presence of standard heparin. Reg Anesth Pain Block 23:157, 1998.
19. Horlocker TT, Wedel DJ: Neuraxial block and low molecular weight heparin: Balancing perioperative analgesia and thromboprophylaxis. Reg Anesth Pain Block 23: 164, 1998.
20. Walker SM, Cousins MJ: Complex regional pain syndromes: Including "reflex sympathetic dystrophy" and "causalgia." Anaesth Intensive Care 25:113, 1997.
21. Bickerstaff DR, Kanis JA: Algodystrophy: An under-recognized complication of minor trauma. Br J Rheumatol 33:240, 1994.

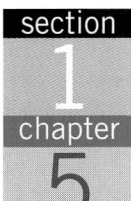

GENERAL ORTHOPAEDIC RADIOLOGY: RADIOGRAPHY, ARTHROGRAPHY, TOMOGRAPHY, MYELOGRAPHY, AND DISKOGRAPHY

William J. Glucksman and Karl B. Coyner

Summary

- A radiograph is produced by passing x-rays from an x-ray tube through filter, collimator, patient, grid, and detector.
- Fluoroscopy differs from standard radiography in that it uses an image intensifier and video detector to create a real-time x-ray image.
- A conventional tomogram is produced by adding motion during an x-ray exposure to blur structures outside the desired focal plane.
- In arthrography, myelography, and diskography, contrast agents are used to outline soft-tissue structures not visible on plain radiographs.

Clinical Relevance

- Plain film radiography remains the primary imaging modality for assessing most musculoskeletal disorders, including trauma, malignancy, infection, metabolic abnormalities, congenital and developmental abnormalities, and arthritis.
- Conventional tomography may be useful in assessing fracture healing in patients with orthopaedic hardware.
- Arthrography is used to evaluate joint abnormalities and is often combined with cross-sectional techniques (magnetic resonance imaging [MRI], computed tomography [CT]).
- Myelography combined with CT can aid in the diagnosis of degenerative disk disease, spinal stenosis, and arachnoiditis.
- Diskography is a targeted examination technique used to evaluate discogenic back pain.

INTRODUCTION

The seminal event in the history of radiology was the discovery of x-rays by William Roentgen on November 8, 1895. Roentgen, a professor of physics at the University of Würzburg in Germany, was investigating the behavior of accelerated electrons, or cathode rays, between metal electrodes in an evacuated glass tube. Roentgen accidentally discovered that his laboratory apparatus produced a previously unrecognized type of electromagnetic radiation with unusual properties: an ability to penetrate solids and an ability to cause fluorescence in certain types of detectors. In addition, a photograph-like image of the penetrated solid could be created by exposing a photographic plate next to the fluorescing detector. While experimenting with various objects in his laboratory, Roentgen found that the fine skeletal detail of his hand could be seen when he placed his hand between the tube and the detector. In the first public demonstration of x-rays (the name suggested by Roentgen for this radiation), he created a sensation by producing skeletal radiographs of audience members. News of his discovery quickly spread, and his methods were widely duplicated. For his efforts, Roentgen was awarded the first Nobel Prize in physics in 1901.

The first documented radiograph used for clinical diagnosis in the United States was obtained at Dartmouth College in 1896 and revealed a Colles fracture.[1] The introduction of radiographic evaluation of fractures led to significant changes in accepted standards of fracture management. The development of a calcium tungstate screen by the Edison laboratories allowed for the x-ray evaluation of patients in real time. This technique was named fluoroscopy by Thomas Edison. Many technical innovations have improved the overall quality and efficacy of the radiographic examination. Standardized radiographic film replaced glass plates in the 1920s. Automatic film processors were introduced in the 1940s. The development of intensifying screens reduced radiation exposure but produced grainy images. These screens were replaced by barium lead sulfate screens and then by rare-earth screens in the 1970s. The advent of digitally formatted imaging has led to the development of picture archiving and communication systems.

THE ROENTGEN IMAGE

A radiograph is produced when x-rays generated from an x-ray tube are passed through a filter, a collimator, the patient, a grid, and finally a detector (Fig. 1). Within the x-ray tube, electrons are created at the cathode (negative electrode) by heating a tungsten wire filament to a high temperature. These negatively charged electrons are accelerated across a large voltage potential applied between the cathode and a tungsten anode (positive electrode). A broad spectrum of electromagnetic radiation containing many different energies is produced. A narrow beam of x-rays is formed by filtering and collimation. A filter is a sheet of metal, usually aluminum, that removes electromagnetic radiation below a chosen threshold energy. The collimator determines the size and shape of the x-ray beam, reducing patient exposure and x-ray scatter.

The x-ray beam then passes through the patient under study. Differential attenuation and scatter of the x-rays occur. Scatter may be reduced with the use of a grid, a plate containing aligned sheets of attenuating lead. Unscattered x-rays that have passed through the patient pass directly through the grid, and scattered x-rays, most of which travel at an angle to the direct path, are attenuated by the lead sheets of the grid.

The radiographic image is formed on a detector system, which can be one of four types. The first is a standard film-intensifying screen cassette. The intensifying screen, which is a plate of fine-grained rare-earth phosphor compounds, spatially fluoresces with an intensity proportional

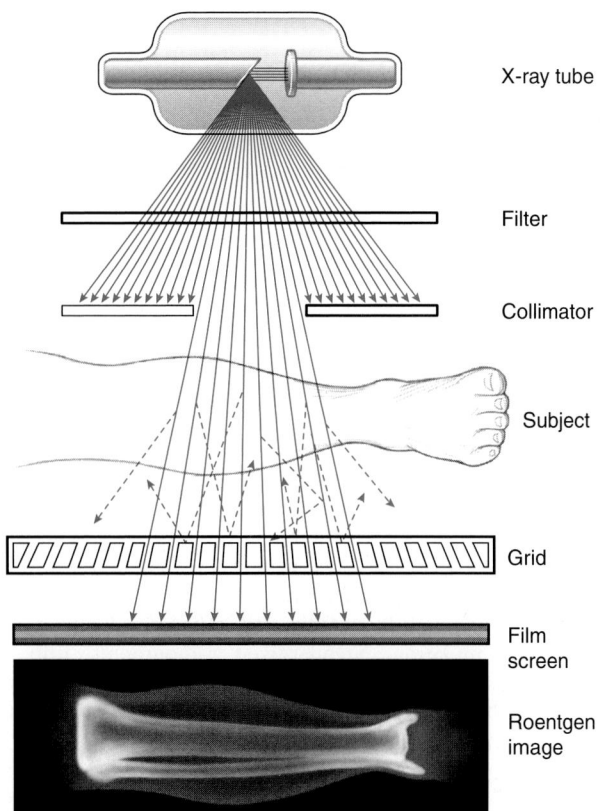

X-ray tube

Filter

Collimator

Subject

Grid

Film screen

Roentgen image

Fig. 1. Production of a radiographic image.

to the incident x-ray intensity. A photographic film placed parallel to the intensifying screen records the visible light pattern produced by the fluorescence. The second type of detector system is used in fluoroscopic units. In this system, the film is replaced by an image intensifier and video camera. A video image is produced that may be displayed on a gray-scale monitor and recorded on tape. The third type of detector system contains multiple small x-ray detectors that directly produce a digital image. The fourth type consists of a photographic plate with light-sensitive phosphor that produces a localized charge proportional to the intensity of incident light. This charge is then translated by a laser into a set of digital pixels that can be imaged on a monitor and stored on a computer. Radiography using the latter two types of detector systems is the basis for computed radiography and is replacing conventional film-screen radiography in some centers.

The roentgen image forms as a result of differing attenuation of the x-ray beam by the various tissues within the patient. Differences in attenuation are roughly determined by tissue density or, more specifically, mass density, atomic number, and electron density of the elements contained in the tissues. Bone attenuates energies because of its calcium content; the principal interaction is the photoelectric effect. Metal is the most attenuating, followed by cortical bone, trabecular bone, water or soft tissue, fat, and air. The detected pattern of differential attenuation may be displayed either directly in standard film radiographs or as

digital gray-scale images in digital detector systems. Highly attenuating objects, such as metal prostheses and cortical bone, appear white. Water and soft tissues appear as various shades of gray, whereas fat is darker gray and air appears black.

FLUOROSCOPY

Fluoroscopy allows for the x-ray examination of a patient in real time. The patient is positioned on a specially designed table, underneath which is an x-ray source. Over the patient is a fluoroscopic screen; this screen is mechanically connected to the x-ray source so that the screen and source can move simultaneously over the area of interest. The fluoroscopic image intensifier converts the x-ray image into a light-source image that, in turn, is recorded on a video camera and displayed on a monitor.

Fluoroscopy may be used in fracture fixation and in a variety of radiological procedures, such as arthrography, myelography, and diskography. It can be helpful in the evaluation of suspected nonunion, abnormal joint motion, and complex bone structures requiring nonstandard views.

COMPUTED RADIOGRAPHY

In computed radiography, the x-ray image is converted into a two-dimensional spatial array of digital pixels that can be processed, displayed, transmitted, and stored in digital format on a computer. This system has several advantages over standard film radiography. Contrast and density can be readily manipulated for optimal display of both bone and soft tissues. Archival storage and retrieval are also easier with computed radiography because images can be conveniently and permanently stored on tape or disk, obviating the need for a large film storage library. Finally, computed radiography images can be electronically transmitted to distant monitors for review and interpretation (teleradiology).

THE RADIOGRAPHIC EXAMINATION

In the radiographic examination, standard views of the body part should be obtained. Routine radiograph protocols may vary among institutions. In Table 1, orthopaedic radiology projections are summarized. Most examinations require two views 90 degrees apart. Oblique views may also be included in a routine examination when areas of complex anatomy such as the spine, ankle, or acetabulum are being imaged. Radiographs of long bones should include the joints proximal and distal to the shaft. Special views can be obtained to ensure proper evaluation of an area not optimally visualized during the routine examination. For example, in the case of a calcaneus fracture, adding Broden's views may permit better evaluation of the subtalar joint.

Radiographs obtained after the application of stress can provide information regarding ligament injury and joint stability. Stress radiographs are used to evaluate instability about the knee, ankle, first metacarpophalangeal joint, acromioclavicular joint, and wrist. Flexion and extension views of the spine permit identification of occult ligamentous

TABLE 1. ORTHOPAEDIC RADIOLOGY PROJECTIONS

Area	Routine View	Additional Views
C-spine	AP, lateral, odontoid	Lateral swimmer's: cervicothoracic junction Obliques: pedicles, foramina Pillar: lateral masses Fuch's: AP projection of dens Flexion/extension views: ligamentous injury
T-spine	AP, lateral, lateral swimmer's	Obliques: facets Lateral cone dorsolumbar junction (as needed)
L-S spine	AP, lateral, lateral cone L5-S1	AP cone L5-S1: lumbar-sacral articulation, transitional vertebra Obliques: posterior elements
Scoliosis series	AP, lateral	Lateral bending
Pelvis	AP	Inlet/outlet: pelvic fractures Judet views: acetabular fractures
Sacrum	AP, lateral	
SI joints	AP, Ferguson outlet	
Hip	AP, frog lateral	Lateral shoot-through (trauma) False profile (arthritis)
Pediatric hip	AP pelvis, AP pelvis in frog position	
Femur	AP, lateral (include both joints)	Obliques (as needed)
Knee	AP, lateral	Obliques: trauma Merchant: patellofemoral joint Sunrise: patellofemoral joint Tunnel: intercondylar notch Weightbearing views: arthritis
Tibia/fibula	AP, lateral	Obliques (as needed)
Ankle	AP, lateral, mortise	Obliques: trauma (as needed) Stress views: ligamentous injury
Foot	AP lateral, oblique	Lateral oblique: trauma (as needed) Weightbearing foot: longitudinal arch
Calcaneus	Axial (Harris Beath), lateral	Broden's views: posterior subtalar joint, calcaneus fracture Isherwood views: anterior, middle, and posterior subtalar joints
Toes	AP, lateral, oblique	
Sesamoids	Tangential view	
Mechanical axis	AP standing, entire lower extremity	
Scanogram	AP hips, knees, ankles with ruler	
Shoulder	AP (IR, ER), axillary, scapular Y	Grashley: GH joint in profile (true AP) Transthoracic lateral: trauma Bicipital groove (tangential): bicipital groove Subacromial outlet: impingement syndrome West Point view: modified axillary Velpeau axillary: modified axillary (patient in sling)
AC joint	AP without and with weights (bilateral exam)	
Clavicle	AP, AP axial (20 degrees)	
SC joint	PA, oblique, lateral	
Humerus	AP, lateral (include both joints)	Oblique (as needed)
Elbow	AP, lateral	Lateral oblique: radial head Medial oblique: coronoid process Radial head: capitellum view, radiohumeral articulation Axial flexion: olecranon process
Radius/ulna	AP, lateral	Obliques (as needed)
Wrist	AP, lateral, oblique	Scaphoid view: trauma Clenched fist: scapholunate dissociation Carpal tunnel: osseous structures of carpal tunnel Semi-supinated oblique: pisiform-triquetral joint
Hand	AP, lateral, oblique	Ball catcher's (bilateral): arthritis
Finger	AP, lateral	First MCP joint stress view: gamekeeper's thumb

AP, anteroposterior; C-spine, cervical spine; T-spine, thoracic spine; L-S spine, lumbar-sacral; SI, sacroiliac; IR, internal rotation; ER, external rotation; GH, glenohumeral; MCP, metacarpophalangeal; AC, acromioclavicular; SC, sternoclavicular.

injury and instability in trauma patients. Weightbearing views, often obtained of the knee, can more accurately demonstrate cartilage loss and abnormal alignment in a patient with arthritis. Traction views are occasionally used for evaluating the hip for subtle subchondral fractures in a patient with suspected osteonecrosis.

Proper technique is necessary to maximize the quality of the examination and minimize x-ray exposure to the patient. Proper positioning is always important. To minimize blurring of the image, there must be adequate immobilization during the exposure. Such immobilization can be difficult to achieve, particularly in patients who find it painful to assume the necessary radiographic position and in those with multiple traumatic injuries. Fast film-screen combinations should be used to shorten exposure time and thus decrease both the potential for motion artifact and the total x-ray dose to the patient. Penetration can be optimized by using a phototiming device or by adjusting exposure to accommodate the size of the patient. Image detail can be improved by decreasing the amount of scattered radiation produced during an exposure; this can be accomplished with the use of grids and collimation. A Bucky grid should be used when obtaining radiographs of thick body parts such as the abdomen or pelvis, because the grid will absorb the increased scatter produced. Collimation, or reducing the size of the exposed area, leads to decreased amounts of scatter.

RADIOGRAPHY: CLINICAL APPLICATIONS

TRAUMA

Radiography is the primary imaging modality used to evaluate orthopaedic trauma. It permits quick and accurate diagnosis of fractures and dislocations as well as characterization of fractures in terms of location, extent, fracture pattern, and alignment. Serial radiographs are used to monitor fracture healing and to detect complications.

Diagnostic accuracy can be improved by carefully assessing the overlying soft tissues, obtaining nonstandard views when indicated, and performing additional imaging

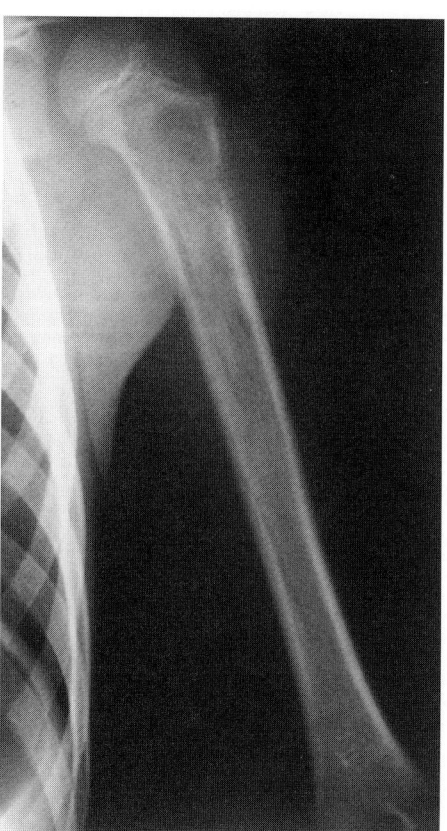

Fig. 3. Acute osteomyelitis of the humerus. Radiograph shows prominent bone destruction and periosteal reaction.

procedures as necessary. Soft-tissue abnormalities such as joint effusions, fat-fluid levels, localized soft-tissue swelling, and fat stripe obliteration may be signs of underlying bone or joint trauma (Fig. 2). Selective use of nonstandard views, tomography, and CT can permit better evaluation of fractures in areas of complex anatomy. MRI and bone scintigraphy are useful for detecting occult stress fractures, nondisplaced acute fractures, and stress fractures.

INFECTION

Radiographic findings of acute osteomyelitis include bone destruction, periosteal reaction, and soft-tissue swelling (Fig. 3). Soft-tissue swelling may be the only finding early in the disease process, because radiographically detectable osteolysis usually does not occur until 7 to 10 days after the onset of symptoms.[2] MRI or bone scanning can be used to detect osteomyelitis earlier in the course of the disease. Radiographic changes in subacute and chronic osteomyelitis reflect the reparative response of bone. The affected bone may become enlarged and sclerotic with a thickened cortex. Abscesses, sinus tracts, and sequestra may be identified (Fig. 4).

In the case of joint sepsis, radiographs may reveal only a nonspecific joint effusion. Joint aspiration is necessary for early diagnosis of joint infection. Late findings include narrowing of the joint space because of articular cartilage loss and subchondral bone destruction.

Spine infections usually originate at the vertebral body end plate; disk and end-plate destruction are hallmarks of such infections. Disk space narrowing, end-plate erosions, and a paraspinal mass may be seen.

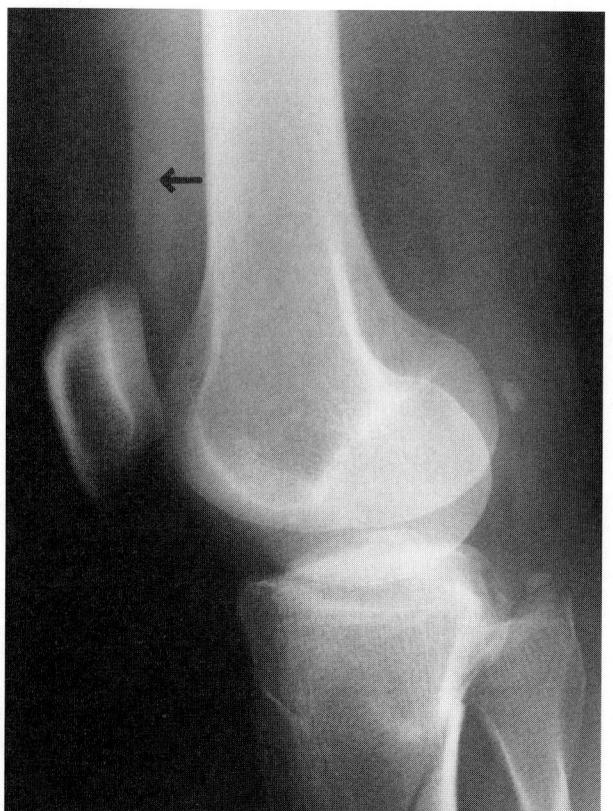

Fig. 2. Cross-table lateral view. Knee shows a fat-fluid level *(arrow)* indicative of fracture extension through an articular surface. A tibial plateau fracture was seen on the anteroposterior view.

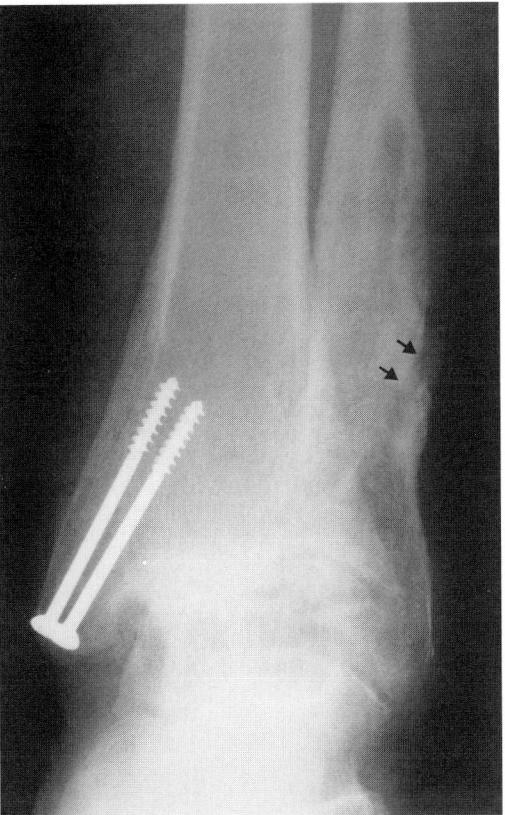

Fig. 4. Chronic osteomyelitis of the distal fibula. The fibula is enlarged with a thickened cortex and a sinus tract *(arrows)* extending outward through the cortex.

The radiographic findings in soft-tissue infection are nonspecific soft-tissue swelling and the obliteration of fat planes, indicative of soft-tissue edema. Radiographs are usually obtained out of concern about underlying osteomyelitis. Soft-tissue air is a specific sign of soft-tissue infec-tion, which results from gas-forming bacteria. Identification of a localized soft-tissue mass in the setting of infection suggests abscess formation. MRI is used for better charac-terization of the type and extent of the inflammatory proc-ess.

TUMOR

Plain radiography is the most specific imaging modality for the evaluation of bone tumors. Radiographic features typi-cal of benign lesions include a geographic pattern of de-struction with a narrow zone of transition and a solid pattern of periosteal reaction (Fig. 5). Features typical of aggressive or malignant lesions include a poorly defined margin with a wide zone of transition, a moth-eaten or permeative pattern of bone destruction, an interrupted pat-tern of periosteal reaction, and a soft-tissue mass (Fig. 6). The location of the lesion within the skeleton as well as within the affected bone can be characteristic of certain types of tumors. For example, a well-defined eccentric le-sion extending from the metaphysis to the subchondral bone plate in a long bone is typical of a giant cell tumor. A visible tumor matrix can be helpful in determining the tissue type of the lesion. For example, calcific density in a pattern of arcs and whorls is typical of a cartilage tumor such as enchondroma or chondrosarcoma. Cloud-like calcific density suggests an osteoid-producing tumor such as osteosarcoma.

CT, MRI, and bone scintigraphy are used primarily for staging purposes. CT-guided needle biopsy has a role in tissue diagnosis of some lesions.

METABOLIC AND ENDOCRINE ABNORMALITIES

Bone tissue has an organic matrix, a crystalline component, and cellular material. Normally, there is a balance between bone resorption and formation. With various endocrine and metabolic conditions, this balance is disrupted and in-creased bone production, increased bone resorption, or in-adequate mineralization occurs. On radiographs, these bone changes are seen as increases or decreases in bone density.

Fig. 5. Nonossifying fibroma. *A* and *B* show a well-defined, sclerotic, lob-ulated border and typical eccentric location.

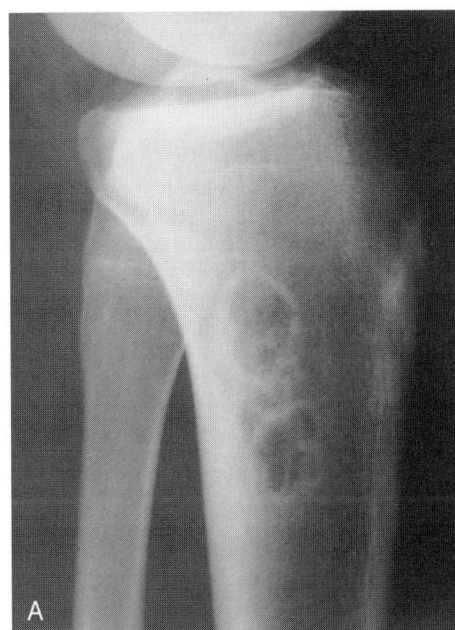

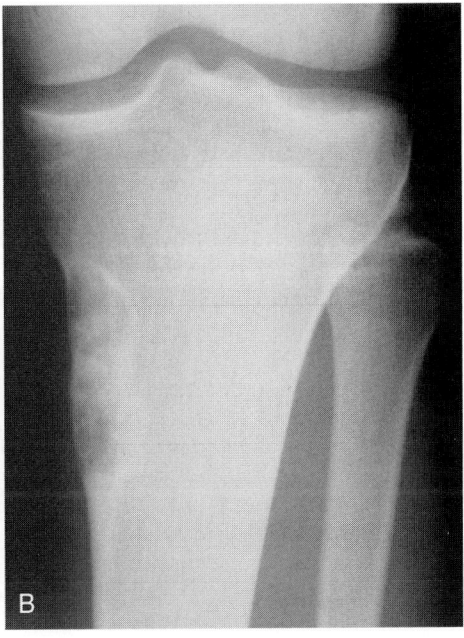

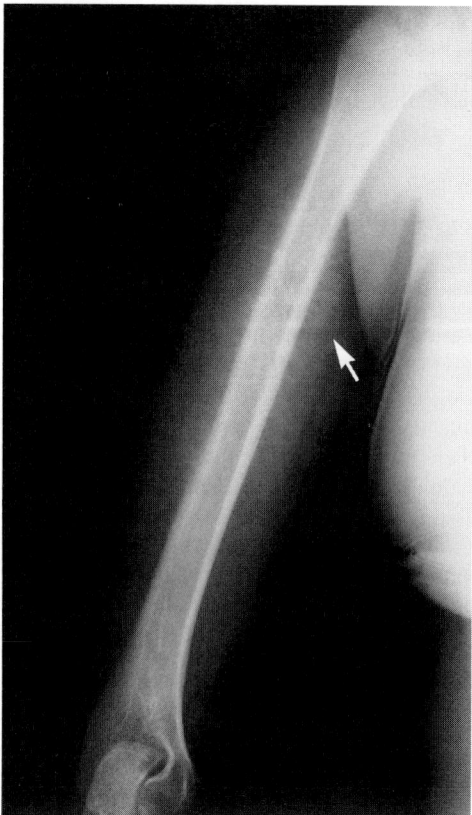

Fig. 6. Osteosarcoma of the humerus. A permeative pattern of bone destruction and an aggressive periosteal reaction (sunburst pattern) are demonstrated.

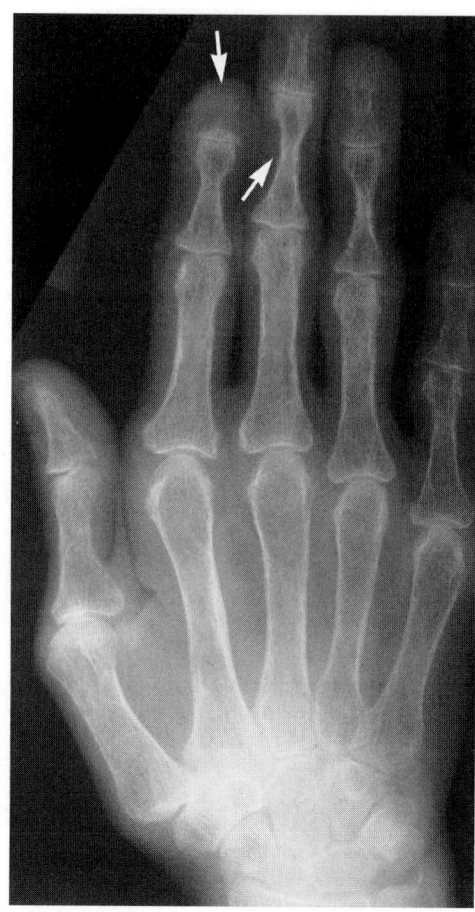

Fig. 7. Bone resorption. Bone resorption *(arrows)* typical of hyperparathyroidism.

Osteopenia is a general term used to describe radiolucent bone. It can be seen in patients with a variety of disorders, including osteoporosis, osteomalacia, and hyperparathyroidism. Examining the radiograph for more specific features can be helpful in making a more specific diagnosis. Looser zones or pseudofractures are seen in patients with osteomalacia. These incomplete fractures typically occur in the pubic rami, proximal femur, and proximal ulna and are usually bilateral and symmetric. Characteristic findings in hyperparathyroidism include subperiosteal, intracortical, endosteal, and subligamentous bone resorption (Fig. 7). Brown tumors and calcification involving the soft tissue and cartilage may also be seen. Multiple compression fractures of varying degrees are often seen in patients with severe osteoporosis. However, because radiographic changes are not apparent until bone mass has decreased by 30% to 50%, radiography is not the optimal imaging modality for detecting osteoporosis.[3]

CONGENITAL AND DEVELOPMENTAL ABNORMALITIES

Radiographs reveal various congenital and developmental conditions and can be essential for diagnosis. Skeletal anomalies range from failure of formation to abnormal growth, development, maturation, and modeling. Conditions of abnormal bone formation such as sacral agenesis, congenital pseudarthrosis, and intercarpal fusions can be

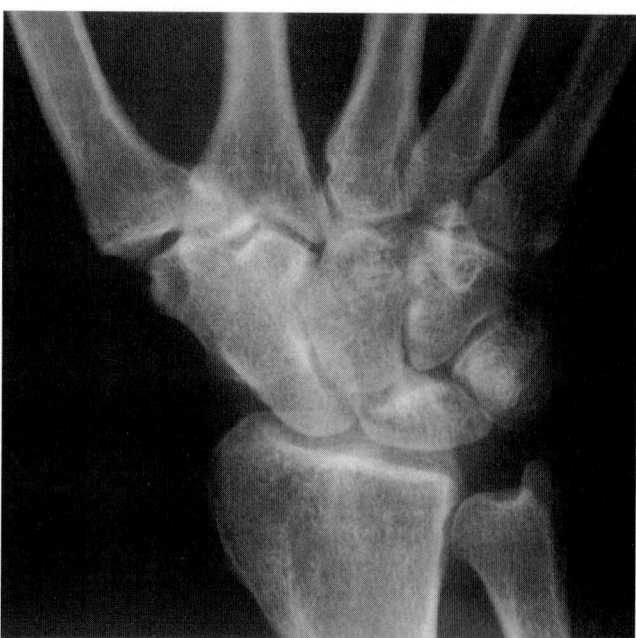

Fig. 8. Congenital fusion. Radiograph shows scaphoid, trapezium, and trapezoid.

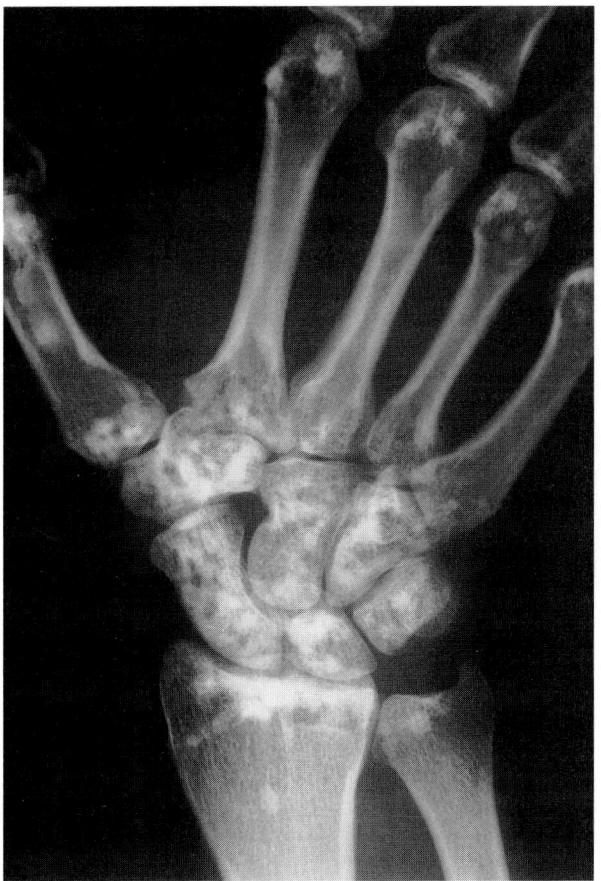

Fig. 9. Multiple periarticular sclerotic densities. They are characteristic of an osteopoikilosis.

diagnosed radiographically (Fig. 8). Skeletal dysplasias are conditions of abnormal maturation and modeling, resulting in increased bone density, and can often be differentiated and classified on the basis of their characteristic radiographic appearance. For example, osteopoikilosis, an asymptomatic disorder caused by failure to resorb coalescent trabeculae, is manifested radiologically by multiple circular areas of increased density in periarticular bone (Fig. 9). Various developmental disorders can be diagnosed and monitored radiographically, including tibia vara, developmental dysplasia of the hip, and Legg-Calvé-Perthes disease.

ARTHRITIS

Arthritides comprise a variety of disorders affecting joints, primarily resulting from degenerative, inflammatory, and metabolic processes. Radiography is the most useful imaging modality for evaluating arthritis. Routine projections can be used for most joints. Weightbearing views permit more accurate definition of the extent of cartilage loss in large joints such as the knee.

Radiographic findings play an integral role in the diagnosis of arthritis and in defining the extent of disease. Radiographs show the morphological abnormality of the joints affected and the skeletal distribution of those changes. Radiologically, osteoarthritis is characterized by localized joint space narrowing, osteophyte formation, subchondral cyst formation, and subchondral sclerosis. It is typically seen in weightbearing joints (Fig. 10). Rheumatoid arthritis, an inflammatory polyarticular arthritis, is characterized by marginal erosions, uniform joint space loss, synovial cyst formation, and subluxation. It has a symmetric, bilateral joint distribution (Fig. 11). Gout, a microcrystalline arthropathy, is caused by the deposition of urate crystals in and around joints. The radiological features of gout include marginated erosions that give the appearance of an overhanging edge, soft-tissue masses (tophi), and asymmetric joint involvement (Fig. 12).

ADDITIONAL RADIOGRAPHIC TECHNIQUES

CONVENTIONAL TOMOGRAPHY

Tomography is a general term used to describe various techniques that produce planar images of sections of the body using x-rays. The term is derived from the Greek noun *tomos,* meaning "section" or "cut."[1] *Conventional tomography* refers to the use of ordinary radiograph and an x-ray tube to generate a sectional image. The addition

Fig. 10. Osteoarthritis. This view shows osteoarthritis of the knee bilaterally with osteophytes about the medial and lateral compartments and prominent joint space narrowing in the lateral compartment of the left knee.

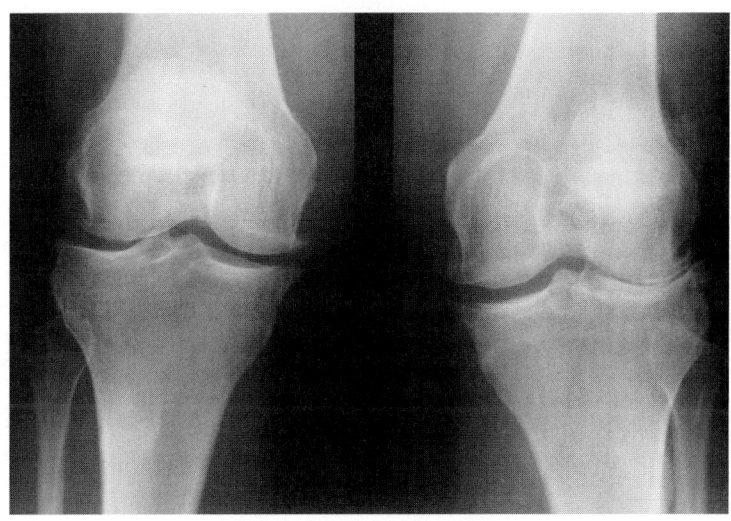

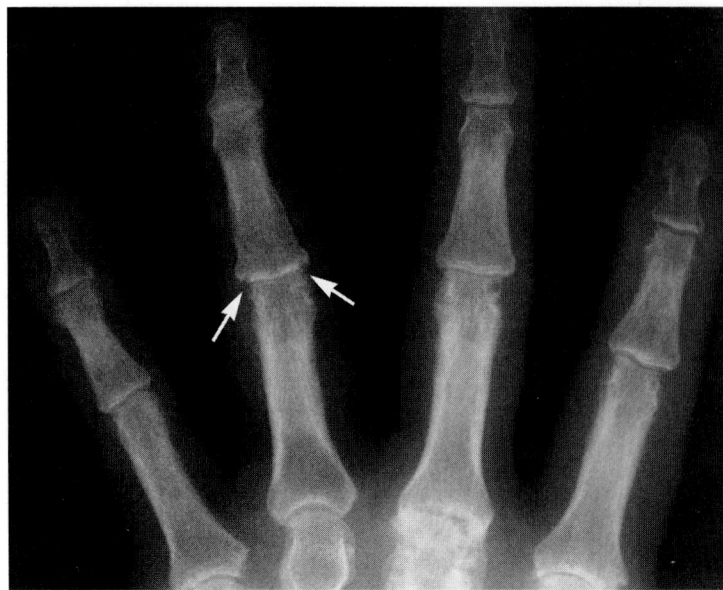

Fig. 11. Rheumatoid arthritis. Marginal erosions *(arrows)* are shown.

of motion during the exposure results in the blurring of structures outside the desired focal plane. The motion can be simple (linear) or complex (circular, spiral, or hypocycloidal). Conventional tomography can be used to detect, define, and characterize bone and joint abnormalities better (such as complex fractures and subtle bone lesions) by eliminating potentially obscuring overlying structures.

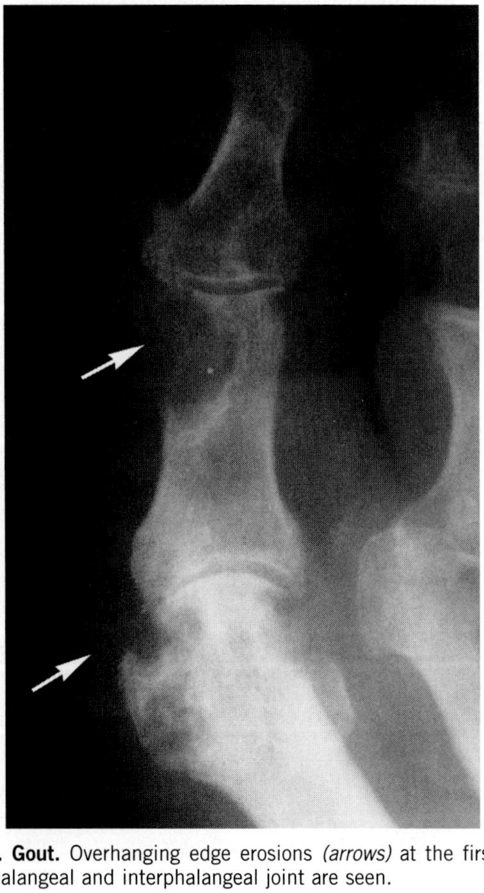

Conventional tomography has been almost completely replaced by CT, which is readily available, fast, and relatively easy to perform and has a lower radiation dose. CT allows for axial imaging, reformation in any plane, and the creation of three-dimensional images. For these reasons, conventional tomography is used only selectively, most commonly in the evaluation of fracture healing in patients with orthopaedic hardware (Fig. 13). The usefulness of CT can be limited in these patients because of "star" artifact produced by the hardware. Star artifact does not occur with conventional tomography.

ARTHROGRAPHY

Arthrography is used to evaluate joint abnormalities not detectable by radiography alone. It involves intra-articular injection of air, contrast media, or a combination of the two. Single-contrast technique involves injection of contrast media alone, whereas double-contrast technique requires injection of contrast media and air. The first arthrographic examination was described in 1905 by Wenoff and Roberson, who created a pneumoarthrographic device using oxygen as the contrast agent.[1] Because of poor soft-tissue contrast, patient discomfort, and crude radiographic technique, this device gained little acceptance. With the development of iodinated contrast agents, the introduction of fluoroscopy, and improvements in radiography, arthrography has become an accepted imaging modality for evaluating internal joint derangements. However, with the development of MRI, the number of arthrographic examinations performed has decreased significantly. Arthrography is used more selectively and is often combined with cross-sectional MRI or CT techniques.

The shoulder and wrist are the joints most commonly studied with arthrography. Shoulder arthrography is usually performed to determine whether the rotator cuff is torn. Extension of contrast or air into the subacromial-subdeltoid

Fig. 12. Gout. Overhanging edge erosions *(arrows)* at the first metacarpophalangeal and interphalangeal joint are seen.

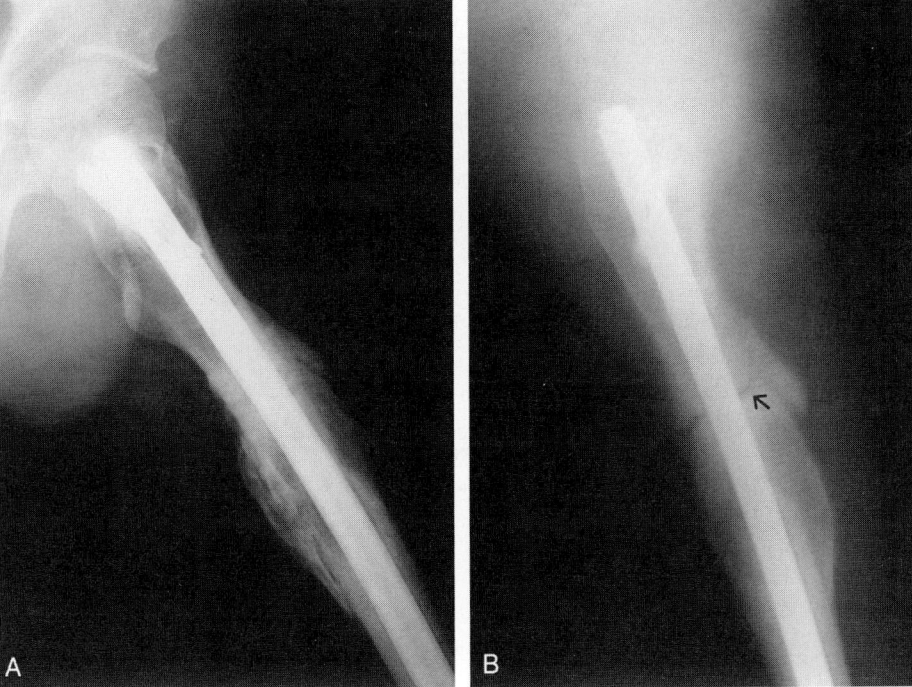

Fig. 13. Nonunion. *A* and *B*, Nonunion *(arrow in B)* of a femur fracture on a lateral tomogram is shown.

bursa after a glenohumeral joint injection indicates a full-thickness tear, whereas extension of contrast into the region of the tendons alone indicates a partial articular side tear (Fig. 14). Chondral defects, labral tears, biceps injury, and loose bodies are difficult to detect with arthrography without the addition of sectional imaging. Arthrography can suggest a diagnosis of adhesive capsulitis by demonstrating an unusually small joint volume.[4] Wrist arthrography is performed to evaluate for tears of the triangular fibrocartilage and the intraosseous ligaments. Abnormal passage of contrast from one joint compartment to an adjacent joint compartment indicates a perforation or tear (Fig. 15). Although MRI can be used to evaluate the wrist, arthrography is still considered the standard technique for diagnosing interosseous ligament tears.[5, 6]

As noted, arthrography is often combined with the cross-sectional imaging techniques MRI and CT. The added joint distention and contrast provided by this combined technique can be helpful in the evaluation of certain capsular, ligamentous, and cartilage abnormalities. In CT arthrography, air or a combination of air and contrast media is injected into the joint before imaging with CT. CT arthrography is commonly used to identify loose bodies and can also be useful in the evaluation of chondral and osteochondral lesions, labral tears, and synovial cysts (Fig. 16).

Magnetic resonance (MR) arthrography is rapidly evolving and involves intra-articular injection of saline or diluted paramagnetic contrast media before MRI. This combined technique may be more accurate than MRI alone in detecting loose bodies and chondral lesions and in assessing osteochondral lesions for stability. Because of its multiplanar imaging capability and superior soft-tissue contrast, MR arthrography is usually the arthrographic technique of choice. CT arthrography may be preferred in the evaluation

of loose bodies because small intra-articular fragments may be less conspicuous on MRI.

Indications for MR arthrography can vary, depending on the joint to be imaged and the clinical questions to be

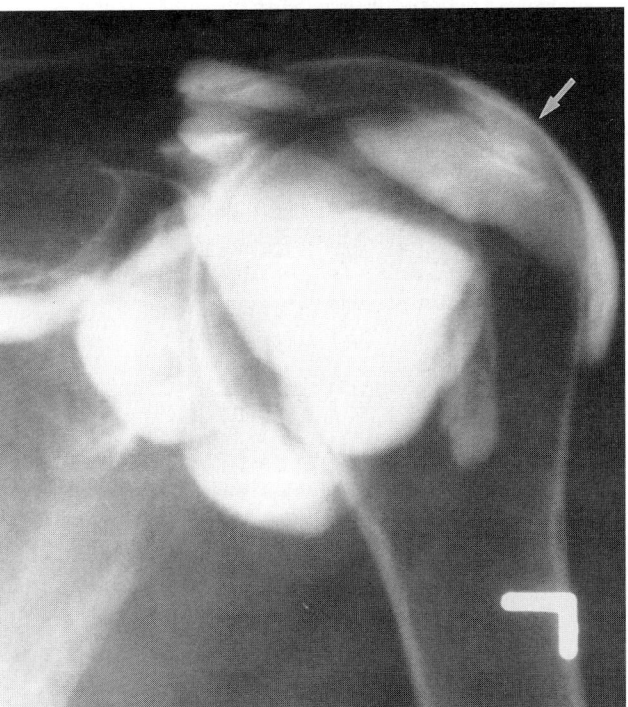

Fig. 14. Full-thickness rotator cuff tear. A shoulder arthrogram is shown. Contrast has extended into the subacromial-subdeltoid bursa *(arrow)*.

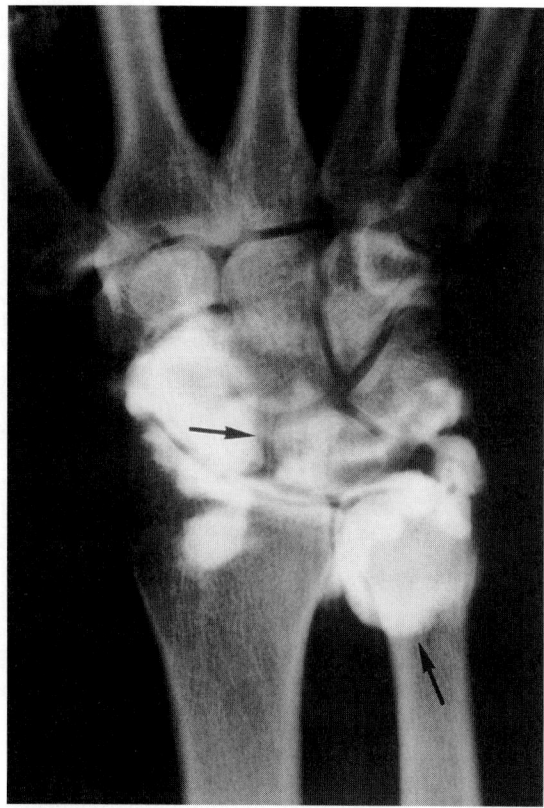

Fig. 15. Wrist arthrogram. This arthrogram shows tears of the scapho-lunate ligament and triangular fibrocartilage *(arrows)* after a single compartment radiocarpal injection.

answered. In the shoulder and hip, MR arthrography may help in the evaluation of labral tears (Fig. 17). In the shoulder, MR arthrography may aid in assessing partial and small full-thickness tears of the rotator cuff and in evaluating the rotator cuff after repair. In the knee, MR arthrography is used to evaluate postmeniscectomy patients for recurrent meniscal tears. In the ankle and elbow, MR

arthrography is used to evaluate suspected ligamentous tears. The disadvantages of MR arthrography include added cost, time, invasiveness, and exposure to ionizing radiation. Although intra-articular injection of paramagnetic contrast material has not been shown to have significant adverse effects, institutional approval is required, because the Federal Drug Administration has not yet approved the use of paramagnetic contrast for intra-articular injection.

ASPIRATION ARTHROGRAPHY

Joint sepsis and component loosening after joint replacement surgery are often as difficult to diagnose as they are to manage. Aspiration arthrography is commonly performed in an attempt to diagnose these complications when they are not obvious clinically or radiographically. The technique consists of placing a needle into the joint under fluoroscopic guidance and aspirating any joint fluid present. Contrast media is then injected to confirm that the needle is properly placed, to identify sinus tracts and periarticular abscess collections, and to identify any extension of contrast along the bone-cement interface, which confirms the presence of loosening.

ANESTHETIC ARTHROGRAPHY

Determining causes of various pain syndromes is often difficult. In a patient with hip pain, it is sometimes unclear whether the pain originates from the spine, the sacroiliac joint, or the hip. In a patient with ankle pain, it may be unclear whether the pain originates from the tibiotalar joint, the subtalar joint, or the surrounding soft tissues. Anesthetic arthrography involves injection of a local anesthetic and corticosteroids, under fluoroscopic control, to identify and facilitate treatment of painful joints.

Under fluoroscopic guidance, a needle is placed into the targeted joint. Next, a small amount of radiopaque contrast is injected to confirm correct needle placement. The anesthetic agent and corticosteroids are then injected. Joints commonly injected are the lumbar facet joints, the sacroiliac joint, and the hip joint. Pain relief, even if temporary, suggests the pain source has been identified. Treatment can then be directed toward that particular joint. Some patients

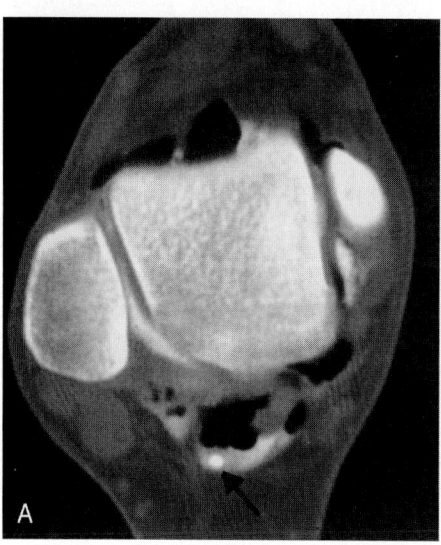
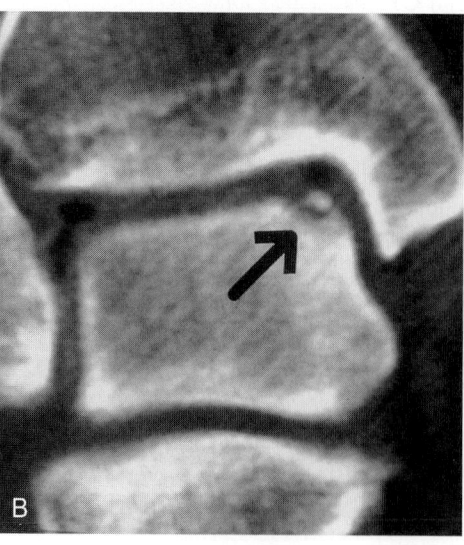

Fig. 16. CT arthrogram of an ankle. A small loose body *(A, arrow)* in a patient with osteochondritis dissecans *(B, arrow)* of the talar dome is shown.

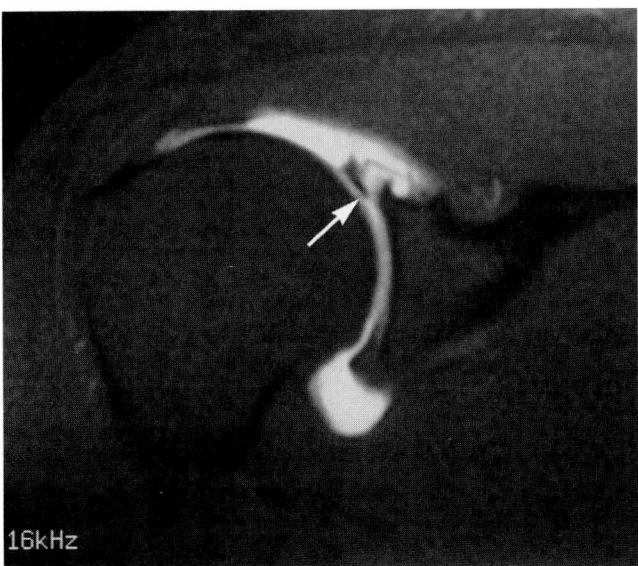

Fig. 17. MR arthrogram of the shoulder. Contrast extends through a superior labral tear *(arrow).*

obtain complete relief of their symptoms with one or more injections and do not require further treatment.

Anesthetic arthrographic technique is also used in other areas of the body. Epidural, spinal nerve sheath, tendon sheath, and bursa injections can be performed in a similar manner.[7–10]

MYELOGRAPHY

Myelography involves injection of contrast solution under fluoroscopic guidance into the subarachnoid space. The contrast outlines the subarachnoid space, spinal cord, and nerve root sheaths. The injection site is usually the lumbar region, normally the L2-3 or L3-4 level. Tilting the patient enables the contrast to fill the thoracic and cervical regions.

Use of myelography has decreased in recent years with the development of CT and MRI. Currently, myelography is almost always performed as a combination study with CT. The axial images obtained with CT can show the morphology of the central canal, foramina, disks, facets, and bone more completely. CT myelography is sometimes considered in cases of suspected spinal stenosis, because the technique permits further assessment of the contribution of the bony and hypertrophic changes. Myelography can also be useful for demonstrating the severity of compression by documenting a functional block in the area of stenosis.[11, 12] In the evaluation of the postoperative spine, myelography is used when MRI is inadvisable, because of the presence of artifact-producing orthopaedic hardware. Myelography may also be helpful in diagnosing arachnoiditis.

DISKOGRAPHY

In diskography, contrast media is injected under fluoroscopic guidance into the nucleus pulposus using a double-needle technique. The patient's symptoms are carefully monitored during the injection. If during the injection the patient experiences pain that mimics his or her usual symptoms, the pathological changes in the disk are considered to be likely responsible for the patient's symptoms. The radiographs and CT scan that follow the injection provide additional morphological information that may be useful in surgical planning (Fig. 18).

Diskography has remained controversial since it was first described by Lindblom in 1948.[13] Advocates stress its utility as an adjunct to the more traditional imaging modalities such as CT and MRI in the evaluation of chronic back pain. MRI and CT function primarily as screening techniques in the evaluation of radicular pain. Diskography is a

Fig. 18. CT image after a lumbar diskogram. Degenerative disk change is evident at L5/S1 with extension of contrast through the periphery of the disk indicative of an annular tear *(A and B, arrow).*

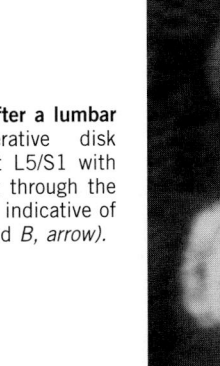

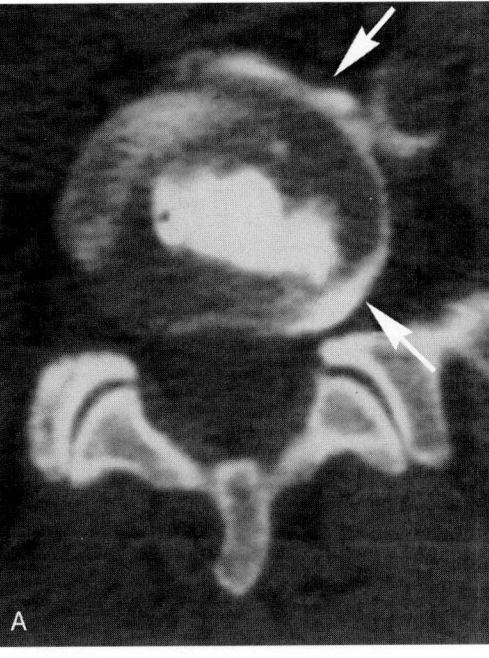

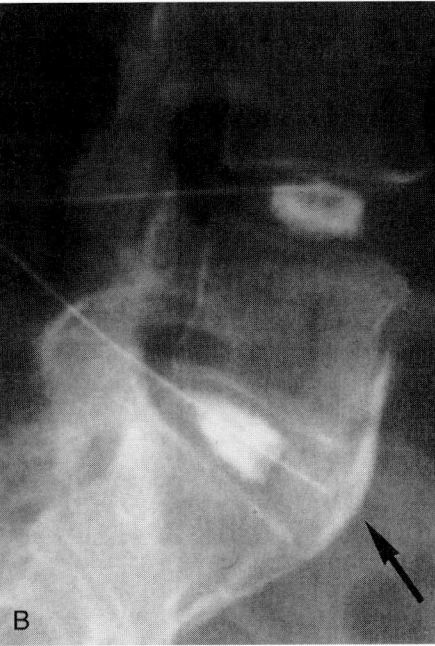

targeted, provocative examination technique that is used primarily to evaluate chronic discogenic back pain with or without radicular symptoms.

Diskography is considered in patients who do not respond to conservative therapy and whose previous diagnostic study findings are normal, equivocal, or inconsistent with the symptoms. Diskography is usually performed only on patients being considered for surgery. Findings can be helpful in deciding whether to operate and, if surgery is deemed necessary, in planning the extent of surgery. Diskography can be particularly useful in determining symptomatic disk levels in patients with multilevel disease.[10, 14]

REFERENCES

1. Eisenberg RL: Radiology: An Illustrated History. St. Louis, Mosby–Year Book, 1992.
2. Greenspan A: Orthopedic Radiology. Philadelphia, Lippincott-Raven, 1997, p 20.1.
3. Chew FS: Skeletal Radiology: The Bare Bones. Baltimore, Williams & Wilkins, 1997, p 276.
4. Freiberger RH, Kaye JJ: Arthrography. New York, Appleton-Century-Crofts, 1979, p 168.
5. Schreibman KL, Freeland A, Gilula LA, et al: Imaging of the hand and wrist. Orthop Clin North Am 1997; 28:537.
6. Gilbert TJ, Cohen M: Imaging of acute injuries to the wrist and hand. Radiol Clin North Am 1997; 35:701.
7. Link S, El-Khoury GY, Guilford WB: Percutaneous epidural and nerve block and percutaneous lumbar sympatholysis. Radiol Clin North Am 1998; 36:509.
8. Resnick D: Arthrography, tenography, and bursography. In Resnick D (ed): Diagnosis of Bone and Joint Disorders. Philadelphia, WB Saunders, 1995, p 277.
9. Schreibman K, Gilula L: Ankle tenography: A therapeutic imaging modality. Radiol Clin North Am 1998; 36:739.
10. El-Khoury GY, Renfrew DL: Percutaneous procedures for the diagnosis and treatment of lower back pain: Discography, facet joint injection and epidural injection. AJR Am J Roentgenol 1991; 157:685.
11. Boden SD: The use of radiologic imaging studies in the evaluation of patients who have degenerative disorders of the lumbar spine. J Bone Joint Surg Am 1996; 78: 114.
12. Haughton V: Imaging techniques in intraspinal diseases. In Resnick D (ed): Diagnosis of Bone and Joint Disorders. Philadelphia, WB Saunders, 1995, p 237.
13. Lindblom K: Diagnostic puncture of intervertebral disks in sciatica. Acta Orthop Scand 1948; 17:231.
14. Horton WC, Daftari TK: Which disc as visualized by magnetic resonance imaging is actually a source of pain? A correlation between magnetic resonance imaging and discography. Spine 1992; 17:S164.

section 1 chapter 6

MUSCULOSKELETAL HELICAL COMPUTED TOMOGRAPHY

Eric A. Brandser

Summary
- Computed tomography (CT) provides excellent osseous tomographic detail.
- Helical CT has fundamentally changed the application of CT to skeletal evaluation.
- Volume averaging and gantry slice limitations can be minimized with attention to positioning and scan parameters.
- Cone-beam CT promises further capabilities for CT evaluation of the skeletal system.

Clinical Relevance
- CT has better osseous detail than other modalities, including magnetic resonance imaging (MRI).
- Fractures in the plane of the CT gantry can be missed, especially with thick slices.
- Optimal imaging requires proper positioning and scan techniques.
- Multiple plane scanning or multiplanar reconstruction extends the clinical utility of CT.

CT is a powerful modality for evaluating the musculoskeletal system. It provides good tissue contrast and excellent definition of bone, making it better than MRI for characterization of fracture lines or exact delineation of processes that affect bones. CT does have limitations, including the fact that cross-sectional images are only acquired in the plane of the CT gantry. Fractures or abnormalities that run in the plane of the gantry can be difficult to detect. However, collection of volumes of data, multiplanar reconstruction capabilities, and attention to patient positioning can minimize the impact of the CT gantry orientation. CT technology continues to evolve, and helical (or spiral) scanners are commonplace. Newer technologies, including limited cone-beam CT, show promise for significantly altering the way physicians use CT to detect and characterize orthopaedic abnormalities.

HELICAL CT

Helical, or spiral, CT has significantly changed the way musculoskeletal diseases are imaged. Conventional CT and helical CT are fundamentally different techniques. Conventional CT scanning involves alternating patient translation and x-ray exposure, whereas helical CT scanning involves simultaneous patient translation and x-ray exposure.[1] Helical CT is so named because the x-ray beam can be thought of as tracing a helix or spiral curve on the patient's skin. With helical CT, patient translation and slice data acquisition occur simultaneously (Fig. 1).[2, 3] Individual slices are reconstructed from the volumetric data.

There are advantages of helical CT over conventional CT. Helical CT is faster, both in the data acquisition phase and in the total time required to complete a patient

Fig. 1. Principles of helical CT. Diagram illustrates how x-ray tube rotation and patient translation occur simultaneously (top row), resulting in a volume of data which can be reconstructed into contiguous slices (middle row). The data can also be reconstructed into multiple overlapping slices at no additional radiation or data collection time cost (bottom row) (From Toshiba America Medical Systems, Inc., Tustin, CA.)

Time

Helical scanning projection data

Projection data extracted for one rotation

study.[2, 3] This is significant when working with patients who are in pain or very ill or who are victims of trauma. The speed of data acquisition is important as it minimizes unintentional intrascan or interscan motion, which can degrade multiplanar and three-dimensional reconstructions. In helical CT, nearly-spaced, overlapping slices can be reconstructed from the basic data set at no additional radiation cost to the patient (see Fig. 1). This differs from conventional CT, in which collecting overlapping slices results in additional radiation dose to the patient.[2, 3] Reconstructing slices at close intervals decreases volume averaging and improves the quality of multiplanar reconstructions, improving detection of lesions or fractures that run parallel to the plane of the CT gantry (Fig. 2).

OPTIMIZING CT STUDIES

A number of parameters under the user's control affect CT image quality (Table 1). Slice thickness can be varied from less than a millimeter to more than a centimeter. Slice thickness should be chosen to best answer a given ques-

tion. If the area in question is an extremity, thinner slices are appropriate to better define subtle fractures. For example, when studying scaphoid and distal radius fractures, slices 2 mm thick, reconstructed at 0.5-mm or 1-mm increments, are appropriate. Overlapping slices improve lesion detection by reducing volume averaging.[3] With conventional CT, overlapping slices increase time to acquire a study and the radiation dose to the patient. With helical CT, overlapping slices are reconstructed from the helical data without increased radiation to the patient. Some authors advocate a large amount of slice overlap, such as five slices per gantry rotation (e.g., 2-mm slices per every 1 mm), especially when multiplanar reconstructions are to be generated.[2, 3] It is common to use a 50% interslice overlap (e.g., 5-mm slices every 2.5 mm) for most orthopaedic CT. When scanning the lumbar spine in large patients where the signal-to-noise ratio would suffer with thin cuts, thicker slices are used. In the lumbar spine, 3- or 5-mm slices are typical, depending on the number of vertebral segments to be covered.

Image display and reconstruction postprocessing filters

Contiguous Slices

Overlapping slices or reconstruction

Fig. 2. Reduced volume averaging with overlapping or reconstructed slices. The left portion of the diagram demonstrates a potential lesion (sphere) only partially imaged on two contiguous slices; volume averaging could render the lesion inconspicuous on CT images, whereas, with overlapping reconstructions or slices, the lesion will be optimally displayed on the image midway between the original images. Overlapping slices with conventional CT increases patient radiation dose, whereas overlapping reconstruction of helical data does not increase dose. (From Toshiba America Medical Systems, Inc., Tustin, CA.)

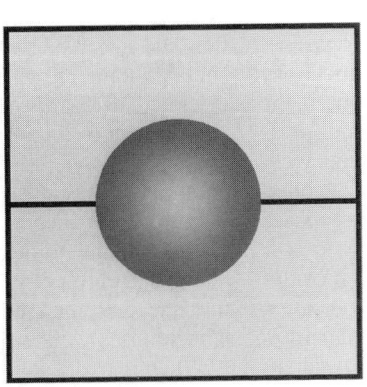
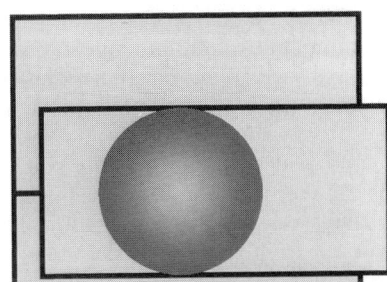

TABLE 1. PARAMETERS AFFECTING CT QUALITY

- Slice thickness
- Slice overlap
- Use of filters
- Pitch of spiral
- Patient positioning

can enhance skeletal CT images.[2] Edge-enhancing, user-defined filters improve edge conspicuity and make fractures more distinct. Use of an edge-enhancing filter is common when scanning the extremities.

In helical CT, pitch is a user-defined parameter that affects image quality and coverage; it represents the amount of patient translation into the gantry per rotation of the CT tube and detectors.[2, 3] It is traditionally represented as a ratio such as 1:1, 1:1.5, 1:2.0, etc. The first number represents the time for a CT acquisition in seconds (1-sec scan time is common), and the second number represents the number of slice thicknesses the patient translates into the gantry during that same amount of time. By convention, most scans use a pitch of 1:1. The main advantage of increasing pitch is increased coverage during a CT scan; patient radiation dose also is lower with increased pitch. The disadvantage is loss of data for image reconstruction. However, slight increases in pitch do not adversely affect image quality. Wang and Vannier[4] have shown that increasing pitch to 1.4 causes no loss of information in the resultant CT image. Most researchers agree that the upper limit for pitch is 1:2.0 with current CT technology (single row detectors, see below).[2] Increasing pitch can improve spatial resolution. If slices 3 mm thick with a pitch of 1:1 are compared with slices 2 mm thick with a pitch of 1:1.5, the distance covered is the same, but longitudinal resolution is better with the 2-mm scan.

Whether to do multiple scans in different planes versus a helical data set in one plane with reconstructions in other planes depends on the institution or scanner's capability. Some machines have excellent software for image reconstruction; on other machines, it is easier and faster to scan in two planes. Single-plane scanning reduces the amount of x-ray exposure and time to complete scanning. However, in some cases, reconstructions from one helical scan take longer to perform and yield less detailed information than acquiring the other plane directly. When maximal spatial detail is needed, the directly acquired two-plane examination may be preferred over multiplanar reconstructions.

Patient Positioning. Patient positioning is critical for high-quality CT examinations. This is especially true if the anatomy to be studied runs in an oblique orientation, as does, for example, the scaphoid or calcaneus. CT can accurately evaluate fractures of the scaphoid if careful attention to patient positioning is maintained. Detecting scaphoid fractures can be notoriously difficult; special views are often used to improve early detection.[5] Helical CT can evaluate occult or complex scaphoid fractures, assess healing fractures, and evaluate the postsurgical wrist.[6, 7] Helical CT yields precise anatomic detail necessary for operative fixation. High-quality CT images provide important informa-

tion regarding fracture plane orientation and location, fracture fragment position, bone resorption, and secondary degenerative changes in adjacent joints. Unlike conventional tomography, CT works equally well with casted and uncasted patients.

Standard axial CT often does not adequately demonstrate a scaphoid fracture. Some authors advocate special positioning to obtain images of the scaphoid.[6, 8–11] When scanning the scaphoid bone, it can be useful to obtain two sets of images. The first image is obtained with the gantry of the CT scanner oriented along the long axis of the scaphoid in an oblique sagittal plane. As for positioning, the patient is placed prone on the gantry with the affected arm overhead, elbow flexed at about 45 degrees, with the volar surface of the hand palm on the table and the wrist in slight ulnar deviation. The thumb is extended, and the orientation of the proximal thumb is used as a guide for aligning the scaphoid bone with the CT gantry. Two-mm slices are obtained with a 1-mm reconstruction interval in this plane.

The other plane for imaging the scaphoid is an oblique coronal plane, which parallels the coronal axis of the scaphoid view. For this view, the patient remains in a position similar to that for the earlier scan but supinates the forearm with the wrist in neutral position so that the palm faces the top of the head. The arm is flexed to approximately 50 degrees, bringing the scaphoid into parallel alignment with the CT gantry. As before, 2-mm slices are obtained with a 1-mm reconstruction interval. Images are photographed in bone detail. Accurate patient positioning also optimizes CT evaluation of fractures of the distal radius and ulna. These are complex injuries and often require operative intervention. Conventional radiographs, although important, often do not yield enough information for surgical planning when fracture lines are complex. The status of the articular surface of the distal radius, as well as the articular surface of the distal radioulnar joint, is important for fracture classification and treatment decisions.[12–15] CT scanning is usually requested for patients with known distal radius fractures to better evaluate the articular surface, the number of fragments, and if the radiocarpal and/or distal radioulnar joints are involved. To perform helical CT of the distal radius and ulna, typically two scans are acquired (Fig. 3). These studies are operator-dependent in terms of optimal scan acquisition.

CT is an important tool for evaluating patients with calcaneal fractures[16, 17]; CT of the calcaneus is another area where correct positioning and scan alignment improve image quality and diagnostic value. The amount of comminution and articular incongruency of the posterior facet of the subtalar joint are the primary determinants of risk for accelerated osteoarthritis.[18] Open reduction and internal fixation to restore alignment of the subtalar joint may decrease the risk. CT yields valuable information as a preoperative planning tool.[16, 17] The goals of operative intervention are to restore the height and congruency of the posterior facet of the subtalar joint and to restore the length of the calcaneus. Therefore, it is important to assess fracture extension into the anterior calcaneus to the level of the calcaneocuboid joint as well as facet involvement.

When performing CT of the calcaneus, two scans are obtained. For the first scan, the patient is positioned so that

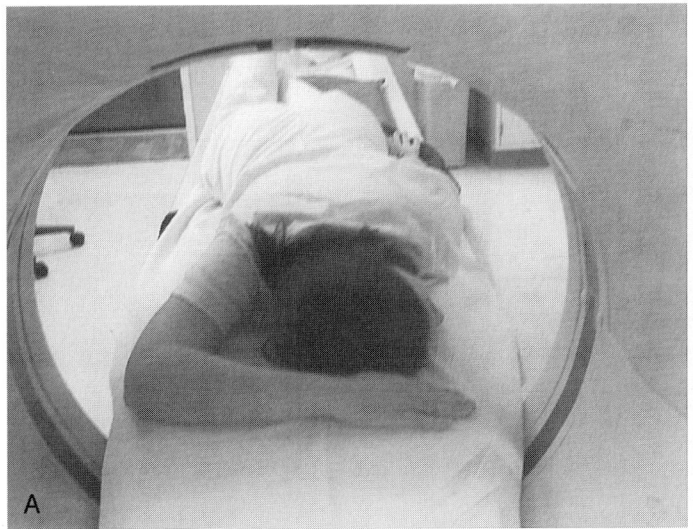

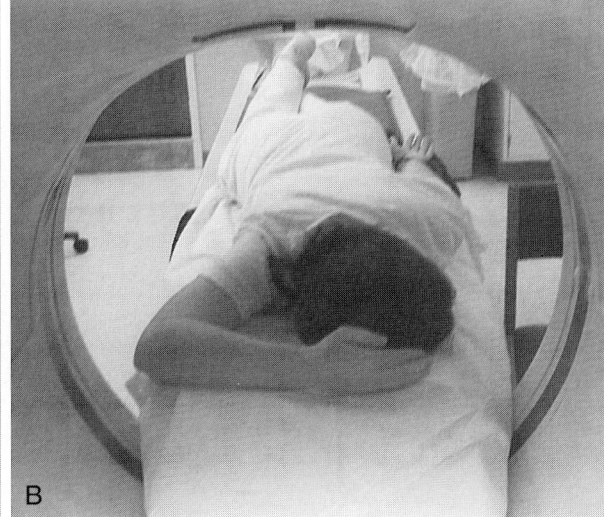

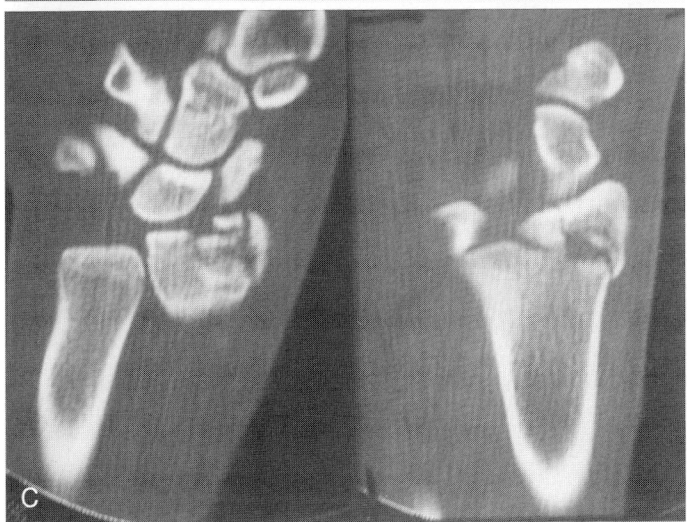

Fig. 3. CT evaluation of distal radius fracture. *A,* Proper patient position for images sagittal to distal radius. Note that the palm is down and the arm is flexed slightly less than 90 degrees to minimize artifacts from the proximal radius, ulna, and elbow. *B,* Proper patient position for images coronal to distal radius. As before, the arm is flexed slightly less than 90 degrees. CT scan shows proper patient orientation. *C,* Coronal images show fracture extension to articular surface with associated depressed fragment and articular incongruity.

an oblique coronal puts the gantry perpendicular to the posterior facet of the subtalar joint, using 3-mm slices with a pitch of 1:1, reconstructed every 1.5 mm. The second scan is in the axial plane, parallel to the longitudinal axis of the os calcis and perpendicular to the calcaneocuboid joint. Scan parameters are the same as the oblique coronal images. From the oblique coronal study, sagittal reconstructions are generated. If needed for preoperative planning, reconstructions can be made parallel to the plane of the posterior facet of the subtalar joint to show any incongruity of the joint en face.

Careful attention to patient positioning will improve the diagnostic utility of images obtained, allowing better decision-making by the orthopaedic surgeon.

CONE-BEAM CT

A development in CT technology that will significantly alter the approach to CT imaging of patients is called limited cone-beam CT.[19] This is a helical CT scanner that obtains multiple slices of information in a single revolution of the x-ray tube. With current scanners, a fan-shaped

beam of x-rays is directed through the patient and collected on a single row of detectors. From these data, individual slices are reconstructed. With cone-beam CT, a cone-shaped beam of x-rays is directed through the patient to multiple rows of detectors, with multiple slices reconstructed from the data (Fig. 4). This promises to dramatically increase the ability to rapidly image patients in the trauma setting or to obtain very thin slices for bone detail.

CONCLUSION

CT scanning provides important diagnostic information regarding the musculoskeletal system. CT provides better osseous anatomic detail than either plain radiography or MRI and is helpful for detecting small fractures and characterizing fracture extent. This is particularly true for injuries of the wrist, scaphoid, and calcaneus. CT scanning can guide operative versus conservative care. If operative treatment is undertaken, CT delineates anatomic detail of fracture fragments as a preoperative map for open reduction and internal fixation.

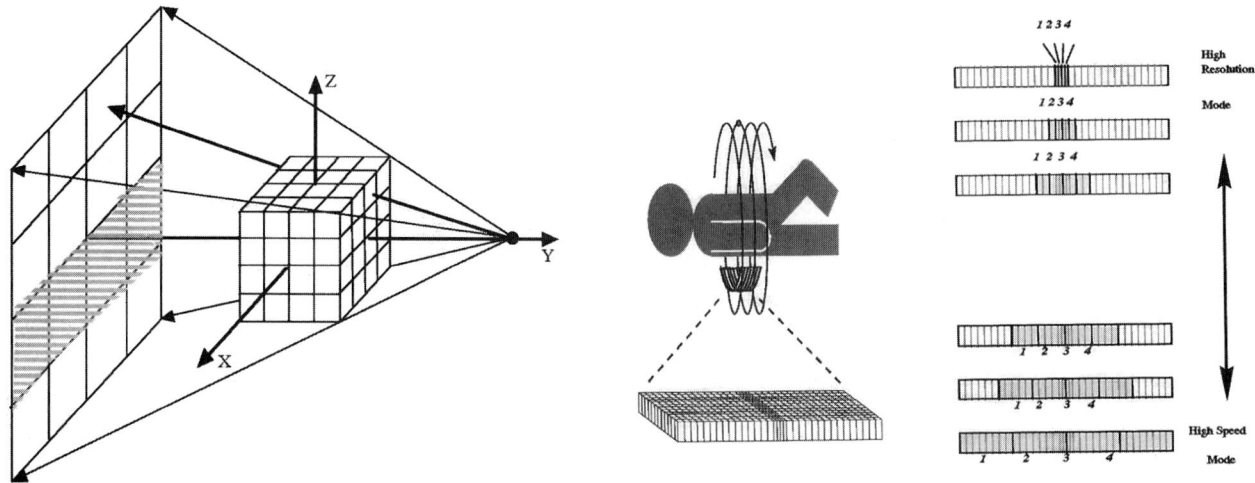

A   B

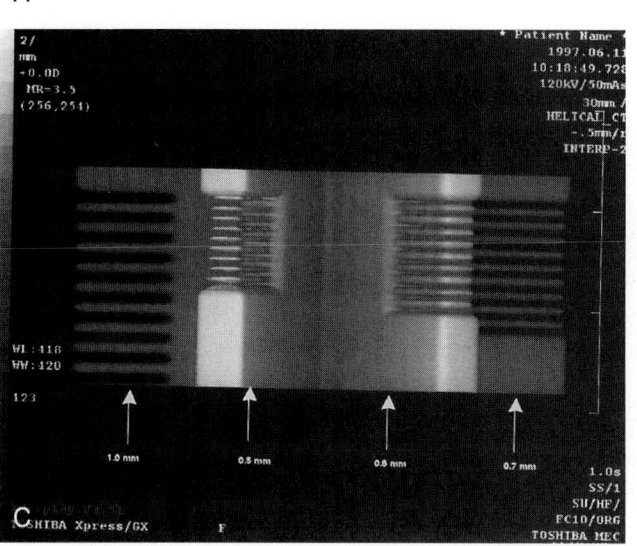

Fig. 4. Principles of cone-beam CT. *A,* A cone-shaped beam of x-rays directed through a patient to multiple rows of detectors allows simultaneous collection of multiple rows of data from the patient. With a fan-shaped beam, used in current CT scanners, only a single row of data is collected at a time (shaded row). *B,* The multirow array of x-ray detectors can be configured to collect very thin slices of data in a high-resolution mode or, by using more of the detector array, collect thicker slices in a high-speed mode. *C,* Three-dimensional reconstructed image of a comb phantom with tines arranged progressively closer to each other. Note excellent separation of tines at even 0.5-mm spacing (Courtesy of Toshiba America Medical Systems, Tustin, CA).

Musculoskeletal CT requires attention to user-controlled parameters if diagnostic utility is to be maximized. Patient position, slice thickness, reconstruction interval, and choice of imaging plane are critical decisions that depend on the patient's particular injury and the area to be imaged.

Technological advances in CT include helical or spiral scanning in which volumetric data collection allows multiplanar reconstructions in virtually any plane. Overlapping reconstructed images or volume averaging reduce missed fractures or abnormalities in the plane of the CT gantry. Limited cone-beam CT shows promise for dramatically increasing the utility of CT in the future.

REFERENCES

1. Crawford C, King K: Computed tomography scanning with simultaneous patient translation. Med Phys 1990; 17:967.
2. Tohki Y: Principles of helical scan. In Kimura K, Koga S (eds): Basic Principles and Clinical Applications of Helical Scan. Tokyo, Iryokagakusha, 1993, p 110.
3. Fishman E: Spiral CT evaluation of the musculoskeletal system. In Fishman EK, Jeffrey RB (eds): Spiral CT: Principles, Techniques and Clinical Application. New York, Raven Press, 1995, p 141.
4. Wang G, Vannier MW: Optimal pitch in spiral computed tomography. Med Phys 1997; 24:1653.
5. Bridgman C: Radiography of the carpal navicular bone. Med Radiogr Photogr 1949; 25:104.
6. Bush C, Gillespy T, Dell P. High resolution CT of the wrist: Initial experience with scaphoid disorders and surgical fusions. AJR 1987; 49:757.
7. Stewart N, Gilula L: CT of the wrist: A tailored approach. Radiology 1992; 183:13.
8. Sanders W: Evaluation of the humpback scaphoid by computed tomography in the longitudinal axial plane of the scaphoid. J Hand Surg Am 1987; 13:182.
9. Biondetti P, Vannier M, Gilula L, et al: Wrist: Coronal and transaxial CT scanning. Radiology 1987; 163:149.
10. Pennes D, Jonsson K, Buckwalter K: Direct coronal CT of the scaphoid bone. Radiology 1989; 171:870.
11. Friedman L, Johnston G, Yong-Hing K: Computed tomography of wrist trauma. J Can Assoc Radiol 1990; 41:141.
12. Frykman G: Fracture of the distal radius including sequelae of shoulder-hand-finger

syndrome, disturbance in the distal radioulnar joint, and impairment of nerve function: A clinical and experimental study. Acta Orthop Scand 1967; 108(S):1.

13. Melone CP: Open treatment for displaced articular fractures of the distal radius. Clin Orthop 1986; 202:103.

14. Missakian M, Cooney WP, Amadio PC, et al: Open reduction and internal fixation for distal radius fractures. J Hand Surg Am 1992; 17:745.

15. Gartland JJ, Werley CW: Evaluation of healed Colles' fractures. J Bone Joint Surg Am 1951; 33:895.

16. Hindman BW, Ross SD, Sowerby MR: Fractures of the talus and calcaneus: Evaluation by computed tomography. J Comput Tomogr 1986; 10:191.

17. Sanders R, Fortin P, DiPasquale T, et al: Operative treatment in 120 displaced intra-articular calcaneal fractures. Clin Orthop 1993; 290:87.

18. Heckman JD: Fractures and dislocations of the foot. In Rockwood CA, Green DP, Bucholz RW (eds): Rockwood and Green's Fractures in Adults. Philadelphia, Lippincott, 1991, p 2041.

19. Silver MD: High-helical-pitch, cone-beam computed tomography. Phys Med Biol 1998; 43:847.

MAGNETIC RESONANCE IMAGING

section 1
chapter 7

Stephen J. Eustace

Summary

- Magnetic resonance generates images with excellent contrast and spatial resolution in multiple planes.
- Three factors directly affect image quality—the field strength of the imaging magnet, the type of pulse sequence used in tissue excitation, and the type of receiver coil used to record signal.
- Fat is hyperintense on T_1-weighted scans; fluid is hyperintense on T_2-weighted scans.

Clinical Relevance

- Magnetic resonance imaging (MRI) improves evaluation of internal joint structures.
- MRI improves evaluation of injury to soft tissues, including injury secondary to trauma, infection, or tumors.
- MRI improves evaluation of disorders involving bone marrow.
- MRI allows optimum evaluation of diseases of the spine.

This chapter discusses basic principles of MRI, practical aspects of MRI that affect image quality, and applications of MRI in the evaluation of the spine and extremities.

CLINICAL RELEVANCE

The development of MRI has dramatically altered our understanding of musculoskeletal disorders. When employed appropriately, it allows noninvasive evaluation of the spine, including the intervertebral disks and spinal cord; the extremities, including internal joint structures (as an alternative to arthrography or arthroscopy); and bone cortex and marrow (as an alternative to computed tomography or scintigraphy). It is the best method for evaluating soft tissues of the extremities (as an alternative to computed tomography or ultrasound) (Figs. 1 and 2).

SEMINAL SCIENTIFIC OBSERVATIONS (HISTORICAL REVIEW)

Bloch and Purcell are credited with the initial description of the principles of nuclear magnetic resonance. They received Nobel prizes for their work in 1948 and 1952, respectively. Through the next two decades, magnetic resonance via spectroscopy was used to study the nature of chemical compounds. It was not until 1973, when three-dimensional magnetic resonance was described by Lauterbur at Harvard, that the medium was first used to create a diagnostic image.[1] The first clinical image of the wrist was published in a 1977 study by investigators at the University of Nottingham.[2]

FUNDAMENTAL SCIENCE

When two poles of a magnet are apposed, they repel and are displaced. In a similar way, protons magnetized within the bore of a magnetized large-bore coil are deflected by the brief application of an electromagnetic field in the form of a radiofrequency pulse. Deflected protons realign with the parent field following cessation or removal of the applied magnetic field. Such movement of protons behaving as small magnets within the parent coil generates current or electromagnetic signal from which the diagnostic image is derived. In sequence, the generated electromagnetic signal is localized in space by rapidly switching three orthogonal magnetic gradients, is converted from the frequency to the digital domain by using a mathematical fourier transform, and is finally converted to a diagnostic image by applying varying shades of grey according to the signal intensity recorded at points in space.[3]

Three physical components directly affect the quality of the derived image. The derived image is affected by the strength of the *parent magnetic field;* the strength, duration, frequency, and pattern (pulse sequence) of the *applied excitatory electromagnetic pulse;* and the size, shape, configuration, and location of the *coil* used to sample generated signal (Fig. 3).

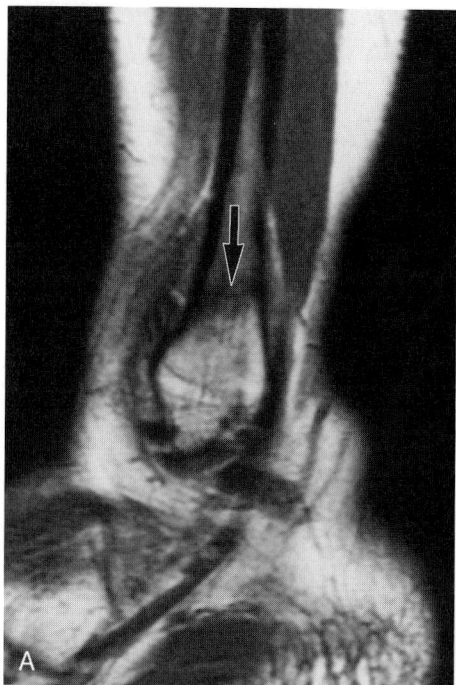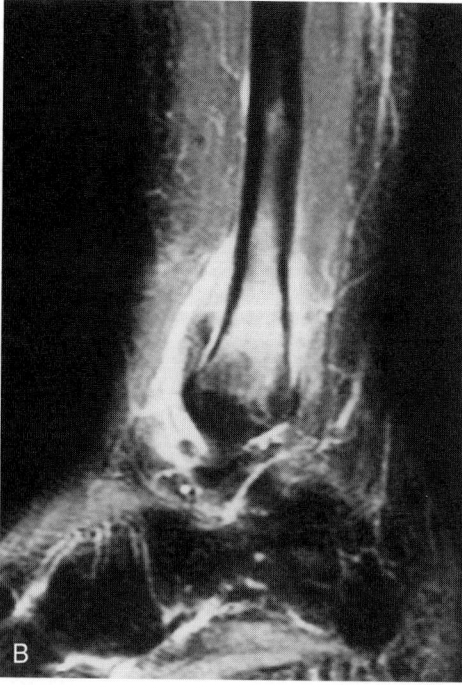

Fig. 1. A female jogger. *A,* Sagittal T_1-weighted image shows a transverse hypointense band through the distal shaft of the fibula *(arrow). B,* Sagittal fat-suppressed image (inversion recovery) in the same patient shows extensive marrow edema throughout the distal fibula, secondary to the presence of a fatigue fracture.

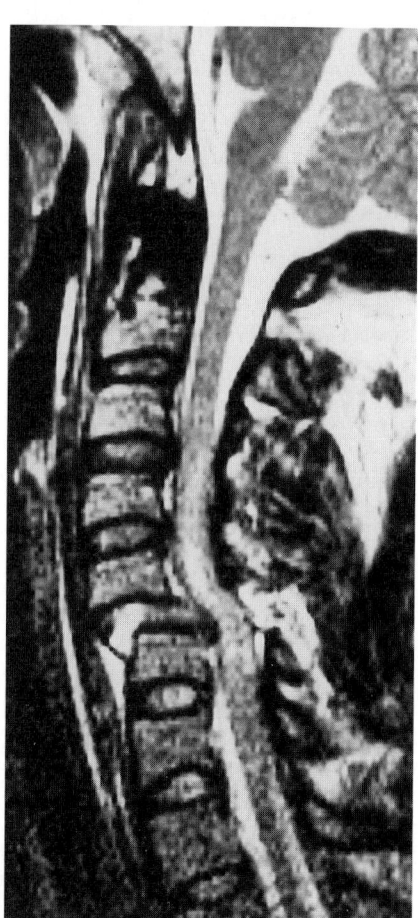

Fig. 2. Adult male patient following hyperflexion sports injury. Sagittal T_2-weighted image shows anterior subluxation at C5–6 with retropulsion of disk and secondary cord contusion.

The Parent Magnetic Field. A strong magnetic field induces greater magnetism in tissue and hence generates greater image signal following tissue excitation. Permanent magnets commonly employed in dedicated extremity MRI systems are relatively weak (0.2 to 0.35 T), limiting the recorded image signal and quality. In contrast, superconducting magnets in all-purpose units are stronger (0.5 to 1.5 T) and generate signal-rich images. Permanent systems are considerably cheaper (approximately $300,000) and incur minimal maintenance costs. Superconducting systems, in contrast, are expensive (ranging from $700,000 to 1.5 million dollars) and incur considerable maintenance costs at up to $100,000 a year.

The Applied Excitatory Electromagnetic Pulse. Tissue excitation derived by an applied electromagnetic pulse may be varied in form by the range of frequencies in the excitatory pulse and by the strength, duration, and pattern of delivery of the pulse. The pattern in which the excitatory pulse is applied is termed the pulse sequence. The *gradient echo pulse sequence* uses a single excitatory pulse that only partially deflects tissue protons before image signal is sampled; rapid acquisition is achieved at the expense of image signal. The *spin echo sequence* uses an excitatory pulse that deflects spins 90 degrees followed by a 180-degree refocusing pulse before the signal is sampled. Such a sequence allows signal-rich image aquisition at the expense of acquisition speed. The *fast spin echo sequence,* which is a modification and is now the foundation for most modern MRI protocols, uses a 90-degree pulse followed by a series of 180-degree pulses, each of which yields an echo or signal. Such a sequence allows rapid acquisition of high-quality images (Fig. 4). Improved image contrast yielded by suppressing signal from fat may be achieved either by the application of a frequency-selective fat suppression pre-pulse or by the application of an inversion

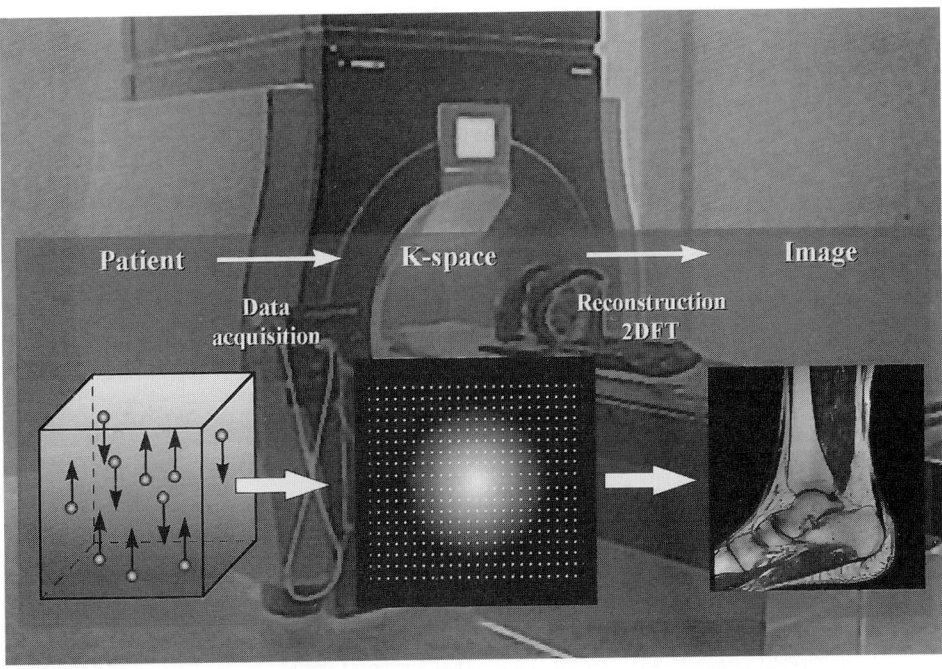

Fig. 3. The mechanics of MRI. The organs of the patient are longitudinally magnetized by a strong and homogeneous magnetic field. An imaging pulse sequence is applied, thus generating detectable transverse magnetization. The generated NMR signals are spatially encoded before measurement and stored in computer memory. The resulting raw data are not interpretable visually because they are scrambled during the application of the MRI pulse sequence by the spatial encoding pulses. The raw data, referred to as k-space data, are computer-reconstructed, thus generating the anatomic image.

pre-pulse (inversion recovery) to any of the above sequences.[4]

Image contrast: before tissue excitation, tissue protons align or rotate around the Z axis of the magnetic field (the parent field) generated by the imaging magnet. Such alignment results in a net magnetization vector in the Z axis, described as longitudinal magnetization. Random rotation around the Z axis (out of phase) results in neutralization of magnetization in the X-Y plane, or absence of transverse magnetization.

Following excitation, spins are deflected to the X-Y plane. Deflected spins now rotate in phase or as a single vector in the X-Y plane, which results in the presence of transverse magnetization. Magnetic vectors oriented in the X-Y plane lack longitudinal magnetization.

Following excitation and removal of the excitatory pulse, spins or in-phase magnetic vectors in the X-Y plane begin to dephase, leading to a loss of transverse magnetization. As protons dephase in the transverse plane, they reorient to

the parent field and regain longitudinal magnetization. Recovery of longitudinal magnetization generates T_1 signal; loss of transverse magnetization generates T_2 signal. If excitatory pulses are applied to tissue repeatedly, movement of induced magnetic vectors becomes negligible, described as steady state. If the excitatory pulse is applied repeatedly immediately following recovery of longitudinal magnetization (short TR), prior to complete loss of transverse magnetization, sequential pulses induce steady state transverse magnetization, and therefore yielded signal is from recovery of longitudinal magnetization (T_1-weighted). In contrast, if sequential excitatory pulses are applied after a delay that allows not only recovery of longitudinal magnetization but also complete loss of transverse magnetization (long TR), tissue weighting in the yielded image is a function of the time at which the signal is sampled (echo time, [TE]). If the signal is sampled early (short TE), it will contain both T_1- and T_2-weighted information (a function of the tissue proton density); if the signal is sampled

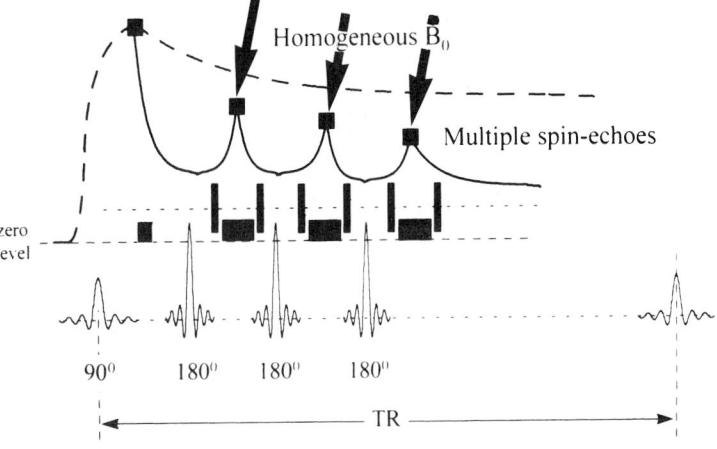

Fig. 4. Diagrammatic representation. The fast spin echo pulse sequence yields multiple echoes for a single excitatory 90-degree pulse by using serial 180-degree refocusing pulses *(arrows)*.

late (long TE), it will contain predominantly T$_2$-weighted information. On T$_1$-weighted images, fat is hyperintense, and fluid is hypointense; on T$_2$-weighted images, fat is hypointense, and fluid is hyperintense.

Receiver Coils. Electromagnetic signal generated by the excitatory pulse sequence is sampled by receiver coils, either body or surface coils. Movement of excited protons behaving as bar magnets within these coils generates image signal.

Surface coils, in contrast to the body coil, are directly apposed to the excited extremity tissues and therefore yield improved image signal. Simple surface coils may be flexi-

ble and conform to the configuration of a joint, thereby improving image signal, although the field of view or coverage is limited. Variations include the quadrature and the phased array coils. The quadrature coil, used routinely to image the knee, simultaneously samples signal in two planes to improve image quality. The phased array coil represents an array of surface coils linked as a single segment, allowing improved coverage without loss of signal.[5]

The ultimate quality of the derived MR image is a function of the type of magnet employed, the method of tissue excitation, and the type of coil used to sample signal.

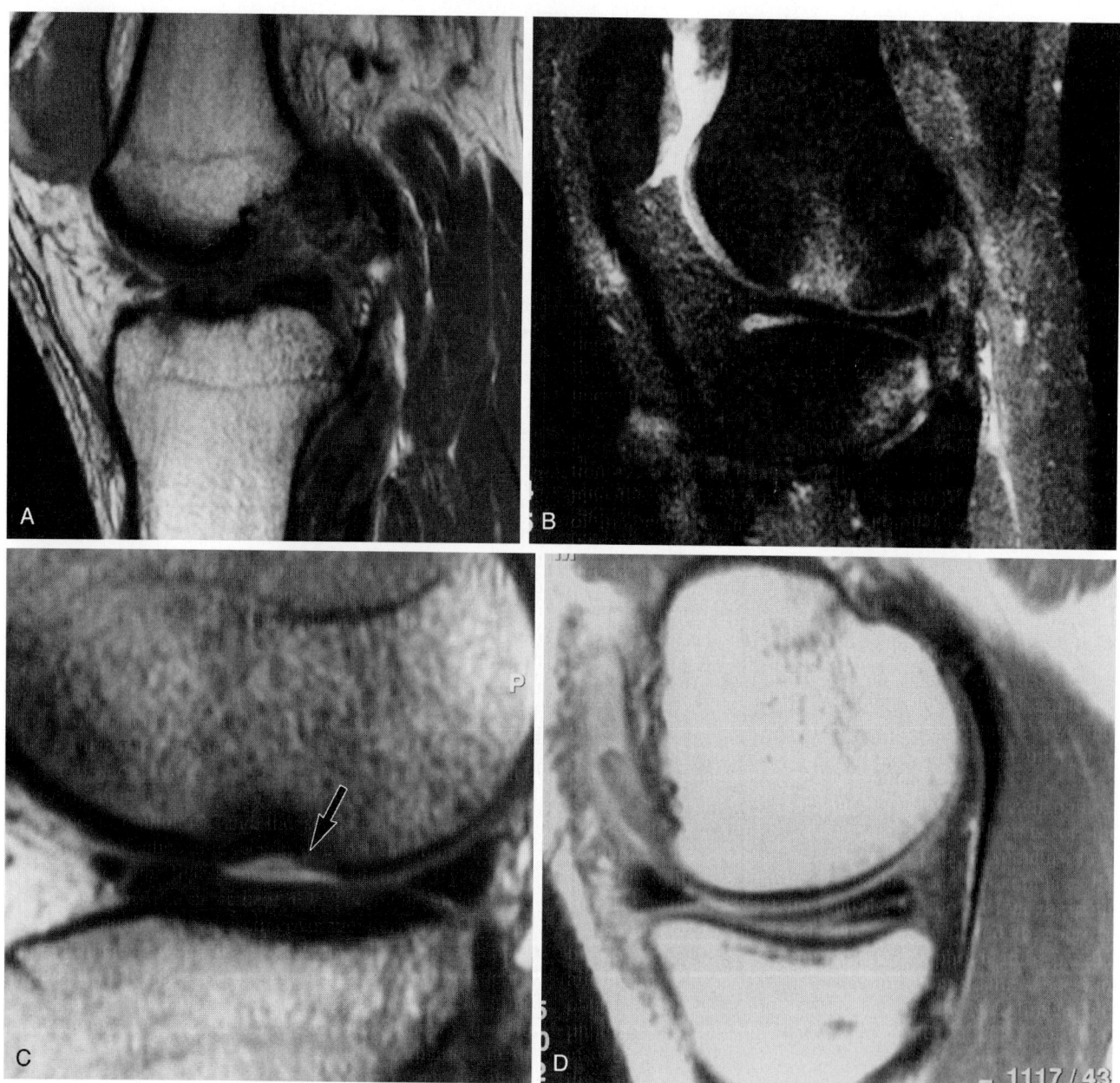

Fig. 5. Young male patient following sports injury. *A,* Sagittal proton density–weighted MR image shows disruption of the anterior cruciate ligament, with secondary alteration in signal and contour. *B,* Fat-suppressed image in the same patient shows characteristic contrecoup bone bruises of the midlateral femoral condyle and of the posterolateral tibial plateau. *C,* Zoomed image of the lateral femoral condyle shows disruption of the articular surface with osteochondral defect *(arrow). D,* Sagittal image of the same patient shows linear signal through the posterior horn of the medial meniscus extending to the inferior surface secondary to medial meniscal tear.

CLINICAL RELEVANCE AND APPLICATIONS

Improved contrast and multiplanar imaging capability afforded by MRI has dramatically altered the understanding and assessment of orthopaedic diseases of the spine and extremities.

THE EXTREMITIES
Intra-Articular Soft Tissues
The Knee

MRI is now routinely used to evaluate suspected meniscal tears, which are characterized by identification of linear signal abnormality extending to a surface; to evaluate suspected cruciate injury, particularly of the anterior cruciate ligament (characterized by primary alteration in the ligament configuration and by secondary signs including contrecoup bone bruises (Fig. 5), and to evaluate the collateral ligaments where edema or discontinuity are used as markers of injury. Less commonly, MRI is used to evaluate the extensor mechanism (for example, the patella tendon commonly injured in adolescent basketball players and the quadriceps tendon injured in the poorly conditioned middle-aged adult). High-resolution imaging affords detailed evaluation of the articular cartilage, particularly at the patellofemoral articulation where a grading system, similar to that at arthroscopy, is employed (grade 1 to 3 cartilage narrowing).[6–8]

The Shoulder

Multiplanar imaging allows detailed evaluation of the rotator cuff and the glenoid labrum. Rotator cuff injury, predominantly of the supraspinatus tendon, ranges from degenerative tendinopathy (signal abnormality on T_1 and proton density scans) to partial tear (signal abnormality on all sequences, with edema on T_2-weighted scans), to full thickness tear (usually of the anterior tendon margin) where fluid (hyperintense on T_2-weighted scan) is identified traversing the tendon, allowing communication between the joint space and the subacromial bursa. The labrum is best identified in the axial plane where it is identified as a hypointense structure marginating the osseous glenoid. Most frequently, evaluation of the labrum is undertaken in patients with persistent unidirectional instability complicating dislocation when injury to the anteroinferior labrum is suspected. Less frequently, MRI is undertaken to evaluate the superior labrum in patients with shoulder pain complicating a fall or throwing patients in whom a superior labral tear is suspected.[9–11]

Other Joints

MRI is now routinely used to evaluate intercarpal ligaments (scapholunate and lunatotriquetral ligaments) and the triangular fibrocartilage in the wrist as well as collateral ligaments; syndesmosis; long flexor, extensor, peroneal, and Achilles tendons in the ankle. MRI is useful in visualizing the labrum in the hip, as well as the collateral ligaments, the biceps, and the brachialis and triceps insertions at the elbow.[12–14]

Intra-articular contrast, introduced either directly (direct arthrography) or by intravenous injection (indirect arthrography), is now commonly used to improve evaluation of joint structures. In this regard, MR arthrography has been shown to improve the evaluation of the glenoid labrum and rotator cuff in the shoulder (Fig. 6), of recurrent meniscal tears in the knee, of the collateral ligaments in the ankle and elbow, of the intercarpal ligaments in the wrist, and of the labrum in the hip.[15, 16]

Extra-Articular Soft Tissues
Muscle Injury

Muscle injury, most frequently involving the calf, may follow a direct contusion or laceration or follow indirect trauma acutely manifested as muscle strain (Fig. 7) or as delayed onset muscle soreness (DOMS).

Muscle strains are graded according to severity. First degree strains are manifest as focal signal abnormality without a tear, on MRI; second degree strains are seen as a partial tear; and third degree strains are characterized by a complete tear with hemorrhage and retraction. Muscle tears most commonly occur during vigorous exercise and most frequently involve muscles that cross two joints, have an abundance of fast twitch fibers, and undergo eccentric muscle contraction, such as the gastrocnemius.

DOMS is also most frequently identified in muscles with eccentric contractions, following chronic overuse. On MRI, DOMS is manifest by local signal abnormality most frequently at muscle or fascial attachments but occasionally at sites remote from the site of tenderness.[17, 18]

Vessels

Both noncontrast "time of flight" and dynamic gadolinium techniques are used to image vascular injury. In this regard, MRI has been used in the evaluation of post-traumatic arterial laceration and thrombosis of deep veins

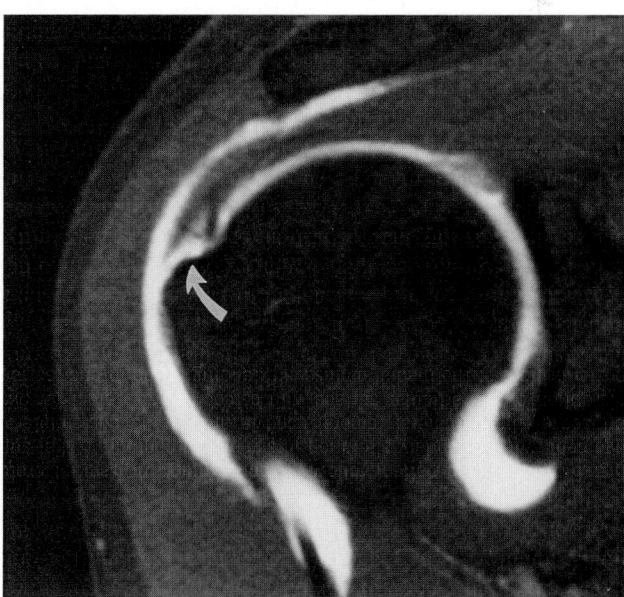

Fig. 6. An elderly patient with shoulder pain following injury. Coronal oblique fat-suppressed T_1-weighted image following gadolinium arthrography shows a full-thickness tear at the insertion of the supraspinatus, allowing communication from the shoulder joint space to the subacromial bursa (arrow).

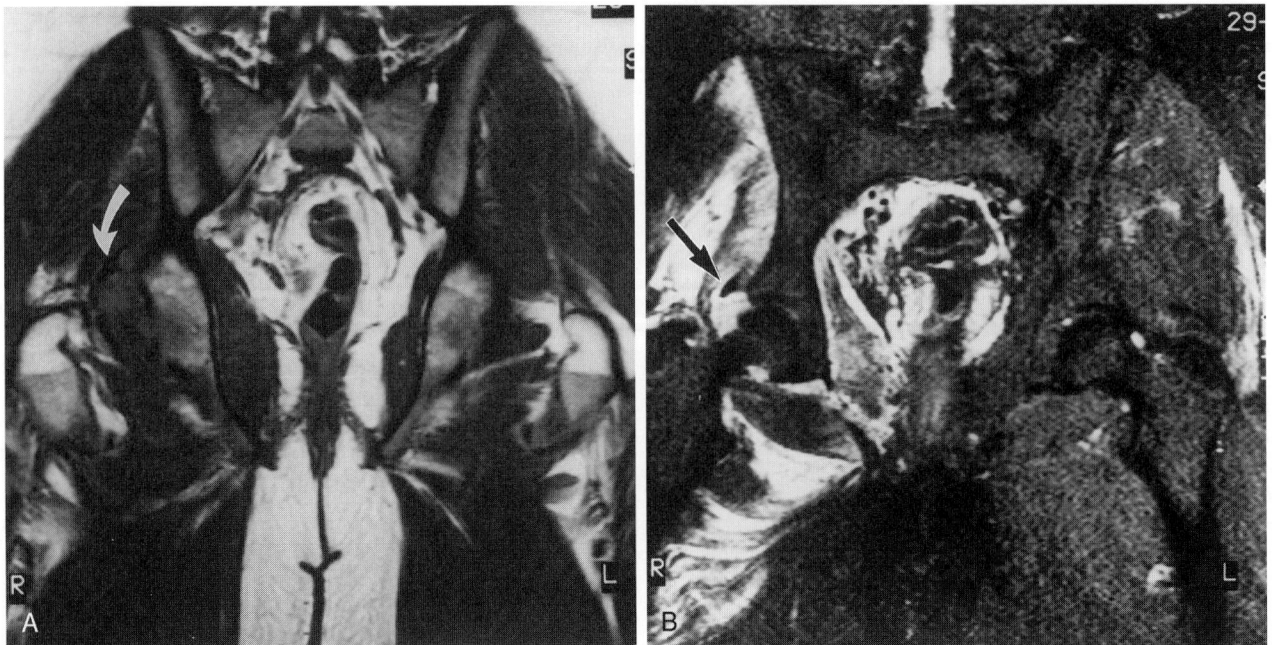

Fig. 7. A young patient following motor vehicle accident and posterior hip subluxation. Coronal T_1 *(A)* and fat-suppressed *(B)* images show extensive edema within the muscles of the right buttock with an associated displaced superior labral fragment *(arrow)*.

within the pelvis (following hip replacement or pelvic trauma).

Infection

The ability of MRI to localize sites of edema identified via signal hyperintensity, particularly on fat-suppressed images, allows noninvasive evaluation of soft-tissue infection, cellulitis, fasciitis, and myositis. Although focal fluid pockets are readily identified on T_2-weighted fat-suppressed images,

gadolinium enhancement may improve the evaluation of the extent of the inflammatory process.

Tumors

Improved contrast resolution on MRI affords rapid localization and tissue characterization of soft-tissue masses. Features suggestive of a malignant soft-tissue mass include signal heterogeneity within the mass, poorly defined margins, extensive poorly marginated edema within the adja-

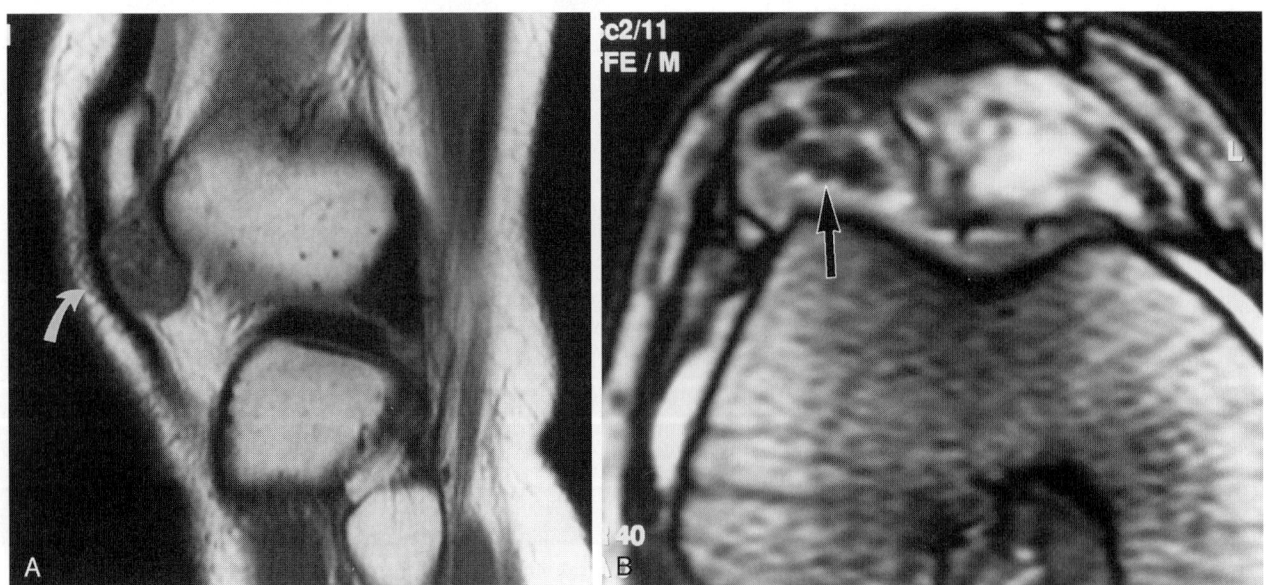

Fig. 8. Young adult with knee pain. *A*, Sagittal proton density–weighted image shows a lobular mass within Hoffa's fat immediately below the patella *(arrow)*. *B*, Axial gradient echo image in the same patient shows susceptibility artifact within the mass, indicating the presence of hemosiderin typical of pigmented villonodular synovitis.

cent soft tissues, and dramatic enhancement (rapid upslope) within the mass following administration of gadolinium (Fig. 8).

Bone Marrow

Unlike conventional radiography, MRI allows detailed evaluation of bone marrow and specifically allows detection of marrow edema. Bone marrow edema may reflect local trauma, the presence of tumor, hyperemia in infection or inflammation, or impaired marrow drainage secondary to venous thrombosis as occurs in avascular necrosis or lymphatic obstruction.[19]

Traumatic bone marrow edema, termed a bone bruise, varies in pattern relative to mechanism. Impaction injury results in poorly marginated marrow edema; distraction injury results in linear marrow edema perpendicular to the axis of stress. Shear injury results in linear bone marrow edema, usually in an oblique orientation[19] (see Figs. 1 and 5B).

THE SPINE

DEGENERATIVE DISK DISEASE

The intervertebral disk is composed predominantly of water and mucopolysaccharide, accounting for T_1 signal hypointensity and T_2 signal hyperintensity in health. In adulthood, as the disk degenerates, it loses water and mucopolysaccharide content, resulting in morphological changes, particularly loss of height of the disk and annular bulging.

The precursor to disk degeneration is thought to be tearing of the outer annular fibers anteriorly, laterally, or posteriorly. In most cases, these annular tears are not identifiable on MRI. Occasionally, tears are conspicuous on heavily T_2-weighted scans as foci of hyperintensity (high intensity zones) secondary to the presence of edema and granulation tissue. Nerve roots apparently exit at the periphery of the annulus and may be irritated, accounting for the correlation between high intensity zones and low back pain. Disk herniations are well visualized on T_1-weighted scans, contrasted against epidural fat. On T_2-weighted scans, the herniated portion is usually slightly hyperintense relative to the rest of the degenerating disk. The compressed nerve root adjacent to the herniated disk may occasionally enhance following the administration of gadolinium.

Using MRI, signal abnormalities are noted in the marrow immediately adjacent to the vertebral body end plate and degenerating disk, preceding radiographic evidence of end-plate sclerosis. Early in discogenic degeneration, end-plate marrow becomes T_1 hypointense and T_2 hyperintense (type 1 change); later, the marrow adjacent to the end plate appears to become fatty and manifests as T_1 signal hyperintensity and persistent although slightly less marked T_2 signal hyperintensity (type 2 change). In end-stage disease, marrow becomes replaced by dense bone, obvious on radiographs and hypointense on both T_1- and T_2-weighted scans at MRI. Both type 1 and type 2 changes enhance following the administration of gadolinium and should not be incorrectly attributed to the presence of local marrow infection.[20, 21]

TRAUMA

Recognizing its ability to visualize soft tissues including the intervertebral disk and the spinal cord, MRI should be considered in patients with neurological impairment, prior to either closed or open reduction, to determine the integrity of intervertebral disks. The presence of cord enhancement suggests the presence of edema rather than hemorrhage; the presence of susceptibility artifact suggests cord hemorrhage rather than edema.[22]

REFERENCES

1. Lauterbur PC: Image formation by induced local interactions: Examples employing nuclear magnetic resonance. Nature 1973; 242:190.
2. Hinshaw WS, Bottomley PA, Holland GN: Radiographic thin section image of the human wrist by nuclear magnetic resonance. Nature 1977; 270:722.
3. Hashemi RH, Bradley WG. MRI: The Basics. Baltimore, Williams & Wilkins, 1997.
4. Hennig J, Nauerth A, Friedburg H: RARE imaging: A fast imaging method for clinical MR. Magn Reson Med 1986; 3:823.
5. Elster AD: Questions and Answers in Magnetic Resonance Imaging. Chicago, Mosby, 1994.
6. Stoller DW, Genant HK: Magnetic resonance imaging of the knee and hip. Arthritis Rheum 1990; 33:441.
7. Mink JH, Deutsch AL: Magnetic resonance imaging of the knee. Clin Orthop 1989; 244:29.
8. Burk DL Jr, Mitchell DG, Rifkin MD, et al: Recent advances in magnetic resonance imaging of the knee. Rad Clin Am 1990; 28:379.
9. Palmer WE, Brown JH, Rosenthal DI. The rotator cuff: Evaluation with fat-suppressed MR arthrography. Radiology 1993; 188:683.
10. Uri DS: MR imaging of shoulder impingement and rotator cuff disease. Radiol Clin N Am 1997; 35:77.
11. Eustace S, Denison B: MR imaging of acute orthopaedic trauma to the upper extremity. Clin Radiol 1997; 52:338.
12. Hodler J, Yu JS, Goodwin D, et al: MR arthrography of the hip: Improved imaging of the acetabular labrum with histologic correlation in cadavers. Am J Roentgenol 1995; 165:887.
13. Fritz RC: MR imaging of the elbow. Semin Roentgenol 1995; 30:241.
14. Binkovitz LA, Ehman RL, Cahill DR, et al: Magnetic resonance imaging of the wrist. Radiographics 1988; 8:1171.
15. Palmer WE, Caslowitz PL, Chew FS: MR arthrography of the shoulder: Normal intra-articular structures and common abnormalities. Am J Roentgenol 1995; 164:141.
16. Tirman PFJ, Stauffer AE, Crues JV III, et al: Saline magnetic resonance arthrography in the evaluation of glenohumeral instability. Arthroscopy 1993; 9:550.
17. Fleckenstein JL, Shellock FG: Exertional muscle injuries: Magnetic resonance evaluation. Top Magn Reson Imaging 1991; 3:50.
18. El Khoury GY, Brandser EA, Kathol MH: Imaging of muscle injuries. Skel Radiol 1996; 25:3.
19. Eustace S: Basic Principles. In Magnetic Resonance Of Orthopedic Trauma. Philadelphia, Lippincott, Williams & Wilkins. 1999, pp 59–76.
20. Czervionke LF: Lumbar intervertebral disc disease. Neuroimaging Clin Am 1993; 4:465.
21. Modic MT, Masaryk TJ, Ross JT: Imaging of degenerative disc disease. Radiology 1988; 168:177.
22. Kulkarni MV, McArdle CB, Kopanicky D: Acute spinal cord injury: MR imaging at 1.5 T. Radiology 1987; 164:837.

section
1
chapter
8

MUSCULOSKELETAL SONOGRAPHY

Jon A. Jacobson

Summary
- Advantages of musculoskeletal sonography, compared with magnetic resonance imaging (MRI), include relative low expense, portability, and improved accessibility.
- Disadvantages of musculoskeletal sonography include operator dependence and long learning curve.
- Sonography results may be equal to those of MRI for many indications when performed by an experienced sonographer.
- When evaluating symptoms or physical findings present only with specific patient movement or positioning, musculoskeletal sonography is the imaging method of choice.

Clinical Relevance
- Musculoskeletal sonography may be considered when investigating a specific soft-tissue abnormality, such as tendon abnormalities, joint effusion, soft-tissue foreign body, developmental dysplasia of the hip, carpal tunnel syndrome, and certain soft-tissue masses such as Baker's cyst and wrist ganglion.
- MRI may be considered when there is a need to evaluate for cartilage and bone marrow abnormalities.

Although first applied in the late 1970s, musculoskeletal sonography is receiving increased interest for two principal reasons. First, improved technology allows depiction of superficial structures with exquisite detail. Second, today's emphasis on cost containment has made musculoskeletal sonography an attractive alternative to MRI.

Several advantages of ultrasonography as compared with MRI include relative low expense, portability, improved access, and ability to evaluate a joint dynamically. The primary disadvantage of ultrasonography is the inherent operator dependence. In addition, the learning process is lengthy, and the resulting images may not be familiar to the referring physician.

Ultrasound images are produced when the sound beam originating from an ultrasound transducer travels through the soft tissues and is reflected back to the transducer. Bright echoes are produced at soft-tissue interfaces where much of the sound beam is reflected. Figure 1 shows an example of this in cortical bone, which is bright or hyperechoic, with posterior shadowing due to sound beam reflection. Normal tendons appear hyperechoic, but to a lesser degree than cortical bone, and demonstrate internal fibrillar echoes. Muscle is relatively hypoechoic, and simple fluid is anechoic. Normal peripheral nerves demonstrate alternating hyperechoic and hypoechoic bundles.

The following sections review several applications of musculoskeletal sonography. These are summarized for each of the major joints. Finally, there is a brief discussion comparing musculoskeletal ultrasonography with MRI.

SHOULDER SONOGRAPHY

One of the initial and most common applications of musculoskeletal sonography is examination of the shoulder; more specifically, that of the rotator cuff. Controversy ex-

SUP

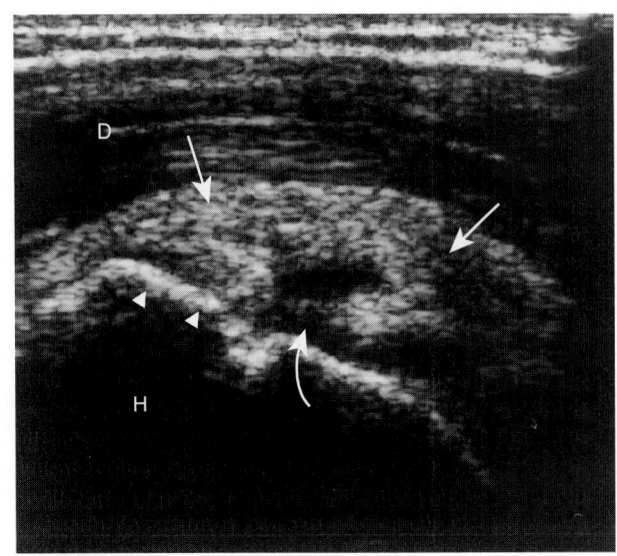

LAT

MED

INF

Fig. 1. Supraspinatus tear: partial thickness, articular. Coronal sonographic image longitudinal to the supraspinatus tendon demonstrates the hypoechoic tendon tear *(curved arrow)*. Note normal surrounding supraspinatus tendon *(arrows)* and cortex of proximal humerus *(arrowheads)*. (D = deltoid muscle; H = humerus; SUP = superior; INF = inferior; LAT = lateral; MED = medial).

POST

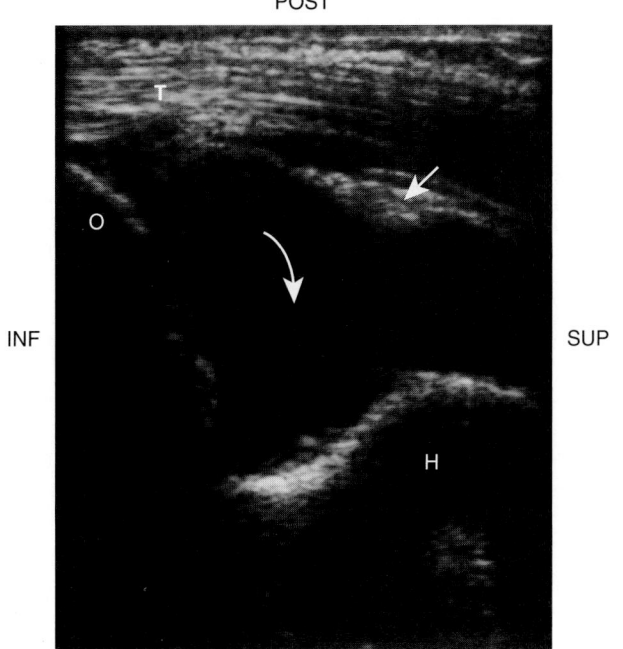

Fig. 2. Elbow effusion: septic, gonococcal. Sagittal sonographic image of the posterior elbow demonstrates the anechoic effusion *(curved arrow)* displacing the hyperechoic olecranon fat pad *(arrow)*. (T = triceps tendon; O = olecranon; H = humerus; SUP = superior; INF = inferior; POST = posterior; ANT = anterior).

ists regarding the effectiveness of ultrasonography in this application as sensitivities for diagnosis of rotator cuff tears have ranged from 33% to 100%.[1] This wide range is likely due to the operator dependence of sonography.

Focal abnormalities of the rotator cuff generally appear hypoechoic, disrupting the normal echotexture (see Fig. 1). Partial-thickness tears extend to one surface of the tendon, and focal full thickness tears extend to the articular and bursal surfaces. Massive tendon tears appear as nonvisualization of the tendon due to tendon retraction. There is difficulty in differentiating a small full-thickness tear from a partial-thickness tear or focal tendinosis as each may

appear hypoechoic. Tendinosis and tendon tear may coexist in the continuum of a diseased tendon, making this differentiation difficult. Sonography is most reliable in diagnosing large full thickness tears and in excluding rotator cuff disorders.

Other tendon abnormalities about the shoulder may be investigated with sonography. Long head of biceps brachii tendon tear, tenosynovitis, and subluxation may be identified.[1] In fact, the ability to evaluate biceps tendon subluxation dynamically is an advantage over MRI. Other sources for shoulder pain may be diagnosed with sonography, including ganglion cysts, bursitis, and calcific tendinitis.[1]

ELBOW SONOGRAPHY

Sonography of the elbow is used primarily to evaluate soft-tissue infection. Sonography can diagnose soft-tissue cellulitis, abscess, bursitis, and joint effusion and then provide immediate guided aspiration for diagnosis. Cellulitis appears as a branching hypoechoic pattern in the subcutaneous tissues. Bursitis, an abscess formation, is usually well-defined hypoechoic or anechoic fluid collections. Joint effusion occurs when hypoechoic or anechoic fluid distends the joint recesses and displaces the intracapsular fat pads (Fig. 2). Sonography is more sensitive than radiography in detecting elbow effusions.[2]

Other potential applications for elbow sonography include evaluating the distal biceps brachii and triceps tendons and evaluating epicondylitis. Although various elbow ligaments can be visualized with sonography, sonography's ability to diagnose ligamentous injury is unproven. Sonography may also be used to evaluate cubital tunnel syndrome.[3] Sonography has an advantage over MRI in diagnosing ulnar nerve subluxation; abnormal nerve position may be present only with elbow flexion and will remain undetected on MRI when the elbow is in extended position.

WRIST SONOGRAPHY

The three most common applications for wrist sonography include evaluation for ganglion cyst, carpal tunnel syn-

Fig. 3. Wrist ganglion. Sagittal sonographic image of the dorsal wrist demonstrates the lobular and septated anechoic ganglion cyst *(curved arrow)*. Note communication to radiocarpal joint (*). (rad = radius; lun = lunate; cap = capitate; ET = extensor tendon; SUP = superior; INF = inferior).

DORSAL

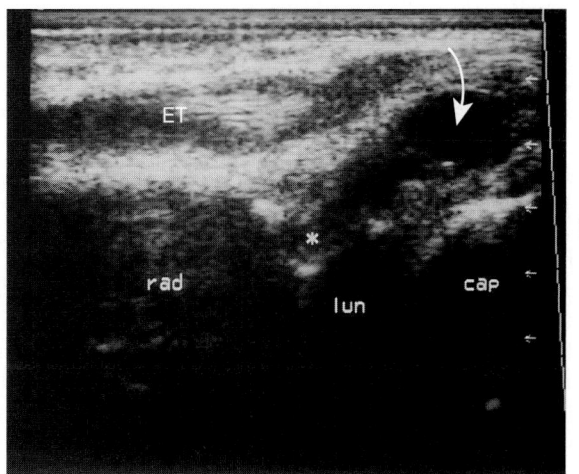

VOLAR

ANT

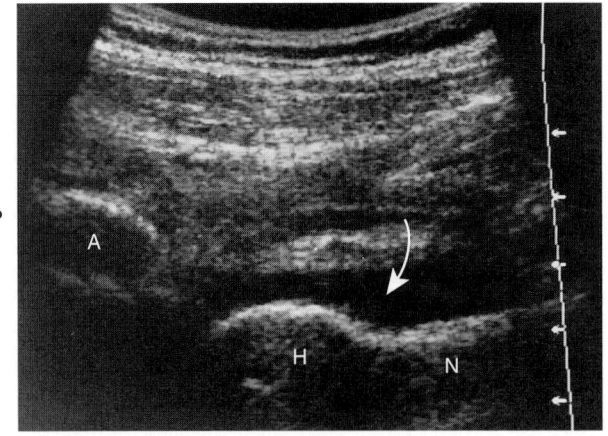

SUP

INF

A

H   N

POST

Fig. 4. Hip effusion: aseptic. Sagittal sonographic image of anterior hip parallel to femoral neck demonstrates the anechoic joint effusion *(curved arrow)* distending the joint capsule. (A = acetabulum; H = femoral head; N = femoral neck; SUP = superior; INF = inferior; ANT = anterior; POST = posterior).

drome, and tendon abnormalities. When a palpable mass about the wrist is anechoic and appears as a cyst by sonography, a benign ganglion cyst is likely (Fig. 3). Sonography and MRI are equally effective in diagnosis of occult wrist ganglion cysts.[4] Evaluation for carpal tunnel syndrome can also be accomplished with sonography as enlargement of the median nerve more than 10 mm^2 at the proximal carpal tunnel is seen with this condition.[5] Various tendon abnormalities may be identified with sonography, such as tendon tear, tendinosis, and tenosynovitis (including inflammatory and de Quervain's tenosynovitis).

HIP SONOGRAPHY

Sonography is effective in evaluating the pediatric hip for developmental dysplasia and joint effusion. Various algorithms employ hip sonography in screening for developmental dysplasia. One such protocol uses sonography at 2 weeks of age if the clinically abnormal hip is unstable and at 4 to 6 weeks of age if the patient has a stable hip click or if significant risk factors are present.[6] Sonography has the benefit of visualizing the unossified hypoechoic femoral heads, which are not visible by radiography. Sonography is also useful in evaluating the painful pediatric hip when there is concern for infection or synovitis.[7] Because the appearance of a joint effusion cannot predict infection, sonography-guided aspiration should then be used to exclude infection (Fig. 4).

In the adult, the application of sonography includes evaluation for joint effusion and tendon/muscle injury. The visualization of joint effusion in large adult patients may prove difficult, however, and fluoroscopic aspiration is often required to exclude infection.

KNEE SONOGRAPHY

A common application for knee sonography is confirmation of Baker's or popliteal cyst. In an older individual, sonography can effectively diagnose Baker's cyst, thereby excluding other diagnoses such as malignant tumor or thrombophlebitis. Baker's cyst is typically anechoic or hypoechoic and demonstrates a communicating neck to the

posterior knee between the semimembranosus and medial gastrocnemius tendons (Fig. 5).[8] Meniscal disorders are better visualized on MRI than sonography.

Other applications of knee sonography include evaluation for quadriceps or patellar tendon tears and patellar tendinosis or jumper's knee.

FOOT AND ANKLE SONOGRAPHY

The most common application for sonography of the foot and ankle is evaluation for tendon abnormalities. Full thickness tears appear as nonvisualization of the involved

POST

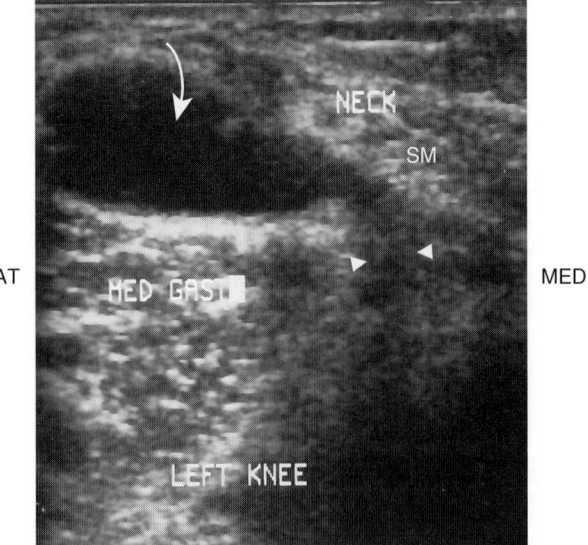

NECK

SM

LAT

MED GAST

MED

LEFT KNEE

ANT

Fig. 5. Baker's cyst. Axial sonographic image of the posterior knee demonstrates an anechoic fluid collection *(curved arrow)* communicating to the posterior knee joint *(arrowheads)* between the medial gastrocnemius muscle/tendon (MED GAST) and the semimembranosus tendon (SM). (POST = posterior; ANT = anterior; MED = medial; LAT = lateral).

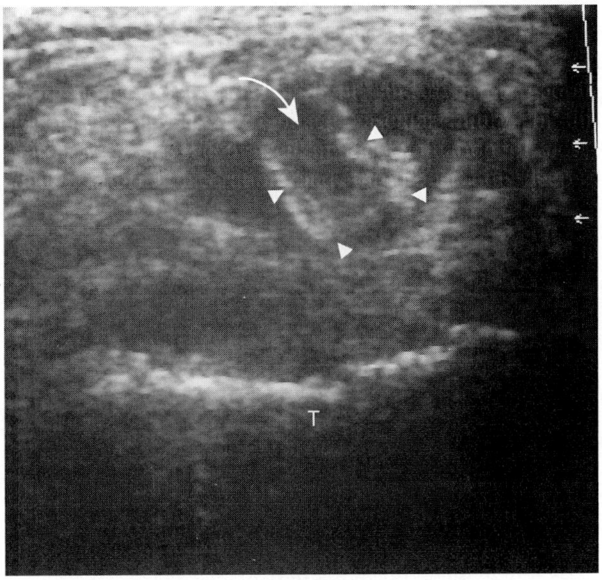

MED

POST   ANT

LAT

Fig. 6. Posterior tibial tendon, partial thickness tear. Axial sonographic image of the posteromedial ankle demonstrates an anechoic cleft *(curved arrow)* of the hyperechoic posterior tibial tendon *(arrowheads)*. Note surrounding tenosynovitis *(arrows)*. (T = tibia; ANT = anterior; POST = posterior; MED = medial; LAT = lateral).

tendon. Partial-thickness tears appear as hypoechoic or anechoic clefts interrupting the hyperechoic fibrillar echotexture of a normal tendon (Fig. 6).[9] Tendinosis can also be diagnosed. One advantage of sonography is the ability to evaluate for transient peroneal tendon subluxation. Such subluxation may occur only during dynamic foot positioning and may remain undetected on MRI when the ankle is in a fixed neutral position.

Another useful application is evaluation for soft-tissue foreign bodies. In particular, radiolucent foreign bodies such as wood, which are not visible with routine radiography, may be visualized. All soft-tissue foreign bodies are hyperechoic and are typically surrounded by a hypoechoic halo representing a foreign body reaction.[10] High-resolution ultrasound transducers are effective in this situation; wooden foreign bodies as small as 2.5 mm can be located with sonography.[10]

Sonography is also useful in evaluation for joint effusion, abscess, and cellulitis when there is concern for soft-tissue infection.

MUSCULOSKELETAL SONOGRAPHY VERSUS MRI

Comparison of these two imaging methods for certain musculoskeletal applications has been inconclusive. Although it is true that MRI is more widely used and accepted, musculoskeletal sonography can demonstrate similar results for specific indications when performed by an experienced sonographer. It is essential that the sonographer understand the advantages and limitations of ultrasound and that the referring physician is familiar with the sonographer's abilities.

Sonography is most successful when evaluating for a specific problem, such as tendon abnormality, ganglion or Baker's cyst, joint effusion, carpal tunnel syndrome, and soft-tissue foreign body. Sonography may also be considered when there is a contraindication for MRI, such as presence of certain metal devices and foreign bodies. MRI should be considered when a global evaluation is required, to include areas such as articular cartilage and bone marrow.

REFERENCES

1. Jacobson JA, van Holsbeeck MT: Musculoskeletal ultrasonography. In Boutin RD, Sartoris DJ, eds: Orthopedic Clinics of North America: Musculoskeletal Imaging Update, vol 29. Philadelphia, W.B. Saunders, 1998, p 135.
2. De Maeseneer M, Jacobson JA, Jaovisidha S, et al: Elbow effusions: Distribution of joint fluid with flexion and extension and imaging implications. Invest Radiol 1998; 33:117.
3. Chiou HJ, Chou YH, Cheng SP, et al: Cubital tunnel syndrome: Diagnosis by high-resolution ultrasonography. J Ultrasound Med 1998; 17:643.
4. Cardinal E, Buckwalter KA, Braunstein EM, et al: Occult dorsal carpal ganglion: Comparison of US and MR imaging. Radiology 1994; 193:259.
5. Chen P, Maklad N, Redwine M, et al: Dynamic high-resolution sonography of the carpal tunnel. Am J Radiol 1997; 168:533.
6. Harcke HT: Screening newborns for developmental dysplasia of the hip: The role of sonography. Am J Radiol 1994; 162:395.
7. Zawin JK, Hoffer FA, Rand FF, et al: Joint effusion in children with an irritable hip: US diagnosis and aspiration. Radiology 1993; 187:459.
8. Helbich TH, Breitenseher M, Trattnig S, et al: Sonomorphologic variants of popliteal cysts. J Clin Ultrasound 1998; 26:171.
9. Waitches GM, Rockett M, Brage M, et al: Ultrasonographic-surgical correlation of ankle tendon tears. J Ultrasound Med 1998; 17:249.
10. Jacobson JA, Powell A, Craig JG, et al: Wooden foreign bodies in soft tissue: Detection at US. Radiology 1998; 206:45.

section
1
chapter
9

NUCLEAR MEDICINE

Christopher J. Palestro and Maria B. Tomas

Summary

- Nuclear medicine is the branch of medicine that makes use of radioactive materials for diagnostic and therapeutic purposes.
- Bone scintigraphy is a very sensitive, whole body screening procedure for a variety of skeletal disorders.
- Uptake of the bone agent, a diphosphonate, is dependent on blood flow and the rate of new bone formation (osteoblastic activity).
- Gallium scintigraphy is used in conjunction with bone scintigraphy to enhance the specificity of the radionuclide diagnosis of osteomyelitis.
- Labeled leukocyte scintigraphy for evaluation of musculoskeletal infection may be used alone or in combination with either bone scintigraphy or bone marrow scintigraphy, depending on the region involved.
- The sensitivity of bone scintigraphy for detecting fractures approaches 100%. Fractures near joints are visualized within 3 days after their occurrence, whereas those in the axial skeleton and shafts of the long bones may not be evident until 10 to 12 days after.
- In the acute phase, avascular necrosis appears as an area of decreased activity on a bone scan, and in the reparative phase it appears as an area of increased uptake.
- Three-phase bone scintigraphy is the radionuclide procedure of choice for diagnosing osteomyelitis in otherwise normal bone.
- Gallium imaging is used in conjunction with bone scintigraphy to enhance the specificity of the radionuclide diagnosis of osteomyelitis, especially for vertebral location.
- Labeled leukocyte imaging has limited use in vertebral osteomyelitis.
- Occasionally, on bone scintigraphy, osteomyelitis may present as an area of decreased rather than increased uptake, especially in children.

FUNDAMENTAL SCIENCE

Nuclear medicine is the branch of medicine that makes use of radioactive materials for both diagnostic and therapeutic purposes. Therapy with unsealed sources is beyond the scope of this review, which focuses on diagnostic nuclear medicine as it pertains to the orthopaedic patient.

Although radionuclide images are interpreted by visual analysis in much the same way as traditional radiographic studies, there are important differences. For radionuclide imaging, the patient is injected with a radioactive material and emits photons, which are electronically transformed into emission images. In traditional radiographs, computed tomography, magnetic resonance imaging (MRI), and ultrasound, an external source of energy is transmitted through the patient, and the resulting images are, therefore, transmission images. Nuclear medicine images are functional, not anatomic studies, and the whole body can be surveyed after a single injection. These studies are, therefore, complementary to anatomic studies.

Three radionuclide studies are especially useful in the orthopaedic patient: bone scintigraphy, gallium scintigraphy, and labeled leukocyte scintigraphy.

Bone scintigraphy, with its ease of administration and high sensitivity, is an excellent screening procedure for a variety of skeletal disorders. The tracer used is a diphosphonate, usually methylenediphosphonate, labeled with technetium 99m (^{99m}Tc). Diphosphonate is adsorbed onto the surface of bone crystal and has an affinity for new bone. Tracer uptake reflects primarily osteoblastic activity but is also dependent on blood flow. Because functional changes generally occur earlier than structural changes in the course of a disease process, bone scans often detect abnormalities before they are radiographically apparent.[1]

A variation of the traditional scan is the three-phase (or triple-phase) bone scan. The patient is injected with the area of interest positioned under the imaging device, known as a gamma camera. The first, or flow, phase is a series of rapid-acquisition images performed as the radionuclide initially passes through the area under investigation. This phase provides information about blood flow to the region of interest. The second or blood pool phase, usually a single image performed immediately after the first phase, provides information about periosseous extracellular fluid alterations. The third or bone phase, performed 2 to 3 hours alter injection, allows assessment of osteoblast uptake of tracer. Three-phase bone scintigraphy is often performed to distinguish between cellulitis and osteomyelitis.

Gallium 67 scintigraphy is used as an adjunct to bone scintigraphy in patients with suspected osteomyelitis. Several factors are responsible for gallium uptake in infection. Some gallium is transported by leukocytes, intracellularly bound to lactoferrin. Most gallium is, however, transported bound to transferrin. It is likely that the gallium-transferrin complex crosses the capillary membrane at sites of inflammation (because of increased permeability); gallium then dissociates from transferrin and binds to the available lactoferrin. Direct uptake of gallium by infective organisms has also been described. Finally, certain microorganisms produce siderophores, low-molecular-weight chelating agents for iron-gathering purposes. Presumably, these siderophores bind with gallium, and the siderophore-gallium complex is incorporated into the microorganism, which is eventually phagocytized by a macrophage.[2]

Imaging is usually performed 48 to 72 hours after injec-

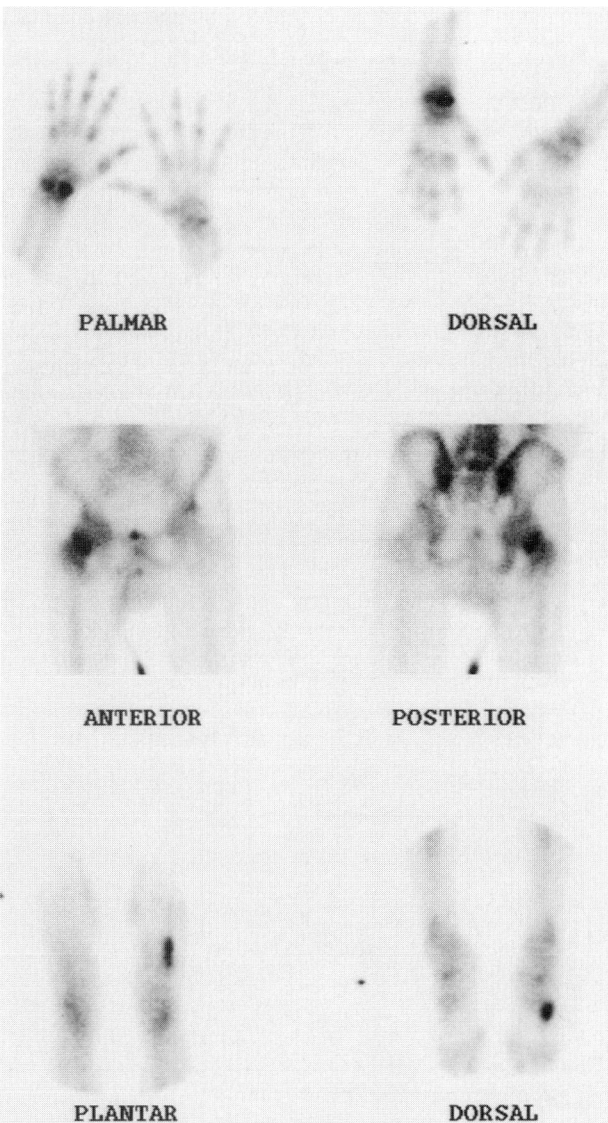

Fig. 1. Scintigraphic fracture detection. Top, Radiographically unde-tected traumatic fractures of the distal right ulna and radius. Middle, Right femoral neck fracture in a patient with equivocal radiograph findings. Bottom, Radiograph-negative stress fracture of the left fourth metatarsal.

Imaging is performed 18 to 24 hours after injection. Ideally, wound dressings should be changed just before imaging to reduce false-positive results.

INDICATIONS FOR SCINTIGRAPHY
Fracture

Radiographs are the modality of choice for diagnosing skeletal trauma. Whole body scintigraphic imaging may be useful in cases of multiple trauma, as well as for regions that are difficult to assess radiographically to rule out oc-cult fractures. For metaphyseal or epiphyseal injuries, nearly all fractures will be scintigraphically visible within 72 hours of their occurrence. In the shaft of long bones and in the axial skeleton, it may take 10 to 12 days before the fracture can be identified. The overall sensitivity of bone scintigraphy for detection of fractures approaches 100%.[4]

In particular circumstances (i.e., wrist and hip), bone scintigraphy is a highly sensitive and specific modality, because scintigraphic changes often precede radiographic changes. Wrist fractures are positive within 3 days after their occurrence; false-negative results have been reported in elderly patients with hip fractures who were studied within 72 hours of injury. Consequently, if the initial study is negative, it should be repeated several days later, or MRI scans should be considered.[5, 6]

Bone scintigraphy is useful for detecting stress fractures of the femoral neck, tibia, and foot (Fig. 1). Fractures of the pars interarticularis (spondylolysis) can also be identi-fied, and the addition of tomographic imaging can precisely localize the abnormality (Fig. 2). Enthesopathies such as shin splints and plantar fasciitis, which may easily be over-looked radiographically, are readily identifiable on bone scan.

tion. Normal large bowel accumulation of gallium can hinder evaluation of the abdomen and pelvis, and addi-tional images at 96 hours or later as well as cathartics may be necessary.

Labeled leukocyte scintigraphy is extremely useful for the evaluation of musculoskeletal infection. Leukocytes are labeled with ⁹⁹ᵐTc, or with indium 111 as the radiolabel. About 40 mL of whole blood is drawn from the patient; the leukocytes are separated from the rest of the blood elements, labeled with radionuclide, and reinjected into the patient, a process that requires 2 to 3 hours. Tracer uptake is dependent on concentration of labeled cells at inflamma-tory foci. A mixed population of leukocytes is usually labeled, the majority of which are neutrophils. Conse-quently, this procedure is most sensitive for detecting neu-trophil-mediated inflammatory conditions.[3]

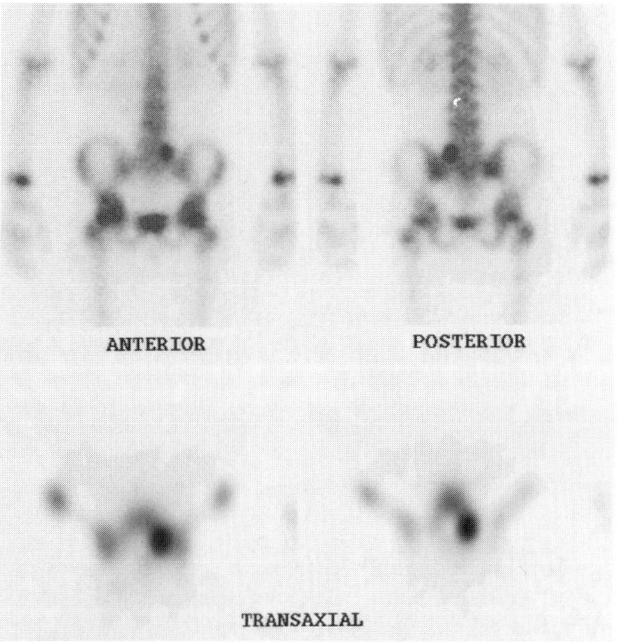

Fig. 2. Spondylolysis. Transaxial tomographic images demonstrate in detail that the intense uptake along the left lateral aspect of the fifth lumbar vertebra is within the posterior elements.

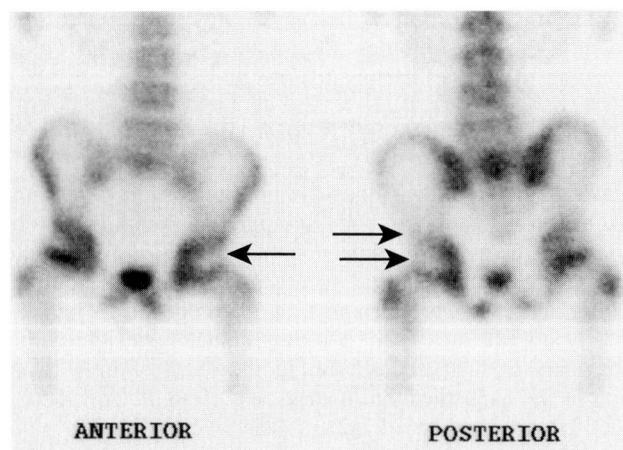

Fig. 3. Avascular necrosis. This shows a photopenic defect (decreased activity) in the left femoral head and growth plate (*arrows*) in a 6-year-old child with Legg-Calvé-Perthes disease.

accumulation, whereas hypertrophic nonunion is characterized by intense uptake at the site.[7]

Osteonecrosis

Scintigraphic findings parallel the two main phases of this condition. Initially, there is interruption of the blood supply, which results in bone necrosis and, therefore, appears as decreased uptake on the bone scan (Fig. 3). In the second, reparative phase, new vessels grow into the avascular area, with deposition of new bone, usually on the trabeculae of necrotic bone; hence, there is increased tracer uptake. As with many other skeletal abnormalities, scintigraphic changes may predate the radiographic changes by weeks to months. For evaluation of postfracture avascular necrosis of the femoral head, normal or increased activity on scans performed within 4 weeks after trauma is a good indication of uncomplicated fracture healing. Decreased uptake, however, does not reliably predict nonunion.

"Spontaneous" osteonecrosis of the medial femoral condyle, a condition of uncertain cause, usually affects women older than 50 years. Radiographs are frequently osteopenic but otherwise normal. Intensely increased uptake in the medial femoral condyle extending into the metaphysis is the classic scintigraphic presentation of this entity.[8]

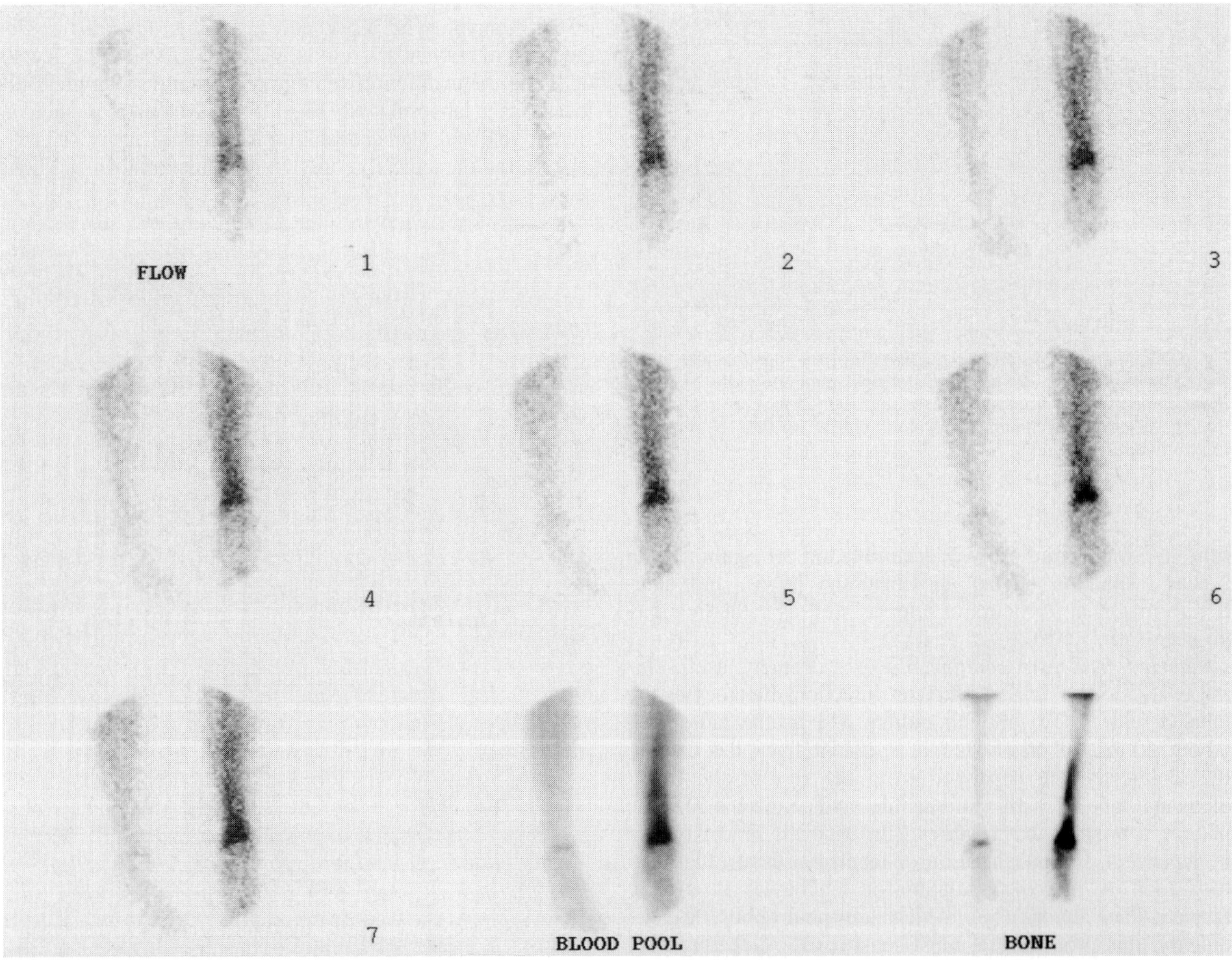

Complications of fracture healing may also be evaluated by bone scintigraphy. Decreased uptake at a fracture site is suggestive of atrophic nonunion, or pseudoarthrosis. Atrophic nonunion is characterized by diminished tracer

Fig. 4. Three-phase bone scan in osteomyelitis. There is focal hyperperfusion, focal hyperemia, and focal bony uptake in osteomyelitis of the distal left tibia. Unfortunately, this same pattern, which can be found in numerous other conditions, is not specific for the diagnosis.

The sensitivity of bone scintigraphy for detecting femoral head avascular necrosis in Legg-Calvé-Perthes disease is about 95%, often predating radiographic changes by a considerable length of time.[9]

Infection

A multitude of nuclear medicine studies are available for the diagnostic work-up of suspected orthopaedic infection; no single procedure is ideal for every situation. Regardless of the radionuclide study used, radiography of the region of interest is a prerequisite. Often the diagnosis can be made radiographically, eliminating or at least reducing the number of ancillary studies needed. Even when nondiagnostic, radiographs provide important information that may not only guide but also facilitate interpretation of subsequent studies.

Three-phase bone scintigraphy is the radionuclide procedure of choice for diagnosing osteomyelitis in otherwise normal bones. The presence of focal hyperperfusion, hyperemia, and bony uptake on delayed images is virtually diagnostic of osteomyelitis (Fig. 4). Tracer uptake by bone

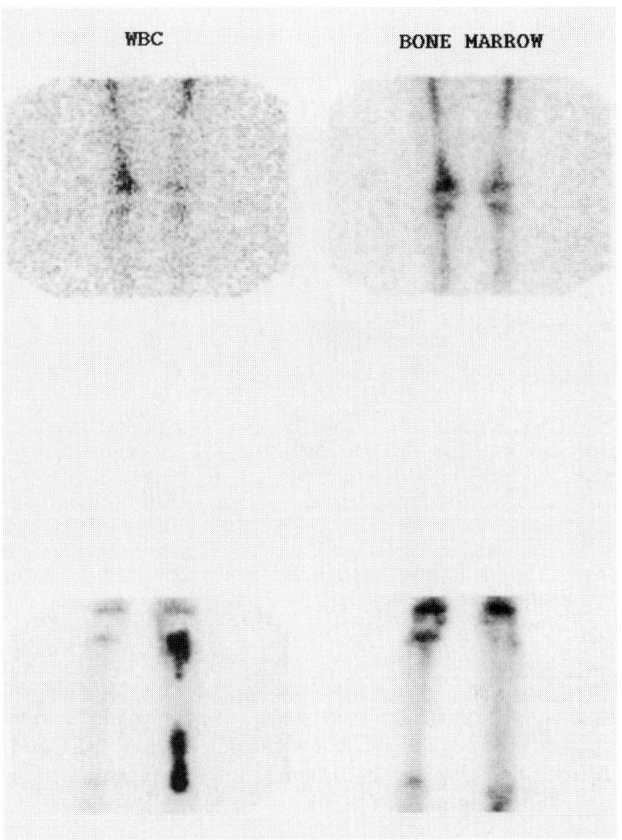

Fig. 6. Leukocyte/marrow imaging in suspected osteomyelitis. Top, There is asymmetric uptake of labeled leukocytes in the distal tibias. The same pattern is present on the marrow scan; hence, the study is negative for osteomyelitis. Bottom, There is intense uptake of labeled leukocytes in the proximal and distal left tibia, whereas there is nearly absent activity in these regions on the marrow scan. Hence, the combined study is positive for osteomyelitis.

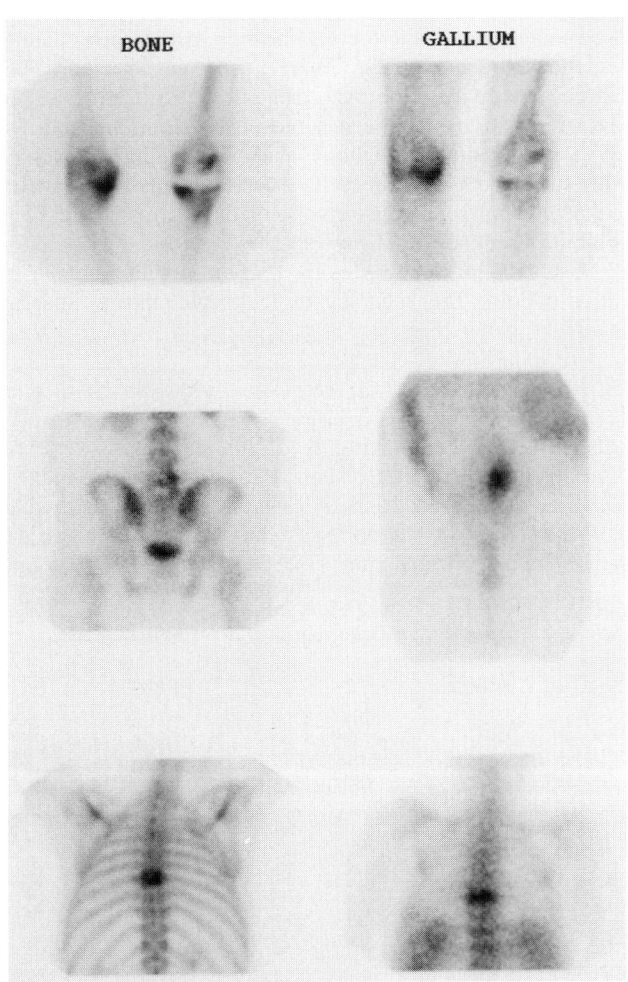

Fig. 5. Bone/gallium imaging in suspected osteomyelitis. Top, The study is negative for infection of the left total knee replacement. Middle, A positive study in lower lumbar spine osteomyelitis. Note the intense uptake of gallium compared with the more subtle changes on the bone scan. Bottom, An equivocal study. The pattern and intensity of the abnormality are virtually identical on both studies.

depends on increased bone mineral turnover; fracture, trauma, and the neuropathic joint, among other conditions, can mimic osteomyelitis, and under these circumstances bone imaging is not specific.[10] The majority of patients referred for radionuclide evaluation of osteomyelitis have underlying bone abnormalities. Attempts at improving the specificity, and hence the accuracy, of the radionuclide diagnosis of osteomyelitis include four-phase bone scintigraphy, gallium scintigraphy, and labeled leukocyte scintigraphy.

Four-phase bone scintigraphy consists of a three-phase bone scan with additional imaging the day after injection. Tracer uptake in normal bone generally ceases by 4 hours after injection, whereas uptake in woven, immature bone continues for several more hours. In osteomyelitis, uptake at 24 hours may be greater than that at 4 hours, in contrast to normal bone in which the uptake remains unchanged. The accuracy of four-phase bone imaging is about 85%, with higher specificity but lower sensitivity than the three-phase bone scan. Although of some value for distinguishing cellulitis from osteomyelitis, there is a relatively high false-positive rate; consequently, this technique has not gained wide acceptance.[11]

Bone/gallium scintigraphy is used in the evaluation of so-called complicated osteomyelitis. Because the uptake

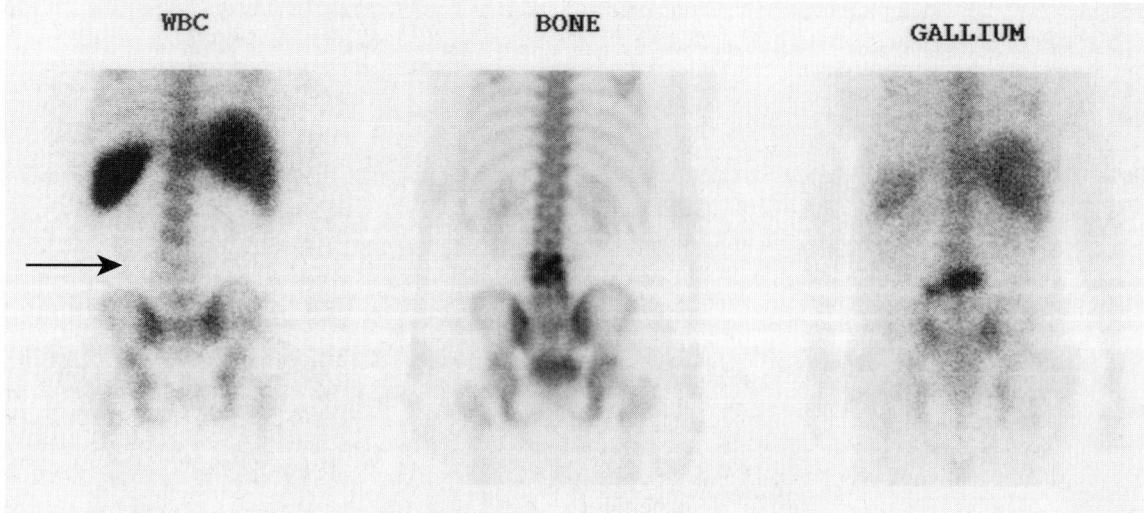

Fig. 7. Vertebral osteomyelitis. Midlumbar spine osteomyelitis presents as nonspecific decreased activity on the labeled leukocyte image (*arrow*). There is intense uptake in two contiguous vertebrae on the bone scan, and the gallium scan shows extension of the abnormality into the surrounding soft tissues.

mechanisms of bone-seeking radiopharmaceuticals and gallium are different, the two studies may provide complementary information about a particular disease process. Illustrated in Figure 5, the criteria[12] for interpretation of the combined study are as follows:

Positive for osteomyelitis: When the distribution of the two radiotracers is spatially incongruent or when their distribution is spatially congruent and the intensity of gallium uptake exceeds that of the bone agent.

Negative for osteomyelitis: When gallium images are normal, regardless of the bone scan results, or when the spatial distribution of the two tracers is congruent and the relative intensity of gallium uptake is less than that of the bone tracer.

Equivocal for osteomyelitis: When the distribution of the two tracers is spatially congruent and the relative intensity of uptake of each is similar.

The fact that leukocytes do not usually accumulate at sites of increased bone mineral turnover in the absence of infection would seem to make labeled leukocyte imaging an ideal procedure for diagnosing complicated osteomyelitis. The results reported, however, have been inconsistent; some studies indicate a high sensitivity and low specificity, and others report just the opposite. False-positive results are associated with fracture, orthopaedic hardware, and the neuropathic joint and have been attributed to "inflammation." Although inflammation may accompany these entities, the usual cellular response is mononuclear, not neutrophilic. Labeled leukocyte uptake in inflammation not mediated by neutrophils is uncommon; therefore, such uptake, in the absence of infection, must be due to something other than inflammation.[3, 11]

The normal distribution of labeled leukocytes includes the liver, spleen, and bone marrow. In adults, hematopoietically active marrow is assumed to be limited to the axial skeleton and proximal 25% to 30% of the humeri and the femora. The real difficulty in interpreting labeled leukocyte images is not nonspecific inflammation but differentiating

marrow from infection. Combining labeled leukocyte and bone imaging and interpreting the two studies in a manner analogous to bone/gallium images improve specificity but reduce sensitivity. Improved specificity with little or no loss in sensitivity has been achieved by combining labeled leukocyte imaging with bone marrow imaging (performed with sulfur colloid). Infection stimulates uptake of labeled leukocytes but suppresses uptake of the marrow tracer. The combined leukocyte/marrow scan is positive for infection when uptake of leukocytes is present without uptake of sulfur colloid. The accuracy of leukocyte/marrow imaging is 90% or better (Fig. 6).[11]

APPLICATIONS
The Spine

Labeled leukocyte imaging is of limited use in vertebral osteomyelitis. Although osteomyelitis typically presents as increased uptake on labeled leukocyte images, more than half the cases of vertebral osteomyelitis present as decreased uptake, which may also be associated with nonin-

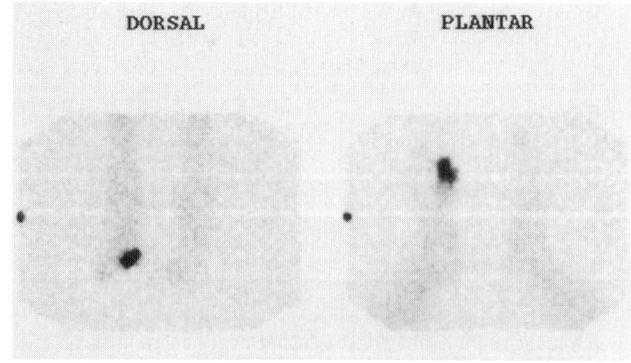

Fig. 8. Diabetic osteomyelitis. Intense focal uptake in the first metatarsal of the right foot of a diabetic patient with a pedal ulcer is virtually diagnostic of osteomyelitis on indium-labeled leukocyte scintigraphy.

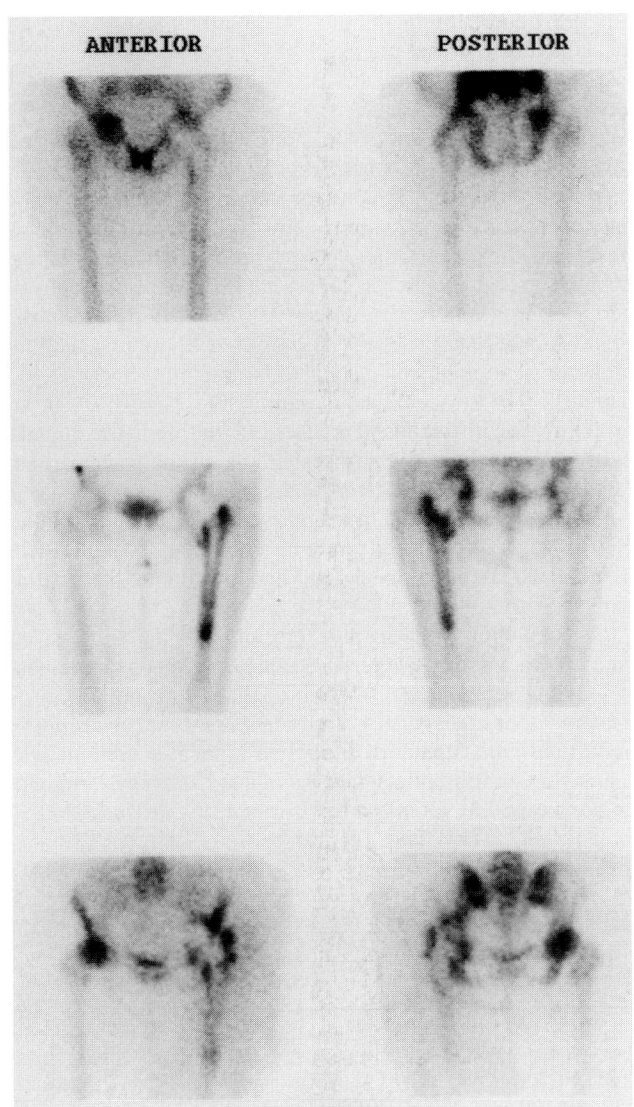

Fig. 9. Bone scintigraphy of hip replacements. Top, Normal bone scan. Middle, Focally increased uptake at the tip of the femoral component of a left total hip replacement most suggestive of loosening. Bottom, Diffusely increased periprosthetic activity around the femoral component of a left hip replacement, most suggestive of infection.

diagnosing this entity is the labeled leukocyte study, with an accuracy of 80% to 90% (Fig. 8).[14]

The major complication of the mid- and hindfoot is the neuropathic, or Charcot, joint. Continued ambulation on an insensate joint leads to instability, which causes joint degeneration, subluxation, and destruction. Although infection is infrequent in the Charcot joint, determining whether or not infection is present is a formidable task. Neither radiography nor bone scintigraphy is particularly useful, and the role of MRI is unclear. Labeled leukocyte uptake in the uninfected Charcot joint has also been described. Originally attributed to inflammation, recent data confirm that such uptake reflects hematopoietically active marrow, and as in other parts of the skeleton, leukocyte/marrow scintigraphy may be useful for determining whether or not infection is present.[15]

The Painful Joint Replacement
The vast majority of the approximately 600,000 total hip and knee replacements performed annually in the United

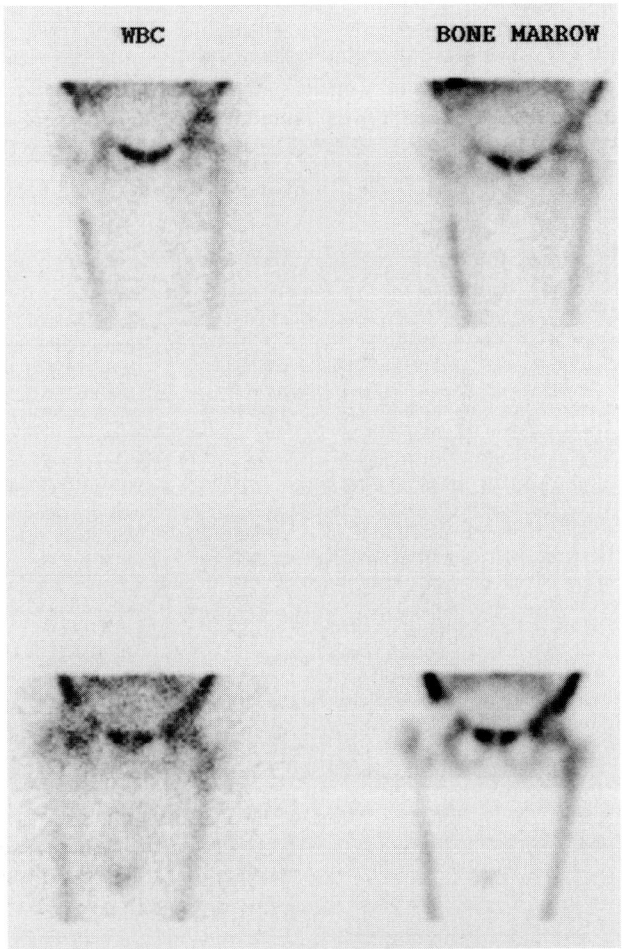

Fig. 10. Leukocyte/marrow imaging of hip replacements. Top, Diffuse periprosthetic activity around the right hip replacement on the labeled leukocyte study is identical to the uptake pattern on the marrow scan. The combined study is negative for infection. Bottom, Although there is uptake around the proximal aspect of the right hip replacement on the leukocyte study, there is no corresponding uptake on the marrow image, and the combined study is positive for infection.

fectious conditions, such as tumor, Paget's disease, and infarction. Labeled leukocyte imaging for vertebral osteomyelitis is, therefore, nonspecific. Although MRI is the current imaging procedure of choice for diagnosing spinal osteomyelitis, bone/gallium scintigraphy is the radionuclide procedure of choice (Fig. 7).[11, 13]

The Diabetic Foot
The foot complications to which the diabetic patient is prone are the most common causes of nontraumatic lower extremity amputation in the United States. Because of poor specificity, bone scintigraphy is not useful for differentiating osteomyelitis from other conditions, such as fracture and the neuropathic joint, which frequently coexist in the diabetic foot. The single most useful radionuclide study for

States are successful in terms of relief of pain and restoration of function. Complications such as loosening and infection do occur, and nuclear medicine is often used to determine the cause of the patient's pain. Bone scanning is used as a screening test for the painful joint replacement. Regardless of the location or type of joint replacement, a normal bone scan is considered strong evidence that the patient's pain is not related to the prosthesis. For cemented hip replacements more than 1 year old, focal uptake at the tip of the femoral component suggests aseptic loosening, whereas diffusely increased periprosthetic uptake suggests infection (Fig. 9). There are numerous caveats, however. For all hip replacements less than 1 year old, periprosthetic uptake patterns are extremely variable, and the significance of the findings on a single scan (unless it is normal) is difficult to assess. In the case of porous-coated hip arthroplasties, periprosthetic uptake in the absence of complications may persist for well beyond 1 year. Similar findings have also been observed in knee replacements. Thus, for porous-coated hip arthroplasties and knee replacements, bone scintigraphy is most valuable when it is negative or when serial studies are available for comparison.[11]

One of the most serious complications of joint replacement surgery is infection. Our work suggests that the current state-of-the-art nuclear medicine procedure for diagnosing this entity is combined leukocyte/marrow scintigraphy (Fig. 10). With a sensitivity and specificity of 90% or better, this technique is superior to any other nuclear medicine procedure available.[16, 17]

The Child

The majority of children who are seen for suspected osteomyelitis present with a hematogenous origin (nonsurgical); therefore, bone scintigraphy is extremely accurate. There has been some controversy, however, about the role of bone imaging in neonates. Initial reports indicated that, in contrast to older children and adults, bone scintigraphy in neonates was relatively insensitive for detecting osteomyelitis. More recent data suggest, however, that the sensitivity of bone scintigraphy in neonates is similar to that in older patients. These seemingly contradictory conclusions are probably due to technical factors. In the pediatric population, osteomyelitis often arises in the metaphysis adjacent to the growth plate, where the normally intense uptake of the bone agent could potentially mask an abnormality. Newer, higher resolution imaging equipment, coupled with meticulous attention to detail, has overcome these problems.[18]

Osteomyelitis occasionally presents as an area of decreased, rather than increased, uptake in the pediatric hip. It must be remembered, therefore, that while photopenia is usually associated with infarction, it may, on occasion, be associated with infection, and when clinical symptoms warrant, additional studies, such as labeled leukocyte imaging and/or aspiration, should be performed.[1]

REFERENCES

1. Fogelman I, Collier BD: An Atlas of Planar and SPECT Bone Scans. St. Louis, MO, CV Mosby, 1989, p 1.
2. Palestro CJ: The current role of gallium imaging in infection. Semin Nucl Med 1994; 24:128.
3. Palestro CJ, Goldsmith SG: The role of gallium and labeled leukocyte scintigraphy in the AIDS patient. Q J Nucl Med 1995; 39:221.
4. Spitz J, Lancer I, Tittle K, et al: Scintimetric evaluation of remodeling after bone fracture in man. J Nucl Med 1993; 34:1403.
5. Holder LE, Schwartz C, Wernicke PG, et al: Radionuclide bone imaging in the early detection of fractures of the proximal femur (hip): Multifactorial analysis. Radiology 1990; 174:509.
6. Slavin JD Jr, Mathews J, Spencer RP: Bone imaging in the diagnosis of fractures of the femur and pelvis in the sixth to tenth decades. Clin Nucl Med 1986; 11:328.
7. Murray IPC: Bone scintigraphy in trauma. In Murray IPC, Ell PJ (eds): Nuclear Medicine in Clinical Diagnosis and Treatment. Edinburgh, Churchill Livingstone, 1994, vol 2, p 1013.
8. Galasko CSB, Weber DA: Radionuclide Scintigraphy in Orthopedics. Edinburgh, Churchill Livingstone, 1984, p 200.
9. Murray IPC: Vascular manifestations. In Murray IPC, Ell PJ (eds): Nuclear Medicine in Clinical Diagnosis and Treatment. Edinburgh, Churchill Livingstone, 1994, vol 2, p 997.
10. Schauwecker DS: The scintigraphic diagnosis of osteomyelitis. Am J Roentgenol 1992; 158:9.
11. Palestro CJ, Torres MA: Radionuclide imaging in orthopedic infections. Semin Nucl Med 1997; 27:334.
12. Seabold JE, Palestro CJ, Brown ML, et al: Procedure guideline for gallium scintigraphy in inflammation. J Nucl Med 1997; 38:994.
13. Palestro CJ, Kim CK, Swyer AJ, et al: Radionuclide diagnosis of vertebral osteomyelitis: Indium-111-leukocyte and technetium-99m-methylene diphosphonate bone scintigraphy. J Nucl Med 1991; 31:1861.
14. Newman LG, Waller J, Palestro CJ, et al: Unsuspected osteomyelitis in diabetic foot ulcers: Diagnosis and monitoring by leukocyte scanning with indium-111 oxyquinoline. JAMA 1991; 266:1246.
15. Palestro CJ, Mehta HH, Patel M, et al: Marrow versus infection in the Charçot joint: Indium-111 leukocyte and technetium-99m sulfur colloid scintigraphy. J Nucl Med 1998; 39:346.
16. Palestro CJ, Kim CK, Swyer AJ, et al: Total hip arthroplasty: Periprosthetic 99mTc sulfur colloid imaging in suspected infection. J Nucl Med 1990; 31:1950.
17. Palestro CJ, Swyer AJ, Kim CK, et al: Infected knee prosthesis: Diagnosis with In-111-leukocyte, Tc-99m-sulfur colloid, and Tc-99m-MDP imaging. Radiology 1991; 179:645.
18. Palestro CJ: Musculoskeletal infection. In Freeman LM (ed): Nuclear Medicine Annual 1994. New York, Raven Press, 1994, p 91.

PRINCIPLES OF NEURO-ORTHOPAEDIC REHABILITATION

Mary Ann Keenan

Summary

- Many orthopaedic principles and techniques have evolved from management of neuro-orthopaedic syndromes. Poliomyelitis alone required a broad array of surgical and nonsurgical treatment modalities in its management.
- Principles of neuro-orthopaedic treatment can be extrapolated to rehabilitation of more common musculoskeletal problems.
- Diagnosis and treatment are dependent on careful physical examination of the patient and instrumented laboratory analysis of function.
- Functional recovery from noninherited problems is generally inversely related to age of onset.
- Prevention of deformity and secondary complications is paramount in the care of neuro-orthopaedic patients.

GENERAL PRINCIPLES OF NEURO-ORTHOPAEDIC REHABILITATION

DEFINITION

Neuro-orthopaedics is the subspecialty that treats the musculoskeletal consequences of complex nervous system disorders and injuries.[1] Because these neurological problems involve the patient in a generalized manner, they are best approached from a broad viewpoint rather than the more traditional orthopaedic perspective of anatomic subspecialties. Rehabilitation is an approach to patient care that focuses on recovering lost function. Rehabilitation utilizes operative and nonoperative techniques. It is important for every orthopaedic subspecialty to apply the appropriate rehabilitation principles to the care of patients. This chapter focuses on the most common disorders treated in neuro-orthopaedics.

Neuro-orthopaedic rehabilitation differs from acute medical care that attempts to cure specific diseases. In neuro-orthopaedic rehabilitation, the goal is to improve function in a person with a permanent disability or chronic disease. This leads to improved quality of life for the patient and his or her caretakers. The disability may be the result of a congenital or an acquired problem. Neuro-orthopaedic rehabilitation views the functional problems of a patient in relation to the entire musculoskeletal system.

RESTORATION OF FUNCTION

Restoring function requires surgical and nonsurgical treatments. Functional restoration involves correcting limb deformities, increasing muscle strength, maximizing motor control, and providing adaptive equipment. It requires that the individual be trained to use residual function most effectively. The patient needs guidance in the challenge of adjusting to an altered lifestyle. It is crucial to prevent complications that impede progress. The needs of the patient are complex. A team approach, utilizing the talents of many disciplines, is the most successful model for rehabilitation.

For the neurological patient, wellness requires maximizing function and mobility and avoiding the complications of chronic inactivity. Complications cause further loss of function in an already compromised person. Potential complications of physical immobility include decubiti, infection, pain, social isolation, and physical and emotional dependence. This results in a costly loss of productivity for patients and their caretakers.

Rehabilitation begins in the acute care setting of both inpatient and outpatient facilities. The fundamentals of good patient care are more difficult and time-consuming to provide to neurologically disabled patients, but they are especially critical. General principles include (1) accurate diagnosis of all current problems, (2) adequate treatment of all medical and orthopaedic problems, (3) adequate nutrition, (4) discontinuance of all invasive tubes and monitoring devices as soon as the condition permits, and (5) early mobilization of the patient. Rehabilitation often requires an aggressive surgical approach to correct musculoskeletal problems.

COMMON PROBLEMS IN THE NEURO-ORTHOPAEDIC PATIENT
Inadequate Nutrition and Dehydration

Inadequate nutrition and dehydration are common issues. Involvement of a dietitian to help monitor and correct these problems is useful. Monitoring of serum albumin levels and total lymphocyte counts is helpful. Good nutritional status is the basis for avoiding many complications. The normal requirement is 30 kcal/kg/day for maintaining body weight. Patients with chronic diseases commonly have poor appetites. The physically handicapped person may have difficulty in obtaining and preparing adequate amounts of food. The other form of malnutrition to be avoided is obesity as relative inactivity leads to diminished caloric requirements.

Spasticity and Upper Motor Neuron Syndrome

Upper motor neuron (UMN) dysfunction occurs following injuries to the brain or spinal cord from stroke, traumatic brain injury, anoxia, infections of the brain, and perinatal trauma (i.e., cerebral palsy or static encephalopathy). Weakness, impaired voluntary and postural motor control, spasticity, and contracture are all components of UMN syndrome. Many complications result from spasticity and UMN (Table 1). The most common complications are extremity contractures, which lead to skin maceration, ulcers,

TABLE 1. COMPLICATIONS OF SPASTICITY
Contractures
Decubitus ulcers
Hygiene difficulties
Fracture malunion
Joint subluxation or dislocation
Heterotopic ossification
Peripheral neuropathy

and difficulty with hygiene. Fractures in the presence of spasticity can lead to malunions. Extremes of limb position cause peripheral nerve lesions such as cubital tunnel or carpal tunnel syndrome. Severe spasticity can cause joint subluxation or dislocation such as hip dislocation, which occurs with severe long-standing adductor spasticity. Posterior subluxation of the knee can occur in the presence of hamstring spasticity. Iatrogenic fractures can occur in the presence of spasticity and contracture; the humerus is vulnerable to spiral fracture when attempting to put the arm in a sleeve if a shoulder adduction and internal rotation contracture are present. Heterotopic ossification is thought to be stimulated in part by the mechanical tension caused by the spasticity.

Spasmolytic Drugs. Drugs can be useful in managing spasticity. Oral medications are used when there is spasticity affecting multiple large muscle groups in the body and when the spasticity is not severe.

Lioresal (baclofen) inhibits both polysynaptic and monosynaptic reflexes at the spinal cord level. It also has general central nervous system depressant actions. Antispastic agents that have sedating properties, such as baclofen, Valium (diazepam), Zanaflex (tizanidine), and clonidine, may compromise patients with attention deficits and/or memory disorders.

Baclofen pump technology has an advantage over oral drug therapy because of the small concentrations it introduces intrathecally. The small intrathecal doses are effective in controlling spasticity while minimizing central side effects. The pump is placed in a subcutaneous pocket in the abdominal wall. A catheter is routed subcutaneously from the intrathecal space to the pump. The pump can be refilled by injecting into the reservoir chamber. The dosage and rate of administration can be easily adjusted using a laptop computer, which sends signals to the pump using radio signals.

Dantrium (dantrolene) produces relaxation by directly affecting the contractile response of skeletal muscle at a site beyond the myoneural junction. It causes dissociation of the excitation-contraction coupling probably by interfering with the release of calcium from the sarcoplasmic reticulum. Dantrolene is helpful in controlling clonus. Although it does not affect the central nervous system directly, it does cause drowsiness, dizziness, and generalized weakness. The most serious potential side effect is hepatotoxicity.

Casts. Casting has been shown to temporarily reduce muscle tone and is frequently used to correct a contracture. Most commonly, casting is used in conjunction with nerve blocks for temporarily reducing spasticity or after surgical release. The cast is changed weekly until the problem has been corrected.

Splints. Anterior and posterior clam-shell splints can be used to control joint position and still allow for active and passive range of motion of the joints in therapy. A splint applied to only one side of an extremity is not sufficient to control excessive spasticity and may result in skin breakdown from motion of the extremity against the splint. A poorly applied splint can also obscure an early contracture.

Nerve Blocking Agents. When a patient has potential for spontaneous improvement but requires control of muscle spasticity for an extended time, temporizing nerve block techniques are used.

Phenol. Phenol exerts two actions on nerves. The first is a short-term effect similar to that of a local anesthetic, which is directly proportional to the thickness of the nerve fibers. The second effect is long term and results from protein denaturation. This leads to wallerian degeneration of the axons. Animal studies have shown that the nerves regenerate completely with time. The direct injection of a nerve using a 5% solution of phenol after surgical exposure gives relief of spasticity for up to 6 months. Mixed nerves containing sensory fibers should not be injected as this could cause unwanted sensory loss or painful dysesthesia. Reduction of spasticity for up to 3 months can also be obtained by percutaneous injection of muscle motor points with an aqueous solution of phenol after localization using a nerve stimulation and needle electrode. Anesthetic and phenol nerve blocks are often combined with a casting or splinting program.

Botulinum Toxin. Ordinarily, an action potential propagating down a motor nerve to the neuromuscular junction triggers the release of acetylcholine (ACh) into the synaptic space. The released ACh causes depolarization of muscle membrane. Botulinum toxin type A is a protein produced by *Clostridium botulinum* that attaches to the presynaptic nerve terminal and inhibits the release of ACh at the neuromuscular junction.

Botulinum toxin is injected directly into a spastic muscle. Clinical benefit lasts 3 to 5 months. Current practice is not to administer a total of more than 400 U in a single treatment session to avoid excessive weakness or paralysis. This upper limit of 400 U may be reached rather quickly when injecting a few large muscles. A 3- to 7-day delay between injection of botulinum toxin A and the onset of clinical effect is typical. Effects are not experienced by the patient immediately; usually, a follow-up visit is arranged to check the result. Because botulinum toxin is the most potent biological toxin known and the cost is relatively high, it is desirable to use the smallest possible dose in order to achieve results.

When muscle spasticity is permanent, and no change in muscle tone is anticipated, then definitive procedures such as dorsal rhizotomy, peripheral neurectomy, tendon lengthening or release, and tendon transfer can be considered. If the spasticity is not severe, orthotic devices along with a daily range-of-motion program may be sufficient to prevent joint contractures.

Contractures

Joint and muscle contractures are the unfortunate result of inactivity and uncontrolled spasticity. They are difficult to correct and greatly extend the rehabilitation program. Contractures may result in problems of positioning an individual in bed, a chair, or in orthotic devices. They can lead to difficulties with hygiene and skin care. Pressure sores may result from extremes in position or the limited positions the patient can assume. Shoe wear may become impossible secondary to foot deformities.

Contractures result in malalignment of a limb, causing the muscles to function at a mechanical disadvantage, which accentuates muscle weakness. Sitting and standing balance are compromised when contractural deformities displace the location of the center of gravity relative to the base of support. Functional use of extremities is severely limited by lack of adequate joint motion. Joint contractures in children can result in structural changes in the skeleton. Muscle growth lags behind skeletal growth, and this discrepancy in growth rates can lead to increasing deformity.

When contractural deformities are long-standing and fixed, surgical release is indicated (Fig. 1). Tendons, ligaments, and joint capsules are involved. If the deformity is severe, complete correction at the time of surgery may be impossible. Neurovascular structures must be protected from excessive traction. Serial casts or drop-out casts may be necessary following surgery to gain the desired limb position.

Pressure Sores

Pressure sores result from poor nutritional status, decreased awareness or sensation, contractures, or decreased mobility. Prevention is crucial. A decubitus ulcer greatly adds to the length and cost of hospital stay. Ulcers are a potential source of sepsis and often require that a flap graft be rotated to cover the defect. The threshold of skin tolerance to breakdown is in inverse ratio of the intensity and duration of the pressure. The clinical rule of protecting the patient's skin is to change position every 2 hours. There is no cushion that completely prevents decubitus ulcers.

Bladder Control and Urinary Tract Infections

Urinary tract infections are a common source of sepsis and prolonged morbidity. An indwelling catheter is the most frequent source of contamination. In an acutely ill or multiply injured patient, an indwelling catheter may be necessary for hemodynamic reasons. As soon as the catheter is not needed for medical problems, it should be removed. Incontinence is not sufficient reason for continued use of an indwelling catheter. Urinary incontinence can be managed in a male with a carefully applied condom catheter. Care must be taken to inspect the penis frequently for signs of skin maceration or pressure. In the female patient, diapering and frequent linen changes are necessary.

Restoring bladder function to achieve adequate reflex voiding or balanced bladder may require the use of an intermittent catheterization program. In a balanced bladder, the residual urine volume should not exceed one-third of the volume of voided urine. In general, an intermittent catheterization program is initiated if the residual volume is greater than 100 mL or if the voided volume exceeds 400 mL. The patient is catheterized every 4 hours, then every 6 hours for 24 hours, and then is reassessed. Good records are necessary throughout the program.

Acquired Deformities

Other acquired musculoskeletal deformities are common and should be avoided when possible. Paralysis or weakness of trunk muscles can result in deformities of the spine. Scoliosis and kyphosis can lead to impaired respiratory function and balance problems both for walking and sitting. External support in the form of bracing or seating modifications can eliminate or minimize this tendency.

Disuse and lack of muscle tone lead to osteoporosis. This predisposes to fractures. Such fractures should be treated aggressively and in a manner that maximizes function and minimizes prolonged immobilization.

Peripheral nerve palsies can result from pressure secondary to decreased bed and chair mobility. Pressure can result from braces, splints, and casts; these require careful monitoring. In those patients who form heterotopic ossification, the new bone formation may also impinge on peripheral nerves.

Muscle Weakness and Physiological Deconditioning

During sustained exercise metabolism is primarily aerobic. The principal fuels for aerobic metabolism are carbohydrates and fats. In aerobic oxidation the substrates are oxi-

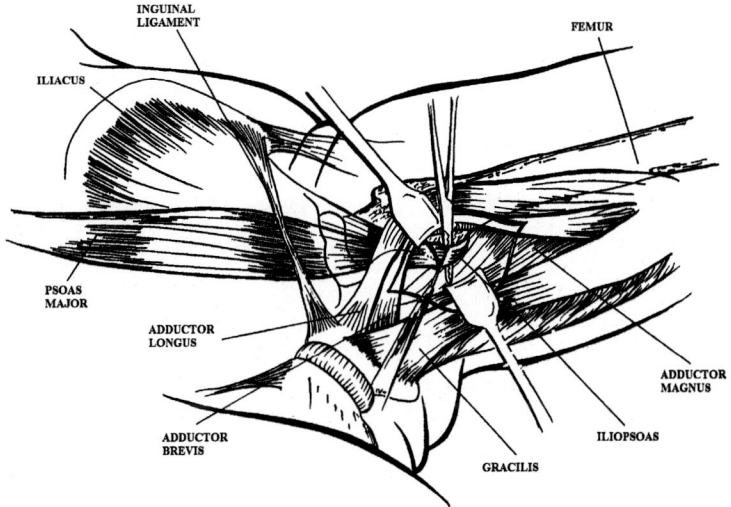

Fig. 1. Recession. This shows recession of the iliopsoas tendon from the lesser trochanter to correct a hip flexion deformity in an ambulatory patient.

dized through a series of enzymatic reactions leading to the production of adenosine triphosphate for muscular contraction. A physical conditioning program can increase aerobic capacity in several ways. The cardiac output is improved, the hemoglobin level is increased, and the cells' capacity to extract oxygen from the blood is enhanced. Finally, the muscle mass is increased by hypertrophy.

Prolonged immobilization of extremities, bedrest, and inactivity lead to pronounced muscle wasting and physiological deconditioning. The disabled patient has increased energy demands over normal individuals to perform many activities of daily living. Therefore, it is important that the disabled patient be mobilized as quickly as possible to prevent unnecessary physiological decline. The patient should also be placed on a daily exercise program to maximize muscle strength and aerobic capacity.

PATTERNS OF NEUROLOGICAL IMPAIRMENT

In diseases affecting the nervous system, the location and size of the primary lesion determine the degree of paralysis and the extent to which motor control is impaired and spasticity is present. Following peripheral nerve injuries or diseases affecting primarily the peripheral nerves, the pathological condition is restricted to the lower motor neuron. Normal motor control from the brain is preserved, spasticity is absent, and the magnitude of disability depends on the amount of weakness and paralysis.

Pathological conditions of the brain cause UMN syndromes, with impairment of motor control, spasticity, and stereotypical patterns of movement (synergy). Cognitive, memory, and sensory deficits are also commonly seen in these patients. Motor activity can be considered a hierarchical system of voluntary and involuntary neurological mechanisms. Motor control is graded in the extremity using a clinical scale (Table 2).[1] The extremity may be hypotonic or flaccid and without any volitional movement. A spastic extremity may be held rigidly without any volitional or reflexive movement. Patterned or synergistic motor control is defined as a mass flexion or extension response involving the entire extremity. Mass flexion in the upper extremity consists of shoulder abduction, forearm pronation, and flexion of the elbow, wrist, and fingers. Mass extension in the lower extremity consists of extension of the hip and knee with equinovarus of the foot and ankle. Synergistic movement may be reflexive, in response to a stimulus, but without volitional control. Some patients can also volitionally initiate synergistic movement. Selective motor control with pattern overlay is defined as the ability to move a

single joint or digit with minimal movement in the adjacent joints when performing an activity slowly. Rapid movements or physiological stress make the mass pattern more pronounced. Selective motor control is the ability to volitionally move a single joint or digit independently of the adjacent joints. Spasticity can mask underlying motor control. Two types of volitional muscular activity are clinically identifiable: selective and pattern control. The highest level of motor activity, selective movement, depends on the integrity of the cerebral cortex.

Spasticity relates to two types of involuntary muscle responses that depend on the sensitivity of the muscle spindle to the rate of stretch. If a muscle is quickly extended above the threshold of the velocity-sensitive receptors of the spindle, a phasic response may be elicited. If spasticity is severe, sudden stretch may trigger clonus, which consists of repeated bursts of "phasic" activity at 6 to 8 cycles/sec. If the muscle is stretched slowly below the threshold of the velocity components of the spindle, a phasic response is not triggered, but the spindle is still capable of detecting changes in length, which may generate a "tonic" response consisting of continuous muscle hypertonus. The tonic muscle activity during slow stretch is called "clasp knife" resistance.

Patients with brain injury involving the brain stem may exhibit severe muscular hypertonus, which is continuously present and is called decorticate or decerebrate rigidity, depending on the posture of the limbs. In decerebrate posturing, the patient's arms are held tightly flexed while the legs are held in extension. In decorticate posturing, both the upper and lower extremities are in rigid extension. Patients with severe muscular rigidity are at extreme risk for developing contractural deformities.

When a spastic patient is sitting or standing, labyrinthine activation increases tone in the extensor muscles of the lower extremity and upper limb flexion. Consequently, when checking for spasticity, the patient should be examined in the upright rather than supine position in order to elicit the maximum stretch response. Conversely, when checking for maximal range of motion, the patient should be tested in the supine position, minimizing muscle tone and enabling maximum joint range.

Limb posture also influences the intensity of reflex and voluntary activity. These patterns of excitation and inhibition are determined by a complex of multisegmented spinal reflexes.

The final steps of sensory integration occur in the cerebral cortex, where basic sensory data are integrated into the more complex sensory phenomena. When central nervous

	Motor Control	Description
	TABLE 2. CLINICAL SCALE OF MOTOR CONTROL	
Grade 1	Flaccid	Hypotonic, no active motion
Grade 2	Rigid	Hypertonic, no active motion
Grade 3	Reflexive mass pattern (synergy)	Mass flexion or extension in response to stimulation
Grade 4	Volitional mass pattern	Patient-initiated mass flexion or extension movement
Grade 5	Selective with pattern overlay	Slow volitional movement of specific joints Physiological stress results in mass action
Grade 6	Selective	Volitional control of individual joints

TABLE 3. MANUAL MUSCLE TESTING SCALE

0   No contraction
1   Trace contraction
2   Active movement with gravity eliminated
3   Active movement against gravity
4   Active movement against gravity and resistance
5   No detectable weakness

system injury involves the cerebral cortex, the patient responds to basic modalities of touch and pain. However, more complex aspects of sensation, such as those of shape, texture, proprioception, and two-point discrimination, may be impaired. These simple tests quickly determine the patient's ability to interpret basic sensory information. Most patients do not routinely use an affected hand unless proprioception is intact and they can discriminate between two points applied simultaneously to the fingers less than 10 mm apart. Patients with absent proprioception across the major lower joints have balance abnormalities or are unable to walk.

Manual muscle testing is often useful for evaluating an individual's ability to perform functional tasks and is used to document progress in the rehabilitation program.[2] The evaluation is subjective, but the use of gravity resistance provides a measure of objective standardization (Table 3). A normal muscle grade as determined by manual testing does not always imply normal strength. A significant amount of weakness must be present to be detected by this method.

SPINAL CORD INJURY

GENERAL CONSIDERATIONS

Trauma to the spinal cord causes dysfunction with nonprogressive loss of sensory and motor function distal to the point of injury. The annual incidence rate is estimated to be approximately 15,000 per year. There are approximately 400,000 spinal-injured patients presently in the United States.[3] The leading causes of spinal cord injury (SCI) are motor vehicle accidents, gunshot wounds, falls, and sports injuries.

Patients usually divide into groups. The first group consists of younger individuals who sustained their injury primarily from high-energy trauma. Gunshot wounds are now the leading cause of spinal injury in many urban centers. The second group consists of older individuals with cervical spinal stenosis who sustain their injury from minor trauma and commonly have no vertebral fracture. With the benefits of an organized program of medical care, the life expectancy of paraplegic and quadriplegic patients is now approaching that of a normal life span.[4]

COMMON TERMS IN SCI

Tetraplegia. Tetraplegia refers to the impairment or loss of motor and sensory function in the cervical nerve segments, resulting in dysfunction in the arms, trunk, pelvic organs, and legs.

Paraplegia. Paraplegia refers to the impairment or loss of motor and sensory function in the thoracic, lumbar, or sacral level, resulting in dysfunction in the trunk (depending on the level of injury), pelvic organs, and legs. The arms are spared.

Complete Injury. A complete SCI means that there is no preservation of sensory or motor function more than three nerve segments below the level of injury.

Incomplete Injury. An incomplete SCI means that there is some preservation of sensory and/or motor function existing more than three nerve segments below the level of injury.

NEUROLOGICAL EXAMINATION

Neurological examination is critical to the classification and treatment of spinal injuries because it determines the patient's potential recovery. The neurological level of lesion refers to the highest neural segment having normal motor and sensory function. Patients are further subdivided according to whether they have complete or incomplete spinal cord function. This is determined by the absence or presence of motor or sensory function in the most distal part of the spinal cord innervating the sacral nerves. The presence of sacral nerve function is critical because patients with incomplete injuries have the potential to recover normal neurological function over a period of up to 2 years.

The diagnosis of complete SCI cannot be made until the period of spinal shock is over, as evidenced by the return of the bulbocavernosus reflex. The bulbocavernosus reflex is determined by digital examination of the rectum, feeling for contraction of the anal sphincter while squeezing the glans penis or clitoris. Spinal shock can be understood on the basis of the monosynaptic stretch reflex. At a given neural segment of the spinal cord, afferent sensory fibers enter the cord and anastomose with the anterior motor neurons at the same level. In a complete injury of the spinal cord, there is no return of reflex activity at the site of injury because the reflex arc is permanently interrupted. However, when spinal shock disappears, there is a return of reflex activity in the distal segments below the level of injury. Spinal shock in a complete spinal injury patient may last as little as several hours or as long as several months. Individuals with complete spinal injury who have recovered from spinal shock have a negligible chance for any useful motor return.

Another important factor is whether the patient is sacral or areflexic. This is simply determined by digital examination of the rectum. If there is reflex contraction in the anal sphincter, it can be inferred that the other sacral reflexes and striated pelvic muscles that are responsible for penile erections and bladder and bowel emptying are also working reflexively. Maneuvers to trigger sacral reflex activity and contraction of the external sphincter are (1) insertion of a digit into the anus, (2) squeezing the glans penis or clitoris (bulbocavernosus reflex) (3) tapping over the suprapubic region, and (4) tugging on a Foley catheter.

INCOMPLETE SCI
Evaluation

The motor pathways descend in the corticospinal tracts in the anterior cord and synapse with the anterior motor neurons. When checking for sacral motor function, it is important to test toe flexion because it is the volitional motor function that is most likely preserved. Pain and temperature ascend in the lateral spinothalamic tract to the brain. It is checked by testing the patient's sharp-dull discrimination. Proprioception, vibration, and two-point discrimination ascend in the posterior columns. Light touch may be carried by a variety of sensory tracts throughout the spinal cord and is tested with a wisp of cotton. When checking for sacral sensation, the skin at the anal mucocutaneous junction, scrotum, and penis should be individually examined because sensation may not be present in all three areas.[4]

Anterior Cord Syndrome

Anterior cord syndrome results from direct contusion to the anterior cord by bone fragments and/or from damage to the anterior spinal artery. Depending on the extent of cord involvement, only posterior column function (proprioception and light touch) may be present. The presence of pain (sharp-dull discrimination) in addition to light touch signifies the entire posterior half of the cord has some intact function and thus a better prognosis for motor recovery. Patients with anterior cord syndrome who have no recovery of motor function and lack pain sensation 4 weeks after injury have a very poor prognosis for significant motor return.

Central Cord Syndrome

The central gray matter cord contains nerve cell bodies and is surrounded by white matter consisting primarily of ascending and descending myelinated tracts. The central gray matter has a higher metabolic requirement and is more susceptible to trauma and ischemia. Central cord syndrome often results from minor injuries, such as from a fall in older patients who have a cervical spinal canal stenosis. Because the central gray region in the cervical spinal canal contains the tracts ascending and descending to the legs, the hands and upper extremities are more severely affected than the lower extremities. The overall prognosis for patients with central cord syndrome is variable. Most patients are able to walk despite severe upper extremity paralysis.

Brown-Séquard Syndrome

Brown-Séquard syndrome refers to hemisection of the cord. These patients have an excellent prognosis and will ambulate.

Mixed Syndrome

Mixed syndrome refers to patients with diffuse involvement of the entire cord. The prognosis for recovery is good. As with all incomplete syndromes, early motor recovery is the best prognostic indicator.

MANAGEMENT
Lower Extremities

Contracture prevention and maintenance of range of motion is important in all SCI patients.[5] Treatment begins immediately following injury. Teaching the patient to sleep in the prone position is the most effective means of preventing hip and knee flexion contractures. Passive hamstring stretching with the knee extended is initiated to prevent shortening from spasticity. The SCI patient must be able to flex the lumbar spine and hips 120 degrees, with the knee extended so as to be able to perform lower extremity dressing independently. If there is a restriction of hip joint flexion, a long spine fusion immobilizing the lumbar spine will prevent the patient from independent dressing.

Patients with extensive lower extremity paralysis need two strong arms to bring themselves to an upright standing position with crutches. Patients lacking at least grade 3 quadriceps strength will require knee-ankle-foot orthoses (KAFO) to stabilize the knee and will require the knee to be locked in extension while walking.[6] Most patients who require bilateral KAFOs utilize a swing-through rather than a reciprocal crutch-assisted gait. Because strenuous upper extremity exertion is required and the rate of energy expenditure is extremely high, this mode of ambulation is not practical for most patients. Most patients prefer to use a wheelchair. Wheelchair propulsion on a level surface requires a much lower expenditure of energy. Paraplegic patients with grade 3 or greater hip flexor and knee extensor strength are able to walk with unsupported knees and only require ankle-foot orthoses to stabilize the foot and ankle. They also usually require crutches because of their absent or impaired hip extensor and adductor muscle strength. They are able to achieve a reciprocal gait pattern. Most are limited, community ambulators because of the added physical exertion caused by crutch assistance. Generally, they prefer a wheelchair for long-distance mobility.

Because most ambulatory SCI patients have weak hip extensor muscles, they learn to hyperextend the lumbar spine. This aligns the center of gravity of the trunk posterior to the hip joint during the stance phase of gait to avoid forward collapse. This posture decreases the demand on the arms during crutch use for weightbearing support. Spine stabilization procedures that decrease lower lumbar spine mobility into lordosis deprive the patient of this important gait maneuver.

Upper Extremities
C4-Level Function

Patients with cervical lesions above C4 may have impairment of respiratory function, depending on the extent of injury, and may require a tracheostomy and mechanical ventilatory assistance. Phrenic nerve stimulation via implanted surgical electrodes enables the patient to ventilate without mechanical assistance using the diaphragm when diaphragmatic paralysis is due to UMN injury. The high tetraplegic patient can operate an electric wheelchair with attached respiratory equipment, using chin or tongue controls. Mouth sticks, which are lightweight rods attached to a dental bite plate, enable the patient to perform desktop skills, operate push-button equipment, and pursue vocational and recreational activities.

Patients with C4 lesions and normal diaphragm function are respirator-independent. With training, the tetraplegic patient should be able to achieve a vital capacity 50% to 60% of normal using only the diaphragm.

C5-Level Function

At the C5 level, the key muscles are the deltoid and elbow flexors. If these muscles are weak, the patient will benefit from assistance from mobile arm supports attached to the wheelchair. Mobile arm supports are balanced to exert a vertical force to counteract gravity, enabling the patient with poor muscle strength to feed independently and perform other functional tasks with the hands. A ratchet wrist-hand orthosis (WHO) with a fixed wrist joint and a passively closing mechanism attached to the thumb and fingers enables the patient to grasp objects between the thumb and fingers.

Surgery can further enhance upper extremity function. The goals of surgery are to provide active elbow extension, active wrist extension, and restoration of key pinch by tenodesis. Transfer of the posterior deltoid to the triceps gains active elbow extension. The brachioradialis is transferred to the extensor carpi radialis brevis muscle to provide active wrist extension. The flexor pollicis longus tendon is attached to the distal radius, and the interphalangeal joint of the thumb is fused. This provides for lateral (key) pinch of the thumb against the index finger by tenodesis when the wrist is extended.

C6-Level Function

Acquisition of key C6 musculature—the wrist extensors—enables the patient to manually propel a wheelchair, transfer, and even live independently. If wrist extensor strength is poor, a WHO with a free wrist joint and a rubber band extensor assist will enable the patient to complete wrist extension. A wrist-driven WHO flexor hinge mechanism links the wrist joint to a finger attachment that causes the metacarpophalangeal joint to flex when the wrist is extended, enabling the patient to actively grasp between the fingers and thumb. Some patients develop a natural tenodesis of their thumb and finger flexor muscles due to myostatic contracture or spasticity, enabling them to grasp without the need of an orthosis. Most patients who have good wrist extensor strength are able to operate a manual wheelchair but may require an electric wheelchair for long distances.

These patients may also be able to transfer independently if there are no elbow flexion contractures and they can passively lock their elbows in extension while transferring.

The goals of surgery in the C6 patient are restoration of lateral pinch and restoration of active grasp. Lateral pinch can be obtained either by tenodesis of the thumb flexor or by transfer of the brachioradialis to the flexor pollicis longus. Transfer of the pronator teres to the deep finger flexors will provide active grasp.

C7-Level Function

The key muscle in C7 tetraplegic patients is the triceps. All C7 tetraplegic patients with intact triceps function should be able to transfer and live independently if there are not other complications. Despite the presence of finger extension, these patients may also require a flexor hinge WHO.

Surgery can enhance function in these patients. The goals of surgery for the C7 tetraplegic patient are active thumb flexion for pinch, active finger flexion for grasp, and hand opening by extensor tenodesis. Transfer of the brachioradialis to the flexor pollicis longus will provide active pinch. Transfer of the pronator teres to the deep finger flexors allows for active finger flexion and grasp. If the finger extensors are weak, tenodesis of these tendons to the radius will provide hand opening with wrist flexion.

C8-Level Function

The key C8 muscles are the finger and thumb flexors, which enable a gross grasp. The presence of the flexor pollicis longus enables the patient to obtain lateral pinch between the thumb and the side of the index finger. Intrinsic muscle function is lacking in these patients, and clawing of the fingers is usually present. A capsulodesis of the metacarpophalangeal joints will correct the clawing and improve hand function. Active intrinsic function can be gained by splitting the superficial finger flexor tendon of the ring finger into four slips and transferring these tendons to the lumbrical insertions of each finger.

Skin

Maintenance of skin integrity is crucial to SCI care. From the moment the patient enters the emergency department, preventive measures must be instituted to avoid skin breakdown even while critical diagnostic procedures and lifesaving measures are performed. Just 4 hours of continuous pressure on the sacrum is sufficient to cause full-thickness skin necrosis. Turning the patient side-back-side every 2 hours will avoid skin ulceration that greatly prolongs the cost and length of rehabilitation treatment. These simple procedures preclude the need for flotation, Stryker's frames, cyclically rotating beds, and similar devices.

When the patient is allowed to sit, a progressive program to increase the time of sitting tolerance is started. Paraplegic patients with normal upper extremities are taught to perform raises in the wheelchair and decompress the skin for approximately 15 seconds every 15 minutes. Tetraplegic patients who are unable to perform raises can lean to either side and/or forward for 1-minute intervals on an hourly basis to achieve decompression. Those patients unable to perform decompressive maneuvers will require assistance from another person or may use an electric wheelchair with a powered recliner that enables them to assume a supine posture every hour.

All patients must be taught to inspect their skin at least twice a day when dressing and undressing. Mirrors attached to a rod enable the paraplegic patient to independently examine skin over the sacrum and ischia. Tetraplegic patients usually require assistance with skin inspection. If there is evidence of chronic skin inflammation over bony prominences or redness persists 30 minutes after removal of pressure, incipient pressure necrosis must be avoided. Pressure transducers placed under the bony prominences will determine if pressure exceeds acceptable levels. Up to 40 mm Hg is well tolerated by most patients. If pressures exceed this amount, then a custom-fitted foam cushion with appropriate cutouts is prescribed.

Development of any open areas in the skin over the ischia or sacrum, even superficially, is an indication to temporarily discontinue sitting. The patient must remain in a prone or side-lying position to avoid pressure until the lesion is healed. Failure to take aggressive steps to eliminate pressure and allow healing will lead to chronic inflammation, scarring, and a loss of elasticity, creating a vicious cycle that further increases susceptibility to pressure necrosis.

Excessive hip and knee flexor spasticity that prevents the patient from lying prone or supine requires the patient to assume a constant side-lying posture when in bed, which leads to excessive pressure over the greater trochanters. Flexor spasticity or contracture that prevents continuous lying prone should be corrected medically before development of pressure sores and before skin flap procedure. Failure to correct flexion deformities inevitably decreases the likelihood of successful skin closure. Surgical tenotomy and myotomy of hip and knee flexors is the most effective surgical method of correcting the problem when nonoperative measures fail. Neurosurgical procedures such as myelotomy or rhizotomy are less effective in our experience and run the risk of interfering with reflexic bladder emptying and penile erections. Intrathecal baclofen pumps may be very useful in controlling lower extremity spasticity.

In the neglected patient with a full-thickness pressure sore, surgery will be necessary. The initial phase consists of débridement of all infected soft tissue and bone as well as treatment of spasticity and contractures that may have prevented the patient from lying prone, predisposing the patient to pressure sores. Once all wounds have a clean granulating base and the patient is able to lie prone 24 hours per day, the patient is a candidate for a rotational flap. In recent years, the myocutaneous gluteus maximus and tensor fascia femoris and other types of myocutaneous flaps have provided the surgeon a superior and reliable method of providing skin coverage. Sitting tolerance must be carefully re-established following flap surgery. Because most pressure sores in chronically injured SCI patients are the result of failure to relieve pressure by appropriate measures, patient education is the key element of a successful rehabilitation outcome.

Ischial or trochanteric pressure sores commonly lead to septic arthritis of the hip. In such cases, femoral head and neck resection is required. In the normal paraplegic patient with an intact hip joint, the passive weight of the limbs cantilevered about the posterior thigh exerts an upward force on the pelvis, decompressing the ischia. Consequently, about 30% of the body weight is supported on the thigh. Femoral head and neck resection disrupts the bony leg of the femur to the pelvis and results in a greater concentration of pressure on the ischia, thereby increasing the chance of recurrence even after successful flap closure.

Pressure sores affecting the ankle commonly occur over the heel or malleoli. Following initial débridement, wound healing can nearly always be obtained by placing the patient in a short leg-healing cast that protects the wound from any external pressure. The cast is changed every 1 or 2 weeks until healing occurs. Rotational flaps are rarely needed.

Bladder Function

Intermittent catheterization has been the single factor most responsible for SCI patients living a near-normal life span.[7] Urinary tract infection is no longer the leading cause of death in SCI patients. Most patients who have intact sacral reflex activity following complete injury will be able to obtain reflex bladder emptying. Some patients with complete SCI will be able to trigger reflex emptying of their bladder by suprapubic tapping, stroking the thighs, performing Valsalva's maneuver of forcibly exhaling against the closed glottis, or using Credé's method of applying external pressure on the bladder. These patients require the use of an external condom catheter. Not all reflex bladders will reflexively empty, and some, despite reflex emptying, will have an excessive residual urine volume. Anticholinergic medication to decrease bladder neck spasm of the

smooth muscle of the internal sphincter or antispasmolytic medications to decrease tone in the striated muscle of the external sphincter may improve bladder emptying. Some patients require surgical sphincterotomy. Patients with areflexic bladders void by the application of pressure on the bladder by Valsalva's or Credé's maneuvers.

Bladder diversion using an ileal conduit as a primary means of achieving bladder drainage is contraindicated. This procedure leads to a chronic acid-base imbalance, osteoporosis and, ultimately, renal failure from secondary infection. The suprapubic catheter is also not used as a means of primary treatment for the same reasons that permanent indwelling catheters are contraindicated. The constant presence of an indwelling catheter leads to bladder constriction and increases the risks of renal calculi, infection and, ultimately, death from renal failure. For men, the external condom catheter is the treatment of choice. For women, padding or diapering is the preferred treatment, although some women aesthetically prefer an indwelling catheter despite the risks of a shortened life span.

Sexual Function

Women can perform coitus and deliver normal children regardless of whether they have preserved reflex activity. Among males with complete spinal cord lesion, the ability to obtain an erection depends on whether they have reflexic or areflexic sacral function. Approximately 90% of patients with complete SCI and sacral reflex activity can be expected to have reflex erections. Most of these men will be able to perform coitus, but less than half will be able to ejaculate. Sacral sparing plays a great role in prognosticating sexual potential in the male. Patients able to distinguish pain (sharp-dull discrimination) are usually able to achieve psychogenic erections.

Autonomic Dysreflexia

Splanchnic outflow conveying sympathetic fibers to the lower body exits at the T8 region. Patients with lesions above T8 are prone to autonomic dysreflexia. They are subject to bouts of hypertension, which may be preceded by dizziness, sweating, and headaches. A plugged catheter is the most common precipitating cause of dysreflexia. The catheter should be carefully checked and the bladder irrigated. Calculi or infection and fecal impaction (of the urinary system) are frequent causes of dysreflexia. Pressure sores or any noxious stimulation may trigger dysreflexia. If the patient's blood pressure does not respond to identification and treatment of the causative disorder, treatment with antihypertensive medication is begun.

RECOVERY OF NEUROLOGICAL FUNCTION

The most reliable tool for assessing neurological status in SCI is the International Standard for Neurologic and Functional Classification of Spinal Cord Injury, published by the American Spinal Injury Association (ASIA) and the International Medical Society of Paraplegia (IMSOP).[8] This instrument provides quantitative measures of sensory and motor function.

Neurological recovery is determined by comparing changes in the ASIA motor score (AMS) in successive neurological examinations.[8] The AMS is the sum of strength grades for each of the 10 key muscles tested bilaterally, which represent the neurological segments from C5 to T1 and from L2 to S1. In a neurologically intact person, the maximum AMS score is 100 points.

The most important prognostic indicators of recovery are completeness and level of injury, using the definition of sacral sparing. Using completeness and level of injury (tetraplegia or paraplegia), patients are divided into four groups: complete paraplegia, incomplete paraplegia, complete tetraplegia, and incomplete tetraplegia. The rate of motor recovery in all groups declines rapidly in the first 6 months following injury, with minimal changes after this time.

Complete Paraplegia. Patients with paraplegia who remain complete 1 month after injury have a 96% chance of remaining complete.[9] Thirty-eight percent of those with injuries at or below T9 will recover some lower extremity function. No patients with a neurological level above T9 regained volitional lower extremity motor function. Only 5% of muscles with a strength of 0/5 at 1 month will recover to 3/5 (see Table 3) or greater strength one year after injury. Furthermore, only 5% of individuals will become independent community ambulators at 1 year.

Incomplete Paraplegia. Motor recovery is better in individuals with incomplete injuries.[10] Between 1 month and 1 year after injury, there is an average increase of 12 points in AMS, regardless of the level of injury. Additionally, there is a 76% chance of becoming a community ambulator.

Complete Tetraplegia. Ninety percent of individuals with complete tetraplegia 1 month after injury will remain complete.[11] Among the 10% who undergo late conversion to incomplete status, lower extremity motor recovery is minimal and inadequate for ambulation. Recovery of AMS points is independent of neurological level. Waters and colleagues[9–12] reported that with the exception of the triceps muscle, all upper extremity muscles with grade of at least 1/5 at 1 month after injury would recover to at least 3/5 by 1 year following injury.

Incomplete Tetraplegia. In patients with incomplete tetraplegia, motor recovery of upper and lower extremity muscles occurs concurrently.[12] Nearly all muscles with at least 1/5 strength 1 month after injury recover to at least 3/5 by 1 year postinjury. Forty-six percent of the patients examined by Waters and colleagues[11] attained independent community ambulation status 1 year after injury. The number of individuals with incomplete tetraplegia who can attain independent community ambulation is lower than for individuals with incomplete paraplegia and comparable lower extremity function. This is because upper extremity function may be insufficient to allow crutch-assisted ambulation for tetraplegic patients, whereas those with incomplete paraplegia have normal upper extremity strength.

A minority of individuals with SCI can ambulate independently after injury.[13] The proportion of patients who can ambulate varies with the level and completeness of the injury. The lower extremity motor score (LEMS), which is the sum of the strength grades of the bilateral key lower extremity muscles, can be used to predict successful ambulation. The motor groups are as follows: L2: hip flexors (iliopsoas), L3: knee extensors (quadriceps), L4: ankle dorsiflexors (tibialis anterior), L5: long toe extensors (extensor hallucis longus), and S1: ankle plantarflexors (gastrocne-

mius, soleus). In an individual with no deficit, the total possible LEMS is 50 points. The LEMS at 30 days is used to predict the chance of successful ambulation in incomplete tetraplegic, incomplete paraplegic, and complete paraplegic patients. All patients with a LEMS of at least 20 and an incomplete injury are expected to be community ambulators by 1 year after injury.

STROKE (BRAIN ATTACK)

GENERAL CONSIDERATIONS

Stroke, also known as brain attack or cerebrovascular accident (CVA), is caused by the cessation of cerebral oxygenation from thrombosis, hemorrhage, or emboli, which results in death of neurons in the brain. This leads to deficits in cognition, motor, and sensory function.

Cerebrovascular accidents are the third leading cause of death in the United States.[3] The incidence rate of stroke is 1 per 1000 each year. Approximately 200,000 persons each year die as the result of stroke, and 250,000 survive. In the United States stroke is the leading cause of hemiplegia in adults, with two million persons with permanent neurological deficits. Cerebral thrombosis causes approximately three-fourths of strokes. The majority of survivors following stroke have the potential for significant function and useful lives if they receive rehabilitation.[14–18] The average life expectancy for patients surviving the first several months is approximately 6 years.

ANATOMY

Infarction of the cerebral cortex in the area of the brain supplied by the middle cerebral artery or one of its branches is most commonly responsible for stroke. The middle cerebral artery supplies the area of the cerebral cortex responsible for hand function. The anterior cerebral artery supplies the area of the cerebral cortex responsible for lower extremity motion. The typical clinical picture following middle cerebral artery stroke is contralateral hemianesthesia (decreased sensation), homonymous hemianopsia (visual field deficit), and spastic hemiplegia with more paralysis in the upper extremity than in the lower extremity. Because hand function requires relatively precise motor control, even for assistive activities, the prognosis for the functional use of the hand and arm is considerably less than for the leg. Return of even gross motor control in the lower extremity may be sufficient for walking.

Infarction in the region of the anterior cerebral artery causes paralysis and sensory loss of the opposite lower limb and, to a lesser degree, the arm. Patients with cerebral arteriosclerosis who have repeated bilateral infarctions are likely to have severe cognitive impairment, which limits their function even when motor function is good.

NEUROLOGICAL RECOVERY

Motor recovery after stroke follows a fairly characteristic pattern. The size of the lesion and the amount of collateral circulation determine the amount of permanent damage. Most recovery occurs within 6 months, although functional improvement may continue as a result of further sensorimotor re-education as the patient learns to cope with disability.

Initially after a stroke, the limbs are completely flaccid.

There is a gradual increase in muscle tone (spasticity) over the next few weeks in the shoulder adductor muscles and the flexor muscles of the elbow, wrist, and fingers. Spasticity also develops in the lower extremity muscles. Most frequently, there is an extensor pattern of spasticity in the leg characterized by hip adduction, knee extension, and equinovarus of the foot and ankle. In some cases, a flexion pattern of spasticity is seen with hip and knee flexion.

Recovery of selective motor control (the ability to move one joint independently of the others) depends on the extent of the cerebral cortical damage (see Table 2).[19, 20] Dependence on the more neurologically primitive mass movement patterns (synergistic motor control) decreases as selective control improves. The extent to which motor impairment restricts function differs between the upper and lower extremities. Synergistic (mass pattern) movement is not functional in the upper extremity, which relies on non-stereotypical movement to perform activities. Mass pattern movement may be useful in the lower extremity, where the patient uses flexion synergy to advance the limb forward and mass extension synergy for limb stability during standing.

The final processes in sensory perception occur in the cerebral cortex, where basic sensory information is integrated into complex sensory phenomena such as proprioception, spacial relationships, shape, sight, and texture. Patients with severe parietal dysfunction and sensory loss may lack sufficient perception of space and awareness of the involved segment of their body to ambulate. Patients with severe perceptual loss may lack balance to sit, stand, or walk. A visual field deficit further interferes with limb use and may cause a patient to be unaware of a limb.

TRAUMATIC BRAIN INJURY

INCIDENCE

Injury to the brain is a leading cause of death and disability.[3] In the United States 410,000 new cases of traumatic brain injury (TBI) cases can be expected each year. Eighty-nine percent of these patients will survive the injury. Approximately 80% of the survivors will have a good or moderate neurological recovery and will have a normal life span despite the injury. Head injury occurs at least twice as commonly in males as in females. It occurs most often in 15-to-24-year-olds. Approximately one-half of these injuries occur as a result of a motor vehicle accident.

PROGNOSIS

Prognosis following TBI has traditionally been predicted relative to the Glasgow Coma Scale (Table 4).[21] The Glasgow Coma Scale evaluates a patient's responses to eye opening, motor responses, and verbal responses. The Glasgow Outcome Scale (Table 5) is frequently used to determine outcome following brain injury. Using the Glasgow Coma Scale within 24 hours of a patient's admission to the hospital, a score of 11 or greater is associated with an 82% probability of moderate or good neurological recovery. Lower scores have a significantly higher incidence rate of severe sequelae.

Although demonstrated to predict mortality accurately, recent studies have suggested the Glasgow Coma Score as a single variable may have limited value as a predictor of

TABLE 4. GLASGOW COMA SCALE		
EYE OPENING:	Spontaneous	4
	Speech	3
	Pain	2
	None	1
MOTOR RESPONSE:	Obeys	6
	Localizes	5
	Withdrawal	4
	Abnormal flexion	3
	Extension	2
	None	1
VERBAL RESPONSE:	Oriented	5
	Confused	4
	Inappropriate	3
	Incomprehensible	2
	None	1

The Glasgow Coma Scale is the total of the eye opening, motor response, and verbal scores.

functional outcome. Many trauma centers are now using the Revised Trauma Score (RTS) to assist with triage of multitrauma patients. The RTS combines the Glasgow Coma Scale as well as the systolic blood pressure and respiratory rate and is used to predict both mortality and disability.

Age is an extremely important determinant for survival and eventual neurological outcome. When age alone is considered, patients younger than 20 years were shown to have a 62% incidence rate of moderate or better recovery; patients from 20 to 29 years of age displayed a 46% chance of moderate or better recovery. The incidence rate of good recovery declines with advancing age.

Duration of coma can be used as an index of the magnitude of the brain injury and can be related to outcome. Patients recovering from coma within the first 2 weeks of injury have a 70% chance of good recovery. The recovery rate drops to 39% in the 3rd week and to 17% in the 4th week. Decerebrate or decorticate posturing indicates a brain-stem injury and is a poor prognostic sign.

PHASES OF NEUROLOGICAL RECOVERY
The Period of Acute Injury

The orthopaedic management of traumatic brain injury (TBI) can be divided into three distinct periods: the period of acute injury, the period of physiological recovery, and the period of functional adaptation to residual deficits.[1, 14, 15]

The initial phase of management occurs in the acute care hospital immediately following injury. The majority of TBIs are the result of motor vehicle accidents. Multiple trauma is common. The orthopaedic surgeon is a consultant with a critical role. Aggressive treatment of orthopaedic

TABLE 5. GLASGOW OUTCOME SCALE
Dead
Persistent vegetative state
Severely disabled
Moderately disabled
Good recovery

Grades long-term recovery following traumatic brain injury.

injuries at an early stage is important to functional outcome.

The first priority is to accurately diagnose all injuries. It is common for injuries such as fractures or major peripheral nerve injuries to go undetected. Garland and Bailey[16] reported an 11% incidence rate of delayed diagnosis of fractures, with an average time to diagnosis of 57 days. In the comatose patient, radiographs of all major joints and any other areas suspect for injury should be obtained. It is important not to assume that all neurological deficits present are from central nervous system injury. Thirty-four percent of TBI patients have missed peripheral nerve injuries.[17] Especially in the presence of a limb fracture, a peripheral nerve injury should be suspected.

The second rule of orthopaedic care is to assume that the patient will make a good neurological recovery. All orthopaedic injuries should be treated promptly and appropriately.[16, 18] When possible, internal fixation is best. Spasticity develops, and casting a spastic joint in a flexed position may result in a joint contracture or an unsatisfactory reduction. Fracture healing is accelerated, presumably by the same humoral factors that contribute to heterotopic bone formation. Fracture malunion is a common and potentially avoidable complication.

The Period of Physiological Recovery

Neurological recovery can proceed for a prolonged time. The majority of improvement in motor control occurs within the first 6 months following injury. Cognitive changes are made most rapidly in the early phases following brain injury but can continue for a very prolonged time, often years. Consequently, definitive surgical procedures are avoided during this transitional stage. There is no exact time that must elapse before considering surgery to improve musculoskeletal function. The orthopaedic surgeon must consider the rate of continued improvement in motor control when deciding at what point to intervene surgically. If the additional improvement in motor control will be overridden by the complications of contracture formation, osteopenia, peripheral nerve compression, and muscle atrophy, then early surgical intervention is appropriate.

The Period of Functional Adaptation to Residual Deficits

When neurological recovery has ceased, the TBI patient is commonly left with residual limb deformities from spasticity, contractures, and muscle imbalance. It is at this time that definitive orthopaedic surgical procedures are performed to rebalance the muscle forces and correct the residual deformities.

The surgical principles and procedures used to treat spastic limb deformities are the same in stroke, brain injury, and other UMN syndromes. There are differences in the frequency of use and expectations for outcomes between diagnostic groups.

Heterotopic Ossification

Heterotopic ossification presents clinically with an intense inflammatory reaction about the joint seen as redness, warmth, severe pain, and rapidly decreasing range of motion. Although the time of initial occurrence is variable, heterotopic ossification is usually detected 2 months following the onset of TBI. Generally, radiographs show evidence of the heterotopic bone in the form of spotty periarticular calcification. The pathoetiology of heterotopic ossification in the head injured patient remains uncertain.

POLIOMYELITIS

ACUTE POLIOMYELITIS

Because of effective immunization programs, acute poliomyelitis has become a rare occurrence in most of the world. The last major epidemics in the developed world occurred during the early 1950s.

Poliomyelitis is the result of a viral infection that attacks the anterior horn cells of the spinal cord. The anterior horn cells control the skeletal muscle cells of the trunk and limbs. All of the anterior horn cells are affected with the acute infection. This accounts for the diffuse severe paralysis seen with the initial infection. A variable number of anterior horn cells survive the initial infection.

Acute polio is characterized by the sudden onset of paralysis accompanied by fever, acute muscle pain, and often a stiff neck. Paralysis of the respiratory muscles is life-threatening in the acute stage. When the shoulder muscles are involved, respiratory compromise should be suspected because of the proximity of the anterior horn cells controlling both respiratory and shoulder muscles in the spinal cord. Mechanical support of ventilation may be required.

Treatment in the acute stage consists of providing the needed respiratory support, decreasing muscle pain, and performing regular range-of-motion exercises to prevent the formation of joint contractures.

SUBACUTE POLIOMYELITIS

The subacute stage of polio is characterized by the recovery of a variable amount of muscle function. Mechanisms of regaining strength include anterior horn cell survival, axon sprouting, and muscle hypertrophy. Although all of the anterior horn cells in the spinal cord are affected by the initial infection, some will survive. The average number of anterior horn cells to survive is 47% (range 12% to 94%) as seen from postmortem studies. The pattern of anterior horn cell survival in the spinal cord is random and does not follow anatomically continuous areas. The distribution of the paralysis is variable, depending on which cells were destroyed.

Additional muscle function is gained during the recovery phase by axon sprouting. Each individual anterior horn cell innervates a group of muscle cells. When muscle cells are "orphaned" by the death of their anterior horn cell, a nearby nerve cell can sprout additional connections (axons) and "adopt" some of these muscle cells. A motor unit is defined as a nerve cell and all of the muscle cells it controls. The axon sprouting that occurs after polio can result in very large motor units.

The other mechanism by which patients regain strength after polio is by muscle hypertrophy. The surviving muscle cells enlarge in an effort to provide additional needed power. During the subacute stage of the disease, which may last from 16 to 24 months following onset, the emphasis is on preventing deformities and preserving function. Splinting and braces are often helpful to maintain joint position and supplement function.

RESIDUAL POLIOMYELITIS

During the residual stage, the orthopaedic surgeon traditionally becomes active, utilizing surgical procedures to restore lost function and provide structural stability. In the growing child, it is important to prevent the formation of skeletal deformities resulting from the muscle imbalance.

The person with compromised function of the diaphragm is taught glossopharyngeal breathing in which air is swallowed into the lungs. This provides sufficient air exchange for light activities performed while sitting. The person often still requires mechanical support of ventilation while sleeping.

POSTPOLIO SYNDROME

It has become common to see individuals who had polio as a child returning to complain of increasing weakness. Many are concerned about loss of function. Polio has always been considered a static disease in that the paralysis is not progressive. The increasing weakness has been attributed to the overuse of muscles already weakened by the polio.[19–20] Often, muscles that were thought unaffected exhibit weakness at a later date. Studies have shown that a muscle must lose 30% to 40% of its strength for weakness to be detected using manual muscle testing.[21] Gait laboratory studies have also demonstrated that activities of daily living require more muscle strength and stamina than were previously appreciated.[20] Polio survivors have traditionally been encouraged to work harder to regain strength. The concept of "no pain, no gain" has proved detrimental to the polio survivor because it has encouraged chronic overuse of muscles and resulted in further deterioration of function.

Most polio survivors begin to notice the deterioration approximately 30 years after the onset of the disease. The combination of symptoms varies slightly among people. The diagnosis of postpolio syndrome is made on the following clinical criteria: a history of poliomyelitis, a pattern of muscle weakness that is random and does not follow any nerve root or peripheral nerve distribution, and a constellation of symptoms indicating decreasing strength and function (Table 6). There are no tests that are diagnostic for postpolio syndrome. Electromyography can demonstrate the presence of large motor units resulting from the previous axon sprouting. These findings are supportive but not diagnostic of polio.

Treatment of Postpolio Syndrome

Treatment is directed at preserving current muscle strength and preventing further weakness. Generally, it is not possi-ble to strengthen a muscle that has been weakened by polio. Some gain in strength can be seen when chronic overuse is corrected. The basic principles of treatment are (1) lifestyle modification to prevent chronic overuse of weak muscles, (2) a limited exercise program incorporating frequent rest periods to prevent disuse atrophy and weakness, (3) use of lightweight orthotics to protect joints and substitute for muscle function, and (4) orthopaedic surgery to correct limb or trunk deformities.

CEREBRAL PALSY

GENERAL CONSIDERATIONS

Cerebral palsy, or static encephalopathy, is a nonprogressive and nonhereditary disease with many diverse neurological findings. The onset may be prenatal, perinatal, or postnatal. An exact cause is not always known, but the condition is associated with prematurity, perinatal hypoxia, cerebral trauma, and neonatal jaundice. It is estimated that over 500,000 persons in the United States are affected by this disorder. The degree of neurological impairment is severe in one-third of cases and mild in approximately one-sixth of cases. Little is credited with the first description of cerebral palsy in 1862, but Dr. Winthrop Phelps coined the term *cerebral palsy* in 1937.

CLASSIFICATION

Because of the diversity of neurological deficits in cerebral palsy, a classification system is essential.[22] The disease can be classified by the pattern of motor involvement and by the topographical distribution of findings.

Motion disorders can be divided into three basic groups: spastic, dyskinetic, and mixed. The spastic group is characterized by clonus and hyperactive deep tendon reflexes. These patients can be helped by orthopaedic intervention. The dyskinetic group consists of a variety of specific motion disorders such as athetosis, ballismus, chorea, dystonia, and ataxia. Each of these conditions represents a precise neurological definition. For practical purposes, however, dyskinetic patients are grouped together because their motion disorders are not amenable to surgical correction. The mixed group usually consists of a combination of spasticity and athetosis with total body involvement.

The geographic distribution of the neurological involvement forms the second classification system.

Monoplegia refers to single limb involvement, usually spastic in nature. This pattern is rare; it is advisable to have the patient run before making the diagnosis. The stress of performing an activity very fast, such as running, often uncovers spasticity in another limb.

Hemiplegia refers to spasticity in the upper and lower extremity ipsilaterally. Equinovarus posturing is common in the lower extremity. The upper extremity is usually held with the elbow, wrist, and fingers flexed and the thumb adducted. The major problem interfering with upper extremity function, however, is a loss of proprioception and stereognosis. Surgery for the upper extremity aims at making the hand assistive and improving cosmesis. An arm, which involuntarily is held severely flexed while walking, can present a major social disadvantage for the patient.

TABLE 6. SYMPTOMS OF POST POLIO SYNDROME
Increasing muscle weakness
Severe fatigue
Muscle pain
Muscle cramping
Muscle fasiculations
Joint pain or instability
Sleep apnea
Intolerance to cold
Depression

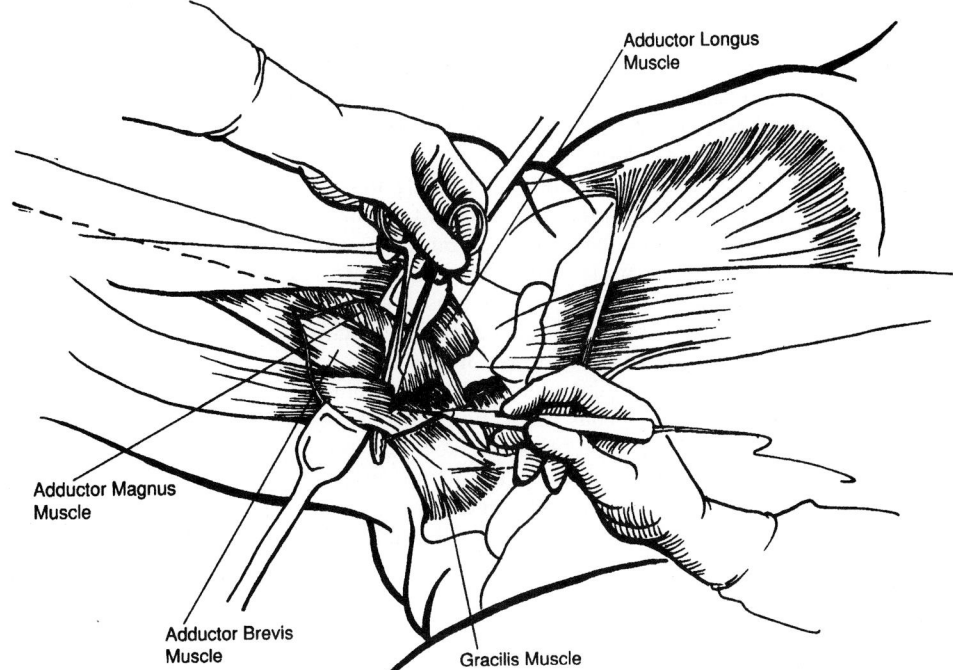

Fig. 2. Hip adductor tenotomy for limb scissoring.

Paraplegia refers to neurological deficits involving both lower extremities only. It is rare in spastic cerebral palsy. When it is encountered, it is important to rule out the existence of a high spinal cord lesion, which could also be responsible for the neurological findings. Bladder problems coexist with spastic paralysis of the lower extremities secondary to spinal cord disorder.

Diplegia is the most common pattern in the spastic patient and refers to a major involvement in both lower extremities with only minor incoordination in the upper extremities. Spastic diplegia accounts for 50% to 60% of the cerebral palsy patients in the United States. The lower extremities exhibit marked spasticity with worse involvement proximally about the hips, hyperactive deep tendon reflexes, and positive Babinski's signs. The hips are commonly held in a position of flexion, adduction, and internal rotation secondary to the spasticity. The knees are in valgus position and may have excessive external rotation of the tibia. The ankles are in equinus position with a valgus attitude of the feet. Speech and intellectual functions are usually normal or only slightly impaired. Esotropia and visual perceptual problems are common. Surgical correction is often necessary (Figs. 2 and 3).

Total body involvement, sometimes referred to as *quadriplegia*, is characterized by involvement of all four extremities, head, and trunk. Sensory deficits are also typical. Speech and swallowing are commonly impaired. The most serious deficit is often the inability to communicate with others. Mental retardation is found in approximately 45% of these patients. Intelligence is often masked by communication dysfunction. Ambulation is not usually a goal because equilibrium reactions are severely impaired or absent. Sitting may require braces or adaptive supportive devices. Scoliosis and dislocated hips may interfere with sitting. The orthopaedic problems in these patients are scoliosis, contractures, and dislocated hips.

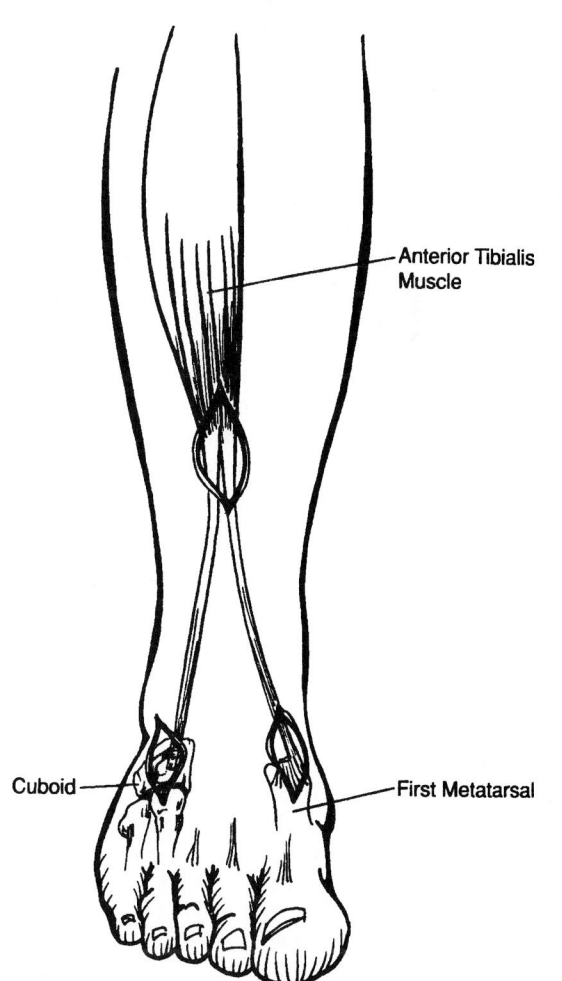

Fig. 3. Split anterior tibialis tendon transfer. This procedure is used to correct a spastic varus foot deformity caused by the tibialis anterior muscle.

NEUROMUSCULAR DISORDERS

GENERAL CONSIDERATIONS

Neuromuscular disorders represent a diverse group of chronic diseases characterized by progressive degeneration of skeletal musculature resulting in weakness, atrophy, joint contractures, and increasing disability. These disorders are best classified as motor unit diseases because the primary abnormality may involve the motor neuron, the neuromuscular junction, or the muscle fiber. Two broad categories are considered. *Myopathy* refers to diseases of the muscle fibers. *Neuropathy* refers to disorders in which muscle degeneration is secondary to lower motor neuron disease. Most of the diseases are hereditary, although point mutations may result in spontaneous cases. Early diagnosis is important for initiation of appropriate therapy and for genetic counseling. Treatment programs are symptomatic and supportive. Appropriate orthopaedic intervention can significantly increase the functional capacity of the individual.

DIAGNOSIS
Clinical Features

Diagnosis is based on many factors. Clinical history and examination will delineate the onset and pattern of muscle involvement. A careful genetic history is important. These diseases have typical clinical patterns.[22-24] Neuropathies generally present with distal involvement. Muscle fasciculation and spasticity are common, and muscle atrophy is in excess of the weakness. Myopathies usually display weakness of the proximal limb musculature initially. Fasciculation and spasticity are not seen. The weakness is more pronounced than atrophy. Disorders of neuromuscular transmission, such as myasthenia gravis, present with fatigue and ptosis.

Muscle Enzymes

Serum muscle enzymes are elevated in myopathies but normal in neuropathies. Muscle enzyme studies involve creatine phosphokinase, lactate dehydrogenase, aldolase, serum glutamic oxaloacetic transaminase, and serum glutamic pyruvic transaminase. Creatine phosphokinase elevation in muscular dystrophy is greatest in the Duchenne type and less prominent in the more slowly progressive disease forms. In Duchenne's muscular dystrophy, the highest enzymes levels occur at birth and during the first few years of life before the disease is clinically apparent. As the disease progresses and the muscle mass deteriorates, the enzyme levels decrease.

Electromyography

Electromyography (EMG) and nerve conduction studies differentiate between primary muscle diseases and neuropathy. EMG shows distinctive differences among muscle disease, peripheral nerve disorders, and anterior horn cell abnormalities. A myopathic electromyograph shows increased frequency, decreased duration, and decreased amplitude of action potentials. Increased insertional activity is also evident with short polyphasic potentials and a retained interference pattern. A neuropathic electromyograph shows an opposite pattern, with decreased frequency but increased duration and increased amplitude of action potentials. In addition, frequent fibrillation potentials, a group polyphasic potential, and a decreased interference pattern can be seen. In myasthenia gravis and the myotonic diseases, the EMG patterns are diagnostic. In myasthenia, the fatigue phenomenon is exhibited. In myotonia the electromyograph is characterized by positive waves and trains of potentials firing at high frequency, which then wax and wane until they slowly disappear.

Muscle Biopsy

Muscle biopsy can distinguish between myopathy, neuropathy, and inflammatory myopathy. The biopsy, however, cannot be used to determine prognosis. Histochemical staining can be used to differentiate between the congenital myopathies. It is important to choose the biopsy site carefully to gain the maximum information.

Histologically, muscle fiber necrosis, fatty degeneration, and proliferation of the connective tissue characterize myopathies. There is an increased number of nuclei evident, and some nuclei migrate from their normal peripheral position to the center of the muscle fiber.

Neuropathies display small angulated muscle fibers. Bundles of atrophic fibers are intermingled with normal bundles. There is no increase in the amount of connective tissue. Biopsies in polymyositis exhibit prominent collections of inflammatory cells. There is segmental necrosis with a mixed pattern of fiber degeneration and regeneration. Edema of the tissues occurs along with perivasculitis.

DUCHENNE'S MUSCULAR DYSTROPHY

Duchenne's muscular dystrophy is a progressive disease that affects males. It is inherited in a sex-linked recessive manner. The clinical onset occurs between 3 to 5 years of age, when sufficient muscle mass has been lost to impair function. Generally, these children have a normal birth and developmental history. Early signs include pseudohypertrophy of the calf, which is the result of the increase in connective tissue, planovalgus feet secondary to heel cord contracture, and proximal muscle weakness. The proximal muscle weakness may be exhibited by Gowers' sign, in which the child uses the arms to support the trunk while attempting to rise from the floor. Other signs are hesitance when climbing stairs, acceleration during the final stage of sitting, and shoulder weakness.

Weakness and contractures prevent independent ambulation in approximately 45% of children by the age of 9 years. The remainder have lost this function by the age of 12 years. The common sequence of lost function is difficulty in rising from the floor, ascending stairs, and then walking. Cardiac involvement is seen in 80% of the children with posterobasal fibrosis of the ventricle and electrocardiographic changes. Clinical evidence of cardiomyopathy may not be obvious secondary to the decreased level of activity. Pulmonary problems are common in the advanced stages of the disease. Periodic evaluation of pulmonary function is required. Mental retardation has been noted in 30% to 50% of patients. The intellectual impairment is present from birth and is not progressive.

Efforts are made to keep the child ambulating for as long as possible to prevent the complications of obesity, osteoporosis, and scoliosis.[22] The hip flexors, tensor fascia lata, and triceps surae develop contractures that limit walking. With progressive weakness and contractures, the base of support decreases, and the patient cannot utilize normal mechanisms to maintain upright balance. The child walks with a wide-based gait, hips flexed and abducted, knees flexed, and the feet in equinus and varus position. Lumbar lordosis becomes exaggerated to compensate for the hip flexion contractures and weak hip extensor musculature.

SPINAL MUSCULAR ATROPHY

Spinal muscular atrophy is a neuropathic disorder in which there are fewer anterior horn cells present in the spinal cord congenitally.[24, 25] The very severe, infantile form of the disease is called the Werdnig-Hoffmann syndrome. The disorder is inherited in an autosomal-recessive pattern. Approximately 20% of patients are ambulatory, and 1% are totally dependent.

The goal of orthopaedic intervention is to prevent collapse of the spine and to prevent contractures. Orthotic support is often needed to stabilize the spine. In the non-ambulatory patient, adaptive seating devices or orthotics may be used. If collapse of the spine occurs, then spinal fusion is indicated. Fractures are also common in these patients secondary to their decreased mobility and function.

CHARCOT-MARIE-TOOTH DISEASE

Charcot-Marie-Tooth disease is the most common of the hereditary degenerative myopathies.[26-29] It is generally inherited in an autosomal-dominant pattern. The EMG shows a neuropathic pattern, and the nerve conduction velocity of the involved nerves is markedly decreased. Muscle enzyme levels are normal. Clinical onset of the disease is most common between the ages of 5 and 15 years.

The peroneal muscles are affected early in the course of the disease; the disorder is therefore sometimes referred to as progressive peroneal atrophy. The intrinsic muscles of the feet and hands are affected later. Patients usually present with progressive claw-toe and cavus deformities of the feet.

REFERENCES

1. Keenan MA, Esquenzai A, and Pelenski J: A neuro-orthopaedic approach to the management of common patterns of upper motoneuron dysfunction after brain injury. J Neuro Rehabil 1999; 12:119.
2. Kendall FPM, Provance PG: Muscles: Testing and Function. Baltimore, Williams & Wilkins, 1993, 4th ed.
3. Anderson DW: The national head and spinal cord injury survey. J Neurosurg 1980; 53, S1.
4. Capen D, Zigler JE: Spinal Cord Injury. In Nickel V, Botte MJ (eds): Orthopaedic Rehabilitation. New York, Churchill Livingstone, 1992, p 411.
5. Botte M: Extremity problems in spinal cord injury. In In Nickel V, Botte MJ (eds): Orthopaedic Rehabilitation. New York, Churchill Livingstone, 1992, p 427.
6. Waters RL, Yakura JS, Adkins R, et al: Determinants of gait performance following spinal cord injury. Arch Phys Med Rehabil 1989; 70:811.
7. Rossier AB, Fam BA, DiBenedetto M, et al: Urethro-vesical function during spinal shock. Urol Res 1980; 8:53.
8. American Spinal Injury Association: International Standards for Neurological and Functional Classification of Spinal Cord Injury. Chicago, American Spinal Injury Association, 1996.
9. Waters RL, Yakura JS, Adkins RH, et al: Recovery following complete paraplegia. Arch Phys Med Rehabil 1992; 73:784.
10. Waters RL, Adkins RH, Yakura JS, et al: Motor and sensory recovery following incomplete paraplegia. Arch Phys Med Rehabil 1994; 75:67.
11. Waters RL, Adkins RH, Yakura JS, et al: Motor and sensory recovery following complete tetraplegia. Arch Phys Med Rehabil 1993; 74:242.
12. Waters RL, Adkins RH, Yakura JS, et al: Motor and sensory recovery following incomplete tetraplegia. Arch Phys Med Rehabil 1994; 75:306.
13. Jennett B, Teasdale G, Braakman R, et al: Prognosis of patients with severe head injury. Neurosurgery 1979; 4:283.
14. Kane RL, Chen Q, Finch M, et al: Functional outcomes of posthospital care for stroke and hip fracture patients under medicare. J Am Geriatr Soc 1998; 46:1525.
15. Keenan MAE: Rehabilitation of the neurologically disabled patient. In Wilkins R (ed): Neurosurgery. New York, McGraw-Hill, 1996, p 445.
16. Garland DE, Bailey S: Undetected injuries in head-injured adults. Clin Orthop 1981; 155: 62.
17. Stone L, Keenan MA: Peripheral nerve injuries in the adult with traumatic brain injury. Clin Orthop 1988; 233:136.
18. Garland DE, Dowling V: Forearm fractures in the head-injured adult. Clin Orthop 1983:190.
19. Halstead LS: Post-polio syndrome. Sci Am 1998; 278:42.
20. Perry J, Mulroy SJ, Renwick SE: The relationship of lower extremity strength and gait parameters in patients with post-polio syndrome. Arch Phys Med Rehabil 1993; 74:165.
21. Beasley WC: Quantitative muscle testing: Principles and applications to research and clinical services. Arch Phys Med Rehabil 1961; 42:398.
22. Roberts A, Evans GA: Orthopedic aspects of neuromuscular disorders in children. Curr Opin Pediatr 1993; 5:379.
23. Fowler WM Jr: Rehabilitation management of muscular dystrophy and related disorders: Comprehensive care. Arch Phys Med Rehabil 1982; 63:322.
24. Birch JG: Orthopedic management of neuromuscular disorders in children. Semin Pediatr Neurol 1998; 5:78.
25. Stewart H, Wallace A, McGaughran J, et al: Molecular diagnosis of spinal muscular atrophy. Arch Dis Child 1998; 78:531.
26. Mann RA, Missirian J: Pathophysiology of Charcot-Marie-Tooth disease. Clin Orthop 1988; 234:221.
27. Martel J, Mierau D, Donat J: Charcot-Marie-Tooth disease. J Manipulative Physiol Ther 1995; 18:168.
28. Mann DC, Hsu JD: Triple arthrodesis in the treatment of fixed cavovarus deformity in adolescent patients with Charcot-Marie-Tooth disease. Foot Ankle 1992; 13:1.
29. Wood VE, Huene D, Nguyen J: Treatment of the upper limb in Charcot-Marie-Tooth disease. J Hand Surg Br 1995; 20:511.

section
1
chapter
11

GAIT ANALYSIS IN ORTHOPAEDICS

Sylvia Õunpuu

Summary
- An understanding of biomechanical principles and typical (normal) gait is fundamental to the understanding and treatment of gait abnormalities.
- Computerized gait analysis is a powerful tool for documenting and determining the cause of gait abnormalities and thus aiding treatment decision-making.
- On completion of this chapter, the reader will have an appreciation for the following:
  - Definition and components of gait analysis.
  - Gait terminology including phases of the gait cycle.
  - Normal gait patterns.
  - Use of gait analysis in diagnosis and treatment planning.
  - Use of gait analysis in outcomes evaluation.

Gait analysis can be defined as the documentation of gait. This is a broad definition for a large assortment of techniques ranging from observational gait analysis to computer-assisted three-dimensional (3D) analysis of movement. Computerized gait analysis, consisting of 3D motion and kinetic analysis, dynamic electromyography (EMG), pedobarography, and oxygen consumption more accurately defines the state of the art in terms of the technology that is available for treatment decision-making today. By providing objective documentation, including a description of how a patient walks (joint kinematics and temporal and stride parameters) and information about the potential causes of movement abnormalities (joint kinetics and EMG data), the clinician can be better equipped to make treatment decisions intended to improve a patient's gait function. Computerized gait analysis does not replace the more traditional tools such as assessments of passive joint range of motion and muscle strength and radiography used in clinical decision-making. It should be used in conjunction with these tools to provide a more complete description of the patient, which cannot be obtained in any other way. Gait analysis, however, does not dictate a specific treatment protocol for a given disease. The ultimate treatment decision depends on the philosophies of the treating physician. Gait analysis allows for more informed treatment decisions and ultimately for more objective documentation of treatment outcomes.

CLINICAL GAIT ANALYSIS METHODS

DEFINITION AND PURPOSE

In this chapter, clinical gait analysis is defined as the systematic assessment of human locomotion through objective documentation of gait patterns. The purposes of gait analysis are to (1) document an individual's gait function, (2) aid in treatment decision-making for the correction of gait abnormalities, helping the clinician differentiate between primary and secondary gait disorders, and (3) aid in treatment evaluation. The most common use of routine clinical gait analysis is in the surgical decision-making process for ambulatory persons with neuromuscular disorders such as cerebral palsy.[1–6] The postoperative gait analysis is probably the next most common use of clinical gait analysis and contributes a significant amount to present knowledge of gait disorders. The information gained in treatment evaluation allows for "fine tuning" of treatment decisions for future patients and over the long-term modification and development in treatment protocols.[7, 8]

APPROPRIATE PATIENT REFERRAL

Computerized gait analysis may be appropriate for any adult or child who has a gait problem that requires treatment, not only for treatment decision-making but also for treatment evaluation. Gait analysis is most commonly used for surgical decision-making for patients with neuromuscular disorders (cerebral palsy, stroke, traumatic brain injury, and myelomeningocele) because of the complexity of the associated gait abnormalities, which may be at multiple joints of the lower extremities and bilaterally. This is particularly important because surgical intervention is generally irreversible. Gait analysis, however, is not limited to patients with neuromuscular disorders and can be applicable to a wide variety of gait problems. Gait analysis techniques are useful in "dissecting" the exact location of malalignment syndromes involving the lower extremities, determining the causes of and compensations for chronic knee pain, diagnosis of limping gait and in the prescription and evaluation of orthoses to name a few.

GAIT ANALYSIS METHODS

The components of a comprehensive gait analysis may include all of the following: (1) videotaping, both before the application of external measurement devices and during the data collection, (2) comprehensive clinical examination (passive joint range of motion and muscle strength), (3) estimation of bony torsions (tibial torsion and femoral anteversion), (4) temporal and stride parameters, (5) 3D joint kinematics (motion), (6) joint kinetics (joint moments and powers), (7) muscle activation patterns (EMG) during gait, (8) oxygen consumption, and (9) foot pressure. Any individual or subset of these components may be requested depending on the nature of the gait disorder. The integration of all this information will provide the most complete picture of an individual's ambulation. The following sections provide brief descriptions of these nine components.

Videotaping

Videotaping provides qualitative documentation about the way a person walks. The additional information gathered from a video record (with slow motion and pause capabilities) in comparison to observation of gait in real time alone can provide a surprising amount of information about the more subtle details of gait disorders. Simultaneous coronal and sagittal plane views with a split screen increases clinicians' appreciation of the degree of "out-of-plane" motion seen in many gait disorders. Furthermore, slow motion and stop-framing enhance video techniques and zooming capabilities, which can provide close-up views of the feet, may be the only means of evaluating the subtleties of motion and position of the hindfoot and forefoot during gait.

Clinical Examination

The clinical examination includes measurement of passive joint range of motion and muscle strength that can be correlated with joint kinematics and kinetics to help determine the potential causes of gait abnormalities. Clinical assessment may also include evaluation of the predominant type of muscle tone if applicable. The specific measures required will depend on the patient's underlying condition. Unfortunately, the clinical examination has many limitations beyond the fact that it is subjective and the variability in results among examiners can be high. In those patients with neuromuscular disorders, the correlation between many clinical examination measures and gait function is quite poor.[9, 10] The poor correlation is generally related to increased tone typically experienced during upright posture and movement as well as the fact that joint range-of-motion limitations on clinical assessment do not fall within the required range of the specific joint during gait. Also, strength measures may be somewhat limited when the specific task is associated with pain, not to mention the difficulty in obtaining reliable strength measures from children. Nevertheless, the clinical examination is an important component of any comprehensive gait analysis.

Bony Abnormalities

Assessment of bony abnormalities such as tibial torsion and femoral anteversion are important in determining the role of abnormal torsions in transverse plane gait abnormalities. Although computerized tomographic and Magilligan's radiographic methods are commonly used to measure femoral anteversion, femoral anteversion may also be estimated by a palpation method as described by Ruwe et al.[11] Estimates of tibial torsion may also be obtained by measuring the foot-thigh angle or bimalleolar axis.[12] Unfortunately, the intraobserver variability for the estimation of tibial torsion is quite high.

Temporal and Stride Variables

These parameters include measures such as velocity, cadence, stride length, step length, and percentage of stance to swing. These measures can provide an indication of the level of function compared with normal values. They can also be compared with previous values from the same patient to evaluate treatment effects. Temporal and stride variables are stature dependent, so stature changes must be taken into account when evaluating treatment over time. When comparing with "normal" temporal and stride values, the values should be matched by height, not age.[13] In persons with stature below typical for their age, an age-matched comparison may result in overestimation of the "expected" values. Conversely, in older patients these measurements decrease with increasing age.[14] Therefore, temporal and stride variables should be matched by age in elderly patients.

Temporal and stride measurements are also referred to as "outcome" measures because they cannot provide any information to support specific treatment requirements (i.e., type of muscle transfer). As a result, their utility as a stand-alone tool is limited for clinical decision-making.

Temporal and stride measurements are typically calculated using the motion measurement system data when 3D motion data are collected. Foot switches may also be used in combination with motion data collection or as a stand-alone tool to calculate temporal information. These are small devices that are applied to the base of the foot in specific locations to indicate when a specific portion of the foot is not in contact with the ground. Many simpler methods of obtaining this information have been developed for use when a motion system is not available. These range from manually measured footprints to automated instrumented walkways.

Joint Kinematics

Joint kinematics include variables used to describe the spatial and temporal movement of the body without considering the forces that cause the movement. These include linear and angular displacements, linear and angular velocities, and linear and angular accelerations in three dimensions. Angular displacements, which describe the motion of the joints (hip, knee, and ankle) and segments (trunk, pelvis, thigh, shank, and foot) in the coronal, sagittal and transverse planes during the gait cycle, are the most commonly reported. The angle definitions (specific orientation of segments for each joint angle) for these variables vary depending on the marker placement and mathematical models used to calculate joint angles. Kinematic data from each patient are compared with laboratory-specific normalized data, thus allowing an objective comparison of how motion in the specific patient deviates from age-matched persons. A kinematic analysis is the only way to provide objective information about 3D joint motion during gait. It is indispensable in understanding gait abnormalities in all planes of motion.

Reflective marker systems are currently the most successful technique for obtaining full body joint motion data. Reflective joint/segment markers are aligned with respect to specific bony landmarks on the trunk, pelvis, and both lower extremities (Fig. 1). The 3D location of each marker is determined within a calibrated space, and joint angle motion is then determined using Euler angles.[15] For more

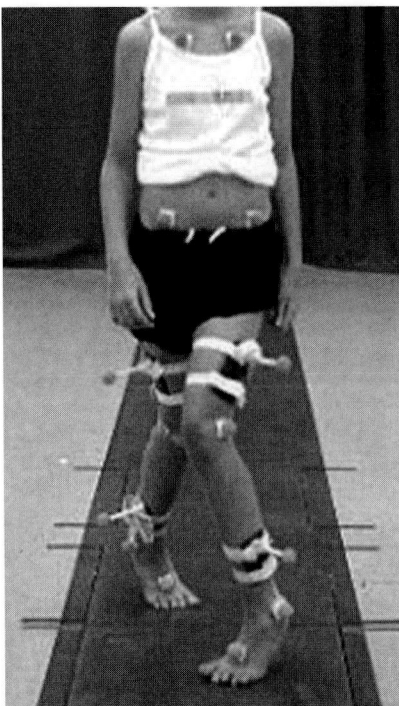

Fig. 1. Typical placement of joint and segment markers for the collection of motion data. Simultaneous force platform contact for both the right foot and left foot will enable calculation of the joint kinetics during this walk.

details on the current methods used, the reader is referred to Davis and DeLuca.[16]

Joint Kinetics

Joint kinetics provide information about the cause of motion abnormalities[5, 17] and are very useful in evaluating orthosis function.[18] Typical joint kinetic patterns are used to document and better understand specific gait abnormali-

ties such as the quadriceps avoidance gait (with no knee extensor moment in stance). Joint kinetics calculations can be made only when ground reaction force and joint kinematic information are obtained simultaneously. Ground reaction forces are measured using force plate data, which may be collected on those patients with sufficient step lengths (one foot contact with an individual force plate).

For clinical gait applications, joint kinetic data are most typically used to calculate joint moments and power. Joint moments refer to a body's response to the external loads associated with gait. The external loads include the forces resulting from the ground, the segment weight, and the segment inertia (resistance to change in motion). The joint moments are produced by any structure that constrains joint motion, such as muscle forces, other soft-tissue structures (ligamentous) and external structures (ankle-foot orthosis). The internal joint moment (represented on the plotted data) also provides an indication of which muscle group is dominant. For example, a person with excessive knee flexion in stance will have a net knee extensor moment with associated knee extensor contractions (Fig. 2). Joint powers refers to the rate at which a moment is being rotated and is the product of the joint moment and the joint angular velocity. Joint powers are related to the type of muscle contraction. A net power generation is typically associated with concentric contraction, and net power absorption is typically associated with eccentric muscle contraction. Power data can provide information about which joint energy is generated for forward progression during gait. As with kinematics, some background knowledge is necessary to interpret joint kinetic data. The reader is referred to publications by Winter[19] and Õunpuu.[5]

Muscle Activity

The muscle activity during locomotion can play an important role in the assessment of a gait disturbance. This is especially true in the cases of neuromuscular disease or suspected muscle imbalance, which can follow nerve in-

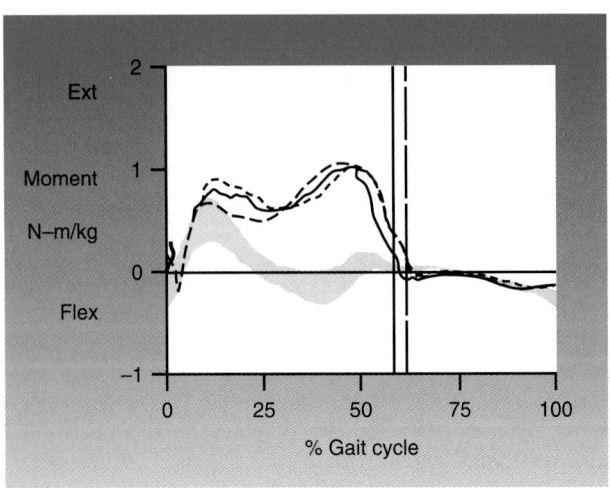

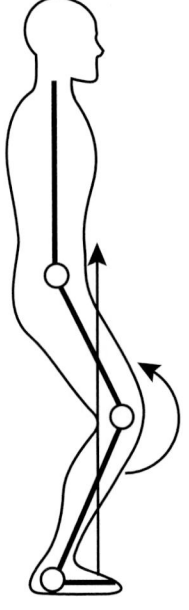

Fig. 2. A net internal knee extensor moment. When standing in knee flexion, the external loads acting on the body tend to flex the knee. The body's response to these loads is a net internal knee extensor moment provided by the quadriceps.

jury. There is no other means of determining which muscles or muscle groups are causing atypical motion. Recommendations for specific muscle transfers can be substantiated based on the knowledge of specific firing patterns of muscles versus the typically expected patterns. Such EMG studies in the patient with cerebral palsy have resulted in improved understanding of the role of the rectus femoris versus the vastus muscles in limiting swing-phase knee flexion, which contributes to clearance problems. Surface electrode studies have specified the pathologic activity of the rectus femoris and have exonerated the remainder of the vastus muscles in cerebral palsy.[20] EMG techniques have also assisted in treatment decision-making for foot and ankle deformities.[21–23]

Performing appropriate muscle transfers is complex, especially in the patient with neuromuscular problems who may not be able to change muscle activity (contractions) during gait voluntarily. In general, if a muscle is to be transferred to perform a different function, it must be active at the phase of the gait cycle when its new function is required. If the muscle is not active to perform the new function, the transfer will be unsuccessful unless the muscle activity pattern can be changed. In the patient with normal control, this may require "reeducation" of the muscle to achieve the desired function in gait. In the patient with abnormal control, reeducation is not normally possible, and the muscle must be transferred with enough tension to create a "tenodesis" effect. This may have functional implications when the joint is required to move in the opposite direction during another point in the gait cycle. Dynamic EMG data collected during gait will assist in selection of the most appropriate muscles to be transferred and ultimately improve consistency of outcome.

Muscle activity during gait and other voluntary activities may be measured using dynamic EMG techniques. Muscle activation is measured by placing electrodes on (surface) or in (fine wire) the particular muscles of interest on both lower extremities (Fig. 3). Surface electrodes are used for individual muscles or muscle groups just under the skin surface. Fine-wire electrodes are typically used for deep muscles such as the posterior tibialis and toe flexors. The advantages of each electrode type have been discussed in detail.[19, 24] Generally, fine-wire electrodes should be used only when necessary, that is, when the muscle of interest is deep (under other surface muscles) or when the surface muscle of interest is very small. Using surface electrodes on "small" muscles poses the risk of "cross-talk": when activity of an adjacent muscle is recorded along with activity from the muscle of interest. The use of fine-wire electrodes for large surface muscles provides no advantage over the surface electrode in the quality of the EMG signal.[25] Fine-wire electrodes may also cause cramping and increase the level of spasticity in patients with tone abnormalities. This may ultimately modify a patient's "typical" walking pattern.

The EMG techniques used in clinical gait analysis provide the clinician with on-off information based on the raw signal. The EMG signal amplitude information is limited if normalization techniques are not used. For quality control, the raw (or original) EMG signal must be examined initially for potential artifacts. Then different techniques such as full-wave rectification, linear enveloping, and

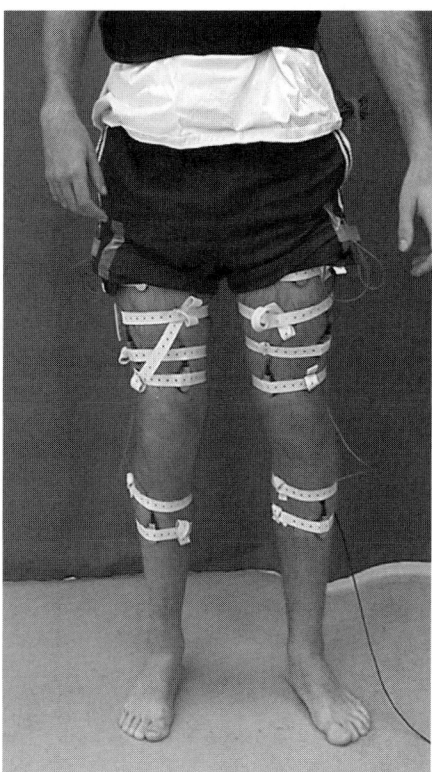

Fig. 3. Set-up for dynamic electromyography data collection. Surface electrodes are placed on both lower extremities.

integration can be used to process the raw EMG signal.[19] Each technique has advantages depending on the application of the EMG data. Some type of processing is necessary if EMG data are to be averaged across strides or patients.

Oxygen Consumption

Many orthopaedic conditions disturb walking to the extent that there is increased consumption of energy.[26] Oxygen consumption (oxygen consumed over period of time, measured in milliliters per kilogram per minute) and cost (oxygen consumed over a specific distance, measured in milliliters per kilogram per meter) are measures of the efficiency of gait. These parameters can be measured using a variety of methods, all of which measure the content and volume of expired air. The patient initially sits quietly to determine resting values and then walks until steady state is reached (Fig. 4). Oxygen consumption and cost values for patients can be compared with normal values as well as between conditions (barefoot vs. brace) in individual patients. The effects of orthopaedic treatment on energy consumption may also be evaluated. Like temporal and stride parameters, however, energy measures have little influence on the specifics of surgical intervention, so as a stand-alone tool their contribution is limited.

Plantar Pressures

The measurement of the foot pressures and center of the pressure path during the stance phase of gait can be made using a variety of techniques that use pressure-sensitive

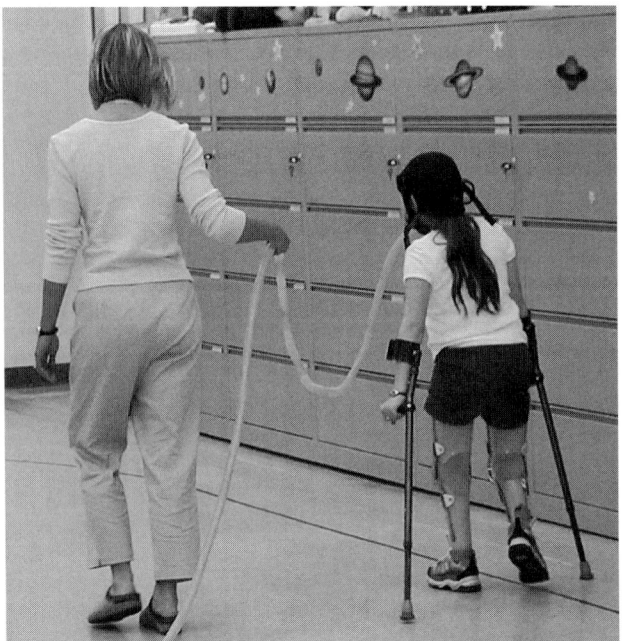

Fig. 4. Collection of oxygen consumption and cost measures during gait. The patient ambulates while breath-by-breath method is used to measure gait efficiency.

cells. Foot pressure measurements can be obtained during barefoot walking on a pressure-sensitive mat or when shod with or without orthoses using a pressure-sensitive insert (Fig. 5). Such data can be useful in clinical situations in which abnormal pressures are specifically problematic such as the insensate foot of the patient with diabetes or other neurologic disturbances. Areas of high pressure can be noted and may influence details in surgical intervention to the foot-ankle and assist in evaluating the effects of bony surgery to the foot. As with all types of gait data, comparison to normal pressure distribution patterns provides a basis for treatment decision-making.

Test Protocol

A gait analysis test may consist of all or a combination of the individual components listed previously. Therefore, the actual time required for a gait analysis assessment (1 to about 4 hours) varies depending on the number of tests performed as well as the level of cooperation of the patient and specific testing conditions (barefoot and brace or walking and running). Gait analysis can be completed with walking aids such as walkers or crutches if these aids do not interfere with the markers or consistently block their view from the cameras.

COMPONENTS OF THE GAIT CYCLE

Important to the description and discussion of pathologic gait among clinicians is a consistent terminology that facilitates communication. The following is a list of the basic terms needed to describe gait and definitions of the phases of the gait cycle.

PLANES OF MOTION

In 3D gait analyses, the planes of motion refer to body-embedded planes (planes defined by the anatomy) and not the observer's perspective from the "front" or "side" of the patient. When out-of-plane motion occurs (e.g., excessive internal hip rotation), the "side" view of the patient will result in an underestimation of the knee flexion-extension angle. Three-dimensional gait analysis will provide the knee flexion-extension angle based on the knee angle definition (long axis of the thigh in relation to the long axis of the shank as viewed along a line connecting the medial and lateral femoral condyles) irrespective of the rotational orientation of the lower extremity. Two-dimensional (2D) gait analyses provide only a "side" view and thus result in errors when out-of-plane motion occurs. Davis et al[27] compared the error associated by applying 2D techniques to 3D motion and found errors in ankle plantar flexion-dorsiflexion of up to 30 degrees.

The planes of motion used in 3D gait analysis are defined as follows:

Coronal plane: the vertical plane that divides the body into anterior and posterior parts.
Sagittal plane: the vertical plane that divides the body into the right and left parts.
Transverse plane: the horizontal plane that divides the body at right angles to the coronal and sagittal planes.
Line of progression: A line that is parallel to the walkway along which the patient proceeds during the data collection.

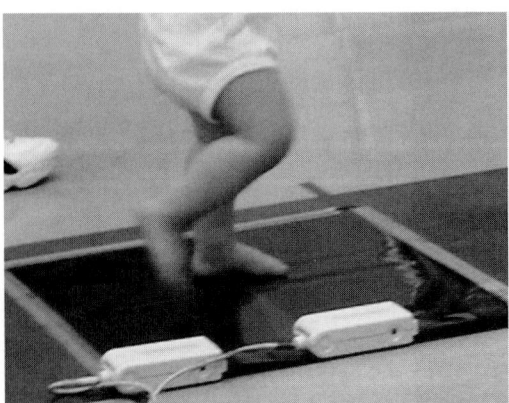
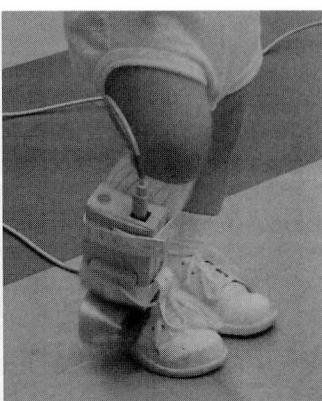

Fig. 5. Foot pressure measurement system. Foot pressure distributions are collected during barefoot walking using a pressure-sensitive mat and while shod using pressure-sensitive inserts.

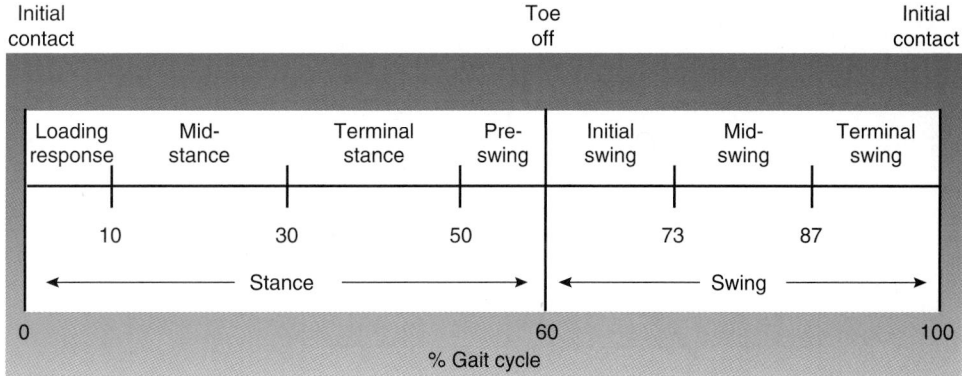

Fig. 6. Phases of the gait cycle.

When describing gait, the gait cycle is used as the primary reference for all measures and allows comparison between measures and data collected from multiple persons. The relevant definitions of the gait cycle are listed next.

Gait cycle: The period of time from one event (usually initial contact) of one foot to the following occurrence of the same event with the same foot.

Normalization of the gait cycle: Initial contact of one foot to the following initial contact of the same foot is unitized and represented as 100% of the gait cycle. This allows averaging of data across patients who may not have similar gait cycle time.

Stance phase (ST): The period of time when the foot is in contact with the ground. In normal gait this represents about 60% of the gait cycle.

Swing phase (SW): The period of time when the foot is not in contact with the ground. In normal gait this represents about 40% of the gait cycle. In those cases in which the foot never leaves the ground (foot drag), it can be defined as the phase when all portions of the lower extremity are in forward motion.

Double support (DS): The period of time when both feet are in contact with the ground. This occurs twice in the gait cycle: at the beginning and end of the stance phase. In normal gait, this represents about 10% of the gait cycle at the beginning and another 10% at the end of the stance phase.

Single support (SS): The period in time when only one foot is in contact with the ground. In walking, this is exactly equal to the swing period of the other limb.

Phases of the gait cycle: The stance and swing phases may be further divided into subphases as described by Perry.[28] This terminology is very useful for referring to specific portions of the gait cycle (Fig. 6).
- Loading response, 0% to 10%/double support.
- Midstance, 10% to 30%.
- Terminal stance, 30% to 50%.
- Preswing, 50% to 60%/double support.
- Initial swing, 60% to 73%.
- Midswing, 73% to 87%.
- Terminal swing, 87% to 100%.

Initial contact: The point in the gait cycle when the foot initially makes contact with the ground; this marks the beginning of the stance phase.

Toe-off: The point in the gait cycle when contact with the ground is terminated; this marks the beginning of swing phase. It typically occurs at 60% of the gait cycle in normal gait. For those cases in which the foot never leaves the ground (foot drag), it is often assumed to be the point when all portions of the lower extremity have achieved forward motion.

Step length: The distance from one event of one foot to the following occurrence of the same event with the other foot. The right step length is the distance from the left heel to the right heel when both feet are in contact with the ground.

Stride length: The distance from initial contact of one foot to the following initial contact of the same foot, sometimes referred to as cycle length.

Velocity: The average horizontal speed along the direction of progression measured over one or more strides (typically reported in centimeters per second).

Cadence: The number of steps per unit time (typically reported in steps per minute).

TYPICAL GAIT

Typical (normal) gait patterns for kinematic, kinetic, and EMG data are used as the reference from which to base treatment decisions and treatment evaluation. It is important to have an understanding of the typical patterns to appreciate what is pathologic. In this section, the 3D kinematics of the trunk, pelvis, and lower extremities are described along with the sagittal plane joint kinematic, moment, and power.

JOINT KINEMATICS
Like most gait variables, joint kinematics are best communicated through the use of plots. Plots are the most efficient way to communicate "time series" data. The timing is as critical as the range of motion when describing pathologic gait and is not easy to appreciate from visual observation alone. All kinematic plots follow the same plotting convention (Fig. 7). The horizontal axis indicates the time line and is represented as percentage of gait cycle, and the vertical axis indicates the degree of joint or segment motion. The stance phase begins at initial contact or 0% of the gait cycle. The vertical line at approximately 60% of

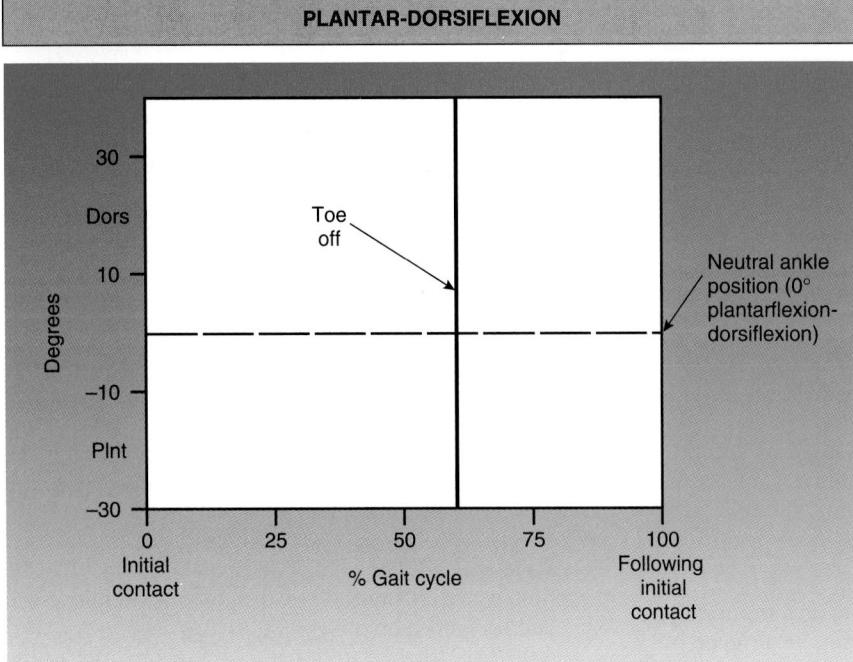

PLANTAR-DORSIFLEXION

Fig. 7. Standard plotting format. All kinematic and kinetic data follow a similar plotting format. The horizontal axis represents 0% to 100% of the gait cycle with the vertical line at about 60% representing toe-off. The horizontal axis represents the joint angle in degrees for the kinematic plot. Computerized gait analysis calculates the joint angle 60 times per second and plots those angles on a graph.

the gait cycle indicates toe-off, which marks the beginning of the swing phase or the last 40% of the gait cycle. The specific angle definitions for each of the kinematic plots have been previously published.[13] In brief, the exact angle is determined by the joint and segment marker locations, which should ultimately relate in some logical way to the anatomy. Unfortunately, joint marker positions vary from laboratory to laboratory because of different alignment protocols. Joint angles (i.e., hip, knee, and ankle) are relative angles and define the motion of the distal segment in relation to the proximal segment. As such, observers should be oriented so that they view the motion of the second segment from the appropriate position on the first segment. The only exception to this is the pelvis and foot progression. Pelvic motion is the motion of the pelvis in relation to the laboratory coordinate system, and foot progression is the orientation of the foot to the line of progression. Unfortunately, differences in marker set placement and thus joint angle definitions limit the ability of data to be compared directly from laboratory to laboratory.

Because of the complexity of hip motion and difficulty of observational interpretation of this joint, the angle definitions for hip motion will be described (Fig. 8). In the coronal plane, the hip joint is defined as the relative angle between a line perpendicular to the pelvic transverse plane and the long axis of the thigh after both lines are projected onto the pelvic coronal plane. In the sagittal plane, the hip joint is defined as the relative angle between a line perpendicular to the pelvic transverse plane and the long axis of the thigh after both lines are projected onto the pelvic sagittal plane. In the transverse plane, the hip joint is defined as the relative angle between a line joining the anterosuperior iliac spine (ASIS) and a line connecting the medial and lateral epicondyles after the latter has been projected onto the pelvic transverse plane. As a result,

absolute position of the thigh (i.e., whether the thigh reaches a vertical position) is not given in any of these definitions. In observational gait analysis, hip angle is typically assumed based on thigh position and not the hip angle, which requires an appreciation for pelvic position as well as thigh position.

During normal gait, the majority of motion occurs in the sagittal plane. Mature gait typically begins at about age 5, after which gait patterns are similar to adults except for temporal and stride parameters.[29] Gait kinematics and kinetics show consistent changes in older adults in comparison to younger adults.[14] These include reductions in range of motion and changes in temporal and stride parameters, which are not consistent in relation to stature as found in younger adults. The following is a description of the typical segment and joint motion (Table 1) by plane seen in young adults.

CORONAL PLANE
Upper Body
There is negligible motion of the upper body with an overall range of motion of 1 degree.

Pelvis
The pelvis rises from midswing and loading response and drops from midstance to initial swing. The overall range of motion of the pelvis is about 8 degrees with the neutral position (pelvis parallel to the floor) occurring in midstance and midswing.

Hip
Hip motion in the coronal plane mimics the motion of the pelvis in the coronal plane. The hip generally reaches peak adduction during loading response and progressively ab-

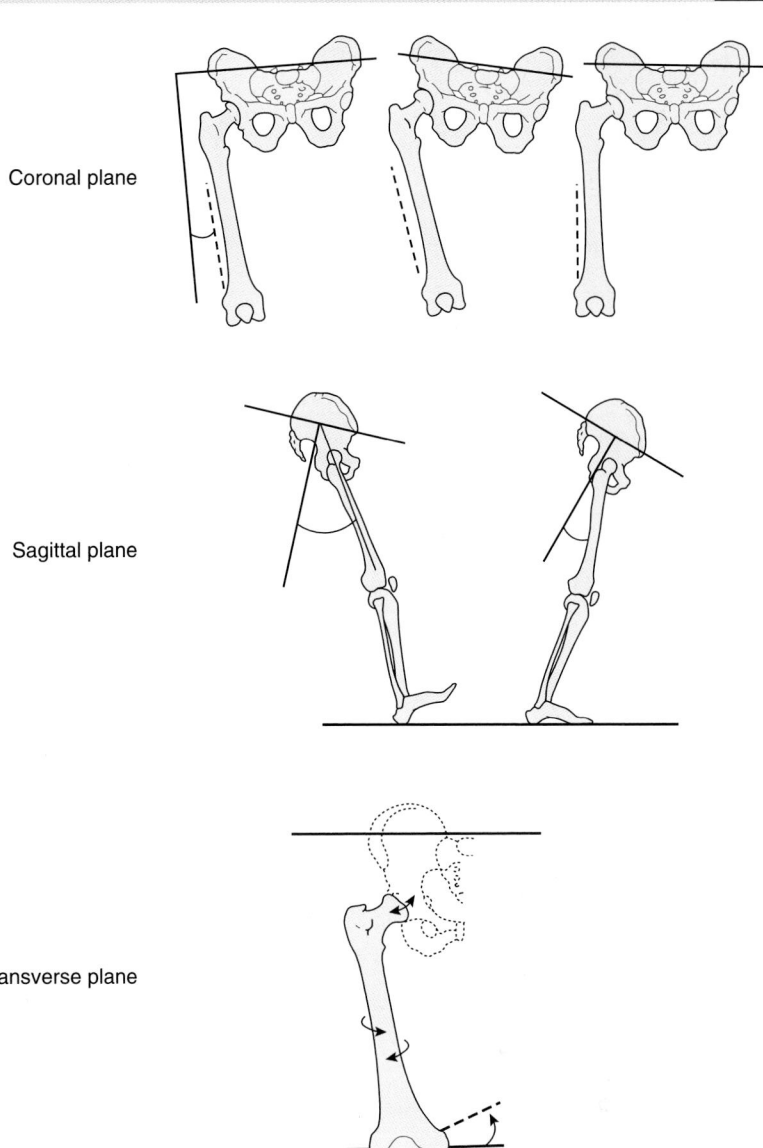

Coronal plane

Sagittal plane

Fig. 8. Joint angle definitions for the hip. The joint angle definitions for the hip represent the relative angle between the pelvis and the femur segment. The arc in each figure indicates the angle of interest for each plane of motion.

Transverse plane

ducts throughout the remainder of stance, reaching peak abduction in initial swing. The overall range of motion for the hip is 13 degrees (see Fig. 8).

Knee
Knee motion in the coronal plane is negligible with the mean position of approximately 1 degree varus.

SAGITTAL PLANE
Upper Body
There is minimal motion of the upper body with a range of approximately 3 degrees in an oscillating pattern similar to the pelvis.

Pelvis
The typical pelvis is usually tilted anteriorly between 4 and 10 degrees. A mild oscillating pattern shows an increasing anterior tilt during midstance and initial swing; the overall range of motion is about 4 degrees. If the line joining the

ASIS to the posterosuperior iliac spine (PSIS) were parallel to the floor, there would be zero tilt (as indicated by the horizontal axis of the plot).

Hip
The hip extends throughout stance phase from maximum flexion (37 degrees), which is attained in terminal swing, to maximum extension in terminal stance (6 degrees); flexion begins in preswing and continues throughout the swing phase. In normal gait, the overall range of motion is about 43 degrees.

Knee
The knee flexes in loading response (20 degrees) and then extends. It begins flexing again in terminal stance, reaching about 45 degrees of flexion at toe-off. The second peak knee flexion (64 degrees) occurs at approximately 33% of the swing phase. This is critical for foot clearance of the swing limb, which is in the range of a few millimeters in

TABLE 1. TYPICAL ACTIVITY PATTERNS FOR THE LOWER EXTREMITY MUSCLES

Hip abductors
- Active during stance for pelvic stability.
- During loading response.
    Controls pelvic drop on swing side by limiting stance side hip adduction.
    Eccentric contraction.
- During midstance.
    Produces pelvis rise on swing side by producing stance side hip abduction.
    Concentric contraction.

Hip adductors
- Individual variation is high.
- Active during toe-off and initial swing.
    Aid in hip flexion.
    Concentric contraction.
- Active during terminal swing.
    Internally rotate femur.

Gluteus maximus
- Active terminal swing and loading response.
    Produces hip extension.
    Concentric contraction.
- Muscle elongated before contraction during hip flexion in swing.

Hip flexors
- Active in terminal preswing and initial swing.
    Initiates hip flexion.
    Concentric contraction.
- Elongation before contraction during hip extension in first half of stance.

Vastus muscles
- Active terminal swing.
    Preparation for initial contact and associated force requirement.
- Active at initial contact and during loading response.
    Initially restricts/controls knee flexion.
    Eccentric contraction.
    Secondarily active knee extension.
    Concentric contraction.

Rectus femoris
- Activity varies with walking velocity.

- Active terminal swing.
    Preparation for initial contact and associated force requirement.
- Active during initial contact and loading response.
    Initially restricts/controls knee flexion.
    Eccentric contraction.
    Secondarily active knee extension.
    Concentric contraction.
- At higher velocities activity is seen at toe-off.
    Slow knee flexion.
    Eccentric contraction.

Hamstrings
- Active during terminal swing.
    Decelerate swinging leg
    Eccentric contraction.
- Active during loading response.
    Hip extension.
    Concentric contraction.
- Elongation before shortening during hip flexion in swing.

Triceps surae
- Active during midstance and beginning of terminal stance (second rocker).
- Controls forward progression of the tibia during ankle dorsiflexion.
    Eccentric contraction.
- Active during terminal stance.
- Ankle plantar flexion.
    Concentric contraction.
- Peroneal muscle action is similar.

Tibialis anterior and toe extensors
- Active during loading response.
    Control lowering of the forefoot to the floor.
    Eccentric contraction.
- Active at toe-off and in-swing.
    Dorsiflexion of the ankle for clearance.
    Concentric contraction.

The typical activity patterns for the major muscles or muscle groups in the lower extremities are described with respect to the phases of the gait cycle. The type of muscle contraction is also indicated. The muscle activity patterns reflect the joint kinetics.

normal gait. The knee normally does not extend fully at initial contact or in terminal stance. Normal range of knee motion is about 60 degrees.

Ankle
The overall range of motion is about 30 degrees with two waves of plantar flexion followed by dorsiflexion. Peak dorsiflexion (12 degrees) is reached in terminal stance followed by peak plantar flexion (18 degrees) in initial swing.

TRANSVERSE PLANE
Upper Body
Motion of the upper body is opposite to the pelvis with internal rotation in stance and external rotation in swing with an overall range of 5 degrees.

Pelvis
The overall range of motion of the pelvis is about 8 degrees consisting of a few degrees of internal rotation at initial contact, external rotation during stance, slight external rotation at toe-off, and internal rotation in swing.

Hip
The thigh in relation to the pelvis is slightly internally rotated throughout the majority of the stance phase and externally rotates in initial swing with an overall range of motion of about 8 degrees.

Knee
The knee shows progressive internal rotation in stance and external rotation in swing. The typical range of motion is 11 degrees.

Foot Progression
The foot progression angle is the angle between the long axis of the foot (as represented by the second metatarsal projected onto the floor) and the line of progression. In normal gait, the foot is rotated slightly external to the direction of progression; however, there is large intrasubject variability. The foot externally rotates in initial swing with an overall range of motion of approximately 6 degrees.

The data on the plots represent the mean (one standard deviation) of normal children ranging in age from 5 to 14 years.

MUSCLE ACTIVITY

Normal muscle activity has been documented by many groups.[19, 24, 28, 30] The work of Sutherland et al[31] on the development of gait includes the changes in muscle activation patterns that occur up until 7 years of age when they approximate normal adult patterns. Most muscles are active at the beginning and end of the swing and the stance phases with minimal muscle activity in midstance and midswing. Generally, during gait, elongation of the muscle occurs through passive stretch or eccentric contraction before shortening contractions occur. The typical activity of the major muscle groups during gait is listed in Table 1.

JOINT KINETICS

Once mature gait patterns have been developed, the joint kinetics assume very specific patterns. These patterns generally remain similar across people, with changes noted only in the peak amplitudes, primarily as a result of changing velocities[19] and body mass. The peak joint moments and powers increase as walking velocity increases. The normal sagittal plane joint kinematics and kinetics for the hip, knee, and ankle are plotted in Figure 10 and were calculated as described by Davis and DeLuca[16] and Kadaba et al.[32] This format was selected so that the motion followed by the moment and then the power could be examined sequentially for a specific phase in the gait cycle. This helps in the interpretation of the gait analysis data. For example, during midstance, the motion of the ankle can be determined on the motion plot (i.e., ankle dorsiflexion). Looking at the moment plot over the same portion of the gait cycle, there is a net ankle plantar flexor moment, which indicates the ankle plantar flexors are active. Finally, looking again at the same portion of the gait cycle in the power plot, there is a net power absorption, which is associated with an eccentric muscular contraction. This is what would be expected as the ankle is dorsiflexing under the control of the ankle plantar flexors; thus, the muscle is lengthening under tension. This step-by-step process can be used to evaluate all the joints at each phase in the gait cycle. A detailed description of the joint kinetics with respect to the phases of the gait cycle is given in the next section. An understanding of typical kinetics is possible only through knowledge of the typical muscle activity patterns (see Table 1), which produce the joint moments.

As with the joint kinematic data, joint moments and powers are best presented in a plot format. Both the joint moments and joint powers are normalized with respect to the body weight (measured in kilograms) to reduce the variability that is related to an individual's body mass. The net muscle moment is generally referred to as extensor (negative) or flexor (positive). The joint powers are labeled as generation (positive) and absorption (negative).

A description of the motion, moment, and power for the hip, knee, and ankle are given next. Specifics are described related to specific phases of the gait cycle as described previously.

Sagittal Plane (Fig. 10)
Hip
1. Loading response/midstance. Hip extension with significant net extensor moment produced by the concentric contraction hip extensors.
   - Pull the body forward (and upward).
   - Counter a ground reaction force that passes well in front of the hip.
   - Posterior tilt of upper body and pelvis reduces magnitude of moment.
2. Terminal stance. Hip continues to extend, but the hip extensors fall silent.
   - Momentum (aided by gravity) carries the body forward.
   - Power "absorption" associated with passive tissue stretch.
   - Increasing anterior tilt of upper body and pelvis reduces magnitude of moment and advances center of gravity.
3. Preswing/initial swing. Hip flexion with net flexor moment produced by concentric contraction of the iliopsoas (and sometimes the rectus femoris).
   - Important net power generation.
   - Thigh (and knee) accelerated forward, producing hip flexion and aiding in knee flexion.
4. Terminal swing. Minimal hip extension with hip extensor moment produced by concentric contraction of the hip extensors.
   - Aids in decelerating the thigh, thereby extending the knee.
   - Knee extension also facilitated by posterior pelvic tilt.

Knee
1. Loading response. Knee flexion with net knee extensor moment produced by eccentric contraction of the knee extensors.
   - Shock absorption during loading response.
2. Midstance/terminal stance. Relatively small moments across the knee during most of stance.
   - Knee stability provided by "plantar flexion–knee extension couple" (i.e., increasing plantar flexor moment during second rocker).
   - Knee flexor moment associated with gastrocnemius activity.
3. Terminal swing. Knee extension with net knee flexor moment produced by eccentric contraction of the knee flexors (hamstrings).
   - To decelerate the extending knee.
   Two-joint muscles (hamstrings) produce:
   - Hip extensor moment to decelerate the thigh (extends the knee).
   - Knee flexor moment to control rate of knee extension.

Ankle
1. Loading response (first rocker). Minimal plantar flexion with small dorsiflexor moment produced by eccentric contraction of the ankle dorsiflexors.
   - Prevent foot slap.
2. Midstance/terminal stance (second rocker). Dorsiflexion with gradually increasing plantar flexor moment as body center of mass moves forward and center of pressure of the ground reaction force moves distally.

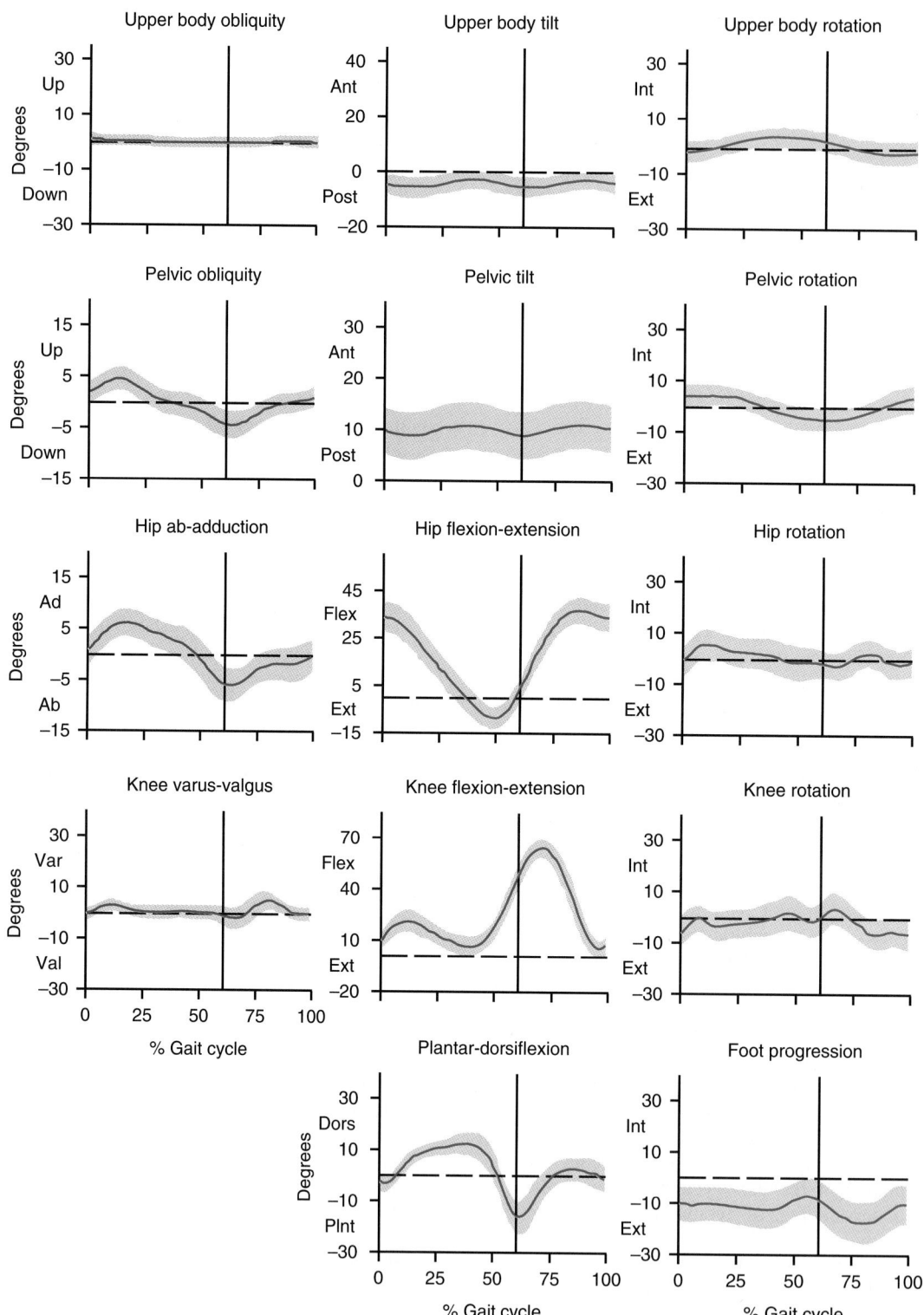

Fig. 9. Normal gait kinematics. The mean (± standard deviation) joint kinematics in the coronal (first column), sagittal (second column), and transverse (third column) planes for the upper body, pelvis, hip, knee, and ankle are plotted. This is a mature gait pattern.

- Controls forward progression of tibia over plantigrade foot.
- Produced by eccentric contraction of the plantar flexors.
- Ankle grows more "rigid."

3. Terminal stance/preswing (third rocker). Ankle begins to plantar flex with increasing plantar flexor moment.
   - Concentric contraction of the ankle plantar flexors.
   - Ankle moment reaches peak value near end of single support.

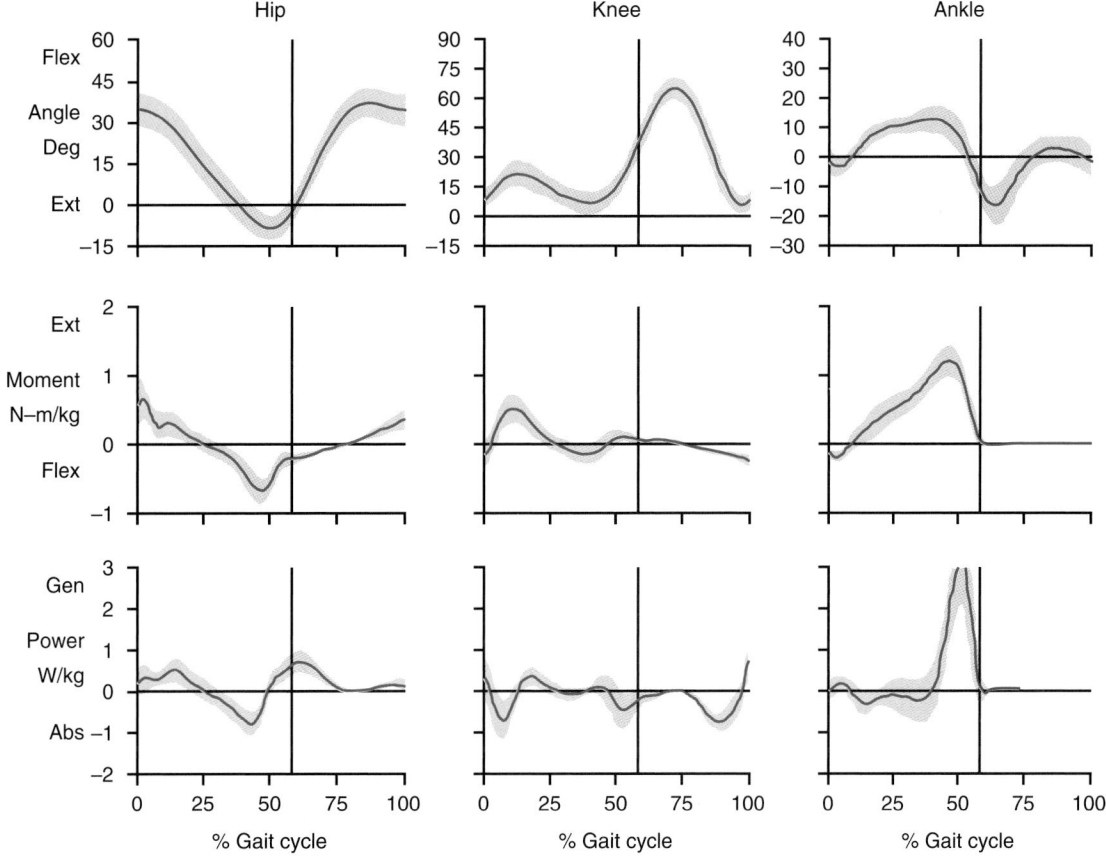

Fig. 10. Sagittal plane joint kinetics. The mean (± standard deviation) joint kinematic (first row), joint moment (second row), and joint power (third row) for the hip, knee, and ankle are plotted. The plotting format in this manner allows interpretation of the joint kinematics and kinetics at a specific phase in the gait cycle.

- Ankle power generation significant during this interval.
- Acceleration of the ankle upward and forward serves to accelerate the knee, aiding in producing knee flexion.

Coronal Plane

Although the majority of motion typically occurs in the sagittal plane, the coronal plane (Fig. 11) is important in typical gait and is often implicated in pathologic gait. In typical gait, the motion, moments, and powers are seen primarily at the hip joint with minimal motion, moments, and powers at the knee and ankle joints.

Hip

1. Loading response.
   - Hip adduction.
   - Net abductor moment.
   - Contralateral pelvic drop must be controlled.
   - Eccentric contraction of abductors.
   - Net power absorption.
2. Midstance/terminal stance and preswing.
   - Hip abduction.
   - Net abductor moment.
   - Contralateral pelvic rise is produced.
   - Concentric contraction of abductors.
   - Net power generation.

PATHOLOGIC GAIT: APPLICATIONS OF CLINICAL GAIT ANALYSIS

Pathologic gait can range from temporary gait deviations in one plane of motion to complex chronic deviations in all planes of motion. In many cases, the clinician may not appreciate how the observation of gait abnormalities alone limits awareness of gait deformity and in some cases may be misleading until interpretation of gait analysis data. The primary reason for misinterpretation of gait disorder on observational assessment alone is that in many cases motion is "out of plane." Pathologic gait is typically characterized by reduced motion in the sagittal plane and increased motion in the coronal and transverse planes. Motion in the coronal and transverse planes may be a compensation or coping response for limited or abnormal motion in the sagittal plane. Abnormal transverse plane motion may also be secondary to torsional body deformity.

In the following section, applications of gait analysis to a variety of pathologies are reviewed.

CEREBRAL PALSY

Of all the neuromuscular disorders, cerebral palsy involves one of the most variable interactions between central motor control and dynamic muscle imbalance, which combines to create complex gait abnormalities. Abnormal motion with

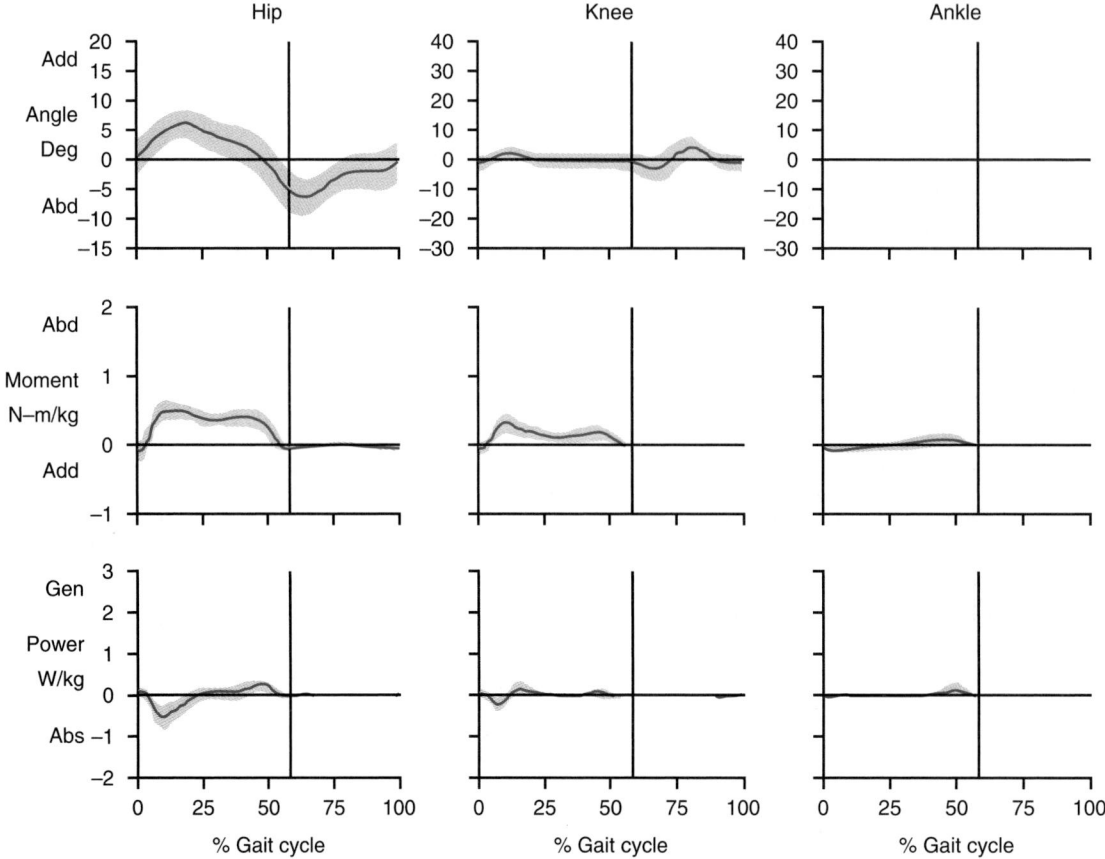

Fig. 11. Coronal plane joint kinetics. The mean (± standard deviation) joint kinematic (first row), joint moment (second row), and joint power (third row) for the hip, knee, and ankle are plotted. Plotting in this manner allows interpretation of the joint kinematics and kinetics at a specific phase in the gait cycle.

respect to timing and degree may occur bilaterally (and asymmetrically) at all levels (trunk, pelvis, hip, knee, and foot/ankle). Gait analysis is a critical component in understanding the primary deviations versus the compensatory mechanisms prior to treatment decision-making. Gait analysis has been shown to impact the clinician's decision-making process by providing data to support, add, or delete surgical procedures recommended using visual and clinical examination information alone.[9] The use of gait analysis has allowed for the development of the single-stage multi-level surgery with simultaneous corrections of joint contractures and skeletal abnormalities. As well, the use of gait analysis has allowed for critical evaluation of these complex surgeries. The following case, involving a patient's rotational profile, is an example of how transverse plane kinematics may be used to provide more accurate information than obtainable through visual observation.

Case 1

A 5-year-old girl with spastic diplegia presented for surgical decision-making. Visual observation suggested a symmetric gait pattern with bilateral internal hip rotation (internally pointing knees) and associated bilateral internal foot progression (Fig. 12). However, transverse plane kinematic data (Fig. 13) revealed significant asymmetries at all levels, which were not appreciated on visual observation alone.

The pelvis showed a fixed symmetric position with the left side externally rotated (retracted) and the right side internally rotated (protracted) throughout the gait cycle. The left hip showed significant internal rotation in relation to the pelvis, and the right hip showed normal rotation with respect to the pelvis. Therefore, the resulting in-pointing knee on the right was a result of the right internally rotated pelvis, not hip. Internal foot progression on the left was a secondary effect of the internal hip rotation, and internal foot progression on the right was a result of excessive internal pelvic rotation on the right. Therefore, gait analysis data would support a decision for femoral derotation osteotomy on the left side only. Visual observation alone would have suggested the need for bilateral procedures.

FOOT AND ANKLE ABNORMALITIES

Equinovarus and supination deformities are common problems in the adult and child with neuromuscular disorders. Effective treatment of the gait disorders must differentiate the role of many muscles that can possibly contribute to these problems. The use of surface and intramuscular electromyography, motion data, close-up, and slow motion video along with specific clinical examination measures can provide a more complete understanding of the cause of abnormal motion and positioning of the foot and ankle during gait. A repeat of these measures after surgery will

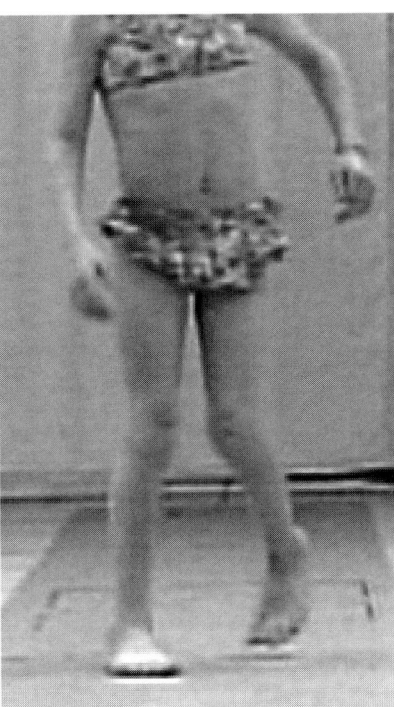

Fig. 12. Frontal view of a child with cerebral palsy (case 1). The frontal view of this child shows in-pointing knees and bilateral internal foot progression. The usual interpretation of this presentation is bilateral internal hip rotation with associated internal foot progression.

also allow critical evaluation of outcomes. Because of limitations in foot modeling, motion analysis data for the foot are usually limited to ankle plantar flexion/dorsiflexion and foot rotation and progression. Therefore, high-quality close-up videotaping of the motion can provide excellent additional information about forefoot and hindfoot positioning during gait, which is difficult to appreciate in "real time" when watching a patient ambulate. Appreciating the presence of a dynamic forefoot adductus versus forefoot supination will indicate the need for different procedures for correction of different problems.

Case 2

A 7-year-old girl with left spastic hemiplegia presented for surgery to correct an equinovarus foot-ankle deformity. Evaluation of the close-up video records of the foot during gait showed a hindfoot varus throughout the gait cycle that was not fixed (correction on Coleman Block test) and a forefoot adductus and supination in terminal swing (Fig. 14). EMG data showed inappropriate activity of the posterior tibialis during swing phase (Fig. 15) and during rapid passive forefoot eversion stretch implicating the posterior tibialis muscle as a possible cause of the hindfoot varus. Based on the supination position of the foot in terminal swing, a split anterior tibial tendon transfer was performed. On the basis of the hindfoot varus position and inappropriate activity of the posterior tibialis during gait and passive stretch, a lengthening of the posterior tibialis was performed. The heel cord contracture was treated with a gastrocnemius lengthening. Postoperative video records

(Fig. 16) and motion data confirmed the positive results reported by the patient.

Case 3

A patient presented with severe pes planus noted bilaterally. This patient had difficulty tolerating braces, and surgery was being considered for correction of the foot deformity. The pedobarograph was used to document the

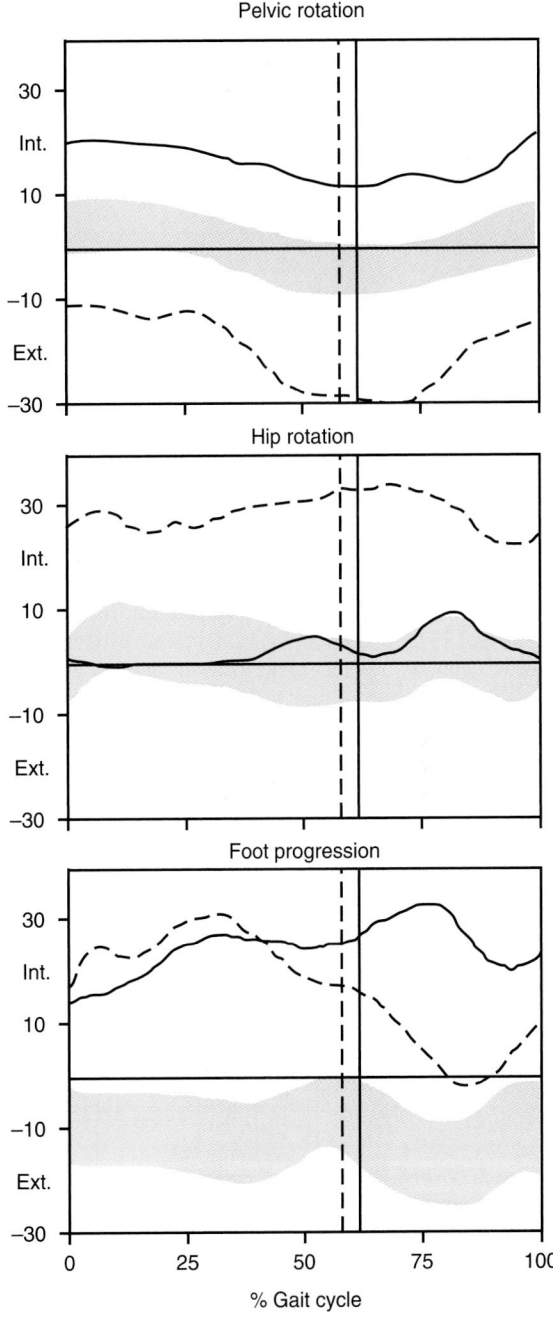

Fig. 13. Transverse plane kinematics for a child with cerebral palsy (case 1). The right (solid line) versus left (dashed line) kinematics for the pelvis, hip, and foot progression for a 7-year-old child with cerebral palsy. There is a consistent asymmetry of the pelvis with internal rotation of the right hemipelvis and associated external rotation of the left hemipelvis. Internal rotation is noted on the left hip with normal rotation on the right. There is bilateral internal foot progression.

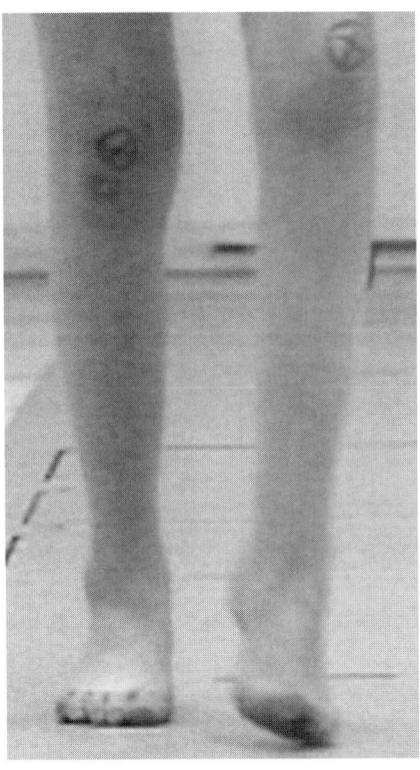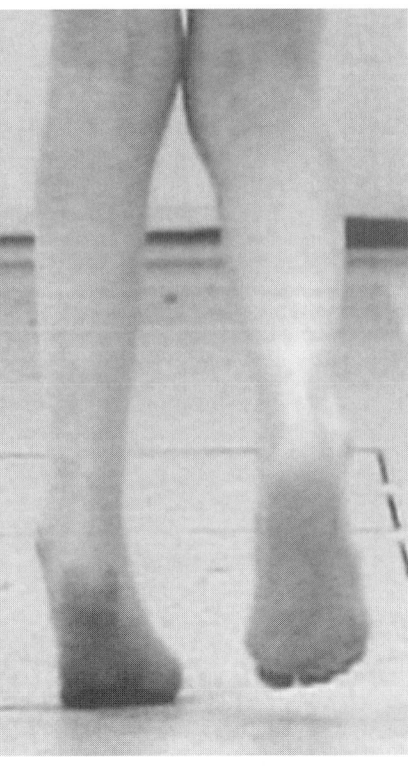

Fig. 14. Close-up view of the foot and ankle before surgery (case 2). These frames are taken from a close-up video record used to document foot position during gait. A close-up position of the forefoot shows excessive supination positioning in terminal swing with associated inappropriate position of the forefoot for initial contact on the lateral border. A close-up view of the hindfoot shows varus and excessive ankle equinus positioning in stance.

pressure distribution under the feet both before and after surgery. Pedobarograph data showed high-pressure areas under first metatarsal head and medial midfoot preoperatively (Fig. 17). The patient underwent bilateral Evans anterior calcaneal advancement osteotomies. Visually this patient appeared to continue to have pes planus postoperatively; however, there was a significant change in her weight distribution postoperatively (see Fig. 17). Weight was more evenly distributed throughout the foot, and there was a significant reduction of weightbearing medially. The pedobarograph was a very valuable instrument in determining the changes in weightbearing pre- versus postoperatively.

POSTPOLIO AND PARALYTIC DISORDERS
Both kinematic and kinetic data can provide insight into the mechanics of walking and ultimately treatment decision-making in patients with paralysis and severe muscle weakness. In the case of muscle weakness or absence, joint kinematics and moments will provide insight into the mechanisms the patient uses to compensate.

Case 4
A patient with postpolio who has 0/5 quadriceps strength reported reduced stability with her solid ankle-foot orthosis (AFO), which was recommended to reduce knee hyperextension. When ambulating barefoot, the patient was able to

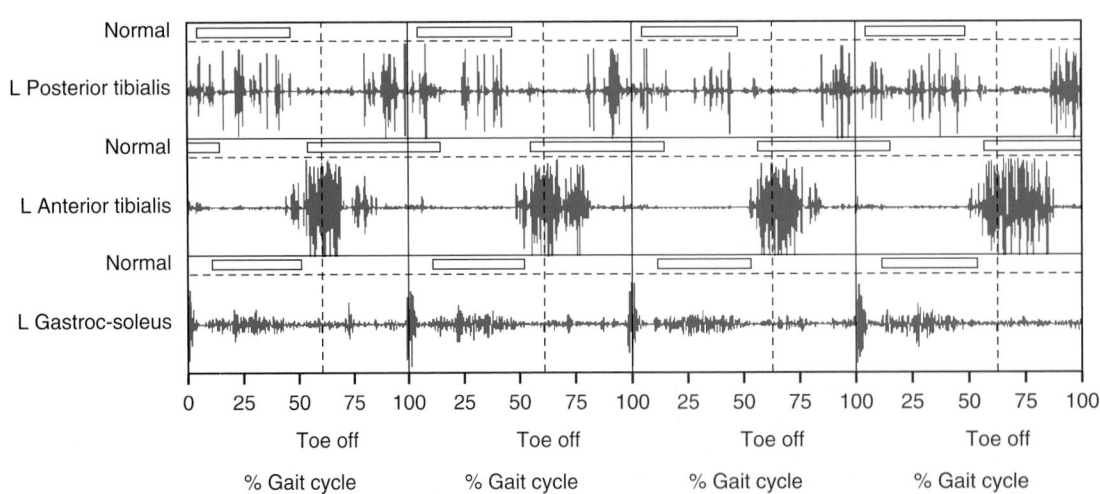

Fig. 15. Dynamic electromyographic data before surgery (case 2). Muscle function for the posterior and anterior tibialis and gastrocnemius are plotted for four gait cycles; the bar above indicates typical function for these muscles. Muscle function of the posterior tibialis (first row) shows inappropriate activity in swing in all four gait cycles.

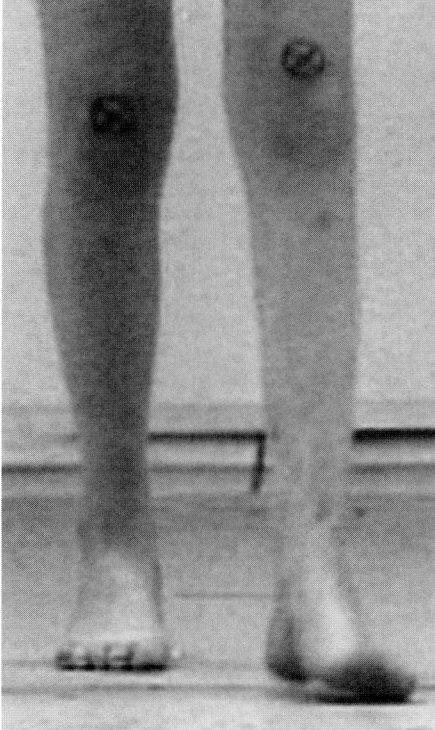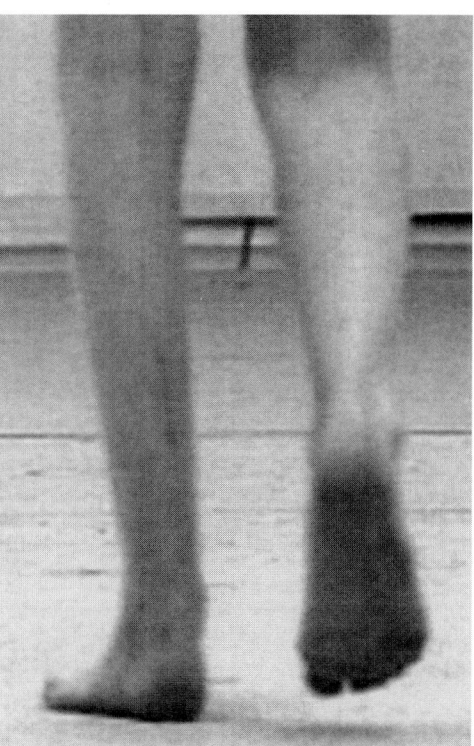

Fig. 16. Close-up view of the foot and ankle after surgery (case 2). Postoperative position of the foot/ankle during gait can be compared with the preoperative position shown in Figure 14. On the left, the forefoot shows typical supination positioning in terminal swing with associated appropriate position of the forefoot for initial contact. On the right, the hindfoot shows normal positioning in stance and a plantigrade foot.

Preoperative foot pressures (right side two gait cycles)

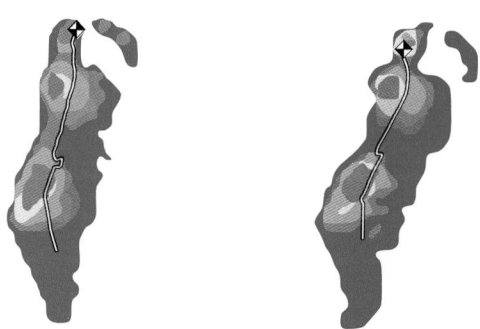

Postoperative foot pressures (right side two gait cycles)

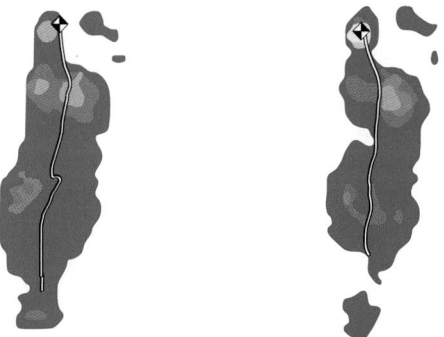

Fig. 17. Pedobarograph results before and after foot surgery (case 3). Presurgery results show large increases in pressure along the medial aspect of the foot with two abnormal peak pressures. After Evans anterior calcaneal advancement osteotomies, the postoperative plantar pressure data reveal a more evenly distributed pressure with a reduction in the peak pressures noted in the area of the arch and first metatarsal head. The center of pressure pattern (indicated with the line) is also more lateral.

maintain stance stability at the knee with knee hyperextension and a net knee flexor moment (Fig. 18), which does not require any quadriceps strength. When ambulating with an AFO, the patient reported increased knee instability and thus was not wearing the AFO. The knee kinetic data when the AFO was worn revealed a reduction of the flexor moment toward a neutral moment (Fig. 19) that provides a mechanical explanation for the patient-reported knee instability. The data suggest the patient would not be able to sustain a knee extensor moment due to the quadriceps strength. The AFO moves the patient closer to that margin.

MYELOMENINGOCELE

The use of gait analysis techniques in the ambulatory patient with myelomeningocele is relatively new in comparison to its use in those with cerebral palsy. The complexity of gait patterns in patients with sacral through L4 level myelomeningocele can only begin to be appreciated through careful examination of the 3D kinematics and kinetics of this patient population. Primary gait deviations are seen at all levels of the lower extremities and secondary compensations at the pelvis in trunk in those patients with L4 and L5 functional lesions. Much of our understanding of how these patients manage to walk with minimal muscular strength has been possible through gait analysis techniques.

In many patients with L4 level myelomeningocele, concern surrounds the deterioration of the knee over time. One of the proposed causes of this concern is the knee "valgus" thrust during loading response, which the clinician can observe when watching the patient from the frontal view. At this point in the gait cycle, there appears to be a rapid medial motion of the knee. Joint kinetic data for the knee in the coronal plane would allow an objective confirmation

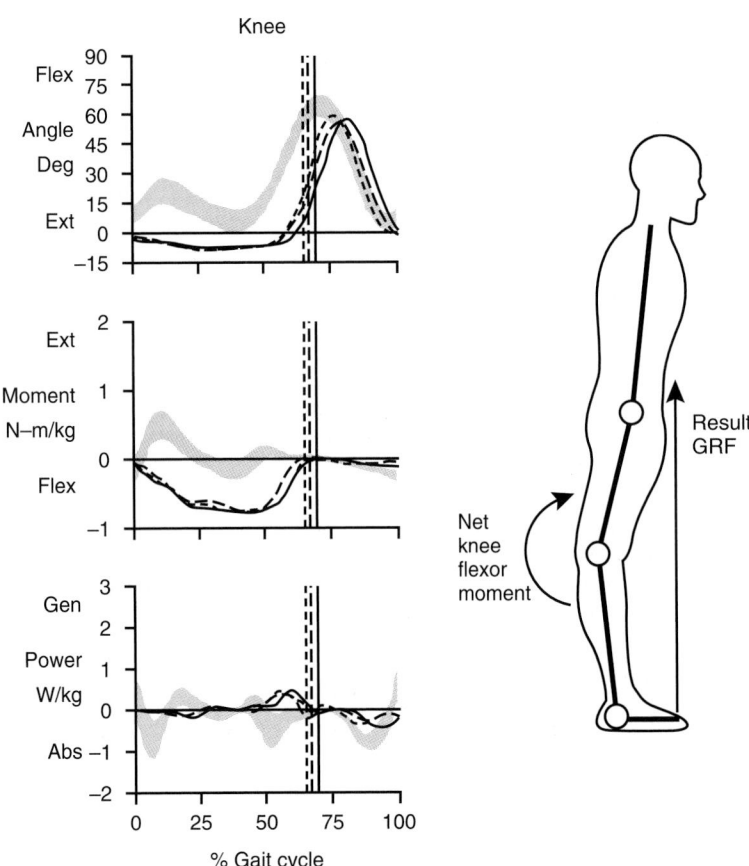

Fig. 18. Barefoot walking in a patient with quadriceps insufficiency (case 4). The knee kinematic, moments, and power data for a patient with 0/5 quadriceps strength reveal knee hyperextension in stance with an associate severe knee flexor moment pattern. The resultant ground reaction force passes anterior to the knee, applying an external load that extends the knee. This provides knee stability in stance because the quadriceps are not required to function.

Fig. 19. Ankle-foot orthosis (AFO) walking in a patient with quadriceps insufficiency (case 4). The knee kinematic, moments, and power data during AFO walking reveal less knee hyperextension in stance than when barefoot with an associated reduction in the knee flexor moment pattern. This results in a reduction in the knee stability in stance as the resultant ground reaction force gets closer to the knee center. If the resultant ground reaction force passes posterior to the knee center, an external flexor load will be applied to the knee. The 0/5 quadriceps will not be able to supply an internal moment and the knee will collapse.

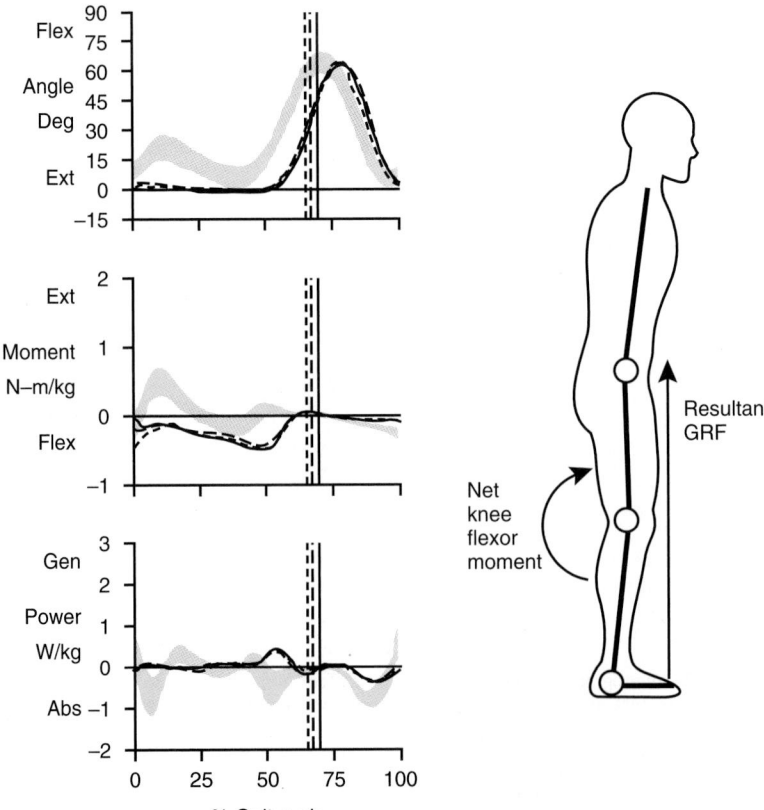

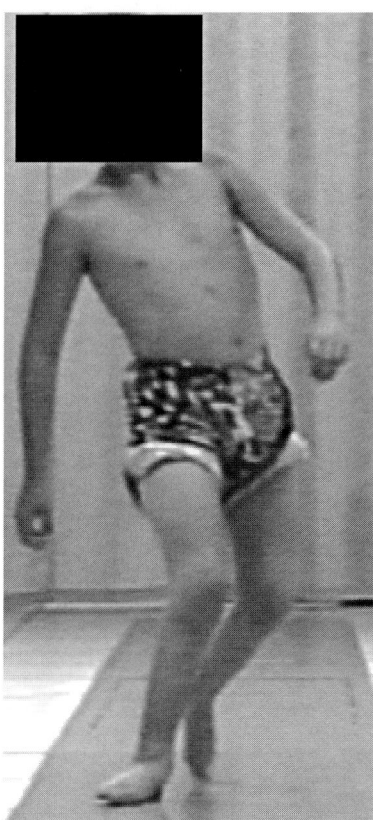

Fig. 20. Visual knee valgus thrust (case 5). An 18-year-old man with L4 functional level myelomeningocele presents with a knee valgus thrust during loading response bilaterally. This photograph was taken during loading response on the right side.

of this problem; that is, the net knee internal moment would be adductor. In many cases, however, an abnormal knee moment is not present in the knee data. This suggests that our visual impression of the knee valgus thrust was not sufficient in determining whether bracing above the knee was necessary to protect the lateral compartment. Research has shown that the presence of a knee valgus thrust confirmed by joint kinetic data is highly correlated with the degree of lateral trunk motion and not on the visual presence of a valgus thrust.[33]

The following case example illustrates the use of knee moment data for the basis of treatment in a child with myelomeningocele.

Case 5

A 10-year-old boy with a diagnosis of L4-level myelome-ningocele presented with a "visual" knee valgus thrust (Fig. 20) for which bracing with a knee-ankle-foot orthosis was being considered to protect the lateral knee compartment. Joint kinetic data for the knee in the coronal plane showed an internal net knee abductor moment within the typical range (Fig. 21), suggesting that the clinician's visual impression of the knee valgus thrust was not consistent with an actual kinetic knee valgus thrust. As a result, solid AFOs were recommended for treatment. A repeat gait analysis was recommended in 2 years to determine whether the status of the knee was unchanged.

TRANSVERSE PLANE ABNORMALITIES

One of the most important roles of gait analysis is in the understanding the various contributions to transverse plane abnormalities. Our visual observation of gait tends to focus on where the knees are pointing and foot progression. Normal foot progression may be possible with a combination of two deformities "canceling" each other out, that is, internal femoral torsion (internal hip rotation) and external tibial torsion. When adding the possibility of asymmetric pelvic rotation, rotation in the transverse plane through the knee, and foot deformity, dissecting the transverse plane visually is nearly impossible. The transverse plane rotation plots for the pelvis, hip, knee, and ankle can assist in comprehending the components of abnormality and ultimately in treatment decision-making. Transverse plane abnormalities are not limited to patients with idiopathic femoral anteversion and tibial torsion with associated knee pain; they also occur in many patients with cerebral palsy. The following example illustrates a case of malignant malalignment.

Case 6

A 16-year-old boy presented with knee pain. Visual evaluation of his gait patterns revealed normal foot progression angles and essentially a normal gait pattern otherwise (Fig. 22). The experienced observer may have observed bilateral in-pointing knees. Evaluation of the transverse plane kinematics (Fig. 23) shows a significant increase in internal hip rotation bilaterally and normal foot progression bilaterally as observed. The only possible combination of deformity to allow this degree of internal hip rotation with a normal foot progression angle is external tibial torsion as well. The standing image with the knees pointed forward highlights a significant external tibial torsion (see Fig. 22). Subsequent clinical examination measures confirmed internal femoral torsion and external tibial torsion. The combination of

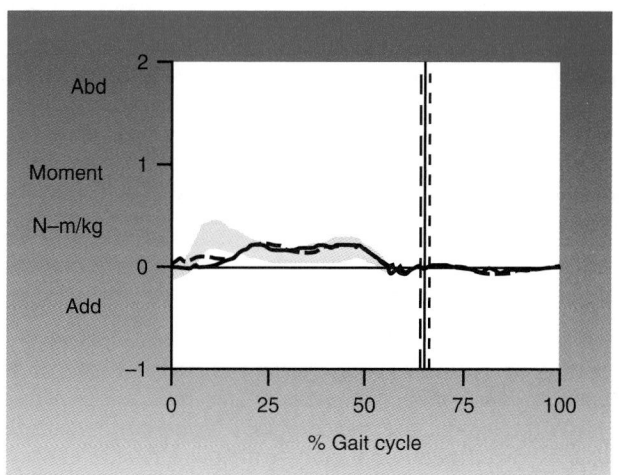

Fig. 21. Coronal plane knee kinetics (case 5). The coronal plane knee kinetics for this patient show a typical knee moment in stance on the right side. The gray band indicates the age-matched normal findings. This suggests that the visual indication of a knee valgus thrust was not predictive of an actual knee valgus thrust.

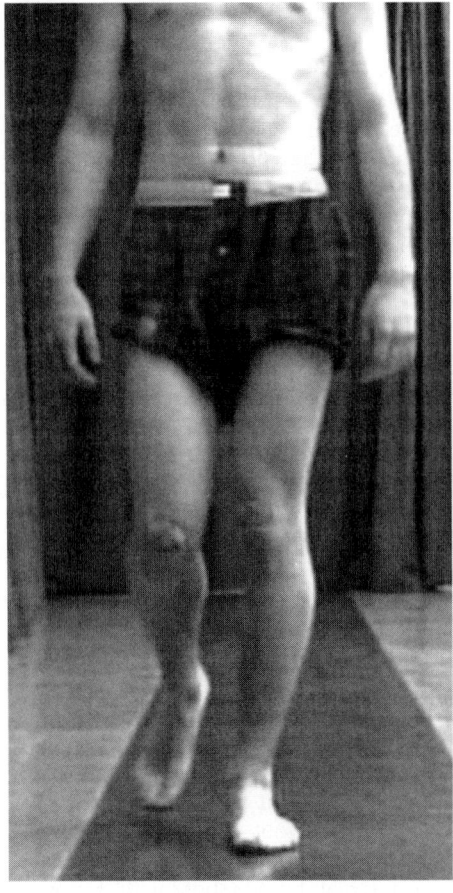

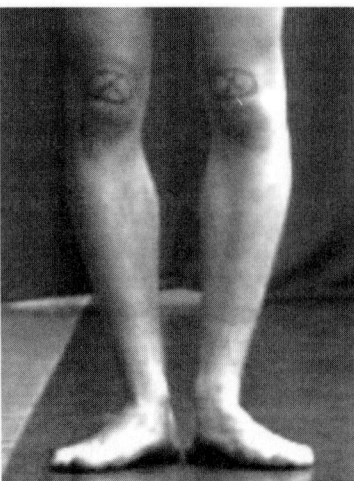

Fig. 22. Frontal view of male patient with knee pain (case 6). The frontal view of this 16-year-old boy with knee pain shows normal foot progression bilaterally and possible in-pointing knees. A close-up frontal view with the patient standing and the knees aligned straightforward reveals a severe knee varus deformity as well as severe external tibial torsion. Observation of this patient alone does not suggest major transverse plane abnormalities.

this malalignment was most likely the cause of the knee pain.

THE "LIMPING" GAIT DISORDERS

In many cases, the cause of a gait disorder is unclear. Diagnosing gait abnormalities can become further complicated when the patient uses voluntary compensations to overcome a primary gait deviation. This is more feasible in patients with normal muscle control. One of the primary purposes of gait analysis, therefore, is to differentiate between primary deviations, secondary abnormalities (gait deviations at an adjacent joint), and voluntary compensations. Frequently, the focus is on the compensation, which, if treated, may take away the patient's mechanism to deal with the primary problem.

Case 7

A 6-year-old girl with normal neuromuscular control presented with a "toe-walking" pattern on the left side of no apparent cause. She exhibited greater than usual plantar flexion throughout the stance phase. Gait analysis data revealed a fixed pelvis obliquity with the left side elevated throughout the gait cycle (Fig. 24). This abnormal pelvic position suggested a left hip abnormality, which was confirmed on radiographs as a hip dislocation. Consequently, there was a severe functional hip abductor weakness. The

excessive equinus of the left ankle was a voluntary compensation to equalize leg lengths because of the functional shortening on the left side as a result of the left pelvic elevation. The equinus would also serve to assist clearance of the contralateral limb in swing (which was functionally long due to the ipsilateral pelvic drop) and minimize the vertical excursion of the center of gravity.

GAIT ANALYSIS AS A RESEARCH TOOL

A natural extension of gait analysis methods for treatment decision-making is in research. Because data are collected and processed by computer, this facilitates the computational and statistical methods that are used in research. Generally, gait analysis research follows one of two related directions: the evaluation of specific treatment protocols and the documentation of a particular gait disorder.

The evaluation of treatment[21, 34–38] has led to the development of new operative procedures, which have ultimately changed the course of treatment. An example of this is the rectus femoris transfer now commonly used in the treatment of stiff-kneed gait in children with cerebral palsy.[7, 8, 35, 36] The study of the gait patterns in patients with myelomeningocele has also led to modifications in the types of orthoses typically prescribed for these

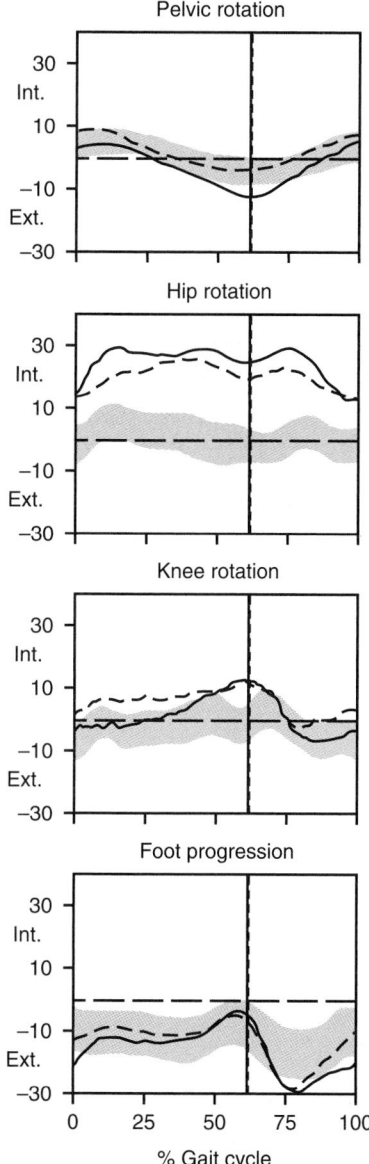

Fig. 23. Transverse plane kinematics (case 6). The bilateral transverse plane kinematics for case 6 reveal a neutral pelvis with bilateral internal hip rotation, normal knee rotation, and foot progression. A neutral foot progression with the degree of hip rotation would only be possible with bilateral external tibial torsion. The significance of the tibial torsion is not appreciated during ambulation but is very apparent in the standing view with the knee aligned forward. The associated kinematic data support the large external tibial torsion noted in the standing picture and suggest that the knee pain may be related to abnormal bony deformity of the femur and tibial and abnormal hip rotations during gait.

patients.[39] Additionally, when treatment is evaluated in groups of patients such as those who have had selective dorsal rhizotomy[40, 41] we can better predict the outcome clinically in similar patients. Research, however, is not limited to neuromuscular disorders. Gait analysis has led to a better understanding of quadriceps avoidance gait in persons with knee pain,[42] the implications of total joint re-

placement,[43, 44] and the biomechanics of running and running injury.[45]

Because gait analysis in many centers has been routinely performed over nearly 20 years, long-term outcomes can now be studied. This is a much-needed addition to the literature that focuses on outcomes at 1 and 2 years after surgery. Research has suggested that the long-term results (6 years postoperatively) of the multilevel surgical approach in the patient with cerebral palsy are positive.[46-48] These studies show the effects of the hamstring lengthening on improved knee function in stance, the gastrocnemius lengthening on ankle function in stance, and femoral derotation osteotomies on hip motion in the transverse plane are all maintained at 6 years after surgery. A comparison to a natural history database shows that patients with cerebral palsy continue to decline over time without treatment.[49]

Systematic review of data collected pre- and post-treatment can provide much information about the impact of the treatment and may allow for "fine tuning" of procedures in the future. One example of this is the study of the impact of unilateral hip fusion on gait. In the patient requiring hip fusion, the gait analysis procedure is not directly involved in the surgical decision-making process; however, it can be a useful procedure for better understanding of the effects and implications of surgical intervention. The patient with hip fusion shows compensations for the inability to flex and extend the hip at the pelvis, lumbar spine, ipsilateral knee and ankle, and contralateral hip.[50] To allow for rotation of the fused side thigh segment, the patient with hip fusion increases pelvic motion in the sagittal plane to a range of 18 to 20 degrees (normal = 3 ± 1 degrees). Because these patients maintain an upright trunk position, the lumbar spine absorbs the increased motion of the pelvis. The ipsilateral knee compensates by showing progressive flexion with an associated increase in knee extensor moment, and the ankle must plantar flex prematurely. On the contralateral side, the opposite hip requires increased sagittal plane range of motion to accommodate the increased range of motion of the pelvis. The compensations described provide a basis for the lower back pain, patellar femoral knee pain, and contralateral hip pain experienced in many of these patients long term.

GAIT ANALYSIS AND ITS ROLE IN OUTCOME MEASURES

Gait analysis plays a significant role in the objective documentation of outcomes. This is of particular importance given the current health care climate. A systematic approach of performing routine pre- and postoperative gait analysis on a patient-by-patient basis can lead to increased comprehension of the mechanics of gait abnormalities and ultimately substantiate individual surgical decisions. Long-term application of this approach can facilitate research such as the study of patient groups based on diagnosis or treatment methods. Ultimately, this type of critical examination of treatment will lead to improved treatment deci-

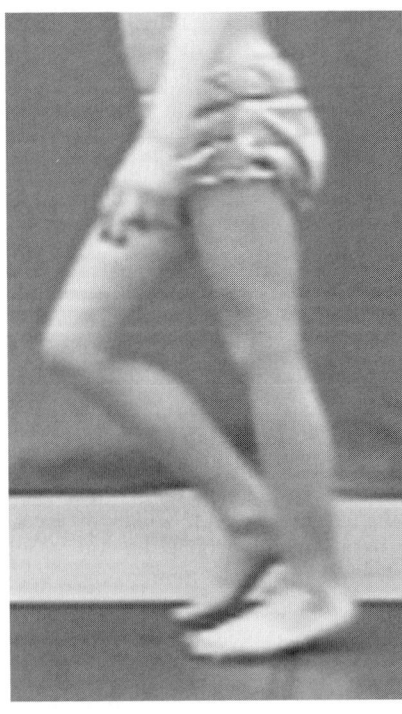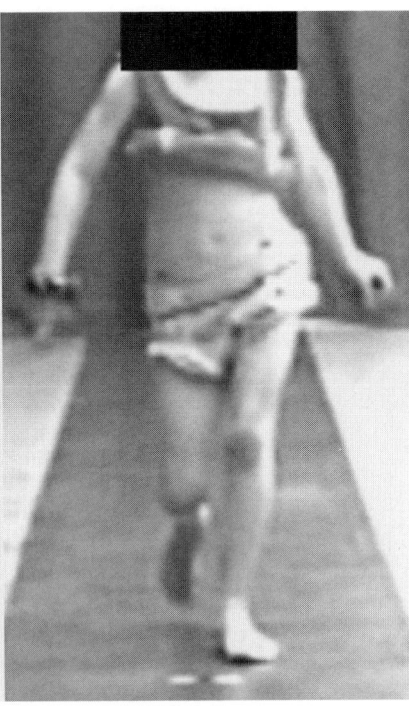

Fig. 24. Toe-walking gait pattern (case 7). The lateral view of this patient reveals an early heel rise in stance, which was the primary gait problem. The frontal view, however, revealed a severe asymmetry at the pelvis with the left side elevated throughout the gait cycle and the associated depression of the opposite pelvis because of hip abductor insufficiency as a result of a dislocated hip.

sion-making. Although the use of computerized gait analysis is a relatively new addition to routine treatment evaluations, it has already had a profound effect on treatment protocols, especially in the area of orthopaedic treatment decisions in patients with neuromuscular disorders. Increased understanding of gait pathomechanics in many different clinical problems has led to more informed treatment decision-making, which is ultimately based on the philosophy of the treating physician.

REFERENCES

1. DeLuca PA: Gait analysis in the treatment of the ambulatory child with cerebral palsy. Clin Orthop 1991; 264:5.
2. Gage JR, Õunpuu S: Gait analysis in clinical practice. Semin Orthop 1989, 4:72.
3. Gage JR, Õunpuu S (eds): Surgical Intervention in the Correction of Primary and Secondary Gait Abnormalities. Amsterdam, the Netherlands, Elsevier Science, 1991.
4. Gage J: The role of gait analysis in the treatment of cerebral palsy. J Pediatr Orthop 1994; 14:701.
5. Õunpuu S: Joint kinetics: Interpretation and clinical decision-making for the treatment of gait abnormalities in children with neuromuscular disorders. In Harris G, Smith P (eds): Human Motion Analysis: Current Applications and Future Directions. Piscataway, NJ, IEEE Press, 1996, p 268.
6. Rose SA, Õunpuu S, DeLuca PA: Strategies for the assessment of pediatric gait in the clinical setting. Phys Ther 1991; 71:961.
7. Gage JR, Perry J, Hicks RR, et al: Rectus femoris transfer to improve knee function of children with cerebral palsy. Dev Med Child Neurol 1987; 29:159.
8. Perry J: Distal rectus femoris transfer. Dev Med Child Neurol 1987; 29:153.
9. DeLuca P, Davis R, Õunpuu S, et al: Alterations in surgical decision making in patients with cerebral palsy based on three-dimensional gait analysis. J Pediatr Orthop 1997; 17:608.
10. Õunpuu S, Davis R, Walsh H, et al: Sagittal plane pelvic motion: Relationship to standing pelvic tilt and clinical measures. Dev Med Child Neurol 1995; 37:25.
11. Ruwe P, Gage J, Ozonoff M, et al: Clinical determination of femoral anteversion. J Bone Joint Surg Am 1992; 74:820.
12. Gage JR: Gait Analysis in Cerebral Palsy. London, MacKeith Press, 1991.
13. Õunpuu S: In Spivack BS (ed): Gait Analysis for the Clinician. New York, Marcel Dekker, 1996.
14. Winter DA: The Biomechanics and Motor Control of Human Gait: Normal, Elderly and Pathological. Waterloo, Ontario, Canada, University of Waterloo Press, 1991.
15. Greenwood DT: Principles of Dynamics. Englewood Cliffs, NJ, Prentice Hall, 1965.
16. Davis R, DeLuca P: In Harris G, Smith P (eds): Clinical Gait Analysis: Current Methods and Future Directions. Piscataway, NJ, IEEE Press, 1996, p 17.
17. Winter DA: Concerning the scientific basis for the diagnosis of pathological gait and for rehabilitation protocols. Physiother Canada 1985; 37:245.
18. Õunpuu S, Bell KJ, Davis RB, et al: An evaluation of the posterior leaf spring orthosis using gait analysis. Dev Med Child Neurol 1993; 35:8.
19. Winter DA: Biomechanics and Motor Control of Human Movement. New York, Wiley, 1990.
20. Õunpuu S, DeLuca PA, Bell KJ, et al: Using surface electrodes for the evaluation of the rectus femoris, vastus medialis and vastus lateralis muscles in children with cerebral palsy. Gait Posture 1997; 5:211.
21. Perry J, Hoffer MM: Preoperative and postoperative dynamic electromyography as an aid in planning tendon transfers in children with cerebral palsy. J Bone Joint Surg 1977; 56:531.
22. Waters R, Frazier J, Garland D: Electromyographic gait analysis before and after operative treatment for hemiplegic equinus and equinovarus deformity. J Bone Joint Surg Am 1982; 64:284.
23. DeLuca PA: The use of gait analysis and dynamic EMG in the assessment of the child with cerebral palsy. Hum Movement Sci 1991; 10:543.
24. Basmajian JV, DeLuca CJ: Muscles Alive: Their Functions Revealed by Electromyography. Baltimore, MD, Williams & Wilkins, 1985, p 380.
25. Kadaba MP, Wooten ME, Gainey J: Repeatability of phasic muscle activity: Performance of surface and intramuscular wire electrodes in gait analysis. J Orthop Res 1985; 3:350.
26. Duffy CM, Hill AE, Cosgrove AP, et al: Energy consumption in children with spina bifida and cerebral palsy. A comparative study. Dev Med Child Neurol 1996; 38:238.

27. Davis RB, Õunpuu S, Tyburski DJ, et al: A comparison of two dimensional and three dimensional techniques for the determination of joint rotation angles. Proceedings: International Symposium on 3-D Analysis of Human Movement. 1991; 67.

28. Perry J: Gait Analysis: Normal and Pathological Function. Thorofare, NJ, Slack, 1992.

29. Õunpuu S, Gage JR, Davis RB: Three-dimensional lower extremity joint kinetics in normal pediatric gait. J Pediatr Orthop 1991; 11:341.

30. Bleck UE: Orthopaedic Management in Cerebral Palsy. Philadelphia, MacKeith Press, 1987.

31. Sutherland DH, Olshen RA, Biden EN, et al: The Development of Mature Walking. London, MacKeith Press, 1988.

32. Kadaba MP, Ramakrishnan HK, Wootten ME: Measurement of lower extremity kinematics during level walking. J Orthop Res 1990; 8:383.

33. Õunpuu S, Thomson JD, Davis RB, et al: An examination of knee function during gait in children with myelomeningocele. J Pediatr Orthop 2000; 20:629.

34. DeLuca P, Õunpuu S, Davis R, et al: Effect of hamstring and psoas lengthening on pelvic tilt in patients with spastic diplegic cerebral palsy. J Pediatr Orthop 1998; 18: 712.

35. Õunpuu S, Muik E, Davis RB, et al: Part I: The effect of the rectus femoris transfer

location on knee motion in children with cerebral palsy. J Pediatr Orthop 1993; 13: 325.

36. Õunpuu S, Muik E, Davis RB, et al: Part II: A comparison of the distal rectus femoris transfer and release on knee motion in children with cerebral palsy. J Pediatr Orthop 1993; 13:331.

37. Rose SA, DeLuca PA, Davis RB, et al: Kinematic and kinetic evaluation of the ankle after lengthening of the gastrocnemius fascia in children with cerebral palsy. J Pediatr Orthop 1993; 13:727.

38. Sutherland DH, Santi M, Abel MF: Treatment of stiff-knee gait in cerebral palsy: A comparison by gait analysis of distal rectus femoris transfer versus proximal rectus release. J Pediatr Orthop 1990; 10:433.

39. Thomson J, Õunpuu S, Davis R, et al: The effects of ankle foot orthoses on the ankle and knee in persons with myelomeningocele: An evaluation using three-dimensional gait analysis. J Pediatr Orthop 1999; 19:27.

40. Boscarino LF, Õunpuu S, Davis RB, et al: The effects of selective dorsal rhizotomy on gait in children with cerebral palsy. J Pediatr Orthop 1993; 13:174.

41. Cahan LD, Adams JM, Perry J, et al: Instrumented gait analysis after selective dorsal rhizotomy. Dev Med Child Neurol 1990; 32:1037.

42. Berchuck M, Andriacchi T, Bach BR, et al: Gait adaptations by patients who have a

deficient anterior cruciate ligament. J Bone Joint Surg Am 1990; 72:871.

43. Berman AT, Zarro VJ, Bosacco SJ, et al: Quantitative gait analysis after unilateral or bilateral total knee replacement. J Bone Joint Surg Am 1987; 69:1340.

44. Dorr LD, Ochsner JL, Gronley J, et al: Functional comparison of posterior cruciate-retained versus cruciate-sacrificed total knee arthoplasty. Clin Orthop 1988; 236: 36.

45. Novacheck TF: The biomechanics of running. Gait Posture 1998; 7:77.

46. Davis RB, Õunpuu S, Bell K, et al: A long-term follow-up of the effects of rectus femoris, hamstring and gastrocnemius surgery on the knee in persons with cerebral palsy. Gait Posture 1996; 4:183.

47. Õunpuu S, Keggi JM, Davis RB, et al: A long-term follow-up of the effects of heel cord surgery on the ankle in persons with cerebral palsy. Gait Posture 1996; 4:184.

48. Õunpuu S, DeLuca PA, Davis RB, et al: The long-term effects of femoral derotation osteotomies: An evaluation using gait analysis. Dev Med Child Neurol 1999; 41:16.

49. Bell KJ, Õunpuu S, Davis RB, et al: An evaluation of the natural progression of gait in children with cerebral palsy. Dev Med Child Neurol 1996; 38:30.

50. Õunpuu S, Davis RB, DeLuca PA, et al: Surgical hip fusion: Gait kinematics and kinetics. Gait Posture 1998; 7:159.

section 1 chapter 12

LOWER EXTREMITY ORTHOTICS AND PROSTHETICS

Christopher J. Aiken and Robert S. Lin

Summary
- Regardless of specific design or construction methodologies, all orthotics should adhere to some basic tenets in order to provide optimum function.
- There should be an intimate fit of the extremity and the orthosis. Even slight anatomic inconsistencies within an orthosis can cause skin irritation and ulceration and enhance any pathological tone.
- Thermoplastic orthotic designs are very effective in controlling a wide range of orthopaedic deformities, but only if total contact is achieved.
- A firm understanding of the functional anatomy of the lower limb is essential for understanding lower extremity orthotics.

Lower limb orthoses are the most common type of orthotic device encountered by health care professionals. This chapter is designed to fulfill the need for a brief, readable summary of clinically relevant lower extremity orthotics. It is intended to help the reader gain a basic understanding of

the fundamentals of lower extremity orthoses and serve as a reference for practitioners. Each section covers orthotic objectives, prescribed use, and design criteria. Fully understanding the information in this chapter should help the physician manage patients with musculoskeletal disorders through employment of an appropriate orthosis.

UNIVERSITY OF CALIFORNIA BIOMECHANICS LABORATORY INSERT

Pathologies and Mechanical Factors. Flexible flatfoot (pes planus), pes planovalgus, valgus instability of subtalar joint, correct excessive eversion/pronation.
Objectives
1. Reduce subtalar joint deformity.
2. Support medial longitudinal arch to relieve ligamentous strain.
3. Maintain optimal position of calcaneus.

Orthotic Prescription. The University of California Biomechanics Laboratory (UCBL) Insert is effective at treating the flexible flatfoot by supporting the medial longitudinal arch (while it helps maintain the optimal position of

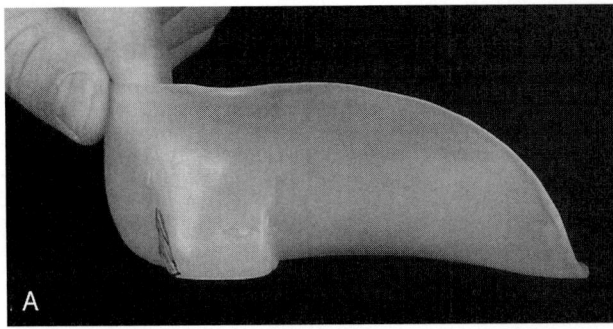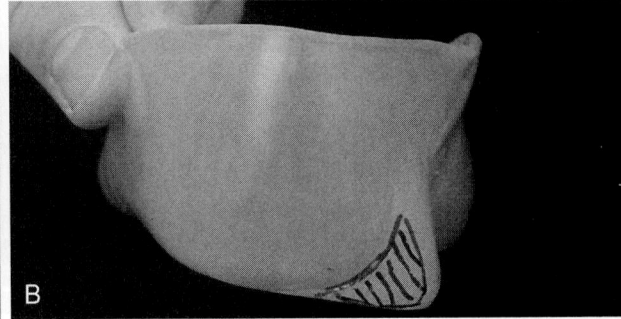

Fig. 1. The UCBL is often used in treatment of pes planovalgus. Posterior *(A)* and medial *(B)* view of the UCBL. Notice medial wedge used to increase the moment arm to resist the foot from collapsing into valgus.

the calcaneus relative to the talus) and by stabilizing the intertarsal and tarsometatarsal joints.[1] In children the treatment should continue until the deforming forces have been alleviated through the end of the growth period. As long as the deformity is flexible, preventing or at least minimizing foot deformities is the long-range goal.[2]

Orthotic Design. The UCBL is a removable orthosis, usually 3/4 of the foot length which is placed in the shoe, extending from the posterior border of the shoe to just proximal to the metatarsal heads (Fig. 1). Typically, it is a rigid plastic orthosis molded over a modified model of the mid- and hindfoot. The foot is casted in maximum manual correction. It has posterior and medial/lateral trimlines covering the heel and both sides of the foot to a level just below the malleoli.[3] A medial heel post is often included to increase the moment arm to provide greater resistance to the foot collapsing into valgus.

ANKLE-FOOT ORTHOSES

Thermoplastic Solid Ankle-Foot Orthosis

Pathologies and Mechanical Factors. Cerebral palsy, stroke, traumatic brain injury, multiple sclerosis, amyotrophic lateral sclerosis, severe spasticity, profound weakness, flaccid paralysis, severe varus/valgus, Charcot's joint, arthritis, spina bifida.

Objectives
1. Control medial/lateral instability at the ankle by providing maximum resistance to varus/valgus of the hindfoot.
2. Provide maximum resistance to plantarflexion, preventing footdrop during swing phase of gait.
3. Provide a rigid lever to facilitate push-off by not collapsing into dorsiflexion.
4. Influence the knee joint indirectly through sufficient lever arms and plantarflexion/dorsiflexion angles. Control the knee by preventing hyperextension or hyperflexion (plantarflexion–knee extension couple).
5. Decrease tone by putting a stretch on the gastrocsoleus complex.
6. Resist forefoot pronation and supination.
7. Control midtarsal joint from abducting or adducting.

Orthotic Prescription. The thermoplastic solid ankle-foot orthosis (AFO) is a versatile design capable of treating a wide variety of disorders. It is very effective at treating the ankle-foot complex when maximum control is needed

in all three planes of motion. One clinical issue to consider is its rigidity, which can impede balance. This AFO may limit too much motion, especially in patients with athetosis or ataxia who depend on some of their movement patterns to function. An AFO affects all three phases of the stance component of gait (rocker) potentially slowing down gait and shortening stride length; and the patient needs at least fair quadriceps strength unless the AFO is set in some plantarflexion.[4–9]

Orthotic Design. The AFO is a removable, rigid thermoplastic orthosis that fits inside a shoe and is typically set in neutral alignment or 3–5 degrees of dorsiflexion. The AFO is set as high as possible without interfering with terminal knee flexion for children and 1.5 inches below the apex of the fibular head for adults. The trimlines are midline of the anteroposterior calf dimension and cross anterior to the apex of the medial and lateral malleoli. The toe plate should extend ⅛ to ¼ inch past the longest toe, especially in children, so that the plate does not influence toe grasp (especially in cerebral palsy) and to allow room for growth. The medial wall of the footplate should be high, encompassing the navicular, following the slope of the shaft of the first metatarsal. This broad total contact surface area helps decrease localized pressure. The lateral wall slopes down from the lateral malleolus to encompass the shaft of the fifth metatarsal. The toe break trimline should be vertical and stop just proximal to the first and fifth metatarsal heads. The footplate also provides support and correct positioning of the arches of the foot (Fig. 2).

Posterior Leaf Spring AFO

Pathologies. CVA, footdrop, peripheral neuropathy, peroneal nerve palsy, weak dorsiflexors, hemiplegia, mild diplegia, mild crouch gait.

Objectives
1. Decelerate plantarflexion at heelstrike and provide swing-phase clearance.
2. Facilitate swing-phase clearance during gait.
3. Allow for increased motion/function.

Orthotic Prescription. The posterior leaf spring (PLS) AFO is effective at compensating for weak dorsiflexors by assisting plantarflexion at heelstrike and swing phase of the gait cycle.[8, 10] With intimate control of the calcaneus and the addition of a Gillette heel wedge, varus/valgus deformities of the calcaneus can be effectively controlled. Contra-

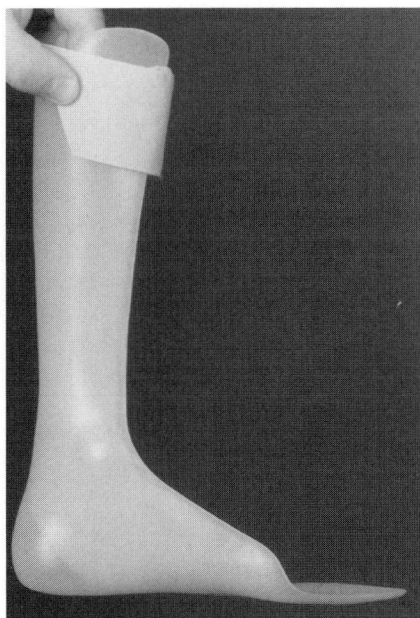

Fig. 2. Lateral view of solid AFO. Thermoplastic AFO has the advantage of lighter weight and improved cosmesis. Solid AFO is very effective at treating the ankle-foot complex when maximum control is needed in all three planes of motion.

indications to the use of a PLS AFO are severe extension or flexor tone, moderate to severe crouch, and severe varus/valgus.

Orthotic Design. The PLS AFO is characterized by narrower trimlines on the calf shell and often lower medial and lateral walls on the footplate. Otherwise, the remaining components are the same as those of the solid AFO. The PLS AFO should be preset at 5 degrees dorsiflexion (Fig. 3). By integrating dorsiflexion into the PLS AFO, the orthosis is being preloaded in anticipation that the weight of the foot and the shoe will plantarflex to approximately 90 degrees for adequate toe clearance in swing. When considering a PLS AFO, it is important to match the patient's needs and deficits to the flexibility of the orthosis. Three determinants of PLS AFO flexibility are plastic thickness, anteroposterior trimlines, and radius at the distal third of the calf shell. These three characteristics are combined empirically by the certified orthotist to obtain an optimally designed AFO.

Articulated/Hinged AFO

Pathologies. Footdrop, hemiplegia, spastic diplegia, postoperative patient with changing clinical picture (soft-tissue surgery: e.g., heel cord lengthening, posterior tibial tendon lengthening) to progressively allow more motion.

Objectives
1. Prevent plantarflexion while allowing some or complete dorsiflexion.
2. Dorsiflexion motion allows forward progression of the body and attempts to place a stretch on the Achilles tendon at the same time.
3. Control medial/lateral stability at the ankle.

Orthotic Prescription. The articulated AFO is the AFO design of choice for the patient who can utilize it. Articulated AFOs can be used effectively when the patient has passive range of motion of at least 5 degrees dorsiflexion (ideally 10 degrees) without compromising the neutral position of the subtalar and midtarsal joints.[8, 9, 11, 12] Articulated AFOs typically incorporate a plantarflexion stop to control genu recurvatum and encourage the progression of the lower extremity over the foot, allowing a stretch of the calf muscles during stance phase. Articulated AFOs should be used with care for patients with severe coronal plane deformities, patients with severe spasticity, and those unable to achieve passive dorsiflexion.

Orthotic Design. Same components and trimlines as those of the solid AFO, with joints made of metal or plastic at the ankle-joint axis (Fig. 4). Metal joints offer a number of options for control of the ankle, ranging from plantarflexion/dorsiflexion stops to plantarflexion/dorsiflexion assist, but are heavier and less cosmetically appealing. Plastic ankle joints such as the Oklahoma and Tammarck joints allow free motion, with plantarflexion stops incorporated into a posterior plastic shelf on the AFO.

Floor Reaction Orthosis

Pathologies and Mechanical Factors. Crouch gait/persistent knee flexion, spastic diplegia, weak quadriceps, overlengthening of Achilles tendon, postpolio paralysis.

Objectives
1. Provide knee extension moment during weightbearing/stance phase.
2. Minimize knee flexion during second rocker.
3. Provide same function as solid AFO in the frontal plane.

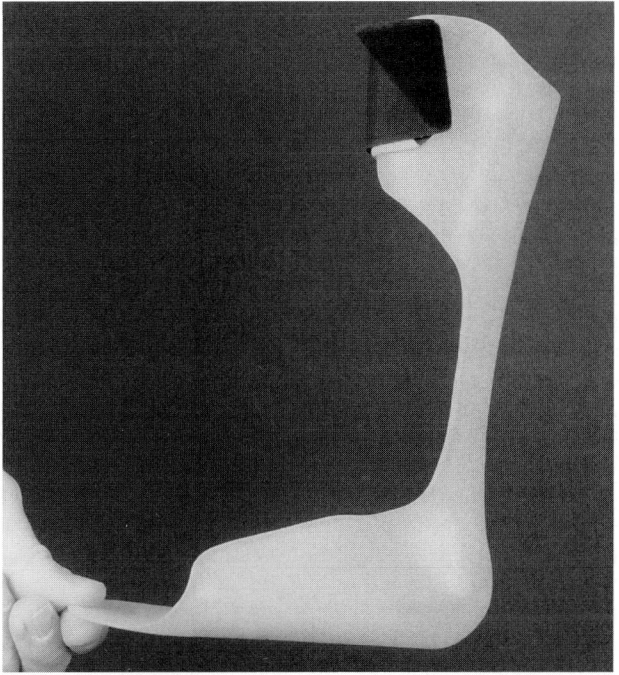

Fig. 3. Lateral view. This is a lateral view of PLS AFO.

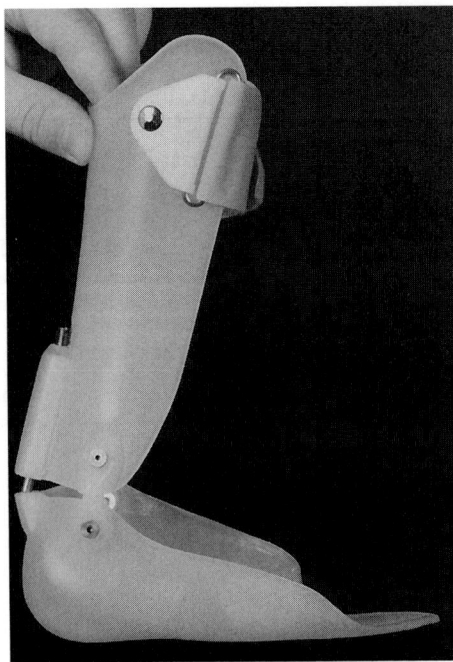

Fig. 4. Articulating AFO. Articulating AFO with plastic Tammarak joints with an adjustable posterior stop varies plantarflexion range as well as the amount of dorsiflexion assist.

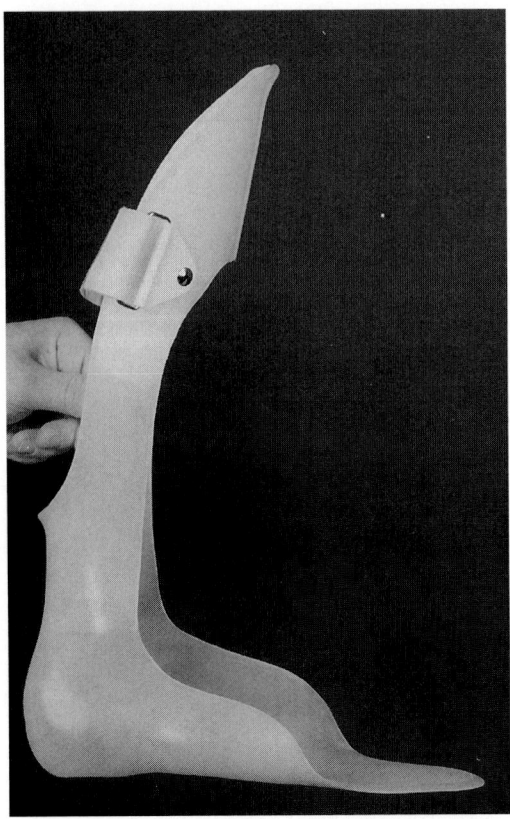

Fig. 5. Lateral view. This is a lateral view of FRO.

Orthotic Prescription. The concept of the floor reaction orthosis (FRO) is the same as that of the solid AFO in the coronal plane: to stabilize the ankle and subtalar motion. The FRO also helps minimize knee flexion as a result of the ground reaction forces onto the knee. The amount of knee extension moment during stance phase of gait depends on the plantarflexion/dorsiflexion angle of the ankle. The greater the plantarflexion angle, the greater the knee extension moment. This biomechanical principle is referred to as the plantarflexion knee extension couple. Contraindications to the use of the FRO are recurvatum or posteriorly unstable knee, external foot rotation in excess of 25 degrees, knee flexion contracture exceeding 15 degrees, or fixed dorsiflexion (must be able to get ankle to neutral or slight plantarflexion).[13–15]

Orthotic Design. There are three types of the FRO: one-piece solid ankle (Fig. 5), two-piece solid ankle, and the articulated FRO (Fig. 6). The one-piece FRO has the same design as that of the solid AFO but also has an anterior pretibial-wrapped trimline. The anterior proximal trimline ends at the tibial tubercle and extends down approximately one-third of the shank of the leg. The anterior aspect is padded with pressure-sensitive foam for comfort and protection. The two-piece FRO has the same trimline as the one-piece except that the anterior tibial shell is removable and fastened to the posterior shell with Velcro closures. The two-piece FRO is much easier to don and doff than the one-piece FRO, but it is cosmetically bulkier. The advantage of this design is that the anterior shell may be replaced by a standard Velcro strap closure if the clinical picture dictates it. The articulated FRO is a rear entry design with a completely solid anterior shell from the tibial tubercle to the ankle joint axis. It minimizes orthotic im-

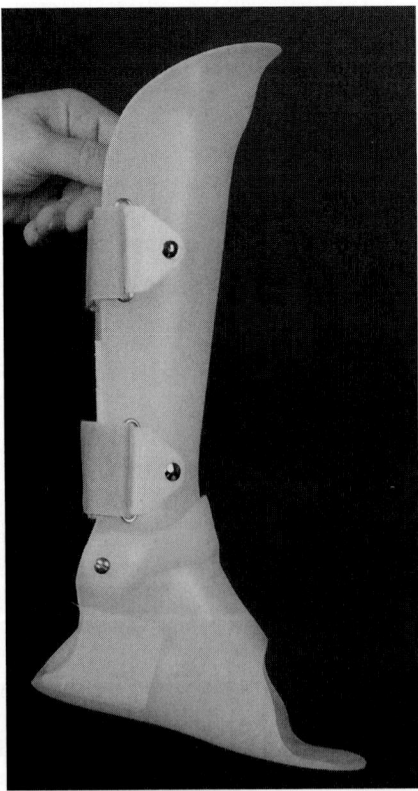

Fig. 6. Lateral view. This is a lateral view of articulated rear-entry FRO with a dorsiflexion stop.

pediment during first and third rockers while still providing a knee extension moment during the second rocker. The articulated FRO allows plantarflexion at the first rocker and prevents dorsiflexion at the second rocker so the tibia cannot progress over the top of the talus. The result is knee extension during stance phase.[14] The ankle joints are typically some type of free motion joint such as Oklahoma joints. The foot piece or FRO is the same as a solid AFO except that it encompasses the dorsum of the foot and overlaps the anterior shell at the ankle joint axis, providing a dorsiflexion stop.

Conventional AFO

Pathologies and Mechanical Factors. CVA, peripheral neuropathy, footdrop, peroneal nerve palsy, poor swing phase clearance, significant fluctuating edema.

Objectives
1. Control or assist plantarflexion or dorsiflexion.
2. Provide a minimum contact brace to allow for fluctuations in edema.

Orthotic Prescription. The conventional AFO is often appropriate when sagittal plane control is needed in the presence of significant fluctuating edema.[11] The minimal contact design is able to effectively accommodate volume changes throughout the course of a day without undue pressure or constriction.

Orthotic Design. There are four basic components to the conventional double upright AFO (Fig. 7). There is the proximal calf band with an anterior closure strap, medial and lateral uprights, ankle joints, and a stirrup to interface with the shoe. The calf band provides proximal control and is located 1½ inches below the apex of the fibula head to avoid impingement of the peroneal nerve. The calf band is

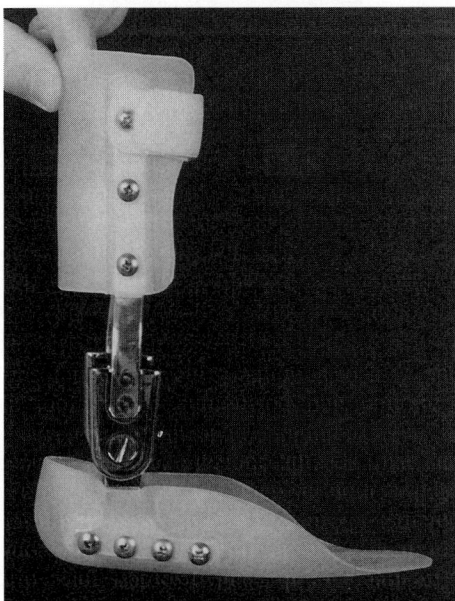

Fig. 7. Hybrid articulating AFO. Hybrid articulating AFO with double action ankle joints used in conjunction with a thermoplastic brace allows for adjustable plantarflexion/dorsiflexion range of motion.

typically made of aluminum and is 1½ to 2 inches wide. The uprights provide medial-lateral stability and attachment for the ankle joints. The uprights should have no contact with the patient's skin and can be made of aluminum or steel. Several categories of ankle joints can be used, depending on the functional deficit and amount of control needed. The solid AFO provides no motion in the sagittal plane, the dorsi assist/Klenzak joint provides swing phase clearance, and the bi-channel adjustable ankle joint can give resistance or assistance to either plantarflexion or dorsiflexion, making this the most versatile design.[16]

TIBIAL FRACTURE ORTHOSIS

Pathologies. Diaphyseal fractures of tibia and fibula.
Objectives
1. Union of the fracture with acceptable alignment.
2. Displacement of vertical forces to the tibia or fibula during ambulation.
3. Promotion of fracture healing while maintaining range of motion and muscle tone and reducing edema.

Orthotic Prescription. Orthotic fracture management is rarely the initial treatment for a fractured limb. Once the acute symptoms of pain and edema have subsided (usually 1 to 3 weeks) and there is acceptable alignment, a fracture orthosis can be applied. At this point, an x-ray film should be taken to assess the alignment of the fractured bone.[17] Contraindications to orthotic management of fractures are severe soft-tissue damage, excessive wound drainage, spastic disorders, and anesthetic limbs.[11] Orthotic fracture management is attributed to soft-tissue attachments and constraints, elastic deformation, and principles of fluid mechanics. In fracture management, soft tissues such as the interosseus membrane act as a rigging that helps maintain bony alignment and prevent unwanted shortening. When enclosed by the fracture orthosis, the soft tissues around the fracture site behave mechanically as fluids, producing lateral and oblique forces that help offset the vertical loads produced during ambulation. According to Pascal's law, 80 percent of the force is absorbed by the soft tissue within the fracture orthosis.[11] Additionally, the controlled movement that occurs at the fracture site (fracture ends telescope up to 2 cm during weightbearing and return to their normal position during swing phase) within the brace actually promotes healing while helping the patient maintain range of motion and muscle tone and reducing edema.

Orthotic Design. Tibial fracture orthoses are typically made out of thermoplastics, making them lightweight, durable, easily adjustable, and simple to apply. Fracture orthoses consist of an anterior and posterior shell as well as a shoe insert with ankle joints. The anterior shell has a patellar-tendon bearing design proximally and extends distally over the malleoli. The posterior shell extends from below the popliteal crease down to just proximal to the malleoli. The shoe insert attaches to the anterior shell and allows dorsiflexion/plantarflexion while resisting inversion/eversion. The two shells are held together with Velcro closures that make for easy application while allowing for swelling and maintaining hydraulic compression for fracture alignment and comfort.

FEMORAL FRACTURE ORTHOSIS

Pathologies. Distal femoral fractures, tibial plateau fractures, postoperative knee ligamentous repairs.

Objectives

1. Fracture healing with acceptable alignment and function.
2. Displacement of vertical forces to the femur during ambulation.
3. Promotion of fracture healing while maintaining range of motion at the knee, minimizing atrophy of thigh, and reducing edema.

Orthotic Prescription. Femoral fracture management, unlike management of tibial fractures, requires stability at the fracture site before orthotic treatment is begun, usually 4 to 6 weeks postinjury. The delay in application of the femoral fracture orthosis allows time for volume changes in the thigh to stabilize. Femoral fractures have a greater tendency to shorten, and they require traction to initiate intrinsic stability at the fracture site.[11, 18] Fractures of the middle and proximal third of the femur do not respond well to fracture orthoses, often developing unacceptable varus angulation. Varus angulation can be the result of difficulty of tissue containment in the thigh, patient obesity, the center of gravity being located medial to the fracture site, or the pull of recovering hip abductors and adductors. Distal femoral fractures respond better because a more effective three-point force system can be applied to resist varus angulation. This three-point force system incorporates a lateral pressure applied to the knee to help stabilize against varus deformation at the fracture site. See the preceding section on tibial fracture orthoses for mechanisms of fracture management.

Orthotic Design. The femoral fracture orthosis is thermoplastic and consists of a femoral shell section, a tibial shell section, knee joints, and a shoe insert with ankle joints. Typically, the femoral and tibial sections are anterior, opening with anterior tongues to provide circumferential pressure. The femoral section's proximal medial edge extends approximately 3 cm below the perineum. The proximal portion of the femoral shell usually incorporates either a quadrilateral brim or an ischial containment brim. Both these brims are designed to help off-weight the lower extremity through the orthosis as well as provide rotational control of the proximal femur. Posteriorly, the femoral and tibia sections are trimmed back to allow 90 degrees of knee flexion. The two shells are attached with double uprights containing either free motion or an adjustable flexion/extension knee joint.

PATELLA TENDON–BEARING ORTHOSIS

Pathologies. Calcaneal fractures, arthritic joints, Charcot's joints, plantar skin, plantar ulcerations.

Objectives

1. Relieve weightbearing below the knee (non-weightbearing).
2. Reduce forces on plantar surface of foot (partial weightbearing).
3. Transmit axial forces from the knee region through the orthosis.

Orthotic Prescription. The patella tendon–bearing (PTB) orthosis is used when non-weightbearing or partial weightbearing is desired below the knee. This reduction or unloading of forces to the plantar surfaces of the foot is achieved through anteroposterior compression at the patella tendon and popliteal fossa, medial-lateral pressure at the medial tibial plateau and shaft of the fibula, and anteroposterior compression down the proximal third of the lower leg from the clam shell design of the orthosis. To achieve total non-weightbearing, a Patten bottom is mounted to the PTB orthosis.[11] This orthosis is contraindicated for people who have unstable knees or who have vascular impairment because of potential excess compression in the popliteal area compromising arterial flow.

Orthotic Design. The PTB orthosis is fabricated with the knee in approximately 10 degrees of flexion; if the ankle is fixed, it should be set at about 7 degrees of dorsiflexion. The proximal third of the orthosis should be total contact to optimally distribute forces over the largest surface area possible. The anterior shell is attached to the posterior shell with Chicago-style screws allowing for articulating anterior opening to the proximal brim. The posterior shell's trimlines are the same as those of the solid AFO except that the posterior proximal edge starts at the popliteal fossa (Fig. 8). If maximum weightbearing elevation is desired, a patten bottom can be mounted to the posterior shell with two steel uprights medially and laterally. The Patten bottom surface pad is rockered to allow for a smooth transition and is typically set in 7 degrees of

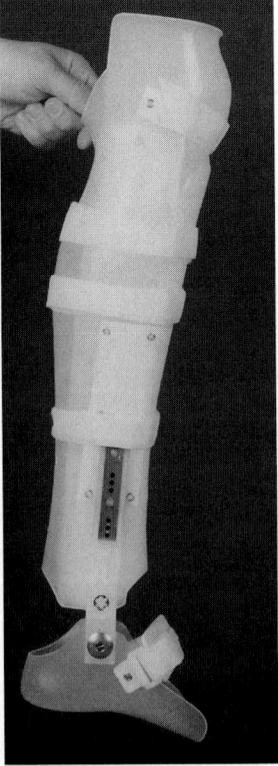

Fig. 8. Prefabricated functional tibial fracture orthosis. Anterior and posterior shells are held together by Velcro straps. The orthosis must be adjusted regularly so the snug compression of soft tissue, which maintains fracture stability and alignment, is not lost.

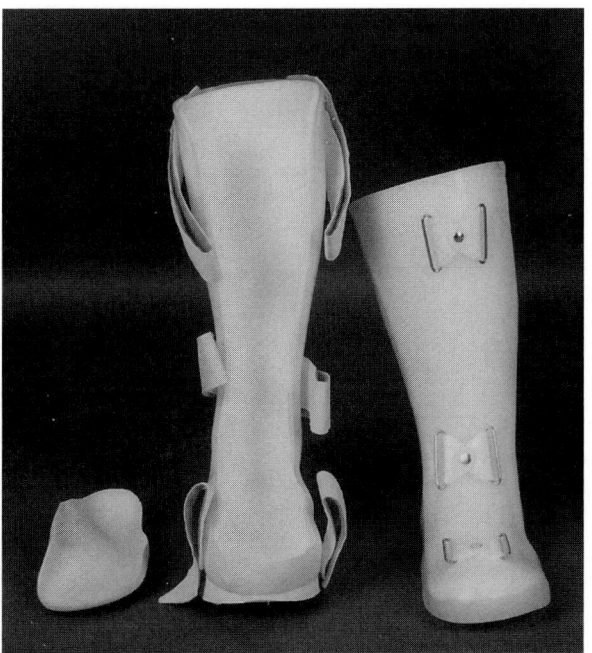

Fig. 9. Anterior view of neuropathic walker (CROW boot). Viewed from right to left are removable Plastazote insert, foam-lined AFO with rockered bottom, and foam-lined anterior tibial shell.

quarter-inch Aliplast foam. The total contact AFO combines a foam-lined AFO (anterior and posterior shell) that is formed over a removable insert. This orthosis must be able to fit in the patient's shoe; typically, the toes are left open, with the anterior shell stopping at midfoot.

KNEE ORTHOSIS

Patients who require support or control of the knee but not the foot and ankle may benefit from a knee orthosis (Table 1). All knee orthoses are designed on the premise that abnormal translation or motion can be restricted by the application of leverage to the knee joint. This can be achieved most effectively when leverage is applied at a distance from the joint. Materials, straps, hinge styles, and patient compliance all determine the effectiveness of orthotic management.[22–26]

Knee-Ankle-Foot Orthosis

Pathologies. Postpolio, cerebral palsy, myelomeningocele, spinal cord injury, genu recurvatum, muscular dystrophy.
Objectives
1. Direct control of the knee in addition to ankle or foot control.[11]
2. Unload the skeletal structures of the lower extremity during weightbearing and transfer those forces directly to the pelvis.

dorsiflexion to allow for a smooth progression through the gait cycle.

NEUROPATHIC WALKER/TOTAL CONTACT AFO

Pathologies. Charcot's joint, chronic ulcerations, chronic Charcot's joint recurrences.
Objectives
1. Total contact design helps reduce excessive vertical forces per unit area.
2. Nearly complete elimination of motion is thought to reduce plantar shear forces.
3. Ankle is locked up to decrease excessive forces through the ankle and midtarsal joint.
4. Protect inadequate subtalar joint stability.

Orthotic Prescription. The neuropathic walker, also known as a CROW (Charcot Restraint Orthotic Walker) boot, is often prescribed after initial total contact casting of a Charcot joint or for an unstable subtalar joint where joint stability has not occurred after fracture healing. The orthosis is easily donned and doffed, which facilitates observation of skin integrity and areas of excessive pressure/friction and maintains proper foot hygiene. The total contact AFO is similar to the neuropathic walker but is used if the affected leg size is near normal. With the total contact AFO, the orthosis fits inside a shoe instead of incorporating a shoe surface on the bottom.[19–21]
Orthotic Design. The neuropathic walker is a bivalved total contact design with a rockered bottom crepe sole (Fig. 9). The footbed is lined with a half-inch Plastazote insert and extends one-half inch past the longest toe on the foot. The anterior and posterior shells are typically lined with

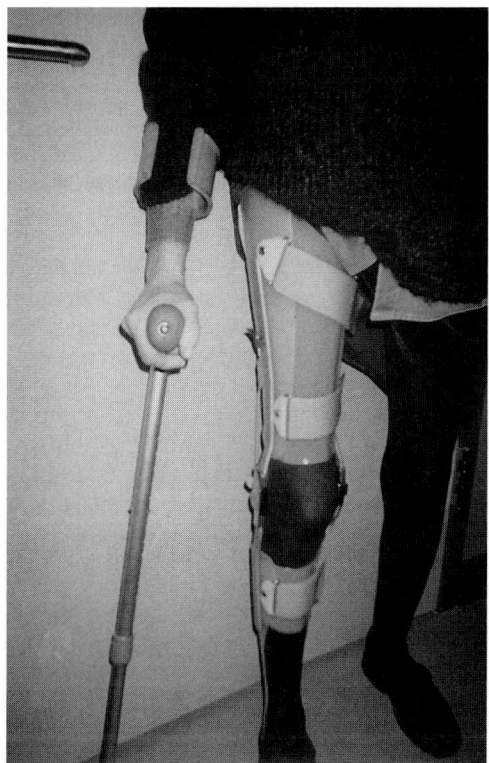

Fig. 10. Anterior view. This is an anterior view of postpolio patient wearing a double upright thermoplastic KAFO with ischial containment brim and triggerlock knee joints.

TABLE 1. KNEE ORTHOSES		
Type of Knee Orthosis	**Pathologies/Objectives**	**Orthotic Design**
Patellar stabilizing orthoses	Recurrent subluxation/dislocation of patella. Chondromalacia patellae. Osgood-Schlatter's disease. Assist patella to track normally. Protect against subluxation/dislocation. Control pain.	Elastic sleeve design with patellar cutout and two circumferentially wrapped rubber arms that apply dynamic tension to a crescent-shaped lateral patella pad. An elastic circumferential counterarm maintains proper positioning of pads and prevents rotation of brace.
Ligamentous instabilities (functional knee orthoses)	Designed to provide mechanical stability to those who have had ligamentous deficiencies or who have had ligament reconstruction without impeding performance. Increase performance in patients with instability and weakness. Decrease pain. Allow patient to return to higher level of activity.	Semirigid or rigid, thigh and calf cuffs, hinges and strap/cuff configurations vary depending on functional control (hinge position critical).
Osteoarthritis (functional knee orthoses)	These braces are indicated for pain relief and joint degeneration associated with medial or lateral unicompartmental osteoarthritis. Depending on which compartment is affected, apply either a varus or valgus force on the knee. Help redistribute weight absorbed by the compressed side of the knee joint.	Rigid thigh and calf cuffs, either single or double uprights with polycentric knee joints. The braces use a three-point pressure system, either varus or valgus corrective force depending on affected compartments, to unload the involved compartment.
Postoperative or rehabilitative	These braces are designed to provide rigid immobilization at selected angles or controlled motion of the injured knee treated surgically or nonsurgically. Decrease load on healing tissue. Adjustable to various leg shapes/sizes (edema).	Large surface area; soft padded thigh and calf cuffs/straps; single axis, polycentric, or posterior offset knee joints with adjustable flexion/extension stops. Easy to don/doff and comfortable.
Prophylactic knee orthoses	These braces are designed to prevent or reduce the severity of knee injury while not inhibiting knee mobility in people without knee injuries. Prevent knee injury from occurring. Protect medial and collateral ligaments from contact injuries.	Single lateral upright, thigh and calf cuff/strap, single axis or polycentric knee joint with or without 180° stop.

Orthotic Prescription. The knee-ankle-foot orthosis (KAFO) is prescribed when there is a need for direct control of the knee in addition to control of the ankle or foot. By encompassing the knee, ankle, and foot, a longer lever arm and better mechanical advantage for controlling the knee complex are gained. The KAFO can also be used when there is a need to unload the skeletal structure of the lower extremity during weightbearing. This unloading is accomplished by incorporating either an ischial containment or quadrilateral brim to the KAFO.[5, 27]

Orthotic Design. The KAFO can be of conventional metal design, thermoplastic, or both (Fig. 10). The conventional KAFO consists of proximal and distal thigh bands, double uprights with knee joints, a calf band, ankle joints, and stirrups to attach to a shoe. The thermoplastic KAFO consists of a plastic thigh shell with an anterior tongue closure, double uprights with knee joints, and a thermoplastic AFO section that fits into a patient's shoe. With either design, there is a variety of knee and ankle joints from which to choose, depending on the biomechanical control needed.

CONCLUSION

As long as the design complements the biomechanical disorder or deficit, it is possible to reduce pain, provide stability, improve function, and reduce fatigue with a well-designed and executed orthosis. This chapter on lower extremity orthotics is intended as an introduction and reference for physicians and health care providers dealing with the biomechanical losses of musculoskeletal disorders.

REFERENCES

1. Colson JM, Berglund G: An effective orthotic design for controlling the unstable subtalar joint. Orthot Prosthet 1979; 33:39.
2. Wenger DR: Corrective shoes and inserts as treatment for flexible flatfoot in infants and children. J Bone Joint Surg Am 1989; 71:800.
3. Henderson WH, Campbell JW: UC-BL shoe insert: Casting and fabrication. Bull Prosthet Res 1969; 10:215.
4. Carlson WE, Vaughan CL, Damiano DL, et al: Orthotic management of gait in spastic diplegia. Am J Phys Med Rehab 1997; 76:219.
5. Clark DR, Perry J, Lunsford TR: Case studies: Orthotic management of the adult postpolio patient. Orthot Prosthet 1986; 40:43.
6. Glancy J, Lindseth RE: The polypropylene solid ankle orthosis. Orthot Prosthet 1972; 26:14.

7. Knutson LM, Clark DE: Orthotic devices for ambulation in children with cerebral palsy and myelomeningocele. Phys Ther 1991; 71:947.

8. Lin RS, Gage JR: The neurological control system for normal gait. J Prosthet Orthot 1989; 2:119.

9. Wilson H, Haideri N, Song K, et al: Ankle-foot orthoses for preambulatory children with spastic diplegia. J Pediatr Orthop 1997; 17:370.

10. Banzinger E, Hewitt C, Ford RL: Dynamic dorsiflexion assists polypropylene ankle foot orthosis. J Assoc Child Prosthet Orthot Clin 1991; 26:65.

11. Weber D, Agro M, Anweiler L, et al: Clinical aspects of lower extremity orthotics. Ontario, Canada, The Canadian Association of Prosthetics and Orthotics, 1993, p 261.

12. Weber D: Use of the hinged AFO for children with spastic cerebral palsy and midfoot instability. J Assoc Child Prosthet Orthot Clin 1991; 25:61.

13. Harrington ED, Lin RS, Gage JR: Use of the anterior floor reaction orthosis in patients with cerebral palsy. Orthot Prosthet 1983; 37:34.

14. Lin RS: Thermoforming plastic improves floor reaction orthoses. Biomechanics, September 1998, p 69.

15. Saltiel J: A one-piece laminated knee-locking short leg brace. Orthot Prosthet 1969; 23:68.

16. Berger N, Edelstein JE, Fishman S, et al (eds): Lower Limb Orthotics. New York, New York University Medical Center, 1986.

17. Sarmiento A, Gersten L, Sobal P: Tibial shaft fractures treated with functional braces: Experience with 780 fractures. J Bone Joint Surg 1989; 71:602.

18. Sarmiento A, Sinclair W: Application of prosthetic-orthotic principles of orthopaedics. Artif Limbs 1967; 11:28.

19. Boninger ML, Leonard JA: Use of bivalved ankle and foot orthosis in neuropathic foot and ankle lesions. J Rehabil Res Dev 1996; 33:16.

20. Gristina AG, Thompson WA, Kester N, et al: Treatment of neuropathic conditions of the foot and ankle with a patellar tendon–bearing brace. Arch Phys Med Rehabil 1973; 54:562.

21. Morgan JM, Biehl WC, Wagner FW: Management of neuropathic arthropathy with Charcot restraint orthotic walker. Clin Orthop 1993; 296:58.

22. Beck C, Drez D: Instrumented testing of functional knee braces. Am J Sports Med 1986; 14:253.

23. Crawley PW: Postoperative knee bracing. Clin Sports Med 1990; 9:763.

24. Grace T: Prophylactic knee braces in injury to the lower extremity. J Bone Surg 1988; 70:422.

25. Horlick SG, Loomer RL: Valgus knee bracing for medial gonarthrosis. Clin J Sports Med 1993; 3:251.

26. Palumbo PM: Dynamic patellar brace: A new orthosis in the management of patellofemoral disorders. Am J Sports Med 1981; 9:45.

27. Hoehne JA: Weightbearing KAFO utilizing modern prosthetic above-knee socket design. J Prosthet Orthot 1989; 2:82.

28. Goldberg B, Hsu JD: Atlas of Orthoses and Assistive Devices, 3rd ed. St. Louis, Mosby, 1997.

29. Shamp JK: Neurophysiologic orthotic designs in the treatment of central nervous system disorders. J Prosthet Orthot 1989; 2:14.

30. Taylor CL, Harris SR: Effects of ankle-foot orthoses on functional motor performance in a child with spastic diplegia. Am J Occup Ther 1986; 40:492.

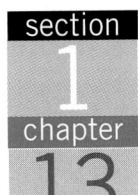

BASIC CONCEPTS OF BIOMECHANICS

David Pienkowski

Summary

- Simple principles of physics and mechanics can be used to calculate the forces exerted on human (or other animal) joints or generated by muscles. Forces usually considered in these calculations are (1) joint reaction forces, (2) ground reaction forces, and (3) muscle forces.
- The magnitude and direction of unknown muscle forces or joint reaction forces can be determined by simple algebraic, vector, or graphic methods.
- Biomechanical analyses often reveal nonintuitive (but experimentally verifiable) results, especially for joint reaction forces. For example, the hip joint reaction force in double-limb stance can be as small as one-third of body weight, but in single-limb stance the hip joint reaction force is approximately three times body weight.

Clinical Relevance

- Optimal healing of traumatized musculoskeletal tissue depends on the restoration of physiologically correct stress and strain in the cells of the tissue. A true understanding of this healing process requires quantitative knowledge of the "correct" levels of stress and strain.
- Biomechanical analysis is a tool for quantifying (1) how the musculoskeletal system works (i.e., what is normal), (2) departures from normal (as a result of trauma, wear, or disease), (3) how well a given therapy returns the system to normal, (4) the mechanical consequences of a new surgical procedure, prosthetic or orthotic device, or rehabilitation regimen.
- Good surgeons teach their patients the basic science underlying their condition and treatment. Biomechanics is an effective tool for communicating quantitative musculoskeletal truths to the patient (e.g., the seesaw model of the hip is a useful device to show how the abductor muscles maintain balance, why joint reaction forces during single-limb stance are large, and how postural swaying, weight loss, and use of a cane are effective means of reducing hip pain during weight-bearing activities).
- Simple biomechanical analyses often ignore the mechanical behavior of musculoskeletal tissue. However, the study of biomechanics is incomplete in the absence of tissue material property considerations (and vice versa).

Biomechanics applies engineering methods to anatomy and physiology to help understand and quantify the relationship among forces and the motion or deformation of musculoskeletal components. DaVinci is credited with the beginning of modern studies in biomechanics.[1]

CLINICAL RELEVANCE

Biomechanical analysis is a powerful tool for understanding how the joints of the body function normally and after trauma, disease, or surgical repair. Biomechanical analyses establish quantitative standards for clinical performance. Calculation of an unknown muscle or joint contact force can provide clinically useful information regarding, for example, the origin and degree of hip disorder and can allow one to predict the outcome if the conditions of the clinical situation change (e.g., weight gain or loss).

RELATION TO OTHER DISCIPLINES

The study of biomechanics is inseparably related to and influenced by anatomy, biology, orthopaedic practice, and materials considerations (Fig. 1). The simplifying assumptions used to formulate biomechanical problems differ from those actually present in the musculoskeletal system and the practice of orthopaedics. Knowledge of these related fields is, therefore, necessary to justify the simplifying assumptions as well as to make subsequent models more sophisticated and reflective of reality. This chapter considers only rigid body mechanics of the human skeleton (dark blue insert region of Fig. 1). Part II briefly considers deformable body (materials) mechanics (dashed outline region of Fig. 1).

THE APPROACH TO BIOMECHANICAL ANALYSIS

Analysis of a musculoskeletal joint begins with anatomic study of the joint followed by representation of this anatomy with engineering equivalents (e.g., rigid beams, cables, hinges, linear forces). A model built with these engineering equivalents can then be subjected to analyses by using simple principles of physics, mechanics, and mathematics.

DIMENSIONAL ANALYSIS

Study of biomechanics begins with an understanding of the units of measurement (Fig. 2), the most important of which are the fundamental units for length, mass, and time.[2] From these are derived specific quantities for torque (moment), speed, and acceleration and derived units with special names for force (newton) and power (watt). The correct scientific units are those of the International System of Units (SI), but the antiquated English system remains in

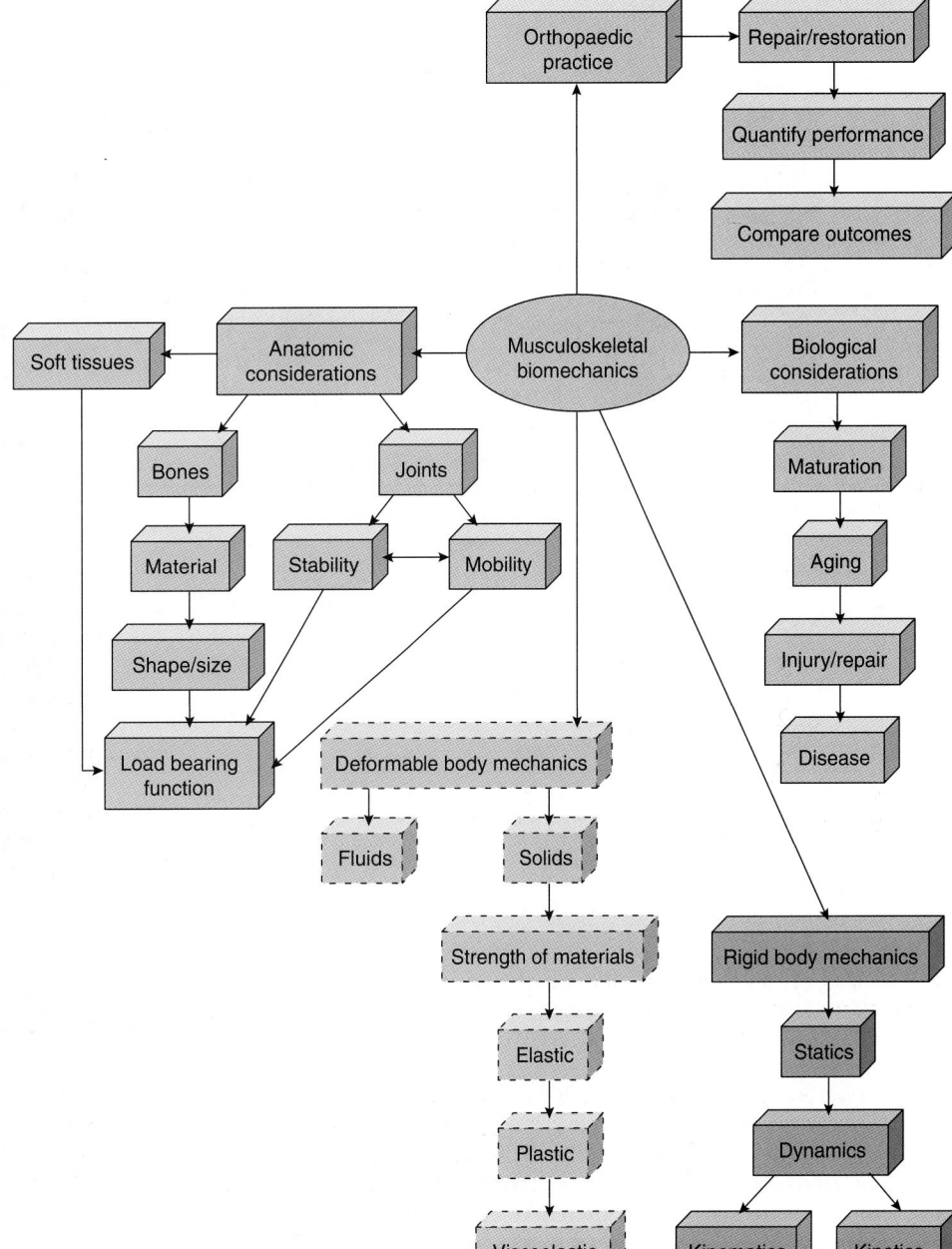

Fig. 1. The related fields of biomechanics. An understanding of musculoskeletal biomechanics requires knowledge of the anatomy and biology of the constituent tissues, material properties (of both rigid and deformable bodies), mechanics, and orthopaedic practice.

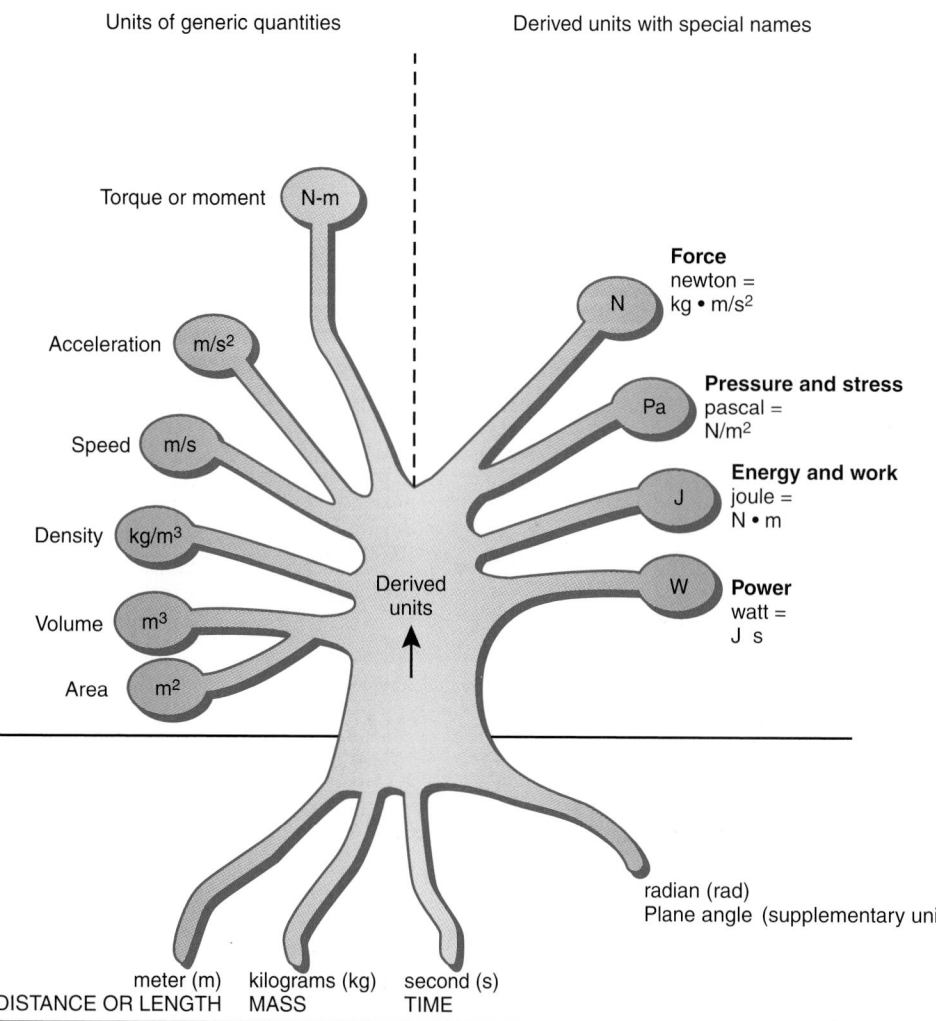

Units of generic quantities | Derived units with special names

Torque or moment   N-m

Acceleration   m/s²

Force
newton =
kg • m/s²

Speed   m/s

Pressure and stress
pascal =
N/m²

Density   kg/m³

Energy and work
joule =
N • m

Derived
units

Power
watt =
J s

Volume   m³

Area   m²

radian (rad)
Plane angle (supplementary unit)

meter (m)   kilograms (kg)   second (s)
DISTANCE OR LENGTH   MASS   TIME

Fundamental units of biomechanics

Fig. 2. The units of biomechanical analyses. Specific and derived units of biomechanical measurements are obtained from the fundamental units of length, mass, and time.

common use. The SI unit for force is the newton (4.448 N = 1 lb). Use of units to check the validity of a problem-solving effort is called dimensional analysis and should be routinely performed.

PART I: RIGID BODY MECHANICS

FUNDAMENTAL PRINCIPLES OF STATIC BIOMECHANICAL ANALYSES

Insight into the working of the musculoskeletal system can be obtained by using simple principles of rigid (nondeforming) body mechanics:

1. Two (the first and the third) of Newton's three laws of mechanics.
2. Three principles of static mechanical analyses (described later).
3. Models using one or more of six simple machines (i.e., lever, pulley, wheel, screw, wedge, inclined plane).
4. Simple algebraic, trigonometric, graphic, or vector analyses.

5. Application and interpretation of the numerical answer to solve the clinical problem and provide insight into how the answer would change if the parameters of the problem change.

Static biomechanical analyses require only Newton's first law of inertia (an object remains at rest or in a uniform state of motion [because of inertia] if it is acted on by zero net external force) and Newton's third law of action-reaction (for an object to remain in equilibrium, each force acting on the object must be balanced by an equal magnitude but oppositely directed reactive force). Dynamic (moving bodies) analyses, discussed in the last section of Part I, will require application of Newton's second law (force = mass times acceleration). Principles of static mechanical analyses needed for biomechanics are (1) bodies in equilibrium are in equilibrium along each of their axes, (2) forces are transmitted from one body to another only by direct contact of bodies, and (3) forces can be mathematically or graphically manipulated according to the principles of vector analysis.

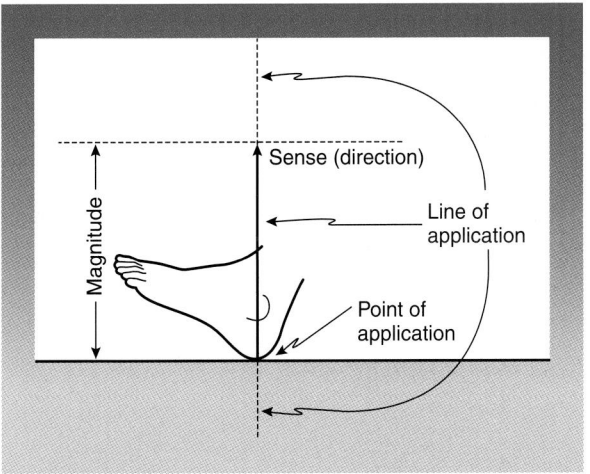

Fig. 3. The four elements of a vector. Considering each vector as being composed of the four elements shown facilitates graphic solution of biomechanical problems.

VECTORS AND VECTOR ANALYSIS

A vector is a quantity (e.g., a muscle force or a joint reaction force) that has both magnitude and direction. The magnitude and direction of a muscle force or a joint reaction force are often of clinical importance. Vector analysis is a convenient means for quantifying these forces. A vector consists of four elements: point of application, line of application, sense (direction), and magnitude (Fig. 3). The first two (point of application and line of application) may be graphically manipulated (i.e., moved along parallel paths) to obtain the solution to a biomechanics problem in which these lines represent musculoskeletal vector quantities. This is commonly done in vector addition (Fig. 4). In this illustration, vector **A** is moved parallel to its original location (dashed lines) to form a parallelogram, which can be resolved trigonometrically. The diagonal of this parallelogram (vector **C**) is the sum of vector **A** and vector **B**. This graphic movement of the point of application and line of application of vector **A** and vector **B** to form a parallelogram stands in sharp contrast to the inviolability of the sense and magnitude of a vector. That is, the sense and magnitude (length of the line) of a vector may never be manipulated. Thus, in Figure 4, dashed **A** can never be longer or shorter than solid **A**, nor can it point in any direction other than the direction of solid **A**.

VECTOR DECOMPOSITION

A vector that does not lie perfectly along one axis but, instead, is pointed in a combination of two directions (i.e., at an angle θ) can be "decomposed" into its components in both of these directions (Fig. 5). This is commonly done by a graphic technique in which the projection of **A** onto the X axis determines the component of **A** along the X axis (i.e., A_X). A similar process is used for the Y axis to calculate the component of **A** in the Y direction (A_Y). Vector decomposition can also be done trigonometrically:

$$A_X = \mathbf{A} \cos \theta$$

$$A_Y = \mathbf{A} \sin \theta$$

Vector decomposition is just the reverse of vector addition. That is,

$$A_X + A_Y = \mathbf{A} \text{ (graphic addition) or}$$

$$\sqrt{(A^2_X + A^2_Y)} = |\mathbf{A}|,$$

where the two vertical lines denote the magnitude of **A**.

CLINICAL IMPORTANCE OF VECTOR DECOMPOSITION

Vector directions are always expressed with respect to a coordinate system, usually the right-hand Cartesian coordinate system with two or three mutually perpendicular axes, each of which are usually oriented vertically and horizontally to the observer. However, there are occasions in which the best coordinate system is one that coincides with the long axis of a bone to facilitate an understanding of the clinical relevance of the vector components. Usefulness of anatomic axes, instead of fixed coordinate axes, is best demonstrated by considering a two-dimensional engineering model of a selected upper extremity muscle.[3] The biceps muscle generates a force $\mathbf{F}_B$ that is vertical and directed upward (Fig. 6). The line of action of this muscle is vertical and parallel to the humerus. The biceps muscle attaches

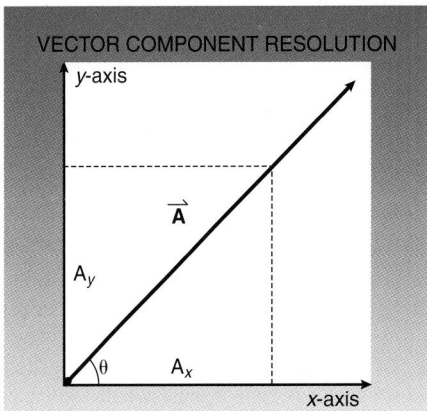

Fig. 5. Decomposition of a vector. A vector at an angle can be "decomposed" into its X-axis and Y-axis components as shown. Vector decomposition is useful for solving problems in biomechanics and for providing a clinically useful interpretation of a vector.

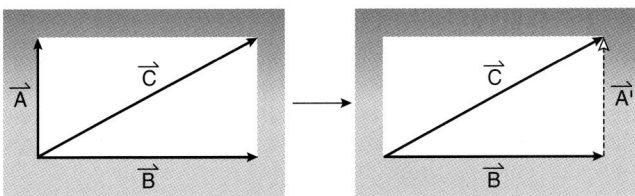

Fig. 4. Graphic addition of two vectors. Vectors **A** and **B** are graphically added to yield vector **C** by completing the parallelogram. This illustration also shows the tip-to-tail method of vector addition and builds on the graphic manipulation of the four vector elements shown in Figure 3.

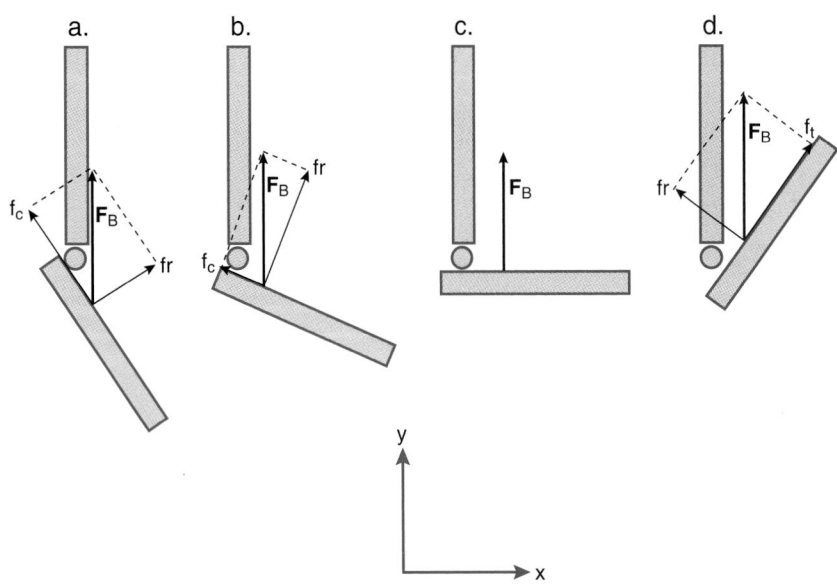

Fig. 6. Decomposition of biceps muscle force in the flexed and extended forearm. Vector decomposition can be used to explain the component of muscle force that causes limb segment motion and the ability to hold weight in the hand and can also provide insights regarding muscle-related joint stability or instability.

to the radius/ulna at a single point. The biceps muscle force $\mathbf{F_B}$ is decomposed not into X- and Y-axis components but components parallel (f_C) and perpendicular (f_R) to the radius/ulna model. Note that

$$\sqrt{(f^2_C + f^2_R)} = |\mathbf{F_B}|$$

where the two vertical lines denote the magnitude of $\mathbf{F_B}$. Note the clinical relevance of these two components: f_C is responsible for generating a compressive force that tends to compress that segment of the ulna/radius that lies between the biceps muscle insertion and the humerus, whereas f_R is the component of the biceps muscle force perpendicular to the long axis of the radius/ulna (this force causes forearm rotation, i.e., flexion). As the forearm flexes (moves from a to d in Fig. 6), notice how the magnitudes of each of the components of $\mathbf{F_B}$ change relative to the moving reference frame (the long axis of the radius/ulna). The component tending to rotate the forearm (f_R) increases with flexion and reaches a maximum when the elbow is at a 90-degree angle (Fig. 6C). At this angle, all of the biceps muscle force tends to flex the forearm in this position. That is,

$$\mathbf{F_B} = f_R$$

and the biceps muscle no longer provides compression of the segment of the ulna/radius that lies between the biceps muscle insertion and the humerus (i.e., $f_C = 0$). As forearm flexion continues, the magnitude of the rotational component f_R decreases, but the other component of $\mathbf{F_B}$ changes sign ($\mathbf{F}$ compression becomes $\mathbf{F}$ tension relative to the long axis of the forearm) and now tends to lengthen the segment of the ulna/radius that lies between the biceps muscle insertion and the humerus.

The preceding demonstrates (1) the usefulness of decomposing vectors relative to a bone's long axis (instead of fixed external X-Y axes) to gain meaningful insights into muscle contributions to joint stability (compression) and

motion (rotation), (2) how the anatomy and point of attachment of varying muscles can provide different contributions to joint stability and motion, and (3) the musculoskeletal importance (and prevalence) of a third-class lever (fulcrum-effort-load) design.[4] This compact (muscles close to bones) third-class lever design allows a large range of high-speed motion as well as great strength despite the apparent mechanical disadvantage. This strength occurs because of the penniform arrangement of muscle fibers in the arm[5] that provides high-force contraction over a small excursion (exactly the demands of this biomechanical design). This underscores the importance of considering both musculoskeletal anatomy and physiology as integral components of every biomechanical analysis (see Fig. 1).

GRAPHIC ANALYSIS OF JOINT BIOMECHANICS

Graphic vector analysis is also useful to obtain quantitative information regarding muscle and joint reaction forces. A classic example of simple graphic analysis is to calculate the forces generated during stair climbing.[2] The specific problem is to determine the magnitude of the knee extensor muscle force and the tibio-femoral joint reaction force (Fig. 7A). This model excludes the femur, upper thigh, and remainder of the upper body because they have no role in modeling the problem in question. It is useful to assume in this and most simple two-dimensional models that only one muscle group is responsible for maintaining the position shown. In this case, the quadriceps group is considered to be the only muscle that extends the knee and is responsible for resisting gravity to maintain the position shown. This single-muscle assumption enables a simple three-force (muscle, joint reaction, and ground reaction) model to be constructed and solved by graphic methods.

Each of these three forces is then decomposed into each of their four vector elements as done previously (see Fig. 3). The ground reaction force has a magnitude equal to and oppositely directed from the body weight $\mathbf{W}$ of the subject (from Newton's third law). Because force is transmitted

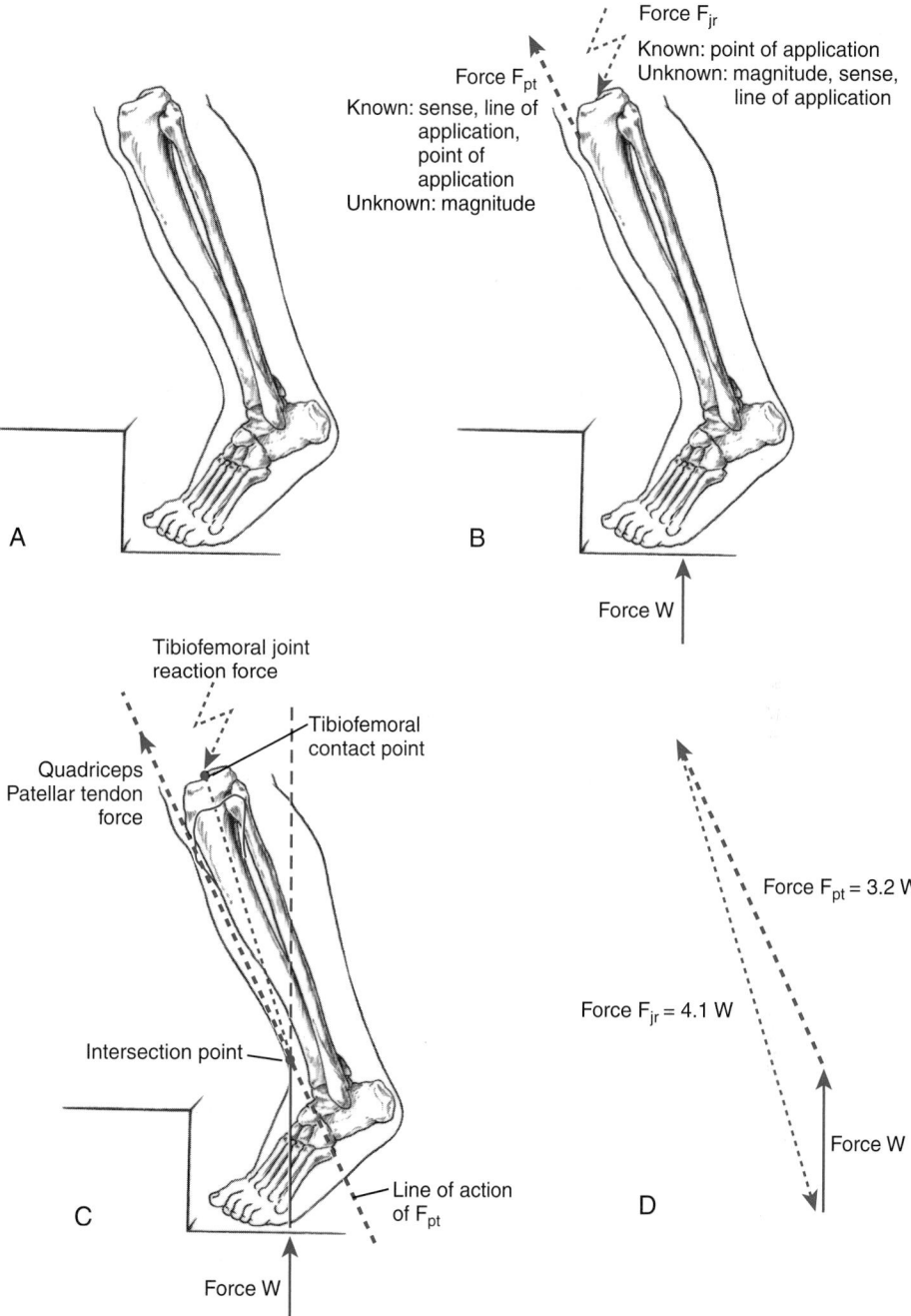

Fig. 7. Static biomechanical analysis of knee forces during stair climbing. The processes of formulating and determining the muscle and joint reaction forces in the knee of a stair climber during single-limb stance are shown.

only by direct contact, the point of application of this force is known, and because gravity is vertical, the line of application is known and so is the sense (upward). Thus, all four elements of the ground reaction force vector **W** are known. The joint reaction force $\mathbf{F}_{jr}$ is of unknown magnitude, sense, and line of application. All that is known of $\mathbf{F}_{jr}$ is its point of application. (It must be the tibio-femoral contact point because of the principle that forces are transmitted only by direct contact.) The quadriceps muscle force ($\mathbf{F}_{pt}$) has a line of action along the patellar tendon and is thus parallel to the long axis of the tibia (not the long axis of the femur). Thus, three elements of this force vector

(point and line of application and sense) are known. Only the magnitude of $\mathbf{F}_{pt}$ remains unknown (Fig. 7B).

To solve for the magnitudes of $\mathbf{F}_{jr}$ and $\mathbf{F}_{pt}$, note that the lines of action of **W** and $\mathbf{F}_{pt}$ intersect at a point just anterior to the ankle (Fig. 7C). Because these three forces are in equilibrium in this two-dimensional model, the line of action of $\mathbf{F}_{jr}$ must also pass through this intersection point. This means that the line of action of $\mathbf{F}_{jr}$ is defined by the intersection point and the tibio-femoral contact point. Three forces in equilibrium in two dimensions are known as *concurrent* forces and must form a closed triangle.[4] To do this, the vector **W** is moved upward along its line of action until its lower end touches the intersection point. This is permissible because neither the magnitude nor the sense of **W** are altered. $\mathbf{F}_{jr}$ is moved to the left, parallel to its original direction, until its lower end touches the lower end of **W** and the upper end touches the point of application of $\mathbf{F}_{pt}$. This completes the triangle (Fig. 7D) and is the hallmark of static equilibrium of three forces in two dimensions. Given a known body weight **W**, the tibiofemoral joint reaction force during single-limb stance of stair climbing is thus 4.1 times the magnitude of **W**, and the quadriceps muscle force required to maintain this position is 3.2 times **W**.

ANALYTIC VERSUS GRAPHIC METHODS

Graphic analysis is simple and easily communicated to patients and students. The accuracy of graphic analysis is surprisingly good, as shown in the following example. Consider a person of weight W standing with heel elevated on one limb (Fig. 8). If the goal is to calculate the muscle force $\mathbf{F}_{ts}$ enabling this position to be maintained, as well as the joint reaction force of the tibia on the talus, $\mathbf{F}_{jt}$, one can take an analytical approach. As before, it is assumed that a single muscle group (the triceps surae) holds the limb in the position shown. On the basis of a study of the pertinent anatomy, one can estimate the angle of the line of action of this muscle with the horizontal (45 degrees) and (as also estimated from anatomy) the line of action of the joint reaction force is 60 degrees with the horizontal. Assuming a two-dimensional problem and that all bodies are rigid (nondeformable), the principles of static biomechani-

cal analyses can be used: if the body under consideration is truly in equilibrium, then it must be in equilibrium in each of its component directions (i.e., the X and Y axes). This principle, which has its origins in Newton's first and third laws, states that the sum (denoted by Σ) of X-axis forces is equal to zero:

$$\Sigma F_X = 0$$

and the sum of Y-axis forces is equal to zero:

$$\Sigma F_Y = 0$$

Replacing forces with their algebraic equivalents (and being careful to associate the correct signs with the directions of these forces) and summing these forces to zero leads to

$$\Sigma F_x = 0 \text{ means that } \mathbf{F}_{jt} \cos \beta = \mathbf{F}_{ts} \cos \alpha$$

and

$$\Sigma F_y = 0 \text{ means that } \mathbf{F}_{jt} \sin \beta = \mathbf{F}_{ts} \sin \alpha + W$$

Because there are two unknowns and two independent equations, the unknowns can be explicitly determined:

$$\mathbf{F}_{ts} = 1.92 \ W$$

$$\mathbf{F}_{jt} = 2.72 \ W$$

Although this analytical approach used many simplifying assumptions, more sophisticated models could use one or more of the following: multiple muscle groups instead of one, distributed instead of point forces, forces in three dimensions instead of two, deformable bodies instead of rigid bodies.

A graphic model of this problem is similar to the knee (see Fig. 7). It is another two-dimensional three-concurrent-force model. The three forces are the ground reaction force (all four vector elements known), the triceps surae muscle force (all but the magnitude known, the other three elements determined from anatomy), and the joint reaction force (only the point of application is known). Extending the lines of action of the joint reaction force and the muscle force, determining the point of intersection, forming the line of action of the joint reaction force by drawing a line containing the point of application of the joint reactive force and this point of intersection, and shifting the line of action of the joint reaction force parallel to form a closed-force triangle (indicative of static equilibrium) yield the results presented in Figure 9. Here, the magnitudes of the two calculated forces ($\mathbf{F}_{ts} = 1.84 \ W$ and $\mathbf{F}_{jt} = 2.62 \ W$) can be compared with those calculated in the preceding paragraphs by using an analytical approach. This comparison shows that the joint reaction and muscle forces calculated by the graphic method are approximately 4% different from those calculated analytically. Given the assumptions made to simplify the model, this is good agreement indeed. Thus, for many purposes, the choice of technique (graphic, analytical, vector) is immaterial with regard to accuracy.

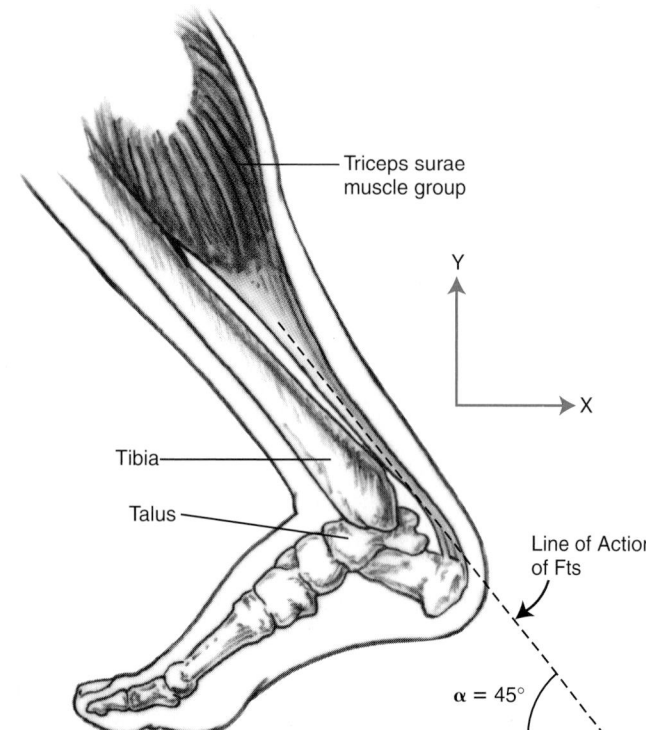

Fig. 8. Static biomechanics of the ankle joint during raised-heel single-leg stance. The components of interest in the early stages of formulating an approach to solving for the magnitude of the triceps surae muscle force and tibio-talar joint reaction force are shown.

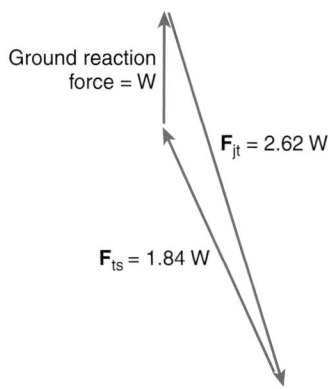

Fig. 9. Graphic solution of ankle joint static biomechanics. A completed triangle is formed from the three concurrent forces (ground reaction force = body weight of the subject, tibio-talar joint reaction force, and triceps surae muscle force) as shown in Figure 8. This closed triangle provides the solution to the desired muscle and joint reaction forces (expressed in body weight [**W**] units).

TORQUE AND LIMB SEGMENT ROTATION

The upper and lower extremities perform their tasks of feeding, grooming, gait, and so on because muscles attached to these limbs (that have a nonzero force component perpendicular to the long axis of the limb) contract and rotate the limb segment (compare with Clinical Importance of Vector Decomposition section). Force generation alone is insufficient to cause limb rotation: force must act at a distance from the center (or axis) of rotation in a direction perpendicular to this distance to generate a torque that produces limb segment rotation. Torque is calculated from the expression

$$\mathbf{T} = \mathbf{r} \times \mathbf{F},$$

where $\mathbf{T}$ is the torque (units of newton-meters), $\mathbf{r}$ is the "lever arm" (i.e., the perpendicular distance of the line of action of the force from the center of rotation), and $\mathbf{F}$ is the muscle force. The "$\times$" here denotes a vector multiplication operation called a cross-product whose magnitude can be expressed as

$$|\mathbf{T}| = |\mathbf{r}|\, |\mathbf{F}|\, \sin\theta$$

The muscle force $\mathbf{F}$ is determined by muscle volume, muscle length, type of muscle, arrangement of muscle fibers, degree of effort, and other factors.[6] Lever arm considerations (i.e., the musculoskeletal implications of r) require further elaboration. In some instances (e.g., the elbow), the lever arm distance changes with elbow flexion such that r increases to aid the muscle force in generating torque for lifting weights (Fig. 10). A weight placed in the hand requires the least counterbalancing torque when the arm is extended and the most counterbalancing torque when the arm is flexed at 90 degrees. The anatomy of the upper extremity helps meet these load-bearing demands by increasing r with increasing elbow flexion.

Similarly, the knee uses the patella (Fig. 11) to vary the lever arm through which the quadriceps muscle creates torque that extends the knee. When the knee of a seated patient is extended (leg horizontal), the torque required to

Fig. 10. Schematic illustration of the extended and flexed upper extremity. The point of attachment of the biceps muscle, in conjunction with the anatomic design of the elbow joint, contributes to lever arm increases that aid muscle force–generated torque that in turn enables limb segment rotation. It is important to note that r_{flexed} is greater than $r_{extended}$.

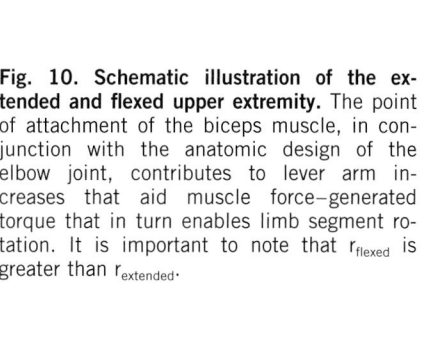
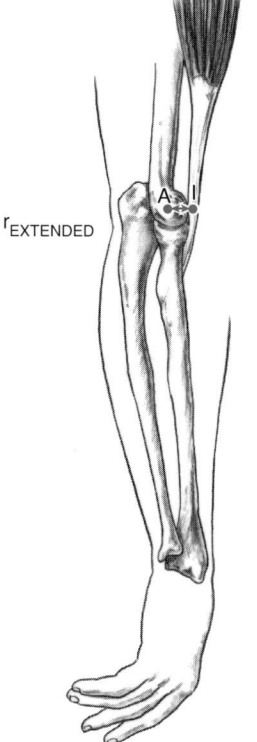
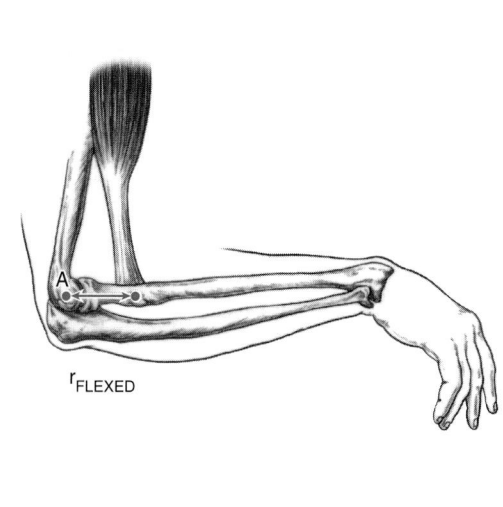

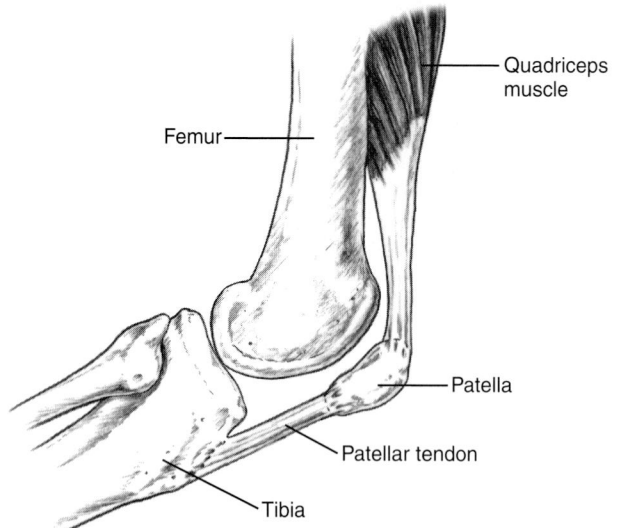

Fig. 11. Sagittal view of the knee. The patella serves as a variable-lever arm for the quadriceps muscle and thereby increases extension torque at the knee.

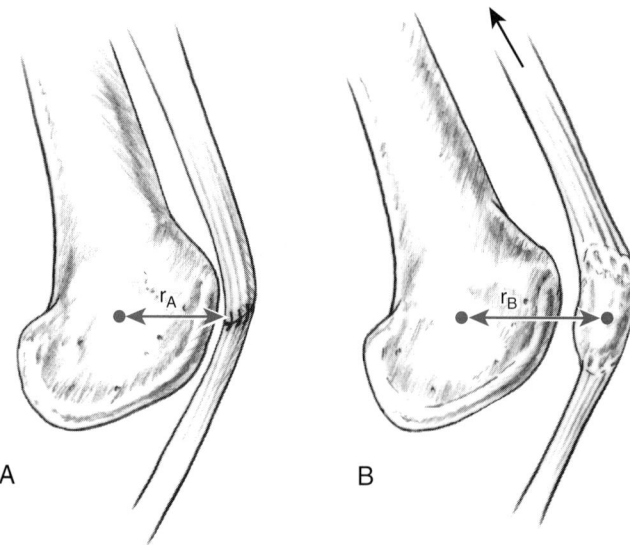

Fig. 13. The effect of patellectomy on the quadriceps lever arm. Patellectomy reduces the lever arm r (from r_B to r_A) of the quadriceps muscle and thereby increases the force required of this muscle to cause the same degree of knee extension.

hold the leg in this position is maximal. To increase the torque required to hold the leg in full extension (horizontal) and decrease the force requirements of the quadriceps muscle, the patella serves as a variable-lever arm. With increasing knee extension, the patella rises up from within the femoral notch to increase the quadriceps lever arm (Fig. 12A). Rotation of the leg from a flexed-knee position (thigh horizontal) requires much less torque, and in this case the patella "sinks" into the femoral notch, thereby

reducing the quadriceps lever arm (Fig. 12B). Treatment of knee pain by patellectomy leads to loss of this variable-lever arm (Fig. 13) and substantially increases the peak magnitude of muscle force required to extend the leg. Surgical elevation of the tibial tubercle (Fig. 14) is another method of increasing the quadriceps lever arm $\mathbf{r}$, thereby decreasing the muscle force $\mathbf{F}_q$ required and subsequently decreasing the joint (patello-femoral) reaction force $\mathbf{F}_{jpf}$ and thus possibly decreasing pain.

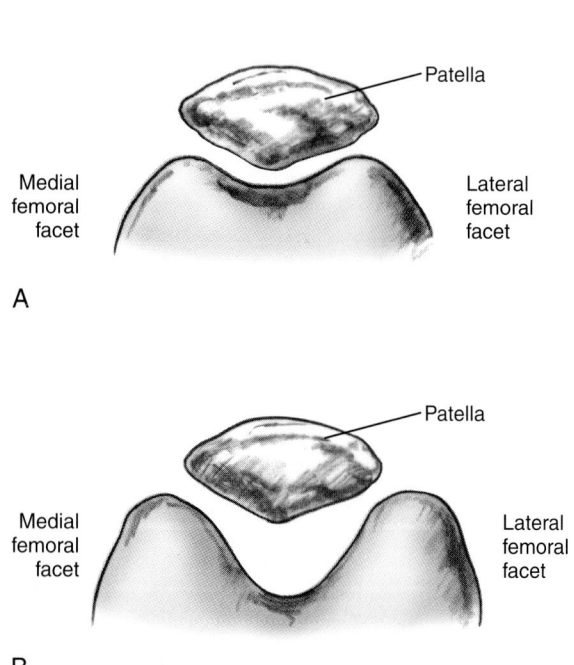

Fig. 12. Transverse view of the patello-femoral joint. The patella "rides up" (superiorly and anteriorly) from the femoral notch during knee extension (B to A) to increase the lever arm of the quadriceps muscle when torque is most needed.

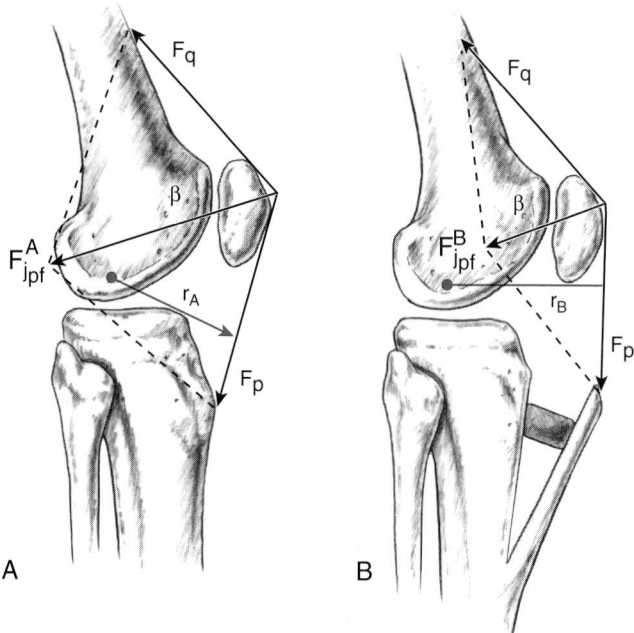

Fig. 14. Elevation of the tibial tubercle. Elevating the tibial tubercle can increase the lever arm of the quadriceps. Less quadriceps muscle force is now needed to generate the same torque, and the magnitude of the patello-femoral contact force (F_{jpp}) is also reduced. (Redrawn from Maquet P: Mechanics and osteoarthritis of the patello-femoral joint. Clin Orthop 1979; 144:70.)

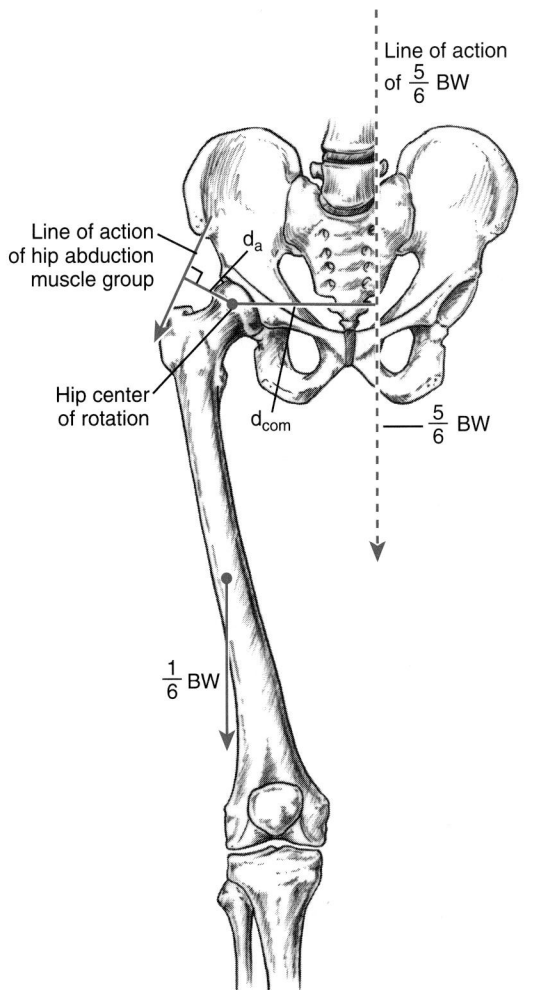

Fig. 15. Diagram of the hip during single-limb stance. The center of rotation of the hip, the lever arm of the abductor muscle forces (d_a), and the lever arm (d_{com}) of the remainder of body weight (5/6 W) that must be balanced by the hip abductor muscles are shown.

TORQUE AND BALANCE ABOUT THE HIP DURING SINGLE-LEG LIMB STANCE

A first-class lever (load-fulcrum-force) is a useful model for understanding body balance during the single-limb stance portion of the gait cycle and also offers insights into how to alleviate hip pain during weightbearing activity.[4] Equilibrium of this model relies on equating the torques generated on each side of the hip (just as would be done for each side of a seesaw). As in all biomechanics problems, we begin with consideration of the anatomy of the hip (Fig. 15). Assuming a fixed hip center of rotation (as shown) located a distance d_a from the line of action of the hip abductor muscle group (this anatomically measured distance is approximately 0.05 m), the force generated by this muscle group must create a torque that counterbalances the torque created in the other direction by the body weight supported by the standing limb acting over the distance d_{com}. Because each lower extremity weighs approximately 1/6 BW, the weight of the body supported by the standing limb is 5/6 BW. Equilibrium during standing and postural balance during the single-limb stance portion of gait occur

because the abductor muscle group creates a torque about the center of rotation of the hip that equals 5/6 BW times the horizontal distance from the center of rotation of the hip to the center of the 5/6 BW body mass (d_{com}). A first-class lever model (Fig. 16) equates the torque created by the hip abductor muscles to the torque created by 5/6 BW. That is,

$$F_{ha} \times d_a = 5/6 \text{ BW} \times d_{com},$$

where F_{ha} is the hip abductor muscle force. Based on anatomic measurements and center-of-mass calculations,[3] the value for d_{com} is typically about 0.11 m. Note carefully that this center of mass of the body in single-limb stance is located to the right (in the diagram) of the anatomic center. This center-of-mass offset occurs because the supporting limb is removed from the center of mass calculation, and thus the center of mass shifts to the side of the limb not touching the ground. Note also that because the lever arm d_a is much shorter than the lever arm d_{com}, the hip abductors must contract with considerably more force (1.83 BW) than might be expected.

Similarly, from the seesaw analogy, the total weight on the fulcrum (in this case the hip) equals the two forces, F_{ha} and 5/6 BW. Thus, the hip joint reaction force is

$$F_{hjr} = F_{ha} + 5/6 \text{ BW}.$$

Typically, for a 734-N (165-lb) adult, the hip abductor muscles must generate 1343 N (302 lb), and this produces a joint reaction force of 1982 N (446 lb, 2.7 W; Fig. 17A). This surprising result is in marked contrast to the hip joint reaction force generated during static dual-limb stance (1/3 W on each hip).

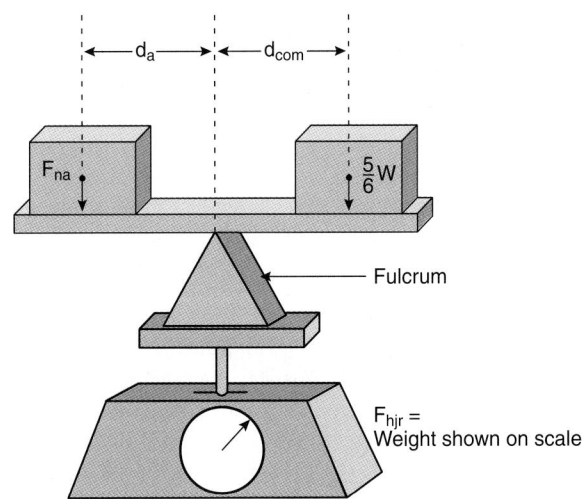

Fig. 16. Torque equivalence of a balanced seesaw. A first-class lever is the model for balance at the hip during the single-limb stance portion of gait and the lumbar spine during lifting. Note that the seesaw balances when

$$F_{na}d_a = \tfrac{5}{6} W d_{com}$$

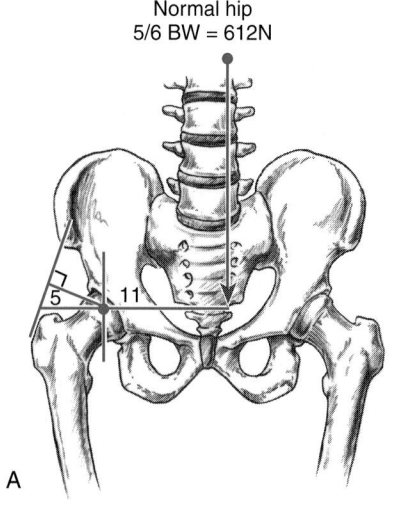

Normal hip
5/6 BW = 612N

A

1 pound
Weight gain
5/6 BW = 616N

B

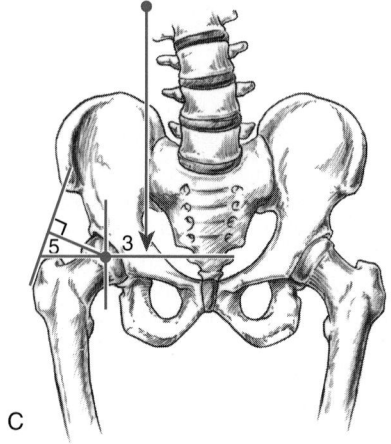

Lateral lean =
5/6 BW lever arm
reduction

C

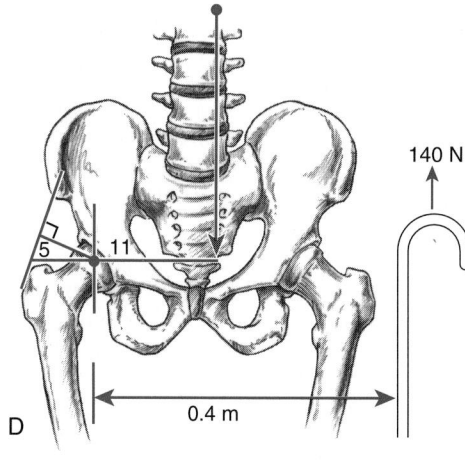

Use of cane =
additional torque
supplementing hip abductors

140 N

0.4 m

D

Fig. 17. Changes in hip joint reaction force as a result of weight gain, lateral leaning, and cane use. By studying Figure 16 and by using the quantitative methods of the simple seesaw model, one can gain an understanding of the variation in forces about the hip that result from variation in the individual's activities, posture, weight, and so on. (Modified from Fung YC: Biomechanics: Mechanical Properties of Living Tissues. New York, Springer-Verlag, 1993.)

Patients with painful hips are well advised to lose weight, because for each pound of body weight lost the hip joint reaction force will decrease by 2.7 lb (Fig. 17B). Changes in the abductor muscle force lever arm should be considered when reducing and fixing femoral neck fractures, because alterations of neck angle can alter the force required of the abductors. Similarly, swaying the upper torso toward the painful hip during single-limb stance on that hip (the lateral lurch shown in Fig. 17C) reduces the lever arm through which 5/6 BW acts, thus reducing the muscle force required and substantially reducing $\mathbf{F}_{hjr}$.[7] The simple lever model of the hip also demonstrates the effectiveness of cane use for reducing hip forces during single-limb stance.[4] The cane's efficacy (Fig. 17D) derives not as much from the modest force exerted on the cane but primarily from the long lever arm through which this modest force acts.

FORCE AND TORQUE CONSIDERATIONS IN THE LUMBAR SPINE

A first-class lever model can also be used to understand the high loads imposed on the lumbar spine during lifting tasks

(Fig. 18). The erector spinae muscles are the primary force-generating muscles that act about a very short lever arm (the distance from the line of action of the erector spinae muscles to the center of the lumbar disk is approximately 3 cm). Considerable muscle force must be exerted to maintain the body in the posture shown because the center of mass of the upper body $\mathbf{W}_B$ (viewed from a sagittal perspective) is anterior to the long axis of the spine. When an object is lifted and held a considerable distance $\mathbf{d}_o$ anterior to the spine, the torque generated by the product of this weight and its large distance from the spine means that, because of the small distance through which they act, the erector spinae muscles must generate a large force to supply the torque needed to maintain an erect posture. That is,

$$\mathbf{F}_{es} \times \mathbf{d}_{es} = \mathbf{W}_B \times \mathbf{d}_B + \mathbf{W}_O \times \mathbf{d}_o.$$

The sum of these forces ($\mathbf{F}_{es} + \mathbf{W}_B + \mathbf{W}_o$) often exceeds 11 times body weight primarily because $\mathbf{F}_{es}$ is large. Such large lumbar spine joint reaction forces, repetitively applied to aging lumbar vertebrae segments, provide insight

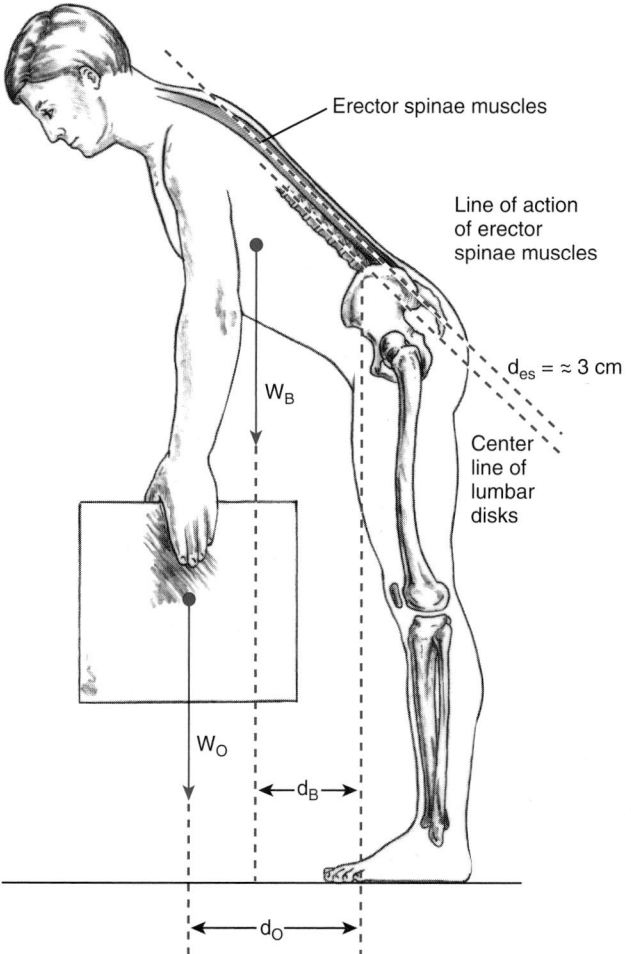

Fig. 18. Forces on the lumbar spine. The erector spinae muscles act over a small lever arm (distance from their insertion to the center of the lumbar vertebral disk) to balance the upper body mass and loads held in the hand that are at a considerable distance from this fulcrum.

into the high incidence of lower back pain and injury, especially during "improper" (excessive lever arms or load magnitudes) lifting.[8]

KINEMATICS OF HUMAN MOTION

Kinematics is the study of body (whole or segment) motion without consideration of the forces that cause the motion. Studies of kinematics are especially important for low-load-bearing/high-mobility joints in the hand and upper extremity but have also found considerable use in understanding human gait. Study of gait kinematics begins with terminology of the gait cycle (Fig. 19). Readers should be aware of the two different sets of terms that exist to describe gait.[9] More advanced study of kinematics frequently involves quantitative descriptions of one body that is translating in three dimensions and simultaneously rotating on three separate axes with respect to a fixed coordinate system. Although study of three-dimensional translation is a comparatively simple endeavor that has been described in many sources,[3] quantitative description of three-dimensional rotation of an object makes use of tools unfamiliar to most. These tools include use of direction cosines, projection angles, Cardan angles, Euler angles, Euler parameters, and helical axes of motion.[10] Each of these represents a specific mathematical approach to quantifying the three-dimensional rotation of one body relative to another fixed body, and each tool has its own advantages and disadvantages for specific circumstances. Further discussion of three-dimensional rotations involves mathematical development beyond the scope of this chapter. The interested reader is referred to other sources.[11]

Dynamics of Musculoskeletal Movement

Static biomechanical analyses of individual joints in equilibrium require an inventory of muscle, gravitational, and joint reaction forces, all of which were added and equated to zero. When bodies are in motion, however, Newton's second law (F = ma) must be considered, and it gives rise to increased amplitudes of existing muscle and joint reaction forces. These increased force amplitudes arise because

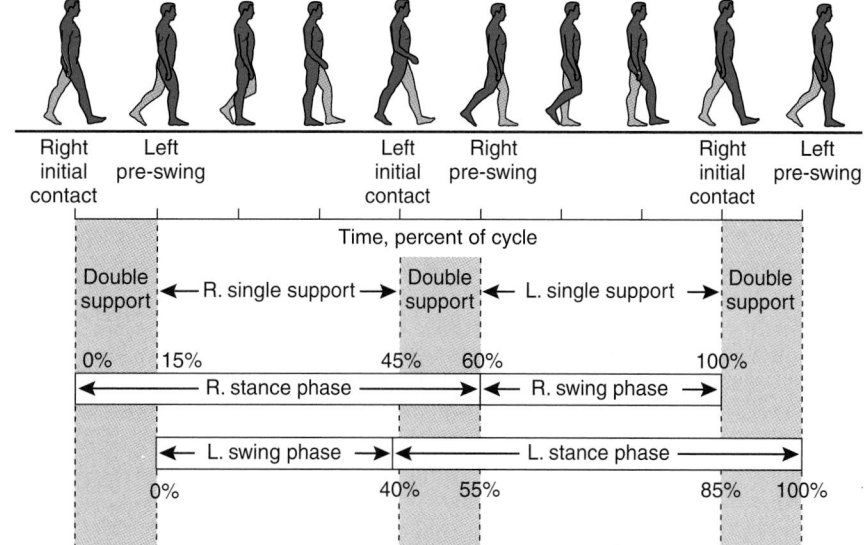

Fig. 19. The human gait cycle. Terminology used to describe gait and the timing of the gait cycle events is shown. (Adapted from Inman VT: Human Walking. Baltimore, Williams & Wilkins, 1981, p 26.)

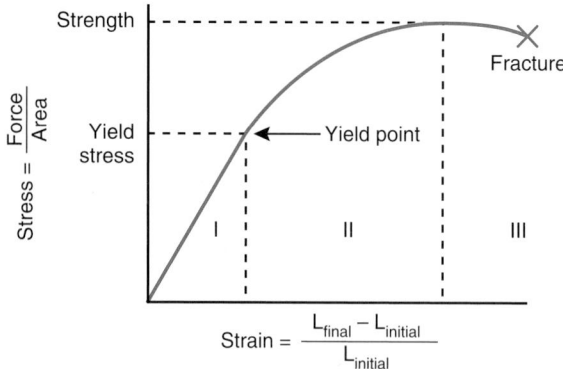

Fig. 20. Stress-strain relationship of human bone in tension. This is the stress-strain relationship of an ideal material when subjected to uniaxial tension.

of the increased muscle forces that cause the motion and the increased joint reaction forces that must oppose these muscle forces.

For example, consider the knee of a seated patient whose thigh is horizontal and the lower limb is flexed at a 60-degree angle to the vertical.[3] To hold this limb steady in this position, a classic static biomechanical analysis shows that the quadriceps muscle must generate a force of 195 N and a tibio-femoral joint reaction force of 158 N is present. If instead of holding the limb motionless at this angle, the individual is now actively engaged in a maximal quadriceps muscle effort to extend the vertically hanging lower limb (i.e., rotate it as rapidly as possible), a dynamic biomechanical analysis must now be performed. If this analysis is done for the instant when the limb is at the same 60-degree angle, inclusion of F = ma terms in the force equilibrium equations reveals that the quadriceps muscle must now generate 1488 N of force and a joint reaction force of 1349 N results. The effect of this maximal muscle contraction and dynamic limb swinging results in muscle and joint reaction forces that increase approximately eightfold. The increased muscle and joint loads resulting from dynamic movements have been confirmed by empirical measurements. More details on musculoskeletal dynamics can be found in other sources.[3, 5, 11]

PART II: DEFORMABLE BODY MECHANICS

LOAD-BEARING ROLE OF MUSCULOSKELETAL TISSUES

Bone and soft tissues that comprise a joint experience the joint reaction forces calculated in Part I. To function well, these tissues must withstand these forces and not fracture or deform excessively while in service. To better understand how the musculoskeletal system performs its load-bearing function, the simplistic rigid body assumptions made in Part I of this chapter are now discarded in favor of a more realistic consideration of the actual mechanical behavior of the solid materials used in the musculoskeletal system. Although the remainder of this section focuses on the load-bearing properties of musculoskeletal tissues, it is

important for the reader to remember that the load-bearing properties of bone are secondary to the organism's need for calcium homeostasis.[12]

STRENGTH OF MATERIALS FUNDAMENTALS

Study of deformable bodies (materials) allows an understanding of how force applied to musculoskeletal parts causes a change in the dimensions of those parts. A commonly used approach for the study of deformable body mechanics is the stress-strain curve (Fig. 20). Stress (force divided by original cross-sectional area of the object to which the force is applied) measured in units of pascals [see Fig. 2]) is plotted as a function of strain (change in length of the object divided by the object's initial length) measured in dimensionless units of meters per meter of a precision machined object being loaded. Note that there are three regions of this stress-strain curve. Region I represents the initial linear portion of the curve, and it is a measure of the elastic properties of the material. Elasticity is a material's property that is defined by Hooke's law[13]:

$$F = kx,$$

where F is the force (or load) applied to deform the material, x is the amount of material deformation caused by the force F, that is,

$$x = l_f - l_i$$

and k is a constant of proportionality (Fig. 21). If force is divided by the object's original cross-sectional area and deformation is divided by the object's initial length (l_i), then the F = kx relationship can be expressed as

$$\sigma = E\epsilon,$$

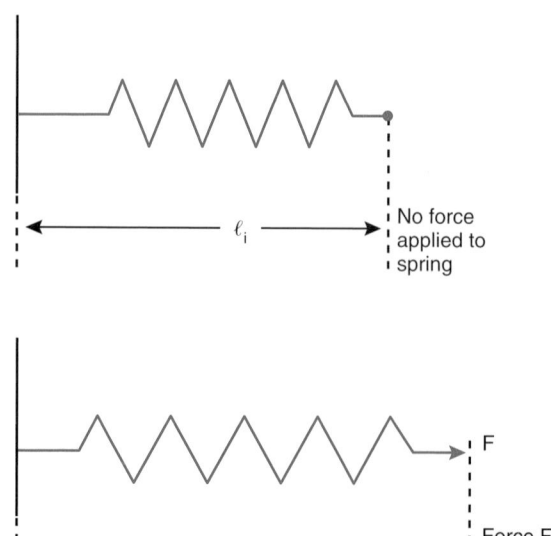

Fig. 21. Linear elastic deformation of a spring. Hooke's law shows how an applied force F causes a linear elastic deformation (x) of a spring according to a proportionality constant (k).

where σ denotes stress and ϵ denotes strain. When the object is subjected to a tensile force (pulled apart), the constant of proportionality k is known as Young's modulus and is commonly given the symbol E. This linearly elastic region represents a nonpermanent, recoverable elastic deformation of the object. During Region I, the total volume of the object increases as a result of this elastic deformation.

Eventually when subjected to a progressively increasing force, the object reaches a point at which the material can no longer withstand the force applied. This point, commonly called the yield point, is the degree of deformation beyond which the material cannot fully recover spontaneously when the deforming force is released. Beyond the yield point, the material begins yielding and undergoes subsequent permanent nonrecoverable plastic deformation. The plastic deformation section of the stress-strain curve, Region II, is characterized by no net change in volume of the material. The maximum stress withstood by the material is called the strength of the material. After the peak of the stress-strain curve has been reached, the material can no longer withstand the increasing applied load and often begins a rapid progression to failure (Region III).

STRESS-STRAIN VERSUS LOAD-DEFORMATION CURVES

Stress-strain curves are independent of the shape of the object being deformed. Load-deformation curves can look very similar to stress-strain curves, but load-deformation curves not only measure the intrinsic material properties of the material but also take into account the shape of the object. This distinction is subtle but important: load-deformation curves define the *extrinsic* mechanical properties of an object and are never to be confused with stress-strain curves, which define the intrinsic material properties of an object.

BONE MATERIAL CHARACTERISTICS, SIZE, AND SHAPE

Shape, size, and material properties all have important roles in the ability of musculoskeletal components to bear load without fracture or excessive deformation. For example, the size of bone will change in response to the loads to which it is exposed. The outer diameter of a normal young adult femur will increase to compensate for increased applied loads (e.g., arising from a newly implemented weightlifting exercise program). Outer femoral cortical diameter will also increase in response to increasing bone porosity (i.e., osteoporosis) in the presence of normal loads. Both shape changes occur so that the femur can meet the loads imposed on it without excessive deformation or fracture.

VISCOELASTICITY

All discussion thus far has assumed that only solid materials are used in the musculoskeletal system. Fluid materials and their influence on the mechanical behavior of actual musculoskeletal components have been ignored. However, actual musculoskeletal tissues are a combination of elastic solids and viscous fluids. This property is referred to as viscoelasticity.

The mechanical behavior of a viscous (fluid) component is, in simplest form, expressed as a linearly proportional relationship between the force applied to this component and the time-dependent rate of the component's deformation, that is,

$$F = k' \dot{x}$$

where $\dot{x}$ is the time rate of change of the deformation of the component and k' is a constant of proportionality. These viscous mechanical properties are modeled by using a dashpot.

The mechanical properties of viscoelastic materials are modeled by using combinations of springs and dashpots (Fig. 22). Although the two-series element (Maxwell) and two-parallel element (Kelvin-Voight) models are simple first-guess choices for modeling the elastic and the viscous elements, neither is adequate to represent the viscoelastic properties of actual musculoskeletal tissues. Instead, the more complicated three-element series-parallel combination of springs and a dashpot, called the standard solid model, is used to model the viscoelastic behavior of cartilage and other biological tissues.[3]

All physiologically moist materials used in the musculoskeletal system display some degree of viscoelastic mechanical properties. This means that the mechanical properties of these tissues depend on the following:

1. Maintenance of physiologically relevant moisture levels in the tissues.
2. Loading history (all prior application of forces).
3. Rate of loading (commonly expressed in units of strain rate).

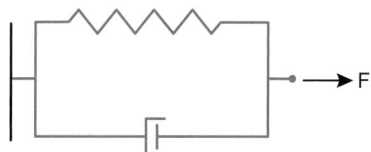

(A) Maxwell model

(B) Kelvin-Voight model

(C) Standard solid model

Fig. 22. Mathematical models of viscoelasticity. Combinations of springs and dashpots are used in series, parallel, and combination to develop models of viscoelastic materials behavior that can be used to quantify the actual materials behavior of musculoskeletal components.

THE VISCOELASTICITY OF CORTICAL BONE

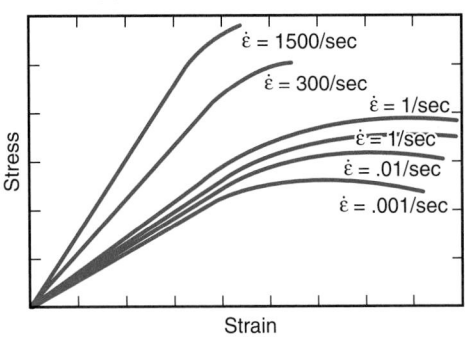

Fig. 23. Strain rate dependence of cortical bone. Stress-strain curves of cortical bone are tested at varying strain rates. Note the increasing slope and strength of bone as strain rate increases.

The first point is important when reading reports describing the in vitro testing of tissues. The second point is more profound: it means that the object's mechanical behavior in the next loading cycle is dependent on all previous loading cycles. The third point is clinically important because the stiffness and strength of the musculoskeletal material depend on the rate at which the load is applied to generate the material's stress-strain curve.

Consider the classic illustration showing that the strength of human cortical bone varies with loading rate in tension (Fig. 23).[14] Note that bone becomes stronger as well as stiffer as the rate of loading increases. Bone has lower strength when subjected to the smaller strain rates accompanying normal gait, but this is acceptable because the mechanical demands on bone are less during this activity. When running, the loads applied to bone increase in magnitude and decrease in time interval over which they are applied (i.e., strain rate increases). Thus, because of the viscoelastic properties of bone, it becomes stronger when added strength is needed. Although a complete mechanical description of the viscoelastic properties of bone is beyond the scope of this discussion, it is important to recognize that these viscoelastic properties enable the tissue to meet the mechanical demands of the skeleton without change in the materials' shape or amount. Bone's viscoelastic properties efficiently meet the demands of the musculoskeletal system and serve a protective function in sports-related activities and subcritical traumatic events. Eventually, however, bone strength increase reaches a limit, and strain rates beyond this point result in decreasing bone strength. The interested reader is encouraged to consult the sources listed next for more information regarding the deformation of bone during physiological loading.[5, 15–18]

REFERENCES

1. Nigg BM, Herzog W: Biomechanics of the Musculoskeletal System. Chichester, Wiley, 1999.
2. Nordin M, Frankel VH: Basic Biomechanics of the Musculoskeletal System. Philadelphia, Lea & Febiger, 1989.
3. Ozkaya N, Margareta N: Fundamentals of Biomechanics. New York, Springer, 1999.
4. Cochran GVB: A Primer of Orthopaedic Biomechanics. New York, Churchill Livingstone, 1982.
5. Mow VC, Hayes WC: Basic Orthopaedic Biomechanics. Philadelphia, Lippincott-Raven, 1997.
6. Garrett WE, Best TM: Anatomy, physiology, and mechanics of skeletal muscle. In Simon SR (ed): Orthopaedic Basic Science. American Academy of Orthopaedic Surgeons, 1994.
7. Black J, Dumbleton JH: Clinical Biomechanics: A Case History Approach. New York, Churchill Livingstone, 1981.
8. Waters TR, Putz-Anderson V, Garg A: Applications Manual for the Revised NIOSH Lifting Equation. Cincinnati, U.S. Department of Health and Human Services, Public Health Service, 1994.
9. Perry J: Gait analysis in sports medicine. Instr Course Lect 1990; 39:319.
10. Andrews JG: Segment and Joint Orientations in Space. Iowa City, IA, University of Iowa, 1993.
11. Ghista DN: Human Body Dynamics: Impact, Occupational, and Athletic Aspects. Oxford Medical Engineering Series. Oxford, England, Clarendon Press, 1982.
12. Broadus AE: Mineral balance and homeostasis. In Favus MJ (ed): Primer on the Metabolic Bone Diseases and Disorders of Mineral Metabolism. Philadelphia, Lippincott-Raven, 1996, p 57.
13. Byars EF, Snyder R: Engineering Mechanics of Deformable Bodies. Scranton, PA, International Textbook Company, 1969.
14. McElhaney JH: Dynamic response of bone and muscle tissue. J Appl Physiol 1966; 21:1231.
15. Cowin SC: Bone Mechanics. Boca Raton, FL, CRC Press, 1989.
16. Fung YC: A First Course in Continuum Mechanics. Englewood Cliffs, NJ, Prentice Hall, 1977.
17. Einhorn TA: Bone strength: The bottom line [editorial]. Calcif Tissue Int 1992; 51:333.
18. Neumann DA, Cook TM: Effect of load and carrying position on the electromyographic activity of the gluteus medius muscle during walking. Phys Ther 1985; 65:305.
19. Maquet P: Mechanics and osteoarthritis of the patellofemoral joint. Clin Orthop 1979; 144:70.

ORTHOPAEDIC BIOMATERIALS

Patrick W. Kwok and Courtland G. Lewis

Summary

- Bone is the basic orthopaedic biomaterial. The use of composites (bone/stainless steel, Vitallium/polyethylene, host bone/allograft bone) requires an understanding of material properties and loading mechanics.
- Methods of fabrication/preparation have profound impact on the resulting material properties and load-bearing potential of biomaterials.
- Fatigue endurance is of primary interest in assessing functional performance of implants.
- Wear of the bearing surface is the principal issue with joint arthroplasty survival.

Over the course of the century, orthopaedic surgeons have used many synthetic materials to replace human tissue and provide improved function. The failures and successes of these biomaterials are well documented, particularly in the total joint replacement literature. Only by understanding the molecular and physical properties of metals, ceramics, polymers, and plastics can one select materials appropriate to the design of an implant. The useful life of an implant depends on its design, biocompatibility with the harsh chemical environment in vivo, and ability to withstand the millions of repetitive cycles imparted by the gait cycle.

In this chapter, the following topics are covered:

- Biomechanics of biomaterials: definition of stress/strain, modulus, and viscoelastic properties.
- Tribology of biomaterials: friction, wear, and lubrication between materials, as well as corrosion.
- Specific comparisons between metals, ceramics, polymers, and plastics: moduli comparisons, material properties, and clinical applications.
- New developments: bioabsorbable materials, cross-linked polyethylene, the persistent problem of polyethylene wear.

BIOMECHANICS/MATERIALS SCIENCE

To be able to discuss the material and physical properties of a biomaterial, one must be familiar with certain terms and definitions.

Stress: internal force acting on an object caused by an external force. Stress equals force imparted to a body, defining the internal resistance of a body to a load. Normal stress is perpendicular to the face of the material, in the form of either compressive or tensile force. Shear stress is applied parallel to the face of the object. Stress is measured in newtons per square meter, or pascals.

Strain: measure of the deformation of a body as a result of loading. Strain equals change in length/original length. Strain is dimensionless and has no units.

Stress/strain curve: depicts the general properties of materials; material dependent (Fig. 1).

Load/deformation curve: similiar to stress/strain but depicts the general properties of a structure; shape-dependent.

The following definitions are based on Figure 1, a stress/strain curve:

Young's modulus of elasticity (E): the ratio of stress to strain or the slope of the stress/strain curve under the elastic portion of the curve. The modulus measures the material stiffness and its ability to resist deformation when a force is applied. Measured in newtons per square meter (pascals), or in the United States pounds per square inch (psi), the modulus can represent resistance to compression, tension, or shear force.

Elastic limit: defined as the maximum stress that a material can withstand without permanent deformation or failure. Energy can be recovered up to this point once the applied force is released, but beyond the elastic limit the length or shape is no longer fully recoverable. It is the same as the yield point for many materials.

Yield point/proportional limit: point of transition from the elastic to plastic region. This is the point at which there is an increase in strain with a proportionally lesser increase in stress.

Yield strength: the amount of stress at which the material deviates from linear proportionality between stress and strain. A specific amount of permanent, or plastic, deformation usually measured at 2% strain is used as a gauge

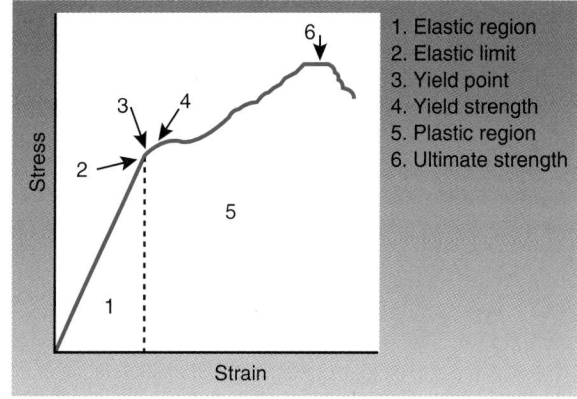

Fig. 1. Typical stress/strain curve. This curve indicates the following biomechanical properties: (1) elastic region; (2) elastic limit; (3) yield point; (4) yield strength; (5) plastic region; (6) ultimate strength. (From Jones RE, Hoffmann A: Implant problems & management of complications. Presented at the Southwestern Orthopaedic Surgery Board Review, 1997.)

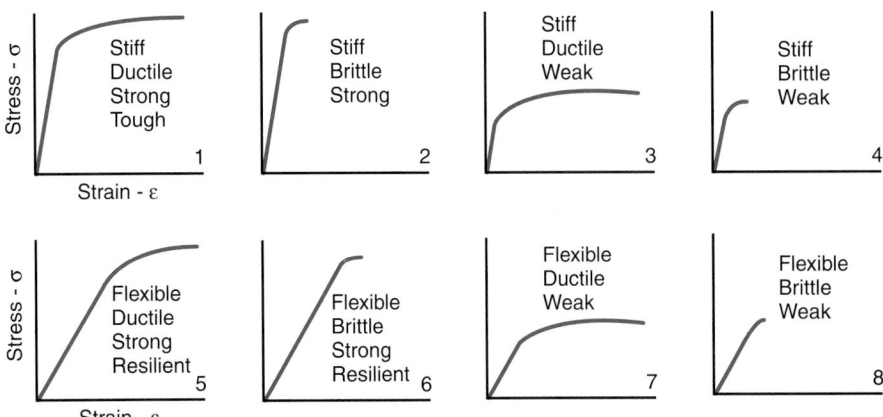

Fig. 2. Outline of relative relationships among elastic modulus, plastic deformation, ultimate strength, and energy to failure. (From Simon, Orthopaedic Basic Science.)

to compare different materials. This line is parallel to the initial slope of the stress/strain curve. Its intersection with the curve represents the yield point, whereas the intersection with the X axis represents 2% strain.

Ultimate strength: maximum stress obtained before failure, typically at the point of rupture of the material.

Breaking point: point at which the material ruptures at a higher strain but lower stress than its ultimate strength (typical of tendons).

Ductility: a property of a material that undergoes significant plastic deformation before fracture (Fig. 2). The degree of a material's permanent deformation beyond the yield point defines that material's ductility. The amount of energy used to plastically deform the material is not recoverable. An example of a ductile material is stainless steel.

Brittle: a property of a material that does not exhibit a significant plastic region and, therefore, has little ability to deform before failure. Brittle materials, such as ceramic, fail within the elastic region and do not have distinguishable yield and ultimate stresses. Unlike the fracture pattern of a ductile material, the rupture of a brittle material results in fragments that resemble their original shape. A material's yield and ultimate strengths can be altered through various manufacturing techniques (see the later section on Metallic Processing). When a material is stressed repeatedly after initial plastic deformation, the result is a material with a different yield strength and ultimate strength. This is called work-hardening. The microstructure of stainless steel can be changed via press machines and result in increased yield stress and decreased ductility. Because the work is completed in a temperature below the steel's melting point, this process is called cold-working.

Toughness: total energy needed to fracture material. This can be quantified as the area under the stress-strain curve. It is important to understand that a brittle material with a high modulus and high ultimate strength can be equally as tough as a ductile material with a high ultimate strain.

Hardness: ability of a material to resist plastic deformation at its surface. Harder surfaces tend to scratch softer surfaces, and the latter can leave films covering the former. Relative hardness, coefficient of friction, and polishing all contribute to the behavior of anticipated couplings in vivo.

Fatigue failure/endurance limit: the number of cycles to material fracture at a specified stress level (Fig. 3). With each cycle, microdamage of the material accumulates until the material fails. Furthermore, the damage accumulates more quickly when each cycle is loaded at a higher stress. The endurance limit on the curve is the level of stress under which a material can be theoretically loaded an infinite number of cycles without failure. In other words, the initiation of fatigue cracks does not exist at this level of stress despite any number of cycles. Fatigue failure can occur as the result of crack initiation followed by crack propagation. About 80% of the cyclic loading involves the initiation of a crack, whereas the last 20% aids in its propagation. If the stress of the material increases to the point exceeding the material's ultimate stress, the material will fail. In the case of some implants, the endurance limit may not be realized in several years of daily use.

Viscoelasticity: a property of a material in which its stress-strain relationship is time dependent (Fig. 4). This entity is the result of internal friction, or resistance, within the material. Examples include all biological tissues, plastics, and most composites. *Creep* is an increase of deforma-

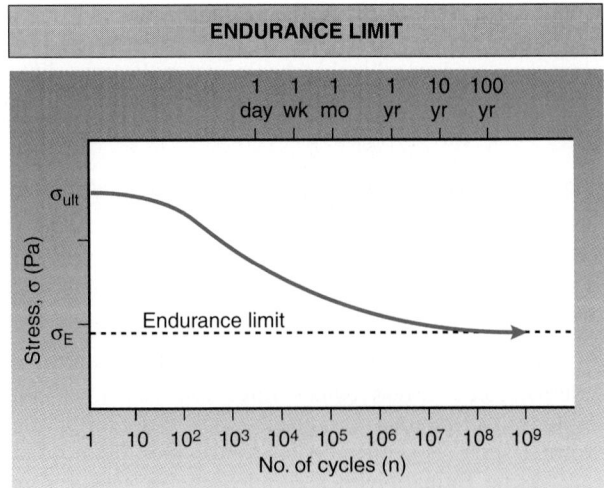

Fig. 3. Endurance limit. The endurance limit is a design-critical parameter in the fabrication of load-bearing implants. (From Simon, Orthopaedic Basic Science.)

VISCOELASTIC PROPERTIES

Fig. 4. Viscoelasticity. Viscoelasticity is related to deformation (strain) under constant load over time. Stress relaxation indicates the load required to maintain constant deformation over time. (From Jones RE, Hoffmann A: Implant problems and management of complications. Presented at the Southwestern Orthopaedic Surgery Board Review, 1997.)

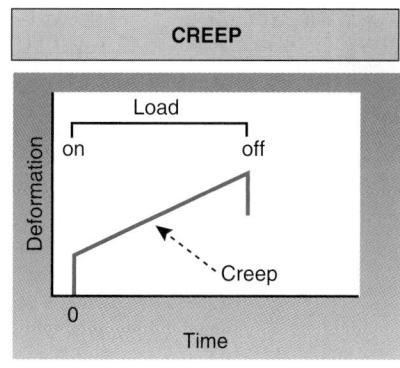

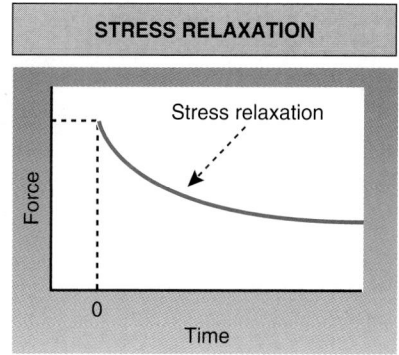

tion (strain) in response to a constant force over time. *Stress relaxation* is a decrease in the amount of force, or stress, needed to maintain a constant deformation over time. At low strain rates (Fig. 5), the material with viscoelastic properties may exhibit viscous behavior, with no appreciable elastic deformation. However, with the increase in strain rate, the modulus of the material as well as the ultimate strength is increased while the ultimate strain is decreased. The same material at high strain rates may act much like a brittle, elastic solid. Because a material may manifest both types of behavior, one must specify the strain rate used during materials testing.

Anisotropy: a characteristic with all biological materials in which mechanical properties vary with orientation of the material.

TRIBOLOGY

When materials, whether like or unlike, come into contact, interactions occur during their relative motions with one another. Tribology is the study of friction, lubrication, and wear of materials. Furthermore, in this section the concept of corrosion, which is particularly important when implanting biomaterials in vivo (subjecting them to the body's harsh chemical environment), is discussed.

FRICTION

Friction is defined as the resistance to motion between two bodies. When a load creates contact between the two bodies, both chemical and mechanical interactions can result. The coefficient of friction, either static or dynamic, can be derived from the ratio between the frictional force and load, independent of the surface area of the interface. Frictional forces are due to the roughness of the contacting surfaces and each interface's chemical composition. Because the surfaces are often not smooth but rather rough (to a relative degree), ultrastructural crystalline "points" increase the stress contact and lead to bonding of the two bodies at these junctions. As a result, a significant initial force is needed to overcome these bonds, as reflected by the static coefficient of friction. Once the two bodies are in relative motion, chemical reactions come into play to further break up these bonds, and subsequently a smaller force is needed to maintain a constant velocity.

The coefficient of friction values can ultimately be used in materials testing to compare different bearing surface combinations. Table 1 shows that the natural hip joint bathed in synovial fluid still has the lowest coefficient of friction, despite attempts to create synthetic substitutes for the normal hip articulation. The combination of cobalt-chromium (Co-Cr), cobalt-chromium-molybdenum (Co-Cr-Mo), and polyethylene, used widely in total joint replacements, has a coefficient 10 times greater than that of the diarthrodial joint.

LUBRICATION

Lubrication implies inserting material between two bodies to decrease the interaction between them. By interposing the lubricant, the frictional resistance and local stress concentrations are decreased, because the contract between the asperites, or areas of micropoint contact, is decreased. Effectiveness of a lubricant depends on the viscosity of the material and, in the case of a synovial joint, the permeability of the cartilage. A lubricant too low in viscosity may be pressed out from between the interfaces. In contrast, a lubricant too high in viscosity may provide increased separation between the two surfaces, but it may create a shearing stress between the asperites and the lubricant rather than within the lubricant's film. Therefore, the most effective lubricant, especially in a joint, is one in which the

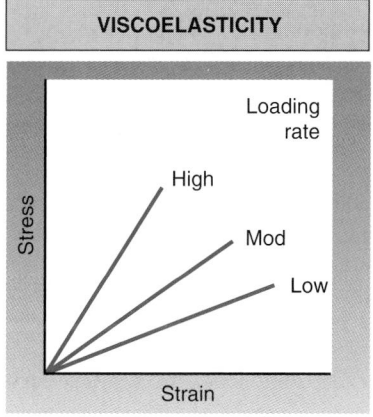

Fig. 5. Viscoelasticity is a rate-dependent function.

TABLE 1. COEFFICIENTS OF FRICTION FOR VARIOUS MATERIAL COMBINATIONS		
	Coefficients	
Material Combination	μ_s	μ_D
Rubber tire/concrete (dry)	1.0	0.7
Rubber tire/concrete (water)	0.7	0.5
Leather/wood	0.5	0.4
Steel/steel		0.5
Co-Cr/Co-Cr (saline)		0.35
UHMWPE/steel (serum)	0.35	0.07–0.12
UHMWPE/steel (synovial fluid)	0.07	0.04–0.05
UHMWPE/Co-Cr (serum)		0.05–0.11
UHMWPE/Ti$_6$Al$_4$V (serum)		0.05–0.12
Al$_2$O$_3$/Al$_2$O$_3$ (saline)		0.09
UHMWPE/Al$_2$O$_3$ (saline)		0.05
Hip joint (natural) (saline)		0.005–0.01
Hip joint (natural) (synovial fluid)		0.002 lowest

The coefficient of friction within a normal diarthrodial joint is among the lowest of any known materials. Co-Cr, cobalt-chromium; UHMWPE, ultra-high molecular weight polyethylene.
From Black J: Orthopaedic Biomaterials in Research and Practice. New York, Churchill Livingstone, 1988.

material is not squeezed out with specific loads and decreases the dynamic coefficient of friction.

The following is a list of lubricating mechanisms or regimens that depend on the relative motion between the two surfaces and the type of material used as lubricant:

1. Hydrodynamic: this can be thought of as hydroplaning, in which the surfaces are completely separated. The relative motion of the surfaces maintains a thick, fluid film such that the interfaces do not contact each other. Therefore, the viscosity of the lubricant is crucial in the success of this mechanism. If external pressure is applied between the two bodies, then it is called hydrostatic lubrication.
2. Squeeze-film: the rigid bearing surfaces provide a direct resistance to prevent the fluid, or lubricant, from extruding from the antisolution but at the same time provide the dynamic pressure necessary to compress the viscous fluid.
3. Elastohydrodynamic: the bearing surfaces are elastic and, under pressure, can deform to accommodate the roughness of the surfaces and maintain a thick, lubricant film throughout. This results in a coefficient of friction only slightly higher than that of hydrostatic lubrication, but it still leads to low wear rates. One valid concern, however, is the subsurface fatigue that can potentially occur if the load, or pressure, exceeds the elasticity of the bearing surface.
4. Weeping: at least one of the bearing surfaces is porous, and relative motion can squeeze fluid out of the deforming surface and contribute to the fluid film of the lubricant. This augmentation to the elastohydrodynamic mechanism creates a pressurized environment, resulting in a highly efficient system with a low coefficient of friction.
5. Boosted: relevant to diarthrodial joints and based on the squeeze-film model, water from the synovial fluid is hydrostatically pressurized into the cartilage matrix, leaving a lubricant now consisting of a concentrated acid-protein complex.

6. Boundary: this mechanism relies on a very thin monolayer of lubricant. This film adheres to each of the surfaces just enough to minimize the contact between the asperites and modify the surface properties through chemical interactions. The coefficient of friction and wear rate are significantly higher compared with the other fluid-film mechanisms. When attempting to characterize the mechanism of lubrication of a typical diarthrodial joint, it is most likely a combination of elastohydrodynamics, weeping, and boundary lubrication. Total joint arthroplasties, alternatively, cannot rely on the weeping mechanism so important in the natural human joint consisting of articular cartilage in contact with synovial fluid.

WEAR

Despite the mechanisms of lubrication as described previously, articulating surfaces that move in relation to one another and contact one another essentially always lose material from those interfaces. This loss of material can be the result of both mechanical and chemical factors, depending on the material properties of the respective interfaces. It is important to understand that an articulating system with a low frictional coefficient does not necessarily lead to a system with a low wear rate, because the factors resulting in frictional forces are different from those that cause wear particles.

The following is a summary of available wear mechanisms:

1. Abrasive: a rough or hard surface can slide in relation to a softer surface and essentially plow through the latter, causing debris in the form of needles and curls. The process usually leads to the lowest wear rate compared with the mechanisms listed next but can still cause significant damage if stress concentrations exist and if there is chemical bonding between the interacting surfaces.
2. Adhesive: fragments of even the smoothest surfaces adhere to each other as a result of atomic affinity. With relative motion, these bonded fragments may not separate at the original interface but rather through one of the bases of the fragments. As a result, a fragment from one surface is transferred to the other surface.
3. Transfer: this mechanism occurs when material from a softer surface fills in the opposing rough, hard surface, forming a smooth film, which essentially alters the interface. This transfer film is potentially unstable, leading to third-body wear.
4. Third-body wear: sometimes this is categorized as a subset of abrasive wear. Either wear debris or foreign particles are introduced between two surfaces, producing local, high-stress concentrations that abrade one or both of the surfaces. This may lead to increased wear rates in the articulating system.
5. Fretting: this occurs when similar or different materials experience interface micromotion and debris generation. Examples include a screw head/plate construct or a femoral head component on the morse taper of the femoral stem.
6. Fatigue: in certain instances, focal cyclic loading of the high-stress concentrations to localized regions may

cause surface cracks or fractures. This mechanism is thought to be the driving force behind polyethylene sub-surface delamination in total knee arthroplasty. Two factors, especially in total joint arthroplasties, may contribute to higher surface stresses and ultimately lead to fatigue wear of polyethylene. First, if the articulating surfaces are incongruent, the poor-fitting construct can increase the contact stresses. Second, if the softer material (in this case, polyethylene) is too thin, then the underlying material (e.g., metal-backed cup or tibial tray) creates an environment of increased contact stresses. As a result of these contributing factors, the surfaces of the thin polymers crack, and further contact stresses cause propagation of these fatigue cracks tangential to the surface, extruding debris into the joint space. Ultimately, wear is accelerated through material loss and third-body wear. For this reason, it is recommended that the thickness of the polyethylene insert, especially in total knee arthroplasties, be a minimum of 8 mm in an attempt to lower contact stresses and decrease fatigue wear. Hence, wear in this scenario is a combined function of material properties, implant design and fabrication, and surgical technique (selection and implantation).

Manufacturers and laboratory scientists continue their search for the optimal material for total joint arthroplasties. At present, material wear represents the principal challenge in total joint arthroplasty. The size of the debris particles is just as important as the amount of wear debris. In general, the softer material involved in the articulation will wear down. For example, in a metal-on-polyethylene pairing, the polyethylene will wear, whereas in a metal-on-ceramic construct, primarily metal debris will be found.

Because many polymers have viscoelastic properties, creep plays a role in implant function. Whereever peak contact stresses occur, "cold flow" can lead to deformation and shape change of components without significant loss of material, and the resulting permanent deformity can still affect mechanical function. Unlike polymers, metals and ceramics do not creep at body temperatures.

When comparing "like" pairs of materials to "unlike" pairs of materials, the former construct tends to have higher wear rates, because similar materials are able to bond more easily. In general, the rates of debris accumulation can be listed in decreasing order: metal/metal > ceramic/polymer > metal/polymer.

MATERIAL PROPERTIES COMPARISON

The graph in Figure 6 compares the moduli of various biomaterials used in orthopaedics.

Presented in descending order of relative ultimate tensile strength are: Co-Cr (wrought), titanium (Ti), stainless steel (wrought), Co-Cr (cast), cortical bone, plaster of Paris or tendon, ultra-high molecular weight polyethylene (UHMWPE) or polymethylmethacrylate (PMMA), fascia, skin, cartilage, cancellous bone, and muscle.

Presented in descending order of relative yield strength (2% strain), the biomaterials used are as follows: Ti, Co-Cr (wrought), stainless steel, Co-Cr (cast), cortical bone, UHMWPE or plaster of Paris, and cartilage.

MATERIAL PROPERTIES

METALS
Metals are the most widely used materials in orthopaedics. Their material characteristics include high strength and

TABLE 2. EFFECTS OF FABRICATION TECHNIQUE ON MATERIAL PROPERTIES OF COMMON ORTHOPAEDIC ALLOYS

Material Type	Elastic Modulus (GPa)	Ultimate Tensile Strength (MPa)
Annealed stainless steel 316 ASTM F55-82	200	515
Annealed stainless steel 316L ASTM F55-82	200	480
Cold-worked stainless steel 316 and 316L ASTM F55-87	200	860
Cast Co-Cr-Mo alloy ASTM F75-87	250	655
Wrought Co-Ni-Cr-Mo alloy ASTM F562-84	240	793–1000
Unalloyed titanium ASTM F67-89	105	240–550
Cast Ti_6Al_4V alloy ASTM F1108-88	110	860
Wrought Ti_6Al_4V ELI alloy ASTM F136-84	110	860–896

Co, cobalt; Cr, chromium; Mo, molybdenum; Ni, nickel; Ti, titanium; Al, aluminum; V, vanadium.

From American Association of Orthopaedic Surgeons: Orthopaedic Knowledge Update: Hip and Knee Reconstruction. Rosemont, IL, AAOS Publications, 2000, 2nd ed.

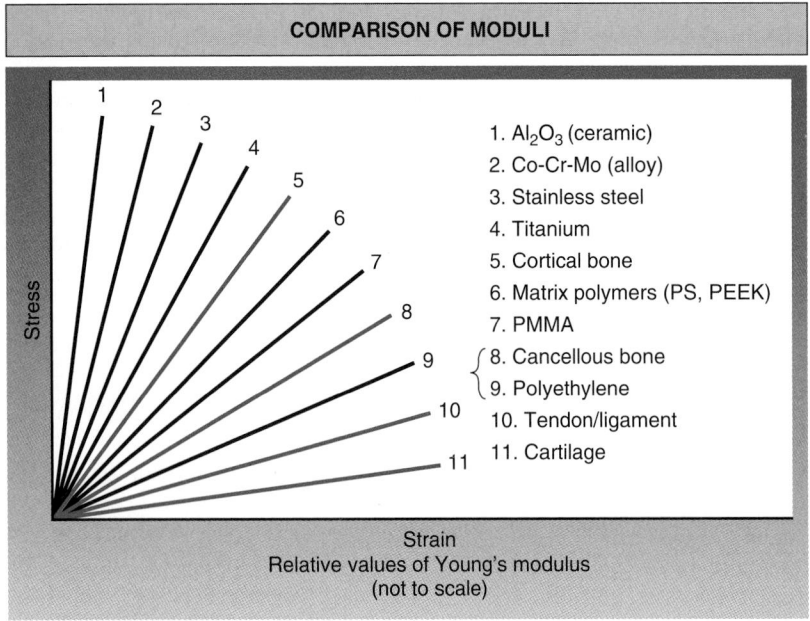

COMPARISON OF MODULI

1. Al$_2$O$_3$ (ceramic)
2. Co-Cr-Mo (alloy)
3. Stainless steel
4. Titanium
5. Cortical bone
6. Matrix polymers (PS, PEEK)
7. PMMA
8. Cancellous bone
9. Polyethylene
10. Tendon/ligament
11. Cartilage

Stress / Strain
Relative values of Young's modulus
(not to scale)

Fig. 6. Orthopaedic biomaterials. Materials such as ceramics, metal alloys, matrix polymers, and polyethylene have elastic moduli that span the range of biomaterials (cortical bone, cancellous bone, tendon/ligament, and cartilage). (From Miller MD: Review of Orthopaedics. Philadelphia, WB Saunders, 1996, 2nd ed.)

ductility, with the capability of withstanding high peak stress and having relatively high fatigue endurance limits. Alloys can now be fabricated to meet the needs of most orthopaedic situations, from fracture fixation to prosthetics/braces to total joint replacement. The three most commonly used metals are stainless steel, Co-Cr-Mo, and Ti-based alloys (Table 2).

Metallic Bonding

The interatomic structure of a metal consists of a grouping of positively charged nuclei, which are surrounded by freely mobile electrons. The nondirectional nature and the freedom of the atoms enable metal constructs to be packed densely, filling in interatomic gaps. As a result, metallic materials are able to undergo significant deformation without fracture and, therefore, tend to be strong and ductile.

As metals solidify from their hot liquid state, the crystals, or grains, are often irregular before they coalesce. Impurities, or "inclusions," can collect between the grains and significantly alter the properties of the resulting metal. A metal can be weakened by stress risers and areas of crevice corrosion if there are inclusions or high concentrations of surface porosity. Furthermore, if the grain size increases significantly, the tensile strength of the metal may decrease.

Metallic Processing

Recrystallinization, or annealing, is a process in which the metal is heated to regain its original lower energy state. The shape and the material properties of the metal can be uniquely altered by cold working and annealing. Cold-working, which includes hammering, forging, rolling, and drawing, involves deforming a metal beyond its yield stress, resulting in the elongation of the grains in the direction of the stress with no change in grain volume. This process elevates the material's internal stresses. Furthermore, by manipulating the grains at an ambient temperature, this "work hardening" leads to increased stiffness.

Overall, the metal changes shape and has a higher yield stress, ultimate stress, and endurance limit. It is, however, less ductile.

Voids and impurities can often result from casting, a process in which hot liquid metal is poured into a mold. The inclusions tend to concentrate along the grain boundaries, causing the material to be less strong.

Alternatively, forging involves heating a metal to submelting temperatures and pressing into a die under very high loads. The resultant metal has fewer voids.

Finally, hot isostatic pressing (HIP) produces a fine-grained material from metallic powder under an environment of high temperature and pressure. This increases the overall strength of the metal. Different manufacturing techniques are used to optimize metals for different implant applications.

CORROSION

Corrosion is a process in which a metal is degraded by electrochemical reactions generated in a physiological environment. As a result, the surface of the metal is altered, and metal ions are extruded into the body's fluids and tissues. By definition, a material that releases a concentration of ions greater than 10^6 per mole is said to be corrosive, whereas one releasing less is said to be immune. All metals corrode, and the degree of corrosion depends on the material's composition.

In general, stainless steel corrodes more readily than cobalt or titanium-based alloys. A corrosion-resistant surface layer can be formed on stainless steel or cobalt-based alloys by immersion in acid solutions. This process of passivation creates a stable oxide or hydroxide layer, which mimics natural corrosion but ultimately protects the metal from the environment. Ti-based alloys create a layer of corrosion resistance through self-passivation. However, any scratch or nick may compromise the oxide layer of a metal and lead to enhanced corrosion; Ti-based alloys are sensitive to notching or surface scratches. Furthermore, any change in the pH and oxygen tension of the surrounding environment may alter the layer's effectiveness against corrosion.

There is a variety of corrosion mechanisms that may occur in vivo:

Uniform attack: the most common type of corrosion that affects all metals in a conductive, electrolyte solution, including bodily fluids. Metal ions are released into an aqueous environment, bonding with either hydrogen or oxygen.

Galvanic attack: occurs when two dissimilar metals, or two areas of a metallic material with different energy levels, are in close proximity. There needs to exist an environment that allows conduction through the metal as well as through a solution. One metal acts as an anode and relinquishes electrons to the other metal, acting as a cathode. As a result, an electric potential is established, creating a corrosive medium in which the metal with the higher free energy, the anode, is oxidized. This process may be clinically significant, especially in today's application of modular components. It has been shown that potentially disastrous corrosion results when stainless steel is mixed with cobalt-based alloys. Alternatively, a modular system consisting of a cobalt-based alloy and a Ti-based alloy has actually led to a stable electrochemical environment. In a system containing Ti_6Al_4V, the Ti alloy resists galvanic corrosion via the process of self-passivation, creating an interface of Ti dioxide, TiO_2. Given the ion interphase potential, orthopaedists are able to use Co-Cr femoral heads with Ti-based femoral stems with little worry about galvanic corrosion.

Crevice corrosion: occurs when crevices or cracks exist in the metal, which creates a localized area of low oxygen tension and increased extrusion of metallic ions. An environment with a high concentration of chloride or hydrogen ions (low pH) further accelerates this corrosive process. Stainless steel is the most affected, especially in areas between a screw head and a plate. Co-Cr alloys and less commonly Ti alloys can also be affected when

scratches compromise the passivation layer and expose the metal to the corrosive chloride-rich medium.

Pitting: a more concentrated, localized area of crevice corrosion in which a portion of the oxide layer is compromised. This localized defect can become a point of high stress, leading to fatigue failure. Stainless steel is again greatly affected, but newer manufacturing processes of vacuum melting and remelting along with the incorporation of chromium, nickel, or molybdenum have significantly protected this metal from pitting corrosion. Much like crevice corrosion, Co-Cr alloys are mildly affected, and Ti-based alloys are relatively resistant.

Intergranular attack: another type of galvanic corrosion in which impurities gathered in an area between grains create an electric potential. This can also occur within alloys in an area exposing two grains with differing energy levels.

Stress corrosion: occurs when a crack forms in an area of tensile stress surrounded by a corrosive environment. The passivating layer may be compromised, accelerating the corrosion. If the crack continues to propagate, the increased stress concentration may lead to implant failure.

Fretting corrosion: occurs between two contacting materials in which there exists motion, damaging the protective oxide layer and releasing metal ions. This corrosive event can occur between a screw head and plate, between an acetabular screw and the metal-backed acetabular cup, or between a femoral head and the stem's morse taper.

By becoming cognizant of the potential pitfalls of mixing implant materials, an orthopaedist can make informed decisions concerning fixation methods and lower the incidence of catastrophic failures.

Stainless Steel

This is an iron-based alloy (Fig. 7). Among the many subtypes, the alloys used in making implants are grades

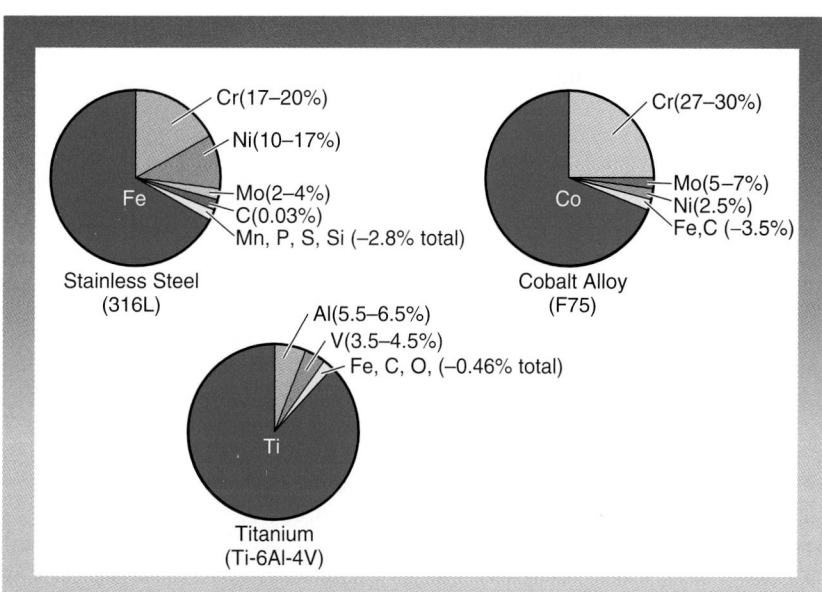

Fig. 7. Elemental composition of common orthopaedic alloys. (From Simon, Orthopaedic Basic Science.)

316 and 316L (ASTM F-55–56). The latter is most commonly used, consisting of 60% to 70% iron, 16% to 20% chromium, 8% to 17% nickel, 2% to 4% molybdenum, less than 0.03% carbon, and a small percentage consisting of manganese and silicon. As stated in the Corrosion section, stainless steel, in general, is vulnerable to processes such as crevice and stress corrosion, which render implants made of stainless steel more or less temporary devices for fracture fixation. Still, chromium and nickel fortify the passivating layer and the molybdenum resists pitting corrosion. Also, limiting the amount of carbon, as with type 316L, prevents the precipitation of chromium and, therefore, minimally compromises the protective layer.

This material is used mainly for devices in fracture fixation, such as plates and screws, although some forged alloys may be used in total joint components. To avoid catastrophic corrosion, stainless steel components should not be in close proximity to implants made of Co-Cr.

Co-Cr Alloys

One type of Co-Cr alloy, ASTM F-75, consists of 60% cobalt, 27% to 30% chromium, 5% to 7% molybdenum, 2.5% nickel, and less than 0.35% carbon. This alloy, also called Vitallium, was originally used as a casting alloy, but its brittle nature left significant casting defects. Therefore, despite its inherent strength, F-75 cannot withstand the high-stress, high-cyclic loading imparted on a casted femoral stem implant. However, through forging and/or hot isostatic pressing, decreased volume of defects/porosities and a smaller grain size led to an 80% increase of yield strength. This changed the mechanical properties of the alloy and, along with its high strength, high wear and corrosion resistance, and biocompatibility, made it much more suitable for load-bearing and articulating applications. This material is second only to Ti in its ability to resist corrosion and fatigue. A large percentage of femoral head implants are made of Co-Cr.

Ti and Ti Alloys

This group of metals is especially attractive as implantable devices because of superior biocompatibility as well as its corrosion resistance from self-passivation. Ti and its alloys are approximately half as stiff as Co-Cr and stainless steel but still five times stiffer than cortical bone. Because the modulus of Ti is closer to that of cortical bone, it has been shown that the use of Ti plates leads to less stress shielding of the cortical bone and ultimately less bone resorption/remodeling underneath the fixation plate.

Commercially pure Ti, or ASTM F-67, can be sintered and therefore applied as a porous layer in cementless total joint components. The Ti-based alloy, Ti_6Al_4V, despite its high strength-weight ratio and its ductility, is notch sensitive. As a result, porous coating made of this Ti alloy cannot be extensively applied without significantly decreasing fatigue strength of the overall implant.

Another well-documented observation with Ti alloy is its poor wear characteristics when articulating with UHMWPE. Poor shear strength of the material leads to adhesive wear, burnishing the Ti surface and disrupting the self-passivating layer. Ultimately, third-body wear accelerates the process. To counteract the wear, manufacturers have attempted to use the processes of nitride implantation to create a harder, smoother metal surface, which in theory can better resist wear and corrosion. These surfaces have largely been abandoned for clinical application.

CERAMICS

This group consists of composite nonmetallic materials, either bioactive or inorganic, hydroxyapatite, aluminum oxide (Al_2O_3) (ZrO_2), and zirconium oxide.

Chemistry

Ceramics are crystalline materials, similar in structure to metals (excepting Ti). As opposed to the primarily ionic bonds found in metals, however, substitution of oxygen moieties results in a charge-neutral material with a densely packed crystal structure. Covalent bonding occurs to a variable degree between molecules.

Fabrication

Structural ceramics are fabricated using techniques similar to hot isostatic pressing for metals. A microgranular slurry is molded, after which, at variable pressures and temperatures, the material is sintered. Prolonged sintering to create maximum density also results in larger grain size; addition of calcium oxide or manganese oxide facilitates fabrication of denser aluminum oxide. Zirconium oxide is difficult to manufacture but has a fracture toughness nearly twice that of aluminum oxide.

Wear

Aluminum oxide and zirconium oxide have hydrophilic surfaces that contribute to a "low contact angle" at a water-based surface and hence high "wettability." This factor, as well as high surface smoothness, contributes to low coefficients of friction. In total joint applications, either one of these materials mated with UHMWPE appears to have volumetric wear on an order of magnitude less than Co-Cr on polyethylene. Nonetheless, improved survivorship of total hip arthroplasty using these articulating surfaces has not been proven. Aluminum oxide and aluminum oxide articulations appear to function well; zirconium oxide against zirconium oxide demonstrates unacceptably high wear.

Bone Substitutes (Ceramic)

Surface Preparations. Hydroxyapatite ($Ca_{10}[PO_4]_6[OH]_2$), the mineralized crystalline structure found in bone, is a ceramic by definition. The use of hydroxyapatite coatings on total hip stems has been a clinical reality for more than 10 years. Plasma-sprayed surfaces have been created that appear to be osteoconductive, although there are significant variations in both chemical composition and stability from application to application. Some preparations have suffered from spalling of the ceramic from the substrate surface, but increased on-growth of bone has been demonstrated in others, driving their continued use by some surgeons.

Bone Graft Substitutes. Hydroxyapatite is relatively nonresorbable in pure form but can also serve as a filler for bone defects such as in tibial plateau or distal radius fractures or benign neoplasms. Other ceramics, such as tricalcium phosphate, which does resorb over time, may also play a role. Further evolution of these materials has resulted in grouts that cure at body temperature and may have a role in initial fracture stabilization. Addition of bioactive molecules, in particular bone growth factors, to these fillers represents an exciting new horizon in orthopaedics.

POLYMERS

Two polymers, PMMA and UHMWPE, remain mainstays in the domain of orthopaedic biomaterials.

Chemistry. Covalently bonded polymers, consisting of repeating carbon-based units, are the building blocks of both UHMWPE and PMMA. Both molecular weight and degree of branching of the polymer determine their structural properties. The structural orientation of molecular strands establishes the crystallinity in which there is ultrastructural heterogeneity within a material consisting of more and less crystalline regions.

Fabrication. UHMWPE has been a single-source material based on resins produced by Hoechst (Frankfurt am Main, Germany) for many years. Variations in fabrication technique, however, have had a profound impact on the resultant material. The two principal forms of implant manufacture are ram extrusion and compression molding; newer milling systems have also allowed for multiradius milling of articulating surfaces. Direct molding of articular surfaces has been performed as well. When only the surface of an implant is heat pressed, however, melting of the surface layer has been found to alter crystallinity and hence material properties, thus creating a stress riser in the subsurface region, leading to mechanical breakdown at this level.

Wear. The simple truth regarding any manufactured bearing is that it will undergo wear. This is as true of total joint articulations as it is of any machine part. Both the formation of wear debris and its effects on surrounding tissue (in this case, bone) are the most troublesome issues in total joint arthroplasty today. In addition to subsurface delamination previously noted, oxidation at the same level has been identified in both polyethylene specimens that have been implanted and those left on the shelf. The principal culprit appears to have been the formation of oxygen free radicals when polyethylene was sterilized via gamma-ray radiation in an air environment. The resultant oxidation effect was that of molecular chain shortening or localized cross-linking, both of which change local material properties and promote implant wear. Most manufacturers have modified acetabular linear fabrication through the use of controlled gamma-ray radiation followed by thermal quenching to dissipate free radicals. Such implants clearly demonstrate increased inter- and intra-acetabular cross-linking and show less wear in hip simulator settings. Whether these findings, with the associated changes in material properties of the implant, result in the projected improved clinical longevity or not remains to be proven in long-term clinical studies.

PMMA. Despite the theoretical deficiencies of PMMA as a grouting agent, it remains the material of choice for fixation of total joint implants within bone. PMMA is strong in compression but much less so in tension and in torsion, arguably the most common loading scenarios in total hip arthroplasty. Furthermore, the elastic modulus of PMMA is far below that of cobalt-based alloys, resulting in a high mismatch in material properties within the bone-PMMA-implant composite.

Although various preparations of PMMA are chemically similar, small variations result in different handling characteristics. The constituents of bone cement include monomeric methacrylate in liquid form (including hydroquinone, which inhibits spontaneous polymerization and toluidine as an accelerant) and polymeric microspheres (with barium or zirconium oxide to create radiopacity and dibenzoyl peroxide as an initiator) in powder form. The rate of the polymerization process depends on temperature, humidity, and handling of the material (Fig. 8). There is a significant exotherm in the formation of cross-linked polymer, with release of 544 J/g of monomer used.

Strength properties can be improved by vacuum or centrifugation mixing, either of which reduces voids in the cement mass. PMMA contracts approximately (1%) on completion of curing. Techniques to provide a dry cement-bone interface, optimize interdigitation at the endosteum, and prevent inclusions in the cement are essential to obtaining the best longevity of PMMA used clinically.

Specific techniques (first, second, and third generation) related to use of PMMA in total hip arthroplasty are discussed elsewhere.

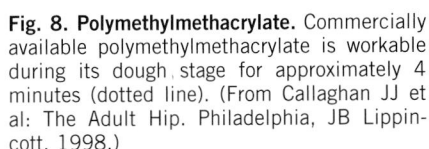

Fig. 8. Polymethylmethacrylate. Commercially available polymethylmethacrylate is workable during its dough stage for approximately 4 minutes (dotted line). (From Callaghan JJ et al: The Adult Hip. Philadelphia, JB Lippincott, 1998.)

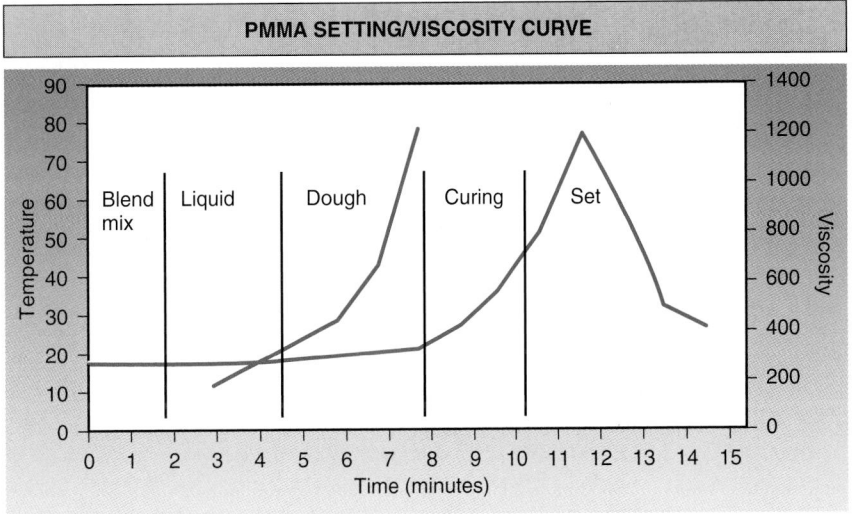

Bioresorbable Polymers. Over the past 20 years, there has been interest in fabricating polymers able to resorb over time. The theoretical advantages of load-bearing implants that are able to serve as a mechanical scaffold for tissue ingrowth and then resorb are considerable. These range from improved loading of the implant (particularly in fracture fixation) to prevention of stress bypass in bone implant constructs.

Most implants to date have been based on polylactic acid or polyglycolic acid; these materials have an extensive track record as resorbable sutures with predictable resorption kinetics and excellent biocompatibility. Aside from orbital fracture fixation, such implants have yet to see practical clinical applications as plates or rods; their performance as screws and fixation pegs appears to be very good.

With the high interest in tissue engineering in the year 2002, these materials have been seen as potential scaffolds for osteoblast and fibroblast ingrowth in bioengineered bone, tendon, and ligament. Angiogenesis and hence cellular nutrition within these devices appear to be the principal constraints to the fabrication of clinically useful intercalary implants at this time.

Biomaterials used in orthopaedic applications are remarkable for both their constancy and their potential. Stainless steel, Vitallium, and titanium alloys as well as UHMWPE and PMMA have stood the test of time and continue to serve patients with musculoskeletal problems well. Ceramics and bioresorbable materials demonstrate increasing application; the latter offer the possibility of providing growth factors and other biomolecules to orthopaedic problems in the years ahead.

BIBLIOGRAPHY

1. Beaty JH (ed): Biomaterials in total joint arthroplasty. In Orthopaedic Knowledge Update 6: Home Study Syllabus. Rosemont, IL, American Association of Orthopaedic Surgeons, 1999.
2. Black J: Orthopaedic Biomaterials in Research and Practice. New York, Churchill Livingstone, 1988.
3. Bradley RJ Jr: Biomechanics and biomaterials. In Dee R (ed): Principles of Orthopaedic Practice. New York, McGraw-Hill, 1997.
4. Buchhorn GH, Willert HG (eds): Technical Principles, Design and Safety of Joint Implants. Seattle, Hogrefe and Huber, 1994.
5. Burstein AH, Wright TM: Fundamentals of Orthopaedic Biomechanics. Baltimore, Williams & Wilkins, 1994.
6. Callaghan JJ, Dermis DA, Rosenberg AG (eds): Orthopaedic Knowledge Update: Hip and Knee Reconstruction. Rosemont, IL, AAOS, 1995.
7. Cholewicki J: Orthopaedic Biomechanics. In Patel TC (ed): Orthopaedic Surgery Board Review Manual. Wayne, PA, Hospital Physician, 1998.
8. Daniels AU: Arthroplasty: Introduction and overview. In Canale ST (ed): Campbell's Operative Orthopaedics. St. Louis, CV Mosby, 1998.
9. Dean DD: The effect of ultra-high molecular weight polyethylene wear debris on mg63 osteosarcoma cells in vitro. J Bone Joint Surg Am 1999; 81:452.
10. Early JS: Biomechanics & Biomaterials. Presented at the Southwestern Orthopaedic Surgery Board Review, Dallas, 1997.
11. Elfick APD: Wear in retrieved acetabular components: Effect of femoral head radius and patient parameters. J Arthroplasty 1998; 13:291.
12. Estok DM II: Factors affecting cement strains near the tip of a cemented femoral component. J Arthroplasty 1997; 12:40.
13. Gilbert JL: Metals. In Callaghan JJ, Rosenberg AG, Rudash HE (eds): The Adult Hip. Philadelphia, Lippincott-Raven, 1998.
14. Jones RE, Hoffmann A: Implant problems & management of complications. Southwestern Orthopaedic Surgery Board Review, Dallas, 1997.
15. Klekamp J: The use of vancomycin and tobramycin in acrylic bone cement. J Arthroplasty 1999; 14:339.
16. Landry ME: Morphology of in vitro generated ultrahigh molecular weight polyethylene wear particles as a function of contact conditions and material parameters. J Biomed Mater Res 1999; 48:61.
17. Lautenschlager EP: Structure and properties of acrylic bone cement. In Functional Behavior of Orthopaedic Biomaterials. Boca Raton, FL, CRC Press, 1984.
18. Litsky AS, Spector M: Biomaterials. In Simon SR (ed): Orthopaedic Basic Science. Rosemont, IL, AAOS, 1994.
19. Miller MD: Review of Orthopaedics. Philadelphia, WB Saunders, 1996, 2nd ed.
20. Mow VC, Flatow EL, Foster RJ: Biomechanics. In Simon SR (ed): Orthopaedic Basic Science. Rosemont, IL, AAOS, 1994.
21. Scott CP: Effectiveness of bone cement containing tobramycin. J Bone Joint Surg Br 1999; 81:440.
22. Sieber HP: Analysis of 118 second-generation metal-on-metal retrieved hip implants. J Bone Joint Surg Br 1999; 80:46.
23. Wirth MA: Isolation and characterization of polyethylene wear debris associated with osteolysis following total shoulder arthroplasty. J Bone Joint Surg Am 1999; 81:29.
24. Wroblewiski BM: Low-friction arthroplasty of the hip using alumina ceramic and cross-linked polyethylene. J Bone Joint Surg Br 1999; 81:54.

section

2

STRUCTURE AND FUNCTION OF THE MUSCULOSKELETAL SYSTEM

**VICTOR GOLDBERG AND
BRIAN JOHNSTONE**

EMBRYOLOGY OF BONE

Richard A. Schneider, Theodore Miclau, and Jill A. Helms

Summary
- Except for small regions of the face, all the human bones are of mesenchymal origin.
- Proximal to distal, anterior to posterior, and dorsal to ventral patterning of limb buds is under the control of various tissue factors.
- Regulation of angiogenesis is essential for both intramembranous and endochondral ossification.
- Mechanical environment influences bone formation, shape, and length.

EVOLUTIONARY ORIGINS OF THE SKELETON

Most members of the animal kingdom have either an exoskeleton or an endoskeleton, depending on whether their skeletal tissues form on the outside or inside of the body. Primitive vertebrates had both a true exoskeleton and an endoskeleton. The exoskeleton is believed to have originated early during vertebrate evolution as a series of dermal plates that covered the entire body and served as protective armor. Internal support for the gills, sense organs, neural tube, appendages, and organs of the trunk was provided by a cartilaginous endoskeleton, which later in evolution also came to use bone.[1] In modern vertebrates, most skeletal elements are part of the endoskeleton; however, vestiges of the exoskeleton are present in the skull and pectoral girdle. Although such exoskeletal derivatives have become thoroughly integrated with elements of the endoskeleton, they still form in a manner that is unlike the endoskeleton and characteristic of the exoskeleton. Bones of the exoskeleton are termed "dermal" on the basis of their historical association with the skin and ectoderm. Endoskeletal elements develop first as cartilage and in most cases are subsequently replaced by bone. Therefore, bones of the endoskeleton are termed "cartilage replacement bones."[2]

ORGANIZATION OF THE SKELETON

Anatomically, vertebrates have cranial, axial, and appendicular skeletons, all of which arose independently during evolution and, consequently, form through different developmental processes. The cranial skeleton is subdivided into three parts: the viscerocranium, which is the cartilaginous skeleton of the jaws and gill arches or their derivatives; the neurocranium, which includes the capsules surrounding the olfactory organs, eyes, and internal ears, as well as the box enclosing the brain; and the dermatocranium, whose parts consist exclusively of dermal bones in the cranial vault and tooth-bearing elements around the mouth (Fig. 1). Both the viscerocranium and neurocranium are preformed in cartilage and typically are replaced by bone. The axial skeleton contains the vertebrae around the neural tube, the ribs that support the body cavity, and the pectoral and pelvic girdles that provide attachment for the appendages. The appendicu-lar skeleton includes the lobed fins of fish and the limbs of those vertebrates that evolved on land.

SKELETOGENIC MESENCHYMA

EMBRYONIC SOURCES OF SKELETAL MESENCHYMA

All skeletal tissues in vertebrates are derived from either ectoderm or mesoderm, which are two of the three embryonic germ layers. Skeletal elements of ectodermal origin are found only in the head and are derived from a population of mesenchymal cells known as the neural crest.[3] Cranial neural crest cells emerge during neurulation along the dorsal margins of the neural tube and migrate into the face and jaws. The remaining skeletal elements in the body come from mesoderm (Fig. 2). The mesoderm that flanks the sides of the neural tube is termed paraxial mesoderm and in the trunk is arranged as individual segmental units called somites. The paraxial mesoderm gives rise to posterior parts of the cranial skeleton as well as the axial skeleton in the trunk. Specifically, the axial skeleton of the trunk originates from a portion of each somite termed the sclerotome. The appendicular skeleton is derived from a ventral population of mesoderm termed the lateral plate.

PATTERNING OF THE SKELETAL ELEMENTS

The molecular basis for skeletal patterning appears to involve multiple signaling centers and reciprocal interactions among various tissues. This process is best understood in the limb and involves the molecular specification of three embryonic axes: proximal-distal (shoulder to digits), an-

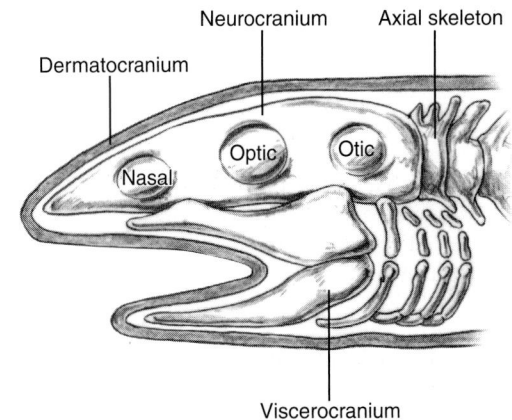

Fig. 1. Organization of the cranial skeleton in a highly schematized and generalized vertebrate head. The cranial skeleton is subdivided into the viscerocranium, which is the cartilaginous skeleton of the jaws and gill arches or their derivatives; the neurocranium, which includes the nasal, optic, and otic capsules, as well as the box enclosing the brain; and the dermatocranium, whose parts consist of dermal bones in the cranial vault and tooth-bearing elements around the mouth. (Modified from Feduccia A, McCrady E: Torrey's Morphogenesis of the Vertebrates. New York, Wiley, 1991. This material is used by permission of John Wiley & Sons, Inc.)

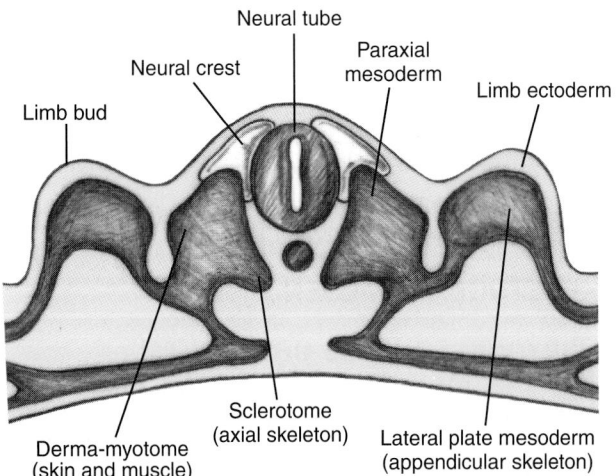

Fig. 2. Origins of skeletal mesenchyma. These origins are shown in transverse section at the level of the limbs through a generalized amniote embryo. In the head, cranial neural crest cells emerge along the dorsal margins of the neural tube and migrate into the face and jaws. The remaining skeletal elements in the body come from mesoderm. The mesoderm that flanks the neural tube is termed paraxial mesoderm. The paraxial mesoderm gives rise to posterior parts of the cranial skeleton as well as the axial skeleton in the trunk. Specifically, the axial skeleton of the trunk originates from a population of cells termed the sclerotome. The appendicular skeleton is derived from a ventral population of mesoderm termed the lateral plate. (Modified from Tabin CJ: The initiation of the limb bud: Growth factors, Hox genes, and retinoids. Cell 1995; 80:671.)

teroposterior (thumb to little finger), and dorsoventral (back of hand to palm). The limb first forms as a mesenchymal cell bud, which originates from the lateral plate and paraxial mesoderm, and is covered by a layer of thick epithelium called the apical ectodermal ridge (AER) (Fig. 3). The AER controls proximal to distal growth of the limb and is induced and maintained by an area of underlying mesoderm at the distal tip called the progress zone. Disrupting the AER during development can result in truncation of skeletal elements. Pattern formation along the anteroposterior axis of the limb bud is dependent on a subpopulation of mesenchymal cells located at the posterior margin of the progress zone, known as the zone of polarizing activity (ZPA). The ZPA establishes skeletal pattern along the anteroposterior axis.[4]

Several molecules have been implicated in limb bud morphogenesis.[5] Members of the fibroblast growth factor (FGF) family such as *FGF2*, *FGF4*, and *FGF8* can substitute for the AER and maintain distal outgrowth of the limb. Other genes, including engrailed-1 and radical fringe, position the AER along the distal margins of the limb bud.[6] Sonic hedgehog *(Shh)* is the principal signal from the ZPA and establishes the anteroposterior axis.[7] A positive feedback loop exists between signals in the ZPA and AER, which enables outgrowth of the limb. Finally, *Wnt7a* and the transcription factor *Lmx-1* are required for dorsoventral patterning.[8] The combined interactions of these tissues and genes provide the developmental framework in which a limb skeleton can be properly patterned.

CONDENSATION OF SKELETAL MESENCHYMA

The onset of skeletogenesis begins with the condensation of mesenchymal cells at future sites of ossification.[9] Mes-

enchymal cell condensation involves the activation of transcription factors such as *Hoxa4*, *Cart1*, *Cbfa1*, and *Sox9*. These genes participate in defining the population of cells that contribute to the condensation, but precisely how this occurs is unclear. Some clues about the function of one of these transcription factors during mesenchymal condensation come from analyses of a *Sox9⁻/⁻* chimeric mouse.[10] *Sox9* regulates *collagen 2a1*, and *Sox9⁻/⁻* cells are excluded from all cartilage but are found adjacent to the condensations in the mesenchyma.[10] These results indicate that *Sox9* is one of the first transcription factors that is essential for chondrocyte differentiation. Other growth factors, including those in the transforming growth factor-β (TGF-β) superfamily, induce mesenchymal and chondrocyte cell proliferation during the condensation step[11] but do not appear to be essential for the process of condensation.

Subsequent to the aggregation of mesenchymal cells in a chondrogenic condensation, structural proteins such as syndecan-3, tenascin, and versican are produced. Shortly thereafter, cells in the central region of the aggregation begin to adopt a cartilaginous phenotype. The sustained expression of *Col2* demarcates this event, followed shortly thereafter by the induction of core binding factor 1 *(Cbfa1)* and Indian hedgehog *(Ihh)* in the same cells. The functions of *Cbfa1* and *Ihh* at this early stage are unknown. Mice carrying null mutations in *Cbfa1* and *Ihh* form normally positioned, albeit smaller, condensations, suggesting that the proteins are not essential for condensation or the initial

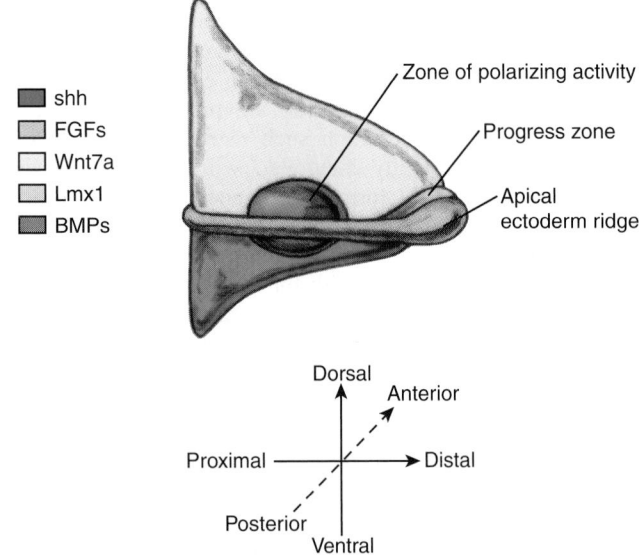

Fig. 3. Embryonic axes and patterns of gene expression in the developing limb. The limb forms as a bud of mesenchyma, which originates from the lateral plate and paraxial mesoderm, and is covered by a layer of thick epithelium called the apical ectodermal ridge (AER). The AER controls proximal to distal growth and is induced and maintained by an area of underlying mesoderm at the distal tip called the progress zone. Pattern formation along the anteroposterior axis is dependent on a subpopulation of mesenchymal cells located at the posterior margin of the progress zone, known as the zone of polarizing activity (ZPA). The ZPA establishes skeletal pattern along the anteroposterior axis. Genes in the fibroblast growth factor (FGF) family are responsible for the function of the AER. Sonic hedgehog *(Shh)* is the principal signal in the ZPA. Members of the bone morphogenetic protein family maintain cell proliferation in the progress zone. *Wnt7a* and *Lmx-1* play a role in dorsoventral patterning. (Modified from Tabin CJ: The initiation of the limb bud: Growth factors, Hox genes, and retinoids. Cell 1995; 80:671.)

commitment to a chondrogenic lineage. However, what is clear from analyses of the *Cbfa1* and *Ihh* null phenotypes is that, in addition to their obvious ossification defects, the process of cartilage maturation is also perturbed.[12, 13]

BONE FORMATION

INTRAMEMBRANOUS AND ENDOCHONDRAL OSSIFICATION

Dermal bones grow through the deposition and calcification of a bone matrix, which replaces interstitial substances within condensed mesenchyma. As a consequence, dermal bones are said to ossify intramembranously, and typically they form in close association with the ectoderm; this is an artifact of their history as components of the exoskeleton.

The growth of cartilage replacement bones occurs in two ways. First, a calcified matrix can be deposited along the external layers of cartilage (a process called perichondral ossification). Second, internal resorption of cartilage and its replacement by bone (endochondral ossification) can occur. Both processes contribute to long bone formation, in which perichondral ossification occurs along the surface of the cartilaginous scaffold and endochondral ossification occurs in the growth plates and at the epiphyses. In the earliest stages of endochondral ossification, mesenchymal cells aggregate and change their phenotype from small fibroblast-like cells to rounded, enlarged cells. These cells differentiate into chondrocytes and mature into hypertrophic chondrocytes. Hypertrophic chondrocytes secrete large amounts of a specialized extracellular matrix (ECM), rich in collagen type X, which becomes calcified and invaded by capillaries. Ossification then occurs as the terminal hypertrophic chondrocytes undergo apoptosis, the cartilage ECM undergoes degradation, and neovascularization accompanies the deposition of bone matrix by osteoblasts. The newly formed bone matrix is later remodeled by bone-resorbing osteoclasts, resulting in vascular channels filled with hematopoietic cells.

The earliest stages of intramembranous ossification are similar to those of endochondral ossification, because mesenchymal cells condense under the influence of specific epithelial signals.[14] Subsequently, endothelial cells invade these condensations to establish a blood supply. Osteoblasts then lay down new bone, which subsequently undergoes remodeling.

Multiple regulatory pathways affect the development of bone. Parathyroid hormone–related peptide *(PTHrP)* and *Ihh* appear to regulate chondrocyte growth and maturation.[15] The transcription factor *Cbfa-1* is necessary for the differentiation of osteoblasts and the formation of bone matrix.[16] Mutations in genes such as *csf-1*, c-*fos*, and c-*src*, which affect the development and function of osteoclasts, lead to defects in bone remodeling with subsequent development of osteopetrosis. Likewise, mutations in osteoprotegerin lead to a phenotype resembling osteoporosis.

THE ROLE OF ANGIOGENESIS IN BONE DEVELOPMENT

Angiogenesis is essential for the formation of bone during both intramembranous and endochondral ossification. In the process of intramembranous ossification, mesenchymal cells aggregate and, concomitantly, endothelial cells invade the tissue to establish a blood supply. During endochondral ossification, chondrocytes proliferate, differentiate, and undergo apoptosis, and the ECM forms and remodels as the blood supply is developed.

The process of endochondral ossification represents a particularly interesting physiological phenomenon because an avascular tissue (cartilage) is converted into a highly vascularized tissue (bone). A critical component in the replacement of cartilage by bone is the regulation of angiogenesis. Initially, capillaries invade the cartilaginous anlage in the central region, where chondrocytes have undergone hypertrophy, thereby establishing the primary ossification center (Fig. 4). The primary ossification center expands, causing the metaphysis and proliferating chondrocytes to be restricted to the epiphyses. Chondrocytes continue to undergo hypertrophy and apoptosis and replacement with bone, thus establishing the growth plates. In humans the growth plate closes at the end of puberty, whereas in mice the growth plates can remain open for life. The secondary ossification center, located at sites of contact between bones, forms later during development and is characterized by the presence of hypertrophic cartilage. This region also undergoes vascularization, but the molecular regulation of this event appears to be distinct from vascularization of the growth plates.[17] Some of the key modulators of angiogenesis during skeletal development include members of the vascular endothelial growth factor family[18] as well as their receptors, *Flt*, *Flk*, and members of the neuropilin gene family.[19]

Fig. 4. Schematic illustration of the role of angiogenesis during endochondral ossification of a long bone. The perichondrium is composed of flattened mesenchymal cells that lie adjacent to the underlying chondrocytes. These perichondrial cells are the first to differentiate into osteoblasts. Shortly after forming a bony collar, vascular endothelial cells invade the hypertrophic cartilage matrix, which is partly remodeled by matrix metalloproteinases. The precise origins of osteoblasts that replace the cartilage template are not known; likely sources include the perichondrium and the surrounding connective tissues. When angiogenesis is perturbed or delayed, ossification of the long bones is also disrupted.[17] (Modified from Netter FH: Musculoskeletal system: Anatomy, physiology, and metabolic disorders. In Woodbine RT, Crelin ES, Kaplan F (eds): The CIBA Collection of Medical Illustrations. New Jersey, CIBA-GEIGY, 1991.)

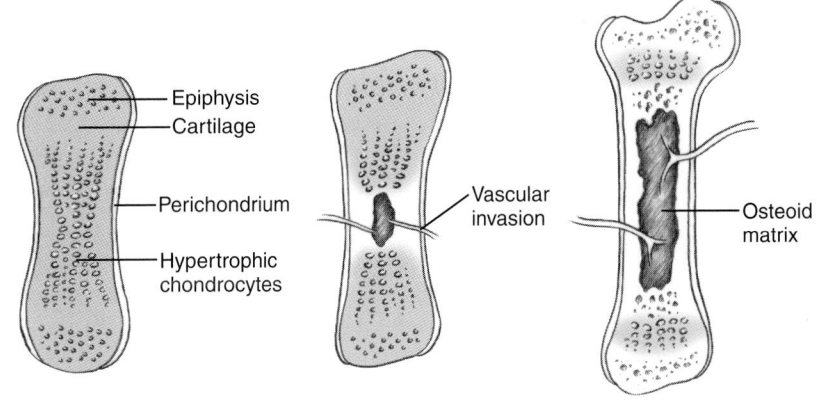

Epiphysis
Cartilage
Perichondrium
Hypertrophic chondrocytes
Vascular invasion
Osteoid matrix

BONE FORMATION AND THE MECHANICAL ENVIRONMENT

Mechanical forces can influence the shape and length of growing bones. Mesenchymal cells can differentiate into bone, cartilage, or fibrous tissue, depending on local mechanical input.[20] Both in vitro and in vivo studies have demonstrated that mechanical factors influence chondrogenesis and bone development during the early stages of endochondral ossification. There is growing evidence that deforming strain favors fibrous tissue or bone formation, whereas hydrostatic compression induces formation of fibrocartilage or cartilage.[21] However, at this time the precise effects of these mechanical stimuli on the cellular and molecular basis of skeletogenesis are poorly understood. This is an exciting area of research for both biologists and bioengineers alike.

REFERENCES

1. Carroll RL: Vertebrate Paleontology and Evolution. New York, WH Freeman, 1988, p 698.
2. Patterson C: Cartilage bones, dermal bones, and membrane bones, or the exoskeleton versus the endoskeleton. In Andrews S, Miles R, Walker A (eds): Problems in Vertebrate Evolution. London, Academic Press, 1977, p 77.
3. Noden DM: Interactions and fates of avian craniofacial mesenchyme. Development 1988; 103:121.
4. Saunders JWJ, Gasseling MT: Ectoderm-mesenchymal interactions in the origin of wing symmetry. In Fleischmajer R, Billingham RE (eds): Epithelial-Mesenchymal Interactions. Baltimore, Williams & Wilkins, 1968, p 78.
5. Johnson RL, Tabin CJ: Molecular models for vertebrate limb development. Cell 1997; 90:979.
6. Laufer E, Dahn R, Orozco OE, et al: Expression of radical fringe in limb-bud ectoderm regulates apical ectodermal ridge formation (see comments). Nature 1997; 386:366.
7. Riddle RD, Johnson RL, Laufer E, et al: Sonic hedgehog mediates the polarizing activity of the ZPA. Cell 1993; 75:1401.
8. Cygan JA, Johnson RL, McMahon AP: Novel regulatory interactions revealed by studies of murine limb pattern in Wnt-7a and En-1 mutants. Development 1997; 124: 5021.
9. Hall BK, Miyake T: Divide, accumulate, differentiate: Cell condensation in skeletal development revisited. Int J Dev Biol 1995; 39:881.
10. Bi W, Deng JM, Zhang Z, et al: Sox9 is required for cartilage formation. Nat Genet 1999; 22:85.
11. Mundlos S, Olsen BR: Heritable diseases of the skeleton: Part I. Molecular insights into skeletal development-transcription factors and signaling pathways. FASEB J 1997; 1:125.
12. St. Jacques BM, Hammerschmidt M, McMahon AP: Indian hedgehog signaling regulates proliferation and differentiation of chondrocytes and is essential for bone formation. Genes Dev 1999; 13:2072.
13. Ferguson C, Alpern E, Miclau T, et al: Does adult fracture repair recapitulate embryonic skeletal formation? Mech Dev 1999; 87:57.
14. Hall BK: The role of tissue interactions in the growth of bone. In Dixon AD, Sarnat BG (eds): Factors and Mechanisms Influencing Bone Growth. New York, Alan R. Liss, 1982, p 205.
15. Vortkamp A, Lee K, Lanske B, et al: Regulation of rate of cartilage differentiation by Indian hedgehog and PTH-related protein. Science 1996; 273:613.
16. Komori T, Yagi H, Nomura S, et al: Targeted disruption of Cbfa1 results in a complete lack of bone formation owing to maturational arrest of osteoblasts (see comments). Cell 1997; 89:755.
17. Vu TH, Shipley JM, Bergers G, et al: MMP-9/gelatinase B is a key regulator of growth plate angiogenesis and apoptosis of hypertrophic chondrocytes. Cell 1998; 93: 411.
18. Gerber H, Vu TH, Ryan AM, et al: VEGF couples hypertrophic cartilage remodeling, ossification and angiogenesis during endochondral bone formation. Nat Med 1999; 5:623.
19. Neufeld G, Cohen T, Gengrinovitch S, et al: Vascular endothelial growth factor (VEGF) and its receptors. FASEB J 1999; 13:9.
20. Ogden JA: Chondro-osseous development and growth. In Fundamental and Clinical Bone Physiology. Philadelphia, JB Lippincott, 1980, p 100.
21. Carter DR, Van Der Meulen MC, Beaupré GS: Mechanical factors in bone growth and development. Bone 1996; 18:5S.

BONE: STRUCTURE, FUNCTION, GROWTH, AND REMODELING

section 2
chapter 2

Natalie Sims and Roland Baron

Summary
- Bones have three major functions: to serve as (1) mechanical support, (2) sites of muscle insertion, and (3) a reserve of calcium and phosphate for the organism.
- The organic matrix of bone is formed mostly of collagen and also of noncollagenous proteins. Hydroxyapatite crystals bind to both types of proteins.
- Most components of the bone matrix are synthesized and secreted by osteoblasts.
- Resorption of the bone matrix is required for adaptation to growth, repair, and mineral mobilization. This process is performed by the macrophage-related osteoclast.
- Bone is remodeled throughout life by the activation-resorption-formation (ARF) sequence by which the coordinated actions of osteoclasts and osteoblasts replace old with new bone.
- In the normal adult skeleton, remodeling is coupled such that the level of resorption is equal to the level of formation, and bone density remains constant.
- Intramembranous ossification is the process by which flat bones are formed. For this process, osteoblasts differentiate directly from mesenchymal cells to form the bone matrix.
- Long bones are formed by endochondral ossification, which is characterized by the presence of a cartilaginous phase modified by chondrocyte differentiation followed by ARF remodeling.

Clinical relevance
- The most common bone diseases arise from disruptions in the process of bone remodeling; osteoporosis occurs when the balance is in favor of bone resorption, and osteopetrosis occurs when the balance is in favor of formation.
- Chondrodysplasias result from defects in endochondral ossification.
- The fracture repair process involves a less organized form of bone histogenesis followed by cycles of bone remodeling.
- Fracture healing rates relate directly to the speed of bone remodeling and can be altered with therapy.

INTRODUCTION

DEFINITION

Bone is a specialized connective tissue that, together with cartilage, makes up the skeletal system. These tissues serve three functions: (1) mechanical: support for and site of muscle attachment for locomotion; (2) protective: for vital organs and bone marrow; and (3) metabolic: as a reserve of ions, especially calcium and phosphate, for the maintenance of serum homeostasis, which is essential to life.

In this chapter, the mechanisms of bone remodeling, histogenesis, and bone growth are described. Remodeling is the process by which old bone is replaced by new bone, characterized by the coordinated actions of osteoclasts and osteoblasts in the ARF sequence. Histogenesis is the formation of new bone during embryonic development; it occurs by two means: intramembranous ossification and endochondral ossification. Bone growth is a term used to describe the changes in bone structure that follow histogenesis during the period of skeletal growth and maturation.

CLINICAL RELEVANCE

An understanding of the basic mechanisms of remodeling, histogenesis, and growth is essential to treating bone disease and accelerating fracture repair.

SEMINAL SCIENTIFIC OBSERVATIONS

The history of bone anatomic research is long and distinguished. Galileo was the first to suggest a biomechanical function for bone, and it was his work, as well as that of Vesalius in the 16th century, that first described the anatomy of the skeleton in detail.

Hunter (1763) was the first to demonstrate the dynamic nature of bone remodeling, using vital staining techniques developed by Belchier in the 1730s. Hunter showed that as bones increase in size, they undergo complex patterns of bone formation and resorption. Hunter also first described the manner in which trabecular bone is laid down along lines of maximal stress. Bougery (1832) carried out detailed architectural studies of the structure of bone and suggested that maximum bone strength was achieved with a minimum of material. This work was further developed by the engineer/anatomist team of Culmann and Meyer (1867), but it is Wolff (1869) who is best remembered for showing mathematically the morphological adaptation of bone structure to its function (resulting in Wolff's Law).

The structure of the epiphyseal growth plate and the organization of chondrocytes within it were first described by Goodsir and Flourens working independently in the 1840s. It was not until 100 years later that the mechanisms of endochondral function were explained in considerably more detail by Bloom and Bloom, and more knowledge was added by the electron microscope studies of the 1950s and 1960s.

Early microscopic studies by Andral (1829) noted the role of vascularization in bone ossification. Bernard (1878) stressed the importance of fluid homeostasis to vitality, but the skeleton was still considered a purely mechanical structure until Bloom's work in 1941, when the role of the skeleton in calcium homeostasis was established.

The presence of bone cells had been described by many

early researchers. In 1911, Dubreuil proposed different roles of osteoclasts and osteoblasts; these roles were not fully accepted until early in vitro studies of the 1930s, when many fundamental regulators of bone cell function, such as parathyroid hormone (PTH), were also noted. Osteoblast function was understood well before that of the osteoclast, with significant advances being made by electron microscope studies in the 1950s. In the 1960s, Owen delineated the osteoblast lineage and its stromal cell origins. In 1966, Frost proposed the model of the basic multicellular unit and described its role in the ARF sequence. Although electron microscopic studies in the 1950s described the basics of osteoclast structure, the mechanisms of osteoclast function remained elusive until detailed electron microscopic and biochemical studies by a number of researchers in the 1960s. In 1975, Walker used marrow transplants to rescue osteopetrosis and thereby revealed the hematopoietic origin of the osteoclast.

During the 1980s, local regulation of bone cell activity was the subject of intense study, and many cytokines were described and found to act as autocrine and paracrine regulators of bone cell function. Advances in bone research in the 1990s focused on the molecular basis of skeletal development and remodeling; they are discussed in more detail in the pages to follow.

FUNDAMENTAL SCIENCE

BONE AS AN ORGAN: MACROSCOPIC ORGANIZATION

Anatomically, two types of bones can be distinguished in the skeleton: flat bones (skull bones, scapula, mandible, and ileum) and long bones (tibia, femur, humerus, etc.). These are derived by two distinct types of development: intramembranous and endochondral, respectively (see the section, Skeletal Development: Histogenesis), although the development and growth of long bones actually involve both processes. The main difference between intramembranous and endochondral bone formation is the presence of a cartilaginous phase in the latter.

External examination of a long bone shows two wider extremities (the epiphyses), a more or less cylindrical tube in the middle (the midshaft or diaphysis), and a developmental zone between them (the metaphysis). In a growing long bone, the epiphysis and the metaphysis, which originate from two independent ossification centers, are separated by a layer of cartilage, the epiphyseal cartilage (also called the growth plate). This layer of proliferative cells and expanding cartilage matrix is responsible for the longitudinal growth of bones; it becomes entirely calcified and remodeled and is replaced by bone by the end of the growth period (see the section, Skeletal Development: Histogenesis). The external part of the bone is formed by a thick and dense layer of calcified tissue, the *cortex* (compact bone), which, in the diaphysis, encloses the medullary cavity where the hematopoietic bone marrow is housed. Toward the metaphysis and the epiphysis, the cortex becomes progressively thinner, and the internal space is filled with a network of thin, calcified trabeculae; this is the *cancellous bone,* also named spongy or *trabecular bone.* The spaces enclosed by these thin trabeculae are also filled with hematopoietic bone marrow and are continuous with the diaphyseal medullary cavity. The outer cortical bone

surfaces at the epiphyses are covered with a layer of articular cartilage that does not calcify.

There are, consequently, two surfaces where bone is in contact with the soft tissues: an external surface (the periosteal surface) and an internal surface (the endosteal surface). These surfaces are lined with osteogenic cells organized in layers, the periosteum and the endosteum.

Cortical bone and trabecular bone are made up of the same cells and the same matrix elements, but there are structural and functional differences. The primary structural difference is quantitative: 80% to 90% of the volume of compact bone is calcified, whereas only 15% to 25% of the trabecular volume is calcified (the remainder being occupied by bone marrow, blood vessels, and connective tissue). The result is that 70% to 85% of the interface with soft tissues is at the endosteal bone surface, including all trabecular surfaces, leading to the functional difference: the cortical bone fulfills mainly a mechanical and protective function, and the trabecular bone serves a metabolic function.

BONE AS A TISSUE: BONE MATRIX AND MINERAL

Approximately 90% of the bone matrix consists of type I collagen fibers. Within lamellar bone, the fibers are usually oriented in a preferential direction for optimal bone strength. This fiber organization allows the highest density of collagen per unit volume of tissue. The lamellae can be parallel to each other if deposited along a flat surface (trabecular bone and periosteum) or concentric if deposited on a surface surrounding a channel centered on a blood vessel (cortical bone haversian system). Spindle or plate-shaped crystals of hydroxyapatite $[3Ca_3(PO_4)_2 \cdot (OH)_2]$ are found on the collagen fibers within them and in the ground substance. They tend to be oriented in the same direction as the collagen fibers.

When bone is formed very rapidly during development and fracture healing or in tumors and some metabolic bone diseases, there is no preferential organization of the collagen fibers. They are then not as tightly packed, and they are found in somewhat randomly oriented bundles: this type of bone is called *woven bone,* as opposed to lamellar bone. Woven bone is characterized by irregular bundles of collagen fibers, large and extremely numerous osteocytes, and delayed, disorderly calcification that occurs in irregularly distributed patches. Woven bone lacks the strength of lamellar bone, and it is for this reason that it is usually replaced by bone remodeling (see later discussion).

Numerous noncollagenous proteins present in bone matrix have been purified and sequenced, but their role has been only partially characterized (Table 1). Most noncollagenous proteins within the bone matrix are synthesized by bone-forming cells, but not all: approximately a quarter of the bone noncollagenous proteins are plasma proteins that are preferentially absorbed by the bone matrix, such as α_2-HS-glycoprotein, which is synthesized in the liver. The major noncollagenous protein produced is osteocalcin, which makes up 1% of the matrix and which may play a role in calcium binding and stabilization of hydroxyapatite in the matrix and/or regulation of bone formation, as suggested by increased bone mass in osteocalcin knockout mice.[1] Another negative regulator of bone formation in the matrix is matrix Gla protein, which appears to inhibit pre-

TABLE 1. NONCOLLAGENOUS PROTEINS IN BONE

Protein	Molecular Weight	Role
Osteonectin	32K	Calcium, apatite, and matrix protein binding[98]
		Modulates cell attachment[99]
α_2-HS-glycoprotein	46–67K	Chemotactic for monocytes[100]
		Mineralization via matrix vesicles[101]
Osteocalcin (bone Gla protein)	6K	Involved in stabilization of hydroxyapatite[102]
		Binding of calcium[102]
		Chemotactic for monocytes[102]
		Regulation of bone formation[1]
Matrix-Gla-protein	9K	Inhibits matrix mineralization[2]
Osteopontin (Bone sialoprotein I)	50K	Cell attachment (via RGD sequence)[103]
		Calcium binding[99]
Bone sialoprotein II	75K	Cell attachment (via RGD sequence)[103]
		Calcium binding[99]
24K phosphoprotein (α-1[I] pro-collagen N-propeptide)	24K	Residue from collagen processing
Biglycan (proteoglycan I)	45K core	Regulation of collagen fiber growth
		Mineralization and bone formation[3]
		Growth factor binding[104]
Decorin (proteoglycan II)	36K core plus side chains	Collagen fibrillogenesis[104]
		Growth factor binding[104]
Thrombospondin and fibronectin		Cell attachment (via RGD sequence)[105]
		Growth factor binding
		Hydroxyapatite formation[106]
Others (including proteolipids)		Mineralization
Growth factors		
IGF-I and IGF-II		Differentiation, proliferation, and activity of osteoblasts[26, 28]
TGF-β		Induction of bone and cartilage in osteogenesis and frac-
Bone morphogenetic proteins		ture repair[32, 90]

IGF, insulin-like growth factor; TGF, transforming growth factor.

mature or inapropriate mineralization, as demonstrated in a knockout mouse model.[2] In contrast to this, biglycan, a proteoglycan, is expressed in the bone matrix; it positively regulates bone formation, as demonstrated by reduced bone formation and bone mass in biglycan knockout mice.[3]

CELLULAR ORGANIZATION WITHIN THE BONE MATRIX: OSTEOCYTES

The calcified bone matrix is not metabolically inert, and cells (osteocytes) are found embedded deep within the bone in small lacunae (Fig. 1). All osteocytes are derived from bone-forming cells (osteoblasts) that have been

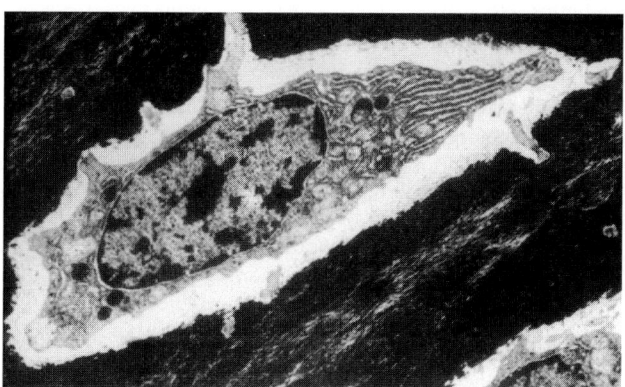

Fig. 1. Osteocyte. This is an electron micrograph of an osteocyte within a lacuna in calcified bone matrix. The cell has a basal nucleus, cytoplasmic extensions, and well-developed Golgi complex and endoplasmic reticulum.

trapped in the bone matrix that they produced and that became calcified. Even though the metabolic activity of the osteoblast decreases dramatically once it is fully encased in bone matrix, these cells still produce matrix proteins. Osteocytes have numerous long cell processes rich in microfilaments, which are in contact with cell processes from other osteocytes (there are frequent gap junctions) or with processes from the cells lining the bone surface (osteoblasts or flat lining cells). These processes are organized during the formation of the matrix and before its calcification; they form a network of thin canaliculi permeating the entire bone matrix. Osteocytic canaliculi are not distributed evenly about the cell but are directed mainly toward the bone surface. Between the osteocyte's plasma membrane and the bone matrix itself is the periosteocytic space. This space exists both in the lacunae and in the canaliculi, and it is filled with extracellular fluid (ECF), the only source of nutrients for the osteocyte. ECF flow through the canalicular network is altered during bone matrix compression and tension.

Osteocyte structure varies according to cell age and functional activity. A young osteocyte has most of the ultrastructural characteristics of the osteoblast from which it was derived, except that there has been a decrease in cell volume and in the importance of the organelles involved in protein synthesis (rough endoplasmic reticulum, Golgi apparatus). An older osteocyte, located deeper within the calcified bone, shows a further decrease in cell volume and organelles and an accumulation of glycogen in the cytoplasm. These cells synthesize small amounts of new bone matrix at the surface of the osteocytic lacunae, which can subsequently calcify. Osteocytes express, in low levels, a number of osteoblast markers, including osteocalcin, osteopontin, osteonectin, and the osteocyte marker E11.[4, 5]

Despite the complex organization of the osteocytic network and its location within the bone matrix, the exact function of these cells remains obscure. Given the structure of the network and the location of osteocytes within lacunae where ECF flow can be detected, it is likely that osteocytes respond to bone tissue strain and influence bone remodeling activity by recruiting osteoclasts to sites where bone remodeling is required.[6] Osteocyte cellular activity is increased after bone loading; studies in cell culture have demonstrated increased calcium influx and prostaglandin production by osteocytes after mechanical stimulation,[7] but there is not yet any direct evidence for osteocytes signaling to cells on the bone surface in response to bone strain or microdamage.

The fate of the osteocyte is to be phagocytosed and digested together with the other components of bone during osteoclastic bone resorption.[8]

THE OSTEOBLAST AND BONE FORMATION

The osteoblast is the bone-lining cell responsible for the production of the bone matrix constituents, collagen, and ground substance (Fig. 2). Osteoblasts never appear or function individually; they are always found in clusters of cuboidal cells along the bone surface (approximately 100 to 400 cells per bone-forming site). At the light microscope level, the osteoblast is characterized morphologically by a round nucleus at the base of the cell (away from the bone surface), an intensely basophilic cytoplasm, and a prominent Golgi complex located between the nucleus and the apex of the cell. Osteoblasts always line the layer of bone matrix that they are producing but before it is calcified (called, at this point, osteoid tissue). Osteoid tissue exists because of a time lag of approximately 10 days between matrix formation and subsequent calcification. Behind the osteoblast is usually one or two layers of cells: activated mesenchymal cells and preosteoblasts (see later). A mature osteoblast does not divide.

At the ultrastructural level, the osteoblast is characterized by the presence of an extremely well-developed rough endoplasmic reticulum with dilated cisternae and a dense granular content and the presence of a large circular Golgi complex comprising multiple Golgi stacks. These organelles are involved in the major activity of the osteoblast: the production and secretion of collagenous and noncollagenous bone matrix proteins, including type I collagen. Osteoblasts also produce a range of growth factors under a variety of stimuli, including the insulin-like growth factors (IGFs),[9] platelet-derived growth factors (PDGFs),[10] basic fibroblast growth factor (bFGF),[11] transforming growth factor-β (TGF-β),[12] a range of cytokines,[13] and bone morphogenetic proteins (BMPs).[14] Osteoblast activity is regulated in an autocrine and paracrine manner by these growth factors, whose receptors can be found on osteoblasts, as well as receptors for a range of endocrine hormones. Classic endocrine receptors include receptors for parathyroid hormone/parathyroid hormone–related protein receptor, thyroid hormone,[15] growth hormone,[16] insulin,[17] progesterone,[18] and prolactin.[19] Osteoblastic nuclear steroid hormone

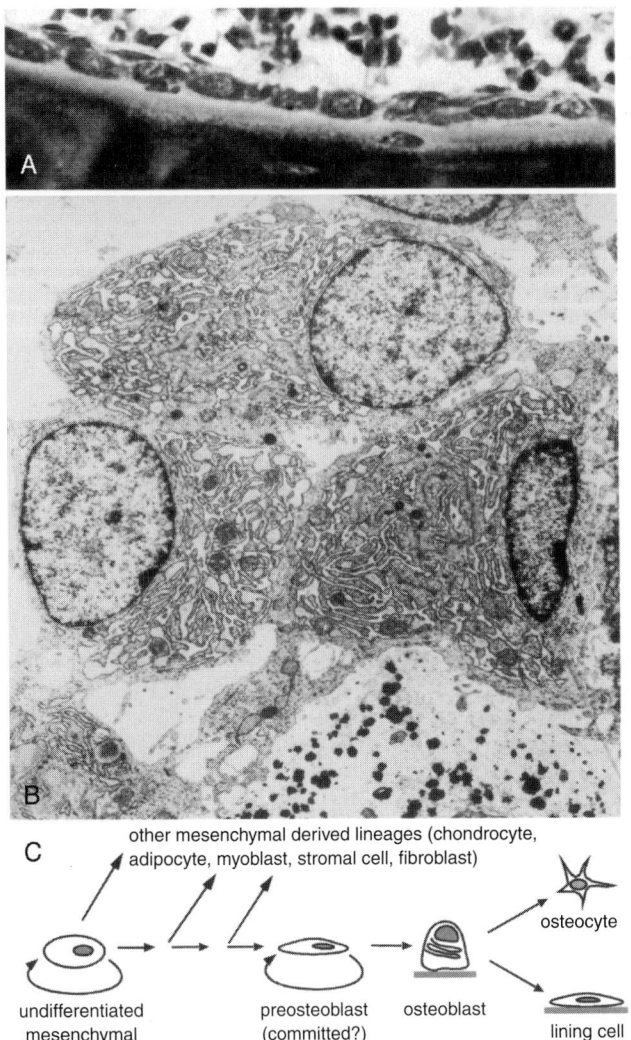

Fig. 2. Osteoblasts and osteoid tissue. *A,* Light micrograph of a group of osteoblasts producing osteoid; note the newly embedded osteocyte. *B,* Electron micrograph of three osteoblasts covering a layer of mineralizing osteoid tissue. Note the prominent Golgi complex and endoplasmic reticulum characteristic of active osteoblasts. The black clusters in the osteoid tissue are deposits of mineral. *C,* Osteoblast lineage. Osteoblasts originate from undifferentiated mesenchymal cells, which are capable of proliferation and may differentiate into one of a range of cell types. The preosteoblast is also capable of proliferation and may be already committed to an osteoblast phenotype. The mature osteoblast no longer proliferates but can differentiate further into an osteocyte once embedded in the bone matrix or to a lining cell on the bone surface.

receptors include receptors for estrogens,[20, 21] androgens,[22] vitamin D₃,[23] and retinoids.[24] Receptors for paracrine and autocrine effectors include those for epidermal growth factor (EGF),[25] IGFs,[26, 27] PDGF,[12] TGF-β,[28] interleukins (ILs),[29, 30] FGFs,[31] and BMPs.[32] Osteoblasts also have receptors for several adhesion molecules (integrins) involved in cell attachment to the bone surface.[33]

Osteoblasts do not operate in isolation; gap junctions often occur between osteoblasts working together on the bone surface. Osteoblasts also appear to communicate with the osteocyte network within the bone matrix (see earlier) as cytoplasmic processes on the secreting side of the osteoblast extend deep into the osteoid matrix and are in contact with processes of the osteocytes dwelling there.

Osteoblasts originate from local pluripotent mesenchymal stem cells, either bone marrow stromal stem cells (endosteum) or connective tissue mesenchymal stem cells (periosteum). These precursors, with the right stimulation, undergo proliferation and differentiate into preosteoblasts, at which point they are committed to differentiate into mature osteoblasts, although evidence suggests preosteoblast commitment may be more fluid than previously understood.[34]

The committed preosteoblast is located in apposition to the bone surface and is usually present in layers below active mature osteoblasts. These preosteoblasts are elliptical cells, with an elongated nucleus, and are still capable of proliferation. Preosteoblasts lack the well-developed protein-synthesizing capability of the mature osteoblast and do not have the characteristically localized, mature, and rough endoplasmic reticulum or Golgi apparatus of the mature cell.

The development of the osteoblast phenotype is gradual, with a defined sequence of gene expression and cell activity during development and maturation. In the early stages of osteoblast proliferation, the proliferative genes c-*myc* and c-*fos* are expressed. As the cell matures, its function and protein production schedule change. When osteoblasts begin to lay down osteoid, type I collagen, fibronectin, and some growth factors are expressed. While cells are still producing type I collagen, they also begin producing alkaline phosphatase and then matrix Gla protein. Later, collagen production slows, and the wave of alkaline phosphatase production is followed by osteocalcin and osteopontin production.[35]

Toward the end of the matrix-secreting period, a further step is involved in osteoblast maturation. Approximately 15% of the mature osteoblasts become encapsulated in the new bone matrix and differentiate into osteocytes. In contrast, some cells remain on the bone surface, becoming flat lining cells. The signaling mechanism that determines which cells become osteocytes is not understood.

There is evidence that after mechanical stimulation, bone lining cells develop ultrastructural features of osteoblastic differentiation and activity without any cell proliferation.[36] By 48 hours after mechanical loading, lining cells became cuboidal, with rounded nuclei and abundant rough endoplasmic reticulum, characteristics of a mature osteoblast. This would provide a mechanism for the rapid osteogenic response after mechanical stimuli and is consistent with earlier studies demonstrating increased osteoblast activity without cell proliferation following PTH treatment.[37]

Mechanism of Bone Formation

Bone formation occurs by three coordinated processes: the production and maturation of the osteoid matrix and the subsequent mineralization of the matrix. In normal adult bone, these processes occur at the same rate so that the balance between matrix production and mineralization is equal. Initially, osteoblasts deposit collagen rapidly, without mineralization, producing a thickening osteoid seam. This is followed by an increase in the mineralization rate to equal the rate of collagen synthesis. In the final stage, the rate of collagen synthesis decreases, and mineralization continues until the osteoid seam is fully mineralized. This

time lag (the mineralization lag time or osteoid maturation period) appears to be required for osteoid to be modified so it is able to support mineralization. Although this delay is not yet understood, it is likely that either collagen cross-linking occurs or an inhibitor of mineralization, such as matrix Gla protein,[38] is removed during this time, thus allowing mineralization to proceed.

To initiate mineralization in woven bone or in growth plate cartilage, high local concentrations of Ca^{2+} and PO_4^{3-} ions must be reached in order to induce their precipitation into amorphous calcium phosphate, leading to hydroxyapatite crystal formation. This is achieved by membrane-bound matrix vesicles, which originate by budding from the cytoplasmic processes of the chondrocyte or the osteoblast and are deposited within the matrix during its formation.[39] In the matrix, these vesicles are the first structure wherein hydroxyapatite crystals are observed. The membranes are very rich in alkaline phosphatases and in acidic phospholipids, which hydrolyze inhibitors of calcification in the matrix, including pyrophosphate and adenosine triphosphate (ATP), allowing condensation of apatite crystals. Once the crystals are in the matrix environment, they will grow in clusters that later coalesce to completely calcify the matrix, filling the spaces between and within the collagen fibers. In adult lamellar bone, matrix vesicles are not present, and mineralization occurs in an orderly manner through progression of the mineralization front into the osteoid tissue.

THE OSTEOCLAST AND BONE RESORPTION

The osteoclast is the bone lining cell responsible for bone resorption (Fig. 3). The osteoclast is a giant multinucleated cell, up to 100 μm in diameter and containing 4 to 20 nuclei. It is usually in contact with a calcified bone surface and within a lacuna (Howship's lacuna) that is the result of its own resorptive activity. It is possible to find up to four or five osteoclasts in the same resorptive site, but there are usually only one or two. Under the light microscope, the nuclei appear to vary within the same cell: some are round and euchromatic, and some are irregular in contour and heterochromatic, possibly reflecting asynchronous fusion of mononuclear precursors. The cytoplasm is "foamy" with many vacuoles. The zone of contact with the bone is characterized by the presence of a ruffled border with dense patches on each side (the sealing zone).

Characteristic ultrastructural features of this cell are abundant Golgi complexes around each nucleus, mitochondria, and transport vesicles loaded with lysosomal enzymes. The most prominent features of the osteoclast are, however, the deep foldings of the plasma membrane in the area facing the bone matrix (ruffled border) and the surrounding zone of attachment (sealing zone). The sealing zone is a ring of contractile proteins that attach the cell to the bone surface, thus sealing off the subosteoclastic bone-resorbing compartment. The attachment of the cell to the matrix is performed via integrin receptors, which bind to specific RGD (arginine-glycine-aspartate) sequences in matrix proteins (see Table 1). The plasma membrane in the ruffled border area contains proteins that are also found at the limiting membrane of lysosomes and related organelles and a specific type of electrogenic vacuolar proton ATPase involved in acidification. The basolateral plasma membrane

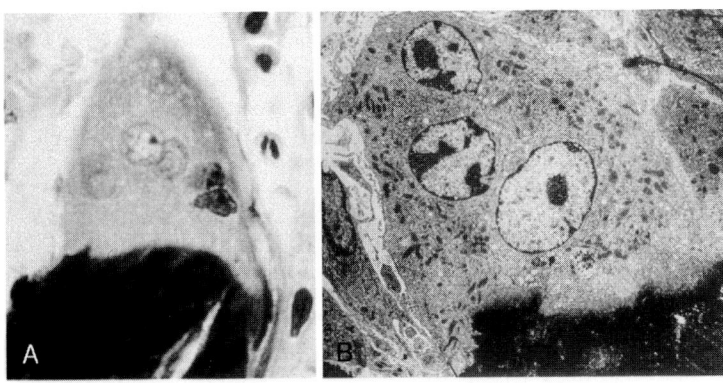

Fig. 3. Osteoclasts and the mechanism of bone resorption. Light micrograph (*A*) and electron micrograph (*B*) of an osteoclast, demonstrating the ruffled border and numerous nuclei. *C*, Osteoclastic resorption. The osteoclast forms a sealing zone via integrin-mediated attachment to specific peptide sequences within the bone matrix, forming a sealed compartment between the cell and the bone surface. This compartment is acidified such that an optimal pH is reached for lysosomal enzyme activity and bone resorption.

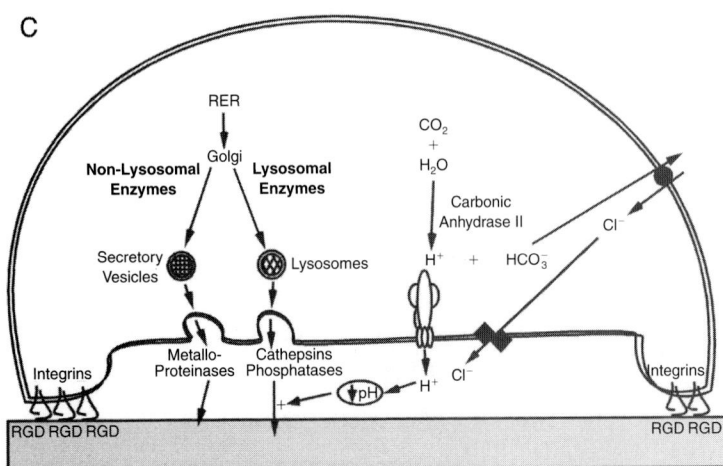

of the osteoclast is specifically enriched in Na^+, K^+-ATPase (sodium pumps), HCO_3^-/Cl^- exchangers, and Na^+/H^+ exchangers[40] and numerous ion channels.[41-43]

Lysosomal enzymes such as tartrate-resistant acid phosphatase and cathepsin K are actively synthesized by the osteoclast and are found in the endoplasmic reticulum, Golgi, and many transport vesicles. The enzymes are secreted, via the ruffled border, into the extracellular bone-resorbing compartment, where they reach a sufficiently high extracellular concentration because this compartment is sealed off. The transport and targeting of these enzymes for secretion at the apical pole of the osteoclast involve mannose-6-phosphate receptors. Furthermore, the cell secretes several metalloproteinases such as collagenase (MMP-13) and gelatinase B (MMP-9),[44] which appear to be involved in preosteoclast migration to the bone surface as well as bone matrix digestion.[45, 46]

Attachment of the osteoclast to the bone surface is essential for bone resorption. This process involves transmembrane adhesion receptors of the integrin.[47] Integrins attach to specific amino acid sequences (mostly RGD sequences) within proteins in or at the surface of the bone matrix. In the osteoclast, $\alpha_v\beta_3$ (vitronectin receptor), $\alpha_2\beta_1$ (collagen receptor), and $\alpha_v\beta_5$ integrins are predominantly expressed.[48] Without cell attachment, the acidified microenvironment cannot be established and the osteoclast cannot be highly motile.

After osteoclast adhesion to the bone matrix, $\alpha_v\beta_3$ binding activates cytoskeletal reorganization within the osteoclast, including cell spreading and polarization.[49] In most cells, cell attachment occurs via focal adhesions, where stress fibers (bundles of microfilaments) anchor the cell to the substrate. In osteoclasts, attachment usually occurs via podosomes, clusters of small focal adhesion-like structures. Podosomes are more dynamic structures than focal adhesions and occur in cells that are highly motile. The continual assembly and disassembly of podosomes allow osteoclast movement across the bone surface during bone resorption. Integrin signaling and subsequent podosome formation are dependent on a number of adhesion kinases, including the proto-oncogene *src*, which, although not required for osteoclast maturation, is required for osteoclast function, as demonstrated by osteopetrosis in the *src* knockout mouse.[50] It has been noted that Pyk2, another member of the focal adhesion kinase family, is also activated by $\alpha_v\beta_3$ during osteoclast attachment and is required for bone resorption.[51]

Osteoclasts resorb bone by acidification and proteolysis of the bone matrix and hydroxyapatite crystals encapsulated within the sealing zone. Carbonic anhydrase type II produces hydrogen ions within the cell, which are then pumped across the ruffled border membrane via proton pumps located in the basolateral membrane, thereby acidifying the extracellular compartment. The protons are highly concentrated in the cytosol of the osteoclast; ATP and CO_2 are provided by the mitochondria. The basolateral membrane activity exchanges bicarbonate for chloride, thereby avoiding alkalinization of the cytosol. K^+ channels in the basolateral domain and Cl^- channels in the apical ruffled border ensure dissipation of the electrogenic gradients generated by the vacuolar H$^+$-ATPase. The basolateral sodium pumps might be involved in secondary active transport of calcium and/or protons in association with an Na$^+$/Ca^{2+} exchanger and/or an Na$^+$/H$^+$ antiport.

The first process during bone matrix resorption is mobilization of the hydroxyapatite crystals by digestion of their link to collagen via the noncollagenous proteins, and the low pH dissolves the hydroxyapatite crystals, exposing the bone matrix. Then the residual collagen fibers are digested either by cathepsins, now at optimal pH, or activated collagenases. The residues from this extracellular digestion are either internalized or transported across the cell and released at the basolateral domain. Residues may also be released during periods of sealing zone relapse, as probably occurs during osteoclast motility, and possibly induced by a calcium sensor responding to the rise of extracellular calcium in the bone-resorbing compartment.

Osteoclast function is regulated by both locally acting cytokines and systemic hormones. Although studies of osteoclastic receptors have been limited by the difficulty in obtaining pure osteoclast preparations, osteoclastic receptors for calcitonin,[52] androgens,[53] thyroid hormone,[54] insulin,[55] and glutamate[56] have been demonstrated. The presence of estrogen receptors in osteoclasts remains controversial.[57, 58] Although PTH receptors have been demonstrated in osteoclasts,[59] the significance of this finding is unclear, because purified osteoclasts do not respond to PTH treatment.[60] Instead, endocrine regulation of bone resorption may be mediated by osteoblasts; for example, PTH can stimulate osteoblastic production of macrophage colony-stimulating factor (CSF) and IL-6, which then act directly on the osteoclast.[61] Other hormones act on osteoclast precursors, such as 1,25-dihydroxyvitamin D$_3$, which affects precursor proliferation but is unlikely to act directly on mature osteoclasts because they do not express vitamin D receptors.[62, 63]

A large number of paracrine regulators of osteoclast function act via osteoblast signaling. Some examples include IL-18, which increases osteoclast proliferation via increased osteoblastic production of granulocyte-macrophage CSF[64] and osteoclast inhibitory factor (OCIF), described next. IL-6 acts in an autocrine manner on osteoclasts via gp130.[65] Nitric oxide is also an autocrine regulator of osteoclast function.[66] Osteoclasts also possess receptors for CSF-1,[67] IGF-1,[68] IL-1,[69] and PDGF.[70]

Origin and Fate of the Osteoclast

The osteoclast derives from hematopoietic cells in the mononuclear/phagocytic lineage (Fig. 4).[71] Precursor cells fuse at the bone surface to form the multinucleated osteoclast.[72] Although this may occur at the early promonocyte stage, monocytes and macrophages already committed to

their own lineage might still be able to form osteoclasts under the right circumstances.

A series of studies have described the importance of OCIF,[73] also known as osteoprotegerin (OPG),[74] as well as this protein's ligand, ODF (also described independently as OPGL, RANKL, and TRANCE)[75, 76] in osteoblast-mediated stimulation of osteoclastogenesis. These two proteins act as competitive regulators of bone resorption. ODF, which is expressed by osteoblasts and stromal cells, induces osteoclast formation by direct contact with ODAR (also known as RANK and TRANCER), a receptor expressed by osteoclast progenitor cells. ODAR is also expressed in mature osteoclasts and has been shown to regulate mature osteoclast function as well. In contrast, ODF can act as a decoy ODAR-type receptor and competitively inhibit the formation of mature, functional osteoclasts.

Despite its mononuclear/phagocytic origin, the osteoclast membrane expresses distinct markers: it is devoid of several macrophage markers, including Fc and C$_3$ receptors; like mononuclear phagocytes, however, the osteoclast is rich in nonspecific esterases, synthesizes lysozymes, and expresses mannose-6-phosphate receptors.[77] The osteoclast, unlike macrophages, also expresses millions of copies of the calcitonin and vitronectin receptors, including the integrin $\alpha_v\beta_3$.[47, 52] Osteoclasts also express high levels of pp60c-src,[78] a nonreceptor tyrosine kinase involved in osteoclast adhesion (see prior discussion).

The osteoclast appears to undergo apoptosis (programmed cell death) after a cycle of resorption,[79] characterized by loss of the ruffled border, detachment from the bone surface, and condensation of the nuclear chromatin.

BONE REMODELING

Bone remodeling is the process by which bone is turned over; it is the result of the activity of the bone cells at the surfaces of bone, mainly the endosteal surface (which includes all trabecular surfaces). Remodeling is traditionally classified into two distinct types: haversian remodeling within the cortical bone and endosteal remodeling along the trabecular bone surface. This distinction is more morphological than physiological because the haversian surface is an extension of the endosteal surface, and the cellular events during these two remodeling processes follow exactly the same sequence.

Remodeling Sequence

Bone formation and bone resorption do not occur along the bone surface at random: they are coordinated as part of the turnover mechanism by which old bone is replaced by new bone. In the normal adult skeleton, bone formation only occurs, for the most part, where bone resorption has al-

Fig. 4. Osteoclast life cycle. The osteoclast is derived from a mononuclear hematopoietic precursor cell that on activation fuses with other precursors to form a multinucleated osteoclast. The osteoclast first attaches to the bone surface and then commences resorption. After a cycle of bone resorption, the osteoclast undergoes apoptosis.

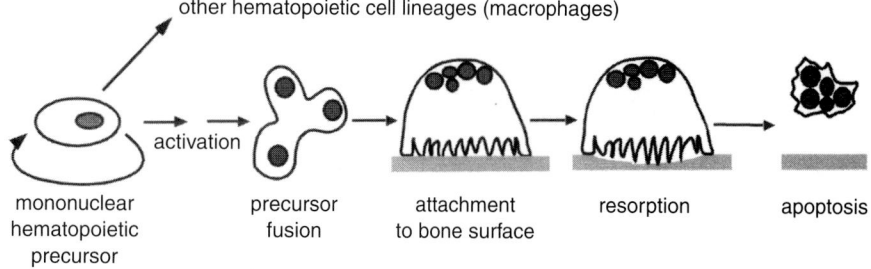

other hematopoietic cell lineages (macrophages)

mononuclear hematopoietic precursor — activation — precursor fusion — attachment to bone surface — resorption — apoptosis

ready occurred. This basic principle of cellular activity at the remodeling site is the ARF sequence (Fig. 5).[80, 81]

Under some signal, a locally acting factor released by lining cells, osteocytes, marrow cells, or in response to bone deformation or fatigue-related microfracture, a group of preosteoclasts are activated. These mononuclear cells attach to the bone via $\alpha_v\beta_3$ integrins and fuse to form a multinucleated osteoclast, which will, in a definite area of the bone surface, resorb the bone matrix. After resorption of the bone and osteoclast detachment, uncharacterized mononuclear cells cover the surface and a cement line is formed. The cement line marks the limit of bone resorption, and acts to cement together the old and the new bone. This is termed the reversal phase and is followed by a period of bone formation. Preosteoblasts are activated, proliferate, and differentiate into osteoblasts, which move onto the bone surface, forming an initial matrix (osteoid), which becomes mineralized after a time lag (the osteoid maturation period). The basic remodeling sequence is therefore ARF; it is performed by a group of cells called the basic multicellular unit (BMU). The complete remodeling cycle takes about 3 months in humans (Fig. 6).

For many years it has been accepted that bone resorption and formation are linked in the same way as bone matrix formation and calcification. In other words, in the normal adult skeleton, the coupling of bone resorption and formation in remodeling results in equal levels of cellular activity so that bone turnover is balanced: the volume of bone resorbed is equal to the volume formed. This paradigm implies that, for example, a reduction in osteoblast activity would effect a similar reduction in osteoclast activity such that bone volume is maintained. However, a 1998 study in which osteoblast ablation was induced in mature transgenic mice demonstrated that the dramatic reduction in bone formation is not associated with a reduction in osteoclast activity.[82] In these mice, the subsequent osteopenia (bone loss) is striking, and it calls our understanding of bone cell coupling into question. Interestingly, it may be also argued that because osteoblasts are completely absent in this model, they are required to modulate osteoclast activity or

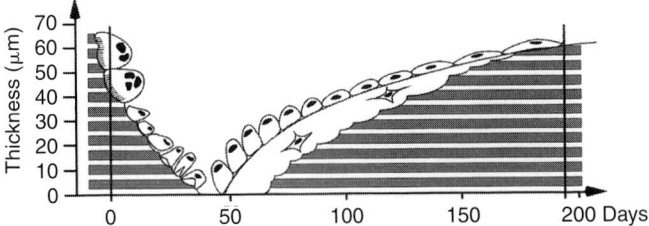

Fig. 6. Normal cancellous bone remodeling sequence. The duration and depth of the phases of the sequence were calculated from histomorphometric analysis of bone biopsy samples from young individuals. (Adapted from Eriksen EF, Axelrod DW, Melsen F: Bone Histomorphometry. New York, Raven Press, 1994, p 13. Used with permission.)

else bone resorption can continue in an unregulated manner, thus causing the bone loss observed. In any case, it is clear that studies are needed to define the potential mechanism of the coupling of bone cell activity.

Haversian Versus Endosteal Bone Remodeling

As mentioned, although cortical bone is anatomically different to trabecular bone, its remodeling occurs after the same sequence of events. The major difference is that, although the average thickness of a trabecula is 150 to 200 μm, the average thickness of the cortex is of the order of 1 to 10 mm. There are no blood vessels in the trabeculae, but the bone envelope system and the osteocyte network are able to carry out enough gaseous exchange, being always relatively close to the surface and the highly vascularized marrow. Consequently, bone remodeling in the trabecular bone will occur along the trabecular surface. Alternatively, the cortical bone itself needs to be vascularized. Blood vessels are first embedded during the histogenesis of cortical bone; the blood vessel and the bone that surround it are then called a primary osteon. Later, cortical bone remodeling is initiated either along the surface of these vascular channels or from the endosteal surface of the cortex. The remodeling process in cortical bone also follows the ARF sequence. Osteoclasts excavate a tunnel, creating a cutting cone. Again, there is a reversal phase in which mononuclear cells attach and lay down a cement line. Osteoblasts are then responsible for closing the cone, leaving a central canal, centered on blood vessels and surrounded by concentric bone lamellae. For mechanical reasons, all these haversian systems are oriented along the longitudinal axis of the bone.

Bone Turnover and Skeletal Homeostasis

In a normal young adult, about 30% of the total skeletal mass is renewed every year (half-life, 20 months). In each remodeling unit, osteoclastic bone resorption lasts about 3 days, the reversal 14 days, and bone formation 70 days (total, 87 days). The linear bone formation rate is 0.5 μm/day. During this process, about 0.01 mm^3 of bone is renewed in one given remodeling unit. Theoretically, with balanced matrix deposition and calcification as well as a balance between osteoclast and osteoblast activity, the amount of bone formed in each remodeling unit (and, therefore, in the total skeleton) equals the amount of bone that was previously resorbed. Thus, the total skeletal mass

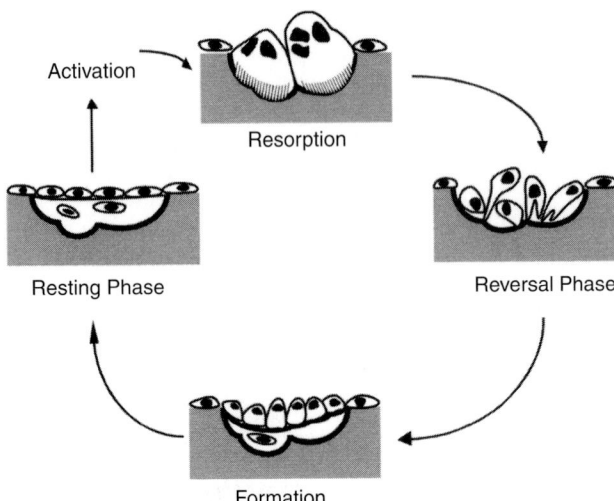

Fig. 5. The bone remodeling sequence. This is the activation-resorption-formation cycle of bone remodeling as it occurs in trabecular bone. See text for details.

remains constant. This skeletal homeostasis relies on a normal remodeling activity. The rate of activation of new remodeling units would then determine only the turnover rate.

SKELETAL DEVELOPMENT: HISTOGENESIS
Intramembranous Ossification

During intramembranous ossification, a group of mesenchymal cells within a highly vascularized area of the embryonic connective tissue proliferates, forming early cell condensations within which cells differentiate directly into osteoblasts. These cells will synthesize a woven bone matrix, while at the periphery mesenchymal cells continue to differentiate into osteoblasts. Blood vessels are incorporated between the woven bone trabeculae and will form the hematopoietic bone marrow. Later this woven bone will be remodeled by the ARF sequence and progressively replaced by mature lamellar bone.

Endochondral Ossification

Development of long bones begins with condensation of the mesenchyme to form a cartilaginous model of the bone to be formed (Fig. 7). Mesenchymal cells undergo division and differentiate into prechondroblasts and then into chondroblasts. These cells secrete the cartilaginous matrix. Like osteoblasts, the chondroblasts become progressively embedded within their own matrix, where they lie within lacunae, and they are then called chondrocytes. Unlike osteocytes, however, chondrocytes continue to proliferate for some time, which is allowed in part by the gel-like consistency of cartilage. At the periphery of this cartilage (the perichondrium), the mesenchymal cells continue to proliferate and differentiate. This is called appositional growth. Another type of growth is observed in the cartilage by cell proliferation and synthesis of new matrix between the chondrocytes (interstitial growth).

Beginning in the center of the cartilage model, at what is to become the primary ossification center, chondrocytes differentiate and become hypertrophic. During this process, hypertrophic cells deposit a mineralized matrix, in which cartilage calcification is initiated by matrix vesicles.[83] Once this matrix is calcified, it is partially resorbed by osteoclasts. After resorption and a reversal phase, osteoblasts differentiate in this area and form a layer of woven bone on top of the remaining cartilage. This woven bone is later remodeled into lamellar bone.

The embryonic cartilage is avascular. During its early development, a ring of woven bone is formed at the periphery by intramembranous ossification in the future midshaft area under the perichondrium (which becomes periosteum). After calcification of this woven bone, blood vessels, preceded by the osteoclasts entering the primary ossification center, will penetrate this bone and the calcified cartilage, forming the blood supply, which will allow seeding of the hematopoietic bone marrow and invasion of osteoclasts to resorb the calcified cartilage, as described previously.

Secondary ossification centers begin to form at the epiphyseal ends of the cartilaginous model; by a similar process, trabecular bone and a marrow space are formed at these ends. Between the primary and secondary ossification centers, epiphyseal cartilage (growth plates) remain until adulthood. The continued differentiation of chondrocytes, cartilage mineralization, and subsequent remodeling cycles allow longitudinal bone growth to occur, such that, as new bone is formed, the bone will reach its final adult shape. There is, however, a progressive decrease in chondrocyte proliferation so that the growth plate becomes progressively thinner, allowing mineralization and resorption to catch up. It is at this point that the growth plates are completely remodeled and longitudinal growth is arrested.

The growth plate demonstrates, from the epiphyseal area to the diaphyseal area, the different stages of chondrocyte differentiation involved in endochondral bone formation (Fig. 8). First is a proliferative zone, in which the chondroblasts divide actively, forming isogenous groups and ac-

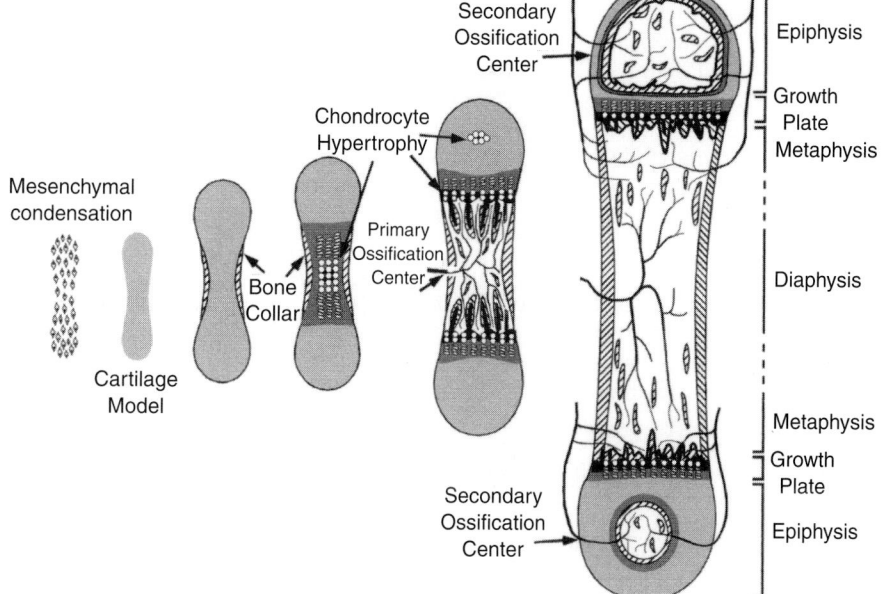

Fig. 7 Bone development. The schematic diagram shows the initial stages of endochondral ossification. Bone development begins with mesenchymal condensation to form a cartilage model of the bone to be formed. After chondrocyte hypertrophy and cartilage matrix mineralization, osteoclast activity and vascularization result in the formation of the primary and then secondary ossification centers. In mature adult bones, the growth plate is fully resorbed, so that one marrow cavity extends the full length of the bone. See text for details.

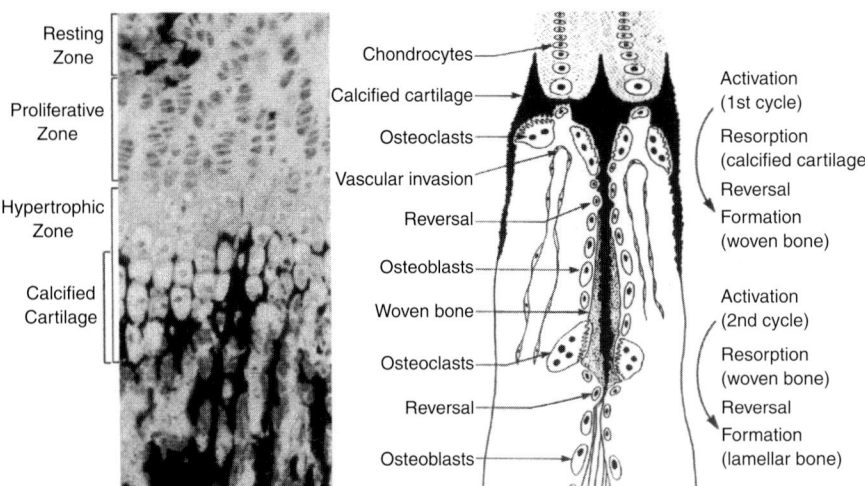

Fig. 8. Bone growth and remodeling at the growth plate. The light micrograph demonstrates the zones of chondrocyte differentiation as well as mineralization (black). The schematic representation shows the cellular events occurring at the growth plate in long bones. Note that bone formation in this process occurs by repeated activation-resorption-formation cycles of bone remodeling beginning with the calcified cartilage matrix.

tively synthesizing the matrix. These cells become progressively larger, enlarging their lacunae in the prehypertrophic and hypertrophic zones. Lower in this area, the matrix of the longitudinal cartilage septa selectively calcifies (zone of provisional calcification). The chondrocytes become highly vacuolated and then die through programmed cell death (apoptosis). Once calcified, the cartilage matrix is resorbed, but only partially, by osteoclasts, leaving the calcified longitudinal septa and blood vessels appear in the zone of invasion. After resorption, osteoblasts differentiate and form a layer of woven bone on top of the cartilaginous remnants of the longitudinal septa. Thus, the first ARF sequence is complete: the cartilage has been remodeled and replaced by woven bone. The resulting trabeculae are called the primary spongiosa. Still lower in the growth plate, this woven bone is subjected to further remodeling (a second ARF sequence) in which the woven bone and the cartilaginous remnants are replaced with lamellar bone, resulting in the mature trabecular bone called secondary spongiosa.

Chondrocyte differentiation is regulated by a number of factors. The first factor shown to control chondrocyte differentiation was PTH-related peptide (PTHrP).[84] This factor prolongs chondrocyte proliferation, and in PTHrP knockout mice, the main phenotype is bone shortening caused by premature chondrocyte hypertrophy.[85] Targeted overexpression of PTHrP results in the opposite phenotype, with a prolonged delay in chondrocyte maturation.[86] PTHrP is part of a genetic signaling cascade, in which it not only is regulated by factors expressed earlier in chondrocyte differentiation, such as Indian hedgehog (Ihh),[87] but also regulates chondrocyte differentiation itself and alters gene expression in more mature chondrocytes. Other factors that regulate chondrocyte differentiation include the FGFs and BMPs.[88–90]

GROWTH IN BONE SHAPE AND DIAMETER (MODELING)

Growth in the diameter of the metaphysis is the result of a deposition of new membranous bone beneath the periosteum that will continue throughout life. In this case, resorption does not immediately precede formation. The midshaft

is narrower than the metaphysis, and the growth of a long bone progressively destroys the lower part of the metaphysis and transforms it into a diaphysis, accomplished by continuous resorption by osteoclasts beneath the periosteum.

CLINICAL RELEVANCE AND APPLICATIONS

BONE REMODELING IN FRACTURE HEALING

Fracture healing involves three phases: inflammation, reparation, and bone remodeling. After coagulation and inflammatory cell response, the inflammation phase ends with the recruitment and proliferation of mesenchymal cells. During the reparation phase, the undifferentiated mesenchyme undergoes rapid chondrogenesis, which is modified by endochondral ossification. The callus is reshaped and strengthened during subsequent cycles of ARF-sequence bone remodeling. The healing process, therefore, follows the same pathway as normal chondrogenesis and osteogenesis described previously.

Early in the reparative phase, new bone formation also occurs adjacent to old bone. This appositional bone growth resembles intramembranous ossification and forms a bridge spanning and surrounding the fracture site and the central cartilaginous callus. Chondrocytes within the callus cartilage mature by the same process as in endochondral bone growth but in a more disorganized manner. Vascularization of the callus and the invasion of osteoclasts in the mineralized cartilage also reflect the processes observed in endochondral bone growth. Osteoclasts degrade cartilage matrix until only thin spicules remain. Osteoblasts migrate to line the cavities formed and produce new woven bone matrix, which is strengthened by subsequent cycles of bone remodeling.

In rigidly fixed fractures, healing occurs without the intermediate cartilage phase and fracture calluses heal more quickly. As noted in the Bone Remodeling section, a completed ARF sequence will take approximately 3 to 6 months in a normal adult. For this reason, fractured bones in general are unlikely to regain their prefractured strength and form until at least 6 months after injury and treatment. During the many stages in fracture healing, several cytokines and growth factors regulate matrix production. Various factors such as BMPs, TGF-β, and PDGF have been successfully used to augment healing in experimental models.[91]

DEFECTS IN BONE REMODELING

The bone remodeling process is precisely controlled, such that the activity of osteoclasts and osteoblasts are coupled and the rates of matrix deposition and mineralization are coupled. Most of the bone diseases involve defects in one and/or the other of these couplings; for example, a decrease or increase in bone mass generally results from an imbalance in the first coupling mechanism. In osteoporosis (see Chapter 2-8), the balance is disrupted, resulting in a relative excess of bone resorption (or deficiency in formation). In contrast, osteopetrosis results from a relative deficiency in bone resorption. A defect in the second form of coupling can be observed in the abnormal increase in osteoid tissue seen in osteomalacia and rickets. Other diseases, such as Paget's disease (Chapter 2-9) and hyperparathyroidism, involve only an abnormal bone turnover rate. Tumorigenesis involves a complete disruption of the normally ordered processes involved in bone remodeling.

DEFECTS IN BONE HISTOGENESIS AND BONE MATRIX PROTEINS

Congenital defects in bone histogenesis include a variety of chondrodysplasias, which generally are not well characterized because of the range of defects and rarity of the disease. There has been considerable success in localizing genes that cause skeletal dysplasias, and comparison with transgenic mouse models has revealed a role for these genes in bone histogenesis. One example is Jansen's osteochondrodysplasia, which occurs because of a mutation in the PTH/PTHrP receptor.[92] Another is cleidocranial dysplasia, which results from a mutation in the *cbfa1* gene[93] which regulates osteoblast maturation. A range of skeletal abnormalities has been assigned to various mutations in the three forms of the FGF receptor[94] and to BMP defects.[95]

A number of bone diseases are also associated with defects in bone matrix proteins. Keutel's syndrome, which is characterized by abnormal cartilage calcification, is associated with a mutation in matrix Gla protein, a matrix protein that inhibits mineralization.[96] Also, osteogenesis imperfecta, an osteopenia associated with reduced matrix collagen quality and quantity, is also associated with reduced levels of the noncollagenous proteins osteonectin, biglycan, and decorin.[97]

REFERENCES

1. Ducy P, Desbois C, Boyce B, et al: Increased bone formation in osteocalcin-deficient mice. Nature 1996;382:448.
2. Luo G, Ducy P, McKee MD, et al: Spontaneous calcification of arteries and cartilage in mice lacking matrix GLA protein. Nature 1997;386:78.
3. Xu T, Bianco P, Fisher LW, et al: Targeted disruption of the biglycan gene leads to an osteoporosis-like phenotype in mice. Nature Genet 1998;20:78.
4. Aarden EM, Wassenaar AM, Alblas MJ, et al: Immunocytochemical demonstration of extracellular matrix proteins in isolated osteocytes. Histochem Cell Biol 1996;106:495.
5. Wetterwald A, Hoffstetter W, Cecchini MG, et al: Characterization and cloning of the e11 antigen, a marker expressed by rat osteoblasts and osteocytes. Bone 1996;18:125.
6. Lanyon LE: Osteocytes, strain detection, bone modeling and remodeling. Calcif Tissue Int 1993;53(suppl 1):S102.
7. Ajubi NE, Klein-Nulend J, Alblas MJ, et al: Signal transduction pathways involved in fluid flow-induced PGE$_2$ production by cultured osteocytes. Am J Physiol 1999; 276:E171.
8. Elmardi AS, Katchburian MV, Katchburian E: Electron microscopy of developing calvaria reveals images that suggest that osteoclasts engulf and destroy osteocytes during bone resorption. Calcif Tissue Int 1990;46:239.
9. Canalis E, Pash J, Gabbitas B, et al: Growth factors regulate the synthesis of insulin-like growth factor-I in bone cell cultures. Endocrinology 1993;133:33.
10. Rydziel S, Shaikh S, Canalis E: Platelet-derived growth factor-aa and -bb (PDGF-aa and -bb) enhance the synthesis of

PDGF-aa in bone cell cultures. Endocrinology 1994;134:2541.
11. Globus RK, Plouet J, Gospodarowicz D: Cultured bovine bone cells synthesize basic fibroblast growth factor and store it in their extracellular matrix. Endocrinology 1989;124:1539.
12. Canalis E, Pash J, Varghese S: Skeletal growth factors. Crit Rev Eukaryot Gene Expr 1993;3:155.
13. Manolagas S, Jilka R: Bone marrow, cytokines, and bone remodeling. N Engl J Med 1995;332:305.
14. Zhou H, Hammonds RG Jr, Findlay DM, et al: Retinoic acid modulation of mRNA levels in malignant, nontransformed, and immortalized osteoblasts. J Bone Miner Res 1991;6:767.
15. Rizzoli R, Poser J, Burgi U: Nuclear thyroid hormone receptors in cultured bone cells. Metabolism 1986;35:71.
16. Barnard R, Ng KW, Martin TJ, et al: Growth hormone (GH) receptors in clonal osteoblast-like cells. Endocrinology 1991;128:1459.
17. Levy JR, Murray E, Manolagas S, et al: Demonstration of insulin receptors and modulation of alkaline phosphatase activity by insulin in rat osteoblastic cells. Endocrinology 1986;119:1786.
18. Wei LL, Leach MW, Miner RS, et al: Evidence for progesterone receptors in human osteoblast-like cells. Biochem Biophys Res Commun 1993;195:525.
19. Clement-Lacroix P, Ormandy C, Lepescheux L, et al: Osteoblasts are a new target for prolactin: Analysis of bone formation in prolactin receptor knockout mice. Endocrinology 1999;140:96.
20. Komm BS, Terpening CM, Benz DJ, et al: Estrogen binding, receptor mRNA,

and biologic response in osteoblast-like osteosarcoma cells. Science 1988;241:81.
21. Eriksen EF, Colvard DS, Nicholas JB, et al: Evidence of estrogen receptors in normal human osteoblast-like cells. Science 1988;241:84.
22. Colvard D, Spelsberg T, Eriksen E, et al: Evidence of steroid receptors in human osteoblast-like cells. Connect Tissue Res 1989;20:33.
23. Darwish HM, DeLuca HF: Recent advances in the molecular biology of vitamin D action. Prog Nucleic Acid Res Mol Biol 1996;53:321.
24. Kindmark A, Torma H, Johansson A, et al: Reverse transcription-polymerase chain reaction assay demonstrates that the 9-cis retinoic acid receptor alpha is expressed in human osteoblasts. Biochem Biophys Res Commun 1993;192:1367.
25. Ng KW, Partridge NC, Niall M, et al: Epidermal growth factor receptors in clonal lines of a rat osteogenic sarcoma and in osteoblast-rich rat bone cells. Calcif Tissue Int 1983;35:298.
26. Bennett A, Chen T, Feldman D, et al: Characterization of insulin-like growth factor I receptors on cultured rat bone cells: Regulation of receptor concentration by glucocorticoids. Endocrinology 1984;115:1577.
27. Mohan S, Linkhart T, Rosenfeld R, et al: Characterization of the receptor for insulin-like growth factor II in bone cells. J Cell Physiol 1989;140:169.
28. Kells AF, Schwartz HS, Bascom CC, et al: Identification and analysis of transforming growth factor beta receptors on primary osteoblast-enriched cultures derived from adult human bone. Connect Tissue Res 1992;27:197.

29. Shelly JA, Laborde AL: Interleukin-1 binding, internalization, and processing in a murine osteoblastic cell line, MC3T3.E1. Eur Cytokine Netw 1992;3:469.

30. Lacey DL, Erdmann JM, Tan HL, et al: Murine osteoblast interleukin 4 receptor expression: Upregulation by 1,25 dihydroxyvitamin D3. J Cell Biochem 1993;53:122.

31. Debiais F, Hott M, Graulet AM, et al: The effects of fibroblast growth factor-2 on human neonatal calvaria. J Bone Miner Res 1998;13:645.

32. Koenig BB, Cook JS, Wolsing DH, et al: Characterization and cloning of a receptor for BMP-2 and BMP-4 from NIH-3T3 cells. Mol Cell Biol 1994;14:5961.

33. Clover J, Dodds RA, Gowen M: Integrin subunit expression by human osteoblasts and osteoclasts in situ and in culture. J Cell Sci 1992;103:267.

34. Liu F, Malaval L, Aubin JE: The mature osteoblast phenotype is characterized by extensive plasticity. Exp Cell Res 1997;232:97.

35. Stein GS, Lian JB: Molecular mechanisms mediating proliferation/differentiation interrelationships during progressive development of the osteoblast phenotype. Endocr Rev 1993;14:424.

36. Chow JW, Wilson AJ, Chambers TJ, et al: Mechanical loading stimulates bone formation by reactivation of bone lining cells in 13 week old rats. J Bone Miner Res 1998;13:1760.

37. Dobnig H, Turner RT: Evidence that intermittent treatment with parathyroid hormone increases bone formation in adult rats by activation of bone lining cells. Endocrinology 1995;136:3632.

38. Luo G, Ducy P, McKee MD, et al: Spontaneous calcification of arteries and cartilage in mice lacking matrix GLA protein. Nature 1997;386:78.

39. Anderson HC: Molecular biology of matrix vesicles. Clin Orthop 1995;314:266.

40. Baron R, Neff L, Roy C, et al: Evidence for a high and specific concentration of (Na^+,K^+)-ATPase in the plasma membrane of the osteoclast. Cell 1986;46:311.

41. Ravesloot JH, Ypey DL, Vrijheid-Lammers T, et al: Voltage-activated K^+ conductances in freshly isolated embryonic chicken osteoclasts. Proc Natl Acad Sci U S A 1989;86:6821.

42. Ypey DL, Weidema AF, Hold KM, et al: Voltage, calcium, and stretch activated ionic channels and intracellular calcium in bone cells. J Bone Miner Res 1992;7 (suppl 2):S377.

43. Miyauchi A, Hruska KA, Greenfield EM, et al: Osteoclast cytosolic calcium, regulated by voltage-gated calcium channels and extracellular calcium, controls podosome assembly and bone resorption. J Cell Biol 1990;111:2543.

44. Sato T, Foged NT, Delaisse JM: The migration of purified osteoclasts through collagen is inhibited by matrix metalloproteinase inhibitors. J Bone Miner Res 1998;13:59.

45. Blavier L, Delaissé JM: Matrix metalloproteinases are obligatory for the migration of preosteoclasts to the developing marrow cavity of primitive long bones. J Cell Sci 1995;108:3649.

46. Everts V, Delaissé JM, Korper W, et al: Degradation of collagen in the bone-resorbing compartment underlying the osteoclast involves both cysteine-proteinases and matrix metalloproteinases. J Cell Physiol 1992;150:221.

47. Davies J, Warwick J, Totty N, et al: The osteoclast functional antigen, implicated in the regulation of bone resorption, is biochemically related to the vitronectin receptor. J Cell Biol 1989;109:1817.

48. Zambonin-Zallone A, Teti A, Grano M, et al: Immunocytochemical distribution of extracellular matrix receptors in human osteoclasts: A beta 3 integrin is colocalized with vinculin and talin in the podosomes of osteoclastoma giant cells. Exp Cell Res 1989;182:645.

49. Reinholt FP, Hultenby K, Oldberg A, et al: Osteopontin—A possible anchor of osteoclasts to bone. Proc Natl Acad Sci U S A 1990;87:4473.

50. Soriano P, Montgomery C, Geske R, et al: Targeted disruption of the c-src proto-oncogene leads to osteopetrosis in mice. Cell 1991;64:693.

51. Duong LT, Lakkakorpi PT, Nakamura I, et al: PYK2 in osteoclasts is an adhesion kinase, localized in the sealing zone, activated by ligation of $\alpha_v\beta_3$ integrin, and phosphorylated by Src kinase. J Clin Invest 1998;102:881.

52. Warshawsky H, Goltzman D, Rouleau MF, et al: Direct in vivo demonstration by radioautography of specific binding sites for calcitonin in skeletal and renal tissues of the rat. J Cell Biol 1980;85:682.

53. Mizuno Y, Hosoi T, Inoue S, et al: Immunocytochemical identification of androgen receptor in mouse osteoclast-like multinucleated cells. Calcif Tissue Int 1994;54:325.

54. Abu EO, Bord S, Horner A, et al: The expression of thyroid hormone receptors in human bone. Bone 1997;21:137.

55. Lee K: Sonic hedgehog. Curr Biol 1998;8:R744.

56. Chenu C, Serre CM, Raynal C, et al: Glutamate receptors are expressed by bone cells and are involved in bone resorption. Bone 1998;22:295.

57. Collier FM, Huang WH, Holloway WR, et al: Osteoclasts from human giant cell tumors of bone lack estrogen. Endocrinology 1998;139:1258.

58. Pederson L, Kremer M, Foged NT, et al: Evidence of a correlation of estrogen receptor level and avian osteoclast estrogen responsiveness. J Bone Miner Res 1997;12:742.

59. Teti A, Rizzoli R, Zambonin Zallone A: Parathyroid hormone binding to cultured avian osteoclasts. Biochem Biophys Res Commun 1991;174:1217.

60. McSheehy PM, Chambers TJ: Osteoblast-like cells in the presence of parathyroid hormone release soluble factor that stimulates osteoclastic bone resorption. Endocrinology 1986;119:1654.

61. Marlin TJ, Ng KW: Mechanisms by which cells of the osteoblast lineage control osteoclast formation and activity. J Cell Biochem 1994;56:357.

62. Kurihara N, Gluck S, Roodman GD: Sequential expression of phenotype markers for osteoclasts during differentiation of precursors for multinucleated cells formed in long term human marrow cultures. Endocrinology 1990;127:3215.

63. Narbaitz R, Stumpf WE, Sar M, et al: Autoradiographic localization of target cells for 1 alpha 25-dihydroxyvitamin D_3 in bones from fetal rats. Calcif Tissue Int 1983;35:177.

64. Udagawa N, Horwood NJ, Elliot J, et al: Interleukin-18 (interferon-gamma-inducing factor) is produced by osteoblasts and acts via granulocyte/macrophage colony-stimulating factor and not via interferon-gamma to inhibit osteoclast formation. J Exp Med 1997;185:1005.

65. Gao Y, Morita I, Maruo N, et al: Expression of IL-6 receptor and gp130 in mouse bone marrow cells. Bone 1998;22:487.

66. Sunyer T, Rothe L, Kirsch D, et al: Ca2+ or phorbol ester but not inflammatory stimuli elevate inducible nitric oxide synthase messenger ribonucleic acid and nitric oxide (NO) release in avian osteoclasts: Autocrine NO mediates Ca2+-inhibited bone resorption. Endocrinology 1997;138:2148.

67. Hofstetter W, Wetterwald A, Cecchini MC, et al: Detection of transcripts for the receptor for macrophage colony-stimulating factor, c-fms, in murine osteoclasts. Proc Natl Acad Sci U S A 1992;89:9637.

68. Hou P, Sato T, Hofstetter W, et al: Identification and characterization of the insulin-like growth factor I receptor in mature rabbit osteoclasts. J Bone Miner Res 1997;12:534.

69. Xu LX, Kukita T, Nakano Y, et al: Osteoclasts in normal and adjuvant arthritis bone tissues express the mRNA for both type I and II interleukin-1 receptors. Lab Invest 1996;75:677.

70. Zhang Z, Chen J, Jin D: Platelet-derived growth factor (PDGF)-BB stimulates osteoclastic bone resorption directly: The role of receptor beta. Biochem Biophys Res Commun 1998;251:190.

71. Walker DG: Bone resorption restored in osteopetrotic mice by transplants of normal bone marrow and spleen cells. Science 1975;190:784.

72. Walker DG: Control of bone resorption by hematopoietic tissue. The induction and reversal of congenital osteopetrosis in mice through use of bone marrow and splenic transplants. J Exp Med 1975;142:651.

73. Tsuda E, Goto M, Mochizuki S, et al: Isolation of a novel cytokine from human fibroblasts that specifically inhibits osteoclastogenesis. Biochem Biophys Res Commun 1997;234:137.

74. Simonet WS, Lacey DL, Dunstan CR, et al: Osteoprotegerin: A novel secreted protein involved in the regulation of bone density. Cell 1997;89:309.

75. Lacey DL, Timms E, Tan HL, et al: Osteoprotegerin ligand is a cytokine that regulates osteoclast differentiation and activation. Cell 1998;93:165.

76. Yasuda H, Shima N, Nakagawa N, et al: Osteoclast differentiation factor is a li-

gand for osteoprotegerin osteoclastogenesis-inhibitory factor and is identical to TRANCE/RANKL. Proc Natl Acad Sci U S A 1998;95:3597.

77. Baron R, Neff L, Brown W, et al: Polarized secretion of lysosomal enzymes: Co-distribution of cation-independent mannose-6-phosphate receptors and lysosomal enzymes along the osteoclast exocytic pathway. J Cell Biol 1988;106:1863.

78. Horne WC, Neff L, Chatterjee D, et al: Osteoclasts express high levels of pp60^{c-src} in association with intracellular membranes. J Cell Biol 1992;119:1003.

79. Kameda T, Ishikawa H, Tsutsui T: Detection and characterization of apoptosis in osteoclasts in vitro. Biochem Biophys Res Commun 1995;207:753.

80. Frost HM: Bone Remodeling and Its Relationship to Metabolic Bone Disease. Springfield, IL, Charles C Thomas, 1973.

81. Parfitt AM: The cellular basis of bone remodeling: The quantum concept reexamined in light of recent advances in the cell biology of bone. Calcif Tissue Int 1984;36(suppl 1):S37.

82. Corral DA, Amling M, Priemel M, et al: Dissociation between bone resorption and bone formation in osteopenic transgenic mice. Proc Natl Acad Sci U S A 1998;95:13835.

83. Shukunami C, Ishizeki K, Atsumi T, et al: Cellular hypertrophy and calcification of embryonal carcinoma-derived chondrogenic cell line ATDC5 in vitro. J Bone Miner Res 1997;12:1174.

84. Vortkamp A, Lee K, Lanske B, et al: Regulation of rate of cartilage differentiation by Indian hedgehog and PTH-related protein. Science 1996;273:613.

85. Amizuka N, Henderson JE, Hoshi K, et al: Programmed cell death of chondrocytes and aberrant chondrogenesis in mice homozygous for parathyroid hormone-related peptide gene deletion. Endocrinology 1996;137:5055.

86. Weir EC, Horowitz MC, Baron R, et al: Macrophage colony-stimulating factor release and receptor expression in bone cells. J Bone Miner Res 1993;8:1507.

87. Lanske B, Karaplis AC, Lee K, et al: PTH/PTHrP receptor in early development and Indian hedgehog-regulated bone growth. Science 1996;273:663.

88. Trippel SB, Wroblewski J, Makower AM, et al: Regulation of growth-plate chondrocytes by insulin-like growth-factor I and basic fibroblast growth factor. J Bone Joint Surg Am 1993;75:177.

89. Kawakami Y, Ishikawa T, Shimabara M, et al: BMP signaling during bone pattern determination in the developing limb. Development 1996;122:3557.

90. Shukunami C, Ohta Y, Sakuda M, et al: Sequential progression of the differentiation program by bone morphogenetic protein-2 in chondrogenic cell line ATDC5. Exp Cell Res 1998;241:1.

91. Sandberg MM, Aro HT, Vuorio EI: Gene expression during bone repair. Clin Orthop Rel Res 1993;289:292.

92. Schipani E, Kruse K, Jüppner H: A constitutively active mutant PTH-PTHrP receptor in Jansen-type metaphyseal chondrodysplasia. Science 1995;268:98.

93. Mundlos S, Otto F, Mundlos C, et al: Mutations involving the transcription factor cbfa1 cause cleidocranial dysplasia. Cell 1997;89:773.

94. Burke D, Wilkes D, Blundell TL, et al: Fibroblast growth factor receptors: Lessons from the genes. Trends Biochem Sci 1998;23:59.

95. Storm EE, Kingsley DM: Joint patterning defects caused by single and double mutations in members of the bone morphogenetic protein (BMP) family. Development 1996;122:3969.

96. Munroe PB, Olgunturk RO, Fryns J-P, et al: Mutations in the gene encoding the human matrix gla protein cause Keutel syndrome. Nature Genet 1999;21:142.

97. Fedarko NS, Gehron Robey P, Vetter UK: Extracellular matrix stoichiometry in osteoblasts from patients with osteogenesis imperfecta. J Bone Miner Res 1995;10:1122.

98. Miyauchi A, Hruska KA, Greenfield EM, et al: Osteoclast cytosolic calcium, regulated by voltage-gated calcium channels and extracellular calcium, controls podosome assembly and bone resorption. J Cell Biol 1990;111:2543.

99. Marie JC, Wakkach A, Coudray AM, et al: Functional expression of receptors for calcitonin gene-related peptide, calcitonin, and vasoactive intestinal peptide in the human thymus and thymomas from myasthenia gravis patients. J Immunol 1999;162:2103.

100. Yamamoto T, Kurihara N, Yamaoka K, et al: Bone marrow-derived osteoclast-like cells from a patient with craniometaphyseal dysplasia lack expression of osteoclast-reactive vacuolar proton pump. J Clin Invest 1993;362:367.

101. Kurihara N, Gluck S, Roodman GD: Sequential expression of phenotype markers for osteoclasts during differentiation of precursors for multinucleated cells formed in long-term human marrow cultures. Endocrinology 1990;127:3215.

102. Warshawsky H, Goltzman D, Rouleau MF, et al: Direct in vivo demonstration by radioautography of specific binding sites for calcitonin in skeletal and renal tissues of the rat. J Cell Biol 1980;85:682.

103. Martin TJ, Ng KW: Mechanisms by which cells of the osteoblast lineage control osteoclast formation and activity. J Cell Biochem 1994;56:357.

104. Sinnett-Smith J, Zachary I, Valverde AM, et al: Bombesin stimulation of p125 focal adhesion kinase tyrosine phosphorylation. Role of protein kinase C, Ca^{2+}, mobilization, and the actin cytoskeleton. J Biol Chem 1993;268:14261.

105. Amizuka N, Henderson JE, Hoshi K, et al: Programmed cell death of chondrocytes and aberrant chondrogenesis in mice homozygous for parathyroid hormone-related peptide gene deletion. Endocrinology 1996;137:5055.

106. Teti A, Marchisio R, Zambonin A: Clear zone in osteoclast function: Role of podosomes in regulation of bone resorbing activity. Am J Physiol 1991;261:1.

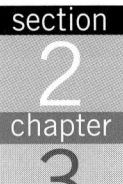

section 2 chapter 3
ARTICULAR CARTILAGE: STRUCTURE, FUNCTION, AND PHYSIOLOGY

Michael T. Bayliss and Jayesh Dudhia

Summary

- Articular cartilage has one of the lowest coefficients of friction of any known substance, not just of biological substances.
- Articular cartilage is an avascular structure; its nutrition is derived from synovial fluid through diffusion.
- In articular cartilage, the ratio of matrix to cells is very high.
- Cartilage matrix protects chondrocytes from host immune defenses, making cartilage a favored tissue for transplantation.
- Articular cartilage extracellular matrix is composed mainly of type II collagen, the proteoglycan aggrecan, noncollagenous matrix proteins, and water.

Clinical Relevance

- Deformation of articular cartilage under load extrudes water from the tissue and thus contributes to the surface lubrication and the extremely low coefficient of friction; the low coefficient of friction facilitates energy-efficient motion and low wear.
- The viscoelasticity of cartilage and subchondral bone contribute to energy absorption at the joint surface.
- Deformation of articular cartilage under load increases joint contact surface area and, therefore, decreases surface stress and protects the joint surface from damage.
- When damaged, articular cartilage has extraordinarily poor reparative/healing properties; serious damage, whether traumatic, infectious, or immunological, usually leads to arthritis.
- Ligament and muscle control of joint motion prevents damage to articular cartilage.

INTRODUCTION

Articular cartilage is not the homogeneous tissue that most people think it is. One of the major functions of articular cartilage is to provide a smooth articulating surface that has a very low coefficient of friction and to distribute load efficiently. The physicochemical properties that are characteristic of the tissue are a consequence of the macromolecular composition of its extracellular matrix.[1, 2] There is variation in cell activity and composition throughout its depth so that the chondrocytes and the extracellular matrix at the surface of the tissue are very different from those in the middle and deep layers of cartilage.[3–5] The composition of the matrix also varies as to the compartment being investigated. For example, in any one zone the pericellular region of the tissue has a composition different from that

of the territorial and interterritorial zone. The age of the individual is the most important factor that influences the structure and composition of the tissue.

Figure 1 shows the relative proportions of matrix components in adult human articular cartilage. There is a great amount of water in the tissue. Without hydration, the specific properties of articular cartilage would be absent. It is also obvious that there is also a very high concentration of the two major organic components, collagen and proteoglycan. Although a number of collagen types have been identified in cartilage, type II is by far the most abundant; it is present throughout the tissue.[6] However, there are differences in its composition and extracellular organization in different zones and compartments (territorial versus interterritorial). Collagen type II provides cartilage with its tensional properties. It controls the swelling and water-imbibing properties of the fixed charge density associated with

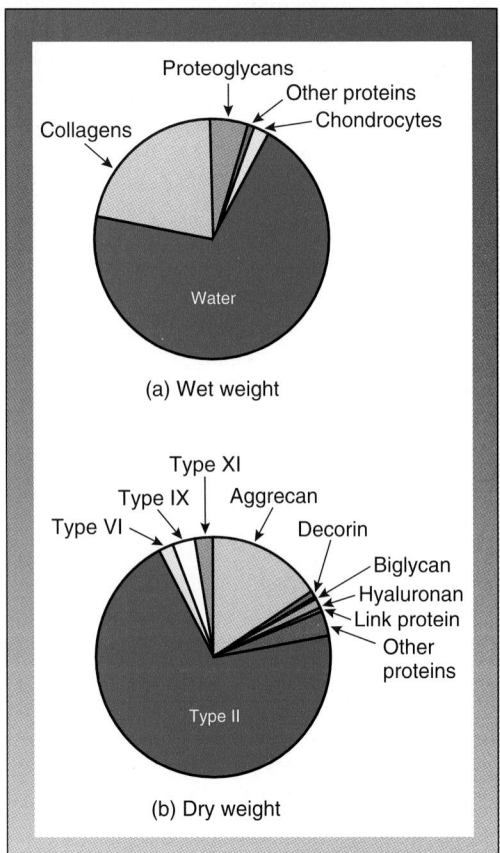

ARTICULAR CARTILAGE COMPOSITION

(a) Wet weight

Collagens · Proteoglycans · Other proteins · Chondrocytes · Water

(b) Dry weight

Type VI · Type IX · Type XI · Aggrecan · Decorin · Biglycan · Hyaluronan · Link protein · Other proteins · Type II

Fig. 1. Matrix constituents. This shows the proportions of macromolecules in the extracellular matrix of adult human articular cartilage.

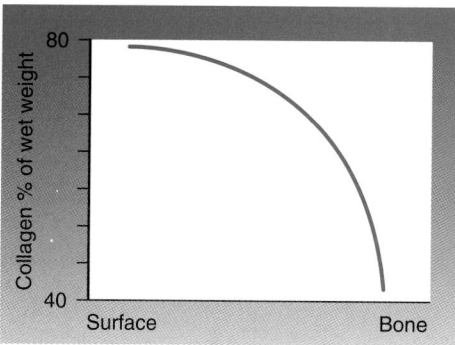

Fig. 2. Type II collagen distribution. This shows distribution of type II collagen content of articular cartilage through the depth of the tissue.

the proteoglycans (mainly aggrecan).[5] The correct organization of collagen type II is, therefore, vital if articular cartilage is to function efficiently. For example, its concentration is very high in the upper zone of cartilage where it is deposited in a parallel arrangement with the surface of the tissue. Its concentration gradually decreases with depth, and its organization becomes perpendicular to the articulating surface in these zones (Fig. 2).

In contrast, the negatively charged proteoglycan, aggrecan, provides cartilage with its water-imbibing properties and enables it to withstand compressive forces. Aggrecan also varies in concentration and structure throughout the depth of the tissue; it is this feature that gives articular cartilage the ability to respond rapidly to changes in the load applied. If the concentration of aggrecan was high throughout the depth of articular cartilage, a sharp boundary would be generated between the synovial space and the tissue when a load was applied. The tissue would, therefore, not be able to distribute the load and would fail to act as an efficient engineering material.[7]

Attention has been focused on the family of low-molecular-weight, leucine-rich proteoglycans (decorin, biglycan, fibromodulin),[8] mainly because they are known to control collagen type II fibril growth, bind growth factors, and undergo extensive post-translational modification that has been associated with the onset of joint disease. For example, Cs-Szabo et al have shown that there is a decrease in the concentration of these molecules in the late stages of osteoarthritis (OA) and also that the age-related increase in the appearance of nonglycosylated forms of the molecules was not observed in the diseased tissue.[9] These findings are consistent with an increase in the biosynthetic activity of the chondrocyte.

Although less is known about the structure and extracellular organization of noncollagenous matrix proteins in articular cartilage, those that have been characterized are proving to be very useful as "markers" of tissue turnover. For example, fibronectin facilitates a number of cell-cell and cell-matrix interactions. Fragments generated during fibronectin's turnover can also activate cartilage turnover.[10] In this respect, it is interesting that the concentration of fibronectin in osteoarthritic cartilage is elevated. Other noncollagenous matrix proteins have been investigated; many of them show aging and compartmental distributions. A protein such as cartilage intermediate layer protein is so named because it is found predominantly in the middle

layers of adult articular cartilage.[11] Similarly, cartilage oligomeric matrix protein changes its tissue concentration with increasing age and its pericellular or intercellular location. There is very little known about the interactions of these last two proteins with other matrix components, but the small amount of information that is available has implicated them in the formation of the collagen type II network. Many other proteins are present in articular cartilage, many of which are still known only by their molecular weights. The importance of these components in the formation of a stable collagen network is still unknown.

PROTEOGLYCANS

There are many types of proteoglycan in articular cartilage, but the one that is associated with the swelling properties of the tissue is aggrecan. The swelling and water-imbibing properties are associated with the glycosaminoglycans that are covalently bound to the protein core.[12] Consequently, the high content of chondroitin and keratan sulfate associated with aggrecan is what most individuals consider to be important in the extracellular organization of the molecule (Fig. 3).

Aggrecan is a very large molecule that consists of a central protein core of some 2000 amino acids with several distinct domains that have different functions.[13] Those domains that are functionally most important are the chondroitin sulfate domains carrying a very large number of negatively charged glycosaminoglycan chains of chondroitin sulfate. There are some 100 such chains, each consisting of an average 40 to 50 disaccharide units with two negatively charged groups, sulfate on the N-acetyl galactosamine and carboxyl on the glucuronic acid residue. These two domains contribute some 8000 to 10,000 negatively charged groups to the molecules, all fixed to the protein core. An extended protein domain next to the chondroitin sulfate–rich region has a specific amino acid repeat structure and carries a number of keratan sulfate chains. This unique domain, as well as increasing the fixed charge density of the molecule, probably confers special properties to it, but these are unknown at the present time. Another domain with important functional properties is the N-terminal hyaluronan-binding domain, G1. This gives the aggrecan molecule the ability to interact specifically with hyaluronan. This mechanism is used to link a large number of aggrecan molecules to one molecule of hyaluronan, forming a very

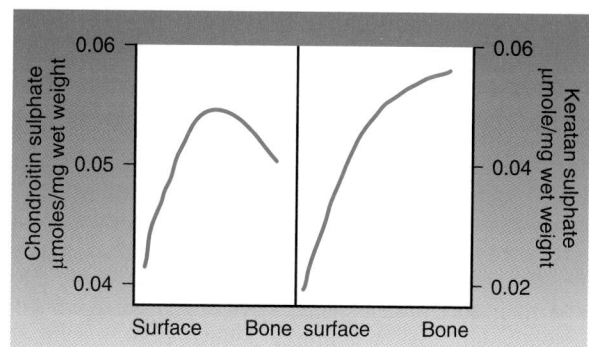

Fig. 3. Glycosaminoglycan distribution. This shows distribution of chondroitin sulfate and keratan sulfate content of articular cartilage throughout the depth of the tissue.

Aggrecan

Aggregate

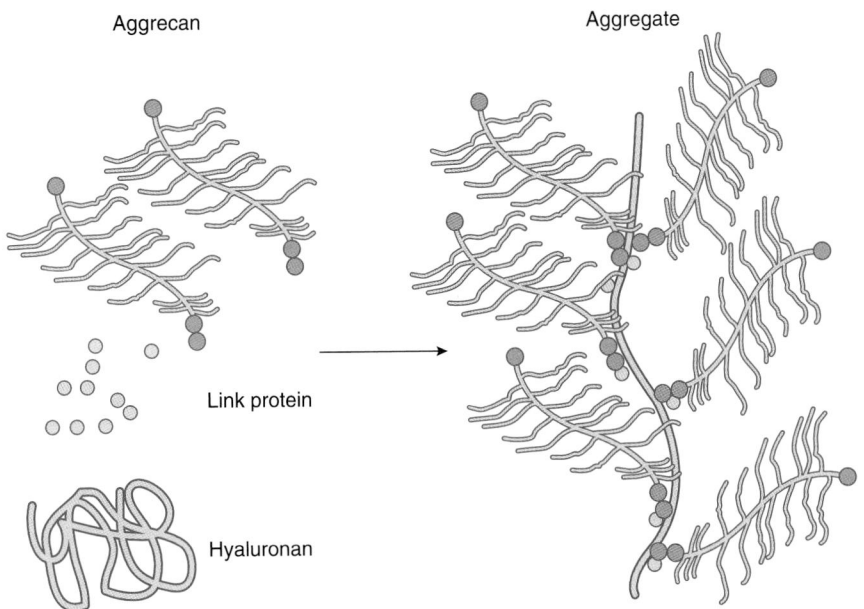

Link protein

Hyaluronan

Fig. 4. Schematic representation of proteoglycan aggregates. This shows three components of proteoglycan aggregates and how they combine to form functional aggregated structures in the extracellular matrix.

high molecular-weight complex. Although the binding of aggrecan to hyaluronan is tight—almost as strong as that between antigen and antibody—an additional protein stabilizes the complex by binding to the hyaluronan and the G1 domain of the aggrecan. Other globular domains of aggrecan have less well-defined properties. For example, the G2 domain is homologous with the major part of the G1 domain, but it cannot bind to hyaluronan, and its function is unknown. Similarly, the C-terminal G3 domain contains sequences homologous to epidermal growth factor, complement regulatory component, and a lectin, but their functions are not yet known (Fig. 4).[14, 15]

The basic structural features of aggrecan described above have been determined largely from studies of molecules purified from young animal cartilage. It is clear that a structure of this kind has the potential to generate aggregates of widely varying composition and molecular weight to suit the mechanical and physicochemical properties of cartilage from different sources. These molecular changes are a consequence of biosynthetic and catabolic events, regulated by many cellular and extracellular processes. The extent to which these occur within articular cartilage, however, is not uniform; factors such as species, site (which joint), zone (through the cartilage depth), tissue compartment (pericellular, territorial, interterritorial), and region of the joint (topographical distribution) determine specific qualitative and quantitative changes in aggrecan structure. However, it is the age of the individual that appears to have the most profound effect on the composition, stoichiometry, and stability of aggregates. Nowhere is this more evident than in normal human articular cartilage.[16] The changes consist mainly of an increased polydispersity and heterogeneity in the molecular size of individual aggrecan molecules, brought about by extracellular proteolytic cleavage of their core proteins (Fig. 5). This may be confined to regions within the chondroitin sulfate–rich domain, but with advancing age an increased concentration of the "free G1" domain is observed, confirming that proteolytic modification of aggrecan can be extensive.[17]

The average size of the hyaluronan polymer decreases with the individual's age[18]; also, studies have indicated that there is an age-related increase in the fragmentation of link protein preparations and a decrease in the concentration of link protein relative to aggrecan, suggesting that aggregation may be less effective in adult cartilage. Although these structural changes may give the impression of a molecular system that is degenerating during aging, this is not the

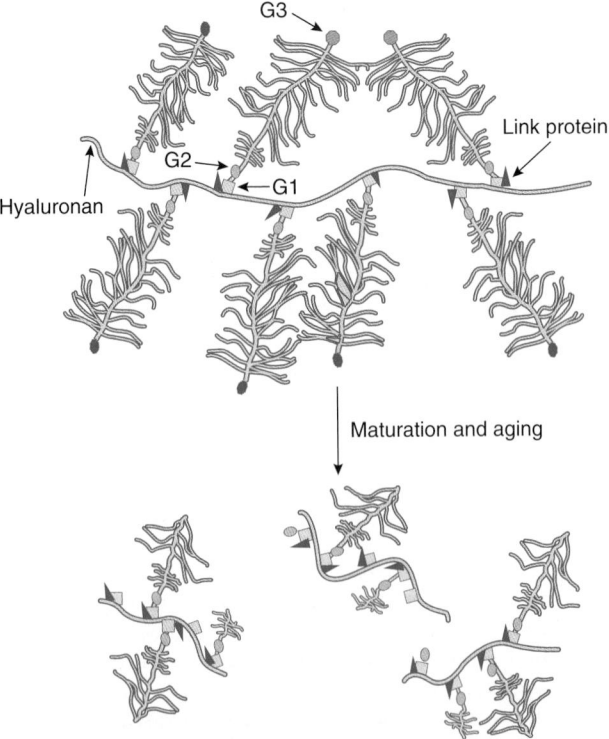

Maturation and aging

Fig. 5. Age-related changes in aggrecan. These are changes that occur in the structure of aggrecan in human articular cartilage as it ages. These changes are unrelated to the observations made of osteoarthritic cartilage.

case. The molecules in normal, mature cartilage provide it with the properties that enable it to survive the changing biochemical and biophysical environment to which it is exposed. The aggregates represent an important structural unit, a key function of which is to provide a stable environment of high fixed-charge density, essential for imbibing and retaining water in the tissue by the high osmotic swelling pressure created.

Other, low-molecular-weight, proteoglycans are also found in articular cartilage. They were originally considered minor components, but it has become increasingly clear that their molar concentration is quite high and that they have very important structural and biological roles in the tissue.[19] Decorin was the first of these to be defined structurally. It contains one side chain of dermatan sulfate, slightly different from the traditional chondroitin sulfate chains found in aggrecan; the glucuronic acid residue is often exchanged for iduronate within the chain sequence. This side chain can adopt more complex secondary structures, and it appears quite likely that it can form specific interactions with other molecules in the tissue. Four members of this family of proteoglycans—decorin, fibromodulin, lumican, and biglycan—have been shown to interact with collagens; they may have a role in regulating the size of the collagen fibrils formed. Decorin, fibromodulin, and lumican can also form specific protein-protein interactions, via the leucine-rich repeat region in their protein core, to various collagens including collagen II. From electron microscopy data as well as from studies in vitro, it appears that they also bind to distinct sites on the collagen and are found localized along the collagen fibers in the tissue.[20]

COLLAGENS

The major structural element of the articular cartilage is the collagen network.[21, 22] A large number of collagen II molecules are assembled into collagen fibers. This is a very tightly regulated assembly process occurring outside the cells and requires a modification of the pro-form of collagen secreted by the chondrocyte. Specific proteolytic enzymes then remove N- and C-terminal extensions. After removal of the extensions, the collagen molecules can associate to form fibers in a very specific manner. The collagen molecule consists of three protein chains, forming a standard triple helical structure. This is a compact, tightly bound, functional molecule, which is some 3000 Å long and only 15 Å thick. The peptide backbone is resistant to proteolysis; it is protected by the side chain constituents of its amino acid residues. Each end of this processed molecule, however, retains a few amino acids, forming a telopeptide structure different from the rest of the molecule (Fig. 6). Lysine residues in this telopeptide participate in cross-link formation between neighboring collagen molecules, which further stabilize the fibers. They constitute new stable derivatives called pyridinolines and are uniquely found in such cross-linked collagen. Also unique to collagens are the hydroxyproline residues. They are essential for the stability of the collagen molecule, as are the hydroxylysine residues. In most mature tissues, collagen molecules, once they are incorporated into the extracellular matrix, have an exceptionally long life (>200 years), making them susceptible to nonenzymatic glycation via the so-called

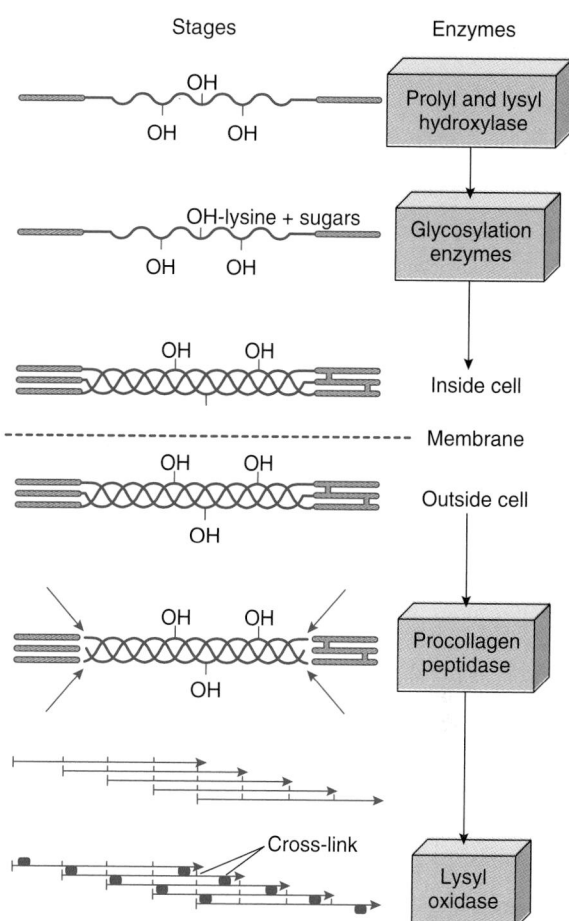

Fig. 6. Fibril assembly. This shows how type II collagen is assembled into cross-linked fibrils.

Maillard reaction. The accumulation of nonenzymatic glycation products is supported by the well-known color change of articular cartilage from bluish in young age to yellow-brown in the elderly. Nonenzymatic glycation results in increased cross-linking, which is of a different nature from the enzymatic cross-links formed during the assembly of collagen. Thus, biochemical changes in the collagen network have a considerable effect on the biomechanical properties, primarily the stiffness, of the cartilage.[23]

The collagen II that makes up the bulk of these fibers is specific for cartilage, but the fibers are more complex than they appear in that they contain an additional collagen—collagen type XI—also unique for cartilage.[24] Current knowledge indicates that collagen type XI, which represents only a small percentage of the total collagen content, may have a role in determining the thickness of the collagen II fibers. It is apparent that the growth of these fibers is very tightly regulated and differs between compartments of the tissue. The thinnest fibers in the tissue occur in the territorial matrix close to the cells in the superficial parts of the articular cartilage. In general, fiber thickness also increases in all compartments, going from the superficial zones of the articular cartilage to the deep zones. For example, the thickness of the fibers actually increases by a factor of about four, from the thinnest fibers found in the superficial territorial compartment to those thickest in the

Type IX Collagen molecules

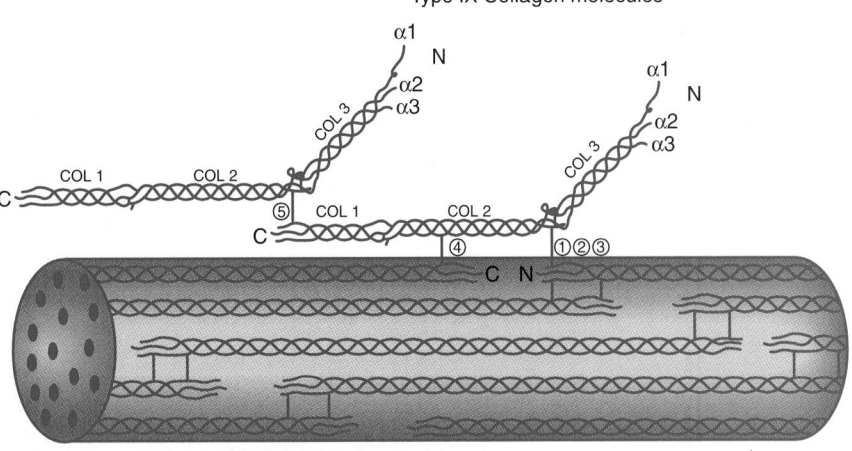

Type II Collagen fibril

Fig. 7. Types II and IX collagen. This shows the relationship between type II collagen and the lower-molecular-weight type IX collagen.

deep interterritorial compartment. The fibers run in preferred directions in different parts of the articular cartilage. Those in the most superficial parts run parallel to the surface, and those in the deep parts run perpendicular. In an intermediate part of the cartilage, fibers run in a random direction.

The factors that govern the assembly of the collagen molecules into fibers, resulting in the specific dimensions, are not known. Assembly may involve a series of other constituents of the collagen fibrillar network, for example, collagen type IX. The collagen IX molecule contains the classic triple helical structure organized into three different collagenous domains, interrupted by nontriple helical domains. It has been shown that the collagen IX molecule is bound to the collagen II fiber surface in the tissue. This binding is stabilized by covalent cross-links, creating a fiber in which no more collagen II molecules can be added to increase the fiber thickness and, thereby, the strength of the collagen II fiber itself—unless the collagen IX is removed by proteolysis (Fig. 7).

MATRIX PROTEINS

A major family of matrix proteins contains leucine-rich repeats; this was discussed in relation to the members of the family that are considered to be proteoglycans (Fig. 8).[8, 19] The protein core of these molecules contains a central domain of characteristic repeats of some 25 amino acids.[25] Thus, 10 to 11 repeats in each matrix protein are surrounded by sets of disulfide loops; in most cases, there is an N-terminal and a C-terminal extension. The central leucine-rich repeat domain exposes a surface of so-called "β-sheet" structures that are known to participate in protein-protein interactions. Indeed, most of the members of this family of proteins bind specifically to other constituents in the matrix and contribute to the structural network. The N-terminal extension peptide in some cases has glycosaminoglycan chains attached to it and can contain repeated tyrosine sulfate residues. In the case of one of these proteins, proline, arginine-rich, leucine-rich repeat protein (PRELP), it has become adapted for interactions with heparin, but it may also lack this terminal extension altogether. Molecules such as chondroadherin may provide feedback conformation to the cells by interacting with the $\alpha_2\beta_1$ inte-

grin receptor on the chondrocyte surface. Chondroadherin also shows high expression in the lower region of the growth plate between the zone of proliferating chondrocytes and the hypertrophic zone. Chondroadherin is also expressed in articular cartilage where it is found primarily in the deeper one-third of the tissue. Another molecule with the potential to interact with the cell surface is PRELP.[26] It contains a domain specifically designed for binding to heparin/heparan sulfate. This could influence interactions at the cell surface of the chondrocyte where heparan sulfate is found, and it could modulate the effects of fibroblast growth factor, which has potent effects on chondrocyte metabolism and which depends on heparin/heparan sulfate chains for its activity.

Another abundant cartilage macromolecule is cartilage oligomeric matrix protein (COMP).[12] The protein is made up of five identical subunits linked together close to their N-terminus, via a so-called heptad repeat, stabilized by disulfide bonds. Each chain is terminated at the C-terminal end with a globular structure. COMP shows a pronounced homology to the thrombospondin family, one of which (the trimeric thrombospondin-1) has been demonstrated as a protein in cartilage. Although very little is known about the function of COMP in cartilage, it is likely that it can interact specifically with other molecules through the five subunits that provide the potential for multimeric interactions. COMP increases in concentration as the articular cartilage develops, but it is deposited in the interterritorial compartment in the superficial zone of the tissue; it may be that COMP is required for appropriate control of cell growth and proliferation.

The 92kDa protein, cartilage intermediate layer protein,[11] is a novel protein with little homology to previously described molecules. It consists of a single polypeptide chain, but the primary sequence of the molecule does not provide any indication of its function. It is interesting, however, that the protein is primarily localized in the midzones of the mature cartilage, in the interterritorial matrix furthest from the chondrocyte. Cartilage matrix protein is also unique for cartilage, albeit not present in normal articular cartilage.[27] This protein contains three identical subunits, and it contains von Willebrand's factor motifs typical for proteins with collagen-binding properties.

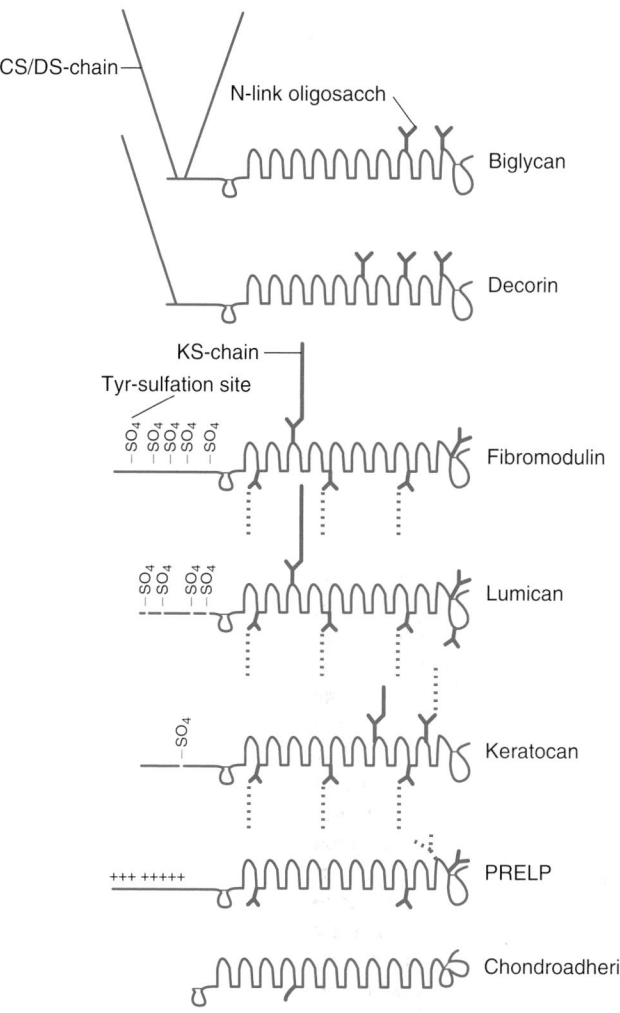

Fig. 8. Leucine-rich matrix proteins. This shows members of the family of leucine-rich, low-molecular-weight proteoglycans (decorin, biglycan, and fibromodulin) and how their core protein is related to the other members of this family of tandem leucine-rich repeat containing extracellular proteins. New members include osteoglycin (mimecan) and osteoadherin.

There are many more matrix proteins in cartilage whose functions have not been clearly defined, such as Matrix-Gla protein, bone sialoprotein, fibronectin, and so on. Many of these proteins are produced in greater amounts by osteoarthritic chondrocytes, and so they have been used as markers of joint disease.

ALTERED EXPRESSION OF MATRIX MACROMOLECULES IN JOINT DISEASE

OA is largely a clinical diagnosis made from patient history, radiograph, joint instability, and pain. Because these features are only present late in the process and only then lead to patient awareness, very little is known about the early events in OA. Many studies of articular cartilage in OA have focused on samples obtained at joint replacement surgery. Unfortunately, a misconception has made several investigators draw erroneous conclusions from studies of the cartilage that is retained in severely affected joints. It is now becoming increasingly accepted that there is no normal cartilage in a diseased joint. An understanding of the early events in human OA, which may be amenable to therapeutic intervention, will only emerge from studies of other sources of diseased cartilage, such as nonsymptomatic joints with very minor, early focal lesions.

Samples from knee joints of patients undergoing amputation due to tumors in the extremities have been obtained. Some of these patients have early fibrillation and, in some cases, slight surface erosion. Of course, it is not known if these individuals would have progressed to clinically defined OA, but these samples have been used to quantitate changes in matrix constituents and to identify altered metabolic events. The tissue with slight surface fibrillation shows metabolic alteration similar to that obtained using normal-looking cartilage from a severely affected joint, indicating that the biochemical abnormality affects all areas of the joint and that these samples represent different stages of the same degenerative process (Lorenzo, Bayliss, and Heinegard, unpublished data).

One of the early events in the OA process appears to be an increased volume of the tissue: it swells. This can only be accomplished if the tensile properties of the collagen network become impaired, thereby preventing this structural element from resisting the swelling pressure generated by the osmotic properties of the proteoglycans. Thus, one of the early events in OA has to involve processes affecting the collagen network, although not necessarily the collagen fibers themselves. This information has been available for some time, yet no one has investigated which of the molecules associated with the collagen network is the first to be affected (Fig. 9).[28]

Early in the development of OA, the level of aggrecan in the tissue also changes. This is mostly inferred from histochemical studies by staining with metachromatic and/or cationic dyes. However, although a pronounced reduction and altered distribution of such staining in the early OA specimens are seen, the total amount of aggrecan in the cartilage does not decrease (Lorenzo, Bayliss, and Heinegard, unpublished data). At the same time, in other studies, Heinegard and his colleagues have shown that there is a substantial release of proteoglycan fragments into synovial fluid in early OA. It seems likely that early in OA the proteoglycans that are lost from the tissue are replaced by the chondrocytes to give an unchanged overall tissue content. The altered histological staining pattern possibly indicates a redistribution of aggrecan in the various compartments as a consequence of different rates of synthesis and degradation in each region of the tissue.[29]

A consistent finding in early cartilage lesions, is increased synthesis of COMP, cartilage intermediate layer protein, and an uncharacterized 39kDa protein (Lorenzo, Bayliss, and Heinegard, unpublished data). Similar observations were made in the late stages of the disease, indicating that early changes are indeed part of the OA process. From studies of the distribution of the proteins in the cartilage, it appears that COMP is expressed by a novel population of cells in the deeper layers of the cartilage and that these cells also express a high level of cartilage intermediate layer protein (Lorenzo, Bayliss, and Heinegard, unpublished data). These findings may, therefore, be an indication that some of the earliest responses in the OA process are initiated in the deeper layers of the cartilage rather than in the superficial zones.[30]

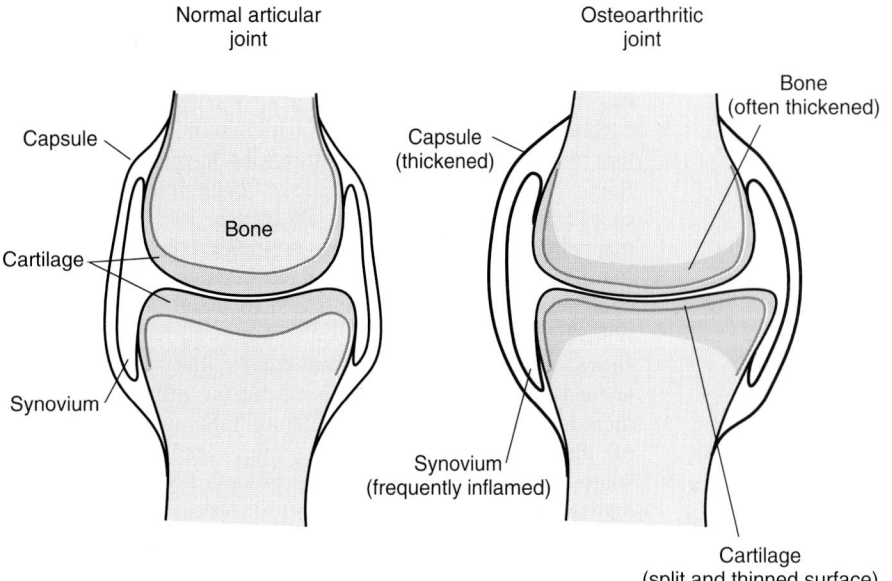

Fig. 9. Normal and osteoarthritic cartilage. This shows the relationship between "normal" articular cartilage and the early and late stages of osteoarthritis.

Normal
- Smooth articulation
- Even load distribution
- Good joint congruity

Early changes
- Cartilage surface damage and cell activation
- Increased bone remodeling
- Synovium mild inflammation
- Capsule thickened

Late changes
- Cartilage extensive damage and eventual loss
- Bone thickening and distortion
- Capsule damaged
- Frequently a distorted joint
- Abnormal load distribution

Outcome
Range of movement with pain and discomfort

We have measured changes in the concentration of several matrix constituents that reside in the cartilage. The level of PRELP decreases, whereas that of fibronectin and decorin increases (Lorenzo, Bayliss, and Heinegard, unpublished data). These changes are consistent with an alteration in the surface of the collagen fibrils and, therefore, alteration of the tensile properties. It may be that their distribution in the tissue is altered and they fail to provide the appropriate mechanical properties for a particular compartment.

One factor that should be considered in terms of modulating the progression of joint disease is the load to which the joint is subjected. It is quite possible that the load produced by normal activity may be harmful to the chondrocyte, when the macromolecular composition and structure has been altered.[31] Many of the "early" OA specimens we have examined also have some surface degradation. This may result from degradation of the molecules linking the collagen fibrils, which interferes with their stability. This would result in a mechanically impaired collagen network, which in turn may yield surface disruption when the tissue is mechanically loaded.

REFERENCES

1. Kempson GE, Muir H, Pollard C, et al: The tensile properties of the cartilage of human femoral condyles related to the content of collagen and glycosaminoglycans. Biochim Biophys Acta 1973; 297: 456.
2. Mow VC, Mak AF, Lai WM, et al: Viscoelastic properties of proteoglycan subunits and aggregates in varying solution concentrations. J Biomech 1984; 17:325.
3. Stockwell RA: The cell density of human articular and costal cartilage. J Anat 1967; 101:753.
4. Bank RA, Bayliss MT, Lafeber FP, et al: Aging and zonal variation in post-translational modification of collagen in normal human articular cartilage: The age-related increase in nonenzymatic glycation affects biomechanical properties of cartilage. Biochem J 1998; 330:345.
5. Muir H: The chondrocyte—architect of cartilage: Biomechanics, structure, function, and molecular biology of cartilage matrix macromolecules. Bioessays 1995; 17:1039.
6. Bruckner P, van der Rest M: Structure and function of cartilage collagens. Microsc Res Tech 1994; 28:378.
7. Kempson GE: The mechanical properties of articular cartilage. In Sokoloff L (ed): The Joints and Synovial Fluids. New York, Academic Press, vol 2, pp 177–238.
8. Rosenberg L: Structure and function of dermatan sulfate proteoglycans in articular cartilage. In Kuettner K (ed): Articular Cartilage and Osteoarthritis. New York, Raven Press, 1992, pp 45–63.
9. Cs-Szabo G, Roughley PJ, Plaas AH, et al: Large and small proteoglycans of osteoarthritic and rheumatoid articular cartilage. Arthritis Rheum 1995; 38:660.
10. Homandberg GA: Potential regulation of cartilage metabolism in osteoarthritis by fibronectin fragments. Front Biosci 1999; 4: 713.
11. Lorenzo P, Bayliss MT, Heinegard D: A novel cartilage protein (CILP) present in the mid-zone of human articular cartilage increases with age. J Biol Chem 1998; 273:234.

12. Maroudas: The role of water, proteoglycan, and collagen in solute transport in cartilage. In Kuettner K (ed): Articular Cartilage and Osteoarthritis. New York, Raven Press, 1992, pp 355–371.

13. Hardingham TE, Fosang AJ, Dudhia J: Aggrecan, the chondroitin sulphate/keratan sulphate proteoglycan from cartilage. In Kuettner K (ed): Articular Cartilage and Osteoarthritis. New York, Raven Press, 1992, pp 5–20.

14. Aspberg A, Miura R, Bourdoulous S, et al: The C-type lectin domains of lecticans, a family of aggregating chondroitin sulfate proteoglycans, bind tenascin-R by protein-protein interactions independent of carbohydrate moiety. Proc Natl Acad Sci USA. 1997; 94:10116.

15. Dudhia J, Flannelly JK, and Bayliss MT: Developmental regulation of the alternatively spliced EGF- and CRP-motifs of aggrecan. Trans Orthop Res Soc 2000; 24:17

16. Hardingham T, Bayliss M: Proteoglycans of articular cartilage: Changes in aging and in joint disease. Semin Arthritis Rheum 1990; 20:12.

17. Maroudas A, Bayliss MT, Uchitel-Kaushansky N, et al: Aggrecan turnover in human articular cartilage: Use of aspartic acid racemization as a marker of molecular age. Arch Biochem Biophys 1998; 350:61.

18. Holmes MW, Bayliss MT, Muir H: Hyaluronic acid in human articular cartilage: Age-related changes in content and size. Biochem J 1988; 250:435.

19. Iozzo RV: The biology of the small leucine-rich proteoglycans: Functional network of interactive proteins. J Biol Chem 1999; 274:18843.

20. Scott JE: Proteodermatan and proteokeratan sulfate (decorin, lumican/fibromodulin) proteins are horseshoe-shaped: Implications for their interactions with collagen. Biochemistry 1996; 35:8795.

21. Eyre DR: The collagens of articular cartilage. Semin Arthritis Rheum 1991; 21:2.

22. Eyre DR: The specificity of collagen cross-links as markers of bone and connective tissue degradation. Acta Orthop Scand 1995; 266:166.

23. Bank RA, Bayliss MT, Lafeber FP, et al: Aging and zonal variation in post-translational modification of collagen in normal human articular cartilage: The age-related increase in nonenzymatic glycation affects biomechanical properties of cartilage. Biochem J 1998; 330:345.

24. Mendler M, Eich-Bender SG, Vaughan L, et al: Cartilage contains mixed fibrils of collagen types II, IX, and XI. J Cell Biol 1998; 108:191.

25. Matsushima N, Ohyanagi T, Tanaka T, et al: Super-motifs and evolution of tandem leucine-rich repeats within the small proteoglycans: Biglycan, decorin, lumican, fibromodulin, PRELP, keratocan, osteoadherin, epiphycan, and osteoglycin. Proteins 2000; 38:210.

26. Bengtsson E, Neame PJ, Heinegard D, et al: The primary structure of a basic leucine-rich repeat protein, PRELP, found in connective tissues. J Biol Chem 1995; 270:25639.

27. Hedbom E, Antonsson P, Hjerpe A, et al: Cartilage matrix proteins: An acidic oligomeric protein (COMP) detected only in cartilage. J Biol Chem 1992; 267:6132.

28. McDevitt CA, Muir H: Biochemical changes in the cartilage of the knee in experimental and natural osteoarthritis in the dog. J Bone Joint Surg Br 1976; 58: 94.

29. Rosenberg L: Chemical basis for the histological use of safranin O in the study of articular cartilage. J Bone Joint Surg Am 1971; 53:69.

30. Hollander AP, Pidoux I, Reiner A, et al: Damage to type II collagen in aging and osteoarthritis starts at the articular surface, originates around chondrocytes, and extends into the cartilage with progressive degeneration. J Clin Invest 1995; 96:2859.

31. Price JS, Till SH, Bickerstaff DR, et al: Degradation of cartilage type II collagen precedes the onset of osteoarthritis following anterior cruciate ligament rupture. Arthritis Rheum 1999; 42:2390.

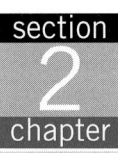

section
2
chapter
4

MUSCLE, TENDON, AND LIGAMENT: STRUCTURE, FUNCTION, AND PHYSIOLOGY

Donald T. Kirkendall and William E. Garrett, Jr

Summary

- The arrangement of myofibrils, the most distinctive feature of skeletal muscle, gives skeletal muscle its characteristic striated appearance. The interdigitated arrangement of thick myosin filaments and thin actin filaments that are connected to the Z disks make up the sarcomere, which is considered the functional unit of the skeletal muscle.
- For the muscle to contract, it must first be excited and that stimulus must pass deep into the fiber to activate the contractile process. The two primary systems for processing this stimulus are the transverse tubule system (T system) and the sacroplasmic reticulum (SR).
- Muscle contraction consists of three steps: muscle excitation, excitation-contraction coupling, and contraction. Isometric contraction force of muscle is length-dependent.
- Tendon and ligament are both classified as dense connective tissues that are similar under both gross and microscopic examination and that consist primarily of collagen fibers.
- In addition to transmitting force, tendon is flexible so that it can bend at joints, dampen shocks, and limit potential damage to muscle. Tendon also shows some degree of extensibility.
- Normal tendon usually does not fail under strain.
- Ligament is a tough, flexible, firm, white, fibrous tissue that connects bones and supports viscera and that varies in thickness, length, and shape. Because tendon and ligament are closely related, many of the features of ligaments are similar to those of tendons.

Any introductory chapter on muscle, tendon, and ligament will present those most basic elements of each tissue so that when factors about these tissues are presented in some depth in subsequent chapters, the reader can return to the introductory chapter for selected basic concepts. With this model in mind, our intent is to present the foundations of each tissue.

SKELETAL MUSCLE

Among the variety of interesting properties of muscle is its amazing adaptability to overload and underload. Much of this plasticity is based on its structural components. The high density of postmitotic nuclei along the length of each muscle fiber, the different isoforms of structural proteins, and the limited space within each cell contribute to the adaptive response.

Embryonic development of the muscle fiber and synapse is a fascinating topic. Lieber[1] presents a concise summary of this feature of muscle development and should be consulted for those interested in this concept.

CONNECTIVE TISSUE

The basic muscle cell is the fiber; a thin, cylindrical cell ranging from 10 to 100 μm. Diameter of the cell is an important feature; diameter is related to force production, and changes in fiber diameter indicate a change in the usage pattern of the fiber. The length of the fiber is highly variable, depending on the architecture of the muscle. Whereas diameter is fundamental to force production, length is related to contraction velocity. The "scaffolding" that surrounds the fiber is the basal lamina, an important component in the recovery of muscle from injury, whether the injury damages the basal lamina or not or if the motor neuron is compromised also. Each fiber is surrounded by the collagenous endomysium. A number of fibers are bundled together to form fascicles, which are surrounded by the more substantial perimysium. Ultimately, the bundles of fascicles are grouped into muscles and surrounded by the epimysium. The simplistic thought is that each cell is connected at each end to tendon; however, the cells seem to be intimately related to this connective tissue network[2,3] that plays a fundamental role in force transmission.

CELLULAR ORGANELLES
Nuclei: Command and Control

The cell is a mosaic of regions, each dominated by its own nucleus.[4] Each region controls the local structural proteins, and more nuclei are necessary as the cell increases in size. Should the development of nuclei be inhibited, subsequent muscle growth is also inhibited.[5] The concept of nuclear domain is under scrutiny: rat muscle that has atrophied as a result of space flight shows reduced density of nuclei,[6] and there is some suggestion of an aging influence when myonuclei do not multiply in hypertrophied aging humans.[7]

Mitochondria: Aerobic Energy Development

The primary noncontractile elements of muscle are the mitochondria, which are responsible for providing energy for aerobic contraction. Mitochondria are located both intermyofibrillar and subsarcolemmal[8] (mostly fiber types I and IIA). There is evidence that mitochondria are not discrete organelles but connected by a reticular network,[9] suggesting some level of communication of this highly adaptable feature of skeletal muscle. The process whereby the mitochondria (or any other aspect of the muscle) generate energy is beyond this brief review.

Myofibrils: Tension Development

The myofibrils are probably the most distinctive feature of skeletal muscle; their arrangement gives skeletal muscle its characteristic striated appearance. The interdigitated arrangement of thick myosin filaments and thin actin filaments that are connected to the Z disks make up the sarcomere and is considered the functional unit of the skeletal muscle. Myosin filaments are arranged hexagonally, and the actin filaments are arranged hexagonally in a 6:1 ratio to myosin; that is, there are 6 actin filaments for about every myosin filament, with obvious sharing of actin by adjacent myosin filaments. Although the sarcomere does appear to be relatively homogeneous, subtle differences exist among the fiber types. For instance, the Z disks are thicker in type I fibers than in types IIA and IIB fibers[10]; a similar pattern has been demonstrated for M-line thickness,[11] the banding of which is a reliable ultrastructural marker of fiber type.[12]

Myosin. The thick myosin filament is a relatively large molecule. The cross-bridge area is arranged in an antiparallel pattern extending toward the actin filament. The myosin filament is composed of two heavy portions and four lighter portions. These heavy chains contain the myosin adenosine triphosphatase (ATPase) necessary for the energy transfer required for the contractile process. Just as the whole fiber can be differentiated into fibers with distinct characteristics, so can the major histocompatibility complexes (MHCs) and are similarly named: MHCI, MHCIIa and MHCIIb. Hybrid fibers that contain coexistent MHCs have also been identified.[13]

Actin. The thin actin filament is a double helix of G-actin molecules (like a strand of pearls twisted along its long axis). At periodic intervals along the actin filament are active sites where the cross-bridges of the myosin filaments will attach to generate tension. Access to these active sites is regulated by the proteins tropomyosin and troponin. Tropomyosin lies in the grooves of the actin filament, and the three-part troponin molecule (troponin T, troponin C, and troponin I) inhibits the potential interaction of the myosin cross-bridge with the active site on the actin filament.

Cytoskeleton: Fiber Integrity

Any structure that is involved in connecting protein filaments with each other is considered to be a part of the subcellular skeleton. Thus, the intermediate filament desmin and cytoskeletal actin maintain the integrity of the myofilaments and connect the fibrils to the sarcolemma via the anchoring protein dystrophin.[14] Any damage to this network leads to cellular disruption. If some components are missing, muscular dystrophy or other muscle disorders can develop.[14]

Muscle Membranes: A Means for Excitation

The contractile elements are not the only well-defined arrangement within skeletal muscle. For the muscle to contract, it must first be excited, as explained at the beginning of this chapter.

The T system is an invagination of the sarcolemma that crosses the long axis of the fiber and is designed to get the electrical signal deep into the fiber to the myofibrils. The T system acts as an intermediary to get the electrical signal on the surface deep into the fiber.

The SR is more complex. It serves to store, release, and take up calcium during rest, contraction, and relaxation. For contraction to occur, calcium must bind with the regulatory protein troponin C along the actin filament to open the active site. The SR network must be extensive so that calcium has a small transit distance to the troponin C molecule. A pouch of the SR is in contact with the T system in the area of the Z disks so that when the fiber is activated and the signal passes down the T system, the SR can then release calcium from this expansive network.

Muscle Fiber Types: Tissue Heterogeneity

Differentiated skeletal muscle and its ability to adapt has been described in the literature.[1,10] In brief, muscle tissue can be distinguished by its contractile properties (e.g., slow or fast twitch), myoglobin content (red or white), some statement of energy sources (SO, FOG, FG), or some arbitrary system (I, IIA, IIB). Table 1 summarizes the various nomenclatures; Table 2 summarizes some of the differences among the main fiber types, which are self-evident and logical.

Muscle Architecture: Structural Organization

Subcellular organization leads to macroscopic organization. The common image of a muscle is that of the fusiform biceps brachii: tendon, muscle belly, tendon. In fact, there are numerous architectures of muscle that dictate function. Muscle architecture is considered "the arrangement of muscle fibers relative to the axis of force generation".[1] Fibers can be arranged with the cells parallel to the force-generating axis (e.g., biceps brachii). If the fibers are at a single angle off the force-generating axis, they are unipennate (e.g., vastus lateralis); muscles that are oriented at several angles to the force-generating axis are multipennate (e.g., gluteus medius). To determine the physiological cross-sectional area (a calculated area that is proportional to the maximal tetanic tension of a muscle and is an important variable in studying muscle function), the pennation angle needs to be known, along with muscle density, mass, and length. Further details on architecture and physiological cross-sectional area can be found in the literature.[1,15,16,17]

It is interesting to realize that muscle comprises similar building blocks, but it has remarkably different contractile characteristics that are largely based on its anatomy. Speed of contraction is related to muscle length and the character-

TABLE 1. COMMON FIBER COMPOSITION NOMENCLATURES		
Slow Twitch	Fast Twitch	
Tonic	Phasic	
Red	Intermediate	White
I	IIa	IIb
S	FOG	FG
S	FR	FF
ST	FTa	FTb

TABLE 2. SELECTED CHARACTERISTICS OF HUMAN SKELETAL MUSCLE FIBER TYPES

Structural Aspects	Type I	Type IIA	Type IIB
Neuron size	Small	Large	Large
Neuron conduction velocity	Slow	Fast	Fast
Neuron recruitment threshold	Low	High	High
Muscle fiber diameter	Small	Larger	Largest
Sarcoplasmic reticulum development	Least	More	Most
Density: mitochondria	Highest	Less	Least
Density: capillaries	Very dense	Less	Poor
Myoglobin content	High	Moderate	Low
Mechanical Aspects			
Time to peak tension	Slow	Faster	Fastest
Twitch tension	Low	Higher	Highest
Fatigue resistance	High	Lower	Lowest
Elasticity	Low	High	High
Metabolic Aspects			
Fuel stores: phosphogens	Low	Higher	Highest
Fuel stores: glycogen	Low	High	High
Fuel stores: triglyceride	High	Moderate	Low
Enzyme activity: ATPase	Low	High	High
Enzyme activity: glycolytic enzymes	Low	High	High
Enzyme activity: oxidative enzymes	High	High	Low

istics of each fiber's ATPase. Strength of contraction is based on the cross-sectional area of a fiber, and the ultimate force output is dependent on the physiological cross-sectional area. Certain muscles are intended to respond in certain ways. Whereas the nervous systems tells which fiber to contract and how often to contract, this impulse does not tell the muscle how to contract.

Muscle Mechanics

Contraction consists of three steps: muscle excitation, excitation-contraction coupling, and contraction. These three processes serve as the basis for any discussion of muscle contraction. Details of the establishment of the membrane potential, action potentials, and propagation of the action potential should be common knowledge to the reader.

Contractile Mechanics: Excitation

When a signal from the central nervous system travels down the axon to the synapse, it stimulates the release of the neurotransmitter acetylcholine, which diffuses across the synapse to receptors on the postsynaptic membrane. This causes a change in sarcolemmal permeability to sodium and leads to depolarization of the sarcolemma that moves away from the synapse in all directions.

Contractile Mechanics: Excitation-Contraction Coupling

At various locations along the sarcolemma, the membrane invaginates deep into the interior of the fiber. The action potential follows the membrane into the cell along the T system. At the bottom of the T tubule, the action potential

stimulates the adjacent sarcoplasmic reticulum to release calcium by a process that is not fully understood. Once released, calcium's high affinity for troponin C causes calcium to rush toward that regulatory protein. This coupling is so named because it couples membrane excitation with eventual muscle contraction.

Contractile Mechanics: Contraction

Once calcium binds the troponin C molecule, the inhibitory effect of the troponin-tropomyosin complex on the active site is removed (tropomyosin "rolls away," taking troponin with it, thus opening up the active site). Now that the active site is opened, the myosin cross-bridges bind the active site. The breakdown of adenosine triphosphate by myosin ATPase releases the energy necessary for the cross-bridge to pull the actin filament toward the center of the sarcomere. Adenosine triphosphate is also needed to break the cross-bridge from the active site so that the cross-bridge will attach to the next active site, thereby "ratcheting" the actin filament more toward the center of the sarcomere, generating more and more tension. This process continues until the sarcolemma ceases to be activated. Once sarcolemmal activation ends, an active SR membrane pump moves calcium back into the SR, and the troponin-tropomyosin inhibition of the active site is reestablished.

Mechanics: The Length-Tension Relationship

It is well known that the isometric contraction of muscle is length-dependent. At short muscle lengths, the tension is low, and it increases with increasing muscle lengths. There is an optimal length, at which peak muscle tension can be seen. When muscle length is further increased, the amount of tension produced begins to decline. The concept is that the amount of force generated is proportional to the degree of shortening as well as the number of active cross-bridges. For example, at short length (the "ascending limb") there is the potential for numerous cross-bridges to be active, but the short length (and thus short sarcomere length) does not allow for much shortening. At long muscle lengths (the "descending limb"), there is plenty of "room" for shortening, but when the length of the sarcomere is great, there are cross-bridges on the myosin filament that do not have any active sites with which to interact. At the plateau portion of the curve is the "optimal" combination of shortening length and cross-bridge interaction.

One other aspect of this isometric preparation is the passive length-tension relationship (Fig. 1). When the muscle is stretched and prepared for excitation, the muscle exerts no tension in the absence of stimulation. However, once the length of the muscle in increased to lengths along the area of the descending limb, the muscle exerts tension prior to stimulation. This passive tension is attributed to structural proteins (titin) within the myofibrils[18] and is an important feature of muscle mechanics, sometimes referred to as the parallel elastic component of muscle.

Mechanics: The Force-Velocity Relationship

The length-tension relationship can be explained by identifiable anatomic features, but this characteristic does not lend itself to a simple structural explanation. In brief, the velocity that a muscle can contract is related to the force resisting the muscle. Experimentally, the muscle is maxi-

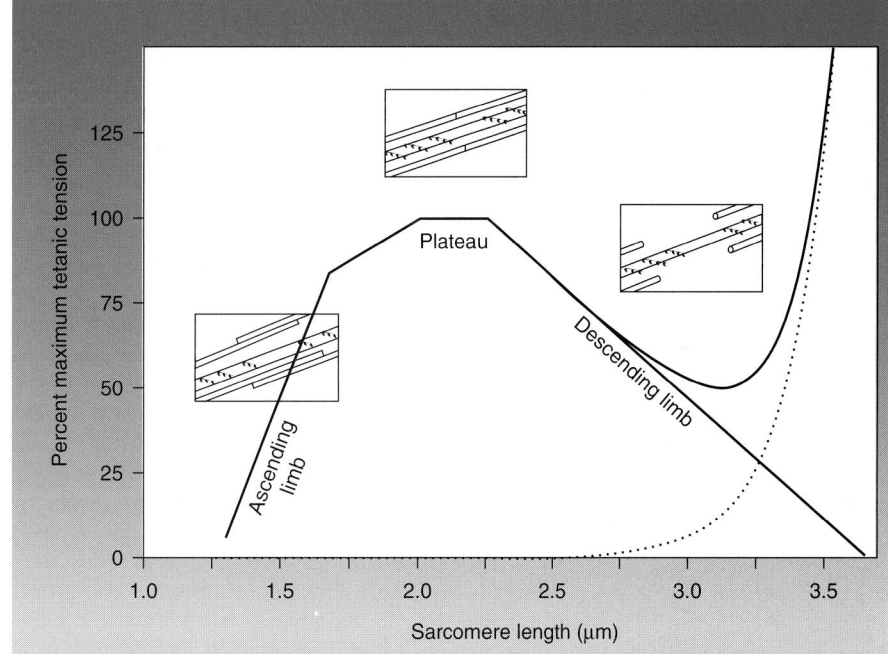

Fig. 1. Length-tension curve of skeletal muscle. (From Lieber RL: Skeletal Muscle Structure and Function. Philadelphia, Williams & Wilkins, 1992.)

mally stimulated against a constant load and the velocity of shortening (or lengthening) measured and plotted for multiple loads. The general shape of the curve is a hyperbola. (Fig. 2). Notice that for shortening contractions, as shortening velocity increases, the tension produced decreases. For lengthening contraction, the relationship is an increase in force with increasing lengths, leading to a plateau. The details of the eccentric (lengthening) force-velocity curve are numerous and can be found in reviews.[19]

What makes skeletal muscle fascinating is the potential interaction of anatomic and mechanical characteristics; for example, determining the force-velocity characteristics of a predominantly type IIA muscle with some physiological cross-sectional area at a preset length after exposure to microgravity, resistance training, or endurance training. The possibilities are almost limitless when involving such elements as hormones, gender, activity, inactivity, immobilization, medication, aging, and so on.

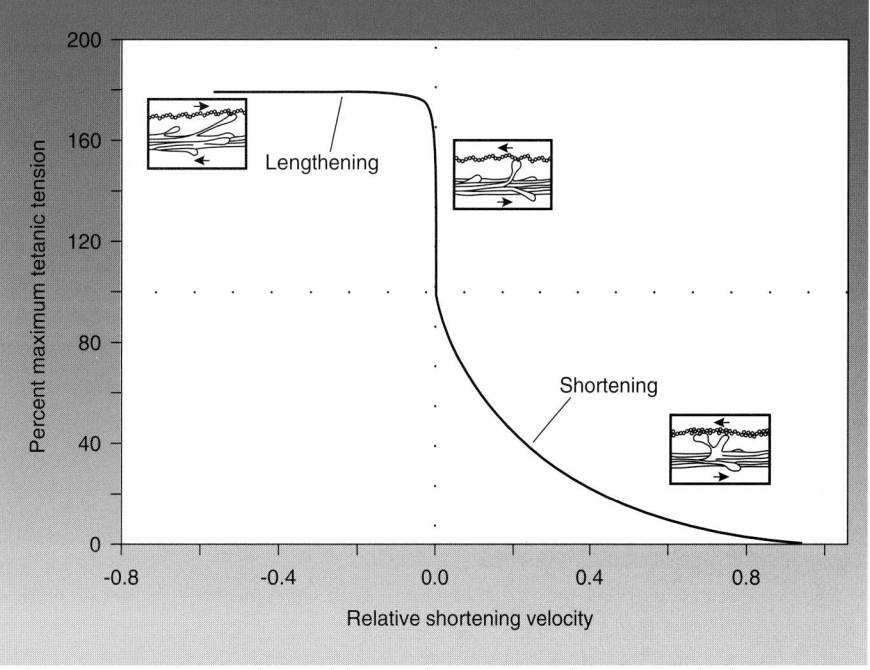

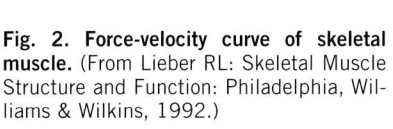

Fig. 2. Force-velocity curve of skeletal muscle. (From Lieber RL: Skeletal Muscle Structure and Function: Philadelphia, Williams & Wilkins, 1992.)

TENDON

Tendon and ligament are both classified as dense connective tissues that are similar under gross and microscopic examination. Although their roles differ, tendon connecting muscle to bone and ligament connecting bone to bone and supporting viscera, their underlying anatomic, physiological, and mechanical features are similar.

The highly organized tendon connects muscle to bone and is very capable of resisting extremely high tensile forces while transmitting forces from muscle to bone. This dense, regularly arranged collagenous tissue comprises fibers, variously shaped cells, and ground substance. Nearly 85% of the dry weight of tendon dictates the mechanical and physiological characteristics and quality of the tendon. In addition to its force transmission duties, tendon is flexible so that it can bend at joints, dampen shocks, and limit potential damage to muscle.[20]

Tendon also shows some degree of extensibility. If the energy from strain used to stretch a tendon could be recovered, a beneficial elastic effect would be achieved. Muscles lengthen and shorten in a cyclic manner. During lengthening, elastic energy can be stored and used as elastic recoil. For example, the Achilles tendon is stretched late in the stance phase when the triceps surae muscles contract and the ankle dorsiflexes. Before plantarflexion, muscle activation ceases, and stored energy helps to initiate plantarflexion.

BASIC STRUCTURE

Tendon (Fig. 3) consists of collagen, which is densely packed fibers that extend the entire length of the tendon. These fibers are arranged in parallel to its long axis. Collagen fibers consist of thinner fibrils and the few centrally located fibroblasts. Fibers are grouped in fascicles; each tendon is made up of multiple fascicles.

Surrounding the tendon is a membrane, called the epitenon, that is similar to the synovium. The inner surface of the epitenon is continuous with the endotenon that binds the collagen and contains neural, vascular, and lymphatic supply. In some tendons, a loose areolar tissue, called paratenon, surrounds the epitenon. The presence of elastic fibers in the paratenon allows for stretch, especially in tendons that do not bend around a joint. The paratenon can be replaced by either a synovial sheath or a bursa and is occasionally referred to as the tenosynovium; e.g., the tendons of the flexor muscles of the wrist and hand. Without this sheath, the paratenon may be termed the tenovagium. The epitenon and paratenon make up the peritenon.

Tendon is fairly well vascularized; more so than cartilage and less so than muscle. Blood arrives at the tendon through connections at the perimysium, periosteum, and other surrounding tissues passing through the paratenon. Tendons may be characterized as being vascular or avascular, with the vascular tendons encased in a paratenon and its accompanying vessels and the avascular tendons enveloped in a sheath that functions as a conduit where diffusion through synovial fluids provides nutrients to tendons.

The nervous innervation of tendon is limited to a sensory role for proprioceptive input from mechanoreceptors found near the muscle-tendon junction. Because tendon has no motor function, it receives no efferent innervation.

The endotenon is continuous with the perimysium and periosteum and forms the connection of tendon to muscle and bone, respectively. At the bony insertion (the osteotendinous junction), the collagen fibers enter as Sharpey's fibers. This simple, yet direct, attachment to bone occurs as the fibrils pass directly into bone and fibrocartilage with minimal contact with the periosteum. A more complex connection involves superficial fibrils inserting into the periosteum, with deeper fibrils inserting directly into bone.

Chemistry

The main fibroblast responsible for the production of tendon collagen and its matrix is the tenocyte, a cylindrically shaped cell capable of producing matrix precursors, elastin, proteoglycans, and collagen. There are few tenocytes, but there are ample ground substance and some elastin.

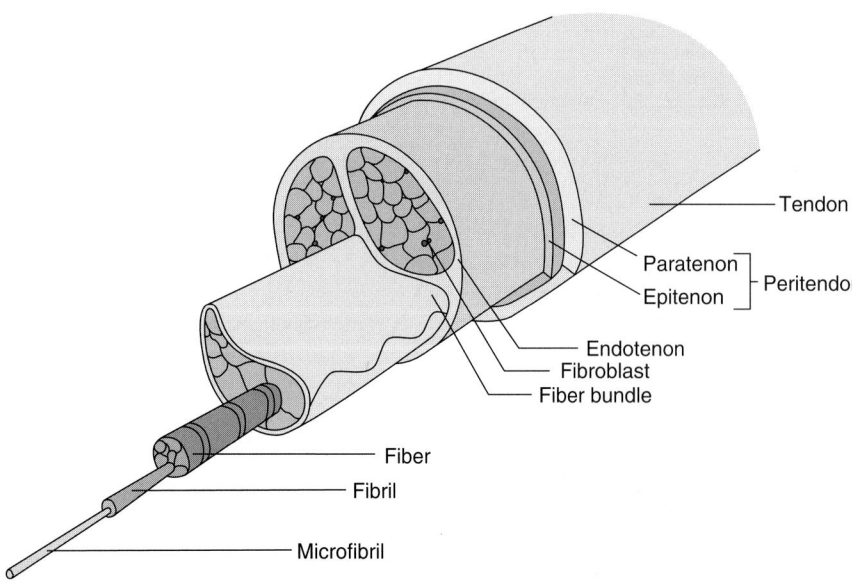

Fig. 3. Structural organization of tendon. (From Best TM, Garrett WE Jr: Muscle and tendon. In DeLee JC, Drez D [eds]: Orthopaedic Sports Medicine: Principles and Practice. Philadelphia, WB Saunders, 1994.)

Collagen

More than 12 different types of collagen have been identified, but it is easiest to think of collagen as either fiber-forming or non–fiber-forming. Types I, II and III are fiber-forming collagens and make up the bulk of the collagen secreted into extracellular spaces, which eventually form fibrils. Type I is the most abundant and makes up about 90% of the collagen in the body; it is also the primary collagen of tendons. The collagen of articular cartilage is primarily type II. The other collagens are non–fiber-forming. Basement membrane collagens are mostly types IV and V.

The tenocyte produces the precursor molecule procollagen that is secreted and cleaved to form tropocollagen. Collagen fibrils then are assembled via non-covalent cross-links. Covalent cross-links then bind fibrils into the typical triple helix that yields this strong protein (Fig. 4).

Elastin

Elastin is required of structures that experience great changes in length in the absence of permanent change in structure. There is a small amount of elastin in the tendons of the extremities, with much more in places like the ligamentum nuchae. In tendons, elastin is less than 1% of dry weight as compared with the aorta, where elastin makes up 30% to 60% of dry weight. The distinctive elastic properties are due to the linkage of unique, copper-dependent amino acids desmosine and isodesmosine to lysine residues.

Ground Substance

Much of the viscoelastic properties of tendon are due to its ground substance. The stability of the collagen skeleton of tendon is largely due to the water-binding capacity of proteoglycans, glycosaminoglycans, plasma proteins, and other

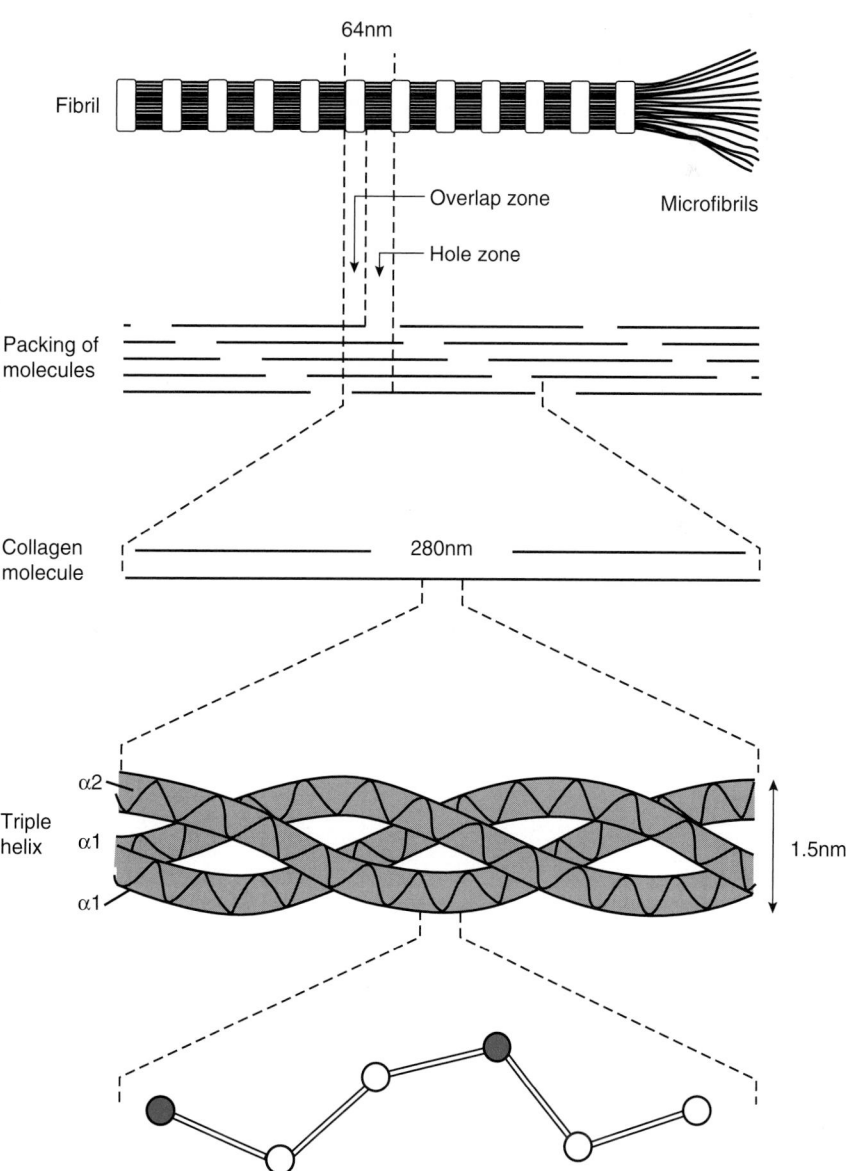

Fig. 4. Collagen microstructure. Three α-chains coil to form a triple-stranded helical rod. (From Best TM, Garrett WE Jr: Muscle and tendon. In DeLee JC, Drez D [eds]: Orthopaedic Sports Medicine: Principles and Practice. Philadelphia, WB Saunders, 1994.)

small molecules. The portions of the tendon that experience the greatest tensile forces have low proteoglycan content and high rates of collagen synthesis as opposed to areas that undergo frictional and compressive forces.[21]

Proteoglycans comprise 1% to 20% of the dry weight of tendon, depending on factors such as age, site, and the history of mechanical loading. Proteoglycans represent an assorted family of glycosylated proteins that contain abundant sulfated polysaccharides (glycosaminoglycans). The principal proteoglycan component in tendon is a low molecular weight dermatan sulfate. Larger molecular weight proteoglycans are present in the fibrocartilaginous regions of the tendon, which are placed under compressive loads in vivo.

The physical properties of proteoglycans are determined by the presence of a large number of negatively charged glycosaminoglycans that attract counter-ions and water molecules in the tissue. These characteristics are believed to contribute to the tissue's compressive properties and viscoelastic behavior.

TENDON BIOMECHANICS

The parallel arrangement of fiber bundles is quite efficient at transmitting high muscle forces to the skeleton for movement. However, tendons do have a low resistance to shear forces; tendons are designed to transmit forces with minimal deformation or energy loss.

Collagenous tissues such as ligament and skin show a stress-strain relationship similar to that of tendon. Two primary characteristics are stress-relaxation (decreased stress over time with constant deformation) and creep (increased length over time with a constant load) (Fig. 5). These properties lead to a load-deformation relationship for tendon that is dependent on tendon's behavior prior to assessment (history-dependent properties).

Figure 6 presents a typical load-deformation curve. Four distinct features of the curve are shown, taking into consideration tendon anatomic microstructure. The initial "toe" region relates to the arrangement of the fibers with the direction of the stress; i.e., straightening out the initial "waviness" of the fiber bundles. The following linear portion of the curve (the elastic stiffness of the tendon) is due to the elongation of the helical structure. At the end of the linear portion, unpredictable failure begins to lead to eventual rupture: a recoil of tendon at the ruptured end. In vivo, there is some protection as the maximum isometric force of a muscle is about one-third that necessary for tendon failure. However, repetitive submaximal loading and fatigue can lead to tendon failure.

Normal tendon usually does not fail in response to

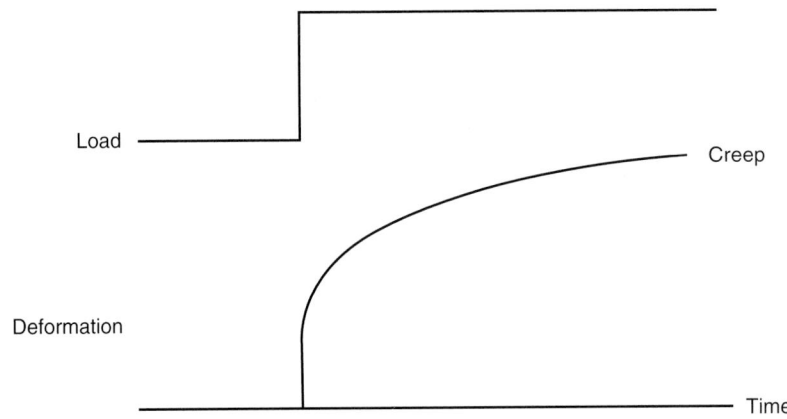

Fig. 5. Graph representation of creep and stress-relaxation in tendon. (From Best TM, Garrett WE Jr: Muscle and tendon. In DeLee JC, Drez D [eds]: Orthopaedic Sports Medicine: Principles and Practice. Philadelphia, WB Saunders, 1994.)

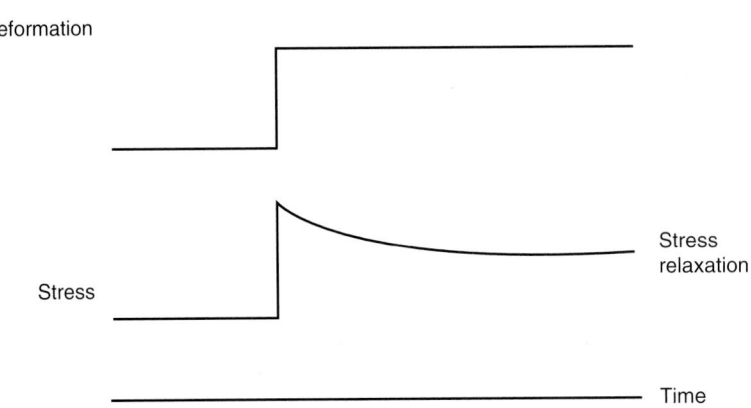

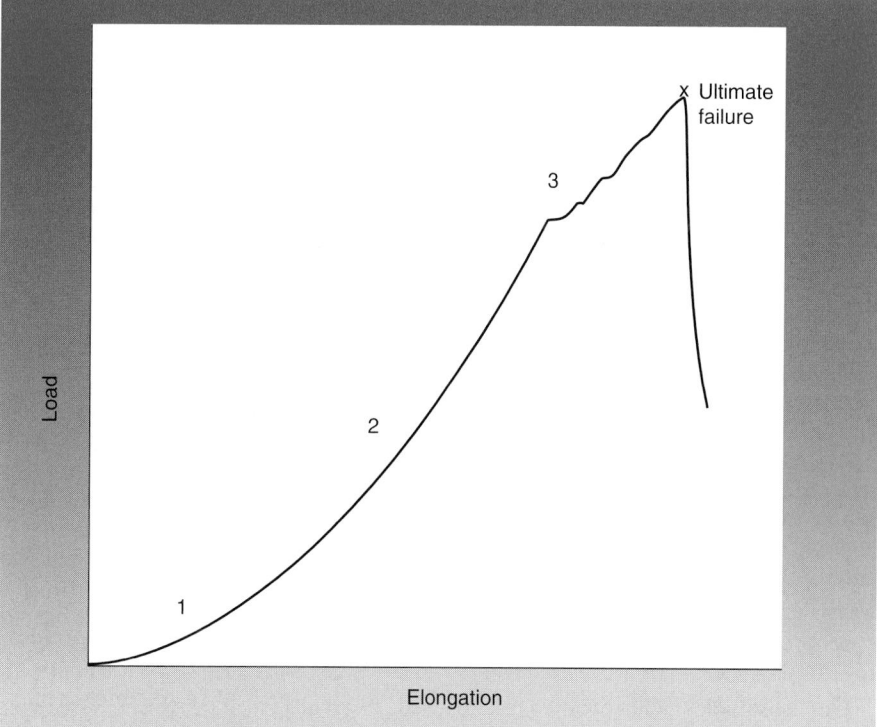

Fig. 6. Representative load-elongation curve. This graph shows[1] the primary region (or region of low stiffness, or "toe"), secondary (or "linear") region,[2] and the region of high stiffness.[3] (From Best TM, Garrett WE Jr: Muscle and tendon. In DeLee JC, Drez D [eds]: Orthopaedic Sports Medicine: Principles and Practice. Philadelphia, WB Saunders, 1994.)

strain. When this muscle-tendon-bone unit fails, the typical location is bone, bone-tendon junction, or muscle-tendon junction. Nonetheless, diseased tendon can fail. Kannus and Jozsa[22] showed that 97% of nearly 900 patients with spontaneous tendon rupture demonstrated degenerative changes in the ruptured tendon (e.g., hypoxic degenerative tendinopathy, mucoid degeneration, tendolipomatosis, or calcifying tendinopathy).

Tendons transfer tension from muscle to bone. According to Cutts et al,[23] when the muscle contracts, the resulting stretch by the tendon leads to three outcomes. First, tendon compliance makes it difficult to maintain joint stability as changes in force lead to changes in tendon length. On the contrary, control of fine motor tasks is simple because the necessary force for change is reduced from small changes in muscle length. Second, a tendon stretch effectively stores elastic energy that is released upon recoil, reducing the work of the muscle. Third, stretching of the tendon determines that the muscle may have to shorten more than it normally might. Therefore, this extensibility can be considered as either advantageous, such as when the tendon acts like a spring, or disadvantageous, as when energy is being transferred to an external system.

Ker et al[24] suggest that the function of a tendon should be considered in combination with the muscle. They describe a combined mass of the muscle and tendon. Thin tendons (those that stretch the most) require longer muscle fibers to yield the ideal ratio of muscle mass to tendon mass. Their optimum ratio of 34 yields a stress of 10 MPa that is well below the 100 MPa breaking point for normal tendon; mammalian tendons are far thicker than necessary.

Ker et al also note that the safety factor (the difference between tendon stress and its breaking point) is reduced in muscles that supply elastic recoil during locomotion. For example, they report that the stress on the Achilles tendon can be as high as 67 MPa, suggesting that the safety factor for this tendon is low in comparison with that of other tendons. The addition of degenerative changes to the tendon will effectively raise the muscle-to-tendon mass ratio, and the breaking force of tendon will approach the stress forces, leading to rupture.

Plasticity Of Tendon

Numerous conditions may alter the normal character of tendon. Common conditions routinely seen by orthopaedists include immobilization, exercise, aging, and medications.

Immobilization

As with ligament, immobilization leads to profound changes in the mechanical properties of tendon. Most importantly, there is a decrease in the strength of tendon plus an increase in collagen turnover.[25, 26] Like so many other tissues, tendon is intimately affected by immobilization.

Exercise

The literature is equivocal about the effects of exercise training on tendon function. Some studies show an increase in tendon strength,[27-29] but a 1-year study of exercise training in pigs showed no changes in tendon mechanical properties, area, or collagen content of flexor tendons,[30] although improvements in strength, area, and collagen content were demonstrated in extensor tendons.[29] Furthermore, although increases in load to failure were found in the tendons of trained animals, no differences were seen for weight, water, or collagen content.[28] There does appear to be an increase in collagen synthesis as smaller fibril bundles have been documented.[31]

Woo and colleagues[32] proposed a model of the mechanical responses of tendon to immobilization and exercise (Fig. 7). The model proposes that tendon undergoes profound insult as a result of immobilization, but training has little or no effect on these mechanical properties.

Aging

Tensile strength reaches a plateau after collagen maturation and then declines with age. This decline is related to decreases in insoluble and total collagen content.[33] The loss of collagen and its cross-linking leads to an increase in tendon stiffness.[34, 35]

A variety of degenerative conditions can affect the function of tendon. Of interest is the absence of spontaneous tendon rupture in the absence of some preexisting histopathological condition.[22] In nearly 900 patients, degenerative changes were seen in practically all those with spontaneous rupture. The most common conditions seen were hypoxic degenerative tendinopathy (44%), mucoid degeneration (21%), tendolipomatosis (8%), and calcifying tendinopathy (5%).

Medication

Corticosteroids. Glucocorticoids are used frequently in the treatment of injuries because of their powerful anti-inflammatory effects. Glucocorticoids inhibit the synthesis of collagen,[36] and local injections around patellar and Achilles tendons can precede a tendon rupture.[37, 38] The systemic effects of oral glucocorticoid treatment has been demonstrated in patients with bilateral Achilles tendon rupture.[39, 40]

Laboratory studies are less conclusive because of the common variables of dosage, duration of therapy, location of injection, or type of drug. For example, local injection of hydrocortisone acetate (20 mg/kg) every 3rd day for 24 days showed increases in peroneal tendon strength in the absence of changes in collagen content, but the same injection schedule into knee joints led to reduced tensile strength of the interface between the posterior cruciate ligament and bone.[41] Daily injections of prednisolone (2 mg/kg) near the peroneal tendons for 2 weeks increased the maximum load, stress, energy absorption, and elastic stiffness, the last owing to more stable cross-linking within the tendon.[42] Long-term injection schedules (10 mg/kg cortisone every 3rd day for 55 days) do not alter mechanical properties, but the hydroxyproline content is reduced.[43]

Corticosteroids impact tendinous tissue in two ways. During the first week or two, corticosteroid injection induces a rapid increase in the tendon's mechanical stability because of a change in the cross-linking pattern. Then, an inhibition of protein synthesis leads to collagen thinning, which in turn leads to a progressive reduction in collagen content.[20, 43]

Nonsteroidal Anti-Inflammatory Agents. It is well known that indomethacin increases the tensile strength of tendons and total collagen content.[44] Similar results were found in tendons undergoing repair,[45] suggesting that much

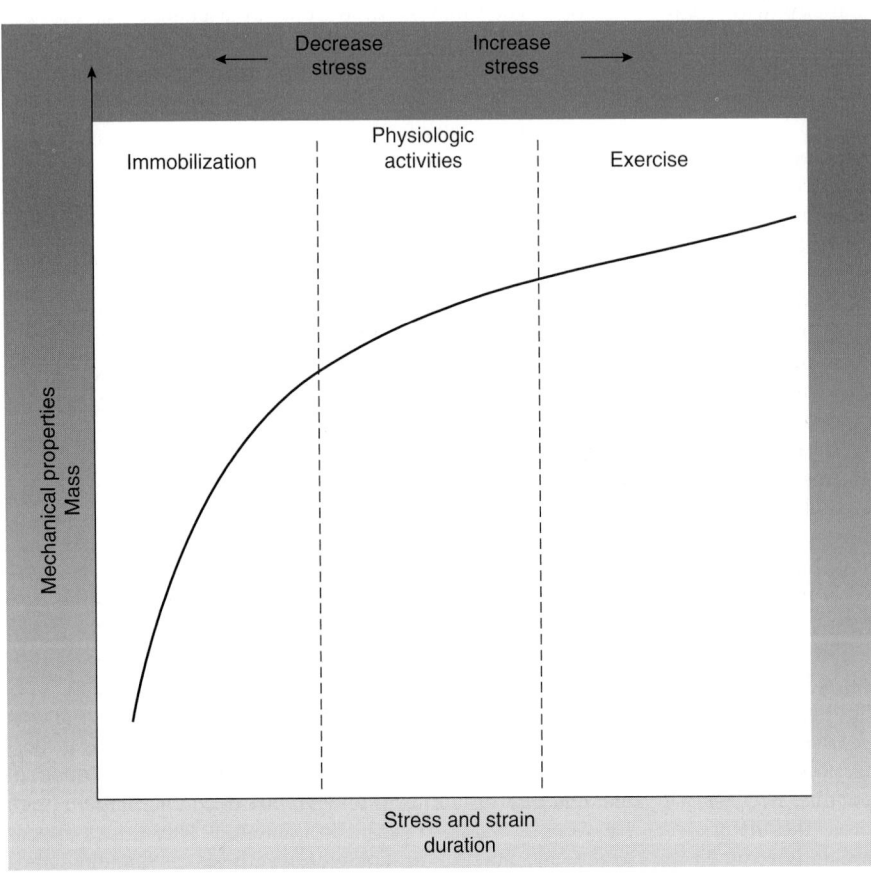

Fig. 7. Hypothetical association of stress and motion on tendon mechanical properties. (From Woo SL-Y, Gomez MA, Woo Y-K, et al: Mechanical properties of tendons and ligaments II: The relationships of immobilization and exercise on tissue remodeling. Biorheology 1982; 19:397.)

of the increase in tendon strength was due to improved collagen cross-linking.[20]

LIGAMENT

Like tendon, ligament is classified as a dense connective tissue and is similar to tendon on gross and microscopic examination. Ligament is a tough, flexible band of firm, white, fibrous bands of connective tissue that connects bones and supports viscera and that varies in thickness, length, and shape. Because tendon and ligament are closely related, many of the features of ligaments are similar to those of tendons.

Hundreds of ligaments have been identified and are generally named according to their bony attachments (e.g., fibulocalcaneal) or their relationship to other ligaments (e.g., lateral collateral). Some are distinct structures with specialized functions (anterior cruciate ligament), whereas the structure and function of others (e.g., hip capsular ligaments) are less clear because they are continuous with the joint capsule. Depending on their location, ligaments may be covered by a thin layer of synovium (intracapsular ligaments), a thin layer of areolar tissue (capsular ligaments), or fat and areolar tissue (extracapsular ligaments). Regardless of their location and other differences, the primary function of ligament is to stabilize the relationship between adjoining bones.

BASIC STRUCTURE

Microscopic views of ligament show a high degree of organization, with several rows of fibroblasts within bundles of a matrix that is primarily type I collagen (70% of dry weight). Elastin, also present, makes up less than 1% of the dry weight.[46, 47] Ligaments that are primarily elastin (flavin, nuchal ligaments) have remarkably different mechanical characteristics from those of more collagen-dominated types.

The fibrils of the collagen matrix are from 150 nm to 250 nm in diameter and are grouped into 1-μm to 20-μm fibers that are themselves bunched into subfascicular elements 100 μm to 250 μm in diameter. Binding around 3 to 20 of these subfascicular bundles with loose connective tissue (epitenon) forms a fascicle, which can be arranged in a spiral array (like the anterior cruciate ligament) or pass straight from bone to bone (like collateral ligaments).[46, 47]

Ligament appears almost hypovascular, especially when compared with surrounding tissues. However, there is a fairly uniform microvascular tree that arises from the insertion sites of the ligament. This arrangement supplies sufficient nutrients to support the cellular network with sufficient needs for maintaining the matrix. Damage to this microvascular network places the ligament at risk for rupture.[46, 47]

Historically, the ligament has been believed to be without neural innervation. However, recent animal and human studies have demonstrated the presence of pain fibers in the capsular ligaments of spinal facets as well as proprioception and nociception in the medial collateral and anterior cruciate ligaments. Unlike tendon, ligaments contain less collagen and more ground substance, and the collagen is in a more random arrangement than in tendon. Furthermore, fibers in ligament are arranged in more of a woven pattern as compared with tendon fibers that are arranged along the long axis of the tissue.[46, 47]

CHEMISTRY

Although there can be subtle intra- and interligament variations in matrix, cell density, and shape, all ligaments consist of fibroblasts surrounded by a matrix of water and macromolecules, mostly type I collagen.[47, 48] As with tendon, the makeup of the water-macromolecular matrix dictates the nature of the ligament.

COLLAGEN

About 70% to 80% of the dry weight of ligament is collagen, with type I collagen being the main component (90%) of the cylindrical, cross-banded fibers. The remaining 10% is made up of type III collagen, which is in contrast to tendons that have less type III collagen.[46]

ELASTIN

Typically, ligaments are less than 5% elastin, but certain ligaments, like the ligamentum flavum, can have a very high (e.g., 75%) concentration of elastin. The random coils of elastin chains allow elastin to endure deformation without damage, then return to its original size and shape once unloaded.[47]

PROTEOGLYCANS

Although they occupy less than 1% of the macromolecular structure of the ligament,[47] proteoglycans play an important role in organizing the extracellular matrix and tissue fluids[49–52] and contain a higher concentration of glycosaminoglycans. For a more detailed discussion of proteoglycans, the reader is referred to published reviews.[51, 53]

LIGAMENT BIOMECHANICS

Mechanical testing of ligaments is usually done in a bone-ligament-bone preparation and typically involves an examination of the load (or force) and elongation. As with tendon, the curve can be described as having an initial region of low stiffness (toe region), followed by a region of high stiffness in a non-linear response. The shape of the curve is related to the crimp of collagen fibrils and a nonuniform use of individual fibers. The low-stiffness region is where the crimp is straightened out, and the high-stiffness region is due to the larger forces required to elongate fibrils (Fig. 8).

The interaction of collagen and ground substance is reflected in the ligament's viscoelasticity (history-dependent). The concept of viscoelasticity is that a tissue's response is based on time as well as strain and evidenced as creep, stress relaxation, and hysteresis. The shape of the load elongation curve will vary according to the prior loading. With ever-increasing loading repetitions on the ligament, there is a reduction in peak load, and there are increases in elongation and a reduction in the energy loss with unloading[54] (area within the hysteresis loop, Fig. 9). These me-

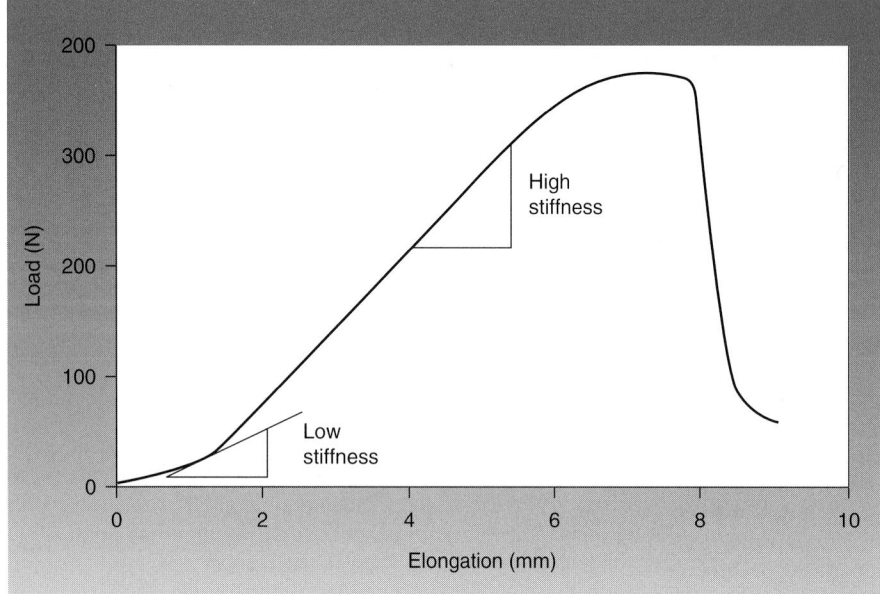

Fig. 8. Load-deformation curve from mechanical tensile testing of ligament. (From Woo SL-Y: Anatomy, biology and biomechanics of tendon, ligament and meniscus. In Simon SR [ed]: Orthopaedic Basic Science. Rosemont, IL, American Academy of Orthopaedic Surgeons, 1994.)

chanical features have direct clinical applications. For example, during reconstruction of the anterior cruciate ligament, stress relaxation can account for reduction of graft forces to around 80% of the initial force within about 1 hour.

When a ligament has been inactive for a long time, fluid is absorbed. The first few applications of force cause some of the extra fluid to be extruded so that in the first few cycles following inactivity there is increased stiffness and energy loss (hysteresis area). Following some preconditioning (initial cycles), the behavior of the ligament becomes more predictable. In any testing of biomechanical proper-

ties, preconditioning is an important feature of testing protocols.[54]

In interpreting any biomechanical data, the profound variations in anatomic location, chemistry, species, prior stress exposure, age, maturation, length of immobilization, testing protocols, methods of gripping ligaments, definitions, and other factors must be taken into account.[55, 56] As such, it is not surprising that no individual mechanical factor can be used as a representative variable for all ligaments. When reading discussions about individual ligament properties within this volume, the reader should consider these factors.

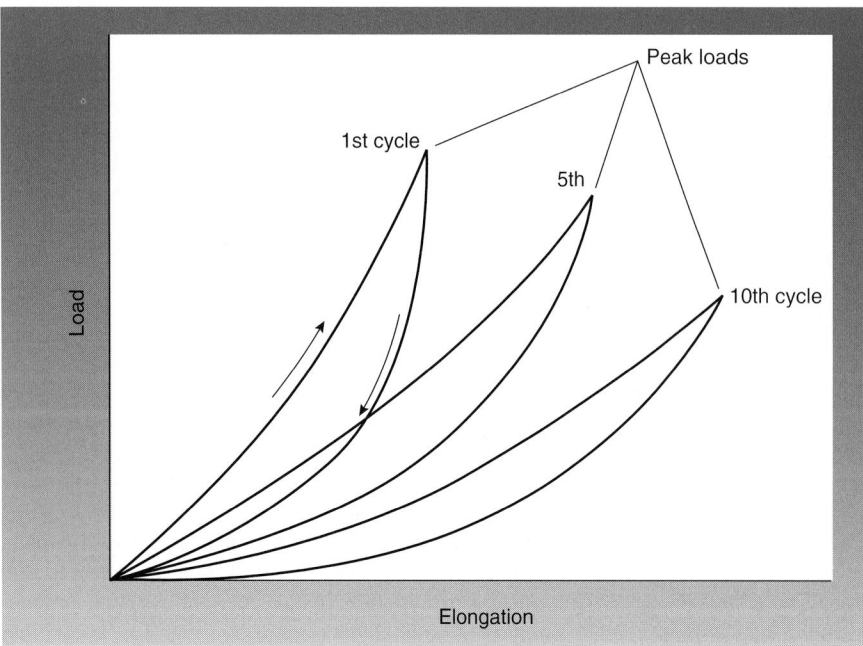

Fig. 9. Hysteresis curves of loading and unloading of ligament over ten cyclic tests.

REFERENCES

1. Lieber RL: Skeletal Muscle Structure and Function. Philadelphia, Williams & Wilkins, 1992.

2. Loeb GE, Pratt CA, Chanaud CM, et al: Distribution and innervation of short, interdigitated muscle fibers in parallel-fibered muscles of the cat hindlimb. J Morphol 1987; 191:1.

3. Ounjian M, Roy RR, Eldred E, et al: Physiological and developmental implication of motor unit anatomy. J Neurobiol 1991; 22:547.

4. Hall ZW, Ralston E: Nuclear domains in muscle cells. Cell 1989; 59:771.

5. Rosenblatt JD, Yong D, Parry DJ: Satellite cell activity is required for hypertrophy of overloaded adult rat skeletal muscle. Muscle Nerve 1994; 17:608.

6. Allen DL, Yasui W, Tanaka T, et al: Myonuclear number and myosin heavy chain expression in rat soleus single muscle fibers after spaceflight. J Appl Physiol 1994; 81:145.

7. Hikida RS, Hagerman FC, Staron RS, et al: Satellite cells and myonuclei in young and elderly muscles: Effect of training. Med Sci Sports Exerc 1997; 29:S290.

8. Ogata T, Yamasaki Y: Ultra-high resolution scanning electron microscopy of mitochondria and sarcoplasmic reticulum arrangement in human red, white, and intermediate muscle fibers. Anat Rec 1997; 248:214.

9. Kayar SR, Hoppeler H, Mermod L, et al: Mitochondrial size and shape in equine skeletal muscle: A 3-dimensional reconstruction study. Anat Rec 1988; 222:333.

10. Prince FP, Hikida RS, Hagerman FC, et al: A morphometric analysis of human muscle fibers with relation to fiber types and adaptations to exercise. J Neurol Sci 1981; 49:165.

11. Payne CM, Stern LZ, Curless RG, et al: Ultrastructural fiber typing in normal and diseased human muscle. J Neurol Sci 1975; 25:99.

12. Sjostrom M, Kidman SIW, Henriksson-Larsen K, et al: Z- and M-appearance in different histochemically defined types of human skeletal muscle fibers. J Histochem Cytochem 1982; 30:1.

13. Staron RS: Correlation between myofibrillar ATPase activity and myosin heavy chain composition in single human muscle fibers. Histochem 1991; 96:21.

14. Brown RH: Dystrophin-associated proteins and the muscular dystrophies. Annu Rev Med 1997; 48:457.

15. Powell PL, Roy RR, Kanim P, et al: Predictability of skeletal msucle tension from architectural determination in guinea pig hindlimbs. J Appl Physiol 1984; 57:1715.

16. Wickiewicz TL, Roy RR, Powell PL, et al: Muscle architecture of the human lower limb. Clin Orthop Rel Res 1983; 179:275.

17. Lieber RL, Fazeli BM, Abrams RA, et al: Architecture of selected wrist flexor and extensor muscle. J Hand Surg 1990; 15:244.

18. Magid A, Law DJ: Myofibrils bear most of the resting tension in frog skeletal muscle. Science 1985; 230:1280.

19. Stauber WT: Eccentric action of muscles: Physiology, injury, and adaptation. Exerc Sport Sci Rev 1989; 17:157.

20. Best TM, Garrett WE Jr: Muscle and tendon. In DeLee JC, Drez D (eds): Orthopaedic Sports Medicine: Principles and Practice. Philadelphia, WB Saunders, 1994.

21. Abrahams M: Mechanical behavior of tendon in vitro: A preliminary report. Med Biol Eng 1967; 5:433.

22. Kannus P, Jozsa L: Histopathological changes preceding spontaneous rupture of a tendon. J Bone Joint Surg Am 1991; 73:1507.

23. Cutts A, Alexander RM, Ker RF: Ratios of cross-sectional areas of muscles and their tendons in a healthy human forearm. J Anat 1991; 176:133.

24. Ker RF, Alexander RM, Bennett MB: Why are mammalian tendons so thick? J Zool 1988; 216:309.

25. Amiel D, Woo SL-Y, Harwood FL, et al: The effect of immobilization on collagen turnover in connective tissue: A biochemical-biomechanical correlation. Acta Orthop Scand 1982; 53:325.

26. Noyes FR: Functional properties of knee ligaments and alterations induced by immobilization. Clin Orthop 1977; 123:210.

27. Tipton CM, Schild RJ, Tomanek RJ: Influence of physical activity on the strength of knee ligaments in rats. Am J Physiol 1967; 212:783.

28. Viidik A: The effects of training on the tensile strength of isolated rabbit tendons. Scand J Plas Reconstr Surg 1967; 1:141.

29. Woo SL-Y, Ritter MA, Amiel D, et al: The biomechanical and biochemical properties of swine tendons: Long-term effects of exercise on the digital extensors. Connect Tissue Res 1980; 7:177.

30. Woo SL-Y, Gomez MA, Amiel D, et al: The effects of exercise on the biomechanical and biochemical properties of swine digital flexor tendons. J Biomech Eng 1981; 103:51.

31. Michna H: Morphometric analysis of loading-induced changes in collagen-fibril populations in young tendons. Cell Tissue Res 1984; 236:465.

32. Woo SL-Y, Gomez MA, Woo Y-K, et al: Mechanical properties of tendons and ligaments II: The relationships of immobilization and exercise on tissue remodeling. Biorheology 1982; 19:397.

33. Vogel HC: Influence of maturation and age on mechanical and biochemical parameters of connective tissue of various organs in the rat. Connect Tissue Res 1978; 6:161.

34. Bailey AJ, Robins SP, Balian G: Biological significance of the intermolecular crosslinks of collagen. Nature 1984; 251:105.

35. Eyre DR: Cross-linking in collagen and elastin. Ann Rev Biochem 1984; 53:717.

36. Nimni ME, Bavetta LA: Collagen synthesis and turnover in the growing rat under the influence of methylprednisolone. Proc Soc Exp Biol Med 1964; 117:618.

37. Lee HB: Avulsion and rupture in the tenocalcaneus after injection of hydrocortisone. Br Med J 1957; 2:395.

38. Oxlund H: Changes in connective tissues during corticotropin and corticosteroid treatment. Thesis. University of Aarchus, Denmark, Institute of Anatomy, 1983.

39. Lee MLH: Bilateral rupture of Achilles tendon. Br Med J 1961; 1:1829.

40. Melmed EP: Spontaneous bilateral rupture of the calcaneal tendon during steroid therapy. J Bone Joint Surg Br 1965; 47:104.

41. Oxlund H: The influence of a local injection of cortisol on the mechanical properties of tendons and ligaments and the indirect effect on skin. Acta Orthop Scand 1980; 51:231.

42. Oxlund H, Manthorpe R, Viidik A: The biomechanical properties of connective tissue in rabbits as influenced by short-term glucocorticoid treatment. J Biomech 1981; 14:129.

43. Oxlund H: Long-term local cortisol treatment of tendons and the indirect effect of skin. Scand J Plast Reconstr Surg 1982; 16:61.

44. Vogel HC: Mechanical and chemical properties of various connective tissue organs in rats as influenced by nonsteroidal antirheumatic drugs. Connect Tissue Res 1977; 5:91.

45. Carlstedt CA, Madsen K, Wredmark T: The influence of indomethecin on tendon healing: A biomechanical and biochemical study. Arch Orthop Trauma Surg 1986; 105:332.

46. Amiel D, Frank C, Harwood F, et al: Tendons and ligaments: A morphological and biochemical comparison. J Orthop Res 1984; 1:257.

47. Frank C, Woo S, Andriacchi T, et al: Normal ligament: Structure, function and composition. In Woo SL-Y, Buckwalter JA (eds): Injury and Repair of Musculoskeletal Soft Tissues. Park Ridge, IL, American Academy of Orthopaedic Surgeons, 1988.

48. Buckwalter JA, Maynard JA, Vailas CA: Skeletal fibrous tissues: Tendon, joint capsule and ligament. In Albright JA, Brand RA (eds): The Scientific Basis of Orthopaedics. Norwalk, CT, Appleton & Lange, 1987.

49. Buckwalter JA: Cartilage. In Delbecco R (ed): Encyclopedia of Human Biology. San Diego, Academic Press, 1990.

50. Hardinham TE: Proteoglycans: Their structure, interactions and molecular organization in cartilage. Biochem Soc Trans 1981; 9:489.

51. Poole AR, Webber C, Pidoux I: Localization of a dermatan sulfate proteoglycan (DS-PGII) in cartilage and the presence of an immunologically related species in other tissues. J Histochem Cytochem 1986; 34:619.

52. Muir H: Proteoglycans as organizers of the extracellular matrix. Biochem Soc Trans 1983; 11:613.

53. Rosenberg L, Choi HU, Neame PJ, et al: Proteoglycans of soft connective tissue. In Leadbetter WB, Buckwalter JA, Gordon SL (eds): Sports-Induced Inflammation: Basic Science and Clincal Concepts. Park Ridge, IL, American Academy of Orthopaedic Surgeons, 1990.

54. Danto MI, Woo SL-Y: The mechanical properties of skeletally mature rabbit anterior cruciate ligament and patellar tendon over a range of strain rates. J Orthop Res 1993; 11:58.

55. Woo SL-Y, Ohland KJ, Weiss JA: Age and sex-related changes in the biomechanical properties of the rabbit medial collateral ligament. Mech Ageing Dev 1990; 56:129.

56. Woo SL-Y, Peterson RH, Ohland KJ: The effects of strain rate on the properties of the medial collateral ligament in skeletally immature rabbits and mature rabbits: A biomechanical and histological study. J Orthop Res 1990; 8:712.

section
2
chapter
5

PERIPHERAL NERVE STRUCTURE: FUNCTION AND PHYSIOLOGY

David C. Preston

Summary

- Somatic motor, somatic sensory, and autonomic fibers are carried within peripheral nerves
- All peripheral nerves are derived from motor and sensory nerve roots in the spine.
- Nerve fibers run in fascicles and are protected by three different layers of connective tissue: epineurium, perineurium, and endoneurium.
- Intraneural topography is not constant and changes as nerve traverses along its distal to proximal axis.
- The axon is a complex structure with structural, metabolic, and electrical properties.
- Nerve transmission along an axon occurs via the propagation of action potentials that result from a positive feedback cycle of intracellular depolarization and the opening of voltage-dependent sodium ion channels.
- Myelin insulation results in saltatory conduction and markedly increases nerve conduction velocity.

Clinical Relevance

- Most nerve entrapment syndromes, both at the root level and in the limbs, can be recognized by their unique patterns of sensory and motor dysfunction.
- Clinical symptoms and signs differ between entrapments at the root level and those in the periphery primarily because of the wide overlap of adjacent myotomes and dermatomes.
- Because of less tensile strength of the nerve roots compared with peripheral nerve in the limbs, severe stretch injuries often result in root avulsion rather than direct peripheral nerve injury.
- The rate of slow axonal transport (1 to 2 mm/day) system is the rate-limiting factor in regrowth of injured nerve that has undergone axonal loss.
- Remyelination does not require axonal transport for recovery and can typically occur over several weeks.
- Certain disorders can preferentially affect large- or small-diameter nerve fibers.

The principal role of the peripheral nervous system is to faithfully transmit information to and from the brain and spinal cord. Within the peripheral nerves are somatic motor, somatic sensory, and autonomic fibers. Somatic sensory fibers convey sensory information from a variety of receptors in the skin and joints to the dorsal horn of the spinal cord, where it is processed segmentally and transmitted rostrally. Somatic motor fibers carry information from the spinal cord and brain stem to muscles throughout the body to effect all types of movement. Similar to the somatic system, most of the information from the autonomic nervous system is ultimately relayed through the peripheral nerves as well. Autonomic fibers carry both afferent and efferent information, supplying blood vessels, sweat glands, and the internal organs. Orthopaedic surgeons commonly are referred patients with a variety of conditions that result in peripheral nerve dysfunction. Most frequent are radiculopathies, spinal stenosis, peripheral entrapments, and trauma, among other conditions. This chapter provides a review of the basic gross and microscopic anatomic structure of peripheral nerves as well as the underlying electrical and chemical events that allow peripheral nerves to function.

ANATOMY

The primary motor neurons, the anterior horn cells, reside in the ventral gray matter of the spinal cord. The axons of these cells ultimately become the motor fibers in peripheral nerves. Their projections first run through the white matter of the anterior spinal cord before exiting ventrally as the motor roots. In contrast to the anterior horn cell, the primary sensory neuron, the dorsal root ganglion, does not reside within the spinal cord itself but lies outside, near the intervertebral foramen. The dorsal root ganglia are bipolar cells with two separate axonal projections. Their central projections form the sensory nerve roots, which enter the spinal cord on the dorsal side either to ascend in the posterior columns or to synapse with sensory neurons in the dorsal horn. The peripheral projections of the dorsal root ganglia ultimately become the sensory fibers in peripheral nerves.

In the adult, the spinal cord is shorter in length than the bony spinal column.[1] Typically, the conus medullaris of the spinal cord lies adjacent to the L1 vertebral body. Thus, below L1, the motor and sensory roots must descend through the thecal sac together before exiting at their appropriate spinal level. In this area, the lumbosacral nerve roots are known as the cauda equina.

At each spinal level, motor and sensory roots unite in the intervertebral foramen just distal to the dorsal root ganglion to form a mixed spinal nerve. There are 31 pairs of spinal nerves (8 cervical, 12 thoracic, 5 lumbar, 5 sacral, 1 coccygeal). Almost immediately, each spinal nerve divides into a dorsal ramus and a ventral ramus. Unlike the dorsal and ventral nerve roots, the dorsal and ventral rami both contain motor and sensory fibers. The dorsal ramus runs posteriorly to supply muscular innervation to the paraspinal muscles at that segment and sensory innervation to the skin adjacent to the spine at that level as well. The ventral ramus differs, however, depending on the segment within the body. In the thoracic region, each ventral ramus continues as an intercostal nerve. In the lower cervical (C5-T1) and lumbosacral regions (L1-S1), the ventral rami unite to form the brachial plexus and lumbosacral plexus, respectively.

Within each brachial and lumbosacral plexus, motor and sensory nerve fibers from different nerve roots intermix to ultimately form individual peripheral nerves. Each peripheral nerve generally supplies muscular innervation to several muscles and cutaneous sensation to a specific area of skin, in addition to sensory innervation to underlying deep structures.

All muscles supplied by one nerve root (i.e., spinal segment) are known as a myotome, whereas all cutaneous areas supplied by a single nerve root are known as a dermatome (Fig. 1). For both myotomes and dermatomes, there is considerable overlap between adjacent segments.[1, 2] Most areas of skin supplied by one dermatome receive partial innervation from both the dermatome above and below. Similarly, most muscles are supplied by at least two or three myotomes (e.g., the triceps is innervated by C7 and partially innervated by C6 and C8). Because of this arrangement, motor fibers from the same nerve root supply muscles innervated by different peripheral nerves, and sensory fibers from the same nerve root supply cutaneous sensation also by way of different nerves. For instance, the C6 motor root supplies the biceps (musculocutaneous nerve), deltoid (axillary nerve), and brachioradialis (radial nerve), among other muscles. Similarly, C6 sensory fibers innervate the lateral forearm (lateral antebrachial cutaneous sensory nerve) and thumb (median and radial nerves).

On the microscopic level, nerve fibers are protected by three different layers of connective tissue: the epineurium, perineurium, and endoneurium (Fig. 2).[3] The thick epineurium surrounds the entire nerve and is in continuity with the dura mater at the spinal cord level. Within the epineurium, axons are grouped into bundles or fascicles, surrounded by a layer of connective tissue known as the perineurium. A final layer of connective tissue, the endoneurium, is present between individual axons. Within each nerve, an effective blood-nerve barrier is formed from the combination of vascular endothelium supplying the nerve and the connective tissue of the perineurium.[3, 4] Together, the three layers of connective tissue give peripheral nerve considerable tensile strength, usually in the range of 20 to 30 kg. However, the weakest point of a nerve occurs where the nerve roots meet the spinal cord, which can only sustain 2 to 3 kg of force.[5, 6]

Within a nerve, nerve fibers do not run in a straight course as might be expected for a wire or cable. Indeed, intraneural topography changes substantially as nerve traverses along its distal to proximal axis (Fig. 3).[7, 8] No constant or characteristic pattern is found for any nerve. Intraneural topography is constantly altered by fascicular

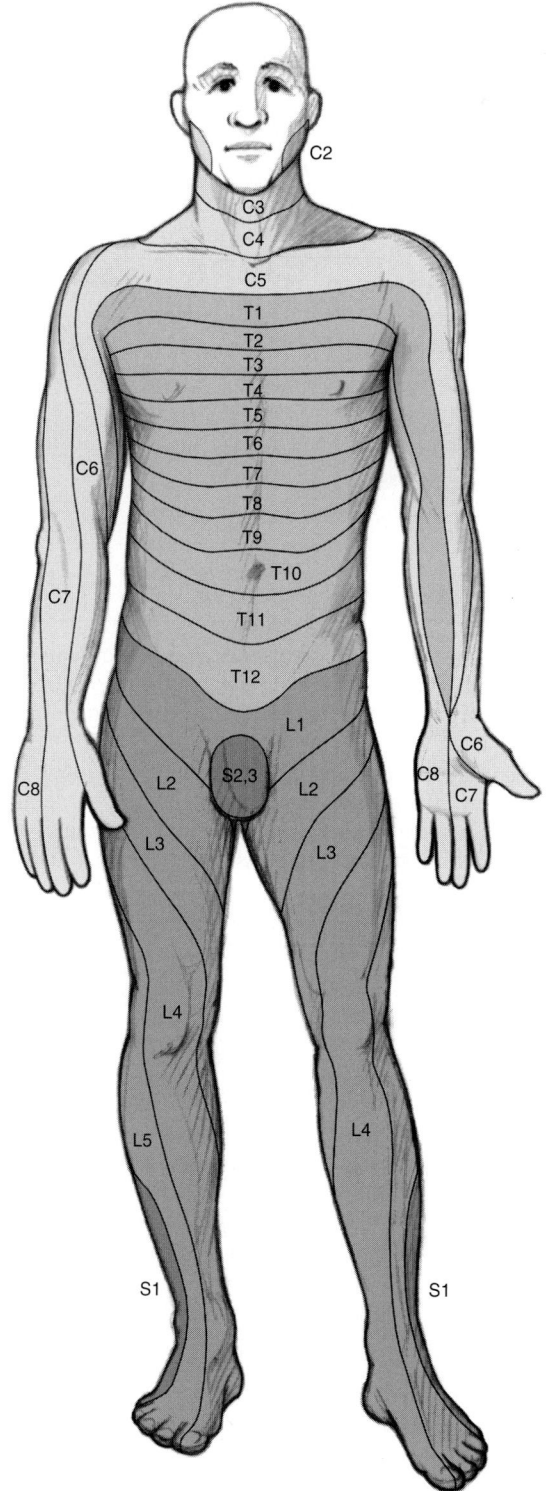

Fig. 1. Dermatomes. The cutaneous area supplied from one spinal segment (i.e., one sensory nerve root) is known as a dermatome. There is wide overlap of adjacent dermatomes above and below. Consequently, a nerve root lesion, even if severe, never results in anesthesia but only altered or decreased sensation. (Redrawn from Gardner E, Gray DJ, O'Rahilly R: Anatomy. Philadelphia, WB Saunders, 1975, 4th ed.)

anastomoses, division, and migration of nerve bundles. Indeed, in microscopic dissections, the longest length of any nerve is approximately 15 mm in which intraneural topography remains uniform.

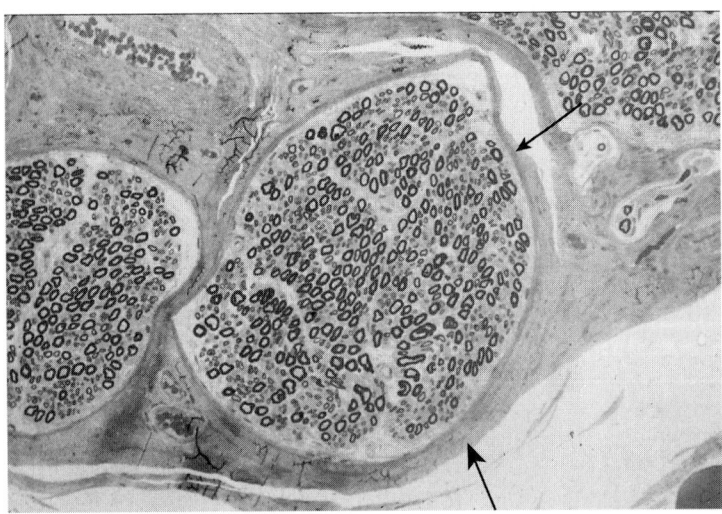

Fig. 2. Internal peripheral nerve anatomy. Myelinated fibers are recognized as small dark rings (myelin) with a central clearing (axon). The endoneurium is present between axons. Axons are grouped into fascicles, surrounded by perineurium *(arrow)*. Surrounding the entire nerve is the last layer of connective tissue: the epineurium *(large arrow)*. (From Preston DC, Shapiro BE: Electromyography and Neuromuscular Disorders. Boston, Butterworth-Heinemann, 1998.)

PHYSIOLOGY

The axon has structural, metabolic, and electrical properties. Indeed, most of the surface area and volume of a nerve cell are contained within the axon. A typical anterior horn cell has a diameter in the range of 50 to 100 μm, yet its axon may be as long as 1 m, in the case of sciatic nerve axons. Each axon is enclosed by the axolemma, a fine trilaminar membrane. The intracellular contents of the axon, the axoplasma, contain cellular organelles and cyto-

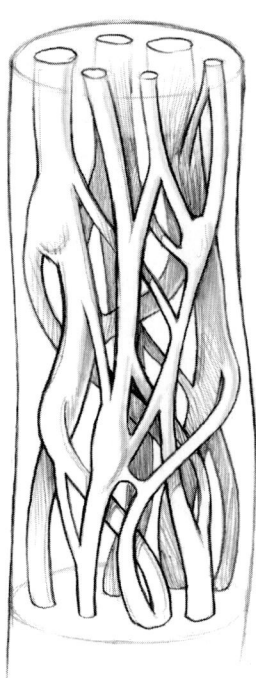

Fig. 3. Substantial intraneural nerve topography changes. Intraneural topography is constantly altered by fascicular anastomoses, division, and migration of nerve bundles. Sunderland illustrated the plexiform character of nerve fascicles with extensive anatomic dissections. No constant or characteristic fascicular pattern was found for any nerve. (Redrawn from Sunderland S: Nerves and Nerve Injuries. Edinburgh, Churchill Livingstone, 1978, 2nd ed, p 27.)

skeletal elements.[9] The internal cytoskeleton is composed mainly of microtubules in the range of 25 nm in diameter and finer neurofilaments in the range of 10 nm in diameter. Microtubules are not only important for the maintenance of the cytoskeleton but are also integral for the process of axonal transport. Both anterograde and retrograde axonal transport systems exist. Glycoproteins, glycolipids, lipids, cholesterol, acetylcholinesterase, and other enzymes are transported down the axon. The rate of axonal transport occurs both at fast (400 mm/day) and slow (1 to 2 mm/day) rates for different agents.[10]

The essential function of peripheral nerve is to transmit information reliably to and from the periphery. Although the function of nerves may superficially appear similar to electrical wires, there are vast differences between them. At the molecular level, a complex set of chemical and electrical events occurs that allows for the creation of the action potential, the response that allows peripheral nerves to transmit information.[11, 12] Each axonal membrane is an electrically active structure. This results from a combination of a specialized membrane and the presence of an intracellular sodium ion (Na^+)/potassium ion (K^+) pump (Fig. 4). The specialized axonal membrane is semipermeable to anions and cations. The membrane is always impermeable to large negatively charged anions and, in addition, is relatively impermeable to Na^+ in the resting state. This semipermeable membrane, in conjunction with an active Na^+/K^+ pump, which pumps Na^+ outside in exchange for K^+, leads to concentration gradients across the membrane: the concentration of Na^+ is larger outside the membrane, whereas the concentration of K^+ and larger anions is greater inside. The combination of these electrical and chemical gradients results in forces that create a resting equilibrium potential. At the nerve cell body, this resting membrane potential is approximately -70 mV inside compared with approximately -90 mV outside and distally in the axon.

Voltage-dependent Na^+ channels line the membrane of the axon. When current is injected into the axon, depolarization occurs (i.e., the axon becomes more positive internally). Depolarization results in opening of the Na^+ channels, allowing Na^+ to rush into the axon, driven both by

Fig. 4. Resting membrane potential. At rest, the axonal membrane is negatively polarized, inside compared with outside. This resting potential results from the combination of a membrane that is semipermeable to charged particles and an NA^+/K^+ pump. At rest, the concentration of Na^+ and chloride (Cl^-) is higher in the extracellular space, with the concentration of K^+ and large anions (A^-) greater inside the axon. (Redrawn from Preston DC, Shapiro BE: Electromyography and Neuromuscular Disorders. Boston, Butterworth-Heinemann, 1998.)

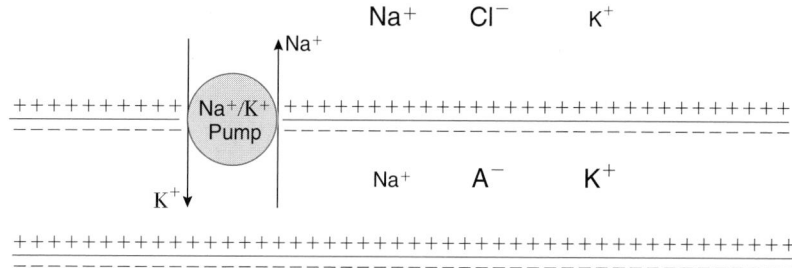

concentration and electrical gradients. Every time a depolarization of 10 to 30 mV occurs above the resting membrane potential (i.e., threshold), an action potential is created from a cycle of positive feedback: more Na^+ channels open, more influx of Na^+, further depolarization, more Na^+ channels open, and so on (Fig. 5). Action potentials are always all-or-none responses, which can then propagate away from the initial site of depolarization down the course of a nerve. However, the depolarization of the axon is short lived, because the opening of the Na^+ channels is time limited. Once activated, Na^+ channels quickly inactivate within 1 to 2 msec. Na^+ channel inactivation along with increased K^+ conduction and the Na^+/K^+ pump then reestablishes the resting membrane potential.

The conduction velocity of the action potential is proportional to the cross-diameter of the axon. The larger the diameter, the less electrical resistance there is and the faster the conduction velocity is.[3] However, even for the largest diameter unmyelinated axons, conduction velocity of an action potential rarely exceeds 3 to 5 m/sec. Conduction velocity can be greatly increased with the addition of myelin. Myelin insulation is present on all fast-conducting

fibers and is derived from Schwann's cells, the major supporting cell in the peripheral nervous system. Myelin is composed of concentric spirals of Schwann's cell membrane. For every myelinated fiber, successive segments are myelinated by single Schwann's cells. Thus, the axonal membrane is exposed only distally near the neuromuscular junction and at the small uninsulated gaps between two adjacent Schwann's cells, known as the nodes of Ranvier. Thus, most of the nerve is effectively insulated with myelin, and depolarization occurs by way of saltatory conduction: depolarization only occurs at each node of Ranvier, with current jumping from node to node (Fig. 6).[13] Although more current is needed for saltatory conduction, much less nerve membrane needs to be depolarized, less time is required, and, subsequently, conduction velocity dramatically increases. In myelinated axons, the density of Na^+ channels is highest in nodal areas, the areas undergoing depolarization. With the addition of myelin, large human peripheral nerve fibers typically conduct in the range of 35 to 75 m/sec, far faster than could be achieved by increasing the diameter of unmyelinated fibers alone. Myelinated fibers are used to transmit all motor information and most touch and discriminative sensory functions.

Not all human peripheral nerve fibers, however, are myelinated. Unmyelinated fibers, which conduct very slowly (<3 m/sec), convey primarily pain, temperature, and autonomic functions. Schwann's cells also support these unmyelinated fibers; however, one Schwann's cell typically surrounds several unmyelinated fibers but without the formation of concentric spirals of myelin.

When an individual axon is depolarized, an action potential propagates down the nerve. Distally, the axon divides into many twigs, with each twig going to a neuromuscular junction and then to an individual muscle fiber. An axon, along with its anterior horn cell and all muscle fibers with which it is connected, is known as a motor unit. When an

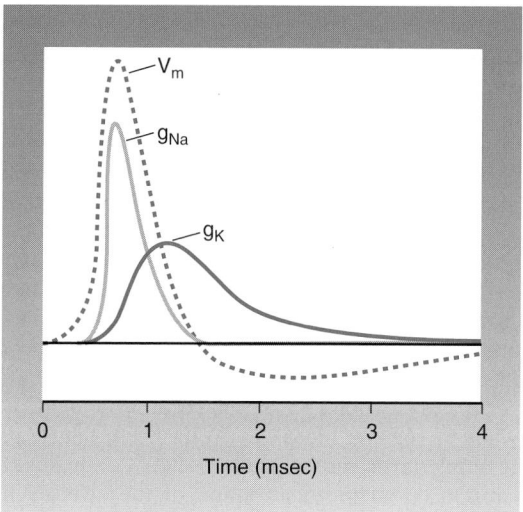

Fig. 5. Action potential. When the resting membrane voltage (V_m) is depolarized to threshold, voltage-dependent sodium ion (Na^+) channels are opened, increasing Na^+ conductance (g_{Na}) and resulting in an influx of Na^+ and further depolarization. The action potential, however, is short lived because of the inactivation of the Na^+ channels within 1 to 2 msec and an increase in potassium ion (K^+) conductance (g_k). These changes, along with the Na^+/K^+ pump, allow the axon to reestablish the resting membrane potential. (Redrawn from Preston DC, Shapiro BE: Electromyography and Neuromuscular Disorders. Boston, Butterworth-Heinemann, 1998.)

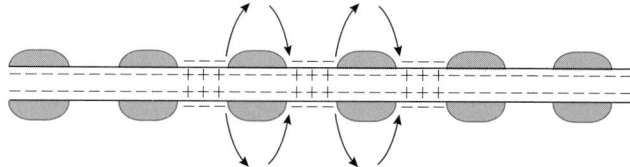

Fig. 6. Saltatory conduction. Myelinated fibers propagate action potentials by way of saltatory conduction. Depolarization only occurs at the small uninsulated areas of membrane between nodes, with the action potential jumping from node to node. Thus, less membrane needs to be depolarized, less time is required, and, consequently, conduction velocity dramatically increases. (Redrawn from Preston DC, Shapiro BE: Electromyography and Neuromuscular Disorders. Boston, Butterworth-Heinemann, 1998.)

Fiber Type	Name	Subtype	Diameter	Conduction Velocity	Alternative Classification
TABLE 1. PERIPHERAL NERVE CLASSIFICATION SCHEMES					
Myelinated Somatic Afferent/Efferent					
Cutaneous afferent	A	β	6–12 μm	35–75 m/s	α
		δ	1–5 μm	5–30 m/s	
Muscle afferent	A	α	12–21 μm	80–120 m/	I Ia, Ib
		β	6–12 μm	s	II
		δ	1–5 μm	35–75 m/s	III
				5–30 m/s	
Muscle efferent Anterior horn cells (α and γ motor neurons)	A		6–12 μm	35–75 m/s	
Myelinated Autonomic Efferent					
Preganglionic efferent	B		3 μm	3–15 m/s	
Unmyelinated Somatic/Autonomic Afferent/Efferent					
Postganglionic efferent Afferent to dorsal root ganglion (pain)	C		0.2–1.5 μm	1–2 m/s	IV
Sensory Receptor					
Hair follicle	Aβ				
Skin follicle	Aβ				
Muscle spindle	Aα				
Joint receptor	Aβ				
Pain, temperature	Aδ, C				

action potential is generated, all muscle fibers in the motor unit are subsequently activated, again an all-or-none response.

Peripheral nerve fibers can be classified in one of several ways (Table 1) based on whether they are (1) myelinated or unmyelinated, (2) somatic or autonomic, (3) motor or sensory, or (4) large or small diameter. On the basis of Table 1, there are several important points to appreciate. First is the direct relationship between fiber diameter and conduction velocity: the larger the diameter, the faster is the conduction velocity. Large-diameter fibers have the most myelin and the least electrical resistance, both of which result in faster conduction velocities. The small myelinated (Aδ, B) and unmyelinated (C) fibers carry autonomic information (afferent and efferent) and somatic pain and temperature sensations. Second, the largest and fastest cutaneous fibers are the Aβ fibers from hair and skin follicles. Note that the size and conduction velocities of these fibers are similar to those of muscle efferent fibers from the anterior horn cells. These myelinated fibers have velocities in the range of 35 to 75 m/sec. Third, the largest and fastest fibers are the muscle afferents, the Aα fibers (also known as Ia fibers), which originate from muscle spindles and mediate the afferent arc of the muscle stretch reflex.

CLINICAL RELEVANCE

Understanding the basics of peripheral nerve function and structure has direct clinical relevance and applications. From knowledge of gross peripheral nerve anatomy, most nerve entrapment syndromes, both at the root level and in the limbs, can be recognized by their unique patterns of sensory and motor dysfunction. For instance, entrapment of the S1 nerve root results in a pattern of sensory disturbance in the S1 dermatome (i.e., posterior lateral thigh and leg, sole of the foot) and weakness in the S1 myotome (e.g., gluteus maximus, lateral hamstrings, gastrocsoleus). However, clinical symptoms and signs differ between entrapments at the root level (i.e., radiculopathy) and those in the periphery. This is due primarily to the wide overlap of adjacent myotomes and dermatomes. Because of this arrangement, a single muscle is usually innervated by two or three myotomes. Similarly, each area of skin receives innervation not only from a single dermatome but from the level above and below as well. Because of the high degree of overlap between spinal segments, a single nerve root lesion seldom results in significant sensory loss and never anesthesia. Similarly, on the motor side, a severe single nerve root lesion usually results in mild or moderate weakness and never paralysis. For instance, a severe lesion of the C5 motor root may cause weakness of the biceps; however, paralysis does not occur because of the C6 motor fibers innervating the biceps as well. Accordingly, patients with a single-level radiculopathy often complain of pain and paresthesias in the distribution of the affected dermatome. However, on clinical testing, most often vague or ill-defined hypoesthesia is present with little or no weakness because of the wide overlap of adjacent dermatomes.

Knowledge of the gross anatomy of the spinal cord and nerve roots is also essential in understanding the entrapment syndromes of the lower lumbosacral spine. Because the spinal cord terminates in the adult at the level of the L1 vertebral body, entrapment syndromes below that level can never result in spinal cord compression but solely compression of the lower lumbosacral nerve roots (i.e., cauda equina). The cauda equina syndrome is a pure lower motor neuron syndrome. No upper motor neuron signs (e.g., spasticity, hyperreflexia, Babinski's signs) occur. Cauda equina syndromes most frequently result from large central disk herniations or tumors or from hemorrhage after trauma. The fact that the spinal cord terminates at the L1 level also allows for the safe introduction of a spinal needle below that level to sample cerebrospinal fluid (i.e., lumbar puncture) or injection of certain drugs or agents (i.e., contrast material for a myelogram) without the risk of possible spinal cord injury.

Knowledge of the tensile strength of nerve has important clinical consequences in patients with trauma. Because the tensile strength of the nerve roots is far less than that of peripheral nerve, severe stretch injuries may more often result in root avulsion than direct peripheral nerve injury. Root avulsion carries a much graver prognosis and usually indicates that surgical exploration and repair of peripheral nerves are not indicated.

In clinical practice, traumatic injuries to a limb often result in neural injury as well as associated orthopaedic injury. Knowledge that intraneural topography is intricate and constantly alternating has direct implications for nerve repair. When the ends of a lacerated nerve are sutured together, it is highly unlikely that individual axons are properly aligned. In such a situation, nerve regrowth is often incomplete or aberrant. Indeed, when nerve injury does occur after axonal loss, axonal regrowth is limited by the normal physiology of the axon. The slower axonal transport (1 to 2 mm/day) system is the rate-limiting factor in normal regrowth of nerve. Thus, a patient with a traumatic brachial plexopathy with complete denervation whose nerve subsequently does regrow may require many months or years to recover.

Knowledge of the role of myelin has important clinical consequences. When myelin is disrupted in a nerve injury, conduction may cease with resulting numbness or weakness depending on whether the nerve fiber is sensory or motor, respectively. However, remyelination does not require axonal transport for recovery and can typically occur over a few weeks. Thus, two patients with severe radial neuropathies at the spinal groove, one resulting from demyelination, the other from axonal loss, may have very similar clinical pictures. However, the patient with demyelination may recovery over several weeks, whereas the patient with an axonal loss lesion may require 12 to 18 months, with the recovery dependent on the rate of slow axonal transport. Of note, nerve conduction and electromyographic studies, the commonly performed electrical tests of peripheral nerve, can usually differentiate between axonal loss and demyelinative lesions.

Knowledge that different modalities are conveyed with different diameter nerve fibers has important clinical relevance. Certain diseases preferentially affect either large- or small-diameter fibers. For instance, diabetes, alcohol, and amyloidosis preferentially affect small-diameter nerve fibers. Because small-diameter nerve fibers mediate pain, temperature, and autonomic sensations, these patients will complain of burning pain and will be found to have decreased pain, temperature, and autonomic function on physical examinations. This is in contrast to peripheral neuropathies, which affect large fibers, such as vitamin B_{12} deficiency, in which patients complain of pins-and-needles paresthesias and are found to have decreased touch and vibration senses on clinical testing.

REFERENCES

1. Gardner E, Gray DJ, O'Rahilly R: Anatomy. Philadelphia, WB Saunders, 1975, 4th ed.
2. Aids to the Examination of the Peripheral Nervous System. London, Baillière Tindall, 1986.
3. Thomas PK, Olsson Y: Microscopic anatomy and function of the connective tissue components of peripheral nerve. In Dyck PJ, Thomas PK (eds): Peripheral Neuropathy. Philadelphia, WB Saunders, 1993, p 97.
4. Preston DC, Shapiro BE: Electromyography and Neuromuscular Disorders. Boston, Butterworth-Heinemann, 1998.
5. Sunderland S, Bradley KC: Stress-strain phenomena in human spinal nerve roots. Brain 1961; 84:120.
6. Sunderland S, Bradley KC: Stress-strain phenomena in human peripheral nerve trunks. Brain 1961; 84:125.
7. Sunderland S: The intraneural topography of radial, median and ulnar nerves. Brain 1945; 68:243.
8. Sunderland S: Nerves and Nerve Injuries. Edinburgh, Churchill Livingstone, 1978, 2nd ed, p 27.
9. Thomas PK: Microscopic anatomy of peripheral nerve fibers. In Dyck PJ, Thomas PK (eds): Peripheral Neuropathy. Philadelphia, WB Saunders, 1993, p 39.
10. Ochs S, Worth RM: Axoplasmic transport in normal and pathologic systems. In Waxman SG (ed): Physiology and Pathobiology of Axons. New York, Raven Press, 1978.
11. Hodgkin AL, Huxley AF: A quantitative description of membrane current and its application to conduction and excitation in nerve. J Physiol (Lond) 1952; 117:500.
12. Koester J: Voltage-gated ion channels and the generation of the action potential. In Kandel ER, Schwartz JH, Jessell TM, (eds): Principles of Neural Science. Norwalk, CT, Appleton & Lange, 1991, 3rd ed, p 104.
13. Huxley AF, Stampfli R: Evidence for saltatory conduction in peripheral myelinated nerve fibers. J Physiol 1972; 227:323.

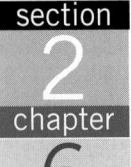

section
2
chapter
6

BONE GRAFTS AND BONE SUBSTITUTES

N. Schachar, C. Fennel, T. Otsuka, and A. Ladd

Summary

- Indications for a bone graft or bone graft substitute are
    To fill a cavity or defect caused by a cyst, a tumor, or trauma.
    To bridge a major defect and reestablish the continuity of a bone.
    To promote union of a fracture, a fracture non-union, or an osteotomy.
    To augment a joint fusion.
    To provide a bone block to limit joint motion.
- Even when using allograft or xenograft, immuno-suppression is not a prerequisite for bone grafting success.
- Fresh autologous bone is the best bone graft material.
- The major problems with autologous bone are limited supply and difficulties encountered at the donor site.
- Vascularized bone grafts heal more rapidly than free bone grafts.
- Bone in continuity with adjacent cartilage (osteo-chondral graft) may be used to replace a damaged or diseased joint surface.
- Bone graft substitute materials contain collagen, bone morphogenic protein (BMP), ceramic, calcium salts, or a polymer or a combination of these.
- Bone graft substitute materials may have both osteoconductive and osteoinductive properties.
- Addition of fresh autologous bone marrow increases the osteoinductivity of all bone graft material and all bone graft substitute materials.

BONE GRAFTS

Bone grafts or substitutes are transplanted frequently for the following reasons:

1. To fill cavities or defects resulting from cysts, tumors, or other bone voids or defects.
2. To bridge major defects or reestablish the continuity of a long bone.
3. To promote union or to fill defects in fresh fractures, malunions, delayed unions, or osteotomies.
4. To bridge joints and thereby provide arthrodesis to eliminate joint motion.
5. To provide bone blocks, which limit joint motion.
6. To establish union in a pseudarthrosis.

Bone grafts have been used for decades, and the incidence of bone transplantation is increasing in current practice (Fig. 1). The principles, indications, and techniques of bone grafting procedures, which were well established before "the metallurgic age" of orthopaedic surgery, are currently evolving and changing.[1] Different from transplantation of other organs and tissues, bone transplantation does not seem to require the maintenance of viability as an indispensable condition to achieve its purpose. When the bone cells, osteocytes, are excluded from the circulation of the graft, they die unless they come in contact with a reestablished blood supply on the surface of the transplant bed. The bone graft or transplant is expected to be incorporated into the graft site after transplantation. Therefore, a transplant substance that does not obstruct or indeed stimulates this incorporation is, in theory, an excellent material.

PROPERTIES OF AN OPTIMAL BONE GRAFT OR BONE SUBSTITUTE

The ideal properties of an optimal graft or substitute material include some or all of the following (Table 1):

1. Is a void filler.
2. Is biocompatible.
3. Is osteoconductive.
4. Is osteoinductive.
5. Provides structural stability.
6. Permits revascularization and new bone formation.

HISTORY OF BONE TRANSPLANTATION
Autologous Bone Grafts

Autologous bone grafts have had years of experience and remain the gold standard in bone transplantation. They were originally used as bone pegs or crude bone plates fixated with wire loops. The originators of internal fixation added osteogenesis to these principles to develop bone grafting for nonunion into a common and practical procedure.

Autologous cancellous bone grafts possess all of the elements of a *gold standard*. That is, they contain (1) hydroxyapatite and collagen, which are well suited to serve as an osteoconductive framework; (2) numerous stromal cells within the tissue, which have osteogenic potential; and (3) cancellous bone and adjacent hematoma, which contain a family of growth factors, most notably BMP and transforming growth factor-β, which induce and augment the regenerative process.[2] Autologous cortical bone is inferior to autologous cancellous bone regarding bioactivity, but it is mechanically strong and can withstand loading. The intact cortex does not stimulate transplantation immunity. The inert cortical transplant is also regarded as a potential source of infection because of foreign body reaction at the graft site.

The disadvantage of an autologous bone graft is its requirement for an operative incision at a healthy donor site with added morbidity, risk of infection, mechanical instability, and fracture (see Younger and Chapman[3]). The added operative time, increased hemorrhage, and potential

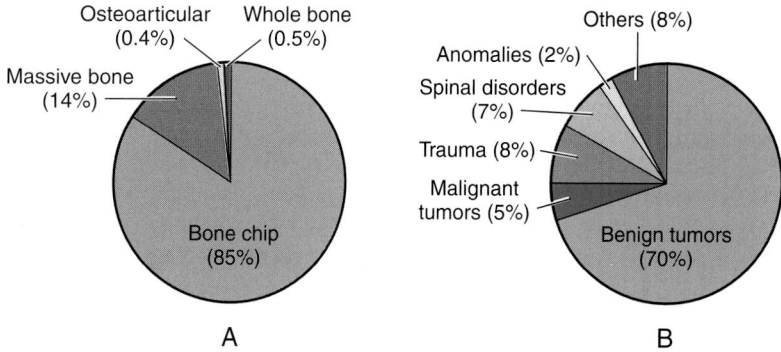

Fig. 1. Bone graft prevalence rate. Bone grafts have been used for decades; the prevalence rate of use has been increasing in current practice. *A,* Frequency of use of various types of bone graft. *B,* Diagnosis for which bone graft was part of the treatment. (Redrawn from Iwamoto Y, Sugioka Y, Chuman H, et al: Nationwide survey of bone grafting performed from 1980 through 1989 in Japan. Clin Orthop 1997; 335:292.)

for persistent pain at the donor site are additional risks. Often the limited availability of donor bone at a single site, dependent on age and sex, is a factor. The donor bone is often not the same type and strength desired for the recipient site. Potential donor sites have historically included the iliac crest, the tibia, the fibula, and the rib.

Patzakis et al[4] advocated the use of vascularized autologous corticocancellous bone grafts to treat infection, particularly infected tibial nonunions. The Ilizarov technique of advancing intercalary bone transplant is a unique type of autologous bone transposition or transplantation. With this technique, a cortical osteotomy is made through healthy bone at a site distant from the defect and the intercalary fragment, between the defect and the corticotomy, and is pulled through the limb with wires until the defect is closed. New autologous bone forms in the widening distraction gap.[5]

Allograft Bone Grafts

Allograft can be chosen of suitable size and shape for the desired purpose or defect to be filled, an advantage over autograft bone.[6] Antigenicity of the donor bone remains theoretically problematic. There is a reported 4% to 5% infection rate as well as a significant fracture rate.[7] Berrey et al[8] described frequent allograft fracture in the case of osteoarticular allografts but argued that this rate does not differ greatly from the incidence for autologous grafts or custom-made metallic implants. When a fracture occurs, continuity and useful function can be restored.[8] Describing the problem of immune reaction, Stevenson and Horowitz[9]

showed that bone grafts and parenchymal organs bear class I and class II antigens. Cell-mediated and antibody-mediated cytotoxicity specific for donor antigens develops after transplantation of bone and parenchymal organs. The mechanism of rejection of bone allografts is less clear. Nonvascularized bone grafts do not contain an intact vascular structure, nor do they often contain living cells, which are the usual targets of rejection. The incorporation of a nonvascularized bone graft depends not only on the biological properties of the graft and the responsiveness of the host bed but also on the stability of fixation and the mechanical loading of the graft.[9]

Allografts can be "banked" or preserved by various preservation and processing methods. Absolute asepsis must be maintained to prevent degeneration and preserve bone formation ability. The type of structural allograft with the best clinical record is the massive segmental intercalary allograft when applied to wide bone loss such as that associated with tumor or, less commonly, trauma.

PRESERVATION METHODS FOR ALLOGRAFTS

The usual methods of preservation of banked bone allografts are fresh frozen bone, freeze-dried bone, and demineralized bone allografts.

Fresh Frozen Bone

The usual method of deep-freezing fresh bone is passively in a −30°C to −80°C freezer in a sterile container. This method is the simplest and most frequently used. Freeze-

Graft	Immunogenicity	Mechanical Properties	Inductiveness	Graft Derived
Autologous cancellous	—	—	+++	+++
Autologous cortical	—	+++	+++	++
Allogeneic fresh cortical	+++	+++	+	—
Allogeneic frozen cortical	++	+++	++	—
Allogeneic freeze-dried cortical	+	++	++	—
Allogeneic irradiated cortical	+	++	++	—
AAA	—	—	++	—
Xenogeneic cortical	++++	+++	—	—

TABLE 1. COMPARATIVE PROPERTIES OF MAMMALIAN BONE GRAFTS

From Goldberg VM, Stevenson S: Bone transplantation. In Evarts CM (ed): Surgery of the Musculoskeletal System. New York, Churchill Livingstone, 1990, p 121.

drying bone, by vacuum desiccation using liquid nitrogen, uses ethylene oxide gas sterilization and allows preservation of the bone at room temperature.

Demineralization of bone represents the other extreme of processing, which attempts to completely remove the mineral phase of bone by the use of hydrochloric acid and ethylenediaminetetraacetic acid. The resultant substrate, which retains bone-forming ability, is retained for transplantation. This process greatly decreases the material strength properties. The enhanced osteoinductive capability is afforded by the BMP. This processing method is said to decrease antigenicity. The clinical results with this method show decreased osteoinductive capacity compared with autograft. This material is frequently used, because there is not an adequate supply of fresh autologous bone graft with its decreased transplant immunity for use. Freezing is known to decrease the immunogenicity of fresh allogeneic bone but not as much as freeze-drying.

Xenograft

Historical experience includes the use of xenograft bone graft. Xenograft stimulates strong antigenicity and processing by which the substrate protein is excluded. If used, the recipient recognizes the xenograft as a foreign body, and incomplete removal of the protein incites a rejection reaction. If the protein has been completely removed, the xenograft can become completely incorporated as inorganic bone. Xenograft is inferior in respect to its organizational adaptability and bone formation ability. Kiel bone, or processed bovine bone, has been compared favorably with frozen allograft.[10] Xenograft bone potentially represents an unlimited supply of available material if it can be rendered safe for transplantation to the human host.[10]

Pyrost bone substitute has been shown to be a promising orthopaedic material.[11] This material not only supports osteoblast attachment but also allows proliferation of osteoblasts.[11] One report cited the successful use of bovine bone graft for occipitocervical fusion for atlantoaxial instability in patients with rheumatoid arthritis.[12]

Composite Grafting

The mixing of autograft with allograft or xenograft is reported to be effective in recruiting the mutual properties of each different type of graft to the benefit of the patient. However, the evidence to support this technique is anecdotal at best.

CLASSIFICATION BY BONE STRUCTURE
Cortical Bone Graft

Cortical bone grafting (Table 2) is infrequently used for osteoinduction or osteoconduction but is often used for augmenting bone biomechanical strength and stability. Cortical onlay strut grafts can be used for augmenting deficient bone in revision total joint surgery. The speed of revascularization is remarkably slow, although the form of incorporation is the same as for cancellous bone. This feature, however, provides the advantage of durability and bone duration, which provides strong and stable reinforcement to deficient autologous cortical bone. Vascular penetration of the graft is primarily the result of peripheral osteoclastic resorption and vascular invasion of Volkmann's and haversian canals. Thus, transplanted bone weakens considerably compared with normal bone. The rate of weakening depends on the rate of revascularization, the size of the transplant, and other environmental factors. This resorption can vary from a period of months to years. If the rates of revascularization and of creeping substitution of new bone into the graft are synchronous, then the mechanical strength of the cortical graft will be restored or maintained. The strength and stability of cortical bone far exceed those of cancellous bone. The transplanted cortical bone is restructured by mechanical stimulation modified by such factors if it is in an orthotopic site. The graft is not completely absorbed or replaced but remains embedded in the cortical bone with a "ghost" of necrotic bone of the graft surrounded by new appositional host bone.

Cancellous Bone Graft

When new bone formation is desired, cancellous bone graft alone is used (see Table 2). Cancellous bone fragments or morcellized cancellous bone alone can be used to fill any bone defect or cavity. Spongy or cancellous bone is usually revascularized rapidly and completely replaced. After implantation, the resulting hemorrhage and inflammation lead to rapid resorption. The surviving osteoblasts on the surface of the transplant survive and make new bone at an early stage, although many die. Host osteoblasts and blood vessels invade the fragments of cancellous bone aided by osteoclasts. During this early phase of inflammation and revascularization, osteoinduction occurs rapidly and new bone formation occurs, usually in dynamic equilibrium. New bone formation occurs on the fragments of cancellous graft material, evidence of osteoconduction, which occurs for several months after transplantation of the cancellous graft material. The final phase of cancellous graft incorpo-

TABLE 2. ATTRIBUTES OF GRAFT TYPES						
Type	Cells	Collagen	Mineral	Growth Factors	Blood Supply	Structure
Cancellous auto-graft	√	√	√	√	—	—
Cancellous allo-graft	—	√	√	?	—	—
Pedicle graft	√	√	√	√	√	√
Osteochondral graft	√	√	√	√	—	√

ration is the integration of the graft into a streamlined mechanical supporting structure, whereby the graft is completely resorbed and replaced by viable host bone. This process is similar to the pathophysiology described for the phased response seen in avascular necrosis of the femoral head.[13]

Bone and Cartilage Graft

Osteochondral or osteoarticular grafts (see Table 2) are frequently used to replace bone and joint tissue for bone and soft-tissue tumors. Osteochondral transplants are also used to resurface joints destroyed by osteoarthritis, fractures, or osteochondritis dissecans. Autologous osteochondral and cartilage grafts are typically not practical. Both fresh and preserved osteochondral allografts are generally used in the form of osteochondral plugs, dowels, wafers, or massive hemiarticular grafts, replacing the bone and cartilage on one or both sides of the joint.

The articular cartilage, successfully transplanted, is nourished by synovial diffusion. The persistence of the cartilage matrix, particularly the proteoglycans and collagen matrix, depends on the viability of the cartilage chondrocytes. The viability of the osteocytes in the supporting bone is not considered essential. It is not clear whether the donor chondrocytes are replaced by the host cartilage cells or whether persistence or replication of the donor chondrocytes sustains articular cartilage function of the grafts. Failure of the osteoarticular allografts has been attributed to the degeneration of the allograft's articular cartilage and fracture of the underlying allograft bone.[14] Tomford et al[15] explained that both fresh and frozen cartilage allografts function well to relieve joint pain resulting from cartilage injury. Fresh cartilage appears to remain viable for many months and be most applicable to small injuries, such as osteochondritis dissecans, traumatic defects, and osteonecrosis. Frozen cartilage allografts appear to survive in massive hemi- or whole joint replacements used for limb salvage surgery after tumor resection and to maintain the joint space for several years.[15]

Vascularized Autograft

The first successfully vascularized bone transplant was performed by Taylor and colleagues in 1975 using vascularized fibula to treat an open fracture of the femur.[16] It is theorized that more than 90% osteocytic survival is achieved with this transplantation procedure. Graft-host union occurs quickly, and resorption is rapidly followed by osteoconduction and remodeling. A fresh vascularized cortical autograft contains active graft-derived bone-inductive factors. The fibula is the most commonly used vascularized autograft.[17] Vascularized grafts can also be obtained from the iliac crest, scapula, and rib. In some cases, growth of transplanted bone with accompanying growth plate can be expected.[18] This technique can be extremely useful for rebuilding bone after injury or for limb salvage surgery after excision of malignant tumors.

TECHNIQUES FOR GATHERING AUTOGRAFT BONE

In general, autograft bone is harvested from the iliac crest, tibia, fibula, or rib. Large amounts of suitable graft material for many purposes can be gathered from the iliac crest. Few functional problems arise as a result of bone harvesting. Cancellous bone is obtained from the medullar cavity of the iliac wing in its anterior or posterior portion. Muscle damage is usually minimal and hemorrhage is minimal when the subperiosteal approach is used. If necessary, full-thickness corticocancellous grafts can be obtained. A variety of techniques can be used to obtain cancellous strips or cancellous chips or morsels. Blood loss can be controlled, and bone wax or other hemostatic agents are easy to use in this location. When gathering large volumes of bone, it may be necessary to use a drain. When obtaining bone from an infant, it is important to leave the epiphyseal plate intact. In most cases, complications are few. In rare cases, an artificial "bridge" is used to reconstruct the line of the crest. A visible deformity and postoperative pain at the donor site have resulted in rare cases. A serious complication is damage to the lateral femoral cutaneous nerve of the thigh at the anterior iliac crest, causing neuralgia, paresthesia, anterolateral thigh numbness, or pain. This is referred to as meralgia paresthetica. It is important to pay attention to the deep circumflex iliac artery in the iliac muscle.

Cortical grafts are often used for support and fixation rather than for stimulating bone formation and can be taken from the tibial crest. The fibular strut graft is also frequently used for structural support and for stability. It is usually obtained from the middle one-third shaft by cylindrical subperiosteal dissection. After harvesting the graft, the periosteum may be resutured with the expected outcome of reformation of the fibula. Attention to the anatomy prevents damage to the peroneal nerve and the lateral compartment musculature. Harvesting of the distal fibula in the vicinity of the distal tibiofibular joint is avoided to prevent valgus deformity and ankle mortise instability, especially in the younger patient.

Rib grafts can be used in spinal fixation or in scoliosis operations involving the thoracic spine. Small amounts of corticocancellous or cancellous bone can be obtained from the greater trochanter, the proximal ulna, and the distal radius.

Bone harvested from the excised femoral head is often used as autograft transplant material around the acetabular prosthesis or the femoral stem in hip surgery. Autograft is used when a femoral head is in situ and available and as allograft when it is not or when there is insufficient material available as autograft.

OPERATIVE CLASSIFICATION OF BONE TRANSPLANTS
Onlay Bone Graft Method

Onlay bone graft may be applied to pseudarthrosis to obtain joint fusions. It can also be used for nonunions of the shaft of any long bone. The graft bed is usually flat and smooth to allow widest contact with the transplanted bone. A full-thickness massive cortical graft from the tibia, long enough and wide enough for firm fixation, may be used to provide an onlay graft. This technique is rarely used in current practice.

The endosteal bone is used for cancellous bone graft and as an adjunctive bone graft around the cortical bone plate, which is secured with screw fixation. Occasionally, dual-onlay bone grafts are applied on opposing cortices. Onlay bone graft may occasionally be used without internal fixation.

Inlay Bone Graft Method

This seldom-used technique combines the osteoinductive/osteoconductive components of bone transplantation with the biomechanical aspects of corticocancellous bone graft transplants by advancing or sliding a plate of full-thickness cortical bone to the marrow aspect, usually from a metaphyseal or diaphyseal location across a joint interval or fracture defect. The transplant is carefully advanced into a prepared trough of the exact size and secured in place with internal fixation. Most commonly used for joint fusion or pseudarthrosis, the donor site may be autologous bone from a local adjacent site or the iliac crest and infrequently the tibial cortex (e.g., Russe operation for scaphoid, Phemister operation).

Intramedullary Graft Method

This method consists of the insertion of cortical, corticocancellous, or cancellous bone graft material into the prepared open ends of the medullary canal at the fractured ends of the bone during reduction. It is usually accompanied by internal fixation.

The Morcellized Cancellous Bone Graft Technique

This is perhaps the most common method applied to transplantation and uses prepared morcellized cancellous bone fragments of a desired size and texture, depending on availability, which is packed closely applied to the prepared graft bed. This technique gives the best osteoconduction and osteoinduction. It does permit structural stability, for which secondary reinforcement or fixation is necessary. This is the most commonly used technique in joint fusion, spinal fixation, or whenever additional osteoinduction and osteoconduction are required to stimulate bone formation. It is also the perferred method for filling defects for benign bone tumors.

Intercalary Graft Method

Intercalary grafts may be used in a middiaphyseal location to replace missing or removed segmental bone often resulting from trauma or secondary to tumor excision. In some cases, this method is used to fill a defect remaining during a leg-lengthening procedure.

Cortical or Cancellous Dowel Method

Cortical dowels or osteochondral dowels of autologous or allogeneic bone are used to replace defects left at the site of an osteochondral fracture, to repair defects such as osteochondritis dissecans, or to reconstruct fractures of the scaphoid bone, much as an intramedullary bone graft is used at a fracture site in the diaphysis of a long bone.

Strut Graft Method

The application of a biomechanically strong, primarily cortical plate of bone, usually with additional fixation aimed at maintaining, reinforcing, or augmenting strength of a construct, is referred to as strut grafting. Strut graft transplants can be fabricated from entire segments of diaphyseal bone, plates of cortical bone, tibial autograft, or allograft bone. These struts can also be fashioned from rib, fibula, or iliac crest. Many applications for strut grafting exist, including reinforcement of revision prostheses and metaphyseal bone adjacent to bone tumors, spinal fixation or fusion, and reinforcement of collapsed femoral heads in the face of avascular necrosis and fibrous dysplasia.

Massive Bone Graft

Massive osteoarticular allograft transplantation is now widely used for reconstruction of joints in which wide excision for tumor or massive bone loss secondary to failed total joint replacement exists. An entire vascularized fibula is used in this setting by some surgeons either instead of the allograft or in place of it. The rate of incorporation may be problematic if it is too rapid, leading to allograft fracture, or may be appropriate if slow, leading to maintained mechanical strength of the transplant.

Some clinicians augment the allograft with autologous cancellous bone. Muscolo et al[19] reported that such massive femoral allografts can function for as long as 36 years. Mankin et al reported a fracture rate of 19%, a nonunion rate of 14%, and an infection rate of 10%. At this time, approximately 17% of osteoarticular allografts in their study have been revised to total joint arthroplasty/allograft composites.

Osteochondral Allograft

Osteochondral allograft wafers of fresh bone and cartilage have been used by Gross et al to resurface half or whole joint surfaces destroyed by primary or secondary osteoarthritis. In this application, consideration has to be given to the alignment and preparation of the joint for transplantation to protect the cartilage on the osteochondral graft. The issue of fixation and the prognosis of these osteochondral allografts remain the subject of debate.[20]

BONE BANKING

Bone banks are indispensable for the provision of allograft bone, often a popular substitute for, or even in preference to, autograft bone. Stringent guidelines exist for safe and reliable bone banking, including standard criteria for acceptable donors, proven techniques for retrieval of tissues, and appropriate storage facilities and conditions. The allograft bone stored must be aseptic and preserved in such a manner as to preserve the bone quality and osteoinductive capacity as much as possible. Banking is also known to decrease the immunogenicity of fresh allograft bone, as do all other treatments.[21]

It is important to be able to obtain allograft bone grafts of the size and shape required for the various applications indicated. Donor selection criteria are essential and are well defined by agencies involved in setting and maintaining standards for tissue banking. Careful screening of donors diminishes the potential for infections, communicable diseases, malignancies, or metabolic bone disease that could endanger the recipient or adversely affect the quality of the transplanted bone tissue.

Bone-banking techniques range widely, from fresh-frozen storage of sterile-procured donor bone to processed bone, including freeze-drying and other methods of preservation, which, although used to sterilize and process bone for storage, are known to affect the osteoinductive capacity of the bone as well as its biochemical properties.

Bone Marrow

Bone marrow is a readily available source of osteoinductive capacity. The osteoinductive capacity of red marrow has been appreciated for some 35 years. Because of the difficulty in obtaining large amounts of marrow, its limited osteoconductive capacity, and lack of biomechanical strength, it is not often used as an adjuvant technique, although the recent emergence of bone substitutes has renewed interest in the use of bone marrow. Marrow can be combined with autograft, allograft, xenograft, and substitutes to increase osteoinductive capacity.[22, 23] Marrow provides mesenchymal stem cells (MSCs), which, depending on the application and environment, can differentiate into osteogenic, chondrogenic, or other cell lines. This differentiation depends on the site of implantation, cell density, and the specific molecular cues received by the implanted marrow. Local bone defects can be repaired through site-directed delivery of MSCs in an appropriate carrier vehicle.[24] In addition, the combination of bone marrow with demineralized bone matrix produces a synergistic response in the defect that is greater than that achieved with either marrow or demineralized bone matrix alone.[25]

Autoclaved Bone

Autoclaving autologous bone from the site of a tumor is another technique used by clinicians.[26, 27] After in bloc excision of a tumorous bone, the segment is autoclaved and reinserted after the tumor is eradicated. This was reported by Thompson in 1956 and is still used, particularly in countries where allografts are unpopular and other techniques of reconstruction are inaccessible.[28] The autoclaved bone is purportedly strong enough to support early weight-bearing or allow the insertion of a joint arthroplasty. Compression strength of such bone is said to be about the same as newborn bone, but it is decreased in strength by about 50% compared with normal bone, with a bending strength about 65% of normal.

Most transplantation antigens are thought to be depleted. When demineralized substrate is added, new bone formation is stimulated. The strength has been reported to be 84% of unprocessed bone.[28] Research is available on the osteoinductive capacity and strength of bone pasteurized by temperatures of 60°C to 70°C. Bone boiled for 10 minutes shows delayed replacement by new bone formation, but normal resorption and new bone formation do occur.

BONE GRAFT SUBSTITUTES

HISTORICAL REVIEW

The progression of orthopaedic operative intervention of acquired bony deformities over the last 40 years has resulted in a need for bone void–filling materials. Traditionally, this has been managed by use of autograft or allograft. There has been a continued desire to develop synthetic substitutes that could take the place of harvested bone.

The ideal bone graft substitute has void-filling capability and bone growth stimulation property and at the same time

	Compression Strength (kg/mm²)	Bend Strength (kg/mm²)	Elasticity
TABLE 3. MECHANICAL INTEGRITY OF VARIOUS BIOMATERIALS			
Material	**Compression Strength (kg/mm²)**	**Bend Strength (kg/mm²)**	**Elasticity**
Human cortex	16–18	10–20	1,800
Vitallium	66–76	66–76	20,000
Aluminum	500	50–130	40,000
Zirconium	800	100–150	21,000
Bioglass	<30	<7	3,500
Ceravital	50	10	6,500
Dense Ha	50–90	10–20	7,800
A-WGC	108	23	11,700
CaPO₄ cements (Norian SRS)	—	—	—

HA, hydroxyapatite; A-WGC, apatite-woolastonite glass ceramic; CaPO₄, calcium hydroxyapatite.

provides structural integrity. To date, the ideal material does not exist.

The earliest forms of synthetic bone substitutes were in non-calcium-based materials. Products such as methylmethacrylate and stainless steel have been used traditionally to bridge defects and apply structural stability to limbs. However, their inherent nonbiological nature has led to the evolution of synthetic substitutes that are designed to be biologically interactive with bone. The earliest of these products became available in 1992. (See Tables 3 and 4.)

FUNDAMENTAL SCIENCE
Bone Substitutes

The variety of products available are primarily calcium-based materials, the high-temperature ceramics using silicone as their keystone element (Table 5).

Nonstructural Substitutes

A variety of graft substitutes have been developed for circumstances that do not require structural stability. This group of materials is characterized by their malleability and their attempt to contain elements that cause osteoconduction or osteoinduction or a combination of both.

The first product of this nature, Collagraft (Zimmer, Warsaw, IN), is a mixture of hydroxyapatite, tricalcium phosphate, and bovine collagen. It was initially approved for the treatment of diaphyseal and metaphyseal defects, requiring the utilization of aspirated autologous bone marrow in an attempt to make the implanted material osteoinductive. Chapman et al[29] conducted a prospective, randomized study using this material in bone fractures that required grafting. Compared with autograft, the product provided healing radiographically on an equivalent basis. It did, however, produce antibodies to the bovine collagen. In 12% of the patients, nonspecific allergic problems were identified. This material did not provide any structural support and required the use of a procedure for harvesting bone marrow.[29] As with other bovine substitutes, concerns about immunogenicity theoretically exist.

Several manufacturers developed lyophilized demineralized human bone allografts in a gel matrix. The human bone is typically granulated and then gamma-ray radiated

TABLE 4. BIOCERAMIC FAMILY AND APPLICATIONS

Material	Artificial Bone	Artificial Prosthesis	Bone Packing Material	Osteosynthetic Material
Hydroxyapatite	√	√	√	√
TCP	√		√	
Bioglass	√			√
CPSA glass fiber compound material	√			√
Ceravital glass ceramic	√			√
A-W glass: ceramic	√	√	√	
TCP glass: ceramic	√	√		
Aluminum	√	√	√	√
Zirconium		√		
Titanium				
Carbon		√		
Composite ceramic	√	√	√	√

TCP, tricalcium phosphate; CPSA, calcium oxide–phosphorus pentoxide–silicon dioxide–aluminum oxide; A-W, apatite–woolastonite.

to prevent infection. The demineralization process results in the presence of structural proteins of the BMP category, which infers an osteoinductive capability but not structural stability. The most long-standing product of this type, Grafton DBM Gel (Osteotech, Eatontown, NJ), has been available since 1991. The manufacturer subsequently developed a semirigid, or putty, form of the material, which has been available since 1996. The Grafton DBM Gel is formulated with glycerol, which has potential neurotoxicity, but there have been no reports of toxicity with this product. GenSci Regeneration Sciences (Mississauga, Ontario) produces a product similar in nature (Dynagraft) with both a gel and putty version using demineralized allograft. This material is suspended in a propylene oxide polymer combined with ethylene oxide. This particular carrier has been used for more than 25 years without evidence of cytotoxicity. Osteoinductive capability of these products has been determined by their ability to form ectopic bone in mouse muscle tissue. These materials have the advantage of filling large bone voids and, in putty form, are capable of contouring to the shape of the bone. Biological capability is likely varied because no assays or standards exist.

Modifications in the science of the construction of the gels have been made by Sofamor Danek Group (Memphis, TN). By using a 17% porcine origin gelatin in aqueous solution (Osteofil), this group created a heat-sensitive material that flows through a syringe at 120°F and hardens to a rubber-like consistency at body temperature. The gelatin material is subsequently degraded by protease. Its bioavailability is measured using the Urist osteoinduction assay (analysis of ectopic bone formation in rat muscle). In an attempt to provide some structural integrity to the same product, Opteform (Exactech Inc., Gainesville, FL) has been developed using the same material as Osteofil but with the addition of compacted corticocancellous human bone chips. Again, the material is fluid when heated and, when cooled to body temperature, produces a rubber-like material. To date, no noncommercial published studies exist on any of these products in orthopaedic usage.

Ceramic Materials

The ceramics currently available can be distinguished as either high-temperature (manufactured) or low-temperature (biological) ceramics. The high-temperature (greater than 100°C) treatment of mineral salts can produce a very solid and stable material that is biologically inert. NovaBone (USBiomaterials, Alachua, FL) is a silicon-based ceramic designed for reconstructive procedures and bone defect–filling applications, but it has not yet received Food and Drug Administration (FDA) approval. The silica breaks down as the sodium is replaced by hydrogen to form $S_i(OH)_4$. Calcium and phosphate combine to form a surface layer that binds proteins. Osteogenic cells then infiltrate and form new bone. Coral has been introduced as an intriguing substitute for human cancellous bone because of the similarity in its ultrastructure to human metaphyseal bone. Investigation of this material has been ongoing for more than 25 years. Coral can act as a substitute in that it can be milled into a variety of shapes to serve as a structural graft. The treatment of the coral with ammonium sulfate transforms the coral tricalcium phosphate into hydroxyapatite. ProOsteon (Interpore Cross, Irvine, CA) is the

TABLE 5. BONE GRAFT PRODUCTS (AND TYPE) AND MANUFACTURERS

Product	Manufacturer
Calcium phosphate	
SRS/CRS	Synthes (Norian)
E-Tex	E-Tex
Calcium sulfate	
Osteoset	Wright Medical Technology
Osteoset-tobramycin	
Calcium sulfate with demineralized human bone	
Allomatrix	Wright Medical Technology
Demineralized human bone	
Grafton DBM	Osteotech
DynaGraft	GenSci Regeneration Sciences
Osteofil	Sofamor Danek
Coral	
ProOsteon	Interpore Cross
Bioactive glass	
NovaBone	USBiomaterials

principal manufacturer of this material. Chapman et al[29] showed that this material is capable of being used for structural defects in metaphyseal areas. Progressively over time, up to about 6 months, native bone is laid down along the porous network of the coral. The material itself is not absorbed by osteoclasts; therefore, the potential for true remodeling of this material is unknown.[29] Prospective studies by Wolfe[30] and Bucholz[31] and their colleagues showed comparable results with these materials versus autograft with substantial cost savings.

Calcium Sulfate

To date, only three manufacturers have used calcium sulfate as a graft substitute: Wright Medical Technology (Arlington, TX), Interpore Cross, and Synthes (Norian, Cupertino, CA). Calcium sulfate's most familiar name, plaster of Paris, has been used since the 19th century, but literature references in the 1950s permitted approval by the FDA to treat bone defects. Each manufacturer has different forms. It is currently available commercially as Osteoset (Wright Medical Technology) and comes in the form of small pill-shaped pellets. A version is available with tobramycin impregnated to assist in filling void defects in infected regions. Pellets are absorbed in 6 to 8 weeks and are designed to act as a gap filler to allow vascular ingrowth and facilitate healing of the bone. These pellets do not provide any structural support and, therefore, do not eliminate the need for either internal or external fixation should it be required.

Calcium Phosphate Cements

In an attempt to mimic the biological nature of human bone more closely, products have been created that have primarily calcium phosphate as their base. The first of these products to market was SRS (Norian). This material consists of tricalcium phosphate and calcium carbonate, which is mixed with a solution of calcium phosphate before use. Once mixed, the material has a working time of approximately 5 minutes. When injected into the bone at body temperature, it hardens and crystallizes, forming dahlite crystalline structure, which is very similar to normal human cancellous bone in its chemical composition. It is not structurally similar to human bone on the surface. Dahlite is 3% to 5% calcium carbonate, which is a significant percentage to permit instability and osteoclastic activity. The material, once fully crystallized by the first 24 hours, can provide structural compression strength equivalent to that of human metaphyseal bone but is weak in torsion and shear.[32] The manufacturer's unpublished prospective, randomized study examines 323 patients with distal radial fractures.[33] One hundred sixty-one patients underwent treatment with the SRS cement. The treated patients regained function earlier compared with controls. The advantages of function were diminished by 3 months, and by the end of the first year there were no functional differences between the control group and the SRS group. Because of its biologically similar nature to bone, this material is remodeled by osteoclast activity. The degree of remodeling depends on the mass of material and its location. Peripheral regions will remodel preferentially to central regions because there are higher levels of stress and more inherent remodeling in those locations. Bone Source

(Howmedica Leibienger, Dallas, TX) and Alpha BSM (E-Tex, Cambridge, MA) are additional calcium phosphate–based materials. They are both liquids that crystallize on introduction into the bone, forming a hard material. E-Tex material is distinguishable from Norian's SRS by its rapid absorbability. All of these products theoretically are able to conform specifically to the shape of the bone void defect and distinguish themselves from the demineralized bone matrix materials by also providing some structural support in compression.

CONCLUSION

The management of a wide variety of orthopaedic problems requires the use of material to either fill a void or provide a structural support to promote adequate healing. The standard by which all of the materials are judged is human autologous bone. Because autologous grafting may be limited, physicians have sought other void-filling materials to substitute for human autograft. Traditionally, this has been in allograft and occasionally in xenograft. However, a variety of products have been developed that may permit wide-scale production and use of synthetic void-filling and structural materials. Harvesting of human autografts is not without inherent costs and morbidity. Synthetic materials, therefore, are a very attractive alternative to autograft and allograft should they stand the tests of rigid clinical scrutiny. The variety of materials available can be loosely grouped into those that are injectable and those that are rigid. In general terms, the injectable forms, with the exception of some of the newer calcium phosphate materials, do not provide structural integrity to the graft site.

To date no prospective analysis has compared the efficacy of a variety of these materials. From what few published data are available, it is apparent that most of these materials, when properly used, are successful alternatives to bone graft. The demineralized matrix forms such as Grafton DBM or DynaGraft can be used to fill bone voids and, in theory, by the presence of their bone proteins can heal a bone defect by osteoinduction. The calcium phosphates and the ceramic materials such as ProOsteon can provide some structural compressive strength in addition to space-filling capability.

When materials that provide structural strength are used, one must carefully analyze the environment in which they are being used. If the bone in question is subject to torsional or shear forces, then typically some other form of more traditional internal or external fixation will be required while the bone is healing. If the forces on the bone are shown to be purely compressive, it may be possible to diminish or eliminate other forms of fixation while the bone is healing. However, in materials that are only providing space-filling capability, more traditional forms of internal or external fixation must be used while the bone is healing.

An experimental variety of synthetic substitutes are becoming available for clinical use as bone graft substitutes. These materials have been evaluated for up to 25 years, and enough evidence has collected to suggest that they will remain in our armamentarium of alternatives. It is yet to be seen whether they will ultimately prove to be effective enough to eliminate the need for autografting procedures.

REFERENCES

1. Iwamoto Y, Sugioka Y, Chuman H, et al: Nationwide survey of bone grafting performed from 1980 through 1989 in Japan. Clin Orthop 1997; 335:292.
2. Lane JM, Bostrom MPG: Bone grafting and new composite biosynthetic graft materials. AAOS Instruct Course Lect 1998; 47:525.
3. Younger EM, Chapman MW: Morbidity at bone graft donor sites. J Orthop Trauma 1989; 3:192.
4. Patzakis MJ, Scilaris TA, Chon J, et al: Results of bone grafting for infected tibial nonunion. Clin Orthop 1995; 315:192.
5. Green SA: Skeletal defects. Clin Orthop 1994; 301:111.
6. Zatsepin ST, Burdygin VN: Replacement of the distal femur and proximal tibia with frozen allografts. Clin Orthop 1994; 303: 95.
7. Tomford WW, Thongphasuk J, Mankin HJ, et al: Frozen musculoskeletal allografts. J Bone Joint Surg Am 1990; 72: 1137.
8. Berrey H, Lord CF, Gebhardt MC, et al: Fractures of allografts. J Bone Joint Surg Am 1990; 72:825.
9. Stevenson S, Horowitz M: The response to bone allografts. J Bone Joint Surg Am 1992; 74:939.
10. Block JE, Poser J: Does xenogenic demineralized bone matrix have clinical unity as a bone graft substitute? Med Hypoth 1995; 45:27.
11. Tsuang Y-H, Lin F-H, Sun J-S, et al: In vitro cell behaviour of osteoblast on pyrost bone substitute. Anat Rec 1997; 247:164.
12. Säveland H, Aspenberg P, Zygmunt S, et al: Bovine bone grafting in occipito-cervical fusion for atlanto-axial instability in rheumatoid arthritis. Acta Neurochir (Wien) 1994; 127:186.
13. Rosenwasser MP, Garino JP, Kiernan HA, et al: Long term followup of thorough debridement and cancellous bone grafting of the femoral head for avascular necrosis. Clin Orthop 1994; 306:17.
14. Flynn JM, Springfield DS, Mankin HJ: Osteoarticular allografts to treat distal femoral osteonecrosis. Clin Orthop 1994; 303: 38.
15. Tomford WW, Springfield DS, Mankin HJ: Fresh and frozen articular cartilage allografts. Cartilage Allografts 1992; 15: 1183.
16. Taylor GE, Miller GDH, Ham FJ: The free vascularized bone graft. Plast Reconst Surg 1975; 55:533.
17. Goldberg VM, Stevenson S: Bone transplantation. In Evarts CM (ed): Surgery of the Musculoskeletal System. New York, Churchill Livingstone, 1990, p 115.
18. Ostrup LT, Fredrickson JM: Distant transfer of a free, living bone graft by microvascular anastomoses. Plast Reconst Surg 1974; 54:274.
19. Muscolo DL, Petracchi LJ, Ayerza MA, et al: Massive femoral allografts followed for 22 to 36 years. J Bone Joint Surg Br 1992; 74:887.
20. Kandel RA, Gross AF, Ganel A, et al: Histopathology of failed osteoarticular shell allografts. Clin Orthop 1985; 197: 103.
21. Friedlaender GE, Strong DM, Tomford WW, et al: Autograft/allograft: Long-term follow-up of patients with osteochondral allografts: A correlation between immunologic responses and clinical outcome. Orthop Clin North Am 1999; 30:583.
22. Burwell RG: The function of bone marrow in the incorporation of a bone graft. Clin Orthop 1985; 200:125.
23. Salama R, Weissman SL: The clinical use of combined xenografts of bone and autologous red marrow. J Bone Joint Surg Br 1978; 60:111.
24. Bruder SP, Fink DJ, Caplan AI: Mesenchymal stem cells in bone development, bone repair and skeletal regeneration therapy. J Cell Biochem 1994; 56:283.
25. Tiedeman JJ, Connoly JF, Strates BS, et al: Treatment of nonunion by percutaneous injection of bone marrow and demineralization bone matrix. Clin Orthop 1991; 268:294.
26. Köhler P, Kreicbergs A, Strömberg L: Physical properties of autoclaved bone. Acta Orthop Scand 1986; 57:141.
27. Johnston JO, Harries TJ, Alexander CE, et al: Limb salvage procedure for neoplasms about the knee by spherocentric total knee arthroplasty and autogenous autoclaved bone grafting. Clin Orthop 1993; 181:137.
28. Köhler P, Glas J-E, Larsson S, et al: Incorporation of nonviable bone grafts. Acta Orthop Scand 1987; 58:54.
29. Chapman MW, Bucholz R, Cornell C: Treatment of acute fractures with a collagen–calcium phosphate graft material: A randomized clinical trial. J Bone Joint Surg Am 1997; 79:495.
30. Wolfe SW, Pike L, Slade JF III, et al: Augmentation of distal radius fracture fixation with coralline hydroxyapatite bone graft substitute. J Hand Surg Am 1999; 24:816.
31. Bucholz RW, Carlton A, Holmes R: Interporous hydroxyapatite as a bone graft substitute in tibial plateau fractures. Clin Orthop 1989; 240:53.
32. Constantz BR, Ison IC, Fulmer MT, et al: Skeletal repair by in situ formation of the mineral phase of bone. Science 1995; 267: 1796.
33. Norian SRS: In Orthopaedic and Rehabilitation Devices (panel transcript document #3463t2.pdf). Available at http://www.fda.gov/ohrms/dockets/ac/cdrh98t.htm#.

CALCIUM HOMEOSTASIS

Edward M. Greenfield and Thomas A. Einhorn

section
2
chapter
7

Summary

- Extracellular calcium homeostasis is tightly controlled in normal conditions.
- Extracellular calcium levels are monitored by a plasma membrane receptor (recently discovered) found in many tissues, including the parathyroid gland, the thyroid gland, the kidney, and the skeleton.
- Altered extracellular calcium levels regulate production of hormones (parathyroid hormone, 1,25-dihydroxyvitamin D_3, and calcitonin) that, in turn, alter calcium fluxes in their target organs (bone, kidney, and intestine).
- Altered extracellular calcium levels also exert direct effects on the target organs.

Clinical Relevance

- Chronically altered production of or responses to parathyroid hormone lead to a number of metabolic bone diseases (hyperparathyroidism, hypoparathyroidism, etc.).
- Chronically altered production of or responses to 1,25-dihydroxyvitamin D_3 lead to osteomalacia.
- Osteomalacia can also be caused by hypophosphatemia or other conditions that impair mineralization.
- Osteoporosis, the most common metabolic bone disease, results from a dysregulation of bone cell function and can be exacerbated by dietary calcium insufficiency. However, in osteoporosis, calcium homeostasis is, for the most part, maintained normally.

The concentration of ionized calcium in extracellular fluid is exquisitely regulated so that normal values are held between 4.5 and 5.0 mg/dL. This ionized calcium level represents about half of the normal total calcium level; the remainder exists either bound to albumin or other serum proteins or complexed to citrate or phosphate ions. The importance of the tight regulation of ionized calcium homeostasis is illustrated by the muscle tetany induced by severe hypocalcemia as well as by the risk of nephrolithiasis, cardiac conduction abnormalities, and nervous system problems induced by hypercalcemia. Calcium homeostasis is controlled by rapid changes in secretion of hormones that regulate calcium fluxes at target tissues, primarily bone, kidney, and intestine. The three major calcium regulating hormones are parathyroid hormone (PTH), 1,25-dihydroxyvitamin D_3 (1,25-D_3), and calcitonin. The physiological importance of these hormones is illustrated by clinical disorders such as hyper- and hypoparathyroidism, rickets, and osteomalacia. Although PTH, 1,25-D_3, and calcitonin also regulate phosphorus and magnesium homeostasis, this chapter focuses on calcium homeostasis. Readers interested in details concerning phosphorus and magnesium homeostasis are referred to reviews of these subjects.[1, 2]

FUNDAMENTAL SCIENCE

The initial response to changes in ionized calcium levels is a rapid change in secretion of PTH and calcitonin by, respectively, the parathyroid and thyroid glands. Thus, lowered calcium levels increase PTH secretion, and elevated calcium levels increase calcitonin secretion (Fig. 1). The resultant changes in PTH and calcitonin levels act together with 1,25-D_3 to rapidly reestablish normal calcium levels. Understanding of the mechanisms involved in regulation of PTH and calcitonin secretion has increased substantially in the last few years with the discovery and characterization of the receptor responsible for sensing extracellular ionized calcium.[3, 4] It is a seven-transmembrane, G-protein–coupled receptor found on many cell types, including parathyroid chief cells and thyroid C cells that, respectively, secrete PTH and calcitonin. The physiological importance of this calcium-sensing receptor is indicated by the finding that mutations in the receptor are responsible for both familial hypocalciuric hypercalcemia and neonatal severe primary hyperparathyroidism.[3, 4] These conditions are characterized by an increase in the calcium "set point" that regulates hormone secretion. Familial hypocalciuric hypercalcemia results from an autosomal-dominant mutation that causes a relatively mild effect on receptor function, leading to mod-

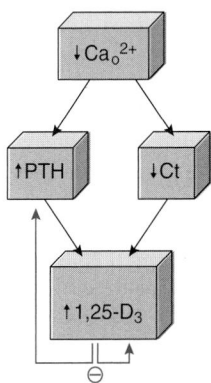

Fig. 1. Extracellular calcium levels and hormone production. Extracellular calcium regulates production of parathyroid hormone (PTH), 1,25-dihydroxyvitamin D_3 (1,25-D_3), and calcitonin (Ct). This figure and Figures 2, 3, and 5 illustrate responses to decreased extracellular calcium. Responses to increased extracellular calcium would therefore be in the opposite direction of those indicated in the figures. Blue arrows denote inhibitory effects. See text for details.

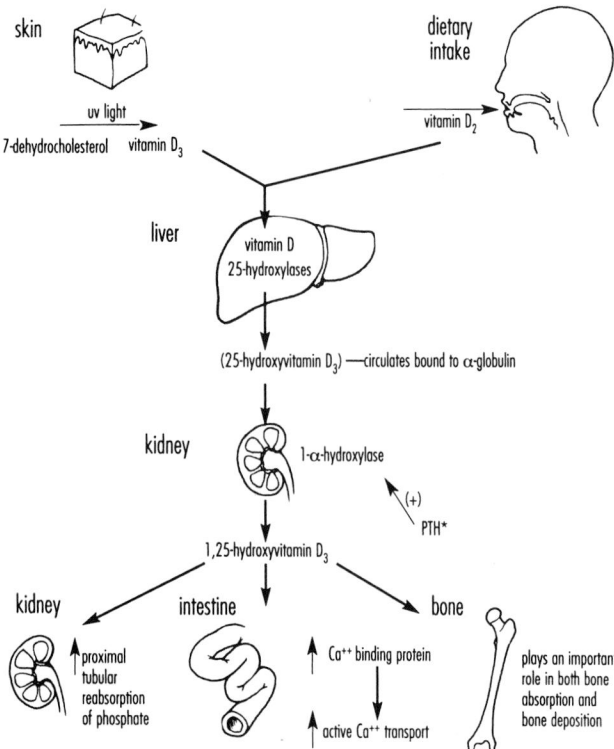

Fig. 2. Vitamin D metabolism. Parathyroid hormone, serum phosphate, ionized calcium, and 1,25-dihydroxyvitamin D₃ all influence 1-α-hydroxylase activity. (From Einhorn TA, Gill SS: Bone metabolism and metabolic bone disease. In Beaty JH [ed]: Orthopaedic Knowledge Update 6. Rosemont, IL, American Academy of Orthopaedic Surgeons, 1999, pp 149–165.)

erate hypercalcemia. In contrast, neonatal severe primary hyperparathyroidism causes a life-threatening hypercalcemia that in individual patients results either from mutations in both alleles of the receptor gene or from a heterozygotic mutation that causes a more severe change in receptor function.

Vitamin D is a fat-soluble steroid hormone that regulates calcium homeostasis either by a direct action on tissues or by indirect effects on various calcium-regulating systems. Endogenous production of vitamin D begins in the skin where 7-dehydrocholesterol is converted to cholecalciferol (vitamin D₃) on exposure to ultraviolet light (Fig. 2). In light-skinned individuals, only 15 minutes of daily bright sunlight or artificial light to the hands and face is required to produce enough vitamin D₃ to undergo further metabolism resulting in the minimum requirement of 10 μg of active metabolite, 1,25-D₃ (calcitriol). Dark-skinned people require longer exposures. Vitamin D₂ (ergocalciferol) may be obtained through the diet (see Fig. 2). These two forms have the same function and both are metabolized to an active 1,25 metabolite. Both metabolites are stored in several tissues throughout the body; adipose tissue and muscle have the highest concentrations. Because there are few dietary sources containing significant amounts of vitamin D, most milk in the United States is supplemented with vitamin D₂. Once ultraviolet light acts to convert 7-dehydrocholesterol to vitamin D₃ in the skin, this metabolite circulates to the liver where it is hydroxylated at its 25th carbon

to produce 25-hydroxyvitamin D₃ (calcifediol) (see Fig. 2). Once formed, 25-hydroxyvitamin D₃ is transported, bound to an α-globulin to undergo 1-α-hydroxylation in the kidney (see Fig. 2). This hydroxylation at the first carbon position occurs in the mitochondria of renal tubular cells, is activated by parathyroid hormone, and is the rate-limiting step in the production of the biologically active 1,25-dihydroxyvitamin D₃. The production of 25-hydroxyvitamin D₃ decreases with age. In addition, the impairment of renal function associated with aging can lead to a reduction in the activity of the 1-α-hydroxylase enzyme. These two effects combine to decrease the production of 1,25-dihydroxyvitamin D₃ in older individuals.

One type of effect of the calcium-regulating hormones is to control production of each other (see Fig. 1). For example, PTH rapidly increases the rate-limiting step in 1,25-D₃ synthesis by up-regulating 1-α-hydroxylase activity in the kidney.[5] Conversely, calcitonin decreases 1-α-hydroxylase activity.[6] Because extracellular calcium is increased by PTH and 1,25-D₃ but decreased by calcitonin, the coordinated changes in levels of the three hormones act together to reestablish normal calcium homeostasis. In addition, there are also negative feedback interactions among the calcium-regulating hormones that dampen the calcium homeostatic mechanisms (see Fig. 1). For example, 1,25-D₃ reduces PTH levels by a transcriptional mechanism[7] and reduces its own production by inhibiting the activity of the 1-α-hydroxylase enzyme.[5]

The calcium-regulating hormones also have effects on the functions of their classical target cells. Thus, PTH increases extracellular calcium levels primarily by increasing calcium reabsorption in the kidney and resorption of bone (Fig. 3). PTH exerts its effects by activating a seven-transmembrane G-protein–coupled receptor.[8] The renal effects occur primarily in the thick ascending limb of the loop of Henle and the distal tubule. As depicted in Figure 4, PTH increases bone resorption indirectly by binding to receptors on osteoblasts and thereby regulating production of secreted and plasma membrane–bound cytokines that, in turn, regulate differentiation and activity of osteoclasts, the cells that resorb bone.[9, 10] The cytokine that is probably most important in this regard is a membrane-bound member of the tumor necrosis factor superfamily known as

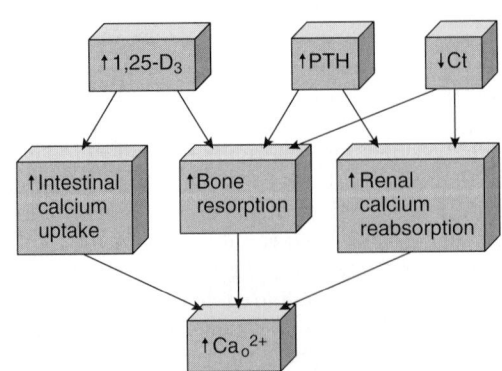

Fig. 3. Hormonal regulation. Parathyroid hormone (PTH), 1,25-dihydroxyvitamin D₃ (1,25-D₃), and calcitonin (Ct) regulate extracellular calcium levels. See text for details.

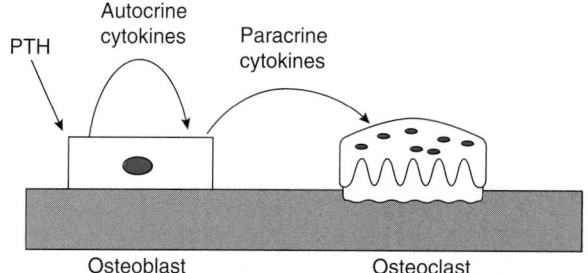

Fig. 4. Parathyroid hormone (PTH) and bone resorption. PTH increases bone resorption indirectly by inducing osteoblasts to produce autocrine and paracrine cytokines. The autocrine cytokines, such as interleukin-6, further increase production of the paracrine cytokines that stimulate osteoclast activity and differentiation. The paracrine cytokine that is probably most important is known as osteoclast differentiation factor, osteoprotegerin ligand, TRANCE, or RANK ligand. See text for details.

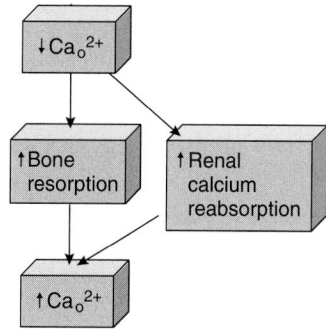

Fig. 5. Extracellular calcium effects on bone and kidney. Extracellular calcium levels also directly regulate bone resorption and renal calcium reabsorption. See text for details.

osteoclast differentiation factor, osteoprotegerin ligand, TRANCE, or RANK ligand.[9]

1,25-D_3 increases extracellular calcium levels primarily by increasing calcium absorption in the intestine and resorption of bone (see Fig. 3). 1,25-D_3 stimulates bone resorption by a mechanism similar to that described previously for PTH.[9, 10] However, unlike the receptors for PTH, calcitonin, and extracellular calcium, the classical 1,25-D_3 receptor is a member of the nuclear steroid receptor family.[7] It has also become clear that some of the effects of 1,25-D_3 are mediated by a second membrane-bound receptor that is as yet uncharacterized.[7] This membrane-bound receptor appears to be most important for the rapid, nongenomic effects of 1,25-D_3. The increased intestinal calcium absorption induced by 1,25-D_3 is due to up-regulation of at least two proteins: calbindin, a calcium-binding protein that facilitates transport of calcium through the cytoplasm of the intestinal cells, and the intestinal plasma membrane calcium pump that transports calcium across the cell membrane against a substantial concentration gradient.[5]

PTH and 1,25-D_3 also increase bone formation by acting directly on osteoblasts and, in certain circumstances, these anabolic effects can predominate over the classical resorptive effects described earlier.[7, 11] The anabolic effects tend to be slower and are, therefore, more important in chronic conditions, whereas the resorptive effects are rapid and more important in acute regulation of calcium homeostasis. For example, the anabolic effects of PTH result in the overproduction of osteoid in chronic hyperparathyroidism. The anabolic effects of PTH and 1,25-D_3 may also be involved in the coupling between bone resorption and bone formation that leads to the filling in of Howship's lacunae generated by active osteoclasts.[7]

Calcitonin decreases extracellular calcium levels primarily by increasing renal calcium excretion and by inhibiting bone resorption (see Fig. 3).[6] Calcitonin inhibits bone resorption by directly inhibiting osteoclast activity and differentiation.[6, 9, 10, 12] Osteoclasts and renal tubule cells express the calcitonin receptor, a seven-transmembrane G protein–coupled receptor, with a relatively high level of similarity to the PTH receptor.[12]

Extracellular calcium not only controls the levels of the hormones that regulate calcium homeostasis but also has direct effects on the target organs themselves (Fig. 5). Thus, elevated extracellular calcium strongly inhibits renal calcium reabsorption[3] and osteoclast activity.[4, 9] These direct effects of calcium are likely to be mediated by the extracellular ionized calcium-sensing receptor discussed above because it is expressed by many renal epithelial cells as well as by osteoclasts.[3, 9]

CLINICAL RELEVANCE AND APPLICATIONS

The mechanisms described in the preceding section act together in a coordinated fashion to rapidly reestablish calcium homeostasis in response to acute changes in extracellular calcium levels. Chronic disturbances in these processes lead to a number of metabolic bone diseases. Two groups of metabolic bone diseases are discussed in this section: those that cause altered levels of PTH-induced cellular responses (Table 1) and those that cause osteomalacia (Table 2). Although osteoporosis, the most prevalent metabolic bone disease, can be associated with chronic dietary calcium insufficiency or mild impaired vitamin D metabolism, calcium homeostasis is usually maintained in this condition.

TABLE 1. CONDITIONS WITH ALTERED CALCIUM HOMEOSTASIS DUE TO ALTERED LEVELS OF PTH-INDUCED CELLULAR RESPONSES

Conditions that cause hypercalcemia:
　Humoral hypercalcemia of malignancy
　Primary hyperparathyroidism
　　Adenoma of a single parathyroid gland
　　Hyperplasia of multiple parathyroid glands
　Secondary hyperparathyroidism
　Familial hypocalciuric hypercalcemia
　Neonatal severe primary hyperparathyroidism
Conditions that cause hypocalcemia:
　Primary hypoparathyroidism
　　Isolated
　　Complexed with other syndromes
　Pseudohypoparathyroidism
　　Type 1a
　　Type 1b
　　Type 1c
　　Type 2

TABLE 2. CONDITIONS THAT CAUSE OSTEOMALACIA

Impaired vitamin D uptake or metabolism:
    Dietary vitamin D deficiency
    Vitamin D–dependent rickets
        Type 1
        Type 2
    Intestinal disease or surgery
    Liver disease
    Insufficient exposure to sunlight
    Renal osteodystrophy
    Anticonvulsants
Hypophosphatemia:
    X-linked hypophosphatemic rickets
    Hereditary hypophosphatemic rickets with hypercalciuria
    Autosomal-dominant hypophosphatemic rickets
    Fanconi's syndrome
    Aluminum-containing antacids
    Oncogenic osteomalacia
Impaired mineralization:
    Hypophosphatasia
    Bisphosphonates
    Aluminum

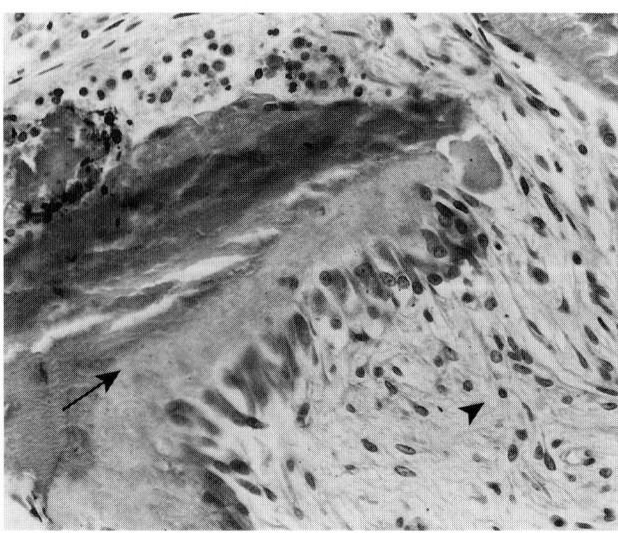

Fig. 6. Osteitis fibrosa cystica. Photomicrograph of bone is from a patient with secondary hyperparathyroidism and osteitis fibrosa cystica. Note extensive osteoblastic osteoid production *(arrow)* and marrow fibrosis *(arrowhead)*. (Hematoxylin and eosin, ×100.)

Hyperparathyroidism and humoral hypercalcemia of malignancy cause more than 90% of all cases of hypercalcemia. Humoral hypercalcemia of malignancy is often caused by secretion by tumors of PTH-related protein.[13] PTH-related protein has effects similar to those of PTH on calcium homeostasis because the two molecules have substantial amino acid identity in their amino terminal domains and, therefore, bind to and activate the same receptor.[8] Humoral hypercalcemia of malignancy is a major clinical problem in patients with late-stage tumors. In contrast, primary hyperparathyroidism is usually asymptomatic in current medical practice, having been discovered when blood calcium levels are measured in patients being evaluated for other reasons.[4, 14] It is usually due to an increased calcium "set point" in the parathyroid chief cells of a single adenomatous parathyroid gland.[14] In this case, the mechanism resembles that described above for familial hypocalciuric hypercalcemia. Most other cases of primary hyperparathyroidism are due to hyperplastic enlargement of the four parathyroid glands.[14] Parathyroid hyperplasia can also present in association with more complex syndromes, such as multiple endocrine neoplasia.

Secondary hyperparathyroidism is a response to chronically disturbed regulation of the calcium homeostatic mechanisms, which results in elevated PTH production. It is usually caused by the phosphate accumulation that results from the loss in functional renal mass in renal osteodystrophy. Phosphate accumulation lowers the serum-ionized calcium level, thereby stimulating the parathyroid gland. In severe cases, parathyroid gland overactivity leads to a substantial secretion of parathyroid hormone and extensive osteoclastic activity, resulting in destruction of the trabecular bone. This condition is known as osteitis fibrosa cystica (Fig. 6). Treatment involves controlling serum phosphate levels through the use of aluminum-containing phosphate-binding antacids or calcium carbonate. Some patients with severe secondary hyperparathyroidism experience severe bone pain if PTH levels are especially difficult to control. In addition, brown tumors can occur in these

patients just as they do in patients with primary hyperparathyroidism. For severe symptomatic secondary hyperparathyroidism, a partial or total parathyroidectomy may be indicated.

In contrast to the hyperparathyroid conditions, hypoparathyroidism causes hypocalcemia and hyperphosphatemia. Impaired PTH secretion in isolated primary hypoparathyroidism is inherited in either a dominant or a recessive fashion. The mutations can be in the PTH gene itself, in the extracellular ionized calcium-sensing receptor, or in an uncharacterized gene on the X chromosome.[15]

Primary hypoparathyroidism, like primary hyperparathyroidism, can also present in association with more complex syndromes.[15] Pseudohypoparathyroidism is due to impaired responsiveness of PTH target cells rather than reduced PTH secretion. As illustrated in Fig. 7, the reduced respon-

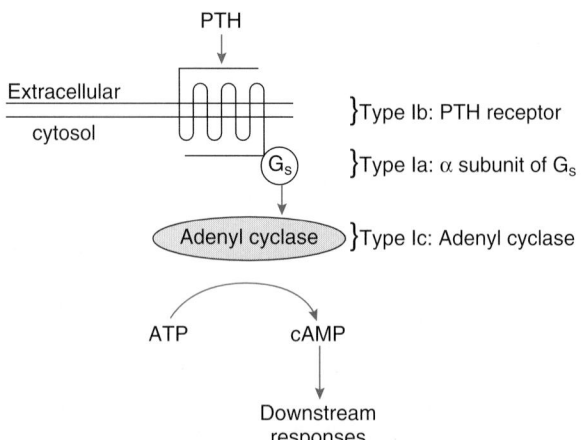

Fig. 7. Pseudohypoparathyroidism. Impaired responsiveness of PTH target cells in pseudohypoparathyroidism types Ia, b, and c. See text for details.

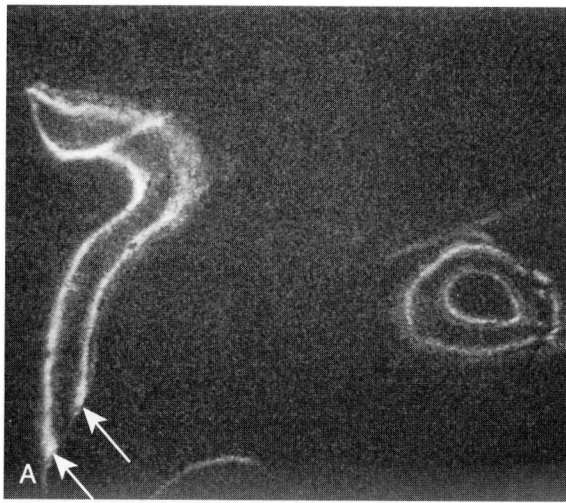 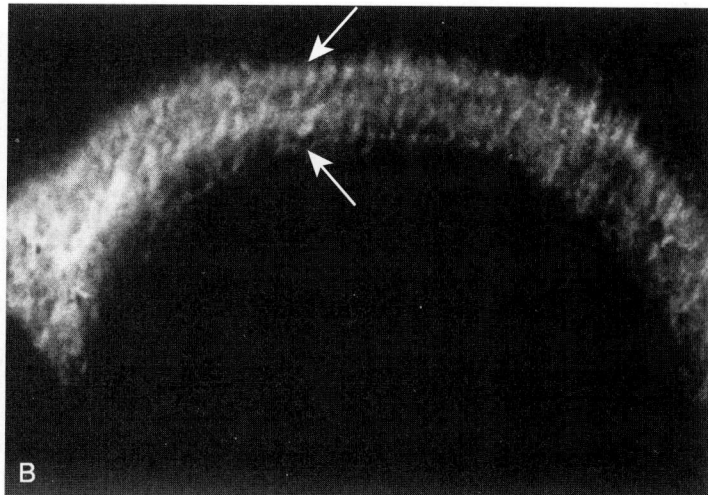

Fig. 8. Osteomalacia. *A,* This is a photomicrograph of fluorescent tetracycline labels *(arrows)* in an unstained bone biopsy section. Each label represents the uptake of tetracycline at mineralization fronts only at the times of oral administration. The distance between the labels (measured in microns) and the numbers of days between times of tetracycline administration are values used to calculate the calcification rate, which is expressed in microns per day. The appearance of the tetracycline labels in this photomicrograph is normal (×100). *B,* Photomicrograph of fluorescent tetracycline labels *(arrows)* of the mineralization front in the bone from a patient with osteomalacia. Note that although the patient adhered to the same tetracycline labeling protocol, slow and abnormal mineralization has caused the two lines to be indistinct and appear "smudged" (×100).

siveness can be due to a variety of mechanisms, including reduced expression of the PTH receptor (pseudohypoparathyroidism type 1b); decreased levels of $G_{s\alpha}$, the G-protein responsible for coupling the receptor to the cAMP signal transduction pathway (type 1a); impaired activity of adenyl cyclase, the enzyme that synthesizes cAMP (type 1c); or some other uncharacterized aspect of PTH-induced signal transduction (type 2).[16] Patients with pseudohypoparathyroidism types 1a and 1c also present with Albright's hereditary osteodystrophy, which is characterized by short stature, shortened limbs, brachydactyly, heterotopic ossification, thickened calvaria, and dental hypoplasia.[16]

Osteomalacia is a metabolic bone disease characterized by impaired mineralization of newly formed osteoid that, on histological examination of bone biopsy samples, leads to an increase in size of osteoid seams and a decrease in the separation of tetracycline labels[17] (Fig. 8). Most cases of osteomalacia are due to low 1,25-D_3 levels in noninherited conditions (intestinal disease or surgery) that reduce vitamin D uptake or to metabolism (liver disease, insufficient exposure to sunlight, renal osteodystrophy, or anticonvulsants that up-regulate liver oxidases that degrade vitamin D).[4, 17–20] The clinical diagnosis of osteomalacia is often challenging because patients usually have nonspecific symptoms such as muscle weakness or diffuse aches and pains. The radiographic appearance of osteomalacia often mimics other osteopenic conditions such as osteoporosis. One distinguishing radiographic feature, however, is the presence of pseudofractures, or Looser's zones. These are radiolucent areas of bone that result from multiple microstress fractures and that heal by the formation of osteomalacic bone which is not sufficiently mineralized (Fig. 9).

Rickets, the childhood form of osteomalacia, particularly affects rapidly growing bones and growth plates.[21] Thus, infants with rickets exhibit widened cranial sutures and wrists as well as frontal bossing. In older children, rickets

affects primarily the appendicular skeleton, leading to varus or valgus deformities of the legs.[21] Classical rickets from dietary vitamin D deficiency has become rare because of vitamin D supplementation of milk. Rickets can also be caused by hereditary deficiency in either production of or responses to 1,25-D_3. Deficiency in production of 1,25-D_3

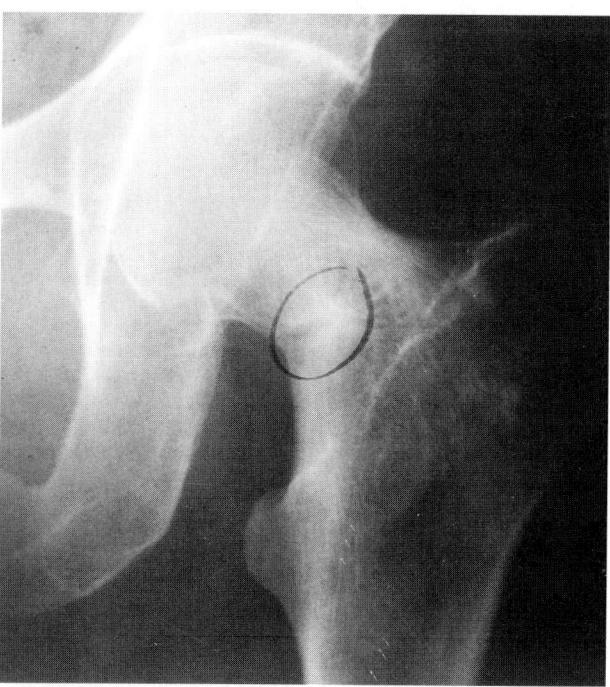

Fig. 9. Looser's zone. This is an anteroposterior radiograph of a proximal femur in a patient with osteomalacia who has a Looser zone on the medial aspect of the femoral neck. These radiolucent areas result from multiple microstress fractures that heal by the formation of osteomalacic bone.

is known as vitamin D–dependent rickets type 1 and is thought to be caused by a lack of renal 1-α-hydroxylase activity.[21] Deficiency in response to 1,25-D$_3$ is a rare condition resulting from mutations in the vitamin D receptor.[21] It is known as vitamin D–dependent rickets type 2 because high-dose vitamin D ameliorates the disease in some cases.[21]

Osteomalacia and rickets can also be caused by hypophosphatemia.[1] Hereditary forms of hypophosphatemic rickets result from impaired renal phosphate reabsorption caused by mutations either in the PEX gene, an X-linked metalloproteinase of unknown function (X-linked hypophosphatemic rickets), or in unidentified autosomal-recessive or -dominant genes (hereditary hypophosphatemic rickets with hypercalciuria or autosomal-dominant hypophosphatemic rickets, respectively).[1] Hypophosphatemia, acting with acidosis, also contributes to the osteomalacia found in Fanconi's syndrome.[1] Noninherited forms of hypophosphatemia can be caused by phosphate malabsorption from aluminum-containing antacids[20] or by tumors that secrete a humoral factor that inhibits renal phosphate reabsorption (oncogenic osteomalacia).[1]

Osteomalacia can also be caused by impaired mineralization. Hypophosphatasia is an inherited form of osteomalacia. It results from mutations in the alkaline phosphatase isoenzyme that is found primarily in liver, bone, and kidney.[22] Impaired enzyme activity leads to accumulation of pyrophosphate as well as other physiological substrates.[22] High levels of pyrophosphate are thought to cause osteomalacia because this compound inhibits hydroxyapatite nucleation and crystal growth.[22] Thus, it is not surprising that osteomalacia can also be caused by bisphosphonates, which are stabilized pyrophosphate analogues.[20] Because aluminum is also a mineralization inhibitor, high aluminum levels resulting from the treatment of hyperparathyroidism in renal osteodystrophy with aluminum-based phosphate binding agents can also cause osteomalacia.

SUMMARY

This chapter has reviewed the mechanisms responsible for control of extracellular calcium homeostasis in normal conditions. Extracellular calcium levels are monitored by a calcium-sensing receptor that regulates production of PTH, 1,25-D$_3$, and calcitonin. These hormones maintain calcium homeostasis by regulating calcium fluxes in bones, kidneys, and intestines. This chapter also reviewed the mechanisms responsible for altered calcium homeostasis in a number of disease conditions, including humoral hypercalcemia of malignancy, hyperparathyroidism, hypoparathyroidism, pseudohypoparathyroidism, osteomalacia, rickets, hypophosphatemia, and hypophosphatasia.

REFERENCES

1. Drezner MK: Phosphorous homeostasis and related disorders. In Bilezikian JP, Raisz LG, Rodan GA (eds): Principles of Bone Biology. San Diego, Academic Press, 1996, p 263.

2. Rude RK: Magnesium homeostasis. In Bilezikian JP, Raisz LG, Rodan GA (eds): Principles of Bone Biology. San Diego, Academic Press, 1996, p 277.

3. Brown EM, Harris HW, Vassilev PM, et al: The biology of the extracellular Ca^{2+}-sensing receptor. In Bilezikian JP, Raisz LG, Rodan GA (eds): Principles of Bone Biology. San Diego, Academic Press, 1996, p 243.

4. Nemeth EF: Calcium receptors as novel drug targets. In Bilezikian JP, Raisz LG, Rodan GA (eds): Principles of Bone Biology. San Diego, Academic Press, 1996, p 1019.

5. Christakos S: Vitamin D gene regulation. In Bilezikian JP, Raisz LG, Rodan GA (eds): Principles of Bone Biology. San Diego, Academic Press, 1996, p 435.

6. Becker KL, Nylen ES, Cohen R, et al: Calcitonin: Structure, molecular biology, and actions. In Bilezikian JP, Raisz LG, Rodan GA (eds): Principles of Bone Biology. San Diego, Academic Press, 1996, p 471.

7. Farach-Carson MC, Ridall AL: Dual 1,25-dihydroxyvitamin D$_3$ signal response pathways in osteoblasts: Cross-talk between genomic and membrane-initiated pathways. Am J Kidney Dis 31:729, 1998.

8. Segre GV: Receptors for parathyroid hormone and parathyroid hormone-related protein. In Bilezikian JP, Raisz LG, Rodan GA (eds): Principles of Bone Biology. San Diego, Academic Press, 1996, p 377.

9. Greenfield EM, Bi Y, Miyauchi A: Regulation of osteoclast activity. Life Sci 65: 1087, 1999.

10. Suda T, Nakamura I, Jimi E, et al: Regulation of osteoclast function. J Bone Miner Res 12: 869, 1997.

11. Dempster DW, Cosman F, Parisien M, et al: Anabolic actions of parathyroid hormone on bone. Endocr Rev 14:690, 1993.

12. Goldring SR: The structure and molecular biology of the calcitonin receptor. In Bilezikian JP, Raisz LG, Rodan GA (eds): Principles of Bone Biology. San Diego, Academic Press, 1996, p 461.

13. Goltzman D, Henderson JE: Expression of PTHrP in disease. In Bilezikian JP, Raisz LG, Rodan GA (eds): Principles of Bone Biology. San Diego, Academic Press, 1996, p 809.

14. Bilezikian JP: Primary hyperparathyroidism. In Favus MJ (ed): Primer on the Metabolic Bone Diseases and Disorders of Mineral Metabolism. Philadelphia, Lippincott-Raven, 1996, p 181.

15. Thakker RV: Molecular basis of PTH underexpression. In Bilezikian JP, Raisz LG, Rodan GA (eds): Principles of Bone Biology. San Diego, Academic Press, 1996, p 837.

16. Levine MA: Pseudohypoparathyroidism. In Bilezikian JP, Raisz LG, Rodan GA (eds): Principles of Bone Biology. San Diego, Academic Press, 1996, p 853.

17. Einhorn TA, Gill SS: Bone metabolism and metabolic bone disease. In Beaty JH (ed): Orthopaedic Knowledge Update 6. Rosemont, IL, American Academy of Orthopaedic Surgeons, 1999, p 149.

18. Goodman WG, Coburn JW, Slatopolsky E, et al: Renal osteodystrophy in adults and children. In Favus MJ (ed): Primer on the Metabolic Bone Diseases and Disorders of Mineral Metabolism. Philadelphia, Lippincott-Raven, 1996, p 341.

19. Rao DS, Honasoge M: Metabolic bone disease in gastrointestinal, hepatobiliary, and pancreatic disorders. In Favus MJ (ed): Primer on the Metabolic Bone Diseases and Disorders of Mineral Metabolism. Philadelphia, Lippincott-Raven, 1996, p 306.

20. Bikle DD: Drug-induced osteomalacia. In Favus MJ (ed): Primer on the Metabolic Bone Diseases and Disorders of Mineral Metabolism. Philadelphia, Lippincott-Raven, 1996, p 333.

21. Liberman VA: Hereditary deficiencies in vitamin D action. In Bilezikian JP, Raisz LG, and Rodan GA (eds): Principles of Bone Biology. San Diego, Academic Press, 1996, p 903.

22. Whyte MP: Hypophosphatasia: Nature's window on alkaline phosphatase function in man. In Bilezikian JP, Raisz LG, Rodan GA (eds): Principles of Bone Biology. San Diego, Academic Press, 1996, p 951.

OSTEOPOROSIS: ETIOLOGY, DIAGNOSIS, AND TREATMENT

Robert R. Recker and M. Janet Barger-Lux

Summary

- Osteoporosis is a skeletal disorder characterized by decreased bone strength predisposing to an increased risk of fracture.
- In the United States, epidemiologists attribute at least 1.3 million fractures per year to osteoporosis.
- Osteoporosis plays a role in 70% of all fractures that occur in people 45 years of age and older.
- Nearly 90% of hip fractures occur in older individuals who fall from no more than standing height.
- Osteoporosis is diagnosed by a dual-energy x-ray absorptiometry (DXA) measurement of bone mineral density (BMD) more than 2.5 standard deviations below the reference mean.
- Each standard deviation decrement in BMD is associated with a 1.5- to 3-fold increase in fracture risk.
- Increased fracture risk in osteoporosis is due not only to decreased bone mass but also to decreased trabecular connectivity. Decreased trabecular connectivity plays a much larger role in fracture causation than is commonly recognized.
- Osteoporosis-related fractures are not limited to low-trauma events.
- For prevention and treatment of osteoporosis, one should include:
    Adequate physical activity.
    Hormone replacement therapy (HRT) for patients with hormone deficiency (e.g., postmenopausal women).
    Antiresorptive medication (e.g., bisphosphonates).
    Calcium intake of 1000–1500 mg/day.
    Sufficient vitamin D to maintain 25-hydroxyvitamin D at about 32 ng/mL.
    Adequate protein intake.

Osteoporosis is a condition leading to structural failure of the human skeleton, often prematurely (i.e., before completion of the prevailing human life span). *Established* or *severe* osteoporosis is characterized by fragility fractures and the distress, deformity, and disabilities (and deaths) that follow them. The most recent National Institutes of Health (NIH) consensus statement on osteoporosis defined osteoporosis simply as "a skeletal disorder characterized by compromised bone strength predisposing to an increased risk of fracture."[1] Most practitioners are familiar with osteoporosis among postmenopausal women, but it also occurs among elderly men. *Secondary* osteoporosis occurs as a complication, often long delayed, of the many conditions, diseases, and medications that over time undermine bone strength.

Although once regarded as a feature of natural aging in women, osteoporosis is no longer considered dependent on either age or sex.[1] Among patients 45 years of age and older, epidemiologists estimate that 70% of fractures involve underlying osteoporosis,[2] although the diagnosis is often missed. Without appropriate assessment and referral, patients with osteoporosis are less likely to receive the follow-up treatment that could prevent their next fracture.

The objectives of this chapter are to (1) outline the effects of osteoporosis on bone; (2) relate etiological factors to the health histories of patients; (3) present diagnostic criteria for osteoporosis; (4) propose that orthopaedists consider osteoporosis in the assessment of every patient who presents with fracture; and (5) outline recommended approaches to the treatment of osteoporosis.

EFFECTS OF OSTEOPOROSIS ON BONE

Osteoporotic bones fracture because their strength has been undermined. As bone fragility increases, the force required to effect fracture decreases. Figure 1 presents a diagram of this relationship and provides a scheme for grouping factors that affect the intrinsic fragility of bone tissue as well as the external force applied to it.[3] In osteoporosis, the skeleton itself is underweight, as evidenced by a low value for total body bone mineral content. Thin, porous cortices account for much of the deficit in bone mass. However, low bone mass does not explain entirely the fragility of osteoporotic bone. Bone quality is also impaired, as evidenced by microscopic abnormalities (e.g., undermineralized matrix, accumulation of fatigue damage, and thinning, perforation, and disruption of trabeculae). The trabecular changes produce a loss of trabecular connectivity that is particularly damaging to bone strength.[4]

The lower part of Figure 1 relates to the forces that originate in falls and other mishaps. Especially among older adults, any impairment of vision, gait, balance, or level of consciousness (whether by condition, disease, or treatment) can increase propensity to fall and the application of force sufficient for the failure of fragile bone. Environmental factors include poor lighting, clutter, and the other household hazards that can increase the risk of falling.

EPIDEMIOLOGY OF FRACTURES

In the United States, epidemiologists attribute at least 1.3 million fractures per year to osteoporosis. This figure is

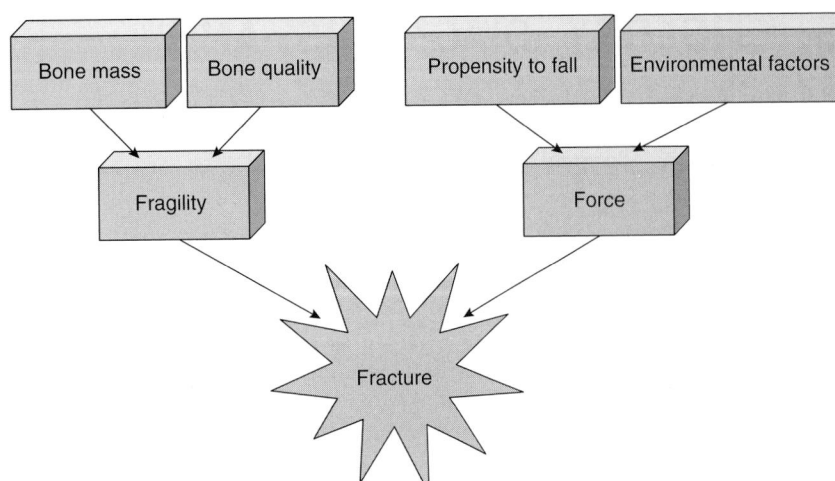

Fig. 1. Fragility, force, and fracture. Schematic representation of some of the factors that affect bone fragility and the force applied to bone in the course of traumatic mishaps. As the skeleton becomes more and more fragile, less and less force is required to produce fracture. (Adapted from Heaney RP, Barger-Lux MJ: Calcium, bone metabolism, and structural failure. Triangle 1985; 24:91–100.)

based on an assumption that 70% of all fractures in persons 45 years of age and older involve underlying bone fragility.[2]

In the United States and in most other populations, the incidence of hip fractures rises exponentially with aging. The sex-specific incidence of hip fracture is about 2:1 women to men; however, about 80% of all hip fractures occur in elderly women, owing to their greater longevity. Available data for the United States indicate that "overwhelming" trauma and local disease account for only a minority of hip fractures (10% and 1%, respectively); the remaining 89% typically involve an older person with osteoporosis who falls from no greater than standing height.[5]

Studies from the United States and Europe report similar findings for the prevalence of vertebral deformities: For adults in their 50s, figures are higher among men than women, and the pattern is reversed among older adults.[6, 7] Table 1 lists the percentages of women and men in whom at least one vertebral deformity was present. The individuals were from two age strata of a rural, noninstitutionalized U.S. population.[6] Available data show that the incidence of distal forearm fractures increases steadily among white women from age 40 to 65 and then levels off. Among men, the incidence is fairly constant from age 20 to 80. The sex-specific incidence of distal forearm fractures is about 4:1, women to men.[2]

The epidemiological data on fractures harbor *some* good news. The variation among Western nations in incidence of hip, vertebral, and distal forearm fractures is nontrivial. These differences suggest that environmental factors might be manipulated to reduce such injuries.[2]

ETIOLOGY AND RISK

Three pathophysiological mechanisms influence risk for eventual osteoporotic fracture. These involve (1) bone mass, which has proved to be the aspect of bone fragility that is most accessible to study; (2) bone geometry and architecture, which influence strength independently of mass; and (3) the mechanisms that lead to falling among older adults. All three probably involve "a varying mixture of inherited and environmental determinants."[2]

Figure 2 presents a schematic diagram of the earlier gain and later loss of bone mass (skeletal weight) as it relates to the human life span. Skeletal growth and consolidation conclude with acquisition of a final increment in bone mass early in adult life, with peak bone mass at about age 30.[8] In healthy adults, bone mass holds steady until, for women, about the time of menopause, when bone loss begins. (However, the effect of estrogen deprivation on bone mass can be postponed for the duration of estrogen replacement therapy.) Some degree of "age-related" bone loss occurs in all older adults, although predictably to a greater extent among those who are physically inactive, poorly nourished, or otherwise in poor health.

Table 2 presents, in broad categories, putative causes of osteoporosis[9] as they relate to the assessment of patients. The greatest risk factor for osteoporotic fracture is having sustained a previous fracture of the same type; persons with at least one vertebral deformity have 7 to 10 times the risk of a new vertebral fracture event than those without, and the risk of a second hip fracture is similarly increased.[2] Exposed to equivalent force, even if that force occurs in the course of a serious fall or a vehicular mishap, fewer persons of any age with healthy skeletons suffer fractures than do those with occult skeletal deterioration. For these reasons, Table 2 associates *any* fracture after age 45 with the possibility that established osteoporosis may be present.

DIAGNOSIS

No aspect of osteoporosis has received more attention than BMD. A search of the National Library of Medicine's on-

TABLE 1. PERCENTAGES OF WOMEN AND MEN WITH AT LEAST ONE VERTEBRAL DEFORMITY[6]		
Variable	50–59 Years	80–89 Years
Women	10%	45%
Men	29%	39%

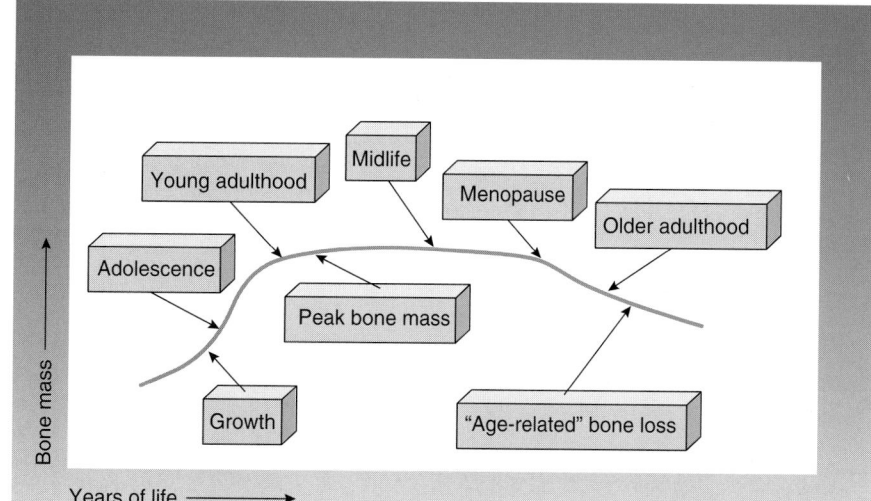

Fig. 2. Schematic diagram of a typical bone mass "lifeline."

TABLE 2. PATIENT ASSESSMENT

Characteristic	Causal Factors								
	Established Osteoporosis	Hereditary Influences	Inadequate Body Weight	Inadequate nutritional status	Hypovitaminosis D	Inadequate Skeletal Loading	Deleterious Effects on Bone	Hypogonadism	High likelihood of falling
All patients									
Osteoporosis, height loss, or fractures in parents, siblings, maternal or paternal relatives		X							
Persistent underweight (e.g., BMI <20, calculated from young adult height and usual adult weight)			X						
For women: anorexia nervosa or female athlete triad				X				X	
Any malabsorption syndrome, chronic or recurrent diarrhea, or long-term GI complaint				X					
Long-term avoidance of calcium-rich foods (e.g., attributed to dislike, milk allergy, or lactose intolerance)				X					
Extended periods of bedrest (e.g., in association with surgery, illness, injury, or pregnancy)						X			
Current or long-term avoidance of (or incapacity for) exercise or physical work						X			

Table continued on following page

TABLE 2. PATIENT ASSESSMENT (Continued)

Characteristic	Causal Factors								
	Established Osteoporosis	Hereditary Influences	Inadequate Body Weight	Inadequate nutritional status	Hypovitaminosis D	Inadequate Skeletal Loading	Deleterious Effects on Bone	Hypogonadism	High likelihood of falling
Exposure to drugs associated with low bone mass (e.g., corticosteroids, anticonvulsants, antimetabolites)							X		
Cigarette smoking or heavy alcohol consumption							X		
Treatment with thyroid hormone without yearly monitoring							X		
For women: late menarche or extended oligomenorrhea or amenorrhea								X	
Mature and older adults Fracture of any bone after age 45, especially if low trauma	X								
Hyperparathyroidism without periodic monitoring of bone mass							X		
Treatment with radiation therapy							X		
For women: menopause or oophorectomy without estrogen replacement								X	
Older adults Height loss of 1 in or more since midlife	X								
Development of posture changes characteristic of osteoporosis	X								
Avoidance of (or lack of opportunity for) sun exposure					X				
For men: thinning of beard or body hair								X	
Frequent falls or current falling hazards in the home									X
Any difficulty with vision, balance, mobility, or level of consciousness									X

A careful review of a patient's health history and current situation can identify putative causes of osteoporosis and osteoporosis-related fractures. Positive responses to items such as those listed here are associated with the causal factors on the right. Occurrences need not be recent to be significant. As appropriate, the patient can be asked to list, identify, describe, or indicate frequency or duration.

BMI, body mass index weight in kg/ht in m²; GI, gastrointestinal.

line database retrieved 11,979 entries with "bone mineral density" in the title. (BMD measured by methods other than quantitative computed tomography is actually "areal" density, a two-dimensional approximation of true density.) BMD accounts for most, but not all (i.e., 75% to 90%), of the variance in bone strength, and the relationship of BMD and fracture parallels that of blood pressure and stroke,[10] as shown in Table 3. Despite efforts over the years to find a "fracture threshold" in the results of BMD measurements, it now seems clear that the inverse relationship between BMD and fracture risk is a continuous one. Each standard deviation decrement in BMD is associated with a 1.5- to 3-

TABLE 3. RELATIONSHIP BETWEEN RISK FACTORS AND CLINICAL OUTCOMES

Parameter	Risk Factor	Clinical Outcome
Blood pressure	Hypertension	Stroke
Bone mineral density	Low bone mass	Fracture

fold increase in fracture risk.[11] In 1994, however, an expert panel under the auspices of the World Health Organization (WHO) proposed criteria for the diagnosis of postmenopausal osteoporosis by use of BMD measurements.[12] Table 4 presents these criteria. The authors of a 2000 position paper noted that validation data for the WHO thresholds are strongest for BMD measurements made by DXA instruments at the hip measurement site.[13]

Table 5 lists situations in which bone mass measurements, preferably by DXA, can facilitate clinical decision-making. DXA instruments are scanning devices that deliver small doses of x-ray radiation; they can generate BMD and bone mineral content (BMC) for sites of interest at the proximal femur, distal forearm, and lumbar spine. A rapid DXA scan of the total body can yield measures of total body BMC and body composition.

Figure 3 presents a diagnostic flow chart geared to orthopaedics practice. It recommends that the practitioner consider osteoporosis in the assessment of every patient who presents with fracture, and presents alternate pathways that terminate in referral for patients in whom a diagnosis of osteoporosis is likely to be confirmed.

In cases of secondary osteoporosis, it is not unusual to find that the primary condition has not been previously identified.[14] The majority of patients with secondary osteoporosis, however, are those who have been treated with corticosteroids, anticonvulsants, antimetabolites, or any of numerous other drugs or in whom osteoporosis has developed as an unfortunate side effect of long survival with another chronic health problem.

APPROACHES TO TREATMENT

Many patients who seek evaluation in the osteoporosis clinic have concerns about osteoporosis without current symptoms. Some of them can be evaluated, informed about effective approaches to prevention, and reassured. Others will be found to have osteopenia, occult osteoporosis, or, not infrequently, established osteoporosis with multiple vertebral deformities. Patients with active complaints commonly have spine fractures with acute or chronic pain, appendicular stress fractures, secondary osteoporosis, or a combination of these.

When fractures have occurred, the first goals of osteoporosis treatment are part of the practice of orthopaedics, namely to relieve pain and discomfort and restore function and mobility. Inadequate attention to these issues can be devastating to the osteoporosis patient in that *any* restriction of bone loading (e.g., bedrest) beyond a matter of days yields rapid loss of bone mass. In addition, every patient who visits the osteoporosis clinic (even the "worried well") can benefit from the other three treatment goals, namely to improve nutritional status, to maintain or increase bone strength, and to prevent future fractures.

Bone health requires good nutrition throughout life but perhaps most acutely in active efforts to prevent or treat osteoporosis. In contrast to the daily calcium intake of 1000 to 1500 mg recommended for adults and used in virtually every treatment regimen, persons who habitually avoid calcium-rich foods have intakes that average only 300 to 500 mg/day.[15] The antiresorptive agents (e.g., estrogen, selective estrogen receptor modulators, and bisphosphonates) used to prevent and treat osteoporosis require adequate supplies of calcium and vitamin D.

Although serum 25-hydroxyvitamin D is useful to evaluate vitamin D status, laboratory reports frequently identify as "low" only the dramatically deficient levels characteristic of osteomalacia. However, it is increasingly clear that correction of subtler effects of hypovitaminosis D (such as osteopenia) requires higher levels of 25-hydroxyvitamin D.[17] Scientists working in this area place the lower limit for optimum 25-hydroxyvitamin D at about 32 ng/mL (80 nmol/L).[18]

A controlled trial from our research unit demonstrated the practical value of attention to calcium and vitamin D. Older women were treated with continuous *low*-dose hormone replacement therapy (HRT) (i.e., conjugated equine estrogen, 0.3 mg/day, plus medroxyprogesterone, 2.5 mg/day), with supplementation as needed to maintain calcium intake and 25-hydroxyvitamin D at or near the levels just

TABLE 4. GENERAL DIAGNOSTIC CATEGORIES FOR ADULTS, BY RESULTS OF BMD MEASUREMENTS, WITH CORRESPONDING DIAGNOSTIC CATEGORIES AS ADOPTED BY THE WORLD HEALTH ORGANIZATION[12]

Diagnostic Category	BMD	T Score[1]
Unaffected	Not more than 1 SD below reference mean[2]	No lower than −1
Osteopenia (low bone mass)	1 to 2.5 SD below reference mean	−1 to −2.5
Osteoporosis	More than 2.5 SD below reference mean	Lower than −2.5
Established osteoporosis	More than 2.5 SD below reference mean and at least one fragility fracture at any site	Lower than −2.5

A 2000 position paper reported that validity of the World Health Organization thresholds is best when hip bone mineral density (BMD) is measured by dual-energy x-ray absorptiometry.[13]

SD, standard deviation.

[1] T scores are SD units from a reference group of young normals; Z scores, which have much less clinical usefulness, are SD units from an age-matched reference group.

[2] Reference data from white females aged 20 to 29 years.

TABLE 5. MEASUREMENT OF BONE MASS

An older adult of either sex has lost height, developed posture changes characteristic of osteoporosis, *or presents with fracture.*

A postmenopausal woman *presents with fracture.*

Starting (or stopping) hormone replacement therapy is being considered.

Treatment with glucocorticoid drugs is being started or continued.

An adult of any age and either sex has had hypogonadism, poor nutritional status, or impaired mobility that lasted for months or years.

Patient history includes a condition that is associated with low bone mass (e.g., hyperparathyroidism, hyperthyroidism, poorly monitored treatment for hypothyroidism, anorexia nervosa, lengthy amenorrhea, bowel disease, or treatment with antiseizure drugs).

The results of bone mass measurements, preferably by dual-energy x-ray absorptiometry (DXA) at the hip,[13] can facilitate decision-making by physicians and patients in the situations outlined here.

cited. A 3.5-year treatment period yielded "a bone-sparing effect that is similar or superior to that provided by other, higher-dose HRT regimens," with HRT-related symptoms that were "mild and short-lived."[18] Numerous studies list poor protein-calorie nutrition as a regular finding among hip fracture patients; in one study, positive outcomes at 6 months were dramatically higher among patients who were fed (not merely *offered*) an oral supplement (20 g protein, 2.50 kcal) daily for the first month after fracture.[19]

Authoritative and comprehensive guides to the treatment of osteoporosis arise from the efforts of periodic consensus conferences and the collaborative efforts of professional societies. Among these, the consensus statement from the NIH conference of March 2000[1] and the *Physician's Guide* from the National Osteoporosis Foundation[20] reflect the best current thinking of scientists and practitioners. Both are available online.

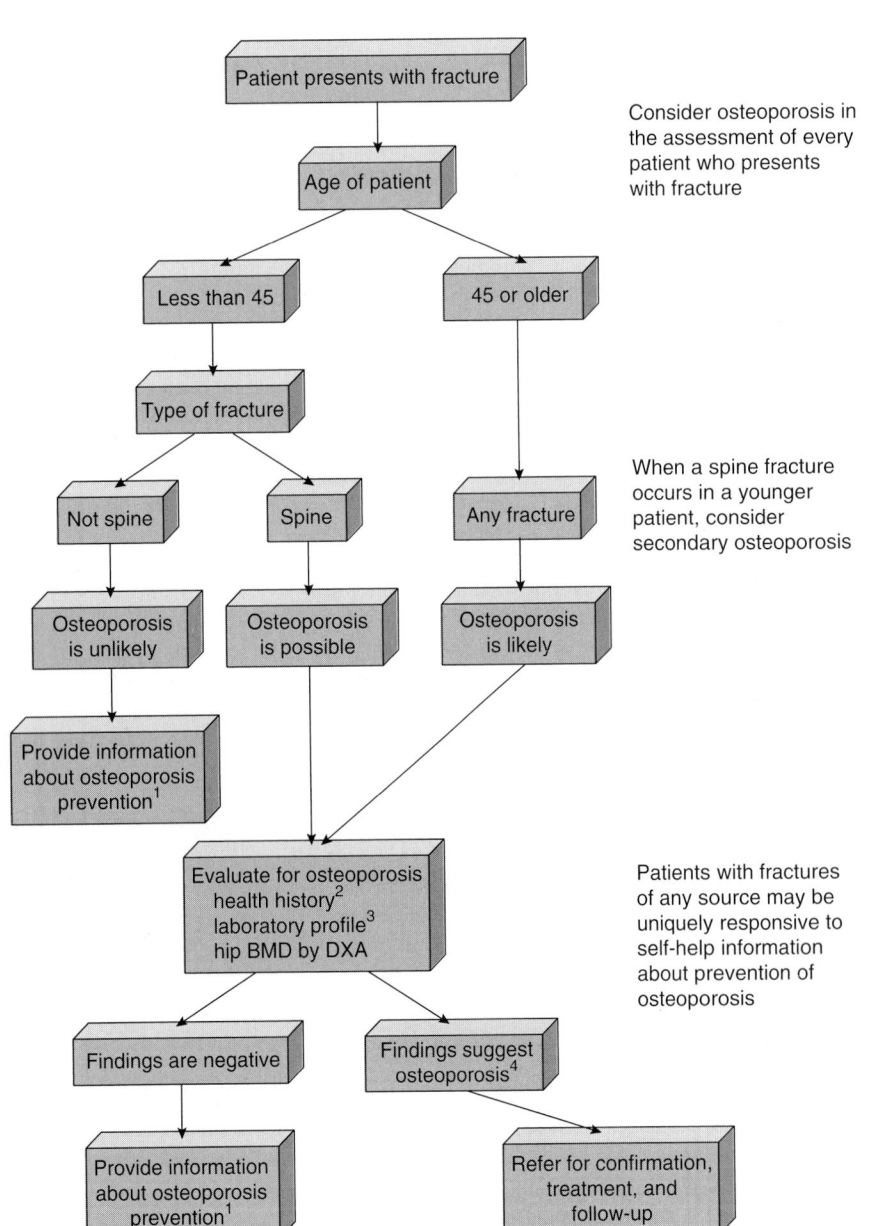

Consider osteoporosis in the assessment of every patient who presents with fracture

When a spine fracture occurs in a younger patient, consider secondary osteoporosis

Patients with fractures of any source may be uniquely responsive to self-help information about prevention of osteoporosis

Fig. 3. Diagnostic flow chart. The flow chart approaches the diagnosis of osteoporosis from the perspective of orthopaedics practice. 1, with attention to maintaining a BMI of 20–24, a calcium intake of 1000–1500 mg/d, regular physical activity, and a reliable source of vitamin D; for details, refer to the current online version of the *Physician's Guide to Prevention and Treatment of Osteoporosis*[14] at www.nof.org; 2, with attention to the items presented in Table 1; 3, CBC, multichannel serum chemistry, ESR, serum protein electrophoresis, 25-hydroxyvitamin D, serum testosterone and FSH (males only), with further analyses as indicated; 4, either primary osteoporosis or osteoporosis secondary to another health problem.

REFERENCES

1. National Institutes of Health: Osteoporosis prevention, diagnosis, and therapy: NIH consensus statement. 2000; 17:1.
2. Cooper C: Epidemiology of osteoporosis. Osteoporosis Int Suppl 1999; 2:S2.
3. Heaney RP, Barger-Lux MJ: Calcium, bone metabolism, and structural failure. Triangle 1985; 24:91.
4. Marcus R: New perspectives on the skeletal role of estrogen [editorial]. J Clin Endocrinol Metab 1998; 83:2236.
5. Gallagher JC, Melton LJ, Riggs BL, et al: Epidemiology of fractures of the proximal femur in Rochester, Minnesota. Clin Orthop 1980; 150:163.
6. Davies KM, Stegman MR, Heaney RP, et al: Prevalence and severity of vertebral fracture: The Saunders County Bone Quality Study. Osteoporosis Int 1996; 6:160.
7. O'Neill TW, Felsenberg D, Varlow J, et al: The prevalence of vertebral deformity in European men and women: The European vertebral osteoporosis study. J Bone Miner Res 1996; 11:1010.
8. Recker RR, Davies KM, Hinders SM, et al: Bone gain in young adult women. JAMA 1992; 268:2403.
9. Rizzoli R, Bonjour J-P: Determinants of peak bone mass and mechanisms of bone loss. Osteoporosis Int Suppl 1999; 2:S17.
10. Lauritzen JB: Hip fractures: Incidence, risk factors, energy absorption, and prevention. Bone 1996; 18:S65.
11. Marshall D, Johnell O, Wedel H: Meta-analysis of how well measures of bone density predict occurrence of osteoporotic fractures. BMJ 1996; 312:1254.
12. World Health Organization: Assessment of Fracture Risk and Its Application to Screening for Postmenopausal Osteoporosis (WHO technical report series 843). Geneva, World Health Organization, 1994.
13. Kanis JA, Gluer C-C for the Committee of Scientific Advisors, International Osteoporosis Foundation: An update of the diagnosis and assessment of osteoporosis with densitometry. Osteoporosis Int 2000; 11:192.
14. Maugars Y, Berthelot JM, Lalande S, et al: Osteoporosis fractures revealing anorexia nervosa in five females. Rev Rheum 1996; 63:201.
15. Heaney RP: Nutrition and risk for osteoporosis. In Marcus R, Feldman D, Kelsey J (eds): Osteoporosis. San Diego, Academic Press (in press).
16. Adams JS, Kantorovich V, Wu C, et al: Resolution of vitamin D insufficiency in osteopenic patients results in rapid recovery of bone mineral density. J Clin Endocrinol Metab 1999; 84:2729.
17. McKenna MJ, Freaney R: Defining hypovitaminosis D in the elderly. In Burckhardt P, Dawson-Hughes B, Heaney RP (eds): Nutritional Aspects of Osteoporosis. New York, Springer-Verlag, 1997, p 268.
18. Recker RR, Davies KM, Dowd RM, et al: The effect of low-dose continuous estrogen and progesterone therapy with calcium and vitamin D on bone in elderly women: A randomized, controlled trial. Ann Intern Med 1999; 130:897.
19. Delmi M, Rapin CH, Bengoa JM, et al: Dietary supplementation in elderly patients with fractured neck of the femur. Lancet 1990; 335:1013.
20. National Osteoporosis Foundation: Physician's Guide to Prevention and Treatment of Osteoporosis. Washington, DC, National Osteoporosis Foundation, 2000.

section 2 chapter 9

MUSCULOSKELETAL TUMORS, PAGET'S DISEASE, AND FIBROUS DYSPLASIA

Joseph M. Lane, Safdar N. Khan, and Margret Lobo

Summary

- A tumor is caused by mutations in genes that control cell replication.
- Treatment of a musculoskeletal tumor is determined in large part by its Musculoskeletal Tumor Society classification.
- Virus and heredity play a likely role in the cause of Paget's disease.
- Paget's disease can usually be controlled medically. Complications of Paget's disease (deformity, fracture, arthritis) are often best treated operatively.
- Second-generation bisphosphonates may be effective therapy for controlling pain and decreasing the frequency of pathological fracture in patients with fibrous dysplasia.

Because many benign tumors are never recognized, the true incidence of musculoskeletal tumors in the United States is unknown. During growth, 43% of children experience at least one hole in a bone. The majority of these spontaneously resolve and disappear by adulthood. Approximately 5000 bone and soft-tissue malignancies occur in the United States each year.[1] Osteogenic sarcoma, the most common malignant bone tumor, occurs once in 2.2 individuals per million per year. Although uncommon, malignant musculoskeletal tumors account for a large portion of the cost of musculoskeletal care, because complex and expensive care is necessary if one attempts to cure the condition.

MUSCULOSKELETAL TUMORS

BASICS OF NEOPLASIA

Tumors are clones of cells induced to aberrancy by mutations in genes that control cell replication.[2] Tumor genesis requires that two highly complex pathways be affected and uncoupled. First, the pathway responsible for DNA transcription, translation, and replication must be inappropriately turned on. Also, the pathway responsible for suppression of cell replication must become ineffective. Genes involved in cell replication that are quantitatively or qualitatively abnormal or hyperfunctional are termed oncogenes. Impaired replication suppression resulting from mutations in genes that inhibit cell proliferation is best illustrated by the growth-suppressing retinoblastoma protein (pRb). The active form of this gene is the unphosphorylated pRb protein. Conversion to the phosphorylated (inactive) form occurs in a cell cycle–dependent fashion. A normal cell cycle is divided into five stages: G_0 phase, which consists of cells that are resting; G_1 phase; S phase; G_2 phase; and M phase.

Inactivation of the pRb protein (pRb-p) occurs at the time of the G_1/S-phase transition. Phosphorylation (inactivation) occurs because of activated (phosphorylated) cyclin/cyclin-dependent kinases, which are the key intracellular regulators of cell cycle progression. Inactivation of pRb-p lasts until the late M phase, when the pRb-p dephosphorylates, thus binding and inactivating S-phase transcription factors. Unphosphorylated pRb stops cell division in the G_1 phase because of its preferential binding to various transcription factors, whereas phosphorylated rBp (pRb-p) does not bind, thus permitting continuation of the cell cycle. Interestingly, the absence of pRb has been associated with malignant phenotype. Because active or unphosphorylated pRb binds and hence inactivates essential transcription factors needed for DNA synthesis, the retinoblastoma gene is considered to be a tumor suppressor gene. Deletion or absence of this gene has been noted in the development of various cancers such as retinoblastoma, osteosarcoma, and small cell lung carcinoma.

Chromosome abnormalities may occur. Chromosomes do not need to be abnormal for the DNA to malfunction enough to produce a neoplasm. Oncogene point mutations are more common than gross chromosomal defects. A group of proteins that control cell growth division is called growth factors. Alternation of growth factors or inappropriate response to growth factors may lead to a neoplasm.

An intracellular metabolic pump known as the p-glycoprotein pump is a normal protective cell mechanism that rids toxins from cells. In addition to pumping natural toxins out of the cytoplasm, this pump eliminates the chemotherapeutic agent doxorubicin hydrochloride and other chemotherapeutic agents from the cell, thus keeping their intracellular concentration low and preventing toxic effects on the tumor cell. This produces resistance to chemotherapeutic agents.

A neoplasm is considered malignant if at least one of its cells can escape from its primary site, travel to a distant site, survive at the distant site, reproduce neoplastic cells at the new site, and attract sufficient blood supply to continue multiplying. Hematogenous metastases occur when a primary neoplasm invades local tissue, and a malignant cell invades a local vessel, comes loose, and is transported to a distant site. The cell then lodges in a capillary of a distant organ, invades the cell wall of the capillary, and enters into the adjacent tissue to produce a metastasis.

MALIGNANT VERSUS BENIGN TUMORS

Malignant tumors have the ability to metastasize (i.e., spread to a distant site and grow), whereas benign tumors do not. Occasionally, however, benign tumors such as giant cell tumor and chondroblastoma transport cells to a distant site (lung). Carcinomas are malignant tumors that arise from cells of endothelial or epithelial origin. Sarcomas are malignant tumors that arise from cells of mesenchymal origin. Tumors are further classified by histological appearance to their tissue of origin. Malignant tumors are graded on their potential for metastasis by the Musculoskeletal Tumor Society staging system.

Musculoskeletal Tumor Society Classification

The Musculoskeletal Tumor Society developed a classification system for both benign and malignant tumors. This classification system considers the histological grade, the anatomic site, and the tumor's ability to spread. Benign bone tumors are classified as stage I, those that are latent and well circumscribed within a bone. Those that demonstrate active growth, often associated with alteration in the contour of the bone in which they reside, are classified stage II. Aggressive lesions that have the potential to penetrate the bone surface and transport to lung or another distant site are classified as stage III.

Malignant tumors classified as stage IA have low-grade histological activity, are localized within an anatomic site, and have no distant spread. Stage IB tumors have low-grade histological activity, are located in more than one anatomic site, and have no evidence of distant spread. A stage IIA tumor has high-grade histological activity, is located within a single anatomic site, and has no distant spread. A stage IIB tumor has high-grade histological activity and extends beyond one anatomic site but has no distant spread. A stage IIIB tumor can be either a low- or high-grade lesion, can be in one or more anatomic sites, and has spread into either regional lymph nodes or lung.[3] Treatment programs are based on the classification and the anatomic location of the tumor.

Clinical Presentation

Benign and malignant bone tumors may be discovered incidentally in the course of evaluating another musculoskeletal disorder, as is often the case with an enchondroma of the proximal humerus. When a tumor presents with pain, the pain is frequently not affected by activity and often is present and more severe at night. The tumor may present as a palpable mass, although this is usually a later finding, except for a soft-tissue tumor. The palpable mass is frequently fixed to adjacent tissue and is often very firm. A tumor may appear to grow rapidly as a consequence of a hemorrhage within the lesion. Finally, a tumor may present as a pathological fracture, which usually occurs at the site of the lesion and after low-force trauma.

Misdiagnosis of a tumor usually occurs for one of two reasons: (1) lack of detection of an abnormality such as a laboratory or radiographic finding that suggests the neoplasm or (2) attribution of an abnormal clinical, laboratory, or radiographic finding to a benign condition. Whenever a new mass develops, it should be considered a tumor until proven otherwise. Hematomas do not occur spontaneously in patients without trauma. Muscle strain develops after an individual has performed a relatively vigorous activity or a muscle contraction sufficient to cause tissue disruption. Isolated muscle hypertrophy is not produced by exercise. Rest pain may be due to tumor, infection, or inflammation. Therefore, tumor is included in the differential diagnosis of pain, especially that occurring at night. If pain does not resolve with the usual conservative management, its diagnosis should be reconsidered because a hidden malignancy may be the cause. One cause of a low-force fracture is an underlying benign or malignant tumor.[4] Laboratory findings associated with a tumor are usually nonspecific. Occasionally, there will be constitutional symptoms or an elevated sedimentation rate. Serum alkaline phosphatase and bone formation markers may be high in bone-forming tumors. Other specific laboratory findings are not commonly abnormal, although collagen breakdown products may be elevated in rapidly growing tumors.

Radiographic evaluation of a tumor not only may lead to a specific diagnosis but is critical for defining the location and extent of the lesion. Plain radiographic images are essential for evaluation because they demonstrate the size and location of the lesion and also show the host response to the lesion. Plain radiographs also may demonstrate specific matrix characteristics of the lesion. Because benign tumors grow slowly, the host has the opportunity to develop changes such as marginal sclerosis or gradual expansion of the cortex in response to the growing tumor. Malignant tumors frequently grow quickly and may outgrow the host response, be permeative or infiltrative, and break through the cortex into adjacent soft-tissue compartments. Bone scintigraphy can indicate whether the lesion is latent or active, can indicate the presence of additional lesions, and can help in identification of skip lesions. A specialized bone scan such as a single-photon emission computed tomography scan functions much like a computed tomography (CT) scan and can give clear definition of a specific lesion. Certain rapidly growing tumors, both benign and malignant, may appear negative on a bone scan, as is sometime seen with histiocytosis X and multiple myeloma.

A CT scan and magnetic resonance imaging (MRI) can produce cross-sectional images. A CT scan demonstrates the location of the lesion and also provides a very clear picture of any ossified or calcified matrix. The MRI is much more sensitive for soft-tissue extension and has greater capability of defining subtle differences within the matrix formed by the lesion. Reactive tissue edema adjacent to the tumor may suggest that the tumor is larger than it appears. A magnetic resonance arteriogram (MRA), a variant of the MRI, can help define the vascular pattern to the lesion.

Specialized studies such as ultrasonography may be helpful in determining cystic lesions. Arteriograms are rarely used today in light of the MRA; however, an arteriogram may be part of therapeutic embolization of the lesion. The positron emission tomography (PET) scan is a measure of the metabolic activity of the tumor and is helpful in determining living versus necrotic tumor and response to preoperative chemotherapy.

Biopsy

Definite diagnosis of a lesion requires histological sampling. A biopsy can be performed by many routes, either open or percutaneously with a needle biopsy or by cytology performed using fine-needle aspiration.

Cytology can differentiate malignant from benign tumors, but it requires close collaboration with the cytology laboratory. Because a very small sample is taken, special studies for tumor activity and subtyping are difficult. Cytology is most effective in soft-tissue lesions. A fine-needle biopsy is a small biopsy. It has more capability for defining the tissue, but it also recovers only a small sample of the lesion. A fine-needle biopsy can be performed with CT guidance. An open biopsy provides a larger sample; therefore, there is greater capability for defining specific activity and special properties of the tumor. An open biopsy is most helpful in determining ossification. The rapidly growing edge of a tumor is often most diagnostic.[5]

To enhance reliability and avoid complications, (1) the biopsy should be performed in a way that does not compromise a subsequent definitive resection; (2) meticulous hemostasis must be achieved; (3) the biopsy should be performed so that it does not spread tumor to compartments that are not involved by the tumor; (4) iatrogenic complications, such as a fracture, should be avoided because of the stress-concentrating effect of the biopsy defect. These recommendations have been espoused by Aboulafia[6] based on careful review of the Musculoskeletal Tumor Society collaborative studies on hazards of biopsy.

Several studies showed that a biopsy performed at an oncology center is much more reliable in terms of the true diagnosis and tumor activity. In this age of preoperative chemotherapy, biopsy-obtained tissue may be most suitable for defining a lesion because at ultimate resection after chemotherapy, much of the tumor may have been modified or become necrotic, thus compromising one's ability to specifically identify and classify the tumor.

Surgical Margins

The treatment of a tumor depends on defining the margins of the lesion and is predicated on achieving specific resection margins determined by the activity of that specific tumor. A resection margin may be intralesional, as is often the case with curettage or piecemeal resection, which leaves tumor at the margin of the resection. A resection margin may be "marginal," as is often the case after en bloc resection or amputation through reactive tissue adjacent to the tumor. With a marginal resection, reactive tissue is left at the margin of the tumor and tumor satellites may be present at that edge. A wide margin can be achieved either by en bloc resection or amputation, which removes the tumor within the compartment by dissection through normal tissue at all sites. There is the potential for a skip lesion or lesions located beyond the resection, even though all resection surfaces consist of normal tissue. A radical resection or amputation removes entire anatomic compartments that contain the tumor and leaves only normal tissue in the patient.

The resection margin indicated for control of a benign stage I tumor is usually intralesional. The resection margin indicated for control of a benign stage II tumor is either marginal or intralesional, plus an effective adjuvant, such as phenol, cryosurgery (liquid nitrogen), or methylmethacrylate. The resection margin indicated for control of a benign stage III tumor is either a wide or marginal resection plus an effective adjuvant. Adjuvant treatment of a benign tumor is usually phenol, cryosurgery, or methylmethacrylate.

For a malignant stage IA or IB tumor, treatment should include wide excision. For a malignant stage IIA or IIB tumor, treatment should include wide excision plus effective adjuvant therapy. For a malignant stage III tumor, with lung involvement, treatment should include a thoracotomy plus wide excision or, in patients with a poor prognosis, just a palliative procedure. An amputation does not produce a better cure rate than a limb salvage operation as long as the resection margins of the two operations are equal.[7] A high-grade malignant tumor will respond to adjuvant preoperative chemotherapy, and local control can be enhanced by radiotherapy preoperatively, postoperatively, or immediately postoperatively using the brachycatheter technique (see Chapter 7–3).

BENIGN BONE TUMORS
Osteoid Osteoma
Osteoid osteoma is a benign tumor that has a richly innervated nidus less than 2 cm in diameter and consists of primitive woven bone and osteoid. It is found in children and young adults and accounts for approximately 1% of benign bone tumors. The diagnosis is suggested by the presence of a lesion causing nighttime pain that is dramatically relieved by nonsteroidal anti-inflammatory medication. Radiographically, one sees a dense sclerotic area in a juxtacortical location with a central lytic nidus (Fig. 1).

If the lesion is in cancellous bone adjacent to a joint, sclerosis may not be present, and there may be clear evidence of associated arthritis with synovial effusion. The lesion is easily identified by radiograph, bone scan, or a thin-cut CT scan through the suspicious area.

Treatment includes long-acting nonsteroidal medication, which yields a cure rate of more than 50%. However, a cure may require 4 years of treatment. Lesions associated with scoliosis or joint disease or that have failed nonoperative management may be suitable for surgical ablation. Preoperative planning should include precise localization of the tumor with a CT scan, planar tomography, and in some cases a Geiger-Mueller counter used intraoperatively after preoperative radioisotope labeling of the lesion or intraoperative fluorescence of preoperatively administered tetracycline in ultraviolet light (Wood's lamp). A new therapeutic modality consists of CT localization of the lesion followed by radiofrequency ablation with a probe inserted percutaneously. Tumor recurrence is possible. An osteoid osteoma produces prostaglandins. Treatment of a recurrent lesion is difficult because these small lesions are often hidden in postoperative bone sclerosis.

Osteoblastoma
Osteoblastoma, a rare bone-forming tumor, accounts for 3% of benign bone tumors. A typical osteoblastoma is larger than 2 cm. Diagnosis of an osteoblastoma should be considered if the lesion is painful but does not have as dramatic a response to nonsteroidal medication as an osteoid osteoma. In addition, an osteoblastoma may not produce nighttime pain. An osteoblastoma has a sclerotic border with a lytic center located in the medullary portion of a bone. An osteoblastoma also can occur in the posterior portion (neural arch) of the spine. Growth of this tumor produces a fusiform expansion of the bone. Radiographs, bone scan, and especially CT scans are very effective in identifying the lesion and demonstrating its matrix, size, shape, and location (Fig. 2).

Recommended treatment of an osteoblastoma is complete marginal resection or an intralesional resection (curettage) plus an effective adjuvant, such as phenol, liquid nitrogen, or methylmethacrylate, or resection of noncritical bones. Cryosurgery, radiation, or chemotherapy may be used on lesions of this kind that are not fully resectable. After radiation, 1% to 2% of osteoblastomas progress to a low-grade osteogenic sarcoma. Whether they were osteogenic sarcoma initially or were converted to a malignancy by the radiation is uncertain. Osteoblastomas account for 3% of benign bone tumors.

Osteochondroma
Osteochondroma is a benign developmental growth located in the metaphyseal area of a long bone. The lesion has an osseous base in continuity with the cortex and the medullary canal of the host bone, and it has a cartilaginous cap. The cartilage cap will continue to grow as long as the adjacent epiphyseal plate or apophyseal plate is open. Osteochondroma is the most common benign skeletal tumor. It usually occurs singly as a random event. However, a relatively rare autosomal-dominant form of osteochondroma has multiple lesions and may cause severe growth deformities, affecting both bone length and alignment.

An osteochondroma may or may not be symptomatic. It usually comes to clinical attention because of its mass, which may cause limitation of motion of an adjacent joint. An osteochondroma can occasionally cause pain by irritating tendons that move over the osteochondral lesion mass. Histologically, an osteochondroma has a cartilaginous cap

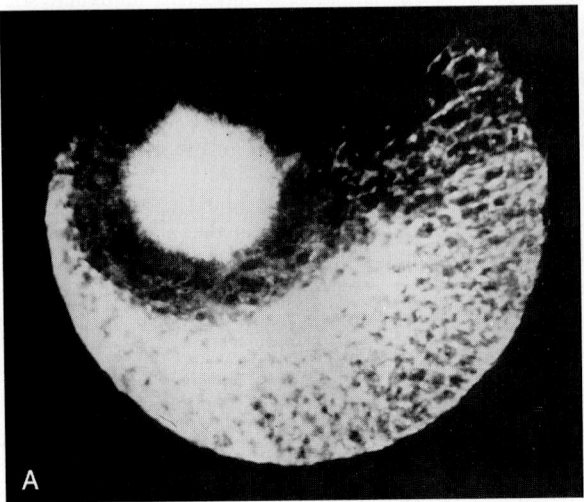 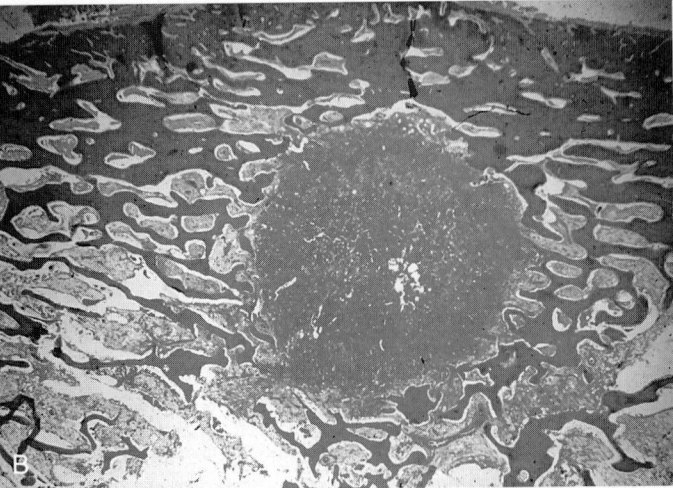

Fig. 1. Osteoid osteoma specimen. *A,* Radiograph of an osteoid osteoma demonstrates the nidus. *B,* Histology of the same specimen is shown.

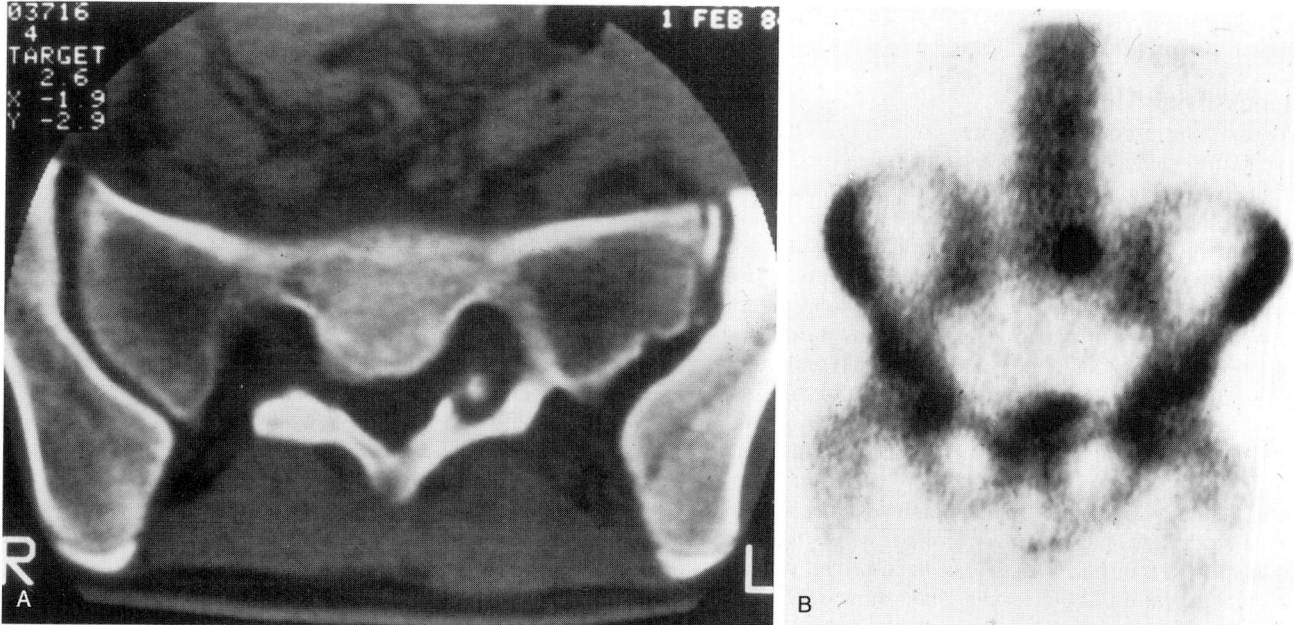

Fig. 2. Osteoblastoma. *A,* CT scan shows an osteoblastoma in the posterior element of the sacrum. *B,* A bone scan demonstrates increased uptake in the sacrum.

and underlying bone that has a direct connection with the adjacent medullary canal.

A plain radiograph is usually sufficient for diagnosis, but a CT scan may be helpful in defining the lesion's orientation to the host bone. An MRI may be helpful in evaluating osteochondroma in adults to determine whether the cartilaginous cap is present and growing. A cartilaginous cap more than 1 cm thick in a skeletally mature individual should be reviewed carefully to be sure that the cartilage is not malignant.

An osteochondroma can be monitored conservatively if the lesion is small and the cartilaginous cap is 0.5 cm thick or less. If the lesion causes complaints because of its size, it should be excised with the perichondrium and periosteum down to the lesion's bony base. If the perichondrium is not removed, recurrence is possible. Other reasons for treatment include tendinitis and growth after skeletal maturity.

Malignant transformation of an osteochondroma is rare, occurring in less than 1% of cases. Malignant transformation is seen most frequently with multiple osteochondromas and is associated with a cartilage cap that is 1 cm thick or more.

Enchondroma

An enchondroma consists of mature benign cartilage. Malignant transformation is rare. Enchondroma, usually a solitary lesion, accounts for 25% of benign bone tumors and is quite common in the small bones of the hands and the feet. Relatively rare multiple enchondromatosis (Ollier's disease) causes bony deformities and has a higher rate of malignant degeneration.

An enchondroma is diagnosed with the aid of a plain radiograph, which demonstrates a long oval lesion in the bone. It is usually lobulated and typically has a sharply

demarcated margin. Calcification may or may not be present within the lesion. However, calcification, when present, is best seen on a CT scan and is highly suggestive of cartilage. Most enchondromas have a positive bone scan. An active bone scan of an enchondroma does not indicate malignancy. Malignant degeneration is suggested if the lesion has marked marginal scalloping or causes expansion of the bone or persistent night pain or if definite growth is noted on serial radiographs.

Recommended treatment is careful observation with serial radiographic examinations to demonstrate that there is little or no growth. If the lesion has scalloping along its edge, a marginal intralesional resection is suggested. Local recurrence after this procedure is extremely uncommon for a true enchondroma, assuming that all lesional cells have been removed.

Multiple enchondromatosis is associated with shortening and angular deformities of the appendicular skeleton. Malignant degeneration occurs in 25% of patients with multiple enchondromatosis. When multiple enchondromatosis is associated with calcified hemangiomas, it is known as Maffucci's syndrome. Malignancy occurs in more than 70% of patients with Maffucci's syndrome.

Chondroblastoma

Chondroblastoma is an epiphyseal tumor that occurs in adolescence. It occurs more frequently in boys than girls. Approximately two-thirds of chondroblastomas occur in the proximal humerus, the distal femur, and the proximal tibia. Chondroblastomas occur in an apophysis or an epiphyseal ossification center. Diagnostic imaging studies show a lucent epiphyseal abnormality with or without fine calcifications within the lesion.

The recommended treatment is intralesional curettage combined with local adjuvant such as phenol or liquid nitrogen. Local recurrence is about 14%. The lesion is known to rarely transport to the lung.

Nonossifying Fibroma

Nonossifying fibroma and fibrous cortical defect lesions are essentially identical except for location. Nonossifying fibroma occurs in bone, whereas fibrous cortical defect occurs on the surface of a bone. They are benign tumors that are usually solitary with a predilection for the diaphysis of long bones. Nonossifying fibroma and fibrous cortical defect lesions are found in up to 30% to 40% of children between the ages of 4 and 8 years. Nonossifying fibromas are most frequently found in the metaphyseal region of a long bone. A nonossifying fibroma may cause pain as a result of weakening of the cortex and may present as a partial fracture. Fibrous cortical defects are found incidentally.

A plain radiograph is usually diagnostic, so that additional studies are not necessary if the lesion is well circumscribed. MRI can help identify an unsuspected partial pathological fracture. A bone scan may show mild increased activity. A fibrous cortical defect usually heals spontaneously. If a nonossifying fibroma is associated with pain or fracture, the physician should wait until the fracture has healed before performing curettage with or without a bone graft. A recurrence is extremely unusual.

Giant Cell Tumor

Giant cell tumor is an aggressive benign tumor that almost always is located in the epiphysis and the metaphysis of a long bone. Giant cell tumor is usually a solitary lesion that becomes symptomatic if enough bone stock has been replaced by the lesion. Most giant cell tumors occur after the epiphyseal plate has closed. Pain without an obvious pathological fracture is the most frequent presenting complaint. Most patients with a giant cell tumor experience local pain, swelling, and tenderness. Calcium levels are normal but must be evaluated to differentiate a giant cell tumor from a brown tumor caused by systemic hyperparathyroidism.

A radiograph usually demonstrates that the lesion has destroyed both medullary and cortical bone. A giant cell tumor is characterized by an expanding zone of radiolucency located in the end of a long bone. Frequently, the tumor presents with expansion of the cortex, and a few may break through the cortex of the bone and the periosteum. The treatment of choice is thorough curettage plus adjuvant therapy. The most frequently used adjuvant therapy is methylmethacrylate packing of the operative defect in bone. Alternative treatments include phenol and cryosurgery. For unresectable giant cell tumors such as those located in the pelvis or spine, radiation therapy can be used but is associated with malignant degeneration. Giant cell tumors that occur in expendable bones can be resected.

Aneurysmal Bone Cyst

An aneurysmal bone cyst is an expansile cyst of bone that has a high rate of local recurrence. Aneurysmal bone cyst occurs throughout childhood and early adulthood. It is frequently encountered in the proximal humerus, the femur, the tibia, and the ileum. An aneurysmal bone cyst may be superimposed on another preexisting lesion such as a chondroblastoma, fibrous dysplasia, or giant cell tumor.

Diagnostic radiographs show an expansile lytic lesion that usually causes cortical thinning. Differential diagnosis includes simple bone cyst and a low-grade malignancy. The diagnosis can be clarified by a CT scan and an MRI. These studies can help determine whether there is soft-tissue extension of the lesion. Treatment of an aneurysmal bone cyst may include curettage and bone grafting. Local adjuvant therapy such as cryosurgery or phenol may decrease recurrences.

Simple Bone Cyst

A simple bone cyst, also called a unicameral bone cyst, usually occurs in a long bone. When located adjacent to an epiphyseal plate, a simple bone cyst may be quite active. When located at a distance from the epiphyseal plate, it is usually inactive. Simple bone cyst occurs in childhood and has a high fracture rate.

Simple bone cyst is diagnosed by visualizing a lytic lesion that expands the bone and is associated with a fracture. An MRI may demonstrate fluid within the lytic lesion. Treatment of a unicameral bone cyst includes steroid injection using two needles. Data suggest that insertion of demineralized bone matrix and marrow into the cyst may help in the healing. The steroid injection treatment is associated with a 60% to 70% cure rate.

Eosinophilic Granuloma

Eosinophilic granuloma is a destructive lesion in bone composed mostly of benign histiocytes as well as a varying number of eosinophils. Eosinophilic granuloma is a common disease usually seen in children between the ages of 2 and 10 years. Fifty percent of patients with eosinophilic granuloma have more than one lesion. When located in the metaphyseal or diaphyseal region, an eosinophilic granuloma can be associated with a vigorous periosteal reaction. Lesions with nearly identical histology are seen in more generalized multisystem disease known as either Hand-Schüller-Christian syndrome or Letterer-Siwe disease. Hand-Schüller-Christian syndrome occurs in children aged 3 through 12 years and is associated with diabetes insipidus, exophthalmos, and hepatosplenomegaly. Letterer-Siwe syndrome is very rare, occurs in much younger children, and has a very poor, often fatal prognosis (see Chapter 9–7).

An eosinophilic granuloma can usually be diagnosed radiographically but should almost always be confirmed histologically. Many of these lesions do not have increased activity on a bone scan. Therefore, plain radiograph images are necessary to stage these lesions. Cross-sectional imaging such as a CT scan and an MRI may be helpful. Recommended treatment is curettage. Treatment using radioablative frequency or percutaneous steroid injection, or both, has been reported. The precise role of these new treatment modalities has yet to be determined.

COMMON BENIGN SOFT-TISSUE TUMORS
Lipoma

Lipoma, the most common soft-tissue tumor, occurs in all age groups and is most frequently found near the shoulder, back, and neck. A lipoma is characteristically soft and grows very slowly.

Imaging studies with an MRI or a CT scan can be helpful in differentiating a benign lipoma from a liposarcoma. A lipoma is best treated by careful observation.

Simple excision, which is almost always successful, should be reserved for lesions that grow or are troublesome because of their location.

COMMON MALIGNANT BONE TUMORS
Osteogenic Sarcoma (Osteosarcoma)

Osteogenic sarcoma is a malignant bone tumor characterized by formation of sarcomatous bone by malignant cells. Most osteosarcomas occur in adolescence with a second peak in late adulthood associated with Paget's disease or previous radiation. At presentation, most osteosarcomas already have micrometastases to the lung. Osteosarcomas occur most often in the metaphyseal area of long bones and can present with a pathological fracture. They are characterized by periosteal elevation, cortical breakthrough, and new bone formation under the periosteum.

An osteosarcoma is usually diagnosed radiographically and is confirmed by a biopsy. MRI best demonstrates the soft-tissue extent of the lesion. CT is most useful for determining whether metastasis to the lung has occurred. A bone scan is the best modality to identify and locate a skip lesion (Fig. 3).

Treatment of osteogenic sarcoma consists of a combination of adjuvant chemotherapy to destroy the micrometastasis and shrink the local tumor. This is followed by either a wide or a radical surgical excision of the lesion, which can be either a limb salvage operation or an amputation. The cure rate for osteogenic sarcoma is the same as for amputation or limb salvage as long as an equally wide margin of normal tissue is removed en bloc on all sides of the tumor in continuity with the tumor.

Currently, the cure rate for osteogenic sarcoma is 60% to 70%. Prognosis is improved in patients who demonstrate a definite favorable response to preoperative chemotherapy.

Ewing's Sarcoma

Ewing's sarcoma is a relatively common tumor occurring in childhood and early adulthood. Ewing's sarcoma is a small cell malignancy whose cause is not clear. The malignant cell has minimal cytoplasm. Ewing's sarcoma can occur in flat bones such as the ileum or the scapula or in the diaphysis of a long bone. Ewing's sarcoma is frequently associated with an elevated sedimentation rate, fever, and a large soft-tissue mass.

The diagnosis can be made by imaging studies. Plain radiographs demonstrate the infiltrative permeative lesion with elevation of the periosteum and a large soft-tissue mass. The large soft-tissue mass is best seen on MRI. This highly malignant lesion is usually treated with a combination of adjuvant chemotherapy and, when possible, resection of the tumor. When adequate resection is not possible, high-dose radiation produces an excellent initial tumor response but has an overall poor prognosis, although it can occasionally produce a cure. Sarcoma can occur in patients treated by radiation.

Chondrosarcoma

Chondrosarcomas commonly affect older adults but can occur, albeit rarely, in younger individuals. Chondrosarcomas are malignant cartilaginous tumors. The most common chondrosarcomas are difficult to differentiate histologically from an enchondroma. Chondrosarcoma is a slow-growing tumor that causes endosteal scalloping and expansion of the cortex. A grade II chondrosarcoma has more histological features of malignancy and more aggressive growth. A grade III chondrosarcoma is a highly malignant tumor. A grade III chondrosarcoma variant known as a dedifferentiated chondrosarcoma has a high rate of metastasis and a very poor prognosis.

On plain radiographs a chondrosarcoma appears as an expansile lesion with internal calcifications. A chondrosarcoma can be differentiated from an enchondroma by endosteal scalloping, cortical breakthrough, and areas of lysis within the tumor. Chondrosarcomas occur in the metaphysis, diaphysis, and occasionally in the epiphysis.

Treatment of a chondrosarcoma should consist of resection of the lesion. Borderline lesions may be treated with curettage and adjuvant therapies, but frank grade II and grade III chondrosarcomas clearly need at least a wide surgical margin. Chondrosarcoma does not respond well to radiotherapy. Only the grade III and dedifferentiated chondrosarcomas have some response to adjuvant chemotherapy. The prognosis of grade III chondrosarcoma is poor; survival rates range from 10% to 40%. Grade I chondrosarcomas have an excellent prognosis, with cure rates of 90% or more and a very low rate of late metastasis.

Malignant Fibrous Histiocytoma

Malignant fibrous histiocytoma is a non-bone-forming malignancy of bone or soft tissue that consists of fibrous tissue and histiocytes. Malignant fibrous histiocytoma occurs in all age groups and is occasionally found in areas adjacent to avascular necrosis or trauma. There is no diagnostic laboratory abnormality. Malignant fibrous histiocytomas are lytic lesions that destroy bone and can broach the cortex.

Diagnostic radiographic images show a lytic lesion with breakthrough and poor margination. MRI is the best method for defining the margins of the tumor. A bone scan is usually positive.

Treatment for a malignant fibrous histiocytoma consists of adjuvant chemotherapy in high-grade lesions and complete surgical resection (at least a wide margin) in all lesions. These tumors may be treated with radiotherapy but with very minimal benefit.

Multiple Myeloma

Multiple myeloma is a primary bone tumor that can occur in multiple locations. It is a tumor of plasma cells that occurs in people older than 40 years. A benign variant, plasmacytoma, does occur, but almost all cases convert to typical malignant multiple myeloma with time. Multiple myeloma is associated with severe osteoporosis and marked fragility of bone. Discrete lytic lesions may occur at multiple sites. Multiple myeloma is usually associated with a high sedimentation rate and anemia, and patients may have a high serum calcium level.

Radiographic evidence of osteopenia is usually diagnostic. One can see multiple active lesions in a bone scan. However, many myeloma sites may be negative on bone scan, whereas the MRI is characteristic of a permeative marrow-packing disorder. The diagnosis of multiple myeloma is assisted by immunoelectrophoresis of the serum or the urine or both. A single narrow spike on immunoelectrophoresis studies is diagnostic, although 2% of patients will have negative results. Bone marrow biopsy is diagnostic and is the gold standard.

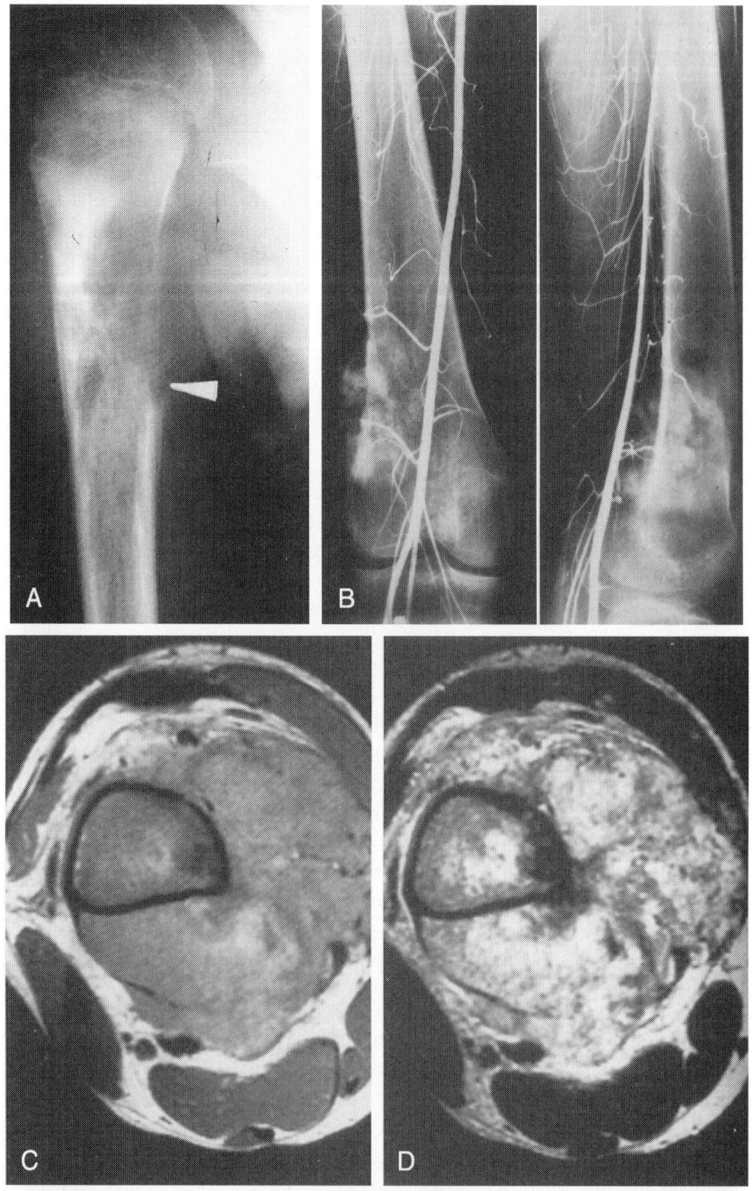

Fig. 3. Osteogenic sarcoma. *A,* An anteroposterior radiograph shows an osteosarcoma of the humerus with a Codman's triangle *(arrowhead). B,* An arteriogram demonstrates an osteosarcoma of the distal femur. *C* and *D,* Axial magnetic resonance images of an osteosarcoma of the distal femur show soft-tissue extent of disease, including association with major neurovascular bundles and muscle groups. (From Stark D, Bradley W: Magnetic Resonance Imaging. Philadelphia, CV Mosby, 1999, 3rd ed, vol 2, p 860.) *E,* This serial bone scan demonstrates a distal femur osteosarcoma: a comparison of technetium bone scan before and after chemotherapy shows mild improvement. *F,* Histology of osteosarcoma with sarcomatous osteoid formation is demonstrated.

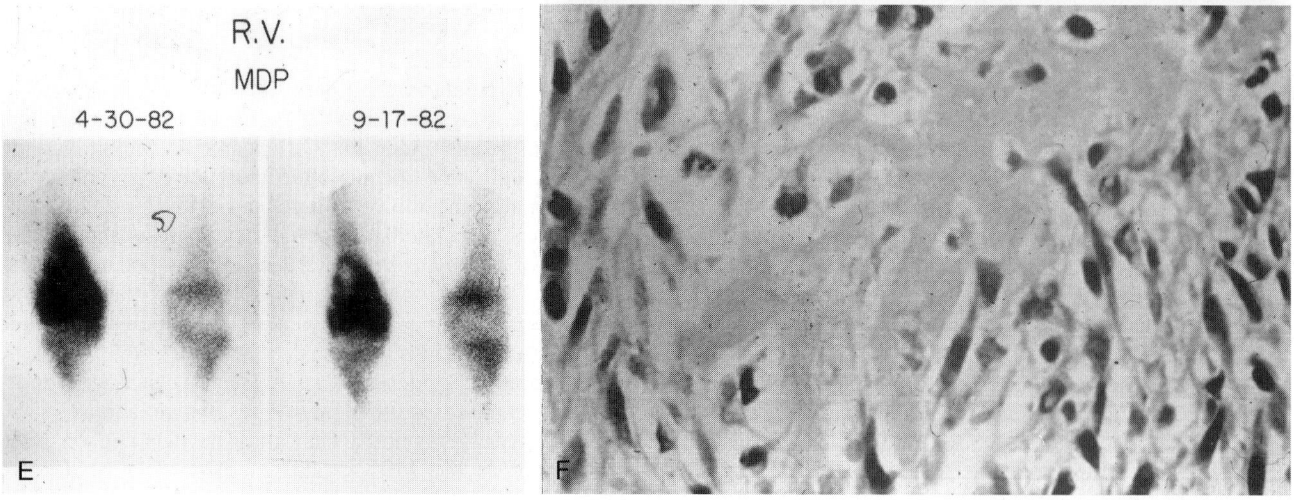

Treatment usually consists of high-dose chemotherapy and selective radiation. Pathological fractures, which are common, are best treated with stabilization of the whole bone from end to end.

COMMON SOFT-TISSUE MALIGNANCIES
Liposarcoma
Liposarcoma is a common disease. Low-grade liposarcoma can be difficult to differentiate from a large benign lipoma. They both occur in superficial and deep soft tissue and in multiple sites, although most liposarcomas arise deep to the investing muscle fascia and most benign lipomas arise superficial to this fascia. A large liposarcoma can have a calcified margin. There are no laboratory abnormalities. The diagnosis is usually suggested by imaging studies of the lesion and is confirmed by biopsy. Liposarcoma is treated with operative resection; one should strive for at least a wide resection margin. If the lesion is high grade and greater than 10 cm in diameter, radiotherapy is an option. The effectiveness of chemotherapy alone as a treatment modality is uncertain at this time.

Synovial Sarcoma
Synovial sarcoma may be either monophasic or biphasic. The monophasic variety is highly lethal with a very poor prognosis. Synovial sarcoma can occur in soft tissues usually adjacent to a joint but outside the joint along tendons and ligaments. A low-grade, slow-growing synovial sarcoma is often seen with internal calcification.

The diagnosis is first suggested by radiographs showing calcification. In addition, MRIs can be used. Lymph node spread can occur, especially in the epithelial variety. A synovial sarcoma is best treated with high-dose chemotherapy, resection, and radiation, either before or after the operative resection. Radiation therapy administered with radiation catheters at surgery is another good treatment option (see Chapter 7–3). Prognosis for the monophasic variety of synovial sarcoma is poor, although there are long-term survivors. Biphasic synovial sarcomas, especially those associated with calcification, have a good prognosis.

SUMMARY
Benign and malignant tumors occur frequently within the musculoskeletal system. Benign tumors are easily treated once diagnosis is made. Some lesions are self-curing, and others require simple curettage or another intralesional procedure. Aggressive benign tumors require either resection or an intralesional operation with an adjuvant. Malignant tumors require at least a wide resection. If they are high grade, they also require adjuvant systemic chemotherapy. Radiotherapy is helpful in the treatment of soft-tissue malignancies, which may have a skip lesion unidentified at surgery. Malignant bone and soft-tissue musculoskeletal tumors are relatively uncommon compared with certain types of carcinomas (e.g., breast, lung, prostate). Unfortunately, malignant bone and soft-tissue musculoskeletal tumors are frequently diagnosed late because of confusion with a common benign orthopaedic disorder. Patients who have nighttime pain or who do not experience the normal pattern of response to treatment should be reevaluated for an underlying malignant tumor that may have been missed. Oncological therapy has led to high cure rates for most tumors, especially in the ability to save an involved limb.

PAGET'S DISEASE

In 1876 Sir James Paget described a disease that begins in middle age or later. Long bones of the lower extremity, the pelvis, and the skull are affected most frequently. Paget noted that the affected bones enlarged and softened, so that those bearing weight yielded and became unnaturally curved and misshapen. Paget identified the condition as a chronic inflammation of bone and named it osteitis deformans. Over the last 125 years, much knowledge about Paget's disease has been gained, including a better understanding of the disorder, characterization of the pathophysiology, and a large array of highly effective treatment modalities.

Paget's disease is a localized, grossly deforming bone-remodeling disorder (Fig. 4). Approximately 3% of the population older than 40 years are afflicted by the disease; diagnosis in individuals younger than 40 years is unusual.

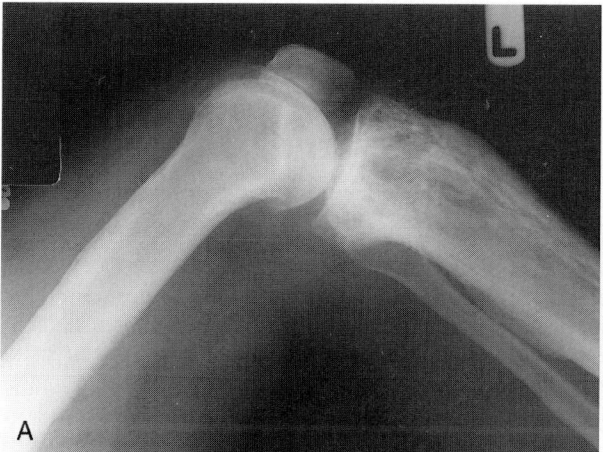
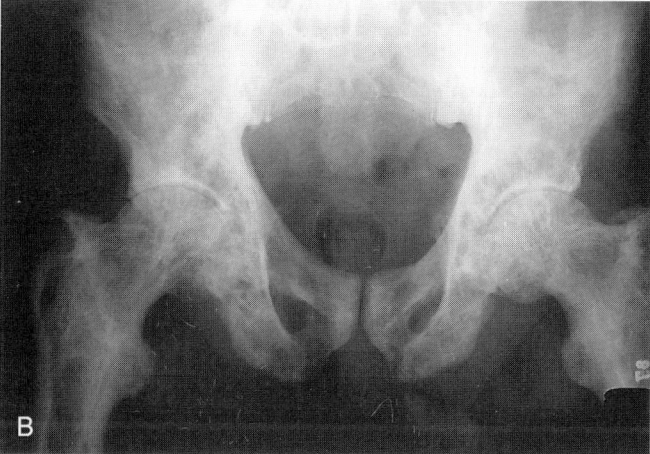

Fig. 4. Paget's disease. *A,* In this view showing Paget's disease of the tibia, expansion and clustered excessive bone formation are evident. *B,* In this patient with Paget's disease of pelvis and femurs, note the distorted remodeled bone. The patient's hips have mild deformity and arthritis with narrowed joint space.

Only 5% of patients present with pain at the abnormal site. The pathophysiology of the disease is unknown, but abnormal osteoclasts are certainly involved and initiate the remodeling event. Osteoblasts then rapidly form new, poor-quality bone in a haphazard fashion. Osteoclasts in diseased bone are markedly increased in number and size and can contain as many as 100 nuclei, and they contain paramyxoviral-like nuclear inclusions. Osteoclast precursors from patients with Paget's disease were found to be hyper-responsive to 1,25-dihydroxyvitamin D_3, and osteoclast-like multinucleated cells formed more rapidly in marrow culture of patients. Additionally, these cells produced increased levels of interleukin-6 (IL-6) and expressed high levels of IL-6 receptors. Increased concentrations of IL-6 are detectable in bone marrow and peripheral blood of patients with Paget's disease. Enhanced IL-6 production and hypersensitivity of osteoclasts to the marrow milieu may partially explain increased bone turnover at sites other than the primary lesion.

Characteristic remodeling in Paget's disease begins at one end of a bone and is associated with increased bone resorption by large abnormal osteoclasts. As the zone of resorption passes along the bone, the affected bone begins to undergo a series of resorption and formation sequences leading to a mosaic pattern of crossed small segments of collagen and woven bone. Although woven bone appears substantial in a radiograph, it is, in fact, weak. Remodeling causes the bone to become enlarged and deformed, extremely brittle, and susceptible to a pathological fracture.

Virus infection of osteoclasts in pagetic bone may be responsible for the remodeling. Microfilaments resembling members of the paramyxoviral nucleocapsid family have been found in most of the diseased osteoclasts. In situ hybridization demonstrated the presence of paramyxoviral antigens in pagetic osteoclasts but not in nonpagetic osteoclasts from the same patient.[8] Viral messenger RNA (mRNA) sequences have been detected in pagetic specimens by some but not all investigators.[9, 10] There is little evidence that the suspected viral agents within the osteoclast are infectious. Cloning of the microfilament is necessary for definite identification of a virus and to demonstrate an etiological relationship to the disease. There is a definite genetic component that predisposes one to Paget's disease. An epidemiological study in Spain observed that more than 40% of their index patients had at least one first-degree relative with Paget's disease. In this cohort, transmission was autosomal dominant.[11] In a U.S. survey, 12% of patients with Paget's disease were noted to have a first-degree relative with the disease. In familial Paget's disease, the disease segregates within chromosome 18. Paget's disease may be produced by a viral infection in a genetically susceptible host.

Paget's disease is a common disorder in certain parts of the world, including England, western Europe, and the United States. Up to 8% to 10% of the elderly population in these countries have Paget's disease. One-third are diagnosed incidentally. One-third are symptomatic from Paget's disease, and one-third have complications of Paget's disease, including deformity and fracture.

Symptomatic individuals may experience deformity, pain, local warmth, tenderness, and swelling. The direct cause of the pain is probably multifactorial. The pain may be due to increased vascularity within the lesion, microfractures from expanding lytic lesions, or abnormal mechanical stresses caused by deformity.

The bones most commonly affected are the femur, pelvis, spine, skull, and tibia. Radiographic findings of Paget's disease include a lytic wedge of resorption followed by osteoblastic widening of the bone with loss of a clear trabecular pattern and associated deformity. A disorganized intramedullary space with widening of the cortex and periosteal enlargement is seen radiographically.

Laboratory findings associated with Paget's disease include elevation of bone-forming markers, such as bone-specific alkaline phosphatase and osteocalcin, and, more importantly, an elevation of collagen breakdown products highlighted by the elevation of N-telopeptide, pyrodinoline peptide, and deoxypyrodinoline peptides. The degree of elevation of these indexes approximates the severity of abnormal bone turnover. Alkaline phosphatase levels greater than 10 times the upper limit of normal typically signify skull involvement.

Treatment with bisphosphonate compounds pamidronate, alendronate, and risedronate achieves approximately 80% reduction in the biochemical indexes of bone turnover compared with 50% reduction achieved with salmon calcitonin and etidronate. Suppression of the remodeling process can ameliorate certain symptoms (pain, warmth, headache, and neural compression) in most patients. The newer agents are also successful in inducing remission of 1 year or longer after a single course of treatment for 50% to 75% of patients. After treatment with the new bisphosphonates the healing bone is lamellar, and it does not have a mineralization defect. With the newer pharmacological agents, it may be possible to arrest progression and prevent long-term complications. Current medical management attempts to obtain normal biochemical indexes after treatment. Once biochemical remission is achieved, serum biochemical indexes should be obtained every 4 to 6 months. Retreatment is recommended if serum biochemical indexes increase 25% above baseline or rise above the upper limit of normal.

Medical management is currently warranted for patients with Paget's disease who have elevation of collagen breakdown products and for those with lower extremity involvement. Although genetic and infectious approaches to prevention and treatment of Paget's disease have promise, the excellent results with bisphosphonates are currently the best treatment for preventing progression or complications of Paget's disease.

Operative treatment of Paget's disease is indicated for complications (deformity, pathological fracture) of the disease. Operations greatly improve the quality of life for these patients. Because of the associated deformity and abnormal intramedullary space, intramedullary devices are seldom applicable for treatment of a pathological fracture in Paget's disease. Single or double plates, or a combination, are usually more effective. Occasionally, an osteotomy may be performed to restore rotatory and angular alignment. Arthritis, although common in Paget's disease, is usually congruent and often responds well to nonsteroidal anti-inflammatory medication. Occasionally, a joint replacement may be necessary. For arthritis in a patient with Paget's disease, joint replacement can produce excellent results with minimal blood loss, because arthritis in Paget's disease usually occurs in "burned-out" areas of the disease. Complications of surgical treatment of pagetic bone include hemorrhage, infection, fracture, delayed union, nonunion, and aseptic loosening of hardware. Sarcomatous change in pagetic bone, particularly in the spine, is associated with a very high mortality rate. Paget's osteosarcoma occurs in the humerus in one-third of cases. Cure, after either amputation or limb salvage and chemotherapy, is much more likely in these cases than in Paget's osteosarcoma located elsewhere.

Paget's disease may have a genetic cause: up to 40% of individuals in a single family have been noted to have Paget's disease. More work is needed to determine the genetic and molecular character of this disease. The intracellular virus particles that have been observed may be etiological or may be a coevent. If a virus does play a role in the pathogenesis of Paget's disease, development of a vaccine or use of antiviral medication is likely to be helpful.

FIBROUS DYSPLASIA

Fibrous dysplasia is a rare, non–gender-selective, noninherited congenital disorder most commonly recognized before the age of 30 years. The hallmark of this disease is extensive proliferation of fibrous tissue and immature woven bone within the bone marrow, causing osteolytic lesions leading to pathological fractures. The proliferative cells in the marrow stroma express alkaline phosphatase. The fibrotic lesions within the bone contain mature, but abnormal, osteoblasts. Fibrous dysplasia represents approximately 2.5% of known bone disorders and comprises about 7% of benign bone tumors.[12] Fibrous dysplasia most commonly occurs in the long bones, the ribs, and the skull. However, any bone may be affected. The symptom complex may include bone pain, localized deformity, and repeated pathological fractures of the affected bone during childhood and adolescence. Fibrous dysplasia occurring in only one location (monostotic) is approximately six times more common than fibrous dysplasia occurring in multiple locations (polyostotic).[13]

The polyostotic form may occur in conjunction with café au lait spots (hyperpigmented macules with rough borders) and multiple endocrinopathy, generally as a result of end-organ hyperactivity. This combination of findings is the McCune-Albright syndrome, a mosaic gene disorder with a G protein dysfunction.[14] Excessive production of IL-6 may be a pathogenic factor, because mesenchymal cells proliferate but do not differentiate into osteoblasts.

The lesions are well defined, characterized by thin cortices and a ground-glass appearance radiographically (Fig. 5). The lesions can be lobulated with trabeculated areas of radiolucency. Laboratory findings of bone remodeling are either normal or slightly elevated. Histologically, the lesions consist of spindle-shaped swirls of fibroblasts within the marrow. Within the well-defined lesion are trabeculae of woven bone, and cystic regions lined by multinucleated

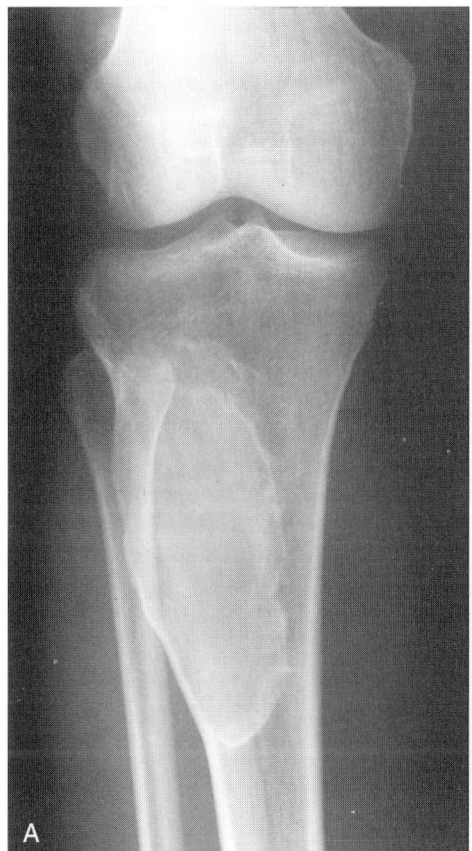
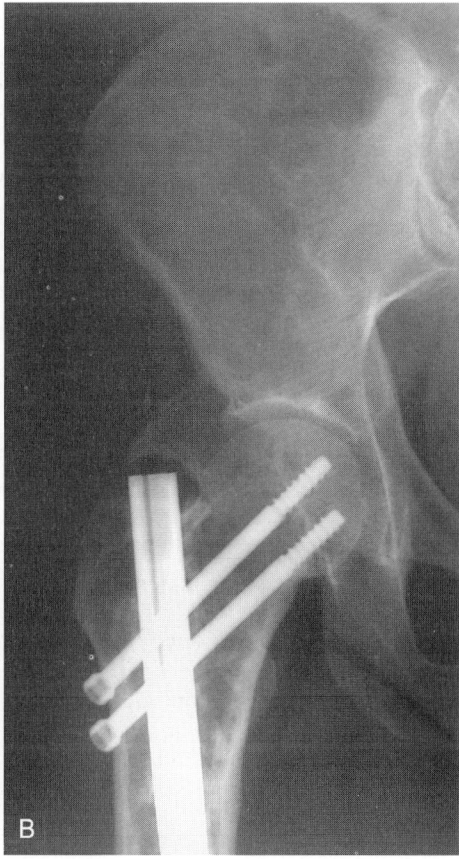

Fig. 5. Fibrous dysplasia. *A,* In this view showing fibrous dysplasia of the proximal tibia, note the expansion and ground-glass appearance of the lesion. *B,* This view shows a patient with fibrous dysplasia of the right hemipelvis and proximal femur. This is a mixed lytic lesion with cortical thinning. The femur has been prophylactically stabilized with a reconstruction intramedullary nail.

giant cells may be present. In the polyostotic form, cartilage is often present within the lesions.

Spontaneous healing of the involved bone does not occur. In severe forms of the disease, untreated lesions progress and new areas of involvement form. The usual treatment options are preventive orthopaedic procedures such as curettage, internal fixation, and bone grafting. These procedures were designed to control the extent of the lesion and to treat pathological fractures that often develop in the affected areas. Medical treatment with calcitonin, etidronate, and mithramycin has achieved poor results.

The use of second-generation bisphosphonates has provided benefit for patients with fibrous dysplasia. It is known that the cause of fibrous dysplasia lesions is an excess of osteoclastic activity with increased bone resorption. Excess osteoclastic activity is also attributed to other metabolic bone diseases such as Paget's disease and high-turnover osteoporosis. Patients with these diseases have been treated successfully using second-generation bisphosphonates. Two European groups reported positive response to intravenous pamidronate therapy for fibrous dysplasia.[12, 15] Chapurlat et al[12] assessed the long-term effects of intravenous pamidronate in patients with fibrous dysplasia. Twenty patients, 11 males and 9 females, received a 180-mg course of intravenous pamidronate every 6 months for a total of 39 months; end points were assessed at these times. The severity of bone pain was significantly reduced, biochemical markers were decreased, and bone formation in preexisting lesions was noted in nine patients.[12] No fractures occurred in the study population, but four patients did experience stress lines during the trial. A similar study by Pfeilschifter and Ziegler[16] reported the results of intravenous infusions of 60 mg of pamidronate in eight patients, five of whom had McCune-Albright syndrome. All patients had pain relief, and two had radiographic evidence of reduced size of some of the osteolytic lesions. Lane et al[17] demonstrated the efficacy of either oral or oral and intravenous bisphosphonates in six patients with fibrous dysplasia. The participants were monitored for changes in N-telopeptide, pain score, and radiographic evidence with a minimum 2-year follow-up. They found that combination bisphosphonate therapy diminishes pain, prevents fractures, lowers N-telopeptide values, and leads to partial resolution of fibrous dysplasia lesions. They determined that, in their population, patients could be maintained on oral therapy after initial intravenous treatment. Current evidence suggests that second-generation bisphosphonates are useful in managing fibrous dysplasia.

REFERENCES

1. Parker SL, Tong T, Bolden S, et al: Cancer Statistics 1997. Cancer J Clin 1997; 47:5.
2. Kumagai SG, McGuire MH: Cellular and molecular biology. In Simon MA, Springfield D (eds): Surgery for Bone and Soft Tumors. Philadelphia, Lippincott-Raven, 1998, p 9.
3. Enneking WF, Spanier SS, Goodman MA: A system for the surgical staging of musculoskeletal sarcoma. Clin Orthop Rel Res 1989; 153:106.
4. Ward WG: Orthopaedic oncology for the nononcologist: Introduction and common errors to avoid. AAOS Instr Course Lect 1999; 48:577.
5. Mankin HJ, Mankin CJ, Simon MA: The hazards of the biopsy revisited: Members of the Musculoskeletal Tumor Society. J Bone Joint Surg Am 1996; 78:656.
6. Aboulafia AJ: Biopsy. AAOS Instr Course Lect 1999; 48:587.
7. Glasser DB, Lane JM, Huvos AG, et al: Survival, prognosis, and therapeutic response in osteogenic sarcoma: The Memorial Hospital experience. Cancer 1992; 69:698.
8. Basle MF, Russell WC, Goswami KA, et al: Paramyxovirus antigens in osteoclasts from Paget's bone tissue detected by monoclonal antibodies. J Gen Virol 1985; 66:2103.
9. Mee AP, Dixon JA, Hoyland JA, et al: Detection of canine distemper virus in 100% of Paget's disease samples by in situ-reverse transcriptase-polymerase reaction. Bone 1998; 23:171.
10. Ralston SH, Digiovine FS, Gallagher SJ, et al: Failure to detect paramyxovirus sequences in Paget's disease of bone using the polymerase chain reaction. J Bone Miner Res 1991; 6:1243.
11. Morales-Piga AA, Rey-Rey JS, Corres-Gonzales J, et al: Frequency and characteristics of familial aggregation in Paget disease of bone. J Bone Miner Res 1995; 10:663.
12. Chapurlat RD, Delmas PD, Leins D, et al: Long term effects of intravenous pamidronate in fibrous dysplasia of bone. J Bone Miner Res 1997; 12:1746.
13. Henry A: Monostotic fibrous dysplasia. J Bone Joint Surg Br 1969; 51:300.
14. Bell NH, Avery S, Johnston CC Jr: Effects of calcitonin in Paget's disease and polyostotic fibrous dysplasia. J Clin Endocrinol Metab 1970; 31:283.
15. Chapurlat RD, Delmas PD, Liens D, et al: Long term effects of intravenous pamidronate in fibrous dysplasia of bone. J Bone Miner Res 1997; 10:1746.
16. Pfeilschifter J, Ziegler R: Effect of pamidronate on clinical symptoms and bone metabolism and McCune-Albright syndrome. Med Klin 1998; 93:352.
17. Lane JM, Khan SN, O'Connor WJ: Bisphosphonate therapy in fibrous dysplasia. Clin Orthop 2001; 382:6.

section

3

TRAUMA

CHRISTOPHER T. BORN

WILLIAM G. DeLONG, JR

PRIORITIZATION AND MANAGEMENT OF THE POLYTRAUMA PATIENT

C. William Schwab and Christopher T. Born

Summary

- Polytrauma remains a leading cause of death in adults younger than 44 years of age.
- Survival can be increased by adherence to established trauma management protocols.
- Trauma-related deaths occur in a trimodal distribution.
- Following resuscitation, trauma patients need continued reassessment and evaluation to identify all injuries.
- Definitive management is best delivered by a coordinated team of traumatologists (surgical and orthopaedic), nursing, and other key subspecialists.

EPIDEMIOLOGY OF TRAUMA CARE

Trauma is the leading cause of death in the first four decades of life and ranks third after cancer and atherosclerosis as the major cause of death in all age groups in the United States. Annually, more than 200,000 deaths occur from injury in our country. For every trauma death, there are two patients who suffer with disability. Permanently disabling brain or spinal cord injuries affect 80,000 people each year. Trauma patients occupy 12% of all hospital beds, and the total cost related to trauma care in the United States is estimated to be 100 billion dollars annually. The amount lost to indirect costs (i.e., lost wages, insurance costs, property damage, employer costs, and production losses) is probably double this amount.[1, 2]

The current trauma systems have developed from our knowledge of the management of the critically injured patient gained during World War II, the Korean conflict, and the Vietnam War. The evolution of the trauma systems within the United States has stimulated us to develop a more rapid and focused team response in addition to correctly utilizing key medical resources to care for the needs of the seriously injured patient. This is irrespective of where the patients are injured or where they might receive definitive care.[3]

The key elements to successful trauma care include the development of a well-organized prehospital system that can rapidly mobilize, evaluate, stabilize, and evacuate the injured patient. In-field advanced resuscitation techniques are a critical element to patient survival. These techniques, linked to accurate triage criteria, allow patients to be brought to specialized centers for trauma care where contemporary diagnostic and therapeutic resources are immediately available and dedicated to the injured.

Deaths from trauma have a trimodal distribution. The first peak (50% of cases) occurs within seconds to minutes of injury. Massive injury and lacerations to the brain, brain stem, spinal cord, heart, aorta, or other large vessels generally cause these fatalities. The second peak of death takes place within minutes to hours, and it is within this "golden hour" that trauma systems have the ability to increase survival by rapid in-field stabilization and transport to a trauma center for surgical intervention. Primary causes of death during this time include subdural hematomas, hemothorax or pneumothorax, splenic rupture, liver lacerations, massive pelvic disruptions, and multiple injuries associated with significant blood loss. The third peak of death (20% of cases) takes place several days to weeks following injury and is primarily caused by multiorgan failure and sepsis. This third peak can be flattened with adequate resuscitation and accurate diagnosis and rapid treatment at the initial event and on hospital arrival.

ASSESSMENT AND MANAGEMENT PRIORITIES OF THE MULTIPLY INJURED PATIENT

Victims of serious blunt or penetrating trauma sustain a significant physiological insult that begins at the time of the injury. They require a directed and precise resuscitation by a surgeon-led trauma team.[3, 4] On arrival at the trauma center, the patient's care is classically divided into four phases, as outlined by the American College of Surgeons Advanced Trauma Life Support educational program.[5] There is an initial rapid **primary survey** designed to assess for immediate life-threatening problems that are managed by a set of primary emergency **resuscitation** measures. This usually occurs within minutes, and it is crucial to further care that the Airway be controlled, Breathing assured, and Circulation supported (the "ABCs"). As the patient is provisionally stabilized, a more thorough **secondary survey** is then performed, during which an evaluation of all body systems is carried out to identify and catalogue all of the patient's injuries. This is used to plan further immediate as well as longer-term care and will help reduce disability. This is most commonly completed in 15 to 20 minutes and guides the setting of diagnostic and therapeutic priorities. A longer period of **definitive care** and continued reevaluation then follows while the patient is either in the intensive care unit or in the hospital. At an early point during this time, a careful and complete **tertiary survey** is performed, followed by serial examinations to help identify new, related problems or unrecognized injuries. This is important for the victim of blunt multisystem trauma, particularly when central nervous system (CNS) injury is involved.[6] The rate of delayed diagnosis for this patient population can be as high as 10%.[7, 8]

Several scoring systems are used to communicate among physicians the injury level and progressive status of the patient. These include the Glasgow Coma Scale (GCS) and

TABLE 1. GLASGOW COMA SCALE: NORMAL = 15		
Criterion	Assessment	Score
Eye Opening	Maximum	4
	Spontaneous	4
	To voice	3
	To pain	2
	None	1
Verbal Response	Maximum	5
	Oriented	5
	Confused	4
	Inappropriate words	3
	Incomprehensible sounds	2
	None	1
Motor Response	Maximum	6
	Obeys commands	6
	Localized pain	5
	Withdrawn to pain	4
	Flexion to pain	3
	Extension to pain	2
	None	1
Total = A + B + C		

the Revised Trauma Score (RTS) (Tables 1 and 2).[9, 10] The GCS is physiologically based and helps assess and quantify the patient's level of consciousness. Values are given to degree of eye opening, verbal response, and motor response. Scores can range from 3 to 15, with 15 being normal. The RTS (0 to 12, normal = 12) incorporates the GCS and other physiological parameters (respiratory rate and systolic blood pressure) and can also be used to monitor and track a patient's progress. Any degree of altered physiology, and therefore a lower score, is a significant predictor of serious injury. Thus, a GCS score of 13 to 14, though seemingly a minor change, is correlated with anatomic brain injury and would require, at a minimum, a computed tomographic scan of the brain or medical observation. Similarly, an RTS score of less than 12 indicates anatomic injury to alter basic cardiopulmonary or brain function. Other anatomic scores (Injury Severity Score

TABLE 2. REVISED TRAUMA SCORE		
Criterion	Assessment	Score
Respiratory rate (breaths/min)	10–29	≥4
	>29	≥3
	6–9	≥2
	1–5	≥1
	0	≥0
Systolic blood pressure (mm Hg)	>89	≥4
	76–89	≥3
	50–75	≥2
	1–49	≥1
	0	≥0
Glasgow Coma Scale Score	13–15	≥4
	9–12	≥3
	6–8	≥2
	4–5	≥1
	3	≥0
Total of A + B + C		

[ISS], Abbreviated Injury Scale [AIS]) and their clinical applications are available but are used more as anatomic injury qualifiers and quantifiers. The ISS and AIS are rarely used as "language" for early communication between physicians,[11, 12] whereas GCS and RTS, in certain regions, are commonly used.

PRIMARY SURVEY AND RESUSCITATION

At the time of the primary survey, the "ABCDE" algorithm of initial assessment is invoked. This consists of Airway, Breathing, Circulation, Disability, and Exposure. A prioritization exists in the body's ability to deliver oxygen and nutrients to the key core organs and that death or permanent injury will follow a logical time progression if this is impaired. A blocked airway will kill more rapidly than a compromised ability to breathe. Accordingly, the latter, breathing impairment, is then more immediately life-threatening than a diminishing blood volume and failing circulation. In addition, the primary survey is conducted in tandem with the initial resuscitative efforts as the immediate life-threatening problems are identified.

Airway management is a fundamental priority in all trauma patients. Noisy breathing, snoring, gurgling, stridor, or dysphonia may signify abnormal airflow and lack of orotracheal patency. The mouth and oropharynx must be assessed and cleared of any obstruction. The presence of facial injury with the potential to block air passage from secondary edema is noted. Supplemental oxygen should always be administered. Airway patency can be assisted by the chin lift or the jaw thrust with use of an oropharyngeal or a nasopharyngeal airway. *The possibility of an unidentified cervical spine injury always exists*, and care must be taken to limit motion and to maintain the in-line neutral position of the neck. In the absence of a frank obstruction, a bag-valve mask with oxygen can be used. Frequent re-evaluation of the airway's patency is mandatory, particularly in the presence of facial injuries or progressive obtundation. Many seriously injured patients require definitive control of the airway (e.g., shock, CNS injury) by endotracheal intubation. This is usually performed by a three-person team using in-line cervical immobilization and orotracheal intubation.[13] Most emergency or trauma center intubations are performed with select pharmacologics used for sedation and ultra-rapid chemical paralysis.

Second, a rapid assessment of the patient's **breathing** is carried out. Altered mental status or abnormal breath sounds suggest the presence of oxygenation or ventilatory compromise. The patient may appear cyanotic or ashen gray. The chest wall should be visualized and its integrity with respect to deformity or penetrating injury should be assessed, along with any kinetic asymmetry. The use of accessory muscles or the presence of suprasternal, supraclavicular, or intercostal retractions may be indicative of respiratory dysfunction. Auscultation will help determine the presence of air (pneumothorax) or blood (hemothorax) in the chest. Immediately life-threatening chest injuries should be identified and treated at this time (Table 3). The most common life-threatening chest injuries identified in the primary survey are tension pneumothorax, massive hemotho-

TABLE 3. LIFE-THREATENING CHEST INJURIES

Injury	Treatment
Tension pneumothorax	Chest decompression—large needle or intravenous catheter in second intercostal space, midclavicular line—followed by decompression by tube thoracostomy
Flail chest with pulmonary contusion	Intubation and ventilatory support with signs of any respiratory dysfunction, analgesics
Hemothorax	Chest tube placement, if >1000 mL immediate blood drainage—operating room/thoracotomy
Pneumothorax	Chest tube placement
Open pneumothorax	Occlusive dressing, chest tube; if >3–4 cm hole into pleural cavity to operating room—débridement, closure
Cardiac tamponade	FAST ultrasound, ECCO for diagnosis; pericardiocentesis/pericardial windows/sternotomy
Agonal	Left anterior thoracotomy to release tamponade or perform open cardiac massage

rax, pericardial tamponade, flail chest, sucking chest wound, and pneumothorax.

Third, an assessment of **circulation** is carried out with concurrent intravenous access and infusion. The presence or absence of pulses at the carotid, femoral, and radial levels can help estimate systolic blood pressures. Palpable pulses at all three points suggest a systolic blood pressure of greater than 80 mm Hg, whereas the absence of the radial pulse but presence of palpable carotid and femoral pulses suggests a systolic pressure of 70 mm Hg. The presence of a carotid pulse alone signifies a systolic pressure of 60 mm Hg. During this time, skin color and temperature are also noted along with the capillary refilling time. Capillary refilling time of greater than 2 seconds is considered abnormal. The presence or level of shock (defined as inadequate tissue/organ perfusion) is assessed by multiple clinical parameters, and the hemorrhage (which can produce or exacerbate shock) is treated accordingly (Table 4). Sources of external hemorrhage are controlled manually or by the application of pressure dressings. Internal bleeding is generally treated in the operating room.

Resuscitation for hemorrhagic shock includes the use of large-bore peripheral venous catheters or 8.5 French femoral or subclavian central lines to maximize flow. A 2 to 3 L bolus of warmed, isotonic electrolyte solution (Ringer's lactate) can be used initially for most patients suspected of blood loss. The patient is continuously monitored to see whether the response is sustained, transient, or minimal. Class I hemorrhage will stabilize and not require immediate transfusion. Class II and III shock may demonstrate a temporary, positive response but then usually deteriorate and requires additional fluid or blood products, or both. Sustained hemorrhage will probably require surgical intervention, and a failure to respond at all will necessitate multiple transfusions. Monitoring should include vital signs, CNS status, skin perfusion, and urine output. In the event of a poorly sustained response or none at all, central venous pressure, monitoring arterial blood gases, and serial transfusions may need to be used, but the patient is usually best served with rapid operation to control bleeding. An electrocardiogram and the use of a Swan-Ganz catheter may be considered in the elderly or if myocardial dysfunction is suspected. Blood products are generally reserved for transient or nonresponders. O-positive uncrossmatched blood can be used for male patients and O-negative for females.[14] Type-specific blood usually can be available in 10 to 20 minutes, whereas crossmatched blood may require 30 minutes or more. In the event of massive shock or exsanguination (systolic blood pressure lower than 80 mm Hg and no response to fluids), the concomitant coagulopathy can be deterred by the contemporaneous use of fresh frozen plasma, platelets, and calcium as well as by keeping the patient and transfusion products warm. All of these maneuvers should be viewed as a means of temporary or transient support of blood pressure, used only to support life until operative control of bleeding is obtained. No attempt should be made to stabilize the bleeding patient by fluid or component therapy alone.

A brief neurological evaluation will record the level of consciousness on admission and thereby determine **disability**. The "AVPU" mnemonic describes whether the patient is Alert and responsive to Vocal or Painful stimuli, or, in the worse case, Unresponsive. As important, a quick peripheral neurological examination assesses the patient's ability to feel and move all *four* extremities.

Exposure in the trauma setting has two meanings. First, all clothing needs to be removed to provide adequate expo-

TABLE 4. CLASSIFICATION OF SHOCK

Class	Blood Volume Lost (%)	Signs and Symptoms	Fluid Therapy
I	10–15 (5–750 mL)	Minimal	Crystalloids required
II	20–30 (800–1500 mL)	Tachycardia, tachypnea, anxiety, decreased pulse pressure, slowed capillary refill	Crystalloids (2–3 liters)
III	30–40 (2000 mL)	Tachycardia, tachypnea, lowered systolic blood pressure, agitation, confusion, diaphoresis, skin pallor	Crystalloids and blood (blood replaced at 3:1 ratio of estimated blood loss)
IV	>40 (>2500 mL)	Immediately life-threatening: marked decrease in or absent blood pressure, coma, tachycardia, tachypnea, cold, clammy skin	Rapid infusion of red blood cells, crystalloids, blood products; probably will require surgery for cavitary bleeding (abdomen, chest, pelvis)

sure for visual inspection of the patient and access for diagnostic and therapeutic procedures. Second, a patient brought in from the field may already be hypothermic from exposure, or, paradoxically, removal of the patient's clothing in the admitting area may induce further hypothermia. Control of the patient's body temperature is critical and can be managed by the application of body warmers, the use of radiant or convected air heaters, and the use of warmed fluids for infusion.

ADDITIONAL DIAGNOSTIC AND RESUSCITATIVE MANEUVERS

In patients with suspicion of or having serious injuries, the placement of a **nasogastric tube**, after it is verified that no skull base fractures are present, may be both diagnostic and therapeutic. By removing stomach contents and reducing gastric volume and pressure, one reduces the risk of gastric aspiration and can assess the presence of blood. **Urinary catheter** placement is carried out after a rectal examination has been performed. It allows for bladder decompression and urinary output monitoring. A urine specimen should be collected and sent for analysis. *In the event of a suspected urethral injury*, Foley catheterization should be held until a retrograde urethrogram has been performed (Table 5). In the event of a disrupted urethra, suprapubic cystostomy should be considered.

Diagnostic peritoneal lavage should be considered in the evaluation of any blunt abdominal trauma, particularly if results of the abdominal examination are equivocal or in the event of unexplained hypotension. Absolute and relative contraindications include the existing need for an exploratory laparotomy, obesity, history or physical examination evidence of prior abdominal surgery, advanced cirrhosis, established coagulopathy, and advanced pregnancy. In the adult, laparotomy is indicated if there is free aspiration of gross blood, gastrointestinal contents, or bile, or if the red cell count is greater than 100,000/mm^3 after lavage with 1000 mL of fluid. Other threshold criteria for laparotomy include the presence of enteric contents or the egress of lavage fluid via the chest tube or Foley catheter.

A newer area of diagnostics available in the admitting of some trauma centers is **focused abdominal sonography for trauma (FAST)**. This allows the evaluating physician to identify fluid in the pelvis, Morrison's pouch, splenic recess, and pericardial sac. Currently, a positive finding for abdominal fluid by focused abdominal sonography for trauma would require exploratory laparotomy (unstable patients) or, at a minimum, a CT scan of abdomen and pelvis (stable patients).[15]

Adjuncts to the initial evaluation and resuscitation of the trauma patient include other invasive and noninvasive monitoring techniques. **Arterial blood gases** can help determine the acid-base status, a low pH indicating hypoperfusion and anaerobic metabolism most commonly from hypovolemic blood loss. Noninvasive **pulse oximetry** measures the oxygen saturation of hemoglobin, with an O_2 saturation of greater than 93% considered acceptable and corresponding with a Po_2 of 75 mm Hg. **End-tidal CO_2 monitoring** (ETCO$_2$) affords the accurate placement of the endotracheal tube by confirming carbon dioxide concentration. **Central venous pressure** may give a gross estimate of a patient's volume status (normal, 2 to 10 mm Hg). Pulmonary artery catheterization can help evaluate cardiac output, left-sided cardiac performance, and pulmonary hypertension as may be related to pulmonary disease. In addition, pulmonary wedge pressures can assess volume status through measurement of the pulmonary artery wedge pressure and ventricular end diastolic pressure.

Consideration may need to be given to **intubation** if a patient cannot be ventilated or oxygenated adequately (Table 6). Any efforts to control the airway must be done with attention to the cervical spine, and care is always taken to prevent any or further spinal cord injury (in the event of an unidentified cervical spine lesion). Of patients with injuries above the clavicles, 5% to 10% may have a cervical spine injury. Intubation techniques include orotracheal, nasotracheal, and cricothyroidotomy. Nasotracheal intubation is appropriate for patients who are spontaneously breathing and obtunded. Difficulty in maintaining cervical spine control and presentation of such a noxious stimulus for the excitable patient presents a significant disadvantage to this technique. It is contraindicated in the presence of suspected mid-face, cribriform plate, or basilar skull injuries. Orotracheal intubation following a rapid induction of sedative and paralytic agents is an acceptable alternative in the hands of a skilled intubator and with proper neck control. In-line immobilization by a skilled and dedicated person and visualization of the vocal cords are required.[16-18] Cricothyroidotomy is considered in the presence of glottal edema, laryngeal fracture, or severe oropharyngeal hemorrhage. It is also the best alternative following failed nasotracheal or orotracheal techniques. The cricothyroid membrane is incised between the thyroid and the cricoid cartilage, in the midline where the skin is very close to the membrane and few vascular structures are present. This affords rapid and safe entry into the tracheal lumen.

During the initial assessment, **radiographs** should in-

TABLE 5. SIGNS OF POSSIBLE URETHRAL INJURY

Pelvic fracture
Blood at the urethral meatus
High-riding prostate on rectal examination
Scrotal hematoma
Perineal lacerations or ecchymosis

TABLE 6. INTUBATION REQUIREMENTS

Nonsecure or unstable airway.
Unconscious patient with a head injury (especially any patient with GCS ≤8).
Patient demonstrating signs of respiratory failure (i.e., inadequate or labored breathing, RR >35, deteriorating blood oxygenation with pulse oximetry <92%, rising Pco$_2$ [>45]).
Flail chest with pulmonary contusion in addition to respiratory failure.
Severe hemorrhagic shock.
Inhalation burns.
Combative patient.

GCS, Glasgow Coma Scale score; RR, respiratory rate.

clude an anteroposterior chest film,[19] a pelvis film, and a lateral cervical spine film when possible. These should not, however, interfere with the emergency resuscitation process, life-saving procedures, or even, at times, surgery to control bleeding.

Blood samples for laboratory analysis and crossmatching can be collected at the time of intravenous line placement. Laboratory tests might include complete blood count, prothrombin time, partial thromboplastin time, platelet count, and glucose measurement. In elderly patients or those with known or suspected premorbid medical conditions, other tests can be selected to monitor electrolytes and renal and liver function. In patients in shock, base deficit (arterial blood gases) and lactate levels are suggested.

SECONDARY SURVEY

Following the recognition and stabilization of the patient's life-threatening injuries, a complete head to toe evaluation is completed. It is important to remember that continued attention must be given to those problems already identified at the time of the primary survey. The overall management of the patient is one of ongoing monitoring, reassessment, and resuscitation carried out in parallel with the secondary survey and eventually definitive care.

From whatever sources are available, as complete a **history** as possible is obtained. This should include the circumstances and mechanism of the current injury; the patient's past medical history, medications, allergies, and vaccinations; time of the patient's last meal; and any other information that might be useful in developing a working composite of the victim's current physiological state. Knowledge of the type, magnitude, and direction of forces acting at the time of injury will help to direct attention to possible injuries and the requirement for additional studies for both blunt and penetrating trauma. Questions might include seatbelt use, airbag deployment, ejection from vehicle, vehicle types and speeds, distance of fall, type and caliber of weapon, number of shots fired, and so on. (Specific concerns regarding burns, electrocution, drowning, environmental or hazardous materials exposure, poisoning, and other types of injury are important but outside the scope of this chapter. A suggested reading of a more comprehensive manual is found at the beginning of the reference section.)

The **physical examination** in the secondary assessment is a thorough one, with the focus being directed to some degree by the circumstances and mechanism of injury. The physical examination for a single gunshot wound to the abdomen might logically center on the trunk and abdomen (while not forgetting the back), whereas a gunshot followed by a fall down a stairwell would mandate a more complete examination of the head and axial and appendicular skeleton. In general, the physical examination of the secondary survey begins with the head and scalp, logically progressing downward to include the eyes, ears, nose, throat, and neck. A maxillofacial examination and a quick visual acuity check should be carried out. The chest and abdomen are reevaluated by inspection, palpation, percussion, and auscultation. In the abdomen, its shape, the presence of tenderness, muscle guarding, and pain are subtle

but important factors. Gross pelvic instability may be noted by manual pressure on the iliac wings. A rectal examination prior to urinary catheter placement and a vaginal examination should be completed, along with an inspection of the genitalia and perineum. The musculoskeletal examination should include palpation of all bones and joints of the appendicular skeleton to assess for crepitation, abnormal motion, and instability. The presence of lacerations, abrasions, and swelling should be noted, and open wounds should be sterilely dressed. The patient should be logrolled with adequate support of the axial skeleton and cervical spine to limit motion. Any limb fracture or joint dislocation should be treated and supported by a single provider to minimize pain when moving. A comprehensive neurological examination is carried out and includes repeat determination of level of consciousness, pupillary size and reactivity, and motor and sensory evaluations. Open fracture wounds or traumatic arthrotomies should *not* be digitized with unsterile gloves or repeatedly inspected, to avoid further contamination. Rather, a single coordinated and clean examination with sterile gloves and analgesis should be considered. Radiographs should be ordered of suspicious areas to include the joint above and below the injury site. Obvious fractures should be splinted. Documentation is particularly important in the presence of suspected head or spinal cord injury as well as fractures or dislocations. The GCS score is recalculated to look for trends of improvement or deterioration.

At the time of the secondary survey, additional diagnostic testing may be considered. In most patients with blunt injury, a three-view cervical spine x-ray series should be completed.[20, 21] For patients at high risk for axial skeleton injury from blunt trauma, pelvic and anteroposterior and lateral thoracic and lumbar spine radiographs should also be obtained.[22, 23] Other diagnostic imaging, including arteriography, CT scanning, additional genitourinary contrast studies, and so on, may be necessary and may require a trip away from the admitting area. Close monitoring is therefore required by experienced personnel, including monitoring of hemodynamic stability. Situations or areas of the hospital must be avoided in which monitoring of vital signs or the ability to employ acute resuscitative measures might be precluded.

DEFINITIVE TREATMENT AND TERTIARY SURVEY

The period of **definitive care** may follow the identification and management of life-threatening injuries, which includes any special studies that might be required. Certainly, some procedures may be carried out as part of resuscitation (e.g., endotracheal tube placement, chest tube insertion, or pelvic external fixation in the admitting area), or the period of definitive care may commence in the operating suite. It is during this time that an overall management plan is enacted, along with prioritizations and appropriate specialty consultations based on the patient's catalogue of injuries. It is critical that a complete transfer of information take place if the patient is transferred to a team of intensivists by the admitting surgeons. In large academic centers, it is also important that the critical care consultants communicate regularly among themselves and with the trauma team to coordinate and facilitate patient management. A **tertiary survey** with careful, serial reassessments and repeat head-to-toe examination should take place within 24 to 48 hours. Ongoing resuscitation may interfere with the thoroughness of the tertiary survey. The survey may also be compromised by other factors such as medication, intoxication, and head injury. Additional studies should be prioritized based on patient stability and the need for ongoing resuscitation.[5]

OTHER CONSIDERATIONS

CENTRAL NERVOUS SYSTEM INJURY

Head injury can be devastating, and steps must be taken to reduce the impact of brain trauma as quickly as possible. The GCS (see Table 1) can be used to quantify the level of consciousness, with a score of 13 to 15 consistent with minor head injury, while a score of 9 to 12 and less than 8 signify moderate to severe levels, respectively. Pupillary function and extremity weakness or lateralization are also important components of the neurological examination in the head-injured patient. Treatment strategies center around the support of cerebral metabolism by providing normal perfusion of oxygen and removal of carbon dioxide. The prevention of increased intracranial pressure should be carried out in consultation with the neurosurgical team. Maintaining systolic blood pressure in the normal range and blood oxygenation will help prevent further or secondary cerebral ischemia. Hypocapnia induced by hyperventilation may transiently reduce cerebral blood volume and pressure through vasoconstriction, whereas fluid restriction and diuretics may limit overhydration and secondary cerebral edema; these sophisticated maneuvers require pulmonary artery catheter monitoring. Pharmacological sedation and paralysis may also be employed. Emergency CT scanning is indicated in all cases with a GCS score of 14 or under and should be used even more liberally in patients older than 55 years of age. Intracranial pressure (ICP) monitoring is a useful adjunct, and efforts are made to keep the ICP in the 4 to 10 mm Hg range. The cerebral perfusion pressure (mean arterial pressure −ICP) is another important parameter to follow and should be maintained at greater than 60 mm Hg by manipulations to lower ICP or raise arterial pressure.[23, 24]

SPINAL CORD INJURY

Spinal cord injury should always be suspected and appropriate radiograph studies carried out as outlined previously. Until spinal injury is proven otherwise, patients with blunt or penetrating injuries are always managed with spinal precautions. High-dose methylprednisolone given within the first 8 hours is currently recommended for the treatment of acute spinal cord injuries.[2] The recommended dosage is 30 mg/kg body weight given over 15 minutes followed by an infusion of 5.4 mg/kg/h for 23 hours. Early neurosurgical and orthopaedic consultation should be sought to assist in the management of these injuries. CT scanning is most helpful in identifying all suspicious areas, and magnetic resonance imaging should be promptly available to delineate any complex cases.

GERIATRIC, PEDIATRIC, AND PREGNANT PATIENTS

Special consideration should be given to geriatric, pediatric, and pregnant patients. For the elderly patient, the risk of death is associated with lesser injury severity than in younger adult patients. The physiological reserves are diminished and response to resuscitative efforts are more unpredictable.[25] In addition, the presence of comorbid medical problems such as cardiac disease, chronic pulmonary conditions, renal insufficiency, and liver disease make the course more complicated and good outcome less predictable.[26] This population is also unique because of very common use of medications: Coumadin, diuretics, β-blockers, and so on.

Pediatric patients have similar management priorities to those of adults. However, therapeutic quantities of blood, fluids, and medications differ, and the patient's size needs to be considered with respect to heat loss. With the significant physiological reserve of pediatric patients, signs of volume depletion may not be recognized until very late, often with catastrophic results. Airway and cervical spine anatomy are unique and require special attention with respect to management.[5] A heightened awareness of the abused child needs to be maintained.[5]

The pregnant patient may have some altered responses to injury because of the requisite anatomic and physiological changes that occur with the gravid state. The response to hypovolemia may be altered secondary to the physiological hypervolemia of pregnancy. Maternal and fetal hypotension should be avoided by the liberal use of fluid and blood product replacement. Adequate treatment of the mother will promote the best chance for fetal survival. Problems unique to the pregnant victim should be considered, including abruptio placentae, premature membrane rupture, amniotic fluid embolism, and isoimmunization. Essential diagnostic x-ray studies should *not* be bypassed, and early consultation with an obstetrician should be sought.[5]

MUSCULOSKELETAL CONSIDERATIONS

Orthopaedic consultation should be obtained when musculoskeletal injury is identified. The orthopaedic team should be able to work in concert with the trauma staff in coordinating the care and the timing of diagnostic and therapeutic interventions. The orthopaedist can assist in the admitting area with the splinting of fractures, provisional reduction of dislocations, identification of additional injuries, and suggestion of additional radiograph studies when appropriate. A provisional treatment plan can be developed in conjunction with traumatologists with respect to the timing and prioritization of surgical procedures. Select pelvic ring injuries that are felt to be the source of hemodynamic instability can be emergently managed in the admitting area with the use of external fixation or pelvic clamps.[2] Open fractures should be inspected and then re-dressed with antiseptic solution until the patient is brought to the operating room. The débridement and stabilization of open fractures and dislocations should be delayed only by the mitigating presence of other, higher priority injuries, usually of a life-threatening nature. Concerns over the effects of intramedullary nailing in the presence of chest and head injury are still not fully resolved.[27] In the majority of scenarios, however, the ability of early stabilization of long bone fractures

TABLE 7. PHYSICAL SIGNS FOR VASCULAR INJURY

Pulse deficit
Ischemia
Hemorrhage
Large/expanding/pulsatile hematoma
Presence of a bruit or thrill
Ankle/brachial index <0.9*
Cadaveric distal extremity

* Doppler-derived systolic ankle pressure divided by the highest brachial artery systolic pressure.

to reduce the mortality rate appears well established.[28] Fracture or dislocation with an associated, isolated arterial injury has a high (>95%) salvage rate. Combined vascular and skeletal extremity trauma involving injury to artery, bone, soft tissue, and nerve has the potential for a high amputation rate.[29] The identification of concomitant vascular injury may at times be at issue. The presence of one or more "hard signs" should mandate further investigation by direct surgical exploration and control and repair or arteriography (Table 7). These injuries are best managed by teamwork between orthopaedic and trauma and vascular surgeons. The most important prognostic factor is the time interval between the index injury (not the time of hospital arrival) and the re-establishment of arterial blood flow to the injured extremity. These patients should be transported to the operating room immediately (again, barring other mitigating priorities) for diagnosis, usually with on-table arteriograms. Definitive revascularization or temporary intraluminal shunting can then begin immediately, with orthopaedic fracture stabilization carried out in conjunction or closely following. Liberal four-compartment fasciotomy should be considered, particularly after prolonged ischemic times. The restoration of perfusion is the sine qua non of limb viability and should take precedence over skeletal repair in the combined-injury patient. Delay in restoration of blood flow is the most commonly identified factor contributing to limb loss.[30] The concern that vascular repair may be disrupted by orthopaedic stabilization does not appear to be real with experienced surgeons.

ANTIBIOTICS AND TETANUS

For most closed injuries, prophylaxis against surface organisms requires only first-generation cephalosporins, whereas in open injuries, gram-negative and anaerobic coverage must be considered depending on wound type and location at the time of injury.[2] An accurate tetanus immunization history is important. With open or penetrating wounds, supplemental immunization is usually recommended.[5]

REFERENCES

1. Committee on Trauma. Trauma Evaluation and Management Program for Medical Students. American College of Surgeons, Chicago, IL, 1999.
2. Kasser JR, Beaty JH, Garfin, SR, et al (eds): Orthopaedic Knowledge Update 5. American Academy of Orthopaedic Surgeons, Rosemont, IL, 1996.
3. Committee on Trauma: Resources for Optimal Care of the Injured Patient: 1999. American College of Surgeons, Chicago, IL, 1999.
4. Hoff WS, Reilly PM, Rotondo MF, et al: The importance of the command-physician in trauma resuscitation. J Trauma 1997; 43(5):772.
5. Committee on Trauma: Advanced Trauma Life Support for Doctors. American College of Surgeons, Chicago, IL, 1997.
6. Grossman MD, Born CT: Tertiary survey of the trauma patient in the ICU. In Schwab CW (ed): Surg Clin North Am. Philadelphia, WB Saunders, 2000, p 805.
7. Born CT, Ross SE, Iannacone WM, et al: Delayed identification of skeletal injury in multisystem trauma: The "missed" fracture. J Trauma 1989; 29(12):1643.
8. Enderson BL, Reath DB, Meadors J, et al: The tertiary trauma survey: A prospective study of missed injury. J Trauma 1990; 30(6):666.
9. Teasdale G, Jennett B: Assessment of coma and impaired consciousness: A practical scale. Lancet 1974; 2:81.
10. Champion HR, Sacco WJ, Copes WS, et al: A revision of the Trauma Score. J Trauma 1989; 29(5):623.
11. Baker SP, O'Neill B, Haddon W, et al: The Injury Severity Score: A method for describing patients with multiple injuries and evaluating emergency care. J Trauma 1974; 14:187.
12. Civil ID, Schwab CW: The abbreviated injury scale, 1985 revision: A condensed chart for clinical use. J Trauma 1988; 28:87.
13. Rotondo MF, McGonigal MD, Schwab CW, et al: Urgent paralysis and intubation of trauma patients: Is it safe? J Trauma 1993; 34(2):242.
14. Schwab CW, Shayne JP, Turner J: Immediate trauma resuscitation with type O uncrossmatched blood: A two-year prospective experience. J Trauma 1986; 26(10):897.
15. Fernandez L, McKenney MG, McKenney KL, et al: Ultrasound in blunt abdominal trauma. J Trauma 1998; 45(4):841.
16. Frankel H, Rozycki G, Champion H, et al: The use of TRISS methodology to validate prehospital intubation by urban EMS providers. Am J Emerg Med 1997; 15(7):630.
17. Sing RF, Reilly PM, Rotondo MF, et al: Out-of-hospital rapid-sequence induction for intubation of the Pediatric Patient. Acad Emerg Med 1996; 3:41.
18. Sing RF, Rotondo MF, Zonies DH, et al: Rapid sequence induction for intubation by an aeromedical transport team: A critical analysis. Am J Emerg Med 1999; 16:598.
19. Schwab CW, Lawson RB, Lind JF, et al: Aortic injury: Comparison of supine and upright portable chest films to evaluate the widened mediastinum. Ann Emerg Med 1984; 13:896.
20. Ross SE, Schwab CW, David ET, et al: Clearing the cervical spine: Initial radiologic evaluation. J Trauma 1987; 27(9):1055.
21. Eastern Association for the Surgery of Trauma: Practice parameters for identifying cervical spine injuries following trauma. Trauma Practice Guidelines 1998. www. EAST. org
22. Frankel HL, Rozycki GS, Ochsner MG, et al: Indications for obtaining surveillance thoracic and lumbar spine radiographs. J Trauma 1994; 37(4):673.
23. Civil ID, Ross SE, Botehlo G, et al: Routine pelvic radiology in severe blunt trauma: Is it necessary? Ann Emerg Med 1988; 17:488.
24. Joint Section on Neurotrauma and Critical Care: Guidelines for the Management of Severe Head Injury. Brain Trauma Foundation, Philadelphia, 1996.
25. McMahon DJ, Schwab CW, Kauder DR: Comorbidity and the elderly trauma patient. World J Surg 1996; 20(8):1113.
26. Schwab CW, Kauder DR: Trauma in the geriatric patient. Arch Surg 1992; 127:701.
27. Scalea TM, Scott JD, Brumback RJ, et al: Early fracture fixation may be "just fine" after head injury: No difference in central nervous system outcomes. J Trauma 1999; 46(5):839.
28. Bone LB, Johnson KD, Weigelt J, et al: Early versus delayed stabilization of femoral fractures: A prospective randomized study. J Bone Joint Surg Am 1989; 71:336.
29. Howe HR, Poole GV, Hansen KJ, et al: Salvage of lower extremities following combined orthopaedic and vascular trauma: A predictive salvage index. Am Surg 1987; 53:205.
30. Atteberry LR, Dennis JW, Russo-Alesi F, et al: Changing patterns of arterial injuries associated with fracture and dislocation. J Am Coll Surg 1996; 183:377.

PRINCIPLES OF OPERATIVE FRACTURE STABILIZATION AND FIXATION

Carl T. Hasselman and Gary S. Gruen

Summary

- Understanding the basic principles of external and internal fixation is mandatory to ensure that the optimal biomechanical and biological milieu exists for osseous union.
- Failure of fracture union can be multifactorial but usually results from inadequate fixation or failure of the biological repair process.
- Screws and plates can be used for interfragmentary compression, splinting, or neutralization.
- Intramedullary nails serve as internal splints in long bone fractures.
- External fixators are mostly used for open fracture care but can also function as external splints in conjunction with limited internal fixation.
- By knowing the strengths and weaknesses of each technique, the optimal environment for fracture union can be ensured.

INTRODUCTION

The primary goals of fracture treatment are to achieve an osseous union and restore function to the injured extremity. Each fracture has a personality of its own (e.g., location, comminution, bone quality, comorbidities, biomechanical demands), which must be considered when choosing a treatment. Thus, a fracture surgeon must understand the strengths and weaknesses of each treatment option before using a bone plate, intramedullary (IM) nail, or external fixator. In this chapter we review the basic concepts of fracture healing and discuss the technical, biological, and biomechanical principles of internal and external fixation.

FRACTURE HEALING

After a fracture, there is a vascular disruption of the bone, which results in the formation of a hematoma.[1–3] Subsequently, revascularization of the area occurs, and the devascularized bone ends are resorbed.[4] Fracture healing then occurs by callus formation or primary bone repair, each of which is dependent on fracture reduction and stabilization.

An anatomically reduced and rigidly held fracture avoids micromotion and results in primary bone healing (Fig. 1). If the bone ends are in direct contact, then cutting cones traverse the fracture site and new haversian canals form without callus.[5, 6] A gap greater than 200 μm at the bone ends causes woven bone to be layed down before haversian remodeling.[5, 6] Primary bone healing is typically seen with an anatomic reduction and rigid plate fixation and may require 18 months for completion.

When micromotion occurs at the fracture site, such as with external fixation, IM fixation, or casting, then healing occurs by callus formation (Fig. 2). Mesenchymal cells from the hematoma and new vascular system lay down a callus of fibrous tissue, cartilage, and woven bone.[4] As time progresses and the biological milieu changes, the callus mineralizes and fracture motion decreases.[7, 8] The woven bone is slowly replaced by lamellar bone, and remodeling of the fracture occurs.[9] Although clinical and radiographic union may take several months, the remodeling process can take up to several years until complete.[10]

Although the two types of fracture healing are described as distinct, both primary and callus repair may be seen within the same fracture, such as a comminuted long bone fracture when several fixation techniques are used. This may become more apparent later in this chapter as the different types of fixation are explored.

When the fractured ends of bones fail to heal, a nonunion is said to occur. Although a number of variables

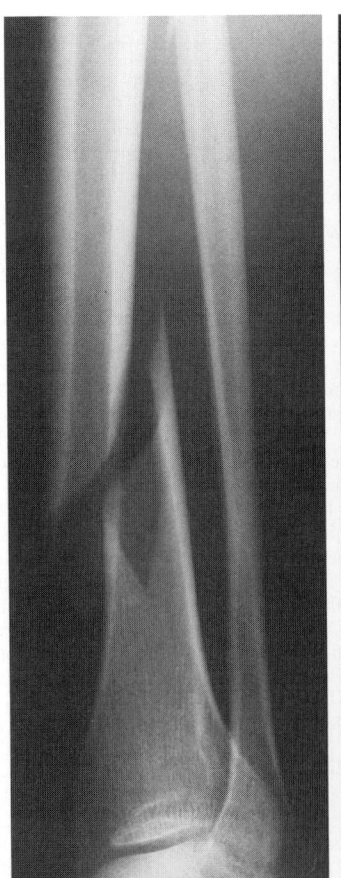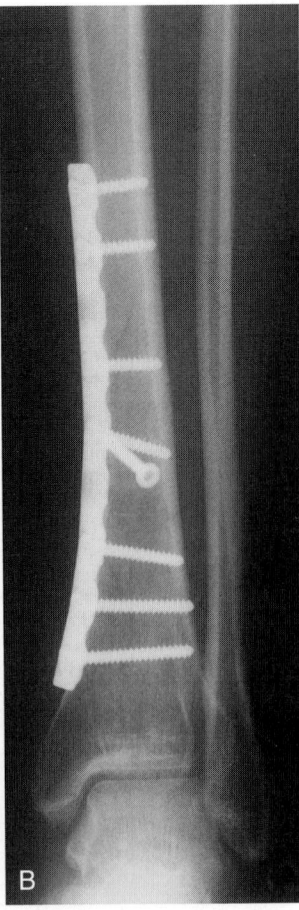

Fig. 1. Primary bone healing. These are (*A*) preoperative and (*B*) 3-month postoperative radiographs of a spiral distal tibial fracture treated with anatomic reduction and rigid fixation. Note that the healing process occurs with no callus formation.

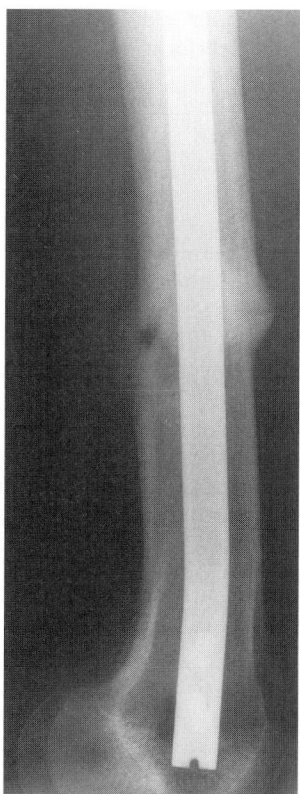

Fig. 2. Callus healing. This is a 10-week postoperative radiograph of a midshaft femur fracture treated with an intramedullary nail. Note the callus formation typical of micromotion at the fracture site.

(e.g., infection, smoking, age, comorbidities) can result in a nonunion, a few generalizations can be made about the failure of bone to heal. Nonunions are categorized as hypertrophic or viable if sufficient vascularity and biology exist in the area for healing; an atrophic or nonviable nonunion exists when there is no evidence of a biological reaction to the fractured area.[11] Viable (hypertrophic) nonunions are characterized by abundant callus formation and failure of the callus between the bone ends to ossify. This type of nonunion typically results from failure to stabilize a fracture adequately, with too much motion occurring between the fractured ends of bone. Viable (hypertrophic) nonunions can be treated by improving the fracture fixation and decreasing the motion within the fracture. In contrast, a nonviable (atrophic) nonunion is characterized by atrophy and resorption of the fracture ends with little or no callus formation. This type of nonunion usually results from a loss of vascularity within the fractured area and requires more complex procedures to induce bone healing.

SCREWS AND PLATES

Screws come in a variety of sizes and types. The screw's size is based on its major diameter (the diameter of the threads), whereas its type (cortical or cancellous) is based on the difference between its major diameter and minor diameter (the diameter of its shaft between threads). Cortical and cancellous screws can be fully threaded, partly threaded, or cannulated. Cortical screws have a smaller difference between their major and minor diameters and are available in sizes ranging from 1.5 to 4.5 mm. Cancellous screws have a larger difference between their major and minor diameters and are available in sizes ranging from 3.0 to 6.5 mm. Cannulated screws come in a number of sizes and allow a guide wire to be placed before screw insertion. This ensures appropriate screw placement and maintains fracture reduction while the screw is being inserted over the guide wire.

Screws are used to secure implants to bone and to achieve interfragmentary compression of the fractured ends (lag screw). Lag screws can be either "by design" or "by intention" (Fig. 3). A lag screw by intention involves overdrilling the near cortex so that the threads only engage the far cortex. By turning the screw, the screw head pulls the

A. LAG SCREW "BY INTENTION"

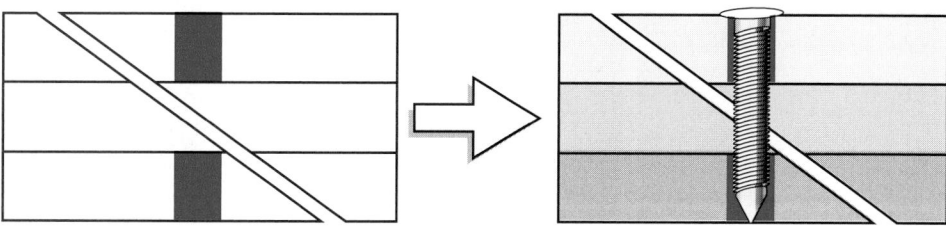

Fig. 3. Lag screws. These diagrams are (*A*) "by intention" and (*B*) "by design."

B. LAG SCREW "BY DESIGN"

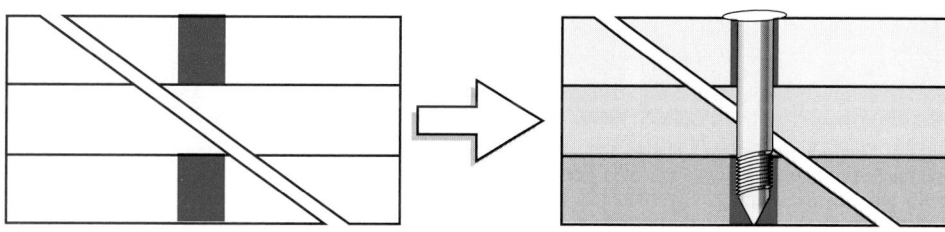

near cortex bone to the far cortex bone, and interfragmentary compression is achieved. This technique is typically used in diaphyseal fractures using cortical screws. A lag screw by design involves a partially threaded screw with a smooth shank. By turning the screw, the screw head pulls the near cortex to the far cortex, and interfragmentary compression is achieved. For this technique to be successful, all of the screw threads must be on one side of the fracture. This technique is particularly useful in epiphyseal and metaphyseal fractures where the bone is spongy.

The optimal lag screw angle for interfragmentary compression is perpendicular to the fracture; however, for resistance to axial compression, the optimal angle is perpendicular to the shaft of the bone. Therefore, the use of a plate or external fixator to resist axial compression and bending is usually used in conjunction with lag screws. The only situation in which lag screw fixation alone is adequate is in long spiral fractures of small non-weightbearing bones.

Plates also are available in a variety of sizes and types. The size of the plate is named for the size of the screw that holds it to the bone and ranges from 2.7 to 4.5 mm; however, newer minifragment sets have even smaller plates and screws. The type of plate is named for its shape or design such as limited contact, dynamic compression, one-third tubular, reconstruction, buttress (cloverleaf, H, L, T),

and so on. The reason for many different plates lies in the various functions they perform.

Plates can achieve static compression to a fracture much like a lag screw. By securing the plate to one side of the reduced fracture and then tensioning the plate with an external device (before securing the plate to the other fragment), compression at the fracture site is achieved (Fig. 4). In addition, plates such as the dynamic compression plate have eccentric holes that allow for compression at the fracture site during plate application without the use of an external tensioning device. When a plate is used to secure a diaphyseal fracture of a long bone, the number of screws recommended to be both above and below the fracture depends on which bone is involved.[12] In the tibia, femur, and humerus, a minimum of eight cortices should be penetrated by screws both above and below the fracture. In the forearm, a minimum of six cortices on each side of the fracture should be secured to the plate by screws.

Plates can also achieve dynamic compression by transforming the normal loads at the involved area into compressive loads at the fracture site. This can be done in one of three ways: the tension band technique, antiglide technique, and hip screw.[13–18] A plate as a tension band is best exemplified by transverse fractures of the femoral shaft (Fig. 5). When walking, the shape of the femur causes an

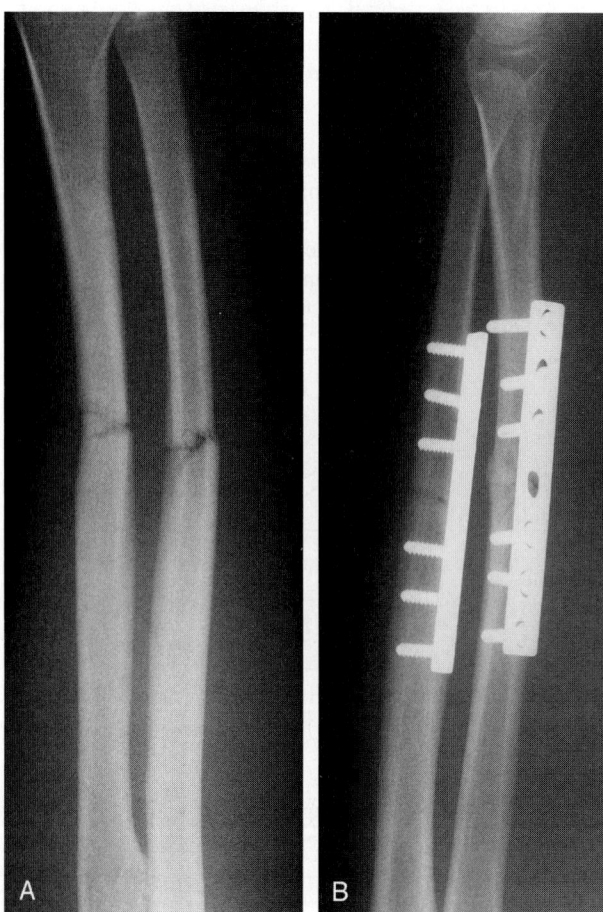

Fig. 4. Compression plate. These are (A) preoperative and (B) 1-month postoperative radiographs of a bone forearm fracture treated with compression plating. There are no lag screws, and the plates provide compression across the fracture site.

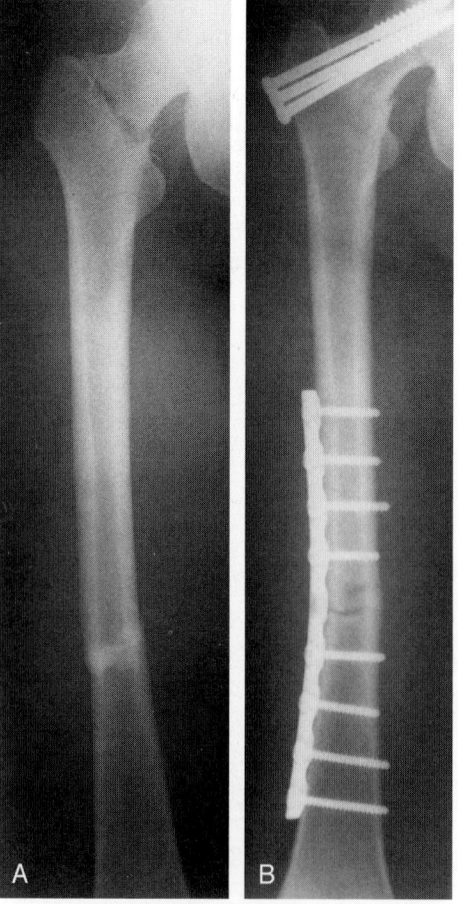

Fig. 5. Tension band. These are (A) preoperative and (B) 3-week postoperative radiographs of ipsilateral femoral neck and shaft fracture in which the shaft was treated with a laterally placed compression plate. This plate will act as a tension band until the fracture unites.

eccentric load to be applied to the bone, so that the lateral side of the femur is in tension while the medial side is in compression. By applying a plate in compression to the lateral cortex, the eccentric load is converted to compressive forces both medially and laterally. However, when no eccentric load is applied, no compressive forces are generated at the fracture site. An antiglide plate is best exemplified by oblique fractures of long bones. By applying the plate to one side of the fractured bone, the plate and bone create an axilla, which prevents displacement of the other fragment along the oblique fracture line when an axial load is applied. By preventing this gliding of the two fragments past each other, shear forces are converted into compressive forces at the fracture site. This technique is most commonly applied to simple oblique fractures of the distal fibula (Fig. 6). The third way a plate can act in the dynamic mode is when a hip screw is used for a peritrochanteric fracture (Fig. 7). A large partially threaded lag screw is used to secure the femoral head and neck to a plate, which is firmly attached to the femoral shaft. When weightbearing is allowed, the weight of the body and the pull of the hip abductors cause the shaft of the lag screw to slide within the barrel of the plate. This results in interfragmentary compression of the fracture fragments.

Plates can also serve as neutralization devices. Although lag screws can provide excellent interfragmentary compression, they cannot resist torsional, axial, or bending forces very well. An external fixator or plate used in conjunction with a lag screw can function to neutralize these forces. In this manner, a plate (or external fixator) secured to the fractured bone will act as a neutralization device (Fig. 8).

Plates can also serve as a buttressing device in a fracture

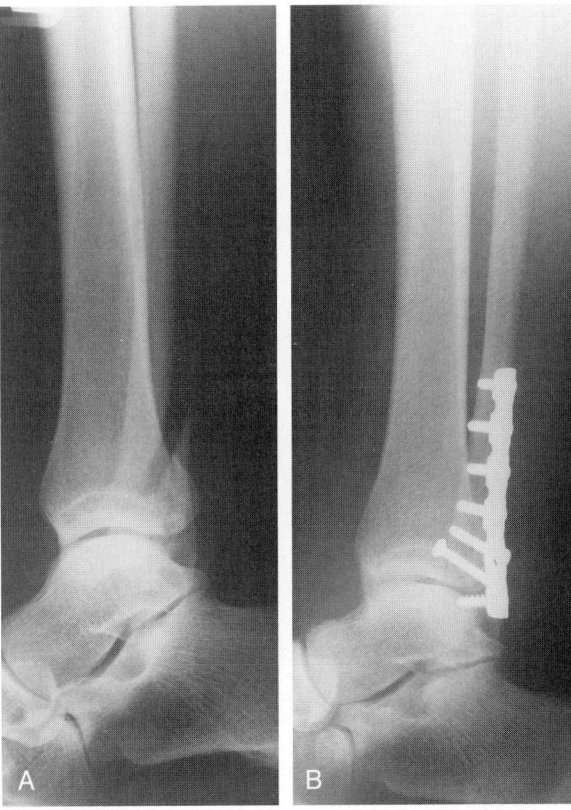

Fig. 6. Antiglide plate. These are (*A*) preoperative and (*B*) 1-month postoperative radiographs of an oblique distal fibula fracture treated with an antiglide plate. Although a lag screw was also placed for interfragmentary compression, the antiglide plate could also serve this purpose.

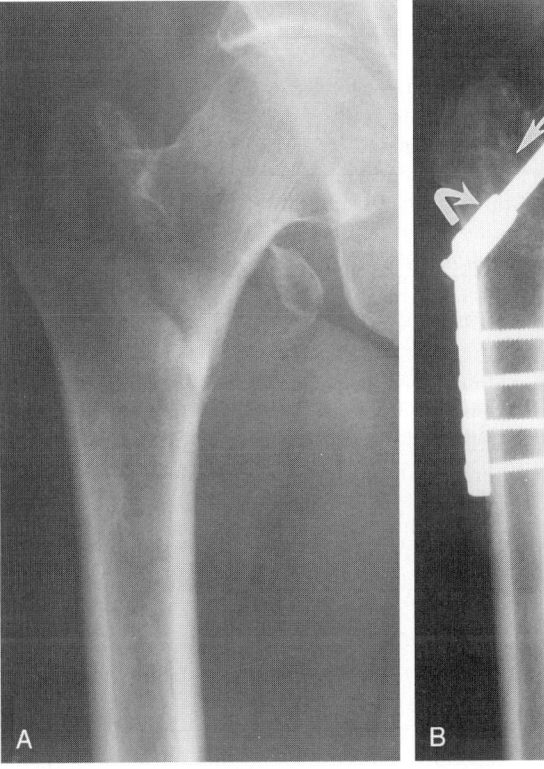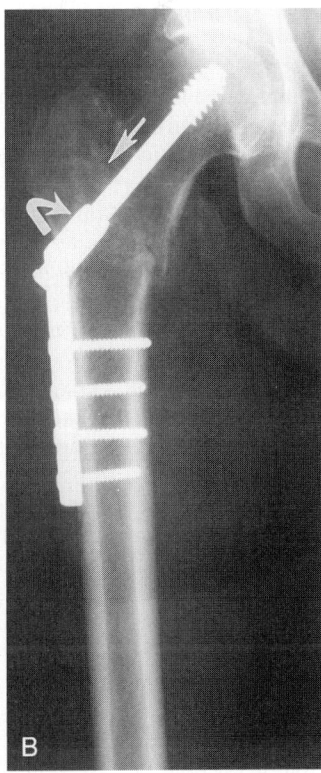

Fig. 7. Hip screw. These are (*A*) preoperative and (*B*) 6-week postoperative radiographs of an intertrochanteric hip fracture treated with a dynamic hip screw. This screw allows for compression at the fracture site with weightbearing. The *straight arrow* above the screw shows the sliding direction of the screw within the barrel of the plate (*curved arrow*).

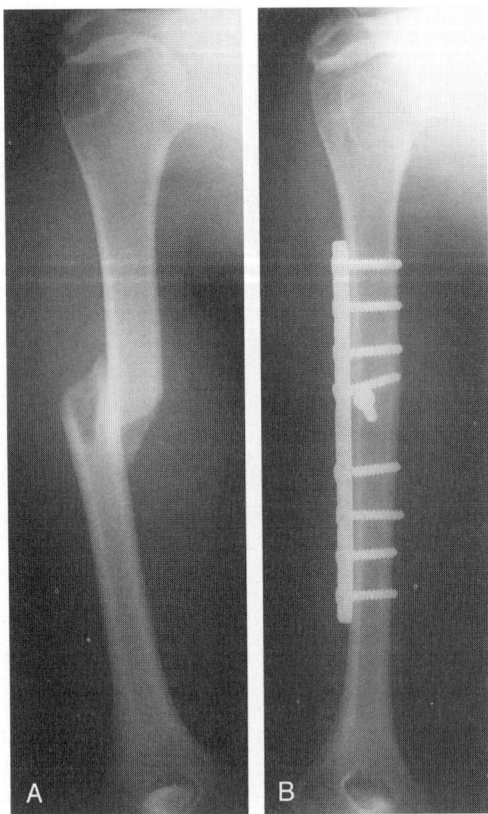

Fig. 8. Neutralization plate. These are (*A*) preoperative and (*B*) 1-month postoperative radiographs of a midshaft humerus fracture treated with a lag screw and plate. The plate serves to neutralize bending forces across the fracture site, which has been initially fixed with an interfragmentary lag screw.

Rigidity of the fixation (and, therefore, motion at the fracture site) is related to the rigidity of the implant and the working length of the implant.[20] This length is the distance between firm fixation points to bone proximally and distally. Torsional rigidity is inversely proportional to the working length, and bending rigidity is inversely proportional to the square of the working length. Therefore, if a longer working length is required, then a stronger implant will be required to prevent failure of the fracture stabilization.

A major drawback to plate fixation is that it requires a stable soft-tissue envelope around the fracture for the incision to heal. In many fractures, the soft tissues are disrupted by the initial injury, and further insult by an incision may lead to poor healing. For example, a comminuted tibial shaft fracture may be stabilized by a plate; however, skin slough and wound dehiscence are not uncommon complications using this technique.[21–23] Also plate fixation in part requires evacuation of the fracture hematoma and stripping of the periosteum. Although the clinical importance of the hematoma to fracture healing is unknown, it is thought to be a source of mesenchymal cells from which osteoblasts arise.[4, 24] Stripping of the periosteal circulation in areas of heavy myofascial attachments does substantially reduce blood flow to the fracture ends.[25, 26] This stripping reduces the bone blood flow significantly more than IM reaming.[27] However, the role of the periosteal circulation in

of metaphyseal bone. This is commonly used in fractures of the tibial plateau. Cancellous lag screws can be placed around or within the plate to achieve interfragmentary compression of the fracture fragments; however, the plate is designed to resist axial loads to the fracture by exerting a force perpendicular to the flat surface of the plate. This is in contrast to the other plate applications in which the force is generated parallel to the plate.

In addition to fixation of a fracture, specialized plates can be used for guiding its reduction. The supracondylar screw and the blade plate are specifically designed to assist in reducing and stabilizing supracondylar, intercondylar, and comminuted subtrochanteric fractures of the femur (Fig. 9).[7] Most of these devices have a fixed angle of 95 degrees between the plate and blade (or screw). By placing the blade (or screw) parallel to the distal joint line of the knee and then securing the plate to the lateral femoral cortex, the correct alignment of the joint line with respect to the femoral shaft can be achieved.

Finally, plates can serve as internal splints for fracture stabilization. The use of bridge plating has emerged in which the plate is placed without stripping the soft tissues from the bone (Fig. 10).[19] In this manner, the plate serves only as a splint to resist axial, torsional, and bending forces much like an IM nail or external fixator. Because bridging of the fracture does not create rigid fixation, motion occurs at the fragments and callus healing ensues.

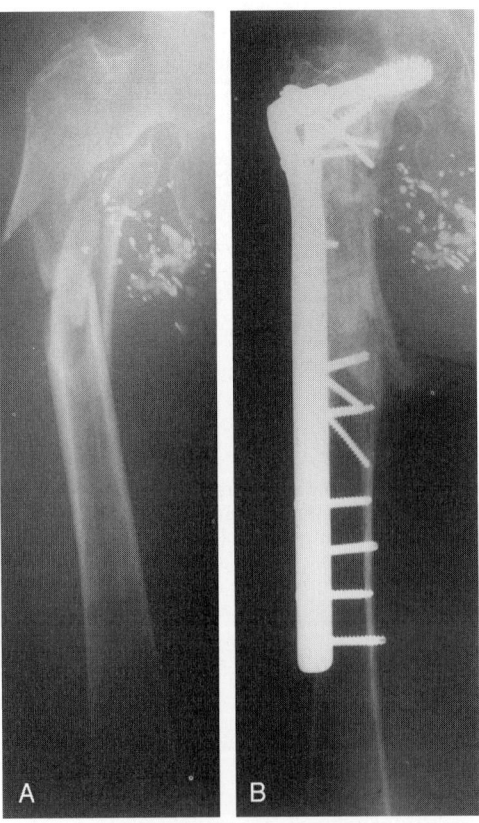

Fig. 9. Condylar screw. These are (*A*) preoperative and (*B*) 8-month postoperative radiographs of a highly comminuted subtrochanteric femur fracture resulting from a gunshot wound. This fracture was treated with a condylar screw to maintain alignment of the femoral head with the shaft.

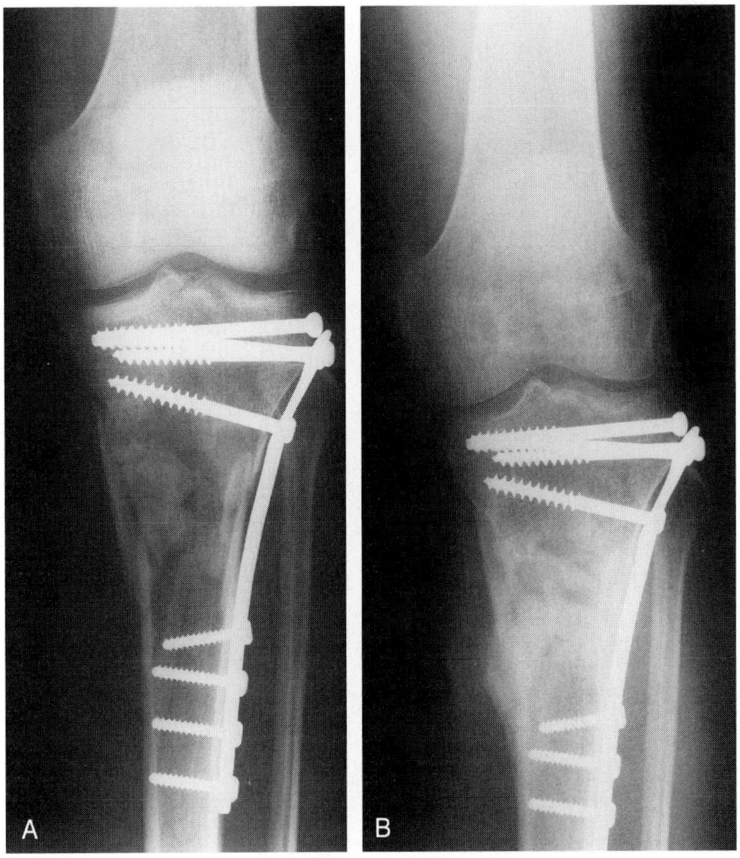

Fig. 10. Bridge plate. These are (A) immediate postoperative and (B) 5-month postoperative radiographs of a highly comminuted tibial plateau fracture treated with a bridge plate. This plate serves as an internal splint only, and no fixation through the fracture site is noted.

areas where no myofascial attachments exist is small, and the critical mount of stripping before fracture healing is impaired is unknown.[28] Nonetheless, one must use caution when using a plate to fix a fracture where little soft-tissue coverage exists and the soft-tissue is moderately or severely damaged, such as the tibial diaphysis.

Plates are made of metal alloys, which are much stiffer and stronger than bone. Furthermore, the neutral axis of the bone-plate construct is along the plate, with little load sharing done by the bone. Therefore, the plate absorbs much of the stress, and the bone beneath it becomes porotic. This process is known as stress shielding (Fig. 11).[29, 30]

INTRAMEDULLARY FIXATION

IM nails have become increasingly popular for fixation of diaphyseal and metadiaphyseal fractures in long bones. Although IM nails come in a variety of designs, size, and types, they all serve as splints for fracture stabilization. IM nails can be solid or can be cannulated to allow for canal enlargement by reaming and insertion over a guide wire. IM nails can also have different cross-sectional shapes, including a longitudinal slot, and are currently manufactured from either stainless steel or titanium.

The insertion of an IM nail can be technically challenging, and several pitfalls must be avoided to ensure adequate fracture alignment and fixation. First, the starting point for the nail should allow straight access to the IM canal. In anterograde femoral nailing this should be slightly

posterior in the piriform fossa, whereas in retrograde femoral nailing the starting point should be slightly anterior (4 mm) and lateral (2 mm) to the posterior cruciate ligament insertion in the intercondylar groove (unpublished data of Gary S. Gruen). For the tibia, the starting point is in line with the tibial spine and behind the patellar ligament. In the humerus, the starting point is at the insertion of the supraspinatus just posterior to the bicipital groove. An improperly placed starting hole may result in malalignment of the fracture fragments as the nail is inserted. In addition, medial placement of the starting point of an IM femoral nail may devascularize the femoral head or create a fracture within the femoral neck. Anterior and lateral placement of the femoral starting hole may also cause further comminution of the fracture site as a result of increased hoop stresses placed on the bone.[31, 32] Hoop stresses are the forces acting on the circumferential shape of the bone and are concentrated at the tip of the rod as it makes contact with the IM canal.[31, 32] If these stresses exceed the strength of the bone, then further comminution of the fracture will occur during nail insertion (Fig. 12).

Another technical consideration is that the fracture should be reduced through longitudinal traction and manual manipulation before reaming or nail insertion. Once the fracture is reduced, a guide wire can be placed into the IM canal through the starting hole to maintain the alignment. If a solid IM nail is chosen, it can be inserted into the proximal fragment and used as a joystick to achieve reduction of the distal fragment before crossing the fractured area. If an adequate reduction of the fracture is not

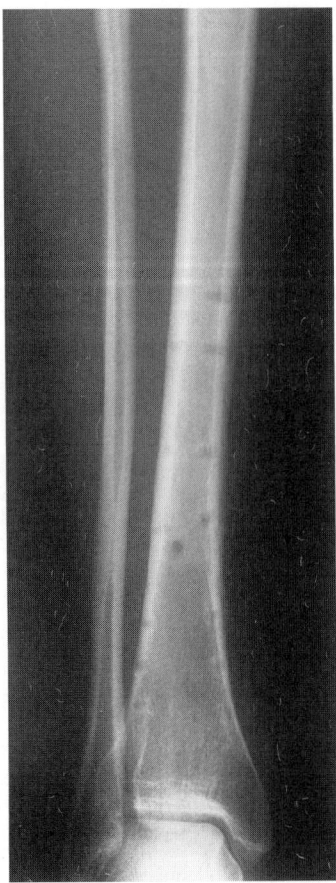

Fig. 11. Plate porosity. This is a radiograph of a distal tibia fracture 3 weeks after removal of the fixation plate. Note the porosity of the bone under the plate.

trol over bending forces with little control over torsional forces and no control of axial forces. Because static locking has reliably led to fracture union, there is little role for dynamic locking at the time of fracture fixation.[33–35] Furthermore, by having several interlocking holes at each end of the nail, the types of fractures treated by IM nailing has increased. This is best exemplified by studies of fractures in the distal femur.[36] When two screws are used at an end of the nail, the fracture can be within 2.5 cm of the more proximal distal locking screw without compromising rotational stability.

IM nails can be placed with or without first reaming the medullary canal before insertion. Whether to ream or not is an issue of debate among trauma surgeons. The benefits of reaming are that a larger IM nail can be placed and the bony contact of the nail is increased.[37] IM nail stiffness is proportional to the fourth power of its radius; therefore, even small changes in its diameter will have dramatic effects on its rigidity,[37, 38] For example, increasing the nail's radius by 25% will double its bending strength. By reaming, the contact length of the IM nail is increased, and this will increase the nail's ability to resist deforming forces and enhance bony contact. A distinct disadvantage to reaming is that the endosteal blood supply is disrupted during the reaming process. Moreover, the endosteal circulation is markedly impaired with a tight-fitting reamed or unreamed IM nail and may not return to normal values over time.[27, 39] In one study, Rhinelander[27] showed a significant

achieved before reaming or nail insertion, either eccentric reaming of the cortices will occur (with weakening of the thinned cortex) or the nail may impinge against the distal cortex and further comminution of the fracture will occur. Finally, proper length, rotation, and varus-valgus alignment should be obtained before interlocking of the IM nail. To choose the proper length of the IM nail, a measurement can be made directly off the fully inserted guide wire when an adequate reduction is achieved. However, in highly comminuted fractures, the appropriate IM nail length may be difficult to determine. In this situation, IM nails of known length may be measured against the uninjured side and the appropriate size nail used for the injured extremity. If both sides are fractured, the size of the IM nail is chosen on the least comminuted side, and the same size is used on both sides. Failure to choose the proper nail length can result in leg length discrepancies, which may be noticed by the patient once ambulation begins.

Although the first IM nails were designed to be used without additional fixation, most IM nails available today have holes at both ends for proximal and distal interlocking screws. This provides an option for inserting screws at one or both ends of the nail. Inserting screws into both ends is called static locking and provides for control of axial, torsional, and bending forces. When no interlocking screws are used or screws are inserted at only one end of the bone, it is called dynamic locking and only provides con-

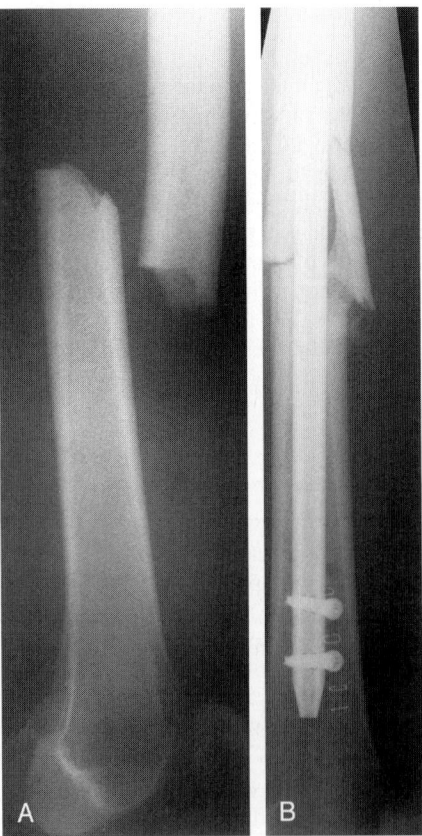

Fig. 12. Further fracture comminution. These are (A) preoperative and (B) immediate postoperative radiographs of a midshaft femur fracture in which the fracture site was comminuted by insertion of the intramedullary nail.

delay in union when a tight-fitting IM nail was inserted. Thermal necrosis and fat embolism are additional concerns and have been attributed to reams. However, newer reamers using deeper cutting flutes and smaller drive shafts have contributed to successful outcomes.[40]

Because of its IM placement, an IM nail acts as a load-sharing device compared with the load bearing of a plate and will tolerate longer periods of loading before failure for a given fracture.[37, 38] Load sharing is best seen with transverse diaphyseal fractures or fractures with minor comminution and some cortical contact between the fracture fragments (Fig. 13). However, in the case of an extensively comminuted diaphyseal fracture treated by a statically locked IM nail, the nail may be completely load bearing until callus formation is well underway, and failure of the nail is a higher concern (Fig. 14).[37, 38]

As with any splint, the working length of an IM nail is the distance between areas of fixation proximally and distally. The bending rigidity of an IM nail is inversely proportional to the square of the working length, whereas the torsional rigidity is inversely proportional to the working length.[20] In severely comminuted fractures of the diaphysis this length may be several inches, whereas in a transverse fracture it may be only a few millimeters. When a highly comminuted diaphyseal fracture is fixed with a statically locked IM nail, the working length is the distance between the proximal and distal locking screws. In this case, the

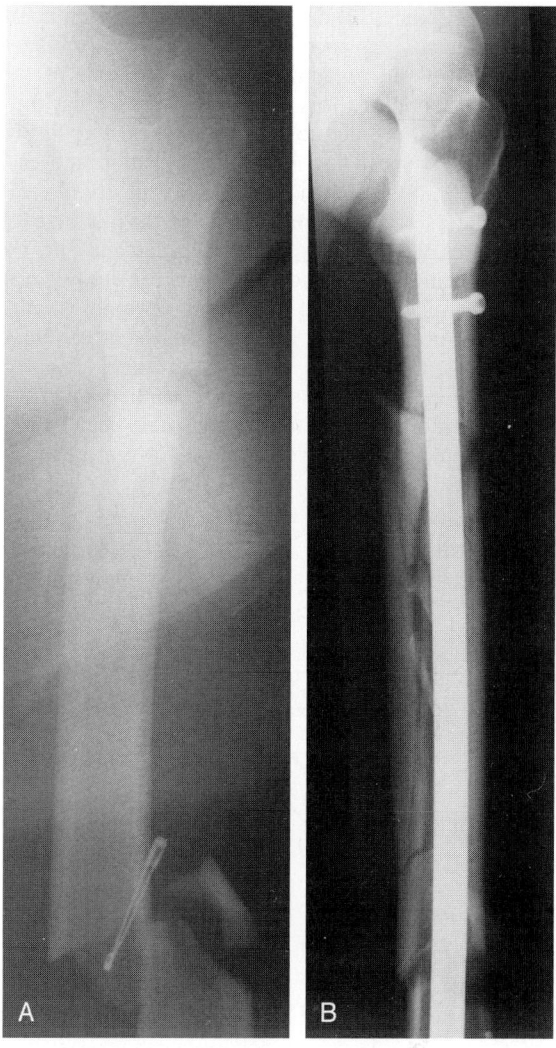

Fig. 14. Intramedullary nail load bearing. These are (A) preoperative and (B) 2-week postoperative radiographs of a segmental femur fracture treated with an intramedullary nail. Because of the significant lack of cortical contact, the nail will serve as a load-bearing device until healing occurs.

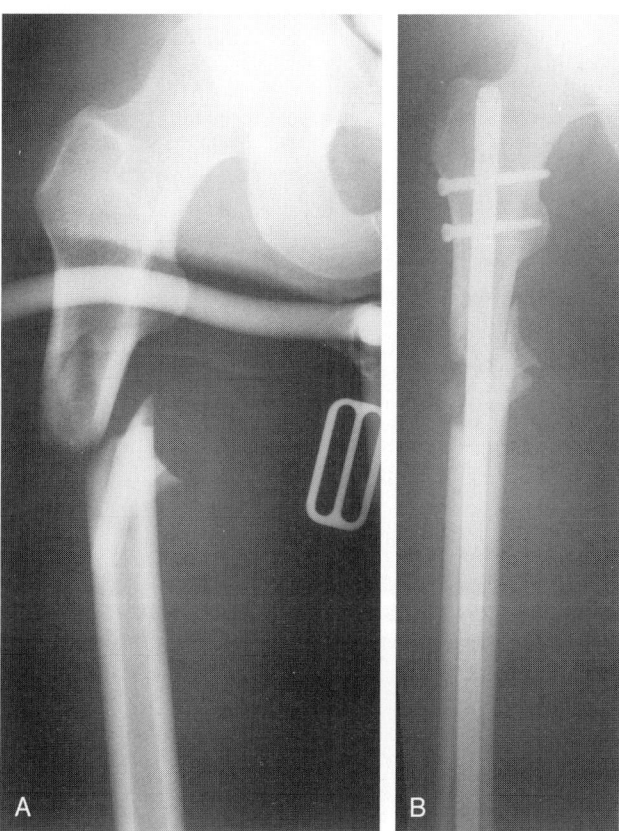

Fig. 13. Intramedullary nail load sharing. These are (A) preoperative and (B) 3-month postoperative radiographs of a subtrochanteric femur fracture treated with an intramedullary nail. Because of the cortical contact at the fracture site, the nail acts as a load-sharing device.

surgeon may opt for a larger nail to ensure adequate fixation that will tolerate longer and higher periods of loading so as to prevent failure of the device before fracture union.

The stiffness or rigidity of the IM nail is dependent on its size, cross-sectional geometry, and material properties. Placing longitudinal slots within the nail will decrease its torsional strength but have no effect on its bending properties.[41] Most IM nails are currently made of stainless steel or titanium. Although titanium is less stiff than stainless steel, both are much stiffer than bone. Titanium has a higher fatigue strength than stainless steel, but it is also more notch sensitive than stainless steel.[37] Notch sensitivity is the sensitivity that a material has to stress concentrations within its structure such as screw holes. This is important because many IM nail failures occur at the locking holes.[42, 43]

EXTERNAL FIXATION

External fixators have been used by orthopaedic surgeons for a long time and continue to be an important part of fracture care. External fixators use a frame, which connects pins percutaneously placed into the bone to stabilize the fracture site without placing metal into the zone of injury. The major attraction to this type of fixation is that the soft tissues around the fracture site are not disturbed by its application. The speed and ease of application and ease of removal are also distinct advantages to its use. In adults, external fixators are commonly used for the stabilization of open fractures with marked soft-tissue damage and as the initial stabilization of pelvic and lower extremity fractures in hemodynamically unstable patients. External fixation is also used as an adjunct to internal fixation in certain fractures such as that of the distal radius and tibial pilon. Although an external fixator can be applied quickly and easily, important biomechanical and biological principles must be adhered to in order to achieve fracture healing.

The configuration of an external fixator assume many designs (Fig. 15). A unilateral external fixator has pins on one side of the fractured bone, whereas a bilateral fixator has pins on two sides of the bone. Unilateral and bilateral designs can also be uniplanar or biplanar. Uniplanar, unilateral fixators are popular because they allow for easy access to wounds. However, in some instances such as severe comminution of the bone, this design may not provide for adequate resistance to torsional and bending forces. Biplanar, unilateral constructs such as a delta or triangular frame will increase the rigidity of the construct but were not effective and are not commonly used.[44] Bilateral fixators were used in the past to increase rigidity of the frame construct but are usually no longer used and are of historical importance only. Currently, most external fixators are designed with pins and frames that are rigid

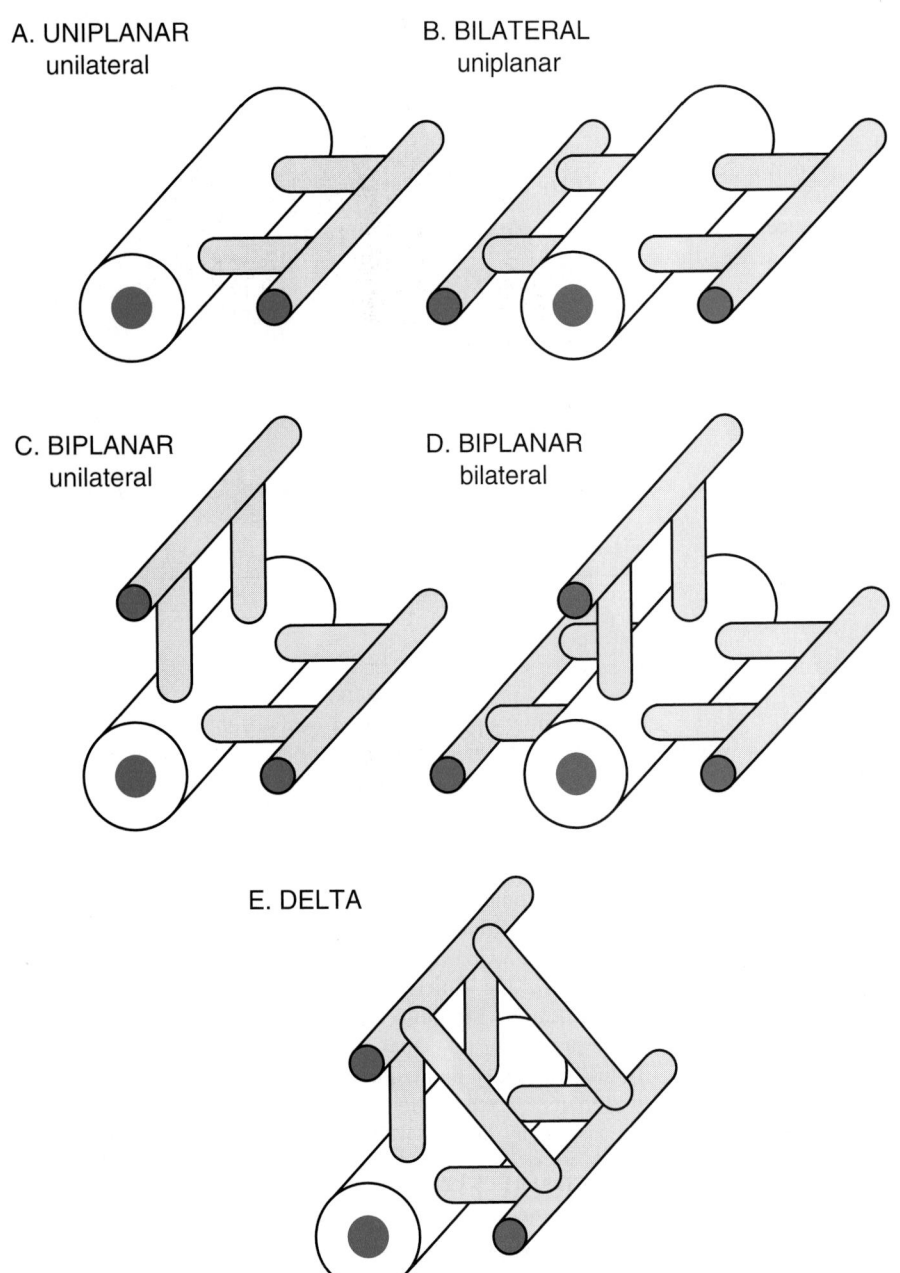

A. UNIPLANAR
unilateral

B. BILATERAL
uniplanar

C. BIPLANAR
unilateral

D. BIPLANAR
bilateral

E. DELTA

Fig. 15. External fixator designs. These show the (*A*) unilateral uniplanar, (*B*) bilateral uniplanar, (*C*) biplanar unilateral, (*D*) biplanar bilateral, and (*E*) delta frame.

enough to allow for unilateral, uniplanar fixation of most fractures. External fixators, which use a ring with tensioned transfixation wires, have become popular for the treatment of proximal and distal tibial metaphyseal/intra-articular fractures.[45]

The fixation bars can be either simple rods made of steel or carbon fiber or elaborate pistons, which allow for compression, distraction, or dynamization of the fractured bone. Most of the articulations used to connect the fixation pins to the bars are universal joints and allow for fracture reduction after application of the frame. However, it is helpful to obtain a preliminary reduction of the fracture with longitudinal traction to visualize better the location for the fixation pins.

The appropriate placement of the fixation pins into the injured extremity is determined by the anatomy of the body part, the amount of soft-tissue injury, and the degree of construct rigidity needed. The pins should be placed in an area that has the least chance of injuring major arteries, veins, and nerves.[46] Pins should not be placed in areas of significant soft-tissue damage because this may result in pin site infection or poor wound healing. The number of pins needed and their spacing are determined by the rigidity of fixation required (see later discussion). Once the site for pin insertion is determined, a small skin incision is made and dissection is carried to the bone. The bone may be predrilled through both cortices, and the depth of the threads needed are determined. Fixation pins are usually half-pins and can be self-drilling, self-tapping, and straight or tapered depending on the manufacturer. The type of pin used will determine the technique of pin insertion. However, if a conical or tapered pin is used, it should not be reversed because pin site loosening may occur. After fixation pin placement, the frame is assembled with connection of the universal joints between the pins and the bars. The fracture is then reduced, and all parts of the frame are tightened (Fig. 16).

The rigidity of an external fixator must be a balance between being stiff enough to maintain fracture reduction while allowing micromotion to occur at the fracture site. An external fixator that is too rigid will prevent callus formation and may require prolonged use of the fixator for fracture fixation. It then becomes a race between fracture healing and failure of the external fixator. In contrast, an external fixator that is not rigid enough will either lose the fracture reduction or allow too much motion at the fracture site, resulting in a delayed union or nonunion.

The rigidity of an external fixator can be most significantly increased by altering the pin size. Increasing the radius of the fixation pin increases its bending strength by a power of four. However, the size increase is limited by the size of the bone diaphysis. Placing a screw hole greater than 20%[47] or 30%[48] of the bone's diameter will significantly weaken it and increase the risk for fracture. Although this weakness will resolve in 6 to 8 weeks through bone remodeling, the removed pin remains a stress riser until remodeling can occur.

Rigidity of the external fixator can also be increased by altering other factors.[49] Increasing the number of pins or bars will increase rigidity, as will increasing the spread of the pins. Applying radial preload to the pins will increase their fixation and prevent loosening. Radial preload is achieved by making

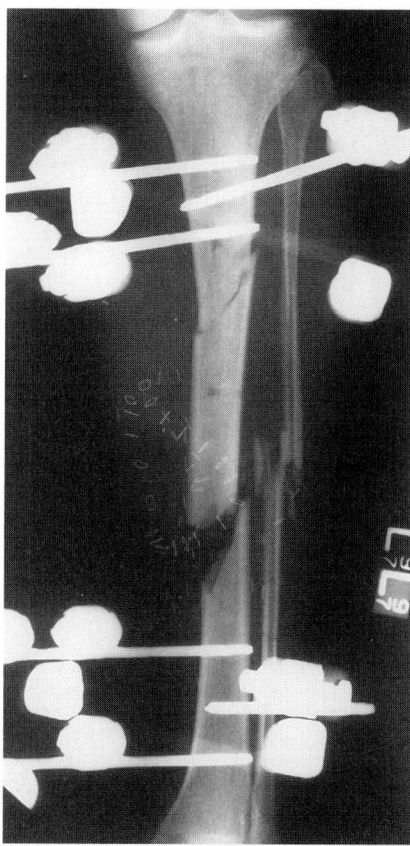

Fig. 16. External fixation. These are immediate postoperative radiographs of an external fixator in a delta configuration used to treat an open segmental tibial fracture with soft-tissue loss.

the pilot hole for the pin smaller than the root diameter of the pin or using a pin with tapered threads.

The complications associated with external fixation are related to the biology and biomechanics associated with its use.[50] Within a short period of time after pin placement, the epidermis will surround the pin site and bacteria will attempt to colonize the tract. A pin tract infection can ensue, leading to deep infection or osteomyelitis. The best treatment for pin site infections is prevention and early intervention. Placing the pin in areas of little soft tissue and preventing the pistoning of soft tissues around the pin are the most important prophylactic methods. If drainage from the pin sites or cellulitis is noted around the pins, then antibiotics to cover skin flora should be initiated along with increased pin site care. If this fails to eradicate the infection, then the pin must be removed and local débridement initiated.

Other potential complications associated with external fixation is pin site loosening or fracture at the pin site. Because fixation pins are screws into bone, the same size restrictions apply in that the pin must not exceed 20%[47] to 30%[48] of the bone's diameter or else the bone will be significantly weakened. Also, as the bone is drilled, heat is generated by the drill bit. If the temperature is allowed to exceed 50°C, cell death of the bone ensues, leading to an increased risk for pin site loosening.[51] The use of a water-cooled sharp drill at lower speeds can decrease the risk of thermal necrosis.

SUMMARY

Although the designs of internal and external fixation are evolving, the basic principles of fracture reduction and stabilization have not changed. By learning these basic concepts and becoming proficient in the techniques outlined in this chapter, the surgeon can effectively plan and carry out the procedure, which will optimize function of the extremity and minimize complications.

REFERENCES

1. Grundes O, Reikeras O: The role of the hematoma and periosteal sealing for fracture healing in rats. Acta Scand Orthop 1993; 64:47.
2. Grundes O, Reikeras O: The importance of the hematoma for fracture healing in rats. Acta Orthop Scand 1993; 64:340.
3. Potts WJ: The role of the hematoma in fracture healing. Surg Gynecol Obstet 1933; 57:318.
4. Buckwalter JA, Cooper RR: Bone structure and function. Instruct Course Lect 1987; 36:27.
5. Schenk R, Willenegger H: Zum Histologischen Bild der Sogenannten Primarheilung der Knochenkompakta Nach Experimentellen Osteotomien am Hund. Experientia 1963; 19:593.
6. Schenk RJ, Willenegger H: Histologie der Primaren Knochenheilung. Langenbecks Arch Klin Chir 1964; 308:440.
7. Perren SM, Boitzy A: Cellular differentiation and bone biomechanics during the consolidation of a fracture. Anat Clin 1978; 1:13.
8. Udupa KN, Pradad GC: Chemical and histochemical studies on the organic constituents in fracture repair in rats. J Bone and Joint Surg Br 1963; 45:770.
9. Frost HM: Skeletal physiology and bone remodeling. In Urist MR (ed): Fundamental and Clinical Bone Physiology. Philadelphia, JB Lippincott, 1980, p 208.
10. Wendeberg B: Mineral metabolism of fractures of the tibia in man studied with external counting strontium 85. Acta Orthop Scand Suppl l961; 52:1.
11. Weber H, Czech O: Pseudarthrosis. Bern, Huber Verlag, 1976.
12. Muller ME, Allgower M, Schneider RW, et al: Manual of Internal Fixation. New York, Springer-Verlag, 1979, 2nd ed.
13. Brunner CF, Weber BG: Special Techniques in Internal Fixation. New York, Springer-Verlag, 1982.
14. Jacobs RR, Armstrong JH, Whittaker JH, et al: Treatment of intertrochanteric hip fractures with a compression hip screw and a nail plate. J Trauma 1976; 16:599.
15. Kaufer H: Mechanics of the injured hip. Clin Orthop 1980; 146:53.
16. Pauwels F: Der Schenkelhaslbruch, ein Mechaniches Problem. Stuttgarte, Enke, 1935.
17. Pauwels F: Gessammelte Abhandlungen Zur Funktionellen Anatomie des Bewegungsapparates. Berlin, Springer-Verlag, 1982.
18. Schaffer JJ, Manoli A: The antiglide plate for distal fibular fixation. J Bone Joint Surg Am 1987; 69:596.
19. Blatter G, Weber BG: Wave plate osteosynthesis as a salvage procedure. Acta Chir Orthop Traumatol Cech 1993; 60:273.
20. Tarr RR, Wiss DA: The mechanics and biology of intramedullary fracture fixation. Clin Orthop 1986; 212:10.
21. Hicks JH: The relationship between metal and infection. Proc R Soc Med 1957; 50:842.
22. Johner R, Wruhs O: Classification of tibial shaft fractures and correlation with results after rigid internal fixation. Clin Orthop 1983; 178:7.
23. Leach RE: Fractures of the tibia and fibula. In Rockwood CA, Green DP (eds): Fractures in Adults. Philadelphia, JB Lippincott, 1984, 2nd ed.
24. Dominguez J, Mundy GR: Monocytes mediate osteoclastic bone resorption by prostaglandin production. Calcif Tissue Res 1980; 31:29.
25. Rand JA, Chao EYS, Kelly PJ: A comparison of the effect of open intramedullary nailing and compression plate fixation on fracture-site blood flow and fracture union. J Bone Joint Surg Am 1981; 63:427.
26. Rhinelander FW: The normal microcirculation of diaphyseal cortex and its response to fracture. J Bone Joint Surg Am 1968; 50:784.
27. Rhinelander, FW: Effects of medullary nailing of the normal blood supply of diaphyseal cortex. Instruct Course Lect 1973; 22:161.
28. Rhinelander FW, Phillips RS, Steel WM, et al: Microangiography in bone healing: II: Displaced closed fractures. J Bone Joint Surg Am 1968; 50:643.
29. Moyen B, Comtet J, Roy JC, et al: Refracture after removal of internal fixation devices: Clinical study of 20 cases and physiopathologic hypothesis. Lyon Chir 1980; 76:153.
30. Moyen BJ, Lahey PJ Jr, Weinberg EH, et al: Effects on intact femora of dogs of the application and removal of metal plates: A metabolic and structural study comparing stiffer and more flexible plates. J Bone Joint Surg Am 1978; 60:940.
31. Johnson, KD, Tencer AF, Blumenthal S, et al: Biomechanical performance of locked intramedullary nail systems in comminuted femoral shaft fractures. Clin Orthop 1986; 206:151.
32. Johnson KD, Tencer AF, Sherman MC: Biomechanical factors affecting fracture stability and femoral bursting in closed intramedullary nailing of femoral shaft fractures with illustrative case presentations. J Orthop Trauma 1987; 1:1.
33. Cross A, Montgomery RJ: The treatment of tibial shaft fractures by the locking medullary nail system. J Bone Joint Surg Br 1987; 69:489.
34. Klemm KW, Borner M: Interlocking nailing of complex fractures of the femur and tibia. Clin Orthop 1986; 212:89.
35. Thoresen BO, Alho A, Ekeland A, et al: Interlocking intramedullary nailing in femoral shaft fractures. A report of forty-eight cases. J Bone Joint Surg Am 1985; 67:1313.
36. Folgar C, Alexander JW, Lindsey R: Comparison of fracture stability in intramedullary nailing of distal femur fractures with one or two distal locking screws. Presented at the 12th annual meeting of the Orthopedic Trauma Association, Boston, MA, 1996.
37. Gustillo RB, Kyle RF, Templeman D: Biomechanics of fracture fixation devices. In Gustillo RB, Kyle RF, Templeman D (eds): Fractures and Dislocations. St. Louis, MO, CV Mosby, 1993.
38. Allen WC, Piotrowski G, Burstein AH, et al: Biomechanical principles of intramedullary fixation. Clin Orthop 1968; 60:13.
39. Hupel TM, Aksenow SA, Schemitsch EN: Cortical bone and soft tissue blood flow in loose and tight fitting locked unreamed nailing. Presented at the 12th annual meeting of the Orthopedic Trauma Association, Boston, MA, 1996.
40. Agnew SG: Intramedullary reamer redesign: The effect on pressure and temperature. Tech Orthop 1998; 13:9.
41. Krettek C, Miclau T, Blauth M, et al: Recurrent rotational deformity of the femur after static locking of intramedullary nails. J Bone Joint Surg Br 1997; 79:4.
42. Browner BD: Pitfalls, errors and complications in the use of locking Küntscher nails. Clin Orthop 1986; 212:192.
43. Bucholz RW, Ross SE, Lawrence KL: Fatigue fracture of the interlocking nail in the treatment of fractures of the distal part of the femoral shaft. J Bone Joint Surg Am 1987; 69:1391.
44. Behrens F, Searls K: External fixation of the tibia. Basic concepts and prospective evaluations. J Bone Joint Surg Br 1986; 66:246.
45. Behrens F: A primer of fixator devices and configurations. Clin Orthop 1989; 245:5.
46. Green S: Complications of External Skeletal Fixation. Springfield, Il, Charles C Thomas, 1981.
47. Bechtol CO, Lepper H Jr: Fundamental studies in the design of metal screws for internal fixation of bone. J Bone Joint Surg Am 1956; 38:1385.
48. Burstein A, Currey J, Frankel VH, et al: Bone strength: The effect of screw holes. J Bone Joint Surg Am 1972; 54:1143.
49. Briggs BT, Chao EYS: The mechanical performance of the standard Hoffmann-Vidal external fixation apparatus. J Bone Joint Surg Am 1982; 64:566.
50. Paley D: Problems, obstacles, and complications of limb lengthening by the Ilizarov technique. Clin Orthop 1990; 250:81.
51. Matthews LS, Green CA, Goldstein SA: The thermal effects of skeletal fixation-pin insertion in bone. J Bone Joint Surg Am 1989;71:835.

COMPLICATIONS OF FRACTURES: ACUTE

E. H. Schemitsch and Markku T. Nousiainen

Summary

- Acute complications of fractures include thromboembolism, fat embolism syndrome (FES), acute respiratory distress syndrome (ARDS), multiple-organ dysfunction syndrome (MODS), hemorrhagic shock and other bleeding disorders, tetanus, gas gangrene, osteomyelitis, implant failure, nervous and vascular injury, and compartment syndrome.
- Each of these complications can have an important impact on the biopsychosocial indexes of personal health.
- Because these complications can occur during all ages, their impact on public health can be significant.
- The natural history, diagnosis, and treatment for each of the complications are varied.
- In all patients, there should be no delay in the diagnosis and treatment.

Fractures may be associated with a variety of acute complications. Because these complications can cause substantial morbidity and even mortality, rapid diagnosis and prevention of their development are essential. In this chapter we summarize the epidemiology, pathophysiology, diagnosis, prevention, and treatment of several important acute complications of fractures. Each is classified with regard to its ability to develop systemic or local (bone and soft-tissue) problems.

SYSTEMIC COMPLICATIONS

THROMBOEMBOLISM: DEEP VENOUS THROMBOSIS AND PULMONARY EMBOLISM

Deep venous thrombosis (DVT) and pulmonary embolism (PE) are among the most common complications of trauma and orthopaedic surgery.[1] Developing in the pre-, intra-, or postoperative period, the clinical signs and symptoms of these thromboembolic events are often difficult to detect. Nevertheless, knowledge of the risk factors that are associated with DVT and PE development can allow the orthopaedic surgeon to better estimate a patient's chance of experiencing either of these problems.

Factors known to increase the risk of DVT and PE development include the following:

Fracture location: patients with fractures of the lower extremities and pelvis are more prone to experience DVT and PE than those with fractures of the upper extremity.[2]

Patient age and health status: the risk of thromboembolism rises with (1) increased age, (2) presence of health problems such as acquired trauma, heart disease, infection, obesity, resistance to activated protein C by factor V Leiden, hyperhomocystinemia, nephrotic syndrome, and

certain cancers, (3) a history of DVT and varicose veins, (4) use of oral contraceptives, and (5) being in the intra- or postpartum phase of pregnancy.[3]

Timing, extent, and duration of fracture surgery: prolonged surgeries, especially those performed a few days after trauma, promote thromboembolism.[4] The nature of injury sustained has little effect on the incidence of DVT formation; rather, it is the presence of the aforementioned risk factors that plays a more significant role.[5]

Degree and length of immobilization: immobilization with calf muscle inactivity sets up the stage for venous stasis, making this risk factor more important to the development of DVT than is injury, anesthesia, or surgery.[6]

Very little information is available about the incidence of DVT and PE in patients with isolated orthopaedic injuries. Nevertheless, one study showed that patients who had early operative fixation (less than 27 hours after injury) of fractures in the lower extremity, distal to the hip, had a 28% chance of experiencing DVT and a 4% chance of experiencing PE.[1] In the general trauma population, clinical factors that predict an increased risk of DVT include increasing age, spinal cord injury, lower extremity and pelvic fracture, direct venous injuries, multiple blood transfusions, and prolonged immobilization.[4] Between 35% and 65% of trauma patients with pelvic fracture experience DVT, whereas 2% to 12% experience PE.[4]

Pathophysiology

Venous stasis, hypercoagulability, and endothelial damage are the three main factors that promote the development of a thrombus.[7] Depending on the degree of collateral drainage, the circulatory system's response to this thrombus can either be benign (up to two-thirds of patients with thrombi can be asymptomatic) or involve a perivascular inflammatory reaction or edema distal to the occlusion.[7] When thrombi form in the larger veins of the leg (popliteal, femoral, and iliac), embolization of the free end of the thrombus to the pulmonary circulation can lead to serious consequences. Occlusion of the pulmonary artery or its major branches can cause acute dilation of the right side of the heart or sudden death as a result of lung ischemia.[7] Obstruction of smaller branches may cause pulmonary infarction or hemorrhage.[7] The pathophysiological response to PE ultimately depends on the extent of obstruction to pulmonary blood flow, size of the occluded vessels, number of emboli, overall status of the cardiovascular system, and local release of vasoactive factors.[7]

It is important to realize that thrombosis usually develops bilaterally, even if one extremity is injured or thrombosis is clinically present in one leg.[7] The location of the DVT is also relevant: approximately 10% of proximal DVTs (thromboses at or above the popliteal fossa) embolize massively or fatally.[8] When DVT occurs below the knee, the risk of significant PE has been found to be minimal.[9]

Diagnosis

The classic presentation of DVT includes calf or thigh discomfort and venous distention and edema distal to the obstruction. A positive Homans's sign, erythema, increased skin temperature, and fever may also be found. These symptoms and signs usually evolve between postoperative days 7 and 10 but can develop later.

Findings indicative of PE relate to the extent of pulmonary arterial tree occlusion, the presence of preexisting cardiopulmonary disease, and whether pulmonary infarction occurs.[7] Common symptoms and signs include dyspnea, pleuritic pain, cough, tachypnea, crackles, and tachycardia.

Because the aforementioned symptoms and signs have low specificity, DVT or PE must be confirmed using one or more diagnostic tests. For DVT, the noninvasive test of choice is color-flow duplex ultrasound (Fig. 1).[10] Venography is the gold standard invasive test but is costly and can induce iatrogenic thrombosis in peripheral veins (Fig. 2).[11]

Diagnostic studies for PE include chest radiographs, electrocardiographic (ECG) monitoring, arterial blood gas measurements, perfusion/ventilation ($\dot{V}/\dot{Q}$) scans, pulmonary angiography, and helical computed tomography (CT) scans.[12] Findings from chest radiographs, such as Hampton's hump (indicating an area of atelectasis or infarction) and Westermark's sign (associated with an area of hypovolemia), are usually nonspecific or absent.[13] Sinus tachycardia and T-wave inversion in the anterior leads are the most common abnormalities on the ECG strip.[13] Arterial blood gases will show a decrease in partial pressures of both arterial oxygen (PaO_2) and arterial carbon dioxide ($PaCO_2$), whereas the $\dot{V}/\dot{Q}$ scan will show a high ventilation/perfusion ratio (with high sensitivity but low specificity) (Fig. 3).[14] Pulmonary angiography is the gold standard test but carries with it important morbidity and mortality risks (Fig. 4).[14] One study suggested that evaluation of symptomatic patients with a combination of CT and duplex Doppler ultrasonography with compression may lead to a substantial improvement in the diagnosis of DVT and PE compared with other imaging combinations.[12]

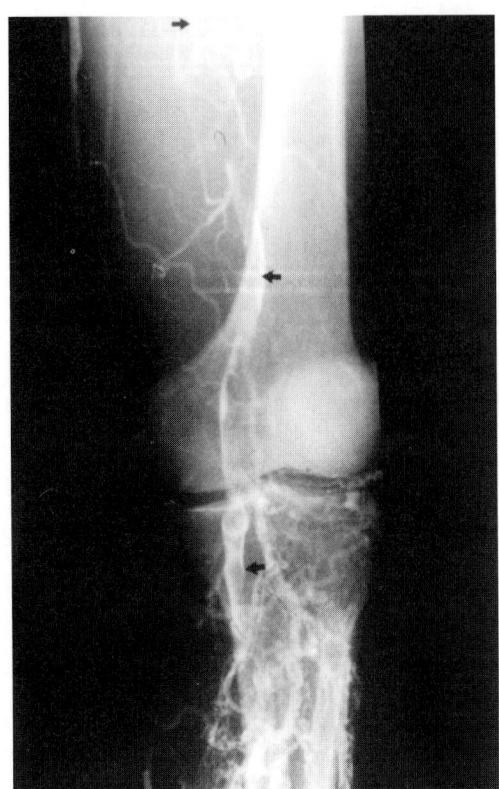

Fig. 2. Deep venous thrombosis. This venogram shows three sites *(arrows)* of thrombosis in an individual who experienced acute swelling and tenderness of the lower leg.

Prevention

Considering the substantial morbidity and mortality that can ensue once DVT or PE has been established, great care must be taken to prevent their development and to identify these events early, if they do occur. General measures include good preoperative conditioning (if possible), careful handling of the lower limbs during surgery, and early postoperative mobilization.

Because of the potential risk for significant bleeding complications, pharmaceutical prophylaxis is usually not used in children and young, healthy adults. Outside of these populations, the evidence for initiating pharmacological prophylaxis against DVT and PE is overwhelming. In one study, medical prophylaxis was found to reduce the incidence of DVT by 50% in patients who undergo surgery for hip fracture.[15]

At this time, evidence suggests that low-molecular-weight heparin (LMWH) is the ideal drug of choice in patients who sustain isolated hip fractures or major trauma.[4] Well-designed studies on these patients showed that LMWH provides superior protection against DVT and PE in the immediate postinjury period compared with low-dose heparin or aspirin.[16, 17]

Ideally, thromboprophylaxis should be started as soon as primary hemostasis has taken place after the original injury (as evidenced by a relatively stable hemoglobin).[4] Except for withholding therapy during perioperative periods, LMWH should be used until the patient no longer requires any further surgeries.[4] LMWH can be continued, or warfarin prophylaxis can be instituted until the patient's high-risk status resolves;

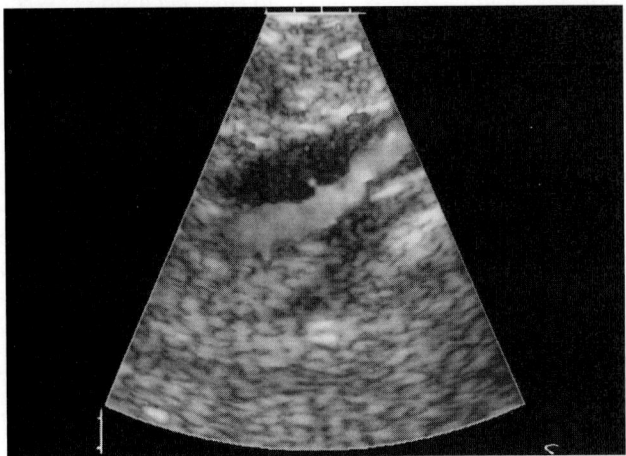

Fig. 1. Deep venous thrombosis (DVT). This Doppler ultrasonogram shows the presence of a DVT in the left iliac vein.

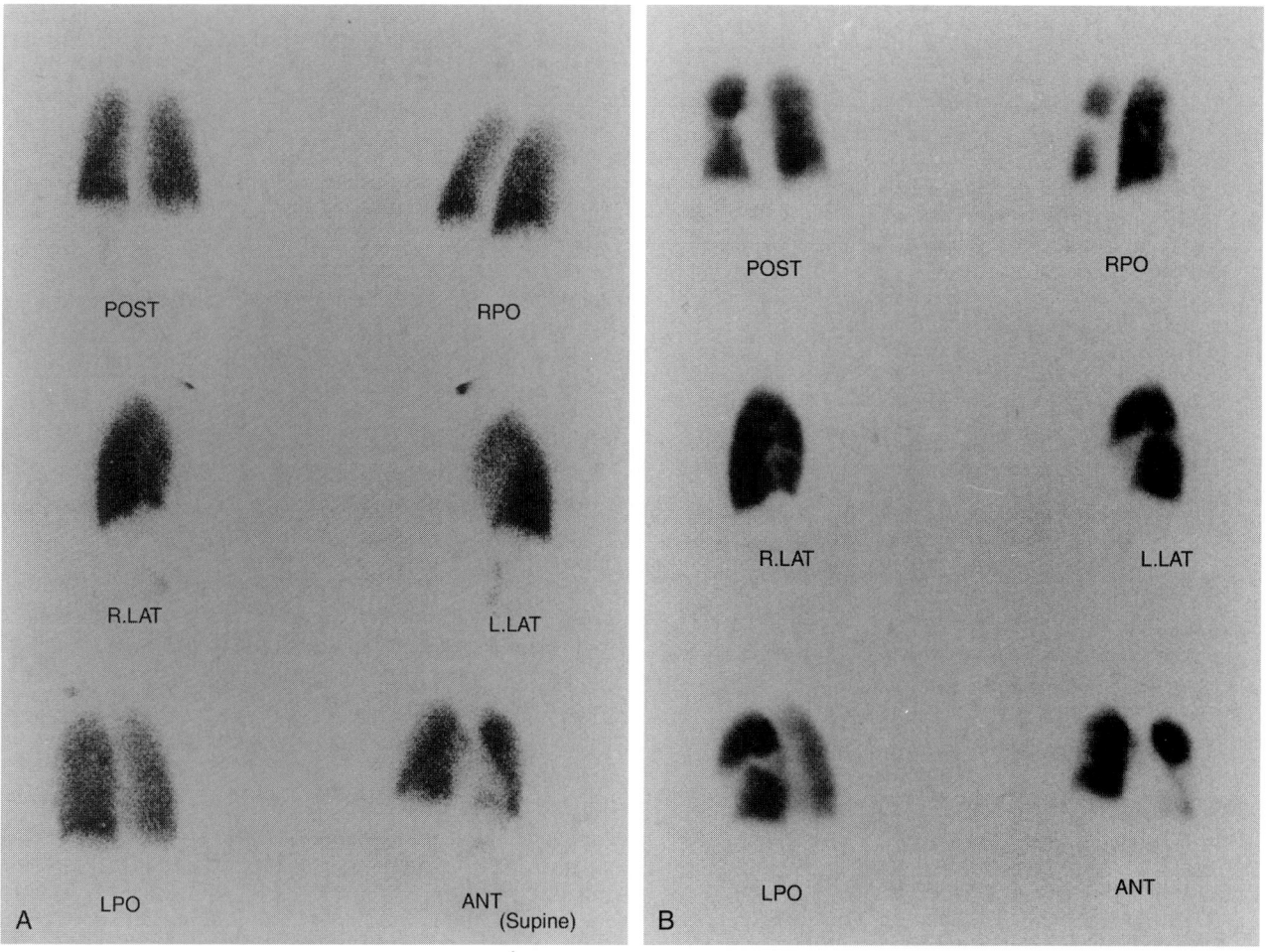

Fig. 3. Pulmonary embolus (PE). *A* and *B,* This perfusion lung scan indicates the presence of a PE in the left lingula and superior segment of the left upper lobe. The ventilation scan was normal.

the goal is to keep the international normalization ratio within the range of 2.0 to 3.0.[4]

Recommendations on the actual duration of warfarin therapy remain controversial.[18] As such, the presence of known risk factors, such as medical illnesses, type of injury and surgery, prolonged immobilization, and estrogen use should be taken into account so as to guide the length of therapy that is needed. It is important to remember that the patient's hydration status should be optimized throughout this postinjury period.

If anticoagulant therapy fails or is contraindicated and the patient is at risk for PE, insertion of a filter into the inferior vena cava may be considered.[13, 19] Selective placement has been shown to minimize the incidence of PE in patients with pelvic fractures and proximal DVT.[20]

Treatment

Once DVT or PE develops or is suspected, the patient should be started on either standard heparin or LMWH (if not contraindicated) until diagnostic testing can prove its presence or absence.[4, 21, 22] If DVT is present, heparin or LMWH administration should continue for 5 to 7 days.

If PE develops, the patient should also be given oxygen and be encouraged to sit up to promote respiratory efforts. An urgent consultation should be made to the internal medicine and general or vascular surgery services. Depending on the patient's health status, these services may suggest that pharmacological thrombolysis or thrombo/embolectomy be performed.[13]

Both the incidence of postdischarge DVT and PE development in orthopaedic surgery patients and the optimal pharmacological prophylaxis for thromboembolic prevention are still unknown.[23] Current recommendations suggest that patients with positive venography should receive heparin or warfarin past the date of discharge.[23] For those patients with reversible risk factors, such as surgery, a short course of anticoagulation (4 to 6 weeks) should be administered.[18] Patients without reversible predisposing factors, such as the presence of cancer, should be considered for long-term (i.e., 6 months or more) pharmacological therapy.[18] An indefinite period of anticoagulation should be considered in patients with recurrent PE if the risk of major bleeding is low.[24]

FAT EMBOLISM SYNDROME

FES, a potentially fatal syndrome, develops when fat globules embolize in the microvasculature of the lungs, brain, kidneys, and skin. It is thought to be a common subclinical event after long bone or pelvic trauma and intramedullary reaming.[25, 26] These findings occur in 0.5% to 2.0% of

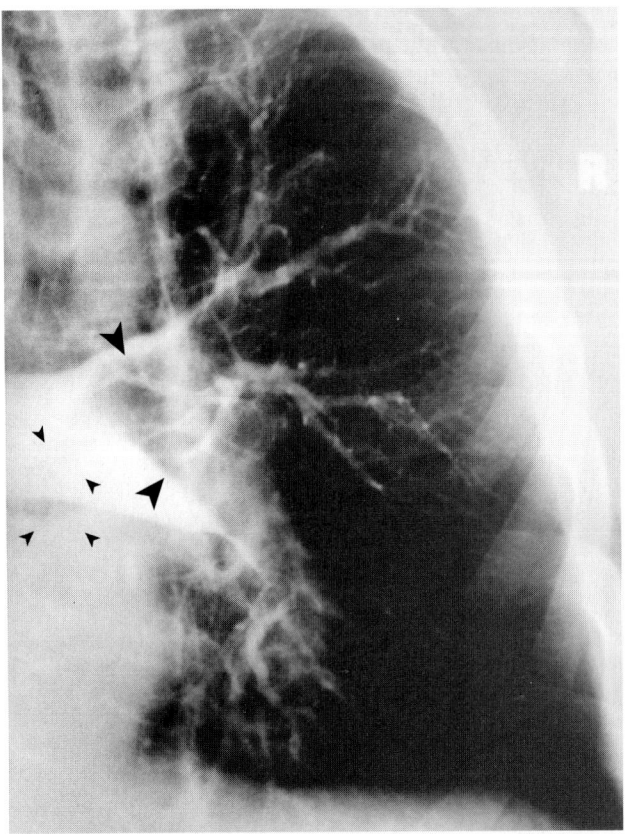

Fig. 4. Massive pulmonary embolus (PE). This section of a chest angiogram shows the presence of a PE in the left pulmonary artery (arrows).

patients with single fractures; this prevalence rises to between 5% and 10% in patients with multiple fractures.[26, 27] Evolution of ARDS is a rare but severe sequela of FES.[25]

Pathophysiology

Two theories, the mechanical and the biochemical, have been proposed to explain how FES develops. The mechanical theory suggests that bone, fat, and marrow emboli cause the symptoms.[28] These particles enter the circulatory system after bone fractures. Larger emboli lodge in the pulmonary arteries, causing respiratory compromise.[28] Smaller emboli pass through pulmonary precapillary shunts or a patent foramen ovale to enter the systemic circulation.[28]

Synthesis of the acute-phase proteins is also thought to be responsible for causing the formation of obstructive fat emboli.[28] In vitro and in vivo studies showed that C-reactive protein agglutinates very low-density lipoproteins, Intralipid, and chylomicrons.[28] Because plasma levels of C-reactive protein rise at the same time as the onset of symptoms of FES, it is theorized that C-reactive protein may play an important role in macroglobule production.[28]

The biochemical theory proposes that free fatty acids are responsible for the damage seen in this syndrome.[28] Mobilized by the lysis of triglycerides or the release of catecholamines secondary to trauma, free fatty acids flow into the pulmonary capillary bed.[28] These compounds cause endothelial damage and are toxic to pneumocytes.[28] Pulmonary edema, hemorrhage, and clot formation ensue, setting the stage for organ dysfunction.[28]

Diagnosis

Two different sets of criteria for the diagnosis of FES have been developed. The first suggests that a diagnosis can be made if one major and four minor signs are present in association with macroglobulinemia.[29] Major signs include respiratory distress (comprising tachypnea, dyspnea, a decrease in PaO_2, an increase in $PaCO_2$, and cyanosis); cerebral involvement (such as confusion, drowsiness, and lethargy leading to convulsions and coma); and petechial rash.[29] Minor signs include fever (greater than 38.5°C), tachycardia, jaundice, a decrease in hematocrit level, and renal and retinal changes.[29]

The other set of criteria is less restrictive. Here, FES can be assumed to have developed if the PaO_2 is less than 60 mm Hg, the $PaCO_2$ is greater than 55 mm Hg, the respiratory rate is greater than 35 breaths per minute, or there is clinical evidence of respiratory distress.[30]

FES can be diagnosed only on the basis of patient history and clinical findings. Adjunctive laboratory tests may be used to evaluate the progression of FES. Blood gas readings will show hypoxemia. Chest radiographs may show multiple bilateral patchy areas of consolidation ("snowstorm" appearance), especially in the upper and middle parts of the lungs.[26] Nonspecific ST-segment changes may be seen on the ECG.[26]

Prevention

General measures that should be taken to prevent the development of FES include proper and early fracture care, maintenance of fluid and electrolyte balance, and oxygen administration.[31] Movement of fracture ends must be controlled with proper splinting to minimize the amount of embolic material that may be spilled into the circulation. Definitive skeletal stabilization should occur within 24 hours after injury. Study outcomes show that early, in comparison to delayed, stabilization minimizes both morbidity and mortality rates in multiply injured patients.[32, 33]

With regard to fixation technique, both intramedullary nailing and plate osteosynthesis have been found to reduce the incidence of several post-traumatic complications of fractures, including FES.[34, 35] Research suggests that the method of fracture fixation plays a minor role in the development of pulmonary dysfunction. The presence of other factors (such as delayed fixation)[32, 33] appears to be more important in promoting the development of pulmonary problems.

Treatment

When FES does develop, immediate steps must be taken to maintain sufficient blood oxygenation. If hypoxemia is severe, endotracheal intubation and mechanical ventilation are indicated. Pulmonary function will usually recover within 3 to 5 days after the onset of symptoms.[28]

A variety of medications, including heparin, ethanol, and corticosteroids, have been suggested to treat FES. None of these agents have been clearly found to have a favorable clinical effect in controlled trials, so their use is not suggested.[28]

Because FES does not occur as an isolated condition, associated mortality rates range from 12% to 87%.[26]

ACUTE RESPIRATORY DISTRESS SYNDROME

Pulmonary compromise is commonly seen in patients who sustain traumatic injuries. Of concern is the development of ARDS.

Pathophysiology, Diagnosis, and Management

ARDS describes the condition in which, subsequent to the release of inflammatory cytokines, the permeability of alveolar and capillary membranes is increased.[36] This increase in permeability leads to the development of acute pulmonary edema with concomitant severe arterial hypoxemia.[36–38] Patients in whom ARDS is developing will initially have an increased respiratory rate. As such, arterial blood gas measurement will show a lowered PO_2 along with a decreased PCO_2. Administration of supplemental oxygen will cause a large rise in PaO_2, indicating the presence of pulmonary ventilation-perfusion mismatching.[36] As the alveolar and capillary changes progressively deteriorate, right-to-left shunting of blood through collapsed or filled alveoli is initiated.[36] As such, the worsening hypoxemia cannot be corrected by supplemental oxygen.[36] Instead, mechanical positive end-expiratory pressure ventilatory support is needed to open the collapsed alveoli and decrease the shunting.[36] Chest radiograph films will show bilateral interstitial infiltrates and characteristic air bronchograms (Fig. 5).

Prevention

Considering the serious consequences of respiratory failure, it is prudent for orthopaedic surgeons to anticipate situations that may induce ARDS and to know preventive measures. Retrospective studies of trauma patients indicate that the strongest determinants of post-traumatic ARDS include hemorrhagic shock at admission to the emergency room, high injury severity scores, significant neurological injury, and fractures that are associated with severe tissue trauma.[37, 38] This body of research shows that the incidence of ARDS can be minimized if early operative stabilization (i.e., less than 24 hours after trauma) of major fractures is performed.[33, 35, 38] A delay in orthopaedic surgery past this period can result in up to a fivefold increase in the incidence of ARDS.[38]

MULTIPLE ORGAN DYSFUNCTION SYNDROME

MODS, or multiple organ system failure, is defined as the failure of two or more organ systems remote from the site of original insult after injury, operation, or sepsis.[39, 40] This syndrome develops mostly in trauma patients who have a high injury severity score (i.e., 25 or higher).[39]

Pathophysiology and Diagnosis

This syndrome is the end result of a sequence of damaging events that are initiated by the normal metabolic response to injury and lead to systemic hypermetabolism and the inability of organs to maintain their functional roles.[39, 40] Two distinct patterns of onset can occur.[41] Early MODS develops within 12 to 36 hours of injury, whereas late MODS becomes clinically overt on postinjury days 6 to 8.[41] In both patterns, it is theorized that the presence of dead tissue produced from multisystem trauma and shock stimulates an inflammatory response, which eventually becomes uncontrolled.[40] The high energy demands of inflammation quickly deprive the body of its energy reserves. Once these reserves become depleted, organs begin failing in a consistent pattern. First, the lung fails, followed by the liver, gastric mucosa, and then the kidneys.[42]

Patients with late-onset MODS usually sustain their injuries quite well in the early post-trauma period.[41] For these individuals, the development of immunosuppression and subsequent infection during the first postinjury days proves to be the instigator of the hyperinflammatory response.[43]

Studies showed that the degree of immunosuppression that develops after trauma can be directly related to the severity of injuries.[43] Aside from the intuitive fact that the trauma patient's condition worsens with increasing number of sustained injuries, this research suggests that fractures play a major role in promoting the evolution of immune dysfunction in multiple-trauma patients. For this reason, it is imperative that fractures be treated along with all other serious injuries in the immediate post-trauma period.

Treatment and Prevention

Important treatment measures that are known to prevent the development of MODS include replacement of lost body fluids, control of hemorrhagic sites, ventilatory support, prevention of sepsis, and supply of adequate nutrition.[40, 44] Early, rigid stabilization of pelvic, spinal, and femoral fractures has been proven to help prevent the onset of pulmonary failure.[45] Fracture fixation minimizes the development of further tissue damage.[45] It also allows the patient to sit upright, thereby promoting pulmonary ventilation.

Concern about the effect of certain kinds of skeletal stabilization on the development of MODS has been raised. Studies suggest that the method of fracture fixation plays a minor role in the development of pulmonary dysfunction in

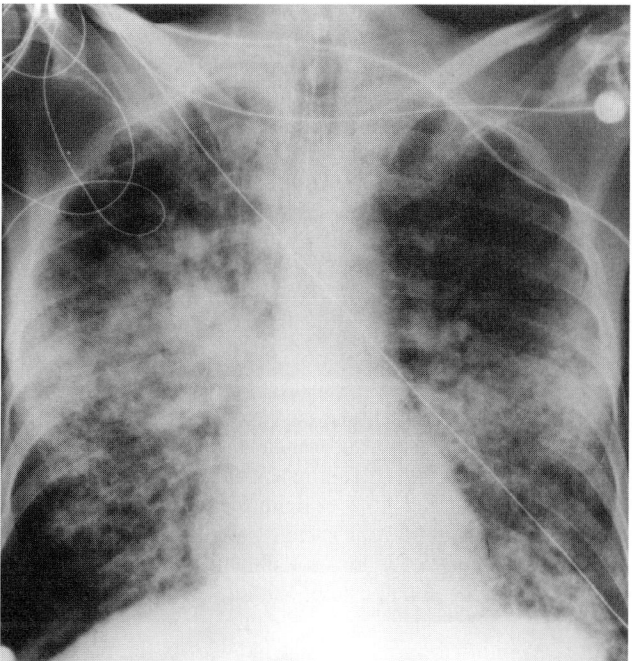

Fig. 5. Adult respiratory distress syndrome (ARDS). This chest radiograph indicates classic air bronchograms in a patient with severe ARDS.

the trauma patient, although this is still controversial.[25, 35] Despite this, the orthopaedist must often have to decide whether to perform a timely, yet nonoptimal stabilization procedure or an amputation to minimize a severely injured trauma patient's risk of MODS.

HEMORRHAGIC SHOCK

Of the various types of shock that can develop, the orthopaedic surgeon should be particularly watchful for hemorrhagic shock in the early post-trauma period. Hemorrhagic shock describes the clinical state in which, as a result of blood loss, capillary blood flow to tissues is reduced to levels below that required for oxidative metabolism.[44] Although all bony fractures induce acute hemorrhage to some degree, fractures involving the pelvis (particularly causing posterior ring disruption) are commonly associated with hemorrhagic shock.[42, 46]

Diagnosis

In response to increasing volumes of blood loss, physiological mechanisms attempt to accommodate the reduction in cardiac output, central venous pressure, and tissue perfusion in varying degrees. Easily monitored clinical signs that indicate how well the body is dealing with hemodynamic instability include the patient's heart rate, blood pressure, respiratory rate, urine output, and mental status.[47] In general, the greater the volume of blood loss, the higher are heart and respiratory rates, the lower are the blood pressure and urine output, and the more confused the patient will become.[47] Any reversal of these signs after resuscitation has begun indicates an improvement in hemodynamic status.

Treatment

As described in the American College of Surgeons Advanced Trauma Life Support Program, management of all trauma patients involves performing primary and secondary surveys.[47] Resuscitative measures are instituted along the "ABCDE" guidelines as indicated.[46, 47]

The majority of hemodynamically unstable patients respond to basic fluid resuscitative measures.[46] For those who remain unstable, treatment options include application of a pneumatic antishock garment, arteriography of the suspected bleeding vessel with subsequent therapeutic embolization, and immediate operation on the exsanguinating site.[46, 48] Indications for and against the use of each of these therapies and their specific outcomes are dependent on the type of fracture, location and severity of vascular damage, and number of other injuries sustained.[46, 48]

BLEEDING DISORDERS

Because blood vessels are commonly damaged with fractures, the orthopaedic surgeon should be knowledgeable of the management of individuals with either acquired or congenital bleeding disorders. Although such patients are rarely seen, they can experience serious hematological and orthopaedic complications if their underlying bleeding problem is not treated appropriately from the time they present in the emergency department.

Pathophysiology

Hemostasis can be conveniently broken down into three interrelated pathways.[49] The primary pathway involves platelet adherence to the collagen of damaged vessel walls and the release of platelet-derived adenosine diphosphate and thromboxane A_2 to promote further platelet adherence.[49] The secondary pathway relates to the interreaction between the various clotting factors to produce fibrin, which acts to hold the platelet plug more firmly together.[49] Once the clot is formed and tissue repair has started, the tertiary pathway is initiated. Here, plasmin is produced; its role is to digest the clot so as to allow for vascular patency.[49]

Of concern to the orthopaedic surgeon are patients who have either congenital or acquired bleeding disorders. Examples of congenital disorders include hemophilia A and B, von Willebrand's disease (deficiencies in factor VIII, IX, and von Willebrand's factor, respectively), and Kasabach-Merritt syndrome (a disease in which thrombocytopenia occurs secondary to platelet sequestration in hemangiomas).[50] Disseminated intravascular coagulation (DIC) is an example of an acquired bleeding disorder that develops secondary to some underlying disease, such as a cancer, or from the way traumatic injuries are treated during hospitalization. In DIC, an overstimulation of the clotting process occurs. This eventually leads to a deficiency of clotting factors; the end result is diffuse hemorrhage secondary to systemic hypocoagulability.[51]

Diagnosis, Treatment, and Prevention

Three basic principles must be adhered to in managing individuals with congenital bleeding disorders: early establishment of hemostasis, immobilization of the fracture using appropriate methods, and maintenance of hemostasis during healing.[52]

To provide early hemostasis, appropriate coagulation studies should be obtained and adequate factor replacement given as soon after the bony injury as possible.[53] Once adequate factor replacement has been achieved, attention should then focus on managing the fracture. Fractures should be treated in the same manner as they would be in patients without bleeding disorders.[53] The only exception involves patients who have antibodies to their deficient factor; elective open reduction and internal fixation of fractures in these individuals are contraindicated.[54]

If closed reduction is performed, special care should be taken to ensure that the postreduction splint is rigid, well padded, and split. This will minimize the risk of any rebleeding and vascular or nerve damage that may ensue from soft-tissue swelling after the reduction.[53] Infusion therapy is not necessary for cast changes unless the affected limb is to be manipulated.[53] Unaffected limbs should always be exercised, because disuse may promote the development of subsequent hemarthroses.[52] Postfixation regimens for weightbearing and physical therapy are no different for patients with bleeding disorders; fracture healing has not been found to be delayed in hemophilia.[52] To minimize the risk of rebleeding, pain management should never include use of nonsteroidal anti-inflammatory drugs or intramuscular analgesics. Rather, intravenous opiates should be used.[55]

If open reduction and internal fixation of the fracture are necessary, use of a pneumatic tourniquet and electrocautery for dissection and coagulation is suggested to minimize blood loss.[53] Postoperatively, compression bandages and a splint will help minimize the formation of a hematoma.[55]

Sutures should be left in for a longer period than usual.[52] If sutures are removed carefully, administration of the deficient factor is unnecessary.[52]

With regard to acquired causes of disorders of secondary hemostasis, DIC is the most worrisome. Although it develops only very rarely during orthopaedic surgeries in healthy patients,[51] it has been noted to occur with higher frequency in cancer patients who sustain pathological bone fractures.[56, 57] In both patient populations, hypotension, tissue trauma with the entrance of procoagulatory material (often of metastatic origin) into the circulation, and transfusion reactions are the most likely causes for the initiation of the bleeding disorder.[51, 57]

To prevent DIC, patients should have their coagulation status worked up and corrected before surgery.[57] If, in the postoperative period, DIC is suspected by either clinical or laboratory investigation, an internal medicine or hematology consult should be made. Reversal of DIC will involve treatment of the underlying pathological disorder, institution of life support measures, and administration of either clotting factors and platelets if the bleeding is minimal or heparin if the bleeding is severe, thereby releasing clotting factors back into the blood.[51]

For patients who sustain pathological fractures, it is suggested that preoperative fibrinogen and fibrin degradation product levels be obtained.[56] If abnormal levels are found, a hematologist should be consulted for advice on correction.[56] If the patient is deemed suitable for surgery, the surgeon must use meticulous surgical technique to minimize release of procoagulatory tumor tissue into the vasculature.[57]

TETANUS

Tetanus is a neurological disorder caused by the release of the exotoxin, tetanospasmin, by *Clostridium tetani*. It is a severe but preventable complication of any wound. As a result of comprehensive toxoid vaccination programs throughout North America, the incidence of tetanus remains low (between 1995 and 1997, 124 cases were reported in the United States). However, because of the considerable morbidity or mortality, it is important that one knows how to manage wounds that are at risk for *C. tetani* infection.

Pathophysiology

The obligate anaerobic, spore-forming bacterium *C. tetani* is a ubiquitous organism in both the environment and humans.[59] As such, spores can easily gain access into human tissue through lesions in the skin. Spore germination and vegetative cell division occur only in wounds that have a low oxidation-reduction potential (i.e., deep puncture wounds or sutured necrotic wounds).[59] In this environment, the toxin that is responsible for the clinical symptoms of this illness, tetanospasmin, is synthesized and released.[59] On release, the toxin blocks the release of inhibitory neurotransmitters such as glycine, and γ-aminobutyric acid is blocked.[59] Unregulated excitatory synaptic activity ensues. Increased muscle tone and spasms initially develop in the muscles affected by the wound. As the toxin is transported retrogradely, muscular changes progressively spread to the masseter (causing trismus, or lockjaw) and other muscles of the face.[59] The muscles of the pharynx, shoulder, back, abdomen, proximal limbs, intercostal space, and diaphragm can also be affected.[59] Unchecked stimulation of the autonomic nervous system can lead to hypertension, tachycardia, hyperpyrexia, diaphoresis, and arrhythmias.[59] In severe cases, the patient may die of asphyxia, pneumonia, or cardiac arrest.

The incubation period for tetanus is variable and ranges from a few days to weeks.[59] The length of this period is dependent on the distance of the primary wound infection from the central nervous system; the retrograde axonal transport rate of tetanospasmin is approximately 250 mm per day.[59]

Diagnosis

The diagnosis of tetanus is based on clinical findings. Wound and cerebrospinal fluid cultures should be taken, but the bacterium is often not isolated.[59] Tetanus is unlikely if the patient has a history of immunization or a serum antitoxin level of 0.01 units/mL or greater.[59]

Prevention

Tetanus toxoid is an effective antigen, providing immunological protection against tetanospasmin for at least 10 years.[60] For this reason, all children should undergo the active immunization protocol appropriate for their health jurisdiction. Booster shots should then be administered every 10 years thereafter. Partially immunized or unimmunized patients older than 7 years who present with clean, minor wounds should receive the tetanus vaccine immediately.[60] For routine wound management in children younger than 7 years who are not adequately vaccinated, the diphtheria-tetanus-pertussis vaccine should be given.[60] Partially immunized or unimmunized patients who present with all other types of wounds should be given the tetanus vaccine and 250 units of tetanus immunoglobulin (from separate syringes and in separate sites).[60] Two follow-up doses should be given, the first at 4 to 8 weeks and the second at 6 to 12 months after the initial vaccination.[60] A booster is appropriate if the patient has not received tetanus toxoid within the preceding 5 years.[60]

Great care should be taken with regard to wound management. All necrotic tissue and foreign bodies must be removed to prevent the development of an environment that promotes spore germination.

Treatment

If the aforementioned preventive measures have been unsuccessful, attempts must be made to minimize the effects of muscular and sympathetic hyperactivity.[59] Heavy sedation and muscle relaxants can be used. Before the development of dysphagia or respiratory compromise, intubation or tracheostomy, with or without mechanical ventilation, should be performed. Because antibiotics do not neutralize tetanospasmin, their use is of questionable benefit. Nevertheless, antibiotic therapy with penicillin is indicated, because these drugs do kill vegetative *C. tetani* cells and other bacteria found in tissue wounds.[59]

GAS GANGRENE (MYONECROSIS)

Gas gangrene refers to the condition that occurs when *Clostridium* species invade healthy muscle from adjacent traumatized and infected tissues. It is an anaerobic infection and usually develops in contaminated, necrotic muscle that has been closed without having undergone adequate débridement.[61] Although up to 50% of deep wounds have been found to be infected, the prevalence of gas gangrene development is low (1.8%).[62]

Pathophysiology

Aside from colonization by *Clostridium* species, an essential factor in the development of gas gangrene is the presence of a deep, necrotic wound that has no communication to the surface.[61, 63] This condition sets up an anaerobic environment, which allows the bacteria to proliferate.[61] Because of the short incubation period of these microbes, clinical features appear within 1 to 3 days after injury.[63] With the release of numerous exotoxins, uncontrolled tissue necrosis develops.[61] Myonecrosis and hemolysis give the affected tissue a soft, friable, and semifluid consistency that is blue-black in color.[61] Bullous vesicles form in the overlying skin because of the production of a hemorrhagic exudate.[61] Gas bubbles caused by bacterial fermentation develop in the necrotic tissue.[61] Hematogenous spread of clostridial exotoxins rapidly leads to organ failure.[61]

Diagnosis

Clinical features of gas gangrene develop within 1 to 3 days after injury.[61, 63] The patient will complain of the sudden sensation of pain in the wound, which quickly increases in severity. Soon after, localized edema and bulla formation may be seen. Torn bullae may exude their contents, which are deep red in color and have an unique sweetish smell.[63] As myonecrosis progresses, renal failure, hypotension, delirium, coma, and, ultimately, death develop within 24 to 48 hours.

Once myonecrosis is suspected, tissue samples from the affected site and Gram stains of the exudate should be taken immediately. Frozen sections of muscle allow for pathological diagnosis of clostridial myonecrosis.[63] Radiographs may be helpful in identifying pockets of gas in muscle or subcutaneous tissues.

The signs and symptoms of myonecrosis are often indistinguishable from another common clostridial soft-tissue complication: anaerobic cellulitis.[63] Shared symptoms include exudate and gas formation, edema, and a foul-smelling discharge.[63] Despite the similarities, the distinction should be made because treatment methods vary. Although tissue affected by gas gangrene needs to be decompressed and excised, areas of cellulitis need only be decompressed.[63] Distinguishing features for myonecrosis versus cellulitis include a shorter period of incubation (up to 3 days versus after 3 days), an acute versus gradual onset, and severe pain versus the absence of pain in the affected area.[63]

Prevention

The most important step to prevent clostridial proliferation is early, meticulous excision of all necrotic tissue. If any nonviable muscle is thought to remain in a wound, closure should be avoided.

Treatment

The only effective, and therefore life-saving, treatment is early diagnosis. On diagnosis, general supportive measures, such as fluid and electrolyte replacement, should be immediately initiated. Broad-spectrum antibiotics such as penicil-

lin G and clindamycin should be administered. Antibiotic therapy can be specifically tailored later, once culture and sensitivity results are reported. Rapid surgical decompression, with deep incisions and fasciotomies, and débridement are then performed. In advanced cases of necrosis, amputation may be the most appropriate surgical procedure. Although the true efficacy of hyperbaric oxygen chambers has not been determined, their use has been found to limit the spread of infection.[64]

LOCAL COMPLICATIONS: SOFT TISSUE

VASCULAR INJURY

Damage to blood vessels is another serious complication of fracture. The overall arterial injury rate in isolated fractures is low and has been determined to be less than 1%. This rate increases to between 2% and 6% in combined fracture/dislocations.[65] As with neurological injury, a thorough examination of the vascular system must be performed at and distal to the site of fracture.

Fractures typically associated with damage to a major artery include those around the knee (popliteal artery) and elbow (brachial artery) and the humeral (brachial artery) and femoral (femoral artery) diaphysis.[66]

Pathophysiology

A variety of injuries can be sustained by arteries either during the initial traumatic event or on subsequent contact with bone fragments. For example, arteries can become compressed, lacerated, or torn when in contact with jagged bone ends. Bleeding from cuts and tears can lead to hematoma formation, which can also cause compression. Contact with bone fragments may induce arterial spasm, aneurysm formation, or intimal injury, resulting in acute vessel blockage. Occlusive thrombi can form as marrow and fat are released from the fractured bone.

Diagnosis and Treatment

Proper history taking, physical examination, and laboratory investigation will usually reveal the presence of vascular injury. Vessel lacerations and tears are diagnosed by observing for bleeding and local swelling. Auscultation and palpation can detect the presence of bruits, thrills, and pulsating hematomas. If arterial occlusion has occurred, any of the classic symptoms of ischemia may develop, among them severe limb pain, pallor and/or coldness of skin, loss of distal pulses, paresthesias, and eventual muscle paralysis. Importantly, although the absence of distal pulses is a good indicator of arterial damage, their presence should never preclude the existence of vascular injury.

Whenever vascular injury is suspected, one should seek consultation with a vascular surgeon immediately. Depending on the circumstance, Doppler ultrasonography and/or angiography will be performed.

In the presence of an active hemorrhage, expanding hematoma, arteriovenous fistula, distal pulseless extremity, or severe ischemia, immediate vascular repair guided by intraoperative arteriography should be planned (Fig. 6).[67, 68] If a dislocation or fracture fragments are thought to be interfering with the integrity of vessel function, a reduction, followed by skeletal stabilization, is necessary. If pulses return to normal after reduction, an arteriogram should be

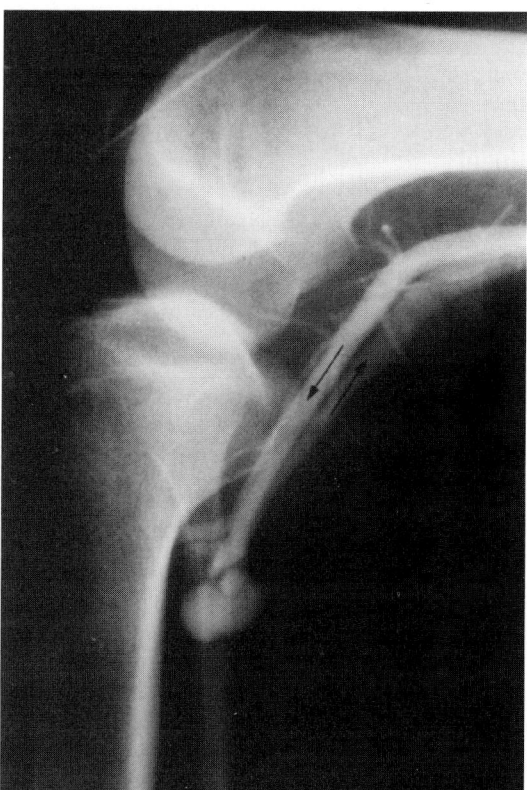

Fig. 6. Traumatic arteriovenous fistula and pseudoaneurysm. This angiogram indicates pseudoaneurysm and fistula *(arrows)* between the femoral artery and vein after deep laceration of the medial upper calf.

obtained.[69] If pulses do not return within 30 minutes (to rule out transient spasm), Doppler ultrasonography should be performed.[67] If the arterial pressure or ankle/brachial index (the systolic arterial pressure in the injured extremity divided by the arterial pressure in an uninvolved arm [ABI]) is 1.00 or greater, the vascular status of the patient should be observed indefinitely.[67, 68] If the ABI is found to be below 1.00, arteriography of the affected vessel should be performed.[67] The presence of a major arterial injury will necessitate operation or embolization.[67] If a minor arterial injury is found, the patient's condition can be observed; serial arteriography or duplex Doppler scanning can be performed to monitor the artery's status.[67] Some authorities suggest that an ABI of 0.90 is as acceptable a cut-off value as 1.00 for performing arteriography.[68] A timely diagnosis is critical, because the window for treatment before irreversible damage occurs in muscle distal to an arterial lesion is between 6 to 8 hours.

COMPARTMENT SYNDROME

Compartment syndrome refers to a condition in which the circulation and function of tissues within a fibro-osseous compartment are compromised by the presence of increased pressure within that space. Increased pressure can develop from either an increase in compartment content (i.e., as a result of bleeding, increased capillary permeability, increased capillary pressure, or inflammation/infection) or decreased compartment size (caused by external pressure such as tight dressings).

All fractures involving the elbow, forearm, and proximal and middle thirds of the tibia have great potential for developing compartment syndrome. Open tibial fractures in adults are associated with the highest prevalence of compartment syndrome; this complication can develop in up to 20% of such fractures.[70]

Pathophysiology

Two complementary theories, the arteriovenous gradient and the ischemia-reperfusion injury, describe the pathophysiology of compartment syndrome. The arteriovenous gradient theory states that compromised blood flow in the arterial, capillary, or venous systems can lead to compartment syndrome.[71] Several causes for reduced blood flow can be identified, among them hypotension, increased vascular resistance secondary to shock or arterial spasm, and increased tissue pressure subsequent to a constrictive dressing or extravasated blood in a compartment.[71]

The ischemia-reperfusion injury theory explains the cause of compartment syndrome as follows. When blood flow to a compartment is compromised, ischemia develops. The presence of ischemia impairs cellular metabolism to the point at which the integrity of cell membranes cannot be maintained. When the capillary endothelium begins to break down, intracellular and intravascular fluids gain access into the interstitial space, leading to interstitial edema and an increased compartmental pressure.[71]

Reperfusion of the affected compartment can have both beneficial and damaging effects. By providing oxygen and other various substrates for cellular metabolism and by washing away metabolic by-products, reperfusion can help restore cellular activity.[71] Nevertheless, new blood flow can worsen preexisting cellular damage. Local vasodilation and hyperemia not only promote compartment edema but also cause important cellular metabolites to be washed away.[71] Reestablished blood flow brings molecules, enzymes, and cells (i.e., neutrophils and leukocytes), which can promote the destruction of already damaged tissues.[71]

Diagnosis

Because the presenting symptoms of compartment syndrome can be so variable and the physical examination is often inconclusive, its diagnosis can be difficult. Nevertheless, a clinical diagnosis can be made with the symptoms and signs of a tense, swollen muscle compartment, pain disproportionate to the clinical situation, pain on passive stretch of the affected muscle bed, hypoesthesia in the distribution of the nerves traversing the compartment, and a suspicious history.[72]

Adjunctive diagnostic aids that may be useful in the diagnosis of compartment syndrome include the slit catheter, side-ported needle, and simple needle. Studies comparing the efficacy of these three tools indicate that side-ported needles are ideal for use in the emergency room setting.[73] They provide accurate readings of compartment pressure and can test multiple compartments at one time.[73] Slit catheters also provide accurate readings but have the advantage of being able to be used as indwelling units.[73] As such, they can measure compartment pressures over a period of time.[73]

Unfortunately, great controversy exists regarding the manner in which these sphygmomanometers should be used and their readings interpreted. Some surgeons suggest that the development of compartment syndrome can be prevented if continuous compartment pressure monitoring is instituted as soon after the traumatic event as possible.[74] This is especially applicable in patients who sustain fractures that commonly develop compartment syndrome (see prior discussion), in young children, and in those who are unconscious, are multiply injured, or have equivocal symptoms in the presence of nerve injury.[74] In such cases, decompression should be performed when the difference between the compartment and diastolic pressures is less than 30 mm Hg or when the compartment pressure exceeds a range of 30 to 45 mm Hg.[72–74] Only when the difference in pressures steadily rises and the compartment pressure drops may the monitoring device be withdrawn.

Because of the variety of guidelines for decompression and the fact that continuous monitoring may often be too cumbersome to perform in some (polytraumatized) patients, it is strongly suggested that the surgeon's decision to monitor for and treat compartment syndrome depend on the clinical context.[75] In all cases, it is better to err on the side of performing a fasciotomy than not to decompress a muscle compartment because of the lack of clear symptoms and signs.[75]

Treatment

Prompt decompression is the only effective treatment for this condition. Initially, all constrictive dressings, including casts and bandages, must be completely removed. The affected limb should be placed at the level of the heart to help promote perfusion. If improvement is seen over the next hour, frequent evaluations should be made until recovery is evident. If conditions deteriorate, emergency fasciotomy of the affected compartment must be performed. Internal fixation of the fracture is essential during this procedure, because casting is contraindicated in the presence of fasciotomy wounds. Such wounds are left open for 7 to 10 days. At this time, closure is then performed with suturing or skin grafting (if the degree of edema makes direct closure of the wound margins impossible).

REFERENCES

1. Abelseth G, Buckley RE, Pineo GE, et al: Incidence of deep vein thrombosis in patients with fractures of the lower extremity distal to the hip. J Orthop Trauma 1996; 10:230.
2. Rogers FB: Venous thromboembolism in trauma patients. Surg Clin North Am 1995; 75:279.
3. Rosendaal FR: Risk factors for venous thrombosis: Prevalence, risk, and interaction. Semin Hematol 1997; 34:171.
4. Montgomery KD, Geerts WH, Potter HG, et al: Practical management of venous thromboembolism following pelvic fractures. Orthop Clin North Am 1997; 28:397.
5. Giachino AA, Desmarais R, Desjardins D, et al: Incidence and prevention of deep venous thrombosis. J Bone Joint Surg Br 1985; 67:675.
6. Freeark RJ, Boswick J, Fardin R: Posttraumatic venous thrombosis. Arch Surg 1967; 95:567.
7. Sevitt S, Gallagher NG: Venous thrombosis and pulmonary embolism: A clinicopathological study in injured and burned patients. Br J Surg 1961; 48:475.
8. Consensus Conference: Prevention of venous thrombosis and pulmonary embolism. JAMA 1988; 256:744.
9. Barnes RW: Current status of noninvasive tests in the diagnosis of venous disease. Surg Clin North Am 1982; 62:489.
10. Rose SC, Zwiebel WJ, Nelson BD, et al: Symptomatic lower extremity deep venous thrombosis: Accuracy, limitations, and role of color duplex flow imaging in diagnosis. Radiology 1990; 175:639.
11. Albrechtsson U, Olsson CG: Thrombotic side-effects of lower limb phlebography. Lancet 1976; 1:723.
12. Goodman LR, Lipchik RJ: Diagnosis of acute pulmonary embolism: Time for a new approach. Radiology 1996; 199:25.
13. Goldhaber SZ: Medical progress: Pulmonary embolism. N Engl J Med 1998; 339:93.

14. Oudkerk M, van Beek EJ, van Putten WK, et al: Cost-effectiveness analysis of various strategies in the diagnostic management of pulmonary embolism. Arch Intern Med 1993; 153:947.
15. Powers PJ, Gent M, Jay RM, et al: A randomized trial of less intense postoperative warfarin or aspirin therapy in the prevention of venous thromboembolism after surgery for fractured hip. Arch Intern Med 1989; 149:771.
16. Geerts WH, Jay R, Code K, et al: A comparison of low-dose heparin with low-molecular-weight heparin as prophylaxis against venous thromboembolism after major trauma. N Engl J Med 1996; 335:701.
17. Gent M, Hirsh J, Ginsberg JS, et al: Low-molecular-weight heparinoid Orgaran is more effective than aspirin in the prevention of venous thromboembolism after surgery for hip fracture. Circulation 1996; 93:80.
18. Hirsh J: The optimal duration of anticoagulant therapy for venous thrombosis. N Engl J Med 1995; 332:1710.
19. Jones TK, Barnes RW, Greenfield LJ: Greenfield vena caval filter: Rationale and current indications. Ann Thorac Surg 1986; 42:48.
20. Headrick JR, Barker DE, Pate LM, et al: The role of ultrasonography and inferior vena caval filter placement in high-risk trauma patients. Am Surg 1997; 63:1.
21. Hyers TM, Hull RD, Weg JC: Antithrombotic therapy for venous thromboembolic disease. Chest 1992; 102:408S.
22. Simmonneau G, Sors H, Charbonnier B, et al: A comparison of low-molecular-weight heparin with unfractionated heparin for acute pulmonary embolism. N Engl J Med 1997; 337:663.
23. Ricotta S, Iorio A, Parise P, et al: Postdischarge clinically overt venous thromboembolism in orthopaedic surgery patients with negative venography: An overview analysis. Thromb Haemost 1996; 76:887.
24. Schulman S, Granqvist S, Holmstrom M,

et al: The duration of oral anticoagulant therapy after a second episode of venous thromboembolism. N Engl J Med 1997; 336:393.
25. Schemitsch EH, Jain R, Turchin DC, et al: Pulmonary effects of fixation of a fracture with a plate compared with intramedullary nailing: A canine model of fat embolism and fracture fixation. J Bone Joint Surg Am 1997; 79:984.
26. Muller C, Rahn B, Pfister U, et al: The incidence, pathogenesis, diagnosis, and treatment of fat embolism. Orthop Rev 1994; 23:107.
27. Eddy A, Rice C, Carrico C: Fat embolism syndrome: Monitoring and management. J Crit Illness 1987; 2:24.
28. Ten Duis HJ: The fat embolism syndrome. Injury 1997; 28:77.
29. Gurd AR, Wilson RI: The fat embolism syndrome. J Bone Joint Surg Br 1974; 56:408.
30. Lindeque BG, Schoeman HS, Dommisse GF, et al: Fat embolism and the fat embolism syndrome: A double-blind therapeutic study. J Bone Joint Surg Br 1987; 69:128.
31. Richards RR: Fat embolism syndrome. Can J Surg 1997; 40:334.
32. Bone LB, McNamara K, Shine B, et al: Mortality in multiple trauma patients with fractures. J Trauma 1994; 37:262.
33. Bone LB, Johnson KD, Weigelt J, et al: Early versus delayed stabilization of fractures: A prospective randomized study. J Bone Joint Surg Am 1989; 71:336.
34. Goris RJ, Gimbrere JS, van Niekerk JL, et al: Early osteosynthesis and prophylactic mechanical ventilation in the multitrauma patient. J Trauma 1982; 22:895.
35. Bosse MJ, MacKenzie EJ, Riemer BL, et al: ARDS, pneumonia, and mortality following thoracic injury and a femoral fracture treated either with intramedullary nailing with reaming or with a plate. J Bone Joint Surg Am 1997; 79:799.
36. Ingram RH: Adult respiratory distress syndrome. In Wilson JD, Braunwald E, Issel-

bacher KJ, et al (eds): Harrison's Principles of Internal Medicine. New York, McGraw-Hill, 1991, 12th ed, p 1122.

37. Modig J, Hedstrand U, Wegenius G: Determinants of early adult respiratory distress syndrome: A retrospective study of 220 patients with major fractures. Acta Chir Scand 1985; 151:413.

38. Johnson KD, Cadambi A, Seibert GB: Incidence of adult respiratory distress syndrome in patients with multiple musculoskeletal injuries: Effect of early operative stabilization of fractures. J Trauma 1985; 25:375.

39. Moore FA, Moore EE: Evolving concepts in the pathogenesis of post injury multiple organ failure. Surg Clin North Am 1995; 75:257.

40. Beal AL, Cerra FB: Multiple organ failure syndrome in the 1990s: Systemic inflammatory response and organ dysfunction. JAMA 1994; 271:226.

41. Moore FA, Sauaia A, Moore EE, et al: Postinjury multiple organ failure: A bimodal phenomenon. J Trauma 1996; 40:501.

42. Fry DE, Pearlstein L, Fulton RL, et al: Multiple system organ failure: The role of uncontrolled infection. Arch Surg 1980; 115:136.

43. Wichmann MW, Ayala A, Chaudry IH: Severe depression of host immune functions following closed-bone fracture, soft-tissue, trauma, and hemorrhagic shock. Crit Care Med 1998; 26:1372.

44. Parrillo JE: Shock. In Wilson JD, Braunwald E, Isselbacher KJ, et al (eds): Harrison's Principles of Internal Medicine. New York, McGraw-Hill, 1991, 12th ed, p 231.

45. Johnson KD, Cadambi A, Seibert GB: Incidence of adult respiratory distress syndrome in patients with multiple musculoskeletal injuries: Effect of early operative stabilization of fractures. J Trauma 1985; 25:375.

46. Mucha P, Welch TJ: Hemorrhage in major pelvic fractures. Surg Clin North Am 1988; 68:757.

47. American College of Surgeons Committee on Trauma: Advanced Trauma Life Support Program 1988 Instructor Manual. Chicago, American College of Surgeons, 1989.

48. Klein SR, Saroyan RM, Baumgartner F, et al: Management strategy of vascular injuries associated with pelvic fractures. J Cardiovasc Surg 1992; 33:349.

49. Handin RI: Bleeding and thrombosis. In Wilson JD, Braunwald E, Isselbacher KJ, et al (eds): Harrison's Principles of Internal Medicine. New York, McGraw-Hill, 1991, 12th ed, p 348.

50. Menendez LR, Thommen VD: Kasabach-Merritt syndrome complicating treatment of a closed femoral fracture. Clin Orthop Rel Res 1995; 316:185.

51. Demirjian Z, Sara M, Stulberg D, et al: Disseminated intravascular coagulation in patients undergoing orthopedic surgery. Clin Orthop Rel Res 1974; 102:174.

52. Kemp HS, Matthews JM: The management of fractures in haemophilia and Christmas disease. J Bone Joint Surg Br 1968; 50:351.

53. Wolff LJ, Lovrien EW: Management of fractures in hemophilia. Pediatrics 1982; 70:431.

54. Feil E, Bentley G, Rizza CR: Fracture management in patients with hemophilia. J Bone Joint Surg Br 1974; 56:643.

55. Houghton GR, Duthie RB: Orthopedic problems in hemophilia. Clin Orthop Rel Res 1979; 138:197.

56. Olson SA, Humphreys WG, Allen WC: Disseminated intravascular coagulation complicating Ender's nailing of a pathologic fracture in prostatic carcinoma: A case report. Clin Orthop Rel Res 1990; 258:242.

57. Nyska M, Klin B, Margulies JY, et al: Disseminated intravascular coagulopathy in patients with cancer undergoing operation for pathological fractures of the hip. Int Orthop 1987; 11:179.

58. Centers for Disease Control and Prevention: Tetanus surveillance: United States, 1995–1997. Mor Mortal Wkly Rep 1998; 47:1.

59. Bartlett JG: Tetanus. In Andreoli TE, Bennett JC, Carpenter CC, ET AL (eds): Cecil Textbook of Medicine. Philadelphia, WB Saunders, 1996, 20th ed, p 1636.

60. Centers for Disease Control and Prevention: Diphtheria, tetanus, and pertussis: Recommendations for vaccine use and other preventive measures. Mor Mortal Wkly Rep 1991; 40:2.

61. Murray PR: Anaerobic Gram-positive spore-forming bacilli. In Murray PR, Kobayashi GS, Pfaller MA, et al (eds): Medical Microbiology. St. Louis, Mosby–Year Book, 1994, 2nd ed, p 294.

62. Altemeier WA, Furste WL: Studies in virulence of *Clostridium welchii*. Surgery 1949; 25:12.

63. deHaven KE, Evarts CM: The continuing problem of gas gangrene: A review and report of illustrative cases. J Trauma 1971; 11:983.

64. Guidi ML, Proietti R, Carducci P, et al: The combined use of hyperbaric oxygen, antibiotics and surgery in the treatment of gas gangrene. Resuscitation 1981; 9:267.

65. Fears RL, Gleis GE, Seligson D: Diagnosis and treatment of complications. In Browner BD, Jupiter JB, Levine AM, et al (eds): Skeletal Trauma: Fractures, Dislocations, Ligamentous Injuries. Philadelphia, WB Saunders, 1998, 2nd ed, p 567.

66. Apley AG: Principles of fractures. In Apley AG (ed): Apley's System of Orthopaedics and Fractures. Oxford, England, Butterworth-Heinemann, 1993, 7th ed, p 544.

67. Modrall JG, Weaver FA, Yellin AE: Diagnosis and management of penetrating vascular trauma and the injured extremity. Emerg Med Clin North Am 1998; 16:129.

68. Johansen K, Lynch K, Paun M, et al: Noninvasive vascular tests reliably exclude occult arterial trauma in injured extremities. J Trauma 1991; 31:515.

69. Merrill KD: Knee dislocations with vascular injuries. Orthop Clin North Am 1994; 25:707.

70. Singer RW, Kellam JF: Open tibial diaphyseal fractures: Results of unreamed locked intramedullary nailing. Clin Orthop Rel Res 1995; 315:114.

71. Tollens T, Janzing H, Broos P: The pathophysiology of acute compartment syndrome. Acta Chir Belg 1998; 98:171.

72. Matsen FA, Winquist RA, Krugmire RB: Diagnosis and management of compartment syndromes. J Bone Joint Surg Am 1980; 62:286.

73. Moed BR, Thorderson PK: Measurement of intracompartmental pressure: A comparison of the slit catheter, side-ported needle, and simple needle. J Bone Joint Surg Am 1993; 75:231.

74. McQueen M: Acute compartment syndrome. Acta Chir Belg 1998; 98:166.

75. Sanders R, Swiontkowski M, Nunley J, et al: The management of fractures with soft-tissue disruptions. J Bone Joint Surg Am 1993; 75:778.

COMPLICATIONS OF FRACTURES: CHRONIC

Matthew D. Pepe and John L. Esterhai

Summary

- Complications following musculoskeletal trauma resulting in fracture are relatively infrequent but can result in significant long-term morbidity.
- This chapter addresses complications that are chronic in nature, including complications associated with prosthetics and orthotics, post-traumatic arthritis, avascular necrosis, heterotopic ossification, implant device complications, and chronic pain.
- Attention to surgical technique and postoperative care are important to avoid complications associated with prostheses.
- Complications associated with orthoses can be avoided by following the basic principles of design to provide an adequate area of compliant pressure distribution with adequate contouring.
- Post-traumatic arthritis may occur following intra-articular fractures and may be a source of joint stiffness and pain, causing long-term disability.
- Heterotopic ossification can occur following fractures of the acetabulum, hip, femoral head, proximal humerus, and elbow region. Surgical excision is recommended for high-grade lesions causing disability.
- Avascular necrosis can occur following fractures of the proximal humerus, scaphoid, femoral neck, and talus and is related to the degree and the duration of displacement. When conservative modalities fail, treatment involves arthroplasty for the hip and shoulder and salvage techniques for the wrist and ankle.

COMPLICATIONS ASSOCIATED WITH PROSTHETICS

The use of prosthetic devices is often necessary following musculoskeletal trauma that results in amputation. Common complications include joint contracture and skin problems.

JOINT CONTRACTURE

Joint contracture may occur in any of the proximal remaining joints after an amputation as a result of the patient's underlying disease, trauma, surgical technique, or postoperative routine. During above-knee amputation, adductor myodesis is important to prevent abduction contracture of the hip. A Lisfranc or Chopart amputation requires reattachment of the tibialis anterior and extensor tendons and can avoid debilitating equinus deformity.

A postoperative stretching routine may be necessary following amputation. To prevent abduction flexion contracture after above-knee amputation, the surgeon must counsel the patient to avoid placing pillows beneath the stump and prescribe a once- or twice-daily prone stretching routine. Postoperative rigid dressings after below-knee amputations help prevent flexion contracture.

SKIN PROBLEMS

Skin problems represent a large percentage of the complications occurring in amputations,[1] even after a patient begins to use a definitive prosthesis. An area of a previous scar may open or blister from prosthetic socket pressure or friction. This can be treated with prosthetic adjustment and a period of several days of rest from the use of the prosthesis to give the area a chance to heal. No further treatment needs to be done if the patient is able to wear the prosthesis without recurrence of the breakdown. If recurrent breakdown occurs that cannot be controlled with prosthetic revision, the area may need to undergo scar revision.

Small areas of split-thickness skin grafts usually do not present a problem for prosthetic usage. However, grafts that are non-mobile and adherent may break down during the initial period of wearing a prosthesis. If these areas cannot be loosened by scar massage or relieved by modification of the prosthesis, revision of the stump or excision and application of a full-thickness graft may be required.

Draining sinuses after amputation may signal a retained foreign body or ring sequestrum. Radiographs should be obtained in cases of persistent drainage and will assist in making the diagnosis. Extensive periosteal stripping of the bone end during amputation can cause devascularization, resulting in a ring sequestrum. The periosteum should be sharply transected at the level of the bone cut to avoid this complication. If drainage persists despite rest, surgical removal of the sequestrum is warranted.

COMPLICATIONS ASSOCIATED WITH ORTHOTICS

Orthoses are mechanical devices used to stabilize joints, to substitute for loss of motion, to protect a healing fracture, to prevent abnormal movement of joints, and to restore the anatomic position of joints.[2] Following the basic principles of design to provide an adequate service area of compliant pressure distribution with adequate contouring is imperative to avoid complications.

Spinal, upper extremity, and lower extremity orthoses can cause pressure sores. The surgeon and the orthotist must work in concert to avoid this complication. It is virtually impossible to avoid points of pressure, especially with lower extremity orthoses. The ischial area, knee region, calf, and ankle are especially vulnerable,[3] and the orthosis should be carefully molded and padded in these areas.

The problems of decreased muscle power and atrophy occur when an orthosis prevents or substitutes for the action of a group of muscles. This can occur in the spine, when a patient becomes "wed" to the orthosis and is unable to function without it. An orthosis that substitutes for a muscle group will cause atrophy of this group unless the muscles are able to function. Patients should be taught exercises to maintain muscle strength when upper and lower extremity orthoses are used. Patients wearing spinal orthoses should be weaned gradually with a program of abdominal and back extensor strengthening.

POST-TRAUMATIC ARTHRITIS

Fractures that involve the articular surface of joints may cause an increased predisposition toward arthritis. Comminution of the articular surface, degree of incongruity, duration of immobilization, and the particular joint involved are factors that help determine the incidence of post-traumatic arthritis.

The extent of comminution of an articular surface after fracture is one of the most important determinants in the development of arthritis. High-energy trauma causes cartilage damage and chondrocyte death at impact, and the resultant comminution of the articular surface makes anatomic fracture reduction difficult, even with open reduction and internal fixation.

Displaced articular fracture fragments with metaphyseal bone loss necessitate bone graft for support. Frequently fracture fragments are small and irreducible, leaving the joint with a loss of articular cartilage and subchondral bone. The amount of acceptable articular incongruity after fracture reduction varies with the joint involved in the fracture but plays an important role in determining post-traumatic arthritis.[4, 5] Unfortunately, there are no accurate data on the amount of articular depression and displacement that leads to degenerative joint disease. For instance, after fracture of the tibial plateau, there is an alteration in the contact relationship between the distal femur and proximal tibia. Beyond a certain critical threshold that is dependent on the joint involved, depression or displacement of the plateau leads to a significant rise in joint "stress" (force per unit area).[6] A greater depth of articular cartilage allows for more displacement of the fracture fragments, and most authors recommend the depth of articular cartilage as the amount of acceptable displacement[7]; for example, in a joint with a 2 mm thickness of cartilage, more than 2 mm of displacement will predispose toward the development of arthritis. Any amount of displacement larger than the depth of cartilage would expose subchondral bone, increasing the predisposition toward arthritis. Therefore, more than this amount of displacement is an indication for open reduction and internal fixation[4, 5, 8, 9] with restoration of the joint surface if possible.

AVASCULAR NECROSIS

Avascular necrosis due to circulatory disruption can be a devastating complication of fracture. Continued pain and disability following healing of fractures of the femoral neck, proximal humerus (Fig. 1), scaphoid, or talus should alert the clinician to the possibility of avascular necrosis. The prevalence has been shown to range from 10% to 63%[10–13] and is related to the degree and duration of fracture displacement and the surgical approach used for reduction. Greater fracture displacement causes more significant disruption of arterial supply and therefore has the highest incidence of post-traumatic necrosis. The anatomy in each of these locations is such that there is a tenuous blood supply, with one main artery that supplies the majority of the bone area, making the blood supply vulnerable to injury at the time of fracture. Avascular necrosis may not become evident until 2 years following the injury[14, 15]; however, it usually becomes apparent within 8 weeks.[16]

It is well known that outcomes following displaced fractures of the proximal humerus, scaphoid, femoral neck, and talus are less than optimal. In 1949, Phemister noticed that union was achieved four times less frequently when avascular necrosis did occur than when it did not occur,[17] probably as a result of callous forming from just one end of the fracture. Rigid internal fixation expedites union and allows for potential revascularization of the avascular segment, without the risk of motion across the fracture site becoming a disrupting force.[18] Anatomic reduction of displaced fractures is associated with a lower incidence of avascular necrosis.[19–22]

The treatment of post-traumatic avascular necrosis differs from the treatment of avascular necrosis of nontraumatic origin. In general, treatment is directed toward controlling symptoms and using supportive measures when there is involvement of the femoral and humeral heads, with activity modification and crutch use as needed.[23] Physical therapy can be an important adjunct to improve existing range of motion of the glenohumeral joint.[24] Although there are no clinical studies, some authors feel that limited weight-bearing in the setting of talar body osteonecrosis reduces the degree of severity and limits progression until reperfusion has a chance to occur.[16]

Core decompression and grafting, while effective in the treatment of osteonecrosis of the femoral head from nontraumatic sources, has no role in the treatment of fracture-induced avascular necrosis.[23] The same principles apply to talar body and glenohumeral avascular necrosis, wherein decompression and grafting are ineffective.[16, 24] Although some authors have found poor outcomes with surgical treatment of the scaphoid when avascular necrosis and nonunion have occurred,[25] bone grafting and internal fixation are recommended before significant arthritis and collapse have occurred,[26] and some authors even recommend a vascularized bone graft.[27] The outcome after avascular necrosis of the humeral head tends to be better than the outcome after avascular necrosis of the femoral head, talus, and scaphoid, perhaps because the glenohumeral joint is a non-weightbearing joint. In the setting of avascular necrosis with extensive involvement, collapse and incongruity can cause significant disability, and prosthetic hemiarthroplasty of the femur[23] and humerus are indicated. If arthritis has involved the acetabulum or glenoid, total hip replacement or total shoulder replacement (in the setting of an intact rotator cuff) is indicated. Significant involvement of the talus is treated with fusion, and extensive involvement of the scaphoid merits a salvage procedure, either limited fusion, proximal row carpectomy, or wrist fusion.[26]

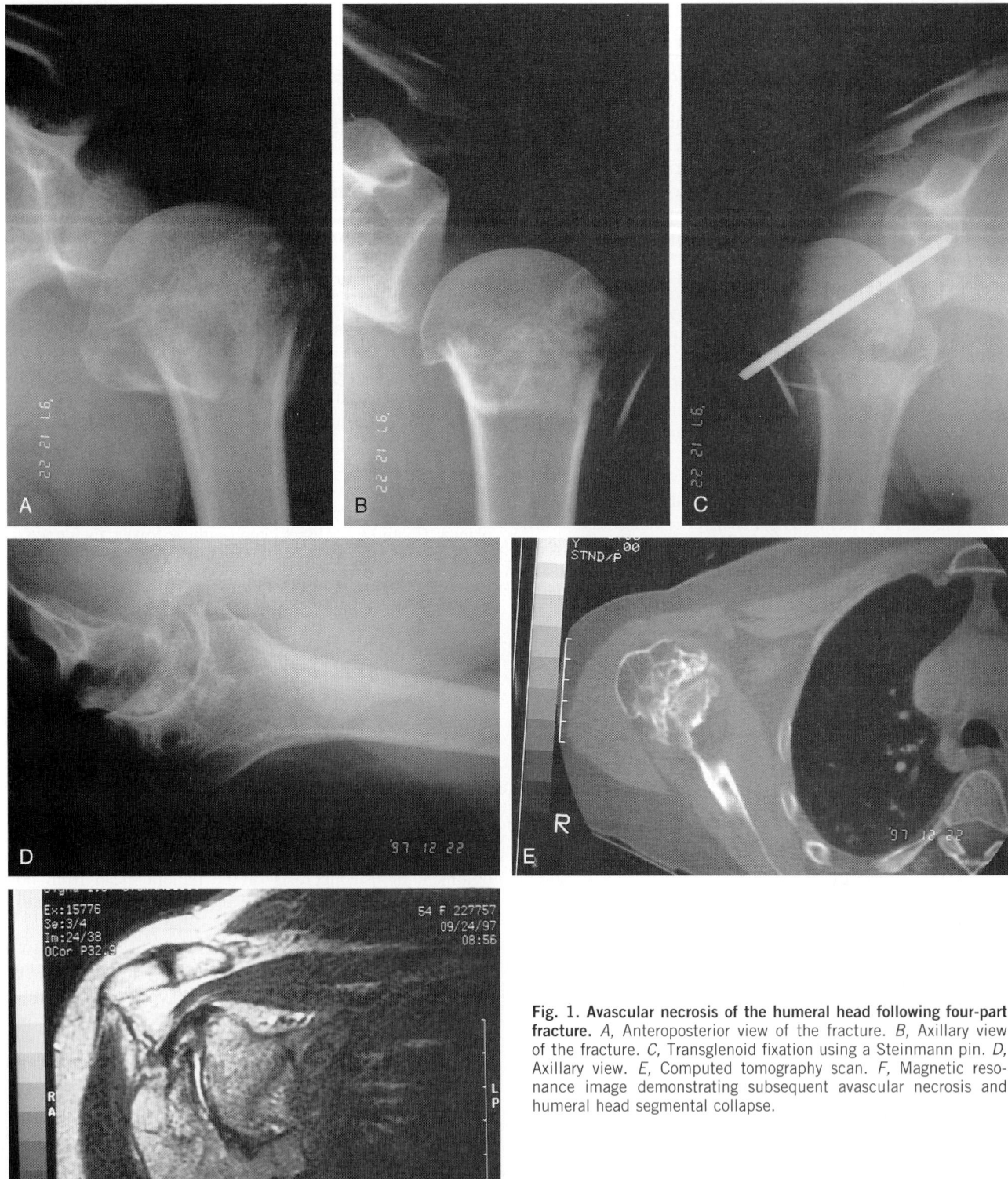

Fig. 1. Avascular necrosis of the humeral head following four-part fracture. *A*, Anteroposterior view of the fracture. *B*, Axillary view of the fracture. *C*, Transglenoid fixation using a Steinmann pin. *D*, Axillary view. *E*, Computed tomography scan. *F*, Magnetic resonance image demonstrating subsequent avascular necrosis and humeral head segmental collapse.

HETEROTOPIC OSSIFICATION

Heterotopic ossification is the formation of bone in periarticular regions and is a well-described but poorly understood complication of fractures and dislocations of the acetabulum (Fig. 2), hip and femoral head, proximal humerus, and elbow regions. Although heterotopic ossification can occur following closed treatment of these fractures, the incidence is higher following open reduction and internal fixation. This increased frequency is perhaps due to the extensive soft tissue dissection and stripping that occurs during surgery. The cause is multifactorial and involves an

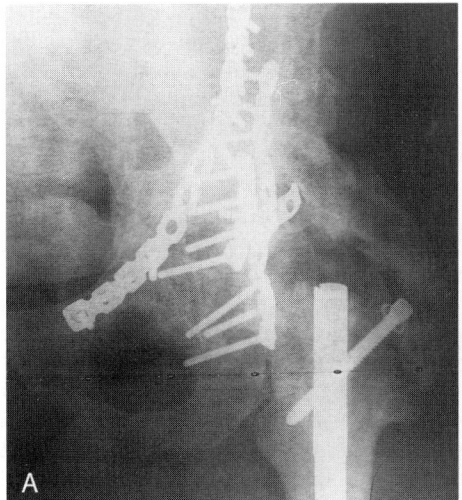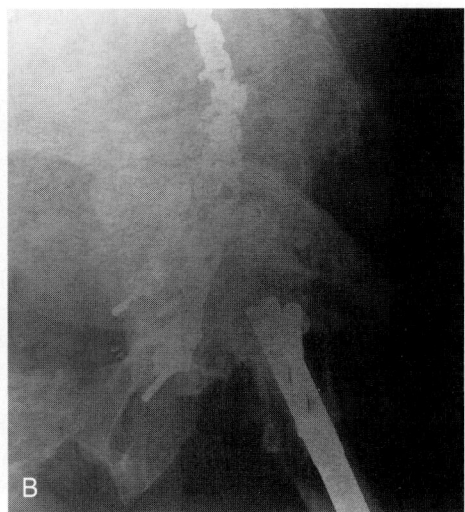

Fig. 2. High-grade heterotopic ossification. This shows ossification following both column acetabular fracture and ipsilateral femoral shaft fracture. *A*, Anteroposterior radiograph. *B*, Iliac oblique radiograph.

inducing agent, osteogenic precursor cells, and an environment that is conducive to bone formation.[28] Risk factors for heterotopic ossification formation include a time delay between injury and surgery,[29] central nervous system injury,[30] previous heterotopic bone formation, and male sex.[28] Heterotopic bone has been reported in as many as 90% of patients undergoing repair for acetabular fracture[31, 32] and up to 89% of patients sustaining elbow trauma with concomitant central nervous system injury.[33] Heterotopic ossification may be seen on plain radiographs by 3 to 6 weeks and usually reaches its maximum by 12 weeks.[32]

A variety of prophylactic treatments have been advocated to reduce the incidence of heterotopic ossification, including diphosphonates, nonsteroidal anti-inflammatory medication, and low-dose radiation.[28, 31, 32, 34, 35] The efficacy of diphosphonates is in question, however, because mineralization of the osteoid resumes after cessation of the medication. Both indomethacin and radiation therapy have been shown to be effective in reducing the incidence of heterotopic ossification. In a randomized, prospective study, Moore et al[32] compared the efficacy of indomethacin and radiation therapy in preventing heterotopic ossification formation after acetabular fractures. They found a 27% prevalence of heterotopic ossification with radiation prophylaxis and a 46% prevalence with indomethacin prophylaxis, with no significant differences between the two groups because of the small sample size.

Excision of the heterotopic ossification has been advocated for high-grade lesions causing restriction of motion and disability.[35–37] Some authors have advocated delaying surgical resection for 12 to 18 months. They have stressed the importance of assessing the patient clinically, radiographically, by monitoring the serum alkaline phosphatase, and by obtaining technetium bone scintigraphy,[36] ascertaining that the heterotopic ossification has reached full maturity. Computed tomography can be a useful adjunct in preoperative planning to assess the exact location of the ossification and the structures that may be at risk during the approach. It can also be used to assess the quality of the joint, which is often obscured by the overlying heterotopic ossification. Recently, McAuliffe and Wolfson[37] advocated early excision (average 7 months) for heterotopic ossification around the elbow, with good functional results.

COMPLICATIONS OF IMPLANT DEVICES USED FOR FRACTURE FIXATION

The use of implants for fracture fixation has increased in recent years with advances in biomaterials, biomechanics, and understanding of fracture healing. The success of using implants in fracture surgery depends on the type and size of the device, the inherent stability of the damaged tissue, the surgical technique, and the postoperative rehabilitation protocol.[38]

The material and method of fabrication of the implant determine its properties. Metals are used for most fracture fixation devices and exhibit high strengths, moderate ductility, and a degree of plastic deformation.[38] The three basic types of metals used in orthopaedics are iron, cobalt-chromium or cobalt-nickel, and titanium alloys.[39, 40] Most implants are manufactured from stainless steel because of its biocompatibility, low cost, ease of fabrication, and combination of mechanics and corrosion resistance.[38] Processing techniques are available, such as powder metallurgy and hot isostatic pressing, that can be used to produce metals with excellent mechanical strength and corrosion resistance.

The design plays an important role in determining the strength of an implant, as even the strongest material cannot make up for a design flaw. Factors such as length, width, and cross-sectional area help determine the mechanical properties of a device.[40] For a uniform structure, the strength in tension or compression is inversely proportional to its diameter squared, and in bending or torsion is inversely proportional to the diameter to the fourth power. Device rigidity is also influenced by implant geometry.

There are three categories of failure of metal implants: brittle failure, plastic failure, and fatigue failure.[39] Implants with low ductility can exhibit brittle failure when loaded beyond the ultimate strength, such as torsionally overloading a screw head during insertion. Plastic deformation, a more common mode of failure of implants, occurs when the yield point of a material is exceeded. In this instance the device permanently bends, causing malalignment of the fracture. The straight-line portion of the stress-strain curve represents the area of elastic behavior beyond which the yield point is exceeded, resulting in plastic changes. To function adequately in the stabilization of fractures, an implant must be able to withstand repeated stresses below the yield point of the material. This can sometimes result in fatigue failure and delayed failure of an implant device. To minimize the possibility of fatigue failure, implants are made of high-strength materials that are corrosion resistant, and implant designs avoid notches or sharp edges that act as stress risers.

SCREWS

Screws are commonly used in fracture fixation both by themselves and in combination with plates. Because they are relatively small, they cause little damage to the periosteal and endosteal blood supply. However, they provide little load-bearing capacity because of their size. Complications related to screw use can come from the mechanics of the screw itself and the principles related to their use.[38]

There have been numerous studies on screw fixation and their effect on bone. Bechtol et al[39] studied the effect of drill holes on bone strength. They found that drill holes of up to 20% of the diameter of the bone decreased the strength of the bone by 40% of its original strength. Even small drill holes acted as stress risers, decreasing the strength of bone significantly. Burstein et al[41] studied the effect of screw holes on the mechanical properties of bone in an animal model. They found that the placement of a screw in the screw hole did not significantly increase the bone strength. As healing progressed, the bone regained its original strength, but when the screw was removed, it was as if a new drill hole had been made. With an empty screw hole, it took 12 weeks for the bone to regain its original strength, and even then the screw hole was still visible on plain radiograph.

In a clinical situation, screws are subject to a complex system of forces, such as extraction forces that tend to pull them out of bone, as well as bending and shearing forces as the plate moves with respect to the bone.[42] Fatigue failure can occur with continued cyclical loads over a period of time. The ability of a screw to maintain compression across a fracture site or to hold a plate to the bone depends on the holding power of the screw in bone, which is in turn dependent on the bone density and quality, and the surface area and configuration of the thread.[38]

PLATES

Plates are commonly used for osteosynthesis, and second to screws are the oldest implants used for fracture fixation. When plates are used, it is important that the cortices be able to withstand compressive forces. When comminution is present or there is a gap in the opposite cortex, micromotion occurs that subjects the plate to bending stresses.[43] This causes the plate to become a load-bearing device and to cycle as load is placed on the extremity, resulting in a race between fracture healing and implant failure.[38]

Soft-tissue problems can arise as a result of plate fixation of fractures and can be due to the surgical approach, host tissue quality, poor soft tissue handling, and the bulk of the plate. During exposure and fracture reduction, the surgeon must maintain soft tissue attachments to the fracture fragments. Devascularization of the bone can lead to a delayed or nonunion.[43] In certain areas of the body, such as the distal tibia, soft-tissue coverage is relatively thin, and wound closure over the plate may be difficult. Even though the wound may close at the time of plate fixation, breakdown occasionally occurs, predisposing to infection. Soft-tissue transfer techniques are then necessary for bone and hardware coverage. Bone grafting is an important adjunct to plate fixation in comminuted fractures or fractures that lack cortical support opposite the plate. This will lead to a cortical buttress opposite the plate as healing occurs, diminishing the bending forces on the plate.[38]

INTRAMEDULLARY FIXATION

Intramedullary nailing is the treatment of choice for diaphyseal fractures of the femur and displaced diaphyseal fractures of the tibia.[44] An intramedullary nail acts as a load-sharing device when cortical apposition is present and can act as a gliding splint if it is not locked.[44] Osteopenia from stress shielding, which is commonly seen with plates, is avoided. Therefore, there is an extremely low rate of refracture after rod removal.

Intramedullary fixation has a significant biological advantage over plate fixation because it can be performed in a closed manner with an image intensifier. This technique maintains soft-tissue attachments at the fracture site, resulting in low rates of infection and nonunion.[44] Early weightbearing in stable fracture patterns is allowable secondary to the favorable biomechanics of intramedullary rods.[38]

Failures of intramedullary devices are usually secondary to the use of small-diameter nails and very proximal or distal fracture patterns.[44] Fatigue failure is the most common form of failure of intramedullary nails, particularly those that are interlocked (Fig. 3). A large working area of the rod, as is seen in comminuted fractures, causes increased bending and rotational forces on the implant.[38] The strength of the nail is proportional to the radius to the third power, so small increases in nail diameter can cause significant increases in strength. Smaller nails may have insufficient metal on the anterior aspect of the rod at the screw holes, causing a weak point in these areas prone to breakage if the fracture is in close proximity.[38, 44] Loss of reduction can occur if the rod is erroneously locked dynamically. Proximal or distal fractures must be locked on at least one end to provide rotational control. Long oblique, spiral, and comminuted fractures must be locked statically.[45] Brumback et al,[45] in a study of 133 dynamic femoral nailings, found a loss of fixation in 10.5% of fractures, which was attributed to fracture lines unseen at the time of surgery.

SLIDING HIP SCREW

The sliding hip screw is the implant of choice in the treatment of intertrochanteric hip fractures.[46] This device functions in a load-sharing capacity, allowing secure fixation of the femoral head and neck to the shaft while impaction occurs at the fracture site. Early patient mobilization and weightbearing can be allowed in stable fracture patterns.

Complications associated with the use of the sliding hip screw in intertrochanteric fractures are few, and when they do occur they are usually related to the fracture pattern or the position of the screw in the femoral head.[46] Comminution of the posteromedial cortical buttress in intertrochanteric fractures causes inherent instability, with a tendency for the fracture to collapse into varus position. Anatomic

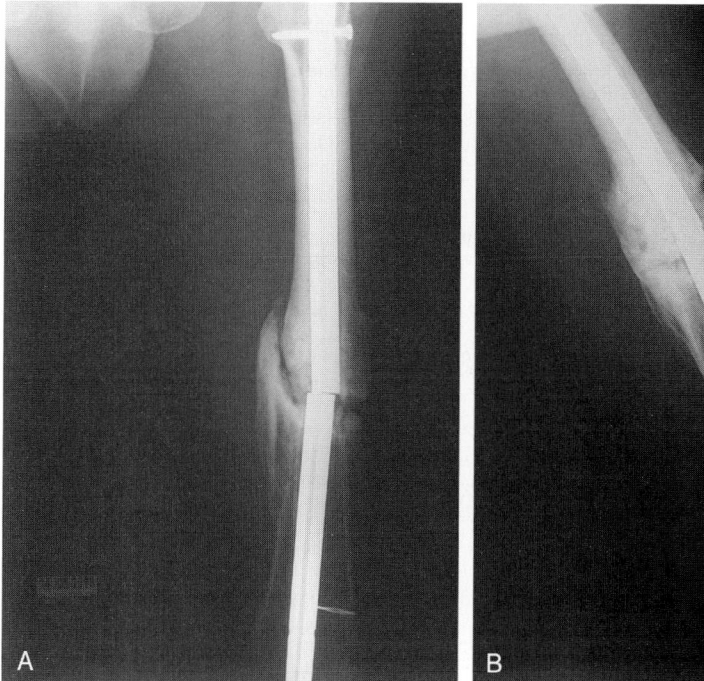
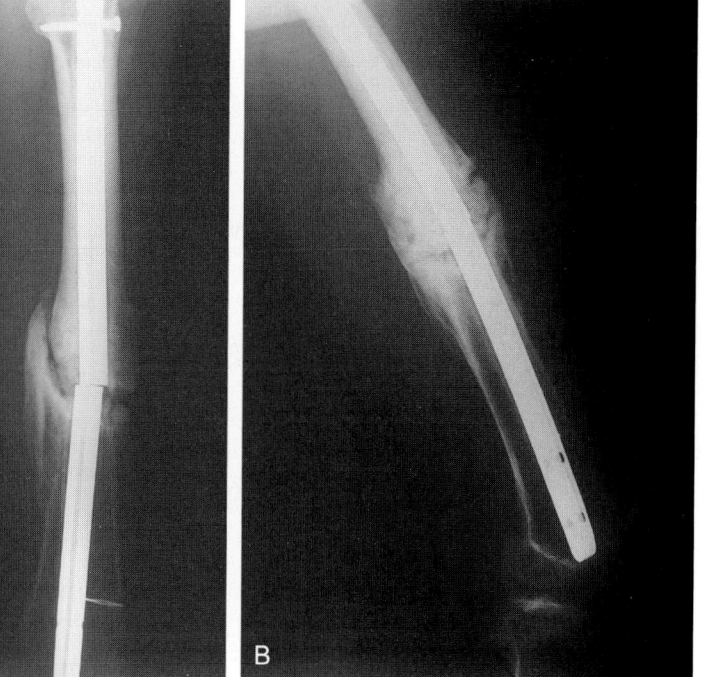

Fig. 3. Fatigue failure of an intramedullary rod secondary to femoral shaft nonunion. *A,* Anteroposterior radiograph. *B,* Lateral radiograph of the nonunion and intramedullary rod failure.

fixation of this fragment has been shown to increase the stability of the fracture complex by as much as 53% in large fragments.[47] Because the sliding hip screw allows controlled impaction at the fracture site, an anatomically reduced unstable fracture can impact spontaneously to a stable, medial position.[38]

The position of the lag screw in the femoral head is important in avoiding cut-out. The optimal position is in the center of the head or slightly inferior and posterior, within 1 cm of the subchondral bone. The highest rates of screw cut-out have occurred with anterior and superior positioning.[38]

Complications can also occur with the hip screw when it loses its sliding capacity, converting to a fixed-angle device.[46] Failure to achieve a stable reduction can result in excessive fracture collapse. This results in excessive sliding of the barrel on the screw, causing the barrel to come in contact with the screw threads. This converts the device into a load-bearing, fixed-angle device that has an increased risk of failure.

CHRONIC PAIN

Chronic pain following fracture healing is a poorly understood problem that may cause significant, long-term disability for the patient. The cause is multifactorial and may involve post-traumatic arthritis, joint stiffness, venous and lymphatic disruption, neuromata, and autonomic dysfunction. There are many psychosocial sequelae that follow chronic pain, and narcotic addiction is not uncommon.

As previously mentioned, post-traumatic arthritis may follow displaced, intra-articular fractures, even those that are anatomically reduced and fixed. Treatment for this condition involves arthroplasty for the knee, hip, shoulder, and elbow, and fusion for most other joints. Joint stiffness and limitation in motion may contribute to post-fracture pain and disability. This may occur as a result of the initial trauma that causes soft tissue injury with resultant scarring, adhesions, and loss of motion. Motion loss may also be caused by treatment, whether it is from long-term casting or a surgical approach for open reduction and internal fixation. The energy that goes into creating a fracture causes a zone of soft-tissue disruption that extends beyond the bony injury. This can cause significant venous and lymphatic disruption, which may lead to chronic swelling and fluid accumulation even after the fracture has healed. Most patients who have sustained a fracture experience weather-related ache. Complex regional pain syndrome may follow a fracture but also commonly occurs following low-energy, minor trauma in which fracture is not sustained. Treatment involves a multidisciplinary approach, and this complication can frequently lead to significant long-term pain and disability.

Patients with chronic, refractory pain following musculoskeletal trauma are frequently addicted to narcotics, disabled, and unable to return to work, which causes serious psychosocial sequelae. A patient with severe post-fracture pain may require narcotic analgesics, which can be habit- and tolerance-forming. Such patients may become anxious over the chronicity of the problem and the inability to work, leading to social and familial dysfunction. Sleep patterns are disrupted by the patient's worrying about the situation, and often hypnotics are prescribed. Depression can follow, which occasionally necessitates treatment with antidepression medication. Patients can go through cycles of severe pain, limited function, and depression. Such problems are best treated by prevention, and at present, by a holistic, multidisciplinary pain treatment approved program.

REFERENCES

1. Thompson R: Complications of lower extremity amputations. Orthop Clin North Am 1972; 3:323.
2. Jordan H: Orthopaedic Appliances. Springfield, IL, Charles C Thomas, 1963.
3. Pierce R Jr, Whitaker J: Complications of traction, plaster casts, and appliances. In: Epps C (ed): Complications in Orthopaedics. Philadelphia: JB Lippincott, 1994, p 69.
4. Bradway J, Amadio P, Cooney W: Open reduction and internal fixation of displaced, comminuted intra-articular fractures of the distal end of the radius. J Bone Joint Surg Am 1989; 71:839.
5. Knirk J, Jupiter J: Intra-articular fractures of the distal end of the radius in young adults. J Bone Joint Surg Am 1986; 68:647.
6. Brown T, Anderson D, Nepola J, et al: Contact stress aberrations following imprecise reduction of simple tibial plateau fracture. J Orthop Res 1988; 6:851.
7. Goss T: Scapular fractures and dislocation: Diagnosis and treatment. J Am Acad Orthop Surg 1995; 3:22.
8. Melcher G, Degonda F, Leutenegger A, et al: Ten year follow up after operative treatment for intra-articular fractures of the calcaneus. J Trauma 1995; 38:713.
9. Thermann H, Krettek C, Hufner T, et al: Management of calcaneal fractures in adults. Clin Orthop 1998; 353:107.
10. Barnes J, Brown J, Garden R, et al: Subcapital fractures of the femur: A prospective view. J Bone Joint Surg Br 1976; 58:2.
11. Hopkins C, Nugent J: Femoral neck fractures is children. Orthop Trans 1986; 10:125.
12. Jaberg H, Warner J, Jakob R: Percutaneous stabilization of unstable fractures of the proximal humerus. J Bone Joint Surg Am 1992; 74:508.
13. Resch H, Povacz P, Frohlich R: Percutaneous fixation of three and four part fractures of the proximal humerus. J Bone Joint Surg Br 1997; 79:295.
14. Norris T: Fractures of the proximal humerus and dislocations of the shoulder. In Browner B, Jupiter J, Levine A, et al (eds): Skeletal Trauma: Fractures, Dislocations, Ligamentous Injuries. Philadelphia: WB Saunders, 1992, p 1201.
15. Connor P, Flatow E: Complications of internal fixation of proximal humerus fractures. Inst Course Lect 1997; 46:25.
16. Adelaar R: Complex fractures of the talus. In Adelaar R (ed): Complex Foot and Ankle Trauma. Philadelphia: Lippincott-Raven, 1999, p 81.
17. Phemister D: Treatment of the necrotic head of the femur in adults. J Bone Joint Surg Am 1949; 31:55.
18. Marsh J, Buckwalter J, Evarts C: Delayed union, nonunion, malunion, and avascular necrosis. In Epps C (ed): Complications in Orthopaedic Surgery, vol. 1. Philadelphia, JB Lippincott, 1994, p 203.
19. Edholm P, Lindblom K, Maurseth K: Angulations in the fractures of the femoral neck with and without subsequent necrosis of the head. Acta Radiol Scand 1967; 6:329.
20. Garden R: Stability and union in subcapital fractures of the femur. J Bone Joint Surg Br 1964; 46:630.
21. Garden R: Malrreduction and avascular necrosis in subcapital fractures of the femur. J Bone Joint Surg Br 1971; 53:183.
22. Smyth E, Shah V: The significance of good reduction and fixation in displaced subcapital fractures of the femur. Injury 1974; 5:197.
23. Steinberg M, Steinberg D: Avascular necrosis of the femoral head. In Steinberg M (ed): The Hip and Its Disorders. Philadelphia, WB Saunders, 1991, p 624.
24. Satterlee C: Osteonecrosis and other non-inflammatory degenerative diseases of the glenohumeral joint. In Norris T (ed): Orthopaedic Knowledge Update: Shoulder and Elbow. Rosemont, IL: American Academy of Orthopaedic Surgeons, 1997: 181.
25. Green D: The effect of avascular necrosis on Russe bone grafting for scaphoid nonunion. J Hand Surg 1985; 10:597.
26. Ruby L: Fractures and dislocations of the carpus. In Browner B, Jupiter J, Levine A, et al (eds): Skeletal Trauma: Fractures, Dislocations, Ligamentous Injuries. Philadelphia, WB Saunders, 1992, p 1025.
27. Yuceturk A, Isiklar Z, Tuncay C, et al: Treatment of scaphoid non-unions with vascularized bone graft based on the first dorsal metacarpal artery. J Hand Surg Br 1997; 22:425.
28. Frassica F, Frassica D, Coventry M: Ectopic bone. In Morrey B (ed): Joint Replacement Arthroplasty. New York, Churchill Livingstone, 1991, p 867.
29. Ilahi O: Post-traumatic heterotopic ossification about the elbow. Orthopedics 1998; 21:265.
30. Garland D: Clinical observations on fractures and heterotopic ossification. Clin Orthop 1988; 233:86.
31. Matta J, Siebenrock K: Does indomethacin reduce heterotopic bone formation after operations for acetabular fractures? J Bone Joint Surg Br 1997; 79:959.
32. Moore K, Goss K, Anglen J: Indomethacin versus radiation therapy for prophylaxis against heterotopic ossification in acetabular fractures. J Bone Joint Surg Br 1998; 80:259.
33. Garland D, O'Halleran R: Fractures and dislocations about the elbow in the head injured adult. Clin Orthop 1982; 168:38.
34. Frassica F, Coventry M, Morrey B: Ectopic ossification about the elbow. In Morrey B (ed): The Elbow and Its Disorders. Philadelphia, WB Saunders, 1993, p 505.
35. Jupiter J: Heterotopic ossification about the elbow. In: Tullos H (ed): Instuctional Course Lectures, vol 40. Rosemont, IL: American Academy of Orthopaedic Surgeons, 1991, p 41.
36. Helfet D, Schmeling G: Fractures of the acetabulum: Complications. In Tile M (ed): Fractures of the Pelvis and Acetabulum. Media, PA: William & Wilkins, 1995, p 461.
37. McAuliffe J, Wolfson A: Early excision of heterotopic ossification about the elbow followed by radiation therapy. J Bone Joint Surg Am 1997; 79:749.
38. Koval K, Frankel V, Kummer F, et al: Complications of fracture fixation devices. In: Epps. C Jr (ed): Complications in Orthopaedic Surgery, vol. 1. Philadelphia, JB Lippincott, 1994, p 131.
39. Bechtol C, Ferguson A, Laing P: Metals and engineering in bone and joint surgery. Baltimore: Williams & Wilkins, 1959.
40. Dumbleton J, Black J: An introduction to orthopaedic materials. Springfield, IL: Charles C Thomas, 1975.
41. Burstein A, Currey J, Frankel V, et al: Bone strength, the effect of screw holes. J Bone Joint Surg Am 1972; 54:1146.
42. Jacobs C: Mechanics of screw fixation. Bull Hosp Joint Dis 1977; 38:94.
43. Muller M, Allgower M, Schneider R, Willenegger H: The manual of internal fixation. Berlin: Springer-Verlag, 1991.
44. Bucholz R, Brumback R: Fractures of the shaft of the femur. In Rockwood C Jr, Green D, Bucholz R (eds): Fractures in Adults. Philadelphia: JB Lippincott, 1991, p 1653.
45. Brumback R, Reilly J, Poka A, et al: Intramedullary nailing of femoral shaft fractures. Part I: Decision-making errors with interlocking fixation. J Bone Joint Surg Am 1988; 70:1441.
46. Zuckerman J, Schon L: Hip fractures. In: Zuckerman J (ed): Comprehensive Care of Orthopaedic Injuries in the Elderly. Baltimore, Urban & Schwarzenberg, 1990, p 23.
47. Apel D, Patwardhan A, Pinzur M, et al: Axial loading studies of unstable intertrochanteric fractures of the femur. Clin Orthop 1989; 246:156.

section
3
chapter
5

SHOULDER GIRDLE AND PROXIMAL HUMERAL FRACTURES

Stephen Kottmeier

Summary

- Fractures of the shoulder girdle and the proximal humerus are quite common in all age groups.
- Fractures of the humerus constitute 5% of all fractures.
- The incidence rate of proximal humeral fractures increases with age.
- Approximately 80% of proximal humeral fractures in the elderly are nondisplaced or minimally displaced and are best managed by closed means.
- Although most displaced unstable proximal humeral fractures are best treated with open reduction and internal fixation, special circumstances may call for either an external fixator or a prosthesis replacement.
- Prosthesis replacement of the humeral head as treatment for an acute fracture produces better results than prosthesis replacement for salvage after failure of open reduction and internal fixation.
- Although postfracture osteonecrosis of the head of the humerus does occur, its impact on clinical outcome is quite variable.
- Clavicle fracture, the most common fracture in childhood, accounts for 5% to 10% of all fractures in adult and for 50% of fractures involving the shoulder girdle.
- Although most clavicle fractures are best treated by closed means, unstable distal clavicle fractures do better if treated with open reduction and internal fixation.
- Fracture of the scapula is uncommon, accounting for 3% to 5% of shoulder girdle injuries and less than 1% of all fractures.
- Because of the proximity of vital structures and the extreme force necessary to fracture the scapula, approximately 90% of patients with fracture of the scapula have significant associated injuries.
- Most scapular fractures are best treated by closed means.
- Some displaced fractures of the scapular neck, the acromion, or the glenoid may do better with operative treatment.

Fractures involving the shoulder girdle may occur in patients of all ages and from injury mechanisms ranging from low to high energy. Effective treatment demands thorough history and physical examination as well as an understanding of regional osseous and soft-tissue anatomy. The proximity of neurovascular and intrathoracic structures may render some of these injuries life- or limb-threatening. Selective imaging studies facilitate characterization of fracture morphology and determination of a fracture classification. The patient's medical status, expectations, and skeletal comorbid conditions must be identified and addressed. Most fractures involving the shoulder girdle can be effectively managed nonoperatively. In surgical management, methods of fixation should be sufficiently rigid to allow immediate postoperative motion. Implant insertion techniques should respect articular, myotendinous, and neurovascular integrity and should involve little or no additional compromise of the osseous blood supply.

PROXIMAL HUMERAL FRACTURES

Fractures of the proximal humerus are diverse with regard to both fracture pattern and patient population. The goal of management for these injuries is restoration of painless satisfactory shoulder function. This is most predictably attained by restoration of osseous anatomy and preservation of soft-tissue integrity. The management plan must be based on an understanding of existing variables and obstacles, including the patient's medical condition, bone quality, and associated lesions as well as the limitations of implants, fixation techniques, and the surgeon's own skills. Successful treatment demands a thorough understanding of regional anatomy and an accurate assessment of fracture morphology. Treatment is highly individualized owing to the multiple variables unique to both the patient and the fracture.

HISTORY AND EPIDEMIOLOGY

Fractures of the proximal humerus constitute 5% of all fractures. The incidence rate increases with advancing age owing to the inferior quality of senescent bone.[1, 2] Reduction in trabecular density and cortical thinning render the elderly population at considerable risk for fracture with low-energy mechanisms of injury. Approximately 80% of proximal humeral fractures in elderly patients are minimally displaced or nondisplaced and respond favorably to conservative treatment with a well-monitored rehabilitation program. Coexistent medical concerns must be appreciated in this patient population. Fractures of the proximal humerus in younger individuals represent high-energy lesions often associated with considerable displacement, comminution, and other traumatic injuries.

In either age group, the patterns of displaced fractures represent a therapeutic challenge. Kocher[3] in 1896 and Codman[4] in 1934 initiated efforts to establish an anatomic classification describing consistently encountered injury patterns. The anatomic four-part classification scheme adopted and modified by Neer[5] in 1970 offers a comprehensive approach to the successful characterization and treatment of these fractures.

PATHOANATOMY AND PATHOGENESIS

The proximal humerus is composed of four well-defined anatomic parts: the greater tuberosity, the lesser tuberosity, the shaft, and the anatomic head. The anatomic neck is the region of the previous epiphyseal plate. The surgical neck is the region distal to the tuberosities and the anatomic neck. It is a region of cortical thinning, rendering it structurally weak and susceptible to fracture. The neck-shaft inclination averages 145 degrees, and humeral head retroversion 30 degrees, with respect to the longitudinal axis.

The shoulder girdle muscles and rotator cuff terminations keep the proximal humerus in a state of equilibrium. Fractures of individual components disturb this balance, exerting deforming forces on fracture fragments. The pectoralis major muscle, via its attachment to the humeral shaft, exerts an anterior and medial deforming force on the shaft. The supraspinatus, infraspinatus, and teres minor, inserting on the greater tuberosity, exert external rotation forces on the humeral head. They are neutralized by the internal rotational force imparted by the subscapularis via its attachment to the lesser tuberosity. The integrity of the rotator cuff, particularly in the elderly population, is often superior to the quality of bone. With a fracture, the position of the articular humeral head component is governed by whatever osseous-tendinous attachments are retained. These deforming forces and subsequent malpositioning of fragments complicate satisfactory reduction with the use of closed methods.

An understanding of intraosseous and extraosseous vascular supply to the proximal humerus is of considerable importance to the assessment and management of fractures involving this region. Avascular necrosis of the articular component can arise from traumatic or surgical violation of blood supply.[6, 7] The impact of necrosis, from the standpoint of perceived shoulder pain and impaired performance, is variable but may be considerable. Treatment efforts are therefore directed toward preservation of remaining blood supply when feasible. The principal blood supply to the articular segment is provided by the arcuate artery.[8] This structure represents the intraosseous termination of the ascending branch of the anterior humeral circumflex artery, which traverses the bicipital groove. Fracture or surgical dissection within this region may, accordingly, jeopardize the remaining blood supply. Limited additional vascular supply is offered by the posterior humeral circumflex artery and rotator cuff insertional vessels.

CLINICAL FEATURES

Inspection of the injured patient often reveals extensive ecchymosis involving the shoulder girdle, periphery of the involved upper extremity, and thoracic region. Assessment of shoulder function may be compromised if range of motion is limited by pain. Skin integrity must be assessed, and the neurovascular status of the limb ascertained. Significant potential for neurovascular deficit exists, particularly in high-energy injuries with considerable displacement or in elderly patients with atherosclerotic vessel disease.[9] The axillary artery is most vulnerable to injury at its junction with the anterior humeral circumflex artery. The presence of a peripheral pulse does not ensure patency of the axillary artery. Asymmetric pulse and a regional expanding hematoma warrant angiographic study. Neurological deficit manifests most commonly in the form of axillary neuropraxia. Sensation impairment within the axillary dermatome ("sergeant's patch") is the most reliable indicator of such a lesion, because motor function status (deltoid) is likely equivocal in the unwilling patient.

INVESTIGATIONS

Accurate radiographic characterization of fracture morphology requires properly oriented projections of acceptable quality (Fig. 1). Evaluation begins with performance of orthogonal scapular views obtained perpendicular and parallel to the longitudinal axis of the scapula. These views are supplemented by an axillary view to assess for dislocation, degree of tuberosity displacement, and glenoid lesions; this view can be achieved in the presence of discomfort, with only minimal abduction. A modified Velpeau axillary view is a less desirable alternative. Articular head splitting and impression lesions are best identified with computed tomography. This technique further serves to quantify comminution, displacement of segments, and extent of articular involvement to both the anatomic head and glenoid.

Recognition of the mechanical and biological consequences of common patterns of injury is achieved only with a clear understanding of the pathoanatomy involved. Effective execution of treatment, whether operative or nonoperative, is predicated upon an accurate characterization of fracture morphology. Any method of classification used must enable reproducible cataloguing of injuries to direct treatment as well as a mechanism by which to predict outcome. Codman observed that fractures of the proximal humerus involved the four anatomic segments in isolation or in various combinations. The clinical relevance of this was appreciated by Neer,[10] who in 1970 established a four-part classification (Fig. 2). Despite concerns regarding reproducibility, the Neer classification remains the standard on which evaluation and treatment are based.[11–13]

In the Neer scheme, the fracture pattern is assigned according to the number of displaced parts (greater tuberosity, lesser tuberosity, anatomic head, shaft). Emphasis is placed on both radiographic pattern and deforming forces. Direction of displacement depends on the net effect of deforming forces exerted by the retained musculotendinous attachments on the individual displaced fracture fragments. Displacement is defined as separation or angulation of a segment from subjacent components by at least 1 cm or 45 degrees, respectively. The presence of nondisplaced fragments or fracture lines does not influence fracture assignment. Eighty-five percent of proximal humeral fractures are nondisplaced regardless of location and number of fracture lines. These accordingly cannot be assigned within the Neer classification, which encompasses only displaced variants.

The AO alphanumeric classification focuses on fracture location and its impact on articular vascular supply.[14] Type A fractures (extra-articular unifocal) offer no significant compromise to vascular supply and are accordingly associated with minimal risk of avascular necrosis. Type B and type C fractures are intra-capsular (extra-articular and intra-articular, respectively) and typically involve three or four segments. Each group is further subdivided numerically. Valgus impacted head fragments may retain considerably

Arm supported in sling.

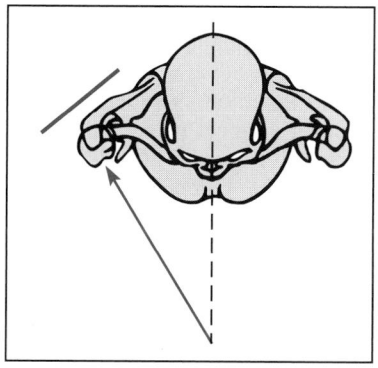

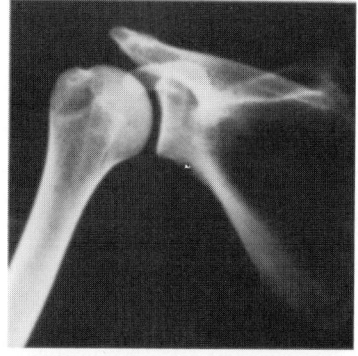

No overlap of head and glenoid.

Lateral in scapular plane.

Arm supported in sling.

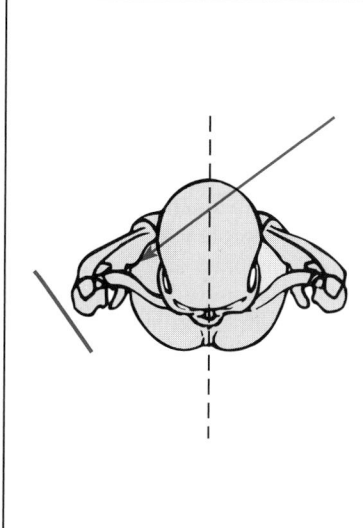

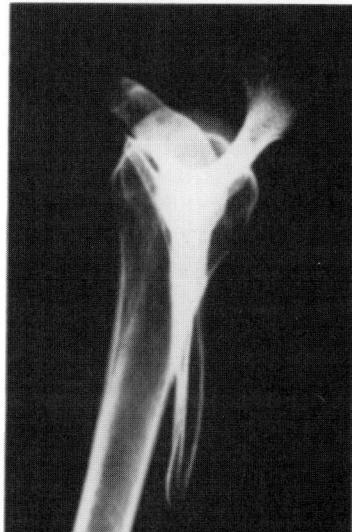

90° to AP.

Head in center of glenoid.

Identify anterior and posterior displacement.

Identify greater tuberosity displacement.

Evaluate shape of acromion for cause of impingement or cuff tears.

Emergency axillary.

Arm is gently abducted.

Tube at the hip.

Involved shoulder supported on pad.

Arm holds IV pole or is supported by assistant.

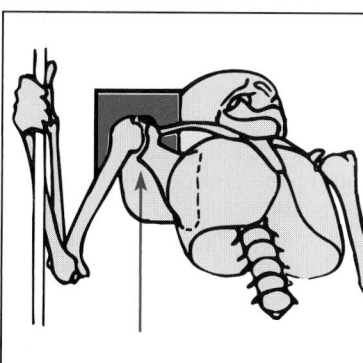

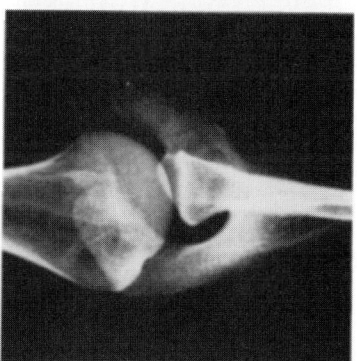

Evaluate glenoid for uneven wear or rim fractures.

Identify anterior and posterior dislocation.

Identify displaced tuberosities.

Identify unfused acromial epiphysis.

Fig. 1. Trauma series views. (Reproduced from Browner BE, Jupiter JB, Levine AM, et al: Skeletal Trauma. Philadelphia, WB Saunders, 1998, 2nd ed, vol 2, p 1558; from Norris TR: In Chapman MW, Madison M [eds]: Operative Orthopaedics. Philadelphia, JB Lippincott, 1988, p 203.)

more blood supply than their varus counterparts. Accordingly, a trend toward preservation rather than replacement has evolved for such lesions.

GOALS, INDICATIONS, AND CONTRAINDICATIONS
Goals
The goal of treatment is to restore painless function by maintaining acceptable fracture alignment while respecting the limitations of bone quality, the patient's compliance, and the osseous vascular supply. The implementation of a rehabilitation protocol that will achieve motion and strength in the long term while respecting the limitations of operative and nonoperative treatment in the short term is essential to the realization of this goal. Restoration of anatomy, achievement of adequate soft-tissue and osseous healing, and preservation of osseous vascular supply and joint motion, both active and passive, maximize shoulder function.

Indications and Contraindications
The majority of proximal humeral fractures are nondisplaced according to Neer's criteria and do not require oper-

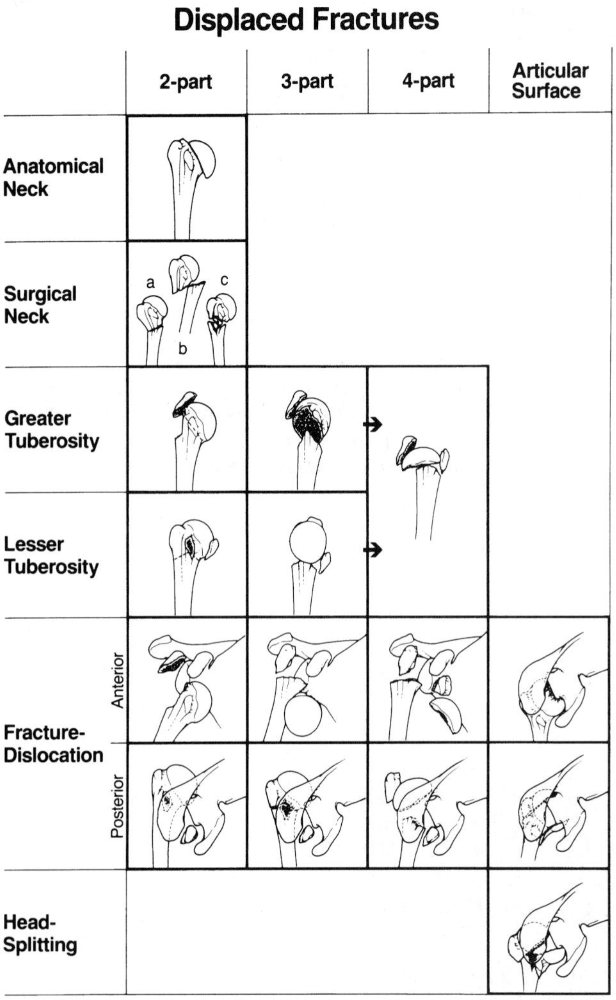

Displaced Fractures

Fig. 2. Neer classification for upper humeral fractures. The most commonly used classification at present, this comprehensive system encompasses anatomy and biomechanical forces that result in the displacement of fracture fragments. The classification is based on accurate identification of the four major fragments and their relationship to one another. A displaced fracture is either two-part, three-part, or four-part. In addition, fracture-dislocations can be either two-part, three-part, or four-part. Fissure lines or hairline fractures are not considered displaced fragments. A fragment is considered displaced only if it is separated by more than 1 cm or is angulated more than 45 degrees from the other fragments. Impression fractures of the articular surface also occur and are usually associated with an anterior or posterior dislocation. Head-splitting fractures are usually associated with fractures of the tuberosities or surgical neck. (From Rockwood CA, Matsen RA: The Shoulder. Philadelphia, WB Saunders 1998, 2nd ed, vol 1, p 342; after Neer CS: Displaced proximal humeral fractures. Part I: Classification and evaluation. J Bone Joint Surg Am 1970; 52:1077.)

ative treatment (Fig. 3). Early introduction of a well-controlled physiotherapy program, within 2 weeks, can yield very acceptable results in the majority of individuals sustaining such lesions. Fracture patterns with little or no displacement are likely stable owing to intact periarticular soft tissues. Treatment consists of short-term sling immobilization with introduction of assisted motion during early phases of clinical union, usually within 3 weeks. Good to excellent results can be expected in more than 75% of such cases.[15]

The remaining 15% of proximal humeral fractures are displaced variants that pose a therapeutic challenge. Considerable residual displacement may have a substantial negative impact on shoulder performance. Tuberosity displacement or surgical neck angulation may result in subacromial impingement in positions of abduction and impaired range of motion.[16] Often, treatment in the form of operative fixation or prosthetic hemiarthroplasty is required to achieve functional recovery. No uniform criteria for surgical indications exist, as no single method of operative treatment is ideal for all fractures in all patients. Operative indications must be highly individualized to meet the demands and limitations of the patient, bone quality, fracture pattern, soft-tissue envelope, and implants and techniques employed. Those patients with displaced patterns who are at considerable medical risk or unlikely to comply with postoperative limitations and postoperative therapy should be considered for nonoperative treatment.

PROCEDURES

Operative treatment requires an accurate characterization of fracture morphology as well as an understanding of regional anatomy and the attributes and limitations of implants and insertion. Traditional principles of rigid fixation that require good quality bone for success may not be applicable. The soft-tissue stripping required for implant insertion with such techniques further jeopardizes remaining blood supply. Older patients with diminished trabecular and thinned cortical bone and comminution are not well suited for such techniques, given concerns about fixation failure. Attention must be directed toward both fixation rigidity and soft-tissue preservation. Maintaining stability at the risk of vascular compromise is undesirable.

Tension band fixation techniques allow incorporation of rotator cuff tissues, which in the elderly serve as a more reliable anchor for implant fixation than adjacent bone.[17, 18] It may be augmented with a single cancellous screw or intramedullary devices for additional control.[19–21] Minimally invasive or percutaneous techniques of fixation deemed "biological" continue to evolve.[22, 23] The additional dissection required for insertion of plates may further compromise blood supply and limit postoperative joint motion. External fixation is best reserved for surgical neck fractures that have extensive cortical comminution or are associated with severe compromise of soft tissues. Complex three- and four-part fractures in older patients are managed with hemiarthroplasty. For such fractures in the younger population, newer techniques of biologically benign fixation continue to evolve, and early results are encouraging.

Two-Part Surgical Neck Fractures

Two-part fractures of the surgical neck region occur in the weak metaphyseal bone inferior to the tuberosities. The humeral head with both tuberosities attached maintains a neutral orientation. Owing to the intact tuberosities and arterial arcade, vascular supply is preserved. Impacted fractures deemed stable are treated nonoperatively with early introduction of controlled mobilization.

Incompletely displaced fractures most commonly manifest with apical anterior angulation because of an intact posterior soft-tissue hinge. Fracture malunion in this position may compromise functional forward flexion of the

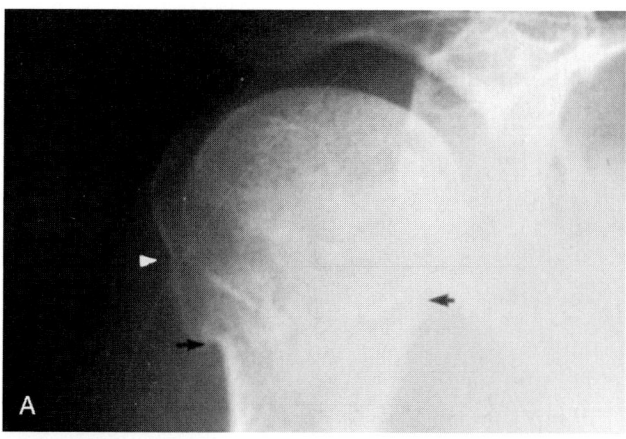
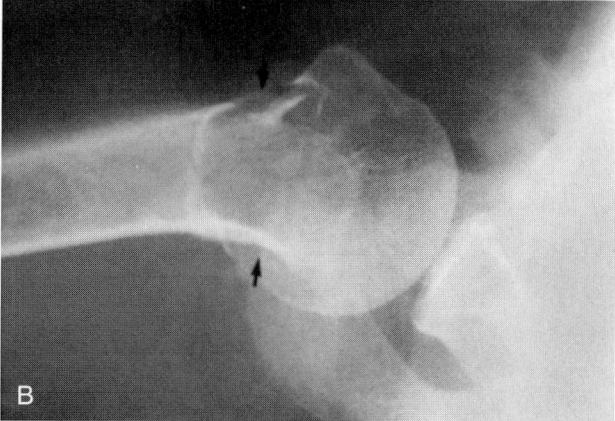

Fig. 3. Views. Anteroposterior (*A*) and axillary (*B*) radiographs of a patient with an undisplaced surgical neck fracture. Fractures of this type are best treated with immobilization in a sling followed by early active and active assisted motions. (From Browner BE, Jupiter JB, Levine AM, et al: Skeletal Trauma. Philadelphia, WB Saunders, 1998, 2nd ed, vol 2, p 1584.)

shoulder. Nonimpacted two-part surgical neck fractures with complete displacement are often unstable. The shaft component is displaced anteriorly and medially by the unopposed force of the pectoralis major. Closed reduction is achieved with application of laterally and posteriorly directed forces to the shaft component with simultaneous correction of apex anterior angulation. Abduction is avoided to lessen deforming forces and the threat to neurovascular structures. Interposed soft tissue (e.g., biceps tendon) may hinder reduction. Reduction, although otherwise easily accomplished, is difficult to maintain with closed treatment techniques. If stable impaction cannot be accomplished, fixation is warranted to preserve the reduction (Fig. 4).

Fixation techniques to address surgical neck fractures range from minimally to considerably invasive. Avoidance of excessive soft-tissue stripping diminishes the potential for motion deficit, infection, and avascular necrosis. No single device can be used for all fracture patterns in all patients. Operative approach, implant selection, fixation construct, and postoperative regimen must be individualized.

Percutaneous insertion of tip-threaded pins offers an attractive minimally invasive method of fixation for fractures amenable to closed or judicious joystick reduction techniques. Pin purchase may be suboptimal in inferior bone, and early postoperative range of motion should be restricted. The application of this approach in the elderly is therefore limited. Alternatively, open fixation with heavy nonabsorbable suture or wire with incorporation of the rotator cuff tendon, particularly in elderly patients, may afford more secure fixation.[24] If the surgical neck is significantly comminuted, the inclusion of vertically oriented pins in a tension band configuration may enhance bending and rotational stability.

Application of extramedullary plates for acute fracture management necessitates soft-tissue stripping, further compromising the existing blood supply to osseous elements.[25–27] Fixation failure, implant-related impingement, and a tendency toward varus alignment limit the utility of this approach. Intramedullary devices have evolved to meet the demands of such fractures and address the limitations

of the tissues. Small-caliber devices alone (Rush pin, Ender nails) inserted antegrade through small wounds achieve insufficient rotational control. Inadequate proximal purchase and prominence within the subacromial space are additional concerns. Innovation in intramedullary implant design and insertion techniques continues in an effort to improve intramedullary fixation (less soft-tissue stripping, biomechanical superiority) for the treatment of proximal humeral fractures.

Two-Part Greater Tuberosity Fractures

Displaced two-part fractures involving the greater tuberosity can result in considerable functional impairment if undertreated. Deforming forces displacing the tuberosity include those exerted by the infraspinatus, teres minor, and supraspinatus muscles. Displacement is dictated by fracture location within the tuberosity. The unopposed pull of the retained cuff tissues (supraspinatus and infraspinatus) displaces the greater tuberosity posteriorly and superiorly within the subacromial space. A traumatic tear of the rotator cuff often exists within the space between the supraspinatus and subscapularis or posteriorly between the supraspinatus and infraspinatus. The retained attachments of the supraspinatus and infraspinatus tendons tend to displace the fragment posterosuperiorly within the subacromial space. The two-part fractures may occur in isolation or in combination with anterior dislocation of the glenohumeral joint. Residual displacement is pathognomonic for a longitudinal tear of the rotator cuff. The extent of displacement is often underappreciated with conventional radiography, particularly on the AP view. A computed tomography (CT) scan may more accurately visualize the displacement, aiding in determination of the indications for fixation.

Left untreated, malunion of the tuberosity and tear of the tendon compromise strength and motion, particularly of external rotation and abduction, because of subacromial encroachment. Open reduction with fixation is required to limit this compromise and restore integrity to the rotator cuff. Lesser degrees of displacement may be poorly tolerated in younger active individuals. The fractured tuberosity can be accessed via a deltoid-splitting approach. Transosseous sutures are incorporated within the fragment and

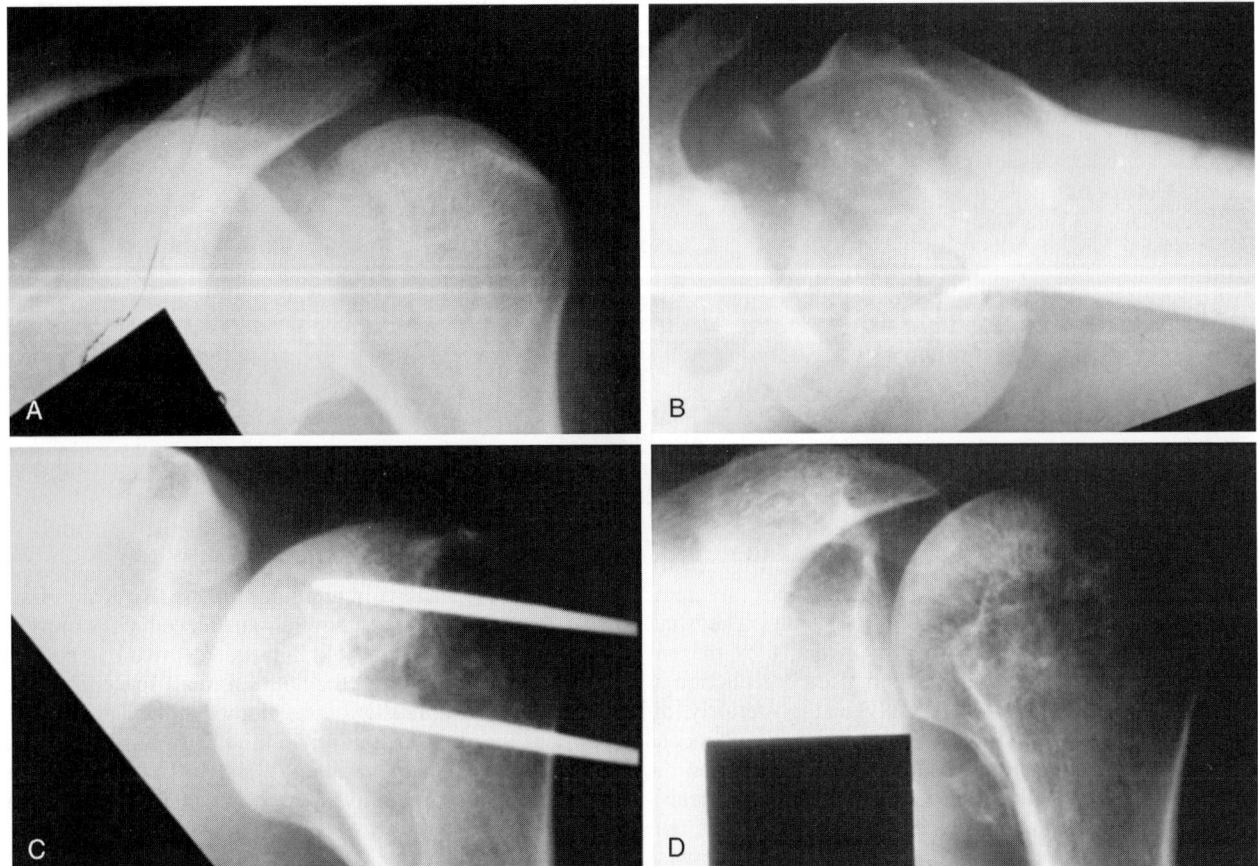

Fig. 4. Posterior dislocation: two-part neck posterior fracture-dislocation. *A*, The AP view was not diagnostic in the opinions of the first three orthopaedic surgeons assessing this fracture-dislocation. *B*, The axillary view demonstrating the posterior head displacement enabled the diagnosis to be established. *C*, Open reduction and internal fixation (ORIF) with two Steinmann pins. *D*, Four-month follow-up, after pin removal at 6 weeks, shows good early healing of the articular segment. A longer follow-up will be needed to ensure that late collapse with avascular necrosis does not occur. (From Browner BE, Jupiter JB, Levine AM, et al: Skeletal Trauma. Philadelphia, WB Saunders, 1998, 2nd ed, vol 2, p 1587; courtesy of Charles A. Rockwood, Jr, MD.)

attached cuff tissues.[28] Adjuvant screw fixation may be considered in patients with good quality bone, thereby avoiding implant impingement within the subacromial space. Screw fixation alone for these fractures is reserved for large fragments of good bone quality. Cuff repair is emphasized regardless of the fixation method elected. The greater tuberosity is restored to a position approximately 5 mm inferior to the articular surface summit.

Two-Part Lesser Tuberosity Fractures

Two-part fractures involving the lesser tuberosity occur most frequently in combination with posterior glenohumeral dislocation. Isolated injuries are rare and may be associated with intra-articular subluxation of the long head of the biceps. The unopposed pull of the subscapularis displaces the fragment medially. An axillary radiograph or axial computed tomography scan is required to adequately define the lesion. Malunion of lesser tuberosity fractures may compromise internal rotation and functional performance of the limb posterior to the body. If the lesion is displaced, involves the articular surface, or obstructs motion, open reduction and fixation should be performed. A deltopectoral approach is selected, and fixation is achieved with a transosseous suture incorporating the rotator cuff.

Two-Part Anatomic Neck/Articular Fractures

Because two-part fractures of the anatomic neck are extremely rare, no meaningful data can be derived from the literature regarding optimum treatment. The absence of soft-tissue attachments devascularizes the segment and does not permit effective closed reduction techniques. Prosthetic hemiarthroplasty is currently the most reasonable option. Preservation of the articular component may be pursued in the younger active patient, with the understanding that prognosis is guarded.

Screw fixation often offers suboptimal purchase, and proximity to of the screws to the joint surface must be considered. Certainly, in the elderly population, prosthetic hemiarthroplasty provides the most predictable and desirable outcome. Similar concerns apply to two-part fractures (or those with more parts) of the articular surface that do not involve the anatomic neck region. Impression lesions of the head region are treated according to the degree of humeral head involvement and the chronicity of dislocation, if present.[29] Acute dislocations reduced concentrically with less than 20% involvement of the articular surface are stable and can be managed nonoperatively. Those with 20% to 45% articular involvement and of less than 6 months in duration can be managed with void-filling procedures (tuberosity and cuff transfer) and osteotomy as necessary to achieve glenohumeral stability. Lesions involving 45% or more of the surface or presence of dislocation that are more than 6 months in duration are best treated by hemiarthroplasty with implant version modification to lessen dislocation recurrence.

Three-Part Fractures

Although occurring in several combinations, three-part fractures of the proximal humerus typically involve a surgical neck component and either the greater or lesser tuberosity. The presence of a single retained tuberosity and rotator cuff attachment imparts an unopposed rotation force on the attached articular component. Untreated fractures with resultant displacement and subsequent malunion will yield inferior results and compromised function. Closed treatment is ineffective, because persistent displacement will compromise rotator cuff efficiency and glenohumeral joint motion. Nonoperative treatment is therefore reserved only for those patients whose medical or mental status does not allow for uncomplicated operative treatment and compliance with the postoperative course of physical therapy.

Operative fixation remains the preferred method of managing displaced three-part fractures. The humeral head retains continuity with a single tuberosity, often ensuring some preservation of blood supply. Prosthetic replacement is justified only for significant articular, soft-tissue, or osseous compromise, which is commonly encountered in older patients. Methods of fixation similar to those for two-part fractures are utilized. The biceps tendon serves to facilitate orientation of the tuberosities. They are secured first to each other, with heavy nonabsorbable suture or wire, and subsequently to the proximal humeral shaft, with intramedullary augmentation as necessary.[30] The inherent advantages and disadvantages of exposure (minimal versus extensile) and implant (percutaneous, wire, plate, rod, composite) must meet the needs and anatomy of the patient.

Four-Part Fractures

Classification as a four-part fracture requires (1) more than 1 cm displacement of each of the four segments or (2) greater than 45 degrees angulation of the fracture components with respect to one another. Four-part fracture patterns typically involve the bicipital groove, compromising the ascending branch of the anterior humeral circumflex artery and, accordingly, the arcuate artery. Rates of vascular necrosis rates between 13% and 34% have been described after closed reduction of three- and four-part fractures of the proximal humerus.[31] Prosthetic replacement remains the treatment of choice for elderly patients because of poor bone stock that would be intolerant of fixation techniques and demands and expectations that may be predictably met with hemiarthroplasty.[10, 32, 33] Patients whose medical or mental status renders them poor candidates for surgical treatment should be treated conservatively.

The notion that delayed hemiarthroplasty may be offered to resolve failure of open fixation or closed treatment is invalid.[34] Interim changes in both osseous and soft tissues preclude the more optimal result that can be achieved with hemiarthroplasty in the acute setting. Successful clinical outcome requires proper implant insertion and selection,

union of the tuberosities, and compliance with a postoperative protocol emphasizing range of motion. Proper height and anatomic humeral head offset restore the normal lever arm, enhancing rotator cuff and deltoid function. The height of the implant must restore myofascial sleeve tension while maintaining the tuberosities inferior to the summit of the implant. Retroversion of 35 to 45 degrees is desired to maintain both functional joint motion and implant stability. Proximal bone deficit compromises implant stability as well as the ability to assess height and version. Cement fixation and implants of modular design facilitate this treatment. Insertion of a cementless, porous-coated device may be considered only if a satisfactory interference fit is achieved. In one study, results were better and the risk of tuberosity nonunion was diminished with cementless insertion than with cementation techniques.[35]

Despite earlier concerns about malunion, nonunion, and fixation failure as well as traumatic and surgically induced avascular necrosis, osteosynthesis of four-part fractures has a role. The extent of avascular necrosis and its impact on outcome are initially indeterminate. Revascularization of the humeral head via creeping substitution has been described and consequently has prompted a trend toward fixation in the younger population. Efforts to retain the humeral head via modified surgical approaches and fixation, described to limit additional vascular compromise, have demonstrated early promise. Valgus-impacted four-part fractures are uniquely amenable to articular segment preservation and fixation (Fig. 5).[36, 37] The presence of intact medial soft tissues in this subgroup may afford cephalic revascularization, accounting for an observed lower rate of avascular necrosis.

COMPLICATIONS AND RESULTS
Complications

Complications arising from fractures of the proximal humerus may result, as previously described, from compromise of myotendinous, osseous, and neurovascular structures. Some of the complications are common to fracture treatment in general, others more unique to proximal humeral fractures.

The likelihood of avascular necrosis depends on fracture pattern, location, degree of displacement, and the status of periarticular soft tissues. The reported incidence rate ranges from 3% to 25% for three-part fractures to greater than 90% for four-part fractures.[10, 31] Radiographically, findings in avascular necrosis may range from transient cyst formation to subtotal or total humeral head collapse. The impact on clinical outcome is variable.

Nonunion of proximal humeral fractures is uncommon regardless of treatment type selected. It may occur secondary to fracture distraction, interposition of soft tissues, or compromise of regional blood supply, or postoperatively as a result of inadequate fixation and excessive imposition of motion.

The consequences of malunion and implant-related pain and motion restriction have been previously described. The most common complications following shoulder hemiarthroplasty are failure of the tuberosities to unite and malposition of components. Both conditions fail to restore the myotendinous balance of the rotator cuff necessary for proper shoulder function.

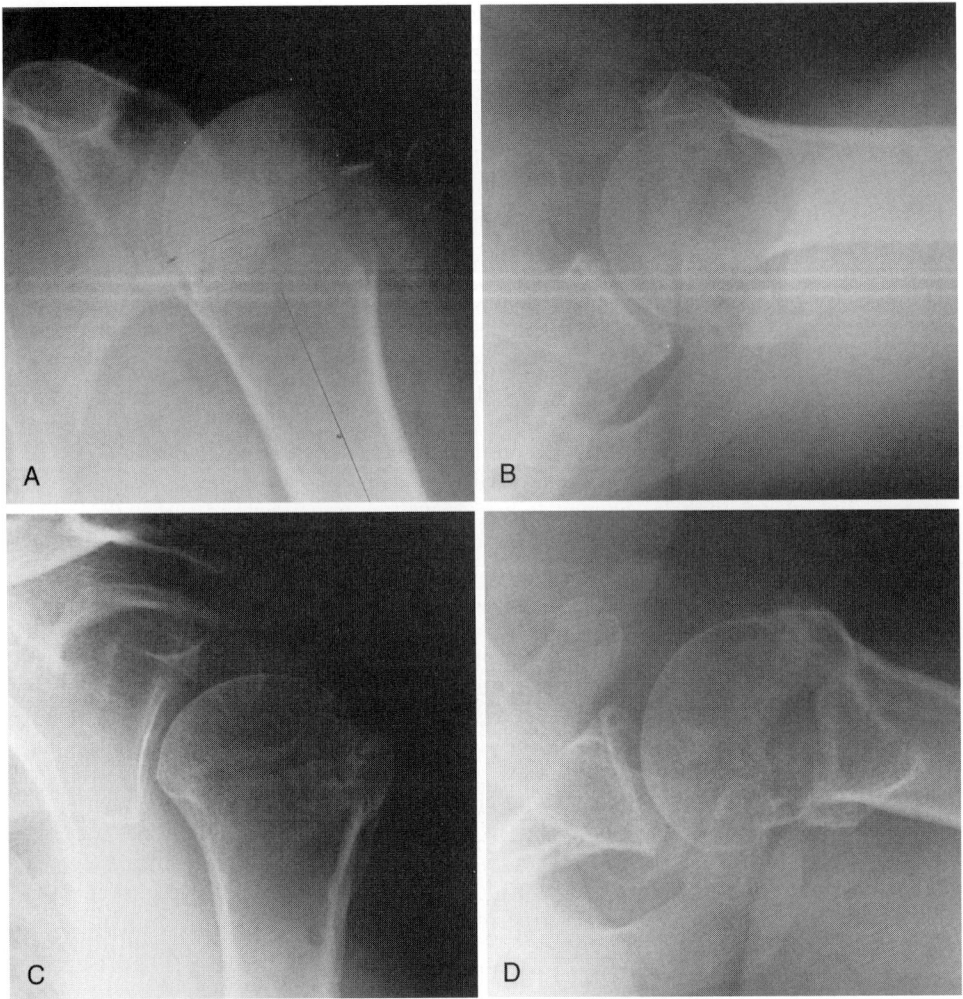

Fig. 5. Views. True AP (*A*) and axillary lateral (*B*) radiographs of a valgus-impacted four-part fracture that occurred in a 67-year-old woman. It was treated with open reduction and limited internal fixation. *C* and *D*, The position of the articular segment was not altered because it was firmly impacted and stable. The tuberosities were reduced and fixed with heavy nonabsorbable suture. (From Browner BE, Jupiter JB, Levine AM, et al: Skeletal Trauma. Philadelphia, WB Saunders, 1998, 2nd ed, vol 2, p 1617.)

Postoperative infection may occur subsequent to any form of operative treatment. Despite the precarious blood supply to the articular segment, the remainder of the shoulder is well-vascularized, conferring a diminished risk of operative wound sepsis. Range-of-motion restriction is not uncommon after either nonoperative or operative treatment. It may arise from soft-tissue injury, malunion, implant position, and adhesion formation. Heterotopic ossification is another potential source of motion deficit, possibly occurring from retained bone debris, repetitive forceful maneuvers, or delayed surgical treatment.

Results

The results of nonoperative treatment for nondisplaced or minimally displaced fractures of the proximal humerus are uniformly favorable if physical therapy is initiated within 2 weeks of injury.[38, 39] Surgical outcomes for displaced lesions parallel the ability to achieve and maintain reduction while preserving range of motion in both the short and the long term.[40, 41] Avoidance of complications is, of course, crucial to the end result. Primary prosthetic replacement for severe fracture of the proximal humerus has yielded 80% to 90% satisfactory results.[42] End-result determinants include proper implant insertion, union of the tuberosities,

and observance of a strict supervised physiotherapy program.

CLAVICLE FRACTURES

Fractures of the clavicle are common in all age groups. Treatment and potential complications, however, differ greatly among them. Although the majority of such fractures typically heal uneventfully, inappropriate or inadequate treatment may generate undesirable results.

The clavicle is subcutaneous along its entire length, rendering it vulnerable to externally applied forces. Anatomic proximity of the clavicle to the first rib and thoracic outlet may result in serious injury to neurovascular and intrathoracic structures. The unique anatomy and kinesiology of the clavicle present significant concerns from the standpoint of treatment, particularly with significantly displaced fracture patterns.

HISTORY AND EPIDEMIOLOGY

Fracture of the clavicle is common, accounting for 5% to 10% of all fractures in the adult population and for approximately 50% of all fractures involving the shoulder girdle.[43] It is the most common fracture in childhood. Methods of reduction and immobilization were reported as early as 3000 B.C., and later by Hippocrates in 400 B.C. Through the years, cumbersome devices designed to maintain reduction have yielded to less constraining methods that encourage limb mobilization. Contemporary techniques of surgical fixation continue to evolve, yet the indications for such treatment remain relatively unresolved.

PATHOANATOMY AND PATHOGENESIS

The clavicle plays an important mechanical role.[44] It serves as an osseous strut interconnecting the forequarter and thorax, maintaining distance between them. It kinematically integrates the complex motions of muscle groups and joints of the shoulder girdle. During abduction, it rotates axially as much as 45 degrees. As evidenced with claviculectomy, the unimpaired presence of the clavicle better ensures strength, stability, and motion of the shoulder. Additionally, the clavicle serves as a site of muscle origin and insertion, enhancing shoulder mobility. Suspension of the scapula is another task of the clavicle, requiring functional integrity of the trapezius superiorly and the coracoclavicular ligaments inferiorly. This structure also offers protection to subjacent nerves and vessels supplying the upper extremity as they traverse the thoracic outlet.

The clavicle, via a central ossification center, is the only long bone to ossify by intramembranous ossification. Epiphyseal centers of ossific growth develop at both ends; the sternal end is the region of dominant longitudinal growth. Injuries displaced to either pole, often deemed "fractures," may actually represent physeal separation.[45] Physeal injuries to the sternoclavicular joint can occur into young adulthood.

The clavicle is a subcutaneous S-shaped structure. From a cephalad perspective, its medial portion is convex anteriorly, and its lateral portion convex posteriorly. Clavicular cross-sectional anatomy ranges from flattened at the lateral end to tubular at the medial end with a weakened central transitional zone. This middle third, devoid of significant muscular attachment, is more susceptible to maximal bending and torsional forces.

The clavicle is anchored securely at both ends by the robust ligaments of the sternoclavicular and acromioclavicular joints. The acromioclavicular ligaments give horizontal stability to the distal pole. The coracoclavicular ligaments (conoid, trapezoid) provide vertical stability to the middle and distal clavicular regions and via the coracoid, scapular suspension. Important neurovascular structures traverse the undersurface of the inner third of the clavicle, which is protected by its thicker tubular cross-section. The relationship of the clavicle to these underlying vital structures is of significance when one considers the potential impact of fracture fragments and fracture callus in acute and chronic injuries. Under such circumstances, the costoclavicular space between the first rib and clavicle may be violated, resulting in neurovascular impairment.[46-48]

The clavicle may be fractured by forces applied indirectly through the outstretched upper extremity or by forced inward rotation of the shoulder. Directly applied force may be responsible for most fractures occurring at either the medial or lateral end. Conflicting data exist regarding the influence of gender, mechanism, and age on fracture pattern. The concept that zone-specific anatomic sites have different mechanisms of injuries is not universally accepted. Clinical observations and biomechanical studies suggest a fall directly onto the shoulder as the most likely mechanism of all fractures.[49] The energy of injury is responsible for the amount of displacement, comminution, and injury to surrounding and underlying soft tissues.

CLINICAL FEATURES

Clinical assessment begins with an adequate history, which details the mechanism of injury and ascertains the presence or absence of additional regional or remote trauma. Energy applied to the shoulder girdle sufficient to fracture the clavicle may result in coexistent injury to the head and cervical regions. The patient typically cradles the arm on the side of fracture at the side of the body and is reluctant to move it owing to discomfort. Observation for deformity, open wounds, and potential impending compromise to overlying skin is performed. The head is typically positioned in a manner to relieve tension on attached musculature contributing to deformity.

With fractures involving the middle third of the clavicle, the weight of limb displaces the lateral fragment inferiorly and the upward pull of sternocleidomastoid and trapezius muscles displaces the medial fragment superiorly. In more distal fracture variants, the coracoclavicular ligaments, if compromised, may not be able to restrain the medial fragment from superior displacement. In general, fracture comminution, location, and associated ligamentous injury dictate the resultant deformity.

Further clinical evaluation must establish the patency of the subclavian vessels.[50, 51] The presence of an asymmetric pulse, bruit, or pulsatile hematoma warrants further vascular assessment. Auscultation of the chest to exclude apical lung injury is recommended, as is detailed neurological examination to identify any existing deficits that imply brachial plexopathy.[52]

INVESTIGATIONS

Radiographic assessment of clavicle fractures is initiated with a conventional AP view to establish the zone of fracture, degree of comminution, and displacement. This view should adequately visualize the proximal humerus and upper lung fields. Injuries of the lateral third of the clavicle are better appreciated on a modified AP projection with 15 degrees of cephalad tilt and reduced penetration (modified Zanca's view). For such fracture patterns, an axillary view delineates displacement in the AP plane. Further cephalad tilt better visualizes both middle- and medial-third injuries otherwise obscured by superimposition of overlying ribs and vertebra.[53]

Stress views with application of weights to the wrist may identify unstable interligamentous injuries. In the presence of comminution, a contralateral comparison view is encouraged to define the presence of appreciable clavicular shortening. Articular fractures involving either the medial or lateral clavicular pole are evaluated with computed tomography. If vascular compromise is suspected, arteriography or venography should be performed. The presence of a first rib fracture implies high-energy injury within the costoclavicular space, and a heightened level of suspicion for such an injury should be maintained.

Most classification schemes are derived from the fracture's location and its role in intrinsic stability. Distinct subgroups exist that differ in presentation and clinical behavior. Allman[54] classified fractures of the clavicle into three categories. Group 1 fractures occur within the middle third and are the most common site of occurrence (80%), representing a region unsupported by ligaments. The majority of these fractures occur medial to the coracoclavicular ligaments. Group 2 fractures account for 10% of all clavicle fractures, occur within the distal third, and are often the result of direct trauma to the region. Group 3 fractures are relatively uncommon (5%), involving the medial end of clavicle. These are often nondisplaced provided the costoclavicular ligament complex remains intact.

In the Neer[55, 56] classification, type 1 distal fractures of the clavicle remain lateral to the intact coracoclavicular ligaments. Because ligamentous attachment remains with the medial fragment no appreciable displacement results. Appreciating the therapeutic challenges inherent to type 2 lesions, Neer subclassified them according to location with respect to the attachment and integrity of the coracoclavicular ligaments. In type 2 distal patterns, the fracture occurs medial to (type 2A) or between (type 2B) the coracoclavicular ligaments. In type 2A lesions, both conoid and trapezoid ligaments maintain attachment to the distal fragment only. Stability of the medial fragment is lost, and displacement is accentuated by the weight of the limb. Type 2B patterns are interligamentous, and the medial fragment is rendered unstable if the attached conoid ligament is disrupted. Type 3 distal clavicular fractures are stable and involve the articular surface of the distal clavicle. If initially unrecognized, they are often incorrectly assigned a diagnosis of "acromioclavicular sprain." Symptomatic manifestations in the form of arthrosis may present in delayed fashion.

GOALS, INDICATIONS, AND CONTRAINDICATIONS
Goals
The clavicle, as described previously, serves many purposes. Treatment goals should be directed toward uncompromised restoration of this important component of the shoulder girdle. The "personality" of both the fracture and the patient must be considered. Immediate concerns involve the status of overlying soft tissues and underlying neurovascular structures. Long-term concerns to be addressed in the early phases of treatment include necessary efforts to achieve painless union while preserving function.

Indications
Most clavicle fractures can be successfully managed with simple support of the shoulder in a sling, with the expectation of painless uncompromised function. Residual deformity and limited shortening are unlikely to impair shoulder performance. Controversy exists regarding the limits of acceptable displacement, because studies have reported conflicting results.[57-59] Several hundred methods of closed treatment have been described, attesting to the absence of universally accepted indications and methods of treatment. These methods either simply support the shoulder to control comfort or attempt to reposition the fracture and maintain alignment. Reduction, when achieved with closed efforts, is hard to sustain because the clavicle is difficult to immobilize and has numerous forces acting directly and indirectly upon it.

Indications for surgical treatment include the presence of neurovascular deficit, compromise of skin integrity in the form of open fracture or impending necrosis due to fracture displacement, and lesions in polytraumatized individuals (surgical treatment would facilitate mobilization). Severe displacement with soft-tissue interposition and fracture instability are relative indications for fixation. Forequarter instability or suspensory injuries of the glenoid are most predictably managed with osteosynthesis. Displaced type 2 (distal) lesions represent a relative indication, because some studies suggest a favorable outcome with conservative treatment.[60, 61]

Contraindications
The few relative and even fewer absolute indications for operative treatment have been described. Surgical management for cosmetic reasons alone is seldom justified. The "unobjectionable bump" associated with successful closed treatment is better tolerated than the potential complications associated with surgical management. In general, a risk-benefit analysis for most fracture patterns in most patients favors conservative treatment.

PROCEDURES
A variety of implants and fixation constructs may be considered for fixation of clavicle fractures. Depending on fracture location and morphology, plates may be easily contoured to meet the wide range of clavicle fractures and the bone's complex shape.[62, 63] Disadvantages include osteoporosis induced by stress shielding and subsequent refracture upon extraction of the plates. Intramedullary devices, despite achieving poor rotational control, have met with considerable clinical success. The absence of a distinct intramedullary canal throughout the course of the clavicle makes application of such techniques difficult. Ease of implant extraction, diminished stress shielding, and limited soft-tissue stripping with insertion are distinct advantages. Disadvantages associated with intramedullary fixation include the potential for implant failure and migration.

Fractures of the middle third of the clavicle are preferentially treated closed. Reports suggest no long-term difference between sling, figure-of-eight, and other commercially available or fabricated device application methods.[64] Despite the deformity, results of conservatively treated middle-third fractures are very satisfying from a functional standpoint.[65] Shortening in excess of 1 cm, according to some investigators, may result in functional sequelae.[57] Type 3 medial-third fractures are usually minimally displaced or nondisplaced and, in the absence of neurovascular deficit, are treated symptomatically with sling application only.

Type 2 distal fractures are often unstable owing to detachment of coracoclavicular ligaments from the medial fragment. If significantly displaced, such fractures are managed with operative stabilization (Fig. 6). Very distal fractures may not be amenable to plate fixation because of the small size of the distal fragment. Modified plates, transacromial fixation, anchorage of the medial fragment to the coracoid, or a combination of these techniques may be

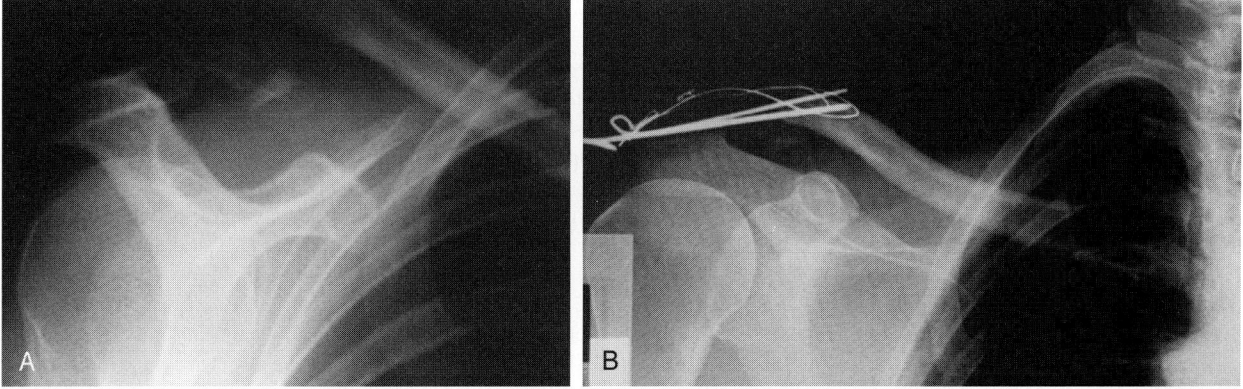

Fig. 6. Views. *A,* A 55-year-old woman sustained a comminuted type 2 fracture of the distal clavicle in a motor vehicle accident. *B,* Fixation was achieved with the use of two transacromial Kirschner wires exiting through the thick dorsal cortex of the medial fragment in combination with a tension band wire. (From Browner BE, Jupiter JB, Levine AM, et al: Skeletal Trauma. Philadelphia, WB Saunders, 1998, 2nd ed, vol 2, p 1684.)

required.[60, 66, 67] Neer,[56] observing a propensity for nonunion and unpredictable outcome for conservative management, encouraged operative stabilization for this distal clavicle fracture subtype.

Type 3 distal clavicle fractures are likely stable and nondisplaced and are often initially unrecognized. They are commonly identified late, manifesting with painful degenerative changes to the distal clavicular articular surface. If symptoms warrant, treatment in the form of distal clavicular resection with preservation of coracoclavicular ligaments is appropriate.

COMPLICATIONS AND RESULTS
Complications
Complications of clavicle fractures may arise when clavicular function or regional anatomy is compromised. The impact of clavicle fracture malunion on shoulder function is incompletely understood. Most malunited fractures are asymptomatic. Significant shortening of the clavicle may impair its kinematic function, resulting in impaired shoulder performance. For patients with functional or neurological impairment, corrective osteotomy may be considered.

Significant injury, fracture displacement, and soft-tissue stripping and interposition may contribute to nonunion. Failure to unite after operative treatment is often secondary to technical inadequacy or to the selection of high-risk displaced fractures for operative intervention. Distal-third fractures constitute only 10% of all clavicle fractures yet represent as much as 50% of all nonunions occurring after closed treatment. Interligamentous type 2 fractures are more prone to nonunion as a result of instability associated with detachment of ligaments from the medial fragment.

Symptoms of nonunion include discomfort, impaired strength and motion, and neurovascular disturbance. In patients with shoulder pain and radiographically confirmed nonunion, the exact source of discomfort must be ascertained, because the nonunion may prove to be an asymptomatic incidental finding. Coexistent sources of pain must be considered, including neurovascular compression and arthrosis.

Operative treatment methods of managing nonunion include intramedullary transacromial fixation, tension band constructs, plates of various design, and coracoclavicular stabilization with screws or slings. Although successful intramedullary techniques have been described, plate fixation may be preferable owing to complex and deformed anatomy.[68–70] An AP radiograph of the contralateral shoulder should be taken to aid in identification of clavicular shortening and the potential need for intercalary bone grafting. Asymptomatic nonunions require no treatment.

Exuberant callus and residual fracture deformity may result in neurological and circulatory disturbance by narrowing the thoracic outlet, thereby compressing the subjacent brachial plexus and subclavian vessels. Depending on the fracture's mechanism and location, injury to the underlying brachial plexus may range from trunk to cord level involvement. It is necessary to clarify the type and mechanism of neurological involvement, because decompression will unlikely remedy traction injuries. Treatment methods for addressing compressive neuropathy include corrective osteotomy and excision of callus or the first rib.[71]

Muscular atrophy of the trapezius or compromise of its attachment may lead to ptosis of the scapula, resulting in neurovascular compression in the absence of clavicular deformity. Patients may present with neurogenic complaints of paresthesia in the neck, shoulder, and ulnar aspect of the forearm and hand, all indicative of a lower trunk lesion of the brachial plexus. A postural reeducation program emphasizing trapezius muscle strengthening may remedy this problem.

Vascular insult may occur acutely or chronically when the configuration of the thoracic outlet is altered. Middle-third fractures may distort the normal anterior convexity of the medial clavicle, resulting in vascular penetration or occlusion. An arteriogram is recommended if asymmetric pulse, pallor, bruit, or a pulsatile hematoma is appreciated. Delayed vascular compromise may manifest as subclavian vein or artery thrombosis and aneurysm formation.

Post-traumatic arthritis may involve either the medial or lateral pole of the clavicle and, accordingly, the sternoclavicular or acromioclavicular joint. This problem is most commonly identified after unrecognized type 3 distal fractures. Computed tomography, bone scanning, and selective injection therapies serve to establish articular sources of pain. Treatment includes activity modification, medicinal agents, injection therapy, and surgical excision of the involved pole with preservation of stability to the resected pole.

RESULTS

The majority of clavicle fractures heal uneventfully. A favorable outcome is more likely ensured if clavicular length is maintained and stability and articular surfaces of both poles are preserved.

Minimally displaced middle-third fractures respond well to closed treatment.[65] Neer[72] reported that less than 1% of such fractures fail to unite. Conversely, a nonunion rate of 22% to 30% was observed for type 2 distal-third fractures that were treated nonoperatively.[56] Factors influencing union include fracture stability, degree of displacement, and soft-tissue stripping and interposition. Approximately 75% of patients with nonunion of the clavicle experience symptoms requiring operative intervention.

SCAPULAR FRACTURES

Shoulder mobility depends on efficient synchronous movement of glenohumeral and scapulothoracic articulations. The scapula offers continuity between the axial skeleton and the upper extremity. In combination with the clavicle, it serves to maximize shoulder motion while offering a foundation for the upper extremity. Injury mechanisms resulting in fracture of the scapula are of high energy and are often responsible for coexistent limb- and life-threatening lesions. The majority of scapular fractures are nondisplaced or minimally displaced and are effectively treated nonoperatively. Significant residual displacement may have very serious functional consequences. Fractures of the scapula can result in considerable morbidity if undetected or improperly managed. Guidelines for treatment continue to evolve, but none is based on controlled studies.

HISTORY AND EPIDEMIOLOGY

Fractures of the scapula are uncommon, accounting for 3% to 5% of shoulder girdle injuries and less than 1% of all fractures. Approximately 90% of patients sustain additional associated injury owing to the considerable violence responsible for generating these fractures. Scapular fractures are often recognized late, being obscured on chest radiographs by the overlying thorax or clinically by more immediate life- or limb-threatening injuries. The distribution of fractures involving the scapula is as follows: fractures of body and spine, 50% of total; fractures of neck, 25%; fractures of glenoid cavity, 10%; fractures of the acromial and coracoid processes, 7% each. One of the earliest descriptions of scapular fractures was published in 1805 by Desault, who described a method of reduction and an immobilization device for managing them. Since that time, nonoperative treatment methods have been advocated and surgical indications have been better defined.[73–76] Classification schemes, surgical approaches, and methods of fixation continue to be developed, yielding predictable and desirable outcomes.

PATHOANATOMY AND PATHOGENESIS

The scapula is invested in multiple muscular layers that convey mobility and offer protection. It is stabilized to the thorax ventrally by the sternoclavicular joint and dorsally by muscular contributions of the serratus and the major and minor rhomboid muscles. The subscapularis and serratus anterior envelop the scapula anteriorly, and the posterior surface is covered by the infraspinatus, supraspinatus, and trapezius muscles. The levator scapulae and rhomboid muscles insert on its medial border; the teres minor and major originate on its lateral border. From the coracoid, the pectoralis minor and the short head of the biceps as well as the coracobrachialis attach. The triceps and long head of the biceps take origin from the inferior and superior glenoid, respectively. The suprascapular notch, located medial to the coracoid, is covered superiorly by the transverse scapular ligament. The suprascapular artery traverses above this ligament; within the notch is the suprascapular nerve. Neurovascular injury can accordingly accompany fractures involving of the notch region. The scapular spine, located posteriorly, continues laterally to form the acromion, from which the deltoid takes origin.

The scapula is irregularly shaped, offering several articulating surfaces (acromioclavicular, glenohumeral, and scapulothoracic). The bursa-lined scapulothoracic interface contributes to scapular and, hence, upper extremity motion and function. Two-thirds of all overhead motion is achieved through the glenohumeral joint, which may experience joint reaction forces in excess of 90% body weight. Joint incongruity may accordingly have a very negative impact on shoulder performance. If these articulations in isolation or combination are traumatically distorted, shoulder function, which depends on simultaneous harmonious interaction of humeral and scapular motions, may be compromised.

In addition to anchoring the forequarter to the thorax, the scapula serves to suspend the upper extremity. Instability of this suspensory linkage can significantly affect upper extremity function. Goss[77] described the superior shoulder suspensory complex (SSC) as a bony/soft-tissue ring at the end of superior and inferior bony struts. Constituents of the ring are the glenoid process, coracoid process, coracoclavicular ligaments, distal clavicle, acromioclavicular joint, and acromial process. The superior strut is defined by the middle clavicle and the inferior strut by the lateral scapular body/spine. Injury to a single component is common but often of minimal consequence. Failure of the ring in two or more places ("double disruption") may yield a potentially unstable anatomic situation. Various combinations of ring and strut injuries have been described.

Scapular fractures are infrequent owing to the protection of the thoracic cavity anteriorly, the thick muscular envelope posteriorly, and its inherent mobility, which allows dissipation of forces. Indirect injuries sustained by axial or torsional loading of the outstretched arm may result in glenoid articular and neck fractures. Direct mechanisms (fall, blow) frequently cause injury to the scapular body and processes (acromion, coracoid). Traction injuries may also occur, imparted by the numerous attached ligaments and muscles.

Fractures of the glenoid rim occur as a result of laterally applied force of high energy that impacts the humeral head against the margin of the glenoid. Glenoid fossa fractures result when a laterally applied force impacts the humeral articular surface directly within the central portion of the glenoid. Fracture orientation is often transverse, with propagation and fracture components depending on the degree and directionality of force. Fractures of the scapular neck may occur by direct or indirect mechanisms. Significant displacement is likely in the event of high-energy mechanisms or coexistent injury to the superior support structures (clavicle, acromioclavicular joint, acromion, coracoid). The combination of a scapular neck fracture with a clavicle fracture or acromioclavicular injury, because of the weight of the upper extremity, may lead to ventral and medial-distal displacement of the glenoid. Fractures of the acromion result most often from direct trauma and occasionally from deltoid avulsion mechanisms.

CLINICAL FEATURES

Fractures of the scapula are often undetected on initial presentation, because gross deformity, ecchymosis, and soft-tissue swelling may be limited. An asymmetric "flattened" appearance may be evident if there is glenoid neck displacement or acromial fracture. The patient typically keeps the arm adducted and resists active motion. Guarding and painful inability to comfortably elevate the arm may be misinterpreted as a rotator cuff tear. Pain with inspiration is commonly a result of associated rib fractures or co-contraction of periscapular respiratory muscles. Owing to the significant level of energy required to generate these fractures, other coexistent injuries must be identified, some of which may prove threatening to life and limb.[78, 79] Of patients with scapular fractures, 98% have associated injuries (approximately 3.9 in total). Auscultation of the chest and review of initial and follow-up chest radiographs should be performed to exclude pneumothorax. Rib fractures and pulmonary contusion are not uncommon associated injuries. Intracranial, cervical, and upper extremity neurovascular lesions must be recognized and appropriately managed.

INVESTIGATIONS

Scapular fractures are often identified incidentally on chest radiographs, frequently in polytraumatized individuals. If such a fracture is suspected clinically or radiographically, true scapular AP, lateral and axillary views ("trauma series") are obtained. This initiates radiographic survey and fracture classification. Systematically, the scapular body and spine, scapular processes (acromial, coracoid, and glenoid), and the articulations (scapulothoracic, glenohumeral, and acromioclavicular) are assessed. Fracture patterns may involve these components in isolation or combination.

An AP view with the arm abducted, if tolerated by the patient, allows visualization of the lateral scapular border and scapular neck. If a displaced scapular neck fracture is identified, radiographic scrutiny of superior support structures (clavicle, acromioclavicular joint, acromion, and coracoid processes) should be performed. Fractures involving the suprascapular notch may herald injury to the suprascapular nerve. With proper positioning of the beam and patient, a true glenohumeral AP view ("Grashey" projection) enables inspection of intra-articular fracture variants. A scapular lateral view serves to identify displaced fractures of the scapular body, coracoid, and acromion.

To further facilitate inspection of glenoid rim, acromial, and coracoid fractures, an axillary view is obtained. It reveals any articular incongruity or rim displacement and any resultant joint instability. "Os acromiale," best visualized on an axillary projection, is the result of failure of adjacent ossification centers to unite. Smooth margins and uniform

space suggest the presence of such a condition rather than a fracture of the acromion. Although occasionally symptomatic, os acromiale may be misinterpreted as a fracture. A prone axillary (West Point) view is performed to identify anterior inferior glenoid avulsion ("bony Bankart") lesions.

Surrounding thoracic structures and the complex osseous anatomy may compromise visualization of the scapula. Other imaging modalities, most often in the form of computed tomography with reformatted images, further and more accurately delineate the extent of injury (Fig. 7). Analysis in this manner serves to quantify fragment size as well as translational and angular displacement, particularly in glenoid cavity and scapular neck fractures.

Several scapular fracture classification schemes exist, most of which are based on anatomic location. Six scapular zones are commonly described:

- Glenoid.
- Scapular neck.
- Scapular body.
- Scapular spine.
- Coracoid.
- Acromion.

Ada and Miller[80] proposed such a classification of scapular fractures on the basis of 113 observed fractures. Type 1 fractures involve the acromion or coracoid; type 2 involve the scapular neck; type 3 are intra-articular glenoid fractures; and type 4 are scapular body fractures. Type IA involves the acromion, type B the base of the acromion or spine, and type C the coracoid. Individual scapular fracture components have been further subclassified to enable more efficient cataloguing of injuries and determination of preferential treatment and prognosis.

Scapular neck fractures are described according to degree and directionality (translational or angulatory) of displacement.[81] This fracture pattern, which does not involve the joint, extends from the suprascapular notch region to the lateral scapular border. Displacement of the neck is often limited in the presence of an intact clavicle and acromioclavicular joint. When combined with displaced fractures of the clavicle and acromioclavicular joint disruption, a functional imbalance often exists.

Ideberg,[82] in 1987, described 200 intra-articular glenoid fractures and offered a classification scheme. The scheme was elaborated upon by Goss,[83] who described nine variants based on fracture locations and combinations. In this scheme of glenoid "cavity" fractures, distinction is made between "fossa" and "rim" fractures as well as proximity and integrity of remaining scapular elements.

Five types of acromial fractures have been identified and classified into three groups.[84] These fractures are not to be confused with os acromiale, which is found in 3% of the population and is bilateral in 62% of cases. Type 1A acromial fractures are avulsion lesions resulting from indirect mechanisms involving muscle (deltoid) contraction. Type 1B injuries are true undisplaced fractures, characterized by direct injury mechanisms resulting in no displacement and no compromise of the subacromial space. Type 2 patterns are displaced without subacromial encroachment. Type 3 fractures result in subacromial space compromise as a result of inferior displacement of the acromial fractures or a vertically displaced scapular neck fracture in the presence of a nondisplaced fracture of the acromion.

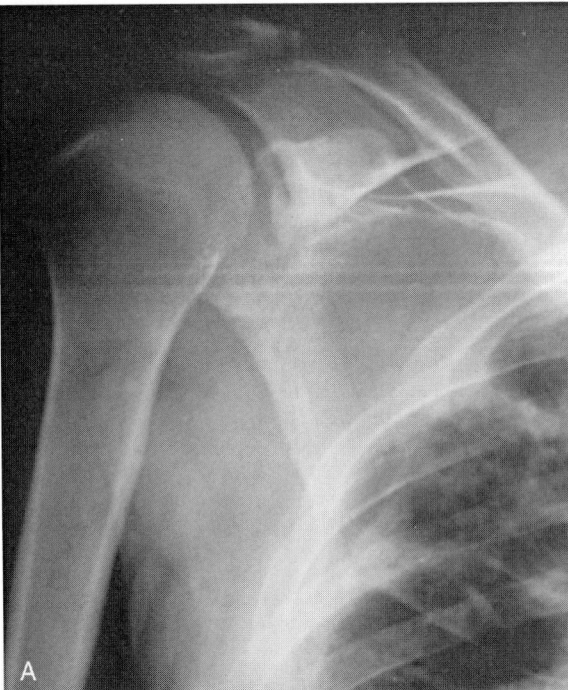

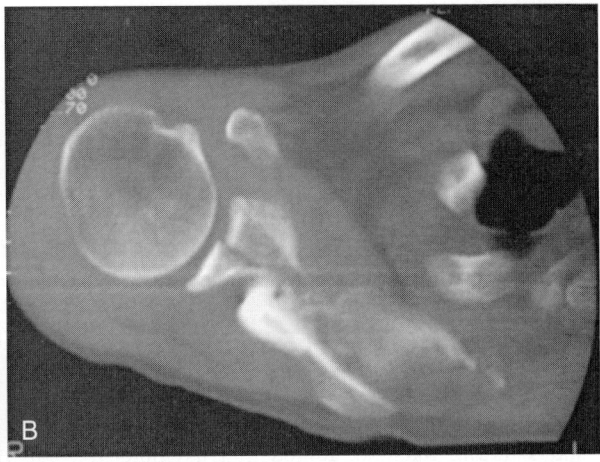

Fig. 7. Impacted glenoid fracture. *A*, AP radiograph fails to define displacement of the articular surface of the glenoid fixation. *B*, CT scan demonstrates displacement (articular step-off). (From Browner BE, Jupiter JB, Levine AM, et al: Skeletal Trauma. Philadelphia, WB Saunders, 1998, 2nd ed, vol 2, p 1660.)

GOALS, INDICATIONS, AND CONTRAINDICATIONS

Goals

The goal of treatment for scapular fractures is restoration of painless effective scapular function. The majority of lesions can be managed nonoperatively with cryotherapy techniques and short-term sling immobilization followed by controlled progressive range-of-motion exercises. Isometric and progressive resistance exercises are introduced as pain and soft-tissue swelling resolve. The goal of management of glenoid cavity lesions is the preservation of joint stability, mobility, and congruence. Treatment of scapular neck fractures should focus on sustaining the rotator cuff abduction lever arm length. In general, the maintenance of efficient scapular function as an effective interface between the upper extremity and thorax should be emphasized.

Indications

A precise algorithm of preferential treatment of scapular fractures, based on results of well-controlled studies, is lacking. The literature is insufficient to substantiate surgical indications and intervention. Most classifications offer an anatomic scheme defining fracture morphology, yet provide no or limited data supporting a plan of treatment or prognosis.

Surgical treatment is rarely indicated for scapular fracture because the majority of patients do well with nonoperative therapy. Significant displacement, however, may have unfavorable long-term consequences affecting function and, accordingly, outcome. Indications for operative treatment continue to be better defined but are based on results of uncontrolled comparisons of operative and nonoperative treatments.

No clear mandates exist for surgical treatment of scapu-

lar body fractures. Severe distortion of the scapular body may compromise the scapulothoracic articulation, resulting in painful crepitation. A relative indication for fixation includes lesions in polytraumatized individuals with pulmonary compromise, who may benefit from mobilization and freedom from external support devices. Additional indications are scapular body fractures with projection of a lateral spike within proximity of the glenohumeral joint and fractures involving the suprascapular notch that threaten the suprascapular nerve.

Scapular neck angulation may compromise range of motion and lead to glenohumeral instability. Medially displaced scapular neck fractures may result in rotator cuff dysfunction if the normal biomechanical abduction lever arm is compromised. Ada and Miller[80] observed disability in patients with displaced scapular neck fractures. Pain at rest and exertional weakness were frequently observed. On the basis of their findings, these researchers encouraged operative fixation for scapular neck fractures with (1) greater than 40 degrees of angulation in either the transverse or coronal plane or (2) more than 1 cm of medial translation. A short period of postoperative observation is encouraged, followed by serial radiography, as some lesions may adopt a more acceptable position with rest and early active motion.

Fixation of an ipsilateral clavicle fracture or acromioclavicular separation should be considered if this component of the injury directly contributes to glenoid neck fracture displacement and instability ("floating shoulder").[85–87] Double disruption injuries of the shoulder suspensory complex are managed operatively. Often, only the suspension lesion (sternoclavicular-acromial linkage) need be addressed, particularly in nonarticular injuries of the neck.

Operative fixation of glenoid rim and fossa fractures is

indicated if subluxation of the humeral head is present or if the humeral head cannot be maintained concentrically within the glenoid fossa and instability is anticipated.[88-90] Significant residual incongruity of the glenoid articular surface may result in arthrosis and motion deficit. Parameters of acceptability, as offered by DePalma,[91] are fracture displacement exceeding 10 mm and involvement of either one-fourth of the anterior or one-third of the posterior articular surface. In the clinical analysis performed by Ideberg,[82] correlation between fragment size and shape and shoulder instability could not be established. No meaningful data exist describing how much articular displacement can be accepted without significant sequelae.

The treatment of acromial fractures is based primarily on the effect of the fracture, if any, on the subacromial space. Operative treatment is reserved for type 3 lesions to allow uncompromised motion and limit impingement-related symptoms. Fractures of the coracoid occur most commonly at the base and are often minimally displaced. Significant instability and displacement may arise if acromial fracture is combined with separation of the acromioclavicular joint in the presence of intact coracoclavicular ligaments. For such injuries, reduction of the acromioclavicular joint component alone may be sufficient.

Contraindications

As mentioned, the majority of scapular fractures can and should be managed nonoperatively. Osteosynthesis of the scapula should not be performed if (1) the patient's medical status does not allow surgery or (2) the fracture and surgeon's skills would not yield the desired results. Type 6 (comminuted) fractures of the glenoid fossa are preferentially managed nonoperatively, because satisfactory reduction and fixation will not likely be achieved and because surgical access may further compromise soft tissues and accordingly jeopardize stability and union.

PROCEDURES

Surgical management of a scapular fracture demands an accurate diagnosis, appropriately selected approach, and well-executed osteosynthesis (Fig. 8). Additionally, a well-formulated and supervised postoperative program is required. The regions of substantial available bone stock include the glenoid neck, coracoid, scapular spine, and lateral scapular border. Available implants are limited to transosseous wire and sutures, interfragmentary screws, and contoured plates, which are chosen according to fracture size and location as well as operative approach.

Scapular body fractures are approached posteriorly. Numerous incisions and approaches have been described, most of which involve detachment of the deltoid from the scapular spine, exploiting the interval between the musculotendinous units of the teres minor and infraspinatus muscles.[89] This approach permits access to the scapular spine, lower lateral scapular border, and inferior portion of the glenoid.

Fractures of the scapular neck are exposed in similar fashion. The lateral scapular border serves as a reference to assess reduction as well as a source of bone of adequate quality for rigid plate fixation along the posterior glenoid. Occasionally, in the presence of shoulder suspensory complex lesions, only the suspensory element (clavicle,

acromioclavicular joint, acromion) needs to be addressed surgically. The adequacy of the indirectly reduced scapular neck component is then assessed radiographically and fixated if necessary.

Anterior rim lesions are approached anteriorly via a deltopectoral approach, and posterior lesions approached posteriorly as described previously. Fixation options include anatomic restoration with screw fixation of the rim component, or surgical excision if sufficiently small, with restoration of soft-tissue attachments to preserve stability and eliminate any resultant osseous voids. The capsular incision is preferentially lateral to the glenoid rim to avoid excessive dissection of the fragment, which may devascularize it. If the fracture is highly comminuted, articular reconstitution with tricortical grafting may be considered.

Glenoid fossa fractures, depending on location and fracture obliquity, are best visualized, reduced, and fixated through a posterior approach. Type 2 lesions are approached in this manner and fixated with interfragmentary screws directed superiorly. A contoured buttress plate is desirable inferiorly to neutralize shear stresses. Lesions involving the superior position of the glenoid may necessitate a more formal superior approach in which both the trapezius and supraspinatus are incised in line with muscular fibers.

Combined posterior and superior approaches are occasionally necessary for type 3 through 5 lesions. These variants are particularly challenging. Emphasis should be placed on articular reconstitution and restoration of superior suspension if compromised. The relationship of the remaining superomedial and inferomedial fragments is of little consequence if they are minimally displaced.

The proximity of the suprascapular nerve must be appreciated in superior or extensile posterior approaches, and the axillary nerve in both anterior and posterior approaches. Fixation of acromial fractures can be accomplished with tension band techniques or plate and screw constructs. Excision is considered only in the event of symptomatic small avulsion lesions.

COMPLICATIONS AND RESULTS
Complications

Complications of nonoperative treatment of scapular fractures depend on fracture location and the degree of comminution and displacement. Motion deficit after scapular fractures is probably the most common complication. Abduction is most often compromised, a finding observed in more subtle nonarticular injuries as well. A functional range is generally maintained, however. Residual displacement of rim fractures can result in joint instability. Joint incongruence from malreduced fossa fractures can lead to arthrosis and motion deficit.

Malreduction of scapular neck fractures, if fragments are displaced medially and inferiorly, will compromise the mechanical advantage of the rotator cuff, resulting in weakness and fatigue. Scapular body malunion may be without consequence. Painful scapulothoracic crepitation may be managed with resection of ventral surface prominences. Displaced type 3 acromial fractures, if unreduced, may result in subacromial space narrowing, generating impingement-like symptoms.

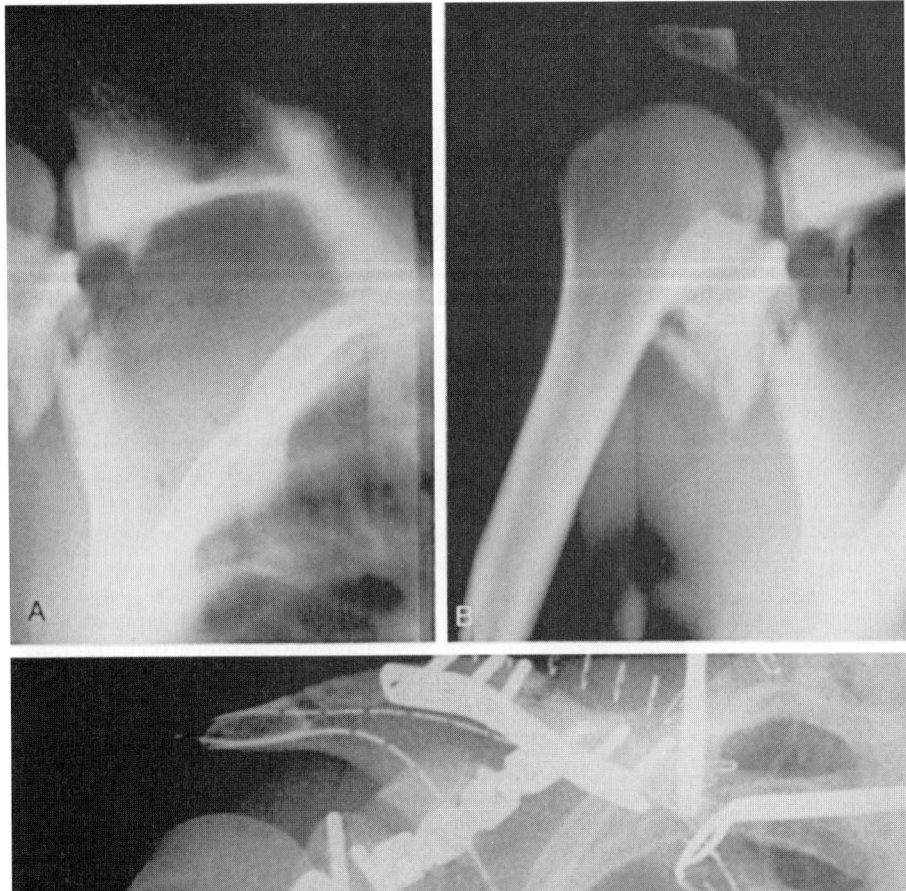

Fig. 8. Views. *A* and *B,* Anteroposterior CT scans show extension of fracture through the scapular spine (*arrow* in *B*) isolating the upper glenoid fragment and coracoid. *C,* Complex fixation was required for stabilization because of clavicle fracture and intra-articular displacement. (From Browner BE, Jupiter JB, Levine AM, et al: Skeletal Trauma. Philadelphia, WB Saunders, 1998, 2nd ed, vol 2, p 1659; courtesy of Dr. Roy Sanders.)

Results

The overwhelming majority of scapular fractures are only minimally displaced, and they respond well to supervised physical therapy and short-term immobilization. Long-term meaningful outcome studies are few, owing to the rarity of the lesion and often-delayed care. Most studies cite good results with nonarticular, minimally displaced fractures of the scapula. Operative indications continue to broaden because of the inferior results observed with conservative management of displaced articular, scapular spine, and neck injuries. Results are often determined by other associated injuries to regional osseous and soft tissues. The combination of these injuries determines the overall functional result.

SCAPULOTHORACIC INJURY

Severe injury to the scapulothoracic articulation may result in "dislocation," in which the inferior angle of the scapula is locked intrathoracically between adjacent ribs.[92, 93] More violent injury may result in "dissociation," with lateral translation of the entire shoulder girdle. This latter injury has been termed a "closed, complete traumatic forequarter amputation of the upper extremity," because it typically manifests with extensive myotendinous and neurovascular disruption.[94] Clinical awareness of this entity is essential to establishing a prompt diagnosis and restoration of vascular continuity.

Scapulothoracic dissociation results from high-energy injuries that exert traction on the upper extremity and shoulder girdle. Compromise of periscapular myotendinous structures and the sternoclavicular-acromial linkage renders the entire forequarter unstable. Complete or partial disruption of the brachial plexus and arterial injury at the subclavian level is common.

Physical examination often demonstrates a patient in cardiovascular collapse with a flail anesthetic limb. Massive soft-tissue swelling and absence of peripheral pulse are characteristic findings in the presence of scapulothoracic dissociation. A spectrum of neurological injury has been described, including cases in which no neurological deficit was identified.[95]

To further establish the diagnosis, a true nonrotated chest radiograph is obtained. Asymmetrically greater distance from the spine to the medial vertebral scapular border suggests traumatic translocation of the shoulder girdle.[96–98] Arteriography to delineate the vascular injury is encouraged. Neurological imaging (myelography, magnetic resonance imaging) and electrophysiological assessment are performed as necessary in later phases of evaluation and treatment.

Because of its infrequent occurrence, awareness of this injury is crucial. Treatment begins with resuscitative efforts, because a mortality rate of 20% has been described.[99] Vascular reconstitution with surgical exploration of the brachial plexus is performed to establish the extent and level of injury. Depending on the muscular, tendinous, and neurovascular injuries present, either early above-elbow amputation or limb salvage efforts may be elected. Shoulder immobilization to allow healing of periscapular muscles is recommended, with consideration given to stabilization of the disrupted sternoclavicular-acromial linkage.

Neurorrhaphy, forequarter stabilization, and musculotendinous transfer techniques may be considered in the later phases of treatment. A poor outcome is expected for those injuries with complete neurological impairment secondary to avulsion lesions. Incomplete and neuropraxic injury patterns have a more favorable albeit guarded prognosis.[100]

REFERENCES

Proximal Humeral Fractures

1. Lind T, Kroner K, Jensen J: The epidemiology of fractures of the proximal humerus. Arch Orthop Trauma Surg 1989; 108:285.
2. Bengner U, Johnell O, Redlund-Johnell I: Changes in incidence of fracture of the upper end of the humerus during a 30 year period: A study of 2,125 fractures. Clin Orthop 1988; (231):179.
3. Kocher T: Beitrage zur kenntnis einer praktisch wichtiger Fracturenformen. Basel, Carl Sallman Verlag, 1896.
4. Codman EA: The Shoulder: Rupture of the Supraspinatus Tendon and Other Lesions In or About the Subacromial Bursa. Boston, Thomas Todd, 1934.
5. Neer CS: Displaced proximal humeral fractures. Part 1: Classification and evaluation. J Bone Joint Surg Am 1970; 52:1077.
6. Lee CK, Hansen AR: Post-traumatic avascular necrosis of the humeral head in displaced proximal humeral fractures. J Trauma 1981; 21:788.
7. Brooks CH, Revell WJ, Heatley FW: Vascularity of the humeral head after proximal humeral fractures. J Bone Joint Surg Br 1993; 75:132.
8. Gerber C, Schneeberger AG, Vinh TS: The arterial vascularization of the humeral head: An anatomic study. J Bone Joint Surg Am 1990; 72:1486.
9. Zuckerman JD, Flugstad DL, Teitz CC, et al: Axillary artery injury as a complication of proximal humeral fractures: Two case reports and a review of the literature. Clin Orthop 1984; (189):234.
10. Neer CS: Displaced proximal humerus fractures. Part 2: Treatment of three-part and four-part displacement. J Bone Joint Surg Am 1970; 52:1090.
11. Bernstein J, Adler LM, Blank JE, et al: Evaluation of the Neer system of classification of proximal humerus fractures with computerized tomographic scans and plain radiographs. J Bone Joint Surg Am 1996; 78:1371.
12. Sidor ML, Zuckerman JD, Lyon T, et al: The Neer classification system for proximal humerus fractures: An assessment of interobserver reliability and intraobserver reproducibility. J Bone Joint Surg Am 1993; 75:1754.
13. Siebenrock KA, Gerber C: The reproducibility of classification of fractures of the proximal end of the humerus. J Bone Joint Surg Am 1993; 75:1751.
14. Mueller ME: The Comprehensive Classification of Fractures of Long Bones. Berlin, Springer-Verlag, 1990.
15. Kristiansen B, Christensen SW: Proximal humeral fractures: Late results in relation to classification and treatment. Acta Orthop Scand 1987; 58:124.
16. Keene JS, Huizenga RE, Engber WD, et al: Proximal humeral fractures: A correlation of residual deformity with long-term function. Orthopedics 1983; 6:173.
17. Darder A, Sanchis V, Gastadi E, et al: Four-part displaced proximal humerus fractures: Operative treatment using Kirschner wires and a tension band. J Orthop Trauma 1993; 7:367.
18. Koval KJ, Sanders R, Zuckerman JD, et al: Modified tension band wiring of displaced surgical neck fractures of the humerus. J Shoulder Elbow Surg 1993; 2:85.
19. Cornell CN, Levine DL, Pagnani MJ: Internal fixation of proximal humerus fractures using the screw–tension band technique. J Orthop Trauma 1994; 8:23.
20. Wheeler DL, Colville MR: Biomechanical comparison of intramedullary and percutaneous pin fixation for proximal humeral fracture fixation. J Orthop Trauma 1997; 11:363.
21. Zifko B, Poigenfurst J, Pezzei C, et al: Flexible intramedullary pins in the treatment of unstable proximal humeral fractures. Injury 1991; 22:60.
22. Jaberg H, Warner JJP, Jakob RP: Percutaneous stabilization of unstable fractures of the humerus. J Bone Joint Surg Am 1992; 74:508.
23. Resch H, Povacz P, Frolich R, et al: Percutaneous fixation of three- and four-part fractures of the proximal humerus. J Bone Joint Surg Br 1997; 79:295.
24. Hawkins RJ, Bell RH, Gurr K: The three part fracture of the proximal part of the humerus. J Bone Joint Surg Am 1986; 68:1410.
25. Esser RD: Treatment of three- and four-part fractures of the proximal humerus with a modified cloverleaf plate. J Orthop Trauma 1994; 8:15.
26. Kristiansen B, Christensen SW: Plate fixation of proximal humeral fractures. Acta Orthop Scand 1986; 57:320.
27. Sehr JR, Szabo RM: Semitubular blade plate for fixation in the proximal humerus. J Orthop Trauma 1989; 2:327.
28. Flatow EL, Cuomo F, Maday MG, et al: Open reduction and internal fixation of two-part displaced fractures of the greater tuberosity of the proximal part of the humerus. J Bone Joint Surg Am 1991; 73:1213.
29. Pritchett JW, Clark JM: Prosthetic replacement for chronic unreduced dislocations of the shoulder. Clin Orthop 1987; (216):89.
30. Cuomo F, Flatow EL, Miller SR, et al: Open reduction and internal fixation of two- and three-part displaced surgical neck fractures of the proximal humerus fractures. J Shoulder Elbow Surg 1992; 1:287.
31. Hagg O, Lundberg B: Aspects of prognostic factors in comminuted and dislocated proximal humeral fractures. In Bateman JE, Welsh RP (eds): Surgery of the Shoulder. Philadelphia, BC Decker, 1984.

32. Hawkins RJ, Switlyk P: Acute prosthetic replacement for severe fractures of the proximal humerus. Clin Orthop 1993; (289):156.

33. Neer CS: Articular replacement for the humeral head. J Bone Joint Surg Am 1955; 37:215.

34. Norris TR, Green A, McGuigan FX: Late shoulder arthroplasty for severe displaced proximal humerus fractures. J Shoulder Elbow Surg 1995; 4:271.

35. Burkhead WZ: Use of porous-coated modular prosthesis in the treatment of complex fractures of the proximal humerus. Tech Orthop 1994; 8:184.

36. Jakob RP, Miniaci A, Anson PS, et al: Four-part valgus impacted fractures of the proximal humerus. J Bone Joint Surg Br 1991; 73:295.

37. Resch H, Beck E, Bayley I: Reconstruction of the valgus-impacted humeral head fracture. J Shoulder Elbow Surg 1995; 4: 73.

38. Koval KJ, Gallagher MA, Marsicano JG, et al: Functional outcome after minimally displaced fractures of the proximal part of the humerus. J Bone Joint Surg Am 1997; 79:203.

39. Kristiansen B, Angerman P, Larsen TK: Functional results following fractures of the proximal humerus. Arch Orthop Trauma Surg 1989; 108:339.

40. Schai P, Imhoff A, Preiss S: Comminuted humeral head fractures: A multicenter analysis. J Shoulder Elbow Surg 1995; 4:319.

41. Rasmussen S, Hvass I, Dalsgaard J, et al: Displaced proximal humeral fractures: Results of conservative treatment. Injury 1992; 23:41.

42. Bigliani LU: Fractures of the proximal humerus. In Rockwood CA, Matsen FA (eds): The Shoulder. Philadelphia, WB Saunders, 1990.

Clavicle Fractures

43. Nordqvist A, Petersson C: The incidence of fractures of the clavicle. Clin Orthop 1994; (300):127.

44. Moseley HF: The clavicle: Its anatomy and function. Clin Orthop 1968; (58):17.

45. Ogden JA: Distal clavicular physeal injury. Clin Orthop 1984; (188):68.

46. Bargar WL, Marcus RE, Ittleman FP: Late thoracic outlet syndrome secondary to pseudoarthrosis of the clavicle. J Trauma 1984; 24:857.

47. Della Santa D, Narakas A, Bonnard C: Late lesions of the brachial plexus after fracture of the clavicle. Ann Hand Surg 1991; 10:531.

48. Kay SP, Eckardt JJ: Brachial plexus palsy secondary to clavicular nonunion: Case report and literature survey. Clin Orthop 1986; (206):219.

49. Stanley D, Trowbridge EA, Norris SH: The mechanism of clavicle fracture. J Bone Joint Surg Br 1988; 70:461.

50. Howard FM, Shafer SJ: Injuries to the clavicle with neurovascular complications. J Bone Joint Surg Am 1965; 47: 1335.

51. Penn I: The vascular complications of fractures of the clavicle. J Trauma 1964; 4:819.

52. Dugdale T, Fulkerson J: Pneumothorax complicating a closed fracture of the clavicle: A case report. Clin Orthop 1987; 221:212.

53. Riemer BL, Butterfield SL, Daffner RH, et al: The abduction lordotic view of the clavicle: A new technique for radiographic visualization. J Orthop Trauma 1991; 5:392.

54. Allman FL: Fractures and ligamentous injuries of the clavicle and its articulation. J Bone Joint Surg Am 1967; 49: 774.

55. Neer CS II: Fractures of the distal clavicle with detachment of the coracoclavicular ligaments in adults. J Trauma 1963; 3:99.

56. Neer CS II: Fractures of the distal third of the clavicle. Clin Orthop 1968; (58): 43.

57. Eskola A, Vainionpaa S, Myllynen P, et al: Surgery for ununited clavicular fracture. Acta Orthop Scand 1986; 57:366.

58. Faithfull DK, Lam P: Dispelling the fears of plating midclavicular fractures. J Shoulder Elbow Surg 1993; 2:314.

59. Poigenfurst J, Rappold G, Fischer W: Plating of fresh clavicular fractures: Results of 122 operations. Injury 1992; 23: 237.

60. Kona J, Bosse MJ, Staeheli JW, et al: Type 2 distal clavicle fractures: A retrospective review of surgical treatment. J Orthop Trauma 1990; 4:115.

61. Nordqvist A, Petersson C, Redlund JI: The natural course of lateral clavicle fracture: 15 (11–21) year follow-up of 110 cases. Acta Orthop Scand 1993; 64: 87.

62. Mullaji AB, Jupiter JB: Low-contact dynamic compression plating of the clavicle. Injury 1994; 25:41.

63. Schwarz N, Hocker K: Osteosynthesis of irreducible fractures of the clavicle with 2.7mm ASIF plates. J Trauma 1992; 33: 179.

64. Anderson K, Jensen P, Lauritzen J: Treatment of clavicle fractures: Figure of eight bandage vs. a simple sling. Acta Orthop Scand 1987; 57:71.

65. Nordqvist A, Petersson CJ, Redlund-Johnell I: Mid-clavicle fractures in adults: End result study after conservative treatment. J Orthop Trauma 1998; 12:572.

66. Ballmer FT, Gerber C: Coracoclavicular screw fixation for unstable fractures of the distal clavicle. J Bone Joint Surg Br 1991; 73:291.

67. Edwards DJ, Kavanagh TG, Flannery MC: Fractures of the distal clavicle: A case for fixation. Injury 1992; 23:44.

68. Boehme D, Curtis RJ, Dehaan JT, et al: Non-union of fractures of the mid-shaft of the clavicle: Treatment with a modified Hagie intramedullary pin and autogenous bone-grafting. J Bone Joint Surg Am 1991; 73:1219.

69. Capicotto PN, Heiple KG, Wilbur JH: Midshaft clavicle nonunion treated with intramedullary Steinmann pin fixation and onlay bone graft J Orthop Trauma 1994; 8:88.

70. Seiler JG, Jupiter JB: Intercalary tricorti-cal iliac bone grafts for the treatment of chronic clavicular nonunion with bony defect. J Orthop Tech 1993; 1:19.

71. Connolly JF, Dehne R: Delayed thoracic outlet syndrome from clavicular non-union: Management by morcelling. Nebr Med J 1986; 71:303.

72. Neer CS II: Nonunion of the clavicle. JAMA 1960; 172:1006.

Scapular Fractures

73. Hardegger FH, Simpson LA, Webber BG: The operative treatment of scapular fractures. J Bone Joint Surg Br 1984; 66: 725.

74. McGinnis M, Denton JR: Fractures of the scapula: A retrospective study of 40 fractures scapulae. J Trauma 1989; 29: 1488.

75. Nordqvist A, Petersson C: Fracture of the body, neck or spine of the scapula. Clin Orthop 1992; 283:139.

76. Wilbur MC, Evans EB: Fractures of the scapula and analysis of forty cases and a review of the literature. J Bone Joint Surg Am 1977; 59:358.

77. Goss TP: Double disruptions of the superior shoulder suspensory complex. J Orthop Trauma 1993; 7:99.

78. Armstrong CP, Van der Spuy J: The fractured scapula: Importance and management based on a series of 62 patients. Injury 1984; 15:324.

79. Thompson DA, Flynn TC, Miller PW, et al: The significance of scapular fractures. J Trauma 1985; 25:974.

80. Ada JR, Miller ME: Scapular fractures: Analysis of 113 cases. Clin Orthop 1991; 269:174.

81. Goss TP: Fractures of the glenoid neck. J Shoulder Elbow Surg 1994; 3:42.

82. Ideberg R: Unusual glenoid fractures: A report of 92 cases. Acta Orthop Scand 1987; 58:191.

83. Goss TP: Fractures of the glenoid cavity (current concepts review). J Bone Joint Surg Am 1992; 74:299.

84. Kuhn JE, Blasier RB, Carpenter JE: Fractures of the acromial process: A proposed classification system. J Orthop Trauma 1994; 8:6.

85. Herscovici D, Fiennes AGT, Allgower M, et al: The floating shoulder: Ipsilateral clavicle and scapular neck fractures. J Bone Joint Surg Br 1992; 74:362.

86. Leung KS, Lam TP: Open reduction and internal fixation of ipsilateral fractures of the scapular neck and clavicle. J Bone Joint Surg 1993; 75:1015.

87. Rikli D, Regazzoni P, Renner N: The unstable shoulder girdle: Early functional treatment utilizing open reduction and internal fixation. J Orthop Trauma 1995; 9: 93.

88. Aulicino PL, Reinert C, Kornberg M, et al: Displaced intra-articular glenoid fractures treated by open reduction and internal fixation. J Trauma 1986; 26:1137.

89. Goss TP: Fractures of the glenoid cavity: Operative principles and techniques. Tech Orthop 1993; 8:199.

90. Kavanagh BF, Bradway JK, Cofield RH: Open reduction and internal fixation of displaced intra-articular fractures of the

glenoid fossa. J Bone Joint Surg Am 1993; 75:479.

91. DePalma AF: Surgery of the Shoulder. Philadelphia, JB Lippincott, 1983, 3rd ed, p 366.

Scapulothoracic Injury

92. Hollinshead R, James KW: Scapulothoracic dislocation (locked scapula). J Bone Joint Surg Am 1979; 61:1102.

93. Nettrour LF, Krufky EL, Mueller RE: Locked scapula: Intrathoracic dislocation of the inferior angle: A case report. J Bone Joint Surg Am 1972; 54:413.

94. Ebraheim NA, Pearlstein SR, Savolaine ER, et al: Scapulothoracic dissociation (closed avulsion of the scapula, subclavian artery, and the brachial plexus): A newly recognized variant, a new classification, and a review of the literature and treatment options. J Orthop Trauma 1987; 1:18.

95. Lange RH, Noel SH: Traumatic lateral scapular displacement: An expanded spectrum of associated neurovascular injury. J Orthop Trauma 1993; 7:361.

96. Kelbel JM, Hardon OM, Huurman WW: Scapulothoracic dissociation: A case report. Clin Orthop 1986; 209:210.

97. Oreck SL, Burgess A, Levine A: Traumatic lateral displacement of the scapula: A radiographic sign of neurovascular disruption. J Bone Joint Surg Am 1984; 66: 758.

98. Rubenstein JD, Ebraheim NA, Kellum JF: Traumatic scapulothoracic dissociation. Radiology. 1985; 157:297.

99. Ebraheim NA, An HS, Jackson WT, et al: Scapulothoracic dissociation. J Bone Joint Surg Am 1988; 70:428.

100. Rorabeck CH: The management of the flail upper extremity in brachial plexus injuries. J Trauma 1980; 20:29.

section **3** chapter **6**

FRACTURES OF THE HUMERAL SHAFT

M. Bradford Henley and Sean Nork

Summary

- Approximately 3% of fractures treated by the orthopaedic surgeon are fractures of the humeral shaft.
- The goals of treatment include osseus union with minimal deformity to restore extremity function.
- Factors influencing treatment are associated injuries (e.g., radial nerve palsy, open fractures), osteoporosis, preexisting deformity, and overall medical comorbidities.
- Nonoperative treatment is indicated in the majority of fractures.
- Indications for operative treatment are fractures with vascular injury, floating elbow or shoulder, failure of closed treatment, open fractures, polytrauma, nonunion, and pathological fractures.
- Operative treatment options consist of open reduction and plating, flexible intramedullary (IM) nailing, locked rigid IM nailing, and external fixation.
- Special consideration is given to patients with concomitant radial nerve injury.

Fractures of the shaft of the humerus account for 1% to 3% of all fractures treated by the orthopaedic surgeon. These fractures occur in every age group, although the cause may differ with age group. Associated neurological injuries occur with these fractures. Therefore, careful history and physical examination are important. The extensive soft-tissue coverage and its abundant blood supply produce a favorable environment for fracture healing. A complex array of forces generated by the muscle attachments to the humerus combine to produce deformity and discomfort for the patient.

In most cases, nonoperative treatment leads to a successful union with an excellent functional result. However, some fractures require operative treatment. Options for surgical treatment include plate fixation, IM stabilization, and external fixation. Surgical approaches may be anterior, anterolateral, lateral, medial, or posterior. Special consideration is always given to patients with a radial nerve palsy that occurs either at the time of fracture or with closed manipulation.

HISTORICAL REVIEW

Traditionally, the treatment for fractures of the humeral shaft has consisted of upper extremity immobilization until fracture union occurs.

- In 1933, JA Caldwell developed the hanging arm cast for treatment of humeral shaft fractures.
- In 1963, Holstein and Lewis emphasized the association of radial nerve paralysis and specific distal fracture patterns.
- In 1977, A Sarmiento introduced the functional brace as the primary nonoperative treatment method and reported a union rate of 100% at an average of 8.5 weeks.
- Between 1975 and 1995, operative management with plate fixation for selected patients yielded union rates of 95% to 100%.
- During the 1990s, locked IM nailing for selected patients produced union rates of 95% to 100%.

Currently, operative treatment has gained popularity for specific indications, because it facilitates earlier functional restoration and enhances comfort.

PATHOGENESIS

The majority of fractures of the humeral shaft are the result of trauma. Most fractures either are due to a fall on the outstretched extremity or occur from low-energy mechanisms relating to athletic activities. Spiral fractures may occur from arm wrestling and pitching. More complex fractures of the shaft of the humerus are associated with higher-energy mechanisms of injury, including motor vehicle accidents, falls from heights, industrial accidents, and gunshot wounds. The cause is important, because high-energy injuries and open fractures are more commonly associated with neurological and vascular injury to the extremity. Radial nerve injury is associated with both distal fracture patterns and open fractures.[1–4] Pathological fractures occur more commonly in the older age groups. They generally result from low-energy mechanisms of injury and usually are associated with metabolic disorders or metastases.

CLINICAL FEATURES

Fractures of the humeral shaft are associated with pain, swelling, and deformity of the upper extremity. They are easily diagnosed except in the unresponsive patient with multiple injuries. The location of the fracture relative to the muscular attachments determines the subsequent deformity and displacement of the fracture fragments (Fig. 1). In fractures proximal to the pectoralis insertion, the proximal fragment is abducted and externally rotated by the rotator cuff, and the distal fragment is displaced medially by the pectoralis major. Fractures that occur between the pectoralis insertion and the deltoid insertion are characterized by adduction and medial displacement of the proximal fragment and proximal and lateral displacement of the distal fragment by the deltoid. For fractures distal to the deltoid insertion, the proximal fragment is pulled into abduction and the distal fragment shortens axially.

The importance of an accurate, well-documented physical examination must be emphasized. A careful soft-tissue and neurological examination should be performed. The radial nerve is at risk of injury because of its close proximity to the humeral diaphysis, especially in its middle and distal thirds. The examination should include both sensory (dorsal first web space) and motor examinations. Injuries of the median and ulnar nerves occur less frequently. If a

closed, manipulative reduction is performed, a second neurological and vascular examination is necessary.

INVESTIGATION

Radiographic evaluation should include two orthogonal radiographic views (anteroposterior [AP] and lateral) of the humeral shaft and adjacent joints. Imaging of the shoulder and elbow should be performed to rule out an associated injury and intra-articular fracture extension. If indicated by the physical examination, radiographic evaluation of the forearm or shoulder is required to rule out a floating elbow or floating shoulder injury complex. Electrodiagnostic studies in patients with neurological deficits are not indicated in the first 7 to 10 days. Computed tomography (CT), magnetic resonance imaging (MRI), and bone scans are unwarranted except in pathological fractures.

GOALS, INDICATIONS, AND CONTRAINDICATIONS

The goals (Table 1) of treatment for fractures of the humerus are to obtain bony union and maximize upper extremity function. Because of the large soft-tissue envelope surrounding the humerus, delayed union and nonunion are uncommon as long as the fracture fragments have not been markedly translated or distracted. Definitive management is nonoperative in the majority of cases. Minor malalignments (20 degrees of sagittal plane angulation, 30 degrees of coronal plane angulation, and 1 inch of shortening) are compensated for easily and are accepted readily.[5, 6]

Initial management is manipulative closed reduction and immobilization of the upper extremity. After reduction, and with the patient under adequate sedation or analgesia, the humerus is immobilized in the reduced position. Coaptation splints, Velpeau's dressings, hanging arm casts, and abduction braces are used commonly. With most midshaft frac-

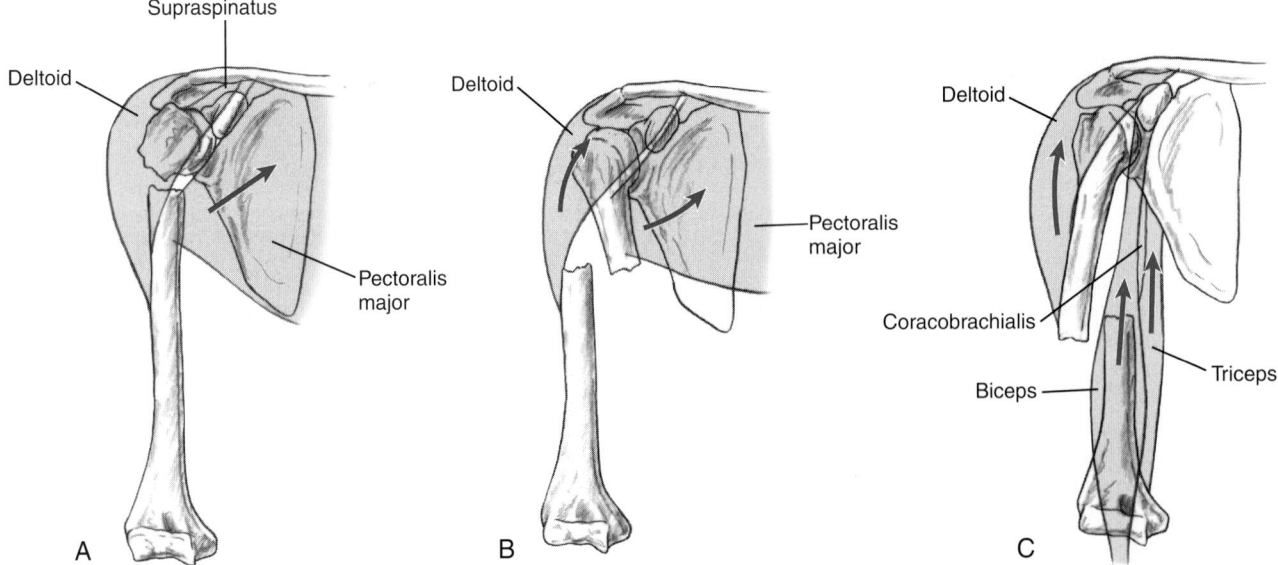

Fig. 1. View. *A,* A fracture above the insertion of the pectoralis major results in abduction and external rotation of the proximal fragment. *B,* A fracture between the insertion of the pectoralis major and the deltoid creates adduction of the proximal fragment, and the deltoid produces shortening and lateral displacement of the shaft fragment. *C,* A fracture below the deltoid insertion results in abduction of the proximal fragment. (Epps H Jr, Grant RE: Fractures of the shaft of the humerus. In Rockwood CA Jr, Green DP, Bucholz RW (eds): Rockwood and Green's Fractures in Adults, ed. 3, Philadelphia, JB Lippincott, 1991, vol 1, pp 843–869.)

TABLE 1. TREATMENT OPTIONS FOR HUMERAL SHAFT FRACTURES	
Nonoperative treatments	Hanging arm cast with avoidance of distraction
	Coaptation splint
	Velpeau's dressing
	Abduction brace
	Functional bracing
	Skeletal traction
Operative treatments	Open reduction and plating
	Antegrade and retrograde locked nailing
	Antegrade and retrograde flexible nailing
	External fixation

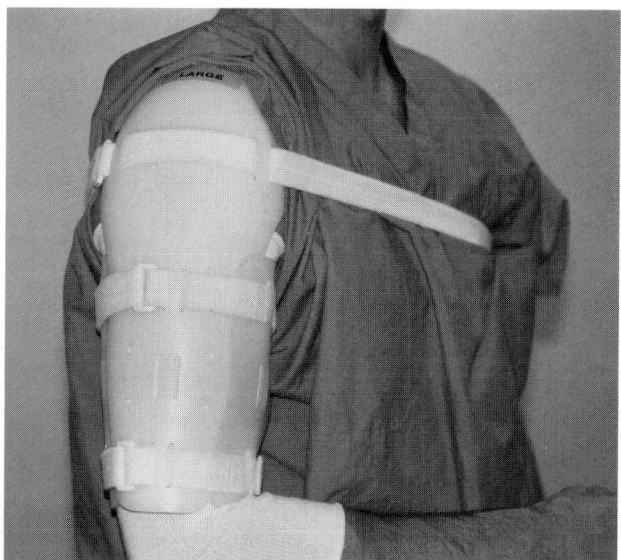

Fig. 2. Custom humeral orthosis.

tures, the arm should be splinted in neutral to a few degrees of valgus. The initial immobilization is removed after resolution of the acute pain and swelling, and a functional humeral brace is applied.[7–9] A union rate of 94% to 100% can be expected with functional bracing.[7–9]

DETAILS ABOUT CLOSED MANAGEMENT

Several alternatives exist for the closed management of humeral shaft fractures. They include hanging arm casts, coaptation splints, specialized abduction splints, Velpeau wraps, and functional bracing. Given the excellent results and patient tolerance, functional bracing is currently the treatment of choice for nonoperative management of fractures of the humerus.

The hanging arm cast was first introduced in 1933 and has been used to treat humeral shaft fractures successfully. The cast should be lightweight, and the elbow is fixed at 90 degrees of flexion. Distraction must be avoided because it has been associated with nonunion.

Hanging arm casts are contraindicated with flail extremities associated with dense brachial plexopathy or high quadriplegia. The use of this technique requires diligence and frequent adjustments to maintain fracture alignment. The location of the forearm suspension loop is adjusted to control angulation of the fracture in both the sagittal and coronal planes. One of the difficulties with the hanging arm cast is that the patient must sleep in the upright position because gravity is used to maintain fracture alignment. Frequent radiographic examination is necessary to confirm maintenance of the reduction. More commonly, the hanging arm cast is used to afford an initial reduction. After the initial pain and swelling subside, a functional brace is applied.

The coaptation splint can be applied as the initial treatment for most closed fractures of the humeral shaft. A U-shaped sugar-tong splint is applied from the axilla, around the apex of the elbow, and terminating over the middle clavicle. Use of an abduction pillow or brace may help avoid the common dependent position of varus and extension.

The functional brace, as described by Sarmiento, relies on compression of the soft tissues surrounding the fractured humerus to maintain fracture alignment. This treatment method is associated with extensive periosteal callus. The arm is initially immobilized in either a hanging arm cast, a Velpeau dressing, or a coaptation splint. Seven to 14 days after injury, and after the initial pain and swelling have subsided, the preliminary immobilization is discontin-

ued. The humeral fracture should be getting "sticky" when the fracture brace is applied. Custom-molded orthoses offer improved hydrodynamic support (Fig. 2). Early exercises (Codman's) and active range-of-motion exercises of the shoulder and elbow are encouraged. The brace is worn until fracture healing occurs, at approximately 8 to 10 weeks. Fracture healing is defined as absence of pain and motion at the fracture site with concomitant radiographic evidence of healing.

Nonoperative treatment should be abandoned in favor of operative management if (1) an acceptable closed reduction cannot be obtained or maintained, (2) the patient cannot or will not comply with nonoperative treatment, or (3) the soft-tissue injury precludes brace immobilization.

DETAILS ABOUT OPERATIVE MANAGEMENT

The indications for operative treatment of humeral shaft fractures are limited (Table 2). They are open fractures, floating elbow or shoulder, vascular injury, polytrauma, segmental fractures, intra-articular extension of the fracture, pathological fractures, radial nerve dysfunction after manipulation, transverse fracture patterns, and failure of closed treatment. The choice of implant depends on surgeon expe-

TABLE 2. RELATIVE INDICATIONS FOR OPERATIVE MANAGEMENT OF ACUTE HUMERAL SHAFT FRACTURES
Open fractures
Floating elbow or shoulder
Vascular injury
Polytrauma (e.g., bilateral humeral fractures)
Segmental fractures
Associated intra-articular extension or fracture
Pathologic fractures
Radial nerve dysfunction after manipulation
Failure of closed treatment
Spinal cord injury (high quadriplegia) or brachial plexopathy

TABLE 3. ADVANTAGES AND DISADVANTAGES OF THE TREATMENT OPTIONS FOR HUMERAL SHAFT FRACTURE		
Technique	**Advantages**	**Disadvantages**
Functional bracing	Simple. Inexpensive. Consistent union rates.	Patient compliance. Frequent follow-up evaluation.
Plating	Rapid. Radial nerve exploration possible. Avoids shoulder and elbow joints. No fluoroscopy needed. Very high union rates.	Open exposure required. Radial nerve exposure and mobilization. Additional stripping required. Poor fixation in osteoporotic bone. Large scar.
Locked intramedullary nailing	Rapid. Allows early weight-bearing. Load-sharing device. Good for osteoporotic bone.	Fluoroscopy required. Affects shoulder (antegrade) or elbow (retrograde) joint.
Bundled flexible nailing	Rapid. High union rates.	No formal locking capability.
External fixation	Rapid skeletal stabilization. Good for massive soft tissue injury.	Pin site inflammation and infection. Motion restricted by soft tissue–pin interface. Lower union rate.

rience, associated injuries, extent and location of the soft-tissue injury, fracture pattern, and location of the fracture. In general, open fractures are treated with plating, although currently, there is growing experience with locked IM nailing of open humeral fractures.

Plate fixation is the standard against which other methods of operative stabilization must be compared. It has consistently produced a predictable rate of union ranging from 95% to 100%.[10–13] The method allows for direct examination of the radial nerve and requires no fluoroscopy. It can be accomplished with the patient in virtually any position. Flexible IM nailing is a rapid and simple technique with high union rates.[14, 15] Use of bundled nails is associated with diminished rotational stability and a higher reoperation rate to achieve healing. The use of locked IM nails has been shown to be associated with a high union rate with both antegrade and retrograde entry portals.[16–19] Concern about damage to the rotator cuff is associated with antegrade nailing, but this issue has not been evaluated definitively. External fixation is reserved for complex fractures with significant soft-tissue loss or contamination (e.g., colonized burns) (Table 3).

CHOICE OF SURGICAL APPROACH

Many surgical approaches to the humeral shaft have been described for open reduction and internal fixation. They include the medial approach,[20] the anterior and anterolateral approaches, the direct lateral approach,[21, 22] and the posterior approach.[23, 24]

In the anterior approach, the humerus can be exposed from the most proximal extent with use of the deltopectoral interval, to a point approximately 5 cm from the distal articulation. It is useful for proximal- and middle-third fractures. The interval between the biceps and the brachialis is used, and the brachialis is split in line with its fibers to expose the anterior aspect of the distal humerus (Fig. 3).

The anterolateral approach can be used to expose the entire shaft of the humerus. It is useful for fractures at any

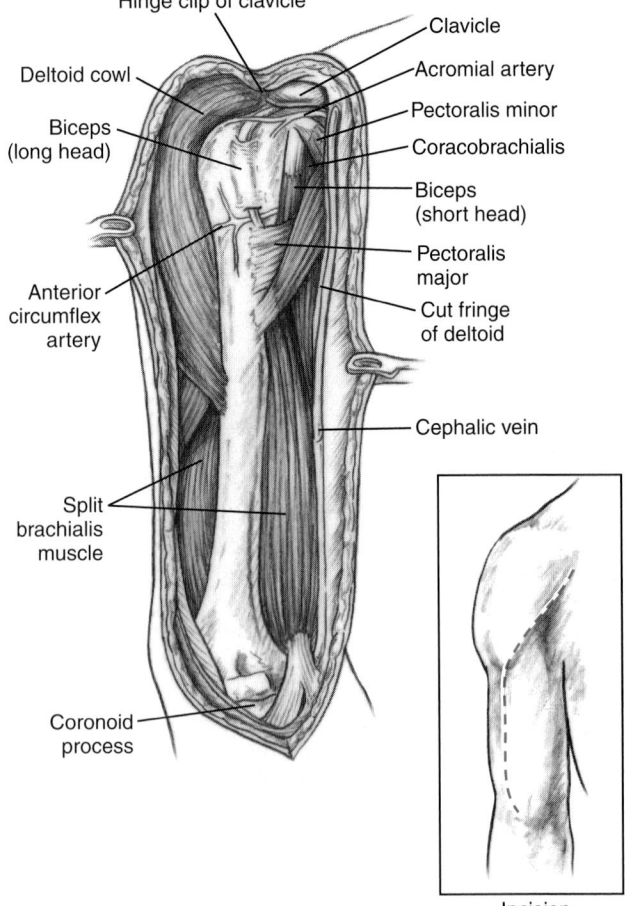

Fig. 3. Anterior approach. This demonstrates interval biceps and brachialis with splitting of brachialis muscle in line with its fibers. (Redrawn from Henry AK: Extensile Exposure. New York, Churchill Livingstone, 1973, 2nd ed, p. 36.)

Labels on figure: Hinge clip of clavicle; Clavicle; Deltoid cowl; Acromial artery; Pectoralis minor; Biceps (long head); Coracobrachialis; Biceps (short head); Pectoralis major; Cut fringe of deltoid; Anterior circumflex artery; Cephalic vein; Split brachialis muscle; Coronoid process; Incision location at the humeral shaft but generally is best for proximal- and middle-third fractures. In proximal-third fractures, the deltopectoral interval is used. Throughout the shaft of the humerus, the intermuscular interval along the lateral septum is used for exposure. The radial nerve must be identified and protected. Distally, dissection continues in the interval between the brachialis and the brachioradialis, where the radial nerve lies. The lateral antebrachial cutaneous nerve is at risk with both the anterolateral and direct lateral approaches.

The direct lateral approach can be used to expose the entire shaft of the humerus.[21] It is generally used for fractures of the middle or distal third, but more proximal fractures can be approached in this manner as well. The major advantages of the lateral exposure are supine positioning of the patient and exploration of the radial nerve along the entire exposure. Proximally, the dissection can be extended through the deltopectoral interval to approach the shoulder anteriorly. Distally, the interval between the triceps and brachioradialis can be developed (Fig. 4). This approach can be modified from the classic Kocher approach by placement of the incision more posteriorly and protection of the origin of the extensor carpi radialis longus and the extensor carpi radialis brevis.[22]

The posterior approach can be modified and extended to expose 94% of the humeral diaphysis.[23] This exposure is most useful for middle and distal fractures, especially when repair of the radial nerve is required. It can be extended proximally as well, though this maneuver is limited by the axillary nerve and accompanying posterior humeral circumflex vessels. The major disadvantages associated with this approach are the requirement for prone or lateral positioning and splitting of the medial head of the triceps (with variable denervation) (Fig. 5). The location of the radial nerve at the posterior aspect of the humerus and at the

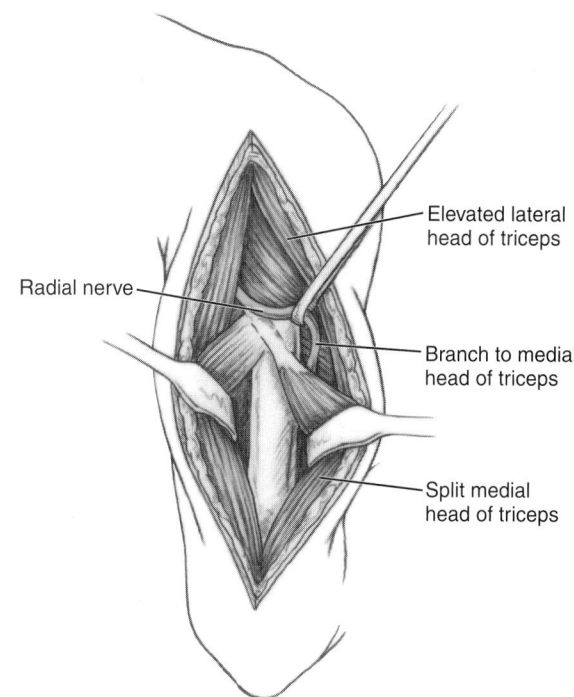

Fig. 5. Posterior triceps-splitting approach. This approach uses mobilization of the radial nerve. (Redrawn from Gerwin M, Hotchkiss RN, Weiland AJ: Alternative operative exposures of the posterior aspect of the humeral diaphysis with reference to the radial nerve. J Bone Joint Surg Am 1996; 78:1691.)

intermuscular septum has been well described.[23, 24] The radial nerve must be mobilized to allow posterior plate placement. On the average, the radial nerve pierces the intermuscular septum approximately 10 cm proximal to the lateral epicondyle and crosses the humerus approximately 13 to 17 cm proximal to the distal articular surface.

The medial approach can be used to expose the humeral shaft from the pectoralis major insertion proximally to the coronoid fossa distally.[20] The exposure produces an excellent cosmetic result and is especially useful for secondary procedure. The exposure uses the intermuscular interval between the anterior and posterior compartments. The ulnar nerve, median nerve, and brachial arteries must be identified in this approach, which is used infrequently except in the patient with a concomitant brachial artery injury.

PROCEDURES

PREOPERATIVE PLANNING

If surgical stabilization is planned, a thoughtful preoperative plan is mandatory. The condition of the patient as well as the associated injuries helps dictate the procedure. Comparison radiographs of the contralateral humerus are often helpful, especially in cases of segmental comminution. The presence of an associated intra-articular injury at the elbow or the shoulder influences the surgical decision, and the intra-articular injury should take priority. The fracture pattern, position of comminution or butterfly fragments, and location of the fracture all contribute to selection of surgical approach and implant.

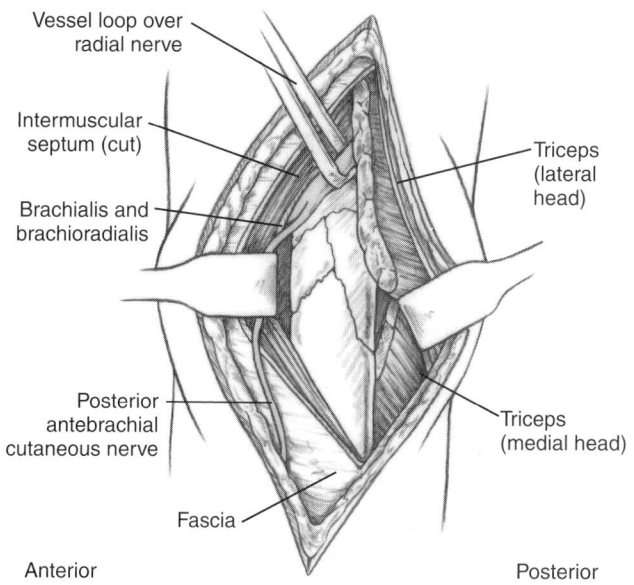

Fig. 4. Direct lateral approach. This uses the interval between triceps and lateral intermuscular septum, brachialis, and brachioradialis. (Redrawn from Mills WJ, Hanel DP, Smith DG: Lateral approach to the humeral shaft: An alternative approach for fracture treatment. J Orthop Trauma 1996; 10:84.)

If rigid IM nailing is chosen, templates should be used to estimate nail length and diameter from the uninjured limb segment. The "isthmus" of the humerus is in the distal third. In many patients, reaming is required, especially if the canal measures less than 7 mm because the smallest locking implants are 7 mm and greater in diameter. Small reamers and guide rods may be required, starting at 5.5 mm and increasing in 0.5-mm increments. Reaming should be limited to the amount needed to fit the smallest-diameter nail available.

Several biomechanical studies have evaluated the fixation strength of constructs used in the treatment of humeral fractures.[25–28] Whether greater resistance to bending or torsion is associated with more rapid healing or a lower rate of malunion remains unknown. It appears, however, that solid nails have higher rigidity in torsion compared with plates and flexible IM nails and that locked IM devices have higher torsional rigidity than unlocked devices. Additionally, plating has the highest bending rigidity, followed by solid nails.

ASSOCIATED RADIAL NERVE INJURY

The common occurrence of radial nerve injury in association with a fracture of the humerus necessitates special consideration.[1, 3, 4, 29–31] Overall, approximately 10% of humeral fractures are associated with a primary injury to the radial nerve.[1, 4, 30, 32] Of these, approximately three-quarters are expected to recover spontaneously, usually within 3 months.[1, 4, 32] Both early[31] and late[4, 29, 30] explorations of the radial nerve have been suggested. Commonly cited indications for early exploration include open fractures, secondary nerve injury (when a previously normal radial nerve loses function after a manipulative reduction), and Holstein-Lewis fracture patterns (distal third, spiral, and long obliquity). In most instances of closed fracture, delaying nerve exploration allows for spontaneous recovery of minimally damaged nerves, which is expected to occur in most cases. A study by Pollock and associates[4] found that only 8% of patients with a radial nerve palsy required exploration, and all the radial nerves recovered. In cases with persistence of radial nerve paralysis after 2 to 3 months, high rates of recovery (up to 91%) can be expected with surgical exploration and treatment. Typically, electromyography should be performed prior to exploration if no spontaneous recovery of nerve function is observed.

In the case of an open humeral fracture with an associated radial nerve palsy, early exploration is unambiguously indicated in the literature. Foster and colleagues[3] reported that in 64% of 14 patients with open humeral shaft fractures with a radial nerve palsy, the radial nerve either was lacerated or was interposed within the fracture site. Of the five patients with complete laceration of the nerve, four had full motor return after primary repair.

TECHNICAL DETAILS

ANTEGRADE NAILING

For antegrade IM nailing, the patient is positioned supine on a radiolucent table with a small rolled towel under the ipsilateral scapula. The C-arm is brought in from the side opposite to the injured extremity, with the cathode rotated 180 degrees so that it is placed under the table and patient.

The injured arm is extended slightly (e.g., 20 degrees), the elbow is flexed to 90 degrees, and the forearm is allowed to rest against the thoracoabdominal wall. This positioning places the distal humerus in approximately 50 to 70 degrees of internal rotation and generally reduces the fracture in rotation. An AP view of the shoulder and humerus can be easily obtained with the C-arm rotated back 45 to 60 degrees (Fig. 6). Similarly, with the arm in the identical position, a transcapular lateral (the "scapular Y view" with superimposed humeral head) can be obtained by rotation of the C-arm over the top of the patient by 20 to 40 degrees. In this way, orthogonal images can be obtained without manipulation of the injured arm. This allows for a perfect starting point on two standard views of the proximal humerus and shoulder.

Alternatively, the C-arm may be brought in from the same side of the table as the injured extremity. It may be positioned either perpendicular to the operating table or at the head of the table parallel to the patient's body. With any of these arrangements, however, the surgeon, assistant, and scrub nurse are crowded by the image intensifier and technician.

If a rigid nail is used, the entry site is just medial to the greater tuberosity in the sulcus seen on the AP image. For flexible nailing, the entry site used is through the lateral portion of the greater tuberosity and distal to the insertion of the rotator cuff.

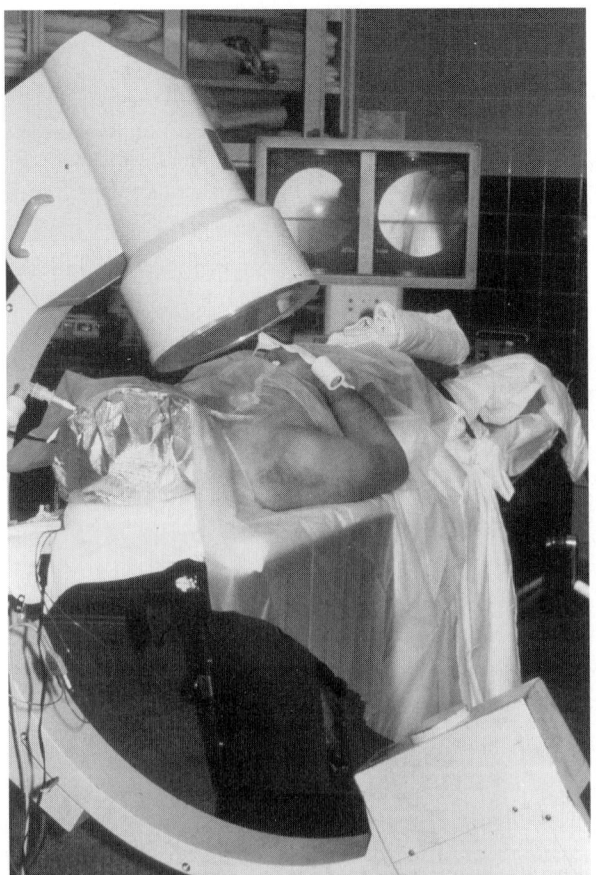

Fig. 6. Intraoperative setup. This is for an AP image of humerus with the image intensifier brought in from the opposite side of the operating table.

An incision in Langer's lines, at the lateral border of the acromion, is cosmetically preferred for the skin, although other surgeons use a skin incision that is perpendicular to Langer's lines and parallel to the fibers of the deltoid. The lateral skin flap is elevated from the deltoid muscle, The starting point for insertion of a terminally threaded Steinmann pin (or awl) is found through imaging of the proximal humerus in both the AP and lateral planes. On the lateral image, the starting point is exactly collinear with the midaxial plane of the humeral diaphysis. On the AP view, the starting point is in the sulcus, just medial to the prominence of the greater tuberosity. Once the entry point is identified, the Steinmann pin is inserted into the proximal humerus at the same angle as the proximal portion of the reamed IM nail (approximately 10 to 15 degrees) (Fig. 7).

The fibers of the deltoid are now split bluntly in line with their orientation and are elevated off of the insertion of the rotator cuff and greater tuberosity. A Gelpi retractor is used to maintain access to the cuff. The rotator cuff is incised sharply, in line with its fibers, just medial to its insertion. Two sutures are placed in each side of the cuff to facilitate retraction and later repair. The terminally threaded guide pin is overreamed with an 8-mm cannulated drill bit, and the Steinmann pin is removed. For a reamed IM nail, a bulb-tipped reaming guide wire is passed into the nail entry site, is manipulated across the fracture with fluoroscopic guidance, and impacted into the center of the distal humerus above the olecranon fossa. A second guide wire of equal length is used to measure the length of the IM portion of the first guide wire, which guides selection of the proper length IM nail.

RETROGRADE NAILING

For retrograde IM nailing, the patient is positioned laterally or prone. A radiolucent armboard is positioned so that the injured arm is abducted at 90 degrees from the body and supported by the armboard. The forearm hangs at 90 degrees over the lateral edge of the armboard. The C-arm is brought in from the head of the operating table bed so that posteroanterior (PA) and lateral views of the entire humerus can be obtained by rotation of the head of the C-arm (Fig. 8).

The entry site is just proximal to the olecranon fossa and is approached through a posterior midline, triceps muscle–splitting approach. An elliptical opening, approximately 1 × 2 cm, is created in the posterior cortex with the use of a drill and bur to gain entry to the medullary canal (Fig. 9). Rotational and axial control is afforded by filling the medullary canal with flexible nails and splaying them within the proximal humeral metaphysis and head (Fig. 10).

PLATING

The choice of the approach for plating is determined by the fracture location, pattern, and comminution (position and size) as well as comorbid conditions (e.g., thoracoabdominal trauma). In the medial, anterior, anterolateral, and direct lateral approaches, supine positioning is used. If a posterior approach is to be used, lateral or prone positioning is advantageous. In general, a 4.5-mm broad or 4.5 narrow dynamic compression plate should be used, depending on the size of the humerus. The broad plate is helpful in neutralizing torsional forces and preventing propagation

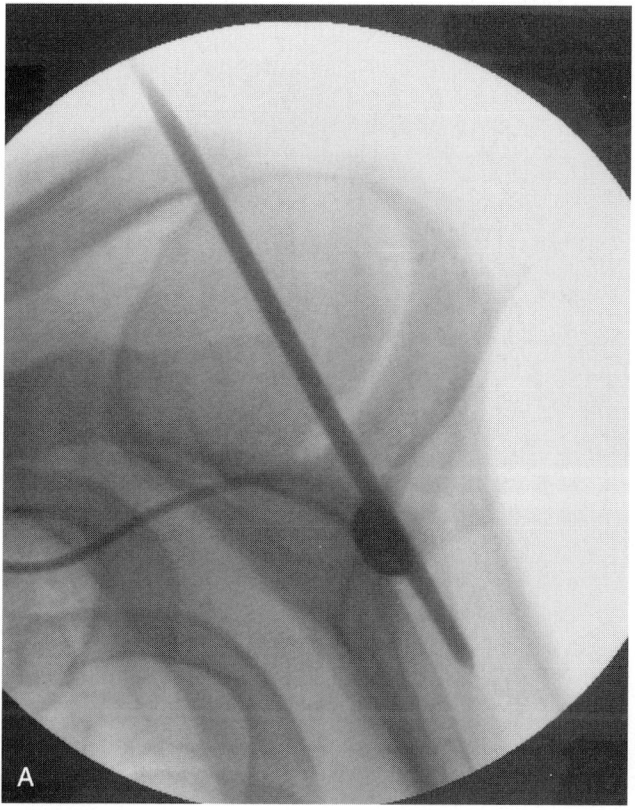 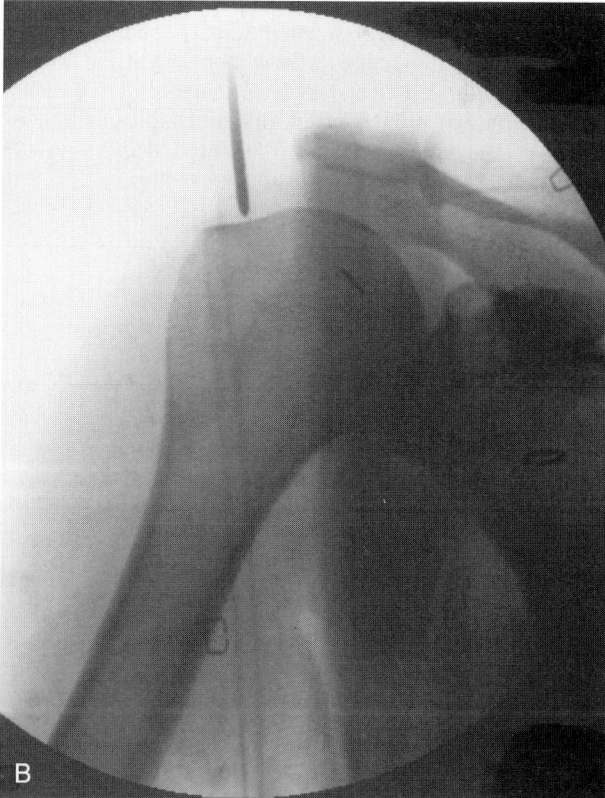

Fig. 7. View. *A*, AP image of insertion site for standard locking IM nails. *B*, Scapular-Y lateral image of the same entry point.

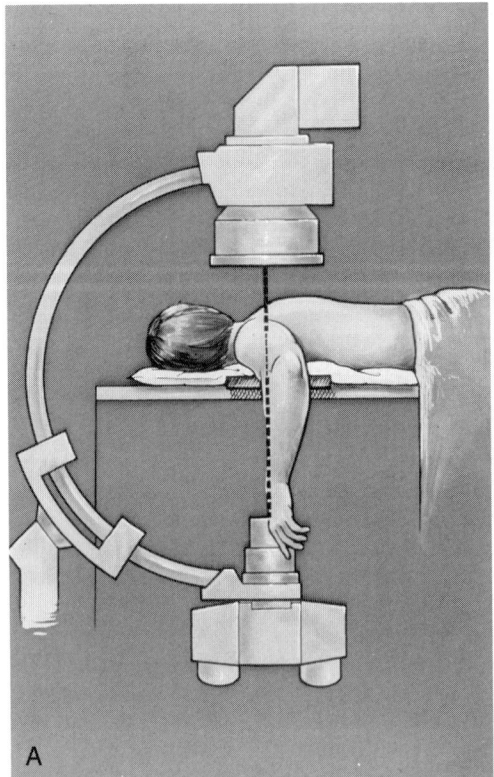

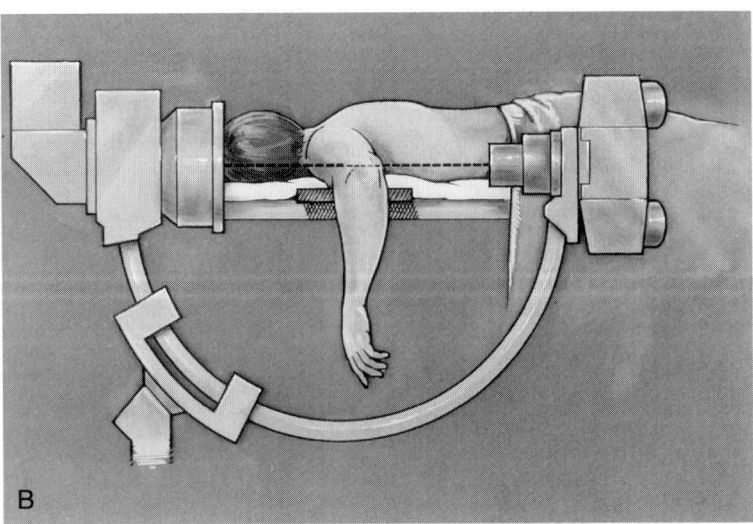

Fig. 8. View. C-arm position for PA image *(A)* and lateral image *(B)* for retrograde flexible IM nailing.

of cracks because its holes are staggered (Fig. 11). The narrow plate may be considered if the broad plate is wider than the humerus. A minimum of seven cortices above and below the fracture site is recommended.[33]

The basic principles of internal fixation should be followed for humeral fractures. They include (1) the use of extensile exposures, (2) avoidance of unnecessary soft-tissue dissection, (3) protection and identification of the neurovascular structures, especially the radial nerve, and (4) rigid internal fixation in compression.

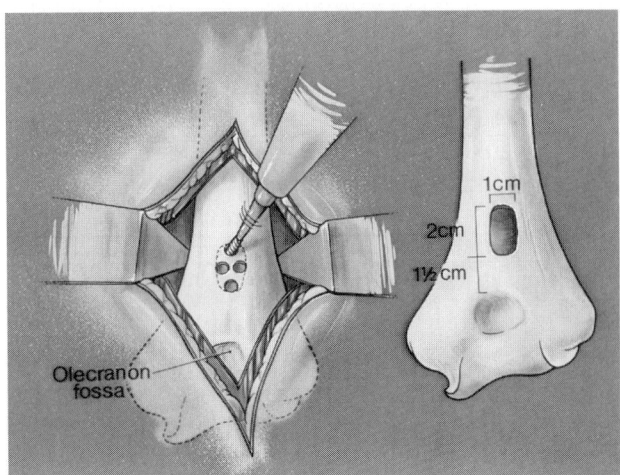

Fig. 9. View. *Left,* Initiation of cortical window with drill and bur. *Right,* Completed cortical window.

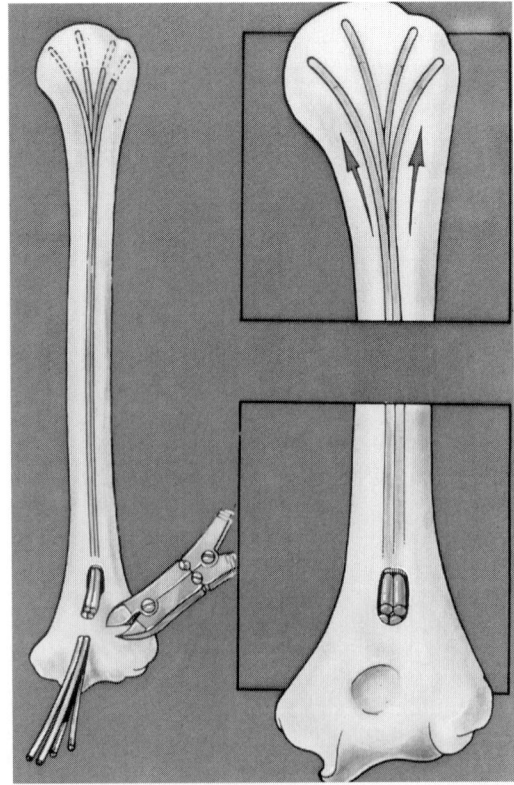

Fig. 10. View. Stabilization of humeral fracture with canal-filling flexible IM nails. Splayed distribution within the humeral head provides rotational control.

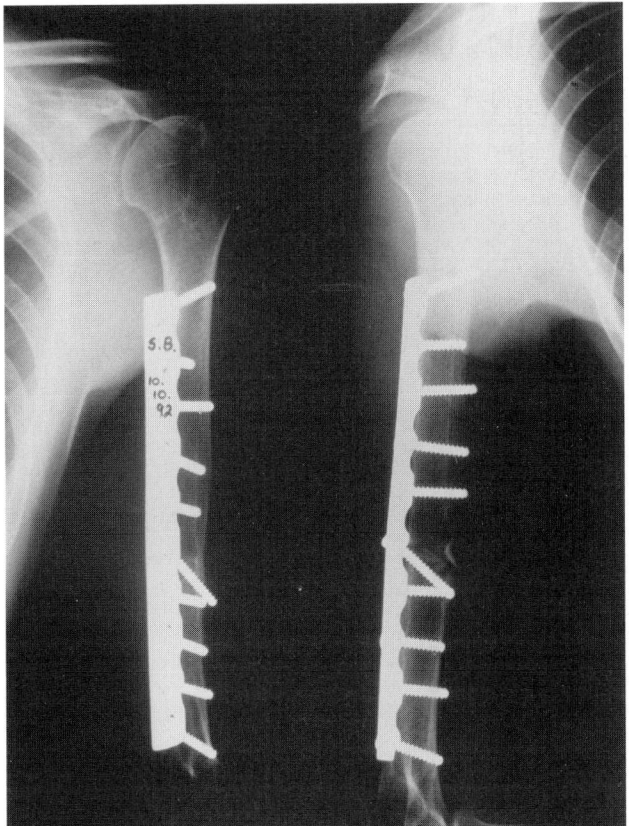

Fig. 11. AP and lateral radiographs. These are radiographs of humeral fracture stabilized by a posteriorly placed 4.5 broad dynamic compression plate.

EXTERNAL FIXATION

External fixation may be performed with the use of either unilateral half-pins or tensioned transfixion wires. Half-pins are generally placed from lateral to medial in the humerus in the proximal third (greater tuberosity and metaphysis), middle third, and distal third (lateral epicondyle and metaphysis). These sites avoid the axillary nerve at the junction of the proximal and middle thirds, and the radial nerve at the junction of the middle and distal thirds of the humerus.

Shortening of the humerus by as much as approximately 3 cm is well tolerated in most patients. In cases of radial nerve injury necessitating neurorrhaphy, the humerus may be shortened to allow for a tension-free primary repair of the nerve. Similarly, in cases of open fractures with a devitalized segment of bone or with segmental bone loss, acute shortening at the time of fixation may be considered.

POSTOPERATIVE MANAGEMENT

Regardless of the treatment modality selected, early active range-of-motion exercise of the affected extremity is expected. With closed management, the initial immobilization is removed, and a functional brace is applied as soon as the pain and swelling subside sufficiently. Early range-of-motion exercise of the shoulder and elbow is encouraged. The patient is instructed to sleep upright to ensure proper alignment of the fracture. The brace is removed after 6 to 10 weeks, when fracture healing has occurred sufficiently to prevent a change in alignment.

The postoperative management of patients who undergo surgical stabilization of an isolated humeral fracture includes early range-of-motion exercise of the shoulder and elbow. No postoperative immobilization is used for patients treated with plates, locked IM nails, or external fixation. Light strengthening exercises may begin after provisional healing, with additional resistance added as the fracture consolidates. If antegrade locked nailing is used, active range-of-motion exercise of the shoulder is delayed while the rotator cuff heals. Patients treated with bundled flexible nails may benefit from the hydrodynamic support afforded by a fracture orthosis during the initial postoperative period.

External fixation requires frequent (twice daily) pin site care with 1% hydrogen peroxide. Patients are told that they will likely have at least one pin site infection. The external fixator is removed after fracture healing (8 to 16 weeks) if status of the pin sites allows the fixator to stay in place for long enough.

COMPLICATIONS AND RESULTS

COMPLICATIONS

The most common complications associated with any form of treatment of a humeral shaft fracture are malunion, nonunion, infection, and radial nerve palsy. Malunion of the humerus is well tolerated.[5, 6] Up to 20 to 25 degrees of angulation, 15 degrees of rotation, and shortening by 2 to 3 cm do not cause any functional limitations.

Nonunion occurs in as many as 6% of closed fractures treated without surgery and 25% of fractures managed surgically. Factors associated with nonunion include segmental fractures, poorly reduced fractures, alcohol abuse, obesity, malnutrition, smoking, and inadequate plate fixation.[33, 34]

TABLE 4. COMPLICATIONS OF TREATMENTS FOR HUMERAL SHAFT FRACTURE				
Technique	Nonunion	Malunion	Infection	Implant Pain
Functional brace	Rare (0–6%)	Rare	0	0
Plate	Rare (0–5%)	Rare	Rare	Rare
Locking nail	Rare (0–5%)	Rare	Rare	Variable
Flexible nails	Rare (0–5%)	Rare	Rare	Variable
External fixation	Common (6–22%)	Variable	Common	Until removal

TABLE 5. SHORT-TERM RESULTS AND UNION RATES OF TREATMENTS FOR HUMERAL SHAFT FRACTURE			
Authors	Year	Treatment	Rate of Union (%)
Sarmiento et al	1977	Functional brace	100
Balfour et al	1982	Functional brace	98
Wallny et al	1997	Functional brace	94
Crolla et al	1993	Locked IM nail (A)	100
Ikpeme et al	1994	Locked IM nail (A)	100
Ingman et al	1994	Locked IM nail (A/R)	95
Lin et al	1997	Locked IM nail (R)	100
Stern et al	1984	Various IM devices*	88
Foster et al	1985	Kuntscher's IM nails	91
Brumback et al	1986	Various IM devices†	94
Hall et al	1987	Enders' nails	99
Rodriguez-Merchan et al	1995	Hackethal's nails	95
Bell et al	1985	Plate	97
Foster et al	1985	Plate	100
Dabezies et al	1992	Plate	97
Rodriguez-Merchan et al	1995	Plate	95
Mostafavi et al	1997	External fixation	94

* Rush's pins (52), Samson's rods (7), Kuntscher's rod (1); antegrade insertions.
† One Rush's rod (21), one Enders' nail (5), two Rush's rods (16), two Enders' nails (18), three Rush's rods (1), three Enders' nails (2); mixture of retrograde, epicondylar, and antegrade insertions.
A = antegrade insertion; IM = intramedullary; R = retrograde insertion.

Fracture union is improved in patients with polytrauma who use crutches to axially load the humeral shaft after IM nailing.[11] Nonunion is usually treated with either compression plate fixation and autogenous bone graft or reamed locked IM nailing. At least seven or eight cortices of fixation should be obtained proximal and distal to the nonunion site. Healing of nonunions is a challenge in smokers and in patients with poor nutrition or systemic disease.

Although infection is uncommon with plating and IM nailing, pin tract inflammation or infection is the rule with external fixation (Table 4). Infected nonunions require aggressive surgical débridement, with resection of all nonviable soft tissues and bone, combined with parenteral antibiotics and stable compressive fixation.

SHORT-TERM RESULTS AND OUTCOMES

The results (Table 5) of closed treatment of humeral shaft fractures with functional braces are excellent.[6–9, 35] Union rates approaching 100% are the rule. The average time to union with bracing is 7 to 9 weeks.[7, 9] Malunion is uncommon; more than 85% of patients demonstrate angulation of less than 10 degrees.[8] Wallny and associates[8] reported that 95% of their 87 patients were content with their treatment, and 80% had good functional results at a minimum follow-up of 2 years.

Compression plating is associated with similarly high rates of union, ranging from 95% to 100%.[10–13] In a prospective study by Rodriguez and colleagues, 100% of patients returned to work and 80% had good functional results after treatment with compression plating. These results were similar to those found in patients treated with Hackethal's nails in the same study.

Small flexible IM nails such as Enders' nails and Rush's rods have been associated historically with a large number of complications and secondary surgical procedures.[14] Stern and associates[14] reported complications in 67% of patients and additional operative procedures in 64% after IM fixation, primarily with Rush's pins and Samson's rods. These findings are in contrast with those of other studies,[15, 36] which demonstrate good results with flexible IM fixation. Hall and Pankovich,[36] prospectively evaluating 86 patients who had been treated with stacked Enders' nails, found rapid union and excellent range of motion at both the shoulder and elbow. Similarly, stacked Hackethal's nails have been shown to produce a high rate of union, good functional results, and few complications.

Locked IM nailing has gained popularity because of a high union rate with few complications.[16–19] Because of concern about shoulder discomfort after an antegrade nailing, however, retrograde nailing has gained popularity.[16, 17] Several studies have demonstrated good return of shoulder and elbow motion after locked nailing.[17, 19]

REFERENCES

1. Amillo S, Barrios RH, Martinez-Peric R, et al: Surgical treatment of the radial nerve lesions associated with fractures of the humerus. J Orthop Trauma 1993; 7:211.
2. Holstein A, Lewis GB: Fractures of the humerus with radial nerve paralysis. J Bone Joint Surg Am 1963; 45:1382.
3. Foster RJ, Swiontkowski MF, Bach AW, et al: Radial nerve palsy caused by open humeral shaft fractures. J Hand Surg [Am] 1993; 18:121.
4. Pollock FH, Drake D, Bovill EG, et al: Treatment of radial neuropathy associated with fractures of the humerus. J Bone Joint Surg Am 1981; 63:239.
5. Klenerman L: Fractures of the shaft of the humerus. J Bone Joint Surg Br 1966; 48:105.
6. Zagorski JB, Latta LL, Zych GA, et al: Diaphyseal fractures of the humerus: Treatment with prefabricated braces. J Bone Joint Surg Am 1988; 70:607.
7. Sarmiento A, Kinman PB, Galvin EG, et

al: Functional bracing of fractures of the shaft of the humerus. J Bone Joint Surg Am 1977; 59:596.

8. Wallny T, Westermann K, Sagebiel C, et al: Functional treatment of humeral shaft fractures: Indications and results. J Orthop Trauma 1997; 11:283.

9. Balfour GW, Mooney V, Ashby ME: Diaphyseal fractures of the humerus treated with a ready-made fracture brace. J Bone Joint Surg Am 1982; 64:11.

10. Bell MJ, Beauchamp CG, Kellam JK, et al: The results of plating humeral shaft fractures in patients with multiple injuries: The Sunnybrook experience. J Bone Joint Surg Br 1985; 67:293.

11. Foster RJ, Dixon GL Jr, Bach AW, et al: Internal fixation of fractures and non-unions of the humeral shaft: Indications and results in a multi-center study. J Bone Joint Surg Am 1985; 67:857.

12. Dabezies EJ, CJD Banta, CP Murphy, et al: Plate fixation of the humeral shaft for acute fractures, with and without radial nerve injuries. J Orthop Trauma 1992; 6:10.

13. Rodriguez-Merchan EC: Compression plating versus Hackethal nailing in closed humeral shaft fractures failing nonoperative reduction. J Orthop Trauma 1995; 9:194.

14. Stern PJ, Mattingly DA, Pomeroy DL, et al: Intramedullary fixation of humeral shaft fractures. J Bone Joint Surg Am 1984; 66:639.

15. Brumback RJ, Bosse MJ, Poka A, et al: Intramedullary stabilization of humeral shaft fractures in patients with multiple trauma. J Bone Joint Surg Am 1986; 68:960.

16. Ingman AM, Waters DA: Locked intramedullary nailing of humeral shaft fractures: Implant design, surgical technique, and clinical results. J Bone Joint Surg Br 1994; 76:23.

17. Lin J, Hou SM, Hang YS, et al: Treatment of humeral shaft fractures by retrograde locked nailing. Clin Orthop 1997; 342:147.

18. Crolla RM, de Vries LS, Clevers GJ: Locked intramedullary nailing of humeral fractures. Injury 1993; 24:403.

19. Ikpeme JO: Intramedullary interlocking nailing for humeral fractures: Experiences with the Russell-Taylor humeral nail. Injury 1994; 25:447.

20. Jupiter JB: Complex non-union of the humeral diaphysis: Treatment with a medial approach, an anterior plate, and a vascularized fibular graft [published erratum appears in J Bone Joint Surg Am 1990; 72:1270]. J Bone Joint Surg Am 1990; 72:701.

21. Mills WJ, Hanel DP, Smith DG: Lateral approach to the humeral shaft: An alternative approach for fracture treatment. J Orthop Trauma 1996; 10:81.

22. Moran MC: Modified lateral approach to the distal humerus for internal fixation. Clin Orthop 1997; 340:190.

23. Gerwin M, Hotchkiss RN, Weiland AJ: Alternative operative exposures of the posterior aspect of the humeral diaphysis with reference to the radial nerve. J Bone Joint Surg Am 1996; 78:1690.

24. Uhl RL, Larosa JM, Sibeni T, et al: Posterior approaches to the humerus: When should you worry about the radial nerve? J Orthop Trauma 1996; 10:338.

25. Henley MB, Monroe M, Tencer AF: Biomechanical comparison of methods of fixation of a midshaft osteotomy of the humerus. J Orthop Trauma 1991; 5:14.

26. Dalton JE, Salkeld SL, Satterwhite YE, et al: A biomechanical comparison of intramedullary nailing systems for the humerus. J Orthop Trauma 1993; 7:367.

27. Zimmerman MC, Waite AM, Deehan M, et al: A biomechanical analysis of four humeral fracture fixation systems. J Orthop Trauma 1994; 8:233.

28. Schopfer A, Hearn TC, Malisano L, et al: Comparison of torsional strength of humeral intramedullary nailing: A cadaveric study. J Orthop Trauma 1994; 8:414.

29. Sonneveld GJ, Patka P, van Mourik JC, et al: Treatment of fractures of the shaft of the humerus accompanied by paralysis of the radial nerve. Injury 1987; 18:404.

30. Samardzic, M, Grujicic D, Milinkovic ZB: Radial nerve lesions associated with fractures of the humeral shaft. Injury 1990; 21:220.

31. Postacchini F, Morace GB: Fractures of the humerus associated with paralysis of the radial nerve. Ital J Orthop Traumatol 1988; 14:455.

32. Mast JW, Spiegel PG, Harvey JP, et al: Fractures of the humeral shaft: A retrospective study of 240 adult fractures. Clin Orthop 1975; 112:254.

33. Healy WL, White GM, Mick CA, et al: Nonunion of the humeral shaft. Clin Orthop 1987; 219:206.

34. Foulk DA, Szabo RM: Diaphyseal humerus fractures: Natural history and occurrence of nonunion. Orthopedics 1995; 18:333.

35. Wallny T, Sagebiel C, Westermann K, et al: Comparative results of bracing and interlocking nailing in the treatment of humeral shaft fractures. Int Orthop 1997; 21:374.

36. Hall RF Jr, Pankovich AM: Ender nailing of acute fractures of the humerus: A study of closed fixation by intramedullary nails without reaming. J Bone Joint Surg Am 1987; 69:558.

section
3
chapter
7

ELBOW

Roman A. Hayda

Summary

- The elbow fracture prevalence rate is about 7% of all fractures, whereas elbow dislocation is the second most common dislocation after that of the shoulder, with a prevalence rate of about 20%.
- Fractures and dislocations are a result of minor falls, sports injury, and high-energy trauma.
- Thirty to forty percent of bicolumnar distal humerus fractures are open.
- Neurovascular injury is most commonly reported in elbow dislocation in up to 20% of cases, with most cases recovering spontaneously. All three major nerves and their branches are at risk at the time of injury and treatment. They all should be evaluated thoroughly before and after treatment.
- Treatment of all fractures and dislocations of the elbow focus on reestablishing early motion.
- Most distal humerus and olecranon fractures require operative fixation, whereas many radial head fractures and elbow dislocations may be treated nonoperatively.
- Satisfactory functional outcome can typically be achieved by restoring stability and allowing early motion. Loss of motion is directly related to injury severity and prolonged immobilization.

The elbow is a critical joint that allows people to interact with the world around them. Injury may result in loss of motion, creating difficulty or inability to perform personal hygiene, to feed oneself, or to pursue vocational and avocational activities. A clear understanding of anatomy and its restoration in case of injury minimizes the sequelae of trauma. Although Lister performed open treatment of closed olecranon fractures in the 1880s, most complex fractures of the elbow were treated closed with the "bag of bones" technique or casting with resultant malunion, nonunion, instability, and loss of function.[1] Improved understanding of the biomechanics of the elbow and the evolution of implants and their application in the last several decades have allowed for more complete restoration of function. Nonetheless, significant challenges remain.

ANATOMY

The difficulty in treating elbow fractures and dislocations lies in the complex surface anatomy of the joint and its tremendous range of motion. Although this highly congruent joint has great stability, accurate reconstruction is necessary to maintain motion.

The articular surface of the distal humerus consists of the spheroidal capitellum and the spool-shaped trochlea. These are supported by two narrow columns that coalesce into the humeral diaphysis above the olecranon and coro-

noid fossae (Fig. 1A). The semilunar (greater sigmoid) notch of the proximal ulna articulates with the trochlea. Its semicircular shape and central longitudinal ridge provides some intrinsic varus-valgus and anteroposterior stability to the ulnohumeral joint. The concave radial head rotates on the capitellum and is buttressed medially by the lateral trochlear ridge and lesser sigmoid notch of the proximal ulna. Failure to maintain mediolateral trochlear width or the length of the semilunar notch restricts motion. Furthermore, malalignment of the center of rotation of the radiocapitellar joint relative to the axis of the trochlea blocks motion.

The carrying angle formed by the ulnohumeral angle in extension is of lesser importance. It has greater cosmetic than functional significance in adults in distinction to children, in whom reduction may lead to increasing deformity and functional problems.

Ligamentous anatomy further adds to the stability of the elbow. Valgus stability is maintained by the anterior band of the medial collateral ligament[2] (see Fig. 1B). The radial head does not significantly contribute to valgus stability except in case of medial collateral ligament compromise. The lateral collateral ligament is less well defined anatomically. Varus instability is prevented principally by the lateral ulnohumeral ligament with contribution from the radiocapitellar ligament (Fig. 1C). Additional dynamic stabilization is offered by opposing muscle forces of the flexor and extensor musculature.

Several neurovascular structures are at risk during the traumatic event and during treatment because of their proximity to the joint. The ulnar nerve winds around the medial epicondyle. The median nerve and brachial artery overlie the brachialis and the anterior capsule. The radial nerve traverses the joint anterolaterally between the brachioradialis and brachialis muscles. Understanding neurovascular anatomy is crucial in evaluating trauma and in preventing iatrogenic injury.

PATHOGENESIS

Fractures and dislocations of the elbow are caused by direct and indirect forces. Fracture patterns are determined by the degree of flexion of the elbow and force vectors. Experimental studies suggest that when the elbow is flexed less than 90 degrees and an indirect axial force is applied to the forearm, fractures of the radial head and coronoid result. Greater degrees of flexion tend to cause fractures of the distal humerus. Olecranon fractures are created by direct impact with the elbow flexed at 90 degrees.[3]

CLINICAL FEATURES

Fractures and dislocations of the elbow are seen in a variety of clinical scenarios ranging from minor falls to high-

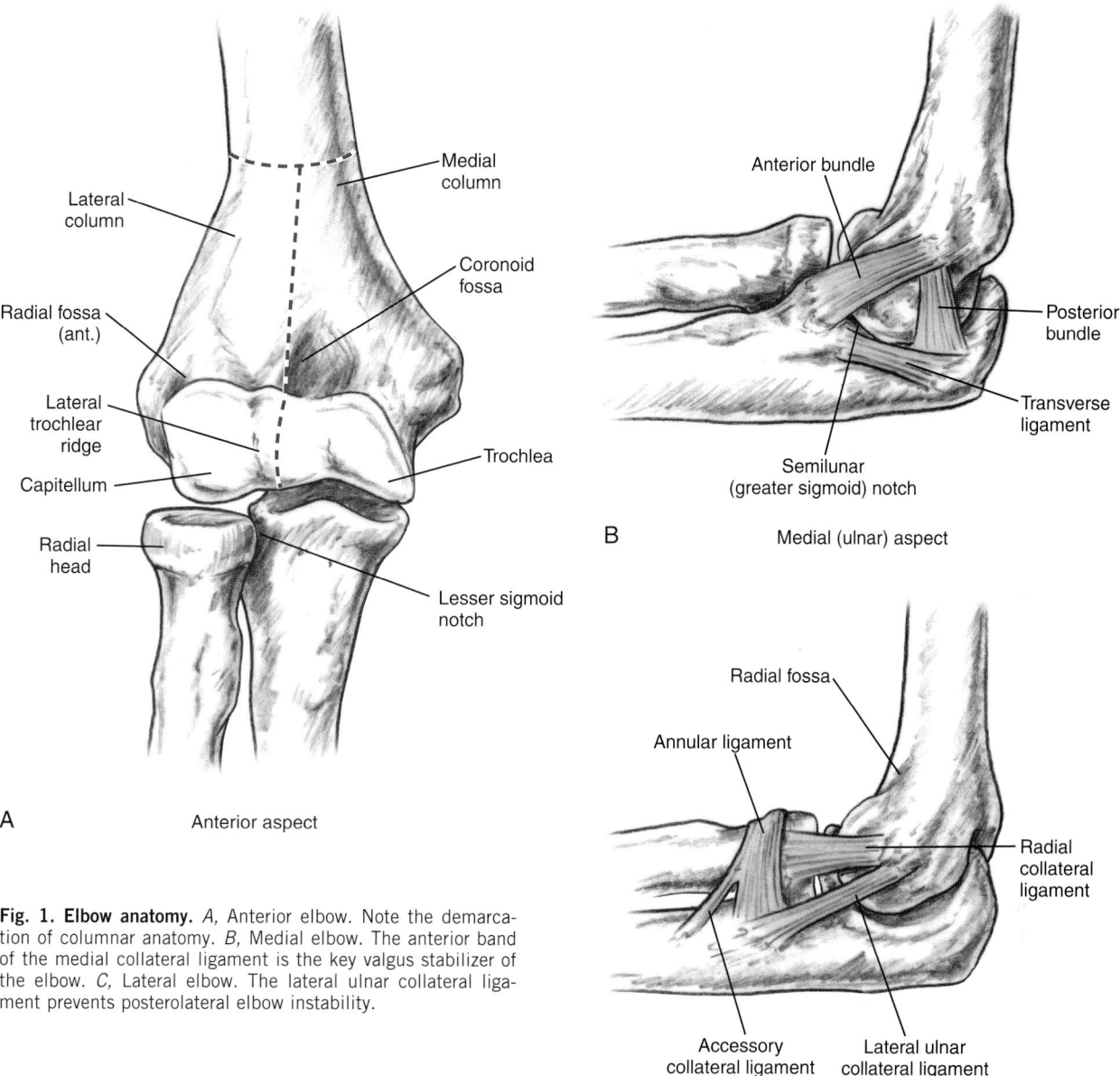

Fig. 1. **Elbow anatomy.** *A,* Anterior elbow. Note the demarcation of columnar anatomy. *B,* Medial elbow. The anterior band of the medial collateral ligament is the key valgus stabilizer of the elbow. *C,* Lateral elbow. The lateral ulnar collateral ligament prevents posterolateral elbow instability.

energy motor vehicle and industrial accidents. Pain and tenderness about the elbow should direct the clinician's examination. Swelling may mask gross deformity, and disruption of the triangular relationship between the olecranon and the medial and lateral epicondyles or loss of motion suggests a significant injury. In addition to a careful neurovascular examination, the wrist, forearm, and shoulder must be carefully evaluated to rule out an associated injury. Anteroposterior and lateral radiographs of the elbow should be obtained in all suspected fractures or dislocations. A posterior fat pad sign, if seen on the lateral radiograph, indicates an effusion and possibly an occult fracture. Oblique radiographs may reveal otherwise occult fractures.

When a diagnosis of elbow trauma is made, it is critical to establish adequate skeletal and soft-tissue stability to

reinstitute motion.[4–6] Immobilization for more than 3 to 4 weeks is associated with increased loss of motion. Therefore, most current treatment plans focus on obtaining rigid internal stabilization to allow rapid initiation of protected motion protocols.

PROCEDURES

DISTAL HUMERUS

Fractures of the distal humerus can be classified broadly as intra- and extra-articular. Early understanding of the pathomechanics of fractures of the distal humerus led to multiple classification schemes, each focusing on a subset of fractures. These were primarily descriptive and did not assist with treatment. Of historical interest is the Milch classifica-

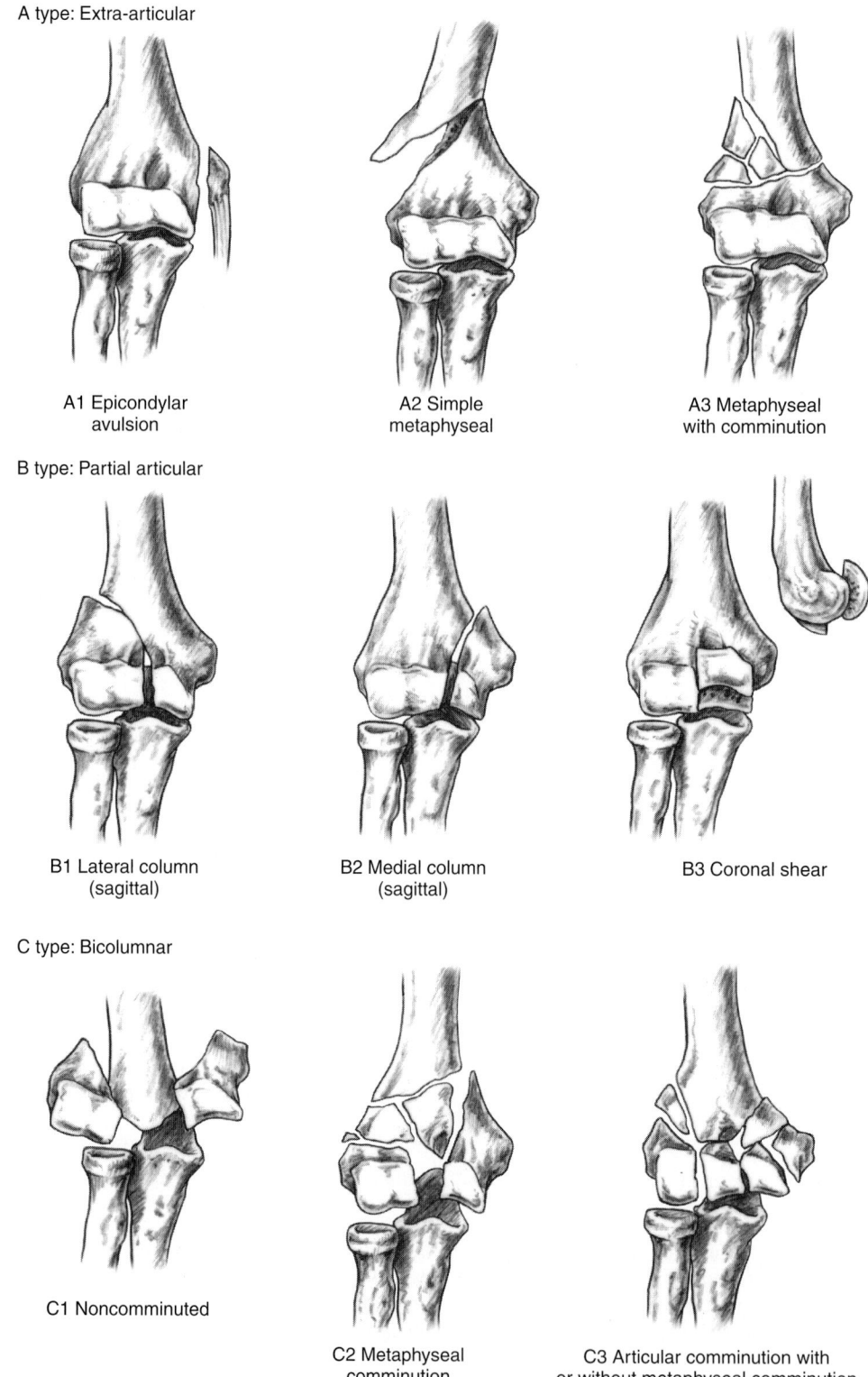

A type: Extra-articular

A1 Epicondylar
avulsion

A2 Simple
metaphyseal

A3 Metaphyseal
with comminution

B type: Partial articular

B1 Lateral column
(sagittal)

B2 Medial column
(sagittal)

B3 Coronal shear

C type: Bicolumnar

C1 Noncomminuted

C2 Metaphyseal
comminution

C3 Articular comminution with
or without metaphyseal comminution

Fig. 2. The Orthopaedic Trauma Association distal humerus fracture classification. (From Orthopaedic Trauma Association Committee for Coding and Classification: Fracture and dislocation compendium. J Orthop Trauma 1996; 10,1.)

tion of single-column injuries, which was well accepted despite its weaknesses. Lateral type 1 fractures, which did not include those of the lateral trochlear ridge, were considered stable; type 2 fractures were unstable due to the inclusion of the ridge. Articular discontinuity is now known to be the critical determinant of the need for surgery.

The universal classification scheme of Müller as adopted by the Orthopaedic Trauma Association (OTA)[7] provides a framework for understanding the injury and planning fixa-

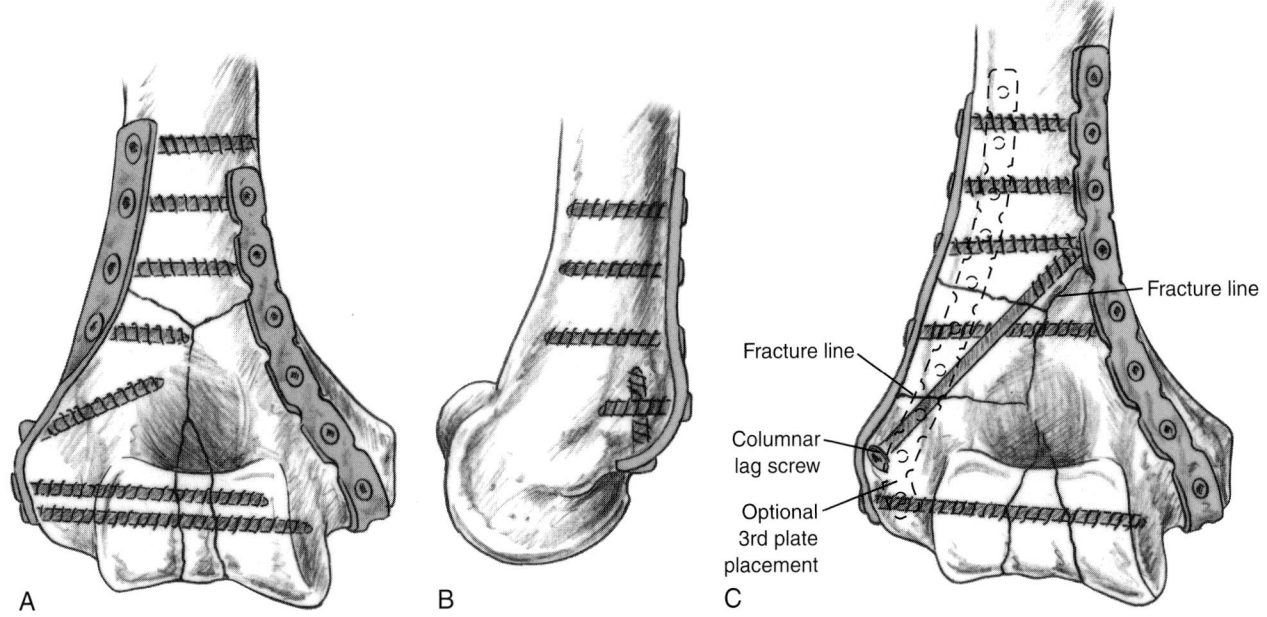

Fig. 3. Distal humerus fracture plating. *A*, Posterior view of the application of medial and lateral plates with a transtrochlear screw. *B*, Medial view. The plate may cradle the medial epicondyle with two distal screws placed 90 degrees to one another. *C*, Alternate placement of plates (dashed lines) and columnar screws.

tion (Fig. 2). In this classification scheme, there are three major divisions. The A types are extra-articular and include epicondylar avulsion (A1) and simple and comminuted transcolumnar fractures (A2 and A3). The B types include single-column intra-articular (B1: lateral column; B2: medial column) and coronal shear fractures (B3). The C types are the bicolumnar intra-articular injuries: noncomminuted (C1), metaphyseal comminution (C2), and articular comminution with or without metaphyseal comminution (C3). A total of 27 subdivisions exist, but these 9 suffice for clinical decision-making.

Extra-Articular Fractures

Fractures of the epicondyles are rare in adults. They represent avulsions of the flexor pronator mass or the ulnar

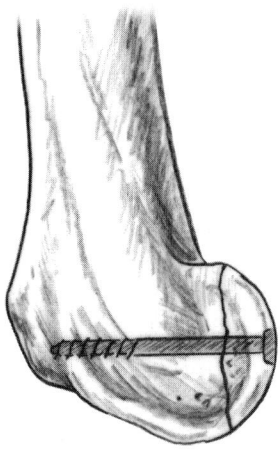

Fig. 4. Capitellar fracture fixation. This is a type 1 fracture fixed with an anterior-to-posterior lag screw with a recessed head.

collateral ligament on the medial side and injury to the extensor group and the lateral collateral ligament on the lateral side. Most are minimally displaced. Usual treatment consists of short-term splinting for 1 to 2 weeks and early motion. Reduction and fixation are required only if the fragment is interposed in the joint or if the soft-tissue injury results in significant instability.

Transcolumnar extra-articular fractures are infrequent injuries in adults. The fracture is typically through a direct anterior or posterior force applied to the distal humerus. If displacement is minimal or nonexistent, satisfactory function can be achieved nonoperatively. In some series,[8, 9] a protocol of immobilization for no more than 3 weeks followed by protected motion in a brace until union was achieved resulted in motion loss of less than 25 degrees of extension or flexion.

Usually these fractures are displaced and/or angulated. Reduction is difficult to achieve and to maintain with casting. Long-term immobilization leads to stiffness. Appropriate operative treatment and early mobilization consistently results in improved function.[4] The most stable construct consists of medial and lateral plates (Fig. 3A). One-third tubular or pelvic reconstruction plates or precontoured plates applied to both columns usually provide adequate stability. The columns usually contain enough cortical bone for secure screw purchase, unless severe comminution exists. No significant difference has been noted in the stability between one-third tubular or pelvic reconstruction plates oriented at 90 degrees to one another.[10] In the case of very distal transverse fractures, the medial plate can be contoured around the medial epicondyle cradling it. Two screws may be placed at 90 degrees to each other through the plate (Fig. 3B). Another means of augmenting stability is placing the screw through the distal end of the plate, directing it into the column proximally across the fracture

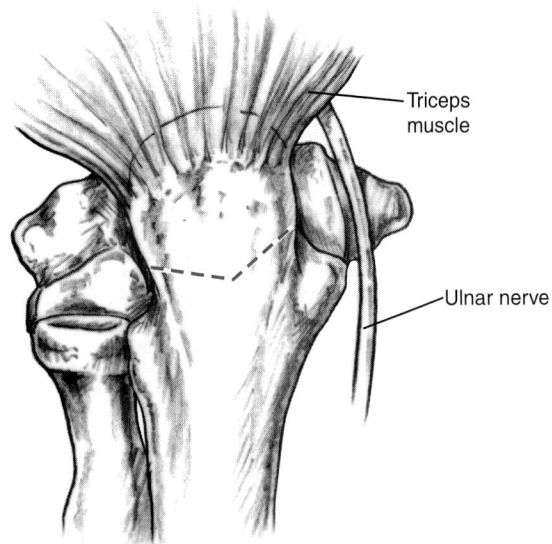

Fig. 5. Olecranon osteotomy. This is a surgeon's end-on view of osteotomy. The ulnar nerve should be protected and the articular surface of the distal humerus visualized and preserved.

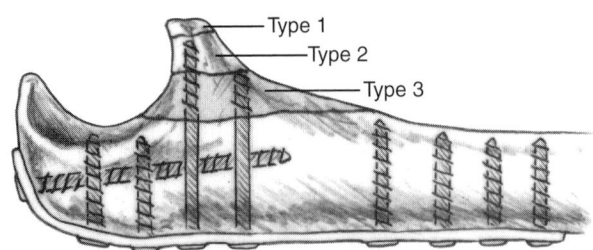

Fig. 7. Coronoid fracture. This is Morrey's classification of coronoid fractures, with posterior plate and lag screw fixation of a type 3 fracture. A contoured plate of this type may also be used for comminuted olecranon and maximal ulnar fractures.

site (Fig. 3C). Percutaneous pinning, which is useful in this pattern of pediatric fracture, is appropriate only in a minority of adult cases. Similarly, use of column screws alone does not provide adequate stability to allow early motion. Situations in which the clinical picture precludes stable fixation and early motion with plate and screws may be treated with pinning. However, infection, stiffness, malunion, and nonunion are more likely with pinning techniques.

Articular Fractures

Single-column injuries are rare and comprise only 3% to 4% of fractures of the distal humerus. However, the intra-

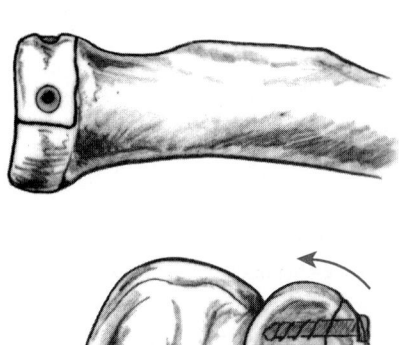

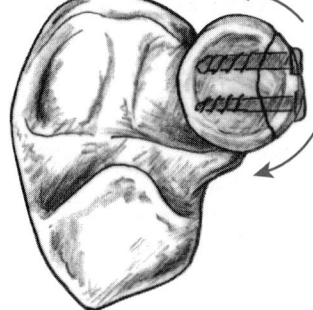

Fig. 6. Radial head fracture. This shows fixation of a type 2 radial head fracture. The screw heads are buried and kept in the "safe zone," which does not articulate with the lesser sigmoid notch in full pronation and supination.

articular nature requires accurate restoration and early motion. Operative management is the treatment of choice unless surgery is contraindicated by factors such as severe polytrauma or soft-tissue injury.[11] The lateral column is most commonly involved. Reduction and fixation can be achieved through a posterior approach with an olecranon osteotomy. The osteotomy allows visualization and restoration of articular continuity. In select cases without comminution, isolated medial or lateral approaches may be utilized. Plating provides optimal stability, although lag screw fixation may be considered if the fracture is a long oblique type with adequate bone quality.

Articular fractures of the capitellum occur as a result of shear forces. Originally described by Hahn and Steinthal in the 19th century, similar patterns have been observed and subsequently classified by Bryan and Morrey.[5] Type 1 fractures involve the articular surface with the underlying bone of the capitellum. Type 2 as observed by Kocher and Lorenz consists of the articular surface with only a thin rim of subchondral bone. Type 3 is a comminuted fracture of the capitellum. Computed tomography scanning or plain radiograph may be useful to distinguish these fracture types and to define the quality of reduction. Type 1 fractures may be treated nonoperatively if not displaced or if closed anatomic reduction is obtained. Anatomy is restored by axial traction in extension and digital manipulation followed by flexion to maintain fracture reduction.[12] Casting for 3 to 4 weeks followed by motion coupled with close radiographic follow-up results in satisfactory function. Displaced, irreducible fractures require open reduction with internal fixation through a posterolateral approach. K-wires, interfragmentary screws, or differential-pitch screws such as the Herbert screw (Zimmer, United States) may be used. Screws may be placed from posterior to anterior; adequate screw purchase without overpenetration must be ensured. Screws may also be placed anterior to posterior, recessing the head (Fig. 4). Regardless of direction, fixation must allow early motion. Type 2 and 3 fractures do not contain adequate bone for fixation. Use of fibrin glue may be considered, but early open or arthroscopic excision leads to a good short-term result. Progressive degenerative changes, instability, and loss of motion may develop over time in these patients and may require secondary treatment.

A rare variant of articular shear fracture traverses the entire articular surface of the distal humerus in the coronal plane.[13] This may consist of a single fragment or be comminuted. The principles of treatment remain the same: restoration of articular anatomy and early motion. Despite the

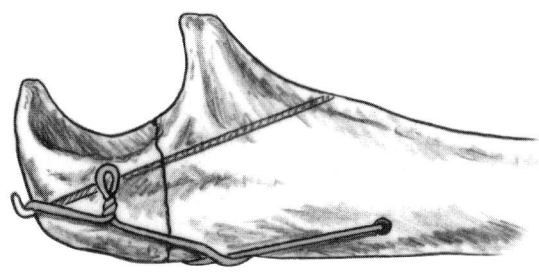

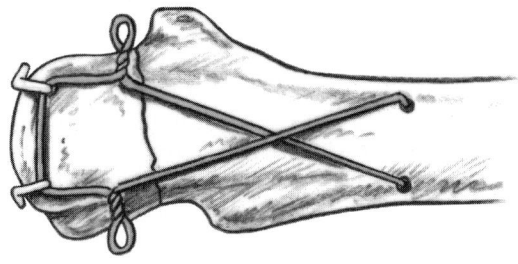

Fig. 8. Olecranon fracture tension band wiring. These are lateral and posterior views of tension band wiring. Note double-knot technique and anchoring of K-wire in the anterior ulnar cortex to improve fixation.

lack of soft-tissue attachments, avascular necrosis is uncommon.

Type C bicolumnar injuries are challenging to treat because the articular surface is both fragmented and dissociated from the humeral shaft. Displacement and instability are always present. Up to 30% to 40% of these are open injuries as a result of high-energy trauma.[4] Analysis of results has demonstrated the superior results of operative treatment over nonoperative management in almost all cases.[14] Nonoperative treatment should be chosen only when there is a contraindication to surgery. Operative treatment allows for accurate articular restoration with secure fixation to the humeral diaphysis.

Surgical reconstruction of this fracture requires a careful preoperative plan. Good quality anteroposterior, lateral, and oblique radiographs will reveal adequate detail to plan reduction and fixation. Radiographs in traction may be necessary to define the components of the fracture. Additional studies such as computed tomography scanning are of little additional value. Typically, pelvic reconstruction plates, one-third tubular plates, and precontoured plates are used. Bone loss should be anticipated; iliac crest or allograft bone should be available during the reconstruction. The preferred surgical approach is posterior, incorporating any posterior wound or previous incision when necessary. A chevron-type olecranon osteotomy allows full visualization of the joint and carries minimal risk of morbidity (Fig. 5). A delayed and nonunion rate of 2% to 5% and hardware prominence have been reported as complications.[4, 9]

Restoration of the articular surface is of paramount importance. In simple noncomminuted fractures, a coronal transtrochlear lag screw will restore and hold the fracture. In the case of comminution, defects should be bone-grafted

with particular attention paid to maintaining trochlear width. Lag screw fixation should be used cautiously, and overcompression should be avoided. The overcompressed, narrowed trochlea impedes motion by impinging on the ridge of the greater sigmoid notch. Comminuted articular segments may be held in place with recessed lag screws or with threaded K-wires cut below the articular surface.[4]

Once the articular surface is reconstructed, it should be reattached to the shaft by restoring the columnar anatomy. Medial and lateral plates applied 90 degrees to one another allow for early motion (see Figs. 5 and 7). Care must be taken not to place screws within the olecranon or coronoid fossae: they will impede motion. Once the construct is completed, the elbow should be placed through a gentle range of motion to rule out impediments to motion and to assess fracture stability. Bone graft should be used liberally to fill any defects. If necessary, three plates may be used: one medially on the medial column and two on the lateral column (one posterior and the other lateral) (see Fig. 7).[4] Screws alone or Y plates do not have adequate rigidity to withstand flexion/extension forces.[10] Open fractures may be fixed definitively at the time of initial débridement unless severe contamination is present.

At the conclusion of the case, the chevron olecranon osteotomy is fixed with a tension band technique. The ulnar nerve is routinely transposed anteriorly subcutaneously, and the wound is closed over a drain.[15] Brief immobilization followed by early motion leads to good or excellent results in 75% of cases. The resultant elbow is stable, with an average range of motion from 15 to 120 degrees allowing return to activities similar to those prior to injury.[16–18] Although passive motion is not advocated, the judicious use of continuous passive-motion devices may assist in restoring motion while not causing heterotopic ossification associated with manipulation.[19]

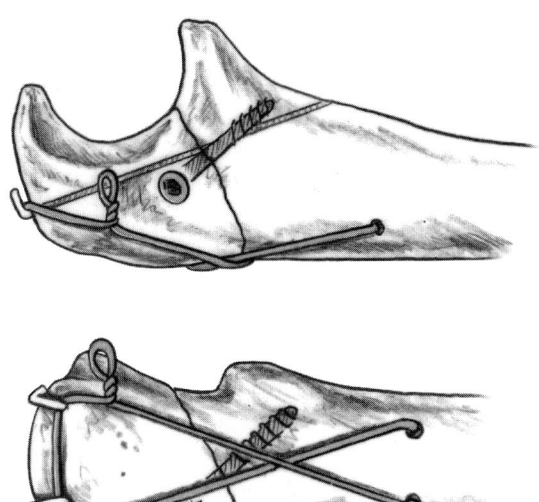

Fig. 9. Oblique olecranon fracture fixation. These are lateral and posterior views of lag screw fixation and tension band wiring of an oblique olecranon fracture.

ELBOW DISLOCATION

Elbow dislocation comprises 20% of all dislocations and is second in frequency to dislocations of the shoulder. Most commonly a hyperextension force levers the olecranon on the distal humerus, resulting in a posterior dislocation. Alternatively, an axial load applied to the forearm in a slightly flexed position has been proposed as a mechanism of injury. Eighty percent of elbow dislocations are posterior or posterolateral. Other forms of dislocation are also seen. These are named by the position of the forearm relative to the arm. The rare medial and lateral dislocations and especially anterior dislocations are associated with greater soft-tissue injury. Divergent dislocations in which all three joints of the elbow are dislocated from one another also have a severe soft-tissue disruption. Five to ten percent of dislocations are associated with radial head and neck fractures, and 10% to 12% may have avulsion fractures of the epicondyles or fracture of the coronoid process. An undefined number have osteochondral injury.

Treatment consists of prompt atraumatic reduction under adequate anesthesia to minimize muscle forces. True lateral radiographs should confirm a concentric reduction. Open reduction is necessary when closed means are not successful. Stability should be carefully assessed following reduction. Elbows that are unstable in 30 degrees of flexion or more should be considered for hinged bracing and fixation of associated fractures. After reduction, care consists of splinting for 7 to 10 days followed by active motion. Lengthy immobilization is associated with increased loss of motion without improved stability.[20] Routine operative repair of ligaments does not improve results.[21] Long-term functional results are good with minimal loss of terminal extension. Radiographs demonstrate mild degenerative changes with preservation of joint space.[22]

Fracture dislocation of the elbow does not carry the same favorable prognosis. Fractures of the radial head and neck, the coronoid, and ulna can be seen in conjunction with elbow dislocation. When these fractures are observed, particularly those of the coronoid, stability assessment following reduction must be carried out.[23] The reader is referred to the sections on these fractures for their management. Radial head excision should not be carried out acutely when the medial collateral ligament is injured because the radial head has secondary function as a valgus restraint.[2] A hinged distractor may be useful to restore stability in highly unstable fracture dislocations.

Anterior dislocation may be associated with olecranon fractures. These transolecranon fracture dislocations should not be confused with Monteggia's fractures because the proximal radioulnar relationship is maintained. In this injury, both the radiocapitellar and the ulnohumeral joints are dislocated. Reduction of the ulnohumeral joint will occur with anatomic restoration of the olecranon fracture and the associated coronoid fragment. Good function can be expected with rigid fixation and early motion.[24]

RADIAL HEAD AND NECK FRACTURES

Radial head fractures are frequently seen as a result of falls on the outstretched hand, with transmission of axial loads from the wrist to the elbow. A fracture is suspected when a fall has occurred resulting in elbow pain. The radial head is often tender. An effusion may be appreciated posterolaterally within the triangle formed by the radial head, the olecranon, and the lateral epicondyle or seen as a posterior fat-pad sign on the lateral radiograph. In addition to anteroposterior and lateral views, an oblique radial head projection may assist with diagnosis. It is important to evaluate the ipsilateral wrist and distal radioulnar joint clinically and radiographically to rule out injury to this area.

The Mason classification is a practical, well-accepted scheme that can guide the clinician. Type 1 fractures are nondisplaced, type 2 are displaced (single fragment), and type 3 are comminuted. Little disagreement exists in the treatment of type 1 injuries. Aspiration of the joint may be considered to relieve a painful hemarthrosis. Early motion is instituted to minimize stiffness. When the fracture fragment exceeds one-third of the radial head surface, displacement may be noted with early motion, leading to poorer results.[25] In these larger nondisplaced fractures, it is unclear whether longer immobilization will lead to superior results.

Treatment of type 2 fractures is more controversial. Options include nonsurgical management, excision, and open reduction and internal fixation. Surgical treatment should be undertaken if there is a block to motion. Instillation of local anesthetic into the joint or an examination under anesthesia may determine restriction of flexion, extension, pronation, or supination. Closed reduction is typically not successful in these cases. Excision or internal fixation should be performed, followed by early motion. Larger fragments can be securely fixed with Herbert's differential pitch screws (Zimmer, United States) or 2.7-mm minifragment screws (Fig. 6). When placed in the lateral nonarticular 90-degree arc of the radius, impingement should not occur. Good-to-excellent results can be expected in most cases. Smaller fragments precluding fixation may be excised. Although a well-controlled prospective study has not been performed, most studies suggest that internal fixation results in better motion with less pain when compared with excision.[26, 27]

Type 3 fractures are comminuted and represent a challenge to treatment. Use of multiple screws, K-wire, or a minifragment T-plate applied laterally may allow for secure fixation of the fracture. In the presence of severe comminution or osteopenia precluding internal fixation, excision may be considered. Many authors have recommended early excision, although some have demonstrated good results with delayed excision.[28] Excision results in satisfactory function for activities of daily living in 92% of cases at long-term follow-up.[29, 30] Before excision, the medial collateral ligament and the distal radioulnar joint must be assessed. In the presence of ligamentous injury, a prosthetic spacer should be placed if excision is performed.[31, 32]

Essex-Lopresti recognized an injury complex consisting of a radial head fracture with disruption of the interosseous ligament and the distal radioulnar joint. A high degree of suspicion must be maintained in all radial head fractures to prevent delayed diagnosis and a poor result. Maintenance of the correct axial relationship of the radius and ulna is important until ligament healing has occurred. The head should be fixed or prosthetically replaced. The distal radioulnar joint is reduced in supination with digital pressure and fixed temporarily with pins.[33]

The surgical approach to most radial head and neck fractures is through the posterolateral Kocher method. Adequate exposure can be obtained for most fracture treatment. The capsulotomy should stay volar to the midcoronal plane to preserve the lateral collateral ligament complex. Rotation of the forearm will expose the remainder of the fracture. Implants should be placed laterally on the radius or buried to preclude impingement within the lesser sigmoid notch.

CORONOID FRACTURES

Coronoid fractures occur infrequently and usually do not require treatment. They have been identified in up to 10% of elbow dislocations. Three basic types have been described. Type 1 fractures are minor tip avulsions. Type 2 may involve up to 50% of the coronoid process, and type 3 consists of more than 50% of the coronoid. Types 1 and 2 are treated nonsurgically with early mobilization. Continued instability may be seen in type 3 injuries because the coronoid process serves as a site of attachment of the medial collateral ligament and the anterior capsule while serving as an anterior buttress for the greater sigmoid notch. The dynamic action of the brachialis will also displace the fragment. Operative fixation may be necessary to preserve elbow stability. When a coronoid fracture is seen in conjunction with an olecranon fracture, lag screw fixation from posterior should be performed during fixation of the olecranon fracture (Fig. 7). Failure to capture the coronoid fragment may lead to significant flexion forces transmitted to the plate construct, increasing the potential for failure. Isolated fractures can be reduced and fixed through an anterior approach. Delayed reconstruction in the face of chronic instability has been described, utilizing the tip of the olecranon or a segment of radial head.[34]

OLECRANON FRACTURES

Olecranon fractures occur as a result of a direct blow to the olecranon in the flexed position. A wide variety of classification schemes have been proposed, reflecting the many patterns encountered. Colton's classification is one of the simplest, describing the displacement and pattern of fracture. Type I fractures are nondisplaced (displaced less than 2 mm) and are stable when gently flexed to 90 degrees. Type II fractures are displaced. The four patterns of type II fractures are A, avulsion; B, transverse; C, comminuted; D, fracture/dislocations. Type I fractures can be treated with splinting or casting in midflexion with protected mobilization at 3 to 4 weeks. Resisted extension or flexion beyond 90 degrees should not be allowed until radiographic union is attained in 6 to 8 weeks. Displaced fractures require operative treatment to overcome the force of the triceps. Casting in extension may affect reduction, but the duration of immobilization required will result in loss of flexion. Fracture pattern is the key determinant in selecting the method of fixation.

Transverse patterns are most commonly seen. The classic *Arbeitsgemeinschaft für Osteosynthesefragen* (AO) tension band technique with two K-wires and double-knot figure-of-eight wire usually results in excellent healing and motion in up to 97% of cases (Fig. 8).[35] However, prominent hardware requiring removal in 50% to 80% of cases has

been cited as a deficiency of this method. An intramedullary lag screw with a tension band has been shown to be marginally biomechanically stronger, but clinical results have not been shown to be superior.[36] Screw failure and fracture fragmentation have been reported with this technique.

Oblique fractures may displace along the obliquity if tension banding alone is used. A lag screw placed perpendicular to the fracture with a tension band wire will overcome this problem (Fig. 9). Alternatively, lag screw fixation through a plate may be utilized.

Comminuted fractures must be fixed rigidly while maintaining the length of the greater sigmoid notch. Tension banding cannot control the comminuted segments adequately. Plating with supplementary lag screw fixation where possible provides the most rigid construct. Although one-third tubular plates have been used, the more rigid pelvic reconstruction plates are easily contoured to fit around the tip of the olecranon and provide stable fixation with less chance of fatigue failure. Judicious use of a distal compression device may further augment stability. A combination of plates, screws, and tension banding may be useful in complex patterns or when the fracture extends beyond the coronoid. Bone grafting should be considered in case of bone loss, particularly if the geometry of the sigmoid notch would be altered. Coronoid fragments should be reduced and incorporated into the construct to withstand compressive forces and to add stability in flexion.

The posterior approach provides ready access to the ulna. The ulnar attachment of the lateral ligament must be preserved to prevent late instability, particularly when the fracture is associated with an elbow dislocation. The plate may be applied medially, laterally, or directly posteriorly, dependent on fracture pattern and soft-tissue coverage. No biomechanical difference has been noted with lateral or posterior plate placement.[37] Dorsal plates may require removal after healing because of subcutaneous position.

Excision of the olecranon may be considered in any fracture pattern requiring surgical management. Instability is not a problem if the triceps is attached level with the articular surface, even if up to 60% of the articular surface is involved.[38, 39] Secure fixation can be achieved with heavy nonabsorbable suture through bone tunnels, allowing early motion. Complications are few, but primary use of this technique is usually reserved for elderly patients with comminuted fractures precluding adequate fixation. Caution is necessary when excision is performed in the presence of elbow dislocation or other fractures, particularly those involving the coronoid.

COMPLICATIONS

NEUROVASCULAR INJURY

Three major nerves—the radial, median, and ulnar nerves—along with the brachial artery cross the elbow joint in close proximity to the osseous structures. All are at risk at the time of injury and during closed or surgical treatment. All should be carefully examined to include their branches before and after treatment. The median and ulnar nerves are at particular risk with elbow dislocations and extra-articular distal humerus fractures. The median nerve has been entrapped within the joint when reducing posterior elbow dislocations. The radial nerve or its branches may be injured with lateral injuries or lateral surgical approaches. The ulnar nerve, because of its superficial location and constrained position within the cubital tunnel, is particularly vulnerable. In all posterior and medial approaches to the elbow, the ulnar nerve should be identified and protected. When plating the medial column of the distal humerus, routine transposition should be performed when the plate is contoured to cradle the medial epicondyle.

Residual nerve deficits following treatment of injuries to the elbow are also treatable. The ulnar nerve is prone to encasement in scar and bone. Surgical decompression with anterior transposition can be successful if nonoperative measures fail.[6]

The brachial artery is rarely injured during elbow trauma. It may be lacerated in extra-articular fractures or high-energy dislocations. Prompt recognition with vascular repair and distal fasciotomy will lead to a satisfactory result. However, severe distal soft-tissue injury, underlying patient factors, or associated trauma may preclude vascular reconstruction and a functional result. Amputation should be considered in these instances.

OPEN FRACTURE

Open fractures of the elbow are common because of the superficial position of this joint. When recognized, appropriate treatment consists of antibiotics, tetanus prophylaxis, and wound débridement. In the absence of gross contamination, definitive internal fixation may be done at the time of initial surgery. Local or free-tissue transfers may be necessary to provide coverage. Results depend on the ability to débride contaminated and devitalized tissue adequately while providing stable osseous fixation. Gross contamination or severe comminution may necessitate external fixation, with resulting imperfect reduction and loss of motion.

LOSS OF MOTION

Loss of motion remains the most common complication of elbow trauma. Even minor trauma may result in loss of terminal extension. A flexion/extension arc of 30 degrees to 130 degrees of flexion, with 50 degrees of pronation and supination, is used in the routine activities of daily living. Restoration of this functional range of motion is the goal of treatment. Loss of motion has been consistently associated with prolonged immobilization. Therefore, internal fixation must be rigid to allow motion within 2 to 3 weeks of injury. Careful treatment with rapid institution of active range of motion usually results in attaining functional motion. However, passive motion, particularly forced manipulation, should be avoided because it prolongs the inflammatory cycle, promoting stiffness and heterotopic ossification. Continuous passive motion machines have been found useful in restoring motion while not inducing abnormal bone formation.[19] Motion gains can be expected, particularly in the first 6 months up to the first year. Dynamic splinting should be considered if the fracture has healed and if functional motion has not been restored within 3 months.

When functional motion loss persists, surgical intervention may be necessary. Morrey[40] facilitated evaluation and decision-making by pointing out intrinsic and extrinsic causes of motion loss. Intrinsic causes are caused by the joint surface itself, such as degenerative change, malunion, and arthrofibrosis. Failure to restore trochlear width and greater sigmoid length will impede motion. Similarly, misplacement of the relative centers of rotation of the trochlea with respect to the capitellum causes a block to motion. Extrinsic causes include muscular and capsular contractures, which restrict motion. Ectopic bone and misplaced hardware block motion. Careful identification of these factors will allow for an appropriate preoperative plan. Posterior, medial, lateral, and combined approaches have been proposed for dealing with this difficult problem. Evaluation of soft tissues and the area of the predominant causative factor will determine the optimal approach in these highly individualized problems. Surgical care of contracture is best left to surgeons familiar with the treatment of elbow contracture. Principles of care are complete capsulectomy, osteophyte excision, and judicious use of distraction arthroplasty, followed by a range-of-motion therapy program. Satisfactory function can be obtained with a stable pain-free joint when patients are selected carefully and surgery is performed correctly.[6, 40]

NONUNION AND MALUNION

Nonunion and malunion are infrequent with carefully planned surgery and well-executed postoperative therapy. When these complications do occur, intervention may improve function. Nonunion is seen in the supracondylar area (2% to 11%) and in the olecranon (2% to 5%). Supracondylar nonunion is associated with significant capsular contracture, with motion occurring through the nonunion site. In the younger patient with reasonable bone stock, union can be achieved by releasing the capsular contracture, removing the fibrous nonunion, bone grafting, and applying rigid internal fixation with two or three plates in a 90-degree orientation as described in the earlier section on distal humerus fractures.[6] Total elbow arthroplasty should be considered in the elderly low-demand patient.

Several options exist in the treatment of olecranon nonunion. Rigid internal fixation with plates and bone-grafting is a highly successful technique, providing that articular congruity can be restored and adequate bone stock remains.[41] Excision is highly reliable in the older patient. It should not be used in case of elbow instability. Otherwise, excellent pain-free motion with good strength can be expected. The triceps should be reattached flush with the articular surface of the olecranon.

When Monteggia's fracture is excluded with its dislocated radial head, problematic malunions about the elbow are isolated to the distal humerus. These malunions may be intra- or extra-articular. Intra-articular malunions are rare and typically involve loss of trochlear width. Osteotomy with placement of intercalary bone graft and stable fixation has been reported but remains a procedure of formidable difficulty and uncertain results.[42, 43] Such a procedure should be carefully considered only by highly experienced surgeons.

Malunion in the supracondylar area may cause a cosmetic deformity in adults and is not usually associated with functional problems. However, significant cubitus valgus may be associated with ulnar neuritis. A carefully planned closing wedge osteotomy with rigid internal fixation can correct the deformity when necessary.

HETEROTOPIC OSSIFICATION AND SYNOSTOSIS

Heterotopic ossification occurs in 3% to 6% of cases of elbow dislocations and fractures. It may block functional motion. Risk factors have not been elaborated, but head-injured patients are at particular risk. No surgical approach is associated with an increased incidence rate. Routine prophylaxis with Indocin has not been advocated but should be considered for head-injured patients. Heterotopic bone may be excised if there is significant motion restriction. Previously, excision was delayed for 12 months until the bone had reached "maturity." More recent reports have suggested that early excision with adjunctive nonsteroidal agents or radiation therapy has resulted in more rapid return to functional motion.[44] There are no prospective randomized studies to confirm this hypothesis.

Synostosis is a rare complication of elbow trauma. Most commonly, the proximal radioulnar joint is involved, although the ulnohumeral and radiocapitellar joint may be affected. Resection with and without interposition restored an average of 139 degrees of forearm rotation in one series. Recurrence was seen in 1 of 18 limbs.[45]

TOTAL ELBOW ARTHROPLASTY, ALLOGRAFT REPLACEMENT, AND ARTHRODESIS

Total elbow arthroplasty has evolved to a degree where a reliable implant is available. When an elderly patient sustains a comminuted fracture of the elbow, which precludes stable reduction and fixation, total elbow arthroplasty using a semiconstrained cemented prosthesis may allow for rapid restoration of function. A recent series reported on use of this technique in 20 elderly patients (average age 72 years, range 48 to 92 years).[46] Complications were few, with a pain-free functional arc of motion in nearly all patients. It must be emphasized that a resurfacing implant is inappropriate as it will lead to elbow instability. Furthermore, replacement arthroplasty should be used only in elderly low-demand individuals. It may also be used in select cases of malunion and nonunion.

Another option for treatment of highly comminuted fractures about the elbow, more applicable to the younger patient, is allograft replacement of the distal humerus, radial head, or olecranon. Dean et al[47] reported on a limited series, with 10 of 20 satisfactory results at an average 7.5 years' follow-up. However, also noted was a complication rate of 70%, limiting indications to select salvage cases. Isolated replacement of the radial head in the treatment of sequelae of head resection in the presence of an Essex-Lopresti lesion demonstrated more uniform improvement with minimal complications.[48]

Fusion is a final option to consider when dealing with a salvage situation in a high-demand patient such as a laborer.[6] Fusion in 90 degrees of flexion with the use of a contoured plate is generally accepted, although individual patient needs should be considered when performing this uncommon procedure. Trial casting may assist in choosing the best degree of flexion. The radiohumeral joint should be spared when possible to allow pronation and supination.

REFERENCES

1. Brown RF, Morgan RG: Intercondylar T-shaped fractures of the humerus: Results in ten cases treated by early mobilization. J Bone Joint Surg Br 1971; 53:425.
2. Morrey BR, Tanaka S, An K-N: Valgus stability of the elbow: A definition of primary and secondary constraints. Clin Orthop 1991; 265:187.
3. Amis AA, Miller JH: The mechanisms of elbow fractures: An investigation using impact tests in vitro. Injury 1995; 26:163.
4. Jupiter JB: Complex fractures of the distal part of the humerus and associated complications. AAOS Instr Course Lect 1995; 44:187.
5. Bryan RS, Morrey BF: Fractures of the distal humerus in the adult. In Morrey BF (ed): The Elbow and Its Disorders, 2nd ed. Philadelphia, WB Saunders, 1993, p 328.
6. Modabber MR, Jupiter JR: Reconstruction for post-traumatic conditions of the elbow joint. J Bone Joint Surg Am 1995; 77:1431.
7. Orthopaedic Trauma Association Committee for Coding and Classification: Fracture and dislocation compendium. J Orthop Trauma 1996; 10:1.
8. Sarmiento A, Horowitch A, Aboulafia A, et al: Functional bracing for comminuted extraarticular fractures of the distal humerus. J Bone Joint Surg Br 1990; 72:283.

9. Aitken GK, Rorabeck CH: Distal humeral fractures in the adult. Clin Orthop 1986; 207:191.
10. Helfet DL, Hotchkiss RN: Internal fixation of the distal humerus: A biomechanical comparison of methods. J Orthop Trauma 1990; 4:260.
11. Jupiter JB, Neff U, Regazzoni P, et al: Unicondylar fractures of the distal humerus: An operative approach. J Orthop Trauma 1988; 2:102.
12. Ochner RS, Bloom H, Palumbo RC, et al: Closed reduction of coronal fractures of the capitellum. J Trauma 1996; 40:199.
13. Jupiter J, McKee M, Toh CL: Coronal shear fracture of the distal humerus. J Shoulder Elbow Surg 1994; 3:70.
14. Zagorski JB, Jennings JJ, Burkhalter WE, et al: Comminuted intraarticular fractures of the distal humeral condyles: Surgical vs nonsurgical treatment. Clin Orthop 1986; 202:197.
15. Wang KC, Shih HN, Hsu KY, et al: Intercondylar fractures of the distal humerus: Routine transposition of the ulnar nerve in a posterior operative approach. J Trauma 1994; 36:270.
16. Helfet DL, Schmeling GJ: Bicondylar intraarticular injuries of the distal humerus in adults. Clin Orthop 1993; 292:26.
17. Holdsworth BJ, Mossad MM: Fractures of

the adult distal humerus: Elbow function after internal fixation. J Bone Joint Surg Br 1990; 72:362.
18. Letsch R, Schmit-Neuerburg KP, Sturmer KM, et al: Intraarticular fractures of the distal humerus: Surgical treatment and results. Clin Orthop 1989; 241:238.
19. Soffer SR, Yahiro MA: Continuous passive motion after internal fixation of distal humeral fractures. Orthop Rev 1990; 19:88.
20. Mehlhoff TL, Noble PC, Bennett JB, et al: Simple dislocation of the elbow in the adult. J Bone Joint Surg Am 1988; 70:244.
21. Josefsson PO, Gentz CF, Johnell O, et al: Surgical versus non-surgical treatment of ligamentous injuries following dislocation of the elbow joint: A prospective randomized study. J Bone Joint Surg Am 1987; 69:605.
22. Josefsson PO, Johnell O, Gentz CF: Long term sequelae of simple dislocation of the elbow. J Bone Joint Surg Am 1984; 66:927.
23. Josefsson PE, Gentz CF, Johnell O, et al: Dislocations of the elbow and intraarticular fractures. Clin Orthop 1989; 246:126.
24. Ring D, Jupiter JB, Saunders RW, et al: Transolecranon fracture dislocations of the elbow. J Orthop Trauma 1997; 11:545.

25. Radin EL, Riseborough EJ: Fractures of the radial head: A review of eighty eight cases and analysis of the indications for excision of the radial head and non-operative treatment. J Bone Joint Surg Am 1966; 48:1055.

26. Geel CW, Palmer AK, Ruedi T, et al: Internal fixation of proximal radial head fractures. J Orthop Trauma 1990; 4:270.

27. Khalfayan EE, Culp RW, Alexander AH: Mason type II radial head fractures: Operative versus nonoperative treatment. J Orthop Trauma 1992; 6:283.

28. Broberg MA, Morrey BF: Results of delayed excision of the radial head after fracture. J Bone Joint Surg Am 1986; 68: 669.

29. Goldberg I, Peylan J, Yosipovitch Z, et al: Late results of excision of the radial head for an isolated closed fracture. J Bone Joint Surg Am 1986; 68:675.

30. Coleman DA, Blair WF, Shurr D: Resection of the radial head for fracture of the radial head: Long term follow-up of seventeen cases. J Bone Joint Surg Am 1987; 69:385.

31. Judet T, Garreau deLoubresse C, Piriou P, et al: A floating prosthesis for radial head fractures. J Bone Joint Surg Br 1996; 78: 244.

32. Harrington J, Tountas AA: Replacement of the radial head in the treatment of unstable elbow fractures. Injury 1981; 12:405.

33. Edwards GS, Jupiter JB: Radial head fractures with acute distal radioulnar dislocation: Essex-Lopresti revisited. Clin Orthop 1988; 234:61.

34. Esser RD: Reconstruction of the coronoid process with a radial head fragment. Orthopedics 1997; 20:169.

35. Wolfgang G, Burke F, Bush D, et al: Surgical treatment of displaced olecranon fractures by tension band wiring technique. Clin Orthop 1987; 224:192.

36. Murphy DF, Greene WB, Gilbert JA, et al: Displaced olecranon fractures in adults: Biomechanical analysis of fixation methods. Clin Orthop 1987; 224:210.

37. King GJ, Lammens PN, Milne AD, et al: Plate fixation of comminuted olecranon fractures: An in vitro biomechanical study. J Shoulder Elbow Surg 1996; 5:437.

38. Inhofe PD, Howard TC: The treatment of olecranon fractures by excision of fragments and repair of the extensor mechanism: A historical review and report of 12 fractures. Orthopedics 1993; 16:1313.

39. Gartsman GM, Sculco TP, Otis JC: Operative treatment of olecranon fractures: Excision or open reduction with internal fixation. J Bone Joint Surg Am 1981; 63:718.

40. Morrey BF: Post-traumatic contracture of the elbow: Operative treatment, including distraction arthroplasty. J Bone Joint Surg Am 1990; 72:601.

41. Papagelopoulos PJ, Morrey BF: Treatment of nonunion of olecranon fractures. J Bone Joint Surg Br 1994; 76:627.

42. McKee M, Jupiter J, Toh CL, et al: Reconstruction after malunion and nonunion of intra-articular fractures of the distal humerus: Methods and results in 13 adults. J Bone Joint Surg Br 1994; 76:614.

43. Cobb TK, Linscheid RL: Late correction of malunited intercondylar humeral fractures: Intra-articular osteotomy and tricortical bone grafting. J Bone Joint Surg Br 1994; 76:622.

44. McAuliffe JA, Wolfson AH: Early excison of heterotopic ossification about the elbow followed by radiation therapy. J Bone Joint Surg Am 1997; 79:749.

45. Jupiter J, Ring D: Operative treatment of post-traumatic radio-ulnar synostosis. J Bone Joint Surg Am 1998; 80:248.

46. Cobb TK, Morrey BF: Total elbow arthroplasty as primary treatment for distal humeral fractures in elderly patients. J Bone Joint Surg Am 1997; 79:826.

47. Dean GS, Hollinger EH, Urbaniak JR: Elbow allograft for reconstruction of the elbow with massive bone loss: Long term results. Clin Orthop 1997; 341:12.

48. Szabo RM, Hotchkiss RN, Slater RR: The use of frozen allograft radial head replacement for treatment of established symptomatic proximal translation of the radius: Preliminary experience in five cases. J Hand Surg Am 1997; 22:269.

section 3 chapter 8

FOREARM FRACTURES

J. David Evanich and Gregory J. Schmeling

Summary

- Forearm fractures disrupt the complex architecture of the forearm: the radius and ulna, their proximal and distal articulations, and the interosseous membrane.
- The goal of treatment is restoration of function, especially forearm rotation.
- Anatomic reduction and rigid fixation are critical to success in the vast majority of forearm fractures.
- Rigid fixation allows early motion and prevents muscle contraction and joint stiffness, thereby improving the functional result.
- Meticulous attention to surgical detail aids in minimizing the complications of infection, neurovascular injury, nonunion, and synostosis.

The unique ability to position the hand in space is greatly affected by the movements of the forearm. This is particularly true for supination and pronation. The forearm axis can be viewed as a joint complex.[1] Any injury to this complex must be aggressively treated to ensure functional forearm motion.

Many treatment options are available to treat forearm fractures. Cast immobilization, fracture bracing, external fixation, plate and screw fixation, and intramedullary nailing have their appropriate indications. The exceedingly high union rate and predictable outcome of compression plate fixation makes it the standard by which all other treatment methods must be measured.[2-8]

HISTORICAL REVIEW

Forearm fractures have provided a challenge to the orthopaedic surgeon for decades. Early management consisted of closed treatment that met with disappointing results.[9-11] This can be understood when considering the unforgiving architecture of the forearm. Maintaining two parallel bones in exact alignment, rotation, and length can be difficult in a plaster cast. Deforming muscular forces and cast loosening that occurs as swelling decreases contribute to this formidable task. A high incidence rate of nonunion and patient dissatisfaction led many practitioners to search for a better solution.

Several intramedullary devices have been introduced and applied to forearm fracture treatment. The use of small, round, and flexible intramedullary wires and rods improved the nonunion rate only slightly compared with closed treatment.[12] Enhancements by Sage[12, 13] led to a rigid, prebent, diamond-shaped nail that significantly decreased the nonunion rate but was technically demanding. More modern nail designs are available with union rates comparable to those of dynamic compression plating but with poorer functional outcome and patient satisfaction rates.[13, 14]

In the 1940s, Eggers[15] introduced a slotted plate that rigidly fixed the fracture ends in opposition. The slots were meant to allow the muscular forces to apply compression across the fracture. Later, the Arbeitsgemeinschaft für Osteosynthesefragen/Association for the Study of Interal Fixation (AO/ASIF) group developed a plate designed for dynamic compression upon plate application. This was the predecessor to the modern AO/ASIF compression plate.[16] Several investigators utilizing this plate have reported excellent union rates, functional outcome, and patient satisfaction rates.[2–7, 17] Initially, 4.5-mm compression plates were used, but they were too rigid for this fracture. High refracture rates were found after the 4.5-mm plate removal.[2, 18–20] A smaller, 3.5-mm compression plate was later used with excellent results.[4, 18–20] The 3.5-mm compression plate has become the standard by which all other treatment methods are measured.

PATHOGENESIS

The majority of forearm fractures result from a single episode of trauma. The mechanism of injury is most likely a direct blow, although many patients are unable to recall the exact course of events resulting in the fracture. Commonly obtained histories leading to a forearm fracture include motor vehicle accidents, athletic endeavors, and falls from a height. Fractures resulting from gunshot wounds carry a higher risk of neurovascular injury and have more extensive soft-tissue destruction. Pathological fractures, albeit uncommon in the forearm, should be considered in cases in which minimal trauma resulted in a fracture or a lesion is apparent on imaging studies.

CLINICAL FEATURES

Initial examination of a forearm fracture often reveals a readily apparent deformity. The deformity results from the high energy required to produce the fracture, coupled with the multitude of deforming muscular forces. The skin should be thoroughly inspected for any breaks that may communicate with the fracture. Associated pain and crepitus are usually present but need not be elicited, as further soft-tissue damage may occur.

Swelling, secondary to fracture hematoma and soft-tissue injury, can be found with most forearm fractures. More severe swelling is seen in high-energy injuries and with delays in clinical presentation. Tense forearm compartments, pain out of proportion to the injury, or pain with passive extension of the fingers may point to compartment syndrome. Any suspicion of compartment syndrome warrants immediate fasciotomy. Suspicion of a compartment syndrome in an unconscious patient or a patient with depressed central nervous system function warrants compartment pressure measurements and fasciotomies as indicated.

The proximal and distal articulations of the forearm must be examined. Pain, deformity, or instability at the elbow or wrist may indicate injury to the respective articulations. A high index of suspicion is needed to diagnosis proximal ulnar fractures associated with radial head dislocations (Monteggia's dislocation) or distal radial shaft fractures associated with distal radioulnar joint disruption (Galeazzi's fracture).[21–25] Variations of these combinations are possible.

Neuromotor examination should include the radial (extensor digitorum communis with a neutral wrist), median (abductor pollicis brevis), posterior interosseous (extensor pollicis longus), and ulnar (first dorsal interosseous) nerves. Sensory examination is accomplished by testing the autonomous zones of the radial (first dorsal web space), median (volar pad index finger), and ulnar (volar pad small finger) nerves. Vascular examination consists of palpation of the brachial, radial, and ulnar pulses, along with examination of distal capillary refill.

INVESTIGATION

Anteroposterior and lateral views of the forearm constitute the minimum radiographic imaging necessary for the evaluation of a suspected forearm fracture. The elbow and wrist must be included on each film to help evaluate the extent of injury. Dedicated views of the elbow and wrist are sometimes needed to further define the fracture and identify dislocations. Classification of the fracture pattern helps to compare outcomes between treatment groups. The Orthopaedic Trauma Association has developed a classification system and has recommended its use for all fractures.[26]

TREATMENT GOALS, INDICATIONS, AND CONTRAINDICATIONS

Goals, indications, and contraindications for treatment are outlined in Table 1.

PROCEDURES

PREOPERATIVE PLANNING
The complex anatomy of the forearm demands careful preoperative planning to obtain a satisfactory operative result. Good orthogonal radiographs of the forearm, including the elbow and wrist, are essential. The injury must be thoroughly assessed to select a fixation type.

In those select cases in which intramedullary nailing is appropriate, several requirements must be met. The fracture pattern must be amenable to the use of an intramedullary nail. This requires the most proximal and distal extent of the fracture to be at least 3 cm from the elbow and wrist joints, respectively.[14] The intramedullary canal must be at least 3 mm in diameter along the entire length. Finally, the length and shape of the rod must be chosen to conform to the anatomy of the reduced fractured forearm bones. The highest rates of union have been seen with rigid, prebent rods with a shape and locking mechanism that helps prevent rotation.[13, 14]

Most forearm fractures requiring internal fixation are treated with plate and screw fixation. Initially, the surgical approach that provides easiest access to the fractures must

TABLE 1. GOALS, INDICATIONS, AND CONTRAINDICATIONS FOR TREATMENT OF FOREARM FRACTURE

Treatment Type	Indications	Specific Treatment	Union Rate	Functional Satisfaction Rate
Nonoperative	Nondisplaced radius and ulna fractures Isolated ulnar shaft fractures with <50% displacement and <10% angulation	Cast immobilization or fracture bracing	85–90%[32]	Not available
External fixation	Severely compromised soft tissues with or without extensive fracture comminution (e.g., burns, GSWs, severe grade II B/C open fractures)	Pin and bar construct spanning fracture site	Temporizing	Not applicable
Intramedullary rodding	Displaced radius and ulna fractures with compromised soft tissues	Rigid intramedullary rod placement after closed or open reduction	94–100%[12, 13, 33]	70–78%[12, 13, 33]
Compression plating	Displaced single bone fractures Vast majority of displaced radius and ulna fractures	Compression plate and screw fixation after open reduction	88–98%[2, 4–7, 17]	80–92%[2, 4–7, 17]
Compression plating with reduction of radial head	Monteggia fracture/dislocations	Compression plate and screw fixation of proximal ulna shaft fracture with reduction of radial head dislocation	90–100%	83–86%[24, 25]
Compression plating with reduction of distal radioulnar joint	Galeazzi fracture/dislocations	Compression plate and screw fixation of distal radial shaft fracture with pinning of distal radioulnar joint in supination	94–100%[23–25]	92–100%[23–25]

GSW, gunshot wound.

be determined. Length and size of the plate must be considered. Our choice most often has been a small-fragment 3.5-mm compression plate that permits at least six cortices on each side of the fracture. The use of six cortices has been shown to decrease loosening and promote union.[16, 27] The 3.5-mm size has been shown to be a nice balance between strength and rigidity.[20] Semitubular plates are too weak and often fail. An increase in refracture has been seen in the use of 4.5-mm plates, most likely secondary to increased rigidity and stress shielding.[19, 20]

TECHNICAL DETAILS

The surgical approach to the forearm fracture is often dictated by the fracture pattern. In plate and screw fixation of both bone forearm fractures, two incisions are recommended to avoid synostosis. Occasionally, both fractures must be exposed before attempted reduction as the reduction of one fracture may inhibit the reduction of the corresponding fracture.

An extraperiosteal dissection is recommended to avoid devascularization of the fracture fragments. This is particularly important in comminuted fractures. In severely comminuted fractures, a bridge plate is preferable to preserve blood supply. A distractor can help align the fracture fragments, and a dental pick may be used to tease them into place. Restoration of length, rotation, axial alignment, and radial bow are the goals of fracture reduction. Reestablishment of the radial bow has been shown to correlate with the preservation of forearm rotation.[8, 9]

In Monteggia's dislocation, anatomic reduction and internal fixation of the proximal ulnar fracture usually reduces the radial head. If the radial head is unstable with elbow and forearm motion, the ulnar reduction must be reassessed first. If the reduction appears anatomic, the examiner should explore the radiocapitellar articulation for soft-tissue interposition or incompetence of the annular ligament. One then removes the soft tissue or reconstructs the annular ligament as appropriate.[9] If the reduction of the radial head is stable, the arm is kept in supination for 3 to 4 weeks. Flexion and extension of the elbow is allowed after the soft tissues have quieted down (3 to 7 days).

In Galeazzi's fracture, anatomic reduction and internal fixation of the distal radius fracture usually reduce the distal radioulnar joint. The stability of the distal radioulnar joint is then assessed with sagittal stress and during forearm and wrist motion. If the distal radial ulnar joint is stable, the arm is splinted for 3 to 7 days, and then motion is allowed. If the distal radial ulnar joint is unstable, the arm is placed in full supination, and the stability is reassessed. If stability is achieved with full supination, the limb is immobilized in supination for 6 weeks. Therapy then begins to regain motion. If the distal radial ulnar joint remains unstable in full supination, the joint is reduced and pinned in full supination. The limb is immobilized for 6 weeks, after which the pins are removed, and therapy to regain motion is allowed.[4]

Fixation is best achieved using a 3.5-mm compression plate with 3.5-mm screws. At least six cortices should be obtained on each side of the fracture. Standard AO compression techniques should be followed (Fig. 1). Reduction and fixation should be confirmed with radiographic images during the procedure. Full-length intraoperative plain films

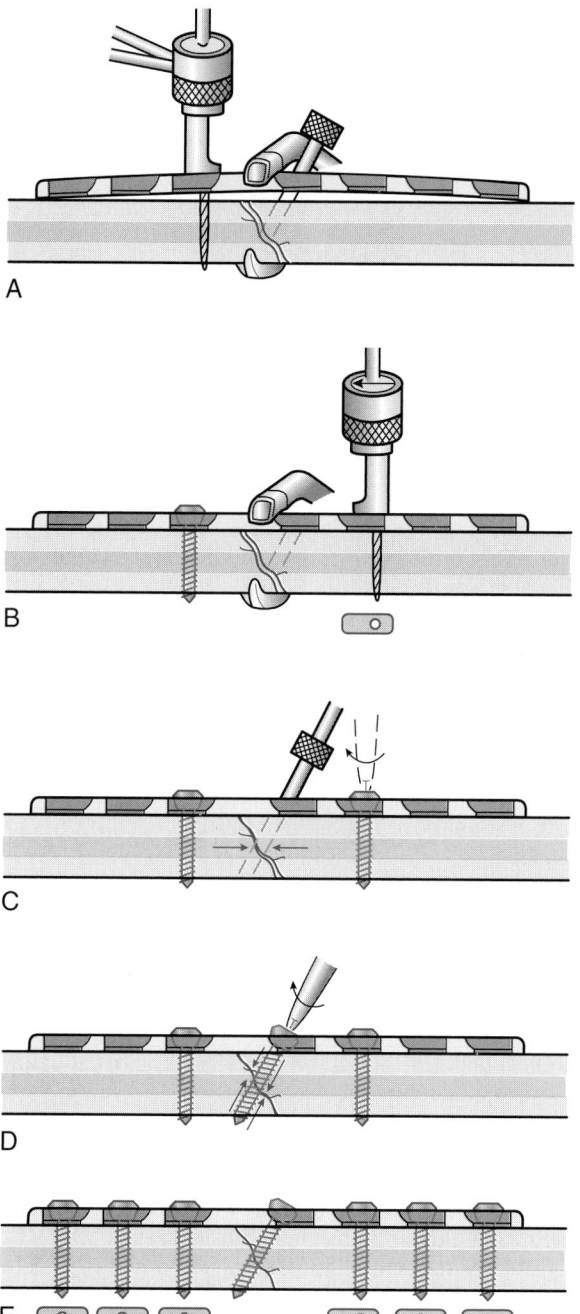

Fig. 1. View. *A,* The fracture is reduced and held with a clamp. The preoperative plan determines the plate position to allow for lag screw placement. A screw is placed in a neutral position. *B,* An eccentrically placed screw is placed on the other side of the fracture. The plate compresses the fracture as the screw is tightened. *C,* A gliding hole and pilot hole are drilled across the fracture. *D,* A lag screw is placed across the fracture and tightened. Compression occurs at the fracture site. *E,* The remaining screws are placed in neutral position to secure the plate to the bone. (Redrawn from Browner BD, Jupiter JB, Levine AM, et al: Skeletal Trauma: Fractures, Dislocations, and Ligamentous Injuries, 2nd ed. Philadelphia, WB Saunders, 1998, p 1433.)

on completion are recommended to ensure adequate reduction and fixation.

Acute bone grafting used to be advocated for comminuted forearm fractures.[1, 2, 4, 11] Most authors cite Anderson et al[2] and Chapman et al[4] when making this recommendation. Anderson et al retrospectively looked at a consecutive series of comminuted forearm fractures that were grafted. Their union rate of comminuted, grafted fractures was identical to that of noncomminuted fractures that were not grafted. They did not compare the comminuted, grafted forearm fractures to a group of comminuted, nongrafted forearm fractures. They assumed that comminuted fractures would have lower rates of union when compared with the noncomminuted, nongrafted fractures. Chapman et al made their recommendation based on the same rationale. Wright et al[28] established the rate of union of comminuted forearm fractures that were not grafted. They excluded open fractures and fractures with segmental bone loss. The union rate of comminuted, nongrafted forearm fractures in the series of Wright et al was 97%. The union rate of comminuted, grafted forearm fractures in the series of Anderson et al and Chapman et al was 98%. Although the three series are not directly comparable, one can safely conclude that routine bone grafting of comminuted forearm fractures is not indicated. Acute bone grafting of forearm fractures should be reserved for those with segmental bone loss and those with open, comminuted fractures in which the local biology predictably needs stimulation.

Segmental bone loss has been treated with interpositional fibular allograft in our hands. A step-cut is made at one junction to provide a greater surface area for integration. The other junction is transverse to allow for rotational correction and then compressed with a plate. Oral antibiotics are used for 6 weeks. Early motion is permitted. Integration with junction obliteration on radiograph usually occurs by 12 weeks, and full rehabilitation begins.

Surgical wounds are closed after copious irrigation. The skin over the radius may be closed alone, but the skin and fascia over the ulna should be closed to prevent muscle herniation. Wounds from open fractures should be thoroughly irrigated and débrided before reduction and internal fixation. The traumatic wounds are left open to drain. The traumatic wounds are closed, or the soft tissue is reconstructed in a delayed fashion after repeat irrigation and débridement at 48 hours. Irrigation and débridement are repeated every 48 hours, if necessary, until wound closure (Fig. 2)

Rigid fixation with a 3.5-mm compression plate remains the mainstay of treatment in open forearm fractures. The concept of biological plating, while important in all fractures, is very important in open fractures. Internal fixation is completed without further injury to the vascular supply of the bone fragments. A bridge plating technique is used to span gaps of segmental bone loss, acting as an "internal external fixator." Bone reconstruction follows soft-tissue reconstruction, as a stable soft-tissue envelope is able to tolerate bone reconstruction.

POSTOPERATIVE MANAGEMENT

Standard monitoring for compartment syndrome should be performed after any forearm injury. Tense compartments and pain out of proportion to the injury are signs and

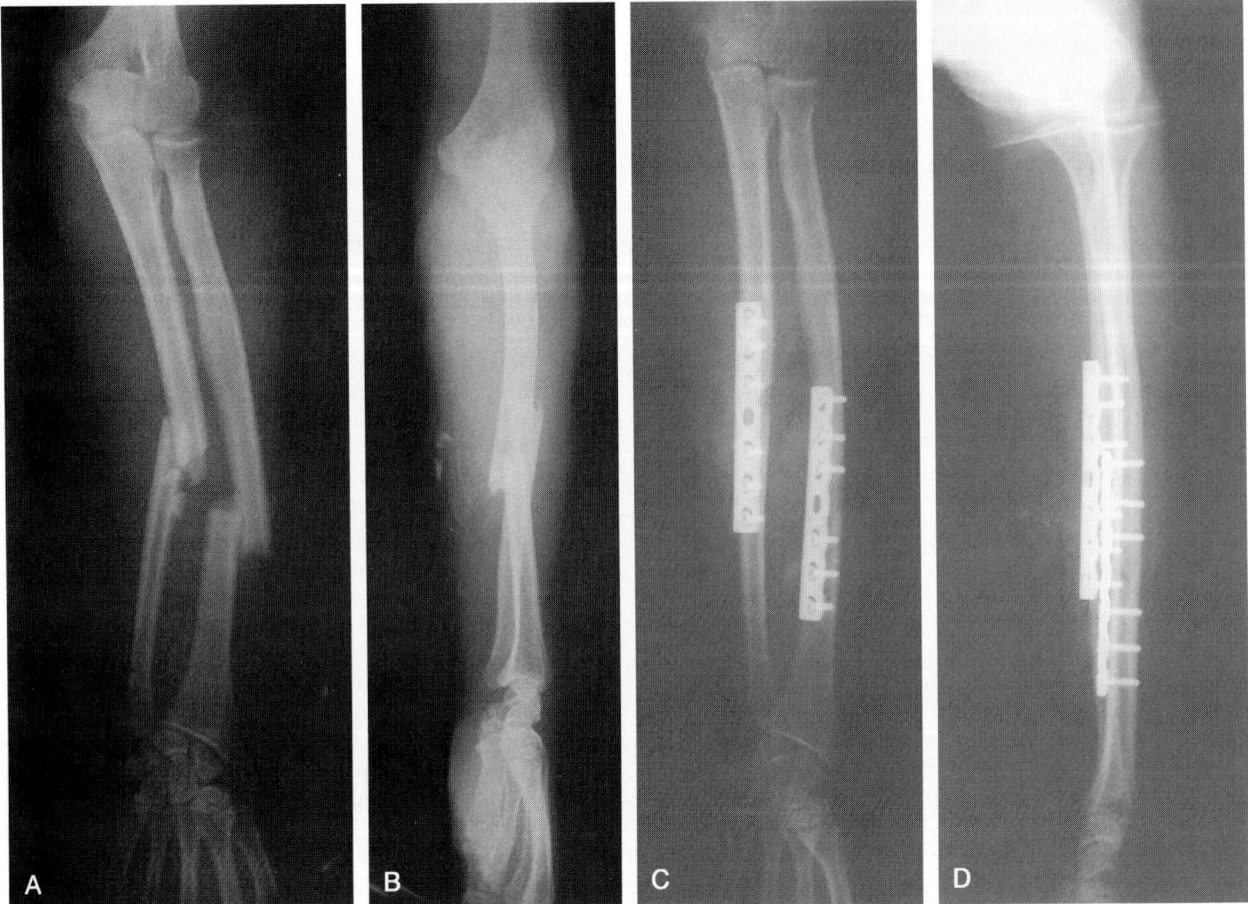

Fig. 2. View. *A,* Anteroposterior radiograph of a 23-year-old male involved in a motor vehicle accident. *B,* Lateral view of the same patient. Bone fragments are visible near the skin. A 3-cm laceration was present at the fracture site. *C,* Postoperative anteroposterior radiograph. *D,* Lateral radiograph. The patient was taken to the operating room for emergency irrigation and débridement. The fracture was reduced and internally fixed with 3.5-mm plates and screws. Healing occurred at 8 weeks. The patient had a full range of motion.

symptoms of an evolving compartment syndrome. As mentioned earlier, a low threshold for performing fasciotomies should be maintained or compartment pressure measurements should be obtained.

Postoperative immobilization depends on the fracture pattern, quality of the fixation achieved, and the reliability of the patient. Initially, all patients are placed in a well-padded, lightly compressive posterior splint for 5 to 7 days. In the reliable patient with a stable fracture and secure fixation, a soft dressing may be used following the initial splint. Patients who are unreliable, have severely comminuted fractures, or have insecure fixation require some type of external immobilization. This consists of a gauntlet cast, long-arm cast, or a functional brace.

Once the patient is comfortable, digital motion is encouraged while in the splint. Sutures are removed at 10 to 14 days. Active-assisted range of motion of the elbow, wrist, and hand is begun once immobilization permits. Activities of daily living are permitted from the onset. No heavy lifting or strenuous activities are allowed until trabeculae cross the fracture site. This radiographic union occurs at approximately 6 to 16 weeks. Persistent pain, abundant callus, and fixation loosening may indicate fixation failure and pseudarthrosis.

COMPLICATIONS AND RESULTS

COMPLICATIONS

As with any surgical procedure, short-term and long-term complications can occur.[18–20, 27, 29–31] The most common early complications include infection, nerve palsy, and compartment syndrome. Late complications include nonunion, synostosis, and refracture after plate removal.

Infection usually presents with erythema, swelling, drainage, and mild pain. Superficial wound infections can be treated with dressing changes and antibiotics. Deep infections usually respond to formal irrigation and débridement, retention of the hardware, and antibiotic therapy.

Nerve palsies in forearm fractures are often secondary to excessive swelling or vigorous retraction. This most often results in a neuropraxia and dysfunction secondary to stretching of the nerve. As there is no anatomic disruption of the involved nerve, return of function is the rule rather than the exception. Treatment consists of functional bracing, range-of-motion exercises, and monitoring for return of function.

The recognition and treatment of compartment syndrome was discussed in the preceding section. An unrecognized compartment syndrome can lead to devastating sequelae, including ischemic muscle contractures. Awareness and a high index of suspicion are mandatory.

The incidence rate of nonunion decreases as the rigidity and security of fixation increases. Nonunion occurs in less than 2% to 5% of the cases treated with compression plating.[2, 4] Persistent pain and lack of radiographic union help identify nonunions. Occasionally, it is difficult to tell if a nonunion exists because of the lack of external callus with open reduction and internal fixation. Treatment consists of autogenous iliac crest bone grafting and replating (if needed).

Synostosis—bony cross union—is a difficult problem.[31] Techniques for preventing synostosis include using two incisions (rather than a single incision) and avoiding placing bone graft along the interosseous membrane. Treatment consists of resection, with overall results being fair. Better results are obtained when the middle third of the forearm is involved, as opposed to the proximal and distal aspects.

Refracture has been documented after plate removal.[18–20, 27] It has occurred more often with removal of a 4.5-mm plate than with removal of a 3.5-mm plate. Greater stress shielding with the 4.5-mm plate may play a role. Plate removal is not routinely recommended. A prominent and irritating ulnar plate is one indication for removal. Avoidance of strenuous activities, with or without external bracing, is recommended for at least 6 weeks after plate removal to help prevent refracture. We recommend replating after refracture. Intramedullary rodding or cast immobilization of nondisplaced fractures has also been suggested.

SHORT-TERM RESULTS AND OUTCOMES

The two primary goals of forearm fracture treatment are union and return of function. Many studies have reported results for treatment with compression plating, which are often difficult to analyze and compare because of uncontrolled variables and lack of study consistency. Anderson et al[2] proposed a simple, objective measure of postfracture function and patient satisfaction to aid in outcome evaluation (Table 2).

Anderson et al[2] retrospectively evaluated 330 acute diaphyseal radius and ulna fractures in 244 patients treated

TABLE 2. OUTCOME EVALUATION AFTER FOREARM FRACTURE TREATMENT

Functional Result	Anderson Criteria
Excellent	Union with <10-degree loss of flexion-extension and <25% loss of pronation-supination
Satisfactory	Union with <20-degree loss of flexion-extension and <50% loss of pronation-supination
Unsatisfactory	Union with >30-degree loss of flexion-extension and >50% loss of pronation-supination
Failure	Nonunion with or without loss of motion

with compression plating. The overall union rate was 97.1%. Radius fracture union occurred in 97.9% of the cases at an average of 7.4 weeks. Ulna fracture union occurred in 96.3% of the cases at an average of 7.3 weeks. Functional results, judged by the above criteria, were excellent or satisfactory in 85% of the cases. Infection rate was 2.9%. Refracture after plate removal occurred in eight bones treated with 4.5-mm plates.

Chapman et al[4] performed a retrospective study of 129 diaphyseal radius and ulna fractures in 87 patients treated with compression plating. Fracture union occurred in 97% and delayed union in 1.5%. The nonunion rate was 1.5%. The average time to union was 12 weeks. Functional results based on the criteria of Anderson et al revealed excellent or satisfactory results in 91%. The majority with unsatisfactory results had more than one injury to the involved extremity. Infection rate was 2.1%. Refracture occurred after removal of two 4.5-mm plates. No refracture occurred after removal of 31 3.5-mm plates.

Many complications related to the treatment of forearm fractures have been attributed to errors in judgment and technique. Meticulous attention to detail including anatomic reduction, rigid internal fixation, limited extraperiosteal dissection, and careful handling of the soft tissues will decrease these complications.

REFERENCES

1. Kellam JF, Jupiter JB: Diaphyseal fractures of the forearm. In Browner BD, Jupiter JB, Levine AM, et al (eds): Skeletal Trauma: Fractures, Dislocations, and Ligamentous Injuries, 2nd ed. Philadelphia, WB Saunders, 1998, p 1421.
2. Anderson LD, Sisk TD, Tooms RE, et al: Compression-plate fixation in acute diaphyseal fractures of the radius and ulna. J Bone Joint Surg Am 1975; 57:287.
3. Burwell HN, Charnley AD: Treatment of forearm fractures in adults with particular reference to plate fixation. J Bone Joint Surg Br 1964; 46:404.
4. Chapman MW, Gordon JE, Zissimos AG: Compression-plate fixation of acute fractures of the diaphyses of the radius and ulna. J Bone Joint Surg Am 1989; 71:159.
5. Dodge HS, Cady GW: Treatment of fractures of the radius and ulna with compression plates. J Bone Joint Surg Am 1972; 54:1167.
6. Duncan R, Geissler W, Freeland AE, et al: Immediate internal fixation of open fractures of the diaphysis of the forearm. J Orthop Trauma 1992; 6:25.
7. Hadden WA, Reschauer R, Seggl W: Results of AO plate fixation of forearm shaft fractures in adults. Injury 1985; 15:44.
8. Schemitsch EH, Richards RR: The effect of malunion on functional outcome after plate fixation of fractures of both bones of the forearm in the adult. J Bone Joint Surg Am 1992; 74:1068.
9. Crenshaw AH Jr: Fractures of the shoulder girdle, arm, and forearm. In Canale ST (ed): Campbell's Operative Orthopaedics, 9th ed. St. Louis, Mosby, 1998, p 2281.
10. Fischer TJ, Lee ML, Rosenwasser MP, et al: Elbow and forearm: Adult trauma. In Beaty JH (ed): Orthopaedic Knowledge Update 6: Home Study Syllabus, 6th ed. Rosemont, IL, American Academy of Orthopaedic Surgeons, 1999, p 232.
11. Richards RR, Corley FG Jr: Fractures of the shafts of the radius and ulna. In Rockwood CA Jr, Green DP, Bucholz RW, et al: Rockwood and Green's Fractures in Adults, 4th ed. Philadelphia, Lippincott-Raven, 1996, p 870.
12. Sage FP: A medullary fixation of fractures of the forearm. J Bone Joint Surg Am 1959; 41:1489.
13. Smith H, Sage FP: Medullary fixation of forearm fractures. J Bone Joint Surg Am 1957; 39:91.
14. Zinar DM: Forearm fractures: Intramedullary nailing. In Wiss DA (ed): Fractures. Philadelphia, Lippincott-Raven, 1998, p 154.

15. Eggers GW: Internal contact splint. J Bone Joint Surg Am 1948; 30:40.
16. Heim U: Forearm and hand/mini-implants. In Müller ME, Allgöwer M, Schneider R, et al (eds): Manual of Internal Fixation, 3rd ed. Berlin, Springer-Verlag, 1991, p 453.
17. Moed BR, Kellam JF, Foster RJ, et al: Immediate internal fixation of open fractures of the diaphysis of the forearm. J Bone Joint Surg Am 1986; 68:1008.
18. Deluca PA, Lindsey RW, Ruwe PA: Refracture of bones of the forearm after removal of compression plates. J Bone Joint Surg Am 1988; 70:1372.
19. Hidaka S, Gustilo RB: Refracture of bones of the forearm after plate removal. J Bone Joint Surg Am 1984; 66:1241.
20. Rosson JW, Shearer JR: Refracture after the removal of plates from the forearm: An avoidable complication. J Bone Joint Surg Br 1991; 73:415.

21. Mikic ZDJ: Galeazzi fracture-dislocations. J Bone Joint Surg Am 1975; 57:1071.
22. Mohan K, Gupta AK, Sharma J, et al: Internal fixation in 50 cases of Galeazzi fracture. Acta Orthop Scand 1988; 59:314.
23. Moore TM, Klein JP, Patzakis MJ, et al: Results of compression-plating of closed Galeazzi fractures. J Bone Joint Surg Am 1985; 67:1015.
24. Reckling FW: Unstable fracture-dislocations of the forearm (Monteggia and Galeazzi lesions). J Bone Joint Surg Am 1982; 64:857.
25. Ring D, Jupiter JB, Simpson NS: Monteggia fractures in adults. J Bone Joint Surg Am 1998; 80:1733.
26. Orthopaedic Trauma Association: Fracture and dislocation compendium. J Orthop Trauma 1996; 10:21.
27. Stern PJ, Drury WJ: Complications of plate fixation of forearm fractures. Clin Orthop 1983; 175:25.

28. Wright RR, Schmeling GJ, Schwab JP: The necessity of acute bone grafting in diaphyseal forearm fractures: A retrospective review. J Orthop Trauma 1997; 11:288.
29. Langkamer VG, Ackroyd CE: Internal fixation of forearm fractures in the 1980s: Lessons to be learnt. Injury 1991; 22:97.
30. Patterson BM: Forearm fractures: Open reduction and internal fixation. In Wiss DA (ed): Fractures. Philadelphia, Lippincott-Raven, 1998, p 143.
31. Vince KG, Miller JE: Cross-union complicating fracture of the forearm. J Bone Joint Surg Am 1987; 69:640.
32. Sarmiento A, Cooper JS, Sinclair WF: Forearm fractures: Early functional bracing: A preliminary report. J Bone Joint Surg Am 1975; 57:297.
33. Marek FM: Axial fixation of forearm fractures. J Bone Joint Surg Am 1961; 43:1099.

section 3 chapter 9

WRIST FRACTURES

Rodrigo Moreno, Rupinder Grewal, and Luis R. Scheker

Summary
- Distal radius fractures, the most common wrist fractures, make up 74% of all forearm fractures.
- The most common mechanism of injury is a fall on a hyperextended, outstretched hand.
- Fractures are diagnosed from physical examination using palpation of the wrist and radiographs.
- Although several classification systems have been developed to identify wrist fractures, the system most commonly used is the Frykman classification.
- Treatment of wrist fractures depends on displacement, comminution, stability, and the site of the fracture. Displaced fractures require anatomic reduction and maintenance of the reduction with appropriate fixation and immobilization.
- Closed reduction with internal or external fixation is the treatment of choice for most fractures. However, if the fracture is unreducible, open reduction must be performed.

Wrist fractures are the result of injury to the interconnecting joints between the carpal bones and the radius and ulna. Distal radius fractures are the most common wrist fractures. An epidemiological study performed in The Netherlands reported the overall incidence of this fracture to be 42 per 10,000 inhabitants.[1] Patients older than 79 years have greater age-specific incidence, and the male-to-female ratio is 1:1.4 in all the age groups. In patients older than 50 years, this ratio changes to 1:6.[1] Seventy-four per-

cent of all the fractures of the forearm occur at the distal radius.[2]

Scaphoid fractures are the second most common fracture of the wrist. A study published in 1999 reported the annual incidence as 4.3 per 10,000 inhabitants.[3] Scaphoid fractures represent 60% of the carpal fractures and 11% of the hand fractures.[3] The most common mechanisms of injury for all types of wrist fractures are accidental falls, sport injuries, and motor vehicle accidents.[1]

HISTORY OF WRIST FRACTURES

Long before the advent of the radiograph, Pouteau[4] in 1783 and Colles[5] in 1814 described wrist fractures and dislocations. They differentiated between fracture of the distal radius and dislocation of the carpus and observed abnormal mobility of the ulna. Sir Astley Cooper[6] published a book entitled *A Treatise on Dislocations and Fractures of Joints* in 1822. Barton,[7] in 1838, described anteroposterior fracture-dislocations of the wrist.

However, Roentgen's discovery of the x-ray in 1895 greatly affected the understanding of fractures. It led Destot[8] to investigate wrist problems, and he was able to combine his studies of wrist anatomy and clinical conditions with radiographic interpretations. Destot recognized the angulatory changes associated with diastasis of the scaphoid and lunate but did not understand their importance.

The concept of carpal instability began to surface again as a number of papers described scaphoid instabilities, although the secondary characteristics of scapholunate diastasis or midcarpal angulatory changes were seldom mentioned. It was not until Fisk[9] described carpal instability from fracture to the scaphoid, in his 1968 Hunterian Lecture, that this condition received serious attention. In 1972, Linscheid and colleagues[10] further described carpal instability as collapse deformities in the sagittal plane, either as dorsal intercalated segment instabilities (DISI) or volar intercalated segment instabilities (VISI). Associated ligament damage with distal radius fractures is not uncommon. Arthroscopic studies have shown a high incidence of ligament injuries.[11]

ANATOMY

The wrist consists of (1) eight carpal bones aligned in proximal and distal rows of four bones each and (2) the distal joint surfaces of the two forearm bones, the radius and the ulna. From radial to ulnar, the carpal bones are as follows: proximally, the scaphoid, lunate, triquetrum, and pisiform (as seen from a palmar view) and distally, the trapezium, trapezoid, capitate, and hamate (Fig. 1). The wrist joints are as follows:

- Radiocarpal joint, which connects the distal radius with the proximal surfaces of the scaphoid and lunate.
- Ulnocarpal joint, which connects the distal ulna via the triangular fibrocartilage (TFC) with the lunate and the triquetrum.
- Joints of the proximal carpal row, which connect the scaphoid, lunate, and triquetrum via the dorsal, palmar, and interosseous ligaments.

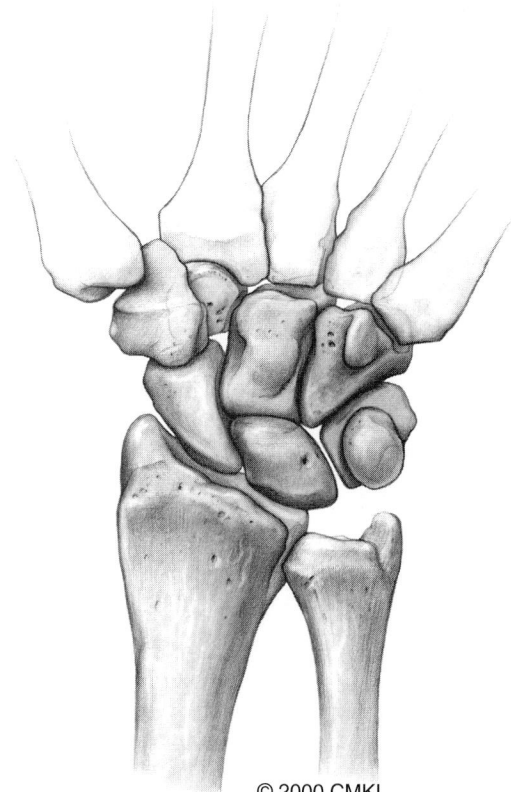

© 2000 CMKI

Fig. 1. Anatomy of the wrist.

- Midcarpal joint, which connects the head of the capitate and hamate with a concavity formed by the scaphoid, lunate, and triquetrum and radially connects the trapezium and trapezoid with the scaphoid.
- Distal radioulnar joint (DRUJ).

The DRUJ also can be considered a part of the forearm joint complex, which consists of the proximal and distal radioulnar joints (which should be regarded as a single joint because they can move only together) and the interosseous membrane. These three structures work together to create joint stability, produce forearm rotation, and provide lifting capabilities.

The distal radial metaphysis is primarily cancellous bone with thin cortices and has three articular surfaces, the scaphoid fossa (articulates radius with scaphoid), the lunate fossa (articulates radius with lunate), and the sigmoid notch (articulates radius with ulnar head).[8] The radial inclination of the distal radius in the anteroposterior (AP) view is 22 degrees (13 to 30 degrees), the volar tilt is 11 degrees (1 to 21 degrees), and the sigmoid notch is inclined distally and medially by approximately 22 degrees. The DRUJ normally has an ulnar variance of +0.14 mm with the elbow flexed 90 degrees and in neutral position of the forearm. In pronation, the ulnar length increases up to 0.69 mm.[12]

The dorsal extensor tendons crossing the wrist run inside the extensor compartments that hold the tendons close to the bone for mechanical advantage. Most of the palmar flexor tendons are constrained within the carpal tunnel, except for the flexor carpi radialis (FCR), flexor carpi ulnaris (FCU), and palmaris longus (PL). The flexor carpi ulnaris is the most powerful wrist muscle because of its short muscle fibers. The lack of soft tissues at the wrist makes the nerves susceptible to injury.

The radiocarpal ligaments run from the radius to lunate and triquetrum dorsally and to the capitate, lunate, and triquetrum palmarly in an arrangement similar to that of the reins on a horse, preventing the carpus from translocating ulnarly. Ulnocarpal ligaments run from the TFC complex (TFCC) and the ulnar styloid to the capitate, lunate, and triquetrum. These ligaments play a role in fracture patterns and intra-articular fragment displacement.

The TFCC is the main stabilizer of the DRUJ.[13] It comprises a fibrocartilage disc, which has a shock-absorbent cartilaginous center, and thickening in the periphery, which consists of the volar radioulnar and dorsal radioulnar ligaments. These ligaments originate from the distal sigmoid notch and gain insertion into the fovea and styloid, actually creating two volar and two dorsal ligaments that lock the DRUJ in full pronation and full supination, providing stability. The other elements of the TFCC are the ulnar collateral ligament, the extensor carpi ulnaris (ECU) tendon sheath, and the DRUJ capsule. The TFCC gives origin to the palmar ulnocarpal ligaments and blends into the palmar and dorsal radioulnar ligaments. It blends distally into the ulnar collateral ligament. The space between the ligament insertion into the fovea and the styloid is called the prestyloid recess, as seen in an arthrogram.

The nerve supply for the wrist comes from the nerves that cross the joint, which include the median nerve, the ulnar nerve, the superficial radial nerve, and the posterior interosseous nerve. Buck-Gramcko[14] identified a total of 13 branches in his 1977 work.

BIOMECHANICS

The wrist transfers force and motion of the hand to the forearm and upper extremity. The wrist has three types of movements: flexion-extension, radial-ulnar deviation, and supination-pronation. Flexion and extension of the wrist occur at the radiocarpal joint and the midcarpal joint. Midcarpal extension involves radial deviation, and midcarpal flexion is associated with some ulnar deviation. The proximal row of the carpal bones flexes during radial deviation and extends during ulnar deviation. Pronation and supination occur when the radius rotates around a fixed ulna through the proximal RUJ and the DRUJ.

During gripping while lifting, two forces pass through the forearm. The forearm muscles generate an axial load, which runs from the hand to the distal radius to the capitellum of the elbow. A transverse force runs from the hand to the radius to the ulnar head and is the force of gravity (resistance) against which the arm has to lift (Fig. 2). A cadaver study published in 1987 found that the axial load transmitted through the ulnocarpal joint was 21%, and through the radiocarpal joint, 79%.[15] When dorsal angulations of the radius increased more than 10 degrees to 45 degrees, the load through the ulna rose from 21% to greater than 67%.

Load also changes with ulnar variance. For example, with ulnar positive variance, the contact area of the lunate changes from the radiolunate to the TFCC. In 1986, Werner and colleagues[16] observed that lengthening of the ulna by 2.5 mm raised the force borne by the ulnocarpal joint from 18.4% to 41.9%.

PATHOGENESIS

The most common mechanism of injury to produce wrist fractures, particularly distal radius fractures, is a fall on a hyperextended, outstretched hand. Sports-related injuries are the second most common, with higher incidences predominantly in adolescents and young adults, and motor

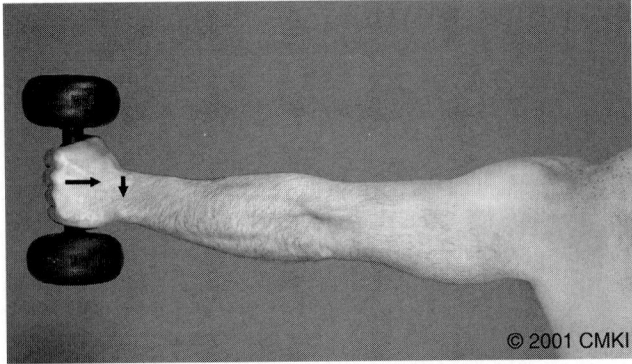

Fig. 2. View. During gripping while lifting, two forces pass through the forearm, as indicated by arrows. The axial load is generated by the forearm muscles. The transverse force is the force of gravity against which the arm must lift. The ulna passively lifts the radius, whereas the humerus is elevated by the deltoid.

vehicle accidents are third.[1] The palmar aspect fails in tension, and the fracture propagates dorsally, causing failure in compression and shear stresses at the dorsal surface. Dorsal and volar Barton's (shearing intra-articular) fractures are commonly associated with high-velocity impacts, such as in motor vehicle accidents.[17]

Richards and associates[11] used arthroscopy to examine the association between distal radius fractures and soft-tissue intra-articular injuries. They found TFCC tears in 35% of intra-articular distal radius fractures and in 53% of extra-articular fractures. Scapholunate injuries were present in 21.5% of intra-articular fractures and in 6.7% of extra-articular fractures. A higher possibility of TFCC tears occurs in fractures with a greater amount of displacement and radial shortening. The amount of energy associated with the injury, extent of ulnar-radial deviation at the time of impact, direction of applied force, its point of application, and the strength of the ligaments and bone determine the extent of displacement and amount of radial shortening.[11]

The most commonly fractured carpal bone is the scaphoid. Generally, scaphoid fractures are caused when a person falls on an outstretched arm with the wrist dorsiflexed or jams the arm into another person (such as while playing football).[18] The distal third of the scaphoid receives a reaction force when the hand contacts the floor in dorsiflexion.[19] Fractures to the hamate usually occur on the hook area. Of the 59 patients with fractures of the hook of the hamate reviewed by Stark and associates,[20] 54 had sports-related injuries that occurred while they were swinging baseball bats, golf clubs, or tennis rackets.

CLINICAL FEATURES

Symptoms commonly associated with a wrist fracture are pain, tenderness, swelling, crepitus, deformity of the wrist (like the dinner fork deformity seen in Colles' fracture), and loss of range of motion. Fractures can show up without evident deformity, as in non-displaced fractures, but with tenderness at the site.

Evaluation of a wrist injury should begin with a detailed history of the incident involving the injury. It should include the time of the injury, the onset and presentation of symptoms, and the position of the wrist at the time of injury. In addition, one should consider the amount of stress to which the wrist was subjected, the activities that aggravate, re-create, or improve pain, and the activity the patient was participating in at the time of the injury. Onset of symptoms can indicate the area of the wrist in which the fracture has occurred; for example, sudden onset and persistence of ulnar-sided wrist pain may indicate a fracture of the hook of the hamate. The time that has elapsed from injury to presentation affects presenting symptoms as well as treatment options.

PHYSICAL EXAMINATION

A visual assessment of pain or limitation of motion should be made before a physical examination. This assessment should include the patient's ability to remove a coat or get out of a chair, willingness to shake hands, and posturing of the extremities. Also, both upper extremities should be observed to assess atrophy (in late presentation), discoloration, and asymmetry. Areas of ecchymosis, erythema, or obvious deformity should be noted. Such symptoms may indicate an underlying fracture that should be assessed radiographically.

Palpation of the wrist may help establish a possible diagnosis. For example, if palpation of the radial styloid reveals tenderness, contusion or fracture of the styloid may be present. Pain upon palpation of the large sulcus just distal to the radial styloid, known as the anatomic snuffbox, or palpation of the scaphoid tubercle (which is located along the distal course of the flexor carpi radialis tendon on the palmar aspect of the wrist) may suggest a scaphoid fracture. The scaphoid can be palpated easily with touch of the distal two-thirds of the bone volarly at the base of the thenar area and dorsally through the snuffbox. The hook of the hamate (which is approximately 1 cm radial and distal to the pisiform and just proximal to the base of the fifth metacarpal) is easily felt, and pain on firm palpation of the area may suggest a fracture or nonunion from a previous injury. Palpation over the volar or dorsal surface of the DRUJ or at the fovea of the ulnar styloid may reveal tenderness and swelling due to acute injury to the DRUJ.

Once palpation has been performed, the patient's range of motion, consisting of flexion, extension, ulnar and radial deviation, and supination and pronation, should be carefully assessed. Active and passive ranges of motion should be compared with those in the contralateral limb. Restriction of motion that is secondary to pain or due to mechanical dysfunction should be noted. Ligamentous injuries can be identified through assessment of the stability of the joint, which is performed by placement of stress on the joint and comparison with the contralateral side. Ligamentous injuries, which cannot be seen on radiographs, can be more detrimental than fractures.

Assessing the neurovascular status of the wrist, principally of the median nerve, is an important aspect of the physical examination. It is common to see median nerve praxis in heavily comminuted and displaced distal radius fractures. Both two-point discrimination and thenar muscle function should be recorded.

INVESTIGATION

Radiographic evaluation routinely includes posteroanterior (PA), lateral, and oblique views. In displaced fractures, the radiographic diagnosis is evident, but fractures are often missed when they manifest without displacement. When scaphoid fractures are suspected, we recommend using a PA view, with the patient's hand making a fist and placing it in ulnar deviation so that the scaphoid extends (Fig. 3). If scapholunate ligament injuries are present, this view makes it possible to see dissociation.

If fracture is suspected but is not seen on plain radiographs, the wrist should be immobilized; if symptoms persist, new radiographs should be obtained within 2 weeks. If no fracture is seen on the second set of radiographs and symptoms persist, a bone scan is useful.[21] Computed tomography (CT) and magnetic resonance imaging (MRI) are helpful in more complex cases. For example, if a subtle subluxation of the DRUJ is suspected, computed tomography of the DRUJ in full supination and pronation may help diagnosis of the injury. Once the existence of a fracture has been confirmed, neurological and vascular deficits

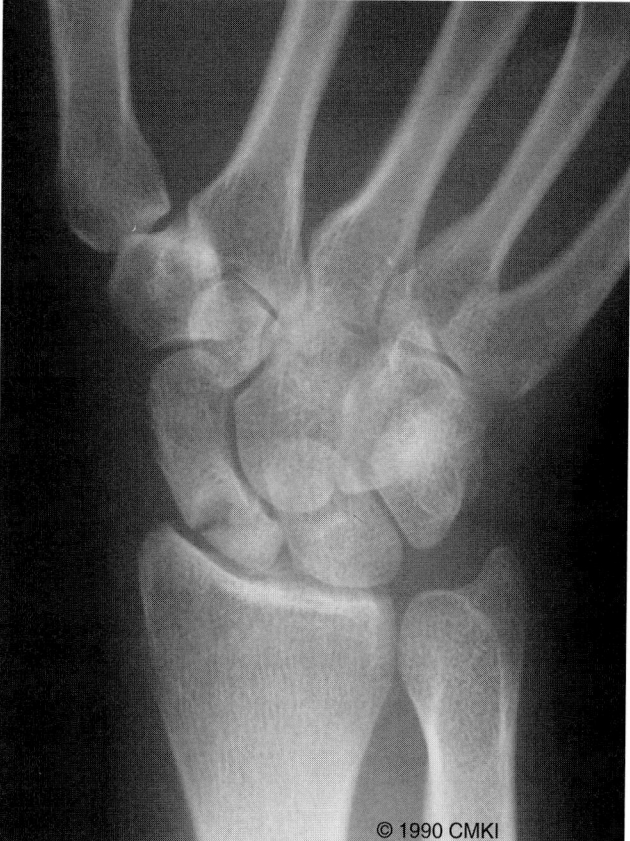

© 1990 CMKI

Fig. 3. PA view. This is a view of a scaphoid fracture with the patient's hand in ulnar deviation so that the scaphoid extends.

should be assessed, along with associated carpal or DRUJ instability.

MANAGEMENT

After the location of the fracture has been determined, the first step in the management of wrist fracture is to classify the type of fracture. Classification helps determine the choice of treatment. Classification systems have been developed for fractures of both the distal radius and the scaphoid.

CLASSIFICATION SYSTEMS FOR DISTAL RADIUS FRACTURES

The numerous classification systems for distal radius fractures are based on eponyms, fracture pattern, or mechanism of injury.

Eponymic Classification

The fracture eponyms were based on clinical deformity only, before the discovery and diagnostic use of radiographs.

Colles' fracture, described in 1814, occurs when a person falls forward on an extended arm and on the palm of the hand (Fig. 4). It is generally extra-articular and occurs within 2 to 5 cm proximal to the wrist joint, with dorsal

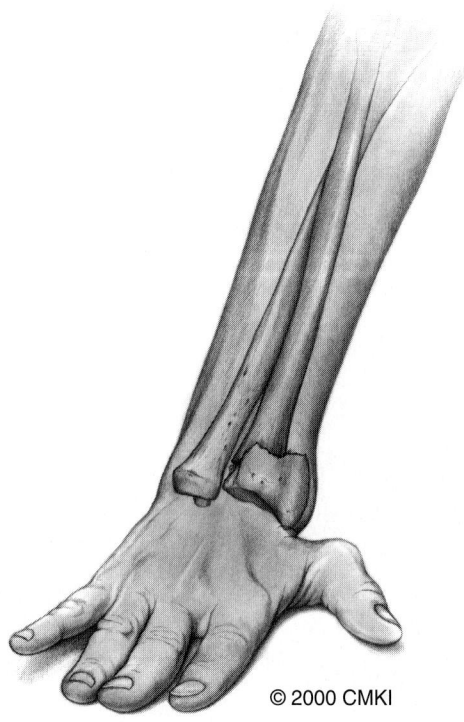

Fig. 4. Colles' fracture.

Other Classification Systems

Other classification systems are the AO, modified Gartland universal, Melone, Mayo Clinic, and Fernandez. The AO classification was developed to aid in the diagnosis of more severe distal radius injuries.[25] It comprises type A (extra-articular), type B (partial articular), and type C (completely articular). These types are further subdivided according to the bone that was fractured and the comminution of the fracture.

The modified Gartland universal classification is treatment-directed and based on fracture location.[26] Type I is an extra-articular nondisplaced fracture; type II is an extra-articular displaced fracture; type III is an intra-articular nondisplaced fracture; and type IV is an intra-articular displaced fracture. These types are further subdivided as A (reducible stable fracture), B (reducible unstable fractures), and C (unreducible unstable fractures).

The Melone and the Mayo Clinic classification systems further describe intra-articular fractures of the radius. Melone[27] classified intra-articular injury by considering the radial articular surfaces as having four components—radial shaft, radial styloid, dorsal medial fragment, and palmar medial fragment. Type I fractures can be either nondisplaced or displaced but are stable after closed reduction, and the joint surfaces have been preserved. Type II fractures are unstable, with comminution and displacement of the medial complex. Type III fractures are unstable, with displacement of the medial complex and an additional spike fragment from the comminuted radial shaft; this additional fragment can project into the flexor compartment of the wrist, damaging the medial nerve or adjacent tendons. Type IV fractures show a wide separation or rotation of dorsal and palmar medial fragments with disruption of distal radial articulations (Fig. 7).

The Mayo Clinic classification further subdivides intra-articular fractures to stress that other surfaces may require

angulation, radial displacement, and shortening with a dinner fork deformity.[22] Colles' fracture is the most common distal radius fracture.

Smith's fracture, which is also called a reverse Colles' fracture, occurs from falling backward on an extended arm and on the palm of the hand.[23] It was first described in 1847. It is in the same area as Colles' fracture but has a palmar displacement with a garden spade deformity.

Barton's fracture is a dorsal or palmar lip fracture of the distal radius with subluxation or dislocation of the carpus (Fig. 5).[23] The dorsal fracture occurs after a fall on an extended arm with the wrist pushed in extreme extension. The palmar fracture is also called a Smith II fracture, because the palmar lip is fractured and the hand is displaced palmarly, as in Smith's fracture.

Frykman Classification

The Frykman classification is the most commonly used system for distal radius fractures.[24] It differentiates extra-articular from intra-articular injuries, but it does not stress fracture stability, comminution, or displacement. The classification types are based on the fracture pattern of the distal radius with or without an accompanying distal ulna fracture (Fig. 6). Types I and II are extra-articular with and without a distal ulna fracture, respectively. Types III and IV involve the radiocarpal joint with and without a distal ulna fracture, respectively. Types V and VI involve the distal radioulnar joint with and without a distal ulna fracture, respectively. Types VII and VIII involve both the radiocarpal and the distal radioulnar joints with and without a distal ulna fracture, respectively.

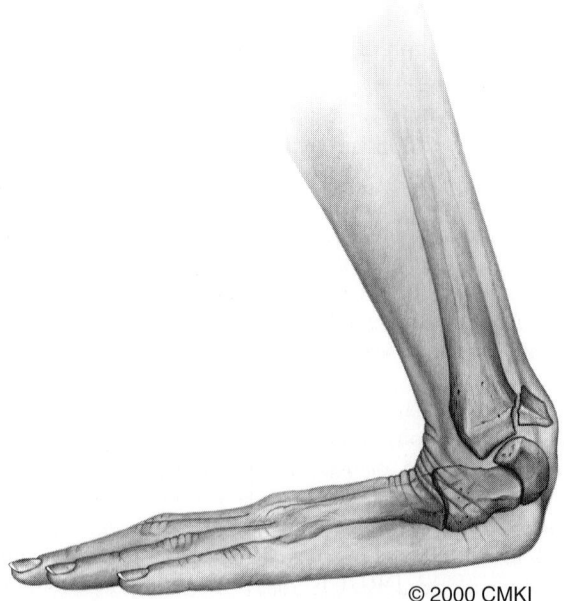

Fig. 5. **Barton's fracture.** (From Orthopaedic Knowledge Update: Spine. Rosemont, IL, AAOS, 1997, p 92. Originally from Cybulski G: Contemp Neurosurg 1992; 14:1.)

the one that caused the injury facilitates treatment.[29] Type I fractures are extra-articular bending fractures of the metaphysis, like Colles' fracture. Type II are shearing fractures of the joint surface, like Barton's fracture. Type III are compression fractures of the joint, like die punch fractures. Type IV are avulsion fractures of the ligamentous attachments, like styloid fractures. Type V are high-velocity injuries with a combination of the preceding types.

Fernandez also developed a prognostic classification of associated DRUJ injury based on the residual DRUJ stability and fracture after reduction of the radial fracture. Type I injuries are stable DRUJ lesions in which the joint is

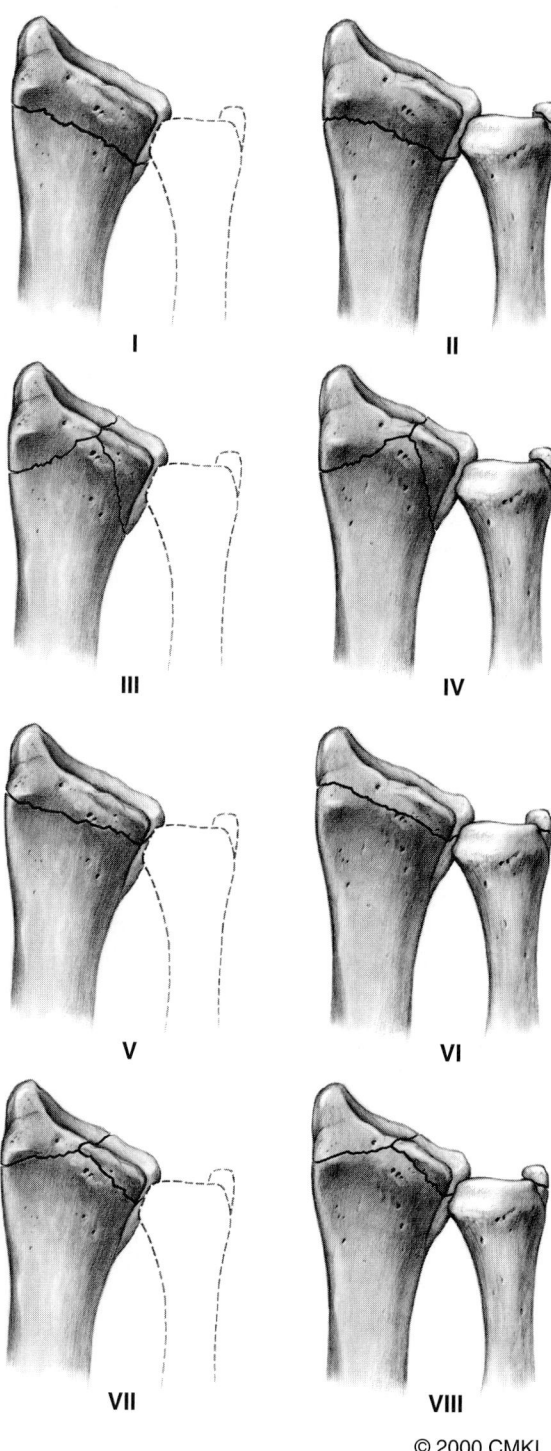

Fig. 6. Frykman's classification of distal radius fractures.

© 2000 CMKI

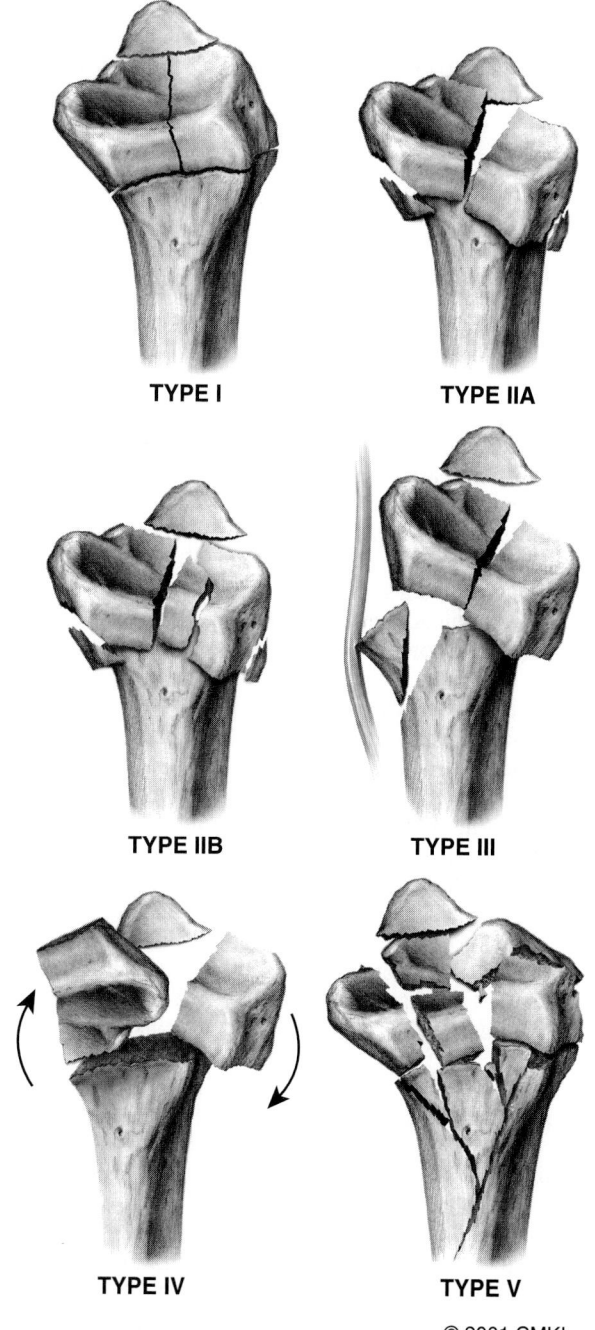

TYPE I   **TYPE IIA**

TYPE IIB   **TYPE III**

TYPE IV   **TYPE V**

© 2001 CMKI

Fig. 7. Melone's classification of distal radius fractures. (From Orthopaedic Knowledge Update: Spine. Rosemont, IL, AAOS, 1997, p 93. Originally from Cybulski G: Contemp Neurosurg 1992; 14:1.)

treatment in addition to the radial metaphysis and the radial shaft.[28] The three articular surfaces of the radius are regarded as separate components: type I fractures are nondisplaced; type II are displaced and involve the radioscaphoid joint; type III are displaced and involve the radiolunate joint; and type IV are displaced and involve both the radiocarpal joints and the sigmoid fossa.

The Fernandez classification is based on the mechanism of injury and the belief that applying a force opposite to

stable and congruent; type IA injuries include avulsion of the ulnar styloid tip, and type IB are stable fractures of the ulnar neck. Type II injuries are unstable DRUJ lesions with subluxation or dislocation of the joint; type IIA include TFCC substance tears, and type IIB are avulsion fractures of the base of the ulnar styloid. Type III injuries are potentially unstable as a result of skeletal disruption of the joint; type IIIA involve the sigmoid notch, and type IIIB involve the ulnar head.[30]

CLASSIFICATION SYSTEMS FOR SCAPHOID FRACTURES

Scaphoid fracture classification systems are the Mayo classification, Rüsse's classification, and Herbert's classification. The Mayo classification is based on location of the fracture.[18] It is divided into tuberosity fractures, distal third fractures, middle third fractures, and proximal pole fractures. Rüsse's classification is based on the direction of the fracture: horizontal oblique, transverse, or vertical oblique.[31]

Herbert's classification is based on stability and is divided into four categories.[32] Type A, stable acute fractures, includes fracture of the tubercle and incomplete waist fracture. Type B, unstable acute fractures, includes distal oblique fracture (B1), complete waist fracture (B2), proximal pole fracture (B3), and trans-scaphoid perilunate fracture (B4). Type C are fractures with delayed union. In type D fractures, nonunion is established, and there may be fibrous and pseudoarthrosis features (Fig. 8).

Cooney and associates[33] defined displaced unstable scaphoid fractures as having (1) more than 1 mm of offset, (2) more than 15 degrees of lunocapitate angulation, or (3) more than 45 degrees of scapholunate angulation. Weber[19] described angulated scaphoid fractures that are hinged open dorsally on the intact palmar lateral ligament, and are associated with mild dorsiflexion instability of the lunate.

TREATMENT OF DISTAL RADIUS FRACTURES

In the choice of treatment for fractures, the patient's age and general medical condition should be considered. Treatment depends on the displacement, comminution, stability, and site of the fracture. DRUJ reduction is a very important component of the fracture reduction. When reduction is inadequate or the intra-articular step-off is greater than 2 mm, results are poor and post-traumatic arthritis may occur.[34]

Fractures can be categorized as nondisplaced (extra- or intra-articular) or displaced. Nondisplaced fractures can be treated initially with a long-arm cast in a neutral position of pronation and supination and volar or dorsal flexion for 4 to 6 weeks. If the ulnar styloid is fractured, it should be immobilized with a long-arm cast in neutral position for 6 weeks and then, if necessary, a short-arm cast for 3 more weeks to limit forearm use and prevent displacement. Extreme flexion should be avoided, because it increases carpal tunnel pressure and limits function of the flexor tendons. To maintain the reduction, three-point fixation should be used during application of the cast. When a DRUJ injury is present, the forearm should be immobilized in supination, if possible.

Displaced fractures require anatomic reduction and maintenance of the reduction with appropriate fixation and immobilization. Altissimi and colleagues[35] found that in 71%

of patients treated with cast only, the initial deformity was reproduced. For this reason, some method of maintaining stability for dorsal cortex strength is necessary. This can be achieved through either closed reduction with internal or external fixators or open reduction.

Percutaneous pinning techniques include those described by Clancey[36] (crossed pins inserted from the radial styloid and from the most ulnar aspect of the dorsal radius), Rayhack[37] (pins inserted from radius to ulna), De Palma[38] (ulnar pinning), and Kapandji[39] (dorsal and radial pins into the fracture site and across to the opposite cortex) as well as the use of intramedullary pins such as the Ulson device[40] (Fig. 9). When closed reduction is achieved by ligamentotaxis, these techniques are very useful. A large percentage of distal radius fractures can be treated through closed reduction and percutaneous pinning. Fractures that usually cannot be fixed adequately are complex articular fractures (AO type C3), volar intra-articular displaced fractures, and marginal shearing fractures of the volar lunate facet. These types of fractures usually require open reduction techniques.

External fixators can be used alone or in combination with percutaneous pinning. If fixators are used alone, excessive distraction is required to maintain reduction, and complications such as disuse atrophy, joint stiffness, and iatrogenic nonunion can develop. When used in unstable fractures, external fixators should be combined with percutaneous pinning and bone grafting.[41] External fixators are contraindicated in patients who have osteoporotic bones, are unable to provide pin care, or are uncooperative or mentally unstable.[42]

Open reduction is indicated when closed methods are unsuccessful in restoring the anatomy of the distal radius. Plating techniques include the use of 3.5-mm T-plates, of PI plates,[43] and of double plating dorsally with two one-quarter tube plates or with 2.0-mm titanium plates.

For volar shearing fractures, 3.5-mm T-plates are useful for reducing the fracture through a buttress effect. In some intra-articular unreducible fractures, such plates could be placed dorsally so that the 3.5-mm screws can securely fix the distal fragments. The disadvantages of these plates are the difficulty in contouring the plate to the dorsal cortex and the relatively large screws. Also, when plates are applied to the dorsal cortex of the distal radius, tendon irritation of the extensor compartments may occur.

The PI plate was designed as a low-profile plate, precontoured distally to the curvatures of the dorsal distal radius. It uses 2.4-mm self-tapping screws or 1.8-mm buttress pins distally and 2.7-mm self-tapping screws proximally.[41] Although the screws and pins were designed to be recessed into the plate to diminish irritation of the overlying extensor tendons, extensor tendon irritation and rupture have been reported in the literature.[44-46]

A third technique for stabilizing distal radius fractures, double plating with the use of two 2.0-mm titanium plates or two quarter-tube plates, has been described. Hahnloser and associates[47] reported fewer complications with double plating than with the PI plate. Further trials involving more cases are necessary.

For intra-articular fractures, arthroscopy-assisted reduction with fixation also has been described. This procedure should be performed 3 to 7 days after injury to avoid swelling and complications from fluid infusion into an

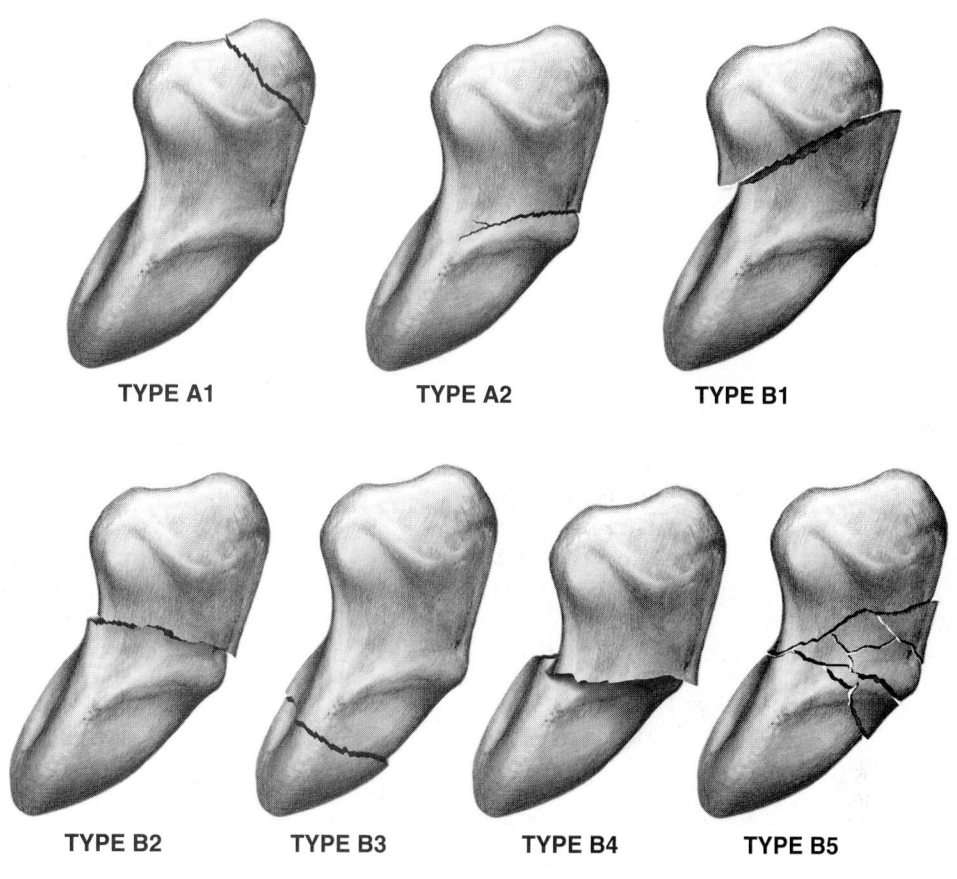

TYPE A1 **TYPE A2** **TYPE B1**

TYPE B2 **TYPE B3** **TYPE B4** **TYPE B5**

Fig. 8. Herbert's and Rüsse's classifications of scaphoid fractures. (From Orthopaedic Knowledge Update: Spine. Rosemont, IL, AAOS, 1997, p 93. Originally from Cybulski G: Contemp Neurosurg 1992; 14:1.)

TYPE C **TYPE D1** **TYPE D2**

HERBERT CLASSIFICATION

© 2001 CMKI

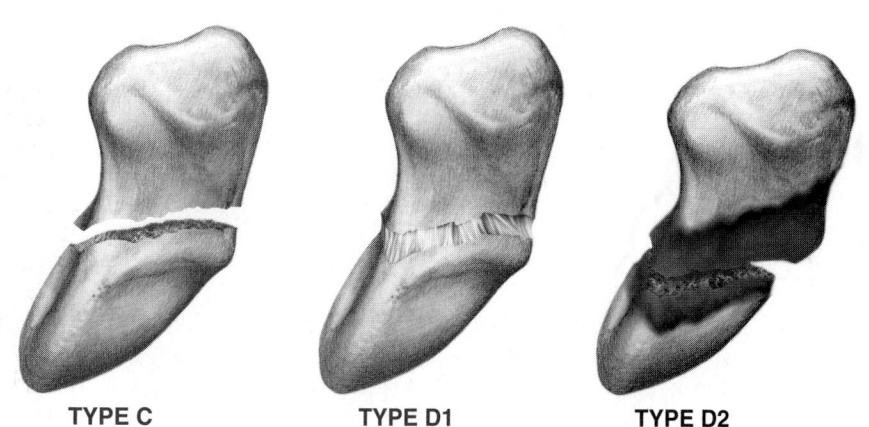

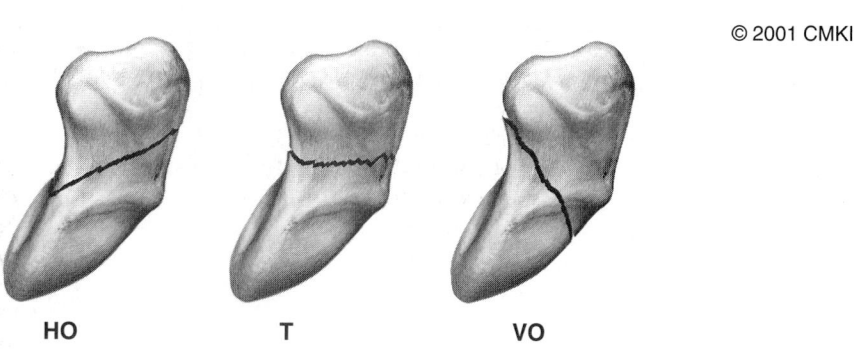

HO **T** **VO**

RUSSE CLASSIFICATION

© 2001 CMKI

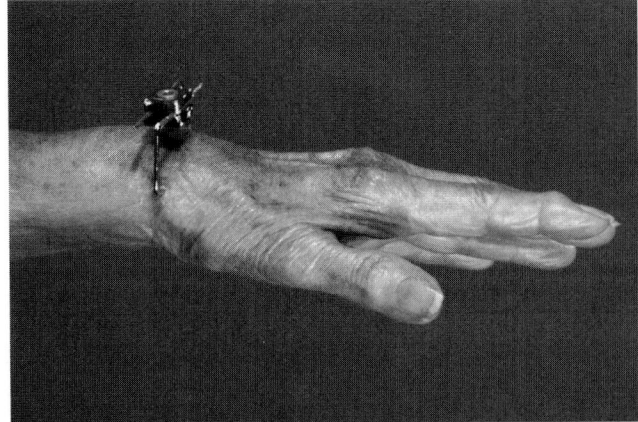

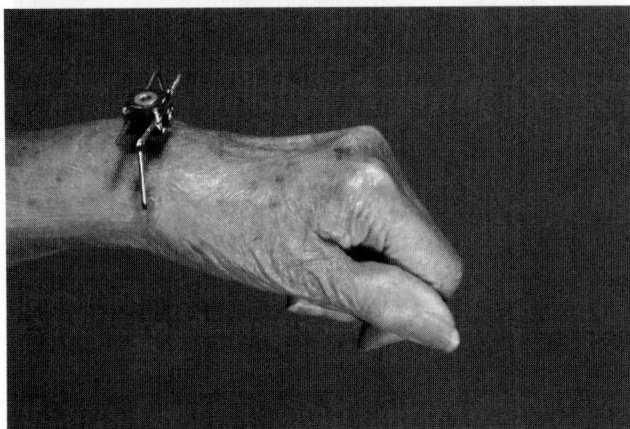

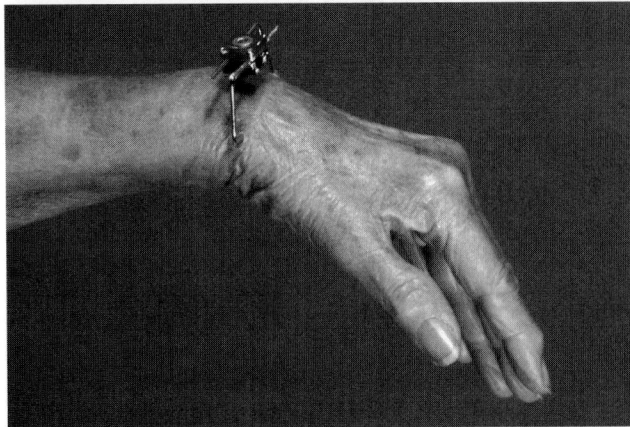

© 1997 CMKI

Fig. 9. The Ulson device. It maintains reduction while enabling mobilization of the wrist. (From Regan JJ, McAfee PC, Mack MJ: Atlas of Endoscopic Spine Surgery. St. Louis, Quality Medical Publishing, Inc., 1995.)

acute fracture. A bone graft may be needed when marked comminution and loss of dorsal support occur.[11] Contraindications to arthroscopy are open fractures and the presence of severe swelling with increased risk of compartment syndrome.

The Authors' Approach to the Treatment of Distal Radius Fractures

We approach treatment progressively, starting with a closed reduction in the operating room with the patient under anesthesia. We perform reduction using finger-traps or longitudinal traction with extension of the wrist and then slight flexion and ulnar deviation. The reduction is evaluated with a scan, and the type of fixation is chosen. The length of the radius is considered to prevent ulnar impaction and incongruity of the DRUJ.[16] Anatomic reduction of intra-articular fragments is essential to diminish the possibility of post-traumatic arthritis.[34] Volar and dorsal angulation must be restored to a slight volar inclination or minimum less than 10 degrees of dorsal angulation[48] to prevent DRUJ incongruity and instability.

Three fracture categories are differentiated: reducible stable, reducible unstable, and unreducible. If the fracture is reducible stable, without or with minimum dorsal comminution, the preferred treatment is to perform a percutaneous pinning technique or intramedullary pinning using the Ulson device. If the fracture is reducible unstable, we evaluate the comminution and the fragments involved. If the fracture is unstable because it has a volar medial facet, as described by Melone,[27] we use a volar approach and stabilize the fragment with a volar plate (Fig. 10).

If the fracture is unreducible, open reduction must be performed. Shearing fractures, such as the Barton volar or dorsal fracture, usually are unstable and difficult to reduce in a closed manner. In these cases, we prefer plating with 3.5-mm T-plates if the fragments are large enough to be

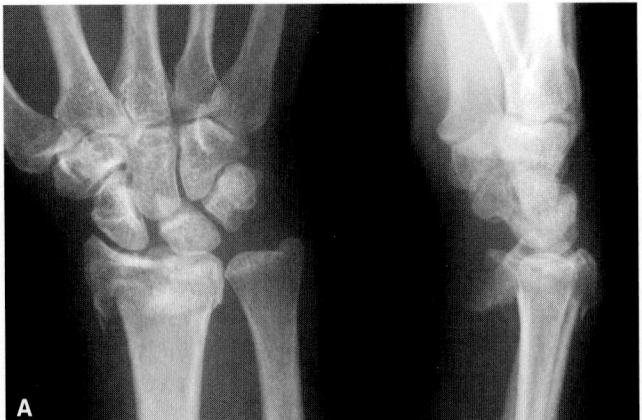

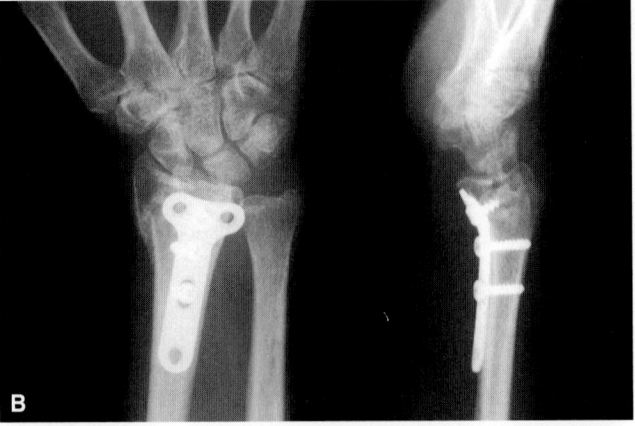

© 1993 CMKI

Fig. 10. View. *A,* Unstable fracture with a displaced volar fragment. *B,* Fixation with a volar 3.5-mm T-plate.

fixed with 3.5-mm screws or with PI plates if small distal fragments are observed. When we use the PI plate, we try to not cut it, and we recommend its early removal (within 5 to 6 months) to diminish the risk of extensor tendon rupture. In addition, when a PI plate is used, part of the extensor retinaculum should be placed between the plate and the tendons to diminish tendon irritation. We believe that the sharp edges observed when plates are cut[49] are important factors in the several extensor tendon ruptures reported in the literature.[44-46] In cases in which both volar and dorsal fragments (coronal fracture) are present, percutaneous pinning can be used to stabilize the displaced fragments dorsally, and bone grafting associated with a volar plate can maintain the reduction volarly.

Complications of Distal Radius Fractures

Malunion is common in complex comminuted distal radius fractures. Pain results from radiocarpal, ulnocarpal, or radioulnar arthritis secondary to malunited fractures. Pin track infections may occur with percutaneous techniques and with external fixators. Superficial nerve injuries may occur, especially with percutaneous pinning or external fixators. Extensor tendinitis of dorsal compartments and tendon ruptures has been described, principally with the use of dorsal plating. Other complications are median nerve neuropathy, reflex sympathetic dystrophy, finger stiffness, and Volkmann's contracture.[24, 27, 34, 38]

TREATMENT OF SCAPHOID FRACTURES

Treatment of scaphoid fractures depends on location and stability (Fig. 11). Cast immobilization is indicated in patients with stable nondisplaced fractures. Controversy exists about the position of the wrist and the joints to be immobilized.[50] Acute, nondisplaced, middle-third scaphoid fractures are usually placed in a long- or short-arm cast until the fracture has healed.[50] The use of a long or short-arm cast also is controversial. Stewart[51] reported a 95% union rate using a short-arm cast, whereas Gellman and associates[50] reported less time required for healing with use of a long-arm cast. We believe that the wrist should be placed in radial deviation with slight extension of the wrist. The thumb should be included in the cast, because free movement of the thumb includes the scaphotrapezial joint. A below-elbow cast that includes the thumb has demonstrated high rates of union in stable nondisplaced fractures.[51]

A study of nondisplaced scaphoid fracture reported a 90% to 100% union rate when the fracture is placed in a traditional cast within 3 weeks of injury; average healing time was 9 to 12 weeks.[52] Stable fractures treated within 6 weeks to 6 months of injury were reported to have a 90% union rate, but the time to union was 20 to 24 weeks, or almost double the time required when treatment was started within 3 weeks.[53] For scaphoid fracture in an athlete, the patient's desires regarding sports participation should be considered. Treatment options are (1) traditional casting with no participation in sports activities until healed, (2) a cast plus use of a playing cast in sports, when applicable, and (3) open reduction and internal fixation of the fracture with immediate return to sports participation as symptoms permit.[18] Acute percutaneous scaphoid fixation is an option for these patients. Haddad and Goddard[54] reported 50 cases treated with acute percutaneous fixation, with 100% healing rate in 55 days in average and immediate active motion.[54]

For an athlete with a stable, nondisplaced acute scaphoid fracture who requests a playing cast, the wrist is kept in a thumb spica cast while the patient is not playing or practicing, and a protective playing cast is applied for participating in sports. Studies have reported a 90% to 92% healing rate and average healing time of 3 to 6 months when a playing cast is used.[55, 56]

For unstable displaced scaphoid fractures, proximal pole fractures, or vertical oblique fractures, open reduction with internal fixation (ORIF) is the treatment of choice.[56-58]

Internal fixation can be performed with K-wires or

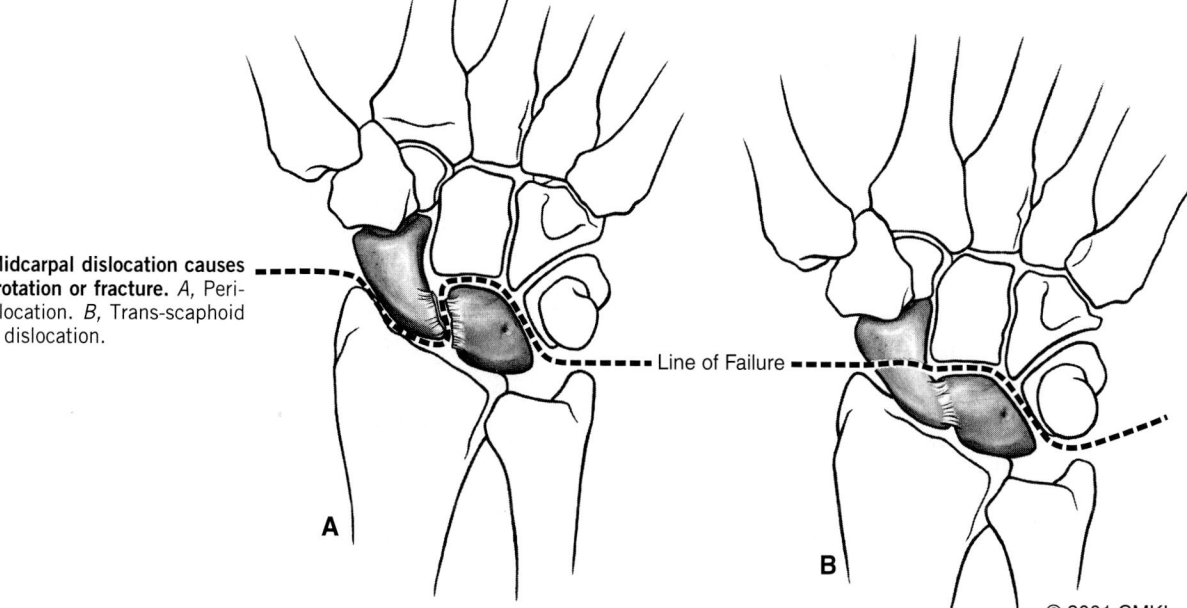

Fig. 11. Midcarpal dislocation causes scaphoid rotation or fracture. *A*, Perilunate dislocation. *B*, Trans-scaphoid perilunate dislocation.

Line of Failure

A

B

© 2001 CMKI

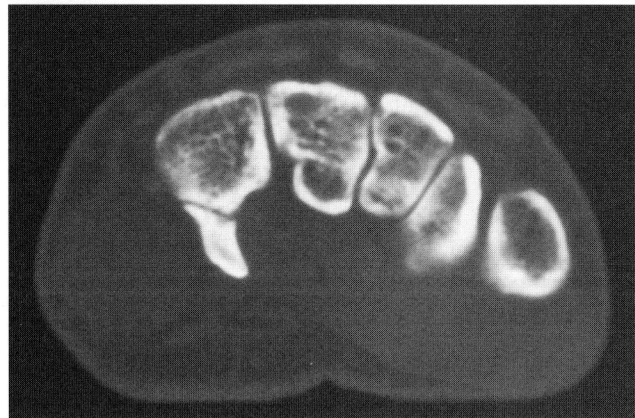

© 1990 CMKI

Fig. 12. A fracture in the hook of the hamate.

screws.[59] Several screws, such as the Herbert, cannulated 3.5-mm AO, and Acutrak, can be used. In a study published in 2000, Trumble and colleagues[59] compared internal fixation with the Herbert screw and with the 3.5-mm cannulated screw and found no statistical difference between the two methods.[59] Currently, we are using the Acutrek screw, which can be placed dorsally and volarly and is buried inside the bone. We use the volar approach when open reduction is needed in waist fractures, and the dorsal approach in proximal pole fractures.

Nonunion of a scaphoid fracture usually occurs because of failed initial diagnosis or because the patient was not seen until several months after injury. Nonunion in a nondisplaced fracture can be managed with immobilization or by open or percutaneous fixation. Nonunion of a displaced fracture must be reduced and must receive bone grafting regardless of the symptoms, to prevent future osteoarthritis. Grafting techniques may use cancellous or corticocancellous bone. Matti,[60] in 1937, described a technique that used cancellous bone through a dorsal approach with filling of both cavities. Rüsse,[31] in 1960, described the use of a corticocancellous grafting through a volar approach. We prefer the volar approach because it allows repair of the scaphoid in a more anatomically correct manner.

Higher rates of nonunion and avascular necrosis are seen when the proximal pole of the scaphoid is involved, because the blood supply to the proximal pole comes from the distal two-thirds of the scaphoid (through one volar and one dorsal branch of the radial artery) and may be poor.[61] When nonunion occurs in a proximal pole fracture, the preferred approach is dorsal. Curettage of the proximal pole must be performed until cancellous bone is seen. Cancellous bone is impacted inside, and fixation with K-wires or screws is performed. Some surgeons have recommended vascularized bone grafts or free vascularized bone grafts when no vascularity is seen at the proximal pole.[62]

TREATMENT OF HAMATE FRACTURES

Fractures of the hamate can occur at the body (which is uncommon) or at the hook area. Nondisplaced fracture of the hamate body must be treated with immobilization. If the fracture is displaced, open reduction and fixation should be performed. Fractures of the hook of the hamate

are more common. They should be suspected when the patient has pain at the base of the hypothenar area distal to the pisiform (Fig. 12). Some cases are diagnosed because the flexor tendons to the small finger have been ruptured.[20] Diagnosis can be performed with carpal tunnel radiographs, but a CT scan is the most reliable diagnostic method.[63]

When diagnosed in the acute stage, hook of the hamate fractures require closed treatment in a short-arm cast; the thumb and the small finger must be included in the cast to relieve the tension on the transverse carpal ligament, which originates in the hook of the hamate. If nonunion develops, excision of the hook is the best option.[20, 63]

TREATMENT OF FRACTURES OF THE TRIQUETRUM, CAPITATE, TRAPEZIUM, AND TRAPEZOID

Triquetrum fractures usually are produced by impingement of the ulnar styloid with dorsiflexion and associated ulnar deviation. They are usually asymptomatic, and if treatment is needed, excision of the fractured fragment can be performed.

Fractures of the capitate are rare and may be associated with scaphoid fractures. With these fractures, the proximal pole of the capitate is rotated 180 degrees, usually without soft-tissue attachment. According to the literature, the mechanism of injury is hyperdorsiflexion of the wrist.[64] However, we have observed a hyper–volar flexion mechanism in a 16-year-old patient with proximal capitate pole fracture and complete scaphoid waist fracture. Closed treatment is indicated in nondisplaced capitate fractures, and open reduction with internal fixation in displaced fractures. Avascular necrosis of the proximal pole may occur.

Isolated fractures of the trapezium also are rare. Usually they are associated with metacarpal fractures (Fig. 13) or with distal radius fractures. Fractures can occur at the body or at the trapezial ridge.[65] Trapezial ridge fractures can be produced by direct trauma or by avulsion of the flexor retinaculum. If the fracture is displaced, open reduction with internal fixation is indicated. If the fractured fragment is very small, the fragment can be excised. Checroun and

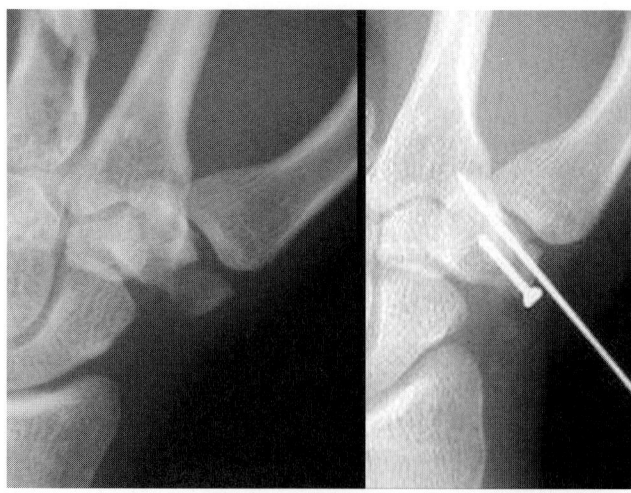

© 2000 Moreno

Fig. 13. Digital radiograph of a trapezium fracture.

associates[66] have reported radial artery injuries to be associated with trapezium fractures.

Fractures of the trapezoid are rare. Because it is fastened to the trapezium, capitate, and scaphoid by strong ligaments, fractures of the trapezoid are limited. They are the result of indirect forces applied to the second metacarpal. When a fracture is suspected but is not confirmed by plain radiographs, computed tomography is useful.[67]

Pisiform fractures also are rare, and half of them are associated with distal radius fractures of the hamate or triquetrum. Diagnosis can be made from 30-degree supination oblique views. Initial treatment is with immobilization, and if painful nonunion is present, excision is indicated, along with repair of the flexor carpi ulnaris.

RESULTS

The outcome of fracture management depends on three factors: (1) ability to properly diagnose the problem, (2) selection of appropriate treatment, and (3) communication between the physician and the patient so that treatment can be carried to fruition in the most expedient manner. Fractures of the distal radius are not simple fractures that can be treated by the most junior staff member, and anatomic reduction achieves the best result. Carpal injuries are more difficult to treat than distal radius fractures, because in addition to the element of bone involvement there is ligament detachment, and the sharpest fibers cannot be reproduced. Early restoration of the relationship of involved structures may allow healing of torn ligaments, but detached ligaments might require additional procedures.

ACKNOWLEDGMENT

We would like to thank Mrs. Patricia E. Killion for her editing skills, research, and perseverance during the preparation of this manuscript.

REFERENCES

1. Oskam J, Kingma J, Klasen HJ: Fracture of the distal forearm: Epidemiological developments in the period 1971–1995. Injury 1988; 29:353.
2. Alfram P, Bauer CH: Epidemiology of fractures of the forearm. J Bone Joint Surg Am 1962; 44.
3. Hove LM: Epidemiology of scaphoid fractures in Bergen, Norway. Scand J Plast Reconstr Surg Hand Surg 1999; 33:423.
4. Pouteau: In Stimson LA (ed): Fractures and Dislocations. New York, Lea & Febiger, 1912, 7th ed, p 310.
5. Colles A: On the fracture of the carpal extremity of the radius. Edin Med Surg J 1814; 182.
6. Cooper Sir A: Treatise on Dislocations and on Fractures of the Joints. London, Longman, Hurst, Rees, Orme, and Brown, 1822.
7. Barton JR: Views and treatment of an important injury of the wrist. Med Exam 1838; 1:365.
8. Destot E: Injuries of the wrist: A radiographic study [translated by FRB Atkinson]. New York, Paul B Hoeber, 1926.
9. Fisk GR: Carpal instability and the fractures scaphoid (Hunterian Lecture 1968). Ann R Coll Surg London 1970; 46:63.
10. Linscheid RL, Dobyns JH, Beabout JW, et al: Traumatic instability of the wrist: Diagnosis, classification, and pathomechanics. J Bone Joint Surg Am 1972; 54:1612.
11. Richards RS, Bennett JD, Roth JH, et al: Arthroscopic diagnosis of intra-articular soft tissue injuries associated with distal radial fractures. J Hand Surg (Am) 1997; 22:772.
12. Palmer AK, Glisson RR, Werner FW: Ulnar variance determination. J Hand Surg (Am) 1982; 7:376.
13. Palmer AK, Werner FW: The triangular fibrocartilage complex of the wrist—anatomy and function. J Hand Surg (Am) 1981; 6:153.
14. Buck-Gramcko D: Denervation of the wrist joint. J Hand Surg (Am) 1977; 2:54.

15. Short WH, Palmer AK, Werner FW, et al: A biomechanical study of distal radial fractures. J Hand Surg (Am) 1987; 12:529.
16. Werner FW, Glisson RR, Murphy DJ, et al: Force transmission through the distal radioulnar carpal joint: Effect of ulnar lengthening and shortening. Handchir Mikrochir Plast Chir 1986; 18:304.
17. Oliveira JC: Barton's fractures. J Bone Joint Surg Am 1973; 55:586.
18. Rettig AC: Management of acute scaphoid fractures. Hand Clin 2000; 16:3:381.
19. Weber ER: Biomechanical implications of scaphoid waist fractures. Clin Orthop 1980; 149:83.
20. Stark HH, Jobe FW, Boyes JH, et al: Fracture of the hook of the hamate in athletes. J Bone Joint Surg Am 1977; 59:575.
21. Stordahl A, Schjoth A, Woxhold G, et al: Bone scanning of fractures of the scaphoid. J Hand Surg (Br) 1984 9:189.
22. Burke FD: Colles' fractures: Conservative treatment. In Barton N (ed): Fractures of the Hand and Wrist. London, Churchill Livingstone, 1988, p 267.
23. Smith RJ, Floyd WE: Smith's and Barton's fractures. In Barton N (ed): Fractures of the Hand and Wrist. London, Churchill Livingstone, 1988, p 252.
24. Frykman G: Fracture of the distal radius including sequelae, shoulder hand finger syndrome, disturbance in the distal radioulnar joint and impairment of nerve function: A clinical and experimental study. Acta Orthop Scand Suppl 1967; 108:1.
25. Muller ME, Nazarian S, Koch P: Classification AO de Fracturen. Berlin, Springer, 1987.
26. Cooney WP, Agee JM, Hastings H, et al: Symposium: Management of intraarticular fractures of the distal radius. Contemp Orthop 1990; 21:71.
27. Melone CP Jr: Unstable fractures of the distal radius. In Lichtman DM (ed): The Wrist and Its Disorders. Philadelphia, WB Saunders, 1988, p 160.

28. Missakian ML, Cooney WP, Amadio PC, et al: Open reduction and internal fixation for distal radius fractures. J Hand Surg (Am) 1992; 17:745.
29. Fernandez DL: A practical, simplified, comprehensive and treatment-oriented classification of fractures of the distal radius. Presented at the Fourth International Federation of Societies for Surgery of the Hand, Bone and Joint Injuries Committee, Paris, May 1992.
30. Green DP, Hotchkiss RN, Pederson WC: Green's Operative Hand Surgery. New York, Churchill Livingstone, 1999, 4th ed, p 940.
31. Rüsse O: Fracture of the carpal navicular: Diagnosis, non-operative treatment, and operative treatment. J Bone Joint Surg Am 1960; 42:759.
32. Amadio PC, Taleisnik J: Fractures of the carpal bones. In Green DP (ed): Operative Hand Surgery. New York, Churchill Livingstone, 1993, 3rd ed, vol 1.
33. Cooney WP, Dobyns JH, Linscheid RL: Fractures of the scaphoid: A rational approach to management. Clin Orthop 1980; 149:90.
34. Knirk JL, Jupiter JB: Intraarticular fractures of the distal end of the radius in young adults. J Bone Joint Surg Am 1986; 68:647.
35. Altissimi M, Marcini GB, Assara A, et al: Early end late displacement of fractures of the distal radius: The prediction of instability. Int Orthop 1994; 18:61.
36. Clancey GJ: Percutaneous Kirschner wire fixation of Colles' fractures: A prospective study of thirty five cases. J Bone Joint Surg Am 1984; 66:1008.
37. Rayhack JM, Langworthy JN, Belsole RJ: Transulnar percutaneous pinning of displaced distal radius fractures: A preliminary report. J Orthop Trauma 1989; 3:107.
38. De Palma AF: Comminuted fractures of the distal end of the radius: By ulnar pinning. J Bone Joint Surg Am 1952; 34:651.
39. Kapandji A: Bone fixation by double per-

cutaneous pinning: Functional treatment of non-articular fractures of the distal radius. Ann Chir Main Memb Super 1976; 6:903.

40. Martello J, Mejia H, Cautilli D, et al: Management of unstable distal radius fractures using the Ulson device. Presented at the American Society for Surgery of the Hand Annual Meeting, Denver, September 1998.

41. Pennig DW: Dynamic external fixators of the distal radius fractures. Hand Clin 1993; 9:587.

42. Frykman G, Peckham RH, Willard K: External fixators for the treatment of unstable wrist fractures: A biomechanical, design feature, and cost comparison. Hand Clin 1993; 9:555.

43. Ring D, Jupiter JB, Brenwald J, et al: Prospective multicenter trial of a plate for dorsal fixation of distal radius fractures. J Hand Surg (Am) 1997; 22:777.

44. Lowry KJ, Gainor BJ, Hoskins JS: Extensor tendon rupture secondary to the AO/ASIF titanium distal radius plate with associated plate failure: A case report. Am J Orthop 2000; 29:789.

45. Kambouroglou GK, Axelrod T: Complications of the AO/ASIF titanium distal radius plate system (PI plate) in internal fixation of the distal radius: A brief report. J Hand Surg (Am) 1998; 23:737.

46. Schnur PP, Chang B: Extensor tendon rupture after internal fixation of a distal radius using a dorsally placed AO/ASIF titanium plate. Ann Plast Surg 2000; 44:564.

47. Hahnloser D, Platz A, Amgwerd M, et al: Internal fixation of distal radius fractures with dorsal dislocation: PI plate or two 1/4 tube plates? A prospective randomized study. J Trauma 1999; 47:760.

48. Short WH, Palmer AK, Werner F, et al: A biomechanical study of distal radial fractures. J Hand Surg (Am) 1987; 12:529.

49. Jacob M, Rikli DA, Regazzoni P: Fractures of the distal radius treated by internal fixation and early function. J Bone Joint Surg Br 2000; 82:340.

50. Gellman H, Caputo RJ, Carter V, et al: Comparison of short and long thumb-spica casts for non-displaced fractures of the carpal scaphoid. J Bone Joint Surg Am 1989; 71:354.

51. Stewart MJ: Fracture of the carpal navicular (scaphoid): A report of 436 cases. J Bone Joint Surg Am 1954; 36:948.

52. Cooney WP III, Dobyns JH, Linscheid RL: Nonunion of the scaphoid: Analysis of the results from bone grafting. J Hand Surg (Am) 1980; 5:343.

53. Mack GR, Wilckens JH, McPherson SA: Subacute scaphoid fractures: A closer look at closed treatment. Am J Sports Med 1998; 26:56.

54. Haddad FS, Goddard NJ: Acute percutaneous fixation using a cannulated screw. Chir Main 1998; 17:119.

55. Riester JN, Baker BE, Mosher JF, et al: A review of scaphoid fracture healing in competitive athletes. Am J Sports Med 1985; 13:159.

56. Rettig AC, Weidenbener EJ, Gloyeske R: Alternative management of midthird scaphoid fractures in the athlete. Am J Sports Med 1994; 22:711.

57. Herbert TJ, Fisher WE, Leicester AW: The Herbert bone screw: A 10-year perspective. J Hand Surg (Br) 1992; 17:415.

58. Rettig AC, Kollias SC: Internal fixation of acute scaphoid fractures in the athlete. Am J Sports Med 1996; 24:182.

59. Trumble TE, Gilbert M, Murray LW, et al: Displaced scaphoid fractures treated with open reduction and internal fixation with a cannulated screw. J Bone Joint Surg Am 2000; 82:633.

60. Matti H: Uber die behandlung der navicular fraktur und der refractura patellae durch plombierung mit spongiosa. Zentralbl Chir 1937; 64:23.

61. Gelberman RH, Menon J: The vascularity of the scaphoid bone. J Hand Surg (Am) 1980; 5:508.

62. Doi K, Oda T, Soo-Heong T, et al: Free vascularized bone graft for nonunion of the scaphoid. J Hand Surg (Am) 2000 25:507.

63. Bishop AT, Beckenbaugh RD: Fracture of the hamate hook. J Hand Surg (Am) 1988; 13:135.

64. Stein F, Siegel MW: Naviculocapitate fracture syndrome: A case report: New thoughts on the mechanism of injury. J Bone Joint Surg Am 1969; 51:391.

65. Binhammer P, Born T: Coronal fracture of the body of the trapezium: A case report. J Hand Surg (Am) 1998; 23:156.

66. Checroun AJ, Mekhail AO, Ebraheim NA: Radial artery injury in association with fractures of the trapezium. J Bone Joint Surg Br 1997; 22:419.

67. Miyawaki T, Kobayashi M, Matsuura S, et al: Trapezoid bone fracture. Ann Plast Surg 2000; 44:444.

HAND FRACTURES

Steven P. Sampson

Summary

- A thorough understanding of regional anatomy of hand is key to the proper treatment of hand fractures.
- Most phalangeal and metacarpal fractures may be successfully treated with closed or percutaneous fracture stabilization.
- Periarticular fractures surrounding the proximal interphalangeal joint are associated with the greatest morbidity; this joint has been called the "most critical" hinge.
- Proper anatomic alignment of articular injuries is essential for reducing stiffness, loss of motion, and post-traumatic arthrosis.

Fractures of the hand are extremely common injuries that lead patients to seek emergency treatment. Proper fracture care may reduce the disability effects of such injuries. Thorough understanding of the regional anatomy of the hand is imperative to both nonsurgical and surgical treatment of these fractures and periarticular trauma.

EXTRA-ARTICULAR FRACTURES: PHALANGES AND METACARPALS

DISTAL PHALANX

Fractures of the distal phalanx are the most common injuries seen in the emergency room. They are usually associated with varying soft-tissue injuries to the fingertip, pulp, and nail bed. Displaced extra-articular injuries of the distal phalanx must be reduced and frequently must be stabilized with Kirschner's (K) wire fixation to allow better postinjury soft-tissue care without the fear of repeated loss of reduction. Nail bed repair aids rotational alignment, and replacement of the sterile nail provides a stent for both the nail bed repair and the distal phalanx fracture. Closed tuft fractures may benefit from subungual hematoma drainage

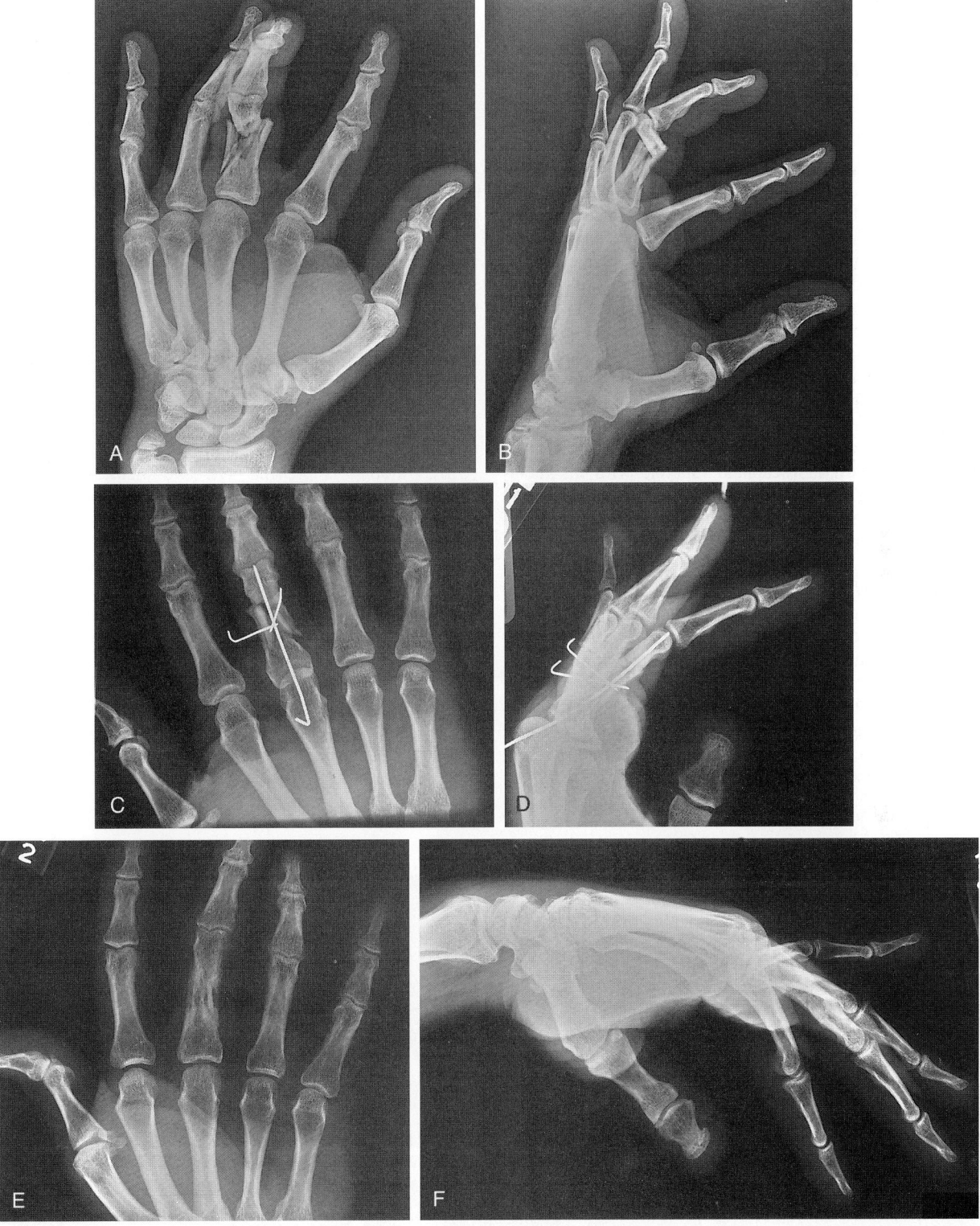

Fig. 1. Proximal phalanx shaft fractures. AP (*A*) and lateral (*B*) radiographs of the long finger reveal an open comminuted extra-articular fracture of the proximal phalanx. One month after SP/CRIF, AP (*C*) and lateral (*D*) radiographs show maintenance of alignment and early fracture healing. Six months after fixation, AP Brewerton (*E*) and lateral (*F*) radiographs show evidence of complete healing and excellent alignment.

through the nail plate to help alleviate severe fingertip pain.

MIDDLE PHALANX

Extra-articular fractures of the middle phalanx are more difficult to treat because of (1) the very high ratio of cortical to trabecular bone (i.e., longer fracture healing time) and (2) the lack of predictability with regard to fracture angulation. Distal-third fractures of the middle phalanx shaft tend to deform with an apex-volar configuration because of the stronger pull of the flexor superficialis insertion on the proximal fragment. In contrast, fractures of the proximal-third middle phalanx shaft tend to deform with the apex dorsal, because the flexor superficialis insertion tends to flex the distal fragment, and the central slip insertion extends the proximal fragment. Closed reduction is necessary for any significant angulation or malrotation. Assessment for rotational malalignment consists of (1) checking for parallel alignment of all fingernails in both finger extension and flexion and (2) noting whether all fingers point toward the scaphoid tubercle with the metacarpophalangeal (MP) and proximal interphalangeal (PIP) joints flexed. Percutaneous K-wire fixation may be required to maintain proper angulation or to correct malrotation.

PROXIMAL PHALANX

Fractures of the proximal phalanx usually angulate apex-volar, with the proximal fragment flexed by the strong pull of the intrinsic muscles (Fig. 1). Closed reduction is performed on the basis of three anatomic concepts. First, three-quarters of the proximal phalangeal circumference is surrounded by the extensor mechanism. Second, because the intrinsic muscle force is pulling the proximal fracture fragment into flexion, the distal fragment must be flexed

after longitudinal traction. Combining these two anatomic facts allows easier maintenance of closed reduction of these fractures. Third, with maximal MP flexion, the proximal fragment can be "locked" if the MP collateral ligaments are made taut. This anatomic feature also simplifies attempted closed reduction. Extra-articular angulated proximal phalangeal fractures are usually treated with percutaneous K-wire fixation. Long oblique fractures may also be treated with limited open reduction and screw fixation as long as the fracture length is at least two times the diameter of the bone. Complications of open reduction in this zone are common and result in the need for hardware removal and tendolysis once the fracture is healed.

METACARPALS

Extra-articular fractures of the metacarpals can angulate, rotate, and shorten (Fig. 2). These fracture displacements are governed by several regional anatomic features. The index and long metacarpals are mechanically part of the fixed unit of the hand, and minimal carpometacarpal (CMC) motion is present. The two metacarpals form the stiffest structural attachment of both the longitudinal and proximal transverse arches. In contrast, the ring and little metacarpals are mobile, allowing 30 to 40 degrees of flexion and extension at their CMC joints as well as supination. Distally, the four metacarpals are firmly tethered together by the deep transverse metacarpal ligament.

Because of the lack of mobility of the index and long metacarpals, only 10 to 15 degrees of fracture angulation is usually acceptable, whereas in the ring and little metacarpals, up to 40 to 50 degrees of apex-dorsal angulation may be tolerated. A 1-degree malrotation of the metacarpal shaft leads to 5-degree malrotation deformity of the involved digit. In vitro studies have shown that 2 mm of metacarpal

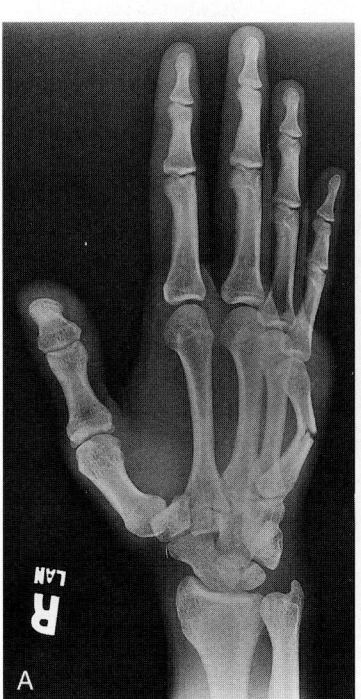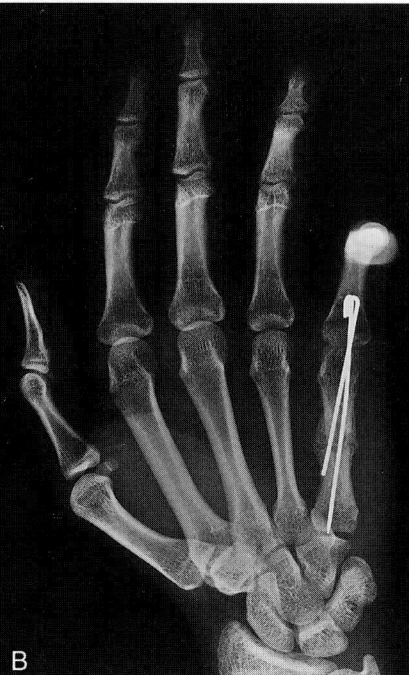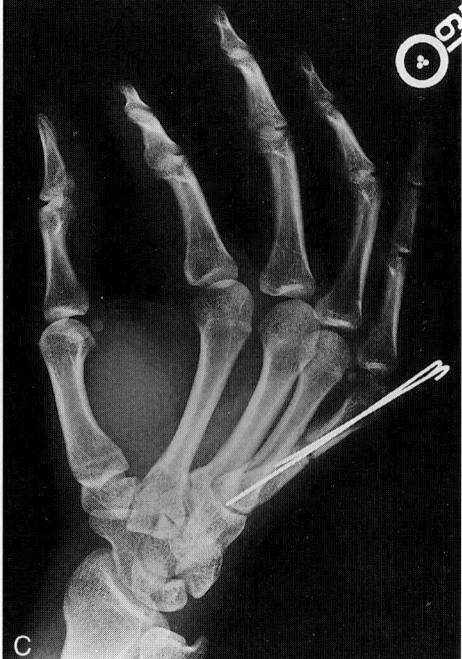

Fig. 2. Metacarpal shaft fractures. *A,* Oblique radiograph reveals a midshaft metacarpal fracture with evidence of MP joint clawing. SP/CRIF was performed. Postoperative AP (*B*) and lateral (*C*) radiographs demonstrate anatomic reduction.

shortening leads to a 7-degree MP joint extensor lag. Likewise, 6 mm of metacarpal shortening results in a 21-degree MP extension lag. Clinically, the effect of even 6 mm of metacarpal shortening is minimized by the fact that the MP usually hyperextends approximately 21 degrees. In general, any metacarpal fracture angulation that significantly shortens enough to produce a clinical pseudo-claw deformity at the MP joint requires closed reduction and percutaneous K-wire fixation.

Fractures of the metacarpal neck usually involve palmar metaphyseal comminution and are typically easy to reduce with a Jahss maneuver, but the reduction is difficult to maintain. The Jahss reduction maneuver involves longitudinal traction and disimpaction of the fracture followed by manipulation of the distal head and neck fragment onto the proximal shaft fragment. Distal control is obtained with maximal flexion of the PIP and MP joints; proximal control is obtained with wrist extension, which "locks in" the involved CMC joint. This reduction maneuver is contraindicated as a holding posture, however, because of the likelihood of skin breakdown over the dorsal PIP joint.

Numerous methods of operative fixation have been proposed for malrotated and angulated metacarpal fractures. I favor percutaneous intramedullary K-wire fixation applied in a retrograde manner. Care is taken to minimize metacarpal head trauma. An attempt is made to place the intramedullary wire along the straight dorsal cortex. Rotational control is obtained by splinting the involved and adjacent MP joints in flexion and then buddy-taping the fingers.

Closed reduction of metacarpal shaft fractures is easier to maintain. Three-point molding is obtained by locking the proximal base in extension, applying a gentle dorsal-apical mold over the reduced fracture site in concert with a palmar-upward mold in the region of the metacarpal head and neck. Follow-up radiographs should be obtained weekly for the first 2 weeks, because fracture reduction may be lost once soft-tissue swelling subsides.

PERIARTICULAR FRACTURES AND DISLOCATIONS

OVERVIEW OF JOINT INJURIES

The hinged joints of the phalanges—the distal interphalangeal (DIP), PIP, and MP joints—are stabilized by four key soft-tissue structures: the two collateral ligaments, the extensor tendon/capsular insertion, and the volar plate. When two of the four soft-tissue restraints are significantly ruptured or avulsed with or without periarticular bone, the joint becomes unstable and may subluxate or dislocate.

DIP JOINT

Jammed fingers are extremely common hyperextension injuries involving sprain of the collateral ligaments, rupture of the volar plate, or both. When severe enough, a dorsal dislocation may occur that many times is open. A thorough irrigation of the open volar wound prior to closed reduction is necessary. These injuries are typically easy to reduce with traction and direct pressure over the dorsally displaced distal phalanx. Complex or irreducible dorsal dislocations may require extraction of various structures, such as the volar plate, the flexor digitorum profundus (FDP) tendon, or an osteochondral fracture. Postreduction stability should be checked with active joint flexion. Dorsal splint-

ing of the DIP joint should be typically limited to 1 week if joint stability is present. Any significant delay in joint mobilization is associated with marked residual stiffness or arthrofibrosis, not instability.

Dorsal chip fracture of the distal phalanx articular surface is associated with "mallet" fractures. These fractures must be splinted for approximately 6 weeks and are much easier to treat than their "nonbony" terminal tendon avulsion counterpart. When a fracture affects 30% to 40% of the dorsal distal phalangeal articular surface, which includes significant involvement of one or both collateral ligaments, volar subluxation of the distal phalanx may result. When the DIP joint subluxes, closed reduction with percutaneous wire fixation is indicated. Rarely, open reduction is required, which may entail internal fixation of a large articular fragment or excision of a small avulsion fragment along with reinsertion of the terminal tendon into the remaining distal phalanx.

Intercondylar injury of the DIP joint is less common than the same injury of the PIP joint. Closed reduction and K-wire fixation should be attempted. However, the condylar process of the middle phalanx may rotate on its collateral ligament in such a way as to mandate open reduction.

Volar marginal avulsion injuries of the distal phalanx may involve avulsion of the FDP tendon in addition to the volar plate. Early repair of the FDP tendon, in the first 10 to 14 days, is required to avoid significant difficulties of tendon repair. Unfortunately, this injury is often regarded as "only a sprain," and the patient presents in delayed fashion for treatment, which then involves much more complexity and potential complications.

PIP JOINT

The PIP joint is the most critical hinge joint. With the MP joints flexed 90 degrees, the PIP joint is responsible for 85% of the remaining flexion cascade of the finger pulp to the distal palmar flexion crease. The direction and rate of the force applied to the PIP joint often dictates the type and location of the injury. Angulatory forces frequently result in damage to collateral ligaments, whereas longitudinal forces cause impact joint surface loading, resulting in intra-articular fractures or fracture-dislocations. In vitro studies have shown that hyperextension forces applied at a rapid rate result in middle phalangeal articular avulsion fractures, whereas those forces applied at a slower rate involve the proximal phalanx (Figs. 3 and 4).

Distal PIP joint injuries involving the middle phalangeal articulation most commonly involve the volar lip. With PIP joint hyperextension, the volar plate may avulse off varying percentages of the middle phalanx. Once 30% to 40% of this surface is involved, the collateral ligaments are ineffective restraints to a dorsal subluxation force of the central slip extensor mechanism. Closed reduction requires traction and varying amounts of PIP flexion to maintain joint congruency, best seen on a true lateral radiograph of the finger. If reduction can be obtained, a PIP extension block-splinting protocol must be carefully followed weekly to void missing resubluxation. Occasionally, when the volar lip fragment is large, open reduction with internal fixation may be indicated. Late presentation of dorsal subluxation or joint incongruity may require a volar plate arthroplasty reconstruction.

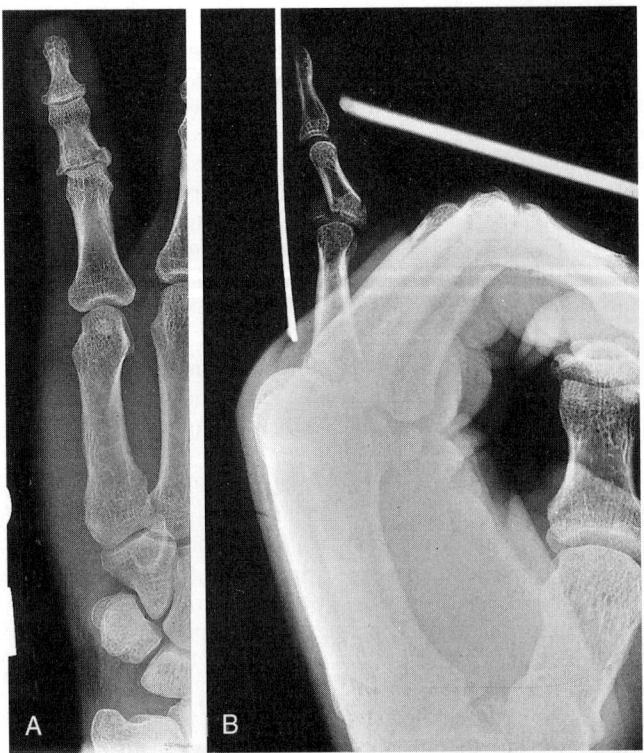

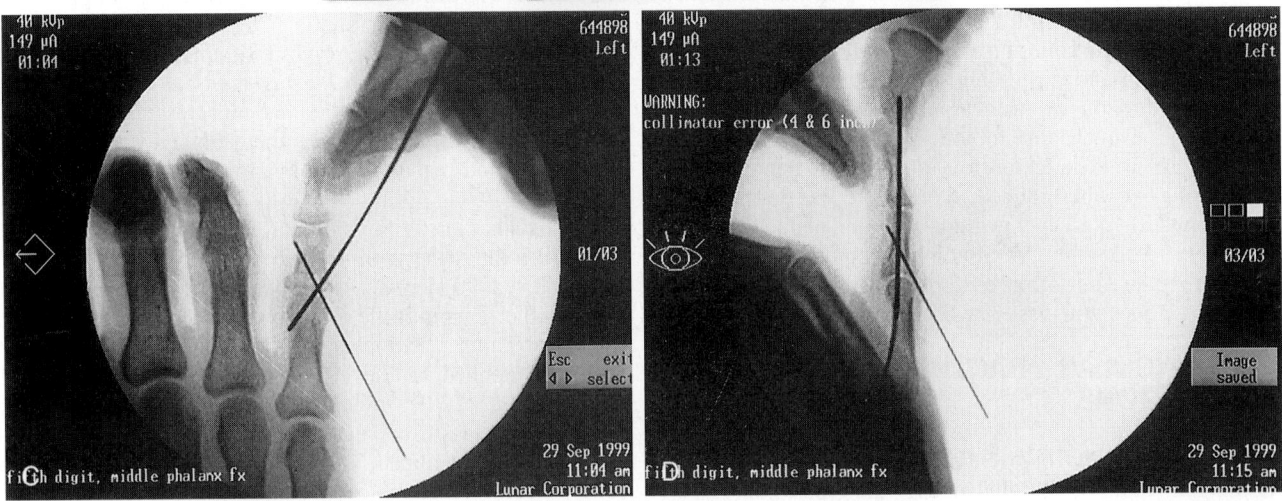

Fig. 3. Middle phalanx PIP joint fractures. AP (*A*) and lateral (*B*) radiographs show a comminuted intra-articular fracture. Open reduction with internal fixation using K-wires was performed. Postoperative AP (*C*) and lateral (*D*) radiographs show restoration with joint congruency, especially the lateral view.

Dorsal lip fractures of the middle phalanx are relatively uncommon injuries and are associated with PIP hyperflexion. When these injuries are nondisplaced, the central slip must be neutralized by placement of the PIP joint in full extension for 6 weeks and mobilization of the DIP joint. Open reduction with internal fixation is required for displaced fractures.

Pilon injuries of the PIP joints are marked impaction forces causing severe comminution and joint depression of the middle phalangeal articular surface. Computed tomography (CT) scanning with 1-mm cuts may be useful to formulation of a surgical plan. The key to a satisfactory clinical outcome is the correction of PIP joint subluxation by way of external traction and carefully controlled joint mobilization.

Proximal phalangeal PIP joint articular injuries may be unicondylar or bicondylar. Closed reduction with wire fixation is frequently required to maintain reduction. Open reduction is necessary when the articular fragment malrotates, hinging on its own collateral ligament.

MP JOINT

Periarticular fractures may involve basilar collateral ligament avulsion injuries of the proximal phalanx or metacarpal head fractures (Fig. 5). Special radiographic evaluation of these injuries may include Brewerton's views and re-

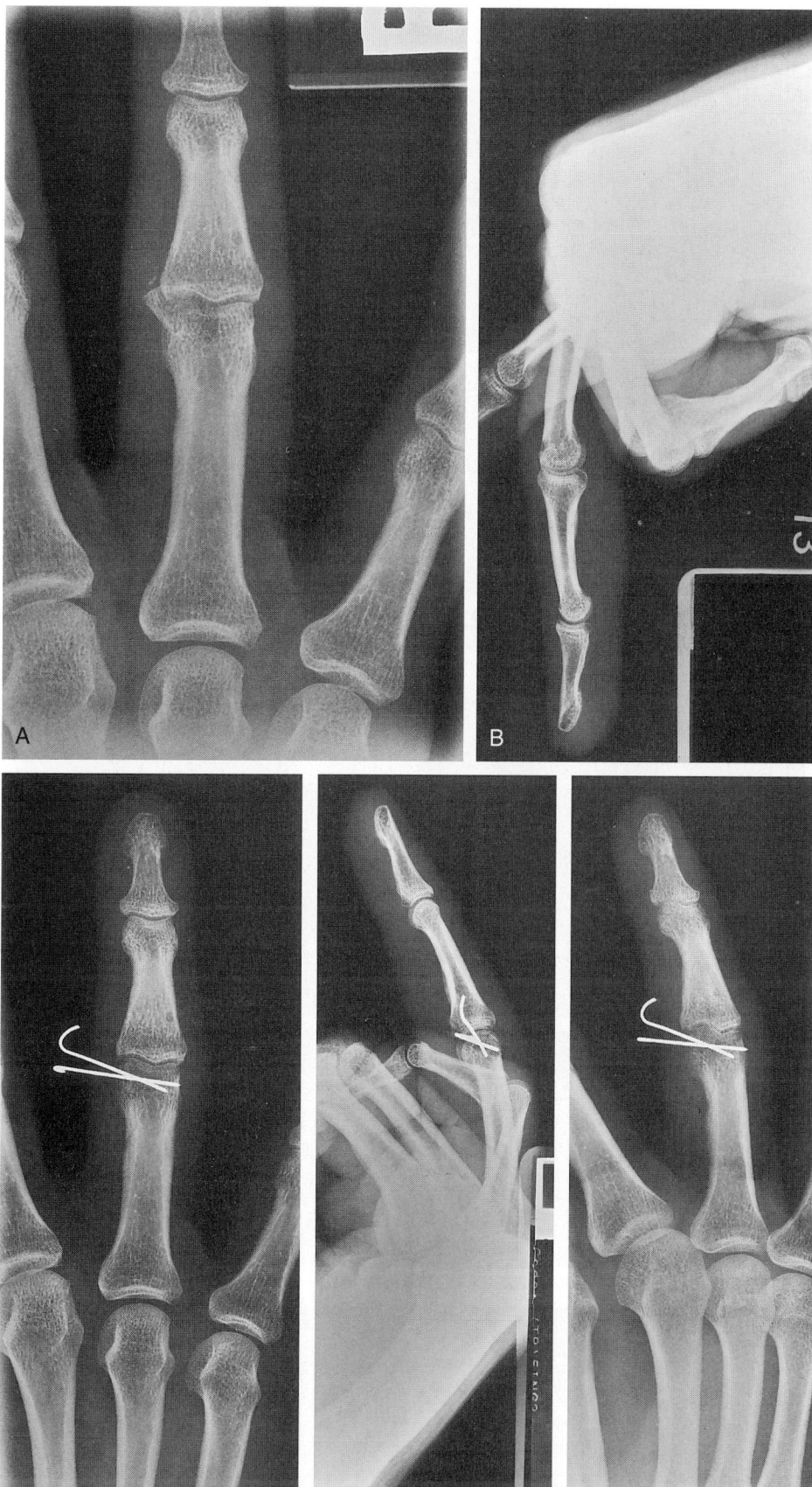

Fig. 4. PIP joint fractures, proximal phalanx. AP (*A*) and lateral (*B*) radiographs show a displaced condylar proximal phalanx fracture. Open reduction with internal fixation was required because the articular surfaces were markedly displaced. Postoperative AP (*C*), lateral (*D*), and oblique (*E*) radiographs of the PIP joint show anatomic joint reduction.

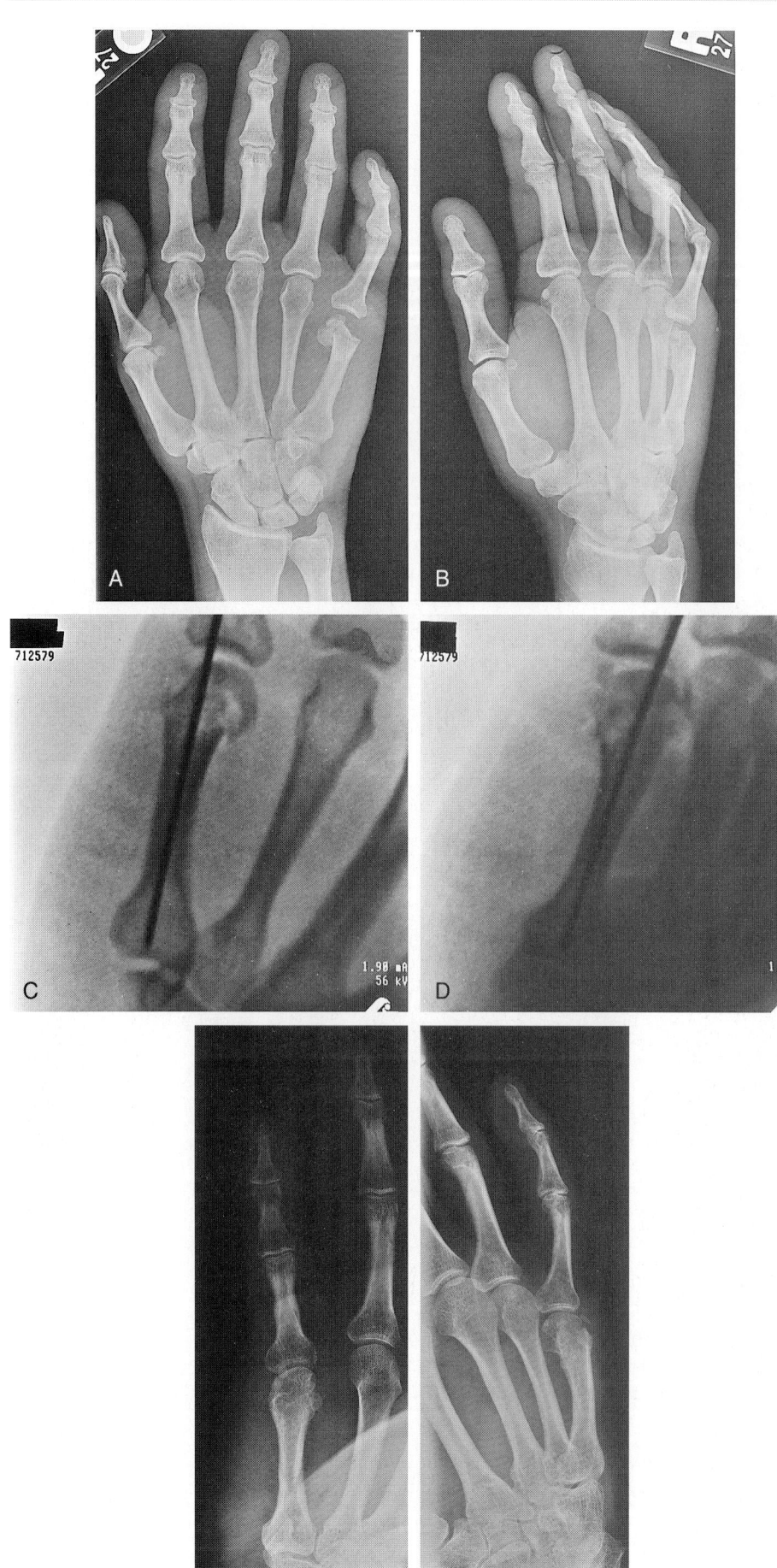

Fig. 5. Metacarpal head fractures. AP (*A*) and oblique (*B*) radiographs reveal a comminuted metacarpal head fracture that was misdiagnosed in the emergency room as a "boxer's fracture." Open reduction with K-wire fixation was able to restore the head onto the neck of the small metacarpal, as shown on postoperative AP (*C*) and oblique (*D*) radiographs. Four months after surgery, AP (*E*) and oblique (*F*) radiographs demonstrate restoration of the joint surface with no evidence of avascular necrosis.

verse oblique views as well as CT evaluation. Stability of the MP joint must be clinically assessed with maximum flexion of the MP joint followed by application of radial and ulnar stress. Displaced or unstable proximal phalangeal articular injuries require open reduction with internal fixation. Metacarpal hand fractures are usually a result of direct or clenched fist trauma. Thorough débridement of open

injuries is mandatory to reduce the possibility of joint sepsis. CT evaluation of head-splitting, closed metatarsal head fractures may reveal fragments of suitable size to allow rigid fixation and early joint mobilization. Severely comminuted head fractures may result in post-traumatic arthrosis and require MP arthroplasty as a salvage procedure.

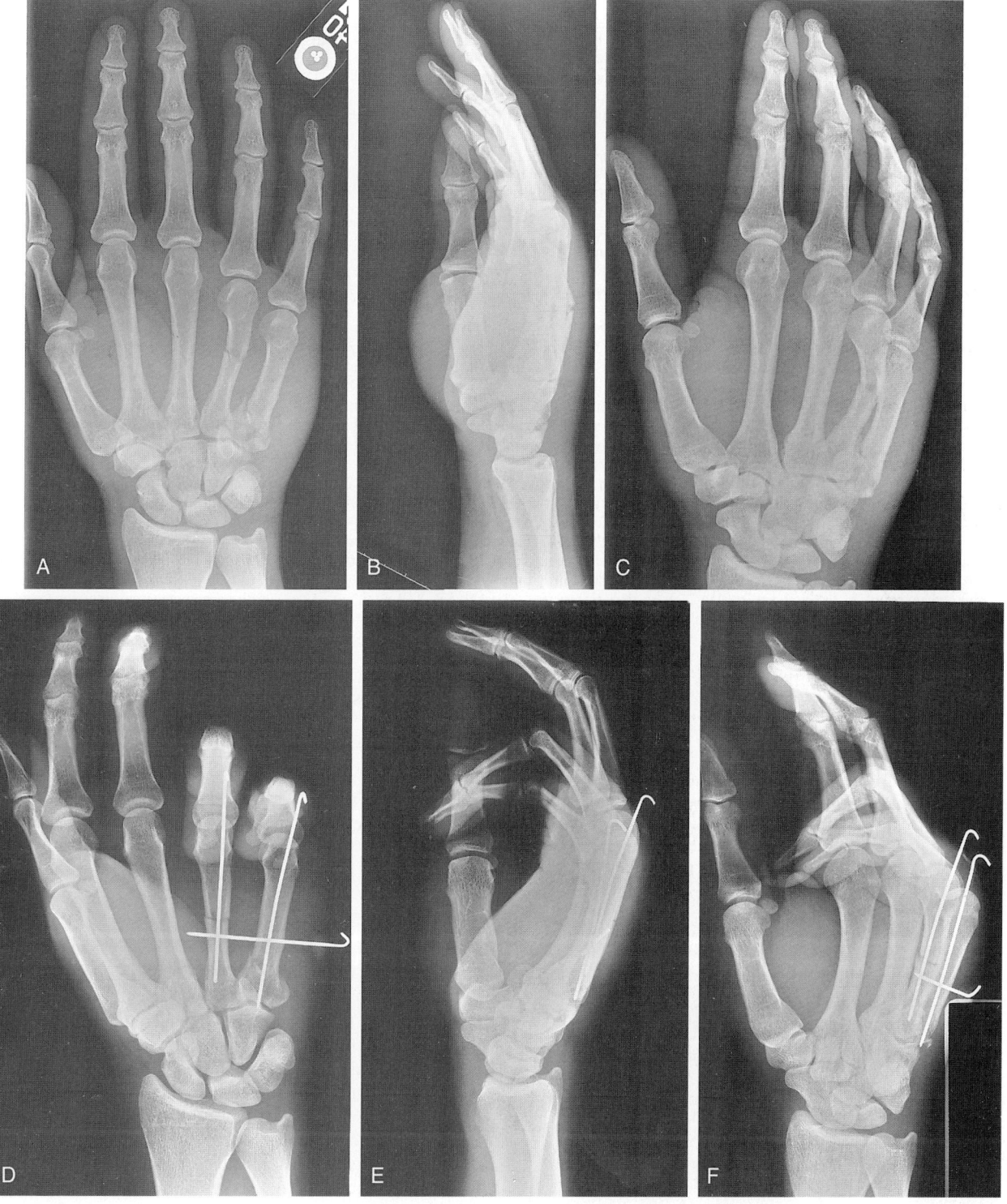

Fig. 6. Views. AP (*A*), lateral (*B*), and oblique (*C*) radiographs of the right hand reveal a mildly angulated shaft fracture of the ring metacarpal and a comminuted dorsal fracture-subluxation of the CMC joint of the little finger. SP/CRIF was performed. Postoperative AP (*D*), oblique (*E*), and lateral (*F*) radiographs show acceptable reduction and alignment of the fracture.

CMC JOINTS

Basilar fractures of the mobile fourth and fifth metacarpals and thumb metacarpal are commonly associated with CMC fracture-dislocations (Fig. 6). Closed or, possibly, open reduction with internal fixation is recommended. Post-traumatic arthrosis is commonly seen as a result of joint incongruency. CMC arthroplasty with ligament reconstruction may be required in late reconstruction. Intra-articular inju-

ries to the "fixed unit" CMC joint of the index and long fingers may be associated with avulsion of the wrist extensor tendinous insertion. Displaced avulsion fractures require reinsertion. Displaced fracture-dislocations of the index and long fingers require closed or, possibly, open reduction of these injuries. Late reconstruction may require arthrodesis of the index and long CMC joints.

BIBLIOGRAPHY

1. Ebinger T, Erhard N, Mentzel M: Dynamic treatment of displaced proximal phalangeal fractures. J Hand Surg Am 1999; 24:1254.
2. Belsky MR, Eaton RG, Lane LB: Closed reduction and internal fixation of proximal phalangeal fractures. J Hand Surg Am 1984; 9:225.
3. Hastings H: Unstable metacarpal and phalangeal fracture treatment with screws and plates. Clin Orthop 1987; 214:37.
4. Strickland JW, Steichen JB, Kleinman WB, et al: Phalangeal fractures: Factors influencing digital performance. Orthop Rev 1982; 11:39.
5. Valey JW, Wagner DA, Hastings H III: Effect of proximal phalangeal fracture deformity on extensor tendon function. J Hand Surg Am 1998; 23:673.
6. Jahss SA: Fractures of the proximal phalanx: A new method of reduction and immobilization. J Bone Joint Surg 1938; 18:726.
7. Strauch RJ, Rosenwasser MP, Lunt JG: Metacarpal shaft fractures: The effect of shortening on the extensor mechanism. J Hand Surg Am 1998; 23:519.
8. Kozin SH, Thoder JJ, Lieberman G: Operative treatment of metacarpal and phalangeal shaft fractures. J Am Acad Orthop Surg 2000; 8:111.
9. Gonzalez MH, Hall RF Jr: Intramedullary fixation of metacarpal and proximal phalangeal fractures of the hand. Clin Orthop 1996; 327:47.
10. Page SM, Stern PJ: Complications and

range of motion following plate fixation of metacarpal and phalangeal fractures. J Hand Surg Am 1998; 23:827.
11. Eaton RG, Littler JW: Joint injuries and their sequelae. Clin Plast Surg 1976; 3:85.
12. Ghobadi F, Anapoole DM: Irreducible distal interphalangeal joint dislocation of the finger: A new cause. J Hand Surg Am 1994; 19:196.
13. Trumble TE, Vedde NB, Benirschke SK: Misleading fractures after profundus tendon avulsions. J Hand Surg Am 1992; 17:902.
14. Bowers WH, Wolf JW Jr, Neh IJ, et al: The proximal interphalangeal joint volar plate. I: An anatomical and biomechanical study. J Hand Surg Am 1980; 5:79.
15. Hastings H III, Carroll C IV: Treatment of closed articular fractures of the metacarpophalangeal and proximal interphalangeal joints. Hand Clin 1988; 4:503.
16. Chin KR, Jupiter JB: Treatment of triplane fracture of the head of the proximal phalanx. J Hand Surg Am 1999; 24:1263.
17. Kiefhaber TR, Stein PJ: Fracture dislocation of the proximal interphalangeal joint. J Hand Surg Am 1998; 23:368.
18. Rosenstaat BE, Glickel SZ, Lane LB, et al: Palmar fracture dislocation of the proximal interphalangeal joint. J Hand Surg Am 1998; 23:811.
19. Eaton RG, Malerich MM: Volar plate arthroplasty of the proximal interphalangeal joint: A review of ten years experience. J Hand Surg 1980; 5:260.

20. McElfresh EC, Dobyns JH, O'Brien ET: Management of fracture-dislocation of the proximal interphalangeal joint by extension block splinting. J Bone Joint Surg Am 1972; 54:1705.
21. Schenck RR: Dynamic traction and early passive movement for fractures of the proximal interphalangeal joint. J Hand Surg Am 1986; 11:850.
22. Wolfe SW, Katz LD: Intra-articular fractures of the phalanges. J Hand Surg Am 1995; 20:327.
23. Stein PJ, Romar RJ, Kiefhaber TR, et al: Pilon fractures of proximal interphalangeal joint. J Hand Surg Am 1991; 16:844.
24. McElfresh EC, Dobyns JH: Intra-articular metacarpal head fractures. J Hand Surg Am 1983; 8:383.
25. Lane CS, Kennedy JF, Kuschner SH: The reverse oblique x-ray film: Metacarpal fractures revisited. J Hand Surg Am 1992; 17:504.
26. Duncan RW, Freeland AE, Jabaley ME, et al: Open hand fractures: An analysis of the recovery of active motion and of complications. J Hand Surg Am 1993; 18:387.
27. Gainor JG, Stark HH, Ashworth CR, et al: Tendon interposition arthroplasty of the fifth carpometacarpal joint for treatment of post-traumatic arthritis. J Hand Surg Am 1991; 16:520.
28. Breen TE, Gelberman RH, Jupiter JB: Intraarticular fractures of the basilar joint of the thumb. Hand Clin 1998; 4:491.

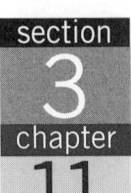

section 3 chapter 11

PELVIS AND SACRUM

Madhav Karunakar and James A. Goulet

Summary
- Pelvic fractures represent 3% of all fractures.
- Determination of pelvic stability is the key to treatment.
- High-energy pelvic fractures may be associated with life-threatening hemorrhage.
- Classification systems can be used to predict stability, associated injuries, and mortality.
- Despite early aggressive resuscitation, including the application of external fixators, a 10% mortality rate persists.

Over the past two decades, the management of pelvic ring injuries has changed dramatically as more patients with pelvic ring injuries survive high-energy automobile accidents and require the attention of orthopaedic surgeons. A host of factors have contributed to the change in approach. Prehospital mortality for polytraumatized patients in general has decreased as advanced trauma and life support (ATLS) protocols have become more routinely applied. Additionally, changes in the use and type of passenger restraints may be facilitating the early survival of individuals with pelvic fractures caused by high-energy motor vehicle accidents, decreasing the likelihood of sudden death from head and chest trauma.

Pelvic fracture management has followed a progression toward increasing intervention and surgical treatment of select pelvic ring injuries. The rationale for intervention initially arose from poor results observed in nonoperative management of displaced pelvic ring injuries. In 1948, Holdsworth[1] studied 27 patients with untreated sacroiliac (SI) dislocations, reporting that only half returned to work. All 27 patients had persistent low back pain. In 1966, Raf[2] reported on 65 patients with double vertical fractures of the pelvis. He found that outcome was worse if SI dislocation was present and noted a high incidence of nerve injury with posterior fractures through the sacrum. In 1972, Slatis and Huittinen[3] reported on the late sequelae of unstable pelvic fractures, noting problems with pelvic obliquity, impaired gait, disabling low back pain and signs of persistent nerve damage to the lumbosacral plexus in 46% of patients. They concluded that, although observation without surgical intervention afforded good results in fractures of moderate severity, obvious shortcomings existed in the management of severe pelvic injuries. In 1988, Tile[4] reviewed 248 patients with pelvic ring injuries and reported that stable injuries resulted in few major long-term problems with only mild to moderate pain. In contrast, vertically unstable injuries in Tile's series resulted in many problems; 60% of patients exhibited continued pain. Since then, renewed interest has developed in the operative management of pelvic fractures. In 1989 Matta published his techniques for the operative fixation of pelvic fractures.[5] More recently, Routt popularized percutaneous methods of fixation.[6] Short-term results suggest that improved outcomes may be achieved with open reduction of unstable pelvic fractures.[7, 8]

Although early mortality rates for patients with pelvic ring injuries has improved dramatically, mortality associated with these injuries remains high, ranging from 9% to 20%.[8] Survival is closely tied to hemodynamic stability. Hemodynamically unstable patients have been reported to have a mortality approaching 50%, whereas hemodynamically stable patients have a mortality of less than 10%.[9, 10] Early and aggressive resuscitation of patients with pelvic ring injuries remains a substantial challenge.

Management of pelvic ring injuries incorporates diverse challenges. The orthopaedic surgeon involved in pelvic fracture management must have knowledge and experience in acute resuscitation of trauma patients, have excellent assessment skills when contemplating surgical intervention, and develop highly specialized technical expertise in the operating suite.

ANATOMY

A knowledge of pelvic anatomy is critical in understanding fracture patterns and in determining treatment goals. The pelvic ring consists of three bones: the sacrum and two innominate bones. Each innominate bone is formed from the fusion of three ossification centers: the ilium, the ischium, and the pubis, which join at the triradiate cartilage of the acetabulum. The innominate bones join the sacrum posteriorly at the SI joints, and anteriorly they join each other at the pubic symphysis.

Ligaments are critical to pelvic stability (Fig. 1). The posterior SI ligaments, running from the sacrum to the posterior iliac spines, are the strongest ligaments in the body. The sacrotuberous ligaments consist of a strong band running from the posterolateral sacrum and dorsal aspect of the posterior iliac spine to the ischial tuberosity. The sacrotuberous ligaments along with the posterior SI ligaments maintain vertical stability of the pelvis. The sacrospinous ligaments run from the lateral edge of the sacrum and coccyx, separating the greater and lesser sciatic notches,

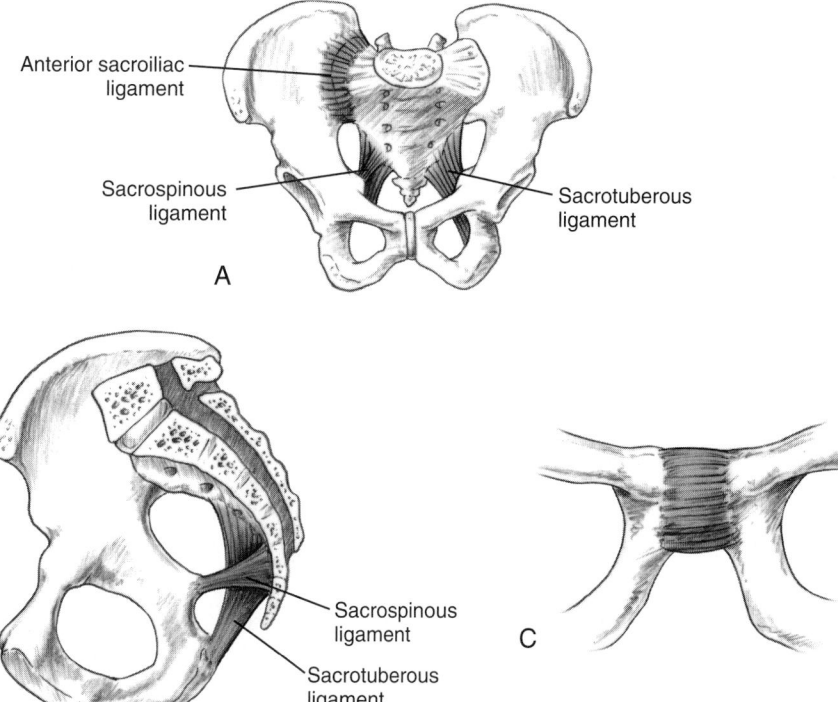

Anterior sacroiliac ligament

Sacrospinous ligament

Sacrotuberous ligament

A

Fig. 1. Views. *A*, Anteroposterior view of pelvic ligaments. *B*, Lateral view of pelvic ligaments. *C*, The symphysis pubis is the main anterior stabilizing ligament.

Sacrospinous ligament

Sacrotuberous ligament

B

C

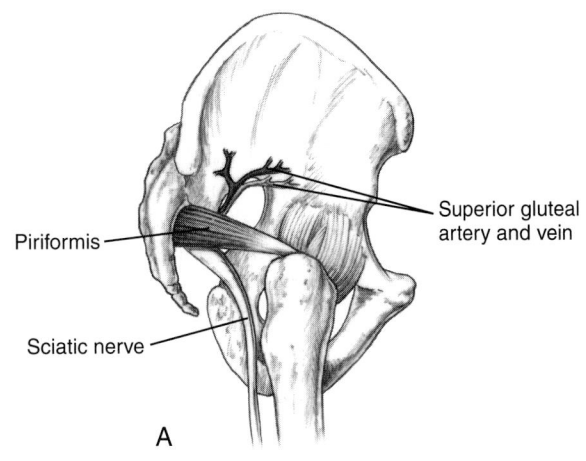

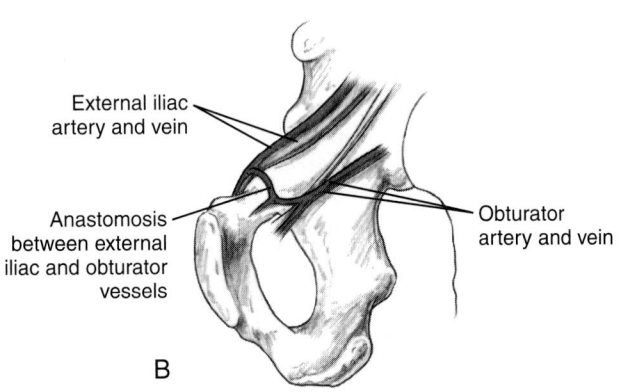

Fig. 2. Views. *A,* Relationship of superior gluteal and sciatic nerve to piriformis tendon. *B,* The corona mortis is an anastomosis between the external iliac and obturator vessels.

and insert on the ischial spine. The iliolumbar ligaments run from the L4 and L5 transverse processes to the posterior iliac crest to provide stability between the spine and the pelvis.

An understanding of the location of major nerves and vessels in relation to bony anatomy is particularly important for the application of percutaneous techniques of achieving pelvic ring stability (Fig. 2). The sciatic nerve is formed by roots from the lumbosacral plexus (L4, L5, S1, S1-3) and exits the pelvis deep to the piriformis muscle. The lumbosacral trunk is formed by the anterior rami of L4 and L5 and crosses the anterior sacral ala and the SI joint. Fractures of the sacral ala or dislocations of the SI joint are most likely to injure the lumbosacral trunk. The L5 nerve root exits below L5 transverse process and crosses the sacral ala 2 cm medial to the SI joint; it may be injured during an anterior approach to the SI joint.

Pelvic fractures are frequently associated with large amounts of blood loss. The internal iliac artery (hypogastric artery) is the most important vascular structure in pelvic trauma. The anterior division consists of the inferior gluteal artery, the internal pudendal artery, obturator artery, and inferior vesicular and middle rectal arteries. The posterior division consists of the superior gluteal artery, iliolumbar artery, and lateral sacral artery. The superior gluteal

artery is the largest branch of the internal iliac artery. It courses along the SI joint and exits through the greater sciatic notch superior to the piriformis. The superior gluteal artery supplies the gluteus medius, gluteus minimus, and tensor fascia lata muscles. The superior gluteal artery is the most commonly injured artery in pelvic fractures. The majority of bleeding after pelvic fracture results from venous injury. The pelvic viscera lie on a large thin-walled venous plexus that drains into the internal iliac vein. Massive bleeding after may result from disruption of this venous plexus.

Other neurovascular structures that lie in close proximity to the bony pelvis may be damaged when a pelvic fracture occurs.

The close relationship of the urogenital tract and the bony pelvis results in a high incidence of urinary tract injuries (Fig. 3). Bladder rupture and posterior urethral injuries are the most common injuries. Signs of bladder injury include inability to void despite a full bladder, blood at the urethral meatus, high riding or abnormally mobile prostate, and an elevated bladder. A retrograde urethrogram should be obtained to rule out urethral injury before insertion of a Foley catheter if an anterior pelvic disruption is present or any sign of urethral injury exists. Anatomic differences between males and females result in a higher incidence of urethral injuries in males. The male urethra has three portions: prostatic, membranous, and bulbous. The bulbous urethra, located inferior to the urogenital diaphragm, is the most common site of injury. In contrast, the female urethra is short, not rigidly fixed to the pubis or pelvic floor, more mobile, and less susceptible to injury from shear forces.[11] If the urethra is ruptured, retrograde urethrogram dye will extravasate into the perineum. Impotence may occur in 25% to 47% of male patients with urethral rupture. Impotence is likely secondary to damage of parasympathetic nerves (S2-4). Absence of meatal blood or high-riding prostate does not rule out a urethral injury.[11]

Bladder injuries may result from bony spicules arising from pubic rami fractures, blunt force causing rupture, or shearing injuries. The superior and upper posterior portions of the bladder are covered by peritoneum. The remainder of the bladder is extraperitoneal and covered with loose areolar tissue. Intraperitoneal ruptures usually require oper-

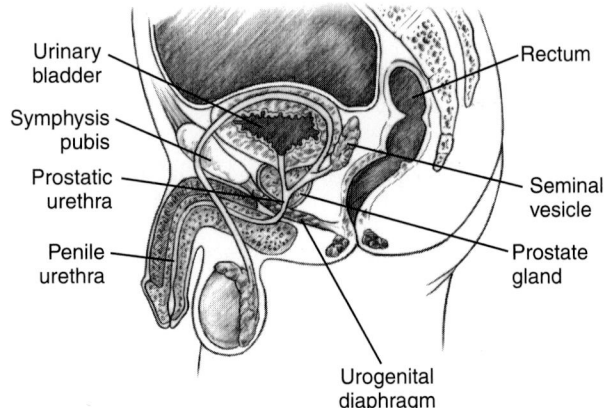

Fig. 3. View. The proximity of the urogenital tract to the bony pelvis results in a high incidence of injuries.

ative repair, whereas extraperitoneal ruptures are managed nonoperatively unless undergoing laparotomy. Extraperitoneal bladder ruptures are typically managed with suprapubic catheter drainage and broad-spectrum antibiotics. A cystogram is performed before catheter removal to verify healing. Eighty-seven percent are healed by 10 days and virtually all are healed by 3 weeks.[12]

PATHOGENESIS

Pelvic fractures range in severity from relatively benign avulsion injuries to massive pelvic disruptions. The mechanism of injury is typically high-energy trauma. Lateral compression injuries are frequently seen in motor vehicle accidents, vertical shear injuries occur with a fall, and anteroposterior (AP) compression injuries occur in pedestrians struck by automobiles. Low-energy fractures include avulsion of the tendon bone complex in younger patients and fractures in elderly patients who have fallen from a standing position.

CLINICAL FEATURES

Most low-energy pelvic fractures can be treated with rest and analgesia until the pain has resolved enough to allow a return to normal activities. In contrast, patients with high-energy pelvic fractures often are critically ill and have other life-threatening injuries.[13–15] The emergency evaluation of the polytrauma patient with a pelvic ring injury involves a multidisciplinary approach, including general surgeons, orthopaedic surgeons, and emergency care personnel. These patients may present with hemodynamic instability or associated major central nervous system, chest, or abdominal injuries.[13–15]

Orthopaedic evaluation should include a determination of the stability of the pelvic fracture. The practice of compressing and distracting the iliac wings and applying manual leg traction to determine instability lacks sensitivity, is nonspecific, and should be avoided. Radiographs are the most useful tools in the diagnosis of pelvic stability. Standard AP pelvis trauma films will show 90% of cases of posterior instability.[16] Stable fractures are characterized by impacted vertical fractures of the sacrum, nondisplaced fractures of the posterior SI complex, or subtle fractures of the upper sacrum, as evidenced by asymmetry of the sacral arcuate lines. Unstable fractures are characterized by cephalad displacement of the hemipelvis exceeding 0.5 cm and SI diastasis exceeding 0.5 cm.[16] Findings suspicious for pelvic instability include cephalad hemipelvic displacement less than 1 cm or a diastatic fracture of the sacrum or ilium less than 0.5 cm. These indeterminate cases may require further imaging to determine stability. Edeiken-Monroe et al[16] found that standard radiographs accurately evaluated pelvic stability in 88% of cases they studied. A fracture of the fifth lumbar transverse process, previously described as a sign of an unstable pelvis, was found in both stable and unstable injuries and was not a reliable sign of pelvic instability.

If the patient is hemodynamically stable, additional radiographs can be obtained to improve the understanding of the fracture. The acute treatment of an unstable pelvic fracture should never be delayed for additional radiographic studies. The inlet pelvis is a 40- to 45-degree caudal tilt view that shows AP displacement. Inward rotation associated with lateral compression injuries can also be identified (Fig. 4). An outlet pelvis is a 40- to 45-degree cephalad tilt view that shows vertical displacement and fractures of the sacral foramina. A computed tomography (CT) scan is particularly useful for sacral fractures and SI joint fractures or dislocations. A lateral sacral view can be important to prevent missing transverse fractures (Fig. 5).

The orthopaedic examination is not complete until a rectal exam is performed. A high-riding prostate may indicate a urethral tear. The sacrum should be palpated for frac-

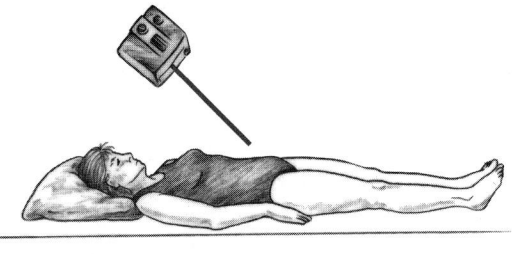 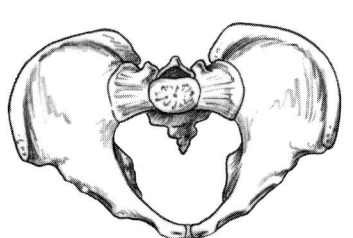

A Inlet view of pelvis

Fig. 4. Views. *A,* An inlet pelvis view with 40- to 45-degree caudal tilt shows AP displacement. *B,* An outlet pelvis view with 40- to 45-degree cephalad tilt shows vertical displacement and sacral foramina fractures.

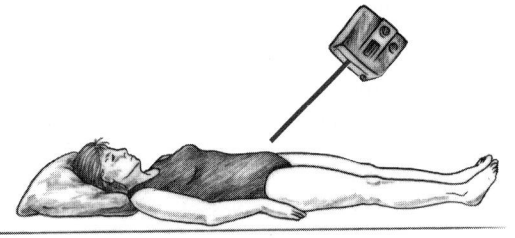 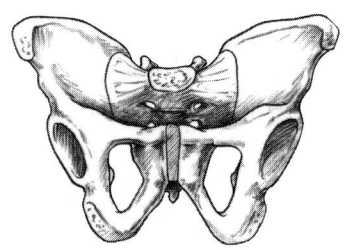

B Outlet view of pelvis

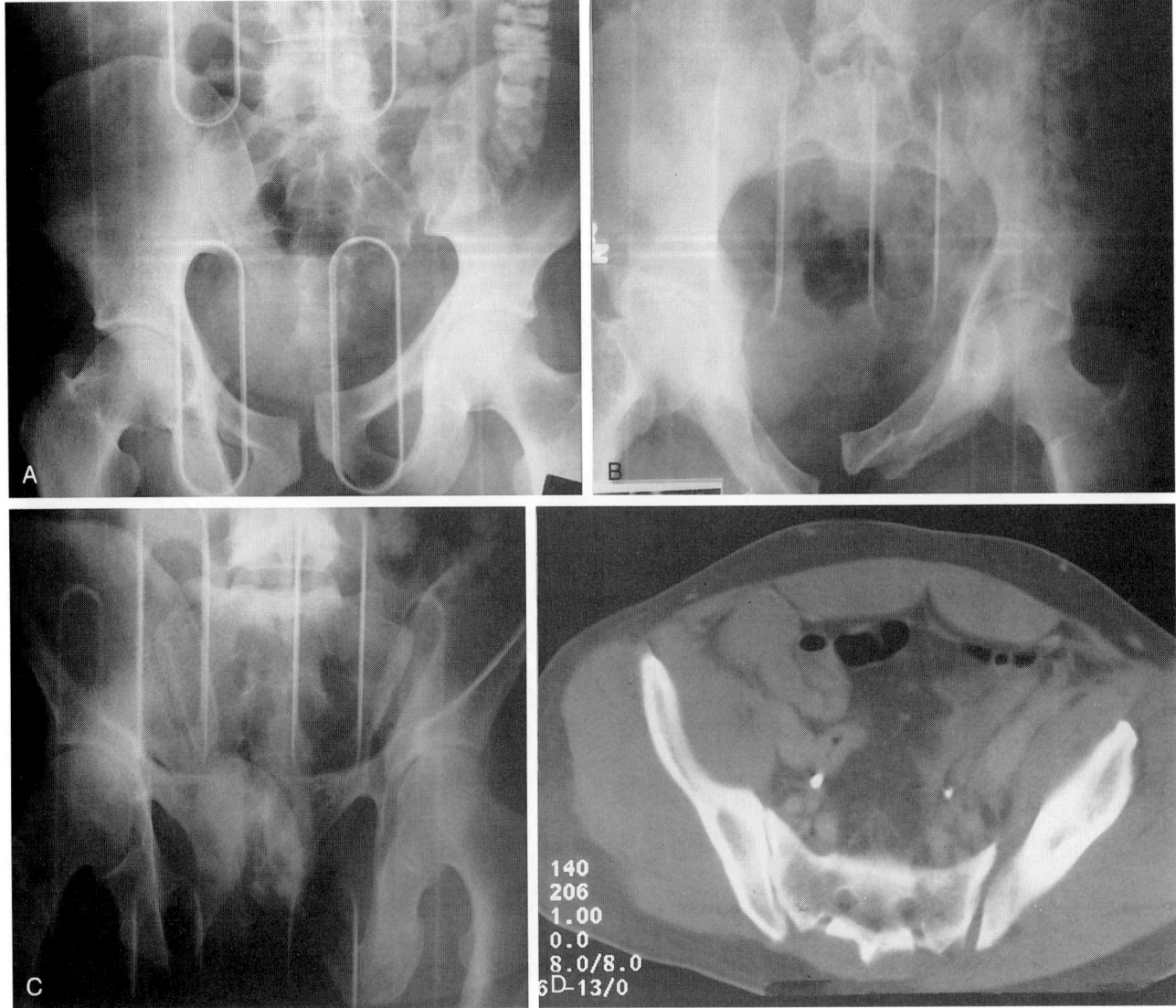

Fig. 5. Views. *A*, AP pelvis. *B*, Inlet pelvis. *C*, Outlet pelvis. *D*, CT scan demonstrates symphyseal disruption and sacroiliac joint widening.

tures. If suspicion for a rectal tear is high, flexible sigmoid-oscopy may be performed to examine for rectal tears. Vaginal bleeding may suggest simply a laceration or may indicate an open fracture. A speculum examination should be performed if vaginal bleeding is found. All perineal skin lacerations should be explored to rule out connection with a fracture site.

Fracture classification is important in determining stability, associated injuries, and resuscitation requirements. Tile[4, 17, 18] proposed a classification based on a continuum of stability. Type A fractures are stable and do not fracture through the pelvic ring or soft tissues (Table 1). The posterior ligamentous arch is intact. These fractures include avulsion-type fractures, iliac wing fractures, and transverse fractures of the sacrum or coccyx. A type B fracture is rotationally unstable. These injuries are partially stable with an incomplete disruption of the posterior arch. This sub-group includes open book and lateral compression injuries. Type C fractures are vertically unstable with complete disruption of the posterior arch and pelvic floor. Posterior

translation and vertical translation are possible. The hemi-pelvis is completely unstable.

The Young and Burgess[14] classification is based on Tile's (Table 2) and includes four injury mechanism sub-types: anterior posterior compression (APC), lateral compression (LC), vertical shear (VS), combined mechanism (CM) (Fig. 6). The subtypes have been closely correlated with resuscitation needs and the patterns of associated injuries. An APC injury results from anterior impact to the pelvis leading to pubic symphysis diastasis or an anterior vertical fracture pattern of the rami without translational realignment of the posterior pelvis. The anterior SI ligaments as well as ipsilateral sacrospinous and sacrotuberous ligaments are disrupted. The pelvis is rotationally unstable. The LC injury results from a lateral impact to innominate bone with rotation of the pelvis toward the midline. The sacrotuberous and sacrospinous ligaments and internal iliac vessels are shortened rather than stretched. A VS injury results in vertical translation of the hemipelvis. This usu-ally occurs as a disruption of the SI joint. A CM injury

TABLE 1. TILE CLASSIFICATION

Type	Description
A	Stable pelvic fractures
A1	Typically an avulsion fracture
	Pelvic ring intact
A2	Nondisplaced ring fracture
A3	Transverse fractures of sacrum and coccyx
	Pelvic ring intact
B	Rotationally unstable, vertically stable
B1	Anteroposterior compression injury
	Open book pelvic fractures
	Divided into three stages: Stage 1, pubic symphysis diastasis <2.5 cm, no involvement of posterior pelvic ring; stage 2, pubic symphysis diastasis >2.5 cm, unilateral posterior pelvic ring injury; stage 3, pubic symphysis diastasis >2.5 cm, bilateral posterior pelvic ring injuries
B2	Lateral compression injury, ipsilateral
	Rami are commonly fractured anteriorly
	Posterior complex is crushed
B3	Lateral compression, contralateral (bucket handle)
	Major anterior lesion is usually on the opposite side of the posterior lesion, but all four rami may be fractured anteriorly
	Affected hemipelvis rotates anteriorly and superiorly (like the handle of a bucket)
	Flexion of hemipelvis results in leg length discrepancy
	Reduction requires derotation of hemipelvis
	Usually caused by a direct blow on the iliac crest
C	Rotationally and vertically unstable
C1	Ipsilateral anterior and posterior pelvic injuries
C2	Bilateral hemipelvic disruptions
C3	Any pelvic fracture with an associated acetabular fracture

The Denis classification is used to describe sacral fractures.[20] The classification is divided into three zones based on the potential for neurological injury (Fig. 7). Zone I involves the alar region. The L5 nerve root is at highest risk but neurological injury is rare (5.9%). Zone II includes the sacral foramina. The risk of neurological injury is 28% with involvement of the L5, S1, S2 nerve roots. A zone III injury involves the central sacral canal. Neurological injury may occur in 56% of patients and frequently involves bowel, bladder, and sexual function (cauda equina). The highest incidence of neurogenic bladder injury occurs with zone III injuries. A cystometrogram should be obtained to evaluate bladder function.[20, 21] Most sacral fractures with the exception of transverse fractures can be classified as pelvic fractures. Transverse sacral fractures may be missed on pelvic radiographs and CT scans. A lateral radiograph of the sacrum is the imaging modality of choice. These fractures should be considered spine injuries and are classified as Denis zone III, because the most significant injury involves the spinal canal. Transverse sacral fractures may also develop late kyphotic deformities.

Patients with high-energy pelvic fractures often have abdominal, head, and thoracic injuries.[9, 10, 14] Sixty percent to 80% of patients have musculoskeletal injuries, 12% have urogenital injuries, and 8% have lumbosacral injuries. Aggressive fluid resuscitation is critical in the hemodynamically unstable patient. The severity of blood loss can be determined by assessing pulse, blood pressure, and capillary refill. These indicators can be used to evaluate a pa-

involves features of both a lateral compression and a vertical shear injury or both a lateral compression and an APC injury.[14]

Burgess et al[13] showed that the transfusion requirements for patients with lateral compression injuries averaged 3.6 units compared with a mean of 14.8 units with APC injuries, 9.2 with VS fractures, and 8.5 units with a CM (Table 3). The overall mortality for pelvic fractures in their study was 8.6%. A higher mortality rate was seen in the APC (20%) and CM (18%) types compared with the LC (7%) and VS (0%) types. Exsanguination from pelvic injuries as a result of LC injuries was rare. The most common identifiable cause of death for patients with LC injuries was a closed head injury, whereas with APC injuries the cause of death was combined pelvic and visceral injury.[13, 14]

The crescent fracture is a posterior fracture dislocation of the SI joint. It is a subset of the LC-type injuries. The injury involves a combination of ligamentous disruption of the inferior portion of the SI joint and a vertical fracture of the posterior ilium extending from the middle of the SI joint and exiting the iliac crest. The posterosuperior iliac spine remains firmly attached to the sacrum via the superior portion of the posterior ligamentous complex. The pattern of associated injuries is similar to that seen with other LC injuries with a significant number of closed head injuries and visceral injuries and a low incidence of life-threatening pelvic bleeding.[19]

TABLE 2. YOUNG AND BURGESS CLASSIFICATION

Subclassification	Anatomic Features
APC	
Type I	Symphysis widened 1–2 cm
	SI ligaments intact
Type II	Symphysis widened >2 cm
	Anterior SI ligaments disrupted
	Sacrospinous ligaments ruptured
	Sacrotuberous ligaments ruptured
	Posterior SI ligaments intact
Type III	Complete separation of hemipelvis from pelvic ring
	No vertical displacement as seen in LC type III
LC	
Type I	Anterior pelvic ring injury
	Impacted sacrum on side of injury
Type II	Anterior pelvic ring injury
	Crescent fracture of iliac wing or near SI joint
Type III	LC type I or II on side of injury
	Addition of open book type injury of SI joint on opposite side
	Pelvic ring internally rotated on injury side; opposite side is externally rotated
VS	Vertical displacement of hemipelvis
	Usually occurs as rupture of SI joint but occasionally occurs as fracture
	Through sacrum or ilium
CM	Combination of LC and VS or LC and APC

SI = sacroiliac; LC = lateral compression; VS = vertical shear; APC = anteroposterior compression; CM = combined mechanism.

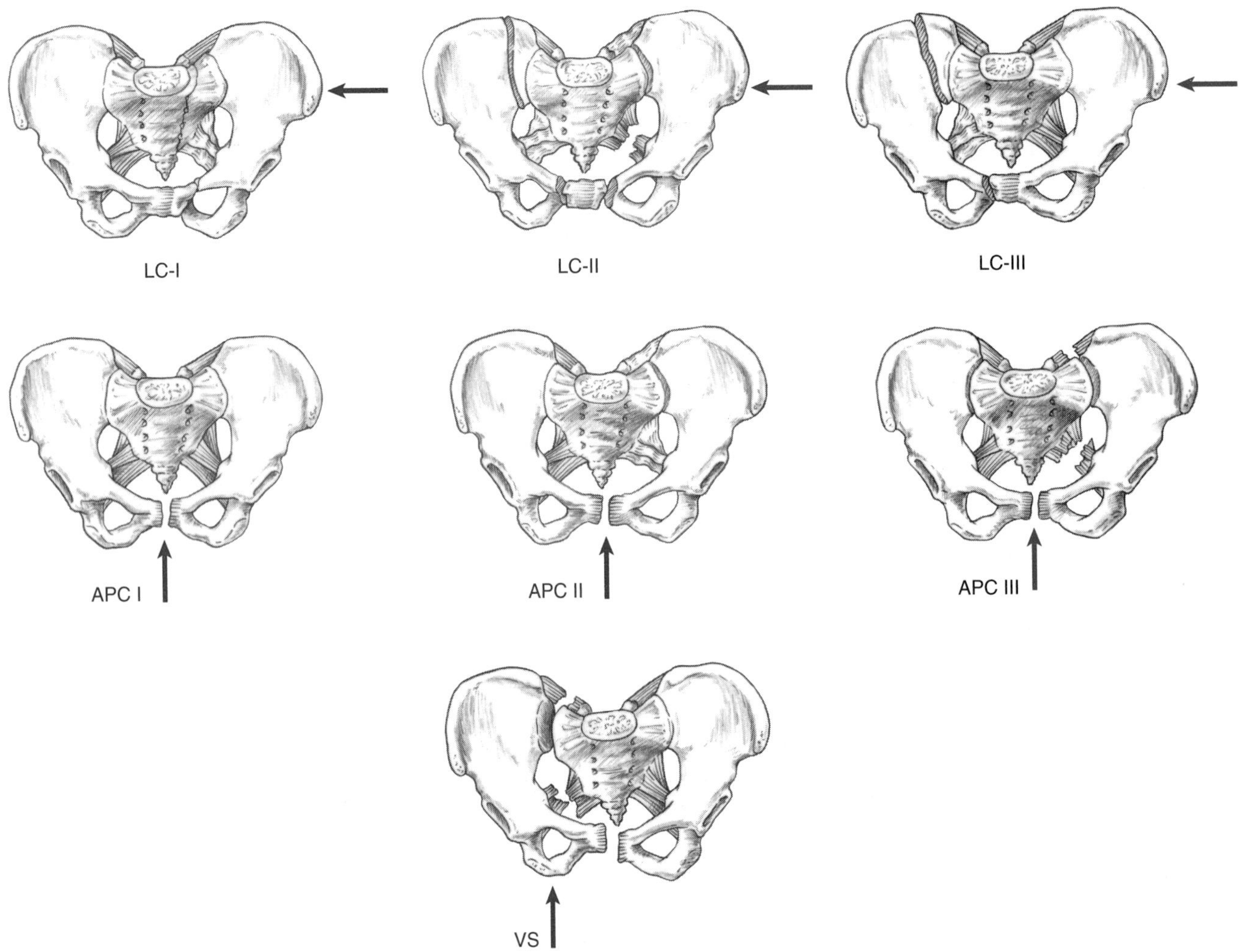

LC-I

LC-II

LC-III

APC I

APC II

APC III

VS

Fig. 6. Views. Lateral compression, anteroposterior compression, and vertical shear mechanism of injury as described in Young and Burgess pelvic fracture classification.

tient's response to the resuscitative effort. Two large (16 gauge or larger) intravenous cannulas should be established. Replacement volume is estimated by using the formula of 3 mL of crystalloid for each 1 mL of blood loss.

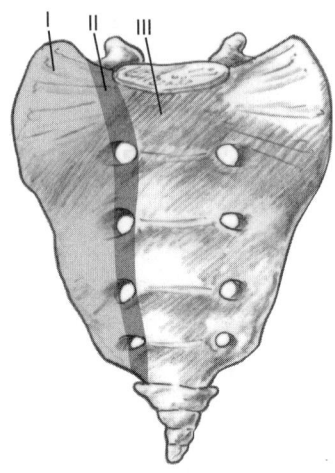

Fig. 7. View. Denis classification of sacral fractures.

A minimum of 2 L of crystalloid solution is given over 20 minutes or more rapidly for patients in shock. If an adequate blood pressure is obtained, crystalloid is administered until type-specific fully matched blood is available. If the response is poor, an additional 2 L of crystalloid is given and type-specific or non–cross-matched universal donor (O negative) blood is prepared[22] (Table 4).

Displaced pelvic fractures can be temporarily stabilized by simple means during the initial evaluation and transportation. These methods rely on immobilization and partial reduction of displacement. A sheet can be tied around the pelvis or the legs can be tied together in an internally rotated position to approximate an anterior pelvic diastasis. Military antishock trousers have proved to be effective in the prehospital treatment of hypotensive patients with pelvic fractures. Their use in the hospital is not common because they limit access to injured areas of the body, decrease expansion of the lungs, and may contribute to the development of compartment syndrome in hypoperfused extremities.[8]

In most cases, blood loss from a pelvic injury occurs from cancellous bone at the fracture site or from a retroperitoneal lumbar plexus venous injury. Only 20% of pel-

		Transfusion Requirement (units)	Mortality (%)	
Type	Description			Associated Injuries
APC	Pubic symphysis diastasis Rotationally unstable	14.8	20	Death usually results from hemorrhage in visceral and pelvic structures
LC	Lateral impact Sacrospinous, sacrotuberous ligaments intact	3.6	7	Death related to brain injury
VS	Vertical translation Hemipelvis unstable	9.2	0	Similar to lateral compression
CM	LC + VS or LC + APC	8.5	18	Variable

TABLE 3. YOUNG AND BURGESS CLASSIFICATION

APC = anteroposterior compression; LC = lateral compression; VS = vertical shear; CM = combined mechanism.

vic hemorrhage deaths are attributed to a major arterial injury. Posterior arterial bleeding is more common in patients with unstable posterior pelvic fractures. Anterior arterial bleeding (pudendal or obturator) is more common in patients with LC injuries. The most frequently injured arterial vessel with a posterior fracture is the superior gluteal artery.[23]

Hemorrhage from a pelvic fracture is seldom the only source of bleeding.[10] Poole et al[24] found, in a large series of polytrauma patients with pelvic fractures, that the major source of bleeding was from nonpelvic sites. The abdomen and bladder are frequently injured and should be evaluated as a source of hemorrhage. A supraumbilical diagnostic peritoneal lavage is recommended to avoid a false-positive result secondary to pelvic hematoma. An emergent laparotomy is indicated if the initial aspirate reveals more than 5 mL gross blood or obvious enteric contents. In hemodynamically stable patients, a CT scan or ultrasonogram can be used to evaluate the abdomen noninvasively.

If diagnostic peritoneal lavage is negative and the patient remains hemodynamically unstable, external fixation may have a role in the patient's acute management. Riemer et al[6] documented an overall decrease in mortality rate from 26% to 6% in patients with pelvic ring injuries after initiating a protocol that included external fixation and early mobilization for pelvic fractures. The mortality for hypotensive patients decreased from 41% to 21%. Benefits of external fixation include immobilization of fractures limiting the clot disruption that may occur during patient movement and transfer. Experimental evidence exists that reduc-

tion of an open book pelvis leads to an increase in retroperitoneal pressure, which may aid in the tamponade of venous bleeding.[25]

Despite this evidence, the use of external fixation remains controversial. Gruen et al[26] reported on 36 hemodynamically unstable multiple-trauma patients whose pelvic fractures were not acutely stabilized by external fixation. These patients received both volume resuscitation and treatment of associated injuries. Thirty-nine percent of the fractures were rotationally unstable, whereas 61% were both rotationally and vertically unstable. The overall mortality rate was 11%. All deaths were attributed to associated injuries and comorbidities.

A continued unexplained blood loss despite fracture stabilization and aggressive resuscitation mandates angiographic exploration to look for continued arterial bleeding. The techniques for arteriography and embolization were developed in the 1970s. Embolization provides the most direct and beneficial means of controlling arterial hemorrhage. It avoids the retroperitoneal contamination associated with operative ligation of bleeding vessels while preserving the tamponade effect in the retroperitoneal space. The timing of arteriography and embolization is controversial. Most authors recommend arteriography after the initial stabilization or laparotomy or both. A skilled radiologist is of critical importance. Aggressive fluid resuscitation must be continued during angiography. Hypothermia may develop during a prolonged radiographic procedure if the patient is not adequately warmed and resuscitated. Complications include necrosis of buttocks after occlusion of the

TABLE 4. SHOCK (CLASSES OF HEMORRHAGE)

Variable	Class I	Class II	Class III	Class IV
Blood loss	Up to 750 mL Up to 15%	750–1500 mL 15%–30%	1500–2000 mL 30%–40%	>2000 mL >40%
Pulse rate (bpm)	<100	>100	>120	>140
Blood pressure	Normal	Normal	Decreased	Decreased
Pulse pressure	Normal	Decreased	Decreased	Decreased
Respiratory rate	14–20	20–30	30–40	>35
Urine output (mL)	>30	20–30	5–15	Negligible
Fluid replacement	Crystalloid	Crystalloid	Crystalloid and blood	Crystalloid and blood

TABLE 5. TRANSFER CRITERIA FOR PELVIC FRACTURES
Persistent hemodynamic instability after initial resuscitation
Bladder/urethral injuries and pelvic fractures
Open pelvic fractures
Laterally directed force causing fractures through iliac wing, sacral ala, or foramina, which are displaced internally
Anteroposterior compression injury with anterior displacement of greater than 2.5 mm
Complete translational instability: sacroiliac joint dislocation, complete displacement of sacral fracture
Acetabular fractures associated with pelvic ring injuries

entire iliac artery, skin slough, paresis of the femoral or sciatic nerve, and necrosis of the bladder.[8] Burgess et al[13] found that embolization was needed in 20% of APC, VS, and complex fractures but in only 1.7% of LC fractures.

Open fractures include direct communication between the pelvic fracture site and a vaginal, rectal, perineal, or other skin laceration. The mortality rate is reported to be up to 50%.[8] Early diagnosis is essential, and a thorough examination must be performed so that these injuries are not missed. Small vaginal or rectal tears that communicate with and contaminate the fracture site may be missed. Radiographs should be checked for air in the soft tissue and retroperitoneum. Rectal and perineal wounds must be treated aggressively. Diverting colostomy is the mainstay of treatment[27] (Table 5).

GOALS, INDICATIONS, AND CONTRAINDICATIONS

The goal of treatment in the hemodynamically unstable patient is resuscitation and prevention of further hemorrhage. The goals of fracture treatment are the same as with other bones: a healed fracture with the prevention of nonunion, malunion, or other complications. External fixation is indicated for the immediate management of patients with hemodynamic instability associated with pelvic fractures.[7, 28] External fixation has also been used in rotationally unstable pelvic fractures.[18] Open reduction and internal fixation is preferred for definitive management and has been shown to give superior results. Operative indications include diastasis of the pubic symphysis greater than 2.5 cm, SI joint dislocations, displaced sacral fractures, crescent fractures, posterior or vertical displacement of hemipelvis (greater than 1 cm), rotationally unstable pelvic ring injuries, sacral fractures in patients with unstable pelvic ring injuries requiring mobilization, and displaced sacral fractures with neurological injury (Table 6).

Contraindications for internal fixation include unstable critically ill patients, severe open fractures with inadequate wound débridement, crushing injuries, Morel-Lavallee lesions, and the placement of a suprapubic tube in the operative field. Specific contraindications for percutaneous fixation include a dysmorphic upper sacrum, obesity, skin compromise, and poor fluoroscopic images.

PROCEDURES

A preoperative plan requires quality radiographs, including an AP pelvis, and inlet and outlet views (Table 7). A CT scan is helpful to evaluate the sacrum for posterior injury and is part of routine preoperative evaluation. The mechanism of injury, soft-tissue condition, and patient positioning should be reviewed. Before the start of a percutaneous procedure, the ability to obtain adequate fluoroscopic images must be confirmed. The need for skeletal traction as a reduction aid should also be determined. Pelvic ring internal fixation is not routinely performed acutely after injury. Definitive stabilization is usually performed 2 to 3 days after stabilization. However, if a laparotomy is performed and an unstable anterior lesion is present, internal fixation of the symphysis may be performed.

TECHNICAL DETAILS

External fixation is indicated for hemodynamically unstable pelvic fractures.[6] External fixation should be avoided in the hemodynamically stable patient unless it will serve as definitive stabilization. Infected or contaminated pin sites may compromise future approaches to the anterior SI joint and the iliac wing. The surgeon should be familiar with the external fixation equipment so that it may be used quickly and efficiently in the critically ill patient. Pins can be placed either along the iliac crest or in the supra-acetabular region. Placement in the iliac crest is simple and direct. This location is most appropriate for rapid pin placement in a hemodynamically unstable patient. The thickest bone for pin insertion is in the anterior pillar of the iliac wing. Anatomically, the iliac crest overhangs laterally. A pin placed in the center of the crest will miss the iliac wing. The best starting position is in the medial one-third of the anterior pillar. Supra-acetabular pins are placed at the level of the anteroinferior iliac spine in a direction perpendicular

TABLE 6. OPERATIVE INDICATIONS	
Treatment	**Indications**
Nonoperative	Nondisplaced fractures
	Minimally displaced fractures
	Most pubic rami fractures
	LC type 1, Tile type B2
	Symphysis disruption <2.5 cm
	APC type 1
External fixation	Acute fixation of open book (Tile type B1, Young and Burgess APC type II, Bucholz II)
	Hemodynamic instability (APC type II and III, LC type II and III, VS, CM)
	Type B2, B3 (rotationally unstable)
ORIF	Symphysis disruption >2.5 cm
	Sacroiliac joint dislocation
	Displaced zone II sacral fracture
	Crescent fracture (LC type II)
	VS fracture

LC = lateral compression; APC = anteroposterior compression; VS = vertical shear; CM = combined mechanism; ORIF = open reduction and internal fixation.

TABLE 7. PREOPERATIVE PLAN		
Pelvic Injury	**Preferred Exposure**	**Implant**
Symphysis disruption	Pfannenstiel	Six-hole 3.5-mm curved reconstruction plate
Pubic rami	Pfannenstiel, Stoppa	3.5-mm lag screw
	Ilioinguinal	3.5-mm reconstruction plate
Iliac wing	Iliac, Iliofemoral	3.5-mm lag screws
	Ilioinguinal	3.5-mm reconstruction plate
Crescent fracture	Posterior	3.5- or 4.5-mm medullary lag screws
		3.5-mm reconstruction plate
		Iliosacral screws
Sacroiliac joint disruption	Iliac	Iliosacral screw
		Dual two-hole 4.5-mm DC plates
	Posterior	Iliosacral screws
Sacral fracture	Posterior	Iliosacral screw
		Tension band plate
		Sacral bars

DC = dynamic compression.

to the floor. This pin is in close proximity to the hip joint and must be inserted with great care, using an image intensifier for guidance. The skin incision is placed at right angles to the pelvic brim in line with the direction of the planned reduction, avoiding the need for additional relaxing incisions. A spinal needle or Kirschner wire can be placed along the inner table of the pelvis to help determine the orientation of the hemipelvis. Frame constructs are varied. The frame should be far enough away from the abdomen to allow for abdominal distention, for future surgical approaches, and for upright positioning.

Symphyseal plating is performed through a Pfannenstiel incision. The superficial transverse incision is converted to a deep longitudinal approach. Transection of the rectus abdominis is unnecessary. The linea alba is split between the two heads of the rectus abdominis. Detachment of one head of the rectus abdominis from the injury is common. The simplest method to achieve a reduction is by placing a large pointed reduction clamp around each side of the symphysis (Fig. 8). The reduction may require the use of a pelvic reduction clamp if the posterior ring is disrupted. The displaced innominate bone is typically externally rotated with posterior and cephalad displacement.[29] A number of different plates have been recommended to stabilize a symphyseal disruption, including two-hole, four-hole, and six-hole plates. Both 3.5-mm and 4.5-mm plates and screws have been recommended. Proponents of the two-hole fixation technique claim the advantage that implant loosening may permit the return of physiological motion of the symphysis after fixation and may avoid late problems of implant fatigue failure.[30] However, fracture reduction is more frequently lost with a two-hole plate. We prefer a six-hole curved 3.5-mm reconstruction plate (Fig. 9).

SI screws can be placed both through open techniques or percutaneously.[31] The procedure can be performed in either the supine or prone position. The technique is technically demanding and requires good C-arm visualization.[32] A thorough understanding of the radiographic anatomy is critical to perform this procedure. The pelvic inlet, outlet, and lateral sacral views must be obtained to define the safe corridor for screw placement (Fig. 10). The ideal pelvic

inlet view should superimpose the upper sacral vertebral bodies as concentric circles. If the anterior cortex of S1 overlies the coccyx, the concavity of the sacrum may not be appreciated. This may result in a screw penetrating the anterior border of the S1 body. The ideal pelvic outlet view is obtained when the symphysis is superimposed on the second sacral vertebral body. The outlet view allows

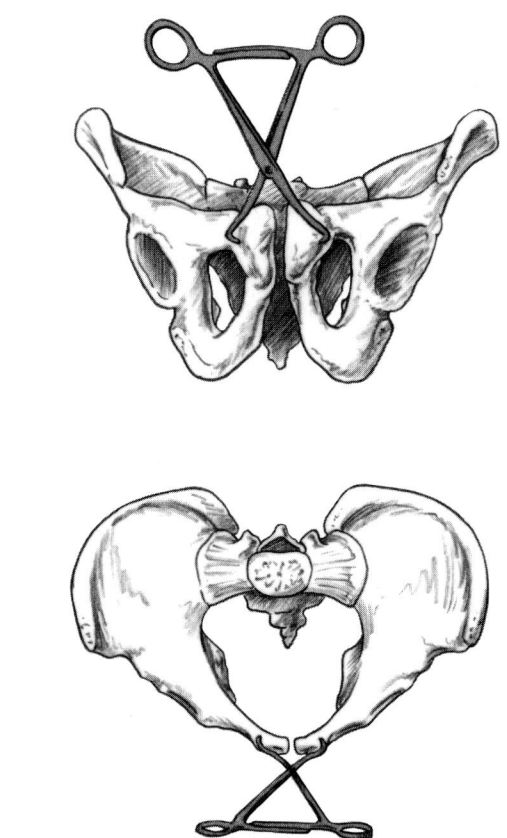

Fig. 8. View. Reduction of symphyseal disruption with pointed reduction clamp.

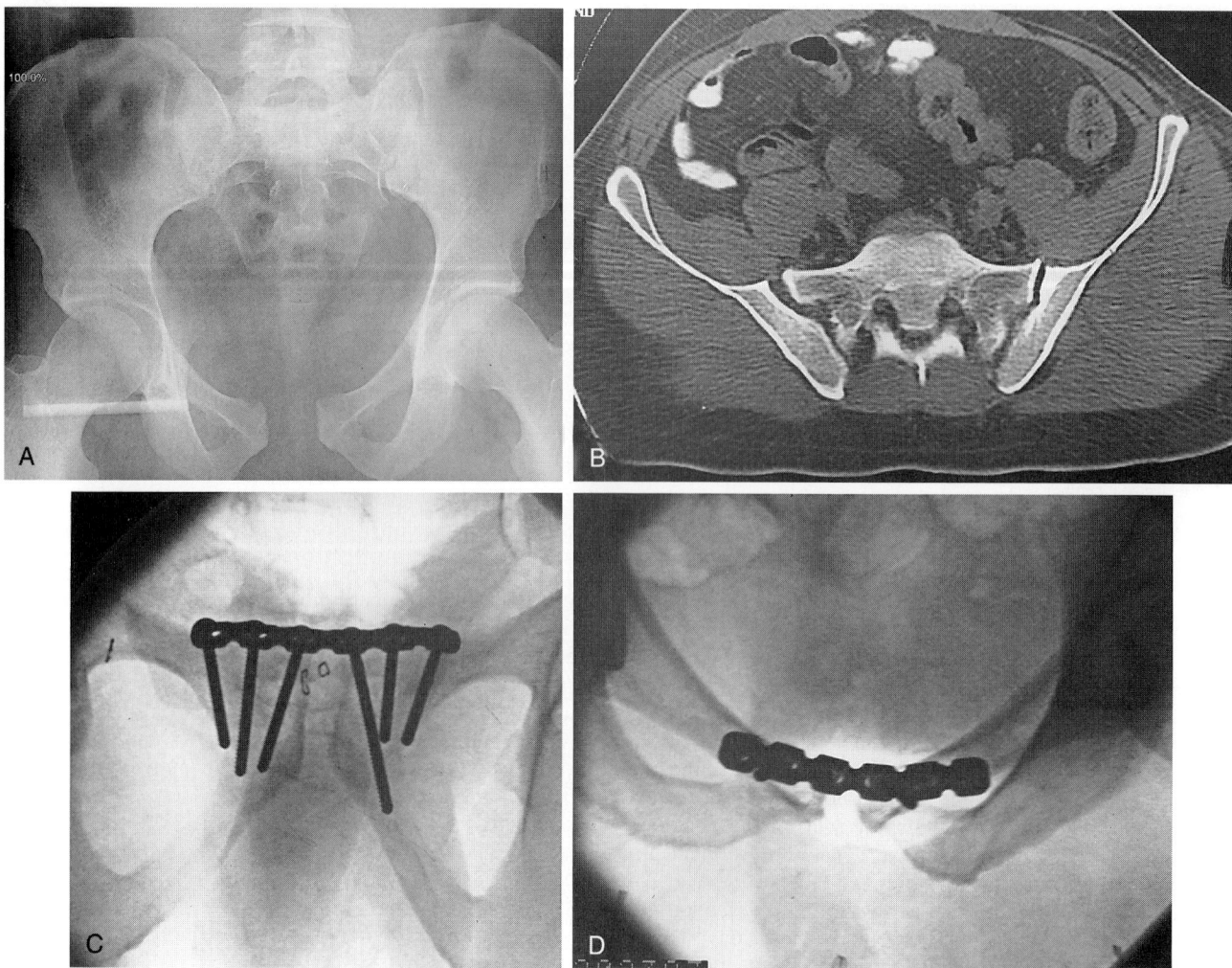

Fig. 9. Radiographs. *A*, AP view of symphyseal disruption. *B*, CT scan with sacroiliac joint widening. *C*, Outlet view postfixation. *D*, Inlet view postfixation.

visualization of the S2 foramina.[31] A lateral sacral view is obtained by superimposing the greater sciatic notch images. The iliac cortical density parallels the sacral alar slope and is almost always caudal and posterior to it. The iliac cortical density denotes the anterior extent for safe SI screw insertion.[33] An anatomic reduction is required to perform this technique, because sacral fracture displacement will narrow the safe corridor for placement of screws. The angle of screw placement may vary between an SI dislocation and a sacral fracture. The screw placement for a sacral fracture must be in a transverse position to allow the screw to achieve fixation in the sacral body. Sacral fractures are treated with a fully threaded cancellous screw to avoid overcompression of the foramina. SI dislocations are compressed with cancellous lag screws (Fig. 11).

SI joint dislocations can be treated by both percutaneous and open techniques.[28, 34] An open approach can be performed either anteriorly or posteriorly. For the posterior approach, a vertical incision is made 2 cm lateral to the posterosuperior spine. The gluteal muscle is reflected from the posterior iliac wing, and the gluteus maximus origin is reflected from the sacrum. The greater sciatic notch must

be exposed for assessment of reduction. For sacral fractures, the multifidus muscle is elevated, providing visualization of the sacral foramina. A Matta angled jaw clamp (Synthes, Paoli, PA) can be used to obtain reduction by placing one tip on the sacrum through the sciatic notch and the other along the outer table of the ilium. Fixation is performed with SI screws. For an anterior approach, the incision is from the anterosuperior iliac spine to the iliac tubercle. The iliac muscle is sharply dissected subperiosteally off of the iliac wing. The L5 nerve root lies 2 cm medial to the SI joint and must be protected during the dissection. Fixation is usually limited to two two-hole plates placed at 90 degrees to each other. Lange et al[35] reported on 27 patients with SI dislocations treated with an anterior approach. Three (11%) incomplete L5 nerve palsies were noted postoperatively with full improvement in two (Fig. 12).

Crescent fractures can be approached either via an anterior or a posterior approach. The posterior approach provides an easier dissection without requiring special care for the L5 nerve root and excellent exposure of the SI joint and iliac wing.[19] The iliac wing fragments can be reduced

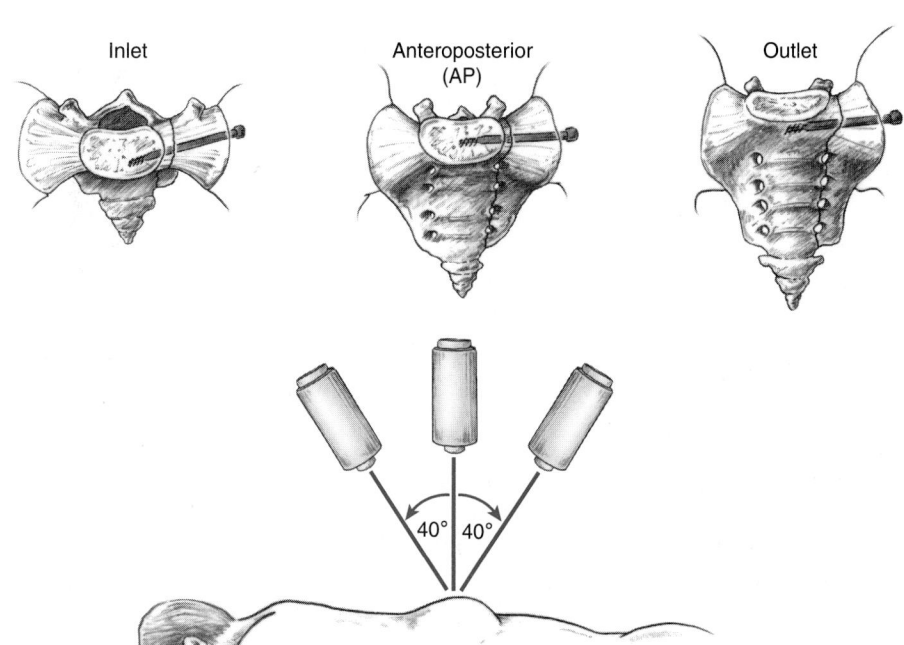

Fig. 10. Safe corridor for iliosacral screw placement.

to the intact posterosuperior iliac spine and fixed in place with one or two 3.5-mm cortical lag screws placed between the pelvic tables from posterior to anterior. A 3.5-mm reconstruction plate can be placed along the outer table to help neutralize the rotational and shear forces across the fracture site. If the intact posterosuperior iliac spine fragment is small, SI screws may be required to stabilize the iliac wing.

POSTOPERATIVE MANAGEMENT

Postoperative weightbearing status depends on fracture pattern and associated injuries. Most unstable fractures require non-weightbearing restrictions for 3 months. Early weightbearing may be allowed in rotationally unstable but vertically stable fractures.

COMPLICATIONS

Complication rates for unstable pelvic injuries are high (Tables 8 and 9). An awareness of complications and adequate preoperative planning can reduce this rate. The Morel-Lavallee lesion is a significant soft-tissue degloving injury associated with pelvic trauma.[36] The subcutaneous tissue is torn away from the underlying fascia, creating a cavity filled with hematoma and liquefied fat. The diagnosis is based on physical examination findings, including a soft fluctuant area that commonly occurs over the greater trochanter but may also occur in the flank and lumbodorsal region. The management is important because the presence of necrotic tissue and hematoma in the subcutaneous tissue increases the risk for infection. Open débridement is the preferred treatment for most Morel-Lavallee lesions. The

TABLE 8. EARLY COMPLICATIONS				
Complication	**Incidence**	**Prevention**	**Features**	**Treatment**
Infection	0.5%–2%	Pin care	Fever	I&D
		Soft tissue	Drainage	
Hematoma	Underreported	Drain	Inadequate hemostasis	Drainage
Bladder injury	Unknown	Blunt retraction	Hematuria	Catheterization repair
DVT	35%–50%	Low-dose heparin	Doppler	Warfarin (Coumadin)
			MRV	Heparin
PE	0.5%–2%	Low-dose heparin	Confusion	Coumadin
		LMW heparin	Hypoxia	Heparin
		Coumadin	Tachycardia	
		SCD	Cardiovascular collapse	
		IVC filter		

I&D = irrigation and débridement; DVT = deep vein thrombosis; MRV = magnetic resonance venography; LMW = low molecular weight; SCD = sequential compression device; IVC = inferior vena cava; PE = pulmonary embolism.

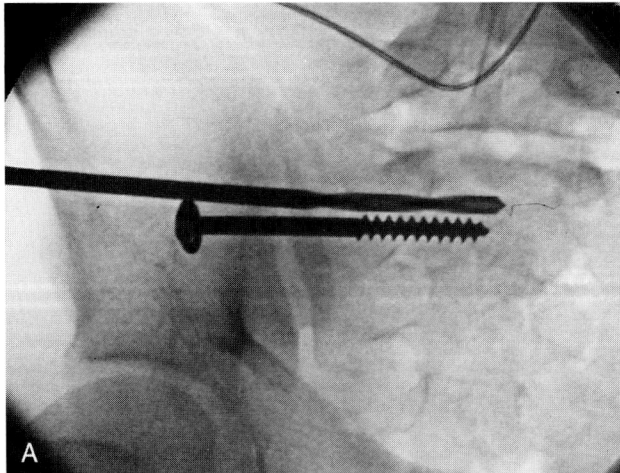
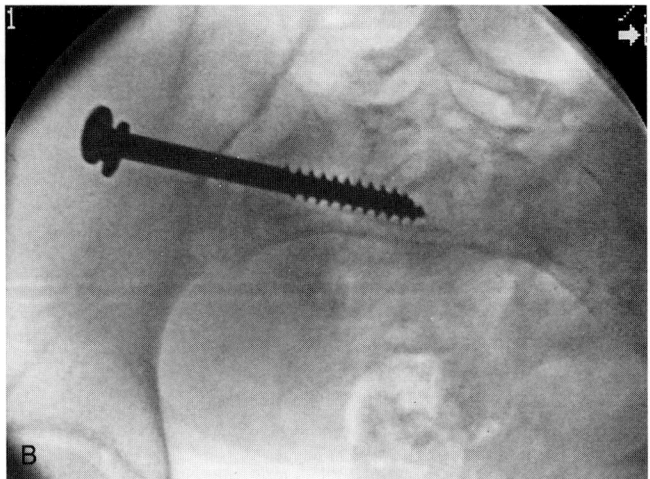
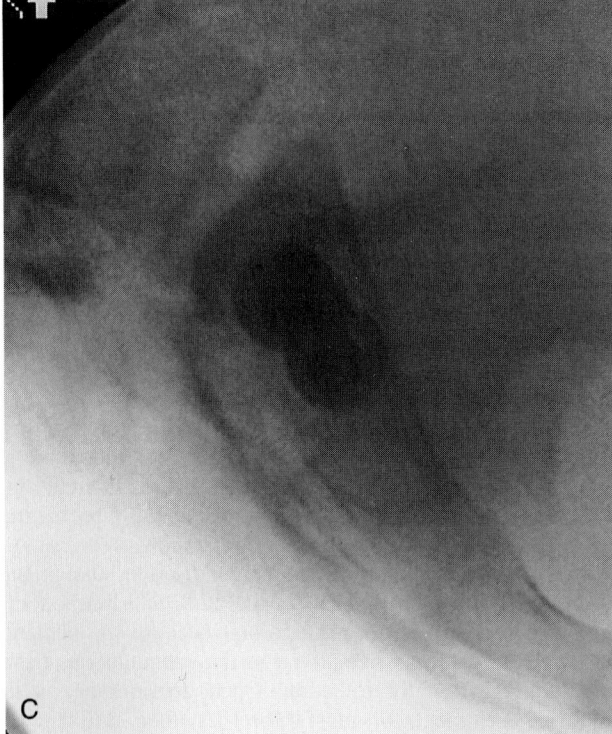

Fig. 11. Radiographs. *A*, Outlet radiograph shows position of iliosacral screw above sacral foramina. *B*, Inlet radiograph shows location of iliosacral screw within sacral body. *C*, Lateral sacral view.

TABLE 9. LATE COMPLICATIONS			
Complication	**Incidence**	**Features**	**Treatment**
Pain	50%	Low back Malunion Nonunion SI joint disease	Treat individually
Nonunion	Uncommon	Pain	Stable fixation Bone grafting
Malunion	Unknown	Unreduced unstable fractures LLD Pelvic obliquity	Pelvic osteotomy Leg lengthening
Nerve injury	10%–15%	Traction injury Iatrogenic	Observation, splint or brace may affect outcome

SI = sacroiliac; LLD = limb length discrepancy.

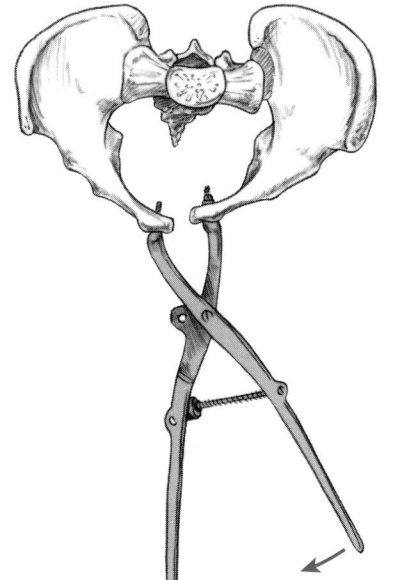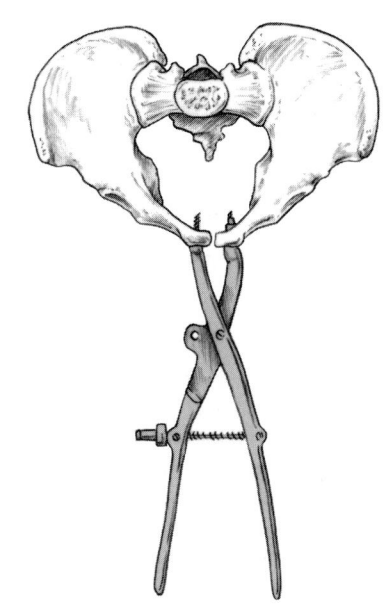

Fig. 12. View. Indirect reduction of sacro-iliac diastasis through an anterior approach.

incision should be placed close to the middle of the degloved area to decrease the risk of flap necrosis. The hematoma should be evacuated and the necrotic fatty and connective tissue sharply débrided. The wounds should be packed with gauze and normal saline-soaked dressing changes performed. Prophylactic antibiotics should cover gram-positive organisms in particular. If the overlying skin is intact, débridement can be performed at fracture fixation. It is important to close the deep fascia tightly and leave the distal portion of the wound open for dressing changes if skin compromise is apparent.

The incidence of deep venous thrombosis in patients with pelvic trauma has been reported to be between 35% and 60%. Geerts et al[37] performed venography on 100 patients with pelvic fractures and found a 61% incidence of deep venous thrombosis and a 29% incidence of proximal deep venous thrombosis. The incidence of symptomatic pulmonary embolism in pelvic trauma is 2% to 10%. Fatal pulmonary embolism occurs in 0.5% to 2% of patients with pelvic trauma. The risk factors most consistently seen with a trauma population are increasing age, spinal cord injury, fractures of the lower extremity and pelvis, and duration of immobilization. The classic clinical findings of deep venous thrombosis include leg tenderness, swelling, and increased temperature. The sensitivity of detecting a deep venous thrombosis in a trauma patient is unreliable because lower extremity fracture, edema, and soft-tissue injury are present. The diagnosis of deep venous thrombosis cannot reliably be made in the trauma patient. Duplex Doppler ultrasonography is the most widely used screening test to evaluate venous thrombosis in trauma patients.

Given the high incidence of deep venous thrombosis in this population, routine prophylaxis is recommended. Common forms of prophylaxis include low-dose heparin, low molecular weight heparin, mechanical devices, and vena caval filters. Knudson et al[38] performed a randomized trial of low-dose heparin and no prophylaxis in 154 trauma patients. Serial duplex Doppler ultrasonography was per-

formed every 3 to 5 days. Low-dose heparin offered no additional protection compared with controls. Intermittent pneumatic compression by itself has been shown to be ineffective prophylaxis for trauma patients. Fisher et al[39] performed a randomized study of intermittent pneumatic compression in patients with pelvic fractures, finding no significant difference with or without pneumatic compression. Low-molecular-weight heparin is a promising prophylactic agent, with almost complete bioavailability after injection, convenient dosage, and no monitoring required. Low molecular weight heparin is more efficacious than low-dose heparin in preventing deep venous thrombosis. Compared with controls, low-dose heparin has reduced the risk of deep venous thrombosis and proximal vein thrombosis in one series by 19% and 12%, respectively, whereas the risk reductions with low molecular weight heparin were 43% and 65%, respectively.[40]

Treatment of deep venous thrombosis in pelvic trauma depends on whether the patient will require surgical reconstruction. Deep venous thrombosis can be identified both preoperatively and postoperatively. The following approach is recommended. In patients who will be treated nonoperatively and in those who have already undergone acute reconstruction, low molecular weight heparin and mechanical prophylaxis (graduated compression stockings and intermittent pneumatic compression) can be used. Within 36 hours, most patients will no longer be actively bleeding; it appears safe to administer low molecular weight heparin prophylaxis at this time. For patients undergoing surgical procedures, the heparin can be discontinued at midnight the evening before surgery. Postoperative prophylaxis is reinitiated with warfarin. Because of the risk of intraoperative embolization during surgical manipulation, preoperative screening with bilateral venous ultrasonography or magnetic resonance venography (MRV) should be performed within 24 hours of surgery on all patients with pelvic trauma who require a delayed surgical reconstruction (more than 4 days after injury). If a proximal deep venous thrombosis is found, a vena caval filter should be placed preoperatively. If no deep venous thrombosis is found, routine postoperative prophylaxis is performed. For patients with contraindications to anticoagulation such as intracranial bleed, prophylactic vena caval filter and screening ultrasonography or MRV should be considered.[5, 31a]

The incidence of sciatic or lumbosacral nerve injury in pelvic trauma is between 10% and 15%. A higher incidence has been noted in fracture dislocations with posterior pelvic instability. Anatomically, this can be explained by the close relationship of the lower lumbar and sacral nerve roots to the sacrum and SI joint (Fig. 13). In 1966, Huittinen and Slatis reviewed the nonoperative treatment of 147 unstable pelvic fractures and found a 46% rate of persistent nerve injury. Helfet et al[41] evaluated 28 patients with 30 vertically unstable fractures of the hemipelvis. Preoperative ipsilateral neurological injury to the sciatic lumbosacral plexus was found in 50% of these fractures. Posterior approaches and reduction led to significant unilateral changes in the somatosensory evoked potentials (SSEPs) concurrent with manipulating the hemipelvis for reduction. Routine careful identification and retraction of the L5 nerve root intraoperatively did not result in SSEP monitoring changes during anterior approaches.

Nonunions and malunions occur as a result of inadequate initial treatment of displaced pelvic fractures. Pain is the most common subjective complaint and is usually related to the posterior pelvic injury. Deformity is also a common complaint and is related to the malunion or malpositioned nonunion. Cranial displacement of the hemipelvis results in shortening of the ipsilateral extremity. The sacrum and coccyx become more prominent with this displacement and can be troublesome when sitting or lying.

Matta et al[29] reported on the operative correction of 37 pelvic nonunions and malunions. The procedures are technically demanding. In their series, the average operating time lasted 7 hours and the average blood loss was 2000 mL with a complication rate of 19%. A three-stage reconstruction is often required. The first stage involves an anterior approach to mobilize structures and perform osteotomies. The patient is then repositioned, and a posterior approach is performed to complete the mobilization or osteotomy. Reduction and internal fixation of the posterior pelvis is performed. The third stage involves a repeat anterior approach for reduction and internal fixation of the anterior pelvis.

RESULTS AND OUTCOMES

Long-term functional outcome after pelvic ring injury has not been adequately documented (Table 10). The natural history of unstable pelvic fractures in all published studies has shown a high incidence of residual disability, severe low back pain, pelvic obliquity, and gait disturbances. Henderson[42] presented 26 patients with nonoperatively treated pelvic fractures with a minimum of 5 years follow-up. Subjective complaints included frequent or daily low back discomfort (50%), localized dysesthesia (46%), and work disability (38%). Objective findings included neurological deficits (42%), motor weakness or abnormal deep tendon reflexes, and persistent limp (32%). Long-term outcome correlated well with both the amount of residual vertical displacement and the stability of the fracture. Semba et al[43] also found a correlation between displacement on the initial film and residual symptoms. Patients with less than 1 cm of combined anterior and posterior vertical displacement at initial injury were asymptomatic, whereas those with more than 1 cm of displacement at injury had an increased frequency of late severe low back pain.

Gruen et al[44] studied outcomes of multiple-injury patients with unstable pelvic ring injuries treated by open reduction and internal fixation. They reported that 62% of patients returned to work full time and that the majority of patients with pelvic fractures (77%) had mild disability (Sickness Impact Profile score = 10) at 1 year. The authors noted that open book injuries tended to have higher individual and total Sickness Impact Profile scores than LC fractures despite similar Injury Severity scores.

Tornetta et al[45] evaluated 29 patients with rotationally unstable but vertically stable pelvic ring injuries treated with open reduction and internal fixation. The primary indication for surgery was symphyseal disruption. All patients were seen 3 years or more after injury. Follow-up evaluation revealed that 96% had no pain or pain only with strenuous activity, 76% ambulated without assistance or limitations, and 76% returned to their preinjury occupation.

Copeland et al[46] found that women with pelvic fractures have higher rates of urinary tract complaints, cesarean section, and gynecological pain than a matched group of female multiple-trauma patients without pelvic fractures. Twenty-one percent of female patients with pelvic fractures in this series had urinary tract symptoms despite a low incidence of frank genitourinary injuries. They postulated that the significant incidence of stress incontinence is due to the disruption of the pelvic floor musculature or interruption of its innervation. Urinary tract complaints were more common in patients with residual pelvic fracture displacement in a lateral or vertical direction as opposed to a medial direction. In LC injuries the pelvic floor becomes redundant, whereas in APC or VS injuries the pelvic floor is placed under tension and can be disrupted. The study also found a significantly higher rate of gynecological pain

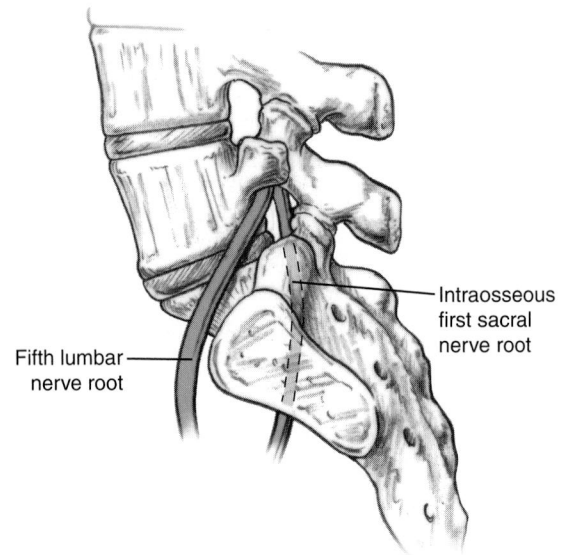

Fifth lumbar nerve root

Intraosseous first sacral nerve root

Fig. 13. View. Relationship of L5 nerve root to sacral body and ala.

TABLE 10. LONG-TERM FUNCTIONAL OUTCOME		
Study	Subject Group	Key Findings
Nonoperative		
Holdsworth[1]	Untreated sacroiliac dislocations	100% low back pain 50% unable to return to work
Slatis and Huittinen[3]	Unstable pelvic fractures	Disabling low back pain Pelvic obliquity Impaired gait 46% lumbosacral nerve damage
Henderson[42]	Unstable pelvic fractures	50% low back pain 46% localized dysesthesia 42% neurological deficits 32% persistent limp
Semba et al[43]	Displaced pelvic fractures	<1-cm displacement asymptomatic >1-cm displacement low back pain
Tile[4]	248 pelvic ring disruptions	Stable injuries, few major long-term problems 60% pain with vertically unstable injuries 5.5% permanent nerve injury 2.5% permanent urethral damage 4% malunion with leg length discrepancy
Operative		
Gruen et al[44]	Unstable pelvic fractures	62% return to work 77% only mild disability
Tornetta et al[45]	Rotationally unstable pelvic fracture	96% no pain or pain only with strenuous activity 76% ambulate without assistance 76% return to preinjury occupation
Copeland et al[46]	Female multitrauma with pelvic fracture	20% gynecological pain Increased rate of cesarean section Increased rate of urinary tract complaints
McCarthy et al[47]	Female multitrauma with pelvic fracture	Lower scores on SF-36 compared with age- and gender-standardized norms

(20%) and a significant increase in the rate of postinjury cesarean section compared with a cohort group. McCarthy et al[47] found that women with pelvic fractures scored lower on all scales of the SF-36 compared with age- and gender-standardized norms.

The outcome of unstable pelvic fractures appears to vary based on the initial displacement, fracture classification, and associated injuries. Long-term studies are required to better determine how operative intervention alters the natural history of these severe injuries.

REFERENCES

1. Holdsworth FW: Dislocation and fracture-dislocation of the pelvis. J Bone Joint Surg Br 1948; 30:461.
2. Raf L: Double vertical fractures of the pelvis. Acta Chir Scand 1966; 131:298.
3. Slatis P, Huittinen VM: Double vertical fractures of the pelvis: A report on 163 patients. Acta Chir Scand 1972; 138:799.
4. Tile M: Pelvic ring fractures: Should they be fixed? J Bone Joint Surg Br 1988; 70:1.
5. Montgomery KD, Geerts WH, Potter HG, et al: Thromboembolic complications in patients with pelvic trauma. Clin Orthop 1996; 329:68.
6. Riemer B, Butterfield SLM, Diamond DL, et al: Acute mortality associated with injuries to the pelvic ring: The role of early patient mobilization and external fixation. J Trauma 1993; 35:671.
7. Bucholz RW: The pathological anatomy of Malgaigne fracture: Dislocations of the pelvis. J Bone Joint Surg Am 1981; 63:400.

8. Falinger MS, McGanity PLJ: Current concepts review. Unstable fractures of the pelvic ring. J Bone Joint Surg Am 1992; 74:781.
9. Gilliland MD, Ward RE, Barton RM, et al: Factors affecting mortality in pelvic fractures. J Trauma 1982; 22:691.
10. Mucha P, Farnell MB: Analysis of pelvic fracture management. J Trauma 1984; 24:379.
11. Colapinto V: Trauma to the pelvis: Urethral injury. Clin Orthop 1980; 151:46.
12. Corriere JN Jr, Sandler CM: Management of the ruptured bladder: Seven years experience with 111 cases. J Trauma 1986; 26:830.
13. Burgess AR, Eastridge BJ, Young JWR, et al: Pelvic ring disruptions: Effective classification system and treatment protocols. J Trauma 1990; 30:848.
14. Dalal SA, Burgess AR, Siegel JH, et al: Pelvic fracture in multiple trauma: Classification by mechanism is key to pattern of

organ injury: Resuscitative requirements and outcome. J Trauma 1989; 29:981.
15. Trunkey DD, Chapman MW, Lim RC, et al: Management of pelvic fractures in blunt trauma injury. J Trauma 1974; 14:912.
16. Edeiken-Monroe BS, Browner BD, Jackson H: The role of standard roentgenograms in the evaluation of instability of pelvic ring disruption. Clin Orthop 1989; 240:63.
17. Tile M: Acute pelvic fracture: I. Causation and classification. J Am Acad Orthop Surg 1996; 4:143.
18. Tile M: Acute pelvic fracture: II. Principles of management. J Am Acad Orthop Surg 1996; 4:152.
19. Borrelli J, Koval KJ, Helfet DL: The crescent fracture: A posterior fracture dislocation of the sacroiliac joint. J Orthop Trauma 1996; 10:165.
20. Denis F, Davis S, Comfort T: Sacral fractures: An important problem: Retrospec-

tive analysis of 236 cases. Clin Orthop 1988; 227:67.

21. Pohlemann T, Tscherne H: Fixation of sacral fractures. Tech Orthop 1995; 9:315.

22. American College of Surgeons: Advanced Trauma and Life Support Manual. Chicago, American College of Surgeons, 1989.

23. O'Neill PA, Riina J, Sclafani S, et al: Angiographic findings in pelvic fractures. Clin Orthop 1996; 329:60.

24. Poole GV, Ward EF, Muakkasa F, et al: Pelvic fracture from major blunt trauma: Outcome is determined by associated injuries. Ann Surg 1991; 213:532.

25. Grimm MR, Vrahas MS, Thomas KA: Pressure-volume characteristics of the intact and disrupted pelvic retroperitoneum. J Trauma 1998; 44:454.

26. Gruen GS, Leit ME, Gruen RJ, et al: The acute management of hemodynamically unstable multiple trauma patients with pelvic ring injuries. J Trauma 1994; 36:706.

27. Hanson PB, Milne JC, Chapman MW: Open fractures of the pelvis. Review of 43 cases. J Bone Joint Surg Br 1991; 73:325.

28. Matta JM, Saucedo T: Internal fixation of pelvic ring fractures. Clin Orthop 1989; 242:83.

29. Matta JM, Dickson KF, Markovich GD: Surgical treatment of pelvic nonunions and malunions. Clin Orthop 1996; 329:199.

30. Lange RH, Hansen ST: Pelvic ring disruptions with symphysis pubis diastasis: Indications, technique, and limitations of anterior internal fixation. Clin Orthop 1985; 201:130.

31. Routt MLC, Meier MC, Kregor PJ, et al: Percutaneous iliosacral screws with the patient supine technique. Oper Tech Orthop 1993; 3:35.

31a. Montgomery KD, Potter HG, Helfet DL: Magnetic resonance venography to evaluate the deep venous system of the pelvis in patients who have an acetabular fracture. J Bone Joint Surg Am 1995; 77: 1639.

32. Routt MLC, Simonian PT, Mills PT: Iliosacral screw fixation: Early complications of percutaneous technique. J Orthop Trauma 1997; 11:584.

33. Routt MLC, Simonian PT, Agnew SG, et al: Radiographic recognition of the sacral alar slope for optimal placement of iliosacral screws: A cadaveric and clinical study. J Orthop Trauma 1996; 10:171.

34. Routt MLC, Simonian PT, Inaba J: Iliosacral screw fixation of the disrupted sacroiliac joint. Tech Orthop 1995; 9:300.

35. Lange RH, Webb LX, Mayo KA: Efficacy of the anterior approach for fixation of sacroiliac dislocations and fracture-dislocations. Presented at the annual meeting of OTA, Seattle, WA, 1991.

36. Hak DJ, Olson SA, Matta JM: Diagnosis and management of closed internal degloving injuries associated with pelvic and acetabular fractures: The Morel-Lavallee lesion. J Trauma 1997; 42:1046.

37. Geerts WH, Code KI, Jay RM, et al: A prospective study of venous thromboembolism after major trauma. N Engl J Med 1994; 331:1601.

38. Knudson MM, Lewis FR, Clinton A, et al: Prevention of venous thromboembolism in trauma patients. J Trauma 1994; 37:480.

39. Fisher CG, Blachut PA, Salvian AJ, et al: Effectiveness of pneumatic leg compression devices for the prevention of thromboembolic disease in orthopaedic trauma patients: A prospective, randomized study of compression alone versus no prophylaxis. J Orthop Trauma 1995; 9:1.

40. Geerts WH, Jay RM, Code KI, et al: A comparison of low-dose heparin with low-molecular-weight heparin as prophylaxis against venous thromboembolism after major trauma. N Engl J Med 1996; 335:701.

41. Helfet DL, Koval KJ, Hissa EA, et al: Intraoperative somatosensory evoked potential monitoring during acute pelvic fracture surgery. J Orthop Trauma 1995; 9:28.

42. Henderson RC: The long-term results of nonoperatively treated major pelvic disruptions. J Orthop Trauma 1989; 3:41.

43. Semba RT, Yasukawa K, Gustilo RB: Critical analysis of results of 53 Malgaigne fractures of the pelvis. J Trauma 1983; 23:535.

44. Gruen GS, Leit ME, Gruen RJ, et al: Functional outcome of patients with unstable pelvic ring fractures stabilized with open reduction and internal fixation. J Trauma 1995; 39:838.

45. Tornetta P, Dickson K, Matta JM: Outcome of rotationally unstable pelvic ring injuries treated operatively. Clin Orthop 1996; 329:147.

46. Copeland CE, Bosse MJ, McCarthy ML, et al: Effect of trauma and pelvic fracture on female genitourinary, sexual, and reproductive function. J Orthop Trauma 1997; 11:73.

47. McCarthy ML, MacKenzie EJ, Bosse MJ, et al: Functional status following orthopaedic trauma in young women. J Trauma 1995; 39:828.

section 3 chapter 12

ACETABULAR FRACTURES

Christopher T. Born, William G. DeLong, Jr, and Patrick J. Brogle

Summary

- Most acetabular fractures occur in conjunction with blunt, high-energy injuries.
- Associated injuries must be addressed, and the timing of surgical treatment adjusted accordingly.
- Careful radiographic evaluation is essential to successful management of these injuries.
- Accurate classification of the fracture type aids the choice of the correct operative approach.
- There is the potential for significant complications, including heterotopic ossification, infection, osteonecrosis, and post-traumatic arthritis.
- These complex cases are best managed by experienced surgeons in centers that are properly staffed and equipped.

Acetabular fractures generally occur as the result of blunt, high-energy injury in which the impact force is transmitted through the femoral head. They are frequently associated with thoracic, abdominal, and head injuries typical to the patient population most commonly affected. Management of acetabular fracture involves (1) stabilization of the patient, (2) adequate radiographic evaluation of the injury, (3) classification of the fracture type, and (4) thoughtful selection of the proper surgical approach.

The decision to treat these fractures operatively is based on the fracture pattern and the extent of injury to the joint. Ultimately, anatomic reduction is achieved through osteosynthesis, which allows for patient mobilization and a return of joint function. In the event that an irreversible chondral injury has occurred, the restoration of local anatomy can improve the results of future reconstructive procedures. The treatment of acetabular fractures is highly specialized and should be carried out by surgeons experienced in the techniques of reduction at centers with the appropriate medical resources and equipment to manage the injuries.

HISTORICAL REVIEW

For many years, acetabular fracture was managed nonoperatively. In the mid-1960s, Professor Robert Judet and associates[1] recognized that optimal results could best be achieved with open reduction and internal fixation techniques. They understood the difficulty of interpreting the three-dimensional topography of the pelvis and acetabulum from standard radiographs and worked to devise more precise imaging techniques. With his protégé, Emil Letournel, Judet developed and refined a systematic approach to the operative management of these injuries.[2] The classification scheme of Judet and Letournel remains the mainstay for categorization of the fracture patterns and, as such, helps the surgeon focus on the appropriate surgical approach.[3]

ANATOMY

The acetabulum is formed by the maturation of the triradiate cartilage with contributions from the ilium, ischium, and pubic bones. These structures coalesce at the time of skeletal maturity to form the innominate bone. There is a central nonarticular fossa filled with a fat pad (the pulvinar) and an outer fibrocartilaginous rim (the labrum). The inferior margin of the acetabulum is notched and is covered by the transverse ligament that completes the ring.

A major contribution by Judet and Letournel was to divide the lateral wall of the iliac wing and the acetabulum into two columns, anterior and posterior (Fig. 1). It is this concept that forms the basis of the classification system for acetabular fracture.

Other significant regional anatomic points must be considered. The superior gluteal artery (SGA) exits the pelvis at the greater sciatic notch, as does the sciatic nerve. The artery is part of the essential blood supply for the gluteal muscles and may be injured either at the time of fracture or iatrogenically during surgery. If extensile posterolateral exposures are considered, an arteriogram to document flow of the SGA should be carried out to avoid ischemic necrosis of the abductor muscle flap. The sciatic nerve may also be injured at the time of impact. At the level of the sciatic notch, the more anterior peroneal component is highly susceptible to injury by posterior dislocation of the hip. The *corona mortis*, an accessory vessel sometimes found between the inferior epigastric and obturator arteries, may be

injured at the time of surgery if an ilioinguinal approach is used. Inadvertent sectioning of this vessel and retropubic retraction of the stump may make for difficulty in controlling the resultant hemorrhage. The rate of presence of this anastomotic variant may be as high as 25%.[4, 5]

PATHOGENESIS

Acetabular fractures usually result from high-energy blunt forces, although central impaction can occur with a low-energy fall directly onto the hip. The amount of displacement is directly related to the force of impact, which is generally transmitted through the femoral head. The position of the leg with respect to the pelvis and the direction of the resultant force vectors at the time of impact determine the primary fracture pattern. Hip flexion with internal rotation commonly produces posterior wall and column injuries. Hip extension with external rotation causes anterior wall and column injuries.

CLINICAL FEATURES

APPEARANCE
Because of the great energy generally required to cause acetabular fractures, there frequently are other, associated injuries. An understanding of the mechanism and force vectors of injury, in conjunction with a thorough physical examination, helps identify concomitant visceral, thoracic, and head trauma as well as other musculoskeletal injuries. The latter often include femoral head fractures, hip dislocations, femoral shaft fractures, and knee and pelvic ring injuries.

From a neurological standpoint, the sciatic nerve and the lumbosacral plexus should be considered "at risk." A detailed neurological assessment of the involved extremity should always be carried out, with particular attention paid to the function of the foot dorsiflexors (peroneal component) and plantiflexors (tibial component). Associated sciatic nerve injury is thought to occur in 10% to 13% of all acetabular fractures.[6] The nerve can be injured by posterior dislocation of the hip or by entrapment within a fracture coursing through the sciatic notch.

If the fracture has occurred with a crush or shearing component to the hip girdle region, an internal degloving injury known as a Morel-Lavallee lesion can result. This lesion may significantly complicate the management options and compromise incisions made in the area. If unsuspected, the presence of this lesion may not become clinically evident for several days and is heralded by local and regional ecchymoses and fluctuance. Bleeding from local soft tissues and the severed subjacent fasciocutaneous vessels can cause a significant, expanding hematoma that can compromise the skin. The infection rate following surgery is higher in the presence of Morel-Lavallee lesions.[7, 8]

CLASSIFICATION
The classification scheme most commonly used for acetabular fractures is that of Judet and Letournel.[2] It is based on their systematic analysis and treatment of several hundred acetabular fractures and their anatomic division of the innominate bone into anterior and posterior columns. They categorized acetabular fractures into five simple (*elemen-*

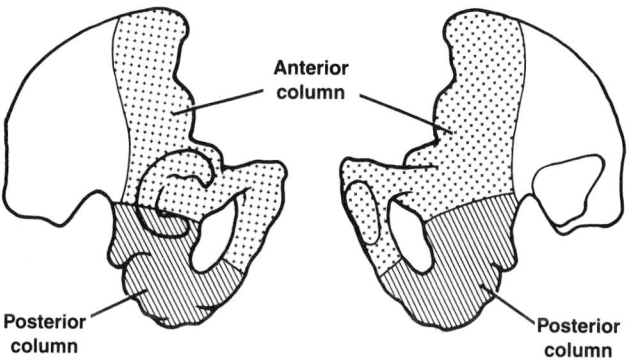

Fig. 1. Anterior and posterior columns of the pelvis. These are viewed from the outer and inner aspects. (Perry DC: Acetabular fractures. Orthop Clin North Am 28:405, 1997.)

tary) and five complex (*associated*) types (Figs. 2 and 3). The elementary types are fracture of the posterior wall, which is the most common, fractures of the posterior column, the anterior wall, and the anterior column, and transverse fractures. The associated types include transverse fractures with associated posterior wall injury, combined posterior column and posterior wall fractures, and T-type injuries. The most complex of the associated injuries are the anterior with posterior hemitransverse fracture and the both-column fracture. By convention in this classification scheme, a *both-column fracture* is one in which the articular segment of the acetabulum is dissociated from the iliac wing, the sacroiliac joint, or both.

The AO Group and the Orthopaedic Trauma Association have modified the Letournel classification to include A, B, and C types signifying severity.[9, 10]

INVESTIGATION

Radiographic evaluation of the acetabulum generally begins with the anteroposterior radiograph obtained in the trauma admitting area. Isolated posterior wall fractures may sometimes be missed because they are minimally displaced or because of interference from overlying bowel gas or

trauma equipment, such as spine boards and traction splints, which can obscure the field. If a hip dislocation has occurred, a posterior wall fracture must at least be suspected in addition to the potential for intra-articular retention of fracture fragments after hip reduction.

Adjunctive 45-degree iliac oblique and 45-degree obturator oblique views complete the series of three radiographs known as the *Judet views*. The six fundamental radiographic landmarks may be identified, and the fracture classification can be defined, from these radiographs. These landmarks are (1) the iliopectineal line, (2) the ilioischial line, (3) the pelvic "teardrop," (4) the trabecular condensation of the acetabular roof, (5) the anterior rim, and (6) the posterior rim. The iliac oblique view provides an en face view of the iliac wing and posterior column, including the greater and lesser sciatic notches. The outline of the anterior rim is rotated into view ahead of the posterior rim. The obturator oblique view best defines the iliopectineal line and fractures of the pubic rami. The posterior rim is brought into view, allowing for visualization of displaced posterior wall fractures (Fig. 4).

An estimation of the amount of the weightbearing dome that is involved can also be made from these three radiographic views through calculation of the *roof arc angle*. If

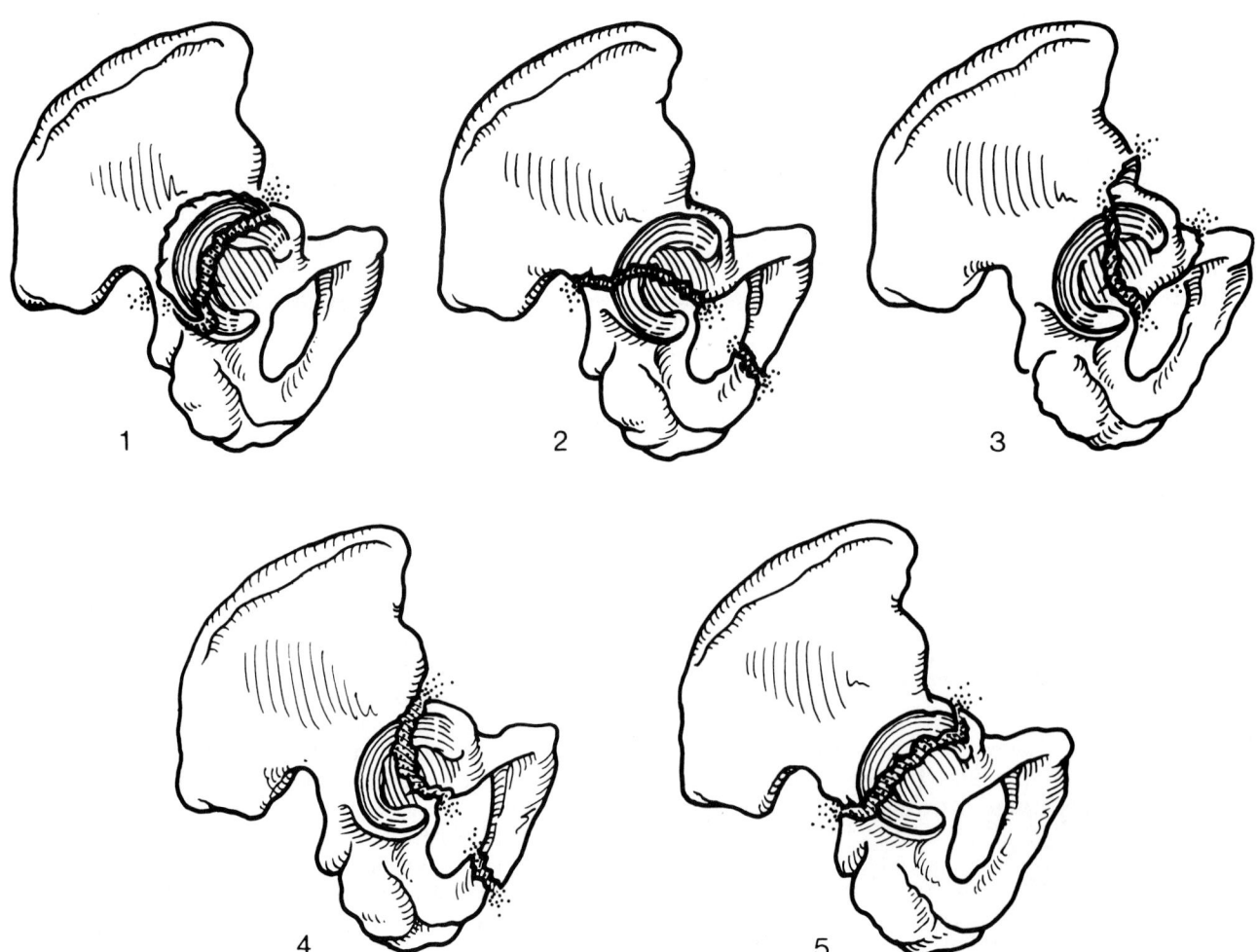

Fig. 2. Judet-Letournel classification of five elementary fractures. 1 = posterior wall fracture; 2 = posterior column fracture; 3 = anterior wall fracture; 4 = anterior column fracture; 5 = transverse fracture. (Perry DC: Acetabular fractures. Orthop Clin North Am 28:405, 1997.)

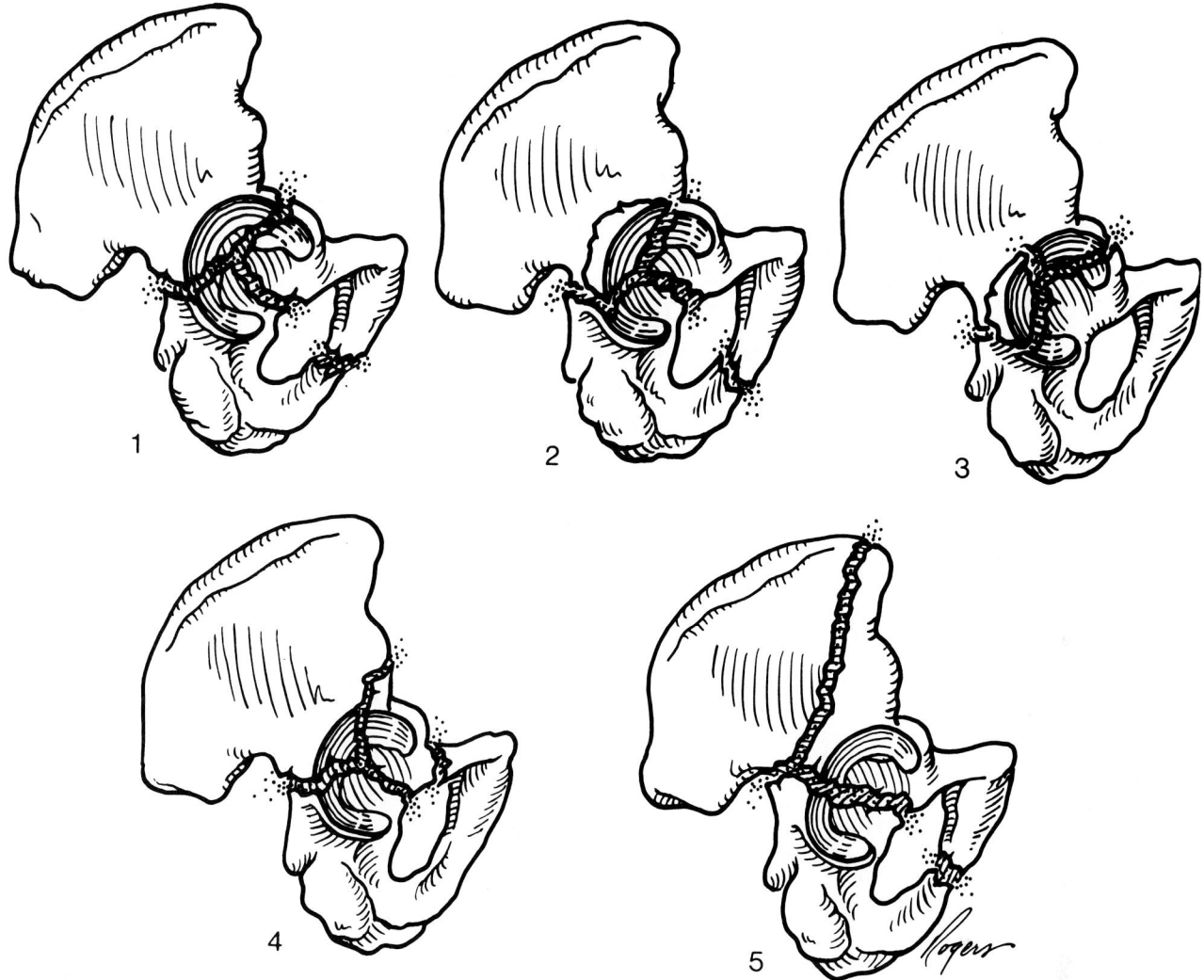

Fig. 3. Judet-Letournel classification of five associated fractures. 1 = T-shaped fracture; 2 = posterior column plus posterior wall fracture; 3 = transverse plus posterior wall fracture; 4 = anterior column plus posterior-hemitransverse fracture; 5 = associated both-column fracture. (Perry DC: Acetabular fractures. Orthop Clin North Am 28:405, 1997.)

the roof arc angle is greater than 45 degrees on the three Judet views, and if there is congruency between the acetabulum and the femoral head, consideration can be given to nonoperative management of the fracture, provided that there is no associated posterior wall injury.[11–13]

Further radiographic investigation of the pelvis should be carried out with thin-cut computed tomography (CT) scans. Some scanners come with software packages that will allow three-dimensional reconstructions of the injury image. CT (with or without three-dimensional reconstruction) is helpful in preoperative planning to better characterize the "personality" of the injury. It allows additional visualization of the spatial relationships of the major fracture components and helps identify subchondral "marginal impaction" that may require elevation and grafting. Further, intra-articular bone fragments that require arthrotomy and retrieval may not be appreciated on plain radiographs. Associated injuries of the posterior pelvic ring are also better visualized with CT.

TREATMENT

The primary goals to be kept in mind when one is dealing with acetabular injuries are (1) to ensure congruency and stability of the joint and (2) to provide for an adequate weightbearing platform and pain-free functional motion of the hip. Surgery should be carried out by a team that is knowledgeable in the techniques of pelvic and acetabular reconstruction and is using appropriate operating room equipment and instrumentation for osteosynthesis. The latter include oversized screws, specialized plates that can be contoured to the unique topology of the pelvis, reduction clamps that have been specifically designed with respect to the local anatomy for this type of surgery, and radiolucent surgical tables and advanced fluoroscopic equipment. The capability for auto-reinfusion of a portion of the patient's intraoperative blood loss should also be available. In addition, an understanding of the unique anatomy and multiple possible approaches is essential.

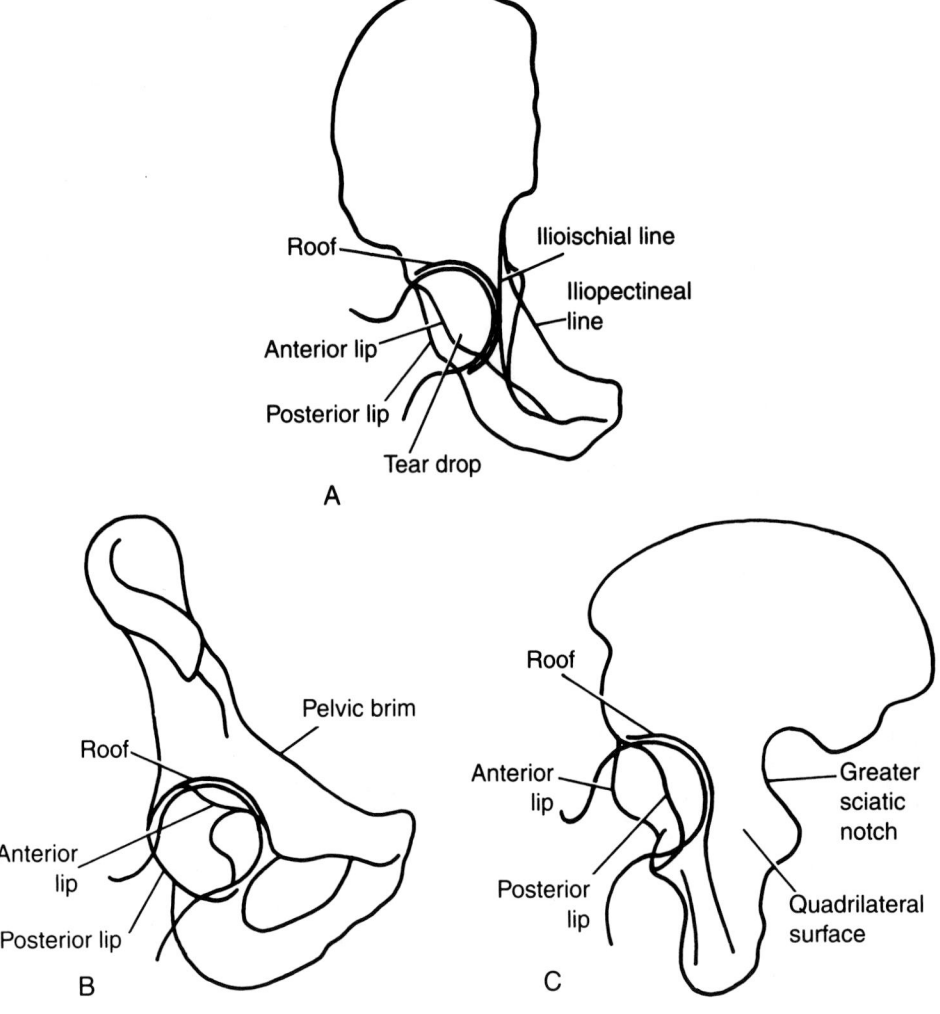

Fig. 4. Radiographic landmarks on the acetabulum. *A*, Anteroposterior view. *B*, Obturator oblique view. *C*, Iliac oblique view. (Perry DC: Acetabular fractures. Orthop Clin North Am 28:405, 1997.)

INDICATIONS

Acetabular fractures can be treated nonsurgically under certain circumstances. They include congruency of the acetabulum on the three Judet views with roof arc angle measurements of greater than 45 degrees on each. *Congruency* is defined as less than 2 mm of articular step-off. There should be no medial femoral head subluxation. Isolated posterior wall fractures should have less than 50% involvement at the level of the fovea when viewed on thin-cut CT scans (Fig. 5). In the case of associated both-column fractures, the acetabular dome fragments may remain congruent about the femoral head despite their separation from the rest of the ilium; this is known as *secondary congruence,* for which nonoperative treatment can also be considered. Other factors to be taken into account are the patient's age and physiological status and the presence or absence of local infection. Severe osteoporosis in the elderly may preclude stable internal fixation, but age itself is not an absolute contraindication to surgery. Many older patients can have a satisfactory outcome with operative treatment (Fig. 6).[14]

Acetabular fractures that are treated nonoperatively may require femoral skeletal traction for 6 weeks and monitoring with serial radiographs to evaluate for subsequent displacement.

Several aspects of patient care must be kept in mind if the decision is made to treat acetabular fractures nonoperatively. Pin care and proper skin precautions should be employed to diminish the chance of infection and decubitus ulcer formation that may occur during the bedrest phase of treatment. Deep venous thrombosis and pulmonary embolism are possible consequences of prolonged immobilization. Pharmacotherapeutic prophylaxis against these two complications should be instituted, along with the adjunctive use of pneumatic compression stockings. Placement of a vena cava filter should also be considered.

The issues in surgical management include availability of an operative team and the necessary equipment. The best time for surgery is generally between about 72 hours and 2 to 3 weeks after injury. This time frame allows for stabilization of intrapelvic and retroperitoneal clot. If too much time is allowed to pass, provisional fracture healing will take place, and it will become increasingly difficult to mobilize fragments for reduction. The rate of "anatomic" reduction (i.e., less than 1 mm of residual displacement) declines as the complexity of the fracture pattern, the age

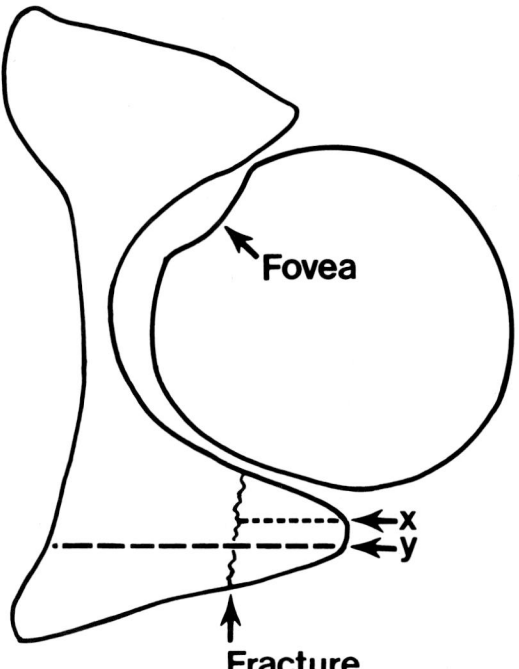

Fig. 5. View. CT scanning can measure the percentage of posterior wall involvement at the level of the fovea. The depth of the fracture is shown by line X. The depth of the posterior wall is shown by line Y. The percentage of posterior wall involvement can be calculated from these two measurements. (From Born CT, Dalton GP: Deconstruction of fractures of the posterior acetabular wall. Operative Tech Orthop 1993; 3:47.)

of the patient, and the interval from injury to surgery increase.

The use of a fracture-type table that allows for intraoperative traction is important, as is the positioning of the patient. The deforming force of femoral head impaction can be neutralized with traction. Prone positioning rather than lateral decubitus positioning for the Kocher-Langenbeck approach diminishes gravitational medialization in some cases with medial wall instability. The supine position for the ilioinguinal approach likewise affords good exposure of the quadrilateral surface and also reduces medial displacement forces.

PROCEDURES

The surgical approaches used for acetabular fractures affecting only one wall or column include the traditional Kocher-Langenbeck approach for posterior injuries and the ilioinguinal or Smith-Peterson approach for anterior injuries.

Posterior wall fractures are most common. They may be complicated by marginal subchondral impaction requiring elevation and grafting of the depressed articular component. Generally, such fractures can be managed with lag screw fixation and the application of a neutralizing posterior buttress plate. In the presence of a very small fragment, a supplementary "spring plate" can be contoured from a section of a 1/3 tubular plate and secured under the main reconstruction plate (see Fig. 6).

Injuries to the posterior column may require manipulation of the posterior component with one of the large pelvic reduction clamps. Control of the proximal and distal fragments can be obtained with large reduction clamps attached to 4.5-mm screws strategically placed so as not to interfere with subsequent plate placement as the fracture is held in the reduced position. The use of a 5.0- or 6.0-mm Schantz screw in the ischium can provide rotational control of the posterior column during fracture reduction.

The ilioinguinal approach is most commonly used for fractures of the anterior wall and anterior column. Fracture lines can be visualized through the three anatomic windows that are created. Supplementary plate or intertable screw fixation can be used for any iliac wing components present.

The most displaced component of the transverse fracture is generally addressed first. Frequently, it is posterior. With the Kocher-Langenbeck approach, the posterior column elements are exposed and the inferior ischiopubic fragment is rotationally manipulated with a Schantz pin. A finger can be placed through the sciatic notch to palpate the medial wall, and the reduction is "docked" and held with one of the large pelvic clamps. A posterior plate is applied after a lag screw has been placed to capture the anterior column component. In some cases, this screw can be directed just inside the acetabulum and run down into the pubic ramus, but good fluoroscopic visualization and knowledge of the three-dimensional anatomy are prerequisites for such a maneuver. If necessary, the anterior component can be addressed through a separate, simultaneously or sequentially performed ilioinguinal incision.

Associated both-column fractures and anterior column fractures with posterior hemitransverse injuries are most frequently managed with anterior ilioinguinal approaches. The iliac wing components are first reduced and fixed; then the pelvic brim components are treated with a long contoured plate placed along the iliopectineal line. A spring plate can be dropped over the pelvic brim to hold the medial, quadrilateral fragments, and a long intrapelvic screw can secure the posterior column. As with procedures described earlier, an understanding of the relevant pelvic anatomy and multiplanar fluoroscopy are prerequisites for safe screw placement.

T-type fractures can sometimes be reduced through a posterior approach. An anteriorly directed screw secures the anterior column, and the posterior component is held with a plate.

Strategies for more complex patterns include using a traditional approach for the more displaced column and attempting an indirect reduction of the other. Alternatively, two approaches can be used sequentially. Care must be taken to avoid inadvertent fixation of fragments in the first approach that need further reduction and fixation in the subsequent approach. A single extensile approach can also be considered, particularly in cases of both-column injuries with comminution of posterior wall column or in fractures that are being addressed late (more than 3 to 4 weeks after injury). The latter include the modified iliofemoral and triradiate techniques.[15]

In some instances, a combined approach using a posterior Kocher-Langenbeck incision simultaneously with the lateral window of the ilioinguinal component ("floppy lateral") allows better manipulation of anterior fracture fragments than can be accomplished through an indirect, purely

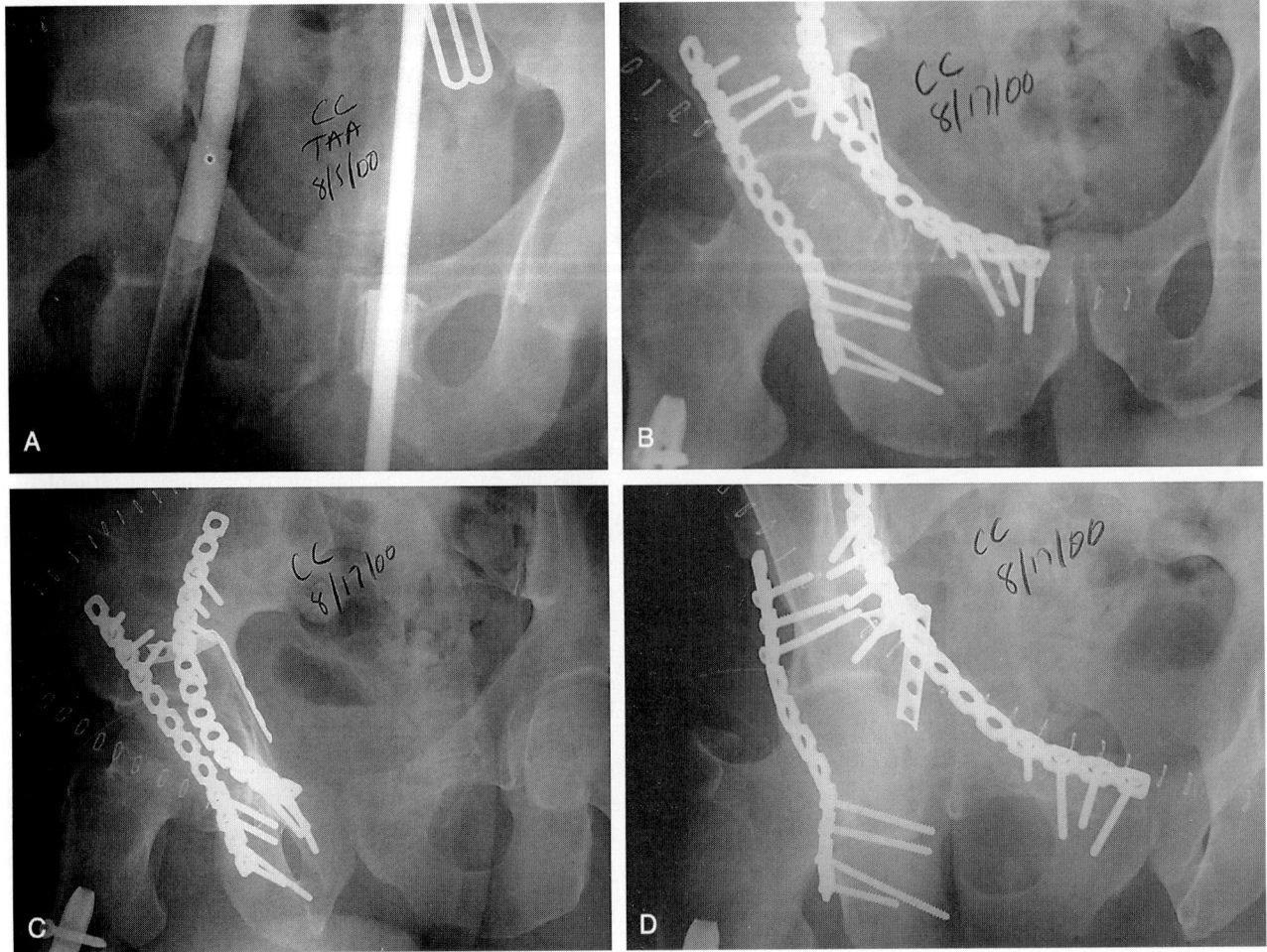

Fig. 6. View. *A,* Preoperative radiograph of a 46-year-old man who was struck by a car shows a displaced transverse fracture of the right acetabulum. Postoperative AP (*B*), iliac oblique (*C*), and obturator oblique (*D*) views show reconstruction carried out through sequential anterior and posterior approaches. A spring plate was used to help maintain the position of the quadrilateral surface.

posterior approach. Ultimately, choosing the correct surgical approach or approaches takes experience and the ability to interpret the preoperative radiographs.

INDIVIDUAL APPROACHES
Kocher-Langenbeck Approach
Whereas the ilioinguinal approach is carried out with the patient in a supine position, the posterior approach requires either a lateral decubitus or prone position. The external rotators must be taken down, a step that may lead to heterotopic ossification. The sciatic nerve can be directly visualized and protected if the hip is kept in extension and the knee in flexion to reduce tension. Access can be gained to the entire posterior column and posterior wall. If required, further superior and anterior exposure can be achieved by carrying out a trochanteric osteotomy, which can be repaired with wires or cannulated screws. Along with the risk of iatrogenic injury to the sciatic nerve and heterotopic ossification, loss of hip adduction strength occurs and may correlate with a lower hip rating score and compromised functional outcome.[16] Further anterior extension of the Kocher-Langenbeck approach to the anterosuperior iliac spine ("triradiate approach") allows even greater access to anterior column structures.

Ilioinguinal Approach
The incision for the ilioinguinal approach begins at the upper portion of the lateral iliac wing and extends down to the anterior superior iliac spine and across to about 1 cm above the pubic symphysis. The lateral femoral cutaneous nerve of the thigh, which is at risk of being transected, should be dissected out and identified. Not infrequently, reduction considerations place this nerve under traction, and patients should be warned in advance of the possibility of sensory deficits to the skin supplied by that structure.

The key to this incision involves gaining access to the fractures through three anatomic windows that are created. Laterally, exposure through the first is gained to the entire iliac wing and fossa posteriorly to the sacroiliac joint and medially to the superior component of the iliopectineal eminence. The second window exposes the pelvic brim and the quadrilateral surface. The third window provides access to the pubic ramus and the symphysis and to the retropubic space of Retzius. During operation, flexion of the hip can facilitate fracture exposure and reduction and can reduce the tension on the neurovascular structures.

This approach requires an intimate understanding of the anatomy of the inguinal canal and ring. It leaves the abductors undisturbed and has a lower rate of heterotopic ossification than the traditional posterior Kocher-Langenbeck approach. The disadvantages are that it does not allow direct intra-articular viewing of the acetabulum and does not enable stabilization of posterior wall fragments to be carried out. The posterior column can be addressed with a posterior column screw that has an intrapelvic starting point and that may obviate a secondary posterior exposure. The quadrilateral surface can be readily accessed, and its stabilization can be obtained by using a spring plate that is anchored under the primary anterior column plate.

Extended Iliofemoral Approach

This approach was developed by Letournel in 1974. It is carried out with the patient in the lateral position. It allows extensive visualization of the entire posterior column, the external ilium, and the anterior column up to the iliopectineal eminence.[15] The tradeoff for this excellent access to the entire hemipelvis relates to the dependence of the gluteal abductor mass on the SGA and the ascending branch to the lateral femoral circumflex artery. If the SGA was damaged at the time of the original injury, the anatomic dissection used in the approach (which requires transection of the lateral femoral circumflex artery) may devascularize the large posterior hip abductor flap.[4, 17] There is also a significant incidence rate of heterotopic ossification with this approach.

Modified Stoppa Approach

Other approaches include the ilioanterior or modified Stoppa approach, which allows excellent intrapelvic exposure through a dissection posterior to the iliac vessels, psoas muscle, and femoral nerve.[18] Ligation of anastomotic vessels found between the iliac and obturator systems allows for exposure to the quadrilateral surface soleus gutter and pelvic brim from the symphysis to the sacroiliac joint. This approach is useful when significant injury has occurred to the quadrilateral surface.

POSTOPERATIVE MANAGEMENT

Considerations for mobilization of the patient are based on associated injuries and the stability of the fracture reduction that has been obtained. A continuous passive motion machine may be used to begin early hip motion once the wound has stabilized. Prophylaxis against deep venous thrombosis may be carried out with a postoperative regimen of warfarin, although some surgeons now favor the use of low molecular weight heparin. The latter may be associated with a slightly higher incidence rate of postoperative hematoma if instituted too soon following surgery. In patients with associated head, thoracic, or abdominal injury that precludes mobilization, an inferior vena caval filter

may be placed. The use of intermittent pneumatic compression boots or stockings may also be useful.

The affected side should not bear weight for a minimum of 8 weeks, and healing should be monitored with radiographs of serial Judet views. Heterotopic ossification can cause severe limitations of joint motion and make future reconstruction difficult. Indomethacin, 25 mg orally three times daily, has been advocated by some investigators, although other studies have not clearly shown the efficacy of this regimen.[19] Alternatively, radiation therapy with single-dose (700 or 800 cGy)[20, 21] or multiple-dose treatments[22] can be considered.

COMPLICATIONS

Acetabular surgery is fraught with the potential for numerous complications. They include deep venous thrombosis and pulmonary embolism, neurological injury, heterotopic ossification, infection, osteonecrosis of the femoral head or acetabular segments, and post-traumatic arthritis. In addition, the potential for intra-articular placement of hardware is always present. Vascular injury may occur. The structures at most risk are the SGA, the femoral artery, and the corona mortis. The lateral femoral cutaneous nerve of the thigh and the femoral nerve are at risk during an ilioinguinal approach, and the sciatic nerve can be injured during reduction or through retractor placement during a posterior approach.

Malreduction is a matter of the clinician's technique. There is significant debate as to what constitutes an acceptable reduction, but ultimately, only an anatomic reduction has the best chance for excellent results.[23]

Post-traumatic arthritis may produce debilitating pain and functional limitations. Conversion of failed surgical repair of an acetabular fracture to total joint arthroplasty is a consideration and is facilitated if the regional anatomy has been restored by the first procedure. Satisfactory outcome of total hip arthroplasty is not automatic, however, and revision surgery reportedly has an appreciably high rate of complications from neurovascular injury and infection. In addition, implant loosening and failure frequently occur, possibly resulting in part from regional acetabular avascular necrosis.[24]

SUMMARY

Acetabular fractures that meet the criteria for surgical treatment present significant challenges. The optimal result allows the patient early mobilization with the best anatomic reduction possible. Preoperative planning is essential, and an understanding of the unique anatomy and topography of the pelvis and the acetabulum is a prerequisite for undertaking this very difficult surgery. The goal is restoration of joint motion and function.

REFERENCES

1. Judet R, Judet J, Letournel E: Fractures of the acetabulum: Classification and surgical approaches for open reduction: Preliminary report. J Bone Joint Surg Am 1964; 46: 1615.
2. Letournel E, Judet R, Elson RA (eds): Fractures of the Acetabulum. Berlin, Springer-Verlag, 1981.
3. Letournel E: Acetabulum fractures: Classification and management. Clin Orthop 1980; 151:81.
4. Bosse MJ, Poka A, Reinert CM, et al: Preoperative angiographic assessment of the superior gluteal artery in acetabular fractures requiring extensile surgical exposures. J Orthop Trauma 1989; 2:303.
5. Juliano PJ, Bosse MJ, Edwards KJ: The superior gluteal artery in complex acetabu-

lar procedures: A cadaveric angiographic study. J Bone Joint Surg Am 1994; 76: 244.

6. Fassler PR, Swiontkowski MF, Kilroy AW, et al: Injury of the sciatic nerve associated with acetabular fracture. J Bone Joint Surg Am 1993; 75:1157.

7. Hak DJ, Olson SA, Matta JM: Diagnosis and management of closed internal degloving injuries associated with pelvic and acetabular fractures: The Morel-Lavallee lesion. J Trauma 1997; 42:1046.

8. Kottmeier SA, Wilson SC, Born CT, et al: The Morel-Lavallee lesion. Orthop Trans 1992; 16:49.

9. Muller ME, Nazarian J, Koch P, et al: Comprehensive Classification of Long Bones. Berlin, Springer-Verlag, 1990.

10. Orthopaedic Trauma Association Committee for Coding and Classification: Fracture and dislocation compendium. J Orthop Trauma 1996; 10(Suppl 1):XX.

11. Olson SA, Matta JM: The computerized tomography of the subchondral arc: A new method of assessing the acetabular articular continuity after fracture: A pre-

liminary report. J Orthop Trauma 1993; 7: 402.

12. Matta JM, Mehne DK, Roffi R: Fractures of the acetabulum: Early results of a prospective study. Clin Orthop 1986; 205: 241.

13. Matta JM, Anderson LM, Epstein HC, et al: Fractures of the acetabulum: A retrospective analysis. Clin Orthop 1986; 205: 230.

14. Helfet DL, Borrelli J, Dipasquale T, et al: Stabilization of acetabular fractures in elderly patients. J Bone Joint Surg Am 1992; 74:753.

15. Alonso JE, Davila R, Bradley E: Extended iliofemoral versus triradiate approaches in management of associated acetabular fracture. Clin Orthop 1994; 305:81.

16. Dickenson WH, Duwelius PJ, Colville MR: Muscle strength testing following surgery for acetabular fractures. J Orthop Trauma 1993; 7:39.

17. Schatzker J, Tile M: The Rationale of Operative Fracture Care. New York, Springer-Verlag, 1987.

18. Cole JD, Bolhofner BR: Acetabular frac-

ture fixation via a modified Stoppa limited intrapelvic approach: Description of operative technique and preliminary treatment results. Clin Orthop 1994; 305:112.

19. Moed BR, Maxey JW: The effect of indomethacin on heterotopic ossification following acetabular fracture surgery. J Orthop Trauma 1993; 7:33.

20. Lo TC, Healy WL, Covall DJ, et al: Heterotopic bone formation after hip surgery: Prevention with single-dose postoperative hip irradiation. Radiology 1988; 168: 851.

21. Anglen JO, Moore KD: Prevention of heterotopic bone formation after acetabular fracture fixation by single-dose radiation therapy: A preliminary report. J Orthop Trauma 1996; 10:258.

22. Moed BR: Complications of acetabular fracture surgery: Prevention and management. Int J Orthop Trauma 1992; 2:68.

23. Matta JM, Helfet DIL, Mears DC: Current concepts in the management of acetabular fractures. Instr Course Lect 1997; 151:151.

24. Born CT (ed): Pelvic trauma: Update. Operative Tech Orthop 1997; 7:72.

section 3 chapter 13

HIP

Daniel S. Horwitz

Summary

- Hip fractures in the United States have an incidence of greater than 250,000 per year, with total costs estimated to exceed 8 billion dollars a year.
- These numbers are expected to triple by the year 2050.
- These fractures occur primarily in the elderly, have multiple associated medical risks, and are usually the result of a simple fall.
- Surgical treatment and rapid mobilization are the primary factors in returning patients to a prefracture level of function.
- Multiple surgical treatments are available, and the timing and choice of treatment must be individualized in each case.

The incidence of hip fractures has been linked to many factors, including age, sex, race, and coexisting medical conditions. In general, increasing age is associated with increasing risk of fracture, with the overall incidence doubling for each decade past 50 years of age. The female to male ratio is approximately 2:1, and the white race to black or Hispanic ratio is approximately 2:1 to 3:1.[1] In general, these fractures are the result of low-energy trauma such as a fall, with the exception being in the younger population, in whom these injuries tend to result from high-energy trauma. Additional risk factors for these fractures include neurological impairment, decreased physical

activity, use of psychotropic medication, malnutrition, malignancy, poor balance, impaired vision, and senile dementia. With a growing recognition of osteoporosis in a large percentage of the general population, many people assume that those patients with osteoporosis would be at significantly higher risk for hip fracture, but this remains a debated topic. In some studies, osteoporosis has been shown to occur no more frequently in patients with a hip fracture than in age-matched patients without fracture,[2] whereas other studies have suggested only a small increased risk in comparison to other factors.[3] Bone quality itself appears to play at most a small role in the occurrence of these fractures.

In contrast to hip fracture in the elderly population, this injury in a younger population is generally associated with high-energy trauma such as motor vehicle accidents. Its diagnosis in this setting can be much more difficult because of associated injuries, and its final outcome may be more devastating. In general, displaced femoral neck fractures in the younger patient (younger than 50 years of age) should be treated on an emergency basis to decrease the incidence of vascular compromise to the femoral head.

In the elderly patient population, the 1-year mortality rate after hip fractures ranges from 14% to 50%. This is significantly higher than in age-matched populations, but by 1 year the mortality rate approaches that for age-matched control subjects. It is believed by many practitioners that those same factors that place a patient at increased risk for a fracture may be partially responsible for this increased mortality. Certainly, addressing the overall health problems and nutritional deficiencies in the elderly can significantly decrease the incidence of hip fracture as well as the rate of mortality following a hip fracture.[4]

HISTORICAL REVIEW

Although hip fractures were described before the 19th century, the primary recognition and initiation of treatment of hip fractures began in the mid 1800s. These fractures were initially treated closed with traction. By the early 1900s, casting had been introduced as a treatment regimen. This resulted in approximately 30 to 40% union rates.[5] The first described application of internal fixation was in the late 1800s. However, this technique did not begin to gain broad acceptance until the 1930s. In 1931, Smith-Peterson introduced the triflanged nail, which was later modified with the addition of a side plate. These early surgical interventions achieved union rates of 60% to 70%. Sliding characteristics

were later introduced between the nail and the side plate and the triflanged nail was ultimately modified to a screw-type device. At about the same time as the introduction of the early nail devices, a multiple pin technique for treating femoral neck fractures was introduced, and hemiarthroplasty was added as a treatment option in the 1940s. Despite the multiple advances in orthopedics over the last 20 to 30 years, the primary treatment modalities for hip fractures remain sliding screw devices, multiple pins or screws, and hemiarthroplasty.

INTRACAPSULAR HIP FRACTURE

PATHOGENESIS

The majority of intracapsular hip fractures are the result of a simple fall. In general, the mechanism of injury is described as a direct blow to the region of the greater trochanter, often associated with forced external rotation of

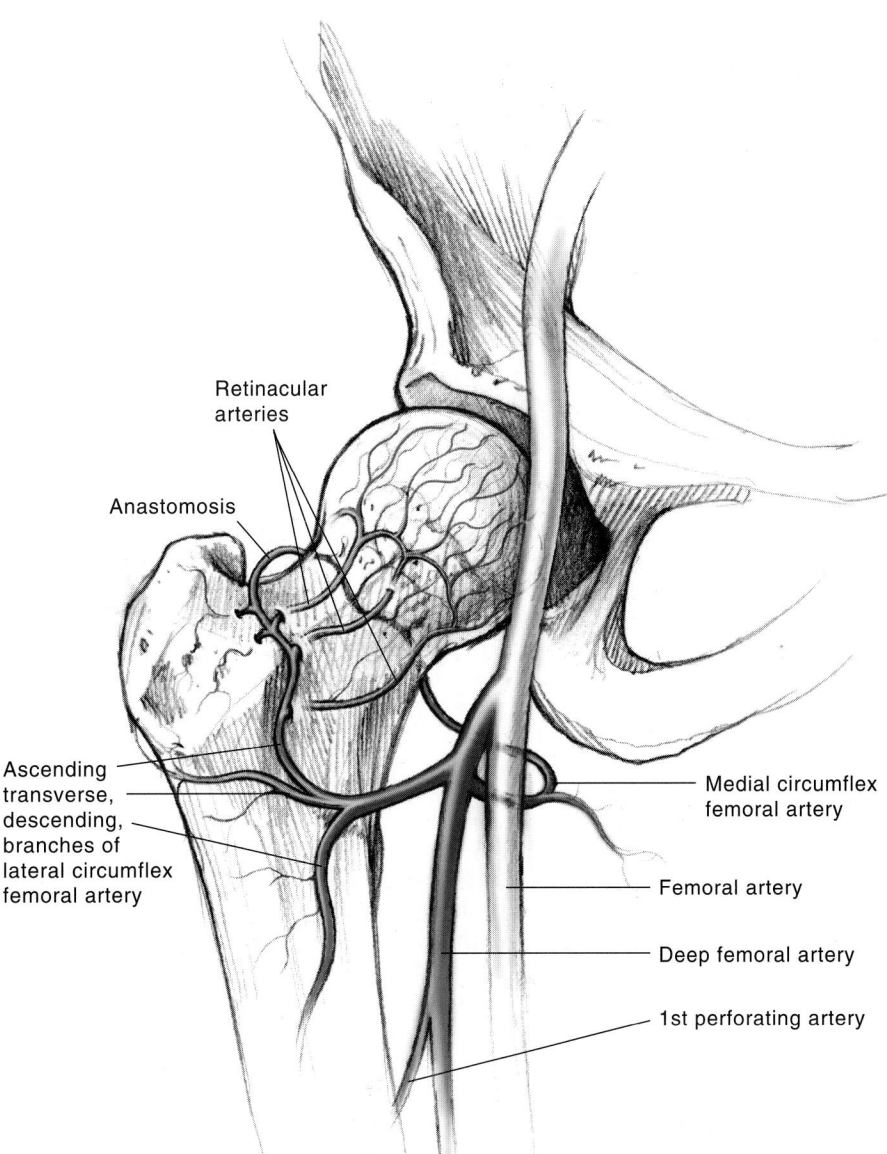

Fig. 1. Vascular supply of the proximal femur and hip.

Retinacular arteries

Anastomosis

Ascending transverse, descending, branches of lateral circumflex femoral artery

Medial circumflex femoral artery

Femoral artery

Deep femoral artery

1st perforating artery

the extremity. A related theory is that in osteopenic bone cyclical loading may result in the production of a stress fracture and, in fact, the femoral neck fracture may be the cause of the patient falling.[6] In general, any associated medical condition that could result in poor balance, poor vision, confusion, or loss of consciousness could potentially contribute to a fall. It has been shown that simple mechanical protection of the lateral aspect of the hip can significantly decrease the incidence of femoral neck fractures in the elderly.[7]

Femoral neck fractures in young adults are generally associated with high-energy trauma such as motor vehicle accidents. In these cases, close attention must be paid to other associated skeletal injuries, with special attention given to the possibility of a concomitant femoral neck/femoral shaft fracture.

ANATOMY

The anatomy of the femoral neck can be divided into two crucial areas: vascular and bony. The vascular supply to the femoral head and neck originates in the medial and lateral femoral circumflex arteries. These arteries form an extracapsular ring and then radiate up the femoral neck as the ascending cervical arteries (Fig. 1). The vascular contribution to the femoral head through the ligamentum teres is believed to be insignificant in the skeletally mature person. On the basis of this vascular anatomy, it is fairly obvious why a displaced fracture of the femoral neck puts the blood supply to the femoral head at such risk.

The bony anatomy of the femoral head and neck is classically divided into five trabecular groups (Fig. 2). Although the quality of the bony trabeculae does not necessarily increase the risk of a fracture, it has been shown that poor bone quality does lead to more fracture comminution, and it has also been shown that the quality of the bone does play an important role in the stability of the fixation.[8]

CLASSIFICATION

The most commonly used classification scheme for femoral neck fractures is that proposed by Garden (Fig. 3). This classification system is based on the degree of displacement shown on the anteroposterior (AP) radiograph, with types I and II representing minimally displaced fractures and types III and IV representing significantly displaced fractures. Although this classification system is helpful in predicting postoperative complications and does help direct surgical intervention, it has not been shown to have good interobserver reliability. Because of this drawback, newer classification schemes have been accepted by the Orthopedic Trauma Association. In its classification of fractures, the number 31 designates the proximal femur and the letter B designates the intracapsular/neck location. The Pauwels classification describes the verticality of the fracture, with type I more horizontal and type III more vertical. This can be helpful when attempting to express the axial instability of a given fracture.

CLINICAL FEATURES

The clinical presentation of intracapsular hip fractures is quite variable. Patients with fractures that are minimally

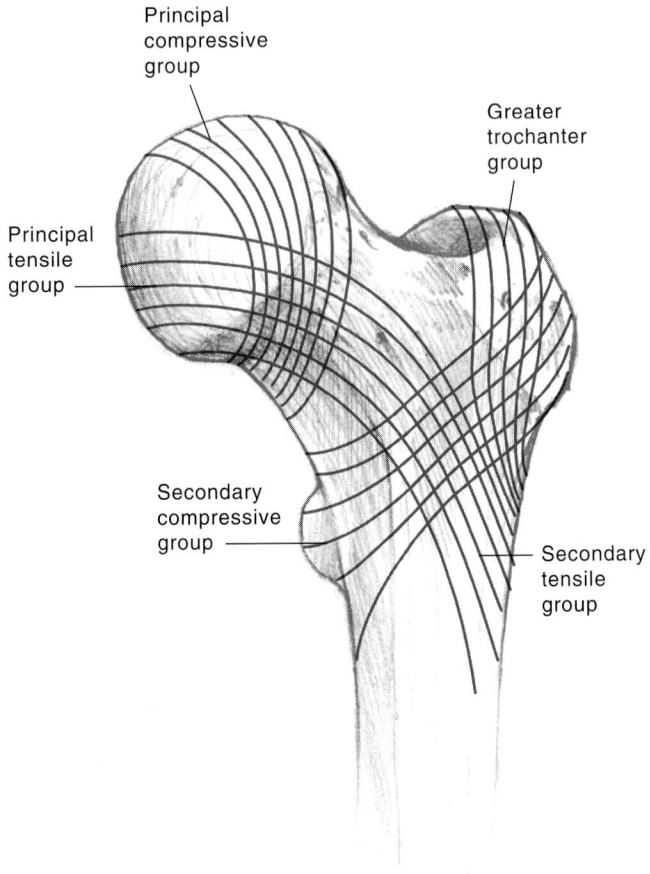

Fig. 2. Bony trabecular anatomy of the proximal femur. All five groups of bony trabeculae are readily evident on radiograph in a nonosteoporotic femur.

displaced or impacted often demonstrate only minimal pain and may, in fact, ambulate independently. Patients with fractures that are displaced classically present with a shortened and externally rotated lower extremity and have significant pain with flexion, extension, and rotation. Femoral neck fractures associated with a high-energy injury or in a multitrauma setting can be very difficult to diagnosis and assess. In these cases, the injury may be masked by associated fractures in the femoral shaft or acetabulum. If the trauma-setting AP pelvis radiograph does not adequately show both femoral necks, it is imperative that the condition of the femoral neck be well documented either preoperatively or intraoperatively.

INVESTIGATION

In general, AP pelvis and cross-table lateral radiographic views of an affected hip will adequately demonstrate significant femoral neck pathology. Care should be taken to avoid the frog-leg lateral radiograph, as the flexion and rotation used could cause a minimally displaced fracture to displace. For those patients in whom a fracture is suspected but plain radiographic findings are negative, the additional methods of investigation used are bone scan and magnetic resonance imaging (MRI). Radionuclide bone scan is usu-

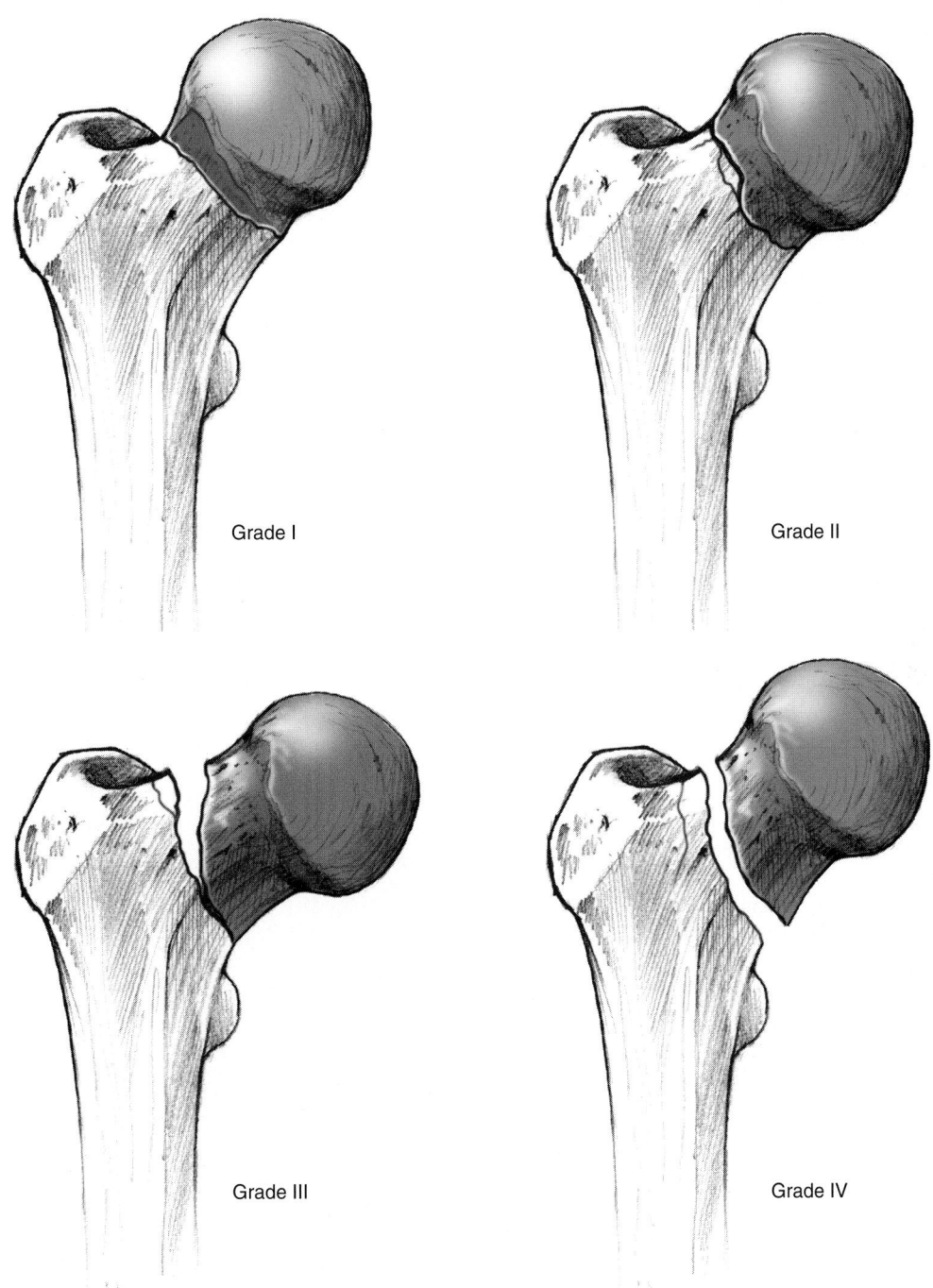

Fig. 3. The Garden classification of femoral neck fractures. Grade I is an incompletely impacted fracture with valgus malalignment. Grade IV is a completely displaced fracture with no engagement of the two fragments, and the compression trabeculae in the femoral head line up with the trabeculae on the acetabular side.

ally not positive until 2 to 3 days after fracture has occurred, and studies that have been performed directly comparing these two techniques have shown that the MRI scan is not only more sensitive but is, in the long run, more cost effective.[9] The appropriate use of MRI in these cases is dependent on communication between the orthopaedic surgeon and the emergency room physician, so that at-risk patients can be identified and screened, hopefully preventing the displacement of an occult fracture.

TREATMENT GOALS, INDICATIONS, AND CONTRAINDICATIONS

Although the nonoperative treatment of intracapsular hip fractures has historically been shown to have some success,

TABLE 1. TREATMENT OPTIONS FOR FEMORAL NECK FRACTURES		
Fracture Type	**Treatment Options**	**Expected Outcomes**
Nondisplaced	Screw fixation	>95% healed, <2% AVN
Impacted valgus	Screw fixation in situ	>95% healed, <2% AVN
Minimally displaced	Reduction and screw fixation	>90% healed, 5% AVN
Moderately displaced	Reduction and internal fixation	80% healed, 10–20% AVN
	Hemiarthroplasty	<2% dislocation
Completely displaced	Reduction and internal fixation	60–70% healed, 20–40% AVN
	Hemiarthroplasty	<2% dislocation

AVN, avascular necrosis.

the only indications for this treatment currently would be near imminent death. Even in those patients who are significant anesthesia risks, percutaneous pinning can be performed with minimal anesthesia and local augmentation. A question has been raised in the past about operative intervention for impacted valgus fractures. Unfortunately, closed treatment of these injuries has resulted in displacement of some of these "stable" fractures, with subsequent need for more significant surgical intervention.[10] Therefore, the current recommendation is that all identifiable femoral neck fractures be stabilized in some fashion. Table 1 outlines the fracture types and different treatment options. The timing of surgical intervention has been debated, and current recommendations are that a patient be brought to medically optimal condition and then treated on an urgent but not emergency basis. The only exception to this remains a younger patient with a displaced fracture, who should be treated on an emergency basis.

PROCEDURES

The different techniques used to treat femoral neck fractures can be generally divided into two approaches: internal fixation and joint replacement. For those fractures in which reduction and internal fixation is appropriate, the most crucial component of the surgery is undoubtedly the reduction. The reduction technique for displaced fractures is most commonly longitudinal traction, often accompanied by gentle internal rotation. It is crucial that a reduction be radiographically evaluated not only on the AP view but also on the lateral view. A true lateral view of the femoral neck should show the femoral neck directly parallel to the femoral shaft; generally, this will not be obtained with the fluoroscopy unit parallel to the floor, but more commonly with fluoroscopy 10 to 20 degrees short of parallel. This position is important not only for obtaining a true lateral view but also for giving the surgeon an excellent reference for estimating the anteversion of the femoral neck when placing screws or a guide wire for a compression screw device. Debate currently remains about the role of capsular decompression in treating femoral neck fractures, and there are those who propose routine decompression of intracapsular hematoma to allow any intact blood vessels to experi-

ence less pressure. When internal fixation has been chosen as the operative treatment, it is essential that a near anatomic reduction be obtained. In many cases, this may mean extending the lateral approach to the femur neck to perform an anterior capsulotomy and palpation of the fracture fragments and/or direct visualization. Deficiency in fracture reduction has been shown to significantly increase implant and postsurgical complications.[11]

The methods of internal fixation most commonly accepted for femoral neck fractures include the use of multiple screws, the use of a compression screw side plate device, and the use of a compression screw intramedullary device. The multiple cannulated screw technique is relatively simple and can be performed either percutaneously or through a small lateral incision. It does require an accurate screw placement in a parallel fashion, with insertion to subchondral bone (Fig. 4). Failure to place the screws into subchondral bone can lead to early implant failure, especially in the osteopenic patient, and failure to place the screws in a parallel position can prevent compression at the fracture sight. Studies looking at the number and orientation of screws have concluded that three screws in an inverted triangle represent the optimal construct.[12, 13]

A compression screw with side plate device requires a more extensive lateral approach and is often considered in

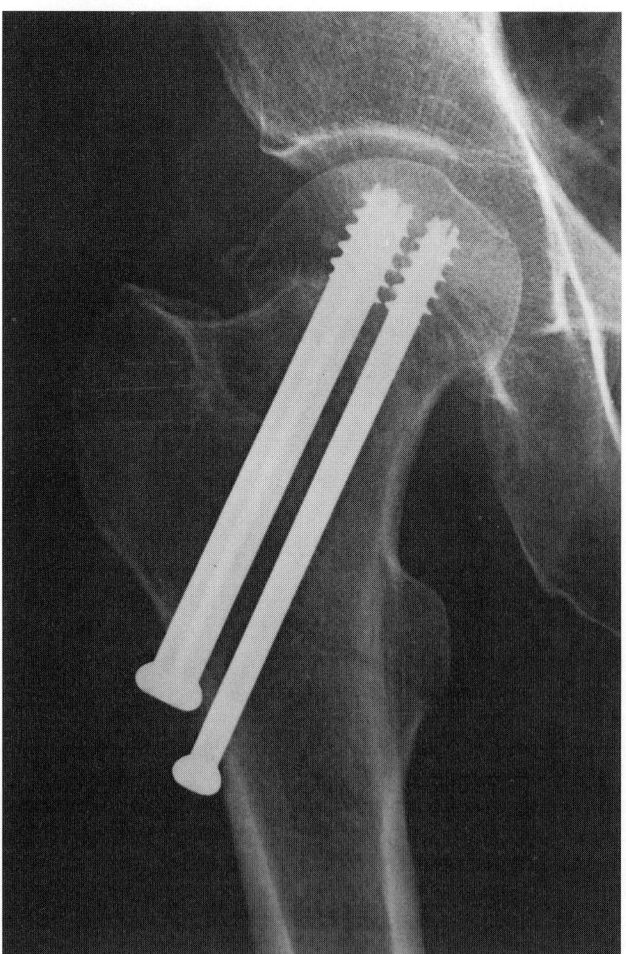

Fig. 4. Parallel placement of cannulated screws for treatment of femoral neck fracture.

those fractures that are extremely vertical and/or in those patients with extremely poor bone quality, in whom the multiple screw technique may not provide adequate stability. It is crucial when using a screw and side plate device that a second derotation screw or guide wire be placed in the femoral neck to avoid rotation through the fracture site during tapping and screw placement. Studies looking at the optimal screw placement in the femoral head have concluded that a central placement into subchondral bone on the AP and lateral radiographic views is the best position for a compression screw.[14, 15] Intramedullary devices have gained in popularity, although their introduction into the United States has been associated with a higher incidence of intraoperative complications. With the exception of a fracture involving both the femoral neck and the femoral shaft, indications for the use of an intramedullary compression screw device for femoral neck fractures is quite limited.

With the successful introduction of hemiarthroplasty in the 1940s, use of this technique has been broadly expanded in treating femoral neck fractures. The first implants introduced were unipolar hemiarthroplasties, later followed by the introduction of the bipolar arthroplasty, which allows motion not only between the prosthetic head and the acetabulum but also between an inner head and an interposed polyethylene shell. To date, most studies comparing the two systems report no advantage with the bipolar device.[16, 17] The surgical approach for either of these implants is identical and involves either a direct posterior approach or a modified anterolateral (Harding) approach. There remain some conditions, although rare, for total joint arthroplasty in the treatment of a femoral neck fracture, including significant prior degenerative changes in the hip, severe rheumatoid arthritis, and salvage for failed open reduction and internal fixation in a middle-aged group. It is essential that whenever replacement of the femoral head is performed, great attention must be paid to the anteversion of the prosthesis to minimize postoperative dislocation. In general, when arthroplasty (total or hemi) is chosen, a cemented technique is most commonly used on the femur.

POSTOPERATIVE CARE

In patients in whom hemiarthroplasty is performed, weightbearing as tolerated is initiated immediately. In patients in whom internal fixation has been performed, there remains some debate about the appropriate weightbearing status. Some studies suggest that patients can be placed on a weightbearing-as-tolerated regimen and that they will regulate themselves, thus avoiding an overload on the implants.[18] Perhaps of greater concern than patients who maintain their cognitive abilities to protect themselves in weightbearing are those patients with dementia, psychiatric problems, or a closed head injury. It is very unlikely that prescribing a protected weightbearing status in these patients will make a significant difference, and these cases are perhaps better addressed by choosing a more biomechanically stable construct.

The risk of deep venous thrombosis and pulmonary embolism has been well documented in patients with hip fractures, even those treated with methods allowing early mobilization. The most common methods of prophylaxis include pneumatic devices, early ambulation, warfarin, heparin, and aspirin. Although no single treatment protocol can be considered a standard of care, it is clear that just as with elective arthroplasty patients, the problem of thromboembolic disease must be addressed in every patient with a hip fracture.

SPECIAL PROBLEMS

One of the classic subsets of hip fracture patients is patients with Parkinson's or related neuromuscular diseases. The historical recommendations adhere to the belief that these patients are at an increased risk of dislocation and therefore an anterior approach should be used if hemiarthroplasty is indicated. More recent studies have shown that the rate of complications and, more specifically, the rate of dislocation in this subset of patients is not greater and does not appear dependent on the approach; therefore, the posterior approach for hemiarthroplasty is acceptable.[19]

As noted earlier, severe dementia, closed head injury, and psychiatric disease may all be indications for the use of more biomechanically stable fixations such as a screw and side plate over the use of cannulated screws. Each case, however, must be individualized based on the likely compliance of the patient as well as overall bone quality and fracture characteristics.

Pathological factors of the femoral neck are most commonly metastatic in nature and are generally an indication for prosthetic replacement. Great care must be taken in choosing a femoral component, as it is often necessary to bypass destructive lesions in the femoral shaft. Incomplete femoral neck fractures that are radiosensitive can often be treated with a reconstruction-type nail and radiation.

Concomitant femoral neck and shaft fractures, although a relatively rare problem, are missed in up to 30% of patients with hip fractures.[20] When these fractures do occur in conjunction, they are generally the result of high-energy trauma, and in the surgical approach to these injuries, the femoral neck takes clear priority. There are multiple techniques for treatment, and again the method used must be individualized to each patient as well as each surgeon. These techniques include placement of cannulated screws in the anterior aspect of the neck followed by the use of a standard antegrade or reconstruction type nail. When using this technique, it is imperative that the neck fracture be reduced and stabilized before nailing begins, and the neck position must be confirmed many times to ensure that reduction has not been lost. A variation on this technique is the use of screws in the femoral neck with a retrograde nail for the femoral shaft fracture. Another option remains: the use of screws or a compression screw/side plate for the femoral neck fracture combined with plating of the femoral shaft. Whichever method of internal fixation is chosen, it is essential that an anatomic reduction of the femoral neck be achieved, either through closed or open methods.

COMPLICATIONS AND RESULTS

The most common complications related to the operative treatment of femoral neck fractures are osteonecrosis, nonunion, and failure of fixation. The rate of osteonecrosis following femoral neck fractures is generally 5% to 8%. The rate for displaced femoral neck fractures ranges from 20% to 35%. Early studies by Garden confirmed that the adequacy of reduction was directly related to osteonecrosis and late segmental collapse.[21] Similarly, early failure of fixation, which occurs in up to 30% of displaced femoral neck fractures, appears directly related to the reduction achieved.[11] The degree of posterior comminution of the femoral neck has also been implicated as a potential cause of early fixation failure.[22]

The incidence of nonunion has also been found to relate to the degree of fracture displacement. In nondisplaced fractures, it ranges from 0% to 5% and in displaced fractures it ranges from 10% to 30%. When nonunion occurs and the femoral head remains viable, a valgus osteotomy and bone grafting remains the treatment of choice to achieve union. In a more elderly patient, conversion to hemiarthroplasty may be the preferred treatment.

Dislocation and infection associated with hemiarthroplasty have been described and both have incidences ranging from 2% to 10%. Late hip pain and protrusio resulting from hemiarthroplasty are rare and generally require conversion to a total hip arthroplasty.

INTERTROCHANTERIC HIP FRACTURES

The demographic distribution of intertrochanteric fractures is similar to that of femoral neck fractures. The same medical problems that put patients at risk for intracapsular fractures also apply to intertrochanteric fractures. Although osteoporosis itself has not been isolated as a risk factor, increased exercise and hormonal supplementation in postmenopausal women, coupled with adequate calcium intake, has been shown to reduce the incidence of intertrochanteric hip fracture.[23] The mechanism of injury is similar to that of femoral neck fractures in that it is usually a direct blow to the greater trochanter as a result of a fall or occasionally a twisting injury to the lower extremity. The bony anatomy of the proximal femur, as has been reviewed, is more important with intertrochanteric fractures than the vascular anatomy. The lesser trochanter and calcar femorale make up a significant medial column of support to the intertrochanteric region, and fractures that disrupt this support tend to be more unstable.

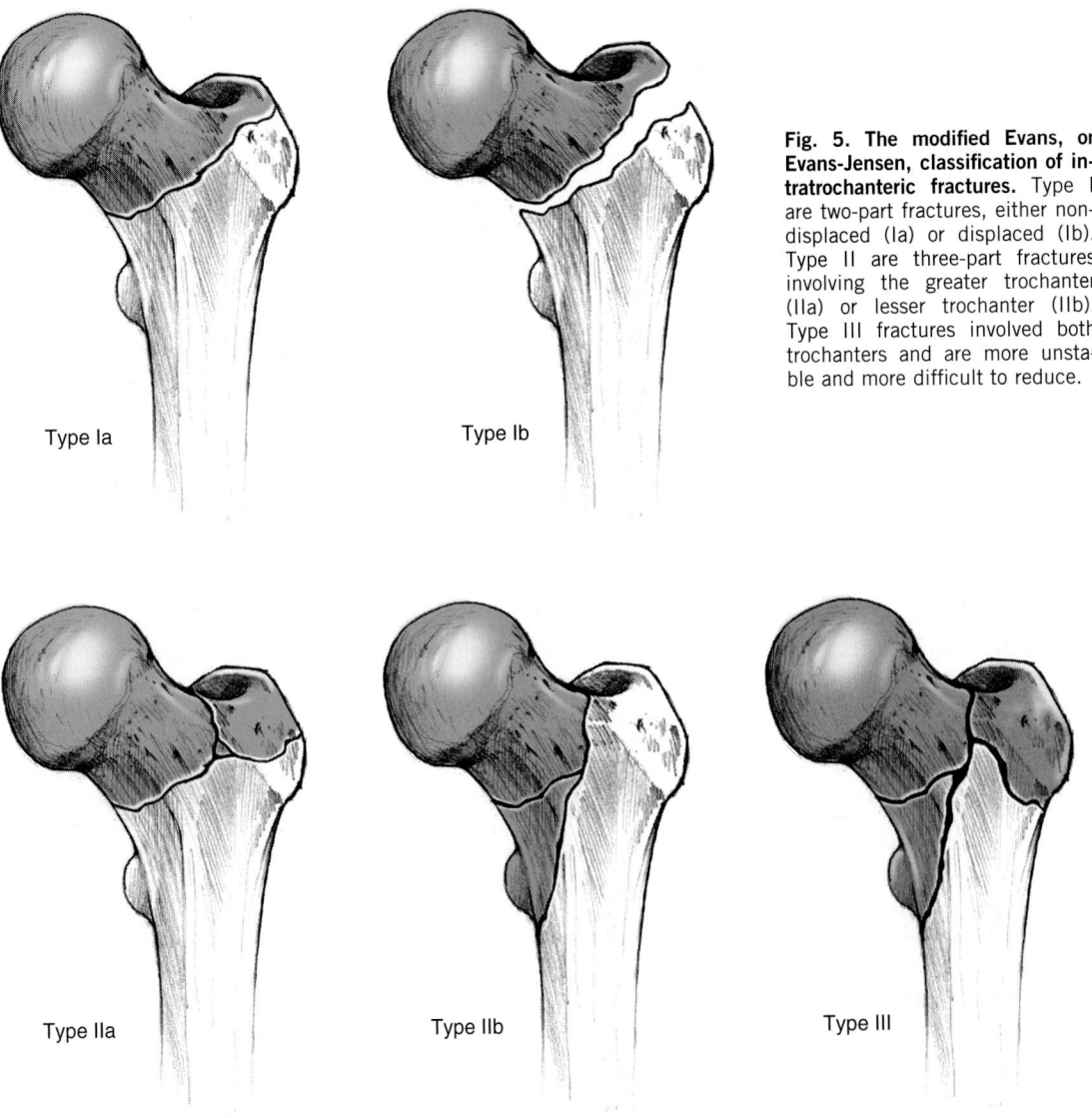

Fig. 5. The modified Evans, or Evans-Jensen, classification of intratrochanteric fractures. Type I are two-part fractures, either nondisplaced (Ia) or displaced (Ib). Type II are three-part fractures involving the greater trochanter (IIa) or lesser trochanter (IIb). Type III fractures involved both trochanters and are more unstable and more difficult to reduce.

Type Ia

Type Ib

Type IIa

Type IIb

Type III

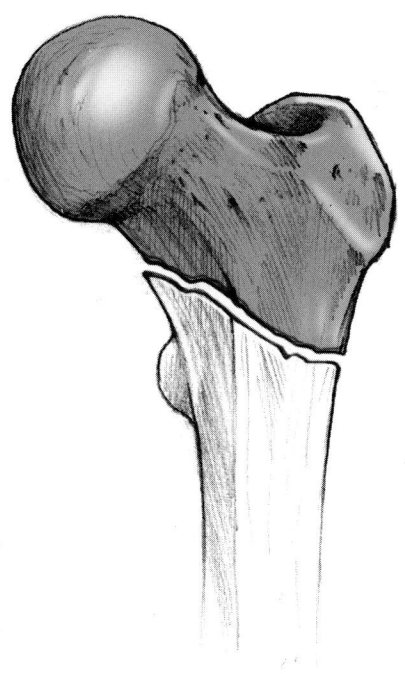

Fig. 6. An intertrochanteric fracture with reversed obliquity. These fractures are unstable because of their tendency toward medial shaft migration.

Another anatomic consideration, which relates to intertrochanteric fractures more so than to femoral neck fractures, is the muscular insertion of the iliopsoas onto the lesser trochanter. This muscular insertion tends to produce a flexion force on the lesser trochanter and can cause it to significantly displace.

CLASSIFICATION

The modified Evans classification system has been shown to be an excellent predictor of post-fixation stability. This classification relies on the intrinsic bony stability of the fracture based on the degree of comminution and the primary fracture orientation (Fig. 5). More recently, the reproducibility of this system has been questioned, and there is a current trend to classify intertrochanteric fractures simply as either stable or unstable, based on the degree of involvement of the posterior medial cortex and lesser trochanter as well as the presence of reverse obliquity.[24] Some surgeons believe that the conversion of an unstable fracture to a stable one requires a reduction of the posterior medial fragment, whereas others believe that this is not necessary if adequate internal fixation is provided.

The concept of reverse obliquity is an important one to understand both in terms of stability, as outlined earlier, and in terms of fixation. The reverse oblique pattern consists of a fracture line extending from proximal-medial to distal-lateral (Fig. 6). This pattern is inherently unstable because the femoral shaft tends to displace in a proximal and medial direction in relation to the hip, and in this case there is no bony anatomy to resist the displacement. This becomes important when choosing fixation devices. The screw and side plate device ideally has the barrel fixed to the femur and the compression screw settling into it, but

with a reverse oblique pattern the barrel is seated in a bony fragment separate from the shaft, and the construct is therefore more likely to fail. Some surgeons suggest that this is the ideal situation for the use of intramedullary fixation, as outlined below.

CLINICAL FEATURES AND INVESTIGATION

The clinical features of these fractures are similar to those of femoral neck fractures in that patients with a displaced fracture usually present with a shortened and externally rotated lower extremity. Plain radiographs consisting of AP pelvis and cross-table lateral views are usually adequate in defining the characteristics of the fracture; however, in patients with significant hip pain and negative radiographic findings, a limited-cut MRI scan should be strongly considered and has been shown to be quite sensitive and specific (Fig. 7).

TREATMENT GOALS, INDICATIONS, AND CONTRAINDICATIONS

As with an intracapsular hip fracture, the primary goal of treatment is to achieve stability so that early weightbearing can begin. The primary methods of fixation all rely on the quality of bone, the quality of reduction, and the characteristics of the fixation device chosen. As with femoral neck

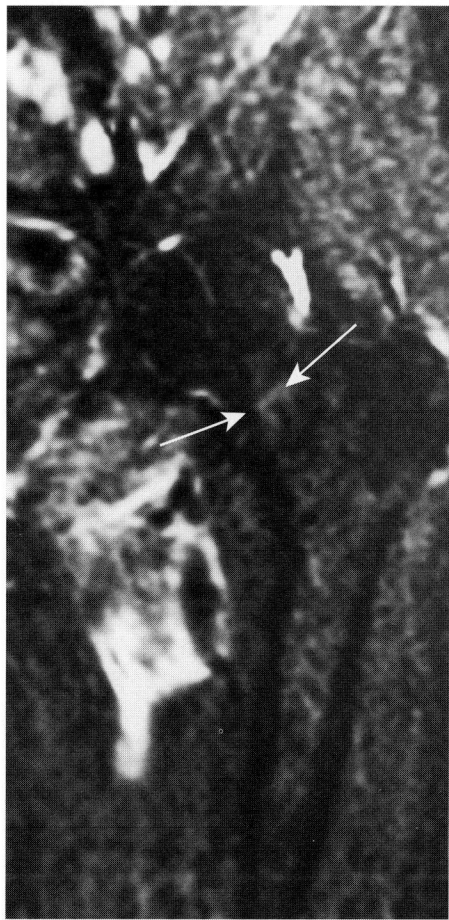

Fig. 7. MRI findings of a nondisplaced/occult femoral neck fracture. The changes here are subtle and can be easily missed even by an experienced radiologist.

fractures, these patients should be surgically stabilized as soon as their overall medical condition has been optimized. A significant delay in surgery has been shown to significantly increase postoperative mortality.[25] Historically, a medial displacement osteotomy was proposed as a method of increasing bony stability, but this has not been shown to be advantageous. An anatomic reduction and stable fixation with proper screw placement in the center of the femoral head appears to have superior results.[26] The role of hemiarthroplasty in treating intertrochanteric hip fractures was recently evaluated, and several studies have been performed that show earlier initiation of weightbearing and no significant increase in complications at 6 months. The overall functional results, however, have been found to be similar to results of open reduction and internal fixation, even in patients with poor bone quality.[27, 28] Based on this, the current recommendation for intertrochanteric hip fractures is open reduction and internal fixation, with the exception of pathological lesions or displaced fractures for which treatment has been significantly delayed (more than 3 weeks).

PROCEDURE

The most common treatments chosen for intertrochanteric hip fractures are the screw and side plate, the short intramedullary hip screw, and fixed angle devices such as the blade plate. Alternative devices such as flexible intramedullary condylocephalic nails have been somewhat successful but with significantly higher complication rates.[29]

All of the primary fixation devices rely on achieving an adequate intraoperative reduction and visualization of the fracture. This is achieved by placing the patient on a fracture table with a perineal post and the effected extremity in foot traction. Under direct fluoroscopic visualization, traction is gently applied so that a reduction is achieved on an AP view. Residual varus deformities should never be accepted and excessive valgus should also be avoided. It is crucial at this point that an adequate lateral view be obtained. In unstable fracture patterns, proximal displacement of the lesser trochanter will generally occur and posterior sag of the femoral shaft is not uncommon. It is important to confirm that the posterior sag can be corrected manually before a surgical approach is performed, and often a crutch can be used outside the operative field as an external support on the femoral shaft to correct the sag. Alternatively, the ability to correct the sag can be confirmed with the plan for interoperative manipulation with an elevator posterior to the femoral shaft, avoiding the use of the external crutch. Rotation should be carefully addressed, with an attempt made to minimize rotational deformity. In comminuted fractures, this can be difficult to estimate and one may have to rely on a lateral view of the femoral neck to estimate anteversion in relation to the distal femur. In such fractures, determining the anteversion of the contralateral femoral neck can be quite helpful in making estimations on the involved side. If an adequate closed reduction cannot be achieved, forceful traction should be avoided and instead a direct open reduction minimizing soft-tissue stripping should be performed.

A screw and side plate construct requires a lateral approach, placement of a guide wire into the femoral head, reaming over the guide wire, placement of the screw, and

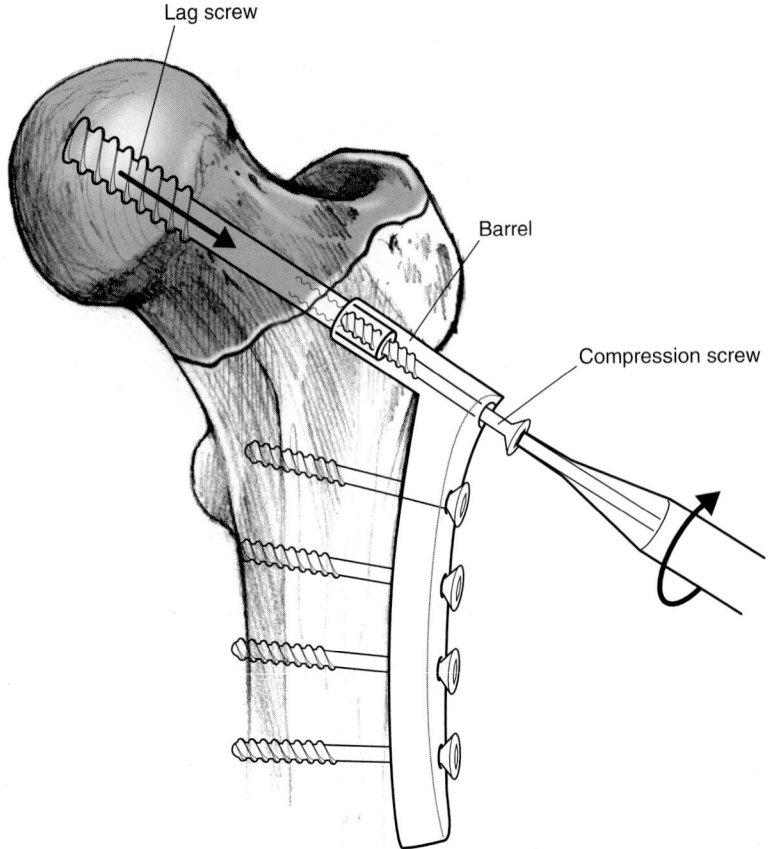

Lag screw

Barrel

Compression screw

Fig. 8. By advancing the compression screw, the lag screw is pulled to the side plate, compressing the fracture. The lag screw must be left short so there is room for compression, and excessive tightening should be avoided, especially in osteoporotic bone.

subsequent placement of a side plate. In general, a 130- or 135-degree side plate is adequate for most fractures, with the exception of those patients with significant varus or valgus deformity. The sliding characteristics of a higher angle side plate construct have not been shown to be of benefit.[30] The compression screw should be placed into subchondral bone in the direct center of the femoral head. A common practice is to use a compression screw that is 10 to 15 mm shorter than the length that has been measured and drilled based on the guide wire. This allows for immediate compression across the fracture site and some increased early stability (Fig. 8). It is essential that the traction be released on the extremity prior to performing this compression.

Many systems offer the option of a long-barreled or short-barreled side plate. The long barrel is generally chosen because it allows more contact with the screw and better stability and sliding characteristics. In patients in whom a compression screw of less than 80 mm is used, however, strong consideration should be given to using the short-barreled side plate so that there is adequate room for compression to occur.

The inherent instability of many intertrochanteric hip fractures has lead to the increased use of short interlocked

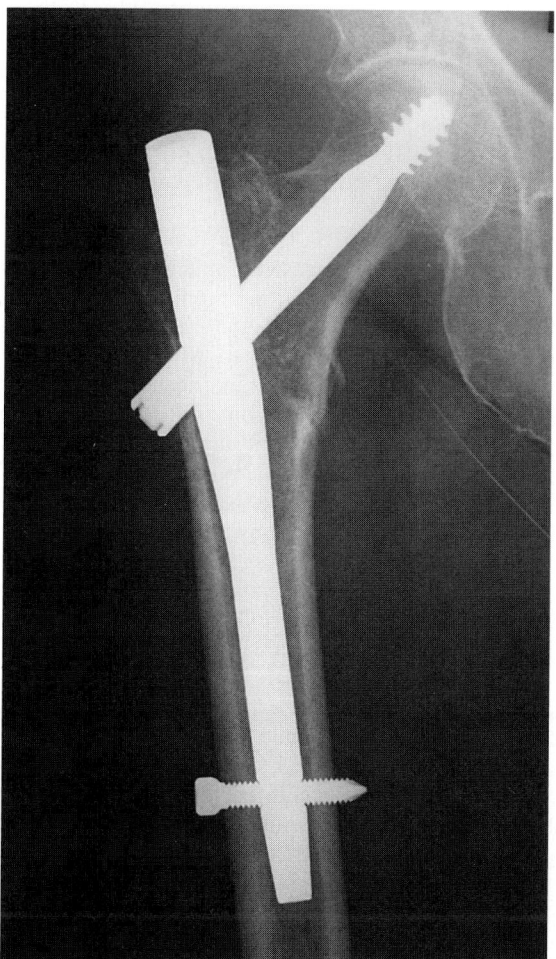

Fig. 9. An intramedullary device used for treating an intertrochanteric fracture. In this case, the device was chosen not for an unstable fracture pattern but to minimize dissection in an elderly immunosuppressed patient.

intramedullary hip screws such as the trochanteric or Gamma nail (Stryker/Howmedica, Rutherford, NJ) (Fig. 9). The advantages of such a construct include intramedullary placement, which provides more effective load sharing and therefore greater stability to the entire construct. These devices are generally placed through the tip of the greater trochanter and require significantly less surgical exposure; however, they too rely on an adequate reduction and correction of posterior sag. There have been multiple reports of complications associated with these devices, and recent changes have been made in product design to minimize the risk of intraoperative problems. Clinical studies have been performed comparing screw and side plate fixation to intramedullary fixation and have failed to show any significant advantage in terms of operating time, complication rate, and functional outcome; therefore, the role of intramedullary devices remains under investigation.[31, 32] Perhaps the most promising use of these devices is in reverse oblique fracture patterns, which, as discussed earlier, are inherently unstable and may be subject to greater failure of screw and side plate devices, especially in osteopenic bone.

Debate remains about operative reduction and fixation of the posterior medial fragment in unstable fraction patterns. Biomechanical studies have shown increased stability with reduction of this fragment, and many surgeons routinely provide fixation with cerclage wiring or an interfragmentary screw.[33] Unfortunately, mobilization of the fragment is quite difficult and often requires release of the psoas insertion. Medial vascular complications have been reported in attempting to mobilize this fragment and reports of excellent results even without reduction have raised questions regarding its role.

POSTOPERATIVE CARE

If the goal of adequate reduction and stable internal fixation has been achieved, most patients can be begin weightbearing as tolerated. If a hip screw device has been used, the sliding characteristics rely on weightbearing to allow the construct to settle to a stable position. If the construct is unstable, most patients will be able to regulate themselves and not initiate full weightbearing until healing has begun. If exceptions such as dementia and psychiatric disease exist, however, the postoperative weightbearing status may have to be modified. Thromboembolic disease should be addressed in all patients, but the role for full anticoagulation with warfarin is minimal in this patient population, who should be rapidly mobilized.

SPECIAL CONSIDERATIONS

The role of open reduction and internal fixation in the treatment of a pathological intertrochanteric fracture is a complex subject. Fixation with cement augmentation has been shown to be somewhat effective but also has a fairly high failure rate and its use remains controversial in a patient with an undetermined life expectancy.[34] Prosthetic replacement has been found to be quite successful but usually requires the use of a calcar replacing stem. The use of a hemiarthroplasty does require careful evaluation of the entire femoral shaft to ensure that there are no additional impending pathological fractures, and many authors recommend the routine use of long-stem prosthesis in patients with multiple bony lesions.

COMPLICATIONS

The most common complications of intertrochanteric femur fractures remain loss of reduction, malreduction, loss of fixation, and nonunion. As noted earlier, limitation of weightbearing has not been shown to reduce the incidence of nonunion or loss of fixation. The occurrence of malreduction is dependent on adequate preoperative planning and achieving adequate reduction intraoperatively. The most common rotational deformity is excessive internal rotation, which is usually the result of intraoperative leg position. Mechanical failure and loss of fixation have been reported in up to 16% of patients and appear partially related to the initial placement of the screw in the femoral head.[35] As noted previously, a central placement of the screw as shown in both AP and lateral views within 1 cm of the subchondral surface has been found to be ideal.

In patients with severely osteopenic bone, some surgeons augment screw fixation with the introduction of cement into the femoral head. This can be technically difficult, and great care should be taken to avoid extravasation of cement into the fracture itself.

Nonunion is an uncommon complication following internal fixation of intertrochanteric fractures with an incidence of less than 2%.[35] In patients who have not lost bone stock and/or are not severely osteopenic, revision open reduction and internal fixation with or without bone grafting is often successful in achieving union. A valgus osteotomy can also be used in combination with revision internal fixation and has been shown to have excellent results.[36] In the elderly, patients with extremely poor bone stock, or those with significant bony destruction, a hemiarthroplasty or a total hip replacement remains an excellent salvage for a nonunion.

HIP DISLOCATION AND FEMORAL HEAD FRACTURES

Dislocation of the hip and femoral head fractures both represent high-energy injuries, which were once thought to be rare but are becoming more common. Associated long bone and abdominal or thoracic trauma often mask these injuries, which emphasize the need to obtain a good AP pelvis radiograph for all trauma patients. The relatively high rate of associated degenerative arthritis has led to more aggressive treatment of femoral head fractures as well as acetabular fractures associated with dislocation. In general, hip dislocation and fracture dislocation are treated as emergency conditions, and controlled reduction with heavy sedation or general anesthesia should be performed as soon as possible. Minor delays in reduction (i.e., 1 hour) have not, however, been shown to be detrimental.[37] These injuries represent a broad and complex topic and what follows is a brief summary of the critical issues.

PATHOGENESIS AND CLASSIFICATION

As both hip dislocations and femoral head fractures generally require a massive amount of energy to occur, there is often fragmentation of surrounding bony and cartilaginous structures. These fragments can become entrapped in the joint and cause significant wear, and interposed bone or a widened joint space are often indications for joint débridement. When the hip is dislocated, the blood supply to the

TABLE 2. THE PIPKIN CLASSIFICATION FOR FEMORAL HEAD FRACTURE		
Type	**Fracture Location**	**Associated Injuries**
I	Fragment below the ligamentum teres	None
II	Fragment above the ligamentum teres	None
III	Either	Femoral neck fracture
IV	Either	Acetabular fracture

femoral head can be compromised, and direct compression of the sciatic nerve is not uncommon in posterior dislocations.[38]

Hip dislocation has recently been organized under the Orthopaedic Trauma Association classification system, which tends to simplify the description but has no prognostic role.[39] In addition, this system does not indicate direction, which can be important if there are associated fractures or neurovascular compromise. In general, anterior dislocations constitute 10 to 15% of these injuries, with the remainder being posterior. The Pipkin classification (Table 2) describes femoral head fractures associated with posterior hip dislocation and is perhaps most useful in its delineation of infratectal and supratectal injuries. A fracture that involves a significant portion of the femoral head above the fovea represents a major disruption of joint congruity, and this often necessitates anatomic reduction and internal fixation. The Pipkin III injury carries an especially poor prognosis.

CLINICAL DIAGNOSIS AND TREATMENT

These injuries are often missed if attention is not given to the AP pelvis radiograph, as the significant discomfort in the hip is often masked by other injuries. High-quality radiographs are generally required to assess fracture patterns in both the femoral head and acetabulum, and computed tomography is usually recommended to further define the injury pattern. Some authors have begun to look at the role of MRI in investigating labral disruptions, microfractures, and interposed cartilaginous structures, and this remains an expanding area of study.[40]

The initial management of these injuries is early reduction through gentle closed means or open means if necessary. Delayed surgical intervention is based on radiographic findings as well as the individual patient. Significantly displaced acetabular fractures are generally treated with attempted anatomic reduction and internal fixation, the specific approach used dictated by the fracture pattern. Similarly, displaced femoral head fractures involving a significant portion of the weightbearing surface are usually treated with reduction and internal fixation to restore joint congruity and begin early motion. As many of these fractures are associated with posterior dislocations, the free fragment is commonly anterior medial in location, and an anterior approach to the hip has been found to be most useful in visualizing, reducing, and fixing the fragment.[41] It is possible, however, to perform a posterior approach for an acetabular fracture and address a femoral head fracture

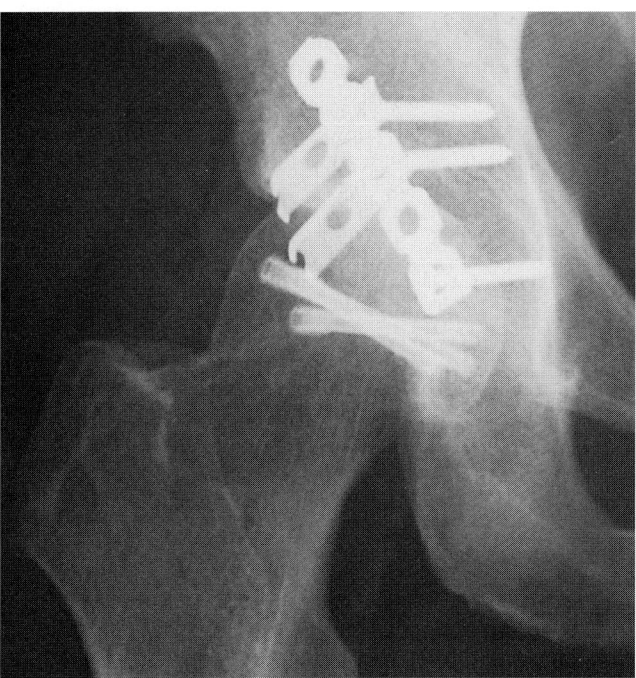

Fig. 10. Postoperative views of a patient with a displaced femoral head fracture, a posterior wall fracture, and posterior instability. A single posterior approach was used here, and a traction pin in the proximal femur allowed adequate visualization to repair both fractures through a single approach.

through the same incision (Fig. 10). There are indications, primarily in the elderly, for immediate total hip arthroplasty, especially if the femoral head is significantly compromised. Gaining adequate stability for the acetabular component may require concurrent internal fixation of acetabular fractures in these cases.

Aseptic necrosis, traumatic arthritis, recurrent dislocation, and sciatic nerve injury are all well described complications of treating hip dislocations and femoral head fractures. Minimizing these complications depends on a prompt recognition of the injury, appropriate early treatment, and operative intervention when indicated. When surgery is

performed, heterotopic ossification and thromboembolic disease become issues that must also be addressed.

GREATER TROCHANTERIC FRACTURES

Isolated injury to the greater trochanter remains an extremely rare problem. Two subsets exist for this injury based on patient characteristics. The first and most common type is an apophyseal separation in the skeletally immature, and the second is a comminuted fracture of the greater trochanter in the skeletally mature, usually the result of a high-energy direct blow.

CLINICAL DIAGNOSIS AND TREATMENT

Significant pain, swelling, and antalgic gait are the most common presentation of an isolated greater trochanteric fracture. Since either the abductor musculature or short external rotators are usually attached to the fracture fragments, the chosen treatment depends on the degree of displacement. Minimally displaced or nondisplaced fractures can usually be successfully treated with protected weight-bearing. Fractures displaced less than 1 cm can also be treated with abduction bracing or casting. In contrast, fractures displaced more than 1 cm in skeletally immature patients are usually treated with open reduction and internal fixation using interfragmentary screws or wires. The role of open reduction and internal fixation in displaced fractures in adults remains controversial and is generally recommended only if a significant portion of the greater trochanter is involved and concern over abductor shortening and permanent abductor weakness exists.

POSTOPERATIVE TREAMENT AND COMPLICATIONS

If open reduction and internal fixation is performed, the postoperative protocol must carefully protect the construct, as the abductors will displace the fragment if overused. The use of crutches for 4 to 6 weeks is recommended in both operative and nonoperative treatment of these fractures, followed by fairly aggressive physical therapy at 6 to 8 weeks to restore abductor strength. The most common complication of these fractures is residual abductor weakness and shortening with a resultant gluteus medius gait.

REFERENCES

1. Hinton RY, Smith GS: The association of age, race, and sex with the location of proximal femoral fractures in the elderly. J Bone Joint Surg Am 1993; 75:752.
2. Aitken JM: Relevance of osteoporosis in women with fracture of the femoral neck. Br Med J 1984; 288:597.
3. Hayes WC, Myers ER: Biomechanical considerations of hip and spine fractures in osteoporotic bone. Inst Course Lect 1997, 46:431.
4. Slemenda C: Prevention of hip fractures: Risk factor modification. Am J Med 1997; 103:65.
5. Fielding JW: A continuing end-result study of intracapsular fracture of the neck of the femur. J Bone Joint Surg Am 1962; 44:965.
6. Urovitz EM: Etiological factors in the pathogenesis of femoral trabecular fatigue fractures. Clin Orthop 1977; 127:275.
7. Wallace RB: Iowa FICSIT trial: The feasibility of elderly wearing a hip joint protective garment to reduce hip fractures. J Am Geriatr Soc 1993; 41(3):338.
8. Swiontowski MF: Intracapsular fractures of the hip. J Bone Joint Surg 1994; 76: 129.
9. Rubin SJ: Magnetic resonance imaging: a cost effective alternative to bone scintography in the evaluation of patients with suspected hip fractures. Skeletal Radiol 1998; 27(4):199.
10. Cserhati P: Nonoperative or operative treatment for undisplaced femoral neck fractures: a comparative study of 122 non-operative and 125 operatively treated cases. Injury 1996; 27(8):583.
11. Chua D, Jaglal SB, Schatzker J: Predictors of early failure of fixation in the treatment of displaced subcapital hip fractures. J Orthop Trauma 1998; 12(4):230.
12. Holmes CA: Biomechanics of pin and screw fixation of femoral neck fractures. J Orthop Trauma 1993; 7:242.
13. Levi N: Fracture of the femoral neck: optimal screw position and bone density determined by computer tomography. Injury 1996; 27(4):287.
14. Den Hartog BD, Bartal E, Cooke F: Treatment of the unstable intertrochanteric fracture: Effect of the placement of the screw, its angle of insertion, and osteotomy. J Bone Joint Surg Am 1991; 73:726.

15. Baumgaertner MR: Awareness of tip-apex distance reduces failure of fixation of trochanteric fractures of the hip. J Bone Joint Surg Br 1997; 79(6):969.

16. Gilbert MS: Unipolar or bipolar prosthesis for the displaced intracapsular hip fracture? An unanswered question. Clin Orthop 1998; 353:81.

17. Cornell CN: Unipolar versus bipolar hemiarthroplasty for the treatment of femoral neck fractures in the elderly. Clin Orthop 1998; 348:67.

18. Koval KJ: Postoperative weight-bearing after a fracture of the femoral neck or an intertrochanteric fracture. J Bone Joint Surg 1998; 80(3):352.

19. Staeheli JW, Frassica FJ, Sim FH: Prosthetic replacement of the femoral head for fracture of the femoral neck in patients who have Parkinson disease. J Bone Joint Surg Am 1988; 70:565.

20. Riemer BL, Butterfield SL, Ray RL, et al: Clandestine femoral neck fractures with ipsilateral diaphyseal fracture. J Orthop Trauma 1993; 7:443.

21. Garden RS: Malreduction and avascular necrosis in subcapital fractures of the femur. J Bone Joint Surg Br 1971; 53:183.

22. Scheck M: The significance of posterior comminution in femoral neck fractures. Clin Orthop 1980; 152:138.

23. Kanis JA: Evidence for efficacy of drugs affecting bone metabolism in preventing hip fracture. Br Med J 1992; 305:1124.

24. Gehrchen PM: Poor reproducibility of Evan's classification of the trochanteric fracture; assessment of 4 observers in 52 cases. Acta Orthop Scand 1993; 64:71.

25. Zuckerman JD: Postoperative complications and mortality associated with operative delay in patients who have a fracture of the hip. J Bone Joint Surg Am 1995; 77:1551.

26. Desjardins AL, Roy A, Paiement G, et al: Unstable inertrochanteric fracture of the femur: A prospective randomized study comparing anatomical reduction and medial displacement osteotomy. J Bone Joint Surg Br 1993; 75:445.

27. Stern MB, Angerman A: Comminuted intertrochanteric fractures treated with a Leinbach prosthesis. Clin Orthop 1987; 218:75.

28. Haentjens P: Treatment of unstable intertrochanteric and subtrochanteric fractures in elderly patients. J Bone Joint Surg Am 1989; 71:1214.

29. Sernbo I: Unstable intertrochanteric fractures of the hip: Treatment with Ender pins compared with a compression hip screw. J Bone Joint Surg Am 1988; 70: 1297.

30. Meislin RJ: A biomechanical analysis of the sliding hip screw: the question of plate angle. J Orthop Trauma 1990; 4(2):130.

31. Madsen JE: Dynamic hip screw with trochanteric stabilizing plate in the treatment of unstable proximal femoral fractures: A comparative study with the Gamma nail and compression hip screw. J Orthop Trauma 1998; 12:241.

32. Goldhagen PR, O'Connor DR, Schwarze E: A prospective comparative study of the compression hip screw and the Gamma nail. J Orthop Trauma 1994; 5:367.

33. Apel DM: Axial loading studies of unstable intertrochanteric fractures of the femur. Clin Orthop 1989; 246:156.

34. Harrington KD, Johnston JO, Turner RH, et al: The use of methylmethacrylate as an adjunct in the internal fixation of malignant neoplastic fractures. J Bone Joint Surg Am 1972; 54:1665.

35. Davis T: Intertrochanteric femoral fractures. J Bone Joint Surg Br 1990; 72:26.

36. Knight WM, Delee JC: Nonunion of intertrochanteric fractures of the hip: A case study and review. Orthop Trans 1982; 16: 438.

37. Dreinhofer KE, Schwarzkopf SR, Haas NP, et al: Isolated traumatic dislocation of the hip: Long-term results in 50 patients. J Bone Joint Surg Br 1994; 76:6.

38. Epstein HC: Traumatic Dislocation of the Hip. Baltimore: Williams & Wilkins, 1980.

39. Levin PE: Hip dislocations. In Browner BD, Jupiter JB, Levine AM, Trafton PG (eds): Skeletal Trauma, vol 2, Philadelphia: WB Saunders, 1992.

40. Laorr A: Traumatic hip dislocation: Early MRI findings. Skeltal Radiol 1995; 24: 239.

41. Thoupe M, Swiontkowski MF, Seiler J, et al: Operative management of femoral head fractures. Orthop Trans 1989; 13:51.

FEMORAL SHAFT FRACTURES

Robert F. Ostrum and Brian L. Davison

Summary
- Most femoral shaft fractures occur in young patients and are the result of high-energy trauma, including motorcycle and other motor vehicle accidents and gunshot wounds. Elderly and osteopenic patients can sustain a femur fracture after low-energy injuries or falls.
- Treatment with intramedullary nails has led to a functional approach with early ambulation and range of motion of the knee and hip. Generally 3 months is needed to obtain fracture union and return to full weightbearing. Normal activities and stair climbing can be achieved at 4 to 6 months, but full return to running and sports can take up to a year.
- Subtrochanteric fractures of the femur are difficult to manage because of the high bending forces on the proximal femur. Complication rates increase when a medial buttress cannot be reconstituted.
- Open fractures of the femur, perhaps with the exception of grade 3B fractures, are amenable to treatment with a reamed intramedullary nail.
- Recent usage of retrograde femoral nailing has been promising in the treatment of selected femur fractures, including bilateral fractures, floating knee injuries, and ipsilateral femoral neck and shaft fractures.

The purpose of this chapter is to familiarize the reader with the management of femoral shaft fractures. Although antegrade nailing has long been considered the gold standard, recent advances in retrograde nailing have led to an increase in its popularity. Special indications for plating of the femoral shaft or external fixation will also be considered. Associated fractures such as ipsilateral femoral neck and shaft fractures as well as floating knee injuries deserve special considerations for their treatment. Open femur fractures are usually treated with reamed nailing as either a primary or delayed procedure. External fixation can be reserved for those fractures with extreme soft-tissue injury or contamination, fractures in ischemic limbs due to vascular injury, and the most severely injured patients who require resuscitation prior to nailing. Because of the large surrounding musculature and stable intramedullary nailing techniques, the union rates for femoral shaft fractures are high. Infections are uncommon and can be dealt with, especially after union. Treatment with good fixation, early motion, quadriceps strengthening, and progressive weightbearing has led to excellent functional results.

HISTORICAL TREATMENTS

Early attempts at treatment of femoral shaft fractures involved splinting with a variety of materials. Mortality rates were high, and patients who did survive had shortened and malaligned extremities. Skin traction was later popularized by Buck in the 1860s, but the limited force that could be applied to the bone made reduction poor in adults. Skeletal traction was the treatment of choice in the early 1900s. Skeletal traction allowed sufficient force to be applied to maintain femoral length and alignment. Union rates with this form of treatment were good, but a minimum of 6 weeks in traction followed by spica casting led to other problems. These included knee stiffness, residual limb shortening, malalignment, and pulmonary complications from prolonged recumbency.

In the last 50 years, the benefits of early functional treatment of fractures have been documented, and enthusiasm for traction techniques has waned. The advent of intramedullary nailing of femoral shaft fractures by Kuntscher in the 1940s was originally met by skepticism in the United States. This technique, along with the evolution of intramedullary implants, has transformed femoral shaft fractures from a disabling injury to a temporary setback with short recovery times and excellent functional results.[1]

ANTEGRADE FEMORAL NAILING

During the last half century, antegrade intramedullary rodding has become the standard of care for most femoral shaft fractures. The concept of intramedullary rod fixation for femur fractures originated in Germany by Gerhard Kuntscher.[2] In the 1970s, Klemm and Schellmann, followed by Kempf and Grosse,[3] disciples of Kuntscher, refined the techniques and popularized it in the United States, Europe, and throughout the world.

The first intramedullary rod designs did not have interlocking capabilities. Maintenance of alignment and length depended on the interference fit between the rod and the cortical bone proximal and distal to the fracture. In comminuted fractures, this interference fit was often not enough to resist shortening and rotational instability. Therefore, these rods were recommended for treatment of femoral shaft fractures in which cortical contact between the fragments would prevent shortening and resist rotation during the healing process. Cerclage wires were used to reconstruct cortical contact between fragments and expand the nail's uses. In the 1980s, femoral rods with the capability of interlocking proximal and distal to the fracture were introduced. This expanded the indications for intramedullary rodding to include femur fractures in which significant

TABLE 1. WINQUIST AND HANSEN CLASSIFICATION OF COMMINUTION

Type	Criteria
I	No comminution or insignificant butterfly fragment. Almost complete cortical contact between proximal and distal fragments following reduction.
II	Comminution or butterfly fragment that involves less than 50% of the femoral circumference. Proximal and distal fragments have greater than 50% cortical contact following reduction.
III	Comminution or butterfly fragment that involves greater than 50% of the femoral circumference. Less than 50% cortical contact following reduction.
IV	Severe comminution with the loss of all cortical contact between main proximal and distal fragments following reduction.

comminution existed (Winquist type III and IV, Table 1). Interlocking of the rod prevented shortening and rotational instability from occurring during the healing process.

Ideally, an interlocking intramedullary rod should have sufficient strength to allow full unrestricted ambulation during fracture healing while preventing significant shortening, angulation, or rotational displacement of the fracture fragments. It would be stiff enough to avoid excessive motion at the fracture site, which can impede healing, yet flexible enough to avoid stress shielding of the femur by allowing appropriate load transfer to the bone. Femoral rods function in a load-sharing capacity with the femur. Each implant has material and structural properties, which predict the ease of insertion, stiffness, and fatigue life of the implant. Several studies of femoral fracture healing have demonstrated union rates of 95% and above with several different implants.[4, 5] With union rates this high, it is difficult to substantiate a clinical advantage of one design over another. It is important that the surgeon understand relative strength, stiffness, and radius of curvature of the rod being inserted. Rods, which are stiffer, require a more precise position of the starting hole and greater overreaming to avoid "bursting" of the femur during insertion.[6] Radius of curvature affects the appropriate position of the starting point to avoid comminution of the shaft. The surgeon should study the features of the rod being used and adhere to good surgical technique to avoid complications.

The biomechanical characteristics of an implant are determined by its materials, shape, and design. Titanium nails have a modulus of elasticity closer to that of cortical bone than stainless steel but are also more sensitive to notching, which can lower the fatigue life of the implant.[7] Slotted implants are significantly less stiff to torsional forces than nonslotted implants.[7] In cannulated nails, increasing the wall thickness increases stiffness and strength. The strength of a nail correlates clinically with its fatigue life, whereas the stiffness determines the force needed for insertion and amount of fracture site motion seen with physiological stresses. The strength is proportional to the third power of the diameter, whereas the stiffness is proportional to the fourth power of the diameter.[7] Currently available unslotted nails have approximately 75% of the bending and 50% of

the torsional stiffness of an intact femur.[8] The axial load to failure is from 100% to 400% of body weight for a 70-kg person.[8]

Patient positioning is also at the discretion of the surgeon, but there are some noted advantages to each position. Lateral positioning allows easier access to the piriformis fossa and facilitates location of the correct starting position. However, it can be difficult to determine the appropriate rotation of the leg during interlocking, and the potential for valgus sag at the fracture site in infraisthmal fractures can be troublesome. Lateral positioning of a patient with chest injuries may lead to increased difficulty with ventilation of the dependent lung and increased pulmonary morbidity. Additionally, patients with multiple orthopaedic injuries require repositioning after the femoral rodding, which increases total operative time and anesthesia. Supine positioning with or without a fracture table makes location of the correct starting point in the piriformis fossa more difficult but decreases the problems of determining correct rotation and eliminates the problems of a dependent lung. Several authors have demonstrated a technique of supine rodding without the use of a fracture table and believe that this decreases set-up time and allows multiple procedures to be performed without moving or repositioning the multiply injured patient.[9]

The correct entry point is essential to minimize the hoop stress in the proximal femur and therefore avoid the complication of "bursting" of the proximal femur during rod insertion. Johnson et al[6] identified the starting point that minimized the hoop stress in the proximal femur during rod insertion to be directly medial to the greater trochanter in the piriformis fossa in a position that is in line with the intramedullary canal of the femur. Positioning the starting hole more than 6 mm anterior or 8 mm posterior to this position resulted in high insertional forces and hoop stress in the proximal fragment, which predispose the proximal femur to bursting (Fig. 1). Overreaming the canal by 1 mm decreases the insertional force and hoop stress.

The incision should start approximately 2 cm proximal and in line with the center of the greater trochanter. Dissection should allow access to the piriformis fossa under fluoroscopic guidance. The starting hole can be made with an awl or a guide pin, which can be overdrilled with a cannulated reamer. Both methods require that the location of the starting hole be appropriately positioned in the piriformis fossa before creating a large perforation in the cortex (Fig. 2). Once the starting hole has been developed, a ball-tipped guide rod is inserted to the level of the fracture. The reduction should be performed by external manipulation for all closed femur fractures owing to the increased rate of delayed union and infection reported with open reduction. Reduction can be obtained with the use of manual or assisted traction, the use of a reduction rod in the proximal fragment, and various "reduction crutches" or bolsters for the distal fragment. A slight bend at the tip of the guide rod will also assist in passing the rod across the fracture.

Reaming of the medullary canal allows for insertion of larger-diameter rods and decreases the force required for insertion.[6] Increasing the rod diameter dramatically increases strength and allows for the use of larger interlocking bolts. Most manufactures recommend reaming the fe-

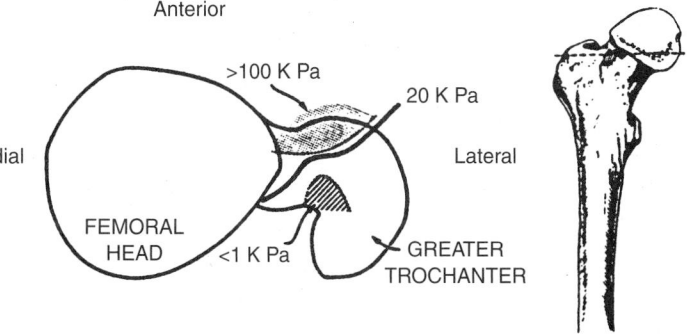

Fig. 1. View. *A,* Coronal view of the proximal femur, with a map of common hoop stresses that are generated distally. *B,* Position of section for part A. (From Johnson KD, Tencer AF, Sherman MC: Biomechanical factors affecting fracture stability and femoral bursting in closed intramedullary nailing of femoral shaft fractures, with illustrative case presentations. J Orthop Trauma 1987; 1:1.)

mur between 1 and 2 mm over the desired rod diameter to minimize the force needed for rod insertion. The amount of overreaming is determined by the relative stiffness of the implant. Fat emboli have been identified as a consequence of entering and reaming the femoral canal, but randomized clinical trials have not found significant differences in patient outcome or pulmonary complications when reamed and unreamed rodding are compared.[10] Recent clinical trials that compared smaller unreamed rods and larger reamed rods noted a higher incidence rate of delayed union and hardware failure in the unreamed group.[11] Therefore, most authors currently recommend reamed intramedullary rods for femur fractures.[10, 11]

The success of reamed antegrade femoral rods in the treatment of femur fractures has made it the gold standard for these injuries to which all other treatment methods must be compared. Union rates in large clinical studies have been from 96% to 99%, with infection and hardware failure rates of only 1%. Winquist and Hansen[5] reported the results of 520 femur fractures treated with reamed in-

tramedullary rods. Of the 420 fractures in patients monitored for at least 1 year, only 4 patients developed a nonunion, and 4 had a deep postoperative infection. Subsequent studies have confirmed these results.

Static interlocking has become the standard of care for all femur fractures as the result of a three-part investigation at the Maryland Shock Trauma Center.[12] The initial phase of the investigation noted a 10% prevalence rate of loss of reduction during the postoperative period in femur fractures treated with a reamed femoral rods that were not statically locked. Shortening or rotation occurred as the result of fracture comminution not recognized at the time of surgery. They subsequently treated all femur fractures with a statically locked rod and reported a 98% union rate without the need for dynamization and significantly decreased the rate of malunion.[4] The final phase of their study attempted to address the concerns of stress shielding of the femur by a static locked intramedullary rod and concerns of possible refracture after hardware removal. In 103 patients who had a statically locked rod removed an average of 14 months

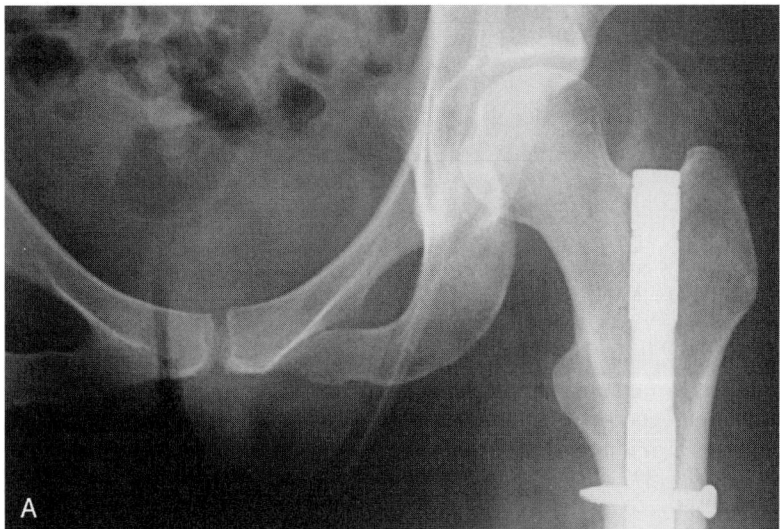

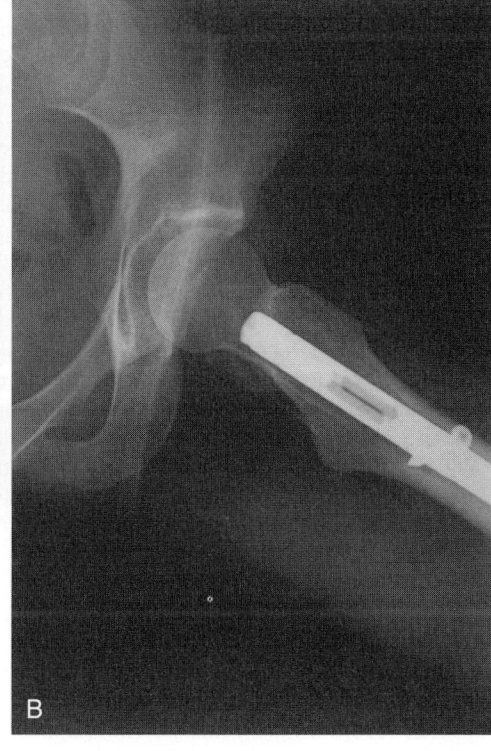

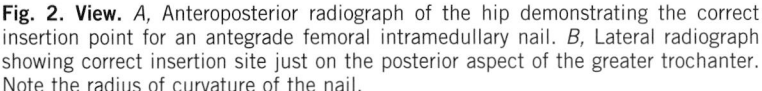

Fig. 2. View. *A,* Anteroposterior radiograph of the hip demonstrating the correct insertion point for an antegrade femoral intramedullary nail. *B,* Lateral radiograph showing correct insertion site just on the posterior aspect of the greater trochanter. Note the radius of curvature of the nail.

after injury, only 1 refracture occurred in a patient who retrospectively had a persistent cortical gap at the time of rod removal.[13] They concluded that routine dynamization is not needed for fracture healing or maturation and that statically locked rods can be removed when desired if fracture callous is present around the entire circumference of the femur. Dynamization should be reserved for fractures that are axially stable but lack signs of healing at 3 to 5 months postoperatively. The indications for rod removal are currently unclear, and no long-term studies have proven removal necessary. Current indications for rod or locking bolt removal are pain located over the tip of the nail and trochanteric bursa region or over the head or tips of the locking bolts.

Biomechanical and clinical testing has been performed to determine the need for one versus two distal locking bolts.[14] These studies demonstrated no significant difference in the rotational and axial load to failure when one versus two locking bolts is used. A difference was noted in the amount of toggle in the anteroposterior plane in infraisthmal fractures, with two screws allowing less motion. The use of two screws is commonly recommended in infraisthmal fractures and severely comminuted fractures and one screw for all other fractures. The one screw is generally placed in the most proximal of the distal screw holes. When one screw is placed in the most distal hole, the hole just proximal to this is a stress-riser in the rod and may lead to increased rod failure.[7]

The proximal locking bolt can be oblique or transverse depending on the rod design and can be routinely placed with the assistance of a targeting guide. Distal targeting guides have not been successful owing to deformation of the rod during insertion and inaccuracy of the targeting device. Most surgeons currently use the free-hand method, in which the image intensifier is positioned with the screw hole perfectly circular. A sharp trocar or drill can then be placed in the center of the hole and drilled parallel to the beam of the image. Care should be taken not to drill forcibly against the rod; notching the rod in this region has been shown to decrease the strength of the rod and may lead to fatigue failure of the rod before union.

Postoperatively, patients should be instructed in knee range-of-motion exercises and quadriceps rehabilitation. Patellofemoral joint symptoms are common in the recovery period, and appropriate terminal knee extensions, quadriceps muscle sets, and straight leg raises are often needed for recovery. The appropriate time to allow full weight-bearing is determined by the strength of the rod and locking bolts used, amount of comminution and callous at the fracture, and status of the quadriceps rehabilitation program. Many current rod designs allow for early weight-bearing in fractures, which have some cortical contact at the fracture site to load-share with the rod. In more unstable fracture patterns, only touch-down or partial weight-bearing is allowed until healing is noted on follow-up radiographs.

RETROGRADE FEMORAL NAILING

Intramedullary nailing of femoral shaft fractures has become the standard of treatment. Antegrade nailing has a long track record with a refined technique over the last 50 years. Problems accessing the correct starting point in large patients as well as the difficulty in treating very distal supracondylar fractures have led some surgeons to use retrograde femoral nails. Retrograde intramedullary nailing of femoral shaft fractures has demonstrated good results and an increase in popularity.

Initial attempts at retrograde femoral intramedullary nailing were performed with the use of an antegrade femoral or tibial nail inserted from a medial femoral condylar approach.[15] This led to an increase in comminution and malunion. Further attempts at using an antegrade nail through an intercondylar approach led to improved results but also concerns about the effects of this starting point on the patellofemoral joint. These initial questions about an intra-articular starting point have been addressed both in the laboratory and clinically. A biomechanical patellofemoral contact pressure study demonstrated no increases in patellofemoral mean pressures, maximum pressures, or contact area with a properly inserted nail[16]; however, when the nail was 1 mm prominent at the intercondylar notch starting point, the mean and maximum pressures increased at 90 and 120 degrees of knee flexion.[16] This study stresses the importance of insertion of the nail below the articular surface. Several clinical series have demonstrated no decreased knee motion or increase in patellofemoral disorders using this approach.[17–19] The average knee score in ambulatory patients was 98 points for pain and 97 points for function.[17] The average knee flexion was 129 degrees (range 60 to 135 degrees), with only three patients who had associated lower extremity trauma having less than 100 degrees.[17] In those patients without associated ipsilateral injuries to the involved limb, the knee extension was normal, and flexion to within 10 degrees of the contralateral limb was seen.[19] Herscovic's[17] study showed that 13 of 41 patients had some knee pain, but only 5 had patellofemoral crepitation. All of these patients had multiple injuries or associated problems. Moed and Watson[18] had two patients with knee pain related to the patellar tendon; however, these authors used a patellar splitting approach. In the series by Ostrum et al,[19] 4 of 57 patients had symptomatic chondromalacia, and 1 had recurrent effusions. All of these series of retrograde nailing demonstrated no significant increase in patellofemoral disorders or a decrease in knee motion.

The best indications for retrograde intramedullary nailing include obesity, pregnancy, bilateral fractures, and the multiply traumatized state (Fig. 3). The piriformis starting point for antegrade nailing is extremely difficult in larger patients, and an incorrect insertion portal can lead to comminution, varus, and proximal femoral bursting.[6] The multiply traumatized patient with thoracic, visceral, or cerebral injuries can be most expediently managed in the supine position on a radiolucent table. Retrograde nailing allows the treatment of multiple fractures with a single preparation and drape. Distal one-third and supracondylar femur fractures are also easily amenable to retrograde nailing. Prevention of recurvatum deformity due to flexion of the distal fragment secondary to the gastrocnemius muscle pull is important and must be done prior to reaming, nail insertion, and interlocking. Intra-articular fractures demand meticulous reduction and fixation of the joint surface. If reaming and insertion of the nail through the intercondylar

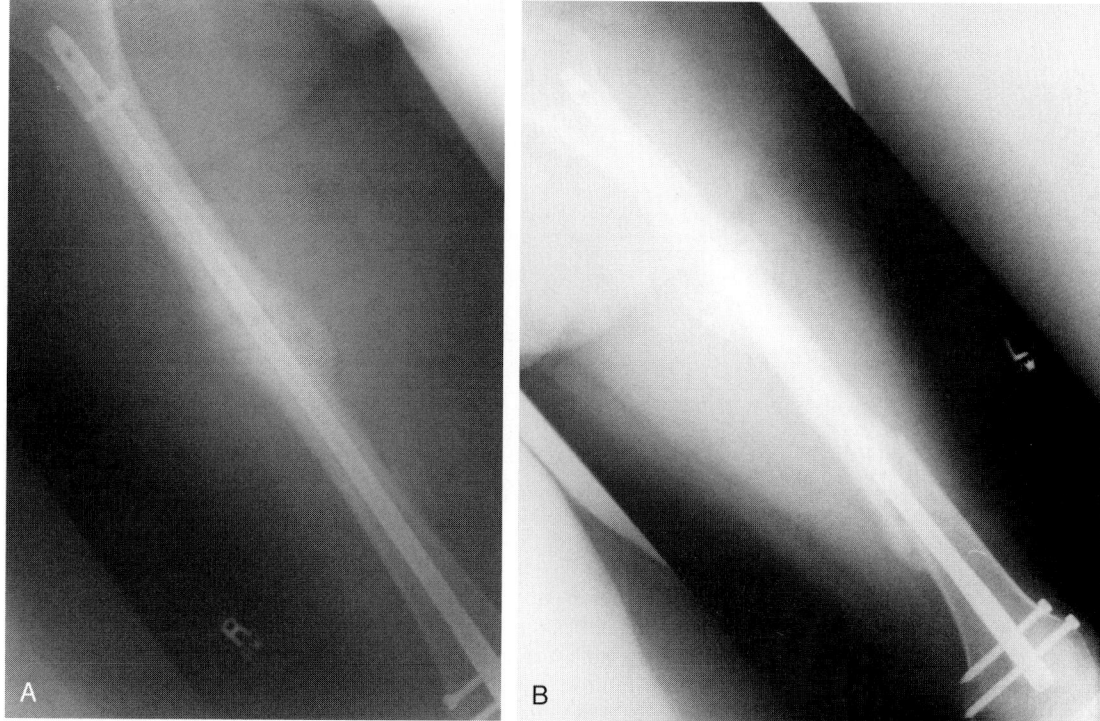

Fig. 3. View. *A*, Bilateral femoral shaft fractures. Anteroposterior radiograph of a right isthmal femoral shaft fracture treated with a retrograde femoral nail. *B*, Left segmental femur fracture. Note the proximal tip of the nail above the lesser trochanter. The stable right femur fracture was nailed first to determine length before treatment of the segmental fracture.

notch compromises the articular surface repair, then plate fixation should be considered.

Other good indications include concomitant fractures of the ipsilateral femoral neck, tibial shaft, acetabulum, and pelvis. Displaced femoral neck fractures can be treated first with either multiple cancellous screws or a sliding hip screw followed by a retrograde nail when seen in combination with an ipsilateral femoral shaft fracture. Floating knee injuries carry a high morbidity and mortality rate. These two fractures can be treated with a single 4-cm medial parapatellar tendon incision and a retrograde femoral nail and an antegrade tibial nail. Acetabulum fractures can be treated with the appropriate approach without compromise or concerns about previous incisions made for antegrade nailing by early use of a retrograde nail. Instability of the anterior or posterior pelvic ring secondary to fractures is a contraindication to use of the fracture table for femoral nailing. Intramedullary nailing, antegrade or retrograde, on a radiolucent table is a preferred method of treatment.

Retrograde femoral intramedullary nailing is performed with the patient in the supine position on a radiolucent operating room table. The entire limb from the toes to the iliac crest is prepared and draped into the sterile field. A bolster is placed under the knee to provide approximately 45 degrees of knee flexion. A 3-cm medial parapatellar tendon approach is used, and the synovium is cleared from the intercondylar notch. A guide pin for the rigid entry reamer is inserted under biplanar fluoroscopy. On the anteroposterior radiograph, the guide pin is centered between the femoral condyles and centered in the metaphysis. On the lateral view, the guide pin should be placed just

above Blumensaat's line at the top of the intercondylar notch (Fig. 4). A rigid reamer is then used over the guide pin to open the insertion site into the metaphysis. A ball-tipped guide rod for diaphyseal reaming is inserted. Reduction of the femoral shaft fracture is accomplished with manual traction and external fragment manipulation. Short-acting chemical muscle paralysis can be helpful at this stage. Reaming to 1 mm above cortical chatter and exchanging of the guide rods is done. A retrograde nail is selected so that the proximal tip of the nail is above the inferior edge of the lesser trochanter. Even in distal femur fractures, the use of a longer nail that fills the isthmus allows for less motion of the nail within the medullary canal. This avoids the problems of instability and excessive motion and maintains axial alignment.

The nail is inserted at least 3 mm deep to the articular surface. Distal locking is done through the attached targeting guide, and proximal locking is usually done free-hand in an anterior-to-posterior direction. Attention should be given to femoral rotation before interlocking. Early knee motion is encouraged, and full knee motion is usually seen by 12 weeks. Weightbearing is progressed depending on the amount of cortical contact and for more unstable fractures as callous appears.

Current results for retrograde intramedullary nailing have demonstrated high union rates and low complication rates. Three series demonstrated union in 95% of fractures treated.[17–19] In two series utilizing smaller-diameter nails, however, dynamization was needed to accomplish union.[18, 19] Two of 45 fractures in another series had nail failure and required revision surgery.[17] Complications in-

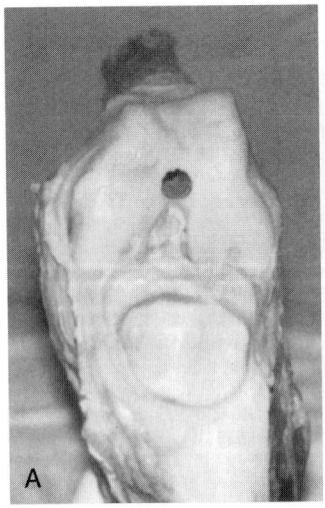 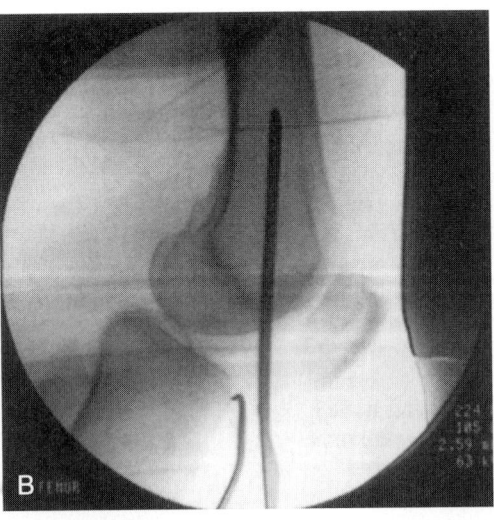

Fig. 4. View. *A,* Cadaveric femur shows an entry portal just superior to the intercondylar notch. *B,* Lateral fluoroscopic view shows the entry point for the retrograde femoral nail at Blumensaat's line. (From Ostrum RF, DeCicco J, Lakatos R, et al: Retrograde intramedullary nailing of femoral diaphyseal fractures. J Orthop Trauma 1998; 12:464.)

clude nonunion and knee pain. Of greater concern is the one patient with an infected retrograde intramedullary nail who developed a septic knee joint. This responded to nail removal, synovectomy, and antibiotic therapy. Distal femoral screws can also be symptomatic owing to the lack of soft tissues covering the screws and rubbing of the screw heads on the iliotibial band. In one series, 21% of patients required screw removal.[19] Delayed unions or nonunions have led to dynamization and exchange nailing, and concerns have been expressed about the use of smaller-diameter nails.[18, 19] Five of seven patients (8% of the series population) healed after dynamization[19] and 30% (10 of 34) of patients with smaller-diameter nails required dynamization in a second series.[18]

The risk of infection and a subsequent septic knee joint make open-grade 3B fractures a contraindication. Retrograde nailing has been used for subtrochanteric fractures, but stretching the indications for this implant can lead to malunion or metal failure. One subtrochanteric fracture had retrograde nail failure and was revised by an antegrade nail with subsequent union.[19]

Retrograde femoral intramedullary nailing is not meant to replace antegrade nailing but to increase the indications for intramedullary fixation. For intra-articular fractures, anatomic restoration of the joint surface is mandatory before retrograde nailing. Attention to the proper entry site is necessary to avoid injury to the posterior cruciate ligament or the patella and to maintain correct axial alignment. The use of retrograde intramedullary nailing has led to good results with few complications and no knee problems and has expanded the techniques for the treatment of difficult femoral shaft fractures.

PLATING OF FEMORAL SHAFT FRACTURES

Open reduction with compression plating has been used for the treatment of femoral shaft fractures for more than three decades. This continues to be a useful technique for certain femur fractures that are not optimal for intramedullary nailing techniques. Some examples include ipsilateral femoral neck and shaft fractures, femurs with an excessively nar-

row intramedullary canal, spinal fractures that require strict supine positioning during fracture care, and in areas of the world where the equipment necessary for intramedullary nailing may not be available.

In the 1960s and 1970s the Arbeitsgemeinschaft für Osteosynthesefragen group popularized the treatment of fractures with open reduction and internal fixation to allow early mobilization of the adjacent joints in an attempt to avoid "fracture disease."[20] The goal of plate osteosynthesis for long-bone fractures was to obtain rigid internal fixation through the use of lag screws, cerclage wires, and compression plates. Primary vascular bone formation was demonstrated in diaphyseal fractures treated with compression and rigid internal fixation. In contrast, fractures without rigid internal fixation healed with fracture callus opposite the plate that was proportional to the amount of motion at the fracture site. The radiographic appearance of this "irritation callus" was believed to demonstrate mechanical instability and the precursor of plate failure unless loading was reduced.[20]

For best results, femoral fractures treated with rigid internal fixation required placement of the plate laterally on the tension side of the bone and an intact medial cortex for compression. If comminution was present, the medial cortex was reconstructed anatomically with lag screws and augmented with bone graft. This technique required dissection of the soft tissues from the edges of fracture fragments to allow for anatomic reduction and lag screw placement.[20]

In 1979, Magerl et al[21] reported the results of 67 diaphyseal fractures of the femur in this manner with the goal of rigid internal fixation using either a straight broad round hole compression plate or a condylar plate. Eleven fractures were bone grafted primarily, and 9 were grafted secondarily to treat cortical defects or delayed healing. Seven plates (10%) required revision before union. Five plate failures occurred, 1 within 8 weeks of injury and 4 later as a result of delayed fracture healing. The other 2 plates bent with 2 weeks of application and required replating.

Bostman et al[22] treated 102 femur fractures treated with a dynamic compression plate over a 10-year period. Primary bone grafting was not routinely performed. Early aseptic loosening occurred in 12 patients following plating of the femur fracture. Five additional patients developed a nonunion, which was manifested by plate failure between 4 and 8 months postoperatively. The overall complication rate for femoral plating was 24% in this series.

Research on the biological nature of fracture healing resulted in the development of indirect reduction techniques and the limited contact dynamic compression plate for treatment of diaphyseal long bone fractures.[23, 24] The earlier goal of anatomic rigid fixation of all fracture fragments has been revised. Currently, many authors advocate restoration of length and axial and rotational alignment of diaphyseal fractures with minimal soft-tissue stripping opposite the implant. Anatomic alignment of extra-articular comminuted fracture fragments through open reduction is discouraged if it requires stripping of the soft-tissue attachments. Bridging of the comminuted segment with stable fixation above and below is recommended. Compression plating is reserved for Winquist type I transverse and short oblique fractures in which the tensioning of the plate will result in load-sharing between the bone and plate.[24]

Reimer et al[23] reported the results of 123 femur fractures treated with indirect reduction techniques and plating with titanium limited-contact dynamic compression plates. The majority of femur fractures in this study were the result of high-energy injuries, with 62% classified as Winquist type III or IV or segmental fractures. Eighty-one fractures were primarily bone-grafted, with the ipsilateral proximal tibia being the most common donor site. Seven plates (6%) failed before union. Two plates failed within 3 weeks of injury in multiply injured patients and required revision of fixation. Four additional plates failed between 3 and 5 weeks, and 1 plate failed 28 weeks postoperatively. Two other plates bent more than 10 degrees but were left intact, and the femur fractures healed in this position. No correlation was found between the Winquist classification and the plate failure. Most fractures healed with abundant callus.

Rozbruch et al[24] reported the results of 25 femur fractures treated with indirect reduction and plating between 1993 and 1994 at Inselspital University in Bern, Switzerland. Only two fractures were bone-grafted primarily. Nineteen fractures were treated with a blade plate and 9 with a limited-contact dynamic compression plate. The rate of implant failure was 13%. Currently, a broad 4.5-mm dynamic compression plate or limited-contact dynamic compression plate is the implant of choice for plating of femoral shaft fractures. Routinely, the plate should be placed on the lateral side of the femur, because this is the tension side of the bone. The optimal plate length as well as the number and arrangement of screws is currently under investigation. Standard technique advises eight cortices of fixation on both sides of the fracture.[24] Biomechanical data support the use of longer plates with bicortical screws placed as close to the fracture as possible and at the end of the plate to obtain the most stability. The remaining screw holes can be filled at the discretion of the surgeon to obtain eight cortices of fixation on each side of the fracture. Indirect reduction techniques, which minimize soft-tissue stripping, especially of comminuted fracture fragments, should be performed.

Postoperatively, the patient should be encouraged to perform knee range-of-motion exercises to regain full motion. Terminal knee extensions without resistance are also needed to regain quadriceps function and leg control. The patient should ambulate with minimal weightbearing on the extremity until signs of fracture healing are seen on follow-up radiographs to prevent failure of fixation. Should irritation callus appear opposite the plate, then weightbearing should be stopped, as this is an indication of motion at the fracture site and possible loosening of the implant. Hardware removal is not routinely recommended and, if desired by the patient, should take place at least 18 months following injury and after all 4 cortices have solid bridging callous.

EXTERNAL FIXATION

External fixators were used previously to treat femoral shaft fractures to union primarily for grade III open fractures or those with severe contamination. This was due to concerns over osteomyelitis with intramedullary nailing of open fractures. However, the rate of complications with external fixation became unacceptable, and other techniques showed improved results. The biggest problems seen with external fixation of the femoral shaft fractures were pin tract infection and decreased knee motion. The knee stiffness was common, and 90 degrees of motion was the usual result after fixator removal and physical therapy.[25, 26] The placement of half pins through the iliotibial band and vastus musculature leads to decreased knee flexion and scarring of the injured muscles to the fracture site. Worse results were seen with distal third fractures as far as knee motion, and early frame removal with cast (or cast brace) application led to malunion. The time in the frame was long, and casting of shaft fractures without a spica is difficult. This often led to frame removal prior to complete union and subsequent angular deformities.

The major indications at the present time for external fixation of femoral shaft fractures are for immediate temporary stabilization of the bone with later intramedullary nailing. Grade IIIB open fractures can be débrided several times until the bone and medullary canal are considered clean. Reamed intramedullary nailing can then be performed. Another indication for temporary external fixation is the multiply injured patient (Fig. 5). Often, simple unilateral frames can be placed on the femur in minutes, without fluoroscopy, as a form of stabilization. This external fixation allows for patient mobilization without traction and improved pulmonary care. It is believed that this minimizes fracture fragment motion and that the patients have fewer pulmonary complications than with traction. When appropriate resuscitation has been performed and the patient's clinical status has improved, reamed intramedullary nailing can be performed easily within the first few weeks after admission. Recent articles have shown temporary external fixation to be a useful technique in patients who present with a femur fracture and an ischemic limb from ipsilateral arterial injuries. The fixator can be placed quickly for bony stabilization and allow emergent vascular repair. In one recent series, the fixators were converted to intramedullary nails at an average of 11 days after injury. There were no failures of the vascular repair, and all fractures united with good functional results.[27]

The technique is simple and can be done at the bedside with sterile technique if necessary. Using the trauma radio-

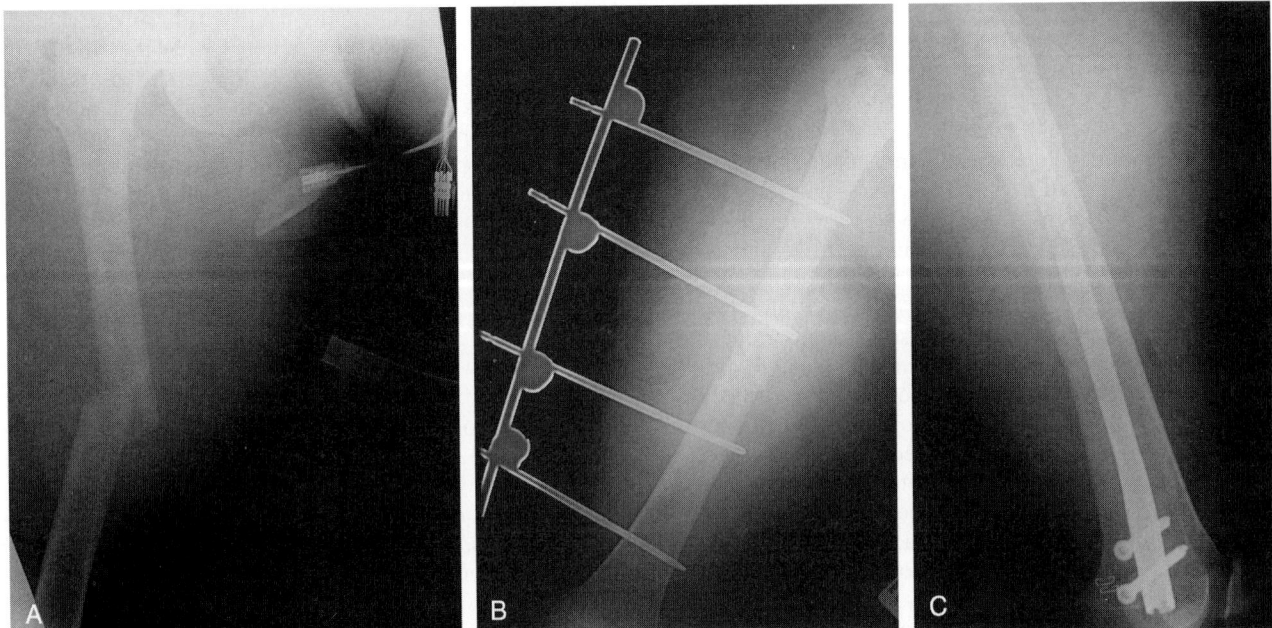

Fig. 5. View. *A,* Midshaft femur fracture in a multiply traumatized patient who was hemodynamically unstable. *B,* Temporary external fixation was applied rapidly at the time of admission. Note the placement of two half pins near the fracture site and two distant. *C,* Lateral radiograph of retrograde femoral nailing performed on day 5 when the patient was stable.

graphs as a template, the goal is to place two half pins proximal and two distal to the fractures site. An incision is made in the midaxial line through the iliotibial band. Blunt dissection is carried out down to the bone, and a triple trocar is inserted through the incision. Five-millimeter pins should be used and inserted bicortically after predrilling. Optimal placement of the pins would include two close to the fracture site and one placed as far proximal and one as far distal as practical to give the frame a greater working length. When fluoroscopy is not available, then axial traction is applied to the limb to get gross alignment and length. Two fixator bars are stacked to form a stable lateral half-pin frame. Skin is released from around the pin sites after traction is applied, and the pin sites are dressed with a bulky sterile wrap dressing. No increase in infection rate or knee complications have been seen after exchange nailing of the femur following temporary external fixation.[27]

SUBTROCHANTERIC FEMUR FRACTURES

The femoral shaft fracture in the subtrochanteric region presents a fixation dilemma owing to multiple factors. The bending moments in the subtrochanteric area are extremely high, and loss of medial cortical bone increases the forces on the implant. A small proximal fragment and marked displacement due to muscular forces add to the reduction and fixation difficulties. Treatment options include intramedullary devices, first or second generation, and proximal plating techniques. The use of a lower-angle, such as a 95-degree, plate has yielded better results with a lower incidence rate of malunion than the conventional sliding hip screw (Fig. 6).

Biomechanical studies have compared different implants to determine their mechanical stiffness in a laboratory model. Tencer et al[28] demonstrated that intramedullary implants were only 5% as stiff in torsion, whereas plated femurs were almost 50% as stiff when compared with an intact femur. Both intramedullary nails and plate constructs were nearly 80% as stiff as controls when tested in bending. The locked nails were found to be able to support up to 300% to 400% of body weight, whereas the plates failed at 100% to 200% of body weight. A recent study by Pugh et al[29] showed that the second-generation nail was stiffer than the first-generation nail in the in vitro testing of these implants, especially in the unstable model.

Intramedullary nailing of these fractures is a technical challenge and, despite proper technique, malunion, nonunion, and implant failure can still be seen. Brien et al[30] compared a Zickel nail, a 95-degree blade plate, and an interlocking nail in the treatment of subtrochanteric femur fractures. The difficulty in treating these fractures is demonstrated by the malunion and nonunion rates. With the Zickel nail, there were 10 malunions and 1 nonunion in 21 patients treated. In the 25 patients treated with a 95-degree blade plate, there were 6 malunions and 2 nonunions. The intramedullary nail group had the best results, with a decrease in operating time and blood loss as well as only 2 malunions and 1 nonunion in these 33 patients.

The small proximal fragment is usually flexed and externally rotated because of the iliopsoas and gluteus medius muscles, respectively, whereas the distal shaft fragment is adducted and shortened from the forces of the adductors and hamstrings. This deformity due to muscle contractions makes the piriformis fossa starting point extremely difficult to find, and if a second-generation nail is contemplated, then a slightly more anterior starting hole is necessary for

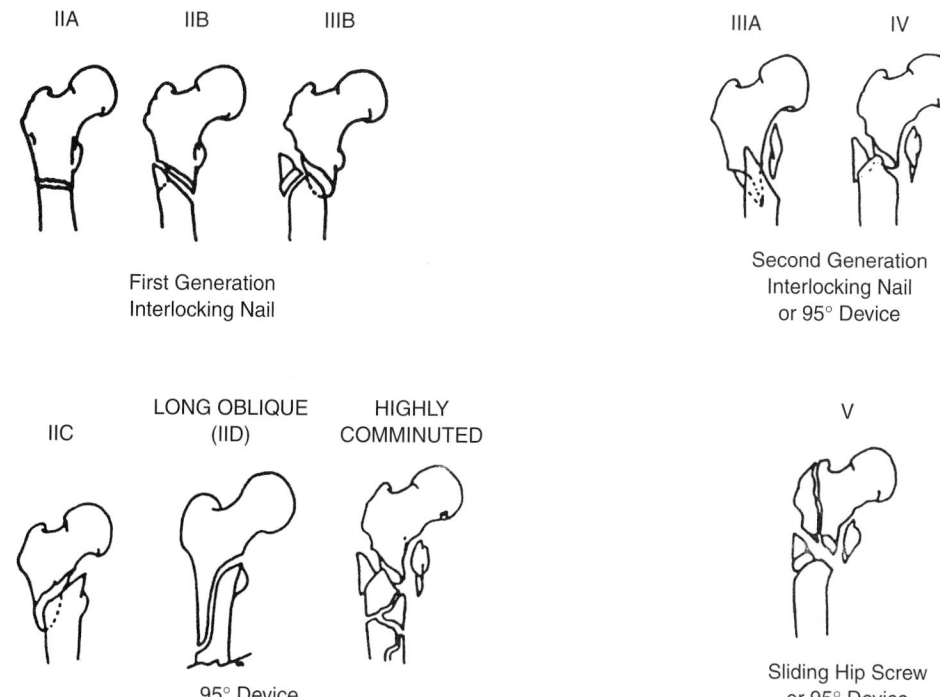

IIA   IIB   IIIB

First Generation
Interlocking Nail

IIIA   IV

Second Generation
Interlocking Nail
or 95° Device

IIC   LONG OBLIQUE (IID)   HIGHLY COMMINUTED

95° Device

V

Sliding Hip Screw
or 95° Device

Fig. 6. View. Implant choices depend on subtrochanteric fracture morphology and comminution. Absence of medial buttress and lesser trochanter is important in the decision-making process. (Modified from Sanders R, Regazzoni P: Treatment of subtrochanteric femur fractures using the dynamic condylar screw. J Orthop Trauma 1989; 3:206.)

the cephalic screws. A more valgus starting point can lead to eccentric reaming and iatrogenic comminution with further medial bone loss and varus angulation.[3] To correct the flexion and abduction of the proximal fragment, often a bone-holding clamp or Schanz's pin must be applied to correct the deformation and allow access to the piriformis fossa. On opening the insertion site, an intramedullary instrument can be inserted to manipulate the proximal fragment toward the distal intramedullary canal and allow passage of the guide wire. The femur should be held in its reduced position during reaming to prevent eccentric reaming of the medial and posterior cortices and a malunion after nail insertion. A slightly more anterior starting hole is required for a second-generation reconstruction nail, and overreaming by 1.5 mm allows for rotation of the nail and easier insertion of the cephalic screws in an anteverted plane into the femoral head.

The choice of nail depends on the fracture configuration. When the lesser trochanter is intact, a first-generation implant is sufficient with an antegrade screw from the greater to the lesser trochanter. A reconstruction nail is used when the medial cortex around the lesser trochanter is not intact (see Fig. 6). The type of femoral head fixation—blades versus screws—is not as important as maintaining an anatomic reduction without varus angulation. A recent report by French and Tornetta[31] demonstrated a 100% union rate without implant failure with the use of a cephalomedullary nail. However, critical analysis of the postoperative radiographs demonstrated that the average femoral neck-shaft angle was 128.9 degrees and that 61% of the fractures were reduced in at least 5 degress of varus.[31] The incidence rate of intraoperative problems is also high, and the

operative times are prolonged with the use of a second-generation nail for subtrochanteric fractures. The presence of an intact piriformis fossa is necessary for an intramedullary device but does not mean that a nail must be used.

The 95-degree condylar blade plates or condylar screw implants have also demonstrated good success in the treatment of these fractures. Although biomechanical studies demonstrate the inferiority of plate constructs versus nails in mechanical testing to failure,[28] the use of good surgical technique has led to acceptable results. Indirect reduction techniques, without medial stripping, or addition of medial bone graft has led to less implant failure and malunion. Kinast et al[32] showed that indirect reduction techiques, when applied to blade plate fixation of subtrochanteric fractures, decreased the time to union (4.2 months versus 5.4 months) and the prevalence rate of nonunions (0% versus 16.6%) when compared with "classic AO/ASIF" technique. Sanders and Regazzoni[33] had similar results using a 95-degree condylar screw; however, the overall union rate was only 77.3%. Five technical failures were seen, and four of these patients had indirect reduction with extensive medial fracture comminution. Those with stable medial bony configurations did better than those with medial comminution. This again stresses the high bending forces on this tension band plate in the subtrochanteric region, especially without a medial buttress. The loss of medial bony contact combined with a varus reduction leads to a high incidence rate of failure. Surgical reconstruction of a medial buttress, indirect reduction, or bone graft should be considered in these comminuted fractures.

The use of a guide pin laid along the femoral neck to determine the degree of anteversion is helpful before in-

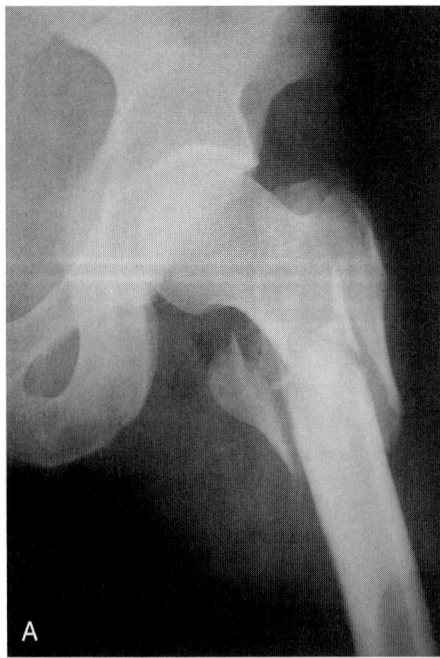
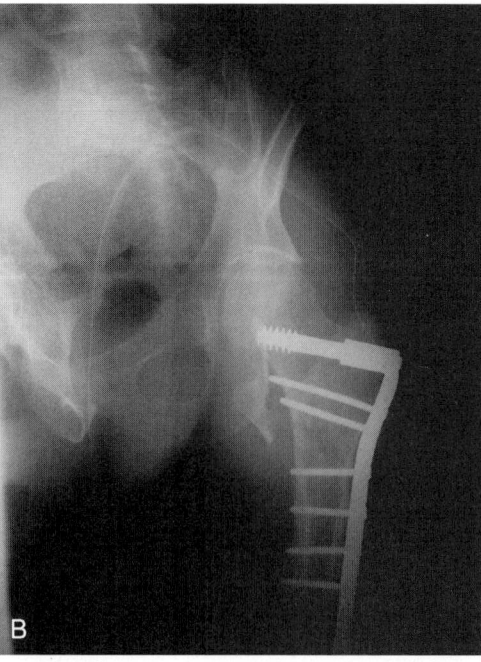

Fig. 7. View. *A,* Anteroposterior radiograph of a subtrochanteric femur fracture with intertrochanteric extension and a displaced fracture of the lesser trochanter. *B,* Fixation with a 95-degree condylar screw and plate with restoration of the neck-shaft angle.

serting the guide pin. The 95-degree angle guide can then be used for placement of the guide pin into the femoral head. Insertion of the 95-degree condylar blade or screw from the midlateral point of the greater trochanter allows for purchase along the compression trabeculae of the medial femoral neck and inferior head. By placing the implant in its appropriate position and using the plate as a reduction device, the incidence rate of varus is less than can be seen with intramedullary nailing. These plating devices also allow for additional screws to be placed in the proximal fragment to correct flexion as well as give excellent proximal fixation (Fig. 7). The advantages of the condylar screw over the blade plate are its ability to allow correction of the plate following the insertion of the screw into the head, the choice of plate lengths independent of the screw, and the possibility of submuscular insertion of the plate before connecting it to the screw. In addition, the 95-degree condylar screw is a more forgiving implant and does not require the precise three-plane insertion that is needed with the blade plate. Despite these fixation advantages, there was still a 23% to 37% complication rate with 95-degree implant fixation for subtrochanteric fractures.[33] Improvements in understanding of soft-tissue handling, indirect reduction, and judicious bone grafting have led to improved results.[32]

Sliding hip screws, such as the 135-degree implants, do not give more than one point of fixation of the proximal fragment. In addition, the sliding mechanism often leads to medial displacement of the distal fragment and shortening. These devices also have a higher incidence rate of malunion and nonunion than do the 95-degree plates or the intramedullary nails. Their use is probably limited to those fractures with intertrochanteric extension, elderly patients without high demands, and patients with subtrochanteric fractures that propogate from proximal laterally to distal medially.[33] Those fractures with a reverse obliquity config-

uration, distal lateral to proximal medial, will not do well with this sliding device and are prone to extreme medialization and shortening of the femoral shaft.

The high concentration of bending forces makes fixation of subtrochanteric fractures a challenge. An understanding of these stresses with careful preoperative planning can lead to good results with the use of any implant. The advantages and disadvantages of intramedullary nailing versus plating of these proximal fractures must be weighed in each case, with consideration given not only to the fracture configuration but also to the patient's demands. Liberal use of bone grafting can decrease the incidence rate of failure with plate fixation, especially when indirect reduction techniques are not employed. Careful attention to reduction of the proximal fragment and avoidance of eccentric reaming is essential for intramedullary nailing of these difficult fractures.

IPSILATERAL HIP AND FEMORAL SHAFT FRACTURES

Concomitant ipsilateral fractures of the femoral hip and shaft present a fixation problem for the treating surgeon. Previous experience has led to less than satisfactory results in the treatment of one or the other fracture. As orthopaedic implants have evolved, so have treatment options. Poor results were seen with operative management of the hip fracture followed by traction or casting of the shaft fracture.[34] Better results were obtained with internal fixation of both fractures, but often one fracture was compromised.

The classification that helps the most in determining treatment options is the one that defines the femoral hip fracture.[35] The overwhelming majority of the femoral shaft fractures associated with these hip fractures are located at the isthmus, making them amenable to intramedullary nailing.

Type 1 fractures are nondisplaced femoral hip fractures with a femoral shaft fracture. The treatment of choice is three cancellous screws for femoral neck fractures and a sliding hip screw for intertrochanteric fractures. The hip fracture is fixed first, often without the need for reduction, because these fractures are nondisplaced. Following hip fixation, a retrograde femoral intramedullary nail is inserted, preferably overlapping with the plate of the hip screw to avoid a potential stress riser (Fig. 8). Although others have advocated use of a second-generation cephalomedullary device for the treatment of these fractures, the results have not been good for the hip, and intraoperative technical problems and operative times have increased.[34]

Type 2 fractures are femoral shaft fractures with a missed femoral neck fracture. The majority of these are nondisplaced or minimally displaced and can be picked up weeks after the femoral nailing. These have been reported with femoral plating as well as retrograde nailing and are most likely not related to the antegrade insertion technique. Fortunately, the prevalence rate of avascular necrosis in these missed fractures is less than that reported for most femoral neck fractures. The prevalence rate in the literature is 3% for the missed versus 10% for solitary fractures.[30] These are most amenable to two or three cancellous screws inserted either around the antegrade nail or above the retrograde nail. Occasionally a reduction must be performed, and with an antegrade nail this can be difficult to reduce and hold fixed. Should varus angulation increase or hip pain commence in the future, an osteotomy can be performed on the hip once the femoral shaft is healed. The results of these proximal hip osteotomies have not been uniformly good, and avascular necrosis has been reported.[36]

Type 3 fractures are displaced femoral neck fractures associated with a femoral shaft fracture. These are often basicervical, vertical, femoral neck, or intertrochanteric hip fractures. These patients must have adequate treatment of their femoral hip fracture performed first as a priority. The implant of choice is the one that would normally be used for that fracture. As comminuted basicervical femoral neck fractures, vertical neck fractures, and intertrochanteric fractures are all optimally treated with a sliding hip screw, this becomes the implant of choice. An open reduction of the hip fracture is carried out by direct manipulation of the floating shaft fragment with an abduction, traction, and internal rotation maneuver. The sliding hip screw is applied with a two- or four-hole side plate, depending on the location of the femoral neck fracture. Following the reduction of the femoral hip fracture, a retrograde intramedullary is inserted, preferably with the implants overlapping. In a recent series, 10 patients were treated for displaced femoral hip fractures associated with a shaft fracture.[35] One of three fractures with a high Pauwel angle was fixed and healed in 5 degrees of varus. In four patients with displaced intertrochanteric hip fractures and three with basicervical femoral neck fractures, the hip fractures healed without varus angulation, and all of the shaft fractures healed. One patient developed an infection of the knee and the retrograde nail and required implant removal and antibiotics, with a good response.

Bose et al[37] attempted to use a second-generation nail to treat ipsilateral femoral neck and shaft fractures and concluded that the technique was demanding and that technical errors with insertion of the reconstruction nail led to fracture complications. Wiss et al[36] attempted a "reverse nail

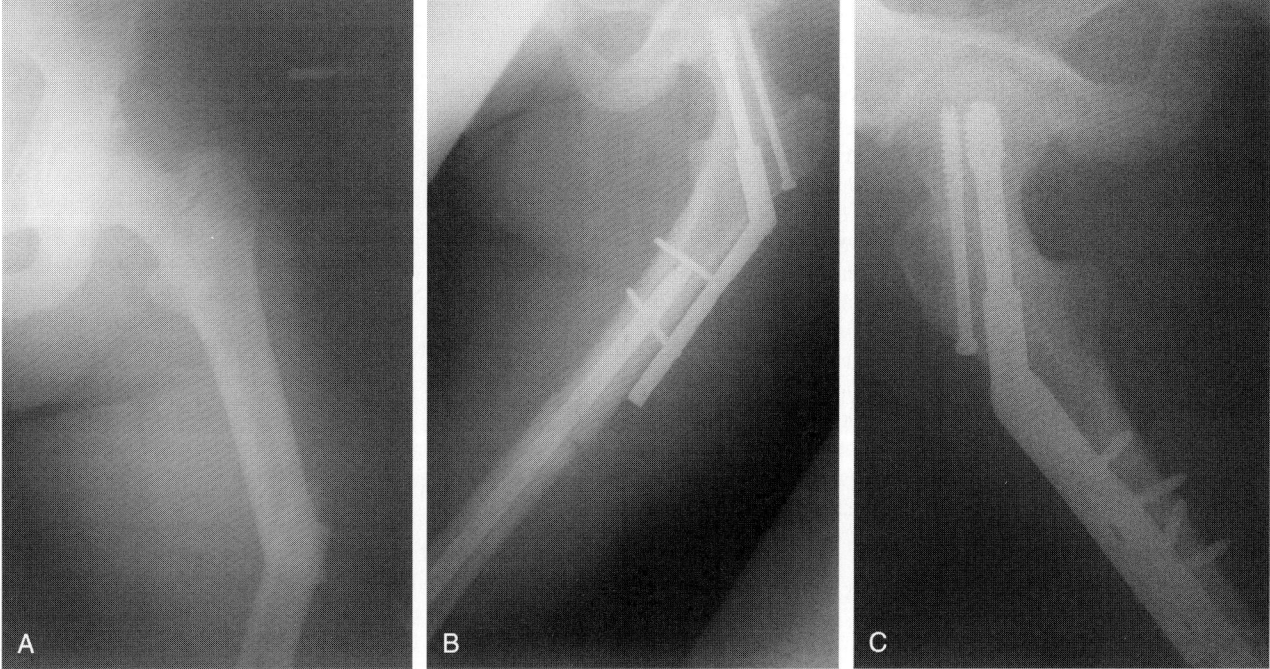

Fig. 8. View. *A*, Radiograph of the femur showing a nondisplaced basicervical femoral neck fracture associated with an isthmal femoral shaft fracture. *B*, Anteroposterior radiograph demonstrating fixation of the femoral hip fracture with a sliding hip screw followed by a retrograde intramedullary nail for the shaft fracture. Note the overlap of the two implants. *C*, Lateral radiograph of the hip showing restoration of the femoral neck angle without displacement.

construct" in 13 patients and a second-generation nail for 14 patients with these combined fractures. Six patients (18%) developed a varus nonunion (2 reconstruction nails and 4 reverse nails). Five of the six hips that had osteotomies healed, but two developed avascular necrosis. The attempted use of a second-generation nail has been shown to have a higher incidence rate of poor results, as has the use of screws around an antegrade femoral nail.[34] Both of these treatments give priority to the femoral shaft by fixing it first, and often the screws provide less than adequate fixation for the hip fracture.

Nondisplaced and missed femoral hip fractures associated with femoral shaft fractures appear to do well. The incidence rate of avascular necrosis is low, and the nondisplaced fractures do not displace. The theory behind these good results appears to be that the majority of the energy of the trauma is dissipated through the femoral shaft fracture. Varus is occasionally seen in the missed fractures, especially when displaced around an antegrade nail. Displaced femoral hip fractures are often vertical in orientation and unstable. Primary treatment of the hip fracture with a sliding hip screw followed by a retrograde intramedullary nail gives priority and optimum fixation to the hip fracture. In addition, there is no compromise in the treatment of the femoral shaft fracture. The use of a single implant, such as a cephalomedullary nail, can lead to compromised fixation of one of the fractures and should be used cautiously.

OPEN FEMORAL SHAFT FRACTURES

The results of primary intramedullary nailing of open femoral shaft fractures have been good. These fractures have been treated by débridement followed by reamed intramedullary nailing. Two prerequisites cited by the authors for this form of treatment were early débridement, within 8 hours, and the ability to accomplish a thorough débridement.[38] The infection rates with early reamed nailing are low, 1.6% to 10%, and the infectious complications were effectively dealt with. The biggest question remains the treatment of open grade 3B open femoral shaft fractures.

Brumback et al[38] reported on 89 open femoral shaft fractures treated with this regimen. All fractures healed in an average of 5 months, and no infections developed in the grade 1, 2, or 3A fractures. In the 27 grade 3B fractures, 1 infection developed after immediate nailing and 2 after delayed nailing. Multiple débridements with interim external fixation are an option for contaminated fractures with extensive soft-tissue injury.

O'Brien et al[39] reviewed 63 open femoral shaft fractures that were treated with primary reamed intramedullary nailing. Despite having 26 grade 2 and 15 grade 3 open fractures, there were only 3 deep infections and only 1 case of osteomyelitis. All complications were treated successfully with standard methods.

Remarkably, these open fractures healed well in several series, and treatment of late infection by nail removal, reaming, and antibiotics was successful.[38, 39] Management of the soft tissues with delayed closure is an extremely important aspect in the management of these fractures, and if the débridement is inadequate, then the results are compromised. Another concern is that should infection develop after retrograde nailing, then the possibility of a septic knee exists. However, the distal locking screws of an antegrade nail are often intra-articular as well. The risks of infection are high with grade 3B fractures, and if a satisfactory soft-tissue envelope or cleansing of the wounds cannot be obtained, then this may be one of the few indications for treating these fractures by union in an external fixator.

The treatment of open grade 1 through 3A femoral shaft fractures with primary reamed intramedullary nailing has been successful. The surgeon must be cautious with the use of this technique in grade 3B open fractures, as the infection rate increases. Thorough and repeated débridement is an essential part of this management protocol, and delayed nailing should be used when questions of contamination arise.

FLOATING KNEES: IPSILATERAL FEMORAL AND TIBIAL SHAFT FRACTURES

Ipsilateral femoral shaft and tibial shaft fractures should perhaps be best recognized for the increased morbidity and mortality associated with this injury. Mortality rates range from 5% to 15%, and amputation has been seen in about 25% of cases.[40] Treatment protocols have varied over the years, and the tibia fracture continues to be associated with a higher incidence rate of problems.[40]

Although protocols have varied, there appears now to be a consensus that intramedullary nailing of the femur is the key to the treatment of this injury complex. Initially, antegrade nailing demonstrated good results, and recently retrograde nailing has been advocated.[40] Initial attempts at conservative fracture care or traction as well as less than adequate fixation techniques led to a 30% deep infection rate and only 28% good results.[41] Anastopoulos et al[42] demonstrated that intramedullary nailing of the femur was an essential part of the treatment of these injuries and increased the incidence of good and excellent results to 81%. The ability to treat both fractures with an intramedullary nail through a single 4-cm incision at the knee, supine position, and a single surgical drape is extremely appealing (Fig. 9). Gregory et al[40] used this technique on 24 patients with 26 fractures. Despite good surgical technique, 18 additional procedures were necessary to obtain union. The majority of these procedures, 13 in 5 complicated tibia fractures, demonstrate the severity of the tibia shaft fracture and the difficulties with its management. Ligamentous injuries to the knee, deep infections, malunions, and amputations have led to poor results in the treatment of these combined fractures.[41, 42] Intramedullary femoral nailing has solved the femoral shaft fracture problem, but despite current surgical techniques, the tibia fracture continues to have an increased morbidity rate because of the nature of its severity. Functional results after the treatment of this fracture complex are good if no other debilitating injury has otherwise affected the patient or limb.

NONUNIONS

The majority of patients treated with intramedullary nailing of a femur fracture will heal without complications as long

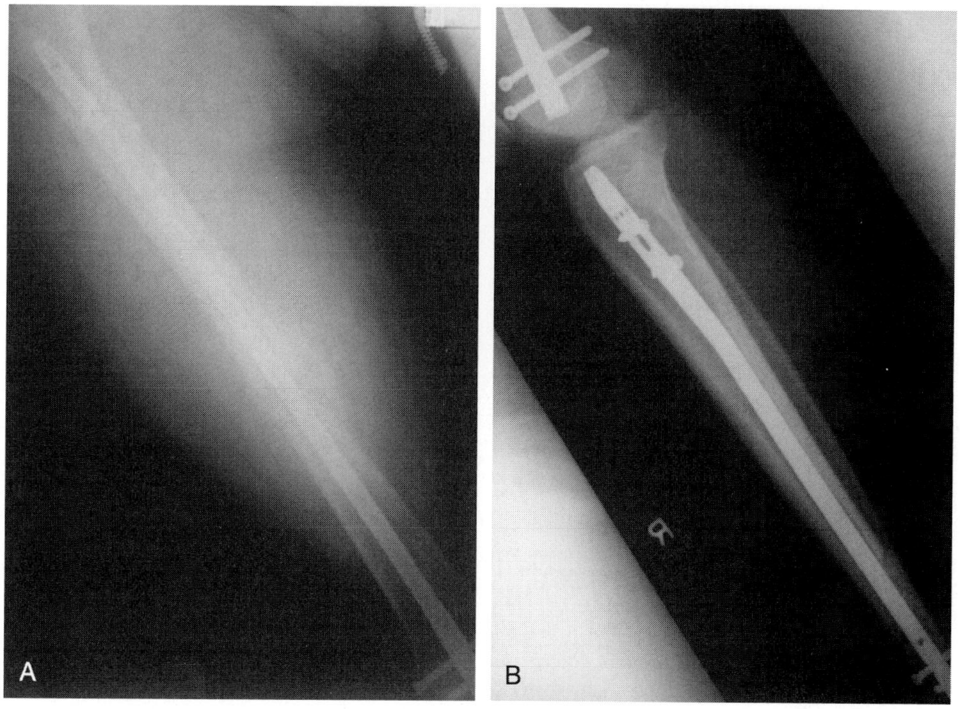

Fig. 9. View. *A*, Management of a floating knee injury. Two-month radiograph of a midshaft femoral shaft fracture treated with a retrograde intramedullary nail. *B*, Lateral radiograph of the distal third tibial shaft fracture treated with an intramedullary nail. Note the retrograde femoral nail in the distal femur. The femoral nailing is performed first, and the entire surgery is done through a parapatellar tendon incision.

as good surgical technique is performed. Fracture union will generally occur within 3 to 6 months. However, a few patients will experience difficulty with fracture union or develop a postoperative deep infection. In these cases, analyzing the fracture and the likely cause for the complication is helpful when planning subsequent treatment.

Axially stable femur fractures treated with an antegrade or retrograde intramedullary rod that are not progressing to union within the 3- to 6-month period are generally candidates for dynamization by removal of either the proximal or the distal locking bolts. Those fractures with bone loss, an atrophic nonunion, or comminution should not be dynamized and are better managed with bone grafting to avoid the shortening that may occur with dynamization. Fractures that do not progress to union after dynamization should be treated with reamed exchange nailing. This technique involves removal of the original implant, reaming of the intramedullary canal until good cortical chatter is encountered, and placement of an intramedullary nail with a larger diameter. If the fracture had previously been open, then intraoperative intramedullary cultures are needed to rule out a low-grade infection (Fig. 10).

Webb et al[43] reported a series of 101 femoral nonunions treated by intramedullary nailing, and union was achieved in 98 femurs at an average of 20 weeks. Only 7 patients were bone-grafted, and the authors suggest that at least 2 mm of additional reaming is necessary to stabilize the bone and stimulate bone regeneration in these nonunions. Although four of eight patients with preexisting osteomyelitis had a flare-up, all went onto union, and three had no drainage after nail removal.

Femur fractures that were originally treated with a plate can be treated with bone grafting 3 to 6 months following injury if an acceptable amount of fracture healing is not progressing and the screws and plate are stable. Fractures without significant bone loss or comminution that do not progress to union in 6 to 9 months are generally treated with either plate removal and revised compression plating or intramedullary nailing.

When a deep infection occurs before fracture union in femurs treated with intramedullary nailing, the infection generally involves the entire intramedullary canal. The intramedullary canal must be débrided to control the infection, and appropriate cultures should be obtained. Many orthopaedic traumatologists recommend removal of the implant, thorough reaming of the intramedullary canal, and primary reimplantation of an appropriately sized nail along with a 6-week course of the appropriate intravenous antibiotic. When the infection is caused by highly virulent organisms, external fixation can be used to stabilize the fracture for several weeks while the infection is treated before a second intramedullary nail is implanted. Deep infection in a femur fracture treated with a retrograde nail has the potential to communicate with the knee joint and cause a septic joint. This must be evaluated and treated at the same time as the infected nail. When the infection involves a fracture treated with a plate, a thorough irrigation and débridement is performed, and the stability of fixation is assessed. Stable implants are generally retained, but loose implants need to be removed. The fracture can then be stabilized with a new plate following débridement, or a temporary external fixator can be used until the infection is controlled.

Using these principles, Cove et al[44] reviewed their series of 13 infected and 33 noninfected femoral shaft nonunions. The patients with infected nonunions were treated with a staged procedure that included removal of hardware, serial débridements, external fixation or traction, antibiotics, and final definitive fixation with bone grafting. Eight of the 13 patients required a free vascularized fibula, and external

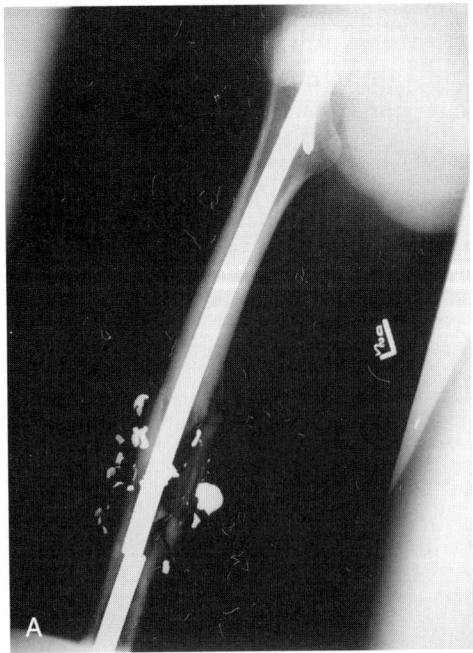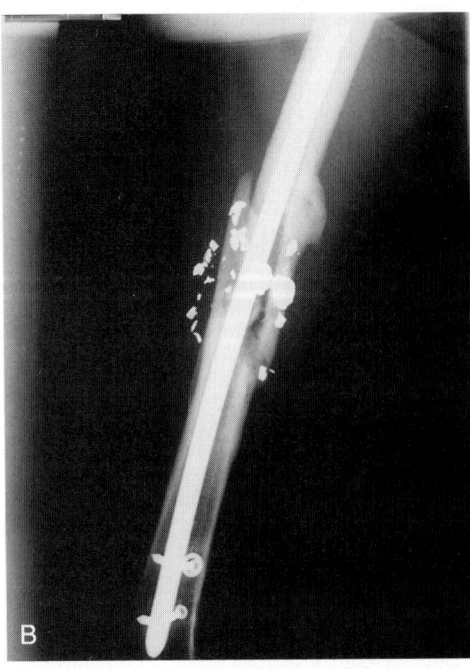

Fig. 10. View. *A*, Lateral radiograph of a femoral shaft nonunion and a broken intramedullary nail 6 months following a gunshot wound to the leg. *B*, Lateral radiograph 3 months after exchange nailing with reaming and insertion of a larger nail. Intramedullary culture results were positive, and the patient was treated with antibiotics for 6 weeks. The distal screws are broken because of immediate weightbearing by the patient following the exchange nail procedure.

fixation or plating was the predominant form of fixation. For the 33 noninfected nonunions, a single-stage fixation/grafting procedure was performed, and 21 patients were treated with plating and bone grafting. Forty-one of the 44 patients achieved union at an average of almost 12 months from fixation. Intramedullary fixation seems to have a shorter time to union but can be extremely challenging if a nail has not previously been in place or an angular deformity is present.[43, 44]

These reports and others demonstrate the complexity of treating these nonunions. Fortunately, axially stable fractures respond well to dynamization. Exchange nailing, with or without bone grafting, is useful for atrophic nonunions. Infected nonunions must be débrided extensively and treated with intravenous antibiotics prior to definitive fixation. Although exchange nailing has been the predominant form of treatment, other methods of fixation such as "wave" plating with bone graft have led to good results.[44]

REFERENCES

1. Bucholz RW, Brumback RJ: Fractures of the shaft of the femur. In Rockwood CA, Green DP, Bucholz RW (eds): Fractures in Adults, vol 2. Philadelphia, JB Lippincott, 1991, p 1653.
2. Kuntscher G: Die Marknagelung von Knochenbruchen. Arch Klin Chir 1940; 200: 443.
3. Kempf H, Grosse A, Beck G: Closed locked intramedullary nailing: Its application to comminuted fractures of the femur. J Bone Joint Surg Am 1985; 67:709.
4. Brumback RJ, Uwagie-Ero S, Lakatos RP, et al: Intramedullary nailing of femoral shaft fractures: Fracture healing with static interlocking fixation. J Bone Joint Surg Am 1988; 70:1453.
5. Winquist RA, Hansen ST, Clawson K: Closed intramedullary nailing of femoral fractures: A report of five hundred and twenty cases. J Bone Joint Surg Am 1984, 66:529.
6. Johnson KD, Tencer AF, Sherman MC: Biomechanical factors affecting fracture stability and femoral bursting in closed intramedullary nailing of femoral shaft fractures, with illustrative case presentations. J Orthop Trauma 1987; 1:1.

7. Russell TA: Biomechanical concepts of femoral intramedullary nailing. Int J Orthop Trauma 1991; 1:35.
8. Johnson KD, Tencer A: Mechanics of intramedullary nails for femoral fractures. Unfallchirug 1990; 93:506.
9. Karpos PA, McFerran MA, Johnson KD: Intramedullary nailing of acute femoral shaft fractures using manual traction without a fracture table. J Orthop Trauma 1995; 9:57.
10. Bone LB, Anders MJ, Rohrbacher BJ: Treatment of femoral fractures in the multiply injured patient with thoracic injury. Clin Orthop 1998; 347:57.
11. Tornetta P, Tiburzi D: The treatment of femoral shaft fractures using intramedullary interlocking nails with and without intramedullary reaming: A preliminary report. J Orthop Trauma 1997; 11:89.
12. Brumback RJ, Reilly JP, Poka A, et al: Intramedullary nailing of femoral shaft fractures: Decision-making errors with interlocking fixation. J Bone Joint Surg Am 1988; 70:1441.
13. Brumback RJ, Ellison TS, Poka A, et al: Intramedullary nailing of femoral shaft fractures: Long-term effects of static inter-

locking fixation. J Bone Joint Surg Am 1992; 74:106.
14. Hajek PD, Bicknell HR, Bronson WE, et al: The use of one compared with two distal screws in the treatment of femoral shaft fractures with interlocking intramedullary nailing. J Bone Joint Surg Am 1993; 75:519.
15. Sanders R, Koval KJ, DiPasquale T, et al: Retrograde reamed femoral nailing. J Orthop Trauma 1993; 7:293.
16. Morgan E, Ostrum R, DiCicco J, et al: The effects of retrograde intramedullary nailing on the patellofemoral articulation. J Orthop Trauma. 1999; 13:13.
17. Herscovici D Jr, Whiteman K: Retrograde nailing of the femur using an intercondylar approach. Clin Orthop 1996; 332:98.
18. Moed BR, Watson JT: Retrograde unreamed intramedullary nailing of fractures of the femoral shaft in the multiply injured patient. J Bone Joint Surg Am 1995; 77: 1520.
19. Ostrum R, DiCicco J, Lakatos R, et al: Retrograde intramedullary nailing of femoral diaphyseal fractures. J Orthop Trauma 1998; 12:464.
20. Muller M, Allgower M, Schneider R, et

al: Manual of Internal Fixation, 2nd ed. New York, Springer-Verlag, 1979, p 228.

21. Magerl F, Wyss A, Brunner CH, et al: Plate osteosynthesis of femoral shaft fractures in adults. Clin Orthop 1979; 138:62.

22. Bostman O, Varjonen L, Vainionpaa S, et al: Incidence of local complications after intramedullary nailing and after plate fixation of femoral shaft fractures. J Trauma 1989; 29:639.

23. Riemer BL, Kelly J, Butterfield S, et al: Titanium LC/DC plates and indirect reduction technique fixation of femoral diaphyseal fractures due to high energy blunt trauma. American Academy of Orthopaedic Surgeons Annual Meeting, February 1996, Anaheim, CA.

24. Rozbruch SR, Muller U, Gautier E, et al: The evolution of femoral shaft plating technique. Clin Orthop 1998; 354:195.

25. Rooser B, Bengston S, Herrlin K, et al: External fixation of femoral fractures: Experience with 15 cases. J Orthop Trauma 1990; 4:70.

26. Dabezies EJ, D'Ambrosia R, Shoji H, et al: Fractures of the femoral shaft treated by external fixation with the Wagner device. J Bone Joint Surg Am 1984; 66:360.

27. Iannacone WM, Taffet R, Delong WG, et al: Early exchange intramedullary nailing of distal femoral fractures with vascular injury initially stabilized with external fixation. J Trauma 1994; 37:446.

28. Tencer AF, Johnson KD, Johnston DWC, et al: A biomechanical comparison of various methods of stabilization of subtrochanteric fractures of the femur. J Orthop Trauma 1984; 2:297.

29. Pugh KJ, Morgan RA, Gorczyca JT, et al: A mechanical comparison of subtrochanteric femur fracture fixation. J Orthop Trauma 1998; 5:324.

30. Brien WW, Wiss DA, Becker V, et al: Subtrochanteric femur fractures: A comparison of the Zickel nail, 95 degree blade plate, and interlocking nail. J Orthop Trauma 1991; 5:458.

31. French BG, Tornetta P: Use of an interlocked cephalomedullary nail for subtrochanteric fracture stabilization. Clin Orthop 1998; 348:95.

32. Kinast C, Bolhofner BR, Mast JW, et al: Subtrochanteric fractures of the femur: Results of treatment with a 95° condylar blade plate. Clin Orthop 1989; 238:122.

33. Sanders R, Regazzoni P: Treatment of subtrochanteric femur fractures using the dynamic condylar screw. J Orthop Trauma 1989; 3:206.

34. Wolinsky PR, Johnson KD: Ipsilateral femoral neck and shaft fractures. Clin Orthop 1995; 318:81.

35. Ostrum R, Poka A: Ipsilateral femoral hip and shaft fractures: A management protocol. Am J Orthop 1999; 28:4.

36. Wiss DA, Sima W, Brien WW: Ipsilateral

fractures of the femoral neck and shaft. J Orthop Trauma 1992; 6:159.

37. Bose WJ, Corces A, Anderson LD: A preliminary experience with the Russell-Taylor reconstruction nail for complex femoral fractures. J Trauma 1992; 32:71.

38. Brumback RJ, Ellison PS, Poka A, et al: Intramedullary nailing of open fractures of the femoral shaft. J Bone Joint Surg Am 1989; 71:1324.

39. O'Brien PJ, Meek RN, Powell JN, et al: Primary intramedullary nailing of open femoral shaft fractures. J Trauma 1991; 31:113.

40. Gregory P, DiCicco J, Karpik K, et al: Ipsilateral fractures of the femur and tibia: Treatment with retrograde femoral nailing and unreamed tibial nailing. J Orthop Trauma 1996; 10:309.

41. Fraser RD, Hunter GA, Waddell JP: Ipsilateral fracture of the femur and tibia. J Bone Joint Surg Br 1978; 60:510.

42. Anastopoulos G, Assimakopoulos A, Exarchou E, et al: Ipsilateral fractures of the femur and tibia. Injury 1992; 23:439.

43. Webb LX, Winquist RA, Hansen ST: Intramedullary nailing and reaming for delayed union or nonunion of the femoral shaft. Clin Orthop 1986; 212:133.

44. Cove JA, Lhowe DW, Jupiter JB, et al: Treatment of femoral diaphyseal nonunions. J Orthop Trauma 1997; 11:513.

FRACTURES OF THE DISTAL FEMUR

Frederick S. Bennett

Summary

- Successful treatment of distal femoral fractures depends on anatomic reduction and stable internal fixation with early mobilization of the knee joint.
- An array of implants are available, including the 95-degree blade plate, the 95-degree condylar screw and side plate, the condylar buttress plate, and the retrograde intramedullary nail.
- Principles of fracture surgery must be meticulously adhered to, including careful preoperative planning, careful handling of the soft tissues, and precise reconstruction of the articular surface.

This chapter addresses treatment of fractures that involve only the most distal portion of the femur. Femoral shaft fractures are discussed in Chapter 3–14. A practical distinction is made between distal diaphyseal fractures that can be stabilized by standard antegrade femoral nailing and more distal metaphyseal or articular fractures for which standard nailing would be impossible or would provide tenuous fixation.

Fractures of the distal femur occur in two generally distinct groups of patients, in both of which the fractures are frequently accompanied by formidable complicating factors. The young patient with high-energy trauma often has an array of life-threatening head, chest, and intra-abdominal injuries. Although stabilization of the femoral fracture within 24 hours is desirable, the definitive reconstruction may need to be delayed until the patient's overall condition permits. Elderly patients are usually injured in simple falls from standing height. They often present with pulmonary, cardiovascular, and other medical conditions that can seriously jeopardize their ability to survive a substantial surgical procedure.

Traditionally, classification systems have considered only the severity of the bony injury. The most widely used is the AO classification, which categorizes the degree of articular and supracondylar comminution (Fig. 1). However, the magnitude of the challenge also escalates with the extent of soft tissue injury, a larger limb, and the presence of osteoporosis.

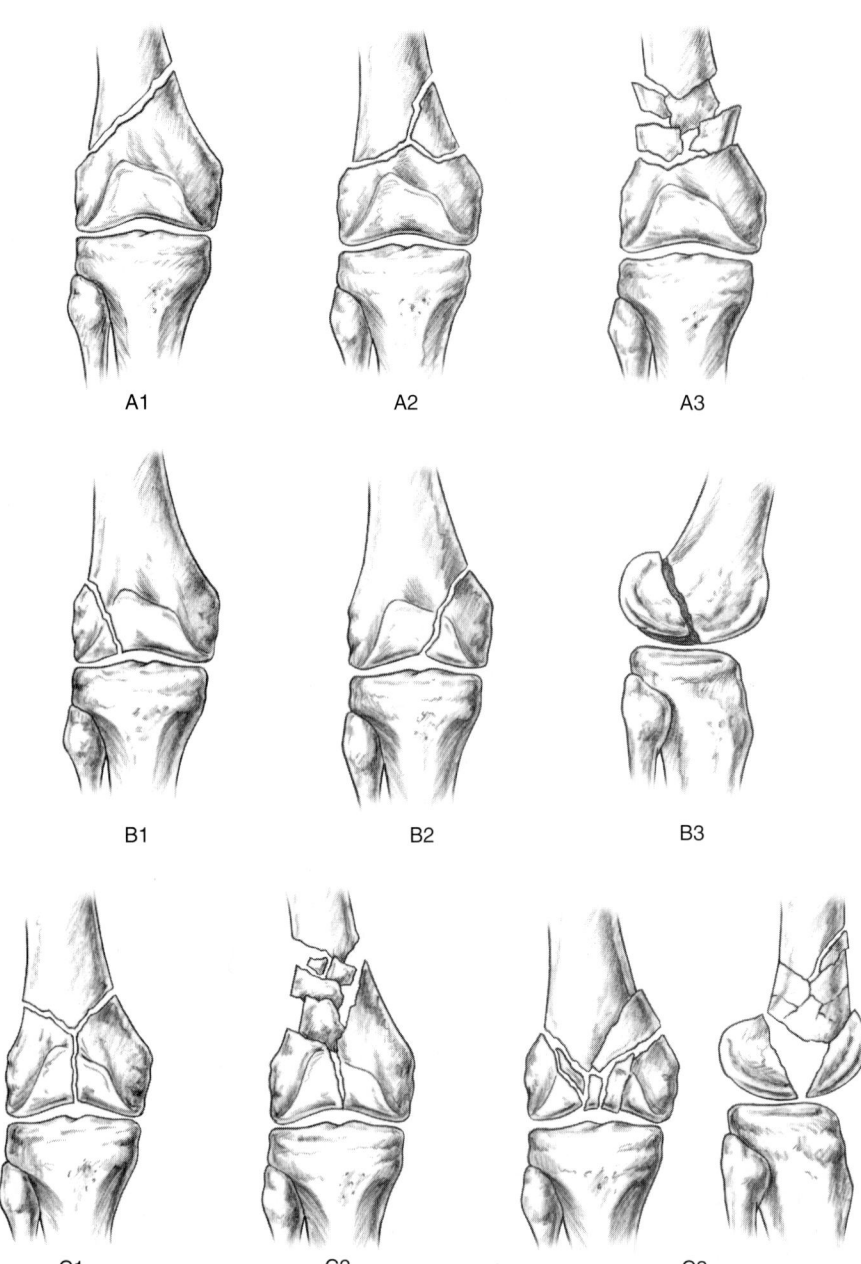

A1 A2 A3

B1 B2 B3

C1 C2 C3

Fig. 1. AO fracture classification. (Redrawn from Helfet D, Lorich D: Fractures of the distal femur. In Browner B, Jupiter J, Levine A, et al [eds]: Skeletal Trauma. Philadelphia, WB Saunders, 1998, 2nd ed, p 2048.)

HISTORICAL REVIEW

The major turning point in the evolution of treatment of distal femoral fractures occurred in 1970, when the Swiss AO Group presented the orthopaedic community with an appropriate device and well-defined goals of treatment as well as important principles of surgical technique and postoperative care. The group recommended anatomic reduction with preservation of the blood supply to the fracture fragments, stable internal fixation with a 95-degree blade plate (Fig. 2), and early mobilization of the knee. Using relatively stringent criteria, Wenzl and associates[1] reported a 73.5% rate of good or excellent results in 112 patients treated according to these principles. As greater experience was gained with the AO blade plate and technique, and with management of severe comminution of the medial buttress with bone grafts, adjunctive medial internal fixa-

tion, or both, the surgical indications broadened. A preponderance of favorable reports with 60% to 85% rates of good to excellent results began to appear in the orthopaedic literature.[2–6]

Another device that achieved widespread and lasting popularity was the 95-degree supracondylar lag screw with side plate (see Fig. 2). Excellent outcomes and greater ease of use compared with the 95-degree blade plate have been noted by numerous investigators.[6, 7] The greater ease of use results from two technical points. First available rotation either of the condylar lag screw within the distal femoral fragment or of the screw with the barrel of the side plate (depending on whether a keyed device or an unkeyed device is used) allows flexion of the distal fragment to be adjusted late in the fixation effort. In contrast, with the blade plate, the entire reduction, including varus-valgus, flexion-extension, and rotation, is determined as soon as

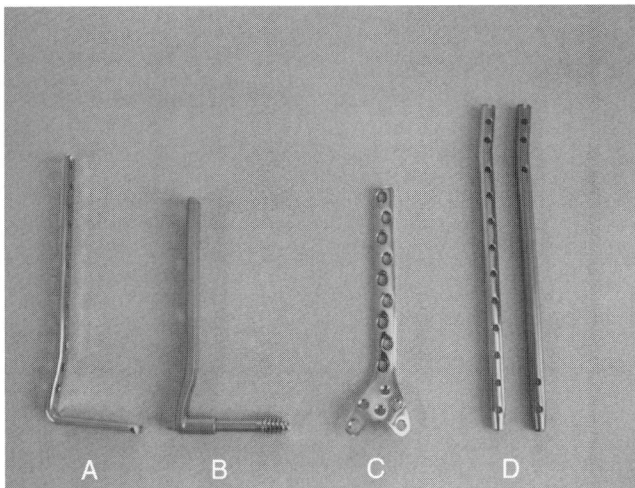

Fig. 2. Fixation devices for the distal femur. *A,* 95-degree blade plate. *B,* 95-degree condylar lag screw and side plate. *C,* Condylar buttress plate. *D,* Retrograde intramedullary nail.

the seating chisel is driven. Second, the path for the lag screw is reamed in a gradual fashion, whereas the path for the blade plate is created by driving a chisel across the reconstructed condyles. Problems arise when the bone is hard, as in young patients, or when one or more of the condylar fragments is small, precluding optimal interfragmentary screw fixation. Even if pilot holes have been drilled, driving a chisel risks disrupting the articular reconstruction.

Various condylar buttress plates have been specifically designed to fit the distal femur (see Fig. 2). They are most useful in fractures with extensive comminution of the condyles. Countersunk anteroposteriorly oriented screws used to fix coronal splits in the condyles may block the intended path of a blade plate or condylar lag screw. Furthermore, the large condylar portion of these implants can act as a central wedge, forcing the various articular fragments apart. Condylar buttress plates, however, have multiple holes at the broad distal end that allow transverse screws to be angled around and between anteroposteriorly oriented screws. Condylar buttress plates should always be available in the operating room to enable salvage of failed attempts to insert a blade plate or condylar lag screw. The primary shortcoming of currently available devices is that the screw-plate junction is not fixed, thus often allowing the condyles to toggle into varus during the healing process.

Improved conceptualization of important elements of technique paralleled the development of better implants. Mast and colleagues[8] clarified the concept and method of indirect fracture reduction with application of the lateral plate devices in essence as extramedullary nails. The goal is to maximally preserve soft-tissue attachments to the fracture fragments. Only the minimal amount of lateral cortex necessary to apply the device is exposed. The condylar blade plate, condylar lag screw with side plate, or buttress plate is then applied to the condyles. Traction is applied across the fracture site to regain length. Length of the bone is then secured with a clamp or one or two screws placed proximal to the comminuted supracondylar region. The intervening comminuted fragments are gently teased into place with sharp-pointed clamps and instruments while

their soft-tissue attachments are maintained. This method has been quite effective in allowing rapid healing through preservation of vascularity around the zone of fracture, thus often eliminating the need for bone grafting.

Henry and associates,[9] in 1991, reported on the use of a retrograde supracondylar nail to stabilize distal femoral fractures (see Fig. 2). This class of implants allowed circumferential preservation of the soft-tissue sleeve around the fracture. Originally designed for use in elderly patients with osteoporotic bone, the supracondylar nail soon proved useful in treatment of young patients with high-energy trauma as well.[10] For example, floating knee injuries, including those with articular comminution of the distal femur, could be treated on the standard operating room table with a single parapatellar incision and the use of tourniquet control, with less dissection, smaller blood loss, and shorter operative time. A retrograde nail, however, provides suboptimal fixation in very distal fractures owing to the inability to achieve solid bicortical purchase with at least two distal locking screws. Furthermore, like the blade plate and condylar lag screw, it can function as a disrupting wedge with AO-type C3 fractures. Although the retrograde supracondylar nail was first touted as providing enhanced fracture stability over laterally applied devices, subsequent bench tests have shown little overall difference.[11, 12]

Hybrid external fixators and Ilizarov segmental bone transport techniques provide additional options in cases in

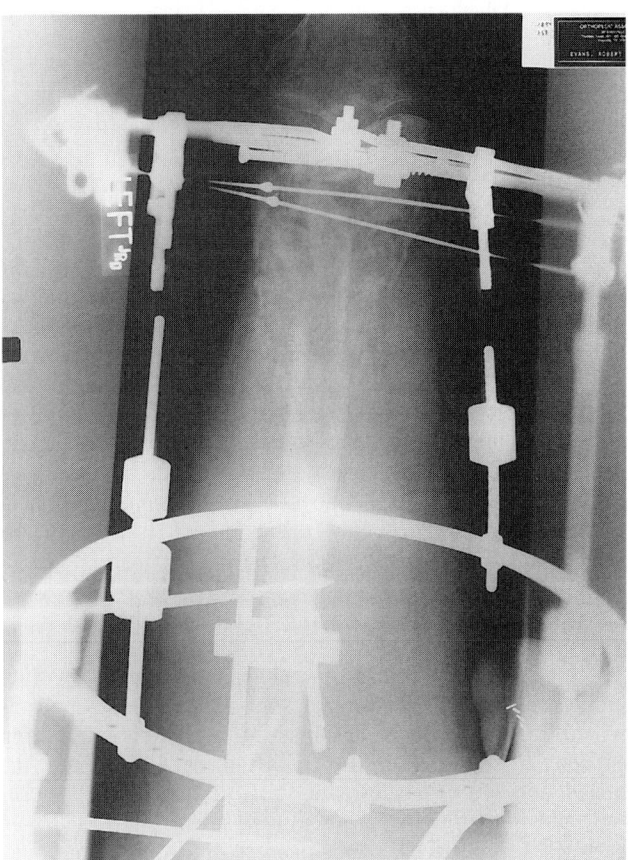

Fig. 3. View. This is a severe distal femur fracture with segmental bone deficit, including partial absence of the femoral condyles, which was treated with tension-wire external fixator and autogenous bone graft.

TABLE 1. DISTAL FEMUR FRACTURES: TREATMENT OPTIONS, CLINICAL INDICATIONS, AND EXPECTED OUTCOMES

Treatment Type	Indications	Outcome
Nonoperative	Moribund, nonambulatory patient	Residual deformity, articular incongruity
Temporary knee-spanning external fixator	Vascular injury; segmental bone loss with large graft anticipated; severe soft-tissue injury; extensive multitrauma	N/A—temporary
Tension-wire external fixator proximal to knee	Segmental bone loss, partial loss of condyles, need to decrease extent of surgery	Loss of knee motion
Blade plate	AO classifications: A1, A2, A3, C1, C2	60%–95% good to excellent
Condylar lag screw	AO classifications: A1, A2, A3, C1, C2; osteoporosis; surgeon's lack of mastery of blade plate	60%–95% good to excellent
Lateral buttress plate	AO classifications: C3 and very low A1, A2, A3, C1, C2; failure of blade plate or condylar lag screw fixation	Possible progressive varus deformity
Retrograde nail	Fracture above TKA, preexistent knee arthritis; lower extremity neurological impairment; obese patient; long segment of comminution; need to decrease extent of surgery; ipsilateral tibia fracture; AO classification: A1, A2, A3, C1, C2	Possible decreased knee function
Knee fusion	Young patient, laborer with unsalvageable knee articulation	Permanent activity limitations inherent to knee fusion
Primary long-stem total knee arthroplasty with allograft or hinged distal femoral replacement	Elderly patient; preexistent severe osteoporosis and/or arthritis; fracture that destabilizes existing TKA	Earlier weightbearing and mobility with decreased morbidity
Supplemental medial plate	Loss of medial buttress and already stripped by trauma	Decreased knee motion; enhanced healing and better alignment through enhanced stability
Supplemental intramedullary plate or cortical allograft	Comminuted medial buttress	Enhanced healing and better alignment through enhanced stability
Bone graft	Comminuted medial buttress; bone loss from trauma or débridement; atrophic nonunion; soft tissues well-controlled	Accelerated healing; improved union rates

TKA = total knee arthroplasty.

which segmental bone loss is greater than 6 to 8 cm or the residual condylar mass is too small to allow fixation by more conventional methods (Fig. 3). Good results have been obtained in elderly patients with severe osteoporosis and preexistent arthritis with the use of long-stem total knee replacement with segmental allograft in order to allow earlier weightbearing.[13] Alternatively, constrained distal femoral replacement total knee arthroplasty can be used.[14, 15] With all these available options taken into consideration, it is rare today to encounter a distal femoral fracture that is not best treated surgically (Table 1).

PATHOGENESIS

The mechanism of injury in young adults usually involves high-energy axial loading of the flexed knee, such as would occur against the dashboard of an automobile during sudden deceleration or as the result of a fall onto the flexed knee from a substantial height. Intercondylar splitting and comminution are common as the shaft is driven between the condyles. With open fractures, the bone surfaces must be carefully inspected for foreign material and thoroughly débrided. Vascular injury must always be suspected. The threshold for angiographic evaluation should

be low. Concomitant knee injuries, such as fracture of the tibial plateau or patella, are common and often require internal fixation.

Distal femoral fractures in the elderly usually result from simple falls from standing height. Torsion and varus-valgus stress produce lower-energy fractures that are closed and do not as often involve splitting of the condyles. Because of fragile osteoporotic bone, however, supracondylar comminution can be similarly severe in elderly patients.

RELEVANT ANATOMY

The geometry of the femoral condyles is important to operative fracture reduction and hardware placement. When viewed from the lateral perspective, the femoral shaft is aligned with the anterior half of the condyles. Fixation devices must be similarly aligned (Fig. 4). An axial cross-section of the condyles shows a trapezoidal configuration, wider medially than laterally, and wider posteriorly than anteriorly. The decrease in width from posterior to anterior on the medial side must be taken into account in the assessment of the depth of hardware penetration toward the medial side; otherwise, extraosseous prominence of hardware would lead to irritation of the medial soft

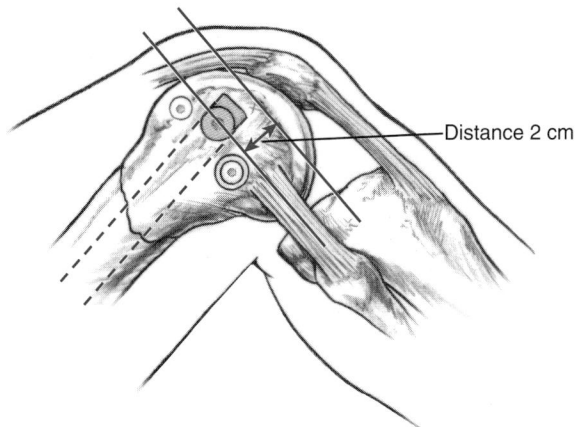

Distance 2 cm

Fig. 4. Appropriate placement of internal fixation devices for the distal femur. Correct starting points are shown for the blade plate (*rectangle*) and condylar lag screw (*circle*). (Redrawn from Helfet D: Fractures of the distal femur. In Browner B, Jupiter J, Levine A, et al [eds]: Skeletal Trauma. Philadelphia, WB Saunders, 1992, p 1665.)

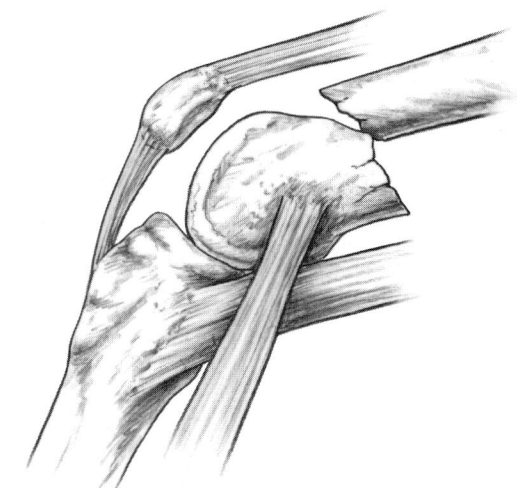

Fig. 6. Pull of the gastrocnemius muscle hyperextends the condyles. Knee flexion and traction force applied anteriorly facilitate reduction. (Redrawn from Green NE, Swiontkowski MF: Fractures of the distal femur. In Browner B, Jupiter J, Levine A, et al [eds]: Skeletal Trauma. Philadelphia, WB Saunders, 1998, 2nd ed, p 1644.)

tissues, with resultant pain and limitation of knee motion (Fig. 5).

Forces imposed on the fracture by the muscles that pull across it produce characteristic deformities. Shortening occurs under the forces of the quadriceps femoris and the hamstrings. The gastrocnemius keeps the knee flexed when the limb is extended, producing an apex-posterior or hyperextension deformity at the fracture site (Fig. 6). Reduction therefore requires some knee flexion and a traction force applied to the anterior aspect of the condyles with either a transfixing pin or a sharp tenaculum. Commonly, when the condyles are split from one another, there is relative malrotation along the sagittal plane as well as toeing in or toeing out because the shaft becomes wedged between the condyles. The shaft must be cleared from the gap between the condyles with adequate longitudinal traction or with temporary medial displacement of the shaft to allow the condyles to be clamped to one another with the shaft out of the way. The latter technique is generally preferred, because traction tightens the extensor mechanism anteriorly against the condyles, making visualization of the articular reduc-

tion quite difficult. Retraction of the patella and extensor mechanism to allow visualization for articular reduction is also greatly enhanced if the limb is kept extended.

PROCEDURE

PREOPERATIVE PLANNING

Plain radiographs of the knee and entire femur in the anteroposterior (AP) and lateral views usually suffice to demonstrate the fracture pattern. The entire femur should be visualized in at least the AP view to rule out more proximal fractures of the hip and femoral shaft. Oblique views of the knee are occasionally helpful in demonstrating coronal fracture lines in the condyles. If the fracture pattern is unclear from immediate postinjury films, radiographs with traction applied either manually or with a tibial pin are usually more interpretable. Close attention should be given to ruling out of coronal fracture lines in the condyles, because they would significantly increase the difficulty of the operative procedure and influence the choice of implants.

Surgery should be performed as soon as the patient is medically stable and a good preoperative plan has been made. When definitive stabilization must be delayed, there are several temporizing measures from which to choose, depending on the individual clinical setting and estimates about when the surgery can be done. A long-leg splint, knee immobilizer, or locked hinged knee brace can be used to protect the limb from further injury if surgery is to be performed within 1 to 2 days. Regaining length is not generally a problem within this time frame. When a longer delay in surgery is anticipated, traction is necessary to prevent soft-tissue contracture and loss of length that would complicate fracture reduction. A tibial pin should be placed several centimeters distal to the tibial tubercle to allow the potentially contaminated pin site to be draped out of the operative field. In patients with vascular injury or heavily contaminated or unstable soft tissues, an external

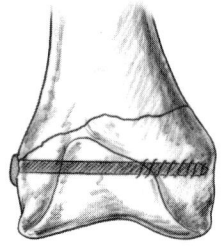
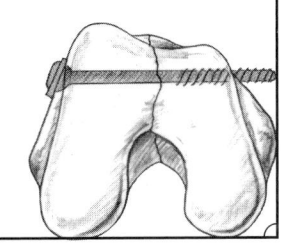

Fig. 5. Distal femoral geometry. Screws that appear to be within bone on an AP projection may protrude medially. (Redrawn from Helfet D: Fractures of the distal femur. In Browner B, Jupiter J, Levine A, et al [eds]: Skeletal Trauma. Philadelphia, WB Saunders, 1992, p 1665.)

fixator spanning the knee serves well as a form of temporary, portable traction.

SURGICAL EXPOSURE

When a laterally applied device is used, the vast majority of distal femoral fractures can be adequately exposed through a standard lateral approach without tibial tubercle osteotomy (Fig. 7).[9] The vastus lateralis is elevated off of the lateral intermuscular septum, and a complete lateral parapatellar arthrotomy is performed. Distally, the skin incision must curve gently anteriorly toward the lateral border of the tibial tubercle so that adequate visualization of the intercondylar region is obtained. Manipulation and reduction of the condylar fragments are facilitated by keeping the knee extended and displacing the condylar mass laterally, thus allowing the fracture to shorten. This maneuver moves the femoral shaft out of the way and relaxes the extensor mechanism, allowing it to be retracted.

Additional exposure is sometimes necessary when there is substantial articular fragmentation of the medial femoral condyle. Excellent visualization can be obtained with a tibial tubercle osteotomy, but this does add time and complexity to the procedure. Complications can be avoided by raising a large enough fragment to allow secure repair (approximately $5 \times 2 \times 1$ cm). Use of a small supplement medial incision should be considered as an alternative to a tibial tubercle osteotomy. Coronal splits in the medial condyle can often be reduced through the standard lateral incision. Small stab wounds in the medial soft tissues suffice to allow interfragmentary screws to be directed percutaneously while they are viewed from the lateral incision. When necessary, longer medial incisions can be used to directly visualize and reduce the comminuted medial femoral condyle. Extension of the medial wound far enough proximally to allow application of a medial plate must be performed, with care taken to avoid the superficial femoral artery at the adductor hiatus.

Retrograde supracondylar nails are inserted through anterior incisions ranging from percutaneous patellar tendon–splitting incisions 2 to 3 cm long to formal wide medial or lateral parapatellar arthrotomies with eversion and displacement of the patella. Percutaneous techniques are applicable only to simple AO A-type fracture patterns and to AO C-type fractures in which the intercondylar split is truly a nondisplaced fissure that can be stabilized with percutaneous, transversely oriented screws. In most cases, however, retrograde supracondylar nailing should be performed through a formal arthrotomy for complete direct visualization and anatomic reduction of the articular surface.

ASSESSING REDUCTION

One of the most difficult but crucial elements in successful management of a distal femoral fracture is intraoperative assessment of the accuracy of reduction. It begins preoperatively with careful examination of the other, uninjured extremity. The surgeon must develop clear goals with regard to the final length and alignment of the fractured limb, because extensive comminution often makes "puzzle-piece" reconstruction of the fragments impossible. Optimally, full-length radiographs of the uninjured leg are obtained to allow measurements of the target anatomic and mechanical axes of the knee. Because such radiographs are not always practical in a multiple-trauma setting, the surgeon should at least visually examine the tibiofemoral angle of the uninjured extremity and the rotational alignment to form a clear mental image of what the injured extremity should look like when the procedure is completed. Before the patient is draped for surgery, the length of the unin-

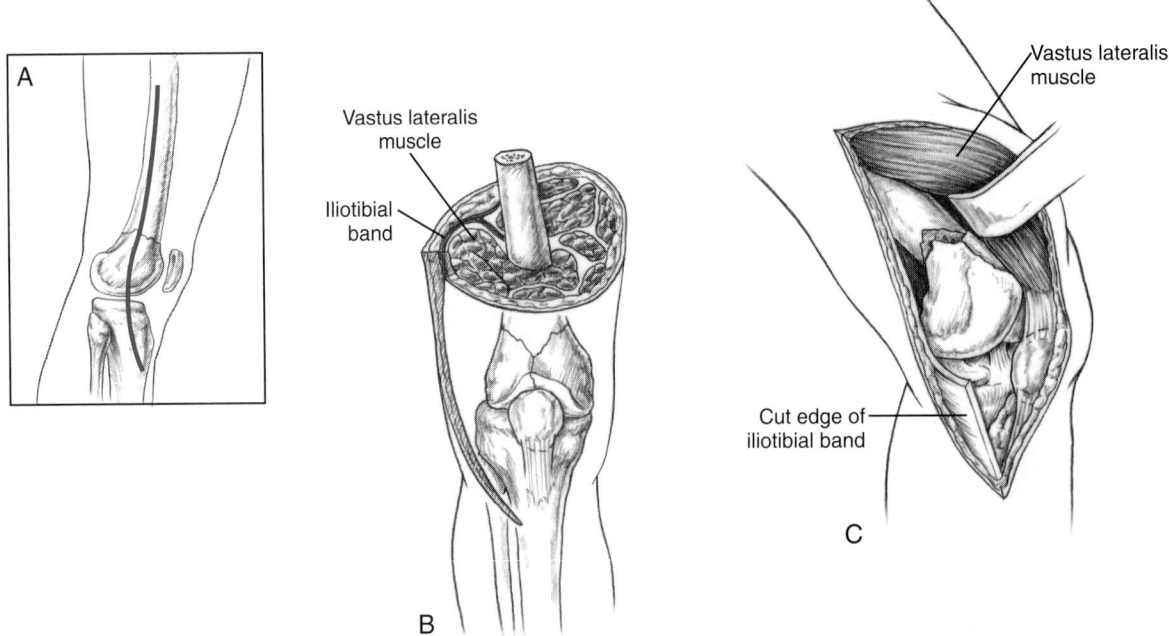

Fig. 7. Standard incision and lateral approach to the distal femur. (Redrawn from Green NE, Swiontkowski MF: Fractures of the distal femur. In Browner B, Jupiter J, Levine A, et al [eds]: Skeletal Trauma. Philadelphia, WB Saunders, 1998, 2nd ed, p 1661.)

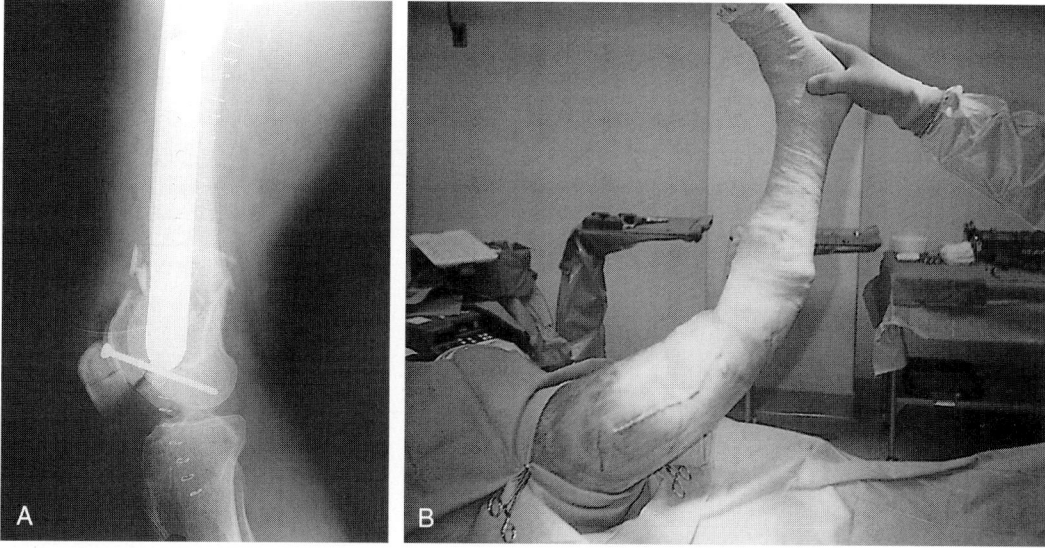

Fig. 8. Views. Lateral radiograph (*A*) and clinical photograph (*B*) of distal femoral fracture stabilized in hyperextension. Hyperextension of the knee was obvious evidence of malreduction.

jured femur can be measured with the C-arm of the image intensifier and a long metal ruler.

Sagittal plane alignment (flexion-extension) of the condyles is particularly difficult to assess intraoperatively with the C-arm. Other supporting clues must therefore be used, particularly when the transmetaphyseal disruption is low and the condylar mass is short. The degree to which the knee can be extended should be precisely matched to the other, normal knee (Fig. 8). Finally, plain radiographs should be obtained in both the AP and lateral views before the wound is closed to allow final confirmation of the accuracy of reduction. The profile on the lateral view of the sturdy posterior cortex can often be used as a key to assess the accuracy of the reduction because this cortex frequently is not comminuted (see Fig. 8).

ARTICULAR REDUCTION

The overall strategy in reduction of comminuted distal femoral fractures is to assemble the fragments in a sequence that progressively simplifies the fracture pattern. In an AO-type C3 fracture, each condyle is first reconstructed individually to obtain separate whole medial and lateral condyles. Countersunk partially threaded 4.0-mm cancellous screws are inserted roughly from anterior to posterior and as perpendicularly as possible to the coronal fracture lines. They should be countersunk completely below the thickness of the articular cartilage. The medial and lateral condyles are then reduced to each other, clamped with large reduction forceps, and fixed provisionally with K-wires or small-diameter Steinmann's pins. Once temporary intercondylar fixation is achieved, one or two large-fragment, partially threaded, 6.25-mm cancellous screws should be inserted from lateral to medial to compress the condyles together, unless there is bone loss or comminution that precludes stable compression. If the latter condition is present, fully threaded screws should be used. These transverse screws should be inserted at a point on the lateral

cortex where they will not interfere with seating of the specific lateral plate device that will be used.

SUPRACONDYLAR REDUCTION

The next step is reduction of the reconstructed condyles to the femoral shaft. The technique differs substantially according to the device being used. The blade plate and condylar lag screw can be used reliably as reduction tools, whereas the condylar buttress plate and supracondylar nail cannot. The fixed-angle relationship of both the blade plate and the condylar lag screw, and the fact that they are usually utilized in cases without severe articular comminution, makes them useful handles to grasp and correct the relationship of the condyles to the shaft. The key to a successful reduction is accurate initial insertion of the blade or lag screw with regard to varus-valgus and rotation and, in the case of the blade plate, with respect to flexion-extension of the condyles as well. Appropriate orientation is achieved through the use of the summation wire technique (Fig. 9). The blade plate or lag screw must be inserted as distally as possible without violating the articular surface.

Type C3 fractures, and all fractures in which buttress plates are used, are best reduced in a more delicate and circumspect manner with application of distraction forces distal to the knee—manually, with a femoral distractor, or with a fracture table—to avoid disruption of the articular reduction. Additionally, because currently available buttress plates are nonlocking, any distraction or compression forces applied with the device are likely to be dissipated as angulation between the screws and the plate, producing varus-valgus malalignment of the fracture instead of achieving the desired length adjustments. Therefore, the push-pull screw technique is not generally useful when a condylar buttress plate is used.

The supracondylar nail is similar to the condylar buttress plate, in that it requires a near anatomic reduction of the condyles to the shaft prior to its application. Distraction

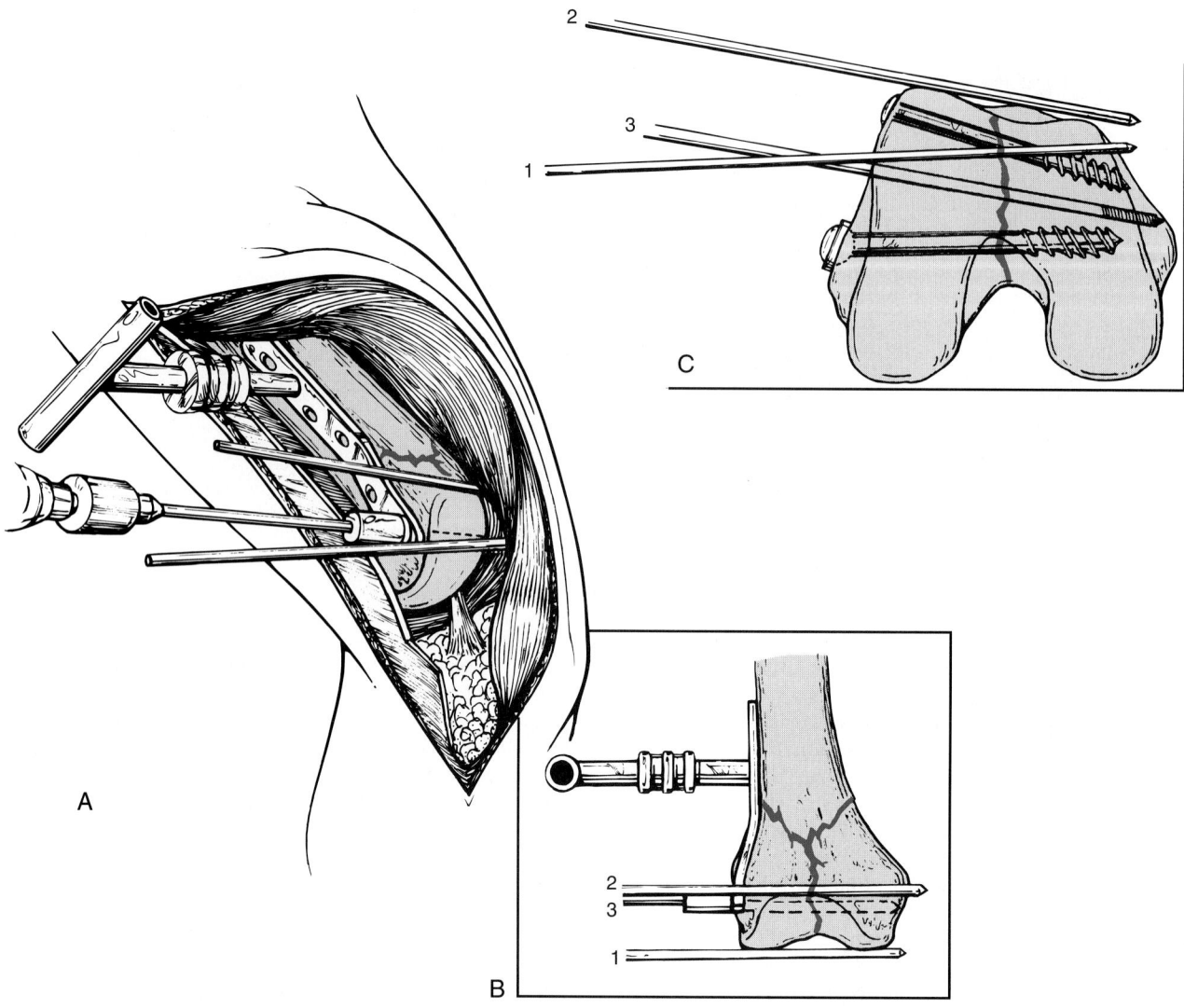

Fig. 9. Summation wire technique. Wire 3 is parallel to the joint line (*wire 1*) and the anterior surface of the femur (*wire 2*). Wire 1 guides varus-valgus alignment. Wire 2 guides rotational alignment. (From Browner B, Jupiter J, Levine A, et al [eds]: Skeletal Trauma. Philadelphia, WB Saunders, 1998, 2nd ed, vol 2, p 2059. From Mize RD: Supracondylar and articular fractures of the distal femur. In Chapman MW [ed]: Operative Orthopaedics. Philadelphia, JB Lippincott, 1988.)

forces are best applied distal to the knee. The starting channel must be oriented precisely along the central axis of the condylar mass as confirmed by use of the C-arm. Over-reaming helps avoid disruption of the articular reduction during nail insertion. The nail must be sunk well below the articular cartilage to avoid destruction of the patellar cartilage when knee motion begins. Distal locking is performed first; length is adjusted with application of either compression or distraction forces. Proximal locking is then completed.

VASCULAR INJURY

Vascular injury accompanying a distal femoral fracture is a complex emergency. Rarely are the fracture patterns sufficiently simple to allow rapid definitive stabilization prior to vascular repair. Open fractures should be rapidly but thoroughly débrided. Temporary knee-spanning external fixation is then performed to preserve length and gross alignment and to protect the vascular repair in the early

postoperative period. Conversion to internal fixation should be performed within 2 weeks.

BONE GRAFT

Indirect reduction techniques have drastically reduced the need for primary bone grafting of distal femoral fractures. Union rates of around 90% without grafting are achievable with good surgical technique.[16, 17] This fact is important because autogenous grafting significantly increases the length and physiological stress of the surgical procedure. Bone grafting remains useful and necessary in severe open fractures with bone loss or extensive periosteal stripping. Autogenous bone is preferred. It is safest to delay the bone graft procedure until all the wounds have healed, soft-tissue reconstructive procedures have been completed, and the limb is completely reepithelialized.

USE OF CEMENT

Several investigators have found cement augmentation of fixation to be highly useful in the management of distal

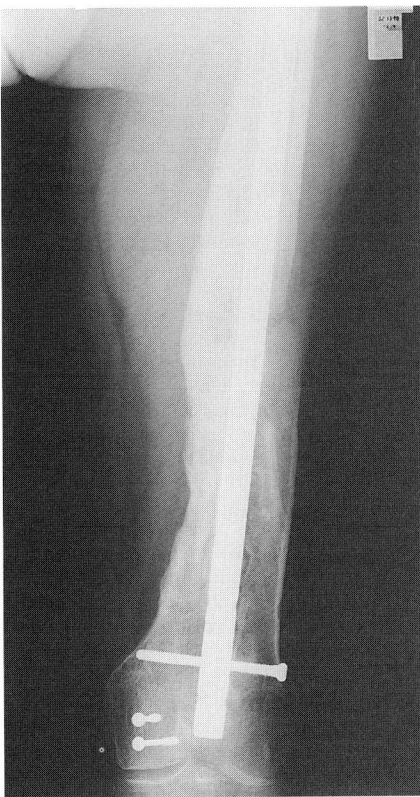

Fig. 10. View. Healing of extensively comminuted fracture of the distal femur through preservation of soft-tissue vascularity without shortening or use of bone graft.

femoral fractures in osteoporotic bone.[5, 18] Although cement can improve early stability of the fixation construct, its use results in a proportional loss of bone stock that can complicate any subsequent procedure that might be necessitated by infection, nonunion, refracture, or malunion. Use of structural allografts or intramedullary plates may provide suitable alternatives to the use of cement.

SHORTENING

Fracture site impaction with intentional primary shortening to improve fracture stability has been suggested and implemented with some success. Unfortunately, it does result in symptomatic limb length discrepancies.[19] Furthermore, this technique cannot be used as a matter of routine, because fracture patterns in which useful improvements in stability can be obtained without major limb shortening are in the minority. Available techniques in the surgical management of distal femoral fractures enable successful treatment without significant shortening, even in the most complex injuries with substantial segmental comminution extending high into the diaphysis (Fig. 10).

POSTOPERATIVE MANAGEMENT

Patients should be mobilized out of bed and should begin gait training as soon as their other injuries and overall medical condition permit. Prophylaxis against deep venous thrombosis should be considered. Postoperative use of con-

tinuous passive motion machines can facilitate return of motion and improve comfort in some patients. Potential benefits of continuous passive motion must be weighed against the risk of increased irritation of severely injured soft tissues and repetitive cycling of osteoporotic, highly comminuted, or tenuously stabilized fractures. Time to full weightbearing is approximately 12 weeks, which can be modified depending on relevant characteristics of the specific fracture and the individual patient. Patient size and the presence of other injuries or impaired agility must be considered.

COMPLICATIONS

Even highly skilled surgeons encounter some very difficult fractures or difficult patients. In the experience of a surgeon who has treated many such cases, some fail to heal, and some have residual angulation. However, as long as the articular surface has been well reduced, further opportunities are available to correct residual problems after the first procedure. Four to six months of healing of the comminuted fragments often allows more stable fixation and facilitates correction and maintenance of alignment. Articular incongruity, however, should be corrected as soon as the condition of the soft tissues and the overall condition of the patient allow.

Supracondylar malunion can be corrected by performance of wedge or dome-shaped osteotomies with revision fixation. Even if a supracondylar nail was used initially, a lateral device is usually employed for revision, because it is difficult to obtain adequate stability with only two distal locking screws after a new, reoriented channel is cut in the short and often osteoporotic distal fragment for a second supracondylar nail.

Treatment of supracondylar nonunion should follow established principles for treatment of nonunions in general. If the nonunion is hypertrophic and residual angulation is mild, the femur with good bone quality can be persuaded into alignment with the use of a femoral distractor, bone clamps, and a lateral compression device and of a blade plate or condylar lag screw with side plate to apply leverage to the distal fragment. The nonunion site can be partially disrupted and loosened with a small osteotome, if necessary, to decrease the correctional force that must be applied. Bone grafting of hypertrophic nonunions is not necessary. Atrophic nonunions should always undergo grafting. Use of retrograde nailing techniques to treat nonunions should be avoided, because of published reports of union rates as low as 25%.[20] Ilizarov techniques should be reserved for extreme situations with extensive bone defects or infection, because the distal wires often remain quite painful and retard knee motion.

Deep infections involving the hardware and the fracture site should be suppressed, if possible, with administration of intravenous or oral antibiotics until adequate healing occurs to allow removal of the fixation device. If the infection remains active with cellulitis of the limb and systemic symptoms, the hardware and bone graft may need to be removed, and an external fixator placed. Once the infection is controlled and good coverage has been obtained, bone grafting can be performed. Revision internal fixation with removal of the external fixator may also be considered.

REFERENCES

1. Wenzl H, Casey PA, Herbert P, et al. Die operative Behandlung der distalen Femur-fraktur. AO Bull 1970; Dec.
2. Chiron JS, Casey P: Fractures of the distal third of the femur treated by internal fixation. Clin Orthop 1974; 100:160.
3. Mize RD, Bucholz RW, Grogan DP: Surgical treatment of displaced, comminuted fractures of the distal end of the femur. J Bone Joint Surg Am 1982; 64:871.
4. Healy WL, Brooker AF Jr: Distal femur fractures: Comparison of open and closed methods of treatment. Clin Orthop 1983; 174:166.
5. Olerud S: Operative treatment of supra-condylar-condylar fractures of the femur: Technique and results in fifteen cases. J Bone Joint Surg Am 1972; 54:1015.
6. Sanders R, Regazzoni P, Revdi TP: Treatment of supracondylar-intracondylar fractures of the femur using the dynamic condylar screw. J Orthop Trauma 1989; 3: 214.
7. Radford PJ, Howell CJ: The AO dynamic condylar screw for fractures of the femur. Br J Accident Surg 1992; 23:89.
8. Mast J, Jakob R, Ganz R: Planning and Reduction Technique in Fracture Surgery. Berlin, Springer-Verlag, 1989.
9. Henry SL, Trager S, Green S, et al: Management of supracondylar fractures of the femur with the GSH intramedullary nail: Preliminary report. Contemp Orthop 1991; 22:631.
10. Iannacone WM, Bennett FS, DeLong WG, et al: Initial experience with the treatment of supracondylar intramedullary nail: A preliminary report. J Orthop Trauma 1994; 8:322.
11. David SM, Harrow ME, Peindl RD, et al: Comparative biomechanical analysis of supracondylar femur fracture fixation: Locked intramedullary nail versus 95-degree angled plate. J Orthop Trauma 1997; 11:344.
12. Firoozbakhsh K, Kambiz B, DeCoster TA, et al: Mechanics of retrograde nail versus plate fixation for supracondylar femur fractures. J Orthop Trauma 1995; 9:152.
13. Kraay MJ, Goldberg VM, Figgie MP, et al: Distal femoral replacement with allo-graft/prosthetic reconstruction for treatment of supracondylar fractures in patients with total knee arthroplasty. J Arthroplasty 1992; 7:7.
14. Bell KM, Johnstone AJ, Court-Brown CM, et al: Primary knee arthroplasty for distal femoral fractures in elderly patients. J Bone Joint Surg Br 1992; 74:400.
15. Freedman EL, Hak DJ, Johnson EE, et al: Total knee replacement including a modular distal femoral component in elderly patients with acute fracture or nonunion. J Orthop Trauma 1995; 9:231.
16. Bolhofner BR, Carmen B, Clifford P: The results of open reduction and internal fixation of distal femur fractures using a biologic (indirect) reduction technique. J Orthop Trauma 1996; 10:372.
17. Ostrum RF, Geel C: Indirect reduction and internal fixation of supracondylar femur fractures without bone graft. J Orthop Trauma 1995; 9:278.
18. Struhl S, Szporn MN, Cobelli NJ, et al: Cemented internal fixation for supracondylar femur fractures in osteoporotic patients. J Orthop Trauma 1990; 4:151.
19. Blatter G, König H, Janssen M, et al: Primary femoral shortening osteosynthesis in the management of comminuted supracondylar femoral fractures. Arch Orthop Trauma Surg 1994; 113:134.
20. Koval KJ, Seligson D, Rosen J, et al: Distal femoral nonunion: Treatment with a retrograde inserted locked intramedullary nail. J Orthop Trauma 1995; 9:285.

TRAUMATIC KNEE INJURIES

section 3
chapter 16

John T. Gorczyca

Summary

- Proper function of the knee is important in walking and in most activities. Injuries to the knee must be treated properly to maintain knee function.
- The vascular and neural structures that cross the knee are very susceptible to injury, and evaluation of the injured knee must start with these structures to detect and treat these injuries promptly.
- Knee injuries occur most commonly in association with other injuries, which must be properly evaluated and treated.
- The goals in treating fractures involving the knee are to restore the joint surface and mechanical alignment of the limb and to achieve optimal healing of bone, tendon, and ligaments, to allow painless function of the knee.
- Decisions regarding surgery for the patient with an injured knee must take into consideration the patient's age, health, and activity level.

TIBIAL PLATEAU FRACTURES

The tibial plateau consists of the medial tibial plateau and the lateral tibial plateau. These two smooth joint surfaces articulate with the respective femoral condyles. The tibial plateau supports forces that are greater than body weight during walking and much greater than body weight during running or when standing from a seated position.

Fractures of the tibial plateau may impair the precision with which the knee functions in several ways.[1] Prolonged immobilization of a tibial plateau fracture can result in significant loss of knee motion.[2] Fractures that heal with displacement at the articular surface are likely to result in degenerative changes of the articular surface.[3] Fractures with significant depression of the articular surface can result in instability of the knee. Fractures that heal in a malaligned position will result in an imbalance of forces at the plateau, with excessive compressive forces applied to the cartilage on one side of the joint and tension applied to the opposite collateral ligaments. This can result in articular degeneration and/or ligamentous laxity.

These fractures are important because improper care can result in significant morbidity, whereas proper diagnosis and treatment can predictably result in good or excellent functional outcomes in most patients.

HISTORICAL REVIEW

In the early 1950s, tibial plateau fractures were treated predominantly by traction or immobilization in splint. In 1958, the Arbeitsgemeinschaft für Osteosynthesefragen group began to study stable fixation techniques for operative stabilization of tibial plateau fractures to allow anatomic reduction and early postoperative knee motion. In 1979, Schatzker, McBroom, and Bruce reported their experience with surgical stabilization of select tibial plateau fractures: 89% of patients had acceptable results. Other authors have reported similar results with internal fixation.[3] There is a trend in the past several years to treat complex tibial plateau fractures with limited internal fixation in conjunction with external fixation.

PATHOGENESIS

Tibial plateau fractures are usually caused by a significant traumatic event resulting in axial load, a bending force, or a combination of the two.[4] Most injuries are caused by violent trauma such as motor vehicle, sporting, or industrial accidents. In elderly patients with osteopenic bone, the traumatic injury may be as insignificant as landing on the leg with the knee fully extended.

CLINICAL FEATURES

The patient with a tibial plateau fracture commonly presents with pain in the region of the knee after a traumatic event. The patient is unable to walk on the affected leg, and the knee appears swollen. A tense knee effusion may be present, but in many cases the hematoma may dissipate through the fracture into the leg compartments and the knee will not have a significant hemarthrosis. The patient may or may not be able to move the knee, depending on the inherent stability of the fracture and the patient's tolerance for pain. Gentle palpation of the knee region in the alert patient will allow localization of the injury to the tibial plateau. Occasionally, crepitation can be appreciated with palpation.

The examination must include thorough assessment of the vascular and neurological function of the extremity. The dorsalis pedis and posterior tibial pulses should be palpated, and capillary perfusion of the skin should be checked and compared with the contralateral side. The patient should be able to demonstrate active flexion and extension of the ankle and digits. Compartment syndrome of the leg must be ruled out at the initial examination and with serial examinations. Severe pain, difficulty with active motion of the ankle or toes, or pain with passive motion of the ankle or toes are early findings of compartment syndrome that cannot be overlooked. If the physical findings are not clear or if the patient cannot comply with the physical examination, then compartment pressure measurement should be performed.

Open wounds should be identified early.[5] Wounds that communicate with the fracture should have a sterile dress-

ing applied. Tetanus booster or immune globulin should be administered (if indicated) and appropriate antibiotic prophylaxis started while arranging for emergency irrigation and débridement of the open fracture.[6]

An extremely useful test on physical examination is stability of the fully extended knee to varus and valgus stress. This is often too uncomfortable for the nonanesthetized patient to tolerate. Varus or valgus laxity of greater than 10 degrees indicates significant articular depression or ligamentous injury, either of which carries a poor prognosis if treated nonoperatively.

The most widely accepted means for describing tibial plateau fractures is the Schatzker Classification (Fig. 1).[1] Type I tibial plateau fractures have a split (wedge) of the lateral tibial plateau. Type II fractures have a split of the lateral tibial plateau with associated depression of the weightbearing articular surface. Type III tibial plateau fractures have depression of the lateral plateau without an associated split (wedge). Type IV fractures involve the medial tibial plateau, and have a higher incidence of associated vascular and/or neural injury. Type V fractures involve both the medial and lateral plateaux, but some part of the articular surface remains in continuity with the tibial shaft. Type VI fractures, in addition to having an intraarticular component, include a fracture component that separates the metaphysis and diaphysis.

INVESTIGATION

Radiographic investigation of tibial plateau fractures must include anteroposterior radiographs of the knee and of the entire tibia. Traction films are also helpful. After viewing the tibial plateau fracture and determining how distal the fracture extends into the tibial shaft, it is important to rule out fracture involving the distal femur.

Anteroposterior and lateral tomography of the proximal tibia will allow accurate measurement of articular depression, if present. Injuries with multiple fractures of the articular surface are best evaluated with computed tomography (CT) scans. Sagittal and coronal plane reconstructions of the CT images will also allow assessment of articular displacement.

If the pedal pulses are diminished or if one has a high index of suspicion for a vascular injury, then an arteriogram of the superficial femoral artery with distal run-off (or, alternatively, the consultation of a vascular surgeon) should be obtained.

TREATMENT GOALS, INDICATIONS, AND CONTRAINDICATIONS

The goals in treating tibial plateau fractures are (1) to allow the fracture to heal in normal alignment with a congruous articular surface, (2) to return the patient to his or her previous level of functioning, and (3) to avoid complication.

In a healthy, active patient, nonoperative treatment is reserved for minimally displaced (<2 mm), stable fractures. In general, as patient age increases and activity level decreases, a larger amount of displacement can be tolerated. However, a tibial plateau fracture that demonstrates significant instability to varus or valgus stress due to displacement of a femoral condyle into a defect in the tibial plateau, almost always requires operative treatment if a

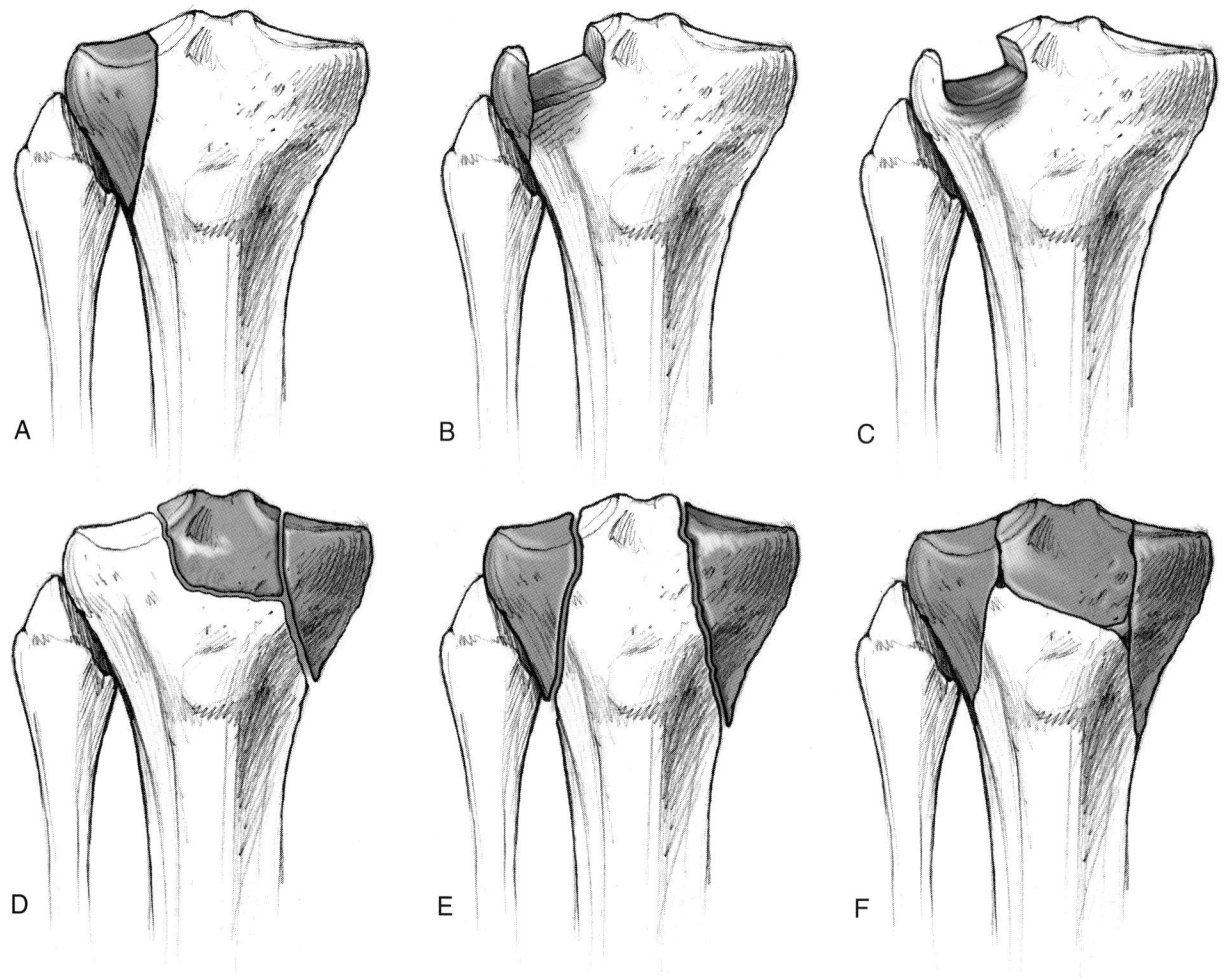

Fig. 1. The Schatzker classification of tibial plateau fractures. *A*, Type I tibial plateau fracture involves a split (wedge) on the lateral tibial plateau without articular depression. *B*, Type II tibial plateau fracture with split-depression involvement of lateral tibial plateau. *C*, Type III tibial plateau fracture involves depression of lateral articular surface and occurs most commonly in osteopenic bone. *D*, Type IV tibial plateau fracture involves the medial tibial plateau and represents high-energy injuries with a higher incidence of neural and vascular injuries. *E*, Type V tibial plateau fractures involve both the medial and lateral plateaux. *F*, Type VI tibial plateau fractures include a fracture component that separates the metaphysis from the diaphysis.

functioning knee is the goal. Nonoperative treatment consists of either traction or splinting initially, and then applying a cast-brace when the swelling diminishes and the patient is comfortable enough to begin protected knee motion.[7] Patients with complex fractures, however, may require long periods of immobilization before joint motion can be safely and comfortably initiated. The patient will begin resistive quadriceps exercises and weightbearing when the healing is sufficient to prevent fracture displacement, generally in 8 to 12 weeks (Table 1).

Tibial plateau fractures with minimal displacement of a large fragment can usually be reduced through percutaneous means. This is often true with type I fractures. These can be treated with percutaneous screw placement using fluoroscopic guidance (Fig. 2A) The percutaneous technique, with fluoroscopic guidance, avoids a larger surgical incision and does not necessitate significant elevation of tissue from the bony surface. Thus, there is minimal additional injury to the circulation of the bone and soft tissues, and consequently minimal impairment of healing. The drawback of this technique is that direct visualization of

the joint structures is not possible unless the surgeon uses an arthroscope.[8]

Tibial plateau fractures with moderate or significant articular depression or comminution cannot be reduced with closed or percutaneous means.[9, 10] These fractures require exposure of the fracture for open reduction and internal fixation. If the fracture involves only the medial or only the lateral tibial plateau (i.e., types I, II, III, and IV), then stabilization of the fracture with a single buttress plate is the preferred method after the joint surface has been reduced (Fig. 2B to D) In most cases that require elevation of a depressed articular surface, the articular surface will sink back into the void if it is not mechanically supported with bone graft[11] or bone graft substitute.

Tibial plateau fractures that involve both of the plateaux (types V and VI) represent a special problem. After reduction and stabilization of the articular surface, the next step is restoration of proper mechanical alignment to the tibia. A single plate, applied medially or laterally, is insufficient to stabilize this alignment. The use of both medial and lateral plates is an option, but it carries a significant risk

TABLE 1. TREATMENT OF TIBIAL PLATEAU FRACTURES

Treatment Type	Indications	Specific Treatment	Outcome
Nonoperative	Nondisplaced, stable fracture *or* very old or nonambulatory patient	Immobilization of knee until sufficient healing has occurred (4–8 weeks) to allow protected knee motion	Healing of fracture with limited but acceptable function
Percutaneous fixation	Schatzker I fractures with minimal, if any, displacement	Multiple lag screws inserted across fracture through small incisions Early, protected knee motion Delayed (6–8 weeks) weight-bearing	Healing of fracture, good function
Open reduction and internal fixation	Schatzker I, II, III, and IV fractures with displacement and/or instability	Large incision, articular surface visualized and reduced, bone grafting (if necessary) used to support articular surface, screws and plate maintain reduction of joint Early, protected knee motion	Healing of fracture with acceptable knee motion and a decreased incidence of post-traumatic articular degeneration (compared with nonoperative treatment of these fractures)
Open reduction with limited internal fixation, ring (hybrid) external fixation	Schatzker V and VI fractures in active patients	Provisional reduction of joint surface through limited incision; stabilization of joint reduction with wires attached to external fixator ring; ring connected by external fixator or Ilizarov device to tibial shaft	Healing of fracture with acceptable motion Decreased incidence of nonunion and wound healing problems; high incidence of pin-track infections

because the dissection required to expose both the medial and lateral surfaces of the proximal tibia can devitalize a significant portion of this bone, making nonunion of the fracture more common.

A better alternative for most Schatzker V and VI tibial plateau fractures is to reduce and stabilize the articular surface after exposing the joint through the fracture line and elevating as little periosteum off the bone as possible. Lag screws can be inserted percutaneously to minimize dissection. Bone graft is inserted and impacted, if indicated. Tensioned wires are used to secure the articular surface of the tibia to an external fixator ring. The ring is connected to one or more bars, which attach to the tibial shaft by half-pins and/or wires. This ring fixator will maintain proper axial alignment until healing has occurred (Fig. 2E and F). The technique requires an accurate knowledge of the fracture pattern and the cross-sectional anatomy of the proximal leg to avoid injuring the neurovascular structures with the wires.[12, 13]

PROCEDURES
Preoperative Planning

As previously mentioned, anteroposterior and lateral radiographs of the proximal tibia are recommended to evaluate the fracture. The complex geometry of multifragmentary fractures is best evaluated with the transverse plane images of a CT scan.[14] If articular depression is present, it can best be quantified by anteroposterior and lateral tomography or with reconstructed images from a CT scan.

More important than the nature of the fracture is the state of the patient. Healthy, young, active patients require a stable knee with full motion, proper mechanical alignment of the extremity, and a congruous articular surface to avoid degeneration of the articular cartilage. Debilitated,

older, sedentary patients can tolerate some mechanical malalignment or articular malreduction if they have a limited life expectancy. This is especially true if there is significant risk associated with surgery because of the patient's medical state. Nonambulatory patients are best treated nonoperatively, if possible.

If surgery is chosen as the treatment method, then a plan for approach to and fixation of the fracture is necessary. A drawing or tracing of the fracture should be made, then redrawn with the fracture in a reduced position. Next, the appropriate implants should be drawn in place. It must be noted that percutaneous reduction of a fracture is sometimes not possible. Thus, the surgeon who plans for percutaneous fixation with cannulated screws must also be prepared to perform open reduction and internal fixation using a buttress plate and screws. The surgeon should also be prepared to harvest iliac crest bone graft in most cases, as this is the most desirable substance for supporting an impacted articular surface after it is reduced.

Technical Details

Percutaneous fixation of a type I tibial plateau fracture is performed after the fracture is anatomically reduced. Usually, longitudinal traction on the leg will align the fracture, and any residual gap can be closed with a large pointed clamp applied percutaneously across the fracture. Care must be taken to avoid applying pressure to the skin with the clamp. Next, two or more guide wires are applied perpendicular to the fracture line, taking care to avoid the articular surface. Fracture reduction and proper wire placement must be confirmed on both anteroposterior and lateral radiographs before the lag screws are inserted. Washers should be used if the bone is osteopenic or weak.

Open reduction is performed through a medial parapatel-

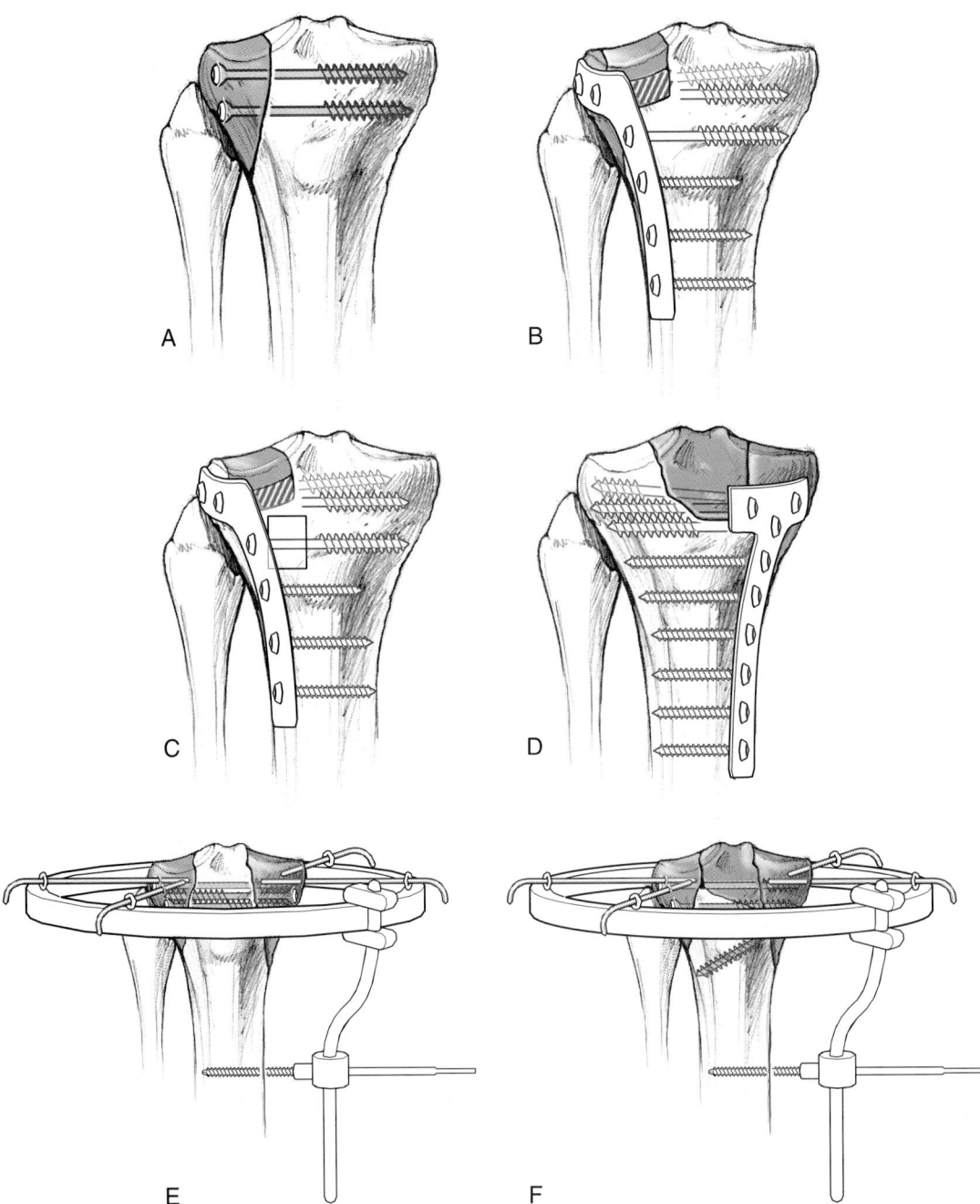

Fig. 2. Types of fixation. *A,* Fixation of a type I tibial fracture using two lag screws, which can be inserted by open or by percutaneous techniques. *B,* Fixation of a type II fracture is achieved by open reduction with elevation of the depressed articular surface, placement of bone graft to maintain articular reduction, and buttress plate stabilization. *C,* Fixation of a type III fracture requires elevation of the articular surface, bone grafting, and a buttress plate to stabilize the weak lateral metaphysis. *D,* Fixation of a type IV fracture using open reduction and a long medial buttress plate. *E,* Fixation of a type V fracture is achieved by limited open reduction, lag screw fixation, and ring fixator stabilization. *F,* Optimal fixation for a type VI fracture requires open reduction, lag screw fixation, and a ring fixator to maintain both length and alignment.

lar, lateral parapatellar, or midline incision, depending on whether the fracture involves the medial plateau, the lateral plateau, or both, respectively. If possible, the dissection should continue down to the fracture line, which can be gently opened to expose the articular fragments. If the bone quality is good, adequate stability of type I fractures can be obtained using lag screws or a buttress plate.[15] If a

buttress plate is to be used to stabilize the fracture, then extraperiosteal or subperiosteal dissection is performed to expose the bone. The meniscotibial attachment can be incised, allowing proximal retraction of the meniscus and excellent visualization of the articular surface. Nonabsorbable suture should be used to repair the meniscotibial attachment.

TABLE 2. COMPLICATIONS OF TIBIAL PLATEAU FRACTURES

Complication	Incidence (%)	Ways to Minimize	How to Treat
Infection	1–5	Perioperative antibiotics Sterile technique Postoperative drain	Emergent irrigation and débridement Intravenous antibiotics
Nonunion	<3	Achieve stable fixation Minimize periosteal stripping during surgery (visualize articular surface through fracture) Avoid elevation of periosteum from both plateaux	Revise fixation if necessary for stability, iliac crest bone grafting[16]
Degenerative knee arthritis	10–30	Aim for perfect articular congruity Reduce and stabilize axial alignment of limb	When severe, knee arthroplasty vs. arthrodesis Best treatment is prevention (Fig. 3)
Knee contracture	5–15	Obtain stable fixation of fracture Begin early, active knee motion	Consider manipulation vs. release of adhesions when fracture healing is complete

If the articular surface is depressed, it should be elevated from the cancellous bone with as much surrounding bone as possible. An osteotome is used to lift the bone en masse and over-reduce it slightly. After bone graft or bone graft substitute is packed beneath the bone, the fracture is closed

and provisionally stabilized with Kirschner's wires. Axial load is applied across the joint to reduce the articular surface and further impact the cancellous bone. Lag screws are then inserted parallel to the articular surface. The articular surface is then aligned to the shaft and stabilized with a lateral plate (Schatzker II and III), a medial plate (Schatzker IV), or a ring fixator (Schatzker V or VI).

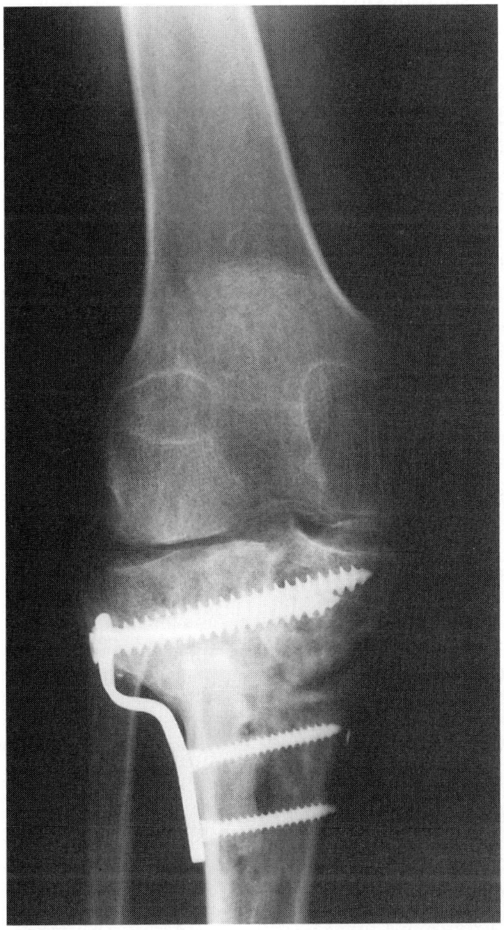

A thigh tourniquet will minimize bleeding during surgery. If a tourniquet is used, it should not remain inflated for longer than 2 hours, and hemostasis should be achieved before definitive wound closure. A large 4.8 mm suction drain placed deep to the fascia will minimize postoperative hematoma formation.

Postoperative Management

The extremity should be splinted with the knee flexed 30 to 40 degrees for 3 to 5 days to protect the soft tissues during the early healing phase. Then, active knee motion can be initiated, but resistive exercises must be avoided during the early postoperative period. The knee should be splinted in full extension during the interim to prevent flexion contracture. Likewise, the patient must not bear weight on the involved extremity until 8 to 12 weeks after surgery, when significant healing of the fracture will have occurred. At this point, physical therapy directed at quadriceps strengthening, overall extremity conditioning, and gait training can be initiated.

Complications and results are summarized in Table 2 and illustrated in Figure 3.

PATELLAR FRACTURES AND EXTENSOR MECHANISM DISRUPTIONS

The patellar tendon, patella, and patellar ligament are three integral components of the extensor mechanism of the knee. Displaced patellar fractures compromise function of the extensor mechanism, resulting in limited and weak knee extension. The joint reaction forces in the patellofemoral joint can approach six to eight times body weight. It follows that significant displacement or malposition of the patella's articular surface can create degenerative changes in the patellofemoral joint. Likewise, disruption of the pa-

Fig. 3. Improper treatment of a type VI tibial plateau fracture. A single plate and an imperfect articular reduction have resulted in malalignment, articular degeneration, and metaphyseal nonunion.

tellar tendon or ligament will result in significant impairment of active knee extension.

The goal in treating fractures of the patella or extensor mechanism is to achieve complete, anatomically correct healing so that the patient can achieve full strength, obtain normal knee motion, and return to previous activity level with minimal discomfort.

PATHOGENESIS

Most patellar fractures and extensor mechanism injuries result from a traumatic event in which the knee is flexed while the quadriceps muscle is forcefully contracting. A direct blow to the anterior knee, such as from a car dashboard or from a baseball bat, can also create a patellar fracture. In general, the greater the force applied to the patella at the time of fracture, the greater the comminution present and the more difficult open reduction and internal fixation of the patellar fracture will be.

CLINICAL FEATURES

Typically, patients have pain in the region of the knee after a traumatic event. Contusions and swelling are usually visible. Most patients are unable to actively extend the knee because of discontinuity of the extensor mechanism. With displaced patellar fractures, a defect is often palpable between the fracture fragments. Likewise, a defect can occasionally be appreciated just superior or inferior to the patella when the patellar tendon or patellar ligament is disrupted, respectively.

A multifragmentary patellar fracture may have palpable crepitation, but the absence of crepitation does not rule out fracture. If a tense knee effusion is present, aspiration will alleviate the patient's pain and provide the opportunity for intra-articular injection of anesthetic for thorough examination of the knee ligaments.

Patellar fractures are best classified by their radiographic appearance. Simple fractures have a single fracture line that can be vertical, horizontal, or oblique in its orientation. The location of the fracture in the inferior pole, mid-patella, or superior pole is helpful in the description. Fractures with comminution are best described by noting the portion of the patella that is comminuted and any other fracture lines (e.g., "a vertical fracture with inferior pole comminution"). Some high-energy fractures are highly comminuted (stellate) and are best described as such.

As important as the fracture type is the amount of displacement present. One must note whether longitudinal displacement between the fragments has occurred. Also, any step between fragments at the articular surface should be noted.

INVESTIGATION

Anteroposterior and lateral radiographs of the knee are necessary to evaluate patellar fractures. Additionally, a Merchant view, or any view taken tangential to the patellofemoral articulation, will provide more information on fractures and displacement in the horizontal and sagittal planes.

Tomography, computed tomography, and bone scanning are usually not required but may reveal nondisplaced fractures that escape detection by standard radiographic analysis.

TREATMENT GOALS, INDICATIONS, AND CONTRAINDICATIONS

As mentioned previously, the goals in treating patellar fractures and extensor mechanism injuries are to regain full, painless function of the knee and to avoid complications.

Nonoperative treatment is reserved for minimally displaced fractures of the patella.[17] In general, a step (articular incongruity) of up to 2 mm and a separation of up to 3 mm can be accepted.[18] The knee should be immobilized in full extension for approximately 6 weeks, after which progressive knee flexion and resistive knee extension exercises can be initiated. If the patient's activities are limited by chronic illness, however, then a greater amount of fracture displacement can be accepted for nonoperative treatment (Table 3).[19]

Operative treatment of patellar fractures is performed if significant displacement or articular incongruity is present and the patient is ambulatory. Simple, horizontal fractures are best treated with tension band wiring. Simple, vertical fractures are best treated with lag screws. Digital palpation of the articular surface should be performed through the retinacular tear (or a limited incision) to ensure accurate reduction before definitive fixation. Fractures with minimal comminution can be stabilized with a combination of lag screws and tension band wiring (Fig. 4.) In some cases, a combination of cerclage wire and a tension wire can be used to reduce and stabilize the fracture. Tension band wiring will provide fixation strong enough to allow early

TABLE 3. TREATMENT OF PATELLAR FRACTURES			
Treatment Type	**Indications**	**Specific Treatment**	**Outcome**
Nonoperative	Nonambulatory patient or minimally displaced fracture	Immobilize knee in extension for at least 6 weeks	Healing
Open reduction and internal fixation	Displaced fracture with minimal, if any, comminution	Lag screw fixation of vertical fracture (if present), tension band wiring of horizontal or oblique fracture	Good to excellent function
			Healed fracture
			Good motion
			Prominent wires
Partial patellectomy	Significant comminution with one or two large fragments remaining	Excision of small fragments, repair of extensor mechanism to retained fragment(s)	Good healing
			Good function
Complete patellectomy	Severely comminuted and displaced fracture	Excision of all bony fragments, repair of extensor mechanism	Fair to good results
			Weak knee extension
			Difficulty descending stairs

active knee motion, but is not strong enough to withstand resistive quadriceps exercises or walking.

If significant comminution has occurred in one part of the patella, occasionally a combination of cerclage wire and tension band wire can be used to reduce and stabilize the fracture. More commonly, however, treatment should consist of excision of the multiple small fragments and retention of one or two large fragments. This will provide good to excellent results in most cases.[20] Meticulous preservation of the soft-tissues and repair of the tendon or ligament to the bone with nonresorbable suture should be performed. A tension band wire or nonresorbable suture or tape fastened to the tibial tuberosity will protect the repair long enough to allow early active knee motion but will not withstand resistive quadriceps exercises. Care should be taken to repair the tissue to the patella as close to the

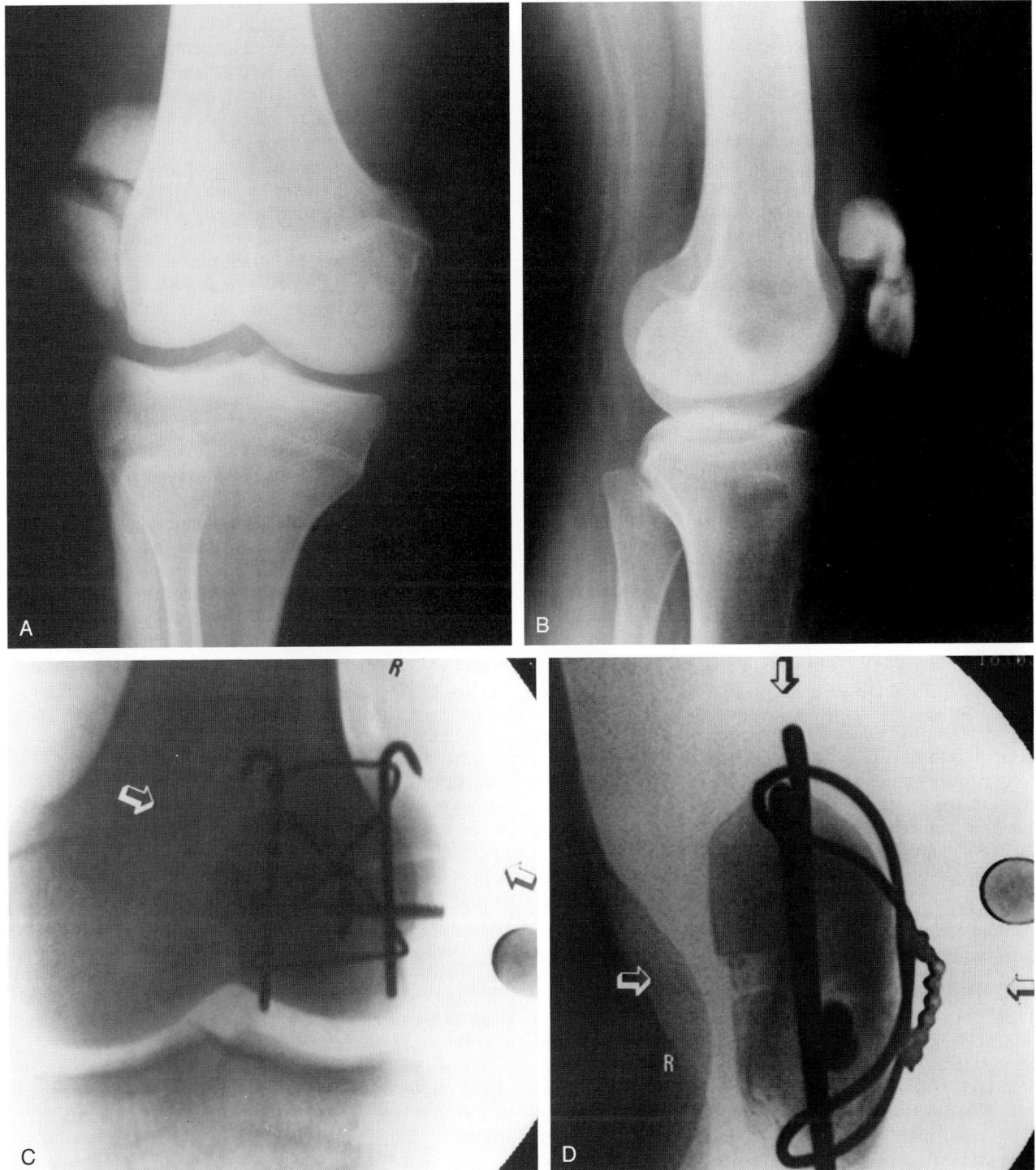

Fig. 4. Radiographs. *A* and *B,* AP and lateral radiographs of the knee demonstrate a multifragmentary patella fracture with three large fragments. *C* and *D,* Postoperative radiographs demonstrate reduction and stabilization with a lag screw, Kirschner wires, and tension band wiring.

articular surface as possible, to prevent patella tilting and abrasion of the femoral articular cartilage by the subchondral bone edge.

Occasionally, the patella has been pulverized so badly that repair is not feasible. It should be noted that when at least 25% of the length of the patella is present, the extensor mechanism will have acceptable function.[21] Complete patellectomy, however, will result in significant loss of knee extension strength.[22–24] Thus, complete patellectomy should be avoided whenever possible. When salvage of a portion of the patella is not possible, resection of the fragments and repair of the retinaculum should be performed. Complete excision of the patella will often result in lengthening of the extensor apparatus, so the retinaculum should be imbricated during the repair to shorten it and prevent extension lag.

After complete patellectomy, protection of the extensor mechanism repair cannot be achieved with a tension band wire or suture, as the patella is no longer present as a fixation point. Thus, early knee motion is usually unsafe. In these instances, knee immobilization in extension should be performed for at least 6 weeks.

If the extensor mechanism injury consists of disruption of the patellar tendon or ligament, repair should be performed with nonresorbable suture to the bone through drill holes. The patellar ligament, when repaired, should not be overtightened, as this will create patella baja. The repair can be protected with wire or Mersilene tape (Mersilene polyester fiber, Johnson and Johnson Ethicon, Somerville, NJ) from the patella to the tibial tuberosity.

PROCEDURES
Preoperative Planning

After analysis of the radiographs, the surgeon should have an understanding of the fracture pattern. The overall health and activity level of the patient should be considered. Even in the sick and elderly patient, however, operative repair of a patellar fracture is usually beneficial in that it will allow the patient to walk or transfer (e.g., from bed to chair).

Surgery can be performed through longitudinal or transverse incisions centered on the anatomic location of the patella. Prior to inflation of the tourniquet, wrapping an esmarch bandage from proximal to distal should lengthen the quadriceps muscle. This will facilitate approximation of the proximal and distal ends during surgery.

A true appreciation for the severity of comminution is often not gained until the fracture is surgically exposed. Thus, the surgeon should be prepared to use all of his or her surgical options—tension band wiring, lag screws, and partial patellectomy—when surgically treating a patellar fracture.

Technical Details

When tension band wiring of a simple fracture is performed, the fracture is initially reduced and stabilized with two parallel 1.6 mm Kirschner's wires. Next, a 1.0- or 1.2-mm cerclage wire is passed through the tendon and ligament posterior to the Kirschner wires. This can be placed in a simple loop or in a figure-of eight fashion, although most often a simple loop will provide more stability. Passage of the wire through the ligament and tendon is facilitated by passing a 14-gauge or 16-gauge angiocatheter in the desired position in the reverse direction, and then pass-

ing the cerclage wire through the Silastic catheter while extracting the needle from the catheter. The catheter is then withdrawn over the wire, and the wire ends are ready for tightening.

The Kirschner wires are bent to 180 degrees on one end, then rotated so that the bend will capture the tension band wire. After final tightening of the cerclage wire, the Kirschner wire is advanced and tapped into bone. The opposite end is cut short, if necessary, to prevent prominence of the hardware. After stabilization of the fracture, the tear in the retinaculum is repaired with a heavy, absorbable suture.

There is laboratory evidence to suggest that interfragmental lag screws used in conjunction with tension band wiring will resist displacement of a transverse fracture better than Kirschner's wires and tension band wiring.[25] A study demonstrating that this is a clinically significant difference has not been performed.

Vertical fractures can be repaired with lag screws after provisional Kirschner wire fixation. To palpate the fracture, the surgeon may need to incise the retinaculum enough to accommodate his or her finger. The patellar cartilage is 6 to 8 mm thick, so an intraoperative Merchant view is necessary to ensure that the screw threads do not protrude beyond the subchondral bone and into the thick articular cartilage.

If partial patellectomy is performed, repair of the patellar tendon or ligament to the remaining patellar fragments will be necessary. A trough should be created in the exposed bone close to the articular surface. Three drill holes should be made from the trough to the anterior surface of the patella, taking care to aim the drill to maximize the distance between the drill holes. Two separate sutures are passed in a modified Bunnell fashion through the tendon or ligament, one located entirely in the medial side and one in the lateral side. The sutures are then passed through the patella and tied. A tension band wire or a Mersilene tape that secures the patella to the tibial tuberosity will protect the repair of the patellar ligament. Such protection is not possible after patellar tendon repair. It is best to place and tie the protecting wire or tape at the appropriate length before tying the tendon repair, as this will help to prevent overtightening and the resultant patella baja.

Postoperative Management

After operative treatment of patellar fracture, the repair is never strong enough to tolerate resistive quadriceps exercises until significant healing has occurred. Thus, if the patient is allowed to bear weight on the extremity, it should be done with the knee immobilized in a brace in full extension. Active motion of the knee against gravity can usually be tolerated, but terminal stretching is prohibited until significant healing of the repair has occurred. This typically takes 6 weeks in a healthy patient with a patellar fracture, and 8 to 12 weeks with patellar tendon or patellar ligament repair.

When the surgeon considers the repair strong enough to allow progressive resistance to the quadriceps muscles, quadriceps sets and gait training without a brace are allowed.

COMPLICATIONS AND RESULTS

The best results in treating patellar fractures are obtained when precise anatomic reduction and stable fixation are achieved.[26] Chronic pain or quadriceps weakness are not uncommon after patellar fractures, particularly when the fracture diastasis is greater than 2 mm or the joint incongruity is greater than 1 mm.[27] It is not clear whether these chronic symptoms are a result of the imperfect reduction, or whether they result from irreversible cartilage injury sustained at the trauma. It is likely that both contribute to the symptoms.

Infection occurs in less than 2% of closed patellar fractures. The incidence can be minimized by providing prophylactic antibiotics and by following sterile technique.

Nonunion of the patella is very uncommon if the bone ends are not widely separated. It can be prevented by minimizing stripping of the patella fragments during open reduction and internal fixation. Excision of small, comminuted fragments will also decrease the incidence of this complication, as these fragments are often devitalized and may not contribute to fracture healing. If the nonunion creates significant symptoms, stable internal fixation or partial patellectomy will usually lead to improvement.[28]

Symptomatic hardware is a common complication because most people have minimal subcutaneous tissue about the patella, so the wires or sutures are often prominent.[29,30] It must be remembered that stable fracture repair is of paramount importance, and that prominent hardware can be removed when healing and remodeling are complete, usually 12 months after surgery. If possible, however, the Kirschner wires should be cut so that they do not protrude, and the cerclage wire twist should not be located anterior to the patella, as in that location it is impossible to bend the wire so that it will not be prominent.

Arthritis after patellar fracture may occur with a large step at the articular surface, but it is not known how large a step can be tolerated without producing articular degeneration. What has been shown is that a patella that is rotated in the sagittal plane due to repair of the tissues too far anteriorly will almost certainly result in patellofemoral arthritis.[31] Repairing the patellar tendon or ligament to the patella as close to the articular surface as possible will help to prevent this complication.

Patella enlargement, caused by aggressive healing after repair of a comminuted fracture, has also been correlated with degenerative arthritis of the patellofemoral joint. For this reason, treatment of symptomatic patella enlargement with patellectomy occasionally improves knee function.

KNEE DISLOCATIONS

Knee dislocation results from a significant traumatic event to the lower extremity. The force must be significant enough to injure several stabilizing structures before the knee dislocates. The popliteal artery, popliteal vein, and sciatic nerve cross the knee and are susceptible to injury when the knee dislocates. Thus, improper treatment can result in a painful, stiff, unstable knee and, in some cases, loss of limb.

CLINICAL FEATURES

Patients who have sustained a knee dislocation will generally have a history of a significant force to the knee, although some cases may occur with a low-energy event, particularly in obese patients. Most often, patients report pain in the knee and inability to walk. The appearance of the extremity can be deceiving, as the knee may spontaneously reduce shortly after the injury, and, because of a tear in the capsule, an appreciable effusion may not be present.

If the knee appears bent or dislocated, the physician must assume that it is dislocated and attempt to reduce it with manual traction. Usually, reduction of the dislocated knee is appreciated and the patient experiences improved comfort. Undue delay should be avoided prior to performing such a maneuver, because emergency reduction of the dislocated knee will improve circulation to the limb and reduce excessive pressure on the soft tissues due to the deformity.

Usually, active knee motion will be limited by the patient's discomfort. It is essential that accurate examination of pedal pulses and distal perfusion be performed. Early detection and repair of an associated vascular injury is essential to maintain limb viability and function.[32] Thorough examination of limb sensory and motor function is essential to identify nerve injury, if present. Compartment syndrome is always a threat and must be ruled out initially and with serial examination.

Stress examination of the dislocated knee will usually reveal multidirectional instability. Knee dislocation usually involves disruption of both cruciate ligaments and at least one of the collateral ligaments. Varus or valgus instability of the fully extended knee indicates that the cruciate ligaments, in addition to the appropriate collateral ligament, have been disrupted. This can be confirmed by gently testing the anterior and posterior stability of the knee at 90 degrees of flexion (anterior and posterior drawer tests) and by testing the anterior and posterior stability with the knee flexed 30 degrees (Lachman's test).

Varus and valgus stability should also be tested at 30 degrees of flexion, which would detect injury to the medial or lateral collateral ligaments if the cruciate ligaments were intact. Isolated ligament injuries do not allow dislocation of the knee and are discussed in depth in Chapters 4-11 and 4-12.

Injury to the posterior cruciate ligament can be diagnosed with the posterior sag sign when the patient relaxes with the hip and knee held in 90 degrees of flexion. Gravity will cause a posterior cruciate ligament–deficient knee to subluxate posteriorly. Additionally, the knee will hyperextend and the femur will externally rotate with respect to the tibia when the extremity is lifted by the great toe (hallux). After complete examination of the involved knee and extremity, it should be splinted with the knee in slight flexion.

Classification of knee dislocation is by direction of displacement of the tibia with respect to the femur.[33] Anterior dislocation and posterior dislocation constitute approximately 75% of all knee dislocations. Anterior dislocation is commonly caused by forceful knee hyperextension (Fig. 5). Posterior dislocation is usually caused by a posteriorly directed force applied to the proximal tibia, as in a dashboard injury in a motor vehicle accident. With anterior and posterior knee dislocation, the popliteal artery can be either avulsed or torn as the knee displaces. Popliteal arterial injury is less common with other types of dislocation.

Medial dislocations are caused by varus force to the knee. Lateral dislocations are caused by valgus force

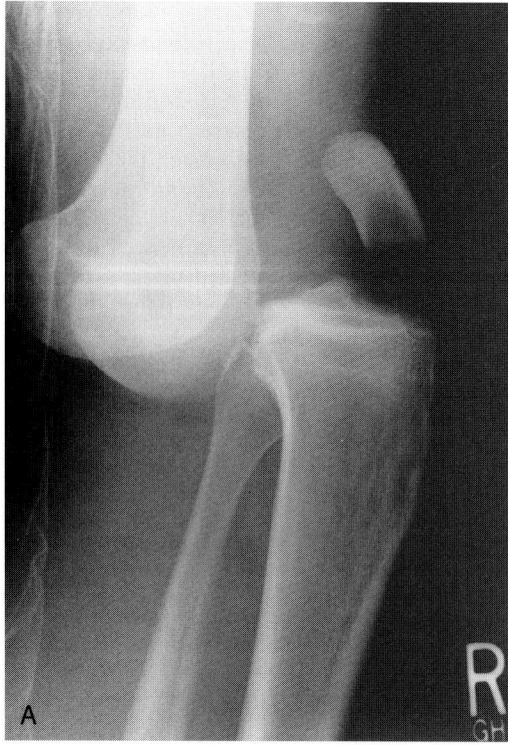
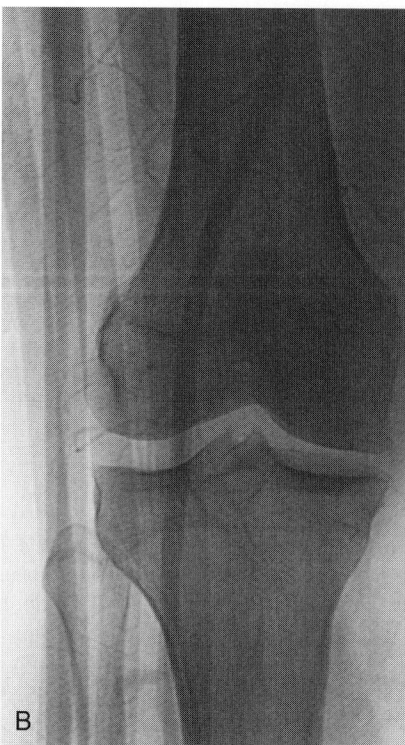

Fig. 5. Views. *A,* Lateral radiograph of the knee shows an anterior dislocation. *B,* After reduction of the dislocation, an arteriogram was obtained. No evidence of arterial injury was visualized.

(Fig. 6). Rotational dislocations are caused by a combination of rotational force and bending force.[34]

INVESTIGATION

Radiographs of the knee must include anteroposterior and lateral views. If radiographs are taken after spontaneous or manual reduction of the dislocation, the alignment of the limb may appear normal but the radiograph may reveal avulsed bone fragments caused by the dislocation (e.g., lateral capsular sign.)

If the mechanism of dislocation is high energy or if any sign of vascular impairment is present, then an emergency arteriogram should be performed to diagnose the lesion early and allow rapid repair of the vascular injury.

TREATMENT GOALS, INDICATIONS, AND CONTRAINDICATIONS

The goal in treating the dislocated knee is to return the limb to normal viability and function. The first priority is to reduce the joint and to detect vascular injury if present.[35] The next priority is to regain knee motion and stability. When ligamentous healing is complete, rehabilitation to restore strength and endurance to the extremity is necessary.

Nonoperative treatment is contraindicated in the healthy person with an active lifestyle. However, an elderly, inactive patient with good perfusion to the distal extremity can be treated nonoperatively. Any resulting knee instability could be treated with a brace, if necessary.

Open reduction of the dislocated knee is rarely necessary, but if the knee cannot be reduced by closed means, an open reduction should be performed on an emergency basis. This occurs most commonly with the posterolateral

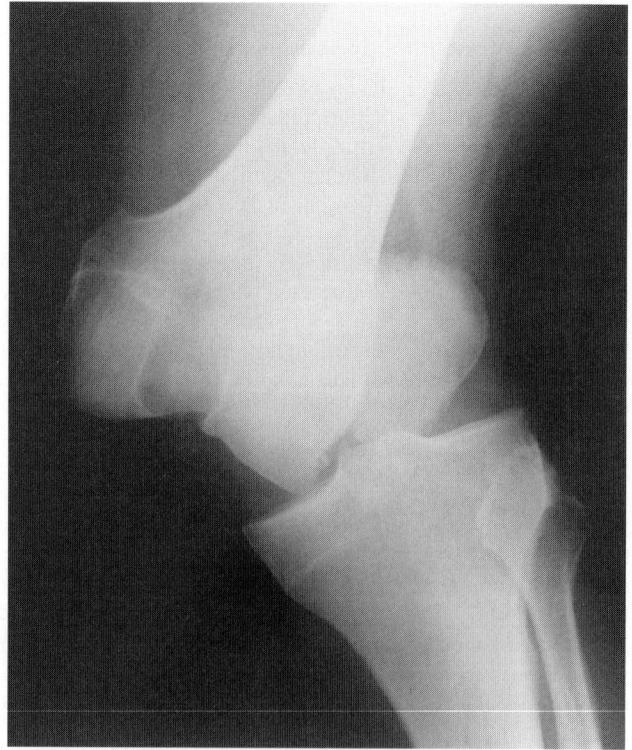

Fig. 6. AP radiograph of the knee. Demonstrates a lateral dislocation of the knee. This injury completely disrupted the anterior cruciate, the posterior cruciate, the medial collateral, and the lateral collateral ligaments.

dislocation of the knee, in which the medial femoral condyle is buttonholed through the capsule.[36] Open treatment is performed through a medial parapatellar incision and the capsular rent is extended longitudinally to allow reduction of the condyle. Any torn structures that are visualized (meniscus, ligaments) are repaired at this time.[37]

Ligamentous reconstruction is commonly used for the healthy, active patient after knee dislocation. It is believed that the knee will function better if the initial swelling of the injury subsides before ligamentous reconstruction is performed. Thus, most surgeons will treat the patient with physical therapy directed at maintaining knee motion and preventing significant muscular atrophy. Reconstruction of all of the torn ligaments is generally performed within 2 to 4 weeks.

RESULTS

After proper treatment of all disrupted ligaments and meniscal tears in a knee that has dislocated, knee instability is not usually a problem. Patients are much more likely to experience knee stiffness and discomfort and must adopt a less active, less strenuous lifestyle. The details of complex ligamentous injuries to the knee are discussed more completely in Chapter 4-13.

REFERENCES

1. Schatzker J, McBroom R, Bruce D: The tibial plateau fracture: The Toronto experience 1968–1975. Clin Orthop 1979, 138:94.
2. Roberts JM: Fractures of the condyles of the tibia. J Bone Joint Surg Am 1968; 50:1505.
3. Blokker CP, Rorabeck CH, Bourne RB: Tibial plateau fractures: An analysis of the results of treatment in 60 patients. Clin Orthop 1984; 182:193.
4. Kennedy JC, Bailey WH: Experimental tibial plateau fractures. J Bone Joint Surg Am 1968; 50:1522.
5. Tscherne H, Lobenhoffer P: Tibial plateau fractures: Management and expected results. Clin Orthop 1993; 292:87.
6. Gustilo RB, Anderson JJ: Prevention of infection in the treatment of one thousand and twenty-five open fractures of long bones. J Bone Joint Surg Am 1976; 58:453.
7. Brown GA, Sprague BL: Cast brace treatment of plateau and bicondylar fractures of the proximal tibia. Clin Orthop 1976; 119:184.
8. Scheerlinck T, Ng CS, Handelberg F, et al: Medium-term results of percutaneous arthroscopically-assisted osteosynthesis of fractures of the tibial plateau. J Bone Joint Surg Br 1998; 80:959.
9. Duwelius PJ, Rangitsch MR, Colville MR, et al: Treatment of tibial plateau fractures by limited internal fixation. Clin Orthop 1997; 339:47.
10. Koval KJ, Sanders R, Borrelli J, et al: Indirect reduction and percutaneous screw fixation of displaced tibial plateau fractures. J Orthop Trauma 1992; 6:340.
11. Lachiewicz PF, Funcik T: Factors influencing the results of open reduction and internal fixation of tibial plateau fractures. Clin Orthop 1990; 257:210.
12. Marsh JT, Smith ST, Do TT: External fixation and limited internal fixation for complex fractures of the tibial plateau. J Bone Joint Surg Am 1995; 77:661.
13. Watson JT: High-energy fractures of the tibial plateau. Orthop Clin North Am 1994; 25:723.
14. Chan PS, Klimkiewicz JJ, Luchetti WT, et al: Impact of CT scan on treatment plan and fracture classification of tibial plateau fractures. J Orthop Trauma 1997; 11:484.
15. Koval KJ, Polatsch D, Kummer FJ, et al: Split fractures of the lateral tibial plateau: Evaluation of three fixation methods. J Orthop Trauma 1996; 10:304.
16. King GJ, Schatzker J: Nonunion of a complex tibial plateau fracture. J Orthop Trauma 1991; 5:209.
17. Braun W, Wiedemann M, Ruter A, et al: Indications and results of nonoperative treatment of patellar fractures. Clin Orthop 1993; 289:197.
18. Sanders R: Patella fractures and extensor mechanism injuries. In Browner BD, Jupiter JB, Levine AM, et al (eds): Skeletal Trauma. Philadelphia: W.B. Saunders, 1992, p 1685.
19. Pritchett JW: Nonoperative treatment of widely displaced patella fractures. Am J Knee Surg 1997; 10:145.
20. Saltzman CL, Goulet JA, McClellan RT, et al: Indications and results of treatment of displaced patellar fractures by partial patellectomy. J Bone Joint Surg 1990; 72:1279.
21. Kaufer H: Mechanical function of the patella. J Bone Joint Surg Am 1971; 53:1551.
22. Jakobsen J, Christensen KS, Rasmussen OS: Patellectomy: A 20-year follow-up. Acta Orthop Scand 1985; 56:430.
23. Sutton FS Jr, Thompson CH, Lipke J, et al: The effect of patellectomy on knee function. J Bone Joint Surg 1976; 58:537.
24. Wilkinson J: Fracture of the patella treated by total excision: A long-term follow-up. J Bone Joint Surg Br 1977; 59(3):352.
25. Burvant JG, Thomas KA, Alexander R, Harris MB: Evaluation of methods of internal fixation of transverse patella fractures: a biomechanical study. J Orthop Trauma 1994; 8(2):147.
26. Levack B, Flannagan JP, Hobbs S: Results of surgical treatment of patellar fractures. J Bone Joint Surg 1985; 67:416.
27. Edwards B, Johnell O, Redlund-Johnell I: Patellar fractures: A 30-year follow-up. Acta Orthop Scand 1989; 60:712.
28. Klassen JF, Trousdale RT: Treatment of delayed and nonunion of the patella. J Orthop Trauma 1997; 11:188.
29. Catalano JB, Iannacone WM, Marczyk S, et al: Open fractures of the patella: Long-term functional outcome. J Trauma 1995; 39:439.
30. Smith ST, Cramer KE, Karges DE, et al: Early complications in the operative treatment of patella fractures. J Orthop Trauma 1997; 11:188.
31. Duthie HL, Hutchinson JR: The results of partial and total patellectomy. J Bone Joint Surg Br 1958; 40:75.
32. Green NE, Allen BL: Vascular injuries associated with dislocation of the knee. J Bone Joint Surg Am 1977; 59:236.
33. Kennedy JC: Complete dislocation of the knee joint. J Bone Joint Surg Am 1963; 45:887.
34. Tornetta P III: Knee dislocation. In Levine AM (ed): Orthopaedic Knowledge Update: Trauma. Rosemont, IL: American Academy of Orthopaedic Surgeons, 1996, p 145.
35. Reckling FW, Peltier LF: Acute knee dislocations and their complications. J Trauma 1969; 9:181.
36. Quinlan AG, Sharrard WJW: Postero-lateral dislocation of the knee with capsular interposition. J Bone Joint Surg Br 1958; 40:660.
37. Meyer MH, Moore TM, Harvey JP Jr: Traumatic dislocation of the knee joint. J Bone Joint Surg Am 1975; 57:430.

TIBIAL SHAFT FRACTURES

A. Paige Whittle and Justin P. Hawes

Summary

- The tibial shaft is the most commonly fractured long bone, resulting in approximately 77,000 hospitalizations per year.[1] Open fractures are more common in the tibial shaft than in any other major long bone.
- Fractures resulting from high-energy mechanisms have higher complication rates. In these fractures, careful attention must be paid to associated soft-tissue injury as well as fracture morphology when planning for fixation.
- Treatment options include casting or functional bracing (stable closed fractures), plate fixation (closed periarticular fractures), reamed or unreamed intramedullary (IM) nailing (unstable closed and most open fractures), external fixation (open periarticular fractures, severe open fractures), and early amputation (mangled extremities).
- Nonunion, malunion, infection, and joint stiffness are common complications of tibial shaft fractures and may be reduced by correctly applying principles of skeletal stabilization and soft-tissue management.

The tibial shaft is the most commonly fractured long bone.[2] Because these fractures have a wide spectrum of patterns and locations, no single ideal treatment exists. Other factors such as stability, displacement, mechanism, associated soft-tissue injury, neurovascular status, age, general medical condition, and functional demands must be considered when planning for fracture treatment. Closed, stable, minimally displaced fractures resulting from a low-energy mechanism are usually amenable to nonoperative treatment with casts or functional braces.[3, 4] Fractures caused by high-energy trauma are frequently unstable, comminuted, and associated with varying degrees of open or closed soft-tissue damage. High-energy fractures usually require operative stabilization to obtain optimal results,[5] and complications are more common. Plate fixation, external fixation, and reamed or unreamed IM nailing have all been advocated for treatment of tibial shaft fractures, and each method has specific, but overlapping indications.[6-9] In severe mangling injuries, early amputation may be the best treatment option.[10]

Soft-tissue assessment is just as important as fracture morphology when developing a treatment strategy. The tibia's subcutaneous anteromedial border makes it more prone to open fractures than any other major long bone.[11] Closed soft-tissue injuries (contusion, muscular crush, closed degloving) can be just as significant as open wounds in outcome and are important to consider when developing a treatment plan.[12] As late as the end of the

19th century, open tibial fractures were associated with such a high mortality rate that they were most likely to be treated with amputation.[13] Over the last 100 years, in particular the last few decades, improved skeletal fixation combined with better open wound management (débridement, antibiotics, early soft-tissue coverage[14]) has enabled the orthopaedic surgeon to salvage all but the most severely traumatized limbs.[15] Currently, the decision to amputate is difficult in many cases. Although it may be technically possible to save the extremity, the patient may have a better functional result with amputation.[16]

PATHOGENESIS

Several mechanisms are responsible for causing tibial shaft fractures. They may be broadly classified as producing direct or indirect (torsional) forces. It is equally important to recognize the degree of energy imparted by the particular mechanism. Fractures caused by a high-energy mechanism are usually more severe. They have a higher degree of comminution and a greater extent of concomitant soft-tissue injury and are associated with a poorer prognosis.

Torsional fractures occur when the body rotates around a fixed foot and result in a typical spiral pattern.[17] These fractures usually are the result of low-energy trauma and consequently are stable and minimally displaced with little soft-tissue damage. Nonoperative interventions are generally sufficient to provide an uncomplicated treatment course. Greater amounts of energy, however, may be involved in certain cases such as high-velocity ski accidents or ground-level falls in an obese individual (energy $\propto$ mass $\times$ velocity^2)[18] (Fig. 1). Direct injuries from three- or four-point bending stresses usually cause transverse or short oblique fractures, often with an associated wedge-shaped butterfly fragment.[17] A greater distance between bending points and increased energy transmission will result in comminuted or segmental fractures with a higher degree of soft-tissue injury (Fig. 2). Direct trauma may also cause a crushing injury when a large force is applied to a relatively small area.[17] Fractures usually are comminuted and associated with significant soft-tissue damage.

Although gunshot wounds are technically open injuries, fractures caused by low-velocity weapons (less than 2000 ft/s [most handguns]) usually are not severe.[19] Comminuted fragments, if present, are often minimally displaced and retain their soft-tissue attachments. High-velocity weapons (greater than 2000 ft/s) and close-range shotgun blasts, however, cause severe open fractures associated with significant soft-tissue loss.[20]

Stress fractures of the tibia are due to repetitive microtrauma, which results in fatigue failure of bone. They frequently occur after a sudden increase in activity and are discussed further in Chapter 4–4. Neoplastic, infectious, iat-

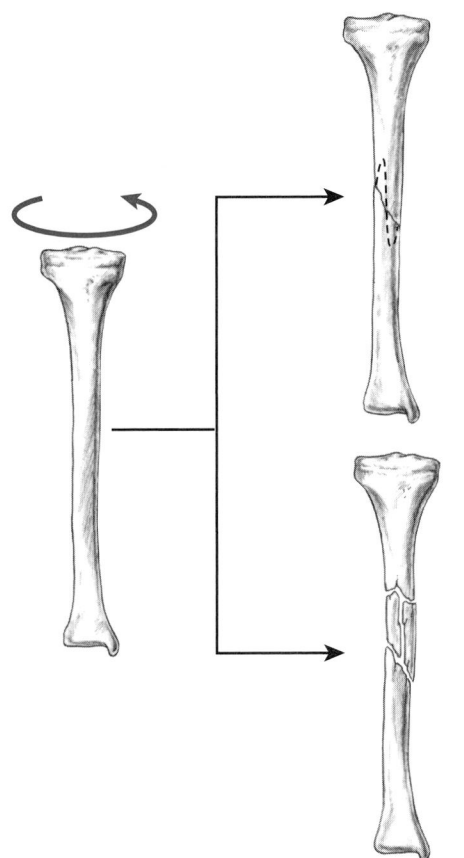

Fig. 1. Torsional fracture. Torsional force leads to a simple or comminuted spiral fracture depending on the energy transferred.

rogenic (i.e., surgery), and metabolic processes have the potential to weaken bone pathologically and make it more prone to fracture,[18] even with normal load-bearing activities. Recognition and treatment of pathological fractures are discussed further in Chapter 7–17.

CLINICAL FEATURES

Most acute tibial shaft fractures can be diagnosed with a good history, physical examination, and routine anteroposterior (AP) and lateral radiographs. Patients present with pain, variable amounts of swelling and deformity, and inability to bear weight. Associated neurological complaints such as tingling, numbness, and weakness may also be present. Fractures resulting from high-energy mechanisms often have open wounds and soft-tissue loss.

It is important to ascertain the details of the traumatic event as accurately as possible. The mechanism points to the amount of energy transmitted, the likely fracture severity, and the potential for associated soft-tissue damage and other injuries. Open fractures that occur in contaminated environments require special consideration regarding choice of antibiotics and method of fixation. Knowing the time that elapsed between injury and treatment is important when the fracture is associated with open wounds, vascular damage, or compartment syndrome.[10, 21] A full medical history should be obtained with emphasis on elements that could impact the patient's acute treatment or long-term

rehabilitation (e.g., previous functional level, previous lower extremity injury, diabetes, peripheral vascular disease, nicotine use).

Initial physical examination should focus on the entire patient and follow advanced trauma life support protocol in polytrauma cases.[22] The skeletal, cutaneous, neurological, vascular, and musculotendinous structures of the entire injured extremity are then examined with a high index of suspicion for associated injuries. The fracture site is tender, often with palpable bony irregularity and crepitation. The presence of deformity is a sign of probable skeletal injury. Boggy soft-tissue swelling could signify an underlying hematoma or a closed degloving injury. Tense swelling should alert the examiner to the potential for compartment syndrome.

Assessment of skin integrity requires circumferential inspection of the leg. Any wound extending through the dermis, regardless of size or distance from the fracture, should be considered an open fracture until proved otherwise. Distant wounds may be caused by initial fracture displacement. Small wounds with persistent bleeding and visible fat droplets are indicative of a communicating fracture. Obvious open wounds should be inspected for anatomic structures and foreign debris and then superficially cleansed and sterilely dressed. Deep wound probing and débridement may cause more harm than good and should

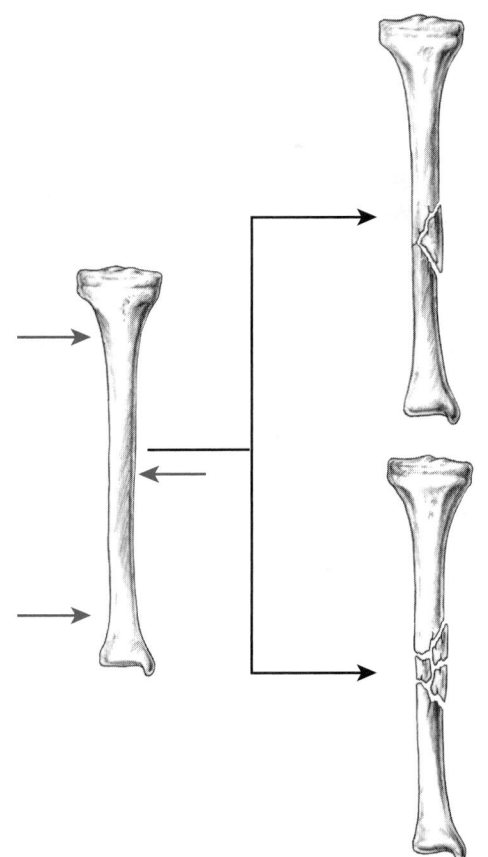

Fig. 2. Segmental fractures. Bending forces cause transverse/oblique fractures with comminution depending on energy and bending point location.

be saved for the operating room. A well-padded splint should be applied to stabilize the leg.

Significant soft-tissue injuries do not necessarily involve open wounds. Abrasions, ecchymoses, and fracture blisters may indicate a significant closed soft-tissue injury.[12] Closed degloving injuries may take several days to manifest their true severity, with gradual loss of perfusion and eschar formation.

The presence and quality of the distal pedal pulses should be documented (using a Doppler device if necessary), as should the color, temperature, and capillary refill of the foot and toes. The function of all nerves that innervate the lower leg (deep peroneal, superficial peroneal, tibial, saphenous, sural) and the strength of the major muscles should be assessed and monitored closely, being aware that sensory and motor deficits may be due to ischemia.

CLASSIFICATION

Numerous classification systems have been proposed for tibial shaft fractures in an attempt to determine prognosis and develop appropriate treatment protocols. Systems like those proposed by Johner and Wruhs (with further development by Müller) focus primarily on fracture morphology and injury mechanism.[17] Soft-tissue injury is most commonly described using the Gustilo-Anderson classification[23, 24] for open fractures and the Tscherne classification for closed soft-tissue injury[12] (Tables 1 and 2). Both Ellis[25] and Nicoll[26] attempted to combine fracture morphology and soft-tissue injury in describing fracture severity. Although of prognostic and statistical value, these classifications do not aid in the selection of treatment.

The Modified Tibial Fracture Classification (Table 3) as described by Trafton combines the Ellis, Gustilo-Anderson, and Tscherne classifications and adds modifications suggested by Leach.[27] The injury characteristic of the highest severity is used to grade the fracture. Although this system is relatively easy to use, it has not yet been clinically proved to be of prognostic value.

INVESTIGATION

Adequate AP and lateral radiographs, including the knee and ankle, provide information about fracture location and

TABLE 1. GUSTILO-ANDERSON CLASSIFICATION OF OPEN FRACTURES[23]

Grade	Description
I	Clean wound <1 cm
II	Laceration >1 cm without extensive soft-tissue damage, flags, or avulsions
IIIa	Extensive laceration (>10 cm) with adequate local soft-tissue coverage available or high-energy trauma regardless of wound size; segmental fractures
IIIb	Extensive soft-tissue loss requiring local or free flap coverage, usually associated with massive contamination
IIIc	Vascular injury requiring repair

From Boynton MD, Schmeling GJ: Nonreamed intramedullary nailing of open tibial fractures. J Am Acad Orthop Surg 1994; 2:107. Copyright 1994 American Academy of Orthopaedic Surgeons.

TABLE 2. TSCHERNE CLASSIFICATION OF CLOSED FRACTURES[12]

Grade	Classification
0	Indirect-force injury with negligible soft-tissue damage
I	Low- to moderate-energy injury with superficial abrasions and contusions
II	High-energy injury with significant muscle contusion and deep contaminated skin abrasions; risk of compartment syndrome
III	High-energy injury with subcutaneous degloving and possible arterial injury of compartment

From Boynton MD, Schmeling GJ: Nonreamed intramedullary nailing of open tibial fractures. J Am Acad Orthop Surg 1994; 2:107. Copyright 1994 American Academy of Orthopaedic Surgeons.

configuration and are usually sufficient to confirm the diagnosis of a suspected tibial shaft fracture. Oblique views of the tibia may be needed to visualize a nondisplaced spiral fracture. Other imaging techniques such as computed tomography, magnetic resonance imaging, and bone scanning are useful in certain situations such as periarticular fractures, infection, stress fractures, and pathological fractures.

Associated injuries may also require further investigation. Arteriography is not necessary when there are obvious signs of vascular injury, but it is useful in evaluating cases with an equivocal vascular examination[28] and in planning soft-tissue coverage. Electromyographic changes after nerve injury are not evident for at least 2 to 3 weeks after the insult but may be used to monitor recovery during rehabilitation. There should be a low threshold for obtaining pressure measurements in patients with tense compartments or altered mental status. There is no clear evidence that the use of routine cultures in open fractures is useful for patient management other than in cases of suspected infection.[29] A Gram stain should be performed in cases of suspected clostridial myonecrosis.

GOALS OF TREATMENT

Generally, the goals of treatment are to obtain a united fracture with minimal deformity or pain while avoiding additional morbidity and returning the patient to his or her previous functional level. Fracture reduction should focus on maintaining limb length and alignment.[30] General guidelines for adequate tibial shaft reduction are 5 degrees or less of coronal angulation, 10 degrees or less of sagittal and rotational deformity, and less than 1.5 cm of shortening.[18] In practice, goals and expectations will differ greatly, and full functional recovery may not always be possible.

INDICATIONS AND CONTRAINDICATIONS

Although general guidelines have been formulated, indications for operative and nonoperative management of tibial shaft fractures overlap to some extent. Choosing a treatment method requires balancing the expected benefits against short- and long-term risks (Table 4).

TABLE 3. MODIFIED TIBIAL FRACTURE CLASSIFICATION

Injury Characteristics	Extent of Injury		
	Minor	*Moderate*	*Major*
Fracture displacement	<50%	50%	Tibial or fibular displacement
Comminution	Minimal	0 or 1 butterfly fragment	>2 free segments or segmental
Wound grade: closed	0	I	II or III
Wound grade: open	I	II	III or IV (Tscherne)
			or
			IIIa-IIIc (Gustilo)
Energy	Low	Moderate	High
Fracture pattern	Spiral	Oblique or transverse	Transverse or fragmented

From Boynton MD, Schmeling GJ: Nonreamed intramedullary nailing of open tibial fractures. J Am Acad Orthop Surg 1994; 2:107. Copyright 1994 American Academy of Orthopaedic Surgeons.

CLOSED TREATMENT

Although improved operative techniques have narrowed the indications,[31–34] many tibial fractures are still amenable to closed reduction and immobilization in a cast or functional brace.[4] Closed treatment is limited primarily to closed, isolated, minimally displaced, axially stable, low-energy tibial shaft fractures[4] or minor open fractures such as those caused by a low-velocity gunshot.[4]

Successful treatment requires acceptable reduction using closed methods and a fracture pattern stable enough to allow early weightbearing[35] (Fig. 3). Features indicative of instability include greater than 50% comminution, more than 50% initial displacement, initial shortening greater than 15 mm, and spiral fractures of the distal third of the tibia. Unstable fractures treated nonoperatively have a higher incidence of malunion than similar fractures treated surgically.[33]

In addition to instability, other contraindications to closed treatment include most open fractures, multiple reduction attempts, periarticular and intra-articular fractures, vascular injury, compartment syndrome, and severe closed soft-tissue injury. Certain patient factors such as noncompliance, impaired sensation, multiple injuries, and obesity will necessitate operative treatment.[30]

PLATING

Plates provide stable fixation, maintain length and alignment, and allow early motion of adjacent joints but require soft-tissue stripping. Plating is primarily indicated for tibial fractures with intra-articular extension and metaphyseal fractures with minimal soft-tissue injury (Fig. 4). Significant open or closed soft-tissue injury is a contraindication to acute tibial plating because of the high risk of infection and wound complications.[36] Some of these injuries may be provisionally stabilized by external fixation and plated after the soft tissues have healed. Plating is also useful for malunions and nonunions.[37] Newer plating techniques emphasizing indirect reduction and minimizing soft-tissue stripping may reduce complications.[38]

INTRAMEDULLARY NAILING

Intramedullary nailing is considered the treatment of choice for closed, unstable fractures and most open fractures (types I, II, and IIIA).[9, 33, 39] The addition of interlocking screws provides control of length, alignment, and rotation in unstable fractures and allows nailing of fractures below the tibial tubercle or 3 to 4 cm proximal to the ankle joint. Numerous studies reported high union rates and a relatively

TABLE 4. GENERAL INDICATIONS/CONTRAINDICATIONS

Treatment	Indications	Contraindications
Closed cast/functional brace	Closed, axially stable fracture with minimal comminution	Most open fractures; multiple reduction attempts; severe soft-tissue injury
Operative plating	Closed fractures with intra-articular extension; nonunion/malunion	Severe open or closed soft tissue injury
Operative reamed IM nailing	Closed, unstable fractures; type I and some type II open fractures	Severe open fractures; intra-articular fractures
Operative unreamed IM nailing	Type II and IIIA open fractures	Type IIIB or IIIC fractures
Operative external fixation	Periarticular fractures; severe open fractures; fractures with vascular injury	
Amputation	Disrupted tibial nerve, warm ischemia time >6 hr	

IM=intramedullary.

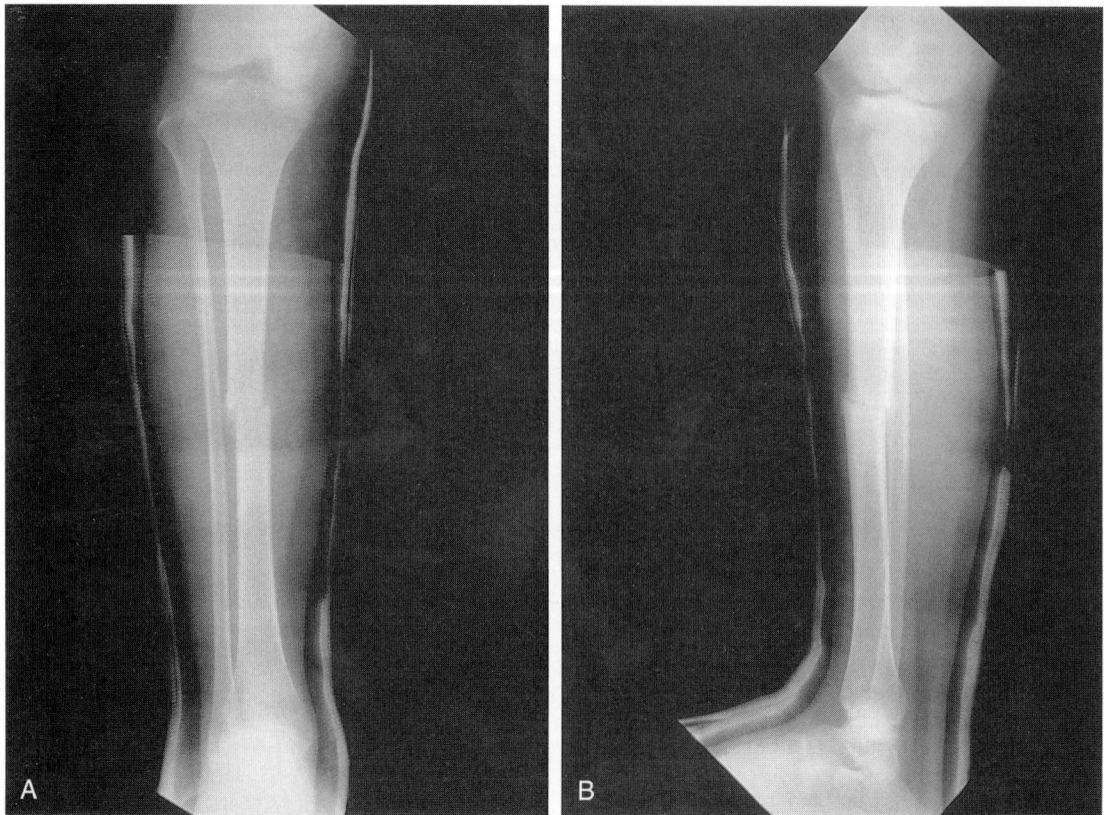

Fig. 3. Closed treatment. *A,* Anteroposterior view of transverse, minimally displaced, axially stable fracture treated with casting. *B,* Lateral view.

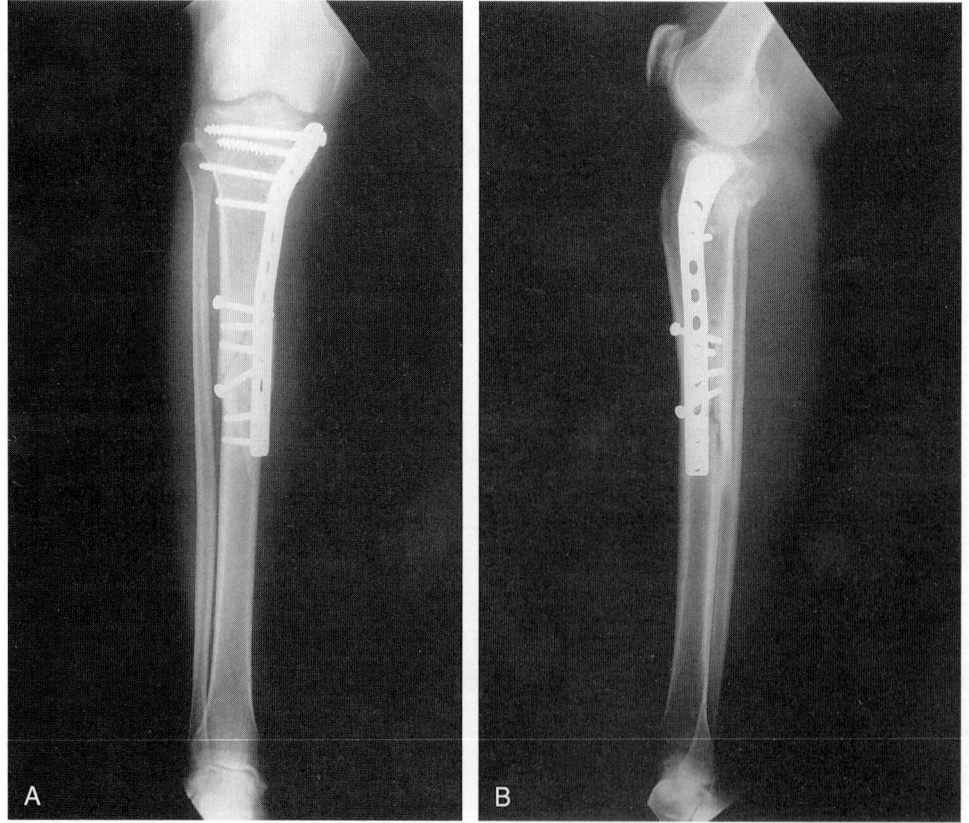

Fig. 4. Plating. *A,* Anteroposterior view of tibial shaft fracture with extension into the tibial plateau treated with plating. Ideally, the plate should be two holes longer. *B,* Lateral view.

low incidence of malunion and infection, even in open fractures. Delayed and nonunions are often easier to treat than with other open techniques, using either dynamization or exchange nailing.

The early use of reamed nails in type II and type III open fractures was associated with an unacceptably high infection rate and led to the belief that their use was contraindicated in higher grade open fractures.[5, 36] With the development of nails that could be inserted without reaming, the indications for IM fixation were broadened to include most open tibial shaft fractures. Subsequent reports examining unreamed locked nailing in open tibial fractures demonstrated high union rates (96% to 100%),[9, 40, 41] an infection rate comparable to or lower than that of other methods (approximately 7%), and a low prevalence of malunion, except in proximal third fractures.

Debate is ongoing concerning the optimal indications for reamed and unreamed IM nailing. Although there is evidence that unreamed nailing entails a lower incidence of infection and comparable healing rates,[42] other studies showed that reaming in open fractures results in a shorter time to union with similar infection rates.[8, 43] Despite these seeming contradictions, certain principles have emerged. Reaming allows the use of larger, stronger implants, which increase stability and decrease the risk of hardware failure; significantly more screws have been shown to fail in unreamed nails.[42] The severity of soft-tissue injury and the adequacy of débridement and soft-tissue coverage are more important in the prevention of infection than the type of implant used. Until larger comparative studies have been performed, however, reamed nailing in severe type II and type III fractures cannot be recommended without reservations.

Intramedullary nailing is not recommended for most fractures with intra-articular extension, although spiral fractures of the distal tibia with nondisplaced intra-articular extension can be treated adequately with IM nailing and supplemental lag screw fixation. In addition, proximal third tibial fractures have been shown to have a high incidence of malunion,[44, 45] require careful attention to entry portal placement, and may necessitate supplemental fixation to ensure a successful outcome. Although some investigators have advocated IM nails for type IIIB fractures,[46] their use in this situation is still not universally accepted. Other contraindications include preexisting deformity, open physes, fractures with very small (less than 8 mm) medullary canals, wounds over the entry portal, open fractures with more than 24 hours delay until treatment, severe contamination, and type IIIC open injuries.

EXTERNAL FIXATION

External fixation provides stable fixation, preserves soft tissues, leaves wounds accessible, minimally disturbs bone vascularity, and causes little blood loss. It can stabilize virtually any fracture, open or closed, throughout the length of the tibia and can be used as either provisional or definitive treatment. Newer frame designs provide uniplanar or multiplanar fixation with half-pins, are less cumbersome, and can be adjusted to allow axial compression (Fig. 5).

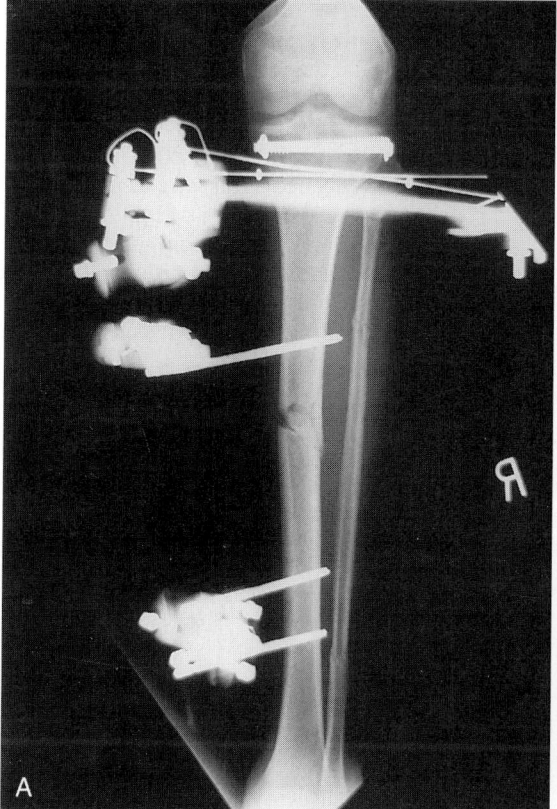 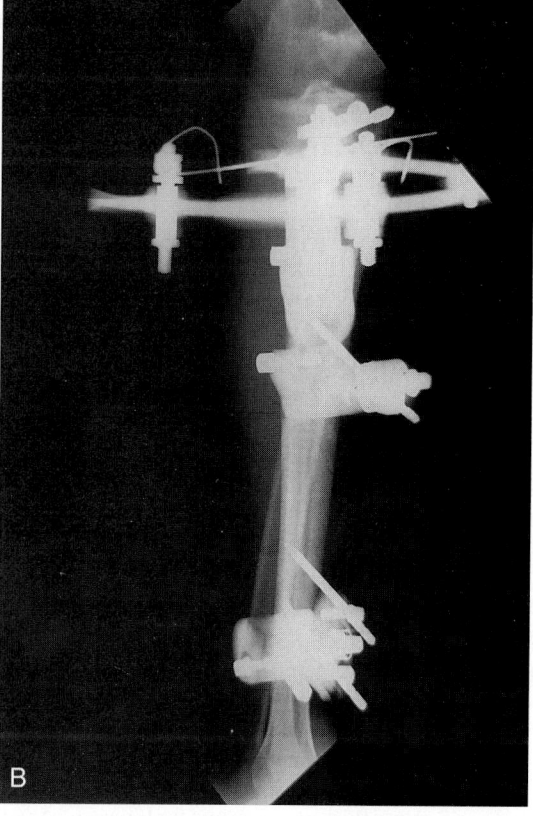

Fig. 5. Two-plane fixation. *A,* Anteroposterior view of ipsilateral tibial plateau and shaft fracture treated with hybrid external fixation. *B,* Lateral view.

TABLE 5. GENERAL RECOMMENDATIONS FOR LOCAL ANTIBIOTIC TREATMENT OF OPEN FRACTURES	
Treatment	Antibiotic "Recipe"
Pulsatile lavage	Polymyxin, 1 million units/L Bacitracin, 50,000 units/L
Antibiotic bead pouch	Tobramycin, 4–9 g/40 g PMMA or Vancomycin, 4–9 g/40 g PMMA

PMMA = polymethylmethacrylate.

Many investigators recommend external fixation as the treatment of choice for periarticular fractures and severe (types IIIB and IIIC) open fractures,[47] particularly those with gross contamination. Other indications include open fractures with delayed treatment (more than 24 hours), fractures with vascular injury, and fractures with segmental bone loss that could be treated by bone transport (see Fig. 4). External fixation can also be used effectively to treat fractures in which IM nailing would otherwise be contraindicated and has potential application with late complications such as nonunion, malunion, or osteomyelitis.

AMPUTATION

Surgeons treating mangling injuries of the tibia face the difficult decision of whether to attempt limb salvage or perform early amputation. Salvage is often technically possible but may result in disastrous medical, social, psychological, and financial consequences. Absolute indications for primary amputation as proposed by Lange et al[10] are complete anatomic disruption of the tibial nerve in adults and crush injuries with a warm ischemia time of more than 6 hours. They also listed relative indications, which include serious associated polytrauma, severe ipsilateral foot trauma, and a projected long course to full recovery. Various other authors have attempted to formulate scores predicting the likelihood of salvage or amputation, but none has proved entirely accurate. Investigation continues into the optimal treatment of mangled extremities.

PROCEDURES

OPEN FRACTURE MANAGEMENT

Open tibial fractures are surgical emergencies and should be treated as soon as possible. In the emergency room, appropriate tetanus prophylaxis is administered, the wound is sterilely dressed, and intravenous antibiotic therapy is initiated. Generally, a first-generation cephalosporin is given for Gustilo type I and type II open fractures. An aminoglycoside is added for larger type II fractures and all type III fractures. Wounds that are heavily contaminated, especially by soil, manure, or sewage, require penicillin.[48]

The best opportunity to obtain a sterile wound is with the initial operative débridement. Wounds should be enlarged to allow exposure of the fracture ends and removal of all debris and nonviable or contaminated tissue. After débridement, the wound is irrigated with 6 to 10 L of sterile saline using pulsatile lavage. Some traumatologists advocate placing bactericidal antibiotics in the last bag of irrigation fluid.[23] Others recommend placing a pouch of antibiotic-impregnated polymethylmethacrylate (PMMA) beads in severe open fractures (Table 5). After débridement and irrigation, the fracture is stabilized by an appropriate method.[49]

Surgical wound extensions can be closed primarily, leaving the traumatic portion open. Small wounds can be left to heal by secondary intention, whereas larger wounds require delayed primary closure or other soft-tissue coverage. Redébridement and irrigation should be performed every 24 to 48 hours until wounds close. Antibiotics are continued for 24 to 48 hours after each surgical procedure. Because delaying soft-tissue coverage longer than 1 week dramatically increases the incidence of infection,[14] definitive wound coverage should be obtained within 5 to 7 days of injury.

NONOPERATIVE TREATMENT
"Preoperative" Planning

The most important determinant of successful nonoperative management is proper patient selection. The criteria have been previously outlined.[3, 30] The necessary equipment includes sufficient cast padding and cast material as well as cool water and a cast saw. Plaster or fiberglass may be used, but plaster allows better molding of the initial cast. Occasionally, a distal tibial or calcaneal traction pin is used to help in the reduction. Medication and equipment to provide safe intravenous sedation are also necessary. As with any procedure, all supplies should be gathered before starting.

Technical Details

Casting a tibial fracture requires two people, one to maintain the reduction and the other to apply the cast. The patient is placed supine with the knee of the injured leg flexed over the end of the table, allowing relaxation of the gastrocnemius. Reduction is usually performed using gravity traction, although skin or skeletal traction may occasionally be necessary. Rotation can be assessed by examining the contralateral extremity or by aligning the second toe with the tibial tubercle. The medial border of the tibia should be somewhat concave to prevent valgus alignment.

While maintaining alignment, a well-padded short-leg cast is applied and then molded along the medial tibial border, behind the malleoli, and under the arch to help maintain reduction. The foot should be maintained in neutral position. Once this cast has hardened, the remainder of the lower extremity is padded with the knee in 5 to 15 degrees of flexion. The cast is then extended two-thirds of the way up the thigh while overlapping the top 6 inches of the initial cast. Supracondylar molding is performed to help prevent rotation, and the cast is then reinforced and trimmed to allow visualization of the toes.

Reduction is assessed with AP and lateral radiographs. Suboptimal alignment can be corrected with a cast change or wedging in a few days when swelling has decreased. An immediate cast change may be necessary if severe malalignment compromises overlying skin. Repeated reduction attempts should prompt consideration of operative stabilization.

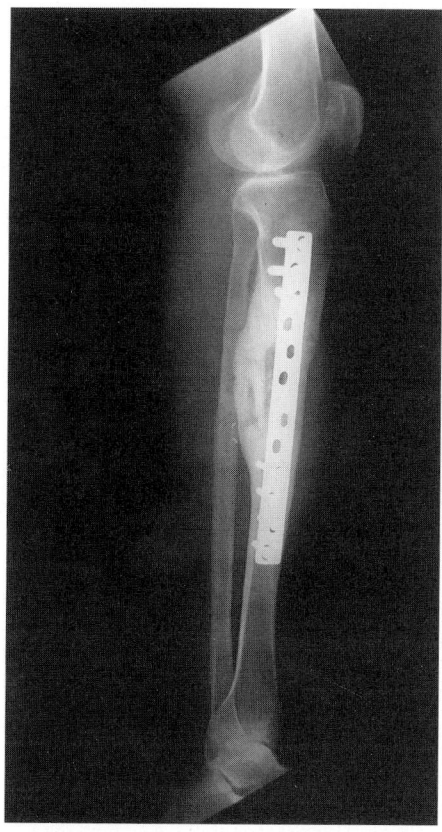

Fig. 6. Comminuted proximal metaphyseal fracture treated with plating and bone grafting.

Postoperative Care

Initial postoperative management centers on prevention of acute complications and usually requires hospitalization. Patients are admitted for extremity elevation, pain control, frequent neurovascular checks, and ambulatory training. There should be a low threshold for dividing the cast or checking compartment pressures. Once discharged, patients should be reexamined weekly with radiographs for the first month to ensure maintenance of alignment. Patients usually can be placed in a patellar tendon-bearing cast or brace 3 to 5 weeks after injury if they are comfortable bearing partial weight and early fracture consolidation is seen on radiographs. Weightbearing is progressed as tolerated, using crutches or a walker as needed.

Casting or bracing is continued until the fracture is clinically and radiographically united, the patient is able to bear full weight without pain, and there is no motion at the fracture site. If there is loss of reduction, a long-leg cast is reapplied and operative treatment considered. After cast removal, the patient is given a program of range-of-motion and strengthening exercises. It generally takes 6 to 12 months before a patient can return to full activity. Contact sports are not permitted until union is solid and full strength and flexibility are regained.

PLATING
Preoperative Planning

Large fragment implants (4.5-mm dynamic compression plates) can provide adequate fixation of tibial shaft and many metaphyseal fractures. Narrow plates are usually suf-

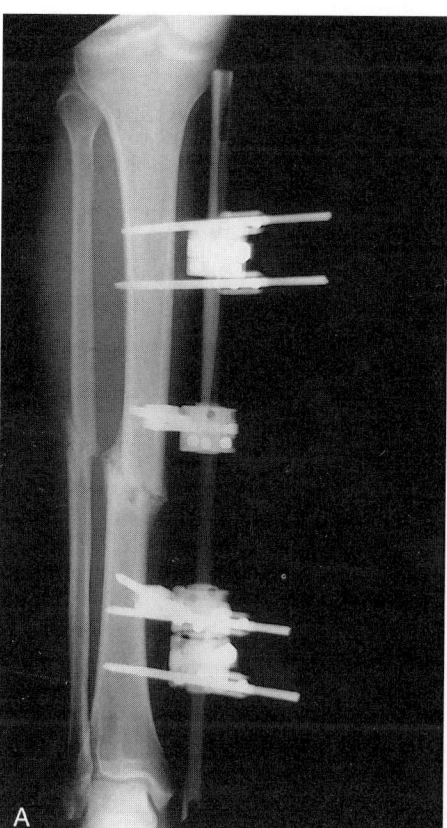
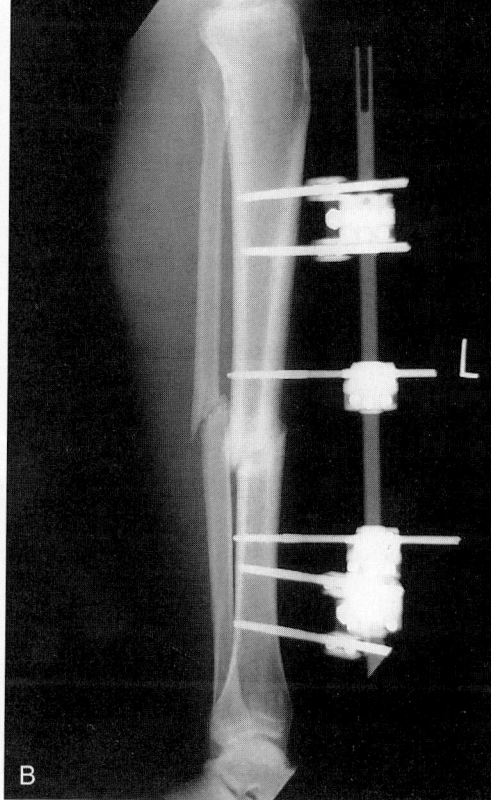

Fig. 7. Open tibial fracture stabilization. *A*, Anteroposterior view of unilateral two-plane external fixator stabilizing open tibial fracture. *B*, Lateral view.

ficient, but broad plates may be required in fractures with bone loss or significant comminution. Stainless steel is preferred because titanium implants have a higher failure rate. Fractures with tibial plateau or pilon extension usually require specifically contoured plates. It is preferable to place at least four screws proximal and distal to the fracture site. Preoperative radiographs should be measured to ensure that a plate of the required length is available. In addition to fracture reduction forceps, an AO femoral distractor can also be a valuable aid. In fractures with significant comminution, bone-grafting instruments should also be available.

Technical Details

Every effort should be made to minimize further soft-tissue damage. Swelling should be allowed to resolve, and the incision and approach should avoid compromised skin and limit soft-tissue stripping. An incision overlying a muscle group has less potential for wound complications than one directly over bone. Although the plate may be placed to buttress the side with greater comminution, medial plates are more prominent and potentially irritating, whereas lateral plates are covered by soft tissue but require muscular stripping. The use of subcutaneous flaps, tourniquets, and forceful retraction can increase soft-tissue complications.

The original AO philosophy recommended anatomic reduction of bony fragments by direct manipulation, lag screw fixation, and application of a neutralization plate but required additional soft-tissue stripping. Mast and others advocate indirect fracture reduction using distraction or a contoured plate, which limits soft-tissue stripping; the plate spans comminuted areas with fragments usually left in situ (Fig. 6). Bone grafting should be performed if there is significant bone loss or if slow healing is expected. Placing bone graft before plate application can avoid additional soft-tissue stripping. Open wounds and severe soft-tissue injuries should be allowed to heal before grafting. Leaving the fascia open will reduce the risk of compartment syndrome.

Postoperative Care

Range of motion of the knee, ankle, and subtalar joints is initiated in the first week if soft tissues permit. Radiographs are taken every 4 to 6 weeks until fracture union. After the first 6 weeks, 15 to 20 pounds of weightbearing is allowed and then progressed over the next 6 weeks if fracture healing is progressing. Most patients will be able to bear full weight without assistance in 4 to 5 months. Unreliable patients should be protected in a cast. Slow healing or hardware failure should prompt early revision. Hardware removal, if desired, is delayed at least 1 year after fracture healing. After hardware removal, weightbearing is protected for 6 to 12 weeks to prevent refracture through screw holes.

EXTERNAL FIXATION
Preoperative Planning

On the basis of the principles of Behrens and Searles,[50, 51] the most commonly used external fixators for tibial shaft fractures are unilateral one-plane or two-plane half-pin constructs. They provide sufficient stability and avoid the po-

tential of soft-tissue tethering and neurovascular injury inherent with transfixion pins. Uncomminuted fractures require a minimum of two pins for each major fragment, and a uniplanar construct usually provides sufficient stability. Comminuted fractures require three pins per major fragment, and two-plane fixation is preferred. Unstable ipsilateral ankle injuries or severe distal soft-tissue wounds require fixation of the foot. The fixator should provide adequate stability, permit progressive weightbearing, and allow dynamization and destabilization as the fracture heals. Systems that accommodate pin placement in more than one plane and have the ability to include the foot are the most useful. In addition to choosing the construct, pin number, and pin placement, preoperative planning should ensure that the power drill, drill bits and sleeves, a radiolucent table, and image intensifier are all available. Reviewing cross-sectional anatomy and "safe zones" for pin placement before surgery will minimize the risk of iatrogenic injury.

Technical Details

Pins are placed through either the anterior or anteromedial cortex along the tibia's subcutaneous border. They should be perpendicular to the long axis and parallel to the joint surfaces. Pins should be less than one-third the diameter of the bone to prevent fracture. Bicortical purchase is necessary to prevent loosening. Optimal pin purchase is obtained at the metaphyseal-diaphyseal junction, and proximal pins should be at least 15 mm from the knee to avoid joint capsule penetration. Some pins have conical rather than cylindrical threaded portions and will loosen if backed out after insertion.

In general, after reduction, the most proximal and distal pins are placed first. The frame is assembled using a bar and the appropriate number of pin clamps and is then attached to the proximal and distal pins. If the fracture reduction is adequate, the clamps are securely tightened. Fracture adjustments are more difficult after the second pin is placed in each segment. The inner pin of each fragment is placed at least 1 cm from the fracture site, and further pins are placed 2 to 3 cm from the fracture if segment length allows. Once all pins are placed and the construct is tightened, reduction is confirmed with full-length AP and lateral radiographs before leaving the operating room.

The initial frame should be rigid enough to minimize fracture motion. Fractures with more inherent instability require stiffer frames. Stability can be increased several ways: increasing pin diameter, increasing the distance between pins, increasing the number of pins or stabilizing bars, decreasing the distance from the bar to the limb, and adding a second plane of fixation. Two-plane fixation can be achieved by connecting pins in different planes to a single bar (Fig. 7), or two bars in separate planes can be connected with bar-to-bar clamps.

Postoperative Care

Daily pin care begins after the initial postoperative dressing change. Patients are examined every 2 to 4 weeks to assess fracture and wound healing and to inspect for pin tract infection. Hip, knee, and ankle range of motion is begun early if these joints are not immobilized as a result of injury. A removable splint should be used to prevent ankle equinus. Bone grafting, if necessary, can be performed once the soft tissues have healed.

Toe-touch weightbearing is allowed for the first 6 weeks and then progressed as callus develops. There is evidence that gradually destabilizing the frame to permit more weightbearing by the bone stimulates fracture healing and may be performed somewhat sooner in axially stable fractures.[52, 53] If callus formation has not increased over 3 months, further intervention is necessary to promote healing. When the fracture is thought to be clinically and radiographically united, the frame can be loosened and stress radiographs obtained. If no motion is detected, the frame can be removed, and the limb is protected in a cast or brace. When full weightbearing is achieved without ambulatory aids, the cast or brace can be removed and formal strengthening exercises begun.

LOCKED IM NAILING
Preoperative Planning

Open fractures can be nailed immediately after appropriate débridement. Closed fractures can be delayed to allow swelling to subside. Radiographs should demonstrate the entire tibia and can be measured to approximate nail length and diameter, an especially important consideration in very tall or short patients. Accurate measurement requires knowing the radiograph magnification. Patients with severely comminuted fractures may require radiographs of the contralateral leg. All necessary equipment (e.g., nail set, reamers, fluoroscopy, radiolucent table) should be available. Additionally, a bone distractor can help obtain and maintain fracture reduction.

Whether to insert the nail with or without reaming should be decided preoperatively. Unreamed insertion usually requires a nail diameter of 8 to 10 mm and cannot be performed when the medullary canal diameter is less than 8 mm.

Most available interlocking systems provide sufficient fixation for diaphyseal fractures. Some proximal and distal fractures, however, require special consideration.[44, 45] Valgus deformity and anterior proximal fragment displacement are common occurrences in proximal third fractures. Nails with a more proximal bend have been shown to decrease anterior translation, and nails with oblique locking screws provide more stability in these fractures. Nail designs with more distally located locking screws have improved the ability to stabilize distal metaphyseal fractures and prevent recurvatum deformity from rotation about a single screw. Occasionally, a small fragment set will be required to provide adjunctive fixation and control rotation in either proximal or distal fractures.

Technical Details

After ensuring that an adequate reduction can be obtained, fluoroscopy should be used to verify correct entry portal placement. The portal should be proximal to the tibial tubercle and in line with the center of the medullary canal on the AP view. The portal is usually created with a curved awl but can also be accomplished by reaming over a Kirschner wire placed in the anterior cortex. Incorrect portal placement increases the risk for iatrogenic injury (i.e., tibial plateau damage, posterior cortex penetration) and malalignment.

Fluoroscopy is used to pass a ball-tipped guide wire across the fracture site and center it approximately 1 cm above the ankle joint. A second guide wire, passed inverted down the reamer, can help prevent guide wire withdrawal during reaming. Flexing the knee will avoid excessive reaming of the anterior cortex and prevent additional soft-tissue damage. Reaming with the tourniquet inflated may lead to thermal necrosis of bone and soft tissue and should be avoided.

After preparing the canal, an appropriate rod diameter is chosen. In reamed nails, a diameter of 1 to 1.5 mm smaller than the last reamer used is appropriate. With an unreamed technique, the canal diameter can then be ascertained by manually passing sounds or reamers across the isthmus; the largest diameter passed without excessive force corresponds to the correct nail size. Nail length can be determined using a radiopaque ruler or by measuring a second guide wire against the one in the canal. Subtracting 5 mm from the measured length will allow the nail to be countersunk and avoid later complaints of anterior knee pain.

After insertion, the nail position (0.5 to 1 cm below the portal and 0.5 to 2 cm above the ankle), fracture reduction, and leg rotation should be checked. Proximal locking screws can be placed using the jig attached to the nail insertion device. Distal screws are placed using a "perfect circle," free-hand technique. AP distal screws should be placed with care to avoid injuring the nearby structures. Fluoroscopy should verify that all screws pass through the nail holes and that they protrude far enough past the far cortex (5 mm) to facilitate removal if broken.

Most nails are statically locked (Fig. 8), although some minimally comminuted transverse diaphyseal fractures are locked dynamically. Distracted fractures should have the distal screws placed first to allow impaction before proximal locking. Because the nail may not prevent malalignment, it is critical to maintain accurate reduction until proximal and distal locking are complete.

Certain technique modifications can decrease the risk of complication associated with nailing proximal and distal fractures. With proximal fractures, accurate reduction can be obtained with a bone distractor or by a limited open reduction and application of a unicortical plate.[54] A lateral or patellar tendon-splitting incision may be required to center the entry portal on the medullary canal and thereby prevent valgus malalignment. Interlocking the proximal nail with the knee in extension relaxes the patellar tendon and prevents anterior angulation. Blocking screws reduce the diameter of the metaphysis and prevent angulation.[55] Distal fractures may require cutting the tip of the nail to allow placement of two distal screws. Associated medial and posterior malleolus fractures can be stabilized with cancellous lag screws. The fibula is plated if it is severely displaced or if plating is necessary for ankle stability.

Assess the muscular compartments by palpation before leaving the operating room. If there is any concern for compartment syndrome, pressures should be measured and fasciotomies performed as indicated.

Postoperative Care

The postoperative regimen varies depending on fracture location, stability, and associated injuries. Use of a removable short-leg brace can help relax healing soft tissues.

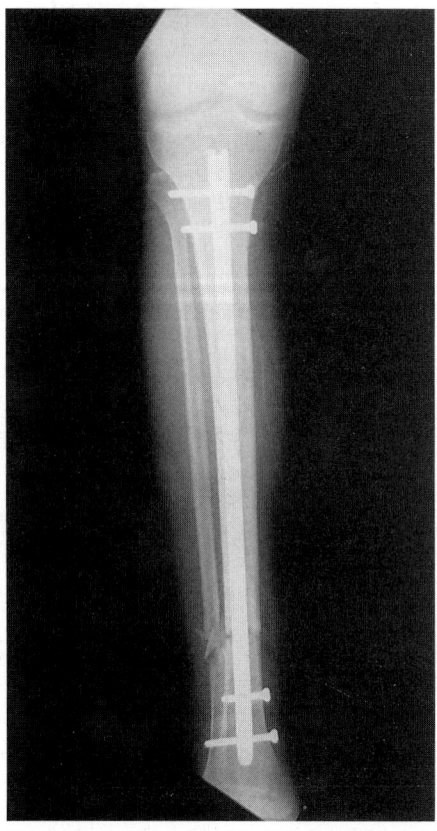

Fig. 8. Interlocking nail inserted without reaming in type III open tibial fracture.

Noncompliant patients and unstable fractures may benefit from supplemental cast immobilization. Partial weightbearing is begun 6 weeks after the injury and is gradually increased as callus formation progresses. Between 3 and 6 months, most fractures have healed and patients are full weightbearing. Most investigators agree that if the fracture is not healed by 6 months and callus formation has not progressed over a 3-month interval, then additional surgery (dynamization, exchange nailing, or bone grafting) is indicated to promote union.

Dynamization is a simple outpatient procedure that allows fracture compression and has a reported 90% success rate.[41] It appears to be most effective when performed within the first 4 months after nailing in axially stable diaphyseal fractures. Exchange nailing has a reported union rate of 93%.[56] It is best suited to fractures with minimal bone loss and can be used in metaphyseal fractures and axially unstable fractures. Bone grafting is indicated for delayed or nonunions associated with significant bone loss and also may be performed after failed dynamization or exchange nailing.

Nail removal is not routinely necessary but may relieve knee pain in patients with prominent hardware. Nails should not be removed until all fracture lines are obliterated and there is full cortical remodeling, a process that usually takes 12 to 18 months. Weightbearing is protected for 6 weeks after nail removal.

COMPLICATIONS

COMPARTMENT SYNDROME

Compartment syndrome is more common in higher energy injuries, with a reported prevalence of 1% in closed fractures[57] and 9% to 19% in open fractures.[21, 58] There is no definitive correlation between method of treatment and development of compartment syndrome. Diagnostic criteria are discussed in Chapter 3–3. Management consists of four-compartment fasciotomies performed through two linear incisions (Fig. 9).

SOFT-TISSUE LOSS

In general, wounds with adequate soft-tissue coverage can be treated with delayed primary closure or split-thickness skin grafting. Two large series reported a 15% and 23%

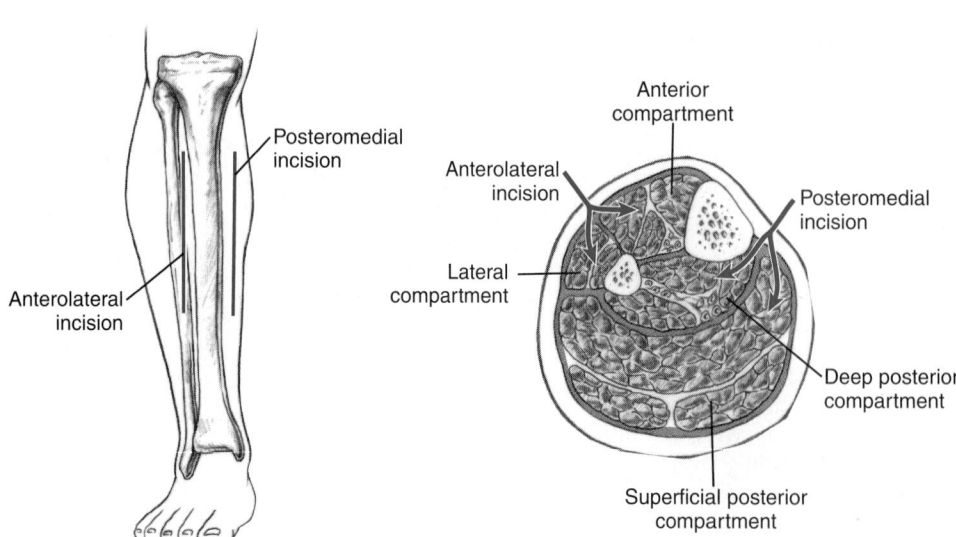

Fig. 9. Four-compartment fasciotomy through anterolateral and posteromedial incisions.

prevalence, respectively, of local or free muscular coverage required in open tibial shaft fractures.[39, 59] Most traumatologists advise obtaining definitive soft-tissue coverage by 7 days, because a longer delay has a significantly higher incidence of infection.

VASCULAR INJURY

Although rare in closed fractures, 6% of open fractures have vascular injury requiring repair (type IIIC).[59] Approximately 60% of type IIIC fractures result in primary amputation.[15] Nonunion and infection are also common in these fractures (25% to 50%).[48] Secondary amputation after prolonged unsuccessful limb salvage has been associated with adverse physical, psychological, social, and economic consequences.[60] Georgiadis and coworkers[61] found that patients with severe open tibial fractures who had successful limb salvage were more likely to consider themselves disabled and less likely to return to work than those treated with amputation.

AMPUTATION

Delayed amputation after attempted limb salvage may be necessary for reasons other than vascular injury. Massive bone and soft-tissue loss, persistent infection, recalcitrant nonunions, and severe ipsilateral foot trauma may obtain a better functional result with early amputation. Delayed amputation has an prevalence of 2.5% to 14% in type IIIA fractures and 5.6% to 16% in type IIIB fractures.[48]

DEEP INFECTION

The risk of infection is determined primarily by the severity of soft-tissue injury and, to a lesser extent, by the surgical procedure. In reviewing open fracture management, Gustilo and coworkers[48] reported an infection prevalence of 0% to 2% in type I fractures, 2% to 7% in type II fractures, and 10% to 25% in type III fractures. Considering type III fractures separately demonstrated an infection rate of 7% in type IIIA fractures, 10% to 50% in type IIIB fractures, and 25% to 50% in type IIIC fractures. Adding an aminoglycoside to the antibiotic regimen for type III fractures[62] and verifying complete débridement of necrotic tissue[7] have been shown to decrease the incidence of infection.

Closed fractures treated with internal fixation have an infection rate ranging from 0% to 3%.[6, 46] The incidence of infection in open fractures has been shown to vary depending on the treatment. Bach and Hansen[60] reported prevalences of wound infection and osteomyelitis of 35% and 19%, respectively, in 26 type II and III fractures treated with plating. The prevalence of infection in series, including all grades of open fractures treated with unreamed IM nailing, ranges from 2.3% to 13%.[9, 40, 43] Although some series reported similar results after reamed nailing, others showed an increased infection rate and discouraged the use of reamed nails in open fractures. The reported prevalence of infection in fractures treated with external fixation is 7% to 14% and comparable to that after unreamed nailing.[7, 39, 63, 64]

Deep infection is treated by surgical drainage, débridement of necrotic tissue, soft-tissue coverage, stable fixation, and appropriate antibiotics. Infections with stable internal fixation can be treated with hardware retention until fracture union. Unstable internal fixation devices should be converted to external fixation.

PIN SITE INFECTION

Pin site infections are common after external fixation, with an prevalence ranging from 10% to 50%.[39, 60, 63] Predrilling pins, bicortical pin purchase, adequate soft-tissue release around the pin, and good pin site care can reduce these complications. Minor infections should respond to oral antibiotics and pin care. Major infections will require intravenous antibiotics with possible pin removal and curettage.

NEUROLOGICAL INJURY

Primary neurological injury as a result of the initial trauma infrequently accompanies tibial shaft fractures. Iatrogenic nerve palsy has a reported prevalence of 4% or less after tibial nailing and most frequently involves the tibial nerve. Neurological dysfunction resolves in more than 90% of cases in 3 to 6 months. Additional iatrogenic injury can be prevented with adequate cast padding and proper pin placement during external fixation.

KNEE LIGAMENT INJURIES

Templeman and Marker[65] found a 22% prevalence of concomitant knee ligamentous laxity in patients with tibial shaft fractures. The medial collateral ligament was involved in all cases, with lower frequencies of posterior cruciate (6%), anterior cruciate (2%), and lateral collateral ligament (2%) involvement. Ligamentous examination should be performed in the operating room after stabilization of the fracture.

MALUNION

Current reports consider fractures with more than 5 degrees of varus or valgus alignment, more than 10 degrees of rotational deformity, and more than 1 to 1.5 cm of shortening to be malunited. Misalignment is more poorly tolerated in the ankle than the knee. Treatment is unnecessary for asymptomatic malunions. Symptomatic malunions are treated with osteotomy and deformity correction.

Malunion after cast or brace treatment ranges from 5% to 55%. The best results were obtained by Sarmiento and coworkers[4] in carefully selected patients. Malunion is more common in series with larger numbers of unstable fractures. Loss of reduction in a cast requiring operative treatment has been reported in 2.4% to 9.3% of cases.[31–33]

Malunion occurs less frequently after plating, with a reported range of 1.7% to 11%.[6, 17] Malunion occurs with greater frequency in comminuted fractures and is most commonly due to poor fracture reduction at surgery.

Malunion after IM nailing has been reported in 0% to 13% of cases and occurs with equal frequency after reamed and unreamed nailing.[9, 41, 42] As with plating, malunion is most frequently caused by accepting an inadequate reduction at surgery. Proximal third fractures have the highest incidence of malunion.

Malunion is more common after external fixation than nailing, with frequencies ranging from 9% to 31%.[7, 21, 39, 63] Loss of reduction after surgery can be treated by remanipu-

TABLE 6. COMPARATIVE RATES OF DELAYED OR NONUNION	
Treatment	Rate of Delayed or Nonunion
Casting[67, 68]	0%–13%
Functional brace[4]	2.5%
Plate[6, 68]	0%–8%
Intramedullary (closed fracture)[32, 33, 69]	0%–5%
Intramedullary (open fracture)[9, 39–41]	0%–8%
External fixation[7, 63, 64]	0%–7%

lation under anesthesia and modifying the fixator to increase stability.

DELAYED AND NONUNION

Although definitions vary, fractures that have not healed by 6 months[23] or do not show progressive healing over a 3-month period[66] can generally be classified as nonunions. Fractures that are healing slowly but are minimally painful and have solid fixation can be observed. Nonunited fractures that are painful after 4 to 6 months or have unstable fixation should be revised. Closed fractures should heal by 16 to 24 weeks, whereas many open fractures will ultimately heal by 9 months without intervention. Fractures with more severe soft-tissue damage have a higher incidence of nonunion. See Table 6 for comparative rates of nonunion.

HARDWARE FAILURE

In any operatively treated fracture, there is a race between fracture union and implant fatigue. Most of the work concerning hardware failure concerns tibial nailing. Nail breakage has been reported in 0% to 6% of cases and screw failure in 6% to 41%.[9, 41, 58] Nail failure nearly always requires revision surgery, whereas screw failure usually does not. Plate fixation has a reported 0.6% prevalence of failure in closed fractures but increases to 10.3% in open fractures.[6] Pin fracture has been reported in 5.9% of cases treated with external fixation.[39]

RESULTS

Functional results after tibial fracture depend significantly on the associated injuries and the degree of soft-tissue damage. Criteria used to determine the successful return of function differ widely, making results among different series difficult to compare.

Ankle stiffness has been reported in 20% to 30%[35, 70] and subtalar stiffness in up to 72% of tibial fractures treated with casting.[71] Tornetta et al[64] reported knee and ankle range of motion after type IIIB fractures treated with IM nailing or external fixation. Knee range of motion was 0 to 130 degrees after nailing compared with 0 to 120 degrees after external fixation. Ankle range of motion after nailing was 0 to 35 degrees and 0 to 30 degrees after external fixation.

Puno and coworkers[32] compared cast with nail treatment for 201 closed, type I, and type II open fractures. Ninety percent of patients treated with nailing returned to work and 90% returned to sports by 12 months after injury. In the group treated with casting, 83% returned to work, and 84% returned to sports 18 to 24 months after injury. Bone and colleagues[33] also compared functional results achieved by nailing or casting isolated displaced tibial fractures. Patients treated with nailing had higher Iowa knee and ankle scores than those treated with casts (96 and 97, respectively, versus 89 and 84). They also scored higher on the SF-36 health profile questionnaire (85 versus 74).

Keating et al[42] reported functional results in 97 patients treated with reamed and unreamed nailing of open tibial shaft fractures. Twenty-six percent of patients treated with reamed nails and 38% with unreamed nails had decreased ankle motion; 19% with reamed nails and 28% with unreamed nails had decreased subtalar motion. Seventy-eight percent of patients with reamed nails returned to their original occupation after isolated fractures, as did 69% of those with unreamed nails. Of patients participating in sporting activities, 66% of those treated with reamed nails and 59% with unreamed nails returned to their preoperative level of participation, whereas 25% of reamed nail patients and 34% of unreamed nail patients had to modify activities.

REFERENCES

1. Pramer A, Furner S, Rice DP: Musculoskeletal Conditions in the United States. Park Ridge, IL, American Academy of Orthopaedic Surgeons, 1992.
2. Puno RM, Vaughan JJ, Stetten ML, et al: Long-term effects of tibial angular malunion on the knee and ankle joints. J Orthop Trauma 1991; 5:247.
3. Sarmiento A, Gertsen LM, Sobol PA, et al: Tibial shaft fractures treated with functional brace. J Bone Joint Surg Br 1989; 71:602.
4. Sarmiento A, Sharpe FE, Ebramzadeh E, et al: Factors influencing the outcome of closed tibial fractures treated with functional bracing. Clin Orthop 1995; 315:8.
5. Bone LB, Johnson KD: Treatment of tibial fractures by reaming and intramedullary nailing. J Bone Joint Surg Am 1986; 68:877.
6. Bilat C, Leutenegger A, Rüedi T: Osteosynthesis of 245 tibial shaft fractures: Early and late complications. Injury 1994; 25:349.
7. Edwards CC, Simmons SC, Browner BD, et al: Severe open tibial fractures. Results treating 202 injuries with external fixation. Clin Orthop 1988; 230:98.
8. Court-Brown CM, Keating JF, McQueen MM: Infection after intramedullary nailing of the tibia. Incidence and protocol for management. J Bone Joint Surg Br 1992; 74:770.
9. Whittle AP, Russell TA, Taylor JC, et al: Treatment of open fractures of the tibial shaft with the use of interlocking nailing without reaming. J Bone Joint Surg Am 1992; 74:1162.
10. Lange RH, Bach AW, Hansen ST, et al: Open tibial fractures with associated vascular injuries: Prognosis for limb salvage. J Orthop Trauma 1985; 25:203.
11. Whittle AP: Fractures of the lower extremity. In Canale ST (ed): Campbell's Operative Orthopaedics. St. Louis, MO, Mosby–Year Book, 1998, 9th ed, p 2067.
12. Oestern HJ, Tscherne H: Pathophysiology and classification of soft tissue injuries associated with fractures. In Tscherne H, Gotzen L (eds): Fractures with Soft Tissue Injuries. Berlin, Springer-Verlag, 1984, p 1.
13. Colton CL: The history of fracture treatment. In Browner BD, Jupiter JB, Levine

AM (eds): Skeletal Trauma. Philadelphia, WB Saunders, 1998.

14. Cierny G III, Bryrd HS, Jones RE: Primary versus delayed soft tissue coverage for severe open tibial fractures: A comparison of results. Clin Orthop 1983; 178:54.

15. Quirke TE, Sharma PK, Boss WK, et al: Are type IIIC lower extremity injuries an indication for primary amputation? J Trauma 1996; 40:992.

16. Georgiadis GM, Ebraheim NA, Hoeflinger MJ: Displacement of the posterior malleolus during intramedullary tibial nailing. J Trauma 1996; 41:1056.

17. Johner R, Wruhs O: Classification of tibial shaft fractures and correlation with results after rigid internal fixation. Clin Orthop 1983; 179:7.

18. Trafton PG: Tibial shaft fractures. In Browner BD, Jupiter JB, Levine AM, et al (eds): Skeletal Trauma: Fractures, Dislocations, Ligamentous Injuries. Philadelphia, WB Saunders, 1992, vol 2.

19. Ferraro SP, Zinar DM: Management of gunshot fractures of the tibia. Orthop Clin North Am 1995; 26:181.

20. Ordog GJ, Wasserburger J, Balesubramaniam S: Shotgun wound ballistics. J Trauma 1988; 28:624.

21. Blick SS, Brumback RJ, Poka A, et al: Compartment syndrome in open tibial fractures. J Bone Joint Surg Am 1986; 68:1348.

22. American College of Surgeons, Committee on Trauma: Advanced Life Support. Chicago, American College of Surgeons, 1993, 5th ed.

23. Gustilo RB, Mendoza R, Williams DN: Problems in the management of type III (severe) open fractures: A classification of type III open fractures. J Trauma 1984; 24:742.

24. Boynton MD, Schmeling GJ: Nonreamed intramedullary nailing of open tibial fractures. J Am Acad Orthop Surg 1994; 2:107.

25. Ellis H: The speed of healing after fractures of the tibial shaft. J Bone Joint Surg Br 1958; 40:42.

26. Nicoll EA: Fractures of the tibia shaft: A survey of 705 cases. J Bone Joint Surg Br 1964; 46:373.

27. Leach RE: Fractures of the tibia and fibula. In Rockwood CA Jr, Green DP (eds): Fractures in Adults. Philadelphia, JB Lippincott, 1984, 2nd ed, p 1593.

28. Applebaum R, Yellin AR, Weaver FA, et al: Role of routine arteriography in blunt lower extremity trauma. Am J Surg 1990; 160:221.

29. Lee J: Efficacy of cultures in the management of open fractures. Clin Orthop 1997; 339:215.

30. Lindsey RW, Blair SR: Closed tibial-shaft fractures: Which ones benefit from surgical treatment? J Am Acad Orthop Surg 1996; 4:35.

31. Hooper GJ, Keddell RG, Penny ID: Conservative management of closed nailing for tibial shaft fractures: A randomised prospective trial. J Bone Joint Surg Br 1991; 73:83.

32. Puno RM, Teynor JT, Nagano J, et al: Critical analysis of results of treatment of 201 tibial shaft fractures. Clin Orthop 1986; 212:113.

33. Bone LB, Sucato D, Stegemann PM, et al: Displaced isolated fractures of the tibial shaft treated with either a cast or intramedullary nailing. J Bone Joint Surg Am 1997; 79:1336.

34. Böstman O, Vainionpää S, Saikku K: Infra-isthmal longitudinal fractures of the tibial diaphysis: Results of treatment using closed intramedullary compression nailing. J Trauma 1984; 24:964.

35. Sarmiento A, Sobol PA, Sewhoy AL: Prefabricated functional braces for the treatment of the tibial diaphysis. J Bone Joint Surg Am 1984; 66:1328.

36. Smith JEM: Results of early and delayed internal fixation for tibial shaft fractures. J Bone Joint Surg Br 1974; 56:469.

37. Mast JW: Preoperative planning in the surgical correction of tibial nonunions and malunions. Clin Orthop 1983; 178:26.

38. Mast J, Jakob R, Ganz R: Planning and Reduction Technique in Fracture Surgery. Berlin, Springer-Verlag, 1989.

39. Henley MB, Chapman JR, Agel J, et al: Treatment of type II, IIIA, and IIIB open fractures of the tibial shaft: A prospective comparison of unreamed interlocking intramedullary nails and half-pin external fixators. J Orthop Trauma 1998; 12:1.

40. Bone LB, Kassman S, Stegemann P, et al: Prospective study of union rate of open tibial fractures treated with locked, unreamed intramedullary nails. J Orthop Trauma 1994; 8:45.

41. Riemer BL, DiChristina DG, Cooper A: Nonreamed nailing of tibial diaphyseal fractures in blunt polytrauma patients. J Orthop Trauma 1995; 9:66.

42. Keating JF, O'Brien PJ, Blachut PA, et al: Locking intramedullary nailing with and without reaming for open fractures of the tibial shaft. J Bone Joint Surg Am 1997; 79:334.

43. Court-Brown CM, Will E, Christie J, et al: Reamed or unreamed nailing for closed tibial fractures. A prospective study in Tscherne C1 fractures. J Bone Joint Surg Br 1996; 78:580.

44. Freedman EL, Johnson EE: Radiographic analysis of tibial fracture malalignment following intramedullary nailing. Clin Orthop 1995; 315:25.

45. Lang GJ, Cohen BE, Bosse MJ, et al: Proximal third tibial shaft fractures. Should they be nailed? Clin Orthop 1995; 315:64.

46. Tornetta P III, Bergman M, Watnik N, et al: Treatment of grade IIIB open tibial fractures. A prospective randomised comparison of external fixation and nonreamed locked nailing. J Bone Joint Surg Br 1993; 75:13.

47. Wiss DA, Stetson WB: Unstable fractures of the tibia treated with a reamed intramedullary interlocking nail. Clin Orthop 1995; 315:56.

48. Gustilo RB, Merkow RL, Templeman D: The management of open fractures. Current concepts review. J Bone Joint Surg Am 1990; 72:299.

49. Ostermann PA, Seligson D, Henry SL: Local antibiotic therapy for severe open fractures. A review of 1085 consecutive cases. J Bone Joint Surg Br 1995; 77:93.

50. Behrens F, Searles K: External fixation of the tibia: Basic concepts and prospective evaluation. J Bone Joint Surg Br 1986; 68:246.

51. Behrens F: A primer of fixator devices and configurations. Clin Orthop 1989; 241:5.

52. Kenwright J, Goodship AR: Controlled mechanical stimulation in the treatment of tibial fractures. Clin Orthop 1989; 241:36.

53. Foxworthy M, Pringle RM: Dynamization timing and its effect on bone healing when using the Orthofix dynamic axial fixator. Injury 1995; 26:117.

54. Benirschke SK, Henely MB, Ott JW: Proximal one-third tibial fracture solution. Orthop Trans 1995; 18:1055.

55. Kretted C, Stephan P, Schandelmaier P, et al: The use of Poller screws as blocking screws in stabilizing tibial fractures treated with small diameter nails. J Bone Joint Surg Br 1999; 81:963.

56. Templeman D, Thomas M, Varecka T, et al: Exchange reamed intramedullary nailing for delayed union and nonunion of the tibia. Clin Orthop 1995; 315:169.

57. DeLee JC, Heckman JD, Lewis AG: Partial fibulectomy for ununited fractures of the tibia. J Bone Joint Surg Am 1981; 63:1390.

58. Singer RW, Kellam JF: Open tibial diaphyseal fractures. Results of unreamed locked intramedullary nailing. Clin Orthop 1995; 315:114.

59. Templeman DC, Gulli B, Tsukayama DT, et al: Update on the management of open fractures of the tibial shaft. Clin Orthop 1998; 350:18.

60. Hansen ST Jr: Overview of the severely traumatized lower limb: Reconstruction versus amputation. Clin Orthop 1989; 243:17.

61. Georgiadis GM, Behrens FF, Joyce MJ: Open tibial fractures with severe soft tissue loss. Limb salvage compared with below-the-knee amputation. J Bone Joint Surg Am 1993; 75:1431.

62. Gustilo RB, Gruninger RP, Davis T: Classification of type III (severe) open fractures relative to treatment and results. Orthopaedics 1987; 10:1781.

63. Marsh JL, Nepola JV, Wuest TK, et al: Unilateral external fixation until healing with the dynamic axial fixator for severe open tibial fractures. J Orthop Trauma 1991; 5:341.

64. Tornetta PI, Bergman M, Watnik N: Treatment of grade IIIB open tibial fractures: A prospective randomized comparison of external fixation and nonreamed locked nailing. J Bone Joint Surg Br 1994; 76:13.

65. Templeman DC, Marker RA: Injuries of the knee associated with fractures of the tibial shaft. Detection by examination under anesthesia: A prospective study. J Bone Joint Surg Am 1989; 71:1392.

66. Russell TA: Fractures of the tibia and fibula. In Rockwood C, Green DP, Bucholz

RW, et al (eds): Rockwood and Green's Fractures in Adults. Philadelphia, Lippin-cott-Raven, 1996, 4th ed, p 2127.

67. Bolhofner BR: Indirect reduction and composite fixation of extra-articular proximal tibial fractures. Clin Orthop 1995; 315:75.

68. Littenberg B, Weinstein LP, McCarren M, et al: Closed fractures of the tibial shaft. J Bone Joint Surg Am 1998; 80:174.

69. Koval KJ, Clapper MF, Brumback RJ, et al: Complications of reamed intramedullary nailing of the tibia. J Orthop Trauma 1991; 5:184.

70. Waddell JP, Reardon GP: Complications of tibial shaft fractures. Clin Orthop 1983; 178:173.

71. McMaster M: Disability of the hind foot after fracture of the tibial shaft. J Bone Joint Surg Br 1976; 58:90.

section
3
chapter
18

DISTAL TIBIA FRACTURES

Bruce French and Paul Tornetta III

Summary

- Distal tibia fractures are relatively infrequent injuries, constituting only a small percentage of all lower extremity fractures.
- Most of these fractures are secondary to high-energy trauma, such as a fall from a height or a motor vehicle accident, resulting in significant bone and soft-tissue damage.
- The goals of treatment of these injuries are reestablishment of articular congruity, stable fixation of the metaphysis to the diaphysis in acceptable alignment, and prevention of complications with rapid return to function. The vast majority of these fractures require surgery to meet these objectives.
- The choice of fixation and the timing of surgery are critical if catastrophic, iatrogenic soft-tissue complications are to be avoided. Acute open reduction and internal fixation of high-energy tibial pilon fractures has led to unacceptably high rates of complications.
- Acute ankle-spanning external fixation followed by delayed reconstruction of the tibial plafond with plating or limited internal fixation combined with external fixation has emerged as the primary treatment option for high-energy fractures.
- Functional recovery depends on the amount of soft-tissue damage and the initial fracture pattern, as well as the quality of the articular reduction. The prognosis for functional recovery in patients with high-energy fractures remains guarded, even if anatomic reduction of the joint surface is achieved.

Distal tibia fractures (fractures within 5 cm of the articular surface of the distal tibia) are relatively infrequent injuries, constituting a small percentage of all lower extremity fractures. Destot, who likened the talus to a pestle (Fr. *pilon*), which drives into the weightbearing surface of the distal tibia, introduced the term "pilon" fracture in 1911. This fracture has also been called a plafond fracture, because of the disruption of the roof of the ankle joint. Kellam and Waddel referred to this injury as the distal tibia "explosion fracture" in deference to the high energy involved and the resultant damage to the bone and soft tissue of the distal tibia.[1]

Historically, many surgeons recommended conservative treatment of pilon fractures, typically resulting in poor functional outcomes. Ruedi and Allgower[2] introduced the modern era of treatment of pilon fractures in 1969 in their landmark article outlining the principles of open reduction and internal fixation. Initial enthusiasm for open reduction and internal fixation of these fractures was tempered by reports of catastrophic complications, particularly in higher-energy fractures. External fixation with limited internal fixation was introduced nearly two decades later as a means to treat these injuries without further disruption of the tenuous soft-tissue envelope of the distal tibia.

Though limited open reduction with external fixation has decreased the complication rate associated with operative treatment, these fractures continue to be problematic in terms of functional outcome and pain. Even with anatomic restoration of the articular surface, early range of motion, and avoidance of iatrogenic complications, satisfactory long-term outcomes can be expected in less than 80% of patients with high-energy fracture patterns. Thus, despite adequate treatment, expectations of functional outcomes for patients with high-energy injuries must be tempered. The possibility of further operative intervention, particularly tibiotalar fusion, must be discussed with each patient prior to embarking on any treatment path.

PATHOGENESIS

Two basic mechanisms account for the vast majority of tibial pilon fractures. Low-energy fracture patterns are generally the product of external rotation, pronation, and dorsiflexion with varying degrees of axial loading. Lauge-Hansen[3] described this injury as having four sequential stages. A vertically oriented medial malleolar fracture is followed by impaction of the anterior lip of the tibia. A supramalleolar fibular fracture precedes a transverse fracture of the posterior malleolus of the tibia. Classically, this injury pattern is associated with a sporting event, such as skiing, and has minimal damage to the surrounding soft-tissue envelope.

High-energy fracture patterns are predominantly the result of axial loading, the talus being driven into the plafond. This implodes the distal tibia articular surface into the metaphysis. The position of the foot at the time of impact determines which part of the plafond will be most affected. High-energy fracture patterns should alert the surgeon to potential soft-tissue compromise.

The wide range of results obtained with treatment of these injuries may be partially explained by these two different mechanisms. Whereas the first is primarily rotational, involving shear forces at the joint, the second involves axial loading, with impaction of the articular cartilage. Axial loading has been shown to cause cartilage damage, and may be responsible for poor outcomes despite anatomic radiographic joint reconstruction.[4]

CLINICAL FEATURES

Pain, swelling, deformity, and crepitus about the ankle, combined with inability to bear weight, are the cardinal signs and symptoms of an acute pilon fracture. In a comatose or multitrauma patient a pilon fracture may be easily overlooked, particularly if there exist more pressing injuries. Thorough examination of the multitrauma patient is essential. Knowledge of the mechanism of injury, such as a fall from a height, may direct the examiner to potential injuries. This may help to avoid missing injuries, which may have a significant impact on the patient's return to function.

Examination of the extremity of a patient with a pilon fracture begins with the skin and soft tissues. Pilon fractures may be associated with marked swelling and the formation of fracture blisters. The amount of soft-tissue damage should be graded according to the Tscherne classification. Marked fracture displacement or tibiotalar dislocation may produce undue tension on the skin and should be reduced immediately by manual reduction. Open fractures should be cleansed and sterilely dressed in the emergency department and represent a surgical emergency. A careful neurologic examination should be undertaken, documenting both motor and sensory findings. In a multitrauma patient this may not be feasible, but attempts must be made, documenting the specific functions that have been tested. Vascular examination should include the posterior tibial and dorsalis pedis pulses as well as capillary refill. A search for signs and symptoms of a compartment syndrome of the lower leg and foot must be undertaken. Concomitant injuries of the foot may also be present and must not be overlooked.

One of the most commonly used classification systems of pilon fractures is that proposed by Ruedi and Allgower.[4] This is a three-part system, based on the amount of comminution of the metaphysis and the articular surface. Type 1 fractures are nondisplaced. Type 2 fractures are displaced, and type 3 fractures feature joint surface comminution and/or impaction. This classification system specifically addresses axial loading injuries as a separate entity and has been shown to have predictive value for clinical outcome. More recently, the Arbeitsgemeinschaft für Osteosynthesefragen/Association for the Study of Internal Fixation and Orthopaedic Trauma Association groups have introduced a classification of distal tibia fractures that is more inclusive than the Ruedi-Allgower scheme (Fig. 1). Type A fractures are distal tibial metaphyseal injuries without intra-articular extension. Type B fractures are partial articular fractures, while type C fractures involve the entire joint surface. These three types are further subclassified according to the amount of comminution and the presence of joint impaction.

INVESTIGATION

Evaluation of the osseous deformity of a pilon fracture begins with good-quality radiographs including the foot, ankle, tibia, and knee. Traction radiographic views in both the anteroposterior and lateral planes, as well as contralateral ankle radiographs, are of particular benefit, particularly if open reduction and internal fixation is being contemplated. These views may be performed after temporary traction is applied, either through a traction pin and a Bohler frame or a spanning external fixator. Even with good-quality radiographs, identification of fracture lines, displaced cortical fragments, and areas of joint impaction is difficult.[5, 6]

Computed tomography (CT) scans have been shown to be a useful adjunct in the evaluation and treatment of pilon fractures and should be considered an essential study.[7] This modality clearly identifies fracture lines and displaced cortical fragments, which may not be apparent even in high-quality radiographs (Fig. 2). The location and extent of joint impaction are clearly delineated (Fig. 3). The surgical approach, particularly if a limited or percutaneous procedure is planned, is greatly facilitated by careful evaluation of the preoperative CT scan. Obtaining the CT scan after temporary external fixation makes the scan easier to evaluate and is more comfortable for the patient.

GOALS, INDICATIONS AND CONTRAINDICATIONS

The goals of treatment of the tibial pilon fracture are threefold: (1) reestablishment of articular surface congruity; (2) stable fixation of the metaphysis to the diaphysis in acceptable alignment; and (3) prevention of iatrogenic complications with rapid return to premorbid lower extremity function. As there is a wide spectrum of severity of both soft-tissue and osseous disruption, no one treatment modality is acceptable for all pilon fractures. Furthermore, each patient must be individually assessed as to an acceptable treatment protocol. Whereas a long-leg cast may be acceptable treatment in a patient with an isolated, nondisplaced fracture, this is not acceptable in a multitrauma patient with concomitant injuries, in whom this modality may preclude adequate mobilization (Table 1).

Nonoperative management in the form of a long-leg cast may have certain limited indications. In fractures without significant metaphyseal comminution, anatomic joint surface alignment, and a congruent mortise, this may be a reasonable treatment alternative. There should be minimal soft-tissue injury, as this cannot be readily evaluated post casting. Closed reduction must be acceptable and, if the joint is involved, its reduction should be confirmed with a CT scan. Finally, the patient must be able to mobilize in the cast.

The majority of pilon fractures will benefit from surgical intervention. There exist a number of surgical options, ranging from open reduction and internal fixation to limited open reduction with external fixation. One of the most

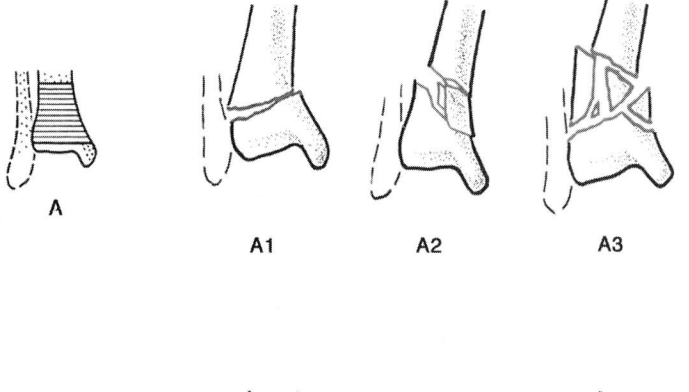

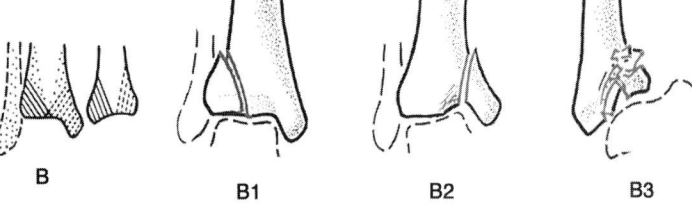

Fig. 1. The AO/OTA classification of distal tibia fractures.

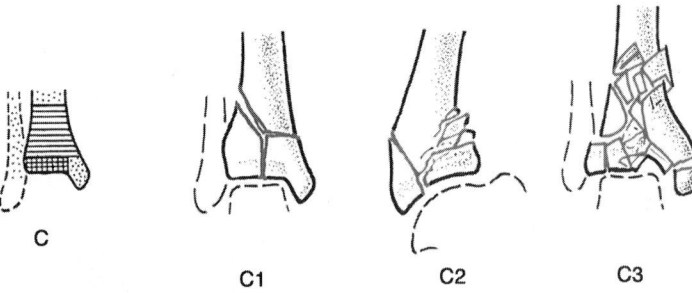

important emerging concepts is that of temporary external fixation (with or without open reduction and internal fixation of the fibula) followed by delayed reconstruction of the tibial plafond. This may be accomplished with either formal open reduction or limited internal fixation with sup-

plementary external fixation when the soft-tissue swelling has normalized. The temporary spanning frame allows for early patient mobilization and easy access to the soft tissues, while maintaining overall length and alignment of the extremity (Fig. 4). Delayed reconstruction of the tibial pi-

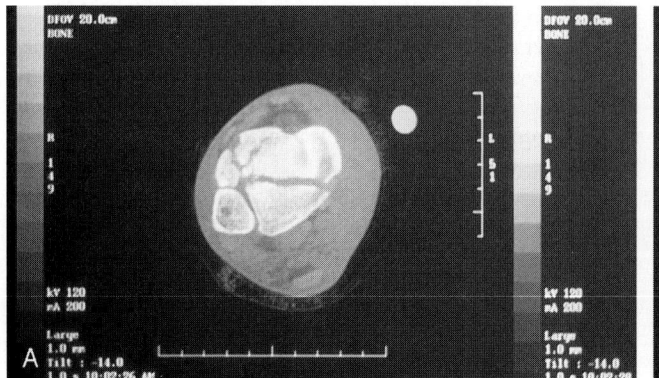

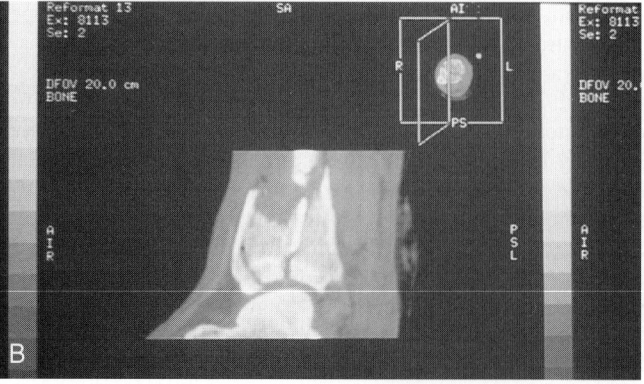

Fig. 2. Examples of fracture characteristics identified by CT scan. *A,* Identification of the number and orientation of the fracture lines at the level of the plafond. *B,* Displaced cortical fragment wedged into the metaphysis. This must be removed before attempts at joint reduction.

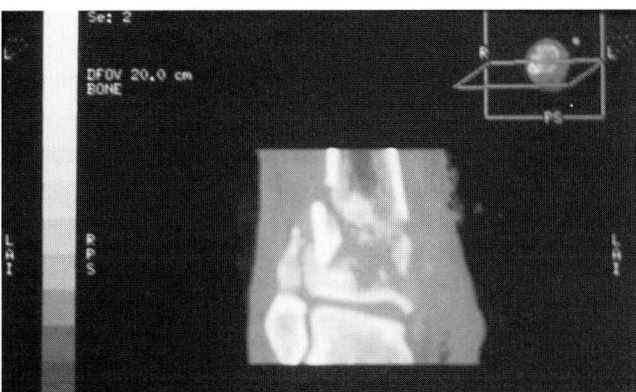

Fig. 3. Examples. These are examples of joint impaction and metaphyseal defect well visualized by the CT scan.

lon can then be based on recovery of the soft tissues and the fracture pattern. In patients with isolated injuries, this may allow for discharge home before formal joint reconstruction.

Acute open reduction and internal fixation of the fibula and tibial plafond through two incisions became a popular treatment option based on the publications of Ruedi and Allgower.[2, 8] As this technique became more prevalent, it became increasingly apparent that failure to achieve stable, anatomic fixation of the pilon and/or compromise of the injured soft tissues by early surgical dissection led to an unacceptably high rate of catastrophic complications. High-energy fracture patterns with soft-tissue compromise are not amenable to acute open reduction and internal fixation for fear of these iatrogenic complications.[9, 10] Though this technique should not be abandoned, acute open reduction and internal fixation should be limited to low-energy fracture patterns with minimal soft-tissue injury and swelling.

External fixation combined with limited open reduction and internal fixation has emerged as the treatment of choice for the vast majority of distal tibia fractures. The versatility of external fixation systems, the convenience of cannulated screws, and the wide availability of intraoperative fluoroscopy have made this technique available to most orthopaedic surgeons. This technique has gained popularity because less surgical dissection and hardware are necessary, making the timing of the surgery less critical.

Although the principles of limited open reduction with external fixation are well outlined, their application has raised considerable debate, particularly surrounding the type of external fixation and the need for concomitant fixation of the fibula. Hybrid external fixation systems, which achieve fixation into the distal fragment with tensioned wires, allow for unrestricted range of motion of the ankle and foot. Articulated frames involve distal fixation into the talus and calcaneus, allowing some ankle motion and no hindfoot motion. Proponents of the hybrid systems point to the unrestricted range of motion of the foot and

TABLE 1. TREATMENT OPTIONS				
Treatment	Indications	Contraindications	Union	Outcome
Cast immobilization	Congruent joint surface; minimal comminution; limited soft-tissue injury; acceptable reduction	Multitrauma; high-energy fracture; open fracture; unacceptable reduction; poor soft tissues	100%	Good functional outcome if reduction is maintained; ankle and hindfoot stiffness common
Temporary external fixation	Open fracture; closed fracture with soft-tissue compromise; hemodynamic compromise	None	N/A	Allows patient mobilization prior to joint reconstruction; good access to soft tissues; may be combined with ORIF of fibula
Acute ORIF	Low-energy fracture; intact soft-tissue envelope; minimal swelling	High-energy fracture; poor soft tissues; high-grade open fracture	90%–100%	80% satisfactory functional outcome with stable, anatomic joint reconstruction; high complication rates in high-energy fracture patterns
Delayed ORIF	Any fracture with intact soft-tissue envelope; treatment 10–14 d after injury	Open, contaminated fractures; poor recovery of soft tissues	90%–100%	Low complication rates in preliminary studies; 80%–90% acceptable outcomes; newer technique not yet evaluated in large series
Limited ORIF with external fixation	Well suited for high-energy fracture patterns; any fracture pattern is amenable	Noncompliant patient; inadequate bone stock for wire purchase	90%–100%	80% acceptable functional results; decreased complication rate vs acute ORIF; pin tract complications common; difficult joint reduction through small incisions
IM nail with internal fixation	Tibial diaphyseal fracture with nondisplaced split through plafond	Inadequate purchase of distal locking screws through IM nail	100%	Satisfactory ankle function to be expected
External fixation without joint reconstruction	Unreconstructable joint surface; salvage for deep infection	Reconstructable joint surface	80%–100%	Poor functional outcome; prelude to tibiotalar fusion; allows for soft tissue care while maintaining limb length and alignment

ORIF, open reduction and internal fixation; IM, intramedullary nail; N/A, not applicable.

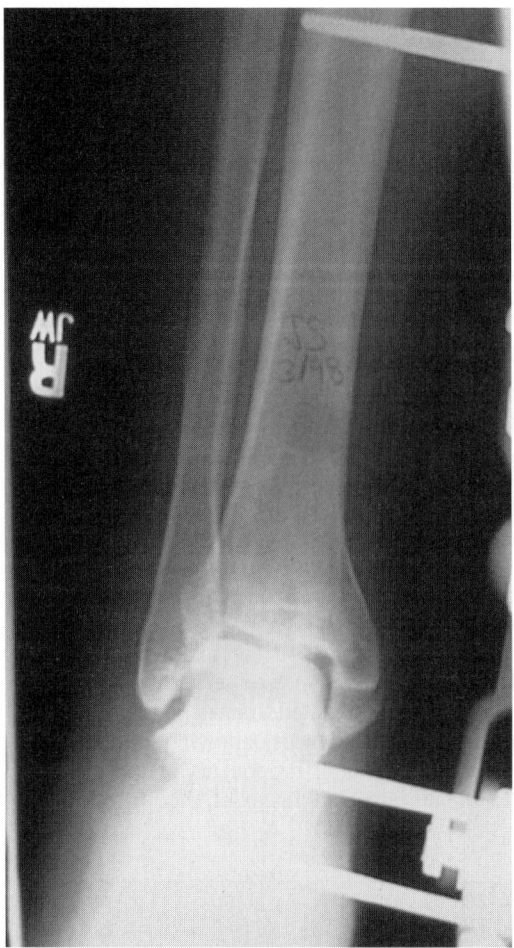

Fig. 4. Temporary spanning external fixation of a pilon fracture.

ing a narrow skin bridge between a potential tibial incision and the fibular incision. Routine plating of the fibula is not indicated in conjunction with limited open reduction and external fixation techniques.

Several authors have recently published protocols for staged reconstruction of tibial pilon fractures.[14, 15] Open reduction and internal fixation of the fibula and spanning or articulated medial external fixation are accomplished within the first 24 hours after the injury. When the soft-tissue envelope has normalized, the articular surface of the distal tibia undergoes formal open reduction and internal fixation with removal of the external fixation device. Preliminary results indicate that this may be a promising technique for prevention of the iatrogenic complications seen with acute open reduction and internal fixation, while avoiding the complications seen with the limited incisions and external fixation techniques. Because this is a new technique, indications are not well delineated. Open, contaminated injuries and injuries in which the soft tissues are slow to recover may not be well suited to this technique. Furthermore, these authors are experienced trauma surgeons, particularly in the evaluation and handling of soft tissues, potentially making their results hard to duplicate by the general orthopaedic population.

Rarely, a diaphyseal tibial fracture will have an extension into the tibial plafond. Typically, the extension is minimally or not displaced. In this situation, the articular surface may be treated with subchondral percutaneous screw fixation perpendicular to the fracture lines as based on the preoperative CT scan, followed by intramedullary nailing of the tibial diaphysis. Using this technique, Konrath et al[16] had no displacement of the articular surface during nail insertion. All patients went on to union without complications associated with the intra-articular fracture extension.

PREOPERATIVE PLANNING

As with any periarticular fracture, preoperative knowledge of the fracture lines and their orientation, as well as any areas of joint impaction, is essential. If open reduction and internal fixation is planned, preoperative templating should be undertaken. If limited open reduction and internal fixation is planned, 4.0-mm partially threaded screws, which may be cannulated, or 3.5-mm screws inserted in lag fashion are adequate for fixation of the joint surface. Complete familiarity with the external fixation system to be used is essential. Good-quality C-arm imaging in both the anteroposterior and lateral planes and a radiolucent operating table are essential. Regardless of the technique chosen, the femoral distractor can be an invaluable tool to help effect the reduction and should therefore be available.

Finally, the need for bone grafting must be determined preoperatively. Fractures with areas of bone impaction will virtually always need a supplemental bone graft. If open reduction of the tibia is undertaken, bone grafting of metaphyseal defects is also recommended. Potential bone graft substitutes and sites should be discussed with the patient in advance. Harvesting of bone graft, particularly from the iliac crest, can add significant length and morbidity to the procedure.

ankle as well as to the benefit of early motion on damaged articular cartilage as the major benefits of these constructs.[11] Advantages of the articulated frames include placement of the frame components outside the zone of injury, maintenance of a plantigrade foot, easier soft-tissue reconstruction, and decreased risk of pyarthrosis. Although the articulated frames do allow for tibiotalar motion, near-normal ankle kinematics can only be achieved if the frame is applied along the ankle axis, which does not correspond to the horizontal axis to which the frame is generally applied.[12] No prospective, randomized studies have been used to compare the two frames. Grade IIIB open fractures and fractures with metaphyseal bone loss or comminution precluding adequate wire purchase are better managed with the spanning frame. Extra-articular pilon fractures and fractures with a stable portion of metaphysis for wire purchase are ideally suited for hybrid frames.

Fibular plating in conjunction with limited open reduction and internal fixation has also been advocated. Studies have not only failed to document the efficacy of this procedure but also have shown increased rates of delayed union, nonunion, infection, and the need for secondary procedures when the fibula has been plated.[13] In addition, fibular plating may limit future surgical options on the tibia by creat-

TECHNICAL DETAILS

Open reduction and internal fixation of pilon fractures should proceed in an orderly fashion in four basic steps. This begins with fibular fixation, generally with a ⅓ tubular plate or a 3.5-mm dynamic compression plate. The incision should be made along the posterior aspect of the fibula, as this allows for a wider skin bridge between the two incisions. Placement of the plate along the posterior aspect of the fibula is also advocated, as this leads to less prominent hardware and easier wound closure. Anatomic fibular reduction typically reduces the anterolateral or Chaput fragment of the distal tibia.

The anteromedial incision extends from the anterior border of the medial malleolus and continues proximally over the anterior border of the tibial crest. Superficial flaps and denuding of the paratenon are avoided. Internal fixation of the tibia can then be accomplished according to the preoperative protocol. Generally, a cloverleaf plate is placed medially, serving as an artificial cortex in the absence of osseous support. Smaller-profile plates may be used to supplement this fixation. If there is a lack of comminution, smaller-profile plates may be used for the primary fixation. Metaphyseal bone defects and defects left by disimpaction

of the articular surface should be grafted with bone or a suitable bone substitute. The wound is closed in layers, first the medial, then the lateral. The wounds should not be closed under tension (Fig. 5).

Limited open reduction and internal fixation combined with external fixation differs from open reduction and internal fixation in that the length and axial alignment of the extremity are controlled by the frame, obviating the need for wide surgical dissection and large plates. Limited incisions are used for joint reduction, bone grafting, and placement of subchondral screws to maintain the joint reduction. Screws should not be used to fix metaphyseal fragments or to fix the metaphysis to the diaphysis, for this requires further periosteal stripping, wider surgical dissection, and may lead to late refracture after removal of the frame (Fig. 6).

In certain fractures anatomic reduction of the joint surface may be obtained by ligamentotaxis applied through the frame or a femoral distraction device. The plafond may then be internally fixed with percutaneously placed subchondral screws perpendicular to the fracture lines as based on the preoperative CT scan. Kirschner's wires or large reduction tenacula may be used to manipulate fragments into position. Areas of joint impaction will never be re-

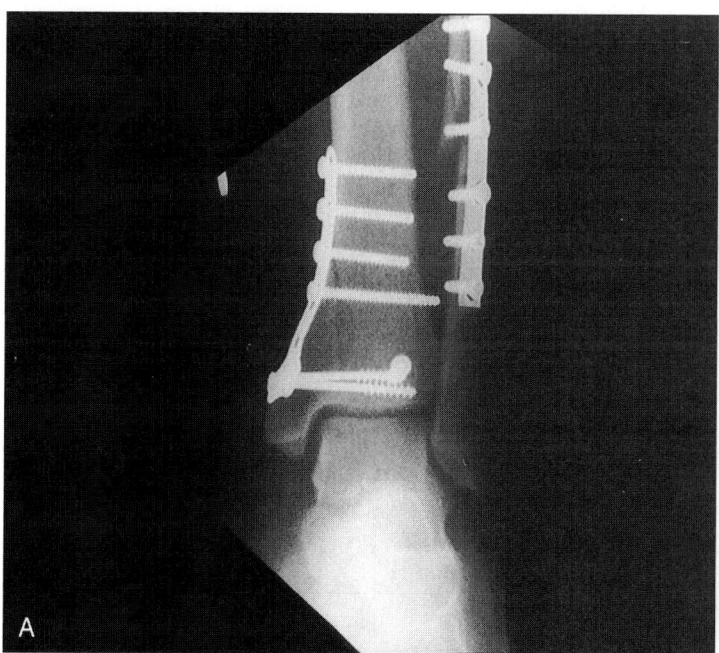

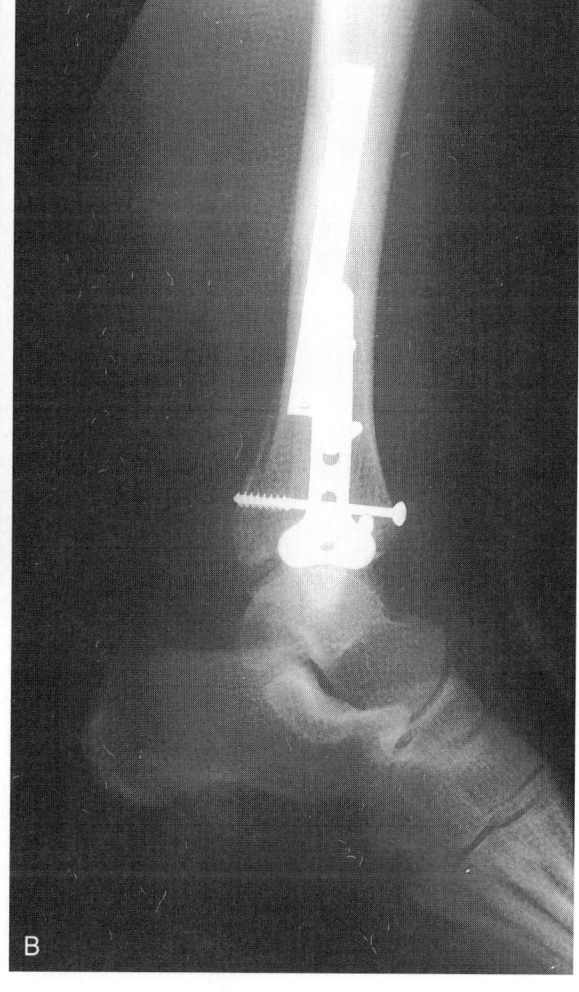

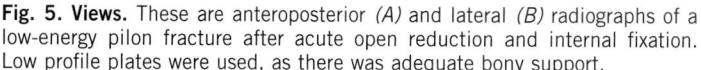

Fig. 5. Views. These are anteroposterior *(A)* and lateral *(B)* radiographs of a low-energy pilon fracture after acute open reduction and internal fixation. Low profile plates were used, as there was adequate bony support.

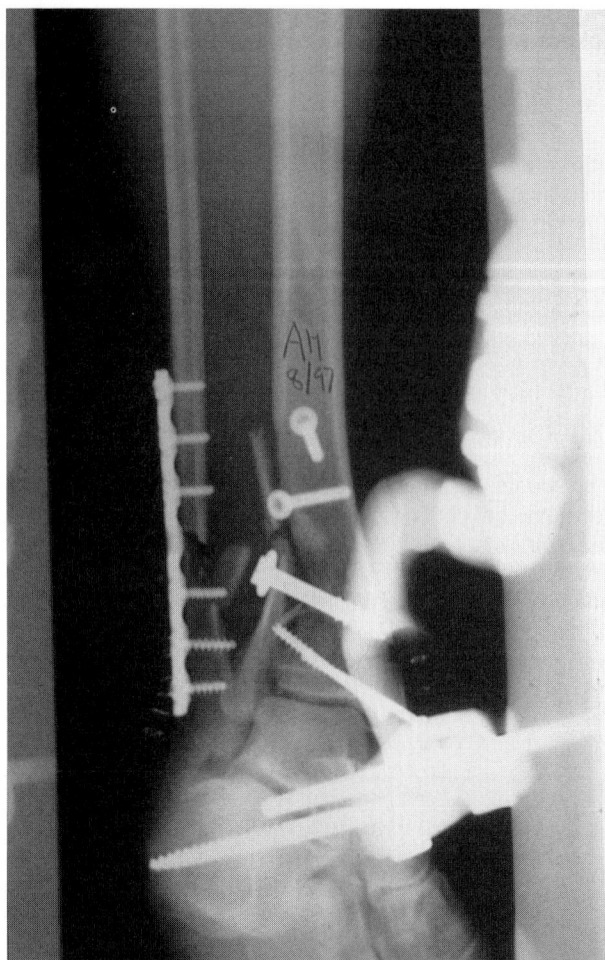

Fig. 6. Anteroposterior radiograph. It shows poor technique of limited open reduction and internal fixation with articulated external fixation. There is inadequate joint reduction, malalignment of the extremity, fixation of diaphyseal fragments and of the metaphysis to the diaphysis with screws, and improper frame application. See Figure 8.

duced in this manner and require an incision for access and disimpaction. This is accomplished through a small longitudinal incision made over the primary fracture line. The fracture is then used as a "trap door," allowing access to the area of impaction as well as visualization of the joint surfaces. The impacted segments are then reduced, followed by bone grafting of the metaphyseal defect to support the reduced segment. After confirming the reduction by intraoperative fluoroscopy, the articular surface is internally fixed with either partially threaded 4.0-mm screws or 3.5-mm screws inserted in lag fashion.

Application of the hybrid external fixation frame requires thorough knowledge of the cross-sectional anatomy of the distal extremity. This type of frame involves placement of narrow tensioned wires in the extracapsular portion of the metaphysis, parallel to the joint line. The technical details have been described.[17] The first wire is placed from posterolateral to anteromedial, beginning in the fibula. The second wire is passed from posteromedial to anterolateral. The wires are then attached to a semicircular frame and tensioned to increase the strength of the construct. Standard 5.0-mm half-pins are then placed proximal to the fracture site into the tibia. Reduction of the metaphysis to the diaphysis is then accomplished under fluoroscopic control using the frame as an indirect reduction tool. Full-length hard copy radiographs should be obtained to verify fracture reduction (Fig. 7). Generally, a third wire or half-pin into the distal fragment is added for further stability.

When using an articulated external fixation frame, the frame may be applied prior to the joint reduction. This type of frame is fixed to two half-pins distally (one in the talus and one in the calcaneus) and two proximal to the fracture into the tibia. As described by Bonar and Marsh,[18] the placement of the first half-pin into the talus is critical. This starting point for the talar pin is in the distal medial neck of the talus, parallel to the dome of the talus as visualized on the anteroposterior fluoroscopic view and perpendicular to the long axis of the talar body on the lateral view. The calcaneal pin is placed next, using the frame as a template. It should be placed superiorly on the

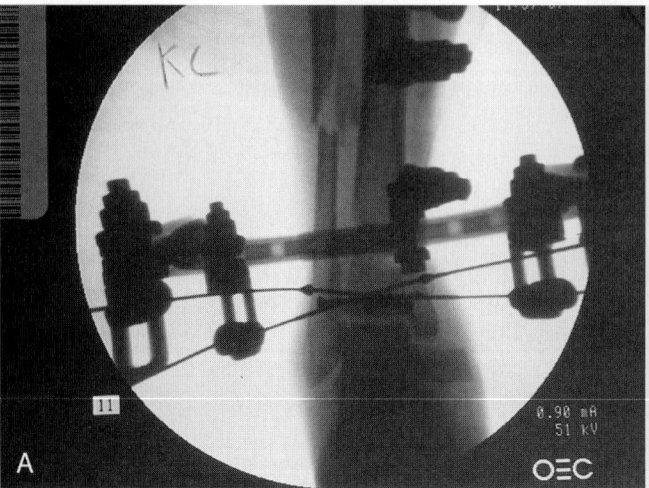
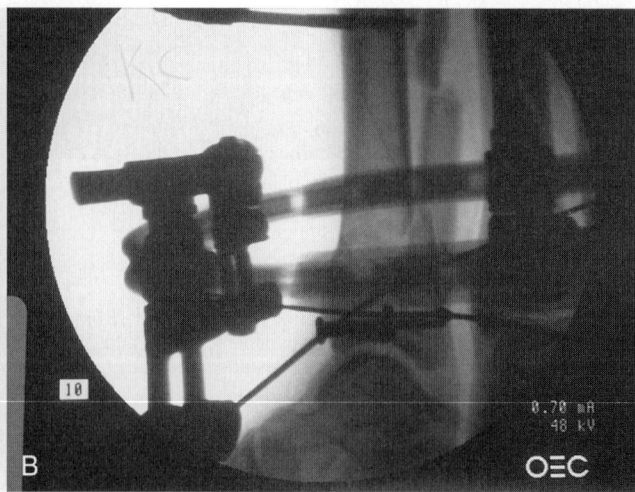

Fig. 7. Views. These are intraoperative fluoroscopic views, *(A)* and *(B)*, of a pilon fracture treated by limited open reduction and hybrid external fixation.

calcaneal tuberosity, as this allows for more postoperative dorsiflexion. The center of the hinge of the articulated fixator should be located near the middle of the talus. Two tibial half-pins are then placed perpendicular to the long axis of the tibia in a medial-to-lateral direction. With the frame as an indirect reduction tool the length, alignment, and rotation of the tibia are reestablished. Further management of the joint surface is then dictated according to the principles outlined previously (Fig. 8).

POSTOPERATIVE MANAGEMENT

Postoperatively, the extremity must be keep elevated to decrease swelling. In bedbound patients, the frame may be suspended from the trapeze bed frame. For pain and soft-tissue considerations, early motion is delayed for 7 to 10 days. Patients in hybrid frames are placed in a footplate or posterior mold during this time. After this period, the mold is worn only at night. Dry dressings are placed over the surgical incisions. Pin sites are cleaned twice daily with saline-impregnated, cotton-tipped applicators until they are free of debris. Dry dressings are wrapped circumferentially around the pins to prevent soft-tissue piston action and pin irritation. The use of bacitracin and other occlusive ointments is discouraged.

In all intra-articular fractures weightbearing is prohibited in the first 8 weeks. At 8 weeks toe-touch weightbearing is started. Full weightbearing is initiated at 3 months. Toe-touch weightbearing may be initiated immediately in extra-articular fractures fixed with a frame.

Depending on the fracture configuration, the frame is typically in place for 3 to 6 months. The status of the pins generally dictates the limit of frame durability. Early, prophylactic bone grafting of the metaphysis, either directly or posterolaterally, should be considered at 10 to 12 weeks if there is no significant callus formation. Early frame re-moval may lead to delayed angular deformity, despite casting, and should be avoided.

RESULTS

Prior to Ruedi and Allgower's[2] series, most authors reported good functional outcomes in less than 50% of cases, most of which were casted. In this series, 74% excellent or good results were obtained with open reduction and internal fixation at 4 years postoperatively. These results were not only maintained at 9-year follow-up, but there were no secondary procedures performed between 5 and 9 years after the primary surgery.[8] The primary criticism of the study is that the patient population included a large proportion of young athletes involved in relatively low-energy injuries. These investigators published another study in which nearly 50% of the fractures were type 3 fractures.[19] At 6-year follow-up 70% of the patients had good-to-excellent results.

A number of subsequent studies have failed to reproduce these results. A dichotomy in complication rates and functional outcomes developed between patients with lower-energy type 1 and 2 fractures treated with acute open reduction and internal fixation versus patients with type 3 fractures similarly treated. A number of authors reported good functional outcomes with low complication rates in nearly 80% of the lower-energy fractures.[9, 20] In type 3 fractures, however, the number of stable and anatomic reductions dropped significantly, while the acute complication rate and the need for subsequent surgery rose alarmingly. Of particular concern were the high rates of skin slough or wound dehiscence with subsequent osteomyelitis, which a number of authors reported to be as high as 50%.[10, 21] Rates for secondary ankle arthrodesis after attempted open reduction and internal fixation of type 3 fractures approached 30% in two separate studies.[20, 22] Early surgical intervention in the form of open reduction

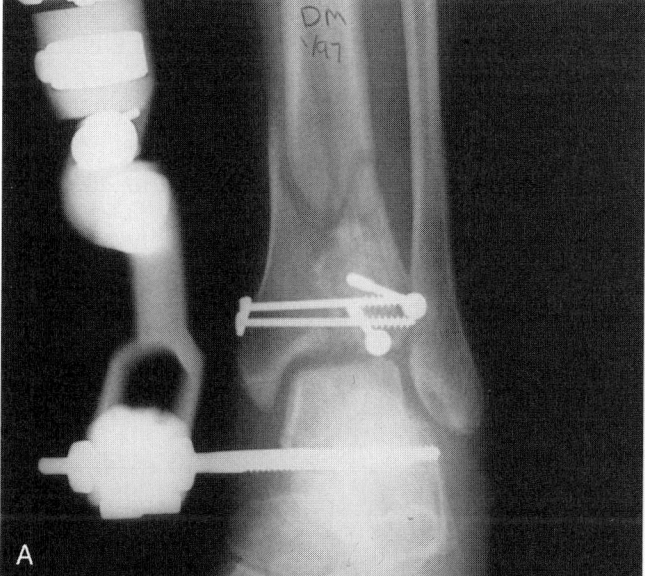
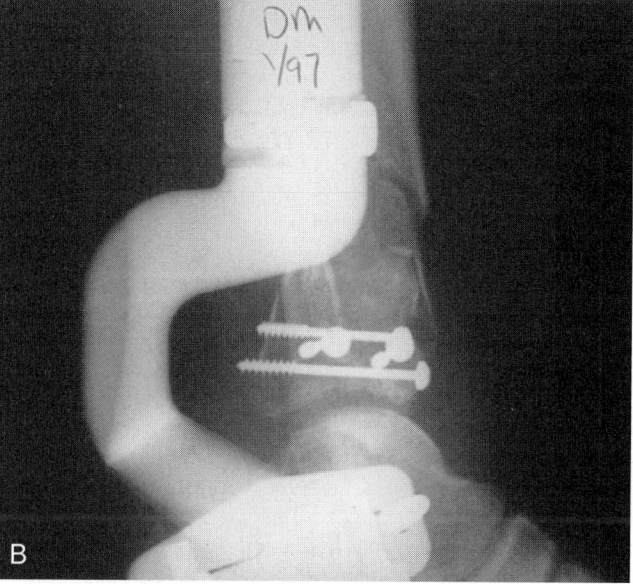

Fig. 8. Radiographs. These are postoperative radiographs, *(A)* and *(B)*, of a pilon fracture treated with limited open reduction and internal fixation and an articulated external fixation device.

and internal fixation through the marginal soft-tissue envelope of the distal tibia was found to result in an unacceptably high rate of soft-tissue complications, resultant infection, and poor outcomes in patients with high-energy fractures.

As early as 1965, Scheck[23] advocated external fixation with limited internal fixation as a means to stabilize comminuted pilon fractures. This technique has emerged as the treatment of choice for most pilon fractures over the last decade. Tornetta et al[24] reported on 26 distal tibia fractures treated with limited open reduction and hybrid external fixation. These authors obtained a 69% good-to-excellent result in their subset of type 3 fractures with short-term follow-up. There were no instances of wound dehiscence and only one deep infection. In another series of pilon fractures treated similarly, the authors reported a 100% union rate with anatomic or good reductions in 97% of the cases.[25] Overall, there was an 82% rate of acceptable results, a number which dropped to 33% for the C2 and C3 fractures. Bone[26] reported on 20 "high-energy" fractures undergoing this technique with a spanning external fixator. Whereas only 30% of the patients had good-to-excellent subjective results, 75% had good-to-excellent range of motion, and complications were minimal. In a study that used the articulated external fixation device on type 2 and 3 fractures, one-third of the patients had good-to-excellent results, with no instances of wound dehiscence or osteomyelitis.[27] Pin tract infections were recorded in 20% of the pins.

In a randomized, prospective study, acute open reduction and internal fixation was compared to limited open reduction with external fixation.[28] Whereas the times to union, radiographic, and clinical outcomes were similar, the open reduction group had a 55% major complication rate compared with 18% in the external fixation group. There was a trend toward fewer anatomic or good reductions in the external fixation group. At the last follow-up, the majority of patients with type 2 and 3 fractures had some degree of radiographic arthrosis. This study helps to confirm that whereas external fixation drastically reduces the number of complications seen with acute open reduction and internal fixation, the prognosis for functional recovery after a pilon fracture remains guarded. A number of authors have applied validated patient outcome measures to patients who have had pilon fractures.[29, 30] These studies have confirmed that there are significant decreases in general health perceptions, physical and emotional role function, and pain and energy levels in patients who have suffered pilon fractures.

Staged protocols that feature acute open reduction of the fibula combined with medially applied spanning or articulated external fixation followed by delayed open reduction and internal fixation with removal of the frame have recently been proposed by a number of authors. Two studies have concluded that this protocol, by avoiding attempts at reconstruction of the tibia during the first 10 to 14 days after the injury, allows for safe open reduction and internal fixation of the tibia.[14, 15] The authors hypothesized that this technique allows for more adequate reduction of the joint than does the limited open reduction technique and avoids the pin tract complications seen with long-term application of the external fixators. The rate of soft-tissue complications and osteomyelitis was low in both series with a high percentage of good-to-excellent clinical and radiographic outcomes. This technique, thus far undertaken by and reported on by experienced orthopaedic traumatologists, has yet to be tested by the general orthopaedic population.

COMPLICATIONS

The most common complication after a pilon fracture is post-traumatic osteoarthritis (Fig. 9). In one study with 3-year follow-up, all type 2 and 3 fractures, regardless of treatment, had some degree of narrowing of the joint space.[28] These changes were noted by 1 year and tended to be progressive. Etter and Ganz[20] found 75% of their type 3 and 53% of their type 2 fractures to have severe-to-moderate osteoarthritis at an average of 10 years after open reduction and internal fixation. These authors, however, found no correlation between radiographic osteoarthritis and subjective results, whereas there was a trend toward poorer objective results with increasing radiographic osteoarthritis. Although a poor reduction virtually guarantees future radiographic osteoarthritis, anatomic reduction does not always protect against it. In all but the most comminuted fractures, some attempt to reconstruct the joint surface is warranted. An ankle arthrodesis is easier to accomplish if the bone stock and alignment of the extremity have been restored. As a salvage procedure, ankle arthrodesis leads to good functional outcomes and effective pain relief (Fig. 10). Patients should be advised as to limitation of activities and the possibility of future surgery, including subtalar fusion, associated with tibiotalar fusion (Table 2).

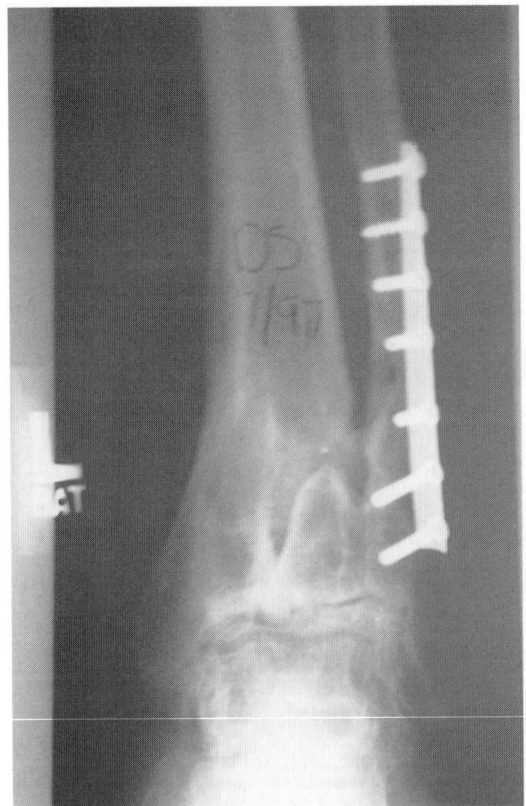

Fig. 9. Severe post-traumatic osteoarthritis. The condition occurred after a high-energy pilon fracture.

TABLE 2. MAJOR COMPLICATIONS

Complication	Rate	Prevention	Treatment
Osteoarthritis	Radiographic OA in up to 100% of pilon fractures; increased rate in high-energy patterns and axial load injuries	Anatomic joint reconstruction and alignment of extremity may occur even if these goals are met	Tibiotalar arthrodesis
Wound dehiscence/delayed wound healing	Reports as high as 50% after acute ORIF; 5% in fractures treated with limited ORIF and Fix external fixation or with delayed ORIF	Maximize skin bridge between incisions; not operative through compromised soft tissue; no tension closure; stable fixation	Wound revision with delayed primary closure; rotational flaps of limited benefit; free flap for exposed bone, tendon, or hardware; STSG for lateral wound possible
Deep infection/pyarthosis	5%–10%; sixfold increased rate with wound dehiscence	Adequate I/D of open fractures; prevent wound-healing complications	Attempt at I/D with hardware retention and IV antibiotics; hardware removal and spanning external fixation ± free flap more common; may require amputation
Delayed/nonunion	5%–10%	Stable fixation if ORIF early; prophylactic bone graft in high-energy fractures with bone loss or comminution	Posterolateral bone graft; direct bone graft with small anterior defect and healthy soft tissues
Malunion	10%–15%	Acceptable initial reduction; stable reduction; ?decreased incidence after ORIF; external fixation in place until fracture union	Reconstruction of joint surface ±/− tibial osteotomy if limited radiographic OA; tibiotalar fusion if radiographic OA present

OA, osteoarthritis; ORIF, open reduction and internal fixation; STSG, split thickness skin graft; I/D, irrigation and débridement; IV, intravenous.

Wound-healing problems represent a serious complication of the treatment of pilon fractures and are best avoided. Careful operative technique and timing are of paramount importance. Operative reconstruction of the high-energy pilon fracture, either by limited incisions or open reduction, is best delayed until the soft-tissue injury and swelling have resolved, typically in 10 to 14 days. The distance between fibular and tibial incisions should be maximized—to at least 5 to 7 cm. Excessive tension on the skin at the time of wound closure should be avoided. The medial wound should be closed prior to the lateral wound to gain coverage of the bone, hardware, and neuro-

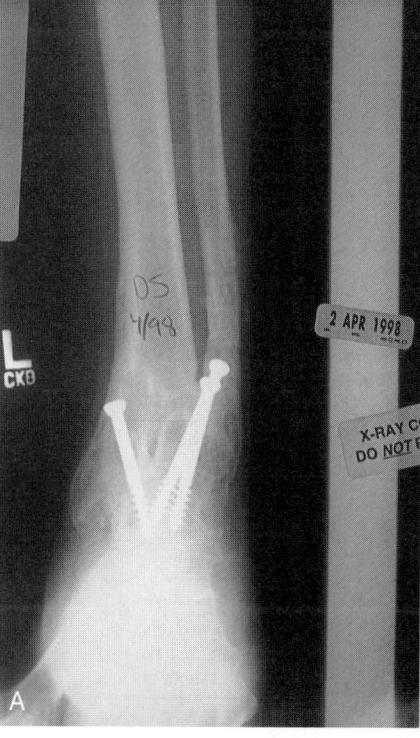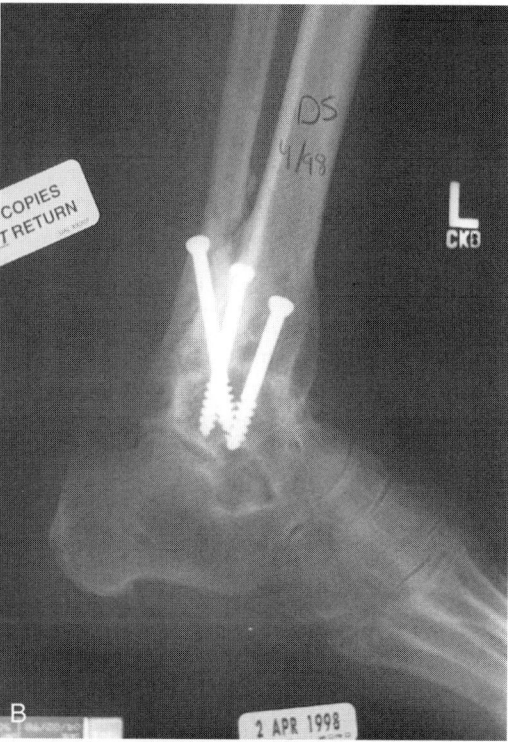

Fig. 10. The same patient from Figure 9. This view is after tibiotalar arthrodesis.

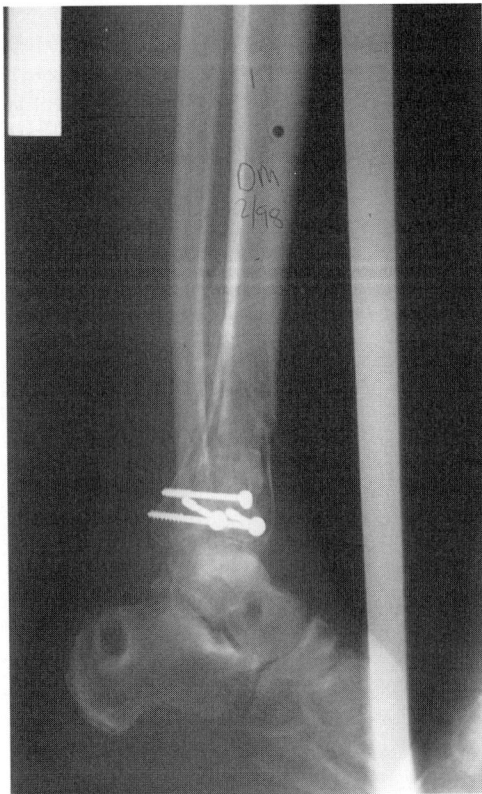

Fig. 11. Example of a pin tract infection. This shows infection of the calcaneus and talus after limited open reduction and articulated external fixation. Note the normal-appearing half-pin tract in the proximal tibia. This patient was immunocompromised, never developing signs of infection while the frame was in place. Recalcitrant osteomyelitis ensued, resulting in a below-knee amputation.

vascular structures. If the lateral wound cannot be easily closed, "pie crusting" with multiple stab incisions parallel to the incision may be effective. If the lateral wound still cannot be closed, it is reasonable to leave it open only to be covered with a split thickness skin graft at a later date.

Should there be failure of the wound closure, either from dehiscence or soft tissue loss (grade 3B fractures), coverage procedures should be undertaken as soon as there is a healthy tissue bed. This typically requires a free muscle flap. Rotational flaps have limited use in this area, particularly if there is a large zone of injury or if two incisions have been used for open reduction and internal fixation. Smaller defects may be covered by split thickness skin grafts, as long as there is no exposed bone or denuded tendon.

Osteomyelitis after the operative treatment of pilon fractures commonly portends a poor prognosis, frequently resulting in ankle arthrodesis or amputation. Prevention begins with aggressive débridement and irrigation of open fractures. Prevention of wound-healing complications and rapid treatment if they do occur is essential. If frank joint sepsis and periarticular infection occur, adequate débridement must be undertaken, even at the expense of the loss of devitalized osteocartilaginous fragments and stabilizing hardware. Pin tract infections must be dealt with aggressively (Fig. 11). At the earliest signs of pin tract infection oral antibiotics should be started. If there is not a favorable, rapid response, intravenous antibiotics are necessary. Pin or wire removal with or without curettage is the final step. Early, prophylactic bone grafting decreases the duration of the time in the external fixation frame, thereby decreasing the rate of pin tract complications.

REFERENCES

1. Kellam J, Waddell J: Fractures of the distal tibial metaphysis with intra-articualr extension—the distal tibial explosion fracture. J Trauma 1979; 19:593.
2. Ruedi T, Allgower M: Fractures of the lower end of the tibia into the ankle joint. Injury 1969; 1:92.
3. Lauge-Hansen N: Fractures of the ankle: 5. Pronation dorsiflextion fractures. Arch Surg 1953; 67:813.
4. Borrelli J, Torzilli S: Effect of impact load on articular cartilage: Development of an intraarticular fracture model. J Orthop Trauma 1997; 11:319.
5. Dirschl D, Adams G: A critical assessment of factors influencing reliability in the classification of fractures, using fractures of the tibial plafond as a model. J Orthop Trauma 1997; 11:471.
6. Martin JS, Marsh JL: Assessment of the AO/ASIF fracture classification for the distal tibia. J Orthop Trauma 1997; 11: 477.
7. Tornetta P III, Gorup J: Axial computed tomography of pilon fractures. Clin Orthop 1996; 323:273.
8. Ruedi T, Allgower M: Fractures of the lower end of the tibia into the ankle joint: Results 9 years after open reduction and internal fixation. Injury 1973; 5:130.

9. Bourne R, Rorabeck C, McNab J: Intra-articular fractures of the distal tibia: The pilon fracture. J Trauma 1983; 23:591.
10. Dillin L, Slabaugh P: Delayed wound healing, infection and nonunion following open reduction and internal fixation of tibial plafond fractures. J Trauma 1986; 26: 1116.
11. Salter R, Simmonds D, Malcom B, et al: The biologic effect of continuous passive motion on the healing of full-thickness defects in articular cartilage. J Bone Joint Surg Am 1980; 62:1232.
12. Fitzpatrick D, Marsh JL, Brown T: Articulated external fixation of pilon fractures: The effects on ankle joint kinematics. J Orthop Trauma 1995; 9:76
13. Williams T, Marsh JL, Nepola J, et al: External fixation of tibial plafond fractures: Is routine plating of the fibula necessary? J Orthop Trauma 1998; 12:16.
14. Sirkin M, Sanders R, DiPasquale T, et al: A staged protocol for sort tissue management in the treatment of complex pilon fractures. J Orthop Trauma 1999; 13:78.
15. Patterson MJ, Cole JD: Two-staged delayed open reduction and internal fixation of severe pilon fractures. J Orthop Trauma 1999; 13:85.
16. Konrath G, Moed B, Watson JT, et al:

Intramedullary nailing of unstable diaphyseal fractures of the tibia with distal intra-articular involvement. J Orthop Trauma 1997; 11:200.
17. Karas E, Weiner L: Displaced pilon fractures: An update. Orthop Clin North Am 1994; 25:651.
18. Bonar S, Marsh JL: Unilateral external fixation for severe pilon fractures. Foot Ankle 1993; 14:57.
19. Ruedi T, Allgower M: The operative treatment of intra-articular fractures of the lower end of the tibia. Clin Orthop 1979; 138:105.
20. Etter C, Ganz R: Long term results of tibial plafond fractures treated with open reduction and internal fixation. Arch Orthop Trauma Surg 1991; 110:277.
21. McFerran M, Smith S, Boulas H, et al: Complications encountered in the treatment of pilon fractures. J Orthop Trauma 1992; 6:195.
22. Teeny S, Wiss D: Open reduction and internal fixation of tibial plafond fractures: Variables contributing to poor results and complications. Clin Orthop 1993; 292:108.
23. Scheck M: Treatment of comminuted distal tibial fractures by combined dual-pin fixation and limited open reduction. J Bone Joint Surg Am 1965; 47:1537.

24. Tornetta P III, Weiner L, Bergman M, et al: Pilon fractures: Treatment with combined internal and external fixation. J Orthop Trauma 1993; 7:489.

25. Barbieri R, Schnek R, Koval K, et al: Hybrid external fixation in the treatment of tibial plafond fractures. Clin Orthop 1996; 332:16.

26. Bone L, Stegemann P, McNamara K, et al: External fixation of severely comminuted and open tibial pilon fractures. Clin Orthop 1993; 292:101.

27. Marsh JL, Bonar S, Nepola J, et al: Use of an articulated external fixator for fractures of the tibial plafond. J Bone Joint Surg Am 1995; 77:1498.

28. Wyrsch B, McFerran M, McAndrew M: Operative treatment of fractures of the tibial plafond: A randomized, prospective study. J Bone Joint Surg Am 1996; 78: 1646.

29. Sands A, Grujic L, Byck D, et al: Clinical and functional outcomes of internal fixation of displaced pilon fractures. Clin Orthop 1998; 347:131.

30. Williams T, Marsh JL, Nepola J, et al: Factors affecting outcome in tibial plafond fractures. Presented at the Orthopedic Trauma Association Meeting, Vancouver, BC, Canada, October 1998.

section 3
chapter 19

FRACTURES AND SOFT-TISSUE INJURIES ABOUT THE ANKLE

Kevin J. Pugh

Summary

- Most malleolar fractures of the ankle are low-energy, rotational injuries.
- The mechanism of injury can give clues to the nature of the injury and the method of reduction.
- The goal of treatment is to restore ankle stability by reconstructing normal anatomic relationships. This restores normal ankle biomechanics and function.
- Anatomic reduction and stable immobilization are the keys to success.
- Preoperative planning should account for injury to the soft tissues as well as to the bone.

INTRODUCTION

The spectrum of injury that can occur to the ankle requires evaluation of the distal tibia and foot as well. This chapter focuses on ligamentous injuries and malleolar fractures of the ankle. Injuries to the distal tibia were discussed separately in Chapter 3–18, and injuries to the hindfoot and the foot will be discussed in Chapters 3–20 and 3–21, respectively.

The ankle is a complex hinge in which both bony and ligamentous structures play important roles in providing stability. Maintenance of ankle function is dependent on maintenance of normal anatomic relationships. Normal gait requires adequate dorsiflexion and plantar flexion of the ankle. The closely related subtalar joint allows the foot to remain plantigrade on uneven surfaces by providing inversion and eversion. The ankle is also a weightbearing joint that must withstand forces that may exceed five times the body weight.

Injuries to the ankle involve more than the bones and ligaments of which the ankle is composed. Soft-tissue coverage of this region is poor, with only a thin layer of skin over the joint. If sufficient energy is imparted to the ankle joint, significant injury can also occur to the skin, resulting in poor healing of both traumatic and surgical wounds. In addition, injuries to the tendons that cross the joint and to the vascular and nervous structures can severely compromise the ability of the ankle and hindfoot to function.

The evaluation of the injured ankle requires a thorough history and a comprehensive examination of the skin and the bony, ligamentous, and neurovascular anatomy of the ankle. Restoration of ankle function is dependent on the ability to restore normal anatomic relationships without causing iatrogenic injury.

PATHOGENESIS

ANATOMY[1, 2]

On the medial side of the distal tibia is the medial malleolus. It is commonly divided into an anterior colliculus—covered on its lateral articular surface with cartilage—and a posterior colliculus. The visible superficial deltoid ligament runs from the anterior colliculus to the talus but is little more than a thickening in the joint capsule and provides very little stability to the joint. The deep deltoid ligament (Fig. 1), the primary medial stabilizer of the joint, is visible only from inside the joint and runs from the posterior colliculus to the talus. It functions to restrain external rotation of the talus in the mortise.

The articular surface of the distal tibia is concave, resulting in large anterior and posterior prominences. The posterior prominence, referred to as the posterior malleolus, is commonly involved in ankle fractures. The fracture is thought to occur as a result of the avulsion of the insertion of the posterior inferior tibiofibular ligament on the posterior lateral surface. Malunion of the posterior malleolus has been shown to result in posterolateral instability of the talus in the mortise. Incongruence of the posterior malleolar fragment can result in decreased contact area and increased contact pressure in the tibiotalar joint.[3]

On the anterolateral side of the tibia lies the incisura, or the groove where the distal fibula articulates with the tibia. The complex distal tibiofibular ligamentous complex called the syndesmosis (Fig. 2) joins these bones. The syndesmosis is composed of several distinct structures that are responsible for the maintenance of the ankle mortise. The

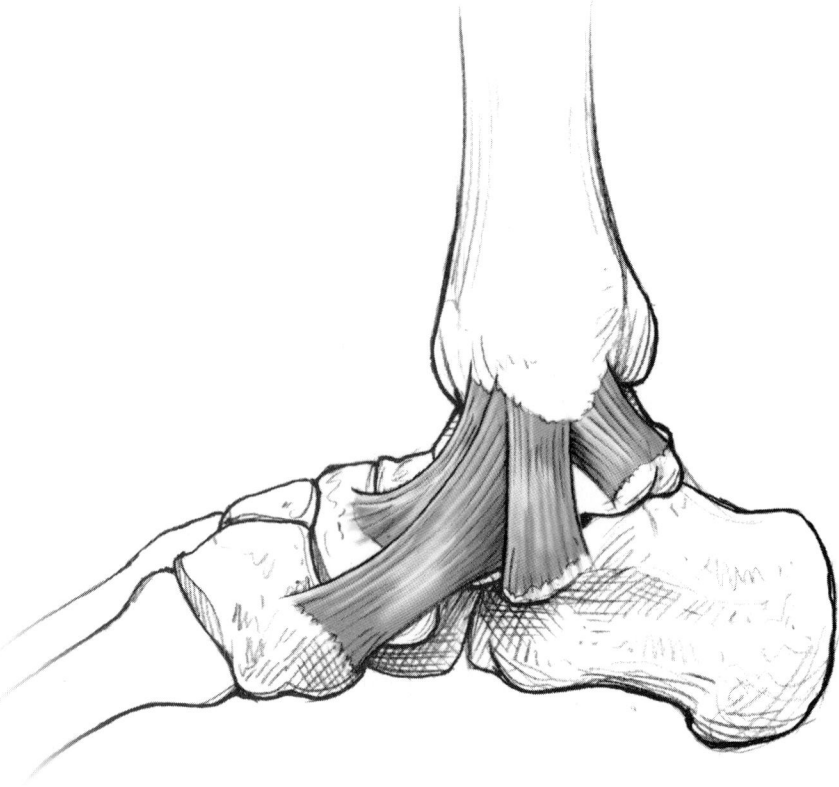

Fig. 1. Medial side of the ankle. The superficial deltoid ligament runs from the medial malleolus to the talus. The deltoid ligament is deep and runs from the posterior colliculus of the medial malleolus to the posterior portion of the talus.

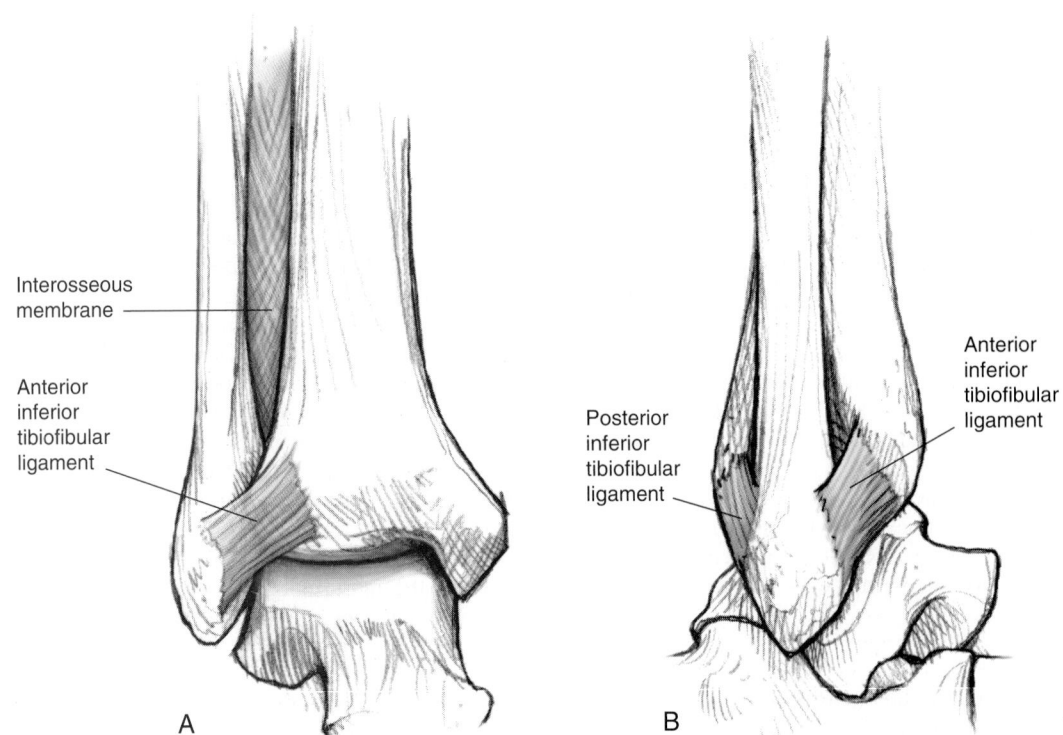

Fig. 2. The ankle syndesmosis. *A,* Anterior view of the ankle syndesmosis demonstrating the anterior inferior talofibular ligament and the interosseous membrane. *B,* Lateral view of the ankle syndesmosis demonstrating both anterior and posterior tibiofibular ligaments.

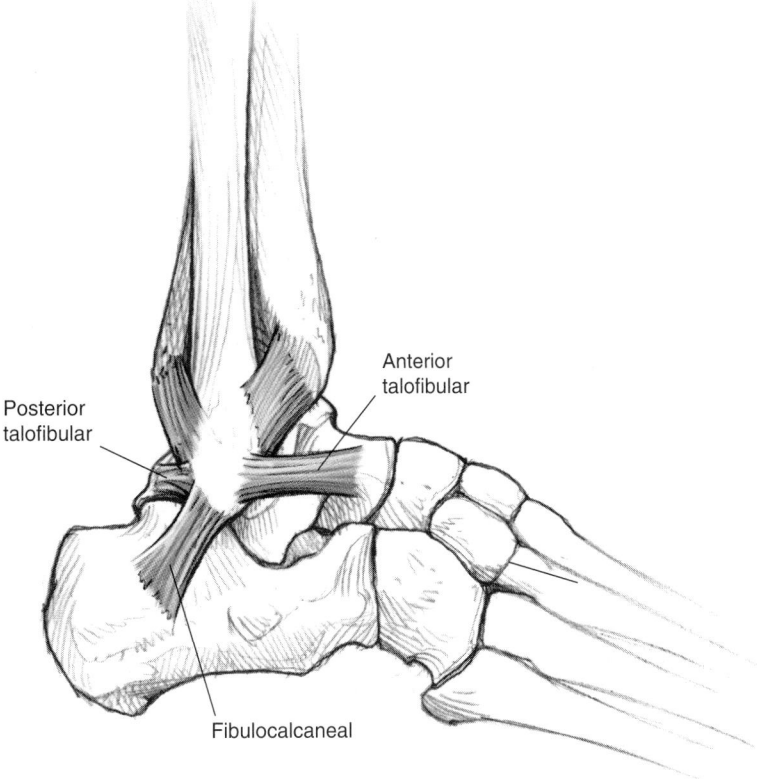

Fig. 3. Lateral ligamentous complex of the ankle. The three components of the lateral complex are the anterior talofibular ligament, the fibulocalcaneal ligament, and the posterior talofibular ligament.

Posterior talofibular

Anterior talofibular

Fibulocalcaneal

anterior inferior tibiofibular ligament runs from the antero-lateral distal tibia to the anterior portion of the lateral malleolus. The posterior inferior tibiofibular ligament runs from the posterolateral portion of the distal tibia to the posterior portion of the distal fibula. Above the incisura, the tibiofibular interosseous membrane thickens to form the interosseous ligament that runs between the tibia and fibula proximally in the thigh. If there is a failure of the syndesmosis, the ankle mortise will widen, allowing the talus to sublux laterally[4] and disrupting the normal weightbearing relationships of the joint. An intact deep deltoid ligament on the medial side does not prevent this lateral shift.

On the lateral aspect of the ankle lies the distal fibula, or lateral malleolus. The medial surface of this bone is covered with articular cartilage and composes the lateral portion of the joint. The lateral ligamentous complex of the ankle has three portions (Fig. 3). The anterior talofibular ligament runs between the anterior fibula and the lateral neck of the talus. In plantar flexion, it lines up with the fibula and functions as a collateral ligament, resisting inversion of the talus. With the ankle in neutral position, it resists anterior translation of the talus relative to the tibia. The fibulocalcaneal ligament lies in the middle and runs distally, beneath the peroneal tendons to the lateral border of the calcaneus. In dorsiflexion, this ligament lines up with the talus and becomes the functional collateral ligament. The posterior talofibular ligament runs from the posterior lateral malleolus to the posterior process of the talus.

There are many important tendinous and neurovascular structures that cross the ankle joint. Medially, on the posterior aspect of the medial malleolus, lie the tendons of the posterior tibialis, the flexor digitorum longus, and the flexor hallucis longus muscles. Posterior to these tendons lie the posterior tibial artery and vein, as well as the posterior tibial nerve. On the superficial anteromedial surface of the ankle lies the saphenous vein and nerve. These structures are at risk during surgical approaches to the medial malleolus.

Posteriorly lies the Achilles tendon, the smaller plantaris tendon, and the sural nerve. On the lateral side, the peroneal tendons course around the posterior aspect of the lateral malleolus and are held in place by a thick retinaculum. On the anterior surface of the ankle lie the tendons of the anterior tibialis, the extensor digitorum longus, and the extensor hallucis longus encased in a thick fibrous retinaculum. The anterior tibial vessels and the deep peroneal nerve also cross the anterior ankle.

BIOMECHANICS

The ankle is a hinge joint whose axis runs posteriorly and inferiorly from the tip of the medial malleolus toward the tip of the lateral malleolus.[5] The obliquity of the ankle joint axis varies but averages 82 degrees, or 8 degrees of varus, when measured from the midline of the tibia in the coronal plane. The tibiotalar articular surface, or plafond, averages 3 degrees of valgus angulation. The angle between the two, or the talocrural angle, measures 83 ± 4 degrees. This angle is comparable from side to side and is a reliable indicator of ankle alignment (Fig. 4).[6]

The fit of the talus in the ankle mortise is precise and remains congruent throughout the entire range of ankle motion. Because of the oblique axis of the ankle joint,

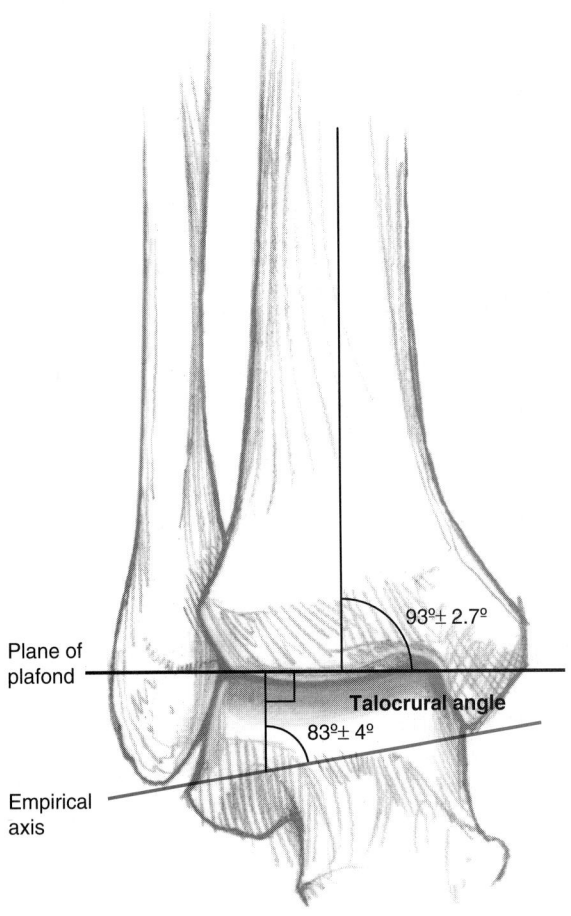

Plane of
plafond

93° ± 2.7°

Talocrural angle

83° ± 4°

Empirical
axis

Fig. 4. Normal ankle relationships. The plane of the tibial plafond is in approximately 3 degrees of lateral tilt. The axis of the ankle joint, as described by the talocrural angle, is in varus alignment. The talocrural angle should be similar to that of the opposite side.

there is an obligatory internal and external rotation of the foot with plantar flexion and dorsiflexion, respectively. It has been reported that the ankle has a mean dorsiflexion of 32 degrees and a mean plantar flexion of 45 degrees when loaded.[7] Normal gait requires at least 10 degrees of active dorsiflexion, whereas athletics requires at least twice that.

CLINICAL FEATURES

HISTORY

The details of how and when the injury occurred, the preexisting medical status, and the functional demands of the injured person allow the treating physician to gain an appreciation of the extent of the injury and to develop a plan of treatment.

The specific mechanism of injury can be helpful in determining the forces involved and can provide clues to the diagnosis. It is helpful to know whether there was a high-energy injury (e.g., a motorcycle accident) or a low-energy injury (e.g., sliding into second base). The location of the

accident is helpful, especially in assessing the degree of contamination present if the fracture is open. It is important to gather details of the medical condition of the patient. Patients having limbs with a history of previous injury or stroke and patients with diabetes or peripheral vascular disease may have unreliable physical examinations because of neurological compromise. A history of smoking, alcohol use, or chronic disease will affect anesthetic management of patients and wound healing and thus will greatly affect preoperative planning. Because the goal of treatment of any ankle injury is to restore the patient to the previous level of function, it is useful to know the preinjury functional status of the patient. The goals of treatment and rehabilitation will be different for the competitive athlete than for the sedentary retiree.

PHYSICAL EXAMINATION

The goal of the physical examination is to rapidly identify those injuries that require urgent treatment, such as open fractures and dislocations, and then to fully characterize the injury. The physical examination begins with an inspection of the skin and the soft tissues, looking for open wounds and other soft-tissue injury, extent of swelling, and obvious deformity. Open wounds are inspected and dressed, and obvious deformities are grossly realigned.

A complete neurovascular examination is a must. The limb should be evaluated for signs of ischemia and capillary refill and for the presence and character of pulses. All the motor units that cross the ankle must be tested, but their strength may be limited by pain. A complete sensory examination is also done. This is important not only to determine if there are associated neurological or vascular injuries, but also to evaluate the limb for an impending compartment syndrome.

In many injuries, the extent of the fracture will be obvious from the initial inspection. In more subtle injuries, each anatomic structure should be palpated and stressed. Localized tenderness over the medial or lateral malleolus may indicate fracture. Tenderness over the lateral ligamentous complex may indicate an ankle sprain, whereas tenderness over the tibiofibular joint may indicate an injury to the syndesmotic ligaments. The proximal tibia and fibula must also be palpated to rule out associated injury. The ankle is put through range-of-motion activities, and the stability of the joint is tested. Because of the function of the lateral ligamentous complex, the stability to inversion stress must be tested in plantar flexion as well as dorsiflexion. Anterior tibiotalar subluxation is indicative of an injury to the anterior fibulotalar ligament.

INVESTIGATIONS

Routine radiograph studies of the injured ankle include an anteroposterior (AP) view, a lateral view, and an oblique internal rotation view called the mortise view (Figs. 5, 6, and 7).[8, 9] The mortise view, a true AP view of the ankle mortise, is obtained by placing the leg in 15 degrees of internal rotation so that the beam is perpendicular to the true axis of ankle rotation. Full-length views of the leg are required if tenderness has been noted in the proximal tibia or fibula. Stress views of the ankle are useful in determining subtle injuries to the syndesmosis and the lateral liga-

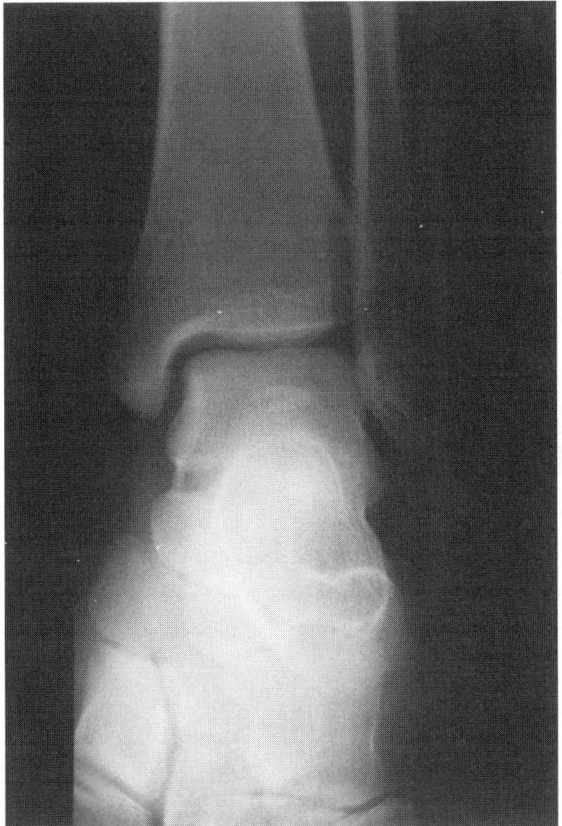

Fig. 5. Normal anteroposterior view of the ankle.

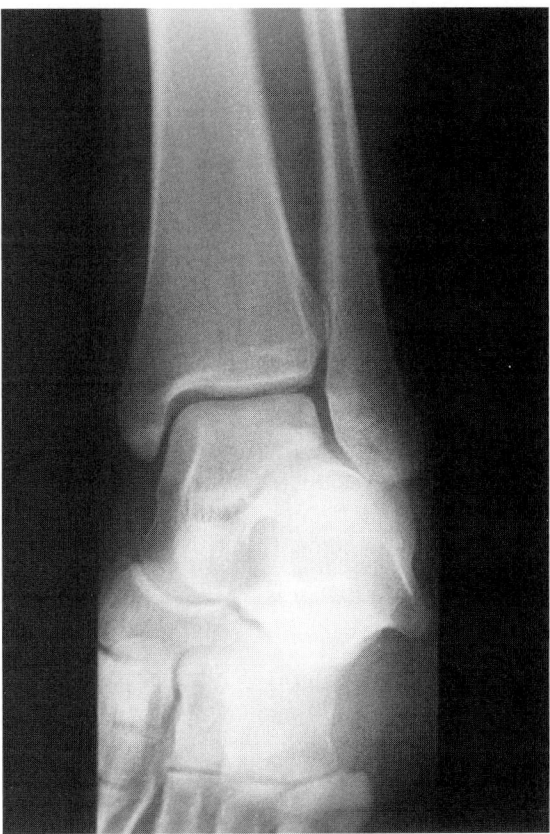

Fig. 7. Mortise view of the ankle.

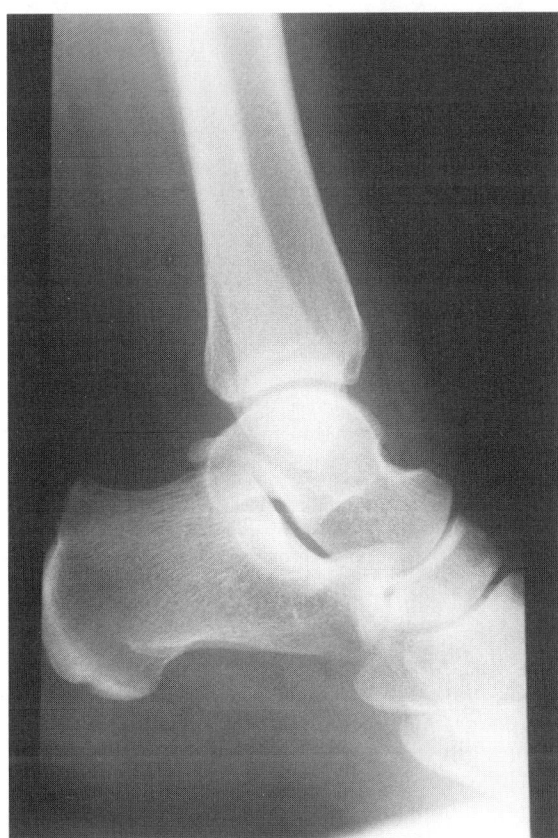

Fig. 6. Normal lateral view of the ankle.

mentous complex. Eversion and external rotation films are helpful in evaluating syndesmotic competence, whereas inversion films can be helpful in evaluating the lateral ligamentous complex. Comparison views of the other side can be helpful in evaluating subtle findings.

Traditional tomography or computed tomography scanning can be helpful in determining the extent and position of articular fragments, the degree of comminution, or the presence of osteochondral lesions on the talus. These studies are not routinely obtained for malleolar injuries but are helpful in specific cases for diagnosis and preoperative planning. Magnetic resonance imaging is useful in evaluating subtle injuries to the articular surfaces of the tibia and the talus, tendons, and ligaments. Technetium bone scanning can be used to look for stress fractures.

CLASSIFICATION

There are two main classification schemes used in describing fractures of the ankle. The Lauge-Hansen system is derived from anatomic studies in cadaveric ankles and is based on the position of the foot at the time of injury and the direction of the deforming force. It is useful in understanding the mechanism of injury and the forces that caused the fracture. An understanding of the Lauge-Hansen scheme (Fig. 8) forms the basis for the rational closed treatment of fractures of the ankle and is fundamental knowledge for all surgeons who treat these injuries. The Danis-Weber classification, based on the injury to the lateral malleolus and the relationship of the fibula to the tibia,

Danis-Weber Classification

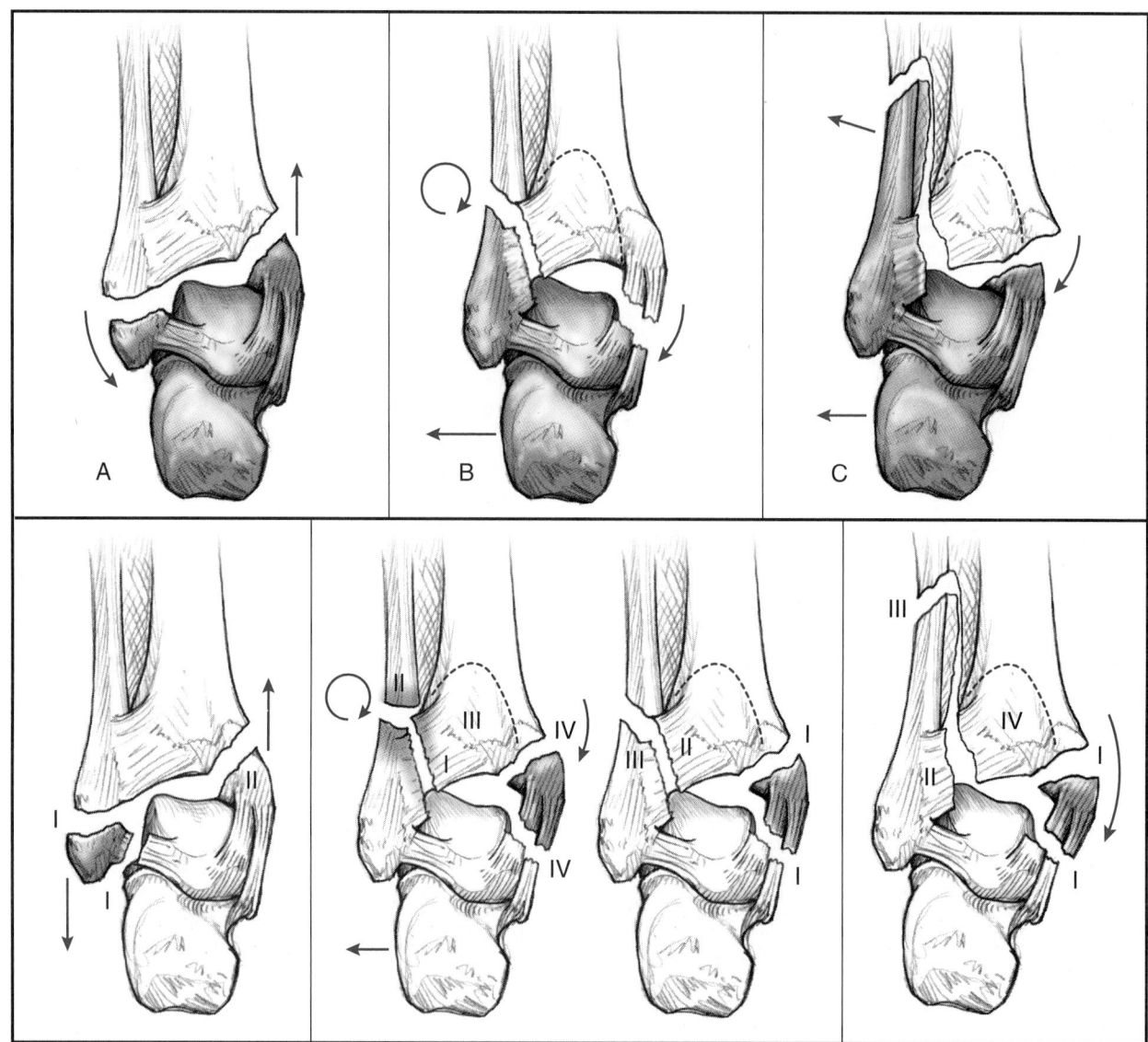

Lauge-Hansen Classification

Fig. 8. Ankle fracture classification schemes. These are the Danis-Weber classification *(above, A–C)* and the corresponding Lauge-Hansen classification *(below).*

is less cumbersome and easier to use. It allows classification of the fracture[10, 11] based on the potential instability of the talus in the mortise and has become the favored scheme as closed management of displaced fractures has fallen out of favor. Although each classification scheme is useful, the actual details of treatment of malleolar fractures are more dependent on the anatomic injury than on the classification of the fracture.

Danis-Weber Classification

Type A: An injury characterized by a transverse fracture of the fibula at or below the level of the plafond, it may be associated with a ligamentous or bony injury to the medial side. It represents a failure of the lateral malleolus

in tension and corresponds to the Lauge-Hansen supination-adduction injury.

Type B: These injuries are characterized by a fracture of the fibula at the level of the plafond, with or without associated injuries to the medial side or syndesmotic ligaments. This corresponds to either a supination–external rotation or a pronation-abduction injury.

Type C: A fracture of the fibula that is proximal to the plafond, this injury corresponds to the pronation–external rotation injury of the Lauge-Hansen classification. It is important to recognize because it signifies a disruption of the syndesmosis that may be more substantial than that seen in the type B injury and thus has a greater potential for instability.

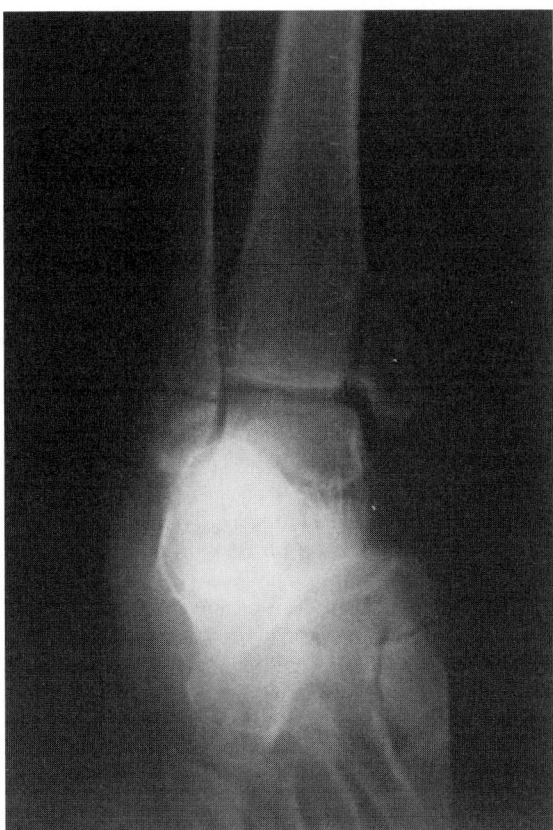

Fig. 9. Supination-adduction fracture. This is a mortise view of a stage II supination-adduction or Danis-Weber type A fracture. There is a tension failure of the fibula with a vertical fracture of the medial malleolus.

Lauge-Hansen Classification System

The first word in each classification corresponds to the position of the foot, and the second word to the force that caused the observed injury.

1. Supination-adduction (Fig. 9): This injury occurs when the inverted foot is adducted and accounts for 10% to 20% of ankle fractures. Stage I is a failure of the lateral ligamentous complex or an avulsion fracture of the lateral malleolus (i.e., a transverse fracture located at or below the level of the plafond). If the adduction continues, stage II of the injury is a vertical, medially displaced fracture of the medial malleolus. Because the mechanism of injury is compression on the medial side, this fracture can be associated with impaction of the medial joint surface.

2. Supination–external rotation (Fig. 10): The external rotation of the inverted foot is the most common mechanism of injury, accounting for 40% to 75% of all malleolar fractures. Stage I is a failure of the anterior inferior tibiofibular ligament, either through the substance of the ligament or by avulsion of its origin on the anterior lateral tibia. Stage II is a rotational, oblique fracture of the lateral malleolus, beginning at the level of the plafond and extending proximally. Stage III is the failure of the posterior inferior tibiofibular ligament, ei-

ther through the ligament or by avulsion of its point of insertion on the posterior tibia, resulting in a posterior malleolus fracture. Though both of the tibiofibular ligaments are disrupted, the distal fracture of the fibula at the level of the plafond should ensure that the more proximal portions of the syndesmosis remain intact. Stage IV of injury is a fracture of the medial malleolus, a rupture of the deep deltoid ligament, or both. Failure to appreciate a medial ligamentous injury may cause the surgeon to confuse a stable stage II injury with an unstable stage IV lesion that requires operative treatment.

3. Pronation-abduction: Forced abduction of the everted foot causes these injuries, which represent 5% to 20% of ankle fractures. Stage I is a tensile failure of the medial side, either through the ligament or with a transverse avulsion fracture of the medial malleolus at the level of the plafond. Stage II is rupture of the anterior and posterior tibiofibular syndesmotic ligaments. As abduction continues, stage III is a bending fracture of the fibula at the level of the plafond. It can be distinguished from a supination–external rotation stage II lesion because the fracture is transverse and can have a marked amount of lateral comminution.

4. Pronation–external rotation (Fig. 11): This injury is

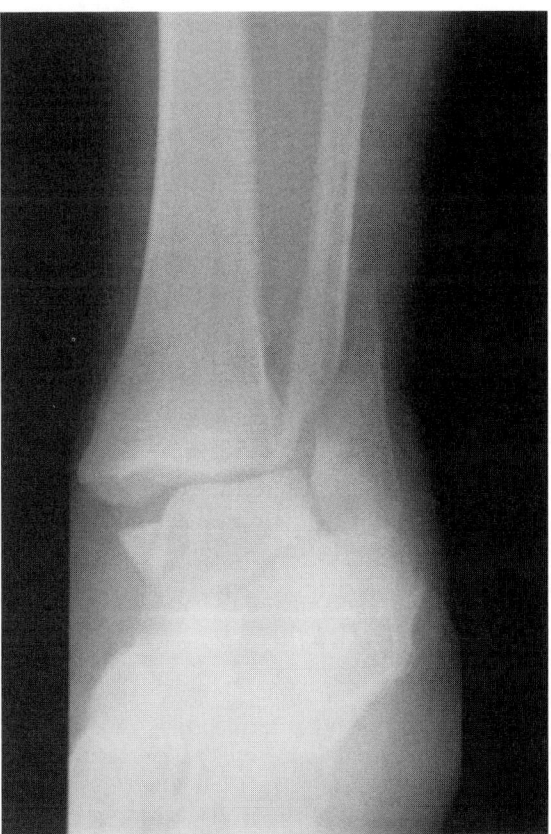

Fig. 10. Supination–external rotation fracture. This is a mortise view of a stage II supination–external rotation or Danis-Weber type B fracture. The fibula fracture is oblique and at the level of the plafond with a tension failure of the medial side.

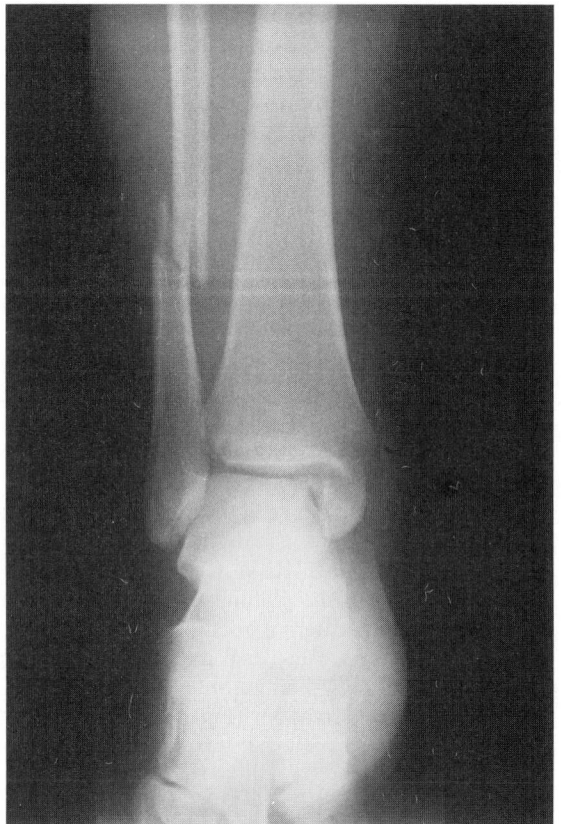

Fig. 11. Pronation–external rotation fracture. This is a mortise view of a pronation–external rotation injury. There is slight widening of the syndesmosis.

caused by the external rotation of the everted foot. Stage I is a rupture of the deltoid ligament or an avulsion fracture of the medial malleolus. Stage II is a failure of the anterior tibiofibular ligament. Stage III is an oblique or spiral fracture of the fibula, which is above the level of the plafond. Stage IV is a disruption of the posterior tibiofibular ligament or a fracture of the posterior malleolus. This mechanism can also cause rotational fractures of the fibula in the proximal leg; thus isolated fractures of the medial or posterior malleolus should be carefully examined for potential instability of the talus in the mortise. This mechanism causes 10% to 20% of malleolar fractures.

GOALS AND INDICATIONS FOR TREATMENT

The goal of treatment for injuries of the ankle is the restoration of normal anatomic relationships. Injuries that are stable can be managed in a closed fashion with casting or bracing and early functional rehabilitation. Unstable or potentially unstable injuries can be managed in a closed manner if the risks of surgery outweigh the benefits to the patient, but they are more reliably managed surgically. It should be stressed, however, that careful closed management is preferable to poorly planned and executed surgical treatment that exposes the patient to the risks of surgery but does not produce the desired benefit.

ANKLE SPRAINS

Most ankle sprains are caused by an inversion injury to the foot and result in injury to the lateral ligamentous complex. They have been classified according to the degree of damage to the ligament. Grade I injuries involve stretching without tearing. Grade II injuries involve partial tearing, whereas grade III injuries involve complete tearing and functional incompetence. Grade I and II injuries are stable and thus have traditionally been treated initially with RICE (rest, ice, compression, and elevation) followed by early motion and functional rehabilitation. Surgical reconstruction of grade III injuries has been advocated in the past; Kannus and Renstrom[12] found that there was no demonstrable difference in results between surgical and nonsurgical care of complete ligamentous injuries and that operative care had a higher complication rate and more cost.

Syndesmosis sprains are unusual but may be differentiated from lateral injuries on physical examination. These patients have pain over the distal tibiofibular joint to palpation or have a positive squeeze test,[13] in which compression of the tibia and fibula at mid-calf causes pain at the syndesmosis. In addition, external rotation stress of the foot may reproduce the pain. Treatment is identical to that of lateral ankle injuries except that the time to full recovery is longer. Surgical stabilization of the syndesmosis is indicated when there is widening of the mortise on plain radiographs.

ANKLE DISLOCATIONS

Ankle dislocations are usually part of a severe ankle fracture. Isolated ankle dislocations are rare and are usually posteromedial. Many of these injuries are open and can be associated with neurovascular injury. Closed reduction and cast immobilization are recommended for closed dislocations.[14] Open dislocations are treated with appropriate wound management and immediate repair of ligamentous structures that are visible in the wound.

ANKLE FRACTURES

The goal of treatment for malleolar fractures is the restoration of the normal tibiotalar relationship. The fibular fracture is extra-articular, but it is the key to restoring ankle congruency because the talus moves with the distal fibular fragment.[15] Reduction of fibular length, rotation, and position in the incisura will reliably place the talar dome under the articular surface of the distal tibia. This fracture must unite in an anatomic position to prevent late lateral subluxation of the talus and early arthrosis. Knowledge of the normal anatomic landmarks is essential to the successful treatment of these injuries.[16, 17]

Type A Injuries

Nondisplaced fractures can be treated by closed methods and do not require surgery. Minimally or moderately displaced fractures can usually be reduced by reversing the mechanism of injury (e.g., abduction of the hindfoot can be managed with a cast).

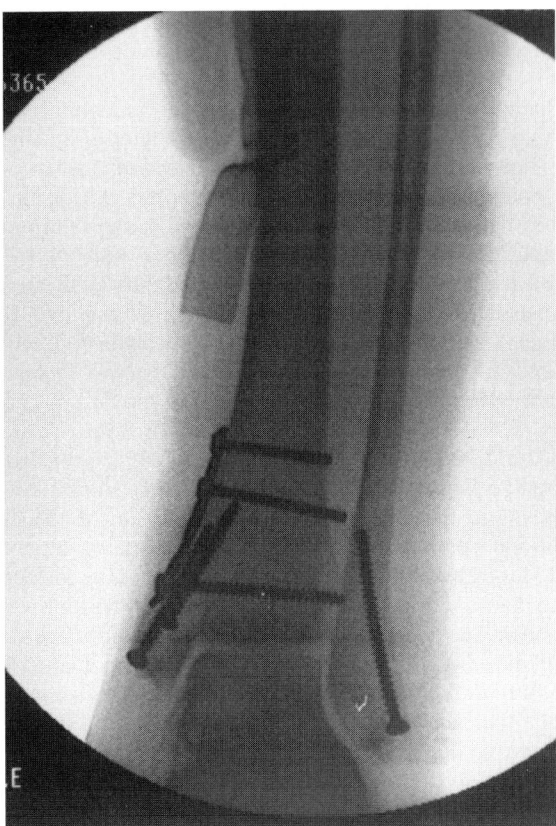

Fig. 12. Operative treatment of a supination-adduction fracture. A vertical screw stabilizes the fibular fracture, and two lag screws and an antiglide plate stabilize the medial malleolus.

Open reduction and internal fixation of type A injuries (Fig. 12) is indicated in fractures that cannot be reduced in an anatomic fashion by closed means or that have lost their initial closed reduction during cast immobilization. Fractures of the medial side with articular impaction should be reduced and possibly bone grafted to restore the weight-bearing surface.

Type B Injuries

Because the fibula fracture is at the level of the plafond, the more proximal soft tissues are usually intact and the potential for syndesmotic disruption is less than that for type C injuries.

The mechanism of injury is important in guiding closed reduction and in identifying all the injured structures. Nondisplaced external rotation type B fractures can be well treated in a cast. It is important to follow these patients closely, however, because stage II injuries can appear radiographically identical to stage IV injuries with a medial ligamentous injury. Any loss of reduction on the follow-up films is an indication for open reduction and internal fixation. Nondisplaced abduction injuries also do well with closed management.

Displaced external rotation injuries can be managed closed if an adequate reduction can be achieved. Closed management may be continued if the talus is restored under the mortise and an anatomic reduction of the lateral

malleolus is achieved. If either of these fails, or if the reduction is lost, open reduction is a must.

If the condition of the soft tissues and the medical status of the patient permit, displaced type B fractures are best treated with open reduction and internal fixation. This ensures accurate reduction of both the talus and the fibula fractures with less risk of late displacement. External rotation fibula fractures are amenable to interfragmentary lag screws and plate fixation (Fig. 13). Abduction fibula fractures are more difficult to stabilize and usually cannot be fixed with lag screws. A spanning plate, with or without bone graft, can be used to restore fibular length and rotation in these comminuted fractures.

After anatomic reduction of the fracture, the stability of the syndesmosis must be tested. Fractures with a medial ligamentous injury are more likely to be unstable than are those with a surgically stabilized medial malleolus. Syndesmotic widening can be seen on plain film, on stress radiographs, or by direct vision. Placement of a syndesmotic screw or direct repair of the ligaments is required to prevent subluxation.

Type C Injuries

These fractures are rarely stable and are suitable for closed treatment only in patients unfit for surgery or with a completely nondisplaced fracture. The first step is to stabilize

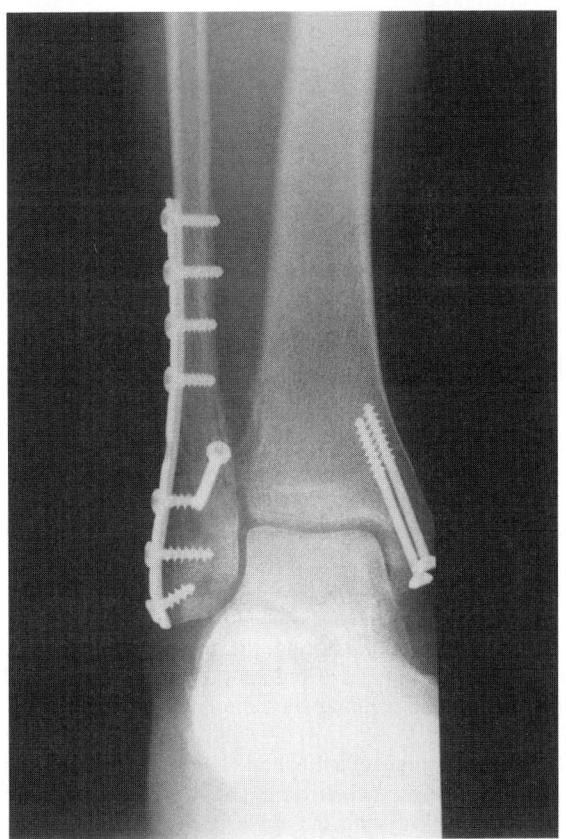

Fig. 13. Operative stabilization of a supination–external rotation injury. This is a medial malleolus fracture repaired with two cancellous lag screws and fibula repaired with an interfragmentary lag screw and a neutralization plate.

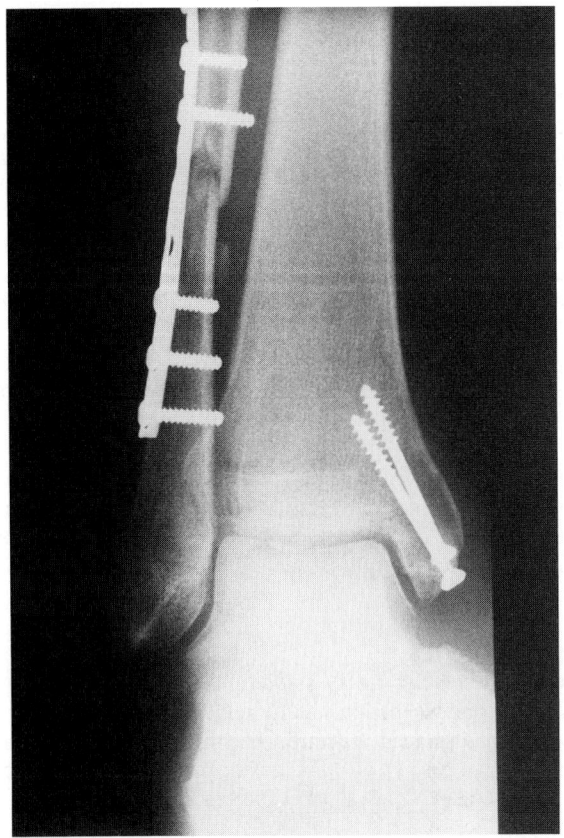

Fig. 14. Operative treatment of a pronation–external rotation injury.

the fibula fracture with a plate and with or without interfragmentary lag screws (Fig. 14). The medial malleolus is then stabilized with lag screws. Posterior malleolus fractures that compose more than 25% of the articular surface are then fixed. Finally, the stability of the syndesmosis is assessed, and it is stabilized as needed.

PROCEDURES

INITIAL TREATMENT

Ankle fractures are often open and involve significant subluxation or dislocation of the ankle joint. After the initial assessment, open wounds should be promptly dressed. Limbs that are deformed because of a displaced fracture should be provisionally reduced to lessen soft-tissue embarrassment, to take pressure off neurovascular structures, and to prevent further damage to the articular surface. Provisional reduction will also reduce patient pain and swelling and aid in accomplishing the complete examination of the ankle.

After a thorough examination, all fractures should have an attempt at closed reduction. The leg is then placed in a well-padded splint with the ankle in the neutral position or in a well-padded, bivalved cast to allow for swelling. Postreduction radiographs are then obtained to assess the reduction. If the ankle is anatomically reduced, the fracture may be treated closed in those injury patterns that are stable. Fractures that are not reducible and in which skin or neu-

rovascular structures are threatened should be taken to the operating room for immediate reduction and stabilization.

Open fractures should be treated as an emergency according to the protocols outlined in Chapters 3–3 and 3–17. Closed injuries may be treated electively early within the postinjury period. One may proceed when the soft tissues can be safely incised, usually with the return of the wrinkles in the skin. The quality of the reduction is affected by the length of time between injury and operative treatment. Fractures should be repaired within two weeks of injury if possible. Konrath and colleagues[18] found that the only difference between early and late fixation was a decreased hospital stay (i.e., 14 days) in the delayed group.

CLOSED REDUCTION

Closed reduction of ankle fractures ideally should be done early in the postinjury course. Organization of the hematoma and contracture of the soft tissues makes ligamentotaxis less effective and closed reduction more difficult if more than a day or two have elapsed since the injury.

Nondisplaced fractures require no reduction but do require a well-molded short-leg plaster cast to maintain the position of the ankle. The key to closed reduction is to reduce the talus to the correct position, not to apply direct pressure on the displaced malleolus. A long-leg cast with the knee flexed 20 degrees is the best choice for the initial period of immobilization because it controls rotation and assists in keeping the patient non-weightbearing.

Patients who are undergoing closed treatment of displaced malleolar fractures need to be followed closely. Patients should have check films made in the cast within 7 to 10 days of the reduction. At this time, the swelling will be reduced and the cast will be looser. If the reduction has been lost, prompt operative treatment can still be done and an excellent result achieved. Patients should be non-weightbearing for a period of 6 to 8 weeks to prevent displacement. If radiographs at this time show sufficient healing, the patient may be changed to a short-leg walking cast or a walking boot. Each patient must be treated individually based on the fracture configuration, reduction, healing, medical status, and functional demands.

PREOPERATIVE PLANNING

Once the decision has been made to operate on the fracture, a thorough preoperative plan must be made that includes patient positioning, type of operative table to be used, surgical approach to be used, how the reduction will be achieved, and implants to be used. A radiolucent table and image intensifier are helpful to check the reduction intraoperatively, as well as to obtain stress views of the syndesmosis. It is helpful on difficult cases to draw the fracture and to do the case on paper before the patient is brought to the operating room.[19] The methods of fixation discussed later are all generally accepted fracture fixation techniques.

FIBULA FIXATION

The accurate anatomic reduction of fibula fractures is very important because the fibula plays a key role in the restoration of the tibiotalar relationship. Distal fibula fractures are approached via a direct lateral approach. Care must be taken to keep soft-tissue flaps thick, to protect the peroneal tendons, and to preserve the superficial peroneal nerve as it runs along the anterior portion of the distal fibula in the distal portion of the wound.

Type A fractures can be fixed with an oblique screw placed longitudinally up the fibular shaft and across the fracture site, a tension band wire, or a plate. Often the end of the plate will need to be modified into a hook to allow more purchase in the distal segment. Type B fractures caused by external rotation are spiral or oblique and are amenable to fixation with interfragmentary lag screws and a one-third tubular or 3.5-mm neutralizing plate. Type B abduction fractures are usually transverse with lateral comminution. They are not normally suitable for lag screw fixation and must be neutralized with a spanning plate. Bone graft may be needed in cases of severe comminution. Type C fractures are best treated with a one-third tubular plate, with or without lag screw fixation. In fibula fractures with significant comminution or shortening, direct reduction of the fracture fragments may be difficult. In these cases, indirect reduction techniques using a small distractor or a plate with the AO tension-distraction device or a lamina spreader can be useful in restoring length.

MEDIAL FIXATION

Displaced fractures of the medial malleolus should be repaired to improve stability and maintain joint congruity. Repair of the deltoid ligament is not usually required. Care must be taken to protect the anteromedial saphenous vein and nerve but allow exposure of the fracture and the medial side of the ankle joint. The flexor tendons, running directly behind the medial malleolus, should be inspected for injury.

Transverse fractures of the medial malleolus at the level of the plafond, consistent with an avulsion mechanism, are best treated with anatomic reduction and cancellous lag screws or tension-banding techniques. Oblique or vertical fractures must be inspected for impaction of the anteromedial portion of the plafond. They are best stabilized with cancellous lag screws or a one-third tubular plate used in an antiglide fashion.

SYNDESMOSIS FIXATION

Stability of the ankle mortise can be determined from the initial plain radiographs, from stress radiographs obtained in the operating room at the time of stabilization, or by direct visualization. The Cotton test[17] for stability is performed by displacing the fibula laterally from the tibia. If there is more than a 3- to 4-mm shift of the talus, instability is present. Laboratory studies show that a disruption of the interosseous ligaments 3.5 to 4.0 cm[21, 22] above the plafond leads to late instability when there is a medial ligamentous injury.

The indications and techniques for stabilization of the syndesmosis are controversial, and there are few data to support any viewpoint. It is clear that widening of the mortise causes pain, instability, and arthritis. There is no clear indication in the literature of when the syndesmosis needs to be stabilized, how much fixation is required, how long the fixation should remain in place, how much activity should be allowed during healing, and if the fixation should be removed.

The syndesmosis should be reduced and fixed with the ankle in a neutral or dorsiflexed position. A large clamp is placed from tibia to fibula to reduce the joint. One or two screws are then placed parallel to the axis of the mortise (i.e., from posterolateral fibula to anteromedial tibia, 2 to 3 cm above the plafond, to stabilize the fibula to the tibia). The optimal screw type to be used is unknown, but most surgeons use a 3.5-mm or 4.5-mm cortical screw (Fig. 15). Patients should be kept non-weightbearing for 6 to 8 weeks; ligamentous healing usually takes this long in adults. The data on advancing the activity level of the patient, as well as the indications for and timing of screw removal, are also poor. Partial weightbearing can begin after 8 weeks. If screw removal is planned, it must be done before breakage, usually at the 12-week mark.

POSTERIOR FIXATION

Indications for operative treatment are posterior talar subluxation, articular incongruity, and syndesmosis instability. Most authors support fixation of the posterior malleolus if it involves more than 25% to 30% of the articular surface as seen on the lateral radiograph.

The method of fixation of posterior fractures is guided by the fracture pattern and the incisions used to treat the associated medial and lateral injuries. If the fracture is exposed through the posterolateral approach used to fix the fibula, it can be reduced by direct visualization and fixed with lag screws or a small fragment buttress plate on the back of the tibia. If the fracture site is not exposed, it can

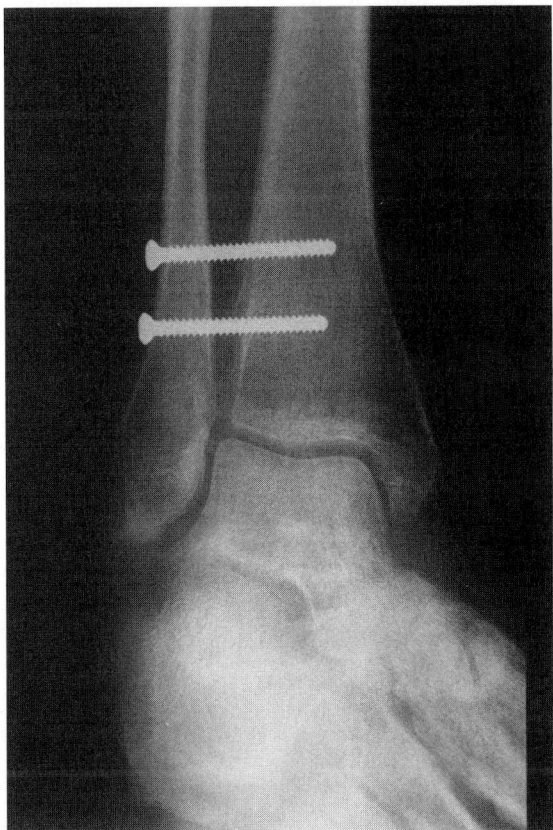

Fig. 15. Ligamentous syndesmosis injury stabilized with two cortical screws.

often be reduced percutaneously and fixed with anterior-to-posterior lag screws placed through small stab incisions from the front.

AFTERCARE

Before the patient leaves the operating room, good-quality mortise and lateral radiographs or C-arm images must be obtained to confirm adequate fracture reduction and hardware placement. The wounds are closed carefully, and the ankle is placed in a well-padded splint with the ankle in neutral position because equinus contractures are easier to prevent than to treat. Patients are given physical therapy for gait training and are discharged when comfortable.

Postoperative immobilization may be a cast, a removable orthosis, or a brace. The weightbearing status of the patient is determined by fracture pattern, quality of fixation, and patient compliance.[23] With malleolar injuries, most patients can be advanced to full weightbearing at the 6- to 8-week point. Physical therapy for range of motion, strengthening, and proprioception is started when the patient is able to fully bear weight and walk comfortably. Persistent swelling of the ankle is common and may persist for several months post union.

COMPLICATIONS AND RESULTS

COMPLICATIONS[24, 25]

Infection after repair of ankle fractures involves not only the wound, but also the joint itself. Infection may present as a wound infection or as an insidious narrowing of the joint space. Infected wounds should be aggressively treated. The ankle joint should be aspirated and cultured, and appropriate antibiotics should be started. Wounds should be closed over suction drains, not left open, to prevent desiccation of the articular surface. Well-fixed hardware should be left in place to provide stability. Retained hardware can be removed after the fracture heals. Unstable fractures with hardware in place should have the hardware removed at the time of débridement and can be stabilized with external fixation.

Nonunions of ankle fractures are rare and can be treated with bone grafting and stable internal fixation. Malunions can be the result of poor initial reduction or failure of fixation. Fractures with more initial instability, comminution, poor bone quality, or bone loss and those that occur in the neuropathic or uncooperative patient are at highest risk for nonunion and implant failure. Post-traumatic arthritis can be caused by malunion or as a result of the initial trauma to the articular surface. It is initially managed with nonsteroidals, activity modification, and orthotics. End-stage degenerative joint disease is best managed with an ankle arthrodesis.[26]

Wound slough and slow-healing wounds are often the result of the initial injury to the soft tissues and are more common after open fractures. A patient with a history of chronic disease or smoking is also at increased risk. Open wounds should be treated aggressively to prevent infection. Definitive closure should be done as soon as the wound is viable, either by split thickness grafting or by tissue transfer. Early consultation with a surgeon skilled in tissue transfers is a must to optimize patient outcome.

RESULTS

The results[6, 27, 28] of treatment of malleolar fractures are dependent on the return of patient function. A variety of scoring systems have been devised, from radiographic criteria to return to work and sports. Predictors of a poor result are severity of the initial injury, talar subluxation, residual fibular shortening, presence of articular impaction, and poor initial reduction. Fractures treated with diligent surgical technique do as well as or better than similar fractures treated with closed methods.[29] In a study that compared open reduction and internal fixation using the AO methodology with closed reduction, operative type A fractures had 78% to 82% good or excellent results, type B fractures had 75% to 83% good to excellent results, and type C fractures had 61% to 85% good to excellent results. Type A fractures treated with closed reduction and casting had 71% to 75% good to excellent results, type B fractures had 35% to 43% good to excellent results, and type C fractures had 22% to 37% good to excellent results.

REFERENCES

1. Sarrafian SK: Anatomy of the Foot and Ankle. Philadelphia, JB Lippincott, 1983.
2. Hamilton WC: Traumatic Disorders of the Ankle. New York, Springer-Verlag, 1984.
3. Macko VW, Matthews LS, Zwerkoski P, et al: The joint contact area of the ankle. The contribution of the posterior malleolus. J Bone Joint Surg Am 1991; 73:347.
4. Leeds HC, Ehrlich MG: Instability of the distal tibiofibular syndesmosis after bimalleolar and trimalleolar ankle fractures. J Bone Joint Surg Am 1984; 66:490.
5. Inman VT: The Joints of the Ankle. Baltimore, Williams and Wilkins, 1976.
6. Phillips WA, Schwartz HS, Kesler CS, et al: A prospective randomized study of the management of severe ankle fractures. J Bone Joint Surg Am 1985; 67:67.
7. Lindsjo U, Danckwardt-Lilliestrom G, Sahlstedt B: Measurement of the range of motion of the loaded ankle. Clin Orthop 1985; 199:68.
8. Mitchell MJ, Ho C, Howard BA: Diagnostic imaging of trauma to the ankle and foot. Part I: Fractures about the ankle. J Foot Surg 1989; 28:174.
9. Mitchell MJ, Ho C, Howard BA: Diagnostic imaging of trauma to the ankle and foot. Part II. J Foot Surg 1989; 28:266.
10. Lindsjo U: Classification of ankle fractures: The Lauge-Hansen or AO system? Clin Orthop 1985; 199:12.
11. Wilson FC: The pathogenesis and treatment of ankle fractures. Classification. Inst Course Lect 1990; 39:79.
12. Kannus P, Renstrom P: Treatment of acute tears of the lateral ligaments of the ankle: Operation, cast, or early controlled mobilization. J Bone Joint Surg Am 1991; 73:30.
13. Hopkinson WJ, St. Pierre P, Ryan JB, et al: Syndesmotic sprains of the ankle. Foot Ankle 1989; 10:36.
14. Toohey JS, Wersing RA: A long-term follow-up study of tibiotalar dislocations without associated fractures. Clin Orthop 1989; 239:207.
15. Yablon IG, Keller FG, Shouse L: The key role of the lateral malleolus in displaced fractures of the ankle. J Bone Joint Surg Am 1977; 59:169.
16. Petrone FA, Gail M, Pee D, et al: Quantitative criteria for prediction of results after displaced ankle fractures. J Bone Joint Surg Am 1983; 65:667.
17. Stiehl JB: Ankle fractures with diastasis. Inst Course Lect 1990; 39:95.
18. Konrath G, Karges D, Watson JT: Early vs. delayed treatment of severe ankle fractures: A comparison of results. J Orthop Trauma 1995; 9:377.

19. Mast JW, Jakob R, Ganz R: Planning and Reduction Technique in Fracture Surgery. New York, Springer-Verlag, 1989.

20. Muller ME, Allgower M, Schneider R, et al: Manual of Internal Fixation, 3rd ed. New York, Springer-Verlag, 1991.

21. Boden SD, Labropoulos PA, McCowin P, et al: Mechanical considerations for the syndesmotic screw. J Bone Joint Surg Am 1989; 71:1548.

22. Burns WC, Prakash K, Adelaar RS, et al: Tibiotalar joint dynamics: Indications for the syndesmotic screw. A cadaver study. Foot Ankle 1993; 14:153.

23. Ahl T, Dalen N, Holmberg S, et al: Early weight bearing of displaced ankle fractures. Acta Orthop Scand 1987; 58:535.

24. Shelton ML, Anderson RL Jr: Complications of fractures and dislocations of the ankle. In Epps CH Jr (ed): Complications in Orthopaedic Surgery. Philadelphia, JB Lippincott, 1986, 2nd ed, vol 1, p 599.

25. Yablon IG: Complications and their management. In Yablon G, Segal D, Leach RE (eds): Ankle Injuries. New York, Churchill Livingstone, 1983, p 103.

26. DeSouza LJ, Gustillo RB, Meyer TJ: Results of operative treatment of displaced external rotation-abduction fractures of the ankle. J Bone Joint Surg Am 1985; 67: 1066.

27. Mazur JM, Schwartz E, Simon SR: Ankle arthrodesis: Long-term follow-up with gait analysis. J Bone Joint Surg Am 1979; 61: 964.

28. Mak KH, Chan KM, Leung PC: Ankle fracture treated with the AO principle— An experience with 116 cases. Injury 1985; 16:265.

29. Hughes JL, Weber H, Willenegger H, et al: Evaluation of ankle fractures: Non-operative and operative treatment. Clin Orthop 1979; 138:111.

section

3

chapter

20

CALCANEUS AND TALUS

Jeff Anglen

Summary

- Fractures of the talus and calcaneus, which may result from a motor vehicle crash or fall from a height, are relatively uncommon injuries.
- Both types of fracture can lead to significant disability and time lost from work.
- Appropriate treatment requires experience, skill, and judgment. Appreciation of the soft-tissue component of the injury is required to avoid complications.
- Successful surgical treatment is dependent upon proper timing, adequate planning, careful, precise reduction, and stable fixation. Failure of any of these components may lead to treatment failure.
- Outcome is dependent upon the severity of the injury as well as on correct treatment.
- Treatment failures may require arthrodesis for salvage.

FRACTURE OF THE TALUS

INTRODUCTION

Fractures of the talus are relatively rare, representing less than 0.5% of all fractures.[1] They represent a challenging problem for the orthopaedist because of their rarity, the high incidence rate of complications, and the significant sequelae of a poor functional outcome.

HISTORICAL REVIEW

Until the late 19th century, talus fracture or dislocation was treated with immobilization and resulted in significant disability. Open injuries were treated with either talectomy or primary amputation because of the high incidence rate of infection, which led to a mortality of 84%.[2] In 1892, Bergmann of Berlin was the first to report open reduction of the

dislocated talus. The term "aviator's astragalus," coined in 1919 by Anderson,[3] reflected the fact that fracture of the neck of the talus was a common injury following crash landings during World War I. The advent of open reduction and internal fixation techniques in the last 40 years has improved outcomes, but certain injuries continue to have a high complication rate and subsequent poor functional results.

PATHOGENESIS

Sixty percent of the talar surface is covered with articular cartilage. There are no muscular or tendinous attachments, and thus no direct muscular motion of the talus. The superior surface articulates with the tibia in the ankle joint, the inferior surface articulates with the calcaneus through the complex subtalar joint, and the distal surface of the talar head articulates with the navicular. Thus, fractures of the talus are commonly intra-articular, and good reduction is necessary. The ligamentous attachments of the talus include the interosseous talocalcaneal ligament, which unites the talus to the calcaneus inferiorly; the deltoid ligament, which connects the talus to the medial malleolus; the anterior talofibular and talocalcaneal ligaments, which join the lateral process of the talus to the fibula and calcaneus; and the posterior talofibular ligament, attaching to the posterior process of the talus.

Vascular anatomy influences the risk of avascular necrosis (AVN) after fracture. All three arteries of the lower limb contribute to vascularization of the talus, but the most important is the artery of the tarsal canal arising from the posterior tibial artery.

Fractures of the talus typically result from high-energy trauma caused by falls or by vehicular violence. Fractures can involve the body (including the posterior process), the lateral process, or the neck. The most common is fracture of the neck, accounting for about 50% of talus fractures. Once widely believed to be caused by forced dorsiflexion, this fracture has not been produced in the laboratory by that mechanism. Rather, a dorsal-to-plantar shear force on the midfoot with the talus compressed into the mortise is required to fracture the talar neck in the cadaver foot. If the force continues, there is medial rotation, displacing the foot through the subtalar joint. Further displacement rotates the talar body around the deltoid ligament and out of the mortise, where it may press on the neurovascular bundle posteromedially. About 50% of talar neck fractures have an associated medial malleolus fracture.

Talar neck fractures have been classified by Hawkins[4] into three types. Type 1 is a nondisplaced fracture of the neck. The subtalar and tibiotalar joints are reduced. Type 2 is a displaced fracture of the neck with a subluxated or dislocated subtalar joint. Type 3 is a displaced fracture with a subluxated or dislocated tibiotalar joint. Some authors consider additional dislocation of the talonavicular joint to represent a separate type, designated type 4.

CLINICAL PRESENTATION

The typical history is that of a fall or crash, with subsequent ankle or foot pain and inability to ambulate. In the intoxicated, obtunded, or intubated patient, swelling, ecchymosis, and/or crepitus on ankle motion should be sought. Approximately 15% of talar fractures are open. In all cases the status of the soft tissues should be carefully assessed. Note is taken of abrasions, blisters, and potential compartment syndrome. Skin that is compromised by displaced fragments should be relieved emergently because of the risk of slough. The most common associated injuries are fractures of the calcaneus and medial malleolus.

INVESTIGATION

In a patient whose history, complaints, or physical examination suggests fracture, anteroposterior and lateral radiographs will reveal the fracture. In most cases, further investigation will not be required. Lateral process fractures, which may result from severe inversion injury, can be mistaken for ankle sprain and thereby missed. Computed tomography (CT) scans may be required to make the diagnosis if it is not evident on plain films.

TREATMENT GOALS, INDICATIONS, AND CONTRAINDICATIONS

The overall goal is to return the patient to pain-free ambulation on a foot that is supple and stable. This requires union in the proper alignment with good joint reduction. Methods for accomplishing these goals depend upon the type of the fracture. Treatment methods are summarized in Table 1.

A reduction with less than 5 mm of displacement and less than 5 degrees of malalignment has been considered adequate,[5] although displacements of as little as 2 mm alter the contact characteristics of the subtalar joint.[6] Perfect reduction should be the goal of an open procedure. A severely mangled foot in the polytrauma patient may require primary amputation.

PROCEDURE

Closed reduction of a displaced type 2 talar neck fracture is attempted by manipulating the head fragment into plan-

TABLE 1. TREATMENT OPTIONS IN FRACTURE OF THE TALUS

Fracture Type	Recommended Treatment
Body fractures—nondisplaced	Immobilization in short cast 6–8 wk
Body fractures—displaced	Open reduction and internal fixation (ORIF)
Posterior process fracture	Short walking cast in 15 degrees equinus 4–6 wk
Lateral process fracture—nondisplaced	Short cast with partial weight-bearing 6 wk
Lateral process fracture—displaced	Large—ORIF; small—excise
Talar neck fracture	
Type 1	Weightbearing cast 6–12 wk, weightbearing at 6 wk
Type 2	Attempted closed reduction; if successful, cast non-weight-bearing; gradually decrease equinus; weightbearing at 3 mo; if unsuccessful, ORIF
Type 3	May attempt closed reduction; but, almost all patients will require ORIF

tar flexion to align it with the body fragment. Varus and valgus deformities must be corrected as well. Verification with radiographs in two planes is required.

When open reduction is required, a medial approach is commonly employed in the interval between the anterior and posterior tibial tendons. A dorsolateral approach may be used to aid reduction in cases of medial comminution, and may provide better screw purchase. Cannulated screws may be placed from anteromedial or anterolateral, or through a separate incision from posterolateral to anteromedial. The posterior approach for fixation permits crossing of the fracture line in a more perpendicular direction, is stronger, and may avoid a tendency toward varus angulation in the face of medial comminution[7, 8] (Fig. 1). If directed from front to back, screw heads should be countersunk below the articular surface. Titanium screws have been recommended to allow magnetic resonance imaging (MRI) evaluation of AVN.

Reduction may be facilitated by the use of traction through the calcaneus with a transverse pin and a femoral distractor or external fixator. Medial malleolus osteotomy is sometimes required and is preferable to incising the deltoid ligament to avoid damage to the medial blood supply. Postoperatively, a short leg non-weightbearing cast is utilized until bony healing is evident. Loading is delayed for about 3 months.

COMPLICATIONS

The complications of talus fracture include infection or soft-tissue slough, nonunion, malunion, post-traumatic arthritis, and AVN. Complications are summarized in Table 2. AVN is caused by damage to the arterial supply and is more common with more displaced fractures. Union may occur in the face of AVN, and only a minority of patients

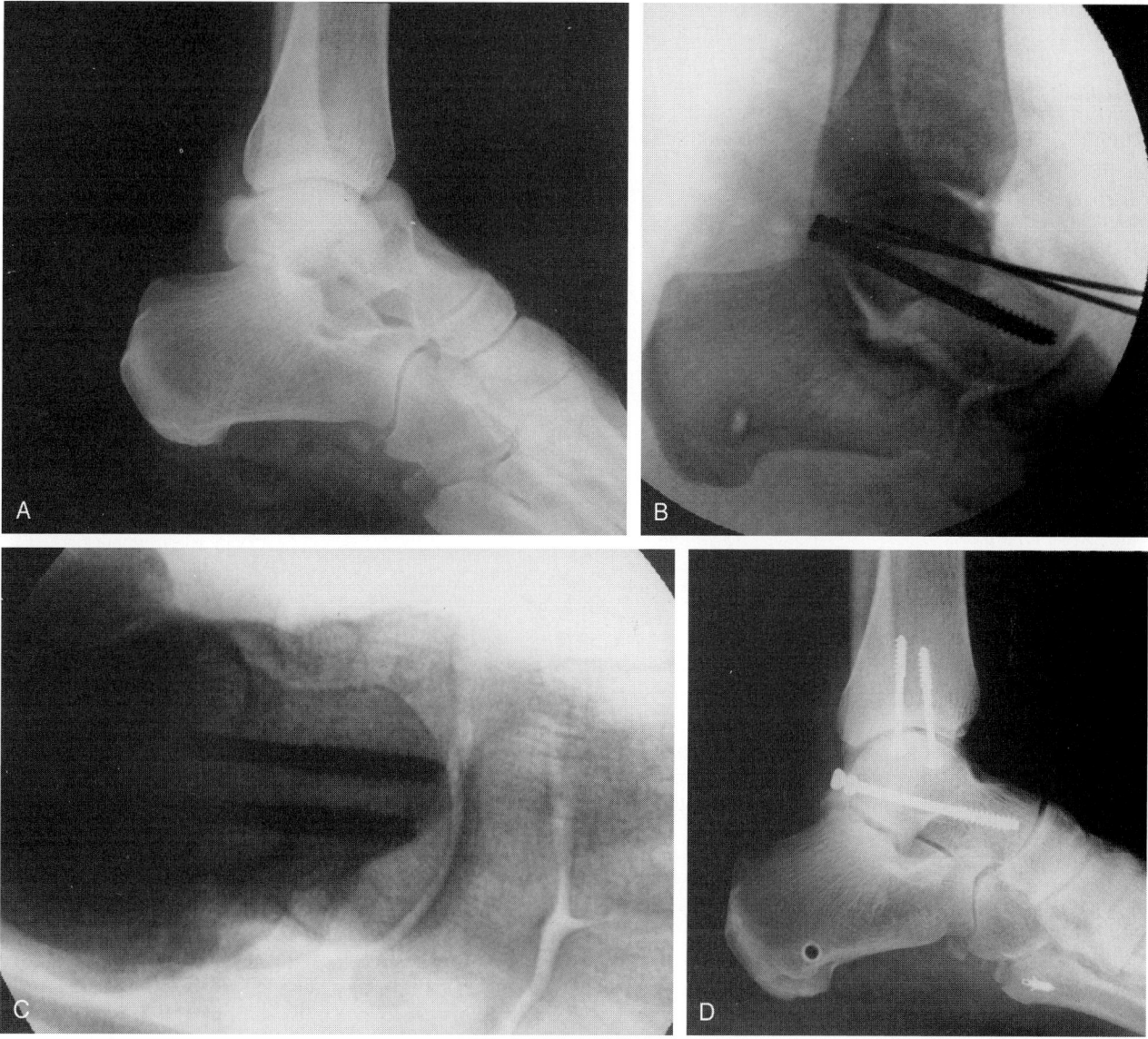

Fig. 1. Reduction and fixation of the talus. *A,* A displaced proximal talar neck fracture at the junction of the neck and body. The subtalar joint is subluxated, making this a Hawkins type 2 fracture. There is an associated medial malleolus fracture and peroneal tendon avulsion. *B,* Fluoroscopic lateral view during open reduction performed through a medial approach with temporary fixation using Kirschner's wires. Screw fixation is placed through a separate posterior approach. *C,* Anteroposterior fluoroscopic view showing screw placement. *D,* Lateral view showing final reduction and fixation.

who develop AVN will have collapse of the dome. The presence of a "Hawkins sign" (subchondral lucency of the talar dome) at 6 weeks post injury is evidence of vascularity of the body, and thus is a good prognostic sign. Persistent sclerosis of the dome on plain radiographs is indicative of AVN. MRI may demonstrate AVN by about 3 weeks. Revascularization of the talus takes a long time. No consensus exists regarding the duration of non-weightbearing for those with AVN.

OUTCOMES
Outcome studies of talar neck fracture treatment have shown clinical ratings of 21% to 35% excellent, 35% to 50% good, and 16% to 41% fair or poor, using the criteria set out by Hawkins.[1, 4, 5] The outcome is related to fracture type: type 1 fractures have relatively good results, type 2 fractures have unsatisfactory outcomes in around 60% of patients, and type 3 fractures have a "universally poor result."[9] The occurrence of complications, particularly AVN, often leads to a poor outcome which requires some type of fusion. Loss of motion is common in both subtalar and ankle joints, often associated with radiographic arthrosis. The incidence rate increases with fracture type. Arthrodesis will often relieve pain significantly, but leads to impaired hindfoot function.[10] It is required in 11.5% to 22% of fractures.[1, 4, 5] Talectomy has been utilized but gives inferior results compared with Blair's tibiotalar or tibiocalcaneal fusion.

Complication	Frequency	Prevention	Treatment
Avascular necrosis	Type 1—0%–13% Type 2—20%–50% Type 3—80%–100%	• Minimize surgical trauma; • Anatomic reduction and stable fixation	Arthrodesis if symptomatic—tibio-calcaneal or Blair's fusion
Infection	More common with type 3 and open fractures	• Early aggressive wound treatment • Prompt reduction of any displacement which threatens skin viability	Usually requires surgical débridement of the sequestered, avascular body and fusion
Nonunion	Rare, except after conservative treatment of displaced fractures (may be as high as 13%)	• Anatomic reduction and stable fixation	Internal fixation, usually with corticocancellous grafting
Delayed union (>6 mo)	4%–6%	• Anatomic reduction and stable fixation	Patience; delay weightbearing until callus seen using a patellar tendon bearing brace
Malunion	28%–47%—more common after comminuted fractures, usually varus, although dorsal displacement of the head also occurs.	• Anatomic reduction and stable fixation • Avoid medial compression due to screw placement	Shoe modification, dorsal talar beak resection, triple arthrodesis
Arthritis	40%–90%	* Anatomic reduction and stable fixation	Conservative: medication, activity modification, orthotics or braces; surgical: fusion

TABLE 2. COMPLICATIONS OF TREATMENT OF FRACTURE OF THE TALUS

FRACTURE OF THE CALCANEUS

INTRODUCTION

Fracture of the calcaneus is the most common tarsal fracture and is a fracture of economic significance, as it often prevents the patient from returning to work. Fracture of the calcaneus is a controversial topic. This stems from the wide variation in fracture severity, the presence of associated injuries, the multiplicity of treatment options, confusing classifications, the subjective nature of the outcome assessment, and confounding causes of disability. Although understanding of the fracture anatomy and disorder has increased greatly in recent years, a consensus on treatment indications has been elusive.

HISTORICAL REVIEW

Fracture of the calcaneus has been recognized to be a severe injury with a high proportion of poor outcomes. Bankart wrote in 1943 that "The results of treatment of crush fractures of the os calcis are rotten. . . ." Four types of treatment have been utilized: (1) conservative, (2) semi-open or minimal incision, (3) open reduction and internal fixation (ORIF) with or without grafting, and (4) primary arthrodesis. From Hippocratic times to the early 20th century, prior to widespread use of radiographs, treatment consisted of rest, foot elevation, and compression bandages. This strategy persists today, coupled with and emphasizing early motion to minimize stiffness.

Although some in the past have reported high percentages of "satisfactory" results with this approach, presently it is most appropriate for nondisplaced fractures, or for patients with high surgical risk of complications. When radiographs came into common use, a variety of semiopen or closed reduction techniques were developed. These methods involved disimpaction of the fracture fragments, reduction of the displacements by manual manipulation or the use of percutaneous spikes (the Essex-Lopresti technique[11]), and maintenance of reduction with plaster, pin traction, or external fixation.

The availability of CT in the 1980s began a period of increased understanding of fracture anatomy,[12] and coupled with new implants and techniques spawned the era of ORIF, which continues to increase in popularity. Although some authors advocate primary arthrodesis in severely comminuted and displaced fractures, the proper role of this strategy is not clear.

PATHOGENESIS

The majority of calcaneal fractures occur in men of working age and the usual cause of the injury is a fall from a height. Between 5% and 9% are bilateral. There are associated compression injuries of the dorsal or lumbar spine in 10%, and associated injuries of the lower extremity are reported in 25% to 70% of patients. The mechanism is axial loading of the hindfoot, driving the talus down into the calcaneus, and producing stereotypic fracture lines and patterns. The "primary" fracture line shears the calcaneus obliquely into anteromedial and posterolateral portions, sometimes splitting the posterior facet. Commonly, secondary fracture lines split the calcaneus more transversely. The posterior facet is driven into the body of the bone and rotated anteriorly around a transverse axis, so that it no longer articulates with the talus. The lateral wall is typically "blown out," accounting for the widening of the heel. The anterior process may be split. The resulting deformity consists of a shortened (both in height and length), widened heel with articular incongruity. Flattening of the calcaneus forces the talus into dorsiflexion, limiting ankle motion.

CLINICAL FEATURES

A history of a fall or axial load and subsequent pain with inability to ambulate should raise the suspicion of calcaneal fracture and the need for radiographs. Patients may complain of ankle pain, and views of the ankle may be read as normal by the inexperienced examiner. A history of diabetes, atherosclerosis, or tobacco addiction should be sought, as these factors may modify the treatment plan. On examination, special attention should be paid to swelling, bruising, blistering, and the overall skin condition. Compartment syndrome of the foot can occur and is probably more common than generally appreciated.

INVESTIGATION

Radiographs routinely obtained include a lateral view of the foot and an axial view of the heel. Anteroposterior and oblique views of the foot may show fracture lines into the calcaneocuboid joint and lateral wall displacement, but add little to the evaluation. Broden's view, taken with the foot dorsiflexed and internally rotated 30 to 40 degrees, and with the x-ray beam angled cephalad between 10 and 40 degrees, is a useful way of visualizing the posterior facet. It is most helpful intraoperatively using portable films or the C-arm to evaluate the reduction of the facet and the position of the hardware. Figure 2 demonstrates this view. CT scanning has become common for intra-articular fractures in patients who are surgical candidates. Both coronal and transverse images are obtained with 3-mm cuts. Sagittal reconstruction may be useful early in the learning curve, but three-dimensional reconstruction is rarely helpful.

Many classification schemes have been developed for these fractures. The first distinction is between intra-articular and extra-articular fractures. The extra-articular fractures make up 15% to 25% of all calcaneal fractures and include tuberosity fractures, Achilles tendon insertion avulsions

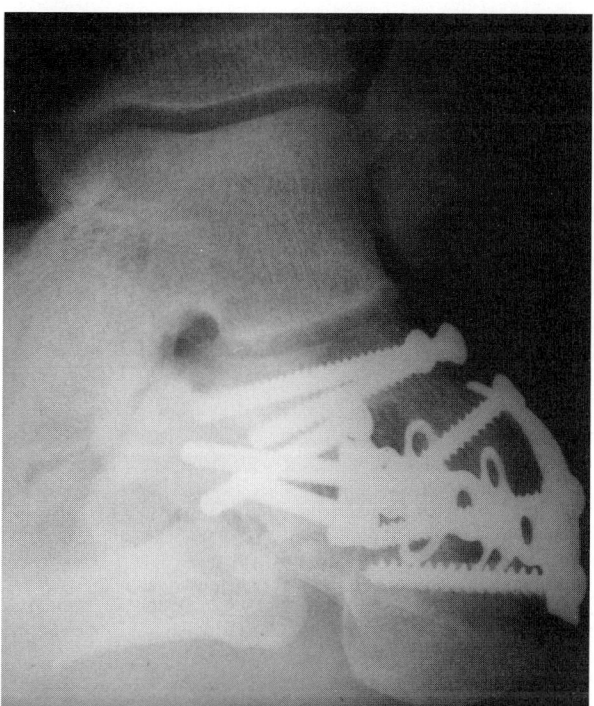

Fig. 2. Broden's view. This postoperative image shows restoration of the articular surface of the posterior facet. (From Sanders R: Intra-articular fractures of the calcaneus; Present state of the art. J Orthop Trauma 1992; 6:252.)

(usually seen in diabetic patients), and fractures of the anterior or sustentacular process. The intra-articular fractures have been divided by Essex-Lopresti into joint depression and tongue types, the distinction being that tongue fractures have the posterior facet and the dorsal surface of the tuberosity on a single piece. This classification is easy to use, but not prognostic. More recently, classifications based on CT findings have proved to be useful.[12, 13] The Sanders classification is based upon the number of fragments seen in the posterior facet on coronal CT imaging, and has proved to be prognostic in the hands of its developers.[14]

TREATMENT GOALS, INDICATIONS, AND CONTRAINDICATIONS

Nonoperative treatment consists of compression wraps, elevation, foot pumps, and early motion. Because nonunion is rarely a problem, the goal is to retain motion and flexibility in the foot. It is appropriate in patients with nondisplaced fractures or those who are not surgical candidates.

Surgical treatment consists of either ORIF or primary subtalar arthrodesis. Primary arthrodesis is controversial, and even its advocates would restrict its use to severely comminuted fractures or to fractures with severe cartilage loss from the posterior facet.[15] Contraindications to surgical treatment include poor skin condition, diabetes, severe osteopenia, poor patient compliance, vascular disease, insensate foot, or nonambulating patient.[13, 16, 17] Heavy tobacco use may be a relative contraindication owing to the detrimental effect on wound healing. Surgery should not be attempted until swelling in the foot has decreased significantly, which may take 7 to 14 days. Absence of pitting edema in the lateral hindfoot, along with the "wrinkle test,"[13] indicates that the skin is ready for surgery (Fig. 3). The goals of ORIF are restoration of calcaneal shape, correction of hind foot varus alignment, and reduction of the posterior facet articular surface.

PROCEDURE

Both lateral and medial approaches have been described. The lateral extensile incision with the patient in the lateral position and with elevation of a full thickness, subperiosteal soft-tissue flap has gained widespread use.[14, 16, 17] Figure 3 also demonstrates the incision. The peroneal tendon sheath is retracted with Kirschner's wires in fibula and talus. The lateral wall piece is removed or retracted. The posterior facet fragments are gently freed and cleaned, and the joint surface is reconstructed. Temporary Kirschner's wire stabilization is used. A Schanz pin in the tuberosity fragment can be used to help reduce the body, correcting height and varus, and may be connected to the femoral distractor. Fluoroscopy verifies the reduction. Bone graft or substitutes are used by some authors in the defect, but not all believe it to be necessary. Fixation is performed using lag screws below the posterior facet, and low-profile plates such as H plates or Y plates (Fig. 4). A careful layered closure is done after portable radiographs verify position, with use of a drain being based on personal preference. Postoperatively, 2 to 3 days of elevation and splinting are followed by early subtalar motion. Sutures are removed at 3 weeks, and weightbearing is avoided for 6 to 8 weeks. Full weightbearing is restricted until 12 weeks.

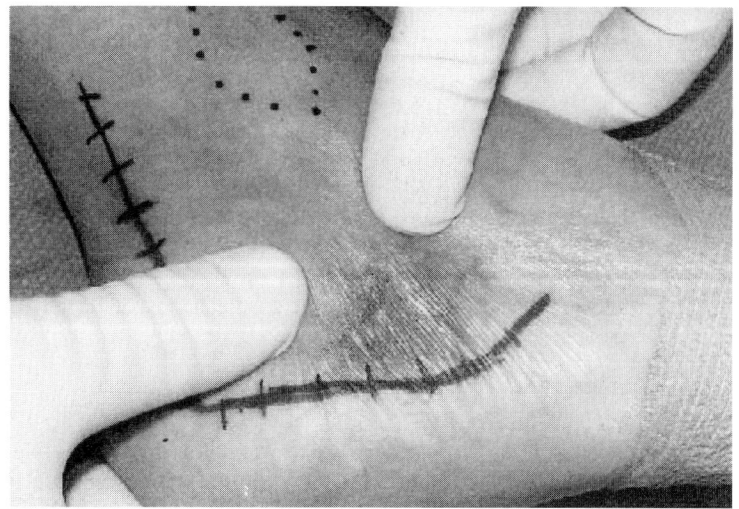

Fig. 3. The wrinkle test. Adequate mobility of the skin to allow wrinkling with gentle squeezing indicates swelling has decreased significantly. The lateral incision for exposure of calcaneus fracture is also shown. The hashed line indicates the incision, which is made down to the bone in the area of the angle, but becomes more superficial proximally and distally. A full-thickness (skin-to-periosteum) flap is carefully and sharply raised from the lateral calcaneus, containing the sural nerve and the peroneal tendons in their sheath. The flap is retracted with Kirschner's wires in fibula, talus, and cuboid. (From Benirschke SK, Sangeorzan BJ: Extensive intraarticular fractures of the foot. Clin Orthop 1993; 296:128.)

The surgical treatment of calcaneus fracture is technically demanding, and requires training and experience. The learning curve requires 30 to 50 procedures or approximately 2 years.[14]

COMPLICATIONS AND RESULTS

The common complications of calcaneus fracture are malunion, wound dehiscence and subsequent osteomyelitis, subtalar arthritis, peroneal tendinitis, and sural nerve paresthesias. These are summarized in Table 3. Malunion, usually following closed treatment, results in a painful, stiff hindfoot, frequently with lateral impingement of the peroneal tendons or fibula. The heel is typically shortened, widened, and in varus alignment. Failure of conservative methods may require surgical treatment, which must be individualized for the particular problem.[18]

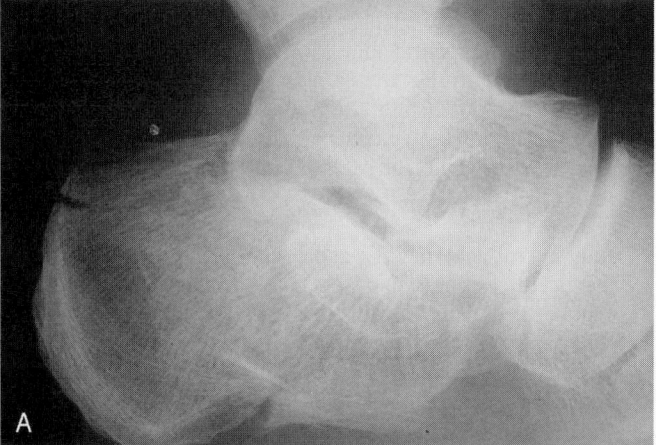

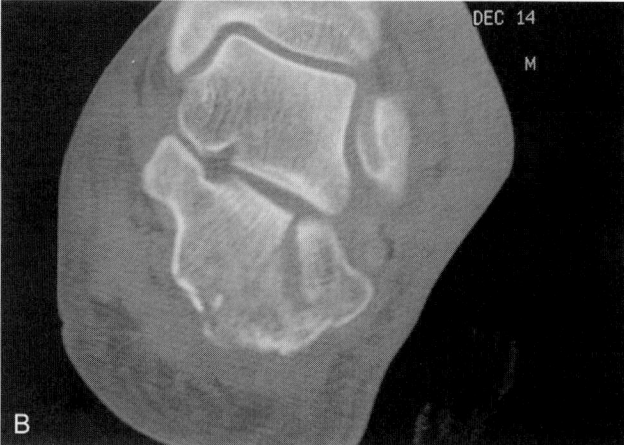

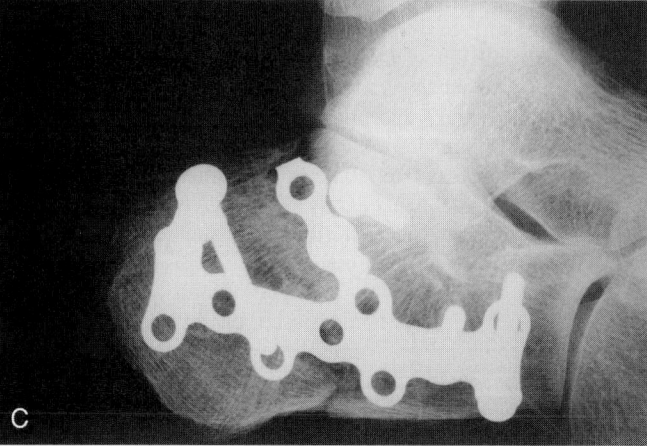

Fig. 4. Fixation of calcaneus fracture. *A,* A preoperative lateral view demonstrates flattening of the calcaneus and impaction of the posterior facet articular surface. *B,* CT scan reveals articular incongruity, lateral wall extrusion, and varus alignment. *C,* Postoperative lateral view shows restoration of calcaneal shape. Note plate position and lag screw placement below the posterior facet.

TABLE 3. COMPLICATIONS OF TREATMENT OF FRACTURES OF THE CALCANEUS			
Complication	**Incidence**	**Prevention**	**Treatment Options**
Malunion	Common following closed treatment of displaced fractures	Anatomic reduction and stable fixation; avoidance of early weightbearing	*Nonoperative:* Padding and elevating the heel with soft heel cups or shoe modification, activity changes, medication *Operative:* Ostectomy for impingement; osteotomy (Dwyer) for malalignment; Subtalar arthrodesis in situ or with subtalar bone block for arthrosis
Wound-healing problems	~ 5%–10%	Patient selection, sufficient delay to surgery, careful handling of tissues, avoidance of nicotine postoperatively	*Nonoperative:* Local débridement, whirlpool, dressing changes *Operative:* Coverage with free tissue transfer
Osteomyelitis	~3%	As above for wound-healing problems and early aggressive treatment of superficial wound problems	*Nonoperative:* Suppressive antibiotics *Operative:* Hardware removal and débridement, local antibiotic administration, IV antibiotics, reconstruction, or amputation
Peroneal tendinitis	5%–20%	Low-profile hardware, gentle intraoperative handling and retraction	*Nonoperative:* Anti-inflammatory medication *Operative:* Hardware removal
Sural nerve paresthesia	0%–20%	Gentle handling and retraction during surgery	*Nonoperative:* Local injection
Arthritis	~ 10% severe enough to require treatment	Anatomic reduction and stable fixation of the articular surface is thought to be helpful but is not a guarantee	*Nonoperative:* Weight reduction, activity modification, orthotics or shoe modification, anti-inflammatory medication *Operative:* Arthrodesis, either subtalar (in situ vs bone block) or triple if calcaneocuboid joint involved

Wound failure and infection are serious problems which may lead to amputation. The risk is higher in patients with diabetes, vascular disease, nicotine addiction, severe soft-tissue injury, or noncompliance. Dehiscence may occur as late as 4 weeks postoperatively. Free flap coverage may be needed because local flaps and skin graft have rarely proved successful. Osteomyelitis usually requires a decision about salvage, fusion, or amputation. Subtalar arthritis may be the result of poor reduction or cartilage necrosis from the injury. Perfect reduction may lessen the risk but is not a guarantee of good results. Subtalar injection can be diagnostic as well as therapeutic. Arthrodesis may be attempted to salvage failures of conservative care.

OUTCOMES

Comparison of outcomes between studies is difficult due to the variation in classification systems, treatment method details, and outcome measurements. Some authors have compared operative with nonoperative treatment and found no difference, but these studies have had significant weaknesses. A prospective randomized trial found a significant advantage to surgical treatment.[19] Most series of operatively treated calcaneus fractures using modern fixation techniques report that anatomic reduction and stable fixation will lead to good or excellent results in 75% or more of cases.[14, 17, 20, 21] However, although anatomic reduction appears to be necessary for a good outcome, it does not guarantee it; anatomically reduced fractures can still have subtalar arthrosis severe enough to warrant fusion. Some degree of subtalar motion is usually lost after calcaneal fracture, and patients should be counseled that the foot will not be normal or asymptomatic even in the best circumstances. Many patients have difficulty on uneven surfaces. However, the majority of patients with reconstructable fractures will return to work and daily activities. Many authors have noted that functional improvement continues slowly for as long as 2 years after injury.

REFERENCES

1. Szyskowitz R, Seggl W, Wildburger R: Late results of fractures and fracture dislocation after ORIF. In Tscherne H, Schatzker J (eds): Major Fractures of the Pilon, the Talus, and the Calcaneus. Berlin, Springer-Verlag, 1993, pp 105–112.
2. Kuner EH, Lindenmaier HL, Münst P: Talus fractures. In Tscherne H, Schatzker J (eds): Major Fractures of the Pilon, the Talus, and the Calcaneus. Berlin, Springer-Verlag, 1993, pp 70–85
3. Anderson HG: The Medical and Surgical Aspects of Aviation. London, Oxford Medical Publications, 1919.
4. Hawkins LG: Fractures of the neck of the talus. J Bone Joint Surg Am 1970; 52:991.
5. Canale ST, Kelly FB: Fractures of the neck of the talus. Long term evaluation of seventy-one cases. J Bone Joint Surg Am 1978; 60:143.
6. Sangeorzan BJ, Wagner WA, Harrington RM, et al: Contact characteristics of the subtalar joint: The effect of talar neck misalignment. J Orthop Res 1992; 10:544.
7. DeCoster TA, McGuire M: Posterior approach for internal fixation of talar neck fractures. Operative Tech Orthopaedics 1994; 4:165.
8. Swanson TV, Bray TJ, Holmes GB Jr: Fractures of the talar neck. A mechanical study of fixation. J Bone Joint Surg Am 1992; 74:544.
9. Daniels TR, Smith JW: Talar neck fractures. Foot Ankle Int 1993; 14:225.
10. Gregory PR, Sanders RW: Ankle and foot injuries. In Levine A (ed): Orthopaedic

Knowledge Updates—Trauma. Rosemont, IL, American Academy of Orthopaedic Surgeons, 1996, pp 198–200.

11. Essex-Lopresti P: The mechanism, reduction technique, and results in fractures of the os calcis. Br J Surg 1952; 39:395.

12. Crosby LA, Fitzgibbons T: Computerized tomography scanning of acute intra-articular fractures of the calcaneus. J Bone Joint Surg Am 1990; 72:852.

13. Sanders R: Intra-articular fractures of the calcaneus: Present state of the art. J. Orthop Trauma 1992; 6:252.

14. Sanders R., Fortin P, DiPasquale T, et al: Operative treatment in 120 displaced intra-articular calcaneal fractures. Clin Orthop 1993; 290:87.

15. Buch BD, Myerson MS, Miller SD: Primary subtalar arthrodesis for the treatment of comminuted calcaneal fractures. Foot Ankle Int 1996; 17:61.

16. Carr JB: Surgical treatment of the intra-articular calcaneus fracture. Orthop Clin North Am 1994; 25:665.

17. Benirschke SK, Sangeorzan BJ: Extensive intra-articular fractures of the foot. Surgical management of calcaneal fractures. Clin Orthop 1993; 292:128.

18. Sangeorzan BJ: Salvage procedures for calcaneus fractures. In: Instr Course Lect 1997; 46:339.

19. Thordarson DB, Krieger LE: Operative vs. nonoperative treatment of intra-articular fractures of the calcaneus. A prospective randomized trial. Foot Ankle Int 1996; 17:2.

20. Zwipp H, Tscherne H, Thermann H, et al: Osteosynthesis of displaced intra-articular fractures of the calcaneus. Results in 123 cases. Clin Orthop 1993; 290:76.

21. Benirschke SK, Mayo KA, Sangeorzan BJ, et al: Results of operative treatment of calcaneal fractures. In Tscherne H, Schatzker J (eds): Major Fractures of the Pilon, the Talus and the Calcaneus. Berlin, Springer-Verlag, 1993, pp 175–185.

section 3 chapter
21 FRACTURES OF THE FOREFOOT AND MIDFOOT

Raymond J. Sullivan and Michael S. Aronow

Summary

- Nondisplaced navicular fractures can be treated with a short-leg cast, whereas displaced avulsion or body fractures will require open reduction and internal fixation in most cases.
- Fractures of the cuboid and cuneiforms can often be treated closed unless there is significant displacement or intra-articular involvement, which requires open reduction and internal fixation.
- Unstable or displaced fractures or dislocations of the tarsometatarsal joints often require open reduction and internal fixation of the first, second, and third tarsometatarsal joints as well as open reduction and percutaneous pinning of the fourth and fifth metatarsocuboid joints when involved.
- The majority of metatarsal shaft fractures can be treated closed with limitations in weightbearing; however, intra-articular involvement or significant displacement, particularly in the sagittal plane, may require open reduction and internal or percutaneous fixation.
- Fractures of the fifth metatarsal base can be treated with a simple hard sole shoe for small avulsion fractures but will require short-leg non-weightbearing cast immobilization or surgery if the fracture is more proximal at the metaphyseal-diaphyseal junction.
- Fractures of the hallux and lesser toes usually require only protection with buddy taping and a hard sole shoe, unless there is significant displacement or intra-articular step-off.

Fractures of the midtarsal bones, including the navicular, cuboid, and cuneiforms, are relatively uncommon injuries. Dislocations or fracture dislocations of the tarsometatarsal joints represent approximately 0.2% of all fractures, with an incidence of approximately 1 per 55,000 individuals per year. Aggressive treatment of these injuries can minimize post-traumatic arthrosis and maintain stable, efficient, non-painful gait. The majority of metatarsal fractures can be treated with closed reduction and short-leg casting with limitation of weightbearing. This is especially true for the first and fifth metatarsals. Residual angulation or shortening may disrupt normal weightbearing across the metatarsal heads and lead to pain and intractable plantar keratoses. Fifth metatarsal base fractures may need extended treatment with non-weightbearing and short-leg casting, especially for those involving the metadiaphyseal junction, because of the increased risk of nonunion. Fractures of the hallux and lesser toe phalanges are the most common fractures seen in the foot. Those fractures that have significant intra-articular displacement may require open reduction and percutaneous pinning to minimize post-traumatic arthrosis. Significant angulation in the dorsal-plantar or mediolateral direction may cause abnormal painful callosities and difficulty with shoe wear. Although sesamoiditis is a common diagnosis, sesamoid fractures are much less common. It is important to differentiate these injuries from the painful bipartite sesamoid that occurs in approximately 10% of the population.

Navicular and fifth metatarsal base fractures as well as Lisfranc's injuries have unique modes of treatment. They can be especially complicated and difficult to treat. This chapter concentrates on the treatment of these injuries with comments on particular issues as they pertain to other midfoot and forefoot fractures.

HISTORICAL REVIEW

- Eichenholtz and Levine[1] in 1964 reported on the largest series of 67 navicular fractures.

- Sangeorzan et al[2] in 1989 classified navicular fractures into three types and stressed the need for anatomic reduction, with many patients requiring open reduction and internal fixation.
- Jacques Lisfranc served as a surgeon in Napoleon's army in the early 1800s. He described an amputation through the tarsometatarsal joints.
- Quénu and Küss in 1909[3] described 30 cases and classified Lisfranc's injuries.
- Hardcastle et al[4] in 1982 further classified Lisfranc's fracture dislocations.
- Myerson[5] and Arntz[6] and their colleagues in the mid-1980s obtained better results with open reduction and internal fixation in patients who had precise anatomic reduction.
- Sir Robert Jones[7] in 1902 described fractures of the base of the fifth metatarsal.
- Stewart[8] in 1960 classified fractures of the base of the fifth metatarsal, noting differences in prognosis and treatment based on location.
- Kavanaugh et al[9] in 1978 described treatment of delayed nonunions of the fifth metatarsal base with intramedullary screw fixation and bone grafting.

PATHOGENESIS

The most common fractures of the navicular result from repetitive stress in running and jumping athletes. Traumatic injuries resulting in avulsion fractures of the tuberosity result from the pull of the posterior tibial tendon or forced eversion, whereas dorsal navicular avulsion fractures result from the pull of the talonavicular or deltoid ligaments with forced plantar flexion. Navicular body fractures result from high axial compression on the forefoot, usually secondary to falls from great heights or motor vehicle accidents.

Cuboid and cuneiform fractures can result from a direct crushing injury or from axially loading a foot in plantar flexion similar to the mechanism described later for Lisfranc's injuries. More commonly, fractures of the cuboid and cuneiforms are seen in conjunction with other fractures of the midtarsus or metatarsals.

Lisfranc's injuries can occur with direct trauma such as a crush injury. In this situation, there is usually plantar displacement of the fractured metatarsals. These injuries can also occur with indirect force such as abduction of a forefoot fixed in an equestrian stirrup or windsurfing board. A second indirect mechanism is seen in extreme plantar flexion of an axially loaded foot. This can occur after a high-energy fall, a motor vehicle accident, an athletic injury, or stepping in a pothole. There is disruption of the weaker dorsal capsule and ligaments, and the associated inversion-eversion forces determine whether there is any medial or lateral displacement of the metatarsals.

A direct crushing force can cause metatarsal shaft fractures. This can often result in open fractures. Metatarsal head and neck fractures, similarly, can be caused by a direct blow to the foot. Fractures of the base of the fifth metatarsal most commonly are secondary to an avulsion force, with the foot being inverted (supinated). Direct compression or a crushing force can also lead to this type of injury, and stress fractures can occur from overuse.

Fractures to the hallux and lesser toe phalanges usually are the result of either stubbing the toe or a dorsal blow to the toe itself. Axially loading the hallux or lesser toe more commonly results in a dislocation in one of the interphalangeal joints. A direct blow to the sesamoid apparatus or avulsion from a hyperplantar flexion injury to the metatarsophalangeal joint can cause sesamoid fractures. Overuse can also result in a stress fracture of the sesamoid.

CLINICAL FEATURES

Midfoot and forefoot fractures usually present with pain on weightbearing, tenderness to palpation of the affected areas, and occasionally obvious deformity. Swelling and ecchymosis are often seen over the entire foot and ankle and are not necessarily isolated to the area of injury. Careful history and detailed physical examination, including neurovascular assessment, should be performed to rule out any other associated injuries. Compartment syndrome of the foot has been reported in severe midtarsal and Lisfranc's injuries and must be identified and treated before fracture fixation.[10] Extensive soft-tissue swelling is common within the first 24 hours in severe injuries. This may preclude acute surgical intervention. A compression foot pump is quite useful in these cases.

Navicular body fractures have been classified by Sangeorzan et al[2] into three types. Type I fractures have a transverse fracture line, and the normal alignment of the foot is maintained. Type II fractures run from dorsolateral to plantar medial and are often comminuted. The dorsal medial fragment is often displaced medially, bringing the forefoot with it. Type III fractures are usually comminuted in the sagittal plane, disrupt the naviculocuneiform and occasionally the calcaneocuboid joints, and are often associated with lateral forefoot displacement (Fig. 1).

The most commonly used classification system for Lisfranc's fracture-dislocations is the Hardcastle et al[4] modification of Quénu and Küss's[3] original classification. In this system, type A is total incongruity in which all five metatarsals are subluxed either medially or laterally relative to the cuneiforms and cuboid. In a type B partial incongruity injury, there is either medial dislocation of the first metatarsal or lateral dislocation of all or some of the second through fifth metatarsals. In type C, divergent dislocations can be either (1) total displacement in which the first metatarsal is displaced medially and the second through fifth metatarsals are displaced laterally or (2) partial displacement in which the first metatarsal displaces medially and the second and third metatarsals are displaced laterally, with no displacement of the fourth and fifth metatarsals. This classification was additionally modified by Myerson et al; type B partial incongruity dislocations are subdivided into type BI for medial dislocations and type BII for lateral dislocations. Type C divergent dislocations are divided into type CI for partial displacement and type CII for total displacement (Fig. 2).

Fifth metatarsal base fractures can be classified according to location.[11] Zone I fractures include fractures through the fifth metatarsal tuberosity and often extend into the fifth metatarsocuboid joint. Zone II fractures, true Jones

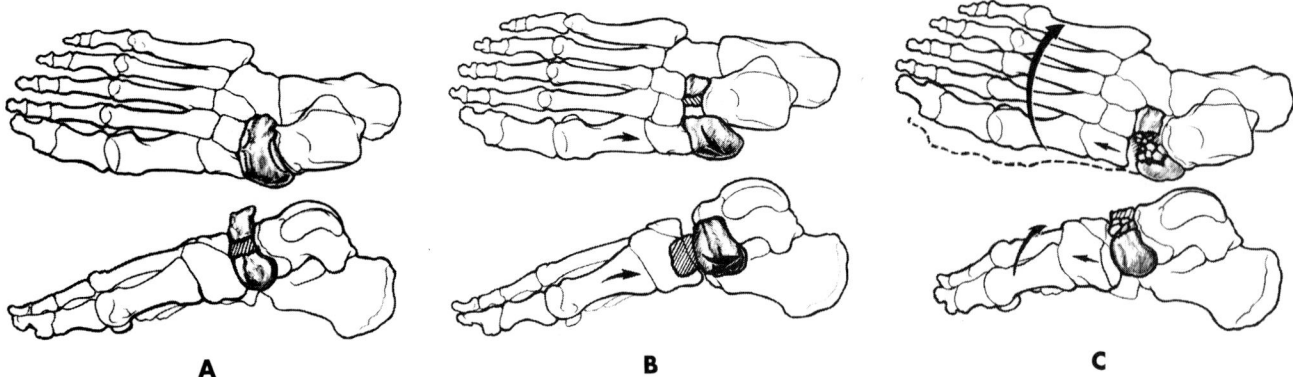

Fig. 1. Classification of navicular fractures. (From Coughlin MJ, Mann RA: Surgery of the Foot and Ankle. St. Louis, Mosby, 1999, 7th ed, vol 2, p 1580; Hansen ST Jr: Swionkowski MF: Orthopaedic Trauma Protocols. New York, Raven, 1993.)

fractures, are located at the metaphyseal-diaphyseal junction. Zone III fractures are distal to the metadiaphyseal junction (Fig. 3).

No distinct classification systems are commonly used in describing cuboid, cuneiform, metatarsal, or phalangeal fractures of the midfoot or forefoot.

INVESTIGATION

Radiographic examination, including anteroposterior (AP), lateral, and oblique radiographs of the foot, is essential in the diagnosis of midfoot and forefoot fractures. Weight-bearing or stress radiographs and 30-degree internal oblique and AP views with 20 degrees of cephalic tilt may be especially useful in evaluating Lisfranc's injuries. Examples of more common Lisfranc's, navicular body, and fifth metatarsal base fractures are seen in Figures 4 to 6. Computed tomographic scanning is often useful in evaluation of navicular, cuneiform, cuboid, and Lisfranc's fractures. Subtle subluxations and intra-articular involvement can be more readily seen with the use of computed tomography.

GOAL

The goal in treatment of all midfoot and forefoot fractures is a painless plantar grade foot that is stable for weight-bearing. This requires anatomic reduction to decrease the incidence of post-traumatic arthrosis deformity.

INDICATIONS

Indications for surgical management of midfoot and forefoot fractures include all open fractures and compartment syndromes. Tarsal fractures with significant intra-articular displacement usually require open reduction and internal

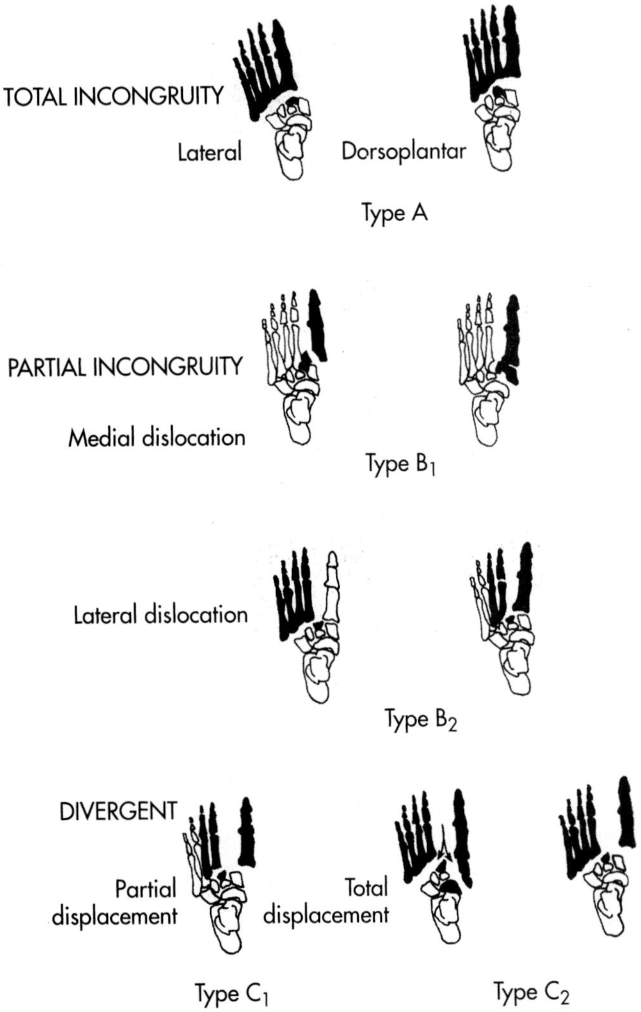

Fig. 2. Lisfranc's injury classification. (From Coughlin, Mann: Surgery of the Foot and Ankle. St. Louis, Mosby, 1999, 7th ed, vol 2, p 1548; From Myerson MS, Fisher RT, Burgess AR, et al: Fracture dislocations of the tarsometatarsal joints: End results correlated with pathology and treatment. Foot Ankle 6:228, 1986.)

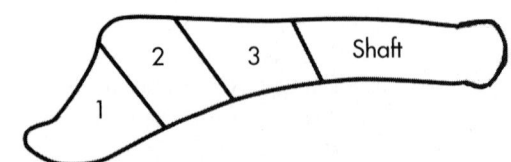

Fig. 3. Fifth metatarsal base fracture classification. (From Coughlin M, Mann R: Surgery of the Foot and Ankle. St. Louis, Mosby, 1999, 7th ed, vol 2, p 1594; Dameron TB: Fractures of the proximal fifth metatarsal: Selecting the best treatment option. J Am Acad Orthop Surg 1995;3:110.)

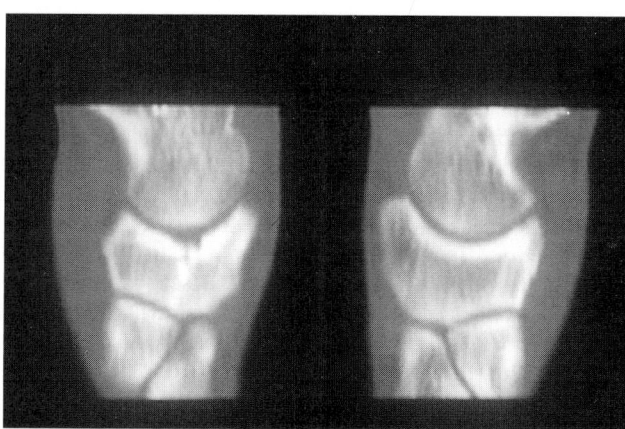

Fig. 4. Computed tomography scan showing type II navicular body fracture.

fixation. Lisfranc's fracture-dislocations with no displacement or subluxation on regular and stress radiographs can be treated with 6 weeks of cast immobilization. Most authors do not believe that cast immobilization by itself is sufficient treatment after closed reduction when there is subluxation on stress radiographs.

Metatarsal shaft fractures that result in significant displacement should be treated with either open reduction and internal fixation or closed reduction and possible percutaneous pinning. Fractures with significant sagittal plane deformity or involving multiple adjacent metatarsals are more likely to require surgery. Phalangeal fractures with a significant intra-articular step-off or angulatory deformity that are unable to be reduced with closed methods should be treated with open reduction and internal fixation or percutaneous pinning. Transverse fractures of the sesamoids with significant fracture gapping and minimal comminution can be treated with open reduction and internal fixation. Significant comminution of the sesamoids may require partial or total excision.

CONTRAINDICATIONS

Surgical intervention in midfoot and forefoot fractures is contraindicated in patients who are medically unfit for surgery. Significant swelling that will not allow for adequate tension-free wound closure is also a contraindication for acute surgical correction unless there is a need for concurrent compartment release. Acute open reduction and inter-

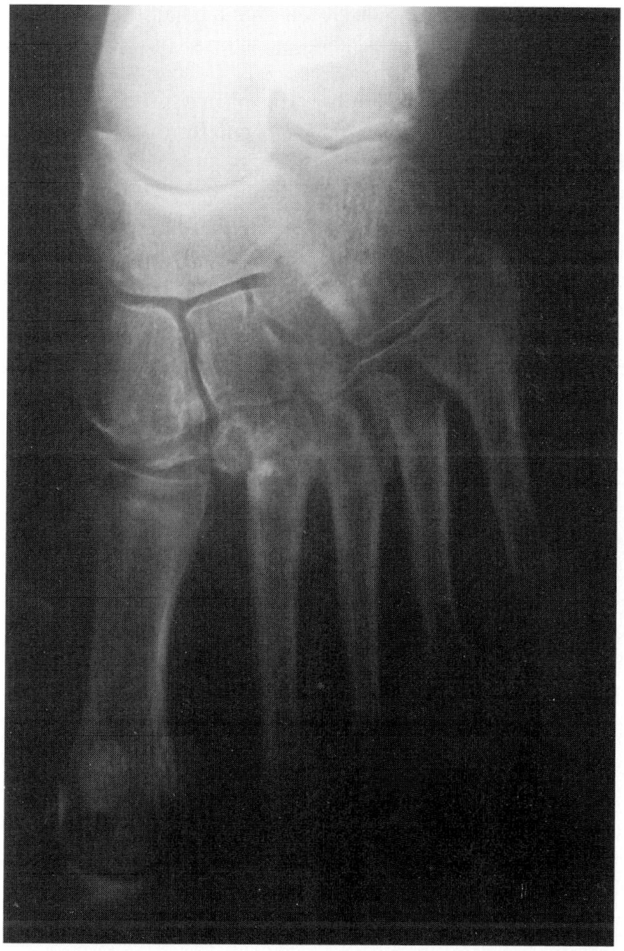

Fig. 5. **Displaced Lisfranc's fracture dislocation type BII.** In this anteroposterior radiograph with 20 degrees of cephalic tilt, note the nondisplaced proximal second metatarsal fragment attached to Lisfranc's ligament.

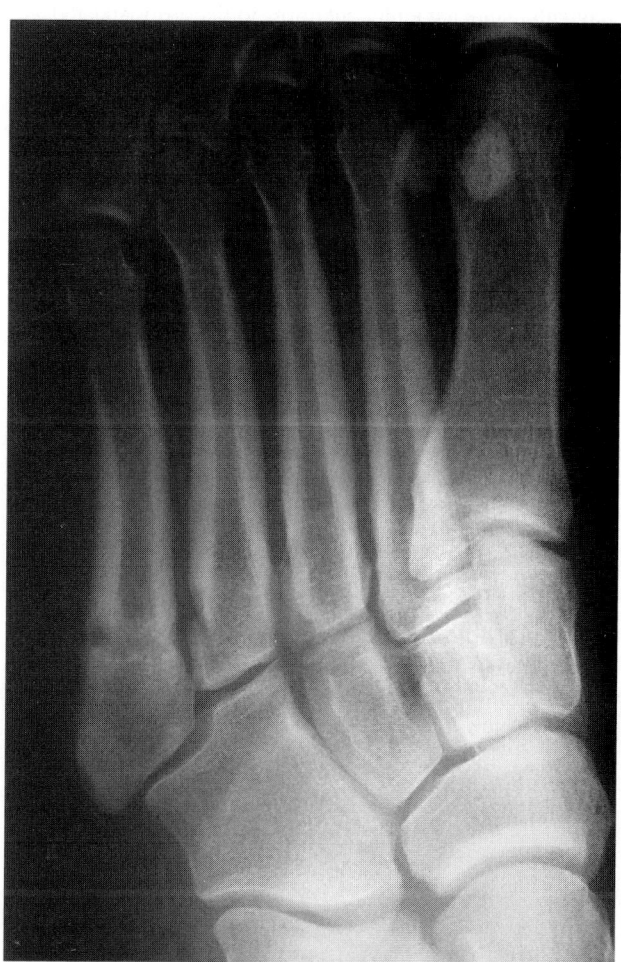

Fig. 6. **Anteroposterior radiograph of a fifth metatarsal base nonunion.**

nal fixation is often contraindicated in patients with active Charcot's fractures or dislocations. Subsequent realignment and fusion may be needed after the patient is safely into the Eichenholtz stage III.

PROCEDURES

PREOPERATIVE PLANNING

In those fractures of the midfoot and forefoot that require surgical intervention, adequate radiographic assessment is mandatory (see the section on Investigation). The patient is placed supine on the operative table. A well-padded non-sterile proximal thigh tourniquet is helpful in maintaining a bloodless field. Small-fragment fracture fixation sets as well as a variety of K-wires and cannulated screw sizes should be available. Cannulated screws are especially useful because of their ability to be used as lag screws and the ease of fluoroscopically guided guide pin insertion. Longitudinal incisions are preferable because of the limitation of injury to crossing neurovascular structures as well as the ability to perform extensile revision surgery.

TECHNICAL DETAILS

Open reduction and internal fixation of displaced navicular fractures is best performed through a dorsomedial incision in the interval between the posterior tibial and anterior tibial tendons. Using minimal soft-tissue stripping, the talonavicular and naviculocuneiform joints are inspected and débrided of loose fragments. Fracture fragments are reduced and held in place with pointed bone-holding clamps or small K-wires. Percutaneous cannulated screw placement can be performed over guide wires fluoroscopically. Two 4.0-mm cannulated screws are ideal (Fig. 7). In comminuted type II and III fractures, a small external fixator from the talar neck or medial malleolus to the first metatarsal can aid in reduction and stabilization of the fracture and the talonavicular joint. In type II fractures with a smaller comminuted plantar lateral fragment and in type III fractures, the lag screws need to cross the naviculocuneiform joint for adequate fixation. The naviculocuneiform screws can be removed after fracture union if desired. Any residual bony defect can be filled in with a lateral calcaneal bone graft in most cases.[12]

Open reduction and internal fixation of Lisfranc's fracture-dislocations is best approached through longitudinal incisions over the dorsal aspect of the midfoot. The first incision is made dorsally between the first and second tarsometatarsal joints. The dissection is carried lateral to the neurovascular bundle to expose the second tarsometatarsal joint and medial to the extensor hallucis longus tendon to expose the first tarsometatarsal joint. The first and second tarsometatarsal joints are débrided of bony fragments to allow for reduction. The first metatarsal is reduced to the medial cuneiform, and provisional fixation is obtained with K-wires. Either cannulated screws or fully threaded cortical screws can be placed in nonlag fashion to avoid compression across the normal articular surfaces. Two parallel 0.045-mm K-wires placed at the medial and lateral aspects of the dorsal first metatarsal can be used to guide the placement of noncannulated screws after checking the adequacy of reduction on fluoroscopy. A large plantar medial fragment is usually attached to the strong Lisfranc ligament at the base of the second metatarsal. Anatomic reduction of the remaining second metatarsal to this fragment is required and can be held in place with a large tenaculum clamp between the medial aspect of the first cuneiform and the second metatarsal base laterally. If the second metatarsal middle cuneiform screw is not sufficient, an additional screw may be placed from the medial cuneiform into either the middle cuneiform or the second metatarsal base. If displacement is noted at the third, fourth, or fifth tarsometatarsal joint, a second incision is made in the interval between the third and fourth tarsometatarsal joints. The third metatarsal is reduced to the lateral cuneiform and stabilized with a single screw. The fourth and fifth metatarsals are reduced to the cuboid and stabilized with percutaneous K-wires from the metaphyseal-diaphyseal junction of the fifth metatarsal and from the

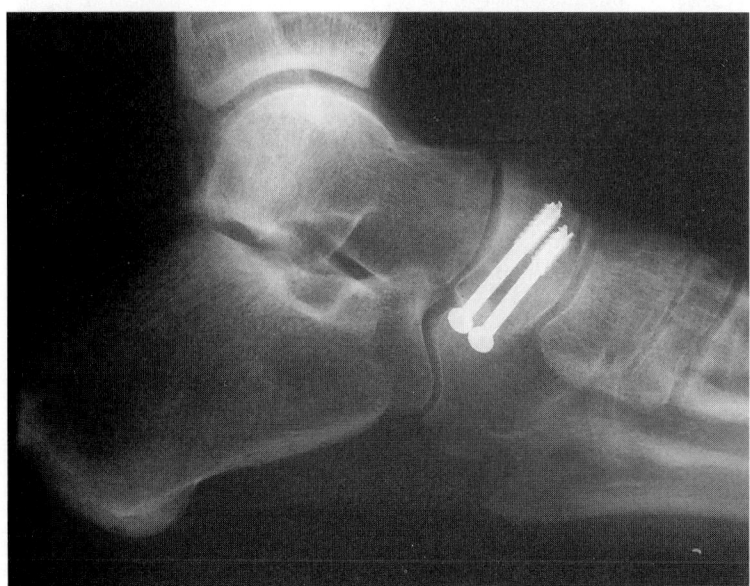

Fig. 7. Cannulated screw placements. This postoperative lateral radiograph shows screw placement within a healed type II navicular body fracture.

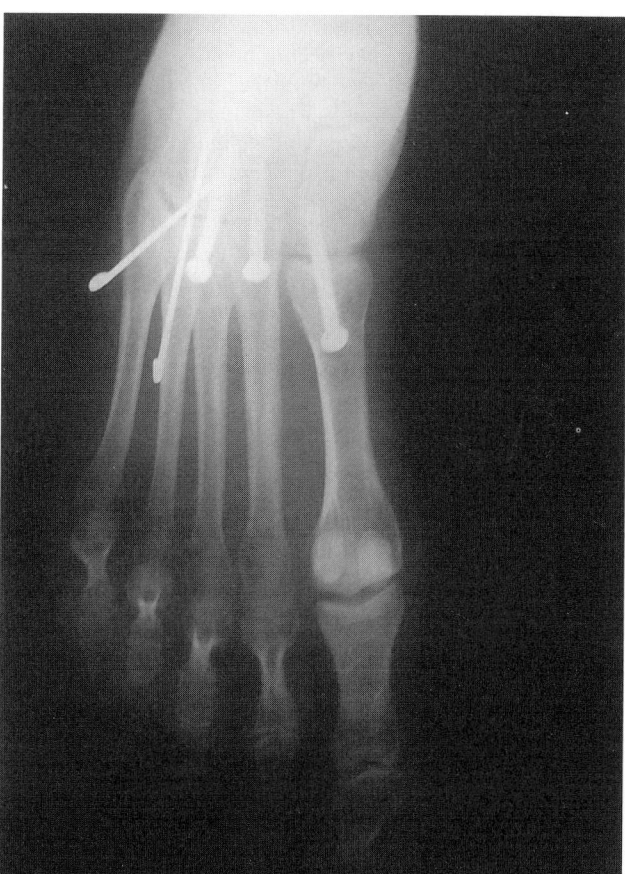

Fig. 8. Lisfranc's open reduction and internal fixation (ORIF). Anteroposterior radiograph shows results after Lisfranc's ORIF with typical screw placement within the first, second, and third metatarsocuneiform joints. Percutaneous pins are used for the fourth and fifth metatarsocuboid joints.

dorsal aspect of the fourth metatarsal into the cuboid (Fig. 8). Any concomitant metatarsal or midfoot fractures are stabilized at the same setting.

Displaced fifth metatarsal base fractures or fifth metatarsal base nonunions that require open reduction and internal fixation are best approached through a longitudinal incision along the lateral aspect of the midfoot centered about the fifth metatarsal tuberosity. Care must be taken during superficial dissection not to injure the distal branch of the sural nerve, which is often found within 2 mm of the tip of the fifth metatarsal tuberosity.[11] A longitudinal split within the peroneus brevis tendon insertion is made for intramedullary screw placement after the fifth metatarsal fracture is reduced (Fig. 9). Lateral calcaneal bone graft can be used to augment fracture healing, particularly if a nonunion is present.

Open reduction and internal fixation of the tibial sesamoid is best approached through a longitudinal medial incision centered about the metatarsophalangeal joint. Excellent visualization of the tibial sesamoid can be obtained through this approach. The fibular sesamoid can be approached through either a dorsal or plantar approach within the first web space. The dorsal approach will eliminate the chance of leaving a painful plantar scar; however, the visualization obtained through this approach is inferior to that obtained

through the plantar approach. Similar approaches can be used for excision of comminuted fractures (Fig. 10). Meticulous dissection should be performed to allow for minimal injury to the flexor hallucis brevis and flexor hallucis longus tendons.

POSTOPERATIVE MANAGEMENT

In general, forefoot and midfoot fractures treated with open reduction and internal fixation require at least 6 weeks of non-weightbearing in a short-leg cast with a toe plate. Strict elevation must be maintained until wound healing is obtained. Percutaneous pins for tarsal and metatarsal fractures may be removed in approximately 6 to 8 weeks. Hallux and lesser toe pins are usually removed at approximately 4 weeks. Range of motion of the ankle and hindfoot are initiated on cast removal at 6 weeks. Radiographic follow-up until clinical healing is mandatory. Midfoot and forefoot range of motion and overall strengthening as well as weightbearing can be initiated on clinical healing.

COMPLICATIONS

The main complication of navicular avulsion fractures is symptomatic nonunion, which, in the case of navicular tuberosity fractures, can lead to posterior tibial tendon dysfunction and an acquired flatfoot deformity. Dorsal avul-

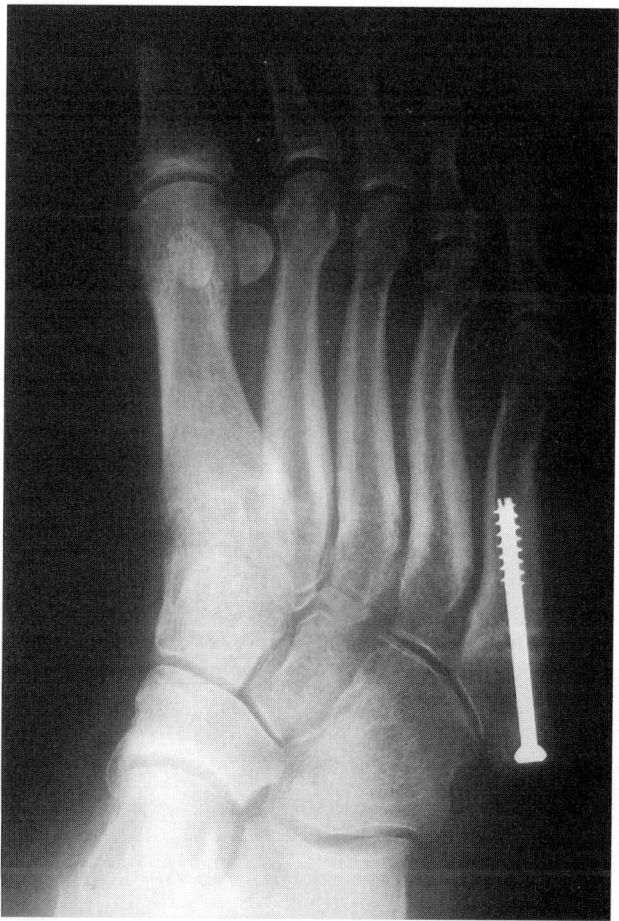

Fig. 9. Healing of a proximal diaphyseal fifth metatarsal nonunion. This anteroposterior radiograph shows healing after bone grafting and intramedullary screw fixation.

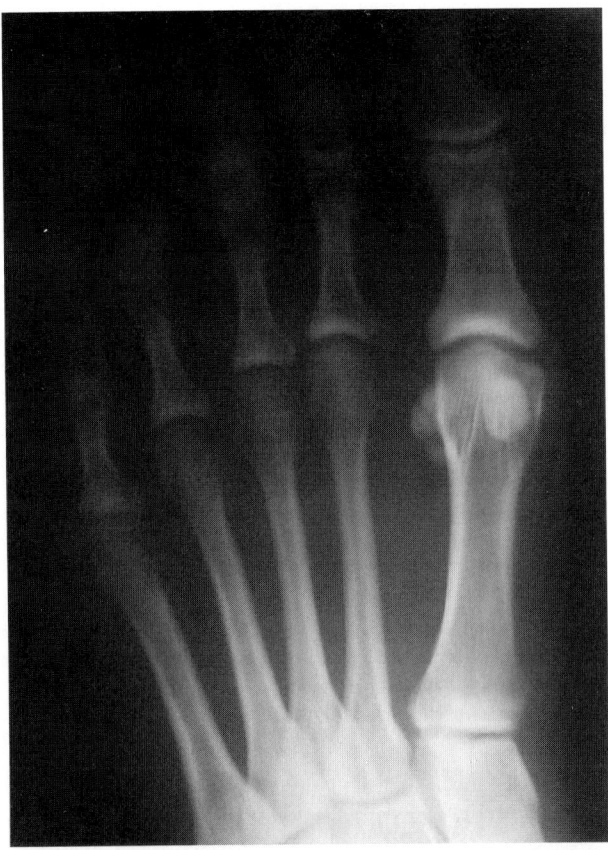

Fig. 10. Comminuted fibular sesamoid fracture. This fracture, as seen on an anteroposterior radiograph, required open excision for a painful nonunion.

sion fracture nonunions are treated with excision of the nonunited fragment. Navicular tuberosity nonunions are treated with delayed open reduction and internal fixation or excision of the nonunited fragment with concomitant posterior tibial tendon advancement. Navicular body fractures can develop post-traumatic deformities and arthritis (Fig. 11). Conservative treatment with anti-inflammatory medications and orthotic arch support can be useful; however, fusion of the involved joint is often required. There is significantly more functional loss with a talonavicular fu-

sion than with a naviculocuneiform fusion. Avascular necrosis of the navicular may occur and was reported in 6 of 21 patients (29%) in the series of Sangeorzan et al.[2] Navicular collapse occurred in only one patient.

The complications of Lisfranc's injuries are post-traumatic arthritis, pain, deformity, activity limitation, and vascular compromise (Fig. 12). The complications of surgical treatment include infection, skin necrosis or wound problems, neurovascular damage, reflex sympathetic dystrophy, post-traumatic arthritis, painful retained hardware, and loss of reduction after K-wire or screw removal. Patients with symptomatic residual arthritis or deformity can be treated with orthotic arch support or tarsometatarsal arthrodesis. Sangeorzan et al[13] reported good or excellent results in 11 of 16 patients with delayed tarsometatarsal arthrodesis using internal fixation. The fourth and fifth metatarsal joints may be incorporated in the arthrodesis if there is significant arthrosis, although many surgeons try to preserve fourth and fifth metatarsal joint motion, which helps maintain a more normal gait.

The incidence of sesamoid nonunion is quite low. Established nonunions have been successfully treated in 19 of 21 patients with open autologous bone grafting, as reported by Anderson and McBryde.[14]

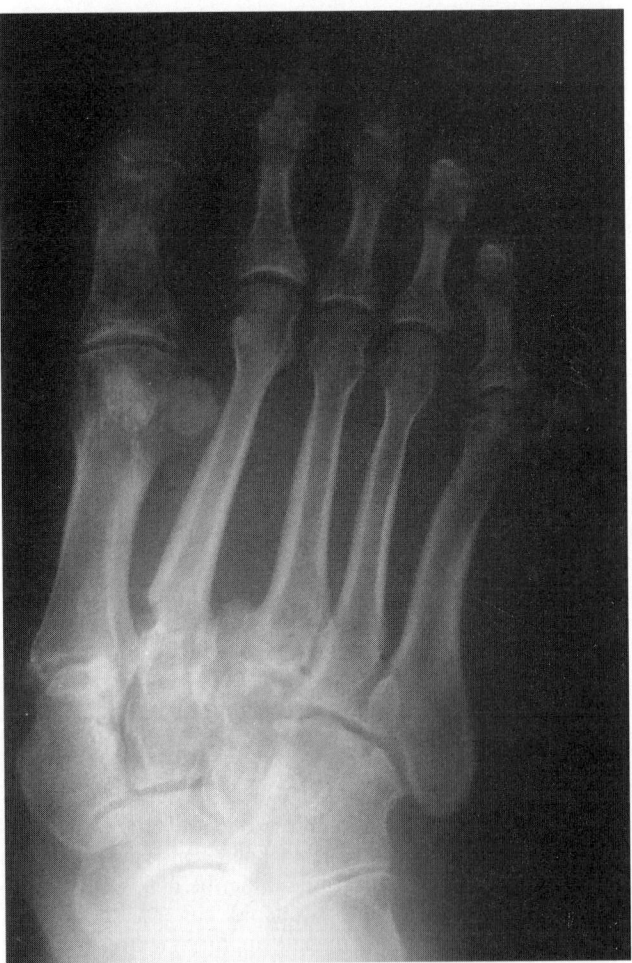

Fig. 12. Severe post-traumatic midfoot after a missed Lisfranc's fracture-dislocation. The patient required open reduction and first, second, and third metatarsocuneiform fusions.

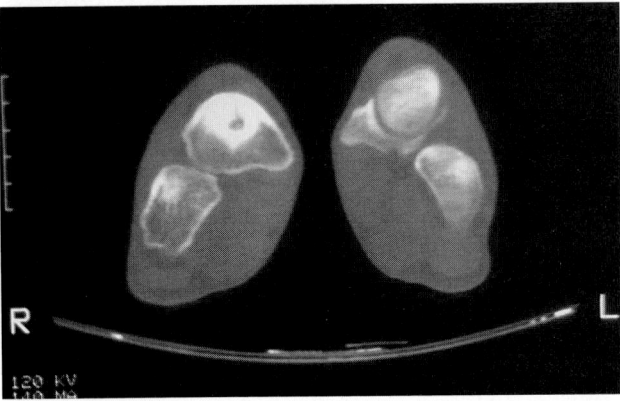

Fig. 11. Navicular nonunion with sclerosis. This computed tomography scan shows nonunion with sclerosis on either side of the fractured navicular body and an intramedullary cyst.

RESULTS

Navicular avulsion fractures tend to do very well when recognized early and properly treated. The results of navicular body fractures are related to the severity of injury and the accuracy of reduction. Sangeorzan et al,[2] in their study of 21 patients with an average 4-month follow-up after open reduction and internal fixation, noted good results in 67%, fair results in 10%, and poor results in 14%. Good results were seen in 100% of type I, 70% of type II, and 25% of type III injuries.

Results after Lisfranc's injuries are correlated with the adequacy of reduction and the amount of initial cartilaginous and soft-tissue injury. Myerson et al[5] noted that patients with a good or excellent result after Lisfranc's injury had a residual distance of 2.9 mm (2 to 5 mm) between the first and second metatarsal bases, whereas those with fair and poor results had an average of 5.8 mm (2 to 14 mm) diastasis. In addition, only one of eight patients who had a direct crush injury had a good or excellent result. Arntz et al[6] found that 28 of 30 patients with a precise anatomic reduction had a good or excellent result, whereas five of six patients who had a fair or poor result had an associated grade II or grade III open injury. Faciszewski et al[15] found no correlation between the amount of diastasis between the first and second metatarsal bases and functional outcome in subtle Lisfranc's injuries. However, six of the seven patients in their study had marked disability and pain and later experienced flattening of the longitudinal arch.

Torg et al[16] reported that acute proximal fifth metatarsal shaft fractures (zone III) without intramedullary sclerosis healed in 14 of 15 cases with 6 to 8 weeks of immobilization in a non-weightbearing cast. Fractures that show delayed union, non-immobilization, or weightbearing also have been reported to have a high healing rate with non-weightbearing short-leg casting.[16] Frank nonunions require open surgical débridement and intramedullary screw fixation with supplemental inlay bone grafting. Avulsion fractures of the base of the fifth metatarsal, including both zone I and zone II fractures, have been shown by Wiener et al[17] to respond to either short-leg casting or soft Jones-type dressing without any evidence of nonunion in 60 patients, although most authors recommend non-weightbearing short-leg cast treatment for zone II fractures. They later reported healing in 19 of 20 patients treated with bone grafting without fixation.

REFERENCES

1. Eichenholtz SN, Levine DB: Fractures of the tarsal navicular bone. Clin Orthop 1964; 34:142.
2. Sangeorzan BJ, Benirschke SK, Mosca V, et al: Displaced intra-articular fractures of the tarsal navicular. J Bone Joint Surg Am 1989; 71:1504.
3. Quénu E, Küss G: Étude sur les luxations du metatarse (luxations métatarsotarsiennes) du diastasis entre le 1er et le 2e metatarsien. Rev Chir 1909; 39:281.
4. Hardcastle PH, Reschauer R, Kutscha-Lissberg E, et al: Injuries to the tarsometatarsal joint. J Bone Joint Surg Br 1982; 64:349.
5. Myerson MS, Fisher RT, Burgess AR, et al: Fracture dislocations of the tarsometatarsal joints: End results correlated with pathology and treatment. Foot Ankle 1986; 6:225.
6. Arntz CT, Veith RG, Hansen ST: Fractures and fracture-dislocations of the tarso-metatarsal joint. J Bone Joint Surg Am 1988; 70:173.
7. Jones R: Fracture of the base of the fifth metatarsal bone by indirect violence. Ann Surg 1992; 35:697.
8. Stewart IM: Jones' fracture: Fracture of base of fifth metatarsal. Clin Orthop 1960; 16:190.
9. Kavanaugh JH, Brower TD, Mann RV: The Jones fracture revisited. J Bone Joint Surg Am 1978; 60:776.
10. Myerson MS: Management of compartment syndromes of the foot. Clin Orthop 1991; 271:239.
11. Donley BG, McCollum MJ, Murphy GA, et al: Risk of sural nerve injury with intramedullary screw fixation of fifth metatarsal fractures: A cadaver study. Foot Ankle Int 1999; 20:182.
12. Biddinger KR, Komenda GA, Schon LC, et al: A new modified technique for harvest of calcaneal bone grafts in surgery on the foot and ankle. Foot Ankle Int 1998; 19:322.
13. Sangeorzan BJ, Veith RG, Hansen ST: Salvage of Lisfranc's tarsometatarsal joint by arthrodesis. Foot Ankle 1990; 10:193.
14. Anderson RB, McBryde AM: Autogenous bone grafting of hallux sesamoid nonunions. Foot Ankle Int 1997; 18:293.
15. Faciszewski T, Burks RT, Manaster BJ: Subtle injuries of the Lisfranc joint. J Bone Joint Surg Am 1990; 72:1519.
16. Torg JS, Balduini FC, Zelko RR, et al: Fractures of the base of the fifth metatarsal distal to the tuberosity. J Bone Joint Surg Am 1984; 66:209.
17. Wiener BD, Linder JF, Giattini JFG: Treatment of fractures of the fifth metatarsal: A prospective study. Foot Ankle 1997; 18:267.

CERVICAL SPINE TRAUMA

Alexander R. Vaccaro, Oren G. Blam, Devry C. Anderson, and Todd J. Albert

Summary

- Cervical spine trauma can be devastating, but the initial steps of management can have a great impact on the long-term functional outcome for the patient.
- Adequate management of cervical spine trauma requires prompt recognition, aggressive resuscitation, and a rapid and accurate diagnostic protocol.
- History, physical examination, plain radiography, and advanced imaging studies are all key components in the diagnostic work-up of cervical spine injuries.
- Both anatomic and mechanistic classification systems for cervical spine injuries help in guiding treatment decisions.
- Acute management of cervical spine trauma seeks to halt the secondary cascade of spinal cord injury by providing pharmacological treatment, achieving spinal realignment, performing spinal cord decompression, and reestablishing spinal stability.
- Nonoperative and operative means to treat cervical spine injuries are chosen based on the injury pattern, injury severity, neurological status, patient's medical condition, and surgeon's experience.

Injury to the cervical spine is an infrequent occurrence fraught with the potential for significant morbidity and at times fatality if not recognized early and managed appropriately. Unfortunately, approximately 40% of cervical spine injuries are associated with a neurological deficit. The reported incidence of hospitalized spinal cord injury cases ranges from 26.6 to 60 per million in the United States, half of which affect the cervical spine.[1] Most of these result from motor vehicle accidents or falls. The typical patient is a young man, although in the elderly the gender frequency is approximately equal. There is a bimodal age distribution that peaks between the ages of 15 to 24 years and over 55 years.[2]

Because early recognition and proper treatment can greatly reduce or avoid devastating long-term sequelae, an understanding of anatomy, pathophysiology, and treatment principles is paramount in obtaining a satisfactory clinical outcome. Diagnosis of a cervical spine injury begins with a patient's complaint of pain (if alert and awake) followed by an accurate physical examination and appropriate plain radiographic examination. When indicated, advanced imaging modalities such as computed tomography (CT) and magnetic resonance imaging (MRI) evaluation of the cervical spine can further delineate the injury profile and direct management decisions. The ultimate goals in the management of these injuries include obtaining appropriate spinal alignment and stability and relieving symptomatic neurological compression.

ANATOMY AND BIOMECHANICS

There are seven cervical vertebrae, which are often divided into two separate anatomic regions because of their differences in morphometry and biomechanics. This includes the upper cervicocranium (occiput to C2) and the subaxial cervical spine (C3-7). The vertebral foramen or canal widens in the cephalad cervical region. The space available for the spinal cord at the C1 level measures approximately 20 mm in the midsagittal plane[3]; this dimension decreases to approximately 14 mm in the subaxial cervical spine.[4] The bony anatomy of the C1 and C2 vertebrae are vastly distinct from that of the subaxial spine. Furthermore, the range of motion of the cervical spine in flexion-extension and rotation are evenly divided between the cervicocranium and subaxial cervical spine.

CERVICOCRANIAL ANATOMY

The atlanto-occipital joints are formed by the two convex occipital condyles articulating with the concave superior facets of C1. The prime ligamentous stabilizer of this joint is the tectorial membrane, a continuation of the posterior longitudinal ligament that extends from the posterior surface of the odontoid process to the posterior surface of the ventral rim of the foramen magnum or clivus. Secondary stabilizers of the atlanto-occipital joint are the articular capsules and the anterior and posterior atlanto-occipital membranes. The anterior atlanto-occipital membrane is a continuation of the anterior longitudinal ligament and inserts onto the anterior surface of the ventral rim of the foramen magnum. The posterior atlanto-occipital membrane extends from the ligamentum flavum to the anterior surface of the dorsal rim of the foramen magnum (Fig. 1). Fifty percent of cervical spine flexion occurs at the atlanto-occipital joint.

The atlas consists of an anterior arch and a posterior arch with two paired lateral masses. The anterior and posterior arches both have midline tubercles that serve as the origins of the longus coli and suboccipital muscles, respectively. Both superior and inferior facets of the atlas arise from the lateral masses and are tilted slightly medially. Just posterior to the C1 lateral mass, the posterior arch is thinned bilaterally by a depression or groove that contains the vertebral artery. The vertebral artery courses from inferior to superior in a posterolateral direction from the foramen transversarium of C2 through the C1 foramen transversarium before it courses medially over the posterior arch of C1 and then cephalad into the foramen magnum.

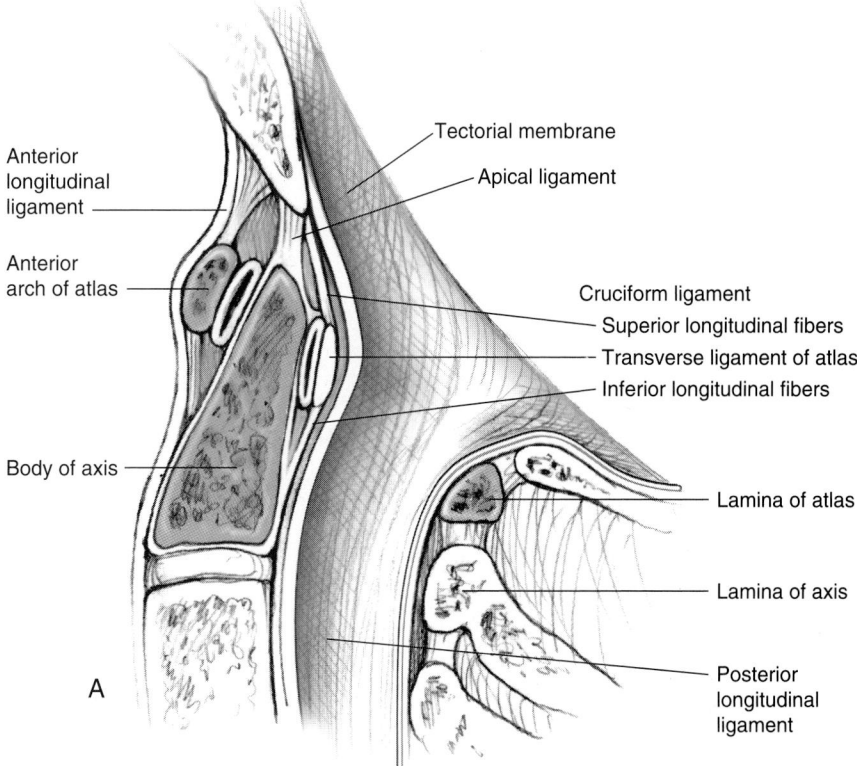

Fig. 1. Cervicocranial junction. *A*, Midsagittal section. The appropriate relationship of the basion or anterior aspect of the foramen magnum to the ring of C1 and the odontoid process is shown. The ligaments at the occipitocervical junction are nicely illustrated. *B*, A coronal section demonstrating the ligaments of the craniocervical junction. Note especially the alar ligaments and the tectorial membrane. (From Martel W: The occipito-atlantoaxial joints of rheumatoid arthritis and ankylosing spondylitis. AJR Am J Rheumatol 1961; 86:223)

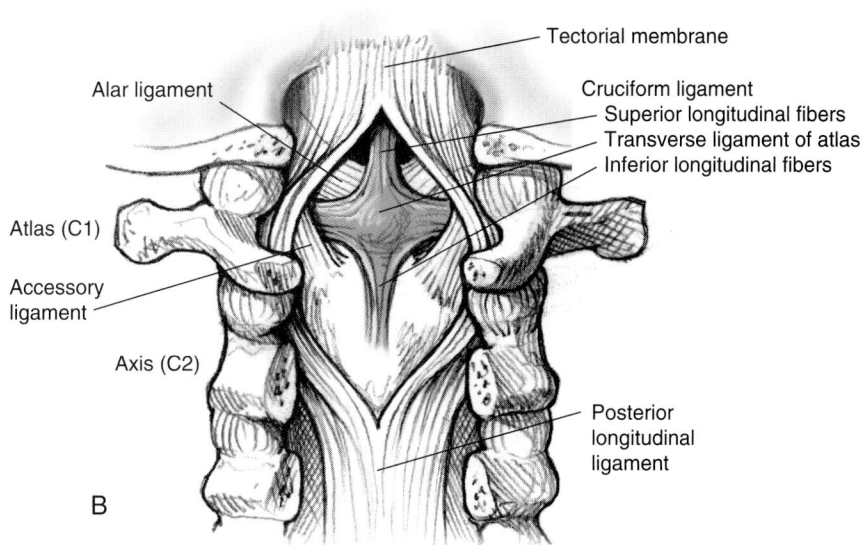

The atlantoaxial joint has three articulations: two saddle-shaped facet joints laterally and the central atlantoaxial joint formed by the odontoid process and the anterior arch of C1. Rotation about this tripartite joint comprises 50% of cervical spine rotation. The transverse (atlantal) ligament, a part of the cruciform complex, is the primary stabilizer of the central atlantoaxial joint. It spans laterally from the posterior surface of the odontoid to attach bilaterally to the medial tubercle on the posterolateral surface of the anterior arch of C1. Two alar ligaments arise from the odontoid tip and transverse ligament and attach superiorly to the lateral rims of the foramen magnum. A midline apical dental ligament connects the tip of the dens to the ventral foramen magnum.

The axis or C2 vertebra is composed of a large vertebral body that has an anterosuperiorly situated bony peg referred to as the odontoid process or dens. Arising from the lateral masses are the superior and inferior articular processes, which project in a vertical direction out of plane with each another: the superior articular process projects

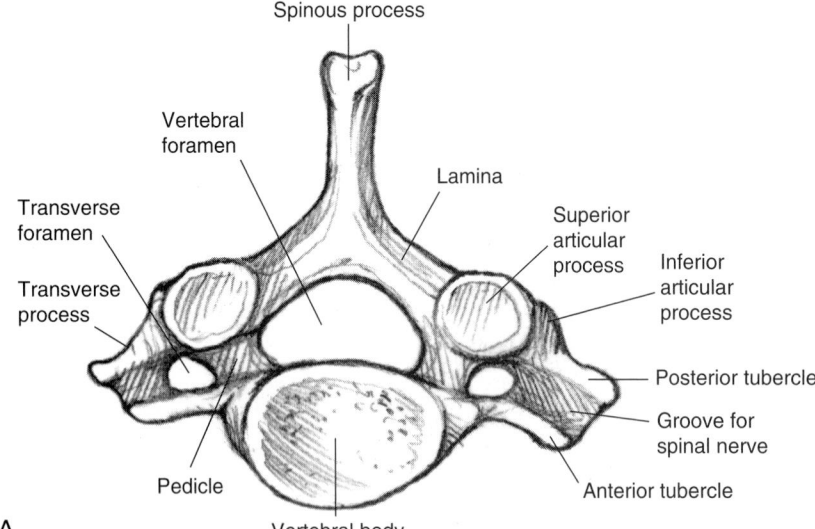

A

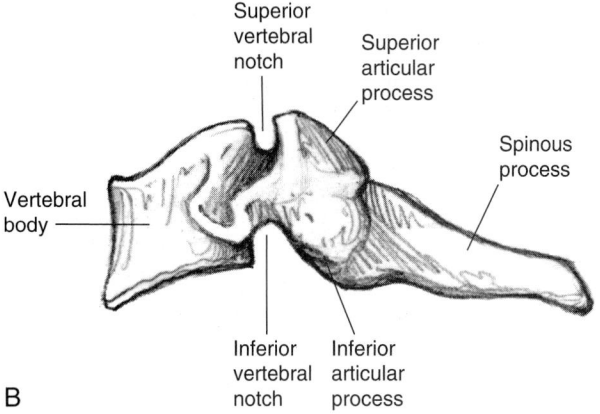

B

Fig. 2. A typical cervical vertebra. *A,* Superior and *B,* lateral views. (From Cramer GD: The Cervical Region in Basic and Clinical Anatomy of the Spine, Spinal Cord, and ANS. St. Louis, Mosby, 1995, p 111.)

more anteriorly than the inferior articular process. The axis does not have a true pedicle or bony connection between the anterior and posterior bony elements like the subaxial cervical vertebrae. Rather, a flat bony isthmus is located medial to the foramen transversarium. The two posterior laminae of C2 connect in the midline and give rise to a bifid spinous process. The odontoid process is a unique structure serving as the origin of the ligamentous stabilizers of upper cervical spine rotation. The base of the dens is surrounded by poorly vascularized ligamentous insertions and a synovial cavity. Fractures in this region are often predisposed to poor healing because of ligamentous distraction and soft-tissue interposition.

SUBAXIAL CERVICAL SPINE ANATOMY

The lower five cervical vertebrae have less variable structures (Fig. 2). Each vertebral body possesses bilateral bony ridges on the posterolateral aspects of the superior end plate called the uncinate processes. These processes articulate with the inferior aspect of the cephalad vertebral body to form the joints of Luschka, or uncovertebral joints. The pedicles anterolaterally and laminae posterolaterally form the bony boundary of the vertebral canal and meet at the pars interarticularis at each level. Projecting laterally from the pars are the lateral processes, which terminate in ante-

rior and posterior tubercles that serve as origins and insertions of the paraspinal muscles. Because the C6 anterior tubercles, also called the carotid tubercles or tubercles of Chassaignac, are large and palpable, they form a convenient landmark during anterior surgical exposures.

Cervical spinal nerve roots exit the spinal canal through the intervertebral foramina, after which they travel a short distance in grooves on the inferior surface of the transverse processes.

The foramen transversarium in the transverse process of C1 through C6 transmits the ascending vertebral artery. Five percent of people will have a vertebral artery coursing through the C7 foramen transversarium as well.[5] Spinous processes project posteriorly from the junction of the laminae and are bifid from C2 through C6. The C7 spinous process, or vertebra prominens, is particularly large and palpable, serving as a landmark for posterior surgical approaches. The superior and inferior articular processes of each facet joint project at a 45-degree angle to the horizontal. This orientation at each level allows for approximately 50% of cervical flexion-extension and rotation.

As elsewhere in the spine, ligamentous constraints to vertebral motion are essential to the stability of the subaxial cervical spine. The anterior ligamentous complex is formed by the anterior longitudinal ligament and the anterior portion of the annulus fibrosis. The posterior longitudinal ligament and the posterior annulus fibrosis form the middle ligamentous complex. The anterior and posterior longitudinal ligaments have strong insertions on the intervertebral disks as well as the vertebral bodies. Posteriorly, the supraspinous ligament connects the tips of the spinous processes. The interspinous ligaments attach along the length of the spinous process and travel vertically to the contiguous spinous process. The ligamentum flavum attaches one lamina to another. The facet joint capsules bind the articulating superior and inferior facets. Together, these posterior ligaments form the posterior ligamentous complex.

INITIAL DIAGNOSIS AND MANAGEMENT

The initial treatment approach of a spinal trauma patient follows the tenets of basic and advanced trauma life support. This involves securing an airway, making sure the patients are oxygenating well, and establishing adequate circulation. Initial assessment and resuscitation measures must be accompanied by proper spinal immobilization in cases of suspected spine injury. The potential presence of cervical spine trauma is suggested by lacerations, abrasions, pain, or deformity in the head or neck region. Unconscious or mentally impaired patients should always be suspected of having a cervical spine injury until proven otherwise. Rapid extrication and transportation to a hospital follows. Important in the initial assessment is the neurological status of the patient because comparison to this baseline later on will affect management decisions.

Appropriate field and then emergency room resuscitation of the patient is crucial for limiting the progression of spinal cord injury. All patients with suspected spinal cord injury should be placed on oxygen, keeping the partial pressure of arterial oxygen (PaO_2) above 100 mm Hg and the partial pressure of arterial carbon dioxide ($PaCO_2$) below 45 mm Hg so that cord hypoxia is minimized. Intubation may be required for proper oxygenation and ventilation if a $PaO_2/PaCO_2$ ratio of 0.75 or a vital capacity of 10 mL/kg cannot otherwise be maintained. In this case, in-line traction of the cervical spine will minimize iatrogenic injury to an unstable neck during the intubation procedure. A cadaveric study with specimens having atlantoaxial instability showed that oral and nasal intubation are equivalent in terms of changing the space available for the cord; chin-lift and jaw-thrust maneuvers compromised canal area the greatest.[6]

Blood pressure must also be maintained, and two large-bore intravenous catheters should be placed as per trauma protocol. A mean diastolic pressure above 70 mm Hg is the goal. Neurogenic shock, present when hypotension accompanies bradycardia in the setting of a spinal cord injury, is treated with fluid replacement first. The neurologically impaired patient, however, may be less able to cope with fluid overload because of respiratory muscle dysfunction; thus, judicious use of vasopressors may be required. The Trendelenburg position may aid in venous return supporting cardiac output and resultant blood pressure.

Cervical spine immobilization is initially addressed with a hard cervical collar. Transfer onto a spinal board and

between stretchers must be done while in-line stabilization is maintained. Two centimeters of occipital elevation through appropriate padding will avoid cervical extension in most adults.

A Foley catheter is important to monitor fluid status as well as to avoid bladder distension, which leads to increased parasympathetic tone potentially compromising spinal cord perfusion. Nasogastric tubes should be placed as needed.

The history taking at this time should focus on the mechanism and severity of injury, neurological symptoms, the presence of spinal pain, and history of neurological dysfunction or underlying spinal disorders. In addition to a careful neurological exam, the entire spine must be visualized and palpated for tenderness or step-offs. Log-rolling the patient again requires in-line stabilization of the neck. Classification of neurological impairment should follow that outlined by the American Spinal Injury Association (ASIA).[7] ASIA A indicates no motor or sensory function distal to the level of injury. ASIA B injuries have preservation of sensory but not motor function below the injury level. With ASIA C injuries there is some remaining weak muscle function distal to the level of injury (graded 1 to 2 of 5), whereas ASIA D patients have weakened but useful muscle strength (grades 3 to 4 of 5) distally. An ASIA E patient has no detectable spinal cord injury.

A patient with a detected spinal cord injury should be treated with intravenous high dose steroids within 8 hours of injury. This consists of methylprednisolone bolused at 30 mg/kg over 15 minutes, followed by a continuous steroid drip set at 5.4 mg/kg/h. When started within 3 hours of injury, the drip should be continued for 24 hours. If begun later, 48 hours of steroid therapy should be considered.[8] Complications such as gastrointestinal bleeding, increased incidence of pneumonia, and difficulty weaning from a ventilator may occur, especially in the 48-hour treatment regimen in otherwise debilitated patients or with high spinal cord injuries. Relative contraindications to high-dose steroid treatment include pregnancy, active infection, penetrating wounds, uncontrolled diabetes, and age younger than 13 years. Steroids may function to stabilize neuronal membranes, decrease inflammation in the cord, bolster spinal cord perfusion, and scavenge free radicals.

Other agents useful in the initial treatment of spinal cord injury are being researched. These include GM_1 gangliosides, prostaglandins, lazaroids, opioid antagonists, thyrotropin-releasing hormone, calcium channel blockers, vitamin E, and others.

Diagnostic imaging begins with a three- or five-view plain radiograph series of the cervical spine. Mandatory are the anteroposterior, lateral, and open mouth anteroposterior or odontoid views. A swimmer's view with one arm fully abducted and the other arm adducted can help image the lower cervical spine in the sagittal view, as can a bilateral shoulder pull-down maneuver. Oblique views of the cervical spine may also be obtained for further inspection of facet joint alignment.

Soft-tissue edema on a lateral radiograph is a common finding in acute cervical trauma: more than 10 mm of soft-tissue shadow anterior to C1, 5 to 7 mm at C4, and 22 mm at C6 may indicate spinal injury. Measurement of residual spinal canal diameter with retropulsed bone after injury does not accurately represent the amount of spinal cord compression that may have occurred during injury. One study of cervical burst fracture morphometry revealed that postinjury canal area measurements are 135% greater than the minimal area occurring during injury.[9] Alignment on the lateral radiograph must also be checked, looking for interruption of imaginary lordotic lines along the anterior vertebral bodies, posterior vertebral bodies, spinous process bases, and spinous process tips. Loss of lordosis itself may indicate paraspinal muscle spasm overlying spinal injury. Severe ligamentous disruption indicative of segmental instability may be inferred from the plain films by certain clues. On the anteroposterior view, angular deformity or spinous process malalignment should alert one to the possibility of injury. On the lateral view vertebral translation of more than 3.5 mm, increased angulation greater than 11 degrees compared with other segmental levels, facet joint widening, a double posterior cervical vertebral body border indicative of rotary malalignment, or interspinous widening are further clues suggesting injury. These radiographic findings, combined with other clinical criteria, comprise a checklist that is useful for determining spinal stability.

Bony injury on plain radiographs or nonvisualization of the entire cervical spine down to the top of the T1 vertebra are indications for CT evaluation with sagittal and coronal reconstructions. MRI studies are required when disk or ligamentous pathology must be ruled out, especially in the setting of a neurological deficit without evidence of bony injury. Magnetic resonance angiography during MRI can evaluate vertebral artery integrity as well.

UPPER CERVICAL SPINE TRAUMA

Despite the larger space available for the cord existing at the cervicocranium, traumatic injury of this region may be associated with catastrophic neurological compromise. In one study of 312 fatal motor vehicle accidents, 93% involved injury to the upper cervical spine.[10] Neurological injury at this level may range from transient loss of distal sensation or motor function to quadriplegia and even death. Clinical vigilance is especially important in the first 24 to 48 hours because cord edema and hemorrhage may result in ascending spinal cord dysfunction.

OCCIPITAL CONDYLE FRACTURES

These rare injuries result from either axial loading that impacts the articular surface or extreme rotation generating tension forces that avulse the insertion of the alar ligaments. Pain is usually located at the base of the skull, and patients may present with slight cervical rotation or head tilt. Concomitant fractures of C1 or other cervical vertebrae should be sought. One study found that 33% of occipital condyle fractures were associated with evidence of atlanto-occipital subluxation.[11] Cranial nerve palsies have also been associated with occipital condyle fractures.[12, 13] A CT scan is often used for precise evaluation of these injuries because radiographs do not demonstrate the occipital condyles well.[14]

Anderson and Montesano[15] classified occipital condyle fractures into three types (Table 1). Type I is a comminuted but nondisplaced impaction fracture (Fig. 3); type II

TABLE 1. OCCIPITAL CONDYLE FRACTURES: CLASSIFICATION OF ANDERSON AND MONTESANO	
Type	**Description**
I	Nondisplaced or minimally displaced and impacted fracture, usually with some comminution
II	Condyle fracture associated with a basilar skull fracture involving the foramen magnum
III	Displaced condylar avulsion fracture through the alar ligament

From Anderson PA, Montesano PX: Morphology and treatment of occipital condyle fractures. Spine 1988; 13:731. Used with permission.

condylar fractures are extensions of basilar skull fractures; and type III injuries are condylar avulsions in which the contralateral alar ligament and tectorial membrane have been compromised. Type I and II occipital condyle fractures are stable and, when not associated with other unstable injuries, may often be treated with immobilization in a hard cervical collar. Type III injuries are associated with extensive ligamentous injury and are best managed with halo immobilization. Persistent or obvious instability is an indication for arthrodesis. Tuli et al[16] presented an alternative classification scheme of occipital condyle fractures using imaging criteria from radiographs, CT, or MRI studies to detect condylar displacement and ligamentous injury to assess stability of the upper cervical spine. Type I fractures are stable and undisplaced; type IIA injuries are stable and

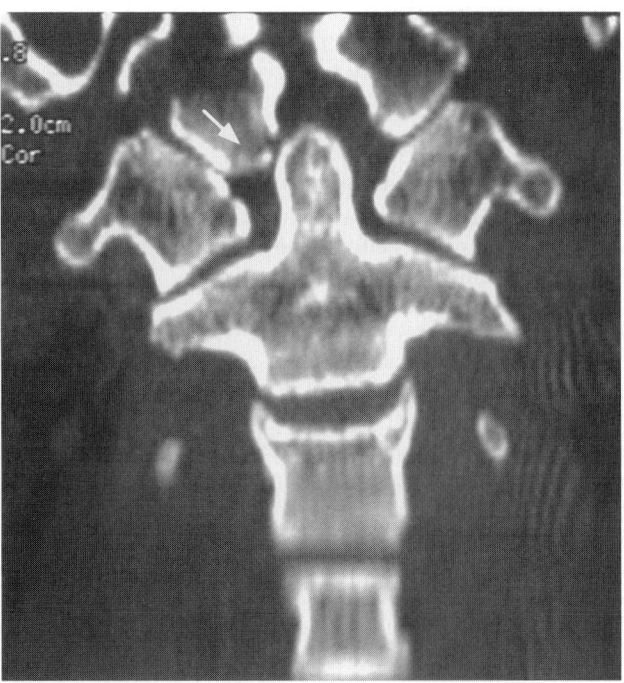

Fig. 3. Upper cervical spine. A coronal reconstruction of a computed tomography scan reveals evidence of a right-sided occipital condyle impaction fracture. This is classified as a type I Anderson and Montesano occipital condyle fracture.

displaced; and type IIB fractures are unstable and displaced.

ATLANTO-OCCIPITAL DISLOCATION

Also known as craniocervical dissociation, this injury is frequently fatal and results from hyperextension, distraction, and rotation forces. Although rare in general, atlanto-occipital dislocation occurs twice as much in children as in adults, likely because the immature atlanto-occipital joint is oriented more horizontally in children.[17] Submental laceration, mandibular fracture, and posterior pharyngeal wall injury are clues for the presence of atlanto-occitpital dislocation given the underlying mechanism of injury.[18] Cranial nerve injuries, especially of the abducens nerve, in addition to brain-stem, proximal spinal cord, and upper cervical spinal nerve root injuries have been reported in association with atlanto-occipital dislocation. Craniocervical junction subarachnoid hemorrhage noted on CT scan is often present.[19] Vertebral artery injuries can occur with this injury mechanism.[20]

The radiographic appearance may be quite dramatic, but often in surviving patients clues to injury are more subtle. The Power's ratio helps detect pathological displacement of the occiput relative to the atlas.[21] It may be calculated from a lateral radiograph, tomograph, or CT sagittal reconstruction. This ratio between the distance from the basion to the posterior arch of C1 and the distance from the opisthion to the anterior arch of C1 is usually 0.8 to 1.0; when greater than 1.0, atlanto-occipital dislocation is suggested. Other radiographic clues to this injury include displacement of Wackenheim's line (which runs along the posterior surface of the clivus and normally intersects the posterior tip of the odontoid), a basion to odontoid tip distance more than 5 mm in adults or 10 mm in children, or a change greater than 1 mm in the horizontal translation of the occiput relative to the atlas between flexion and extension.[22] Other radiographic measurements have been devised as well.[21, 23–25]

The direction of dislocation of the occiput relative to the axis defines the type of dislocation as either pure distraction, anterior, or posterior[26] (Table 2). All three types involve severe ligamentous injury that destabilize the atlanto-occipital joint and make halo immobilization crucial in the initial management. Traction is usually contraindicated, although some authors suggested that minimal traction of up to 5 pounds may be useful to reduce an anterior or posterior dislocation.[27] Posterior atlanto-occipital fusion with autologous bone graft and instrumentation is the standard of care for definitive treatment (Fig. 4).

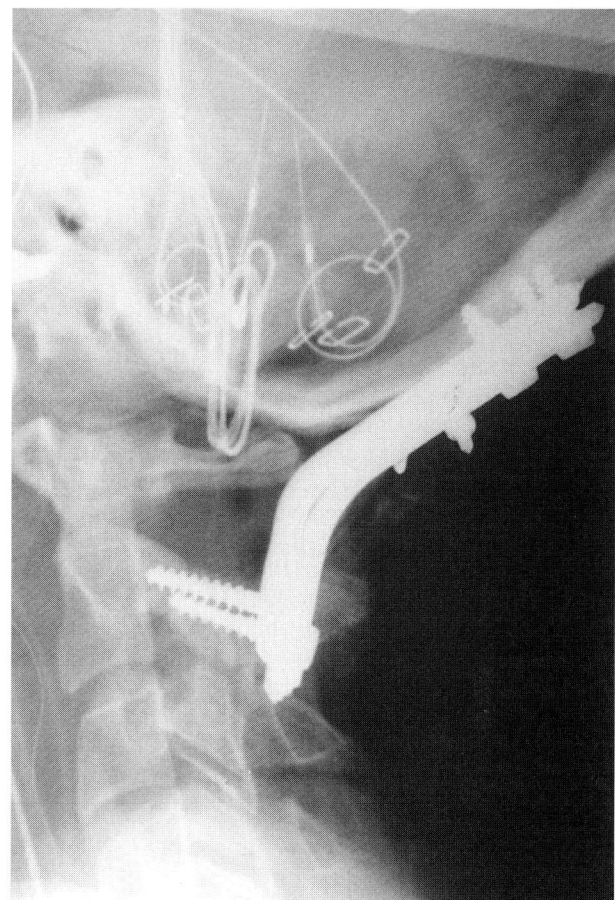

Fig. 4. Occipitocervical fusion. This is a lateral plain roentgenograph of an occipitocervical fusion using plates and screws.

FRACTURES OF THE ATLAS

In contrast to other upper cervical spine traumatic injuries, solitary atlas fractures are uncommonly associated with neurological deficit because they inherently decompress the C1 vertebral canal. A result of primarily axial compression with or without a lateral bending moment, patients with atlas fractures usually present with complaints of upper neck or suboccipital pain. As many as 50% of these fractures are associated with other cervical spine injuries that may themselves result in spinal cord injury.[28] Atlas fractures have been associated with injuries to the suboccipital or greater occipital nerves, lower cranial nerves, and vertebral arteries. Lateral displacement of the lateral masses on the anteroposterior radiograph may be the first radiographic clue for these fractures; CT scanning delineates the extent of bony injury.

Jefferson initially proposed a comprehensive classification scheme of these injuries, which was later modified by Levine and Edwards.[29] Axial compression alone tends to result in a burst pattern with displacement and fracture of both anterior and posterior arches. This injury, named the "Jefferson fracture," breaks the C1 ring in three or four locations and spreads apart the lateral masses. A hyperextension moment may instead lead to a posterior arch fracture without anterior injury. Alternatively, with hyperextension, the anterior arch of C1 may compress against the

TABLE 2. ATLANTO-OCCIPITAL INJURIES: CLASSIFICATION OF TRAYNELIS ET AL	
Type	**Description**
I	Longitudinal distraction
II	Anterior subluxation
III	Posterior subluxation

From Traynelis VC, Marano GD, Dunker RO, et al: Traumatic atlanto-occipital dislocation. J Neurosurg 1986; 65:863.

odontoid process leading to an isolated anterior C1 arch fracture. Hyperextension without axial compression may simply lead to an avulsion of the longus coli muscle and thus a fracture of the anterior tubercle. A lateral bending force in combination with axial compression could lead to a lateral mass fracture in which ipsilateral anterior and posterior arch fractures separate the lateral mass from the remaining atlas ring. Lateral mass fractures may also occur as a result of bony avulsion of the transverse atlantal ligament. Finally, lateral bending may result in a C1 transverse process fracture.

Stability of the atlantoaxial joint is paramount in considering the treatment of atlas fractures. Stable C1 fractures occur when the transverse atlantal ligament remains intact. Spence et al[30] studied the presence of such stability. They found in experimentally contrived atlas fractures that atlantoaxial offset, or total combined lateral overhang of C1 on C2 on an anterposterior radiograph projection, indicates rupture of the transverse ligament when greater than 6.9 mm. Radiograph magnification may complicate this measurement, and others recommend 8 mm as the critical value indicating atlantoaxial instability.[31] CT scan may also suggest a transverse ligament rupture by revealing a bony avulsion at the transverse ligament's insertion laterally. The atlantodens interval, as measured on lateral projections of the cervical spine, is usually less than 3 mm in adults. It is suggestive of transverse ligament rupture when greater than 4 mm.[32] MRI can directly demonstrate the ligament's integrity.[33]

Stable atlas fractures such as posterior ring, anterior tubercle, and transverse process fractures are usually treated with a course of hard cervical collar immobilization. Lateral mass and Jefferson burst fractures without evidence of atlantoaxial instability may occassionally require halo immobilization,[29] although one retrospective study suggested that a rigid cervical collar alone for 10 to 12 weeks may be sufficient to achieve a stable union.[34] Rupture of the transverse atlantal ligament can be treated with a trial of halo immobilization alone if occurring through a bony avulsion. After a period of immobilization, flexion-extension radiographs should be obtained to assess atlantoaxial stability. Nonunion associated with pain or with gross atlantoaxial instability should then be addressed with surgery. Atlas fractures occurring with a midsubstance transverse ligament tear should be treated with an atlantoaxial fusion.[35] Operative treatment at times may be indicated for some atlas fractures because of the morbidity of immobilization in a halo device, especially in the elderly patient with multiple medical comorbidities.[36] When surgical stabilization is opted, fusion may be carried out from C2 to the occiput if there is a concomitant atlanto-occipital injury, if marked degenerative disease is present in the upper cervical spine, or if nonunion develops in the axis ring. C2-1 facet screw fixation and fusion may be effective if adequate alignment can be obtained intraoperatively. This avoids the need to include the occiput in the fusion mass.

ATLANTOAXIAL ROTARY SUBLUXATION

Distinct from solitary transverse ligament insufficiency resulting in traumatic C1-2 instability, atlantoaxial rotary subluxation also involves a facet subluxation at the C1-2 articulation. A flexion-extension and rotation mechanism

asymmetrically loads the ligamentous stabilizers of the atlantoaxial joint, resulting in this injury profile. Patients complain of pain in the upper neck or suboccipital region, and decreased neck rotation can be noted on physical exam. In severe injury, a patient may present with the head tilted one way and chin rotated in the opposite direction. The relationship of the odontoid to the atlantal lateral masses will be asymmetric on an open-mouth odontoid view radiograph. This asymmetry persists in chronic situations despite head rotation 15 degrees to either side as documented by plain radiography or CT scan.[37] Other clues to rotary instability on a plain open-mouth odontoid view radiograph include overlapping of the articulating C1 and C2 facets on the side that is rotated posteriorly and a broader, more midline C1 lateral mass on the side that is rotated anteriorly.

The Fielding and Hawkins classification[38] divides these injuries according to the amount of anterior displacement of the atlas (Table 3). With type I injuries no such displacement occurs and the intact transverse atlantal ligament serves as the pivot for rotation. Type II rotary fixation involves rupture of the transverse ligament so that rotation occurs about one facet joint, with 3 to 5 mm of anterior displacement of C1 on C2. Further atlantoaxial ligament disruption in type III injuries allows more than 5 mm of anterior subluxation of C1 on C2, with rotation bringing one facet more anterior than the other (Fig. 5). Type IV rotary fixation is defined as posterior subluxation of the atlas on the axis and implies a fractured or absent odontoid process.

Rotary subluxations of type II or greater have the potential to cause spinal cord impingement and vertebral artery injury. Halo traction to achieve reduction is usually warranted in unstable traumatic cases, with subsequent halo immobilization. If the transverse ligament is disrupted, when recurrent subluxation occurs or if there is a failure of closed reduction, posterior open reduction and atlantoaxial fusion are recommended.

ODONTOID FRACTURES

Fractures of the odontoid process are ominous injuries associated with a 25% incidence of neurological deficit and a 5 to 10% mortality rate. Craniocervical as well as subaxial cervical spine injuries may accompany these injuries be-

TABLE 3. FIXED ATLANTOAXIAL ROTATORY SUBLUXATION: CLASSIFICATION OF FIELDING AND HAWKINS

Type	Description
I	Rotatory fixation with less than 3 mm of anterior displacement of C1 on C2
II	Rotatory fixation with 3 to 5 mm of anterior displacement of C1 on C2
III	Rotatory fixation with more than 5 mm of anterior displacement of C1 on C2
IV	Rotatory fixation with posterior displacement of C1 on C2

From Fielding JW, Hawkins RJ: Atlanto-axial rotatory fixation (fixed rotatory subluxation of the atlanto-axial joint). J Bone Joint Surg Am 1977; 59a:37. Used with permission.

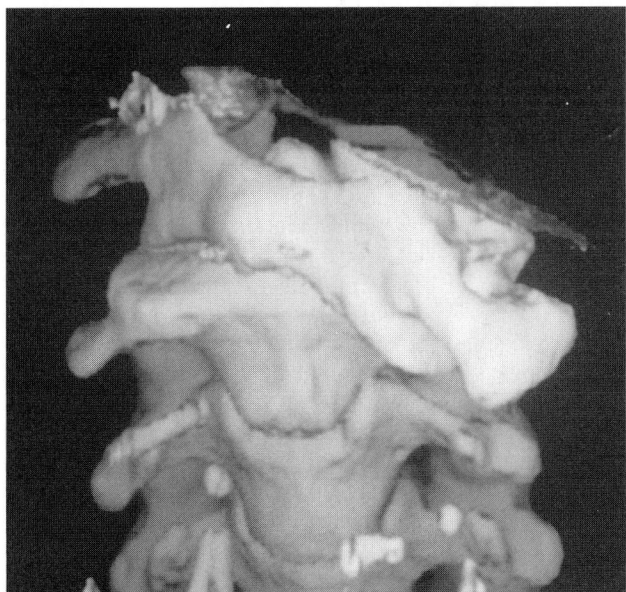

Fig. 5. Type III Fielding rotatory fixation of the atlantoaxial joint. Shown is a three-dimensional computed tomography reconstruction.

cause the mechanism likely involves flexion, extension, and rotation.

The classification scheme of Anderson and D'Alonzo takes note of the position of the fracture line[32] (Table 4). Oblique fractures at the tip of the dens, probably avulsions of the alar ligament, are type I injuries. Type II odontoid fractures occur at the base of the odontoid process, whereas type III fractures extend into the cancellous body of the axis. A type IIA fracture has been defined as well in which the dens fracture is comminuted.[39]

Type I injuries, if they truly exist, do not destabilize the atlantoaxial joint and may be treated with a course of hard collar or halo immobilization. However, care should be taken not to miss an unstable primary injury to the occipito-cervical complex manifested only as an alar avulsion fracture radiographically. Treatment of type II fractures is more controversial. Closed skeletal traction reduction followed by halo immobilization for fractures with less than 6 mm of displacement may achieve union in up to 80% of nonelderly patients,[40–42] whereas surgical fusion can achieve 96% fusion rates in selected patients.[43] Risk factors for nonunion of type II odontoid fractures include age older than 40 years, displacement greater than 6 mm, fail-

ure to maintain a reduction, and angulation greater than 10 degrees.[41, 43] With these risk factors surgery is often recommended. Posterior atlantoaxial fusion or anterior odontoid screw fixation are the two choices for surgical stabilization. Although the odontoid screw procedure is appealing in that it potentially avoids a decrease in postoperative neck motion, it requires a relatively transverse and noncomminuted fracture (Fig. 6). Type III fractures have an 87% union rate with nonoperative measures.[43] Halo rather than hard collar immobilization has been frequently recommended in the nonelderly patient to improve the potential for bony healing.

TRAUMATIC SPONDYLOLISTHESIS OF THE AXIS

With extension, axial compression, and flexion, the C2 pars interarticularis can fail, leading to anterolisthesis of the body of C2 on C3. Hangman's fracture refers to the similar radiographic appearance of this injury to the hyperextension-distraction injury occurring in judicial hangings. Traumatic spondylolisthesis of the axis alone is usually not associated with neurological injury because of decompression of the spinal canal resulting from bilateral pars fracture at the C2 level. Associated cervical spine injuries such as atlas posterior arch or burst fracture, C1 lateral mass fracture, or odontoid fracture frequently occur with this injury. Vertebral artery and cranial nerve injuries also have been reported with this fracture subtype.

The Levine and Edwards classification system describes these injuries with data from lateral plain radiography[44]

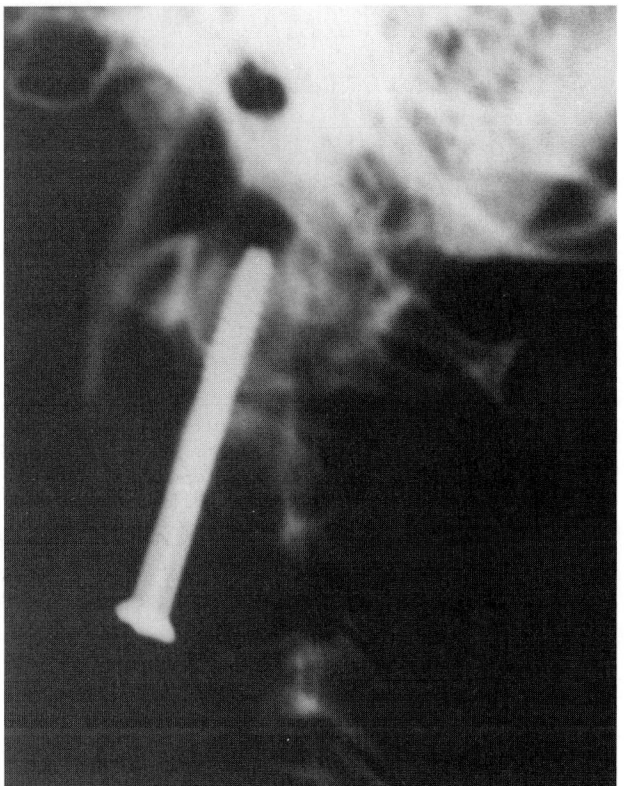

TABLE 4. ODONTOID FRACTURES: CLASSIFICATION OF ANDERSON AND D'ALONZO	
Type	**Description**
I	Oblique avulsion fracture through the alar ligament of the superior third of the dens
II	Fracture at the base of the odontoid
III	Fracture extending into the C2 body and into one or both of the articular processes

From Anderson LD, D'Alonzo RT: Fractures of the odontoid process of the axis. J Bone Joint Surg Am 1974; 56a:1663.

Fig. 6. Screw placement in a type II odontoid fracture. A lateral plain roentgenograph illustrates placement of two 3.5-mm AO lag screws.

TABLE 5. TRAUMATIC SPONDYLOLISTHESIS OF THE AXIS: CLASSIFICATION OF LEVINE AND EDWARDS	
Type	**Description**
I	Less than 3 mm of displacement with no angulation
II	More than 3 mm of displacement and significant angulation
IIA	Minimal displacement with significant angulation
III	C2 pars interarticularis fracture with unilateral or bilateral facet dislocation

From Levine AM, Edwards CC: The management of traumatic spondylolisthesis of the axis. J Bone Joint Surg Am 1985; 67a:217.

(Table 5). Type I injuries are nondisplaced with no angulation and less than 3 mm of displacement. The axis isthmus fails under a compressive extension load. Type II injuries are angulated and have more than 3 mm of displacement. After the compressive extension load causes bilateral pars fractures, a compressive flexion force results in anterolisthesis of C2 on C3. A wedge compression fracture of the anterosuperior aspect of C3 or avulsion fracture of the posteroinferior C2 body may also result. Type IIA injuries exhibit extreme angulation but little displacement, probably because the secondary force vector is a distraction-flexion force that disrupts the posterior longitudinal ligament and posterior disk of C2-3 (Fig. 7). Traction with this injury leads to displacement of the fracture and should be avoided. Type III injuries involve facet dislocations and anterior and posterior ligamentous disruption.

Type I fractures often do not displace with physician-guided flexion-extension radiographs.[44] They are thus stable injuries and can be treated with collar or halo immobilization. The greater instability and displacement seen with type II injuries are usually addressed with halo traction for reduction followed by halo immobilization.[41] One study of 39 patients suggested, however, that hangman's fractures with up to 6 mm of anterior displacement may be treated with hard collars alone.[45] Type IIA injuries require the opposite: manipulation with an extension compression moment followed by halo immobilization. Type III injuries require open reduction and C2-3 fusion, because closed reduction of the facet dislocation may be impossible as a result of displacement or force dissipation through the isthmus fractures. Continued halo treatment postoperatively is often adequate for the management of the isthmus fractures.

AXIS BODY FRACTURES

Various patterns of axis body fractures occur with or without associated injuries. Benzel et al[46] classified C2 body fractures into three types depending on the plane of the vertebral body split (Table 6). Called an atypical or unusual hangman's fracture in other reports,[47–49] type I coronal fractures involve displacement of the posterior vertebral body fragment and result from either an extension-compression force or a flexion-compression or flexion-distraction force. Thirty-three percent may be associated with neurological deficit.[49] When referred to as an atypical hangman's fracture, the isthmus fracture on one side courses into the posterior vertebral body and then through the posterior cortex. With anterior translation of the C2 body, the posterior fractured vertebral cortex is left behind with the posterior elements and may impinge into the anterior thecal sac. Type II sagittal fractures are burst fractures occurring with axial loading and can have some degree of retropulsion into the spinal canal. The horizontal type III C2 body fractures are equivalent to Anderson and D'Alonzo's type III odontoid fractures.

Alternatively, Fujimura et al[50] distinguished four types of axis body fractures: avulsion fractures of the anterior longitudinal ligament, transverse splits of the C2 body, burst fractures of the C2 body associated with bilateral pars fractures and traumatic spondylolisthesis, and sagittal splits

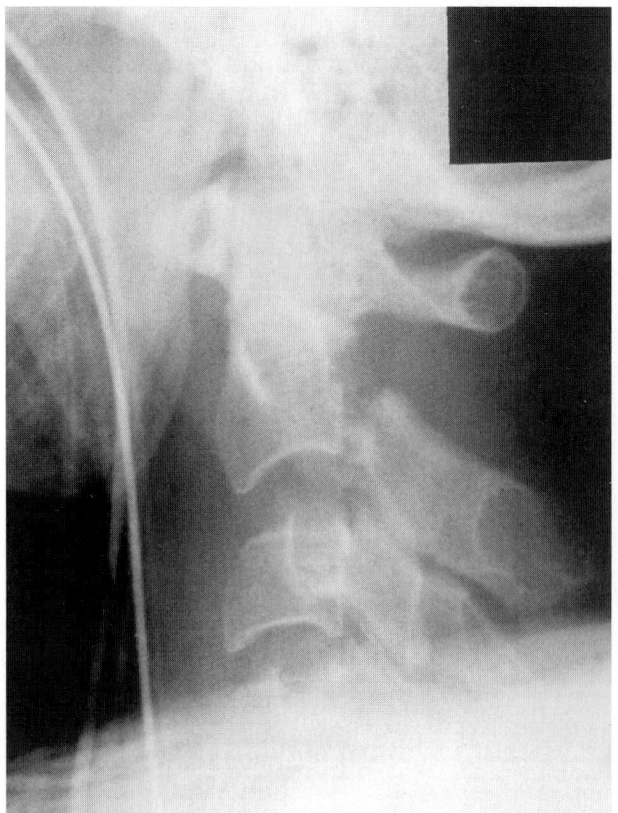

Fig. 7. Type IIA hangman's fracture. Note the angulation without translation.

TABLE 6. AXIS BODY FRACTURES: CLASSIFICATION OF BENZEL ET AL	
Type	**Description**
I	Coronal plane fracture with posterior displacement of the posterior vertebral body fragment; also called atypical hangman's fracture
II	Sagittal plane fracture with a burst pattern and retropulsion into the vertebral canal
III	Horizontal plane fracture equivalent to Anderson and D'Alonzo type III odontoid fracture

From Benzel EC, Hart BL, Ball PA, et al: Fractures of the C-2 vertebral body. J Neurosurg 1994; 81:206.

of the C2 body. In their study of 31 patients, Fujimura and Nishi recommended nonoperative management for types I and II fractures and anterior C2-3 interbody fusion for types III and IV fractures.

SUBAXIAL CERVICAL SPINE TRAUMA

Injury to the subaxial cervical spine may result from myriad forces producing either isolated or multiple noncontiguous fractures in up to 10% of cases. Despite a multitude of possible force vectors causing injury, most can be described mechanistically into the six categories or phylogenies originally described by Allen et al[51] in the early 1980s (Table 7). The direction of traumatic force and position of the neck at the time of injury are considered in this classification; the resultant bony and ligamentous deficiencies are subdivided into stages. Injuries from multiple force directions may not easily fit into the Allen and Fergusson scheme, but an understanding of how the individual forces may lead to specific fracture patterns may help in the comprehension and treatment of these complex bony and soft-tissue disruptions.

COMPRESSION-FLEXION INJURIES

Compression-flexion injuries occur most commonly at the C4, C5, and C6 levels. The five stages of this injury mechanism involve progressive failure of the anterior followed by the posterior cervical columns. In the first two stages, blunting and rounding of the anterior vertebral body and then beaking with loss of vertebral height occur without posterior ligamentous disruption. Treatment is aimed at preventing late deformity and pain; usually a course of hard collar immobilization is sufficient. Stage III injuries have a fracture line extending from the anterosuperior vertebral margin posteriorly through the inferior end plate. Stage IV compressive flexion fractures have less than 3 mm retrolisthesis of the fractured vertebral body segment. These latter two stages of higher energy may occur with posterior ligamentous injury, so MRI evaluation is helpful in evaluating stability. Halo immobilization is effective unless significant ligamentous deficiency is discovered; otherwise, an anterior cervical reconstruction may be necessary to prevent late kyphotic collapse. Retrolisthesis of more than 3 mm into the vertebral canal in stage V injuries usually occurs with significant posterior ligamentous disruption, so consideration for circumferential stabilization is often required (Fig. 8). Surgical intervention in stages III and higher is frequently performed with an anterior approach in the setting of neurological compromise and thecal sac compression.

VERTICAL COMPRESSION INJURIES

These injuries occur most commonly at the C6 and C7 levels. A pure axial load usually results initially in cupping of either vertebral end plate (stage I) followed by frank fracture of the end plates (stage II). Stage III involves peripheral displacement of fragmented vertebral bone. Hard collar immobilization for stage I or halo immobilization for stage II injuries without neurological deficit is often adequate. A neurological deficit in the setting of a stage III injury is preferably managed with an anterior corpectomy and fusion.

Type	Description
TABLE 7. SUBAXIAL CERVICAL SPINE FRACTURES: CLASSIFICATION OF ALLEN ET AL	
Compression-Flexion	
I	Blunting of the anterosuperior vertebral margin
II	Beaking of the anteroinferior vertebral body with decreased vertebral body height
III	Fracture of the anteroinferior vertebral body without retropulsion of fragments into the vertebral canal
IV	Compression-flexion fracture as above with retropulsion into the vertebral canal of less than 3 mm
V	Compression-flexion fracture as above with retropulsion into the vertebral canal of more than 3 mm
Vertical Compression	
I	Central vertebral body cupping with fracture at either the superior or inferior vertebral body end plate
II	Fracture extends through both end plates with minimal displacement
III	Vertical compression fracture with significant displacement
Distraction-Flexion	
I	Facet subluxation with divergent spinous processes
II	Unilateral facet dislocation with approximately 25% anterolisthesis of the cephalad on caudal vertebral body
III	Bilateral facet dislocation with approximately 50% to 100% anterolisthesis of the cephalad on caudal vertebral body
IV	Bilateral facet dislocation with approximately spondylolisthesis of the cephalad on caudal vertebral body
Compression-Extension	
I	Unilateral laminar fracture without displacement
II	Bilateral laminar fractures without displacement
III	Bilateral laminar fractures without displacement with associated articular process or pedicle fractures
IV	Bilateral laminar fractures with less than 100% anterior vertebral body displacement
V	Bilateral laminar fractures with 100% or more anterior vertebral body displacement
Distraction-Extension	
I	Disk space widening with or without a transverse body fracture
II	Retrolisthesis of the cephalad on caudal vertebral body
Lateral Flexion	
I	Nondisplaced unilateral pedicle or laminar fracture with an asymmetric vertebral body compression injury
II	Displaced unilateral pedicle or laminar fracture with an asymmetric vertebral body compression injury

From Allen BL, Fergusson RL, Lehman TR, et al: A mechanistic classification of closed, indirect fractures and dislocations of the cervical spine. Spine 1982; 7:1. Used with permission.

DISTRACTION-FLEXION INJURIES

A stage I distraction-flexion injury involves facet subluxation with subtle spinous process divergence. Stage II injuries describe a unilateral facet dislocation with approximately 25% anterolisthesis of the cephalad vertebral body on the inferior vertebral body (Fig. 9). Stage III injuries describe a bilateral facet dislocation noted by 50% anterolisthesis of the cephalad vertebral body on the inferior vertebral body (Fig. 10). One hundred percent anterior displacement of one vertebral body on the other describes a stage III injury.

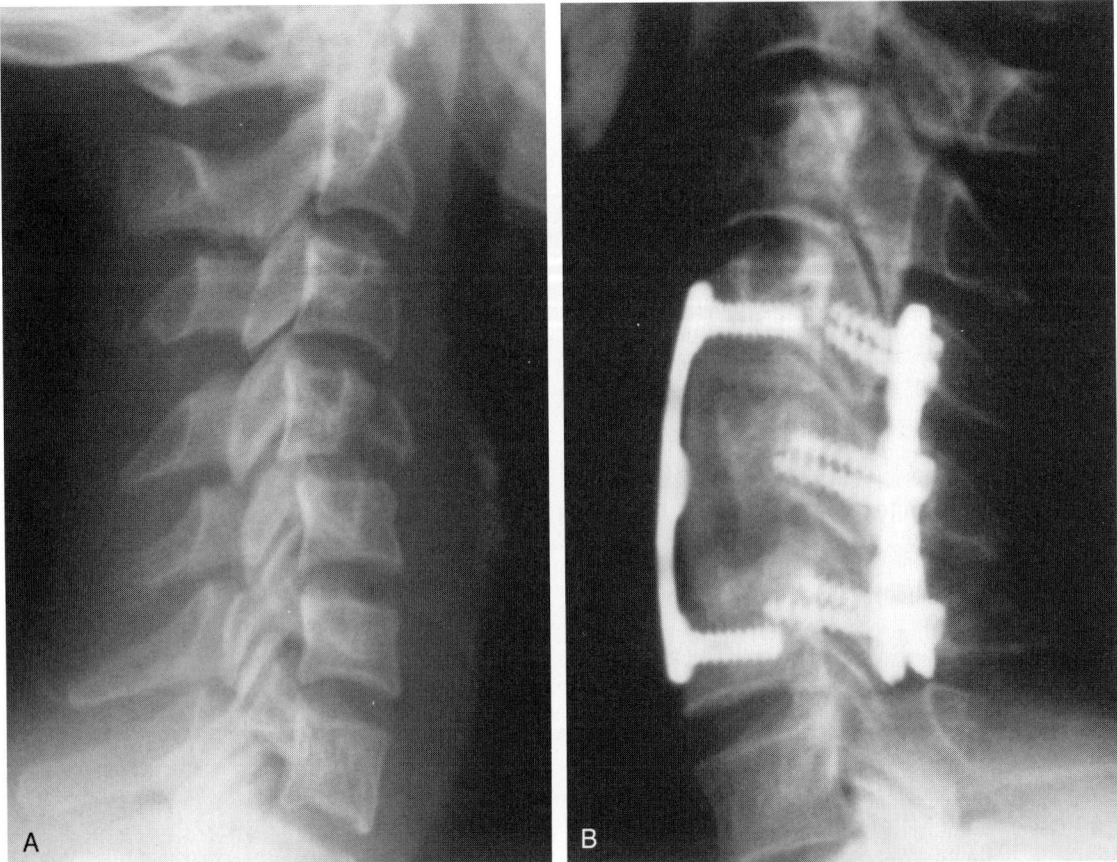

Fig. 8. Compression-flexion injury. *A,* A lateral plain roentgenograph illustrates evidence of a flexion-compression stage III-IV injury at the C4 level. *B,* A lateral plain roentgenogram of an anterior-posterior cervical decompression and stabilization procedure with the use of an anterior plate spanning from C4 to C6 with additional posterolateral mass plates and screws with bone graft used to stabilize a stage V compression-flexion injury.

Although there are rare reports of neurological deterioration during closed manipulative reduction of facet dislocations because of the presence of an extruded disk herniation, all such cases involved intubated, anesthetized patients who were not monitored with voluntary neurological testing.[52, 53] Closed reduction with skeletal traction can be safely performed in the awake, alert patient with weights of up to 160 pounds.[54, 55] Occasionally, gentle manipulation of the cervical spine may be required in the setting of a perched facet injury after traction.[55] Any worsening in the neurological profile of a patient is determined by a careful, unimpaired neurological examination after incremental weight (10 pounds) application. Any change for the worse in the neurological examination should signal the halt of the reduction maneuver with subsequent decrease in the traction weights. An MRI should be obtained after successful or unsuccessful closed reduction or in the nonalert patient before reduction to rule out the presence of a herniated disk, which may occur in 11% to 54% of facet dislocations[56] (Fig. 11). A CT scan may detect an undiagnosed bony injury in distractive flexion injuries in as much as 50% of patients[75] (Fig. 12).

Surgical stabilization is indicated in all distraction-flexion injuries given the loss of ligamentous stability. With successful closed reduction and the absence of a herniated disk, posterior fusion should be performed. Unsuccessful closed reduction without herniated disks require an open posterior reduction and fusion. The presence of a herniated disk requires anterior diskectomy. An anterior fusion should follow an anterior diskectomy when the closed preoperative reduction was successful in obtaining spinal alignment. Otherwise, an anterior reduction maneuver with gentle distraction and a posterior rotatory maneuver through Caspar distraction pins may be attempted. If this is unsuccessful or undesirable, the anterior procedure may be temporarily closed, followed by a posterior reduction and fusion and followed again by a final anterior fusion. Some surgeons may attempt to place an undersized anterior Smith-Robinson graft in a slightly exaggerated anterior position in a dislocated spine with hopes that, with an open posterior reduction, the graft will occupy an acceptable position supporting the anterior column. This may prevent the need to revisit the anterior exposure. The open posterior reduction involves a posterior distraction maneuver to the listhesed vertebra through bony tenaculums clamped at the spinolaminar junction in conjunction with a Penfield or nerve hook manipulating the dislocated facet from its medial aspect. To assist in the reduction, a Kerrison punch may be used to shorten the caudal superior articular process to aid in the reduction maneuver.

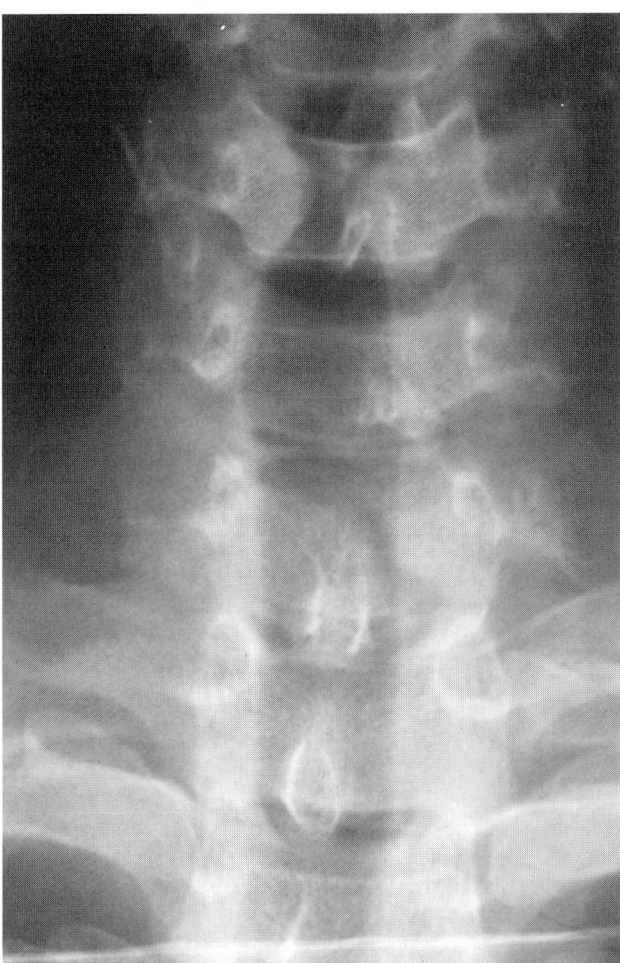

Fig. 9. Distraction-flexion injury. An anteroposterior plain roentgenograph illustrates malalignment of the C6 and C7 spinous processes in the setting of a unilateral facet dislocation.

COMPRESSION-EXTENSION INJURIES

Stage I and II compressive extension fractures describe unilateral or bilateral laminar fractures without displacement. They are usually treated with a hard cervical collar. Progressive disruption of the posterior elements with eventual anterior column failure occurs as one proceeds from a stage III to stage IV injury. Complete (100%) anterior displacement of the cephalad on caudal vertebral body occurs in the stage IV injury pattern and must be approached initially with a posterior open reduction and stabilization procedure. With higher stage injuries, neurological impairment is frequent, but uncommon reports of neurological sparing have been identified.[57]

DISTRACTION-EXTENSION INJURIES

One must be suspicious for the presence of this injury in patients with ankylosing spondylitis or diffuse idiopathic skeletal hyperostosis who complain of cervical pain after trauma. A distraction-extension stage I injury places the anterior spinal ligamentous complex in tension, leading to either solitary anterior ligamentous failure or an undisplaced transverse body fracture. Disk space widening may be seen on plain radiographs. Posterior ligamentous failure occurs in stage II injuries and often leads to retrolisthesis of the cephalad vertebral segment on the inferior vertebral level (Fig. 13). Without displacement in an adult patient, halo immobilization may be adequate in pure bony injuries. Consideration should be given to surgery in injuries involving the disk space because of their unpredictable healing in the adult patient. The surgical treatment of choice is a standard anterior diskectomy and fusion with instrumentation acting as a tension band. Stage II fractures universally require surgical stabilization.

LATERAL FLEXION INJURIES

Lateral flexion stage I injuries involve a nondisplaced unilateral pedicle or lamina fracture with an ipsilateral asymmetric vertebral body compression fracture. Stage II injuries describe the contralateral failure of the bony and ligamentous complex of the involved level in tension, resulting in displacement at the fracture site. For stage II injuries posterior surgical stabilization with segmental fixation is recommended. A hard collar is acceptable treatment for the majority of stage I injuries.

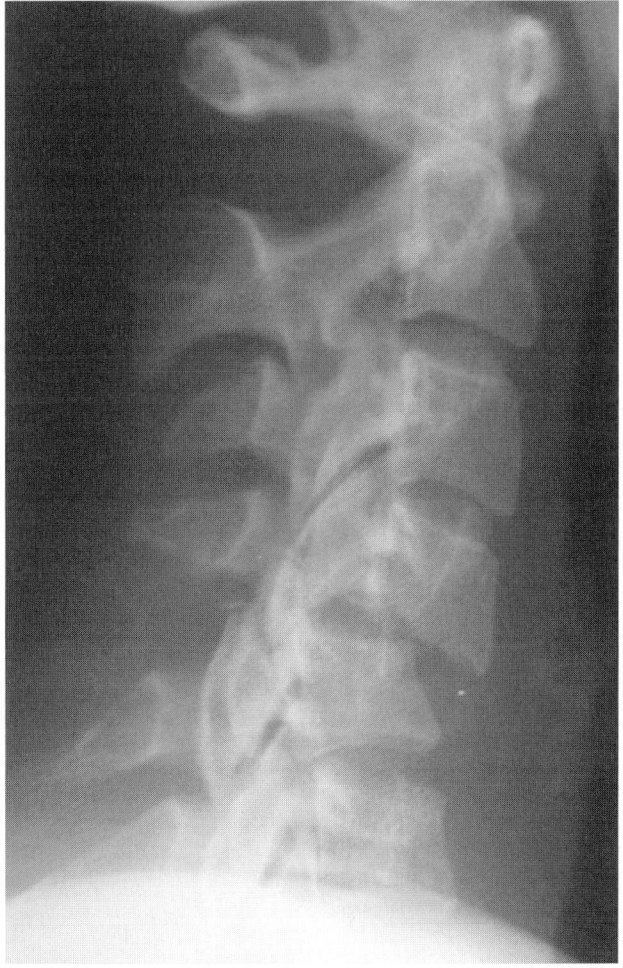

Fig. 10. Distraction-flexion injury. A lateral plain roentgenograph illustrates a stage III distraction-flexion injury at the C4-5 level (i.e., a bilateral facet dislocation). Note the anterosuperior wedging of the C5 vertebral body as the result of the compression-flexion force.

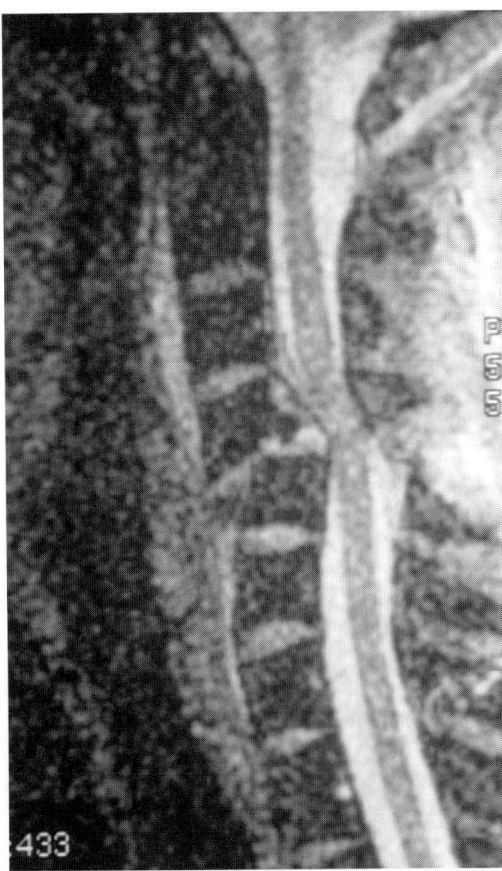

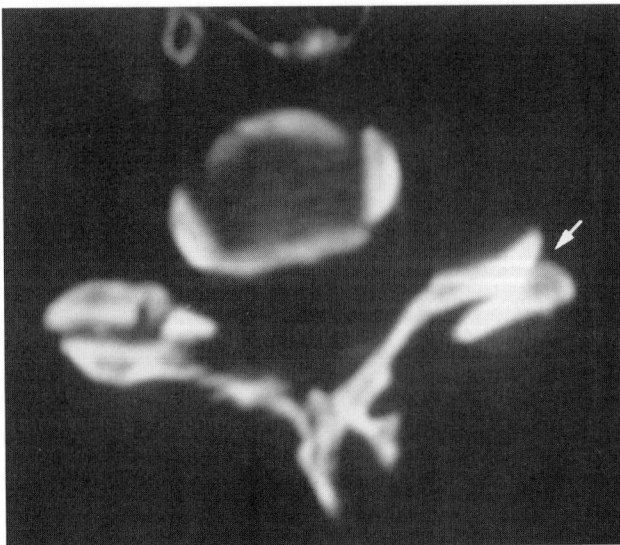

Fig. 12. Distraction-flexion injury. A transaxial computed tomography scan of a unilateral facet dislocation illustrates the right inferior articular process lying anterior to the superior articular process.

Fig. 11. Distraction-flexion injury. A sagittal magnetic resonance imaging scan reveals evidence of a disk extrusion at the level of the cervical dislocation.

Lateral mass and articular process fractures are usually the result of a combined rotatory, anterior shear force in a flexed cervical spine. Superior articular process fractures are more common than inferior articular process fractures. These injuries are usually evident on plain radiography; in addition to an obvious fracture line on a lateral plain radiograph, there may be rotation and lengthening of the cephalad vertebral body. Alternatively, ipsilateral pedicle and lamina fractures can allow the lateral mass to rotate, producing a horizontal appearance of the lateral mass on the anteroposterior and lateral plain radiographs. CT scanning is the imaging study of choice in detecting more subtle injuries. Closed reduction with skeletal traction often is required to obtain adequate spinal alignment. In the absence of a neurological deficit, halo immobilization may be adequate to obtain stable healing, although minimal translation (less than 2 to 3 mm) may be seen on follow-up lateral plain radiography. With significant weakness, radicular pain, or marked initial displacement, operative stabilization by lateral mass plating is preferred.

SURGICAL TECHNIQUES

The guiding principles of operative management of cervical spine trauma are to obtain a stable arthrodesis in appropri-

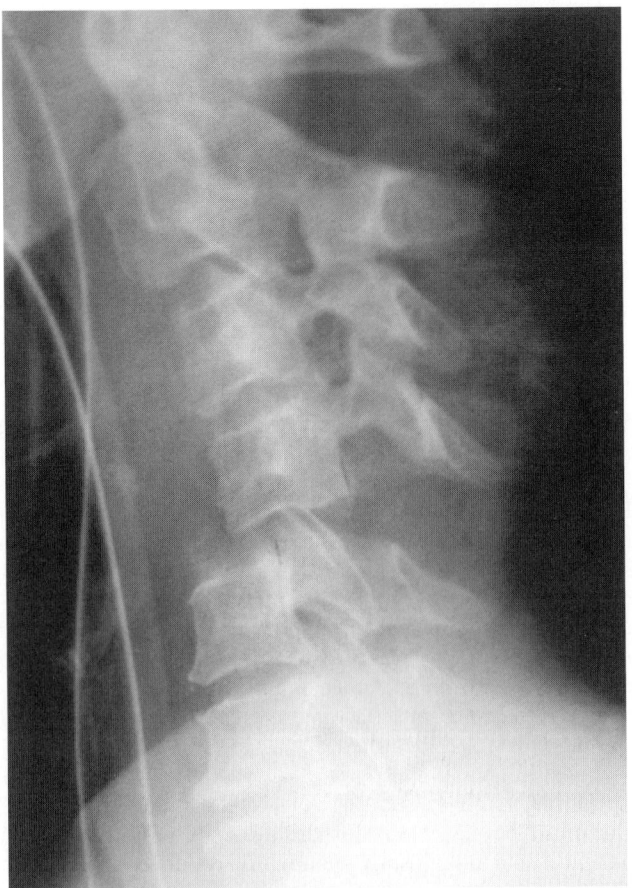

Fig. 13. Distraction-extension injury. A lateral plain roentgenograph of a high-grade distraction-extension injury reveals complete circumferential soft-tissue disruption at the C4-5 level. Note the retrolisthesis at the C4 vertebral body within the canal behind the C5 vertebral body.

ate alignment and to relieve neural compression in the setting of a neurological deficit. Adequate decompression of the spinal cord may be achieved from the anterior or posterior approach. Regardless of the approach, a concomitant stabilization procedure should be performed to prevent a late deformity or instability. In rare situations, circumferential reconstruction of the spine may be necessary in three column injuries at high risk for surgical failure. Basic biomechanical considerations as well as patient age, comorbidities, and surgeon experience will determine the optimal surgical approach.[58]

There is no clear consensus as to the optimal timing of surgical intervention. Early decompression and fusion allow for early patient mobilization and theoretically decrease the extent of the secondary cascade of spinal cord injury (i.e., tissue hypoxia, edema, hemorrhage, and inflammation leading to neuronal damage). A retrospective review of 138 patients requiring operative management suggested improved outcomes in the more severely injured patients.[54] Delayed surgery, however, allows for full medical optimization; and edema subsidence may make surgical decompression procedures less hazardous. A prospective, randomized study of 64 patients comparing early (before 72 hours) versus late (after 5 days) surgery for cervical spinal cord injuries found no significant difference in length of hospitalization, duration of rehabilitation, and neurological improvement.[60]

OCCIPITOCERVICAL ARTHRODESIS

The optimal surgical approach to stabilize and decompress the cervicocranium is posterior. Several surgical methods to achieve fusion have been described. Wiring techniques have been devised to affix sections of iliac crest bone graft decorticated posterior spinal elements. Wires are passed through bur holes in the skull and under the upper cervical laminae or around the C2 spinous process. Use of a contoured Steinmann pin secured with sublaminar and suboccipital wires also has been described with some success. The most rigid and successful form of fixation, however, is with plates or rods and screws, which attach segmentally to the occiput and upper cervical spinal elements. This form

of fixation does not rely on the posterior elements for wire fixation and, therefore, should not pose any difficulties if a posterior decompression is necessary.[61–63]

ATLANTOAXIAL ARTHRODESIS

Atlantoaxial fusions are most frequently performed with a posterior approach. The most popular technique is a Brooks fusion using C2-1 sublaminar wires secured around two wedge-shaped bone grafts. The Gallie fusion, although rarely used, is somewhat safer because the cable is passed through the base of the C2 spinous process rather than beneath the lamina. This technique, however, provides less rotational stability than does the Brooks technique.[64]

The most rigid means of stabilizing the C1-2 articulation is with transarticular screws through the Magerl approach[65, 66] (Fig. 14). The screws are driven from the inferomedial portion of the C2 inferior articular process through the C2 isthmus and the facet joint and into the C1 lateral mass. A supplementary Brooks fusion has been recommended to stabilize the C2-1 articulation further and rigidly attach the added bone graft. The rigidity of this technique often obviates the need for postoperative halo immobilization.[36] Preoperative studies such as conventional or magnetic resonance angiography to locate the course of the vertebral arteries as well as reconstructed CT images to evaluate the size of the C2 isthmus are extremely important for proper screw placement. Research has found that 18% to 23% of people have vertebral artery positions that preclude Magerl screw technique.[67] Incomplete atlantoaxial joint reduction has been identified as the major risk factor for screw misplacement.[68]

ANTERIOR ODONTOID SCREW FIXATION

The major advantage of the odontoid screw fixation technique in the surgical management of odontoid fractures is to avoid the morbidity of decreased cervical range of motion experienced after a C1-2 fusion. This technique only is useful in fracture configurations that are perpendicular to the axis of screw placement. Through an anterior approach, one or two screws are placed from inferior to superior. The use of two anterior odontoid screws may

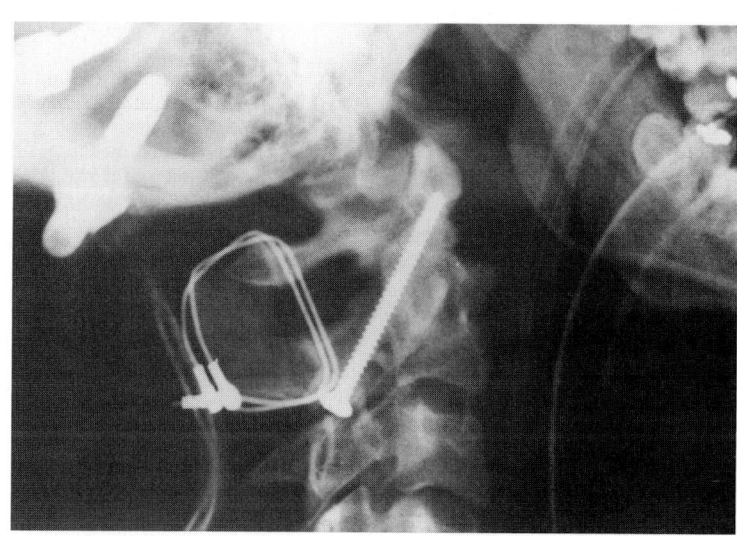

Fig. 14. Atlantoaxial arthrodesis. A lateral plain roentgenograph illustrates C2-1 transarticular screw fixation as well as a supplementary Brooks fusion with autologous iliac crest bone graft. This patient was noted to have an unstable os odontoideum, which was causing neurological compromise.

increase the stiffness to extension loading,[69] but fusion rates as high as 100% have been reported with a single screw technique.[70]

ANTERIOR CERVICAL FUSION

The Smith-Robinson surgical exposure is the standard approach in accessing the anterior cervical elements. This allows adequate visualization to perform a cervical decompression and stabilization procedure. After a decompression, decortication of the exposed end plates is followed by insertion of tricortical iliac crest bone graft, fibular strut graft, or cervical cage packed with autologous cancellous bone graft. The choice of grafting technique depends on surgeon preference. However, consistently acceptable results have been reported with autologous anterior iliac crest and fibular strut graft sources.

Instrumentation should always be used to supplement the anterior fusion to maintain alignment, confer adequate stability, and improve the healing success rate. An anterior cervical plate functions as a tension band in extension and a buttress in flexion. Because of its inherent rigidity, anterior instrumentation may obviate the need for posterior stabilization in some cases of anterior and posterior instability.[71] Anterior plates are often contoured to achieve maximum bone-plate contact as well as to recreate the desired amount of cervical lordosis.

POSTERIOR CERVICAL FUSION

Various methods of posterior cervical stabilization have been described. Wiring techniques may be sublaminar, oblique through the inferior articular process, or interspinous. They afford stability in flexion but less so in extension or rotation. Because cyclical torsional loading leads to significant loosening in cadaver studies, postoperative halo immobilization is often required.

More rigid posterior fixation is accomplished with the use of lateral mass plates. This form of fixation has been found to be extremely safe as long as an understanding of the location of the vertebral artery and nerve root is appreciated. One study has demonstrated a 1.8% risk of radiculopathy per screw placed.[72]

The C7 lateral masses are relatively thin, and often pedicle screw fixation is desired at this level in the absence of a traversing vertebral artery in the foramen transversarium. A mini-laminotomy to allow tactile appreciation of the orientation of the pedicles during pedicle screw placement may help avoid spinal canal encroachment.[73] C2 isthmus screws have also been described. Elsewhere in the cervical spine pedicle anatomy is less consistent, so pedicle screws have not been proven to be safe and effective at the C3 though C6 levels.[74]

CONCLUSION

Improper management of cervical spine trauma patients may be associated with acute or late onset of progressive pain, neurological decline, or deformity. Early recognition, stable immobilization, timely diagnosis, early pharmacological intervention, and appropriate timely definitive treatment are crucial to obtaining an optimal outcome. Both nonoperative and surgical means to manage the spinal cord–injured patient have greatly improved over the past decade. The choice of treatment depends on the severity of injury, presence of neurological compromise, type and location of injury, patient's underlying medical condition, and, most importantly, surgeon's experience and training.

REFERENCES

1. Go BK, De Vivo MJ, Richards JS: The epidemiology of spinal cord injury. In Stover SL, DeLisa JA, Whiteneck GG (eds): Spinal Cord Injury: Clinical Outcomes From the Model Systems. Gaithersburg MD, Aspen, 1995, p 21.
2. Kraus JF, Franti CE, Riggins RS, et al: Incidence of traumatic spinal cord lesions. J Chronic Dis 1975; 28:471.
3. Ebraheim NA, Lu J, Young H: The effect of translation of C1-C2 on the spinal canal. Clin Orthop 1998; 351:222.
4. Matsura P, Waters RL, Adkins RH, et al: Comparison of computerized tomography parameters of the cervical spine in normal control subjects and spinal cord-injured patients. J Bone Joint Surg Am 1989; 71:183.
5. Jovanovich MS: A comparative study of the foramen transversarium of the sixth and seventh vertebra. Surg Radiol Anat 1990; 12:167.
6. Donaldson WF, Heil BV, Donaldson VP, et al: The effect of airway maneuvers on the unstable C1-C2 segment. Spine 1997; 11:1215.
7. American Spinal Injury Association: Standards for Neurologic and Functional Classification of Spinal Cord Injury (rev. ed.) Chicago, IL, American Spinal Injury Association, 1992.
8. Bracken MB, Shepard MJ, Holford TR, et al: Administration of methylprednisolone for 24 or 48 hours or tirilazad mesylate for 48 hours in the treatment of acute spinal cord injury: Results of the Third National Acute Spinal Cord Injury Randomized Control Trial. National Acute Spinal Cord Injury study. JAMA 1997; 277:1597.
9. Chang DG, Tencer AF, Ching RP, et al: Geometric changes in the cervical spinal during impact. Spine 1994; 19:973.
10. Alker G, Oh YS, Leslie IV: High cervical spine and craniocervical junction injuries in fatal traffic accidents: A radiologic study. Orthop Clin North Am 1978; 9:1003.
11. Goldstein SJ, Woodring JA, Young AB: Occipital condyle fracture associated with cervical spine injury. Surg Neurol 1982; 17:350.
12. Levine AM, Edwards CC: Traumatic lesions of the occipito-atlanto-axial complex. Clin Orthop 1989; 239:53.
13. Demisch S, Lindner A, Beck R, et al: The forgotten condyle: Delayed hypoglossal nerve palsy caused by fracture of the occipital condyle. Clin Neurol Neurosurg 1998; 100:44.
14. Bloom AI, Neeman Z, Simon-Slasky B, et al: Fracture of the occipital condyles and associated craniocervical ligament injury: Incidence, CT imaging and implications. Clin Radiol 1997; 52:198.
15. Anderson PA, Montesano PX: Morphology and treatment of occipital condyle fractures. Spine 1988; 13:731.
16. Tuli S, Tator CH, Fehling MG, et al: Occipital condyle fractures. Neurosurgery 1992; 41:368.
17. Bucholz RW, Burkhead WZ: The pathologic anatomy of fatal atlanto-occipital dislocations. J Bone Joint Surg Am 1979; 61:248.
18. Collato PM, DeMuth WW, Schwentker EP, et al: Traumatic atlanto-occipital dislocations. J Bone Joint Surg Am 1986; 67:1106.
19. Przybyliski GJ, Clyde BL, Fitz CR: Craniocervical junction subarachnoid hemorrhage associated with atlanto-occipital dislocation. Spine 1996; 21:1761.
20. Finney HC, Roberts TS: Atlanto-occipital instability. J Neurosurg 1978; 48:636.
21. Lee C, Woodring JH, Goldstein SJ, et al: Evaluation of traumatic atlanto-occipital dislocations. Am J Neuroradiol 1987; 8:19.
22. Wiesel SW, Rothman RH: Occipitoatlantal hypermobility. Spine 1979; 4:187.
23. Dublin AB, Marks WM, Weinstock D, et al: Traumatic dislocation of the atlanto-occipital articulation (AOA) with short-

term survival, with a radiographic method of measuring AOA. J Neurosurg 1980; 52: 514.

24. Harris JH, Carson GC, Wagner LK, et al: Radiologic diagnosis of traumatic occipitovertebral dislocation: 2. Comparison of three methods of detecting occipitovertebral relationships on lateral radiographs of the supine subject. AJR Am J Roentgenol 1994; 162:887.

25. Wholey MH, Brumer AJ, Baker HL: The lateral roentgenogram of the neck. Radiology 1958; 71:350.

26. Dickman CA, Papadopoulos SM, Sonntag VKH, et al: Traumatic occipitoatlantal dislocations. J Spinal Disord 1993; 6:300.

27. Traynelis VC, Marano GD, Dunker RO, et al: Traumatic atlanto-occipital dislocation. J Neurosurg 1986; 65:863.

28. Levine AM, Edwards CC: Treatment of injuries in the C1-C2 complex. Orthop Clin North Am 1986; 17:31.

29. Levine AM, Edwards CC: Fractures of the atlas. J Bone Joint Surg Am 1991; 73:680.

30. Spence KF, Decker S, Sell KW: Bursting atlantal fracture associated with rupture of the transverse ligament. J Bone Joint Surg Am 1970; 52:543.

31. Heller JG, Viroslav S, Hudson J: Jefferson fractures: The role of magnification artifact in assessing transverse ligament integrity. J Spinal Disord 1993; 6:392.

32. Anderson LD, D'Alonzo RT: Fractures of the odontoid process of the axis. J Bone Joint Surg Am 1974; 56:1663.

33. Dickman CA, Mamourian A, Sonntag VKH, et al: Magnetic resonance imaging of the transverse atlantal ligament for the evaluation of atlantoaxial instability. J Neurosurg 1991; 75:221.

34. Lee T, Green BA, Petrin DR: Treatment of stable burst fracture of the atlas (Jefferson fracture) with rigid cervical collar. Spine 1998; 23:1963.

35. Dickman CA, Greene KA, Sonntag VKH: Injuries involving the transverse atlantal ligament: Classification and guidelines based on experience with 39 injuries. Neurosurgery 1996; 38:44.

36. McGuire RA, Harkey HL: Primary treatment of unstable Jefferson's fractures. J Spinal Disord 1995; 8:233.

37. Wortzman G, Dewar FP: Rotary fixation of the atlantoaxial joint: Rotational atlantoaxial subluxation. Radiology 1968; 90: 479.

38. Fielding JW, Hawkins RJ: Atlanto-axial rotatory fixation (fixed rotatory subluxation of the atlanto-axial joint). J Bone Joint Surg Am 1977; 59:37.

39. Hadley MN, Browner CM, Liu SS, et al: New subtype of acute odontoid fractures (type IIA). Neurosurgery 1988; 22:67.

40. Cooper PR, Maravilla KR, Sklar FH, et al: Halo immobilization of cervical spine fractures: Indications and results. J Neurosurg 1979; 50:603.

41. Greene KA, Dickman CA, Marciano FF, et al: Acute axis fractures: Analysis of management and outcome in 340 consecutive cases. Spine 1997; 22:1843.

42. Stoney J, O'Brien J, Wilde P: Treatment of type-two odontoid fractures in halothoracic vests. J Bone Joint Surg Br 1998; 80:4525.

43. Clark CR, White AA: Fractures of the dens: A multicenter study. J Bone Joint Surg Am 1985; 67:1340.

44. Levine AM, Edwards CC: The management of traumatic spondylolisthesis of the axis. J Bone Joint Surg Am 1985; 67:217.

45. Coric D, Wilson JA, Kelly DL Jr: Treatment of traumatic spondylolisthesis of the axis with nonrigid immobilization: A review of 64 cases. J Neurosurg 1996; 85: 550.

46. Benzel EC, Hart BL, Ball PA, et al: Fractures of the C-2 vertebral body. J Neurosurg 1994; 81:206.

47. Effendi B, Roy D, Cornish B, et al: Fractures of the ring of the axis, a classification based on the analysis of 131 cases. J Bone Joint Surg Br 1981; 63:319.

48. Marotta TR, White L, Terbrugge KG, et al: An unusual type of hangman's fracture. Neurosurgery 1990; 26:848.

49. Starr JK, Eismont CC: Atypical hangman's fractures. Spine 1993; 18:1954.

50. Fujimura Y, Nishi Y, Kobayashi K: Classification and treatment of axis body fractures. J Orthop Trauma 1996; 10:536.

51. Allen BL, Fergusson RL, Lehman TR, et al: A mechanistic classification of closed, indirect fractures and dislocations of the cervical spine. Spine 1982; 7:1.

52. Eismont FJ, Arena MJ, Green BA: Extrusion of an intervertebral disc associated with traumatic subluxation or dislocation of cervical facets. J Bone Joint Surg Am 1991; 73:1555.

53. Robertson PA, Ryan MD: Neurologic deterioration after reduction of cervical subluxation. J Bone Joint Surg Br 1992; 74: 224.

54. Cotler JM, Herbison GJ, Nasuti JF, et al: Closed reduction of traumatic cervical spine dislocation using traction weights up to 140 pounds. Spine 1993; 18:386.

55. Starr AM, Cotler JM, Balderston RA, et al: Immediate closed reduction of cervical spine dislocations using traction. Spine 1990; 15:1068.

56. Rizzolo SJ, Vaccaro AR, Cotler JM: Cervical spine trauma. Spine 1997; 19:2288.

57. Jenis LG, Dann EJ, Teebag AK: Complete vertebral fracture/dislocation of the cervical spine with minimal neurologic deficit. J Orthop Trauma 1996; 10:123.

58. Vaccaro AR, Cook CM, McCullen G, et al: Cervical trauma: Rationale for selecting the appropriate fusion technique. Orthop Clin North Am 1998; 29:745.

59. Schlegel J, Bayley J, Yuan H, et al: Timing of surgical decompression and fixation of acute spinal fractures. J Orthop Trauma 1996; 10:323.

60. Vaccaro AR, Daugherty RJ, Sheehan TP, et al: Neurologic outcome of early versus late surgery for cervical spinal cord injury. Spine 1997; 22:2609.

61. Grob D, Dvorak J, Panjabi M, et al: Posterior occipitocervical fusion: A case report of a new technique. Spine 1991; 16(Suppl):S17.

62. Sasso RC, Jeanneret B, Fischer K, et al: Occipitocervical fusion with posterior plate and screw instrumentation: A long term follow-up study. Spine 1994; 19:2364.

63. Smith MD, Anderson P, Grady S: Occipitocervical arthrodesis using contoured plate fixation. Spine 1993; 18:1984.

64. Dickman CA, Crawford NR, Paramore CG: Biomechanical characteristics of C1-2 cable fixations. J Neurosurg 1996; 85:316.

65. Jeanneret B, Magerl F: Primary posterior fusion C1/2 in odontoid fractures: Indications, technique, and results of transarticular screw fixation. J Spinal Disord 1992; 5:464.

66. Magerl F, Seeman PS: Stable posterior fusion of the atlas and axis by transarticular screw fixation. In Kehr P, Weidner A (eds): Cervical Spine. Wien, Springer Verlag, 1987, p 322.

67. Paramore CG, Dickman CA, Sonntag VK: The anatomical suitability of the C1-2 complex for transarticular screw fixation. J Neursurg 1996; 85:221.

68. Madawi AB, Casey ATH, Solanki GA, et al: Radiological and anatomical evaluation of the atlantoaxial transarticular screw fixation technique. J Neurosurg 1997; 86: 961.

69. Sasso R, Doherty BJ, Crawford MJ, et al: Biomechanics of odontoid fixation: Comparison of the one- and two-screw technique. Spine 1993; 18:1950.

70. Chang KW, Liu YW, Cheng PG, et al: One Herbert double-threaded compression screw fixation of displaced type II odontoid fractures. J Spinal Disord 1994; 7:62.

71. Vaccaro AR, Balderston RA: Anterior plate instrumentation for disorders of the subaxial cervical spine. Clin Orthop 1997; 335:112.

72. Graham AW, Swank ML, Kinard RE, et al: Posterior cervical arthrodesis and stabilization with a lateral mass plate. Spine 1996; 21:323.

73. Miller RM, Ebraheim NA, Xu R, et al: Anatomic consideration of transpedicular screw placement in the cervical spine. Spine 1996; 21:2317.

74. Kramer DL, Ludwig SC, Balderston RA, et al: Morphometry of subaxial cervical pedicles: Anatomical considerations related to three techniques of pedicle screw insertion. Presented at the annual meeting of the Cervical Spine Research Society. Palm Beach, FL, 1996.

75. Shapiro SA: Management of unilateral locked facet of the cervical spine. Neurosurgery 1993; 33:832.

section
3
chapter
23

THORACOLUMBAR SPINE INJURIES

Paul E. Savas, Alexander R. Vaccaro, and Todd J. Albert

Summary
- The thoracolumbar spine is the most common site of vertebral column injuries.
- Appropriate treatment of thoracolumbar injuries should be guided by a thorough understanding of spinal anatomy, spinal mechanics, and injury mechanisms.
- Early medical management and early surgical decompression, although still debated, may prove beneficial in preserving and improving neurological function.
- Whether through nonoperative or surgical intervention, the goals of treatment of thoracolumbar injuries are to maximize neurological recovery and maintain or enhance stabilization of the spine for return to satisfactory function.

The majority of thoracolumbar injuries are caused by high-energy trauma. Less common are isolated thoracolumbar fractures that occur from low-energy injuries and from metabolic causes such as osteoporosis.

In patients with traumatic thoracolumbar injuries, associated injuries are not uncommon. Depending on the type of spine fracture, up to 50% of these patients may have multisystem trauma.[1] Intra-abdominal injury can occur in almost 50% of patients suffering from a distraction-type spinal fracture.[2] Concomitant, noncontiguous spine fractures may occur in 5% to 20% of patients having traumatic spine injuries.[3]

PATIENT EVALUATION

CLINICAL EXAMINATION

A complete, documented patient history and physical examination are essential. Spine injuries may be missed in the initial emergency room evaluation because of diverting factors such as multiple injuries and/or lack of cooperation of a patient with a head injury.

Initial evaluation should include a history of the circumstances of the accident, position of the patient when found, whether the patient was wearing a seat belt, and the type of treatment that was performed at the scene of the accident. This information may provide insight as to the possible mechanism of injury.

The physical examination should begin with careful visual inspection followed by systematic palpation. Tissue abrasions, lacerations, and contusions should be investigated. An abdominal contusion from a lap belt, a seat belt sign, may be a diagnostic clue for a flexion-distraction injury of the spine and associated intra-abdominal injuries. Each spinous process should be palpated, noting tenderness, asymmetry, alignment, and interspinous widening.

Care must be exercised during the log-roll maneuver because neurological compromise may potentially result from displacement of an unstable spine injury. A low pulse rate with low blood pressure may represent a sympathectomy resulting from a spinal cord injury rather than hypovolemic shock.

A complete neurological examination can determine the anatomic level of the spinal injury. The neurological examination includes evaluation of sensation, motor function, and reflex function. Evaluation of sensation can assess the anterolateral and the posterior column function of the spinal cord. The anterolateral column, or the spinothalamic tract, can be evaluated by detecting differences in light touch and deep pressure, in sharp or dull discrimination, and in temperature. The posterior column can be tested by detecting differences in vibration and proprioception. Evaluation of specific dermatomal regions should begin in the cervical region and then systematically proceed distally. Evaluation of motor function should include root-specific muscle strength testing of both the upper and lower extremities. Muscle grading can help monitor the improvement or deterioration of motor function. The evaluation of reflex function can help determine the extent of spinal injury and spinal shock. Spinal shock (spinal cord concussion) usually involves a 24- to 72-hour period of paralysis, hypotonia, and areflexia. At the conclusion of spinal shock, there may be hyperreflexia, hypertonicity, and clonus. The bulbocavernosus reflex can facilitate the determination of a complete or incomplete neurological deficit. Other pathological reflexes are significant because their presence or absence can be indicative of an upper or lower motor neuron lesion (Table 1).

RADIOGRAPHIC EVALUATION

Cross-table lateral and anteroposterior (AP) radiographs should be the initial radiographs used for determining spinal abnormalities in patients with acute spinal injury. After the level of injury is determined, greater detail of the injury pattern can be defined by computed tomography (CT) or magnetic resonance imaging (MRI) scans. In every patient with spinal cord injury, the entire spine should be evaluated radiographically to rule out additional spinal injuries, which, if missed, could lead to neurological injury.

From the lateral radiograph, alignment of the vertebral bodies, pedicles, facet joints, spinous processes, and intervertebral foramina can be assessed. Signs indicative of compression-type injuries include buckling of the cortical margins and loss of vertebral body height. Vertebral body cortical disruption from a lateral compression fracture missed on the lateral view may be detected more reliably on the AP view. Disruption of the midline alignment of the spinous processes, disruption of the pedicles, and widening of the interradicular line may represent posterior element

TABLE 1. REFLEX TESTING IN THORACOLUMBAR SPINAL INJURIES	
Reflex	**Levels**
Superficial abdominal reflex above the umbilicus	T7–10
Superficial abdominal reflex below the umbilicus	T11–L1
Cremasteric reflex	T12–L1
Knee jerk reflex	L3–4
Ankle jerk reflex	S1
Anal wink reflex	S2–4
Bulbocavernosus reflex	S3–4

injury and may indicate spinal instability. Displacement or widening of the paraspinal soft-tissue line observed on an AP radiograph of the thoracic spine or an irregularity of the margins of the psoas shadow on the AP radiograph of the lumbar spine may be indicative of an acute spinal fracture.

It may be difficult to obtain satisfactory views of the cervicothoracic junction on the lateral radiograph because of interference by the superimposed shoulders. A swimmer's view or an oblique view of this region may define the vertebral anatomy more clearly. Overpenetrated views may be helpful for assessing the upper two or three thoracic vertebrae.

CT is indicated for further evaluation of thoracolumbar injuries, particularly compression-type fractures. On plain radiographs, approximately 25% of burst fractures may be misdiagnosed as stable wedge fractures.[4] CT, with sagittal and coronal reconstruction, is useful for imaging areas such as the cervicothoracic junction.[5]

MRI provides more distinct visualization of the spinal cord and the surrounding soft tissues. The integrity of the posterior longitudinal ligament, necessary for indirect reduction techniques for burst fractures, can be visualized and evaluated. MRI is useful in the evaluation of acute traumatic disk disruptions and facet dislocations. In the thoracic and lumbar spine, MRI can identify a disk fragment not detected on plain radiographs that might hinder indirect reduction.

MRI is indicated in all cases of neurological deficit and in cases of preexisting neurological injury with progressive deterioration. MRI can provide prognostic information that may help in the treatment of spinal cord injury. Patterns of injury seen within the cord parenchyma can be correlated with neurological outcome. In the evaluation of late spine trauma, MRI can detect post-traumatic syringomyelia and myelomalacia.

MRI is useful in the evaluation of spinal cord injury without radiographic abnormalities. This occurs more commonly in children younger than 8 years and may be attributable to the biomechanical features of the spine in this age group, cord ischemia, and subluxation of the spine.[6]

If MRI is not available, myelography, not routinely used to evaluate spinal trauma, may be selected to complement CT scans. Intraoperative spinal myelography or ultrasonography can be used to evaluate spinal canal patency after indirect reduction of a burst fracture with posterior distraction instrumentation.[7]

Occasionally, bone scans may be useful in ruling out occult acute injuries and fractures in patients who have complete neurological injury, who are uncooperative, who have prolonged symptoms, or who have a negative radiographic evaluation.

ANATOMIC CHARACTERISTICS OF THE THORACOLUMBAR SPINE

Regional anatomic characteristics and differences in the thoracic and lumbar spine may contribute to the pattern of spinal injury in the thoracolumbar spine.

The thoracolumbar junction is a transitional region in the spine between the stable, less mobile thoracic spine and the more flexible lumbar spine. In this junctional region, the rib cage no longer provides protection and support to the vertebral column. The smaller thoracic vertebrae, compared with the larger lumbar vertebrae, are less able to resist deformity. These factors render the thoracolumbar spine more vulnerable to injury and make it the most common location for burst fractures.

Spinal Stability

Various definitions and classifications of spinal (in)stability exist. The integrity of both the skeletal and the neural structures should be considered influential because both are integral components of spinal function.

The anatomical components contributing to the inherent stability of the spine have been grouped into load-bearing columns: anterior, middle, and posterior (Fig. 1).[8–11] The anterior column contains the anterior longitudinal ligament and the anterior half of the vertebral body and annulus fibrosis. The middle column contains the posterior half of the vertebral body and annulus fibrosus and the posterior longitudinal ligament. The posterior column includes all structures posterior to the posterior longitudinal ligament. The anterior and middle vertebral columns provide the majority of the axial load-bearing capacity of the spine. The posterior column resists tension and stabilizes the load shared by the anterior column.[9, 12, 13] Disruption of two columns can indicate instability. Each column, however, does not contribute equally to spinal stability.[14]

The Denis classification[8, 9] of acute thoracolumbar injuries, based on the three-column concept of spinal stability, is probably the most widely accepted (Table 2). Thoracolumbar injuries are divided into minor and major injuries. Minor injuries include fractures of the spinous and transverse processes, the pars interarticularis, and the facet joints. Major spinal injuries include compression fractures, burst fractures, shear fractures (seat belt injuries), and fracture-dislocations. Burst fractures are further categorized into five subtypes based on anatomic variations in an effort to focus on the area of greatest neurological compression.

Criteria for spinal instability have been established to also include neurological deficit, posterior ligamentous complex disruption, deformity, canal compromise, and the mode of failure of the middle column.[14] Stable burst fractures include both anterior-column and middle-column compression failure. Unstable burst fractures can develop when failure of the posterior column occurs in addition to anterior-column and middle-column failure. Instability in compression burst fractures may be revealed by progressive neurological deficit, progression of kyphosis by more than

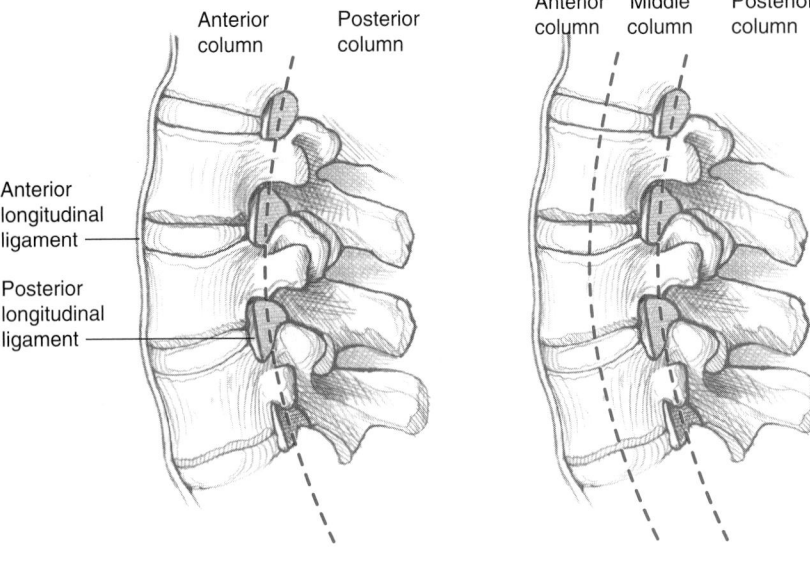

Fig. 1. The columns of the spine.[8–10]

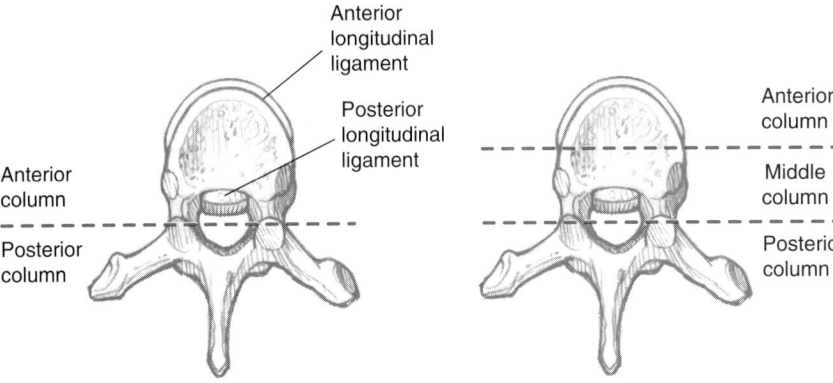

20 degrees, loss of vertebral body height greater than 50%, and the presence of spinal canal occlusion from comminuted, retropulsed middle-column bony fragments.

A mechanistic classification system, based on the three-column concept of spinal stability and the deforming forces that cause these fracture patterns, has been proposed.[11] Insight into the pathogenesis of the thoracolumbar injury may more accurately guide intervention.

In compression-flexion injuries, loading of the flexed spine causes compressive stress through the anterior col-

Type of Fracture	Effect on Spinal Columns			Mechanism
	Anterior	*Middle*	*Posterior*	
Compression				
Type A	Compression	None	None-distraction	Anterior flexion
Type B	Compression	None	None/distraction	Lateral flexion
Burst				
Type A	Compression	Compression	None	Axial load
Type B	Compression	Compression	None	Axial load/flexion
Type C	Compression	Compression	None	Axial load/flexion
Type D	Compression	Compression	None	Axial/rotation
Type E	Compression	Compression	None	Axial/lateral flexion
Seat Belt	None	Distraction	Distraction	Flexion/distraction
Fracture/Dislocation				
Type A	Compression	Distraction	Distraction	Flexion/rotation
Type B	Shear	Shear	Shear	Shear
Type C	Compression	Distraction	Distraction	Flexion/distraction

TABLE 2. THE DENIS CLASSIFICATION OF SPINAL FRACTURES (8, 9)

umn and tension strain through the middle and posterior columns.

Distraction injuries are less common than compression-flexion injuries. They may occur in conjunction with flexion, extension, and lateral deforming forces. This injury pattern should be carefully evaluated because approximately 50% of these injuries have associated intra-abdominal injuries and an increased incidence of concomitant non-contiguous spine fractures.[2]

The fracture pattern in flexion-distraction injuries is determined in part by the location of the axis of rotation at the time of injury. When the axis of rotation is in the vertebral body, a compression fracture of the anterior vertebral body occurs in combination with posterior ligament disruption and facet joint dislocation. When the axis of rotation is anterior to the vertebral column, all three spinal columns fail under tension.

Tensile failure of the vertebral elements can occur in various patterns and may result in the Chance-type fracture or variations thereof.[2] Tension failure can occur through the bony spine only, through the ligamentous structures only (pure dislocation with no bony injury), or through a combination of these two patterns (Fig. 2).

Distraction-extension injuries are rare. They result from tension failure of the anterior column and compression failure of the posterior column.[15] There is a small propensity for progression of deformity or neurological injury. These fractures may be difficult to appreciate on plain radiographs because they may completely reduce after injury. Lateral distraction injuries are uncommon and can have life-threatening injuries associated with them.

Lateral flexion injuries occur when a compressive force from lateral bending of the spine causes an asymmetric compression of the vertebral body and of the posterior elements. Two fracture patterns may occur. In one pattern, the anterior and the middle vertebral columns fail unilaterally. This type of fracture is unlikely to exhibit progressive deformity. In the other pattern, failure of the posterior elements occurs with compression on one side and with tension on the contralateral side. A unilateral articular process dislocation is usually present on the side of tension failure. If posterior-element failure occurs, the incidence of progressive pain and deformity increases.

Translational injuries occur when shear forces cause displacement of the vertebral body anteriorly, posteriorly, or laterally (Fig. 3). The facet joints and all ligamentous structures, including the anterior longitudinal ligament, are often disrupted, with displacements greater than 25%. This injury mechanism is the most destabilizing and has the highest risk of associated neurological injury.[16] Few or no stabilizing structures remain, and acute and chronic deformities may result.

In torsion-flexion injuries, the anterior column fails in compression and rotation, whereas the posterior column fails in tension and rotation. Because of the combined flexion component, the anterior longitudinal ligament, although not ruptured, is usually stripped off the involved vertebrae, and all other ligaments are usually ruptured. The facet joints are usually fractured and/or dislocated. A slice of the superior vertebral body is fractured and translated anteriorly. If not surgically stabilized, almost 75% of patients with this injury type experience progressive defor-

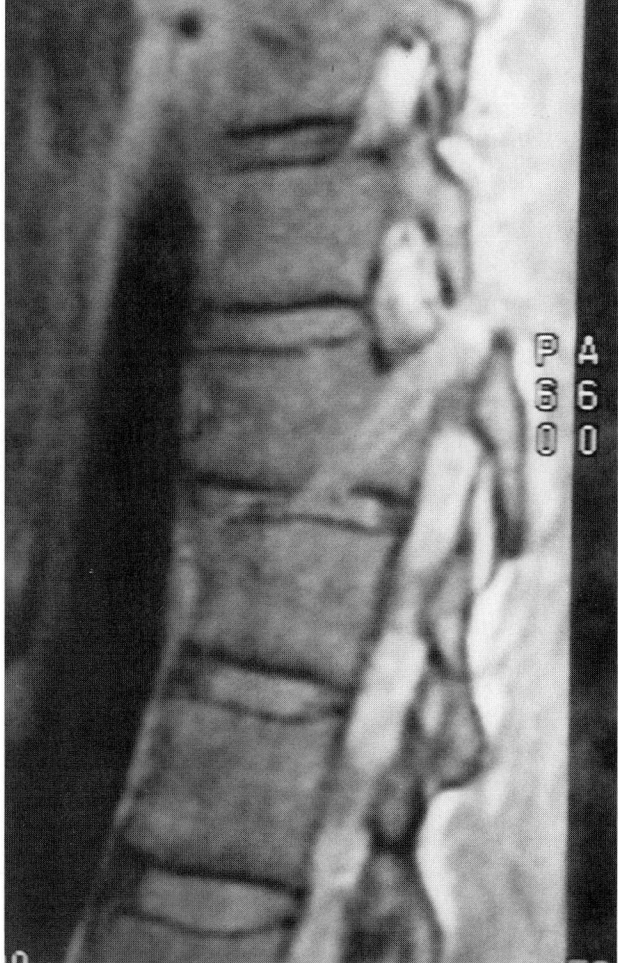

Fig. 2. A flexion distraction injury. A sagittal magnetic resonance imaging scan shows disruption of the posterior interspinous ligaments with propagation of the injury through the posterior and middle vertebral columns and into the anterior disk space. This type of fracture pattern results when the axis of rotation is anterior to the anterior longitudinal ligament.

mity. These fractures are almost invariably associated with paraplegia. Neurological decline after hospital admission occurs more often with this injury mechanism.[16]

Neurological Injury

For adult thoracolumbar injuries, the incidence of neurological damage to the spinal cord or to the cauda equina is 10% to 38%.[4] The incidence of neurological injury can be related to the anatomic characteristics of the spine at the level of injury and to the type of deforming mechanism.

In the thoracic region, root injury is less consequential because the intercostal nerves serve a relatively lesser function than do the lumbar nerve roots. Above the level of the cauda equina, significant neurological deficit may occur from direct injury to the spinal cord.

The segmental arterial network is relatively sparse in the T5 to T9 area of the spinal cord. This renders the spinal cord more vulnerable to injury from vascular ischemia and infarct.

On the basis of clinical evaluation, neurological injuries may be classified as complete, incomplete, or progressive.

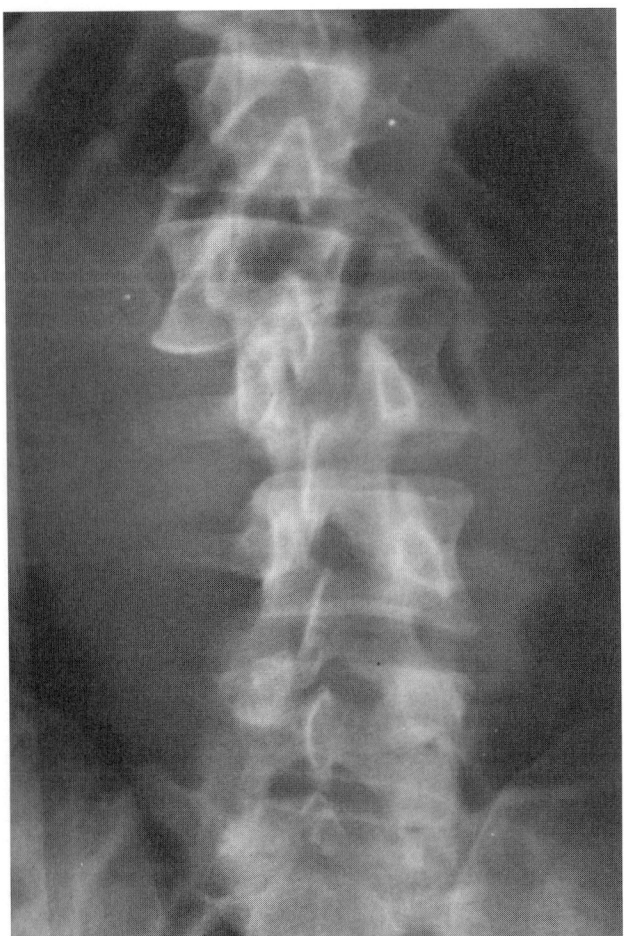

Fig. 3. Translational injury. Unstable rotational-flexion spinal injury with lateral displacement of L2 on L3 is demonstrated on an antero-posterior roentgenogram. Disruption occurs in all three spinal columns. Fracture-dislocation may occur through the facet joints, allowing the vertebral body to translate in an unstable manner.

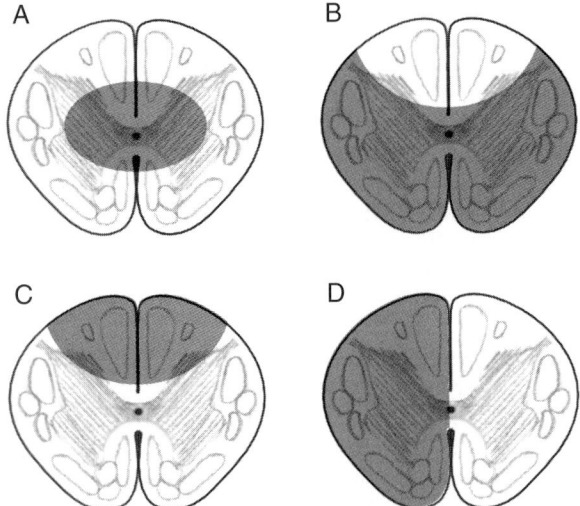

Fig. 4. Specific syndromes of incomplete spinal cord injury. Zones of injury produce the main incomplete injury patterns manifested clinically. *A*, Central cord syndrome. *B*, Anterior cord syndrome. *C*, Posterior cord syndrome. *D*, Brown-Séquard syndrome.

A spinal injury may be considered complete in the absence of spinal shock if there is no definable functional motor or sensory activity below the anatomic level of injury. The prognosis for neurological recovery is poor. Priapism and slow flexion of the great toe are poor prognostic indicators.[17] In patients with complete neurological injuries, improvement of one nerve root level may occur in 80% and two root levels in 20%.[18]

In incomplete spinal injuries, with sparing of the lower sacral segments, there is some preservation of sensory or voluntary motor function below the anatomic level of injury.[19] Sacral sparing is often the only indication that a spinal cord injury is incomplete. Sacral sparing indicates at least some structural continuity of the long spinal tracts and the possibility for functional recovery. The Frankel classification and American Spinal Injury Association classification provide a standardized method of evaluation of motor and sensory function, which may be useful in determining functional recovery in spinal cord injury patients.

Several specific syndromes of incomplete spinal cord injury may occur. They are based on the location of neural damage within the spinal cord (Fig. 4).

The central cord syndrome is the most common incomplete thoracic cord syndrome. There may be complete motor paralysis below the zone of injury, with perianal sensibility sparing and sharp/dull discrimination. With this syndrome, there is a 50% to 75% chance of good functional recovery. Motor recovery usually begins distally and proceeds proximally; the flexors are the first voluntary motor power to be regained.

Anterior cord syndrome is characterized by dorsal column sensibility function only and by complete motor paralysis. Only touch and deep-pressure sensibility are perceived. There is no sharp/dull discrimination below the level of injury. Its prognosis is the worst (10% to 15%) of all incomplete spinal cord injury syndromes. The key to differentiating it from the central cord syndrome is the presence of sacral sparing. Any voluntary sacral motor function or toe flexor control places the patient in the central cord syndrome and provides a better prognosis. Posterior cord syndrome is rare. There is isolated loss of vibration, proprioception, and light-touch sensation and preservation of motor function.

In Brown-Séquard syndrome, injury is limited to one side of the spinal cord. Motor paralysis and loss of proprioception develop on the injury side, and loss of sensibility to pain and temperature develops on the contralateral side. Stab wounds are the most common traumatic cause. This syndrome has the most favorable prognosis for partial or complete neurological recovery.

NONOPERATIVE TREATMENT
Medical Management
Early medical management plays a critical role in the treatment of acute thoracolumbar injuries with neurological deficit. Aggressive medical resuscitation techniques can favorably influence neurological recovery. By maintaining optimal spinal perfusion, a proper environment for maximal neural recovery is provided.[20]

Neurological deficit after traumatic spinal cord injury is related not only to structural damage of the neural elements but also to complex molecular and cellular mechanisms that can lead to secondary neural tissue degeneration. Acutely, local edema, thrombosis, and microvascular disruption propagate the release of various neurotoxic and inflammatory mediators, which damage the blood-brain barrier and neural elements.[19, 21]

Pharmacological agents can protect the neural tissues from the deleterious effects of neurotoxic mediators that are released at the time of injury. Although various pharmacological therapies have been suggested, none have unequivocally demonstrated reversal of spinal cord injury, especially complete neurological injuries.

Intravenous steroids can contribute to cellular membrane stabilization, reduce edema, and buffer electrolyte imbalances. For patients with complete or incomplete neurological lesions, intravenous methylprednisolone (bolus dose: 30 mg/kg followed by 5.4 mg/kg/hour for 23 to 48 hours) should be started only within the first 8 hours of injury. Treatment should persist for 24 hours if initiated within the first 3 hours and for 48 hours when administered between 3 to 8 hours after injury. When compared with naloxone and/or placebo, methylprednisolone is more effective in altering the secondary cascade of neural injury and in enhancing neurological recovery.[19, 22, 23]

Other pharmacological agents, monosialotetrahexosyl ganglioside (GM$_1$), thyrotropin-releasing hormone (TRH), mannitol, and nimodipine have been investigated as to their benefit in promoting neurological recovery. It is suggested that GM$_1$ may enhance neurological recovery by limiting wallerian degeneration and augmenting neurite outgrowth. Even if the administration of GM$_1$ is delayed for 48 hours, it may still be effective. It may antagonistically limit the neuroprotective effect of methylprednisolone.[24]

Closed Reduction and Immobilization

The majority of stable thoracolumbar fractures without neurological deficit can be treated nonoperatively. Nonoperative treatment may be considered when there is adequate post-traumatic spinal stability and when there is limited potential for progressive kyphosis and neurological compromise.[25]

Minor spine fractures, such as transverse process, spinous process, and articular process fractures, are considered stable. They may be treated symptomatically with or without bracing. These fractures should not be ignored. They may be harbingers for more significant associated injuries.

Flexion-compression type fractures with intact posterior elements, loss of vertebral body height less than 50%, and initial kyphosis of less than 30 degrees can be treated with closed reduction and immobilization by casting or bracing with a thoracolumbar orthosis (TLSO). Early ambulation can be initiated with the orthosis. It is usually worn for 3 to 6 months.[26]

The effective type of immobilization should be so fashioned as to provide a corrective force vector opposite the initial primary injury vector. For fractures at or above T7, a cervicothoracolumbar orthosis should be worn. For injuries below T7, a thoracolumbar orthosis should be used.

For low lumbar and lumbosacral injuries, inclusion of one thigh should be considered.[27]

Nonoperative treatment of unstable burst fractures without neurological deficit remains controversial. The controversy centers on the initial degree of mechanical instability, kyphosis, and canal occlusion that can be managed nonoperatively. The relationship between these parameters and the long-term functional outcome of the patient remain unclear.

Burst fractures with less than 30 degrees of kyphosis, less than 50% loss of vertebral body height, and less than 50% canal compromise may be considered stable.[28] For stable thoracolumbar burst fractures without neurological deficit, no significant difference in functional outcome was observed in patients treated nonoperatively compared with those treated operatively.[29] For unstable thoracolumbar burst fractures without neurological deficit treated nonoperatively, functional outcomes appear favorable in some cases.[30, 31]

The technique of recumbent management and bracing of thoracolumbar fractures, however, is not entirely benign. Various complications have been reported, including neurological deterioration, decubitus ulcers, deep venous thrombosis, cord infarction, painful gibbus, late progression of kyphosis, and spinal stenosis.[27]

Neurological decline has been observed in 2% to 21% of patients with thoracolumbar injuries treated nonoperatively.[27] This may be related to the development of late progression of a kyphotic deformity and/or late spinal stenosis. Although canal occlusion may spontaneously decrease by remodeling, canal stenosis and kyphosis may additively cause neural compression.

Neurological recovery can occur for patients with thoracolumbar injuries treated nonoperatively. In patients with incomplete neurological deficit, improvement of at least one Frankel grade has been observed in up to 95% of the patients.[27] Neurological recovery may partially be attributed to the spontaneous remodeling of impinging bony fragments within the spinal canal during the healing process.[30]

Nonoperative treatment is less commonly used for other types of thoracolumbar injuries, such as flexion-distraction injuries and fracture-dislocations; however, results of nonoperative treatment are poor.[30] After 12 to 24 weeks of immobilization in a hyperextension cast or brace, dynamic flexion-extension radiographs should be used to determine residual instability.

For patients with complete neurological injury with fracture-dislocations of the thoracolumbar junction, treatment with 4 to 6 weeks of bedrest can yield satisfactory results. However, surgical stabilization is often preferred to facilitate early immobilization and rehabilitation and to prevent late post-traumatic deformity.[33]

OPERATIVE TREATMENT
Indications for Surgery

The indications for surgical intervention depend on the alignment and stability of the fracture, neurological status of the patient, and overall medical condition of the patient. In patients with an incomplete neurological deficit, significant improvement in neurological function has been observed after surgical reduction and stabilization.[34] For patients with a complete neurological deficit and/or unstable thoracolumbar fractures, surgical stabilization has decreased hospitalization and rehabilitation time and the number of reported complications.[33, 35]

Timing of Surgery

In patients with spinal cord or cauda equina injury, the optimal timing for medical and/or surgical intervention (decompression and stabilization) is unclear.[36]

Although not demonstrated in human clinical studies, a critical window of opportunity (possibly less than 3 hours) may exist by which the decompression of extrinsic pressure on the spinal cord may enhance functional neurological outcome. The reperfusion of the spinal cord after early decompression may be a critical factor in the potential for neurological recovery. Decompression performed within 1 to 3 hours of spinal injury led to recovery of electrophysiological function.[37] Some clinical studies suggest that early decompression, less than 24 hours, may be optimal.[19, 38] In other cases, early surgical intervention has been discouraged because of an increase in neurological deterioration and an increase in morbidity.[39] In the only controlled, prospective, randomized study, no significant differences in functional neurological recovery were detected in patients when operated on either early or late.[40]

Role of Surgical Spinal Decompression

In thoracolumbar injuries with neurological deficit, the complete role and benefit of surgical decompression are still undetermined.[16] Despite varied opinions, there is no direct correlation between the percentage of canal occlusion demonstrated radiographically and the signs and severity of neurological deficit after burst fractures.[41, 42] Instead, the initial maximal amount of contusion of the spinal cord or the cauda equina, along with hematoma, edema, and vascular ischemia perpetuated by various neurotrophic and vasoactive agents, may be the underlying cause of neurological injury.

Although approximately 60% of patients with neurological injury below T12 will gain some return of neurological function with nonoperative treatment, neurological recovery is more predictable in certain cases via anterior decompression.[43] Late decompression, even several years after injury, may enhance neurological recovery at the cord level, the conus medullaris, and the cauda equina.[43, 44]

Surgical Approaches for Decompression of the Spine

Spinal decompression is performed in conjunction with reconstruction of the spine. It may play a major role in surgical decision-making.

Decompression procedures may be performed posteriorly, posterolaterally, or anteriorly.

A posterior decompressive laminectomy for thoracolumbar injuries is destabilizing and should be avoided. A laminectomy in the upper thoracic region and thoracolumbar junction can lead to postlaminectomy kyphosis and progressive neurological deficit. The risk of progressive deformity from a laminectomy may be reduced by the addition of posterior instrumentation.[45, 46] In thoracolumbar injuries, a laminectomy should be performed in only selected cases: repair of dural tears caused by posterior-element fracture,

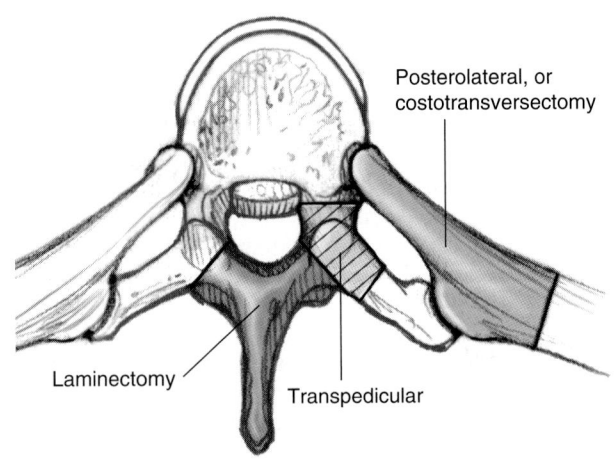

Fig. 5. Approaches for posterior decompression. Laminectomy, transpedicular, posterolateral, and costotransversectomy approaches are shown.

evacuation of an epidural hematoma, and direct neural compression from displaced posterior vertebral fracture fragments.[47]

Posterolateral approaches include costotransversectomy, posterolateral transpedicular decompression, lateral extracavitary decompression, and lateral extrapleural parascapular decompression.[48–50] These approaches allow access to the anterior thecal sac and anterolateral vertebral elements throughout the thoracic and lumbar spine (Fig. 5).

The posterolateral transpedicular approach and the lateral extracavitary approach may be useful when there is significantly lateralized or asymmetric anterior canal occlusion with symptomatic neural compression. These approaches may be more advantageous in the lower lumbar regions, where anterior instrumentation and reconstructive procedures pose a risk to the great vessels.

The posterolateral approach allows access through the pedicle of the respective vertebra to the anterior thecal sac and retropulsed middle-column bony fragments. The exposure with the lateral extracavitary approach may be hindered by the presence of the scapula above the level of T2 and the iliac crest below the level of L4.

The lateral extrapleural parascapular approach is useful for operating on lesions in the upper thoracic spine, T2 to T4. It is a modification of the lateral extracavitary approach.

The anterior approach is the most direct and reliable method for visualizing and decompressing the affected neural tissues. With the anterior approach, there is less manipulation of the neural elements.

Posterior Spinal Surgery

Posterior spinal surgery is the most common method of operative management of thoracolumbar injuries. The mainstay of posterior operative intervention has been the application of distraction instrumentation.[51]

With posterior distraction rod techniques, restoration of vertebral body height and partial clearance of bony fragments from the spinal canal by ligamentotaxis can be achieved. During ligamentotaxis, the posterior annulus fibrosis and the posterior longitudinal ligament, if intact, become taut and push the retropulsed fragments of bone anteriorly away from the spinal cord or the cauda equina. By indirect reduction and ligamentotaxis, posterior distraction techniques may enlarge the compromised spinal canal from 40% to 75% in burst fractures.[52] The more effective clearance of the spinal canal is thought to be related to the greater degree of comminution and the relative mobility of the bony fragments. If the retropulsed fragment is rotated or if spinal canal occlusion is greater than 50%, ligamentotaxis is less effective. Intraoperative ultrasonography may be used to assess spinal canal patency if reduction and distraction are insufficient to relieve cord or cauda equina compression.[7]

Effective spinal canal clearance by distraction methods may be achieved only if the operative correction is performed within the first 3 to 4 days after injury. When operative correction is delayed more than 3 days, only a small decrease in spinal canal encroachment occurs.[53]

When using posterior rod-hook distraction systems, the appropriate rod length and the number of vertebral motion segments to be fused are important factors. Longer rods exhibit certain biomechanical advantages. By increasing the distance from the fracture site, the force on the hooks is decreased. This reduces the risk of hook dislodgment.[54] Contouring of longer rods to the preferred sagittal alignment of the spine allows for earlier contact with the laminae and enhances three-point fixation. Application of high-density polyethylene sleeves to the contoured rods posterior to the fractured vertebrae has been shown to increase the stability and the corrective moments imparted by this type of instrumentation.

To obtain a stable reduction and maintain correction of thoracolumbar injuries, fusion of at least two levels above and two levels below the fracture has been recommended.[55] From a biomechanical analysis of rod fixation of thoracolumbar fractures, the most stable construct involves applying instrumentation to three vertebrae above the fracture and two vertebrae below the fracture. Inclusion of the additional vertebra above the fracture increased the failure moment significantly compared with a two-above/two-below instrumentation technique.[56]

The primary disadvantages of the posterior rod-hook distraction-instrumentation technique are related to the length of the implanted instrumentation. Often five to six uninjured motion segments are immobilized. This can lead to painful degenerative changes of the immobilized facet joints. In an attempt to preserve uninjured motion segments, the rod long-fuse short technique was introduced.[57] With this method, only one level above and one level below the fracture are fused, and three levels above and three levels below the injury are spanned by the instrumentation. The rods are removed at 1 year to regain motion of the unfused joints. Examination of the facet cartilage of the instrumented unfused vertebrae revealed gross and histological findings typical of osteoarthritis.[58, 59] These degenerative changes may lead to chronic pain.

Other shortcomings of the distraction rod-hook technique include hook dislodgment, late vertebral collapse, and progressive kyphosis after rod removal. Overdistraction with long rods may lead to iatrogenic loss of lumbar lordosis and the development of a painful disabling flat-back deformity.[54]

To help circumvent these potential complications, various modifications to the rod-hook system were developed. Square hooks allow for a more gentle contouring of the rod and decrease hook cut-out. The stability of the rod-hook construct can be enhanced with the addition of sublaminar wire segmental fixation. Supplemental sublaminar wire fixation can restore approximately 50% of the rotational stiffness of the intact spine, but it is limited in restoring axial load stability.[60, 61] Augmentation with pedicle screw fixation and use of multiple hooks to apply segmental distraction and/or compression to selected motion segments also increase stability and provide versatility to the rod-hook construct.

The development of pedicle screw fixation has provided an additional tool for the stabilization of unstable spine fractures.[62, 63] The primary advantage of pedicle screw constructs is rigid three-column purchase. It allows for shorter fixation and preservation of motion segments. This ability to include only the immediately adjacent vertebral levels in the fixation construct is of particular advantage in the lumbar spine.

Experimental data in acute-injury models demonstrate that short-segment pedicle screw constructs provide torsional, flexural, and compressive rigidity comparable to longer rod-hook constructs. It has been demonstrated that rotational stability is more effectively controlled by single-level pedicle screw fixation, whereas axial instability is best controlled by a two-level pedicle screw construct.[61]

The stiffness of the short-segment pedicle screw construct can be significantly increased by supplemental, offset, laminar hooks. The offset hooks absorb some of the construct strain. This reduces pedicle screw-bending moments and the likelihood of deformation and clinical failure.[64]

Despite the increased rigidity of pedicle screw systems, posterior short-segment fixation of unstable thoracolumbar fractures has resulted in high failure rates. In one study, 13 of 19 patients with unstable thoracolumbar burst fractures treated with short-segment pedicle screw fixation experienced early progressive kyphosis with angulation greater than 10 degrees. In six patients, instrumentation failure occurred. In those patients in whom the short-segment fixation did not fail, the anterior spinal column was either surgically reconstructed or was not disrupted.[65]

In another study, all failures of short-segment pedicle screw fixation occurred in patients who did not undergo anterior grafting, and no patient with grafting of the anterior spinal column experienced construct failure.[66] Even long posterior rod constructs experience failure if a significant gap or deficiency remains in the reduced vertebral body fracture. From these observations, it appears that instrumentation failures are related to the fracture pattern and to the inability of the injured vertebral bodies to load-share.

McCormack developed a load-sharing classification system of spinal fractures to demonstrate a relationship between the characteristics of the vertebral body fracture pattern and the failure of posterior short-segment pedicle screw fixation and to predict circumstances in which these fractures might occur. Using plain radiographs and CT scans of the fractures, a severity scoring system was formulated based on the degree of comminution, the amount of displacement between vertebral body fracture fragments, and the amount of correction required to realign the deformity. According to this classification, short-segment hardware failure is more likely to occur if there is greater than 30% vertebral body comminution on sagittal CT images, greater than 2-mm displacement between fracture fragments, and greater than 10 degrees of kyphosis correction required.[67]

The best candidates for posterior short-segment fixation by this classification system are those with flexion-distraction injuries, those with minimal burst fractures, and those with fracture-dislocations having low severity scores (less than 6). For patients with burst fractures having high severity scores (greater than 7), a second-stage anterior reconstruction procedure, in addition to the posterior short-segment fusion, is recommended.

This classification system does not take into account ligamentous injuries. Therefore, it may not be useful in all cases when deciding between operative and nonoperative treatment. If surgical treatment is elected, this system is useful in determining which operative approach and fixation method is advantageous.

Anterior Spinal Surgery

Indications for anterior spinal surgery in patients with acute thoracolumbar injuries include unstable fractures with neurological injury, burst injuries detected 5 to 10 days after initial injury, and burst injuries with three-column disruption and deficient anterior column support.[68]

The anterior approach allows direct and more predictable spinal canal decompression compared with indirect decompression by ligamentotaxis via the posterior approach. With anterior decompression, in one study, spinal canal occlusion improved from 58% preoperatively to 4% postoperatively. With posterior indirect reduction, spinal canal patency improved from 45% preoperatively to 16.5% postoperatively.[43]

Anterior surgery also provides the opportunity for the restoration of the load-bearing capacity of the anterior spine. After an anterior column fracture, the load-sharing and the load-transferring ability of the anterior column is decreased. An implant inserted in an anterior intracolumnar position functions as an interbody spacer and load-sharing device and restores axial stability until arthrodesis occurs. Anterior plates alone cannot prevent a vertebrectomy site or an unstable burst fracture from collapsing. With the inclusion of an interbody load-sharing device, the stability of the anterior plate construct is enhanced.[69]

With a deficient anterior spinal column and no structural interbody spacer, a posterior stand-alone cantilever beam construct bears the majority of the load. In this situation, posterior load-bearing implants are prone to early failure.[65, 67]

With the continued refinement of anterior fixation devices, supplementary posterior fixation and fusion may no longer be necessary in select cases of thoracolumbar injuries when the posterior elements are intact. If, however, significant posterior instability exists or if more than one vertebral body has been resected, a second-stage posterior stabilization and fusion procedure is usually recommended.[70]

Interbody devices include autologous or allograft bone grafts, cages, and synthetic materials. When possible, the anterior spinal column should be reconstructed with a biologically active graft to optimize incorporation and long-term stability. Used alone, iliac crest interbody grafts are unable to withstand physiological loads in the erect spine, whereas fibular strut grafts can withstand these loads.

Different anterior surgical approaches can be used to reach the fractured thoracolumbar spine.[71] The approach selected should depend on the location of the fracture.

A transthoracic approach is useful for fractures of T4 to T9. For access to the upper and midthoracic spine, a thoracotomy is usually performed from the right side to avoid injury to the more left-sided cardiac structures. Generally, an incision is made at a level two ribs above the desired vertebral level.

A thoracoabdominal approach, occasionally combined with a subphrenic approach, can be used for fractures of T10 to L1. Limited takedown of the diaphragm avoids a thoracotomy but may not allow for adequate exposure above T12. A subpleural retroperitoneal approach is used for fractures of T12 to L5.

The most difficult area of the spine to approach anteriorly is the upper thoracic spine. Although visualization can be achieved via a thoracotomy, surgical manipulation of the fracture may be limited. For access to T2, T3, and T4, the lateral extrapleural parascapular approach may be useful.[50]

If anterior access is required at the cervicothoracic junction, T2 or T3, an extension of the anterior cervical approach with partial manubriectomy and partial resection of the medial third of the clavicle may be performed. Direct anterior access may also be gained via a sternotomy.

Complications related to anterior thoracolumbar procedures may occur in 11% to 30% of cases.[72] Common complications are pulmonary dysfunction, vascular injury, and blood loss. Sequential same-day anterior and posterior procedures may contribute to increased blood loss compared with these procedures performed alone.[73] Other less common complications include paraplegia, deep wound infection, and death.

There are also specific complications inherent to these surgical approaches. Retroperitoneal approaches may be associated with neurological sequelae, most commonly dysfunction of the sympathetic chain or the ilioinguinal, iliofemoral, and lateral femoral cutaneous nerves. Necessary ligation of segmental vessels may adversely affect spinal cord perfusion, although no cases of related paralysis have been reported.[74] In an attempt to minimize exposure-related pain and pulmonary complications and to expedite rehabilitation, minimally invasive open and endoscopic techniques are being developed.[75]

Combined Anterior and Posterior Surgical Procedures

A circumferential surgical approach may be necessary in certain thoracolumbar injuries (Fig. 6). The sequence of surgical techniques is dependent on the fracture pattern and the neurological status of the patient.

An anterior approach followed by a posterior approach is useful in the stabilization of three-column spinal injuries with symptomatic canal occlusion. If posterior instability is present after anterior decompression and reconstruction, supplemental posterior stabilization is recommended. This

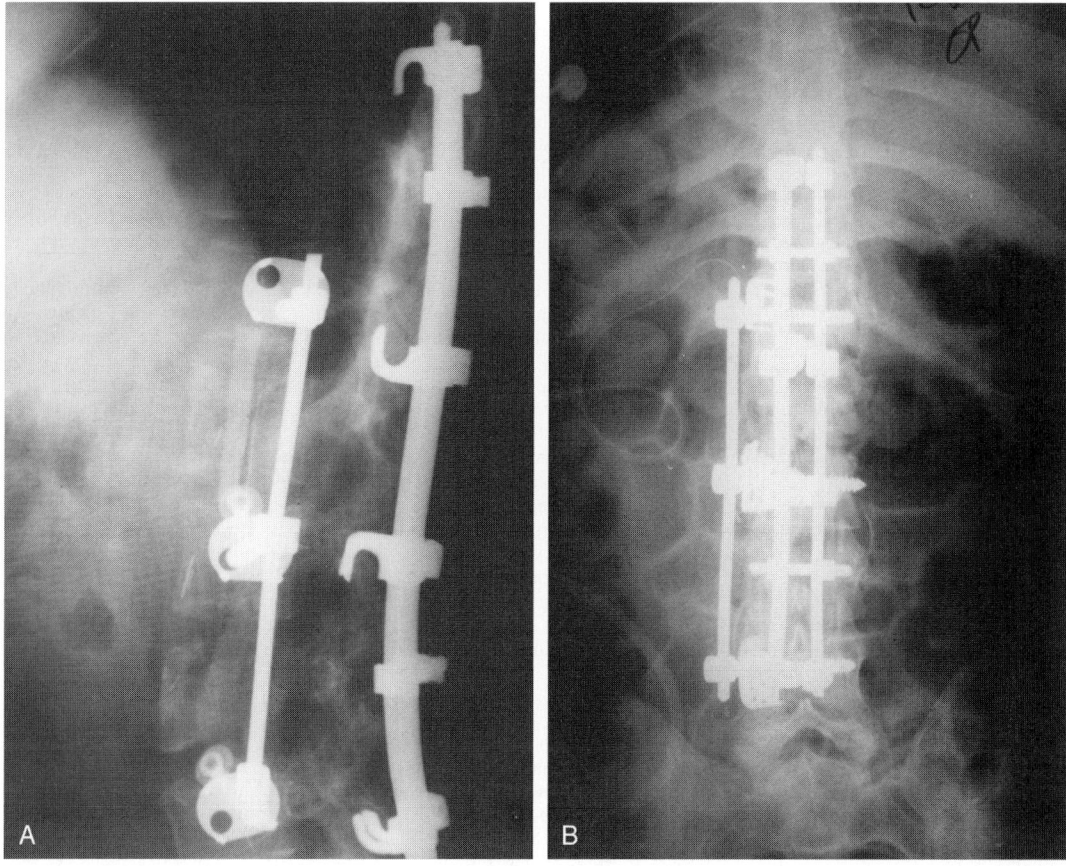

Fig. 6. Results after a circumferential surgical approach. *A,* A lateral roentgenogram after L1 and L3 corpectomies and anterior iliac crest strut graft placement and stabilization with anterior instrumentation and a posterior rod construct. *B,* An anteroposterior view of the constructs and reduction.

technique is also useful when anterior instrumentation poses a risk to the great vessels.

A posterior approach followed by an anterior approach may be useful in the treatment of displaced fracture-dislocations of the thoracolumbar spine with incomplete neurological deficit and spinal canal occlusion. To realign the spine properly, initial reduction is performed through the posterior approach. If, after realignment, residual neural compression is detected, anterior decompression and fusion can then be performed. This technique can also be used less commonly in cases without spinal dislocation in which posterior indirect reduction fails to provide adequate neural decompression and neurological deficit persists.

A posterior-then-anterior surgical procedure may be necessary in patients who suffer a traumatic distraction-extension spinal injury and have ankylosing spondylitis or diffuse idiopathic skeletal hyperostosis. After posterior reduction and stabilization, an anterior column deficiency may remain. This may result in late instability if supplemental anterior reconstruction is not performed.

The posterior/anterior technique may be useful in the management of an open spinal fracture with posterior soft-tissue damage. After initial posterior débridement, anterior stabilization with instrumentation can restore spinal stability. This may help prevent contamination of posterior instrumentation and may decrease the risk of postoperative infection.

A simultaneous anterior/posterior spinal approach may be useful in the treatment of thoracolumbar injuries that do not contain a coronal plane deformity.[76] A one-stage simultaneous procedure results in less operative time, less blood loss, and fewer complications compared with a two-stage procedure.[77]

CONCLUSION

Despite advances in various spinal surgical techniques, appropriate treatment of thoracolumbar spinal injuries should be guided by an understanding of spinal anatomy, of spinal mechanics, of injury mechanisms, and by a detailed examination and neurological assessment of the patient. Although the timing of intervention for spinal injury is debated, early medical management and early surgical decompression may prove beneficial in preserving and improving neurological function. Nonoperative treatment or surgical stabilization can provide satisfactory outcomes in the appropriately selected patient. Stable thoracolumbar injuries without neurological deficit can be treated nonoperatively. For unstable spinal fractures, with or without neurological deficit, surgical treatment is indicated. In the treatment of thoracolumbar injuries, the goals are to maximize neurological recovery and to maintain or enhance stabilization of the spine for early rehabilitation and return to satisfactory function.

REFERENCES

1. Savitsky E, Votey S: Emergency department approach to acute thoracolumbar spine injury. J Emerg Med 1997; 15(1):49.

2. Gumley G, Taylor TKF, Ryan MD: Distraction fractures of the lumbar spine. J Bone Joint Surg Br 1982; 64(5):520.

3. Albert TJ: Concomitant noncontiguous thoracolumbar and sacral fractures. Spine 1993; 18(10):1285.

4. Saboe LA, Reid DC, Davis LA: Spine trauma and associated injuries. J Trauma 1991; 31(1):43.

5. Takada M, Wu CY, Lang TF: Vertebral fracture assessment using the lateral scout-view of computed tomography in comparison with radiographs. Osteoporos Int 1998; 8(3):197.

6. Pang D, Wilberger JE Jr: Spinal cord injury without radiographic abnormalities in children. J Neurosurg 1982; 57:114.

7. Esimont FJ, Green BA, Berkowitz BM: The role of intraoperative ultrasonography in the treatment of thoracic and lumbar spine fractures. Spine 1984; 9:782.

8. Denis F: Spinal stability as defined by the three-column spine concept in acute spinal trauma. Clin Orthop 1984; 189:65.

9. Denis F: The three-column spine and its significance in the classification of acute thoracolumbar spinal injuries. Spine 1983; 8(8):817.

10. Holdsworth FW: Fractures, dislocations, and fracture-dislocations of the spine. J Bone Joint Surg Am 1970; 52(8);1534.

11. Ferguson RL, Allen BL: A mechanistic classification of thoracolumbar spine fractures. Clin Orthop Rel Res 1984; 189:77.

12. James KS, Wenger KH, Schlegel JA: Biomechanical evaluation of the stability of thoracolumbar burst fractures. Spine 1994; 19(15):1731.

13. Panjabi MM, Kifune M, Liu W: Graded thoracolumbar spinal injuries: Development of multidirectional instability. Eur Spine J 1998; 7(4):332.

14. McAfee PC, Yuan HA, Lasda NA: The unstable burst fracture. Spine 1982; 7:365.

15. Mabeshima Y, Iguchi T, Mastubara N: Extension injury of the thoracolumbar spine. Spine 1997; 22(13):1522.

16. Gertzbein SD: Neurologic deterioration in patients with thoracic and lumbar fractures after admission to the hospital. Spine 1994; 19(15):1723.

17. Braakman R, Penning L: Injuries of the Cervical Spine. Amsterdam, Excerpta Medica, 1971.

18. Ducker TB, Russo GL, Bellegarrique R: Complete sensorimotor paralysis after cord injury: Mortality, recovery, and therapeutic implications. J Trauma 1979; 19:837.

19. Bracken MB, Shephard MJ, Collins WF: A randomized, controlled trial of methylprednisolone or naloxone in the treatment of acute spinal-cord injury: Results of the Second National Acute Spinal Cord Study. N Engl J Med 1990; 322:1405.

20. Vale FL, Burns J, Jackson AB: Combined medical and surgical treatment after acute spinal cord injury: Results of a prospective pilot study to assess the merits of aggressive medical resuscitation and blood pressure management. J Neurosurg 1997; 87(2):239.

21. Delamarter RB, Sherman J, Carr JB: Pathophysiology of spinal cord injury: Recovery after immediate and delayed decompression. J Bone Joint Surg Am 1995; 77: 1042.

22. Bracken MB, Shephard MJ, Holford TR: Administration of methylprednisolone for 24 or 48 hours of tirilazad mesylate for 48 hours in the treatment of acute spinal cord injury. Results of the Third National Acute Spinal Cord Injury Randomized Controlled Trial. National Acute Spinal Cord Injury Study. JAMA 1997; 277(20):1597.

23. Bracken MB, Holford TR: Effects of timing of methylprednisolone or naloxone administration on recovery of segmented and long-tract neurological function in NASCIS II. J Neurosurg 1993; 79:500.

24. Geisler FH, Dorsey FC, Coleman WP: Recovery of motor function after spinal-cord injury: A randomized, placebo-controlled trial with GM-1 ganglioside. N Engl J Med 1991; 324(26):1829.

25. Vanichkachorn JS, Vaccaro AR: Nonoperative treatment of thoracolumbar fractures. Orthopedics 1997; 20:948.

26. Cantor JB, Lebwohl NH, Garvey T: Nonoperative treatment of stable thoracolumbar burst fractures with early ambulation and bracing. Spine 1993; 18:971.

27. Fredrickson BE, Yuan HA, Miller HM: Burst fractures of the fifth lumbar vertebra. J Bone Joint Surg Am 1982; 64(7): 1088.

28. Fredrickson BE, Yuan HA, Bayley JC: The nonsurgical treatment of thoracolumbar injuries. Semin Spine Surg 1990; 2:70.

29. Kraemer WJ, Schemitsch EH, Lever J, et al: Functional outcome of thoracolumbar burst fractures without neurological deficit. J Orthop Trauma 1996; 10:541.

30. de Klerk LW, Fontijne WP, Stijnen T: Spontaneous remodeling of the spinal canal after conservative management of thoracolumbar burst fractures. Spine 1998; 23(9):1057.

31. Shen WJ, Shen YS: Nonsurgical treatment of three-column thoracolumbar junction fractures without neurologic deficit. Spine 1999; 24(4):412.

32. Anderson PA, Henley MB, Rivara FP: Flexion-distraction injuries to the thoracolumbar spine. J Orthop Trauma 1991; 5: 153.

33. Bohlman HH, Freehafer A, Dejak J: The results of treatment of acute injuries of the upper thoracic spine with paralysis. J Bone Joint Surg Am 1985; 67:360.

34. McEvoy RD, Bradford DS: The management of burst fractures of the thoracic and lumbar spine: Experience in 53 patients. Spine 1985; 10:631.

35. Wilmont CB, Hall KM: Evaluation of acute surgical intervention in traumatic paraplegia. Paraplegia 1986; 24:71.

36. Glaser JA, Jaworski BA, Cuddy BG: Variation in surgical opinion regarding management of selected cervical spine injuries. A preliminary study. Spine 1998; 23(9): 975.

37. Carlson GD, Minato Y, Okada A: Early time-dependent decompression for spinal cord injury: Vascular mechanisms of recovery. J Neurotrauma 1997; 14(12):951.

38. Levi L, Wolf A, Riagamonti D: Anterior decompression in cervical spine trauma: Does the timing of surgery affect the outcome. Neurosurgery 1991; 29:216.

39. Sonntag VK, Francis PM: Patient selection and timing of surgery. In Benzel EC, Tator CH (eds): Contemporary Management of Spinal Cord Injury. Park Ridge, IL, American Association of Neurologic Surgeons, 1995, p 97.

40. Vaccaro AR, Daugherty RJ, Sheehan TP: Neurologic outcome of early versus late surgery for cervical spinal cord injury. Spine 1997; 22(22):2609.

41. McCullen G, Vaccaro AR, Garfin SR: Thoracic and lumbar trauma: Rationale for selecting the appropriate fusion technique. Orthop Clin North Am 1998; 29(4):819.

42. Kim NH, Lee HM, Chun IM: Neurologic injury and recovery in patients with burst fracture of the thoracolumbar spine. Spine 1999; 24(3):290.

43. Esses SI, Botsford DJ, Kostuick JP: Evaluation of surgical treatment of burst fractures. Spine 1990; 15:667.

44. Bohlman HH, Kirkpatrick JS, Delamarter RB: Anterior decompression for late pain and paralysis after fractures of the thoracolumbar spine. Clin Orthop Rel Res 1994; 300:24.

45. Cotler JM, Vernace JV, Michalski JA: The use of Harrington rods in thoracolumbar fractures. Orthop Clin North Am 1986; 17(1):87.

46. Whitesides TE: Traumatic kyphosis of the thoracolumbar spine. Clin Orthop Rel Res 1977; 128:78.

47. Cammisa FP, Eismont FJ, Green BA: Dural laceration occurring with burst fractures and associated laminar fractures. J Bone Joint Surg Am 1989; 71:1044.

48. Hardaker WT, Cook WA, Friedman AH: Bilateral transpedicular decompression and Harrington rod stabilization in the management of severe thoracolumbar burst fractures. Spine 1992; 17(2):162.

49. Graham AW, MacMillan M, Fessler RG: Lateral extracavitary approach to the thoracic and thoracolumbar spine. Orthopedics 1997; 20(7):605.

50. Fessler RG, Dietz DD: Lateral parascapular extrapleural approach to the upper thoracic spine. J Neurosurg 1991; 75:349.

51. Harrington PR: Treatment of scoliosis: Correction and internal fixation by spine instrumentation. J Bone Joint Surg Am 1962; 44:591.

52. Gertzbein SD, Court-Brown CM, Jacobs RR: Decompression and circumferential stabilization of unstable spinal fractures. Spine 1988; 13:892.

53. Edwards CC, Levine AM: Early rod-sleeve stabilization of the injured thoracic and lumbar spine. Orthop Clin North Am 1986; 17:121.

54. Krag MH: Biomechanics of thoracolumbar spinal fixation: A review. Spine 1991; 16(suppl):S84.

55. Dickson JH, Harrington PR, Erwin WD: Results of reduction and stabilization of

the severely fractured thoracic and lumbar spine. J Bone Joint Surg Am 1978; 60: 799.

56. Purcell GA, Markolf KL, Dawson EG: Twelfth thoracic-first lumbar vertebral mechanical stability of fractures after Harrington rod instrumentation. J Bone Joint Surg Am 1981; 63:71.

57. Stauffer ES: Current concepts review: Internal fixation of fractures of the thoracolumbar spine. J Bone Joint Surg Am 1984; 66:1136.

58. Kahanovitz N: The effect of internal fixation without arthrodesis on human facet joint cartilage. Orthop Trans 1983; 7:14.

59. Kahanovitz N, Arnoczky SP, Levine DB: The effects of internal fixation on the cartilage of unfused facet joints in dogs. Orthop Trans 1982; 6:10.

60. Sullivan JA: Sublaminar wiring of Harrington distraction rods for unstable thoracolumbar spine fractures. Clin Orthop 1984; 189:178.

61. Gurr KR, McAfee PC, Shih C: Biomechanical analysis of anterior and posterior instrumentation systems after corpectomy. J Bone Joint Surg Am 1988; 70:1182.

62. Roy-Camille R, Saillant G, Mazel C: Plating of thoracic, thoracolumbar, and lumbar injuries with pedicle screw plates. Orthop Clin North Am 1986; 17:147.

63. Dick W: The Fixatuer Interne as a versatile implant for spine surgery. Spine 1987; 12(9):882.

64. Chiba M, McLain RF, Yerby SA: Short-segment pedicle instrumentation. Biomechanical analysis of supplemental hook fixation. Spine 1996; 21(3):288.

65. McClain RF, Sparling E, Benson DR: Early failure of short-segment pedicle instrumentation for thoracolumbar fractures. J Bone Joint Surg Am 1993; 75(2):162.

66. Ebelke DK, Asher MA, Neff JR: Survivorship analysis of VSP spine instrumentation in the treatment of thoracolumbar and lumbar burst fractures. Spine 1991; 16:428.

67. McCormack T, Karaikovic E, Gaines RW: The load-sharing classification of spine fractures. Spine 1994; 19(15):1741.

68. Ghanayem AJ, Zdeblick TA: Anterior instrumentation in the management of thoracolumbar burst fractures. Clin Orthop 1997; 335:89.

69. An HS, Lim TH, You JW: Biomechanical evaluation of anterior thoracolumbar spinal instrumentation. Spine 1995; 20: 1979.

70. Mann KA, McGowan DP, Fredrickson BE: A biomechanical investigation of short segment spinal fixation for burst

fractures with varying degrees of posterior disruption. Spine 1990; 15(6):470.

71. Naunheim KS, Barnett MG, Crandall DG: Anterior exposure of the thoracic spine. Ann Thorac Surg 1994; 57:1436.

72. McDonnell MF, Glassman SD, Dimar JR II: Perioperative complications of anterior procedures of the spine. J Bone Joint Surg Am 1996; 78:839.

73. Dansia OA, Shaffrey CI, Jane JA: Surgical approaches for the correction of unstable thoracolumbar burst fractures: A retrospective analysis of treatment outcomes. J Neurosurg 1995; 83(6):997.

74. Winter RB, Lonstein JE, Denis F: Paraplegia resulting from vessel ligation. Spine 1996; 21:1232.

75. McAfee PC, Regan JR, Fedder IL: Anterior thoracic corpectomy for spinal cord decompression performed endoscopically. Surg Laparosc Endosc 1995; 5:339.

76. Acaraglu ER, Schwab FJ, Farcy JP: Simultaneous anterior and posterior approaches for correction of late deformity due to thoracolumbar fractures. Eur Spine J 1996; 5:55.

77. Spivak JM, Neuwirth MG, Giordano CP: The perioperative course of combined anterior and posterior spinal fusion. Spine 1994; 19:520.

section
3
chapter
24

PRINCIPLES OF PEDIATRIC FRACTURES

Peter F. Armstrong

Summary
- There are unique anatomic and biomechanical differences in the child's musculoskeletal system.
- The thick periosteum plays a major role in healing and remodeling and can be useful in providing stability to a fracture reduction.
- Children's bone is more porous and more flexible than adult bone.
- Injuries to the physis (growth plate) can lead to significant growth disturbances.
- It is critical for the protection of a child to recognize the signs suggestive of child abuse.

INTRODUCTION

Children have sometimes been referred to as "accidents waiting to happen." They are constantly on the go and seem to have no fear. It is not surprising, therefore, that fractures occur. This chapter is designed to give you some of the basic principles of pediatric fractures and their management. Entire textbooks are devoted to pediatric fractures, and so the material presented in this and subsequent chapters will only give you a taste of the subject. Those wanting further information are referred to other excellent texts included in the reference list.[1-5]

EPIDEMIOLOGY

It is estimated[6] that each year 1.5% to 2% of children will sustain a fracture of some sort. Landin[7] reported that by the age of 16, 42% of boys and 27% of girls will have sustained at least one fracture. Generally, it seems that the incidence of fractures rises with increasing age.[8-13] In the 6- to 7-year-old group, the prevalence of fractures is about 16% of all injuries. This increases to 24% of injuries in the 14- to 15-year-old group. It is probably not surprising that upper extremity fractures occur three times more commonly than lower extremity fractures. Eighteen percent to 30% of children's fractures will affect the growth plate (physis). The incidence of physeal fractures also seems to rise with increasing age.

ETIOLOGY

The most common cause of pediatric fractures is a fall either on a level surface or from a height. Vehicular accidents of one type or another are the second most common cause, and sports and recreation comprise the third.

ANATOMIC DIFFERENCES

The pediatric skeleton is in a constant state of change as the result of the growth and maturation process. In the infant, there is a considerable amount of cartilage of various types. One of the most important types is found in the growth plate or physis (see Chapters 2-2 and 2-3). The growth plate or physis is the site of longitudinal bone growth and, if injured, has the potential for significant growth disturbances.

The epiphyses are mostly cartilage in the infant. Gradually, various ossification centers appear, and eventually the epiphyses become bone. It is very helpful to be aware of the age when the various ossific nuclei appear and also when the various physes close.[14]

Another significant difference in the child is the presence of a thick, biologically very active periosteum. In the fracture-healing process, it plays a major role as a producer of new bone through membranous ossification. It can be both an obstacle and an aid to obtaining and maintaining a reduction, as is seen in the Management Principles for Pediatric Fractures section.

The periosteum may also contribute to the development of deformity. The periosteum attaches to the epiphysis at either end of a long bone. As longitudinal growth continues, the periosteum both grows and stretches. There is some tension in the periosteum as a result, which may have a slight retardant effect on the longitudinal growth of the bone. When fractures occur, the periosteum is often only partially torn. This releases the tension in part of the periosteum and, therefore, the growth-retardant effect on the physis nearest the tear. Asymmetric growth occurs in that particular physis with resultant deformity. A good example of this is the seemingly innocent fracture in the metaphysis of the proximal tibia. This fracture is notorious for producing a significant valgus deformity (see Chapter 3-26).

Complete tearing of the periosteum may contribute to the phenomenon of "overgrowth," which is seen particularly after femur fractures in children (see Overgrowth section).

BIOMECHANICAL DIFFERENCES

The bone of a child is less dense, more porous, and more vascular than adult bone.[15] The fact that it has a lower modulus of elasticity results in some interesting fracture patterns that are not seen in the adult.

HEALING

In general, the rate of healing of fractures decreases with increasing age. It is also closely related to the level of osteogenic activity in the periosteum and endosteum. As an example, a fractured femur in a 3-week-old child may be solidly healed by 3 weeks. In an adolescent or young adult, it may take up to 20 weeks.[15]

REMODELING

Remodeling is a biological process during which certain bony deformities gradually correct to restore alignment of the long bone. Remodeling should not be relied on to correct a malalignment resulting from careless reduction. Instead, every effort should be made to obtain and maintain an accurate reduction. Remodeling is most helpful clinically in fractures of the distal radius, proximal humerus, and distal clavicle, where it may be difficult to achieve an accurate reduction.

The correction is achieved through a combination of at least three biological activities (Fig. 1):

1. New bone is laid down on the concave surface. This may be due largely to the intact periosteum on that side. It is also influenced by the biomechanical stresses applied to the bone.
2. Bone resorption occurs on the convex side of the bone.
3. There is asymmetric growth in the physis nearest the fracture, resulting in a realignment of the physis to a position perpendicular to the joint reaction forces across the physis.

Certain factors influence the degree of remodeling that occurs.

1. The age of the patient. The younger the patient, the greater is the potential for remodeling.
2. The proximity of the fracture to a physis. The closer the fracture to an actively growing physis, the better is the remodeling. Mid-diaphyseal deformities do not remodel well.
3. The degree of deformity. Lesser deformities have the potential to correct more completely.
4. The plane of the deformity. A deformity that is in the same plane as the plane of motion of the closest joint remodels better than other deformities. There is minimal to no remodeling for rotational deformities.

Remodeling will not help with displaced intra-articular fractures or fractures crossing the physis.

The details of remodeling have been extensively studied after fractures of the distal radius in children. Friberg[16] showed that an angular deformity at this site corrects at a rate of about 0.9 degrees a month or 10 degrees per year.[16–19]

OVERGROWTH

Increased longitudinal growth[20–22] occurs after significant long bone fractures. However, this actually only becomes clinically significant in femur fractures. The potential role of the completely torn periosteum has already been discussed. Another contributing factor is the increased vascularity of the limb during the healing of a major long bone fracture, with resultant growth stimulation. This temporary growth acceleration reaches a maximum at approximately 3 months after the fracture and returns to normal after about 40 months in the tibia and 50 to 60 months in the femur. The average overgrowth in the femur is 0.7 to 0.8 mm and in the tibia 0.3 to 0.4 mm. Slight overgrowth can be seen in an uninjured tibia on the same side as a femoral fracture. The reverse has not been seen.

MANAGEMENT PRINCIPLES FOR PEDIATRIC FRACTURES

1. Perform a thorough examination of the child so nothing is missed.

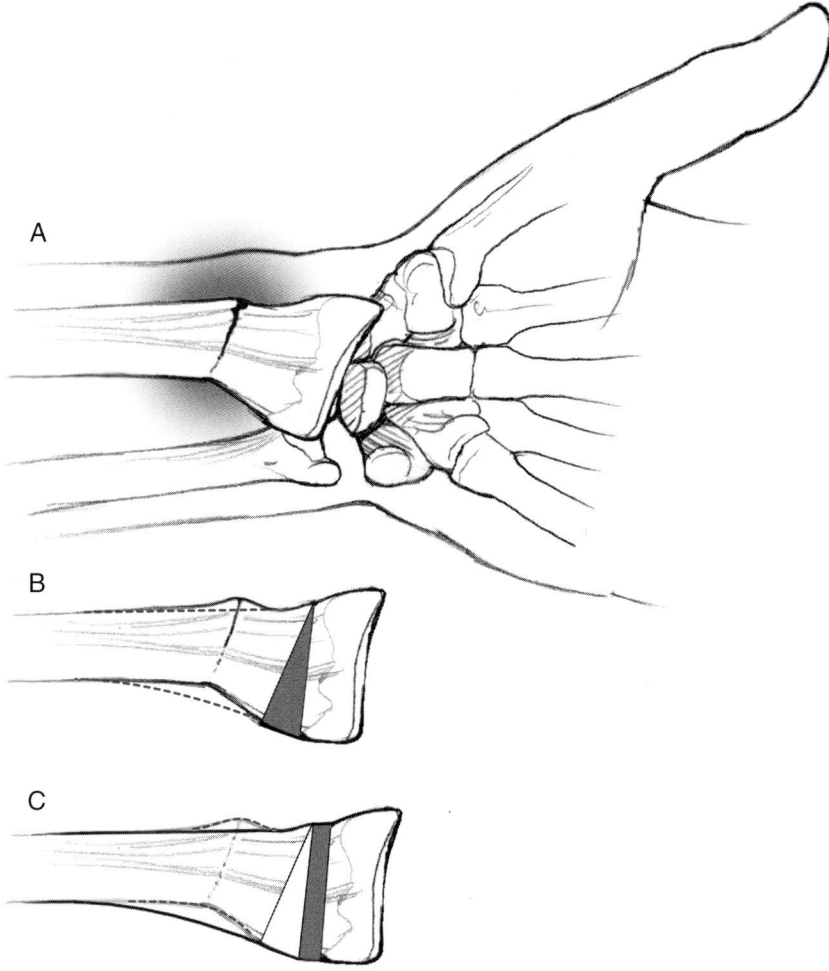

Fig. 1. Remodeling. *A,* Simulated distal radial fracture with apex volar angulation in the plain of motion of the joint. *B,* New bone is laid down on the concave side, and resorption occurs on the convex side. Asymmetric growth has occurred in the physis to align it perpendicular to the long axis. *C,* Fully remodeled bone.

2. Check the neurovascular status of a limb carefully before performing any manipulation of the limb.
3. Radiographs should include the joint above and joint below the fracture.
4. Comparative views of the uninjured side are often useful in the child.
5. Use appropriate analgesia and/or anesthesia.
6. Perform a careful, accurate reduction.
7. Use effective, safe immobilization.
8. Check the neurovascular status after any manipulation.
9. Close follow-up is an important key to success.

CLASSIFICATION OF PEDIATRIC FRACTURES

There are six general types of pediatric fractures: plastic deformation, torus (buckle or compression) fracture, greenstick fracture, complete fracture, physeal fractures (fractures affecting the growth plate), and osteochondral and avulsion fractures (fractures involving epiphyses and apophyses). Some of these injuries may be made more complex if they are open fractures.

PLASTIC DEFORMATION

Pediatric bone has a much greater capacity than adult bone to undergo plastic deformation (Fig. 2) before complete failure (Fig. 3). Bone is able to absorb a certain amount of energy through elastic deformation. When the force or load is removed, the bone returns to its original shape. When the elastic limit is exceeded, the bone then undergoes plastic deformation that does not recover. Of course, if the load continues, the bone will proceed to complete failure.[23] The forearm is the most common site for plastic deformation to occur. They can be very difficult to realign properly. The management of these fractures is discussed in Chapter 3–25.

BUCKLE OR COMPRESSION FRACTURE

Buckle or compression fracture (Fig. 4) is a failure in compression and usually occurs at the junction of metaphyseal (thin cortex) and diaphyseal (thick cortex) bone. The fracture is relatively stable but usually requires splinting to reduce discomfort.

GREENSTICK FRACTURE

A greenstick fracture (Fig. 5) is a more advanced type of plastic deformation. In this case, the load causes a complete fracture on the tension side of the bone. The fracture does not propagate across the bone. The compression side of the bone undergoes plastic deformation. It may be necessary to complete the fracture through the plastic deformity to achieve an adequate reduction.

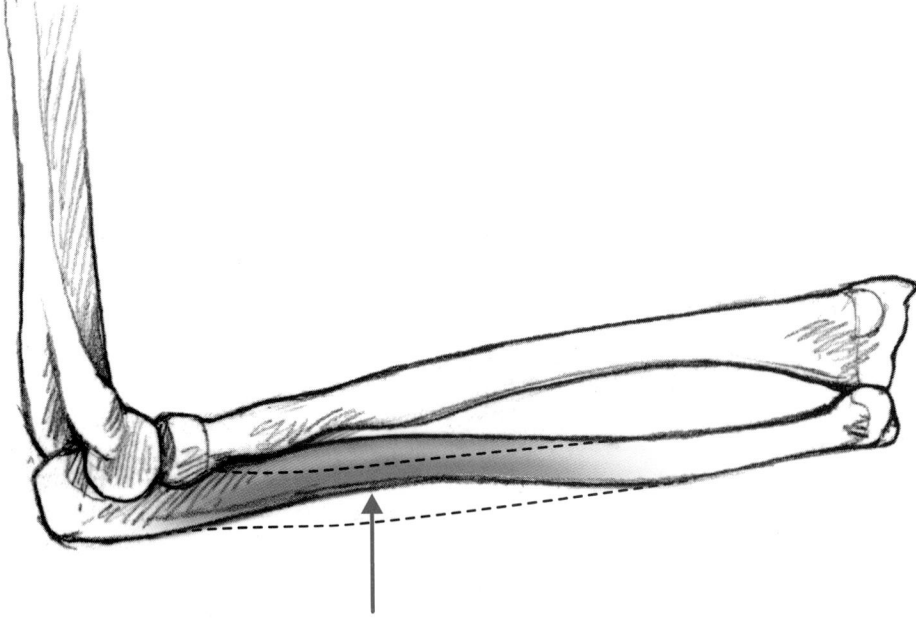

Fig. 2. Plastic deformation.

COMPLETE FRACTURES

Complete fractures can be further subdivided into four groups based on the fracture pattern: transverse, oblique, spiral, and comminuted. The pattern usually is indicative of the type of force that created the fracture.

Transverse

This fracture is usually caused by an angulation type of force or a direct blow applied perpendicularly to the long axis of the bone. Most commonly, the periosteum is torn on the "convex" side of the fracture with one of the bone ends "buttonholed" through the rent in the periosteum. Figure 6A shows a simulated fracture with bayonet apposition and an intact segment of periosteum. If traction alone is used in an attempt to reduce the fracture (Fig. 6B), the periosteum prevents reduction. The proper method of reduction is to recreate the deforming force by increasing the angulation, applying a distal push on the displaced fragment (Fig. 6C), and, finally, correcting the angulation (Fig. 6D). Using the principle of three-point fixation, the periosteum can be used to help stabilize the reduction (Fig. 6E).

Oblique

The mechanism of injury is usually an axial overload that produces a shear failure at an angle of 30 to 45 degrees.

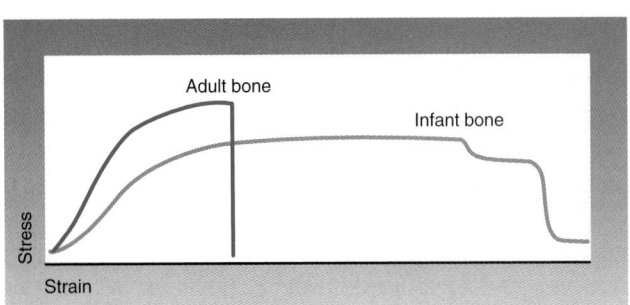

Fig. 3. Comparative stress/strain curves for adult and infant bone. Note the significantly greater elastic then plastic deformation possible in the infant bone before failure compared with the adult bone.

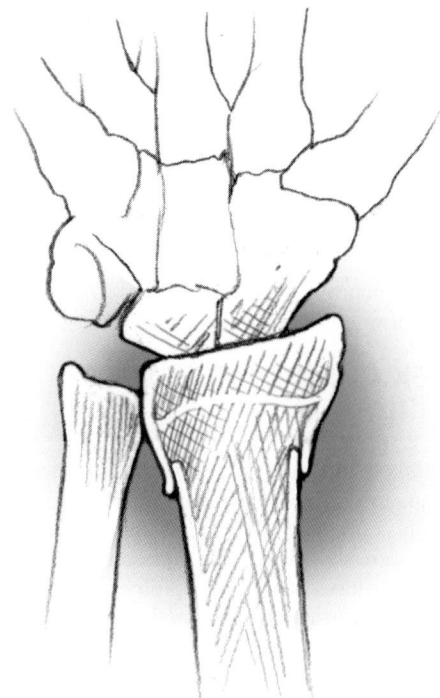

Fig. 4. Buckle fracture.

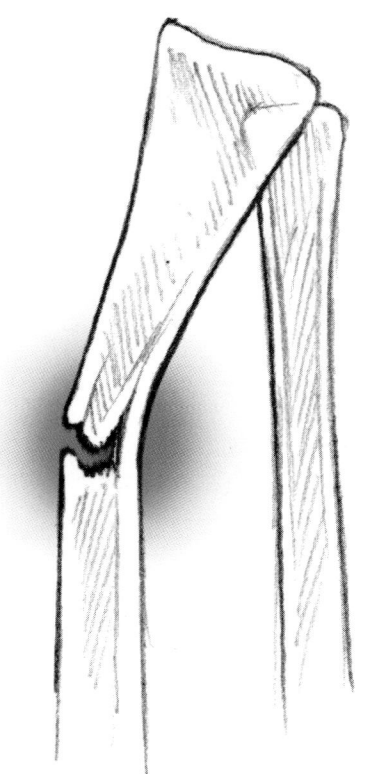

Fig. 5. Greenstick fracture. Note the complete fracture on the convex (tension) side and plastic deformation on the concave (compression) side.

There is often greater periosteal damage with this type of fracture, and, consequently, it is more unstable. The reduction is usually accomplished by longitudinal traction. Achieving stability can be difficult because any axial load such as muscle pull tends to cause the two oblique surfaces to slide on one another. In some instances, this instability may require internal stabilization.

Spiral

A twisting force usually produces this fracture. There is often a considerable amount of intact periosteum. The fracture pattern will indicate whether a clockwise or counter-clockwise force produced the fracture. Obviously, reducing this fracture involves longitudinal traction and rotation in the opposite direction to the one, which produced the fracture. The periosteum can be used to help stabilize the fracture but not by using the three-point principle. A "90-90" type of cast in which the joint above and the joint below are held at an angle to the long axis of the injured bone is effective in preventing rotation at the fracture site (Fig. 7). An example is a spiral tibial fracture that is reduced and held in an above-knee cast with the knee and ankle held at 90 degrees. An axial load will potentially displace this type of fracture.

Comminuted

This type of fracture is very uncommon in children. It is usually due to a combination of angulation plus an axial

load. The periosteum is usually torn on the side opposite the "butterfly" fragment. Because of the high energy involved in creating the fracture, it may be torn completely. If it is intact, it may be helpful in stabilizing the fracture. A very unstable fracture in which the reduction cannot be maintained will require internal fixation.

OPEN FRACTURES

The management of open fractures in a child does not differ from that established for the adult. A fracture with a puncture wound is an open fracture and needs to be treated as such!

PHYSEAL INJURIES

Injuries affecting the growth plate comprise about 15% of all fractures in children. In long bones, the distal physis is more commonly injured than the proximal physis; the distal radial growth plate is injured most frequently. Any injury that involves the physis has the potential for growth disturbances, particularly if it is not recognized and treated appropriately.

There are several classifications of injuries involving the physis. The best known is the Salter-Harris classification.[24] Both Ogden[25] and Peterson[26] expanded on this classification. In this chapter, we focus on the Salter-Harris classification (Fig. 8), but readers are encouraged to look at the other modifications. The types are classified as I to V; the potential for significant complications generally increases as the type designation increases. All of these injuries need to be treated with respect because it is definitely possible to damage the physis further by using inappropriate reduction techniques.

TYPE I

In this fracture, an intact epiphysis is detached from the metaphysis. It is most often the result of a shearing, torsional, or avulsion force. The fracture usually passes through the hypertrophic zone of the physis. In the smaller epiphyses, there can be anywhere from no displacement to complete displacement. If treated early, these patterns can usually be reduced relatively easily and the reduction maintained. Healing usually takes place in 3 to 4 weeks. The incidence of complications, such as growth arrest in the smaller bones, is very low. If the injury is through the capital femoral epiphysis, there is a very high incidence of osseous necrosis of the femoral head. This is a very serious complication with major long-term implications.

TYPE II

This fracture type is very similar to type I except that a small metaphyseal fragment (Thurston-Holland sign) stays with the epiphysis. This is the most common growth plate injury. The metaphyseal fragment usually indicates the side of the intact periosteum. Generally, this type of injury is relatively easy to reduce. In the larger epiphyses, it may be necessary to provide some form of internal fixation to maintain the reduction. The incidence of growth arrest increases proportionally with the cross-sectional area of the physis. The distal femoral growth plate is undulating. Ob-

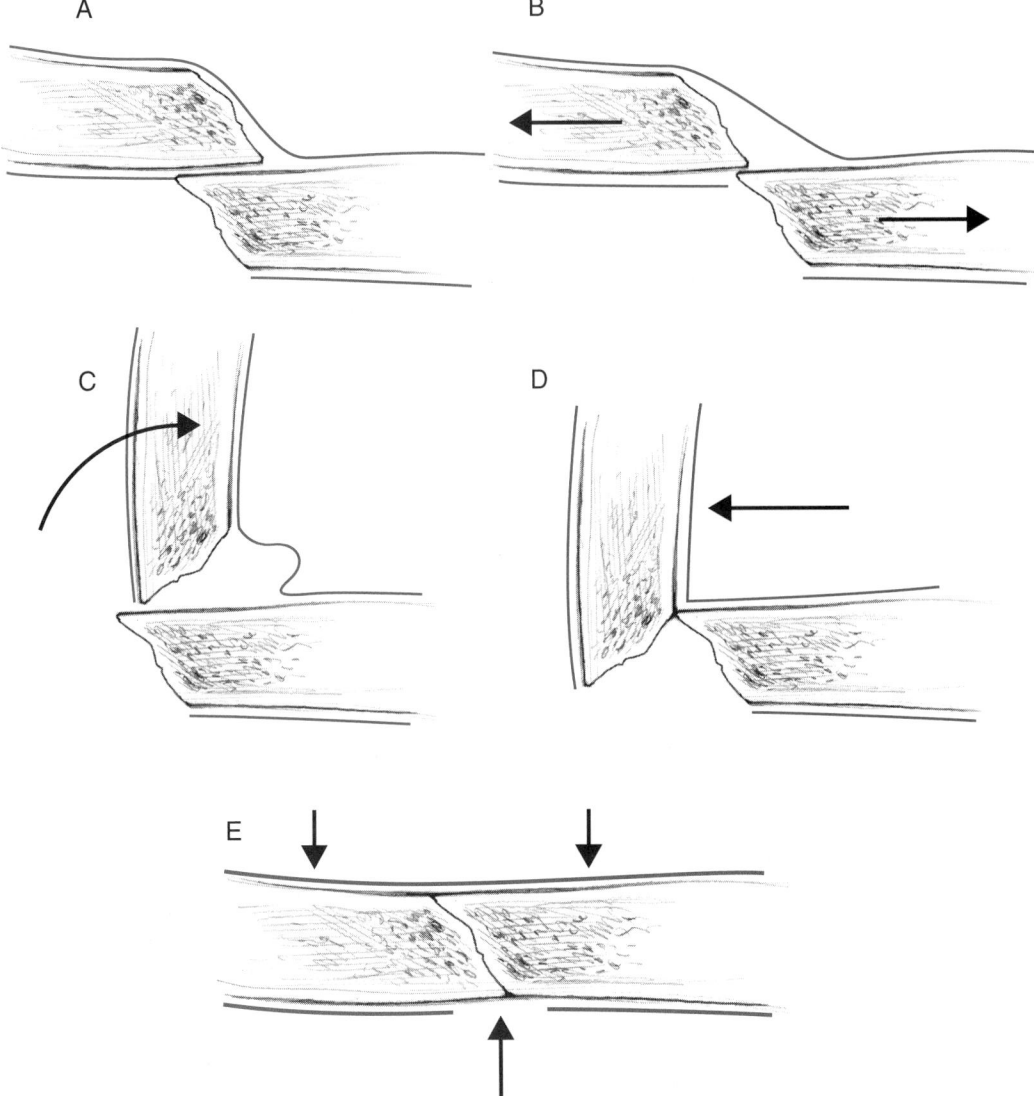

Fig. 6. Reduction using intact periosteal hinge. *A*, Complete fracture with bayonet apposition and intact periosteum. *B*, Longitudinal traction alone does not allow reduction. *C*, Deformity is increased, and a push is applied to the distal fragment. *D*, Once out to length, fracture is reduced. *E*, Three-point fixation is applied through proper molding of cast to hold reduction.

viously, it takes a considerable force to create this injury. Because of the breadth and morphologic features of the plate, there is greater potential for damage to the physis during displacement or reduction.

TYPE III

This type of injury is most commonly seen in growth plates that are partially closed. A common site is the distal tibia (Tillaux's fracture). The fracture line passes through the hypertrophic zone for a variable extent before fracturing through the epiphysis and into the joint. Accurate reduction is necessary to restore the congruity of the joint surface and the position of the growth plate. Some form of fixation is usually required. The consequences of a growth arrest are insignificant if the injury occurs in a plate that is already partially closed. It is a completely different matter if the injury involves the distal femur with a completely open growth plate.

TYPE IV

The fracture line in this type passes through the joint surface, across the epiphysis and physis, and out through the metaphysis. A common site for this injury to occur is in the region of the medial malleolus. This injury has a relatively high incidence of growth arrest, particularly if it is not recognized or treated inappropriately. Another example with a different result is a fracture through the lateral condyle of the humerus. If this is not managed correctly, there is the possibility of a nonunion, with slow, progressive proximal migration of the fragment resulting in a valgus deformity of the elbow.

TYPE V

There are differing opinions as to the actual existence of an isolated type V injury. The original description was of a crushing injury to all or part of a plate with a resultant growth arrest. There is the feeling that crushing of the

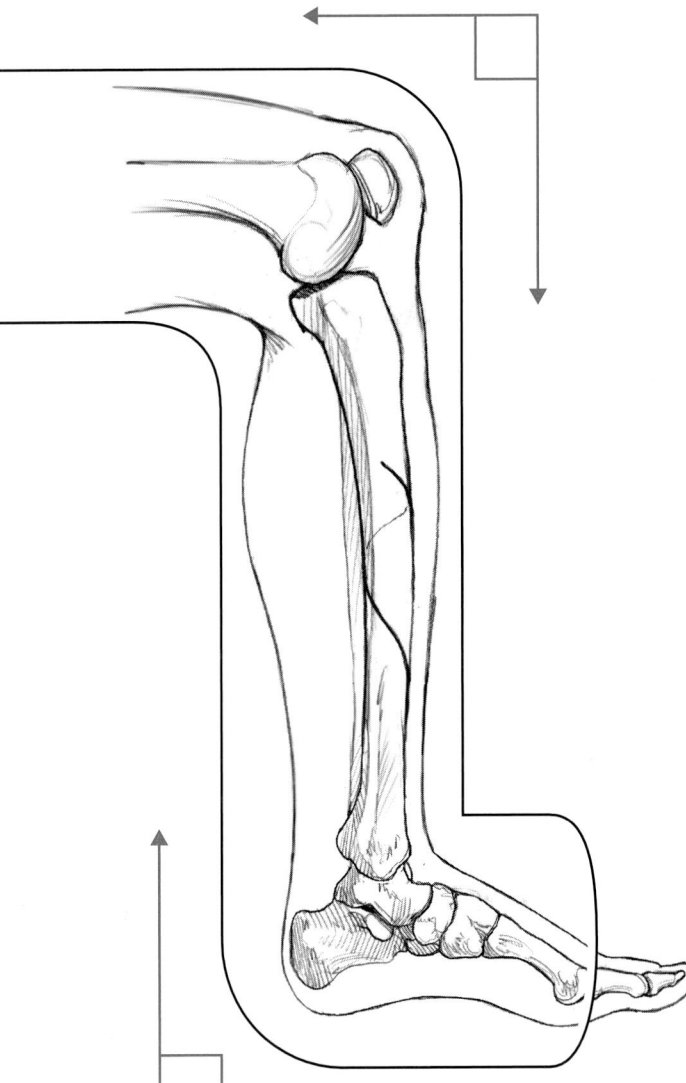

Fig. 7. Casting for a spiral fracture. Diagram shows a spiral fracture of the tibia in a "90-90" cast (the knee and foot are at 90 degrees to the long axis of the tibia). This helps prevent derotation in the cast after reduction.

plate likely occurs with other types of growth plate injury. Type V physeal damage is virtually impossible to detect at the time of injury and only manifests itself as a growth arrest.

GENERAL MANAGEMENT PRINCIPLES FOR PHYSEAL INJURIES

1. Understand the morphology of each fracture. Use multiple radiographic views, comparative views of the other limb, arthrograms, computed tomography (CT) scans, and occasionally stress films.
2. Know the potential long-term implications of each fracture and explain them carefully to the parents.
3. Determine, if possible, the location of intact periosteum.
4. Perform an appropriate, early, gentle reduction. In some instances, a closed reduction will be perfectly adequate. In others, it will be necessary to perform an open reduction. Know the optimal surgical approach that provides good exposure without jeopardizing the blood supply to

the fragment. Avoid trying to reduce a growth plate injury that is more than 1 week old.
5. Use fixation when necessary. Percutaneous pins will suffice for some. Internal fixation with screws may be more appropriate in others.
6. Ensure careful, long-term follow-up to allow early detection of growth disturbances.

GROWTH ARREST

Growth arrests are considered to be complete or partial. The partial ones are further subdivided into peripheral, central, and linear (combined) (Fig. 9).[27]

COMPLETE

Complete growth arrests, if they occur in a young child, can result in a significant limb length inequality. Early detection of growth arrests is critical. One must understand how to predict a future growth discrepancy. It is important

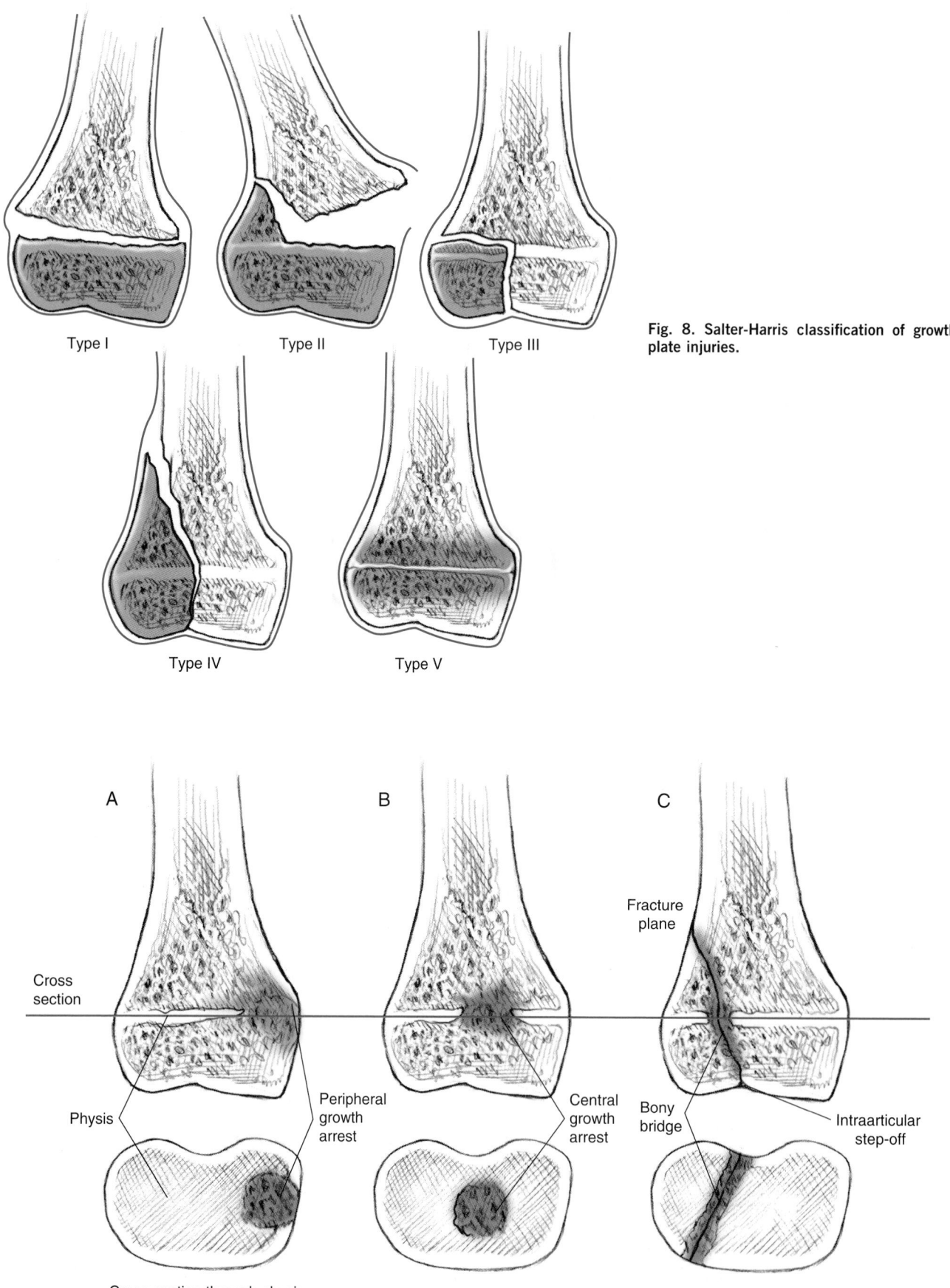

Fig. 8. Salter-Harris classification of growth plate injuries.

Type I

Type II

Type III

Type IV

Type V

A

B

C

Cross section

Fracture plane

Physis

Peripheral growth arrest

Central growth arrest

Bony bridge

Intraarticular step-off

Cross-section through physis

Fig. 9. Partial growth arrests. *A*, Central. *B*, Peripheral (linear).

to know the growth rates of the major long bone physes. For example, the distal femoral physis normally grows at a rate of 9 mm per year and the proximal tibia at 6 mm per year. A predicted discrepancy of 2 cm or less can be ignored in most instances. Those that are predicted to be between 2 and 5 cm are most frequently treated by stopping the growth on the long side. If the discrepancy is predicted to exceed 5 cm, limb lengthening may be indicated.

Example. A 6-year-old boy sustains an injury to his distal femoral physis, resulting in a complete arrest. What will be the most appropriate management of that child's situation? Boys will generally grow until they are 16 years of age. The uninjured side will, therefore, grow an additional $10 \times 0.9 = 9$ cm compared with the arrested side. The options include a 9-cm lengthening of the short femur at 10 to 12 years of age. Another option is a 5-cm lengthening with an epiphyseodesis of the distal femur on the long side at approximately 11 to 12 years of age. If he were 12 years old at the time of the injury, the discrepancy should be approximately $4 \times 0.9 = 3.6$ cm. An immediate epiphyseodesis or stapling of the unaffected distal femoral physis would result in fairly equal leg lengths.

PARTIAL
Peripheral
Damage to the perichondrial ring and peripheral physis can result in a growth arrest. Obviously, if untreated, an angular deformity will develop.

Central
Central bars usually result in a "tenting" of the central portion of the epiphysis, with possible retardation of growth if the bony bridge is large enough.

Linear
A good example of this type of bar is that produced by a type IV medial malleolar fracture. The bar runs in a linear fashion at the site of the old fracture, from the front of the tibia to the back. This type can also result in a significant angular deformity.

MANAGEMENT PRINCIPLES FOR PARTIAL GROWTH ARREST (PHYSEAL BARS)

As mentioned, partial growth arrests or transphyseal bars can be very difficult to treat.[27–29] Before embarking on any surgical treatment, the knowledge of certain facts influences the choice of management.

1. The age of the patient and, therefore, the amount of growth remaining in that physis.
2. The degree of deformity produced by the bar.
3. The location, type, and size of the bar (expressed as a percentage of the total area of the physis). The size is usually determined by biplane polytomography, CT scan, or, more recently, by magnetic resonance imaging (MRI).[30]

For example, if the bar affects less than 30% of the total area of the physis, there are at least 2 years of growth remaining in that physis, and the deformity is less than 20 degrees, a bar resection may result in resumption of normal growth and gradual correction of the deformity. Several other possible treatment plans exist depending on the parameters just listed.

1. If there is little remaining growth, no treatment may be necessary.
2. Arrest growth of the remaining injured physis with or without epiphyseodesis of the contralateral physis depending on the amount of growth remaining.
3. In two bone limb segments, the approach would be the same as in plan 2 with the addition of epiphyseodesis of one or both of the adjacent bones.
4. Perform bar resection or completion of epiphyseodesis with osteotomies to correct angular deformities greater than 20 degrees.
5. Perform limb lengthening in addition to other procedures.

OSTEOCHONDRAL AND AVULSION FRACTURES

OSTEOCHONDRAL FRACTURES
Osteochondral fractures (Fig. 10) are not common in children. There are two areas in which this may occasionally occur. Traumatic dislocations of the patella may result in an osteochondral fragment being sheared off the patella or the lateral femoral condyle. The plain films may reveal the fragment. If they are negative but suspicion is high, a plain or CT arthrogram may be helpful. If possible, the piece should be reduced and fixed.

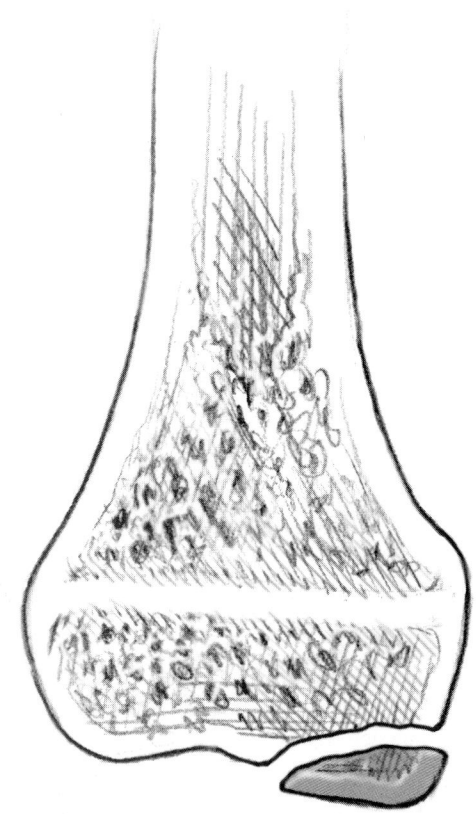

Fig. 10. Osteochondral fracture. Note that the fracture extends across articular cartilage and through epiphyseal bone.

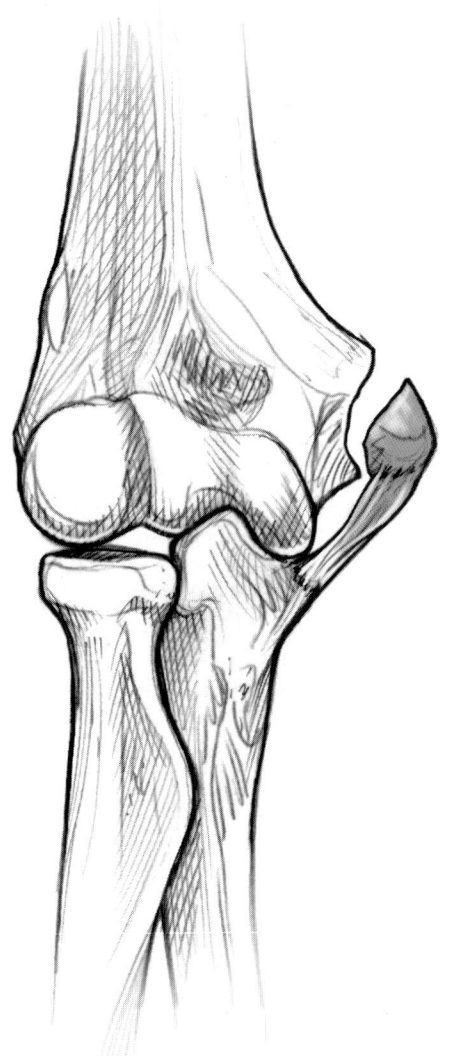

Fig. 11. Avulsion fracture. Note the avulsion of the medial epicondyle at the elbow.

The other situation in which this can occur is after a traumatic posterior dislocation of the hip. In this injury, the posterior lip of the acetabulum can be knocked off. Occasionally, after closed reduction of the hip, the piece can become entrapped in the joint. If a widened medial joint space is shown to exist on an anteroposterior radiograph of the pelvis compared with the other side, further investigation is warranted. A CT arthrogram is often helpful. Obviously, if an entrapped fragment is confirmed, it needs to be openly reduced and fixed.

This subject is covered in more detail in other chapters.

AVULSION FRACTURES

Many of these injuries involve an apophysis, which is a bony prominence to which muscles or tendons are attached. The interface between the apophysis and the main bone segment is through a physis. Some, such as the tibial tubercle, the medial epicondyle, or the greater trochanter, are contiguous with longitudinal growth plates. Growth at these sites occurs at the physis and also by appositional growth. This latter type of growth corresponds directly to the force exerted by the muscles and tendons. These injuries can be classified as acute and chronic. An example of an acute injury is the avulsion of the medial epicondyle around the elbow (Fig. 11). Similarly, the ischial tuberosity can be avulsed. These injuries may require open reduction and internal fixation.

Another type of avulsion fracture does not involve an apophysis but rather involves a ligamentous insertion. The childhood equivalent to the anterior cruciate tear is an avulsion of the anterior tibial spine (Fig. 12). This is an intra-articular osteochondral fracture that may need open reduction and internal fixation.

Osgood-Schlatter disease of the tibial tubercle and Sever's disease of the calcaneal apophysis are both good examples of chronic, repetitive, apophyseal injury. Apophysitis is the general term used for chronic conditions such as these. In most cases, these injuries heal over time. Surgery is rarely required for a painful, nonunited ossicle in the tibial tubercle.

CHILD ABUSE

Unfortunately, this is a medical and social problem with an incidence that continues to escalate. The Children's Bureau

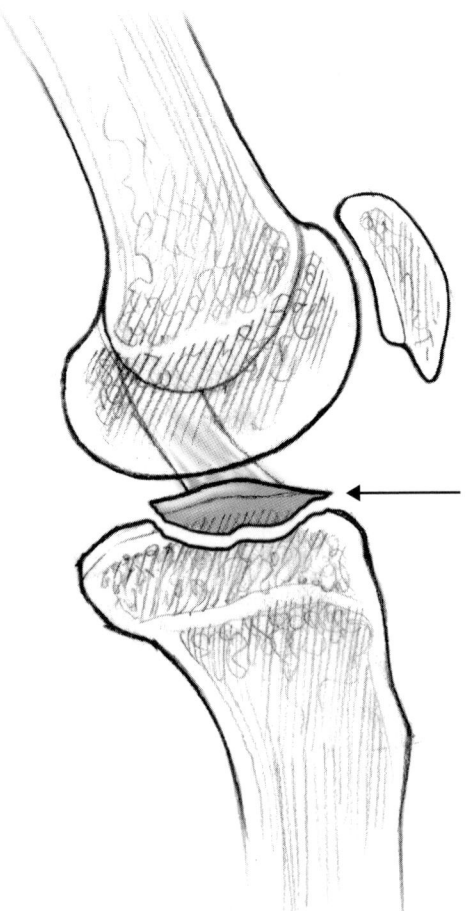

Fig. 12. Avulsion fracture. Note the avulsion of tibial spine in the knee. This is also an osteochondral fracture.

of the U.S. Department of Health, Education, and Welfare enacted a law that requires mandatory reporting by physicians and other health care workers of real or suspected child abuse. It is critical, in the interest of the health and safety of the child, for all physicians to be able to recognize the skeletal and soft-tissue injuries suggestive of child abuse. According to Cramer and Green,[31] soft-tissue injuries are the most common presentation in child abuse. Nevertheless, 10% to 70% of physically abused children demonstrate evidence of bony injury. Thirty to 50% of physically abused children are seen by orthopaedists for fractures or other orthopaedic problems. If there is no intervention and the child is returned to an abusive home, 35% to 50% will be abused again, and the second incident may be fatal in 5% to 10% of the cases.

The signs, on physical examination, that might be indicative of abuse are as follows:

1. Soft-tissue injuries such as bruises, welts, lacerations, and burns on multiple areas of the body.
2. Evidence of significant central nervous system injury. This could be due to blunt trauma or violent shaking.
3. Evidence of acute or healing fractures by clinical or radiographic exam. Of particular significance is evidence of multiple fractures at different stages of healing.

The plain film is the standard for searching for evidence of fractures. It may be supplemented in some cases by ultrasonography, bone scan, or MRI. Any bone could be fractured, but the extremities, skull, and ribs are the most frequently injured. There is no particular fracture pattern that is unequivocally a result of abuse. Nevertheless, certain patterns are seen more frequently than others. Cramer and Green[31] listed them as "metaphyseal or epiphyseal fractures (corner fractures, bucket-handle fractures, chip fractures); posterior rib fractures; multiple or wide, complex skull fractures; scapular and sternal fractures; multiple fractures; and unreported fractures." Transverse fractures are now believed to be more commonly associated with abuse than spiral fractures, although they are not specific for abuse.

To be fair to the parents or guardians, it is important to also know the other nonabuse conditions that may result in frequent fractures or subperiosteal new bone formation. The classic one is, of course, osteogenesis imperfecta.

This is such an important subject, and the reader is strongly encouraged to read other, more detailed resources.

REFERENCES

1. Green NE, Swiontkowski MF: Skeletal Trauma in Children. Vol. 3. Philadelphia, WB Saunders, 1998, p 608.
2. Letts RM: Management of Pediatric Fractures. New York, Churchill Livingstone, 1994, p 1243.
3. Ogden JE: Skeletal Injury in the Child. Philadelphia, WB Saunders, 1990, p 930.
4. Rang M: Children's Fractures. Toronto, JB Lippincott, 1983, p 365.
5. Rockwood C, Wilkens K, Beaty J: Fractures in Children. Vol. 3. Philadelphia, Lippincott-Raven, 1996, p 1531.
6. Reed MH: Epidemiology of children's fractures. In Letts RM, (ed): Management of Pediatric Fractures. New York, Churchill Livingstone, 1994, p 1.
7. Landin LA: Fracture patterns in children. Acta Orthop Scand Suppl 1983; 202:1.
8. Langley J, Dodge J, Silva P: Accidents in the first five years of life: A report from the Dunedin Multidisciplinary Child Development Study. Aust Paediatr J 1979; 15:255.
9. Langley J, Silva P, Williams S: Accidental injuries in the sixth and seventh years of life: A report from the Dunedin Multidisciplinary Child Development Study. Aust N Z J Med 1981; 93:344.
10. Langley J, Silva P: Injuries in the eighth and ninth years of life. Aust Paediatr J 1985; 21:51.
11. Langley J, Cecchi J, Silva P: Injuries in the tenth and eleventh years of life. Aust Paediatr J 1987; 23:35.
12. Chalmers D, Cecchi J, Langley J, et al: Injuries in the 12th and 13th years of life. Aust Paediatr J 1989; 25:14.
13. Lodge J, Langley J, Begg D: Injuries in the 14th and 15th years of life. J Paediatr Child Health 1990; 26:316.
14. Ogden J: Radiologic aspects. In Ogden J (ed): Skeletal Injury in the Child. Philadelphia, WB Saunders, 1990, p 65.
15. Ogden J: General Principles. Skeletal Injury in the Child. Philadelphia, WB Saunders, 1990, p 1.
16. Friberg K: Remodelling after distal forearm fractures in children: The effect of residual angulation on the spatial orientation of the epiphyseal plates. Acta Orthop Scand 1979; 50:537.
17. Friberg K: Remodelling after distal forearm fractures in children: The final orientation of the distal and proximal epiphyseal plates of the radius. Acta Orthop Scand 1979; 50:731.
18. Friberg K: Remodelling after distal forearm fractures in children: Correction of residual angulation in fractures of the radius. Acta Orthop Scand 1979; 50:741.
19. Friberg S: Remodelling after fractures with residual angulation. In Houghton G, Thompson G (eds): Problematic Musculoskeletal Injuries in Children. London, Butterworths, 1983, p 77.
20. Shapiro F: Fractures of the femoral shaft in children. The overgrowth phenomenon. Acta Orthop Scand 1981; 52:649.
21. Staheli L: Femoral and tibial growth following femoral shaft fracture in childhood. Clin Orthop 1967; 55:159.
22. Stephens M, Hsu L, Leong J: Leg length discrepancy after femoral shaft fractures in children. Review after skeletal maturity. J Bone Joint Surg Br 1989; 71:615.
23. Currey J, Butler G: Mechanical properties of bone tissue in children. J Bone Joint Surg Am 1975; 57:810.
24. Salter R, Harris W: Injuries involving the epiphyseal plate. J Bone Joint Surg Am 1963; 45:587.
25. Ogden J: Skeletal growth mechanism injury patterns. J Pediatr Orthop 1982; 2:371.
26. Peterson H: Physeal fractures. Part 3. Classification. J Pediatr Orthop 1994; 14:439.
27. Peterson H: Partial growth plate arrest and its treatment. J Pediatr Orthop 1984; 4:246.
28. Birch J: Posttraumatic physeal arrest. In Letts R (ed): Management of Pediatric Fractures. New York, Churchill Livingstone, 1994, p 1139.
29. Canale S: Physeal injuries. In Green N, Swiontkowski M (eds): Skeletal Trauma in Children. Vol. 3. Philadelphia, WB Saunders, 1998, p 17.
30. Carlson W, Wenger D: A mapping method to prepare for surgical excision of a partial physeal arrest. J Pediatr Orthop 1984; 4:232.
31. Cramer K, Green N: Child abuse. In Green N, Swiontkowski M (eds): Skeletal Trauma in Children. Vol. 3. Philadelphia, WB Saunders, 1998, p 577.

UPPER EXTREMITY

Lawrence L. Haber and George H. Thompson

Summary
- Fractures of the upper extremity are common injuries in children.
- Diagnosis is confirmed by clinical examination and appropriate radiographs.
- Treatment is usually nonoperative, although some fractures, such as displaced supracondylar fractures of the distal humerus, are best managed operatively.
- The goal of operative treatment is restoration and maintenance of acceptable alignment, not rigid fixation. Postoperatively, the extremity is protected with a cast until satisfactory healing has occurred.

Upper extremity fractures in children are extremely common. Diagnosis is suspected by the mechanism of injury and physical examination and is confirmed radiographically. The presence of preosseous cartilage and physes can occasionally make the diagnosis difficult. Most pediatric upper extremity fractures are treated nonoperatively, but occasionally surgery is necessary. Surgery usually involves simple internal fixation to maintain alignment, supplemented by a plaster cast until satisfactory healing has occurred. The indications and techniques for surgical intervention can be found in detail in recent textbooks.[1–5]

Upper extremity fractures commonly involve adjacent epiphyses.[6] Physeal fractures are classified using the Salter-Harris classification because it yields both prognostic information and treatment guidelines.[7] Type I fractures are an epiphyseal separation without a metaphyseal fragment, type II fractures have a metaphyseal fragment. These fractures have a good prognosis with respect to continued growth. The germinal cell layer is usually not involved, and anatomic alignment is not necessary as the remodeling potential is excellent. Type III fractures represent an epiphyseal separation but with a fracture extending through the epiphysis into the joint. Type IV fractures extend across the metaphysis, physis, and epiphysis into the joint. These two fracture types involve the germinal cell layer of the physis and the articular surface of the joint. Anatomic realignment is necessary to minimize the risk for premature or asymmetric physeal closure and degenerative osteoarthritis of the involved joint. Type V injuries represent a crush injury to the physes. A fracture is not visible radiographically, but there will be a growth disturbance in the succeeding months. This type is usually recognized retrospectively. The Salter-Harris classification system is applicable to lower extremity epiphyseal fractures as well.

SHOULDER FRACTURES

Fractures about the shoulder involve the clavicle, the scapula, and the proximal humerus and shaft.

CLAVICLE FRACTURES
Shaft Fractures
The clavicle is the most commonly fractured bone in childhood. The shaft is involved in approximately 85% of clavicle fractures. The usual mechanism of injury is a fall onto the shoulder. The fracture tends to occur at the transition from concavity to convexity and from the round to flat cross-sectional area. Clinically, the child will have direct tenderness, and there may be an obvious deformity. Open fractures are uncommon. A careful neurovascular examination is important, as brachial plexus and axillary artery injuries can occur. An anteroposterior radiograph usually demonstrates the fracture. In difficult cases, a "serendipity" or Hobbs' view with the tube angled 40 degrees cephalad may be helpful.[5]

Except in cases in which the injury is open or a spiked fragment is threatening the skin integrity or neurovascular structures, treatment is nonoperative. Treatment usually consists of a sling or commercial figure-of-eight harness for 2 to 3 weeks until the patient is comfortable. Motion is begun as tolerated. Most fractures heal uneventfully. There is frequently a residual bump, but this will satisfactorily remodel in younger children.

Distal Clavicle Fractures
The second most common clavicle fracture involves the distal end of the clavicle. This usually occurs from a fall or direct blow to the acromioclavicular area.[8] The distal end of the clavicle is an epiphysis, which ossifies as late as 19 years of age. Radiographically, this fracture can appear as an acromioclavicular separation. However, an acromioclavicular separation is a rare injury in childhood. An anteroposterior radiograph will usually show the fracture and possible superior displacement of the distal clavicle on the acromion. These fractures have been classified into three types: type 1, nondisplaced; type 2, displaced; and type 3, extending into the joint. The pediatric clavicle is covered by a thick periosteum. The conoid and trapezoid ligaments insert into this periosteum and not the clavicle. This anatomic relationship secures the integrity of the periosteal tube, thereby allowing even displaced fractures to heal and remodel satisfactorily.

Treatment consists of a sling for 2 to 3 weeks followed by mobilization as tolerated. The only indications for operative treatment are an open injury or severe tenting of the skin. These rarely occur.

Medial Clavicle Fractures

Fractures at the medial or sternal end of the clavicle are very uncommon. This end is also an epiphysis, which does not close until 24 or 25 years of age. This fracture also represents an epiphyseal separation and can mimic a sternoclavicular separation. A force compressing the shoulder toward the midline is the usual mechanism. Shaft displacement can be either anterior or posterior. Local swelling and tenderness are noted on clinical examination. The "serendipity" view or computed tomography scan may be required for diagnosis.

Treatment is typically nonoperative with a sling for 2 to 3 weeks followed by mobilization as tolerated. Closed reduction may be necessary for displaced fractures. Posteriorly displaced fractures are usually stable following reduction and will remodel in young children. Persistent posterior displacement may compromise the mediastinal structures and may need to be treated operatively. Open reduction and internal fixation with sutures is the procedure of choice. Metallic internal fixation may damage the mediastinal structures and should be avoided.

SCAPULA FRACTURES
Body Fractures

Fractures of the scapula in children are uncommon. Most occur as a result of a direct blow. Because these are usually high-energy fractures, the possibility of thoracic or abdominal injuries should be considered. Radiographs include anteroposterior, transcapular lateral, and axillary views. Not only do these characterize the fracture, but they also assess the glenohumeral joint. Glenoid cavity involvement is best seen on the axillary view. Computed tomography may also be useful in evaluating displacement.

Fractures that do not involve the glenoid cavity can be treated in a sling or shoulder immobilizer for 2 to 3 weeks followed by mobilization as tolerated. Nondisplaced fractures extending into the glenoid cavity may be treated in the same manner. Displaced fractures of the glenoid cavity with more than 2 to 3 mm of displacement require open reduction and internal fixation.

Coracoid Fractures

Coracoid fractures are rare in children and are usually the result of an avulsion injury. Traction on the coracoacromial ligaments may cause a fracture of the epiphysis in the upper one-fourth of the coracoid. Traction on the conjoined tendon will cause a fracture of the tip of the coracoid. Because there may be an associated distal clavicle fracture or shoulder dislocation, shoulder radiographs are important. In the absence of other injuries, treatment is conservative.

HUMERUS FRACTURES
Proximal Humerus Fractures

Fractures of the proximal humerus account for less than 1% of all childhood fractures.[9, 10] In children younger than 5 years of age, these are typically Salter-Harris type I fractures; metaphyseal fractures are common between 5 and 10 years of age; and Salter-Harris type II fractures are common in children 11 years of age and older. The mechanism of injury is usually a fall on an outstretched arm or a direct blow to the posterolateral upper arm. Anteroposterior and lateral radiographs of the proximal humerus are obtained for diagnosis. Additional views to assess the glenohumeral joint are performed, if necessary.

The most important issues in treatment are stability and amount of displacement and angulation.[9, 10] In a child younger than 10 years of age, almost any alignment is acceptable, even in completely displaced and angulated fractures. In older children, fractures that overlap and angulation less than 45 degrees are usually acceptable. In a recent study, the only patients with poor results were those who underwent surgery regardless of the amount of displacement.[9] The proximal humeral physis contributes 80% of the growth of the humerus. This affords great remodeling potential. In addition, the universal motion of the glenohumeral joint compensates for mild residual deformities.

Proximal humerus fractures that are stable or have acceptable alignment can be treated with a Velpeau sling. In an unstable fracture with unacceptable angulation, a hanging long-arm cast may provide improved alignment. If reduction is deemed necessary, it should be performed under general anesthesia with muscle relaxation. A shoulder spica in the "salute" position may be necessary to maintain reduction. If the reduction is unstable, then reduction and stabilization with percutaneous Kirschner's wires can be attempted. Open reduction and internal fixation is indicated only for severely displaced fractures in adolescents.

Shaft Fractures

Humeral shaft fractures account for 2% to 5% of fractures in children. They occur most commonly before 3 and after 12 years of age. The mechanism of injury is either a direct blow causing a short oblique or transverse fracture or an indirect twisting mechanism producing a long spiral fracture. Neurological examination is important, as a radial nerve injury may occur with fractures at the junction of the middle and distal one-third of the shaft.[10, 11] Anteroposterior and lateral radiographs will demonstrate the fracture and any displacement or angulation.

Unless an open injury exists, closed treatment is most always acceptable.[10] At least 15 degrees of angulation can be accepted in any plane. Bayonet position is also acceptable. Treatment involves splinting in a favorable position. Usually, a coaptation splint is sufficient. A hanging-arm cast applies gentle traction to gain alignment and is useful for angulated fractures. In a nondisplaced stable fracture, a Velpeau sling may be sufficient. These fractures usually heal in 4 to 8 weeks.

The treatment for an associated radial nerve injury is observation for 16 to 20 weeks. If clinical recovery is not evident at that point, electromyography may be useful.[11] Immediate exploration for a radial nerve injured at the time of reduction is necessary, as the nerve may have been entrapped in the fracture site.

ELBOW FRACTURES

Elbow fractures in children are a frequent source of confusion because of the six growth centers and their various times of ossification and fusion (Table 1).[5] The trochlea and capitellum fuse between 10 and 12 years of age. They

TABLE 1. APPEARANCE OF OSSIFICATION CENTERS ABOUT THE ELBOW

Ossification Center	Age at Appearance
Metaphysis	Birth
Capitellum	0.5–2 years
Radial head	2–4 years
Medial epicondyle	5–9 years
Trochlea	7–9 years
Olecranon	9–11 years
Lateral condyle	10–11 years

then fuse with the lateral condyle to form the distal humeral epiphysis, which closes between 12 and 13 years of age. The medial epicondyle is the last to fuse to the metaphysis, as late as 17 years of age.

The elbow also has three fat pads that may be seen radiographically. The anterior fat pad overlies the coronoid fossa. Deep in the olecranon fossa is the posterior fat pad. The third fat pad is anterior to the supinator muscle. Any of these fat pads can be elevated in an injured elbow, provided the elbow capsule remains intact. Fat pad elevation represents the accumulation of blood in the elbow joint. A torn capsule may prevent these pads from being elevated. However, there is a significant incidence of radiographically visible fat pads in normal elbows. The anterior fat pad is the least reliable. The posterior fat pad is usually deep enough that its elevation truly represents blood in the joint and a possible fracture. The supinator pad may indicate a fracture of the radial head or neck. Regardless of the presence of a fat pad sign, tenderness over a specific area is the most reliable finding in an occult fracture.

Anteroposterior and lateral radiographs are necessary for assessment. There are several radiographic lines that can be used to evaluate the alignment of the distal humerus. Baumann's angle is the intersection of a line drawn along the physis of the capitellum and a line drawn perpendicular to the axis of the distal humerus. A true anteroposterior radiograph of the distal humerus is needed for accuracy. The normal angle is approximately 15 degrees. The carrying angle of the elbow measures the intersecting lines drawn through the shafts of the humerus and the ulna. It is also important to measure alignment on the lateral view. A true lateral radiograph is necessary to judge anterior and posterior displacement. The simplest method is to draw a line down the anterior aspect of the humerus. This line should bisect the middle one-third of the capitellum.

Elbow fractures are divided into those involving the distal humerus and those involving the proximal radius and ulna.

DISTAL HUMERUS FRACTURES
Supracondylar Fractures

The supracondylar fracture of the distal humerus is the most common elbow fracture in children.[1-5] It occurs most commonly in children younger than 10 years of age but can occur at any age. These fractures are classified as a flexion or extension fracture depending on the position of the distal fragment. The latter is most common, accounting

for 96% of fractures. Supracondylar fractures occur by a fall on an outstretched hand with the elbow hyperextended. The Wilkins modification of the Gartland classification is used to classify extension fractures: grade 1, a nondisplaced fracture; grade 2, the anterior cortex opens and the distal fragment begins to hinge posteriorly; and grade 3, displaced.[5] The high incidence of this fracture is due to the thinness of the bone between the olecranon and the coronoid fossa. These fractures are usually easy to diagnose by routine radiographs.

There is a high incidence rate of neurovascular injuries in displaced supracondylar fractures. The anterior interosseous branch of the median nerve and the radial nerves are the most commonly injured.[12, 13] The brachial artery can also be damaged.[12, 14] Disagreements exist regarding management of the "pink" but pulseless hand. Most practitioners feel that a well-vascularized hand with or without a pulse can be observed.[14] The collateral circulation is usually adequate for normal perfusion. In addition, there is a low rate of patency in arteries that have been repaired or bypassed. Exploration is not indicated for neurological deficits, as they are invariably a neurapraxia. The exception is a neurological deficit that is incurred during a closed reduction. In these cases, the fracture should be explored to rule out nerve entrapment in the fracture site.

Nonoperative treatment is indicated for grade 1 fractures. A long-arm posterior splint or a long-arm cast for 3 weeks usually is sufficient. In grade 2 fractures, determine the amount of displacement on the lateral radiographs. The capitellum should make a 30-degree angle with the shaft. This angle decreases as the posterior fragment hinges posteriorly. Some authors recommend closed reduction of grade 2 injuries and immobilization in a long-arm cast with the elbow flexed 90 degrees. However, swelling may ensue and compromise the circulation to the forearm and hand. In general, fracture alignment should be accepted if there is minimal angulation. Closed reduction can be performed if there is near complete loss of the anterior tilt of the distal fragment. If there is any instability, percutaneous pinning with Kirschner's wires should be performed. Two lateral pins can be used to avoid a potential injury to the ulnar nerve.

Grade 3 fractures should always be reduced and stabilized.[15, 16] This is usually done with percutaneous Kirschner's wires (Fig. 1). Fractures treated by closed reduction with less than anatomic alignment risk displacement owing to the very low bone surface area at the fracture fragments. Open reduction is indicated for open or irreducible fractures and for those with vascular insufficiency. An anterior incision is most frequently used. It allows excellent exposure of the fracture site and the neurovascular structures. Postoperatively, the elbow is immobilized in a long-arm posterior splint in 40 to 60 degrees of flexion to minimize the effects of soft-tissue swelling.

In general, supracondylar fractures are not difficult to reduce. Failure to achieve a satisfactory alignment indicates either soft-tissue or muscle entrapment. The entrapped soft tissue may also include neurovascular structures. Therefore, multiple or forced reductions must be avoided. If the distal end of the humeral shaft is trapped in the brachialis muscle, it can sometimes be freed by milking the muscle.[16] Grade 3 fractures are usually cross-pinned for greater sta-

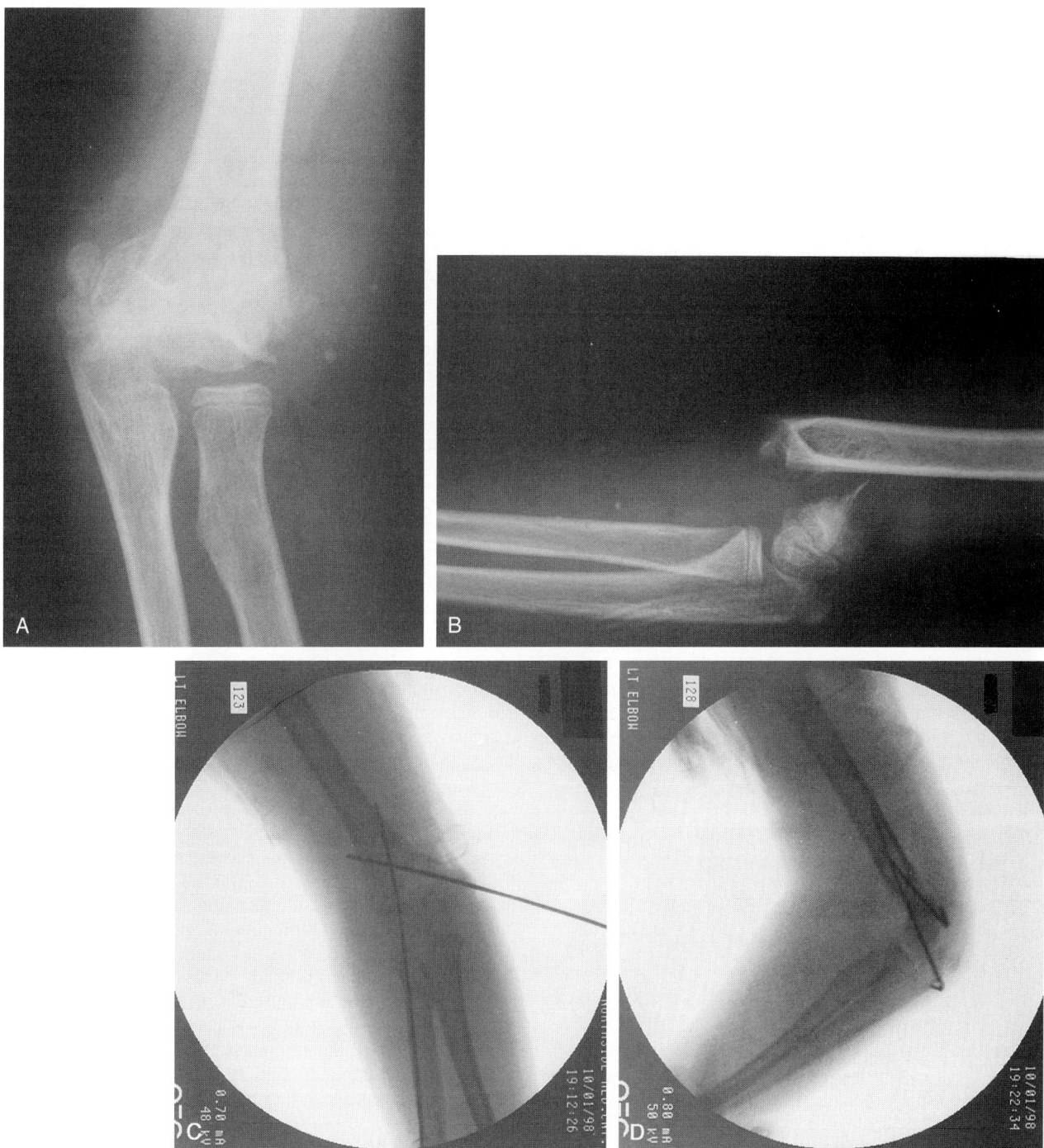

Fig. 1. Radiographs. *A*, Anteroposterior radiograph of the left elbow of an 8-year-old male with a displaced supracondylar fracture. *B*, Lateral radiograph demonstrates extension at the distal fracture fragments (type III). *C*, Intraoperative fluoroscopy following closed reduction and percutaneous cross-pinning. The .062 Kirschner wires pass through the medial and lateral columns, avoiding the olecranon and coronoid fossae. *D*, Lateral view demonstrates restoration of the anterior tilt between the capitellum and distal humerus.

bility.[17] Careful palpation of the medial epicondyle and avoiding a posterior starting point will avoid the ulnar nerve. A small medial incision in very swollen elbows allows direct visualization.[13] Most nerve injuries recover if the pin is removed. However, recovery typically occurs even if the pin is left in 3 weeks.[18]

The most common complication of supracondylar fracture is cubitus varus.[1–5] This occurs as a result of collapse of the medial metaphysis due to comminution, poor apposition, or varus alignment following fixation. Volkmann's ischemic contracture is related to an unrecognized, untreated acute vascular injury.

Fracture-Separation of the Distal Humeral Epiphysis

This uncommon fracture occurs in young children.[19, 20] It is usually due to a birth injury, child abuse, or fall from a height onto an extended elbow. It can be difficult to distinguish from a supracondylar fracture or elbow dislocation. The clinical examination is usually not helpful. Radiographically, it is important to assess the relationship between capitellum and the radial head. This distal humerus is not well ossified in these young children. The relationship between the capitellum and radial head is normal while the humeral and forearm axes are displaced. Displaced fractures require reduction and, frequently, pin fixation because these fracture-separations may be unstable. Cubitus varus is the most common complication.

Lateral Condyle Fractures

The second most common elbow fracture is the lateral condyle fracture (Fig. 2).[1–5] It accounts for approximately 18% of elbow fractures.[21] An avulsion mechanism based on forced varus and an axial loading has been suggested. The Milch classification defines the location of the distal fracture line.[22] In a Milch 1 fracture, the fracture is lateral to the trochlear groove. This fracture is more stable, and the elbow is less likely to dislocate. In a Milch 2 fracture, the fracture line is medial to the trochlear groove and can result in elbow instability. This classification offers no information about the risk for displacement and therefore offers no guidance for treatment. Jakob et al[23] classified this fracture based on displacement: type 1, the fracture is incomplete and nondisplaced; type 2, the fracture extends through the epiphysis, potentially allowing the fragment to

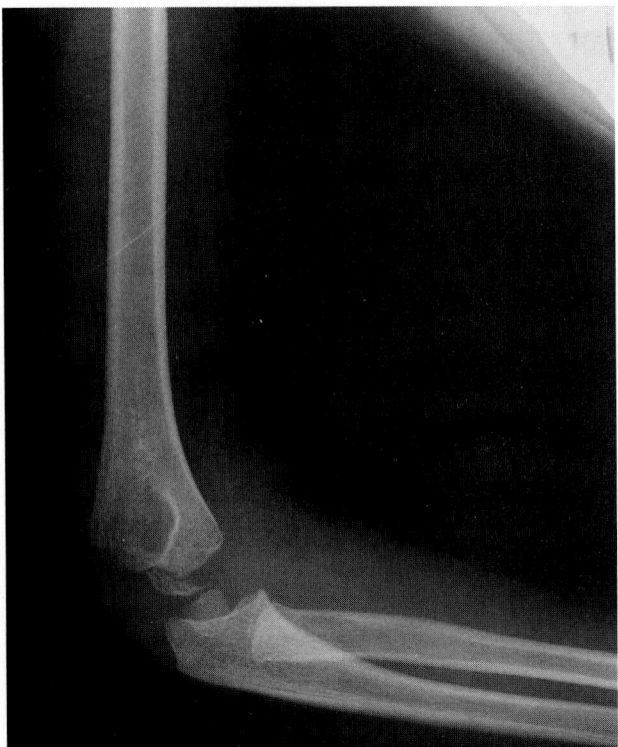

Fig. 2. Lateral radiograph. It shows a displaced fracture of the lateral condyle fracture of the distal humerus.

laterally displace, but not rotate; and type 3, a fracture in which the lateral condyle rotates or is completely displaced.

Type 1 fractures can be treated in a posterior splint or long-arm cast. Type 2 and 3 fractures require reduction and stabilization. Closed percutaneous methods of reduction maneuvers have been described.[24] In type 2 fractures that fail closed reduction and all type 3 fractures, an open reduction and internal fixation with two Kirschner's wires is required. At times, a third wire placed parallel to the joint line may be helpful. The anterior aspect of the joint is exposed carefully so as not to strip the posterior soft tissue from the distal fragment, thereby preserving the blood supply to the capitellum.

Complications of lateral condyle fractures include nonunion and malunion. These may lead to cubitus valgus and possible tardy ulnar nerve palsy. Avascular necrosis is usually the result of iatrogenic soft-tissue stripping or the injury itself.[23] Cubitus valgus is the result of nonunion, malunion, or growth disturbance.

Medial Epicondyle Fractures

Medial epicondyle fractures represent about 10% of elbow fractures in children.[1–5] These are caused by a varus force on an extended arm similar to the mechanism of an ulnar collateral ligament injury in the adult. Anteroposterior and lateral elbow radiographs are necessary for diagnosis. This fracture may be difficult to diagnose in a young child before ossification. An ultrasonogram, computed tomographic scan, examination under anesthesia, or arthrogram may be useful.[25] Classification is based on displacement: type 1, the fracture is nondisplaced; type 2, the fracture is displaced less than 5 mm; and type 3, the fracture is completely displaced and may become trapped in the joint.[24]

Treatment is based on displacement. Treatment of type 1 fractures is nonoperative with immobilization in a long-arm cast for 1 to 2 weeks. Treatment of type 2 fractures is controversial. Closed reduction is performed if the fragment is displaced more than 5 mm and if the elbow is stable. Open reduction and internal fixation is recommended, if the elbow is unstable (Fig. 3). The instability is caused by the avulsion of the ulnar collateral ligament that attaches to the medial epicondyle. In type 3 fractures, open reduction and internal fixation with Kirschner's wires is preferred. The results are usually excellent. However, instability and stiffness can occur.

Medial Condyle Fractures

Medial condyle fractures are uncommon and account for only 2% of elbow fractures.[1–5] They are avulsion injuries caused by forced varus, as well as a direct impact on the flexed elbow. Kilfoyle[27] described a classification based on displacement. It is identical to the classification by Jakob et al of lateral condyle fractures. Diagnosis is frequently difficult in children with an unossified trochlea. Radiographically, there may be a "fleck" of metaphyseal bone. Clinically, the medial aspect of the distal humerus is tender and swollen. Examination under anesthesia can be useful. In a medial condyle fracture, there will be varus instability. This is the opposite of a medial epicondyle injury, which will allow the elbow to open in valgus position.

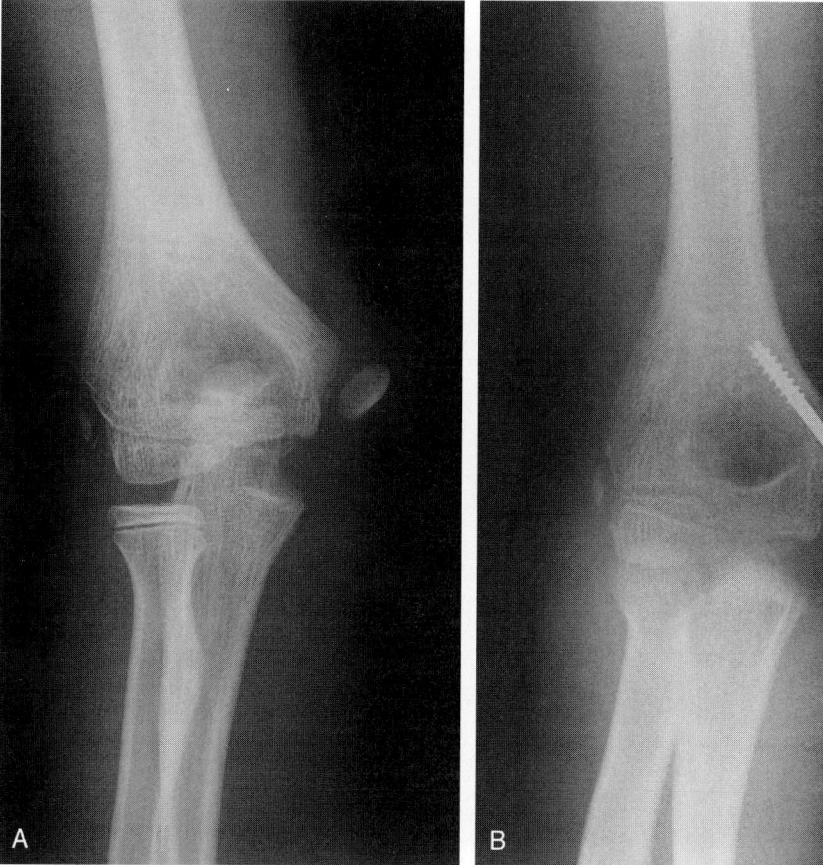

Fig. 3. Radiographs. *A,* Antero-posterior radiograph of the left el-bow of a 10-year-old male with displaced fracture of the medial epicondyle. The elbow was unsta-ble with stress examination under anesthesia. *B,* Anteroposterior ra-diograph 2 months following open reduction and internal fixation.

Treatment is similar to that for lateral condyle frac-tures.[27, 28] Immobilization in a long-arm cast is used for nondisplaced fractures. Minimally displaced fractures can be percutaneously pinned following anatomic reduction with Kirschner's wires. Displaced fractures require open reduction and internal fixation. These fractures are usually healed in 3 weeks.

Other Distal Humerus Fractures
The less common distal humerus fractures include the T-condylar fracture and the lateral epicondyle fracture. The T-condylar fracture is a supracondylar fracture with exten-sion into the joint. It usually occurs in older children. When displaced, open reduction and internal fixation is needed. Fixation depends on comminution and may range from Kirschner's wires to plates and screws. Exposure is controversial. A medial or lateral approach preserves blood supply in a child with open physis but limits the options for fixation to pins and screws. An olecranon osteotomy and posterior approach allows better access by allowing plating, but theoretically will devascularize the capitellum in a child with an open physis. In highly comminuted fractures, olecranon traction may be required, possibly in combination with or before internal fixation. Regardless, these cases are difficult.

The lateral epicondyle fracture is another rare injury. It is thought to occur as the result of an avulsion of the extensor mass. It is usually treated in a posterior splint with early mobilization.

PROXIMAL RADIUS AND ULNA FRACTURES
Radial Head and Neck Fractures
Fractures of the proximal radius account for about 8% of elbow fractures.[1-5] They usually involve either the physis or the neck of the radius rather than the head.[29-32] There is a normal lateral angulation of approximately 15 degrees between the radial neck and the shaft. The proposed mech-anism of fracture is forced valgus and dislocation.

Treatment is based more on displacement and angula-tion. Indications for surgery are controversial. Typically, a fracture that is angulated more than 30 degrees or one that is completely displaced should be reduced and pinned with Kirschner's wires (Fig. 4). Several methods have been de-rived to reduce the fracture percutaneously.[29-31] If this can-not be accomplished, then an open reduction and Kirsch-ner's wire fixation is necessary, usually through a lateral approach, or closed intramedullary pinning can be per-formed.[32] Open percutaneous pinning should be done through the edge of the radial head and the pins left percutaneous. The use of transcapitellar pins should be avoided.

Olecranon Fractures
Fractures of the olecranon in children represent about 5% of elbow fractures. They result from a fall onto a flexed elbow or as the result of a varus or valgus hyperextension injury. Most of these fractures are nondisplaced and do not require operative treatment. If they are displaced and in-

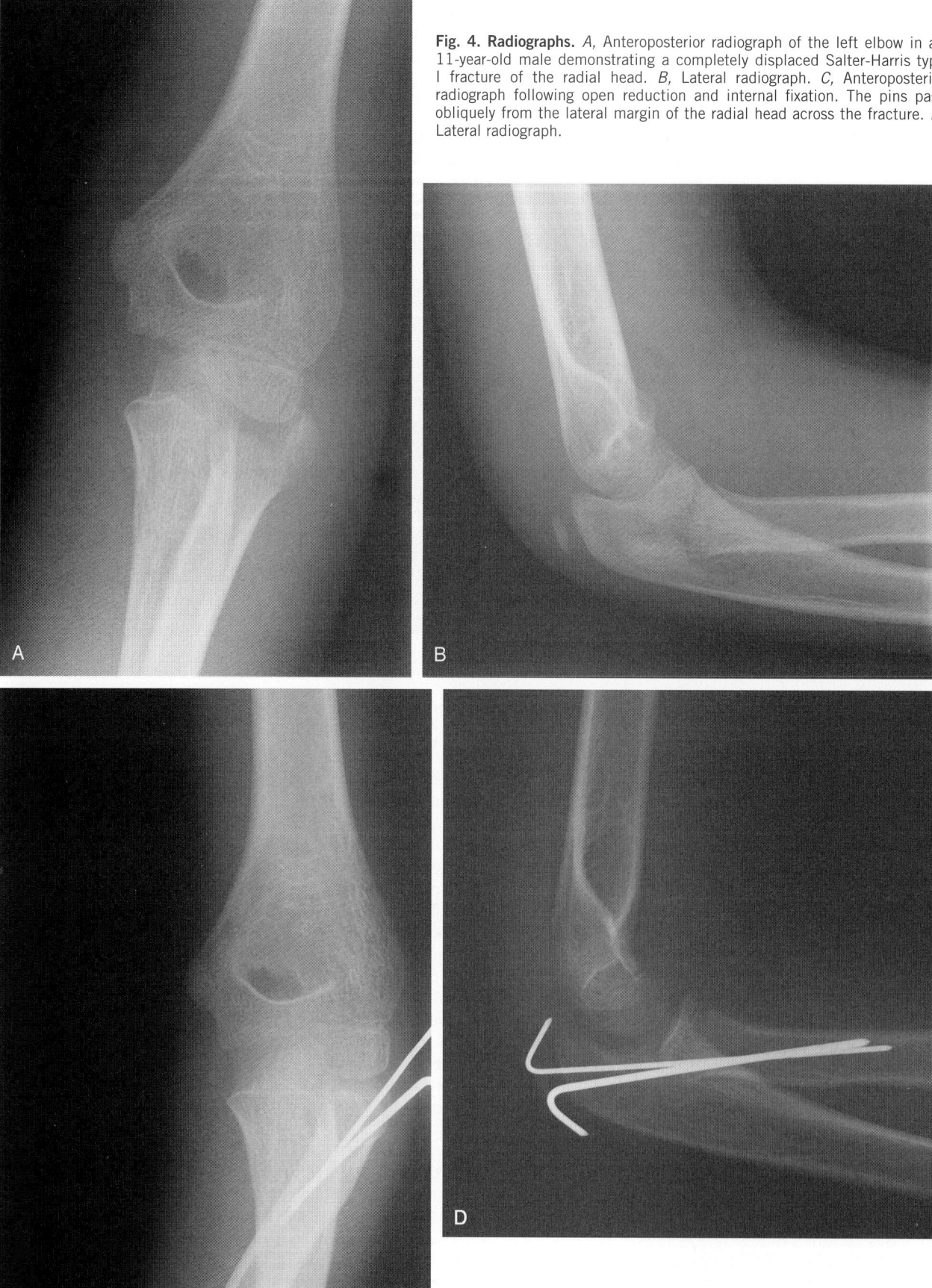

Fig. 4. Radiographs. *A*, Anteroposterior radiograph of the left elbow in an 11-year-old male demonstrating a completely displaced Salter-Harris type I fracture of the radial head. *B*, Lateral radiograph. *C*, Anteroposterior radiograph following open reduction and internal fixation. The pins pass obliquely from the lateral margin of the radial head across the fracture. *D*, Lateral radiograph.

volve the joint, then anatomic alignment by open reduction and internal fixation must be achieved.[33] Assess for other concomitant fractures, such as a radial neck fracture.

Monteggia's Fractures

This is a fracture of the ulna in association with a dislocation of the radial head.[34–36] Bado[34] classified these into four types: type 1, an anterior dislocation of the radial head with anteriorly angulated diaphyseal ulna fracture; type 2, a posterior or posterolateral dislocation of the radial head with a posteriorly angulated ulnar fracture; type 3, a metaphyseal ulnar fracture and anterior dislocation of the radial head; and, type 4, an anterior dislocation of the radius with a proximal one-third fracture of the radius and ulna. Several injuries have been termed Monteggia-equivalent. These include ulnar fractures with radial neck, shaft, and proximal physeal fractures. Also included are anterior radial head dislocations associated with a plastically deformed ulna. In children, closed reduction is usually adequate. If satisfactory alignment cannot be achieved, open reduction and internal fixation will be necessary.

FOREARM AND WRIST FRACTURES

Forearm and wrist fractures are extremely common in children.[1–5] They account for approximately 45% of all pediatric fractures and 62% of upper limb fractures. The majority, 75% to 84%, occur in the distal third, 15% to 18% in the middle third (shaft), and only 1% to 7% in the proximal third. Fracture patterns include plastic deformations, "buckle" or torus fractures, greenstick fractures, and incomplete and complete fractures. Complete fractures may be transverse, short oblique, comminuted, or long spiral fractures. Physeal fractures of the distal radius and ulna are common. Most fractures occur by a fall onto an extended arm. In this instance, the hand is fully pronated until it strikes the ground. At that moment, it is forcefully supinated and axially loaded, causing most forearm fractures. Forced pronation occurs less commonly and may cause Galeazzi's and Monteggia's fracture-dislocations. Other mechanisms include a direct blow, bending force, and axial compression.

RADIUS AND ULNAR SHAFT FRACTURES

Complete fractures of the radius and ulnar shaft are relatively common. The most common mechanism is a fall onto a pronated extended arm that is forcefully supinated upon striking the ground. Anteroposterior and lateral radiographs are necessary to establish the diagnosis. When describing these fractures, it is important to consider displacement, angulation, overlap and rotation. Rotation is the most difficult to judge. As there is very little remodeling of a rotational malunion, careful evaluation is necessary. Many methods have been described. The simplest method to ensure rotation is to anatomically align the fracture. Since this is not always possible, familiarity with the shapes of the bones in the different thirds of the forearm will provide useful information.

Treatment of these fractures depends on displacement and angulation. Closed reduction and immobilization is usually successful, especially in younger children. In children younger than 5 years of age, angulation in the plane of motion up to 20 degrees is acceptable as long as there is no loss of the interosseous space and the fracture is rotationally aligned. In children older than 10 years of age, no more than 10 degrees of angulation should be accepted, assuming that the rotational alignment and the interosseous space are maintained. Although up to 1.0 cm of overlap may be acceptable in children younger than 10 years of age, some would argue that this makes judgment of rotation impossible and should be avoided. If a fracture requires reduction, conscious sedation or general anesthesia is required. At times, traction is useful; however, it can also hinder the reduction of overlapping fragments by trapping them between periosteum under tension. In these cases, it is frequently useful to start with an exaggeration of the deformity. Once the fracture is reduced, it should be placed in a long-arm posterior or sugar-tong splint that will allow for swelling while holding the reduction. This may also be a bivalved long-arm cast. There is controversy over the position of the hand after reduction. Traditional thinking was to supinate proximal fractures and pronate distal fractures to balance the rotational muscular forces. In general, the most stable position at reduction should be chosen. This is usually a neutral position. If a satisfactory closed reduction cannot be achieved or maintained, then open reduction and internal fixation is necessary. Redisplacement is common during the next week.[36] The fracture can then be held by several methods, including plates and screws (Fig. 5) of one or both bones, depending on stability, or flexible rodding (Fig. 6).[37–39] Open fractures need appropriate débridement and management.[40]

DISTAL RADIUS AND ULNA FRACTURES
Torus Fractures

Nondisplaced compression fractures have been called "buckle," or torus, fractures. They are extremely common, particularly in young children. One or both bones may be involved. The mechanism of injury is usually axial loading during a fall onto an outstretched arm. These are low-energy injuries and usually have only mild swelling. Casting is required for 2 to 4 weeks depending on the age of the child. As long as rotation does not cause pain, a short-arm cast can be used. If pain with rotation occurs, a long-arm cast should be used for comfort. These fractures heal uneventfully.

Galeazzi's Fractures

A fracture of the distal radius in association with a dislocation of the distal radioulnar joint is termed a Galeazzi fracture.[41] The fracture is usually at the junction of the middle and distal third of the radius, although any fracture in the distal third of the radius may cause this lesion. Other variations include fractures of both the radius and ulna and segmental fractures of the radius with dislocation of the radioulnar joint. A radius fracture with a physeal fracture of the ulna is most common in children. The injury usually occurs from a fall onto an extended arm with the wrist in full pronation.

Most Galeazzi's fractures can be treated by closed reduction. After the fracture is reduced, it is immobilized in a long-arm cast in full supination for 4 to 6 weeks depending on the age of the child. The extensors can become entrapped and impede reduction, necessitating open reduction. Oblique fractures of the radius can be unstable and require

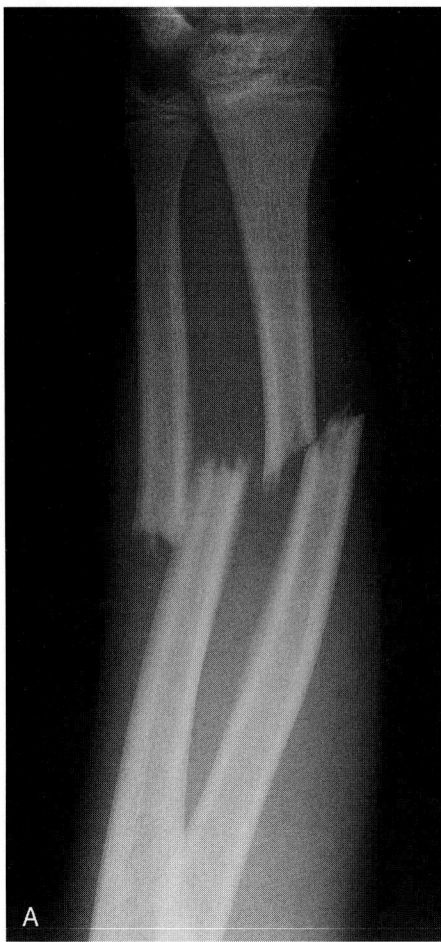
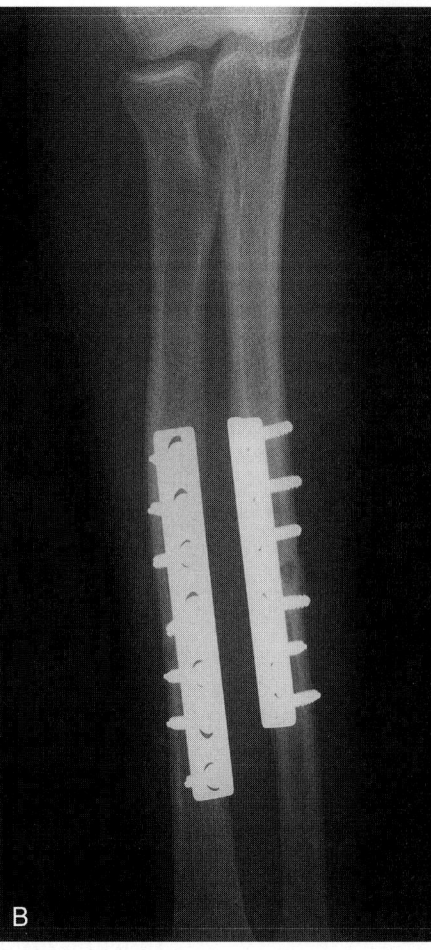

Fig. 5. Radiographs. *A*, Anteroposterior radiograph of the right forearm of a 13-year-old male with a displaced radius and ulnar shaft fracture. *B*, Repeat radiograph 2 months following open reduction and internal fixation with compression plates and screws. Anatomic alignment has been restored.

open reduction and internal pin fixation to maintain reduction.

Complications following a Galeazzi fracture are uncommon. Malunion of the radius can lead to instability and may require reconstruction.

Physeal Fractures

Physeal fractures of the distal radius are the most common growth plate injury.[1, 42] Most Salter-Harris type I fractures are nondisplaced and require a short-arm cast for 2 weeks in young children. In children 4 years of age and older, casting should be for 3 weeks. Some type I and many type II fractures are displaced. Sedation and reduction should be attempted. If alignment and rotation are acceptable, a 50% displacement can be accepted, especially in young children. This is more favorable than repeat reductions that may cause damage to the physis. Immobilization in a long-arm cast for 2 weeks followed by short-arm cast for 2 to 4 weeks is recommended until the fracture is healed. Type III fractures are less common and require internal fixation with either buttress plating or pinning. Type IV fractures are uncommon and frequently require open reduction and internal fixation. Anatomic reduction is important to avoid growth arrest. Type V fractures are rare.

Complications of all distal radius physeal fractures include loss of reduction, growth disturbance, and loss of motion. Frequent follow-up 1 and 2 weeks after reduction

should be performed. Loss of reduction during this time can easily be corrected. Loss of rotation usually involves poor reduction.

HAND FRACTURES

Hand fractures in children are common.[1–5] They usually involve the metacarpals and phalanges.[43, 44]

CARPAL FRACTURES

Carpal fractures, other than of the scaphoid, in children are rare.[45] They usually occur in adolescents approaching maturity. The scaphoid is the most commonly fractured carpal bone in children; such fractures usually occur between 10 and 15 years of age. As a general rule, carpal fractures are treated in a similar fashion to those in adults.

METACARPAL FRACTURES

Metacarpal fractures are common in children and adolescents. Fractures of the metacarpal neck are most frequent, especially of the fourth and fifth metacarpal. As much as 30 degrees of angulation can be accepted with little or no cosmetic deformity or functional impairment. The other metacarpal neck fractures require more exact reduction. Ten degrees of angulation is acceptable. Physeal fractures, usually Salter-Harris type III fractures, are uncommon and should be treated using the same guidelines. Reduction is

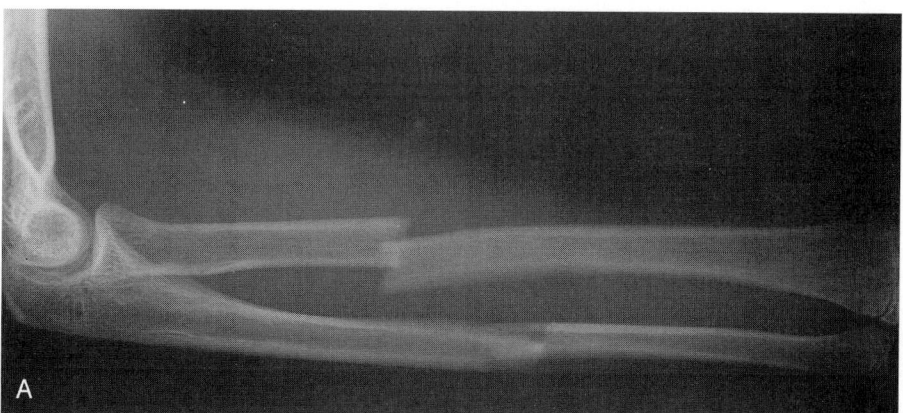

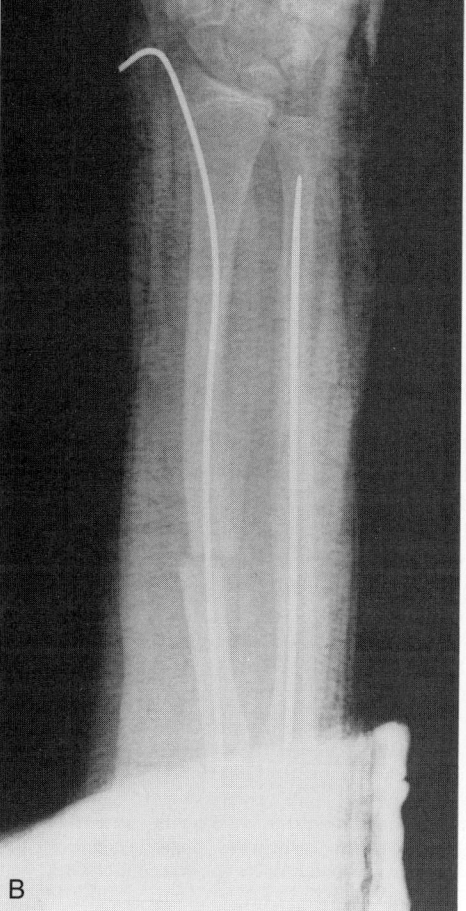
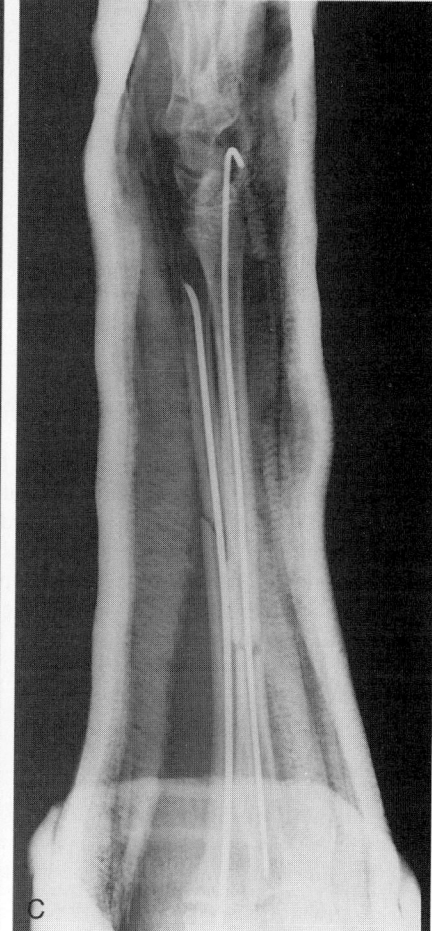

Fig. 6. Radiographs. *A,* Anteroposterior radiograph of the left forearm of an 11-year-old female with a displaced radius and ulnar shaft fracture. *B,* Repeat radiograph following closed reduction and percutaneous intramedullary fixation. Close to anatomic alignment has been restored. *C,* Lateral radiograph.

achieved by holding the metacarpophalangeal joint flexed with pressure over the convexity of the fracture. The metacarpophalangeal joint should remained flexed in the splint. If reduction cannot be maintained, percutaneous pinning may be necessary. Open reduction is rarely needed. Fractures at the base of the metacarpals rarely displace and are usually stable. When displacement occurs, closed reduction is required. Percutaneous pinning may be necessary if unstable. Three weeks of immobilization in a cast or splint is usually sufficient.

Fractures of the first metacarpal usually occur at the base (Salter-Harris type II) or just distal to the physis. These are treated by closed reduction. Up to 30 degrees of angulation in the radial direction can be accepted.

PHALANGEAL FRACTURES
Phalangeal injuries in children commonly involve the physis.[46] Displaced fractures can usually be reduced with digital blocks and manipulation. A young child may require sedation. It is important to correct rotational and angular deformities, especially in the radial and ulnar planes. Deformity in the plane of motion has a high potential for remodeling. Phalangeal fractures are splinted, usually for 2 to 3 weeks, then allowed gentle range of motion.

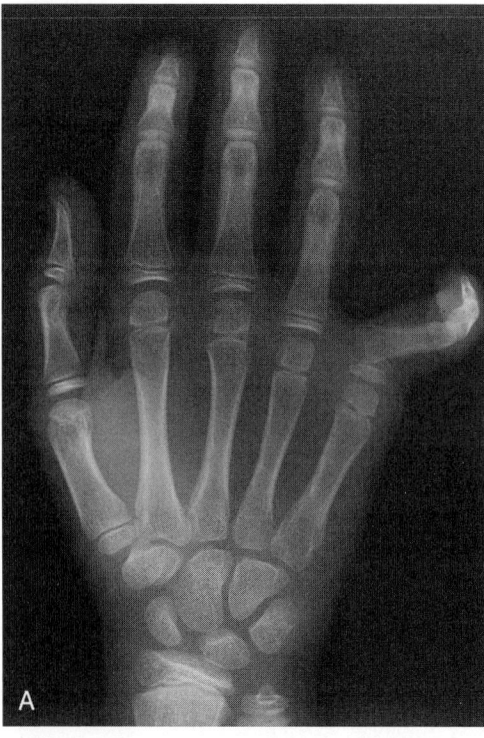

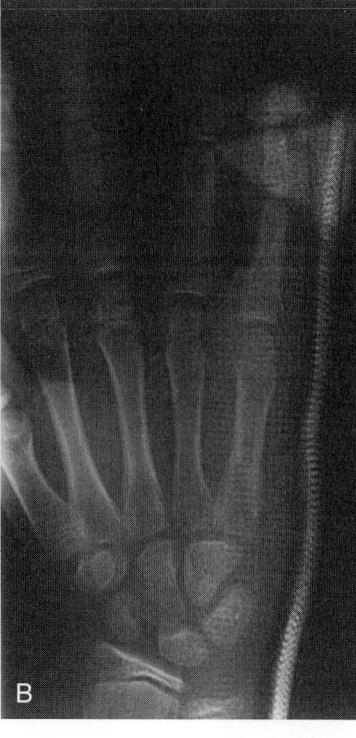

Fig. 7. Radiographs. *A,* Anteroposterior radiograph of the right hand of a 10-year-old male with an angulated Salter-Harris type II fracture of the proximal phalanx of the fifth finger. *B,* Repeat radiograph following closed reduction showing restoration of anatomic alignment.

"Buddy" taping may be useful immediately after the splint is discontinued.

Tuft fractures and Salter-Harris type I and II fractures are common in the distal phalanx. The latter can produce a mallet finger. These can usually be treated by closed reduction and splinting in extension. If the nail bed is disrupted, this is considered an open fracture. This may require surgical exploration. Fractures of the middle phalanx usually involve the body. However, distal intra-articular and proximal physeal fractures can occur. Most can be managed by closed reduction. Oblique fractures of the distal middle phalanx may require stabilization with a percutaneous pin. Fractures of the proximal phalanx are typically physeal and most are treated by closed reduction (Fig. 7). Intra-articular fractures require restoration of articular alignment, usually by open reduction and internal fixation.[44]

REFERENCES

1. Green NE, Swintkowki MF: Skeletal Trauma in Children, 2nd ed. Philadelphia, WB Saunders, 1998.
2. Letts RM: Management of Pediatric Fractures. New York, Churchill Livingstone, 1994.
3. Ogden JA: Skeletal Injury in the Child, 2nd ed. Philadelphia, WB Saunders, 1990, p 327.
4. Rockwood CA Jr, Wilkins KE, Beaty JH: Fractures in Children, 4th ed. Philadelphia, Lippincott-Raven, 1996.
5. Wilkins K: Operative Management of Upper Extremity Fractures in Children. Rosemont, IL, American Academy of Orthopaedic Surgeons, 1994.
6. Peterson CA, Peterson HA: Analysis of the incidence of injuries to the epiphyseal growth plate. J Trauma 1972; 12: 275.
7. Salter RB, Harris WR: Injuries involving the epiphyseal plate. J Bone Joint Surg 1963; 45-A:587.
8. Eidman DK, Siff SJ, Tullos HS: Acromioclavicular lesions in children. Am J Sports Med 1981; 9:150.
9. Berringer DC, Weiner DS, Noble JS, et al: Severely displaced proximal humeral epiphyseal fractures. J Pediatr Orthop 1998; 18:31.
10. Beaty JH: Fractures of the proximal humerus and shaft in children. In Eilert RE, ed: AAOS Instructional Course Lectures. Rosemont, IL: American Academy of Orthopaedics, 1992; 41:369.
11. Shaw JL, Sakellarides H: Radial-nerve paralysis associated with fractures of the humerus: A review of 45 cases. J Bone Joint Surg Am 1967; 49:899.
12. Campbell CC, Waters PM, Emans JB, et al: Neurovascular injury and displacement in type III supracondylar fractures. J Pediatr Orthop 1995; 15:47.
13. Brown IC, Zinar DM: Traumatic and iatrogenic neurologic complications after supracondylar humerus fractures in children. J Pediatr Orthop 1995; 15:440.
14. Sabharwal S, Tredwell SJ, Beauchamp RD, et al: Management of pulseless pink hand in pediatric supracondylar fractures of the humerus. J Pediatr Orthop 1997; 17:303.
15. Pirone AM, Graham HK, Krajbich JI: Management of displaced extension-type supracondylar fractures of humerus in children. J Bone Joint Surg Am 1988; 70: 641.
16. Archibeck M.J, Scott SM, Peters CL: Brachialis muscle entrapment in displaced supracondylar humerus fractures. J Pediatr Orthop 1992; 17:298.
17. Zoints LE, McKellop HA, Hathaway R: Torsional strength of pin configurations used to fix supracondylar fractures of the humerus in children. J Bone Joint Surg Am 1994; 76:253.
18. Lyons JP, Ashley E, Hoffer MM: Ulnar nerve palsies after percutaneous cross-pinning of supracondylar fractures in children's elbow. J Pediatr Orthop 1998; 18: 43.
19. DeLee JC, Wilkins KE, Rogers LF, et al: Fracture-separation of the distal humeral epiphysis. J Bone Joint Surg Am 1980; 62:46.
20. Holda ME, Manoli A, LaMont RL: Epiphyseal separation of the distal end of the humerus with medial displacement. J Bone Joint Surg Am 1980; 62:52.
21. Mirsky EC, Karas EH, Weiner LS: Lateral condyle fractures in children: Evaluation

of classification and treatment. J Orthop Trauma 1997; 11:117.

22. Milch H: Fractures and fracture dislocations of the humeral condyles. J Trauma 1964; 4:592.
23. Jakob R, Fowles JV, Rang M, et al: Observations concerning fractures of the lateral humeral condyles in children. J Bone Joint Surg Br 1975; 57:430.
24. Mintzer CM, Waters PM, Brown DJ, et al: Percutaneous pinning in the treatment of displaced lateral condyle fractures. J Pediatr Orthop 1994; 14:462.
25. Davidson RS, Markowitz RJ, Dormans J, et al: Ultrasonographic evaluation of the elbow in infants and young children after suspected trauma. J Bone Joint Surg Am 1994; 76:1804.
26. Fowles JV, Slimane N, Kassab MT: Elbow dislocation with avulsion of the medial humeral epicondyle. J Bone Joint Surg Br 1990; 72:102.
27. Kilfoyle RM: Fractures of the medial condyle and epicondyle of the elbow in children. Clin Orthop 1965; 41:43.
28. Papavasiliou V, Nenopoulos S, Venturis T: Fractures of the medial condyle of the humerus in childhood. J Pediatr Orthop 1987; 7:421.
29. Bernstein SM, McKeever P, Bernstein L: Percutaneous reduction of displaced radial

neck fractures in children. J Pediatr Orthop 1993; 13:85.
30. D'Souza S, Vaishya R, Klenerman L: Management of radial neck fractures in children: A retrospective analysis of one hundred patients. J Pediatr Orthop 1993; 13:232.
31. Steele JA, Graham HK: Angulated radial neck fractures in children: A prospective study of percutaneous reduction. J Bone Joint Surg Br 1992; 74:760.
32. Gonzalez-Herranz P, Alvarez-Romara A, Burgos J, et al: Displaced radial neck fractures in children treated by closed intramedullary pinning (Metaizeau technique). J Pediatr Orthop 1997; 17:325.
33. Gaddy BC, Strecker WB, Schoenecker PL: Surgical treatment of displaced olecranon fractures in children. J Pediatr Orthop 1997; 17:321.
34. Bado JL: The Monteggia lesion. Clin Orthop 1967; 50:71.
35. Olney BW, Menelaus MB: Monteggia and equivalent lesions in childhood. J Pediatr Orthop 1989; 9:219.
36. Voto SJ, Weiner DS, Leighley B: Redisplacement after closed reduction of forearm fractures in children. J Pediatr Orthop 1990; 10:79.
37. Wyrsch B, Mencio GA, Green NE: Open reduction and internal fixation of pediatric

forearm fractures. J Pediatr Orthop 1996; 16:644.
38. Flynn JM, Waters PM: Single bone fixation of both bone forearm fractures. J Pediatr Orthop 1996; 16:655.
39. Vanderreis WL, Otsuka NY, Moroz P, et al: Intramedullary nailing vs. plate fixation for unstable forearm fractures in children. J Pediatr Orthop 1998; 18:9.
40. Haasbeek JF, Cole WG: Open fractures of the arm in children. J Bone Joint Surg 1995; 77-B:576.
41. Letts M, Rowhani H: Galeazzi equivalent injuries of the wrist in children. J Pediatr Orthop 1993; 13:561.
42. Lee BS, Esterhai JL, Das M: Fracture of the distal radius epiphysis. Clin Orthop 1984; 185:90.
43. Campbell RM Jr: Operative treatment of fractures and dislocations of the hand and wrist region in children. Orthop Clin North Am 1990; 21:217.
44. Hastings H II, Simmons BP: Hand fractures in children. Clin Orthop 1984; 188: 120.
45. Christodoulou AG, Colton CL: Scaphoid fractures in children. J Pediatr Orthop 1986; 6:37.
46. Leonard MH, Dabravcik P: Management of fractured fingers in the child. Clin Orthop 1970; 73:160.

section 3
chapter
26

LOWER EXTREMITY

Peter F. Sturm

Summary

- Lower extremity fractures are extremely common.
- A thickened periosteum with increased osteogenic potential and actively growing physis makes children's bone distinctly different from adults' bone.
- Many fractures can be treated nonoperatively and remodeling is common.
- Physeal fractures may lead to longitudinal and angular growth disturbances.
- Treatment protocols are based on the location of the fracture, the mechanism of the injury, and the age of the child.

Lower extremity injuries in children are exceedingly common. Dislocations and ligamentous injuries are unusual, with forces much more likely to be concentrated through the physis or bone. The mechanisms of injury range from trivial falls (toddler fractures), to severe trauma.

Growing bone is distinctly different from mature adult bone. A much more dynamic situation exists. Longitudinal growth occurs from the physis. Especially in younger children, the periosteum is thickened, exhibiting markedly increased osteogenic potential. Nonunions are extremely un-

common in children's fractures. Remodeling frequently can be expected, especially if the deformity is in the plane of motion. Because of the increased elasticity of young bone, incomplete failure is common, resulting in torus and greenstick fractures.

Physeal fractures present a different set of considerations. Injuries to the physis can cause significant long-term sequelae. Growth disturbances, both longitudinal and angular, may occur. Depending on the child's age, these may progressively worsen over time.

A thorough understanding of the biological and mechanical differences of growing bone is necessary before treatment of these fractures can be undertaken. In an attempt to give some clarity to a rather wide range of fractures, this chapter is organized into four sections: (1) hip fractures, (2) femur fractures, (3) injuries about the knee, and (4) tibial shaft, ankle, and foot injuries.

HIP FRACTURES

Hip fractures are uncommon in children, accounting for less than 1% of all pediatric fractures.[1] They have historically been associated with a high incidence rate of disabling sequelae, however, with the reported incidence being as high as 60%.[2, 3] Newer treatment methods have been

TABLE 1. DELBET CLASSIFICATION

Type	Fracture Location
I	Transepiphyseal
II	Transcervical
III	Cervicotrochanteric
IV	Intertrochanteric

successful in reducing some of these complications.[4, 5] Unlike adults, in whom an underlying pathological process (osteoporosis) makes the femoral neck vulnerable to fracture, significant trauma is required to cause this injury in children. Severe, high-velocity trauma has been implicated in 85% of all injuries.[3, 4]

CLINICAL FEATURES

Children with hip fractures are usually seen in an emergency setting after having been involved in high-velocity trauma. The hip is exceedingly painful and the extremity is shortened and externally rotated. In intertrochanteric fractures, external rotation may not be present. The anatomy and blood supply of the child's hip are distinctive and have a significant impact on complications associated with these injuries. The single physis, which is present at birth, becomes two separate centers, the capital epiphysis with its physis, and the trochanteric apophysis. The capital femoral epiphysis ossifies between the ages of 4 and 6 months, and the trochanteric apophysis at 4 years of age. Between birth and 4 years of age, the blood supply to the head is derived from metaphyseal vessels that arise from the medial and lateral circumflex arteries. After the age of 4, the main blood supply comes from the posterosuperior and posteroinferior retinacular branches of the medial circumflex artery. The metaphyseal contribution becomes insignificant and no clinically important anastomosis exists.[6, 7]

Femoral neck fractures are classified according to the system proposed by Delbet[8] (Table 1). Type I is a transepiphyseal separation with or without dislocation of the femoral head. This is the least common fracture and is usually seen in younger children than the subsequent types. Type II fractures are transcervical. This is the most common type, accounting for approximately 50% of all pediatric hip fractures.[2] Type III fractures are cervicotrochanteric. Type IV are intertrochanteric fractures. The classification is extremely important, as treatment methods and long-term results correlate with fracture location.

INVESTIGATION

Plain radiographs are sufficient to establish the diagnosis of a hip fracture. An anteroposterior view of the pelvis and a cross-table lateral view of the involved hip should be obtained. A technetium bone scan may be helpful later in the course of treatment to document the extent of avascular necrosis (see Complications).

TREATMENT GOALS, INDICATIONS, AND CONTRAINDICATIONS

Treatment is aimed at achieving a stable anatomic reduction by either closed or open means. Internal fixation is usually required to maintain the reduction, and external immobilization (spica cast) is frequently needed as well, especially in younger children. Specific treatment protocols are based on fracture classification (Delbet), whether or not there is displacement, and the age of the child (Table 2).

PROCEDURE
Preoperative Planning

The proximal femoral physis accounts for 15% of the overall growth of the lower extremity. In younger children, every effort should be made to stop internal fixation short of the physis. Unlike in adults, the bone of the femoral neck is not osteoporotic, and good fixation can be obtained even without crossing the physis.

Technical Details

The treatment approach is determined by the fracture classification. In type I fractures without dislocation of the femoral epiphysis, an attempt at closed reduction using traction, abduction, and internal rotation should be made. If this is unsuccessful, an anterior approach should be used to achieve reduction. In children younger than 2 years of age, these reductions are usually stable and a spica cast alone is sufficient for immobilization. In children older than 2 years of age, internal fixation will be required. Obviously, the fixation will need to cross the physis. In those patients with sufficient growth remaining, two smooth Kirschner's wires into the femoral head should be used. The pins can then be bent down and held onto the femur with a semitubular plate. This should be supplemented with a spica cast. In older children and adolescents who do not have significant growth remaining, cannulated screws may be used across the physis.

In type I fractures with dislocation of the femoral head, an open reduction followed by internal fixation and external immobilization should be performed. Anterior dislocations should be approached anteriorly. A posterior approach should be used for posterior dislocation.

In type II and type III fractures, an attempt at closed reduction via longitudinal traction should be made. If this is unsuccessful, an open reduction via an anterior or anterolateral approach is used. Internal fixation should consist of cannulated screws. Ideally two screws should be used, but owing to the narrow diameter of the neck in younger chil-

TABLE 2. FRACTURE TREATMENT BY DELBET TYPE

Fracture Type	Treatment
I	Closed/open reduction Internal fixation >2 years Spica cast <2 years
I (dislocation)	Open reduction Internal fixation
II/III	Closed/open reduction Internal fixation Single-leg spica cast (children) No external immobilization (adolescents)
IV	Traction/spica cast <8 years Closed/open reduction Internal fixation >8 years

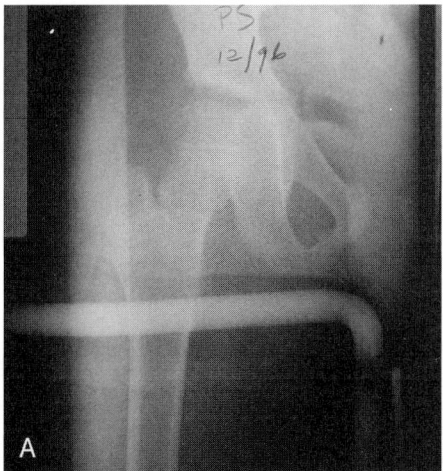

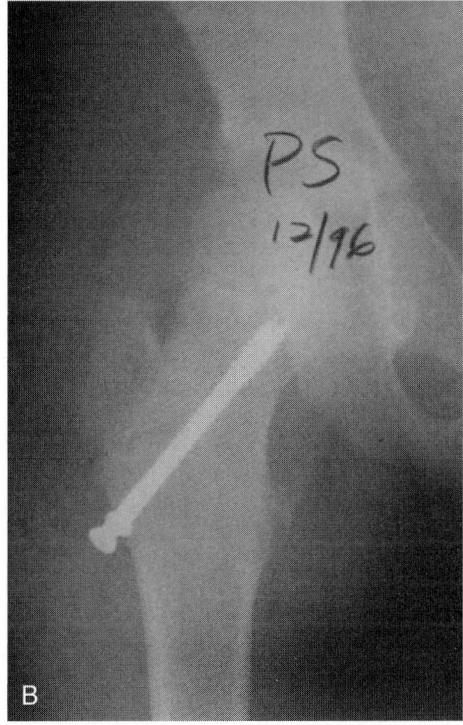

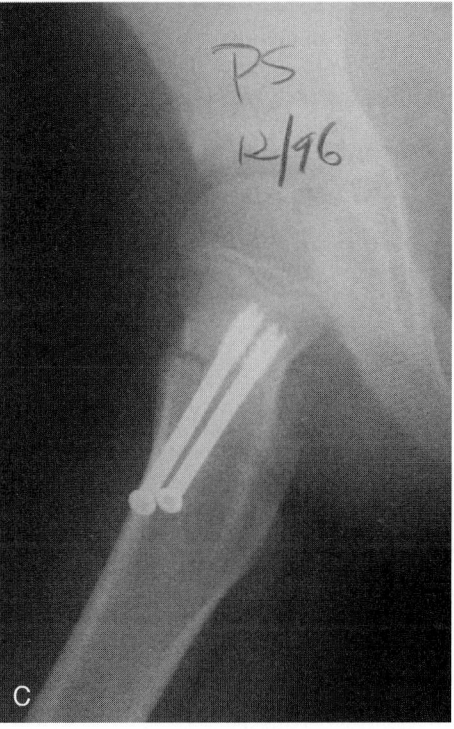

Fig. 1. Radiographs. This is a 7-year-old female with a type II transcervical hip fracture sustained in a motor accident. *A,* Anteroposterior radiography showing minimally displaced type II fracture. *B* and *C,* Anteroposterior and lateral radiograph after closed reduction and fixation with two 4.5 mm cannulated screws.

dren, this is not always possible. In younger children, 4.5 mm screws are sufficient (Fig. 1). In older children and adolescents, 6.5 mm screws are appropriate. Except in adolescents, external immobilization consisting of a single-leg spica cast is added. In type II fractures, there is some evidence that early evacuation of the capsular hematoma by either capsulotomy or aspiration may decrease the risk of avascular necrosis.[9] This remains controversial, and the author does not routinely aspirate the hematoma. Nondisplaced fractures can be managed in a spica cast alone, although because of the risk of late displacement and coxa vara, internal fixation should still be considered.

In children less than 8 years of age, stable reductions can be obtained in type IV fractures with traction followed by spica casting with the leg abducted. In children older than 8 years, an open reduction with fixation with a screw and sideplate is warranted. These come in pediatric and intermediate as well as adult sizes. Again, all attempts should be made to stop short of the physis in children with significant growth remaining.

COMPLICATIONS

The complication rate associated with femoral neck fractures in children is exceedingly high.[3, 4] Avascular necrosis (AVN) is the most common and feared complication, occurring in 31% of all fractures.[3] It is associated with a poor outcome in a large percentage of cases.[5] Unfortunately, the development of AVN is directly related to the fracture type, degree of displacement, and the age of the patient (more common in children older than 10 years) (Table 3). Its occurrence appears to be unaffected by the type of treatment. Radiographic signs and clinical symptoms may appear as early as 6 weeks after injury. A technetium bone scan will show the extent of head involvement early on.

TABLE 3. INCIDENCE OF AVASCULAR NECROSIS (AVN) BY DELBET FRACTURE TYPE	
Fracture Type	% AVN
I	100
II	50
III	25
IV	Minimal

Once AVN is established, there is little evidence that any treatment will alter the natural history.[10]

Premature physeal closure occurs in 28% of patients.[3] The incidence is higher in patients who have internal fixation that crosses the physis, although it has been reported in patients who had external immobilization alone[5] and in patients whose fixation did not penetrate the growth plate.[2] Because the proximal femoral physis contributes only 15% to the overall length of the extremity, severe shortening is a problem only in extremely young children.

Coxa vara has been reported in 19% of patients with femoral neck fractures.[3] Its incidence can be lowered by the use of internal fixation.[4, 5] Although it can lead to relative abductor weakness, a Trendelenburg gait, and potential degenerative joint disease, its occurrence alone has not necessarily been linked to poor results.[5]

Nonunion is extremely unusual.[3] Its incidence is effectively decreased by the use of stable internal fixation.

RESULTS AND OUTCOMES

Results are based on fracture type and displacement. Type I fractures have uniformly poor results, whereas the sequelae of type IV fractures are minimal. At long-term follow-up, Leung and Lam[11] found that 24% of patients had pain, a limp, or significant shortening of the extremity. Radiographic abnormalities occurred in 83% of patients.

FEMORAL SHAFT FRACTURES

Fractures of the femoral shaft are among the most common pediatric injuries requiring hospital admission. The pathogenesis of the injury varies widely depending on the age of the patient. High-speed trauma is the usual cause of injury in children over 6 years of age, with motor vehicle accidents and pedestrians struck by vehicles predominating. Associated head, intra-abdominal, and other skeletal injuries must be carefully looked for. In children younger than 1 year of age, child abuse must be suspected. Beals reported an incidence rate of 70% in his series.[12] In the 1- to 6-year-old age group, moderate trauma during normal play is most often implicated. Pathological fractures may occur. Underlying causes such as unicameral bone cysts, fibrous dysplasia, and osteogenesis imperfecta must be kept in mind. Healing readily occurs in all age groups. Significant complications are rare. Multiple treatment options are available.

CLINICAL FEATURES

The child will present with severe pain and deformity. In subtrochanteric fractures, the proximal fragment will be flexed, abducted, and externally rotated. In children under 1 year of age, child abuse must be strongly suspected. If there is a history of minor trauma in older children, a pathological lesion must be looked for.

INVESTIGATION

Plain anteroposterior and lateral radiographs are all that is needed to make a diagnosis and plan treatment.

TREATMENT GOALS, INDICATIONS, AND CONTRAINDICATIONS

The goal of treatment in femoral shaft fractures is to achieve union with acceptable length and alignment. Treatment guidelines are based on the patient's age, fracture pattern, the presence or absence of associated injuries, and social circumstances. Because of concerns about health care costs in the current medical environment, there has been a strong push to shorten hospitalization time. This has had a significant influence on the treatment of these fractures.

Immediate casting with a spica cast is the treatment of choice for children younger than 8 years of age. This should be done in the operating room at the earliest, safest, and most convenient time. If overnight admission is required prior to casting, the child can be kept comfortable in skin traction with 5 to 10 lb of weight until a cast is placed. Children younger than 2 years of age should be placed in a double spica cast. A one and a half spica with a bar between the legs should be applied in children older than 2 years of age. The author's preferred casting method is as follows[7]: After induction of anesthesia, a short-leg well-padded cast is placed while the child is still in bed. While traction is applied, the cast is extended to a long-leg with the knee in 70 to 90 degrees of flexion. A valgus mold is placed to achieve reduction. The child is then transferred to a spica table while the cast is completed, with continued gentle traction applied (Fig. 2). Plain radiographs are obtained prior to waking the patient and alteration of the cast is then done if necessary. Alignment is deemed acceptable if less than 5 degrees of varus and 15 degrees of valgus is present. The fragments should be overlapped. Shortening of 1.5 cm is optimal, as this will compensate for expected overgrowth.[14]

Weekly follow-up radiographs should be obtained for the first 2 to 3 weeks, as this is the time when shortening and angulation are most likely to occur. Greater than 2 cm of shortening should not be accepted. The cast should be kept on for 4 to 6 weeks depending on the age of the child. Excellent results have been reported using this method.[15-17] Cost savings as compared to traction followed by casting has been shown to be substantial.[15, 18] There is some controversy as to whether fractures with greater than 2 cm of initial shortening should be treated in this manner, although reasonable results have been reported.[16] It is the author's opinion that the advantages of this method are such that even in this circumstance, an attempt at spica casting is worthwhile. If unacceptable shortening is noted, the cast can be removed and the child placed in traction at that time. The only real contraindications to this treatment method are multiple trauma and significant soft tissue injuries. If traction is used for management, a distal femoral pin should be placed under fluoroscopic control in the operating room. Great care should be taken to avoid the

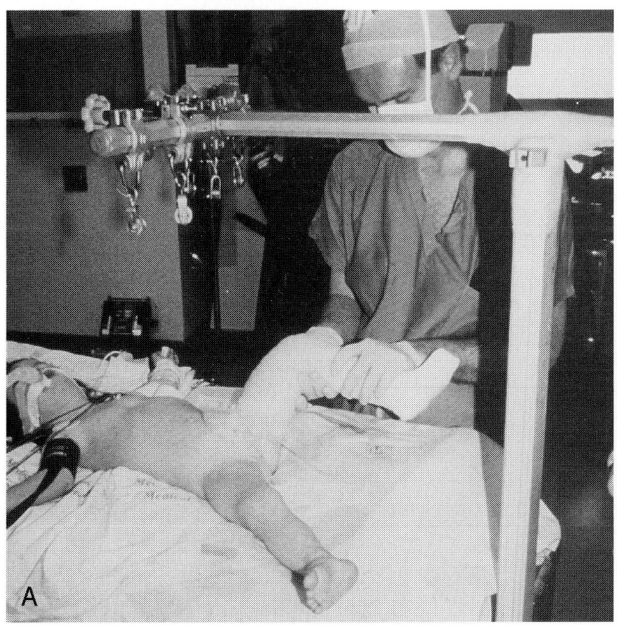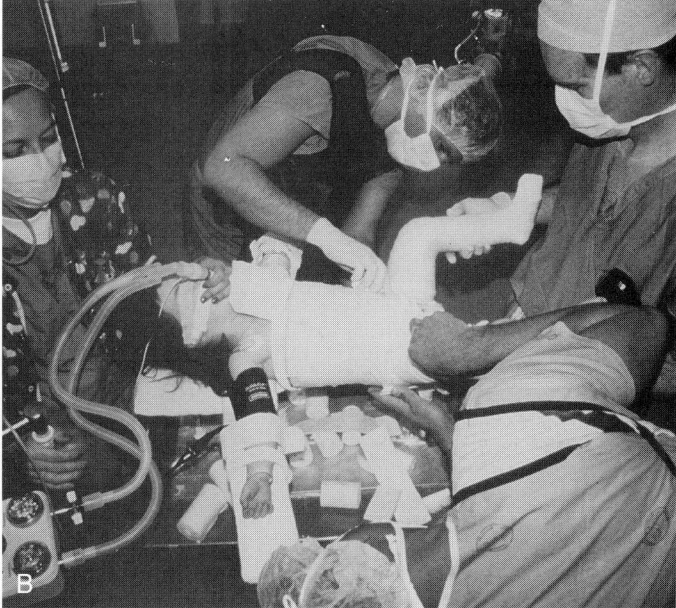

Fig. 2. Application of spica cast. *A,* Long-leg portion of cast being applied with patient in bed. *B,* Patient transferred to spica table for completion of cast. (From Buckley SL: Current trends in the treatment of femoral shaft fractures in children and adolescents. Clin Orthop 1997; 338:60.)

distal femoral growth plate. The child should then be placed in 90/90 traction.

Treatment remains somewhat controversial in the 8- to 12-year-old age group. The traditional method of treatment has been 90/90 traction for 2 to 3 weeks, followed by spica casting. Good results have been reported.[19] The technique does require frequent radiographs, adjustment in traction, and prolonged hospitalization. The financial cost is high,[18] and the patient must spend 6 to 8 weeks in bed. This will also require home tutoring and, in this age of two-career families and single-parent households, a signifi-

cant amount of missed parental work. In addition, in children older than 10 years of age, the incidence of shortening and angulation has been found to be unacceptable.[19, 20]

Surgical treatment in this age group offers a reasonable alternative to traction and casting. Primary indications formerly included polytrauma, severe associated head injuries, and open fractures.[21] More recently, the indications have been expanded to isolated femoral shaft fractures. Good results have been reported with external fixation,[22] flexible intramedullary nails,[23] and compression plating (Fig. 3).[21, 24] Each treatment method has its advantages and disadvan-

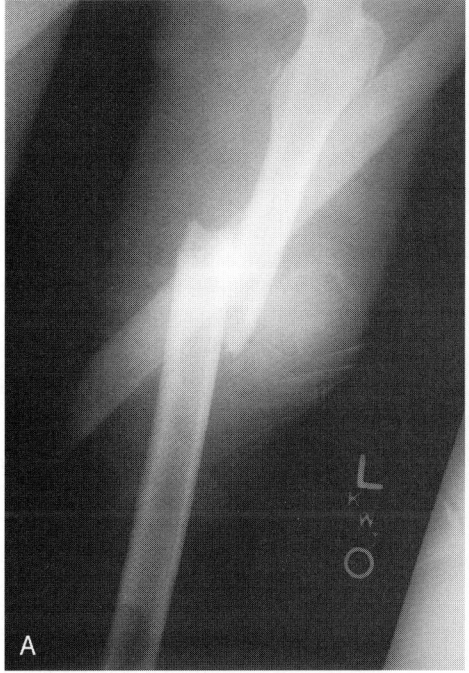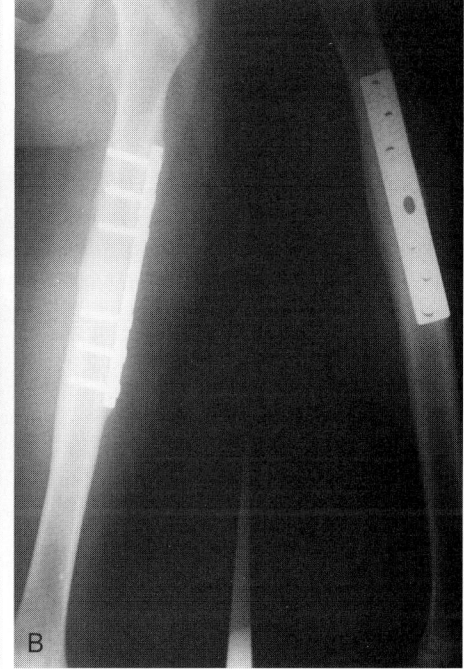

Fig. 3. An isolated left femur fracture in an 11-year-old girl struck by a car. *A,* AP radiograph at the time of injury. *B,* AP and lateral radiograph 6 months after open reduction and internal fixation with a 7-hole 4.5 mm plate. (From Rockwood CA: Fractures in children. J Pediatr Orthop.)

Age (years)	Operative Treatment	Contraindications	Postoperative Treatment	Results
<8	Immediate spica	Multiple injuries Severe soft tissue injury	Bedrest	Good—excellent
8–12	90/90 traction spica cast		Bedrest	Good—excellent Shortening Angulation in children >10 years
	Flexible IM rods		PWB crutches	Good—excellent Occasional rotational malalignment
	External fixation		PWB crutches	Good—excellent Occasional pin site infections
	Compression plating		NWB crutches	Good—excellent Occasional hardware failure
>12	IM rod		WB crutches	Good—excellent Occasional AVN

TABLE 4. TREATMENT OF FEMORAL SHAFT FRACTURES

AVN, avascular necrosis; IM, intramedullary; NWB, non-weightbearing; PWB, partial weightbearing; WB, weightbearing.

tages, and they all allow early mobilization with protected weightbearing and shorter hospitalization. In our study using compression plates, the average hospital stay for isolated femoral shaft fractures was 3.3 days.[24]

Treatment in the 12-year-old and older age group is similar to treatment in adults. Intramedullary rodding is the method of choice. Excellent results have been reported.[25] The potential for AVN secondary to rod placement is a real concern.[25] Rods should not be placed in the piriformis fossa in adolescents to avoid damage to the posterosuperior retinacular branch of the medial circumflex artery. The starting point should be lateralized to the greater trochanter. This tends to aim the guide wire and rod toward the medial cortex. The surgeon must make a conscious effort to adduct the hand as much as possible as the guide wire and rod are being passed. Rods are now available in 8 and 9 mm diameters to fit the smaller canals in this age group (Table 4).

COMPLICATIONS

Complications in the treatment of femoral shaft fracture are unusual. Malunion and shortening are the most common, although significant problems are unusual no matter what

treatment is used. Less than 10 degrees of varus, 15 degrees of valgus, and 20 degrees of anterior or posterior bowing will all tend to remodel with growth. Rotational malalignment does occur but does not appear to be problematic. AVN can occur in adolescents who undergo intramedullary rodding (Table 5).

INJURIES AROUND THE KNEE

The pattern of injury around the knee in children differs significantly from that in adults. While the incidence of ligamentous injuries in adolescents has increased (especially in girls), physeal fractures are much more common. Because ligaments of the knee arise from the epiphysis of the distal femur, the proximal tibia, and the proximal fibula, stresses across the knee joint tend to be concentrated in the open physes (Table 6).

The distal femoral physis accounts for 70% of the growth of the femur and 37% of the growth of the lower extremity.[26] It contributes approximately 1 cm of growth per year. The proximal tibial physis accounts for 53% of the length of the tibia and 25% of the length of the lower extremity and contributes approximately 0.66 cm growth per year.[26] Obviously, damage to either growth plate will have significant long-term sequelae, especially in younger children.

The anatomic relationship of the neurovascular structures around the knee must also be kept in mind. The popliteal artery is adjacent to the posterior surface of the proximal tibial epiphysis. It is tethered by the anterior tibial artery

TABLE 5. COMPLICATIONS IN TREATMENT FEMORAL SHAFT FRACTURES

Complication	Association	Avoidance
Shortening	Spica cast, 90/90 traction	>2 cm shortening unacceptable at any time in treatment
Malunion	Spica cast, 90/90 traction	>10 varus >10 valgus >20 anteroposterior
Avascular necrosis	Intramedullary rods	Avoid piriformis fossa
Hardware failure	Compression plates	Avoid early weight-bearing
Pin site infection	External fixation	Meticulous pin care

TABLE 6. INJURIES AROUND THE KNEE IN CHILDREN

Distal femoral physeal fractures
Proximal tibial physeal fractures
Tibial tubercle fractures
Patella sleeve fractures
Osteochondral fractures
Tibial eminence fractures
Ligamentous/meniscal injuries

running forward to the interosseous membrane and the posterior tibial artery passing under the soleus. The artery is potentially at risk when an injury is caused by sufficient force.

PATHOGENESIS

The type of injury seen is based on both the mechanism and the age of the child. The periosteum is thicker in younger children than in adolescents. Consequently, in younger children, significant trauma is required to produce a fracture, and motor vehicle accidents predominate as the cause of such injuries. In older children and adolescents, many injuries occur during sports activities.

Hyperextension is the usual mechanism of injury in distal femoral and proximal tibial physeal fractures. Tibial tuberosity fractures are thought to occur as a result of a flexion force against a contracted quadriceps. These occur in adolescents at a time of major histological change in the structure of the distal portion of the tubercle.[27] Finally, anterior cruciate ligament tears and tibial eminence fractures are caused by external rotation and deceleration forces.

CLINICAL FEATURES

A careful physical examination will help differentiate the area of involvement. Swelling and tenderness may be diffuse or may be localized to the level of the physis. Gross deformity will exist with a displaced distal femoral or proximal tibial physeal fracture. In these cases, pulses should be carefully palpated, as displaced proximal tibial fractures can be associated with popliteal artery compromise. Marked fullness over the tibial tubercle is suggestive of a fracture at this level. Inability to extend the knee will be present in displaced patella fractures. Patients with anterior cruciate injuries and tibial eminence fractures will have a positive finding on Lachman and anterior drawer tests. Varus and valgus instability is more suggestive of a distal femoral physeal fracture than a collateral ligament tear in children with open physis, especially in younger age groups.

INVESTIGATION

Plain anteroposterior and lateral radiographs will identify most bony injuries about the knee. In cases of suspected Salter-Harris fractures of the distal femur and proximal tibia, varus and valgus stress films may be necessary. Arteriograms are indicated in children with a displaced proximal tibial epiphysis if the pulse is absent or the foot is cool and pale. A magnetic resonance imaging scan may be helpful in confirming suspected meniscal or ligamentous injury.

TREATMENT GOALS, INDICATIONS, AND CONTRAINDICATIONS

Treatment is very much dependent on the location of the injury and the age of the child (Table 7). In fractures involving the femoral or tibial physis, accurate anatomic alignment is mandatory. Salter-Harris fractures of the distal femur can be treated with closed reduction. Traction should be the major component of the reduction maneuver.[28] If there is any question of instability, crossed smooth pins across the fracture may be used. In Salter-Harris fractures

with a large metaphyseal fragment, 4.0 or 6.5 mm cannulated screws placed transversely across the metaphyseal fragment should be considered (Fig. 4). In Salter-Harris fractures, open reduction is required. Fixation again may consist of crossed smooth pins or transversely placed cannulated screws.

Closed reduction can usually be used in Salter-Harris fractures of the proximal tibia. Crossed smooth pins should be used if there is a question of stability. An attempt at closed reduction should be made in Salter-Harris injuries, but open reduction may be necessary

The treatment of tibial tubercle fractures depends on their classification. In type I fractures, in which only the distal portion of the tubercle is involved, closed reduction with casting in extension usually suffices. In type II fractures in which the fracture runs to the junction of the tuberosity and the physis, and in type III fractures in which the fracture crosses the epiphysis into the articular surface, open reduction and fixation with a screw across the tibial tubercle into the metaphysis is required. Genu recurvatum does not occur, as these fractures occur in children close to the end of growth.

Tibial eminence fractures are also treated based on their classification. Type I and II fractures, nondisplaced and hinged, respectively, can be treated with casting in extension. Conscious sedation may be required to achieve full extension due to hamstring spasm. Type III, completely displaced fractures should be treated with either open fixation or arthroscopically, the fragment held down with either a suture or a screw. The physis should not be crossed with the fixation in younger children.

Anterior cruciate ligament reconstruction is dependent on the level of skeletal maturity of the child. The physis should be avoided in younger children. The results of extra-articular repairs are poor.[29]

TABLE 7. TREATMENT OF INJURIES AROUND THE KNEE	
Type	**Treatment**
Distal femoral physeal	Closed reduction
Salter-Harris	Smooth crossed pins if unstable
Salter-Harris	Closed reduction
	Smooth crossed pins
	Metaphyseal cannulated screw
Salter-Harris	Open reduction
	Crossed smooth pins or transverse screws
Proximal tibial physeal	Closed reduction
Salter-Harris	Crossed pins if unstable
Salter-Harris	Closed/open reduction
	Crossed pins if unstable or transverse screws
Patella sleeve	Tension band wiring
Tibial tubercle	Closed reduction
Type I	Casting in extension
Type II, III	Open reduction
	Screw fixation
Tibial eminence	Closed reduction
Type I, II	Casting in extension
Type III	Open/arthroscopic reduction
	Suture/screw fixation

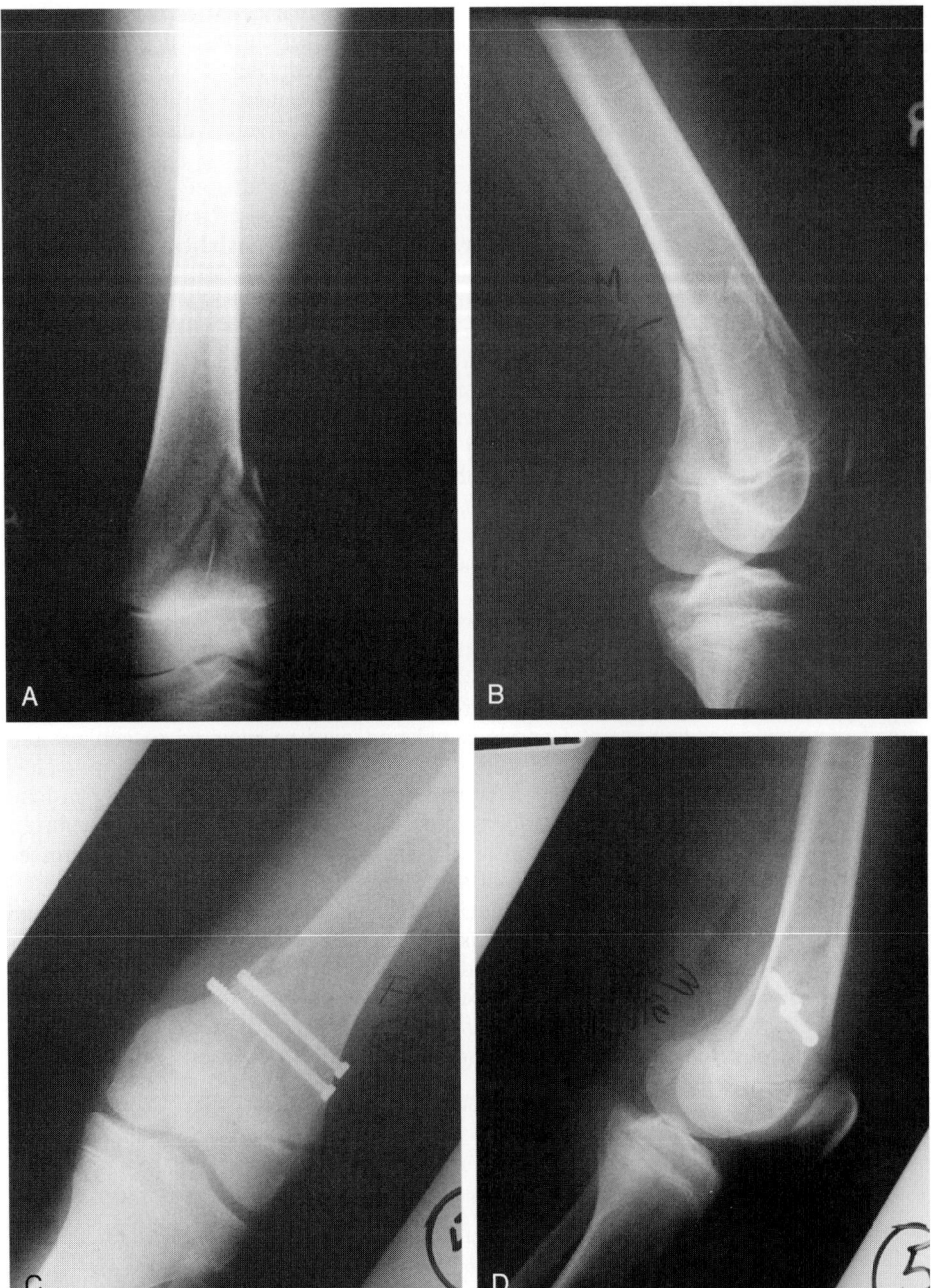

Fig. 4. Radiographs. This is a 13-year-old male with a Salter-Harris type II fracture of his distal femur sustained when his bicycle was struck by a car. *A* and *B*, Anteroposterior and lateral radiographs showing slightly displaced Salter-Harris II fracture. *C* and *D*, Anteroposterior and lateral radiographs after closed reduction and fixation with two cannulated screws.

COMPLICATIONS

The anatomy of the distal femoral physis is distinctive. It is characterized by a series of undulations and four separate mammillary bodies. Owing to this arrangement, the rate of growth arrest after distal femoral physeal fractures is extremely high. Riseborough et al[30] reported a 56% incidence of leg length discrepancy and a 26% incidence of angular deformity in their series. Unfortunately, the prognosis is not dependent on the Salter-Harris grade of the fracture, but rather on the amount of displacement.[31] Even anatomic reduction does not guarantee a good result, and families must be informed of the high risk of long-term problems.

Similarly, in proximal tibial physeal fractures, angular deformity and leg length discrepancy have been reported even in Salter-Harris fractures.[32, 33] In addition, the risks of vascular injury and compartment syndrome, while small, are real, and the treating surgeon must have a high index of suspicion.

Complications in the treatment of tibial tuberosity and tibial eminence fractures are unusual. Fixation crossing the physis in tibial eminence fractures can lead to premature growth arrest in young children. Anterior cruciate ligament laxity is common after type III fractures no matter what type of treatment is used, but it is rarely symptomatic.[34]

TABLE 8. TIBIA/ANKLE/FOOT INJURIES IN CHILDREN
Tibial metaphyseal
Tibial diaphyseal
Greenstick
Complete
Tibia isolated
Tibia with fibula
Open
Tibial physeal
Transitional fractures
Juvenile Tillaux
Triplane
Talus
Calcaneus
Metatarsal
Midfoot

TIBIA, ANKLE, AND FOOT FRACTURES

Injuries to the lower leg and foot are extremely common in children. In younger children, thickened periosteum and excellent remodeling potential usually allow for adequate closed treatment. Injuries involving the physis at the distal tibia carry the possibility of growth arrest, and anatomic reduction is important. Fracture patterns in older adolescents are similar to those in adults and usually should be treated in a similar fashion (Table 8).

PATHOGENESIS

The mechanism of these injuries varies from simple falls (toddler fractures) to sports injuries, to high-velocity trauma (open tibia, talus). Lawn mower injuries can be a treatment nightmare. In these injuries, fractures are usually associated with severe soft tissue injuries and massive wound contamination. Aggressive treatment of these injuries is a necessity.

INVESTIGATION

Plain radiographs are sufficient to identify most tibial diaphyseal and foot injuries. Technetium bone scans may help diagnose stress fractures of the tibial shaft or foot (metatarsals, calcaneus) in young athletes.

The role of bone scans in toddler fractures is somewhat controversial. Toddler fracture should always be considered in children under 4 years of age who present with a limp, even if no definitive history of trauma can be elicited. Plain radiographic films are usually diagnostic. Treatment should consist of a long-leg walking cast for 3 to 4 weeks. If radiographs are normal but the child has tenderness over the tibial crest and pain can be produced by upward compression on the heel, the child should be treated in a similar manner. It is the author's belief that bone scans are rarely if ever indicated in the treatment of these fractures.

Computed tomographic scans are helpful for diagnosing and planning treatment for displaced physeal fractures and transitional fractures. They should be used as an adjunct to plain radiographic films to determine fracture pattern, the amount of displacement, and the degree of joint step-off.

TREATMENT GOALS, INDICATIONS, AND CONTRAINDICATIONS

Closed treatment is usually adequate for closed tibial shaft fractures in children and young adolescents (Table 9). Up to 1.5 cm of shortening can be accepted in children younger than 10 years of age, as approximately 5 mm of overgrowth can be expected. Angulation of up to 10 degrees in children and 5 degrees in adolescents is acceptable. Shannack[35] reported few complications and an average healing time of 5 weeks with closed treatment.

The principle of soft tissue management in open fractures in children is the same as in adults. Adequate irrigation and débridement in the operating room and appropriate antibiotic therapy (cephalosporin in type I and II; cephalosporin and aminoglycoside in type III) is necessary. The need for fasciotomies and vascular repairs is similar to that in adults.[36] Type I fractures heal quickly and can be treated with closed reduction and casting. Most type II fractures are also amenable to casting, although external fixation may be considered. External fixation should be used in type III fractures. Buckley et al[36] reported an average time to healing of 5 months. They also noted spontaneous correction of angular malunion of greater than 10 degrees in three of four patients.

As is true in injuries around the knee, the distal tibial physis is more likely to fail than surrounding ligamentous structures. Salter-Harris I and II fractures have a good prognosis and can be treated with closed reduction and casting. An anatomic reduction is necessary in Salter-Harris fractures to avoid long-term complications.[37] Reduction should be either closed if possible or open if necessary. Physeal malalignment and 2 mm displacement at the fracture site are indications for internal fixation.[37] Fixation should then consist of Kirschner's wires or cannulated screws, parallel to the physis.

Transitional fractures occur in adolescents undergoing physiological closure of the distal tibial physis. The process

TABLE 9. TREATMENT OF TIBIA/ANKLE/FOOT FRACTURES		
Fracture	Treatment	Goals
Tibial diaphyseal		
Closed	Closed reduction, cast	<1.5 cm shortening <10 degrees angulation
Open		
Type I/II	Irrigation, débridement Closed reduction, cast	Same as closed
Type III	Irrigation, débridement External fixation	Soft tissue healing Anatomic alignment
Distal physeal		
Salter-Harris	Closed reduction, cast	<2 mm displacement
Salter-Harris	Closed/open reduction Internal fixation	Anatomic alignment
Transitional fractures	Closed/open reduction Internal fixation	Open reduction and internal fixation for >2 mm displacement

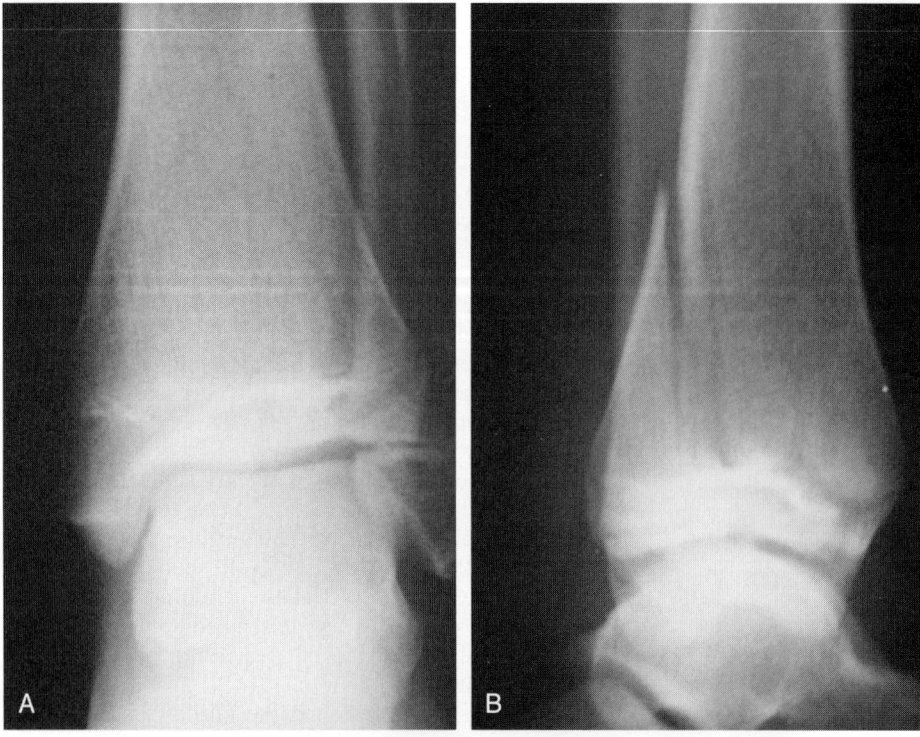

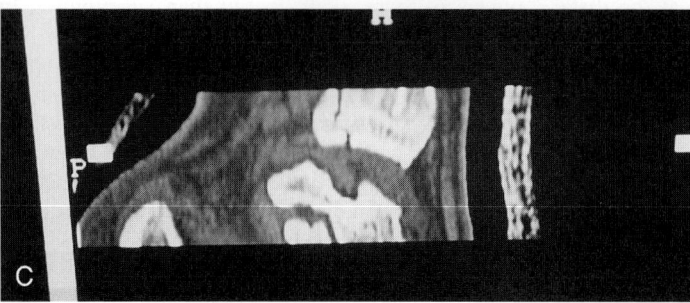

Fig. 5. Radiographs. This is a 14-year-old boy with a triplane fracture sustained falling down a flight of stairs. *A*, Anteroposterior radiograph. Note the faintly visible fracture line running obliquely across the distal tibial metaphysis and a second line at the midpoint of the epiphysis. *B*, Later view. *C*, Sagittal reconstruction of the CT scan clearly showing the Salter-Harris components of the posterior fragment.

starts eccentrically and the anterolateral quadrant is the last to close.[38] The fracture line deviates from the unmineralized area into the joint space when an adequate eversion, external rotation force is applied.[38] Three types of transitional fractures have been described: a biplane or juvenile Tillaux fracture, in which the lateral fragment remains attached to the fibula, and two- and three-part triplane fractures. The latter two characteristically appear as Salter-Harris fractures on anteroposterior radiographs and Salter-Harris fractures on lateral radiographic films (Fig. 5). For fractures with less than 2 mm displacement, a closed reduction consisting of internal rotation of the foot with forward traction on the heel is adequate. The leg should be immobilized in a long-leg cast with the knee flexed 30 degrees. Open reduction and internal fixation is indicated for fractures with greater than 2 mm displacement.[38] Since growth disturbance is not an issue in these patients because of their degree of skeletal maturity, fixation may cross the physis.

Significant foot injuries in children are unusual. As in adults, falls are the most common cause of calcaneal fractures. A higher incidence of associated lower extremity injuries has been reported than in adults,[39] and these must be looked for. Fractures tend to be extra-articular in younger children.[39] Closed treatment is usually sufficient. Open reduction and internal fixation should be reserved for a large displaced fragment (Fig. 6) or displaced intra-articular fractures.

Fractures of the talus and subtalar dislocations are extremely unusual and are usually associated with high-velocity trauma. The treatment of these injuries should be similar to that in adults. Tarsometatarsal joint injuries do occur in children. Surgical reduction is indicated in displaced fractures and instability is best managed with pin fixation across the tarsometatarsal joint. Good long-term results have been reported.[40] Metatarsal fractures are common. Closed treatment is sufficient and long-term problems are rare. Jones fractures (fifth metatarsal) are extremely unusual in younger children but may occur in adolescents. They should be treated as in adults, with open reduction and internal fixation for displaced fractures.

COMPLICATIONS

Complications are unusual in all of these fractures in children. Shannak[35] reported few complications in a series of closed tibial diaphyseal fractures treated by closed methods in 117 children. A rate of infection and delayed union

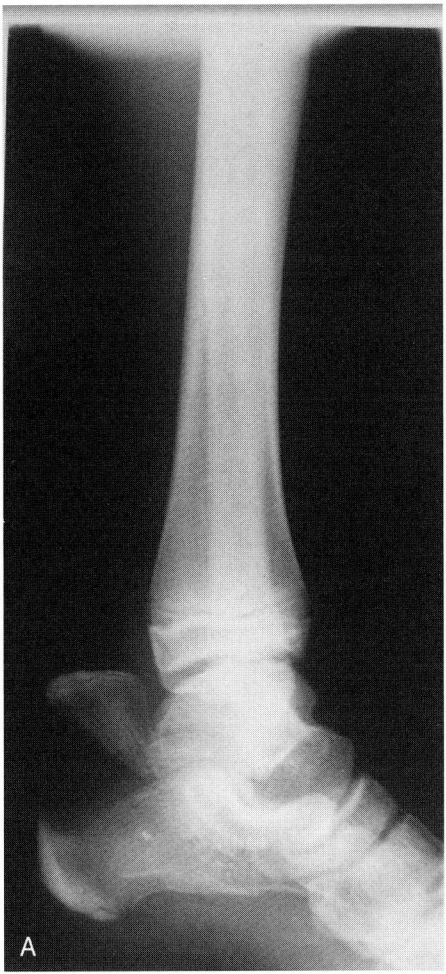
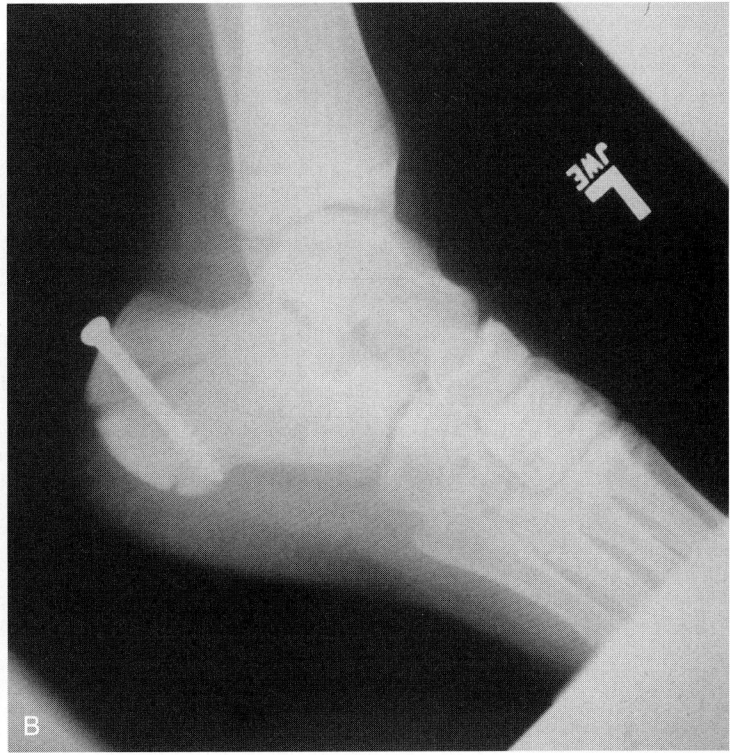

Fig. 6. Radiographs. This is a 15-year-old male with a displaced calcaneal fracture sustained when he landed during a gymnastics routine. *A,* Lateral radiograph showing large displaced extra-articular fragment. *B,* Lateral radiograph after open reduction and fixation with 6.5 mm cannulated screw.

similar to that in adults was reported in a series of open tibia fractures.[36] No children in this series went on to amputation. Overgrowth of greater than 1 cm was noted in 20% of children with severe fractures treated with external fixation. As is expected, displaced distal tibial physeal fractures have been associated with growth disturbances. Anatomic reduction, especially in Salter-Harris fractures, should lower the incidence of this complication.[37]

REFERENCES

1. Ratleff AHC: Fractures of the neck of the femur in children. J Bone Joint Surg Br 1962; 44:528.
2. Canale ST, Bourland WL: Fracture of the neck and intertrochanteric region of the femur in children. J Bone Joint Surg Am 1977; 59:431.
3. Hughes LO, Beaty JH: Fractures of the head and neck of the femur in children. J Bone Joint Surg Am 1994; 76:283.
4. Canale ST: Fractures of the hip in children and adolescents. Orthop Clin N Am 1990; 21:341.
5. Forlin E, Guille JT, Kumar SJ, et al: Complications associated with fractures of the neck of the femur in children. J Pediatr Orthop 1992; 12:503.
6. Chung SMK: The arterial supply of the developing proximal end of the human femur. J Bone Joint Surg Am 1976; 58:961.
7. Ogden JA: Changing patterns of proximal femoral vascularity. J Bone Joint Surg Am 1974; 56:941.
8. Colonna PC: Fractures of the neck of the femur in children. Am J Surg 1929; 6:193.
9. Swiontowski MF, Winquist RA: Displaced hip fractures in children and adolescents. J Trauma 1986; 26:384.
10. Morrissy R: Hip fractures in children. Clin Orthop 1980; 152:202.
11. Leung PC, Lam SF: Long term follow up of children with femoral neck fractures. J Bone Joint Surg Br 1986; 68:537.
12. Beals RK, Tufts E: Fractured femur in infancy: The role of child abuse. J Pediatr Orthop 1983; 3:583.
13. Buckley SL, Sturm PF, Buck BD, et al: Upper extremity restraint during hip spica cast application. J Pediatr Orthop 1993; 13:529.
14. Staheli LT: Femoral and tibial growth following femoral shaft fractures in childhood. Clin Orthop 1967; 55:159.
15. Henderson OL, Morrissy RT, Gerdes MH, et al: Early casting of femoral shaft fractures in children. J Pediatr Orthop 1984; 4:16.
16. Irani RN, Nicholson JT, Chung SMK: Long term results in the treatment of femoral shaft fractures in young children by immediate spica immobilization. J Bone Joint Surg Am 1976; 58:945.
17. Martinez AG, Carroll NC, Sarwark JF, et al: Femoral shaft fractures in children treated with early spica cast. J Pediatr Orthop 1991; 11:712.
18. Newton PO, Mubarak SJ: Financial aspects of femoral shaft fractures in children and adolescents. J Pediatr Orthop 1994; 14:508.
19. Aronson DD, Singer RM, Higgins PF: Skeletal traction for fractures of the femo-

ral shaft in children. J Bone Joint Surg Am 1987; 69:1435.

20. Kirby RM, Winquist RA, Hansen ST: Femoral shaft fractures in adolescents: A comparison between traction plus cast treatment and closed intramedullary nailing. J Pediatr Orthop 1981; 1:193.

21. Ward WT, Levy J, Kaye A: Compression plating for child and adolescent femur fractures. J Pediatr Orthop 1992; 12:626.

22. Aronson J, Tursky EA: External fixation of femur fractures in children. J Pediatr Orthop 1992; 12:157.

23. Heinrich SD, Dvaric DM, Darr K, et al: The operative stabilization of pediatric diaphyseal femur fractures with flexible intramedullary nails: A prospective analysis. J Pediatr Orthop 1994; 14:501.

24. Fyodorov I, Sturm PF, Robertson WW Jr: Compression plate fixation of femoral shaft fractures in children ages eight to twelve. J Pediatr Orthop. (accepted for publication).

25. Beaty JH, Austin SM, Warner WC, et al: Interlocking intramedullary nailing of femoral shaft fractures in adolescents: Preliminary results and complications. J Pediatr Orthop 1994; 14:178.

26. Pritchett JW: Longitudinal growth and growth plate activity in the lower extremity. Clin Orthop 1992; 275:274.

27. Ogden JA, Tross RB, Murphy MJ: Fractures of the tibial tuberosity in adolescents. J Bone Joint Surg Am 1980; 62:205.

28. Beaty JH, Kumar A: Fractures about the knee in children. J Bone Joint Surg Am 1994; 76:1870.

29. Stanitski CL: Anterior cruciate ligament injury in the skeletally immature patient: Diagnosis and treatment. J Am Acad Orthop Surg 1995; 3:146.

30. Riseborough EJ, Barrett IR, Shapiro F: Growth disturbances following distal femoral physeal fracture-separations. J Bone Joint Surg Am 1983; 85:885.

31. Lombardo SJ, Harvey JP Jr: Fractures of the distal femoral epiphysis. J Bone Joint Surg Am 1977; 59:742.

32. Burkart SS, Peterson HA: Fractures of the proximal tibial epiphysis. J Bone Joint Surg Am 1979; 61:996.

33. Shelton WR, Canale ST: Fractures of the tibia through the proximal tibial epiphyseal cartilage. J Bone Joint Surg Am 1979; 61:167.

34. Janarv PM, Westblad P, Johansson C: Long-term follow-up of anterior tibial spine fractures in children. J Pediatr Orthop 1995; 15:63.

35. Shannak AO: Tibial fractures in children: Follow-up study. J Pediatr Orthop 1988; 8:306.

36. Buckley SL, Smith G, Sponseller PD, et al: Open fractures of the tibia in children. J Bone Joint Surg Am 1990; 72:1462.

37. Kling TF, Bright RW, Hensinger RN: Distal tibial physeal fractures in children that may require open reduction. J Bone Joint Surg Am 1984; 66:647.

38. Von Laer L: Classification, diagnosis, and treatment of transitional fractures of the distal part of the tibia. J Bone Joint Surg Am 1985; 67:687.

39. Schmidt TL, Weiner DS: Calcaneal fractures in children: An evaluation of the nature of injury in 56 children. Clin Orthop 1982; 171:150.

40. Wiley JJ: Tarsometatarsal joint injuries in children. J Pediatr Orthop 1981; 1:255.

section
3
chapter
27

SPINE AND PELVIS

John M. Flynn and John Dormans

Summary

- Cervical spine anatomy, mechanism of injury, evaluation, and treatment are different in children. In children, upper cervical spine injuries predominate, with odontoid fractures being the most common.

- Spinal cord injury without radiographic abnormality (SCIWORA) occurs because the spinal column can stretch more than the spinal cord before sustaining damage. Magnetic resonance imaging (MRI) is a key tool to evaluate SCIWORA, as well as possible occult spinal column injuries.

- Many cervical and thoracolumbar fractures in children are adequately treated with immobilization alone. When surgery is necessary, simple posterior tension band fixation is sufficient in most cases.

- Pediatric pelvic and acetabular fractures, while uncommon, are different with respect to presentation, pathoanatomy, and treatment as compared with similar injuries in adults.

- Most pediatric pelvic and acetabular fractures can be classified according to the mechanism of injury, with corresponding pathoanatomy and treatment.

- Most children with pelvic and acetabular fractures can be treated without surgery; there are specific injuries in children that do require a surgical approach to avoid serious long-term problems and complications.

SPINE FRACTURES

Pediatric spinal injuries are uncommon. However, some unique mechanisms of injury, subtleties of evaluation, and potentially serious consequences can make their management challenging. Treatment is based both on the ability of the injured tissue to heal and on biomechanical considerations that determine stability. The continued growth and maturation of the child with the spinal injury can lead to future improvement, as occurs with vertebral body reconstitution after a compression injury, or to further problems, such as the scoliosis that occurs frequently after neurological or growth plate injuries.[1, 2]

The cervical spine changes substantially from birth through adolescence. Young children have physes and apophyses, increased ligamentous laxity, and more horizontally oriented facets.[3] These differences typically resolve by 8 to 10 years of age. McGrory et al[4] found that 90% of cervical spine injuries were between C1 and C3 in the younger children, whereas 60% were below C3 in older children. Likewise, there are also important differences in the thoracolumbar spine. With growth, vertebral bodies that are compressed in injury can regain height. Ring apophyses provide a site of separation and in the thoracolumbar spine can cause a syndrome that is clinically similar to a herniated intervertebral disc.

Historically, the care of pediatric spine injuries has been advanced primarily by an improved understanding of injury

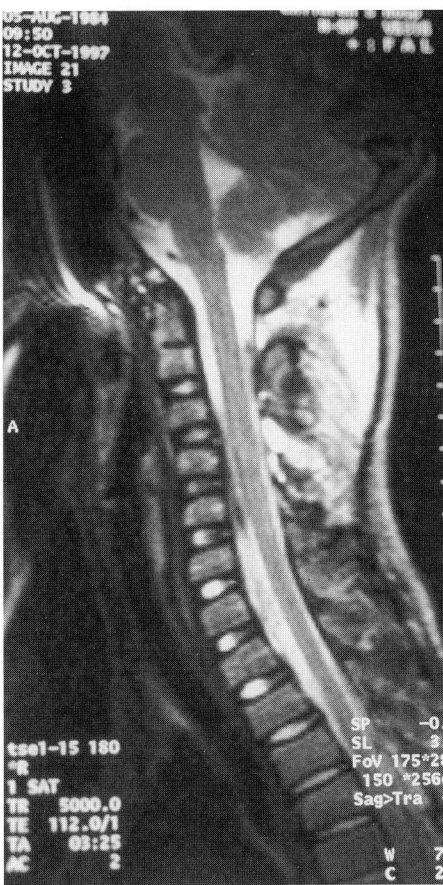

Fig. 1. Magnetic resonance imaging (MRI) scan. A 12-year-old with spinal cord injury without radiographic abnormality had a central cord syndrome and normal findings on plain radiographs. MRI shows edema in the cord and injury to the C3–C4 posterior spinal ligaments, which were unstable and required fusion.

mechanisms and biomechanics, as discussed later. The entity SCIWORA (Fig. 1) was introduced by Pang and Wilberger in 1982.[5] MRI has improved the awareness and treatment of SCIWORA and occult pediatric spine injuries. Halo ring and vest immobilization for pediatric cervical spine fractures has become safer since surgeons have adopted the practice of using more halo pins tightened with less pressure.[6]

PATHOGENESIS

The mechanisms of spinal injuries in children differ from the mechanisms in adults. Falls, birth injuries, and injuries that occur in motor vehicle accidents are most common among infants and young children.[7] Injuries from diving, riding a bicycle, or playing sports are more common in adolescents. Child abuse should be considered as the possible cause of spine injuries in children. The predominant area injured in child abuse is the thoracolumbar junction.[8] Birth trauma may cause spinal injury and should be considered during the work-up of the infant with unexplained decreased muscle tone (the "floppy baby"). Seat-belt injuries are probably the most common cause of pediatric lumbar spine fractures. Airbags have also contributed to spine injuries. Diving accidents remain a common cause of pediatric neck injuries, particularly in adolescents. These inju-

ries tend to be localized to the lower cervical spine and usually result from a combination of compression with either flexion or extension.

CLINICAL FEATURES

The evaluation of spinal injuries is often more difficult in children than in adults. The injuries are less frequent, the patterns are unique, and an adult approach to imaging may overlook injury to unossified tissue. The evaluating surgeon must also recognize the potential for injury at multiple sites. In one series, 16% of patients had more than one site of injury.[9]

The thorough physical examination should focus particular attention on the upper cervical spine. Children often find it difficult to localize their pain to a precise site. Torticollis is an important sign after trauma and may indicate a C1-2 rotary subluxation. Given the predominance of the upper cervical spine injuries in children, signs of head and face trauma warrant a very careful spinal evaluation. The "seat-belt sign," a transverse patch of skin contusion across the abdomen, should alert the surgeon that there may be an injury to the lumbar spine. A detailed neurological examination is always mandatory and should include a test for the bulbocavernosus reflex when neurologic injury is suspected.

INVESTIGATION

Although the imaging of children with suspected spine trauma should always begin with plain radiographs, these studies alone will miss up to 50% of the injuries.[10] The surgeon caring for these injured children should have a thorough understanding of the many factors that make the radiographic interpretation of the pediatric spine different (Table 1). Because upper cervical spine injuries predominate, high-quality radiographs of this area are important. Computed tomography (CT) gives excellent resolution in bone and is ideal for identifying fractures. Unfortunately, a standard CT scan done in the plane of the fracture (e.g., odontoid or Chance's fractures) may miss the injury. Reconstructions are helpful. A dynamic CT scan is the study of choice to evaluate rotary subluxation or fixation of C1-2. As advancing technology improves the image qual-

TABLE 1. UNIQUE FEATURES OF THE PEDIATRIC SPINE

General features
Secondary centers of ossification of the spinous processes can mimic fractures.
Rounding of anterior vertebral body may appear to be wedge compression fractures.
Horizontal facets and ligamentous laxity permit greater intersegment mobility.
Decreased cervical lordosis exists.
Wider prevertebral soft tissues during crying may mimic swelling.

Specific features

C1	Multiple ossification centers may mimic fractures.
C1-2	ADI may be up to 4.5 mm in normal children.
C2	Normal posterior angulation of odontiod (4% of children) may mimic fractures.
	Ossiculum terminale can be confused with fracture.
	Basilar synchondrosis can be confused with fracture.
C2-3	Pseudosubluxation can be mistaken for instability.

ity, MRI is increasingly recognized for its ability to evaluate spinal cord injury, ligament injury, and injuries to unossified tissue (see Fig. 1).

TREATMENT GOALS, INDICATIONS, AND CONTRAINDICATIONS

Many pediatric spinal injuries can be treated with immobilization alone. The care of specific injuries is outlined in Table 2.

PROCEDURES

Pediatric Halo Vest Application

In contrast to application in adults, halo ring and vest application in children is usually performed under general anesthesia, using more pins tightened with less force (Fig. 2). Mubarek et al[6] recommend a head CT scan to find the thickest bone, then sizing of the ring 2 cm bigger than the head circumference. The head should be supported without excessive flexion. Since children are usually under general anesthesia for the halo ring application, the surgeon can ensure that the local anesthetic is placed exactly at the pin site by waiting until the end of the procedure to inject. The ring is placed just below the largest diameter of the head, 1 cm above the ears. Anterior pins are placed just above the lateral two thirds of the orbit, avoiding the temporal muscle. The posterior pins are placed diagonally across the head from the anterior pins. With the patient's eyes closed, the surgeon alternately tightens the anterior and posterior pins to finger tight (~2 inch/lb) for infants or young children, 2 to 4 inch/lb for older children, and 6 to 8 inch/lb for adolescents. An appropriately sized vest is applied. The pins are cleaned daily with saline solution.

Posterior Fusion of the Cervical Spine

As C1-2 is the most commonly injured site in children, it is the most common level requiring fusion. Although there is a variety of fusion techniques for the posterior cervical spine, the Gallie technique[11] is probably the most

		TABLE 2. STANDARD TREATMENT FOR VARIOUS PEDIATRIC SPINAL INJURIES			
Injury	Preferred Treatment	Immobilization Recommended	Indications for Operative Treatment	Procedure Recommended	Outcome
SCIWORA	Immobilization	Hard collar or cervicothoracic orthosis, depending on injury	Unstable injury	Short posterior fusion	Dependent on extent of neurologic injury
Occiput-C1 dislocation	Occiput to C2 posterior fusion	Postoperative halo-vest immobilization	Unstable injury	Occiput-C2 posterior fusion, postoperative halo-vest immobilization	Many die of injury
Atlantoaxial rotary subluxation	Soft collar × 1 week. If unresolved after 1 week, traction followed by hard collar or corrective cervicothoracic orthosis	Soft collar. If later than 1 week, hard collar or corrective cervicothoracic orthosis	Subluxation or dislocation for more than 8–12 weeks (failure to reduce with traction or failure to maintain reduction)	In situ C1-2 fusion	Good if successfully diagnosed and treated early
Odontoid fracture	Reduction. Immobilization × 6 weeks	Halo vest or minerva cast	Nonunion or os odontoideum with instability (rare)	C1-2 fusion	Good. Non-union of odontoid rare in children
Hangman's fracture	Reduction. Immobilization × 6 weeks	Halo vest or minerva cast	Instability after 6 weeks of immobilization (rare)		Good
C3-7 compression fractures and ligamentous injuries	Stable injuries: immobilization × 4 weeks	Hard collar	Unstable injuries	Posterior fusion (anterior decompression and fusion rarely needed in children)	Good
C3-7 facet dislocation	MRI, closed reduction by halo traction, fusion	Halo vest	Unstable injuries (most cases)	Posterior fusion	Neurologic injury is common in bilateral facet dislocation
Chance fractures	Bony Chance fracture: TLSO for 8–12 weeks. Isolated ligament injury: posterior fusion	Thoracolumbar orthosis	Isolated ligament injury. Kyphosis in a brace >25 degrees. Neurologic injury	Posterior fusion (spinous process wiring or compression construct)	Good
Slipped vertebral apophyses	Excision of displaced apophysis if there is neural compression	N/A	Nerve root compression, persistent pain or neurologic symptoms	Excision of displaced apophysis	Generally good. Symptoms typically will not resolve as with a herniated disc

MRI, magnetic resonance imaging; N/A, not XXX; SCIWORA, spinal cord injury without radiographic abnormality; TLSO, thoracolumbosacral orthosis.

widely used. If the spine is unstable, a halo is applied first. A lateral radiograph of the cervical spine should be obtained to ensure reduction. The subfascial dissection is limited to the unstable level to prevent the fusion from occurring at unintended levels. The patient wears the halo vest for 2 months and then spends a few weeks in a hard collar. Most adolescents can be immobilized effectively with a hard collar alone for 3 months.

Posterior Fusion for Chance Fractures

Since Chance fractures are flexion-distraction injuries, the goal of surgical treatment is to re-establish the posterior tension band that has been broken by ligamentous disruption. Posterior wiring and fusion work well for younger children; in older, larger children, a claw compression construct using hook-rod posterior instrumentation gives better fixation. It may be necessary to stagger the hook level to decrease the hardware in the canal at any one level.

Neurological monitoring during surgery is recommended. After positioning, the surgeon should check a preoperative lateral radiograph to ensure proper positioning. Deep dissection should be performed with care; there may be a large hematoma, and the tear may disrupt all posterior structures, including the ligamentum flavum. A construct employing sublaminar titanium cables is strong, safe, and easy to use and will not interfere later with MRI (Fig. 3). Alternatively, spinous process button wires can be used. After passing wires or cables, the facets are prepared. The wires or cables are tightened until visual inspection and the lateral radiograph confirm that the sagittal contour is restored. The local bone is decorticated, and the iliac crest graft is placed. After posterior wiring, a brace is worn until the fusion is solid. A hook-rod construct is usually stable enough to obviate the need for bracing.

COMPLICATIONS AND RESULTS

Complications occur commonly with halo immobilization in children.[12] Pin drainage is managed with antibiotics and local pin care. If there is no response, or if cellulitis or an abscess develops, the pin should be removed and a new

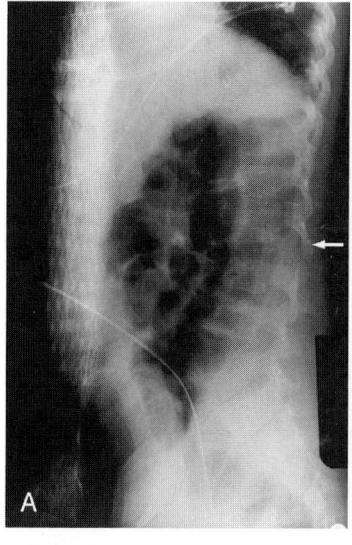
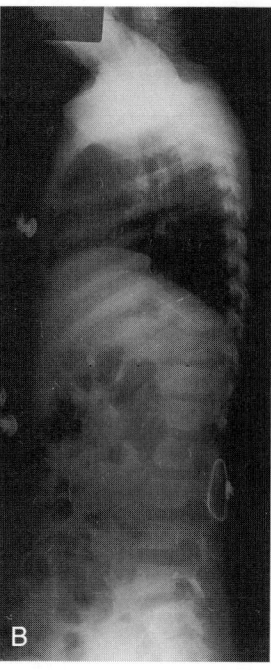

Fig. 3. Radiographs. These are preoperative (*A*) and postoperative (*B*) radiographs of a ligamentous Chance fracture in a 6-year-old treated with posterior tension band wiring. The arrow in *A* shows the site of injury. (From Flynn J, Dormans J: Spine trauma in children. Semin Spine Surg 1998; 10:7.)

pin placed at another site. Sometimes a pin will penetrate the thin inner table of a child's skull. Dural fluid may begin leaking from around the pin. In this situation, the pin should be moved to another site and prophylactic antibiotics should be given until the drainage stops.

After fusing the cervical spine in children, the surgeon may note that the fusion mass has extended to additional levels. This extension can be avoided by taking great care to limit the subperiosteal dissection to the levels to be fused. Pseudoarthrosis is rarely seen in children (except in children with Down's syndrome when allograft is used).

PELVIC AND ACETABULAR FRACTURES

The true prevalence rate of pelvic fractures is difficult to determine but has been estimated to occur in 0.5% to 1% of children with musculoskeletal injuries treated at regional trauma centers.[13–17] In general, acetabular fractures account for 1% to 15% of fractures of the pelvis in children.[16, 18, 19] At our center (a pediatric trauma center), we see approximately 20 children with pelvic fractures per year and 90% of these are the stable types; acetabular fractures are rare. The mortality rate from major pelvic fractures in children, reported to be 0.5% to 9%,[13–17] has declined as intensive care has improved.

PATHOGENESIS

The child's pelvis differs from that of adults in several ways: there are epiphyseal and apophyseal growth centers (with the potential for growth disturbance after fractures), and the pelvis—bone, joints, and ligaments—is more flexible, giving it a greater capacity to absorb energy.

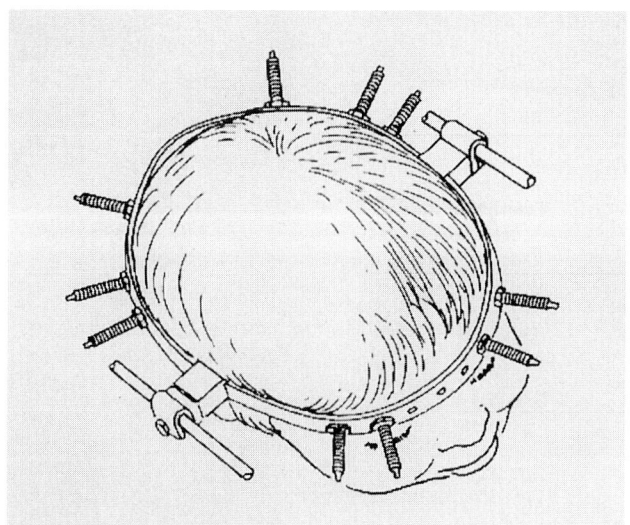

Fig. 2. Typical pin positions. The positions are for use of the halo in a toddler. (Adapted from Mubarak SJ, Camp JF, Vuletich W, et al: Halo application in the infant. J Pediatr Orthop 1989; 9:612.)

TABLE 3. PELVIS FRACTURES: CLASSIFICATION OF TORODE AND ZIEG

Type	Description
I	Avulsion of bony elements
II	Iliac wing fractures
III	Simple ring fractures
IV	Ring disruption fractures

CLASSIFICATION

There are several classification systems for pediatric pelvic fractures. The Pennal-Tile classification is based on mechanism of injury and the presence or absence of stability. Recently, Tile's system has been placed into the Arbeitsgemeinschast für Osteosynthesefragen/Association for the Study of Internal Fixation A, B, C code system of increasing severity.[16] This detailed classification is particularly useful in the management of adult-like adolescent pelvic fractures. Torode and Zieg's classification[17] better emphasizes the injuries seen in younger children, such as isolated iliac wing fractures (Table 3). Acetabular fractures are well described in the classification of Letournel and Judet (Table 4).[16]

Clinical Features

Apophyseal avulsion injuries are generally caused by athletic injury and occur in children 12 to 15 years of age.[13, 14, 20] Pelvic fractures in children are usually the result of high-energy trauma (e.g., motor vehicle trauma). Child abuse should be considered.

The initial steps involved in the care of a child with a major pelvic fracture have been outlined by the American College of Surgeons and necessitate emergency medical teams instituting primary and secondary surveys, large-bore venous access, and other life support measures.[21] Evaluation includes inspection of the body surfaces and coordinated log-rolling to examine for lacerations of the perineum (resulting from open fractures). Pelvic stability, limb temperature, and arterial circulation are evaluated. Doppler ultrasonographic examination may be useful. Gross motor function and sensation (including the perirectal sensation) are assessed. A pelvic examination should be done with the patient under sedation or anesthesia if a vaginal laceration is suspected. Rectal examination is done to check for gross blood (indicating a rectal laceration or sphincter injury) and rectal tone. Associated injuries may include intracranial, intrathoracic, intra-abdominal, lower urinary tract, neurological, and soft-tissue injuries.

Investigation

Anteroposterior, "inlet," and "outlet" radiographs of the pelvis (without gonadal shielding) are obtained to evaluate pelvic injury.[16] When the anteroposterior pelvis film demonstrates involvement of the acetabulum, 45-degree oblique views should be obtained, as described by Letournel and Judet.[19] CT scanning (with soft tissue and bone window technique and cut intervals of 2.5 to 3 mm) may give additional information, particularly in adult-like fractures in adolescents. It is especially helpful for detecting intra-articular loose fragments.

TREATMENT GOALS, INDICATIONS, AND CONTRAINDICATIONS
Hemorrhage

Significant hemorrhage from bleeding bone is rare in young children. Several different methods can be used to

TABLE 4. CLASSIFICATION AND MANAGEMENT OF PELVIC DISRUPTIONS AND FRACTURES

Type	Subtype	Description	Treatment
A		Stable	
	A1	Fracture of the pelvis not involving the ring Isolated avulsions (ASIS, AIIS, ischium, ilium)	Conservative management
	A2	Stable minimally displaced fracture of the ring Isolated pubic rami fractures	Conservative management
B		Rotationally unstable, vertically stable	
	B1	Open-book, isolated	Conservative management *Exception:* Major hemorrhage, laparotomy, or displacement >3 mm External fixation vs. ORIF
	B2	Lateral compression, ipsilateral	Conservative management *Exception:* When associated with laparotomy: ORIF (if anterior ring is amenable)
	B3	Lateral compression, contralateral (buck handle)	Conservative management *Exception:* When widely (>1 cm) displaced: attempted closed reduction; ORIF if not reducible
C		Rotationally and vertically unstable	
	C	Unilateral Vertical shear, displaced	Traction or ORIF of posterior complex with or without internal or external fixation anteriorly
	C2	Bilateral	
	C3	Associated with acetabular fracture	See below
Acetabular		Displaced <2 mm	Conservative management
		Displaced ≥2 mm	ORIF

ORIF, open reduction and internal fixation.

close down pelvic volume and prevent shock.[15, 16, 22] Anterior external fixation with simple fixation can be helpful in reducing pelvic volume.

Fractures of the Pelvis

Most pediatric pelvic fractures are stable. Avulsion fractures of the anterosuperior (sartorius origin) and anteroinferior (rectus femoris origin) iliac spines, the iliac apophysis (external oblique origin), and the ischial rami (hamstring origin) or fractures with single breaks in pelvic ring (including isolated or bilateral pubic rami fractures) are treated with symptomatic measures (bedrest with advancement to protected ambulation). Children with minimally displaced open-book injury (<3 cm) can also be treated in this manner. Patients with displaced ischial rami (hamstring origin) avulsion fractures may have a higher incidence of symptoms after healing.[20]

Closed Reduction

The two indications for closed reduction without internal fixation are a lateral compression injury with a locked symphysis and the tilt fracture described by Tile.[16] Vertical shear or anteroposterior compression injuries are generally unstable, so closed reduction is not recommended.

Skeletal Traction

Skeletal traction (with a distal femoral pin) is indicated for vertical shear injury through the iliac wing, sacroiliac joint, or sacrum that reduces in traction. This generally occurs in children younger than 7 to 10 years. Contraindications for this treatment are lateral compression injuries, open-book A2 injuries, and stable avulsion-type fractures. Fractures that do not reduce in traction should not be maintained in traction.

Spica Cast

The spica cast may be helpful for children with minimally displaced pelvic fractures or avulsion injuries to allow the patient to be treated at home; most of these children can be treated without casting, however. Casting will generally not reduce or hold a reduction of a displaced pelvic fracture. If the displacement is not acceptable, another form of treatment should be selected.

External Fixation

External fixation is useful for open pelvic fractures and for patients who are hemodynamically unstable (to reduce intrapelvic volume). External fixation provides definitive treatment only for B1 open-book injuries and usually cannot hold reductions of displaced posterior ring injuries. The optimal treatment for displaced fractures of the sacroiliac joint, posterior iliac ring, and sacrum is now considered to be accurate reduction (closed, if possible with traction) or open reduction and internal fixation (ORIF).

For the vertical shear pelvic fracture, past literature has recommended skeletal traction with a traction pin through the distal femur.[13–17] Malgaigne fractures (double vertical fractures or fracture-dislocations) with hemodynamic instability should be treated with external or internal fixation of the symphysis diastasis. Skeletal traction may be a good alternative for those who are hemodynamically stable. ORIF is occasionally needed for children with unstable displaced fractures, especially older children, or those with sacroiliac joint disruption.[23]

Internal Fixation of Pelvic Fractures

Occasionally, ORIF may be indicated for children with open fracture with massive displacement of the fragments (e.g., widely displaced fractures of the A2, B1, B2, C1, and C2 type).[14, 23] Failed closed reduction (including traction) may be a relative indication for open reduction, especially if the fracture is widely displaced and the injury is more than 5 to 6 days old. When laparotomy is necessary in children with a concomitant open-book pelvic fracture with diastasis of 3 cm or more, a simple ORIF can be done with a two-hole 3.5-mm dynamic compression plate and cortical screws. Closed or open reduction of displaced pelvic fractures is optimally done at 48 to 72 hours after injury.

Acetabular Fractures

For the most part, acetabular fractures in children historically have also been treated conservatively. However, poor results have been reported for children with comminuted fractures, for which traction did not improve the position of the fragments.[16, 18, 19]

Children with stable, nondisplaced, or minimally displaced (1 mm or less) fractures should be treated with bedrest initially, then toe-touch weightbearing with crutches. Children with significant displacement of fractures or instability of the hip may require skeletal traction for accurate reduction of fracture fragments; traction treatment is appropriate only for fractures that are reducible to less than 2 mm of displacement, however. Children with central fracture-dislocations require prompt reduction, skeletal traction, or ORIF.

Open Reduction and Internal Fixation

Currently, ORIF is indicated for fractures involving the major weightbearing surface with greater than 2 mm displacement and for unstable posterior wall fracture-dislocations.[16, 18, 19] The surgical approach varies according to the pattern of the fracture. Posterior wall injuries are managed best through the Kocher-Langenbeck approach. Anterior column injuries are managed with ilioinguinal approach of Letournel (lower incidence of heterotopic ossification). Reconstruction plates (3.5 or 2.7 mm) are used for posterior wall fractures. Many children's fractures can be treated with lag screws alone. Acetabular fractures should be managed, with a short delay (1 to 2 days), to optimize preoperative planning.

COMPLICATIONS AND RESULTS

The results for children with pelvic and acetabular fractures are better in general than those for adults. Complications of pelvic fractures in children include leg length discrepancy and pelvic obliquity (malunion), sacroiliac fusion, delayed union, heterotopic ossification, and infection following open fractures that involve the perineum, rectum, or vagina.

Complications of acetabular fractures in children include growth arrest of the triradiate cartilage, which can lead to a shallow, dysplastic acetabulum and femoral head subluxation, heterotopic ossification, avascular necrosis of the femoral head, and post-traumatic arthritis.[16, 18, 19, 24] Acceptance of no more than 2 mm of displacement in the acetabulum and careful surgical exposure minimize the incidence of these complications. Up to one-third of patients have residual limp and pain and have had to alter their activities.

Nonunion as a complication is rare; malunion is more common. Fusion of the sacroiliac joint is probably a result of the severe trauma producing the fracture. There is a poor correlation between the anatomic or radiographic appearance and the functional outcome.

REFERENCES

1. Flynn JM, Dormans JP: Spine trauma in children. Semin Spine Surg 1998; 10:7.
2. Murphy MJ, Ogden JA, Bucholz RW: Cervical spine injury in the child. Contemp Orthop 1981; 3:615.
3. Copley LA, Dormans JP: Cervical spine disorders in infants and children. J Am Acad Orthop Surg 1998; 6:204.
4. McGrory BJ, Klassen RA, Chao EY, et al: Acute fractures and dislocations of the cervical spine in children and adolescents. J Bone Joint Surg Am 1993; 75:988.
5. Pang D, Wilberger JE: Spinal cord injury without radiographic abnormality in children. J Neurosurg 1982; 57:114.
6. Mubarak SJ, Camp JF, Vuletich W, et al: Halo application in the infant. J Pediatr Orthop 1989; 9:612.
7. Birney TJ, Hanley EDN: Traumatic cervical spine injuries in childhood and adolescence. Spine 1989; 14:127.
8. Cullen JC: Spinal lesions in battered babies. J Bone Joint Surg Br 1975; 57:364.
9. Hadley MN, Zabramski JM, Browner CM, et al: Pediatric spinal trauma: Review of 122 cases of spinal cord and vertebral column injuries. J Neurosurg 1988; 68:18.
10. Anderson LD, Smith BL, DeTorre J, et al: The role of polytomography in the diagnosis and treatment of cervical spine injuries. Clin Orthop Rel Res 1982; 165:64.
11. Gallie WE: Fracture and dislocations of the cervical spine. Am J Surg 1939; 46:495.
12. Dormans JP, Criscitiello AA, Drummond DS, et al: Complications in children managed with immobilization in a halo vest. J Bone Joint Surg Am 1995; 77:1370.
13. Canale SR, Beaty JH: Pelvic and hip fractures. In Rockwood CA, Wilkins KE, Beaty JH (eds): Fractures in Children, 4th ed. Philadelphia, Lippincott-Raven, 1996, p 1109.
14. Swiontkowski MF: Fractures and dislocations about the hip and pelvis. In Green NE, Swiontkowski MF (eds): Skeletal Trauma in Children, 2nd ed, vol. 3. Philadelphia, WB Saunders, 1998; p 69.
15. McIntyre RC, Bensard DD, Moore EE, et al: Pelvic fracture geometry predicts risk of life threatening hemorrhage in children. J Trauma 1993; 35:423.
16. Tile M: Fractures of the Pelvis and Acetabulum. Baltimore, Williams & Wilkins, 1984, p 1.
17. Torode I, Zieg D: Pelvic fractures in children. J Pediatr Orthop 1985; 5:76.
18. Heeg M, Klasen HJ, Visser JD: Acetabular fractures in children and adolescents. J Bone Joint Surg 1989; 71-B:418.
19. Letournel E, Judet R: Fractures of the Acetabulum. Berlin, Springer-Verlag, 1981.
20. Sundar M, Carty H: Avulsion fracture of the pelvis in children: A report of 32 fractures and their outcome. Skel Radiol 1994; 23:85.
21. American College of Surgeons Committee on Trauma: Advance Trauma Life Support Course: Instruction Manual. Chicago, American College of Surgeons, 1993.
22. Bond SI, Gotschall CS, Eichelberger MR: Predictors of abdominal injury in children with pelvic fracture. J Trauma 1991; 31:1169.
23. Routt ML, Kregor PJ, Simonian PT, et al: Early results of percutaneous iliosacral screws with the patient in the supine position. J Orthop Trauma 1995; 9:207.
24. Rodrigues KF: Injury of the acetabular epiphysis. Injury 1973; 4:258.

ORTHOPAEDIC SPORTS MEDICINE

DARREN L. JOHNSON

MEDICAL ASPECTS OF SPORTS: EPIDEMIOLOGY OF INJURIES, PREPARTICIPATION PHYSICAL EXAMINATION, AND DRUGS IN SPORTS

Thomas D. Armsey and Robert G. Hosey

Summary
- The epidemiology of sports injuries helps identify the necessity for medical event coverage, injury risk factors, and potential prevention strategies.
- The preparticipation examination provides an opportunity for the team physician to identify athletes at risk of injury, to teach injury prevention, and to address athlete wellness.
- Knowledge of performance-enhancing drugs, nutritional supplements, and banned and legal medications is critical in caring for athletes.

Sports medicine as a discipline is a relative newcomer to the medical profession. As the worldwide interest in sports has boomed this past century, it seems natural that a specific niche in the medical world has evolved to provide specialized care for athletes. This branch of the medical community includes a wide range of health care professionals, including orthopaedists, primary care physicians, athletic trainers, physical therapists, and dentists, to name a few. The medical aspects of sports medicine encompass a wide spectrum of topics, including the diagnosis, management, and prevention of illness and injury in an athletic population. As can be imagined, this summarizes a rather expansive list of disease processes, from neurological injuries such as concussions to musculoskeletal injuries to the use of ergogenic aids. This chapter focuses on three rather broad topics that constitute a cornerstone of the practice of sports medicine. Specifically, we examine the epidemiology of sports injuries, the preparticipation physical examination, and the use of drugs in sports.

EPIDEMIOLOGY OF SPORTS INJURIES

In the medical literature, epidemiology is the study of the distribution and determinants of disease.[1] In sports medicine, most epidemiological studies regard acute and chronic injuries as "disease," and the results have broadened our current knowledge in many ways. Specifically, these studies have helped identify causes of injuries, determined the effectiveness of preventative measures, quantified the risks of various sport activities, and identified long-term injury trends in sport.[2] With these data, improved management and treatment plans for common injuries can be developed, and proactive measures can be designed to prevent common and catastrophic injuries to this population.

The injuries sustained in athletics are widely varied but commonly delineated into two distinct categories: acute traumatic injuries ("macrotrauma") and insidious overuse injuries ("microtrauma"). As one would imagine, the proportion of injuries in each of these categories is dependent mainly on the sport in question. For example, in contact sports, such as football, there is a higher proportion of acute traumatic injuries, whereas in noncontact sports, such

as track and field, there is a higher proportion of overuse injuries. Although these types of injuries are inherently different, they both result in debilitation of an athlete's performance and are therefore considered significant by most epidemiological studies.

INJURY DEFINITION AND REPORTING

The current epidemiological data are limited by the lack of a standardized nomenclature among studies. Because the published studies have reported data with different denominators, different definitions of injury, and different selection criteria, each study must be viewed as a separate case report, making it impossible to generalize the results on a broader scale. To remedy this, an attempt is being made to provide all injury data as case rates per 1000 athlete-exposure. An "athlete-exposure" is defined as one athlete's participation in one practice or game in which there is a possibility of sustaining an athletic injury. The current definition of a "reportable injury" is still under question but should include all of the following to allow valid comparison: (1) the injury occurs in a scheduled practice or game; (2) the injury requires medical attention; and (3) the injury results in restriction or exclusion of the athlete from the remaining practice or competition or the following 1 or more days.[3] Currently, several computer software companies are promoting standardized reporting systems, using this standardized nomenclature, which may provide insight into the causes of injuries that can be confirmed by consistent results from numerous investigators.

To date, most studies involving athletic injuries are reported as a cumulative incidence of injury. This is the number of injuries among a specific group of athletes (i.e., "team") followed for a defined period of time (i.e., "season"). Although there are inherent problems with these data, the following discussion reports these data unless otherwise noted. Injuries are classified as "mild" if the athlete was out of competition for less than 7 days, or "significant" if the athlete was disabled for 7 days or more. As mentioned previously, good data are not always available, but the most consistent data from well designed studies are reported.

Although sports medicine is a relatively new field, epidemiological data have already made an impact. Based on the literature to date, athletics has evolved into a less dangerous activity. This is most evident in football, in which drastic equipment improvements, such as improved helmet strength and face-masks, are now standard in hopes of decreasing brain and facial injuries. Rule changes, including the banning of "spear tackling" and "chop blocking" have occurred as a means to decrease cervical spine and knee injuries. The current debate is whether artificial turf is a predisposing factor for injuries and if so, this too may be eradicated in the name of medical science. But football is not the only sport that is evolving. Similar efforts are being made in other sports to create a "safer enviroment." It will be the current and future epidemiological data that will continue to identify high-risk activities and provide the impetus for change.

Unfortunately, all physical activity has an inherent risk of injury. According to the 1992 National Institute of Health report, there are approximately 3 million injuries annually in the United States that are directly related to organized sports. Of these, approximately 770,000 require physician visits and up to 90,000 require hospitalization.[4] In 1996, an estimated $1.3 billion was spent for acute management of these athletes.[5] If these injuries were catalogued as diseases, these figures would be unacceptable to the general public and the medical community. But, because of the incredible popularity of athletes and athletics, most individuals blindly accept injuries as a risk of participation. This may not necessarily be the case, and it is imperative that objective data be generated to determine factors that may potentially improve the injury rates in competitive and recreational sporting activities.

As previously mentioned, all sports have an inherent risk of injury. But which sport is the most dangerous? Overwhelmingly, football has the highest rate of reportable injuries among all organized sports, with injuries occurring in up to 81% of participants per year.[6,7] Football also has the distinction of leading all sports in the absolute number of catastrophic injuries and fatalities in the United States. Over a 6-year period (1982–1988), 187 high school athletes and 50 collegiate athletes were catastrophically injured and 73 of these injuries were fatal.[8] Although impressive on paper, these numbers do not adequately reflect the injury rates among different sports, unless reported in a standard unit. In the case of catastrophic injury and fatalities, when calculated as a rate per 100,000 participants per year, football was surpassed by both ice hockey and gymnastics. Furthermore, if the incidence of injury in football were reported as a percentage of the 1.8 million participants in the United States annual injury rates as low as 35.2% have resulted. It is therefore obvious that most of the current epidemiological data suffer from poor generalizability, and any interstudy comparisons must be critically analyzed for valid conclusions.

INJURY RATES AND SEVERITY

Two well-designed studies have reported injury rates that allow broad comparisons among many different sports. In an extensive study by Rice,[3] 18 intercollegiate sports were prospectively studied and the results reported so that comparisons between each sport are valid. According to Rice, female cross-country running has the highest injury rate per 1000 athlete-exposures (15.9), followed by wrestling (12.8), female soccer (12.6), football (12.2), and female gymnastics (10.2). From these data, it is apparent that several sports have a disproportionately higher rate of injuries compared with other sports. Except for some minor differences, these conclusions are consistent with the National Collegiate Athletic Association (NCAA) injury reports.[9] In these reports, spring football was found to have the highest rate of injury per 1000 athlete-exposures (9.8), followed by wrestling (9.6), female gymnastics (9.3), and female soccer (8.6). These two independent studies correlate very well and should prompt further investigations into the reasons

that a disproportionate number of athletes are being injured during participation in these sports.

As well as describing the number of injuries in sports, epidemiological studies also describe the severity of the injury. Although there are numerous ways to describe the severity of injury in sport, the most common method is reporting severity as a function of time lost from participation. "Mild" is anecdotally used to describe injuries from which it takes less than 7 days for the athlete to return to participation, versus "severe" injuries, from which it takes the athlete more than 7 days to return to sport. When the NCAA analyzed its most current data,[9] it was reported that spring football resulted in the highest percentage of severe injuries. In spring football, 43% of all injuries result in the athletes taking more than 7 days to return to sport. This translates into an injury rate of 4.1 severe injuries per 1000 athlete-exposures. Another means of categorizing injuries as severe is if the injury requires surgical intervention. When reported as such, female gymnastics had the highest percentage of severe injuries, with 8.9% of all surgery-requiring injuries occurring to female gymnasts. Furthermore, female gymnasts have the highest rate of surgery-requiring injuries per 1000 athlete-exposures. The rate is estimated at 0.84 injuries that will require surgery for every 1000 athlete-exposures. This certainly shows that spring football and female gymnastics are high-risk activities that may need to be modified to enhance their safety. The most apparent means to decrease the rates of severe injuries in these sports would be to decrease the number of athlete-exposures. Recently, the NCAA has addressed this issue in spring football by decreasing the contact days allowed, and future data will determine whether this modification will significantly decrease the rate of severe injuries occurring in this select population.

INJURY DEMOGRAPHICS

Characteristic injuries in different sports have been objectively documented by epidemiological studies. Retrospective analysis consistently reports that the knee is the most common site of injury in the sport of football. Of these knee injuries, the medial collateral ligament is the most common structure involved.[10] Few other sports have the amount of data available to make valid conclusions, but certainly trends can be observed. Eighty-four percent of the injuries in soccer involve the lower extremity, with ankle sprains being the most common.[11] In a 12-year prospective study of high school athletes participating in 32 different sports, the knee and ankle were the most common sites of injury in both men and women.[12] When reported as a percentage of all injuries sustained by intercollegiate athletes, the knee is injured about 25% of the time, making it the most common site of injury.[13] Halpern et al[14] reported similar results in high school athletes, noting that 25% of all injuries in this population occurred about the knee and ankle, and that these injuries accounted for 33% of all medical costs. Therefore, any modifications that could decrease the number of knee and ankle injuries in high school and collegiate athletics would have a profound impact on the health of millions of athletes.

Several confounding variables have been recognized in these studies that need to be addressed. First is the level of play, which may influence the injury incidence and patterns. In a large population of Danish soccer players, it was found that the more experienced athletes suffered fewer injuries than the less experienced athletes, with incidence rates of 11.9 versus 18.9 injuries per 1000 athlete exposures. It was also reported that the elite athletes suffered most injuries during competition, whereas the more novice players sustained most injuries during practice.[15] Age and gender of the athlete may also affect injury incidence. In a 7-year prospective study, it was found that males were most likely to sustain an injury during athletic activity between the ages of 10 to 19, whereas females suffered most injuries between 20 and 29 years of age.[11] It seems that the most likely explanation of these results is that more experienced athletes have superior body control and therefore put themselves at risk for injury less than novice athletes. Anecdotally, boys spend more time playing sports at a younger age than females, and therefore succumb to injury at a higher rate as teenagers simply because of increased exposure. But, because of this increased exposure, the males may gain more proprioceptive skills necessary to prevent injuries as they mature, making the rates decrease as they age. If this theory is true, then as females continue to participate in competitive athletics at earlier ages, their injury rates should begin to mirror those of males. Therefore, it remains to be seen whether gender has any intrinsic effect on injury rates in sporting activities.

CONCLUSION

Although this type of data is useful in preparticipation counseling with parents and athletes, the ultimate goal should be to reduce the risk of injury. With the current data, this is quite a difficult task. Therefore, future epidemiological studies must standardize research design, data collection, definitions and terminology, and reporting systems.

PREPARTICIPATION PHYSICAL EXAMINATION

The preparticipation physical examination (PPE) has become an annual undertaking in the sports medicine community. Most sports medicine physicians know all too well the countless hours of preparation, examination, and paper work required to get athletes "cleared" to participate in the upcoming season. At last count there were approximately 6 million high school athletes and over 300,000 collegiate athletes participating in some form of organized sport.[16,17] Most if not all of these athletes were required to a have a PPE prior to engaging in athletic activity. At the high school level, 50 out of 51 (District of Columbia included) interscholastic sports governing bodies require athletes to have some form of a medical evaluation before they can participate in high school sports.[18] Many states have also made the PPE a legal requirement for athletes at the high school level.[19] This means millions of athletes each year are required to undergo a PPE.

For approximately the past 30 years, the PPE has played a role in the evaluation of prospective athletes. At the outset, this may have entailed only a brief visit to the physician's office concluded with a cursory examination and the mandatory heart and hernia check. All that has changed. The PPE has evolved in part because of increased legal pressure, greater public awareness and interest in athletic injuries, and the development of sports medicine organizations. The year 1992 saw the development of a standardized PPE, through the combined effort of the American Academy of Family Physicians, American Academy of Pediatrics, American Medical Society for Sports Medicine, and the American Orthopedic Society for Sports Medicine.

This monograph was updated in 1996 and provides a template for the preparticipation history and physical examination.[20] Although these documents have been widely accepted and used, a standardized PPE has not been adopted on the national level.

OBJECTIVES OF THE PREPARTICIPATION PHYSICAL EXAMINATION

As sports medicine physicians, one of our roles is to encourage safe activity for all individuals. Similarly, the major goal of the PPE is to enssure the health and safety of athletes participating in organized sports (to the best of our capabilities).[21,22] To this extent, the PPE examination should accomplish several objectives.

- Detection of any underlying condition that would restrict athletic participation.
- Identification and evaluation of potential problems (including previous injuries)
- Injury prevention evaluation
- Fulfillment of legal and insurance requirements
- Establishing physician rapport with athletes
- Providing counseling to athletes
- Establishing a database and record-keeping system

Detection of medical problems such as a heart murmur that increases in intensity with Valsalva maneuver or in the standing position (suggestive of hypertrophic cardiomyopathy) is an example of an underlying condition that would restrict participation. Potential problems that may be elucidated during the PPE include pre-existing musculoskeletal injuries that have not been completely rehabilitated, congenital anomalies (alantoaxial instability in Down's syndrome patients), and an overall low level of fitness that may be seen in obese individuals. Injury prevention includes assessment of the student's level of maturity. Individuals with delayed growth and physical maturity may be at increased risk of injury participating in collision sports. In addition to assessing the physical health of students, the PPE also satisfies any legal or insurance requirements as mandated by a scholastic institution or the state government. Beyond the practical aspects of the PPE, this time spent with the athlete is important in developing a trusting relationship with the athlete. This in turn may increase the likelihood of the athlete's discussing an injury or illness with the physician. It may also allow the physician to note changes in behavior in athletes dealing with such struggles as eating disorders or symptoms that can accompany a post-concussive state. Knowing that the PPE may be the only time all year that the athlete sees a physician, some physicians have argued that the PPE is the optimal time to counsel individuals and perform a general health maintenance examination. Topics such as smoking, alcohol and drug use, seat belt use, and violence can be addressed. This may also be an opportune time to teach adolescents self-breast and self-testicular examination. While these efforts should be applauded, the PPE is not meant to take the place of a yearly health maintenance examination performed by the individual's primary care physician.

Another purpose of the PPE is to establish a database and record keeping system. Ideally, each athlete should have a chart maintained in the training room that contains his or her PPE form, consent for emergency treatment, and emergency contact information. These charts could also be used to house injury report forms and subsequent treatment regimens. This system allows tracking of individual injuries and can be maintained throughout the student's academic career. Injury tracking systems, once established, also provide the framework for possible future research endeavors.

FORMAT, TIMING, AND FREQUENCY OF THE PREPARTICIPATION EXAMINATION

As the PPE has evolved, so has the format and the setting in which the examinations are performed. Traditionally, a single physician would be responsible for conducting individual examinations for a large number of athletes, either on an individual basis or through a mass screening. Mass screenings may encounter several problems. They often take place in the school gymnasium or the locker room, where lack of privacy is an issue. Physician burnout is a strong possibility as well. As an alternative, the concept of the sports medicine team approach using PPE stations has come into favor.[23,24] The team approach includes participation from the athletic training staff, team orthopaedists, and team medical staff, thus allowing the work to be broken up among all the staff. This group effort also fosters a line of communication between the members of the sports medicine team. In a group PPE using a station set-up, the athletes progress through a series of approximately six stations where the full examination is carried out in a piece-work fashion. This approach facilitates screening of a large number of people in a relatively efficient manner. (A sample of how the stations may be arranged is shown in Figure 1).

The frequency at which the PPE should be performed has met with varying opinions. One thought is that a full PPE should be performed every 3 to 4 years with interim updating of the athlete's medical history on a yearly basis.[25] The NCAA has endorsed a similar approach, requiring a PPE only on the athlete's initial entrance into college and recommending yearly follow-up.[26] At the time of follow-up, a focused examination can be conducted, directed by any problems divulged in the interim history. Many states and universities, however, require an annual physical examination for high school and collegiate athletes.[27] As a general rule of thumb, the PPE should be conducted 4 to 6 weeks prior to the start of the athletic season. This time lag allows time for follow-up on abnormal findings and rehabilitation of any injuries.[22,28]

PRE-PARTICIPATION HISTORY AND EXAMINATION

A comprehensive medical history is an essential part of the PPE. In fact, most conditions that restrict athletic participation are identified in the history portion of the PPE.[29] The history should divulge previous disease processes, injuries, surgeries, and possible cardiovascular problems. The history portion of PPE should be completed with the help of the athlete's parents in school-aged individuals to provide the most accurate information. The physician may then review this sheet and investigate any potential problems. The examination focuses on the musculoskeletal and cardiovascular systems and can be further directed by any abnormalities uncovered during the history. A standardized history and physical examination form has been developed and gained wide acceptance in the sports medicine community (Figures 2 and 3.)

Although the physical examination is not limited to the musculoskeletal and cardiovascular systems, these certainly are the focal points in asymptomatic individuals with an unremarkable medical history. The musculoskeletal screening examination can generally be accomplished in a short period of time using the 90-second orthopaedic screening examination.[20] This screening examination consists of observing the athlete perform a series of maneuvers and assessing overall musculoskeletal health. Starting at the top, the athlete is asked to

1. Look up, side to side, and down, touch ears to shoulders (cervical spine range of motion).

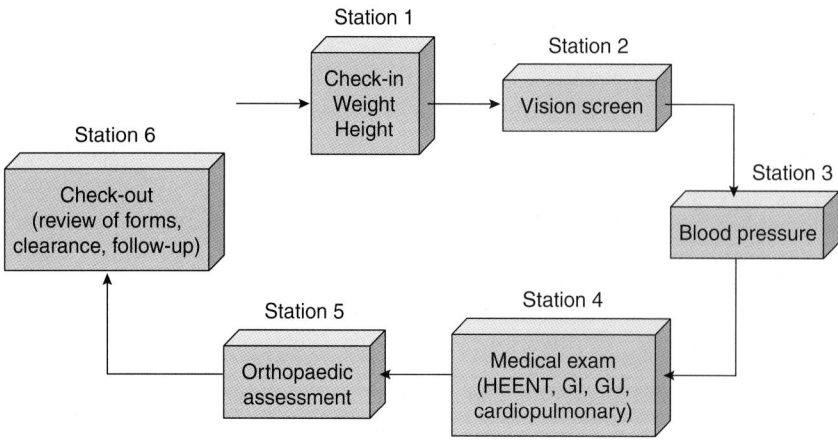

Fig. 1. Station format for performing the preparticipation examination. This schematic depicts a blueprint for setting up stations for performing a large volume of preparticipation examinations. The number and type of staffing members at each station will depend on the number of expected athletes to be screened. Physician staff members should be located at stations 4 through 6 with the head team physician at station 6.

Station 1
Check-in Weight Height

Station 2
Vision screen

Station 3
Blood pressure

Station 4
Medical exam (HEENT, GI, GU, cardiopulmonary)

Station 5
Orthopaedic assessment

Station 6
Check-out (review of forms, clearance, follow-up)

Preparticipation Physical Evaluation

HISTORY

DATE OF EXAM _____

Name _____ Sex _____ Age _____ Date of birth _____
Grade ____ School _____ Sport(s) _____
Address _____ Phone _____
Personal physician _____
In case of emergency, contact _____
Name _____ Relationship _____ Phone (H) _____ (W) _____

Explain "Yes" answers below.
Circle questions you don't know the answers to.

	Yes	No
1. Have you had a medical illness or injury since your last check up or sports physical?	☐	☐
Do you have an ongoing or chronic illness?	☐	☐
2. Have you ever been hospitalized overnight?	☐	☐
Have you ever had surgery?	☐	☐
3. Are you currently taking any prescription or nonprescription (over-the-counter) medications or pills or using an inhaler?	☐	☐
Have you ever taken any supplements or vitamins to help you gain or lose weight or improve your performance?	☐	☐
4. Do you have any allergies (for example, to pollen, medicine, food, or stinging insects)?	☐	☐
Have you ever had a rash or hives develop during or after exercise?	☐	☐
5. Have you ever passed out during or after exercise?	☐	☐
Have you ever been dizzy during or after exercise?	☐	☐
Have you ever had chest pain during or after exercise?	☐	☐
Do you get tired more quickly than your friends do during exercise?	☐	☐
Have you ever had racing of your heart or skipped heartbeats?	☐	☐
Have you had high blood pressure or high cholesterol?	☐	☐
Have you ever been told you have a heart murmur?	☐	☐
Has any family member or relative died of heart problems or of sudden death before age 50?	☐	☐
Have you had a severe viral infection (for example, myocarditis or mononucleosis) within the last month?	☐	☐
Has a physician ever denied or restricted your participation in sports for any heart problems?	☐	☐
6. Do you have any current skin problems (for example, itching, rashes, acne, warts, fungus, or blisters)?	☐	☐
7. Have you ever had a head injury or concussion?	☐	☐
Have you ever been knocked out, become unconscious, or lost your memory?	☐	☐
Have you ever had a seizure?	☐	☐
Do you have frequent or severe headaches?	☐	☐
Have you ever had numbness or tingling in your arms, hands, legs, or feet?	☐	☐
Have you ever had a stinger, burner, or pinched nerve?	☐	☐
8. Have you ever become ill from exercising in the heat?	☐	☐
9. Do you cough, wheeze, or have trouble breathing during or after activity?	☐	☐
Do you have asthma?	☐	☐
Do you have seasonal allergies that require medical treatment?	☐	☐

	Yes	No
10. Do you use any special protective or corrective equipment or devices that aren't usually used for your sport or position (for example, knee brace, special neck roll, foot orthotics, retainer on your teeth, hearing aid)?	☐	☐
11. Have you had any problems with your eyes or vision?	☐	☐
Do you wear glasses, contacts, or protective eyewear?	☐	☐
12. Have you ever had a sprain, strain, or swelling after injury?	☐	☐
Have you broken or fractured any bones or dislocated any joints?	☐	☐
Have you had any other problems with pain or swelling in muscles, tendons, bones, or joints?	☐	☐

If yes, check appropriate box and explain below

☐ Head	☐ Elbow	☐ Hip
☐ Neck	☐ Forearm	☐ Thigh
☐ Back	☐ Wrist	☐ Knee
☐ Chest	☐ Hand	☐ Shin/calf
☐ Shoulder	☐ Finger	☐ Ankle
☐ Upper arm		☐ Foot

	Yes	No
13. Do you want to weigh more or less than you do now?	☐	☐
Do you lose weight regularly to meet weight requirements for your sport?	☐	☐
14. Do you feel stressed out?	☐	☐

15. Record the dates of your most recent immunizations (shots) for:

Tetanus _____ Measles _____
Hepatitis B _____ Chickenpox _____

FEMALES ONLY

16. When was your first menstrual period? _____
When was your most recent menstrual period? _____
How much time do you usually have from the start of one period to the start of another? _____
How many periods have you had in the last year? _____
What was the longest time between periods in the last year? ___

Explain "Yes" answers here: _____
_____
_____
_____
_____
_____
_____
_____
_____
_____

I hereby state that, to the best of my knowledge, my answers to the above questions are complete and correct.

Signature of athlete _____ Signature of parent/gaurdian _____ Date _____

Fig. 2. Preparticipation medical history. This is the sample form to be used for obtaining the preparticipation medical history. (Leawood KS: American Academy of Family Physicians, American Academy of Pediatrics, American Medical Society for Sports Medicine, American Orthopaedic Society for Sports Medicine, American Osteopathic Academy of Sports Medicine, 1992, 1996.)

2. Shrug shoulders against resistance, adduct shoulders to 90 degrees (hold against resistance), followed by internal and external rotation of shoulders at 90 degrees (trapezius and deltoid strength, shoulder range of motion).

3. Flex and extend elbows, pronate and supinate with elbows flexed to 90 degrees with arms at side (elbow and wrist range of motion).

4. Spread fingers apart, make a fist (hand function, any rotational deformities).

Preparticipation Physical Evaluation

PHYSICAL EXAMINATION

Name _____ Date of birth _____

Height _____ Weight _____ % Body fat (optional) _____ Pulse _____ BP___ / ___ / (___ / ___ , ___ / ___)

Vision R 20/ ____ L 20/ ____   Corrected: Y N   Pupils: Equal ____ Unequal ____

	NORMAL	ABNORMAL FINDINGS	INITIALS*
MEDICAL			
Appearance			
Eyes/Ears/Nose/Throat			
Lymph Nodes			
Heart			
Pulses			
Lungs			
Abdomen			
Genitalia (males only)			
Skin			
MUSCULOSKELETAL			
Neck			
Back			
Shoulder/arm			
Elbow/forearm			
Wrist/hand			
Hip/thigh			
Knee			
Leg/ankle			
Foot			

*Station-based examination only

CLEARANCE

☐ Cleared
☐ Cleared after completing evaluation/rehabilitation for: _____
_____
_____
_____

☐ Not cleared for: _____ Reason: _____
Recommendations _____
_____
_____
_____

Name of physician (print/type) _____ Date _____
Address _____ Phone _____
Signature of physician _____ MD or DO

Fig. 3. Preparticipation physical examination. This is the sample form to be used for recording the physical evaluation part of the preparticipation examination. (Leawood KS: American Academy of Family Physicians, American Academy of Pediatrics, American Medical Society for Sports Medicine, American Orthopaedic Society for Sports Medicine, American Osteopathic Academy of Sports Medicine, 1992, 1996.)

5. Contract and relax quadriceps muscles (knee symmetry, patellar function, quadriceps mechanism).
6. Duck-walk away from and toward examiner (hip, knee, and ankle function).
7. Touch toes with legs straight (scoliosis evaluation, hamstring flexibility).
8. Stand on toes, stand on heels (leg and foot strength, calf symmetry).

Any abnormalities of motion or maneuvers that elicit pain should prompt further focused examination. This examination serves as a good screening tool when doing mass screening PPEs, but it may not be sufficient for all populations of athletes (e.g., professional athletes).

In addition to assessing cardiovascular health, the cardiovascular history and examination is aimed at identifying individuals who may be at increased risk of sudden cardiac death. In the United States, the leading causes of sudden cardiac death in high school and collegiate athletes are hypertrophic cardiomyopathy, coronary artery anomalies, myocarditis, and aortic stenosis.[30] Athletes with a history of exercise-related chest discomfort, syncope or near syncope, unexplained shortness of breath or fatigue, a past history of a heart murmur, or a family history of premature death should raise the suspicion of a potential problem. The American Heart Association's (AHA) scientific statement on cardiovascular preparticipation screening of competitive athletes recommends that cardiac evaluation include (but not be limited to) (1) precordial auscultation in both the standing and supine position, (2) assessment of the femoral pulses to exclude coarctation of the aorta, (3) brachial blood pressure measured in the seated position, and (4) evaluation for physical signs of Marfan's syndrome.[31] Detection of a cardiac murmur that is a grade III/VI or louder, a diastolic murmur, or a murmur that increases in intensity with Valsalva maneuver or in the standing position should prompt further evaluation by a cardiologist. Likewise, athletes with blood pressures greater than 135/85 need further follow-up with repeated blood pressure measurements. At this point in time, further cardiovascular screening with either electrocardiogram or echocardiogram is not cost efficient on a large-scale basis.[31,32] The remainder of the physical examination may be used to focus on any complaints noted in the history but also should include examination of the head, ears, eyes, nose, and throat structures, pulmonary examination and abdominal examination including a hernia check. A general assessment of the young athlete's physical maturity should be noted, and testicular examination performed on collegiate males.

Additional testing that may be conducted during the PPE includes measurement of flexibility and percentage of body fat. Although these may provide useful information, they are time and staff intensive.

DETERMINATION OF CLEARANCE

Determination of clearance status is arguably the most important purpose of the PPE. The physician's role is to make a decision regarding clearance based on the safety of the athlete and other participants who may come into contact with the athlete. To this extent, several questions must be answered. Does the athlete's condition put himself or herself, teammates, or competitors at increased risk of injury or illness? Is treatment available for the athlete's condition that will allow him or her to participate after treatment or once treatment is initiated? Is there protective gear that would allow the athlete to participate safely? Can the athlete participate on a limited basis? Is there an alternative sport that the athlete can participate in safely? Based on the answers to these questions the athlete may be (1)

cleared without restriction, (2) cleared after completing further evaluation or rehabilitation for a specific injury or illness, or (3) not cleared for participation (in a particular sport). If the athlete is not cleared, the reasoning leading to that decision should be discussed with the individual, the coaching and training staff, and, for school-aged athletes, the individual's parents. Often a conference involving all of these parties and the physician allows for the best exchange of information.

DISQUALIFYING CONDITIONS

Certain medical conditions warrant restriction from specific types of sports. However, most of these disqualifying conditions do allow for participation in some form of athletic activity. For example, an athlete with a poorly controlled seizure disorder should not be allowed to participate in contact sports, whereas it would be appropriate to allow participation in certain noncontact sports. The American Academy of Pediatrics Committee on Sports Medicine classified individual sports based on the amount of contact and level of strenuousness (Tables 1 and 2).[33] In addition, a list of potential disqualifying conditions based on these parameters has been generated and may assist team physicians in determining clearance.[20] Athletes with cardiovascular abnormalities present a complex situation regarding medical clearance. In 1994, a multidisciplinary task force developed guidelines that were based on the most up-to-date scientific data as well as years of anecdotal experience.[34] Although these guidelines are helpful in determining eligibility, each athlete's case should be considered individually. This year, many athletes will be cleared to play sports with conditions that were once considered disqualifying. For example, an athlete with Marfan's disease may be cleared to participate in highly strenuous sports by an experienced team physician who is comfortable that the athlete understands the risks involved and agrees to serial cardiac, opthomalogical, and musculoskeletal evaluations. Furthermore, in these types of situations it is a good idea to obtain written consent or a legal waiver to be signed by the athlete and parent (if the athlete is a minor). The legal counsel for any academic institution may provide useful information regarding legal issues related to athletic participation or disqualification.

The PPE is an opportune time to address the issue of supplement or drug use in the athlete. Education regarding the potential side effects or legal ramifications may also be discussed. Use of prescription and over-the-counter medications should also be reviewed, as many of these medications appear on the "banned" list and require a physician's note for approved usage. A more detailed account of commonly used performance-enhancing drugs is covered in the next section.

DRUGS IN SPORTS

In 1968, formal drug testing was adopted for the Summer and Winter Olympics in an attempt to maintain the integrity of sports by enforcing compliance with the "banned-substance list." Banned substances are ergogenic in nature and used with the sole intention of increasing in an artificial and unfair manner the athlete's performance in compe-

TABLE 1. CLASSIFICATION OF SPORTS

| | | Noncontact | | |
Contact/Collision	Limited Contact/ Impact	Strenuous	Moderately Strenuous	Nonstrenuous
Boxing	Baseball	Aerobic dancing	Badminton	Archery
Field hockey	Basketball	Crew	Curling	Golf
Football	Bicycling	Fencing	Table tennis	Riflery
Ice hockey	Diving	Field		
Lacrosse	Field	Discus		
Martial arts	High jump	Javelin		
Rodeo	Pole vault	Shot put		
Soccer	Gymnastics	Running		
Wrestling	Horseback riding	Swimming		
	Skating	Tennis		
	Ice	Track		
	Roller	Weight lifting		
	Skiing			
	Cross-country			
	Downhill			
	Water			
	Softball			
	Squash, handball			
	Volleyball			

From American Academy of Pediatrics Committee on Sports Medicine: Recommendations for participation in competitive sports. Pediatrics 1988, 81:737.

tition. Since the commencement of testing by the International Olympic Committee (IOC), numerous elite athletes have been sanctioned for "doping" and subjected to the predetermined penalties. In 1986, after the highly publicized cocaine-related death of a collegiate student-athlete, the NCAA adopted drug testing. Currently, every major sports governing body has adopted a plan to combat drug use among its athletes. But, owing to the lack of uniformity in banned substances across sports, it is essential for every team physician to prescribe and council athletes according to each governing body's specified regulations.

BANNED SUBSTANCES

Generally, banned substances fall into several categories: stimulants, narcotics, anabolic steroids, beta-blockers, diuretics, and growth hormones. Certain restrictions are in place for other medications, including alcohol, local anesthetics, corticosteroids, and beta-agonists. For a complete listing of the NCAA and United States Olympic Committee (USOC) banned and restricted drug list, refer to the Athletic Drug Reference '99.[35]

NUTRITIONAL SUPPLEMENTS

Recently, athletes have attempted to gain a competitive edge through over-the-counter "natural" preparations, known as nutritional supplements. As defined, nutritional supplements are any foodstuff or dietary procedure that either improves or is thought to improve ones' health (dietary aids) or physical performance (ergogenic aids). Because of this nebulous definition, nutritional supplements fall outside of the Food and Drug Administration's umbrella of jurisdiction and are therefore largely unregulated. Because of the lack of federal regulation, the manufacturers of these compounds may advertise unsubstantiated claims

as to their effectiveness. In the United States, more than 12 billion dollars was spent on supplements in 1997 and an estimated 15 billion dollars in 1999.[36] Because of the obvious popularity of these substances and the potential effects on one's health, it is essential for allopathic physicians to be knowledgeable in this arena. Therefore, to counsel potential consumers, physicians must be adequately educated to the risks and benefits of these nutritional supplements.

It is important to remember that competitive athletes must scrutinize all over-the-counter supplements for any substances that may be banned by their governing bodies. Since the USOC (1983) and the NCAA (1986) began random drug testing, many athletes have claimed that an over-the-counter supplement caused them to test "positive" for banned substances. This may well be the truth, since various preparations do contain chemicals that are prohibited by the USOC and the NCAA.

Creatine

Creatine (methylguanide-acetic acid) is an amino acid identified in 1835 by Chevreul. It is naturally synthesized in the human liver, pancreas, and kidneys and is available from a normal diet in meats and fish.[37] In 1993, creatine monohydrate was introduced to the American public as a "safe" nutritional supplement that provides enormous strength gains when taken in conjunction with resistive exercise.

Theoretically, there are two major physiological benefits of creatine supplementation. The first benefit is the fact that increased creatine intake enhances the bioavailability of phosphocreatine in skeletal muscle cells. This, in turn, allows faster resynthesis of adenosine triphosphate from adenosine diphosphate and results in quicker recovery from brief, high-intensity exercise.[38–40] The second theoretical

TABLE 2. RECOMMENDATIONS FOR PARTICIPATION IN COMPETITIVE SPORTS

	Contact/ Collision	Limited Contact/Impact	Noncontact		
			Strenuous	*Moderately Strenuous*	*Nonstrenuous*
Atlantoaxial instability	No	No	Yes*	Yes	Yes
* *Swimming: no butterfly, breast stroke, or diving starts*					
Acute illnesses	*	*	*	*	*
* *Needs individual assessment, eg, contagiousness to others, risk of worsening illness*					
Cardiovascular					
Carditis	No	No	No	No	No
Hypertension					
Mild	Yes	Yes	Yes	Yes	Yes
Moderate	*	*	*	*	*
	*	*	*	*	*
Severe	†	†	†	†	†
Congenital heart disease					
* *Needs individual assessment.*					
† *Patients with mild forms can be allowed a full range of physical activities; patients with moderate or severe forms, or who are postoperative, should be evaluated by a cardiologist before athletic participation.*					
Eyes					
Absence or loss of function of one eye	*	*	*	*	*
Detached retina	†	†	†	†	†
* *Availability of American Society for Testing and Materials (ASTM)-approved eye guards may allow competitor to participate in most sports, but this must be judged on an individual basis.*					
† *Consult ophthalmologist*					
Inguinal hernia	Yes	Yes	Yes	Yes	Yes
Kidney: Absence of one	No	Yes	Yes	Yes	Yes
Liver: Enlarged	No	No	Yes	Yes	Yes
Musculoskeletal disorders	*	*	*	*	*
* *Needs individual assessment*					
Neurologic					
History of serious head or spine trauma, repeated concussions, or craniotomy	*	*	Yes	Yes	Yes
Convulsive disorder					
Well controlled	Yes	Yes	Yes	Yes	Yes
Poorly controlled	No	No	Yes†	Yes	Yes†
* *Needs individual assessment*					
† *No swimming or weight lifting*					
‡ *No archery or riflery*					
Ovary: Absence of one	Yes	Yes	Yes	Yes	Yes
Respiratory					
Pulmonary insufficiency	*	*	*	*	Yes
Asthma	Yes	Yes	Yes	Yes	Yes
* *May be allowed to compete if oxygenation remains satisfactory during a graded stress test*					
Sickle cell trait	Yes	Yes	Yes	Yes	Yes
Skin: Boils, herpes, impetigo, scabies	*	*	Yes	Yes	Yes
* *No gymnastics with mats, martial arts, wrestling, or contact sports until not contagious*					
Spleen: Enlarged	No	No	No	Yes	Yes
Testicle: Absence or undescended	Yes*	Yes*	Yes	Yes	Yes
* *Certain sports may require protective cup.*					

From American Academy of Pediatrics Committee on Sports Medicine: Recommendations for participation in competitive sports. Pediatrics 1988, 81:737.

benefit of creatine supplementation is its ability to delay fatigue. Phosphocreatine, as well as acting as an energy source for working muscle, also buffers the intracellular hydrogen ions that occur during exercise. It is thought that these hydrogen ions contribute to fatigue. Therefore, elevated intracellular phosphocreatine levels should enhance

performance by delaying muscle fatigue and prolonging time to exhaustion.

Numerous laboratory and field studies have demonstrated significant performance enhancement in athletic males, in both brief, high-intensity work output and total time to exhaustion, with creatine supplementation of 20 to 30 g per day.[41-43] Currently, no clinical studies have reported a direct improvement in athletic performance due to creatine supplementation, but in strength athletes, this supplement must be seriously considered as a potential ergogenic aid. Some of the ambiguity of scientific data concerning creatine supplementation may be due to large variation in intracellular creatine concentrations among athletes. Many athletes naturally exhibit concentrations above the mean because of higher rates of endogenous synthesis or elevated intake of creatine in food sources. Further supplementation by these athletes may result in no significant improvements in strength or stamina. On the other hand, athletes with lower than average intracellular creatine levels (e.g., females and vegetarians), may demonstrate significant improvements if creatine is added to their normal diets.

Although creatine monohydrate is considered a nutritional supplement with potential ergogenic effects, some investigators are concerned about its side-effect profile. The potential hazards of this supplement include severe muscle cramping and possible kidney damage when used in a dehydrated state. In 1997, creatine supplementation was blamed for the deaths of two NCAA wrestlers, but autopsy results proved that severe dehydration, not supplemental creatine, was instrumental in their deaths. Currently, there are no data regarding the use of creatine in adolescents and no studies to evaluate the effects of long-term creatine supplementation. Therefore, according to the current scientific data, creatine monohydrate may be a safe and effective ergogenic aid when taken in recommended amounts for short durations in healthy individuals.

Dehydroepiandrosterone

Dehydroepiandrosterone (DHEA) is touted as a "fountain of youth" supplement by marketers and consumed by millions of Americans because of the reported anti-obesity, anti-aging, and anti-cancer effects. In 1985, DHEA was taken off the market by the Food and Drug Administration (FDA) because of a potential association with liver damage. But with the passage of the federal "Dietary Supplement Health and Education Act" in 1994, the supplement industry was able to reclassify this substance as a "nutritional supplement," and DHEA was released to the public as an over-the-counter preparation. Since its introduction, the popularity of this supplement has continued to grow in the United States, and with the recent admission of use by prominent athletes, this growth is certain to increase.

DHEA was first identified in 1934 as an androgen produced in the adrenal glands. It is a precursor to the endogenous production of both androgens and estrogens. As an androgenic precursor, DHEA is thought to increase the production of testosterone and provide an anabolic steroid effect. Popularity for supplementation of DHEA stems from the observation that concentrations of this endogenous hormone steadily decline after approximately 20 years of age,[44] propagating the theory that DHEA may play a role in the aging process. Currently, well-designed published studies regarding the efficacy of DHEA have been scarce. Investigators have determined that DHEA supplementation in doses of 50 to 100 mg/day will significantly increase androgenic steroid plasma levels as well as subjective improvements in physical and psychological well-being.[45,46] Currently, there is no literature to show the effect of DHEA on body composition, fat distribution, strength, or athletic performance. It is also unknown what effect, if any, DHEA would have on a young, healthy individual, since all research participants have been mature adults (>40 years old) with chronic illness.

Although few adverse effects of DHEA supplementation have been reported, there is the potential for serious irreversible morphogenic changes.[47] These include virilization in women, hirsutism, voice deepening, and alopecia. Once again, long-term effects are unknown, but theoretically, DHEA has the potential to increase the risk of uterine and prostate cancer because of the prolonged elevation of estrogens and testosterone. DHEA may also have a feminizing effect with prolonged use by competing with testosterone for receptor binding sites. Although unreported, there are concerns that prolonged use may lead to insulin resistance, decreased levels of high density lipoprotien cholesterol, and potentially liver cancer.

DHEA is a banned substance according to the NCAA and the USOC, falling under the heading of an androgenic-anabolic agent. Therefore, the use of this supplement may lead to disqualification from competitive athletics. Given the sparsity of information, DHEA supplementation must be viewed with caution and skepticism. The use of this agent should be discouraged until scientific studies determine whether it is safe and effective.

Androstenedione

Androstenendione, which is chemically related to DHEA, has recently overwhelmed the nutritional supplement market. As a precursor to endogenous testosterone, this supplement is thought to enhance testosterone levels and therefore provide significant gains in fat-free muscle mass. To date, little research has been completed on this supplement. One prospective study showed no improvement in strength or fat-free muscle mass with androstenedione supplementation in dosages of 100 and 300 mg per day over an 8-week period, but this study had multiple design flaws and therefore may not have achieved valid results.[48] The most current data show that oral androstenedione administration at dosages of 300 mg/day will significantly increase serum testosterone and estradiol levels.[49] This increase in serum sex hormones is short-lived and nomalizes within 24 hours. Therefore, to observe androgenic benefits, a much more frequent dosing schedule may be necessary.

Side effects similar to those of DHEA should be expected (e.g., virilization, hirsuitism, uterine and prostate cancer, gynecomastia, and liver damage) and no data on long-term use have been published. Androstenedione use is prohibited by the NCAA and the USOC, and if detected will potentially lead to disqualification. Therefore, the use of this agent for unsubstantiated gains in strength must be cautioned until further research can be completed.

Beta-hydroxy-beta-methylbutyrate

Beta-hydroxy-beta-methylbutyrate (HMB) is one of the most recent additions to the "nutritional supplement" armamentarium. HMB is a metabolite of the essential amino acid leucine and is produced in small amounts endogenously. It is found in the normal diet in catfish, citrus fruits, and breast milk. HMB was introduced as an ergogenic aid by investigators at Iowa State University, who believe that it may participate in the regulation of protein metabolism. Promoters hypothesize that HMB regulates the enzymes responsible for protein breakdown, and with supplementation muscle mass may increase by slowing muscle degradation.

Currently, researchers have concluded that HMB supplementation may increase muscle mass and strength in livestock and humans. The literature regarding this supplement is sparse, but several randomized, placebo-controlled studies have produced promising results.[50] These studies have yet to be duplicated by anyone besides the original investigators, who hold the patent on the supplement; therefore, the results have met with much scientific scrutiny. Although supplementation with HMB may produce significant increases in muscle mass and strength, it is too early to recommend this agent because of the limited knowledge available regarding its safety profile and mechanism of action.

CONCLUSION

Most nutritional supplements sold in the United States are considered safe by consumers, if taken in appropriate doses and in a pure formulation. But, owing to the lack of quality control in the supplement industry, it is difficult to determine the levels of active ingredients in each tablet or capsule. In a recent consumer report, it was found that there was significant brand-to-brand as well as dose-to-dose variation among the concentrations of supposed active ingredients.[51] Therefore, consumers may be over- or underestimating the doses of these preparations, even when taken according to labeled instructions. From January 1993 to October 1998, the Food and Drug Administration received 2621 reports of serious problems, including 101 deaths, linked to supplements. Furthermore, contaminants have been found in supplement preparations. The most remarkable case resulted in 32 deaths from eosinophilia-myalgia syndrome that were directly linked to the use of the popular nutritional supplement L-tryptophan.[52] The contaminant responsible was formed during the process of purifying L-tryptophan. Also of note are the numerous reports of hepatotoxicity associated with "health food" products (jin bu huan, germander, chaparral, senna, mistletoe, skullcap, comfrey, and crotolaria).[53–55] This is an important reminder that "natural" or "herbal" on a product label does not ensure safety. With these substantial risks and the paucity of scientifically proven benefits, it would seem that nutritional supplementation is unnecessary and potentially dangerous.

REFERENCES

1. Morton RF, Hebel JR: Study Guide to Epidemiology and Biostatics. Baltimore, University Park Press, 1979, p 1.
2. McKeag DB, Hough DO: Epidemiology of Athletic Injuries: Primary Care Sports Medicine. Dubuque, IA, Brown and Benchmark, 1993, p. 63.
3. Rice SG: Epidemiology and mechanisms of sports injuries. In: Teitz CC, Decker BC (eds): Scientific Foundations of Sports Medicine. Philadelphia, WB Saunders, 1989, p 3.
4. Conference on Sports Injuries in Youth. Bethesda, MD, National Institute of Health; 1992. NIH Publication No 93-3444.
5. Hergenroeder AC: Prevention of sports injuries. Pediatrics 1998; 101(6):1057.
6. Garrick JG, Requa RK: Injuries in high school sports. Pediatrics 1989, 84:446.
7. Meeuwisse WH, Fowler PJ: Frequency and predictability of sports injuries in intercollegiate athletes. Can J Spt Sci 1988; 13:35.
8. Mueller FO, Cantu RC: Catastrophic injuries and fatalities in high school and college sports, fall 1982–spring 1988. Med Sci Sports Exerc 1990; 22:737.
9. National Collegiate Athletic Association: Injury Surveillance System: 1997–1998. Overland Park, KS, National Collegiate Athletic Association, 1998.
10. Fetto JF, Marshall JL: Medial collateral ligament injuries of the knee: A rationale for treatment. Clin Orthop 1978; 132:206.
11. Tenvergent EM, Ten Duis HF, Clasen HJ: Trends in sports injuries 1982–1988: An in depth study on four types of sports. J Sports Med Phys Fitness 1992; 32:214.
12. Beachy G, Akau CK, Martinson M, Olderr TF: High school sports injuries: A longitudinal study at Panahou school: 1988 to 1996. Am J Sports Med 1997; 25(5):675.
13. Fowler, PJ: Injuries to university athletes: A challenge for all of us. Paper presented at FISU Sports Medicine Conference in Edmonton, Alberta, 1996.
14. Halpern B, Thompson N, Curl WW, et al: High school football injuries: Identifying the risk factors. Am J Sports Med 1987; 15:316.
15. Nielsen AB, Yde J: Epidemiology in traumatology of injuries in soccer. Am J Sports Med 1989; 7:803.
16. National Federation of State High School Associations: 1995–96 Athletics Participation Survey. Kansas City, MO, National Federation of State High School Associations, 1996.
17. National Collegiate Athletic Association: Participation Statistics Report, 1982–1996. Overland Park, KS, National Collegiate Athletic Association, 1995.
18. Glover DW, Maron BJ. Profile of preparticipation cardiovascular screening for high school athletes. JAMA 1998; 279(22):1817.
19. Feinstein RA, Soileau EJ, Daniel WA: A National survey of preparticipation physical examination requirements. Phys Sports Med 1988; 16(5):51.
20. American Academy of Family Physicians, American Academy of Pediatrics, American Medical Society for Sports Medicine, et al: Preparticiptation Physical Evaluation. Kansas City, MO: American Academy of Family Physicians, 1997.
21. Nichols AW, Buxton BP, Ho KW: Preparticipation examination: A new form in Hawaii. Hawaiian Med J 1995; 54:434.
22. Grafe MW, Paul GR, Foster TE: The preparticipation sports examination for high school and college athletes. Clin Sports Med 1997; 16(4):569.
23. Garrick JG: Sports medicine. Pediatric Clin North Am 1977; 24:737.
24. Linder CW, Du Rant RH, Seklecki RM, et al: Preparticipation health screening of young athletes. Am J Sports Med 1981; 9: 187.
25. Ham JH, Puffer JC: The preparticipation physical examination. In Mellion MS (ed): Office Management of Sports Injuries and Athletic Problems. Philadelphia, Hanley and Belfus, 1987.
26. National Collegiate Athletic Association: 1995–996 Sports Medicine Handbook. Overland Park, KS, National Collegiate Athletic Association, 1995.
27. Feinstein RA, Sorlean EJ, Daniel WA: A national survey of preparticipation physical examination requirements. Phys Sports Med 1988; 16:51–59.
28. McKeag DB: Preseason physical examination for the prevention of sports injuries. Sports Med 1985; 2:413–431.
29. Rifat SF, Ruffin MT, Gorenflo DW: Disqualifying criteria in preparticipation sports evaluation. J Fam Pract 1995; 41: 42–50.
30. Van Camp SP, Bloor CM, Meuller FO, et al: Nontraumatic sports death in high school and college athletes. Med Sci Sport Exer 1995; 27(5):641.
31. Maron BJ, Thompson PD, Puffer JC, et al: Cardiovascular preparticipation screening of competitive athletes. Circulation 1996; 94:850.
32. Glover DW, Maron BJ, Matheson GO: The preparticipation physical examination. Phys Sports Med 1999; 27(8):29.
33. American Academy of Pediatrics Committee on Sports Medicine: Recommendations

for participation in competitive sports. Pediatrics 1988; 81:737.

34. Maron BJ, Mitchell JH: 26th Bethesda Conference: Recommendations for determining eligibility for competition in athletes with cardiovascular abnormalities. J Am Coll Cardiol 1994; 24(4):846.

35. Fuentes RJ, Rosenberg JM: Athletic Drug Reference '99. Durham, NC, Clean Data Inc. 1999, p 314.

36. Dickinson A: 1999 Expo West Presentation: Regulation of dietary supplements. Council for Responsible Nutrition.

37. Walker JB: Creatine: Biosynthesis, regulation, and function. Adv Enzymol Relat Areas Mol Med 1979; 50:177.

38. Greenhaff PL, Bodin K, Soderlund K, et al: The effect of oral creatine supplementation on skeletal muscle phosphocreatine resynthesis. Am J Physiol 1994; 266:E725.

39. Mujika I, Padilla S, Ibanez J, et al: Creatine supplementation and sprint performance in soccer players. Med Sci Sports Exert 2000; 32(2):518.

40. Vandenberghe K, Van Hecke P, Van Leemputte M, et al: Phosphocreatine resynthesis is not affected by creatine loading. Med Sci Sports Exerc 1999; 31(2): 236.

41. Maughan RJ: Creatine supplementation and exercise performance. Int J Sport Nutr 1995; 5(2):94.

42. Birch R, Noble D, Greenhaff PL: The influence of dietary creatine supplementation on performance during repeated bouts of maximal isokinetic cycling in man. Eur J Appl Phys 1996.

43. Harris RC, Soderlund K, Hultman E: Elevation of creatine in resting and exercised muscle of normal subjects by creatine supplementation. Clin Sci 1992; 83:367.

44. Herbert J: The age of dehydroepiandrosterone. Lancet 1995; 345:1193.

45. Morales AJ, Nolan JJ, Yen SS: Effects of replacement dose dehydroepiandrosterone in men and women of advancing age. J Clin Endocrinol Metab 1994; 78(6):1360.

46. Yen SS, Morales AJ, Khorram O: Replacement of DHEA in aging men and women: Potential remedial effects. Ann N Y Acad Sci 1995; 774:128.

47. Dehydroepiandrosterone. Medical Letter 1996; 38:91.

48. King DS, Sharp RL, Vukovich MD, et al: Effect of oral androstenedione on serum testosterone and adaptations to resistance training in young men. JAMA 1999; 281: 2020.

49. Leder BZ, Longcope C, Catlin DH, et al: Oral androstenedione administration and serum testosterone concentrations in young men. JAMA 2000; 283:779.

50. Nissen S, Sharp R, Ray M, et al: Effect of leucine metabolite beta-hydroxy-beta-methylbutyrate on muscle metabolism during resistance exercise training J Appl Physiol 1996; 81(5):2095.

51. Kagan J (ed): Herbal Rx: The promises and pitfalls. Consumer Reports March, 1999, p 44.

52. Teman AJ, Hainline B: Eosinophilia-myalgia syndrome. Phys Sport Med 1991; 19: 81.

53. Gordon DW, Rosenthal G, Hart J, et al: Chaparral ingestion. The broadening spectrum of liver injury caused by herbal medications. JAMA 1995; 273(6):489.

54. Koff RS: Herbal hepatotoxicity: Revisiting a dangerous alternative. JAMA 1995; 273(6):502.

55. Woolf GM, Petrovic LM, Rojter SE, et al: Acute hepatitis associated with the chinese herbal product jin bu huan. Ann Intern Med 1994; 121(10):729.

section 4 chapter 2

SPECIAL CONCERNS OF THE FEMALE ATHLETE

Mary Lloyd Ireland and Susan M. Ott

Summary

- The majority of injuries sustained by female athletes are due to participation in sports rather than their sex.
- Anatomic, hormonal, and functional differences should be understood when treating the female athlete.
- Screening should be done for eating disorders and the female athlete triad.
- Female athletes have increased rates of injury to the anterior cruciate ligament and patellofemoral disorders compared with their male counterparts.

INTRODUCTION

Since the adoption of Title IX in the early 1970s women's sports participation has dramatically increased. The majority of the injuries sustained by female athletes are due to participation in the sport rather their sex, but there are anatomic, hormonal, and functional differences between the sexes which must be considered when caring for the female athlete. Differences between men's and women's versions of sports such as lacrosse and gymnastics and similarities between sports such as men's and women's basketball and soccer should also be understood.

The benefits of exercise are extensive. Females involved in sports are less likely to become pregnant during the teenage years, less likely to become involved in an abusive relationship, and more likely to finish high school and to go on to college. Women involved in sports have better self-esteem and self image.[1] Weightbearing exercise has a positive effect on bone mass in participants of all ages. There are also the cardiovascular and weight control benefits of exercise to be considered, especially in older athletes.

SEX DIFFERENCES

After age 10 to 12 years there are significant differences in all aspects of physical performance when comparing males with females. Females reach physiological and skeletal maturity and achieve peak height velocity before males. Women have more body fat and less lean body mass than males, a difference that can be attributed to increased estrogens in the female and increased androgens in the male.[2] Females have less upper body strength, which even with training remains 30% to 50% less than that of males. Lower extremity strength is much closer in parity.[3] Men also have higher red blood cell counts and hemoglobin

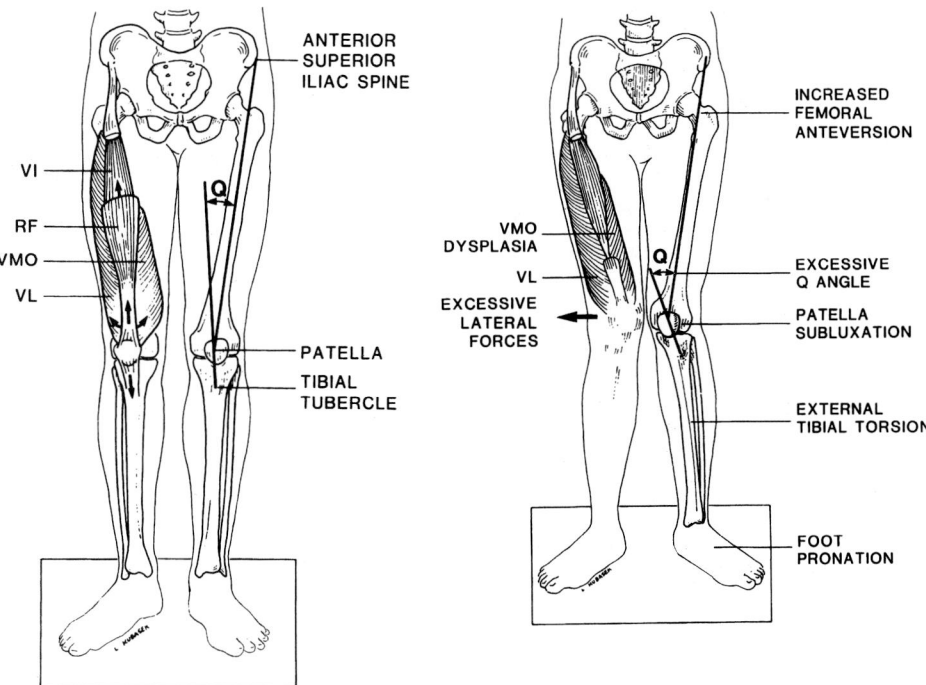

Fig. 1. Normal and miserable malalignment lower extremities. In well-developed quadriceps, lower Q angle, and neutral tibial torsion, there is a superior patellofemoral biomechanical pattern. Miserable malalignment syndrome creates rotatory and laterally directed forces on the patella.

levels than women. Work capacity studies show that there is only a slight difference between males and females in oxygen uptake when the data are expressed relative to body size and composition.[4] Despite these differences women show the same physiological training changes as males and experience significant increases in strength, power, and muscular endurance.[5]

Women have a wider pelvis, are more flexible, and have less developed musculature than men. Lower extremity alignment differs in the female and may predispose to injury. The so-called miserable malalignment syndrome of excessive forefoot pronation, pes planus, external tibial torsion, quadriceps angle of greater than 15 degrees, increased femoral anteversion, hypoplastic vastus medialis obliquus, and heel valgus angulation demonstrates the extreme of lower extremity differences between males and females (Fig. 1). Women have shorter limbs relative to body length. However, the center of gravity of men and women is only slightly different. This difference may account for differences in upper limb musculature with a shorter lever arm for movement and power.[6]

INJURY RATES

There have been many studies comparing injury rates between male and female athletes.[7–10] Studies comparing males and females have been done at the military academies.[11] The National Collegiate Athletic Association (NCAA) has collected data on injury rates for 16 sports since 1982 and for 21 sports since 1997. Soccer, lacrosse, gymnastics, and basketball are the four NCAA sports for which data were collected and in which both males and females compete. The data are reported as the number of

injuries per 1000 athletic exposures. Due to differences in equipment and rules for competition in lacrosse and gymnastics, comparisons of injury rates between men and women in these two sports must be made carefully. Arendt and Dick[12] and Arendt et al[13] reported anterior cruciate ligament (ACL) injury rates for soccer and basketball over a total 10-year period (1989–1993, 1994–1998). The rates of injury in females compared with males were 2.6 times greater in soccer and 3.6 times greater in basketball.

Using the 1997–1998 data, for women the highest rate of injury in collegiate sports was in soccer followed by spring soccer, gymnastics, lacrosse, basketball, fall lacrosse, softball, field hockey, volleyball, and spring volleyball (Table 1). Men's spring football and lacrosse had the highest overall injury rates for men or women. There appears to be a trend in most sports toward more injuries occurring during practices than during games. However, more knee injuries, and ACL, collateral ligament, and meniscus tears occur in games. Compared with males, females sustained greater rates of knee injuries involving the ACL (4.9 times greater), collateral ligament (2.5 times), and meniscus (1.9 times) (Fig. 2). The NCAA classification combines patella and patellar tendon; therefore, no specific diagnosis is documented. The ankle is the most commonly injured body part for both males and females.[9]

Certain injuries are more common in females, although most sports medicine research has been done on males. More research with female athletes needs to be done to prevent injury in the future and to answer the question of why certain injuries are more common in females. Only one long-term study has been done to date on female athletes. The majority of these athletes had continuing problems related to injuries sustained during their collegiate athletic careers. This is of concern. This indicates that we

	Women				Men			
	Injury Rate	**Total Injuries**	**Practice**	**Game**	**Injury Rate**	**Total Injuries**	**Practice**	**Game**
Gymnastics	6.79	258	87%	13%	1.44	6	83%	17%
Fall lacrosse	5.04	11	100%	0%	4.97	44	95%	5%
Lacrosse	5.56	234	68%	32%	5.63	505	57%	43%
Basketball	5.37	721	68%	32%	4.42	648	66%	34%
Spring soccer	8.11	82	54%	46%	10.9	94	74%	26%
Soccer	8.17	919	50%	50%	6.95	1098	49%	51%
Spring volleyball	2.98	42	88%	12%	—	—	—	—
Volleyball	3.84	327	62%	38%	—	—	—	—
Field hockey	3.99	209	62%	28%	—	—	—	—
Softball	4.27	308	54%	46%	—	—	—	—
Wrestling	—	—	—	—	9.42	972	68%	32%
Spring football	—	—	—	—	11.2	1274	100%	0%
Football	—	—	—	—	6.1	4210	57%	43%
Baseball	—	—	—	—	3.34	605	52%	48%
Ice hockey	—	—	—	—	5.79	514	30%	70%

TABLE 1. INJURY RATES PER 1000 ATHLETIC EXPOSURES AND PERCENTAGE IN PRACTICE AND GAMES 1997–1998

Data from NCAA Injury Surveillance System. Overland Park, KS, National Collegiate Athletic Association, 1991–1998.

do not know the long-term effects of athletic injuries on women and more research in this area need to be done.[14]

LOWER EXTREMITY

ANKLE INJURIES

The ankle remains the most frequently injured joint in both male and female athletes. Osteochondritis dissecans of the talus, tibiotalar impingement syndrome, high ankle sprain, chronically subluxating peroneal tendons, and posterior impingement should be included in the differential diagnosis of ankle sprains failing to respond to conservative care.

Stress fractures of the tarsal navicular should be ruled out in athletes at risk with foot pain. Medial tibial stress syndrome or shin splints are a common complaint among athletes and should be differentiated from exertional compartment syndrome and stress fracture.[15]

KNEE INJURIES

Compared with males, females have an increased rate of anterior knee pain, patellofemoral disorders, and ACL injuries.[16–18] Dynamic movement patterns, core stability, and hip strength are different in males and females (Fig. 3). In our experience, anterior knee pain is more common in

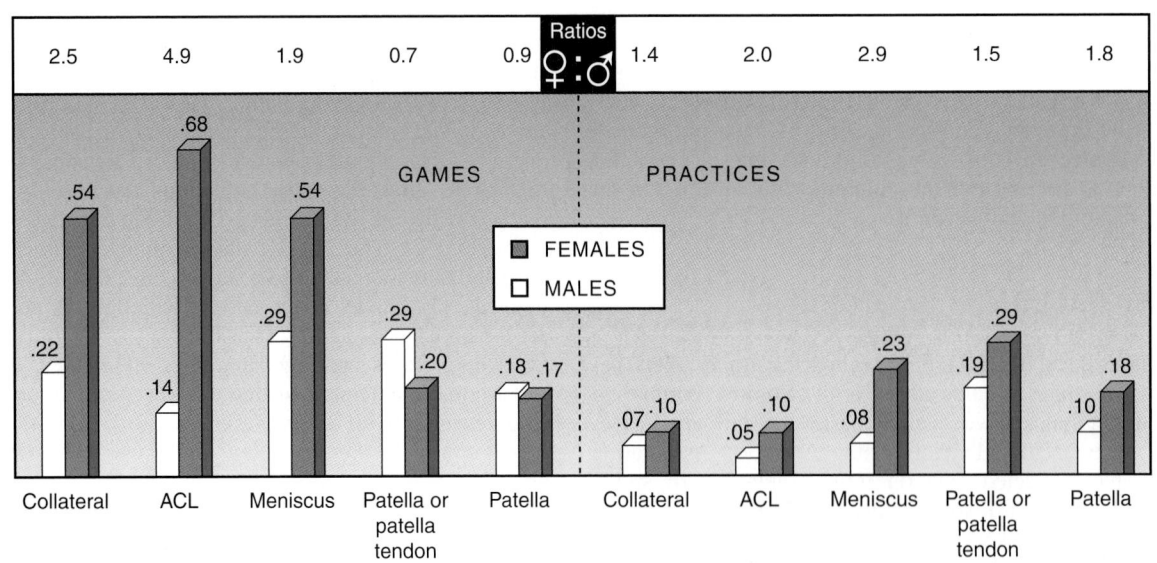

Fig. 2. Knee structure injury rates in basketball. Data are from the NCAA Injury Surveillance System, 1997–1998.[9] Injury rates are expressed as injuries per 1000 athletic exposures.

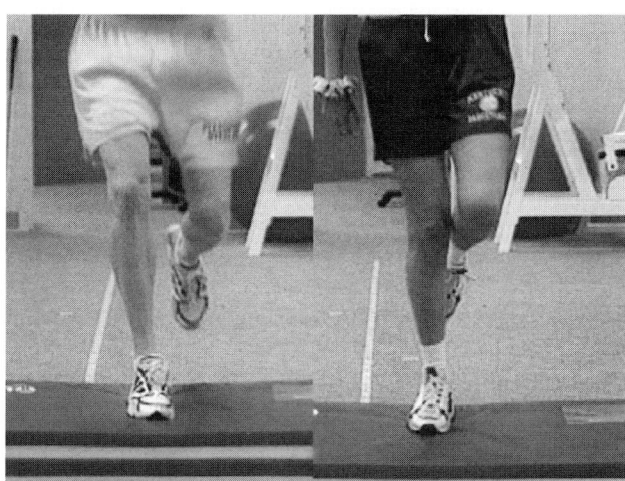

Fig. 3. Dynamics of landing. This photograph demonstrates some of the dynamic differences between males and females. The male (*yellow shorts*) has more flexion at the knee and hip with his body weight back and his knee in less valgus angulation. The female (*blue shorts*) has less knee and hip flexion with her body weight more forward and her knee in more valgus angulation. (Copyright 1999 by Mary Lloyd Ireland, MD)

women and has an extensive differential diagnosis, which is summarized in Table 2. A specific diagnosis should be made in patients with anterior knee pain.

It has been well established that females have a higher rate of ACL injury than males. The reason is most likely multifactorial. Differences in training, neuromuscular responses, laxity, hormonal influences, and anatomic differences all play a role. Hip weakness, anterior hip tightness, and quality of pattern of movement are other contributing

factors. The elastin and collagen tissue in females may contribute to the completeness of ACL tears and scar formation. Due to their lesser muscular development and lower extremity alignment differences, females rely more on the ACL and less on hamstring control. Ligamentous reconstruction should be considered in the ACL-dominant female as she is at high risk for significant meniscal and articular surface injury.[3, 10]

Review of video footage reveals that compared with males, females tend to be in a more upright position, with less hip and knee flexion and their knees in more valgus angulation when landing from jumps as demonstrated in (Figure 4). This "point of no return" with the athlete more upright with an externally rotated pronated lower extremity may predispose to injury. Isokinetic strength testing has revealed a higher hamstring-to-quadriceps peak torque ratio in the trail leg at 60 degrees per second in volleyball players, which is the one statistically significant difference that has been found between males and females. A plyometric jump training program was done in female volleyball players. After training, females showed increased jump heights, increased hamstring strength, decreased peak landing forces, and decreased knee abduction and adduction moments. The females also showed peak torque ratios similar to males athletes after training.[19] This is significant inasmuch as the hamstring strength is increased, there is less strain on the ACL, and this strengthening program could affect the number of ACL injuries in female athletes.

There have been studies showing that there are estrogen receptors within ligamentous structures, including the ACL. Estrogen inhibits type I procollagen synthesis and proliferation fibroblasts in vitro at physiological estradiol concentrations, but the in vivo function of these receptors has yet to be elucidated.[20] There have been further studies linking phase of menstrual cycle to the risk of injury to the

Fig. 4. This diagram shows the "position of no return." The position, which places the anterior cruciate ligament at risk, is an awkward out-of-control landing with the leg pronated in valgus angulation, the body more upright and the leg in pronation and rotation, and the knee in valgus angulation. The safety position is more flexed, body over legs, and more balanced. (Copyright 1998 by Mary Lloyd Ireland, MD)

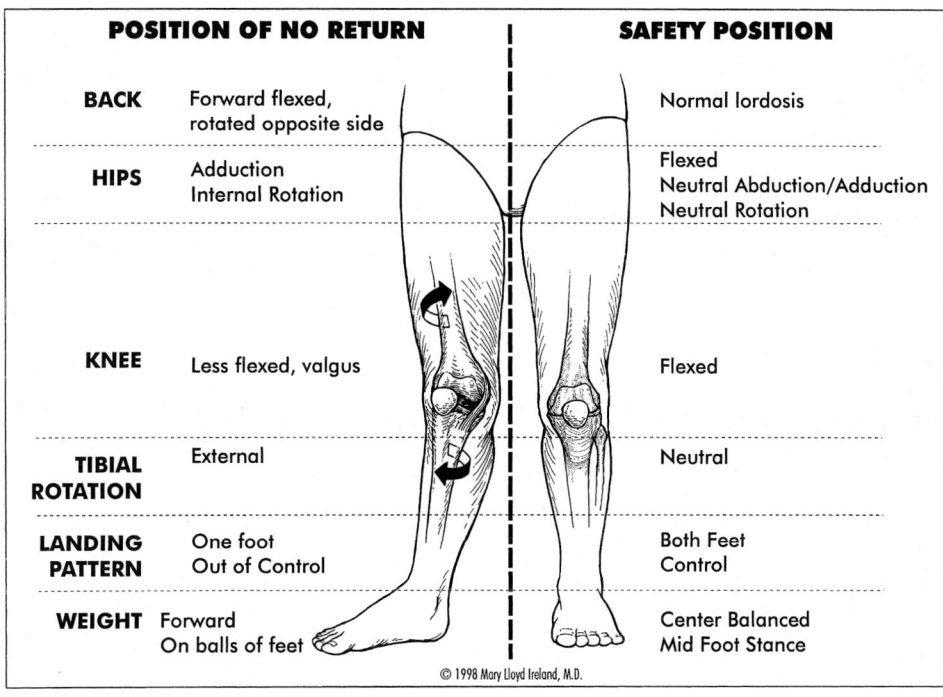

	POSITION OF NO RETURN	SAFETY POSITION
BACK	Forward flexed, rotated opposite side	Normal lordosis
HIPS	Adduction Internal Rotation	Flexed Neutral Abduction/Adduction Neutral Rotation
KNEE	Less flexed, valgus	Flexed
TIBIAL ROTATION	External	Neutral
LANDING PATTERN	One foot Out of Control	Both Feet Control
WEIGHT	Forward On balls of feet	Center Balanced Mid Foot Stance

© 1998 Mary Lloyd Ireland, M.D.

TABLE 2. ANTERIOR KNEE PAIN: DIFFERENTIAL DIAGNOSIS		
Mechanical	**Inflammatory**	**Other**
Repetitive Microtraumatic	Bursitis	Referred pain
Patella	Prepatellar	Lumbar disk herniation
Stability	Retropatellar	Others
Subluxation	Semimembranosus	Reflex sympathetic dystrophy
Dislocation	Pes anserinus	(regional pain syndrome)
Tilt	Tendinitis	Tumors
Rotation	Quadriceps patella	Benign
Malalignment	Pes anserinus	Malignant
Stress fracture	Semimembranosus	
Bipartite	Patella tendinitis	
Fibrous union	Pigmented villonodular synovitis	
Acute fracture	Neuromas/retinacular pain	
Pathological medial plica	Arthritis	
Patellofemoral stress syndrome	Osteoarthritis	
Osteochondral fracture	Rheumatoid arthritis	
Trochlear groove	Psoriatic arthritis	
Patella	Others	
Loose bodies	Reiter's syndrome	
Cartilaginous		
Osteochondral		
Osteochondritis dissecans		
Patella		
Trochlear groove		
Skeletally immature		
Osgood-Schlatter's disease		
Sinding-Larsen-Johansson syndrome		
Acute Macrotraumatic Injury		
Extensor mechanism disruption		
Quadriceps rupture		
Patellar tendon rupture		
Inferior avulsion fracture		
Interstitial		
Skeletally immature		
Tibial tubercle fracture		
Patellar fracture		
Transverse		
Displaced/nondisplaced		
Comminuted		
Status post–anterior cruciate ligament reconstruction		
with central third patellar tendon bone		

ACL. In one study there appeared to be more ACL tears during the ovulatory phase of the menstrual cycle.[21] More work in this area needs to be done with a larger series of athletes.

The majority of ACL injuries sustained by females are of a noncontact mechanism. The American Orthopedic Society for Sports Medicine, the National Athletic Trainers Association, the NCAA, and the Orthopedic Research and Education Foundation sponsored a consensus conference to address the issue of noncontact ACL injuries and define risk factors and directions for future research.[22] The members of the symposium concluded that at-risk situations for noncontact ACL injury include deceleration, cutting or changing directions, and landing. The shoe surface coefficient of friction may increase the risk of ACL injury. There is no evidence that knee braces prevent ACL injury. There is no consensus regarding the role of the notch in ACL injury owing to difficulties in obtaining reliable and reproducible measurements. There are insufficient data on ACL size as measured by notch size to support ligament

size related to risk of injury. There is no consensus regarding hormonal influences on the ACL and risk of ACL injury. There is no basis for modification of participation during various phases of the menstrual cycle or manipulation of sex-specific hormones to prevent ACL injuries.[22]

UPPER EXTREMITY

SHOULDER INJURIES

In younger females, joint laxity and decreased strength can cause shoulder problems. With generalized laxity, sport-dependent problems involving the shoulder can occur. The vicious cycle of physiological instability, rotator cuff weakness, pain, posterior tightness, and further imbalance results in persistent pain and dysfunction in overhead activities. Care should be taken to address scapular dysfunction. A specific diagnosis of the cause of the pain should be made. Restoration of normal range of motion and strength with proper sport biomechanics should be the goal.[23] The cheerleader shown in Figure 5 has bilateral multidirectional

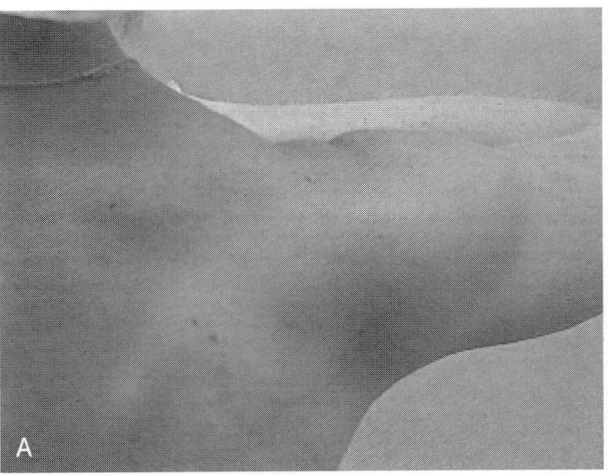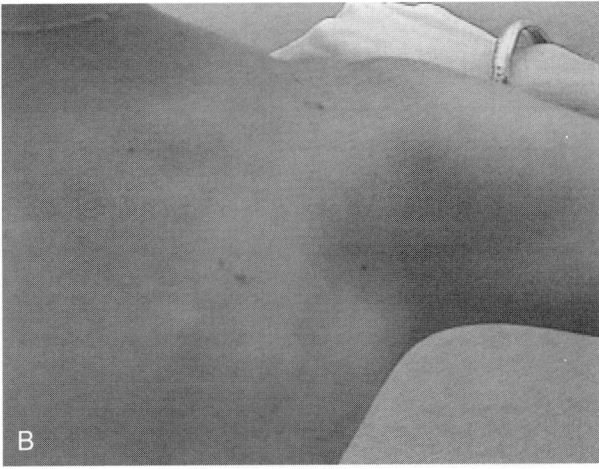

Fig. 5. Voluntary shoulder dislocation. The cheerleader is able to dislocate her glenohumeral joint posteriorly as she moves into horizontal adduction (*A*) and reduce as she externally rotates and abducts (*B*). (Copyright 1999 by Mary Lloyd Ireland, MD)

shoulder laxity. She can voluntarily posteriorly subluxate her glenohumeral joint (Fig. 5*A*) as she moves into horizontal adduction and reduce moving into external rotation (Fig. 5*B*).

ELBOW INJURIES

Females have shorter upper extremities, an increased valgus-carrying angle, decreased upper extremity strength, and increased ligamentous laxity compared with males. Osteochondritis dissecans of the elbow with possible loose body formation should be considered as a diagnosis in axially loading sports such as gymnastics, diving, cheerleading, and tumbling. Elbow dislocations are not infrequent in sports requiring aerial maneuvers.[3] A cheerleader sustained an elbow dislocation when she fell attempting a double back stunt (Fig. 6). Repeated attempts at reduction by bystanders were unsuccessful. An arterial injury occurred as well. Despite counseling, she returned to cheerleading 6 months after the injury with a range of motion of 10 to 140 degrees and full pronation and supination.

HAND AND WRIST INJURIES

Contact injuries in sports such as ice or field hockey or lacrosse can result in fractures to the hand or wrist. Overuse injuries to the wrist are common in gymnastics, golf, weightlifting, racquet sports, and bicycling. In gymnastics the upper extremity becomes a weightbearing limb and studies indicate the incidence of wrist pain in gymnasts to be as high of 73%.[24] The differential diagnosis in chronic wrist pain in any athlete should include triangular fibrocartilage tears, injury to the distal radial physis, ulnar impaction syndrome, dorsal wrist ganglion, dorsal wrist capsulitis, and carpal instability. Other possible sources of wrist pain are hamate fracture, carpal tunnel syndrome, tendinitis, and ulnar nerve compression.

STRESS FRACTURES

There are several populations of female athletes at increased risk for stress fracture. There is a high association between menstrual irregularities and stress fracture which

is discussed below.[25-27] Distance runners, ballet dancers, gymnasts, and those with poor nutrition and menstrual irregularities are at increased risk.[3] A detailed nutritional and gynecological history should be obtained in female athletes presenting with stress fracture.

THE SPINE IN THE FEMALE ATHLETE

Scoliosis is more common in females than males. Early screening with appropriate intervention should be done as part of the preparticipation physical examination. Spondylolisthesis and spondylolysis should be considered in athletes who perform repetitive flexion and extension activities. The radiographic examination should include oblique and standing lateral views. Back pain with a negative radiographic examination should be evaluated with a single-photon emission computed tomography (SPECT) bone scan to rule out fracture. Sciatica can occur with or without spondylolisthesis or lysis and should be evaluated accordingly. Vertebral body fractures, pedicle stress fractures, and multiple compression fractures have also been reported in female athletes and should be in the differential diagnosis of an athlete complaining of back pain.[3] Figure 7 demonstrates a case of spondylolysis.

THE FEMALE ATHLETE TRIAD

The female athlete triad is defined as amenorrhea, disordered eating, and osteoporosis. The triad is a multifactorial problem. The earlier the diagnosis, the better the chance for establishment of normality. Activities such as dancing, cheerleading, gymnastics, figure skating, and distance running, which emphasize a prepubertal body type, perfectionism, thinness, have revealing clothing, and are subjectively judged place women at increased risk for developing this disorder.[28] Other risk factors include a drive to excel at any cost, pressure from coaches and/or parents, lack of knowledge regarding nutrition, a family history of eating disorders, and a history of abuse. Young athletes who are approaching puberty appear to be at increased risk as well. When evaluating an athlete suspected of having the triad it

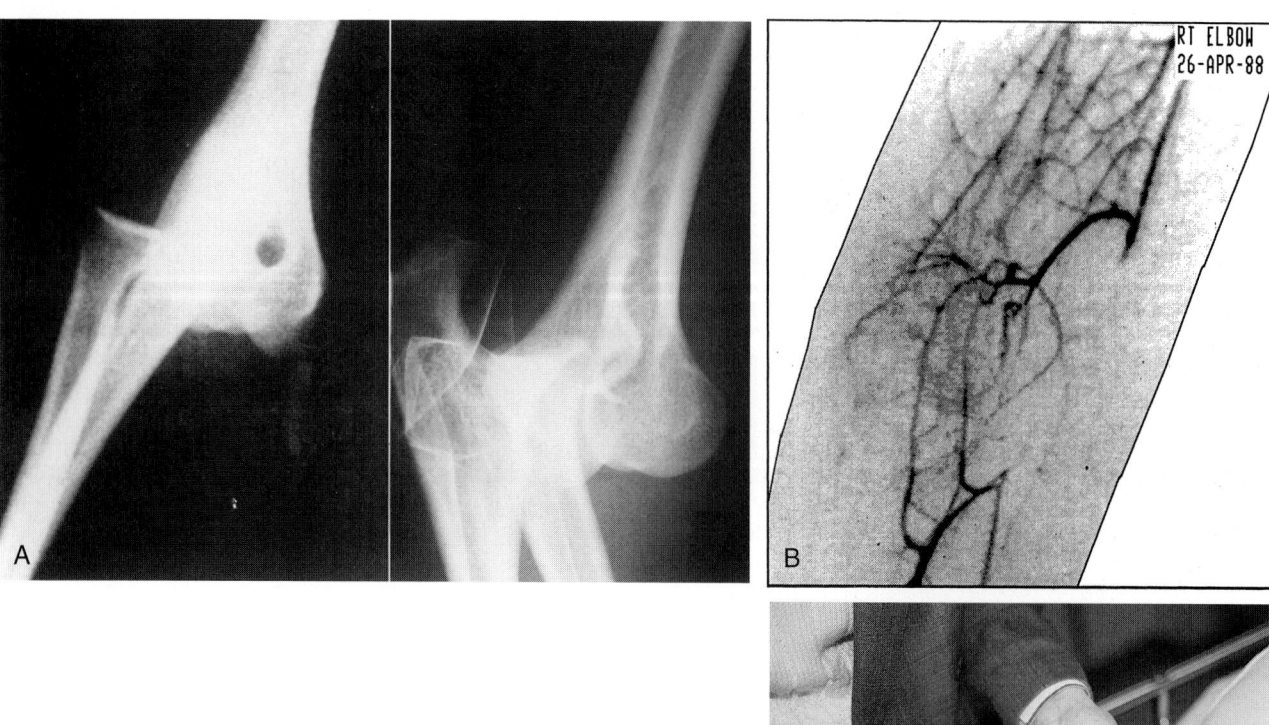

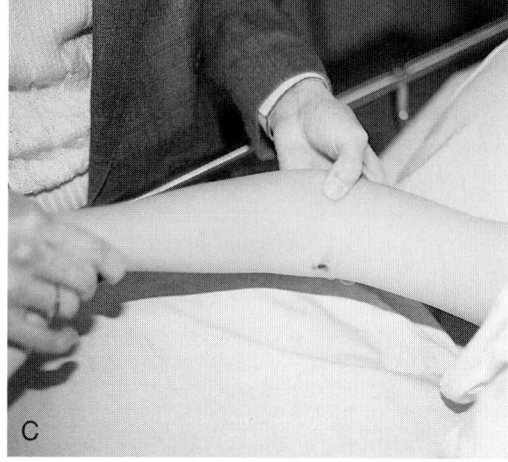

Fig. 6. Elbow dislocation. *A,* Anteroposterior and lateral radiographs show a posterolateral elbow dislocation. Examination revealed a pulseless upper extremity and an ecchymotic area anteromedially. *B,* Arteriogram shows no filling of the brachial artery. *C,* Cephalic vein patch was done to restore normal vascularity to the upper extremity.

is of utmost importance to take a detailed nutritional and menstrual history.[29] The true prevalence of the female athlete triad is unknown. The best treatment for the female athlete triad is prevention through preparticipation physical examination, education, nutritional counseling, and screening. If the triad is already established, the treatment is multidisciplinary with a physician, psychiatrist or psychologist, and nutritionist involved in the care of the athlete.[30] Cure is rare. Educational programs are available.[31] This 22-year-old gymnast died of starvation or nutritional deficiencies (Fig. 8).[31a]

DISORDERED EATING

There is a wide spectrum of eating disorders among athletes, ranging from anorexia nervosa and bulimia, to restrictive eating behaviors, to poor nutritional habits. The risk factors for disordered eating are the same as those listed earlier under The Female Athlete Triad. Those athletes with anorexia nervosa or bulimia are of obvious concern but athletes with less extreme disordered eating pat-

terns are at risk for certain endocrine, skeletal, and psychiatric problems.[32] Eating disorders are 10 times more prevalent in women than in men. The exact prevalence in athletes is unknown but ranges from 15% to 62% of athletes depending on the sport. The prevalence of eating disorders in the nonathlete is estimated at between 1% and 3%. The prognosis for eating disorders is poor. Among nonathletes, 50% do well, 30% struggle and relapse, and there is a 10% to 20% mortality rate. There have been no published studies to date regarding the prognosis of eating disorders in female athletes and it is unknown how often disordered eating patterns resolve after college or competitive athletics. Many continue to struggle with weight concerns and body image after their athletic careers are over.[33]

Anorexia nervosa is defined by the *Diagnostic and Statistical Manual of Mental Disorders,* 4th edition (DSM-IV) as refusal to maintain minimal body weight for height (less than 85% of expected weight), intense fear of weight gain, disturbed body image, and three consecutive months of

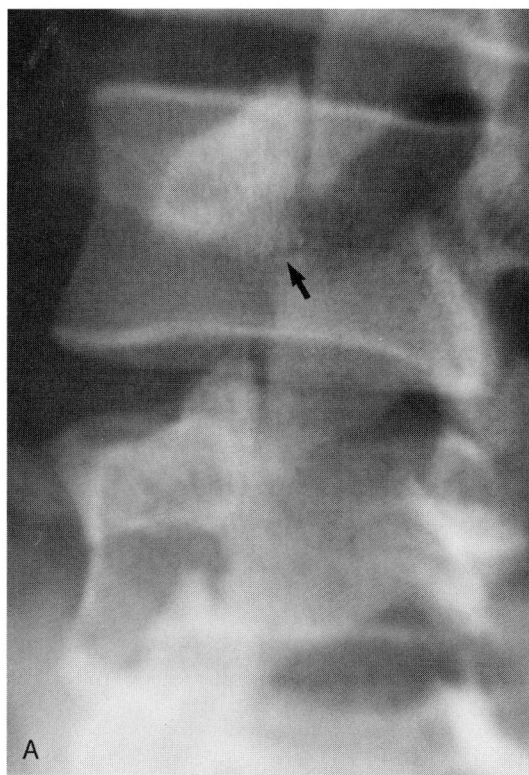

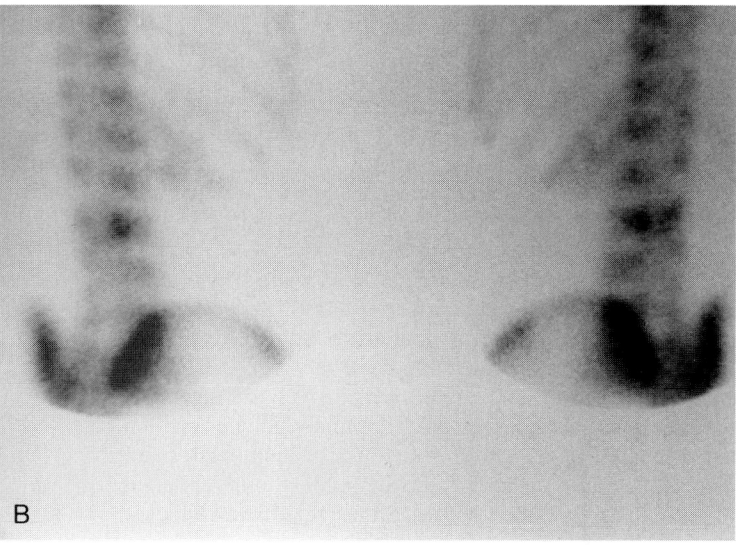

Fig. 7. Spondylolysis. *A,* In this athlete with pain on hyperextension, an acute pars interarticularis defect is seen on oblique views. *B,* The acuteness of the injury is demonstrated on bone scan with increased activity in the L-4 area. (From Fu FH, Stone DA: Sports Injuries: Mechanisms, Prevention, and Treatment, 2nd ed. Philadelphia, Lippincott Williams & Wilkins, 2001.)

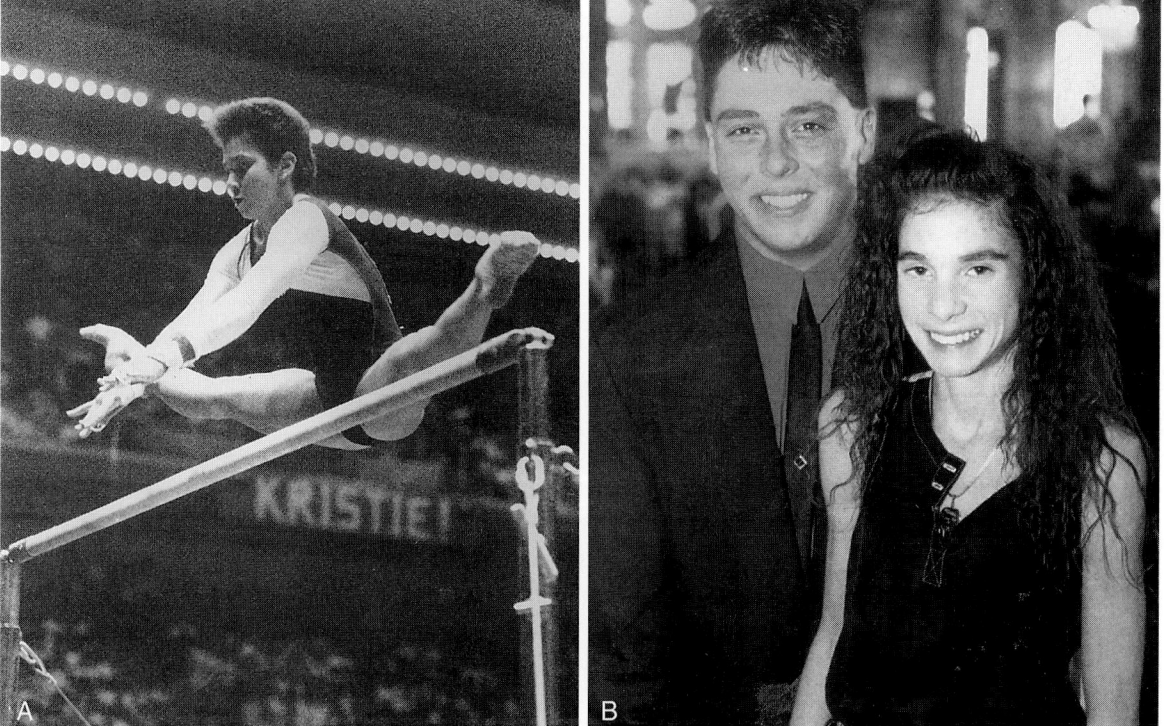

Fig. 8. *A,* Christy Henrich is shown when she was competing at the elite level in gymnastics. *B,* She did not make the Olympic Team. She died of anorexia nervosa. Her picture several months before her death is shown. (Reprinted with permission from API Wide World Photos, 50 Rockefeller Plaza, New York, NY 10020.)

amenorrhea in postmenarchal females or failure to begin menstruating by age 16. Signs and symptoms of anorexia include amenorrhea, fat loss, muscle loss, dry hair, dry skin, cold and discolored extremities, decreased body temperature, lanugo, lightheadedness, decreased ability to concentrate, and bradycardia.[34]

Bulimia nervosa is defined by the DSM-IV as recurrent binge eating within any 2-hour period; overeating; a sense of lack of control over eating during any 2-hour period; recurring behavior compensation for overeating by vomiting, abuse of laxatives, or other drugs; fasting or excessive exercise; binge eating and purging at least twice weekly for 3 months; and negative self–body image and self-image. Disturbed behavior does not occur exclusively during times of anorexia nervosa. Signs and symptoms include swollen parotid glands, chest pain, sore throat, abdominal pain, erosion of tooth enamel, face edema, extremity edema, diarrhea, constipation, menstrual irregularities, knuckle scars, nail changes, and bloodshot eyes.[34]

MENSTRUAL IRREGULARITIES

Primary amenorrhea is defined as absence of menstruation by age 16 in a girl with secondary sex characteristics. Secondary amenorrhea is absence of three of more consecutive menstrual cycles after menarche. Oligomenorrhea is a menstrual cycle greater than 36 days. The prevalence of amenorrhea in the general population is 2% to 6% and in athletic populations, between 3.4% and 66%. All three of these disorders can result in decreased bone mineral density (BMD) and put the patient at risk for early osteoporosis and stress fracture. The exact cause of amenorrhea in athletes is unknown, but it most likely has a hypothalamic origin and results in decreased ovarian hormone production and hypoestrogenemia similar to menopause.[35, 35a–c]

The significance of athletic amenorrhea is the observed skeletal demineralization seen in nonmenstruating athletes which predisposes them to injury, especially stress fracture and early osteoporosis.[36] The long-term effects to bone health caused by athletic amenorrhea are unknown. The danger is that these women are losing bone at a time in their lives when they should be laying it down and they may never achieve peak bone mass.[35] There is also a theoretical risk of increased incidence of cardiovascular disease, infertility, reproductive system cancer, and osteoporosis. Athletic amenorrhea is a symptom of an underlying problem and should be treated in the first 3 months. After ruling out other causes of amenorrhea, treatment of athletic amenorrhea in a woman who has been menstruating for less than 3 years is to decrease exercise intensity and improve nutrition.[37] For an athlete who is more than 3 years post-menarche, treatment is low-dose oral contraceptives.[35]

OSTEOPOROSIS

Osteoporosis is a disease characterized by low bone mass and microarchitectural deterioration of bone tissue leading to enhanced skeletal fragility and increased risk of fracture. Women are four times more likely to develop osteoporosis than men.[38] Osteoporosis is defined in terms of BMD. Bone densitometry by dual photon radiographic absorptiometery is the modality of choice to evaluate BMD.

Weightbearing exercise has a positive effect on bone mass and may reduce the rate of bone loss in adult women but it will not produce a large increase.[39] In the face of athletic amenorrhea, the positive effects of weightbearing exercise are negated. This method is quicker, less expensive, and can image specific body sites more easily than previous scanning methods.[35] Athletes suspected of early osteoporosis, the female athlete triad, and those with oligomenorrhea or amenorrhea should undergo bone densitometry. Educational programs are available.[40, 41]

TABLE 3. SUMMARY OF THE AMERICAN COLLEGE OF OBSTETRICIANS AND GYNECOLOGISTS CONTRAINDICATIONS TO AND RECOMMENDATIONS FOR EXERCISE DURING PREGNANCY

Contraindications
- Pregnancy-induced hypertension.
- Preterm rupture of membranes.
- Preterm labor during the prior or current pregnancy or both.
- Incompetent cervix/cerclage.
- Persistent second- or third-trimester bleeding.
- Intrauterine growth retardation.

1. During pregnancy, women can continue to exercise and derive health benefits even from mild-to-moderate exercise routines. Regular exercise (at least 3 times per week) is preferable to intermittent activity.
2. Women should avoid exercise in the supine position after the first trimester. Such a position is associated with decreased cardiac output in most pregnant women; because the remaining cardiac output will be preferentially distributed away from splanchnic beds (including the uterus) during vigorous exercise, such regimens are best avoided during pregnancy. Prolonged periods of motionless standing should also be avoided.
3. Women should be aware of the decreased oxygen available for aerobic exercise during pregnancy. They should be encouraged to modify the intensity of their exercise according to maternal symptoms. Pregnant women should stop exercising when fatigued and not exercise to exhaustion. Weightbearing exercises may under some circumstances be continued at intensities similar to those prior to pregnancy throughout pregnancy. Nonweightbearing exercises such as cycling or swimming will minimize the risk of injury and facilitate the continuation of exercise during pregnancy.
4. Morphologic changes in pregnancy should serve as a relative contraindication to types of exercise in which loss of balance could be detrimental to maternal or fetal well-being, especially in the third trimester. Further, any type of exercise involving the potential for even mild abdominal trauma should be avoided.
5. Pregnancy requires an additional 300 kcal/d to maintain metabolic homeostasis. Thus, women who exercise during pregnancy should be particularly careful to ensure an adequate diet.
6. Pregnant women who exercise in the first trimester should augment heat dissipation by ensuring adequate hydration, appropriate clothing, and optimal environmental surroundings during exercise.
7. Many of the physiological and morphological changes of pregnancy persist 4–6 wks postpartum. Thus, prepregnancy exercise routines should be resumed gradually based on a woman's physical capability.

Modified from Exercise During Pregnancy and the Postpartum Period, ACOG Technical Bulletin, 89. Washington, DC, American College of Obstetricians and Gynecologists, 1994, pp 3–4.

IRON DEFICIENCY ANEMIA

Women are at greater risk than men for anemia. Forty percent to 50% of adolescent female athletes demonstrate some degree of iron depletion or decreased iron stores without overt anemia.[42] Twenty percent to 30% of female adolescents and young adults (athletes and nonathletes) demonstrate iron deficiency.[32] Runners appear to be at increased risk for iron deficiency anemia during their training season. Black adolescent female runners have twice the incidence of iron deficiency anemia of white adolescent female runners. True iron deficiency anemia should be differentiated from pseudoanemia or sports anemia which results from expanded plasma volume with a normal red blood cell count.[1] Only those athletes at high risk for anemia or those with a previous history of iron deficiency anemia should be screened.

THE AGING FEMALE ATHLETE

As our society becomes more fitness-oriented it has become more acceptable for older women to pursue exercise. Women are continuing to be active in sports which they enjoy and some of those who have never before exercised are beginning fitness programs. Most information on the aging female athlete has been extrapolated from male data, but there have been a few studies suggesting the following positive aspects of exercise in the aging female athlete. As we age we lose muscle mass, flexibility, and bone mass, and aerobic capacity declines.[43] Body weight decreases due to loss of muscle mass while the percentage of body fat increases. Despite these changes, exercise training can still increase the size and strength of conditioned muscle. Exercise programs should take into account prior fitness levels, bone demineralization, and type of exercise. In addition to increased muscle strength, cardiovascular benefits, increase in lean body mass, and increased bone mineralization are other positive outcomes of exercise. Treatment of injuries in older females should be based on activity level and physiological age rather than chronological age.

THE PREGNANT ATHLETE

As women's sports participation increases, so too will the number of women who wish to continue their exercise programs throughout their pregnancy. Of importance is the physical fitness level of the patient prior to conception. In most cases women can safely continue an exercise program during their pregnancy. This should be done in coordination with the athlete's obstetrician. The major concerns for pregnant athletes are the effects of elevated maternal temperature on the fetus, the effect of exercise on blood flow to the fetus, and the effects of exercise on the weight of the fetus.[38] The American College of Obstetricians and Gynecologists guidelines for exercise during pregnancy and contraindications to exercise during pregnancy are summarized in Table 3.[44, 45] The benefits of exercise during pregnancy include weight control, improved muscle tone, improved self-esteem, decreased incidence of varicosities, decreased incidence of back pain, and decreased incidence of sleep disturbance.[46]

CONCLUSION

Appreciation of the unique situations that exist for female athletes will improve their care and treatment. Medical personnel who have added these insights to their armamentarium can make diagnoses more efficiently and institute treatment earlier. The epidemic of knee injuries in females is of concern and requires further research. Very important factors in prevention are strengthening of the trunk and core, low back, and hip musculature and analysis of dynamic movement patterns. The high incidence of eating disorders and hormonal and nutritional imbalances increases the risk for stress fracture. Treatment of eating disorders and menstrual irregularities should be instituted quickly to avoid adverse sequelae to the bone. Exercise can be carried out safely in most pregnant patients in conjunction with their obstetrician and in keeping with their pre-pregnancy level of fitness. Sports participation and physical fitness should be encouraged in women of all ages.

ACKNOWLEDGMENTS

We thank Tom Adler, Ph.D., Carolyn Large, transcriptionist, and Cathy Truda, educational assistant, for their help in the preparation of this manuscript.

REFERENCES

1. Sandborn CF, Jankowski CM: Physiologic considerations for women in sport. Clin Sports Med 1994; 13:315.
2. Wilmore JH: The application of science to sport: Physiological profiles of male and female athletes. Can J Appl Sport Sci. 1979; 4:103.
3. Ireland ML: Special concerns of the female athlete. In Fu FU, Stone DA (eds): Sports Injuries: Mechanisms, Prevention and Treatment. Philadelphia, Lippincott Williams & Wilkins, 1994, pp 153–187.
4. Berg K: Aerobic function in female athletes. Clin Sports Med 1983; 3:779.
5. Baechle TR: Women in resistance training. Clin Sports Med 1984; 3:791.
6. Acurater AE: Biomechanics and the female athlete. In Puhl J, Brown CH, Vox RO (eds): Sports Perspectives for Women. Champaign, IL, Human Kinetics, 1988, p 1.
7. DeHaven KE, Linter DM: Athletic injuries: Comparison by age, sport and gender. Am J Sports Med 1986; 14:218.
8. Whiteside PA: Men's and women's injuries in comparable sports. Phys Sportsmed 1980; 8:130.
9. NCAA Injury Surveillance System.
Overland Park, KS, National Collegiate Athletic Association, 1991–1998.
10. Ireland ML: Anterior cruciate ligament injury in female athletes: Epidemiology. Athletic Training 1999; 34:150.
11. Good JE, Klein KM: Women in the military academies: US Navy (part 1 of 3). Phys Sportsmed 1989; 17:99.
12. Arendt E, Dick R: Knee injury patterns among men and women in collegiate basketball and soccer: NCAA data and review of literature. Am J Sports Med 1995; 23: 694.
13. Arendt EA, Agel J, Dick R: Anterior cru-

ciate ligament injury patterns among collegiate men and women. J Athletic Training 1999; 34:86.

14. Wadley GH, Albright JP: Womens' intercollegiate gymnastics: Injury patterns and "permanent" medical disability. Am J Sports Med 1993; 21:314.

15. Blank S: Transverse tibial stress fracture: A special problem. Am J Sports Med 1987; 15:597.

16. Ireland ML, Wall C: Epidemiology and comparison of knee injuries in elite male and female United States basketball athletes (abstract). Med Sci Sports Exerc 1990; 22:582.

17. Ireland ML: Problems facing the athletic female. In: Pearl AJ (ed): The Athletic Female. Champaign, IL, Human Kinetics P, 1993, pp 11.

18. Zelisko JA, Noble HB, Porter M: A comparison of men's and women's professional basketball injuries. Am J Sports Med 1982; 10:297.

19. Hewett TE, Stroupe AL, Nance TA, N et al: Plyometric training in female athletes: Decreased impact forces and increased hamstring torques. Am J Sports Med 1996; 24:765.

20. Liu SH, Al-Shaikh RA, Panossian V, et al: Estrogen affects the cellular metabolism of the anterior cruciate ligament: A potential explanation for female ahtletic injury. Am J Sports Med 1997; 25:704.

21. Wojtys EM, Huston LJ, Lindenfeld TN, et al: Association between menstrual cycle and anterior cruciate ligament injuries in female athletes. Am J Sports Med 1998; 26:614.

22. Agel J, Albolhm M, Arendt EA, et al: Non-contact ACL Presented at Consensus Symposium of the American Orthopedic Society for Sports Medicine, National Athletic Trainers Association, National Collegiate Athletic Association, and Orthopedic Research and Education Foundation, Hunt Valley, MD, June 1999.

23. Hunter LY, Andrews JR, Clancy WG, et al: Common orthopedic problems of female athletes. Instruct Course Lect 1982; 31:126.

24. Difiorri JP, Puffer JC, Mandelbaum BR, et al: Factors associated with wrist pain in the young gymnast. Am J Sports Med 1996; 24:9.

25. Barrow GW, Saha S: Menstrual irregularity and stress fractures in collegiate female runners. Am J Sports Med 1988; 16:209.

26. Lloyd T, Buchanan JR, Bitzer S, et al: Interrelationships of diet, athletic activity, menstrual status and bone density in collegiate women. Am J Clin Nutr 1987; 46: 681.

27. Matheson GO, Clement DB, McKenzie DC, et al: Stress fractures in athletes: A study of 320 cases. Am J Sports Med 1987; 15:43.

28. Berning JR, Steen SN (eds): Sports Nutrition for the 90s: The Health Professional's Handbook. Aspen, CO, Gaithersburg, 1991.

29. Nattiv A, Agnosti R, Drinkwater B, et al: The female athlete triad: The inter-relatedness of disordered eating, amenorrhea and osteoporosis. Clin Sports Med 1994; 13: 405.

30. Tanner SM: Preparticipation examination targeted for the female athlete. Clin Sports Med 1994; 13:337.

31. ACSM's Hot Topics and Fundamentals of Sports Medicine Series. A Physician's Guide: The Female Athlete Triad (videotape). Indianapolis, American College of Sports Medicine, 1996.

31a. Ryan J: Little Girls in Pretty Boxes. New York, Warner Books, 1995.

32. Nattiv A, Ireland ML: Special concerns of the female athlete. In Safran MR, McKeag DB, Van Camp SP (eds): Manual of Sports Medicine. Philadelphia, Lippencott-Raven, 1998, pp 171.

33. Johnson MD: Disordered eating in active and athletic women. Clin Sports Med 1994; 13:355.

34. American Psychiatric Association: Diagnostic and Statistical Manual of Mental Disorders. 4th ed. Washington, DC, American Psychiatric Association, 1995.

35. Arendt EA: Osteoporosis in the athletic female: Amenorrhea and amenorrheic osteoporosis. In Pearl AJ (ed): The Athletic Female. Champaign, IL, Human Kinetics, 1993, pp 41–60.

35a. Nattiv A, Yeager K, Drinkwater B, et al: The female triad. In Agortini R (ed): Medical and Orthopedic Issues of Active and Athletic Women. Philadelphia, Lippincott Williams & Wilkins, 1994.

35b. Otis CL: Exercise associated amenorrhea. Clin Sports Med 1992; 11:351.

35c. Shangold M: Menstruation. In Shangold M, Mirkin G (eds): Women and Exercise. Philadelphia, FA Davis, 1988, p 129.

36. Gadpaille WJ, Sanborn CF, Wagner WW: Athletic amenorrhea, major affective disorders and eating disorders. Am J Psychiatry 1987; 144:939.

37. Marshall LA: Clinical evaluation of amenorrhea in active and athletic women. Clin Sports Med 1994; 13:371.

38. Snow-Harter CM: Bone health and prevention of osteoporosis in active and athletic women. Clin Sports Med 1994; 13: 389.

39. Dalsky GP: The role of exercise in prevention of osteoporosis. Compr Ther 1989; 15:30.

40. Campbell B, Morwessel R: Osteoporosis . . . Time to Bone up! (Slide Kit). Rosemont, IL, Ruth Jackson Orthopaedic Society.

41. NOF's Physician's Guide to Osteoporosis: Prevention and Treatment. Washington, DC, National Osteoporosis Foundation.

42. Squire DL: Issues specific to the preadolescent and adolescent athletic female. In Pearl AJ (ed): The Athletic Female. Champaign, IL, Human Kinetics, 1993, p. 113.

43. Peters GA: Conditioning the aging female. In Pearl AJ (ed). The Athletic Female. Champaign, IL, Human Kinetics, 1993, p. 185.

44. Heckman JD, Sassard R: Musculoskeletal considerations in pregnancy. J Bone Joint Surg Am 1994; 76-:1720.

45. Exercise During Pregnancy and the Postpartum Period. ACOG Technical Bulletin 189. Washington, DC, American College of Obstetricians and Gynecologists, 1994.

46. Agnosti R: The athletic woman. In Mellion MB (ed): Office Management of Sports Injuries and Athletic Problems. Philadelphia, Hanley & Belfus, 1988, pp 76–88.

THERAPEUTIC MODALITY: REHABILITATION OF THE INJURED ATHLETE

section 4

chapter 3

John Nyland and Michael F. Nolan

Summary
- Traditional therapeutic modalities include cryotherapy, sonotherapy, pulsed electrical stimulation, transcutaneous electrical nerve stimulation, high-volt pulsed current, and iotopheresis.
- Alternative modalities include acupuncture, magnetic field therapy, biofeedback, and massage.
- All therapeutic modalities should be considered adjuncts to progressive functional exercise.
- Controlled studies rarely reach consensus regarding the efficacy of therapeutic modalities, so their use should be individualized to the patient.

This chapter reviews traditional and alternative therapeutic modalities for the treatment of injuries commonly seen in an orthopaedic sports medicine practice. The reader is reminded that active progressive functional exercises are considered the ultimate modality and that other relatively "passive" modalities should be incorporated in a manner that best serves patient advancement toward more independent functional exercise participation.

CRYOTHERAPY

Using an animal model, Dolan et al[1] reported that post-trauma limb volumes following blunt injury were smaller for a group that received cold water immersion (12.8°–15.5°C) compared with untreated control subjects. Myrer et al,[2] in comparing the effects of 20 minutes of ice pack application with those of cold whirlpool immersion (10°C) reported no differences in intra-calf muscle temperature decreases; however, ice packs decreased subcutaneous tissue temperature more than the cold whirlpool, and the cold whirlpool was superior for prolonged temperature reduction. Zemke et al[3] reported that ice massage provided more rapid deep muscular cooling than an ice pack following 15-minute applications. Kuligowski et al[4] reported that cold whirlpool and contrast therapy enabled earlier return to both baseline resting elbow flexion angle and perceived pain level following exercise-induced delayed onset muscle soreness (DOMS) than warm whirlpool or no treatment at all.

Speer et al[5] reported that shoulder surgery patients who received cryotherapy had less pain, slept better, used less pain medication, and had greater overall satisfaction than subjects in a non-cryotherapy control group. Lessard et al[6] reported that knee arthroscopy patients who received a 1-week cryotherapy program in conjunction with exercises had increased exercise compliance, improved weight-bearing status, and reduced pain medication consumption compared with patients who received exercises alone. In comparing a combined cold and compression cryotherapy

system with conventional ice packs among 44 anterior cruciate ligament (ACL) reconstruction patients, Schroder and Passler[7] reported less pain, less swelling, reduced pain medication comsumption, increased active range of motion (AROM), and superior functional scores for the cold-compression system group. In a study of post-unilateral total knee replacement patients, Walker et al[8] reported that patients who used a continuous cooling pad in addition to a continuous passive motion device had decreased pain medication consumption compared with patients who received continuous passive motion either with or without transcutaneous electrical nerve stimulation. Ohkoshi et al,[9] in using implanted thermosensors, reported that ACL reconstruction patients who received cryotherapy had less pain, required less pain medication, had less blood loss, and had lower suprapatellar pouch and intercondylar notch temperatures than the control group.

In contrast to reports supporting cryotherapy, Konrath et al,[10] in studying 103 consecutive ACL reconstruction patients, failed to find objective benefits early in the postoperative course, suggesting that joint compression and/or a placebo effect may be the more beneficial factors. Dervin et al,[11] in assessing 78 ACL reconstruction patients, reported no differences in pain between those who received either circulating ice water or room temperature water in a cold-compression device. In assessing 131 ACL reconstruction patients for the effectiveness of postoperative cooling at 4.4°, 7.2°, 12.8°, or 21°C, Daniel et al[12] reported that all of the cooling pads lowered skin temperature; however, differences were not found between groups for perceived pain, pain medication use, swelling, or AROM.

SONOTHERAPY

In a comparison of the tissue heating effects of 1 MHz and 45 kHz frequency continuous ultrasound using a non-living animal model, Ward and Robertson[13] reported that the heating provided by the 45 kHz ultrasound was very superficial, whereas 1 MHz ultrasound heated both superficial and deep tissues. In using an animal model to assess deep tissue heating differences between ultrasound with coupling gel and underwater ultrasound at 2 cm from the skin surface, Forrest and Rosen[14] reported that only the direct method using coupling gel produced therapeutic temperature increases. In using an animal model to study Achilles tendon healing, Jackson et al[15] reported that the continuous ultrasound group (1.5 W/cm², 4 min) had improved collagen synthesis and greater mechanical strength than a control group.

In assessing the effect of continuous ultrasound to the volar forearm (1.5 W/cm², 5 min) on human skeletal muscle blood flow, Robinson and Buono[16] reported no differences for up to 30 minutes post-treatment, concluding that muscle hyperemia was probably not the primary mechanism responsible for the clinical benefits seen following ultrasound therapy. In contrast to this study, Fabrizio et al[17] reported that ultrasound (1.0 MHz, 1.0 and 1.5 W/cm^2) increased triceps surae blood flow velocity. Ward and Robertson,[18] in assessing continuous 1 MHz ultrasound at three intensity levels (0.5, 1.0, and 2.0 W/cm^2) when delivered underwater reported that increasing the applicator–skin surface distance resulted in progressive and significantly lower tissue temperature increases. From these data, they designed dosage correction factors to provide equivalencies for ultrasound provided away from the skin surface.

Stay et al[19] reported no differences in upper arm swelling, relaxed-elbow extension angle, strength, or soreness between female subjects with exercise-induced DOMS who were treated with pulsed ultrasound (20% duty cycle, 1 MHz, 1.5 W/cm^2, 7 min) and untreated control subjects. Rose et al[20] reported that 1 MHz continuous ultrasound at 1.5 W/cm^2 to the human calf (4°C tissue temperature increase) produced a slower thermal decay and slower deep tissue cooling than 3 MHz ultrasound. From these data they concluded that the effective stretching window following ultrasound therapy was greater for deeper tissues. Draper et al[21] reported that 3 MHz ultrasound heated tissues at 0.8 cm and 1.6 cm depths faster than 1 MHz ultrasound (2.5 and 5 cm^2 sound head sizes). Chan et al[22] reported that continuous ultrasound (3 MHz, 1 W/cm^2, 4 min) increased human patellar tendon temperature at both two times and four times the effective radiating area of a 4.5 cm^2 sound head, but two times the effective radiating area provided greater heating of longer duration. Draper et al,[23] in comparing the deep heating effect of ultrasound (1 MHz, 1.5 W/cm^2, 10 min) on human calf muscle that had been treated with either a real or sham hot pack (75°C) reported that greater temperature increases (>4°C) could be attained with 2 to 3 minutes less total ultrasound time when preheating with a hot pack. Rimington et al[24] reported that ultrasound alone (1 MHz, 1.5 W/cm^2) provided a greater heating effect at a depth of 3 cm in human calf muscle than ultrasound preceded by cryotherapy.

In assessing the effect of phonophoresis (1.5 W/cm^2, 1.0 MHz, 8 min) with 0.33% dexamethasone on adrenal function, Franklin et al[25] reported no evidence of systemic effects. Bare et al[26] failed to find elevated levels of serum cortisol following phonophoresis (1.0 MHz, 1.0 W/cm^2, 5 min) of a 10% hydrocortisone solution to the volar forearm of 16 subjects. Klaiman et al[27] failed to distinguish differences in pain level or pressure tolerance between 49 patients with soft-tissue injuries who were treated with fluocinonide phonophoresis or ultrasound. Ciccone et al[28] reported that phonophoresis with trolamine salicylate was more effective than ultrasound alone in decreasing the effects of DOMS. In an excellent review of phonophoresis, Byl[29] reported that maximal treatment effectiveness requires topical agents that transmit ultrasound, moist skin that is pretreated with ultrasound, heating or shaving, patient positioning that maximizes circulation to the treated area, continuous ultrasound within the thermal ranges ($\geq$ 1.5 W/cm^2) unless there are contraindications for heating based on patient condition (acute injury, open wound), and leaving the drug on the skin with an occlusive dressing after treatment. For acute injury or open wound treatment,

pulsed ultrasound (0.5 to 1.0 W/cm^2) should be used. All patients should be monitored for systemic drug side effects, especially when a large area is treated or when there is a loss of continuity of the stratum corneum (higher diffusion rate for open wounds).

PULSED ELECTRICAL STIMULATION (MOTOR RESPONSE)

In exploring the effect of various combinations of burst and carrier frequencies of neuromuscular electrical stimulation (NMES) pain perception during 50% maximal voluntary isometric quadriceps femoris muscle contractions, Rooney et al[30] reported that burst frequencies of 50, 70, and 90 bps at carrier frequencies of 2500 and 5000 Hz did not differ in perceived pain intensity and that greater pain was reported at 10,000 Hz regardless of burst frequency. They recommended that different burst and carrier frequency combinations be tried on a client-by-client basis (to determine the most comfortable, yet greatest torque-producing stimulus). In a comparison of console and portable battery-powered NMES units for the treatment of the quadriceps femoris of 52 ACL reconstruction patients, Snyder-Mackler et al[31] reported that subjects who trained with console-style clinical stimulators (Fig. 1) had greater training intensities and quadriceps torque than subjects who used battery-powered units. Draper and Ballard[32] compared electromyographic biofeedback and portable NMES used in conjunction with quadriceps setting and straight-leg raises (3 times/day, 30-min sessions, for 4 weeks). They reported that the biofeedback group recovered to 46% of the contralateral quadriceps maximal voluntary isometric contraction, whereas the portable NMES group recovered to 38%.

TRANSCUTANEOUS ELECTRICAL NERVE STIMULATION

Fundamentally, transcutaneous electrical nerve stimulation (TENS) alters the pattern and frequency of nerve action potentials transmitted toward the central nervous system along the stimulated nerve fibers.[33–35] Animal studies using intracellular neurophysiological recording techniques have led to theories related to the ability of TENS to close a theoretical "gate" to nociceptive impulses associated with tissue injury.[36] TENS is also associated with theories of pain relief linked to the activation of a primitive endogenous pain relief system housed in the reticular core of the brain stem. Some investigators have reported that TENS increases endorphin levels,[37] whereas others found no change in circulating endorphins[38] following TENS application. TENS can be viewed as altering the perceptual pain component and being of little value in managing problems related to the other four components (physiological, affective, cognitive, and behavioral).[39] Patients with acute pain that produces frequent nociceptive impulses are likely to benefit more from TENS than patients with chronic pain in whom some tissue repair has occurred. TENS is likely to be more helpful for patients with localized tissue damage and pain than for patients with diffuse pain that is difficult to localize and characterize.

Jensen et al,[40] in studying the effects of TENS, placebo

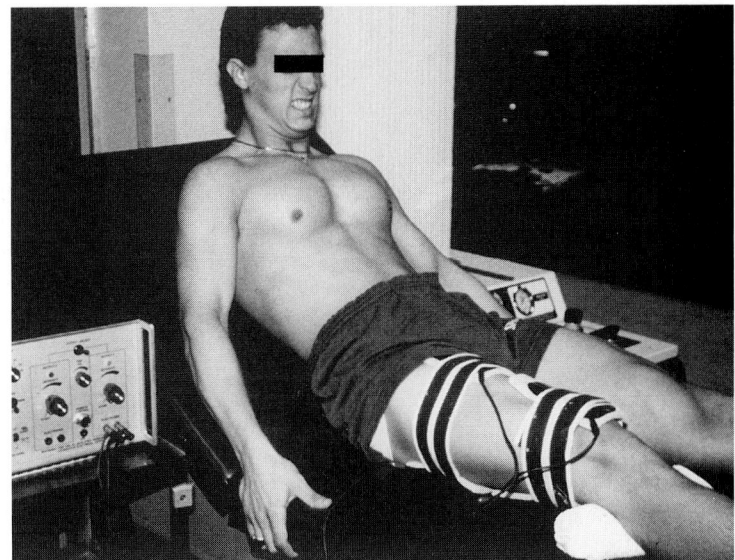

Fig. 1. Console electrical neuromuscular stimulation of the quadriceps femoris.

TENS, and no TENS on 90 patients following arthroscopic knee surgery reported that the TENS group had less pain, required less pain medication, and re-attained preoperative knee muscle strength earlier than the other two groups. Meyler,[41] in evaluating TENS use among 211 patients with differing pain syndromes, reported that TENS was associated with a favorable response in the majority of patients with pain caused by peripheral nerve damage (53%) and musculoskeletal pain due to mechanical causes (69%). Hidderley and Weinel[42] reported that TENS applied to true acupuncture points remote from the pain site of 14 patients undergoing herniorrhaphy reduced their pain level and morphine use compared with patients who received TENS at non-true acupuncture points. Lein et al[43] reported equal increases in wrist pain threshold for auricular, somatic, and combined TENS treatment groups of nonimpaired subjects compared with a control group.

HIGH-VOLT PULSED CURRENT (EDEMA CONTROL)

Whereas evidence for the efficacy of using motor level electrical stimulation ("muscle pumping") for edema reduction is considerable, evidence for edema reduction using sensory level stimulation is less abundant. Michlovitz et al[44] reported no differences in edema control when high-volt pulsed current (HVPC) was added to the ice, compression, elevation treatment of acute ankle sprain patients. Cosgrove et al,[45] using an animal model, reported no differences in edema reduction following blunt trauma between HVPC, symmetrical, biphasic pulsed current, and sham electrical stimulation for edema control.

Using an animal model, Taylor et al[46] reported that cathodal and anodal HVPC, but not alternating current, decreased macromolecular leakage from microvessels following histamine treatment. Based on the results of several experiments using animal models, Mendel and Fish[47] proposed a tentative edema management protocol using cath-

ode HVPC at 120 pps and 90% of visible motor threshold using a water immersion technique. They recommended 30-minute treatments every 4 hours beginning as soon after the injury as possible, or as long as edema is still likely to be forming. They speculated that whatever HVPC was doing to curb edema formation was induced by non-neurological factors, such as affecting microvacular permeability. These studies suggest that the effects of muscle pumping (motor response) may resolve edema once it is formed and that sensory-level cathodal stimulation with HVPC may retard edema formation.

IONTOPHORESIS

Li et al[48] reported that patients with rheumatoid arthritis of the knee who were treated with iontophoresis-delivered dexamethasone had less pain at rest and greater AROM than patients who received placebo treatments. Pellecchia et al[49] reported that patients with infrapatellar tendinitis who were treated with iontophoresis-delivered dexamethasone and lidocaine had less pain, less tenderness with palpation, and better functional scores than patients who received traditional treatment modalities. Gudeman et al[50] reported greater symptom relief and function for plantar fasciitis patients who received iontophoresis with dexamethasone in conjunction with standard modalities than patients who received standard modalities alone. Wieder[51] reported increased knee AROM and a 98.9% decrease in the myositis ossificans mass of a 16-year-old male using iontophoresis-delivered 2% acetic acid solution followed by pulsed ultrasound (three treatments for 3 weeks). Perron and Malouin,[52] in assessing the efficacy of using acetic acid iontophoresis and ultrasound (0.8 W/cm², 1 MHz, 5 min) in the treatment of patients with calcifying shoulder tendinitis failed to report differences between treatment and control groups. Lark[53] advised using the pain-relieving effects of iontophoresis-delivered lidocaine to assess whether the target painful sites are reachable by iontophoresis.

ACUPUNCTURE

Repetitive acupoint stimulation by "needling" is believed to cause repetitive neuronal firing, thereby altering the anatomic, physiological, and chemical components of the synaptic junctions and creating neuronal memory circuits.[54] A National Institutes of Health sponsored panel reported that acupuncture produces equivocal results because of poor study designs, small sample sizes, and inherent difficulties in the use of placebo or sham controls.[55] Currently, there is a wide variation in the practice of acupuncture, with the number of points represented on various training charts ranging from 365 to more than 2000.[56] Based on reports of promising results among large and diverse patient populations, the panel concluded that acupuncture may be useful as a component of a comprehensive patient management program but strongly recommended further research.

Using animal dissections, Egerbacher and Layroutz[57] reported that acupuncture points resembled either neurovascular bundles or cutaneous spinal nerve branches penetrating fascia or dermis, respectively. Tillu and Gupta,[58] in treating 18 patients with a 25-month mean duration of recalcitrant plantar fasciitis symptoms, reported significant pain reduction following acupuncture. Based on a multicenter study of seven practitioners and 58 patients, Macpherson and Fitter[59] reported that acupuncture effectiveness started to plateau after the first seven treatments and that patients with more severe initial conditions (particularly bodily pain) tended to make more rapid improvements. They also reported that patients with "less chronic" symptoms displayed more rapid recoveries. Gaw et al[60] reported similar improvements between patients with osteoarthritis who were treated with either "real" or sham acupuncture. Johnson et al[61] reported no differences in sensation or pain threshold between nonimpaired subjects who received acupuncture at sites that were either related or unrelated to sites of electrically induced finger pain. Takeda and Wessel[62] reported that "real" and sham acupuncture produced similar pain relief for patients with osteoarthritic knee pain.

MAGNETIC FIELD THERAPY

Introducing efficacious electrical changes into the cellular microenvironment may have a beneficial effect on tissue growth and repair. The anti-inflammatory effect and enhanced microcirculation of pulsed magnetic fields (PMF) and pulsed electromagnetic fields (PEMF) are believed to be due to their magnetic and/or electromagnetic field action, independent of any heat produced by the fields themselves, probably via the alterations they induce in cell membrane potentials and ionic fluxes.[63] Using an animal model, Lee et al[63] studied the effects of PMF (17 or 50 Hz) and PEMF (15 or 45 Hz) compared with control in treating Achilles tendon inflammation. They reported that the group treated with a 17 Hz PMF had better collagen alignment and less inflammation than groups treated with other PMF or PEMF frequencies or control by 30 days postinjury. In a study using PEMF for treating 29 patients with persistent rotator cuff tendinitis ($\geq$ 3 months), Binder et al[64] reported that the treated group had less pain and greater AROM following 4 weeks of treatment. In a com-parison of 34 patients with heel pain, Caselli et al[65] reported no differences between patients treated for 4 weeks with either molded insoles with continuous magnetic field foil heel inserts or standard insoles. Foley-Nolan et al[66] in a study of 40 patients with acute whiplash reported less pain and greater AROM among patients who received active PEMF therapy via their soft cervical collars than patients who received collars without an active PEMF. Borsa and Liggett[67] reported no pre- or post-treatment differences between subjects who received "real" CMF, placebo CMF, or no CMF among 45 nonimpaired subjects following an exercise-induced DOMS.

BIOFEEDBACK

Biofeedback provides a method of bioelectrical monitoring and amplifying the physiological processes that are ordinarily not within a patient's awareness or control. Biofeedback can be provided by console (Fig. 2) and portable devices (Fig. 3), in single and multichannel configurations. Using radiographic techniques, Ingersoll and Knight[68] reported that nonimpaired subjects who used electromyographic biofeedback in combination with vastus medialis exercises improved their patellofemoral congruence angle compared with patients who used standard exercise and with control subjects. Draper and Ballard,[32] in studying 30 ACL reconstruction patients, reported that biofeedback was superior to portable NMES for improving knee extensor torque. Levitt et al,[69] in studying 51 patients following knee arthroscopy, reported that patients treated with exercise and biofeedback had greater knee extensor torque than those treated with exercise alone. In treating three patients with volitional posterior glenohumeral joint instability who were treated with exercise and biofeedback at the posterior head of the deltoid muscle, Beall et al[70] reported decreased pain, decreased dislocation episodes, and a successful return to athletic activities following 4 weeks of therapy. In a case study involving a 15-year-old female with volitional posterior glenohumeral joint dislocation, Young[71] reported good results using a dual-channel biofeedback unit (anterior, posterior deltoid heads) for clinical sessions, and a single-

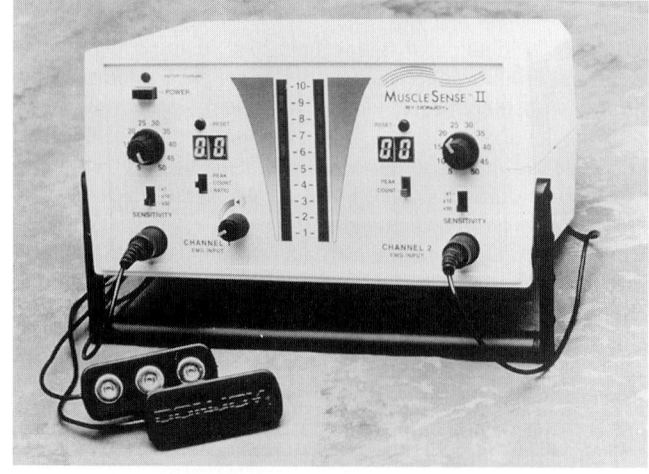

Fig. 2. Console biofeedback device.

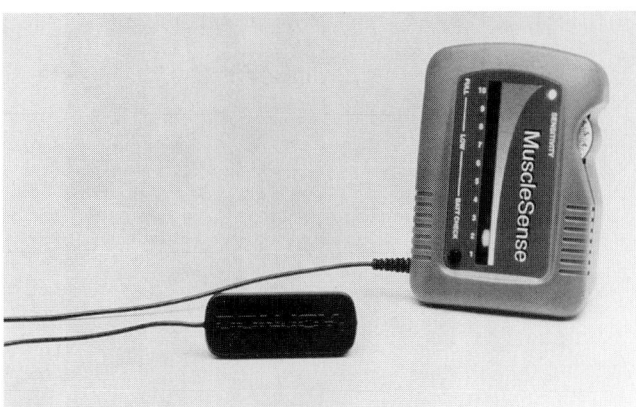

Fig. 3. Portable biofeedback device.

channel unit during home program exercises, which progressed from isometric to AROM to retrain voluntary glenohumeral joint control. Reid et al[72] reported that patients with symptomatic subluxing shoulders who used biofeedback and motor control–based exercises showed greater improvement in work and sport function and had less pain over time than patients who performed an isokinetic exercise strength program. Farmer[73] reviewed the use of biofeedback in combination with visualization to enhance athletic and exercise performance.

MASSAGE

Martin et al,[74] in comparing the effect of a single 20-minute lower extremity massage, active recovery (stationary cycling for 20 minutes at 80 RPM and at 40% VO^2 peak) or rest in supine (20 minutes) on blood lactate clearance following maximal anaerobic leg exercise among 10 cyclists, reported that only the active recovery group had significant decreases in blood lactate measurements. Ti-idus[75] reported that there is little evidence that massage has any significant effect on the physiological factors associated with the exercise recovery process, deeming light exercise of the affected muscles preferable to improve muscle blood flow (thereby enhancing healing). Shoemaker et al[76] compared the effects of forearm and thigh effleurage, petrissage, and tapotement with mild active exercise among 10 nonimpaired subjects. Active exercise increased mean blood flow velocity and vessel diameter, and massage did not. Sullivan et al[77] reported reduced triceps surae H-reflex amplitudes among subjects who received ipsilateral calf petrissage compared with control subjects. In a comparison between massage (2 hours postexercise) and control groups following exercise-induced elbow flexor/extensor DOMS, Smith et al[78] reported reduced serum creatine kinase levels, prolonged neutrophil elevation, and diminished diurnal cortisol reduction for the massage group. Goldberg et al,[79] in assessing the effect of manual massage pressure levels on triceps surae H-reflex amplitude reported decreased amplitudes during deeper massage compared with control conditions, suggesting that inhibitory responses were pressure sensitive.

EXERCISE

Functionally relevant movements (or components thereof) should be included in the exercise prescription as early as possible with consideration for patient safety and tissue healing status. Within any exercise prescription, the clinician needs to decide what percentage of the program will concentrate on isolated deficiencies (Fig. 4) and what percentage will concentrate on integrated multiple joint and multiple neuromuscular component activities (functional tasks) (Fig 5). Clinicians also must weigh the relative client needs regarding the primary energy system demands of the task (adenosine triphosphate–creatine phosphate, anaerobic glycolysis, aerobic) by manipulating training variables (e.g.,

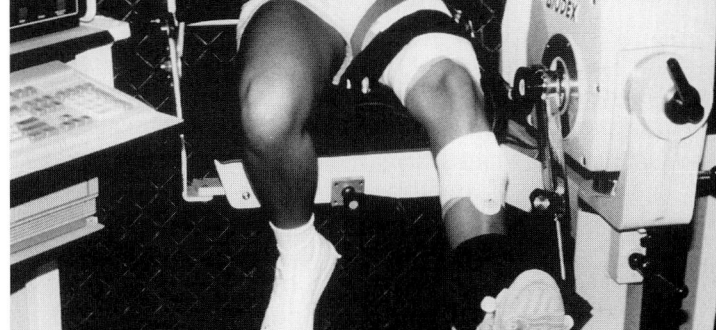

Fig. 4. Conventional isokinetic rehabilitation.

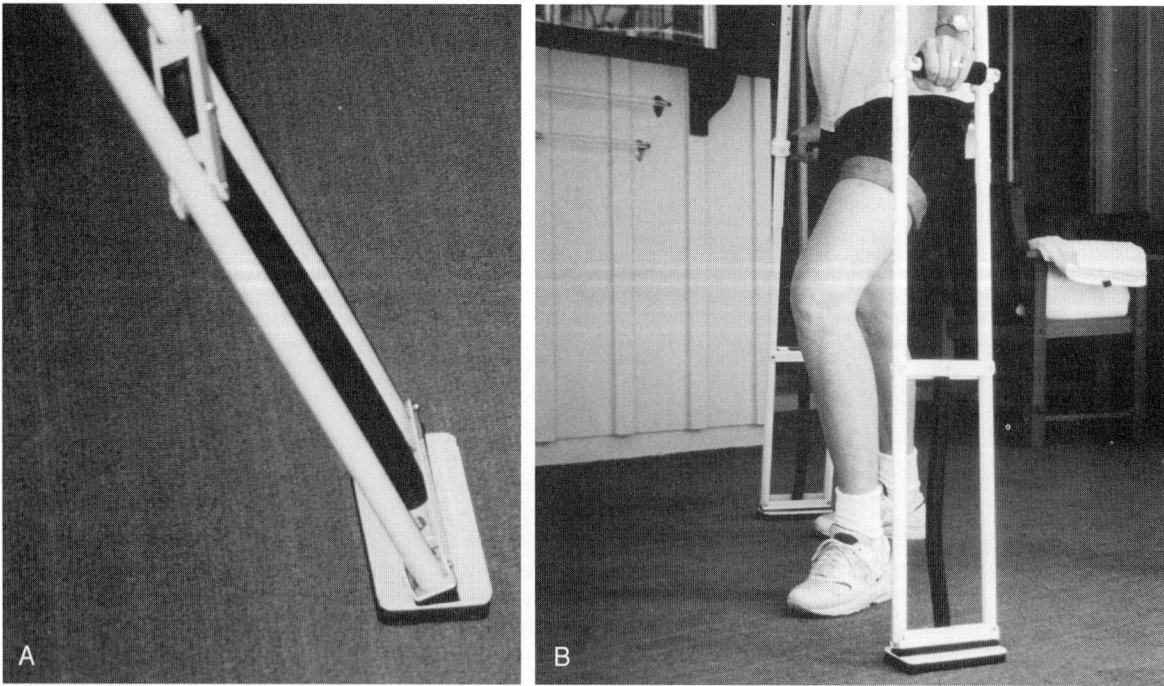

Fig. 5. Views. *A*, Adapted assistive device "3D Foot." *B*, Protected closed kinetic chain functional exercise.

sets, repetitions, recovery time, frequency, exercise choice, exercise order). Similarly, exercise programs should combine the positive attributes of both closed kinetic chain and open kinetic chain function (particularly as they relate to position-specific joint stresses), with progressions toward performance at neuromuscular contraction velocities and modes that simulate performance demands). Client needs regarding the restoration of normal coordination, proprioception, and kinesthesia are of particular importance among the athletic community. Modalities other than exercise should be incorporated in a manner that is considered to be most efficacious for catalyzing specific tissue responses (e.g., control of pain, inflammation, edema, torque increases). To achieve this, clinicians must continually evaluate the effect of their interventions and manipulate all treatment modalities to effect the desired changes, facilitate patient progress, and avoid the likelihood of the patient's "plateauing" at a point far short of the desired outcome.

REFERENCES

1. Dolan MG, Thornton RM, Fish DR, Mendel FC: Effects of cold water immersion on edema formation after blunt injury to the hind limbs of rats. J Athl Train 1997; 32(3):233.
2. Myrer JW, Measom G, Fellingham GW: Temperature changes in the human leg during and after two methods of cryotherapy. J Athl Train 1998; 33:25.
3. Zemke JE, Andersen JC, Guion WK, et al: Intramuscular temperature responses in the human leg to two forms of cryotherapy: Ice massage and ice bag. J Orthop Sports Phys Ther 1998; 27(4):301.
4. Kuligowski LA, Lephart SM, Giannantonio FP, Blanc RO: Effect of whirlpool therapy on signs and symptoms of delayed-onset muscle soreness. J Athl Train 1998; 33(3):222.
5. Speer KP, Warren RF, Horowitz L: The efficacy of cryotherapy in the postoperative shoulder. J Shoulder Elbow Surg 1996; 5(1):62.
6. Lessard LA, Scudds RA, Amendola A, Vaz MD: The efficacy of cryotherapy following arthroscopic knee surgery. J Orthop Sports Phys Ther 1997; 26(1):14.
7. Schroder D, Passler HH: Combination of cold and compression after knee surgery: A prospective randomized study. Knee Surg Sports Traumatol Arthrosc 1994; 2(3):158.
8. Walker RH, Morris BA, Angulo DL, et al: Postoperative use of continuous passive motion, transcutaneous electrical nerve stimulation, and continuous cooling pad following total knee arthroplasty. J Arthroplasty 1991; 6(2):151.
9. Ohkoshi Y, Ohkoshi M, Nagasaki S, et al: The effect of cryotherapy on intraarticular temperature and postoperative care after anterior cruciate ligament reconstruction. Am J Sports Med 1999; 27(3):357.
10. Konrath GA, Lock T, Goitz HT, Schiedler J: The use of cold therapy after anterior cruciate ligament reconstruction. A prospective, randomized study and literature review. Am J Sports Med 1996; 24(5):629.
11. Dervin GF, Taylor DE, Keene GC. Effects of cold and compression dressings on early postoperative outcomes for the arthroscopic anterior cruciate ligament reconstruction patient. J Orthop Sports Phys Ther 1998; 27(6):403.
12. Daniel DM, Stone ML, Arendt DI: The effect of cold therapy on pain, swelling, and range of motion after anterior cruciate ligament reconstructive surgery. Arthroscopy 1994; 10(5):530.
13. Ward AR, Robertson VJ: Comparison of heating of nonliving soft tissue produced by 45 kHz and 1 MHz frequency ultrasound machines. J Orthop Sports Phys Ther 1996; 23(4):258.
14. Forrest G, Rosen K: Ultrasound: Effectiveness of treatments given under water. Arch Phys Med Rehabil 1989; 70(1):28.
15. Jackson BA, Schwane JA, Starcher BC:

Effect of ultrasound therapy on the repair of achilles tendon injuries in rats. Med Sci Sports Exerc 1991; 23(2):171.

16. Robinson SE, Buono MJ: Effect of continuous-wave ultrasound on blood flow in skeletal muscle. Phys Ther 1995; 75(2): 145.

17. Fabrizio PA, Schmidt JA, Clemente FR, et al: Acute effects of therapeutic ultrasound delivered at varying parameters on the blood flow velocity in a muscular distribution artery. J Orthop Sports Phys Ther 1996; 24(5):294.

18. Ward AR, Robertson VJ: Dosage factors for the subaqueous application of 1 MHz ultrasound. Arch Phys Med Rehabil 1996; 77(11):1167.

19. Stay JC, Ricard MD, Draper DO, et al: Pulsed ultrasound fails to diminish delayed-onset muscle soreness symptoms. J Athl Train 1998; 33(4):341.

20. Rose S, Draper DO, Schulthies SS, Durrant E: The stretching window part two: Rate of thermal decay in deep muscle following 1-MHz ultrasound. J Athl Train 1996; 31(2):139.

21. Draper DO, Castel JC, Castel D: Rate of temperature increase in human muscle during 1 MHz and 3 MHz continuous ultrasound. J Orthop Sports Phys Ther 1995; 22(4):142.

22. Chan AK, Myrer JW, Measom GJ, Draper DO: Temperature changes in human patellar tendon in response to therapeutic ultrasound. J Athl Train 1998; 33(2):130.

23. Draper DO, Harris ST, Schulthies S, et al: Hot-pack and 1-MHz ultrasound treatments have an additive effect on muscle temperature increase. J Athl Train 1998; 33:21.

24. Rimington SJ, Draper DO, Durrant E, Fellingham G: Temperature changes during therapeutic ultrasound in the precooled human gastrocnemius muscle. J Athl Train 1994; 29(4):325.

25. Franklin ME, Smith ST, Chenier TC, Franklin RC: Effect of phonophoresis with dexamethasone on adrenal function. J Orthop Sports Phys Ther 1995; 22(3):103.

26. Bare AC, McAnaw MB, Pritchard AE, et al: Phonophoretic delivery of 10% hydrocortisone through the epidermis of humans as determined by serum cortisol concentrations. Phys Ther 1996; 76:738.

27. Klaiman MD, Shrader JA, Danoff JV, et al: Phonophoresis versus ultrasound in the treatment of common musculoskeletal conditions. Med Sci Sports Exerc 1998; 30(9): 1349.

28. Ciccone CD, Leggin BG, Callamaro JJ: Effects of ultrasound and trolamine salicylate phonophoresis on delayed-onset muscle soreness. Phys Ther 1991; 71:666.

29. Byl N: The use of ultrasound as an enhancer for transcutaneous drug delivery: Phonophoresis. Phys Ther 1995; 75(6): 539.

30. Rooney JG, Currier DP, Nitz AJ: Effect of variation in the burst and carrier frequency modes of neuro-muscular electrical stimulation on pain perception in healthy subjects. Phys Ther 1992; 72(11):800.

31. Snyder-Mackler L, Delitto A, Stralka SW, Bailey SL: Use of electrical stimulation to enhance recovery of quadriceps femoris muscle force production in patients following anterior cruciate ligament reconstruction. Phys Ther 1994; 74:901.

32. Draper V, Ballard L: Electrical stimulation versus electromyographic biofeedback in the recovery of quadriceps femoris muscle function following anterior cruciate ligament surgery. Phys Ther 1991; 71:455.

33. Barr JO: Transcutaneous electrical nerve stimulation for pain management. In Nelson RM, Hayes KW, Currier DP (eds): Clinical Electrotherapy, 3rd ed. Stamford, CT: Appleton Lange; 1999:291.

34. Walsh DM, Lowe AS, McCormack K, et al: Transcutaneous electrical nerve stimulation: Effects on peripheral nerve conduction, mechanical pain threshold and tactile threshold in humans. Arch Phys Med Rehab 1998; 9:1051.

35. Robinson AJ: Transcutaneous electrical nerve stimulation for the control of pain in musculoskeletal disorders. J Orthop Sports Phys Ther 1996; 24(4):208.

36. Garrison DW, Foreman RD: Effects of transcutaneous electrical nerve stimulation (TENS) on spontaneous and noxiously evoked dorsal horn cell activity in cats with transected spinal cords. Neurosci Lett 1996; 216:125.

37. Han JS, Chen XH, Sun XI, et al: Effect of low and high frequency TENS on met-enkephalin-Arg-Phe and dynorphin A immunoreactivity in human lumbar CSF. Pain 1991; 47:295.

38. Honig S, Zeale P, Mason A, Fitzgerald D: High frequency transcutaneous electrical nerve stimulation: Lack of correlation with serum beta-endorphin levels and failure of analgesia reversal with naloxone. Clin J Pain 1987; 2:215.

39. Nolan MF: Contemporary perspectives on pain and discomfort. Phys Ther Pract 1993; 2(3):1.

40. Jensen JE, Conn RR, Hazelrigg G, Hewett JE: The use of transcutaneous neural stimulation and isokinetic testing in arthroscopic knee surgery. Am J Sports Med 1985; 13(1):27.

41. Meyler WJ, deJongste MJ, Rolf CA: Clinical evaluation of pain treatment with electrostimulation: a study on TENS in patients with different pain syndromes. Clin J Pain 1994; 10(1):22.

42. Hidderley M, Weinel E: Clinical practice: Effects of TENS applied to acupuncture points distal to a pain site. Int J Pall Nursing 1997; 3(4):185.

43. Lein DH, Clelland JA, Knowles CJ, Jackson JR: Comparison of effects of transcutaneous electrical nerve stimulation of auricular, somatic, and the combination of auricular and somatic acupuncture points on experimental pain threshold. Phys Ther 1989; 69(8):671.

44. Michlovitz S, Smith W, Watkins M: Ice and high voltage pulsed stimulation in treatment of lateral ankle sprains. J Orthop Sports Phys Ther 1988; 9:301.

45. Cosgrove KA, Alon G, Bell SF, et al: The electrical effect of two commonly used clinical stimulators on traumatic edema in rats. Phys Ther 1992; 72:227.

46. Taylor K, Mendel FC, Fish DR, et al: Effect of high-voltage pulsed current and alternating current on macro-molecular leakage in hamster cheek pouch microcirculation. Phys Ther 1997; 77:1729.

47. Mendel FC, Fish DR: New perspectives in edema control via electrical stimulation. J Athl Train 1993; 28(1):63.

48. Li LC, Scudds RA, Heck CS, Harth M: The efficacy of dexamethasone iontophoresis for the treatment of rheumatoid arthritic knees: a pilot study. Arth Care Res 1996; 9(2):126.

49. Pellecchia GL, Hamel H, Behnke P: Treatment of infrapatellar tendinitis: A combination of modalities and transverse friction massage versus iontophoresis. J Sport Rehabil 1994; 3(2):135.

50. Gudeman SD, Eisele SA, Heidt RS, et al: Treatment of plantar fasciitis by iontophoresis of 0.4% dexamethasone: A randomized, double-blind, placebo-controlled study. Am J Sports Med 1997; 25(3):312.

51. Weider DL: Treatment of traumatic myositis ossificans with acetic acid iontophoresis. Phys Ther 1992; 72:133.

52. Perron M, Malouin F: Acetic acid iontophoresis and ultrasound for the treatment of calcifying tendinitis of the shoulder: A randomized control trial. Arch Phys Med Rehabil 1997; 78(4):379.

53. Lark MR, Gangarosa LP: Iontophoresis: an effective modality for the treatment of inflammatory disorders of the temporomandibular joint and myofascial pain. Cranio 1990; 8:108.

54. Chan K-M, Lai J-S, Wong AMK, et al: Scientific basis of traditional medicine and practice in the management of sports injuries. In Chan KM, Maffuli N, Kurosaka M, (eds): Controversies in Sports Medicine. Philadelphia, Williams & Wilkins, 1998.

55. NIH Consensus Conference: Acupuncture. JAMA 1998; 280(17):1518.

56. Points of contention: Acupuncture enters the mainstream. Biomechanics 1996; 3(5): 12.

57. Egerbacher M, Layroutz A: Acupuncture points: Macroscopic and microscopic findings in body- and ear-acupuncture points. Wiener Tierarztliche Monatsschrift 1996; 83(12):359.

58. Tillu A, Gupta S: Effect of acupuncture treatment on heel pain due to plantar fasciitis. Accupunct Med 1998; 16(2):66.

59. Macpherson H, Fitter M: Factors that influence outcome: An evaluation of change with acupuncture. Acupunct Med 1998; 16(1):33.

60. Gaw AC, Chang LW, Shaw L-C: Efficacy of acupuncture on osteoarthritic pain. A controlled, double-blind study. N Engl J Med 1975; 293(8):375.

61. Johnson MI, Kundu S, Ashton CH, et al: The analgesic effects of acupuncture on experimental pain threshold and somatosensory evoked potentials in healthy volunteers. Complement Ther Med 1996; 4(4):219.

62. Takeda W, Wessel J: Acupuncture for the treatment of pain of osteoarthritic knees. Arthritis Care Res 1994; 7(3):118.

63. Lee EW, Maffulli N, Li CK, Chan KM: Pulsed magnetic and electromagnetic fields in experimental achilles tendonitis in the rat: A propective randomized study. Arch Phys Med Rehabil 1997; 78(4):399.

64. Binder A, Parr G, Hazleman B, Fitton-Jackson S: Pulsed electromagnetic field therapy of persistent rotator cuff tendinitis. A double-blind controlled assessment. Lancet 1984; 1(8379):695.

65. Caselli MA, Clark N, Lazarus S, et al: Evaluation of magnetic foil and PPT insoles in the treatment of heel pain. J Am Pod Med Assoc 1997; 87(1):11.

66. Foley-Nolan D, Moore K, Codd M, et al: Low energy high frequency pulsed electromagnetic therapy for acute whiplash injuries: A double blind randomized controlled study. Scand J Rehab Med 1992; 24(1):51.

67. Borsa PA, Liggett CL: Flexible magnets are not effective in decreasing pain perception and recovery time after muscle microinjury. J Athl Train 1998; 33(2):150.

68. Ingersoll CD, Knight KL: Patellar location changes following EMG biofeedback or progressive resistive exercises. Med Sci Sports Exerc 1991; 23(1):1122.

69. Levitt R, Deisinger JA, Remondet Wall J, et al: EMG feedback-assisted postoperative rehabilitation of minor arthroscopic knee surgeries. J Sports Med Phys Fitness 1995; 35(3):218.

70. Beall MS, Diefenbach G, Allen A: Electromyographic biofeedback in the treatment of voluntary posterior instability of the shoulder. Am J Sports Med 1987; 15(2):175.

71. Young MS: Electromyographic biofeedback use in the treatment of voluntary posterior dislocation of the shoulder: A case study. J Orthop Sports Phys Ther 1994; 20(3):171.

72. Reid DC, Saboe LA, Chepeha JC: Anterior shoulder instability in athletes: Comparison of isokinetic resistance exercises and an electromyographic biofeedback re-education program—a pilot program. Physiother Can 1996; 48(4):251.

73. Farmer KU: Biofeedback and visualization for peak performance. J Sports Rehabil 1995; 4(1):59.

74. Martin NA, Zoeller RF, Robertson RJ, Lephart SM: The comparative effects of sports massage, active recovery, and rest in promoting blood lactate clearance after supramaximal leg exercise. J Athl Train 1998; 33:30.

75. Tiidus PM: Manual massage and recovery of muscle function following exercise: A literature review. J Orthop Sports Phys Ther 1997; 25(2):107.

76. Shoemaker JK, Tiidus PM, Mader R: Failure of manual massage alter limb blood flow: Measures by Doppler ultrasound. Med Sci Sports Exer 1997; 29(5):610.

77. Sullivan SJ, Seguin S, Seaborne D, Goldberg J: Reduction of H-reflex amplitude during the application of effleurage to the triceps surae in neurologically healthy subjects. Physiother Theory Prac 1993; 9(1):25.

78. Smith LL, Keating MN, Holbert D, et al: The effects of athletic massage on delayed onset muscle soreness, creatine kinase, and neutrophil count: A preliminary report. J Orthop Sports Phys Ther 1994; 19(2):93.

79. Goldberg J, Sullivan SJ, Seaborne DE: The effect of two intensities of massage on H-reflex amplitude. Phys Ther 1992; 72(6):449.

INJURIES TO THE MUSCLE-TENDON UNIT

section 4 chapter 4

Donald T. Kirkendall and William E. Garrett, Jr.

Summary
- Muscle strains (i.e., stretch-induced injuries) may account for 30% of cases in a typical sports medicine practice.
- Stretch-induced injuries occur at the muscle-tendon junction, usually the distal junction.
- The rectus femoris, gastrocnemius, hamstring, and adductor longus muscles seem most susceptible to stretch-induced injuries, based on their architecture.
- Cyclic stretching and warm-up prior to exercise are preventative.
- Nonsteroidal anti-inflammatory drugs are useful for early treatment of muscle strains but may delay histological repair.

Both the primary care physician and the orthopaedic surgeon frequently see common acute skeletal muscle injuries, including contusions, lacerations, strains, ischemia, and complete ruptures. Significant pain and disability can result from any of these injuries, leading to time lost from participation in occupational and leisure activities. Muscle strains, or stretch-induced injuries, are an important injury to the clinician in either occupational or sports medicine settings because stretch-induced injuries can account for nearly 30% of the typical sports medicine practice.[1, 2] The purpose of this article is to review the mechanism of muscle strain injury, apply the basic research to the clinical case, discuss preventative strategies, and examine current methods of treating muscle strains.

A variety of indirect or noncontact injuries can affect muscle function. Examples of such indirect injuries include delayed onset muscle soreness (DOMS), partial strain injury, and complete rupture of the muscle. These represent a continuum of injuries that have one common denominator: eccentric exercise. When muscle develops tension, the muscle is lengthening.[2, 3] When compared with concentric action, eccentric action can develop high forces while recruiting fewer active motor units,[4] leading to higher tension output per active muscle fiber.

During unaccustomed exercise, eccentric loading leads to microscopic damage to the contractile element of muscle, which appears as random disruptions of the Z-lines.[5] Reversible pain (DOMS), weakness, and limited range of motion are the common signs and symptoms of DOMS. Pain is usually at its peak in the 1 to 2 days following exercise.[6] Weakness and limited range of motion can last for more than a week.[7, 8] A fascinating aspect of DOMS is the rapid adaptation of muscle, as demonstrated by successive bouts of the unaccustomed exercise producing progressively less perceived soreness and less tissue damage.[6] This adaptation is attributed to an increase of sarcomeres in series.

In a muscle strain injury, there is damage to the muscle-tendon unit.[9] When the patient tries to perform physical activity that recruits the damaged muscle, local pain and general weakness of the muscle are reported. Improper rest and rehabilitation of a minor skeletal muscle strain frequently proceeds to a more disabling injury, which further increases the time lost from work and athletics.

We know that muscle strains are a common injury seen in the clinician's office. When one compares our understanding of damage to ligament, tendon, and bone with our understanding of damage to muscle, the basic knowledge of the pathophysiology, treatment, and recovery of the strained muscle is limited. We seem to know very little about that which we see the most. Perhaps the natural history, the self-limiting nature, and the minimal surgical requirements has made stretch-induced injuries of less interest to clinicians. This brief review re-examines the stretch-induced injuries, including the mechanism, location, treatment, and some observations on prevention of these nagging injuries.

MECHANISM OF INJURY

The first step is to develop a method to reproduce the injury in the laboratory. To do this, the simple understanding of just how skeletal muscle is injured in sport or occupational settings is essential. Most clinicians would agree that muscle strain injuries occur when the muscle is passively stretched or activated during stretch.[1, 3, 10] Not surprisingly, eccentric action of the muscle occurs frequently.[2, 3, 11] Eccentric action is a very important factor because muscle forces per active muscle fiber can be very high during lengthening,[4] which adds to the forces by the passive, connective tissue element.[12] In sport, not only are stretch-induced strain injuries seen in "speed athletes" (e.g., sprinters) and American football, basketball, soccer, and rugby athletes, among others, but, as will be shown subsequently, certain muscles seem to be more prone to injury than others.

We applied standard techniques of muscle mechanics and electrophysiology to study rabbit hindlimb muscles, most often the tibialis anterior and the extensor digitorum longus. The first task was to develop a model for the reproducible production of strain injury. The first observation was that activation alone failed to cause either a partial or complete strain injury.[13] Stretch was necessary to obtain an injury. The force necessary for muscle failure was several times the force produced actively during a maximal isometric contraction,[14] which suggested that passive forces must be considered. Therefore, the model of a strain injury was defined. Intact muscle of the rabbit hindlimb, with neural and vascular supply intact, could be stretched to failure or activated during stretch.

PASSIVE STRETCH INJURY

The first concern was the anatomy of the injury. Would the injury be different if the muscle was stretched from the proximal or distal tendon? Would the rate of strain or muscle architecture (pennation) influence the mechanical properties of muscle? Regardless of the strain rate (1, 10, and 100 cm/sec^{-1}) or architecture, or the location of the stretch, the muscle failed predictably at the muscle-tendon junction (MTJ) (Fig. 1), usually the distal junction, leaving a small, variable amount of muscle tissue still attached to the tendon (Fig. 2).[13] Thus, the site of stretched-induced injury was consistently near the muscle-tendon junction. This injury was not an avulsion because a small,

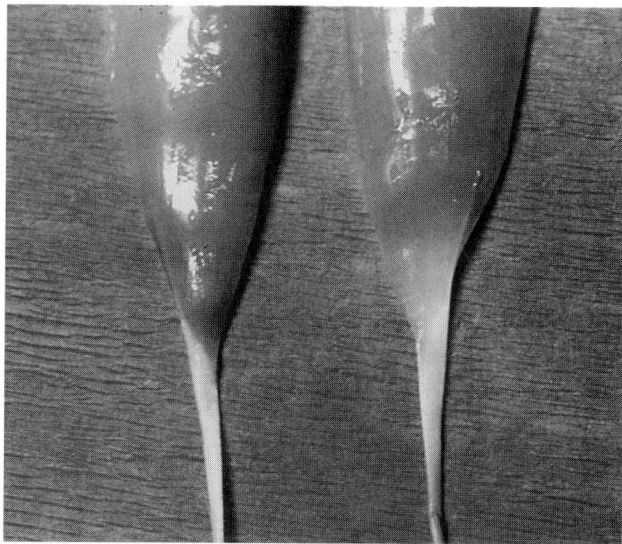

Fig. 1. Note the small hemorrhage at the distal tip of the injured tibialis anterior muscle on the left. This photograph was taken 24 hours after the strain injury. (From Nikolaou PK, MacDonald BL, Glisson RR, et al: Biomechanical and histological evaluation of muscle after controlled strain injury. Am J Sports Med 1987; 15:9.)

variable amount of muscle remained connected to the tendon.

ACTIVE STRETCH INJURY

Clinical observation suggests that most strain injuries occur during powerful eccentric contractions, so a laboratory condition to mimic that which was seen clinically was devised. The same rabbit hindlimb muscles were isolated as before and stretched to failure; however, during stretch, one of three conditions of activation were applied: unstimulated, submaximal stimulation, and tetanic stimulation.[15] The location of the failure was uniformly the MTJ, and the total strain at failure was similar among the three conditions. Interestingly, the force generated at failure was only 15% greater in the activated muscles. However, the energy absorbed (the difference in strain energy between passive and active conditions) was nearly double in the activated condition (Fig. 3). This indicated that although passive elements of muscle can absorb energy, the amount of energy absorbed was enhanced when the muscle was activated.

This may indicate how muscles are able to protect themselves and joint structures from injury. The more energy absorbed by muscle, the more resistant the muscle is to injury. Energy is absorbed by both the passive and the contractile elements of muscle. The passive elements include connective tissue and the fibers themselves and are not dependent on activation. The contractile element of the muscle also participates, because activation of the muscle increases the ability to absorb energy (see Fig. 2).

The increase in energy absorbed due to contraction was found to be around 100%. Any condition that limits the ability of the muscle to contract limits the ability of the muscle to absorb energy, leaving the muscle more susceptible to injury. Two variables that are commonly cited in muscle strain injuries are fatigue and weakness.

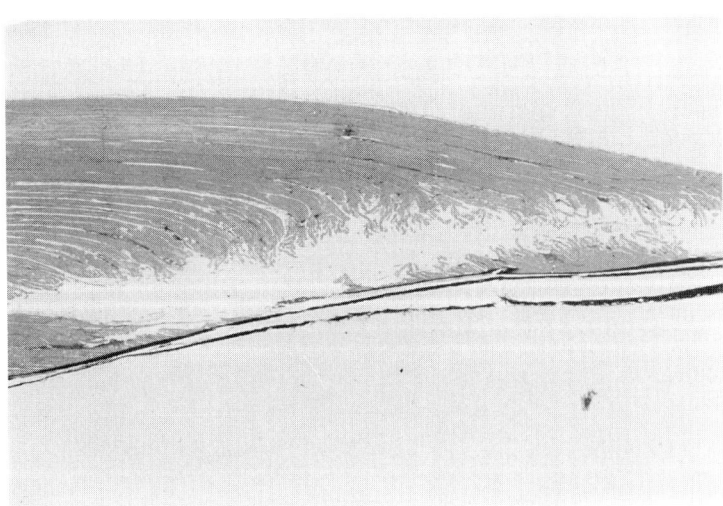

Fig. 2. From the extensor digitorum longus of rabbit. Note the tear of muscle tissue from the tendon. Also note the small but variable amount of muscle tissue still attached to the tendon. (From Taylor DC, Dalton JD, Seaber AV, Garret WE Jr: Experimental muscle strain injury: Early functional and structural deficits and the increased risk for reinjury. Am J Sports Med 1993; 21:190.)

NONDISRUPTIVE INJURIES

So far, this discussion has been directed toward injuries that lead to a complete disruption of the muscle-tendon unit. When there is a change in the linearity of the force-displacement curve of a stretched, inactivated muscle, a "plastic" deformation has occurred, indicating some alteration to the material structure. Using the model of the rabbit hindlimb, physiological, mechanical, and histological characteristics of muscle can be observed.

This model results in a nondisruptive injury, but ultrastructural damage does still occur. Histological section of this injury shows damage near the muscle-tendon junction with a variable amount of muscle tissue attached to the tendon. Some hemorrhaging occurs. A pronounced local inflammatory response is seen 1 to 2 days after the injury. By the 7th day, fibrous tissue begins to replace the inflammatory reaction, leading to scar tissue formation.[15]

Physical damage to the tissue should alter the ability of the muscle to develop tension. Immediately after the injury, the muscle can develop only to 70% of the normal amount of tension. One day later, the muscle's ability to generate tension declines further to 50% of that of the contralateral control muscle. Thereafter, tension production improves and by the seventh day, the muscle is able to develop 90% of the tension produced by the contralateral control muscle.

Contrast this with a muscle having a 7-day-old nondisruptive injury. When this muscle is stretched, the tensile strength is only 77% of that of the control muscle.[16] This is well below the 90% of tension developed that was just mentioned. As strains are in part caused by stretch, this loss of tensile strength may make the muscle more susceptible to a second injury, a scenario frequently seen by clinicians.

VISCOELASTICITY OF SKELETAL MUSCLE

Important preventive strategies against strain injuries include flexibility, warm-up, and pre-exercise stretching. The beneficial adaptation due to stretching has most frequently been linked to stretch-reflex mechanisms. But an additional

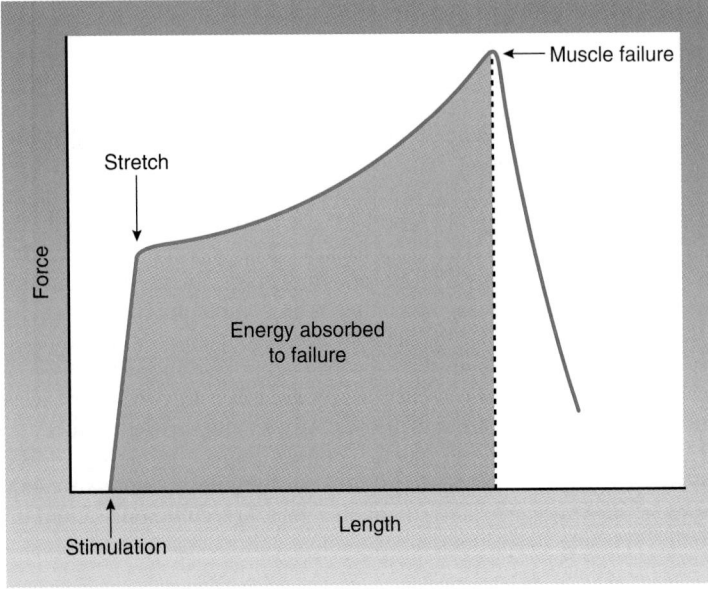

Fig. 3. The area under the length-deformation curve represents the energy absorbed.

feature of muscle, viscoelasticity, needs to be considered. One can visualize viscoelasticity if one imagines hanging a weight on a muscle and noting its new length, then watching the muscle slowly continue to increase in length with time. For tendons and ligaments, if the tissue is stretched to a constant length, its tension gradually decreases with time. This is referred to as stress-relaxation. When multiple cycles are performed a gradual decrease in tension occurs with each successive stretch.[17]

A series of studies was designed to determine whether similar features were prevalent in the muscle-tendon unit. Rabbit hindlimb muscle was repeatedly stretched from an initial force of 1.96 N to 78.4 N, held for 30 seconds, then returned to the initial 1.96 N force. This process was repeated 10 times (Fig. 4). The length needed to obtain the predetermined tension increased 3.45% over the 10 cycles, and 80% of the length change occurred in the first four stretches.[18]

To look at similar properties another way, the muscle was stretched to 10% above its resting length, the tension noted, then the muscle allowed to return to its resting length. This cycle also was repeated 10 times (Fig. 5). Tension fell by nearly 17% over the 10 cycles, with most of the reduction occurring, again, in the first four cycles.[19]

It should be obvious that repetitive stretching attenuates the load on the muscle-tendon unit at any given length. Of particular interest was the absence of reflex effects or other central nervous system mediation. Both innervated and denervated muscle were studied with no apparent differences for the two conditions. These data clearly show that muscle is capable of changes due to stretching and that such changes are a result of inherent muscle-tendon viscoelasticity. Certainly during physiological movement there are additional reflex and central nervous system effects influencing muscle during stretch.

APPLICATION TO THE CLINIC

It is critical that laboratory findings be applied to the clinical setting. The rabbit model showed that muscle strain injuries occur at the MTJ. Would the results of a controlled strain injury be the same finding in athletes injured in the uncontrolled setting of competitive sports? Acute hamstring

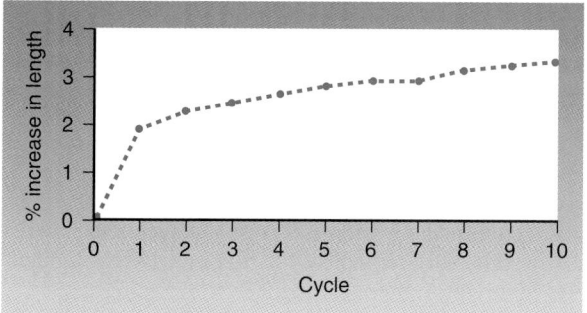

Fig. 4. Relative increase in the length of an extensor digitorum longus when repeatedly lengthened to a constant tension. (From Taylor DC, Dalton JD, Seaber AV, Garrett WE Jr: Experimental muscle strain injury: Early functional and structural deficits and the increased risk for reinjury. Am J Sports Med 1990; 18:300.)

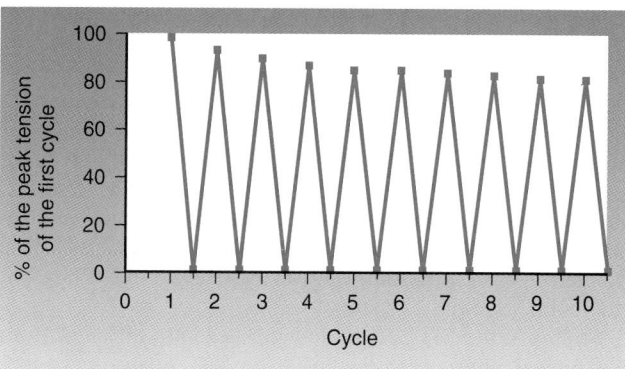

Fig. 5. The muscle tension of an extensor digitorum longus when repeatedly stretched to 10% beyond resting length. (From Taylor DC, Dalton JD, Seaber AV, Garrett WE Jr: Experimental muscle strain injury: Early functional and structural deficits and the increased risk for reinjury. Am J Sports Med 1990; 18:300.)

strain injuries were evaluated within 48 hours of the injury in 10 college athletes.[20] All were examined clinically to determine the mechanism of injury and then imaged with computed tomography (CT) to determine the location of the injury. All the injuries happened while the subject was sprinting or kicking a soccer ball. The injuries were generally proximal and lateral, typically in the biceps femoris. The typical mechanism involved ballistic hip flexion and knee extension. By CT scanning, the injured area appeared as a region of hypodensity, suggesting inflammation and edema in the absence of localized bleeding. It seemed that the long head of the biceps femoris was most frequently injured in our sample (9 of 10) and the injury was focussed on the MTJ of the common tendon of the hamstrings. The 10th patient (a soccer player) injured his semimembranosus while performing an overhead kick, suggesting a different mechanism than that seen in the sprinters.

We expanded our sample base and imaged a larger sample of athletes who were injured through a variety of mechanisms.[21] Fifty patients underwent CT (n = 27) or magnetic resonance imaging (MRI; n = 23) to image their strain injury. Injuries were localized to the quadriceps, hamstrings, adductors, and triceps surae groups. T_2-weighted images were preferred for visualizing the edema, inflammation, and possible hemorrhage of muscle strain injuries. The expected areas of low density were found with CT scanning. The rectus femoris was the location of quadriceps strains, and adductor strains were isolated to the adductor longus. Eleven of the 17 hamstring strain injuries were to the biceps femoris, 4 were to the semimembranosus, and 2 were to the semitendinosus. In the triceps surae group, all strain injuries were located at the distal MTJ of the medial head of the gastrocnemius. Both CT and MRI were effective in locating the injury. More importantly, particular muscles were noted to be susceptible to strain injuries. The muscles were either two-joint muscles (e.g., rectus femoris, gastrocnemius, hamstrings) or of a complex architecture (e.g., adductor longus) and occurred, as can best be determined by CT and MRI imaging, at the MTJ.

Clinicians often see curious, unexplained muscle injuries like the persistent strain of the rectus femoris. To understand the nature of this strain injury, the pertinent anatomy seemed to be an appropriate place to begin.[22] Dissection of cadaveric rectus femoris muscle indicates a direct head originating at the anterior inferior iliac spine, as expected. In addition, an indirect head originating from the superior acetabular ridge was also found. The tendon of this indirect head extended well into the mass of the rectus femoris. Prior laboratory work suggested that most strain injuries occur superficially at the MTJ. However, clinical evidence pointed to a strain at the MTJ of the deep, indirect head of the rectus femoris.

Strains at the MTJ of the indirect head are different from the typical injury near the distal tendon because asymmetry, chronic pain, and anterior thigh masses are evident. Ten patients had their incomplete intrasubstance strain of the proximal, deep tendon of the rectus femoris evaluated with physical examination and imaging studies. Patients were evaluated anywhere from 4 to 156 weeks after injury. Sprinting or kicking was the mechanism in 8 of the 10 injuries (2 patients were unable to recall the mechanism). All but one patient had pain with running. Imaging studies detected the strain to be isolated to the area of the tendon of the indirect head of the rectus femoris. Surgery was performed on two patients; one had the muscle removed and the other had a fibrotic mass excised. Both were asymptomatic and returned to full activity. The explanation for chronic pain in these subjects was unknown, but might be due to differential activation of the superficial and deep portions of the muscle.

So many strain injuries seem to be dependent on the architecture of the muscle. After our experiences noted in Hughes et al,[22] a detailed study of the architecture of the rectus femoris was performed to determine whether these persistent strains were related to some peculiar architectural feature.[23] The rectus femoris of fresh or embalmed cadavers was dissected. Superficial and deep tendons were confirmed. The tendon of the deep component was continuous through nearly the entire length of the muscle arising from the superior acetabular ridge and coursed medially throughout the muscle. It began as a rounded, flattened tissue and migrated laterally, becoming nearly vertical in the distal third of the muscle (Fig. 6). The pennation of the muscle was far more complex than the simple bipennate arrangement normally mentioned. The proximal third appeared to be unipennate and the distal two-thirds was bipennate. The deep tendon and the bipennate arrangement of the distal portion of the muscle created what appeared to be "a muscle within a muscle." Exploration of three chronic strain injuries revealed a pseudocyst consisting of vascular, fibrotic loose connective tissue surrounding the deep tendon with a serous fluid between the connective tissue and the tendon. The anatomic findings were consistent with CT or MRI images of vascular fibrotic processes of the deep tendon of the indirect head.

A most common hamstring strain seen clinically involves one muscle, usually the biceps femoris. More extensive injuries involve more muscles, typically at the common origin of the hamstrings. A unique mechanism of severe hamstring strain injury happens during water skiing.[24] The novice skier crouches prior to being pulled into a standing position by the boat. If the skier's knees are extended too soon, the ski tips are forced down into the

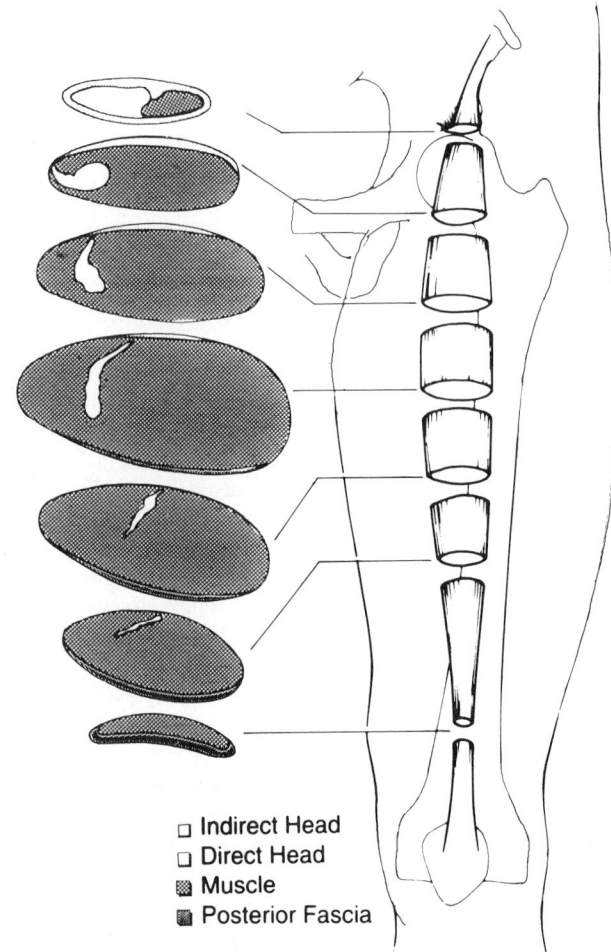

□ Indirect Head
□ Direct Head
▨ Muscle
▩ Posterior Fascia

Fig. 6. The architecture of the indirect head of the rectus femoris muscle. (From Hasselman CT, Best TM, Hughes C, et al: An explanation for various rectus femoris strain injuries using previously undescribed muscle architecture. Am J Sports Med 1995; 23:493.)

water. The pull of the boat pulls the skier forward into excessive hip flexion with the knees extended. Such powerful stretch can lead to a muscle-tendon junction injury or the more disabling avulsion injury of the tendinous origin from the ischial tuberosity. Hamstring strains can also occur in experienced skiers while falling forward on a single slalom ski. Twelve water skiers who suffered a skiing-induced hamstring injury were followed for 0.5 and 18 years after the injury. All the patients realized they had suffered a significant injury when the accident occurred. Complete or partial avulsion had occurred at the proximal tendon. The seriousness of the injury was obvious immediately on physical examination, revealing distal tendon retraction of the hamstring muscles and a visible asymmetry. Conservative management of this injury leads to poor prognosis, so surgical repair is an alternative. Of the 12 patients, 7 returned to prior sports at a lower level, whereas the rest, all with complete disruptions, were limited in sports involving running or agility.

Acute groin injuries are also common in sports, especially in soccer.[25] The adductor longus is injured most commonly during hip abduction, leading to direct and indirect hernias. However, there is an abnormality in the lower abdominal wall musculature that can lead to vague, poorly localized pain in the groin. Players note that the pain is most noticeable during high-intensity, ballistic motions, as in kicking or sprinting. This is very unusual in recreational players and is most often seen in very high caliber athletes doing intense training and competition. "Athletic pubalgia" presents with pain and muscle-tendon injury in the inguinal area near the origination of the rectus abdominis to the pubis and in the adjacent internal oblique muscles near the region of abdominal wall weakness most often associated with direct inguinal hernias. This pain may exist in the absence of any evidence of herniation. When conservative measures fail, a herniorrhaphy procedure reinforcing the abdominal wall musculature can provide excellent relief.

These clinical investigations should be interpreted in light of the basic science studies. Imaging studies and direct observation show muscle disruption near the MTJ in predictable muscles. Disruption does not occur in the midsubstance of the muscle fibers. The muscle-tendon unit could also be injured within the tendon or at the tendon-bone junction. Eccentric activation was the common mechanism of injury, as the basic studies suggested.

PREVENTIVE STRATEGIES

CYCLIC STRETCHING

In the laboratory, studies on rabbits indicate that viscoelastic properties of muscle are responsible in part for great changes in muscle length and that this increased length can decrease strain in a muscle. On the field, a more pressing question is whether stretching, a commonly used method to prevent muscle strains, is effective. To study stretching in a controlled environment, repeated stretch-release cycles were applied to the rabbit model.[26] First, the force to failure of a hindlimb muscle had to be determined. Then the contralateral muscles were cyclically stretched to 50% or 70% of the force to failure. Ten cycles to 50% of failure force resulted in an increase in muscle length at failure with no change in the force at failure or energy absorbed. When muscles were cyclically stretched to 70% of failure force, macroscopic evidence of failure was seen even before the 10 cycles were completed. Thus, cyclic stretching appears to be beneficial because cyclic stretching leads to an increase in muscle length. Further, stretching that leads to forces exceeding 70% may make the muscle more, rather than less, likely for injury.

WARM-UP

Warm-up is considered to be protective against muscle strains, but the mechanism by which warm-up protects against muscle strains intrigued us. Viscoelasticity is known to be temperature dependent. Warm-up through prior activity was mimicked in the laboratory.[27] This method was different than simply using external heating. Rabbit hindlimb muscle was held isometrically and then stimulated tetanically for 10 to 15 seconds, leading a 1°C rise in muscle temperature. Following the repetitive stretch cycling, the muscle was able to stretch more prior to failure and was capable of more force production. Although the changes might be due to temperature elevation, the effects of stretch cannot be discounted despite the muscle being held isometrically. The constant length must allow

for some stretch of the muscle-tendon unit as the fibers contract and elastic components become stretched.

PRIOR INJURY

Previously strained muscle seems to be at risk of another injury. In the clinical setting, patients with a major muscle strain can usually describe a prior minor injury. This would suggest that after a minor injury, mechanical characteristics of the muscle altered. Such alterations might precipitate a more major injury. To test whether mechanical characteristics of muscle were different after a minor strain, investigators applied a nondisruptive strain to the extensor digitorum longus of rabbit by stretching the muscle just short of tissue rupture.[18] Contractile properties of the contralateral control muscle were used for comparison. Finally, failure load of the muscle was determined through passive stretch to failure at a rate of 10 cm/min. The peak tensile load and length at that load were derived for use on the experimental contralateral limb. The change of length to the peak load (of the control limb) was duplicated in the experimental muscle, just short of a disruptive injury. The injured muscle was then passively stretched to failure. Histology was performed on the minor injuries in a small sample of rabbits. The minor strain injury caused incomplete disruptions along the MTJ. In the experimental muscles, the peak load to rupture was 63% of control and the length at rupture was 79% of control. Isotonic shortening velocity was reduced by 51% for the 100 g weight and 6% for the 1000 g weight. Thus, it appeared that a minor injury made the muscle more susceptible to another injury because the muscle ruptured at a reduced load at a reduced length. Thus, return to activity prior to complete healing heightens the risk for a more major injury. In addition, although many patients with sports injuries do quite well with accelerated rehabilitation, early and aggressive rehabilitation may be too stressful for the muscle, thereby risking further injury. Injection for local pain relief while the muscle is still injured may not be appropriate because the lack of inhibition due to pain could result in excessive stress on the muscle, also increasing the risk of further injury.

FATIGUE

Clinical observations and the sports medicine literature suggest that muscle strain injuries occur late in either training sessions or competitive settings. This leads one to conclude that fatigue must play some role in the risk of muscle injury. Mair et al[28] fatigued the EDL of rabbits to 25% or 50% of the contralateral control force using cycles of 5-second isometric tetanic contractions followed by 1-second rest. The muscle was activated while being pulled (at 1, 10, or 50 cm/sec) to failure. Similar data were collected on the nonfatigued contralateral control muscle. The force at failure, length at failure, and energy absorbed prior to failure were determined. There was a trend toward a reduction in force for all groups (i.e., strain rates) tested, but the rate of strain did not influence force at failure. There was no change in muscle length at any of the strain rates; however, significantly less energy was absorbed in both fatigue conditions, with the greatest loss occurring in the most fatigued muscle. The slower the rate at which the muscle was stretched, the greater the energy that was absorbed. Muscles absorb energy while controlling and regulating limb movement. These data indicate that muscles were damaged at similar lengths regardless of fatigue. In contrast, fatigued muscle was unable to absorb energy prior to reaching the amount of stretch that causes injuries. Proper conditioning to delay fatigue is seen as a part of the rationale for the preventing muscle strain injury.

TREATMENT OF MUSCLE STRAIN INJURIES

The pain of a strain injury may prompt physicians to prescribe anti-inflammatory drugs in response to the inflammatory responses known to occur following an injury. Before routine use of anti-inflammatory drugs can be accepted in the treatment of muscle strain injuries, the effects of such medications on muscle recovering from an injury need to be evaluated. Obremskey et al[16] produced a strain injury of the tibialis anterior muscle in 50 rabbits (at a strain rate of 10 cm/min). The animals were subsequently administered piroxicam (16 mg/kg) within 6 hours plus 13 mg/kg every 6 hours. Piroxicam is an anti-inflammatory agent that inhibits the biosynthesis of prostaglandins, which are known mediators of inflammation. Forty control rabbits received no medications. Contractile properties and histology were determined at 1, 2, 4, or 7 days after the injury. On day 1, there was a significantly greater contractile force in the treated animals; however, there was no difference between the treated and untreated animals on days 2, 4, or 7. The animals treated with piroxicam showed a delay in the repair process as determined histologically. The muscles of treated rabbits showed delayed inflammatory cell infiltration, necrosis, myotube regeneration, and collagen deposition. Based on these findings, nonsteroidal anti-inflammatory drugs may be of some benefit for the early treatment of pain control and functional improvement. However, the delay in the repair process seen histologically raises concern regarding their use for long-term treatment.

CONCLUSION

Of the musculoskeletal injuries seen in the office of the practicing physician, muscle strain is one of the most common. Until recently, few data were available about the basic science of muscle strain, the clinical application of this basic science, and the treatment and prevention of muscle strain injuries.

Findings from the laboratory show that certain muscles are susceptible to strain injury (muscles that cross multiple joints or have complex architecture). There is a strain threshold for both passive and active injury. Strain injury is not solely the result of muscle contraction. Rather, strains result from excess stretch or stretch during muscle activation. When the muscle tears, the damage is consistently near the MTJ. After an injury, the muscle is weak and is at risk for further injury. The tension output of the injured muscle returns over the following days as the muscle undergoes predictable progression toward tissue healing.

In the clinic, current imaging methods have been used to confirm the site of injury as the MTJ. The commonly injured muscles include the hamstrings, the rectus femoris, the gastrocnemius, and the adductor longus. Injuries whose clinical presentation was inconsistent with involvement of a single MTJ proved to be at tendinous origins that extended well into the belly of the muscle rather than within the muscle belly itself. There are some unique injuries with a poor prognosis that are potentially repairable surgically. These include injuries to the rectus femoris, to the origin of the hamstrings, and in the abdominal wall.

We have reviewed the literature on the proper management of common muscle injuries and the risks of reinjury. Nonsteroidal anti-inflammatory drugs may have some place early in pain management but show potential for long-term risks in delaying healing of the muscle.

Prevention of injuries is an important obligation of the primary care and sports medicine physician. Data demonstrate the beneficial effects of warm-up, elevated temperature, and stretching on the mechanical properties of muscle. These benefits show that the risk of strain injury to skeletal muscle can be reduced with proper preventative measures. It is good that many of the factors protecting muscle such as strength, endurance, and flexibility are also essential for maximum performance, so physical training in preparation for athletic performance helps to reduce the risk of strain injury. Future research directions should attempt to delineate the repair and recovery process, emphasizing not only recovery of muscle function, but also the susceptibility to reinjury in the recovery phase.

ACKNOWLEDGMENTS

A research agenda as expansive as this requires the assistance of many able colleagues. This direction of research was made possible by the valuable contributions of outstanding collaborators: Louie Almekinders, Frank Bassett, Tom Best, James Dalton, Rich Glisson, Leonard Goldner, Carl Hasselman, Chad Hughes, John Lohnes, Scott Mair, Pantelis Nickolaou, Tom Noonan, William Obremskey, Ross Rich, Marc Safran, Peter Sallay, Tony Seaber, Kevin Speer, and Dean Taylor.

REFERENCES

1. Krejci V, Koch P: Muscle and Tendon Injuries in Athletes. Chicago, Yearbook Medical Publishers, 1979.
2. Peterson L, Renstrom P: Sports Injuries: Their Prevention and Treatment. William E. Grana (ed). Chicago, Yearbook Medical Publishers, 1986.
3. Zarins B, Ciullo JV: Acute muscle and tendon injuries in athletes. Clin Sports Med 1983; 2:167.
4. Stauber WT: Eccentric action of muscles: Physiology, injury and adaptation. Exerc Sports Sci Rev 1989; 17:157.
5. Friden J, Lieber RL: Structural and mechanical basis of exercise-induced muscle injury. Med Sci Sports Exerc 1992; 24: 521.
6. Clarkson PM, Newham DJ: Associations between muscle soreness, damage, and fatigue. Adv Exp Med Biol 1995; 384: 457.

7. Howell JN, Chila AG, Ford G, et al: An electromyographic study of elbow motion during postexercise muscle soreness. J Appl Physiol 1985; 58:1713.

8. Sherman WM, Armstrong LE, Murray TM, et al: Effect of a 42.2-km footrace and subsequent rest or exercise on muscular strength and work capacity. J Appl Physiol 1984; 57:1668.

9. Garrett WE Jr: Muscle strain injuries: Clinical and basic aspects. Med Sci Sports Exerc 1990; 22:436.

10. Radin EL, Simon, SR, Rose RM, Paul IL: Practical Biomechanics for the Orthopaedic Surgeon. New York, Wiley Medical, 1979.

11. Glick JM: Muscle strains: Prevention and treatment. Phys Sports Med 1980; 8:73.

12. Elftman H: Biomechanics of muscle. J Bone Joint Surg Am 1966; 48:363.

13. Garrett WE Jr, Almekinders L, Seaver AV: Biomechanics of muscle tears and stretching injuries. Trans Orthop Res Soc 1984; 9:384.

14. Garrett WE Jr, Nikolaou PK, Ribbeck BM, et al: The effect of muscle architecture on the biomechanical failure properties of skeletal muscle under passive extension. Am J Sports Med 1988; 16:7.

15. Nikolaou PK, MacDonald BL, Glisson RR, et al: Biomechanical and histological evaluation of muscle after controlled strain injury. Am J Sports Med 1987; 15:9.

16. Obremskey WT, Seaber AV, Ribbeck BM, Garrett WE Jr: Biomechanical and histological assessment of a controlled muscle strain injury treated with piroxicam. Am J Sports Med 1994; 22:558.

17. Abbott BC, Lowy J: Stress relaxation in muscle. Proc R Soc Lond 1956; 146:281.

18. Taylor DC, Dalton JD, Seaber AV, Garrett WE Jr: Experimental muscle strain injury: Early functional and structural deficits and the increased risk for reinjury. Am J Sports Med 1993; 21:190.

19. Taylor DC, Seaber AV, Garrett WE: Response of muscle tendon units to cyclic repetitive stretching. Trans Orthop Res Soc 1985; 10:84.

20. Garrett WE Jr, Rich FR, Nikolaou PK, Vogler JB III: Computed tomography of hamstring muscle strains. Med Sci Sports Exer 1989; 21:506.

21. Speer KP, Lohnes J, Garrett WE Jr: Radiographic imaging of muscle strain injury. Am J Sports Med 1993; 21:89.

22. Hughes C, Hasselman CT, Best TM, et al: Incomplete, intrasubstance strain injuries

of the rectus femoris. Am J Sports Med 1995; 23:500.

23. Hasselman CT, Best TM, Hughes C, et al: An explanation for various rectus femoris strain injuries using previously undescribed muscle architecture. Am J Sports Med 1995; 23:493.

24. Sallay PI, Friedman RL, Coogan PG, Garrett WE Jr: Hamstring injuries among water skiers: Functional outcome and prevention. Am J Sports Med 1996; 24:130.

25. Taylor DC, Meyers WC, Moylan JA, et al: Abdominal musculature abnormalities as a cause of groin pain in athletes: Inguinal hernias and pubalgia. Am J Sports Med 1991; 19:239.

26. Taylor DC, Dalton JD Jr, Seaber AV, Garrett WE Jr: Viscoelastic properties of muscle-tendon units: The biomechanical effects of stretching. Am J Sports Med 1990; 18:300.

27. Safron MR, Garrett WE Jr, Seaber AV, et al: The role of warm-up in musclular injury prevention. Am J Sports Med 1988; 16:123.

28. Mair SD, Seaber AV, Glisson RR, Garrett WE Jr: The role of fatigue in susceptibility to acute muscle strain injury. Am J Sports Med 1996; 24:137.

section 4 chapter 5

OVERUSE INJURIES

Delmas J. Bolin and David A. Stone

Summary
- Among the many causes of overuse injuries, probably the most prominent is "transition," a change in mode or use of a particular part of the body.
- The only accepted treatment for chronic exertional compartment syndrome is surgical release.
- Tendon overuse injuries are common; rehabilitation programs can manage pain and restore strength and flexibility.
- Patellofemoral pain is also best treated with rehabilitation programs; bracing may be a useful adjuvant therapy.
- The most common sites for stress fractures are the tibia, the metatarsals, and the fibula.

INTRODUCTION

As the importance of regular aerobic exercise throughout life has become more obvious to the medical and sports medicine communities, the number of people who begin exercise programs or alter them to accommodate such disease states as diabetes, hypertension, and osteoarthritis will increase. These people, as well as the many athletes at all levels of sports aggressively training to improve athletic performances, are all at risk for overuse injuries. The exact

incidence of overuse injuries in sport is not known. Herring and Nilson[1] estimated that approximately 30% to 50% of all sports injuries were due to overuse, but that estimate does not take into account the sports-specific nature of many overuse injuries or the level of play. For example, Priest et al[2] noted a 47% incidence rate of just lateral epicondylitis in recreational tennis players and a 45% incidence rate in professional players, but medial epicondylitis was thought to be more common in high-level players because of the service and forehand motions. The Bureau of Labor Statistics[3] indicates that chronic injuries account for 48% of reported occupational illnesses.

Risk factors for overuse injuries are generally divided into two categories. Intrinsic factors include age, flexibility, strength, alignment of the limb, and previous injury. Extrinsic factors include aspects of the sport (such as biomechanical factors, equipment, field conditions, practice, and game schedules) and demands of the sport. Determining which of these risk factors is important in establishing a treatment program but, as noted by Meeuwisse,[4] often extremely difficult. The tendency to "shotgun" treatment in overuse injuries—by treating as many risk factors as possible as quickly as possible—is tempting, especially when an athlete is in the middle of training and the injury disrupts a training schedule. However, both practitioner and athlete may be confused about what treatment works best.

Of all these risk factors, perhaps the most controversial

are limb alignment and aging. Limb alignment has often been addressed in case control and retrospective studies, but large randomized studies are lacking. Wen et al[5] prospectively evaluated a small group of runners training for a marathon and could not demonstrate a correlation with lower extremity alignment and injury. They noted that static measurements do not correlate with dynamic loading of the lower extremity.

Aging appears to be an important risk factor with significant implications in overuse injuries. Both maximal running and swimming velocities for sprint and endurance events decline from the 3rd to the 8th decades. The decline parallels the decrease in muscle mass, generally quoted as about 7% per decade.[6] Not all muscles atrophy at the same rate, and physical activity is believed to affect this process. Remodeling of motor units also occurs with aging. This process appears to selectively affect type II muscle fibers, resulting in aggregates of type I fibers.[7]

One of the important principles in overuse injuries is "transition." As noted by Leadbetter,[8] "the principle of transition states that sports injury is most likely to occur when the athlete experiences any change in mode or use of the involved part." The transition concept states that tissue homeostasis is disrupted, resulting in the breakdown of cell matrix with an inadequate healing response. The affected structure fails to adapt to the insult and, over time, is more susceptible to injury. The onset of pain may occur at the time of the injury or later, depending on the severity of the insult. The theory of transition implies that a well-designed training program will allow recovery from intense training sessions and maintain tissue homeostasis and, at the same time, provide a stimulus for muscle growth, allow skill acquisition, and improve aerobic and anaerobic performance. It also implies that a rehabilitation program to treat an overuse injury should address these performance parameters in order to prevent reinjury or injury secondary to deconditioning.

CHRONIC EXERTIONAL COMPARTMENT SYNDROME

Chronic exertional compartment syndrome (CECS) is a poorly understood condition; it is characterized by pain brought on by exercise. The most common location is the lower leg, but any compartment can, in theory, be involved. In comparison with acute compartment syndromes, the cause remains unknown. Theories about the cause of CECS include Martens' and Meyersoons'[9] belief that a noncompliant fascia produces a stiff compartment that does not accommodate the increase in blood volume and the muscle volume that occurs with exercise. In support of this theory, Detmer et al[10] demonstrated increased fascial thickness in 25 of 36 fascial biopsies in patients with CECS. Qvarfordt et al[11] measured muscle blood flow during exercise by the xenon 133 clearance technique and found it was decreased. Other theories have included arterial[12] or venous[13] obstruction and elevated intramuscular pressure resulting in capillary occlusions and increased interstitial fluid secondary to increased hyperosmolarity.[14]

Clinically, the symptoms of CECS are pain—achy, sharp, or dull—cramping, swelling, weakness, and numbness or paresthesias. Symptoms increase with exercise and

resolve or reduce with rest. Although earlier studies produced a distinct male predilection, more recent studies have not confirmed this finding. Rampersaud and Amendola[14] believe that younger age (<30 years) and sport activity that involves repetitive stress or running have a high predictive value. The physical examination results may be normal or may demonstrate some stiffness and discomfort over the affected compartments. Although Varelas et al[15] were able to demonstrate lower peak torque and relative peak torque in patients with CECS as compared with control patients, several authors[10, 16] have commented on the lack of physical examination findings. After exercise, the examination may demonstrate substantial weakness and, occasionally, sensory changes. The presence of muscle herniation is noted 20% to 60% of the time.[14]

The lack of physical examination findings to confirm a suspected diagnosis results in the need for a confirmatory test. Before testing, conflicting diagnoses should be ruled out. The differential diagnosis of CECS is complex and is listed in Table 1. The authors usually recommend a trial of stretching and strengthening exercises to resolve strength deficits if present and, in some cases, to recommend a period of rest, usually 2 to 3 weeks, followed by a return to sports. If patients remain symptomatic, testing is arranged. Our present testing protocol is to use a slit catheter to measure pressures (Fig. 1). This allows us to obtain pre- and postexercise pressures. Moed[17] studied the difference among slit catheters, side-ported needles, and simple needles and demonstrated that use of a simple 18-gauge needle was not as accurate as use of a side-ported needle or the slit catheter, with the 18-gauge needle yielding consistently high pressures. We generally use a treadmill for exercise tests, although some studies have used isokinetic exercise[18] or hopping.[19] Whereas varying criteria exist to define positive test results, we prefer the criteria of Pedowitz,[16] which includes an evaluation of resting and postexercise pressures. Various authors[11, 20] have used other criteria, and the specific definition of abnormal pressure is subject to debate. We have had no complications performing deep compartment pressure tests using blind catheter placement.

Currently, there are no clear alternatives to compartment pressure testing. Amendola et al[21] performed a double-blind prospective study to assess the usefulness of magnetic resonance imaging (MRI) in the diagnosis of CECS. They used

---

TABLE 1. DIFFERENTIAL DIAGNOSIS OF COMPARTMENT SYNDROME

Muscle strain
Periostitis
Stress fracture of tibia
Stress fracture of fibula
Peroneal nerve neurapraxia
Popliteal artery entrapment
Posterior tibial tendinitis
Medial tibial stress syndrome
Deep vein thrombosis
Spinal stenosis
Lumbar herniated nucleus pulposis
Diabetic peripheral neuropathy
Peripheral vascular disease

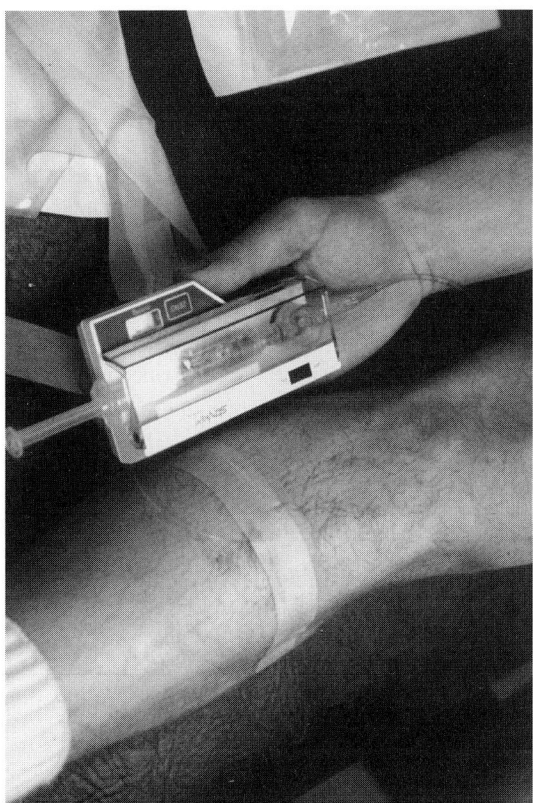

Fig. 1. Determining compartment pressures. This photograph shows a hand-held pressure catheter.

a radiopharmaceutical that is taken up by muscle: methoxy-isobutyl-isonitrile. Of the five patients who had abnormal pressures, four had an abnormal MRI, with abnormal T_1 remaining abnormal. Amendola believed the value of MRI was not clear and, therefore, not indicated. Hayes et al[22] used thallium-201 to demonstrate reversible compartment ischemia. They obtained pressure measurements in eight of the patients studied. Pressure measurements were elevated in four patients, borderline in three, and normal in one. All patients with elevated compartment pressures had positive thallium scan results. For the three patients who were borderline, reversible compartment ischemia was found. As preliminary data, Hayes et al believed thallium testing was encouraging. Mohler et al[23] used near-infrared spectroscopy to diagnose CECS. They found that patients who had CECS of the anterior compartment of the leg had greater relative deoxygenation during exercise as well as delayed reoxygenation after exercise, suggesting that ischemia plays an important role in the pathophysiology of CECS. They did not think they could develop diagnostic criteria because the values obtained were not absolute values of oxygenation; they were encouraged that near-infrared spectroscopy might be useful as a noninvasive diagnostic tool.

Currently, the only accepted treatment of CECS is surgical release. Christensen et al[24] used the diuretic bendroflumethiazide 5 mg daily for 2 to 3 weeks in five middle-aged men and demonstrated a decrease in compartment pressures, as well as symptoms. A larger follow-up study was not performed, and diuretics are not routinely used.

Results of surgical release are varied and limited to some degree because some studies report only on the anterior compartment, and different criteria for a positive test are used. Reneman,[25] for example, limited his study to patients with symptoms in the anterior or lateral compartments. He used a weighted exercise to induce pressure elevations, and his definition of a positive test was a pressure exceeding 15 cm H_2O above the baseline pressure at 6 minutes after exercise. The results of the study were remarkable, with 36 out of 40 patients returning to activities they had been unable to perform before the operation. Three patients were lost to follow-up. Schepsis et al[26] compared results of fasciotomy in patients with anterior compartment release with those of patients with deep posterior compartment release. The groups were not homogeneous in that patients with deep compartment symptoms had been symptomatic for a substantially longer time (16 months versus 6.8 months), and there was a higher percentage of women with deep compartment symptoms (37.5% with anterior compartment symptoms versus 58% with deep compartment symptoms). Exercise tests were performed with an isokinetic exercise machine. Results for the anterior compartment were also excellent, with 96% reporting full unlimited activity at 4.2 years. However, for the patients with deep posterior compartment involvement, results were only 65% good or excellent, with 35% of patients reporting only fair or poor results. Similar results were also obtained by Wallensten,[27] in that only five of nine patients with deep compartment releases had excellent results. All of Wallensten's patients reported improvement. Micheli et al[28] reported on the results of compartment release in 47 young female athletes and noted a lower success rate than studies combining men and women. When the anterior compartment alone was released, the success rate was 89%. However, when other procedures were performed, the success rate was only 76%. Micheli et al noted that time elapsed from onset of symptoms to surgery correlated significantly with outcome, but they did not provide a specific period when results deteriorated.

Failure of compartment release can be multifactorial. As noted by Schepsis et al,[26] catheter placement is critical. Because the soleus bridge overlies the deep posterior compartment proximally, the placement of the catheter should be in the distal third of the compartment. At the time of testing, compression of the superficial posterior compartment will alter pressure readings if the catheter is placed incorrectly, and confirmation of catheter placement is important in all tests. Wiley et al[19] recommended use of ultrasound to provide continuous monitoring of catheter placement, although at present the authors of this chapter have no experience with this technique. Finally, some researchers believe there are as many as seven separate compartments in the lower leg[10]; others[18, 26] test only four, and still others believe the tibialis posterior has its own compartment.[22] Detmer[29] noted a 2% to 10% recurrence rate, with recurrences occurring either early (within 2 months of surgery) or later (up to 2 years after surgery). He believed that a symptom-free interval was an indication that repeat and/or more complete fasciotomy would yield a good result. Because nerve and muscle injury can occur with CECS, a search for these conditions is an important part of postoperative management.

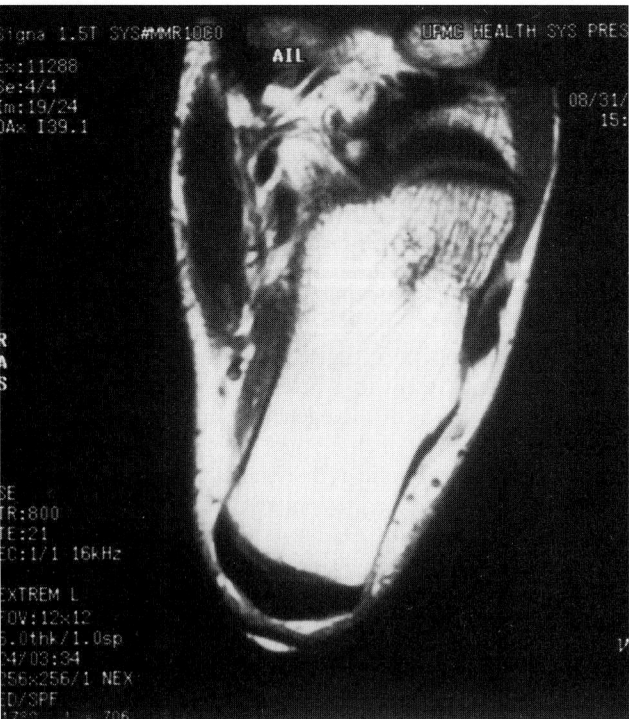

Fig. 2. MRI of Achilles tendon. This MRI demonstrates tendonosis with focal thickening of tendon.

TENDON OVERUSE INJURIES

Overuse injuries of tendons are common. James et al[30] found that approximately 30% of all running injuries were chronic tendon problems. Kannus et al[31] noted a high incidence rate of rotator cuff and Achilles tendon problems in older athletes (Fig. 2). Currently, the cause of these tendon injuries is unknown. Clement et al[32] theorized that tendon injuries were caused by microtrauma produced by eccentric loading of tendon by fatigued muscle, vascular blanching related to limb position, or excess loading of tendon due to limb position. Kraus-Hansen et al[33] performed preliminary work on horse tendons in support of a vascular origin for overuse tendon injury.

Many recent authors have noted that the nomenclature for tendon injuries is confusing and does not reflect the pathologic features of the tendon injury.[34–37] These authors found that an inflammatory response is rarely seen in overuse tendon injuries unless a partial tear is present. Alfredson et al[38] used a microdialysis technique and confirmed that there were no signs of inflammation in the tendons they studied. Thus, the term "tendinitis," although often used, is inaccurate. Tendon disease in cases of intractable overuse injuries is variable with multiple histologic findings, including myxoid degeneration, fibrocartilaginous metaplasia, calcification, hyaline degeneration, and fatty degeneration. In these tendons, the normal type I collagen is replaced by type II or type III collagen resulting in a tissue with altered loading characteristics.[39] Unfortunately, tendon pathology studies represent the findings of those cases that come to surgery, not the cases that resolve with nonsurgical management. In the latter cases, tissue specimens are unavailable. Stone et al[40] found that histology does not correlate with biomechanical properties in a rabbit model of tendon injury.

Currently, the pathologic factors of chronic tendon overuse injuries are not clear. Whereas Fritschy and de Gautard[41] proposed that indications for surgery be based on the presence of morphologic changes seen on imaging studies, Cook et al[42] demonstrated that hypoechoic areas were present in the tendons of elite athletes but were not always symptomatic; in the same study, they were rarely present in control subjects. Khan et al[43] prospectively evaluated patella tendons undergoing surgery and found that neither ultrasonography nor MRI predicted a poor from a good clinical result. Treatment has therefore focused on management of pain and empiric restoration of strength and flexibility patterns of the muscle affecting the injured tendon. Curwin and Stanish[44] initially described eccentric exercise programs for the management of tendinitis. However, rehabilitation programs treating chronic tendon pain are generally successful even without the emphasis on eccentric exercise. Ferretti et al[36] operated on only 18 knees of 150 athletes in their study of patellar tendon histology. Martens et al[35] performed surgery on only 16 of 102 knees in their study. In studies on Achilles tendon pain, Clement et al[32] reported 85 good or excellent results in 109 runners on nonsurgical management. The principles of management in the treatment of overuse tendon injuries have consisted largely of minimizing atrophy by avoiding immobilization and gently progressing a therapeutic exercise program to prevent atrophy and restore strength and flexibility patterns.

Within this framework, specificity of training, maximizing loading, and progression of loading of the tendon are all considered cornerstones of successful treatment.[45] Emphasis on modalities such as heat, ice, ultrasound, and electrical stimulation is not considered important, although they may, in some cases, improve symptoms. Education regarding intrinsic and extrinsic risk factors should be addressed during treatment, and decisions regarding treatment should be based on patient response. Controversy regarding when an athlete has failed rehabilitation and should be considered for surgery is difficult to assess. In a small study, Alfredson et al[46] compared the results of an eccentric rehabilitation program with those of a standard rehabilitation program in older (mean age 44.3 years) patients with long-standing Achilles tendon pain (18.3 months) and found excellent short-term results within a 3-month period. Patients were pushed to perform exercises despite pain and at a slow pace. Follow-up of these patients at 2 years indicated a long-term benefit.[47]

Medical management of tendon overuse is also controversial. Because these conditions are rarely inflammatory, use of nonsteroidal anti-inflammatory medications are not clearly indicated, but they are often used. We recommend they be used for pain control along with acetaminophen. Injection or use of oral steroids is more controversial. Although guidelines for steroid injection in sports have been published,[48] data supporting these guidelines are minimal.

PATELLOFEMORAL PAIN SYNDROME

Patellofemoral pain syndrome is a common source of anterior knee pain frequently associated with overuse. In a survey of runners, Clement et al[49] found patellofemoral problems to be the most common injury. Both Fairbank et al[50] and Thomee et al[51] noted an associated increase in activity in patients suffering from patellofemoral pain. However, not all studies on patellofemoral pain clearly list overuse as the primary cause. Insall et al[52] stated that patella-tracking abnormalities could produce pain in the absence of instability, and several authors have emphasized the relationship of malalignment with patellofemoral pain.[53, 54] As with other overuse conditions, the cause of pain in patellofemoral problems is unclear in many patients. Fulkerson[55] has shown that lateral retinaculum tenderness is common in patients with patellofemoral pain and that in biopsy specimens of patients with malalignment of the patellofemoral joint, injury to small nerve fibers in the retinaculum is present.[56] Other theories on the cause of pain in the patellofemoral joint refer to subchondral bone of the patella,[57] synovitis or synovial irritation,[58] and maldistribution of compressive contact loads.[59]

The clinical features of patellofemoral pain are generally described as dull, aching anterior knee pain provoked by physical activity. Symptoms are also provoked by sitting with the knee in a flexed position for a long time (theatergoers' sign) and by squatting. Crepitus is generally noted and can be audible. Giving way is also noted, but it can be distinguished from the giving way of meniscal and ligamentous injuries if it is associated with ascending or descending stairs, as compared with turning movements.[59] Swelling is not a common physical examination finding, but a mild effusion may be transiently present when significant malalignment is present.

Physical examination findings are considered extremely important. Symptoms are often reproduced by flexing the knee slightly to ensure articular contact and moving the patella proximally and distally. The retinaculum should be examined completely; maneuvers to tilt the patella medially and laterally to palpate peripatellar retinaculum should be included.[60] Displacement of the patella laterally demonstrates tightness of the lateral retinacular structures and apprehension in cases of lateral instability. Desio et al[61] studied the soft-tissue restraints of the patella and found that the medial patellofemoral ligament was the primary restraint to lateral patellar translation, contributing 60% of the restraining force. However, a surprising finding of their study was the contribution of the lateral retinaculum, which was found to be a small but significant restraint to lateral patellar translation. The patella should be observed throughout the entire range of motion of the knee, beginning with the knee in 90 degrees of flexion looking at exit from and reentry into the trochlear sulcus. The Q angle should be measured with the quadriceps relaxed and the patella localized in the trochlea. The orientation of the patellar tendon with the knee flexed 90 degrees should also be observed. The differential diagnosis of anterior knee pain is listed in Table 2.

In addition to the evaluation of the patellofemoral joint,

TABLE 2. DIFFERENTIAL DIAGNOSIS OF ANTERIOR KNEE PAIN
Patellofemoral pain syndrome
Bursitis
Patellar tendinitis
Osteochondritis dissecans of the femoral condyles
Meniscal injury
Sinding-Larsen-Johansson syndrome
Patellar fat-pad inflammation
Medial synovial plica syndrome
Inflammatory or degenerative arthritis
Tumors (e.g., osteoid osteoma)

an evaluation of strength and flexibility patterns around the knee should be performed. Muscle imbalances have long been considered an underlying source of patellofemoral pain, and management of patellofemoral disorders almost always begins with a rehabilitation program. Whereas some authors have found decreases in eccentric quadriceps strength,[57, 62, 63] others have found abnormal activation of the vastus medialis obliquus (VMO) and the vastus lateralis (VL).[64] These findings are not universal in all studies.[65, 66] It is not clear if such activation is a cause or an effect of patellofemoral pain, as pain has been shown to have an inhibitory effect on the quadriceps.[67] Anatomic evidence that the VMO partly originates from the adductor muscles[68] and studies of the nerve supply to the VMO demonstrating a branch of the saphenous nerve could stimulate VMO contraction[69] have altered the basic approach to patellofemoral rehabilitation. Hodges and Richardson[70] were able to demonstrate a greater VMO:VL ratio with weightbearing exercises when adductor activity was added to the exercise. Currently, clinical outcome data demonstrating superior outcomes with this type of exercise is lacking. Hamstring, gastrocnemius, soleus, and iliotibial band stretching may also contribute to altered patellofemoral loading patterns and should be considered part of the rehabilitation prescription.

Radiographs can be helpful in diagnosing patellofemoral pain. A 45-degree weightbearing film is useful in assessing joint space and eliminating tumors and inflammatory or degenerative changes as possible contributors. Patellar positioning (alta, baja) and length of the trochlear groove can be assessed by lateral film. A Merchant view demonstrates patellar forms, positioning, and topography of the trochlear notch (Fig. 3). MRI and computed tomography are usually not necessary unless ligamentous, meniscal, or chondral injuries are suspected.

Rehabilitation of patellofemoral pain has an excellent prognosis. Insall[71] noted that the effect of rehabilitation was "unquestionable," and Tria et al[72] described a 95% success rate for nonsurgical management. However, many questions about optimal management exist. McConnell[73] described patella taping to reduce pain in the management of patellofemoral pain, and Werner et al[74] demonstrated an improvement in quadriceps torque with taping. However, several studies[75–77] performed without tape also demonstrated a high rate of recovery, with complete return to sports. These studies also used a wide variety of quadri-

Fig. 3. Axial radiograph of patella at 45 degrees flexion. This demonstrates tilt and subluxation.

ceps exercise techniques, making the type of quadriceps exercise performed appear less important than other factors, such as the range of motion the exercise was performed through, the intensity and frequency of the exercises, and management of pain. Studies on various types of quadriceps exercise have focused predominantly on quadriceps activation patterns; very few studies have compared outcomes on patellofemoral pain.[78] At present, quadriceps exercises include isometrics, straight-leg-raising exercises, open chain (foot is free to move and does not contact the floor or exercise device; e.g., knee extensions) exercises, and closed chain (foot is fixed to ground; e.g., squat or leg-press exercises). Steinkamp et al[78a] used a mathematical model to estimate patellofemoral joint loading and found that forces on the patellofemoral joint increase as one goes deeper into a squat, whereas joint stress increases in open chain exercises as one goes from 90 degrees of flexion to full extension. Long-term outcomes on the treatment of patellofemoral pain are lacking, but intermediate outcome has been good. Jensen and Albrektsen[79] noted over 80% of patients treated without surgery for patellofemoral pain without malalignment had mild or no pain at a 12 year follow-up.

Taping and bracing has been recommended as an adjuvant treatment for patellofemoral pain. McConnell[73] introduced taping to control patellar motion and pain during exercise. Although taping is used widely, there is little clear data on the effectiveness of the treatment or its purported mechanism of action. The study itself was limited by the absence of a control group. Bockrath et al[80] found a 50% reduction in subjective anterior knee pain symptoms during a 0.2-m step-down exercise when McConnell taping was applied. They noted no difference in patellar motion or positioning. In contrast, Larsen et al[81] found that McConnell taping altered initial positioning of the patella but did not alter its motion during exercise. Long-term outcome data are lacking.

A variety of knee sleeves and braces have been recommended. The design varies from the simple patellar cutout to more elaborate braces with counterbalancing straps. Finestone et al[82] prospectively studied the use of knee sleeves in military recruits with anterior knee pain. A simple knee sleeve offered a nonsignificant decrease in symptoms when compared with more elaborate knee braces, but neither treatment group result was superior to that of the no-brace group. BenGal et al[83] demonstrated that prophylactic knee bracing diminished the development of anterior knee pain in a randomized group of athletes in a strenuous exercise protocol. Knee bracing does not protect against knee injury.[84] Data to date do not clearly define the role of knee bracing. It should be considered adjuvant therapy, not to be substituted for an appropriate rehabilitation program.

STRESS FRACTURES

Stress or "march" fractures were first described in Prussian Army recruits by Breithaupt in 1855.[85] However, the topic received little attention in the orthopaedic literature until the development of the technetium bone scan in the early 1970s.[86] As the popularity of running for personal fitness surged, the diagnosis became more common and led to refocused attention on the problem of fatigue fractures. Stress fractures are now considered the ultimate overuse injury; they affect the physically active, particularly military recruits; track and field athletes; and ballet dancers. In the following sections, the epidemiology, pathophysiology, risk factors, and evaluation and management of common stress fractures are reviewed.

DEFINITION AND RISK FACTORS

A stress fracture results when bone fails to withstand repeated rhythmic subthreshold stress.[87] Numerous theories have been advanced to explain the origin of stress fractures. The earliest model suggests that repetitive stress causes an imbalance in bone remodeling in which periosteal resorption occurs faster than bone formation, leading to weakened cortex that fails under stress.[88] Repetitive strains are necessary for the development of strong bones and are associated with adaptive increases in bone mass.[89] However, a threshold exists above which more repetitive stress leads to the development of microscopic cracks and decreased bone strength.[90] If microscopically damaged bone is continually loaded repetitively, the damage propagates, overwhelming bone remodeling, resulting in a frank stress fracture.

Certain characteristics of bone may predispose to stress fractures. The ability of bone to withstand fracture is dependent on the density of the bone, with higher-density bones being more resistant.[91] The size of bone is also an important risk factor. In a prospective study of 600 military recruits undergoing 12 weeks of basic training, recruits who developed tibial stress fractures had significantly smaller tibial widths and cross-sectional areas.[92] There is evidence to suggest that smaller bone is an important risk factor in athletes. A cross-sectional study of 46 runners, examining the relationship between tibial cross-sectional area and stress fracture, found those with a history of stress fracture had smaller tibial cross-sections than those runners without a history of stress fracture.[93]

In addition to the characteristics of bone, muscle plays an important but often overlooked role in development of stress fractures. Muscle contraction plays a protective role in attenuating ground reactive forces developed at impact during running and jumping. Increased bone strain has been associated with muscle fatigue.[94] Specific manual muscle testing should be performed to identify weakness. Rehabilitation with focus on increasing muscle strength and endurance may be helpful in preventing recurrence but is underutilized in the evaluation and management of stress fractures. More study is needed to define the contribution of muscle fatigue, and there is currently no definitive support for a relationship between stress fracture and muscle size or flexibility.[95] There is, however, evidence to support the role of general fitness in protecting against stress fractures. A study of military recruits found that recruits who had higher weekly levels of activity before enlistment had a significantly lower incidence of stress fracture during basic training than those that did not exercise.[96]

Numerous studies have examined the relationship between stress fractures and intrinsic properties of the patients, such as biomechanics, alignment, and foot structure. The relationship of alignment and stress fractures remains controversial. Genu valgum, genu varum, and tibial torsion have not been associated with increased risk of stress fracture. One study demonstrated 5.4 times increased relative risk of stress fracture in male recruits with a Q angle greater than 15 degrees.[97] Other research failed to demonstrate a relationship between Q angle and stress fracture.[98]

There may be a relationship between foot type and stress fracture. The type of arch is an important determinant of how much ground reactive force is transferred to bone during impact. The high arched (pes cavus) foot is more rigid and therefore transfers more force to the tibia and fibula. By contrast, the flat foot (pes planus) is better able to absorb shock but is associated with prolonged pronation and may promote increased muscle fatigue.[95] In a prospective cohort study examining the relationship between foot type and stress fracture, the group with high arches had four times the incidence of stress fractures compared with the low-arch group.[99] The relative protection may depend on type of fracture. Tibial and fibular stress fractures were more prevalent in higher-arched feet, whereas metatarsal stress fractures were more prevalent in lower-arched feet.[100]

Leg length differences seem to be associated with increased risk of stress fracture. In a case series of 130 stress fractures in military recruits, Freiberg found 73% of tibial, metatarsal, and femoral stress fractures were associated with the longer leg, and 60% of fibular stress fractures were associated with the shorter leg. Although no statistical analysis was done, there was an interesting trend reported

of increasing incidence associated with greater degree of leg length discrepancy.[101]

There are several external factors, such as shoe type and training surface, that are commonly thought to contribute to stress fracture. Both are thought to play a role in determining the ground reactive force, which is transmitted to the body during impact. Running surface properties include its structure and compliance. Cambered track surfaces may unmask underlying anatomic or biomechanical problems. Hard surfaces increase ground reactive forces; soft surfaces require greater muscle activity and may lead to early fatigue. No studies have looked at stress fractures and running surface specifically, but a large epidemiological study failed to detect a contribution of running surface independent of training time.[102]

Running shoes function to cushion the foot during impact. In obtaining a detailed history from a runner, it is important to know the age and mileage of the running shoes. Older shoes do not cushion as well, and a higher rate of stress fracture has been reported in military recruits wearing older running shoes.[103]

In addition, training errors can be an important contribution. In one series, more than 60% of stress injuries were attributable to training errors.[104] Common errors include increasing training by more than 30% over a single season, recent changes in training terrain, and running in worn shoes. Freshman runners experienced nearly two-thirds of the stress injuries in the above study[104] and should be considered at risk because of unrealistic expectations of their training capacity. Proper education and vigilance may help protect this high-risk group.

Female athletes have unique risk factors that should be addressed in the management of any stress injury. Abnormal menstruation is common in female athletes who train at high intensity. More than 50% of athletes involved in ballet, gymnastics, and distance running reported irregular menses.[105] It is now well established that irregular menses are associated with higher risk of stress fracture.[95] Two prospective studies failed to demonstrate a protective effect of oral contraceptive pills (OCP) on stress fracture,[98, 106] but runners using OCP for more than 1 year had significantly fewer stress fractures than nonusers.[107] Regulating menstruation with OCP is probably reasonable adjuvant treatment.

SITE SPECIFICITY

Stress fractures develop at sites that are mechanically loaded repetitively during a particular activity. The most common sites of stress fracture are in the lower extremity, but they have been reported in non-weightbearing sites including the pelvis, upper limbs, and ribs.[108] A number of studies have looked at the site distribution for stress factors. The literature has been reviewed[106] and shows wide variations in site specificity, but the most common sites are the tibia, metatarsals, and fibula (Fig. 4). Several factors seem to be important to distribution, including type and level of activity, age and gender of participants, and diagnostic algorithm.

The majority of site-specificity studies have been retrospective reviews. Prospective studies have appeared, which illustrates the importance of the type of activity on site distribution. A 1-year prospective study of competitive male and female athletes showed that stress fractures ac-

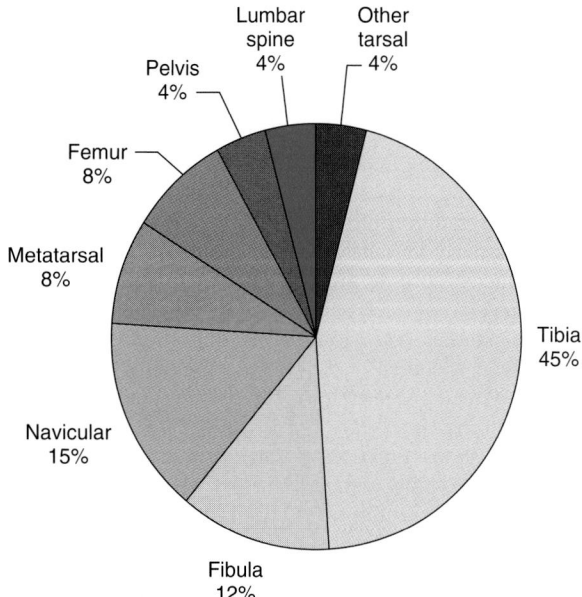

Fig. 4. Site distribution of stress fractures. This diagram is from a prospective study of runners. (Adapted from Bennell KL: The incidence and distribution of stress fractures in competitive track and field athletes: A 12-month prospective study. Am J Sports Med 1996; 24:211).

counted for 20% of the musculoskeletal injuries of the year.[110] Interestingly, there was no difference in the incidence of stress fracture by event, but those participating in sprints, hurdles, and jumps had a higher percentage of metatarsal stress fractures, and those who participated in distance events had higher percentages of tibia, fibula, femur, and pelvis stress fractures.

TIBIAL STRESS FRACTURES

Stress injuries of the tibia represent a difficult management problem in sports medicine. Tibial stress fractures are most commonly associated with runners.[111] As with other stress injuries, they are generally thought to exist as a continuum from stress injury (medial tibial stress syndrome, "shin splints") to frank fracture.[112] The difficulty lies in making an early diagnosis. Generally, most patients complain of insidious onset midtibial medial shin pain that comes on with exertion and that is better after rest. However, with continued training, the pain persists and can be present during daily activities. On examination, there is usually medial tibial pain on palpation. This is the most typical presentation and accounted for 75% of 465 cases of exertional leg pain in a sports medicine clinic.[113] It is important to distinguish this pain from anterior tibial pain. Anterior tibial stress fractures have a separate prognosis and are discussed below. The differential diagnosis includes exertional compartment syndrome, Ewing's sarcoma, osteoid osteoma, periostitis, and fascial herniation.[114] Saphenous nerve entrapment mimicking tibial stress fracture has also been reported.[115]

Radiographs are relatively insensitive. Radiographs will initially be negative in two-thirds of symptomatic patients; half of these will never show radiographic evidence of stress reaction.[116,116a] Oblique views of the tibia can be helpful in demonstrating a fracture line that is otherwise missed on anteroposterior and lateral films.[112] They are helpful in ruling out nonstress injuries and disorders. Bone scan is sensitive but not specific and has been used to diagnose the injury within 3 to 5 days on symptom onset. Negative bone scans have been reported in symptomatic military recruits who subsequently developed stress fractures.[117] Bone scans can remain positive as long as 2 years after a stress fracture, rendering them useless for following clinical course or investigating suspected reinjury.[118] MRI has been increasingly used for early diagnosis. The strength of MRI is its ability to view multiple planes and detect bone marrow edema, an early sign of bone stress often present before stress fracture lines become apparent.

A grading system based on bone scan[119] and MRI[104] is presented in Table 3. The authors used this system to guide treatment and rehabilitation for return to play.[104] Grade 1 injuries (shin splints) were treated with temporary cessation of impact activity, with return to running in 2 to 3 weeks. Grade 2 returned in 4 to 6 weeks. Grade 3 patients had pain with ambulation and did not return for 6 to 9 weeks. Most patients who had pain with exercise and daily activities had a grade 3 injury by MRI. Grade 4 injuries were casted for 6 weeks and then monitored with 6 weeks of nonimpact activity. Success of this rehabilitation regimen relative to other protocols was not reported.

Anterior tibial stress fractures are particularly frustrating injuries most commonly seen in runners and dancers.

TABLE 3. BONE SCAN COMPARED WITH MRI FOR GRADING TIBIAL STRESS INJURIES[1]		
Grade	Bone Scan	MRI
1	Small, ill-defined cortical area of mildly increased activity.	Periosteal edema: mild/moderate on T_2 images. Marrow: Normal on T_1/T_2 images.
2	Better-defined cortical area of moderately increased activity.	Periosteal edema: Moderate/severe on T_2 images. Marrow: edema on T_2 images.
3	Wide to fusiform, cortical-medullary area of highly increased activity.	Periosteal edema: Moderate/severe on T_2 images. Marrow: edema on T_1 and T_2 images.
4	Transcortical area of intensely increased activity.	Periosteal edema: Moderate/severe on T_2 images. Marrow: edema on T_1 and T_2 images. Fracture line clearly visible.

[1] Adapted from Fredericson M: Tibial stress reaction in runners: Correlation of clinical symptoms and scintigraphy with a new MRI grading system. Am J Sports Med 1995; 23:472

These injuries are prone to nonunion because the anterior tibia is under tension as a result of the imbalance of anterior and posterior muscle groups.[120] Our experience has been that these athletes often rush their return to training and so prolong their disability and increase the morbidity rate. Conservative treatments have the greatest chance of success when instituted early, but they are often prolonged and result in nonunion. Casting has been used with little success.[121] Surgical intervention with plate and bone grafting or intramedullary screw fixation may be necessary.[114]

FEMORAL STRESS FRACTURES

Stress injuries of the femur are important clinical problems because, in the absence of a clinician's high index of suspicion, they may be unrecognized, leading to delays in diagnosis and increased morbidity rates.[122] Early studies in military recruits suggested an overall incidence of femoral stress of 22.5%.[123] In athletes, the overall incidence rate is likely similar,[124] although it was previously reported between 2% and 7%.[109, 125]

As with tibial stress fractures, the femoral stress fracture site determines management and prognosis (see Fig. 4). The most common areas of stress fracture are the shaft, the intertrochanteric area, and the neck.[126] Fractures of the lateral neck are in tension and are prone to nonunion and displacement; compression side fractures usually heal. Femoral shaft stress fractures can become complete and displaced if the diagnosis is missed. These injuries can be career-ending for elite athletes.[122]

The typical history is usually vague thigh or groin pain. The diagnosis is typically delayed up to 6 weeks.[126] In a series of 54 military recruits with femoral neck stress fractures, nearly 90% complained of anterior groin pain. The onset in 40% was after a long march in the sixth to eighth week of basic training. On examination, the most frequent finding was pain on palpation of the inguinal area and pain at the extremes of internal and external rotation of the hip. Heel percussion reproduced symptoms in only three patients.[127] In femoral shaft stress fractures, the history is poorly localized thigh or knee pain.[128] Although there are usually few physical findings, the fulcrum test can be helpful in early diagnosis of femoral shaft stress fractures.[124] The hop test has also been reported as positive in 70% of femoral stress fractures.[126]

Radiographic work-up is similar to that of tibial stress fractures and includes radiographs and bone scan. Initial radiographs are often false-negative, and bone scan should be used early (Fig. 5). Femoral stress fractures with negative bone scans have been reported.[129]

Management depends on the site of the fracture and the time of diagnosis. Early diagnosis permits conservative management with athletes returning in 10 to 12 weeks.[126] Conservative treatment involves graduated return to activity after 14 days of being pain-free in daily activities. Exercise prescription should emphasize weightbearing activity modification, aerobic fitness, muscle strength, and proprioception. Nonimpact activities such as cycling, swimming, and running in water should be utilized.[126] Before return to impact activity, the muscles need appropriate rehabilitation to maximize endurance and strength for shock absorption. Conservative management protocols have also been published for compression-sided stress fractures of the femoral neck.[127] If displacement occurs, the incidence rate of complications—including avascular necrosis, nonunion, and varus deformity—is high. In cases of displacement or conservative treatment failures, surgical management with internal fixation may be necessary.[122, 128]

METATARSAL STRESS FRACTURES

Fractures of the metatarsals are seen frequently in dancers, gymnasts, and runners. Several structural characteristics of the foot may predispose to stress injury. As discussed above, there is a relationship between low-arch and metatarsal stress fractures.[100] During the gait cycle, the low-arched foot has prolonged pronation. Hyperpronation is associated with stress injury of the first metatarsal. In the same study, Simkin showed the use of orthotic support decreased the incidence of metatarsal stress fracture, presumably by a cushioning effect, decreasing the forces transmitted to the metatarsals. In studying metatarsal

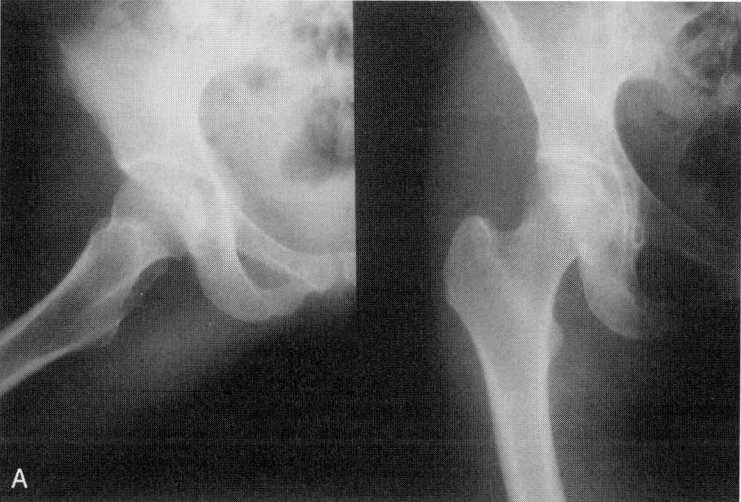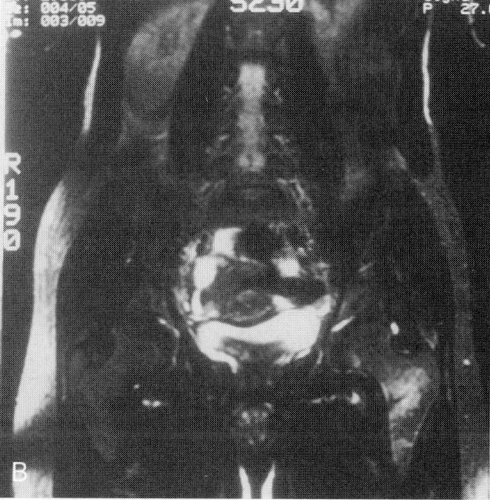

Fig. 5. Views. *A,* Radiograph of the hip demonstrating no evidence of stress fracture in a patient with groin pain. *B,* MRI of the same patient with obvious compression-sided stress fracture of the femur.

length, no relationship was noted between length of the first and second metatarsals and stress fracture incidence.[130] Motion of the metatarsals may contribute to their risk of stress injury. The second and third metatarsals are rigid, and the fourth and fifth have mobility. The fifth has limited motion in abduction and adduction. The relative fixed position of the second metatarsal exposes it to the greatest bending and shear forces during running, contributing to its higher incidence rate of stress fractures.[131] The blood supply of the fifth metatarsal can contribute to complications in stress injury. The proximal third of the fifth metatarsal is supplied by a single nutrient vessel that arises at the junction of the middle and proximal diaphysis. Stress fractures of the proximal diaphysis are therefore at risk for avascularity.[132]

Diagnosis is usually made by clinical history of vague forefoot pain in the absence of a history of trauma; pain increases with activity and decreases with rest. On physical examination, there may be global tenderness, but dorsal motion of the affected metatarsal may reproduce the pain.[133]

Usually, clinical suspicion alone is necessary to make the diagnosis. Judicious use of radiographs can be helpful. On plain radiograph, cortical hypertrophy is present at 2 weeks, with the fracture usually visible at 3 weeks. In cases of competitive athletes where rapid definitive diagnosis is sometimes required, the technetium bone scan is a sensitive but nonspecific way to confirm the diagnosis and may be positive as early as 24 hours after the onset of symptoms.[118]

First-metatarsal stress fractures constitute 10% of metatarsal stress fractures. Occasionally the diagnosis is delayed because, radiographically, one-third heal with minimal intramedullary callus.[134] Treatment is usually for 4 weeks, with the patient in a hard-soled shoe with limited weightbearing. During this time, the majority of the weight is borne on the heel. If the fracture is displaced dorsally, the foot is casted with dorsally applied pressure to prevent dorsal malunion and lateral metatarsalgia.[133]

Fractures of the middle metatarsals constitute 90% of metatarsal stress fractures. Treatment is typically rest or activity modification and 4 weeks in a hard-soled shoe or removable boot. The sole should be stiff to prevent motion (extension) of the metatarsals during the toe-off phase of gait. After cast removal, gentle stretching and nongravity pool exercises can be instituted for 2 weeks, with gradual return to activity including progression from biking to running.[133]

Fifth-metatarsal stress fractures are less common, and a careful history must be obtained to distinguish them from the "Jones fracture," which is an acute injury of the proximal fifth metatarsal. A high index of suspicion and aggressive early work-up is warranted for patients who have lateral foot pain. If the injury is detected as a stress reaction, nonoperative treatment with casting for 3 to 4 weeks may be successful in resolving symptoms and permitting the patient to return to play.

The description and management of stress fractures of the fifth metatarsal are determined by the location of the fracture. Fifth-metatarsal fractures have been described by zone.[135, 136] Zone 1 applies to avulsion fractures. Zone 2 describes fractures at the metaphyseal-diaphyseal junction,

which are always acute injuries. Zone 3 describes fractures of the proximal 1.5 cm of the shaft of the fifth metatarsal. The majority of zone 3 injuries are stress fractures, with patient history and radiographic changes consistent with repetitive injury. Of 237 fifth-metatarsal fractures seen in an office setting over 5 years, 3% were zone 3 fractures.[135] As with other stress fractures, more than 80% of zone 3 fractures are seen in athletes involved in running and jumping activity.[137]

Whereas fractures in zones 1 and 2 rarely fail to heal, zone 3 fractures are often associated with prolonged pain and nonunion. In one series, conservative treatment with elastic wrap and full weightbearing led to nonunion or refracture in 9 of 40 patients.[111] Successful treatment with strict non-weightbearing casting for 6 to 8 weeks has been reported.[139, 140] If conservative measures fail, surgical repair with intramedullary screw fixation[141] or bone grafting[142] has been reported. Screw fixation often leads to symptom resolution by 3 months.[143]

TARSAL NAVICULAR STRESS FRACTURES

Before 1970, tarsal navicular stress fractures in people were thought to be rare. In 1970, the first description of this injury appeared in the literature.[144] In the past 20 years, however, the diagnosis has been much more common. Unfortunately, the diagnosis is often delayed an average of 4 months because of vague symptoms.[145] Patients often present with insidious onset of forefoot pain. This pain is ill-defined, usually localized to the medial aspect of the midfoot or radiating to the first and second rays. It is usually worse with sprinting and jumping and resolves with rest. A history of the patient's activities should be taken. Athletes participating in track and field, football (including Australian rules, soccer, and rugby), and basketball were at highest risk of navicular stress fracture.[146] As with other stress fractures, changes in training regimen may lead to symptoms.[147] On examination, there is usually no discoloration or edema, and there is tenderness over the proximal aspect of the navicular. The patient's inability to hop in the equinus position is a functional test that can reproduce the pain.[148] A thorough physical examination is necessary, including careful observation of gait, range of motion, and strength to rule out posterior tibialis tendonitis. Other differential diagnosis includes talar stress fracture, tarsal tunnel syndrome, and ligamentous injury.

Torg[149] demonstrated that most fatigue fractures of the navicular occur in the sagittal plane in the central third. This area is relatively avascular, providing an explanation for the association of these fractures with nonunion. In a review of published cases, 114 of 137 (83%) navicular stress fractures were partial-thickness fractures.[146] In a smaller series of 12 patients, these fractures usually occurred on the dorsal surface and extended less than 5 mm plantarward.[146a]

Diagnostic evaluation begins with plain radiographs, which are usually normal. In 128 radiographs for suspected navicular stress fracture, 86 were false-negative.[146] Bone scanning has much greater sensitivity for stress reactions. However, in cases where the diagnosis needs to be clarified, CT[145] and MRI offer better anatomic resolution.

Complications of tarsal navicular stress fractures include nonunion and chronic pain that limits or precludes athletic activity. Optimal treatment is paramount to prevent adverse outcomes. The initial treatment reported was for two patients with tarsal navicular stress fractures, one of which was repaired with autologous bone grafting and the other treated with a non-weightbearing cast.[144] Torg recommended treating nondisplaced complete fractures with non-weightbearing casting for 6 to 8 weeks. Displaced complete fractures were treated with open reduction and internal fixation followed by a non-weightbearing cast for 6 weeks.[149] Non-weightbearing casting is now first-line treatment in cases of partial fracture. In 22 patients treated with a non-weightbearing cast immobilization for at least 6 weeks, 86% returned to sports, whereas only 26% of 34 patients were able to return when treated with limited activity with continued weightbearing. Of those patients who failed weightbearing, 6 of 7 were subsequently treated with a non-weightbearing cast for 6 weeks and returned to sports. These results compare favorably with surgery; 11 of 15 patients who failed weightbearing were subsequently

treated with one surgical procedure, and 73% could ultimately return.[145]

Healing of the fracture is usually monitored by clinical examination. The patient should be seen at 3 weeks to reemphasize the importance of strict non-weightbearing.[146] At 6 weeks, if pain persists over the navicular, an additional 2 weeks of non-weightbearing casting should be instituted. Computed tomography scan has not been shown to be more helpful than clinical examination in determining healing. If pain-free at the navicular after casting, the patient can begin weightbearing rehabilitation. Khan suggests a supervised 6-week rehabilitation program that begins with 2 weeks of normal activities of daily living, water running, and soft-tissue stretching and strengthening. If there is no navicular pain, the patient can begin jogging on alternate days for 5 minutes on grass, advancing time and distance gradually. If after 6 weeks, there is no recurrent navicular pain, the patient can gradually return to full training.[146]

REFERENCES

1. Herring SA, Nilson KL: Introduction to overuse injuries. Clin Sports Med 1987; 6:225.
2. Priest JD, Braden V, Gerbierich JG: The elbow and tennis I. Phys Sports Med 1980; 8:80.
3. Counts, Rates, and Characteristics: Occupational Injuries and Illness. Washington, DC, Government Printing Office, 1997.
4. Meeuwisse WH: Athletic injury etiology: Distinguishing between interaction and confounding. Clin J Sports Med 1994; 4:171.
5. Wen DY, Puffer JC, Schmalzried TP: Injuries in runners: A prospective study of alignment. Clin J Sports Med 1998; 8:187.
6. Grimby G, Saltin B: The aging muscle. Clin Physiol 1983; 3:209.
7. Brown MC, Holland RL, Hopkins WG: Motor nerve sprouting. Ann Rev Neurosci 1981; 4:17.
8. Leadbetter WB: Cell-matrix response in tendon injury. Clin Sports Med 1992; 11:533.
9. Martens MA, Meyersoons JP: Acute and effort-related compartment syndrome in sports. Sports Med 1990; 9:62.
10. Detmer DE, Sharpe K, Sufit RL, et al: Chronic compartment syndrome: Diagnosis, management, and outcomes. Am J Sports Med 1985; 13:162.
11. Qvarfordt P, Christenson JT: Intramuscular pressure, muscle blood flow, and skeletal muscle metabolism in anterior tibial compartment syndrome. Clin Orthop Rel Res 1990; 179:284.
12. Freedman BJ, Knowles CH: Anterior tibial syndrome due to arterial embolism and thrombosis: Ischemic necrosis of anterior crural muscles. Br Med J 1959; 2:270.
13. Leach RE, Hammond G, Stryker WS: Anterior tibial compartment syndrome: Acute and chronic. J Bone Joint Surg Am 1967; 49:451.

14. Rampersaud YR, Amendola A: The evaluation of treatment of exertional compartment syndrome: Operative techniques. Sports Med 1995; 3:267.
15. Varelas FL, Wessel J, Clement DB, et al: Muscle function in chronic compartment syndrome of the leg. J Orthop Sports Phys Ther 1993; 18:586.
16. Pedowitz RA, Gershuni DH: Pathophysiology and diagnosis of chronic compartment syndrome. Operative techniques. Sports Med 1995; 3:230.
17. Moed BR, Thorderson PK: Measurement of intracompartmental pressure: A comparison of the slit catheter, side-ported needle, and simple needle. J Bone Joint Surg Am 1993; 75:231.
18. Pedowitz RA, Hargens AR, Mubarak SJ, et al: Modified criteria for the objective diagnosis of chronic compartment syndrome of the leg. Am J Sports Med 1990; 18:35.
19. Wiley JP, Short WB, Wiseman DA, et al: Ultrasound catheter placement for deep posterior compartment syndrome. Am J Sports Med 1990; 18:74.
20. Rorabeck CH, Bourne RB, Fowler PJ, et al: The role of tissue pressure measurement in diagnosing chronic anterior compartment syndrome. Am J Sports Med 1988; 16:143.
21. Amendola A, Rorabeck CH, Vellet D, et al: The use of magnetic resonance imaging in exertional compartment syndromes. Am J Sports Med 1990; 18:29.
22. Hayes AA, Bower GD, Pitscock KL: Chronic (exertional) compartment syndrome of the legs diagnosed with thallous chloride scintigraphy. J Nucl Med 1995; 36:1618.
23. Mohler LR, Styf JR, Pedowitz RA, et al: Intramuscular deoxygenation during exercise in patients who have chronic anterior compartment syndrome of the leg. J Bone Joint Surg 1997; 79:844.
24. Christensen JT, Eklof B, Wulff K: The

chronic compartment syndrome and response to diuretic treatment. Act Chir Scand 1983; 149:249.
25. Reneman RS: The anterior and the lateral compartmental syndrome of the leg due to intensive use of muscles. Clin Orthop Rel Res 1975; 113:69.
26. Schepsis AA, Martini D, Corbett M: Surgical management of exertional compartment syndrome of the lower leg. Am J Sports Med 1993; 21:811.
27. Wallensten R: Results of fasciotomy in patients with medial tibial syndrome of chronic anterior compartment syndrome. J Bone Joint Surg 1983; 65:1252.
28. Micheli LJ, Solomon R, Solomon J, et al: Surgical treatment for chronic lower-leg compartment syndrome in young female athletes. Am J Sports Med 1999; 27:197.
29. Detmer DE: Diagnosis and management of chronic compartment syndrome of the leg. Semin Orthop 1988; 3:223.
30. James SL, Bates BT, Osternig LR: Injuries to runners. Am J Sports Med 1978; 6:40.
31. Kannus P, Nittymake S, Jarvinen M, et al: Sports injuries in elderly athletes: A 3-year prospective controlled study. Age Ageing 1989; 18:263.
32. Clement DB, Taunton JE, Smart GW: Achilles tendinitis and peritendinitis: Etiology and treatment. Am J Sports Med 1984; 12:179.
33. Kraus-Hansen AE, Fackelman GE, Becker C, et al: Preliminary studies on the vascular anatomy of equine superficial digital flexor tendon. Equine Vet J 1992; 24:46.
34. Astrom M, Rausing A: Chronic achilles tendinopathy: A survey of surgical and histopathologic findings. Clin Orthop 1995; 316:151.
35. Martens M, Wouter P, Burssens A, et al: Patellar tendinitis: Pathology and results of treatment. Acta Orthop Scand 1982; 53:445.

36. Ferretti A, Ippolito E, Mariani P, et al: Jumper's knee. Am J Sports Med 1983; 11:58.

37. Khan KM, Cook JL, Bonar F, et al: Histopathology of common tendinopathies: Update and implications for clinical management. Sports Med 1999; 27:393.

38. Alfredson H, Thorsen K, Lorentzon R, et al: In situ microdialysis in tendon tissue: High levels of glutamate but not prostaglandin E2 in chronic achilles tendon pain. Knee Surg Sports Traumatol Arthrosc 1999; 7:378.

39. Khan KM, Maffulli N: Tendinopathy: An Achilles' heel for athletes and clinicians. Clin J Sports Med 1998; 8:151.

40. Stone D, Green C, Rao U, et al: Cytokine-induced tendinitis: A preliminary study in rabbits. J Orthop Res 1999; 17: 168.

41. Fritschy D, de Gautard R: Jumper's knee and ultrasonography. Am J Sports Med 1988; 16:637.

42. Cook JL, Khan KM, Harcourt PR, et al: Patellar tendon ultrasonography in asymptomatic active athletes reveals hypoechoic regions: A study of 320 tendons. Clin J Sports Med 1998; 8:73.

43. Khan KM, Viscentini PJ, Kiss ZS, et al: Correlation of ultrasound and magnetic resonance imaging with clinical outcome after patellar tenotomy: Prospective and retrospective studies. Clin J Sports Med 1999; 9:129.

44. Curwin SL, Stanish WD: Tendinitis: Its Etiology and Treatment. Lexington, MA, Collamore Press, 1984.

45. El-Hawary R, Stanish WD, Curwin SL: Rehabilitation of tendon injuries in sport. Sports Med 1997; 24:347.

46. Alfredson H, Pietila T, Jonsson P, et al: Heavy-load eccentric calf muscle training for the treatment of chronic Achilles tendonosis. Am J Sports Med 1998; 26:360.

47. Alfredson H, Lorentzon R: Chronic achilles tendinosis: Recommendations for treatment and prevention. Sports Med 2000; 29:135.

48. Fredberg U: Local corticosteroid injection in sport: Review of literature and guidelines for treatment. Scan J Med Sci Sports 1997; 7:131.

49. Clement DB, Taunton JE, Smart GW, et al: A survey of running injuries. Phys Sports Med 1981; 9:47.

50. Fairbank JC, Pynsent PB, van Poortvliet JA, et al: Mechanical factors in the incidence of knee pain in adolescent and young adults. J Bone Joint Surg 1984; 66:685.

51. Thomee R, Renstrom P, Karlsson J, et al: Patellofemoral pain syndrome in young women I: A clinical analysis of alignment common symptoms and functional activity level. Scand J Med Sci Sports 1995; 5:237.

52. Insall J, Falvo KA, Wise DW: Chondromalacia patellae: A prospective study. J Bone Joint Surg 1976; 58:1.

53. Vahasarja V, Kinnunen P, Lanning P, et al: Operative realignment of patellar malalignment in children. J Ped Orthop 1995; 15:281.

54. Martinea S, Korobkin M, Fondren FB: Diagnosis of patellofemoral malalignment by computed tomography. J Comput Assist Tomogr 1983; 7:1050.

55. Fulkerson JP: Awareness of the retinaculum in evaluating patellofemoral pain. Am J Sports Med 1982; 10:147.

56. Fulkerson JP, Tennant R, Jaivin JS, et al: Histologic evidence of retinacular nerve injury associated with patellofemoral malalignment. Clin Orthop 1985; 197: 196.

57. Kennedy JC, Alexander IJ, Hayes KC: Nerve supply of the human knee and its functional importance. Am J Sports Med 1982; 10:329.

58. Thomee R, Augustsson J, Karlsson J: Patellofemoral pain syndrome: A review of current issues. Sports Med 1999; 28:245.

59. Bellemans J, Cauwenberghs F, Witvrouw E, et al: Anteromedial tibial tubercle transfer in patients with chronic anterior knee pain and subluxation-type patellar malalignment. Am J Sports Med 1997; 25:375.

60. Fulkerson JP, Hungerford DS: Disorders of the Patellofemoral Joint. Baltimore, Williams and Wilkins, 1990, 2nd ed.

61. Desio SM, Burks RT, Bachus KN: Soft tissue restraints to lateral patellar translation in the human knee. Am J Sports Med 1998; 26:59.

62. Bennet JG, Stauber WT: Evaluation and treatment of anterior knee pain using eccentric exercise. Med Sci Sports Exerc 1986; 18:526.

63. Werner S: An evaluation of knee extensor and knee flexor torques and EMGs in patients with patellofemoral pain syndrome in comparison with matched controls. Knee Surg Sports Traumatol Arthrosc 1995; 3:89.

64. Souza DR, Gross MT: Comparison of vastus medialis obliquus: Vastus lateralis muscle–integrated electromyographic ratios between healthy subjects and patients with patellofemoral pain. J Orthop Sports Phys Ther 1991; 71:310.

65. Macintyre D, Wessel J: Knee muscle torques in patellofemoral pain syndrome. Physiother Can 1988; 40:20.

66. Karst GM, Willet GM: Onset timing of electromyographic activity in the vastus medialis obliquus and vastus lateralis muscles in subjects with and without patellofemoral pain syndrome. Phys Ther 1995; 75:813.

67. Stokes M, Young A: Investigations of quadriceps inhibition: Implications for clinical practice. Physiotherapy 1984; 70: 425.

68. Javadpour SM, Finegan PJ, O'Brien M: The anatomy of the extensor mechanism and its clinical relevance. Clin J Sports Med 1991; 1:229.

69. Gunal I, Arac S, Sahinoglu K, et al: The innervation of vastus medialis obliquus. J Bone Joint Surg 1992; 74:624.

70. Hodges PW, Richardson CA: The influence of isometric hip adduction on quadriceps femoris activity. Scan J Rehabil Med 1993; 25:57.

71. Insall J: Current concepts review: Patellar pain. J Bone Joint Surg 1982; 64:147.

72. Tria AJ, Palumbo RC, Alicea JA: Conservative care of patellofemoral pain. Orthop Clin North Am 1992; 23:545.

73. McConnell J: The management of chondromalacia patellae: A long-term solution. Aust J Phys Ther 1986; 32:215.

74. Werner S, Knutsson E, Erickson E: The effects of taping the patella on concentric and eccentric torque and EMG of the knee extensor and flexor muscles in patients with patellofemoral pain syndrome. Knee Surg Sports Traumatol Arthrosc 1993; 1:169.

75. DeHaven KE, Dolan WA, Mayer PJ: Chondromalacia patellae in athletes. Am J Sports Med 1979; 7:5.

76. McMullen W, Roncarati A, Koval P: Static and isokinetic treatments of chondromalacia patella: A comparative investigation. J Orthop Sports Phys Ther 1990; 12:256.

77. Kannus P, Niittymaki S: Which factors predict outcome in the nonoperative treatment of patellofemoral pain syndrome: A prospective follow-up study. Med Sci Sports Exerc 1994; 26:289.

78. Callaghan MJ, Oldham JA: The role of quadriceps exercise in the treatment of patellofemoral pain syndrome. Sports Med 1996; 21:384.

78a. Steinkamp LA, Billingham MF, Markel DM, et al: Biomechanical consideration in patellofemoral joint rehabilitation. Am J Sports Med 1993; 21:438.

79. Jensen DB, Albrektsen SB: The natural history of chondromalacia patellae: A 12-year follow-up. Acta Orthop Belg 1990; 56:503.

80. Bockrath K, Wooden C, Worrell T, et al: Effects of patella taping on patella position and perceived pain. Med Sci Sports Exerc 1993; 25:989.

81. Larsen B, Andreasen E, Urfer A, et al: Patellar taping: A radiographic examination of the medial glide technique. Am J Sports Med 1995; 23:465.

82. Finestone A, Radin E, Lev B, et al: Treatment of overuse patellofemoral pain: Prospective randomized controlled clinical trial in a military setting. Clin Orthop 1993; 293:208.

83. BenGal S, Lowe J, Mann G, et al: The role of the knee brace in the prevention of anterior knee pain syndrome. Am J Sports Med 1997; 25:118.

84. Tietz CC, Hermanson BK, Kronmal RA: Evaluation of the use of braces to prevent injury to the knee in college football players. J Bone Joint Surg 1987; 69:1.

85. Breithaupt MD: Zur pathologie des menschlichen fusses. Med Zeitung 1855; 24:169.

86. Subramanian G, McAfee J: A new complex of 99m Tc for skeletal imaging. Radiology 1971; 99:192.

87. McBryde AM: Stress fractures in runners. Clin Sports Med 1985; 4:737.

88. Pentecost RL: Fatigue, insufficiency and pathologic fractures. JAMA 1964; 187: 1001.

89. Bass S, Pearce G, Bradney M: Exercise before puberty may confer residual benefits in bone density in adulthood: Studies in active prepubertal and retired female gymnasts. Bone Miner Res 1998; 13:500.

90. Mori S, Burr, DB: Increased intracortical remodeling following fatigue damage. Bone 1993; 14:103.

91. Alho A, Husby T, Hoiseth A: Bone mineral content and strength: An ex vivo study on human femora at autopsy. Clin Orthop Rel Res 1986; 227:292.

92. Beck TJ, Ruff CB, Mourtada FA: Dual-energy x-ray absorptiometry-derived structural geometry for stress fracture prediction in male US Marine Corps recruits. J Bone Miner Res 1996; 11:645.

93. Crossley K: Ground reaction forces, bone characteristics, and tibial stress fractures in male runners. Med Sci Sports Exerc 1999; 31:1088.

94. Yoshikawa T, Mori S, Santiesteban AJ: The effects of muscle fatigue on bone strain. J Exp Biol 1994; 188:217.

95. Bennell K: Risk factors for stress fractures. Sports Med 1999; 28:91.

96. Montgomery LC: Orthopaedic history and examination in the etiology of overuse injuries. Med Sci Sports Exerc 1989; 21:237.

97. Cowan DN: Lower limb morphology and risk of overuse injury among male infantry trainees. Med Sci Sports Exerc 1996; 28:945.

98. Winfield AC: Risk factors associated with stress reactions in female marines. Mil Med 1997; 162:168.

99. Giladi M: The low arch: A protective factor in stress fractures. Orthop Rev 1985; 14:709.

100. Simkin A: Combined effect of foot arch structure and an orthotic device on stress fractures. Foot Ankle 1989; 10:25.

101. Freiberg O: Leg length asymmetry in stress fractures: A clinical and radiological study. J Sports Med 1982; 22:485.

102. Walter SD: The Ontario cohort study of running-related injuries. Arch Intern Med 1989; 149:2561.

103. Gardner LI: Prevention of lower extremity stress fractures: A controlled trial of a shock-absorbent insole. Am J Public Health 1988; 78:236.

104. Fredericson M: Tibial stress reaction in runners: Correlation of clinical symptoms and scintigraphy with a new MRI grading system. Am J Sports Med 1995; 23: 472.

105. Wolman RL, Harries MG: Menstrual abnormalities in elite athletes. Clin Sports Med 1989; 1:95.

106. Bennell KL: Risk factors for stress fractures in track and field athletes: A 12-month prospective study. Am J Sports Med 1996; 24:810.

107. Barrow GW, Saha S: Menstrual irregularity and stress fractures in collegiate female distance runners. Am J Sports Med 1988; 16:209.

108. Lord MJ, Ha KI, Song KS: Stress fractures of the ribs in golfers. Am J Sports Med 1996; 24:118.

109. Bennell KL, Bruckner PD: Epidemiology and site specificity of stress fractures. Clin Sports Med 1997; 16:179.

110. Bennell KL: The incidence and distribution of stress fractures in competitive track and field athletes: A 12-month prospective study. Am J Sports Med 1996; 24:211.

111. Hulkko H, Orava S: Stress fractures in athletes. Int J Sports Med 1987; 8:221.

112. Roub LW, Gumerman LW, Hanley EN: Bone stress: A radionuclide imaging perspective. Radiology 1979; 132:431.

113. Orava S. Puranen J: Athlete's leg pains. Br J Sports Med 1979; 13:92.

114. Chang PS, Harris RM: Intramedullary nailing for chronic tibial stress fractures. Am J Sports Med 1996; 24:688.

115. Hemler DE: Saphenous nerve entrapment caused by pes anserine bursitis mimicking stress fracture of the tibia. Arch Phys Med Rehabil 1991; 72:336.

116. Savoca CJ: Stress fractures: A classification of the earliest radiographic signs. Radiology 1971; 100:519.

116a. Daffner RH, Pavlov H: Stress fractures: Current concepts. Am J Rheum 1992; 159:245.

117. Milgrom C: Negative bone scans in impending tibial stress fractures: A report of three cases. Am J Sports Med 1984; 12:488.

118. Matin P: The appearance of bone scans following fractures, including immediate and long-term studies. J Nucl Med 1979; 20:1227.

119. Zwas ST, Elkanovitch R, Rank G: Interpretation and classification of bone scintigraphic findings in stress fracture. J Nucl Med 1987; 28:452.

120. Blank S: Transverse tibial stress fractures: A special problem. Am J Sports Med 1987; 15:597.

121. Green NE, Rogers RA, Lipscomb AB: Nonunions of the stress fractures of the tibia. Am J Sports Med 1985; 13:171.

122. Johansson C: Stress fractures of the femoral neck in athletes: The consequences of a delay in diagnosis. Am J Sports Med 1990; 18:524.

123. Volpin G: Stress fractures of the femoral neck following strenuous activity. J Orthop Trauma 1990; 4:394.

124. Johnson AW, Weiss CB, Wheeler DL: Stress fractures of the femoral shaft in athletes: More common than expected. Am J Sports Med 1994; 22:248.

125. Matheson GO: Stress fractures in athletes. Am J Sports Med 1987; 15:46.

126. Clement DB: Exercise-induced stress injuries to the femur. Int J Sports Med 1993; 14:347.

127. Fullerton LR, Snowdy HA: Femoral neck stress fractures. Am J Sports Med 1988; 16:365.

128. Lombardo SJ, Benson DW: Stress fractures of the femur in runners. Am J Sports Med 1982; 10:219.

129. Keene JS, Lash EG: Negative bone scan in a femoral neck stress fracture. Am J Sports Med 1992; 20:234.

130. Drez D: Metatarsal stress fractures. Am J Sports Med 1980; 8:123.

131. Gross TS, Bunch RP: A mechanical model of metatarsal stress fracture during distance running. Am J Sports Med 1989; 17:669.

132. Sherref MJ: Vascular anatomy of the fifth metatarsal. Foot Ankle 1991; 11: 350.

133. Weinfeld SB, Haddad SL, Myerson MS: Metatarsal stress fractures. Clin Sports Med 1997; 16:319.

134. Meurman KO: Less common stress fractures in the foot. Br J Radiol 1981; 54:1.

135. Dameron TB: Fractures of the proximal fifth metatarsal: Selecting the best treatment option. J Am Acad Orthop Surg 1995; 3:110.

136. Lawrence SJ, Botte MJ: Jones' fractures and related fractures of the proximal fifth metatarsal. Foot Ankle 1993; 14:358.

137. Torg JS: Fractures of the base of the fifth metatarsal distal to the tuberosity: Classification and guidelies for non-surgical and surgical management. J Bone Joint Surg Am 1984; 66:209.

138. Josefsson PO: Closed treatment of Jones fracture: Good results in 40 cases after 11–26 years. Acta Orthop Scand 1994; 65:545.

139. Acker JH, Drez DJ: Nonoperative treatment of stress fractures of the proximal shaft of the fifth metatarsal (Jones' fracture). Foot Ankle 1986; 7:152.

140. Torg JS: Fractures of the base of the fifth metatarsal distal to the tuberosity: A review. Contemp Orthop 1989; 19:497.

141. DeLee JC, Evans JP, Julian J: Stress fracture of the fifth metatarsal. Am J Sports Med 1983; 11:349.

142. Zelko RR, Torg JS, Rachun A: Proximal diaphyseal fractures of the fifth metatarsal: Treatment of the fractures and their complications in athletes. Am J Sports Med 1979; 7:95.

143. Mindrebo N: Outpatient percutaneous screw fixation of the acute Jones fracture. Am J Sports Med 1993; 21:720.

144. Towne LC, Blazina ME, Cozen LN: Fatigue fractures of the tarsal navicular. J Bone Joint Surg Am 1970; 52:376.

145. Khan KM: Outcome of conservative and surgical management of navicular stress fractures in athletes. Am J Sports Med 1992; 20:657.

146. Khan KM: Tarsal navicular stress fractures in athletes. Sports Med 1994; 17: 65.

146a. Pavlov H, Torg JS, Freiberger RH: Tarsalnavicular stress fractures: Radiographic evaluation. Radiology 1983; 148:641.

147. Bolin DJ, Nelson T: Tarsal navicular stress fracture in a soccer player (abstract). Med Sci Sports Exerc 1999; 31: 343.

148. Fitch KD, Blackwell JD, Gilmour WN: Operation for non-union of navicular stress fracture of the tarsal navicular. J Bone Joint Surg 1989; 71:105.

149. Torg JS: Stress fractures of the tarsal navicular. J Bone Joint Surg 1982; 64:700.

SHOULDER INJURIES IN ATHLETES

Freddie H. Fu, James A. O'Leary, Marc W. Urquhart, and Mark W. Rodosky

Summary
- Shoulder injuries are commonly seen in the athletic population and may result from acute trauma or overuse syndromes.
- Shoulder injuries account for approximately 8% to 13% of all sports-related injuries.
- Overhead sports such as baseball, tennis, swimming, and volleyball frequently produce overuse syndromes, whereas contact sports such as football, hockey, and wrestling often result in direct traumatic injuries to the shoulder.
- Common sites of injury include the rotator cuff, acromioclavicular (AC) joint, biceps tendon, and scapulothoracic (ST) articulation.
- The keys to treatment of the athletic shoulder include knowledge of the mechanics of the sport and mechanism of the injury, accurate anatomic diagnosis, and a multidisciplinary approach to treat the athlete's current condition and modify the causative factors to prevent future injuries.

Successful participation in sporting activities such as baseball, tennis, swimming, and volleyball requires a fluid kinetic chain of highly coordinated overhead movements performed at the extremes of shoulder motion. Effective shoulder function relies on the precise balance between shoulder mobility and joint stability. It is this fragile dichotomy of shoulder motion and stability that is tested by the repetitive demands of overhead sport and frequently leaves the shoulder vulnerable to injury. Injuries involving the shoulder are a common consequence of sports participation and have been estimated to comprise between 8% and 13% of all athletic injuries.[1] Sports with significant overhead demands such as tennis, baseball, volleyball, and swimming often produce repetitive overuse syndromes. In contrast, the injuries encountered in contact sports such as football, lacrosse, hockey, and wrestling are commonly the result of direct trauma.

FUNCTIONAL ANATOMY OF THE SHOULDER GIRDLE

BONY ANATOMY

Knowledge of the normal functional anatomy of the shoulder is critical for the effective care of the injured athlete. The shoulder girdle consists of three bones: the scapula, the clavicle, and the humerus, which form an intercalated complex and work in concert during shoulder motion (Fig. 1). These bones are linked to form four joints: glenohumeral (GH), AC, sternoclavicular (SC), and ST. Normal motion of the shoulder is a complex combination of motion at these four joints. As the arm is abducted in the

plane of the scapula, the initial 120 degrees of motion occurs at the GH joint, and the remaining 60 degrees is the result of motion at the ST articulation. Rotation of the upper extremity occurs primarily at the GH joint.[2] The SC joint allows 40 degrees of rotation in all directions, whereas the coracoclavicular ligaments limit the AC joint motion to approximately 20 degrees.

The scapula overlies ribs 2 through 7 on the posterior thorax and contributes to a pseudoarticulation with the chest wall at the ST joint. The scapula lies 30 degrees anterior to the coronal plane of the body and is tilted 3 degrees medially from the sagittal plane, which facilitates overhead motion and extends the reach of the hand (Fig. 2). Laterally, the scapula expands to form the glenoid, which articulates with the proximal humerus at the GH joint. To increase inferior stability, the glenoid has an average superior tilt of 5 degrees and is retroverted with respect to the body of the scapula by an average of 7 degrees. Two important bony prominences arise from the scapula: the coracoid and the acromion. The coracoid serves as the attachment site for the coracoacromial (CA) and coracohumeral (CH) ligaments and for the conjoined (coracobrachialis and short head of biceps) and pectoralis minor tendons (Fig. 3). The acromion projects from the scapular spine over the head of the humerus and serves as the primary origin of the deltoid muscle.

The proximal humerus consists of the articular surface, the anatomic neck, and the metaphysis. The humeral head is retroverted 30 to 40 degrees relative to the axis of elbow flexion. The normal neck-shaft angle of the humerus is 130 to 140 degrees (Fig. 4). The supraspinatus, infraspinatus, and teres minor tendons of the rotator cuff insert onto the greater tuberosity, whereas the subscapularis tendon inserts onto the lesser tuberosity. The long head of the biceps tendon traverses the bicipital groove to enter the GH joint and insert onto the supraglenoid tubercle.

The GH joint is the primary articulation of the shoulder girdle complex and is formed by the hemispherical humeral head and the shallow glenoid fossa. The radius of curvature of the two surfaces is nearly identical. However, the significant size mismatch and limited glenoid coverage of the head produce inherent joint instability. This unique joint architecture affords maximal mobility, at the expense of stability, which is provided by the static and dynamic restraints of the surrounding capsuloligamentous and muscular structures.

SOFT-TISSUE ANATOMY

The static restraints of the GH joint include the glenoid labrum, joint capsule, GH ligaments, and CH ligament. The glenoid labrum is a fibrocartilaginous structure surrounding the glenoid rim, which acts to deepen the glenoid fossa, provides a load-absorbing function for the humeral head,

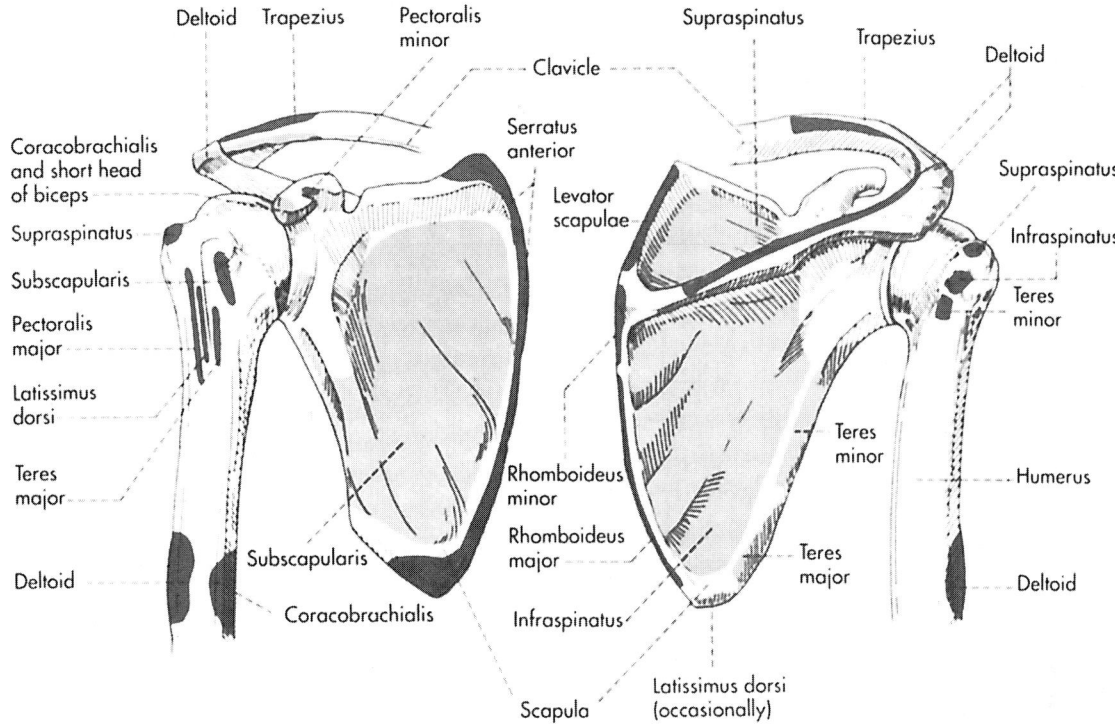

Fig. 1. Muscles of the shoulder and shoulder girdle. (In Miller MD, Cooper DE, Warnder JJP [eds]: Review of Sports Medicine and Arthroscopy. Philadelphia, WB Saunders, 1995, p 115. From Jenkins DB: Hollinshead's Functional Anatomy of the Limbs and Back, 6th ed. Philadelphia, WB Saunders, 1991, Fig. 5–3.)

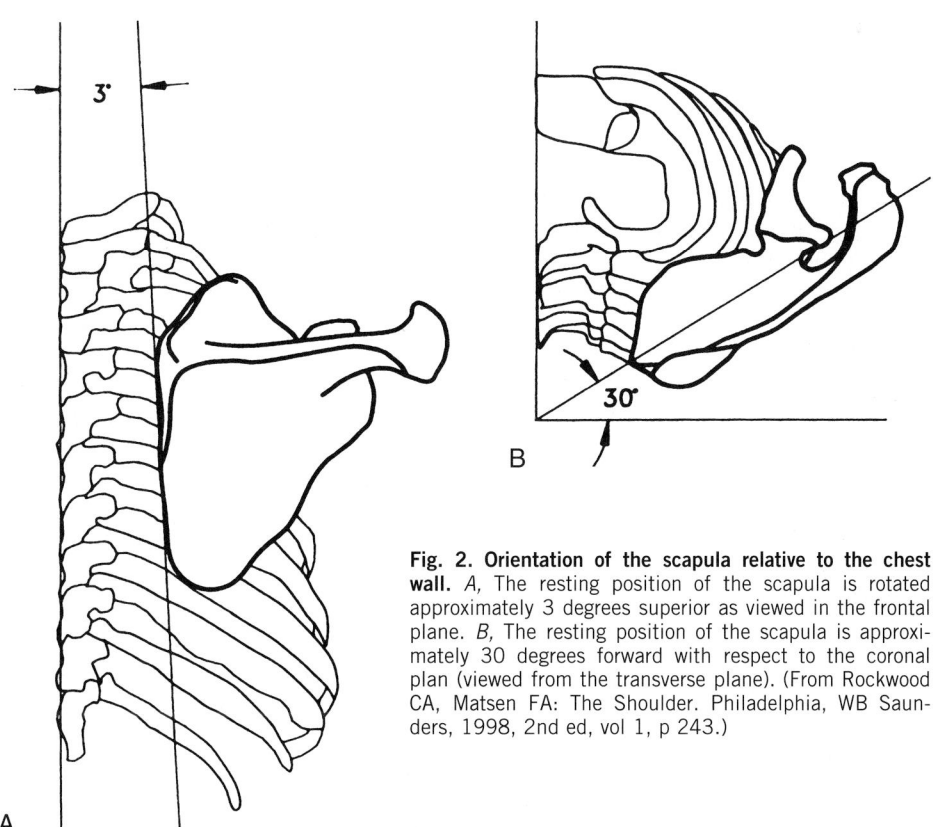

Fig. 2. Orientation of the scapula relative to the chest wall. *A,* The resting position of the scapula is rotated approximately 3 degrees superior as viewed in the frontal plane. *B,* The resting position of the scapula is approximately 30 degrees forward with respect to the coronal plan (viewed from the transverse plane). (From Rockwood CA, Matsen FA: The Shoulder. Philadelphia, WB Saunders, 1998, 2nd ed, vol 1, p 243.)

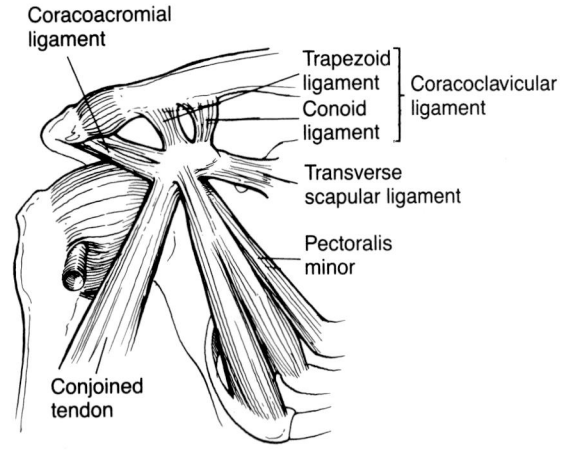

Fig. 3. Muscle and ligament attachments to the coracoid process. (In Miller MD, Cooper DE, Warnder JJP [eds]: Review of Sports Medicine and Arthroscopy. Philadelphia, WB Saunders, 1995, p 115.)

often loosely attached to the periphery. Detachment in an anteroinferior location is frequently associated with instability as a result of disruption of the attachment of the inferior glenohumeral ligament (IGHL) complex.

The GH joint is surrounded by a loose and redundant capsule, which allows maximum joint motion. Thickenings of the joint capsule contribute to joint stability and include the superior glenohumeral ligament (SGHL), middle glenohumeral ligament (MGHL), IGHL, and the rotator interval (see Fig. 5). The rotator interval is the triangular area superior to the subscapularis tendon, inferior to the supraspinatus tendon, and medial to the bicipital groove.

The SGHL originates from the superior labrum anterior to the biceps tendon and inserts onto the humerus with the CH ligament in the region of the bicipital groove on the lesser tuberosity. Both ligaments, but primarily the SGHL, act to control inferior translation of the dependent arm and posterior translation when the joint is adducted, flexed, and internally rotated. The MGHL is a more variable structure that provides a secondary restraint to anterior translation of the head when the shoulder is abducted 45 degrees and externally rotated.[3] The IGHL is a hammock-like structure composed of discrete anterior and posterior bands divided by an intervening inferior capsule. The IGHL complex is the most important static stabilizer of the GH joint, with the anterior band serving as the primary anterior stabilizer of the abducted, externally rotated shoulder. A secondary role of the IGHL is to prevent inferior translation of the abducted shoulder.[4]

Whereas the static capsuloligamentous structures serve as passive "checkreins" at the extremes of motion, the dy-

serves as an attachment for the GH ligaments, and anchors the long head of the biceps tendon (Fig. 5). The anatomy of the labrum and the glenoid rim is highly variable, particularly in the anterosuperior region, where the labrum is

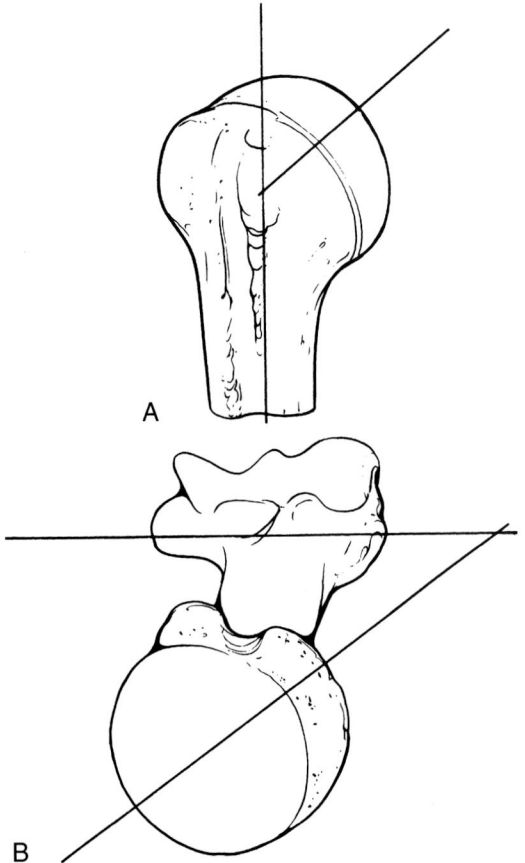

Fig. 4. The proximal humerus. The neck and head of the humerus have an angle of inclination of 130 to 150 degrees in relation to the shaft *(A)* and a retrotorsion angle of 20 to 30 degrees *(B)*. (From Rockwood CA, Matsen FA: The Shoulder. Philadelphia, WB Saunders, 1998, 2nd ed, vol 1, p 13.)

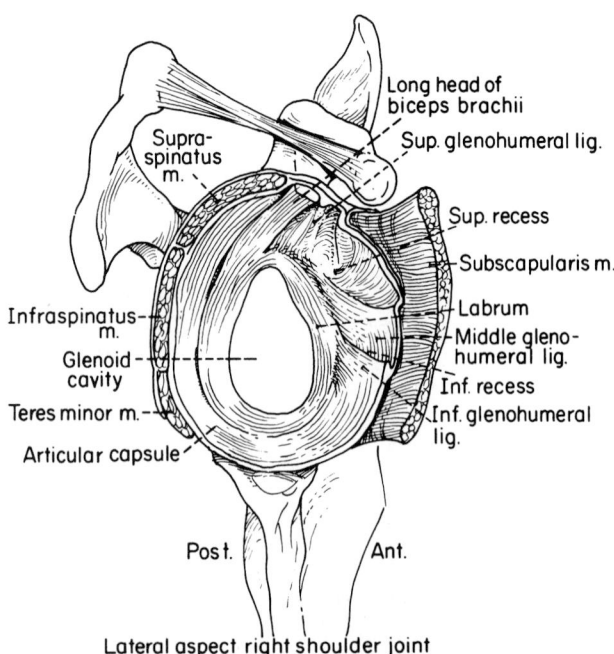

Lateral aspect right shoulder joint

Fig. 5. Schematic representation of the glenohumeral ligaments and the rotator cuff stabilizers of the glenohumeral joint. (In Rockwood CA, Matsen FA: The Shoulder. Philadelphia, WB Saunders, 1998, 2nd ed, vol 1, p 255; From Morrey BF, Cahey EYS: Recurrent anterior dislocation of the shoulder. In Black J, Dumbleton JH [eds]: Clinical Biomechanics. New York, Churchill Livingstone, 1981.)

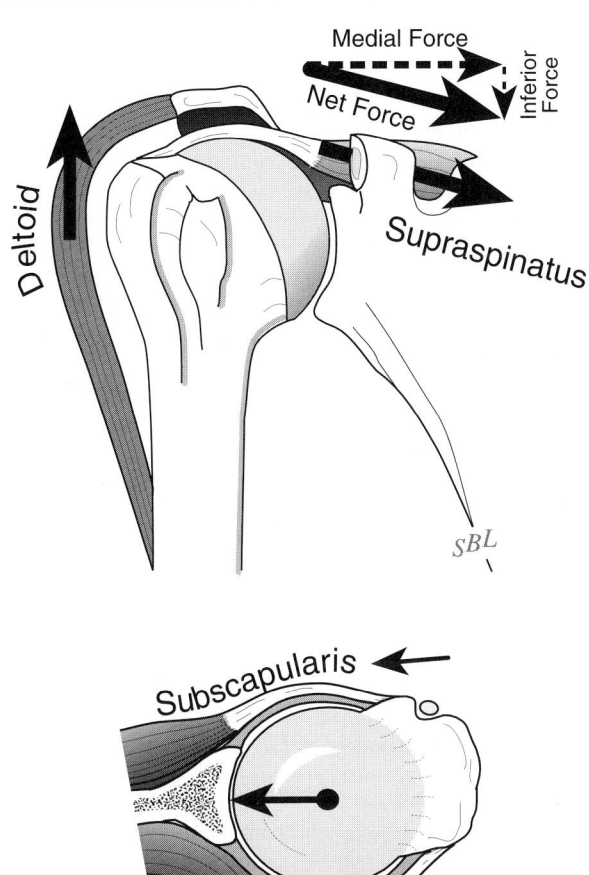

Fig. 6. Dynamic stability of the glenohumeral joint provided by the shoulder musculature. (In Rockwood CA, Matsen FA: The Shoulder. Philadelphia, WB Saunders, 1998, 2nd ed, vol 1, p 55; modified from Matsen FA III, Lippitt SB, Sidles JA, et al: Practical Evaluation and Management of the Shoulder. Philadelphia, WB Saunders, 1994.)

namic stabilizers of the GH joint play a vital role throughout the midrange arc of motion. The dynamic stabilizers of the GH joint include the rotator cuff musculature and the long head of the biceps tendon (Fig. 6). The primary function of the rotator cuff is to maintain and control the humeral head within the glenoid cavity throughout the arc of motion via a "concavity-compression" mechanism. This is enhanced by a steering effect, which directs the compressive forces toward the center of the glenoid.[6] Finally, the dynamic restraints are hypothesized to serve as a physical barrier to translation as they tighten and become rigid. This may also increase the tension on surrounding labral or capsuloligamentous structures, further enhancing joint stability.[7]

BIOMECHANICS

Overuse injuries to the shoulder are common in overhead sports such as baseball, swimming, and volleyball. The three-dimensional biomechanics of throwing have been studied extensively and have been used as a common prototype to better understand the spectrum of overhead shoulder injuries.[8–10] Four primary biomechanical stages of throwing have been described: wind-up, cocking, acceleration, and follow-through (Fig. 7). Studies have shown that the shoulder remains abducted approximately 100 degrees throughout the arc of motion, with maximal external rotation of 175 degrees seen before the acceleration stage. In the horizontal plane, the shoulder goes from 30 degrees of abduction in late cocking to 10 degrees of adduction at the completion of follow-through.[8] Arm speed has been measured at more than 7000 degrees per second as the shoulder rotates from 175 degrees of maximal external rotation to 105 degrees of internal rotation. Peak shoulder torque of up to 52 newton-meters has been measured during the rapid deceleration of the follow-through stage.[9]

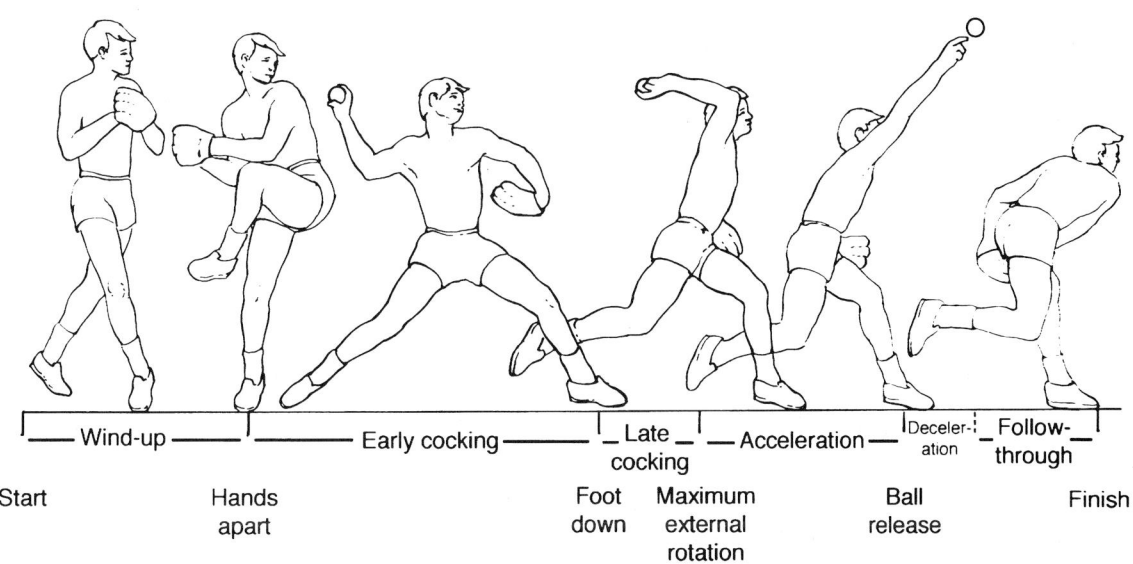

Fig. 7. Phases of the baseball pitch. (In Rockwood CA, Matsen FA: The Shoulder. Philadelphia, WB Saunders, 1998, 2nd ed, vol 1, p 1215; From Pink MM, Perry J: Biomechanics. In Jobe FW, et al [eds]: Operative Techniques in Upper Extremity Sports Injuries. St. Louis, MO, Mosby–Year Book, 1996.)

Electromyographic studies demonstrated the quiescent activity of the rotator cuff musculature during the cocking and acceleration phases of the throw.[10] For most throwing athletes, these early stages are dominated by the activity of the pectoralis major, serratus anterior, latissimus dorsi, and subscapularis muscles. However, it is the rapid deceleration of the follow-through that produces peak eccentric contractions in the rotator cuff musculature as it acts synergistically with the larger trunk muscles to dissipate the kinetic energy of the throw.[10] Therefore, pitching form, technique, and mechanics are vital to the prevention of shoulder injury in the throwing athlete.

The swimming stroke shares many biomechanical principles with the act of throwing and consists of two phases: pull-through and recovery. The pull-through phase is the power-generating event of the stroke and is characterized by the activity of the propulsive forces of the latissimus dorsi and pectoralis major muscles. The recovery phase is analogous to the cocking stage of throwing as the humerus is externally rotated and abducted to clear the greater tuberosity from beneath the acromion. This complex motion is controlled primarily by the supraspinatus, infraspinatus, and middle deltoid muscles. It is during this phase that symptoms of subacromial impingement are most commonly encountered.[11]

IMPINGEMENT SYNDROME AND ROTATOR CUFF DISEASE

HISTORY

Rotator cuff disease has been recognized for more than 150 years. The first report of a rotator cuff tear was by English anatomist J. G. Smith in 1834. Ernest A. Codman, one of the fathers of shoulder surgery, presented his first report of a rotator cuff repair in 1911.[12] In 1934 Codman published his landmark textbook *The Shoulder: Rupture of the Supraspinatus Tendon and Other Lesions in or about the Subacromial Bursa.*[13] Since Codman's classic work, knowledge of the incidence, cause, and treatment of rotator cuff disease has grown steadily. The success of surgical treatment has improved significantly over the past several decades largely as a result of the work of Charles Neer and the addition of anterior acromioplasty to rotator cuff repair.[14] More recently, the advent of shoulder arthroscopy has revolutionized the diagnosis and treatment of rotator cuff disease.

PRIMARY SUBACROMIAL IMPINGEMENT

A common site of disease associated with overuse syndromes in athletes involves the area beneath the acromial arch, which is occupied by the rotator cuff tendons and associated bursa. Primary subacromial impingement results when the rotator cuff and the overlying bursal tissue are compromised by narrowing of this space with forward flexion of the humerus. In the early 1970s, Neer classified subacromial impingement into three stages. Stage I is marked by edema and hemorrhage in the subacromial bursa and supraspinatus tendon as a result of repetitive microtrauma. In stage II, this inflammatory process produces fibrosis and tendinitis in the distal tendon insertion. Finally, stage III is characterized by tendon failure and tearing of the rotator cuff.[15]

The clinical syndrome of subacromial impingement can be further classified as outlet (primary) or nonoutlet (secondary) impingement. Outlet, or primary, impingement involves encroachment on the rotator cuff tendons by a narrowed CA arch. This condition can be precipitated by thickening of the CA ligament, the shape of the acromion, or a prominent AC joint. Bigliani et al[16] demonstrated a direct relationship between acromial morphology and tears of the rotator cuff. Acromial shape was classified into three types, and the incidence of each in the normal population was reported: type I, flat (18%); type II, curved (41%); and type III, hooked (41%) (Fig. 8). Patients with a type III acromion were more likely to experience rotator cuff disease than those with a type I acromial shape.[16] Although it is the most common type of impingement overall, primary impingement is infrequently seen in the younger, athletic population.

SECONDARY IMPINGEMENT

Impingement in the young athlete is frequently due to nonoutlet disease, such as occult instability of the glenohumeral joint, contracture of the posterior capsule, bursal thickening, or rotator cuff dysfunction. Secondary impingement is a very common cause of shoulder pain in the overhead athlete and often results from preexisting ligamentous laxity or acquired traumatic capsular laxity. As previously described, the demands of overhead sports can produce attenuation of the capsular ligaments and injury to the rotator cuff or biceps tendon. Loss or dysfunction of these stabilizing structures results in pathological laxity of the shoulder. The humeral head translates anteriorly, pro-

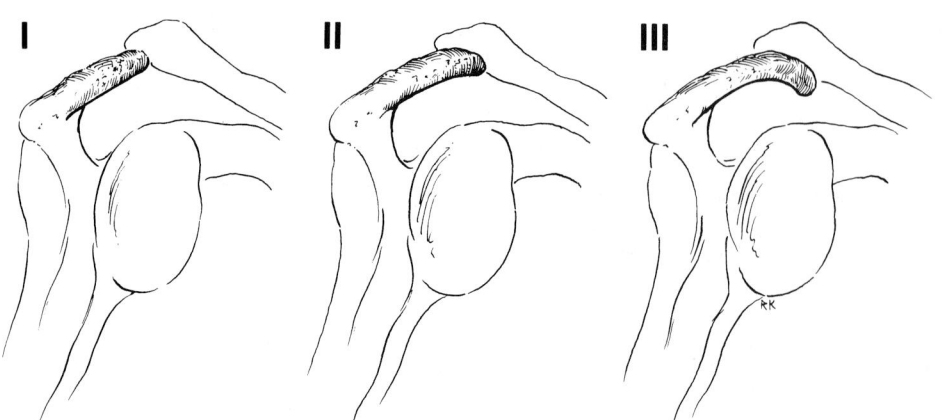

Fig. 8. Three types of acromion morphology as defined by Bigliani and Morrison. Type I, with its flat surface, provided the least compromise of the supraspinatus outlet, whereas the sudden discontinuity or hook in type III was associated with the highest rate of rotator cuff disease in a series of cadaver dissections. (From Rockwood CA, Matsen FA: The Shoulder. Philadelphia, WB Saunders, 1998, 2nd ed, vol 1, p 45.)

ducing impingement of the supraspinatus tendon on the CA arch. This occult instability pattern can result in secondary impingement, rotator cuff fatigue, and tissue failure. Treatment of secondary impingement should include stabilization of the humeral head through exercises, modification of the activity, or surgical intervention.[17, 18]

INTERNAL IMPINGEMENT AND CORACOID IMPINGEMENT

A syndrome of internal impingement has been described in a series of throwing athletes with symptoms of posterior shoulder pain caused by repetitive contact between the undersurface of the supraspinatus tendon and the posterosuperior glenoid.[19, 20] The symptoms of internal impingement are most pronounced during the late cocking phase of the throwing motion. These individuals are thought to be vulnerable to impingement because of repetitive stretching and attenuation of the anterior capsule, which allows excessive external rotation and anterior subluxation of the humeral head. The result is impingement of the rotator cuff on the posterior glenoid rim, which can produce undersurface tears of the cuff and deterioration of the posterior labrum. A less commonly encountered form of impingement that occurs with forward flexion, internal rotation, and adduction of the shoulder has also been described. This is referred to as coracoid impingement syndrome and occurs with mechanical abutment of the lesser tuberosity with the coracoid process.[21] The primary cause of this syndrome is also thought to be chronic force overload, which results in occult instability.

PHYSICAL EXAMINATION

Impingement syndrome can be differentiated from other causes of shoulder pain by the detection of impingement signs on physical examination and by the impingement test. The impingement sign, as described by Neer, is performed by forward flexion of the humerus while the scapula is stabilized with the opposite hand (Fig. 9). This maneuver produces abutment of the greater tuberosity on the undersurface of the CA arch and is considered positive when pain is elicited. A second impingement sign, as described by Hawkins, is performed by internally rotating the shoulder while flexed to 90 degrees in the plane of the scapula. To increase the specificity of the physical examination and to exclude other diagnoses, an impingement test can be performed. The subacromial space is injected with 10 mL of 1% lidocaine, and the patient is asked to assess the percentage of decrease in symptoms as the shoulder is taken through a range of motion and the provocative tests are repeated. If pain relief is absent or incomplete, other diagnoses should be considered.

ROTATOR CUFF DISEASE

Most authors agree that the cause of rotator cuff disease is multifactorial and includes extrinsic factors such bony impingement and intrinsic factors such as tissue degeneration, diminished blood supply, and decreased healing capacity. Injury to the rotator cuff in the younger athlete typically results from chronic microtrauma as a result of overuse or occasionally from acute traumatic disruption of the tendon. Repetitive stress and subacute injury from the throwing motion can lead to diminished tensile strength and elasticity of the cuff tendons with inflammation, degeneration, calcification, and tearing of the cuff. The eccentric phase of throwing, which involves deceleration of the arm during the follow-through, produces peak stress on the cuff and can lead to tearing of a chronically injured tendon. Infrequently, acute rotator cuff tears occur as a result of direct trauma to the shoulder from contact sports or from a fall onto the shoulder.

Aside from an isolated traumatic injury, full-thickness rotator cuff tears are unusual in the younger, athletic population. Rather, rotator cuff tears in this population are frequently partial-thickness lesions of the articular surface of

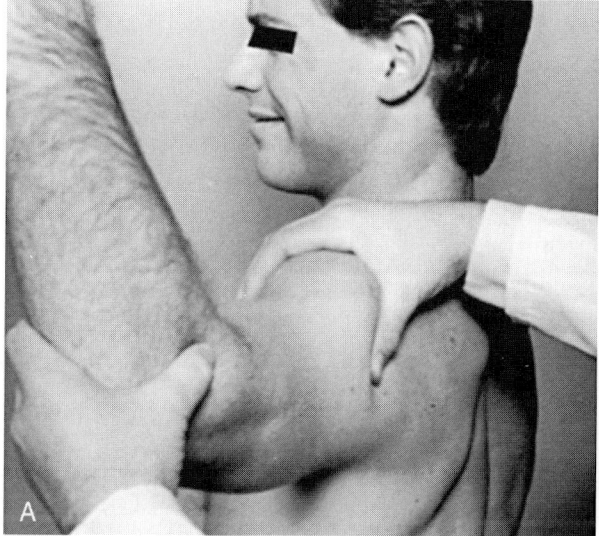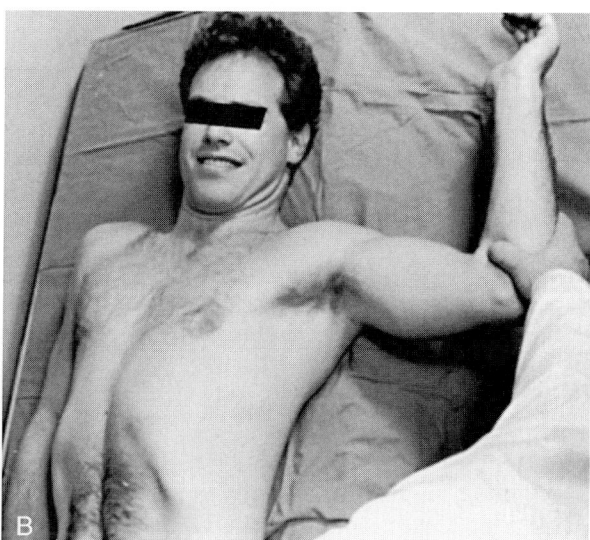

Fig. 9. Impingement signs. *A*, Apprehension test (sitting position) (crank test). The examiner's right thumb applies anterior leverage as the patient's arm is abducted and externally rotated. *B*, Apprehension test (supine position) (fulcrum test). The patient is positioned with the scapula supported by the edge of the examining table. The arm is in abduction and external rotation, producing a feeling of impending anterior instability. (From Rockwood CA, Matsen FA: The Shoulder. Philadelphia, WB Saunders, 1998, 2nd ed, vol 1, p 187.)

the supraspinatus tendon and may be associated with occult instability. Most reports found articular surface tears to be two to three times more common than bursa-sided tears.[22] The cause of this predilection for the articular surface is thought to be multifactorial, including increased shear forces, poor vascularity, and mechanical internal impingement. In contrast, bursa-sided tears are commonly related to acromial disease with direct abrasion and trauma to the cuff tendons.

PHYSICAL EXAMINATION

The physical examination of a patient with suspected rotator cuff disease should include the "drop arm" test, in which the patient is asked slowly lower the arm from an abducted position. A positive test is seen when the patient is unable to smoothly and slowly lower the arm to the side. The examination should also include thorough manual muscle testing of the specific muscles of the rotator cuff. The supraspinatus is tested by abducting both shoulders 90 degrees in the scapular plane with the thumbs pointed in a cranial direction ("full can") while a downward force is applied to both arms by the examiner. The infraspinatus is tested by resisting external rotation with the elbows at the side. Gerber's lift-off test is a very sensitive indicator for subscapularis weakness[23] (Fig. 10). It is performed by having the patient place the dorsum of the hand against his or her back and then lift the hand away from the spine while resistance is applied to the palm by the examiner. The patient with subscapularis incompetency will be unable to lift the hand away from the back.

IMAGING STUDIES

An impingement series of plain radiographs should include a true anteroposterior (AP) view of the glenohumeral joint, axillary lateral, and supraspinatus outlet. The true AP of the shoulder is performed by angling the beam 30 to 45 degrees from the plane of the thorax and toward the affected side. This view should superimpose the anterior and posterior rims of the glenoid. The axillary lateral is per-

formed by abducting the shoulder up to 90 degrees, if tolerated, while the beam is projected in a cranial direction through the axilla. An os acromiale has been associated with impingement syndrome and can be detected on the axillary lateral view. The supraspinatus outlet view delineates the acromial morphology and is performed by directing the beam parallel to the spine of the scapula in a posterior to anterior direction with 5 to 10 degrees of caudal tilt (Fig. 11).

Magnetic resonance imaging (MRI) has been established as the study of choice to detect soft-tissue disease about the shoulder. MRI has several advantages over traditional arthrography, including absence of radiation exposure, ability to detect partial- and full-thickness cuff tears, and sensitivity to determine tear size, tissue quality, and degree of tendon retraction. Magnetic resonance arthrography with gadolinium contrast placed into the joint can further enhance the diagnostic utility of MRI in the setting of rotator cuff disease.

TREATMENT

The initial treatment of impingement syndrome, rotator cuff tendinitis, and partial-thickness cuff tear is typically nonoperative. The goals are to decrease pain and restore strength and motion. Symptomatic relief can often be achieved with modification of activities to avoid aggravating activities, administration of nonsteroidal anti-inflammatory medications, and application of local modalities such as cryotherapy.

Formal physical therapy can be useful during the initial treatment phase of impingement syndrome. Throwing athletes commonly have loss of internal rotation of the dominant extremity as a result of contracture of the posterior capsule, which can exacerbate subacromial impingement. Exercises should include stretching in adduction and internal rotation to achieve symmetric motion. The strengthening phase of therapy should address all muscles groups used in overhead sports, including the trunk and lower extremity musculature. Painful, repetitive overhead activities are avoided while the goals of normal capsular laxity

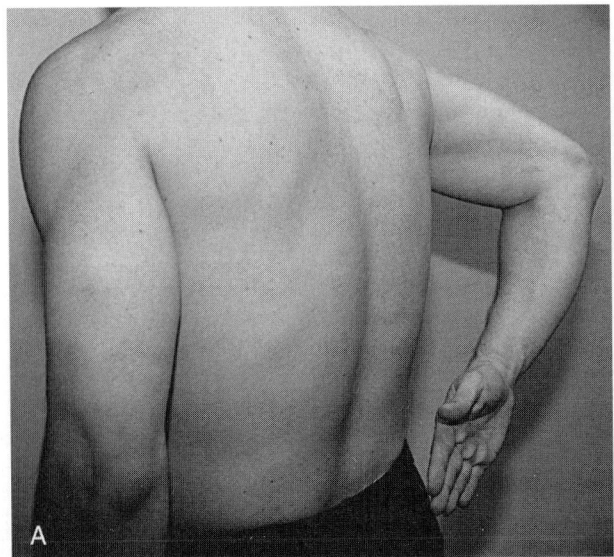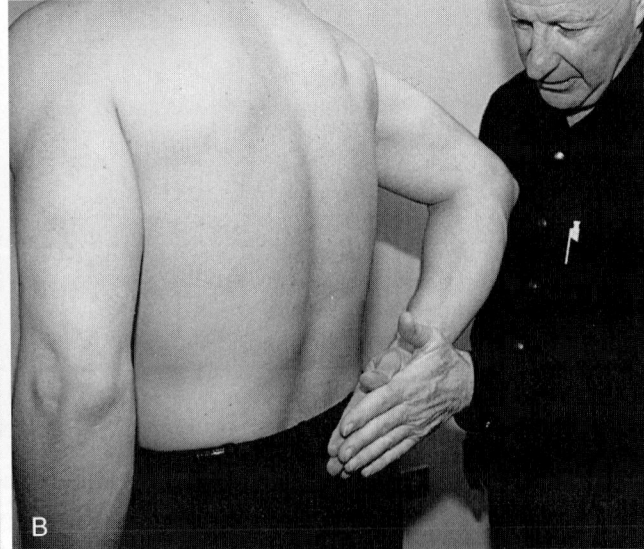

Fig. 10. The lift-off test. (From Rockwood CA, Matsen FA: The Shoulder. Philadelphia, WB Saunders, 1998, 2nd ed, vol 1, p 192.)

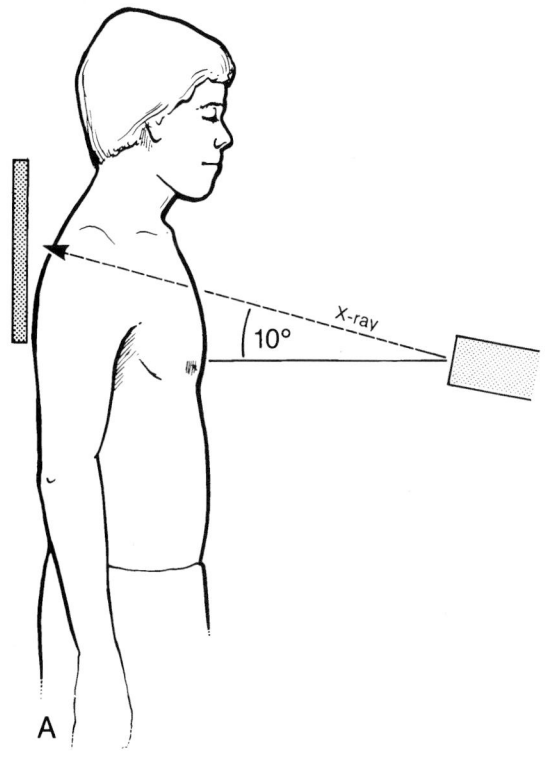

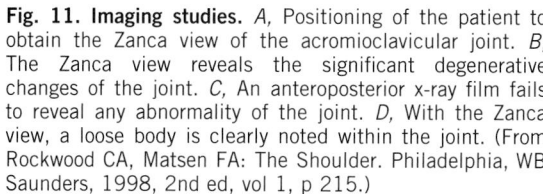

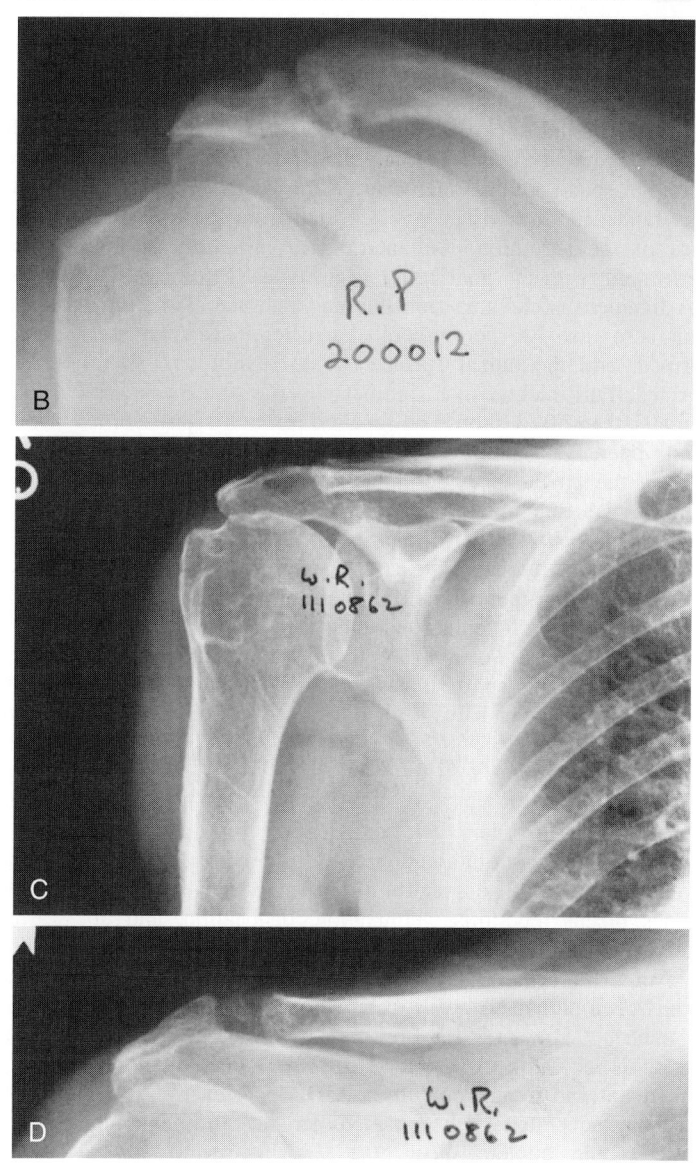

Fig. 11. Imaging studies. *A,* Positioning of the patient to obtain the Zanca view of the acromioclavicular joint. *B,* The Zanca view reveals the significant degenerative changes of the joint. *C,* An anteroposterior x-ray film fails to reveal any abnormality of the joint. *D,* With the Zanca view, a loose body is clearly noted within the joint. (From Rockwood CA, Matsen FA: The Shoulder. Philadelphia, WB Saunders, 1998, 2nd ed, vol 1, p 215.)

and cuff strength are being achieved. Attention is then directed at rotator cuff strengthening to enhance the dynamic stabilizing effect on the glenohumeral joint. This is accomplished through the use of light weights or elastic bands. Finally, the development of the periscapular musculature is important to diminish any secondary ST dyskinesis and to improve the mechanics of the athlete's motion. As symptoms diminish, sport-specific activities are added, such as exercises to enhance the eccentric firing of the cuff during the follow-through phase of the throwing sequence. The limited use of subacromial steroid injections in the refractory case may enhance the success of nonoperative therapy but remains controversial in the younger, athletic population.

Surgical intervention is considered if significant progress is not achieved after a treatment period of approximately 6 to 12 weeks of nonoperative therapy or earlier if evidence of a full-thickness rotator cuff tear is detected. However, the specific length of nonoperative treatment may vary depending on the underlying diagnosis. Younger patients with

full-thickness cuff tears should be considered for early operative intervention to avoid tissue retraction, scarring, or extension of the tear.

Operative treatment may be divided into arthroscopic and open procedures. Arthroscopy has become an essential tool in the diagnosis and treatment of impingement syndrome and rotator cuff disease. The surgical treatment plan can be influenced by the findings of a thorough diagnostic arthroscopy, which may reveal biceps tendinitis, labral disease, glenohumeral arthritis, and rotator cuff disease. Arthroscopic subacromial decompression has become the cornerstone of treatment for patients with primary impingement in whom nonoperative treatment has failed. Most published series demonstrate more than 85% to 90% satisfactory results.[24, 25] The procedure routinely begins with an examination under anesthesia to identify any pathological laxity or loss of motion. If the impingement syndrome is secondary to occult instability, a glenohumeral stabilization procedure should be considered as a vital component of the surgical management.

After the examination of the anesthetized shoulder, a diagnostic arthroscopy is performed to identify any intra-articular disease and to assess the undersurface of the rotator cuff. Partial-thickness tears of less than 50% tendon thickness may benefit from careful débridement. The subacromial space is then entered to perform a decompression. The bursa and soft tissue are débrided from the undersurface of the acromion. An anterior acromioplasty is then performed, with the goal being a flat, type I acromion. The CA ligament is elevated from the undersurface of the anterior acromion. A perihumeral bursectomy is then performed, and the bursal surface of the rotator cuff is inspected. Full-thickness or significant partial-thickness tears (greater than 50%) should be repaired through arthroscopic, "mini-open," or standard open techniques. Rotator cuff repair in the athlete provides reliable relief of pain but can compromise functional status. Therefore, the rate of return to the same level of performance in sports after cuff repair is variable.[27] After surgery, early passive motion is critical with active-assisted isometric exercises beginning at 6 weeks. Exercises to enhance rotator cuff strength are performed between 6 weeks and 3 months after surgery. Final return to overhead sports is achieved typically between 4 to 6 months postoperatively.

BICEPS TENDON DISORDERS

A variety of disorders involving the biceps tendon have been identified as common sources of shoulder pain in the overhead athlete. The spectrum of pathological entities includes biceps tendinitis, subluxation, dislocation, and abnormalities at the biceps anchor and superior labrum. The role of the biceps tendon remains controversial. However, it has been shown to act as a humeral head depressor and to contribute to anterior stability of the shoulder.[7] Biceps tendinitis is frequently associated with concomitant impingement and rotator cuff disease. During elevation of the arm, the biceps tendon becomes vulnerable to impingement between the humeral head, the CA ligament, and the acromial arch.

BICEPS TENDINITIS

The athlete with biceps disease will usually complain of anterior shoulder pain, which is exacerbated by overhead activities and diminished with rest. The symptoms may be masked by coexisting impingement. The physical examination is remarkable for pain with palpation of the tendon in the bicipital groove. The speed test is performed by resist-

ing forward elevation of the arm with the hand held in supination and the elbow extended (Fig. 12). The Yergason test has the patient supinate the forearm against resistance with the elbow flexed at 90 degrees. A positive test produces pain localized to the long head of the biceps tendon.[28]

The most common cause of biceps tendinitis in the athlete is subacromial impingement. Therefore, the initial treatment is directed at eliminating the impingement syndrome. This is accomplished as previously outlined in this chapter. Steroid injection into the bicipital sheath may be of use in the refractory case of biceps tendinitis. Should nonoperative treatment fail, surgical intervention may be considered. The surgical treatment options include tendon débridement, release, or tenodesis.

BICEPS SUBLUXATION

Subluxation of the biceps tendon is occasionally seen in the overhead athlete and most commonly occurs in the setting of subscapularis disruption from the lesser tuberosity. The mechanism of injury can involve forceful extension or external rotation of the abducted shoulder. A tear of the subscapularis insertion may violate the transverse humeral ligament, allowing the biceps tendon to subluxate or dislocate from the bicipital groove. The patient with a suspected biceps tendon subluxation should be carefully assessed for subscapularis rupture with the Gerber "lift-off" test (see Fig. 10).[23] A test for biceps instability can be performed by palpating the tendon in the groove while the arm is held in an abducted/externally rotated position. The arm is subsequently internally rotated and a painful click may be noted as the tendon subluxates over the lesser tuberosity.[29] Operative treatment is generally indicated in the patient with an associated subscapularis tear or chronic, refractory symptoms associated with subluxation.

SUPERIOR LABRAL LESIONS

The superior labrum and biceps anchor are frequent sites of disease in the overhead throwing athlete. A superior labral lesion was found by Andrews et al[30] during an arthroscopic evaluation of throwing athletes with symptoms of shoulder pain, clicking, and popping. This pathological entity has been termed a SLAP lesion because it involves the glenoid attachment of the superior labrum posteriorly and extends anteriorly to the biceps anchor and anterosuperior labrum.[31] This lesion can result from repetitive microtrauma as in a throwing athlete, an eccentric load to the extremity, or the direct trauma of the humeral head being driven up into the

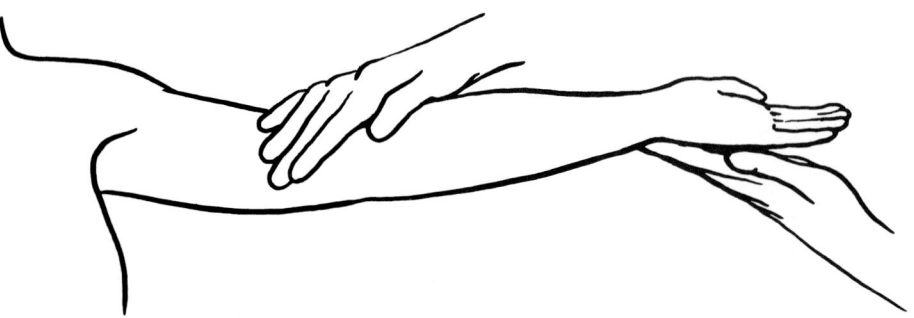

Fig. 12. Speed test. The biceps resistance test is performed with the patient flexing the shoulder against resistance, with the elbow extended and the forearm supinated. Pain referred to the biceps tendon area constitutes a positive test. (From Rockwood CA, Matsen FA: The Shoulder. Philadelphia, WB Saunders, 1998, 2nd ed, vol 1, p 1035.)

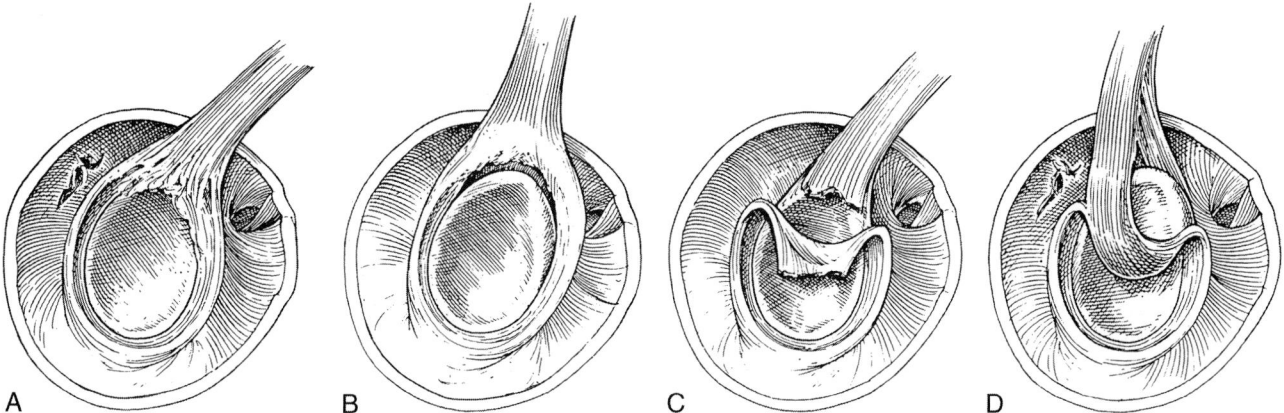

Fig. 13. SLAP lesion classification. *A,* Type I, fraying with intact anchor; *B,* Type II, pathological detachment of the biceps anchor; *C,* Type III, bucket-handle tear with biceps intact; *D,* Type IV, bucket-handle tear into biceps. (In Rockwood CA, Matsen FA: The Shoulder. Philadelphia, WB Saunders, 1998, 2nd ed, vol 1, p 302. From Snyder SJ, Karzel RP, Del Pizzo W, et al: SLAP lesions of the shoulder. Arthroscopy 1990; 6:274.)

superior labrum. SLAP lesions have been associated with partial-thickness tears of the rotator cuff and anterior shoulder instability. Snyder et al[31] classified SLAP lesions into four types based on the anatomic appearance of the lesion, as shown in Figure 13. A type I SLAP lesion involves fraying and degeneration of the labrum with an intact attachment of the superior labrum and biceps anchor to the glenoid. Type II lesions demonstrate detachment of the superior labrum and biceps anchor from the superior rim of the glenoid. A type III SLAP lesion is characterized by a bucket-handle tear of the labrum, with the biceps anchor remaining intact and stable. A type IV lesion has a similar bucket-handle tear of the labrum but also extends into the substance of the biceps tendon with detachment of the biceps anchor.[31]

The clinical presentation of a patient with a SLAP lesion can be variable but typically involves complaints of pain, clicking, or popping felt deep in the shoulder with overhead use of the arm. The physical examination may demonstrate a positive speed or Yergason test. O'Brien et al[32] described a test to differentiate between a SLAP lesion and AC joint disease. The O'Brien active compression test is performed by having the standing patient forward flex the arm to 90 degrees with the elbow in full extension. The arm is then adducted 10 to 15 degrees and internally rotated so that the thumb points toward the floor. The examiner stands behind the patient and applies a downward force to the arm while the patient resists. The maneuver is then repeated with the arm in the same position but the palm fully supinated. The test is considered positive for a SLAP lesion when pain is worse with the first maneuver and is felt "inside" the shoulder. AC disease is suspected when the pain is "on top" of the shoulder.[32] MRI and particularly MR arthrography can be helpful in the diagnosis of a SLAP lesion. However, the gold standard for diagnosis remains the arthroscopic examination with direct inspection and probing.

The indications for surgical management of superior labral lesions remain controversial. However, depending on the type of lesion, associated injuries, and the specific demands of the athlete, most authors recommend an initial trial of nonoperative management. This regimen should include activity modification and strengthening of the rotator cuff, biceps, deltoid, and periscapular muscles. Surgical treatment options include débridement of a frayed labrum and tendon in type I and type III lesions, repair of the biceps anchor in type II lesions, and biceps tenodesis for type IV SLAP lesions.

INJURIES TO THE ACROMIOCLAVICULAR JOINT

ACUTE INJURIES
Acute injuries to the AC joint are very common in a variety of contact sports such as football, ice hockey, and rugby. These injuries can be the result of either direct, acute trauma or chronic repetitive microtrauma, which produces degenerative joint changes. The most common mechanisms for an acute traumatic injury are a fall onto the shoulder or a direct blow to the acromion. This results in the "separated" shoulder, which accounts for 12% of the dislocations of the shoulder girdle.[33] As previously discussed, the AC ligaments provide horizontal stability to the joint, whereas the coracoclavicular ligaments are responsible for vertical stability. The Rockwood modification of the classic Allman-Tossy classification of AC joint injuries includes six types and is based on the extent and pattern of the ligamentous injury[33–35] (Fig. 14).

Type I AC separation involves a sprain or incomplete injury to the AC ligaments, whereas the coracoclavicular ligaments remain intact. The physical examination reveals focal tenderness over the joint and pain with cross-body adduction. The radiographic examination demonstrates no displacement of the distal clavicle, and the coracoclavicular interval is equal to the opposite side. Type II AC separations are characterized by disruption of the AC ligament, whereas the coracoclavicular ligaments remain intact. Radiographs may reveal up to 50% displacement of the distal clavicle and a similar increase in the coracoclavicular distance. Type I and type II injuries are treated symptomatically in the acute setting with ice and a shoulder sling followed by therapy to regain motion and strength. Chronic

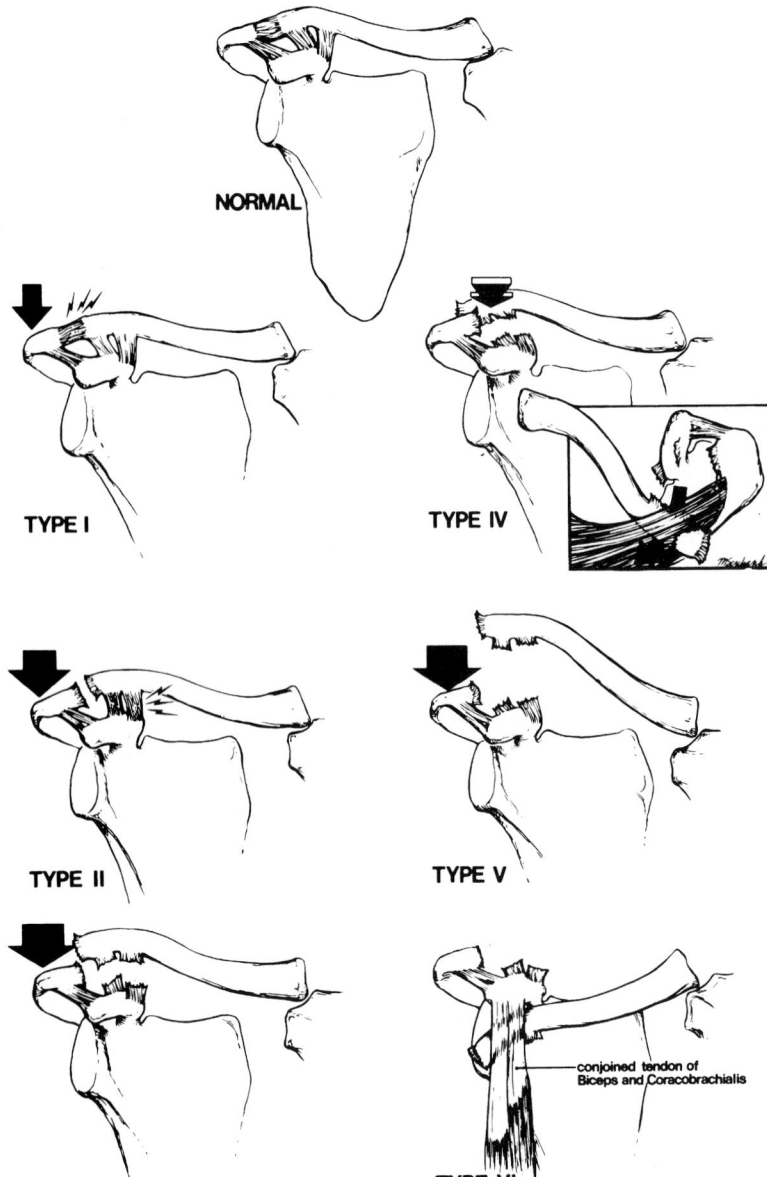

NORMAL

TYPE I

TYPE II

TYPE III

TYPE IV

TYPE V

TYPE VI

conjoined tendon of Biceps and Coracobrachialis

Fig. 14. Schematic drawings of acromioclavicular ligament injuries. (From Rockwood CA, Matsen FA: The Shoulder. Philadelphia, WB Saunders, 1998, 2nd ed, vol 1, p 495.)

symptoms after a type I or II AC joint injury may require distal clavicle resection with formal coracoclavicular stabilization.[37]

In type III injuries, both the AC and the coracoclavicular ligaments are disrupted. On physical examination, deformity and tenderness of the AC joint are noted. Displacement in type III injuries can range from 50% to 100%. Stress views with 10- to 15-lb weights in each hand may be helpful to compare the coracoclavicular distance of the injured shoulder to the normal side. Treatment of type III injuries remains controversial. Most authors advocate nonoperative treatment, consisting of ice and a period of immobilization followed by exercises to regain motion and strength. The most common complication of nonoperative treatment is a cosmetic deformity. Several studies demonstrated no significant difference in pain, strength, or function compared with surgical results.

However, concern over residual symptoms in the athletic population has led some authors to advocate surgical management of acute grade III injuries in the competitive athlete or manual laborer.[38] Others recommend surgical intervention only for patients with persistent symptoms refractory to rehabilitation.[39] Popular surgical treatment options include coracoclavicular fixation with the use of screws or a modified Weaver-Dunn procedure, which involves limited distal clavicle resection, transfer of the CA ligament, and stabilization of the coracoclavicular interval with suture, soft tissue, or hardware. Complications of surgical treatment are common and include postoperative loss of reduction and hardware failure. More favorable results have been reported after acute surgical reconstruction when performed within 3 months after the injury.[38]

Type IV AC dislocations involve complete dislocation of the distal clavicle with posterior displacement penetrating the trapezius muscle. A type V injury is defined by dislocation of the AC joint with a coracoclavicular interval more than twice normal (greater than 100% displacement). A type VI dislocation is a rare injury involving inferior dislocation of the distal clavicle into a subcoracoid position. Because of the severe nature of type IV, V, and VI injuries, initial surgical intervention is usually indicated. Surgical options include AC fixation or coracoclavicular interval fixation, or a combination. The most recent trend favors coracoclavicular fixation with braided suture or screws. The postoperative regimen for these patients may include up to 6 weeks in a sling to prevent displacement followed by motion and strengthening exercises.

CHRONIC INJURIES

The AC joint is the frequent site of disease related to repetitive, overuse injuries in the athletic population. With chronic loading or after a traumatic injury, degenerative changes can occur within the AC joint, which may produce symptoms in the active patient. Joint space narrowing, cysts, and osteophytes may result. A related condition involves osteolysis of the distal clavicle, which is seen predominantly in weight lifters.[40] Symptoms are isolated to the AC joint and are exacerbated with activities that load the joint. An AC joint injection with lidocaine may assist in confirmation of the diagnosis. Initial treatment of both degenerative AC joint disease and osteolysis may include activity modification, nonsteroidal anti-inflammatory medications, and a steroid injection. In the refractory case, distal clavicle resection can provide reliable results and allow return to overhead sports.

INJURIES TO THE SC JOINT

Injury to SC joint is an uncommon but potentially significant occurrence in the athletic population and can result from either direct or indirect trauma. The SC joint is stabilized by the SC and costoclavicular ligaments, which may be sprained during a traumatic injury. Dislocations of the SC joint are rare and account for only 3% of all fractures or dislocations of the shoulder girdle.[33] In the skeletally

immature patient, epiphyseal fractures are more common than ligamentous disruption or dislocation and should be considered in the differential diagnosis.

The majority of traumatic SC dislocations are anterior and are easily detected by noting the prominent medial end of the clavicle lying anterior to the sternum. A posterior SC dislocation is a potentially life-threatening injury resulting from compromise of the trachea, esophagus, or adjacent large vessels (Fig. 15). Signs of dyspnea, dysphagia, venous congestion, or hemodynamic instability should alert the physician to the possibility of these injuries and should be considered a surgical emergency. The diagnosis of an SC dislocation can be facilitated by a radiographic examination, which may include an AP and lateral chest radiograph and a serendipity view (30- to 40-degree cephalic tilt). The radiographs may demonstrate asymmetry of the SC on the AP view and AP displacement on the serendipity image. Computed tomography can be used to confirm a suspected dislocation.

Therapy for minor SC joint injuries without instability, subluxation, or dislocation involves symptomatic treatment with ice, brief immobilization, and gradual return to activities as strength and motion return. Joint subluxation can be treated with reduction, if necessary, followed by a similar but often more prolonged period of immobilization. For anterior dislocation of the SC joint, reduction may be attempted with adequate anesthesia followed by lateral traction and manual pressure on the medial clavicle. Immobilization is usually continued for a minimum of 2 to 3 weeks. Loss of reduction is common and typically does not require surgical intervention.

A posterior SC dislocation may be reduced by abduction and extension of the shoulder over a posterior fulcrum such as rolled towels or a sandbag placed along the thoracic spine. Reduction may require careful grasping of the clavicle manually or with an instrument such as a towel clip. As stated previously, any signs of hemodynamic or airway compromise require emergent reduction in consultation with a cardiothoracic specialist. If closed reduction fails, consideration may be given to open reduction and stabilization of the joint. Symptomatic, chronic instability of the

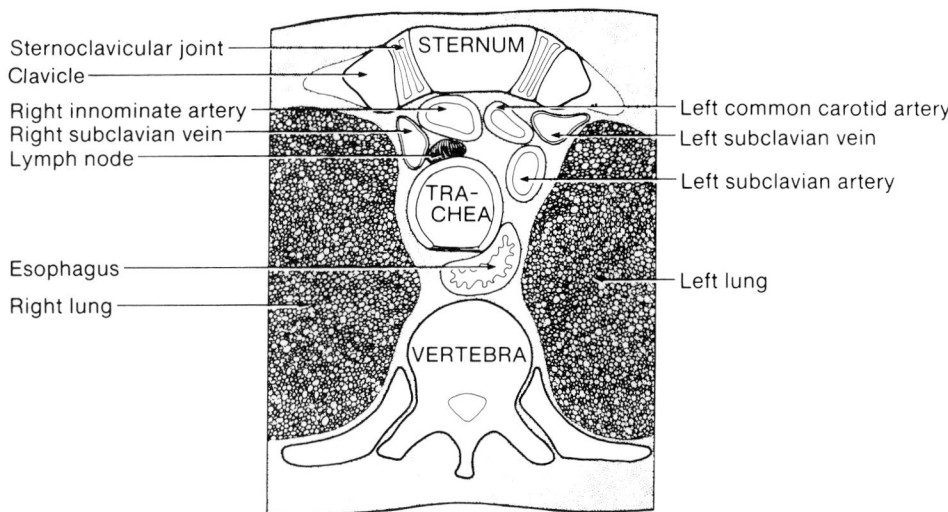

Fig. 15. Applied anatomy of the vital structures posterior to the sternoclavicular joint. Sagittal view in cross-section demonstrates the structures posterior to the sternoclavicular joint. (From Rockwood CA, Matsen FA: The Shoulder. Philadelphia, WB Saunders, 1998, 2nd ed, vol 1, p 560.)

Labels in figure:
Sternoclavicular joint
Clavicle
Right innominate artery
Right subclavian vein
Lymph node
Esophagus
Right lung
STERNUM
Left common carotid artery
Left subclavian vein
Left subclavian artery
Left lung
TRACHEA
VERTEBRA

SC joint may require surgical intervention with the options of stabilization versus medial clavicle resection proximal to the costoclavicular ligaments to avoid clavicular instability.[42]

ST INJURIES

The ST articulation is an infrequent but potentially disabling source of pain and dysfunction in the athletic population. The most common conditions include ST bursitis and crepitus. The anatomy of the ST articulation is marked by the presence of a complex series of bursae lying between the chest wall, the subscapularis muscle, and the serratus anterior muscle. The most common sites of clinical symptoms in this region are the superomedial border and the inferior angle of the scapula.[43] Bursitis in these regions can arise from overuse or dyskinetic shoulder mechanics and may be associated with audible or palpable crepitus. Crepitus may be related to the associated inflammatory bursitis or to an underlying bony abnormality. Numerous structures can produce ST crepitus, including, for example, osteochondromas, bone spurs, rib fractures, hooked scapulae, fibrotic or anomalous muscles, incongruent ST articulations, and elastofibromas.

Physical examination of a patient with ST bursitis may reveal focal tenderness over a region of the scapula or chest wall, mild fullness over the bursa, palpable crepitus with motion, and scapular winging or dyskinesis. Radiographs may be obtained to evaluate the articulation and to rule out underlying bony abnormalities. CT scan is useful to further define the bony anatomy and to enhance findings not well visualized by plain radiography. MRI may assist in the evaluation of the location and size of the affected bursa.

The initial treatment of ST bursitis is nonoperative and includes activity modification, rest, and nonsteroidal antiinflammatory medications. Secondary treatment may include formal physical therapy for periscapular exercises, local modalities such as ultrasonography, and a carefully placed corticosteroid injection into the inflamed bursa. Physical therapy should focus on postural changes to decrease thoracic kyphosis and strengthening of the serratus anterior and subscapularis musculature to enhance soft-tissue interposition between the scapula and the chest wall.

Patients with refractory symptoms may be candidates for surgical intervention. Both open and arthroscopic techniques for bursectomy and scapular resection have been described. Sisto and Jobe[44] reported the results of open bursectomy with bony resection at the inferior border of the scapula in four major league baseball pitchers, all of whom returned to competition at the professional level. For bursitis at the superomedial border of the scapula, McCluskey and Bigliani described a similar procedure of open bursectomy and bony resection with 89% good or excellent results.[45] Arthroscopic management of ST bursitis has been reported by Ciullo and Jones[46] in a series of 13 patients who underwent bursectomy and scapuloplasty. Satisfactory results were reported in all cases.[46]

REFERENCES

1. Hill JA: Epidemiological perspective on shoulder injuries. Clin Sports Med 1983; 2:24.
2. Saha AK: Mechanics of elevation of the glenohumeral joint. Acta Orthop Scand 1973; 44:668.
3. O'Brien SJ, Neves MC, Arnoczky SP, et al: The anatomy and histology of the inferior glenohumeral ligament complex of the shoulder. Am J Sports Med 1990; 18:449.
4. Warner JJP, Flatow EL: Anatomy and biomechanics. In Bigliani LU (ed): The Unstable Shoulder. Rosemont, IL, American Academy of Orthopaedic Surgeons, 1995, p 1.
5. Warner JJP: The gross anatomy of the joint surfaces, ligaments, labrum, and capsule. In Matsen FA III, Fu FH, Hawkins RJ (eds): The Shoulder: A Balance of Mobility and Stability. Rosemont, IL, American Academy of Orthopaedic Surgeons, 1993, p 7.
6. Cain PR, Mutschler TA, Fu FH, et al: Anterior stability of the glenohumeral joint: A dynamic model. Am J Sports Med 1987; 15:144.
7. Rodosky MW, Harner CD, Fu FH: The role of the long head of the biceps muscle and superior glenoid labrum in anterior stability of the shoulder. Am J Sports Med 1994; 22:121.
8. Dillman CJ, Fleisig GS, Werner SL, et al: Biomechanics of the shoulder in sports: Throwing activities. In Matsen FA III, Fu FH, Hawkins RJ (eds): The Shoulder: A Balance of Mobility and Stability. Rosemont, IL, American Academy of Orthopaedic Surgeons, 1993, p 621.
9. Pappas ZM, Zawacki RM, Sullivan TJ: Biomechanics of baseball pitching: A preliminary report. Am J Sports Med 1985; 13:216.
10. Jobe FW, Moynes DR, Tibone JE: An EMG analysis of the shoulder in pitching: A second report. Am J Sports Med 1984; 12:218.
11. Richardson AB, Jobe FW, Collins HR: The shoulder in swimming competition. Am J Sports Med 1980; 81:159.
12. Codman EA: Complete rupture of the supraspinatus tendon: Operative treatment with report of two successful cases. Boston Med Surg J 1911; 164:708.
13. Codman EA: The Shoulder: Rupture of the Supraspinatus Tendon and Other Lesions in or about the Subacromial Bursa. Boston, Thomas Todd, 1934.
14. Neer CS II: Anterior acromioplasty for the chronic impingement syndrome of the shoulder: A preliminary report. J Bone Joint Surg Am 1972; 54:41.
15. Neer CS II: Impingement lesions. Clin Orthop 1983; 173:70.
16. Bigliani LU, Ticker JB, Flatow EL, et al: The relationship of acromial architecture to rotator cuff disease. Clin Sports Med 1991; 10:823.
17. Fu FH, Harner CD, Klein AH: Shoulder impingement syndrome. Clin Orthop 1991; 269:162.
18. Jobe FW, Tibone JE, Jobe CM, et al: The shoulder in sports. In Rockwood CA, Matsen FA III (eds): The Shoulder. Philadelphia, WB Saunders, 1990, p 961.
19. Walch G, Boileau P, Noel E, et al: Impingement of the deep surface of the supraspinatus tendon on the posterior-superior rim: An arthroscopic study. J Shoulder Elbow Surg 1992; 1:238.
20. Jobe CM: Superior glenoid impingement. Orthop Clin North Am 1992; 28:137.
21. Dines DM, Warren RF, Inglis AE, et al: The coracoid impingement syndrome. J Bone Joint Surg Br 1990; 72:314.
22. Gartsman GM: Arthroscopic treatment of rotator cuff disease. J Shoulder Elbow Surg 1995; 4:228.
23. Gerber C, Krushell RJ: Isolated rupture of the tendon of the subscapularis muscle: Clinical features in 16 cases. J Bone Joint Surg Br 1991; 73:389.
24. Paulos LE, Franklin JL: Arthroscopic shoulder development and application: A five-year experience. Am J Sports Med 1990; 18:235.
25. Gartsman GM: Arthroscopic acromioplasty for lesions of the rotator cuff. J Bone Joint Surg Am 1990; 72:169.
26. Olsewski JM, Depew AD: Arthroscopic subacromial decompression and rotator cuff debridement for stage II and III impingement. Arthroscopy 1994; 10:61.
27. Tibone JE, Elrod B, Jobe FW, et al: Surgical treatment of tears of the rotator cuff in athletes. J Bone Joint Surg Am 1986; 68:887.
28. Yergason RM: Supination sign. J Bone Joint Surg 1931; 13:160.

29. Burkhead WZ: The biceps tendon. In Rockwood CA Jr, Matsen FA III (eds): The Shoulder. Philadelphia, WB Saunders, 1990, p 791.
30. Andrews JR, Carson WG, McLeod WD: Glenoid labrum tears related to the long head of the biceps. Am J Sports Med 1985; 13:337.
31. Snyder SJ, Kanzel RP, Del Pizzo W, et al: SLAP lesions of the shoulder. Arthroscopy 1990; 6:274.
32. O'Brien SJ, Pagnani MJ: The active compression test: A new and effective test for diagnosing labral tears and acromioclavicular joint abnormality. Am J Sports Med 1998; 26:610.
33. Cave EM: Fractures and Other Injuries. Chicago, Year Book, 1958.
34. Allman FL Jr: Fractures and injuries of the clavicle and its articulation. J Bone Joint Surg Am 1967; 49:774.
35. Tossy JD, Mead NC, Sigmond HM: Acromioclavicular separations: Useful and practical classification for treatment. Clin Orthop 1963; 28:111.
36. Williams GR, Nguyen VD, Rockwood CA Jr: Classification and radiographic analysis of acromioclavicular dislocations. Appl Radiol 1989; 18:29.
37. Flatow EL, Duralde XA, Nicholson GP, et al: Arthroscopic resection of the distal clavicle with a superior approach. J Shoulder Elbow Surg 1995; 4:41.
38. Weinstein DM, McCann DM, McIlveen SJ, et al: Surgical treatment of complete acromioclavicular dislocations. Am J Sports Med 1995; 23:324.
39. Rowes ML, Dias JJ: Long term results of conservative treatment of acromioclavicular dislocation. J Bone Joint Surg Br 1996; 78:410.
40. Madsen B: Osteolysis of the acromial end of the clavicle following trauma. Br J Radiol 1963; 36:822.
41. Cook F, Tibone JE: The Mumford procedure in athletes. Am J Sports Med 1988; 16:97.
42. Rockwood CA Jr, Grohl GL, Wirth MA, et al: Resection arthroplasty of the sternoclavicular joint. Journal of Bone Joint Surg Am 1997; 79:387.
43. Kuhn JE, Hawkins RJ: Evaluation and treatment of scapular disorders. In Warner JJP, Ianotti JP, Gerber C (eds): Complex and Revision Problems in Shoulder Surgery. Philadelphia, Lippincott-Raven, 1997, p 357.
44. Sisto DJ, Jobe FW: The operative treatment of scapulothoracic bursitis in professional pitchers. Am J Sports Med 1986; 14:192.
45. McCluskey GM III, Bigliani LU: Surgical management of refractory scapulothoracic bursitis. Orthop Trans 1991; 15:801.
46. Ciullo JV, Jones E: Subscapular bursitis: Conservative and endoscopic treatment of "snapping scapula" or "washboard syndrome." Orthop Trans 1992-1993; 16:740.

section
4
chapter
7

DIAGNOSIS OF SHOULDER INSTABILITY AND LABRUM INJURIES

Henry T. Leis and Mark D. Miller

Summary
- The shoulder is the most commonly dislocated major joint in the body.
- Anterior dislocation represents 84% of all shoulder dislocations.
- In patients in whom initial shoulder dislocation occurs before age 20 years, the rate of recurrence is 90%.
- The inferior glenohumeral ligament is the primary restraint to anterior and posterior translation.
- The advances in magnetic resonance imaging (MRI) technology have led to an 88% to 100% sensitivity for diagnosis of labral injury.

HISTORICAL PERSPECTIVE

Shoulder instability and its sequelae have a long history in the annals of medical practice, dating back as far as 300 BC, as recorded in the Edwin Smith Papyrus.[1] Hippocrates described reduction of anterior dislocations in which the physician places a foot upon the chest wall in the axilla.[1] In addition, he described the standard of care in 400 BC for anterior instability, including surgical treatment that utilized a hot poker to scarify the anterior capsule and soft tissues.[2, 3] Modern medicine has expanded our understanding of the anatomy, pathology, and biomechanics of the shoulder. With technological advances, such as shoulder arthroscopy, we are constantly pushing the boundaries of treatment in search of the definitive treatment of shoulder instability and its related sequelae. Understanding the relationships among biomechanics, function, injury, and stability has become more critical with modern technology and the greater prevalence rate of high-demand activities in recreational athletes.

CLASSIFICATION

Several schemes have been developed to classify acute shoulder dislocations and shoulder instability. The most useful are those that help the surgeon determine the optimal treatment for the given pathological condition. Common classifications for shoulder dislocations are those based on the direction of instability. Anterior dislocations are subdivided into (1) subcoracoid, (2) subglenoid, (3) subclavicular, and (4) intrathoracic types. Posterior dislocations have been subdivided into (1) subacromial, (2) subglenoid, and (3) subspinous varieties. The remaining dislocations are superior and inferior (luxatio erecta). In addition, acute shoulder dislocations can be classified according to the extent of instability: that is, subluxation versus dislocation.

A more widely accepted classification of shoulder instability is employed by two commonly used systems, those of Matsen[4] and Warren.[5] Matsen and colleagues[4] described two broad categories of pathology that do not depend on the specific structures injured. The two categories are traumatic unidirectional instability and atraumatic multidirectional instability, usually bilateral. Mnemonics that are useful for treatment are as follows:

- TUBS: *T*raumatic *U*nidirectional instability with a *B*ankart lesion, which usually requires *S*urgery for correction.
- AMBRI: *A*traumatic *M*ultidirectional instability usually involving *B*ilateral shoulders, which is treated with *R*ehabilitation or, if surgery is required, an *I*nferior capsular shift.

The useful characteristic of this system is that the origins, pathological findings, and treatment are included within the classification.[4]

The Warren scheme is more complex. In an attempt to determine optimal treatment modalities, the scheme focuses on (1) direction, (2) frequency, (3) cause, and (4) degree of instability.[5] There currently is no universally accepted classification for instability of the glenohumeral joint.

NATURAL HISTORY

The shoulder is the most commonly dislocated major joint in the body.[6] Anterior glenohumeral dislocations represent 84% of all dislocations about the shoulder, acromioclavicular dislocations 12%, sternoclavicular dislocations 2.5%, and posterior glenohumeral dislocations only 1.5%.[7] The most common complication following traumatic anterior shoulder dislocation and instability is recurrence of instability. Patient age has been shown to be inversely proportional to the rate of recurrence. Debaradino and associates,[8] in a study of U.S. Military Academy cadets, demonstrated a recurrence rate of 87% after nonsurgical treatment, which consisted of closed reduction, immobilization for 3 to 6 weeks, activity restriction, and supervised physical therapy.

Patients older than 40 years at the time of shoulder dislocation have a lower recurrence rate. However, complications after dislocations are more common in this age group. The complications include, but are not limited to, rotator cuff tears and neurological injury. Neviaser and Neviaser[9] reported on 12 patients, all older than 40 years, with recurrent instability. Eleven of the 12 had anterior instability, and all of those with anterior instability had ruptures of both the subscapularis muscle and the anterior capsule.

ANATOMY AND BIOMECHANICS

The shoulder "joint" is actually composed of four separate articulations moving in an intercalary manner. The four joints are the sternoclavicular (SC) joint, the acromioclavicular (AC) joint, the glenohumeral (GH) joint, and the scapulothoracic (ST) joint. They work synergistically to allow extensive range of motion of the shoulder. The articulation between the glenoid and the humeral head allows for 120 degrees of passive motion. The scapulothoracic articulation allows for 60 degrees of outward rotation of the scapula in full abduction and flexion. The joint moves 1 degree for every 2 degrees of movement of the GH joint. Forward flexion is increased by sternoclavicular joint rotation of 45 to 50 degrees and elevation of 35 degrees. A variable amount of elevation is reported in the literature for the AC joint, from 5 to 20 degrees of elevation.

Stability of the shoulder joint is inversely proportional to the range of motion. Thus, stability is sacrificed to allow for circumduction of the joint. Although most joints have a stable bony architecture that provides primary stability, the GH joint has very little inherent stability from bony anatomy. The articular surface of the humeral head is extremely large in comparison with the glenoid. The humeral head is spherical, but the glenoid is oval and does not exactly match the humeral head. The glenohumeral index, which represents the diameter of the glenoid divided by the diameter of the humeral head, is approximately 0.75 in the sagittal plane and 0.6 in the transverse plane.[10] This GH mismatch, in addition to a low radius of curvature of the glenoid fossa, allows for translation of the humeral head on the glenoid that may represent an important factor in both normal and pathological motion of the shoulder.[11] In addition, the orientation of the articular surfaces of the glenoid and the humeral head may contribute to instability.

The humeral head is retroverted 30 degrees in relation to the shaft of the humerus. The glenoid is 7 degrees retroverted in relation to the body of the scapula and tilted superiorly 5 degrees. The scapula is oriented 45 degrees anterior in relation to the sagittal plane; this amounts to 35 to 40 degrees of anteversion of the glenoid.[12]

Stability of the GH joint is influenced most by the surrounding soft tissues, including the labrum, capsule, ligaments, and shoulder muscles, especially the rotator cuff. The labrum is composed of a cartilaginous ring attached to the bony rim of the glenoid. The labrum, which effectively doubles the depth of the glenoid, functions to maintain the humeral head in the glenoid.[13] The labrum functions to block the humeral head from anterior and posterior translation on the glenoid fossa. In addition, the labrum serves as an anchor for the glenoid origin of the inferior GH ligament. The inferior aspect of the labrum is the key to anterior stability of the GH joint.[14] The superior labrum does not seem to play as important a role in stability and often exhibits a normal defect at the superior margin.[15] Stability is also aided statically by a vacuum phenomenon created by the relative negative pressure within the joint in relation to outside atmospheric pressure. The negative pressure creates a "suction effect" when the GH joint is distracted, helping to keep the humeral head contained within the glenoid.[16, 17]

The three GH ligaments, in close association with the capsule, are more accurately described as capsuloligamentous structures. The *superior glenohumeral ligament* (SGHL) and *coracohumeral ligament* (CHL) are important static stabilizers of the shoulder. They are located between the superior surface of the subscapularis and the biceps tendon (Fig. 1).

Boardman and colleagues[18] found that in comparison with the SGHL, the CHL is four times larger in cross-sectional area, is twice as stiff, and can withstand three times the ultimate load before failure.[18] Together, the SGHL and CHL act to decrease inferior translation in forward flexion, adduction, and internal rotation. The SGHL takes origin from the supraglenoid tubercle, anterior to the origin of the long head of the biceps, and inserts onto the anterior anatomic neck, near the lesser tuberosity.

The *middle glenohumeral ligament* (MGHL) also takes origin from the supraglenoid tubercle and joins the posterior tendon of the subscapularis before inserting on the lesser tuberosity. The MGHL resists anterior translation of

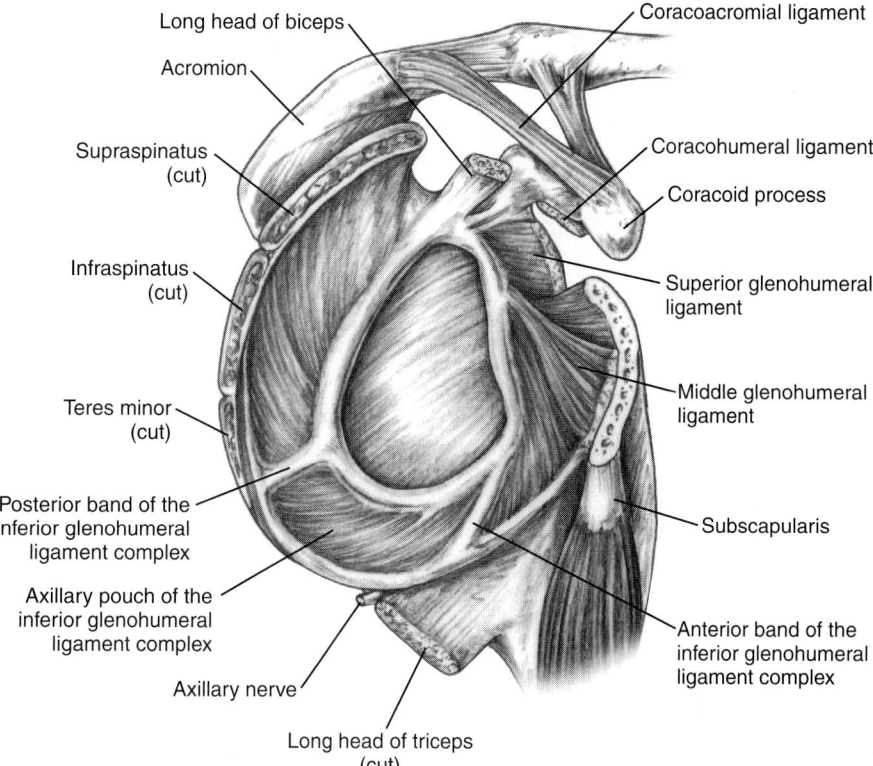

Fig. 1. Glenohumeral ligaments. Note the relationships of the superior, middle, and inferior ligaments, which are intimately related to the shoulder capsule. (From Turkel SJ, Panio MW, Marshall JL, et al: Stabilizing mechanisms preventing anterior dislocation of the glenohumeral joint. J Bone Joint Surg Am 1981; 63:1209.)

Long head of biceps

Acromion

Supraspinatus (cut)

Infraspinatus (cut)

Teres minor (cut)

Posterior band of the inferior glenohumeral ligament complex

Axillary pouch of the inferior glenohumeral ligament complex

Axillary nerve

Long head of triceps (cut)

Coracoacromial ligament

Coracohumeral ligament

Coracoid process

Superior glenohumeral ligament

Middle glenohumeral ligament

Subscapularis

Anterior band of the inferior glenohumeral ligament complex

the humerus, especially when the arm is abducted and externally rotated. The most variable in size of the glenohumeral ligaments, the MGHL is absent or poorly defined in 40% of patients. The MGHL can be extraordinarily thickened into a cordlike structure; when this is the case, it has been referred to as a Buford complex.[19]

The *inferior glenohumeral ligament* (IGHL) is actually a complex composed of three segments: (1) the anterior band, (2) a smaller posterior band, and (3) an axillary pouch between the two bands. The IGHL is considered the largest and most important ligament. It serves as the primary restraint to anterior and posterior translation in external and internal rotation. In abduction, the ligament serves as a secondary restraint to inferior translation. The findings of studies in which cadaveric specimens were tested to quantitate the contribution of capsular structures to stability indicate that the primary anteroposterior (AP) stabilizer of the abducted shoulder is the IGHL.[20] The anterior band was found to be stiffest and to serve as the primary stabilizer at 30 degrees of horizontal extension and at neutral. The posterior band was found to be the primary stabilizer in 30 degrees of horizontal flexion. The IGHL functions as a supportive structure for the humeral head, analogous to a sling. The supportive function of the IGHL is accentuated in abduction and external rotation, in which it functions as the primary ligamentous stabilizer in the shoulder (Fig. 2).[16, 20–22]

The *rotator cuff* comprises four muscles: supraspinatus, infraspinatus, teres minor, and subscapularis (SITS). The rotator cuff and the long head of the biceps tendon together provide dynamic stability to the GH joint. The supraspinatus is the primary abductor and, with the biceps

tendon, it resists inferior translation and superior migration of the humeral head. The infraspinatus is the primary external rotator of the shoulder. The teres minor is a secondary external rotator of the shoulder. The subscapularis is the primary internal rotator of the shoulder; along with the MGHL and IGHL, this muscle acts as a buttress resisting subluxation and dislocation of the humeral head. The rotator cuff muscles are critical in providing stability during dynamic phases of shoulder motion. The rotator cuff acts to center the humeral head on the glenoid; these muscles also help to actively contain the humeral head. During abduction, the other rotator cuff muscles act as depressors, and the supraspinatus and deltoid muscles act as primary abductors; this antagonistic action by the infraspinatus, teres minor, and subscapularis muscles helps prevent impingement of the humeral head.[16, 22]

PATHOLOGICAL FEATURES

The pathological condition associated with anterior instability is often multifactorial; however, certain lesions manifest as more constant findings. The following three classic lesions are associated with anterior instability:

- Detachment of the labrum from the anterior inferior glenoid (Bankart's essential lesion), the most common finding with anterior instability.
- Capsular injury with increased capsular volume.[23, 24]
- Posterosuperior humeral head impression fracture (Hill-Sachs lesion).

The Hill-Sachs lesion should not be confused with flattening of the posterolateral humeral head that is normal.

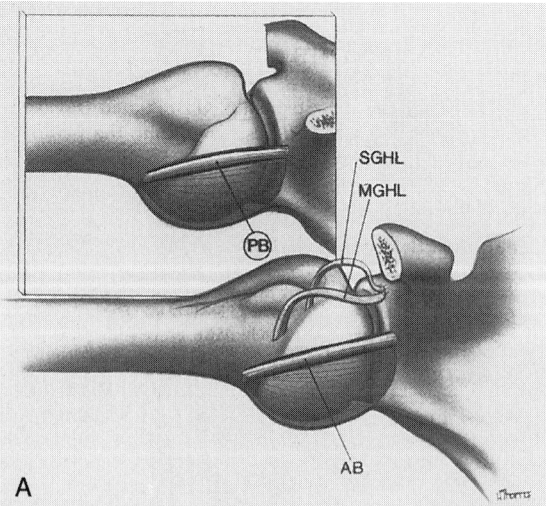
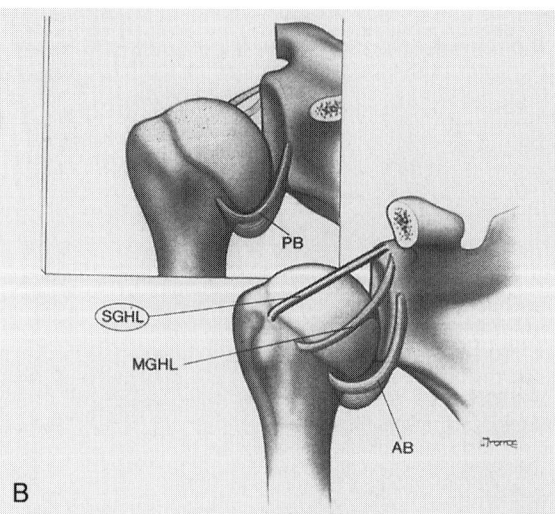

Fig. 2. View. The superior and middle glenohumeral ligaments tighten with adduction and external rotation. (SGHL = superior glenohumeral ligament; MGHL = middle glenohumeral ligament; AB = anterior band [of the inferior glenohumeral ligament complex]; PB = posterior band [of the inferior glenohumeral ligament complex].) (From Warner JJP, Deng X-H, Warren RF, et al: Static capsuloligamentous restraints to superior-inferior translation of the glenohumeral joint. Am J Sports Med 1992; 20:682.)

This flattening is seen below the level of the coracoid, and a Hill-Sachs lesion is seen above the level of the coracoid (Figs. 3 to 5).

Bankart's lesions are defined as involving any disruption of the attachment of the anterior labrum to the glenoid rim. Historically, Perthes[25] was actually the first to recognize that damage to the anterior labrum often led to chronic anterior instability. The "essential lesion" that Bankart[26] later described is classically defined as labral detachment of the IGHL complex from the bony glenoid. Bankart's lesions are commonly associated with traumatic anterior shoulder dislocations. Although this lesion has been recognized as the main source of anterior instability after acute traumatic injury, other injuries may contribute to recurrent shoulder instability. An example would be injury to the anterior capsular ligament. The presence of a Bankart lesion alone is not sufficient to cause shoulder dislocation; therefore, there must be at least one other concomitant injury.[11] Capsular injury or injury to the IGHL most commonly occurs with labral tears and leads to residual instability.

Diagnostic arthroscopy has become exceedingly helpful in localizing the associated injury with anterior instability. Arthroscopy has further expanded the available information about the pathology of capsular injuries, ligamentous injuries, and labral injuries. Capsuloligamentous laxity and its contribution as a cause of multidirectional instability have been increasingly recognized over the past decade.[27] Special effort should be made to determine whether there is a predominant direction to the instability, and surgery should

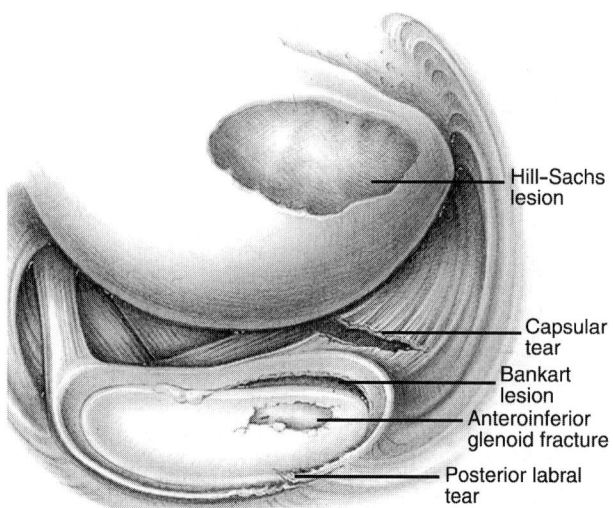

Hill-Sachs lesion

Capsular tear

Bankart lesion

Anteroinferior glenoid fracture

Posterior labral tear

Fig. 3. Hill-Sachs lesion. This radiograph demonstrates the posterolateral humeral head impaction fracture secondary to anterior dislocation. The Hill-Sachs lesion should not be confused with the normal flattening of the humeral head seen at the level of the coracoid.

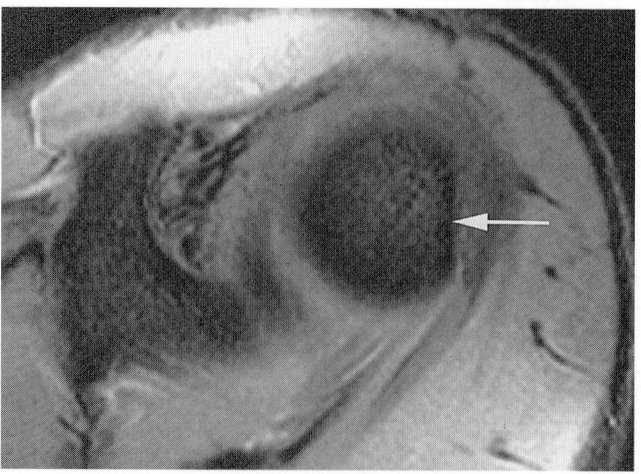

Fig. 4. MRI view. This demonstrates the posterolateral humeral head impression fracture seen with a Hill-Sachs lesion (*white arrow*).

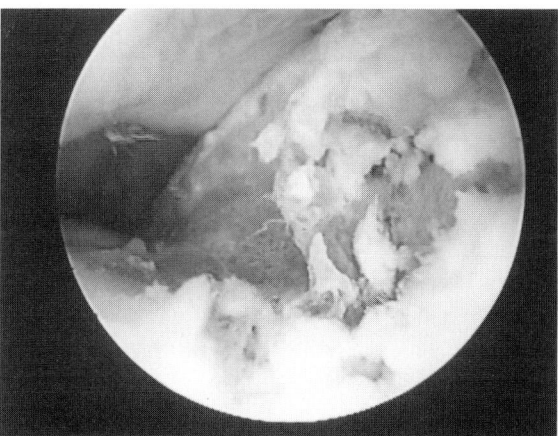

Fig. 5. View. Arthroscopic evaluation reveals a Hill-Sachs lesion of the posterolateral humeral head.

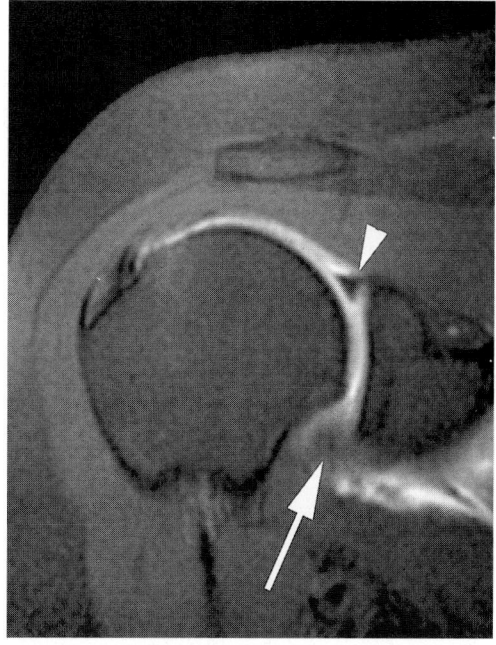

Fig. 7. View. An axial, T_2-weighted, fat-suppressed magnetic resonance image with intra-articular administration of gadolinium demonstrates a focal area of bright signal (*large white arrow*) between the anteroinferior labrum and the glenoid. Note superior labrum (*arrowhead*).

be considered only after conservative means have failed. In addition, biceps tendon subluxation is often associated with a tear of the subscapularis muscle and is also associated with instability and medial displacement of the tendon out of its groove (Figs. 6 to 8).

Superior labral lesions, specifically *superior labral anteroposterior* (SLAP) injuries, have been classified by Snyder and associates[28-30] into four separate lesions and further subdivided by Maffet and colleagues[31] to include three more types (Fig. 9). A SLAP lesion begins in the posterior aspect of the labrum and extends anteriorly to the anchor of the biceps tendon. The classic mechanism of injury is a fall on the outstretched arm with the shoulder held in abduction and forward flexion at the time of im-

pact, which exerts a compression force on the shoulder. The injuries can also be a result of traction injuries. The patient presents with shoulder pain that is exacerbated by overhead activity and occasionally notes a "catching" or "popping" sensation.

Initially, Snyder and associates[28-30] described four types of SLAP tears, as follows:

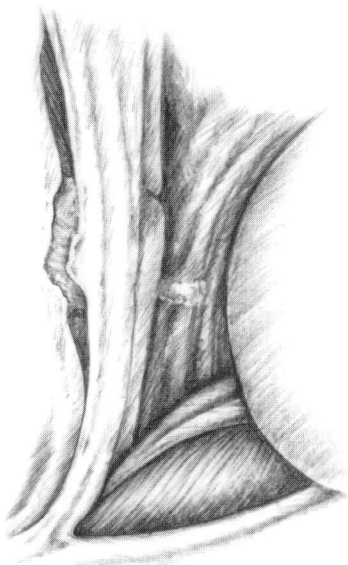

Fig. 6. Bankart lesion, left shoulder. This arthroscopic image demonstrates a large anterior Bankart lesion with displacement of the inferior labrum and inferior glenohumeral ligament complex from the labrum. (Redrawn from Miller MD, Osborne JR, Cooper DE, et al: MRI-Arthroscopy Correlative Atlas. Philadelphia, WB Saunders, 1997.)

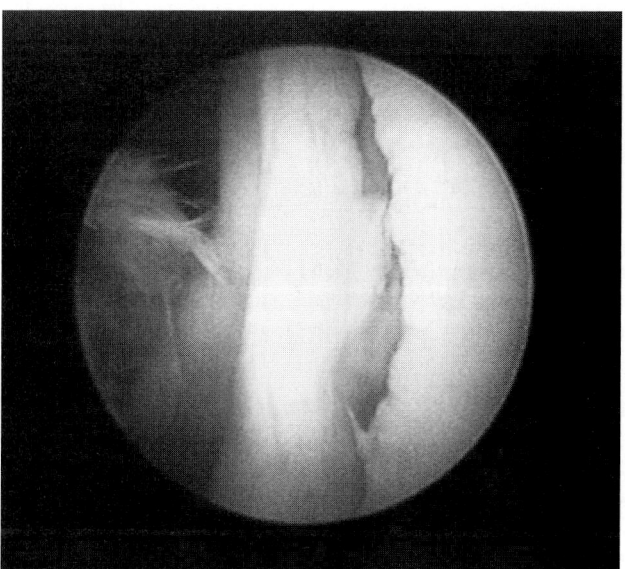

Fig. 8. Arthroscopic image. This demonstrates a large anterior Bankart lesion with displacement of the inferior labrum and inferior glenohumeral ligament complex from the labrum.

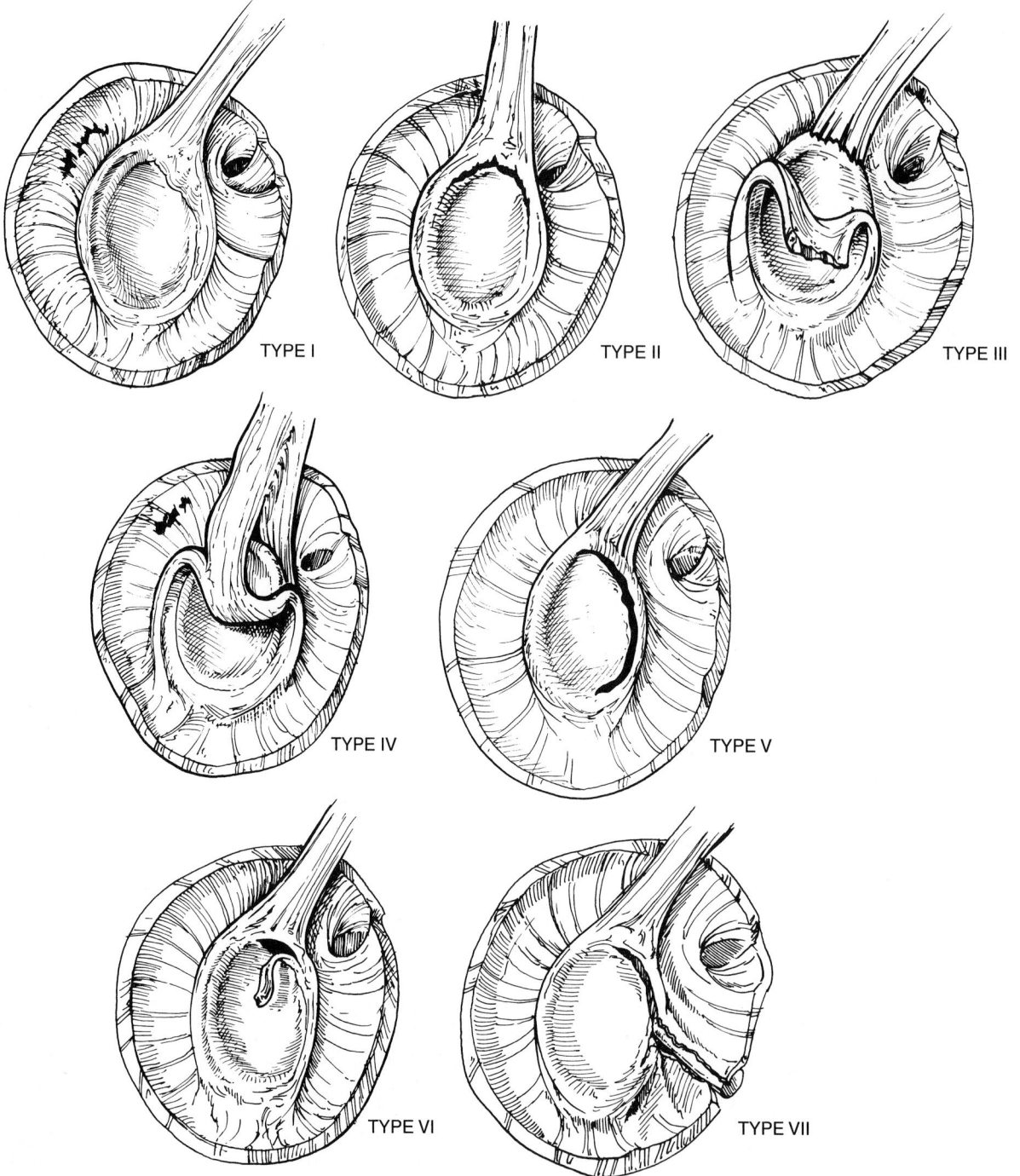

Fig. 9. SLAP lesions. Superior labral anteroposterior lesions, types I through IV as described by Snyder and colleagues[28–30] and types V through VII as described by Maffet and associates.[31] (From Miller MD, Osborne JR, Cooper DE, et al: MRI–Arthroscopy Correlative Atlas. Philadelphia, WB Saunders, 1997.)

- Type I tears involve fraying of the biceps tendon, with the biceps anchor intact on the superior labrum; they require arthroscopic débridement.
- Type II tears involve detachment of the biceps tendon anchor, which requires reattachment and stabilization.
- Type III tears involve bucket-handle superior labral tears with the biceps anchor intact; they are also treated with arthroscopic débridement.
- Type IV tears involve bucket-handle tears of the superior

labrum extending into the biceps tendon; they require either tendon repair or tenodesis, depending on symptoms and the condition of the remaining tendon.

The classification system was expanded by Maffet and colleagues[31] to include types V through VII, as follows:

- Type V tears involve anterior-to-inferior progression of the tear with separation of the biceps tendon, requiring repair or tenodesis of the biceps tendon.

- Type VI tears are similar to type IV tears, with the addition of an anterior-to-posterior flap with separation of the biceps tendon.
- Type VII tears involve capsular extension continuing to the MGHL.

Neviaser[32] has described another variation of the Bankart lesion, the *anterior labroligamentous periosteal sleeve avulsion* (ALPSA) lesion. It is distinct from a Bankart lesion, in that the anterior scapular periosteum in ALPSA is intact and pulls the avulsed anterior labroligamentous structures medially. The injury can then heal in this abnormal position, leading to an incompetent anterior IGHL. This lesion has also been called a "medialized Bankart lesion." It is especially important to recognize the ALPSA lesion during arthroscopy, because the labrum and attached ligaments may heal in a synovial sheath and may not be as easily identified as if they were unattached at one end. The lesion may be revealed on magnetic resonance arthrography (MRA) by the medialized position of the labrum.

Another occult instability lesion is *humeral avulsion of the glenohumeral ligament* (HAGL). Studies have shown that such lesions fail under tension at the glenoid attachment in 40% of cases, in midsubstance in 35%, and at the humeral attachment in 25%.[33] The most common site for the GH ligament to fail is at the labral attachment.[34] However, studies have shown that rupture of the GH ligament may occur at the humeral attachment or in midsubstance.[35] The HAGL lesion has been identified as the sole abnormality in 35% of patients with recurrent instability. Like the ALPSA, this lesion may be difficult to identify at the time of arthroscopy, and surgical repair of the ligament is critical to restoring shoulder stability.[36]

The *glenolabral articular disruption* (GLAD) lesion was first reported by Neviaser,[37] who described a superficial tear of the anteroinferior labrum with an associated injury of the glenoid articular cartilage. The GLAD lesion is different from a classic Bankart lesion, which results from anterior dislocation or subluxation that leads to a tear of the anterior labroligamentous complex with resultant instability. The mechanism of injury in a GLAD lesion is an impaction of the humeral head against the glenoid fossa resulting from a forced adduction with the arm in abduction and external rotation. The main symptomatology is persistent anterior shoulder pain without evidence of instability on examination. Differential diagnosis of a GLAD lesion is based on the mechanism of injury and complete lack of instability on physical examination.

Superior glenoid impingement and glenoid labral cysts may also be encountered during the evaluation and arthrography of the shoulder. Superior glenoid impingement usually occurs in throwing athletes who experience repetitive impingement of the undersurface of the rotator cuff between the greater tuberosity of the humeral head and the superior labrum. The impingement occurs during the late cocking phase of throwing and seems to be related to anterior instability.[38-41] The five structures at risk with this type of impingement are the rotator cuff, the superior labrum and biceps anchor, the greater tuberosity of the humerus, the posterosuperior glenoid, and the anterior labroligamentous structures.[38] The initial treatment of superior glenoid impingement is nonsurgical, involving rest of the injured structures and physical therapy to restore normal biomechanics.

Superior glenoid impingement can also be caused by glenoid labral cysts. The cysts arise from the extrusion of fluid through the labral tears and into the surrounding soft tissues. Cysts can be associated with shoulder pain and may cause a compression neuropathy of the suprascapular or axillary nerves.[42] A cyst that extends into the spinoglenoid notch can compress the distal suprascapular nerve, causing atrophy of the infraspinatus muscle. A cyst that arises from the anteroinferior labrum can cause quadrilateral space syndrome as the cyst compresses the axillary nerve. The end result is pain and atrophy of the teres minor and deltoid muscles.[43]

DIAGNOSIS

HISTORY

The classic history for a patient who presents with an anterior GH dislocation is that of a blow to the anterior brachium that "fulcrums" the shoulder anteriorly with the arm abducted and externally rotated. Posterior instability, which is extremely rare (reported incidence rate of 1.5% of all dislocations about the shoulder), can occur with seizures and electrocution. It results when the external rotators overpower the internal rotators.

Acute dislocations must be documented accurately. The activity at time of injury, the time and place of injury, and the treatment history must be noted. Radiographs and any other diagnostic studies, such as MRI and MRA, should be reviewed.

If the dislocation is associated with a traumatic event, the possibility of Bankart's lesion should be considered.[44-47] In a dislocation associated with a sport, it is important to note the sport involved and the position of the extremity when injured. Atraumatic anterior subluxation of the GH joint usually occurs in athletes who perform a lot of overhead throwing. Anterior instability is symptomatic during the late cocking phase of throwing, whereas posterior instability is more symptomatic during the follow-through phase. Posterior subluxation can occur in athletes whose shoulders are often subjected to posteriorly directed forces, such as interior lineman in football. Subluxation can cause subtle symptoms, including easy fatigue of the arm, loss of throwing velocity, pain during the late cocking phase, and shoulder pain without any sense of instability.

PHYSICAL EXAMINATION

Physical examination should be directed toward reproducing the position and symptoms of the shoulder at time of injury, to determine which structures are injured. It should also include a careful neurovascular examination, with specific attention given to the axillary nerve and brachial plexus. The range of motion must be carefully evaluated, including forward flexion, abduction, external rotation, and internal rotation with the arm adducted and abducted 90 degrees. Laxity of the GH joint must be evaluated in the anterior, posterior, and inferior directions while the scapula is stabilized with the forearm or opposite hand. Inferior laxity is evaluated by testing for the *sulcus sign*. Presence of the sulcus sign indicates multidirectional instability.

If the patient can voluntarily subluxate or dislocate the GH joint, surgery should be delayed. A psychiatric referral is appropriate, because voluntary shoulder dislocation is associated with psychiatric disorders.[3, 48]

Anterior instability is evaluated by testing for the *apprehension sign*. This sign is defined as discomfort produced when the arm is abducted 90 degrees and externally rotated. The apprehension sign is evaluated for at 0, 45, 90, and 120 degrees of abduction. The patient experiences pain or a sensation of the shoulder subluxating at 90 degrees.

The *relocation test*, described by Jobe and associates,[39, 49–51] consists of the application of a posteriorly directed force on the front of the shoulder. If such a force decreases the apprehension sign, the relocation test result is positive. A positive result is suggestive of anterior instability and may indicate the presence of a Bankart lesion (Fig. 10).

Impingement syndrome and rotator cuff disease are commonly found in older patients; however, these disorders can also be associated with throwing activities and repetitive overuse. Neer and Welsh[52] described three stages of subacromial impingement syndrome. Patients usually present with pain during arm-overhead activities and have pain with forward flexion. The *Neer impingement sign*, pain with forward flexion greater than 90 degrees, and positive result of the *Hawkins impingement test*, pain with forward flexion and internal rotation, are further indications of rotator cuff injury. In addition, the patient with rotator cuff injury may have (1) weakness with abduction and external rotation and (2) infraspinatus atrophy.[16] In cases in which the diagnosis of instability versus subacromial impingement is unclear, the type of impingement may be useful to help differentiate between the two entities. The

impingement test consists of the subacromial injection of lidocaine, followed by a second examination; if the pain is resolved after subacromial injection, the diagnosis of impingement is warranted.

Posterior instability may be difficult to evaluate because a posterior dislocation may lack the dramatic deformity found with anterior dislocations. Several key features of a posterior dislocation should be sought: (1) limited external rotation (often 0), (2) limited forward elevation of the arm (often less than 90 degrees), and (3) posterior prominence and rounding of the shoulder accompanied by a flattening of the anterior shoulder and prominence of the coracoid process. The range of motion may be limited because the humeral head is being held on the glenoid rim, either by muscle forces or from mechanical impalement on the glenoid rim.

Proper physical examination is critical in evaluating the patient with posterior dislocation, as studies have shown this injury to be the one most often missed, with an average of 8 months from time of injury to diagnosis.[53] Evaluation should include the posterior apprehension test, the drawer test, the jerk test, and the push-pull test. The examiner performs the *posterior apprehension test* by holding the arm in a position of forward flexion to 90 degrees and internally rotating it while applying a posterior force to the humerus. If the patient demonstrates apprehension as the posteriorly directed force is increased, posterior instability may be present.

The *drawer test* is performed with the patient seated and the forearm resting in the lap. The examiner uses one forearm and hand to stabilize the patient's scapula and clavicle and the other hand to grasp the humeral head. When anterior and posterior forces are applied to the hu-

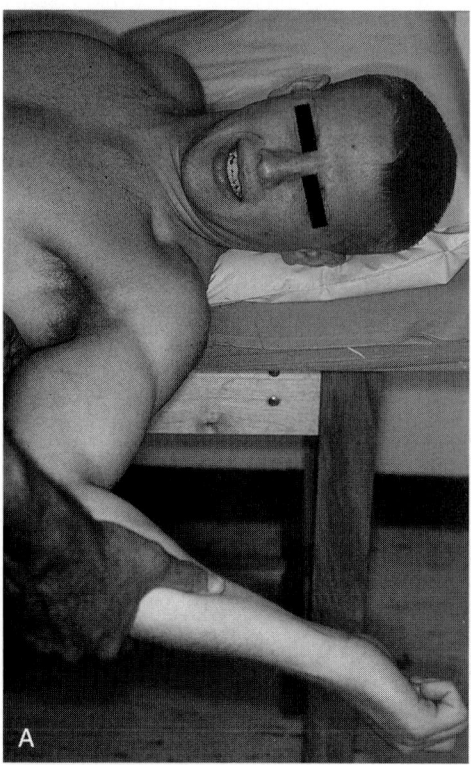 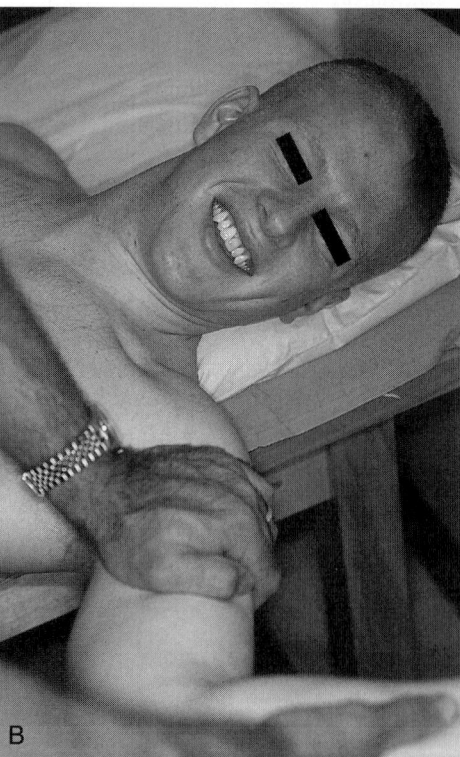

Fig. 10. Views. *A*, This patient clearly demonstrates the apprehension sign. With the arm abducted 90 degrees and externally rotated, the patient experiences discomfort and a sensation of impending subluxation or dislocation. *B*, The relocation test is performed with a posteriorly directed force on the front of the shoulder. As is evident, this maneuver decreases the apprehension sign.

meral head, a normal shoulder has a firm end point, with slight anterior translation and posterior translation up to one-half the diameter of the humeral head. Abnormal findings include increased anterior or posterior translation, "clunking," pain, and apprehension.

The *jerk test* is performed with the patient seated and the arm internally rotated and forward-flexed to 90 degrees. The examiner applies a posteriorly directed force at the elbow, thereby axially loading the humerus. Maintaining the axial load on the humerus, the examiner then moves the patient's arm horizontally across the body. In patients with recurrent posterior instability, this maneuver causes a sudden "jerk" as the humeral head slides off the back of the glenoid. When the arm is moved back to the starting position of 90 degrees abduction, a "jerk" may again be encountered as the humeral head returns to its position within the glenoid rim.

In the *push-pull test*, the patient lies supine with one shoulder off the edge of the table and the arm held in 90 degrees of abduction and 30 degrees of flexion. The examiner applies an axially directed distraction by pulling on the wrist with one hand and pushing down on the humerus with the other hand. The normal shoulder accommodates approximately one-half the diameter of the humeral head in regard to posterior translation. Increased translation, pain, or apprehension with this maneuver is suggestive of posterior instability (Fig. 11).

Labral injury, especially the SLAP lesion, has received greater attention and research in the literature. The evaluation of a possible SLAP lesion should include the following examinations: (1) direct palpation of the biceps tendon and bicipital groove, (2) Speed's test, (3) Yergason's test, (4) the crank test, and (5) O'Brien's test (the active compression test). Direct palpation of the biceps tendon and bicipital groove indicate injury localized to the biceps tendon, its insertion, or both. This injury can be secondary either to bicipital tendinitis or to labral injury at the insertion of the biceps tendon into the glenoid labrum (a SLAP lesion).

Speed's test is performed by means of resisted forward elevation of the supinated arm. Pain with the maneuver is indicative of either bicipital tendinitis or a SLAP lesion.

In *Yergason's test*, the arm is adducted to the patient's side and the elbow is flexed to 90 degrees. The examiner attempts to supinate the forearm as the patient resists. Like direct palpation, this maneuver localizes the problem to the biceps tendon, its insertion, or both.

The *crank test* is performed with the patient seated and the arm held in 90 degrees of abduction and external rotation. The examiner uses one hand to pull back on the patient's wrist while using the other hand to stabilize the shoulder girdle. This test is analogous to the McMurray test for the knee. The patient with anterior instability or anterior labral injury demonstrates apprehension with this maneuver.

O'Brien's test, or the *active compression test*, is utilized for evaluation of SLAP lesions and is also useful for evaluation of AC joint injury.[54] To perform the active compression test the patient maximally internally rotates the arm, with 10 degrees of adduction, 90 degrees of flexion, and the thumb down. The examiner applies a downward force and the patient resists. This maneuver is repeated with the palm up and the arm in maximal external rotation. The active compression test is positive if pain is produced dur-

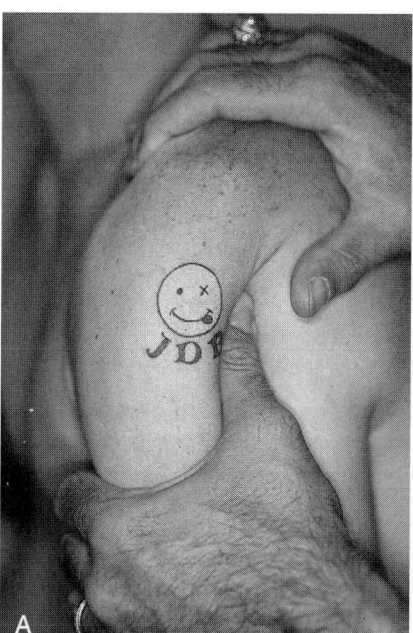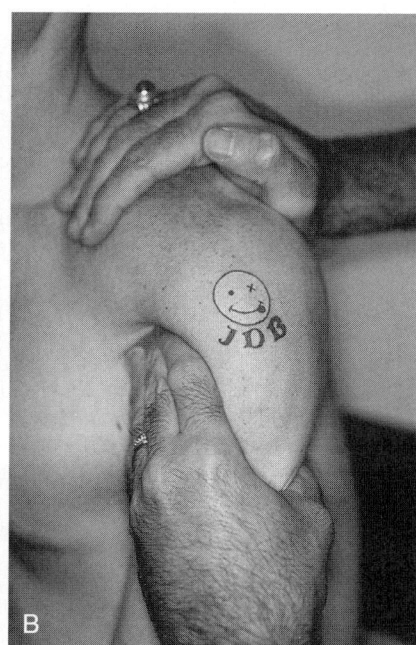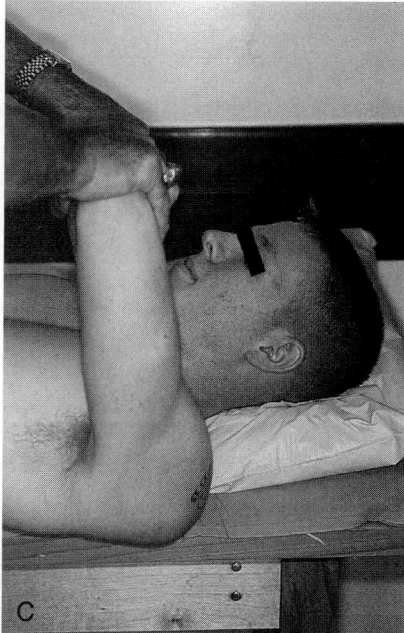

Fig. 11. Tests. *A*, The anterior drawer test is demonstrated. When an anterior force is applied to the humeral head, the increased anterior translation of the humeral head on the glenoid reveals anterior instability. *B*, The posterior drawer test is demonstrated. When a posterior force is applied to the humeral head, the increased posterior translation of the humeral head on the glenoid reveals posterior instability. *C*, The jerk test is performed with the arm internally rotated and forward-flexed. A posterior force is applied at the elbow, axially loading the humerus; the arm is then moved across the body. In patients with recurrent posterior instability, this movement causes a sudden "jerk" as the humeral head slides off the back of the glenoid.

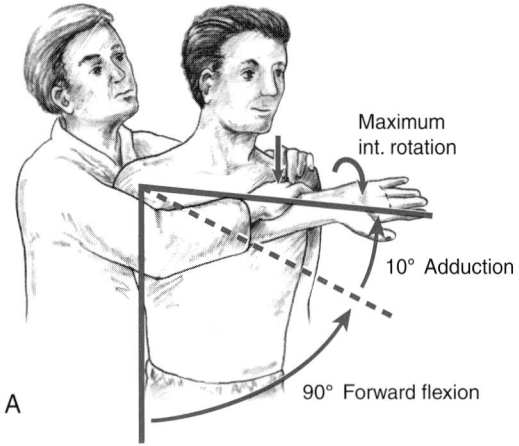

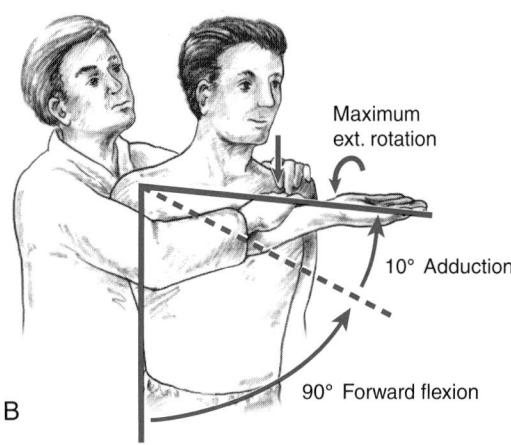

Fig. 12. O'Brien's test. In the active compression test, the patient's arm is forward-flexed to 90 degrees, adducted 10 to 15 degrees, and maximally internally rotated. The patient is instructed to resist as the examiner applies a uniform downward force (*A*). The patient then maximally supinates the arm, and the maneuver is repeated (*B*). (From O'Brien SJ, Pagnani MJ, Fealy S, et al: The active compression test: A new and effective test for diagnosing labral tears and acromio-clavicular joint abnormality. Am J Sports Med 1998; 5:610.)

ing the first maneuver and decreased or relieved during the second. If the pain is localized "on top" of the shoulder, overlying the AC joint, this was shown to correlate with 88% positive findings for AC injury. If pain was localized to "inside" the shoulder or a painful click was encountered, this was shown to correlate with 96% positive findings for labral tears at diagnostic arthroscopy.[54]

The O'Brien test was first described in 1998. We have not found the test to be helpful in making the diagnosis of a SLAP lesion (Fig. 12).[54]

The painful shoulder presents a diagnostic dilemma to the orthopaedic surgeon determining a diagnostic and therapeutic plan. Pain can be nonspecific, and multifactorial causes may be creating symptomatology. Sequential injections of the AC joint, the subacromial space, and the GH joint may help localize the source of injury. This simple course of differential injections can have a profound impact on the diagnosis and treatment of shoulder pain.

RADIOGRAPHS

Radiographs should be obtained to document acute traumatic injury to the shoulder as well as to evaluate chronic instability. Standard AP, axillary lateral, and scapular lateral radiographs should constitute the minimum radiographic evaluation for acute trauma; taken together, these three views are commonly referred to as the "trauma series." The importance of the axillary lateral view cannot be overemphasized, especially in cases of posterior instability.

Additional views may be helpful in making a diagnosis. They are as follows (Table 1):

- For aid in diagnosis of impingement syndrome: the 30-degree caudal tilt to evaluate for subacromial spurring and the supraspinatus outlet view to assess acromial structure.
- To better demonstrate an anteroinferior glenoid injury, a West Point axillary view and a Garth view.
- To reveal a Hill-Sachs lesion, an AP view of the shoulder in internal rotation and the Stryker-notch view.

SOFT-TISSUE IMAGING

MRI of the shoulder has undergone technological advances that have increased the amount of information available to aid the orthopaedic surgeon in making diagnostic and therapeutic interventions in shoulder instability. Routine MRI of the shoulder is performed with a dedicated shoulder coil and the arm positioned by the patient's side in slight external rotation.

Use of intra-articular contrast agents, including saline and gadolinium, has advanced MRA past the level of conventional arthrography. Multiple studies in the literature have shown correlation of the magnetic resonance arthrogram with surgical findings to be as high as 88% in sensitivity and 100% in specificity for diagnosis of tears of the IGHL.[55] For the diagnosis of superior labral tears, studies report sensitivity to be greater than 86% and specificity to be greater than 95% for unenhanced MRI with high-resolution fast spin and gradient echo images.[56] MRA is beneficial in making the diagnosis of a SLAP tear but may lack the sensitivity necessary to differentiate the various types of SLAP lesions.[57–59]

Coronal imaging sequences are most helpful for visualization of SLAP lesions. In the shoulder with such a lesion contrast medium is seen extending into the area of the superior labrum, which normally appears as a dark triangular area. The normal anatomic variation of the superior labral recess that occurs in the anterior superior quadrant of

	TABLE 1. RADIOGRAPHIC CORRELATION IN SHOULDER INSTABILITY	
	View	**Significance**
A	True AP	Post-traumatic arthritis
B	Axillary lateral	Direction of instability
C	Scapular lateral Y view	Direction of instability
D	Stryker notch	Hill-Sachs defect
E	AP-internal rotation	Hill-Sachs defect
F	West Point view	Bankart
G	(Garth view) Apical oblique	Bankart

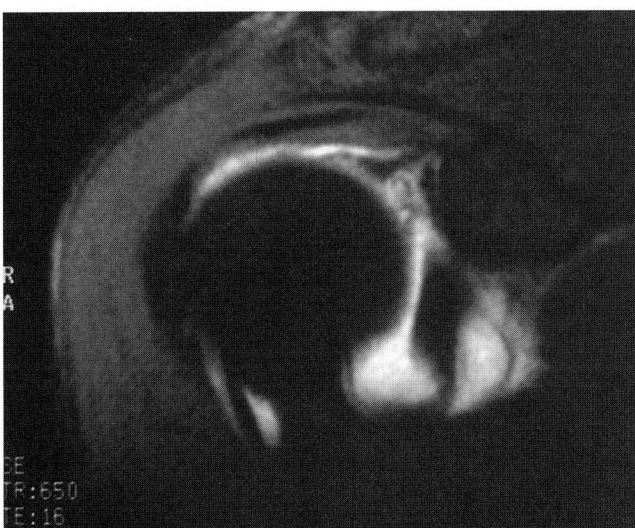

Fig. 13. MRI view. Oblique coronal, fat-suppressed echo, T_2-weighted magnetic resonance image after intra-articular administration of gadolinium reveals a large superior labral lesion surrounded by fluid.

the glenoid labrum can be confused with a SLAP lesion. SLAP lesions can be differentiated from the normal variation, in that a tear is usually irregular in appearance and the labrum may be pulled off of the glenoid. In type III and type IV SLAP lesions, a fragment of the labrum may be visualized hanging from the superior labrum and is outlined by intra-articular contrast agent.

Osseous defects of the glenoid and the humeral head are best visualized with computed tomography scanning (Figs. 13 and 14).[16]

MRA of the HAGL lesion reveals a disruption of the IGHL with subsequent extravasation of contrast agent through the capsular defect at or very near the humeral attachment. In addition, the subscapularis muscle may be disrupted, and a Hill-Sachs lesion may frequently be seen associated with the HAGL lesion.[60]

MRA of a GLAD lesion demonstrates a superficial tear of the anterior inferior labrum with an intact IGHL. The findings consist of a high signal contrast filling a gap between the labrum and the glenoid fossa, with the labrum remaining attached at some point to the glenoid by way of an intact anterior glenoid periosteum. The lesion is best identified with the arm in abduction and external rotation. Along with the labral lesion, there exists an adjacent articular cartilage injury, which must be present for definitive diagnosis of a GLAD lesion. On MRA, the lesion may mimic a chronic Bankart lesion with an associated chondral injury. The GLAD lesion reveals an area of contrast agent undermining a chondral flap tear.[61]

MRA of superior glenoid impingement may reveal a constellation of findings, including partial undersurface fraying or tearing of the rotator cuff, cystic changes in the greater tuberosity below the level of the rotator cuff insertion, high signal consistent with fraying or tearing of the posterosuperior labrum, and partial tearing of the anterior inferior labroligamentous complex.[62]

Glenoid labral cysts arise adjacent to the glenoid labrum and are frequently associated with labral tears and GH instability.[63] With MRI, the cystic lesions can be seen as areas of bright fluid on T_2-weighted images.

EXAMINATION WITH ANESTHESIA

Examination of the shoulder with the use of anesthesia is critical in making the diagnosis of GH instability prior to diagnostic arthroscopy or any planned operative reconstruction. The examination should be performed on both the involved shoulder and the uninvolved shoulder in the operating room. The starting position for each maneuver should be with the humeral head centered in the glenoid. Attention should be given to anatomic landmarks, the coracoid, acromion, and humeral head specifically. Instability maneuvers should be performed with the arm in several different positions.

The examination with anesthesia can be helpful in muscular athletic patients who have a difficult time relaxing during routine physical examination. In addition, the examination may contribute useful information to clarify the degree and direction of instability. Studies have shown this examination to have a sensitivity of 100% and a specificity and positive predictive value of 93%.[64] Several schemes have been utilized to quantify the amount of translation and how it correlates with instability (Fig. 15).

ARTHROSCOPY

Arthroscopy of the GH joint has evolved from a diagnostic to a therapeutic modality. There are numerous advantages to arthroscopic over open treatment for many lesions involving the shoulder; they include (1) less morbidity, (2) preservation of the muscles of the shoulder girdle, (3) smaller incisions with less surgical invasiveness, (4) decreased intraoperative blood loss, (5) improved access to and visualization of the entire GH joint, and (6) shorter postoperative rehabilitation time. Diagnostic arthroscopy has contributed greatly to the orthopaedic surgeon's understanding of the normal and pathological anatomy of the shoulder. Arthroscopic acromioplasty has gained wide acceptance, and the treatment of instability as well as treat-

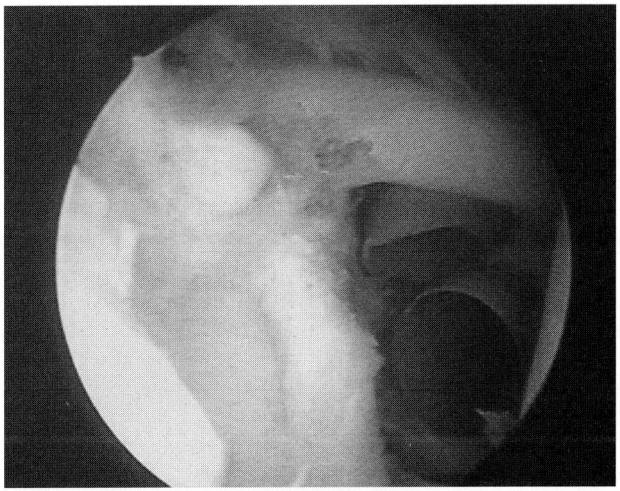

Fig. 14. Arthroscopic view. This demonstrates detachment of the superior labrum and biceps with the lesion extending from the superior to the inferior labrum.

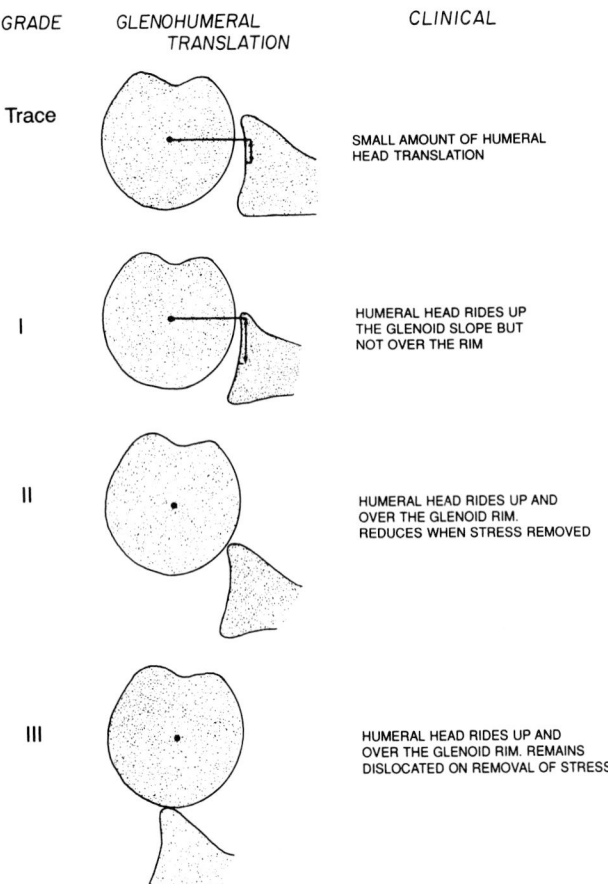

GRADE   GLENOHUMERAL   CLINICAL
            TRANSLATION

Trace

SMALL AMOUNT OF HUMERAL
HEAD TRANSLATION

I

HUMERAL HEAD RIDES UP
THE GLENOID SLOPE BUT
NOT OVER THE RIM

II

HUMERAL HEAD RIDES UP AND
OVER THE GLENOID RIM.
REDUCES WHEN STRESS REMOVED

III

HUMERAL HEAD RIDES UP AND
OVER THE GLENOID RIM. REMAINS
DISLOCATED ON REMOVAL OF STRESS.

Fig. 15. Translation scheme. Translation of the shoulder has been classified by many schemes, including the one shown here. All schemes quantify the amount of translation in relation to the glenoid. (From Hawkins RJ, Bokor DJ: Clinical evaluation of shoulder problems. In Rockwood CA Jr, Matsen FA III [eds]: The Shoulder. Philadelphia, WB Saunders, 1990, p 168.)

ment of labral injuries, including SLAP lesions, has proved invaluable.

The beach chair position has been especially useful. Because it provides a more normal orientation of the GH anatomy than the previously used lateral decubitus position, the beach chair position is now the standard for arthroscopy of the shoulder.

Standard portals utilized for shoulder arthroscopy are the posterior portal, the anterior portal, the lateral portal, the anteroinferior portal, the supraspinatus (Neviaser) portal, and the posterolateral portal (of Wilmington). The posterior portal is the first portal placed, and it is established 2 cm distal and 2 cm medial to the posterolateral corner of the acromion. Local anesthetic with epinephrine is usually injected at the portal site and is helpful to decrease intraoperative bleeding. Sterile saline can be injected into the joint in an effort to distend the joint capsule and to prevent iatrogenic injury to the articular cartilage. After injection of saline with a spinal needle, the surgeon can disconnect the needle to check for free flowback through the needle, which confirms proper placement. The posterior portal and introduction of the arthroscope should be oriented from the starting point of the portal and directed anteromedially

toward the coracoid, which serves as a good aiming point and can be palpated with the surgeon's other hand during placement of the trocar. During placement of the arthroscope, it is sometimes helpful for the assistant to exert a lateral force on the humerus.

The anterosuperior portal, the main working portal for shoulder arthroscopy, is used for instrumentation. The anterior portal is established by placement of a spinal needle directly into the GH joint, just inferior to the biceps tendon, just lateral to the coracoid, and just distal to the acromion. The location can be verified with direct arthroscopic visualization. Placing the arm in adduction decreases the risk of injury to the musculocutaneous nerve. The cannula for the anterior portal can be introduced just under the biceps tendon.

The lateral portal is utilized for arthroscopic acromioplasty. It is located at the lateral margin of the acromion. As for the anterior portal, a spinal needle and cannula are useful in establishing the lateral portal.

The anteroinferior portal is utilized for arthroscopic Bankart's repairs. The anteroinferior portal is placed approximately 2 cm distal to the anterior portal and is established like the anterior portal, with entry of the cannula just superior to the subscapularis tendon. For optimal usefulness, this portal should be placed as low as possible to allow for entry into the joint just superior to the subscapularis tendon.

The supraspinatus portal (Neviaser) is used by some surgeons for inflow and for visualization of the anterior glenoid. This portal is placed in the apex of the supraspinatus fossa with a slight anterior and lateral orientation. The

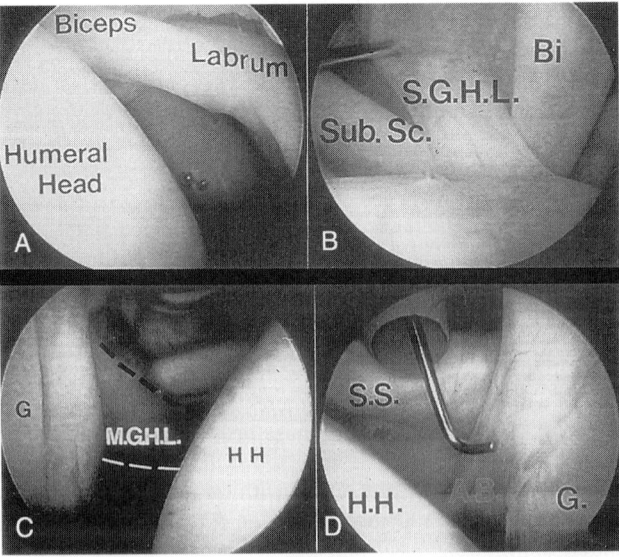

Fig. 16. Views. A and B, Arthroscopic views of the superior aspect of the glenohumeral joint. Note the normal relationship of the biceps tendon and labrum in A and the position of the superior glenohumeral ligament (SGHL) between the biceps tendon (Bi) and the subscapularis tendon (Sub Sc) in B. C, The middle glenohumeral ligament (MGHL) drapes over the subscapularis tendon between the glenoid (G) and the humeral head (HH). D, The anterior band (AB) of the inferior glenohumeral ligament complex attaches to the labrum and glenoid (G). (From Miller MD, Cooper DE, Warner JJP: Review of Sports Medicine and Arthroscopy. Philadelphia, WB Saunders, 1995.)

portal should also be placed with the arm adducted and with the trocar angled posteriorly to avoid injury to the rotator cuff tendons.

The posterolateral portal (of Wilmington) is placed at the posterolateral aspect of the acromion, approximately 1 cm distal to the margin of the acromion. This portal is useful in the arthroscopic treatment of SLAP lesions (Fig. 16).

The sequence for arthroscopic examination of the shoulder is as follows:

1. Visualize the biceps tendon.
2. Visualize the superior labrum.
3. Sweep inferiorly and, in a clockwise fashion, inspect the anteroinferior labrum.
4. Inspect the axillary pouch.
5. Inspect the articular surface of the glenoid and humeral head.

The arm is then externally rotated, and an orderly inspection of the rotator cuff is performed. Placing the arm in external rotation also allows for visualization of the posterior labrum and the posterior aspect of the humeral head. Finally, the GH ligaments can be visualized and probed to assess the integrity of the capsuloligamentous structures. The labrum is then probed and evaluated for the presence of a Bankart lesion or SLAP lesion. Hintermann and Gachter[65] reported their findings at arthroscopy after first-time shoulder dislocation. At the time of arthroscopy, 87% of their patients had Bankart's lesions, 79% had capsular insufficiency, 68% had Hill-Sachs lesions, and 55% had GH ligament injuries.[65]

TREATMENT

In general, treatment of labral injuries involves direct repair of the injured tissues. Capsular tightening procedures are often necessary for chronic injuries. Additional discussion of the treatment of labral injuries can be found in subsequent chapters.

REFERENCES

1. Zimmerman LM, Veith I: Great Ideas in the History of Surgery: Clavicle, Shoulder, Shoulder Amputations. Baltimore, Williams & Wilkins, 1961.
2. Hippocrates: Works of Hippocrates: With an English translation by WHS James and ET Withington. London, William Heinemann, 1927.
3. Rockwood CA, Wirth MA: Subluxations and dislocations about the glenohumeral joint. In Rockwood CA, Green DP, Buchholz RW, et al (eds): Fractures in Adults. Philadelphia, JB Lippincott, 1996, p 1193.
4. Matsen FA, Thomas SC, Rockwood CA: Glenohumeral instability. In Rockwood CA, Matsen FA (eds): The Shoulder. Philadelphia, WB Saunders, 1990, p 526.
5. Galinat BJ, Warren RF, Buss DD: Pathophysiology of shoulder instability. In McGinty JB (ed): Operative Arthroscopy. New York, Raven Press, 1991, p 501.
6. Kazar B, Relovszky E: Prognosis of primary dislocation of the shoulder. Acta Orthop Scand 1969; 40:224.
7. Cave EF (ed): Fractures and Other Injuries. Chicago, Year Book, 1961.
8. Debaradino TM, Arciero RA, Taylor DC: Arthroscopic stabilization of acute initial anterior shoulder dislocation: The West Point experience. J South Orthop Assoc 1996; 5:262.
9. Neviaser RJ, Neviaser TJ: Recurrent instability of the shoulder after age 40. J Shoulder Elbow Surg 1995; 4:416.
10. Saha AK: Dynamic stability of the glenohumeral joint. Acta Orthop Scand 1971; 42:491.
11. Harryman DT, Siddles JA, Clark JM, et al: Translation of the humeral head on the glenoid with passive glenohumeral motion. J Bone Joint Surg Am 1990; 72:1334.
12. Randelli M, Gambrioli PL: Glenohumeral osteometry by computed tomography in normal and unstable shoulders. Clin Orthop 1986; 208:151.
13. Howell SM, Galinat BJ, Renzi AJ, et al: Normal and abnormal mechanics of the glenohumeral joint in the horizontal plane. J Bone Joint Surg Am 1988; 70:227.
14. Turkel SJ, Panio MW, Marshall JL, et al: Stabilizing mechanisms preventing anterior dislocation of the glenohumeral joint. J Bone Joint Surg Am 1981; 63:1208.
15. Cooper DE, Arnoczky SP, O'Brien SJ, et al: Anatomy, histology, and vascularity of the glenoid labrum. J Bone Joint Surg Am 1992; 74:46.
16. Warner JJP, Carbon DN: Overview of shoulder instability. Crit Rev Phys Rehab Med 1992; 4:145.
17. Kumar VP, Balasubramanium P: The role of atmospheric pressure in stabilizing the shoulder: An experimental study. J Bone Joint Surg Br 1985; 67:719.
18. Boardman ND, Debski RE, Warner JP, et al: Tensile properties of the superior glenohumeral and coracohumeral ligaments. J Shoulder Elbow Surg 1996; 5:249.
19. Williams MM, Snyder SS, Buford D: The Buford complex—the "cord-like" middle glenohumeral ligament and advent anterosuperior labrum complex: A normal anatomic capsulolabral variant. Arthroscopy 1994; 10:241.
20. Fu FH, Seel MJ, Berger RA: Relevant shoulder biomechanics. Oper Tech Orthop 1991; 1:134.
21. O'Brien SJ, Schwartz RS, Warren RF, et al: Capsular restraints to anterior-posterior motion of the abducted shoulder: A biomechanical study. J Shoulder Elbow Surg 1995; 4:298.
22. O'Brien SJ, Neves MC, Arnoczky SP, et al: The anatomy and histology of the inferior glenohumeral ligament complex of the shoulder. Am J Sports Med 1990; 5:449.
23. Ticker JB, Bigliani LU, Soslowsky LJ, et al: Inferior glenohumeral ligament: Geometric and strain-rate dependent properties. J Shoulder Elbow Surg 1996; 5:269.
24. Pollock RG, Bigliani LU: Glenohumeral instability: Evaluation and treatment. J Am Acad Orthop Surg 1993; 1:24.
25. Perthes G: Ueber Operationen bei habitueller Schulterluxationen. Dtsch Z Chir 1906; 85:199.
26. Bankart ASB: Recurrent or habitual dislocation of the shoulder joint. BMJ 1932; 2:1132.
27. Baker CL, Uribe JW, Whitman C: Arthroscopic evaluation of acute initial anterior shoulder dislocations. Am J Sports Med 1990; 1:25.
28. Snyder SJ, Wuh HCK: Arthroscopic evaluation and treatment of the rotator cuff and superior labrum anterior posterior lesion. Oper Tech Orthop 1991; 1:207.
29. Snyder SJ, Karzel RP, Del Pizzo W, et al: SLAP lesions of the shoulder. Arthroscopy 1990; 6:274.
30. Mileski RA, Snyder SJ: Superior labral lesions in the shoulder: Pathoanatomy and surgical management. J Am Acad Orthop Surg 1998; 6:121.
31. Maffet MW, Gartsman GM, Moseley B: Superior labrum–biceps tendon complex lesions of the shoulder. Am J Sports Med 1995; 23:93.
32. Neviaser TJ: The anterior labroligamentous periosteal sleeve avulsion lesion: A cause of anterior instability of the shoulder. Arthroscopy 1993; 9:17.
33. Bigliani LU, Pollock RG, Soslowsky LJ, et al: Tensile properties of the inferior glenohumeral ligament. J Orthop Res 1992; 10:187.
34. Rowe CR, Zarins B, Ciullo JV: Recurrent anterior dislocation of the shoulder after surgical repair. J Bone Joint Surg Am 1984; 66:159.
35. Nicola T: Anterior dislocation of the shoulder: The role of the articular capsule. J Bone Joint Surg 1942; 25:614.
36. Wolf EM, Cheng JC, Dickson K: Humeral avulsion of glenohumeral ligaments as a cause of anterior shoulder instability. Arthroscopy 1995; 11:600.
37. Neviaser TJ: The GLAD lesion: Another cause of anterior shoulder pain. Arthroscopy 1993; 9:22.

38. Jobe FW: Superior glenoid impingement. Orthop Clin North Am 1997; 28:137.
39. Kvitne RS, Jobe FW: The diagnosis and treatment of anterior instability in the throwing athlete. Clin Orthop 1993; 291: 107.
40. Liu SH, Boynton E: Posterior superior impingement of the rotator cuff on the glenoid rim as a cause of shoulder pain in the overhead athlete. Arthroscopy 1993; 9: 697.
41. Walch G, Boileau P, Noel E, et al: Impingement of the deep surface of the supraspinatus tendon on the posterosuperior glenoid rim: An arthroscopic study. J Shoulder Elbow Surg 1992; 1:238.
42. Schulte KR, Warner JJP: Uncommon causes of shoulder pain in the athlete. Orthop Clin North Am 1995; 26:505.
43. Cahill BR, Palmer RE: Quadrilateral space syndrome. J Hand Surg 1983; 8:65.
44. Rowe CB, Zarins B: Recurrent transient subluxation of the shoulder. J Bone Joint Surg Am 1981; 63:863.
45. Mok DWH, Fogg AJB, Bayley JIL: The diagnostic value of arthroscopy in glenohumeral instability. J Bone Joint Surg Br 1990; 72:698.
46. Hurley JA, Anderson TE: Shoulder arthroscopy: Its role in evaluating shoulder disorders in the athlete. Am J Sports Med 1990; 18:480.
47. O'Brien SJ, Warren RF, Schwartz E: Anterior shoulder instability. Orthop Clin North Am 1987; 18:395.
48. Rowe CB, Pierce DS, Clark JG: Voluntary dislocation of the shoulder: A preliminary report on a clinical, electromyographic and psychiatric study of twenty-six patients. J Bone Joint Surg Am 1973; 55:445.
49. Jobe FW, Moynes DR: Delineation of diagnostic criteria and a rehabilitation program for rotator cuff injuries. Am J Sports Med 1982; 10:336.
50. Jobe FW, Moynes DR, Brewster CE: Rehabilitation of shoulder joint instabilities. Orthop Clin North Am 1987; 18:473.
51. Hawkins RJ, Bokor DJ: Clinical evaluation of shoulder problems. In Rockwood CA, Matsen FA (eds): The Shoulder. Philadelphia, WB Saunders, 1990, p 149.
52. Neer CS, Welsh RP: The shoulder in sports. Orthop Clin North Am 1977; 8: 583.
53. Hill NA, McLaughlin HL: Locked posterior dislocation simulating a "frozen shoulder." J Trauma 1963; 3:225.
54. O'Brien SJ, Pagnani MJ, Fealy S, et al: The active compression test: A new and effective test for diagnosing labral tears and acromioclavicular joint abnormality. Am J Sports Med 1998; 5:610.
55. Chandnani VP, Gagliardi JA, Murnane TG, et al: Glenohumeral ligaments and shoulder capsular mechanism: Evaluation with MR arthrography. Radiology 1995; 196:27.
56. Gusmer PB, Potter HG, Schatz JA, et al: Labral injuries: Accuracy of detection with unenhanced MR imaging of the shoulder. Radiology 1996; 200:519.
57. Cartland JP, Crues JV III, Stauffer A, et al: MR imaging in the evaluation of SLAP injuries of the shoulder: Findings in 10 patients. AJR Am J Roentgenol 1992; 159: 787.
58. Hunter JC, Blatz DJ, Escobedo EM: SLAP lesions of the glenoid labrum: CT arthrographic and arthroscopic correlation. Radiology 1992; 184:513.
59. Hodler J, Kursunoglu-Brahme S, Flannigan B, et al: Injuries of the superior portion of the glenoid labrum involving the insertion of the biceps tendon: MR imaging findings in nine cases. AJR Am J Roentgenol 1992; 159:565.
60. Tirman PFJ, Steinbach LS, Feller FJ: Humeral avulsion of the anterior shoulder stabilizing structures after anterior shoulder dislocation: Demonstration by MRI and MR arthrography. Skeletal Radiol 1996; 25:743.
61. Sanders TG, Tirman PFJ, Linares R: The glenolabral articular disruption lesion: MR arthrography with arthroscopic correlation. AJR Am J Roentgenol 1999; 172:171.
62. Tirman PFJ, Bost FW, Garvin GJ, et al: Posterosuperior glenoid impingement of the shoulder: Findings at MR arthrography and MR arthrography with arthroscopic correlation. Radiology 1994; 193:431.
63. Tirman PFJ, Feller JF, Jansen DL, et al: Association of glenoid labral cysts with labral tears and glenohumeral instability: Radiographic findings and clinical significance. Radiology 1994; 190:653.
64. Cofield RH, Nessler JP, Weinstable R: Diagnosis of shoulder instability by examination under anesthesia. Clin Orthop 1993; 291:45.
65. Hintermann B, Gachter A: Arthroscopic findings after shoulder dislocation. Am J Sports Med 1995; 23:545.

section
4
chapter
8

SHOULDER INSTABILITY AND LABRAL INJURIES: SURGICAL INDICATIONS AND TECHNIQUES

Scott D. Mair, Brad E. Brautigan, and David N. M. Caborn

Summary

- The goal of treatment of glenohumeral instability is the restoration of stability without compromising shoulder function.
- An accurate diagnosis is essential in planning treatment.
- Indications for surgery are subjective and must be individualized to the patient.
- Surgical options include open and arthroscopic techniques.
- Surgery is generally successful when indications are appropriate and technical essentials are followed.
- Potential complications of surgery include recurrent instability, compromised shoulder motion or function, late glenohumeral arthritis, neurological injury, hardware complications, and infection.

Over the past quarter century, there have been many changes in the operative indications and techniques for treating shoulder instability. The advent of shoulder arthroscopy has resulted in an improved understanding of pathological lesions that lead to instability and pain. Classically, failure of a surgical stabilization procedure has been defined as recurrence of instability. More recently, emphasis has been placed on achieving stability while maintaining range of motion and maximizing shoulder function. Thus, the challenge for the surgeon in treating glenohumeral instability is to achieve a delicate balance, stabilizing the shoulder without compromising function. An accurate diagnosis, as emphasized in Chapter 7, is essential if a satisfactory outcome is to be obtained.

HISTORICAL REVIEW

Hippocrates, in the 5th century B.C., described the difficulties that existed for people suffering from recurrent anterior shoulder dislocations. He spoke of how these people were "obliged to abandon gymnastic exercises" and became "inept in warlike practices, and . . . thus perished."[1] Hippocrates also described the first interventional treatment designed to prevent recurrent dislocations. He advocated placement of a white-hot poker in the axilla to promote scarring of the anteroinferior capsule. His rehabilitation protocol consisted of a lengthy period with the arm bound at the side to promote "cicatrization." It was not until the late 1800s that surgical procedures directed at repair of the anterior structures were described. In 1906, Perthes reported on a direct repair of the lesion associated with recurrent anterior instability.[2] He repaired the detached glenoid labrum and capsule to the glenoid rim with sutures through drill holes, reporting excellent results in patients monitored as long as 17 years. Bankart popularized a similar approach with reports in 1923 and 1939, advocating repair of the "essential lesion," detachment of the glenoid ligament from the bone. Overall, more than 150 open procedures have been described to treat glenohumeral instability. The number of procedures continues to rise as arthroscopic procedures are developed. The first arthroscopic treatment of anterior instability was described by Johnson in the 1980s, who used a 4-mm staple to secure the ligamentous complex.[3] This method was associated with an unacceptable failure rate. Caspari then popularized a technique using a suture punch to place multiple sutures in the capsulolabral complex, advancing it superiorly and then passing the sutures through transglenoid drill holes and tying them over the infraspinatus fascia.[4] Subsequently, Warren developed a bioabsorbable tack to allow fixation of the anterior structures, and Wolf popularized the use of suture anchors and arthroscopically tied knots for repair of the anterior capsule and labrum.[5, 6]

CLINICAL FEATURES AND INVESTIGATION

The history, physical examination, and utility of imaging studies are covered in Chapter 7. The importance of a proper diagnosis in planning treatment options cannot be overemphasized.

GOALS, INDICATIONS, AND CONTRAINDICATIONS

The primary goal in treating glenohumeral instability is the restoration of stability and return of shoulder function. For patients who have suffered an anterior shoulder dislocation, the initial treatment is immobilization with a sling. The duration of immobilization is controversial, because conflicting data exist regarding the role of immobilization and its effect on the rate of subsequent redislocation. In general, rehabilitation is initiated once the patient is comfortable. The initial focus is on restoring range of motion, followed by a progression of strengthening exercises, beginning with isometric exercises. Once these are achieved without pain, strengthening of the periscapular musculature and rotator cuff is instituted.

Patients with anterior subluxation generally respond well to a rehabilitation program similar to that described previously. Management of multidirectional instability, in which the primary pathology is capsular laxity and redundancy, can be a more difficult problem. A prolonged course of rehabilitation involving strengthening of the deltoid, scapular stabilizers, and rotator cuff is instituted. A focus on improvement of proprioception of the shoulder is also important. Patients with posterior instability also are initially treated with rehabilitation. An appropriate rehabilitation program is often successful in significantly improving the symptoms of instability. With all of these entities, patients who have suffered a traumatic event are generally less likely to respond to an exercise program, and surgical intervention may be considered after a shorter period of physical therapy.

The indications for surgical treatment of patients with recurrent anterior shoulder instability are subjective and must be individualized. Many patients choose to live with occasional episodes of subluxation or frank dislocation, and few data support operative intervention to prevent future complications, such as arthritis or rotator cuff injury. The patient who has undergone an appropriate period of rehabilitation and is not satisfied with his or her shoulder function is a candidate for surgery. This includes those who suffer frequent painful dislocations or subluxations and those who are unable to participate in desired activities to protect from episodes of instability. There are patients who live an "apprehensive life," avoiding positions that result in instability, and surgical stabilization can significantly improve their shoulder function and allow resumption of a more active lifestyle.

Because the patient's age is the most important factor in predicting the likelihood of redislocation, surgery is generally considered earlier in younger patients. Significant controversy exists as to the role of surgery, specifically arthroscopic stabilization, in patients younger than 30 years who have suffered a single traumatic anterior dislocation. The high recurrence rate in this age group, as high as 92% in a population of active military personnel, has led some surgeons to recommend surgical treatment after a first dislocation in young, active patients.[7] In the first prospective study addressing this issue, Arciero et al[8] found an 80% incidence of instability in military personnel treated nonoperatively compared with 14% in those treated with arthroscopic Bankart's repair.

Surgical treatment of multidirectional instability or posterior instability, unless preceded by a significant traumatic event, is considered only after failure of a course of physical therapy. With continued symptoms of pain or instability despite a concerted effort at rehabilitation, surgery may be recommended. Results of surgery are reasonably good but generally less predictable than in patients with recurrent anterior instability.

There are several contraindications to surgical treatment of glenohumeral instability. Patients who have not undergone an adequate course of rehabilitation are not surgical candidates. Surgery is also contraindicated in the patient with a seizure disorder that has not been medically controlled, because a seizure postoperatively will almost certainly result in redislocation and failure of the repair. A documented period of approximately 6 months without a seizure after medical intervention is required before surgical intervention. Patients who voluntarily or habitually dislocate their shoulder often have psychological problems or produce dislocations for secondary gain (e.g., attention, narcotic medication, or issues of compensation). They are poor surgical candidates, as are those who are unable or unwilling to comply with a postoperative rehabilitation program and those with a significant history of alcohol or drug abuse.

TABLE 1. DATA ON VARIOUS TREATMENTS FOR SHOULDER INSTABILITY				
Treatment Type	Indications	Specific Treatment	Redislocation Rate	Typical Outcome
Nonoperative	Stability achieved after rehabilitation	Periscapular and rotator cuff strengthening	Range = 20–92%, age dependent	Variable, excellent if no further instability
Arthroscopic	Bankart lesion, few dislocations, throwing athlete	Repair of Bankart lesion	Approximately 10–15%	Full motion, maintained function
Open	Capsular laxity, multiple dislocations, contact athlete	Repair of Bankart lesion, capsular shift if indicated	Range = 3–5%	Stable, 10-degree loss of external rotation

OPEN VERSUS ARTHROSCOPIC SURGICAL TREATMENT

Open techniques have historically been quite successful in achieving shoulder stability and preventing redislocation. However, complications such as loss of motion (primarily external rotation) and imperfect function have led to the development of arthroscopic stabilization techniques, with a goal of providing stability while maximizing function. The role of arthroscopic stabilization, compared with open techniques, is an area of extreme controversy. Theoretical advantages of arthroscopy include less damage to the anterior tissues, particularly the subscapularis tendon, and less postoperative scarring, which may contribute to loss of external rotation. Postoperative pain and bleeding are reduced, by minimizing soft-tissue dissection. Arthroscopic surgery is more likely to be performed on an outpatient basis, and rehabilitation time may be reduced. Arthroscopy allows improved visualization of the labrum and ligamentous structures and improves accuracy in identifying other intra-articular pathological lesions. Although arthroscopy allows precise repair of the Bankart lesion, it may be more difficult to address capsular laxity compared with open techniques. Redislocation rates have been generally higher in reports involving arthroscopic stabilization, and only relatively short-term follow-up is available. As arthroscopic techniques continue to evolve, results may compare favorably with those of open procedures. Currently, arthroscopic stabilization is more commonly performed in patients with a low number of dislocations, a Bankart lesion, and healthy capsuloligamentous structures. It also may be preferable in throwing athletes, in whom minor loss of function or motion can significantly compromise performance. Open techniques are often recommended in patients with multiple dislocations or capsular laxity and in contact athletes, in whom ultimate stability is of primary importance (Table 1).

SURGICAL TECHNIQUES

LABRAL TEARS

Tears of the labrum can occur at any position on the glenoid. In theory, these lesions can result in a mechanical source of pain, analogous to a torn meniscus in the knee, and arthroscopic débridement is expected to produce excellent long-term results. Nevaiser[9] reported uniformly good results with débridement of the labral tear and chondral injury found in glenolabral articular disruption lesions (described in Chapter 7), which by definition occur in shoulders without instability (Fig. 1).

However, labral tears most commonly occur in shoulders with underlying glenohumeral instability. Several studies found that simple débridement of labral tears yields symptomatic relief and early return to activities. However, these results have been found to deteriorate with increasing follow-up time.[10] Multiple authors postulated that the most common source of failure after labral débridement is failure to address concomitant glenohumeral instability. A careful history and examination (including exam under anesthesia) is essential in attempting to determine whether underlying instability is present. In the stable shoulder, arthroscopic labral débridement with a motorized shaver is performed. If concomitant glenohumeral instability is present, it must be addressed using techniques described later in this chapter.

SUPERIOR LABRUM ANTERIOR POSTERIOR LESIONS

Tears or detachment of the superior labrum are evaluated and treated arthroscopically. Type I lesions are treated by débridement of the frayed portion of the labrum and biceps anchor. Care must be taken to avoid overly aggressive débridement of healthy uninvolved tissue, which can progress to biceps tendon rupture. Iatrogenic extension of the superior labrum anterior posterior (SLAP) lesion may create or aggravate preexisting glenohumeral instability. A careful assessment of glenohumeral stability must be performed, because failure to address instability will result in a poor outcome.

The first step in appropriate treatment of type II SLAP lesions is a thorough arthroscopic evaluation to determine whether pathology is truly present. Normal anatomic variants, such as the sublabral hole at the 2 o'clock position and the Buford complex (middle glenohumeral attachment to the biceps anchor and the absence of the anterosuperior labrum) must be recognized. These lesions do not require surgical repair, and fixation will often result in undesired limitation in shoulder motion. Through a standard anterosuperior portal, the superior labrum and biceps anchor are evaluated with an arthroscopic probe. The normal superior labrum may have a "meniscal" appearance, with a free central edge. As the labrum is lifted superiorly with the probe, hemorrhage or inflammatory tissue may be visualized in an acute lesion. However, the majority of these lesions do not come to surgery until they are relatively chronic. In a normal shoulder, the articular cartilage extends to the edge of the labral attachment. With type II SLAP lesions, cancellous bone or fibrous tissue will be visualized as the superior labrum is elevated. Another clue in determining whether pathology exists lies in the degree to which the labrum can be pulled superiorly; more than 3 to 4 mm is likely pathological[11] (Fig. 2).

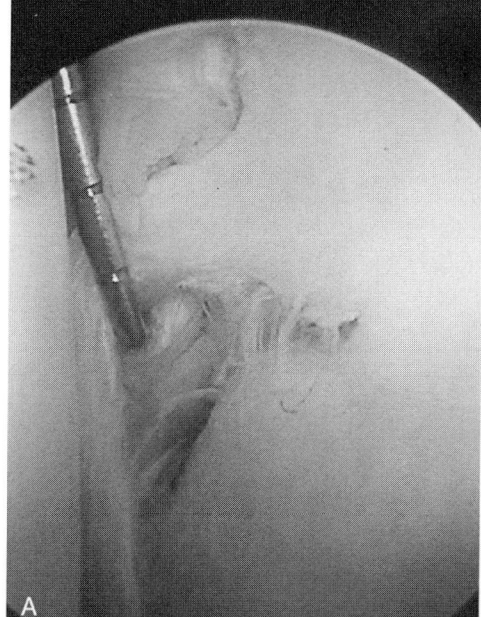 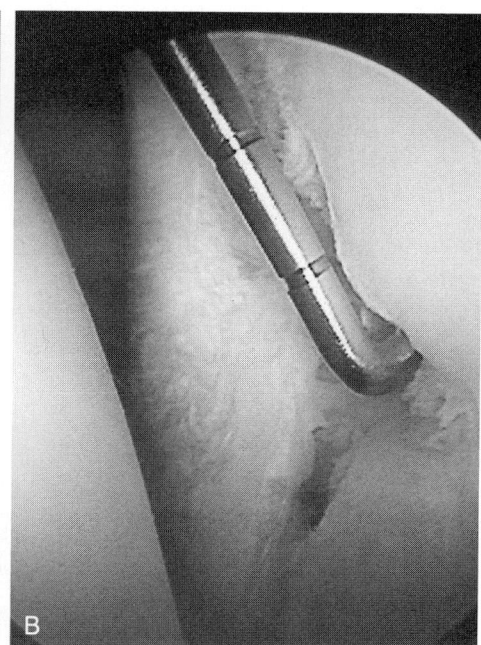

Fig. 1. Glenolabral articular disruption. *A*, Arthroscopic view of anteroinferior labral tear and chondral injury. The patient complained of anterior shoulder pain and had no evidence of instability at examination. The patient is in the beach chair position. *B*, The labral tear and chondral flap have been débrided. The probe is used to confirm that the chondral edge is stable.

Treatment of type II SLAP lesions requires secure fixation of the labrum to the superior glenoid. This is generally accomplished with suture anchors and arthroscopic suture repair of the labral tissue or through the use of bioabsorbable tacks. We prefer the security and versatility of suture repair. The superior glenoid is prepared with a shaver or bur to remove fibrous tissue and provide a bed of vascular, cancellous bone for healing. Lesions that do not extend significantly posterior to the biceps anchor can be repaired through the anterosuperior portal. A drill guide is introduced and placed in position under the detached biceps anchor. After drilling a hole in the cancellous bone through the guide, the suture anchor is deployed by passing it down the same drill guide. The suture must then be passed through the labral tissue. Several variations of "suture passers" are available, which can be pushed through the labrum and allow the suture to be grasped and pulled back through in one step. A knot may then be tied, or if a mattress suture is desired, the second limb of the suture is passed through the labral tissue, approximately 8 mm from the first suture.[11] A knot is tied outside the shoulder, then pushed down the cannula until the labral tissue is firmly secured. This step is repeated several times to lock and secure the knot, the security of the repair is tested with a probe, and the ends of the sutures are cut near the knot with arthroscopic scissors (Fig. 3).

Repair of a type II SLAP lesion that extends significantly posterior to the biceps anchor is more difficult, because the acromion lies above the lesion, making it difficult to gain direct access. Repair of a posterior SLAP lesion often requires the use of an accessory portal. The supraspinatus (Nevaiser) portal, or the "port of Wilmington" lateral to the acromion, may be used, and both are described in Chapter 7. Others advocated the use of a transacromial portal, drilling a hole through the acromion to gain more direct access.[12]

The type III SLAP lesion is encountered relatively infrequently. By definition, the biceps anchor remains intact, so fixation of the anchor back to the glenoid is not required. The bucket-handle–type tear of the labrum is excised using a standard arthroscopic basket punch, followed by débridement of the edge of the tear with a motorized shaver. A probe is then used to palpate the biceps anchor, ensuring that it is securely attached.

Type IV SLAP lesions involve a bucket-handle tear of the superior labrum, which extends into the biceps tendon. Repair of these lesions requires passage of sutures across

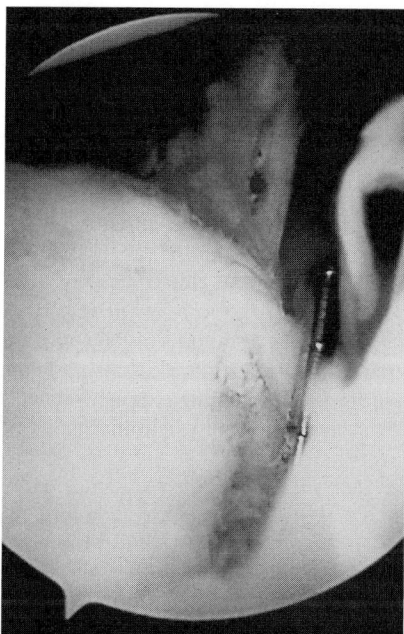

Fig. 2. Type II SLAP lesion. The patient is in the lateral position. With traction applied via the probe, cancellous bone is seen under the biceps anchor, and the biceps pulls away approximately 5 mm.

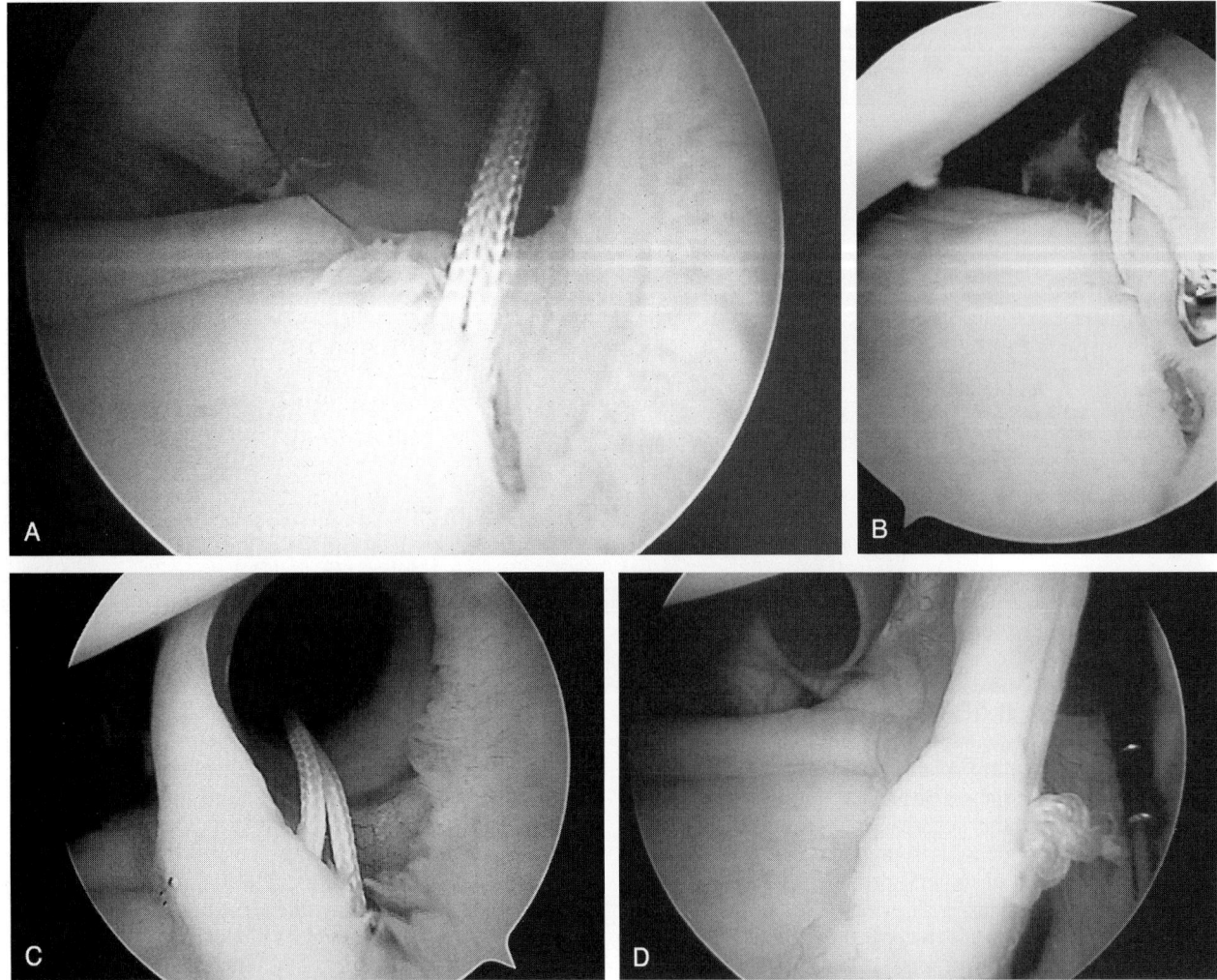

Fig. 3. Repair of SLAP lesion. *A,* The suture anchor has been deployed in the bone. The two limbs of suture exit the anterosuperior portal. *B,* The suture is grasped after passing the grasping device through the labral tissue. *C,* Both limbs of the suture have been passed through the labral tissue to allow an arthroscopic knot to be tied for mattress repair. *D,* An arthroscopic knot has been tied, securing the biceps anchor to the superior glenoid.

the torn biceps tendon as well as the labral tear (Fig. 4). If the biceps anchor is also detached, this must be repaired back to bone as described for type II lesions. If the extension into the biceps tendon is minimal, involving up to approximately 30% of the tendon, excision of the tear may be considered. Although efforts are made to repair these lesions in young, athletic patients, in patients with lower functional demands, the method of biceps excision and tenodesis is a reasonable option, particularly when the lesion is complex or degenerative.

Postoperative Management

In patients with SLAP lesions treated with simple débridement, range-of-motion exercises are initiated as soon as the patient is comfortable. Once a complete range of motion has been regained, strengthening exercises are initiated. When repair of the SLAP lesion has been performed, patients are commonly immobilized in a sling for 2 to 4 weeks, although elbow, wrist, and hand exercises are allowed during this time. In particular, shoulder external rotation and extension are limited, often for 4 weeks to allow

early healing. Burkhart and Morgan[13] emphasized that external rotation beyond neutral places undue stress on repairs of posterior SLAP lesions, and these authors do not allow external rotation for 3 weeks. Limitations to motion should be determined at surgery when the lesion and the repair are assessed. A graduated program of increasing motion is used; full motion is generally gained and strengthening initiated at about 6 weeks postoperatively. Regular activities and sports are usually allowed at 3 to 4 months, again dependent on the extent of the lesion as well as the patient's progress in physical therapy.

INTERNAL IMPINGEMENT

Impingement of the posterosuperior glenoid on the posterior aspect of the supraspinatus tendon or the infraspinatus tendon as a source of pain has been described. It occurs with the shoulder in the abducted, externally rotated position, primarily in overhead athletes. Controversy exists as to the degree to which anterior instability contributes to this phenomenon. Simple débridement of the worn area of the posterosuperior labrum and the undersurface rotator

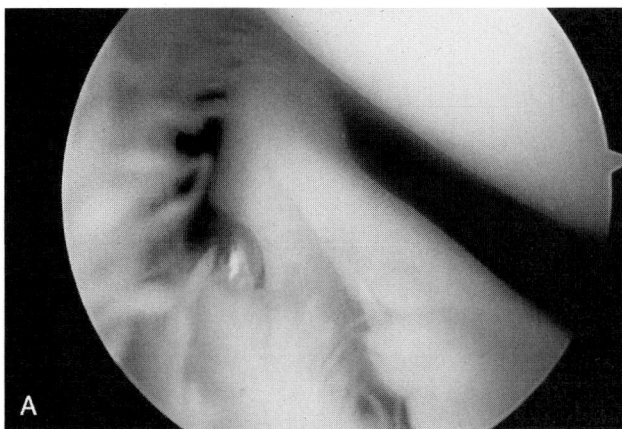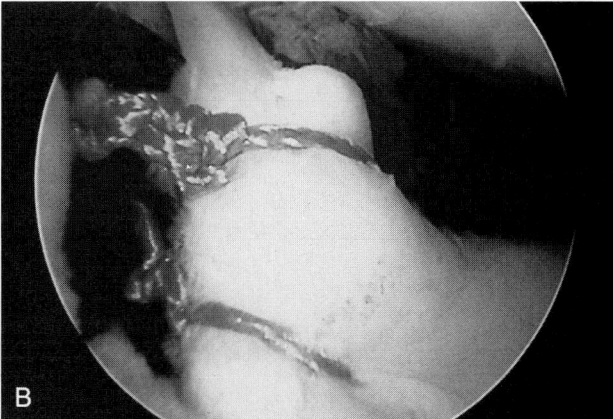

Fig. 4. Type IV SLAP. *A*, Bucket-handle tear extends into the biceps. *B*, Lesion repaired.

cuff generally produces relief of symptoms in the short term. As with other lesions described previously, if anterior instability is contributing to the pathology it must be addressed or recurrence of symptoms can be expected. In patients who have had recurrence of pain, Riand et al[14] described a humeral osteotomy to increase retrotorsion of the proximal humerus in an attempt to allow increased external rotation at the shoulder without internal impingement. This is an extensive procedure, but these authors reported generally good results in overhead athletes who were otherwise unable to perform their sports after failure of simple débridement.

ANTERIOR INSTABILITY

The most consistent finding in traumatic anterior shoulder instability is the detachment of the glenoid labrum from the anterior glenoid rim, which is known as the Bankart lesion. This lesion has been observed to occur in 85% to 100% of patients undergoing surgery after anterior dislocation.[15] The goal of treatment of anterior instability is the reattachment of the Bankart lesion to its normal anatomic location, along with restoration of appropriate tension to the inferior glenohumeral ligamentous complex. The gold standard for comparison is the open Bankart's repair popularized by Rowe et al.[16] Other surgical techniques for restoring stability, which often involve alteration of anatomy, have become less accepted because of a higher incidence of recurrent instability or unacceptable rates of restriction of motion.

Before making the incision, a diagnostic arthroscopy is helpful in confirming the presence of a Bankart lesion as well as identifying any other pathology in the joint that must be addressed. The open Bankart repair is accomplished through an anterior approach to the shoulder. The patient is positioned supine, with the head elevated 30 degrees. An incision is made from just lateral to the coracoid, inferiorly toward the anterior axillary fold. This incision may be made more inferiorly, in the axilla, for cosmetic purposes, with subcutaneous flaps then undermined superiorly. The cephalic vein is identified as the landmark between the deltoid and pectoralis major muscles. The vein can be reflected laterally or medially. We generally prefer to take the vein laterally, with the deltoid: less bleeding is encountered because the majority of feeding vessels to the

vein come from the deltoid. The deltoid is then retracted laterally and the pectoralis medially. The clavipectoral fascia is incised over the subscapularis tendon, and the medial retractor is then replaced under the lateral border of the conjoined tendon.

One of the keys to a successful open Bankart repair is adequate exposure. The deltoid muscle is undermined to allow it to be retracted well laterally. Excessive medial retraction is to be avoided, because the brachial plexus is medial to the coracoid, and injury to the axillary or musculocutaneous nerve can occur with improper placement or overzealous use of the retractor. To prevent iatrogenic injury, the musculocutaneous nerve is palpated as it enters the medial aspect of the coracobrachialis muscle. The axillary nerve is palpated by placing a finger on the lower anterior surface of the subscapularis muscle, which it traverses under before traveling posteriorly below the inferior capsule. If necessary to gain medial exposure, a portion of the conjoined tendon can be divided transversely and repaired at closure. Improved inferior exposure can be achieved by carefully dividing the upper 1 cm of the pectoralis tendon, and superior exposure by dividing the coracoacromial ligament (Fig. 5).

With retractors in place, the subscapularis tendon is inspected. External rotation of the arm helps bring it into the field. The remainder of the procedure involves division of the subscapularis tendon, opening of the capsule to enter the joint, followed by repair of the Bankart lesion. Numerous techniques have been described to accomplish the repair, which fall generally under three categories (Fig. 6).

The first technique involves a vertical division of the subscapularis tendon. The lower one-fourth of the tendon is often left intact to prevent dissection near the axillary nerve. The tendon is then peeled off the underlying capsule, and the capsule opened with a separate incision. The joint is entered, and a humeral head retractor placed over the posterior glenoid, pushing the humeral head in a posterolateral direction. A second retractor is placed medial to the anterior glenoid margin to allow visualization of the Bankart lesion at the anteroinferior aspect of the glenoid. With chronic lesions, the Bankart often "heals" medially, off the glenoid rim, where it does not provide proper ten-

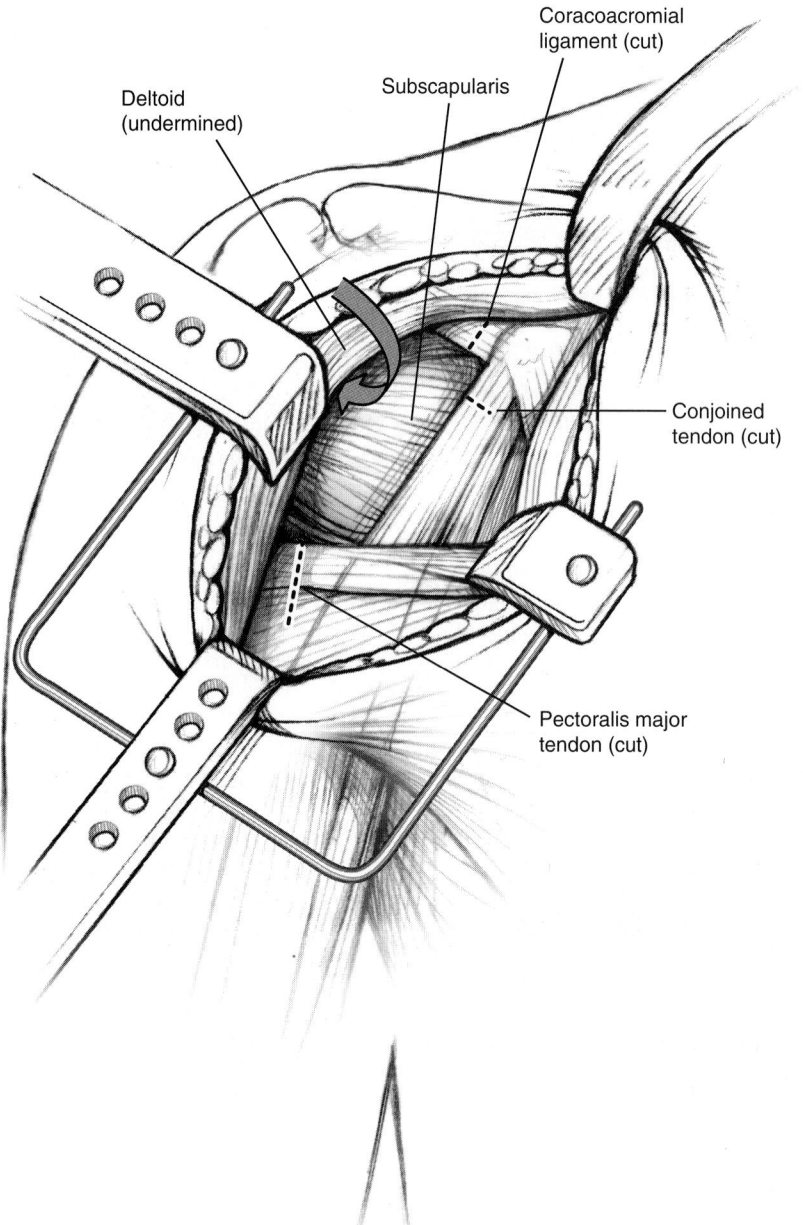

Deltoid
(undermined)

Subscapularis

Coracoacromial
ligament (cut)

Conjoined
tendon (cut)

Pectoralis major
tendon (cut)

Fig. 5. Anterior deltopectoral approach. Exposure can be improved by undermining the deltoid and dividing the coracoacromial ligament and the upper centimeter of the pectoralis major tendon. If necessary to gain medial exposure, a portion of the conjoined tendon may be divided.

sion to the glenohumeral ligaments and the anterior "bumper" is not present. The labrum must be sharply dissected off the medial glenoid to allow anatomic repair. The anterior glenoid margin is then prepared with a rongeur or bur to provide a bleeding surface of cancellous bone to promote healing. Three to four suture anchors are then placed at the anterior glenoid rim. Alternatively, sutures may be passed through drill holes. Again, care must be taken to repair the labrum to the rim of the glenoid, because medialization of the repair will likely result in failure to provide stability. The sutures are taken through the capsule at the point where it attaches to the labrum and are tied over the capsule in mattress fashion, securing the labrum to the anterior glenoid (Fig. 7).

If it is determined that capsular laxity exists in addition to the Bankart lesion, the capsule may be divided in the shape of a T. The inferior leaf is then shifted superiorly

and repaired, whereas the superior leaf is taken inferiorly. Such a shift can correct excessive capsular laxity, but care must be taken not to overly tighten the capsule, which will result in the loss of shoulder motion, most commonly external rotation. The subscapularis tendon is then repaired anatomically before final wound closure.

A second strategy for Bankart's repair is the anterior capsulolabral reconstruction popularized by Jobe et al.[17] This is most commonly advocated for throwing athletes, in whom vertical division of the subscapularis tendon can produce sufficient anterior scarring or motion loss that performance is commonly hindered. The primary difference in this technique is that the subscapularis is divided transversely, in line with its fibers, potentially allowing for a more precise anatomic repair of the subscapularis. The remainder of the procedure is generally similar to that described previously. A potential disadvantage is that expo-

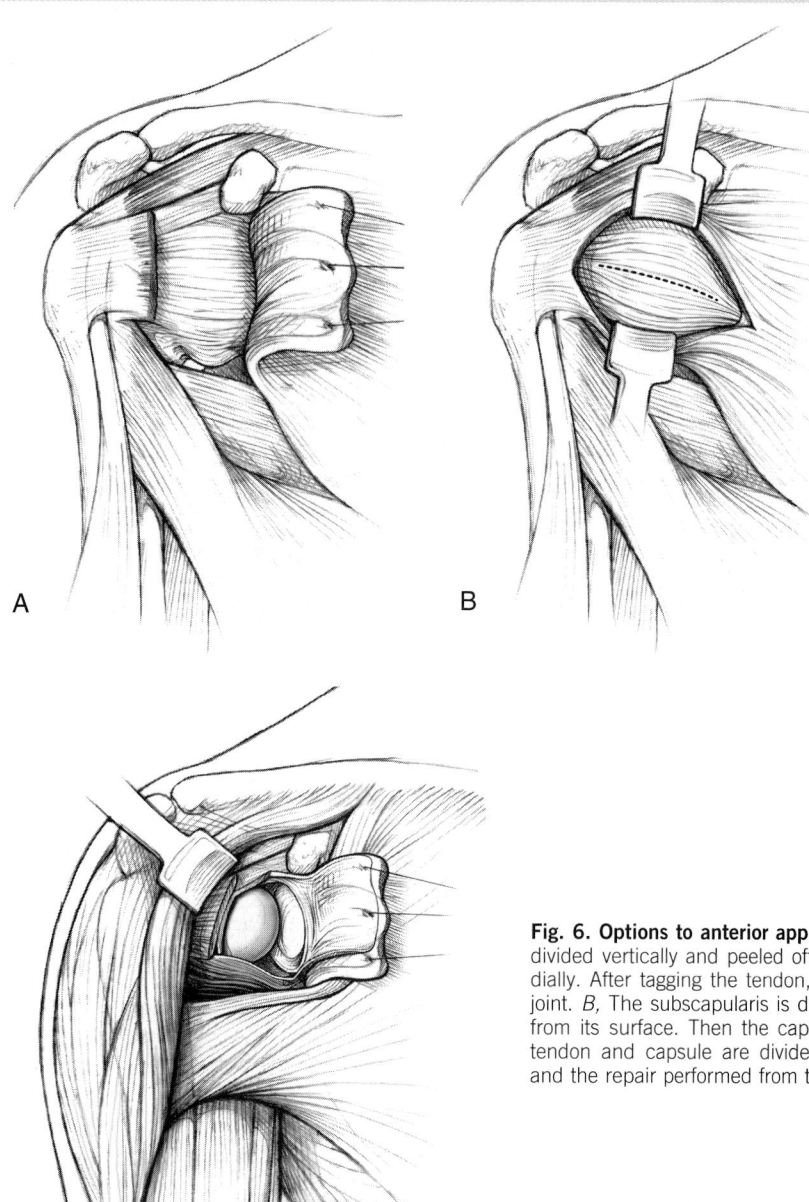

Fig. 6. Options to anterior approach. *A,* The subscapularis tendon is divided vertically and peeled off the underlying capsule, working medially. After tagging the tendon, the capsule is opened to expose the joint. *B,* The subscapularis is divided vertically and the capsule freed from its surface. Then the capsule is opened. *C,* The subscapularis tendon and capsule are divided as one layer. The joint is exposed and the repair performed from the inside.

sure can be more difficult, unless the surgeon is experienced in this technique.

A third option for repair has been popularized by Matsen et al.[1] They advocated vertical division of the subscapularis and capsule together in one layer, which obviates the need for separation of the two layers. The Bankart lesion is then repaired from inside the capsule; sutures are taken around the labrum and tied inside the joint. This does not allow the surgeon to shift the capsule directly, although some capsular laxity may be addressed by taking capsule with the labrum while passing the sutures.

In cases of anterior or anteroinferior instability in which a Bankart lesion is not present, a capsular shift is performed. The approach is similar to that described previously, with flaps of inferior and superior capsule shifted and sutured in pants-over-vest fashion.

ARTHROSCOPIC BANKART'S REPAIR

Arthroscopic Bankart's repair may be performed in the "beach chair" or lateral decubitus position. Use of the beach chair position prevents potential distortion of normal anatomy, allows the arm to be free to dynamically evaluate the glenohumeral ligaments throughout a range of motion, and provides for easier conversion to an open procedure.

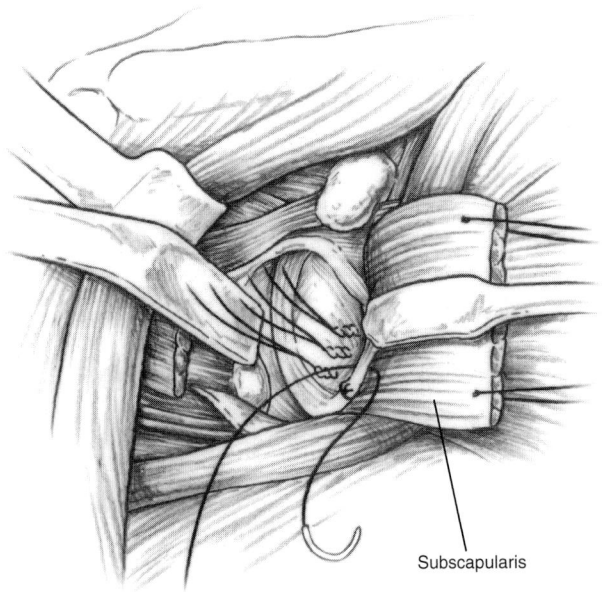

Fig. 7. Bankart's repair. The suture anchors are placed along the anterior glenoid rim. The sutures are then passed through the labral tissue and tied to secure the lesion back to the anterior glenoid margin.

The primary advantage of the lateral position is that distraction of the joint is obtained, allowing easier access to the inferior aspect of the anterior labrum and glenoid, the most important part of the repair. Visualization from the posterior portal, with a standard anterosuperior portal and a second anterior portal placed just above the subscapularis

tendon, is generally used. After inspection of the Bankart lesion, an arthroscopic rasp or knife is used to mobilize the capsuloligamentous complex down to near the 6 o'clock position on the glenoid. This allows for vertical shift of the capsule to address laxity, and prevents medialization of the repair. The anterior glenoid rim is abraded with a shaver or rasp to expose bleeding bone. A drill guide is placed, a hole drilled, and suture anchor positioned at the 5 o'clock position (right shoulder). The suture from the anchor is passed through the capsulolabral interface as described previously in the treatment of SLAP lesions. An arthroscopic knot is then tied. This process is repeated, moving superiorly, with three anchors commonly placed (Fig. 8).

MULTIDIRECTIONAL INSTABILITY

Patients with multidirectional instability (MDI) generally do not have a Bankart lesion, and the primary problem to be addressed is excessive global laxity of the capsule. This entity is most commonly treated with an open inferior capsular shift procedure, attributed to Neer and Foster.[18] In the majority of cases, the capsular shift is performed through an anterior approach, with the initial dissection similar to that of an open Bankart procedure. If the primary direction of instability is clearly posterior, the capsular shift may be performed through the posterior approach. In either case, the capsule is shifted to the degree necessary to address the redundant inferior capsular pouch.

After the initial anterior approach, the subscapularis tendon is divided vertically and elevated off the underlying capsule. The capsule is freed inferiorly; care is taken to protect the underlying axillary nerve. The capsule is then

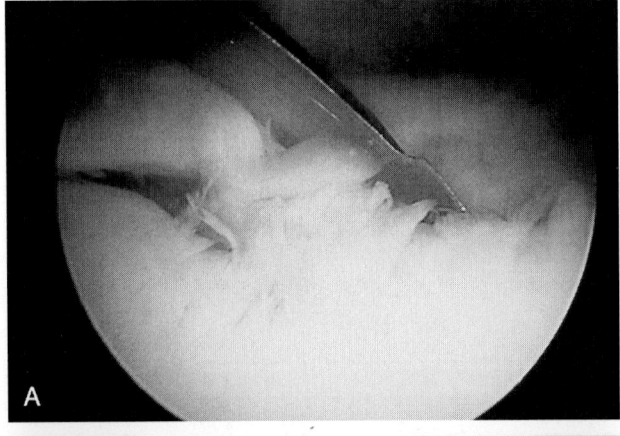

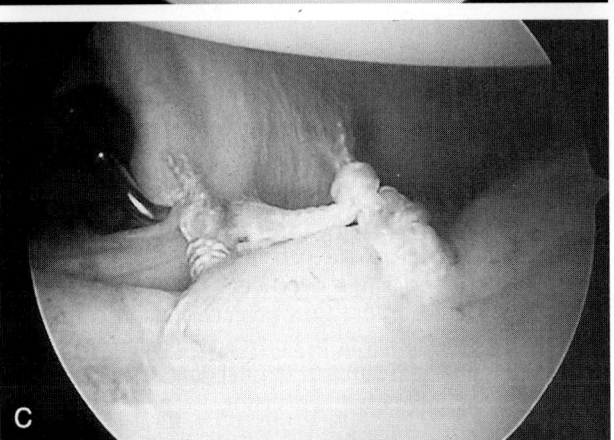

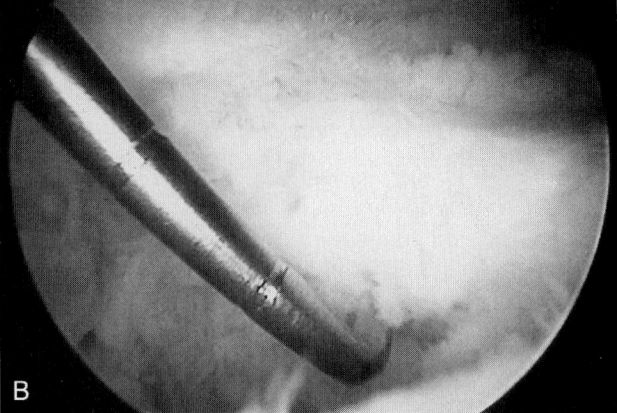

Fig. 8. Arthroscopic Bankart's repair. *A*, Bankart's lesion freed from where it has "healed" medially. *B*, Bankart's lesion after it has been mobilized. *C*, Bankart's lesion repaired with arthroscopically placed sutures.

incised in a vertical direction laterally near the humeral neck, and the incision carried well posteriorly if a large shift is necessary. The capsule is opened in a T shape with a horizontal limb extending to the glenoid, between the inferior and middle glenohumeral ligaments. The inferior limb is then shifted superiorly and repaired to bone with suture anchors or to the remaining lateral stump of capsule. This effectively diminishes the size of the inferior capsular pouch. The rotator interval capsule between the subscapularis and supraspinatus tendons is closed, and the superior flap is taken inferiorly and repaired over the inferior flap. The subscapularis tendon is repaired anatomically (Fig. 9).

POSTERIOR INSTABILITY

Posterior instability is encountered less frequently than anterior instability and is more likely to present as frequent subluxation episodes than recurrent dislocations. It is also less commonly traumatic in origin, although it does occur in certain sports, such as in offensive linemen in football. Posterior labral injury without evidence of instability can also occur in contact athletes, and repair of the labral injury produces good results.[19] In cases of traumatic posterior instability, a posterior capsulolabral detachment, a "reverse Bankart lesion," may be present, and surgical treatment is analogous to that described previously for the Bankart repair. If necessary, some of the posterior capsule can be imbricated in the repair to treat capsular laxity.[20] In cases of atraumatic instability, the underlying pathology is a redundant capsule, usually manifesting with a component of inferior instability as well.

The posterior approach to the shoulder begins with a vertical incision extending approximately 1 cm medial to the posterolateral corner of the acromion down toward the posterior axillary fold. Dissection is carried down to the deltoid muscle, which is split in line with its fibers from the scapular spine extending inferiorly. Classically, the approach was then continued in the internervous plane between the infraspinatus and teres minor, dividing this interval transversely to expose the underlying posterior capsule. Care must be taken not to stray inferiorly, because the axillary nerve and posterior humeral circumflex artery exit the quadrilateral space below the teres minor. An alternative approach involves splitting the infraspinatus in line with its fibers.[21] This allows for a more direct approach to the posterior capsule, but the split must not be carried more than 1.5 cm medial to the glenoid to avoid injury to the suprascapular nerve.

The capsule is opened and retractors are placed to expose the posterior glenoid. If a reverse Bankart lesion is present, it is repaired with suture anchors as described for the anterior Bankart repair. A posterior capsular shift is then performed to address capsular laxity. Because the posterior capsule is quite thin, this repair can appear to be somewhat tenuous. To combat this, some surgeons prefer to divide the infraspinatus tendon vertically, incorporating this tendon into the repair by repairing the lateral flap to the glenoid, then taking the medial flap and suturing it over the top of the lateral flap[22] (Fig. 10).

Posterior instability can also be addressed arthroscopically in much the same manner as described for anterior

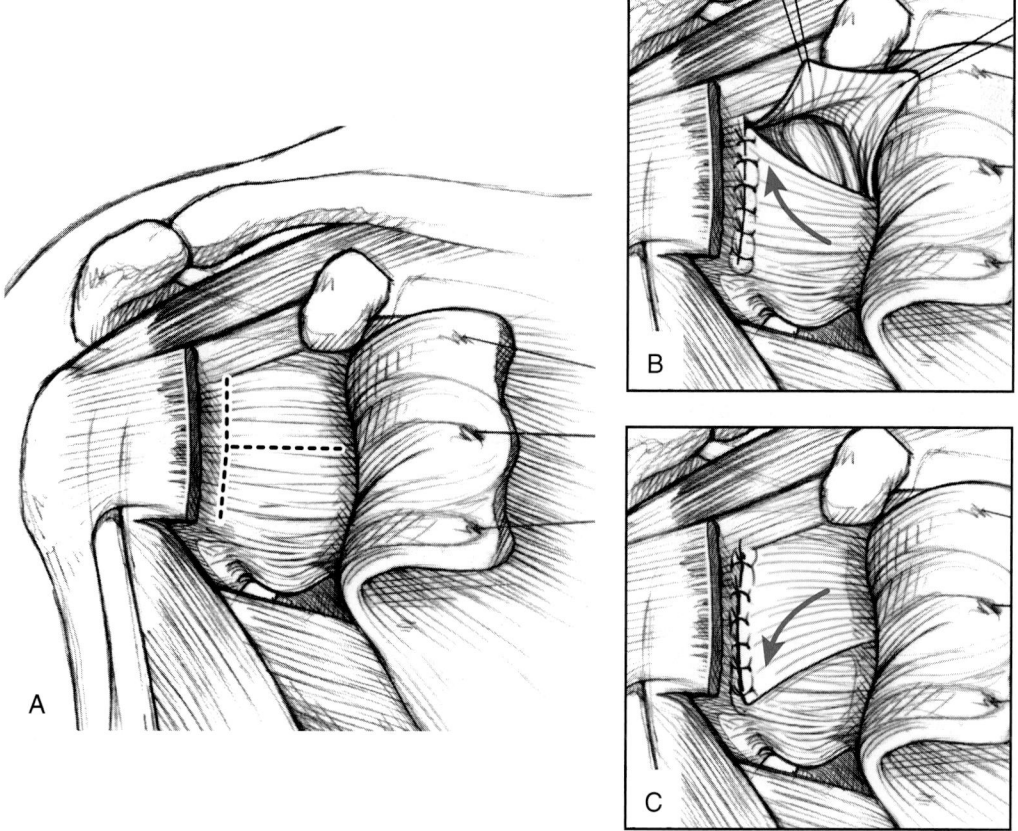

Fig. 9. Inferior capsular shift. The capsule is divided in the shape of a T, inferior leaf shifted superiorly, superior leaf taken inferiorly.

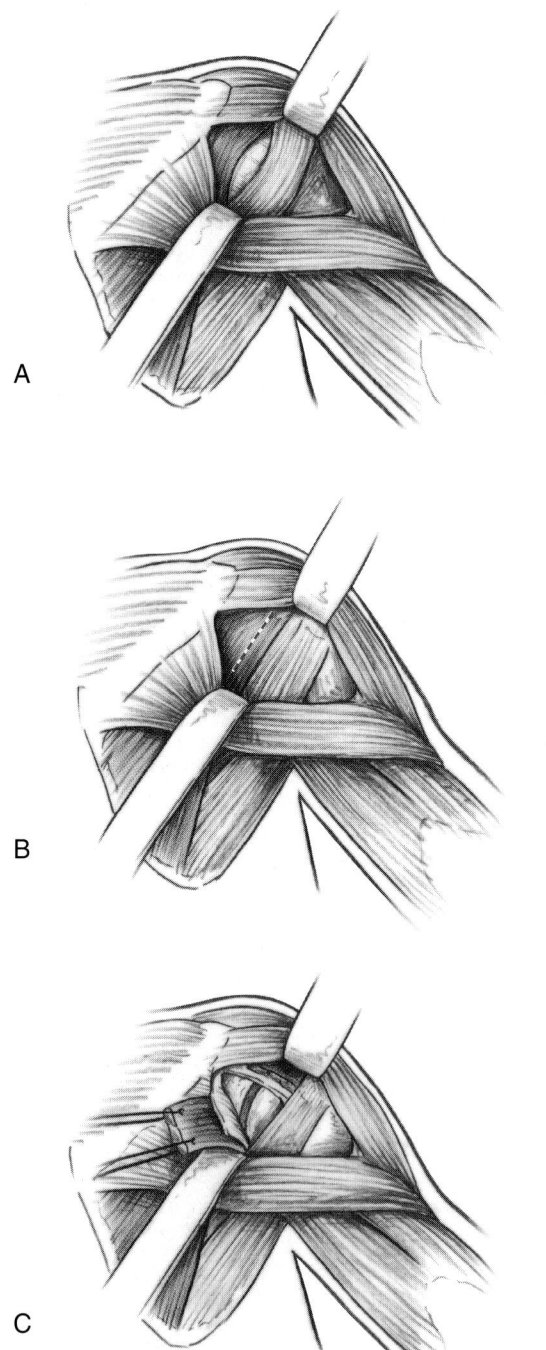

Fig. 10. Posterior approaches. *A,* The capsule is approached between the infraspinatus and teres minor. *B,* The capsule is approached by splitting the infraspinatus. *C,* The infraspinatus and capsule are divided vertically as one layer; the infraspinatus tendon is used to bolster repair.

instability. A reverse Bankart lesion can be repaired with suture anchors and arthroscopically tied knots. The posterior capsule may be incorporated into this repair to tighten the capsule[20] (Fig. 11).

THERMAL CAPSULORRAPHY
Enthusiasm has been growing for treatment of capsular laxity with heat, which results in denaturing of collagen fibers and "shrinking" of the capsule. Thermal probes have been developed, which are used arthroscopically to heat the capsule. The optimal temperature to shrink the capsule without causing excessive thermal injury appears to be about 67°C. The visual effect is often quite dramatic, with the capsule and glenohumeral ligaments clearly tightening as the probe is moved over the tissue (Fig. 12).

This method has been advocated for a wide range of patients, from throwers with subtle anterior instability to patients with severe MDI. Although good results of this technique have been reported in several short-term reports, it must be cautioned that the long-term outcomes are not yet known. Basic science research has shown that tissue can stretch after thermal treatment, and the implications for rehabilitation are not yet well defined.[23] A period of immobilization, from 1 to 3 weeks, is often recommended after thermal capsulorraphy to allow the capsule to begin reconstituting before subjecting it to tensile forces. Certainly, this technique holds promise, but there is much to learn about its indications and long-term effectiveness.

SPECIAL CIRCUMSTANCES
Several circumstances can exist that complicate the surgical management of glenohumeral instability. Details of treatment of these problems fall beyond the scope of this chapter. In the patient with recurrent or continued instability after surgical treatment, the principles of revision surgery are much the same as those described previously, but surgery is technically more difficult secondary to scarring from the prior procedure. If significant bony deficiency of the anterior glenoid exists, reconstitution of bone stock is performed using a transfer of the coracoid process or with a bone graft from the iliac crest. Large Hill-Sachs lesions (posterior humeral head defect from anterior dislocation) may require allograft reconstruction or transfer of the infraspinatus muscle into the defect. Deficiency of the anterior capsule or inferior glenohumeral ligament may require the surgeon to transfer tissue, such as the semitendinosus and gracilis tendons, weaving them into the anterior aspect of the shoulder as a salvage procedure. In severe refractory cases of recurrent instability, glenohumeral arthrodesis may be required as a last resort.

Postoperative Management
After surgery for anterior instability, patients are placed in a sling for 2 to 3 weeks. During this time, passive and active assisted flexion to 90 degrees is initiated, with external rotation limited to neutral. After 3 weeks, active elevation is initiated and external rotation gradually progressed to achieve full motion by 6 to 8 weeks. Periscapular and rotator cuff strengthening are initiated at 6 weeks. Emphasis is also placed on regaining neuromuscular control and proprioception. Unrestricted sports activity is not allowed until 4 months after surgery.

Patients undergoing surgery for MDI or posterior instability are immobilized in a "gunslinger" brace, which keeps the shoulder at neutral rotation, for 4 to 6 weeks, depending on the degree of instability. Range-of-motion exercises are then introduced, and strengthening and neuromuscular exercises are initiated once motion is regained. Return to sports is generally allowed at 6 months postoperatively.

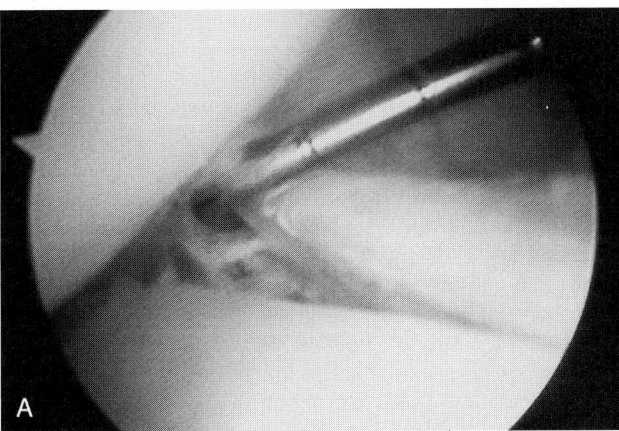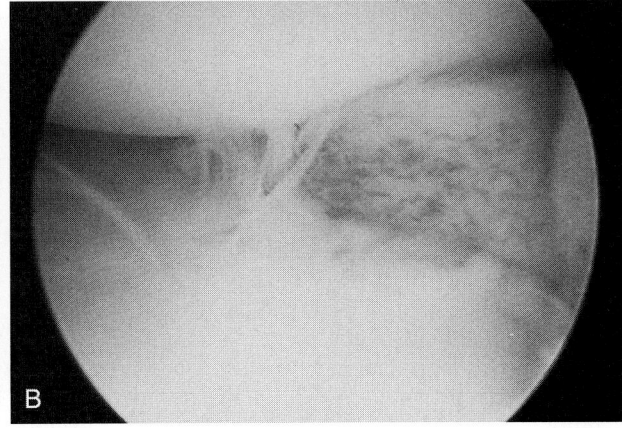

Fig. 11. Arthroscopic posterior repair. *A,* This view shows a "reverse" Bankart lesion. *B,* This view shows repair of the posterior Bankart lesion with capsular imbrication to tighten capsule.

COMPLICATIONS

The most common complications of glenohumeral instability surgery are recurrence of instability and loss of shoulder motion. The rates of these occurring are discussed in the Results and Outcomes section. An overly tight anterior reconstruction, with resultant loss of external rotation, has been implicated in the development of glenohumeral arthritis. The biomechanical effect of overconstraining the anterior aspect of the joint is to force the humeral head posteriorly and increase contact pressures on the glenoid surface. In a 15-year follow-up study of Bankart's reconstruction, restriction of external rotation was found to correlate with degree of degenerative change.[24] Degenerative changes have also been noted after posterior stabilization procedures.

Injuries to the axillary, musculocutaneous, median, ulnar, and radial nerve have been reported after instability surgery. Fortunately, the majority of these reports have involved neurapraxias, which resolved without intervention. To prevent neurological complications, an understanding of anatomy and adequate exposure are required during instability surgery. The axillary and musculocutaneous nerves are most at risk during anterior instability surgery. The axillary nerve is particularly at risk when an inferior capsular shift is performed. The nerve passes 1 to 1.5 cm below the capsule, and effort must be made to identify and protect it when working inferiorly. The musculocutaneous nerve penetrates the coracobrachialis muscle at an average of 5.6 cm below the coracoid, but has been found to penetrate as close as 2 cm.[25] Failure to identify the nerve and placement of a retractor directly on it or overzealous retraction of the conjoined tendon can result in injury to the nerve. Neurological injury can also occur during arthroscopic stabilization procedures. Excessive traction while using the lateral position has been implicated in some cases. Anterior portals placed below the superior border of the subscapularis tendon place the axillary nerve at risk. Injury to the axillary nerve with thermal capsulorraphy to the axillary pouch has also been described. The suprascapular nerve may be injured if the Nevaiser portal is used and the portal placed too far medially.

Migration or inappropriate placement of hardware has resulted in pain or articular cartilage injury to the glenoid or humerus from the implant. Zuckerman and Matsen[26] reported on 37 patients with complications related to screws and staples placed about the glenohumeral joint, with articular cartilage injury occurring in 41% of these cases. A resurgence in the use of implants has occurred with the popularity of suture anchors. Although the pull-out strengths of these anchors is generally quite good, loosening of metallic implants with resultant articular injury has been reported.[27] Postoperative infection requiring removal of metallic suture anchors has also been described.[28] Bioabsorbable anchors have been developed. Loosening of these anchors may result in less articular injury, but they may also go undetected within the joint, because they are not seen radiographically.

Disruption of the subscapularis tendon repair after anterior stabilization can occur, and early detection and revision repair are essential to prevent instability and functional loss.[29] Infection rates after open instability surgery are approximately 0.3% for deep infection and 1.4% when superficial infections are included.[30]

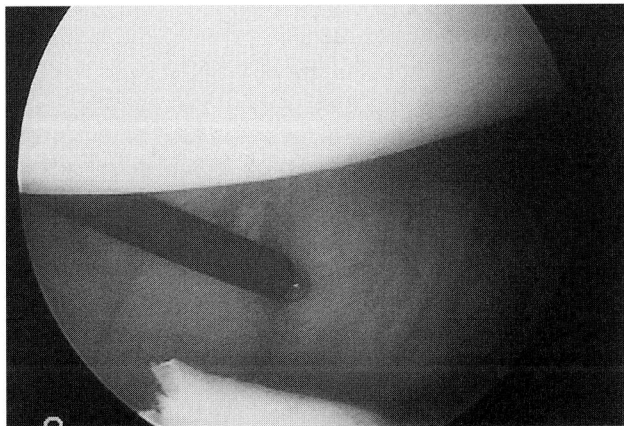

Fig. 12. Thermal capsulorraphy. A thermal probe is used to heat the capsule, thereby "shrinking" it.

RESULTS AND OUTCOMES

SLAP LESIONS

Outcome data after treatment of SLAP lesions are generally lacking, because these lesions were described in the last decade and most reports consist of small series. Significant relief of pain and return to activities after repair of type II lesions has been reported to occur in about 80% of patients.[31, 32] Difficulty in the interpretation of results also stems from the fact that SLAP lesions often occur in the presence of other concomitant pathology. In the largest series of SLAP lesions in the literature, only 28% of 140 lesions occurred in isolation.[33] Another study found that 43% of 84 patients with SLAP lesions had documented instability compared to the opposite shoulder during examination under anesthesia.[34] A careful preoperative history and examination are essential, as is examination under anesthesia, and at the time of arthroscopy the entire joint must be inspected. Failure to address concomitant instability, Bankart's lesions, partial- or full-thickness rotator cuff tears, or other pathology will result in a compromised outcome for the patient.

INSTABILITY

Stabilization procedures are generally quite successful in preventing recurrence of anterior dislocations. In a review of the literature, data were compiled on 3187 patients, in whom a wide variety of surgical procedures for anterior reconstruction had been used. The rate of dislocation ranged from 0% to 18%, with an overall average of 3%.[35] It is important to realize that recurrence rates can increase with length of follow-up. In a long-term series in which 20 patients suffered recurrent dislocation, seven of these first occurred more than 2 years after surgery.[36] Recurrence rates after arthroscopic stabilization are difficult to interpret, because length of follow-up is consistently shorter and techniques continue to evolve. Recurrence rates with arthroscopic stabilization for anterior instability range from 0% to 45%.[37] Currently, redislocation rates are believed to be higher than with open surgery; a general rate of 5% to 15% is common in larger series. As techniques evolve to resemble open repairs more closely and as methods of addressing capsular laxity improve, many arthroscopists believe that long-term results comparable to those seen with open surgery can be achieved.

Recurrent instability after surgery for MDI is more difficult to interpret, because fewer large series exist and follow-up is generally shorter. Definition of recurrence is also more difficult; many of these patients do not experience dislocation but subluxation and pain. In the initial report on inferior capsular shift, Neer and Foster[18] found recurrence of subluxation in one of 40 shoulders, but only 17 patients were monitored for more than 2 years. Cooper and Brems[38] reported recurrence in four of 43 shoulders treated with inferior capsular shift and monitored for a minimum of 2 years. These authors found no deterioration of results in those patients followed up for 6 years.

Recurrence rates after open surgery for posterior instability have been less predictable. Again, the majority of these patients suffer from recurrent episodes of subluxation without dislocation. Some early reports cited recurrence rates greater than 50%. More recent studies reported greater rates of success, with recurrence rates of 12% or less.

Results of revision surgery have been more successful in patients revised for anterior instability than in those with MDI. At an average of 6.5 years after surgery, Zabinski et al[39] found good or excellent results in 78% of patients undergoing revision anterior reconstruction, but good or excellent results were found in only 39% of those undergoing revision for MDI.

Limitations of shoulder function, in particular loss of motion, can occur after instability surgery. It is not uncommon to find series with average loss of external rotation ranging from 10 to 20 degrees after anterior stabilization. A long-term outcome report on the Bankart procedure found that the most common complaint of patients was not recurrent instability but decreased range of motion and intermittent pain; patients placed a high value on full mobility, even to the exclusion of absolute stability.[40] For this reason, current techniques place emphasis on restoration of normal anatomy and prevention of overtightening of the capsuloligamentous structures. The ultimate goal of surgical stabilization is a return to a preinjury level of functional activity. A review of the literature found a rate of return to work ranging from 85% to 98% after Bankart's or capsular shift procedures for anterior instability.[30] Return to sports at a preinjury level has been most problematic. This is particularly true in throwing athletes, among whom only approximately 50% undergoing open surgery achieved their former level of ability. Arthroscopic techniques have been advocated as a method of preserving function while obtaining stability. Enthusiasm exists for arthroscopic treatment of instability in throwing athletes; short-term results show promise for improved function. Currently, long-term outcome data are lacking in this area.

REFERENCES

1. Matsen FA, Thomas SC, Rockwood CA, et al: Glenohumeral instability. In Rockwood CA, Matsen FA, Wirth MA, et al (eds): The Shoulder. Philadelphia, WB Saunders, 1999, p 611.
2. Perthes G: Uber operationen bei habitueller schulterluxation. Dtsch Ztschr Chir 1906; 85:199.
3. Johnson LL: Shoulder arthroscopy. In Johnson LL (ed): Arthroscopic Surgery: Principles and Practice. St. Louis, MO, CV Mosby, 1986, p 1301.
4. Caspari RB, Savoie FH, Meyers JF: Arthroscopic shoulder reconstruction. Orthop Trans 1989; 13:559.
5. Wolf EM: Arthroscopic capsulolabral repair using suture anchors. Orthop Clin North Am 1993; 24:59.
6. Speer KP, Warren RF, Pagnani M, et al: An arthroscopic technique for anterior stabilization of the shoulder with a bioabsorbable tack. J Bone Joint Surg Am 1996; 78:1801.
7. Wheeler JH, Ryan JB, Arciero RA, et al: Arthroscopic versus nonoperative treatment of acute shoulder dislocations in young athletes. Arthroscopy 1989; 5:213.
8. Arciero RA, Wheeler JH, Ryan JB, et al: Arthroscopic Bankart repair versus nonoperative treatment for acute, initial anterior shoulder dislocations. Am J Sports Med 1994; 22:589.
9. Nevaiser TJ: The GLAD lesion: Another cause of anterior shoulder pain. Arthroscopy 1993; 9:22.
10. Altchek DA, Warren RF, Wickiewicz TL,

et al: Arthroscopic labral debridement: A three-year follow-up study. Am J Sports Med 1992; 20:702.

11. Mileski RA, Snyder SJ: Superior labrum lesions in the shoulder: Pathoanatomy and surgical management. J Am Acad Orthop Surg 1998; 6:121.

12. Golser K, Wambacher M, Resch H: Arthroscopic treatment of SLAP lesions: Transacromial approach. In Fu FH, Ticker JB, Imhoff AB (eds): An Atlas of Shoulder Surgery. London, Martin Dimitz, 1998, p 105.

13. Burkhart SS, Morgan CD: The peel-back mechanism: Its role in producing and extending posterior type II SLAP lesions and its effect on SLAP repair rehabilitation. Arthroscopy 1998; 14:637.

14. Riand N, Levigne C, Renaud E, et al: Results of derotational humeral osteotomy in posterosuperior glenoid impingement. Am J Sports Med 1998; 26:453.

15. Maitra RS, Caborn DNM, Johnson DL: Arthroscopic Bankart repair. Curr Opin Orthop 1997; 8:59.

16. Rowe CR, Patel D, Southmayd WW: The Bankart procedure: A long term end-result study. J Bone Joint Surg Am 1978; 60:1.

17. Jobe FW, Giangarra CE, Kvitne RS, et al: Anterior capsulolabral reconstruction of the shoulder in overhand sports. Am J Sports Med 1991; 19:428.

18. Neer CS, Foster CR: Inferior capsular shift for involuntary inferior and multidirectional instability of the shoulder: A preliminary report. J Bone Joint Surg Am 1980; 62:897.

19. Mair SD, Zarzour RH, Speer KP: Posterior labral injury in contact athletes. Am J Sports Med 1998; 26:753.

20. Wolf EM, Eakin CL: Arthroscopic capsular plication for posterior shoulder instability. Am J Sports Med 1998; 26:247.

21. Shaffer BS, Conway J, Jobe FW: Infraspi-natus muscle-splitting incision in posterior shoulder surgery: An anatomic and electromyographic study. Am J Sports Med 1994; 22:113.

22. Hawkins RJ, Janda DH: Posterior instability of the glenohumeral joint: A technique of repair. Am J Sports Med 1996; 24:275.

23. Schaefer SL, Ciarelli MJ, Arnoczky SP, et al: Tissue shrinkage with the holmium: yttrium aluminum garnet laser: A postoperative assessment of tissue length, stiffness, and structure. Am J Sports Med 1997; 25:841.

24. Rosenberg BN, Richmond JC, Levine WN: Long-term followup of Bankart reconstruction: Incidence of late degenerative arthrosis. Am J Sports Med 1995; 23:538.

25. Flatow E, Bigliani L, April E: An anatomic study of the musculocutaneous nerve and its relationship to the coracoid process. Clin Orthop 1989; 244:166.

26. Zuckerman JD, Matsen FA: Complications about the glenohumeral joint related to the use of screws and staples. J Bone Joint Surg Am 1984; 66:175.

27. Behr C, Altchek D: Complications, failed repairs, and revision surgery. In Norris T (ed): Orthopaedic Knowledge Update: Shoulder and Elbow. Rosemont, IL, American Academy of Orthopaedic Surgeons, 1997, p 111.

28. Ticker JB, Lippe RJ, Barkin DE: Infected suture anchors in the shoulder. Arthroscopy 1996; 12:613.

29. Greis PE, Dean M, Hawkins RJ: Subscapularis tendon disruption after Bankart reconstruction for anterior instability. J Shoulder Elbow Surg 1996; 5:219.

30. LaPrade R, Brown G: Recurrent anterior glenohumeral instability: Open surgical treatment. In Warren R, Craig E, Altchek D (eds): The Unstable Shoulder. Philadelphia, Lippincott-Raven, 1999, p 205.

31. Resch H, Golser K, Theoni H, et al: Arthroscopic repair of superior glenoid labral detachment (the SLAP lesion). J Shoulder Elbow Surg 1993; 2:147.

32. Field L, Savoie F: Arthroscopic suture repair of superior labral detachment lesions of the shoulder. Am J Sports Med 1993; 21:783.

33. Snyder SJ, Banas MP, Karzel RP: An analysis of 140 injuries to the superior glenoid labrum. J Shoulder Elbow Surg 1995; 4:243.

34. Maffet MW, Gartsman GM, Moseley B: Superior labrum-biceps tendon complex lesions of the shoulder. Am J Sports Med 1995; 23:93.

35. Rockwood C, Thomas S, Matsen F: Subluxations and dislocations about the glenohumeral joint. In Rockwood C, Green D, Bucholz R (eds): Fractures in Adults. Philadelphia, JB Lippincott, 1991, 3rd ed, p 1021.

36. Morrey B, Janes J: Recurrent anterior dislocation of the shoulder: Long-term follow-up of the Putti-Platt and Bankart procedures. J Bone Joint Surg Am 1976; 58:252.

37. Shaffer BS, Tibone JE: Arthroscopic shoulder instability surgery: Complications. Clin Sports Med 1999; 18:737.

38. Cooper RA, Brems JJ: The inferior capsular-shift procedure for multidirectional instability. Op Tech Sports Med 1992; 1:293.

39. Zabinski SJ, Callaway GH, Cohen S, et al: Revision shoulder stabilization: 2- to 10-year results. J Shoulder Elbow Surg 1999; 8:58.

40. Gill TJ, Micheli LJ, Gebhard F, et al: Bankart repair for anterior instability of the shoulder: Long-term outcome. J Bone Joint Surg Am 1997; 79:850.

section 4 chapter 9

PAINFUL ELBOW ENTHESOPATHY, ENTRAPMENT, AND NEUROPATHY

M. Ramin Modabber and Bert R. Mandelbaum

Summary

- This chapter focuses on lateral epicondylitis, medial epicondylitis, cubital tunnel syndrome, pronator syndrome, and radial tunnel syndrome.
- The section on entrapment neuropathies focuses on the three major nerves that cross the elbow: the ulnar nerve and cubital tunnel syndrome, the median nerve and pronator syndrome, and the posterior interosseous nerve/radial nerve and radial tunnel syndrome.
- Pertinent anatomy, epidemiology, pathophysiology, clinical diagnosis, electromyographic diagnosis, and surgical and nonsurgical treatment are discussed.

LATERAL EPICONDYLITIS

ANATOMY

The musculotendinous origin of the common extensor muscles, including the extensor carpi radialis longus (ECRL) and brevis (ECRB), the extensor digitorum communis, and the extensor carpi ulnaris, is the lateral epicondyle. The most commonly involved musculotendinous origin is that of the ECRB, lying deep to the ECRL (Fig. 1). The lateral collateral ligamentous complex including the annular ligament of the elbow can also be involved.

The biomechanics of the extensor origin have been studied well. Morris et al,[1] via an electromyographic technique,

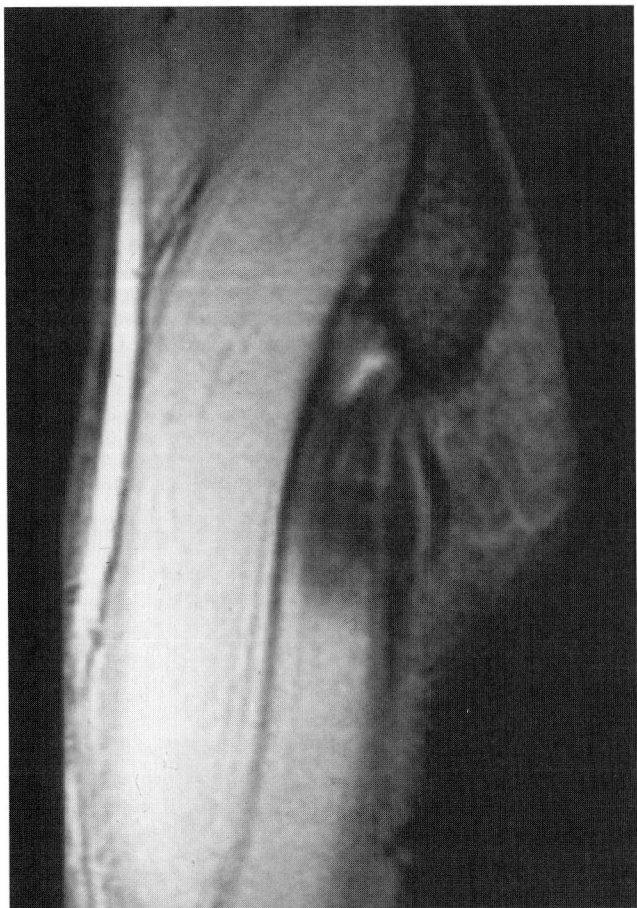

Fig. 1. View. This magnetic resonance image demonstrates an altered signal with likely tear of the ECRB origin.

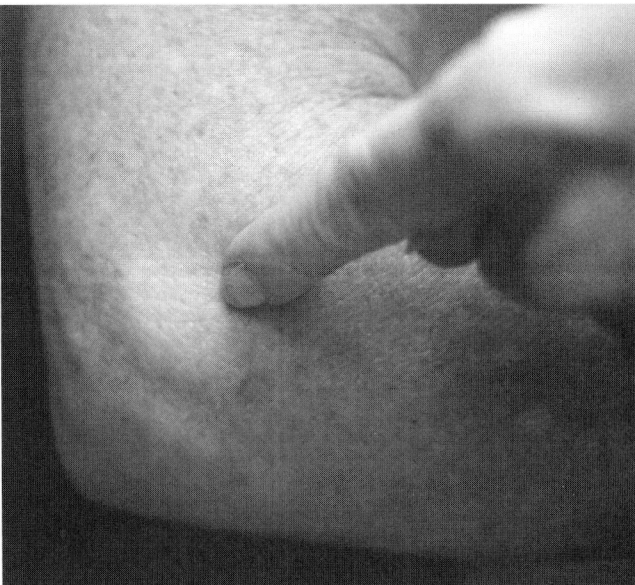

Fig. 2. View. This area of maximal tenderness is just distal and anterior to the lateral epicondyle.

studied the extensor origin and found the greatest muscular activity of all muscles tested was that of the ECRB. During the tennis stroke, the greatest activity occurred during acceleration and early follow-through phases.

EPIDEMIOLOGY

Although the age range for patients with epicondylitis is variable, the majority present in the 4th and 5th decades of life. Male and female prevalence is roughly equal. Dominant versus nondominant arm involvement occurs at a rate of 3:1, respectively.

In tennis, increased number of racquet hours per week, age older than 40 years, poor stroke mechanics, improper grip size, racquet weight, and racquet stringing techniques have all been implicated in the cause of this common condition.

Although tennis has been studied most extensively for this condition, a variety of recreational and occupational activities have also been implicated.

PATHOPHYSIOLOGY

The prevailing opinion, based on clinical, surgical, and pathologic evidence, reveals the most common pathologic finding being microscopic tears within the origin of the ECRB. On gross inspection, the tendon origin of the

ECRB appears abnormal as an inflamed, friable, and pinkish-grey tissue. Often, extension into the radiocapitellar joint is noted. Nirschl and Pettrone[2] demonstrated a near 100% prevalence of this gross pathologic tissue at the ECRB origin. Approximately one-third of those studied were also noted to have gross evidence of tendon rupture. The characteristic microscopic appearance of "angiofibroblastic hyperplasia" was characterized by Nirschl.

DIAGNOSIS

A careful history and physical examination will often allow easy diagnosis of lateral epicondylitis. A history of repetitive activity or overuse is often noted. Patients may also describe a direct blow to the extensor origin or lateral epicondyle as a single event initiating their symptoms. Physical examination reveals tenderness typically at, just distal to, or just anterior to the lateral epicondyle (Fig. 2).

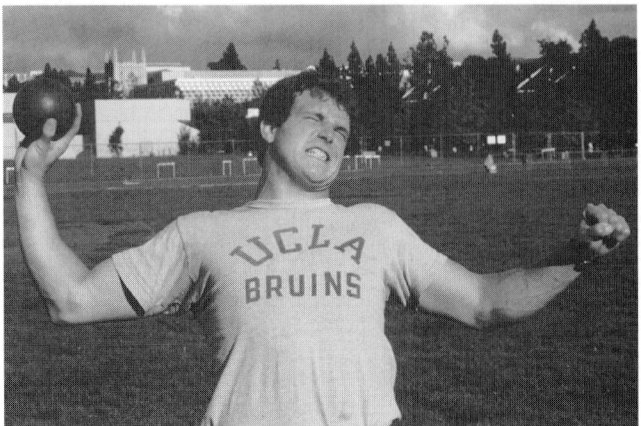

Fig. 3. View. This is an example of valgus overload of the elbow in throwing athletes.

With the elbow held in full extension, resisted wrist and digital extension will reproduce the patient's pain. Typically, range of motion of the elbow, forearm, wrist, and hand is within normal limits. However, in acute inflammatory processes, incomplete elbow extension is often noted.

In the majority of patients, radiographs of the involved elbow show no evidence of any significant bony or joint abnormalities. However, up to one in four patients may have calcification within the soft tissues around the lateral epicondyle.

Related conditions, which should be ruled out in all cases, include cervical disc disease; radial nerve entrapment at the elbow, i.e., radial tunnel syndrome; and intra-articular processes about the elbow.

Diagnosis of lateral epicondylitis is predominantly a clinical one; in the majority of cases, further diagnostic studies are not of significant value.

NONSURGICAL TREATMENT

Although reports in series vary, more than 90% of patients can be successfully managed nonoperatively. Nonoperative management is most successful when a multimodal treatment plan is initiated at the time of diagnosis. The plan may consist of nonsteroidal anti-inflammatory medication (oral or topical), relative rest from activities that produce symptoms, ice application, and counterforce bracing. A directed physical therapy program including stretching, balanced strengthening, and modalities such as ultrasonography and iontophoresis is essential. In more refractory cases, corticosteroid injections may be utilized. Further evaluation may include appropriate grip size in racquet-sport athletes and technique management. Equipment modifications such as lighter racquets with newer composites, low-vibration materials, and stringing with less tension have all been noted to be potentially helpful for racquet sport athletes.

SURGICAL TREATMENT

For maximal success, indications for surgical treatment should be monitored closely. A patient's failure to respond to an appropriate nonoperative treatment program for a minimum of 6 months is appropriate.

Numerous surgical treatments have been advocated. The authors' preferred treatment includes complete débridement of involved tissue from the lateral epicondyle and reattachment through bone holes or suture anchors. This classic surgical treatment has been well described by numerous authors.[2, 3] Recent techniques, including arthroscopic débridement/release, are awaiting long-term outcome analysis.

Postoperative management should include a posterior splint for 7 to 10 days. A progressive mobilization program should follow that includes passive and active assisted elbow and wrist and hand motion. Resisted exercises including strengthening should be postponed until a minimum of 6 weeks postsurgery. In most cases, full athletic activities are permissible at 3 months postsurgery.

Results of these techniques have been successful in 85% to 90% of cases. Postsurgery, up to 10% of patients have persistent pain during athletic activity. The patient should be counseled about this preoperatively, in addition to the possibility of having persistent strength deficits, most notably in wrist extension and grip strength.

MEDIAL EPICONDYLITIS

ANATOMY

Anatomy of the medial aspect of the elbow includes the flexor pronator originating from the medial epicondyle. From proximal to distal, this includes the pronator teres, the flexor carpi radialis, the palmaris longus, the flexor digitorum superficialis, and the flexor carpi ulnaris. The more proximal aspect of the flexor pronator origin is the most commonly involved. These muscles arise from an area superior to the medial epicondyle known as the medial supracondylar ridge.

EPIDEMIOLOGY AND ETIOLOGY

Medial epicondylitis is considerably more rare than lateral epicondylitis, occurring approximately 10 to 20 times less frequently. There is similar age grouping, with patients in their 30s and 40s and with roughly equal male/female distribution. This condition is seen most commonly in throwing athletes despite its common term, "golfer's elbow." The early acceleration phase of throwing transmits the greatest forces to the medial structures of the elbow, including the deeper capsuloligamentous structures (Figs. 3 and 4).[1] Racquet sport athletes as well as golfers also show considerable involvement.

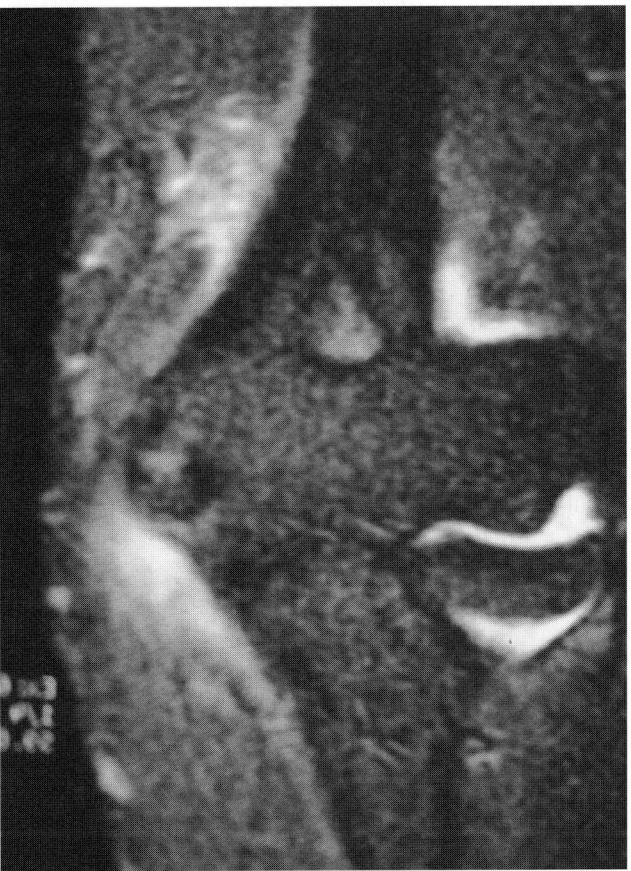

Fig. 4. View. This is a magnetic resonance image of the medial epicondyle showing altered signal within the flexor pronator origin.

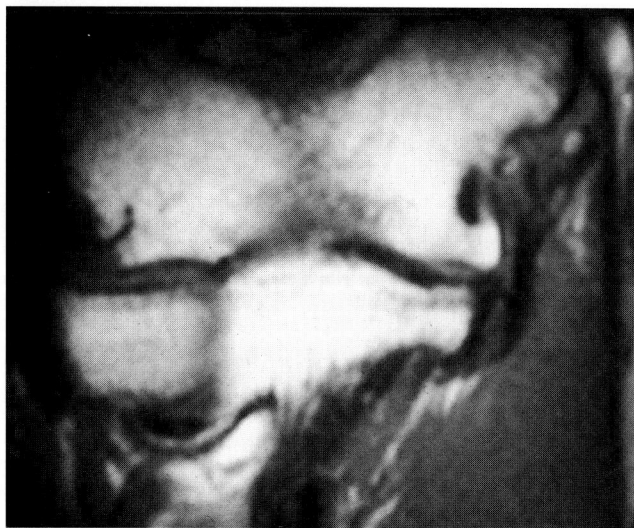

Fig. 5. View. This is a magnetic resonance image of the medial epicondyle showing altered signal within the flexor pronator origin.

PATHOPHYSIOLOGY

Degenerative changes within the tendon may predispose patients with improper technique, inadequate warm-up activities, poor conditioning, or repetitive microtrauma to develop continuing symptoms of medial epicondylitis (Fig. 5). Vangsness and Jobe[4] noted macroscopic tears in the flexor pronator origin in 100% of patients undergoing surgical treatment for chronic medial epicondylitis. There is substantial evidence that progressive medial epicondylitis can lead to adjacent injury in the medial capsuloligamentous structures, including the ulnar collateral ligament complex. Glousman et al[5] demonstrated this with cinematographic and indwelling electromyographic data.

DIAGNOSIS

Just as with lateral epicondylitis, a careful history and physical examination clearly delineate patients with medial epicondylitis. Tenderness is located usually distal and anterior to the medial epicondyle, most notably over the flexor carpi radialis and pronator teres origins. Resisted wrist flexion and forearm pronation with the elbow extended typically exacerbate the patient's pain. Range of motion is usually complete; however, slight flexion deformities at the elbow are not uncommon. Careful ulnar nerve examination is imperative as concomitant ulnar neuropathy is often demonstrated by decreased sensibility in the ulnar half of the ring finger and the palmar aspect of the small finger. A positive elbow flexion test and Tinel's sign in the region of the cubital tunnel may also provide evidence of ongoing ulnar neuritis/neuropathy.

Plain radiographs are typically normal; however, calcification within the structure of the ulnar collateral ligament complex, with or without associated traction spurs, can often be seen. Nevertheless, range of motion, collateral ligament integrity, ulnar nerve function, musculotendinous palpation, and provocative testing should be assessed for all patients with medial elbow pain to determine each of the potential sources discussed above.

NONSURGICAL TREATMENT

Principles similar to those for lateral epicondylitis may be applied to medial epicondylitis. Relative rest, nonsteroidal anti-inflammatory medication, counterforce bracing, a directed physical therapy program toward a balanced stretching and strengthening program, and adjuvant corticosteroid injections may also be beneficial.

As with lateral epicondylitis, a directed nonoperative treatment program for at least 6 months is often successful in the majority of cases.

SURGICAL TREATMENT

Indications for surgery include failure of a directed nonoperative treatment program for a minimum of 6 and often up to 12 months. Careful assessment for adjacent pathologic features is essential in making an accurate diagnosis and successful treatment.

Surgical technique involves a medial incision centered over the medial epicondyle. Subcutaneous flaps should be developed in order to identify and protect the medial antebrachial cutaneous nerves branching from the proximal aspect of the ulnar nerve, and the ulnar nerve posteriorly should be identified and protected throughout the procedure. Ulnar nerve subluxation and stability within the cubital tunnel should be assessed prior to directing attention to the medial epicondyle. The musculotendinous origin should be reflected carefully to identify the disorder, which is typically at the undersurface of the proximal aspect of the flexor pronator origin at the level of the flexor carpi radialis and pronator teres muscles. Pathologic tissue should be débrided, and healthy adjacent tissue should be reattached through drill holes into a bleeding surface of bone in the underlying medial epicondyle. After routine closure, appropriate immobilization requires a posterior plaster splint.

POSTOPERATIVE MANAGEMENT

Immediately after surgery, patients should be instructed on wrist and hand range-of-motion exercises. Sutures and splint can be removed 7 to 10 days postoperatively. Initial therapy should be directed at gentle active and passive elbow, forearm, wrist, and hand range-of-motion exercises. Resisted exercises should be held off for 6 weeks, followed by a strengthening program directed toward the patient's recreational activities. Patients can be returned to athletic activities 3 months postsurgery.

RESULTS

Vangsness and Jobe[4] noted good to excellent results in 97% of patients, more than 85% of patients having no limitations in elbow use. Strength assessment did not reveal any difference between elbows treated surgically and nonsurgically. All athletic patients returned to their original sports despite residual strength deficits noted.

SUMMARY

Despite infrequent reports in the literature and a variety of surgical techniques used for treatment, medial epicondylitis, albeit rarer than its lateral counterpart, can have good results from nonoperative treatment. In refractory cases, surgical treatment can return the majority of active patients to their recreational activities.

COMPRESSION NEUROPATHIES

Compression neuropathies occur about the elbow. By far, the most common is compression of the ulnar nerve. For the sake of completeness, a brief discussion of median nerve compression and radial nerve compression about the elbow are also presented.

ULNAR NEUROPATHY

Ulnar neuropathy about the elbow can be separated into compression ulnar neuropathy and irritative ulnar neuritis. As its name implies, ulnar neuritis may be an inflammatory reaction either within or around the ulnar nerve that can give the same clinical picture as an ulnar neuropathy from compression. However, because ulnar neuritis is not a true compression neuropathy, electrical studies may often be normal, and diagnosis can sometimes be elusive. In cases where ulnar neuropathy is suspected and physical findings are consistent with a subluxing ulnar nerve and/or an active Tinel sign in the ulnar nerve about the elbow, ulnar neuritis should be considered and treatment rendered despite normal electromyographic and nerve conduction studies.

Discussion regarding the compressive ulnar neuropathies at the elbow hinges essentially on anatomic structures proximal and distal to the elbow joint that can cause compression on the ulnar nerve.

Five major sites have been identified.[6] From proximal to distal, these include the following:

The medial intermuscular septum, with compression being caused by the septum itself or Struthers' arcade or by hypertrophy or snapping of the medial head of the triceps muscle.

The medial epicondyle itself, where supracondylar malunions with valgus deformity can cause a stretching/ scarring or compression of the ulnar nerve in this region.

The epicondylar groove, where compression is typically caused by subluxation or dislocation of the nerve in and out of the epicondylar groove. In rare cases, lesions within the groove can put pressure directly on the ulnar nerve.

The true cubital tunnel, where compression is caused by a thickened Osborne's ligament.

The area where the ulnar nerve enters the two heads of the flexor carpi ulnaris muscle in the region where the deep flexor pronator aponeurosis can cause compression.

An essential understanding of these anatomic structures is critical to identifying and treating compression ulnar neuropathies about the elbow.[7]

Diagnosis

As is always the case, a complete history, including work and recreational activities and activities that aggravate or alleviate the condition, is essential. A physical examination beginning in the cervical region, including range of motion of the shoulder, elbow, forearm, wrist, and hand, will often allow one to clinically localize potential concomitant or confusing concurrent diagnosis including thoracic outlet syndrome, brachial plexopathy, cervical disc disease, and nerve compression at additional sites. Inspection of the elbow for deformity and assessment of carrying angle is often an important step in identifying cases of traction or compression neuropathy. Active and passive range of motion of all upper extremity joints is then performed, followed by special tests focusing on the ulnar nerve. Examination for thoracic outlet syndrome, including Adson's maneuver, Wright's maneuver, and Roos' test, may be nonspecific but helpful if the patient's clinical picture is obscure. Palpating along the course of the ulnar nerve is helpful both statically and during flexion and extension cycles to assess for any subluxation, dislocation, or snapping medial head of the triceps muscle. Local tenderness as well as a Tinel sign is often indicative of a compression site. A provocative test, such as the elbow flexion test performed with the elbow in full flexion and the wrist in full extension for 1 minute, can be considered positive if paresthesias or numbness occur in the ulnar innervated digits/ulnar nerve distribution. Involvement within the distribution of the dorsal sensory branch of the ulnar nerve can often distinguish between ulnar nerve compression at or about the elbow versus more distal compression at the level of Guyon's canal at the wrist. Confrontational strength testing in the ulnar innervated digits as well as Semmes-Weinstein monofilament testing for sensation provide additional information about ulnar nerve function.

Typically, sensory findings precede motor involvement, although a positive Wartenberg sign can often be an early presenting sign of ulnar neuropathy, demonstrated by an inability to adduct the small finger. Froment's sign, in which the interphalangeal joint of the thumb is flexed in forceful pinching activities to obviate the use of the adductor pollicis muscle by utilizing the flexor pollicis longus muscle, is also present with more advanced ulnar neuropathy. A positive Jeanne's sign, which involves hyperextension of the metacarpophalangeal joint of the thumb, similarly points to a more advanced ulnar neuropathy. In addition to intrinsic muscle weakness in the hand, extrinsic muscle weakness specifically involving the flexor digitorum profundus to the little finger can be noted. The flexor digitorum profundus to the ring finger is often duly innervated and does not share the weakness often seen in the flexor digitorum profundus to the small finger when motor involvement is noted.

Staging by McGowan in 1950 proved simple and useful in grading ulnar neuropathy.[8] Grade I involvement is sensory involvement including paresthesias and numbness, but no motor weakness is noted. Grade II involvement shows wasting of the interosseous muscles and weakness in ulnar innervated motor units. Grade III involvement includes severe ulnar neuropathy, with complete intrinsic muscle paralysis.

Imaging and Electrodiagnostic Studies

Plain radiographs of the elbow should be taken. An additional view profiling the epicondylar groove is often useful for patients with post-traumatic deformities or arthritic conditions about the elbow. Magnetic resonance imaging has been helpful in identifying compressive ulnar neuropathy from lesions producing a mass effect or identifying accessory muscles such as an anconeus epitrochlearis. Similarly, swelling within the ulnar nerve is often identified, and frank dislocation of the ulnar nerve from the epicondylar groove can be noted as well.

Electrodiagnostic studies are often positive when a compressive ulnar neuropathy is present; it is demonstrated by decreased conduction velocity of the ulnar nerve across the elbow. Additionally, electromyography and nerve conduction studies may elucidate double- or triple-crush lesions or may demonstrate signs of systemic neuropathy, giving the clinician additional diagnostic and prognostic information. It should be noted that in cases of inflammation of the ulnar nerve, i.e., ulnar neuritis, electrical studies may be within normal limits; this does not necessarily indicate normal ulnar nerve function during all activities.

Treatment

Initial treatment for ulnar neuropathy at the elbow in nearly all cases should begin with nonoperative management, which should include relative rest, avoidance of prolonged elbow flexion and, in some cases, immobilization of the elbow and/or wrist. If persistence or progression of symptoms occurs despite an appropriate nonoperative treatment plan, surgical treatment is warranted. In some cases, initial treatment for severely involved ulnar neuropathy of a prolonged nature may indicate more urgent surgical treatment.

Operative procedures for ulnar neuropathy at the elbow are widely varied; a thorough discussion of each is beyond the scope of this chapter. In general, treatment consists of decompression with or without transposition of the nerve. Decompression can be performed within the cubital tunnel and performed with or without a medial epicondylectomy. When a decompression with transposition of the nerve is carried out, subcutaneous, intramuscular, and submuscular techniques have all been described. For primary ulnar neuropathy at the elbow, the authors' preferred choice is a thorough decompression including neurolysis from the most proximal area of the medial intermuscular septum, with an excision of a portion of the medial intermuscular septum, and decompression of each of the anatomic structures mentioned earlier to the level of the two heads of the flexor carpi ulnaris muscle, gaining as much mobilization of the nerve for a tension-free straight line anterior to the medial epicondyle in a subcutaneous fashion. For revision surgery, a submuscular transposition is preferred.

RADIAL TUNNEL AND PRONATOR SYNDROMES

Although far less common than ulnar neuropathy of the elbow, the radial and median nerves can be involved with compression neuropathies at the level of the elbow from a variety of sources. Each of the compression points for both the median and radial nerves is discussed here. In the case of a posterior interosseous nerve syndrome (radial tunnel syndrome), the posterior interosseous nerve can be compressed in several locations.[6] The most proximal region of vulnerability is at the level of the lateral head of the triceps through the region of the elbow and proximal forearm. The classic area of posterior interosseous nerve compression is at the proximal edge of the supinator muscle, i.e., Frohse's arcade. Compression at the supinator muscle midportion as well as through the distal end of the supinator muscle can also be found. The typical clinical presentation is an essentially purely motor neuropathy involving the extensor digitorum communis, extensor digiti minimi, extensor carpi ulnaris, abductor pollicis longus, ECRL and ECRB, and extensor indicis proprius. The pattern of involvement often depends on the amount and the exact location of compression. The dorsal sensory branch of the radial nerve, which branches more proximally, having a higher separation and lying anterior to the lateral intermuscular septum, is seldom involved.

Electrical studies that demonstrate involvement of the supinator muscle may help localize the area of most significant compression lying more proximally prior to the branches to the supinator muscle.

Distinguishing recalcitrant lateral epicondylitis from radial tunnel syndrome can often be difficult. Physical findings of tenderness more distally and anteriorly along the course of the nerve in patients with refractory lateral epicondylitis may often indicate a concomitant posterior interosseous nerve compression. Pain in the elbow on resisted extension of the long finger with the elbow held extended is a common finding in patients with posterior interosseous nerve syndrome. Sensory abnormalities in the hands should be absent in these cases.

Treatment for true posterior interosseous nerve compression that is unresponsive to immobilization, anti-inflammatory medication, and a period of observation should include a thorough decompression of the nerve. Surgical management should include an area of decompression approximately 5 cm proximal to the lateral epicondyle and through the entire course of the supinator muscle. This dissection should be meticulous as numerous vascular branches and musculotendinous origins may need to be disrupted and, when necessary, reattached to ensure complete decompression.

With respect to compression neuropathy of the median nerve at the elbow, the pronator syndrome is the most common clinical presentation. The level of compression is typically from the level of the supracondyloid process superiorly to the flexor digitorum superficialis arch distally.[6] Between these two structures, additional points of compression include the Struthers' ligament, the lacertus fibrosus, and the deep head of the pronator teres muscle. Anomalous muscles, vascular malformations, and distended bursae may also produce symptomatic median nerve compression about the elbow. Post-traumatic deformities in the region of the elbow have also been known to cause compressive median neuropathy.

Clinically, symptoms are often vague, consisting of proximal forearm pain with occasional radiation proximal and distal to the elbow. Numbness of the hand in the median nerve distribution, including the distribution of the palmar cutaneous nerve, should alert the clinician to a pronator syndrome. Repetitive, strenuous motions involving forearm rotation may also alert the clinician to a pronator syndrome. Nocturnal symptoms are typically less common than in more distal compression, i.e., carpal tunnel syndrome.

Pronator syndrome appears to be more common in women than in men. A specific event is often associated with onset, although insidious onset is not infrequent. Diagnosis is often delayed due to vague symptoms, poorly detailed history, difficulty making the clinical diagnosis, and common association with workers' compensation evaluations.

Physical examination can reveal an indentation of the flexor pronator mass below the medial epicondyle, suggesting a constrictive effect of the lacertus fibrosus. Often, swelling in the region of the flexor pronator origin, when compared with the opposite side, is suggestive of a nerve compression in this area. Provocative testing, such as resisted pronation for 90 seconds, can initiate the patient's symptoms. The most common physical examination includes direct palpation with pressure over the proximal portion of the pronator teres approximately 3 to 5 cm distal to the antebrachial flexion crease while the patient exerts resistance to pronation. This should always be compared to the asymptomatic forearm for accuracy of diagnosis.

Electromyographic findings can aid in the diagnosis of pronator syndrome; however, they are often inconclusive. Slowed conduction velocity across the elbow for the median nerve is not commonly seen. However, a significant difference in conduction velocity with the forearm in supination versus pronation can be suggestive of nerve compression in this region.

Treatment should initially consist of nonoperative management, including avoidance of exacerbating activities, a course of nonsteroidal anti-inflammatory medication, and a period of immobilization. If persistence or progression of symptoms occurs despite an appropriate nonoperative management plan, surgical decompression is indicated.

Similar to the previously noted compression neuropathies, a thorough decompression should be performed. Decompression proximal to the elbow in the supracondylar region should be performed with neurolysis through the level of lacertus fibrosus and pronator teres muscle heads. The dissection should continue to the level of the fibrous arch of the origin of the flexor digitorum superficialis muscle. This typically is present 1 to 2 cm distal to the deep head of the pronator muscle. At the time of surgical dissection, aberrant musculature, including Gantzer's muscle, palmaris profundus muscle, or flexor carpi radialis brevis muscle, should be considered as additional sources of compression. Additionally, bicipital bursa and aberrant branches of the radial artery and vena comitans can also cause local nerve compression.

Nevertheless, similar to the previously discussed nerve compression syndromes, a detailed knowledge of the normal and anatomic variations around the elbow is essential to successful surgical management.

REFERENCES

1. Morris M, Jobe FW, Perry J, et al: Electromyographic analysis of elbow function in tennis players. Am J Sports Med 1989; 17: 241.
2. Nirschl RP, Pettrone FA: Tennis elbow: The surgical treatment of lateral epicondylitis. J Bone Joint Surg Am 1979; 61:832.
3. Jobe FW, Ciccotti MG: Lateral and medial epicondylitis of the elbow. J Am Acad Orthop Surg 1994; 2:1.
4. Vangsness CT Jr, Jobe FW: Surgical treatment of medial epicondylitis: Results in 35 elbows. J Bone Joint Surg Br 1991; 73:409.
5. Glousman RE, Barron J, Jobe FW, et al: An electromyographic analysis of the elbow in normal and injured pitchers with medial collateral ligament insufficiency. Am J Sports Med 1992; 20:311.
6. Eversmann WW Jr: Entrapment and compression neuropathies. In Green DP (ed): Operative Hand Surgery. Churchill Livingstone, New York, 1993, 3rd ed, p 1341.
7. Posner MA: Compressive ulnar neuropathies at the elbow. J Am Acad Orthop Surg 1998; 6:282.
8. McGowan AJ: The results of transposition of the ulnar nerve for traumatic ulnar neuritis. J Bone Joint Surg Br 1950; 32:293.

section
4
chapter
10

ELBOW INJURIES IN THE THROWING ATHLETES, INCLUDING INSTABILITY AND OSTEOCHONDRAL/ CHONDRAL LESIONS

Shinji Kashiwagucgi and Takaaki Ikata

Summary

- Although acute elbow injuries are common, repetitive stress causes most symptomatic conditions unique to the elbow.
- Elbow joint stability is provided by the geometry of its joint surfaces, its ligament-capsule complex, and neuromuscular control.
- During the acceleration phase of throwing, tensile loads in the medial collateral ligament (MCL) of the elbow and compressive loads in the lateral column of the joint can be of sufficient magnitude to damage the loaded structures and cause pain, tenderness, and swelling, especially at the medial aspect of the joint.
- The anterior bundle of the elbow's MCL is its primary restraint to valgus strain.
- In an elbow with valgus laxity, repeated forceful throwing can cause widening of the medial joint space and increased tension on the ulnar nerve, resulting in neuropathy.
- While the medial aspect of the elbow is experiencing large tension loads, the lateral compartment is simultaneously experiencing large compression and shear loads that can result in an osteochondral lesion.
- During the deceleration phase of throwing, at terminal elbow extension, large compression loads are generated in the elbow's posterior compartment that can lead to olecranon osteophyte formation, loose bodies, or an olecranon fatigue fracture.
- Posterolateral rotatory instability of the elbow can be identified on physical examination by the lateral pivot shift test.
- Posterolateral rotatory instability of the elbow can be due to either an acute injury or developmental laxity of the ulnar portion of its lateral collateral ligament (LCL).
- A treatment regimen that includes avoidance of the inciting activity, physical therapy modalities, and oral nonsteroidal medication will successfully control symptoms in almost all cases.
- Operative treatment of elbow symptoms related to throwing is indicated in patients with persistent pain and instability who fail to achieve adequate relief of symptoms or disability after a trial of nonoperative treatment as outlined previously.

The elbow joint is susceptible to a variety of injuries as a result of either acute traumatic events or chronic repetitive overuse. In athletes, the incidence of injury is related directly to the duration of exposure and intensity of athletic participation. Although sudden traumatic injuries are common, most symptomatic conditions unique to the elbow result from chronic, excessive, and repetitive stress. These injuries are classified based on mechanism of injury: type 1, tension overload of the medial structures; type 2, compression and shearing injuries of the lateral structures; type 3, extension overload within the posterior compartment; type 4, a combination of these injuries; type 5, laxity of the ulnar part of the LCL, resulting in posterolateral rotatory instability of the elbow.[1, 2] To successfully manage these injuries, a thorough understanding of pertinent regional anatomy, pathophysiology, normal bone development, and biomechanics of the elbow is essential.

FUNCTIONAL ANATOMY

The bony articulations include both a hinge joint and a rotational joint. The three articulations of the elbow are the humeroulnar, humeroradial, and proximal radioulnar. Motion of the elbow occurs in two planes: flexion-extension and pronation-supination.[3] The complex MCL and LCL provide stability to the elbow. Muscle groups emanating principally from the medial and lateral humeral epicondyles control the wrist and fingers. In throwing athletes, rotation of the forearm and rotatory forces at the proximal radioulnar joint are used to help maintain throwing accuracy and precise delivery.

Elbow stability is maintained by the bony configuration, ligamentous capsular complex, and surrounding musculature. The MCL is the primary stabilizer of the medial elbow. Sectioning studies in cadaver elbows have analyzed the relative contribution of elbow structure to valgus stability. Morrey and An[4] showed that, in full extension, valgus stability was equally conferred by the MCL, anterior capsule, and bony articulation. At 90 degrees of flexion, the MCL provided 55% of valgus stability and the articular restraints provided 45%. They also showed biomechanically that the anterior bundle of the MCL is the primary stabilizer in resisting valgus stress.[5, 6] The bony articulation of the radiocapitellar joint is a secondary stabilizer that resists valgus and rotatory stress and is significant only when the anterior bundle of the MCL is absent.

The MCL consists of three bands: anterior, posterior, and transverse (Fig. 1). The anterior band is well defined and distinguished from the anterior portion of the medial joint capsule. It arises from the midportion of the medial epicondyle and inserts onto the coronoid tubercle. Its humeral origin is eccentrically located with respect to the axis of elbow flexion and extension, thus providing stability throughout a full range of elbow motion.[5] The posterior band is a fan-shaped thickening of the posterior capsule and is poorly defined. It inserts onto the medial and posterior aspects of the olecranon. The transverse segment consists of horizontally oriented fibers between the coronoid and the tip of the olecranon and is poorly separated from the capsule.

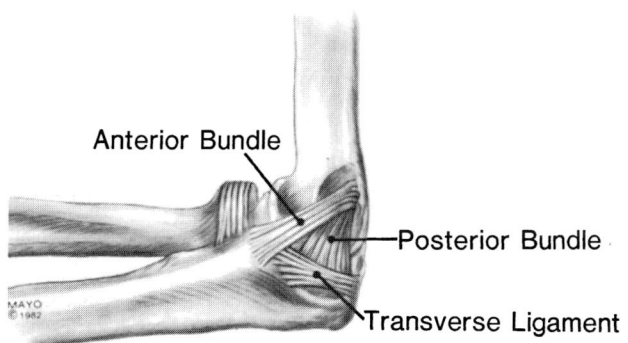

Fig. 1. Orientation of the medial collateral ligament. Included are the anterior and posterior bundles and the transverse ligament. This last structure contributes relatively little to elbow stability. (From Morrey BF: The Elbow and Its Disorders. Philadelphia, WB Saunders, 2000, 3rd ed, p 23.)

The LCL complex is less consistent and not as well understood as the MCL.[7] The annular part of the LCL originates from the lateral epicondyle and blends with the fibers of the annular ligament (Fig. 2). The ulnar band of the LCL originates from the anteroinferior portion of the lateral epicondyle, crosses the radiocapitellar joint, and inserts onto the tubercle of the supinator crest. Additionally, there is a fan-shaped portion that inserts onto the ulna proximal to the supinator crest.

LIGAMENT INSTABILITY

MEDIAL ULNAR COLLATERAL LIGAMENT INJURIES
Injury Mechanism and Pathophysiology
The physical stresses associated with throwing create compression, shear, and distraction on the medial, lateral, anterior, and posterior aspects of the elbow joint. Injury patterns should be described at the each site of the elbow joint. In throwing, the maximum valgus force is encountered across the medial elbow during the acceleration phase of pitching. This provides both a distraction load to the

MCL and a compressive load to the lateral column. Distraction load is transmitted primarily to the MCL complex, the flexor carpi ulnaris, and the medial flexor-pronator musculature. As long as athletes demonstrate proper throwing mechanics, conditioning, and warm-up, these forces are well tolerated. However, factors such as immature bones, poor throwing mechanics, inflexibility, and fatigue can have a cumulative effect that leads to muscle strain, allowing further stress to the MCL. If these loads are applied at a rate that exceeds that of tissue repair, progressive microscopic damage can occur. Initially, this damage appears as edema and inflammation within the MCL. Pain, tenderness, and swelling about the medial aspect of the elbow joint may then arise. Additional stress from continued throwing may result in attenuation of the ligament or degeneration of the ligament fibers themselves. Subsequently, calcification or ossification may occur adjacent to the coronoid tubercle.[8] Ultimately, the ligament can rupture in its midsubstance. Occasionally, it can become avulsed from its proximal origin or distal insertion.[8–10]

Diagnosis
The diagnosis should be based on the athlete's history and physical examination. Patients with a history of repetitive throwing experience pain localized to the medial aspect of the elbow, particularly during the late cocking and acceleration phases of pitching. The pain has a gradual onset and is exacerbated with throwing. On occasion, patients may experience a sudden popping or sharp pain along the medial aspect of the elbow joint as a traumatic event. They are unable to continue throwing at the previous level of performance.

Depending on the location and amount of inflammation within the medial soft tissues, patients may exhibit tenderness over the medial epicondyle, midsubstance of the MCL, or tubercle on the medial aspect of the coronoid process. Injuries in the area of the medial epicondyle may be difficult to differentiate from each other because of the proximity of the adjacent structures. Palpation with the elbow flexed to 100 degrees is recommended.[11] With concomitant ulnar neuropathy, however, varying degrees of

Fig. 2. Radial collateral ligament complex. The radial collateral ligament extends from the humerus to the annular ligament, which is the portion most commonly meant when referring to the radial or lateral collateral ligament. (From Morrey BF: The Elbow and Its Disorders. Philadelphia, WB Saunders, 2000, 3rd ed, p 24.)

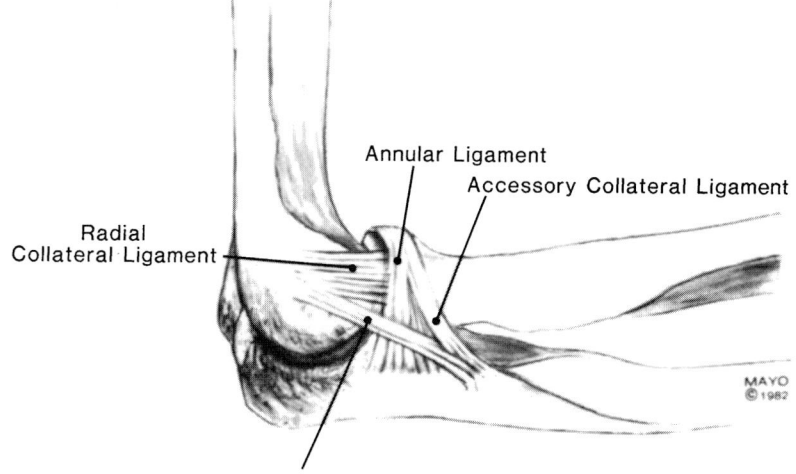

diminished sensibility in the ring and little fingers may be present.

For patients with pain in the area of the medial aspect, a medial instability test is needed to evaluate the MCL further. Valgus instability is tested with the athlete seated, the elbow flexed about 25 degrees to unlock the olecranon from its fossa, and the patient's hand and wrist held securely between the examiner's elbow and trunk.[8] The examiner firmly grasps the patient's elbow and proximal forearm while simultaneously palpating the ulnar collateral ligament along the medial joint line. Varus and valgus stress can then be applied to determine whether there is an increased opening and assess end-point laxity compared with the contralateral elbow.[12, 13] Radiographic studies are also beneficial, including stress x-ray films, saline magnetic resonance imaging (MRI), and computed tomography (CT) arthrograms. In some cases, the T sign described by Timmerman and Andrews[14] is seen on saline MRI or CT arthrogram, confirming the diagnosis.

Treatment

Nonoperative treatment for the throwing athlete with MCL injuries is controversial. Initially, a conservative, nonsurgical treatment program is recommended, with the primary goals being relief of pain and inflammation. Avoidance of the offending activity is required. In addition, cryotherapy, contrast baths, and other physical therapy modalities applied to the affected area may reduce inflammation and pain. The use of nonsteroidal oral anti-inflammatory medications is also beneficial, although corticosteroid injections are generally not recommended. The elbow is placed in a range-of-motion (ROM) brace to prevent a valgus stress. ROM exercise, initially 20 to 90 degrees, is started as soon as tolerated and is increased by 5 to 10 degrees per day. After relief of initial pain and inflammation, a guided rehabilitation program for all muscles surrounding the elbow is essential to restore the muscle tone and endurance needed for dynamic support to the elbow joint. Strengthening exercises can be performed isometrically, isotonically, or isokinetically.

Surgical treatment is necessary for the patient with acute complete disruption of the ulnar collateral ligament or with persistent pain and instability who shows little or no improvement with conservative management.[8, 9, 15] Primary reduction and fixation is indicated for an acute avulsion of the ulnar collateral ligament from its proximal humeral attachment or distal ulnar insertion.[10] Because of attenuation, scarring, or disruption of the MCL, primary repair is unreasonable, and reconstruction with an autologous graft is necessary.

Our technique is a modification of the procedure described by Jobe et al[8, 16] The goal is to reconstruct the anterior bundle of MCL. The graft source is the ipsilateral or contralateral palmaris longus tendon. It is essential to document the presence of this tendon before surgery. Alternate sources of tendon include plantaris tendon, a 3- to 5-mm medial strip of Achilles tendon, or an extensor tendon from the fourth toe. Under tourniquet control, an incision is made over the medial epicondyle, extending both proximally and distally about 5 cm. Care should be taken to protect the ulnar nerve and the medial antebrachial cutaneous nerve. The flexor-pronator muscle is split longitudi-

nally, and the muscle fibers are retracted anteriorly and posteriorly, exposing the MCL. It is important to preserve the origin on the medial epicondyle. After exposure of the MCL, the defect in the ligament can be assessed, especially the anterior bundle. Soft-tissue calcification and degeneration, attenuation, or complete disruption of the ligament may be evident. A longitudinal incision made in line with the fiber may reveal internal degeneration or undersurface detachment of the ligament. After débridement of degenerated tissue, the remnants should be preserved and augmented with the substitute tissue. Opening the capsule allows inspection of the underlying joint. Synovitis, osteochondral loose bodies, osteophytes, or degenerative changes may be identified and débrided. If posterior compartment impingement is present, osteophytes about the olecranon and its fossa are débrided.

Next, bone tunnels are created within the medial epicondyle and proximal ulna with a 3.2-mm drill. The convergent drill holes placed in the proximal ulna are oriented vertically and placed at the level of the coronoid tubercle, approximately 5 mm distal to the articular surface. It is more secure to connect drill holes with a curet or a towel clip.[17] Two convergent bone tunnels drilled within the medial epicondyle meet at the level of the anatomic origin of the anterior bundle.

The palmaris tendon is then harvested via a 2-cm transverse skin incision within the distal flexor crease of the wrist. The median nerve and its palmar cutaneous branch are identified, and the tendon is isolated. Using a tendon stripper, the entire palmaris longus is proximally divided and detached at its musculotendinous junction. Approximately 15 to 17 cm of tendon length is necessary for reconstruction of the MCL. Muscle is stripped off of the tendon graft, a single no. 1 nonabsorbable suture is then placed in both ends with a locking stitch.

The graft is passed through the ulna and crossed in a figure-of-eight fashion using the flexible suture passer. With the elbow held in a neutral varus-valgus position with 45 degrees of elbow, the graft is pulled taut and sutured to itself with no. 1 nonabsorbable sutures (Fig. 3). Additional sutures are used to reattach any remnants of the original MCL to the graft. The elbow is then brought through a full passive ROM to verify the isometry and stability of the ligament reconstruction. The wound is closed over a surgical drain. The elbow is immobilized in a long-arm posterior plaster splint in 90 degrees of flexion and neutral forearm rotation, leaving the hand and wrist free, for 1 week. At week 2, the brace is altered to allow 30 to 90 degrees ROM, which is gradually increased until full ROM is achieved by week 8.

POSTEROLATERAL ROTATORY INSTABILITY

Varus instability and recurrent posterolateral rotatory instability of the elbow joint have been unrecognized clinical conditions. Descriptions of these instability patterns by Morrey et al[1, 18] aided in their diagnosis and treatment. Posterolateral rotatory instability may result from an acute injury to or developmental laxity of the ulnar part of the LCL. This may then allow transient rotatory subluxation of the humeroulnar joint and a secondary subluxation or dislocation of the humeroradial joint. This condition usually follows a significant injury to the elbow joint, such as

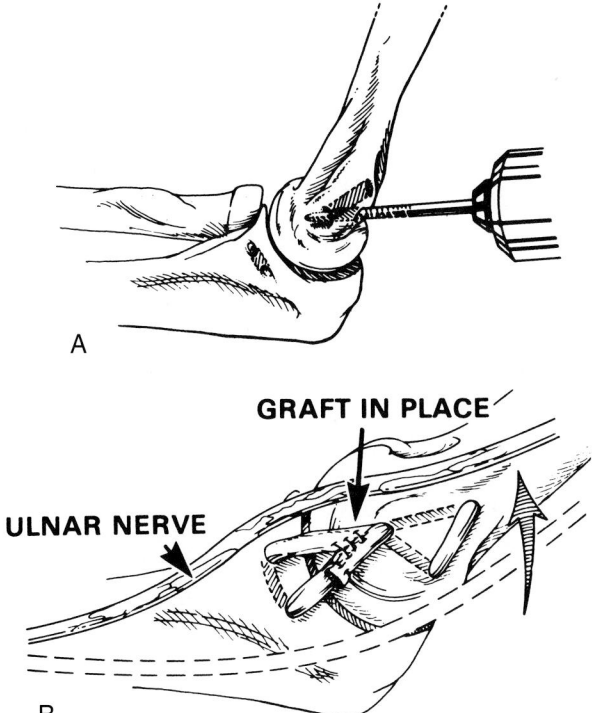

Fig. 3. Surgical technique for medial ulnar collateral ligament injury. *A,* Holes are placed in the anatomic site of origin and insertion of the anterior bundle of the medial ulnar collateral ligament. *B,* The free tendon graft forms a figure-of-eight. (Reproduced from Jobe FW, Stark H, Lombardo SJ: Reconstruction of the ulnar collateral ligament in athletes. J Bone Joint Surg Am 1986; 68:1158.)

elbow dislocation, hyperextension injury, or acute varus stress applied to the elbow joint in a position of extension and forearm pronation. Patients with recurrent posterolateral rotatory instability of the elbow may complain of pain, tenderness, catching, snapping, or gross instability of the elbow joint. O'Driscoll et al[1] reported that the lateral pivot-shift test can be used to diagnose posterolateral rotatory instability.

ENTHESOPATHY AND NEURITIS

MEDIAL EPICONDYLITIS
Injury Mechanism and Pathophysiology
During the acceleration phase of throwing, maximum tensile loads are being applied to the medial aspect of the elbow joint. These forces are transmitted initially to the flexor-pronator musculature originating at the medial epicondyle and subsequently to the deeper MCL.[8, 19, 20] Improper technique, poor conditioning, inadequate warm-up, and fatigue may lead to inflammation of the flexor-pronator mass. Vascular compromise, an altered nutritional state, and tissue overload may result initially in the microscopic histological changes of angiofibroblastic hyperplasia and ultimately in macroscopic tissue disruption.[21] Vangsness and Jobe[22] identified macroscopic rupture of the flexor-pronator origin in 100% of their patients undergoing surgical treatment for medial epicondylitis. These pathological changes are commonly identified in the pronator teres and flexor carpi radialis.[19, 23] Such changes in the flexor-pro-

nator mass and MCLs may cause a cascade of events, including ulnar traction neuropathy, radiocapitellar joint compression overload, and posteromedial olecranon impingement.[19, 24]

Diagnosis
Patients with medial epicondylitis may exhibit pain within the muscle origin with resisted wrist palmar flexion, resisted forearm pronation, and maximum finger flexion. Pain may be localized to the medial aspect of the elbow during the late cocking and acceleration phases of pitching and has a gradual onset exacerbated by overhead activities. Tenderness over the flexor-pronator radial to the medial epicondyle and most often over the pronator teres and flexor carpi radialis is a typical finding. Plain radiographs of the elbow often show hypertrophy of the medial epicondyle. Some patients with medial epicondylitis may have traction spurs, ossicles, and calcification within the medial ligament associated with chronic ligament strain. Concomitant ulnar neuropathy may be present, causing the ulnar nerve to stretch and develop secondary inflammatory changes.

Treatment
Relief of pain and inflammation is the primary goal of nonsurgical treatment. Avoidance of the offending activity is essential; throwing must be stopped until symptoms resolve during daily activities. If batting or fielding produces only minimal pain that does not increase, then monitored participation may be continued during treatment, with ice packs applied for its transient local vasoconstrictive and analgesic effects. Oral nonsteroidal anti-inflammatory medication and galvanic stimulation should be initiated for 1 to 3 weeks. If these initial therapeutic measures have no effect, two or three corticosteroid injections can be given.[19, 25]

After relief of initial pain and inflammation, a rehabilitation program is started, beginning with wrist flexor and forearm pronator stretching and progressive isometric exercises. As flexibility, strength, and endurance improve, eccentric and concentric resistive exercises are added. Medial epicondylitis often responds successfully to a nonsurgical treatment[19, 22, 23]

The indication for surgical treatment of medial epicondylitis is persistent pain in spite of a well-managed nonoperative program for at least 6 to 12 months and exclusion of any other pathological causes of the pain. Surgical treatment is resection of all pathological tissue and firm reattachment of the flexor-pronator mass.[22]

ULNAR NEUROPATHY
Injury Mechanism and Pathophysiology
In throwers with the MCL insufficiency, valgus laxity increases tension on the ulnar nerve as the medial joint space widens. This laxity also produces posteromedial impingement between the olecranon and its fossa. Secondary degenerative changes, including spur formation and loose bodies, also may irritate the nerve. Muscle hypertrophy of the medial head of the triceps and flexor carpi ulnaris has been reported to cause ulnar nerve compression at this level.[24, 26] The nerve may be entrapped between the two heads of the flexor carpi ulnaris. Subluxation or dislocation from the ulnar groove may lead to a friction neuritis.

Diagnosis

Patients with ulnar neuropathy complain of posteromedial elbow pain, radiating to the forearm and hand. Physical examination reveals tenderness of the ulnar nerve, within the cubital tunnel, and along its course. There is diminished sensibility in the ring and little fingers and a positive Tinel sign. The elbow flexion test, which evaluates the condition of the ulnar nerve while maximally flexing the elbow and extending the wrist for 3 minutes, may help confirm the diagnosis of ulnar neuropathy within the cubital tunnel. Patients with ulnar neuropathy feel pain, numbness, and tingling along the ulnar nerve distribution. Nerve conduction speed and electromyography are helpful when positive, but a normal test does not rule out neuropathy.

Treatment

The treatment of ulnar compressive neuropathy at the elbow depends on the degree of motor and sensory impairment. According to McGowen's classification, a "minimal lesion" has no motor weakness for which nonoperative treatment is indicated.[22] As with other medial tension overload injuries, relief of pain and inflammation is the primary goal of nonoperative treatment. Avoidance of the offending activity is essential. Splinting the elbow at 90 degrees with the forearm in neutral position can be instituted for 2 to 3 weeks. Oral nonsteroidal anti-inflammatory medication is administered. However, local injection of a corticosteroid into the medial aspect of the elbow is not recommended.[12] After relief of initial pain and inflammation, a rehabilitation program is started, beginning with a strengthening program for the wrist flexor and forearm pronator, isometric exercise, endurance exercise, and eccentric and concentric resistive exercises. Flexibility exercises also are initiated to prevent muscular tightness.

Although in situ decompression, removal of the medial epicondyle, subcutaneous anterior transposition, and intramuscular anterior transposition are reported, anterior submuscular transposition of the ulnar nerve is commonly recommended for throwing athletes.[12, 28, 29] Submuscular placement protects the ulnar nerve from direct trauma and creates a nearly straight route from arm to forearm in the acceleration phase of throwing.

Patients with chronic ulnar neuropathy often have concomitant medial instability. Anterior submuscular transposition in conjunction with MCL reconstruction is indicated. The nerve is positioned anterior to the medial epicondyle and submuscularly beneath the flexor-pronator mass. A portion of the intermuscular septum and muscle fibers of the flexor-pronator group should be cut out to prevent tethering or nerve impingement.

OSTEOCHONDRAL LESION

LATERAL COMPRESSION INJURIES

When large tensile loads are being applied to the medial aspect of the elbow joint during the acceleration phase, the lateral compartment is simultaneously experiencing strong compressive and shearing forces.[2, 30–32] Acute or chronic repetitive, excessive force predisposes the radiocapitellar

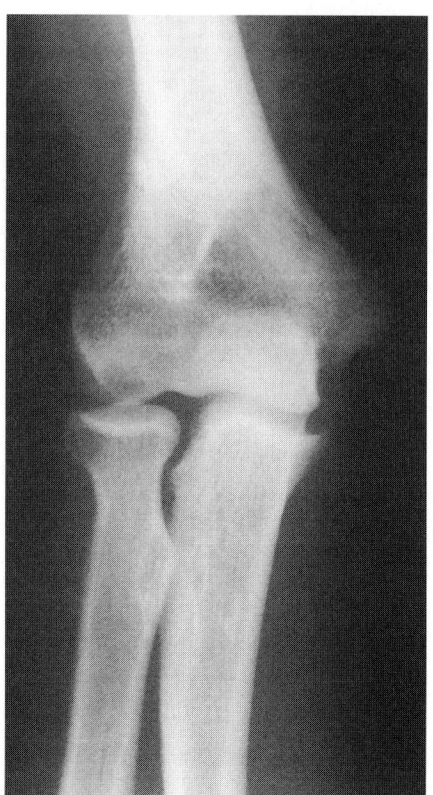

Fig. 4. Radiographic appearance of osteochondritis dissecans of the capitellum. (From Jones RB, Miller RH III: Bone overuse injuries about the elbow. Oper Tech Orthop 2001; 11:56.)

joint to synovitis, osteochondral fracture, osteochondritis dissecans, and degenerative arthritis (Fig. 4). Usually patients have signs and symptoms of medial tension overload. In addition, they may exhibit swelling, tenderness, or palpable crepitus laterally around the radiocapitellar joint.

Lateral compression injuries can be treated surgically or endoscopically.[33, 34] Advances in endoscopic technique have allowed improved visualization, decreased morbidity, and a reduced risk of complications.[33, 35, 36] Use of proper arthroscopic portals, maintenance of maximum elbow distension, and careful attention to detail help minimize the risk of major neurovascular complications. Standard arthroscopic portals are created. Two portals—one superomedial, the other anterolateral—are made, the former for viewing (Fig. 5) and the latter for repair work. Additional midlateral and posterolateral portals can be created as necessary to allow visualization and treatment of the lateral and posterior compartments (Fig. 6). Active elbow ROM exercises are initiated as soon as pain and swelling subside. The strengthening exercises are then begun and progressed as tolerated until full elbow and shoulder motion, strength, and endurance have been regained.

POSTERIOR EXTENSION OVERLOAD INJURIES

Posterior extension overload injuries occur during the acceleration and deceleration phases of throwing. The elbow

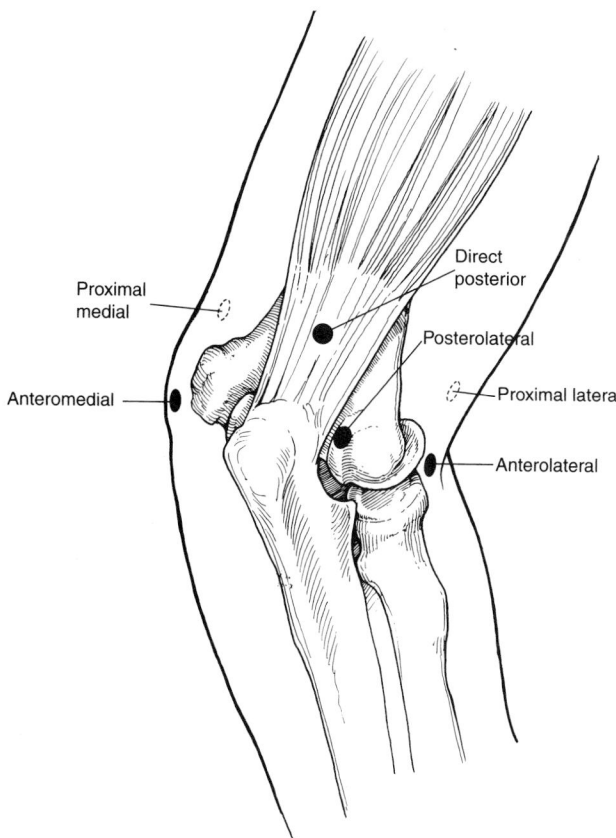

Fig. 5. Arthroscopic portals. (From Miller MD, Osborne JR, Warner JJP, et al: MRI-Arthroscopy Correlative Atlas. Philadelphia, WB Saunders, 1997, p 197.)

rapidly extends during the acceleration phase, and, after the ball is released, the upper extremity is rapidly decelerated. Maximum compressive load to the posterior compartment is created in terminal extension during deceleration. The

elbow flexors contract to slow the rapidly extending elbow, and the ligamentous and bony structures absorb the kinetic energy that is not tempered by these eccentric contractions. The olecranon impacts against the posteromedial aspect of the fossa. Focal inflammation, chondromalacia, and osteophyte formation may result from an acute injury or from chronic, repetitive elbow extension. Posterior extension overload injuries include triceps muscle strain, hypertrophic osteophyte formation, fracture of the tip of the osteophyte, stress fracture of the olecranon, loose-body formation, medial joint laxity with posteromedial impingement, and posterior compartment impingement with scar tissue[30, 31, 37, 38, 39] (Fig. 7). These injuries may be seen with or without an associated medial tension overload injury. Patients with extension overload injuries may exhibit tenderness around the posterior compartment or distal triceps insertion. Loss of extension and pain with valgus stress testing or pain at the extreme ranges of elbow extension may also be present.[30, 31]

Advances in endoscopic surgical technique have also allowed improved visualization, decreased morbidity, and a reduced risk of complications in the assessment and treatment of posterior impaction injuries. Although patient positioning during arthroscopy of the elbow joint is subject to surgeon preference, the lateral decubitus position or the prone position is recommended for these injuries.[40, 41] As with lateral compression injuries, two portals are created: a midlateral portal for viewing and a posterolateral portal for repair work. Additional posterior and posteromedial portals can be created as necessary to allow visualization and treatment of the posterior compartment. After débridement of the olecranon fossa, the posterior compartment is evaluated for signs of hypertrophic spur formation and impingement. An abrasion bur is used to resect bone bulge encroaching on the olecranon fossa. An abrasion bur or an osteotome is used to resect hypertrophic olecranon spurs, eliminating the bony impingement posteromedially.[30, 31, 39]

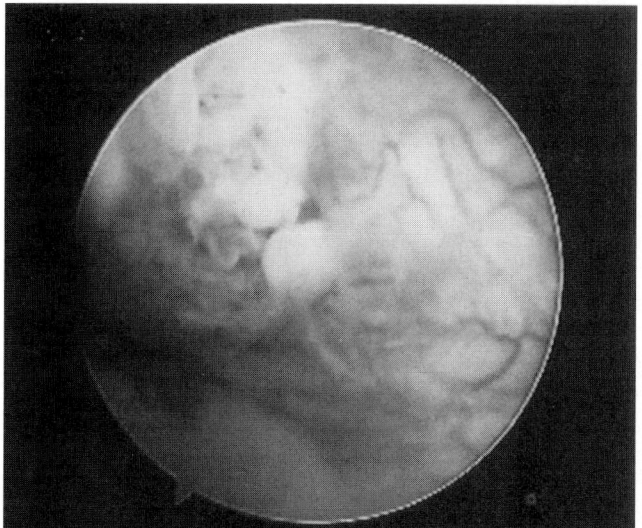

Fig. 6. Medial capsule of the elbow. In this arthroscopic view from the anterolateral portal, inflammatory changes are seen. (From Andrews JR, Timmerman LA: Diagnostic and Operative Arthroscopy. Philadelphia, WB Saunders, 1997, p 186.)

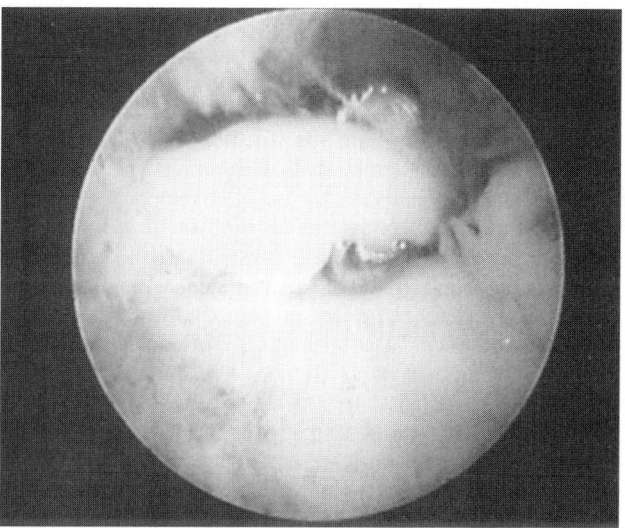

Fig. 7. Arthroscopic view of a loose body in the anterior compartment of the elbow. (From Andrews JR, Timmerman LA: Diagnostic and Operative Arthroscopy. Philadelphia, WB Saunders, 1997, p 183.)

Postoperatively, active ROM exercises are initiated as soon as pain and swelling subside. Strengthening exercises are begun and progressed as tolerated until full elbow and shoulder motion, strength, and endurance are regained. Within 8 to 12 weeks, a progressive throwing program is permitted, with a return to athletic activities approximately 3 to 6 months after surgery.

NORMAL DEVELOPMENT AND INJURY IN THE SKELETALLY IMMATURE ATHLETE

Discussion of the normal growth of ossification centers and maturation patterns is important to understand injuries common in skeletally immature athletes. The maturation sequence at the elbow is more variable than for other joints. In the skeletally immature person, the ligaments and soft tissues withstand stress better than the epiphyseal growth plates. The skeletally immature throwing athlete may present with injuries ranging from apophyseal inflammation, fragmentation, and delayed epiphyseal closure to epiphyseal plate separation.

LATERAL COMPARTMENT INJURY

The capitellum is the first of the six elbow ossification centers to appear. Its pattern of ossification and timing of appearance vary. It is visualized radiographically at 1 to 2 years of age.[42] The central and lateral aspects of the capitellum are frequently the sites of osteochondrosis. The presenting complaint is pain, joint line tenderness, effusion, grating, a decreased motion, or locking if the fragment is free or loose. Plain radiographs in tangential and oblique views can identify the lesion. The capitellum osteochondrosis may be staged anatomically based on progression of the lesion. In the literature, three different stages were described.[43, 44] Treatment options depend on the clinical and radiographic findings. The early-stage lesion is a variant of normal ossification and is subsequently associated with an area of focal radiolucency with or without limited ROM. The average age of this group is 10 years. The recommended treatment is restriction of throwing, and this should be continued until the radiolucent area has disappeared. Usually a cast or posterior splint is not necessary. The capitellum fuses with the trochlea or with the lateral epicondyle before it unites with the humeral shaft. Natural healing of capitellar osteochondrosis is sometimes observed while the lateral epicondyle unites with the humeral shaft.

The progressive-stage lesion presents as an osteocartilaginous osteochondritis dissecans fragment with subchondral radiolucency. The complaint is pain and restricted ROM. These lesions occur at an average age of 12 years. The first choice of treatment is restriction of throwing. If no response to conservative treatment is seen, surgery is indicated, which involves bone peg graft to the affected area.

Terminal-stage lesions present at an average age of 15 years. Surgery or endoscopic treatment is indicated. The osteocartilaginous fragments are removed, the fibrillated cartilage is shaved, or a partially detached fragment is repaired with bone graft fixation.[45] However, long-term follow-up has not demonstrated a favorable outcome in terms of symptoms or radiographic changes.[46, 47] Prevention and early detection comprise the best form of treatment.

The cause of osteochondritis dissecans has been debated for over a century.[48] The term is attributed to Konig,[49] who hypothesized that trauma produced osseous necrosis followed by dissecting inflammation. Some authors took exception to the older term, preferring instead osteochondrosis dissecans, because it is a reparative rather than an inflammatory process.[13, 50–53] The commonly considered theories of cause are direct trauma, indirect trauma, ischemia, and constitutional factors. During acceleration and deceleration phases, strong compressive and shearing forces are created about the radiocapitellar joint as well as distraction forces to the medial aspect of the elbow joint. This repetitive force may be considered a major factor. In addition, the capitellum receives end arteries that terminate in the subchondral plate and are vulnerable to disruption.[54] Panner[55] described osteochondrosis of the entire capitellum, the clinical presentation of which is somewhat different. The average age of onset is 8 years. Some of Panner's cases were simultaneous, and another occurred in the femoral head and the patella. If further trauma is avoided, this type of osteochondrosis will most likely have a benign course, and epiphyseal regeneration will occur in 1 to 3 years; insignificant or mild deformity will be the final result.

The ossification center of the radial head is visualized at 5 years and fuses at 14 to 16 years.[42] During the development of the secondary ossification center, irregular patterns of ossification (segmentation) and secondary pain from stress are seen, which can be classified as osteochondrosis[56] (Fig. 8). The complaints, pathophysiology, and treatment are similar to those of other osteochondroses. The course of radial head osteochondrosis is usually benign, and epiphyseal regeneration occurs in 1 to 2 years; insignificant or mild deformity are the final result. It is sometimes accompanied by capitellum osteochondrosis.

MEDIAL COMPARTMENT INJURY

The medial epicondyle is the second ossification center to appear, usually at 4 to 5 years.[42] It develops slowly, uniting with the humeral shaft at about 15 to 16 years and with the trochlea before that. Repetitive valgus force at the medial epicondyle may stress the normal chondro-osseous

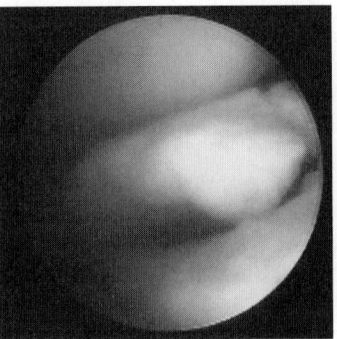

Fig. 8. Arthroscopic view of osteochondritis dissecans. (From Morrey BF: The Elbow and Its Disorders. Philadelphia, WB Saunders, 2000, 3rd ed, p 566.)

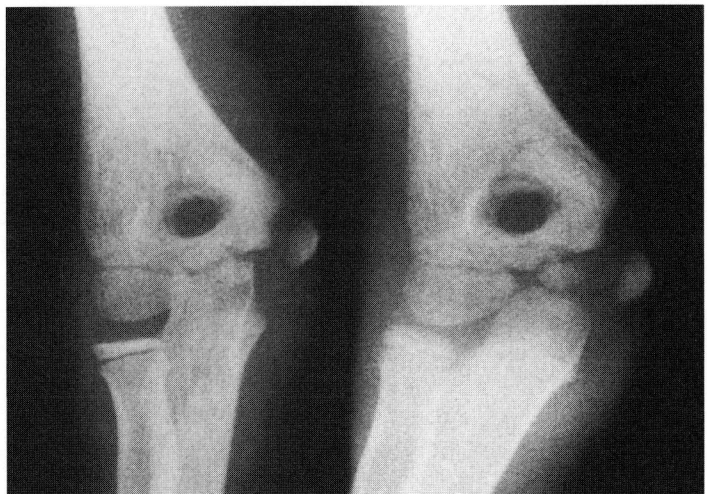

Fig. 9. Normal alignment of the medial epicondyle. The medial epicondyle displaces when valgus stress is impaired to the joint. (From Schwab GH, Bennet JB, Woods GW, et al: Biomechanics of elbow instability: The role of the medial collateral ligament. Clin Orthop 1980; 146:42.)

transformation, resulting in an irregular ossification pattern on roentgenogram, segmentation, and separation[55] (Fig. 9). Such a spectrum of injuries has been broadly termed "little leaguer's elbow."[57] Osteochondrosis of the medial epicondyle is usually self-limiting and heals without major deformity or disability. In the athlete entering adolescence, both muscle mass and muscle strength are increasing rapidly. Bone fragments should be replaced anatomically and fixed by open reduction. The valgus force and sudden contraction of the flexors may be strong enough to cause separation of the entire medial epicondyle. In the final stages of medial epicondyle-humerus fusion, the forces are generally not distributed to the entire medial epicondyle but to one point of muscle origin. A small fragment can be avulsed and may heal as a bony spur on the inferior surface of the medial epicondyle or as ossicle below it (Fig. 10).

The ossification center of the trochlea appears at 8 to 12 years, possibly with several centers, and usually fuses at 14 to 16 years.[42] With maturation, an irregular outline sometimes appears and may be confused with such abnormal processes as avascular necrosis. Osteochondrosis of the trochlea is sometimes recognized, although it rarely results in joint deformity.

POSTERIOR COMPARTMENT INJURY

The olecranon ossification center appears between 8 and 10 years, with fusion to the ulnar shaft at 14 to 15 years.[42] During the development of the secondary ossification center, irregular patterns of ossification and secondary pain from stress are seen, which can be classified either as overuse syndrome or osteochondrosis. Sometimes there are two or more nuclei. An asymmetric pattern of ossification is indicative of osteochondrosis. Fusion proceeds posteriorly from the joint, or anterior side, and, in the throwing athlete, earlier in the throwing arm than in the contralateral arm. During adolescence, persistent pain is indicative of a lack of fusion between the ossified secondary center and the olecranon.[58] In some cases, the physis does not close and causes a delayed union or nonunion of the olecranon, resulting in persistent elbow pain.[9] Bone grafting may be required to induce union across the physis.

TREATMENT PRINCIPLE FOR THE SKELETALLY IMMATURE ATHLETE

Nonsurgical therapy should be considered the primary treatment option, with relief of pain and inflammation as the primary goal. Patients should avoid the offending activ-

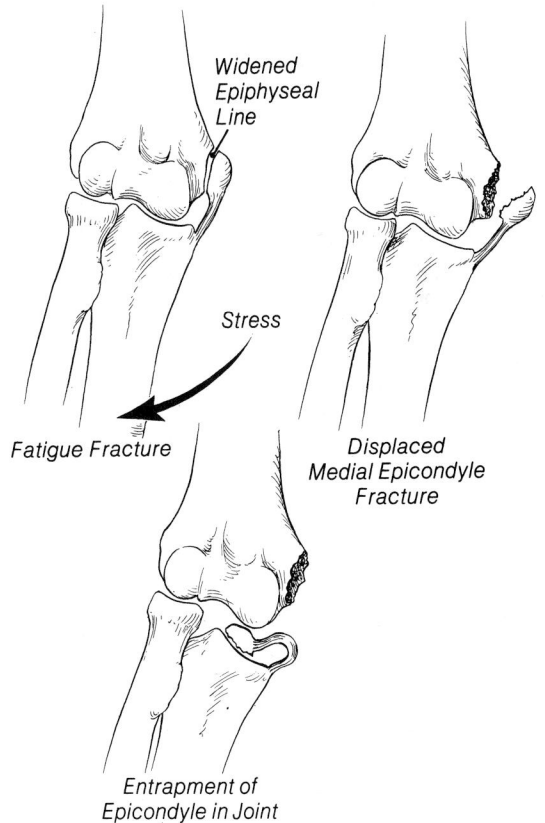

Fig. 10. Role of the physis in displacement and retraction. Continued valgus stress may cause a progressive widening of the physis in the growing individual. The physis may separate, resulting in displacement and distal retraction. In some instances, the medial epicondyle may become entrapped in the joint. (From Schwab GH, Bennet JB, Woods GW, et al: Biomechanics of elbow instability: The role of the medial collateral ligament. Clin Orthop 1980; 146:42.)

ity as well as any other activities that aggravate the condition. Throwing must be stopped until symptoms resolve during daily activities. If playing produces only minimal pain that does not increase, then batting and fielding may be continued during treatment. Any anti-inflammatory agent, cast, or brace is not necessary. An osteochondral lesion in the skeletally immature athlete often responds successfully to nonsurgical treatment.

Surgical treatment should be considered an option only in patients with injuries resulting from a single traumatic event or with refractory symptoms despite 6 to 12 months of conservative management. An avulsion fracture of the medial epicondyle or acute separation of the epiphyseal plate of the medial epicondyle may be surgically reattached. Nonunion of the olecranon is fixed with bone graft. Fragment fixation or débridement is indicated in capitellum osteochondrosis with a dissecting fragment or loose body.

REFERENCES

1. O'Driscoll SW, Bell DF, Morrey BF: Posterolateral rotatory instability of the elbow. J Bone Joint Surg Am 1991; 73:440.
2. Slocum DB: Classification of elbow injuries from baseball pitching. Tex Med 1968; 64:48.
3. Kapandi IA: The Physiology of the Joints: Annotated Diagrams of the Mechanics of the Human Joints: Vol. 1. Upper Limb. Edinburgh, Livingstone, 2nd ed, 1970.
4. Morrey BF, An KN: Articular and ligamentous contributions to the stability of the elbow joint. Am J Sports Med 1983; 11:315.
5. Schwab GH, Bennett JB, Woods GW, et al: Biomechanics of elbow instability: The role of the medial collateral ligament. Clin Orthop 1980; 146:42.
6. Sojbjerg JO, Ovesen J, Nielsen S: Experimental elbow instability after transection of the medial collateral ligament. Clin Orthop 1986; 218:186.
7. O'Driscoll SW, Horii E, Morrey BF, et al: Anatomy of the ulnar part of the lateral collateral ligament of the elbow. Clin Anat 1992; 5:296.
8. Jobe FW, Kvitne RS: Elbow instability in the athlete. Am Acad Orthop Surg Instruct Course Lect 1991; 40:17.
9. Conway JE, Jobe FW, Glousman RE: Medial instability of the elbow in the throwing athlete. J Bone Joint Surg Am 1992; 74:67.
10. Woods GW, Tullos HS: Elbow instability and medial epicondyle fractures. Am J Sports Med 1977; 5:23.
11. Andrews JA, Whiteside JA, Buettner CM: Clinical evaluation of the elbow in the throwers. Op Tech Sports Med 1996; 4:77.
12. Del Pizzo W, Jobe FW, Norwood L: Ulnar nerve entrapment syndrome in baseball players. Am J Sports Med 1977; 5:182.
13. Kenneth MS, Steven PR: Osteochondrosis of the humeral capitellum. Am J Sports Med 1984; 12:351.
14. Timmerman LA, Andrews JR: Undersurface tear of ulnar collateral ligament in baseball players. A newly recognized lesion. Am J Sports Med 1994; 22:33.
15. Benuett JB, Green MS, Tullos HS: Surgical management of chronic medial elbow instability. Clin Orthop 1992; 278:62.
16. Jobe FW, Stark H, Lonibardo SJ: Reconstruction of the ulnar collateral ligament in athletes. J Bone Joint Surg Am 1986; 68:1158.
17. Andrews JA, Jelsma RD, Joyce ME, et al: Open surgical procedures for injuries to the elbow in throwers. Op Tech Sports Med 1996; 4:109.
18. Nestor BJ, O'Driscoll SW, Morrey BF: Ligamentous reconstruction for posterolateral rotatory instability of the elbow, J Bone Joint Surg Am 1992; 74:1235.
19. Leach RE, Miller JK: Lateral and medial epicondylitis of the elbow. Clin Sports Med 1987; 6:259.
20. Woods GW, Tullos HS, King JW: The throwing arm-elbow joint injuries. J Sports Med 1973; 1:43.
21. Nirschl RP: Muscle and tendon trauma, tennis elbow, the elbow and its disorder. In Morrey BF (ed): The Elbow and Its Disorders. Philadelphia, WB Saunders, 1985, p 481.
22. Vangsness CT, Jobe FW: Surgical treatment of medial epicondylitis. J Bone Joint Surg Br 1991; 73:409.
23. Coonrad RW: Tendinopathies at the elbow. Am Acad Orthop Surg Instr Course Lect 1991;40:25.
24. Glousman RE, Barron J, Jobe FW, et al: An electromyographic analysis of the elbow in normal and injured pitchers with medial collateral ligament insufficiency. Am J Sports Med 1992; 20:311.
25. Price R: Local injection treatment of tennis elbow: Hydrocortisone triamcinolone and lignocaine compared. Br J Rheumatol 1991; 30:39.
26. Dangles CJ, Bilos ZJ: Ulnar nerve neuritis in a world champion weight lifter. Am J Sports Med 1980; 8:443.
27. Glousman RE: Ulnar nerve problems in athlete's elbow. Clin Sports Med 1990; 9:365.
28. Dellon AL: Review of treatment results for ulnar nerve entrapments at the elbow. J Hand Surg 1989; 14:688.
29. Janes PC, Mann RJ, Farnworth TK: Submuscular transposition of the ulnar nerve. Clin Orthop 1989; 238:225.
30. Andrews JR: Bony injuries about the elbow in the throwing athlete. Am Acad Orthop Surg Instruct Course Lect 1985; 34:323.
31. Andrews JR, Craven WM: Lesions of the posterior compartment of the elbow. Clin Sports Med 1991; 10:637.
32. Pappas AM: Elbow problems associated with baseball during childhood and adolescence. Clin Orthop 1982; 164:30.
33. Andrews JR: Arthroscopy of the elbow. Am Acad Orthop Surg Instruct Course Lect 1988; 37:195.
34. McManama GB Jr, Michaeli LJ, Berry MY, et al: The surgical treatment of osteochondritis of the capitellum. Am J Sports Med 1985; 13:11.
35. Carson WG Jr, Meyers JF: Diagnostic arthroscopy of the elbow: Surgical technique and arthroscopic and portal anatomy. In McGinty JB (ed): Operative Arthroscopy. New York, 1991, Raven Press.
36. Lindenfeld TN: Medial approach to elbow arthroscopy. Am J Sports Med 1990; 18:413.
37. King JW, Brelsford HJ, Tullos HS: Analysis of the pitching arm of the professional baseball pitcher. Clin Orthop 1969; 67:67.
38. Nuber GW, Diment MT: Olecranon stress fractures in throwers: A report of two cases and a review of the literature. Clin Orthop 1992; 278:58.
39. Wilson FD, Andrews JR, Blackburn TA, et al: Valgus extension overload in the pitching elbow. Am J Sports Med 1983; 11:83.
40. O'Driscoll SW, Morrey BF: Arthroscopy of the elbow. J Bone Joint Surg Am 1992; 74:84.
41. Baker CL, Shalvoy RM: The prone position for elbow arthroscopy. Clin Sports Med 1991; 10:623.
42. Hoffman AD: Radiography of the pediatric elbow. In Morrey BF (ed): The elbow and Its Disorders. Philadelphia, WB Saunders, 1985, p 153.
43. Iwase T, Ikata T: Baseball elbow of young players. Tokushima J Exp Med 1985; 32:57.
44. Conway FM: Osteochondritis dissecans: Description of the stages of the condition and its probable traumatic etiology. Am J Surg 1937; 38:691.
45. Kashiwagucgi S, Ikata T: Conservative treatment of the osteochondrosis of the humeral capitellum. MB Orthop 1997; 10:67.
46. Baur M, Jonsson K, Josefsson PO, et al: Osteochondritis dissecans of the elbow: A long-term follow up study. Clin Orthop 1992; 284:156.
47. Woodward AH, Bianco AJ Jr: Osteochondritis dissecans of the elbow. Clin Orthop 1975; 110:35.
48. Nagura S: The so called osteochondritis dissecans of Konig. Clin Orthop 1960; 18:100.
49. Konig F: Ueber freie Korper in den Gelenken. Dtsch Zchir 1887; 27:90.
50. Litchman HM, McCullough RW, Gandsman EJ, et al: Computerized blood flow analysis for decision making in the treatment of osteochondritis dissecans. J Pediatr Orthop 1988; 8:208.
51. Mau H: Juvenile osteochondroses-enchondral dysostoses. Clin Orthop 1958; 11:154.
52. Novotny H: Preventive and conservative treatment of osteochondritis dissecans. Acta Orthop Scand 1951; 21:40.

53. Pappas AM: Osteochondritis dissecans. Clin Orthop 1981; 158:57.
54. Haraldsson S: On osteochondritis deformans juvenile capitula humeri including investigation of intra-osseous vasculature on distal humerus. Acta Orthop Scand 1959; 38:1.
55. Panner HJ: A peculiar affection of the ca-pitulum humeri, resembling Calvé-Perthes disease of the hip. Acta Radiol 1929; 10: 234.
56. Trias A, Ray RD: Juvenile osteochondritis of the radial head. J Bone Joint Surg Am 1963; 45:576.
57. Brogdon BG, Crow WM: Little leaguer's elbow. AJR Am J Roentgenol 1960; 83; 671.
58. Torg JS, Moyer RA: Non-union of a stress fracture through the olecranon epiphyseal plate observed in an adolescent baseball pitcher. J Bone Joint Surg Am 1977; 59: 264.

section 4 chapter 11

KNEE LIGAMENT INJURIES: EPIDEMIOLOGY, MECHANISM, DIAGNOSIS, AND NATURAL HISTORY

Gregory C. Fanelli and David R. Maish

Summary
- Knee ligament injuries are characterized by the ligaments involved, the chronicity of the injury, the degree and quality of laxity, tear morphology, and the physiological demands that the patient will place on the injured knee.
- An experienced orthopaedic surgeon who takes an accurate history and performs a physical examination can diagnose most knee ligament injuries accurately.
- Arthrometers and stress radiography are used to quantify knee ligament laxity.
- Magnetic resonance imaging (MRI) and diagnostic arthroscopy are very accurate at diagnosing knee ligament injuries and their associated injuries, but they should be reserved for cases with equivocal physical examinations.
- It is important to identify all the individual ligament injuries in an injured knee because combined ligament injuries have a poor prognosis when managed nonoperatively.

DEFINITIONS

The osseous structures of the knee are stabilized and guided by ligaments as they rotate about the three axes that provide the six degrees of freedom of knee motion. Knee motion is not limited to a single degree of freedom. For example, when an anterior force is applied to the tibia of an intact knee, the tibia rotates internally. Conversely, when a posterior force is applied to the tibia of an intact knee, the tibia rotates externally. These predictable rotations are referred to as coupled rotations.

Although ligaments were once thought to be static structures, they are actually physiologically active bands of tough connective tissue that exhibit complex mechanical behavior while providing stabilization to the knee joint. The terms insufficiency, deficiency, and laxity describe a decrease in the functional integrity and the normal restraining forces of a ligament. Ligament insufficiency can be the result of microscopic structural damage, a partial tear, or a complete tear. Isolated ligament injuries involve only one ligamentous structure, whereas combined ligament injuries involve two or more. Knee instability refers to the failure of the knee ligaments to maintain the normal anatomic structural relationships.

A ligament is considered to be a primary restraint when it accounts for the majority of force resisting an externally applied force. Sectioning a primary restraint will increase joint motion. If a secondary restraint is additionally sectioned, joint motion will increase further. However, sectioning a secondary restraint will not alter the limits of joint motion while the primary restraint is intact. A ligament may serve as both a primary restraint to motion in one direction and a secondary restraint to motion in a different direction.

HISTORICAL REVIEW

170: Galen described the presence of the genu cruciata.[1]
1850: Stark wrote the first recorded description of cruciate ligament disruption.[2]
1900: Battle described a surgical repair of the anterior cruciate ligament (ACL).[3]
1903: Mayo Robson described the first operative repair of an acutely torn posterior cruciate ligament (PCL).[4]
1917: Hey-Groves reported the first ACL reconstruction.[5]
1936: Campbell was the first to describe the triad of an injured ACL, medial collateral ligament (MCL), and medial meniscus, but credit for this description has been given to O'Donoghue.[6]
1950: O'Donoghue reported on the repair of knee ligament injuries.[7]
1976: Hughston et al emphasized the importance of the PCL as the basic stabilizer of the knee joint, thereby renewing interest in reconstructive methods to restore its function.[8]
1983: Clancy et al reported that the majority of their PCL reconstruction results were good or excellent when using the medial one-third patellar tendon autograft.[9]
1980s: Arthroscopically assisted cruciate ligament reconstruction techniques were developed.

GENERAL APPROACH TO KNEE LIGAMENT INJURIES

Characterization of knee ligament injuries is essential to determining the optimal form of treatment. Knee ligament injuries are characterized by the ligaments involved, the chronicity of the injury, the degree of laxity, tear morphology, and the physiological demands that the patient will place on the injured knee.

In acute cases, the mechanism of injury is the most important information to be obtained. It is critical to know the setting in which the injury was sustained and to assess the risk of associated injuries. The examiner should inquire about prior knee injuries, duration of injury, knee buckling, sensation of instability, an audible pop, pain (location, severity, time of onset), ability to walk after the injury, freedom of motion, and swelling (rate of onset and size).

The best time to examine the patient is within the first hour after injury prior to knee swelling. It is crucial to achieve relaxation in the painful knee with muscle spasm. A systematic, complete examination consists of inspection, palpation, tests for range of motion, tests for mechanical or meniscal problems, and assessment of ligament stability. Both lower extremities should be completely undressed to allow for comparison. The least painful tests should be performed first; then proceed in a logical fashion. By examining the normal knee first, the individual's baseline laxity can be evaluated while instilling confidence in the patient that the examination is careful and concise.

Examination of the knee begins with assessing the neurovascular status of the limb. In acute knee dislocations with spontaneous reduction, examiners should maintain a high index of suspicion for popliteal artery injury (prevalence 16% to 64%) and peroneal nerve injury (prevalence 14% to 35%).

Then the overlying skin and soft-tissue structures are inspected. Lacerations, ecchymosis, effusions, variation in patellar position, or other deformities should be noted. Hemarthrosis suggests rupture of a cruciate ligament, osteochondral fracture, patellar dislocation, a tear in the vascularized peripheral third of a meniscus, or a tear in the deep portion of the joint capsule. However, the absence of hemarthrosis does not necessarily indicate a less severe ligament injury because disruption of the joint capsule results in blood extravasating into the surrounding tissues. The circumference of the thighs should be compared because the quadriceps undergoes a rapid, reflex atrophy after a significant disorder of the knee.

All palpable structures are gently assessed for tenderness while trying to minimize muscle spasm secondary to pain. The range of motion in both knees should be evaluated. Gait assessment and weightbearing should be observed as well. Meniscal injuries should be assessed (see the section on meniscal injuries). Stress tests to evaluate ligamentous laxity should be performed last. When muscle spasm prevents adequate evaluation of ligamentous laxity, examination under anesthesia is preferable to uncertainty.

Plain radiographs should be obtained to evaluate the injured knee for signs of fracture, avulsion fracture, and degenerative changes (osteophytes, subchondral sclerosis, or joint space narrowing) in the tibiofemoral and patellofemoral joints. Routine studies include standing anteroposterior (AP) views of both knees, a tunnel view, a 30-degree flexion lateral view, and a 30-degree AP axial view of both patellas. The tangential views of the patella are necessary because of the frequent association of acute patelloquadriceps instability with acute medial ligamentous disruptions. Avulsion fractures do not necessarily involve damage to the substance of the ligament itself, but they do result in similar symptoms and physical examination findings. With plain radiographs, these injuries are easily differentiated from ligamentous injury. In children, avulsions of the osteocartilaginous portions of the intercondylar eminences and disruptions of the physis are more common than isolated ligamentous injury.

The KT-1000 (Medmetric, San Diego, CA) and the Stryker Knee Laxity Tester (Stryker Co, Kalamazoo, MI) are instrumented measurement systems that are used to evaluate tibial translation on the femur quantitatively. The side-to-side difference is calculated by subtracting translation of the normal knee from the translation of the injured knee. Arthrometers quantitatively grade the severity of ligament insufficiency and are useful for following the progress of a patient postoperatively.

Potential problems with arthrometers include (1) low intertester reliability secondary to muscle spasm in combined ligament injuries and subsequent incorrect determination of the quadriceps neutral angle, (2) inaccurate measurement of tibial translation secondary to tibial external/internal rotation, (3) changes in the interposed soft tissue over time, and (4) movement of the apparatus during measurement. Knee effusions should be aspirated before KT-1000 arthrometry if they are large enough to cause a ballotable patella or a 1.0-cm increase in midpatellar circumference in comparison with the contralateral knee.

Varus/valgus stress radiography differentiates knee instability caused by physeal separation or tibial plateau fractures from knee instability secondary to ligamentous injury. Therefore, when knee instability is identified on physical examination, stress radiographs should be obtained for patients whose distal femoral and proximal tibial physes are still open and for patients with tibial plateau fractures.

Stress radiographs are used to measure knee ligament laxity quantitatively (Fig. 1). Stress radiographs appear to be advantageous because (1) skeletal displacement is measured without including the variable thickness of interposed soft tissue as in arthrometric measurements, (2) medial and lateral compartments can be measured separately for rotational data, (3) radiography yields reproducible results, (4) radiography is noninvasive, and 5) radiography's measurements are quantified objectively. Disadvantages of stress radiography include its learning curve, difficulty eliminating rotation, and potential for patient variability from guarding when the displacing force is applied. The specific methods of stress radiography are described later for each ligament.

Computed tomography scanning is not used routinely for knee injuries, but MRI has become increasingly important in evaluating ligament injuries. Advantages of MRI include the facts that (1) it is noninvasive, (2) it lacks ionizing radiation, (3) it has the ability to detect disorders of nonosseous structures such as ligaments, menisci, articular cartilage, and (4) it has the ability to image in any plane. The main disadvantage of MRI is its expense.

Diagnostic arthroscopy remains the preeminent standard for diagnosing the presence of cruciate ligament injuries. Arthroscopic assessment of a partial tear can be quantified based only on the tearing that can be observed (one-fourth, one-half, etc.). However, such estimates do not define the actual damage sustained because the ligament may incur

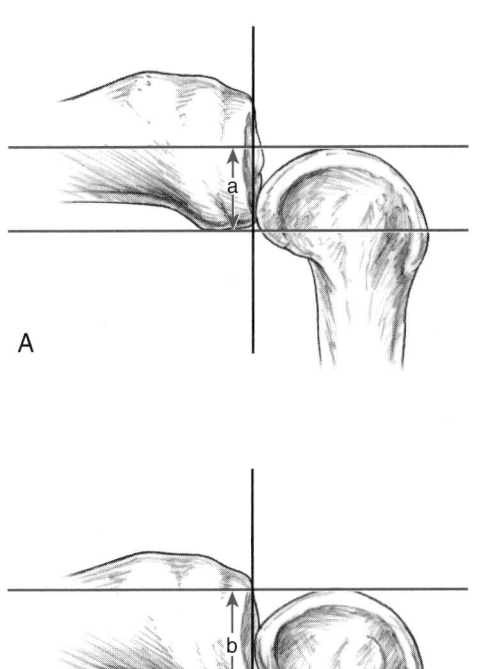

Fig. 1. Measurement of lateral tibial translation on lateral radiograph. This measurement is with 90 degrees of flexion, before and after a posteriorly directed force is applied. Tangents to the anterior aspect of the lateral femoral condyle and the posterior aspect of the tibia are drawn, and the distance between these two tangents is measured. The amount of posterior translation can be determined by subtracting the original distance (a) from the distance after the posterior force is applied (b).

microscopic injury without gross disruption. Furthermore, diagnostic arthroscopy is invasive and expensive. Therefore, it should be used only when physical examination yields equivocal results. In patients who have been selected for surgical management, physical examination under anesthesia and diagnostic arthroscopy are essential for confirmation of the preoperative diagnosis and for excluding other ligamentous injuries.

DIFFERENTIAL DIAGNOSIS

Injuries of the knee include fractures, avulsion fractures, extensor mechanism injuries, patellar disorders, chondral and osteochondral injuries, meniscal injuries, injuries of the collateral ligaments of the knee, injuries of the cruciate ligaments, dislocations of the proximal tibiofibular joint, and traumatic knee dislocations. It is imperative to maintain a high index of suspicion when diagnosing knee ligament injuries because findings are sometimes subtle, masked by soft-tissue swelling, or simply overlooked because more obvious concurrent injuries are present.

TREATMENT

Knee ligaments vary in their capacity to heal. Specifically, the MCL heals rapidly without repair, whereas the cruciate

ligaments have shown a poor capacity to heal even after primary surgical repair. Factors that impair cruciate ligament healing include the complex geometry of the cruciate ligaments, the biomechanical roles of the cruciate ligaments during knee motion, the harsh intra-articular environment that occurs after knee injury, and the intrinsically poor regenerative capacity of the cells in the cruciate ligaments. Therefore, various surgical techniques for cruciate ligament reconstruction have been developed to restore knee stability. The goals of surgical ligament reconstruction are to restore joint stability, to prevent secondary damage to other knee structures, and to maintain full range of knee motion. Treatment is discussed in detail in Chapter 4–12.

ISOLATED ACL INJURIES

EPIDEMIOLOGY

The occurrence rate of ACL injuries in the United States is approximately 250,000 per year. In the general population, the incidence each year is 1 in 3000. The ACL is injured nine times more frequently than the PCL. In one study of acute knee ligament injuries with pathological motion, 48% of the injuries were isolated ACL injuries, and 63% of the injuries involved the ACL. Approximately 70% of ACL injuries are sports-related. Approximately half of adolescent patients with acute traumatic hemarthrosis of the knee will have ACL insufficiency.[10]

Female participation in collegiate athletics has risen dramatically since the passage of the Title IX Education Assistance Act of 1972, but clinicians have noticed a disproportionately high rate of incidence of ACL injuries among women as compared with their male counterparts. Theories proposed to explain this female predilection for ACL injuries are divided into extrinsic and intrinsic categories. Extrinsic factors include body movement during sport participation, muscular strength, coordination, shoe-surface interface, and conditioning. Intrinsic factors include joint laxity, limb alignment, notch dimensions, and ligament size.[11]

The notch width index is defined as the ratio of the width of the intercondylar notch to the width of the distal femur at the level of the popliteal groove on a tunnel view radiograph. The average notch width index of athletes with acute ACL injuries (mean = 0.189) is lower than the average notch width indices of males (mean = 0.239) and females (mean = 0.217). Patients with a notch width index below the critical notch width index (men = 0.20, women = 0.18) are 25 times more likely to develop an ACL injury.

ANATOMY

The ACL is first observed as a condensation of vascular synovial mesenchyme at about 7 to 8 weeks of embryonic development and structurally resembles the adult form by 22 weeks. The ACL is an intra-articular yet extrasynovial structure that extends 38 mm in length from the lateral femoral condyle to its tibial attachment. The tibial attachment is larger than the femoral attachment, which confers a fan-shaped appearance to the ACL. The ACL attaches to the medial aspect of the lateral femoral condyle posterior to the intercondylar notch and to the tibial plateau anterolateral to the anterior tibial spine.

The ACL receives its blood supply primarily from the middle genicular artery and secondarily from the lateral inferior genicular artery via small periligamentous vessels that transversely penetrate the ACL. These vessels branch into a network of longitudinal vessels that run parallel to the collagen bundles within the ligament. Soft-tissue structures supply most of the vessels to the ACL; the bone-ligament junctions are not a significant source of blood.

The ACL is innervated by nerve endings originating from the tibial nerve. Histological studies of the ACL have identified Ruffini's corpuscles (type I, pressure receptors), Vater-Pacini corpuscles (type II, velocity receptors), and free nerve endings (type IV, pain receptors). The paucity of free nerve endings in the ACL might explain the absence of pain at the moment of injury and the development of severe pain only after the joint capsule becomes distended with blood. Also, the type I and II receptors might be responsible for the sensation of instability.[12]

The ACL microstructural hierarchy represents multiple levels of collagen organization. Like other ligaments, the ACL consists of closely packed collagen fiber bundles that are arranged in a parallel fashion along the longitudinal axis of the ligament. The cells populating the ACL resemble fibrocartilage cells, whereas the cells of the MCL resemble fibroblasts. These histological differences might explain the difference between the healing capacities of these two ligaments.[13]

The fibers of the femoral and tibial attachment sites pass through four morphological zones (Fig. 2).[14] Within 1 mm, the tissue morphology changes from flexible tissue to rigid bone. This microstructure is mechanically advantageous because the gradual transition from flexible to rigid tissue allows for dissipation of shearing forces.

BIOMECHANICS

The ACL is the primary restraint to anterior tibial translation with respect to the femur at knee flexion angles greater than 30 degrees. The ACL also provides resistance to internal tibial rotation and varus-valgus angulation. The ACL acts as a collection of individual fascicles constituting two main functional units, the anteromedial bundle and the posterolateral bundle. The anteromedial bundle is taut in flexion, whereas the posterolateral bundle is taut in extension (Fig. 3). This anatomic relationship ensures that a component of the ACL is taut and therefore functional at all degrees of knee flexion. The anteromedial bundle accounts for 95% of the restraining force at 30 degrees of knee flexion and is superior to the posterolateral bundle in terms of modulus, ultimate tensile strength, and strain energy density.

Ligament isometry has been defined as equal length and tension of a ligament throughout the full range of joint motion. The term isometry applies to surgical ligament reconstruction when a graft with uniform kinematic properties and simple geometry is used. Thus, methods to determine the isometric points of the ACL have been investigated. However, there is probably no true isometry in the native ACL due to its complex geometry and the kinematic property variations between the anteromedial and posterolateral bundles.

Normal kinematic knee function requires an intact ACL. Investigators have found that isolated sectioning of the ACL results in increased anterior motion limits, which is more evident at 30 degrees than 90 degrees of knee flexion. Muscles crossing the knee also play a significant role in maintaining physiological kinematics. For example, hamstring activation significantly reduces anterior translation in the ACL-deficient knee, which may explain the usefulness of closed-chain kinetic exercises during rehabilitation following ACL reconstruction.[15]

PATHOGENESIS: MECHANISMS OF INJURY

The most common mechanism of injury is noncontact, decelerating valgus angulation with external rotation. Other mechanisms include hyperextension with torsion, valgus angulation caused by a force applied to the lateral aspect of the knee, and hyperflexion. In soccer, football, and downhill skiing, the most frequent mechanism of injury is val-

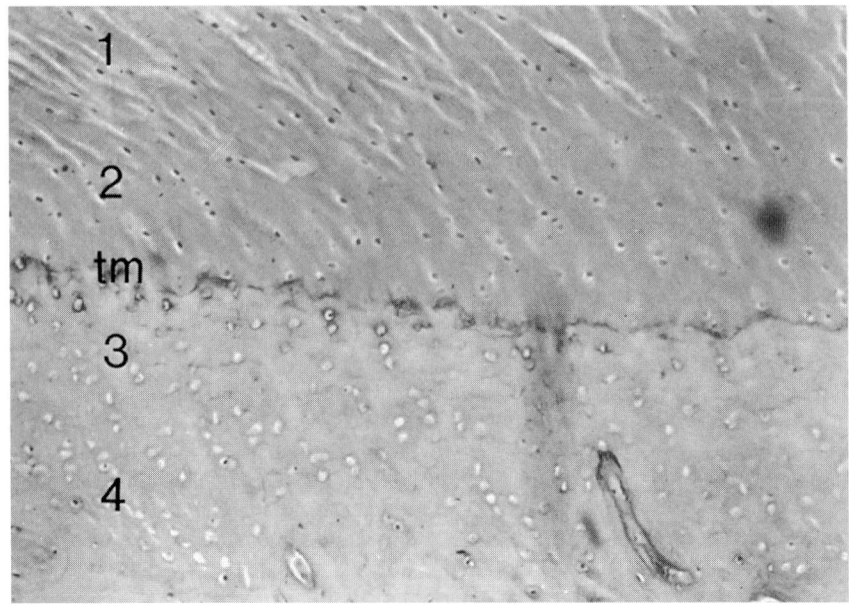

Fig. 2. The morphologic zones of ligament attachment sites. Zone 1 is the ligament substance. Zone 2 represents a region of fibrocartilage separated from zone 3 by a prominent tidemark (tm) that distinguishes mineralized fibrocartilage. Zone 4 represents bone. (From Feagin JA Jr [ed]: The Cruciate Ligaments: Diagnosis and Treatment of Ligamentous Injuries About the Knee. New York, Churchill Livingstone, 1994.)

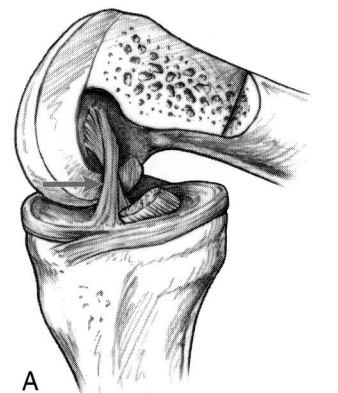
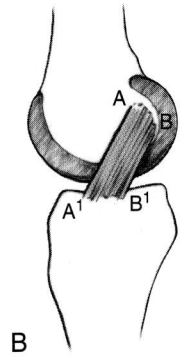
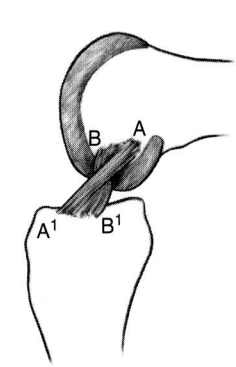

Fig. 3. View. *A,* The ACL in a specimen with the medial femoral condyle resected. The anteromedial bundle *(arrow)* is taut in flexion. *B,* The changes in the shape and tension of the anteromedial band (A-A¹) and posterolateral band (B-B¹) are shown schematically in knee extension and flexion. (Redrawn from Girgis FG, Marshal JL, Monajem AA: The cruciate ligaments of the knee joint. Clin Orthop Rel Res 1975; 106:227, 229.)

gus angulation with external rotation. Due to the biomechanical interdependence of the ACL, MCL, and menisci, valgus angulation with external rotation often produces concurrent damage to these structures. In basketball, the most common mechanism of injury involves hyperextension with internal rotation of the tibia as the player lands from jumping.

CLINICAL FEATURES: HISTORY

Patients with ACL injuries usually complain of pain, instability, and swelling. Their pain is severe and related to activity. The activities that elicit pain vary from intense athletic activity to activities of daily living. Also, the patient claims that the knee gave way, buckled, or popped at the time of injury and may present with immediate and profound disability. However, the ability to continue sports activity does not exclude a knee ligament injury. Finally, patients with ACL injuries complain of significant knee swelling that developed within the first several hours after injury.

CLINICAL FEATURES: PHYSICAL EXAMINATION

On inspection, a large, tense effusion is usually present. More than 70% of patients with an acute traumatic knee hemarthrosis have an ACL injury. However, ACL injury should still be suspected after a violent injury even if an effusion is not present because disruption of the joint capsule allows blood to extravasate into the surrounding soft tissues rather than accumulate in the joint space. Quadriceps atrophy may develop within several days of the injury. Palpation of the posterior aspect of the knee may reveal hamstring spasm. Meniscal tears, cyclops lesions, and hamstring spasm may prevent knee extension; cyclops lesions are formed by contraction of the ACL at the tibial attachment site following rupture of the ACL at the femoral attachment site. Large effusions may inhibit knee flexion. Gait assessment often reveals inability to bear weight on the affected extremity.

Excessive anterior tibial translation is pathognomonic for ACL deficiency and best elicited with the Lachman and anterior drawer tests. The Lachman test is the most reliable test for diagnosing ACL injury, having a reported sensitivity of 87% to 98%. In this test, an anteriorly directed force

is applied to the posterior proximal tibia at 20 to 30 degrees of knee flexion while stabilizing the femur[16] (Fig. 4). The examiner measures the displacement of the tibia and the firmness of the displacement endpoint. If both measurements are normal when compared with that of the contralateral knee, then the test result is negative. If either is abnormal, the test result is positive and graded as 1+ (0 to 5 mm), 2+ (5 to 10 mm), or 3+ (>10 mm). The Lachman test assesses ACL laxity, not instability. False-positive results are obtained when a posteriorly subluxated, PCL-deficient knee is reduced to its normal position. Therefore, it is important to establish the integrity of the PCL and

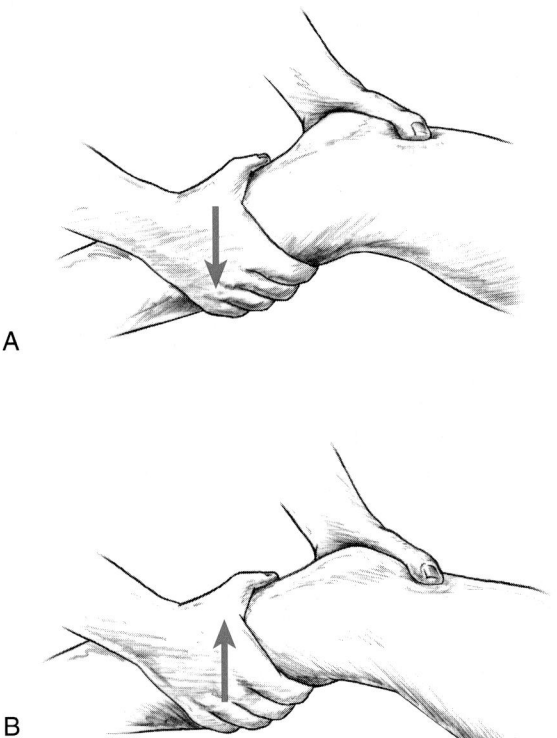

Fig. 4. **Lachman's test for anterior cruciate ligament laxity.** *A,* A posterior force is applied to the tibia, resulting in a normal patellar tendon slope. *B,* Application of an anterior force results in anterior tibial translation that diminishes the patellar tendon slope.

start from the normal anatomic position when performing the Lachman test. Displaced bucket-handle meniscal tears, hamstring spasm, and third-degree MCL tears with extension into the posteromedial corner may cause false-negative results.

The anterior drawer test is less reliable in the acute setting but is highly reliable for chronic injuries. In this test, the hip is flexed to 45 degrees, and the knee is flexed to 90 degrees while a smooth, steady anterior force is applied to the proximal tibia in neutral rotation. The examiner sits on the foot to stabilize the distal lower extremity, palpates behind the knee for hamstring contraction, and places the thumbs over the joint line to assess the step-off between the femoral condyles and the tibial plateau. PCL insufficiency can cause a false-positive result as described above for the Lachman test.

Anterolateral rotary instability can be assessed by tests designed to elicit the pivot-shift phenomenon. Slocum's anterior rotary drawer test, the Hughston-Losee jerk test, and MacIntosh's lateral pivot shift test are all performed by providing a valgus force to the knee during flexion and extension to accentuate the subluxation or reduction of the tibia. In the acute setting, these tests may be difficult to perform secondary to pain and spasm. These tests should be used cautiously because vigorous testing may result in additional iatrogenic trauma.

ACL insufficiency disrupts the normal translation-rotation mechanism of the knee. As the knee is brought from flexion into extension, the iliotibial band eventually moves anterior to the joint's center of rotation, producing an anteriorly directed force on the tibia. This force results in anterior subluxation of the lateral tibial plateau in the ACL-deficient knee. Conversely, as the knee is brought from extension into flexion, the iliotibial band moves posterior to the joint's center of rotation and pulls the tibia posteriorly, which results in reduction of the tibia.

MacIntosh's lateral pivot shift test is graded according to the reduction: 0 (absent), 1+ (rolling), 2+ (moderate), or 3+ (momentary locking). Any laxity in the iliotibial band can produce false-negative results. Posterolateral insuffi-

ciency can result in false-positive results if the examiner does not distinguish the pivot shift test from the reverse pivot shift test (see the later section on PCL physical examination).

In the Hughston-Losee jerk test (Fig. 5), the patient is supine with the knee flexed to 90 degrees as the examiner exerts a valgus stress at the proximal fibula with one hand and internally rotates the tibia by grasping the foot with the other hand. The knee is gradually extended, which causes the lateral tibia to abruptly subluxate anteriorly, or jerk, at about 30 degrees of flexion.

Similarly, in MacIntosh's lateral pivot shift test, the patient is supine with the knee extended as the examiner exerts a valgus stress at the proximal fibula with one hand and rotates the tibia internally by grasping the foot with the other hand. In the ACL-deficient knee, the tibia is subluxated anteriorly in the starting position. Gradual flexion abruptly reduces the tibia at about 30 degrees of flexion.

Slocum's anterior rotary drawer test is performed in neutral rotation as previously described, then performed with the tibia rotated internally 15 degrees, and finally performed with the tibia rotated externally 30 degrees. A positive anterior drawer test in neutral tibial rotation that is accentuated when the test is repeated in 30 degrees of external tibial rotation and reduced when performed in 15 degrees of internal rotation indicates anteromedial instability. Conversely, a positive anterior drawer test in neutral tibial rotation that is reduced when the test is repeated in 30 degrees of external tibial rotation and accentuated when performed in 15 degrees of internal rotation indicates anterolateral rotatory instability.

The flexion rotation drawer test described by Noyes combines elements of the Lachman and pivot shift tests. With the patient supine and the knee neutral (not hyperextended), the leg is lifted upward, allowing the femur to fall posteriorly and externally rotate in the ACL-deficient knee (Fig. 6). The lateral tibia is thereby subluxated anteriorly. Then, the knee is gradually flexed while applying a mild valgus stress and an anterior force to the proximal tibia.

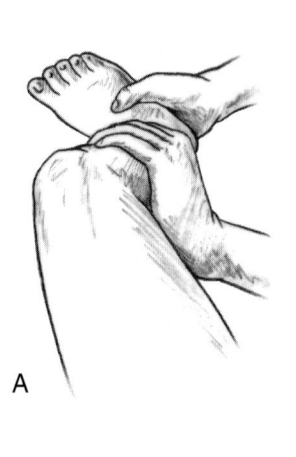
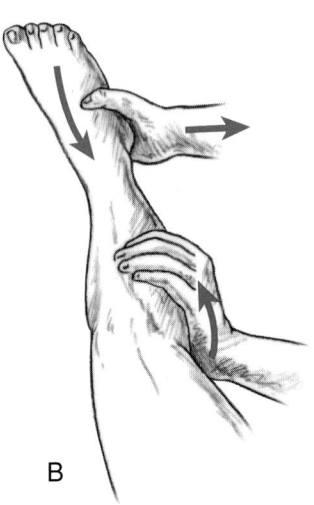
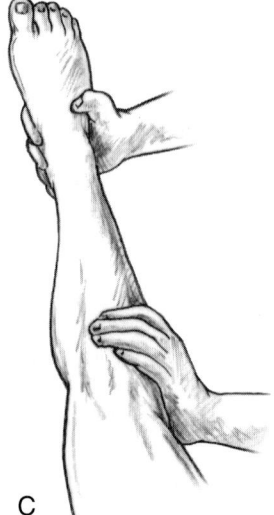

Fig. 5. Jerk test, or lateral pivot shift test. (Redrawn, courtesy JC Hughston, MD.)

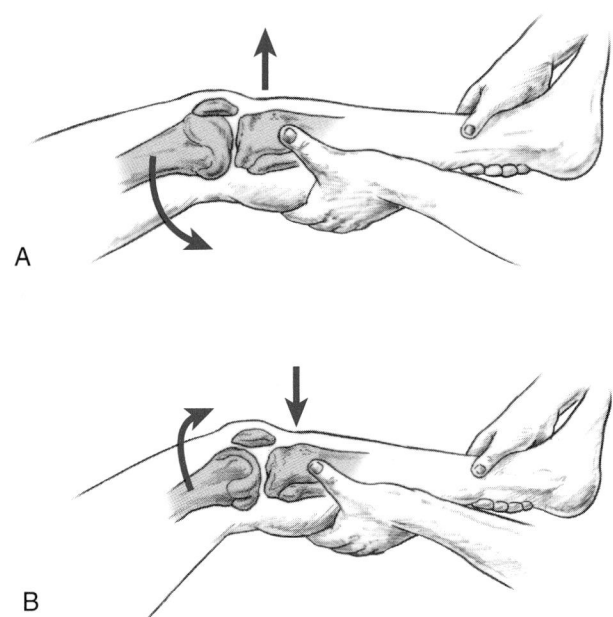

Fig. 6. Flexion rotation drawer test for anterior cruciate insufficiency. (Redrawn, courtesy FR Noyes, MD.)

The tibia moves posteriorly while the femur rotates internally, resulting in reduction of the subluxated tibia.

CLINICAL FEATURES: CLASSIFICATION
ACL laxity is graded on a scale of 0 to 3 by the Lachman test, as described for the MacIntosh test.

INVESTIGATION
An experienced clinician can diagnose ACL injuries by history and physical examination with greater than 90% accuracy. Further investigation should be used to clarify equivocal physical examination results. In a skeletally immature patient with apparent ACL insufficiency, physiological laxity, congenital absence of the ACL, and tibial tubercle avulsion fractures must be ruled out.

On plain radiographs, the lateral capsular sign represents a bony avulsion of the tibial attachment of the lateral capsule. Also known as Segond's fracture, this finding is present in about 6% of ACL injuries and is highly suggestive of ACL injury. The presence of osteophytes along the intercondylar notch, tibial spines, and joint margins are signs of chronic ACL deficiency. A deep lateral femoral notch on the lateral radiograph may suggest chronic ligamentous laxity. The notch view identifies loose bodies and femoral osteochondral lesions while assessing the notch width index for ACL reconstruction. ACL avulsion fractures are uncommon and usually occur in children. ACL avulsion fractures occur almost exclusively at the tibial attachment site.

More than 90% of patients with unilateral disruption of the ACL have side-to-side differences greater than 3 mm when assessed with KT-1000 arthrometry. In addition to diagnosing the presence of ACL injuries, the KT-1000 arthrometer can also accurately differentiate partial from complete tears.[17]

Lateral stress radiographs with an anteriorly directed force applied to the tibia by a Telos device have been used to quantify ACL laxity. Stress radiography appears to be more sensitive and specific than clinical examination and helps to distinguish partial and complete ACL tears.

On MRI, a normal ACL appears as a band of low signal intensity composed of two or three separate fibers at its tibial attachments. Direct evidence of complete tears visualized on T_1- and T_2-weighted images include inability to visualize the ACL, discontinuity in ACL fibers, and abnormal orientation of the remaining ACL fibers. Acute ACL tears appear as diffuse or focal increased signal within the ligament. Chronic ACL tears appear as either a fragmented ligament or an intact band of low signal with an abnormal orientation. Indirect evidence of complete tears includes anterior displacement of the tibia on the femur and excessive posterior bowing of the PCL. Using these findings, complete ACL tears can be diagnosed with an accuracy of up to 100%. Partial tears are more difficult to assess with MRI.

MRI is also useful for diagnosing concomitant injuries to the articular cartilage and subchondral bone such as trabecular microfractures. Also known as bone bruises, these occult bone injuries usually involve the lateral compartment of the knee and are present in the majority of patients with complete ACL tears. Meniscal injuries are found in 70% of acute ACL tears and can be diagnosed by MRI with 90% accuracy.[18]

Occasionally, arthroscopy may confirm and characterize an ACL tear when a definitive clinical diagnosis cannot be made. Examination under anesthesia allows thorough physical examination of the knee to detect multidirectional instabilities. Diagnostic arthroscopy provides visualization of the intra-articular disorder, including meniscal tears and articular cartilage damage. However, arthroscopy cannot evaluate intrasubstance ligament injuries. ACL injury is assessed by placing the knee in a figure-of-four position and looking for the empty lateral wall and vertical strut signs.

NATURAL HISTORY
Nonoperative treatment appears to lead to knee instability, secondary damage to other knee structures including the menisci, and early development of degenerative joint disease. Some investigators believe that the most important factor influencing the prognosis of ACL injuries is meniscal involvement. In contrast with earlier ideas, several studies have shown that ACL tears are significant injuries. Yet, the precise natural history of ACL injury remains controversial. No prospective studies that evaluate all types of patients with various activity levels have been performed; it is unlikely that one will be performed since reliable methods of ACL reconstruction have been developed.[19]

ISOLATED PCL INJURIES

EPIDEMIOLOGY
The prevalence of PCL injury in acute knee injuries reported in the literature varies from 1% to 40%, depending on the patient population being studied by the investigator. The prevalence is approximately 3% in the general population and 38% in reports from regional trauma centers. In

the National Football League, 2% of players had signs of PCL instability. In one study of acute knee ligament injuries with pathological motion, 4% of the injuries were isolated PCL injuries, and 7% of the injuries involved the PCL. Athletic activity and motor vehicle accidents are the most common modes of injury. Ninety-seven percent of PCL injuries in trauma patients are associated with other ligamentous injuries. Isolated PCL injuries are more difficult to detect than combined PCL injuries initially. Approximately 40% of PCL injuries are isolated PCL tears. There does not appear to be any difference in the prevalence of these injuries between males and females.[20, 21]

ANATOMY

The PCL is first observed as a condensation of vascular synovial mesenchyme at about 7 to 8 weeks of embryonic development and structurally resembles the adult form by 22 weeks. The PCL is an intra-articular yet extrasynovial ligament because it lies within its own synovial sheath reflected from the posterior capsule. The average PCL is 38 mm in length and expands in width from 12 mm at the posterior aspect of the tibial plateau to 32 mm at the medial femoral condyle.

The middle genicular artery supplies blood to the PCL and its synovial sheath. The inferior genicular arteries also contribute to the blood supply of the distal segment of the PCL. The vessels in the synovium surrounding the PCL branch anastomose to form a network of periligamentous vessels. These vessels penetrate the ligament transversely and conjoin with a network of longitudinal endoligamentous vessels.

The tibial nerve innervates the PCL and its surrounding synovium via the posterior articular nerve and the popliteal plexus. Similar to those of the ACL, histological studies of the PCL have identified Ruffini corpuscles (type I, pressure receptors), Vater-Pacini corpuscles (type II, velocity receptors), and free nerve endings (type IV, pain receptors).

The meniscofemoral ligaments are intra-articular accessory ligaments of the PCL that extend from the posterior horn of the lateral meniscus to the medial femoral condyle near the origin of the PCL. If the meniscofemoral ligament passes anterior to the PCL, it is referred to as Humphrey's ligament; if it passes posterior to the PCL, it is called Wrisberg's ligament[22] (Fig. 7). These two variations occur in equal frequency. In one cadaveric study, 71% of the knees had one meniscofemoral ligament, and only 6% of the knees had both Wrisberg's and Humphrey's ligaments. Although the meniscofemoral ligaments have significant mechanical strength, their role in knee stability has not been clearly defined. The meniscofemoral ligaments may increase the congruity between the meniscotibial socket and the lateral femoral condyle during knee flexion. Alternatively, they may serve as secondary restraints to posterior tibial translation. Interestingly, all acutely injured knees and the majority of chronically injured knees have at least one meniscofemoral ligament intact at the time of surgery.

BIOMECHANICS

The PCL is the primary restraint to posterior translation of the tibia at knee flexion angles greater than 30 degrees. Although the PCL serves as a secondary restraint to exter-

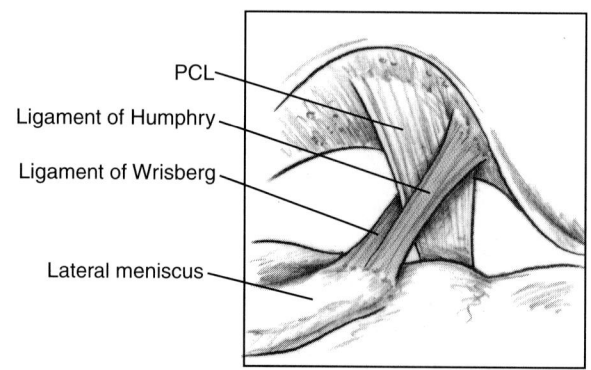

Fig. 7. Anterior view of the knee with soft tissue, joint capsule, and ACL removed. Humphrey's ligament passes anterior to the PCL, and Wrisberg's ligament passes posterior to the PCL. Both meniscofemoral ligaments attach to the lateral meniscus.

nal rotation, isolated rupture of the PCL has little effect on tibial rotational laxity or varus/valgus angulation. The PCL has traditionally been described as consisting of two main structural components, including an anterolateral bundle that tightens with knee flexion and a posteromedial bundle that tightens in knee extension. The anterolateral bundle is superior to the posteromedial bundle in terms of cross-sectional area, stiffness, and ultimate strength. In knee flexion, the PCL tightens to prevent posterior translation while the secondary restraints become slack.

Some investigators have suggested that this description oversimplifies the biomechanics of the PCL. It appears more accurate to describe the PCL as a fiber continuum rather than as morphologically distinct bands or bundles. Different portions of the continuum have been demarcated and identified as the anterior, central, posterior longitudinal, and posterior oblique fiber regions, based on their osseous attachment sites, spatial orientation of their fibers, and mechanical behavior during joint motion[23] (Fig. 8). Comprising the bulk of the PCL, the anterior and central fiber regions have been shown to be highly nonisometric, with maximum tension at 90 degrees of flexion.

Normal kinematic knee function requires an intact PCL. Isolated sectioning of the PCL increases medial compartment pressures by shifting the center of rotation medially and altering the tibiofemoral contact areas. Furthermore, the increased posterior tibial translation decreases the angle between the quadriceps tendon and the patellar tendon, producing greater patellofemoral joint contact forces.

PATHOGENESIS: MECHANISMS OF INJURY

The most common mechanism of PCL injury is a posterior force on the proximal tibia when the knee is flexed, resulting in posterior translation of the tibia on the femur. This mechanism can occur in motor vehicle trauma (e.g., dashboard injury) or noncontact sports injuries (falling on a flexed knee with the foot plantarflexed). Interestingly, falling on a flexed knee with the foot in dorsiflexion does not injure the PCL because the traumatic forces bypass the PCL as they are transferred to the shaft of the femur (Fig. 9). Another mechanism of PCL injury is forced knee hyperflexion. With sudden, severe hyperflexion, the tension

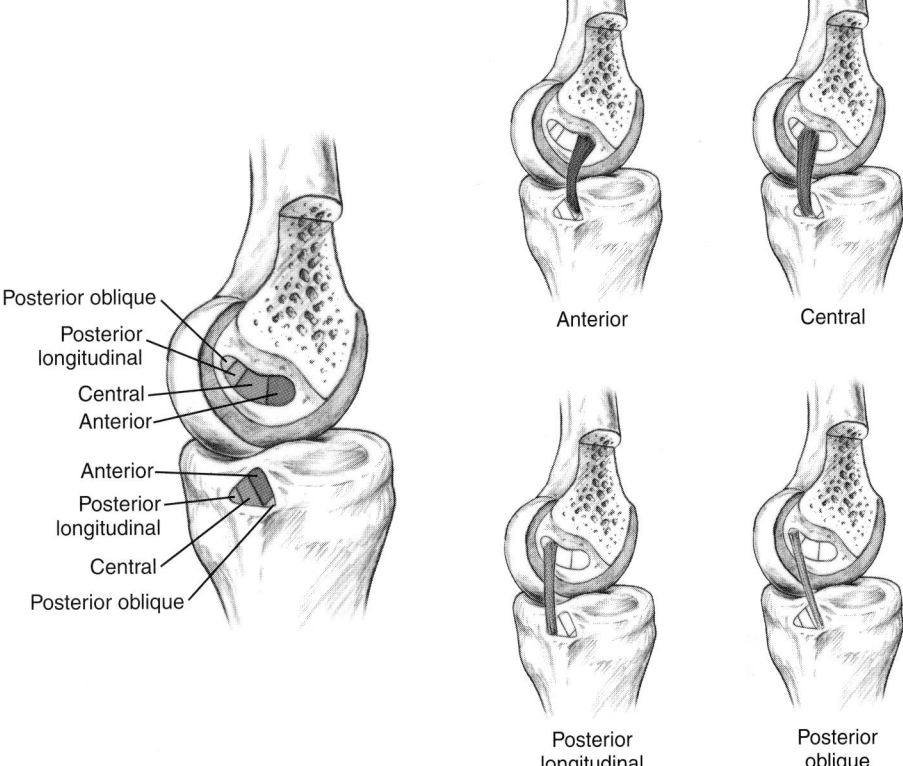

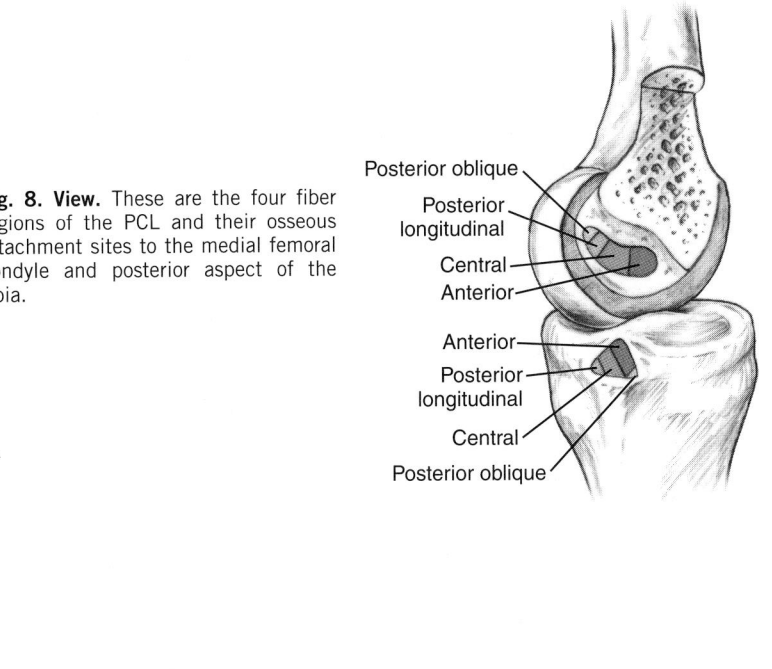

Fig. 8. View. These are the four fiber regions of the PCL and their osseous attachment sites to the medial femoral condyle and posterior aspect of the tibia.

Posterior oblique
Posterior longitudinal
Central
Anterior
Anterior
Posterior longitudinal
Central
Posterior oblique

Anterior

Central

Posterior longitudinal

Posterior oblique

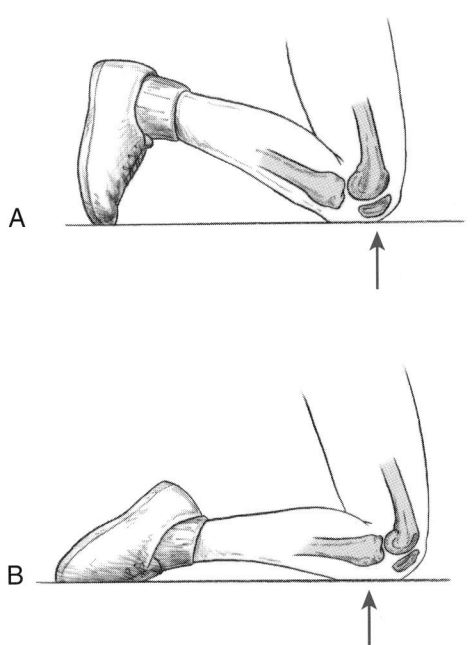

Fig. 9. Fall on a flexed knee. *A,* With the foot dorsiflexed, the traumatic forces are placed on the patellofemoral joint and transferred up the shaft of the femur. *B,* With the foot plantarflexed, the forces are directed at the tibial tuberosity, and the PCL may be injured. (Redrawn from Duri ZA, Aichroth MS, Zorrilla P: The posterior cruciate ligament: A review. Am J Knee Surg 1997; 10:149.)

in the anterolateral band increases beyond its elastic limit, and either plastic deformation or continuity failure can occur. Interstitial failure appears more common with this type of injury. Sudden, violent hyperextension of the knee will injure the PCL and usually cause concomitant tearing of the posterior capsule and disruption of the ACL.

CLINICAL FEATURES: HISTORY

With PCL injury, patients describe experiencing a substantial knee injury, but they are usually able to bear weight. Patients with an acutely injured PCL may complain of pain, mild swelling, or inability to bear weight. Patients with chronic injuries complain of difficulty ambulating with knee extended in the midstance phase, pain or instability while descending stairs, and knee pain on long distance ambulation. In contrast to ACL injuries, gross instability, hearing or feeling a pop, and large, tense effusions are not likely to be experienced in the isolated PCL injury.

CLINICAL FEATURES: PHYSICAL EXAMINATION

Ecchymosis or lacerations over the tibial tuberosity may be present. Quadriceps atrophy and pain with patellar compression may also be present. Swelling is mild and develops slowly in isolated PCL tears. The posterior sag sign is observed when the patient is supine and the knee is flexed to 90 degrees with the foot planted. When the posterior restraint of the PCL is lost, gravity pulls the tibia posteriorly. The lateral contour of the knee is observed for loss of normal prominence of the proximal tibia. Godfrey's test is a variation of the posterior sag sign in which the patient's hips and knees are flexed at 90 degrees, thereby increasing the ability of gravity to elicit posterior tibial subluxation. Passive range of motion from 0 to 90 degrees of flexion produces little discomfort in the isolated PCL tear. Flexion beyond 90 degrees produces increasing pain. Examination of the patient should include gait assessment for lateral thrust and signs of genu varum.

There are several clinical tests that evaluate integrity of the PCL. In the posterior drawer test, the examiner applies a posteriorly directed force to the proximal tibia and notes any decrease in the amount of anterior tibial step-off. However, if there is no quadriceps spasm, the tibia will already be subluxated posteriorly, and there may be no posterior drawer. In fact, a false-positive anterior drawer result could

be elicited in this circumstance. Therefore, it is important to identify the normal anatomic position prior to administering the posterior drawer test.

Some authors believe that the most reliable test for PCL insufficiency is the anterior tibial step-off test. The anterior border of the tibial plateau normally lies approximately 10 mm anterior to the lateral femoral condyle. A decrease in the anterior tibial step-off indicates posterior tibial translation. This test is the basis of the PCL laxity classification system.

The quadriceps active test relies on the identification of the quadriceps neutral angle (Fig. 10). The quadriceps neutral angle is defined as the angle at which the shear component of patellar tendon force is eliminated during a quadriceps contraction. Thus, an isometric quadriceps con-

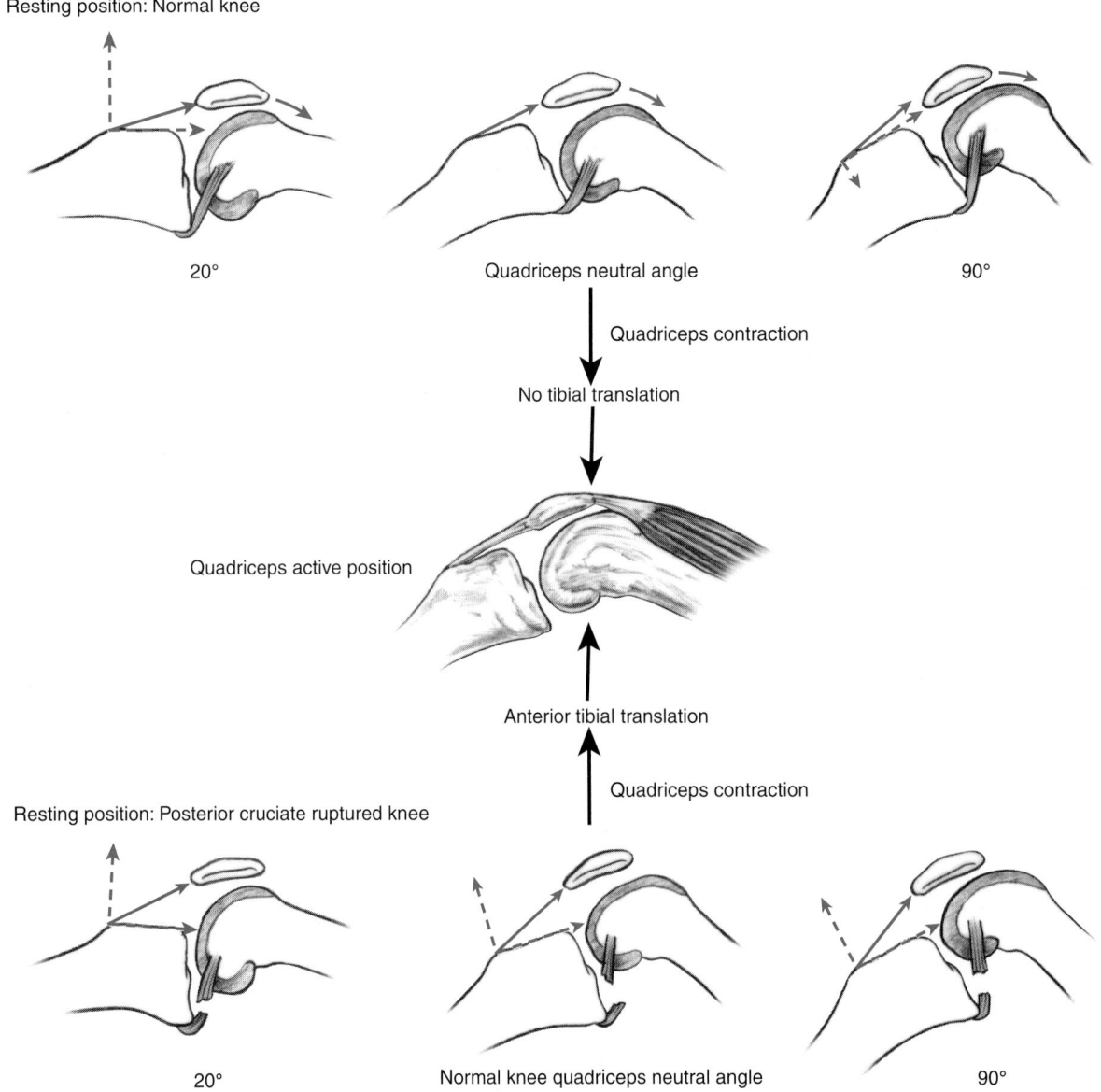

Fig. 10. The quadriceps active test. In the presence of PCL injury, quadriceps contraction at the normal knee's quadriceps neutral angle causes a visible and palpable anterior tibial shift because of the anterior orientation of the patellar tendon. (Redrawn from Daniel D, Stone ML, Barnett P, et al: Use of quadriceps active test to diagnose posterior cruciate ligament disruption and measure posterior laxity of the knee. J Bone Joint Surg Am 1988; 70:387.)

traction does not induce a tibial shift anteriorly or posteriorly at the quadriceps neutral angle. Once the quadriceps neutral angle is identified in the normal knee, the injured knee is positioned at this angle, and the quadriceps is contracted. In the presence of PCL injury, this contraction will cause a visible and palpable anterior tibial shift because of an abnormal anterior orientation of the patellar tendon.[24]

CLINICAL FEATURES: CLASSIFICATION

PCL laxity is graded on a scale of 1 to 3, based on the difference in anterior step-off between that of the injured knee and that of the contralateral normal knee. Grade 1 laxity is defined as a side-to-side difference of 0 to 5 mm, with the tibial plateau prominence remaining anterior to the femoral condyles. Grade 2 laxity is a side-to-side difference of 5 to 10 mm, with the anterior tibia lying anterior to or flush with the femoral condyles. When the side-to-side difference is greater than 10 mm, Grade 3 laxity is present, and combined ligamentous injury should be thoroughly investigated.

INVESTIGATION

In the chronic PCL-deficient knee, the medial compartment and patellofemoral joint are most likely to show evidence of degenerative changes on plain radiographs. Lateral radiographs identify PCL avulsion fractures. In contrast to ACL avulsions, both femoral and tibial avulsions of the PCL have occurred.

The KT-1000 arthrometer is a moderately reliable tool for the investigation of PCL injuries; it is not as useful as it is in ACL injuries. Using 40 pounds of posteriorly directed force and a 3-mm side-to-side difference as the minimal detection of PCL injury results in arthrometer sensitivity of 90% for detecting PCL insufficiency. Although larger side-to-side differences correspond loosely with higher grade tears, the KT-1000 does not appear to be helpful for differentiating the sequential grades of PCL injury.[25]

Lateral stress radiography can be used to evaluate PCL insufficiency with the knee in 90 degrees of flexion using a posteriorly directed force at the level of the tibial tubercle (see Fig. 1). Posterior tibial displacement of the injured knee can then be measured on the lateral radiograph and compared with the normal knee. Stress radiography is superior to both arthrometry and posterior drawer testing for determining PCL status and differentiating complete from partial ruptures.[26]

MRI accuracy for diagnosis of PCL injury ranges from 96% to 100%. The orientation of the PCL is near vertical in the frontal plane and therefore can be visualized in its entirety on a single sagittal projection. On a T_1-weighted image, the normal PCL is distinctly visualized as a homogeneous dark band with a curvilinear appearance. An increase in signal intensity on T_1- or T_2-weighted images should be interpreted as abnormal and consistent with injury.[27] MRI is also very beneficial for diagnosing associated knee injuries such as ligament injuries, meniscal tears, and subchondral bone injuries.

Baseline and serial technetium bone scans may be helpful in evaluating chronic PCL insufficiency by adding information on the status of the joint surfaces. Increased

uptake in the medial compartment and patellofemoral joint may represent the development of degenerative changes and indicate that surgical intervention is warranted.

The role of arthroscopy in diagnosing PCL rupture is controversial. Examination under anesthesia allows thorough physical examination of the knee in order to detect occult posterolateral or posteromedial instability. Diagnostic arthroscopy provides visualization of the intra-articular disorder, including meniscal tears and articular cartilage damage.

Arthroscopic findings of PCL injury consist of direct and indirect findings. Direct findings represent damage to the PCL itself and include midsubstance tears, interstitial tears with ligament stretching, and avulsions. Indirect findings represent damage resulting from PCL insufficiency and include specking and ecchymosis of the synovium overlying the PCL attachment to the medial femoral condyle, the sloppy ACL sign, altered tibiofemoral contact points, and degenerative changes of the patellofemoral joint and medial compartment.

The sloppy ACL sign refers to the relative laxity of the ACL secondary to posterior tibial subluxation in PCL insufficiency. When the tibia is reduced, the normal ACL tension returns. Altered tibiofemoral contact points occur as a result of posterior tibial subluxation. For example, the anterior portion of the menisci will lie closer to the articular surfaces of the femoral condyles.

NATURAL HISTORY

Studies regarding the natural history of the PCL tears have been retrospective, and results have varied. The natural history of isolated PCL tears remains controversial. Some isolated PCL injuries are not even diagnosed, and the outcome is still benign. However, recent studies demonstrate that isolated PCL tears may develop early degenerative changes and increased pain when managed nonoperatively. On the basis of long-term evaluation, investigators have described the natural history of isolated rupture of the PCL in three phases: (1) functional adaptation, from 3 to 18 months after injury, (2) functional tolerance, from 1 to 20 years after injury, (and 3) disabling osteoarthritic deterioration, 25 years after injury. In contrast to isolated PCL injuries, combined ligament injuries involving the PCL have a consistently poor outcome. Knees with combined ligament injuries involving the PCL develop early degenerative changes and progressive functional deterioration when managed nonoperatively.[28, 29]

ISOLATED POSTEROLATERAL COMPLEX INJURIES

EPIDEMIOLOGY

Isolated posterolateral complex (PLC) instability is rare. PLC insufficiency is more commonly associated with an injury to the ACL or PCL.

ANATOMY

The principal anatomic structures at the posterolateral corner of the knee include the lateral collateral ligament (LCL), the arcuate ligament, the popliteal tendon, the popliteofibular ligament, the short lateral ligament (SLL), the fabellofibular ligament, and the posterolateral capsule. The terminology used to describe these PCL structures has been inconsistent. Furthermore, the intricate anatomy of the PLC is complicated further by the variability of these structures.

The anatomy of the PLC can be organized into three layers as described by Seebacher et al[30] (Fig. 11). Layer I, which is the most superficial, consists of the iliotibial tract, including its anterior expansion, and the superficial portion of the biceps, including its posterior expansion. The peroneal nerve lies deep to layer I and posterior to the biceps tendon. Layer II has anterior and posterior components. The quadriceps retinaculum descends adjacent to the patella and forms layer II anteriorly. Posteriorly, layer II is incomplete and is represented by the two patellofemoral ligaments. Layer III forms the lateral part of the joint capsule. Posterior to the overlying iliotibial tract, the capsule divides into two laminae, which are separated by the inferior lateral geniculate vessels. The more superficial lamina encompasses the LCL and ends posteriorly at the SLL or fabellofibular ligament. The deeper lamina passes along the edge of the lateral meniscus and forms both the coronary ligament and the popliteal tendon hiatus.

The LCL is approximately 6 cm in length as it extends posteroinferiorly from the superior aspect of the lateral femoral condyle to the fibular head. The LCL attaches to one of the three fovea lying posterior to the prominent ridge of the lateral epicondyle. The LCL fovea lies between the fovea of the lateral head of the gastrocnemius and the fovea of the origin of the popliteus tendon. The LCL merges with the biceps femoris tendon, and this conjoined tendon inserts on the lateral aspect of the fibular head. When a fabella is present, the fabellofibular ligament will be found running parallel to the LCL from the fabella to insert on the fibula posterior to the insertion of the biceps tendon. When the fabella is absent, the SLL extends from the fibula to the origin of the lateral head of the gastrocnemius adjacent to the lateral limb of the arcuate ligament.

When present, the arcuate ligament consists of a medial limb that arises from the posterior capsule at the distal femur and extends medially to the oblique popliteal ligament over the popliteus muscle. The lateral limb arises from the posterior capsule and courses laterally over the popliteus muscle deep to the lateral inferior geniculate vessels to insert on the posterior fibula.

The final component of layer III is the popliteofibular ligament. Lying deep to the lateral limb of the arcuate ligament, the popliteofibular ligament arises from the fibula posterior to the biceps insertion and joins the popliteal tendon just above the popliteus musculotendinous junction. Thus, the popliteus unit is a Y-shaped structure with a muscular origin from the posterior tibia and a ligamentous origin from the fibula that join together and insert on the femur.

BIOMECHANICS

As well as anatomic dissections, biomechanical analysis of the PLC structures has helped determine their role in knee stability. Multiple investigators have used selective cutting techniques to examine the static contributions to knee stability of the PCL, LCL, popliteal tendon, and arcuate ligament. In all of the studies, PLC sectioning resulted in increased posterior translation, varus rotation, external rotation, and coupled posterior translation–external rotation.

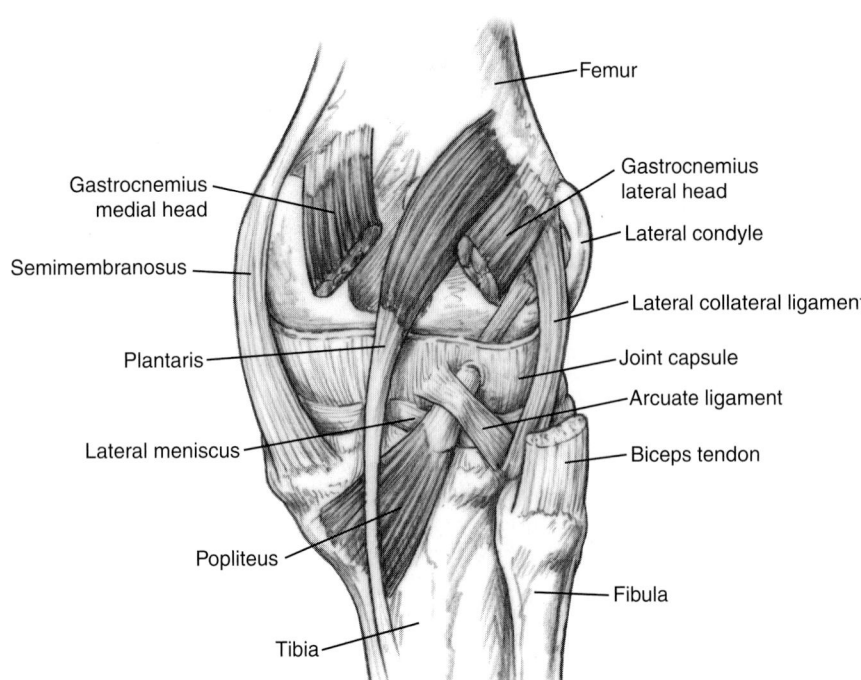

Fig. 11. View. This shows the structure of the posterolateral aspect of the knee.

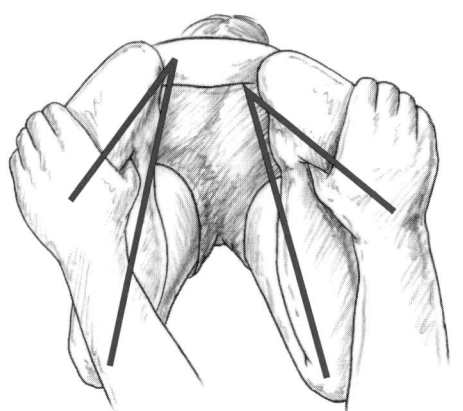

Fig. 12. The external rotation thigh-foot angle test. (Redrawn from Veltri DM, Warren RF: Isolated and combined posterior cruciate ligament injuries. J Am Acad Orthop Surg 1993; 1:67.)

PATHOGENESIS: MECHANISMS OF INJURY

Noncontact hyperextension is usually the mechanism for isolated posterolateral rotatory instability. Also, a blow to the anteromedial aspect of the tibia with the knee near full extension has been implicated as a cause of arcuate ligament complex disruption and posterolateral instability (PLI). A less common mechanism of injury is hyperflexion. Mechanisms that produce injury to the cruciate ligaments can also cause PLC injury.

CLINICAL FEATURES: HISTORY

In the patient with acute isolated PLI, the major complaint is pain in the posterolateral aspect. In chronic injuries, pain may be present along the medial and lateral joint lines. In addition, the patient may complain of dysesthesias or weakness of the leg and foot due to associated injury of the peroneal nerve. The patient may note instability of the knee in extension, with buckling into hyperextension. To avoid this instability, some patients walk with the knee in flexion.

CLINICAL FEATURES: PHYSICAL EXAMINATION

In the acutely injured knee, swelling, tenderness, ecchymosis, or induration may present at the anteromedial or posterolateral aspect. Evidence of peroneal nerve dysfunction, including foot drop and decreased sensation along the dorsum of the foot, may be present. No swelling or limitation of movement is usually found. Minimal disability while walking or running may be noted. Specifically, gait evaluation may demonstrate a varus thrust or hyperextension varus thrust in the injured knee during the stance phase. Similarly, varus knee alignment may be visible with the patient standing.

Isolated complete PLC injury demonstrates maximal increases in posterior translation, varus angulation, and external rotation at 30 degrees of knee flexion, whereas combined PCL-PLC injuries demonstrate increases at both 30 and 90 degrees. The most useful tests for PLI are the prone external rotation test and the varus stress test. The reverse pivot shift, posterolateral drawer, and external recurvatum tests are not specific for PLI injury but are used to supple-

ment the diagnosis. The Lachman test, pivot shift, posterior drawer, and quadriceps active tests are used to elicit combined ligament injuries involving the cruciate ligaments.

Assessment of tibial external rotation can be performed in the prone or supine position. When performed in the prone position, it is referred to as the external rotation thigh-foot angle test (Fig. 12). At both 30 and 90 degrees of knee flexion, the external rotation of the foot relative to the axis of the femur is assessed and compared with that of the contralateral side. The tibial plateaus are palpated to determine their position relative to the femoral condyles. Palpation of the tibial plateaus differentiates whether the external rotation is a result of PLI causing the lateral tibial plateau to move posteriorly or anteromedial instability causing the medial tibial plateau to move anteriorly.

In the dial test, the patient is supine. The examiner places the thumbs on the medial side of both feet and simultaneously externally rotates both lower extremities while maintaining 30 degrees of knee flexion. In either of these tests, disorder is present when the side-to-side difference is greater than 10 degrees.

Varus stress testing is performed with the knee in 0, 30, and 90 degrees of flexion. Isolated PLC injuries have maximal instability at 30 degrees.

In isolated PLC injuries, the Lachman test result is false-positive, and the anterior drawer test result is negative. If the anterior drawer test result is positive, then a combined injury involving the ACL is present.

The external rotation recurvatum test described by Hughston identifies PLI (Fig. 13). With the patient supine, the examiner grasps the great toes of both feet and lifts the legs off the table. Hyperextension at the lateral aspect of the knee, varus angulation, and tibial external rotation indicate PLI.

The posterolateral drawer test is performed with the patient supine and the hip flexed 45 degrees, the knee flexed 80 degrees, and the tibia in 15 degrees of external rotation. In the normal knee, the endpoint to posterior translation is firm, but the endpoint to external rotation is variable. When the lateral tibial condyle rotates externally relative to the lateral femoral condyle, the test result is positive. The posterolateral drawer test is not specific for PLC injury, and comparison with the contralateral knee is necessary to assess qualitatively any increase in external rotation. If the external rotation result is grossly positive or increased at 90 degrees of knee flexion, combined injury involving the PCL is present.

The reverse pivot shift test is performed by bringing the

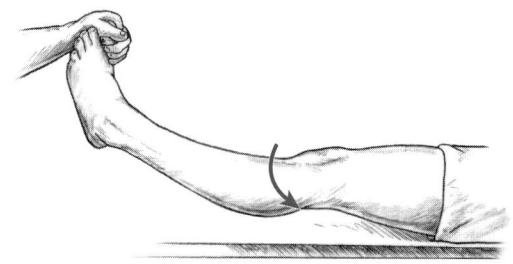

Fig. 13. External rotation recurvatum test. (Courtesy JC Hughston, MD.)

knee from 90 degrees of knee flexion to full extension while a valgus force is applied to the lateral knee with one hand and the foot is externally rotated with the other hand. In the knee with PLI, the lateral tibia plateau is subluxated posteriorly relative to the lateral femoral condyle in flexion. As the knee is extended, the lateral tibial plateau is reduced with a palpable shift or jerk.[31]

CLINICAL FEATURES: CLASSIFICATION

There are three types of PLI: A, B, and C. PLI is defined as a side-to-side difference of at least 10 degrees on the dial test or external rotation thigh-foot angle test with variable degrees of varus instability. PLI type A presents with increased external rotation without varus instability consistent with injury to the popliteofibular ligament and popliteus tendon. PLI type B presents with increased external rotation as well as grade I to II varus laxity, which occurs with damage to the popliteofibular ligament, popliteus tendon, and attenuation of the fibular collateral ligament. PLI type C presents with increased external rotation and grade III varus laxity, which occurs with injury to the popliteofibular ligament, popliteus tendon, fibular collateral ligament, lateral capsule, and cruciate ligaments.[32]

INVESTIGATION

Plain radiographs may demonstrate fractures of the fibular head, displaced medial tibial plateau fractures, or Segond's fractures. Fibular head avulsion fractures are highly suggestive of lateral ligament injury.

Stress radiography for posterior and varus displacement can be utilized to quantify the laxity identified on physical examination. Also, a new device, the Lars Rotational Laxiometer (Lars Inc., Dijon, France), assigns a quantitative value for tibial external rotation. Side-to-side differences greater than 7 degrees suggest PLC laxity.[33]

MRI can reveal injury to the PLC that was missed during physical examination. Partial tears appear as soft-tissue edema adjacent to a continuous ligament or tendon. Complete tears appear as discontinuity in the structure. On T_2-weighted sequences, a partial tear of the musculotendinous junction is visualized as amorphous high signal intensity within the parenchyma of the muscle, high signal intensity extending into the tendon, disruption of the fibers, and possible enlargement of the muscle.[34]

The LCL and fabellofibular, arcuate, and popliteofibular ligaments are extracapsular, precluding arthroscopic assessment of the PLC.

NATURAL HISTORY

When managed nonoperatively, partial tears of the arcuate complex have mild residual laxity but good functional outcomes. However, ruptures lead to poor functional results, including severe instability, muscle weakness, and premature degenerative arthritis.

ISOLATED LCL (FIBULAR) INJURIES

EPIDEMIOLOGY

In one study of acute knee ligament injuries with pathological motion, 2% of the injuries were isolated LCL injuries, and 4% of the injuries involved the LCL.

ANATOMY

See the earlier sections for the anatomy of the lateral aspect of the knee.

BIOMECHANICS

The LCL acts as the primary restraint to varus angulation and contributes to the PLC as the primary restraint to external rotation. Isolated injury to the LCL results in subtle increases in varus and external rotation that are maximal at 30 degrees of knee flexion.

PATHOGENESIS: MECHANISMS OF INJURY

A blow to the medial aspect of the knee is the usual mechanism of injury. If the knee is in full extension when the varus force is applied, the PCL may also be involved, resulting in straight lateral instability. Straight lateral instability is the result of severe trauma and involves disruption of all of the lateral compartment ligaments, the PCL, and frequently the ACL.

CLINICAL FEATURES: HISTORY

The patient with an LCL injury may complain of pain and instability. Complaints of rapid swelling, gross instability, hearing a pop, or inability to bear weight should raise the clinician's suspicion for concomitant cruciate ligament injury.

CLINICAL FEATURES: PHYSICAL EXAMINATION

Abrasions or ecchymosis over the medial aspect of the knee may be present. In order to palpate the LCL, the hip is abducted and externally rotated while the knee is flexed in order to place the heel on the contralateral knee. When the LCL is torn, the taut, narrow band will not be as prominent as it is on the normal side. Some swelling in the lateral aspect of the knee may be present, but an effusion usually suggests concomitant intra-articular injury. Varus alignment and medial thrust on weightbearing may be present. Evidence of injury to the peroneal nerve may be present.

The adduction, or varus, stress test is performed with the patient supine and the knee flexed to 30 degrees in order to eliminate resistance from secondary restraints. With one hand on the medial aspect of the knee and the other hand at the ankle, an adduction force is gently applied. The test is repeated until it produces mild pain; the results are compared with those of the contralateral knee. When the adduction stress test is performed in extension, the intact cruciate ligaments and posterior capsule prevent instability. Therefore, when this test reveals instability in extension, combined injury involving the cruciate ligaments is present.[35]

CLINICAL FEATURES: CLASSIFICATION

Collateral ligament injuries are categorized into three grades. Grade I injury is defined by local tenderness but no clinical instability and represents stretching of the ligament. Grade II injury is characterized by localized tenderness and mild-to-moderate laxity (5 to 10 mm), with a firm endpoint on stress tests at 30 degrees of knee flexion. Grade II injury indicates partial disruption of the ligament. Grade III injury is distinguished by significant instability (>10 mm medial opening), with an indistinct endpoint on stress tests, and signifies complete disruption of the ligament. Injuries associated with clinically detectable lateral opening on varus stress tests or medial opening on valgus stress tests are classified as grade III and involve concomitant cruciate injury.

INVESTIGATION

Plain radiographs may demonstrate fractures of the fibular head, displaced medial tibial plateau fractures, or Segond's fractures. Fibular head avulsion fractures are highly suggestive of lateral ligament injury.

Varus stress radiographs may demonstrate fracture through the distal femoral physis in a skeletally immature patient. The examiner should maintain a high index of suspicion for this injury if there is considerable pain, hemorrhage, and swelling in a young patient.

The LCL is visualized most clearly on coronal images and appears as a thin, dark cord on all sequences. T_2-weighted images of an injured FCL may show interruption of the normally low signal ligament, a serpiginous morphology, or increased signal within and around the ligament. MRI also identifies associated injuries including medial compartment bone bruises, meniscal tears, and muscle tendon tears.

NATURAL HISTORY

Similar to the MCL, the LCL appears to heal well with nonoperative management. The small amount of data on isolated LCL injuries seems to confirm that nonoperative management results in excellent knee function.

ISOLATED MCL (TIBIAL) INJURIES

EPIDEMIOLOGY

MCL tears are common knee injuries in sports. The prevalence of MCL injuries among Division I college football players is approximately 5% to 10%. In one study of acute knee ligament injuries with pathological motion,[36] 29% of the injuries were isolated MCL injuries, and 44% of the injuries involved the MCL. Complete MCL tears rarely occur without involvement of the ACL. Reports on the efficacy of prophylactic knee braces continue to present conflicting evidence.

ANATOMY

The MCL extends 10 to 11 cm between its attachments on the adductor tubercle of the medial femoral condyle and the medial aspect of the tibia 5 to 7 cm below the joint line. Whereas the anterior portion of the MCL is straight, the posterior portion runs posteriorly from its femoral attachment to the medial meniscus and then anteriorly to its tibial attachment so that the ligament is widest at the level of the medial meniscus. The average thickness is 4.3 mm at the femoral attachment and 2.3 mm at the tibial attachment.

Three basic layers incorporate all of the important stabilizing structures on the medial side of the knee (Fig. 14). An injury to the MCL involves structures in any or all of the three layers. Layer 1 is a superficial investing fascia that encases the entire medial aspect of the knee and coalesces with the posteromedial capsule and hamstring muscles. Layer 2 lies deep to this layer and includes the superficial MCL, which has a distal insertion on the medial aspect of the tibia at the level of the pes anserinus tendon. The origin of the superficial MCL is thought to be rein-

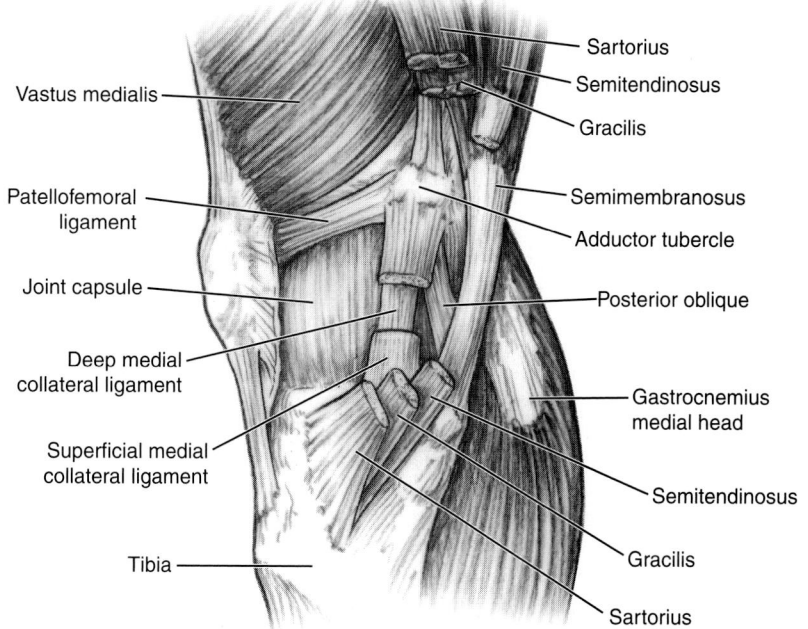

Fig. 14. Structure of the medial aspect of the knee. (Redrawn from Warren LF, Marshall JL: The supporting structures and layers on the medial side of the knee. J Bone Joint Surg Am 1979; 61:56.)

Labels: Vastus medialis — Patellofemoral ligament — Joint capsule — Deep medial collateral ligament — Superficial medial collateral ligament — Tibia — Sartorius — Semitendinosus — Gracilis — Semimembranosus — Adductor tubercle — Posterior oblique — Gastrocnemius medial head — Semitendinosus — Gracilis — Sartorius

forced by a contribution from the vastus medialis. Layer 3 consists of the deep MCL and extends posteriorly as the posteromedial capsule, which includes the posterior oblique ligament.

Cells populating the MCL have morphological characteristics similar to those of fibroblasts. Specifically, spindle-shaped fibroblasts are interspersed along the large-diameter collagen fibrils, which are in direct contact with cellular membranes. These cells may be responsible for the ability of the MCL to heal rapidly and predictably.

BIOMECHANICS

The MCL is the primary medial stabilizer at 30 degrees of flexion and a secondary contributor at full extension. The posterior part of the MCL relaxes during flexion, but the anterior portion remains taut in all positions of knee flexion. The MCL also serves as the primary restraint to internal tibial rotation and anterior tibial displacement. Isolated sectioning of either the superficial or deep MCL results in very small increases in valgus and internal rotation limits. However, when both the superficial and deep MCL are injured, appreciable increases in valgus limits are noted, but changes in anterior translation and internal rotation remain small. The medial capsular layers also contribute to resistance to valgus stresses at the knee.

PATHOGENESIS: MECHANISMS OF INJURY

The most common mechanism of MCL injury is the sudden application of a valgus torque to the knee. The classic example is a direct blow to the lateral aspect of the knee while the foot is planted. MCL overuse injuries can be caused by the whipkick used by swimmers for breaststroke. Noncontact injuries usually involve the same mechanisms of injury that result in ACL injury.

CLINICAL FEATURES: HISTORY

Patients with an MCL injury describe immediate medial knee pain following the traumatic event. In milder injuries, the pain may resolve within a few minutes, and the athlete may return to competition for a short time before onset of tenderness. Patients complain of at least a transient inability to walk. Patients often complain of swelling and sometimes hear a pop.

CLINICAL FEATURES: PHYSICAL EXAMINATION

On inspection, the lateral aspect of the knee may have lacerations or ecchymosis from the direct blow mechanism of injury. In a lean individual, localized swelling can be seen over the injured portion of the superficial MCL. On palpation, localized tenderness and spongy swelling will be present at the site of the injury about 60 minutes after the traumatic event. A mild effusion may gradually accumulate. A large effusion suggests concomitant cruciate ligament injury. Valgus alignment and medial thrust on load bearing may be present.

The abduction, or valgus, stress test is performed with patient supine and the knee flexed at 30 degrees in order to eliminate secondary restraints. With one hand on the lateral aspect of the knee and the other hand at the ankle, an abduction force is applied gently with the leg in slight external rotation. The test is repeated until it produces mild pain, and the results are compared with those of the contralateral knee. When the abduction stress test is performed in extension, the intact cruciate ligaments and posterior capsule prevent instability. Therefore, when this test reveals instability in extension, combined injury involving the cruciate ligaments is present. When an MCL injury is suspected, the ACL should be carefully assessed with the Lachman and anterior drawer tests because of the biomechanical interdependence of these two structures.[37]

CLINICAL FEATURES: CLASSIFICATION

See the earlier classification of LCL injuries.

INVESTIGATION

Routine radiographs have usually normal results in acute MCL injuries. MCL injury rarely produces avulsion fractures, but radiographs are important for ruling out fractures. Ectopic calcification at the proximal femoral attachment, also known as the Pellegrini-Stieda lesion, may develop after MCL injury.

Valgus stress radiographs may demonstrate fracture through the distal femoral physis in a skeletally immature patient. The examiner should maintain a high index of suspicion for this injury if there is considerable pain, hemorrhage, and swelling in a young patient.

MRI is normally unnecessary for the diagnosis of MCL injuries. However, MRI is useful for identification of associated injuries. On T_2-weighted sequences, grade 1 injuries show an intact MCL with periligamentous increased signal that represents edema. On coronal images of more severe injuries, there is increased signal, deformity, and loss of continuity of the fibers. Edema or hemorrhage may cause the MCL to separate from the adjacent bone.

NATURAL HISTORY

Nonoperative management of isolated partial MCL injuries results in excellent knee function without major signs of joint remodeling or radiographic signs of osteoarthritis up to 10 years after injury.[38]

COMBINED LIGAMENT INJURIES

In general, combined ligamentous disruption results from higher energy trauma. Motor vehicle accidents account for 50% of these injuries, and sporting activities account for 40%. It is important to differentiate between isolated and combined ligamentous injuries, because there is general agreement that combined ligamentous injuries require surgical reconstruction. The salient diagnostic features of the most common ligament injury combinations are listed in the following sections.[39, 40]

ACL-MCL

ACL-MCL injuries are the most common knee ligament injury combination and account for approximately 13% of knee injuries with pathological motion. Meniscal injuries are frequently associated with ACL-MCL injuries. Diagnostic features of ACL-MCL injuries include the following:

Increased anterior displacement.
Increased valgus angulation at 0 and 30 degrees of flexion

(isolated MCL: increased at 30 degrees only; isolated ACL: minimal increase).

Increased internal rotation (isolated ACL: minimal increase; isolated MCL: small increase).

ACL-PCL

Acute knee dislocation with spontaneous reduction should be suspected for combined injury to the ACL and PCL. Diagnostic features of ACL-PCL injuries include the following:

Popliteal artery and peroneal nerve injury.

Grossly abnormal anterior-posterior tibiofemoral laxity at 20 degrees and 90 degrees of flexion.

Positive Lachman's test results.

Pivot shift present.

Posterior sag sign.

Increased varus/valgus laxity in extension.

Associated PLC or MCL instability.

ACL-PLC

Combined disruption of the ACL and PLC with the LCL intact may occur with a purely anteriorly directed force. In this situation, the intact LCL prevents external rotation, and an increase in anterior tibial translation is the only clinical finding. Diagnostic features of ACL-PLC injuries include the following:

Positive Lachman's and anterior drawer test results (isolated PLC: pseudo-Lachman only).

Increased varus laxity at 0 and 30 degrees of flexion (isolated LCL: varus laxity at 30 degrees only).

Increased external rotation.

Increased coupled posterior translation–external rotation between 0 and 30 degrees of flexion.

Increased coupled anterior translation–internal rotation between 30 and 60 degrees of flexion (isolated PLC: coupled anterior translation–internal rotation only).

MCL-PCL

MCL-PCL injuries account for 2% of knee injuries with pathological motion. Diagnostic features of MCL-PCL include the following:

Valgus laxity at both 0 and 30 degrees of flexion (isolated MCL: valgus laxity at 30 degrees only)

Positive posterior drawer test result.

Increased external rotation from anterior subluxation of medial tibial plateau.

PCL-PLC

Although injury to the lateral structures is less common in PCL injuries than injury to the medial structures, it is imperative to diagnose PLC injuries for successful PCL reconstruction. As a general rule, involvement of the posterolateral corner must be ruled out when the posterior tibial translation is greater than 10 mm. This assessment may be difficult because posterior tibial subluxation diminishes posterolateral corner laxity. Therefore, it is critical to reduce the tibia to the normal anatomic position and then test the posterolateral corner at both 90 degrees and 30 degrees of flexion.

Furthermore, injury to the PLC should be based on the final position of the lateral tibial plateau and not the amount of increased external tibial rotation alone. An increase in external rotation can occur secondary to anterior subluxation of the medial tibial plateau, posterior subluxation of the lateral tibial plateau, or both. Diagnostic features of PCL-PLC injuries include the following:

Increased posterior laxity more than 20 to 25 mm (isolated PCL: usually less than 10 to 15 mm).

Increased varus rotation (isolated PCL: no increase).

Increased external rotation more than 15 degrees at both 30 and 90 degrees of flexion (isolated PCL: greater than 5 degrees at 30 degrees; isolated PLC: no increase at 90 degrees).

Increased coupled posterior translation–external rotation.

REFERENCES

1. Galen C: On the usefulness of the parts of the body. Ithaca, NY, Cornell University Press, 1968.
2. Stark J: Two cases of rupture of the crucial ligaments of the knee joint. Edinb Med Surg 1850; 74:267.
3. Battle WH: A case after open section of the knee joint for irreversible traumatic dislocation. Clin Soc Lond 1900; 33:232.
4. Mayo Robson AW: Ruptured cruciate ligaments and their repair by operation. Ann Surg 1903; 37:716.
5. Hey-Groves EW: Operation for repair of cruciate ligaments. Lancet 1917; 2:674.
6. Campbell WC: Repair of the ligaments of the knee. Surg Gynecol Obstet 1936; 62:964.
7. O'Donoghue DH: Surgical treatment of fresh injuries to the major ligaments of the knee. J Bone Joint Surg Am 1950; 32:721.
8. Hughston JC, Andrews JR, Cross MJ, et al: Classification of knee ligament instabilities I: The medial compartment and cruciate ligaments. J Bone Joint Surg Am 1976; 58:159.
9. Clancy WG, Shelbourne KD, Zoellner GB, et al: Treatment of knee joint instability secondary to rupture of the posterior cruciate ligament. J Bone Joint Surg Am 1983; 65:310.
10. Stanitski CL, Harvell JC, Fu F: Observations on acute knee hemarthrosis in children and adolescents. J Pediatr Orthop 1993; 13:506.
11. Traina SM, Bromberg DC: ACL injury patterns in women. Orthopaedics 1997; 20:545.
12. Arnockzy SP: Anatomy of the anterior cruciate ligament. Clin Orthop Rel Res 1983; 172:19.
13. Lyon RM, Akeson WH, Amiel D, et al: Ultrastructural differences between the cells of the medial collateral and anterior cruciate ligaments. Clin Orthop Rel Res 1991; 272:279.
14. Cooper RR, Misol S: Tendon and ligament insertion: A light and electron microscopic study. J Bone Joint Surg Am 1970; 52:1.
15. Smith BA, Livesay GA, Woo S: Biology and biomechanics of the anterior cruciate ligament. Clin Sports Med 1993; 12:637.
16. Torg JS, Conrad W, Kalen V: Clinical diagnosis of anterior cruciate ligament instability in athletes. Am J Sports Med 1976; 4:84.
17. Rijke AM, Perrin DH, Goitz HT, et al: Instrumented arthrometry for diagnosing partial versus complete anterior cruciate ligament tears. Am J Sports Med 1994; 22:294.
18. Vahey TN, Meyer SF, Shelbourne KD, et al: MRI imaging of anterior cruciate ligament injuries. MRI Clin North Am 1994; 2:365.
19. Shirakura K, Terauchi M, Kizuki S, et al: The natural history of untreated anterior cruciate ligament tears in recreational athletes. Clin Orthop Rel Res 1995; 317:227.
20. Fanelli GC: Posterior cruciate ligament injuries in trauma patients. Arthroscopy 1993; 9:291.
21. Fanelli GC, Edson CJ: Posterior cruciate ligament injuries in trauma patients II. Arthroscopy 1995; 11:526.

22. Harner CD, Xerogeanes JW, Livesay GA, et al: The human posterior cruciate ligament complex—an interdisciplinary study: Ligament morphology and biomechanical evaluation. Am J Sports Med 1995; 23: 736.

23. Covey DC, Sapega AA: Current concepts review: Injuries of the posterior cruciate ligament. J Bone Joint Surg Am 1993; 75: 1376.

24. Fanelli, GC, Giannotti BF, Edson CJ: Current concepts review: The posterior cruciate ligament arthroscopic evaluation and treatment. Arthroscopy 1994; 10:673.

25. Eakin CL, Cannon WD: Arthrometric evaluation of posterior cruciate ligament injuries. Am J Sports Med 1998; 26:96.

26. Hewett TE, Noyes FR, Lee MD: Diagnosis of complete and partial posterior cruciate ligament ruptures. Am J Sports Med 1997; 25:648.

27. Harner CD, Hoher J: Current concepts: Evaluation and treatment of posterior cruciate ligament injuries. Am J Sports Med 1998; 26:471.

28. Boynton MD, Tietjens BR: Long-term followup of the untreated isolated posterior cruciate ligament–deficient knee. Am J Sports Med 1996; 24:306.

29. Torg JS, Barton TM, Pavlov H, et al: Natural history of the posterior cruciate ligament–deficient knee. Clin Orthop Rel Res 1989; 246:208.

30. Seebacher JR, Inglis AE, Marshall JL, et al: The structure of the posterolateral aspect of the knee. J Bone Joint Surg Am 1982; 64:536.

31. Veltri DM, Warren RF: Anatomy, biomechanics, and physical findings in posterolateral knee instability. Clin Sports Med 1994; 13:599.

32. Fanelli GC, Feldman DD: Management of combined ACL/PCL/PLC injuries of the knee. In Harner CD: Operative Techniques In Sports Medicine: The Posterior Cruciate Ligament. Philadelphia, WB Saunders, in press.

33. Bleday RM, Fanelli GC, Giannotti BF, et al: Instrumented measurement of the posterolateral corner. Arthroscopy 1998; 14: 489.

34. Miller TT, Gladden P, Staron RB, et al: Posterolateral stabilizers of the knee: Anatomy and injuries assessed with MR imaging. AJR Am J Radiol 1997; 169: 1641.

35. Hughston JC, Andrews JR, Cross MJ, et al: Classification of knee ligament instabilities. I. The medial compartment and cruciate ligaments. J Bone Joint Surg Am 1976; 58:159.

36. Albright JP, Powell JW, Smith W: Medial collateral ligament knee sprains in college football: Effectiveness of preventive braces. Am J Sports Med 1994; 22:12.

37. Indelicato PA: Isolated medial collateral ligament injuries of the knee. J Am Acad Orthop Surg 1995; 3:9.

38. Lundberg M, Messner K: Long-term prognosis of isolated partial medial collateral ligament ruptures. Am J Sports Med 1996; 24:160.

39. Fanelli GC, Giannotti BF, Edson CJ: Arthroscopically assisted combined posterior cruciate ligament/posterior lateral complex reconstruction. Arthroscopy 1996; 12:521.

40. Fanelli GC, Giannotti BF, Edson CJ: Arthoscopically assisted combined anterior and posterior cruciate ligament reconstruction. Arthroscopy 1996; 12:5.

section

TECHNIQUES IN KNEE LIGAMENT SURGERY

4

chapter

12

Jeff Brand, Jr, and Darren L. Johnson

Summary

- Approximately 75,000 anterior cruciate ligament (ACL) reconstructions are performed in the United States each year.
- The popularity of soft-tissue grafts, particularly multiple-stranded hamstring grafts, emphasizes the interplay of strong and stiff initial graft fixation and the rehabilitative loads to which the graft and fixation will have to respond and react.
- It has been suggested that treatment of a chronic medial collateral ligament (MCL) injury nonoperatively with operative treatment of the ACL may result in more laxity after reconstruction.
- Failure to discriminate between an isolated lateral collateral ligament (LCL) injury and a combined injury of the LCL and the posterolateral corner results in residual laxity.
- Endoscopic placement of the femoral tunnel in ACL reconstruction is similar in all outcome parameters to the traditional arthroscopic two-incision technique.
- The best results in the literature have combined ACL and posterior cruciate ligament (PCL) reconstruction for the multiple ligament–injured knee.

comitant injuries, technique, and rehabilitation have improved many lives and careers. Careful planning, knowledge of normal and injured patient anatomy, awareness of demands on the knee, attention to surgical detail, and appropriate postoperative care lead to a successful outcome from an often disabling condition.

HISTORY

Although the ACL was described in 170 AD by Galen, more than 1700 years passed before the first surgical repair of the ACL was attempted, by Mayo Robson in 1903. Hey-Groves, in 1917, was credited with performing the first intra-articular reconstruction with the proximally based iliotibial band (ITB) placed through drill holes in the femur and tibia, thus ushering in the era of ligament reconstruction. Building on the work of Hey-Groves and Smith the following year, O'Donoghue in 1963 used the distally based ITB in another intra-articular reconstruction of the ACL.[3] The poor biomechanical properties of the ITB led to its demise as a widely used graft choice in ligament reconstruction.

In 1939 Campbell used the medial strip of the patellar tendon for intra-articular reconstruction. The tendon maintained its distal attachment and was then passed through drill holes and anchored proximally with suture to the periosteum and fascia lata. Also in 1939, Macy reconstructed the ACL with a distally based semitendinosus muscle that was passed through tibial and femoral bone

Approximately 75,000 ACL reconstructions are performed in the United States each year,[1] but PCL injuries represent from 3.4% to 20% of all reported ligament injuries.[2] Advances in graft selection, graft fixation, recognition of con-

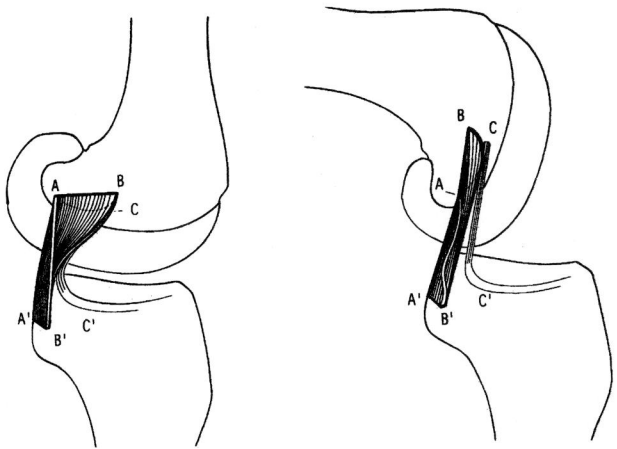

Fig. 1. Independent functioning of the PCL bands. This shows the posterior cruciate ligament in flexion and extension. *A,* Posterior fibers. *B,* More anterior fibers. *C,* Anterior meniscal femoral ligament. Note that the anterior meniscal femoral ligament tightens as the knee is flexed. Its opposite, the posterior meniscal femoral ligament or ligament of Wrisberg, tends to be tighter in extension, such as is seen in the Wrisberg ligament type of discoid meniscus. (Reproduced with permission from Girgis FG, Marshall JL, Al Monajem ARS: The cruciate ligament of the knee joint. Clin Orthop 1975; 106:229.)

tunnels.[3] Zaricznyj,[4] in 1983, introduced the concept of a free semitendinosus graft, which was successful in his reported series of ACL reconstructions. The use of a single-stranded hamstring tendon has evolved into the present triple- and quadruple-stranded grafts and their techniques of fixation.[4] In 1979, Marshall et al[5] reported on the use of the quadriceps tendon for ACL stabilization.

Understanding and treatment of the PCL have lagged those of its more recognized sibling throughout its history. Instead, the same conceptual framework has been applied to the PCL that has been gleaned from ACL research. In 1950, Lindeman suggested the use of the semitendinosus muscle from the tibial attachment to a bony canal on the femur. Hughston et al, in their 1976 report, described the use of medial gastrocnemius muscle following the intra-articular course of the PCL.[6] In 1983 Clancy, borrowing from his work on the ACL, published the results of his technique of free patellar tendon graft intra-articular reconstruction of the PCL. Many principles espoused in this work have been applied to present arthroscopic reconstructions.[7]

Since 1824, the dislocated knee has been appreciated as a severe injury that may be life threatening if not addressed. Among the first writers on this topic were Cooper and Gibson. The first open reduction, involving an 8-week-old dislocation, was attempted in 1881 by Annandale.[8] Because of the rarity of this phenomenon, little consensus has been reached regarding its treatment.

ANATOMY

The cruciate ligaments consist of isolated bands that act as a functional composite of the entire cruciate ligament (Fig. 1). This is particularly true in the PCL. The anterolateral band provides stability of the knee in flexion to posterior tibial translation. It is six times stronger than the postero-

medial band, which diminishes posterior translation of the tibia with respect to the femur when the knee is in the extended position.[9] The two PCL bands have separate femoral insertions, giving the composite PCL a broad femoral insertion: approximately 3 cm from cephalad to caudad and a full 1 cm in depth (Fig. 2). Currently, PCL reconstruction replicates the anterolateral band, possibly at the cost of knee stability throughout the entire range of knee motion. A single-band reconstructed ligament cannot be isometric through the entire arc of knee motion. As the graft experiences cyclic tensile loads with knee motion, it will stretch and relax, perhaps causing graft laxity in the PCL reconstruction.

The ACL consists of two bands: the anteromedial, which tightens in flexion, and the posterolateral, which tightens in extension (Fig. 3). They do not mimic the level of independent function seen in the PCL bands. Although the ligament is hourglass shaped, the insertion sites are smaller and lend themselves better to a single-band reconstruction.

Isometry has proved difficult to measure and interpret in the reconstruction of the ACL. Given two cruciate ligament bands, a single isometric point on the femur and tibia is not possible. Graft impingement and the confines of the notch dictate a more posteromedial position to the tibial tunnel than has been previously advocated. Medial positioning of the tibial tunnel avoids lateral wall impingement and restores tension to the PCL. Posterior tibial tunnel position dictates femoral tunnel position when ACL reconstruction is performed endoscopically, which is currently the most frequent technique.

Failure to recognize and address damage to secondary restraints is a frequent cause of failure in ACL reconstruction and is currently being recognized as the leading cause of PCL postreconstruction laxity. In decreasing order of importance, the secondary restraints of the ACL are the

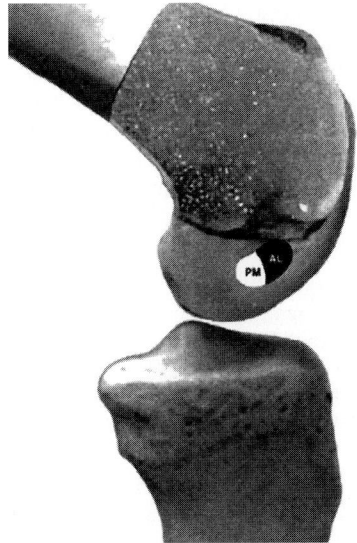

Fig. 2. Posterior cruciate ligament (PCL) femoral insertion. PM = posteromedial band; AL = anterolateral band of the PCL. (Reprinted from Miller MD, Bergfeld JA, Fowler PJ, et al: The posterior cruciate ligament injured knee: Principles of evaluation and treatment. Am Acad Orthop Surg Instr Course Lect 1999; 48:199.)

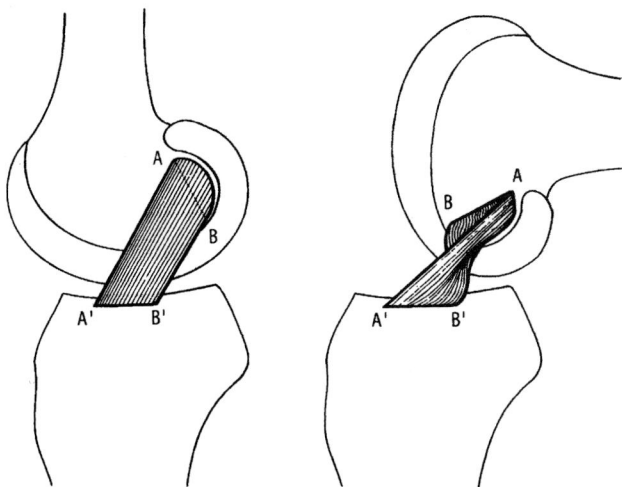

Fig. 3. The anterior cruciate ligament with flexion and extension. This shows the anterior cruciate ligament in flexion and extension, the orientations of the fibers of the ligament relative to each other, and laxity of posterior lateral fibers in flexion. (Reproduced with permission from Girgis FG, Marshall JL, Al Monajem ARS: The cruciate ligament of the knee joint. Clin Orthop 1975; 106:229.)

MCL, ITB, midmedial capsule, midlateral capsule, and LCL.[10] Similarly, the secondary restraints to the PCL in decreasing order of importance are the posterolateral capsule and popliteus, MCL, posteromedial capsule, LCL, and the midmedial capsule.[10] Unrecognized posterolateral corner damage is implicated in PCL graft laxity after reconstruction. Therefore, meticulous evaluation of this structure at reconstruction is mandatory. If damage is suspected, the posterolateral corner must be repaired or reconstructed at PCL reconstruction.

GRAFT SELECTION

Arguably, there are now more choices for graft selection than at any previous time in the history of ligament reconstruction. The popularity of soft-tissue grafts, particularly multiple-stranded hamstring grafts, emphasizes the interplay of strong and stiff initial graft fixation and the rehabilitative loads to which the graft and fixation will have to respond and react. Fixation methods must be rigid and stiff to allow current rehabilitation principles. Current fixation techniques involve soft tissue and bone within a bone tunnel or periosteal fixation away from joint surfaces. Current rehabilitation protocols after knee ligament surgery stress immediate full range of motion, return of neuromuscular function, proprioception, and early weightbearing forces up the kinetic chain. In the early postoperative period, graft fixation is the weak link within the entire system.

BIOMECHANICAL PROPERTIES

Although considered the gold standard in ACL reconstruction, the strength and stiffness of the patella tendon may not be significantly greater than that of the ACL and PCL (Table 1). Initially, the strength of the bone–patella tendon–bone (BPTB) was estimated to be approximately 150% that of the native ACL.[11] However, this was a 14-mm strip of patella tendon, and a 10-mm strip of patella tendon may have less strength at failure (see Table 1). The strength of the ACL is stronger than initially measured by Noyes et al in their landmark study, and the importance of aging on the degradation of material properties of ligaments has come to be appreciated.[12] In fact, the patella tendon may approximate the strength of the native ACL.

The quadrupled hamstring (QH), however, may have nearly double the failure strength of the native ACL (see Table 1). Soft-tissue grafts, those without bone plugs on each end, may actually be stronger than the biomechanical data suggest, because it is difficult to grip soft tissue without grip failures or slippage given the level of force that is applied. If grip fixation could be improved, the failure load may be higher for the soft-tissue grafts. For example, the quadriceps tendon has a large cross-sectional area and yet a relatively low ultimate failure given its large cross-sectional area. The large cross-sectional area and short length of the quadriceps tendon do not allow immobilization of independent fibers in current cryogrip systems.

DONOR SITE MORBIDITY

Harvest site complications with the use of BPTB, like patella fracture, patella tendon rupture, fat pad herniation, arthrofibrosis, anterior knee pain, and the ever-present thigh atrophy, drive the search for new graft choices. The prevalent directions researchers have taken are the use of allograft tissue and QH grafts. Other autologous tissue such as the quadriceps tendon have been reported; however, the data, especially from comparative studies of different graft choices, are not adequate to allow significant analysis of donor site morbidity.

The incidence of anterior knee pain and patellofemoral crepitation after cruciate ligament reconstruction persists even with allograft use.[13, 14] This suggests that factors such as the injury mechanism, surgical insult, and concomitant muscle atrophy help determine the presence of anterior knee pain. Use of QH grafts has diminished the incidence of extension loss and patellar crepitation compared with the

Graft Selection	Ultimate Strength to Failure	Stiffness
Native ACL[12]	2160 N	242 N/mm
Native PCL[9]	1867 N	
Quadrupled hamstrings (semitendinosus and gracilis)[46]	4140 N	807 N/mm
Quadriceps tendon[78]	2353 N	326 N/mm
Patella tendon (10 mm)[79]	2977 N	455 N/mm
Autograft patella tendon (14 mm)[11]	2900 N ± 260 N 160% of native ACL	

TABLE 1. COMPARISON OF ULTIMATE LOAD TO FAILURE AND STIFFNESS OF CRUCIATE LIGAMENT TO THE QUADRUPLED HAMSTRING AND QUADRICEPS TENDON GRAFT IN CRUCIATE LIGAMENT SURGERY

ACL = anterior cruciate ligament; PCL = posterior cruciate ligament.

BPTB.[15] In a similar comparative study of QH and BPTB autografts, the BPTB group tended to experience more anterior knee pain but not to a level of statistical significance. In the BPTB group, five patients had tenderness of the inferior pole of the patella and pain with activity. This finding did not occur with the QH grafts.[16] It is interesting, however, that when the contralateral BPTB is used for a graft source, the incidence of patellar pain and crepitation in the donor knee has not been reported to increase after surgery.[17] In a comparative series of BPTB autografts and BPTB allografts, patellofemoral crepitation and pain were similar in both groups at 1-year and 2-year follow-up.[14] Therefore, anterior knee complaints cannot be eliminated with alteration of graft selection. However, QH grafts in two comparative studies decreased the incidence of these complaints.

A comparative study that evaluated quadriceps atrophy in patients reconstructed with patella tendon grafts or QH grafts demonstrated more rapid quadriceps activation and return of quadriceps strength with a QH graft.[18] Intuitively, it appears that maintence of thigh circumference is an advantage of allograft tissue compared with autograft BPTB. This may be accurate early in the rehabilitative course (e.g., the first 6 months), but the difference in thigh circumference tends toward equalization between these two graft choices at the 2-year postoperative mark.[19] Shelton et al[14] noted that the difference in thigh atrophy between BPTB allograft and autograft at 2 years was slight: 0.6 cm compared with 0.8 cm.

Current investigations suggest that donor site morbidity is slight with the QH grafts. The hamstring tendons regenerate with tendon-like tissue when evaluated with magnetic resonance imaging. Hamstring strength returns, although probably over the course of a year, to near-normal levels. However, the hamstrings are an agonist of ACL function and protective against its injury. Harvesting these tendons alters the proprioceptive loop, and these effects have not been fully evaluated. In comparative studies, however, the QH grafts have not been associated with a higher rate of graft rupture compared with BPTB grafts.

GRAFT LAXITY

Although donor site morbidity favors QH grafts and allografts, postreconstruction graft laxity concerns BPTB graft advocates. Only one comparative study documents this concern to a level of statistical significance[20]; two other investigations compare QH and BPTB grafts have found a trend toward increasing laxity with QH grafts as measured with the KT-1000 and a clinical examination.[15, 16] Rupture rates have been comparable, but study numbers are not high enough to detect slight differences.

Early reports of allograft use, primarily with irradiated patella tendons, suggested that graft laxity after reconstruction may not meet the current standards of BPTB autograft. Knee laxity after cruciate ligament reconstruction does not progress as once suspected.[13, 14] Often patient demands require a stable knee for active sports participation. Concerns persist as to whether these requisites are met by allograft tissue. Several, but not all, studies comparing allograft and autograft tissue found similar levels of knee stability after reconstruction. Although the KT-1000 data were comparable between allograft and autograft tissue in a comparative

series, the pivot glide and Lachman data indicated significant improved stability in the BPTB autograft-reconstructed knee compared with the BPTB allograft-reconstructed knee.[14]

RETURN TO ACTIVITIES

Return to normal activities, particularly in competitive sports, seems to be the ultimate criterion for success of cruciate ligament reconstruction; the patient either can participate or cannot participate. However, graft laxity, giving way, anterior knee pain, muscle weakness, proprioceptive response, age, and motivation to return to sporting and competitive activities also determine the patient's eventual activity level. Aglietti et al[15] noted this to be one of two statistically significant outcomes in their comparative evaluation of BPTB and QH graft: the patella tendon patients were almost twice as likely to return to athletics. Yet to date in comparative studies, the patella tendon autograft has not been superior to allografts regarding return to normal or athletic play.[21]

DISEASE TRANSMISSION

Although all clinicians are concerned about AIDS and HIV, statistically the odds against acquiring these from a soft-tissue graft are staggering. The estimated risk of disease transmission from an allograft is approximately 1 per 1,667,600 or 1 per 8,000,000 if the allograft is deep frozen.[22, 23]

Allografts are usually prepared after harvest from the donor in one of three ways: fresh frozen, deep frozen, or irradiated. Fresh ligament allografts are not performed because of the risk of disease transmission, which is approximately 1:161.[22, 23] Fresh-frozen grafts contain viral contaminants that are potentially active. Prevention of disease transmission rests primarily with donor screening and testing of the tissue for the AIDS and hepatitis viruses. Donors are screened for lifestyle, vocational and recreational pursuits, and general state of health. Donors who are high risk in any area are excluded. Serological testing of prospective donors is another means of graft exclusion. In addition to testing for the HIV antibody, antigen testing can be performed. The antibody does not appear until 3 months after infection, allowing a window for a false-negative test. Antigen testing eliminates this window.

Viruses are inactivated at extremely cold temperatures; this is the principle behind deep-freezing tissue. However, the mechanical properties are slightly altered by the process of deep freezing.[24, 25] Also, a few viral particles may survive the freezing process, which can allow them to still be infectious. Freezing alone is not sufficient protection against the AIDS virus.

Finally, the allograft tissue may be irradiated to sterilize it. Again, however, this weakens the graft. The dose recommended by the American Association of Tissue Banks is 15 to 25 Gy gamma radiation. However, sterilization of all viral particles requires at least 30 Gy,[26] and greater than 30 Gy will alter collagen structure and tensile strength.[24, 25]

Allografts are typically obtained from bone banks that were set up to procure, process, test, and distribute cadaver specimens. Variability exists between bone banks regarding the manner in which they harvest, sterilize, and test tissue samples.

COSMESIS

Patients have limited means with which to evaluate their surgeon's skills. The incision site allows a patient to form an opinion regarding the surgeon's skill level and carries more weight than is often appreciated. Patients rarely fail to be impressed by the small incision that is necessary for a QH graft or an allograft. A small scar not only is more pleasing to the eye but implies a high degree of performance skill to carry out intricate surgery to provide bathing suit–compatible incisions (Fig. 4). Undeniably, the edge in cosmesis has to be given to hamstring and allograft reconstructions.

SUMMARY

Our approach has attempted to individualize graft selection to the patient and the clinical situation. Clinical studies and our experience indicate the patella tendon with interference fixation reliably restores knee stability, improves function, and returns motivated patients to preinjury levels of activities. In young active patients in whom this is a primary concern, the patella tendon is our graft of choice.

When preexisting patellofemoral complaints or risk factors argue against patella tendon harvest, an allograft or a QH graft represents an alternative. In the skeletally immature patient, placement of a soft-tissue graft through smaller bone tunnels may decrease the possibility of a femoral or tibial growth disturbance. Cosmesis is improved with either a QH graft or an allograft, and in appropriate patients it may be the tiebreaker. However, although not clearly demonstrated in the cited clinical studies, postreconstruction laxity dictates a lower level of activity after surgery. These choices, the QH or an allograft, may not allow competitive elite-level athletics in all patients.

The QH graft has biomechanical advantages compared with the patella tendon: specifically, it improves strength, stiffness, and cross-sectional area. The most compelling reason for patella tendon autograft or allograft may be interference fixation and bone-to-bone healing in the tun-

nel. Conventional hamstring fixation may result in residual laxity after reconstruction.

GRAFT FIXATION

Consideration of the anatomic placement of ligament substitutes has fostered rehabilitation efforts that stress immediate full range of motion, immediate weightbearing, neuromuscular strength and coordination, and an early return to athletic competition (3 months). This has placed crucial importance on secure graft fixation at the time of ligament reconstruction. Fixation devices have progressed from metal to biodegradable and from far to near native ligament attachment site. Ideally, the biomechanical properties of the entire graft construct should approach those of the native ligament and facilitate biological incorporation of the graft. Fixation should be done at the normal anatomic attachment site of the native ligament (aperture fixation) and over time allow the biological return of the histological transition zone from ligament to fibrocartilage to calcified fibrocartilage to bone. No commonly used graft fixation provides ultimate failure strength or stiffness comparable to that of the native cruciate ligament (Tables 1–5).

It is important for the surgeon to be aware of the difference in fixation techniques and their associated biological consequences. Different graft substitutes may require different fixation techniques that have direct biological and outcome implications. Knowledge of graft fixation variables will aid the clinician in making the necessary intraoperative and postoperative decisions in cruciate ligament reconstruction.

BIOMECHANICAL PROPERTIES

The majority of tendon fixation constructs are mechanically less stiff than an interference screw against a bone plug, which has been considered to be the gold standard in fixation (see Tables 2–5). Thus, given that ultimate failure strength is comparable between the two given fixation choices, tendon constructs may displace or slip more before they fail, creating greater laxity in the graft reconstruction.

Many tendon fixation devices are considered indirect. They rely on linkage material to connect the tendon to the fixation device. These linkage materials and their junction with the graft are less stiff and strong than the grafts themselves. If creep or laxity is in line with the linkage, it is referred to as the bungee cord effect.[27] These shearing forces may be responsible for tunnel expansion, also known as the windshield wiper effect.

In the native cruciate ligament, the point of fixation is at the joint surface. However, many tendon fixation constructs are placed at a distance from the joint surface with a staple, screw and suture, or soft-tissue washer. When interference fixation is placed closer to the joint surface, increased knee stability at a variety of flexion angles was found and also improved graft isometry.[28, 29]

FEMORAL AND TIBIAL FIXATION

Two key differences between femoral and tibial fixation need to be considered: bone density and the angle at which force is applied to the graft attachment. The bone quality and geometry of the tibia are different from those of the

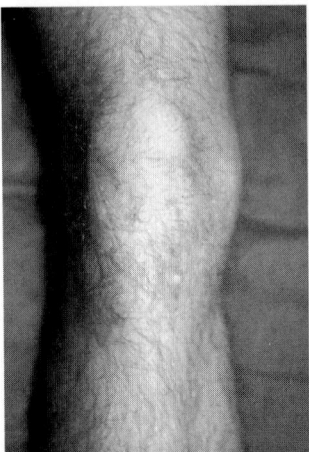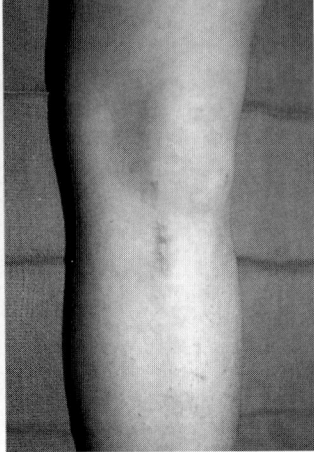

Fig. 4. Skin incisions. The skin incisions for the bone–patella tendon–bone anterior cruciate ligament (ACL) reconstruction (left) and the incision for the harvest and reconstruction of the ACL utilize the quadrupled hamstring tendon (right).

TABLE 2. TIBIAL FIXATION OPTIONS FOR BONE–PATELLAR TENDON–BONE PLUG IN A BONE TUNNEL

Construct	Failure (N)	Stiff (N/mm)	Failure Mode
Suture (no. 5) to button[35]	248 (40.2)	12.8 (2.0)	Button failed; suture pulled through the bone plug
Doubled staples on patella tendon in trough[34]	588	86.3	Graft slipped under staple; 27% bone block breakage
Suture and post[41]	396 (124)	27 (13)	Bone-tendon rupture, bone plug fracture, tibial post pull-out
9-mm interference screw[35]	476 (110.9)	57.9 (3.9)	Grafts pulled out of the tunnel
Interference screw and suture with post[41]	674 (206)	50 (21)	Bone plug fractured, pull-out around tibial screw and suture rupture
7-mm interference screw[30]	461 (230–631)	47 (28–73)	Tendon tearing, slipping of the bone plug
9-mm interference screw[30]	678 (394–947)	68 (32–84)	Tendon tearing, slipping of the bone plug
9 × 25 mm biodegradable screw[72]	293 (156–458)	42 (14–67)	Bone plug slipped, tendon tearing

Values represent means followed by standard deviation or range of variability in parentheses.

femur.[30] The dual photon absorptiometry of the tibial metaphysis was determined to be less than the femoral metaphysis in the same knee of elderly cadavers[31] and in young females.[32] The line of force on the graft is directly in line with the tibial tunnel. The line of applied force to the graft is obliquely oriented to the femoral tunnel in the weightbearing position, which is extension. Based on radiographic studies, the femoral tunnel does not become colinear with the ligament graft until approximately 100 degrees of knee flexion.[33] Given these two factors, one would predict inferior fixation on the tibia. Indeed, Kohn and Rose[30] found a lower rate of tibial failure when using interference fixation for bone plug fixation.

BONE PLUG GRAFT FIXATION: TIBIAL FIXATION STAPLES

Graft tunnel length mismatch is considered the primary indication for staple fixation. In a study by Gerich et al,[34] a set of double staples in a shallow trough (588 N) compared favorably with interference screw fixation (506–758 N) in failure, and the staples were significantly stiffer (86.3 N/

mm) than interference fixation (49.2–54.9 N/mm) in young (mean age, 44 years) human cadaver models. Unfortunately, the incidence of bone block breakage (27%) was greater than the interference screw fixation (0%).[34]

Interference Fixation

Kurosaka et al[35] in 1987 demonstrated superior strength with a larger diameter screw (9 mm) as an interference fixation. In cases of poor bone stock as a result of revision or tunnel widening, graft tunnel length mismatch, or when additional fixation strength is needed for large or noncompliant patients, interference fixation may be backed up with other fixation methods such as a suture and post, Endo-Button, or screw and washer.

Currently, a screw with a 9-mm diameter and at least 20 mm in length is the standard. The difference between outside diameter of the screw and core diameter is the most important consideration.[36] A 9-mm tibial interference screw disengaged from the bone tunnel at significantly more maximum tensile strength and linear load to failure compared with a 7-mm screw[30] (see Table 2).[30] Screw length beyond

TABLE 3. FEMORAL FIXATION OPTIONS FOR BONE–PATELLAR TENDON–BONE PLUG IN A BONE TUNNEL

Construct	Failure (N)	Stiff (N/mm)	Failure Mode
EndoButton[80]	554 (276)	27.0 (13.5)	Tibial bone block fracture or suture breakage; tibial side fixation failure
Press Fit[80]	350 (48)	36.8 (16.3)	Tibial bone plug pulled out; fracture tibial bone block; patellar tendon failed
Interference screw from outside-in[41]	423 (175)	46 (24)	Pull-out around the screw
Endoscopic interference screw[41]	588 (282)	33 (14)	Bone plug fractured; femoral screw pull-out; bone tendon rupture
Metal endoscopic interference screw[81]	558.3 (67.9)	No stiffness reported	Femoral fixation failure; fracture of bone plug; tearing of graft
BioScrew endoscopic interference screw[81]	552.5 (56.4)	No stiffness reported	Femoral fixation failure; fracture of bone plug; tearing of graft

Values represent means followed by standard deviation in parentheses.

TABLE 4. TIBIAL FIXATION OPTIONS FOR A SOFT-TISSUE GRAFT IN A BONE TUNNEL			
Construct	Failure (N)	Stiff (N/mm)	Failure Mode
Stapled semitendinosus[35]	137 (22.6)	8.8 (1.0)	Tendon pulled out of staple
QHT with suture and post[41]	573 (109)	18 (5)	Suture tendon stretches; post pull-out
QHT with screw and soft-tissue washer[41]	821 (219)	29 (7)	Tendon stretches or tibial screw pulls out
QHT with a washer plate[44]	905 (291)	273 (56)	No failure mode given
QHT with RCI titanium screw[44]	350 (134)	248 (52)	No failure mode given

Values represent mean followed by standard deviation in parentheses. QHT = quadrupled hamstring tendon.

20 mm in conjunction with a bone plug does not appear necessary.[37]

The gap between the bone plug and bone tunnel along with the interaction with screw diameter influences the fixation strength. Brown et al[38] suggested that interference (screw outer diameter minus tunnel bone block gap) is correlated with failure, but gap size alone is not.

Despite the clinical success of interference fixation, largely preventable complications have been reported. Countertension through the bone plug sutures can reduce graft advancement as the interference screw is placed.[39] Screw laceration of either the bone plug suture or the graft itself is a clinical concern. If the sutures that are attached to the bone plug are lacerated by the threads from the screw, then poor graft fixation cannot be salvaged with a suture and post construct. Graft laceration may require another graft option.[39] Two cases of bone plug comminution have been reported. Reversing the graft, placing the fractured bone plug in the tibial bone tunnel, salvaged one instance of bone plug comminution. Fixation of the fractured bone plug was obtained with a suture and post. The other instance had to be revised to another graft choice.[40] Painful hardware uncommonly occurs in the area of the tibial screw, and screw removal is effective in relieving this pain.

BONE PLUG GRAFT FIXATION: FEMORAL FIXATION ENDOBUTTON

Primarily, the EndoButton is used with bone plug fixation in femoral tunnel blow-out, which can occur with endo-

scopic techniques. However, interference fixation is preferable in routine femoral bone plug fixation.

The EndoButton was designed for use in the endoscopic ACL reconstruction for femoral fixation and now has been described for use in PCL reconstruction as well.

Interference Fixation

Two studies with human tissue compared a metal 7-mm-diameter screw placed intra-articularly as in endoscopic ACL reconstruction with an outside-in technique using a 9-mm screw. Similar strength and stiffness were found[37, 41] (see Table 3).

Although screw divergence from the bone plug is common when postoperative radiographs are evaluated critically, it is not considered a clinical concern. Dworsky et al[42] described the endoscopically placed interference screw as an active "wedge" effectively blocking the femoral bone plug from being displaced into the joint. In the clinical situation, Fanelli et al[43] showed no increase in fixation failure with divergent interference screws placed endoscopically at angles greater than 20 degrees.

SOFT-TISSUE FIXATION: TIBIAL FIXATION STAPLES

A single staple used with the semitendinosus muscle is neither strong nor stiff[35] (see Table 4). Looping the tendon graft over a second staple, the "belt-buckle" technique, markedly improved fixation in a porcine model. The failure load was 705 N with a stiffness of 174 N/mm.[44] Frequently, staples cause pain at the site of implantation and

TABLE 5. FEMORAL FIXATION OPTIONS FOR A SOFT-TISSUE GRAFT IN A BONE TUNNEL			
Construct	Failure (N)	Stiff (N/mm)	Failure Mode
QHT with Semifix[80]	523 (263)	34.2 (14.3)	Cross-pin toggled; graft slipped off; tibial fixation failure
QHT with Bone Mulch screw[80]	583 (108)	24.4 (4.17)	Tibial fixation failure; implant failure
QHT with an EndoButton, mersilene tape[80]	520 (50)	34.8 (22.3)	Tape broke
QHT with EndoButton and endotape[80]	618 (242)	22.4 (6.9)	Tape broke; tibial fixation failure; tendon failure; implant pulled through bone
	663 (211)	18.1 (6.9)	
	678 (179)	20.6 (7.8)	
QHT with RCI titanium screw[51]	242 (90.7)	No stiffness reported	Failed by graft slipping
QHT with BioScrew[51]	341 (162.9)	No stiffness reported	Failed by graft slipping
QHT BioScrew, 0.5-mm graft sleeves[55]	530 (186)	No stiffness reported	Failed by graft slipping

Values represent mean followed by standard deviation in parentheses. QHT = quadrupled hamstring tendon.

have to be removed. Although the belt-buckle technique has been used successfully, fixation is periosteal and at a distance from joint surfaces.

SCREWS USED AS A POST

A screw can be used with a standard metal washer as a post to tie suture around, or it can be used with a soft-tissue washer against tendon. A screw with a soft-tissue washer placed directly against quadrupled tendon graft is slightly stronger and stiffer than the screw used as a post with suture[41] (Table 4). A screw with a soft-tissue washer is preferable to tibial soft-tissue fixation with a post linked with suture because it avoids the more elastic suture, thereby improving stiffness.

WASHER PLATE

The washer plate, WasherLoc (Arthrotek, Warsaw, IN), is a multipronged washer and screw used to fix the tibial end of the QH graft. It is placed at the distal end of the tibial tunnel and can be recessed to diminish the prominence of the screw head. The ultimate failure load and the stiffness were similar to that of the native ACL[44] (see Table 4). Biomechanically, this is the only tibial soft-tissue fixation device that approximates the ACL in strength and stiffness.

SOFT-TISSUE FIXATION: FEMORAL FIXATION DEVICES
Transfixion Fixation

In cyclic biomechanical testing, both the Trans-fix (Arthrex, Naples, FL) (238 N/mm) and the Bone Mulch Screw (Arthrotek) (257 N/mm) possessed superior stiffness compared with the EndoButton linked with either the endotape (183 N/mm) or the closed loop (179 N/mm). The Trans-fix (1042 N) and the Bone Mulch Screw (978 N) also demonstrated greater ultimate tensile failure than the Endobutton linked with endotape (644 N). However, the highest level of failure was reported with the EndoButton linked with a closed loop (1342 N)[45] (see Table 5). In addition to a favorable strength at failure and stiffness, transfixion devices may allow independent tensioning of the four strands of the QH tendon. In the laboratory, this resulted in a statistically significant increased ultimate tensile strength of the QH graft and an 89% increase in stiffness.[46]

The device does require a second counterincision to deploy the cross pin. Fixation by this device is deeper in the tunnel, allowing for the graft motion in the tunnel, which has been associated with tunnel expansion.

Patients who have had ACL reconstruction with transfixion devices have experienced outcomes similar to those previously cited in the literature. Two patients in a series had the pin repositioned after migration. One of those patients and another patient later had the pin removed because of ITB irritation. This device has since been modified to address the prominence of the pinhead.[47]

EndoButton

A biomechanical study in young human cadavers found that a hamstring construct fixed with an EndoButton and a tibial post failed at 612 N ± 73 N compared with 416 N ± 66 N in the patellar tendon group with interference fixation. The stiffness did not significantly vary between groups. The study noted that either construct represented only 20% to 30% of the failure strength of the native ACL: 2195 N ± 427 N[48] (see Table 5). Direct biomechanical comparison between an EndoButton linked with a closed loop or linked with endotape revealed similar stiffness data, but a much higher ultimate tensile testing was demonstrated with the closed loop: 1345 N versus 644 N for the endotape-linked EndoButton.[45]

Biomechanically, the EndoButton linked with tape has motion of the graft in the tunnel of up to 3 mm, creating shear forces under physiological cyclic loads.[49] This longitudinal motion or bungee effect has been associated with tunnel expansion in clinical trials.[50] The natural history of tunnel expansion is undetermined at present but of obvious concern to surgeons using hamstring fixation with linked devices. Extensive tunnel expansion complicates revision surgery as a result of bone loss and may jeopardize fixation of the graft. Despite this reservation, the EndoButton is still a widely used and a clinically successful form of femoral hamstring fixation.

Interference Fixation

QH grafts offer superior strength and stiffness and decreased harvest morbidity. Conventional means of fixation, however, are positioned periosteally, whereas ideal fixation is at joint surfaces. Interference fixation positions graft fixation at joint surfaces and directly against the graft. Controversy revolves around several issues regarding soft-tissue interference fixation. Is this means of fixation secure, strong, and stiff enough for a progressive rehabilitation so that a patella tendon reconstruction patient benefits? Does the bone tunnel graft interface sufficiently stabilize in the same time frame as the patella tendon bone plug, or does rehabilitation need to be delayed until healing occurs? Are clinical results comparable to reported QH with conventional forms of fixation and BPTB-reconstructed patients?

Initial fixation strength of soft-tissue interference fixation in biomechanical testing appears comparable between a blunt threaded metal screw (RCI; Smith & Nephew DonJoy, Carlsbad, CA) or a biodegradable interference screw for tibial fixation, and a biodegradable screw may be superior in femoral fixation.[51–53] Screw degradation may not compromise graft incorporation and diminish fixation strength.[54] However, these levels of fixation are less than conventional means of QH fixation in the majority of biomechanical testing. Stiffness, or the movement of the graft under load, is superior with soft-tissue interference fixation compared with conventional soft-tissue graft fixation (see Tables 4 and 5). Possibly at the loads seen by the graft during rehabilitation, stiffness determines graft behavior to a greater extent than ultimate load at failure.

Means to improve fixation, particularly tibial fixation, are avidly pursued. Improving the fit of the tendon graft in a bone tunnel with 0.5-mm-sized graft sleeves increased fixation, particularly on the femur, compared with 1-mm-sized graft sleeves.[55] Screw length was increased from 23 to 28 mm.[56] A further increase to 35 mm in length in the tibial tunnel increased the load at failure in a young cadaver bone biomechanical study.[57] A group from Memphis improved load at failure by 40% in a controlled study with tunnel impaction to match graft diameter.[58] Unfortunately, the biological effect of these measures is undecided. Increased pressure on the graft-bone tunnel interface may adversely affect biological graft incorporation or lead to graft necrosis.

Combining the tendon graft with either a free bone plug or an attached bone plug has been explored to increase fixation strength. An attached bone plug harvested with the semitendinosus fixed with a biodegradable screw compared favorably to a BPTB with the same fixation.[59]

Two clinical studies showed an increase in anterior tibial translation measured from the time of operative fixation to later follow-up in some patients. One group is considered back-up fixation to the interference screw in patients with lower bone mineral density or with poor screw purchase.[60] The second group reported a reverse thread screw for the right knee in male patients; this was a group of patients who had residual postreconstruction laxity, and the reverse thread screw did decrease laxity.[61]

SUMMARY

Graft fixation remains the weak link in the early postoperative period after ligament reconstruction, although technological advancements in surgical techniques have allowed for immediate return of neuromuscular function within the extremity. Fixation must not only withstand these early physiological forces but must also facilitate biological incorporation of the graft construct in its entirety. The specific anatomic location of the attachment site will have profound effects on fiber recruitment patterns within the ligament substitute. Fixation of a bone plug in a bone tunnel with a metal or bioabsorbable interference screw appears to uphold our current surgical or rehabilitative demands. Present soft-tissue fixation within a bone tunnel or extra tunnel may not possess the same biomechanical or biological properties as a bone plug in a bone tunnel fixed with an interference screw. Devices that are linked to the graft or placed nonanatomically have been associated with motion through the graft construct and have spurred the search for direct fixation at the joint surface. Controversy remains as to the suitability of soft-tissue fixation for progressive rehabilitation. Other fixation devices are used and have been tested, such as transfixion femoral fixation, hybrid fixation, and tibial washer plate fixation to achieve the normal mechanical characteristics of the native ligament graft more closely.

MCL

The MCL is the most commonly injured knee ligament (Fig. 5). Fortunately, isolated injury treated nonoperatively promotes rapid, secure healing and reliable return to sporting activity.[62] Availability of instrumented laxity of either the MCL or the LCL does not allow rigorous objective outcome analysis. Rather, knee evaluation is dependent on subjective patient reporting and observer examination of the knee, which is inherently variable. Any residual laxity, although well tolerated clinically, has unknown long-term consequences.

As the primary secondary stabilizer to the ACL, the role of the MCL in ACL reconstruction is of obvious importance. Given our inability to rigorously test for laxity of the MCL and to a lesser extent the ACL, treatment of the MCL injury in combination with the cruciate ligament is

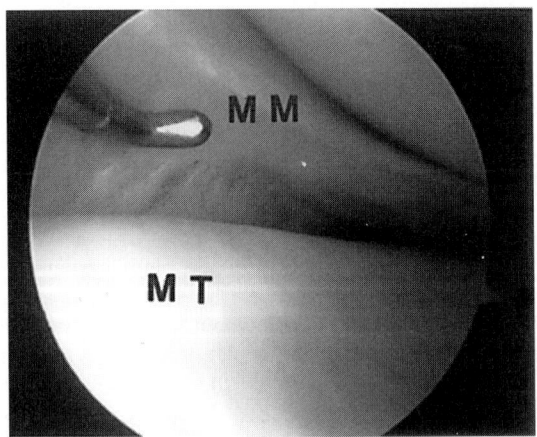

Fig. 5. A meniscocapsular separation. This shows a meniscocapsular separation associated with a medial collateral injury in a knee with a concomitant anterior cruciate ligament injury. MT = medial tibial plateau; MM = medial meniscus.

unsettled. Outcomes in several studies demonstrated that nonoperative treatment of the MCL in combination with operative reconstruction of the ACL results in a well-functioning knee. Association of MCL injury with PCL injury, although not common, has been evaluated even less frequently. Combined operative reconstruction of the ACL and PCL injuries and bracing of the MCL have resulted in excellent functional results in the small number of patients reported.[63] However, it has been suggested that treatment of a chronic MCL injury nonoperatively and operative treatment of the ACL may result in more laxity after reconstruction. This report had a small number of patients, and the impact on outcome in individual patients was not clear.[64]

For the chronic MCL-injured knee, several operative choices exist, suggesting a lack of a standard, time-proven approach. The chronically lax ligament has been imbricated with suture in the past. Thermal shrinkage has been proposed to duplicate this historical surgical approach with current technology. Controlled thermal imbrication of the tissues has been effective in restoring stability to the chronically unstable shoulder. This technology offers similar advantages for the chronically lax MCL. The MCL is anatomically divided into two layers, and this tissue depth may be a problem for the present thermal devices, which by design have a limited depth of penetration.

As an alternative to suture or thermal imbrication of the MCL, the ligament can be advanced through a recession of the femoral insertion. The femoral insertion is isolated with osteotomes, creating a block of bone on which the MCL is inserted. This bone block can be rotated 90 degrees in the coronal plane, increasing the tension in the MCL by displacing the insertion proximally. A screw through the bone block into the lateral femoral condyle with a soft-tissue washer provides secure fixation (Fig. 6).

A BPTB allograft can be fixed with interference screws. The isometric point of the MCL on the femur is located slightly distal to the medial femoral epicondyle. Therefore, a tunnel placed on the femoral epicondyle allows the graft to move to the inferior or distal portion of the tunnel,

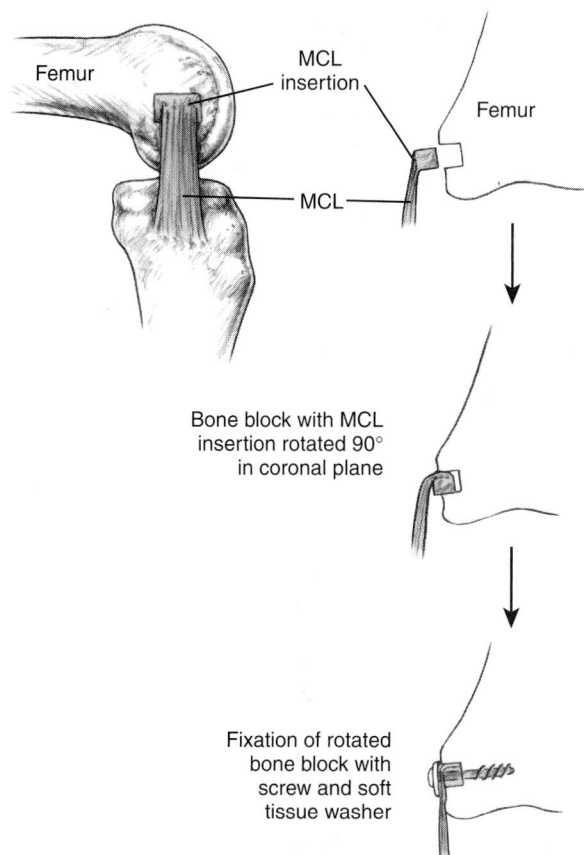

Fig. 6. Recession of the medial cruciate ligament (MCL) femoral insertion. This is the technique of recession of the femoral insertion of the MCL.

which is the femoral origin isometric point. The tibial insertion of the deep fibers of the MCL is broad. Using a Kirschner wire with a suture through a full-knee range of motion will approximate the tibial isometric point and allow correct placement of the tibial tunnel. Because of the scarcity of BPTB, a soft-tissue graft such as the anterior tibialis or the semitendinosus can be looped around the screw and a soft-tissue washer placed at the isometric points of the femur and tibia.

LCL AND POSTEROLATERAL CORNER

Failure to discriminate between an isolated LCL injury and a combined injury of the LCL and the posterolateral corner results in residual laxity. The association of posterolateral corner injuries with cruciate ligament damage is well chronicled, and failure to recognize the posterolateral corner laxity has been implicated in postreconstruction cruciate laxity, particularly the PCL. In fact, some authors suggested that there is no isolated PCL injury, and all are combined with another knee ligament injury. Given that nonoperative treatment of the posterolateral corner combined with ACL reconstruction leads to failure of the ACL by stretch of the graft, similar results are expected with isolated PCL reconstruction and nonoperative treatment of the posterolateral corner.

Surgical anatomy has been detailed by Terry and La-Prade.[65] We refer readers to this excellent investigational anatomic study.

Isolated complete LCL injuries, although less common than MCL injuries, also have been treated successfully nonoperatively. Bracing with a hinged-knee functional brace diminishes forces across the healing ligament and allows for gradual resumption of rehabilitation loads. This approach facilitates rapid return to activities. An operative approach is favored in LCL injuries associated with complete posterolateral corner injuries in active patients.

Operative repair or reconstruction offers many options for surgical redress of this underappreciated common knee injury. Again, the number of procedures suggests there is not a consensus of opinion on the correct management of this enigmatic condition. Surgical choices can be divided into those that anatomically address the major components of the posterolateral corner: the LCL, the arcuate ligament, the popliteus, and the popliteal-fibular ligament. The second group of procedures addresses primarily the LCL and may remove a deforming muscle force.

Traditional operative treatment, although not an anatomic reconstruction of the posterolateral corner, results in improved knee stability. The Clancy biceps tenodesis to the isometric femoral attachment has proved to be simple and reliable. A lateral hockey-stick incision allows the biceps to be exposed and separated from the peroneal nerve. Care must be taken with the peroneal nerve because of the association of peroneal nerve injury with lateral knee injuries and the susceptibility of this nerve to stretch injury. The damaged LCL is explored through its length and the femoral epicondyle exposed through a split in the ITB. The ligament can be sutured if it is acutely torn. The common biceps tendon is separated from the muscle fibers of the short head of the biceps. A Kirschner wire or guide wire for a cannulated screw can be positioned in the superior insertional fibers of the LCL. A 1.2 × 2.5-cm trough is created at the insertion of the LCL fibers. A 6.5-mm screw with a soft-tissue washer is then placed just superior to the lateral femoral epicondyle at the center of the trough, securing biceps tendon and attached muscle to the epicondyle. This reconstruction restores lateral stability and removes a portion of the external rotation force on the proximal tibia. The biceps tenodesis restored knee stability and returned patients with the multiple ligament–injured knee or the PCL-injured knee to activities with intermediate follow-up.[63, 66]

Alternatively, a portion of the biceps tendon can be transferred to the lateral femoral condyle, leaving the remaining portion of the biceps tendon attached to the biceps muscle (Fig. 7). This approach leaves the remaining tendon attached at its insertion on the posterior aspect of the proximal fibula. A third of the biceps tendon is isolated from the surrounding tendon after separating the tendon from the peroneal nerve. The tendon is passed under the ITB to the area of the lateral femoral epicondyle. The isometric point of the lateral femoral epicondyle determines the position of fixation (see Fig. 7). Fixation is provided with a screw and soft-tissue washer. This technique provides reliable restoration of lateral stability and maintains biceps attachment on the proximal fibula, a source of knee proprioceptive protection.

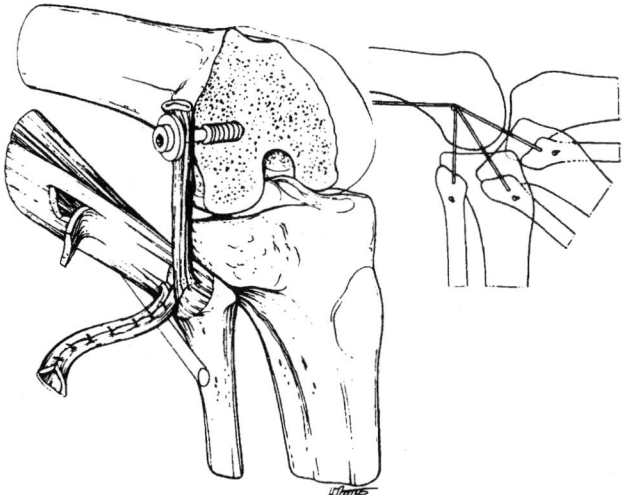

Fig. 7. The tenodesis of the biceps tendon to the lateral femoral epicondyle. The central third of the biceps tendon can be used to anatomically reconstruct the lateral cruciate ligament (LCL). Isometric femoral placement is achieved by examining graft position relative to a Kirschner wire placed at the proposed ligament fixation site. (Reprinted with permission from Veltri DM, Warren RF: Treatment of acute and chronic injuries to the posterolateral and lateral knee. Op Tech Sports Med 1996; 4:174.)

Similarly, the lateral collateral portion of the PLC can be reconstructed with the BPTB allograft, which in one series effectively improved knee function and patient outlook. The isometric area of the lateral epicondyle is selected for a femoral tunnel, and the bone plug is placed in the femoral tunnel and fixed with an interference screw. The proximal fibula is cleared of soft tissue and a tunnel is created. The distal end of the graft is impacted in the proximal fibula and fixed with an interference screw. A 0.0062-inch diameter Kirschner wire can be used as a joy stick to control the bone plugs and properly place them in the bone tunnels.[67]

The anatomic reconstructions attempt to add an oblique vector to the reconstruction in addition to restoring lateral stability. A typical reconstruction uses the isometric point on the femoral epicondyle for proximal location of the graft. The distal insertion of the graft is bifed: one distal limb of the graft attaches to the proximal anterior fibula and the other limb attaches to the posterolateral tibia or posterior fibula, giving the graft an inverted-Y appearance.[68] The majority of grafts can be split into limbs to accommodate an anatomic reconstruction; therefore, graft choices include allograft and autograft tissue.

Comparative prospectively randomized studies are not available, so definitive conclusions regarding treatment of the lateral-sided injuries are not possible. Rather than including comparative studies of two or three different techniques of surgical reconstruction or repair, the reported series involves only one technique in intermediate follow-up. Thus, it is not possible to contrast the results of surgery in different areas such as post-treatment laxity, return to activities, and speed of neuromuscular function.

ACL RECONSTRUCTION

Our technique of transtibial ACL reconstruction, which has evolved from Darren L. Johnson's experience at the University of Pittsburgh, is suitable for all available graft choices. Endoscopic placement of the femoral tunnel is similar in all outcome parameters compared with the traditional arthroscopic two-incision technique. Variation in incision is required for access to different graft choices (see Fig. 4). An endoscopic approach improves cosmesis and avoids a second incision in the area of the quadriceps muscle, speeding neuromuscular return and decreasing muscle atrophy.

Alignment of the limb is of obvious importance, and Noyes et al[69] in particular are responsible for this emphasis. Knees with dynamic varus thrust and specifically those with deficient posterolateral structures should be considered for either staged or concomitant high tibial osteotomy. Failure to address this clinical constellation results in ACL graft failure.

BPTB GRAFT

With the patient in the supine position, a tourniquet is placed around the upper thigh as close to the groin as possible. The leg holder is placed over the tourniquet in a slightly angled position to provide flexion to the pelvis. The well leg is positioned in hip abduction and flexion, which also provides pelvic flexion to avoid back strain during surgical reconstruction (Fig. 8).

The patella tendon harvest incision parallels and is placed at the medial border of the patella tendon. Through that same incision, the anterior medial portal and the tibial tunnel can be drilled. Note that the incision can be moved proximally and distally to harvest the bone plugs so as to minimize the length of incision. Extension of the knee allows skin mobility while the patella tendon is harvested.

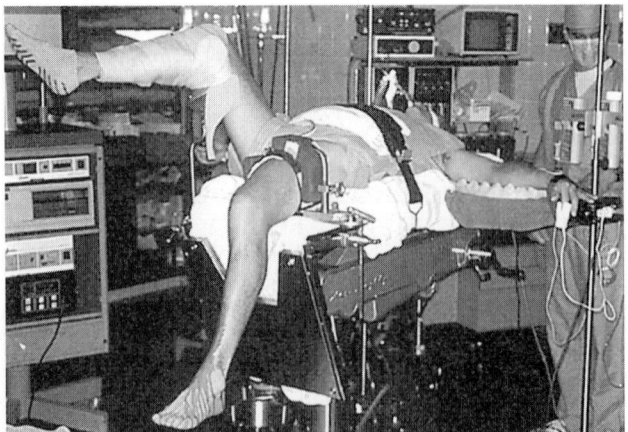

Fig. 8. Patient positioning. This is appropriate patient positioning for knee reconstructive surgery. Note the padding of the uninjured right leg and positioning of the injured left lower extremity. (Reprinted with permission from Miller MD, Harner CD, Koshiwaguchi S: Acute posterior cruciate ligament injuries. The dislocated knee. In Fu FH, Harner CD, Vince KG (eds): Knee Surgery. Baltimore, Williams & Wilkins, p 749.)

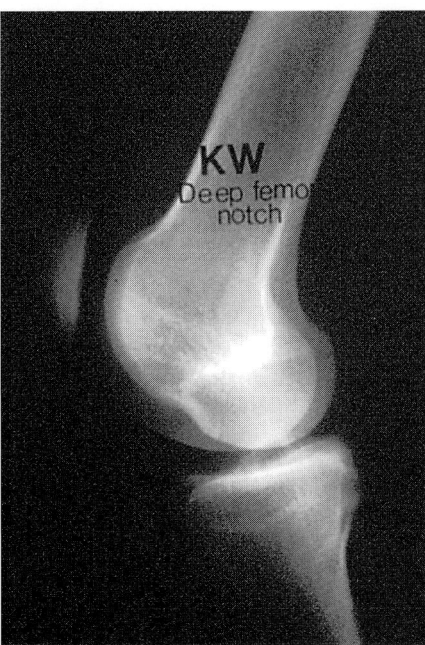

Fig. 9. Deepened femoral sulcus. The deepened femoral sulcus provides radiographic evidence of anterior cruciate ligament rupture. This finding results from repeated knee subluxation.

Pain on kneeling with this incision probably has been overstated, because after BPTB the majority of patients are able to kneel comfortably. These findings are documented in a study involving Muslim culture, for which daily kneeling is required.

If the diagnosis of anterolateral instability is not in doubt, the graft is harvested before the diagnostic arthroscopy is performed. This will shorten operating time and allow graft preparation by a second surgeon while the operating surgeon proceeds with arthroscopy. The tibial bone plug is harvested after the middle third of the patella tendon has been isolated. A small air-powered saw can be used on the cortical bone, and the cancellous portion of the bone plug can be completed with a narrow osteotome. The tibial bone plug and the tendon can be held with a moist sponge to move the patella distally and place the harvest site in the proximal aspect of the wound. The same steps are used to harvest the patella bone plug, and the defect is filled with bone graft from the tibial tunnel. Bone plugs are contoured to fit in 10-mm bone tunnels; however, 9-mm tunnels can be used in small knees. The tibial bone plug usually has a bone step-off where the patella tendon attaches to the tibial tubercle. We prefer to put this step-off in the femoral socket and delineate the bone plug–tendon junction with a skin marker line. The intended femoral bone plug is then contoured to a tapered tip to slide easily into the bone socket. Holes (0.0062 inch) are drilled to pass suture through the bone plug. Sutures are passed with the lead suture as close to the tapered tip of the bone plug as possible to ease graft passage. After the graft passes easily through the appropriate graft sleeves, it is placed on a moist saline sponge until ready for passage.

As an alternative to passing with a lead suture and a Beath pin, a joystick is simple to construct and avoids passing the Beath pin through the vastus lateralis. In patients with a short, thick thigh, the pin exits close to the leg holder, a situation that is avoided with the joystick. A 0.0062-inch Kirschner wire is then drilled into the tendon side of the intended femoral bone plug. To avoid splitting the bone plug lengthwise, one is advised to make a pilot hole with a small rongeur.

After graft preparation, diagnostic arthroscopy is performed via the anteromedial portal placement through the harvest incision, which will eliminate a separate skin incision. Both the anteromedial and anterolateral incisions should be placed at the same level as the inferior pole of the patella and adjacent to the patella tendon. By using an arthroscopy cannula with two ports, a separate inflow portal through the quadriceps muscle can be avoided. Meniscus disorder is addressed first, favoring repair over resection because of the favorable results of meniscus-sparing techniques in concert with ACL reconstruction. As chondral replacement and regenerative techniques are simplified and efficacy is documented, these procedures will be done concomitantly with ligament reconstruction. However, at this time débridement and microfracture may be preferred, with staging chondral reconstruction as a second procedure after knee stabilization.

Controversy exists regarding the residual ACL tissue. Those who advocate maintaining the stump propose it is a source of vascularity and proprioceptive fibers to the newly implanted graft. However, the residual ACL may not adhere to the graft and instead become loose fibrous material in the anterior aspect of the notch, leading to a cyclops lesion (Figs. 9–12).

Other than the A-frame or the stenotic notch (Fig. 13), notchplasty is performed to improve visualization rather than to reduce graft impingement. It is imperative that the surgeon understand how graft impingment relates to proper tunnel position rather than rely solely on notchplasty for relief of graft impingement. Excessive notchplasty will alter tunnel position and remove articular cartilage. Notch-

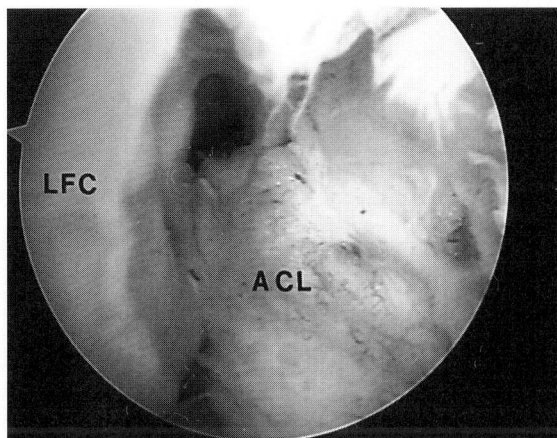

Fig. 10. Empty lateral wall sign. The attachment of the anterior cruciate ligament (ACL) is absent from its insertion on the lateral femoral condyle (LFC).

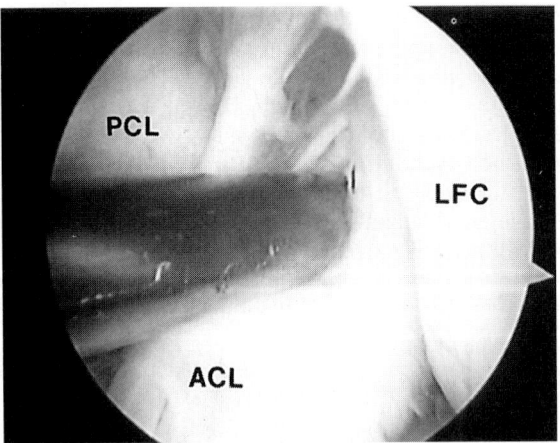

Fig. 11. Abnormal insertion of the anterior cruciate ligament (ACL). The ACL insertion does not normally allow passage of the smooth trocar through its insertion.

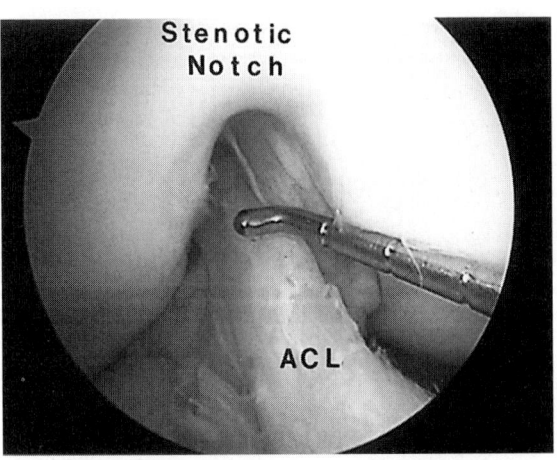

Fig. 13. Stenotic notch. This picture is representative of an A-frame notch, which will require a more complete notchplasty than is typically performed. The tip of the probe is 3 mm in length.

plasty regrowth has been noted on second-look arthroscopy. Hamstring grafts require less bone removal than the patella tendon grafts because of the smaller tunnel diameters. At our institution, a powered shaver with a 5.5-mm full-radius resector at 3 to 5000 rpm allows controlled removal of bone. Metal debris has occurred with this technique in very hard bone, and in this instance one can switch to a high-speed bone bur.

The tibial tunnel is created in the posterior medial aspect of the ACL. The tibial tunnel guide should be positioned at 55 degrees because a flat or horizontal tibial tunnel will lead to posterior femoral blow-out. The ideal location is 6 to 7 mm anterior to the PCL, with the guide pin entering the knee on the lateral downslope of the medial tibial eminence (Fig. 14A). Posterior position is confirmed by extending the knee to evaluate notch impingement on the guide pin. The entrance of the tibial tunnel should be located midway between the tibial tubercle and posterior margin of the medial face of the tibia. Fatal flaws include a tibial tunnel positioned too anteriorly and laterally. Anterior tibial tunnels allow the graft to be guillotined by the notch

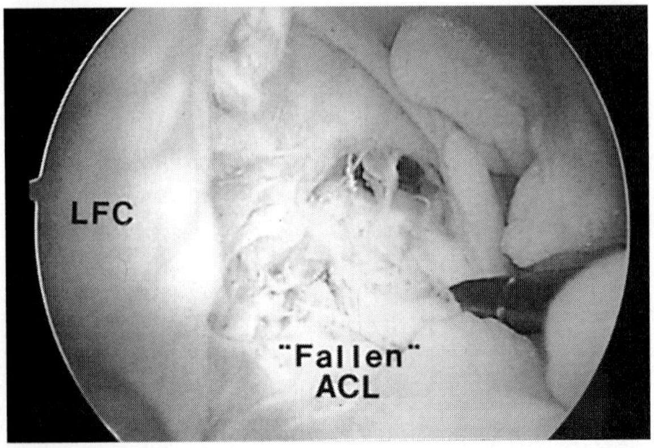

and do not provide a posterior femoral tunnel placement. Lateral tibial positions impinge on the notch and do not restore tension to the PCL. Tibial tunnel position dictates femoral tunnel location, and tunnel malposition is the most common cause of ACL graft failure.[70]

A Beath pin through the tibial tunnel can be used to locate the center of the intended femoral tunnel (see Fig. 14B). A femoral guide is not necessary and orients the femoral tunnel more vertically than is desired. The usual error is anterior placement of the femoral tunnel, and one avoids this by removing the resident's ridge to ensure posterior placement of the femoral tunnel. The adequacy of notchplasty is best evaluated by the visualization of the over-the-top position, and the posterior edge of the femoral tunnel should abut the over-the-top position (see Fig. 14C). The center position of the tunnel is then placed at the 1:30 mark for a left knee or the 10:30 mark for a right knee. Tunnel depth should be approximately 35 mm to allow for seating of the bone plug (see Fig. 14D). The anterior edge of the tunnel is then chamfered and smoothed with a powered shaver and a 5.5-mm full-radius resector at 3 to 5000 rpm. Passage of the Beath pin through the skin precedes graft passage. Again, excessive bone removal during notchplasty positions the graft too proximal on the femur, and care should be taken to avoid this.

The lead sutures are passed through the eyelet of the Beath pin, and the pin is advanced out through the skin. The graft advances into the tibial tunnel by tensile load to the lead sutures with a Kocher clamp applied to the sutures. Once the graft is in the knee, an arthroscopic probe can be used to direct the graft into the femoral tunnel. Note that the edge of the bone plug should be even with the edge of the femoral tunnel. Interference screws, either biodegradable or metal, provide adequate fixation for early weightbearing and rehabilitative loads. Smooth passage of the screw through the anteromedial portal is ensured by passing a no. 11 blade via the portal to its intended destination at the anterior edge of the femoral tunnel. The cannulated screw guide wire precedes the interference screw (see Fig. 14E). The femoral tunnel can be notched to accommodate the screw, but this is not usually necessary.

Fig. 12. Fallen anterior cruciate ligament (ACL). The injured ACL has lost the normal tension in the ligament and is not normally inserted on the lateral wall of the notch.

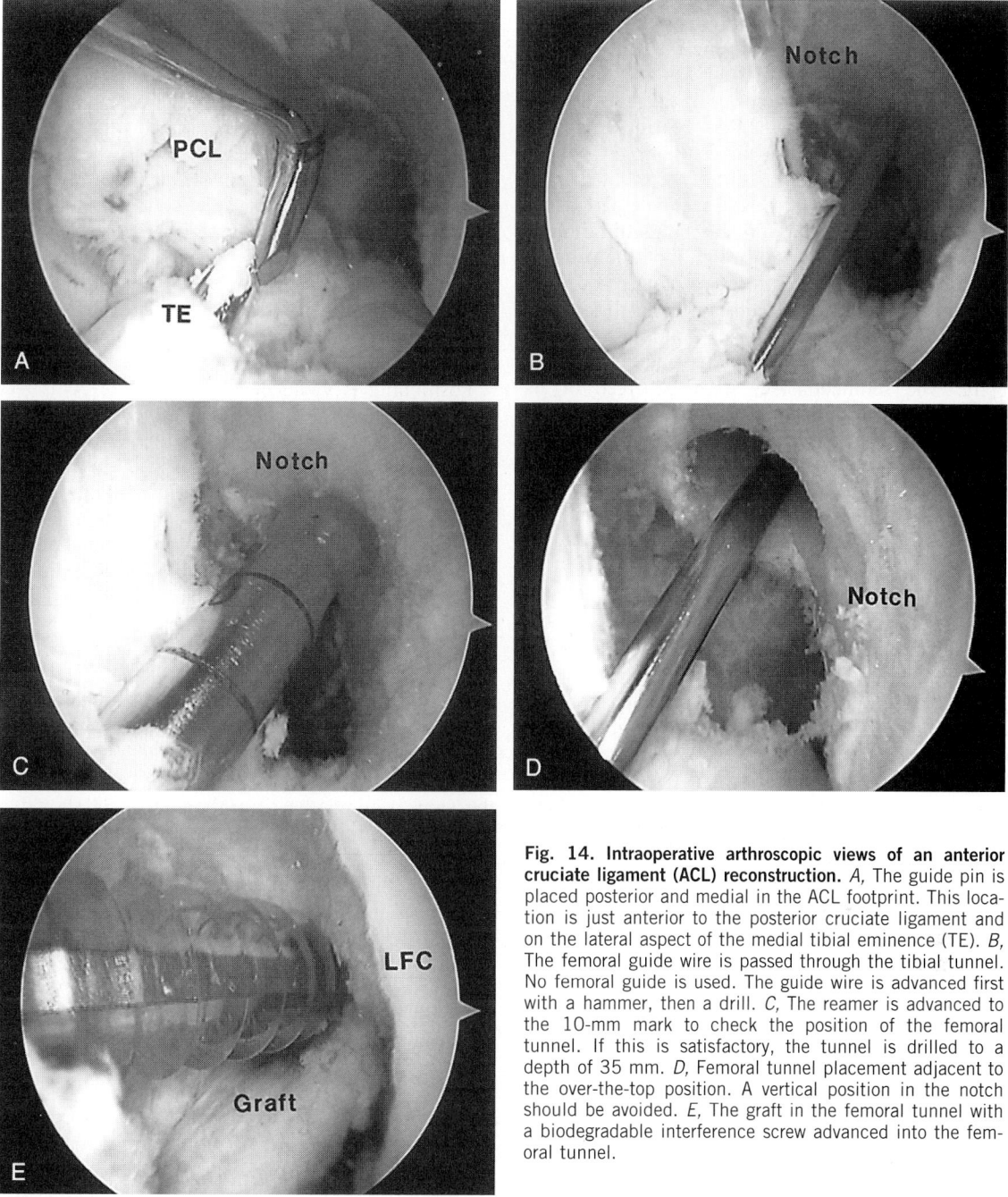

Fig. 14. Intraoperative arthroscopic views of an anterior cruciate ligament (ACL) reconstruction. *A,* The guide pin is placed posterior and medial in the ACL footprint. This location is just anterior to the posterior cruciate ligament and on the lateral aspect of the medial tibial eminence (TE). *B,* The femoral guide wire is passed through the tibial tunnel. No femoral guide is used. The guide wire is advanced first with a hammer, then a drill. *C,* The reamer is advanced to the 10-mm mark to check the position of the femoral tunnel. If this is satisfactory, the tunnel is drilled to a depth of 35 mm. *D,* Femoral tunnel placement adjacent to the over-the-top position. A vertical position in the notch should be avoided. *E,* The graft in the femoral tunnel with a biodegradable interference screw advanced into the femoral tunnel.

After the femoral fixation is deemed secure, the surgeon cycles the knee through an arc of 0 to 120 degrees to check isometry and prestretch the graft. Isometry of less than 3 mm is desired. Preloading the graft removes creep, which may create knee laxity with rehabilitation. Tension should be applied to the graft through the bone plug suture as tibial fixation with an interference screw is performed.

Graft impingement, either superiorly or laterally, is excluded with arthroscopic evaluation before wound closure. A hinged brace will provide stability while quadriceps and hamstring strength return and yet protect from unplanned or sudden movements. A progressive rehabilitation protocol with emphasis on functional activities and neuromuscular exercises will significantly speed return to sporting activities.

QH GRAFT

Contrasting the QH grafts with the BPTB will involve graft harvest, preparation, and fixation. The described technique for ACL reconstruction is adaptable to either graft choice.

A small longitudinal incision, 3 to 4 cm in length, located 1 cm medial to the border of the tibial tubercle and centered three fingerbreadths below the medial joint line will access the pes anserine. The gracilis and semitendinosus are palpable under the skin in thin patients. Subcutaneous fat needs to be separated after opening the incision.

The pes anserine veils the hamstring tendons with thick fascia, which is split parallel to the length of the tibia to release the fascia and the hamstring tendons at their insertion in the medial tibia. An incision in the fascia parallel to the gracilis and semitendinosus, at the superior border of the gracilis, exposes them on the undersurface of the pes anserine fascia. The superior of the two tendons, the gracilis, is rounder and smaller than its counterpart. Both are harvested in the same fashion. A baseball whipstitch of no. 5 Ethibond will secure the distal end of the tendon. Soft-tissue attachments should give way to finger and scissor dissection, until the gracilis protrudes from the wound and moves with a characteristic muscle bounce. A closed-end tendon harvester can then strip the tendon from the muscle belly. The semitendinosus must be freed of its constant attachment to the medial head of the gastrocnemius or the tendon stripper will make a false passage prematurely, amputating the tendon and occasioning a review of other graft options. Pes fascia closure with 2-0 Vicryl facilitates reconstitution of the hamstring tendons, which has been verified with imaging studies.

Muscle from the soft-tissue grafts is removed with an osteotome or knife and forceps. A baseball whipstitch with a no. 5 braided nonabsorbable suture secures each of the four ends of the hamstring grafts. The double-stranded grafts are then quadrupled over a no. 5 braided nonabsorbable suture or a closed-loop EndoButton under tension on a graft board. We use the same suture with a whipstitch on the quadrupled end of the graft.

The controversy surrounding graft fixation of soft-tissue grafts is summarized in the graft fixation section. Currently, soft-tissue fixation is characterized by a series of trade-offs that often are individualized to surgeon and patient demands.

QUADRICEPS TENDON

The quadriceps tendon is harvested through a short longitudinal incision directly over the tendon and proximal pole of the tendon. Fulkerson and Langelan[71] preserved the deep lamina of the tendon and harvested the two superficial lamina of the tendon. The deep lamina maintained joint distention through knee capsule integrity. The bone plug harvest differed little from that of the patella tendon. The tendon of the graft is usually 8 to 9 cm in length, limited by the transition to quadriceps muscle. The defect in the tendon should be closed with absorbable suture.

After stripping the muscle, a baseball whipstitch is placed on each side of the tendon. By placing the tendon end of the graft in the femoral socket and the bone plug in the tibial tunnel, a better match of fixation stiffness at time zero occurs.[72] Because this is not a looped soft-tissue graft, fixation options are limited to those in which suture is linked to a fixation device or interference fixation. Transfixion devices or a closed-loop EndoButton will not suit the quadriceps tendon. Its relatively short length will not allow for a device such as the WasherLoc. Fortunately, the ultimate failure has proved similar between soft-tissue interference fixation and a bone plug interference fixation, although the soft-tissue interference fixation fared poorly under cyclic loads that occur with rehabilitation in this elderly cadaver study.[72]

PCL RECONSTRUCTION

Because of residual postreconstruction laxity, controversy abounds in all aspects of surgical care. Our approach to operative management is emphasized with a discussion of rationale and pertinent options.

Examination under anesthesia determines extent and direction of knee laxity (Fig. 15). Grade II isolated posterior laxity may not be restored to normal knee kinematics given current techniques. A frank discussion with the patient preoperatively will avoid uncomfortable confrontation over persistent symptoms after reconstruction. Concomitant instability must not be ignored; in particular, lateral and PCL instability may be prevalent to the point of being universal.

Positioning is identical to the knee for ACL reconstruction. Coexisting knee disease treatment follows the guidelines discussed for ACL reconstruction. The PCL is débrided to the tibial attachment; care is taken to avoid stripping the posterior capsule from the tibia, allowing fluid extravasation into the posterior calf. Although this can be accomplished through the usual anteromedial and anterolateral portals, most authors advocate shaver placement through an accessory posteromedial portal. The Accufex (Smith & Nephew DonJoy) (Fig. 16) tibial ACL reconstruction guide allows for proper orientation and position of the PCL tibial tunnel. The skin incision is located by trial placement of the guide through the anteromedial portal and scope placement through the anterolateral portal. The tibial tunnel can be performed through a small 4- to 5-cm tibial skin incision. If an ACL reconstruction is planned at the same setting, the tibial bone tunnels should be separated by a 1.5-cm bone bridge. From medial to lateral, the tibial tunnel entrance is midway between the anterior tibial crest and the posteromedial border of the tibia. Posterior and lateral positioning is selected on the tibial footprint of the PCL to replicate the anterolateral bundle, which is five-sixths of the mechanical strength of the PCL (see Fig. 16). Visualization of the guide wire on entry into the joint precludes arterial or neural damage, which presents the most morbid complication of this procedure. A large-an-

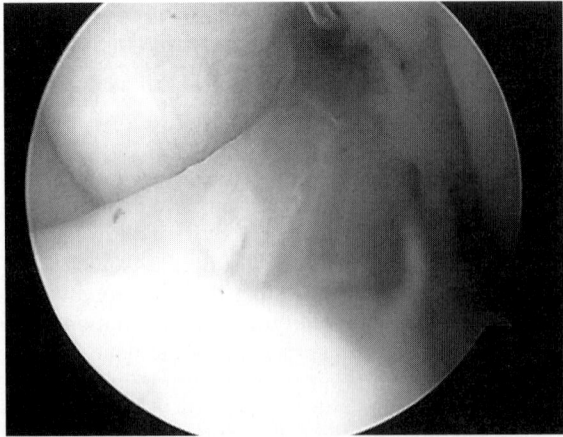

Fig. 15. Pseudolaxity of the anterior cruciate ligament (ACL). Because of the posterior subluxation of the tibia with respect to the femur, the ACL appears to have laxity. This does not represent a tear of the ACL.

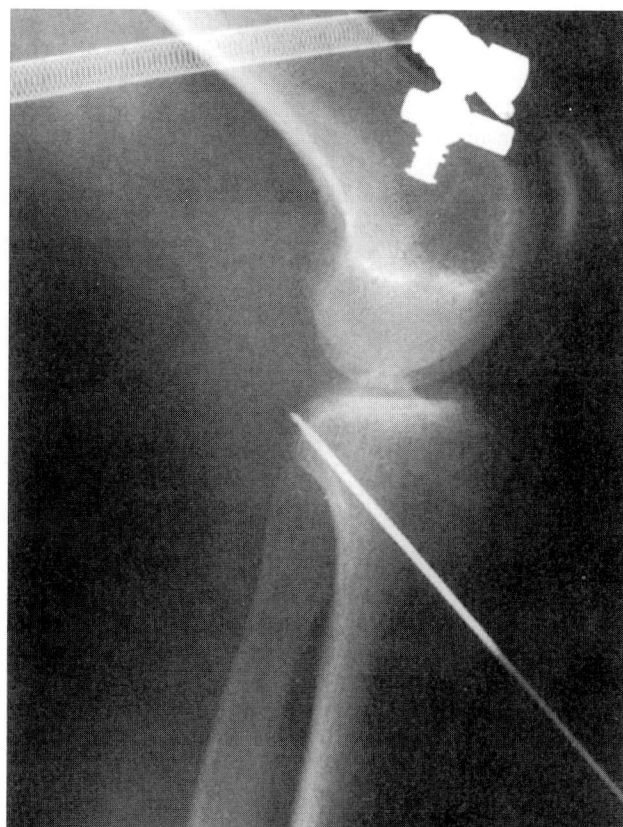

Fig. 16. Posterior cruciate ligament (PCL) tibial tunnel position. A lateral radiograph showing the guide pin located in the distal portion of the PCL tibial insertion.

gled curet through the posteromedial portal protects the posterior capsule from damage as the large-bore reamer advanced by hand creates the tibial tunnel. Graft selection determines tunnel diameter.

An outside-in technique avoids a vastus medialis incision which is particularly important in rehabilitation post-PCL reconstruction. A lack of consensus defines PCL femoral tunnel position. The tunnel for the anterolateral band ideally is reamed at the 1:30/10:30 position with the anterior edge of the tunnel at the margin of the articular cartilage. If a second tunnel for the posteromedial band of the PCL is selected, 3:00/9:00 and 5- to 6-mm posterior to the first tunnel are the desired coordinates. The arthroscope must be switched to the anteromedial portal, and the reamer approaches the medial femoral condyle through the anterolateral portal. Tunnel depth matches graft choice but is not usually bicortical.

Arguably, graft passage represents the technical challenge of this procedure. Use of the arthroscope blunt trocar inserted through the posteromedial portal serves as a pulley to improve passage of the graft through the tibial tunnel into the knee by diminishing the acute angle between the tibial tunnel and the intercondylar notch. The graft is passed in two stages. The first involves passage through the tibial tunnel around the arthroscopic trocar pulley into the knee (Fig. 17). Second, the Beath passing pin through the anterolateral portal and out the femoral tunnel will

allow passage of the graft from the knee into the femoral tunnel. If a double femoral tunnel socket technique is selected, the steps are repeated for each tail of the two-tailed graft.

Interference fixation of the femoral end of the graft, either bone plug or soft tissue, through the anterolateral portal is technically simple and, because of the deadman's angle of the graft entry into the femoral socket, secure as well. When interference fixation of the tibial end of the graft is used, the advantage lies with the biodegradable screw. Tibial interference fixation screws are often placed deep in the tibia because of graft length, which complicates future hardware extrication. Tibial interference screws have complicated secondary reconstructive procedures such as high tibial osteotomy. The tibial screw position against the graft can be confirmed by placing the arthroscope in the tibial tunnel. We recommend back-up fixation to the soft-tissue interference screws with soft-tissue grafts such as post and suture or, if graft length allows, post with a soft-tissue washer. The anterolateral bundle is tensioned in 90 degrees of knee flexion and the posteromedial bundle in 30 degrees of knee flexion to replicate the positions of maximum bundle tension in the native ligament.

A rehabilitative hinged-knee brace allows early protected weightbearing. Rehabilitation protocols lag those of the ACL reconstruction, with emphasis on neuromuscular return and patellar mobility.

Because of postreconstructive knee laxity, research efforts have focused on technical aspects of the procedure. Tibial onlay of patella tendon bone plug has been proposed to reduce the angle at which the graft enters the knee at the posterior tibia, the so-called "killer turn," and ensure posterior placement of the graft. This technique reduces the risk associated with creating a tunnel on the posterior aspect of the tibia but does require an additional incision for

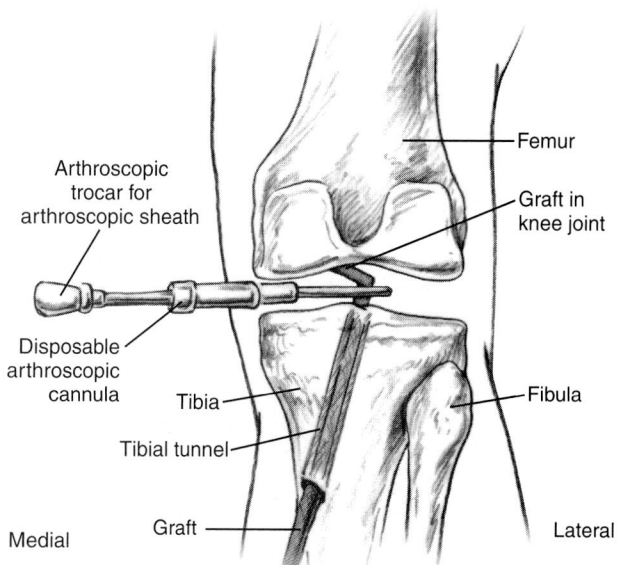

Fig. 17. Graft passage. A blunt trocar passed through the posteromedial arthroscopic portal under the graft will diminish the acute angle at which the graft enters the knee from the tibial tunnel.

graft placement.[40] The PCL femoral attachment approximates 3 cm from proximal to distal, which is poorly replicated by the present reconstructive techniques of the anterolateral bundle. Biomechanically, two bundle techniques provide superior isometry with an expected reduction in graft motion compared with one-bundle techniques.[73] Allograft tissue historically has been more popular in PCL surgery than ACL reconstruction. In ACL reconstruction, allografts in some reports have increased postreconstruction laxity compared with autograft tissue and may play a role in knee laxity after PCL reconstruction. Finally, failure to address concomitant knee instability, particularly the posterolateral corner, will lead to laxity after the "isolated" PCL has been reconstructed.

MULTIPLE LIGAMENT–INJURED KNEE

Generally considered rare, the multiple ligament–injured knee may be more common than we appreciate. A spectrum exists between the high-velocity knee dislocation and the low-velocity or sports-related multiple ligament–injured knee (Fig. 18). The multiple ligament–injured knee can be missed, particularly by primary care physicians who increasingly provide care to this patient population.

Although a knee dislocation usually represents substantial damage to the ACL, PCL, and one of the collaterals, case reports have detailed injuries of only two ligaments.[8] The multiple ligament–injured knee should raise the suspicion of vascular injury, which occurs in up to one-third of dislocations, and neural injury, which may be up to 40% with the peroneal nerve the most commonly affected. Anterior and posterior dislocations are the most common and the most commonly associated with vascular injury. Arteriogram indications have diminished. If the pulses are absent and the foot is frankly ischemic, operative repair in 6 to 8 hours by a trained vascular surgeon is mandatory and the arteriogram causes a delay in this treatment plan. If ischemic time is prolonged, fasciotomies must accompany the vascular repair or grafting. At the other end of the spectrum is the patient with normal pulses, healthy-appearing foot, Doppler's signals that are of normal amplitude, and vascular consultation. This situation can be safely observed with little or no chance of vascular occlusion. In between these two extremes in the clinical spectrum, the arteriogram may be of benefit.

Neural injuries are managed expectantly; serial electromyograms give information regarding extent of damage and prognosis. However, with or without surgical repair, functional return may not be much better than a 50% chance.

A knee dislocation should be reduced on an emergent basis using traction and countertraction. The indications for emergent surgery are an open dislocation, vascular injury, and an irreducible dislocation. The hallmark of the irreducible dislocation is a "dimple sign," created in a lateral or posterolateral dislocation by the medial femoral condyle buttonholed through the capsule with the MCL trapped in the knee joint. In this case, an attempt at a closed reduction should be deferred to an open reduction in the operating room. If the patient is in the operating room, primary ligament suture of the collaterals, the joint capsule, and tagging of damaged nerve ends is prudent. Primary reconstruction of the cruciate ligaments awaits elective scheduling to avoid arthrofibrosis.

"In all studies, however, it is clear that nonoperative treatment can result in a very functional knee joint."[8] The operative treatment one selects must meet this high standard. Treatment options, including bracing, cruciate ligament suture, isolated PCL reconstruction, and reconstruction of both cruciate ligaments, have never been evaluated in a comparative trial, much less a prospective randomized study. Older comparative trials compared older techniques without current rehabilitative methods. Maintenance of knee extension, by whatever means of treatment, must be a priority and occurs more reliably with bracing in extension. A significant persistent flexion contracture retards quadriceps function, leads to anterior knee pain, precludes a normal gait, and diminishes the return to activities.

As in traumatic injuries, timing of ligament reconstruction determines outcome. Although this has not been scientifically validated, the knee capsule heals at 7 to 10 days, allowing arthroscopy without fluid extravasation. Reconstruction within 3 to 4 weeks usually allows return of neuromuscular function, yet does not significantly add to the recovery time after reconstruction. This represents a window for ligament reconstruction. The benefit of acute ACL reconstruction compared with chronic ligament reconstruction has been well accepted. This approach avoids duplicating rehabilitation periods—one from the injury and one from the surgery—and may improve postreconstruction knee laxity.

Preoperative planning trumps surgical execution in most operative situations. Graft selection, choice of which ligaments and structures to address, and technique of surgical approach are among issues to consider. Allografts hasten operating time, decrease additional trauma, and represent our preference in graft selection for this difficult reconstructive problem. In the acute situation, the MCL can be treated as it is in ACL reconstruction.[63] All agree that

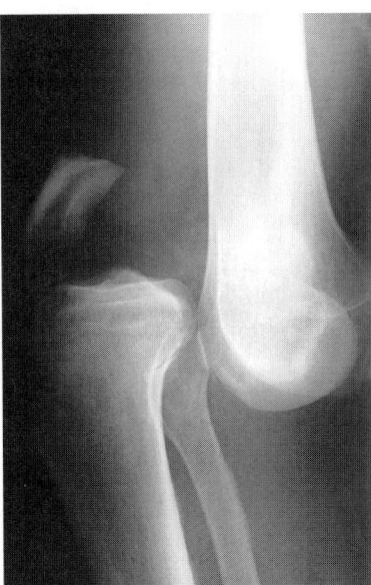

Fig. 18. Radiograph of a knee dislocation. This is an unreduced anterior knee dislocation, named for the position of the tibia with respect to the femur.

significant lateral and posterolateral corner instability should be surgically stabilized; however, the choice of technique to this end is not as unanimous. More controversy yet surrounds the approach to the cruciate ligament reconstruction. Repair of PCL bony avulsions resulted in satisfactory results in a 1985 report, as opposed to ACL bony avulsion repairs. The repair of ACL avulsions was not as successful in return of objective knee stability.[74] Isolated PCL reconstruction to center the knee has been proposed and reported in three patients with short-term good results; two of these patients returned to athletics.[75]

The best results in the literature have combined ACL and PCL reconstruction, with a high return to sporting activities, excellent objective knee stability, and gratifying patient satisfaction.[63] Twenty patients were included in this series. MCL injury treatment consisted of bracing, the biceps tenodesis as described by Clancy stabilized the PLC, 14 of 20 grafts used for PCL reconstruction were allografts, and 16 of the 20 grafts were autografts for the ACL reconstruction. The two tibial tunnels are separated by a bone bridge of at least 1.5 cm. Graft tensioning progresses sequentially with the posterolateral corner first at 30 degrees, followed by the PCL at 70 degrees to restore the normal tibial step, and finally the ACL at 70 degrees. Postoperatively, a hinged-knee rehabilitative brace protects the reconstructions for 10 weeks. For the first 3 weeks the knee is maintained in extension. A posterior calf pad in the brace diminishes the posterior-directed forces on the tibia and preserves reduction of the knee. Progressive knee range of motion is initiated at 4 to 6 weeks postoperatively. By 9 months, depending on rehabilitation progress, the patient is cleared for athletic participation and all patients participate in sporting activities without restriction. Following this program, excellent knee stability was realized; 75% of the patients had a normal Lachman's test, 85% had a normal pivot shift, and 55% had grade I posterior laxity.[63] These results rival those of isolated ligament reconstruction.

CONCLUSIONS

Sound preoperative decision making, graft selection, fixation, and addressing concomitant instability arguably impact outcome to a greater extent than intraoperative choices. For example, patella tendon grafting of the ACL with preexisting patella chondromalacia affects outcome more than minor tunnel malposition. Principles of graft selection and fixation have been discussed. Collateral ligament principles and treatment often determine results of cruciate ligament surgery. The outlined techniques of cruciate ligament surgery adapt to different graft choices and fixation without a substantive change in approach. Finally, surgical repair and reconstruction of damaged structures early in the recovery process may improve outcome in the multiple ligament–injured knee.

REFERENCES

1. Frank C, Jackson D: The science of reconstruction of the anterior cruciate ligament. J Bone Joint Surg Am 1997; 79:1556.
2. Van Dommelen B, Fowler P: Anatomy of the posterior cruciate ligament: A review. Am J Sports Med 1989; 17:24.
3. Naranja R, Corsetti J, Kuhlman J, et al: The search for the holy grail: A century of anterior cruciate ligament reconstruction. Am J Orthop 1997; 26:743.
4. Zaricznyj B: Reconstruction of the anterior cruciate ligament using free tendon graft. Am J Sports Med 1983; 11:164.
5. Marshall J, Warren R, Wickiewicz T, et al: Reconstruction of the ACL: Preliminary report using a quadriceps tendon. Orthop Rev 1979; 8:49.
6. Eriksson E, Haggmark T, Johnson R: Reconstruction of the posterior cruciate ligament. Orthopaedics 1986; 9:217.
7. Clancy W, Shelbourne K, Zoellner G, et al: Treatment of knee joint instability secondary to rupture of the posterior cruciate ligament: Report of a new procedure. J Bone Joint Surg Am 1983; 65:310.
8. Taft T, Almkinders L (eds): The Dislocated Knee. Baltimore, Williams & Wilkins, 1995.
9. Race A, Amis A: The mechanical properties of the two bundles of the human posterior cruciate ligament. J Biomech 1994; 27:13.
10. Fu F, Harner C, Johnson D, et al: Biomechanics of knee ligaments: Basic concepts and clinical application. J Bone Joint Surg Am 1993; 75:1716.

11. Noyes F, Butler D, Grood E: Biomechanical analysis of human ligament grafts used in knee-ligament repairs and reconstructions. J Bone Joint Surg Am 1984; 66:344.
12. Woo S, Hollis J, Adams D, et al: Tensile properties of the human femur-anterior cruciate ligament-tibia complex: The effects of specimen age and orientation. Am J Sports Med 1991; 19:217.
13. Noyes F, Barber-Westin S: Reconstruction of the anterior cruciate ligament with human allograft: Comparison of early and late results. J Bone Joint Surg Am 1996; 78:524.
14. Shelton W, Papendick L, Dukes A: Autograft versus allograft anterior cruciate ligament reconstruction. Arthroscopy 1997; 13:446.
15. Aglietti P, Buzzi B, Zaccherotti G, et al: Patellar tendon versus doubled semitendinosus and gracilis tendons for anterior cruciate ligament reconstruction. Am J Sports Med 1994; 22:211.
16. Marder R, Raskind J, Carroll M: Prospective evaluation of arthroscopically assisted anterior cruciate ligament reconstruction: Patellar tendon versus semitendinosus and gracilis tendons. Am J Sports Med 1991; 19:478.
17. Shelbourne K, Gray T: Anterior cruciate ligament reconstruction with autogenous patellar tendon graft followed by accelerated rehabilitation: A two- to nine-year follow-up. Am J Sports Med 1997; 25:786.
18. Snyder-Mackler L, Deltto A, Bailey S, et

al: Strength of the quadriceps femoris muscle and functional recovery after reconstruction of the anterior cruciate ligament: A prospective, randomized clinical trial of electrical stimulation. J Bone Joint Surg Am 1995; 77:1166.
19. Victor J, Bellemans J, Witvrouw E, et al: Graft selection in anterior cruciate ligament reconstruction—Prospective analysis of patellar tendon autografts compared with allografts. Int Orthop 1997; 21:93.
20. Otero A, Hutcheson L: A comparison of the doubled semitendinosus/gracilis and central third of the patella tendon autografts in arthroscopic anterior cruciate ligament reconstruction. Arthroscopy 1993; 9:143.
21. Harner C, Olson E, Irrgang J, et al: Allograft versus autograft anterior cruciate ligament reconstruction: 3- to 5-year outcome. Clin Orthop 1996; 324:134.
22. Buck B, Malinin T, Brown M: Bone transplantation and human immunodeficiency virus: An estimated risk of acquired immunodeficiency syndrome (AIDS). Clin Orthop 1989; 240:129.
23. Buck B, Resnick L, Shah S, et al: Human immunodeficiency virus cultured from bone. Clin Orthop 1990; 251:249.
24. Butler D, Noyes F, Walz K, et al: Biomechanics of human knee ligament allograft treatment. Trans Orthop Res Soc 1987; 12:128.
25. Noyes F, Barber S, Mangine R: Bone-patellar ligament-bone and fascia-lata allografts for reconstruction of the anterior

cruciate ligament. J Bone Joint Surg Am 1990; 72:1125.

26. Bright R, Green W: Freeze-dried fascia lata allografts: A review of 47 cases. J Pediatr Orthop 1981; 1:13.

27. Fu F: Using bioabsorbable interference screw fixation for hamstring ACL-reconstruction. Orthop Today 1997; 16:36.

28. Ishibashi Y, Rudy T, Kim H, et al: The effect of the ACL graft fixation level on knee stability. Arthroscopy 1997; 13:177.

29. Morgan C: The bone-hamstring-bone composite autograft for the ACL reconstruction. Presented at the 61st Annual Meeting of the American Academy of Orthopaedic Surgeons, New Orleans, LA, 1994.

30. Kohn D, Rose C: Primary stability of interference screw fixation: Influence of screw diameter and insertion torque. Am J Sports Med 1994; 22:334.

31. Brand J, Pienkowski D, Steenlage E, et al: Interference screw fixation strength of quadrupled hamstring tendon graft is directly related to bone mineral density and insertion torque. Am J Sports Med 2000; 28:705.

32. Vuori I, Heinonen A, Sievanen H: Effects of unilateral strength training and detraining on bone mineral density and content in young women: A study of mechanical loading and deloading on human bones. Calcif Tissue Int 1994; 55:59.

33. Malek M, Deluca J, Verch D, et al: Arthroscopically assisted ACL reconstruction using central third patellar tendon autograft with press fit femoral fixation. Am Acad Orthop Surg Instr Course Lect 1996; 45:287.

34. Gerich T, Cassim A, Latterman C, et al: Pullout strength of tibial graft fixation in anterior cruciate ligament replacement with a patellar tendon graft: Interference screw versus staple fixation in human knees. Knee Surg Sports Traumatol Arthrosc 1997; 5:84.

35. Kurosaka M, Yoshiya S, Andrish J: A biomechanical comparison of different surgical techniques of graft fixation of anterior cruciate ligament reconstruction. Am J Sports Med 1987; 15:225.

36. Weiler A, Windhagen H, Raschke M, et al: Biodegradable interference screw fixation exhibits pull-out force and stiffness similar to titanium screws. Am J Sports Med 1998; 26:119.

37. Brown C, Hecker A, Hipp J: The biomechanics of interference screw fixation of patellar tendon anterior cruciate ligament grafts. Am J Sports Med 1993; 21:880.

38. Brown G, Pena F, Grontvedt T, et al: Fixation strength of interference screw fixation in bovine, young human, and elderly human cadaver knees: Influence of insertion torque, tunnel-bone block gap, and interference. Knee Surg Sports Traumatol Arthrosc 1996; 3:238.

39. Matthews L, Soffer S: Pitfalls in the use of interference screws for anterior cruciate ligament reconstruction: Brief report. Arthroscopy 1989; 5:225.

40. Berg E: Autograft bone-patella tendon-bone plug comminution with loss of ligament fixation and stability. Arthroscopy 1996; 12:232.

41. Steiner M, Hecker A, Brown C, et al: Anterior cruciate ligament graft fixation: Comparison of hamstring and patellar tendon grafts. Am J Sports Med 1994; 22:240.

42. Dworsky B, Jewell B, Bach B: Interference screw divergence in endoscopic anterior cruciate ligament reconstruction. Arthroscopy 1996; 12:45.

43. Fanelli G, Desai B, Cummings P, et al: Divergent alignment of the femoral interference screw in single incision endoscopic reconstruction of the anterior cruciate ligament. Contemp Orthop 1994; 28:21.

44. Magen H, Howell S, Hull M: Structural properties of six tibial fixation methods for anterior cruciate ligament soft tissue grafts. Am J Sports Med 1999; 27:35.

45. Brown CH, Hecker AT, Ferragamo M: Comparison of hamstrings and patellar tendon femoral fixation: Cyclic load. Presented at the 25th Annual Meeting of the Academy of Orthopaedic Sports Medicine, Traverse City, MI, 1999.

46. Hamner D, Brown C, Steiner M, et al: Hamstring tendon grafts for reconstruction of the anterior cruciate ligament: Biomechanical evaluation of the use of multiple strands and tensioning techniques. J Bone Joint Surg Am 1999; 81:549.

47. Clark R, Olsen R, Larson B, et al: Cross-pin femoral fixation: A new technique for hamstring anterior cruciate ligament reconstruction of the knee. Arthroscopy 1998; 14:258.

48. Rowden N, Sher D, Rogers G, et al: Anterior cruciate ligament graft fixation: Initial comparison of patellar tendon and semitendinosus autografts in young fresh cadavers. Am J Sports Med 1997; 25:472.

49. Hoher J, Withrow J, Livesay G, et al: Early stress causes graft-tunnel motion in hamstring grafts. Presented at the 44th Annual Meeting of the Orthopaedic Research Society, New Orleans, LA, 1998.

50. L'Insalata J, Klatt F, Fu F, et al: Tunnel expansion following anterior cruciate ligament reconstruction: A comparison of hamstring and patellar tendon autografts. Knee Surg Sports Traumat Arthrosc 1997; 5:234.

51. Caborn D, Coen M, Neef R, et al: Quadrupled semitendinosus-gracilis autograft fixation in the femoral tunnel: A comparison between a metal and a bioabsorbable interference screw. Arthroscopy 1998; 14:241.

52. Weiler A, Hoffman R, Stahelin A, et al: Hamstring tendon fixation using interference screws—A biomechanical study in calf tibial bone. Arthroscopy 1998; 14:29.

53. Brand JC, Caborn DNM, Johnson DL: Is a biodegradable screw comparable to a metal screw for soft tissue interference fixation? Presented at the Meeting of the International Society of Arthroscopy, Knee Surgery and Orthopaedic Sports Medicine, Montreaux, Switzerland, 2001.

54. Weiler A, Hoffman R, Bail HJ: Tendon healing in a bone tunnel—Histological analysis after biodegradable interference fit fixation. Presented at the 18th Annual Meeting of the Arthroscopy Association of North America, Vancouver, British Columbia, 1999.

55. Steenlage E, Brand J, Caborn D, et al: Interference screw fixation of a quadrupled hamstring graft is improved with precise match of tunnel to graft diameter. Arthroscopy 1999; 15:S9.

56. Weiler A, Hoffman R, Siepe C, et al: The influence of screw geometry on hamstring tendon interference fit fixation. Am J Sports Med 2000; 28:356.

57. Selby J, Johnson DL, Hester P, et al: Bioabsorbable interference screw fixation in a bone tunnel: 28 millimeter versus tapered 35 millimeter length screw. Presented at the Annual Meeting of the American Academy of Orthopaedic Surgeons, Orlando, FL, 2000.

58. Cain EL, Phillips BB, Charlepois SB, et al: Effect of tibial tunnel dilation of pullout strength of quadrupled semitendinosus/gracilis autografts in ACL reconstruction secured with bioabsorbable interference screws. Presented at the 25th Annual Meeting of the American Orthopaedic Society for Sports Medicine, Traverse City, MI, 1999.

59. Weiler A, Hoffman R, Sudkamp N, et al: Biomechanical evaluation of patellar and hamstring tendon graft fixation for anterior cruciate ligament reconstruction using a poly-(D,L-lactide) interference screw. Unfallchirurg 1999; 102:115.

60. Liew A, Johnson D: Efficacy of bioabsorbable interference fit screws for hamstring fixation in ACL reconstruction. Presented at the 18th Annual Meeting of the Arthroscopy Association of North America, Vancouver, British Columbia, 1999.

61. Musgrove T, Salmon L, Burt C, et al: The influence of reverse-thread screw femoral fixation on laxity measurements after anterior cruciate ligament reconstruction with hamstring tendon. Am J Sports Med 2000; 28:695.

62. Indelicato P: Non-operative treatment of complete tears of the medial collateral ligament of the knee. J Bone Joint Surg Am 1983; 65:323.

63. Fanelli G, Gianotti B, Edson C: Arthroscopically assisted combined anterior and posterior cruciate ligament reconstruction. Arthroscopy 1996; 12:5.

64. Fealy S, Cavanaugh J, Behr CT, et al: Combined anterior cruciate and medial collateral ligament injuries: An analysis of chronic vs. acute medial ligament laxity. Presented at the 18th Annual Meeting of the Arthroscopy Association of North America, Vancouver, British Columbia, 1999.

65. Terry G, LaPrade R: The posterolateral aspect of the knee: Anatomy and surgical approach. Am J Sports Med 1996; 24:732.

66. Fanelli G, Gianotti B, Edson C: Arthroscopically assisted combined PCL/posterolateral complex reconstruction. Arthroscopy 1996; 12:521.

67. Noyes F, Barber-Westin S: Reconstruction of the lateral collateral ligament of the knee with patellar tendon allograft: Report of a new technique in combined ligament injuries. Am J Sports Med 1999; 27:269.

68. Veltri D, Warren R: Posterolateral instability of the knee. J Bone Joint Surg Am 1994; 76:460.

69. Noyes F, Barber S, Simon R: High tibial osteotomy and ligament reconstruction in

varus angulated, anterior cruciate ligament-deficient knees: A two- to seven-year follow-up study. Am J Sports Med 1993; 21:2.

70. Johnson D, Harner C, Maday M, et al: Revision ACL surgery. In Fu F, Harner C, Vince K (eds): Knee Surgery. Baltimore, Williams & Wilkins, 1994, p 877.

71. Fulkerson J, Langelan R: An alternative cruciate reconstruction graft: The central quadriceps tendon. Arthroscopy 1995; 11: 252.

72. Brand J, Danaceau S, Hamilton D, et al: Comparison of interference fixation of tendon and bone plug for the quadriceps tendon in cruciate ligament reconstruction. Arthroscopy 1999; 15:548.

73. Mannor DA, Shearn JT, Grood ES, et al: Biomechanics of two bundle posterior cruciate ligament reconstruction. Presented at

the International Society of Arthroscopy, Knee Surgery and Orthopaedic Sports Medicine, Washington, DC, 1999.

74. Sisto D, Warren R: Complete knee dislocation: A follow-up study of operative treatment. Clin Orthop 1985; 198:94.

75. Shelbourne K, Porter D, Clingman J, et al: Low-velocity knee dislocation. Orthop Rev 1991; 20:995.

76. Girgis F, Marshall JL, Al Monajem ARS: The cruciate ligament of the knee joint. Clin Orthop 1975; 106:229.

77. Miller M, Bergfeld J, Fowler P, et al: The posterior cruciate ligament injured knee: Principles of evaluation and treatment. Am Acad Orthop Surg Instr Course Lect 1999; 48:199.

78. Staubli H, Schatzmann L, Brunner P, et al: Quadriceps tendon and patellar ligament: Cryosectional anatomy and structural prop-

erties in young adults. Knee Surg Sports Traumatol Arthrosc 1996; 4:100.

79. Cooper D, Deng X, Burstein A, et al: The strength of the central third patellar tendon graft: A biomechanical study. Am J Sports Med 1993; 21:818.

80. Brown CH, Sklar JH, Hecker AT, et al: Biomechanics of endoscopic anterior cruciate ligament graft fixation. Presented at the 2nd World Congress on Sports Trauma/22nd Annual Meeting of the American Orthopaedic Society of Sports Medicine, Buena Vista, FL, 1996.

81. Caborn D, Urban W, Johnson D, et al: Biomechanical comparison between bioscrew and titanium alloy interference screws for bone-patellar tendon-bone graft fixation in anterior cruciate ligament reconstruction. Arthroscopy 1997; 13:229.

section 4

chapter 13

ARTICULAR CARTILAGE INJURIES OF THE KNEE

Peter S. Borden, Scott D. Mair, Vladimir Bobic, and Darren L. Johnson

Summary
- Traumatic injury to the articular cartilage of the knee can produce significant symptoms.
- These injuries are diagnosed on the basis of history, physical examination, magnetic resonance imaging (MRI), and arthroscopy.
- Common signs and symptoms include pain in the area of the lesion, mechanical symptoms secondary to a loose body, and knee effusion.
- Nonoperative treatment options include nonsteroidal anti-inflammatory medications, corticosteroid injections, chondroprotective agents, and viscosupplementation.
- If nonoperative treatment is unsuccessful, multiple arthroscopic procedures are available.
- Current surgical treatment methods are often successful in improving symptoms but cannot produce cartilage equal to native articular cartilage with regard to mechanical properties and durability.
- Current research focuses on achieving a method of restoration of normal articular cartilage after injury.

In 1743, Hunter[1] stated, "From Hippocrates to the present age, it is universally allowed that ulcerated cartilage is a troublesome thing and that once destroyed, it is not repaired." The treatment of traumatic injury to the articular cartilage of the knee continues to be problematic. It has been established that the reparative process of cartilage depends on the biological response of the injured tissue and the ability to produce a substitute tissue to replace the articular surface deficit. Evidence of some form of cartilage healing has been demonstrated under certain conditions;

however, the terms "healing" and "repair" have become rather nonspecific. Repaired articular cartilage generally fails to replicate the structure, composition, and function of normal articular cartilage. Various surgical procedures currently exist for the treatment of articular injuries refractory to nonoperative management, and reasonable success in alleviating patient symptoms has been demonstrated. However, the ability to replace damaged cartilage with tissue that replicates the original articular cartilage remains elusive. Achieving this goal is one of the most important areas of current research in musculoskeletal medicine.

PATHOGENESIS

Mechanical injuries to articular cartilage occur when repetitive and prolonged joint overloading or sudden-impact forces produce high compressive stresses throughout the superficial articular tissue and high shear stresses at the subchondral bone junction. These stresses can cause injuries that can be categorized into three distinct types: (1) microdamage to the cells and matrix without visible disruption of the articular surface, (2) macrodisruption of the articular surface alone (chondral fracture), and (3) fracture of the articular surface and subchondral bone (osteochondral fracture) (Fig. 1). The response of the tissue depends on the extent of injury and depth of penetration as well as the size and location of articular injury.

It is well established that partial-thickness defects of articular cartilage do not undergo spontaneous healing.[2] The reasons for this phenomenon are not completely understood. The most frequent explanation is that mature articular cartilage is avascular and that cells from perivascular mesenchymal pools cannot enter the injured area. It has been proposed that, under appropriate conditions, mesen-

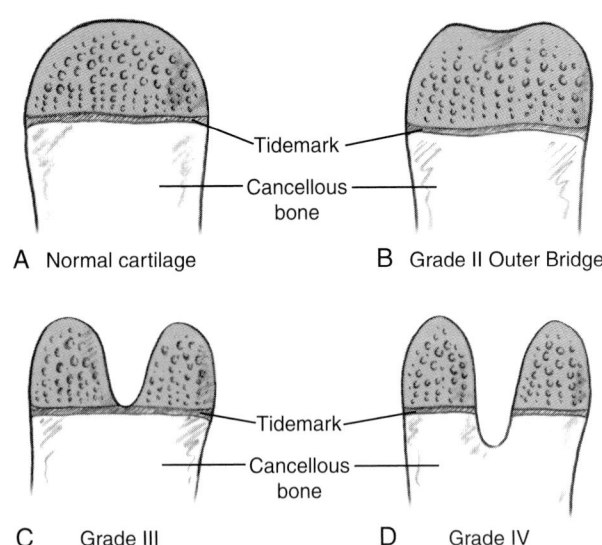

Fig. 1. Classification of injuries. *A*, Normal cartilage. *B*, Grade II. *C*, Grade III. *D*, Grade IV.

Grade	Description
TABLE 1. OUTERBRIDGE CLASSIFICATION OF ARTICULAR CARTILAGE INJGURY	
I	Softening and swelling
II	Fragmentation and fissuring less than one-half inch in diameter
III	Fragmentation and fissuring more than one-half inch in diameter
IV	Subchondral bone exposure

chymal cells can be induced to migrate from the synovial membrane across the articular surface and into the defect. Further research in this area is needed to substantiate this theory.[3] The transient proliferation of chondrocytes to the edges of partial-thickness articular defects has also been reported, but without the capacity to proliferate into the defect and fill the articular void.[4]

Full-thickness articular cartilage lesions have been shown to behave differently than partial-thickness lesions with regard to capacity for spontaneous healing. Penetration of the subchondral bone allows for a reparative process involving fibrin clot formation, cell migration from the bone marrow, and vascular ingrowth of the involved area. It is the violation of the tidemark and subchondral bone that allows for this repair process to be facilitated.

In full-thickness chondral injuries in which the subchondral plate has been penetrated, healing can occur. The reparative tissue infiltrates the defect and covers the subchondral bone, allowing for the ability to decrease or eliminate pain. However, histological studies indicate that the reparative tissue is biomechanically inferior to the original articular hyaline cartilage.[3] The repair tissue is composed of a mixture of fibrous, fibrocartilaginous, and hyalinized tissues, which produces an articular tissue that is less organized and less structurally sound than healthy intact articular cartilage.[3] As a result, the repair tissue may be less durable and more prone to reinjury or early degeneration.

Several major systems have been used to classify the extent of articular cartilage injury on the basis of arthroscopic appearance. In 1961, Outerbridge described a method of grading articular cartilage injury (Table 1) that remains the most commonly used system[5] (Fig. 2). Since then, numerous authors described variations to this classification.[6-12] Despite attempts to provide an ideal classification system, assessment of damaged articular cartilage remains difficult and somewhat subjective. Most systems are insufficient for contemporary clinical requirements for qualitative and quantitative evaluation of articular cartilage damage and repair. A universally accepted grading system

of articular damage is still needed to facilitate a better clinical and scientific understanding of the unsolved problem of cartilage disease.

The ability of articular cartilage to resist stresses and mechanical forces of a minor degree can depend on the physiological health of the preinjury articular tissue and biomechanical quality of the cartilage. In normal adult cartilage, a steady state exists in which the rate of synthesis of matrix components is equal to the rate of degradation of the matrix. Any change in this balance can rapidly affect the condition of articular cartilage. The primary cause, apart from direct mechanical damage, is the degradation of proteoglycans and collagens by active proteinases. Proinflammatory cytokines released within the joint act on the different cells to produce these enzymes. The specific source of these proteinases is dependent on the type of disease. In osteoarthritis, the chondrocytes are the most probable source. However, in rheumatoid arthritis, synovial fibroblasts, macrophages, and chondrocytes play a role in tissue destruction. Although proteoglycans can readily be synthesized, the replacement of collagen after its destruction is rare. Thus, the natural biochemical degradation of joint surfaces, which occurs as an irreversible phenomenon, may predispose certain diseased articular cartilage to injury with stresses that would not normally cause injury in healthy articular cartilage.

CLINICAL FEATURES

The patient with an articular cartilage defect may present after an acute injury, but in many cases pain develops insidiously and may be progressive. Common settings in which acute injury occurs include patellar dislocation (lateral femoral condyle and medial patellar facet), dashboard injuries in which the patella is driven into the trochlea, and sports injuries to the medial or lateral femoral condyle, often associated with ligamentous disruption. Physical examination is often relatively nonspecific. Patients may have pain and tenderness localized to the area of the lesion. Mechanical symptoms such as a catching or locking sensation are common when the injury results in the presence of a loose body or displaced flap of articular cartilage (Fig. 3). Knee effusion is present in many cases and may occur intermittently, particularly with activity. Plain radiographs are generally normal, unless an osteochondral loose body is present or in cases of chronic degenerative changes of the articular cartilage (Fig. 4).

MRI has been extensively researched and used in clinical practice. However, there is considerable disagreement

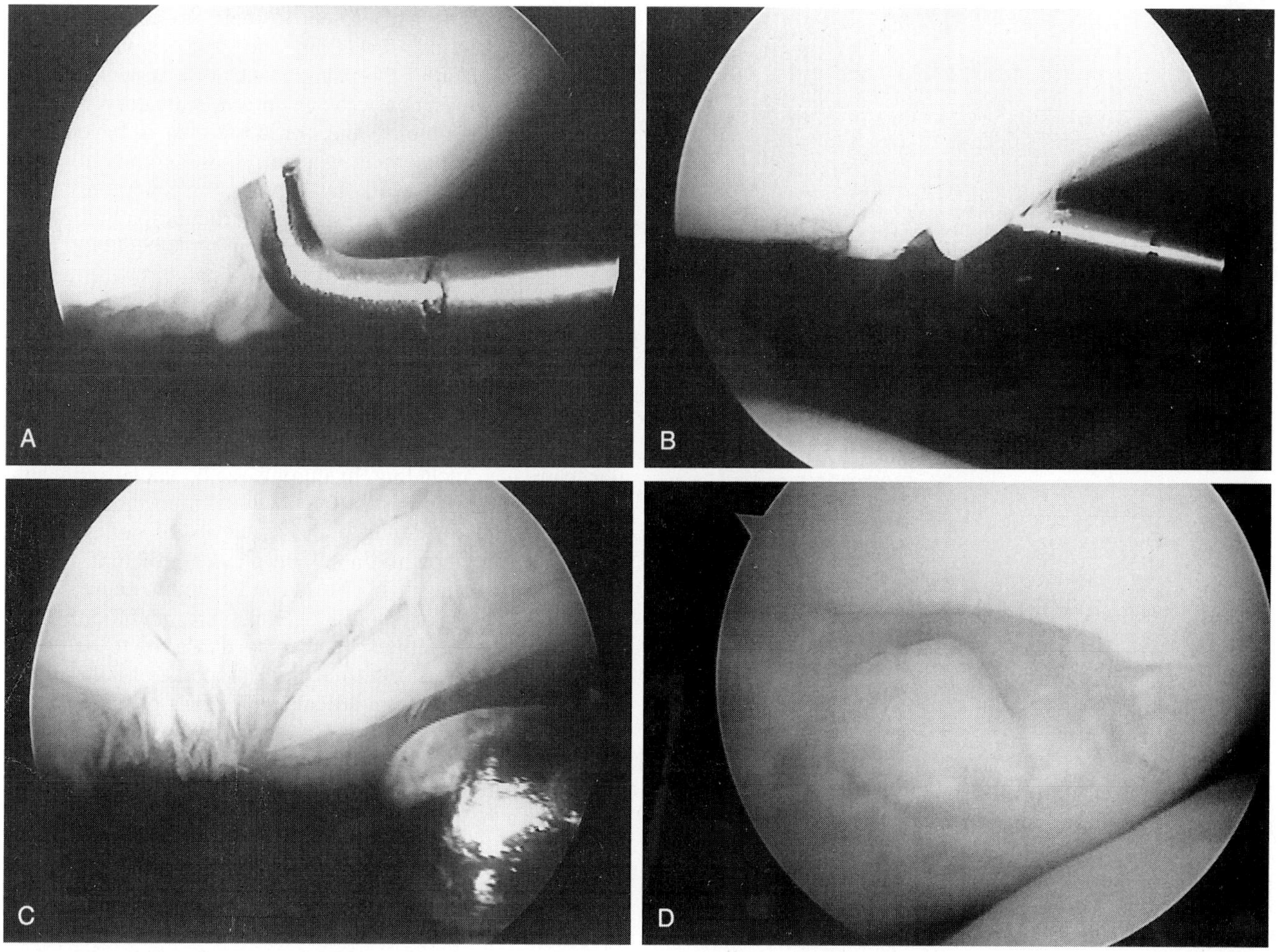

Fig. 2. Arthroscopic view of four grades of articular cartilage injury (Outerbridge's classification). *A,* Grade I. *B,* Grade II. *C,* Grade III. *D,* Grade IV.

with regard to the MRI appearance of normal articular cartilage, the best technique for imaging cartilage abnormalities, and the accuracy of these techniques in the detection of abnormalities. A standard MRI has low sensitivity in diagnosing isolated chondral delamination compared with arthroscopic findings.[13] Standard MRI can, however, frequently diagnose bone bruises or marrow edema, which is an indicator of severe injury to the articular cartilage[14] (Fig. 5). Newer and more advanced MRI techniques, with special articular scanning protocols providing an increased awareness of chondral injury, have begun to replace the standard MRI as a nonsurgical diagnostic tool. The most commonly advocated MRI technique for demonstrating articular cartilage injury is a fat-suppressed three-dimensional T_1-weighted gradient echo technique. Reported sensitivities for the detection of chondral lesions range from 75% to 93%. However, this technique has several limitations, including a prolonged imaging time and inadequate visualization of ligamentous and meniscal pathology, necessitating additional sequences. Use of intra-articular gadolinium enhancement with standard MRI has also been proposed for detection of chondral flap tears and osteoarticular lesions, but it involves an invasive procedure and remains imperfect with regard to sensitivity.

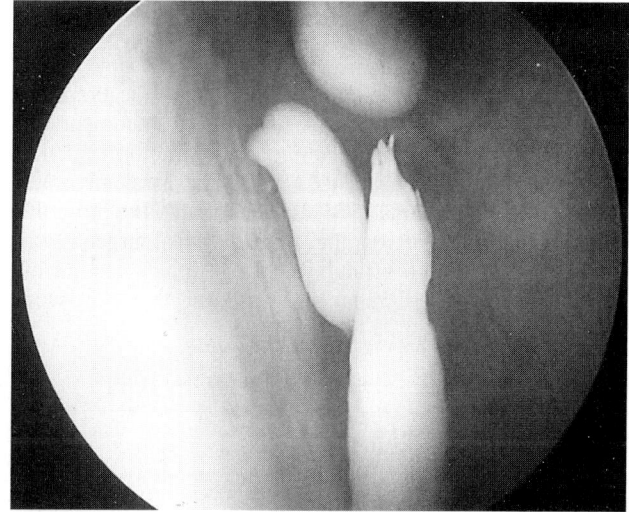

Fig. 3. Arthroscopic view of loose bodies found in lateral gutter of knee.

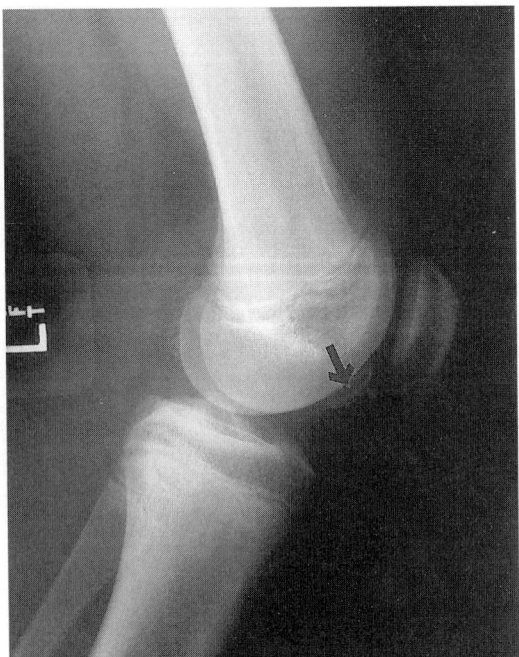

Fig. 4. Osteochondral loose body.

Early diagnosis and treatment of articular cartilage injury can be important in avoiding propagation of injury and worsening of the initial surface defect. Unfortunately, the diagnosis of articular cartilage injury is often difficult. Clinical history and physical examination, standard radiography, and standard clinical MRI generally provide relatively low sensitivity and moderate diagnostic accuracy. Currently, arthroscopy is still the most informative diagnostic tool. Careful visual inspection and probing of articular surfaces are essential. Large osteochondral defects can be covered with a thick layer of fibrocartilage that can go unnoticed without probing and a high index of suspicion. This tissue is usually very soft, is semidetached from subchondral bone, and does not have the glossy appearance of normal hyaline cartilage. Delaminated and semidetached chondral flaps also may become visible only when adequately probed (Fig. 6). Articular injury should be accurately described and recorded in the arthroscopy report, with specific attention paid to size, depth, location, and condition of the opposing articular surface. Documentation of associated injuries to other important structures such as the ligaments and menisci, as well as the axial alignment of the involved extremity, is also important. By providing a detailed description of the findings, the surgeon who treats the patient with articular cartilage injury can formulate an appropriate treatment plan based on the arthroscopy findings.

NONOPERATIVE TREATMENT OPTIONS

It is generally assumed that untreated focal defects of articular cartilage will lead to symptomatic progessive arthrosis. This may be true, but the number of patients with articular injury who live normal lives, free of knee symptoms and without functional problems, is unknown. Many patients slowly experience symptoms from articular degeneration or chronic joint injury and present to their physician in hopes of alleviating the pain, swelling, and progression of symptoms. A discussion of the pharmaceutical treatment of these symptoms such as nonsteroidal anti-inflammatory medications, COX-2 inhibitors, and corticosteroids is beyond the scope of this chapter. In general, these commonly prescribed medications work by suppressing symptoms indirectly, not by directly addressing the articular pathology.

Chondroprotective agents and viscosupplementation have received attention in hopes of treating patients with articular injuries without surgery. Chondroprotective agents are compounds that stimulate chondrocyte synthesis of collagen and proteoglycans as well as synoviocyte production of hyaluronic acid and have been proposed to inhibit cartilage degradation. Examples of compounds that exhibit some of these characteristics are the endogenous molecules of articular cartilage, including hyaluronic acid, chondroitin sulfate, and glucosamine sulfate. Glucosamine sulfate has been proposed to stimulate the synthesis of collagen and proteoglycans. Chondroitin sulfate plays a structural role in binding with collagen fibrils and may inhibit many degradative enzymes by methods of competitive inhibition.[15]

Viscosupplementation is a therapy that aims to be chondroprotective by restoring the fluid properties of the tissue matrix by means of intra-articular injections of highly purified "viscoelastic" solutions of sodium hyaluronate. The proposed function of hyaluronate is to provide lubrication and shock absorption in the compromised knee joint, resulting in a protective effect on the already-diseased cartilage.[16, 17] A series of three to five weekly injections is usually given. Currently, this treatment method is relatively expensive.

Both chondroprotective agents and viscosupplementation have demonstrated favorable results in clinical trials with regard to symptomatic improvement and delayed progression of degenerative changes.[18–21] Further study is necessary to better analyze the efficacy of these compounds with regard to clinical outcomes, particularly in the long term.

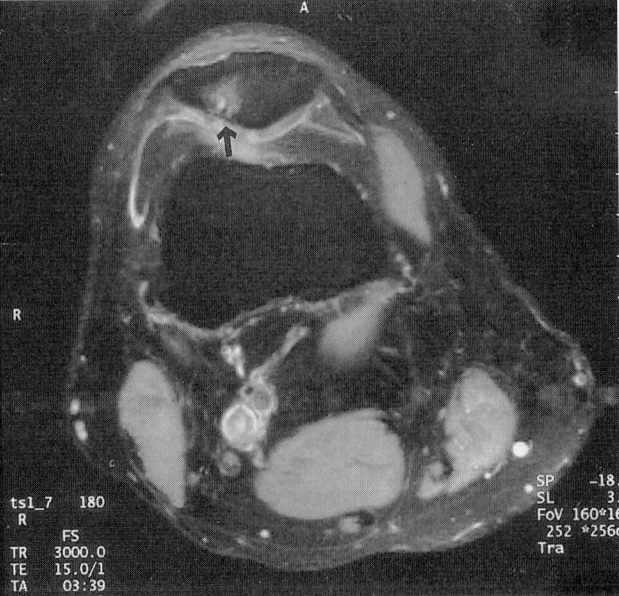

Fig. 5. Bone marrow edema on undersurface of patella. At arthroscopy, overlying articular cartilage had a full-thickness injury.

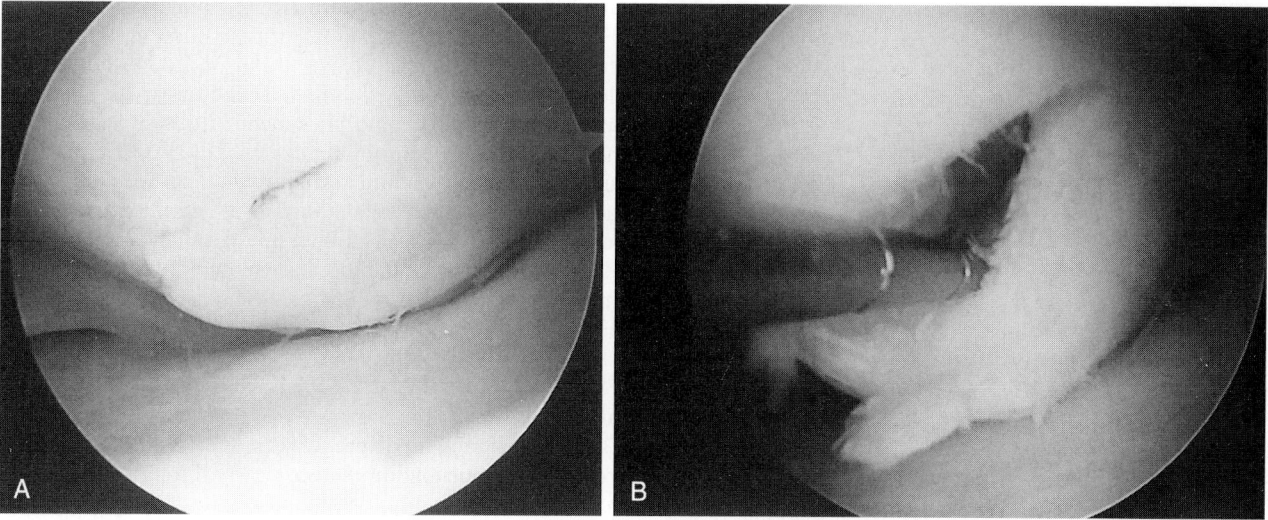

Fig. 6. Articular injury. *A,* The articular surface of the distal femur appears to be a simple fissure. *B,* However, probing the lesion demonstrates true extent of articular injury.

GOALS, INDICATIONS, AND CONTRAINDICATIONS FOR SURGICAL TREATMENT

Candidates for surgical treatment of articular injuries are patients in whom nonsurgical treatment has failed, those with obvious articular injury seen on standard radiographs or MRI, those who remain symptomatic after prior arthroscopy with documented articular damage, and patients with associated ligamentous or meniscal injury requiring operative treatment. The current realistic surgical goals of treating articular cartilage pathology are to decrease symptoms associated with the pathology, halt the progression of articular damage, restore articular surface anatomy, and facilitate a healing or repair process that will replace the damaged tissue with healthier new tissue. Most surgical procedures currently result in the formation of a fibrocartilage tissue replacement that has an inferior biomechanical composition to normal hyaline cartilage. The ultimate goal of surgically treating these articular lesions is to replace the damaged tissue with normal hyaline cartilage equal in composition to the preexisting tissue. As research in this field of orthopaedics continues to advance, an answer to this problem will likely be achieved, providing an exciting future for treatment of articular cartilage injuries.

The only absolute contradiction to any articular cartilage surgery is infection. Relative contradictions depend on the specific procedure performed but generally include advanced or post-traumatic osteoarthritis, rheumatological disease, malalignment of the extremity, and severe medical illness.

SURGICAL TREATMENT OPTIONS AND RESULTS

ARTHROSCOPIC LAVAGE

The mechanism by which arthroscopic lavage and débridement may help the symptoms of articular cartilage injuries is not entirely clear. Removal of loose intra-articular tissue debris and inflammatory mediators generated by the synovial lining generally provides good short-term results for both acute and degenerative chondral lesions. However, lavage generally provides short-term symptomatic relief without correction of the underlying disease. If predisposing malalignment is also present, the beneficial effects of lavage seem to be minimized. Although this simple procedure works well in older sedentary patients, the outcome is generally insufficient for an active population.[22]

ARTHROSCOPIC DÉBRIDEMENT AND ABRASION ARTHROPLASTY

Abrasion arthroplasty of articular lesions was introduced by Johnson[23] in the early 1980s. This technique involves débridement of the articular defect circumferentially to a normal tissue edge and down to bleeding subchondral bone to stimulate a vascular response and fibrin clot formation. The goal is to form a fibrocartilage articular replacement. There has been some degree of disagreement as to the depth of drilling and whether débridement of the subchondral bone should be intracortical or cancellous. It is recommended that the immature repair tissue be protected from excessive loading after the procedure for a minimum of 6 to 8 weeks. At second-look arthroscopy up to 6 years later, Johnson[24] described an intact fibrocartilage tissue with maintained structural integrity. Several studies showed favorable results for short-term relief of pain and swelling. A 5-year follow-up study demonstrated better clinical results with abrasion arthroplasty and débridement versus arthroscopic débridement alone. However, of the patients who had poor results with abrasion arthroplasty (33%), worsening of symptoms occurred.[25] Questions remain concerning the efficacy and long-term results of this procedure.

SUBCHONDRAL DRILLING

This procedure is an extension of the abrasion arthroplasty technique in which the subchondral bone is drilled with multiple drill holes penetrating into the bone marrow for the purpose of stimulating a vascular response. The results of this additional procedure are unknown.

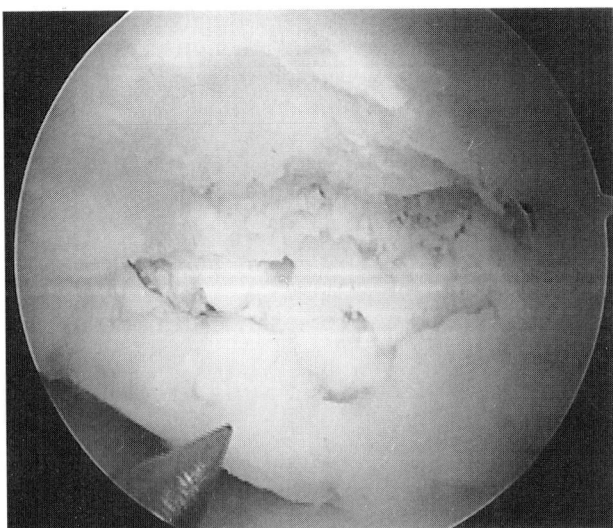

Fig. 7. Microfracture technique. Holes on the femoral condyle made with an awl are evident.

MICROFRACTURE

This procedure was developed by Steadman in the 1980s. It involves arthroscopic débridement of the cartilage defect down to subchondral bone but not through it. Damage to the subchondral bone should be avoided in overaggressive shaving of the soft articular cartilage. Once the subchondral bone has been identified, an arthroscopic awl is carefully used to make multiple drill holes approximately 3 to 4 mm apart and 4 mm in depth across the exposed surface of the lesion. The concept of subchondral penetration and fibrocartilage formation associated with this technique is not new; however, maintaining the integrity of the subchondral bone between the holes is believed to be important for joint surface shape. The use of arthroscopic awls as opposed to subchondral drilling is thought to produce less thermal necrosis in creating the holes.[21] The awls also allow the surgeon improved access to all areas of the joint,

which can be difficult with a straight pin used for drilling (Fig. 7).Use of a continuous passive motion (CPM) machine is recommended for 6 to 8 weeks postoperatively along with non-weightbearing of the affected extremity. Second-look arthroscopy has shown visual improvement of the lesions after microfracture and CPM, and clinical results demonstrate significant improvements in patient satisfaction among both recreational and competitive athletic populations at a mean follow-up of 3.7 years.[26, 27] Currently, microfracture is the most commonly performed first-line treatment for traumatic articular cartilage injuries (Fig. 8).

PERIOSTEAL AND PERICHONDRAL AUTOGRAFTS

These techniques involve excavating the pathological tissue from the osteochondral defect down through subchondral bone and preparing an area for autograft transplantation of either perichondral or periosteal grafts. It is believed that the transplanted tissue can differentiate into tissue closely resembling hyaline tissue.[28] Although animal studies have been encouraging in this area and limited short-term results show promise, long-term results have been limited. In an early study performed with perichondral grafting, 72% of patients were symptom free 1 year postoperatively. At 5 to 7 years, 60% of these patients experienced graft failure with degeneration of the articular surface and painful symptoms.[29] In general, outcomes of these techniques are not better than those of other techniques that allow for fibrocartilage replacement tissue.

OSTEOCHONDRAL AUTOGRAFTS AND ALLOGRAFTS

Replacement of the articular defect with human articular cartilage tissue has become a popular technique with use of autograft tissue or allograft tissue. Autograft harvesting and transplantation techniques have the advantages of using the patient's own tissue and immediate transplantation from donor site to recipient site without additional cost to the patient. However, disadvantages primarily involve donor

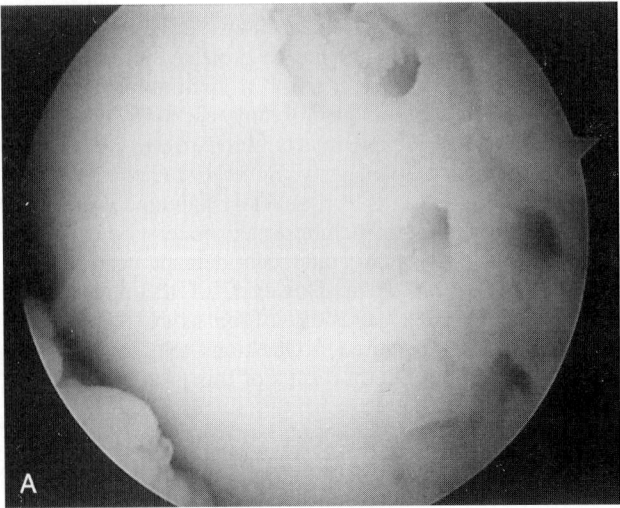
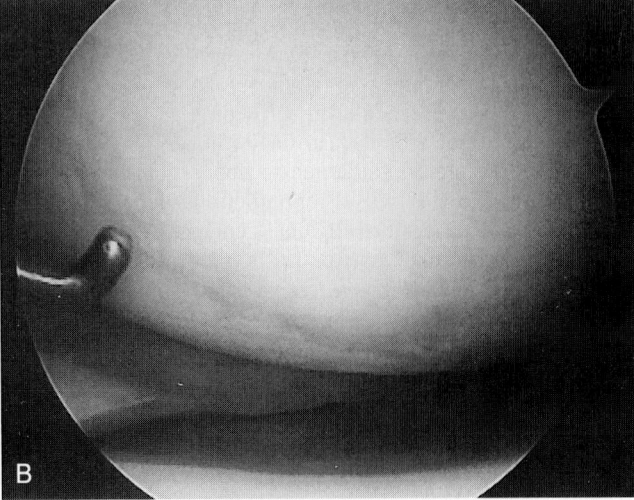

Fig. 8. Microfracture technique. *A,* Femoral lesion treated with microfracture technique. *B,* Same lesion 1 year later at second-look arthroscopy; probe points to repair tissue.

site morbidity and limited amount of donor tissue availability. Also, this technique often involves using multiple small plugs, which increases the likelihood for articular surface height mismatch of the plugs as well as limiting the size of the defect to be treated in this manner. Allograft transplantation has received increased attention for the treatment of osteochondral articular lesions as methods of donor tissue preservation have advanced. Donors are matched according to size of the defect, as determined preoperatively by imaging studies, and more accurately assessed during transplantation before internally fixing the graft to the host site. It is believed that allograft articular cartilage is "immunologically privileged" and rejection of these tissue grafts is minimal, precluding the need for tissue typing and immunological suppression.[30, 31] Patients who receive allograft osteochondral tissue should have acceptable mechanical alignment before transplantation with no evidence of inflammatory conditions or diffuse preoperative arthrosis. In addition, they should be closely monitored after surgery to prevent stiffness of the knee joint.[32, 33] A 2-year follow-up study demonstrated an 86% success rate for allograft treatment of monopolar femoral lesions and a 53% success rate for bipolar lesions.[34] Although clinical results show good short-term success up to 5 years postoperatively, a significant percentage of these patients experience symptoms in the years to follow.

AUTOLOGOUS CHONDROCYTE IMPLANTATION

This procedure involves autologous harvesting of hyaline cartilage chondrocytes, which are then expanded in a cell culture over a specific period of time and implanted into the articular defect with a second surgical procedure. The theoretical advantage of this procedure is the ability to produce a more hyaline-like cartilage.[35] During the second procedure, the transplanted tissue is covered with a periosteal flap, which aids in sealing the new tissue in place and also acts as a mechanical barrier. Preservation of the subchondral bone is emphasized for higher success rates.[36] The current indications for this procedure involve an articular lesion of the distal femur refractory to a prior arthroscopic or surgical cartilage procedure. It is not indicated for patients with osteoarthritis, malalignment, or ligamentous instability associated with the affected extremity.[37] Limited experience with this procedure has shown favorable results, and interest in this treatment as a salvage procedure remains high. Disadvantages of this treatment include the need for two surgical procedures as well as a high cost for the cell culture technique.

OSTEOTOMY AND MECHANICAL REALIGNMENT

In cases of articular damage, malalignment can exist, which tends to place increased stress on the pathological articular region. In such cases, the mechanical axis of the limb passes through the area of diseased cartilage (Fig. 9). An osteotomy of either the proximal tibia or distal femur can help unload the stress and realign the mechanical axis of the extremity, shifting the weightbearing load to the healthy articular bone. The osteotomy indirectly halts the progression of articular degeneration but does not directly address the articular lesion. In cases of significant malalignment, these procedures are quite effective in improving symptoms for up to 10 years or more. In general, clinical results tend to deteriorate after that period of time.[38–40]

COMPLICATIONS

The most common reason for any of these procedures to be considered unsuccessful is the failure to relieve symptoms. In a low percentage of patients, pain and effusion may be increased after surgery. Other complications inherent to any arthroscopic procedure are rare, including knee stiffness, infection, nerve injury, and complications of anesthesia. Certain complications are procedure specific. With osteochondral autograft transfer, mismatch of the level of the cartilage can occur secondary to either overimpaction or inadequate recession of the graft. Symptoms can also develop at the donor site with this procedure. A late hypertrophic response of the regenerate can occur in 10% to 15% of patients undergoing autologous chondrocyte implantation.[41] When osteotomy is performed, malunion can occur as a result of improper correction of the deformity or loss of fixation. Nonunion at the osteotomy site may also occur. In all of the procedures just discussed, late deterioration of results as a consequence of breakdown of the regenerated cartilage has been described.

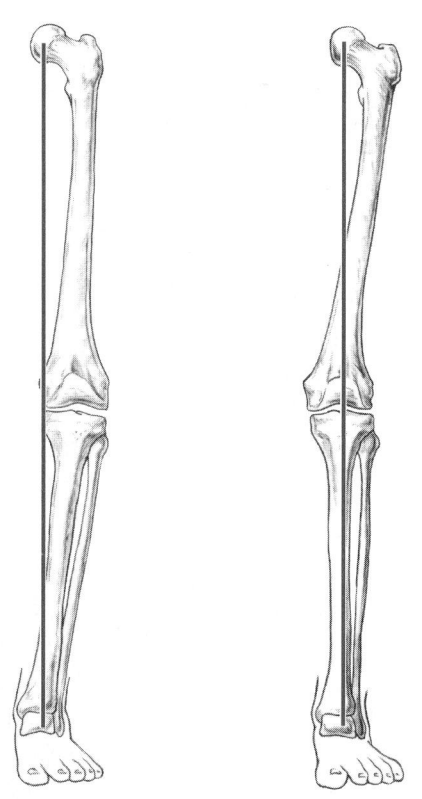

Fig. 9. Mechanical alignment. Varus alignment of lower extremity; normal mechanical alignment.

Varus malalignment   Normal mechanical axis

SUMMARY

Treatment of articular cartilage injuries to the knee continues to present a significant challenge. Current treatment options focus on alleviating symptoms and improving quality of life. Numerous arthroscopic procedures have been developed that are often successful in achieving these goals. However, results remain imperfect, and controversy exists as to which procedures are appropriate, particularly with respect to full-thickness chondral defects. Further, long-term clinical outcome studies are necessary to better understand which methods of treatment are most appropriate for the varied lesions encountered. Current procedures, although often successful in providing relief of symptoms, are unable to produce a regenerated cartilage that is the equal of the native articular surface. Ultimately, the goal in treating this difficult problem is to establish a method of replacing damaged articular tissue with new tissue having the same biomechanical properties and long-term durability of normal hyaline cartilage. This is an area of very active research, and it is anticipated that advancements in gene therapy will bring about a solution for treatment of the articular cartilage defect.

REFERENCES

1. Hunter W: On the structure and disease of articular cartilages. Philos Trans R Soc London Biol 1943; 42:514.

2. Buckwalter JA, Mankin HJ: Articular cartilage. J Bone Joint Surg Am 1997; 79:600.

3. Hunziker EB, Rosenberg LC: Repair of partial-thickness defects in articular cartilage: Cell recruitment from the synovial membrane. J Bone Joint Surg Am 1996; 78:721.

4. Martin JA, Buckwalter JA: Articular cartilage ageing and degeneration. Sports Med Arthrosc Rev 1996; 4:263.

5. Outerbridge HK, Outerbridge AR, Outerbridge RE: The use of a lateral patellar autologous graft for the repair of a large osteochondral defect in the knee. J Bone Joint Surg Am 1995; 77:65.

6. Insall J, Falvo KA, Wise DW: Chondromalacia patellae. A prospective study. J Bone Joint Surg Am 1976; 58:1.

7. Ficat RP, Hungerford DS: Disorder of the PATELLO-FEMORAL Joint. Baltimore, MD, Williams & Wilkins, 1977, p 194.

8. Ogilvie-Harris DJ, Jackson RW: The arthroscopic treatment of chondromalacia patellae. J Bone Joint Surg Br 1984; 66:660.

9. Bentley G, Dowd G: Current concepts of etiology and treatment of chondromalacia patellae. Clin Orthop 1984; 27:209.

10. Johnson-Nurse C, Dandy DJ: Fracture-separation of articular cartilage in the adult knee. J Bone Joint Surg Br 1985; 67:42.

11. Bauer M, Jackson RW: Chondral lesions of the femoral condyles: A system of arthroscopic classification. Arthroscopy 1988; 4:97.

12. Noyes FR, Stabler CL: A system for grading articular cartilage lesions at arthroscopy. Am J Sports Med 1989; 17:505.

13. Kneeland JB: MRI of articular cartilage and cartilage degeneration. In Stoller DW (ed): Magnetic Resonance Imaging in Orthopaedics and Sports Medicine. Philadelphia, Lippincott-Raven, 1997, 2nd ed.

14. Levy AS, Lohnes J, Sculley S, et al: Chondral delamination of the knee in soccer players. Am J Sports Med 1996; 24:634.

15. Hungerford DS: Treating osteoarthritis with chondroprotective agents. Orthop Spec Ed 1998; 4:1.

16. Balazs EA: The physical prospective of synovial fluid and the special role of hyaluronic acid. In Helfet AJ (ed): Disorders of the Knee. Philadelphia, JB Lippincott, 1982, 2nd ed, p 6.

17. Balazs EA, Denlinger JL: Viscosupplementation: A new concept in the treatment of osteoarthritis. J Rheumatol Suppl 1993; 39:3.

18. Delafuente JC: Glucosamine in the treatment of osteoarthritis. Rheum Dis Clin North Am 2000; 26:1.

19. Watterson JR, Esdaile JM: Viscosupplementation: Therapeutic mechanisms and clinical potential in osteoarthritis of the knee. J Am Acad Orthop Surg 2000; 5:277.

20. Rosier RN, O'Keefe RJ: Hyaluronic acid therapy. Instr Course Lect 2000; 5:495.

21. Reginster JY, Deroisy R, Rovati LC, et al: Long-term effects of glucosamine sulphate on osteoarthritis progression: A randomised, placebo-controlled clinical trial. Lancet 2001; 9252:251.

22. Kruger T, Wohlrab D, Birke A, et al: Results of arthroscopic joint debridement in different stages of chondromalacia of the knee joint. Arch Orthop Trauma Surg 2000; 120:338.

23. Johnson LL: Arthroscopic abrasion arthroplasty: Historical and pathologic perspective: Present status. Arthroscopy 1986; 2:54.

24. Johnson LL: Abrasive arthroplasty. In Gintz JB (ed): Operative Arthroscopy. New York, Raven Press, 1991, p 341.

25. Bert JM, Maschka K: The arthroscopic treatment of unicompartmental gonarthrosis: A five-year follow-up study of abrasion arthroplasty plus arthroscopic debridement and arthroscopic debridement alone. Arthroscopy 1989; 5:25.

26. Rodrigo JJ, Steadman RJ, Silliman JF, et al: Improvement of full thickness chondral defect healing in the human knee after debridement and microfracture using continuous passive motion. Am J Knee Surg 1994; 7:109.

27. Blevins FT, Steadman JR, Rodrigo JJ, et al: Treatment of articular cartilage defects in athletes: An analysis of functional outcome and lesion appearance. Orthopedics 1998; 21:761; discussion, 767.

28. O'Driscoll SW, Keeley FW, Salter RB: Durability of regenerated articular cartilage produced by free autogenous periosteal grafts in major full-thickness defects in joint surfaces under the influence of continuous passive motion. A follow-up report at one year. J Bone Joint Surg Am 1988; 70:595.

29. Homminga GN, Bulstra SK, Bouwmeester PS, et al: Perichondral grafting for cartilage lesions of the knee. J Bone Joint Surg Br 1990; 72:1003.

30. Langer F, Gross AE: Immunogenicity of allograft articular cartilage. J Bone Joint Surg Am 1974; 56:297.

31. Zukos DJ, Oakeshott RD, Gross AE: Osteochondral allograft reconstruction of the knee: II. Experience with successful and failed fresh osteochondral allografts. Am J Knee Surg 1989; 2:182.

32. Ghazavi MT, Visrain F, Davis AM: Long-term results of fresh osteochondral allografts for posttraumatic osteochondral defects of the knee. Orthop Trans 1995; 19:454.

33. Gross AE: Use of fresh osteochondral allografts to replace traumatic joint defects. In Gross AE (ed): Allografts in Orthopaedic Practice. Baltimore, MD, Williams & Wilkins, 1992, p 67.

34. Bugbee WD, Convery FR: Osteochondral allograft transplantation. Clin Sports Med 1999; 18:67.

35. Brittberg M, Undahl A, Nilsson A, et al: Treatment of deep cartilage defects in the knee with autologous chondrocyte transplantation. N Engl J Med 1994; 331:889.

36. Mandelbaum BR, Browne JE, Fu F, et al: Articular cartilage lesions of the knee. Am J Sports Med 1998; 26:853.

37. Jackson DW, Scheer MJ, Simon TM: Cartilage substitute: Overview of basic science and treatment options. J Am Acad Orthop Surg 2001; 9:37.

38. Berman AT, Bosacco SJ, Kirshner S, et al: Factors influencing long-term results in high tibial osteotomy. Clin Orthop 1991; 34:192.

39. Insall JN, Joseph DM, Msika C: High tibial osteotomy for varus gonarthrosis: A long-term follow-up study. J Bone Joint Surg Am 1984; 66:1040.

40. Matthews LS, Goldstein SA, Malvitz TA, et al: Proximal tibial osteotomy: Factors that influence the duration of satisfactory function. Clin Orthop 1988; 30:193.

41. Minas T, Peterson L: Advanced techniques in autologous chondrocyte transplantation. Clin Sports Med 1999; 18:13.

MENISCAL INJURY

Emin Taskiran and M. Hakan Özsoy

section 4 chapter 14

Summary

- Meniscal injury mostly occurs in the young population and in those participating actively in sports.
- The injured patient carries some risk of secondary osteoarthritis regardless of the treatment applied, but this may be minimized with appropriate management.
- Its natural history is mainly affected by associated lesions such as anterior cruciate ligament (ACL) injury, chondral lesions, and localization and extent of the lesion in the meniscal body.
- In most cases accurate diagnosis can be made on the basis of the patient's history and proper physical examination.
- Among the investigational procedures, magnetic resonance imaging (MRI) is the most accurate noninvasive diagnostic method, but arthroscopy is still the gold standard.
- Associated lesions, tear pattern of the meniscus, and patient's expectations are the major determinants of treatment in the decision-making process.
- Arthroscopic partial meniscectomy (APM) is still primarily used; however, meniscal repair is becoming the most preferable surgical technique to meet patients' short- and long-term expectations.

MENISCAL INJURY

DEFINITION

The term "meniscal injury" covers the disorders of knee joint meniscus that have mostly traumatic origin.

HISTORICAL REVIEW

The treatment of meniscal lesion has changed considerably in last 30 years as a result of a better understanding of the meniscal function in joint biomechanics.

Thomas Annandale was reportedly the first surgeon who attempted excising and repairing in the 1880s.[1]

In the first half of the 20th century, total meniscectomy became widespread throughout the world in the belief that menisci were unnecessary extensions of tibia.

In 1936, King demonstrated the reparative response of meniscal lesions extending to the vascular area.[1]

Postmeniscectomy radiological changes were described by Fairbank[2] in 1948. These findings were not different from those of secondary osteoarthritis, as would be well understood later. Postmeniscectomy changes were confirmed by other studies.[3, 4]

Both APM and arthroscopic meniscal repair were first introduced in Japan in the 1960s by Watanabe and Ikeuchi.[5]

APM became a widespread procedure in the 1970s after O'Connor's development of the operating arthroscope.[6]

The number of biomechanical studies investigating meniscal function gradually increased during 1970s. It was shown that a small amount of meniscal excision causes an abnormal increase in contact pressure and in the load transmitted through the joint.[7, 8]

DeHaven developed the open meniscal repair technique in 1976.[1]

Henning improved the arthroscopic repair technique in the early 1980s, and the technique gained widespread acceptance shortly thereafter.[1]

Different arthroscopic suture and fixation techniques for meniscal repair were described to reduce morbidity and to improve technique during the 1980s and 1990s.[1]

Several attempts to improve meniscal transplantation, including clinical trials and animal experiments, have been made, but expected results could not be obtained.[9, 10]

A detrimental effect of partial meniscus resection to the articular cartilage was well clarified in long-term follow-up studies.[6, 11]

Long-term results of meniscal repair are encouraging regarding the survival rate of repair and the prevention of articular cartilage degeneration.[1, 12-14]

Meniscal transplantation is still considered an investigational procedure[9, 10]

FUNCTIONAL ANATOMY

Menisci are semilunar-shaped fibrocartilages interposed between the articular surfaces of the femur and tibia. Thus, conformity (joint congruency function) is provided between them (Fig. 1).

Although medial meniscus is firmly attached to the joint capsule throughout its periphery, lateral meniscus has a gap for passage of the popliteal tendon. This difference makes the lateral meniscus more mobile than the medial meniscus. Both menisci are inserted into the intercondylar area of tibia with their anterior and posterior horns. Lateral meniscus may also attach to the intercondylar area of femur by way of the meniscofemoral ligaments. The anterior horn of the medial meniscus and the posterior horn of the lateral meniscus may show some variability with respect to their insertion site and consistency of meniscofemoral ligaments.[15, 16]

Menisci are poorly vascularized structures in an adult, although they are rich in vessels and more cellular during the prenatal period. Microinjection technique demonstrated that vascular structures coming from the perimeniscal capillary plexus penetrate about 10% to 30% of the medial menisci and 10% to 25% of the lateral menisci. This is the reason for their poor healing capacity.[15]

The extracellular matrix of menisci consists mainly of type I collagen (up to 60% to 70% of dry weight). A small

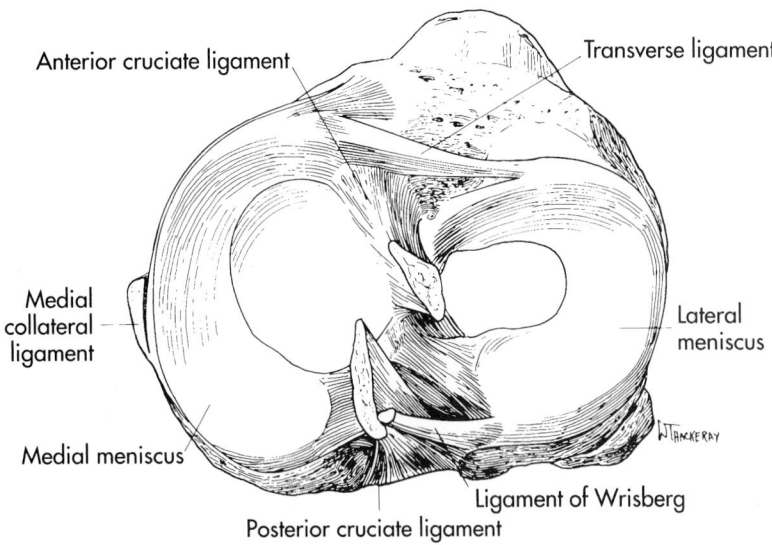

Fig. 1. Gross anatomy of menisci. (From Warren R, Arnoczky SP, Wickiewicz TL: Anatomy of the knee. In Nicholas JA, Hershman EB [eds]: The Lower Extremity and Spine in Sports Medicine. St. Louis, MO, CV Mosby, 1995, p 592.)

amount of proteoglycans is among the constituents of the matrix. Small numbers of fibrochondrocytes found in the matrix are responsible for production of the matrix.[15] The collagen fibers, which are mostly arranged in circumferential fashion, provide the main functions of the menisci (Fig. 2). In a loaded joint, healthy meniscal tissue tends to extrude between the condyles of the tibia and femur. Further extrusion is prevented by circumferential fibers inserting to the bone through the anterior and posterior horns (hoop tension effect) (Fig. 3). Thus, shock absorption and load-distributing functions are achieved.[8, 15, 17]

Several mechanoreceptors have been identified, particularly in the posterior and anterior horns of the menisci.[18] Therefore, menisci protect the joint not only with their mechanical characteristics but also with their proprioceptive capability (proprioceptive function).

Menisci can absorb and secrete synovial fluid during unloading and loading because of the hydrophilic capability of proteoglycans. This fluid lubricates the joint surfaces and facilitates movement (lubricating function).[15]

Medial menisci were also shown to prevent further ante-

rior translation of the femur as a secondary restraint in the absence of the ACL (stabilizing function).[19]

EPIDEMIOLOGY

The function of menisci is primarily mechanical. Therefore, they are readily injured under abnormal strain. Injury is more frequent in the younger population and in those who are active. In Poehling's[20] study, the age range for which meniscal injury frequency reaches its peak is 31 to 40 years in men and 11 to 20 years in women. Medial meniscal lesions are four to five times more frequent than lateral meniscal lesions.[6] Injuries are also more frequent in contact sports that involve pivoting, cutting, and jumping. Meniscal lesions are mostly associated with ACL injury and deficiency. Although the lateral meniscus is more frequently injured with acute ACL disruption, the incidence of medial meniscus injury increases with the chronicity of ACL deficiency.[20, 21]

Isolated lesions are rare in the younger population, and most patients do not have a history of major trauma.[22] The morphology and microstructural status of the meniscal lesions may be different as a result of the presence or absence of major trauma.[22] Accordingly, whereas horizontal flap lesions are mostly degenerative, vertical-longitudinal and radial tears are of traumatic origin.[20]

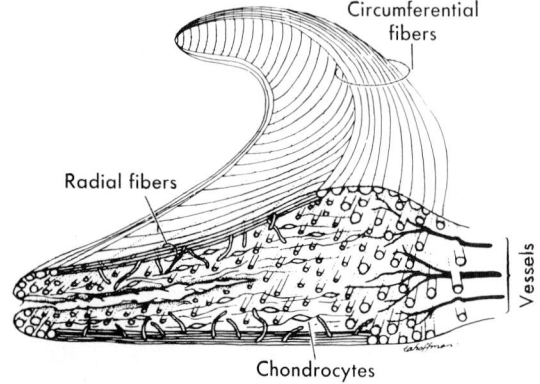

Fig. 2. Orientation of the radial and circumferential fibers in the meniscus. (From Shahriaree H: O'Connor's Textbook of Arthroscopic Surgery. Philadelphia, JB Lippincott, 1984; and Campbell's Operative Orthopedics, St. Louis, CV Mosby, 1992, 8th ed, p 1506.)

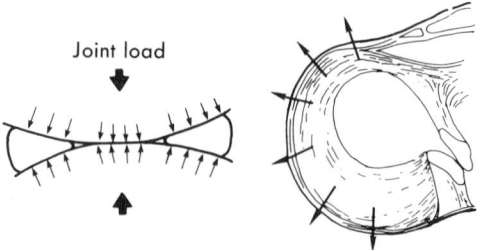

Fig. 3. Hoop-tension effect of the normal meniscus. (From Grood ES: Adv Orthop Surg 1984; 7:193; and from Campbell's Operative Orthopedics, St. Louis, CV Mosby, 1992, 8th ed, p 1507.)

PATHOGENESIS

A history of major trauma is mostly present in the young population, and lesions are associated with ligament injuries. Patients with this condition describe an immediate swelling, possibly a hemarthrosis, after a major twisting injury. In an ACL-deficient knee, anterior subluxation of the tibia exposes the posterior horn of the medial meniscus to a shearing force produced by the femoral condyle.

Peripheral meniscal tears can also cause hemarthrosis even when no ligament lesion is present. However, hemarthrosis is not a common finding in isolated meniscus lesions.

In some cases, there is no history of trauma or only a minor trauma history can be obtained. Therefore, two different origins of tears can be distinguished with regard to patient history: traumatic and degenerative.[20, 22]

In traumatic tears, the microstructure of the meniscus is largely not affected, and such lesions are more amenable to repair. In degenerative tears, however, the collagen structure is often destroyed, and even though repair can be made, the meniscus can hardly function properly afterward.[22] In a stable knee, an intact meniscus tissue is not squeezed between tibial and femoral condyles so as to be torn. For this reason, when no trauma is reported for a tear in a stable knee, a structural defect within the meniscus itself should be suspected.

CLINICAL FEATURES

Meniscal lesions are usually diagnosed clinically. Advanced radiological examinations and arthroscopy are helpful in doubtful cases.

Pain and locking after a twisting injury in a young athlete are typical complaints. If the injury is severe and prevents participation in sports, an accompanying ACL lesion should be suspected. If several injuries have been described, a meniscus lesion developing with chronic ACL deficiency should be suspected.

In individuals of middle and advanced age, degenerative tears are more common, and injury can result from daily activities such as squatting and bending the knees. The patient describes clicking, locking, and swelling along with pain localized to the joint line as the most prominent complaint.

Pain is possibly produced as a result of the meniscus being caught between the condyles. It is not persistent and arises mainly during such activities as stair climbing and squatting. Pain is usually well localized and may be persistent in cases of secondary synovitis and locked menisci. It is severe and does not respond to simple analgesics.

Locking is an inability to extend the knee completely because of a real mechanical block resulting from displacement of the meniscal fragment into the intercondylar groove (Fig. 4). In the chronically locked knee, extension loss may be diminished considerably and is likely to be missed unless compared with the contralateral knee.

Giving way may be experienced in many internal knee pathologies; thus, it is not a valuable sign.

Swelling is not a frequent finding and possibly develops as a result of synovial irritation. Swelling arising shortly after the trauma is an indicator of hemarthrosis, which is not a common finding except in a peripheral meniscal tear.

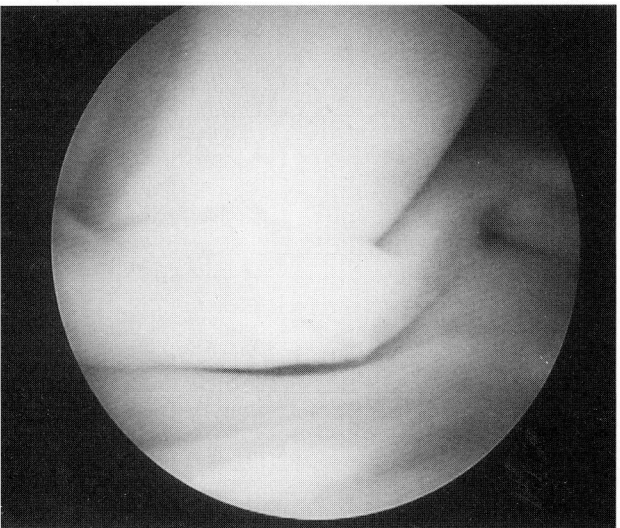

Fig. 4. Arthroscopic view of a bucket-handle tear of the medial meniscus.

Thigh muscle atrophy, especially of the quadriceps and vastus medialis, does occur but is not specific to meniscal lesions.

PHYSICAL EXAMINATION

Local tenderness on the joint line over the torn meniscus on palpation is very helpful in the diagnosis. Occasionally, protruded torn meniscus can be felt when compared with the asymptomatic knee. Sometimes a mass from meniscal cysts, more often over the lateral joint line, can be palpated.

SPECIAL TESTS

Because menisci are located within the joint, they cannot be palpated completely. Several tests have been introduced to detect lesions of menisci. Their main philosophy is to grind or to squeeze the unstable fragment between the femoral and tibial condyles.

McMurray's Test

First, the knee is brought to full flexion while the patient lies in supine position (Fig. 5). Then it is brought to extension while being forced to external and internal rotations. During this maneuver, the index finger and the thumb are placed over the lateral and medial joint spaces to feel a snapping sound.[23]

Apley's Test

While the patient lies in the prone position, the knee is brought to 90 degrees of flexion, and it is subjected to rotatory movements, simultaneously compressing and distracting it from the heel. Pain is localized to the site of the meniscal lesion.[23] The most notable advantage of this test is that it can be applied in patients who cannot move their hips comfortably (Fig. 6).

Steinmann's Test

This test is applied while the patient's legs are hanging from the edge of a high bench (knees flexed 90 degrees).

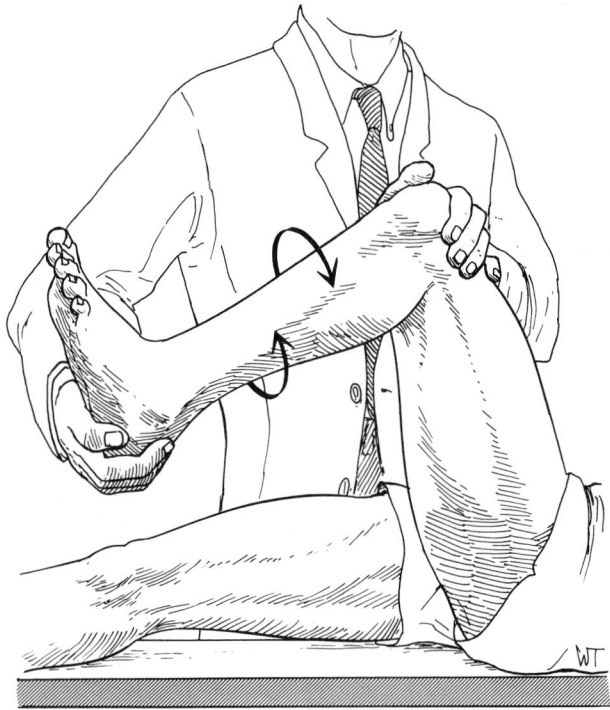

Fig. 5. The McMurray test. (From Kelly MA, Insall JN: Clinical examination. In Insall JN, Windsor RE, Scott WN, et al [eds]: Surgery of the Knee. New York, Churchill Livingstone, 1993, 2nd ed, vol 1, p 63.)

The leg is forced into external and internal rotations at the foot. Pain during external rotation suggests a medial meniscus lesion, whereas pain during internal rotation suggests a lateral meniscus lesion.[23]

Hyperextension Test

Pain localized to the joint space produced during forceful extension is informative. However, a locked meniscus may not be distinguished from an acute ACL lesion.

INVESTIGATION
Plain Radiograph

Anteroposterior, lateral, patellofemoral, and 45-degree knee flexion posteroanterior weightbearing (Rosenberg's view) radiographs should be obtained routinely. Joint space narrowing in the involved compartment is meaningful.

Arthrography

Arthrography is obtained by injecting a radiopaque compound or air, or both (double contrast), into the joint with the knee in a special position. Meniscal tears are detected as fissures, which form as a result of the radiopaque substance leaking into the torn fragments. Only surfaces of the internal joint structures can be imaged. The diagnostic reliability of arthrography ranges between 76% and 95%. Routine use of arthrography is diminishing because of its invasiveness, its requirement of expertise in interpreting the results, and recent developments in MRI. However, currently, arthrography is the most recommended technique in the follow-up of meniscal repairs and their evaluations.[1]

MRI

MRI can show meniscal surfaces and changes in the internal structure of menisci. Menisci appear in the shape of wedges of low signal intensity in the coronal and sagittal planes in all sequences. Peripheral and vascular regions have higher signal intensity. Regardless of whether or not there is a general morphological change in meniscus integrity, increased signal intensity indicates abnormal histological structure of the meniscus. In a classification based on meniscal signal changes, lesions are graded into four grades.[24] Grade 1 indicates the presence of round small hyperintense areas not extending to the surface of the meniscus. Grade 2 is characterized by a linear increase in signal intensity not involving the meniscal surface. During these two phases, meniscal laceration in arthroscopy has not been detected in 80% of the cases. Grade 3 lesions are characterized by global increase of signal intensity in the meniscus with an extension to the upper or lower surface of the meniscus (Fig. 7). These lesions compose 80% of meniscal lacerations in arthroscopy. Grade 4 lesions, differing from Grade 3 lesions, demonstrate loss of wedge shape and fragmentation of the meniscal body, which is consistent with 90% of meniscal lacerations in arthroscopy.[25]

Loss of thickness in cross-section, surface irregularity, disappearance of sharp meniscal edge, and the double posterior cruciate ligament sign are the other findings of a meniscal lesion (Fig. 8). Overall, MRI demonstrates about 93% sensitivity, 84% specificity, and 90% accuracy for medial meniscus and slightly lower specificity for lateral meniscus lesions.[26]

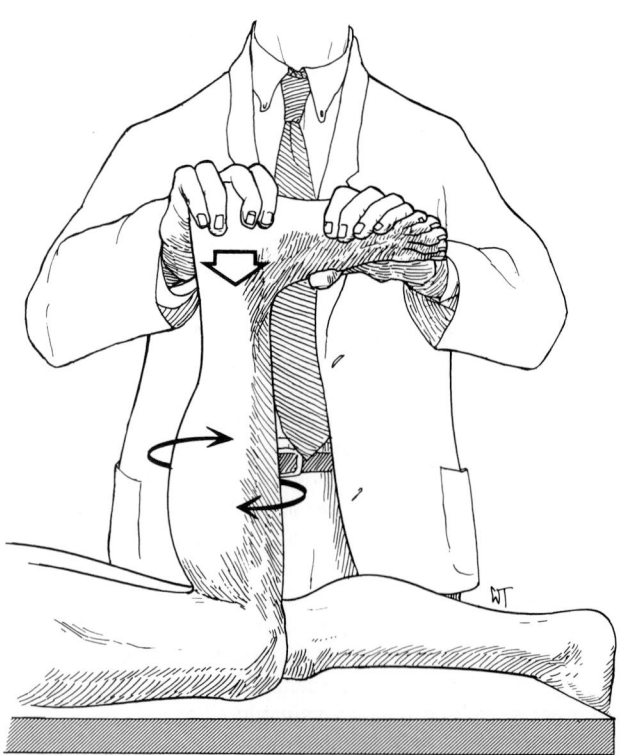

Fig. 6. The Apley test. (From Kelly MA, Insall JN: Clinical examination. In Insall JN, Windsor RE, Scott WN, et al [eds]: Surgery of the Knee. New York, Churchill Livingstone, 1993, 2nd ed, vol 1, p 63.)

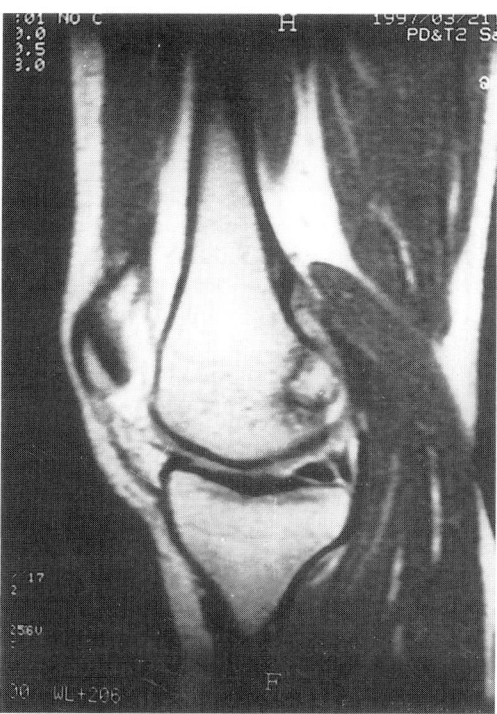

Fig. 7. Grade 3 tear of the posterior horn of the medial meniscus. The view that is presented is a T_1-weighted MRI.

Current MRI techniques do not allow an accurate evaluation of the repaired meniscus as in primary lesions. However, in addition to arthroscopic MRI, noninvasive MRI techniques are also used to fill this gap.[27]

DIFFERENTIAL DIAGNOSIS

One disorder should be distinguished from all other disorders causing knee pain. In an anterior knee pain syndrome, pain is localized anteriorly and not to the joint line, and it increases with prolonged sitting. True locking episodes are not described, and meniscus tests are negative.

Patients with medial and anteromedial knee pain compose the most problematic group. Most have degenerative meniscal disorder as a result of underlying osteoarthritis. Weightbearing radiographs can detect osteoarthritis early. Therefore, these knees cannot be treated as having a discrete meniscal disorder. The patient should be informed about the treatment plan, which should address all pathological conditions.

Osteochondritis dissecans in adolescents and young adults and osteonecrosis in the elderly may show a similar clinical picture to the meniscal injury, and plain radiographs are usually sufficient to differentiate these pathologies.

Other lesions, such as localized villonodular synovitis, imitate meniscal pathology, but most of them are reported as case presentations. In these kinds of rare lesions, arthroscopy is the principal technique to diagnose the pathology.

MANAGEMENT

Nonspecific conservative treatment, including use of nonsteroidal anti-inflammatory drugs, isometric quadriceps exercises, and limitation of bending activities of the knee should be attempted first in most cases. Patients with discrete meniscal symptoms and failed conservative treatments are candidates for surgical intervention (Fig. 9).

The first step of treatment is to distinguish between lesions that should be left alone and those that should be managed by surgical intervention. The basic goal is to restore and protect the anatomic and functional integrity of the meniscus. If this does not succeed, maximum meniscal tissue should be preserved.

There are different options for surgical treatment, which can be classified into two main groups: excisional procedures and meniscal repair.

Regarding excisional procedures, several variables should be considered while deciding on proper treatment. The most significant factors are the localization and extent of lesion; associated ligament injury; patient's activity level, age, profession, and expectations; and microstructural status of the meniscus. Among these factors, the morphology and localization of tear in the meniscal body appear to be the most significant (Fig. 10).[1, 13, 22]

Oblique tears are the most commonly seen lesions. Because total loss of meniscal function may occur with a long tear, repair should be attempted. Partial meniscectomy is an appropriate procedure for short flap lesions.

Vertical-longitudinal tears, the second most common morphological type, together with oblique tears compose about 80% of all meniscal lesions. These are mostly encountered in knees with chronic ACL deficiency. Meniscal repair appears to be a leading choice of treatment, even in lesions of the avascular area.

Horizontal tears encountered mostly in degenerative knees are best treated by partial meniscectomy. If a lesion extends to the meniscocapsular junction, near-total excision may be indispensable.[6]

Radial split tears have mostly a traumatic origin. If a radial lesion extends to the meniscocapsular junction, meniscal function is lost totally. Even though suture placement to hold the fragments together seems difficult, repair should be attempted in young individuals.[28]

Degenerative lesions, which are subjects of debate, are seen in patients older than 40 years without a major trauma history. Partial meniscectomy should be considered first in these patients.

The second classification accounts for meniscal repair of certain localizations of lesion. The meniscus is divided into three circumferential zones from periphery to the central part with respect to the vascularity.[29]

1. Red-to-red zone: This completely vascular area, which has the best healing capacity, consists of about 10% to 30% of the outer part of the meniscus. Successful repair with simple suturing can be obtained in about 90% of vertical-longitudinal tears in this zone.[1, 22]
2. Red-to-white zone: This is an incompletely vascularized area between the vascular and the avascular zone. Lesions in this area show generally good healing, but healing-enhancement techniques should be used.[1]

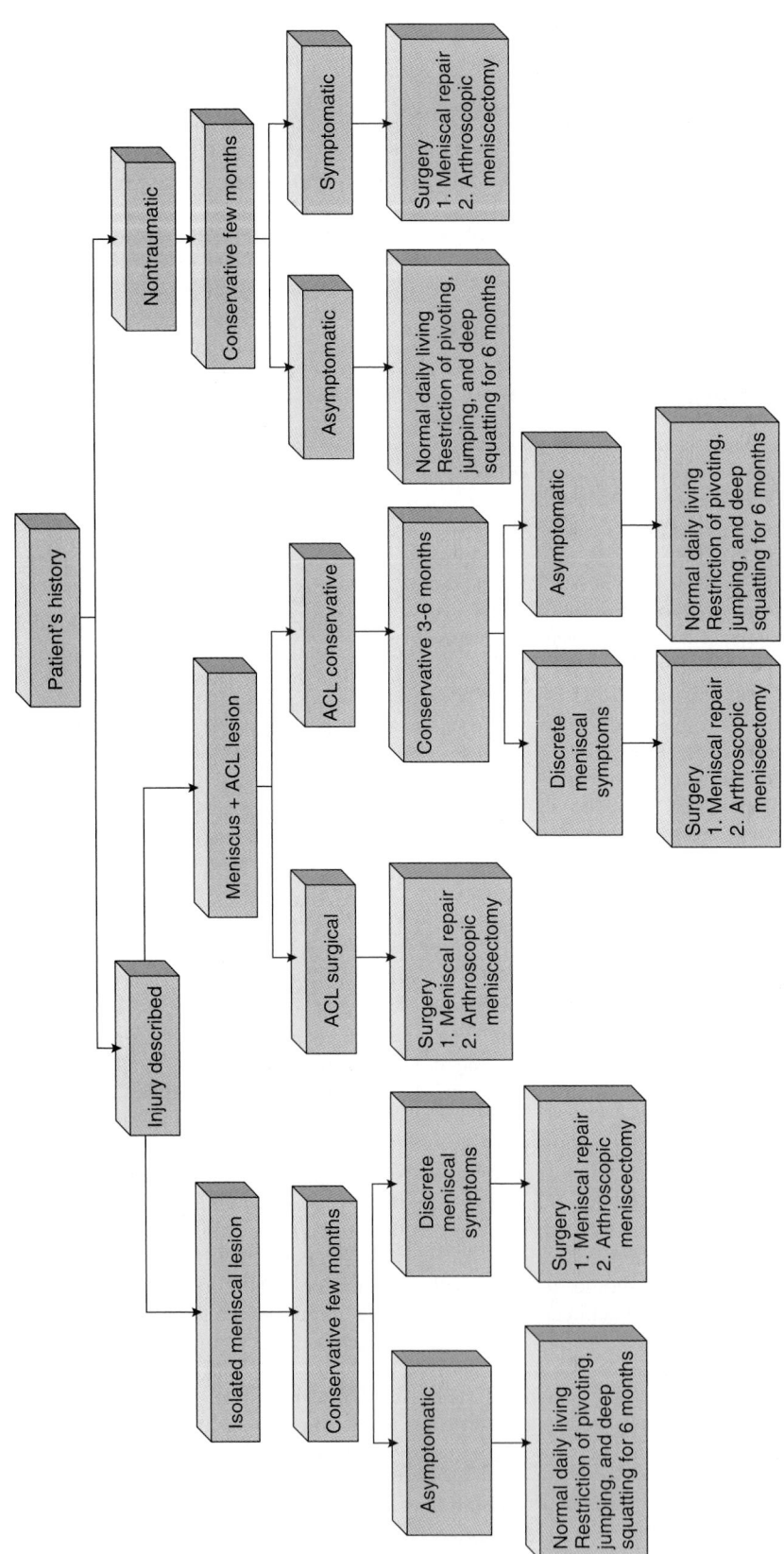

Fig. 8. Algorithm for management of meniscal lesions.

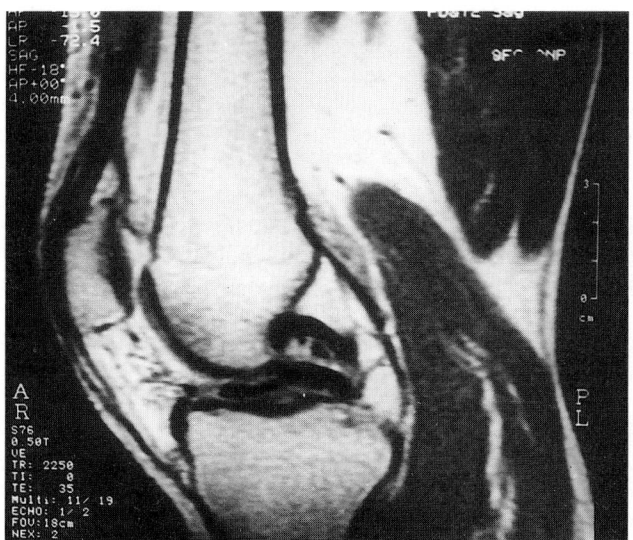

Fig. 9. Double PCL sign of medial meniscus representing a bucket-handle tear.

3. White-to-white zone: This is the completely avascular central portion of the meniscus. Lesions in this zone demonstrate poor healing capacity and high failure rate. Healing-enhancement techniques must be used to increase the success rate.[1, 21, 30]

This classification is a simplistic approach to understanding meniscal healing. In clinical situations, lesions frequently involve more than one zone.

EXCISIONAL PROCEDURES

Menisci have limited intrinsic healing capacity. Repair of torn meniscus cannot be achieved in all cases. Therefore, torn fragments should be removed to alleviate the clinical symptoms. Partial meniscectomy can be successfully applied in most lesions, but total meniscectomy may be indispensable in rare cases.

Total Meniscectomy

Total meniscectomy is the complete removal of the meniscal body. In 1948 Fairbank described postmeniscectomy radiological changes[2]: ridge or osteophyte formation along the periphery of the tibia, flattening of the femoral condyles, and joint space narrowing.

The same findings after meniscectomy were confirmed by other investigators who found a rate of secondary osteoarthritis up to 80%.[3, 4, 31]

Total meniscectomy can be performed via open or arthroscopic techniques. The preservation of meniscocapsular junction cannot be guaranteed by open procedure, and it can be best achieved by arthroscopic techniques.

In view of the current high rates of osteoarthritis, indications for total meniscectomy are limited to lesions that cannot be managed with meniscal repair and partial meniscectomy.

APM

APM is the removal of a minimum amount of meniscal tissue, which can alleviate patients' symptoms.

As in any endoscopic procedure, special surgical equipment is required. Although APM has been accepted as a basic arthroscopic technique, surgeons should familiarize themselves with the technique by taking special instructional courses.

This technique has the advantages of lower surgical morbidity and early return to daily life and sports activities compared with other treatment options.[31, 32] However, it should be kept in mind that APM is a surgical procedure; hence, all steps of surgical principles should be followed properly.

Indications

After the advent of arthroscopy, APM became the most widespread arthroscopic procedure.[34] Irreparable complex tears, degenerative meniscal lesions, and small flap tears, which do not largely impair meniscal function, are the appropriate lesions for APM. In any meniscus lesion that is

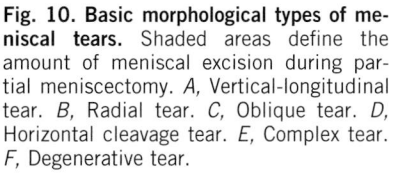

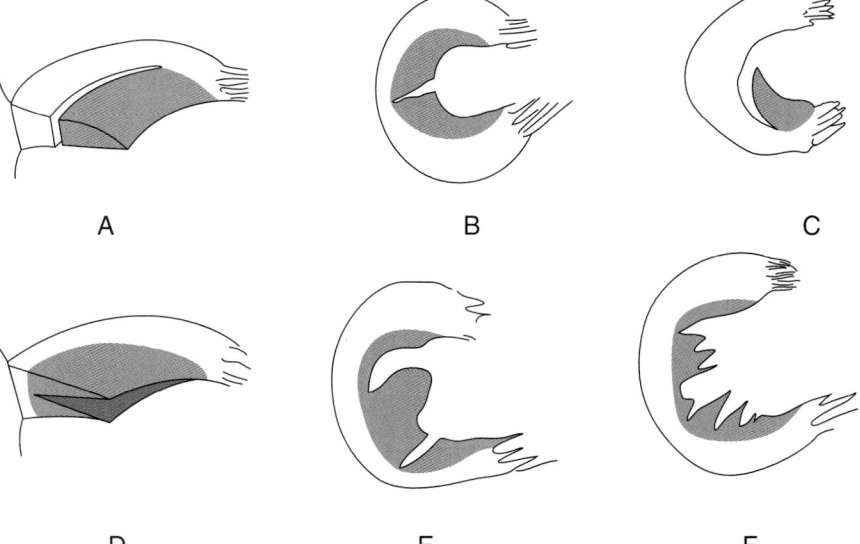

Fig. 10. Basic morphological types of meniscal tears. Shaded areas define the amount of meniscal excision during partial meniscectomy. *A,* Vertical-longitudinal tear. *B,* Radial tear. *C,* Oblique tear. *D,* Horizontal cleavage tear. *E,* Complex tear. *F,* Degenerative tear.

even amenable for repair, APM should be introduced to patients as a therapeutic alternative because of its short-term benefits. In elderly patients, it is preferable to meniscal repair because of lower surgical morbidity and early return to daily activities. Because sports activities can be resumed earlier, APM may also be the treatment of choice among professional athletes.

Advances in meniscal repair techniques and their long-term benefits with regard to articular cartilage protection have decreased the relative indications for APM.

Preoperative Preparation

A proper preoperative planning prevents unnecessary meniscus removal and shortens the operating time. All meniscal lacerations encountered during arthroscopy may not require surgical intervention.

In the presence of associated lesions such as ACL injury, operative planning should be done accordingly. APM is performed as an outpatient procedure in several centers.

Anesthesia

General and regional anesthesia methods are the most widely used. General anesthesia provides complete motor block, thereby allowing easy joint opening. Administration of an intra-articular opiate significantly decreases the post-operative pain and the need for analgesics.[35]

Spinal anesthesia also provides good muscle relaxation, but it may cause severe headache postoperatively. This complication can be avoided by epidural anesthesia, which is more technically demanding. However, desired muscle relaxation may not be accomplished in all cases.

Local anesthesia requires an experienced surgeon and good patient cooperation. Because motor block does not occur, even basic surgery may be difficult in tight knees.

Operating Room Set-Up

Basic endoscopic equipment, including a video camera, 30 to 70-degree optical lenses, light source, video recorder, and a video printer should be present in the operating room.

Arthroscopic Instruments

Basic hand-operated instruments for excisional meniscal surgery include a probe, straight and angled basket forceps, a grasper, low-profile posterior punches, knives, and rasps.

A motorized shaver is an integral part of the excisional procedure. Although meniscal excision can be performed by these classic hardware instruments, lasers and thermal cutters can also be used for the same purpose.

Pneumatic Tourniquet, Leg Holder, Side Support

A bloodless joint increases surgical comfort. In elderly patients and those with a history of thromboembolic disease and circulatory problems, tourniquet use is not advisable. In the case of intra-articular opiate administration for postoperative analgesia, the tourniquet should not be released for 10 minutes after the injection.

The use of a leg holder facilitates the joint opening and allows the surgeon to manipulate the extremity more easily without an assistant. One should be careful not to apply

excessive valgus force in a tight medial compartment because of the risk of medial collateral ligament injury.[5]

Although a simple side support provides less rotational control of the extremity, it is sufficient to obtain good visualization in most cases.

Irrigation Fluids

Ringer's lactate solution is the generally recommended irrigation fluid. Gravity fluid systems generally provide a clear image. A pressurized irrigation system is an alternative way to obtain bloodless field even in a complicated procedure, but the danger of fluid extravasation, particularly after an acute injury, should be kept in mind.

Basic Principles of APM

Although each lesion should be assessed according to its own special features, some basic principles should be remembered in all cases.[5]

All mobile and unstable fragments should be removed.

The meniscocapsular junction should always be preserved, and anatomic orientation of the circumferential collagen fibers should be taken into account during resection.

Sharp edges in rim contour should not be left.

Unnecessary effort should not be spent to obtain a perfectly smooth margin.

Resection should be continued until the healthy meniscal tissue becomes visible.

If one is unsure, less meniscal tissue should be removed.

Hand instruments and a motorized shaver should be used interchangeably, and meniscus should be probed often so as not to remove healthy meniscal tissue.

Surgical Technique

Surgery can be achieved through appropriately localized anterolateral and anteromedial portals in most cases. An accessory portal is rarely required. After the inflow cannula is inserted through the superomedial or superolateral portals, an optic lens is classically put into the joint through the anterolateral portal. A spinal needle should be used to localize the anteromedial portal perfectly. First, a complete arthroscopic examination of the joint should be done with the aid of a probe inserted through the anteromedial portal. Current lens and camera systems and hand instruments allow to the surgeon to use the triangulation technique.

Medial Meniscus. Initially, arthroscope and basket forceps are placed in anterolateral and anteromedial portals, respectively. Medial joint space can be best opened at a knee flexion of 15 to 20 degrees while applying a valgus and external rotation force at the ankle. According to the morphology of the lesion, the fragment can be removed as a block or in small pieces. In a bucket-handle tear (see Fig. 4A), the posterior horn is cut incompletely, and then the anterior horn is punched completely (Fig. 11). The fragment, which is caught through the anterior horn with a grasper, is then turned around and broken through the posterior horn. If the fragment cannot be detached from the posterior horn, an accessory portal is created to cut through the remaining part of the meniscus.[5]

If the anterior horn of the medial meniscus cannot be reached through the anteromedial portal, the arthroscope and hand instruments should be changed to the anterome-

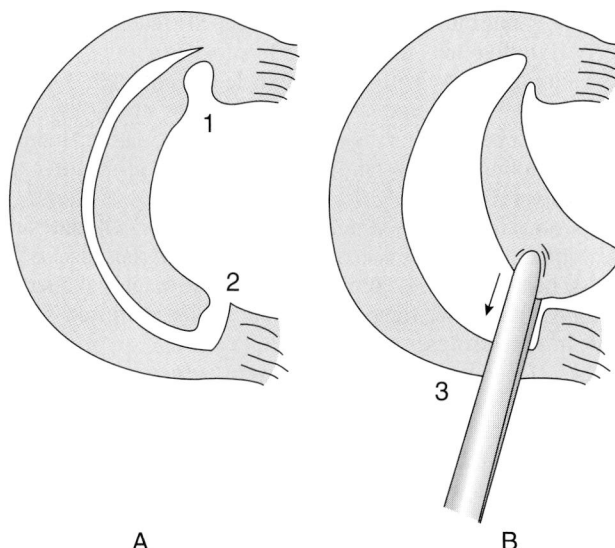

Fig. 11. Technique of meniscal removal for a bucket-handle tear. *A,* Step 1: incomplete cut of posterior horn. Step 2: complete cut of anterior horn. *B,* Step 3: removal of the fragment with a grasper by breaking it off.

dial and anterolateral portals, respectively. The different morphological types should be resected following the same basic principles (see Fig. 10).

Peripheral margins of the posterior horn of the medial meniscus may not be observed during routine arthroscopic examination but can be palpated with a probe. In uncertain situations, a 70-degree scope can be placed through the notch or, alternatively, a posteromedial portal can be created. Another option is to use a 2.7-mm scope through the anteromedial portal.

Lateral Meniscus. The same steps and principles are followed as in medial meniscus resection. The lateral joint space is larger and allows a complete observation and easier manipulation for the surgeon. The anterior horn of the lateral meniscus may not be easily manipulated through the anteromedial portal, and specially angled instruments and accessory portals may be necessary. A meniscal rim in front of the popliteal hiatus should be preserved to maintain the meniscal function properly.

Technical Difficulties
Every effort should be made and great care taken to avoid damaging the articular cartilage. Particularly, the posterior horn of the medial meniscus and the anterior horn of the lateral meniscus may be difficult to reach. Low-profile instruments are necessary to apply safe resection in most circumstances.

Postoperative Care
Once a planned excision procedure is completed, all debris and punched meniscal fragments should be washed out with a cannula and negative aspiration. This will prevent possible debris-related synovitis. Portal incisions are closed with adhesive skin strip or suture or may be left open. Compressive dressing or elastic bandage is applied to the joint.

Isometric quadriceps exercises are started immediately after surgery, and the patient is encouraged to ambulate on the operation day without any support unless additional surgery is done for an associated lesion.[5]

It seems more advisable to start range of motion (ROM) exercises the day after the operation so as not to cause intra-articular bleeding.

The patient can be discharged from the hospital on the day of surgery. At the end of the second week, nearly full ROM and good isometric quadriceps contraction can be obtained with a home exercise program in most cases.

Isotonic and isokinetic exercises can be started at the end of the second week unless any major cartilage pathology exists. Light sports such as bicycling, swimming, and jogging can be resumed at the end of the third week. Strenuous activities are allowed between the fourth and eighth week postoperatively according to the performance of the athlete.[5]

Complications of APM
APM is a more conservative surgery compared with an open meniscectomy. Reported complications are also much lower than with the open technique.[32–34] Damage to the vital structures such as popliteal artery and peroneal nerve is very rare, and those are the only case reports.

The most common complication is postoperative synovial effusion. If effusion persists more than 2 weeks, nonsteroidal anti-inflammatory drugs should be administered. In the case of prolonged effusion, such as that lasting 2 to 3 months, a repeat arthroscopy may be required to remove possible retear or residual fragments.[5]

Swelling immediately postoperatively is an indication of hemarthrosis. It generally occurs as a result of excessive resection of Hoffa's pad or synovial débridement with a motorized shaver. If it does not regress in a few days, joint aspiration should be performed and a Jones compressive dressing should be applied.

Articular cartilage damage may be an inevitable complication of arthroscopic meniscal surgery in the initial learning steps. The majority are incomplete lesions and possibly are not well documented. Their contribution to the degenerative changes is unknown. Articular cartilage damage can be reduced by selecting appropriate portals and creating accessory portals to inaccessible lesions through classic portals.

Instrument breakage can be caused by forceful manipulation in narrow joints and with improper portal placement. It can be prevented by following the same measures just mentioned.

Postmeniscectomy osteonecrosis may appear after an APM procedure. The majority of patients are older than 50 years. Patients generally have a few months without symptoms after the operation, and they describe sudden and severe pain, which may not be well localized. Its etiopathogenesis is unknown. Prospective studies are required.[36, 37]

Other complications that may be encountered in any arthroscopic procedure, such as deep venous thrombosis, synovial fistula, and fluid extravasation, were also seen after partial meniscectomy.

Results of Partial Meniscectomy
The advantages of APM over open meniscectomy such as low surgical morbidity, quick recovery period, short hospi-

talization, and lower complication rate have been well documented by previous studies.[32, 33]

Short-term results demonstrated perfect functional recovery and a very low rate of rerupture of the meniscal rim. One of the most important variables influencing early and late results after partial meniscectomy is the status of articular cartilage at operation, particularly in patients older than 40 years.[38, 39] However, only age does not appear to be a factor that affects the results adversely, and men seem to have better results than women.[39]

Associated ACL deficiency, as well as articular cartilage status, affects the results unfavorably, and reconstruction of the ACL cannot contribute to the prevention of the degenerative process.[39]

Varus malalignment with a tibia-femoral angle less than 4 degrees accelerates the degenerative process in women after partial medial meniscectomy.[39]

Increasing numbers of long-term follow-up studies demonstrated that degenerative changes do occur after partial meniscectomy, although they are less severe and have lower morbidity than after total meniscectomy.[38, 40]

MENISCAL REPAIR

In meniscal repair, the disrupted edges of the meniscus are fixed by sutures or other materials. It was not until the repair techniques improved during the last two decades that meniscal repair gained great attention. It is a more complicated surgery compared with partial meniscectomy. The ultimate goals of meniscus repair should be to obtain a symptom-free knee and prevent secondary osteoarthrosis.

Indications

The question as to which meniscal lesions should be repaired remains unanswered. The menisci have poor intrinsic healing capacity because of insufficient vascularity. The vascular peripheral part shows a remarkably higher healing rate than the central avascular part. Therefore, the localization of the lesion is of prime importance, and the repair should be considered first for lesions located in the red to red zone. Vertical-longitudinal lesions show the highest rate of healing: up to 90% in this zone.[1, 21, 22, 29]

Meniscal repair should also be primarily attempted for the lesion extending through the red to white area together with exogenous fibrin clot. In the young and active populations, the lesions in the totally avascular area should also be considered for a repair using healing-enhancement techniques such as fibrin clot, abrasion of synovial fringe, and creation of vascular access channels.[1] Because of the high success rate of the tears concurrently managed with ACL deficiency, meniscal repair should be the first surgery of choice regardless of lesion localization and size.[1] However, the success and survival rates are lower in the ACL-deficient knee.[1, 21, 22]

In complex, long oblique and radial tears extending to the periphery of the meniscus, excision may cause complete loss of meniscal function. Therefore, in these lesions, repair is advisable, but alternative techniques should be used to promote healing.[1, 28, 30]

Repair is not recommended in degenerative tears and osteoarthritic knees. Although chronological age does not seem to be a factor influencing healing adversely, partial meniscectomy, which provides a shorter recovery period

and lower morbidity, is the recommended treatment, particularly in individuals older than 50 years.[1]

Meniscal lesions with tear length less than 1 cm, incomplete stabile tears, and asymptomatic tears should be left alone. In spite of poor healing capacity, the lateral meniscus, in particular, may show spontaneous healing after an acute injury.

No objective data demonstrate lower healing and survival rates in high-level athletes. However, because of a longer healing period compared with that of partial meniscectomy, meniscus repair may not be the preferred treatment in elite professionals.[1]

The effect of period from injury to surgery on the healing process is another subject of debate. Although fresh lesions, those within 8 weeks after the trauma, have more ability for healing, chronicity of a lesion should not discourage the surgeon from attempting a repair.

For a successful repair, all preparations should be completed, taking into account all the possibilities that might arise during arthroscopy. The patient should be aware of the treatment alternatives and state clearly the preferred treatment. However, the final decision for the most appropriate treatment can be made by the surgeon after considering the patient's expectation upon completion of diagnostic arthroscopy.

Surgical Technique

Once a decision is made for a repair, localization and size of the tear is determined. Then the surgeon attempts to reduce the fragment completely. Subsequently, both sides of the tear and perimeniscal synovium are refreshed by a meniscal rasp. The next step is to fix the lesion, for which there are two main alternatives: open repair and arthroscopic repair. Successful results have been reported with both techniques.

Open Repair

DeHaven[1] first described and developed open repair. A tear localized within 2 to 3 mm of the peripheral margins of the meniscus is accessible with this technique. Lesions limited to the posterior horn are more convenient for open repair. Otherwise, an accessory incision or longer incision may be needed for lesions extending to the middle and anterior thirds.

Posteromedial vertical skin incisions 5 to 6 cm long are used at 90 degrees of flexion of knee for medial meniscus repair. The capsule should be opened just posterior to the medial collateral ligament. Vital structures should be protected with a retractor placed between the capsule and the gastrocnemius (Fig. 12). After refreshing the meniscal edge, vertical mattress sutures are placed and tied over inside or outside the capsule. Different suture materials have been recommended, ranging from absorbable (4-0 polyglactin suture) to nonabsorbable materials (2-0 polyester suture).

Exogenous fibrin clot is recommended for an isolated repair. If repair is combined with ACL reconstruction, the sutures are tied after the tourniquet release to allow fibrin clot formation between the lips of the tear.[1]

The popliteal tendon may hinder manipulation and optimal suture placement on the lateral side. Care should be taken not to pass the sutures through the popliteal tendon, because the stability of the sutures may be diminished.

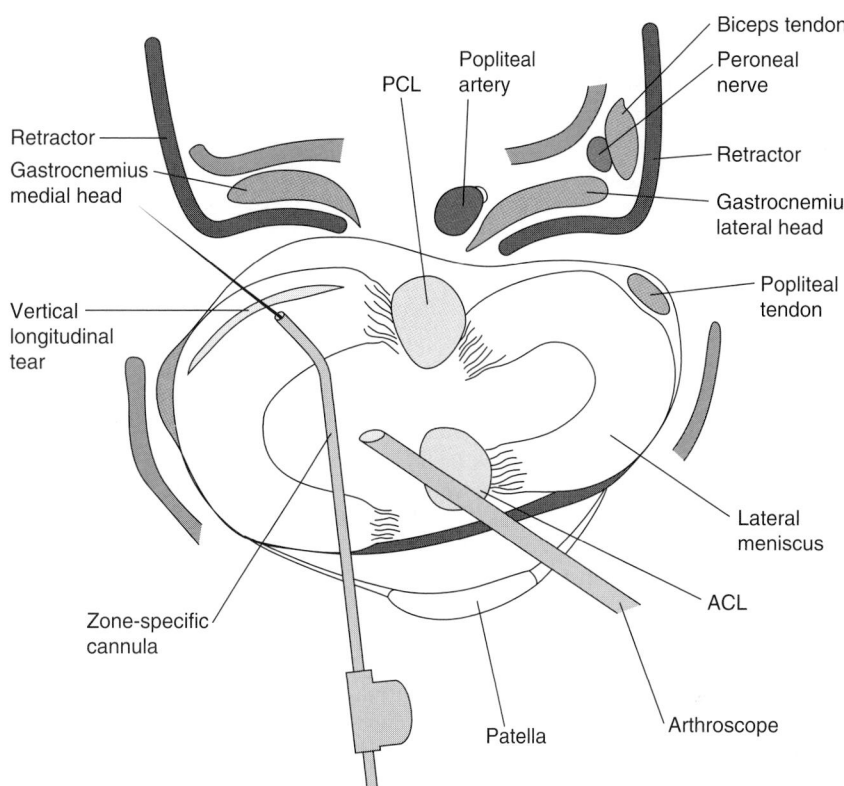

Biceps tendon
Peroneal nerve
Retractor
Gastrocnemius lateral head
Popliteal tendon
Lateral meniscus
ACL
Arthroscope
Patella
Zone-specific cannula
Vertical longitudinal tear
Gastrocnemius medial head
Retractor
PCL
Popliteal artery

Fig. 12. Suture of posterior horn of the medial meniscus. The technique is performed with a zone-specific cannula. The posterior vital structures are protected.

Optimal and reliable suture orientation has been stated as the major advantage of the open technique.[1, 14]

Arthroscopic Techniques

Arthroscopic techniques have some advantages over open repair, but special equipment is required as in other arthroscopic procedures. Although use of meniscal arrow and staple has been described, suture technique is still more widely used in most centers. There are three different techniques based on the direction of the needle and the method by which it is passed: outside-in, inside-out, and all-inside.[1, 29]

Outside-In

A spinal needle (18 gauge) is passed through the capsule and meniscus from outside to the inside of the joint after the capsule is exposed by a vertical incision over the joint line. The main advantages of the technique are its lower complication rate of pericapsular structures and lack of special equipment. However, suture orientation may not be achieved as desired, and a high failure rate has been reported in posterior horn tears of the medial meniscus.[41]

Inside-Out

The special sutures, absorbable or nonabsorbable (commercially available polyglyconate or polyester sutures), long and double-armed, are passed through the meniscus and then the capsule and then are tied over the capsule. The knot is outside the joint.

The technique can be best applied using a zone-specific cannula system or double-barrel cannula system, both of which allow desired suture orientation.[1]

Surgical Technique (Inside-Out)

Medial Meniscus. A vertical skin incision, about 5 to 6 cm long, is made on the posteromedial corner of the knee. Care is taken to protect the saphenous nerve, which crosses the incision line in most cases. The dissection should continue down to the capsule, passing through the deep fascia. The vital popliteal structures should be protected while a special retractor is placed between the capsule and the medial head of gastrocnemius (Fig. 12). After the meniscal fragments and meniscosynovial junctions are refreshed with a rasp, sutures are inserted through the anteromedial or anterolateral portals depending on the suture system used and are taken out through the posteromedial skin incision.[22]

A second skin incision in front of the medial collateral ligament may be required to take out the suture passed for lesions extending through the anterior horn of the meniscus.

Both upper and lower surfaces of the meniscus can be used to insert the sutures. Vertical sutures provide the strongest initial fixation and grasp the circumferential fibers well.[1, 22] The more divergent placement of the suture holds more circumferential fibers and provides better stability.[21] Horizontal- and vertical-oriented sutures can be used according to the tear pattern (Figs. 13 and 14). The sutures should be tied over the capsule after tourniquet release. Exogenous fibrin clot should be placed between the tear edges in an isolated repair. During this step, inflow should be stopped and fluid evacuated. This will enhance the healing ability of the repair. There is no need to replace fibrin clot for a repair combined with an ACL reconstruction.

Lateral Meniscus. After the same initial steps are followed, a posterolateral vertical skin incision is made, and

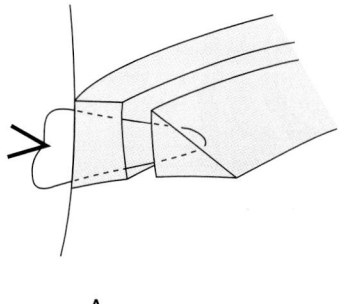

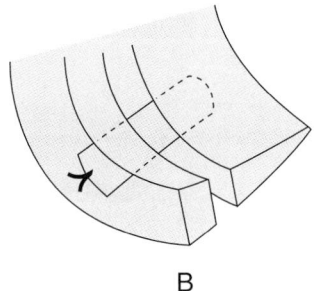

Fig. 13. Commonly used sutures. *A*, Vertical mattress suture. *B*, Horizontal mattress suture.

A

B

the dissection is made deeper down to the capsule, taking the iliotibial band and lateral collateral ligament anteriorly and biceps tendon posteriorly. After considering the proximity of the posterior horn of the lateral meniscus to the popliteal artery, dissection should be made deep enough medially between the capsule and lateral head of the gastrocnemius (see Fig. 12).

Postoperative Care and Rehabilitation

Currently, there are two general tendencies related to postoperative care. One is a classic, more conservative approach,[1, 22] and the other is aggressive and more recent.[42]

DeHaven recommended immobilization of the knee in a hinged brace for the first 2 weeks and then limited motion between 10 and 80 degrees. The brace is abandoned at the end of the fourth week, and the patient is permitted only touch-down walking with double crutches until the end of the sixth week. Full weightbearing is started at the end of the seventh or eighth week. Strenuous activities are restricted for 6 months. A high long-term success rate (79%) was reported in patients following this regimen.[1]

Cannon[22] advocated a similar approach in arthroscopic repair, except the knee is immobilized even longer (3 weeks at 30 degrees of flexion). Partial and total weightbearing is allowed at 4 and 6 weeks, respectively. Contact sports are restricted for about 9 months.

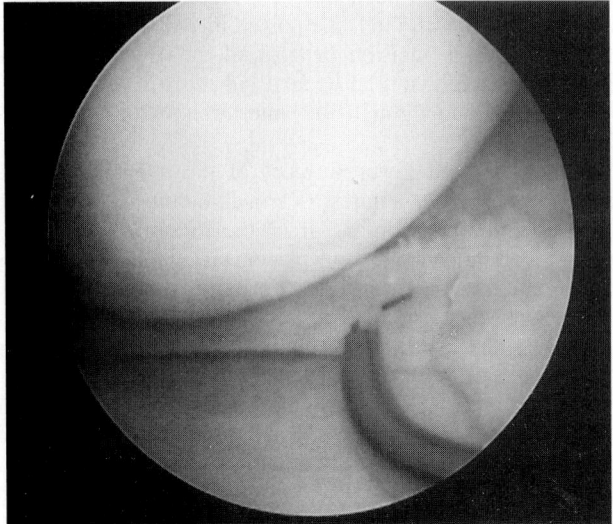

Fig. 14. Arthroscopic view of inside-out meniscal repair.

An accelerated rehabilitation program was attempted in an effort to overcome the problems of slow return to daily life and sports, but it was not highly accepted by patients.

Unrestricted, early, full-motion, immediate weightbearing and return to agility activities as early as 3 months are considered not to decrease the repair success. Early results seem to be comparable to those of conservative approaches.[42]

If a meniscal repair has been done with ACL reconstruction, immediate active or passive motion is recommended to prevent arthrofibrosis. Most surgeons advocate the classic ligament protocol.[1]

All-Inside

The all-inside approach was first described by Morgan in 1991.[1, 29] Special instruments such as a suture passer and a knot pusher are required. Posteromedial and posterolateral portals are used as instrumentation portals, and a 70-degree scope is introduced through the intercondylar notch. It is a technically demanding procedure and is limited to posterior horn peripheral lesions within a margin less than 3 mm for both menisci. Because posterolateral and posteromedial incisions are avoided, its main advantage is cosmetic.

Other techniques such as the T-fix suture system and meniscal arrows are more easily applicable to any part of the meniscus.[1] The short-term results seem acceptable. The complication rate may be lower than in other techniques, but all are technically demanding procedures with unproved benefits.

Complications of Meniscal Repair

The overall complication rate shows great variability. Although Small[34] reported a very low complication rate compared with that of partial meniscectomy, this study included cases of experienced surgeons at the different centers. In a study that focused on any complication from the procedure, Austin and Sherman[43] demonstrated a high complication rate (18%). The most frequent complication encountered in medial meniscal repair is saphenous neuropathy. The branches of the saphenous nerve are highly variable, and they cross the possible incision line in most circumstances. Risk can be eliminated using all-inside repair techniques. Fortunately, high spontaneous healing is observed after a saphenous neuropathy, and a few months should be allowed to pass before surgical exploration.

Another frequent complication is arthrofibrosis, which generally occurs with a simultaneous ACL reconstruction. A ligament rehabilitation program is recommended for postoperative care. Another option is to follow a two-stage operation.

Damage to vital structures such as the popliteal artery and peroneal nerve may occur during the procedure. The surgeon can avoid these complications by using prudent dissection, properly placing the retractors between the capsule and head of the gastrocnemius muscle, and holding the knee in about 90 degrees of flexion. Deep infection has also been reported as a cause of failure. Prophylactic antibiotics and appropriate management of the wound can eliminate this risk.[44] Osteonecrosis is also seen after medial meniscal repair. The same clinical picture occurs as in osteonecrosis after partial meniscectomy.[36] All other complications that may be encountered during or after any arthroscopic procedure may also be experienced during and after meniscal repair. Meniscal repair is an advanced arthroscopic procedure, and most of the complications can be best avoided with proper preoperative planning and proper surgical technique.

Results of Meniscal Repair

Short-term studies focused on healing rate, considering the resolution of the symptoms and clinical signs. Several reported successful results up to 90%.[1] However, the best objective argument could be obtained with second-look arthroscopy.[21, 22] Repaired menisci were roughly graded into three levels based on healing quality.

1. Completely healed meniscus demonstrates incorporation of torn fragment without any cleft.
2. Incompletely healed meniscus demonstrates a cleft between the torn fragment and meniscal body.
3. Unhealed meniscus represents a lack of any repaired tissue with an unstable fragment.

It was observed that most of the incompletely healed lesions showed no symptoms of failure, and most were mentioned as successful repairs.[22] Do these menisci function properly? Are these menisci susceptible to rerupture? Long-term studies in which the average follow-up period varies between 10 and 13 years demonstrated that the involved compartments show insignificant degenerative changes compared with partial meniscectomy.[1, 13, 14] Clinical success and survival rates similar to those of short-term studies, in which incompletely healed lesions are also included, seem to be maintained in these long-term studies. These findings suggest that both completely and incompletely healed menisci function well 10 to 13 years postoperatively, and survival rate does not change significantly during this period.

Distance of the lesion to the vascular area seems to be the major determinant of healing. Although lesions within the 3-mm peripheral part demonstrate a healing rate of about 90%, this drops to 50% to 60% in other lesions with a distance of 5 mm or more.[22] Rubman et al[30] attempted to repair all meniscal lesions in the avascular area using healing-enhancement techniques. Even in complex tears, they reported a high success rate of about 63%. Some authors recommend the meniscal repair as a first choice of treatment in the young population regardless the lesion type. In another study, encouraging results were obtained even in radial tears.[28]

The reconstruction of ACL and repair of the meniscus in one stage gives better results than isolated repairs.[1] This may be attributed to more inflammation and more fibrin clot formation in the joint. In contrast, ACL deficiency appears to decrease both healing and survival rate.[1, 22]

Lesions with tear lengths less than 2 cm demonstrate a lower failure rate than those with longer tear lengths.[22, 29]

Suture preference (absorbable versus nonabsorbable) does not seem to be a factor influencing healing success. However, possible weakening of the tensile strength of an absorbable suture, particularly after the third week, should be considered in postoperative care.

On the basis of the short-term healing success rates, there appears to be no difference between the accelerated and conservative rehabilitation programs. However, no data exist demonstrating long-term results obtained with accelerated rehabilitation. Controlled, prospective clinical trials are needed to elaborate this point.

Because of the unexpectedly bad results of meniscal transplantation and failure to prevent the secondary degenerative changes even after partial meniscectomy, meniscal repair is becoming the treatment of choice in a traumatic meniscal laceration, even in lesions previously regarded as unrepairable.[1, 28, 30]

MENISCAL SUBSTITUTION

In this procedure, the surgeon attempts to replace the resected meniscus with a biological or a synthetic material. Although several clinical trials and experimental studies were conducted, no remarkable progress has been made within the last 15 years.[9] In a great majority of such efforts, allografts were used as graft materials. A few attempts have been made using tendon autografts and synthetic materials.[45]

Indications

Young and mature patients with completely resected menisci as a result of trauma are the foremost candidates for the procedure.

Because ligamentous instability and mechanical axis deviation may endanger the healing process, these disorders should be corrected simultaneously with or before the procedure. In degenerative knees with a resected meniscus, transplantation is contraindicated, considering the risk of the same degenerative events for the transplanted meniscus.

Results

Meniscal substitution allows reduction of pain and relief of symptoms in patients in whom graft incorporation occurs. However, the progression of degenerative radiological findings cannot be prevented with current techniques.[9]

This is a very technically demanding procedure. Graft mismatch and improper fixation of the anterior and posterior horns are still major problems.[10, 45]

Graft shrinkage, which is mostly encountered in freeze-dried allografts, may occur during the cellular regrowth and remodeling phase and causes failure of the meniscal function.[9] Fresh and cryopreserved allografts perform better, but the risk of disease transmission cannot be eliminated.

Meniscal transplantation is still an investigational procedure with several unsolved problems. More clinical trials and animal experiments are required in a carefully selected homogeneous population.

DISCOID MENISCUS

DEFINITION

Discoid meniscus is a morphological anomaly in which the normally semilunar-shaped meniscus is in the shape of a disk.

HISTORICAL OVERVIEW

Discoid meniscus was first described by Young in 1889.

In 1910, Kroiss described "the snapping knee syndrome" and explained its relation to discoid meniscus.[46]

In 1979, Watanabe et al[47] developed a new classification system that is widely accepted today.

EPIDEMIOLOGY

In studies from Scandinavian countries, the United States, and Europe, the disorder has rarely been encountered during arthroscopy, with rates ranging from 0.4% to 3.5%. In the Far East countries, disorder rates as high as 26% in arthroscopic series have been demonstrated.[47]

There is no gender difference and lesions were bilateral in about 10% of cases. Discoid meniscus is mostly found laterally. Discoid meniscus medially is quite rare. Smillie reported only seven cases of discoid meniscus among 10,000 meniscectomy cases. This disorder has been encountered mostly in late childhood and adolescence.[47]

PATHOGENESIS

The cause of discoid meniscus is unknown. Neither the theory of "arrest of fetal development of meniscus" nor the mechanical theory has been explained by further studies.

Currently, the most widely accepted classification scheme, which was described by Watanabe, is as follows: complete type, incomplete type, Wrisberg's variant.

Although first two are described on the basis of the coverage area of the lateral tibial plateau, the Wrisberg type is defined as a normal meniscus with the absence of posterior meniscotibial attachment. The Wrisberg variant, which is not observed by some authors, is a subject of debate.[47]

CLINICAL FEATURES

The main complaint of the patient is joint line pain. A classic finding is a palpable "clunk" felt on the joint line during terminal 15 to 20 degrees of extension. Extension loss, snapping, giving way, joint line tenderness, and a palpable mass at the joint line are the other diagnostic findings. Classic snapping knee syndrome is mostly encountered with the Wrisberg type. Lesions are generally localized in the middle and posterior segments of the meniscus with a horizontal tear.[47]

INVESTIGATION

Findings on plain radiograph can be realized only with comparative films. Such findings include widening of the joint space, hypoplasia of the lateral femoral condyle, and squared-off and cupping of the lateral tibial plateau. Ar-

throgrophy is a valuable diagnostic tool, but it is an invasive procedure.

MRI is an expensive, but the most acceptable, diagnostic technique. A bow-tie view in three consecutive frontal images, increased thickness of the meniscus, and continuity of the anterior and posterior horns of the meniscus in three 5-mm thick sequential images are the radiographic findings.[48]

DIFFERENTIAL DIAGNOSIS

In adolescents, osteochondritis dissecans can be differentiated by anteroposterior, lateral, and tunnel radiographic films. In adults, all meniscal disorders present similar findings. MRI or arthrography may help to clarify the diagnosis.

MANAGEMENT

Conservative measures are advised for rarely symptomatic knees without effusion and mechanical blockage. Patients with extension deficits and prolonged effusion are candidates for surgery. Although some controversy exists regarding the amount of meniscus to be removed, the general tendency is to preserve the sufficient meniscal margin to prevent secondary osteoarthritis.[49] Meniscal repair or reattachment of the posterior horn should be considered for Wrisberg's type to avoid secondary degenerative changes.[50]

MENISCUS CYST

Meniscus cysts are quite rare. Although the overall rate is about 7% in surgically removed menisci, Mills and Henderson[51] found only 20 (0.3%) medial meniscus cysts in 7435 knee arthroscopies. Most of the meniscus cysts were located at the lateral meniscus with horizontal cleavage tears. This pathology is more frequent in males, and a wide age range was reported.

PATHOGENESIS

The etiopathogenesis of the meniscus cyst is not clearly understood. Barrie,[52] in 1979, observed that all meniscal cysts communicated with a torn meniscus. Meniscal cysts are also identified with discoid menisci. Mills and Henderson[51] reported knee trauma in 80% of their patients.

CLINICAL FEATURES

A palpable mass in the joint line along with pain may be diagnostic. The palpable cysts are more prominent at 15 to 30 degrees of flexion, and they disappear at full extension and flexion greater than 90 degrees.

INVESTIGATION

Plain radiographs are generally normal, but in long-lasting untreated cases defects in the tibial plate can be observed that are secondary to the erosion of the cyst. MRI can clearly show the meniscus cyst and the concomitant tear.[53]

DIFFERENTIAL DIAGNOSIS

A differential diagnosis should be performed for all disorders that may cause any mass lesion around the joint line. Pes anserinus bursitis, bursitis of the medial and lateral collateral ligaments, and other types of inflamed bursa should be considered in the differential diagnosis.

MANAGEMENT

Lesions may be left alone in asymptomatic patients. Surgery is a leading choice of treatment in a symptomatic meniscus cyst. APM along with decompression of cyst via arthroscopic or open excision is the most commonly recommended method.[54]

McLaughlin and Noyes advised extra-articular cyst excision and open or arthroscopic meniscal repair to preserve more of the structural integrity and function of the meniscus.[55]

REFERENCES

1. DeHaven KE: Meniscus repair. Am J Sports Med 1999; 27:242.
2. Fairbank TJ: Knee joint changes after meniscectomy. J Bone Joint Surg Br 1948; 30:664.
3. Tapper EM, Hoover NW: Late results after meniscectomy. J Bone Joint Surg Am 1969; 51:517.
4. Johnson RJ, Kettelkamp DB, Clark W, et al: Factors affecting late results after meniscectomy. J Bone Joint Surg Am 1974; 56:719.
5. Ikeuchi H: The early days of arthroscopic surgery in Japan. Arthroscopy 1988; 4:222.
6. Metcalf RW, Burks RT, Metcalf MS, et al: Arthroscopic meniscectomy. In McGinty JB, Caspari RB, Jackson RW, et al (eds): Operative Arthroscopy. Philadelphia, Lippincott-Raven, 1996, p 263.
7. Cox JS, Nye CE, Schaffer WW, et al: The degenerative effects of partial and total resection of the medial meniscus in dogs' knees. Clin Orthop 1975; 109;178.
8. Shrive NG, O'Connor JJ, Goodfellow JW: Load bearing in the knee joint. Clin Orthop 1978; 131:279.
9. Goble EM, Kane SM, Wilcox TR, et al: Meniscal allografts. In McGinty JB, Caspari RB, et al (eds): Operative Arthroscopy. Philadelphia, Lippincott-Raven, 1996, p 317.
10. Messner K: Meniscal regeneration or meniscal transplantation? Scand J Med Sci Sports 1999; 9:162.
11. Neyret P, Donell ST, Dejour H: Results of partial meniscectomy related to the state of the anterior cruciate ligament. Review at 20 to 35 years. J Bone Joint Surg Br 1993; 75:36.
12. Eggli S, Wegmüller H, Kosina J, et al: Long-term results of arthroscopic meniscal repair. An analysis of isolated tears. Am J Sports Med 1995; 23:715.
13. Johnson MJ, Lucas GL, Dusek JK, et al: Isolated arthroscopic meniscal repair: A long-term outcome study (more than 10 years). Am J Sports Med 1999; 27:44.
14. Muellner T, Egkher A, Nikolic A, et al: Open meniscal repair: Clinical and magnetic resonance imaging findings after twelve years. Am J Sports Med 1999; 27:16.
15. Arnoczky SP: Meniscus. In Fu FH, Harner CD, Vince KG (eds): Knee Surgery. Baltimore, Williams & Wilkins, 1994, vol 1, p 131.
16. Berlet GC, Fowler PJ: The anterior horn of the medial meniscus: An anatomic study of its insertion. Am J Sports Med 1998; 26:540.
17. Seedholm BB, Hargreaves DJ: Transmission of load in the knee joint with special

reference to the role of menisci. II. English Med 1979; 8:220.
18. Gray JC: Neural and vascular anatomy of the menisci of the human knee. J Orthop Sports Phys Ther 1999; 29:23.
19. Levy I, Torzilli P, Warren R: The effect of medial meniscectomy on anterior posterior motion of the knee. J Bone Joint Surg Am 1982; 64:883.
20. Poehling GG, Ruch DS, Chalsan SJ: The landscape of meniscal injuries. Clin Sports Med 1990: 9:539.
21. Henning CE: Current status of meniscus salvage. Clin Sports Med 1990; 9:567.
22. Cannon WD Jr: Arthroscopic meniscal repair. In McGinty JB, Caspari RB, Jackson RW, et al (eds): Operative Arthroscopy. Philadelphia, Lippincott-Raven, 1996, p 299.
23. Kelly MA, Insall JN: Clinical examination. In Insall JN, Windsor RE, Scott WN, et al (eds): Surgery of the Knee. New York, Churchill Livingstone, 1993, 2nd ed, vol 1, p 63.
24. Beltran J: MRI of the problem knee. In Taveras JM, Ferrucci JT (eds): Radiology: Diagnosis-Imaging-Intervention. Philadelphia, Lippincott-Raven.
25. Munk B, Madsen F, Lundorf E, et al: Clinical magnetic resonance imaging and arthroscopic findings in knees: A comparative prospective study of meniscus, anterior cruciate ligament and cartilage lesions. Arthroscopy 1998; 14:171.
26. Mackenzie R, Palmer CR, Lomas DJ, et al: Magnetic resonance imaging of the knee: Diagnostic performance studies. Clin Radiol 1996; 51:251.
27. van Trommel MF, Potter HG, Ernberg LA, et al: The use of noncontrast magnetic resonance imaging in evaluating meniscal repair: Comparison with conventional arthrography. Arthroscopy 1998; 14:2.
28. van Trommel MF, Simonian PT, Potter HG, et al: Arthroscopic meniscal repair with fibrin clot of complete radial tears of the lateral meniscus in the avascular zone. Arthroscopy 1998; 14:360.
29. Miller MD, Warner JJP, Harner CD: In Fu FH, Harner CD, Vince KG (eds): Knee Surgery. Baltimore, MD, Williams & Wilkins, 1994, vol 1, p 615.
30. Rubman MH, Noyes FR, Barber-Westin SD: Arthroscopic repair of meniscal tears that extend into the avascular zone: A review of 198 single and complex tears. Am J Sports Med 1998; 26:87.
31. Allen PR, Denham RA, Swan AV: Late degenerative changes after meniscectomy: Factors affecting the knee after operation. J Bone Joint Surg Br 1984; 66:666.
32. McGinty JB, Geuss LF, Marvin LA: Par-

tial or total meniscectomy: A comparative analysis. J Bone Joint Surg Am 1977; 59: 763.
33. Dandy DJ, Jackson RW: Partial meniscectomy. J Bone Joint Surg 1976; 58:142.
34. Small NC: Complications in arthroscopic surgery performed by experienced arthroscopists. Arthroscopy 1988; 4:215.
35. Dalsgaard J, Felsby S, Juelsgaard P, et al: Low-dose intra-articular morphine analgesia in day case knee arthroscopy: A randomized double-blind prospective study. Pain 1994; 56:151.
36. Brahme SK, Fox JM, Ferkel RD, et al: Osteonecrosis of the knee after arthroscopic surgery: Diagnosis with MR imaging. Radiology 1991; 178:851.
37. Prues-Latour V, Bonvin JC, Fritschy D: Nine cases of osteonecrosis in elderly patients following arthroscopic meniscectomy. Knee Surg Sports Traumatol Arthrosc 1998; 6:142.
38. Schimmer RC, Brulhart KB, Duff C, et al: Arthroscopic partial meniscectomy: A 12 year follow-up and two-step evaluation of the long-term course. Arthroscopy 1998; 14:136.
39. Burks RT, Metcalf MH, Metcalf RW: Fifteen year follow-up of arthroscopic partial meniscectomy. Arthroscopy 1997; 13: 673.
40. Rockborn P, Gillquist J: Long-term results after arthroscopic partial meniscectomy: The role of preexisting cartilage fibrillation in a 13 year follow-up of 60 patients. Int J Sports Med 1996; 17:608.
41. van Trommel MF, Simonian PT, Potter HG, et al: Different regional healing rates with the outside-in technique for meniscal repair. Am J Sports Med 1998; 26:446.
42. Barber FA: Accelerated rehabilitation for meniscus repairs. Arthroscopy 1994; 10: 206.
43. Austin KS, Sherman OH: Complications of arthroscopic meniscal repair. Am J Sports Med 1993; 21:864.
44. Blevins FT, Salgado J, Wascher DC, et al: Septic arthritis following meniscus repair: A cluster of three cases. Arthroscopy 1999; 15:35.
45. Kohn D, Verdonk R, Aagaard H, et al: Meniscal substitutes: Animal experience. Scand J Med Sci Sports 1999; 9:141.
46. Aicroth PM, Patel DV, Marx CL: Congenital discoid lateral meniscus in children: A follow-up study and evaluation of management. J Bone Joint Surg Br 1991; 73: 932.
47. Neuschwander DC: Discoid lateral meniscus. In Fu FH, Harner CD, Vince KG (eds): Knee Surgery. Baltimore, MD, Williams & Wilkins, 1994, vol 1, p 393.
48. Ryu KN, Kim IS, Kim EJ, et al: MR im-

aging of tears of discoid lateral menisci. AJR Am J Roentgenol 1998; 171:963.

49. Räber DA, Friedrich NF, Hefti F: Discoid lateral meniscus in children: Long-term follow-up after total meniscectomy. J Bone Joint Surg Am 1998; 80:1579.

50. Rosenberg TD, Paulos LE, Parker RD, et al: Discoid lateral meniscus: Case report of arthroscopic attachment of a symptomatic Wrisberg-ligament type. Arthroscopy 1987; 3:227.

51. Mills CA, Henderson IJ: Cysts of the medial meniscus. Arthroscopic diagnosis and management. J Bone Joint Surg Br 1993; 75:293.

52. Barrie HJ: The pathogenesis and significance of meniscal cysts. J Bone Joint Surg Br 1979; 61:184.

53. Tasker AD, Ostlere SJ: Relative incidence and morphology of lateral and medial meniscal cysts detected by magnetic resonance imaging. Clin Radiol 1995; 50:778.

54. Ryu RK, Ting AJ: Arthroscopic treatment of meniscal cysts. Arthroscopy 1993; 9: 591.

55. Miller RH: Knee injuries. In Canale TS (ed): Campbell's Operative Orthopaedics. St. Louis, MO, CV Mosby, 1998, 9th ed, vol 2, p 1150.

section 4
chapter 15

ANTERIOR KNEE PAIN AND PATELLOFEMORAL JOINT INSTABILITY

Alexander Kalenak

Summary

- Anterior knee pain is often of patellofemoral origin, frequently with no objective abnormality.
- Anterior knee pain may originate from either the patellofemoral joint or from adjacent soft tissues.
- The patella increases the quadriceps moment arm.
- The location and size of the patella articular contact area and the magnitude of the patella's contact stress vary with knee flexion angle.
- Patellar tracking is determined by interplay between the articular surfaces, soft-tissue restraints, and neuromuscular control.
- An isolated patellofemoral disorder rarely produces an effusion. An effusion is more likely due to a meniscal tear, chondral fracture, or anterior cruciate ligament (ACL) injury, but can be associated with a frank patella dislocation or severe patellofemoral arthrosis.
- Radionuclide imaging is useful to confirm the diagnosis in patients with anterior knee pain who have no objective abnormality.
- The vast majority of patients with anterior knee pain or a patellofemoral disorder can be successfully treated nonoperatively.
- Operative treatment should be reserved for those who do not respond to a good nonoperative regimen and in whom a frank patella dislocation, repeated patella subluxations, or severe patellofemoral arthrosis are factors in causing the pain.
- An effective proximal patella realignment operation should be a quadricepsplasty designed to alter the direction of quadriceps pull rather than a mere capsular plication.
- A distal patella realignment operation can alter quadriceps tracking or increase the quadriceps moment arm.

One of the most vexing clinical challenges in orthopaedic surgery is anterior knee pain. This clinical conundrum, according to Dye, was characterized by Stanley James as "the black hole of orthopedics," implying an enigma for which there is no single explanation or therapeutic approach that universally or consistently identifies the problem and is successful in alleviating the problem.

Part of the enigma is the inherent subjectivity of the complaints without easily identifiable, objective findings or abnormalities. Symptoms often are debilitating, interfering seriously with everyday activities or athletic activities. Quite naturally, parents are often distressed to see their child in pain or tears. This presents a major practical problem in the management of anterior knee pain: the anxiety and plaintive perplexity expressed by both parent and child. Often the patient has seen other primary care physicians before seeing the orthopaedic surgeon. The patient is frustrated with repeated visits and sees no light at the end of the tunnel as far as finding pain relief. Without a firm diagnosis, the patient may feel that management lacks direction.

Patients with patellofemoral pain often have no clearly identifiable, objective abnormality. As many as 20% of teenage girls have some or all of the clinical criteria for patellofemoral malalignment, yet only a small percentage ever become symptomatic.[1] Conversely, many patients have patellofemoral crepitus on range of motion but do not have anterior knee pain. Anterior knee pain can be patellofemoral in origin without any objective findings. How does one formulate a rational treatment regimen? Essentially, the development of rational therapy for these patients is an appreciation and understanding of the genesis and pathophysiology of patellofemoral pain. Anterior knee pain has many different causes, some related to the patellofemoral joint, and others related to the joint tissue structures about the patellofemoral joint.[2] It is critical to be deliberate and methodical in evaluating the cause of anterior knee pain. A complete history and a thorough physical examination are crucial. Nonoperative medical treatment (e.g., nonsteroidal, anti-inflammatory medication, ice, physical therapy) for an extended period of time is indicated. Arthroscopy can be a valuable asset in this setting. Coupled with patient education on the pathophysiology of anterior knee pain, it can be a source of reassurance to know that there is no major anatomic abnormality within the knee joint and that the treatment plan continues to be nonoperative management based on arthroscopic findings. It should be good news that there are no torn cartilages, ligaments, or arthritis in the knee and that the inside of the joint is absolutely perfect in appearance. Using video images or photographic images can be quite reassuring. It is imperative that the orthopaedic surgeon and staff explain the cause of pain as arising from soft tissue around the joint as well as pressure that is transmitted through to the subchondral cortical bone. Attempts to alter the mechanical aberrations should be the goal of treatment.

The majority of patients with anterior knee pain and patellofemoral disorders can be treated nonoperatively. Henry and Crosland[3] found that 76% of their patients with patellofemoral disorders could be treated successfully without an operation, and DeHaven et al[4] found this in 82% of their patients. More recently, McConnell[5] stated that 96% of patients can be treated successfully with a closed-chain patellofemoral rehabilitation regimen.

Frustration in regard to the diagnosis and treatment methods, overwork, and "a chance to cut is a chance to cure" mentality can lead to a premature decision for surgery. Orthopaedic surgery training attunes orthopaedic surgeons to use orthopaedic surgical procedures for musculoskeletal disorders, including patellofemoral. This attitude can lead to disaster. The message to orthopaedic surgeons, patients, and rehabilitation personnel should be to emphasize a deliberate, methodical approach to anterior knee pain and patellofemoral disorders, one that takes time and patience and that leads to resolution of symptoms in the majority of patients with patellofemoral disorders.

ANATOMY

The articular surface of the patella has two major facets—medial and lateral—separated by a median ridge (Fig. 1). The medial facet often features a smaller facet called the odd facet at its extreme medial portion that, when present, articulates with the medial condyle in maximum flexion. The articulation between the patella and the trochlea in the axial plane is relatively congruent, whereas that in the sagittal plane (lateral view) is quite incongruent. The transverse congruency ensures mediolateral stability, whereas the sagittal incongruency provides freedom of motion for

the patella in the trochlea, permits sliding articulation, and promotes lubrication. The quadriceps mechanism is composed of four muscles: rectus femoris, vastus intermedius, vastus lateralis, and vastus medialis/vastus medialis obliquus (VMO). The vastus intermedius runs parallel to the femur, but the other muscles insert at an angle. The vastus medialis has a line of action 15 to 18 degrees medial to the long axis of the femur in the frontal plane, the vastus lateralis 20 to 45 degrees lateral, and the VMO 50 to 70 degrees medial to the long axis. The quadriceps mechanism does not function in a straight line but rather at an angle. The quadriceps angle (Q angle) is defined as the angle subtended by the patella tendon and by a line from the center of the patella through the anterosuperior iliac crest. As the quadriceps contracts, the bolstering effect displaces the patella laterally. This may account in part for the fact that the lateral wall of the trochlea is higher and more prominent than its medial counterpart. The VMO is a muscular restraint. The VMO originates from the distal tendinous portion of the abductor magnus and from the adductor longus and medial intermuscular septum and has its own nerve supply. The VMO normally inserts into the superior medial aspect of the patella as far as one-half of the patella length, but in many patients with malalignment the VMO may barely reach the top of the patella, and the fibers are likely to be vertical rather than the normal oblique angle. Therefore, the VMO is a major focus for patella rehabilitation.

Q ANGLE

A Q angle of 10 or 15 degrees is considered normal. The Q angle decreases with flexion as a result of the internal rotation of the tibia relative to the femur.

PATELLOFEMORAL CONTACT AREA

Grelsamer and others[6] noted that only one part of the patella articulates with the trochlea at any given time (Fig. 2). In early degrees of flexion, the distal portion of the patella articulates with the proximal trochlea. As the knee flexes, the contact area moves proximally on the patella. At 90 degrees the superior portion of the patella is in contact with the trochlea. With further flexion, the contact area moves back toward the center of the patella. At full flexion, the medial facet no longer touches the medial trochlea. The odd facet, if present, will articulate with the medial border of the medial femoral condyle in deep flexion. Magnitude of contact increases as the knee flexes. The area quadruples as the knee flexes from 0 to 60 degrees. Some investigators believe the magnitude of contact remains constant between 60 and 90 degrees, whereas others have seen a continued rise in this range. Others have seen a peak of maximum magnitude of contact at 60 degrees. Tracking of the patella has been a subject of debate. Soft-tissue restraints and bony and cartilaginous anatomy play a role. The importance of these structures in patella kinematics still have to be elucidated. It appears in most studies that the normal patella is centered in the trochlea when the knee is flexed. Investigators have found that the patella normally lies in the lateral position at extension.

The patella increases the mechanical efficiency of the quadriceps extensor mechanism. The presence of the patella allows knee flexion and extension to occur with a

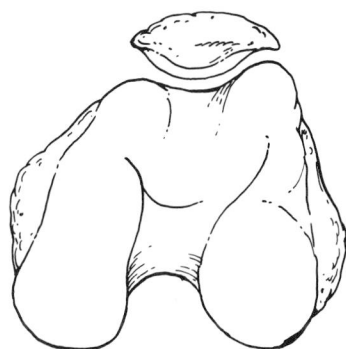

Fig. 1. View. The articular surface of the patella has two major facets, medial and lateral, separated by a median ridge. (From Krackow KA: The Technique of Total Knee Arthroplasty. St. Louis, Mosby, 1990, p 159.)

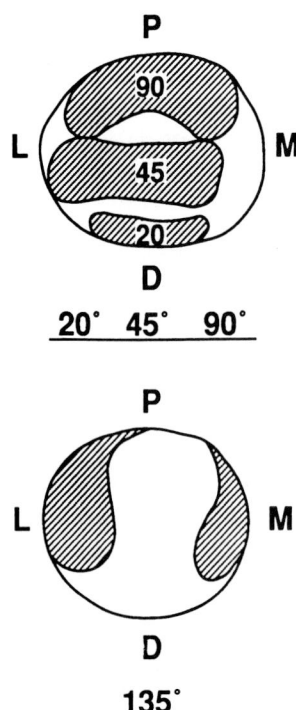

Fig. 2. View. Contact areas of the patella in various positions of knee flexion. (From Ho SSW, Jaureguito JW: Functional anatomy and biomechanics of the patellofemoral joint. Op Tech Sports Med 1994; 2: 243.)

of any one part of this complex can alter normal patella kinematics. This interaction must be taken into account when evaluating and treating anterior knee pain and patellofemoral disorders. The patella should track smoothly within the groove of the femoral trochlea, remaining centered and balanced. Normal patella motion is, in fact, complex with many subtle shifts and rotations.[11–18] The patella has a complex motion arc involving coincident translation and rotation.[13–15, 20] As the knee is extended from the flexed position, the patella translates anteriorly 19 mm me-

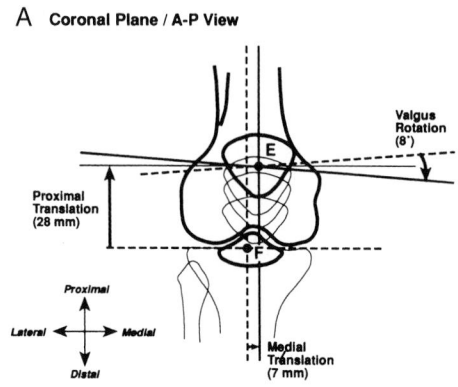

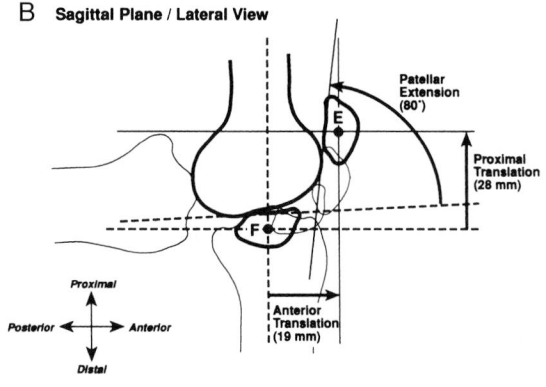

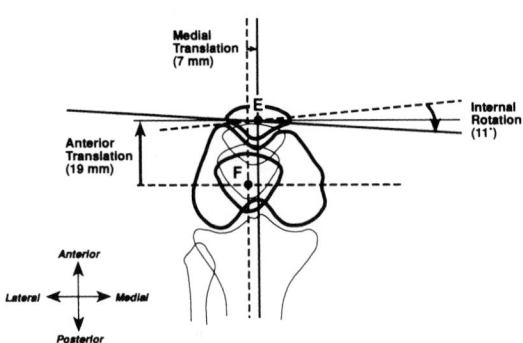

Fig. 3. View. Orthogonal motion of the patella in 6 DOF, relative to a fixed femur, coincident with knee extension. Two translations and one rotation can be measured in each of three standard planes/views: A, Coronal plane/AP view; B, Sagittal plane/lateral view; C, Transverse plane/axial view. Values as reported by Kelman et al: Transactions of the 35th Annual Meeting, Orthopaedic Research Society, 1989. (From Ho SSW, Jaureguito JW: Functional anatomy and biomechanics of the patellofemoral joint. Op Tech Sports Med 1994; 2:242.)

lesser amount of quadriceps force (i.e., the mechanism functions like a lever). In addition to increasing the lever arm of the quadriceps, the patella redirects the force exerted by the quadriceps. As such, it can be considered a pulley. However, in the case of the patellofemoral mechanism, Grelsamer et al[6] suggested that the tension of the quadriceps tendon is generally different from that of the patella tendon. Thus, the patella tendon can be considered an eccentric pulley or cam in that it redirects the force as well as changes its magnitude. The patella and surrounding soft tissue were described by Reider et al.[7] He and his coinvestigators measured 12 parameters of the quadriceps mechanism (Fig. 3). Several were found to correlate significantly with patella shape. In particular, a wider lateral patellofemoral ligament was found to correlate with a Wiberg-type patella. There is great variability in the lateral structures of the quadriceps complex. The most commonly used classification of transverse planes was developed by Wiberg[8] in 1941 (Fig. 4).

The sagittal plane shape of the patella as been described by Grelsamer et al.[9] Conlan et al[10] found that the medial patellofemoral ligament contributes 53% of the restraint of the lateral displacement of the patella, whereas the patella meniscal ligament and associated retinacular fibers of the deep capsule layer contribute an average of 22%.

The goal of the treating physician is to restore and maintain normal kinematics. Patella motion is the result of interaction of three bones (femur, tibia, patella), two articulations (patellofemoral and femoral tibial), one bone-tendon-bone unit (patella–patella tendon–tibia), and one muscle complex (the quadriceps). Injury to or abnormality

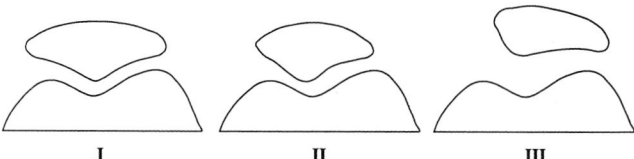

Fig. 4. View. Wiberg's classification of patellar shapes in axial plane. (From Ho SSW, Jaureguito JW: Functional anatomy and biomechanics of the patellofemoral joint. Op Tech Sports Med 1994; 2:240.)

dially (a peak of 7 mm or 30 degrees of flexion) and proximally 28 mm. At the same time, it rotates into valgus in the coronal plane (peak of 8 degrees at 30 degrees of knee flexion), rotates internally in the axial plane (peak of 11 degrees at 15 degrees of knee flexion), and rotates into extension in the sagittal plane.

The relationship between patella and tibia is not fixed. Three-dimensional patella motion relative to the tibia occurs with flexion and extension.[11, 18–22] For instance, as the knee extends, the patella shifts anteriorly 35 to 40 mm relative to the tibia.

Patellofemoral contact increases by more than one-third in size with knee flexion and moves from the distal third to the proximal half as the knee flexes from 20 to 90 degrees. Patellofemoral contact force in the sagittal plane is maximum between 16 and 110 degrees of knee flexion. Forces across the patellofemoral joint have a laterally directed coronal plane component, and the angle of the component vector forces is commonly measured as a Q angle. Neutralizing this coronal plane force is the goal of patella tracking braces, patella taping methods, vastus medialis obliquus strengthening programs, surgical lateral release, and medial reefing or medialization of the tibial tubercle. Anterior tibial tubercle elevation addresses sagittal plane contact forces only. Because of this knowledge and understanding, the coronal component has led to modification such as tibial tubercle anteromedialization, which addresses both sagittal and coronal plane forces.

Patellofemoral contact pressure is maximal between 60 and 90 degrees of knee flexion. Patella tendon tension force is greater than quadriceps tendon force at low knee flexion angles (45 degrees or less), and quadriceps tendon force is greater than patella tendon force at higher flexion angles (greater than 45 degrees).

The Outerbridge classification is crucial in identifying articular cartilages. Outerbridge grade I means that articular cartilage is soft. Grade II articular cartilage has fibrillation less than 0.5 inches in diameter. Grade III has articular cartilage fibrillation greater than 0.5 inches in diameter, and grade IV denotes erosion of articular cartilage with exposed bone.

The anteroposterior thickness of the patella contributes about one-third of the moment arm of the quadriceps in the sagittal plane during knee extension and transmits mechanical loading to subchondral cortical bone. Dye and Vaupel,[23] on the pathophysiology of patellofemoral pain, showed that the origin of patellofemoral pain can be directly traced to supraphysiological mechanical loading and chemical irritation of nerve endings in subchondral and cancellous bone, denoting loss of tissue homeostasis. They stated that the primary factor differentiating this clinical entity from other

knee conditions is inherent subjectivity and that the major problem with primarily subjective conditions is that the final common pathways are central nervous system events. Complex central processing of peripheral nociceptive neurological signals occurs during the perception of pain, allowing various subjective differences among individuals. Patients can also report false symptoms that may be for secondary gain in medicolegal cases or give false symptoms to please the physician. (With these caveats, the presence of patellofemoral pain can be considered a result of nociceptive peripheral nerve irritation and a fundamental reflection of loss of tissue homeostasis.)

According to Dye, the human knee is one of the most complex systems in the biological realm. The knee is composed of 100 billion vertebrate cells. The multiple asymmetric subsystems of the knee are of ancient origin and function in concert as a type of biological transmission. Dye also states that patellofemoral components are routinely subjected to the highest compressive forces of any in the knee, frequently approaching and often exceeding the limits of load acceptance of biological tissue. The peripheral neurological complex is intimately associated with the overall homeostasis of the musculoskeletal system. Pain, pressure, and proprioceptive nerve endings about the knee function as sensitive telemetry devices encoding data to be processed centrally. Neurological components have been demonstrated in all the complex anatomic structures of the patellofemoral system except articular cartilage. It is believed that all patellofemoral tissues have the potential for nociceptive output through substance P fibers. Localized alteration of the neurological telemetry system also can result in patellofemoral pain absent any associated disease of external tissues.

Excessive mechanical overload, either extrinsic or intrinsic, commonly causes patellofemoral nociceptive output. Direct trauma, such as a fall on a flexed knee or a dashboard injury, can result in transient or persistent pain depending on the severity of tissue damage. Excessive intrinsic mechanical loads exceeding tissue acceptance capacity may develop with jumping, hiking, or stair climbing and are common sources of transient, often persistent anterior knee discomfort.

Increased intraosseous pressure of the patella can result in pain directly from bone secondary to transient venous outflow obstruction. This may explain the phenomenon of patella discomfort with prolonged knee flexion in some patients. Dye, on the basis of experimental work, is convinced that the intraosseous environment of the patella can be a nociceptive source in the genesis of anterior knee symptoms. In the case of painful chondromalacia of the patella, part of the nociceptive output may be secondary to excessive load transference to innervated subchondral and cancellous bone. The common experience of patellofemoral pain in some patients with changes of weather may be related to increased barometric sensitivity of nerve endings.

Shifting and transference of load within the patellofemoral system believed to occur in patients with malalignment syndrome can result in excessive mechanical forces, either compression or tension, of a variety of tissues.

Trauma to tissues, either acutely or with repetitive submaximal loading beyond the limits of physiological load acceptance, usually induces a biological cascade of cytokine production.

Cytokines, exemplified by prostaglandins, cathepsins, interleukins, tumor necrosis factors, collagenases, and so on, are chemical hallmarks of musculoskeletal inflammations seen in tendinitis, myositis, and synovitis. Cytokines in tissues produce a chemical irritation in nerve endings, resulting in perception of pain. Dye believed that the pain-producing phenomenon of cytokines has evolved over eons as a type of negative feedback mechanism to alert the chordate to the condition of loss of tissue homeostasis. If the load acceptance capacity of the damaged inflamed tissue is less than that required for activities of daily living, normal activities easily withstood by the system now become superphysiological loads with daily reactivation on the cytokine cascade. Chronic retriggering of the cytokine cascade then becomes a vicious cycle of tissue irritation and continued inflammation manifested by chronic pain. In Dye's experience, more than half of patients with chronic patellofemoral pain have, as part of their mosaic of disease, painful increased osseous remodeling of the patella. He found that reversal of abnormal scintigraphic findings and symptoms in anatomically normal patellofemoral joints takes on average 6 to 9 months with appropriate conservative treatment. His therapeutic approach to patients with chronic patellofemoral pain is threefold and similar to other treatment regimens: addressing pathomechanics, administering appropriate anti-inflammatory therapy, and initiating rehabilitation. The principle is to protect the internal environment to allow the patient's cellular and molecular mechanisms of homeostasis to proceed with tissue healing without further subversion. In conclusion, Dye believed that patients with patellofemoral pain with no overly identifiable structural pathological process have altered tissue homeostasis and that the genesis of chronic pain lies in supraphysiological loading of the patellofemoral components. Such loading is sufficient to reactivate nerve irritation through mechanical or chemical factors.

CLINICAL PRESENTATION/HISTORY

Arriving at an exact diagnosis is a challenge and may be elusive. Historical facts and physical examination findings are fundamental in making a diagnosis. History and physical examination should not be relegated to positions of lesser importance because of modern imaging techniques. Historical facts such as onset of pain (insidious, acute, or related to an incident), relationship to activity (e.g., sports, activities of daily living, night, morning), relationship to repetitive activities or rest, swelling, catching, giving way, redness, and heat should be recorded as part of the historical record. The presence of an effusion is significant in that effusions are unusual in true patellofemoral disorders. Effusions usually point to meniscal tear, chondral fracture, ACL tears, and so on but can be associated with frank patella dislocations and significant patella arthrosis. The pain is often diffuse and difficult to localize. Usually the patient points to the anterior aspect of the knee as the area of pain. Climbing stairs and symptoms after arising from a seated position also correlate with pain related to the patella. Giving way occurs because of quadriceps inhibition

secondary to pain. Symptoms are definitely activity related, such as climbing, squatting, and crawling. Progressive resistive exercises can also provoke pain.

Physical examination should include both lower extremities in the standing, supine, and prone positions. The patellofemoral joint is suspect if observation reveals ambulation with external rotation of the foot. Walking with the foot externally rotated relieves stress on the lateral retinaculum. Observe the knee with the patient standing with the feet straight ahead. In that position, the patella may turn in or "squint," providing some clue that there may be excessive anteversion of the femur or external rotation of the tibia or both creating some dynamic malalignment component. Distally, the more lateral the tibial tubercle is placed (creating external tibial torsion), the greater is the lateral force on the patella. As previously noted, the Q angle should be 15 degrees or less. In addition to measuring the Q angle in complete extension, a 90-degree knee flexion Q angle will provide additional assessment of distal malalignment. Another method of measuring distal malalignment is the tibial sulcus angle, as described by Kolowich et al.[24] Hip rotation for femoral anterversion, foot pronation, and positioning are also important to note.

Examining the peripatella tissues may indicate whether or not there is a tight retinaculum by observing for tilting. The path the patella takes in range of motion in the trochlea should be assessed. Normally, the patella starts laterally in full extension and then moves medially with the knee flexed as it engages the trochlea. If the patella continues to move laterally with progressive knee flexion (the so-called J sign), more evidence of patella malalignment is noted. The other soft tissues, including the patella tendon and quadriceps tendon, iliotibial band, lateral retinaculum, and vastus medialis, should be examined. The girth of the thigh at the VMO should be measured. The VMO is often dramatically atrophic. The medial retinaculum may be exquisitely tender as it inserts in the inferior medial aspect of the patella secondary to the recurrent instability. The tibial tubercle should be examined for apophysitis and bursitis. The inferior pole of the patella may be tender in chronic patella tendinopathy. Atrophy or discoloration of the skin or changes in skin temperature may be indicative of reflex sympathetic dystrophy. Passive patella motion should be assessed. Patella alta and patella baja are most often radiographic, rather than clinical, diagnoses. The passive patella test or medial patellar compression test measures excessive patellar tilt. An inability to rotate the patella to a height above the medial side in the coronal plane is abnormal.[24, 25]

The medial and lateral glide test measures the amount of soft tissue that restricts medial and lateral motion of the patella. The patella is divided into fourths. The knee is flexed approximately 20 to 30 degrees, and the examiner measures how many quadrants the patella is able to be passively displaced medially and laterally. Normally, the patella should be easily displaced medially by two to three quadrants. Inability to immediately displace the patella more than one quadrant suggests excessive tightness in the lateral retinaculum.

Flexibility and strength also are crucial in the work-up of patellofemoral pain. Hamstring tightness is often found, which then contributes to an increase in pressure in the anterior compartment of the knee. Flexibility of the iliotibial band may also be a factor in provocation of anterior knee pain. In the prone position, the knee is flexed maximally; the positioning of the heel in relationship to the buttock gives some indication of quadriceps tightness. This maneuver may be provoke pain. Restoration of the patient's ability to bring the heel to within 6 inches of the buttock is often successful in eliminating pain in the anterior aspect of the knee. Iliotibial band flexibility is also important.

As stated previously, the VMO may be profoundly atrophic. Classification of strength deficits through isokinetic testing can often aggravate symptoms. Manual muscle testing may be normal.

Other areas of disease to be ruled out are meniscal tears, collateral ligament strains, pes anserinus bursitis, iliotibial band flexion syndrome, cruciate instability, osteochondritis dissecans, and arthrosis.

IMAGING

Imaging techniques are used to confirm the physician's clinical suspicion of patellofemoral disorders. The physician should be aware of the indications and limitations of the various imaging techniques used to investigate the patellofemoral joint. All imaging studies should be correlated with history and physical examination to diagnose and treat anterior knee pain and patellofemoral instability successfully.

RADIOGRAPHY

Anteroposterior and lateral views are helpful in identifying loose bodies, bipartite patella, degenerative joint changes, fractures, chondrocalcinosis, and other nonpatellofemoral joint disease.

Tangential views (skyline/sunrise view) of the patella, with the knee flexed often between 60 and 90 degrees, are used to image the surface of the patellofemoral mechanism and the trochlea. The two most popular views are Merchant's view[26] and Laurin's view.[27] As noted previously, patella positioning changes with flexion. Schutzer et al[28] showed that the patella becomes fully engaged in the femoral trochlea between 15 and 20 degrees of flexion and that the position of the patella at 0 to 20 degrees of flexion is usually lateral. Excessive patella tilt increases on average with progressive knee flexion to 30 degrees. Subluxation of the patella in the trochlea groove decreases with progressive knee flexion up to 30 degrees. The relationship between the patella and trochlea in normal or malaligned knees after 30 degrees of flexion is unknown. Therefore, the degree of knee flexion in which the patellofemoral joint is imaged is critical to roentgenographic interpretation. For the Merchant view, the patient lies on the table supine with the knee flexed 45 degrees. For the Laurin view, the patient is seated with the knees flexed 20 degrees. It was Laurin's opinion that knee flexion beyond 20 degrees allows the patella to center passively in the femoral trochlea. It was believed that Merchant's view was easily performed in an office and easily interpreted, whereas Laurin's view is difficult to obtain accurately and somewhat difficult to interpret. The prognostic value of these tangential views in projecting outcome after surgical procedures has not been proved. One should consider obtaining flexed-knee, midpatella computed tomography (CT) scans to define the relationship between the patella and the femoral trochlea more accurately. Schutzer et al again advocated transverse patella CTs in that they allow several positions of knee flexion, are easily reproduced in a clinical setting, can be interpreted easily, and are of prognostic value in projecting outcome after lateral release.

Shellock and colleagues[29] reported on the use of kinematic transverse manipulative midpatella magnetic resonance imaging (MRI) to evaluate the relationship between the patella and the trochlea. Transverse cuts through the midpatella femoral joint were imaged from 0 degrees of flexion to 30 degrees of flexion every 5 degrees. They described four categories of malalignment: lateral subluxation, excessive lateral pressure syndrome, medial subluxation, and lateral to medial subluxation. This technique has not yet been proved to predict the outcome after surgical procedures. It should be noted that the MRI remains investigational but offers the prospect of noninvasive evaluation of patella articular cartilage.

Radionuclide imaging has been advocated by Dye and Boll[30] in the work-up of patients with chronic patellofemoral pain. They suggested that radionuclide scanning can be useful to confirm the presence of actual patella injury in the patient who has anterior knee pain with no evidence of clinical radiographic malalignment and when the diagnosis is in doubt because of a failure to respond to extensive conservative treatment. Radionuclide imaging is useful to confirm that the continuing patella pain is genuine.

DIFFERENTIAL DIAGNOSES

Differential diagnoses are listed in Table 1.

TREATMENT

A well-defined nonoperative treatment regimen designed to correct patellofemoral mechanics by way of strengthening exercises, stretching, brace, taping, and so on is of primary importance. The first goal is to increase strength and bulk

TABLE 1. DIFFERENTIAL DIAGNOSES	
Plica	Prepatella bursitis
Fat pad syndrome	Pes anserinus bursitis
Synovitis	Iliotibial band syndrome
Chondrocalcinosis	Tumors
Osteochondritis dissecans	Referred pain
Bipartite patella	Hip disorders
Cruciate instability	Sinding-Larsen-Johansson disease
Patellofemoral instability	
Patellofemoral malalignment	Osgood-Schlatter disease
Anterior knee pain	Muscle imbalance
Excessive lateral pressure syndrome	Collagen abnormalities (looseness vs. tightness)
Patella alta	Saphenous nerve entrapment
Patella baja	Reflex sympathetic dystrophy
Extra-articular quadriceps tendinopathy	Tumors

of an atrophic VMO. Simple isometrics, straight lifting exercises, and terminal knee extensions done in sets of 10 at least once or twice a day comprise the first strengthening regimen. Weight is added to the foot or ankle in graduated increments of 1 pound up to a total of 15 to 20 pounds. This open-chain exercise program may then be supplemented with extensions on an isokinetic machine or with rubber tubing as the source of resistance. Concomitant with a strengthening regimen is a stretching regimen for the hamstrings. Hamstring tightness has been shown to be a factor in provocation of anterior knee pain symptoms. Therefore, simultaneous strengthening of the VMO and stretching the hamstrings in the initial treatment regimen is mandatory. A closed-chain regimen as described by Mc-Connell[5] may also be incorporated. McConnell popularized the closed-chain exercise regimen as well as patella taping. External support in the form of a felt pad about the patella with a hole cut out for relief is an alternative external support. A commercial elastic or neoprene sleeve with a patella relief may also be prescribed. Lateral buttress is often incorporated into the sleeve and has been popularized by several braces such as the Palumbo. Ice applications three to four times daily, or more frequently if possible, is important. Nonsteroidal anti-inflammatory medication should be a part of all treatment regimens unless there are gastrointestinal contraindications. Formal physical therapy with applications of ultrasonography, iontophoresis, phonophoresis, and transcutaneous electrical nerve stimulation for pain relief are also incorporated in the regimen. Close observation and coaching in the appropriate closed-chain exercises and patella taping are crucial. A regular regimen of visits to a physical therapist can be helpful in that the therapist acts as a coach in counseling the patient and determining whether or not exercises are being performed appropriately. Foot orthotics can be prescribed if there is a gait abnormality. Simple orthotic devices can be fabricated in the office, or a custom-fitted rigid or semirigid orthotic device may be fabricated at an outside facility for a longer lasting orthosis.

As stated previously, McConnell found her treatment regimen to be successful in more than 96% of patients. In addition, DeHaven achieved a success rate of 82% and Henry and Crosland a success rate of 76%. Operative treatment should be reserved for those who do not respond to this nonoperative regimen and in whom a frank dislocation, patella subluxation phenomenon, patella tilt, and chondrosis are factors in the cause of the pain. The proximal realignment options are vastus medialis advancement (popularized by Hughston and Walsh[31] and revised more extensively by Insall et al[32]), lateral retinacular release, and distal realignment procedures such as the Maquet and Fulkerson procedures. Proximal realignment and lateral retinacular release

may be indicated for isolated patella tilt. If there is profound atrophy, advancement of the vastus medialis most likely is indicated. Hughston and Walsh[31] emphasize the importance of proximal extensor mechanism reconstruction as a surgical option for patella subluxation. They often combine this with a distal realignment. Insall and colleagues,[32] in 1979, described a proximal realignment for patellofemoral disorders, which has undergone modification up to now. The alignment involves a lengthy lateral release into the fibers of the vastus lateralis and a straight medial capsular incision into the quadriceps expansion. The medial capsule is tightened by overlapping the medial flap, and the procedure evolved into the proximal "tube" realignment of the patella. This was subsequently modified in 1983.[33] Proximal realignment, according to Kelly,[34] is not a capsular or mere plication but rather a quadricepsplasty designed to alter the pull of the quadriceps. The vastus lateralis and vastus medialis are separated from the quadriceps tendon. The quadriceps must then be reconstructed to redirect the subsequent line of pull in a more medial direction. This is the purpose of the operative procedure: to alter the quadriceps line of pull, restore patella congruence, and prevent patella instability. The functional quadriceps angle is decreased by altering the proximal limb of the quad mechanism.

Several procedures exist for distal patella realignment[35]: the 1904 Goldthwaite procedure, the 1938 Houser tibial tubercle operation, the 1964 Trillat technique, the Elmslie-Trillat method described by Cox in 1976, the 1976 Maquet procedure, and the 1983 Fulkerson anteromedialization procedure. The Fulkerson procedure combines the best features of the Trillat procedure (for treatment of malalignment) and the best features of the Maquet procedure for the treatment of osteoarthritis. The Fulkerson procedure transfers, via anterior medial tubercle transfer, the load from off the critical areas of the patella facets and femoral sulcus. An oblique osteotomy of the tibial tubercle permits the anterior tubercle fragment to slide anteriorly and medially. The obliquity of the osteotomy determines the primary direction to be anterior or medial. Osteotomy is tailored to suit the degree of malalignment and articular damage.

Incorporating a deliberate and methodical approach to anterior knee pain into one's practice will, in most cases, provide the appropriate diagnosis. With patience and persistence, the vast majority of patients will find success in alleviating the pain with nonoperative management. Operative management should be reserved for those patients who have completed a course of nonoperative management for at least 6 months and have demonstrated abnormal patellofemoral mechanics along with the patellofemoral symptom complex.

REFERENCES

1. Shea KP, Fulkerson JP: Rehabilitation of the patellofemoral joint. In Griffin LY (ed): Rehabilitation of the Injured Knee. St. Louis, Mosby–Year Book, in press.
2. Fulkerson JP: The etiology of patellofemoral pain in young, active patients. Clin Orthop 1983; 179:129.
3. Henry JH, Crosland JW: Conservative treatment of patellofemoral subluxation. Am J Sports Med 1979; 7:12.
4. DeHaven KE, Dolan WA, Mayer PJ: Chondromalacia patellae in athletes. Clinical presentation and conservative management. Am J Sports Med 1979; 7:5.
5. McConnell J: The management of chondromalacia patellae. A long term solution. Aust J Physiother 1986; 32:215.
6. Grelsamer RP, Colman WW, Mow VC: Anatomy and mechanics of the patellofemoral joint. Sports Med Arthrosc Rev 1994; 2:178.

7. Reider B, Marshall JL, Koslin B, et al: The anterior aspect of the knee joint. J Bone Joint Surg Am 1981; 63:351.
8. Wiberg G: Roentgenographic and anatomic studies on the femoropatellar joint with special reference to chondromalacia patellae. Acta Orthop Scand 1941; 23:319.
9. Grelsamer RP, Proctor CS, Bazos AN: Evaluation of patellar shape in the sagittal plane. Am J Sports Med 1994; 22:61.
10. Conlan T, Garth WP, Lemons JE: Evaluation of the medial soft tissue restraints of the extensor mechanism of the knee. J Bone Joint Surg Am 1993; 75:682.
11. Reider B, Marshall JL, Ring B: Patellar tracking. Clin Orthop 1981; 157:143.
12. Daniel DM, Teitge RA, Grana WA, et al: Knee and leg: Soft tissue trauma. In Daniel DM, Pellicci PM, Winquist RA (eds): Orthopaedic Knowledge Update 3. Rosemont, IL, American Academy of Orthopaedic Surgeons, 1990, p 564.
13. Kelman GJ, Focht L, Krakauer JD, et al: A cadaveric study of patello-femoral kinematics using a biomechanical testing rig and gait laboratory motion analysis. In Transactions of the 35th Annual Meeting, Orthopaedic Research Society, 1989, p 2.
14. Minns RJ, Walsh WK, Clarke JA: Techniques for measuring the static and dynamic properties of the patella. J Biomed Eng 1989; 11:209.
15. van Kampen A, Huiskes R: The three-dimensional tracking pattern of the human patella. J Orthop Res 1990; 8:372.
16. Dass AG, Adrish JT, Kambic HE: Biomechanical analysis of transfixation of the patella to the tibia. In Transactions of the 37th Annual Meeting, Orthopaedic Research Society, 1991, p 605.

17. Nagamine R: Patellar tracking measurement study in normal knees. In Transactions of the 38th Annual Meeting, Orthopaedic Research Society, 1992, p 479.
18. Heegaard JH, Leyvraz PF, Cumier A, et al: A computer model for analyzing the patellofemoral joint mechanism. In Transactions of the 37th Annual Meeting, Orthopaedic Research Society, 1991, p 571.
19. Rungee JL, Fay MJ, DeBerardino T: Biomechanical implications of olecranization of the patella. Am J Sports Med 1991; 19:542.
20. Williams C, McLean CA, Ahmed AM: Dynamic in vitro simulation of walking gait and corresponding biomechanical characteristics of the human knee. In Transactions of the 37th Annual Meeting, Orthopaedic Research Society, 1991, p 626.
21. Merchant AC: Patellofemoral disorders: Biomechanics, diagnosis, and nonoperative treatment. In McGinty JB (ed): Operative Arthroscopy. New York, Raven, 1991, p 261.
22. van Eijden TMGJ, De Boer W, Weijs WA: The orientation of the distal part of the quadriceps femoris muscle as a function of the knee flexion-extension angle. J Biomech 1985; 18:803.
23. Dye SF, Vaupel GL: The pathology of patellofemoral pain. Sports Med Arthrosc Rev 1994; 2:203.
24. Kolowich PA, Paulos LE, Rosenbeg TD, et al: Lateral release of the patella: Indications and contraindications. Am J Sports Med 1990; 18:359.
25. Fulkerson JP, Kalenak A, Rosenbeg TD, et al: Patellofemoral pain. Am Acad Orthop Surg Instr Course Lect 1992; 41:57.

26. Merchant AC, Mercer RL, Jacobsen RH, et al: Roentgenographic analysis of patellofemoral congruence. J Bone Joint Surg Am 1974; 56:1391.
27. Laurin CA, Dussault R, Levesques HP: The tangential x-ray investigation of the patellofemoral joint. Clin Orthop 1979; 144:16.
28. Schutzer SF, Ramsby GR, Fulkerson JP: Computed tomographic classification of patellofemoral pain patients. Orthop Clin North Am 1986; 17:235.
29. Shellock FG, Mink JH, Deutch A, et al: Evaluation of patients with persistent symptoms after lateral retinacular release by kinematic magnetic resonance imaging of the patellofemoral joint. Arthroscopy 1990; 6:226.
30. Dye SF, Boll DA: Radionuclide imaging of the patellofemoral joint in young adults with anterior knee pain. Orthop Clin North Am 1986; 17:249.
31. Hughston JC, Walsh WM: Proximal and distal reconstruction of the extensor mechanism for patellar subluxation. Clin Orthop 1979; 144:36.
32. Insall J, Bullough PG, Burstein AH: Proximal "tube" realignment of the patella for chondromalacia patellae. Clin Orthop 1979; 144:63.
33. Insall JN, Aglietti P, Tria AJ: Patella pain and incongruence: II. Clinical application. Clin Orthop 1983; 176:225.
34. Kelly MA: Operative treatment: Proximal realignment. Sports Med Arthrosc Rev 1994; 2:243.
35. Cox JS, Cooper PS: Patellofemoral instability in knee surgery. In Fu F, Harner C, Vince K (eds): Knee Surgery. Baltimore, Williams & Wilkins, 1994, p 953.

THE ARTHROSCOPIC MANAGEMENT OF ANKLE INJURIES IN ATHLETES

Champ L. Baker, Jr. and W. David Bruce

Summary

- The most common injuries in athletes are ankle injuries.
- Arthroscopy of the ankle allows a thorough evaluation of the joint and successful treatment of persistent problems in the athlete's ankle.
- Arthroscopic surgery affords the athlete a quicker return to play than open techniques.
- Indications include chondral fractures and loose bodies, osteochondritis dissecans and osteochondral fractures, soft-tissue or bony impingement, and symptomatic syndesmotic instability.
- The anterolateral, anteromedial, and posterolateral portals provide nearly complete visualization of the ankle joint and allow treatment of most lesions.
- Postoperative management focuses on returning the athlete to his or her sport.
- The most common complication is a transient or permanent sensory cutaneous nerve injury about the portal sites. However, careful technique and appropriate portal placement help prevent this complication.

Ankle injuries are among the most common injuries seen in sports medicine. The incidence of ankle injuries in the general population is estimated at one inversion injury per 10,000 persons per day.[1, 2] Ankle injuries compose 45% of basketball injuries, 25% of volleyball injuries, and 31% of soccer injuries.[3] Syndesmotic injury occurs in as many as 10% of all ankle sprains. Concomitant deltoid injury occurs in 3% of lateral ankle sprains.[3]

After the athlete sustains an ankle injury, appropriate nonoperative treatment is directed to returning him or her to the previous level of competition. Management of acute ankle injuries focuses on rest, ice, compression, and elevation (RICE). After the acute symptoms of inflammation, pain, and edema have resolved, the patient begins physical therapy. Rehabilitation consists of active range of motion, strengthening, and proprioceptive training. Unfortunately, residual symptoms are reported in 33% to 40% of patients.[4] If symptoms persist after rehabilitation, diagnostic and therapeutic ankle arthroscopy may be considered.

Arthroscopy of many different joints is currently being performed with great success. Arthroscopic surgery has gained wide acceptance as an effective method for treating persistent problems related to the athlete's ankle. The major indications for diagnostic and therapeutic arthroscopy are (1) articular lesions including chondral fractures and loose bodies, (2) osteochondritis dissecans and osteochondral fractures, (3) soft-tissue or bony impingement syndrome, and (4) symptomatic syndesmotic instability including persistent pain associated with interosseous ligament

injury and associated chondral fracture of the tibial plafond.[5–7] Except when used to fuse the joint, arthroscopy of the arthritic ankle has not been found to be beneficial.[6] Arthroscopic surgery can be used to treat articular pathological lesions associated with instability, but it is not used to treat the instability itself. Otherwise, tibiotalar ankle arthroscopy can be used to successfully treat persistent pain in the athlete's injured ankle. Although it is invasive, arthroscopy provides a more thorough view of intra-articular pathological lesions and a quicker return to sport than most open techniques can offer.

HISTORICAL REVIEW

Arthroscopy was first performed by the Japanese in 1918. In 1931, Burman performed cadaveric studies with ankle arthroscopy and concluded that arthroscopy was unsuitable for the ankle secondary to its narrow joint and convex talar anatomy.[8] In 1939, Tagaki described a reproducible arthroscopic examination of the ankle.[9] During the 1970s, Watanabe[10] and Chen and Wertheimer[11] reported their series of successful ankle arthroscopies. Standard ankle arthroscopic portals were described in the 1970s.

With the introduction of the reliable arthroscopic cameras and instruments in the 1980s and 1990s, many authors reported diagnostic and therapeutic success with the use of arthroscopy in the ankle joint.[5–7]

SPECIFIC INDICATIONS IN THE ATHLETE

ARTICULAR LESIONS: CHONDRAL FRACTURES AND LOOSE BODIES

Loose bodies and chondral fractures result from shear forces about the ankle joint. The surgeon needs to determine if the suspected injury is isolated or if an associated ankle instability, i.e., lateral ankle complex injury, exists. Typically, the patient presents with a history of clicking or locking of the ankle. The presentation is nonspecific other than swelling about the ankle. Usually, the source of pain cannot be pinpointed. An instability examination should be performed because patients with concomitant instability may require open ankle ligament reconstruction. Anteroposterior (AP), lateral, and mortise radiographic views should be obtained. If these views do not identify a specific lesion and if the patient remains symptomatic, magnetic resonance imaging (MRI) and bone scans can help the examiner localize the lesion.

Diagnostic arthroscopy should be considered in patients who do not improve with nonoperative management. Loose bodies and articular surfaces are addressed easily by arthroscopic means (Fig. 1). Persistent instability can be treated easily by open reconstruction after intra-articular arthro-

TABLE 1. STAGES OF TRANSCHONDRAL FRACTURES	
Stage	Description
1	Small area of compressed subchondral bone
2	Incompletely detached osteochondral fragment
3	Completely detached osteochondral fragment without displacement
4	Displaced osteochondral fragment

scopic evaluation. Authors have reported excellent results with arthroscopic surgery when isolated chondral injury or loose bodies are present.[7] Ogilvie-Harris et al reported 75% good to excellent results and an 84% return to previous level of competition in athletes treated arthroscopically for articular injury without associated instability.[7] However, the results are poorer when concomitant instability is present.[7]

OSTEOCHONDRITIS DISSECANS

In 1922, Kappis described loose bodies in the ankle and coined the term "osteochondritis dissecans" of the ankle.[12] In 1959, Berndt and Harty popularized the term "transchondral talar dome fractures" for the same process that Kappis described.[13] These transchondral talar dome fractures occur on the posteromedial and anterolateral talar dome. Using cadaveric specimens, Berndt and Harty demonstrated a traumatic origin for these lesions, with posteromedial lesions resulting from plantar flexion and ankle inversion and with anterolateral lesions resulting from dorsiflexion and ankle inversion. These transchondral fractures are grouped into four stages (Table 1).[14]

Patients often present several weeks after an ankle injury. They report pain with weight bearing and report catching, snapping, and swelling about the ankle joint. On physical examination, the patient often has a mild effusion and tenderness over the anterolateral or anteromedial portion of the joint line. Routine AP, lateral, and mortise radiographs can demonstrate the talar lesion (Fig. 2). Some lesions can be missed secondary to the convexity of the

talus and angle of radiographic projection. Tomograms, computed tomography scans, and MRI are helpful when plain radiographs do not demonstrate the lesion (Fig. 3).

Nonoperative management is recommended for stage 1 and 2 lesions. Rehabilitation is directed at progressing the patient from protected mobilization and partial weightbearing to full weightbearing with strengthening and proprioceptive activity. The need for operative treatment is dictated by the patient's response to physical therapy. If the patient has not improved with 10 to 12 weeks of physical therapy, the surgeon should consider arthroscopic treatment. Stage 3 can be managed similarly to stage 1 and 2 lesions; however, the surgeon should be willing to use operative treatment sooner with this stage than with the other two stages. Stage 4 lesions usually require surgical management. Arthroscopic excision has been effective in the management of these osteochondral lesions (Fig. 4). Baker and Morales showed good-to-excellent results at an average 10-year follow-up in 84% of their patients who had arthroscopic excision of talar osteochondral lesions.[14]

ANKLE IMPINGEMENT

Several distinct sources of ankle impingement are described. The impingement can be hypertrophic soft-tissue or bony. The sites of soft-tissue ankle impingement include

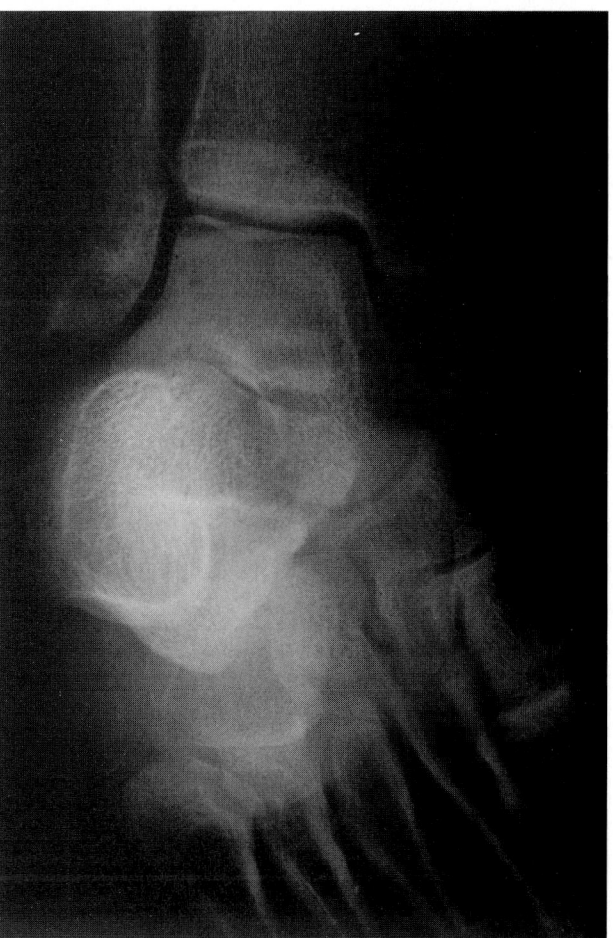

Fig. 2. Mortise view of osteochondritis dissecans of the ankle. This view confirms the presence of the stage 3 talar lesion.

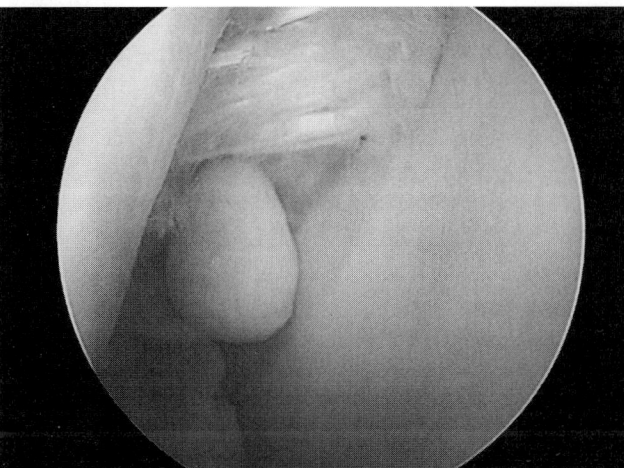

Fig. 1. Articular lesions. Using arthroscopic surgery to treat articular lesions enables the surgeon to easily address loose bodies and the articular surface of the joint.

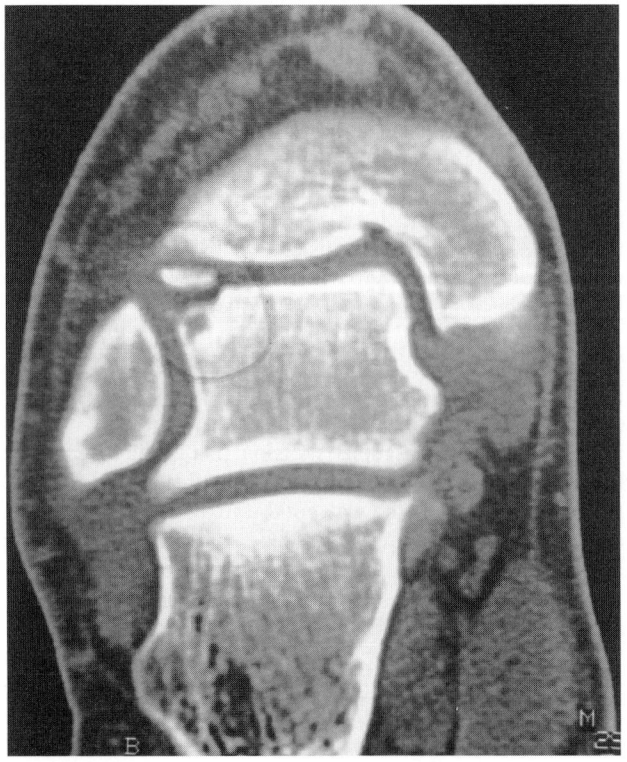

Fig. 3. CT scan of osteochondritis dissecans of the ankle. This imaging technique demonstrates the stage 4 talar lesion if radiographs do not reveal it.

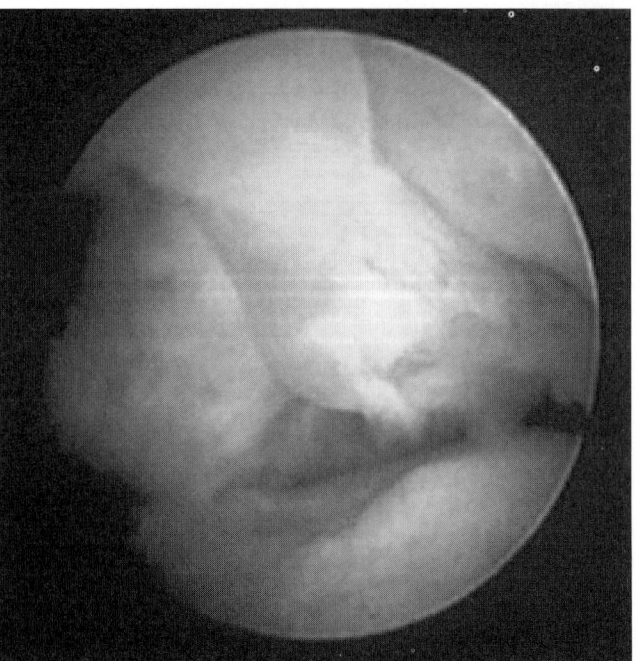

Fig. 5. Anterolateral soft-tissue impingement. Scar tissue can form in the anterolateral portion of the ankle after an ankle inversion injury. Arthroscopic excision of the scar tissue is an effective treatment for most patients.

(1) anterolateral meniscoid tissue, (2) the inferior fascicle of the anteroinferior tibiofibular ligament (or Bassett's ligament),[15] and (3) anteromedial meniscoid tissue.

Soft-Tissue Impingement

Wolin et al[16] originally described a "meniscoid mass" in the lateral gutter following ankle inversion injuries (Fig. 5). Characteristically, a patient with this injury does not have demonstrable instability by examination; however, significant pain is elicited over the anterolateral portion of the joint by forced plantar flexion of the ankle. Liu et al[17] showed that, for the diagnosis of anterolateral soft-tissue impingement, physical examination is 94% sensitive and 75% specific while MRI is only 39% sensitive and 50% specific. Arthroscopic excision of this anterolateral scar tissue has afforded good to excellent results for most patients.[5, 7, 17]

Bassett et al[15] demonstrated a thickened fascicle of the distal anteroinferior tibiofibular ligament (Fig. 6). They be-

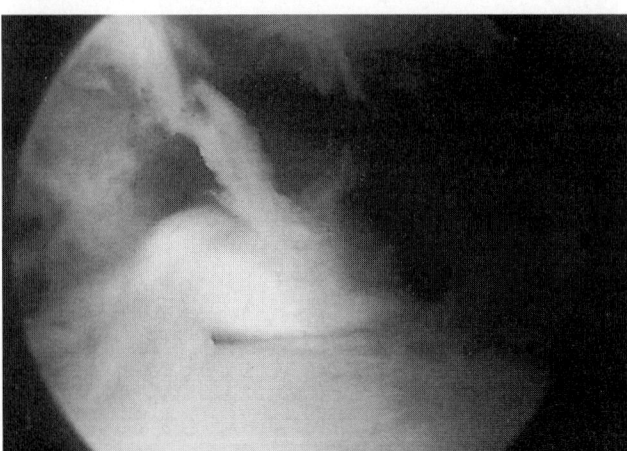

Fig. 4. Arthroscopic excision of stage 4 osteochondral lesion.

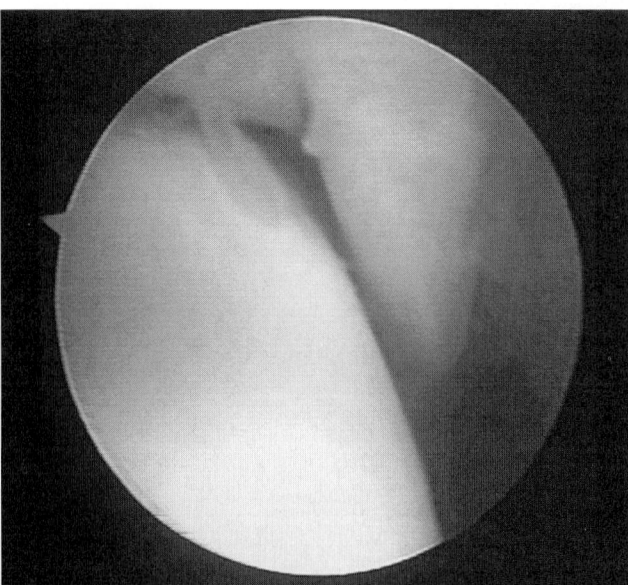

Fig. 6. Bassett's lesion. After an inversion injury to the ankle, the naturally occurring fascicle of the distal anteroinferior tibiofibular ligament can become enlarged and can impinge on the anterolateral talar dome.

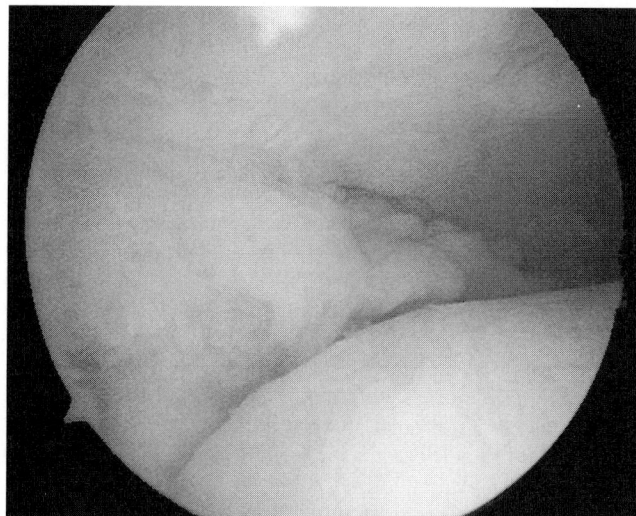

Fig. 7. Medial meniscoid lesion. After a deltoid ligament injury, medial meniscoid scar tissue can impinge on the anteromedial portion of the ankle.

lieved that the fascicle itself is a normal component of the distal anteroinferior tibiofibular ligament; however, after inversion injury to the ankle, the fascicle can become enlarged and can impinge on the anterolateral talar dome. The diagnosis is made by physical examination because radiographs are usually normal and arthrograms have not proved useful. The patient usually experiences full relief of symptoms after excision of this enlarged distal fascicle and débridement of the corresponding talar dome chondral injury that often accompanies this process.[15]

Similar soft-tissue impingement has been described on the anteromedial portion of the ankle.[18] Egol and Parisien[18] described a medial meniscoid lesion associated with previous deltoid ligament injury that resulted in anteromedial impingement (Fig. 7).

Soft-tissue impingement about the ankle should be evaluated with AP, lateral, and mortise radiographs and even with MRI when an articular pathological lesion is sus-

pected. However, physical examination enables the examiner to make the most accurate diagnosis, and injecting the patient's ankle with anesthetic can help him or her determine the source of pain. Arthroscopy has led to good to excellent results for diagnosis and treatment of soft-tissue impingement about the ankle.[17, 19, 20]

Bony Impingement

Anterior impingement syndrome was first described by Morris[21] in 1943, then by McMurray[22] in 1950. They coined the term "athlete's" or "footballer's ankle." This ankle condition probably results from repetitive microtrauma to the anterior ankle capsule. Long-term microtrauma results in the formation of spurs on the anterior-inferior tibial plafond and on the neck of the talus at the capsular attachment. Runners, high jumpers, gymnasts, and dancers are prone to develop this ankle condition. The patient often presents with pain on dorsiflexion of the ankle because these exostoses on the tibia and talus are forced together by this maneuver. Usually, an acute episode precedes these symptoms because the spurs are most often an asymptomatic long-standing condition. Lateral radiographs can demonstrate the presence of these anterior ankle spurs (Fig. 8). Arthroscopic excision of these spurs can successfully alleviate symptoms and can enable the athlete to return to his or her previous level of competition. However, concomitant arthrosis within the joint probably represents a different cause and is associated with much poorer outcomes.[6, 7]

SYMPTOMATIC SYNDESMOTIC INSTABILITY

Ogilvie-Harris et al[7] have demonstrated good success in the management of patients who have persistent pain following a history of syndesmotic disruption. These patients present with a history of an external rotation injury and unresolved pain over the lateral portion of the ankle. Physical examination demonstrates a positive external rotation stress test, a positive compression or squeeze test, and pain with translation of the distal tibiofibular joint. Plain radiographs are

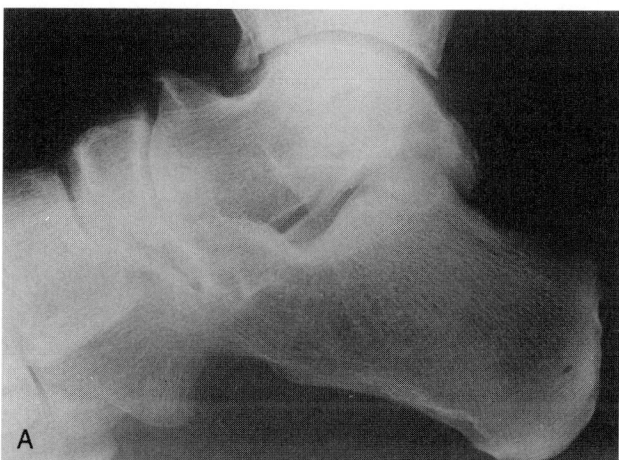
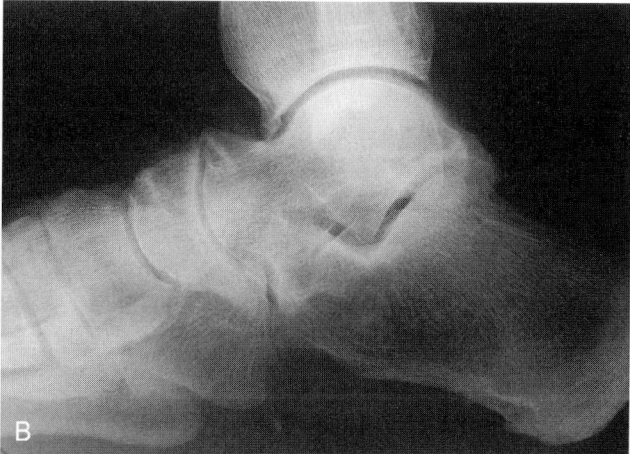

Fig. 8. Radiographs of an anterior tibial spur. *A,* The neutral lateral view and *B,* dorsiflexion view can reveal the presence of a spur that results from repetitive microtrauma to the anterior ankle capsule. Treatment involves arthroscopic excision of the spur.

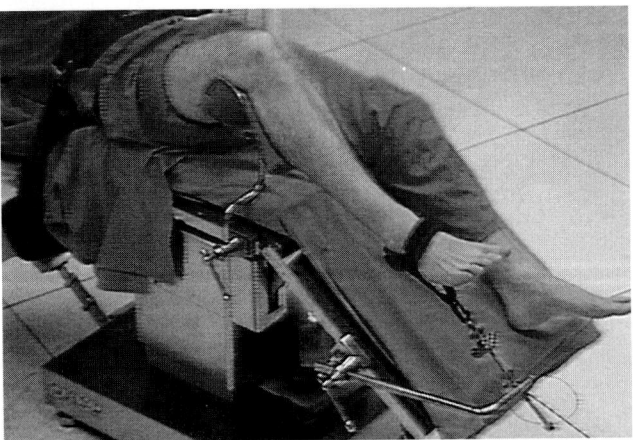

Fig. 9. Noninvasive external distraction. With the patient supine and a bolster placed under the knee, the surgeon flexes the patient's hip to 90 degrees and the knee to 90 degrees as traction is applied by an outrigger attached to the end of the table.

usually normal. MRI and bone scans are moderately successful in localizing the source of pain.

Ogilvie-Harris et al[7] described a triad of lesions that occur with these patients. Typically, rupture of the interosseous ligament, rupture of the posterior-inferior tibiofibular ligament, and chondral fracture of the posterolateral tibial plafond are present. They reported excellent results with arthroscopic excision of this damaged tissue despite persistent instability in the tibiofibular joint. The triad of damaged tissue in the lateral portion of the ankle, rather than the instability itself, seems to be the source of pain associated with syndesmotic instability.

PROCEDURE

The 2.7-mm and 4-mm 30-degree arthroscopes are used. Most anterior lesions can be addressed with the 4-mm arthroscope, which allows for a larger and clearer picture of the ankle joint. The surgeon may need to use the 2.7-mm arthroscope for more posterior lesions. The use of a small or large shaving system depends on the specific procedure. Ankle arthroscopy is performed under sterile conditions with the patient under general anesthesia. Local and regional, instead of general, anesthesia can be used, but they do not offer the complete muscle relaxation that general anesthesia offers. The patient should be positioned so that 360-degree access is available to the ankle. Position the patient supine either with the knee flexed 90 degrees and the foot dangling or, preferably, with a bolster or urology holder placed under the knee, flexing the hip to 90 degrees, and flexing the knee to 90 degrees as traction is brought from an outrigger on the end of the table (Fig. 9). Distraction can be applied with external noninvasive devices or through an invasive pin distractor (Fig. 10). The pin distractor rarely is needed with athletes because noninvasive distractors are usually adequate. In addition, the pin holes left by the invasive distractors serve as stress risers for fracture that slow the return of the athlete to sport.

The three most common portals used are the anterolateral, the anteromedial, and the posterolateral portals (Fig. 11). The anterolateral and anteromedial portals are the only

portals needed in more than 90% of ankle arthroscopies. The anterolateral portal is in close proximity to the intermediate dorsal cutaneous branch of the superficial peroneal nerve. This nerve can be avoided by accurate placement of the anterolateral portal at the medial or lateral edge of the peroneus tertius muscle. To avoid injury to the saphenous vein and nerve, place the anteromedial portal at the medial border of the tibialis anterior and lateral to the visible saphenous vein. If needed, the posterolateral portal is established just lateral to the Achilles tendon and medial to the small saphenous vein, sural nerve, and peroneal tendons.

After positioning the patient and applying the distraction, the surgeon identifies the ankle landmarks including the saphenous vein, tibialis anterior tendon, peroneus tertius, intermediate dorsal cutaneous branch of the superficial peroneal nerve, and malleoli. A thigh tourniquet may be used. The capsule is distended with 20 to 30 mL of irrigation fluid from a syringe and an 18-gauge needle in the anteromedial portal. The needle should be parallel to the tibial plafond, and the fluid should flow with little resistance until the capsule is distended. The anteromedial portal is established by incising only the skin with a No. 11 or No. 15 blade then by blunt hemostat spreading and insertion of a dull trocar. With the arthroscope in the joint, the anterolateral portal is established using a similar needle technique.

The three described portals allow nearly complete visualization of the ankle joint and allow treatment of most

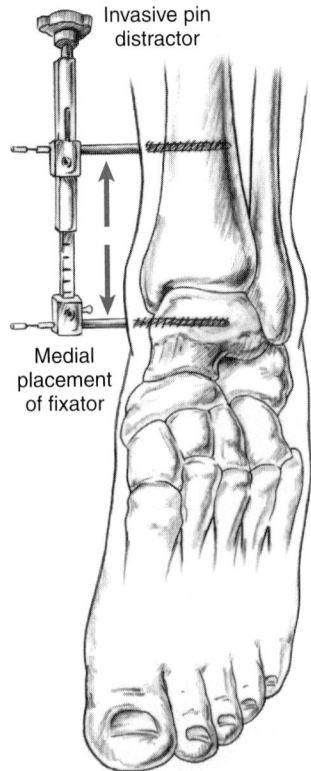

Fig. 10. Invasive pin distraction. Distraction is brought about through either the medial or lateral portion of the ankle. In the medial portion, one pin is placed in the tibia, and one pin is placed in the talus. In the lateral portion, one pin is placed in the tibia, and one pin is placed in the calcaneus. (Redrawn from Hughston Sports Medicine Foundation, Inc.)

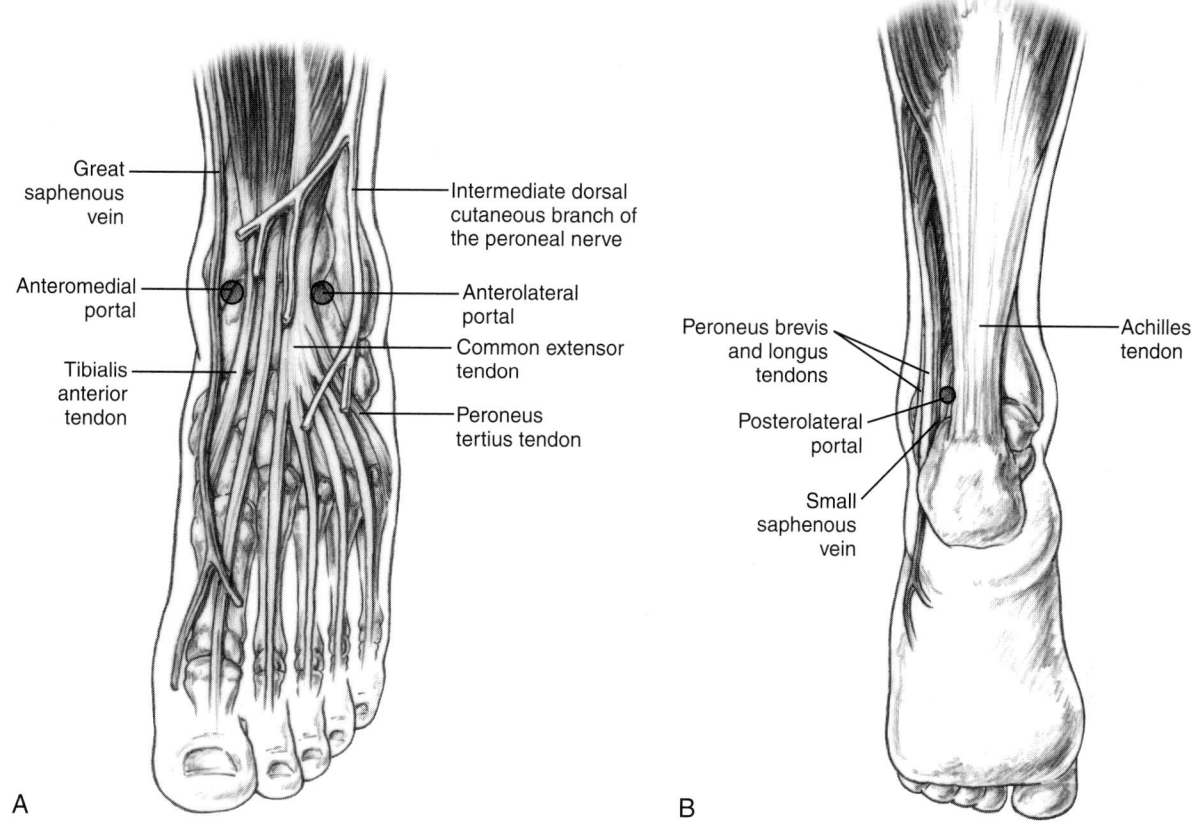

Fig. 11. Arthroscopic portals. *A*, For most arthroscopic surgery of the ankle, only the anterolateral and anteromedial portals are needed. The anterolateral portal is established at the medial or lateral edge of the peroneus tertius muscle. The anteromedial portal is established at the medial border of the tibialis anterior and lateral to the visible saphenous vein. *B*, The posterolateral portal is placed lateral to the Achilles tendon and medial to the small saphenous vein, sural nerve, and peroneal tendons. (Redrawn from Hughston Sports Medicine Foundation, Inc.)

lesions. After the arthroscopic work is finished, the tourniquet is released and hemostasis is obtained. The joint is injected with an anesthetic compound, and the portals are either taped or sutured. A bulky dressing is applied, and the patient is discharged from the hospital the same day.

POSTOPERATIVE MANAGEMENT

During the immediate postoperative period, the patient is instructed on measures to reduce edema and inflammation. When comfortable, the patient begins active-assisted range-of-motion exercises. Weightbearing is protected until full motion has returned. Depending on the status of the articular surface, the patient may begin unprotected weightbearing. Once the patient begins unprotected weightbearing, the rehabilitation program progresses to strengthening and proprioceptive activity. The athlete is allowed to return to sport when he or she has achieved full active motion and strength (usually 6 to 8 weeks provided that the athlete did not have significant chondral injuries).

COMPLICATIONS

Complications of ankle arthroscopy range from 3% to 5%.[5, 6, 14, 19] The most common complication is transient or permanent sensory cutaneous nerve injury about the portal sites. Appropriate portal placement and blunt technique can decrease these inherent risks. The surgeon also must take care when débriding around the anterior capsule of the ankle because of the close proximity of neurovascular structures.

Postoperative use of bulky dressings and portal closure should decrease the risk of postoperative drainage, sinus formation, and deep infection. When closing the portals, the surgeon must be careful to not catch sensory nerves with the suture. Releasing the tourniquet allows adequate hemostasis before the bandages are placed.

As stated earlier, the drill holes created with invasive distractors can serve as stress risers for fracture. Therefore, the surgeon should not use invasive distractors when accomplishing arthroscopy of the ankle.

REFERENCES

1. Brooks SC, Potter BT, Rainey JB: Treatment for partial tears of the lateral ligament of the ankle: A prospective trial. Br Med J 1981; 282:606.

2. Ruth CJ: The surgical treatment of injuries of the fibular collateral ligaments of the ankle. J Bone Joint Surg Am 1961; 43:229.

3. Garrick JG: The frequency of injury, mechanism of injury, and epidemiology of ankle sprains. Am J Sports Med 1977; 5:241.

4. Bosien WR, Staples OS, Russell SW: Residual disability following acute ankle sprains. J Bone Joint Surg Am 1955; 37: 1237.

5. Ewing JW, Tasto JA, Tippett JW: Arthroscopic surgery of the ankle. Instr Course Lect 1995; 44:325.

6. Fitzgibbons TC: Arthroscopic ankle debridement and fusion: Indications, techniques, and results. Instr Course Lect 1999; 48:243.

7. Ogilvie-Harris DJ, Gilbart MK, Chorney K: Chronic pain following ankle sprains in athletes: The role of arthroscopic surgery. Arthroscopy 1997; 13:564.

8. Burman MS: Arthroscopy of direct visualization of joints: An experimental cadaver study. J Bone Joint Surg 1931; 13:669.

9. Tagaki K: The arthroscope. Jpn J Orthop Assn 1939; 14:359.

10. Watanabe M: Selfoc-Arthroscope (Watanabe no. 24 arthroscope). Monograph. Tokyo: Teishin Hospital, 1972.

11. Chen DS, Wertheimer SJ: Centrally located osteochondral fracture of the talus. J Foot Surg 1992; 31:134.

12. Kappis M: Weitere Beitrage zur traumatisch-mechanischen Enstehung der "spontanen" Knorpelabiosungen. Dtsch Z Chir 1922; 171:13.

13. Berndt AL, Harty M: Transchondral fractures (osteochondritis dissecans) of the talus. J Bone Joint Surg Am 1959; 41:988.

14. Baker CL Jr, Morales RW: Arthroscopic treatment of transchondral talar dome fractures: A long-term follow-up study. Arthroscopy 1999; 15:197.

15. Bassett FH III, Gates HS, Billys JB, et al: Talar impingement by the anteroinferior tibiofibular ligament. J Bone Joint Surg Am 1990; 72:55.

16. Wolin I, Glassman F, Sideman S, et al: Internal derangement of the talofibular component of the ankle. Surg Gynecol Obstet 1950; 91:193.

17. Liu SH, Nuccion SL, Finerman G: Diagnosis of anterolateral ankle impingement. Comparison between magnetic resonance imaging and clinical examination. Am J Sports Med 1997; 25:389.

18. Egol KA, Parisien JS: Impingement syndrome of the ankle caused by a medial meniscoid lesion. Arthroscopy 1997; 13: 522.

19. van Dijk CN, Scholte D: Arthroscopy of the ankle joint. Arthroscopy 1997; 13:90.

20. Ferkel RD, Karzel RP, Del Pizzo W, et al: Arthroscopic treatment of anterolateral impingement of the ankle. Am J Sports Med 1991; 19:440.

21. Morris LH: Athlete's ankle. J Bone Joint Surg 1943; 25:220.

22. McMurray TP: Footballer's ankle. J Bone Joint Surg Br 1950; 32:68.

INFECTION

ARLEN D. HANSSEN

DIAGNOSIS AND MANAGEMENT OF MUSCULOSKELETAL INFECTION

Douglas R. Osmon

Summary

- Accurate diagnosis and expedient treatment represent the cornerstone of successful outcome for musculoskeletal infection.
- Multidisciplinary cooperation to obtain and process proper samples for culture and in vitro susceptibility testing is extremely important.
- Antimicrobial therapy should be based on safety and efficacy issues after careful assessment of multiple variables.
- A careful history and examination to assess and obtain proper information pertaining to musculoskeletal infection is helpful in determining the necessary laboratory tests and imaging studies required for establishing the correct diagnosis.

The diagnosis and treatment of musculoskeletal infections require the expertise of many medical and surgical specialties. The purpose of this chapter is to familiarize the reader with certain principles useful in the diagnosis and medical management of osteomyelitis, infectious arthritis, and prosthetic joint infection. In particular, this chapter reviews the microbiology, history, and examination findings, utility of various laboratory and radiographic studies used in the diagnosis, and management of these musculoskeletal infections. Finally, the author's recommendations regarding empiric and directed antimicrobial therapy for the treatment of these infections are discussed. The reader is referred to other chapters in this text for details on the surgical management of these diseases.

MICROBIOLOGY

Accurate information concerning the microbiology of musculoskeletal infections is difficult to obtain from the medical literature. Reasons for this problem include no standard definitions of what constitutes infection, variable methods of intraoperative culture ascertainment and techniques among physicians and microbiology laboratories, and the lack of national and international surveillance mechanisms to help collect and report the microbiology of musculoskeletal infection similar to data collected on antimicrobial resistance and nosocomial infections by others.[1]

OSTEOMYELITIS

Although several classification schemes have been proposed, the classification scheme of Waldvogel is useful when describing the etiology and microbiology of osteomyelitis.[2, 3] Waldvogel classifies osteomyelitis as hematogenous or due to a contiguous focus of infection. Contiguous focus osteomyelitis is further subdivided into osteomyelitis with or without vascular insufficiency. Each type of osteomyelitis can be acute (less than 10 days' duration) or chronic (relapse of osteomyelitis at the same site or disease of more than 10 days in duration). Other classification schemes, particularly the Cierny-Mader classification scheme, is most useful from the surgeon's perspective and is discussed in later chapters.[2]

Hematogenous osteomyelitis in children and adults is most often due to *Staphylococcus aureus* and beta-hemolytic streptococci, whereas aerobic gram-negative bacilli are less common. Some patient groups are predisposed to hematogenous infection due to specific organisms (Table 1). Osteomyelitis due to *Haemophilus influenzae* also causes infection in infants and children, but the incidence of *H. influenzae* osteomyelitis is decreasing because of the *H. influenzae* b conjugated vaccine that is now routinely administered to children.[4] Hematogenous osteomyelitis due to anaerobes and polymicrobial infection is unusual.[5]

Vertebral osteomyelitis, disk space infection, and epidural abscesses can be due to hematogenous seeding or a contiguous focus of infection. *S. aureus* is the most common cause of vertebral osteomyelitis.[6–8] If the infection is caused by hematogenous seeding from the urinary tract, aerobic gram-negative bacilli and enterococci must be considered potential pathogens. Hematogenous seeding of the spinal column by *Pseudomonas aeruginosa* and *S. aureus* is more prevalent among injection drug users. Coagulase-negative staphylococci, *S. aureus,* and aerobic gram-negative bacilli and other common causes of surgical wound infection can cause vertebral osteomyelitis following spine surgery with or without spinal hardware implantation.[1] Candidal infection may occur following candidemia because of infections of intravascular devices. Infection by *Mycobacterium tuberculosis* and *Brucella* spp., among other more unusual pathogens, should be considered in those patients with an exposure history to these pathogens.

Specific clinical situations often predispose to contiguous focus osteomyelitis due to certain pathogens (see Table 1). Contiguous focus osteomyelitis of the foot bones, in patients with diabetes mellitus and/or arterial insufficiency, is polymicrobial in 45% to 85% of cases.[9] The predominant pathogens are *S. aureus*, streptococci, and aerobic gram-negative bacilli. *P. aeruginosa* is typically isolated in cases in which the patient has been soaking foot ulcers or using wet dressings.[9, 10] Anaerobes are present in up to 40% of cases and are more common in severe cases. Organisms often thought to be contaminants, such as coagulase-negative staphylococci and *Corynebacterium* spp. are often pathogens in the setting of diabetic foot bone osteomyelitis.[9] There is often a weak correlation between adequately obtained bone cultures and surrounding soft-tissue cultures.[11]

Following contamination of an open fracture by soil, in addition to *S. aureus,* beta-hemolytic streptococci and aerobic gram-negative bacilli, *Clostridium* spp., *Bacillus* spp., *Stenotrophomonas maltophilia*, *Nocardia* spp., and, rarely,

TABLE 1. MICROBIOLOGY OF OSTEOMYELITIS IN UNIQUE CLINICAL CIRCUMSTANCES

Clinical Situation	Pathogen
Contiguous Osteomyelitis	
Presence of a foreign body	Coagulase-negative staphylococci, *Staphylococcus aureus*
Dog or cat bite	Polymicrobial including *Pasteurella* spp.
Human bite	*Eikenenella corrodens,* oral flora
Puncture injury with sharp object to foot	*Pseudomonas aeruginosa*
Malignant external otitis	*P. aeruginosa*
Skull or mandibular osteomyelitis following periodontal infection	Normal oral flora and *Actinomyces* spp.
Soil contamination	*S. aureus, Enterobacteriaceae, Clostridium* spp., *Bacillus* spp., *Nocardia* spp., atypical mycobacteria
Decubitus ulcer and diabetic foot bone	Polymicrobial including anaerobes
Hematogenous Osteomyelitis	
Neonates	*S. aureus, Enterobacteriaceae,* group B Streptococci
Sickle cell disease	*Salmonella* spp., *S. aureus, Streptococcus pneumoniae*
Injection drug users Hemodialysis	*P. aeruginosa, S. aureus*
Immunocompromise including HIV infection	*Aspergillus, Mycobacterium avium* complex, *Candida albicans, Bartonella henselae*
Population in which organism is endemic or in which there has been significant exposure	*Mycobacterium tuberculosis, Coxiella burnetii, Brucella* spp.

Data from Lew and Waldvogel,[3] Haas and McAndrew,[5] and Nolan and Chapman.[85]

atypical mycobacteria and fungi may also be pathogens.[5] Bacteria in soil where animals are housed may be resistant to antimicrobials used for open fracture prophylaxis because of exposure to antibiotics used in animal feed to enhance animal growth.[12] Osteomyelitis following fixation of an open or closed fracture with an internal orthopaedic fixation device is usually due to *S. aureus* or coagulase-negative staphylococci.

INFECTIOUS ARTHRITIS

A variety of pathogens can cause infectious arthritis, although bacteria cause the majority of cases. When describing the microbiology of infectious arthritis, it is useful to classify the disease into acute and chronic monoarticular disease and a polyarticular presentation. In neonates, acute monoarticular infectious arthritis is caused by group B streptococci and gonococci in 95% of cases. The major pathogens in children are *S. aureus, H. influenzae,* and streptococci. Owing to the introduction of the *H. influenzae* b conjugated vaccine, the incidence of *H. influenzae* infectious arthritis is decreasing. It is believed that peripartum penicillin G prophylaxis for invasive group B streptococcal disease will also decrease the incidence of group B streptococcal neonatal infectious arthritis.[13]

The most common pathogens of acute infectious arthritis among adults are shown in Table 2. In young sexually active adults, infection is most often due to *Neisseria gonorrhoeae*.[14–16] Although certain bacteria cause polyarticular syndromes more commonly (*S. aureus, N. gonorrhoeae* and viruses), reactive arthritis, rheumatic fever, and rheumatoid arthritis are also a common cause of polyarticular arthritis. Infectious arthritis in patients with rheumatoid arthritis is often polyarticular and caused by *S. aureus*.[17] Infectious arthritis in the elderly or in patients with comorbid illnesses is more often due to aerobic gram-negative bacilli.[18] Enterococcal or polymicrobial infectious arthritis is uncommon. Anaerobic infection is also unusual except for foot infections in patients with diabetes mellitus or vascular insufficiency or in the hand following human or animal bites. *Propionibacterium acnes* is a common cause of septic arthritis of the shoulder following rotator cuff repair.[19] *P. aeruginosa* and *S. aureus* are common pathogens among injection drug users. Coagulase-negative staphylococci and *S. aureus* are the most common infections following arthroscopy. *Mycoplasma* spp. can cause infection in patients who are postpartum or hypogammaglobulinemic.[20]

Chronic and indolent monoarticular arthritis is often due to mycobacteria (*Mycobacterium tuberculosis, M. kansasii, M. marinum, M. avium* complex, *M. fortuitum, M. haemophilum, M. leprae*), fungi (*Candida* spp., *Sporothrix schenckii, Coccidioides immitis, Blastomyces dermatitidis, Pseudallescheria boydii*) *Brucella* spp., *Nocardia* spp., *Trophedema whippelii,* and *Borrelia burgdorferi.*

PROSTHETIC JOINT INFECTION

The microbiology of cases of prosthetic joint infection seen at a large tertiary referral center between 1992 and 1997 is shown in Table 3.[21] Aerobic gram-positive cocci (*S. aureus*), coagulase-negative staphylococci, and enterococci are the pathogens in the majority (65%) of these infections. Aerobic gram-negative bacilli such as the Enterobacteriaceae (*Escherichia coli, Proteus mirabilis,* and others) and *P. aeruginosa* are less common, and polymicrobial infections account for 14% of cases. Anaerobic infection is rare but when it occurs is more often caused by gram-positive anaerobes such as peptostreptococci and *P. acnes*. A variety of rare causes of prosthetic joint infection have also been reported.[21]

TABLE 2. FREQUENCY OF COMMON BACTERIA CAUSING SEPTIC ARTHRITIS IN ADULTS*

Microorganisms	Frequency, %
Staphylococcus aureus	68
Streptococci†	20
Haemophilus influenzae	1
Aerobic gram-negative bacilli	10
Miscellaneous and polymicrobial	1

* Excluding *Neisseria gonorrhea.*
† Includes β-hemolytic streptococci, viridans group streptococci, and *Streptococcus pneumoniae.*
From Roberts and Mock.[86]

TABLE 3. MICROBIOLOGY OF 578 PROSTHETIC JOINT INFECTIONS SEEN AT MAYO CLINIC BETWEEN 1992 AND 1997

Microorganism(s)	Prosthetic Joint Infections, n(%)	Microorganism(s)	Prosthetic Joint Infections, n(%)
Coagulase-negative staphylococci	172 (30)	Unknown*	64(11)
Staphylococcus aureus	135 (23)	Streptococci	51 (9)
Polymicrobial	71 (12)	Group B streptococci	20
Coagulase-negative staphylococci	51	Viridans group streptococci	19
S. aureus	26	Group G streptococci	7
Propionibacterium sp.	15	Group C streptococci	2
Enterococci	13	Nutritionally variant streptococci	2
Corynebacterium sp.	12	*Streptococcus pneumoniae*	1
Peptostreptococci	11	Gram-negative bacilli	32 (6)
Viridans group streptococci	7	*Pseudomonas aeruginosa*	11
Bacteroides sp.	5	*Escherichia coli*	8
Group B streptococci	4	*Enterobacter* sp.	5
Aspergillus sp.	3	*Proteus mirabilis*	4
Penicillium sp.	2	*Klebsiella* sp.	2
Actinomyces sp.	2	*Serratia marcescens*	2
Anaerobic gram-positive cocci (not otherwise specified)	2	*Morganella morganii*	1
Enterobacter cloacae	2	*Salmonella* sp.	
Candida albicans	2	Anaerobes	231(4)
Group D streptococci	1	*Propionibacterium* sp.	9
β-hemolytic streptococci (not otherwise specified)	1	Peptostreptococci	8
Pseudomonas aeruginosa	1	*Bacteroides* sp.	5
Pseudomonas picketti	1	Anaerobic gram-positive cocci (not otherwise specified)	1
Citrobacter freundii	1	*Prevotella melaninogenica*	1
Morganella morganii	1	*Veillonella parvula*	1
Clostridium subterminale	1	Enterococci	16 (3)
Serratia marcescens	1	Other microorganisms	14 (2)
Gram-positive bacillus (not otherwise specified)	1	*Candida albicans*	5
Gram-positive cocci (not otherwise specified)	1	*Corynebacterium* sp.	3
Prevotella bivia	1	*Neisseria meningitides*	2
Alcaligenes xylosoxidans	1	*Brucella* spp.	1
Stenotrophomonas maltophilia	1	*Mycobacterium genavensae*	1
Acinetobacter sp.	1	*Mycobacterium fortuitum*	1
		Haemophilus influenzae	1
		Total	578 (100)

* Includes cases in which there was no growth on routine bacterial cultures, routine bacterial cultures were not obtained, or microbiological information was not available.

Adapted from Steckelberg J, Osmon D: Prosthetic joint infections. In Bisno A, Waldvogel F (eds): Infections Associated with Indwelling Devices. Washington, D.C., ASM Press, 2000.

DIAGNOSIS

HISTORY AND PHYSICAL EXAMINATION
General Considerations

Optimal diagnosis and management of musculoskeletal infection begins with a thorough history and physical examination. Assessment prior to initiation of any medical or surgical therapy allows the infectious diseases physician to give advice to the surgeon regarding culture ascertainment, to arrange for specialized cultures to be performed in the microbiology laboratory, and to select the optimal type and dose of empiric and directed antimicrobial therapy. Details regarding prior microbiology as well as medical and surgical therapy of the specific musculoskeletal infection being evaluated should be obtained from the patient, the medical record, or previous health care providers. Any pertinent history concerning a potential hematogenous source of infection, antimicrobial allergies, current medications, coexisting renal and hepatic disease, current or past tobacco abuse, and coexisting comorbidities that may affect the systemic or local immune status of the patient and thus the prognosis of the musculoskeletal infection should be elicited and documented in the medical record. Many of these comorbidities are the same factors that by the Cierny and Mader system classify patients as B or compromised hosts (Table 4).[2]

Osteomyelitis

Hematogenous osteomyelitis in children often occurs after minor trauma, and areas that are typically involved are the metaphyseal regions.

Children with hematogenous osteomyelitis of the long bones typically present with the acute to subacute onset of bone pain, limitation of motion of the extremity, fever, and chills.[22] These symptoms are usually present for several days to weeks prior to presentation. There may be soft-tissue edema, erythema, and tenderness of the involved area. The differential diagnoses of these symptoms include fracture, rheumatic fever, septic arthritis, toxic synovitis, cellulitis, bone infarction in patients with a hemoglobinopa-

TABLE 4. SYSTEMIC AND LOCAL FACTORS IN THE PREOPERATIVE ASSESSMENT OF THE PATIENT WITH A MUSCULOSKELETAL INFECTION

Type of Factor	Factors
Systemic	Malnutrition
	Renal, hepatic failure
	Diabetes mellitus
	Chronic hypoxia
	Immune disease
	Malignancy
	Extremes of age
	Immunosuppression or immune deficiency
Local	Chronic lymphedema
	Venous stasis
	Major-vessel compromise
	Arteritis
	Extensive scarring
	Radiation fibrosis
	Small-vessel disease
	Neuropathy
	Tobacco abuse ($\geq$ 2 packs/day)

Adapted from Mader JT, Shirtliff M, Calhoun JH: Staging and staging application in osteomyelitis. Clin Infect Dis 1997; 25:1303.

thy, leukemia, and bony neoplasms.[22] Neonates often have very few signs and symptoms and can present with only irritability, poor feeding, and decreased range of motion of the involved limb with localized tenderness and swelling or pseudoparalysis. Contiguous septic arthritis in the adjacent joint has been reported to occur in approximately 60% of neonatal cases.[23]

Vertebral osteomyelitis, diskitis, and epidural abscess in adults are typically related to hematogenous seeding or a postoperative complication of spine surgery. These patients typically have associated comorbid conditions and are often elderly, with the exception of injection drug users.[7] The demographic characteristics and presenting signs and symptoms of patients with vertebral osteomyelitis in three recent case series are shown in Table 5.[7, 8, 24] It is clear that the

signs and symptoms of vertebral osteomyelitis are not specific, and appropriate diagnostic testing to distinguish infection from malignancy, osteoarthritis, compression fracture, and other causes of subacute or chronic spine pain in the adult is mandatory.

The lumbar spine is the most commonly involved site, followed by the thoracic and cervical regions. The source of infection is most often from the urinary tract, respiratory tract, skin and soft-tissue infections, injection drug use, infective endocarditis, and intravascular lines. Pain of several days' to months' duration is the most common presenting symptom. Movement, coughing, or straining may exacerbate the pain. Lower extremity weakness, paresthesias, and bowel and bladder dysfunction may occasionally be the most prominent clinical features and are caused by nerve root or spinal cord compromise. Dysphagia and persistent sore throat may be seen in patients with cervical spine involvement.[25] On physical examination, a draining sinus or wound is extremely rare unless the infection is secondary to recent surgery. Fever is present in 26% to 65% of patients, and paraspinal muscle spasm and percussion tenderness of the spine are often present.

Localized long bone pain and/or drainage from a wound or sinus tract of several weeks' to months' duration is a typical presentation of the patient with osteomyelitis without vascular insufficiency. Typically, the tibia or femur is most commonly affected, often due to trauma or prior surgery.[3] Fever and constitutional symptoms are rare unless concomitant soft-tissue infection with cellulitis is present. Risk of pathological fracture is rare, occurring only when extensive disease is present.

Osteomyelitis with associated vascular insufficiency typically involves the bones of the foot in patients with arterial insufficiency. Diabetes mellitus complicated by sensorimotor neuropathy is the most common comorbid condition. A non-healing ulcer represents the portal of entry into the adjacent bone in most cases. Pain may not be present because of the presence of neuropathy, and pedal pulses are usually diminished or absent (Table 6). Cellulitis, deep space infection in the foot, or gangrene often coexists with osteomyelitis of the foot bones. It is often difficult to

TABLE 5. DEMOGRAPHIC CHARACTERISTICS AND RESULTS OF SELECTED DIAGNOSTIC TESTS IN THREE RECENT CASE SERIES OF VERTEBRAL OSTEOMYELITIS

Characteristic	Caragee[7] (1997) (N = 111)	Chelsom & Solberg[8] (1998) (N = 40)	Rezai et al[24] (1999) (N = 57)
Age in years, mean (range)	60 (18–84)	58 (13–91)	48 (24–74)
Gender, % male	60	52	82
Pain, %	91	100	98
Fever, %	16	65	46
Neurologic involvement, %	30	48	68
Location of infection, %			
Cervical	0	10	44
Thoracic	54	33	30
Lumbar	46	57	30
Elevated WBC, % tested	41	58	Not available
Elevated ESR, % tested	95	95	96
Elevated C-reactive protein, % tested	Not available	98	Not available
Positive blood cultures, % tested	59	43	77

ESR, erythrocyte sedimentation rate; WBC, white blood cell count.

TABLE 6. CLINICAL CHARACTERISTICS OF PATIENTS WITH DIABETIC FOOT INFECTION*

Feature	Result
Age, years	59
Duration of diabetes mellitus, years	17
Pedal pulses nonpalpable, %	62
Peripheral neuropathy present, %	84
Foot ulcer present, %	83
Duration of infection > 1 month, %	33
Recent antimicrobial therapy, %	45†
Diagnosis of osteomyelitis‡	29†

* Based on data reported in 24 published studies from 1976 to 1998.
† Highly variable percentages in different studies.
‡ Studies used different criteria; most were not microbiologically or histologically proven.
Adapted from Lipsky BA: A current approach to diabetic foot infections. Curr Infect Dis Rep 1999; 1:253.

determine the presence of osteomyelitis in these patients, but the larger and deeper the overlying skin ulceration is, the more likely there is underlying osteomyelitis. In one study, a skin ulcer of greater than 2 cm^2 had a sensitivity of 56% and a specificity of 92% in diagnosing contiguous osteomyelitis.[26] Other investigators have found that contacting bone at the depth of a foot ulcer using a metal probe ("probe to bone test") has a sensitivity of 66% a specificity of 85%, a positive predictive value of 85%, and a negative predictive value of 56%.[27]

Infectious Arthritis

The typical clinical presentation of bacterial infectious arthritis in the adult is the acute onset over hours to days of pain, swelling, and limitation of motion of a weightbearing joint. Pain and limitation of the joint are present in more than 90% of cases.[15] Fever has been reported to be present in 78% of cases.[28] The knee, ankle, wrist, and shoulder were involved in 81% of the cases in a recent case series of adults.[29] The knee joint is the most common location, followed by the hip joint. Unexplained knee pain should alert the clinician that the knee pain may be referred from the hip, particularly in children. Sacroiliac or sternoclavicular joint infection is more common among injection drug users. Polyarticular infection occurs in approximately 15% of patients and occurs more often among patients with comorbid illnesses such as rheumatoid arthritis.

A large effusion and a marked decrease in range of motion of the joint are typically present on physical examination, although these findings may be minimal or absent in the elderly, in patients taking corticosteroids, or in patients with rheumatoid arthritis. Tenosynovitis, a macular, vesicular, pustular, or petechial rash, and polyarticular involvement is seen with disseminated gonococcal infection whereas monoarticular involvement without rash or tenosynovial involvement is common in later stages of the disease.

Prosthetic Joint Infection

Patients with prosthetic joint infection may present with a range of clinical signs and symptoms. Sudden onset of fever, pain, and swelling of the involved joint similar to native joint infectious arthritis occurs more often with virulent organisms such as *S. aureus* or beta-hemolytic streptococci. A chronic pain syndrome without constitutional symptoms is typical for less virulent microorganisms such as coagulase-negative staphylococci. Many patients with this condition will have constant pain present at rest throughout the day, not just with motion of the joint. In addition, wound healing problems or superficial wound infections have often occurred at the time of prosthesis implantation. Limitation of the joint range of motion may be present, or a draining sinus tract is present in 30% to 40% of patients.

LABORATORY AND RADIOGRAPHIC TESTS
Osteomyelitis

In infants and children with long bone hematogenous osteomyelitis an elevated erythrocyte sedimentation rate (ESR) or C-reactive protein (CRP) is present in more than 90% of cases.[30] A leukocytosis is present in approximately one third of patients. The lack of specificity of these tests, however, does not allow the clinician to diagnose acute osteomyelitis with these tests alone. Blood cultures should also be obtained and are positive in 36% to 76% of cases.[31–33]

Aspiration of associated soft-tissue or subperiosteal abscesses or biopsy of involved bone for appropriate cultures and pathological testing is diagnostic and helps guide antimicrobial therapy. Arthrocentesis should be performed if a joint effusion is present, but in the presence of adjacent cellulitis, one must take care to avoid inoculation of the joint by avoiding needle entry through the cellulitis.

Plain radiographs may be negative early in the disease. Soft tissue swelling and subperiosteal elevations are the earliest abnormalities and may not be seen for several weeks. Thirty percent to 50% of the bone must be destroyed before lytic lesions appear, and typically they do not appear for 2 to 6 weeks after the onset of the illness. Sclerotic changes occur later and when seen in association with periosteal new bone formation suggest chronicity of the infection.[34]

Radionuclide scanning is more sensitive than plain radiographs and may be helpful early in the course of the disease, but its usefulness is often limited by a lack of specificity. Computed tomography (CT) scans and magnetic resonance imaging (MRI) are better able to distinguish soft-tissue infection from osteomyelitis, are more sensitive than plain radiographs, and allow better identification of optimal areas for needle aspiration or biopsy.[35] Radionuclide scanning is advantageous when there are multiple potential areas of involvement.[22]

The ESR and CRP are elevated in as many as 95% of patients with vertebral osteomyelitis (see Table 4). In these recent case series, blood cultures were positive in 40% to 77% of cases. If blood cultures yield a pathogenic organism and there is definitive radiographic evidence of vertebral osteomyelitis, there is usually no need for a biopsy of the involved vertebrae and intervertebral disk space.[25] Needle biopsy of the involved intervertebral disk, vertebrae, or associated epidural abscess or phlegmon under radiographic guidance is the diagnostic procedure of choice. In cases in which the cultures from the initial needle biopsy are negative, a second needle biopsy and/or open biopsy should then be performed to establish the diagnosis.

Although some investigators have reported that plain anterior and posterior radiographs of the spine reveal erosive irregularities of vertebral end plates, with or without disk space narrowing in 95% of cases, others report that the sensitivity of plain radiographs is significantly less.[25, 36] Discrepancies between studies may be due to differences in inclusion criteria, duration of symptoms, or the presence of concomitant spinal pathological lesions such as severe osteoporosis or osteoarthritis. A combination of a gallium scan and a three-phase technetium (^{99}Tc) bone scan is more sensitive and specific than a three-phase ^{99}Tc bone scan alone or in combination with a indium-labeled leukocyte scan for the diagnosis of vertebral osteomyelitis.[37, 38] MRI is the most sensitive and diagnostic imaging technique and provides the best anatomic detail.[39] A gallium scan in combination with a three-phase ^{99}Tc bone scan should be used when spinal hardware degrades the MRI images.

In patients with chronic osteomyelitis of the foot, leukocyte count is not of diagnostic utility.[9] The ESR is nonspecific, but the greater the increase in the ESR is, the greater the risk of osteomyelitis.[9, 26] Blood cultures are usually negative. A bone biopsy is diagnostic and is usually obtained at the time of surgical débridement. Noninvasive testing of the arterial blood supply should be performed to determine the adequacy of blood flow to the foot and whether evaluation by a vascular surgeon is warranted.[40]

Because the infection in patients with contiguous focus osteomyelitis with or without vascular insufficiency is chronic, plain radiographs often show abnormalities. Plain radiography may be definitive in selected patients when associated with the presence of a draining sinus tract or contiguous foot ulcer. However, in cases in which surgery may or may not be necessary, the plain radiographic findings may be confused with other processes difficult to distinguish from osteomyelitis (e.g., neuropathic bone disease). Orthopaedic fixation devices often limit the usefulness of plain radiography, so radionuclide studies, CT scans, or MRI are often used to diagnose osteomyelitis.[41, 42] MRI and CT scans are more helpful than radionuclide scanning in distinguishing soft-tissue infection from osteomyelitis and they also aid preoperative surgical planning. MRI is thought to be the most sensitive and specific test for the diagnosis of foot bone osteomyelitis (Table 7). An

exception is in cases in which neuropathic osteoarthropathy and osteomyelitis coexist.[43, 44] Orthopaedic hardware can interfere with CT or MRI examinations of potential long-bone osteomyelitis. In these instances, the combination of a three-phase ^{99}Tc bone scan and indium-labeled leukocyte scan is often useful. Radionuclide scanning is more efficient when evaluating for osteomyelitis of multiple noncontiguous bones.

Infectious Arthritis

The ESR, CRP, and leukocyte count are elevated in the majority of cases of pyogenic arthritis but are nonspecific and can be elevated in other inflammatory arthropathies. Blood cultures are positive in up to 70% of patients.[17, 45] The diagnostic procedure of choice is arthrocentesis, which should be done as soon as the diagnosis of infection is suspected. Synovial fluid can be cloudy and the leukocyte count is usually between 50,000/mm³ and 100,000/mm³, with more than 75% polymorphonuclear leukocytes. Unfortunately, patients with rheumatoid arthritis and crystal deposition arthritis can have a synovial fluid analysis similar to that of pyogenic arthritis. A low synovial fluid glucose level is not specific for infection. The synovial fluid Gram stain will be positive in 50% to 90% of patients with nongonococcal infective arthritis with no prior antimicrobial therapy.[14, 28] All synovial fluid from adults should also be examined for uric acid and calcium pyrophosphate dihydrate crystals. The polymerase chain reaction detects the nucleic acid of bacterial pathogens and seems to be a promising tool for the detection of infectious arthritis due to *B. burgdorferi, N. gonorrhoeae,* and other pathogens.[46, 47] Synovial tissue cultures are indicated only for patients with chronic inflammatory arthritis when mycobacterial or fungal arthritis is suspected. In disseminated gonococcal disease, the blood cultures and/or cultures from the urethra, cervix, rectum, or pharynx can be positive even when synovial fluid cultures are negative. In monoarticular gonococcal arthritis, the synovial fluid cultures are usually positive and the blood cultures are usually negative.[16]

Plain radiographs are often not helpful in establishing the diagnosis of bacterial arthritis because the most common finding of periarticular soft-tissue swelling and even joint space narrowing due to cartilage destruction are nonspecific and take time to develop. CT scans and MRI and radionuclide studies can identify concomitant periarticular osteomyelitis. It should be emphasized that plain radio-

TABLE 7. COMPARISON OF VARIOUS IMAGING STUDIES IN IDENTIFYING FOOT BONE OSTEOMYELITIS IN DIABETIC PATIENTS*

| Test Modality | Approximate Mean (Range) | | Positive Predictive Value, % |
	Sensitivity, %	Specificity, %	
Plain radiography	60 (28–93)	66 (50–92)	74–87
Technetium-99m bone scan	86 (68–100)	45 (0–79)	43–87
Indium-111 WBC scan	89 (45–100)	78 (29–100)	75–85
MRI	99 (29–100)	83 (71–100)	50–100

* Comparison is based on five to eight studies of each modality (13–88 patients per study).
Adapted from Lipsky BA: Osteomyelitis of the foot in diabetic patients. Clin Infect Dis 1997; 25:1318.
Data from Grayson et al,[27] Eckman et al,[87] Newman,[88] Levine et al.[89]

graphs should always be obtained to establish a baseline and to rule out the presence of fracture or malignancy.

Prosthetic Joint Infection

Routine preoperative testing to diagnose prosthetic joint infection prior to revision arthroplasty includes use of the leukocyte count, ESR, CRP, preoperative plain radiographs, and joint aspiration. An elevated leukocyte count, ESR, or CRP is often present but is not sufficient to diagnose prosthetic joint infection.[48] The CRP was a more sensitive and specific test than the ESR for the diagnosis of total hip arthroplasty (THA) infection in a recent study of 178 patients (202 revision hip replacements).[49] Blood cultures should be obtained only if fever is present.

Plain radiographs, aspiration, and radionuclide studies are most useful in diagnosing prosthetic joint infection.[21] Plain radiographs should be performed in all patients. Radionuclide studies should be reserved for selected patients in whom the diagnosis of infection or periprosthetic loosening is in question. Loosening of the prosthesis, periostitis, or other evidence of osteomyelitis may be seen on plain radiographs. A hip arthrogram of a THA can confirm prosthesis loosening and joint aspiration can be done simultaneously. Sequential technetium and indium-111–labeled leukocyte scans in combination with sulfur colloid marrow scintigraphy is currently the most reliable radionuclide test for the presence of prosthetic joint infection.

The reported sensitivity and specificity of preoperative joint aspiration for THA infection is extremely variable.[48] Different definitions of a positive and negative result, the number of samples taken during aspiration, the inclusion of results of repeat aspiration in some studies, and the unrecognized or unreported use of antibiotics prior to aspiration were thought to account for the differences among the studies. The sensitivity and specificity of aspiration were reported to be 86% and 94%, respectively. In a prospective study of 180 aspirations prior to revision hip replacement in which patients with prior use of antibiotics were excluded from the analysis,[49] Barrack et al found similar results for preoperative aspiration prior to total knee arthroplasty.[50]

Histopathological examination of frozen section periprosthetic tissue is currently the only accurate way to identify prosthetic joint infection intraoperatively at the time of revision surgery. The results of frozen section histopathological sampling are dependent on the definition of acute inflammation, and the experience of the pathologist. In rare circumstances, the pathologist may also find evidence of specific types of inflammation (e.g., necrotizing granulomas) that may indicate mycobacterial or fungal infection. If this situation occurs, it is useful to perform tissue stains for fungi (methenamine silver stain) or mycobacteria (auramine rhodamine stain).

MICROBIOLOGY TESTS

To facilitate obtaining a specific microbiological diagnosis, empiric antimicrobial therapy for osteomyelitis, infective arthritis, or prosthetic joint infection should usually be withheld until all blood cultures, aspirates, and/or intraoperative cultures have been obtained by the surgeon or other health care providers. If there is significant concomitant soft-tissue infection or hemodynamic instability thought to

be due to infection, blood cultures and aspiration of any infected material from affected joints, abscesses, or bones should be taken urgently and empiric antimicrobial therapy initiated promptly. If antimicrobial therapy has already been started and the patient is not systemically ill or soft-tissue infection is not present, antimicrobial therapy should be stopped for 10 to 14 days prior to any diagnostic procedure performed to obtain a microbiological diagnosis.

At the time of diagnostic aspiration of a joint or needle biopsy of bone or disk space, as much fluid or tissue for culture as possible should be obtained by the person performing the procedure. If saline solutions are used at the time of aspiration, the saline should be nonbacteriostatic. Multiple intraoperative tissue samples should be obtained to facilitate the distinction between an intraoperative contaminant and true pathogen, particularly in the setting of foreign bodies such as fracture fixation devices and joint prostheses.[51, 52] Ultrasonification of foreign bodies such as joint prostheses may increase the detection of infection.[53] Cultures of superficial ulcers or sinus tracts should not be the basis for antimicrobial therapy, as they do not reliably predict the organisms subsequently obtained from bone specimens.[11, 54] Every effort should be made to appropriately label specimens and to send them to the microbiology laboratory in appropriate containers. The microbiology laboratory should make every effort to process specimens in a prompt and efficient manner.

A Gram stain should be performed on all specimens submitted for the diagnosis of osteomyelitis or infective arthritis. Intraoperative Gram stains are not useful for the diagnosis of prosthetic joint infection.[48] At least three cultures for aerobes and anaerobes should be obtained intraoperatively in most clinical situations. When the history, physical examination, or intraoperative findings suggest the possibility of unusual infection, special staining or culturing techniques for unusual organisms (e.g., fungi, mycobacteria, *Mycoplasma* spp., *Brucella* spp., *S. aureus,* or *E. coli*), small colony variants, or other organisms can be performed by the microbiology laboratory.[55, 56] There are not enough data to recommend routine use of molecular diagnostic techniques for the diagnosis of most musculoskeletal infections.[47, 57]

Antimicrobial susceptibility tests should be performed if possible on all bacterial isolates thought to be pathogens.[58] A minimal inhibitory concentration (MIC) obtained by broth or agar dilution as opposed to disc diffusion (Kirby-Bauer disc sensitivities) is the best in vitro susceptibility test.[58] Many laboratories do not report the actual or true MIC of an organism but rather report only a breakpoint MIC below which the organism is deemed to be susceptible. The actual MIC may be considerably lower, but this should not generally affect the choice of antimicrobial therapy. Comparison of the breakpoint or actual MICs of various antimicrobials for a given microorganism without taking into account achievable tissue concentrations of a specific antimicrobial is not advisable and may lead to inappropriate antimicrobial choices. For example, the breakpoint MIC of ciprofloxacin for *S. aureus* is 2.0 μg/mL and for cefazolin is 8 μg/mL. These results should not be interpreted by the clinician to suggest that ciprofloxacin has more in vitro activity against staphylococci then cefazolin. In fact the opposite is the case.

Some investigators also advocate performing serum bactericidal titers to monitor the antimicrobial therapy of patients with bone and joint infections.[59, 60] The results of this test represent the dilution of patient's serum, which shows greater than or equal to 99.9% killing of the organism in vitro. These tests are difficult to reproduce within and among laboratories.[58] More recently, investigators have advocated measuring newer pharmacodynamic parameters in selected patients with serious infections (e.g., peak serum concentration of a fluoroquinolone/true MIC ratio) to help predict therapeutic efficacy of a given antimicrobial agent against a specific organism.[61]

ANTIMICROBIAL THERAPY

GENERAL CONSIDERATIONS

The selection of a specific type, route, and dosage of an antimicrobial agent for a given infection in a specific patient requires the integration of knowledge regarding the severity and microbiology of the clinical syndrome being treated, the mechanism of action, the spectrum of activity, the pharmacokinetic properties and potential toxicities of the possible antibiotics to be utilized, and key patient-specific information obtained at the time of the history and physical examination.[62] The cost of an antimicrobial agent is a secondary consideration when two or more antimicrobials are equivalent in terms of safety and efficacy.

Dosages of specific antimicrobials are dictated by the pharmacokinetic properties of each individual drug and the patient's renal and/or hepatic function. For example, vancomycin has a normal serum half-life of 6 hours and is usually administered every 12 hours in patients with normal renal function. However, in the setting of anuria, vancomycin has a serum half-life of 7.5 days.[63] A specific dose of an antimicrobial is chosen to achieve serum concentrations throughout the dosing interval that have eradicated infection and avoided toxicity in experimental models and clinical trials.[61]

The serum concentration of an antimicrobial should be measured when the antimicrobial has a narrow therapeutic range between an effective dose and a dose that causes excess toxicity (e.g., aminoglycosides or vancomycin) or when there is a question of drug absorption when the antibiotic is being given by the oral route. Serum antimicrobial concentrations should be measured at steady state. For most clinical situations, this occurs after four to five half-lives of the drug.

If a serum gentamicin or vancomycin level is reported as too high or low, there are several potential explanations. If the pre-dose serum concentration (trough) is too high, the clearance of the drug is lower than anticipated based on predicted clearance calculated from the age, sex, weight, and creatinine serum concentration in that particular patient. This situation frequently happens in elderly patients with diminished muscle mass. The interval between doses should be increased to correct this problem.

If the post-dose serum concentration (peak) is too high, the clinician should ensure that the timing of the measurement of the vancomycin or gentamicin concentration to the administration of the antimicrobial was correct and that the serum used to measure the drug concentration was not withdrawn through the intravenous line where the drug was infused. Antibiotic remaining in the line can artificially increase the serum concentration. Assuming these problems are not present, a high post-dose serum concentration requires a decrease in the dosage of the gentamicin or vancomycin.

Noncompliance, missed doses, poor oral absorption, measurement of the serum concentration before complete oral absorption, or a better than predicted clearance needs to be considered when serum concentrations are too low. Reviews of serum antimicrobial assay techniques and their interpretation have recently been published.[58, 61]

Duration of therapy and the setting in which the patient will receive treatment (i.e., inpatient or outpatient, home or at an infusion center) are also considerations in choosing an antimicrobial agent. Duration of therapy for specific clinical syndromes is discussed later. Home intravenous antimicrobial therapy for selected patients has become a viable alternative in the last decade.[64–66] Proper selection of patients for participation, patient compliance, and careful monitoring by a treatment team consisting of physicians, pharmacists, and nurses is essential. Semipermanent catheters such as peripherally inserted central catheters or Hickman's or Broviac's catheters can be inserted in the hospital prior to discharge. The importance of frequent nursing and physician evaluation as well as laboratory monitoring of outpatient antimicrobial therapy cannot be overemphasized. In a recent review of the complications of outpatient antimicrobial therapy, access problems, rash, diarrhea, nephrotoxicity, leukopenia, neutropenia, or thrombocytopenia occurred in 11%, 4%, 7%, 8%, 16%, 7%, and 4% of treatment courses, respectively.[65] Recent guidelines have been written.[64] Guidelines for monitoring of laboratory parameters while receiving outpatient antimicrobial therapy are shown in Table 8.

Despite several recent articles suggesting the efficacy of oral antimicrobial therapy with highly bioavailable agents that achieve the same tissue concentrations whether given orally or intravenously,[67–71] the author does not routinely recommend oral therapy as initial therapy for staphylococcal bone and joint infection but reserves it for follow-up therapy after initial intravenous therapy or for chronic suppression of infection. The author does use oral fluoroquinolones to treat osteomyelitis due to susceptible non-pseudomonal aerobic gram-negative bacteria in situations in which impairment of potential fracture healing is not an issue.[72] Further studies to define the role of oral agents in the treatment of bone and joint infection are warranted.

ANTIMICROBIAL THERAPY OF SPECIFIC MUSCULOSKELETAL INFECTIONS
Osteomyelitis

Surgical therapy of acute osteomyelitis in children is not always required and is reviewed elsewhere. Initial empiric therapy of acute hematogenous osteomyelitis is typically administered by the intravenous route. An antistaphylococcal penicillin (e.g., nafcillin, oxacillin), cefuroxime, ampicillin-sulbactam, cefazolin, or other first-generation cephalosporin is appropriate. Vancomycin should be used if methicillin-resistant S. aureus is the suspected pathogen.[22]

TABLE 8. LABORATORY PARAMETERS THAT SHOULD BE MONITORED ON A WEEKLY BASIS DURING COMMUNITY-BASED PARENTERAL ANTIMICROBIAL THERAPY

Antimicrobial	Complete Blood Count	Creatinine Level	Potassium Level	Magnesium Level	Other
β-lactams	1	1			
Aztreonam					
Cephalosporins*					
Carbapenems					
Penicillins*					
Antipseudomonal penicillins*	1	1	2		
Ticarcillin					
Piperacillin					
Ticarcillin/clavulanate†					
Piperacillin-tazobactam†					
Aminoglycosides	1	2			Blood levels as clinically indicated Consider audiogram
Miscellaneous					
Clindamycin	1	1			
Vancomycin	1	2			Blood levels as clinically indicated
Trimethoprim-sulfamethoxazole	1	1	1		
Quinupristin-dalfopristin†	1	1			
Antifungals					
Amphotericin B	1	2	2	2	
Fluconazole	1	1			

Note: Data are number of times per week that test should be done and represent minimal criteria for patients with normal or stable renal function.
* For patients receiving nafcillin, oxacillin, or ceftriaxone, monitoring of liver function tests may be indicated.
† Opinion of the author.
Adapted from Williams D, Rehm S, Tice A, et al: Practice guidelines for community-based parenteral anti-infective therapy. Clin Infect Dis 1997; 25:787.

Therapy can be modified once culture and sensitivity results become available. The duration of intravenous antimicrobial therapy is typically 4 to 6 weeks. The risk of treatment failure is as high as 19% when the duration of therapy is reduced to 3 weeks or less.[22, 34] Oral antimicrobial therapy is controversial but is often prescribed once the patient is afebrile, local signs of inflammation have decreased, the patient is taking medicines by mouth, and patient compliance and follow-up is assured. It requires two to four times the usually recommended doses of the oral antimicrobial, which may lead to an increased incidence of adverse side effects. Oral fluoroquinolones are not routinely recommended in the pediatric population. Close monitoring of the ESR and CRP during the first several weeks following the initiation of therapy may allow the detection of complications from the osteomyelitis.[22, 34, 73, 74]

The surgical indications for vertebral osteomyelitis are reviewed elsewhere. The intravenous route is typically the route chosen for initial empiric therapy of vertebral osteomyelitis. An antistaphylococcal penicillin (e.g., nafcillin, oxacillin) or cefazolin (or other first-generation cephalosporin) is appropriate when staphylococci are thought to be the pathogen. Vancomycin should be used if methicillin-resistant S. aureus is the suspected pathogen. If there is concern about aerobic gram-negative bacteria or if neurologic impairment or hemodynamic instability is present, broad aerobic gram-positive and gram-negative coverage with the combination of vancomycin and cefepime with or without an aminoglycoside is warranted while awaiting the results of blood, biopsy, or intraoperative culture tests. Therapy should be narrowed once the results of in vitro sensitivity testing are available (Table 9). The typical duration of intravenous antimicrobial therapy for vertebral osteomyeli-

tis is 4 to 6 weeks, although longer durations of therapy may be necessary in cases of severe disease, if epidural abscesses are treated with medical therapy alone or if the ESR has not significantly decreased after the completion of therapy.[6] Serial ESR and CRP determinations and MRI scans are often used to guide continued antimicrobial therapy; however, the response of MRI to effective antimicrobial therapy may lag resolution of clinical symptoms. If the patient's symptoms are significantly improved and a standard course of therapy has been administered, the results of these tests alone should not prompt continuation of intravenous or oral antimicrobial therapy.[75, 76]

The standard treatment of chronic contiguous osteomyelitis without vascular insufficiency is 4 to 6 weeks of directed intravenous antimicrobial therapy after surgical débridement and removal of any foreign material with or without additional oral antimicrobial therapy (see Table 9).[3, 5, 77] There have been few comparative clinical trials of different medical regimens for the treatment of osteomyelitis and they all suffer from methodological problems. The combined risk of failure in five comparative studies with 154 evaluable patients was 22%, with variable periods of follow-up.[5] Oral therapy with fluoroquinolones for nonpseudomonal aerobic gram-negative osteomyelitis seems reasonable.[71, 78] The efficacy of rifampin and clindamycin for susceptible staphylococcal osteomyelitis has been shown in experimental models.[78-81] Definitive proof of their benefit in clinical practice is lacking. The topics of local antimicrobial therapy with antibiotic-impregnated beads and hyperbaric oxygen therapy have been recently reviewed.[77, 82]

The surgical therapy of contiguous osteomyelitis with vascular insufficiency requires optimization of hyperglyce-

TABLE 9. ANTIBIOTIC THERAPY OF CHRONIC OSTEOMYELITIS, SEPTIC ARTHRITIS, AND PROSTHETIC JOINT INFECTION DUE TO SELECTED MICROORGANISMS

Microorganisms	Antibiotic Therapy*	Alternative Therapy*
Staphylococcus aureus Methicillin-sensitive	Nafcillin sodium or oxacillin sodium, 1.5–2.0 g IV every 4 h **or** Cefazolin (or other first-generation cephalosporins in equivalent dosages) 1 g IV every 8 h (cephalosporins should be avoided in patients with immediate-type hypersensitivity to penicillin)	Vancomycin,† 30 mg/kg IV in two equally divided doses, not to exceed 2 g/24 h unless serum levels are monitored.
Methicillin-resistant	Vancomycin,† 30 mg/kg IV in two equally divided doses, not to exceed 2 g/24 h unless serum levels are monitored.	Consult Infectious Diseases specialist
Penicillin sensitive streptococci or pneumococci (MIC ≤ 0.1 μg/mL)	Aqueous crystalline penicillin G, 20 × 10⁶ U/24 h IV either continuously or in six equally divided doses **or** Ceftriaxone 2 g IV or IM for 4–6 wk† **or** Cefazolin (or other first-generation cephalosporins in equivalent dosages) 1 g IV every 8 h (cephalosporins should be avoided in patients with immediate-type hypersensitivity to penicillin)	Vancomycin,† 30 mg/kg IV in two equally divided doses, not to exceed 2 g/24 h unless serum levels are monitored (vancomycin therapy is recommended for patients allergic to β-lactams [immediate-type hypersensitivity])
Enterococci or streptococci with MIC ≥ 0.5 μg/mL or nutritionally variant streptococci (All enterococci causing osteomyelitis must be tested for antimicrobial susceptibility to select optimal therapy.)	Aqueous crystalline penicillin G, 20 × 10⁶ U/24 h IV either continuously or in six equally divided doses **or** Ampicillin sodium 12 g/24 h IV either continuously or in six equally divided doses The addition of gentamicin sulfate,‡ 1 mg/kg IV or IM every 8 h for 1–2 wk is optional	Vancomycin,† 30 mg/kg IV in two equally divided doses, not to exceed 2 g/24 h unless serum levels are monitored The addition of gentamicin sulfate,‡ 1 mg/kg IV or IM every 8 h for 1–2 wk is optional
Enterobacteriaciae (based on in vitro susceptibility)	Ceftriaxone 2 g IV q day	Ciprofloxacin 500–750 mg PO bid or levofloxacin 500 mg PO q day for 4–6 weeks
Pseudomonas aeruginosa or *Enterobacter* spp.	Cefepime 2 g IV every 12 h plus ciprofloxacin 750 mg PO bid **or** Gentamicin sulfate‡ 1.5–mg/kg IV or IM every 8 h for 1–2 wk is day is optional	

* Dosages recommended are for patients with normal renal function.

† Vancomycin therapy is recommended for patients allergic to β-lactams (immediate-type hypersensitivity); serum concentration of vancomycin should be obtained prior to and 1 hour after completion of the infusion and should be in the range of 20–40 μg/mL for a peak and 5–10 μg/mL for a trough for twice-daily dosing. Vancomycin should be infused over at least 1 hour to reduce the risk of the "red man" syndrome.

‡ Serum concentration of gentamicin should be obtained prior to and 30 minutes after completion of the infusion and should be in the range of 3–4 μg/mL for a peak and 0.5–1 μg/mL for a trough for synergistic therapy for enterococci. Relative contraindications to the use of gentamicin are age >65 y, renal impairment, or impairment of the eighth cranial nerve. Other potentially nephrotoxic agents should be used cautiously in patients receiving gentamicin.

mia and revascularization when necessary and technically possible.[40] Empiric antimicrobial therapy often must begin prior to the ascertainment of bone cultures because of the presence of concomitant soft-tissue infection. Clinical characteristics that help to define the severity of infection and dictate empiric antimicrobial therapy are shown in Table 10 and potential empiric antimicrobial regimens in Table 11. The duration of therapy for diabetic foot infections is controversial. The type and duration of directed antimicrobial therapy should follow the principles outlined for chronic osteomyelitis without vascular insufficiency (see Table 9). If the osteomyelitic bone is amputated, prolonged antimicrobial therapy is not necessary. The roles of recombinant granulocyte colony-stimulating factor and hyperbaric oxygen therapy remain controversial.[77, 83]

Infectious Arthritis

The optimal method of drainage of an infected joint remains controversial. Empiric antimicrobial therapy similar to that discussed for vertebral osteomyelitis should be begun as soon as possible after culture ascertainment. In the young sexually active adult, empiric therapy should be active against *N. gonorrhoeae*. There are no randomized controlled trials to guide the selection of the type, route, or duration of directed antimicrobial therapy of infectious arthritis. Two to 4 weeks of intravenous therapy is adminis-

TABLE 10. CLINICAL CHARACTERISTICS THAT HELP DEFINE THE SEVERITY OF A DIABETIC FOOT INFECTION

Feature	Mild Infection	Serious Infection
Presentation	Slowly progressive	Acute or rapidly progressive
Ulceration	Involves skin only	Penetrates to subcutaneous tissue
Tissues involved	Epidermis and dermis	Fascia, muscle, joint, bone
Cellulitis	Minimal (<2 cm rim)	Extensive or distant from ulceration
Local signs	Slight inflammation	Severe inflammation, crepitus, bullae
Systemic signs	None or minimal	Fever, chills, hypotension, confusion, volume depletion, leukocytosis
Metabolic control	Mildly abnormal (hyperglycemia)	Severe hyperglycemia, acidosis, azotemia, electrolyte abnormalities
Foot vasculature	Minimally impaired (normal/reduced pulses)	Absent pulses, reduced ankle or toe blood pressure
Complicating features	None or minimal (callus, ulcer)	Gangrene, eschar, foreign body, abscess, marked edema

Adapted from Lipsky BA: A current approach to diabetic foot infections. Curr Infect Dis Rep 1999; 1:253.

tered by most experts.[14, 15] Specific regimens for common pathogens are shown in Table 9. Oral therapy with a highly bioavailable agent such as a fluoroquinolone is reasonable, particularly after the patient has improved on initial intravenous therapy.

Prosthetic Joint Infection

Considerations regarding empiric antimicrobial therapy are similar to those discussed for vertebral osteomyelitis. When removal of the prosthesis is possible, then 4 to 6 weeks of directed intravenous antimicrobial therapy is typically administered.[21] The author knows of no data that would support one duration of therapy over another as long as 4 weeks of therapy is administered for patients undergoing a two-stage exchange procedure. Six weeks of antimicrobial therapy has been successful in eradicating infection in ap-

proximately 90% of patients.[84] Specific regimens can be found in Table 9.

Similar intravenous antimicrobial regimens are utilized initially when the prosthesis is débrided and the components retained. Recent data would suggest that some patients with susceptible staphylococcal prosthetic joint infections can be cured with the administration of the combination of a fluoroquinolone and rifampin, but more studies are needed before this can be recommended as standard therapy.[70] Suppressive antimicrobial therapy may be attempted in the compliant patient with a well-fixed prosthesis who is an unacceptable surgical risk or declines surgery in whom the infection is caused by a low-virulence organism (e.g., coagulase-negative staphylococci) that is known to be susceptible to safe and efficacious oral antimicrobials.

TABLE 11. SUGGESTED ANTIMICROBIAL REGIMENS FOR THE EMPIRIC TREATMENT OF DIABETIC FOOT INFECTIONS*

Severity of Infection	Recommended†	Alternative‡
Mild/moderate (oral therapy)	Cephalexin 500 mg PO qid **or** Amoxicillin-clavulanate 500 mg PO tid **or** Clindamycin 300 mg PO qid	Levofloxacin 500 mg PO q day with or without metronidazole 7.5 mg/kg PO tid
Moderate/severe (intravenous until stable then switch to oral equivalent)	Piperacillin-tazobactam§ 3.375 g IV q 6 h **or** Cefepime 1 g IV q 12 h plus metronidazole 7.5 mg/kg IV q 8 h	Levofloxacin 500 mg IV q day plus metronidazole 7.5 mg/kg IV q 8 h
Life threatening	Imipenem-cilastin§ 500 mg IV q 6 h	Vancomycin,¶ 30 mg/kg IV in two equally divided doses (not to exceed 2 g/24 h unless serum levels are monitored) plus ciprofloxacin 400 mg IV q 12 h plus metronidazole 7.5 mg/kg IV q 8 h

* At usual recommended doses for serious infections; modify based on renal function and body mass.
† Based on theoretical considerations, clinical trials, and expert opinion.
‡ Prescribed in special circumstances, e.g., patient allergies, recent treatment with recommended agent, local antibiotic resistance patterns, regimen compliance, and cost.
§ A similar agent of the same class or generation may be substituted.
¶ Vancomycin therapy is recommended for patients allergic to β-lactams (immediate-type hypersensitivity); serum concentration of vancomycin should be obtained prior to and 1 h after completion of the infusion and should be in the range of 20–40 µg/mL for a peak and 5–10 µg/mL for a trough for twice-daily dosing. Vancomycin should be infused over at least 1 hour to reduce the risk of the "red neck" syndrome.
Adapted from Lipsky BA: A current approach to diabetic foot infection. Curr Infect Dis 1999; 1:253.

REFERENCES

1. Mangram AJ, Horan TC, Pearson ML, et al: Guidelines for the prevention of surgical site infection, 1999. Infect Control Hosp Epidemiol 1999; 20:247.
2. Mader JT, Shirtliff M, Calhoun JH: Staging and staging application in osteomyelitis. Clin Infect Dis 1997; 25:1303.
3. Lew DP, Waldvogel FA: Osteomyelitis [see comments]. N Engl J Med 1997; 336: 999.
4. Howard AW, Viskontas D, Sabbagh C: Reduction in osteomyelitis and septic arthritis related to *Haemophilus influenzae* type B vaccination. J Pediatr Orthop 1999; 19:705.
5. Haas DW, McAndrew MP: Bacterial osteomyelitis in adults: Evolving considerations in diagnosis and treatment. Am J Med 1996; 101:550.
6. Sapico FL: Microbiology and antimicrobial therapy of spinal infections. Orthop Clin North Am 1996; 27:9.
7. Carragee EJ: Pyogenic vertebral osteomyelitis [see comments]. J Bone Joint Surg Am 1997; 79:874.
8. Chelsom J, Solberg CO: Vertebral osteomyelitis at a Norwegian university hospital 1987–97: Clinical features, laboratory findings and outcome. Scand J Infect Dis 1998; 30:147.
9. Lipsky BA: Osteomyelitis of the foot in diabetic patients. Clin Infect Dis 1997; 25: 1318.
10. Lipsky BA: A current approach to diabetic foot infections. Curr Infect Dis Rep 1999; 1:253.
11. Lavery LA, Sariaya M, Ashry H, Harkless LB: Microbiology of osteomyelitis in diabetic foot infections. J Foot Ankle Surg 1995; 34:61.
12. van den Bogaard AE, Stobberingh EE: Antibiotic usage in animals: Impact on bacterial resistance and public health. Drugs 1999; 58:589.
13. Osmon DR: Antimicrobial prophylaxis in adults [review]. Mayo Clin Proc 2000; 75: 98.
14. Goldenberg DL: Septic arthritis [see comments]. Lancet 1998; 351:197.
15. Smith JW, Piercy EA: Infectious arthritis. Clin Infect Dis 1995; 20:225.
16. Cucurull E, Espinnoza LR: Gonococcal arthritis. Rheum Dis Clin North Am 1998; 24:305.
17. Dubost JJ, Fis I, Denis P, et al: Polyarticular septic arthritis. Medicine 1993; 72: 296.
18. McGuire NM, Kauffman CA: Septic arthritis in the elderly. J Am Geriatr Soc 1985; 33:170.
19. Settecerri JJ, Pitner MA, Rock MG, et al: Infection after rotator cuff repair. J Shoulder Elbow Surg 1999; 8:1.
20. Furr PM, Taylor-Robinson D, Webster AD: Mycoplasmas and ureaplasmas in patients with hypogammaglobulinaemia and their role in arthritis: Microbiological observations over twenty years. Ann Rheum Dis 1994; 53:183.
21. Steckelberg J, Osmon D: Prosthetic joint infections. In Bisno A, Waldvogel F (eds): Infections Associated with Indwelling Devices. Washington DC: ASM Press, In press.
22. Sonnen GM, Henry NK: Pediatric bone and joint infections: Diagnosis and antimicrobial management. Pediatr Clin North Am 1996; 43:933.
23. Knudsen CJ, Hoffman EB: Neonatal osteomyelitis. J Bone Joint Surg Br 1990; 72: 846.
24. Rezai AR, Woo HH, Errico TJ, Cooper PR: Contemporary management of spinal osteomyelitis. Neurosurgery 1999; 44: 1018; discussion 1025.
25. Sapico FL, Montgomerie JZ: Vertebral osteomyelitis. Infect Dis Clin North Am 1990; 4:539.
26. Newman LG, Waller J, Palestro CJ, et al: Unsuspected osteomyelitis in diabetic foot ulcers. Diagnosis and monitoring by leukocyte scanning with indium in 111 oxyquinoline [see comments]. JAMA 1991; 266:1246.
27. Grayson ML, Gibbons GW, Balogh K, et al: Probing to bone in infected pedal ulcers: A clinical sign of underlying osteomyelitis in diabetic patients [see comments]. JAMA 1995; 273:721.
28. Goldenberg DL, Reed JI: Bacterial arthritis. N Engl J Med 1985; 312:764.
29. Kaandorp CJ, Dinant HJ, van de Laar MA, et al: Incidence and sources of native and prosthetic joint infection: A community based prospective survey. Ann Rheum Dis 1997; 56:470.
30. Unkila-Kallio L, Kallio MJ, Eskola J, Peltola H: Serum C-reactive protein, erythrocyte sedimentation rate, and white blood cell count in acute hematogenous osteomyelitis of children. Pediatrics 1994; 93: 59.
31. Dich VQ, Nelson JD, Haltalin KC: Osteomyelitis in infants and children: A review of 163 cases. Am J Dis Child 1975; 129: 1273.
32. Nelson JD: Acute osteomyelitis in children. Infect Dis Clin North Am 1990; 4: 513.
33. Unkila-Kallio L, Kallio MJ, Peltola H: Acute haematogenous osteomyelitis in children in Finland. Finnish Study Group. Ann Med 1993; 25:545.
34. Krogstad P, Smith A: Osteomyelitis and septic arthritis. In Feigin RD, Cherry JD (eds): Textbook of Pediatric Infectious Diseases, Vol. 1. Philadelphia: W.B. Saunders, 1998:683.
35. Mazur JM, Ross G, Cummings J, et al: Usefulness of magnetic resonance imaging for the diagnosis of acute musculoskeletal infections in children. J Pediatr Orthop 1995; 15:144.
36. Abbey DM, Hosea SW: Diagnosis of vertebral osteomyelitis in a community hospital by using computed tomography. Arch Intern Med 1989; 149:2029.
37. Palestro CJ, Torres MA: Radionuclide imaging in orthopedic infections. Semin Nuclear Med 1997; 27:334.
38. Hadjipavlou AG, Cesani-Vazquez F, Villanueva-Meyer J, et al: The effectiveness of gallium citrate Ga 67 radionuclide imaging in vertebral osteomyelitis revisited. Am J Orthop 1998; 27:179.
39. Dagirmanjian A, Schils J, McHenry MC: MR imaging of spinal infections. Magn Resonance Imag Clin North Am 1999; 7: 525.
40. Caputo GM, Cavanagh PR, Ulbrecht JS, et al: Assessment and management of foot disease in patients with diabetes [see comments]. N Engl J Med 1994; 331:854.
41. Ma LD, Frassica FJ, Bluemke DA, Fishman EK: CT and MRI evaluation of musculoskeletal infection. Crit Rev Diagn Imaging 1997; 38:535.
42. Boutin RD, Brossmann J, Sartoris DJ, et al: Update on imaging of orthopedic infections. Orthop Clin North Am 1998; 29:41.
43. Lipman BT, Collier BD, Carrera GF, et al: Detection of osteomyelitis in the neuropathic foot: nuclear medicine, MRI and conventional radiography. Clin Nuclear Med 1998; 23:77.
44. Vesco L, Boulahdour H, Hamissa S, et al: The value of combined radionuclide and magnetic resonance imaging in the diagnosis and conservative management of minimal or localized osteomyelitis of the foot in diabetic patients. Metab Clin Exp 1999; 48:922.
45. Ryan MJ, Kavanagh R, Wall PG, Hazleman BL: Bacterial joint infections in England and Wales: Analysis of bacterial isolates over a four year period. Br J Rheumatol 1997; 36:370.
46. Nocton JJ, Dressler F, Rutledge BJ, et al: Detection of *Borrelia burgdorferi* DNA by polymerase chain reaction in synovial fluid from patients with Lyme arthritis. N Engl J Med 1994; 330:229.
47. Li F, Bulbul R, Schumacher HR Jr, et al: Molecular detection of bacterial DNA in venereal-associated arthritis. Arthritis Rheum 1996; 39:950.
48. Spangehl M, Younger A, Masri B, Duncan C: Diagnosis of infection following total hip arthroplasty. J Bone Joint Surg Am 1997; 79:1578.
49. Spangehl M, Masri B, O'Connell J, Duncan C: Prospective analysis of preoperative and intraoperative investigations for the diagnosis of infection at the sites of 202 revision total hip arthroplasties. J Bone Joint Surg Am 1999; 81:672.
50. Barrack RL, Jennings RW, Wolfe MW, Bertot AJ: The Coventry Award. The value of preoperative aspiration before total knee revision. Clin Orthop Rel Res 1997; 345:8.
51. Atkins B, Athanasou N, Deeks J, et al: Prospective evaluation of criteria for microbiological diagnosis of prosthetic joint infection at revision arthroplasty. J Clin Microbiol 1998; 36:2932.
52. Padgett DE, Silverman A, Sachjowicz F, et al: Efficacy of intraoperative cultures obtained during revision total hip arthroplasty. J Arthroplast 1995; 10:420.
53. Tunney MM, Patrick S, Gorman SP, et al: Improved detection of infection in hip replacements: A currently underestimated problem. J Bone Joint Surg Br 1998; 80: 568.

54. Patzakis MJ, Wilkins J, Kumar J, et al: Comparison of the results of bacterial cultures from multiple sites in chronic osteomyelitis of long bones: A prospective study. J Bone Joint Surg Am 1994; 76: 664.

55. Berbari EF, Hanssen AD, Duffy MC, et al: Prosthetic joint infection due to *Mycobacterium tuberculosis*: A case series and review of the literature. Am J Orthop 1998; 27:219.

56. Proctor R, Peters G: Small colony variants in staphylococcal infections: Diagnostic and therapeutic implications. Clin Infect Dis 1998; 27:419.

57. Mariani BD, Tuan RS: Advances in the diagnosis of infection in prosthetic joint implants. Molec Med Today 1998; 4:207.

58. Cockerill FR III: Conventional and genetic laboratory tests used to guide antimicrobial therapy. Mayo Clin Proc 1998; 73: 1007.

59. Weinstein MP, Stratton CW, Hawley HB, et al: Multicenter collaborative evaluation of a standardized serum bactericidal test as a predictor of therapeutic efficacy in acute and chronic osteomyelitis. Am J Med 1987; 83:218.

60. Windsor RE, Insall JN, Urs WK, et al: Two-stage reimplantation for the salvage of total knee arthroplasty complicated by infection: Further follow-up and refinement of indications. J Bone Joint Surg Am 1990; 72:272.

61. Estes L: Review of pharmacokinetics and pharmacodynamics of antimicrobial agents. Mayo Clin Proc 1998; 73:1114.

62. Thompson RL, Wright AJ: General principles of antimicrobial therapy. Mayo Clin Proc 1998; 73:995.

63. Wilhelm MP, Estes L: Vancomycin. Mayo Clin Proc 1999; 74:928.

64. Williams D, Rehm S, Tice A, et al: Practice guidelines for community-based parenteral anti-infective therapy. Clin Infect Dis 1997; 25:787.

65. Hoffman-Terry ML, Fraimow HS, Fox TR, et al: Adverse effects of outpatient parenteral antibiotic therapy. Am J Med 1999; 106:44.

66. Williams DN, Raymond JL: Community-based parenteral anti-infective therapy (CoPAT). Pharmacokinetic and monitoring issues. Clin Pharmacokinet 1998; 35:65.

67. Mader JT, Cantrell JS, Calhoun J: Oral ciprofloxacin compared with standard parenteral antibiotic therapy for chronic osteomyelitis in adults. J Bone Joint Surg Am 1990; 72:104.

68. Gentry LO, Rodriguez-Gomez G: Ofloxacin versus parenteral therapy for chronic osteomyelitis. Antimicrob Agents Chemother 1991; 35:538.

69. Drancourt M, Stein A, Argenson J, et al: Oral treatment of *Staphylococcus* spp. infected orthopaedic implants with fusidic acid or ofloxacin in combination with rifampicin. J Antimicrob Chemother 1997; 39:235.

70. Zimmerli W, Widmer AF, Blatter M, et al: Role of rifampin for treatment of orthopedic implant-related staphylococcal infections: a randomized controlled trial. Foreign-Body Infection (FBI) Study Group. JAMA 1998; 279:1537.

71. Rissing JP: Antimicrobial therapy for chronic osteomyelitis in adults: role of the quinolones. Clin Infect Dis 1997; 25: 1327.

72. Huddleston PM, Steckelberg JM, Hanssen AD, et al: Ciprofloxacin inhibition of experimental fracture healing. J Bone Joint Surg Am 2000; 82:161.

73. Roine I, Faingezicht I, Arguedas A, et al: Serial serum C-reactive protein to monitor recovery from acute hematogenous osteomyelitis in children. Pediatr Infect Dis J 1995; 14:40.

74. Roine I, Arguedas A, Faingezicht I, Rodriguez F: Early detection of sequela-prone osteomyelitis in children with use of simple clinical and laboratory criteria. Clin Infect Dis 1997; 24:849.

75. Carragee EJ: The clinical use of magnetic resonance imaging in pyogenic vertebral osteomyelitis. Spine 1997; 22:780.

76. Carragee EJ, Kim D, van der Vlugt T, Vittum D: The clinical use of erythrocyte sedimentation rate in pyogenic vertebral osteomyelitis. Spine 1997; 22:2089.

77. Mader JT, Shirtliff ME, Bergquist SC, Calhoun J: Antimicrobial treatment of chronic osteomyelitis. Clin Orthop Rel Res 1999; 360:47.

78. Lew DP, Waldvogel FA: Use of quinolones in osteomyelitis and infected orthopaedic prosthesis. Drugs 1999; 58:85.

79. Norden CW: Lessons learned from animal models of osteomyelitis. Rev Infect Dis 1988; 10:103.

80. Shirtliff ME, Mader JT, Calhoun J: Oral rifampin plus azithromycin or clarithromycin to treat osteomyelitis in rabbits. Clin Orthop Rel Res 1999; 359:229.

81. Rissing JP: Animal models of osteomyelitis: Knowledge, hypothesis, and speculation. Infect Dis Clin North Am 1990; 4: 377.

82. Wininger DA, Fass RJ: Antibiotic-impregnated cement and beads for orthopedic infections. Antimicrob Agents Chemother 1996; 40:2675.

83. Gough A, Clapperton M, Rolando N, et al: Randomised placebo-controlled trial of granulocyte-colony stimulating factor in diabetic foot infection [see comments]. Lancet 1997; 350:855.

84. Tsukayama DT, Estrada R, Gustilo RB: Infection after total hip arthroplasty: A study of the treatment of one hundred and six infections. J Bone Joint Surg Am 1996; 78:512.

85. Nolan RL, Chapman SW: Osteomyelitis and diabetic foot infections. In Reese RE, Betts RF (eds): A Practical Approach to Infectious Diseases. Boston: Little, Brown and Company, 1996:606.

86. Roberts NJ, Mock DJ: Joint infections. In Reese RE, Betts RF (eds): A Practical Approach to Infectious Diseases. Boston: Little, Brown and Company, 1996:578.

87. Eckman MH, Greenfield S, Mackey WC, et al: Foot infections in diabetic patients: Decision and cost-effectiveness analyses [see comments]. JAMA 1995; 273:712.

88. Newman LG: Imaging techniques in the diabetic foot. Clin Pediatr Med Surg 1995; 12:75.

89. Levine SE, Neagle CE, Esterhai JL, et al: Magnetic resonance imaging for the diagnosis of osteomyelitis in the diabetic patient with a foot ulcer. Foot Ankle Int 1994; 15:151.

section
5
chapter
2

PEDIATRIC OSTEOMYELITIS AND SEPTIC ARTHRITIS

William J. Shaughnessy

Summary

- Bone and joint infections among children are common.
- Early diagnosis and treatment are critical to achieve good results.
- The differential diagnosis for osteomyelitis and septic arthritis is extensive.
- Needle aspiration of the infected bone or joint is essential to make the correct diagnosis and to begin early treatment.
- Radiographic changes occur only after 1 to 2 weeks and are therefore not reliable in the acute setting.
- Bone scan, computed tomography, ultrasonography, and magnetic resonance imaging are useful in appropriate circumstances.
- Treatment involves early initiation of appropriate intravenous antibiotic therapy in all cases and surgery when frank pus is present.
- Potential complications are serious and include growth arrest, deformity, and joint destruction.

Bone and joint infections represent a challenging and common problem for the orthopaedic surgeon. The frequency of such infections is greater in infants and toddlers than in older children. Virtually all pediatric orthopaedic infections can be cured with early diagnosis and appropriate treatment. Delays in diagnosis and treatment often lead to significant problems caused by damage to the physis and articular cartilage.

DEFINITIONS

Osteomyelitis is an inflammation of the bone. Septic or suppurative arthritis is an inflammation of the joint. Both result from an infection by microscopic bacterial, fungal, or viral organisms. A microbial organism is identified in two thirds of patients with septic arthritis and in 75% of patients with osteomyelitis. In the absence of an identified organism, criteria are required to establish and define the diagnosis of septic arthritis or osteomyelitis. The diagnosis is confirmed when two of the following four criteria are met[1]:

- The aspiration of purulent material.
- Positive results of blood or aspiration cultures.
- The presence of localized pain, swelling, warmth, and decreased range of motion.
- Radiographic changes consistent with infection.

Morrey and Peterson[2] defined the diagnosis of osteomyelitis and septic arthritis as "definite" when an organism was isolated from the bone or joint or when there was histo-

logic evidence of osteomyelitis; as "probable" when blood culture results were positive and there were clinical symptoms and radiographic signs; and "likely" when there were clinical symptoms, radiographic signs, and a positive response to antibiotics.

EPIDEMIOLOGY

The majority of musculoskeletal infections in children are of hematogenous origin. Osteomyelitis is more prevalent in children than in adults. Septic arthritis is more common than osteomyelitis among children, but the incidence of septic arthritis is greatest in older adults.[3, 4] There is evidence that the incidence of acute hematogenous osteomyelitis varies according to race and with seasons of the year.[4]

Musculoskeletal infections can follow surgery or injury, especially penetrating wounds. Impairment of immune defenses is associated with increased risks of osteomyelitis and septic arthritis.

PATHOGENESIS

Bacteria are the usual cause of osteomyelitis and septic arthritis in children. Fungal infections occur most commonly in neonates and in people with immune deficiencies. Primary viral infections are rare.

Staphylococcus aureus is the most common source of osteomyelitis and septic arthritis in children. Gram-negative enteric bacilli and group B streptococci are *common pathogens among neonates. Among older children,* Pseudomonas aeruginosa *is a common finding, particularly after puncture wounds in the foot.* Historically, *Haemophilus influenzae* was a common pathogen in the development of septic arthritis. Widespread vaccination has decreased or eliminated the incidence of joint sepsis related to this last organism.[5]

Bacteremia, trauma, and immune system–mediated conditions each play a role in the development of osteomyelitis and septic arthritis. Bacteremia occurs daily in children.[6] Preceding trauma has been noted in up to 50% of children with osteomyelitis.[7, 8] Animal models have demonstrated development of osteomyelitis following trauma to the physis or metaphysis in the presence of bacteremia.[9] Trauma is less important in the development of septic arthritis, but existing animal models have demonstrated the role of joint injury.[10]

The unique anatomy of the epiphysis, physis, and metaphysis plays an important role in the pathogenesis of osteomyelitis in children. In most cases, osteomyelitis develops in the metaphysis, adjacent to the physis. Metaphyseal capillaries and local histology in this area presumably provide a favorable environment for bacterial multiplication.[11] Although the mechanism is unclear, the relative absence of reticuloendothelial cells in the metaphysis compared with the diaphysis may allow bacterial proliferation. These phagocytic cells of the reticuloendothelial system form a relative barrier, preventing the spread of inflammation and infection from the metaphysis into the medullary canal.[12] Similarly, the physis forms an anatomic barrier to spread of infection into the epiphysis.

This physeal barrier is not present in newborns and young infants, because transepiphyseal blood vessels cross from the metaphysis into the cartilaginous anlage of the epiphysis, and it is common for infections in such patients to spread into the epiphysis and adjacent joint.[13] Such a process is rarely seen after the first several months of life. During the first year of life, most of the epiphyseal secondary centers of ossification form, the physis becomes a distinct structure, and the transepiphyseal vessels disappear.

With effective barriers preventing the spread of the infectious process proximally and distally, the bacteria and immune response products accumulate in the metaphysis. This collection of purulent material is often referred to as "pus." Under pressure, the pus migrates through the thin cortex of the metaphysis, forming a subperiosteal abscess.[14] Because the periosteum is loosely adherent to the cortex and the periosteal blood supply is derived from superficial soft tissues, the periosteum remains viable when elevated. The periosteum continues to form new bone adjacent to the cortex, known as the involucrum. If the infectious process continues, the periosteum may be stripped circumferentially, leaving the underlying cortical bone avascular. This ischemic bone, the sequestrum, allows bacterial proliferation to continue (Fig. 1).

If the metaphysis is intra-articular, such as in the proximal femur or humerus, coexisting septic arthritis develops after the pus exits the metaphysis and enters the intra-articular subperiosteal space (Fig. 2). The speed of this process is related to the age of the child, the immune response, and the microorganism's virulence.

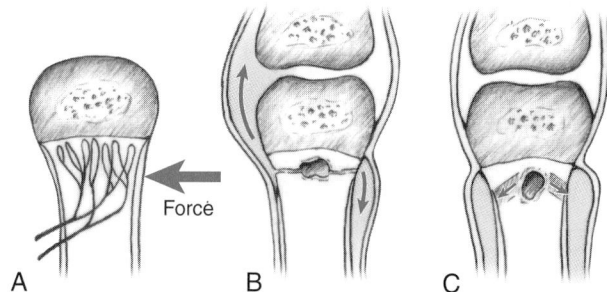

Fig. 1. The pathophysiology of pediatric osteomyelitis and septic arthritis. *A,* The combination of bacteremia and trauma leads to the development of an infection in the metaphysis. *B,* The infection eventually migrates through the porous metaphyseal cortical surface and elevates the surrounding periosteum. If the metaphysis is intra-articular, the infection breaks into the joint and causes concurrent septic arthritis. *C,* The elevated periosteum produces new bone (the involucrum). The devascularized, necrotic cortical bone becomes the sequestrum. (From Dormans JP, Drummon DS: Pediatric hematogenous osteomyelitis: New trends in presentation, diagnosis, and treatment. J Am Acad Orthop Surg 1994; 2:333.)

The pathophysiology of septic arthritis is not as well understood as that of osteomyelitis. Preceding trauma is less common as a precipitating event. Transient bacteremia facilitates bacterial entrance into the synovium and subsequently the joint. Although the presence of some bacteria within the joint is usually controlled by the immune system, uncontrolled bacterial proliferation produces an inflammatory response, which ultimately results in the destruction of articular cartilage. The inflammatory response involves the migration of leukocytes into the joint fluid. The leukocytes, synovial cells, and chondrocytes produce a large variety of enzymes and toxic products. Bacterial breakdown products and proteolytic enzymes liberated by the organisms initiate a process of articular cartilage degra-

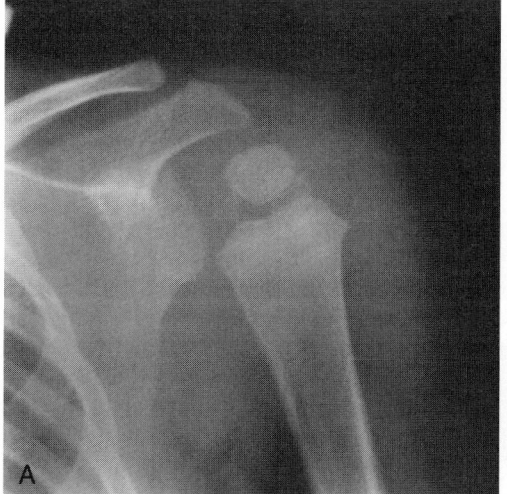
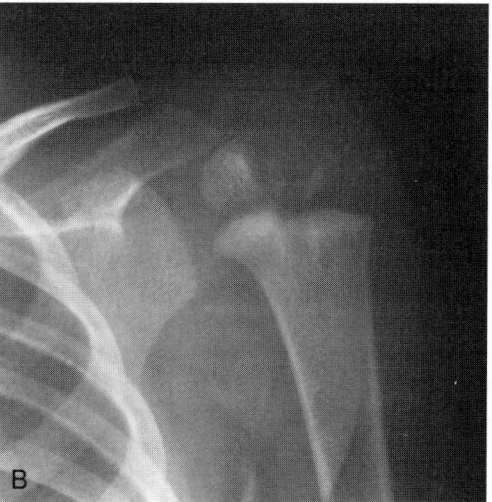

Fig. 2. Pediatric osteomyelitis and septic arthritis in the proximal humerus. *A,* One-year-old girl who had pain and swelling about the left shoulder for 24 hours. Radiographs show superficial soft tissue swelling but no bony changes. Aspiration of the shoulder joint and metaphysis was carried out, followed by operative débridement and irrigation. *B,* Radiograph of left shoulder 1 year after treatment indicates destruction of portions of the metaphysis, physis, and epiphysis by the infectious process. Osteomyelitis of the proximal humerus, proximal femur, and proximal radius often leads to septic arthritis, because the metaphysis is intra-articular. Migration of pus from the metaphysis into the subperiosteal space infects the adjacent joint. Despite the radiographic changes, the patient is asymptomatic and has full range of motion. Observation until skeletal maturity is necessary to ensure that a growth arrest, limb length deformity, or joint abnormality does not develop.

dation, beginning with loss of glucosaminoglycan. This process starts during the first several hours, may lead to irreversible loss of articular cartilage in 24 to 48 hours, and may continue despite the absence of viable microbial organisms.[15–17] In septic arthritis and osteomyelitis, leukocytes and macrophages produce interleukin-1, which mediates the inflammatory response and the production of prostaglandin E.[18]

CLINICAL FEATURES

Children with osteomyelitis or septic arthritis exhibit symptoms such as pain, refusal to walk or bear weight, a limp, local swelling, erythema, and local tenderness. Decreased range of joint motion may be one of the earliest signs.

Nearly half of children with musculoskeletal infections have a history of recent or ongoing infection, such as otitis media or upper respiratory infection. Many children have a history of recent trauma. In most children, if the infectious process has been present more than 24 hours, a fever develops; neonates, however, often do not appear ill, and 50% of neonates do not have a febrile response. Children with "subacute hematogenous osteomyelitis" have few symptoms, and the condition is characterized by an insidious onset and inconclusive laboratory data.[19] Systemic signs of an infection, such as nausea, diarrhea, and malaise, are often not present unless the infection is well established and is associated with bacteremia.

The hip joint is a unique clinical situation because of its deep anatomic location. Because signs and symptoms such as local swelling, erythema, and synovitis are not readily detectable, it is important to assess for decreased range of motion. The hip is particularly prone to loss of internal rotation with almost any effusion or infectious process.

INVESTIGATION

The definitive test for osteomyelitis and septic arthritis is aspiration of the affected bone or joint. The aspirate should be submitted for Gram stain, culture, and antibiotic sensitivity testing. In the case of suspected osteomyelitis, the aspiration should be performed at the site of maximal symptoms, usually along the metaphysis, adjacent to the physis. Aspiration of the subperiosteal space should be performed first. If no material is obtained, the needle is advanced through the thin metaphyseal cortex into the bone. The aspirate should be sent for studies even if only a few drops of bloody fluid are obtained.

In the patient with septic arthritis, aspiration of an infected joint is relatively simple, often accomplished with the use of intravenous or oral sedatives. Aspiration of the hip joint is more difficult and may require an anesthetic. If no joint fluid is obtained from the hip, an arthrogram should be performed to document that the needle entered the joint.

Aspiration of purulent material from the subperiosteal space, bone, or joint confirms the diagnosis of infection and immediately provides a specimen for a Gram stain and culture. Aspiration and culture are essential for the selection of correct antibiotics and to determine whether surgical treatment is necessary (Fig. 3).

In septic arthritis, the aspirated joint fluid is usually cloudy with a leukocyte count exceeding 50.0×10^9/L and a preponderance of polymorphonuclear cells. Although analysis of the cell count is useful, inflammatory diseases such as rheumatoid arthritis can also produce cell counts in excess of 80.0×10^9/L.[20] Conversely, relatively low leukocyte counts, of 50.0×10^9/L or less, are present in 55% of joint aspirates from children with bacteriologically proven septic arthritis.[21] This finding is particularly common early in the course of septic arthritis. Neonates, infants, and patients taking immunosuppressive medications often show little ability to mount an immune response. Therefore, the leukocyte count is often less elevated in joint aspirates from these patients.

Aspirates of bone in cases of presumed osteomyelitis produce positive culture results in 51% to 73% of cases.[22] Aspirates from infected joints yield positive culture results in 54% to 68% of cases. Aspiration of the bone or joint does not alter subsequent bone scans.[23]

Routine laboratory testing other than aspiration is considerably less useful in the determination of pediatric osteomyelitis or septic arthritis. Specifically, the peripheral blood leukocyte count may be elevated in only 25% of children with musculoskeletal infections. The differential blood cell count may be abnormal in only 65%.[2, 24]

The erythrocyte sedimentation rate (ESR) is much more useful than the leukocyte count. The sedimentation rate is elevated in more than 90% of patients with osteomyelitis or septic arthritis, although this elevation may lag behind the onset of symptoms by 48 to 72 hours. The sedimentation rate is typically more elevated with septic arthritis than with osteomyelitis. Patients with both conditions have the highest elevation of the sedimentation rate. Neonates, children who are taking immunosuppressive medications and those who have sickle cell anemia may not show typical elevations in ESR in the presence of a musculoskeletal infection.

C-reactive protein (CRP) is a substance produced by the liver in response to inflammation and tissue necrosis. Although not specific for infection, the C-reactive protein level in the blood is more useful and more sensitive than the sedimentation rate for determination of musculoskeletal infections. Comparisons of the sedimentation rate and C-reactive protein level have shown the CRP to be more sensitive and to respond more rapidly to infections than the sedimentation rate.[25] CRP may be elevated in as many as 98% of patients with osteomyelitis.

Blood cultures should be performed for all patients with suspected osteomyelitis or septic arthritis. Blood culture results will be positive for as many as 50% of patients with bone or joint infections.[2] Children younger than 4 years who are at risk of *H. influenzae* type B septic arthritis, largely those who have not been immunized, are also at risk for development of meningitis. Spinal fluid examination should be considered before starting antibiotic therapy in this group of young patients.

Although plain radiographs are commonly normal in children with septic arthritis and osteomyelitis, radiographs are useful to limit the differential diagnosis and to exclude other conditions. Radiographic evidence of bone destruction is typically delayed by as much as 7 to 14 days and, prior to such changes, may show only soft tissue swelling and obliteration of normal fat planes. In septic arthritis,

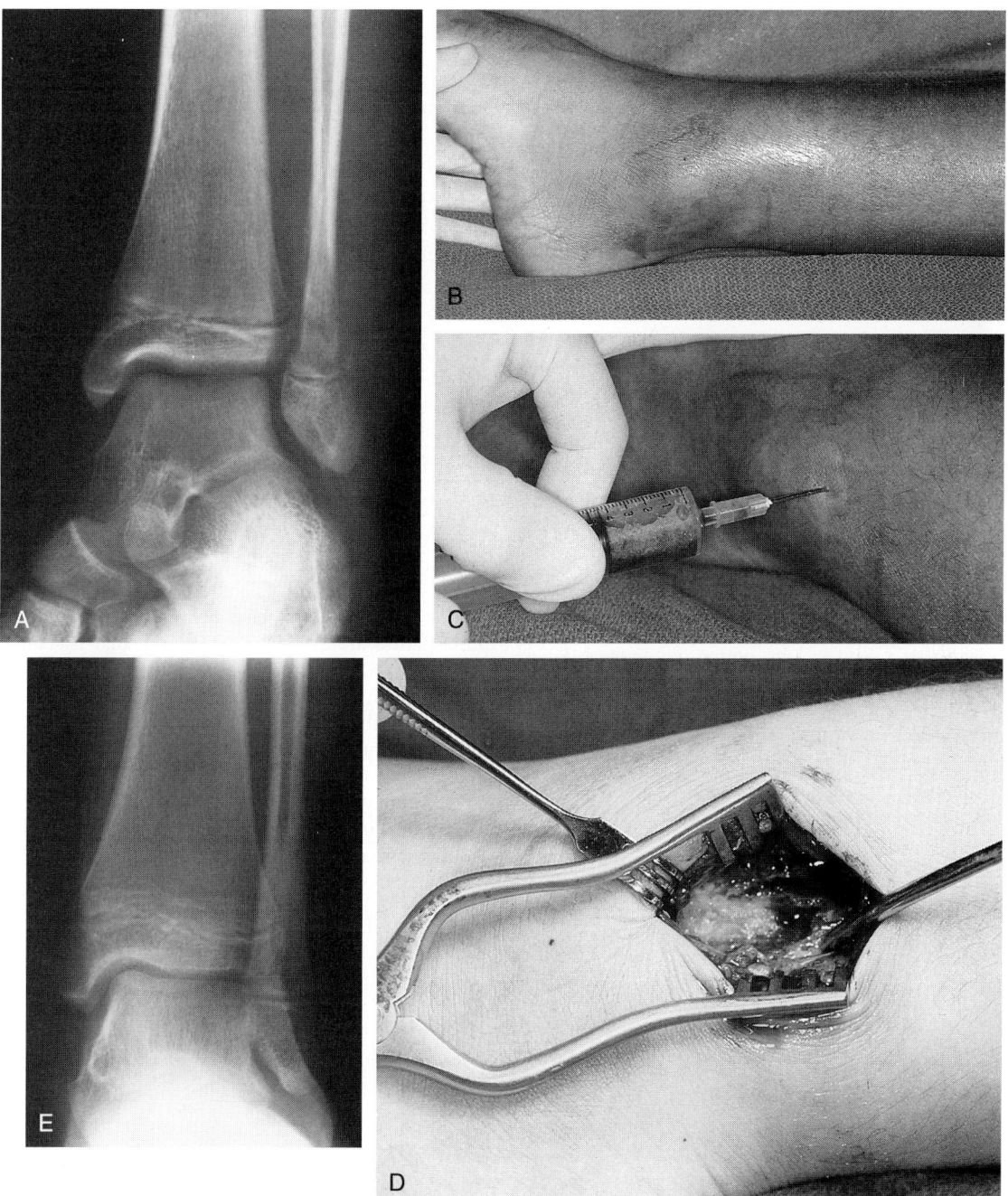

Fig. 3. 14-year-old with hematogenous osteomyelitis of the left distal fibula. *A*, Anteroposterior radiograph taken 12 days after football injury, showing superiosteal new bone formation and bone destruction in the distal metaphysis of the left fibula. The radiology report indicated the possibility of Ewing's sarcoma, emphasizing the broad differential diagnosis. *B*, Examination revealed pain, swelling, erythema, and decreased motion at the level of the lateral left ankle, consistent with osteomyelitis. *C*, Aspiration of the left distal fibula metaphysis produced subperiosteal pus. This finding led to the identification of gram-positive cocci resembling *Staphylococcus aureus*. Appropriate antibiotic therapy was started immediately after Gram's stain results were known. Culture results confirmed the presence of this organism 24 hours later. *D*, Operative débridement was carried out immediately after the aspiration. The subperiosteal abscess was drained, and the necrotic metaphyseal bone was débrided. *E*, Anteroposterior radiograph of left ankle, 10 months after operative débridement, showing complete resolution of the infectious process and healing of the metaphysis.

joint space widening, subluxation, or dislocation is a late finding, and in the hip joint, joint space widening is less sensitive than internal and external rotation ranges of motion. After 1 to 2 weeks, plain radiographic findings are easily recognized; they include periosteal new bone formation, bone destruction, joint space widening, and, ultimately, septic bone necrosis.[26]

Radionuclide imaging is usually not necessary but can be performed when there is doubt about the diagnosis or the site of infection. This evaluation is most commonly necessary in younger children and infants, who have difficulty communicating. Technetium 99m diphosphonate bone scans show increased uptake in 75% of children with osteomyelitis during the first week. Radionuclide imaging is sensitive but not specific, and the technique is limited in its ability to differentiate between septic arthritis and adjacent osteomyelitis. In advanced cases of osteomyelitis, particularly when periosteal abscess formation has stripped the vascular supply from the underlying cortex, decreased uptake, rather than increased uptake, may be seen. This finding is pathognomonic of a large subperiosteal abscess and devascularization of the adjacent bone (Fig. 4). Like the sedimentation rate, bone scans may be of limited usefulness in neonates. Because aspiration of bone and joints does not affect the results of bone scans, aspiration should not be delayed until after bone scanning.

Computed tomography (CT) is useful in the evaluation of subperiosteal and soft tissue abscesses (Fig. 5). Localization and evaluation of bony destruction is facilitated, particularly for lesions of the spine, pelvis, and epiphysis. Ultrasound can be helpful in locating and determining the presence of subperiosteal pus, increased joint fluid, and synovial and capsular thickening. Currently, ultrasound is useful in the detection of pelvic osteomyelitis, subperiosteal abscesses, and soft tissue swelling.[27]

Magnetic resonance imaging (MRI) is very sensitive and specific, with superb depiction of anatomic detail. Unfortunately, use of the technique is limited by cost, availability, and the need for anesthesia in young patients. MRI is probably best utilized for those unusual cases in which conflicting data are present or more simple testing has not confirmed the diagnosis or led to clear treatment options.[28]

The child presenting with possible septic arthritis or osteomyelitis should undergo the following initial studies: plain radiographs, complete blood count with differential,

TABLE 1. INITIAL INVESTIGATIONS FOR CHILDREN WITH POSSIBLE SEPTIC ARTHRITIS OR OSTEOMYELITIS
Plain radiographs Complete blood count with differential count Sedimentation rate C-reactive protein measurement Lyme disease titer Blood cultures

ESR, CRP, serologic test for Lyme disease, and blood cultures. If these studies suggest an infection, aspiration of the affected bone or joint should be performed (Table 1).

DIFFERENTIAL DIAGNOSIS

OSTEOMYELITIS

The differential diagnosis for osteomyelitis in children is extensive, because a variety of noninfectious conditions can mimic osteomyelitis (Table 2). The most common are trauma and fractures in which the symptoms and clinical presentation are similar to infection, that is, pain, swelling, and localized tenderness. Fractures are usually apparent radiographically, the sedimentation rate is usually not elevated, and the symptoms associated with trauma gradually improve, whereas infectious symptoms usually worsen over time.

Children with acute leukemia may present with bone or joint pain similar to that with osteomyelitis. Characteristic features include lethargy, fevers, and abnormal blood test results, including elevated sedimentation rates.[29] Anemia, thrombocytopenia, multifocal pain, the absence of a positive aspirate and culture, or failure to respond to antibiotics should prompt further evaluation. A bone marrow biopsy is usually diagnostic for leukemia. Other primary malignan-

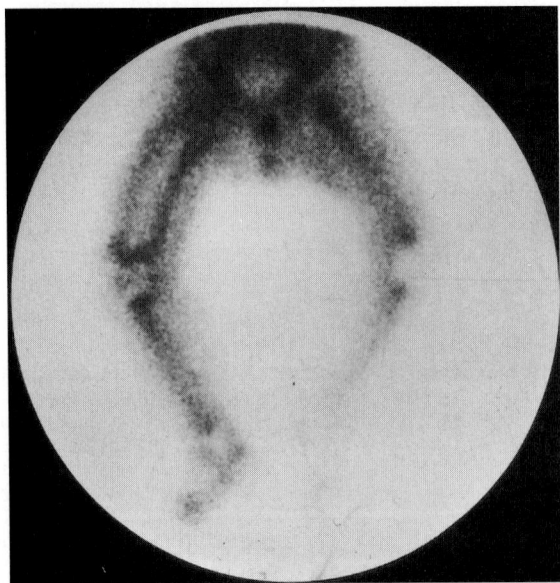

Fig. 4. Bone scan of a 3-week-old child with osteomyelitis of the right femur. This child had swelling and pseudoparalysis of the right lower extremity. Initial radiographs were normal. The bone scan shows a "cold" right femur with decreased uptake along the entire diaphysis. Decreased uptake on bone scan suggests a circumferential subperiosteal abscess extending along the length of the femur. This process strips the vascular supply from the bone, leaving the diaphysis as a sequestrum. Surgical treatment drained the subperiosteal abscess and removed the sequestrum. The intact, viable periosteum "re-formed" a new diaphysis within 3 months.

TABLE 2. DIFFERENTIAL DIAGNOSIS OF PEDIATRIC OSTEOMYELITIS AND SEPTIC ARTHRITIS

Trauma
Acute leukemia
Malignancy
    Ewing's sarcoma
    Osteosarcoma
    Neuroblastoma
Benign lesion
    Eosinophilic granuloma
    Aneurysmal bone cyst
    Unicameral bone cyst
Chronic recurrent multifocal osteomyelitis
Thrombophlebitis
Cellulitis
Toxic or transient synovitis
Juvenile rheumatoid arthritis
Rheumatic fever
Sickle cell disease
Hemophilia
Lyme disease
Henoch-Schönlein purpura
Legg-Calvé-Perthes disease
Slipped capital femoral epiphysis

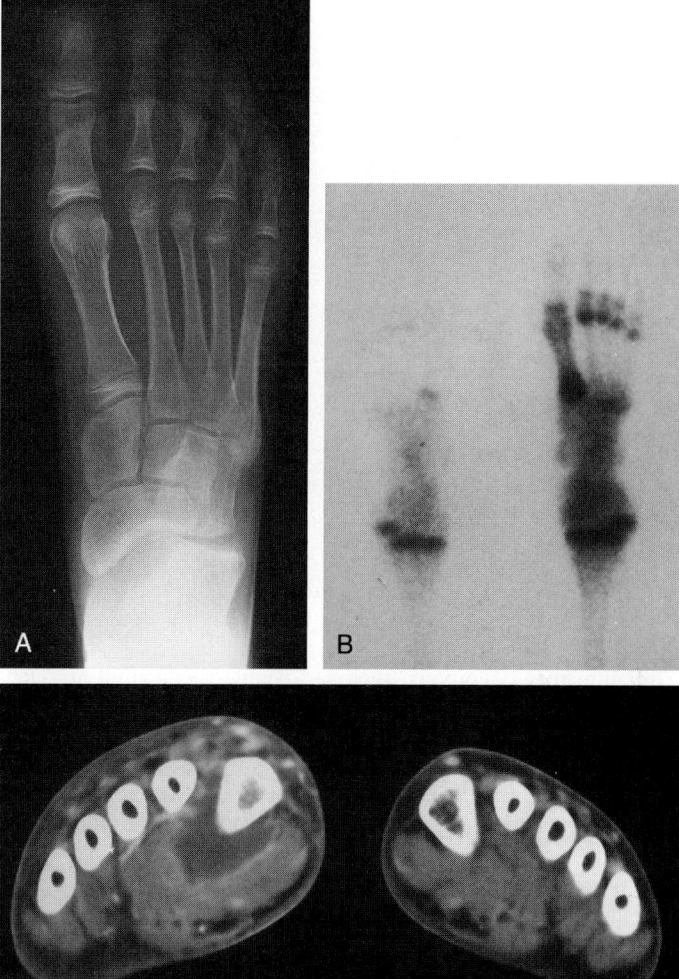

Fig. 5. 11-year-old with osteomyelitis of the right first metatarsal base showing the utility of different imaging modalities. *A,* 72 hours after the onset of right medial foot pain, swelling, and erythema, plain radiographs show no significant abnormalities except for a hint of periosteal elevation along the lateral cortex of the right first metatarsal base. *B,* Bone scan shows dramatically increased uptake in the right foot and specifically along the proximal metaphysis of the right first metatarsal, consistent with osteomyelitis. *C,* CT scan performed the same day as radiographs and bone scan shows a large plantar subperiosteal abscess adjacent to the right first metatarsal base. The abscess was not apparent on other studies and led to immediate surgical irrigation and débridement. Cultures grew *staphylococcus aureus.*

cies often mistaken for osteomyelitis are malignant neuroblastoma, Ewing's sarcoma, and osteosarcoma. Benign tumors such as eosinophilic granuloma (Langerhans' cell histiocytosis) can mimic both osteomyelitis and malignant neoplasia.

Chronic recurrent multifocal osteomyelitis is a noninfectious inflammatory syndrome of unknown etiology. Affected patients, most often adolescent females, present with pain, swelling, erythema, and tenderness suggesting an infectious process. Symptoms are often multifocal and migratory. The condition is characterized by intermittent debilitating symptoms, occasionally lasting weeks at a time. Remissions may last for months or years. Commonly affected sites are the distal femur, proximal tibia, distal tibia, and medial clavicle (Fig. 6). Findings often include lethargy and a mildly elevated sedimentation rate. Plain radiographs show diffuse sclerotic and lytic changes in the metaphysis adjacent to the physis.[30] Culture results are invariably negative. Histologically, the appearance is consistent with acute and chronic inflammation suggesting osteomyelitis. No treatment has been demonstrated to be efficacious. Nonsteroidal anti-inflammatory medications may provide symptomatic relief. Antibiotics are not indicated. The condition may persist for 2 to 5 years.

In addition to the conditions already noted, the differential diagnosis of osteomyelitis includes septic arthritis, thrombophlebitis, and cellulitis.

SEPTIC ARTHRITIS

The differential diagnosis of septic arthritis is more vast than that for osteomyelitis, and because early treatment of septic arthritis is critical, the need to rapidly exclude septic arthritis from the differential diagnosis becomes important.

The most common condition simulating septic arthritis is toxic or transient synovitis. The presentation is similar to that of septic arthritis of the hip, knee or ankle, that is, a young child with a limp of several days' duration. Most children with transient or toxic synovitis, however, have no other findings. Specifically, malaise, fever, loss of appetite, and other constitutional symptoms are absent. There is limited swelling or erythema, and laboratory tests are usually negative. As many as 28% of patients, however, have an elevated sedimentation rate (above 20 to 30 mm per hour). This group is extremely difficult to differentiate from patients with septic arthritis, and joint aspiration is usually necessary and should be performed to differentiate such cases.[31] Most children with toxic or transient synovitis improve dramatically over the course of several days without treatment.

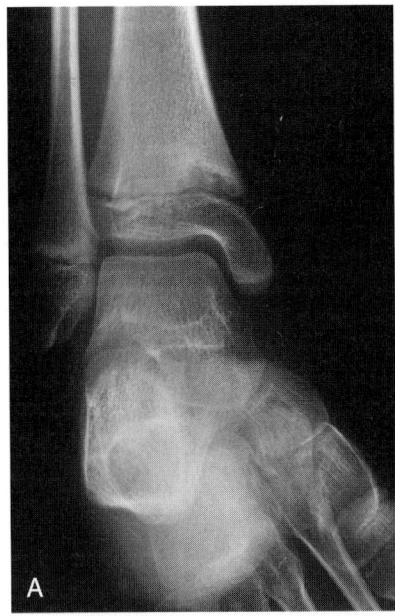
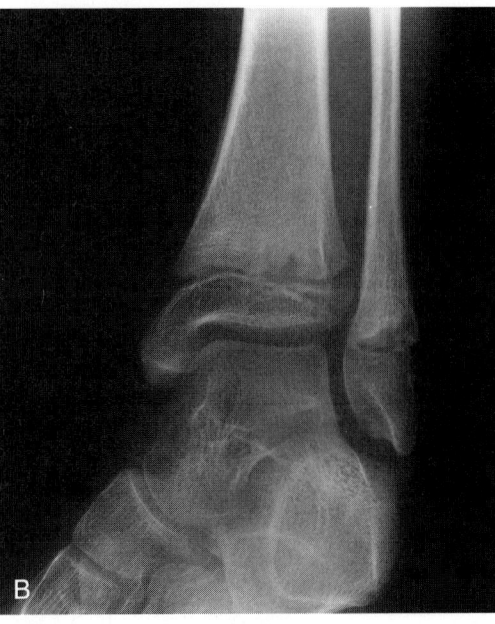

Fig. 6. Chronic recurrent multifocal osteomyelitis in a 9-year-old girl. *A,* Anteroposterior radiograph of the right ankle in this child with recurrent limp, pain, ankle swelling, and tenderness. The radiograph shows metaphyseal irregularity with mixed sclerotic and radiolucent lesions. *B,* Anteroposterior radiograph of the patient's left ankle shows similar findings. She also had radiographic lesions in the medial clavicle, proximal tibia, and distal radius. Treatment was with nonsteroidal anti-inflammatory medications. Symptoms resolved over 2 years.

Inflammatory conditions, such as juvenile rheumatoid arthritis, rheumatic fever, osteomyelitis, sickle cell disease, hemophilia, trauma, Lyme disease, collagen vascular disease and Henoch-Schönlein purpura, are also considerations. The patient with Legg-Calvé-Perthes disease or slipped capital femoral epiphysis may present with a painful, immobile hip joint that is difficult to distinguish clinically from septic arthritis. Radiographs of the hip are diagnostic for these two noninfectious conditions.

MANAGEMENT

Antibiotics represent the primary treatment for children with musculoskeletal infections. Initial treatment is with intravenous antibiotics and should be started as soon as possible after all culture specimens have been obtained. If the causative organism is not identified on Gram stain, the initial intravenous antibiotic treatment is empiric, being based upon the age of the child and other factors. The selection of antibiotics is described in this section for each of three age groups of children: (1) neonates (birth to 4 weeks), (2) young children (4 weeks to 4 years), and (3) older children (older than 4 years). Antibiotic treatment for

children with musculoskeletal infections is summarized in Table 3.

NEONATES

The neonatal period is defined as the first 4 weeks of life. Unique characteristics of the neonate include an immature immune system, the presence of invasive neonatal monitoring, and the unique vascular anatomy of the metaphysis and epiphysis. Lacking a mature immune system, the neonate does not exhibit the usual inflammatory response that characterizes the presence of septic arthritis or osteomyelitis in older children. Neonates with infections may demonstrate only mild swelling, pseudoparalysis of the affected limb, and tenderness. Disuse, tenderness to palpation, and discomfort with joint motion should raise suspicions of an infectious process. Routine laboratory studies, including the leukocyte count, differential count, and sedimentation rate, are of little value. As in older children, blood culture results are positive in 50% of musculoskeletal infections in neonates. Given the paucity of clinical, radiographic, and laboratory findings, aspiration is both mandatory and critical. Multiple sites of infection are observed in nearly 40% of cases.[32]

TABLE 3. COMMON ORGANISMS AND INTRAVENOUS ANTIBIOTIC THERAPY FOR OSTEOMYELITIS AND SEPTIC ARTHRITIS IN CHILDREN

Age	Common Organisms	Empiric Antibiotic(s)	Alternative(s)
Neonate (birth–4 wk)	*Staphylococcus aureus* *Group B streptococci* Gram-negative bacilli	Oxacillin and cefotaxime	Oxacillin and gentamicin
Child 4 wk–4 yr	*S. aureus* *Streptococcus* species *Haemophilus influenzae B*	Oxacillin and cefotaxime	Cefuroxime or ceftriaxone
>4 years	*S. aureus* For penicillin allergy For methicillin-resistant staphylococci	Oxacillin Clindamycin Vancomycin	Cefazolin or cefuroxime

Because the metaphyseal vessels traverse the physis and communicate with the epiphyseal vessels, osteomyelitis in the neonate easily spreads to the epiphysis. As the child matures, the epiphysis develops a separate blood supply, and the vessels traversing the physis disappear. The transient presence of an epiphyseal-metaphyseal vascular communication in the neonate allows metaphyseal osteomyelitis to damage the physis, epiphyseal ossification center, and articular cartilage. As a result, septic arthritis and hematogenous osteomyelitis often occur simultaneously in the neonate. Injury to the physis and articular cartilage can lead to permanent and early disturbances of growth and joint destruction. It is therefore important to perform a thorough search for associated osteomyelitis when septic arthritis is diagnosed in the neonate.

Most cases of neonatal osteomyelitis and septic arthritis in the neonate are due to *S. aureus,* group B streptococci, or gram-negative enteric bacilli. Empiric treatment usually involves an antistaphylococcal penicillin, such as oxacillin and gentamicin, or a broad-spectrum third-generation cephalosporin, such as cefotaxime.[33]

INFANTS AND CHILDREN (4 WEEKS TO 4 YEARS)

For infants and children between 4 weeks and 4 years of age, the principal organisms that cause musculoskeletal infections are *S. aureus*, streptococci, and *H. influenzae* type B in children who have not received the vaccine. For those who have received the influenza vaccine, treatment can be with an antistaphylococcal penicillin, such as oxacillin, methicillin, or a first- or second-generation cephalosporin. For those who have not been immunized against *H. influenzae* or for whom the vaccination history is unknown, a second-generation cephalosporin such as cefuroxime is recommended. Young children, particularly those younger than 2 years, who are at risk for *H. influenza* type B septic arthritis are also at risk for coexisting meningitis. Spinal fluid examination and culture should be considered before antibiotics are started in this population.

CHILDREN OLDER THAN 4 YEARS

In children older than 4 years, most musculoskeletal infections are the result of *S. aureus*. Recommendations for initial treatment begin with an antistaphylococcal penicillin, such as oxacillin, nafcillin, or methicillin. Clindamycin is useful for patients allergic to penicillin and cephalosporins. Vancomycin should be reserved for those situations involving methicillin-resistant staphylococcal infections. Immunocompromised patients require combination therapy, which is best carried out with the assistance of an infectious disease specialist.

Once the principal pathogen is identified, appropriate adjustments in intravenous antibiotic coverage are made. When no pathogen is identified, the empirically chosen antibiotic therapy is continued provided that the patient shows improvement. Under these circumstances, the possibility of a noninfectious cause should also be considered. If the patient shows no improvement after 24 to 36 hours of empiric treatment, consideration should be given to further investigation, surgery, or alterations in the antibiotic regimen.

Limited data are available to provide guidance for the correct duration of antibiotic treatment. Historical recommendations suggest 6 weeks of intravenous antibiotics. Factors utilized to decide upon treatment duration include the virulence of the organism involved, the extent of bony involvement, and the length of time the infection was present prior to treatment. Patients with a prompt response to treatment or those whose infection is caused by sensitive organisms and in whom there is little bone involvement require shorter duration of antibiotic treatment than patients with well-established infections involving large segments of bone caused by unusual organisms. In general, infections caused by group A streptococci or *H. influenzae* type B should be treated for a minimum of 10 to 14 days. Infections caused by *S. aureus* or gram-negative bacilli should be treated for a minimum of 3 weeks.[34] In all circumstances, the patient should show clinical signs of continuous improvement (decreasing pain, swelling, erythema, and fever). Likewise, laboratory evidence, such as a decreasing or normalized C-reactive protein level and sedimentation rate, must be present before antibiotic treatment is discontinued.

Oral antibiotics can often be substituted for intravenously administered medications after 5 to 7 days of treatment, provided that an oral form of the medication is available, the infection is resolving, the medication is tolerated, and adequate serum levels of antibiotic have been demonstrated after compliant administration of the oral medication.[35, 36]

Surgical treatment of osteomyelitis and septic arthritis is indicated when frank pus is aspirated from a joint, subperiosteal space, or bony lesion. Treatment is directed at removal of the purulent material, which is necessary to stop the inflammatory process and tissue destruction. Treatment comprises drainage of subperiosteal abscesses, irrigation and débridement of septic joints, and removal of avascular and necrotic bone. Surgical specimens should be obtained for both culture and histologic examination, because malignant tumors may be mistaken for infection. Surgery is also indicated for patients who are initially treated with intravenous antibiotics but whose disease shows no improvement within 24 to 72 hours.[37] Treatment of several specific infectious conditions warrants mention.

DISKITIS

Diskitis is an inflammatory disorder of the intravertebral disk, probably the result of a hematogenous infection. Patients typically present with a 2- to 4-week history of symptoms involving hip irritability, back, or abdominal pain. Constitutional signs and symptoms of an infection are usually lacking. Although the sedimentation rate and C-reactive protein level are elevated in almost all cases, other laboratory test results are typically negative. Radiographic findings develop only late in the disease process. Disk space narrowing and irregularity of the bony end plates may be present 2 to 6 weeks after the infection begins. Virtually all of these infections are caused by *S. aureus*. Accordingly, biopsy is rarely indicated; rather, the use of empiric antibiotics is advocated. Most patients show improvement with rest, immobilization, or antibiotics.[38]

SICKLE CELL ANEMIA

Patients with sickle cell disease may experience infections due to *Staphylococcus* species, pneumococci, *H. influenzae*,

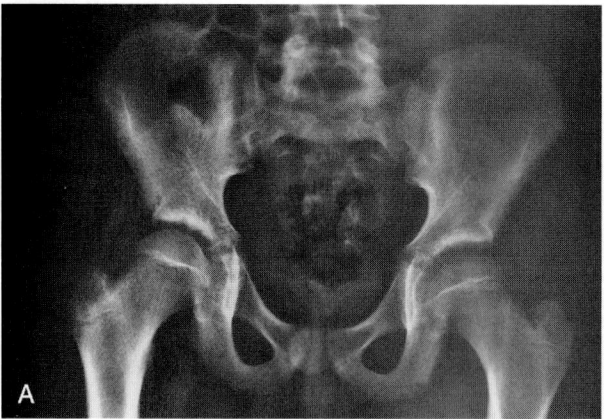 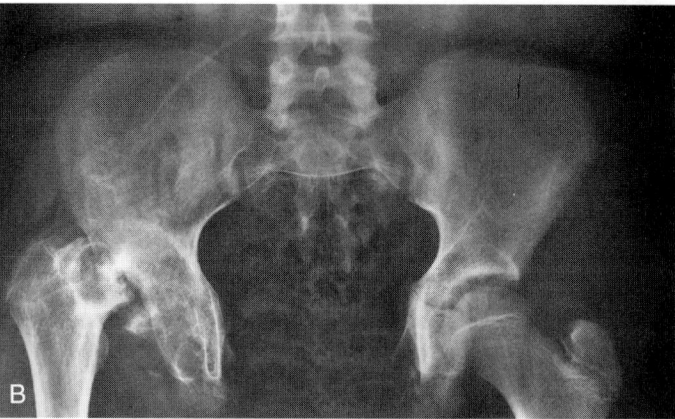

Fig. 7. Septic arthritis of the right hip resulting in septic necrosis after a delay in diagnosis. *A,* Anteroposterior radiograph of a 10-year-old boy with 1 week of pain and decreased range of motion of the right hip. He was unable to bear weight on the right leg. The sedimentation rate was elevated, but other laboratory findings were normal. The radiograph shows no significant abnormalities. Aspiration of right hip revealed frank pus, which grew *Staphylococcus aureus* on culture. Surgical irrigation and débridement of the right hip was carried out, but symptoms had been present for more than 1 week by the time the procedure was performed. *B,* Anterioposterior pelvis radiograph of the same patient at 12 years of age shows septic necrosis of the right hip with advanced destructive changes as a result of the septic arthritis 2 years earlier. The capital femoral physis is no longer present, resulting in a leg length discrepancy. Ultimately, the patient underwent hip arthrodesis. Complications in this case were related to the delay in diagnosis and the presence of *S. aureus* septic arthritis.

or *Salmonella* species. Antibiotic treatment includes a broad-spectrum cephalosporin, such as cefotaxime or ceftriaxone, in addition to an antistaphylococcal drug.[39]

PUNCTURE WOUNDS OF THE FOOT

Puncture wounds of the foot in children are usually associated with *P. aeruginosa,* which accounts for as many as 93% of all cases of osteomyelitis related to foot puncture wounds. Because infection does not develop in most puncture wounds, initial treatment should consist of superficial débridement, tetanus prophylaxis, and patient education regarding the need to return for treatment if signs of infection appear. Antibiotic therapy is reserved for children with cellulitis, osteomyelitis, or septic arthritis. Surgery is indicated for the removal of foreign bodies, débridement of necrotic tissue, drainage of an abscess, or irrigation of an infected joint.[40]

COMPLICATIONS

The majority of children with septic arthritis or osteomyelitis do well following treatment and recover without adverse

sequelae. The complications that occur are typically related to one of the risk factors for a poor prognosis. These factors are premature birth, age of onset less than 6 months, *S. aureus* as the infecting organism, and delay in diagnosis and treatment (Fig. 7).[41]

Complications that may occur as a result of musculoskeletal infections include recurrent infection, late destructive arthritis due to articular cartilage damage, and growth abnormalities due to physeal injury or premature physeal arrest. Some of these complications, including growth arrest, may not be clinically apparent for years after the initial infection has been treated. Therefore, children with osteomyelitis should be followed until they reach skeletal maturity so that the physis may be observed for growth-related abnormalities.[42]

RESULTS

In most cases, musculoskeletal infections in children have no adverse sequelae and are readily treated. Complications are relatively rare and can often be avoided with early detection and initiation of appropriate treatment.

REFERENCES

1. Peltola H, Vahvanen V: A comparative study of osteomyelitis and purulent arthritis with special reference to aetiology and recovery. Infection 1984; 12:75.
2. Morrey BF, Peterson HA: Hematogenous pyogenic osteomyelitis in children. Orthop Clin North Am 1975; 6:935.
3. Gillespie WJ: Epidemiology in bone and joint infections. Infect Dis Clin North Am 1990; 4:361.
4. Gillespie WJ: The epidemiology of acute haematogenous osteomyelitis of childhood. Int J Epidemiol 1985; 14:600.
5. Howard AW, Viskontas D, Sabbagh C: Reduction in osteomyelitis and septic arthritis

related to *Haemophilus influenzae* type B vaccination. J Pediatr Orthop 1999; 19:705.
6. Everett ED, Hirschmann JV: Transient bacteremia and endocarditis prophylaxis: A review. Medicine 1977; 56:61.
7. Dich VQ, Nelson JD, Haltalin KC: Osteomyelitis in infants and children. Am J Dis Child 1975; 129:1273.
8. Manche E, Rombouts GV, Rombouts JJ: Acute hematogenous osteomyelitis due to ordinary germs in children with closed injuries: Study of a series of 44 cases. Acta Orthop Belg 1991; 57:91.
9. Morrissy RT, Haynes DW: Acute hematogenous osteomyelitis: A model with

trauma as an etiology. J Pediatr Orthop 1989; 9:447.
10. Olney BW, Papasian CJ, Jacobs RR: Risk of iatrogenic septic arthritis in the presence of bacteremia: A rabbit study. J Pediatr Orthop 187; 7:524.
11. Speers DJ, Nade SML: Ultrastructural studies of *Staphylococcus aureus* in experimental acute haematogenous osteomyelitis. Infect Immun 1985; 49:443.
12. Whalen JL, Fitzgerald RH, Morrissy RT: A histologic study of acute hematogenous osteomyelitis following physeal injuries in rabbits. J Bone Joint Surg Am 1988; 70:1383.

13. Trueta J: The three types of acute hematogenous osteomyelitis: A clinical and vascular study. J Bone Joint Surg Br 1959; 41:671.

14. Dormans JP, Drummond DS: Pediatric hematogenous osteomyelitis: New trends in presentation, diagnosis and treatment. J Am Acad Orthop Surg 1994; 2:333.

15. Smith L, Schurman DJ, Kajiyama G, et al: The effect of antibiotics on the destruction of cartilage in experimental infectious arthritis. J Bone Joint Surg Am 1987; 69: 1063.

16. Curtiss PHJ, Klein L: Destruction of articular cartilage in septic arthritis. I: In vitro studies. J Bone Joint Surg Am 1963; 45: 797.

17. Curtiss PHJ, Klein L: Destruction of articular cartilage in septic arthritis. II: In vivo studies. J Bone Joint Surg Am 1965; 47: 1595.

18. Tiku K, Tiku ML, Skosey JL: Interleukin-1 production by human polymorphonuclear neutrophils. J Immunol 1986; 136: 3677.

19. Ezra E, Khermosh O, Assia A, et al: Primary subacute osteomyelitis of the axial and appendicular skeleton. J Pediatr Orthop B 1993; 1:148.

20. Baldassare AR, Chang F, Zuckner J: Markedly raised synovial fluid leucocyte counts not associated with infectious arthritis in children. Ann Rheum Dis 1978; 37:404.

21. Fink CW, Nelson JD: Septic arthritis and osteomyelitis in children. Clin Rheum Dis 1986; 12:423.

22. Faden H, Grossi M: Acute osteomyelitis in children: Reassessment of etiologic agents and their clinical characteristics. Am J Dis Child 1991; 145:65.

23. McCoy JR, Morrissy RT, Siebert J: Clinical experience with the technetium-99 scan in children. Clin Orthop 1981; 154: 175.

24. Morrey BF, Bianco AJ, Rhodes KH: Septic arthritis in children. Orthop Clin North Am 1975; 6:923.

25. Unkila-Kallio L, Kallio MJ, Eskola J, et al: Serum C-reactive protein, erythrocyte sedimentation rate, and white blood cell count in acute hematogenous osteomyelitis of children. Pediatrics 1994; 93:59.

26. Jaramillo D, Treves ST, Kasser JR, et al: Osteomyelitis and septic arthritis in children: Appropriate use of imaging to guide treatment. AJR Am J Roentgenol 1995; 165:399.

27. Howard CB, Einhorn M, Dagan R, et al: Ultrasound in diagnosis and management of acute hematogenous osteomyelitis in children. J Bone Joint Surg Br 1993; 75: 79.

28. Mazur JM, Ross G, Cummings J, et al: Usefulness of magnetic resonance imaging for the diagnosis of acute musculoskeletal infections in children. J Pediatr Orthop 1995; 15:144.

29. Kai T, Ishii E, Matsuzaki A, et al: Clinical and prognostic implications of bone lesions in childhood leukemia at diagnosis. Leuk Lymphoma 1996; 23:119.

30. Carr AJ, Cole WG, Roberton DM, et al: Chronic multifocal osteomyelitis. J Bone Joint Surg Br 1993; 75:582.

31. Del Beccaro MA, Champoux AN, Bockers T, et al: Septic arthritis versus transient synovitis of the hip: The value of screening laboratory tests. Ann Emerg Med 1992; 21:1418.

32. Wong M, Isaacs D, Howman-Giles R, et al: Clinical and diagnostic features of osteomyelitis in the first three months of life. Pediatr Infect Dis J 1995; 14:1047.

33. Nelson JD: Skeletal infections in children. Adv Pediatr Infect Dis 1991; 6:59.

34. Nelson JD: Bugs, drugs and bones: A pediatric infectious disease specialist reflects on management of musculoskeletal infections. J Pediatr Orthop 1999; 19:141.

35. Peltola H, Unkila-Kallio L, Kallio MJ: Simplified treatment of acute staphylococcal osteomyelitis of childhood. Pediatrics 1997; 99:846.

36. Nelson JD: Toward simple but safe management of osteomyelitis. Pediatrics 1997; 99:883.

37. LaMont RL, Anderson PA, Dajani AS, et al: Acute hematogenous osteomyelitis in children. J Pediatr Orthop 1987; 7:579.

38. Crawford AH, Kucharzyk DW, Ruda R, et al: Diskitis in children. Clinical Orthop 1991; 266:70.

39. Epps CH Jr, Bryant DD 3d, Coles MJ, et al: Osteomyelitis in patients who have sickle-cell disease: Diagnosis and management. J Bone Joint Surg Am 1991; 73: 1281.

40. Jacobs RF, McCarthy RE, Elser JM: *Pseudomonas* osteochondritis complicating puncture wounds of the foot in children: A 10-year evaluation. J Infect Dis 1989; 160: 657.

41. Betz RR, Cooperman DR, Wopperer JM, et al: Late sequelae of septic arthritis of the hip in infancy and childhood. J Pediatr Orthop 1990; 10:365.

42. Peters W, Irving J, Letts M: Long-term effects of neonatal bone and joint infection on adjacent growth plates. J Pediatr Orthop 1992; 12:806.

ADULT OSTEOMYELITIS AND SEPTIC ARTHRITIS

Robert H. Fitzgerald, Jr. and George Cierny III

Summary

- Chronic osteomyelitis is the common form of osteomyelitis in adult patients and is usually the sequela of trauma.
- Resistant causal organisms are frequently isolated from clinical material obtained during surgical débridement. Isolation of the causal organism and performance of susceptibility studies are critical in the selection of antimicrobial therapy.
- Improved patient selection (normal host defense system) and radical surgical débridement have been responsible for the significant improvement in the successful treatment of chronic osteomyelitis.
- Local muscle flaps, free tissue flaps (microvascular transfer), and bone transportation techniques (Ilizarov's) have made radical débridement possible.
- Septic arthritis occurs in adult patients with compromised host defense mechanisms.
- Septic arthritis in adult patients is associated with a limited clinical response and has a poor prognosis.

Osteomyelitis occurs in a variety of clinical settings, afflicting patients of all ages. The most common forms of osteomyelitis include acute hematogenous osteomyelitis in the pediatric patient and chronic, post-traumatic osteomyelitis in the adult patient. Both forms occur in adult and pediatric patients, but chronic osteomyelitis is uncommon in the child, and acute hematogenous osteomyelitis occurs predominantly in adult patients who have a compromised immune system or who abuse intravenously administered drugs. Chronic osteomyelitis in adult patients is most frequently the sequela of trauma and occasionally recurrent infection following acute hematogenous osteomyelitis during childhood. Infections following orthopaedic implants, in particular total joint arthroplasty, are covered in Chapter 5-7 as they are a unique group of infections. Osteomyelitis of the foot and ankle is commonly the result of vascular compromise and therefore in essence a vascular disease rather than an infectious disease.

HISTORY

The Smith Papyrus (5000–3000 BC) refers to purulent bones and caries. Thus, osteomyelitis was recorded in what is often called the first textbook of surgery. Fossils have been recovered from Java man (*Pithecanthropus erectus*) and Neanderthal man with evidence of osteomyelitis, making it one of the oldest maladies known. A variety of treatments, often conflicting in nature, have been advocated over time (Table 1). Hippocrates promoted rest and immo-

bilization of the afflicted limb. He recommended against removal of necrotic portions of bone, dead tendons, and soft tissues. Galen introduced the term "laudable pus" (pus bonum et laudabie), which influenced treatment for several centuries. Celsus introduced the application of the red-hot iron to infected tissues and bone. Antyllus stressed the importance of resection of diseased bone and surrounding soft tissues. Theoderich introduced the use of compresses soaked with wine. It was Paré who educated physicians about the harmful practice of prolonged conservative treatment with the application of noxious ointments and bandages. He established the importance of surgical extirpation of diseased bone and tissues. The subsequent discovery of bacteria and the establishment of the relationship between bacteria and osteomyelitis provided the foundation for the dramatic improvement in treatment with the introduction of sulfonamides, penicillin, and more potent antimicrobial agents. Orr introduced the combination of wide surgical débridement followed by immobilization. The introduction of local muscle flaps, free vascularized tissue transfers, and tissue transport are the more recent innovations that have changed the treatment and outcome of osteomyelitis.

HEMATOGENOUS OSTEOMYELITIS

PATHOPHYSIOLOGY

The pathophysiology of hematogenous osteomyelitis has as yet to be fully elucidated. Two theories have been accepted: (1) the sluggish circulation in certain anatomic locations within bone, which favors the deposition of bacteria, and (2) a deficiency of tissue-base macrophages for phagocytosis of bacteria. Investigations by Anderson and Parker,[1] utilizing ultrastructural analysis, altered the theories advanced by Hobo[2] in 1921. Hobo, using light microscopy, suggested that the vascular supply to the epiphysis was composed of an arterial side and a venous side connected through a hairpin loop that created sluggish blood flow. Hobo's conclusion of a sluggish blood flow was correct. Anderson and Parker demonstrated that the arterial capillaries are connected to venous lakes that coalesce into venules. Whalen and coworkers[3] also employed ultrastructural techniques to demonstrate that minor trauma to the metaphysis was important in the development of hematogenous osteomyelitis in an animal model. Furthermore, these investigators demonstrated a paucity of circulating polymorphonuclear leukocytes in the epiphysis/metaphysis and that the tissue-base macrophages did not phagocytosize bacteria that migrated into the area (Fig. 1).

Yoon and coworkers[3a] further elucidated the pathophysiology of osteomyelitis through the study of T-cell receptors with reverse transcription-polymerase chain reaction in a murine model of osteomyelitis. These investigators observed that the activation and proliferation of T-cell subsets

TABLE 1. HISTORY OF OSTEOMYELITIS		
1.8 million BC	Java Man (Pithecanthropus erectus)	Osteomyelitic fossils
230,000 BC	Neanderthal Man	Osteomyelitic fossils
1–2 centuries BC	Hippocrates	Rest and immobilization
131 BC	Galen	Pus bonum et laudabile
First century BC	Celsus	Red-hot iron on infected bone; then resect diseased bone
Third century BC	Antyllus	Remove surrounding tissues and drill medullary canal
1266	Theoderich	Wine compresses
1545	Paré	Extirpation of diseased bone
1835	Hunter	Described formation of a sequestrum
1869	Pasteur	Discovered bacteria
1894	Lister	Described relationship of bacteria and osteomyelitis
1927	Orr	Recommended wide drainage, dressing, and immobilization
1935	Dogmagk	Drainage and sulfonamide
1935	Trefouel	Drainage and sulfonamide
1944	Mowlem	Introduced cancellous bone graft
1970	West	Recommended 4 weeks of parenteral antibiotics
1971	Ger	Application of a local muscle flap
1980	Serafin	Application of vascularized composite tissue flap
1985	Cierny	Clinical classification of osteomyelitis
1989	Ilizarov	Tissue transport with external fixator

(notably V_β 14 T cells) was followed by apoptosis (programmed cell death), suggesting that staphylococcal osteomyelitis resulted in superantigenic-like effects on the mouse immune system. Analysis of the local tissue cytokine response revealed that the T-cell cytokines and IL-2 and γIFN showed a late and a relatively short activation pattern compared with that of the inflammatory cytokines IL-1, IL-6, and TNF-α. They hypothesized that downregulation of T-cell immunity and immune cytokines within the osteomyelitic bone may undermine T-cell immunity to *Staphylococcus aureus* and thereby play a key role in the severity of the systemic infection and the local osseous destruction in acute osteomyelitis.

Trueta[4] demonstrated that chronic osteomyelitis is more an ischemic disease of bone than an infectious process.

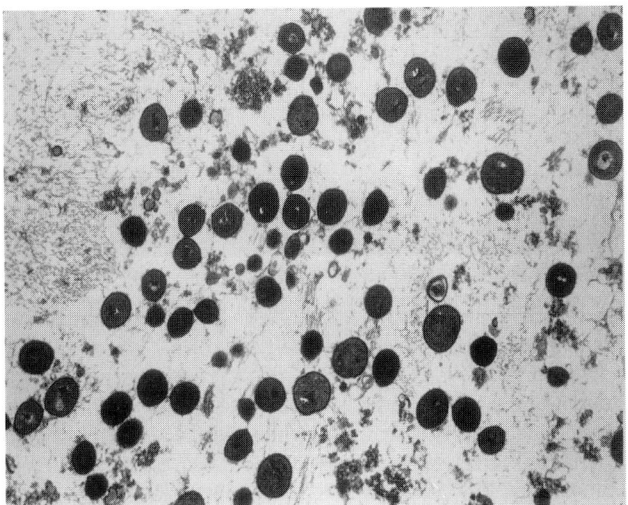

Fig. 1. Transmission electron microscopy of a traumatized growth plate. This was taken 24 hours following a bacteremia. Bacteria are within the cartilaginous defect with nearby phagosomes that are ignoring the bacteria.

Histological examination of osseous specimens demonstrates a predominance of fibrotic scar with minimal vascular tissue. Intramedullary oxygen tension measurements are markedly decreased in osseous sepsis, suggesting that an unfavorable environment may be responsible for the chronicity of osseous infections, because the causal microorganisms are known to survive in avascular and marginally vascularized tissues. The vascularity of bone appears to be a critical factor influencing the outcome of any therapy for osseous infections.

CHRONIC OSTEOMYELITIS

CLASSIFICATIONS

Cierny and Mader[5] introduced the most comprehensive and clinically useful classification (Fig. 2). The emphasis on the patient's generalized health by this classification demonstrates the importance of the patient's immune system in the treatment of this condition. It also permits the surgeon to make some judgment about the type of surgical treatment that might be most appropriate for an individual patient. Older classifications such as that described by Kelly and coworkers[6] are more descriptive but have little value in the management of individual patients. Unfortunately, no classification system addresses the importance of the causal microorganism and its susceptibility. With the emergence of multidrug, resistant causal organisms, some of which are resistant to all currently approved agents, this information can be critical in treatment paradigms, especially in the treatment of nosocomial infections. Unfortunately, inclusion of such information in a classification scheme only makes the classification more complex and less useful in a clinical setting.

The Cierny-Mader Classification system includes four anatomic types of osteomyelitis (I, II, III, IV) and two different physiologic host subtypes (A-host is normal; B-host is compromised). In type I infections the nidus of the

Anatomic type		
Type I	Medullary osteomyelitis	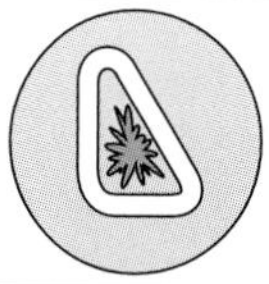
Type II	Superficial osteomyelitis	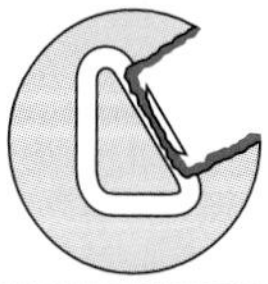
Type III	Localized osteomyelitis	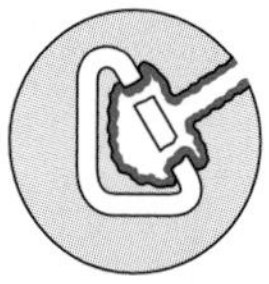
Type IV	Diffuse osteomyelitis	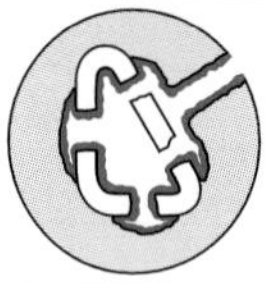

Fig. 2. Cierny and Mader classification of adult osteomyelitis.

Physiology class	
A-Host	Good immune system and delivery
B-Host	Compromised locally
BS-Host	Compromised systematically
C-Host	Requires suppressive or no treatment; minimal disability; treatment worse than disease; not a surgical candidate

infection is located on the endosteal surface of the osseous structure. In type II osteomyelitis, superficial osteomyelitis, there is a primary defect in the soft tisssues, exposing the superficial aspects of the involved long bone. Type III lesions or localized osteomyelitis is a well-marginated sequestration of cortical bone, often combining the features of type I and type II. The osteomyelitic focus can be surgically excised without compromising the integrity of the skeletal segment. The osteomyelitic process in type IV lesions is permeative, involving an entire segment of bone. The lesion may portray characteristics of the other three types and is unstable either before or after surgical débridement.

The staging system also stratifies the host with regard to the patient's physiological capacity to withstand infection, treatment, and the morbidity of the disease. A patient categorized as an A-host is normal, i.e., has excellent health. The patient classified as a B-host has a local (BL), systemic (BS), or a combined local and systemic (BL/S) compromise. Circulatory, hematopoietic, metabolic, immunological, and nutritional status of the patient plays an important role in establishing the host category. The C-host is a patient who is not a treatment candidate; e.g., the disability of the disease is either minimal or the potential morbidity of therapy is too great to justify intervention.

The Cierny-Mader clinical stage of osteomyelitis couples the general and local condition of the host with the extent of the disease. The anatomic site, the extent of tissue necrosis, the condition of the host, and the disability resulting from the disease determine whether treatment should be simple or complex, palliative or curative, ablative or limb-sparing. The clinical stage determines the prognosis and treatment format for each patient. Cierny categorized 1224 patients with refractory long-bone infections he treated over two decades (Fig. 3). The majority of the patients (702 or 57%) were B-hosts.

In a longitudinal study of chronic osteomyelitis of the femur and tibia by Kelly and coworkers,[7] chronic osteomyelitis after fracture of the femur or tibia accounted for 73% of the 425 patients treated. Chronic osteomyelitis in a united fracture was more common in the tibia. However, it occurred with equal frequency in fractures with or without union of the femur.

MICROBIOLOGY

The identification of the causal microorganism(s) and its susceptibility pattern are essential in the treatment of a patient with osteomyelitis.[8, 9] Identification of the causal organism(s) necessitates that antimicrobial therapy be discontinued at least 2 weeks before surgery. The use of a "swab culture" of clinical material from a sinus tract has proved to be unacceptable. The true causal organisms can only be identified from tissue obtained deep within the osteomyelitic cavity through surgical débridement. Multiple tissue specimens should be submitted to the microbiology laboratory for aerobic and anaerobic incubation as well as for analysis of fungal organisms and mycobacteria.

There has been a major change in the microbiology isolated from the wounds of chronic osteomyelitis patients over the past three decades. The initial clinical literature on the microbiology of this disease process reported the predominance of penicillin-susceptible *S. aureus*. Subsequent communications reported the emergence of penicillin-resistant *S. aureus*. More recent studies have reported the emergence of gram-negative bacilli in pure or mixed cultures as the most common causal organisms isolated from osteomyelitic lesions. *Pseudomonas aeruginosa* has become a frequent gram-negative bacillus isolated from clinical material obtained at the time of surgery in patients with osteomyelitis. A concomitant decrease in the recovery of pure *S. aureus* isolates has been reported. Although those *S. aureus* isolates have demonstrated a propensity to be penicillin-resistant, the isolates remained susceptible to the semisynthetic penicillinase-resistant penicillins. However, there has been a new form of resistance that has been common among staphylococcal isolates from patients with musculoskeletal infections: elaboration of B-lactamase. This enzyme obviously renders the staphylococcal isolate resistant to all antimicrobial agents containing a B-lactam ring. Thus, both the cephalosporins and the semisynthetic penicillinase-resistant penicillins are contraindicated in the treatment of a patient from whom a staphylococcal isolate that elaborates B-lactamase is isolated. More recently, multidrug-resistant streptococci have been isolated from musculoskeletal infections. In fact, vancomycin-resistant streptococci have become all too common in major referral centers. A similar pattern of multiple-drug resistance has been observed among the gram-negative bacilli recovered from patients with osteomyelitis. The clinical implications of this change in the microbiology has necessitated major alterations in the antimicrobial therapy for the patients with chronic osteomyelitis. The administration of potentially

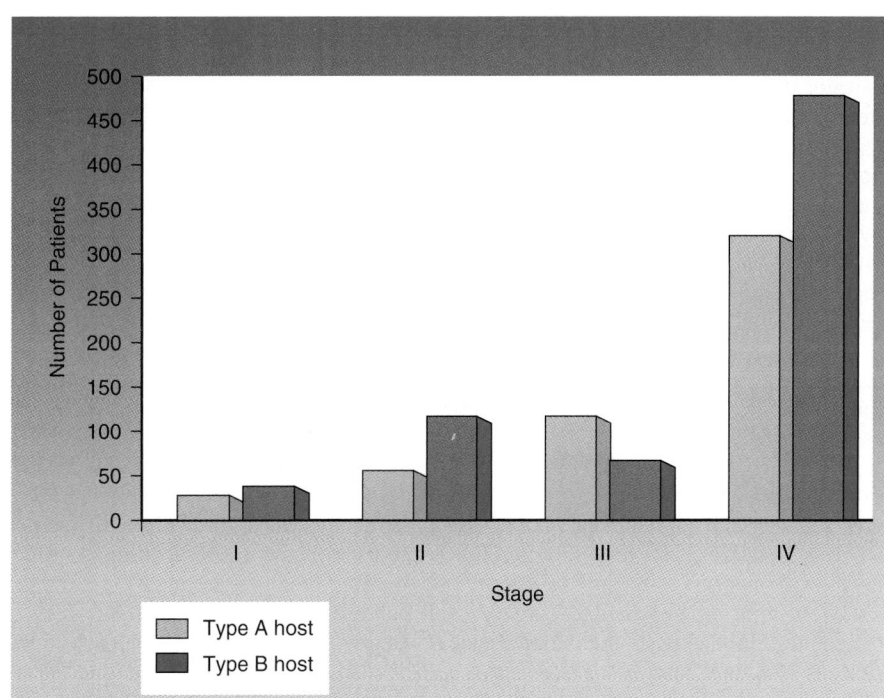

Fig. 3. Stages of osteomyelitis.

toxic antimicrobial agents has become routine in the treatment of the patient, necessitating frequent monitoring of serum peak and trough levels as well as renal, otological, and hematopoetic functions.

Anaerobic microorganisms are frequently ignored during the treatment of chronic osteomyelitis, especially when the infection is polymicrobial. The pathogenicity of anaerobic organisms in musculoskeletal infections was not appreciated until their role in other infections was documented and this information transferred to the musculoskeletal system.[10] Hall and coworkers[11] reported failure in treatment of chronic osteomyelitis in patients with mixed aerobic and anaerobic infections who received only antimicrobial therapy directed against the aerobic causal organisms.

With the efficacy of the depot administration of antimicrobial therapy through the use of antibiotic-loaded polymethyl methacrylate beads, Cierny[5] proposed the administration of antimicrobial therapy before débridement if the causal organism has been identified and susceptibility studies have been performed.

MANAGEMENT

SURGICAL TREATMENT

Osteomyelitis was once considered to be incurable. The prognosis for the afflicted patient has dramatically improved over the past three decades. Application of modern orthopaedic oncological surgical principles have permitted the orthopaedic surgeon to radically excise the infected tissues, improving on the older techniques of débridement and open management of osteomyelitis introduced by Orr. These radical en bloc–type débridements were made possible by modern soft-tissue procedures, e.g., local muscle flaps and free-tissue transfers.[12–15] The efficacy of depot administration of antimicrobial therapy in the treatment of musculoskeletal infections was established during this same period. Subsequently, it has been documented that it is possible to sterilize the local tissues through the introduction of antibiotic-impregnated polymethyl methacrylate beads.[1, 16] The implantation of antibiotic-impregnated beads permits wound closure with local tissues, regional flaps, or free-tissue transfers. This technique obviates the need for repeated open débridements and permits earlier reconstruction with the implantation of foreign bodies if needed. Technological advances in bone transportation introduced by Ilizarov further modified the treatment philosophy and improved outcomes. During bone transportation, osseous segments and their adjacent soft tissues are moved into the defect created during the surgical débridement. Advances in the pharmacological treatment of osteomyelitis with more effective antimicrobial agents have also significantly improved the prognosis for adult patients with chronic osteomyelitis.

The major change in the surgical management of osteomyelitis patients over the past three decades has been aggressive surgical débridement of the osseous structures and adjacent soft tissues. Limb salvage, following these resections, was made possible by soft-tissue and osseous reconstruction with microvascular surgery and bone transport techniques. In the past, the biomechanical integrity of the osseous structures and the need to leave sufficient soft tissue to preserve a regional blood supply limited the amount of débridement the surgeon could perform. With newer surgical techniques, as long as the surgeon protects the neurovascular structures, the remainder of the tissues involved by the infectious process can be excised. Once all the potentially or possibly infected soft tissue has been excised, the wound can be closed by either a local flap or a free-tissue transfer. Once the infectious process is under control, the biomechanical integrity of the osseous structures can be temporarily preserved with an external fixation device and restored with a free osseous tissue transfer. The need to leave potentially or possibly infected soft tissue in the field to preserve blood supply for healing is no longer an issue.

The first surgical procedure should be an extensive surgical excision of all the tissues that are obviously infected (Fig. 4). Marginally vascularized tissues are usually also excised. If the patient has a draining sinus, it can be helpful if methylene blue is injected through a small catheter the night before surgery. The methylene blue permits easy identification of the dead and infected tissue during surgical débridement. Multiple tissue specimens should be submitted to the pathology and the microbiology laboratories for histological examination with special stains and aerobic and anaerobic incubation. There are advantages to adjacent specimens being submitted for analysis, as they should confirm one another. Once the débridement is thorough, flourescence can be injected by the anesthesiologist. A Wood lamp can be used to identify those tissues that are avascular by their failure to fluoresce. If the resection of the osseous tissue compromises the biomechanical support for the extremity, an external fixator can effectively stabilize the extremity. The patient may need one to three subsequent relatively minor surgical débridements performed in the operating room before a second major surgical procedure to achieve wound closure. Depending on the size of the wound and the location, a local muscle flap may permit wound closure.[12, 13] If the wound is too large or in a location precluding a local muscle flap, a free muscle flap can be used. Once the wound heals and the infection is controlled, a free vascularized osseous flap or bone transportation can be performed to reconstitute the biomechanical integrity of the extremity.

A local muscle flap is used most frequently in managing osteomyelitis of the proximal tibia and the distal femur.[12, 13] The medial head of the gastrocnemius muscle is the muscle flap most commonly utilized to achieve wound closure following débridement of an osteomyelitic lesion about the knee, in particular about the proximal tibia. Occasionally, a medial head of the gastrocnemius muscle and the soleus muscle are combined to form a local muscle flap to fill a large dead space. Usually, a split-thickness skin graft is applied to the muscle flap to complete the closure. Initially, the split-thickness skin graft was applied at a subsequent operation. In recent years, the split-thickness skin graft has been applied successfully at the time of the muscle flap procedure. This procedure has given the highest rate of eradication of osteomyelitis. Ger[13] reported only 4 failures among 43 patients treated with débridement and a local muscle flap.[12] The follow-up was less than 2 years in many of his patients. Thus, there remained questions concerning this technique. However, subsequent reports with 2 or more

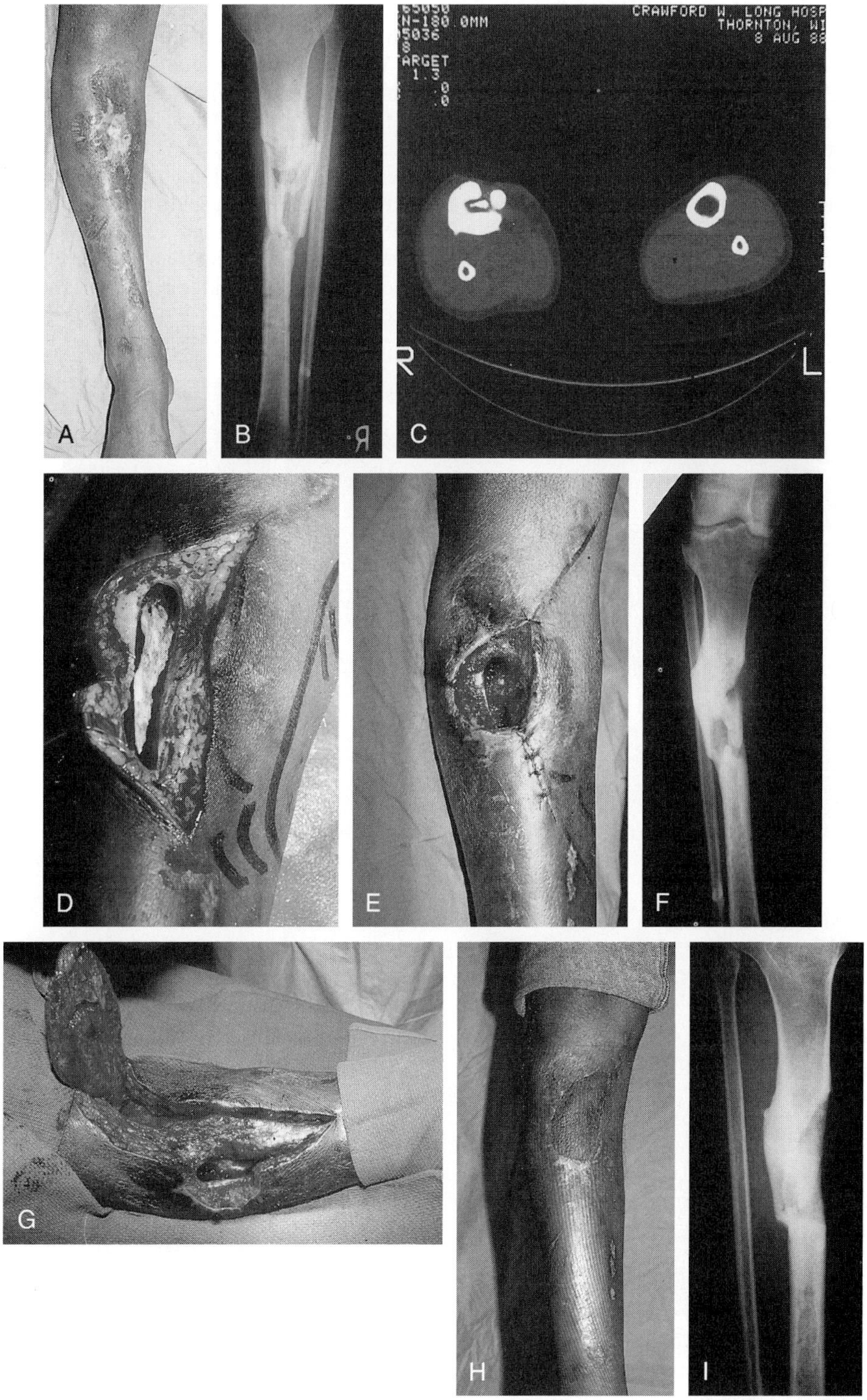

Fig. 4. Views. *A,* Stage IIIA osteomyelitis (tibia), intermittently draining through the atrophic and adherent (immobile) scar on the anterior tibial surface. *B,* Infected tibial union with diaphyseal sequestration and slight tibia vara. *C,* CAT scan illustrating the sequestered cortical fracture fragment, two drainage cloacae, and oedema in the soft tissues anteromedially. *D,* Soft tissues are resected to healthy planes, periosteum excised just to the edge of the cotrical entry to unroof and remove the sequestered fragments *(arrow),* endosteal scar, granulation tissue, and nonviable bone surfaces. *E,* The extended wound as seen 5 days postoperatively; viable margins were approximated, and the defect was dressed open. *F,* The ossesous débridement left less than 60% tibial volume, leaving the maligned tibia at risk for fracture. Cancellous bone grafts were recommended at the second-look débridement. *G,* Revitalization of the combined, type-II and type-III defect (day 5) with a simultaneous transposition myoplasty (gastrocnemius) and cancellous graft. *H,* Soft-tissue reconstruction healed, supple and drainage free, 1 year following coverage/grafting. *I,* One year post–coverage/grafting, the consolidation is complete, the construct stable, and the patient weightbearing without restrictions.

years' follow-up have demonstrated this technique to successfully eradicate the osteomyelitic process in up to 94% of the patients treated.[12]

A benefit of local muscle flaps is improvement of the local blood supply. During the acute stages of the infectious process, the flow of blood through the osteomyelitic bone increases. Subsequently, varying amounts of reduced blood flow have been reported. Although successful treatment of osteomyelitis with surgery and antimicrobial therapy restores the blood flow, blood flow never returns to normal levels. The addition of a local muscle flap to the surgical therapy enhances a local bone-blood flow, which can improve the local host defense and the delivery of antimicrobial therapy.

Free muscle flaps are associated with increased technical difficulty. The failure rate was initially as high as 25% in those patients monitored for 2 or more years.[15] With refinement in the technical aspects of the procedure and improvement in patient selection, the results of free flaps have been improved. In fact, the current success rate is so high that the procedure is routine in many centers.

Because many patients who are B-hosts are also poor candidates for free-tissue transfers, use of external fixation devices (Ilizarov's) that permit bone transportation have yielded great success. Furthermore, there are considerable

cost savings with this technique through reduction in operating room time and hospitalization. Concomitantly, there is a considerable reduction in morbidity rates for the patient (Fig. 5).

Some centers do not have the expertise to perform free vascular flaps. Also, there are patients who have chronic osteomyelitis in anatomic locations not amenable to a local muscle flap and where peripheral vascular disease precludes a free tissue transfer. Such patients can be treated with Papineau's technique.[12] Following the first major débridement, the wound is packed repeatedly with wet-to-dry

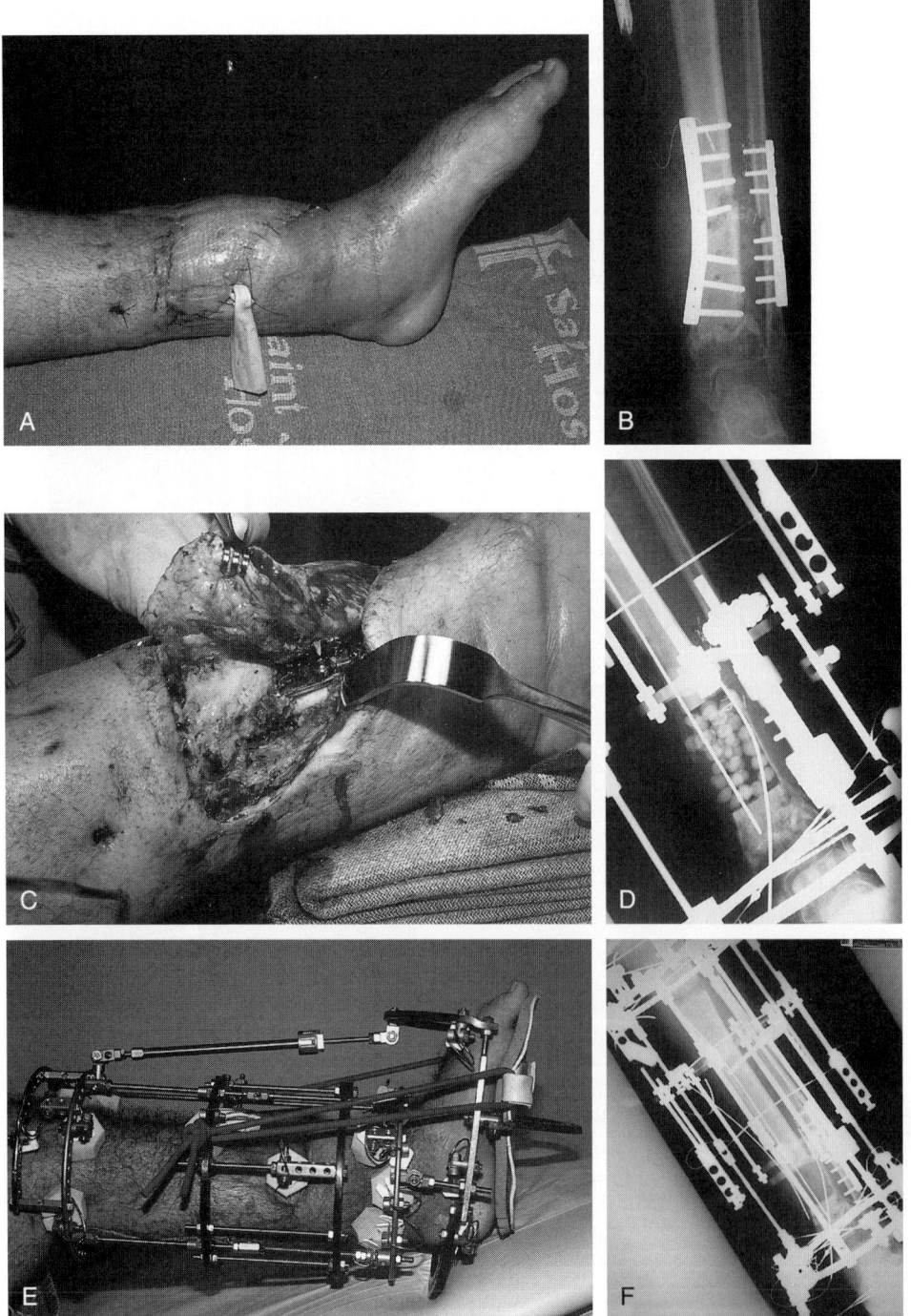

Fig. 5. Views. *A*, Late sepsis (recently drained) following internal fixation/free flap coverage of a IIIB open tibial fracture. *B*, Infected, segmental tibial nonunion with retained hardware, failed stabilization with external fixation, and valgus malignment. *C*, Free flap lifted to reveal dead bone and purulent granulation tissues beneath the plate. *D*, Segmental (4.5 cm) osseous resection with squared docking site surfaces, antibiotic beads within the defect (transport), realignment, and stent wires to hold the soft tissues out to profile. *E*, Trifocal Ilizarov frame for bone transport (T) with correction of valgus and foot/ankle equinovarus deformities. *F*, Antibiotic bead removal/corticotomy performed at 5 weeks; regenerate seen at 4 weeks with stent wires preserving the transport channel to the docking surface of the distal tibia.

dressing until granulation tissue covers the exposed surfaces. Then cancellous bone grafts are packed into the wound. The superficial aspects of the graft will need minor débridement of the superficial layers 2 to 3 weeks later. Further wet-to-dry dressings can lead to secondary epithelialization, or a split-thickness skin graft can be applied.

As mentioned, depot administration of antibiotic delivery systems has been efficacious. Antibiotic-impregnated polymethyl methacrylate beads have been used most often.[18] After débridement, the technique has been used for those wounds that can be closed but have residual dead space. The dead space is obliterated by implanting polymethyl methacrylate beads containing antimicrobial agents specific against the causal organisms isolated from deep tissue specimens obtained from the initial débridement. Preliminary experience comparing this technique with more traditional techniques in a randomized prospective study revealed it to be as effective. Unfortunately, polymethyl methacrylate beads are difficult to excise at a later date when it is necessary to perform a bone-grafting procedure. Thus, a number of surgeons are attempting to develop a biodegradable bead that can deliver high local levels of potentially toxic antimicrobial agents as the beads are resorbed by local tissues. This area of research offers promising new technology. Other surgeons are leaving the polymethyl methacrylate beads in situ unless they must be removed for limb reconstruction.

MEDICAL TREATMENT

Even though lessons learned over the past four decades have dictated the importance of both medical and surgical treatment of the patient with chronic osteomyelitis, there are surgeons who suggest that patients only need a short exposure to antibiotic treatment. Some physicians have suggested that polymicrobic infections are caused primarily by one organism that requires specific antimicrobial therapy while ignoring the other organisms isolated from deep-tissue specimens. The duration of antimicrobial therapy has

remained controversial, with different authorities suggesting a variety of durations.

Many patients with chronic osteomyelitis have polymicrobic infections. It is common for mixed aerobic and anaerobic microorganisms to be isolated from tissue specimens. It is impossible to identify one microorganism as more important than another microorganism. Antimicrobial agents should be selected that will be bactericidal against all of the microorganisms isolated.

Four weeks of antimicrobial therapy became the standard for patients with osteomyelitis, following the recommendation of Kelly and co-workers in 1970.[6] Over the past two decades, the recommendations of infectious disease consultants for the treatment of subacute bacterial endocarditis of 6 weeks of parenteral antimicrobial therapy has been transferred to the treatment of osteomyelitis. There is little conclusive evidence that 6 weeks of therapy has been more effective than 4 weeks. As previously mentioned, antimicrobial therapy before the initial débridement has been proposed. With the depot administration of antimicrobial therapy, the duration of parenteral therapy has been dramatically reduced to 1 to 2 weeks without compromise of the results.

The use of oral therapy following parenteral therapy has also been controversial. Oral therapy has been utilized for patients who have had infections with gram-positive microorganisms but not for patients with gram-negative microorganisms; agents active against gram-negative bacilli have not been available. Recently, European physicians have suggested that a combination of rifampin and a fluoroquinolone can be successfully administered for 6 months in the treatment of infected orthopaedic implants.[7, 19] Unfortunately, reports of patients with osteomyelitis treated with this combination of oral antimicrobial therapy had an unacceptably short follow-up examination. However, this technique warrants evaluation in the treatment of patients with osteomyelitis as it appears to have applicability.

With the increasing use of potentially toxic antimicrobial agents, it is important to monitor the serum peak and trough levels of the agent being administered. Characteristically, the serum peak levels are drawn 1 hour after administration. The serum trough levels are drawn 1 hour before the next scheduled dose. With the emergence of gram-negative bacilli as common causal organisms, monitoring for nephrotoxicity and ototoxicity has become commonplace. The serum creatinine level needs to be monitored at least twice weekly with the administration of aminoglycosides. Similarly, aminoglycoside therapy necessitates weekly audiograms and caloric testing.

RESULTS

Before the development of modern surgical techniques, the success rate of treatment of osteomyelitis was 70%.[14] The success of treatment dramatically improved to 93% with the introduction of local muscle flaps. Unfortunately, the use of this technique is limited to patients with osteomyelitis in anatomic areas where it has its greatest application. The use of free vascularized flaps is technically more challenging and associated with an increased incidence rate of failure.[18] However, in institutions where they are routinely performed, the success rate is high (90%+). Again, this procedure has its limitations. The overall success rate ap-

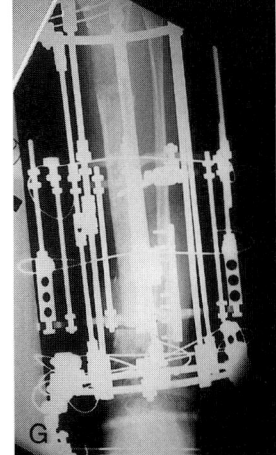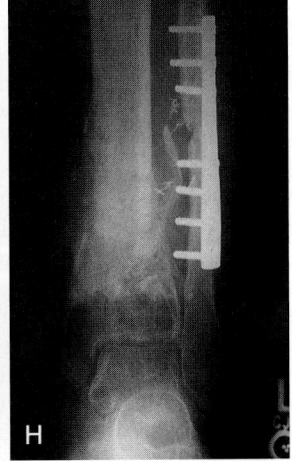

Fig. 5. Views. *Continued. G,* Transport of tibial segment now complete with docking surfaces flush and compressed; the regenerate is 50% consolidated. Marrow was injected into the docking osteosynthesis to augment healing. *H,* Film taken 1 year following débridement with ankle function preserved and the limb aligned, at length and infection-free.

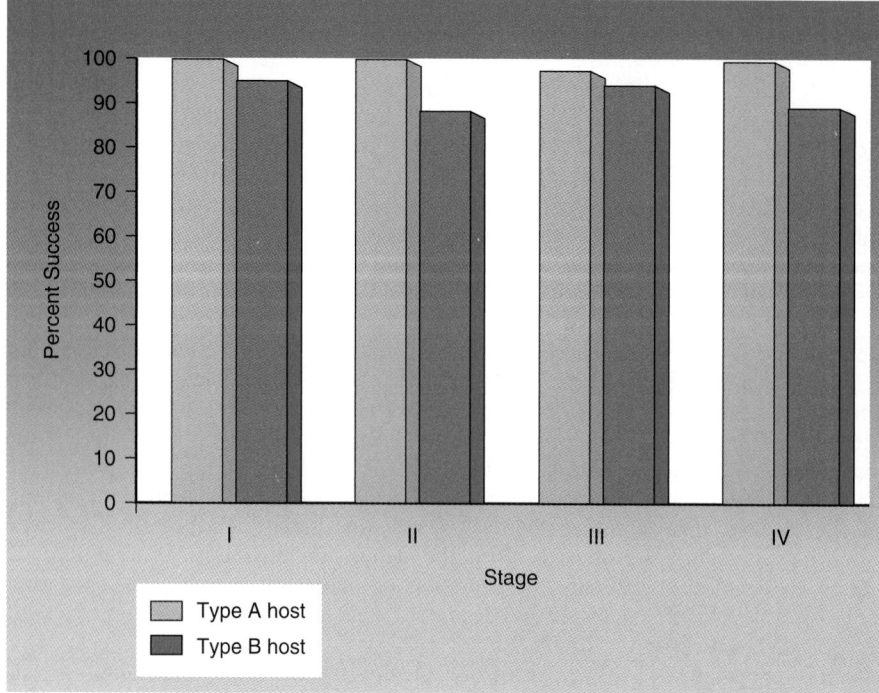

Fig. 6. Results of treatment.

plying modern oncogenic principles and utilizing a variety of techniques for reconstruction depending on the patient and the anatomic location of the septic focus in over 1224 patients treated by one of the authors (GC) is 94% with 2-year follow-up evaluation (Fig. 6). In 522 patients who are type A hosts, the success rate was 99%. In contrast, the success rate for 702 type B hosts was 90%. Patients with stage I or II lesions experienced a higher success rate than patients with stage III and IV lesions.

SEPTIC ARTHRITIS

Septic arthritis afflicts both pediatric and adult patients. Although the pathophysiology is identical in both groups of patients, the clinical findings are quite different. Septic arthritis is twice as common as osteomyelitis during infancy but only as common as osteomyelitis during childhood. In adult patients septic arthritis is distinctly less common than osteomyelitis secondary to open fractures or that complicating intra-articular surgery. The microbiology of septic arthritis varies with the patient population afflicted. Early diagnosis and institution of treatment is critical to the successful treatment of septic arthritis, irrespective of the age group afflicted.

ADULT SEPTIC ARTHRITIS

Septic arthritis in adult patients is uncommon and occurs in patients with compromise of their host defense mechanisms. The patients are usually elderly, chronically ill, or are receiving medications that lower their resistance. It commonly afflicts joints that have early degenerative joint disease. In the elderly patient or the patient with suppression of the immune system, the clinical findings are quite

minimal, similar to those of the neonate with septic arthritis, i.e., a painful, swollen joint may be the only findings. A febrile response and elevation of the peripheral leukocyte count has been found in only a quarter of the patients. The erythrocyte sedimentation rate is customarily elevated. A slight-to-moderate anemia is common. The knee, hip, and shoulder are the most common joints afflicted. The differential diagnosis should include rheumatoid arthritis, monarticular arthritis with internal derangement, crystalline arthropathy, and inflammatory osteoarthritis.

S. aureus is overwhelmingly the common causal organism recovered from clinical material obtained with aspiration or arthrotomy. Blood cultures are rarely of value in the diagnosis of septic arthritis in adult patients. Infections with gram-negative bacillary organisms are fortunately rare as they have been associated with a poor prognosis.

Treatment of septic arthritis in adult patients has included decompression of the joint with repetitive aspirations, arthrotomy, or arthroscopy in addition to parenteral antimicrobial therapy. If the infection is hospital-acquired, the causal organism will invariably be resistant to the common antimicrobial agents, e.g., methicillin-resistant *S. aureus.* Community-acquired infections are associated with the isolation of methicillin-susceptible *S. aureus.* The duration of parenteral therapy will depend on the clinical response of the patient. It is usually a minimum of 3 weeks followed by oral therapy for an additional 3 to 4 weeks. The prognosis of septic arthritis in adult patients is poor. Historically, the infectious process leads to death in one-sixth of patients. Functional joints are the exception rather than the rule following septic arthritis. Many of the patients experience spontaneous fusion or will require surgical arthrodesis of the involved joint.

REFERENCES

1. Anderson CE, Parker J: Invasion and re-sorption in endochondral ossification: An electron microscopic study. J Bone Joint Surg Am 1966; 48:899.
2. Hobo T: Zur Pathogeneses der akuten Haematogenen Osteomyeliti. Acta Schol, Med. Univ. Imper. Kioto 1921; 4:129.
3. Whalen JL, Fitzgerald RH Jr, Morrissy RT: A histological study of acute hematogenous osteomyelitis following physeal injuries in rabbits. J Bone Joint Surg Am 1988; 70:1383.
3a. Yoon KS, Sud S, Song Z, et al: Experimental and hematogenous osteomyelitis: Influence of *Staphylococcus aureus* upon T-cell immunity. J Orthop Res 1999; 17:382.
4. Trueta J: Acute hematogenous osteomyelitis: Its pathology and treatment. Bull Hosp Joint Dis 1953; 14:5.
5. Cierny G, Mader JT, Penninck JJ: A clinical staging system for adult osteomyelitis. Contemp Orthop 1985; 10:17.
6. Kelly PJ, Martin WJ, Coventry MB: Chronic osteomyelitis: Treatment with closed irrigation and suction JAMA 1970; 213:1843.

7. Kelly PJ, Fitzgerald RH Jr, Cabenela ME, et al: Results of treatment of tibial and femoral osteomyelitis in adults. Clin Orthop Rel Res 1990; 259:295.
8. Waldvoger FA Medoff G Schwartz MN: Osteomyelitis: A review of clinical features, therapeutic considerations and unusual aspects. N Engl J Med 1970; 282:198.
9. Waldvogel FA, Vasey H: Osteomyelitis: The past decade. N Eng J Med 1980; 303:360.
10. Fitzgerald RH Jr, Rosenblatt JE, Tenny JH et al: Anaerobic septic arthritis. Clin Orthop Rel Res 1982; 164:141.
11. Hall BB, Fitzgerald RH Jr, Rosenblatt JE: Anaerobic osteomyelitis. J Bone Joint Surg Am 1983; 65:30.
12. Fitzgerald RH Jr, Ruttle PE, Arnold PG, et al: Local muscle flaps in the treatment of chronic osteomyelitis. J Bone Joint Surg Am 1985; 67:175.
13. Ger R: Muscle transposition for treatment and prevention of chronic posts traumatic osteomyelitis of the tibia. J Bone Joint Surg Am 1977; 59:784.

14. May JW Jr, Gallico GG III, Lukash FN: Microvascular transfer of free tissue for closure of bone wounds of the distal lower extremity. N Engl J Med 1982; 306:253.
15. Weiland AJ, Moore JR, Daniel RK: The efficacy of free tissue transfer in the treatment of osteomyelitis. J Bone Joint Surg Am 1984; 66:181.
16. Gillespie WJ, Mayo KM: The management of acute haematogenous osteomyelitis in the antibiotic era: A study of outcome. J Bone Joint Surg Br 1981; 63:126.
17. Papineau LJ: Excision graft with deliberately delayed closure in chronic osteomyelitis. Nouvelle Presse Medicale 1973; 2:2753.
18. Klemm KW: Treatment of infected pseudoarthrosis of the femur and tibia with an interlocking nail. Clin Orthop Rel Res 1986; 212:174.
19. Howard CB, Einhorn M, Dagan R, et al: Ultrasound in the diagnosis and management of acute hematogenous osteomyelitis in children. J Bone Joint Surg Br 1993; 75:79.

section 5 chapter 4 INFECTED FRACTURES AND NONUNIONS

Declan J.M. Bowler and Peter Keogh

Summary

- Infection in an acute fracture or a nonunion is a disaster for the patient. The most important concept in treatment is prevention.
- The single most important factor in reducing the incidence of wound infection and subsequent bone infection in open fractures is the early administration of broad-spectrum antibiotics.
- Clostridial infection is rare but remains the most dreaded complication of open wounds.
- Deep tissue specimens for cultures are mandatory for accurate identification of pathogens.
- Nosocomial infection is a common cause of failure after initial management.
- In infected nonunions, the critical decision for the orthopaedist and patient is whether to opt for limb salvage or amputation.
- The Ilizarov method of treatment is a versatile solution to many of these fractures but is not a panacea.

Infection associated with acute fractures or established nonunions portends increased morbidity and potential for a lifetime of difficulties. Persistent infection, impaired function, socioeconomic and psychological decline, and loss of limb or life are real possibilities. Treatment of these patients remains a formidable challenge for the orthopaedic surgeon and other medical personnel.

The infection arises most commonly from a wound infection in an open fracture or a postoperative consequence of open reduction and internal fixation of a closed fracture (Fig. 1).

The exact incidence of infection in fresh fractures or nonunions is unknown. Factors associated with an increased incidence of infection include (1) surgical fracture treatment, (2) high-energy trauma, (3) sophisticated methods of patient and limb salvage in complex injuries, and (4) the emergence of resistant bacteria. Factors associated with a decreased incidence include (1) an emphasis on infection prevention and (2) advances in surgical techniques of bone and soft-tissue reconstruction.

DEFINITIONS

An infected wound can be defined as one with a purulent discharge from which bacteria can be cultured.[1] Infection of a fracture occurs when pathogens invade and establish a focus of infection in the bone. Nonunion is defined as when all the bone healing processes have ceased and union has not occurred.[2] Infected nonunion is simply nonunion with persisting infection.

HISTORICAL PERSPECTIVE

For most of recorded history, bacterial infection of bone was considered potentially lethal. When amputation became

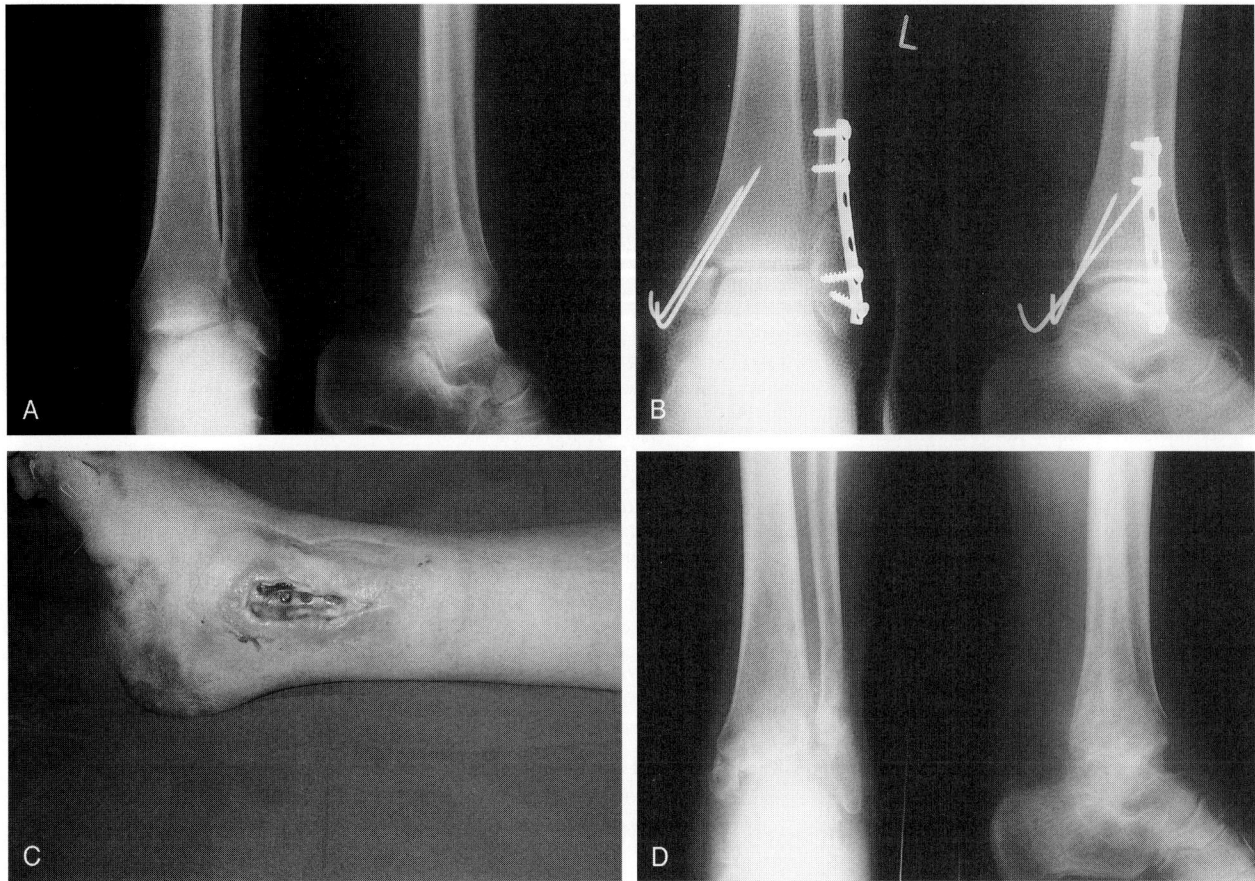

Fig. 1. A 73-year-old man with diabetes mellitus and peripheral vascular disease. He sustained a closed left bimalleolar ankle fracture (A). He was treated conservatively initially because of poor skin condition but then underwent open reduction with internal fixation at 10 days (B). The fibular plate became infected 3 weeks later (C). Despite plate removal and débridement, he developed osteomyelitis/septic arthritis (D). General systemic deterioration necessitated an above-knee amputation at 4 months.

safe and humane, it was considered the treatment of choice for infected open fractures.[3] In the early 20th century, foundations were laid for the currently accepted concepts relating to infected fracture and nonunion management. These include antibiotics, débridement, and repair of the soft-tissue envelope to combat infection, combined with bone grafting and stabilization to promote bone union.

Since the discovery of penicillin, antibiotic therapy has evolved dramatically. However, development has slowed recently and this has unfortunately coincided with the emergence of resistant bacteria. Wound débridement performed on open fracture wounds since World War I[4] is now universally accepted as a keystone of treatment. The importance of the adjacent soft-tissue structures in the prevention of infection has been recognized only recently.

Cortical onlay bone grafting, introduced and popularized by Campbell in 1927 and Phemister in 1947, has been superseded by the current emphasis on cancellous grafting. Vascularized bone grafting was developed in tandem with microsurgical techniques in the 1970s and 1980s. Current methods of stabilization for infected fractures and nonunions include intramedullary nailing and external fixation. Ilizarov introduced the revolutionary technique of distraction osteogenesis in 1951 and this technique is now an extremely useful tool in the surgical armamentarium.

Increasing interest and expertise in the prevention and treatment of infected fractures and nonunions has resulted in the emergence of a subspecialty interest.

PATHOGENESIS

INFECTED FRACTURES

The mere presence of bacteria in bone is not sufficient to produce osteomyelitis. Established infections occur when a sufficient number of virulent organisms, facilitated by certain factors in the local environment, overcome the host defenses. Every open fracture is considered to be contaminated from the time of injury. Gustilo and Anderson[5] showed that 70% of grade 3 open fractures had positive cultures on admission or at wound closure. The organisms gain access to the bone via the open wound. The first 6 hours are called the "golden period" for treatment, as the numbers of bacteria subsequently will multiply exponentially. Antibiotics expand the golden period, thus increasing the operative window of opportunity.

If untreated, the infection progresses and pus elevates the periosteum, which eventually causes necrosis of cortical bone, thereby forming a sequestrum. A sequestrum is a piece of dead bone surrounded by granulation tissue and a layer of living bone, the involucrum. The sequestrum acts as a foreign body and a passive substrate for bacterial colonization and proliferation.[6] Antibiotics, white blood cells, and macrophages cannot be delivered effectively to this avascular region.

The goal of early débridement is to sterilize the wound by reducing the inoculum and removing necrotic bone and soft tissues and harmful bacterial products. It is difficult to maintain sterility in large open wounds for long periods of time, and secondary contaminants such as *Pseudomonas* and *Enterobacter* species eventually appear and become pathogenic. This process of secondary infection within the hospital is called nosocomial infection.[7, 8]

INFECTED NONUNION

Failure of union may be due to a suboptimal mechanical environment, poor vascularity, and possibly infection. Frequent interruption of fracture immobilization for wound care when fractures were treated by casts was historically a predisposing factor toward nonunion. Currently, most fractures are treated with either internal or external fixation devices. The benefits of fracture stability achieved by metallic fixation outweigh the disadvantages of the foreign body effect.[9] Infection should be more properly regarded as one of the complicating factors that can accompany nonunion rather than a direct causative factor.

CLINICAL FEATURES

The diagnosis of infection in a fracture may be obvious or obscure. The symptoms and signs can vary with the rate, duration, and extent of the bone involvement and with the patient's age. The classical triad of infection is fever, swelling, and localized tenderness. Other characteristic features include chills, rigors, nausea, vomiting, malaise, and erythema. The onset may be indolent. The elderly or the very young patient may present in an atypical manner with confusion, irrational behavior, lethargy, or loss of appetite. Early diagnosis is important. An immediate aggressive approach is necessary to prevent a soft-tissue wound infection from becoming an infected fracture.

HISTORY

Historical details ascertained concerning the initial trauma should include how, when, and where the injury occurred. It is important to determine whether the injury was low- or high-energy. The location of the injury is important in determining the degree of potential contamination. Farmyard injuries have a notorious reputation for heavy bacterial contamination, particularly with clostridial species. Another consideration is the timing of any pyrexias, as temperature elevation from wound infection typically occurs on the third or fourth day after injury. In addition to the details of the original injury, previous surgeries and assessment of risk factors for poor bone healing and infection include alcohol abuse, nicotine consumption, diabetes, and drug therapies such as nonsteroidal anti-inflammatory drugs, cytotoxic agents, and corticosteroids.[10] The Cierny-Maders classification of osteomyelitis is useful to stratify the physiological status of the host.[11] The patient's socioeconomic and psychological status may significantly influence the management options.

TABLE 1. SIGNS OF WOUND INFECTION	
Local	**Systemic**
Pain	Pyrexia
Edema	Tachycardia
Erythema	Anorexia
Purulent exudate	Lethargy
Tenderness	Leukocytosis
Odor	Generalized lymphadenopathy
Cellulitis	
Localized lymphadenopathy	

EXAMINATION

Wound infection is usually accompanied by local and systemic signs of infection (Table 1). In infected nonunions, there may be no local signs, especially with low-grade infection associated with a stiff fibrous union. Swelling, induration, erythema, and tenderness represent the typical symptoms. Serosanguineous or purulent drainage from a sinus tract facilitates an easy diagnosis. The infection can be graded clinically into the following categories:

1. Severe: Extensive inflammation and purulent discharge.
2. Mild: Moderate inflammation only.
3. Subclinical: Infection is detected only on culture of operative specimens.

Clinical examination should document any coexisting problems such as soft-tissue scarring or cicatrization, limited joint motion, muscle atrophy, deformity, and leg length discrepancy. It is critical to assess the neurovascular status of the limb, as this has serious implications for the management plan. The nonunion site also may be categorized as stiff or mobile.

INVESTIGATIONS

LABORATORY STUDIES

Hematological studies, including a differential white blood cell count, the erythrocyte sedimentation rate, and the C-reactive protein, are the baseline investigations for evaluation. Neutrophilia and a left shift are the classic responses to acute infection, but frequently the white blood cell count is not elevated. The erythrocyte sedimentation rate is often elevated but is nonspecific. Peak elevation occurs on the third to fifth day and takes many weeks to return to normal. The C-reactive protein level returns to normal more quickly and is a more useful monitor to assess the clinical response to treatment.

Patients with a chronic infected nonunion may have a normochromic normocytic anemia. Nutritional assessment and immune function should be assessed with serum albumin level and total lymphocyte count. Metabolic parameters including glucose tolerance and hepatic and renal profiles should be evaluated and if necessary corrected preoperatively.

MICROBIOLOGY

During an acute infective episode, blood cultures may reveal the causative organism. Aspiration at the site of maximal tenderness or wound swabs are diagnostic and essential for accurate antibiotic treatment. Deep wound cultures are required for correct pathogen identification. Cultures should be sent for Gram stain and for aerobic and anaerobic culture for 7 and 14 days, respectively.

IMAGING STUDIES

Plain radiographs frequently show normal findings in acute infection but may reveal swelling or gas in the soft tissues.

Bone destruction with radiolucency is not apparent until bone mineral loss of approximately 30% to 50% has occurred.[12] The initial changes include subtle loss of cortical density at the fracture site, radiolucency adjacent to metal implants, "scalloping" due to endosteal lysis, and periosteal reaction, which may extend a variable distance beyond the fracture site. In chronic cases, plain radiographs may show sequestra or involucra. Nonunions can be classified as either atrophic or hypertrophic. Tomograms are useful when

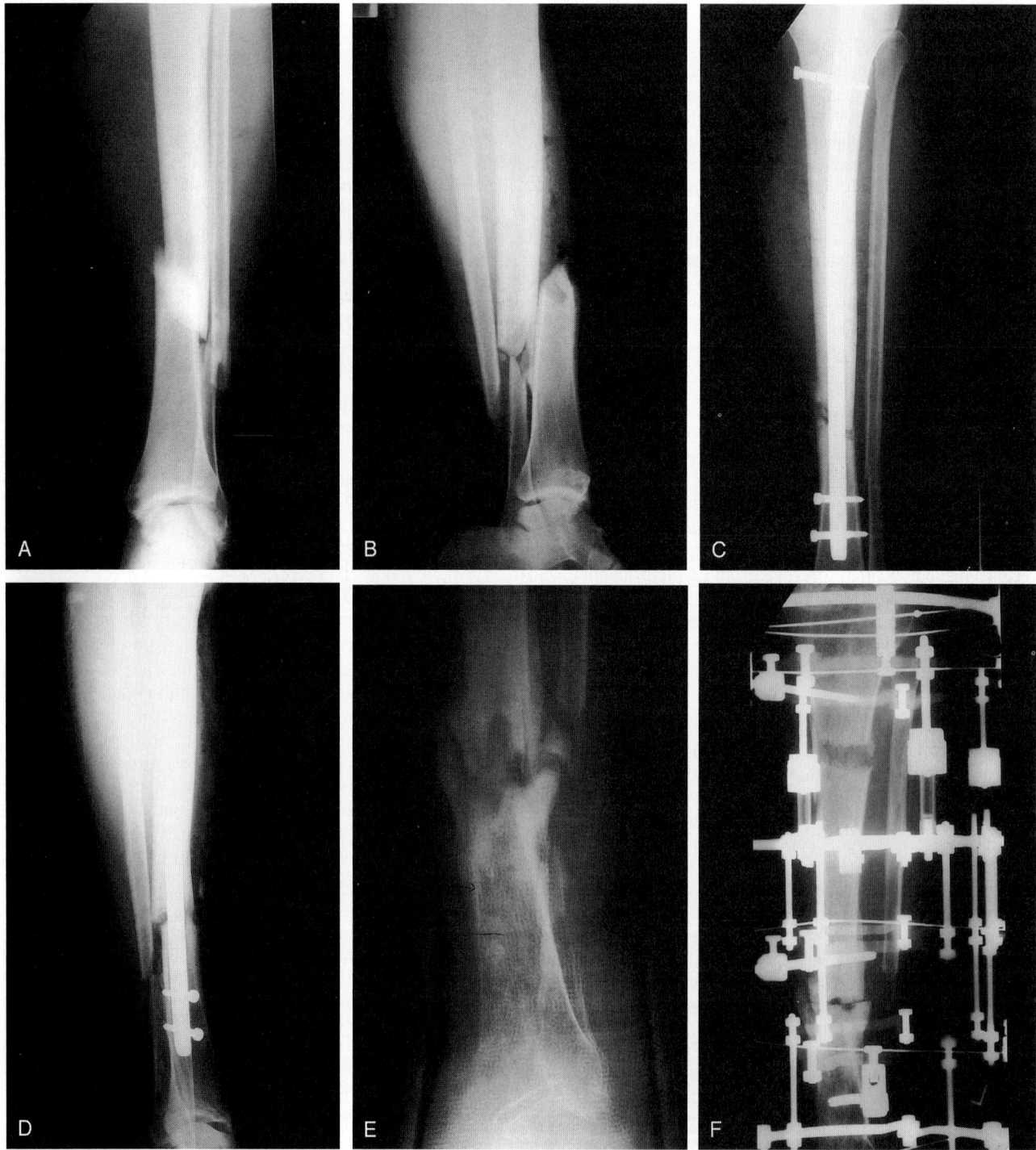

Fig. 2. *See legend on opposite page*

the diagnosis of nonunion is uncertain. A sinogram can potentially outline the extent of an abscess cavity. Sequestra are best delineated with computed tomography. The combinations of technetium 99m methylene diphosphonate with gallium-67 citrate or indium-111–labeled leukocyte scans have added increased sophistication to the imaging of bone infection, but the sensitivity and specificity are 86% and 93%, respectively.[12, 13] Magnetic resonance imaging can demonstrate the extent and anatomic location of osteomyelitis[14] and has a reported sensitivity of 82% to 100%.

Magnetic resonance imaging lacks specificity, with a range of 53% to 94%,[12] and may be subject to image distortion in the presence of metallic implants.

TISSUE BIOPSY

Tissue biopsy remains the gold standard in the diagnosis of deep infection. The specimens obtained at bone biopsy should be ground with a sterile pestle in a mortar to release as many organisms as possible[15] and then cultured aerobically and anaerobically, as described previously.

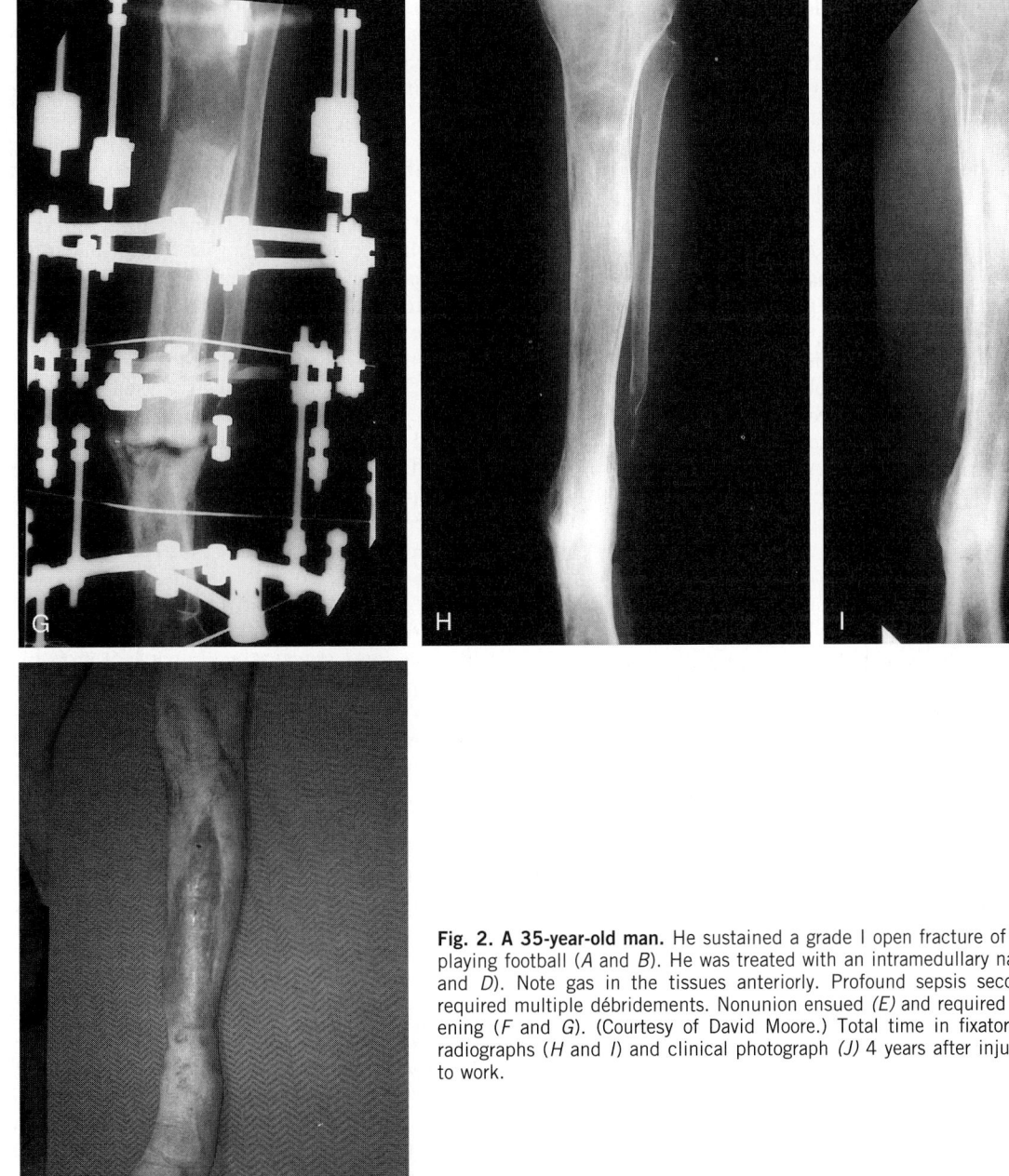

Fig. 2. A 35-year-old man. He sustained a grade I open fracture of the left tibia and fibula playing football (*A* and *B*). He was treated with an intramedullary nail and cephalosporin (*C* and *D*). Note gas in the tissues anteriorly. Profound sepsis secondary to gas gangrene required multiple débridements. Nonunion ensued *(E)* and required Ilizarov unifocal lengthening (*F* and *G*). (Courtesy of David Moore.) Total time in fixator was 12 months. Final radiographs (*H* and *I*) and clinical photograph *(J)* 4 years after injury. Patient has returned to work.

TREATMENT GOALS

The primary objective in the treatment of open contaminated fractures is to prevent wound infection and subsequent spread of infection to bone. If the bone becomes contaminated, treatment is directed to prevent chronic osteomyelitis and promote bone union.

In infected nonunions, the treatment goal is limb salvage. Limb salvage includes eradication of infection, achievement of bony union, and creation of an aligned limb that functions better than amputation and prosthetic fitting. In general, lower limb shortening of more than 2 cm, varus or valgus angulation of more than 15 degrees, and malrotation of more than 10 or 15 degrees may lead to long-term functional disability.

The decision to attempt limb salvage rather than amputation is a fundamental question. Factors to be considered include the patient's age, metabolic status, mobility of the adjacent joints, the neurovascular integrity of the limb, and finally and perhaps most importantly the patient's motivation and socioeconomic status. When informed of the duration of rehabilitation and the possibility of multiple operations in the reconstructive pathway, some patients may elect for amputation. It should be emphasized that a lower limb prosthesis, especially below-knee weightbearing, can function satisfactorily.

Infection prevention starts on the patient's arrival at the hospital. Restoration of intravascular volume increases tissue perfusion and oxygenation of the wound, which helps combat infection. Emergency care of the limb should consist of brief wound inspection, application of a sterile dressing, fracture splinting, tetanus prophylaxis, and intravenous antibiotic administration.

ANTIBIOTICS

Antibiotic therapy should be commenced immediately and, ultimately, should be culture-directed. The early administration of antibiotics that are active against both gram-positive and gram-negative organisms is the single most important factor in reducing the infection rate in open fracture wounds.[8] A combination of a cephalosporin and an aminoglycoside is initially most commonly prescribed for the patient. Length of therapy remains controversial and arbitrary. It is interesting to note that Ilizarov did not use antibiotics in treating osteomyelitis or infected nonunion. He relied on the increased metabolic activity in the limb and that "osteomyelitis burns in the flames of the regenerate."[16]

Gas gangrene is a rare but dreaded complication of open fractures and is frequently fatal.[5, 8, 17] Gas gangrene occurs almost exclusively in wounds that are closed primarily. However, the authors have encountered one patient with gas gangrene in a type I open tibial fracture in which the wound was left open and the patient was treated with a cephalosporin (Fig. 2). Clostridial contamination is likely in farmyard or soil-related injuries and in injuries with a severe crush or vascular compromise. In these situations, penicillin G should be added to the antibiotic regimen. Cephalosporins have an unpredictable activity against many anaerobes, including clostridia.

ANTIBIOTIC BEAD POUCHES

Antibiotic-loaded cement in the form of beads can be used as an adjunct to prevent infection in open fractures.[18] Numerous studies show that gentamicin and other antibiotics will elute from beads in concentrations far above the mean inhibitory concentration of most common pathogens, and this method is superior to any form of systemic therapy in terms of efficacy and safety.[9] In infected nonunions, the beads can be left in place for several weeks to fill and sterilize the dead space prior to cancellous bone grafting.

DÉBRIDEMENT

There is universal agreement that thorough débridement and copious wound irrigation are important factors in the prevention and treatment of chronic infection in open fractures, infected fractures, and infected nonunions. Débridement reduces the inoculum and removes necrotic avascular bone and harmful bacterial products. Inadequate débridement is a common cause of failure.[14]

Patzakis and Wilkins[8] showed that the time elapsed from injury to surgical débridement was not a critical determinant of subsequent infection in the presence of appropriate antibiotics. Nevertheless, most authors advocate undertaking débridement as soon as possible. The initial débridement must be performed with subsequent reconstruction in mind. The placement of incisions should avoid unnecessary soft-tissue compromise. Effective and efficient wound irrigation can be achieved with a pulse lavage system.

Débridement in the acute fracture begins at the outer edge of the wound and proceeds inward. Generous longitudinal extensions of the wound are required. All nonviable soft tissues are removed. In the acutely traumatized limb, muscle viability can be assessed by the four Cs as described by Scully.[19] These are *c*olor, *c*apacity to bleed, *c*ontractility when stimulated, and *c*onsistency. Grossly contaminated and small avascular bone segments that do not contribute to fracture stability are removed. Large devitalized pieces that are structurally important probably should also be removed, as their importance for fracture stability is outweighed by their potential role as nonviable surfaces for bacterial colonization.[20] If there is any doubt about the adequacy of the débridement, it should be repeated within 2 to 3 days and repeated again as necessary.

Débridement of the infected nonunion includes excision of the sinus tract, the avascular scarred soft tissues, and the intervening scar between the bone ends. Saucerization converts the bone cylinder to a saucer and permits drainage and removal of trapped granulation tissue and sequestra. The main disadvantage is that this procedure may severely weaken the bone.[21]

Débridement is technically difficult, as it is not easy to distinguish dead bone from viable bone. Additionally, orthopaedic surgeons have traditionally been apprehensive about creating large bony and soft-tissue defects that will be difficult to reconstruct. During bone débridement, the paprika sign indicates punctate bleeding from live bone.[22] Magnification loupes are of limited value, as cortical bone blood flow is only 1 to 2 mL per 100 g of tissue per minute.[21] When a tourniquet is used, it is impossible to identify viable tissue by this method. The routine use of a tourniquet in débriding acute fractures is inadvisable. The tourniquet adds further ischemia to an already compromised limb. Magnetic resonance imaging and laser flow Doppler ultrasonography are potentially useful adjuncts to aid débridement.[12, 20] Despite these techniques, the final extent of bone débridement is largely based on surgical experience and is best determined at operation.

Apprehension regarding the ability to reconstruct bone or soft-tissue defects, the dead space, must not be a determining factor in the extent of débridement. Serial débridements with intervals of observation periods are helpful to determine tissue viability and also facilitate consultation with colleagues.

PROCEDURES

WOUND COVERAGE

Protracted open wound care techniques have been the standard of care for severe open lower limb injuries. There has been a recent trend toward earlier coverage of the bone.[23] Cole et al[24] reported excellent results in treating 50 consecutive open tibial fractures with immediate wound coverage. It is important to distinguish between coverage of bone and skin closure. In general, bone should be covered as quickly as possible to avoid secondary infection.

Numerous procedures are available, but O'Brien and Morrison's principle[24] is that the simplest procedure that will provide aesthetic coverage of the defect is the wisest approach to minimize patient morbidity (Table 2).

Skin Grafting

Small wounds can be covered by split-skin grafts. The main limitation is that orthopaedic implants and exposed cortical bone, tendon, or cartilage should not be covered with these grafts as the primary mode of coverage.

Fasciocutaneous Flaps

The fasciocutaneous or adipofascial flap is an excellent technique for the open tibial fracture,[24] being both effective and reliable in lower limb reconstruction.[25] The most important principle of flap design is that the flap base should overlie the lateral intermuscular septum or posterior tibial artery to ensure capturing a fascial perforator (Fig. 3). Advantages include extreme versatility; dissection and insetting are simple and quick, and the nonsegmental blood supply is reliable and easily definable, causing minimal donor site morbidity. We believe this flap should be in the armamentarium of the modern orthopaedic traumatologist. The main disadvantages are lack of bulk to fill dead space and a relatively poor improvement in vascularity at the recipient site.

Myocutaneous Flaps

The lateral or medial heads of the gastrocnemius are the most commonly used local muscle flaps in the lower limb. The main indication is to fill a dead space in the proximal two thirds of the leg following débridement of an infected nonunion. The muscle obliterates the dead space, thereby making subsequent cancellous grafting to the area difficult. For this reason, some authors recommend that antibiotic-impregnated cement beads be placed beneath the flap to maintain a sterile dead space for later cancellous grafting.[26]

Free Flaps

Microvascular free flaps are extremely versatile.[27] The latissimus dorsi and rectus abdominis flaps are most commonly used in the lower limb. They are indicated primarily in defects involving the distal one third of the tibia due to the inability to use local flaps in these areas. These flaps improve the local biological environment by bringing in additional blood supply, which theoretically augments host defense mechanisms and promotes osseous and soft-tissue healing. The disadvantages include prolonged operating times, donor site morbidity, and the need for an available microsurgical service. The procedure is contraindicated in polytrauma and hypovolemic patients.

TABLE 2. TREATMENT OPTIONS			
Treatment	Options	Indications	Contraindications
Soft-tissue coverage	Split-skin graft	Limited	Not on exposed bone, metal, or tendon
	Fasciocutaneous flap	Most open acute fractures	Few
	Pedicle muscle flap	Proximal two-thirds of tibia to fill defect in infected nonunion after débridement or acute open fracture	Poor vascular inflow
	Free flap	Distal third of tibia to fill defect in infected nonunion after débridement or acute open fracture	Specialized microsurgical skills required, hypovolemia, active sepsis
Stabilization	External fixator	All infected fractures and nonunions	None
	Intramedullary nails	Acute open fractures	Most infected fractures and nonunions, absolute after infected plating
Bone grafting	Conventional	Delayed and nonunions	Active sepsis
	Papineau	Subcutaneous locations, infected nonunions, small defect <3 cm, metaphyseal	Massive defect, bone loss >3 cm
	Microvascular	Infected nonunions after débridement, defect >6 cm	Active sepsis
Distraction osteogenesis	Ilizarov	All infected fractures and nonunions	Nerve injury, noncompliant patient, smoking

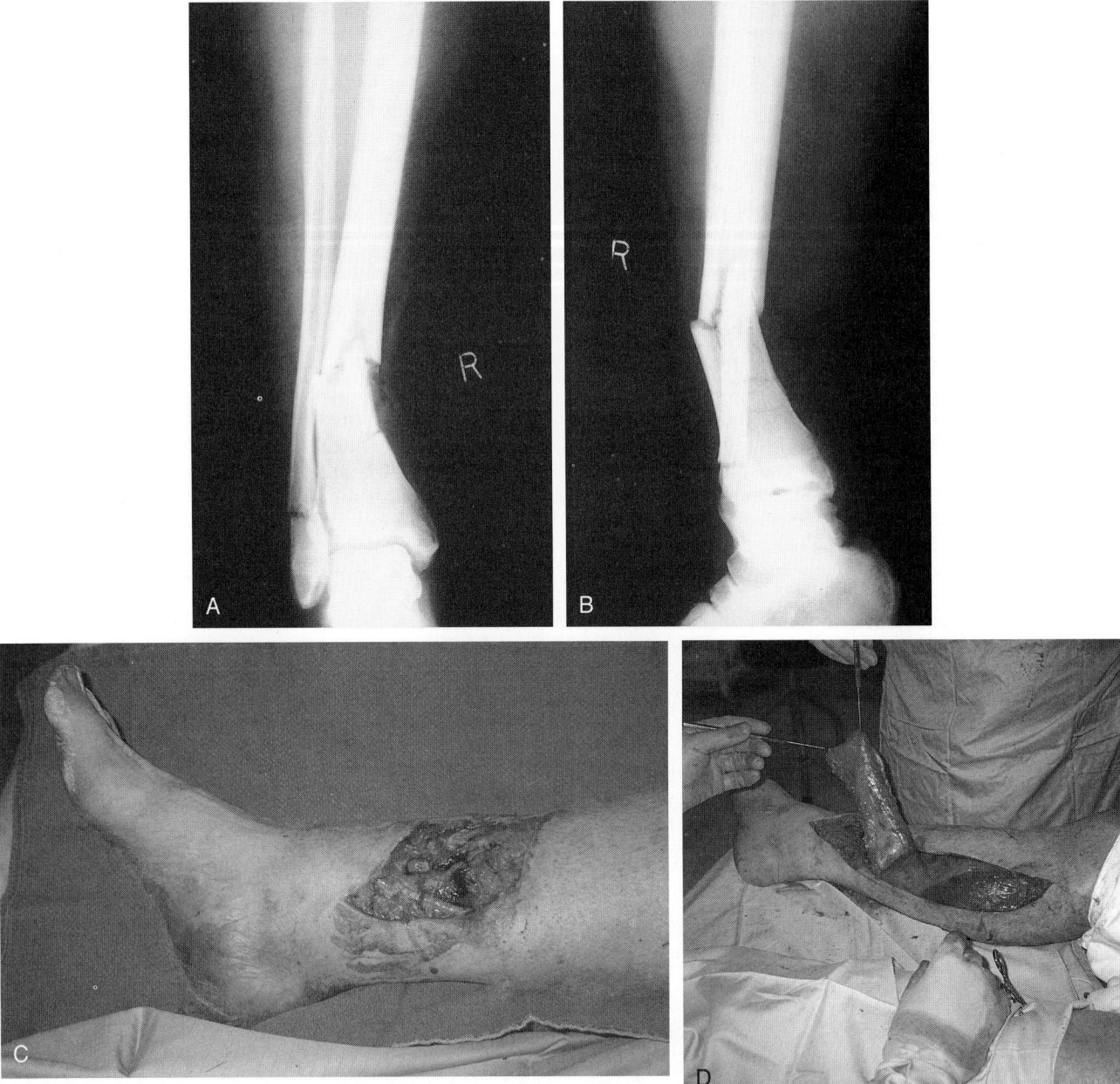

Fig. 3. A 57-year-old man. He was involved in an industrial accident with a grade III B open fracture of the right tibia and fibula (*A* and *B*). Wound at presentation with large defect anteromedially *(C)*. Operative photograph showing adipofascial flap for soft-tissue reconstruction *(D)*.

Acute Shortening

Acute shortening of the bone is a relatively recent concept. Shortening facilitates coverage with available soft tissues when other techniques are impossible or inadvisable. The maximum acute shortening is approximately 5 to 6 cm; otherwise, vessel kinking and vascular compromise are likely. This technique relies on the concept that bone length must be restored at a later date.

STABILIZATION
General

There is experimental and some clinical evidence that stabilization of fractures can decrease the severity of infection.[28]

External Fixator

An external fixator can be used to achieve stability in almost all open fractures, acutely infected fractures, and infected nonunions. The advantages include ease of application, achievement of stability without extensive soft-tissue stripping, a minimum of foreign material in the nonunion zone, and correction of displacement and angulation with minimal surgical trauma. External fixation is the standard treatment for stabilization of active diaphyseal infection. The major disadvantage of conventional external fixators is pin loosening. This is especially true in diseased bone. Other disadvantages are pin tract infection and secondary infection when intramedullary nailing is attempted later. Access to the wound has been cited as one of the advantages, but poorly designed frames and awkward pin placement can hinder access and interfere with flap advancement.

Intramedullary Nailing

Intramedullary nailing is now an accepted alternative in achieving and maintaining stable fixation in many fresh open fractures.[1, 24] Until recently, it was believed to be contraindicated because the infection rate was high and infection was often pandiaphyseal and, once established, was difficult to eradicate.[29] Recent experience suggests that panosseous infection is very rare and the presence of a nail in an infected fracture does not necessarily give rise to widespread osteomyelitis, even when pus tracks along the nail. Treatment of deep infection following nailing is relatively straightforward and generally successful. Options include exchange nailing with reaming of the infected intramedullary rind or conversion to an external fixator.[1, 30, 31]

Intramedullary nailing of established infection in the infected diaphyseal fracture or infected nonunion, especially of the tibia, is controversial. Exacerbation of infection can threaten limb survival; however, the flagrant infections are rare. Lottes[32] reported a series of infected tibial nonunions treated with an intramedullary nail with a subsequent amputation rate of 12.5%. Intramedullary nailing was recommended by Papineau[33] as the preferred method of stabilization with open cancellous grafting. Other proponents stress that nailing in the presence of established infections is a salvage procedure and that patients must be counseled preoperatively that ultimate amputation may be the outcome.[28, 34, 35] The treatment involves inserting the nail into a completely débrided granulating wound, followed by an open wound management policy. The main advantage of the method is that it permits early functional weightbearing, which is important physically and psychologically to this group of chronically debilitated and frequently depressed patients. The procedure is absolutely contraindicated in an infected nonunion resulting from failed plate osteosynthesis because of the precarious blood supply and is generally more suitable for use in the femur than the tibia.

BONE GRAFTING
General

Historically, the most frequently used method of treating nonunions has been bone grafting with a variety of different methods. The primary function of bone graft is to alter local biology at the nonunion site. Autogenous cancellous bone, usually harvested from the ilium, has been the gold standard for most nonstructural applications. Disadvantages of autogenous bone include the limited supply of graft material and the donor site morbidity. Advantages include osteoconductive (protein) and osteoinductive (matrix) properties in the presence of osteoprogenitor cells. For large defects, many authors use a mixture of autogenous and allograft bone and may admix antibiotics into the bone graft.

Conventional Bone Grafting

Conventional or closed cancellous bone grafting often is recommended in infected fresh fractures 4 to 6 weeks after the wound has healed, to prevent nonunion. If flap closure has been employed, the graft can be inserted by lifting the flap edge distant from the vascular pedicle.

Posterolateral bone grafting and other techniques used to create a tibiofibular synostosis[36] also are effective in the treatment of infected tibial nonunions. Advantages of posterolateral grafting include avoidance of the typical anteromedial open wound and zone of injury while placing the bone graft in the most vascular portion of the leg. The disadvantages include potential vascular injury, especially when used in the proximal third of the tibia. Many of these limbs have only one remaining arterial pedicle and a preoperative angiogram is advisable.

Open Cancellous Grafting

Open cancellous bone grafting is often called the Papineau technique.[26, 37] The skeletal defect is first débrided, kept moist, and allowed to granulate, a process that may take 4 weeks. The wound is then packed with cancellous bone chips level with the skin and is left exposed for subsequent wound care. Daily dressing changes are required to prevent desiccation of the bone graft. After about 3 weeks, the graft is overgrown with granulation tissue and can be skin-grafted, allowed to epithelialize, or closed with a rotation flap.

The advantage of the method is its simplicity, but meticulous attention to wound care is essential for success. Disadvantages include unstable skin, graft shrinkage, and the need for a prolonged period of protected weightbearing to allow the graft to corticalize to withstand functional loading. Papineau[33] advocated the use of an intramedullary nail for fracture stability and to prevent the graft from collapsing inward. This technique is most applicable to a limited metaphyseal defect or may be used in patients who are not candidates for flap coverage because of age or concomitant peripheral vascular disease.

Vascularized Bone Grafting

Since the initial descriptions by Taylor in 1975 and Gilbert in 1979, the free vascularized transfer has become a reliable source of living bone for difficult reconstructions in septic nonunions. Various donor sites are available, but the fibula is most suitable for lower limb transplantation.[27] Unlike conventional grafts, vascularized bone transfers are not limited by the defect size or the soft-tissue milieu, and they heal quickly, often within 6 months. In general, vascularized bone grafts are applicable to defects greater than 6 cm in septic nonunions refractory to treatment by more conventional methods.

The fibula has a maximum length of 26 cm with an anatomic structure and shape that is excellent for fixation and resistance to angular and torsional forces. Additionally, when harvested as a composite flap with overlying skin and subcutaneous tissue, bone and soft-tissue defects can be addressed simultaneously. The skin portion can be used as an indicator of anastomotic patency in the postoperative time period.

Preoperative angiograms of donor and recipient sites are useful to identify the vascular anatomy and help preoperative planning. Active infection or an abnormal popliteal bifurcation, present in 5% of patients, are contraindications. Postoperatively, the patient is kept on strict bedrest with limb elevation for 2 weeks. Weightbearing is not allowed until bone union occurs, usually at 6 months. Gradual weightbearing progresses until the graft hypertrophies. The disadvantages are the time-consuming nature and complexity of the technique, which limits application to centers with an experienced microvascular service.[38] Donor site morbidity with ankle stiffness and restricted motion of the great toe are frequently observed.

THE ILIZAROV TECHNIQUE

Gavriil Ilizarov, from Kurgan in Russia, introduced perhaps the most revolutionary idea in orthopaedics this century by demonstrating fracture healing with callus distraction. The Ilizarov method has been increasingly used to treat infected fractures and nonunions. The Ilizarov method involves radical débridement, application of a ring external fixator, and bone lengthening through a corticotomy (specialized osteotomy) by gradual distraction after a latency period of 5 to 7 days. The gradual distraction causes angiogenesis and formation of fibrous tissue at the distraction site. Fibrous tissue is replaced by woven and lamellar bone in the ensuing months and the maintained endosteal and periosteal blood flow increases the extremity blood supply during the treatment. This profound biological stimulus eradicates the infection and hastens bone union.[16]

An accurate clinical and radiological assessment of the extent of the infection and anticipated resection of bone is necessary before débridement. Preoperative planning includes frame preconstruction and assurance of an adequate stock of hardware. The Ilizarov fixator rings are connected to the bone with transfixing 1.5 mm Kirschner wires inserted percutaneously and fixed to the rings under tension by a calibrated wire-tensioning device. Limb deformity can be corrected with hinges strategically placed to produce compression, distraction, rotation, angulation, or translation of the bone segments.

A thorough and extensive débridement with resection of segmental infected bone and adjacent tissues is performed to remove all nonviable tissue. A proximal or distal corticotomy creates the viable bone fragment for transport. The recommended distraction rate is 1 mm/day at a rhythm of 0.25 mm four times daily. The wires slowly cut through the skin and soft tissues of the leg during distraction. Early soft-tissue coverage with rotation or free muscle flaps is widely accepted as the best means of preventing deep infection.[39] The transported bone segment moves along the limb until contact is made with the other major bone segment (docking). Compression is then used to achieve final union, but this may require additional cancellous bone grafting.

An alternative method is to acutely shorten the bone at the infected nonunion site after débridement. This is followed by lengthening at the corticotomy site. Acute shortening of up to 6 cm is possible without significant risk of vessel kinking and vascular compromise.

The advantages of the Ilizarov method are numerous, as it is the only comprehensive approach that simultaneously addresses all factors commonly associated with an infected nonunion. These include infection, nonunion, deformity, length discrepancy, soft-tissue defects, joint stiffness, and osteoporosis. The method is semi-invasive in nature, requiring few blood transfusions or ancillary procedures. The regenerate bone is a living graft that is exactly the right size for the anatomic site and obviates the need to harvest bone graft from other anatomic sites. The disadvantages include lengthy treatment time and delayed healing at the docking site. Pin tract infections are common. This specialized technique requires a skilled multidisciplinary team. Although defects of up to 6 or 7 cm may be reliably treated,[40] the frequency of complications increases with larger defects. The method is contraindicated in limbs with severe posterior tibial nerve damage or in noncompliant patients. Smoking is a relative contraindication.

COMPLICATIONS

SOFT-TISSUE COVERAGE

Complications with myocutaneous or free flaps in the setting of chronic infection are rare. Flap failure is more likely in subacute reconstruction (more than 7 to 15 days) of open tibial fractures.[23, 41]

STABILIZATION

Pin tract infections are common with external fixators. Other complications include neurovascular injury from pin placement and an increased infection rate if the bone is subsequently treated with an intramedullary nail. Stiffness of the knee joint may occur with thigh external fixators if the pins transfix a musculotendinous unit.[42]

The main complication following intramedullary nailing is infection, which can occur in 9.5% of type III open tibial fractures.[1]

BONE GRAFTING

In general, complications from bone grafting are uncommon. In Papineau-type grafting of the diaphysis, refracture may occur during graft maturation[43] and healed scar may be unstable with a tendency to recurrent ulceration.[44] In vascularized bone grafting, stress fracture of the graft up to 2 years postoperatively and donor site ankle stiffness are fairly common complications.

ILIZAROV

True complications of Ilizarov treatment include all intraoperative injuries and all problems occurring during limb lengthening that are not resolved before the end of treatment.[45] These include vascular or nerve damage during pin/wire placement, which is rare. Pin site infections are very common. Fracture of the regenerated bone may occur for up to 1 year following removal of the frame. Joint contractures, particularly of the toes, can be significant and are best avoided by physiotherapy surveillance.

RESULTS

Outcome refers to all possible effects of a disease or intervention. The results and outcomes of various treatment methods for infected fractures and nonunions are difficult to compare. Various combinations of treatments are used, and clearly not all infected fractures and nonunions are the same. In particular, it is not known which outcome measures are the most important or valid in defining success or failure. The traditionally cited outcome measures are confined to the rate of bone union and infection eradication. The amputation rate is also frequently reported but is often emphasized as a treatment failure. Amputation may not reflect treatment failure but may indicate good judgment. More recently, attention has been focused on quality of life parameters like limb function and cosmesis, late symptoms or complications, hospitalization time, speed of recovery, return to work, and overall patient satisfaction.[46]

SOFT-TISSUE COVERAGE

Early coverage significantly improves the union rate and the prevention or eradication of infection. Cierny et al[41] showed that early as compared with late soft-tissue coverage improved the time to union (4 months versus 6.4 months) in 36 type III open tibial fractures.

STABILIZATION

The incidence of infection of the wound after external fixation of a type III open fracture has been reported to range from 7% to 14%.[47]

Intramedullary nailing of infected tibial fractures gives only fair results. Lottes reported a 70% union rate but a 12.5% amputation rate.[32] Miller achieved union in 18 of 19 infected tibial nonunions with open wound management after an average of 6.6 months.[28] Klemm reported a union rate in infected femoral and tibial pseudoarthroses of 89.5% and 62.5%, respectively.[34]

BONE GRAFTING

Emami et al[43] reported 100% union success in 37 infected tibial nonunions after an average of 11 months with open cancellous grafting. With a combination of muscle flaps, both free and local, and bone grafting, both anterior and posterolateral, in 32 patients with infected tibial nonunion, Patzakis showed a 91% union rate in an average of 5.5 months.[22] Green and Dlabal[37] used open anterior bone grafting and external fixation for 7.5 months for infected tibial nonunions and reported success in 13 of 15 patients. In a study of tibial nonunion and segmental defects, Esterhai et al[14] showed that the rate of union and infection eradication for posterolateral bone grafting and microvascular soft-tissue transfer with subsequent bone grafting was 87.5%, compared with 66% for open cancellous grafting. Reckling and Waters[48] had a good to excellent functional result in nine infected tibial nonunions treated by posterolateral grafting.

Bowen et al[46] described the outcome of microsurgical soft-tissue reconstruction of infected tibial nonunions in 15 patients. The mean time to union after bone grafting was 6.5 months and patients reported that satisfaction was related to preservation of the affected limb.

Using vascularized fibular grafts, Yajima et al[49] reported a mean of 6.2 months to radiographic union of infected leg (femur and tibia) fractures and a success rate of 88%. The success rate for microvascular transfers is now over 90%.[23]

ILIZAROV

Success rates in infected nonunions of 85% to 100% have been reported in Russia and Italy.[35, 50] DiPasquale[40] reported a 94% union rate in 11 infected nonunions. Dendrinos et al[51] eradicated infection in all 28 patients with tibial nonunion, with mean duration of treatment being 10 months. Cattaneo et al[52] reported treating 28 infected tibial nonunions with 100% success during a mean treatment time of 9 months.

REFERENCES

1. Court-Brown CM, Keating JF, McQueen MM: Infection after intramedullary nailing of the tibia. Incidence and protocol for management. J Bone Joint Surg Br 1992; 74:770.
2. Einhorn TA: Breakout session 1: Definitions of fracture repair. Clin Orthop 1998; 355S:S353.
3. Kirk NT: Amputations. 1943. Clin Orthop 1989; 243:3.
4. Ostermann PA, Henry SL, Seligson D: The role of local antibiotic therapy in the management of compound fractures. Clin Orthop 1993; 295:102.
5. Gustilo RB, Anderson JT: Prevention of infection in the treatment of one thousand and twenty-five open fractures of long bones: Retrospective and prospective analyses. J Bone Joint Surg Am 1976; 58:453.
6. Gristina AG, Costerton JW: Bacterial adherence and the glycocalyx and their role in musculoskeletal infection. Orthop Clin North Am 1984; 15:517.
7. Gustilo RB: Management of infected fractures. Instr Course Lect 1982; 31:18.
8. Patzakis MJ, Wilkins J: Factors influencing infection rate in open fracture wounds. Clin Orthop 1989; 243:36.
9. Gustilo RB: Management of infected nonunion. In Evarts CM (ed): Surgery of the Musculoskeletal System, 2nd ed. New York, Churchill Livingstone, 1990, p 4455.
10. Christian CA: General principles of fracture treatment. In Canale ST (ed): Campbell's Operative Orthopaedics, 9th ed. St. Louis, Mosby, 1998, p 1993.
11. Cierny G III: The classification and treatment of adult osteomyelitis. In: Evarts CM (ed): Surgery of the Musculoskeletal System. 2nd ed. New York, Churchill Livingstone, 1990, p 4337.
12. Boutin RD, Brossmann J, Sartoris DJ, et al: Update on imaging of orthopedic infections. Orthop Clin North Am 1998; 29:41.
13. Nepola JV, Seabold JE, Marsh JL, et al: Diagnosis of infection in ununited fractures. Combined imaging with indium-111-labeled leukocytes and technetium-99m methylene diphosphonate. J Bone Joint Surg Am 1993; 75:1816.
14. Esterhai J Jr, Sennett B, Gelb H, et al: Treatment of chronic osteomyelitis complicating nonunion and segmental defects of the tibia with open cancellous bone graft, posterolateral bone graft, and soft-tissue transfer. J Trauma 1990; 30:49.
15. Marsh DR, Shah S, Elliott J, et al: The Ilizarov method in nonunion, malunion and infection of fractures. J Bone Joint Surg Br 1997; 79:273.
16. Green SA: Osteomyelitis: The Ilizarov perspective. Orthop Clin North Am 1991; 22:515.
17. Darke SG, King AM, Slack WK: Gas gangrene and related infection: Classification, clinical features and aetiology, management and mortality: A report of 88 cases. Br J Surg 1977; 64:104.
18. Keating JF, Blachut PA, O'Brien PJ, et al: Reamed nailing of open tibial fractures: Does the antibiotic bead pouch reduce the deep infection rate? J Orthop Trauma 1996; 10:298.
19. Scully RE, Artz CP, Sako Y: An evaluation of the surgeon's criteria for determining viability of muscle during debridement. Arch Surg 1956; 73:1031.
20. Swiontkowski MF: Criteria for bone debridement in massive lower limb trauma. Clin Orthop 1989; 243:41.
21. Kelly PJ: Infected nonunion of the femur and tibia. Orthop Clin North Am 1984; 15:481.
22. Patzakis MJ, Scilaris TA, Chon J, et al: Results of bone grafting for infected tibial nonunion. Clin Orthop 1995; 315:192.
23. Tomaino M, Bowen V: Reconstructive surgery for lower limb salvage. Can J Surg 1995; 38:221.
24. Cole JD, Ansel LJ, Schwartzberg R: A sequential protocol for management of severe open tibial fractures. Clin Orthop 1995; 315:84.
25. Stewart KJ, Tytherleigh-Strong G, Baharathwaj S, et al: The soft tissue manage-

ment of children's open tibial fractures. J R Coll Surg Edinb 1999; 44:24.

26. Toh CL, Jupiter JB: The infected nonunion of the tibia. Clin Orthop 1995; 315: 176.

27. Nusbickel FR, Dell PC, McAndrew MP, et al: Vascularized autografts for reconstruction of skeletal defects following lower extremity trauma: A review. Clin Orthop 1989; 243:65.

28. Miller ME, Ada JR, Webb LX: Treatment of infected nonunion and delayed union of tibia fractures with locking intramedullary nails. Clin Orthop 1989; 245:233.

29. Chapman MW: The role of intramedullary fixation in open fractures. Clin Orthop 1986; 212:26.

30. Zych GA, Hutson JJ Jr: Diagnosis and management of infection after tibial intramedullary nailing. Clin Orthop 1995; 315: 153.

31. Patzakis MJ, Wilkins J, Wiss DA: Infection following intramedullary nailing of long bones: Diagnosis and management. Clin Orthop 1986; 212:182.

32. Lottes JO: Medullary nailing of infected fractures of the tibia. J Bone Joint Surg Am 1963; 45:1548.

33. Papineau LJ: [Excision-graft with deliberately delayed closing in chronic osteomyelitis]. Nouv Presse Med 1973; 2:2753.

34. Klemm KW: Treatment of infected pseudarthrosis of the femur and tibia with an interlocking nail. Clin Orthop 1986; 212: 174.

35. Connolly JF: Tibial Nonunion: Diagnosis and Treatment. Illinois, American Academy of Orthopaedic Surgeons, 1991.

36. Rijnberg WJ, van Linge B: Central grafting for persistent nonunion of the tibia. A lateral approach to the tibia, creating a central compartment. J Bone Joint Surg Br 1993; 756:926.

37. Green SA, Dlabal TA: The open bone graft for septic nonunion. Clin Orthop 1983; 180:117.

38. Han CS, Wood MB, Bishop AT, et al: Vascularized bone transfer. J Bone Joint Surg Am 1992; 74:1441.

39. Lowenberg DW, Feibel RJ, Louie KW, et al: Combined muscle flap and Ilizarov reconstruction for bone and soft tissue defects. Clin Orthop 1996; 332:37.

40. DiPasquale D, Ochsner MG, Kelly AM, et al: The Ilizarov method for complex fracture nonunions. J Trauma 1994; 37:629.

41. Cierny G III, Byrd HS, Jones RE: Primary versus delayed soft tissue coverage for severe open tibial fractures. A comparison of results. Clin Orthop 1983; 178:54.

42. Yokoyama K, Itoman M, Shindo M, et al: Contributing factors influencing type III open tibial fractures. J Trauma 1995; 38: 788.

43. Emami A, Mjoberg B, Larsson S: Infected tibial nonunion: Good results after open cancellous bone grafting in 37 cases. Acta Orthop Scand 1995; 66:447.

44. Fleischmann W, Suger G, Kinzl L: Treatment of bone and soft tissue defects in infected nonunion. Acta Orthop Belg 1992; 58:227.

45. Paley D: Problems, obstacles, and complications of limb lengthening by the Ilizarov technique. Clin Orthop 1990; 250:81.

46. Bowen CV, Botsford DJ, Hudak PL, et al: Microsurgical treatment of septic nonunion of the tibia: Quality of life results. Clin Orthop 1996; 332:52.

47. Gustilo RB, Merkow RL, Templeman D: Current concepts review: The management of open fractures. J Bone Joint Surg Am 1990; 72:299.

48. Reckling FW, Waters CH III: Treatment of non-unions of fractures of the tibial diaphysis by posterolateral cortical cancellous bone-grafting. J Bone Joint Surg Am 1980; 62:936.

49. Yajima H, Tamai S, Mizumoto S, et al: Vascularized fibular grafts in the treatment of osteomyelitis and infected nonunion. Clin Orthop 1993; 293:256.

50. Paley D, Catagni MA, Argnani F, et al: Ilizarov treatment of tibial nonunions with bone loss. Clin Orthop 1989; 241:146.

51. Dendrinos GK, Kontos S, Lyritsis E: Use of the Ilizarov technique for treatment of nonunion of the tibia associated with infection. J Bone Joint Surg Am 1995; 77: 835.

52. Cattaneo R, Catagni M, Johnson EE: The treatment of infected nonunions and segmental defects of the tibia by the methods of Ilizarov. Clin Orthop 1992; 280:143.

section 5

chapter 5

HAND INFECTIONS

Stephen B. Schnall and Scott Waller

Summary

- Surgical management of hand infections requires thorough irrigation and débridement through incisions that permit exposure of the entire infected area.
- Coordination of treatment with an infectious disease specialist is particularly helpful.
- Worldwide, tuberculosis is the most common chronic infection of the hand; presentation can be insidious.
- Virtually any structure in the hand can become infected, from paronychia to bones and joints.

INTRODUCTION

Although the topic of hand infections is often given little attention, it is imperative that the physician have a clear understanding of these problems because their impact on the individual patient and overall health costs can be significant.[1-3]

Infection rates greater than 10% have been reported for open fractures of the hand,[4] and it has been reported that nearly 30% of admissions to hospital musculoskeletal infection wards are for infections of the hand.[2] Delays in appropriate treatment have been shown to correlate directly with slower resolution of the infection[5] and higher complication rates.

One must perform a complete history and physical examination, because infections may be related to underlying systemic conditions such as diabetes, rheumatological disorders, and immunocompromised states,[6-9] and the outcome of treatment may depend on control of the underlying disease. Other conditions such as gout, metastatic lesions, and factitious injuries may simulate infections[10] and need to be considered in the differential diagnosis of the patient who presents with an "infection."

A close working relationship with an infectious disease specialist is helpful in dealing with these problems, because the bacteriological flora of hand infections has been noted to change over recent decades.[11] A prevalence of mixed aerobic and anaerobic organisms of nearly 30% has also been reported.[12] However, *Staphylococcus aureus* and a *Streptococcus* species remain the most likely organisms causing hand infections.[13]

GENERAL MANAGEMENT PRINCIPLES

An assessment of the patient's tetanus immunization status must be included in the history. With patterns in our current culture such as increased travel, job relocation, and immigration, it is necessary to check when the last tetanus booster injection was given and to inquire about childhood immunizations if the patient was not born in or did not attend school in the United States. Elderly patients also should be carefully queried, because their attendance at U.S. public schools may have been before the initiation of required immunizations. A booster shot of 0.5 mL of tetanus toxoid should be administered when the patient's last immunization was more than 5 years before the injury. Hyperimmunoglobulin, in addition to the tetanus toxoid booster, should be administered when an initial series of tetanus immunizations has not been given.

Surgical management requires drainage of the infection and débridement through incisions adequate to allow exposure of the infected area in its entirety. In addition to delay in treatment, inadequate initial irrigation and insufficient débridement are significant factors in the failure to eradicate infections of the upper extremity. Initially, the majority of infected wounds that have been débrided should be left open. Primary closure over drains for joint infections can be considered, particularly with elbow and shoulder infections. Although primary closure of débrided infected tissue has been reported, this approach is not universally accepted and should be reserved only for very specific situations.[14] Delayed closure and skin grafting are performed once the wound develops healthy granulation tissue and the wound shows no evidence of continued contamination based on negative wound cultures.[2] In most cases, however, unless flap coverage or skin grafting is deemed necessary, the wounds should be allowed to remain open and heal by secondary intention.

Cultures of infected wounds can be quite helpful in choosing the appropriate antibiotics, but for greatest relevance the cultures should be obtained before the initiation of antibiotic therapy. Patients with persistent infection who received antibiotics before cultures were taken have been shown to have an increased number of mixed flora infections, including anaerobic, mycobacterial, and fungal species.[11] If the offending agent or organism can be anticipated with a high degree of certainty, as in cat bite wounds, cultures may not be necessary,[15] although the general rule of always obtaining a culture is usually the most prudent course.

It should also be mentioned that the treating physician should also observe the type of material expressed from an infected wound. Variations in the consistency, color, and odor of the material can be quite helpful. Viral lesions are vesicular, with more "watery" fluid; purulent abscesses have thicker more "creamy" material; and fungal infections generally are described as more like "cottage cheese." These observations may help the physician in choosing the initial antibiotic regimen.

After cultures are taken, empiric antibiotic coverage can be instituted in an attempt to cover the most likely infecting organisms for the wound based on the mechanism and location of injury. Table 1 outlines the organism coverage that generally can be expected for the individual pharmaco-

TABLE 1. GENERAL ANTIBIOTIC COVERAGE

Antibiotic	Description
Penicillins	
Penicillin G	Anaerobes: streptococci, enterococci
	Facultative anaerobes: *Eikenella corrodens*, *Pasteurella multocida*, anaerobes
Ampicillin	General anaerobic plus anaerobic coverage
Oxacillin	Staphylococci, streptococci
Piperacillin	Streptococci, enterobacteriaceae, *Pseudomonas aeruginosa*, anaerobes
Ampicillin/sulbactam	Streptococci, *Staphylococcus aureus*, *Enterobacteriaceae*, anaerobes
Cephalosporins	
First generation	
Cefazolin	*Staphylococcus aureus*, streptococci, few gram-negative species
Second generation	
Cefotaxime or ceftriaxone	Streptococci, *Haemophilus influenzae*, *Staphylococcus aureus*, Enterobacteriaceae, *Neisseria gonorrhoeae*
Cefoxitin	Anaerobes, *Enterobacteriaceae*, *Neisseria gonorrhoeae*
Third generation	
Ceftazidime	Excellent coverage for *Pseudomonas aeruginosa*
Imipenem	Good general coverage
Aztreonam	Gram-negative coverage only
Gentamicin ⎫ Tobramycin ⎭	Anaerobic and facultative anaerobic gram-negative bacilli, tobramycin best against *Pseudomonas*
Quinolones	
Ciprofloxacin	Most gram-positive and gram-negative but poor anaerobic coverage
Levofloxacin	Same as ciprofloxacin but better *Staphylococcus* coverage
Vancomycin	Gram-positive with excellent coverage for *Staphylococcus aureus*, *Staphylococcus epidermidis*, streptococci, enterococci, clostridia
Clindamycin	*Staphylococcus aureus*, streptococci, clostridia
Metronidazole	Anaerobic bacteria

TABLE 2. SUGGESTED ANTIBIOTICS FOR SPECIFIC INFECTIONS

Infection	Antibiotic
Felon	Penicillins, clindamycin, cephalosporin
Purulent flexor	Cephalosporins, ampicillin/sulbactam; vancomycin quinolone; ceftriaxone
Fungal	Oral potassium iodide (SSKI) for subcutaneous *Sporothrix schenckii*
	Topical fungal cream
	Amphotericin B
Intravenous drug abuse	Penicillins plus aminoglycosides, ampicillin/sulbactam
	Vancomycin plus aminoglycoside
Bite wounds	Penicillins plus cephalosporins, ampicillin/sulbactam
	Clindamycin plus quinolones
Pyarthrosis	Cephalosporins plus aminoglycoside, penicillins; vancomycin, clindamycin
Osteomyelitis	Penicillins plus quinolones
	Cephalosporins plus aminoglycoside
	Vancomycin (particularly if there is retained metal fixation from prior surgery and *Staphylococcus epidermidis* is considered)
Necrotizing fasciitis	Piperacillin plus quinolone, imipenem
Gangrenous infections	Penicillin, hyperbaric oxygen
Atypical mycobacterial	Tetracycline or minocycline plus antituberculosis medication
Tuberculosis	Isoniazid, ethambutol, rifampin

logical agents, and Table 2 provides some empiric coverage suggestions. Final antibiotic coverage should be altered according to the culture sensitivities of the particular organism obtained from the area of infection. Availability of newer drugs and increasing microbial resistance to various antibiotics make coordination of treatment with infectious disease specialists particularly helpful.

Radiographs should be taken as part of the evaluation of an upper extremity infection. Any foreign bodies, fractures, gas in the tissues, or osseous changes consistent with osteomyelitis should be noted (Fig. 1).

Initial dressings and splinting of the wrists and digits must be applied appropriately to avoid stiffness and contractures. The initiation of motion exercises as soon as is possible is critical to ensure maximal recovery of function. Coordination of care with an appropriately trained hand therapist is suggested.

SPECIFIC ANATOMIC LOCATIONS

The unique anatomy of the hand with its various true and potential spaces suggests that the discussion of the surgical treatment of hand infections be anatomically based.

PULP SPACE INFECTIONS (FELONS)

The pulps of the fingers have fibrous septa that lend structural support for the pinching and grasping integral in all daily activities. These bands create many small compartments in which infection may occur. Most often, a history of a penetrating injury can be documented.

A pulp space infection is manifested by severe pain, tenderness, and swelling of the pulp. Aspiration of the pulp may yield a false-negative result, because an isolated compartment with pus may not specifically be entered with the needle. Tenderness of the pulp is usually present from the onset of the infection, but obvious "pointing" of the abscess may not be seen. Osteomyelitis of the adjacent distal phalanx occurs, because the distal phalanx is intimately related to the pulp, but rarely does the infection lead to a purulent flexor tenosynovitis.[16]

Surgical drainage can be accomplished by various incisions, including a longitudinal incision directly over the area of "pointing," or incision on the border of the digit just below the nail and extending distally to the midline[16, 17] of the fingertip. "Fish mouth" incisions, those extending from one border to the other across the hyponychium, are to be condemned, because they frequently lead to unsightly, painful scars. Attention must be directed toward ensuring that all compartments are decompressed. The distal phalanx should be palpated to evaluate for the presence of soft bone, which might indicate osteomyelitis. The wound should be packed open to allow for continued drainage; the packing should be removed after 24 to 48 hours to allow for healing by secondary intention. Daily soaks in saline or irrigation of the wounds should be done during the early postoperative course. If the bone is also involved, then débridement or amputation of the distal phalanx is necessary, depending on the extent of the bone involvement. Disarticulation through the distal interphalangeal joint may provide a more functional digit in very advanced cases.

The usual infecting organism in a pulp space infection is a *Staphylococcus* species, and antibiotics should be selected accordingly.

PARONYCHIAL INFECTIONS

Paronychial infections are the most common infections of the upper extremity. Most often, the infection occurs as a

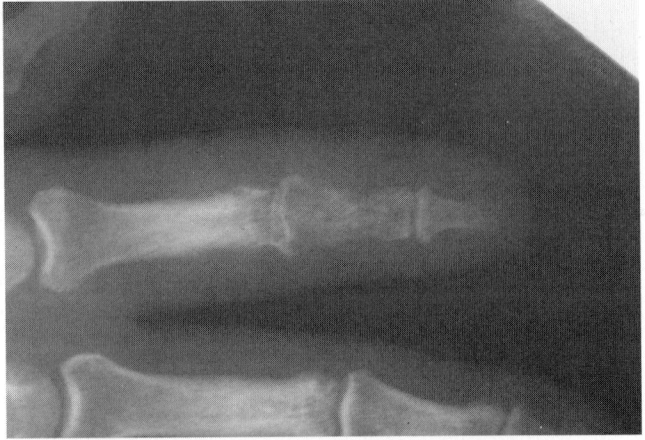

Fig. 1. Osteomyelitis in the index finger. A 60-year-old man had chronic drainage from the finger for 3 months after lacerating it in a fall in brackish water. Before presenting at our facility, he was treated with oral and long-term intravenous antibiotics. On presentation to us, his finger was swollen, erythematous, and painful. A radiograph (the first one in his clinical course) revealed osteomyelitis of the middle phalanx. Cultures grew *Aeromonas hydrophila.*

result of minor trauma in this area from a hangnail, poorly performed manicure, or fingernail biting.[17, 18] The paronychia is the region immediately radial and ulnar to the fingernail, and the eponychium is just proximal to the nail. Infections in these areas can be isolated to either side of the nail or confluent to span both sides of the nail involving the eponychium. Early treatment of an acute paronychial infection begins with warm soaks and oral antibiotics that cover the most likely organism, usually a *Staphylococcus* species. In chronic cases, the microbial flora may be different, and cultures may yield gram-negative bacteria and/or fungal species such as *Candida albicans.*[18] Surgical drainage is necessary if more conservative measures fail to resolve the infection. Partial nail excision or careful incision at the paronychial-eponychial junction should be used. Care is necessary to avoid injury to the underlying nail matrix. An alternative surgical treatment particularly useful in chronic infections is marsupialization of a portion of the skin just proximal to the distal eponychium and wound granulation.[18, 19]

Because paronychial infections are common and usually easily treated, a chronic paronychial infection or one that appears difficult to control should raise suspicion of underlying disease entities such as diabetes that render the host immunocompromised.[7]

HERPETIC INFECTIONS OF THE DIGITS

This infection is a superficial viral infection caused by the herpes simplex virus and does not represent a deep pulp space bacterial infection of the hand. These infections occur in both adult and pediatric populations. Medical and dental personnel are at higher risk in the adult population.[13, 20, 21]

This type of infection presents as a vesicular lesion containing clear to turbid fluid. If turbid, the fluid might resemble pus, but generally the fluid is less viscous in consistency than pus. Local erythema and tenderness may be present but generally to a lesser degree than in bacterial infections.[4] These patients may present with fever, lymphadenopathy, and lymphangitis.[22] The signs and symptoms of infection generally run their course over a 10- to 21-day period, but shedding of the virus may continue for about 2 weeks after the initial signs and symptoms have subsided. The diagnosis can usually be made clinically. Occasionally, however, a Tzanck smear or viral culture may prove helpful.

Nonsurgical management is the treatment of choice, because incision and drainage of these lesions can lead to secondary bacterial infections.[13, 21] Topical acyclovir is not necessary or indicated; however, it can be used intravenously for severe cases and for the immunocompromised patient. Cross-contamination among patients, with hospital personnel serving as the vector, has been observed.[7, 23] Thus, attention to prevention is essential.

PALMAR SPACE INFECTIONS

The palm of the hand has three potential spaces that are commonly involved with infections: the thenar, hypothenar, and midpalmar spaces (Fig. 2). Two other areas in the hand, the dorsal subaponeurotic space and the web spaces, are often confused with palmar spaces. A more proximally located potential space, Parona's space, occupies the distal forearm between the flexor profundus tendons volar and the dorsal pronator quadratus muscle.

The hypothenar space is that potential space between the hypothenar musculature and fascia overlying the hypothenar muscles. Drainage incisions should be placed to avoid the ulnar border of the hand and the hypothenar eminence, because both locations have significant contact with surfaces in daily activities. The incision is best placed on the radial aspect of the hypothenar eminence.[24, 25]

The thenar space is bound on the ulnar border by a fascial band from the palmar aspect of the third metacarpal to the palmar fascia and on the radial border by the fascia and musculature inserting on the proximal phalanx of the thumb. Dorsally, the space is bounded by the adductor pollicis muscle. Volarly, the space is bounded by the flexor pollicis longus and flexor digitorum profundus to the index finger. Surgical drainage can be achieved by a volar incision in line with the thenar crease (making sure to avoid

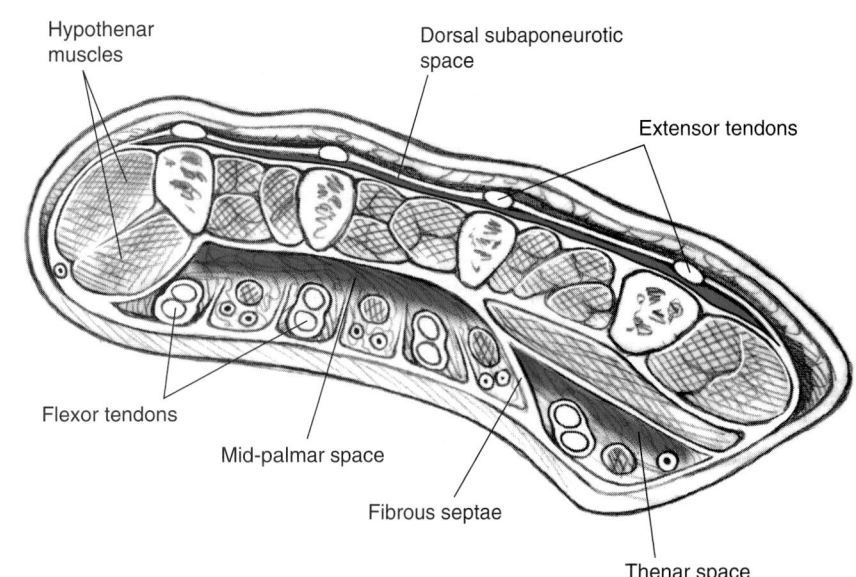

Fig. 2. Palmar spaces.

Hypothenar muscles

Dorsal subaponeurotic space

Extensor tendons

Flexor tendons

Mid-palmar space

Fibrous septae

Thenar space

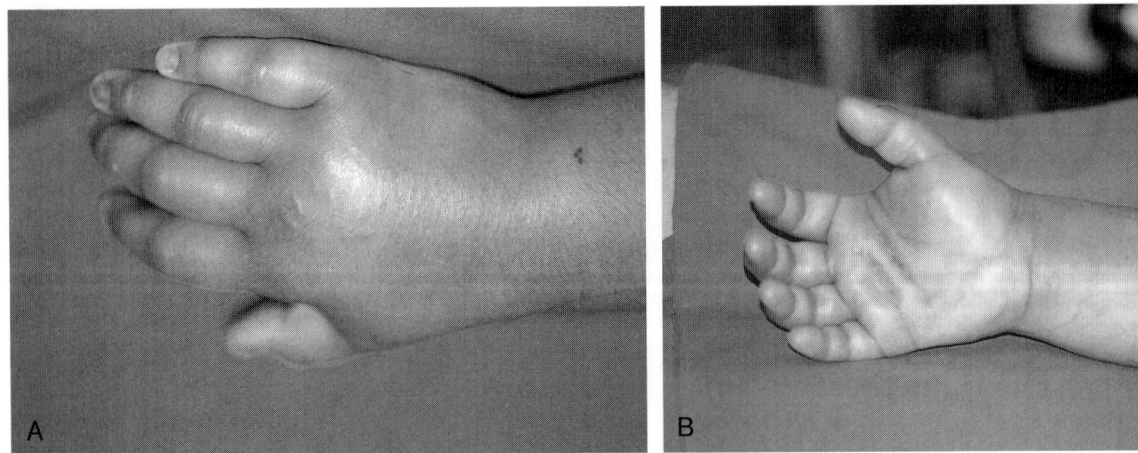

Figure 3. Midpalmar space infection. *A* and *B*, This is a photograph of a 15-year-old girl with a 2-week history of pain and swelling of her hand. She had been treated with intravenous antibiotics for 3 days with little improvement (note the swelling dorsally and loss of the palmar contour of the hand).

the recurrent branch of the median nerve). A dorsal straight line incision over the first dorsal web space is a good alternative, and this incision can be used in combination with the volar incision to obtain adequate drainage.

The midpalmar space is located deep to the flexor tendons and is bound radially by the same fascia forming the ulnar border of the thenar space. The ulnar border of the midpalmar space is the hypothenar musculature. Palmar incisions should be used for drainage.

The diagnosis of palmar space infections may be delayed, because the spaces lie deep to much of the soft-tissue structures in the palm. Although the palmar contour of the hand is usually lost,[25] there may be swelling including or restricted to the dorsum of the hand (Figs. 3 and 4). Therefore, a high index of suspicion must be present to avoid delays in diagnosis, because these delays frequently occur with false-negative aspirations through the dorsum of the hand.

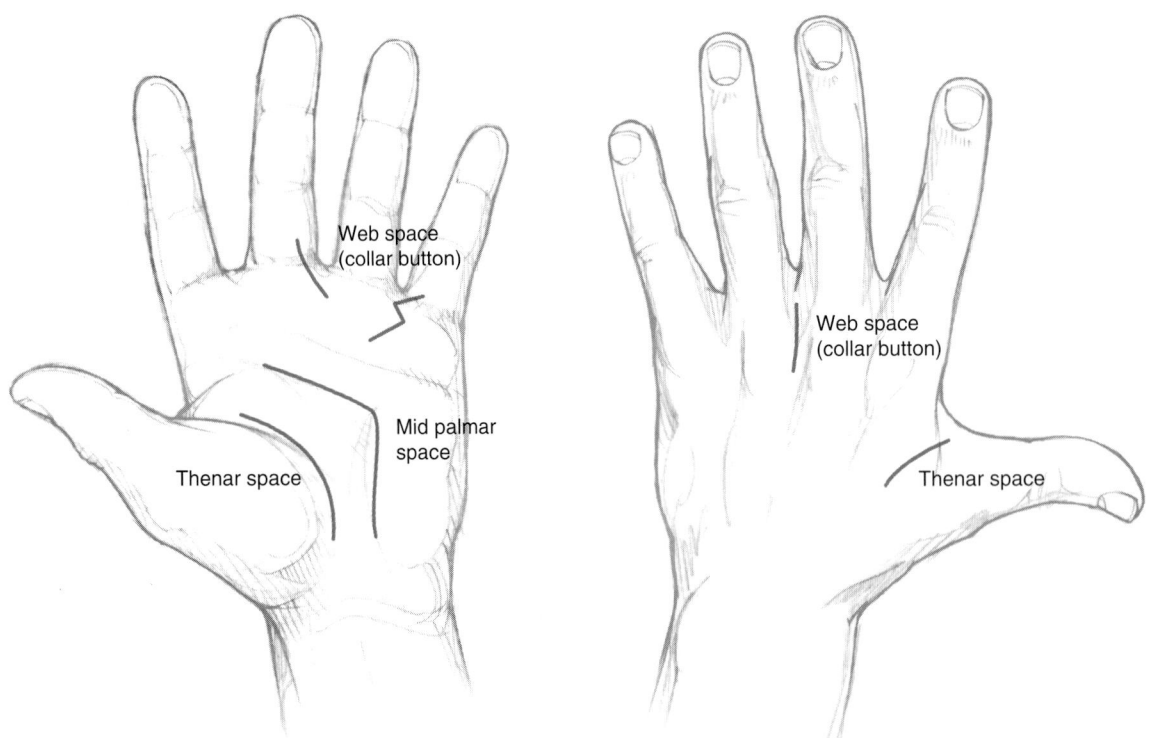

Web space
(collar button)

Mid palmar
space

Thenar space

Web space
(collar button)

Thenar space

Fig. 4. Suggested incisions for drainage of palmar space infections.

WEB SPACE (COLLAR BUTTON) ABSCESSES

The palmar fascia and its attachments to the skin at the level of the web spaces permit infections to begin superficially on the palm and then dissect through a small opening in the fascia to migrate dorsally.[26, 27] These infections present with either a tender palmar abscess pointing in the palm or relatively minimal swelling in the palm but are associated with marked swelling on the dorsum of the web space. In either presentation, purulence should be suspected both dorsally and volarly. Therefore, both dorsal and volar incisions are recommended for appropriate surgical drainage.[24, 25] The volar incision in the web should never be oriented transversely, because this leads to web space contractures. Oblique or zigzag incisions are thus recommended on the volar surface, whereas straight longitudinal incisions should be used on the dorsum of the hand (Fig. 5).

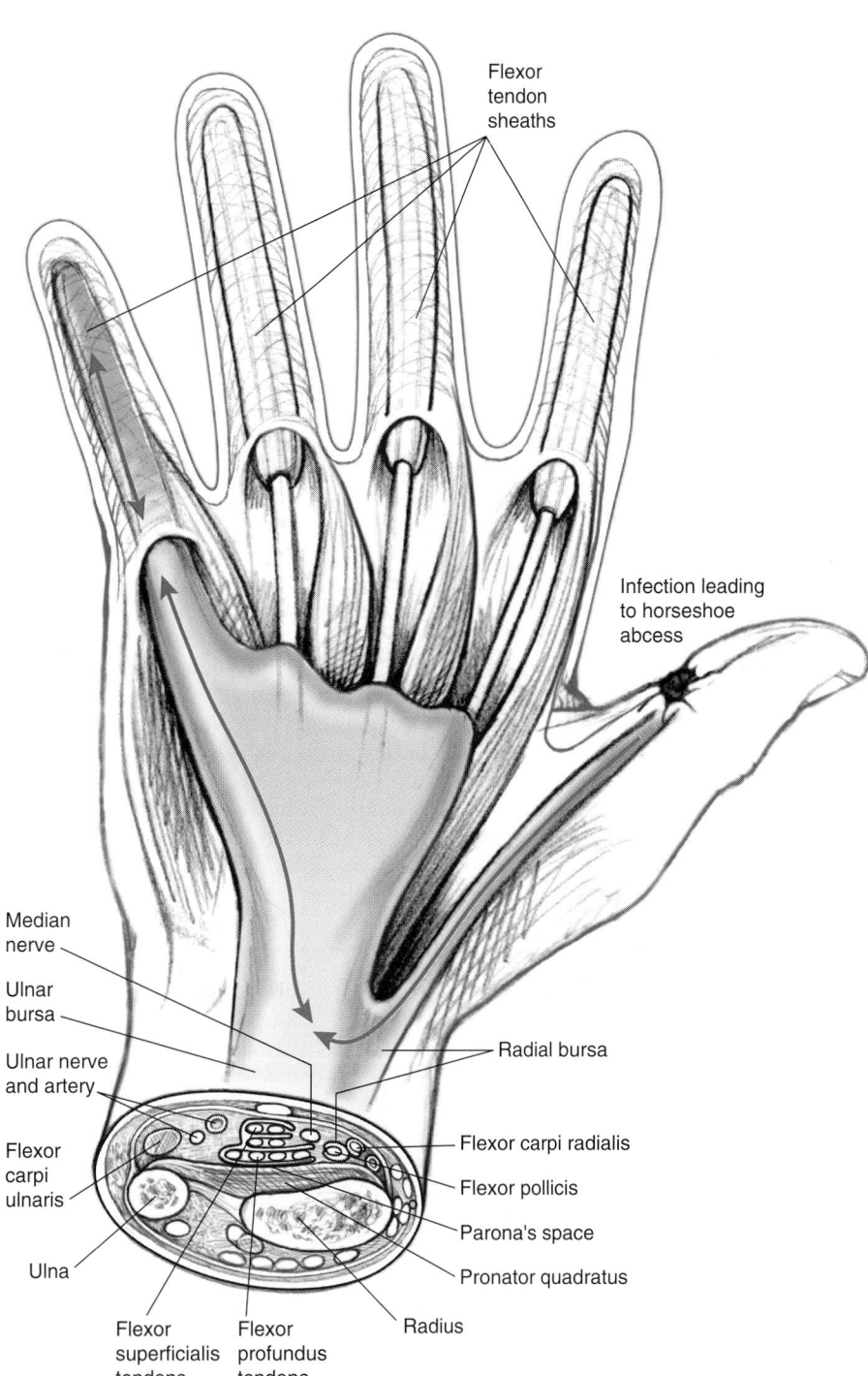

Fig. 5. "Horseshoe" abscess.

PURULENT FLEXOR TENOSYNOVITIS

The flexor tendon sheaths provide nutrition of the tendons and a gliding surface facilitating functional tendon excursion. The flexor tendon sheaths of the index, long, and ring fingers begin proximal to the proximal border of the deep transverse metacarpal ligaments[28] and extend to the level of the distal interphalangeal joints. The tendon sheaths of the little finger and thumb are confluent with the ulnar and radial bursae, respectively, and, therefore, have the potential for extension proximally to the forearm level via the radial and ulnar bursal communications. Additionally, communication between the radial and ulnar bursae is possible via Parona's space (the potential space in the forearm between the pronator quadratus muscle and the flexor profundus tendons). Involvement of the radial and ulnar bursae via Parona's space represents the "horseshoe abscess" (see Fig. 5).

Penetrating trauma is the most common cause of purulent infection involving the tendon sheaths.[24, 29] However, hematogenous spread from other infected regions has also been reported.

The classic "four signs of Kanavel" have been the foundation for the clinical diagnosis of purulent flexor tenosynovitis: tenderness to palpation along the flexor sheath, slightly flexed posture of the involved digit, fusiform (diffuse) swelling of the digit, and excruciating pain with passive extension of the digit (Fig. 6).[30] One must distinguish localized swelling observed with a subcutaneous abscess from the true fusiform swelling of purulent flexor tenosynovitis. To establish true pain with passive extension of the digit, it is useful to stabilize the finger while manipulating only the distal interphalangeal joint. This helps isolate flexor tendon motion and differentiates pain of purulent flexor tenosynovitis from more proximal joint pyarthrosis or local wound pain.

Although some early cases may be treated solely with parenteral antibiotics, very rapid improvement must occur or surgical intervention is necessary. In fact, because of the minimum of space within the tendon sheaths, increased sheath pressure may be a likely factor in the development of tendon necrosis.[25, 31] Partial treatment complicates decision making and often delays the proper diagnosis, thereby contributing to additional tendon and sheath injury. Prompt surgical drainage is, therefore, the prudent course when treating purulent flexor tenosynovitis. Surgical management requires adequate drainage of the sheaths. Neviaser[29] popularized the concept of "closed tendon sheath irrigation," which accomplishes drainage and allows for rapid wound healing and early motion. An incision is made in the palm just proximal to the A1 pulley of the involved digit. A small midlateral incision is made distally in the finger, and the tendon sheath is entered just distal to the A4 pulley at the middle phalanx. A 16- or 18-gauge angiocatheter is inserted approximately 1 to 2 inches into the proximal end of the tendon sheath, and a small drain is placed in the distal incision. Irrigation with sterile saline is continued until the effluent is clear. Sterile dressings and splints are then applied. Postoperatively, the system is irrigated with 50 mL of saline every 2 hours, and at 48 hours the catheter and drains are removed and an exercise program is begun. This method has proved quite successful and enables rapid healing of the wounds. It requires the cooperation of the patient and good ancillary care to ensure that the catheter remains patent and that irrigation is performed properly. Modifications of the closed sheath irrigation technique have been described[25, 31, 32] and share certain similarities. Common to all of these methods is the principle of instituting early range-of-motion exercises.

PYARTHROSIS (INFECTION OF THE JOINTS)

Traumatic injuries are the most common cause of pyarthrosis in the hand. *S. aureus* and *Streptococcus* species remain the most common causative organisms,[33] with the exception of infection arising from bite wounds. Erythema, swelling, and pain (particularly with joint motion) are the cardinal signs of joint infection. Pain not related to joint motion may indicate a local abscess rather than a septic joint.

When there is no identifiable traumatic insult, the immune status of the patient should be investigated. In the young adult, a sexual history should be obtained, with an awareness that gonococcal septic arthritis or tenosynovitis can occur. Rheumatoid variants and the crystalline deposition diseases need to be considered in the differential diagnosis of septic arthritis of the hand.[33]

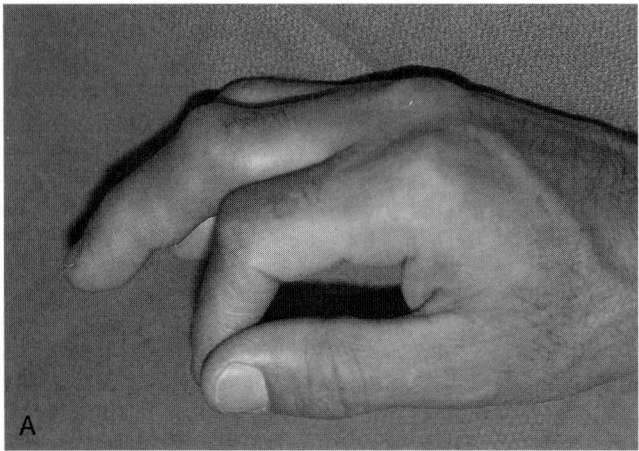
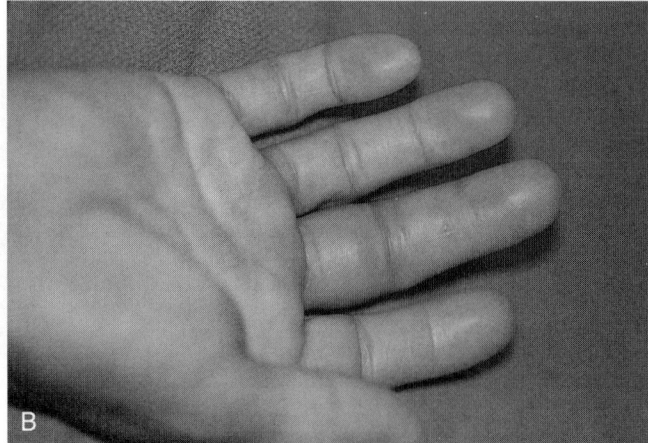

Fig. 6. Purulent flexor tenosynovitis.

Management of septic arthritis includes surgical débridement, with carefully planned surgical incisions. The goal of this approach is preserving the extensor mechanism to prevent late deformity, such as a "septic boutonnière" deformity of the proximal interphalangeal joints.[34] Intravenous antibiotics should be continued for at least 2 to 4 weeks followed by oral administration of antibiotics for a total of 6 weeks of antibiotics after the surgical débridement.

OSTEOMYELITIS (INFECTION OF THE BONES)

Infection of the osseous structures of the upper extremity is most often caused by penetrating trauma or by predisposing conditions such as vascular disease, connective tissue disease, or diabetes.[33] Chronic intravenous drug abuse has also been known to lead to osteomyelitis. When resulting from direct trauma, osteomyelitis is usually secondary to *S. aureus* or *Streptococcus* species. However, mutilating injuries may be associated with mixed gram-positive and gram-negative species.[35] Human bite wounds are predisposed to infections with skin and oral flora. *Staphylococcus epidermidis* osteomyelitis usually occurs after fracture management and is often associated with foreign body internal fixation devices.

Clinically, erythema and tenderness are present. However, the initial diagnosis is generally made with radiographs. Therefore, radiographs should always be obtained to evaluate for the presence of bone involvement.

Surgical débridement of necrotic bone and tissue is the mainstay of treatment, because antibiotic agents cannot penetrate devitalized tissue. Infection in the setting of recent internal fixation requires that the integrity of the fixation be evaluated. If rigid fixation is lost, removal of the implant and alternative stabilization become necessary. If the fixation is secure, then it should be maintained. Widely infected bone needs to be excised, often necessitating extensive reconstructive procedures.

Intravenous antibiotics should be given for at least 4 to 6 weeks, with continued oral antibiotics for suppressive therapy as indicated by the clinical setting.

SPECIFIC INFECTIOUS PROCESSES BY DISEASE PROCESS

TUBERCULOSIS

During the last 10 years, tuberculosis has had a resurgence in the United States in both the pulmonary and musculoskeletal systems.[36] Because of the increasing numbers of immunocompromised patients, a growing population of elderly individuals, and increased travel among nations, there are now an estimated 10 million persons with mycobacterial tuberculosis in the United States. One-fifth of the newly diagnosed cases are associated with extrapulmonary disease.[36] Involvement of the elbow, wrist, and hand represents 2% of those with musculoskeletal involvement. Worldwide, tuberculosis is the most common chronic infection of the hand.[36]

The clinical presentation can be quite insidious, because only one-third of patients with bone involvement have a history of pulmonary disease.[16, 36] Swelling without erythema or increased warmth might indicate a "cold abscess." Radiographs are notable for their distinct lack of bone destruction. Osteopenia, minimal periosteal reaction, and joint narrowing may be subtle findings indicating tubercular joint involvement.[36] The false-negative rates of skin testing for tuberculosis are reportedly as high as 20%.

Aspiration is often nondiagnostic; therefore, it is imperative that tissue biopsy and culture samples be taken. Aerobic, anaerobic, fungal, and mycobacterial cultures should be taken if there is any doubt about the type of infecting organism. Biopsy specimens are performed in these suspected mycobacterial or fungal infections, because cultures take an extended period of time, causing a delay in appropriate treatment when cultures are solely relied on. Specific culture conditions should be requested, because *Mycobacterium tuberculosis* is best grown on Löwenstein-Jensen medium at 37°C, whereas some atypical mycobacteria grow at cooler (30°C to 32°C) temperatures.

Aggressive débridement of all infected tissues is essential. As opposed to purulent bacterial infections, primary wound closure is acceptable when treating mycobacterial infections, although inadequate débridement can lead to wound dehiscence. Appropriate pharmacological agents are necessary, and coordination of patient management with infectious disease consultants is strongly recommended.

ATYPICAL MYCOBACTERIA

Despite the increasing incidence of atypical mycobacterial infections, delay in diagnosis remains frequent[37] because of the indolent nature of these infections. A history of exposure to environments in which these organisms are prevalent should be pursued. Examples include *Mycobacterium marinum* in wounds with aquatic exposure and *Mycobacterium terrae* in wounds with farm exposure.[37] *Mycobacterium avium* complex has an increased prevalence in the immunocompromised population, particularly those with HIV infection.[37]

Skin tests and acid-fast smears are unreliable; therefore, as with tuberculosis, biopsy may be necessary to confirm the diagnosis. Appropriate culture conditions for atypical mycobacteria are performed at a temperature of 30°C to 32°C on Löwenstein-Jensen medium. Aggressive surgical débridement and proper pharmacological agents should be instituted based on history, clinical presentation, and biopsy specimen, because culture identification may take 3 to 6 weeks.[37] Antibiotic therapy is given for at least 4 months. Tetracycline or minocycline are primary drugs of choice; however, combination therapy may be necessary, including antituberculosis medications. Coordination of patient management with infectious disease consultants is again recommended.

INFECTIONS RESULTING FROM PARENTERAL DRUG ABUSE

There is a high prevalence of gram-positive organisms, especially *Staphylococcus* and *Streptococcus* species, in patients with a history of intravenous drug abuse.[1, 38, 39] Gram-negative organisms are also observed in patients older than 40 years.[1] This may be due to changes related to chronic drug use resulting in destruction of peripheral lymphatics.[40] Wide débridement and aggressive wound care are the mainstays of treatment. Antibiotics should provide good aerobic, anaerobic, gram-positive, and gram-negative cover-

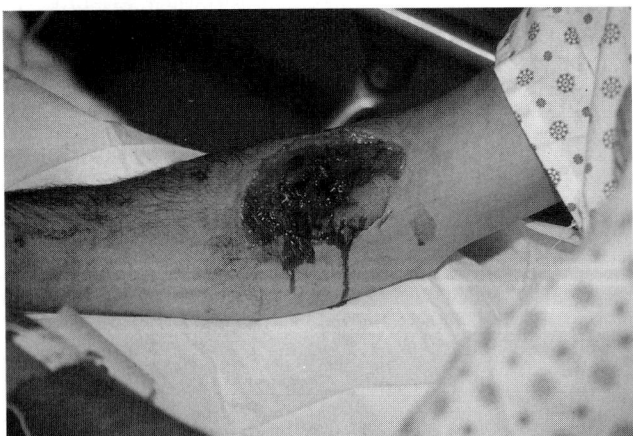

Fig. 7. Large wound caused by dog bite.

age. Associated underlying diseases such as hepatitis and HIV must be considered in this patient population.

BITE WOUNDS

Approximately 1 to 2 million animal bites are treated by physicians per year; dog, cat, and human bites are responsible for 1% of all emergency room visits.[15, 41, 42]

Dog and Cat Bites

Dog and cat bites tend to be seasonal, with a greater incidence in warmer weather. Dog bites represent 80% of all animal bites. In nearly 70% of cases, the dog is known to the victim.[15] Despite the significant pressure exerted during dog bites (up to 450 psi),[41] only 15% to 20% of dog bites become infected.[15] This may be due to the blunt nature of canine teeth and the fact that the wounds inflicted are large, tearing lacerations (Fig. 7). Cat bites, in contrast, have greater than 50% incidence of infection,[15] most likely because of their sharp, needle-like teeth. Because of the nature of feline teeth, they essentially "inject" bacteria into the wound. The bacteriology of dog and cat bites is similar with a combination of aerobic and anaerobic bacteria.[41–43] *Pasteurella multocida* is a gram-negative aerobic and facultative anaerobic organism, is sensitive to penicillin, and is identified in 50% of cat bite infections and in some dog bite infections.[44]

Human Bites

True human bite wounds occur at the fingertips, phalangeal, or metacarpophalangeal level in approximately 85% of cases. In clenched-fist injuries, the joint is violated in 68% of cases. Tendon and bone injuries occur in 20% and 17% of cases, respectively.[45] These wounds should be thoroughly explored, with an awareness that the extensor tendon injury may lie at a more proximal level than the skin wound because of the distal excursion of the tendon that occurs in the clenched fist. Ample incisions should be made both proximal and distal to the skin wound to facilitate proper exploration.[45, 46] Bites inflicted by humans have a mixture of aerobic and anaerobic organisms.[15, 43, 45–48]

One common mouth flora organism is *Eikenella corrodens*, a gram-negative facultative anaerobe.[15, 49] Cultures for aerobic and anaerobic organisms should be requested to maximize the potential of identification of this species.

Human bites, when seen early before established infection and in the absence of bone or joint violation, may potentially be treated on an outpatient basis. This is true only if adequate wound lavage can be performed, broad-spectrum antibiotics are used, and the patient is clearly compliant and reliable.[47, 50] Late presentation,[47] established infection, or bone or joint violation associated with a human bite warrants hospitalization for débridement and intravenous antibiotics.

Combinations of cephalosporins and penicillins or ampicillin/sulbactam should be used. Patients allergic to these drugs should receive either clindamycin or vancomycin.

FUNGAL INFECTIONS

The most common fungal infections of the hand involve the skin and nail. As mentioned, *C. albicans* is usually the pathogen isolated in chronic paronychial infections. *Sporothrix schenckii,* however, remains the most frequent isolate in fungal infections, other than paronychial infections, of the hand. This saprophyte is found in soil and plant materials and can exist in essentially any climate. Those who work in an environment where they are susceptible to penetration by thorns or dirt (gardeners) are at risk. An isolated ulceration may develop at the site of injury initially, but subsequently with lymphatic spread the lymphatics become indurated with subcutaneous nodules along the path. These nodules may ulcerate, giving a violaceous appearance. Treatment has previously included saturated solutions of potassium iodide, although newer orally absorbable agents such as itraconazole may be more efficacious in treating this and other fungi.[51] Treatment should continue for at least 6 weeks.

Other infections include coccidioidomycosis, histoplasmosis, mucormycosis, aspergillosis, and candidiasis. A careful history must include data on travel, birthplace, and a possible immunocompromised status (Fig. 8). Débridement is necessary. However, the mainstay of treatment of fungal infections of the upper extremity is the appropriate use of pharmacological agents.

NECROTIZING SOFT-TISSUE INFECTIONS

Necrotizing soft-tissue infections are characterized by the rapid progression of necrosis of skin, subcutaneous fat, and

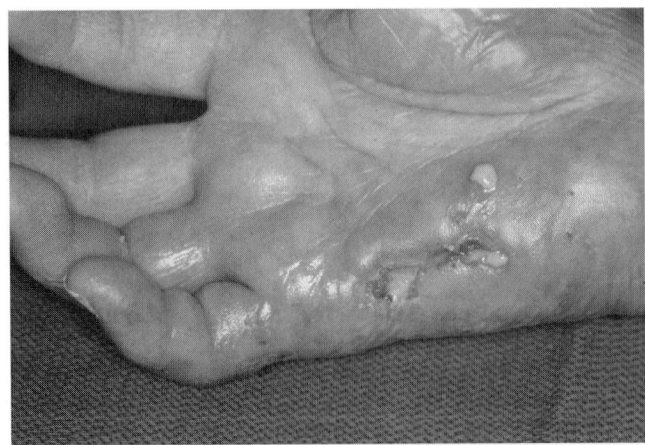

Fig. 8. Mucormycosis in a patient with diabetes.

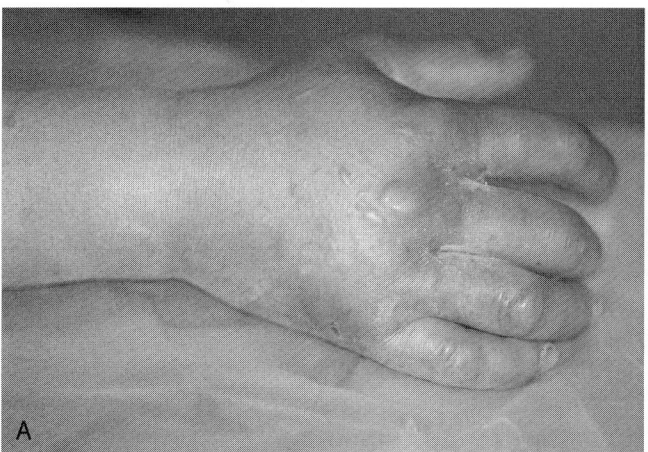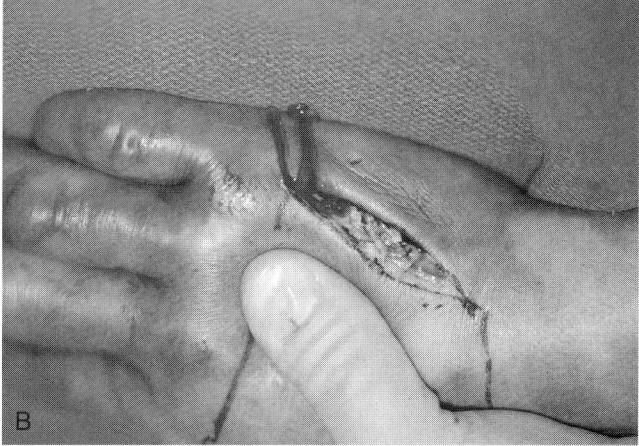

Fig. 9. Early necrotizing fasciitis. *A* and *B,* This man had fallen and suffered a small puncture wound to his hand 16 hours before presentation. Admission temperature was 102°F, and his white blood cell count was greater than 16,000. Note the marked edema and early vesicle formation of the hand and "dishwater" fluid rather than frank purulence noted on initial incision.

fascia. Muscle is not involved. Since the first description in 1871 by Joseph Jones, several terms have been used to describe this entity, including Fournier's disease, Meleney's gangrene, hemolytic streptococcal gangrene, and, most recently in the media, "flesh-eating disease."

Clinically, there is a history of trauma and the onset may mimic cellulitis in its early stages. However, the rapid clinical progression and the significant morbidity and mortality rates associated with the disease require a high index of suspicion and early diagnosis crucial. The condition is generally characterized by edema extending beyond the zone of erythema. Skin vesicles, bullae, and subcutaneous gas may be present; however, lymphangitis is absent. Progression of the disease leads to skin anesthesia, ecchymosis, induration, and necrosis as well as fever, hypotension, and eventually septic shock. The diagnosis may be easily missed when the aspiration does not return frank pus for the unsuspecting physician. At surgery, gray necrotic fascia is noted (Fig. 9). With frozen-section histopathological analysis, there is thrombosis of the small arteries and veins, fascial necrosis, and bacteria. These bacteria are usually polymicrobial combinations of non–group A streptococci, *Staphylococcus* species, gram-negative aerobes, including *Proteus, Pseudomonas, Enterobacter, Escherichia coli,* and *Klebsiella* in addition to various anaerobes.

Treatment requires aggressive fluid and blood product resuscitation, electrolyte monitoring, and broad-spectrum antibiotics with triple pharmacological agents such as the combination of penicillin, aminoglycoside, and clindamycin or ampicillin, piperacillin, and imipenem. However, the most important aspect of the treatment of the condition remains immediate diagnosis and adequate extensive surgical débridement of all necrotic and indurated tissue. Multiple débridements may be necessary.[52] Overall mortality rates have been as high as 38% but can be reduced to less than 15% if managed appropriately. A high index of suspicion and aggressive surgical and intravenous antibiotic management cannot be overemphasized.

Management of these patients is analogous to that of the severely burned patient, making a team effort by surgeons, infectious disease specialists, nutritionists, and therapists mandatory.

REFERENCES

1. Schnall SB, Holtom PD, Lilley JC: Abscesses secondary to parenteral abuse of drugs. J Bone Joint Surg Am 1994; 76: 1526.
2. Schnall SB, Thommen V, Holtom P, et al: Delayed primary closure of infections. Clin Orthop Rel Res 1997; 335:286.
3. Senay EC: Drug abuse and public health a global perspective. Drug Safety 1991; 6:1.
4. McLain RF, Steyers C, Stoddard M: Infections in open fractures of the hand. J Hand Surg Am 1991; 16:108.
5. Glass KD: Factors related to the resolution of treated hand infections. J Hand Surg Am 1982; 7:388.
6. Francel TJ, Marshall KA, Savage RC: Hand infections in the diabetic and the diabetic renal transplant recipient. Ann Plast Surg 1990; 24:304.

7. Glickel SZ: Hand infections in patients with acquired immunodeficiency syndrome. J Hand Surg Am 1988; 13:770.
8. Mandel M: Immune competence and diabetes mellitus: Pyogenic human hand infections. J Hand Surg Am 1978; 3:458.
9. Mann RJ, Peacock JM: Hand infections in patients with diabetes mellitus. J Trauma 1977; 17:376.
10. Kann SE, Jacquemin JB, Stern PJ: Simulators of hand infections. J Bone Joint Surg Am 1996; 78:1114.
11. Stromberg BV: Retreatment of previously treated hand infections. J Trauma 1985; 25:163.
12. Spiegel JD, Szabo RM: A protocol for the treatment of severe infections of the hand. J Hand Surg Am 1988; 13:254.
13. Hurst LC, Gluck R, Sampson SP, et al:

Herpetic whitlow with bacterial abscess. J Hand Surg Am 1991; 16:311.
14. Scott JC, Jones BV: Results of treatment of infections of the hand. J Bone Joint Surg Br 1952; 34:581.
15. Goldstein EJC: Bite wounds and infection. Clin Infect Dis 1992; 14:633.
16. Bolton H, Fowler PJ, Manchester J: Natural history and treatment of pulp space infection and osteomyelitis of the terminal phalanx. Orthop Clin North Am 1949; 31: 499.
17. Canales FL, Newmeyer WL III, Kilgore ES Jr: The treatment of felons and paronychias. Hand Clin 1989; 5:515.
18. Bednar MS, Lane LB: Eponychial marsupialization and nail removal for surgical treatment of chronic paronychia. J Hand Surg Am 1991; 16:314.

19. Keyser JJ, Eaton RG: Surgical cure of chronic paronychia by eponychial marsupialization. Plast Reconstr Surg 1976; 58: 66.

20. Bleicher JN, Blinn DL, Massop D: Hand infections in dental personnel. Plast Reconstr Surg 1987; 80:420.

21. Louis DS, Silva J: Herpetic whitlow: Herpetic infections of the digits. J Hand Surg Am 1979; 4:90.

22. Walker LG, Simmons BP, Lovallo JL: Pediatric herpetic hand infections. J Hand Surg Am 1990; 15:176.

23. Stern H, Elek SD, Millar DM, et al: Herpetic whitlow: A form of cross infection in hospitals. Lancet 1959; 2:871.

24. Neviaser RJ, Green DP (eds): Operative Hand Surgery. New York, Churchill Livingstone, 1988, 2nd ed, vol 3.

25. Floyd WE III, Troum S, Frankle MA: Acute and chronic sepsis. In Peimer C (ed): Surgery of the Hand and Upper Extremity. New York, McGraw-Hill, 1996, p 1731.

26. Bunnell S: Surgery of the Hand. Philadelphia, JB Lippincott, 1948, 2nd ed.

27. Linscheid RL, Dobyns JH: Common and uncommon infections of the hand. Orthop Clin North Am 1975; 6:1063.

28. Kaplan EB: Functional and Surgical Anatomy of the Hand. Philadelphia, JB Lippincott, 1953.

29. Neviaser RJ: Closed tendon sheath irrigation for pyogenic flexor tenosynovitis. J Hand Surg Am 1978; 3:462.

30. Kanavel AB: Infections of the Hand. Philadelphia, Lea & Febiger, 1925, 5th ed, p 201.

31. Schnall SB, Vu-Rose T, Holtom PD, et al: Tissue pressures in pyogenic flexor tenosynovitis of the finger. J Bone Joint Surg Br 1996; 78:793.

32. Juliano PJ, Eglseder WA: Limited open-tendon-sheath irrigation in the treatment of pyogenic flexor tenosynovitis. Orthop Rev 1991; 20:1065.

33. Freeland AE, Senter BS: Septic arthritis and osteomyelitis. Hand Clin 1989; 5:533.

34. Wittels NP, Donley JM, Burkhalter WE: A functional treatment method for interphalangeal pyogenic arthritis. J Hand Surg Am 1984; 9:894.

35. Fitzgerald RH, Cooney WP, Washington JA, et al: Bacterial colonization of mutilating hand injuries and its treatment. J Hand Surg Am 1977; 2:85.

36. Watts HG, Lifeso RM: Current concepts review: Tuberculosis of bones and joints. J Bone Joint Surg Am 1966; 78:288.

37. Kozin SH, Bishop AT: Atypical mycobacterium infections of the upper extremity. J Hand Surg Am 1994; 19:480.

38. Biederman P, Hiatt JR: Management of soft-tissue infections of the upper extremity in parenteral drug abusers. Am J Surg 1987; 154:526.

39. Orangio GR, Pitlick SD, Della-Latta P, et al: Soft-tissue infections in parenteral drug abusers. Ann Surg 1984; 99:97.

40. Neviaser RJ, Butterfield WC, Wieche DR: The puffy hand of drug addiction. J Bone Joint Surg Am 1972; 54:629.

41. Anderson CR: Animal bites. Postgrad Med 1992; 92:134.

42. Wiggins ME, Akelman E, Weiss APC: The management of dog bites and dog bite infections to the hand. Orthopedics 1994; 17:617.

43. Goldstein EJ, Citron DM: Comparative susceptibilities of 173 aerobic and anaerobic bite wound isolates to sparfloxacin, temafloxacin, clarithromycin, and older agents. Antimicrob Agents Chemother 1993; 37:1150.

44. Arons MS, Fernando L, Polayes IM: *Pasteurella multocida:* The major cause of hand infections following domestic animal bites. J Hand Surg Am 1982; 7:47.

45. Patzakis MJ, Wilkins J, Bassett RL: Surgical findings in clenched-fist injuries. Clin Orthop 1987; 220:247.

46. Mann RJ, Hoffeld TA, Farmer CB: Human bites of the hand: Twenty years of experience. J Hand Surg Am 1977; 2:97.

47. Dreyfuss UY, Singer M: Human bites of the hand: A study of 106 patients. J Hand Surg Am 1985; 10:884.

48. Shields C, Patzakis MJ, Meyers MH, et al: Hand infections secondary to human bites. J Trauma 1975; 15:235.

49. Rayan GM, Putnam JL, Cahill SL, et al: *Eikenella corrodens* in human mouth flora. J Hand Surg Am 1988; 13:953.

50. Zubowicz VN, Gravier M: Management of early human bites of the hand: A prospective randomized study. Plast Reconstr Surg 1991; 88:111.

51. Amadio P: Fungal infections of the hand. Hand Clin 1998; 14:607.

52. Gonzales MH, Thomas K, Weinzweig N, et al: Necrotizing fasciitis of the upper extremity. J Hand Surg Am 1996; 21:689.

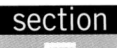

section **5** chapter **6**

SPINAL INFECTIONS

Mark B. Dekutoski

Summary
- Hematogenous and postoperative infections of the spine remain a significant cause of morbidity. Early recognition, diagnostic confirmation, and initiation of appropriate therapy are critical to effective management.
- Postoperative infections require complete débridement of necrotic tissues.
- Instrumentation may need to be maintained until definitive stability via fusion is achieved.
- Antimicrobial management must be tailored to clinical response.
- Definitive long-term follow-up is required. Delaying removal of hardware eliminates residual microbial colonization.

Infection of the spine has been noted throughout history. Tuberculous spondylitis was discovered in the remains of a human from 7000 B.C. Percifal Pott's description of the natural history of tubercular spondylitis in 1779 resulted in recognition of the world's most common infectious disease of the spine, known as Pott's disease. In the preantibiotic era, pyogenic and granulomatous diseases of the spine carried a grim prognosis, but with advances in treatment, mortality is now an uncommon outcome. Vertebral osteomyelitis has also become less common, currently accounting for 2% to 4% of all cases of osteomyelitis.[1]

Infection of the spine is classified according to location, pathogen, cause, and temporal relationship to surgery. Because most spinal infections are hematogenous or occur from direct contamination during surgical exposure, it seems logical to organize the evaluation and management as a function of etiological factors and then timing of presentation relative to surgery. Hematogenous infections of the bone, disk, and epidural space include diseases due to pyogenic, granulomatous, and fungal pathogens. Adult hematogenous infection of the disk originates at the subchondral end plate. Hence, the term "disk space infection" is used interchangeably with "vertebral osteomyelitis."

TABLE 1. CLASSIFICATION OF SPINAL INFECTIONS	
Hematogenous	
Pyogenic	Aerobic and anaerobic organisms.
Granulomatous	Pathological response characterized by formation of Langerhans' giant cells and, usually, caseation.
Direct contamination/Postoperative	
Acute	<3 weeks after surgery.
Subacute	>3 and <12 weeks after surgery.
Delayed	>12 weeks after surgery.

Postoperative disk space infection due to local contamination is discussed in the section on postoperative factors (Table 1).

Definitive diagnosis of osteomyelitis in the pediatric and adult populations is commonly delayed. The average time from onset of symptoms to diagnosis ranges from 8 to 12 weeks.[2] Awareness of the syndrome in the working differential diagnosis for abdominal pain, chest pain, and back pain enhances the likelihood of diagnosis. Consideration of the syndrome early in evaluations for fever, combined with an adequate level of familiarity, also reduces delay. It is hoped that advances in diagnostic testing and physician education will further reduce delays in diagnosis.

PATHOGENESIS

Why does an infection of the spine occur? Vertebral bone remains hematopoietically active throughout adulthood and contains the largest volume of cancellous bone. Ten percent of adult cardiac output at rest is directed to the osseous skeleton. Osseous sinuses and the potential for stasis create an environment for bacterial seeding and proliferation of microorganisms.

The association of venous anatomy with the development of hematogenous osteomyelitis was first described in 1819 and was confirmed in 1884 by Rodet. Current understanding suggests that variation in intra-abdominal pressure affects vertebral fluid dynamics and the vertebral body biomechanical behavior that encourages venous stasis and altered vertebral circulation. These conditions facilitate bacterial seeding and proliferation.

Postoperative infections are related to the balance between bacterial contamination of the wound and the presence of residual necrotic tissue. Excessive handling of soft tissues and prolonged use of retractors, resulting in "crush injury," can cause decreased perfusion and tissue necrosis, which contribute significantly to wound infection. Hematoma and bone graft material, which are essential for the development of fusion, are also available as media for bacterial proliferation. A fresh postoperative fusion mass is in essence a "sequestrum." Without vascular invasion, the bone graft remains dead bone that, in the presence of bacteria, can serve as the nidus for infectious proliferation.

Granulomatous disease is the most common cause of vertebral osteomyelitis worldwide. Tuberculosis caused by *Mycobacterium tuberculosis* is the most common form of the disease. This category comprises all bacterial and fungal organisms that also create a granulomatous response with central caseation and peripheral formation of Langerhans giant cells. The fungal infections include coccidioidomycosis, blastomycosis, histoplasmosis, cryptococcosis, and sporotrichosis.

Granulomatous disease causes an indolent and progressive destruction of osseous structures and ligaments that results in spinal column deformity. The resulting kyphosis and scoliosis can cause neurological compromise. Abscess formation also can cause necrosis of arterial supply to the cord, resulting in ischemic paralysis. Early treatment is imperative to avoid these late sequelae.

CLINICAL FEATURES

In both children and adults, the definitive diagnosis of osteomyelitis is commonly delayed. Awareness of the syndrome and its inclusion in the working differential diagnosis of abdominal, chest, or back pain increase the likelihood of diagnosis. Early consideration of the syndrome in the evaluation of fever, combined with an adequate level of familiarity with the disease entity, helps reduce delays in diagnosis.[2] The specific characteristics of clinical presentation for the various types of spinal infection are discussed here.

HEMATOGENOUS INFECTIONS
Pyogenic Infection
Pyogenic infection of the spine occurs most commonly in the lumbar spine and thoracolumbar spine as a result of the greater volume of bone mass. Typically, patients present with subacute symptoms such as localized back pain or neck pain, chest wall pain, abdominal pain, malaise, weight loss, and fever. The presentation can mimic that of a spinal tumor if night pain is the prominent symptom. Neurological symptoms are usually late manifestations. Groin, retroperitoneal, pleural, or retropharyngeal abscess is potentially the initial presenting symptom.

Patients at risk for hematogenous infection include those with immunocompromise and those with a significant episode of bacteremia. Surgical or endoscopic manipulation of the genitourinary or gastrointestinal tract as well as a higher incidence rate of risk-related procedures that cause bacteremia potentially can seed the vertebral cancellous bone. Direct contamination by a puncture wound to the neck or mouth can result in osteomyelitis. The immunocompromised patient presents an additional challenge because such a patient's relative anergy mutes the inflammatory response and associated pain. Presentation may also be delayed in diabetic patients because of the presence of a neuropathy. Predisposition to vertebral disease may also occur in patients who use intravenous drugs, who lack a spleen, or who have sickle cell disease or an immune deficiency syndrome (from the use of steroids or chemotherapy, the presence of human immunodeficiency virus [HIV], or acquired immunodeficiency syndrome [AIDS]).

In summary, pain, limited spinal motion, and fever are frequently seen in the subacute phase of the disease. Neurological deficit typically manifests late because of associated paraspinous abscess, epidural abscess, or vertebral collapse, which can proceed to establish kyphosis or scoliosis deformities.

Epidural Abscess

Although rare, symptomatic epidural abscess is a surgical emergency. Immunocompromise is a primary risk factor. Patients with epidural abscess present with significant axial back pain with or without radicular features and often go on to have neurological symptoms. Progressive neurological deficit has been attributed to local cord vascular changes and cord compression by an expanding abscess. Unless treatment is initiated, neurological symptoms are progressive and frequently permanent.

Granulomatous Infections of the Spine

Clinical manifestations of tuberculous spondylosis are variable, resulting in delayed diagnosis. Patients frequently present with generalized symptoms such as malaise, chronic fatigue, weight loss, and intermittent fever. Axial pain is common and should direct the evaluation for spondylitis. The thoracic spine is most commonly involved, and organisms initially spread in a subperiosteal fashion, sparing the disks. The disease spreads to contiguous vertebra via the anterior longitudinal ligament.

Patients may present with subcutaneous abscess or fistula. Less than half of the patients experience neurological symptoms; if present, such symptoms are most common with cervical disease. Immunocompromised patients are at particular risk for development of granulomatous infections.

POSTOPERATIVE SPINE WOUND INFECTIONS
Early and Subacute Infections

Early or acute postoperative wound infections occur during the first 3 weeks after surgery. Subacute infections become evident during the 3rd to 12th weeks. Infection in the postoperative period may lead to significant disability, morbidity, and medical expenditure.

The overall prevalence rate of postoperative wound infection often ranges from 0.5% to 15%. For lumbar diskectomy, the prevalence rate is 0.5% to 1%.[3] Spinal fusions without instrumentation have a moderately increased prevalence rate of postoperative wound infection, ranging from 3% to 5%.[4] The prevalence rate of infection of the iliac crest donor site is reported to range from 1% to 20%. When instrumentation is used, the prevalence rate increases to 3.6% to 8%. This higher prevalence rate is likely due to the increased dissection and dead space created by surgery, longer duration of surgery, and greater blood loss.[4–6] Surgery performed to correct deformities in healthy children and adolescents with idiopathic scoliosis has a reported postoperative infection prevalence rate of 0.5% to 5%.[7–9] The prevalence rate dramatically increases to 5% to 15% in the patient with neuromuscular deformity, because of associated preoperative malnutrition, diminished hygiene, and skin or genitourinary tract colonization. Deformity surgery in the adult has a higher prevalence rate of postoperative wound infection than the typical degenerative procedure, with a reported rate of 0.5% to 5%.[10] In contrast to posterior approaches to the spine, anterior approaches are associated with a dramatically lower prevalence rate of infection, 0.6%.[11]

The diagnosis of malnutrition can be confirmed by assessment of an index of protein mass. Serum albumin levels should be greater than 3.5 g/dL, because lower levels are associated with poor wound healing, postoperative infection, and immunosuppression.[12] Prealbumin measurements and total lymphocyte counts also are used as markers of immune competence. The absolute lymphocyte count should be greater than 1500 cells per cubic millimeter. Zinc levels are also important to wound healing, with normal reference ranges from 670 to 1240 mg per liter area.

Neurologically impaired patients are also at greater risk for infection because of poor nutritional status, bladder and bowel incontinence, increased skin colonization with gram-negative microorganisms, and colonization of the genitourinary tract. A classic example is the patient with myelomeningocele. When such a patient is treated preoperatively for urinary tract infections, the risk of postoperative wound infection is reduced dramatically. Difficulty with skin closure in the patient with myelomeningocele can predispose to wound infection after surgery for spinal deformity.

Immunocompromised patients are at risk for postoperative wound infection. They include patients with positive HIV status, sickle cell disease, intravenous drug abuse, tuberculosis, alcohol use, diabetes, and rheumatoid arthritis as well as those who undergo long-term steroid therapy or abuse intravenous drugs or alcohol. Obesity and smoking are believed to independently increase the prevalence of wound infection.[13] Revision surgery is associated with soft tissue devitalization, increased soft tissue tension at closure, and ischemia within retracted soft tissues, which also increases the risk of wound infection. Additional intraoperative risk factors are a longer operative time and greater blood loss. The learning curve required for spinal instrumentation has been correlated with the prevalence of postoperative wound infection in patients undergoing spinal surgery.

Postoperative factors that raise the risk of infection include the development of a wound hematoma. Although controversial, the use of drains seems helpful in minimizing deep infections in patients undergoing extensive reconstruction, but there is no difference in infection rate between single-level lumbar laminectomies with and without the use of drains.[14, 15] Prolonged preoperative hospitalization in patients undergoing halo traction or two-stage spinal procedures is associated with an increased risk of infection.[16]

Diagnosis of postoperative infection is primarily conducted on a clinical basis with confirmation by cultures and laboratory studies. Successful treatment depends on prompt recognition, diagnosis, and initiation of treatment. Delay in diagnosis can increase the morbidity rate significantly. There should be a high index of suspicion for infection when a patient has nonspecific complaints, such as malaise or increased back pain, and the situation warrants further investigation. Unexplained temperatures exceeding 39°C should be thoroughly investigated, and other sites of potential infection, specifically the urinary and pulmonary systems, must be assessed. Erythema, tenderness, fluctuance, pain to deep percussion, and drainage are the signs of early infection.

INVESTIGATIONS

Laboratory evaluation of the patient with suspicion of vertebral osteomyelitis includes complete blood count with differential, measurements of erythrocyte sedimentation rate

(ESR) and C-reactive protein (CRP) level, serum protein electrophoresis to evaluate for myeloma, and urinanalysis to look for a urinary tract infection. A more generalized elevation of serum globulins has been noted in patients with infections.[17] The white blood cell count is nonspecific. Elevations of ESR and CRP are potentially helpful but, again, not specific. The ESR was elevated in 100% of patients with vertebral osteomyelitis reviewed in one large series.[18]

Destructive changes to the vertebra and disk occur progressively throughout the course of the disease. Disk space narrowing, with end-plate lucency, lytic changes, sclerosis, and new bone formation, begins at 2 to 3 weeks. Computed tomography (CT) discerns the early changes to the paravertebral tissues. Later on, the sclerotic bone remodeling changes or pathological fracture become apparent on plain radiographs. Studies have noted abscess formation with vertebral osteomyelitis in more than 80% of cases at presentation.[19]

Nuclear and axial imaging studies have enhanced the potential for early diagnosis. Technetium bone scans are very sensitive, but their specificity is compromised by the prevalence rate of osteopenic compression fractures in the same at-risk cohort. The addition of gallium scanning has significantly enhanced the diagnostic specificity to between 70% and 80%.[20] Indium scans in the axial skeleton lack sensitivity and specificity.[6] Magnetic resonance imaging (MRI) as a noninvasive, nonionizing imaging modality has largely supplanted nuclear imaging studies as a screening or diagnostic tool.

MRI is one of the most valuable evaluations for patients with suspected vertebral osteomyelitis. Decreased signal intensity on T_1-weighted images and increased T_2 signal in the vertebral body and adjacent disk with associated soft tissue mass are characteristic. Sensitivity and specificity of MRI for diagnosis of disk space infection has been reported to reach 96%.[21] Many of the reporting studies, however, do not include pathological confirmation. Furthermore, there is a significant delay between response to treatment and the corresponding resolution on MRI of the changes induced by inflammation and infection; this delay must be kept in mind when one is evaluating the clinical response to treatment (Table 2).

It is imperative that culture specimens be obtained in a sterile fashion. Culture of superficial wound swabs collected in the emergency room or outpatient setting can frequently be misleading. Sterile aspirates of wound seroma or deep wound drainage can be helpful. Obtaining culture specimens before oral antibiotic therapy starts is imperative for guiding definitive therapy. The radiologist or the surgeon performing the biopsy must make active efforts to avoid the "routine" use of preoperative antibiotics as well as the use of antibiotics in injectable fluids.

The CRP level is useful because in a patient without infection, it reaches maximal elevation in 2 to 3 days postoperatively and normalizes by the 5th to 14th day. These characteristics establish the CRP as the optimal serological test for early diagnosis and follow-up of postoperative infection. The ESR peaks much later and often can normalize by the 2nd postoperative week, but in patients who have undergone a spinal fusion procedure, the ESR remains elevated for 3 to 6 weeks. The CRP normalizes earlier in the noninfected patient who has undergone spinal fusion surgery.

Ultrasound can be helpful in guiding aspiration but does not differentiate hematoma from purulence. MRI, CT, and radiography are potentially helpful in diagnosis of late non-postoperative infections but are of limited value in the immediate postoperative period. Gadolinium-enhanced MRI can be helpful in evaluating postoperative epidural abscess, because an air-fluid level within hematoma distinguishes infection from seroma.

GOALS, INDICATIONS, AND CONTRAINDICATIONS

The principles of treatment for hematogenous osteomyelitis are early recognition and institution of effective therapy, which can be monitored for clinical and serological response. In patients with positive results of blood culture, laboratory studies, and imaging studies, a working diagnosis of vertebral osteomyelitis can be made, early treatment can be initiated, and these parameters can be monitored closely for clinical and laboratory response to treatment. ESR and CRP values should both decrease by 50% early in the treatment course. The CRP should decrease within a week, and the ESR within 2 weeks. Although reduction of ESR has correlated with clinical response, the association is not absolute, so the response to therapy should be evaluated clinically from resolution of bacteremia and reductions in fever, myalgia, and pain.[22] If the clinical response wanes and markers of infection remain elevated, reassessment and biopsy should be conducted.

		Signal Intensity				
Process	Pathology	Marrow T_1	Marrow T_2	Disk T_1	Disk T_2	w/Gad. T_1
Acute discitis osteomyelitis	Edema and inflammatory cells	Low	High	nL	High	Bright disk margin
Active rheumatoid arthritis	Inflammatory changes	Low	High	nL	nL	
Degenerative disk disease	Disk dehydration, Inflammation	Low	Intermediate	nL	Low	
Compression fracture	Hematoma	Low	Inhomogenous/increased			
Pathological fracture	Tumor infiltration, Hematoma	Low	Homogenous/increased			
Solid tumors	Tumor Infiltration	Increased	Variable	Do not involve disk		

TABLE 2. MRI CHANGES

When diagnosis is uncertain owing to absence of an organism on culture, inconclusive imaging results, or uncertain clinical findings, a biopsy should be performed. Fine-needle, CT-guided biopsy has not been as effective as one would wish in the clinical setting, in that positive findings and definitive pathological determination are available in less than 50% of clinical cases. The use of a larger-core needle for CT-guided biopsy and transpedicular placement of the needle and core have significantly improved the clinical yield of diagnostic tissue. Open biopsy or Craig's needle biopsy remains another option, but because of potential wound and anesthesia complications, initial attempts at closed-needle biopsy are warranted. Tissue specimens for histopathological evaluation should always be sent with the culture specimens to avoid missing a necrotic tumor. One must always bear in mind, during an open approach to infection diagnosis, that precautions should be taken to use an incision that would not compromise a surgical resection that would be required if a malignancy were found.

The principles of treatment for hematogenous pyogenic osteomyelitis include immobilization and focused antimicrobial therapy. Patients with cervical osteomyelitis are in greater need of immobilization, and many researchers rely on halo immobilization because of the risk of cervical collapse and spinal cord compression. In general, an external orthosis is adequate for both control of pain and reduction of cervical spinal motion. Autofusion (spontaneous fusion) of the lumbar spine with resolution of osteomyelitis occurs in 40% to 60% of cases. Intravenous antibiotic therapy for 6 weeks with close observation of ESR and CRP is usually sufficient, but if the clinical course and laboratory indices do not improve, abscess drainage should be considered.

Progressive kyphosis, the appearance of neurological deficit, or persistent pain with or without radiographic instability may indicate abscess débridement and surgical reconstruction. Anterior débridement and surgical reconstruction with autograft bone is typically necessary, and metal cages for anterior reconstruction should *not* be used. Anterior instrumentation is avoided because of (1) the difficulty of access for its removal and also (2) its relative mechanical disadvantage as buttress fixation in osteopenic or pathological vertebral bodies. Use of posterior spinal instrumentation in the acute pyogenic abscess has been reported. When posterior instrumentation has been used in the setting of acute infection, titanium implants have been found to have less bacterial adherence; they also allow for further imaging of the spine. Although reports of "cured infections with implants" exist, we recommend staged removal of posterior implants after fusion has occurred at the 18- to 24-month postoperative poinbt (Table 3).

TREATMENT FOR EPIDURAL ABSCESS (HEMATOGENOUS INFECTION)

Symptomatic epidural abscess is a surgical emergency but is extremely rare in patients with nonsurgical or hematogenous spinal infections. Immunocompromised patients are the typical patient population at risk, and diagnosis is affirmed by MRI. Careful inspection for the nidus of infection and evidence of cord edema and gliosis is important. Progressive neurological deficit should prompt consideration of surgical decompression and débridement. Careful

TABLE 3. DEEP WOUND INFECTION AFTER SPINAL FUSION FOR ADULT DEFORMITY; RESULTS AT INTERMEDIATE FOLLOW-UP*

Timing of Infection	Total No. Cases	No. Failures†
<3 weeks after operation	11	7
>3 weeks after operation	16	16

* Experience at Mayo Clinic, 1970 to 1994. Intermediate follow-up defined as a minimum of 5 years.
† Failure = recurrence of infection or symptomatic pseudoarthrosis that required reoperation.

attention to drainage of the nidus of purulence is critical and is often overlooked. Progressive neurological deficit has been attributed to local cord vascular changes and expansion of the abscess.

Unfortunately, patients with epidural abscess often undergo laminectomy, which further destabilizes the spine. Instability following laminectomy is an underrecognized cause of progressive neurological deficit in the epidural abscess patient. Fortunately, with initiation of appropriate antimicrobial agents and immobilization, ankylosis of the spine occurs frequently. Nonoperative treatment with antimicrobial therapy and close observation can be considered for the patient presenting with neurological deficit of more than 3 days' duration, the patient without nonprogressive neurological deficit, and the patient who is an extremely poor surgical candidate.

TREATMENT FOR EARLY POSTOPERATIVE INFECTION

Isolated medical management has an extremely limited role and is most commonly utilized for sterile wound dehiscence or wound separation. This situation requires careful attention, because continued drainage is frequently due either to inadequate fascial closure or to fascial dehiscence with hematoma leakage. Isolated medical management for a true postoperative wound infection is not effective.

Surgical management of early postoperative wound infections is mandatory for patients with persistent drainage, recurrent hematoma, or a positive result of aspirate culture. Patients who have suspicious wounds, increasing pain, persistent temperature elevation, and CRP elevation beyond the 2- to 4-day postoperative period should be considered candidates for wound exploration, irrigation, and débridement. A low threshold for surgical intervention in suspicious postoperative wounds is warranted, because the morbidity of untreated infections is significant.

TREATMENT FOR DELAYED WOUND INFECTIONS

Delayed wound infections manifest more than 16 to 20 weeks postoperatively. The average presentation has been 25 months postoperatively.[23–27] Symptoms are generally mild, being poorly localized for 1 to 6 months before the diagnosis is established. Occasionally, wound fluctuance with spontaneous drainage or a deep sinus tract may be present. Mild elevation of the ESR is common, and usually, cultures demonstrate no growth or growth of low virulent organisms such as *Propionibacterium acnes*, *Staphylococcus epidermidis*, or *Micrococcus* species.

TREATMENT FOR GRANULOMATOUS INFECTIONS

Treatment of granulomatous disease of the spinal column centers on early diagnosis, immobilization of the spine, and initiation of effective chemotherapy. Abscess drainage is the typical means of pathological and microbial confirmation. Abscess drainage should be initiated when neurological deficit is present, because neurological recovery is more predictable with surgical intervention.[28] Definitive surgical intervention has an enhanced role in socioeconomically deprived areas, where the direct and indirect costs of prolonged medical therapy are prohibitive. Static or progressive neurological deficit, progressive deformity, and lack of clinical response to medical therapy are all indications for operative intervention. Chemotherapy should be initiated several weeks before surgical débridement and reconstruction to facilitate stabilization of systemic disease.

Definitive management of chemotherapy for granulomatous and fungal disease of the spine should be directed or overseen by a specialist in infectious disease. Because of the small number of cases in North America, most surgical specialists have very limited experience with these conditions. Toxicity of antifungal and antituberculous medications can be life threatening, so treatment must be directed by a specialist who can devote adequate time and appropriate expertise to the management of these cases.

PROCEDURES

POSTOPERATIVE WOUND DRAINAGE

Two patterns or philosophies of postoperative wound débridement are described. The first involves (1) a layer-by-layer débridement, (2) inspection and irrigation of the subcutaneous tissues, and (3) aspiration of the deep fascial tissues if the fascia is intact. This philosophy of wound débridement is based on several assumptions, including the belief that postoperative infection can be isolated to the superficial tissues and that opening of deep tissues, even after irrigation, causes contamination. The alternative technique of wound débridement involves (1) layered débridement of the subcutaneous tissues, (2) irrigation, and (3) opening of the fascia with inspection of and collection of culture specimens from deep tissues. If the deep tissues appear to be uninvolved, the fascia is reapproximated with a monofilament, absorbable suture.

Principles of wound débridement include débridement of all necrotic tissues, use of pulsatile lavage, and removal of loose bone graft. Some surgeons recommend washing the loose bone graft thoroughly and replacing it, but others believe that any bone graft that is floating free should be discarded.[29] One of the principles of early postoperative infection in patients with instrumented fusion is that the instrumentation should be maintained to allow for maintenance of reduction and stabilization. With effective antimicrobial treatment, definitive fusion can occur, and hardware then can be removed.

Wound management after débridement of early infection depends on the time to presentation, the extent of tissue necrosis, and the status of the wound after débridement. Options include single or staged débridement followed by primary wound closure over suction drains. Several surgeons have advocated primary wound closure over irrigation-suction systems continued for 3 to 4 days until the fever and CRP decrease. In the presence of severe soft-tissue necrosis or a polymicrobial infection, multiple débridements should be considered.

The deep and superficial wounds should be packed open. Débridement should be repeated 48 hours later, at which time delayed primary closure over drains is performed. A final option involves leaving the wound open and allowing the wound edges to granulate with dressing changes. This method is best used in refractory infections. With open wound packing, granulation of the wound generally takes several months but can lead to very satisfactory wound closure and infection resolution. All operative wound management should be accompanied by adequate attention to systemic antimicrobial treatment and nutritional management.

Patients with deficiency of posterior soft tissues present an extremely difficult problem, and their infections are often managed with local muscle flaps.[8, 30, 31] The cornerstone of soft tissue transposition is to provide soft tissue coverage and obliterate dead space in order to maintain a vascular tissue bed. This approach creates a local condition that may allow for salvage of hardware. Tissue expanders have been used in some situations but have a limited role, particularly in those patients who have previously irradiated tissues.

Initial antimicrobial management following wound débridement is based on coverage of common organisms. Use of a first-generation cephalosporin with an aminoglycoside is usually sufficient until culture results are available. Routine use of vancomycin is discouraged because of the potential for development of resistant organisms. Antimicrobial agents and dosages are adjusted on the basis of sensitivity results obtained from the cultures. Infectious disease specialists' review of management has significantly enhanced the care of patients with postoperative wound infections requiring débridement. Clinical response, which is evaluated from the wound appearance, signs of systemic illness, and pain, is monitored along with the white blood cell count, ESR, and CRP. When these parameters show a favorable response, the patient is switched to oral antibiotics for 6 to 12 weeks longer. Patients are followed clinically for at least 6 months.

For patients in whom instrumentation is retained, there is a concern about whether an infection can truly be eradicated. Therefore, the principle of treating the infection until fusion is obtained and then removing the retained implants has been followed by some surgeons, with good success.

Treatment of delayed wound infection requires removal of all instrumentation and exploration of the fusion mass. Patients often have a thin sheet of bone overlying the pseudoarthrosis in the fusion mass. If a pseudoarthrosis is present, a second débridement is often conducted 48 hours later with primary closure, followed by antimicrobial therapy for 6 to 12 weeks.

TECHNICAL DETAILS

Expected microorganisms in early postoperative wound infections include *S. aureus* as well as *Staphylococcus epidermis*, which constitutes 50% to 79% of pathogens in

TABLE 4. CURRENT MEDICAL RECOMMENDATIONS FOR GRANULOMATOUS, PARASITIC, AND FUNGAL DISEASES

Tuberculosis	Isoniazid (INH), rifampin, ethambutol, pyrazinamide, streptomycin
Coccidiodomycosis	Fluconazole, itraconazole, or amphotericin B
Blastomycosis	Itraconazole, ketonazole, or amphotericin B
Cryptococcosis	Parenteral amphotericin B followed by fluconazole
Aspergillosis	Amphotericin B or itraconazole
Brucellosis	Doxycycline and gentamicin or doxycycline and rifampin
Actinomycosis	Penicillin or doxycycline and ceftriaxone
Echinococcosis	Mebendazole and surgical débridement

most series. Gram-negative and polymicrobial infections are being observed with greater frequency. Gram-negative infections are particularly noted in the immunocompromised patient, the patient with urinary incontinence, and the patient with wounds that extend into the sacral region. Low-virulence organisms, such as *P. acnes*, *S. epidermidis*, and *Micrococcus varians coxa* are more common in the delayed infections (Table 4).

COMPLICATIONS

Recurrent or residual infection of the spine can lead to spinal instability, deformity, neurological deficit, often associated with disabling pain and functional limitations, or a combination of these conditions. Differentiating chronic infection from severe degenerative changes in the postoperative spine is enhanced by advanced MRI and, when necessary, a CT-guided biopsy. Inadequate treatment can result in persistent infection, which must be differentiated from pseudoarthrosis and segmental instability. Flexion and extension radiographs can be helpful but are usually nondiagnostic. Second serological evaluation and biopsy may be necessary.

Renal, hepatic, and auditory complications of antimicrobial management can create lifelong disability. Although close management of aminoglycoside and vancomycin peak and trough values is well known, the renal toxicity of cephalosporins often is underappreciated. Consultation with and management of such cases by a specialist in infectious diseases helps significantly.

When initial débridement and antimicrobial management of the deep wound infection and disk space infection fails, a more complete "tumor-like" débridement of the tissues is necessary. One approach is to utilize vascularized autograft tissue to optimize osseous healing, local delivery of antimicrobial agents, and dead space management. This extensive reconstructive effort requires an experienced treatment team, because the nutritional systemic and technical complications of this effort can contribute significantly to patient morbidity or mortality.

OUTCOMES

Adequate treatment of vertebral osteomyelitis is accomplished when the infection has resolved, all osseous and soft tissues have been revascularized, and structural and neurological stability is achieved. This end point is very poorly defined in most series studying osteomyelitis in the axial and appendicular skeleton. Recurrence of vertebral osteomyelitis in the immunocompromised patient is common. Colonization of implants or residual necrotic bone remains as a nidus for this secondary event, and long-term surveillance and follow-up are imperative for the treated patient.

Prevention of postoperative wound infections is helped by clear identification and treatment of high-risk patients preoperatively. The malnourished patient should undergo dietary assessment and supplementation for improvement of serum albumin level, total lymphocyte count, and zinc levels. In patients with neuromuscular disorders, treatment of urinary tract infections and administration of preoperative antibiotic coverage for gram-negative organisms are helpful.

Prophylactic antibiotic therapy should be utilized for all spine operations. Intraoperative blood loss of up to 1200 mL does not decrease serum antibiotic levels below therapeutic range. In practice, antibiotics are typically continued for 48 hours, and many surgeons continue antibiotics until drains are removed. A combination of gentamicin and a second-generation cephalosporin should be considered if violation of the dura is encountered during surgery.

Subcutaneous drains should be used to decrease postoperative wound hematoma. Use of intraoperative skin surface barriers, such as sterile drapes impregnated with povidone-iodine, and wound irrigation with saline have been advocated.

REFERENCES

1. Stauffer RN: Pyogenic vertebral osteomyelitis. Orthop Clin North Am 1975; 6:1015.
2. Digby JM, Kersley JB: Pyogenic non-tuberculous spinal infection: An analysis of thirty cases. J Bone Joint Surg 1979; 61B:47.
3. Ozuna RM, Delamarter RB: Pyogenic vertebral osteomyelitis and postsurgical disc space infections. Orthop Clin North Am 1996; 27:87.
4. Massie JB, Heller JG, Abitbol JJ, et al: Postoperative posterior spinal wound infections. Clin Orthop 1992; 284:99.
5. Abbey DM, Turner DM, Warson JS, et al: Treatment of postoperative wound infections following spinal fusion with instrumentation. J Spinal Dis 1995; 8:278.
6. Whalen JL, Brown ML, McLeod R, et al: Limitations of indium leukocyte imaging for the diagnosis of spine infections. Spine 1991; 16:193.
7. Glazer PA, Hu SS: Pediatric spinal infections. Orthop Clin North Am 1996; 27:111.
8. Theiss SM, Lonstein JE, Winter RB: Wound infections in reconstructive spine surgery. Orthop Clin North Am 1996; 27:105.
9. Wenger DR, Mubarak SJ, Leach J: Managing complications of posterior spinal instrumentation and fusion. Clin Orthop 1992; (284):24.
10. Szoke G, Lipton G, Miller F, et al: Wound infection after spinal fusion in children with cerebral palsy. J Pediatr Orthop 1998; 18:727.
11. Faciszewski T, Winter RB, Lonstein JE, et al: The surgical and medical perioperative complications of anterior spinal fusion surgery in the thoracic and lumbar spine in adults: A review of 1223 procedures. Spine 1995; 20:1592.

12. Klein JD, Garfin SR: Nutritional status in the patient with spinal infection. Orthop Clin North Am 1996; 27:33.

13. Andreshak TG, An HS, Hall J, et al: Lumbar spine surgery in the obese patient. J Spinal Dis 1997; 10:376.

14. Payne DH, Fischgrund JS, Herkowitz HN, et al: Efficacy of closed wound suction drainage after single-level lumbar laminectomy. J Spinal Dis 1996; 9:401.

15. Sasso RC, Williams JI, Dimasi N, et al: Postoperative drains at the donor sites of iliac-crest bone grafts: A prospective, randomized study of morbidity at the donor site in patients who had a traumatic injury of the spine. J Bone Joint Surg Am 1998; 80:631.

16. Stambough JL, Beringer D: Postoperative wound infections complicating adult spine surgery. J Spinal Disord 1992; 5:277.

17. Stone DB, Bondiglio M: Pyogenic vertebral osteomyelitis: A diagnostic pitfall for the internist. Arch Intern Med 1963; 112: 491.

18. Carragee EJ, Kim D, van der Vlugt T, et al: The clinical use of erythrocyte sedimentation rate in pyogenic vertebral osteomyelitis. Spine 1997; 22:2089.

19. Larde D, Mathieu D, Frija J, et al: Vertebral osteomyelitis: Disk hypodensity on CT. AJR Am J Roentgenol 1982; 139:963.

20. Sypryt EP, Hardy JG, Hinton CE, et al: A comparison between magnetic resonance imaging and scintigraphic bone imaging in the diagnosis of disc space infection in an animal model. Spine 1988; 13:1042.

21. Modic MT, Feiglin DH, Piraino DW, et al: Vertebral osteomyelitis: Assessment using MR. Radiology 1985; 157:157.

22. Carragee EJ: Pyogenic vertebral osteomyelitis. J Bone Joint Surg Am 1997; 79:874.

23. Heggeness MH, Esses SI, Errico T, et al: Late infection of spinal instrumentation by hematogenous seeding. Spine 1993; 18: 492.

24. Richards BS: Delayed infections following posterior spinal instrumentation for treatment of idiopathic scoliosis. J Bone Joint Surg Am 1995; 77:524.

25. Schofferman L, Zucherman J, Schofferman J, et al: Diphtheroids and associated infections as a cause of failed instrument stabi-

lization procedures in the lumbar spine. Spine 1991; 16:356.

26. Viola RW, King HA, Adler SM, et al: Delayed infection after elective spinal instrumentation and fusion: A retrospective analysis of eight cases. Spine 1997; 22: 2444.

27. Wimmer C, Gluch H: Management of postoperative wound infection in posterior spinal fusion with instrumentation. J Spinal Disord 1996; 9:505.

28. Martin NS: Tuberculosis of the spine: A study of the results of treatment during the last 25 years. J Bone Joint Surg 1970; 52B:613.

29. Rothman SLG: The diagnosis of infections of the spine by modern imaging techniques. Orthop Clin North Am 1996; 27: 15.

30. Manstein ME, Manstein CH, Manstein G: Paraspinous muscle flaps. Ann Plast Surg 1998; 40:458.

31. Stern WE, Balch RE: Surgical aspects of nonspecific inflammatory and suppurative disease of the vertebral column. Am J Surg 1966; 112:314.

section 5 chapter 7

INFECTED TOTAL HIP ARTHROPLASTY

Joshua A. Urban and Kevin L. Garvin

Summary

- The current incidence of deep infection in total hip arthroplasty is approximately 1%.
- Estimates of the total cost of treatment for one infected total hip arthroplasty is $50,000.
- Gram-positive bacteria, especially *Staphylococcus epidermidis* and *Staphylococcus aureus*, are the most common offending organisms.
- Perioperative antibiotics are the most effective prophylactic measure in the prevention of periprosthetic infections.
- Two-stage reimplantation is the gold standard for treatment of infected total hip arthroplasty; success rates average 92.3%.

INTRODUCTION

Periprosthetic infection remains a dreaded complication of total hip arthroplasty (THA). Although more than 90% of these infections can be successfully eradicated and a good functional outcome can be obtained, treatment regimens can be extensive. Often the patient must withstand staged operative procedures, prolonged intravenous antibiotic courses, and extended periods of hospitalization. Estimates of the total cost of treatment have been as high as $50,000 per case. Fortunately, improvements in operative technique and prophylactic methods have decreased the prevalence of

this complication from 9% in the early experience to 1% currently. High-volume centers reported prevalence rates as low as 0.6%.[1]

PATHOGENESIS

Periprosthetic infections develop after pathogens contaminate the joint by one of two routes: direct or hematogenous seeding. Direct seeding of pathogens into the joint can occur at surgery from pathogens originating from the patient, the operating room environment, or the operating room personnel. Direct contamination of the joint can also occur in the immediate postoperative period as a result of contiguous spread from a superficial wound infection, suture abscess, or delayed wound healing.[2, 3] Hematogenous seeding of the joint can occur at any time throughout the life of the prosthesis from transient bacteremia associated with remote infections or invasive procedures of the oral, gastrointestinal, genitourinary, or pulmonary tracts. Direct contamination reportedly represents 51% of periprosthetic infections, whereas 34% are hematogenous in origin, and 14% are unknown (Fig. 1).[2]

S. epidermidis and *S. aureus* are the first and second most commonly isolated pathogens, respectively. The streptococci, enterococci, and gram-positive anaerobes are also frequent pathogens, whereas gram-negative bacteria and mixed organisms are less common causes of infection (Table 1). Infections with the isolation of fungi and mycobacteria have been reported.[2, 3, 5]

FREQUENCY OF ROUTES OF INFECTION OF TOTAL JOINT PROSTHESES

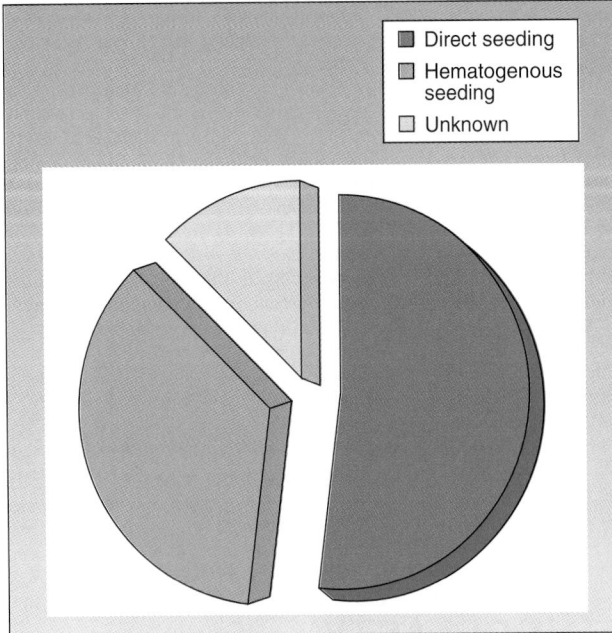

- ■ Direct seeding
- ■ Hematogenous seeding
- □ Unknown

Fig. 1. Frequency of routes of infection of total joint prostheses. (From Brause BD: Sepsis: The Rational Use of Antimicrobials. In Callaghan J et al (ed): The Adult Hip. Philadelphia, Lippincott-Raven, 1998, p 1343.)

TABLE 1. BACTERIOLOGY OF TOTAL HIP INFECTIONS

Pathogen	Frequency of Isolates (%)	
	HSS/Mayo[4]	Fitzgerald[39]
Gram-positive aerobes	76	64
Staphylococcus epidermidis	37	29
Staphylococcus aureus	19	19
Enterococcus	4	5
Streptococcus viridans	7	1
Streptococcus groups A, B, G	3	9
Diphtheroids	4	—
Micrococcus	—	1
Unknown	2	—
Gram-negative aerobes	11	18
Anaerobes	12	14
Fungus	—	5

HSS, Hospital for Special Surgery.
Copyright American Academy of Orthopaedic Surgeons. Reprinted from J Am Acad Orthop Surg X; 3:249.

The large amount of foreign body used in THA predisposes patients to infection. It has been shown that fewer bacteria are required to establish an infection in the presence of a foreign body.[6] Additionally, intrinsic surface properties of each specific biomaterial preferentially attracts certain bacterial species. A retrieval of 171 infected biomaterials revealed *S. epidermidis* as the principal isolate in wounds containing polymers and *S. aureus* predominating

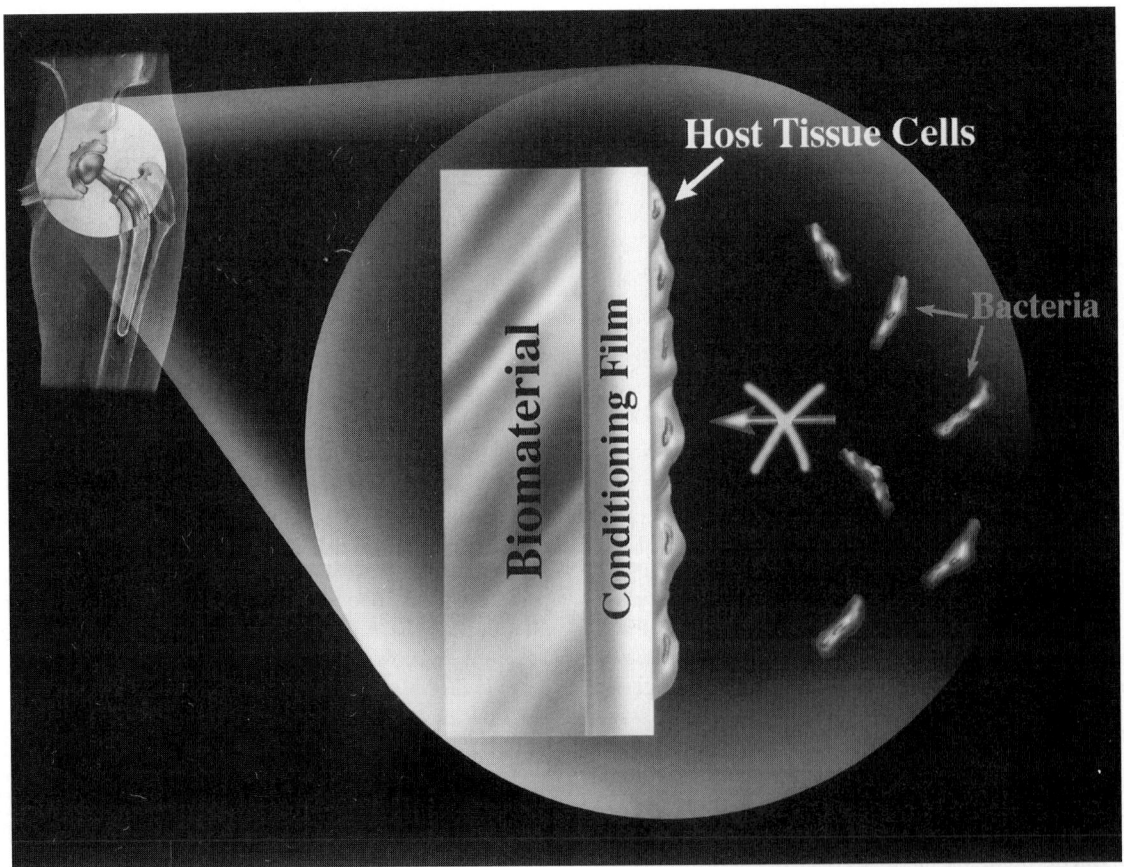

Fig. 2. Race for the surface. The host tissue cells have colonized the biomaterial and established a surface resistant to bacteria.

in wounds with metals. In vitro investigations also demonstrated the preferential adhesion of *S. epidermidis* and *S. aureus* to polymers and metals, respectively.[7] The large surface area of polymers and porous structures and the surface oxide layer of metals are reactive interfaces with which the bacteria interact.

The concept of the "race for the surface" describes the microenvironment of the newly inserted prosthesis.[7] When prosthetic components are implanted into a biological environment, they are immediately coated with a "conditioning film" consisting of host proteins, macromolecules, and cellular elements. This conditioning film becomes colonized by either host tissue cells or bacteria, depending on which arrive first. When tissue cells arrive first and a secure bond is established, a new surface highly resistant to infection confronts incoming bacteria (Fig. 2). When bacteria arrive first, they may produce exopolysaccharide barriers known as the biofilm or glycocalyx within 3 to 4 hours. The glycocalix is a sequestered microenvironment in which the bacteria can grow and propagate, provide additional adhesion for new bacteria, confer resistance to host defense mechanisms, and possibly impede antibiotic penetration (Fig. 3).

The "race for the surface" concept does not adequately explain late hematogenous seeding of previously well-functioning joints. Wear and corrosion have been associated with microenvironmental conditions promoting the establishment of late infection (Fig. 4). Ions released from metal corrosion may stabilize glycocalyx, leading to increased adhesion and antagonist resistance. An immunoincompetent fibroinflammatory zone also develops at the biomaterial-host tissue interface over time as a result of the host's attempt to eradicate the foreign body. This macrophage-mediated inflammatory reaction results in a chronic inflammatory reaction with a self-perpetuating cascade of cytokine and superoxide radical release. Over time the macrophages' oxidative and killing potential becomes exhausted, resulting in a microenvironment vulnerable to infection. Particulate debris generated by wear and corrosion accelerate this chronic inflammatory reaction, leading to expansion of the immunoincompetent fibroinflammatory zone and an increased susceptibility to infection.

PROPHYLAXIS

Prophylactic measures may be used in both the perioperative and postoperative periods. Perioperative prophylactic measures act to diminish the degree of bacterial contamination that inevitably occurs at surgery. Postoperative prophylaxis aims to decrease the consequences of the transient bacteremias associated with infections or manipulations of remote sites.

Perioperative Prophylaxis

Prophylactic measures in the perioperative period include (1) optimizing patient risk factors, (2) administering antibiotic prophylaxis, (3) minimizing intraoperative airborne contamination, and (4) performing surgical techniques that reduce contamination.

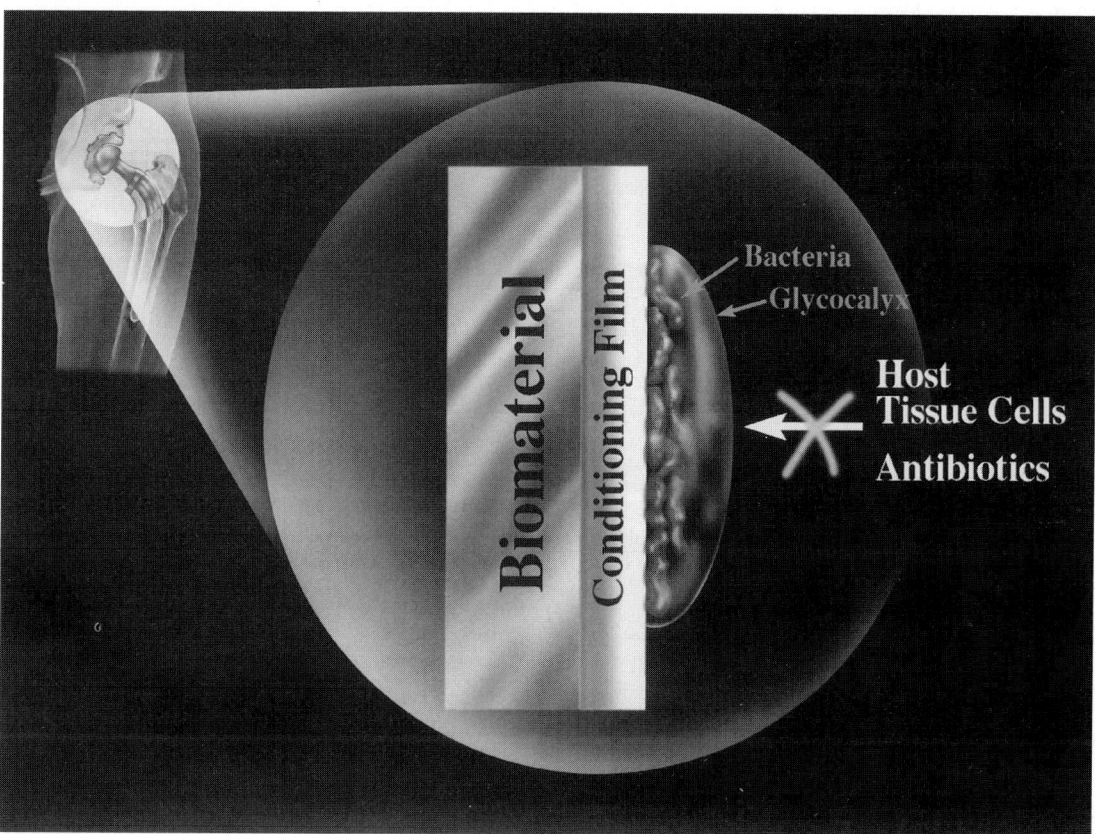

Fig. 3. The race for the surface. When bacteria are able to colonize the surface of the biomaterial, they produce a biofilm, the glycocalix, which provides protection against host defense mechanisms and antibiotics.

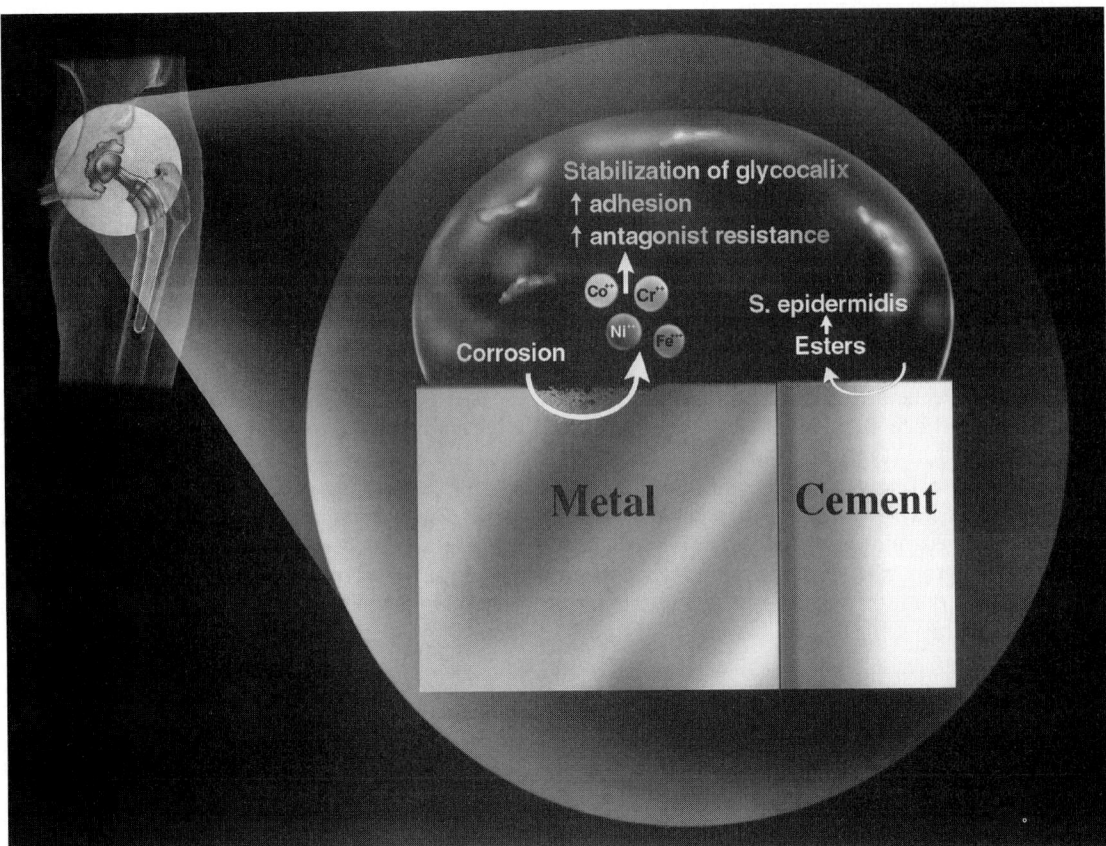

Fig. 4. Conditions promoting the establishment of infections. Ions released from metals stabilize the glycocalix, leading to increased adhesion and antagonist resistance. Esters released from polymethylmethacrylate may be metabolized *by Staphylococcus epidermidis.* (Modified from Gristina AG: Current concepts review: Infection after total hip arthroplasty. J Bone Joint Surg Am 1995; 77(10):1576.)

Optimization of Patient Risk Factors

Patients undergoing THA must have preoperative identification and correction, if possible, of infection risk factors such as conditions associated with immune system impairment, prolonged hospital stay before arthroplasty, psoriatic plaques or thin atrophic skin at the intended operative site, and remote foci of infection (Table 2).[8]

Impairment of the Immune System. This has been associated with advanced age, malnutrition, obesity, use of immunosuppressive drugs, chronic diseases (diabetes melli-

TABLE 2. RISK FACTORS ASSOCIATED WITH AN INCREASED RISK OF POSTOPERATIVE INFECTIONS, THE MECHANISMS BY WHICH THEY EXERT THEIR EFFECT, AND METHODS TO OPTIMIZE THESE RISKS

Risk Factors	Mechanism	Goal
Impairment of the Immune System		
Advanced age	Decreased humoral plus cell-mediated immunity	—
Malnutrition	Most host defenses impaired	Correct nutritional deficiencies
Obesity	Impaired phagocytosis?	Weight loss?
Chronic diseases		
Diabetes mellitus	Decreased chemotaxis/phagocytosis/T-cell response	Serum glucose <220 mg/dL
Rheumatoid arthritis	Decreased chemotaxis/phagocytosis	Temporary cessation of immunosuppressants
Allogenic blood transfusion	Decreased cell-mediated immunity	Autologous/hemodilution/perioperative salvage
Prolonged Hospitalization Before Surgery	Nosocomial colonization?	Avoid prehospitalization
Operative Site		
Psoriatic plaques	Higher incidence of wound infection?	Treat before surgery
Thin, atrophic skin	Higher incidence of wound infection	Careful handling of tissue
Remote Foci of Infection	Transient bacteremias, ? seeding of the joint	Eradication of infections before surgery
Prolonged Wound Drainage	Increased exposure to skin flora	Appropriate surgical technique promoting wound healing

tus and rheumatoid arthritis), and allogenic blood transfusions.[3,8,9] Advanced age, in the absence of disease, has been associated with a diminished humoral (B cell) and cell-mediated (T cell) immune response, resulting in decreased antibody formation, depressed delayed-type hypersensitivity (DTH) responses, decreased proliferative response, and an altered helper-suppressor activity ratio.[9] Decreased thymic activity and constant antigenic pressure throughout life may cause this impaired immunity.

Malnutrition and obesity may adversely affect the immune system. Malnutrition, present in as many as 48% of surgical patients, results in impairment of many host defense mechanisms, including humoral and cell-mediated immunity, phagocyte function, physical barriers (skin and mucous membranes), and other nonspecific defenses (interferon, lysozymes, and complement).[9] No universally accepted definition of malnutrition in patients undergoing total joint arthroplasty has been established. Preoperative total lymphocyte count of less than 1500 cells/mm, an albumin level of less than 3.5 g/dL, and a low serum transferrin level have been shown to predict wound complications.[3,8,10] The Rainey-McDonald nutritional index (Fig. 5) may identify patients who are at increased risk for postoperative infection. Correction of micronutrient deficiencies improves immune indices and reduces the rate of wound complications.

Obesity has also been associated with an increased risk of wound infection.[8,11] The exact influence of obesity on the immune system has not been qualified, although impairment of phagocytosis has been suggested. Attempts at weight loss in the preoperative period may worsen the immunodeficiency because the humoral and cellular responses remain impaired long after the diet has ended.[11]

Certain chronic diseases are associated with an acquired reduction of immune response. Abnormalities of neutrophil chemotaxis and phagocytosis occur in patients with diabetes mellitus and rheumatoid arthritis, and depressed T-cell response is also seen in diabetic patients.[3] Immunosuppressive medications also increase the risk of postoperative wound infection.[12] Accordingly, efforts to decrease the risk of infection in rheumatoid patients have included adjustment of immunosuppressant agents in the perioperative period. The temporary cessation of methotrexate 2 weeks before and after surgery has been associated with decreased infection in rheumatoid patients after total joint arthroplasty.[13] Optimization of immune function in diabetic patients may be achieved by controlling serum glucose levels to less than 220 mg/dL.[14]

Blood transfusions in the early postoperative period may be necessary in as many as 57% of patients after THA.[15] The use of allogenic blood has been associated with impairment of cellular immunity, resulting in an increased risk of postoperative infection.[16] Conservative transfusion practices, such as autologous blood donation, hemodilution, and perioperative blood salvage, reduce the need for allogenic blood.

Prolonged Hospitalization Before Arthroplasty. This has been associated with an increased risk of wound infection. In a review of 23,649 surgical wounds, the prevalence of deep infection was 1.1%, 1.6%, 2.0%, and 4.3% for patients who were hospitalized for 1 day or less, 2 to 6 days, 7 to 13 days, and more than 14 days, respectively.[17] It is unclear whether this relationship is due to skin colonization by resistant nosocomial organisms or a selection bias for high-risk patients with other serious medical conditions.

Operative Site. The condition of the skin at the intended operative site should be assessed preoperatively. The presence of psoriatic plaques has been associated with an increased prevalence of wound infection.[18] It is recommended that treatment of these plaques by a dermatologist be completed before THA to minimize risk of an infection. Thin, atrophic skin has also been associated with higher rates of wound infection.[8] Careful handling of tissue and meticulous wound closure maximizes the wound's healing potential.

Remote Infections. Remote foci of infection in the oral cavity, the genitourinary tract, pulmonary system, and skin have been associated with an increased risk of postoperative infection.[19] A thorough preoperative history and physical examination should be performed to identify and eliminate these foci. Necessary procedures for these areas should be completed before THA.

Minimizing Intraoperative Airborne Contamination

Airborne bacteria in the operating room are almost exclusively gram-positive microorganisms. Individually, these bacteria range in size from 0.3 to 10 μm and, when airborne, usually reside on droplets, dust, and shed epithelial cells ranging in size from 8 to 14 μm.[20] The majority of airborne bacteria are derived from the skin and hair of individuals in the operating room, including the patient, surgeons, nurses, anesthesiologists, and circulating personnel. As many as 5000 to 55,000 organisms are shed per minute by the surgeon, depending on the type of clothing and how recently the individual has showered (most particles are shed immediately after showering). Some individuals, known as dispersers, shed substantially more bacteria than normal. The presence of these dispersers among operating room personnel has been associated with an increase risk of wound infection.[21,22]

Clean-air rooms decrease the number of airborne bacteria by frequent air exchange (up to 300 air changes per hour), filtration, and laminar flow of the operating room air. Laminar flow involves air moving at a uniform velocity along parallel lines in a confined space. Vertical laminar airflow is more effective in reducing airborne contamination than horizontal airflow, particularly if body exhaust suits are not worn. The use of horizontal airflow has been associated with an increased prevalence of infection, which is believed to be due to increased air turbulence at the surgical site from improper positioning of personnel between the airflow unit and the patient.[23]

Charnley[24] attributed most of the 9% to 1% decrease of infection in his patients to the use of clean-air rooms. Universal acceptance of the use of clean-air rooms in

---

Nutritional Index of Rainey-McDonald

$$= [(1.2 \times \text{serum albumin}) + (0.0013 \times \text{serum transferrin})] - 6.43$$

Fig. 5. Rainey-McDonald's nutritional index. Values less than or equal to 0 are consistent with nutritional depletion.

TABLE 3. INDEPENDENT AND COMBINED EFFECTS OF CLEAN-AIR AND PROPHYLACTIC ANTIBIOTICS ON THE RATE OF INFECTION AFTER TOTAL JOINT ARTHROPLASTY[1, 8]

Prophylactic Antibiotics	Laminar Airflow		
	No	*Yes*	f
No	39 of 1161 (3.4%)	13 of 1060 (1.2%)	<.01
Yes	24 of 2968 (0.8%)	10 of 2863 (0.3%)	<.1
p	<.001	<.01	

THA, however, has not occurred subsequently. Although studies confirmed that clean-air rooms significantly reduce the rate of infections, the use of prophylactic antibiotics also results in low rates of infection. When both clean-air rooms and prophylactic antibiotics were used, the decreased prevalence could not be solely attributed to clean air. The Medical Research Council of Great Britain's large multicenter prospective clinical trial reported a prevalence of infection of 1.5% in conventional rooms and 0.6% in clean-air rooms ($p < .001$).[1] Critics pointed out the lack of control for prophylactic antibiotics, and when prophylaxis was accounted for, clean-air rooms did have a significant independent effect. Without the use of antibiotics, the rate of infection decreased from 3.4% in conventional rooms to 1.2% in clean-air rooms (Table 3). When antibiotic prophylaxis was used, clean-air rooms decreased the prevalence of infection from 0.8% to 0.3%, but this effect was not significant ($p < .1$). Other studies[3, 8, 25] suggested a synergistic effect of clean-air rooms in the presence of antibiotic prophylaxis.

Ultraviolet light has also been used intraoperatively to sterilize bacteria present on airborne particles.[26] Although this method is a relatively inexpensive alternative to laminar airflow systems, the lack of definitive studies and concerns about the exposure of the operating room personnel have prevented widespread acceptance.

Limiting operating room traffic, wearing surgical face masks under an overlapping hood, and minimizing conversation during the procedure have also been associated with decreased levels of airborne contamination.[8]

Antibiotic Prophylaxis

Antibiotic prophylaxis is probably the most effective prevention measure reducing periprosthetic infections. Hill et al[27] reported a decrease from 3.3% to 0.9% with the use of prophylactic cefazolin, and others found similar results, with decreased infection rates ranging from 3.1% to 0.9%.[1, 25] Although the effectiveness of antibiotic prophylaxis has led to routine use before total joint replacement, controversy still exists regarding the optimum antibiotic and the duration of prophylaxis. The optimal antibiotic would demonstrate activity against the organisms common to periprosthetic infection (staphylococcus and streptococcus), have adequate bone and soft-tissue penetration, have low toxicity, be inexpensive, and have a long half-life to provide coverage throughout the procedure. The first-generation cephalosporin, cefazolin, has been the most exten-

sively studied agent and is the most commonly used because it meets all of the optimum criteria. Other broad-spectrum agents such as second- and third-generation cephalosporins have been investigated but have not demonstrated improved efficacy. The optimum choice of antibiotic may evolve as new patterns of resistance emerge. One prospective study of preoperative skin swabs from patients about to undergo THA showed a 25% prevalence of cephalosporin-resistant *S. epidermidis*.[28] As the prevalence of these resistant patterns increases, reassessment of the approach to antibiotic prophylaxis will be required.

Prophylactic antibiotics should be given 30 to 60 minutes before surgery. Administration of an antibiotic 1 or more days preoperatively provides no additional protection and may alter the patient's flora and be detrimental.[3] Initiating prophylaxis after the skin is incised is ineffective. Additional doses are recommended if the duration of the procedure exceeds one to two times the half-life of the antibiotic used or if blood loss is significant.[8]

The optimum duration of antibiotic prophylaxis has yet to be determined. Several studies reported no additional benefit when antibiotic prophylaxis was continued beyond 24 hours postoperatively.[29] In a study of 466 joint replacements, no differences were noted among 7-day, 3-day, and 24-hour antibiotic regimens.[26] The increased cost, selection of resistant organisms, concern of antibiotic toxicity, and lack of benefit of longer regimens has led most authorities to recommend a single preoperative dose followed by two or three postoperative doses.

The use of antibiotic-impregnated bone cement as a prophylactic measure is also controversial. Prophylactic antibiotic-impregnated cement has been shown to be effective in reducing the prevalence of infection after THA. Among 476 THA patients, the infection rate for those using gentamicin-impregnated cement was 1.1% and for those using no prophylactic antibiotics, 5.9%.[30] Concerns of the routine use of antibiotic in bone cement have included the possibility of an allergic reaction that may necessitate a second operation to remove the components and all of the cement, the selection for resistant organisms, and weakening of the bone cement. In addition, in a prospective, randomized, consecutive series of 1688 THAs in which antibiotic-impregnated cement and systemic antibiotic prophylaxis were compared, the authors found no difference in infection rates.[31] Thus, the use of antibiotic-impregnated cement may be reasonable in high-risk patients, but its exact role in the prevention of THA infection awaits further study.

Surgical Techniques

Adherence to optimum surgical techniques, such as shorter operating times, gentle handling of tissue, elimination of dead space, and hemostasis, reduces the amount of contamination, necrotic tissue, and hematoma size, factors that are known to promote infection.

Preparation of the operative site includes shaving the area just before surgery and using a preparatory scrub. Shaving the night before can cause soft-tissue injury, which may lead to folliculitis and dermatitis, thereby increasing the number of bacteria present at surgery.[3, 26] Regardless of the antiseptic agent used, it is impossible to sterilize the skin completely. Although bacteria are easily removed from the skin surface, the sequestered oily environments of the hair follicles and subcutaneous glands are not sufficiently infiltrated by these disinfectants. Within 30 minutes bacteria begin to recolonize the surface, and within 3 hours the counts can reach normal levels.[32] The use of a simple adhesive plastic surgical drape reduces wound contamination by decreasing lateral migration of skin bacteria but does not prevent skin recolonization. A plastic drape impregnated with slow-release iodophor prevents skin colonization for up to 3 hours. One disadvantage of adhesive draping is the possibility of damaging or avulsing thin friable skin on removal.

The suction tip may also be a source of contamination. Large volumes of air passing through the tip allow airborne bacteria to accumulate. Up to 55% of suction tips are contaminated after 100 minutes of operative time.[33] Placement of the suction tip into the femoral canal for extended periods also should be avoided because this may draw airborne bacteria directly into the wound. Similarly, the splash basin may be a source of contamination; 74% of splash basins can become contaminated by the end of orthopaedic procedures.[34] It has been recommended that placement of any instrument from the splash basin to the wound be avoided.

Postoperative Prophylaxis

Periprosthetic infections can occur years after the index procedure in previously well-functioning prostheses as a result of hematogenous seeding from transient episodes of bacteremia. Although documenting that the bacteremia is responsible for seeding of the joint has been difficult, late periprosthetic infections have been associated with remote infections of the skin, oral cavity, respiratory tract, gastrointestinal tract, and genitourinary tract (Table 4). Such events have compelled some authors to advocate antibiotic treatment of these remote infections.[2]

The use of prophylactic antibiotics in patients with THA undergoing iatrogenic manipulation of the oral cavity (den-

TABLE 5. INDIVIDUALS AT AN INCREASED RISK OF HEMATOGENOUS PERIPROSTHETIC INFECTIONS

A. Immunocompromised Patients

Inflammatory arthropathies; rheumatoid arthritis, systemic lupus erythematosus
Disease, drug, or radiation-induced immunosuppression

B. Other Patients

Insulin-dependent (type I) diabetes
First 2 years following joint replacement
Previous prosthetic joint infections
Malnourishment
Hemophilia

From Antibiotic prophylaxis for dental patients with total joint replacements. American Dental Association. American Academy of Orthopaedic Surgeons. J Kans Dent Assoc 1997; 82:14.

tal procedures), genitourinary tract (e.g., cystoscopy), or gastrointestinal tract (e.g., endoscopy) is also controversial. Bacteremia can occur with procedures involving these sites and is generally higher in oral manipulations, lower in genitourinary manipulations, and lowest in gastrointestinal manipulations.[8] Some periprosthetic infections have been directly associated with the bacteremia caused by these invasive procedures.[2, 8] The controversy focuses on whether prophylaxis is indicated at all, and if so, whether there is a time in the life of the prosthesis when the risk of prophylaxis (toxicity, cost, selection of resistant organisms) outweighs the risk of developing infection. Currently, the incidence of hematogenous seeding after these procedures and the efficacy of prophylactic antibiotics in preventing this seeding is essentially unknown, especially with respect to genitourinary and gastrointestinal procedures. With regard to dental procedure prophylaxis, it has been demonstrated that the rate of periprosthetic infections from *Streptococcus viridans* originating from the oral cavity is higher in the first 2 years after arthroplasty.[35] The frequency of infection was 0.14 cases per 1000 joint-years in the first 2 years and 0.03 cases per 1000 joint-years afterward. These preliminary data suggest antibiotic prophylaxis for dental procedures may be appropriate within the first 2 years after surgery. In 1997, the American Dental Association and the American Academy of Orthopaedic Surgeons released a joint advisory statement addressing the appropriate use of antibiotic prophylaxis in dental patients with total joint replacements (Tables 5 to 7).[36] Whether antibiotic prophylaxis is indicated for genitourinary and gastrointestinal procedures has yet to be determined.

CLINICAL FEATURES

The clinical picture of an infected THA can be variable and is dependent on several factors, including the virulence of the offending pathogen, immunocompetence of the patient, and timing of surgery. Pain in the groin or thigh, varying in severity from indolent to severe, is the most common presenting symptom in both early postoperative

TABLE 4. ATTRIBUTED PATHOGENIC EVENTS IN PROSTHETIC JOINT INFECTIONS

Clinical Event	Organism (*N*)
Dental	
Manipulation/abscess	*Streptococcus viridans* (4)
Infected wisdom tooth	*Peptostreptococcus* (1)
Capping	*Peptococcus* (1)
Genitourinary	
Urinary tract infection	*Pseudomonas mirablis* (6)
	Escherichia coli (4)
Cervical polypectomy	*Lactobacillus* (1)
Proctitis	*Peptococcus* (1)
Skin	
Abscess/dermatitis/cellulitis	*Staphylococcus aureus* (9)
Cellulitis	Group G streptococci (2)
Desquamative dermatitis	*Staphylococcus epidermidis* (1)
Gastrointestinal	
Tumor/colitis/dermatitis	*S. viridans* (4)
Diverticulitis	*E. coli* (1)
Enteritis	*Salmonella* (1)

Modified from Brause BD: Sepsis: The rational use of antimicrobials. In Callaghan JJ, Rosenberg AG, Rubash HE (eds): The Adult Hip. Philadelphia, Lippincott-Raven, 1998, p 1343.

TABLE 6. INCIDENCE STRATIFICATION OF BACTEREMIC DENTAL PROCEDURES

Higher Incidence[1]

Dental extractions
Periodontal procedures including surgery, subgingival placement of antibiotic fibers/strips, scaling and root planing, probing, recall maintenance
Dental implant placement and reimplantation of avulsed teeth
Endodontic (root canal) instrumentation or surgery only beyond the apex
Initial placement of orthodontic bands but not brackets
Intraligamentary local anesthetic injections
Prophylactic cleaning of teeth or implants where bleeding is anticipated

Lower Incidence

Restorative dentistry[3] (operative and prosthodontic) with/without retraction cord
Local anesthetic injections (nonintraligamentary)
Intracanal endodontic treatment; postplacement and buildup
Placement of rubber dam
Postoperative suture removal
Placement of removable prosthodontic/orthodontic appliances
Taking of oral impressions
Fluoride treatments
Taking of oral radiographs
Orthodontic appliance adjustment

[1] Prophylaxis should be considered for patients with total joint replacement that meet the criteria in Table 5. No other patients with orthopaedic implants should be considered for antibiotic prophylaxis prior to dental treatment/procedures.
[2] Prophylaxis not indicated.
[3] This includes restoration of carious (decayed) or missing teeth.
[4] Clinical judgment may indicate antibiotic use in selected circumstances that may create significant bleeding

From AAOS and ADA Expert Panel: Advisory statement. Antibiotic prophylaxis for dental patients with total joint replacements. AAOS Bull 1997;9.

infections and late hematogenous infections. Wound drainage is the second most common symptom. Drainage occurring within the first few days after surgery can be normal and is typically either sanguineous from a resorbing hematoma or serous from inflamed subcutaneous tissue. Persist-

TABLE 7. SUGGESTED ANTIBIOTIC PROPHYLAXIS REGIMENS IN PATIENTS WITH TOTAL JOINT REPLACEMENT UNDERGOING DENTAL PROCEDURES

1. Patients not allergic to penicillin: cephalexin, cephradine, or amoxicillin 2 g orally 1 hour before dental procedure
2. Patients not allergic to penicillin but unable to take oral medications: cefazolin 1 g or ampicillin 2 g IM/IV 1 hour before the procedure
3. Patients allergic to penicillin: clindamycin 600 mg orally 1 hour before the dental procedure
4. Patients allergic to penicillin and unable to take oral medications: clindamycin 600 mg IM/IV 1 hour before the procedure

No second doses are recommended for any of these dosing regimens.
Adapted from Antibiotic prophylaxis for dental patients with total joint replacements. American Dental Association. American Academy of Orthopaedic Surgeons. J Kans Dent Assoc 1997: 82:14.

ent wound drainage, however, has been associated with a 3.2 times increased risk for periprosthetic infection.[37] Wound drainage of several weeks' duration may result in the formation of a sinus tract and confirms the presence of infection. Fever, chills, and other systemic symptoms can be present in fulminating infections, but they are infrequent in the more common indolent infections.

CLASSIFICATION

The traditional classification of infections in total hip arthroplasty was presented by Coventry[38] in 1975.[3, 4, 39] Periprosthetic infections were divided into three stages based on when the symptoms began after surgery. Stage I infections (acute postoperative) are acute fulminating infections that present within 3 months after the arthroplasty. These infections are the result of direct seeding of the prosthetic joint during the procedure, early postoperative seeding from an infected wound or hematoma, or hematogenous seeding from a remote site early in the postoperative course. Systemic symptoms are common, and the patient usually has an inordinate amount of pain. Persistent wound drainage is often present in these infections. Stage II infections (delayed deep) are more indolent and present from 3 months to 2 years after surgery. These patients often have never had a pain-free interval after surgery and often pose a diagnostic dilemma. Stage III infections (late hematogenous) present with increasing pain and decreased function in a previously well-functioning arthroplasty. A history of a recent remote infection or procedure involving the skin, oral cavity, urinary tract, respiratory tract, or gastrointestinal tract often precedes the infection by days to weeks.

A newer classification, introduced in 1996 to facilitate the management, is an expansion of the traditional system and consists of four categories:[40]

1. Positive intraoperative cultures: at least two intraoperative cultures obtained at the time of revision are positive. Often these results are known only after the revision is performed because these cases typically had no preoperative signs or symptoms suggesting infection. Recommended treatment consists of 6 weeks of intravenous antibiotics and may not require further operative treatment.
2. Early postoperative infection: symptoms develop within 1 month after implantation. Treatment of these infections may consist of débridement, exchange of the polyethylene liner, retention of the components, and intravenous antibiotics for at least 4 weeks.
3. Late chronic infection: symptoms develop insidiously 1 month or more after implantation. Recommended treatment is a two-stage reimplantation.
4. Acute hematogenous infection: symptoms develop acutely in a previously well-functioning hip. If the prosthesis is well fixed and the duration of symptoms is short, the infection is treated in the same manner as for early postoperative infection. If the prosthesis is loose, it should be treated as a late chronic infection.

INVESTIGATION

The diagnosis of a fulminant infection with wound drainage, erythema, swelling, and systemic symptoms is rela-

TABLE 8. SENSITIVITIES AND SPECIFICITIES OF VARIOUS NUCLEAR IMAGING, LABORATORY, AND INTRAOPERATIVE MODALITIES IN THE DIAGNOSIS OF PERIPROSTHETIC INFECTION

Method	Sensitivity	Specificity
Radionucleotide Imaging		
Technetium/gallium	0.38–0.50	0.78–1.00
Technetium/indium 111-WBC	0.89–1.00	0.95–0.98
Indium 111-IgG	0.91–0.97	0.85–1.00
Laboratory Test		
ESR	0.61–0.88	0.79–1.00
CRP	0.91–0.96	0.88–0.92
ESR plus CRP	0.83–0.96	0.96–1.00
Hip aspiration	0.50–0.93	0.82–0.97
Intraoperative Techniques		
Gram stain	0–0.23	0.95–1.00
Intraoperative cultures	0.71–1.00	0.93–0.99
Frozen sections		
5 PMNs/hpf	0.63–0.91	0.89–0.97
10 PMNs/hpf	0.84	0.99

WBC, white blood cell; PMNs, polymorphonuclear leukocytes; hpf, high-power field; IgG, immunoglobulin G; ESR, erythrocyte sedimentation rate; CRP, C-reactive protein.

From Spangehl MJ, Younger SE, Masri BA, et al: Diagnosis of infection following total hip arthroplasty. J Bone Joint Surg Am 1997; 79:1478.

tively straightforward, whereas the more common low-grade infections present more of a diagnostic challenge. Although no currently available test is 100% sensitive or specific, many methods of detection exist and, when used concurrently, will add to the diagnostic certainty (Table 8). After a thorough history and physical examination, the available diagnostic options include (1) radiographic evaluation; (2) serum laboratory tests; (3) hip aspiration; (4) intraoperative Gram's stain, culture, frozen sections, and surgeon's assessment; and (5) polymerase chain reaction (PCR). A common approach for the diagnosis of infection after THA is shown in Figure 6.

RADIOGRAPHIC EVALUATION
Plain Radiographs

Plain radiographs of the entire prosthesis are necessary. Although several findings such as periostitis, rapidly progressive and diffuse osteolysis, and endosteal scalloping may suggest a deep infection, these are also found in aseptic loosening. Periosteal new bone formation is strongly associated with deep infection and is considered to be pathognomonic.[39]

Ultrasonography

Ultrasonography can be used to assess capsular thickness and fluid collections in the hip region. A thickened capsule (greater than 10.2 mm) with marked intracapsular effusion has been associated with deep infection.[41] Few studies investigated this diagnostic method; therefore, it is not widely used, and its role has yet to be defined.

Arthography

Arthrography of the hip is usually performed simultaneously with aspiration because it is of limited predictive value independently. The injection of dye into the joint confirms intra-articular placement of the needle and can detect abnormal bursae and sinuses, which can be suggestive of infection.

Fig. 6. Protocol for the diagnosis of infection after total hip arthroplasty. *Repeat aspiration should be performed before the procedure if clinical suspicion is high or if the erythrocyte sedimentation rate (ESR) and C-reactive protein (CRP) are elevated for another reason. †Consider performing sequential technetium 99m and indium-labeled white blood cell scanning. ‡Frozen sections should be obtained if ESR and CRP are not elevated. (From Spangehl MJ, Younger SE, Masri BA, et al: Diagnosis of infection following total hip arthroplasty. J Bone Joint Surg Am 1997; 79:14787.)

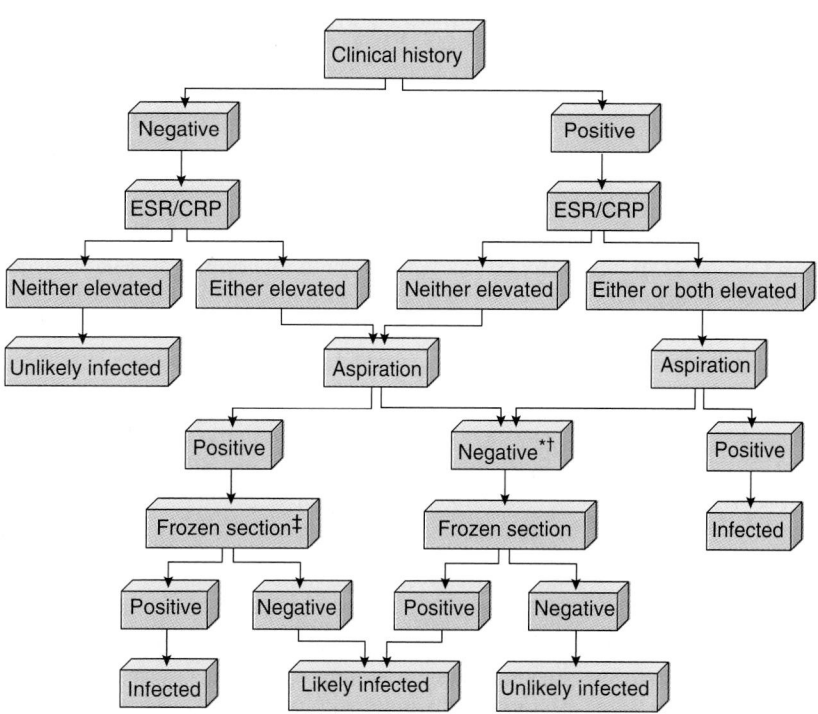

Radionucleotide Imaging

Three-phase bone scans using technetium 99m (^{99m}Tc) methylene diphosphonate are highly sensitive but lack specificity for periprosthetic infections. Increased uptake normally occurs more than 1 year after THA, and the patterns of ^{99m}Tc uptake in aseptic and septic loosening are similar.[41] The combination of gallium 67 citrate and technetium scans, although more accurate, still lacks sufficient accuracy. The combination of indium 111–labeled white blood cell scans (In-WBC) with technetium scans, however, has resulted in improved accuracy; sensitivities and specificities range from 0.89 to 1.00 and 0.95 to 0.98, respectively.

New scintigraphy modalities involving the use of indium 111–labeled nonspecific polyclonal immunoglobulin G and ^{99m}Tc-labeled monoclonal antigranulocytic antibody are being investigated. Few published reports exist, but preliminary data suggest that these new modalities may be preferable to leukocyte scans with a reported higher accuracy.[39, 41] On the basis of available data, sequential ^{99m}Tc and In-WBC scans are the imaging method of choice. It should be noted that nuclear imaging tests are only occasionally required to establish the diagnosis.

SERUM LABORATORY TESTS

The complete blood cell count with differential (CBC), erythrocyte sedimentation rate (ESR), and C-reactive protein level (CRP) are tests that should be routinely ordered. In the absence of a flagrant infection, the CBC is usually nondiagnostic. The ESR is an indirect indicator of acute-phase reactants present in response to inflammation, infections, and neoplastic processes. Several studies showed an association between deep infection and increased ESR values of greater than 30 to 35 mm. However, in uncomplicated THA, the ESR does not return to baseline levels until at least 6 months after surgery and can remain elevated for as long as 1 year, making this an unreliable test in the early postoperative period.[42] The ability of ESR to be influenced by other inflammatory conditions also decreases its specificity and limits its predictive value when used independently. CRP is another acute-phase and nonspecific indicator. In contrast to the ESR, CRP levels return to baseline quickly. After primary and revision THA, CRP levels normalize by 3 weeks (range, 2 to 8 weeks).[43, 44] The reported sensitivity (0.96) and specificity (0.92) of CRP in diagnosing deep infections are superior to those of ESR. Most authors currently support the combination of ESR and CRP in diagnosing infection because sensitivities and specificities of this combination have been reported at 0.96 and 1.00, respectively.[41]

HIP ASPIRATION

Hip aspiration should be performed with fluoroscopy under sterile conditions. If no joint fluid is obtained, injecting nonbacteriostatic saline and respirating may yield a viable sample, which should be analyzed with a cell count and differential, glucose and protein levels, Gram's stain, and cultures. Accepted joint fluid indices consistent with infection include a WBC count greater than 50,000, a differential count of greater than 80% polymorphonuclear leukocytes (PMNs), and low glucose and high protein levels.[3]

Until recently, hip aspiration was routinely performed preoperatively in all THA failures to rule out infection. Its role as a routine screening tool has been questioned because of variable sensitivity and specificity, ranging from 0.50 to 0.93 and 0.82 to 0.97, respectively. Most investigators now favor a more limited role and reserve aspiration to confirm clinical or laboratory suspicion of infection, such as an elevated ESR or CRP.[41]

Various methods have been recommended to increase the accuracy of hip aspiration, including (1) discontinuing antibiotic use 2 to 3 weeks before aspiration; (2) using local bacteriostatic anesthetics only in the superficial tissues; (3) confirming intra-articular position on arthrogram; (4) obtaining multiple samples during the same aspiration; and (5) obtaining a fine-needle biopsy of synovial tissue during aspiration.

INTRAOPERATIVE STUDIES
Gram's Stain

Gram's stain is a simple method used to ascertain the presence of bacteria in the periprosthetic environment. The reported sensitivity of this method is unacceptably low, ranging from 0 to 0.23, leading some authors to abandon it completely.[41] If used, the results of Gram's stain testing should not be the sole basis for determining treatment.

Cultures

A minimum of three intraoperative tissue samples should be sent to the laboratory for culture on both solid and liquid media. Samples should be taken from inflamed tissue adjacent to the prosthesis. Cultures are considered negative when no growth is evident on the final results of the broth subcultures. Intraoperative cultures, however, are not completely reliable because false-positive rates have ranged from 6% to 29%. Techniques advocated to improve the accuracy of cultures include (1) withholding antibiotics until specimens have been obtained, (2) preventing instruments used to obtain the cultures from touching the skin of the patient, and (3) obtaining the specimens immediately after the pseudocapsule is opened from an area not previously cauterized, before any irrigation has been used.

Frozen Sections

Intraoperative frozen histopathology sections can aid in the diagnosis of infection by determining the amount of inflammatory cells present in periprosthetic tissue. More than five PMNs per high-power field (5 PMN/hpf) has been associated with infection.[41] Most studies reported sensitivities and specificities of greater than 0.80 and 0.90, respectively.[41, 45] Specimens should be taken from the most inflamed tissue and analyzed by a pathologist experienced in interpretation of periprosthetic tissue.

Surgeon's Assessment

Occasionally, the periprosthetic environment may appear to the surgeon to be infected despite negative preoperative studies, Gram's stain, and frozen sections. The presence of an abscess, frank purulence, diffuse synovitis, and turbid joint fluid may indicate infection; the tissue's reaction to wear debris may result in similar appearances.[41] Although highly reliant on experience and subject to false interpretation, the surgeon's assessment of the periprosthetic tissues adds diagnostic information in equivocal cases.

Polymerase Chain Reaction

The technique of PCR shows promise in diagnosing periprosthetic infections. The PCR technique begins with the extraction of nucleic acid from a sample of periprosthetic synovial fluid. Multiple copies of this original nucleic acid are made to provide a sufficient volume of DNA for analysis. This amplified nucleic acid is then screened for the presence of bacterial DNA.[46] PCR had improved sensitivity in comparison to the traditional bacteriological studies in a series of 50 total knee replacements.[47] PCR's ability to diagnose infection from small quantities of bacterial DNA makes this technique vulnerable to contamination, and nucleic acid from bacteria killed by antibiotics may yield a positive result for infection when, in fact, the joint is sterile. Any bacterial nucleic acid that falls into the wound from the skin during surgery or is introduced from the skin into the joint during aspiration could also potentially yield a false-positive result. Although bacterial species-specific PCR primers have been designed to minimize the false-positive rate, the role of this technique has yet to be defined.

GOALS, INDICATIONS, AND CONTRAINDICATIONS

The optimum treatment result is eradication of the offending pathogen and restoration of function. Surgical intervention and antibiotic therapy are the primary methods used to achieve these goals. The exact choice of treatment depends on many variables, including type of infection, virulence of the offending pathogen, quality of bone and surrounding soft tissues, implant stability, and patient's medical condition and willingness to undergo further procedures (Table 9).

TWO-STAGE REIMPLANTATION

This method entails the complete removal of all foreign material (prosthesis, polyethylene, and cement), in combination with thorough débridement of all involved tissue. The wound is closed, and the patient begins an interval of intravenous antibiotic treatment lasting at least 6 weeks. New prosthetic components are implanted after the antibiotic regimen has been completed. Two-stage reimplantation is the gold standard for treatment of infected THA, because the highest success rates (average, 92.3%) have been reported with this treatment approach. Medically fit and willing patients with bone stock or a bone stock deficiency amenable to reconstruction are candidates for this procedure.

ONE-STAGE REIMPLANTATION

One-stage reimplantation consists of the resection of all prosthetic components and débridement of all involved tissue with reimplantation of new components at the same surgical setting. After surgery, the patient undergoes a 6-week antibiotic regimen similar to that for a two-stage procedure. A review of multiple studies reported an average success rate of 82% when one-stage reimplantation was performed.[5] This success, coupled with the decreased cost and morbidity associated with the need for less procedures, has established one-stage reimplantation as the pro-

TABLE 9. METHODS OF TREATMENT AVAILABLE AND THE INDICATIONS FOR EACH

Method	Indications
Two-stage reimplantation	Adequate bone stock
	Medically fit for multiple surgeries
One-stage reimplantation	Sensitive organism
	Non–glycocalix-producing organism
	Few or no risk factors for infection
	Adequate bone stock
	Medically unfit for multiple surgeries
Resection arthroplasty	Highly resistant organism
	Multiple risk factors for infection
	Poor bone/soft tissue quality
	Medically unfit for multiple surgeries
Débridement with retention	Less than 3 to 4 weeks of symptoms
	Sensitive organism
	Few or no risk factors for infection
	Well-fixed prosthesis
Chronic suppressive therapy	Sensitive organism
	Treatable with oral antibiotics
	Medically unfit for surgery
	Patient refusal of further surgery
Hip arthrodesis	Refractory infections
	Adequate bone stock
Hip disarticulation	Life-threatening or refractory infections
	Severe loss of bone/soft tissue tissue

cedure of choice for late chronic infections in some European centers. Most centers, however, advocate the two-stage procedure, citing the superior success rates of the two-stage reimplantation. Generally accepted criteria for one-stage reimplantation include (1) a pathogen sensitive to antibiotics, (2) non–glycocalix-producing bacteria, (3) a patient with few or no risk factors for infection (e.g., rheumatoid arthritis, diabetes mellitus), (4) adequate bone and soft tissue, and (5) comorbid medical conditions that place the patient at increased risk with a second major procedure.[5]

RESECTION ARTHROPLASTY (GIRDLESTONE ARTHROPLASTY)

This procedure involves the removal of all foreign bodies and débridement of all involved tissue with no subsequent reimplantation. Postoperatively, the patient undergoes an antibiotic regimen of at least 6 weeks' duration. Although this technique is highly effective at eradicating infection and relieving pain, the functional result is inferior to reimplantation techniques. Some patients function adequately with this technique but will require ambulatory aids and shoe lifts, invariably have a noticeable limp, and their energy expenditure is increased significantly during gait. The indications for resection arthroplasty include (1) a highly resistant pathogen, (2) poor quality of bone and soft tissues, (3) risk factors predisposing to recurrent infections (e.g., chronic immunosuppression, intravenous drug abuse), (4) patient inability or unwillingness to cooperate with the postoperative regimen of reimplantation techniques, and (5) a medically unfit patient.

DÉBRIDEMENT WITH RETENTION OF PROSTHESIS

This method consists of aggressive débridement of all infected and necrotic tissue, exchange of the polyethylene insert, and a postoperative course of intravenous antibiotics. Despite the presence of the retained cement and prosthesis, this method has been successful when instituted within 2 or 3 weeks of infection onset. Indolent infections that become symptomatic or are detected long after seeding (late chronic infections and some acute hematogenous infections) are not amenable to this method and require removal of all prosthetic components. Late chronic infections treated with débridement and retention have had poor results and should be treated with prosthesis removal.

One difficulty with this treatment approach is determining the time limit beyond which recurrence of infection is likely without removal of the prosthesis. For early postoperative infections, a threshold of 1 month is suggested because infections present for longer than 1 month are not as likely to be eradicated without removal of the prosthesis.[40] In this study, 25 of 35 patients (71%) with early postoperative infections were successfully treated with débridement and prosthesis retention. Because no temporal limit has been established in the treatment of acute hematogenous infections, the 1-month threshold has been extrapolated to these infections. Using this threshold, successful eradication of infection occurred in only 50% (3 of 6) of patients with acute hematogenous infections.[40]

Another difficulty when treating acute hematogenous infections is the determination of bacterial seeding timing. Occasionally, the infection can be linked to a bacteremia just days to weeks before onset of symptoms, yet often the onset of symptoms cannot be linked to a precise event. The issue then is whether the onset of symptoms resulted from an acute bacterial seeding or from a subacute indolent infection that has been present for weeks to months. Débridement with retention may be appropriate in the former but not the latter.

The use of additional criteria to improve patient selection will likely improve the success rate of this technique. Suggested criteria include (1) a short duration of symptoms (less than 3 to 4 weeks), (2) a pathogen sensitive to antibiotics, (3) absence of extensive scar tissue, (4) minimal or no risk factors for infection, and (5) a well-fixed prosthesis.[5, 40]

CHRONIC SUPPRESSIVE THERAPY

Chronic suppressive therapy refers to an antibiotic regimen without surgical intervention. The goal of this method is to control the infection by inhibiting the growth and proliferation of the offending bacteria. This method of treatment is most commonly used when the patient's medical condition precludes surgery or when the patient refuses further surgical intervention. For this method to be effective, the infecting organism must be identified and sensitive to antibiotics. The antibiotic of choice should be effective orally and have minimal side effects. A disadvantage of chronic suppressive therapy is the potential for the emergence of resistant organisms. Emergence of bacteria capable of producing

glycocalix is believed to contribute to the failures associated with this treatment. Successful results have been reported with the use of an oral fluoroquinolone and rifampin.[48, 49] Drancourt et al[49] reported successful treatment in 8 of 12 periprosthetic infections after a 6-month course of ofloxacin and rifampin with a follow-up of 12 to 57 months. Although complete eradication of the infection was claimed in the eight successfully treated joints, most patients were monitored for less than 2 years after completion of antibiotic therapy. Longer follow-up of this patient group is necessary because previous studies showed high rates of failure with longer follow-up after chronic suppressive therapy.[39]

OTHER TREATMENT OPTIONS

Hip arthrodesis can be used to treat periprosthetic hip infections. One study of seven patients reported acceptable results.[50] This method is rarely indicated because of the deficiency of bone and poor quality of soft tissues often present after a periprosthetic infection. Life-threatening infection, severe loss of soft tissues and bone stock, and vascular injury may necessitate hip disarticulation. Although this method is rarely indicated, acceptable results of infection control have been reported.[51]

PROCEDURE

TECHNICAL DETAILS

If prosthetic infection is suspected preoperatively, antibiotics are withheld until tissue cultures have been obtained. A cephalosporin is recommended for initial coverage postoperatively until the organism and its sensitivities are identified. Débridement of all inflamed and necrotic tissue, including any involved intrapelvic tissue, is essential. Excision of all foreign bodies is crucial in decreasing the risk of recurrence. The proximity to major visceral and neurovascular structures may necessitate additional preoperative work-up such as a computed tomography scan, an arteriogram, and vascular or urological consultation. Occasionally, an additional exposure through the retroperitoneum is needed.

At reimplantation, cementless acetabular fixation is preferred, and antibiotic-impregnated cement is recommended for femoral fixation. High rates of loosening (18%) and recurrence of infection (18%) have been reported with cementless femoral fixation.[52] Superior success rates have been achieved with one- or two-stage reimplantations using antibiotic-impregnated cement compared with cement not incorporating antibiotics. In two-stage procedures the success rates improve from 85.6% to 92.3%, whereas in one-stage procedures the success rates improve from 55% to 82%. Antibiotic-impregnated cement results in higher local levels of antibiotic than those achieved with intravenous therapy. Additionally, antibiotics within cement elute over time, providing a prolonged duration of effect. The addition of antibiotics theoretically weakens the cement. However, 2 g of antibiotic powder per 40 g of cement is considered safe for the demands of a functional hip prosthesis.

The local benefits of antibiotics in cement have led to interest in antibiotic-impregnated spacers placed within the wound at the time of resection and removed at reimplantation. Antibiotic-impregnated acrylic cement fashioned into the shape of beads has also been used as spacers. These beads are placed in contact with the bone of the acetabulum and medullary canal. Because they serve no mechanical function, greater amounts of antibiotic can be added to the cement without fear of mechanical failure. The beads can be threaded together to facilitate removal. The temporary functional spacer PROSTALAC (*pros*thesis of *a*ntibiotic-*l*oaded *a*crylic *c*ement) consists of a modular stainless steel endoskeleton coated with antibiotic cement and a thin polyethylene cup loosely cemented with a large amount of antibiotic cement. The advantages of this system include the avoidance of a period of poor function and soft-tissue contractures, which can occur during the interval period of traditional two-stage reimplantation. Although early results of the PROSTALAC system yield encouraging cure rates of 93%, dislocation occurred in 8.4% (5 of 60).[53] Additional studies are needed to determine the role of PROSTALAC in infected THA.

POSTOPERATIVE MANAGEMENT

The postoperative antibiotic regimen should be under the supervision of an infectious disease consultant, and sufficient doses must be given to achieve a minimum serum bactericidal titer (SBT) of 1:8. Lieberman et al[54] reported recurrent infection in one of 28 hips; an SBT of at least 1:8 was achieved. In contrast, two of four hips experienced recurrence with inadequate SBT levels of less than 1:8. It should be noted that both of these patients had significant risk factors for recurrent infection. If the titer is less than 1:8, then the antibiotic doses are adjusted and the titers are repeated.[5] Most centers found this method difficult to perform and instead rely on more conventional methods.

The exact duration of the interval between stages is controversial and has ranged from a few weeks to at least 1 year. Most authors recommend a minimum of 6 weeks of intravenous antibiotics.[5] In one study, three of seven infected THAs had recurrence after an antibiotic regimen of less than 28 days. In comparison, only one of 13 infected THAs recurred after more than 28 days of antibiotics.

Response to therapy may be monitored by serial serum ESR and CRP levels. Persistent elevations or increases in both of these indices are suspicious of persistent infection. An aspiration performed at least 4 weeks after the cessation of antibiotics may potentially aid in the diagnosis of persistent infection. If the joint aspirate reveals infection, a second débridement procedure is indicated to excise any retained foreign body and necrotic tissue.

Patients treated with two-stage reimplantation undergo progressive advancement in ambulatory status during the interval period. Immediately after resection, the patient is allowed partial weightbearing ambulation with the support of a walker, which is eventually advanced to crutches as tolerated. Some authors recommended skeletal traction for the initial 2 weeks to allow for the formation of scar tissue and stabilization of the pseudoarthrosis.[55]

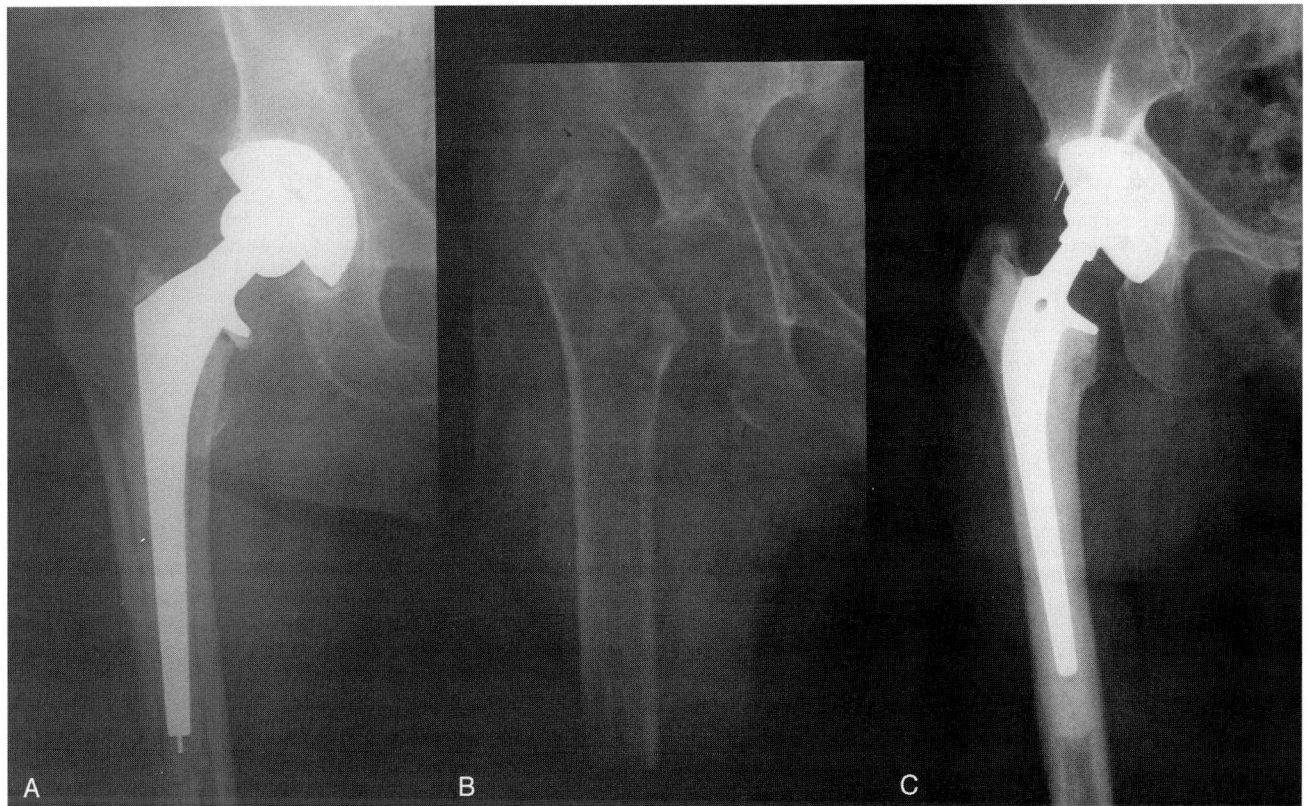

Fig. 7. Sequential roentgenograms of a patient with an infected THA. *A*, Anteroposterior radiograph of a late chronic infection of a total hip arthroplasty. *B*, Anteroposterior radiograph of the resection arthroplasty in the interim period while the patient is receiving antibiotics. *C*, Anteroposterior radiograph of a patient after reimplantation using an uncemented acetabular component and a femoral stem fixed with antibiotic-impregnated bone cement.

In two-stage procedures, if the infectious process has been effectively treated during the interval period, the patient may be reimplanted (Fig. 7). During the second stage, if the intraoperative indices of infection are negative (Gram's stain, frozen section, surgeon's assessment), reimplantation is performed. The patient should remain on intravenous antibiotics after the reimplantation until the intraoperative culture results are determined.

REFERENCES

1. Lidwell OM, Lowbury EJ, Whyte W, et al: Effect of ultraclean air in operating rooms on deep sepsis in the joint after total hip or knee replacement: A randomised study. BMJ 1982; 285:10.
2. Brause BD: Sepsis: The rational use of antimicrobials. In Callaghan JJ, Rosenberg AG, Rubash HE (eds): The Adult Hip. Philadelphia, Lippincott-Raven, 1982, p 1343.
3. McAuley JP, Moreau G: Sepsis: Etiology, prophylaxis and diagnosis. In Callaghan JJ, Rosenberg AG, Rubash HE (eds): The Adult Hip. Philadelphia, Lippincott-Raven, 1982, p 1295.
4. Garvin KL, Fitzgerald RH Jr, Salvati EA, et al: Reconstruction of the infected total hip and knee arthroplasty with gentamicin-impregnated Palacos bone cement. Am Acad Orthop Surg Instr Course Lect 1993; 42:293.
5. Garvin KL, Hanssen AD: Current concepts review: Infection after total hip arthroplasty. J Bone Joint Surg Am 1995; 77:1576.
6. Elek SD, Conen PE: The virulence of Staphylococcus pyogenes for man. A study of the problems of wound infection. Br J Exp Pathol 1957; 38:573.
7. Gristina AG, Barth E, Webb LX: Microbial adhesion and the pathogenesis of biomaterial centered infections. In Gustillo R (eds): Orthopaedic Infection, Diagnosis and Treatment. Philadelphia, WB Saunders, 1989, p 3.
8. Hanssen AD, Osmon DR, Nelson CL: Prevention of deep periprosthetic joint infection. J Bone Joint Surg Am 1996; 78(3):458.
9. Marshall JC, Meakins JL: Immune responses and musculoskeletal disease. In Evarts MC (ed): Surgery of the Musculoskeletal System. New York, Churchill Livingston, 1990, p 4381.
10. Gherini S, Vaughn BK, Lombardi AV, et al: Delayed wound healing and nutritional deficiencies after total hip arthroplasty. Clin Orthop 1993; 293:188.
11. Stallone DD: The influence of obesity and its treatment on the immune system. Nutr Rev 1994; 52:37.
12. Greene KA, Wilde AH, Stulberg BN: Preoperative nutritional status of total joint patients. J Arthroplasty 1991; 6(4):321.
13. Bridges SL Jr, Moreland LW: Perioperative use of methotrexate in patients with rheumatoid arthritis undergoing orthopaedic surgery. Rheum Dis Clin North Am 1997; 23(4):981.
14. Pomposelli JJ, Bacter JK III, Babineau TJ, et al: Early postoperative glucose control predicts nosocomial infection rate in diabetic patients. J Parenter Enteral Nutr 1998; 22(2):77.
15. Bierbaum BE, Callaghan JJ, Galante JO, et al: An analysis of blood management in

patients having a total hip or knee arthroplasty. J Bone Joint Surg 1999; 1:2.
16. Blumberg N, Heal JM: Immunomodulation by blood transfusion: An evolving scientific and clinical challenge. Am J Med 1996; 101:299.
17. Cruse PJ, Foord R: A five-year prospective study of 23,649 surgical wounds. Arch Surg 1973; 107:206.
18. Beyer CA, Hanssen AD, Lewallen DG, et al: Primary total knee arthroplasty in patients with psoriasis. J Bone Joint Surg Br 1991; 73:258.
19. Nelson CL: Prevention of sepsis. Clin Orthop 1987; 222:66.
20. Anspach WE Jr: Barrier materials and special air-handling systems for bacteriologic control in the operating room. Am Acad Orthop Surg Instr Course Lect 1977; 26:47.
21. Davies RR, Noble WC: Dispersal of bacteria on desquamated skin. Lancet 1962; 2:1295.
22. Walter CW, Kundsin KA: Persistent wound drainage after primary total knee arthroplasty. J Arthroplasty 1993; 8:285.
23. Salvati EA, Robinson RP, Zeno SM, et al: Infection rate after 3175 total hip and total knee replacements performed with and without a horizontal unidirectional filtered air-flow system. J Bone Joint Surg Am 1982; 64:525.
24. Charnley J: Postoperative infection after total hip total replacement with special reference to air contamination in the operating room. Clin Orthop 1972; 87:167.
25. Marotte JH, Lord GA, Blanchard JP, et al: Infection rate in total hip arthroplasty as a function of air cleanliness and antibiotic prophylaxis: 10 year experience with 2,384 cementless Lord Madreporic prostheses. J Arthroplasty 1987; 2:77.
26. Nelson CL: Prevention of infection. In Evarts MC (ed): Surgery of the Musculoskeletal System. New York, Churchill Livingstone, 1990, p 4313.
27. Hill C, Flamant R, Mazas F, et al: Prophylactic cefazolin versus placebo in total hip replacement. Report of a multicentre double-blind randomised trial. Lancet 1981; 1:795.
28. James PJ, Butcher IA, Gardner ER, et al: Methicillin resistant Staphylococcus epidermidis in infection of total hip arthroplasties. J Bone Joint Surg Br 1994; 76(5):725.
29. Mauerhan DR, Nelson CL, Smith DL, et al: Prophylaxis against infection in total joint arthroplasty. J Bone Joint Surg Am 1994; 76(1):39.
30. Wannske M, Tscherne H: Results of prophylactic use of Refobacin-Palacos in implantation of endoprostheses of the hip joint in Hannover. Aktuelle Probl Chir Orthop 1979; 12:201.
31. Josefesson G, Komert L: Prophylaxis with

systemic antibiotics versus gentamicin bone cement in total hip arthroplasty. A ten year surgery of 1,688 hips. Clin Orthop 1993; 292:210.
32. Johnston DH, Fairclough JA, Brown EM, et al: Rate of bacterial recolonization of the skin after preparation: Four methods compared. J Surg 1987; 74:64.
33. Strange-Vongnsen HH, Klareskov B: Bacteriologic contamination of suction tips during hip arthroplasty. Acta Orthop Scand 1988; 59:410.
34. Baird RA, Nickel FR, Thrupp LD, et al: Splash basin contamination in orthopaedic surgery. Clin Orthop 1984; 187:129.
35. Osmon DR, Steckelberg JM, Hanssen AD: Incidence of prosthetic joint infection due to viridans streptococci. Presented at the annual meeting of the Musculoskeletal Infection Society, Snowmass, CO, 1993.
36. Advisory statement. Antibiotic prophylaxis for dental patients with total joint replacements. American Dental Association. American Academy of Orthopaedic Surgeons. J Am Dent Assoc 1997; 128:1004.
37. Surin VV, Sundhold K, Bäckman L: Infection after total hip replacement. J Bone Joint Surg Br 1983; 65:412.
38. Coventry MB: Treatment of infections occurring in total hip surgery. Orthop Clin North Am 1975; 6(4)991.
39. Fitzgerald RH Jr: Infected total hip arthroplasty: Diagnosis and treatment. J Am Acad Orthop Surg 1995; 3(5):249.
40. Tsukayama DT, Estrada R, Gustilo RB: Infection after total hip arthroplasty. A study of the treatment of one hundred and six infections. J Bone Joint Surg Am 1996; 78:512.
41. Spangehl MJ, Younger SE, Masri BA, et al: Diagnosis of infection following total hip arthroplasty. J Bone Joint Surg Am 1997; 79:1478.
42. Forster IW, Crawford R: Sedimentation rate in infected and uninfected total hip arthroplasty. Clin Orthop 1982; 168:48.
43. Aalto K, Österman K, Peltola H, et al: Changes in erythrocyte sedimentation rate and c-reactive protein after total hip arthroplasty. Clin Orthop 1984; 184:118.
44. Choudhry RR, Rice RP, Triffitt PD, et al: Plasma viscosity and c-reactive protein after total hip and knee arthroplasty. J Bone Joint Surg Br 1992; 74:523.
45. Lonner JH, Desai P, DiCesare PE, et al: The reliability of analysis of intraoperative frozen sections for identifying active infection during revision hip or knee arthroplasty. J Bone Joint Surg Am 1996; 78:1553.
46. Hoeffel DP, Hinrichs SH, Garvin KL: Molecular diagnosis of infection. Semin Arthroplasty 1998; 9(4):281.
47. Mariana BD, Martin DS, Levine MJ, et al: Polymerase chain reaction detection of

bacterial infection in total knee arthroplasty. Clin Orthop 1996; 331:11.

48. Widmer AF,. Gacchter A, Ochsner PE, et al: Antimicrobial treatment of orthopaedic implant related infections with rifampin combinations. Clin Infect Dis 1992; 14: 1251.

49. Drancourt M, Stein A, Argenson JN, et al: Oral rifampin plus ofloxacin for treatment of staphylococcus-infected orthopaedic implants. Antimicrob Agents Chemother 1993; 37:1214.

50. Kostuik J, Alexander D: Arthrodesis for

failed arthroplasty of the hip. Clin Orthop 1984; 188:173.

51. Fenelon GCC, von Foerster G, Engelbrecht E: Disarticulation of the hip as a result of failed arthroplasty. A series of 11 cases. J Bone Joint Surg Br 1980; 62:441.

52. Nestor BJ, Hanssen AD, Ferrer-Gonzales R, et al: The use of porous prostheses in delayed reconstruction of total hip replacements that have failed because of infection. J Bone Joint Surg Am 1994; 76:349.

53. Masri BA, Duncan CP: Sepsis: Antibiotic-loaded implants. In Callaghan JJ, Rosen-

berg AG, Rubash HE (eds): The Adult Hip. Philadelphia, Lippincott-Raven, 1998, p 1331.

54. Lieberman JR, Callaway GH, Salvati EA, et al: Treatment of the infected total hip arthroplasty with a two-stage reimplantation protocol. Clin Orthop 1994; 301:205.

55. Masri BA, Salvati EA: Two-stage exchange. In Callaghan JJ, Rosenberg AG, Rubash HE (eds): Philadelphia, Lippincott-Raven, 1998, p 1317.

section 5 chapter 8

INFECTED TOTAL KNEE ARTHROPLASTY

Henry D. Clarke, Giles R. Scuderi, and Arlen D. Hanssen

Summary

- Deep infection of a total knee replacement occurs in approximately 1% to 2% of cases.
- Arthrocentesis for culture and sensitivity testing and synovial fluid analysis represent the gold standard of diagnosis. Erythrocyte sedimentation rates, C-reactive protein tests, and radionuclide imaging can provide additional information in some cases.
- Acute postoperative infections or events of late hematogenous seeding, diagnosed within 2 to 3 weeks of onset, may be potentially treated successfully by urgent open débridement and component retention.
- Two-stage reimplantation, incorporating 4 to 6 weeks of intravenous antibiotics and reinsertion of another prosthesis, is currently considered the treatment of choice for chronic infections, with contemporary success rates averaging 90 to 95%.

Deep infection remains one of the most severe complications of total knee arthroplasty. During the 1970s, the overall infection rate following total knee arthroplasty was approximately 5%[1] and with certain early hinged designs exceeded 12%.[2] Treatment of infection in this era included attempts at débridement, resection arthroplasty, or arthrodesis and were associated with high failure rates and poor functional results.[3, 4] Reinsertion of a second prosthesis was usually unsuccessful.[5]

During the 1980s, infection rates in primary total knee arthroplasty decreased to approximately 1% to 2%.[6, 7] Simultaneously, recognition of the importance of the duration of the infection, need for complete débridement, use of adjunctive intravenous antibiotics, and application of optimal soft-tissue coverage increased treatment success rates. Despite modern advances in prevention, instances of deep infection inevitably occur and, although rarely life-threatening, are associated with high morbidity.

The contemporary multidisciplinary treatment approach has considerably improved the prognosis, but successful salvage of a functional extremity still involves costly and time-consuming use of health care resources. The physical, emotional, and financial consequences for the patient, surgeon, and society can often be severe. Two-stage reimplantation techniques are associated with long-term eradication of infection and good functional results in approximately 90% to 95% of patients.[8, 9] During the 1990s, increased focus has been on minimizing the patient's disability and decreasing the costs of treatment of the patient with an infected total knee arthroplasty without compromising long-term success rates.[10, 11]

PATHOGENESIS

With contemporary surgical techniques and perioperative management strategies, the incidence of deep infection after total knee replacement is approximately 1% to 2%.[6, 7] The risk factors predisposing to infection can be broadly grouped into three categories related to the host, bacteria, and the wound environment.[12] Interventions designed to improve the host response, decrease bacterial contamination, and optimize the local wound environment should be systematically considered in the preoperative, intraoperative, and postoperative periods.[12] A disciplined team approach directed toward these three broad elements facilitates the implementation of preventive measures.

Host factors predisposing to an increased risk of infection have been documented in patients with rheumatoid arthritis,[13, 14] patients who use immunosuppressive drugs,[14, 15] and those who have other systemic conditions that affect the immune system such as diabetes,[16] malnourishment,[15, 17] or advanced age.[17] Preoperative evaluation to identify any of these host factors allows medical optimization during the entire perioperative period.

Established bacterial infections at remote sites, including skin lesions,[13, 14, 18] urinary tract infections,[18] and dental abscesses[18] increase the risk of hematogenous seeding of a prosthetic joint and should be treated prior to surgery or aggressively with appropriate antibiotics if they occur postoperatively.[19] The use of prophylactic perioperative antibiotics has been an important preventive advancement. Preoperative systemic antibiotics with excellent antistaphylococcal and antistreptococcal activity should be given within 30 minutes of the skin incision and no later than 5 to 10 minutes before the tourniquet is inflated.[12] Postoperatively, two or three doses of intravenous antibiotics are sufficient.[12] Currently, the use of perioperative antimicrobial prophylaxis is considered the cornerstone of infection prevention.

The clinical significance of technical advances designed to reduce intraoperative airborne bacterial contamination, including laminar flow systems, ultraviolet light, and personnel isolator suits are controversial if perioperative antibiotics are used.[12] Some evidence suggests that horizontal laminar airflow may actually increase infection rates in total knee arthroplasty when used without body exhaust suits, most likely because of the placement of unprotected personnel between the laminar flow source and the operative site.[20] The multiple factors involved in the development of postoperative infection and the vast numbers of patients required to gain the statistical power to enable significant differences between treatment groups has prevented completion of definitive studies. Reasonable conclusions from published reports are that vertical laminar flow is superior to horizontal laminar flow in reducing airborne contamination, and personnel isolator suits should probably be used in conjunction with clean air technology.

The local wound environment can also affect healing. Specific risk factors for deep infection related to the wound include a history of prior surgery or infection of the involved knee joint.[14] Poor-quality surrounding soft tissues or vascular compromise of the extremity should also be carefully heeded; occasionally, soft-tissue coverage procedures or the use of tissue expanders prior to arthroplasty may reduce postoperative wound complications.[21] Intraoperatively, careful tissue handling helps optimize the local wound environment and may prevent marginal skin necrosis or full-thickness sloughing.

The nature of the implanted prosthesis is an important variable in the development of postoperative infection. The concept of bacterial interaction with biomaterials is extensively discussed in Chapter 5–7. Hinged prostheses and other prosthetic surfaces that create large volumes of particulate debris have been implicated in the development of late infection.[13, 22] Postoperative wound complications including hematomas, skin necrosis, and wound drainage contribute to the development of subsequent infection.[13, 23] Whereas early wound drainage can be managed with immobilization and compression, persistent drainage is best treated with early exploration and débridement.[23]

After total joint replacement, antibiotic prophylaxis prior to invasive procedures, such as dental work or cystoscopy, potentially reduces the risk of hematogenous seeding by the bacteremia associated with the invasive procedure. Guidelines issued in 1997 by the American Dental Association and American Academy of Orthopaedic Surgeons regarding the use of antibiotics prior to dental procedures are outlined in Chapter 5–7.[19]

Despite diligent preventive efforts, infection will still occasionally occur. The duration of the infection is an important variable determining effective treatment. In acute postoperative or late infections due to hematogenous seeding, if the suspected duration of the infection exceeds 2 to 3 weeks, the infection should be considered and treated as a chronic infection. The type of infecting microorganism also potentially influences the management of the infection, and at a minimum guides the selection of appropriate antibiotics. In circumstances in which no organism is identified, empiric antibiotics should be selected based on the microorganisms most likely present. In several large studies, the most commonly identified bacteria were *Staphylococcus aureus* and coagulase-negative staphylococcus.[4, 8, 9, 13, 14] Among 357 deep infections that occurred in a group of over 12,000 total knee replacements, 42% were due to *S. aureus,* and 17% were due to coagulase-negative staphylococcus.[13]

CLINICAL FEATURES

Early postoperative infection, although infrequent, is rarely difficult to recognize unless prolonged perioperative antibiotics mask the initial signs. The wound may be erythematous and often has or has had persistent drainage. The patient may fail to proceed with rehabilitation in the expected manner, with persistent pain and swelling. Fever and systemic illness are uncommon. Acute hematogenous infections typically present with a sudden increase in swelling, pain, and erythema in a previously well-functioning prosthesis. Often, a source of bacteremia can be identified through careful questioning. Chronic infections are notoriously more difficult to diagnose, as signs and symptoms are often masked or modified by indiscriminate use of antibiotics. Persistent pain, especially at night or at rest, and recurrent swelling should always raise the suspicion of deep infection. Physical examination may reveal a small eschar occluding a sinus tract, and erythema, edema, warmth, or tenderness of the overlying skin may also be noted (Fig. 1). An effusion and poor range of motion may be indicative of a persistent reactive synovitis. In many cases, however, the outward appearance of a chronically infected knee can be surprisingly unremarkable and the patient's only complaint is a painful arthroplasty.

INVESTIGATIONS

In the event of suspected infection, aspiration of joint fluid should be performed expediently. The synovial fluid obtained should be sent for aerobic and anaerobic incubation and sensitivity testing, Gram's stain, and analysis for total leukocyte count and differential testing. The presence of more than 25,000 leukocytes per cubic millimeter or greater than 75% polymorphonuclear neutrophil leukocytes is evidence of infection.[24] In several large series of infected knee arthroplasties, 94% to 100% of results of preoperative aspirations were positive.[9, 25] False-negative results may be due to recent or concurrent antibiotic treatment and therefore all antibiotics should be discontinued 2 to 3 weeks before an aspiration attempt in the chronic setting. Reaspiration after a 4-week interval without antibiotic treatment has been shown to significantly improve sensitivity and speci-

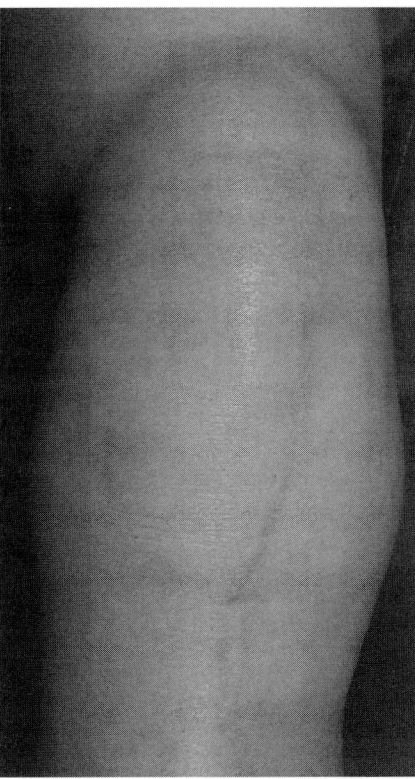

Fig. 1. Photograph demonstrating erythema and swelling. This shows a patient with a chronic infection of a total knee arthroplasty.

ficity.[26] If débridement and prosthesis retention are being considered for treatment of an acute postoperative or late hematogenous infection, one should not wait for final culture results before proceeding with débridement if the clinical signs and symptoms and synovial fluid analysis support the diagnosis. Any time delay only diminishes the success of a débridement with prosthesis retention.

Hematological tests, such as the erythrocyte sedimentation rate and C-reactive protein, often show elevations, but their results are relatively nonspecific for infection. These results may also be difficult to interpret in patients with rheumatoid arthritis or other systemic diseases. An erythrocyte sedimentation rate of greater than 30 mm/h (Westergren) has been reported to have a sensitivity of 80% and a specificity of 62.5% for infection.[26] Normal hematological test results should not rule out the diagnosis of a deep periprosthetic infection, and, in the presence of unexplained pain, additional tests should be considered.

Radiographs should always be obtained and examined for component loosening, osteolysis, and new periosteal reaction that may be suggestive of chronic infection (Fig. 2). Comparison of new radiographs with previous studies may show rapid and dramatic changes. The use of radionuclide scans for the detection of infected total knee replacements is also a consideration. In low-grade chronic infections, or in patients with inflammatory arthritis, the accuracy of these tests may be reduced. When used alone, the accuracy of indium-111–labeled leukocyte scans has been reported to be approximately 78%, and technetium bone scans are even less accurate.[5, 27] When indium-111–labeled leukocyte scans are used in conjunction with tech-

netium-99 sulfur colloid marrow scans to determine areas of incongruent uptake, the combined accuracy is reported to be 95%.[27]

The accuracy of intraoperative frozen section histological analysis to support the diagnosis of infection may also be helpful. The presence of 10 polymorphonuclear neutrophil leukocytes per high-power field has been considered indicative of infection, with a reported sensitivity of 84% and specificity of 99%, when compared with results of intraoperative cultures.[28] The recent application of molecular biological techniques to aid in the detection of infection has led to the development of highly sensitive polymerase chain reaction tests for bacterial DNA.[29] These tests may be potentially useful in situations in which culture results are equivocal and infection is clinically suspected, and they are discussed in more detail in Chapter 5–7. In the final analysis, the practitioner must be able to select appropriate tests and synthesize sometimes conflicting information to diagnose the presence of deep infection and then define an appropriate treatment strategy.

TREATMENT GOALS, INDICATIONS, AND CONTRAINDICATIONS

The treatment goals of the infected total knee arthroplasty include eradication of infection, elimination of pain, and restoration of extremity function. The six basic treatment strategies are (1) chronic antibiotic suppression, (2) débridement with prosthesis retention, (3) resection arthroplasty, (4) arthrodesis, (5) amputation, and (6) reimplanta-

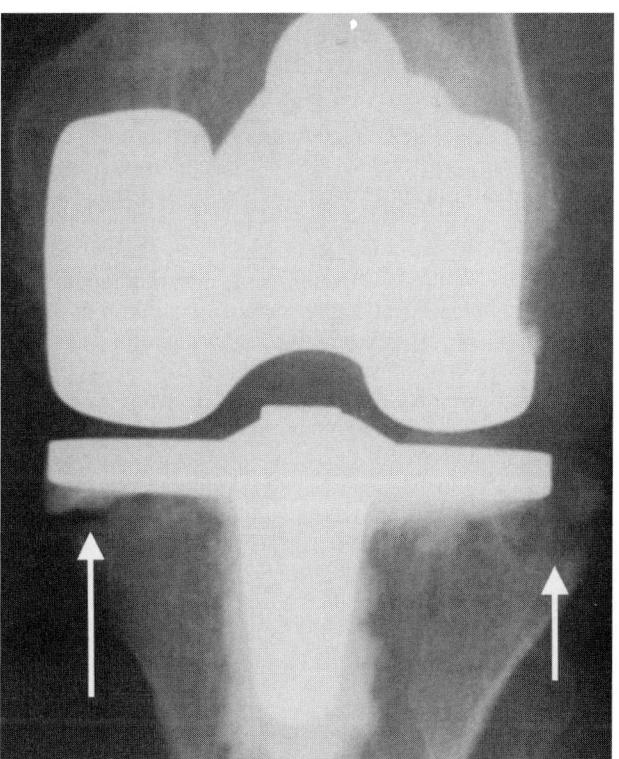

Fig. 2. Anteroposterior radiograph of a total knee arthroplasty. Osteolysis and peripheral bone erosion due to chronic infection are revealed (*arrows*).

TABLE 1. TREATMENT INDICATIONS AND CONTRAINDICATIONS FOR INFECTED TOTAL KNEE ARTHROPLASTY		
Treatment	**Indications**	**Contraindications**
Antibiotic suppression	Patient's medical condition precludes surgery Organism susceptible to oral antibiotics Antibiotic has low toxicity Prosthesis well fixed	Patient with other total joint replacements Young patient High-virulence organism
Débridement and prosthesis retention	Acute infection with duration <2–3 weeks Well-fixed components Low-virulence gram-positive bacteria	Failed prior attempt at prosthesis retention Hinged prosthesis Draining sinus
Resection arthroplasty	Patient with limited activity demands and severe polyarticular involvement Medically compromised patient	Extensive bone loss Arthrodesis of ipsilateral hip or contralateral hip or knee
Arthrodesis	Disrupted extensor mechanism Resistant bacteria Poor soft tissue envelope Young patient	Contralateral amputation Ipsilateral hip or contralateral hip or knee disease Severe segmental bone loss
Direct-exchange arthroplasty	Low-virulence gram-positive bacteria	
Two-stage reimplantation	Patient with high functional expectations and little prior disability	Persistent infection Disrupted extensor mechanism Medical condition precludes multiple operations Poor soft tissue coverage Immunocompromised patient
Amputation	Life-threatening sepsis Persistent infection with severe bone loss	Arthrodesis of ipsilateral hip or contralateral hip or knee

tion of a new prosthesis. Except for the first option, which does not eradicate the infection, the principal concept is extensive surgical débridement with adjunctive use of antibiotics. The specific indications and contraindications for each treatment plan are presented in Table 1.

PROCEDURES

PREOPERATIVE PLANNING

When the diagnosis of infection has been established, the host, bacteria, and wound factors should be considered while an appropriate treatment plan is formulated. A treatment algorithm incorporating specific treatment variables to arrive at the proper treatment strategy is presented in Figure 3. It is important to emphasize that the duration of infection has significant implications in determining appropriate treatment. A preoperative assessment of the adjacent soft tissues is important, and the need for adjunctive soft-tissue procedures at the time of débridement or reimplantation should be coordinated with plastic surgeons.[21, 30] When component removal is anticipated, specific technical details should be reviewed. For example, the presence of well-fixed, long-stemmed components whose removal might seriously compromise the ability to reconstruct the joint may affect treatment decisions. When long stems or intramedullary cement need to be removed, the appropriate equipment should be available, such as specialized osteotomes, high-speed drills, and ultrasonic cement removal equipment.

TECHNICAL DETAILS
Exposure
The fundamental premise of all management techniques, except chronic antibiotic suppression alone, is eradication

of the infection through extensive surgical débridement. To accomplish this goal, adequate exposure is required. The placement of incisions is crucial to wound viability, and if multiple prior incisions are present, the most lateral, midline longitudinal skin incision should be selected. Skin bridges of less than 5 to 7 cm should be avoided. Arthrotomy is usually performed through a medial parapatellar capsulotomy. Mobilization and eversion of the patella may initially be difficult, but a number of techniques, when applied in a systematic fashion, will facilitate exposure. A subperiosteal dissection of the medial collateral ligament and semimembranosus insertion enables external rotation and anterolateral displacement of the tibia. This allows the patella to be subluxed laterally and provides adequate exposure for débridement and component removal. Once the femoral and tibial components are removed, eversion of the patella can usually be accomplished, but this maneuver is best avoided. On occasion, either at the time of component removal or, more commonly, at the time of reimplantation, further exposure is occasionally required. A number of specialized exposure techniques have been utilized effectively.[31] We favor the use of a quadriceps snip as the first option to relieve tension on the extensor mechanism, as this does not have any detrimental impact on postoperative rehabilitation. The snip can be used in conjunction with an anchor pin, drill bit, or suture placed through the distal patellar tendon insertion into the tibial bone. Release of the lateral retinaculum during exposure and reestablishment of the medial and lateral gutters also facilitate exposure. We avoid the use of a tibial tubercle osteotomy or quadriceps turndown during surgical exposure if at all possible and have only rarely used these exposure techniques. Beyond the surgical exposure, technical details of each management option are technique specific.

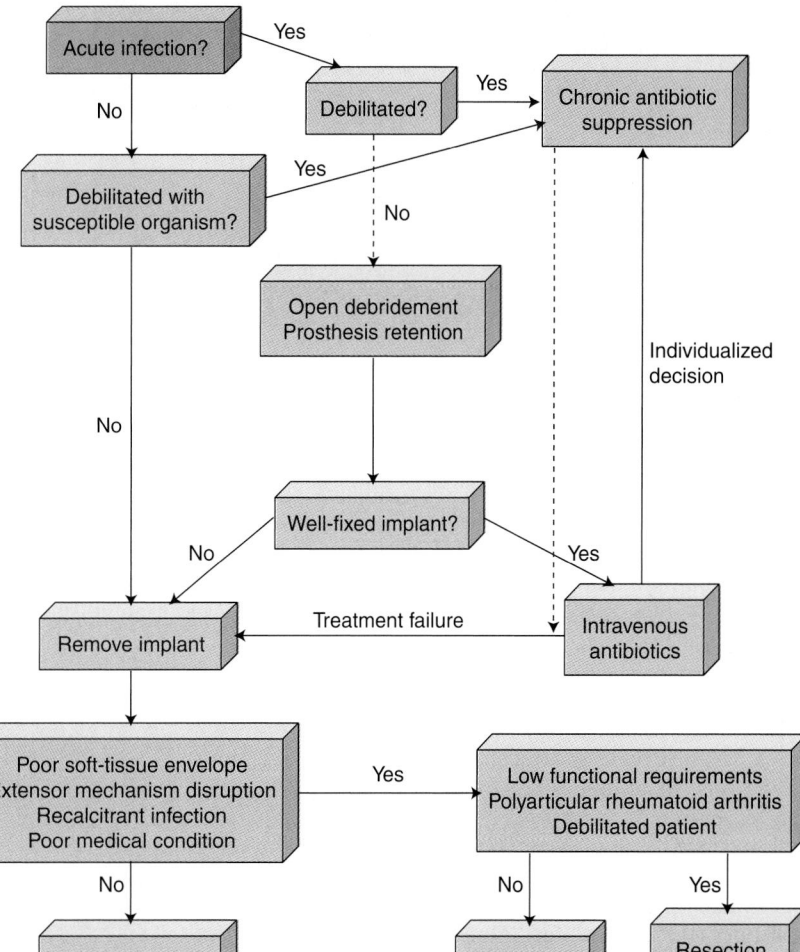

Fig. 3. A treatment algorithm.

Débridement and Prosthesis Retention

Although successful arthroscopic débridement has been reported, we recommend against this treatment approach and instead use an open technique.[32] One-stage open débridement includes a complete synovectomy, removal of modular polyethylene inserts, and débridement of all interfaces. After three to five tissue specimens have been obtained for culture testing, a complete synovectomy is performed and includes débridement of the suprapatellar pouch, medial and lateral gutters, and posterior capsular region. The joint is copiously irrigated, a new polyethylene insert is implanted, and the joint is closed with monofilament suture in the fascia and skin. Two deep drains are inserted to minimize hematoma accumulation, which may act as a growth medium. Two-stage débridement involves the same initial steps as described earlier for a one-stage technique. However, after the initial débridement has been performed, antibiotic-impregnated cement beads, 4 to 5 mm in diameter, containing a combination of 4 to 6 g of vancomycin and tobramycin per 40-g batch of cement are prepared and placed into the joint. More than 50 to 75 beads can be

accommodated without compromising wound closure. The fascia and skin are then closed with monofilament sutures and the knee is immobilized. After 4 to 5 days of empiric intravenous antibiotics and when the results of culture and sensitivity tests are available, the wound is reopened, the beads are removed, another débridement is performed, a new polyethylene insert is implanted, and the wound is again closed.

Definitive Resection Arthroplasty

Following component removal and débridement of all infected tissue and foreign material, several large absorbable monofilament sutures can be used to align the tibial and femoral surfaces. Postoperative cast immobilization with protective weight-bearing for up to 6 months can create enough inherent fibrous stability to avoid the need for external extremity support yet still allow sufficient flexion to facilitate sitting. The stability gained through the fibrous union may allow the patient to ambulate independently with the use of a gait aid.

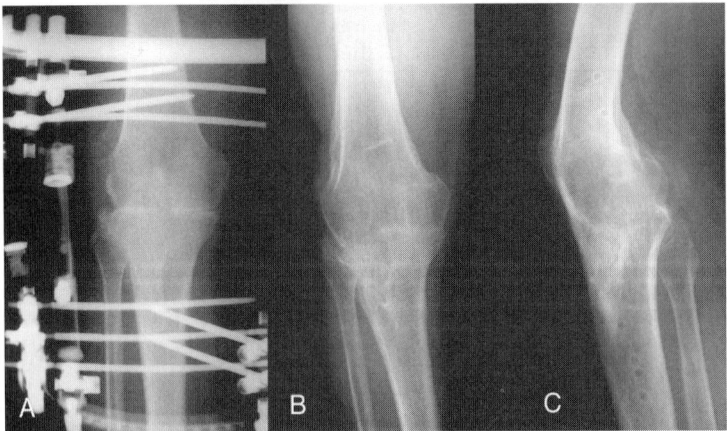

Fig. 4. Radiographs of a patient with an infected total knee arthroplasty treated with excisional arthroplasty and arthrodesis. *A,* This is an anteroposterior radiograph of knee arthrodesis achieved with a multiplanar external fixator. *B* and *C,* These are anteroposterior and lateral radiographs of same patient with a solid knee arthrodesis in neutral coronal alignment and 15 degrees of flexion.

Arthrodesis

Although exposure should allow the complete removal of all infected and foreign material and more than one débridement may be required, collateral dissection of the soft tissues should be minimized to preserve bone vascularity. Removal of bone at the time of débridement should be limited to necrotic material only. Key steps at the time of delayed arthrodesis include preparation of the bone ends, rigid immobilization of the opposed bony surfaces, and bone grafting if necessary. Adequate opposition of vascular, cancellous bone is critical to obtaining osseous union. At the time of arthrodesis, it is often necessary to remove only a few millimeters of bone from previous cuts to achieve good bone-to-bone contact and restore limb alignment. If less than 50% opposition is achieved, bone grafting should be considered.[6] In the absence of significant bone loss, the optimal fusion position is 10 to 20 degrees of flexion, which allows swing-through of the affected extremity during ambulation (Fig. 4).[6] In the presence of bone loss encountered after removal of most total knee arthroplasties, fusion close to full extension can maximize limb length without compromising foot clearance. Optimal limb alignment of 0 to 5 degrees valgus can be achieved with the use of the intramedullary and extramedullary instrumentation used in total knee replacement to create the distal femoral and proximal tibial cuts.

Rigid immobilization can be accomplished with external fixation or intramedullary nailing. External fixation may be performed in the presence of active infection[3] or ipsilateral hip implants. Multiplanar devices with transfixing pins placed medial to lateral in the femur and placed lateral to medial in the tibia, supplemented by additional anterior half-pins placed in both the femur and tibia, provide excellent rigidity (Fig. 5). Alternatively, two uniplane fixators can be placed at 90 degrees to each other with half-pins inserted anteromedially and anterolaterally. It is rare that the use of a single uniplane fixator provides adequate stability. The use of two uniplanar fixators has numerous advantages about the knee, as these devices are easy to apply and also allow placement that minimizes problems with soft-tissue impingement, especially in obese patients. External fixation is typically required for extended periods of up to 10 to 16 weeks. Following removal of the fixation

device, cast immobilization, often 4 to 6 months, should be used until radiographic union occurs.

Arthrodesis with a long intramedullary nail should be avoided in the presence of active infection and is best reserved for the management of aseptic nonunions after failed attempts at external fixation, or when a staged arthrodesis is performed after infection has been eradicated.[33]

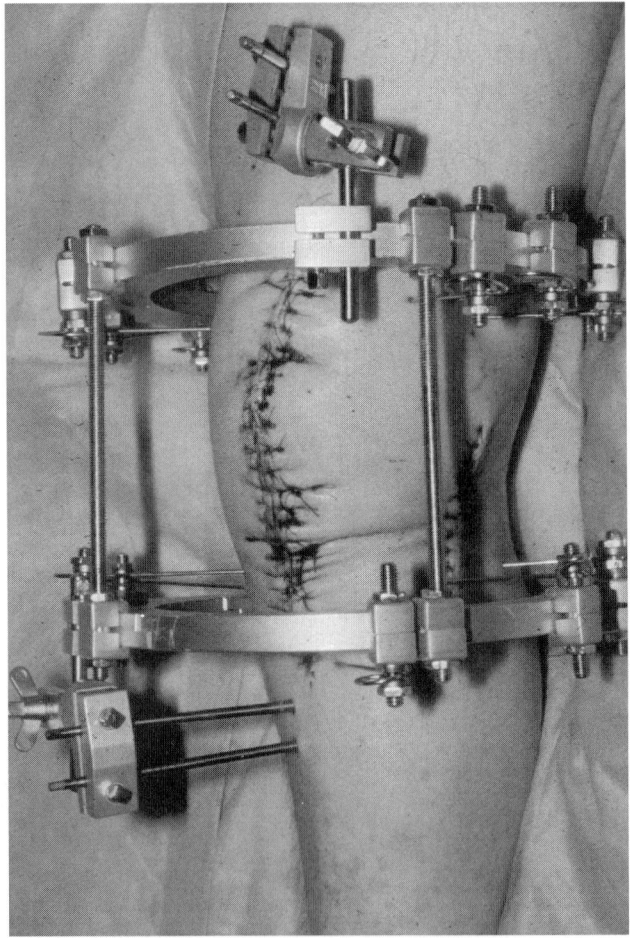

Fig. 5. Photograph of patient with a multiplanar ring fixation device.

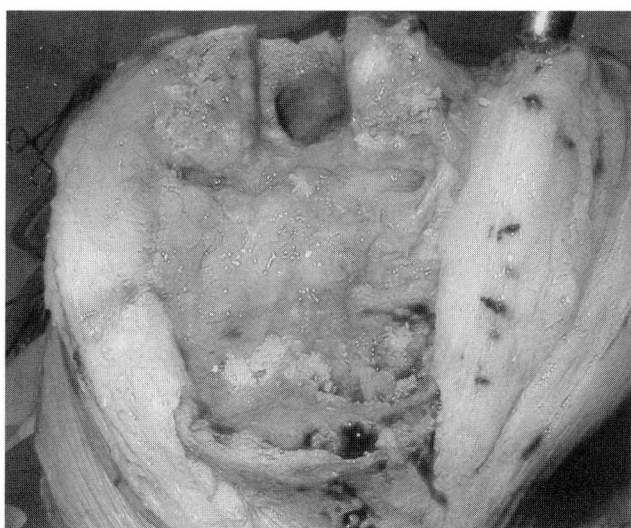

Fig. 6. Intraoperative photograph. This shows a knee joint with proliferative scar, synovitis, and frank purulence.

The tibia should be reamed until contact is established with the isthmus of the canal and then the femur is reamed in a retrograde fashion. To allow passage of the intramedullary nail, bone preparation should create a tibial-femoral angle of 0 degrees.[6] Prior to introduction of the nail, bone graft should be packed posteriorly. During nail introduction, distraction at the joint surfaces should be avoided. The use of proximal and distal locking screws provides rotational stability and reduces the risk of proximal nail migration.

Reimplantation

There have been some advocates for a direct exchange operation whereby a new prosthesis is inserted at the time of débridement and removal of the infected prosthesis. This approach has been rare in the treatment of the infected total knee arthroplasty when compared with the hip joint. The disadvantages of a direct exchange operation in the knee joint are particularly pertinent when one considers the fragile nature of the surrounding soft-tissue envelope of the

knee joint. We currently advise a two-stage reimplantation, which has become the treatment of choice for most patients.[24]

At the time of component removal, care should be taken to preserve as much viable bone as possible. The presence of chronic infection creates formation of abundant synovitis and scar tissue (Fig. 6). Complete débridement and synovectomy are crucial, and the posterior capsular region is frequently débrided inadequately owing to the proximity of the neurovascular structures. In particular, all bone cement should be removed, and careful search for any cement filling drill holes produced at the initial arthroplasty is recommended. Typically, one complete and thorough débridement is sufficient, as multiple sequential débridements predispose toward superinfection with nosocomial organisms.

The insertion of antibiotic-impregnated cement beads or spacer blocks allows local delivery of high concentrations of antibiotics. Although the larger surface area of multiple beads may theoretically provide increased elution of local antibiotics when compared with a single spacer block, no definite clinical advantage has been proven. Block spacers confer definite mechanical advantages over beads by facilitating joint stability and ambulation prior to staged reimplantation. Spacers also allow easier exposure at the time of reimplantation.[34] In most cases, a spacer block is fashioned using two 40-g batches of polymethylmethacrylate cement mixed with 4 to 6 g of antibiotics, but in some patients with severe bone loss, larger spacers are required. We typically use at least 2.4 g of tobramycin and 2 g of vancomycin per pack of cement. When one mixes the antibiotics, the lumps in the crystalline vancomycin should not be crushed, as these facilitate higher elution of local antibiotic. Once the cement has reached a doughy consistency, it is placed into the tibial-femoral space during the final stages of polymerization, and slight longitudinal distraction is intermittently applied to the extremity (Fig. 7). This maneuver helps prevent cement interdigitation into the bone and enables easy removal at the time of reimplantation.

If large spacers are used, the heat generated by the exothermic reaction can be significant. Irrigation can be

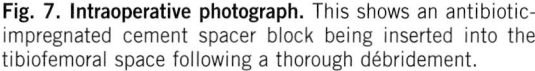

Fig. 7. Intraoperative photograph. This shows an antibiotic-impregnated cement spacer block being inserted into the tibiofemoral space following a thorough débridement.

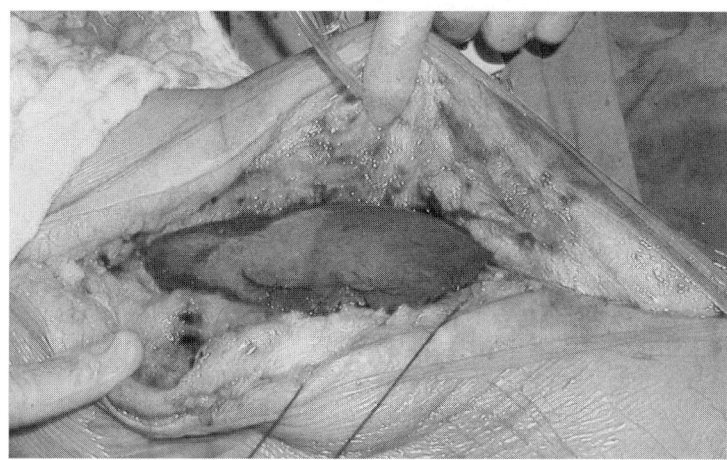

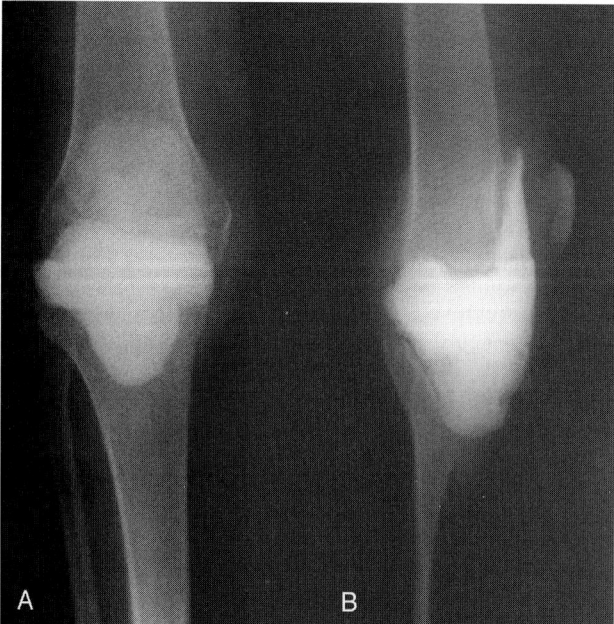

Fig. 8. Radiographs following excisional arthroplasty and the introduction of spacer block. These are anteroposterior *(A)* and lateral radiographs *(B)* of an antibiotic-impregnated cement spacer block with a femoral flange and a tibial peg.

used to cool the block and may prevent damage to the neurovascular structures that lie only millimeters from the posterior capsule. Short pegs or stems can be fashioned to help provide stability. Extending the spacer anteriorly over the distal femur and into the patellofemoral joint also helps with stability and acts to maintain a plane between the patella and femur (Fig. 8). The block should be suitably large to sit on cortical bone and provide stability in extension. If the block is too small and has contact predominantly with cancellous bone or is insufficient to maintain stability, further bone erosion can occur. If the intramedul-

lary canal is opened to remove stemmed components, antibiotic-impregnated cement rods can be placed inside the canals. Use of a cement spacer usually provides enough stability to the knee to allow the patient to walk for short distances in an immobilizer or cast, which facilitates care at home prior to reimplantation.

During the 1990s, functional temporary spacers were developed that incorporate small metallic femoral runners and polyethylene inserts into molded polymethylmethacrylate components. One such device, the PROSTALAC (prosthesis of antibiotic-loaded acrylic cement) allows joint motion and weightbearing during the period prior to reimplantation.[11] A range of motion up to 75 degrees has been reported with the use of this temporary functional spacer.[11] In a similar manner, some surgeons have sterilized the extracted femoral component and reinserted it temporarily using a small polyethylene insert on a cement block.[10] Again, this can potentially reduce the patient's disability between débridement and staged reimplantation, particularly in the patient being treated for simultaneous infected total knee arthroplasties. If an articulating spacer is used, then attention must be paid to equalizing the flexion and extension space or dislocation may occur. We have not been able to demonstrate any improvement in the final functional outcome of reimplantation when using these devices and currently prefer the use of rigid block spacers.

Aspiration prior to reimplantation may be considered if there is clinical suspicion of persistent infection. In most cases, however, our decision to proceed with reimplantation is determined intraoperatively based on the appearance of the tissues and an evaluation of histological frozen section specimens. At the time of reimplantation, adequate surgical exposure must be obtained and the use of one of the previously discussed techniques such as the quadriceps snip may be required in addition to reestablishing the medial and lateral gutters. Although uncemented prostheses with bone graft soaked in antibiotic solution have been successfully used in reimplantation, we favor the use of cemented prostheses.[35] The use of antibiotic-impregnated

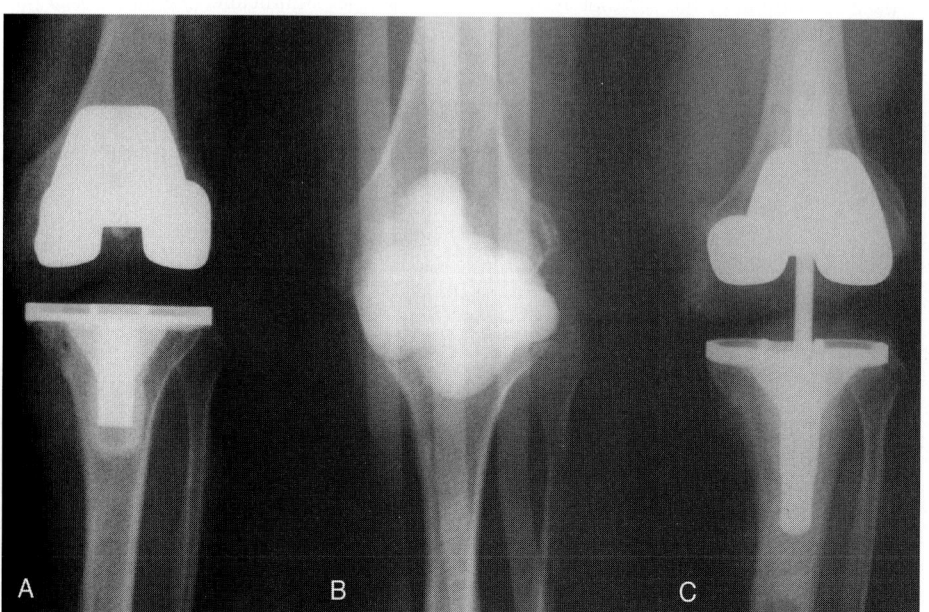

Fig. 9. Sequential radiographs of a patient with an infected total knee arthroplasty treated with a two-stage exchange arthroplasty. These are an *(A)* anteroposterior radiograph of an infected total knee arthroplasty; *(B)* anteroposterior radiograph of same patient with an antibiotic-impregnated cement spacer block in a knee immobilizer; and *(C)* anteroposterior radiograph of same patient following two-stage reimplantation with a posterior stabilized prosthesis augmented with stems and fixed with antibiotic-impregnated cement.

TABLE 2. COMPLICATIONS IN INFECTED TOTAL KNEE ARTHROPLASTY*

Treatment	Complication
Antibiotic suppression	Antibiotic toxicity
	Prosthesis loosening
	Bacterial resistance
Débridement and prosthesis retention	Wound healing problems
	Prosthesis loosening
Resection arthroplasty	20% persistent pain[37]
	13% >20 degrees varus/valgus instability[37]
Arthrodesis	
External fixation	Overall complication rate 20–65%[6,38,39]
	14% painful fibrous nonunion[39]
	3–11% pin site infection[38,39]
	8% painless fibrous nonunion[39]
	7% pin site fracture[39]
	4% amputation[39]
	3–4% wound healing problems[38,39]
Intramedullary nail	Overall complication rate 40–55%[6,33]
	11% hardware failure[33]
	11% painful nonunion[33]
	6–10% proximal migration nail[33,38]
	6–10% wound breakdown[33,38]
	11% amputation[33]
Reimplantation	Overall complication rate 23%[9]
	11–20% wound healing problems[9,34]
	3% knee dislocation[9]
	2–3% patella fracture[8,9]
	2% patella dislocation[9]
	1–2% extensor mechanism rupture[8,9]
Amputation	Wound breakdown
	Persistent infection

* Excluding recurrent infection.

cement at the time of reimplantation has been shown to significantly lower the risk of recurrent infection.[9]

Significant bone loss is often encountered at the time of reimplantation, which may require the use of modular wedges or blocks. Therefore, a prosthesis system, which has a full range of augments, should be available at reimplantation, and these blocks and wedges should be used in conjunction with extended-length stems. In the majority of reimplantations, we currently use a cemented posterior stabilized prosthesis with wedges, blocks, and stems where required (Fig. 9). The use of more constrained designs is reserved for cases with ligamentous insufficiency or iatrogenic instability. One of the authors (G.R.S.) cements only the core prosthesis and avoids introduction of cement into the canal when stem extensions are used. This facilitates removal of the stems if subsequent prosthesis removal is required. Rarely, in cases with severe bone loss, custom prostheses or modular tumor prostheses may be required, and the need for these devices must be anticipated preoperatively.

The postoperative management of individual patients is dependent on numerous variables, including the status of the soft-tissue coverage, the type of exposure required, and whether structural bone grafts were utilized. In general, antibiotics are administered intravenously until final intraoperative culture results and tissue section evaluations have been obtained. If all results are negative for infection, then antibiotics are discontinued

COMPLICATIONS AND RESULTS

COMPLICATIONS

Excluding recurrent infection, the most severe complications following attempts at débridement, resection arthroplasty, arthrodesis, and reimplantation for infected total knee replacements include intraoperative nerve or vascular injury and soft-tissue complications. The proximity of the neurovascular bundle to the posterior capsule places the popliteal structures at risk during the extensive débridements that are crucial in all surgical options. Blunt periosteal elevators can be used to elevate the posterior capsule off the femur to recreate the posterior capsular space. Soft-tissue problems, including marginal skin necrosis and full-thickness slough, may be prevented through careful intraoperative tissue handling, and with the use of tissue expanders or muscle flaps. When problems occur postoperatively, soft-tissue débridement and coverage are required as soon as demarcation occurs. Traumatic avulsion or rupture of the patella tendon is a devastating complication without a reliable solution in these circumstances. If infection is eradicated, then reconstruction with an extensor mechanism or Achilles tendon allograft may be considered; alternatively, bracing or arthrodesis should be considered.

TABLE 3. RESULTS OF TREATMENT OF INFECTED TOTAL KNEE ARTHROPLASTY

Treatment	Result
Antibiotic suppression	27% successful suppression[6]
Débridement and prosthesis retention	23–29% successful eradication of infection (all patients)[4,6,40]
	60–100% success in acute postoperative setting[40,41]
	71–83% success in hematogenous seeding <2 to 4 weeks[41,42]
Resection arthroplasty	50–89% successful eradication of infection[6,13,43]
Arthrodesis	Overall, 84% eradication of infection and 66% fusion on first attempt[13]
	47–81% fusion after resurfacing implants[3,38]
	39–56% fusion after hinged implants[3,38]
External fixation	84–93% eradication of infection[3,39]
	48–84% surgical fusion[3,38,39]
Intramedullary nail	91% successful fusion after infection eradicated[6]
Reimplantation	
One stage with antibiotic cement	70–94% eradication of infection[44,45]
Two stage with antibiotic cement and 4–6 weeks IV antibiotics	91–100% eradication of infection[8,46]
Functional spacer	92–100% eradication of infection[10,11]

Persistent pain or instability after resection arthroplasty may be relieved by arthrodesis. In circumstances in which persistent infection follows a staged reimplantation, arthrodesis may also be attempted as a salvage procedure. However, even arthrodesis is not a reliable solution in some situations, such as in the presence of severe bone loss resulting from the extraction of a hinged prosthesis. In these circumstances, osseous union can be difficult to obtain. When a nonunion is associated with persistent pain, another arthrodesis may be performed with the use of an intramedullary nail and bone grafting. Prior to further attempts to achieve a bony arthrodesis, all infection should be thoroughly eradicated.

In a small number of cases, the final common pathway for patients who have failed one or more treatment modalities is above-knee amputation. This has been reported to occur in approximately 6% of patients with infected total knee replacements because of persistent infection, intractable pain, or inability to obtain a stable fusion.[6, 13] Unfortunately, this outcome is associated with significant persistent disability. Specific complication data for each modality are detailed in Table 2.

RESULTS

Eradication of infection is the primary goal of all treatment strategies except chronic antibiotic suppression. Specific success rates for each modality are quite variable between surgeons, but representative data are given in Table 3.

OUTCOMES

Information regarding the functional outcome of patients treated with each treatment strategy is somewhat limited, especially for techniques such as suppression and arthrodesis. (Specific results are presented in Table 4.) Owing to the increasing emphasis on outcome data during the 1990s, more detailed results of two-staged reimplantations have been reported. Using the standardized Western Ontario and McMaster OA index questionnaire, 23 of 40 patients (58%) with a reimplanted knee believed they were doing better than before their original total knee arthroplasty, whereas 12 of 40 patients (30%) believed they were somewhat better, and only 5 of 40 patients (13%) believed they were somewhat worse.[8] Overall, 78% of the patients who underwent two-stage reimplantation were very satisfied or somewhat satisfied, and 95% felt that they had made the correct decision regarding undergoing the original total knee replacement.[8] Unfortunately, these good overall outcomes following infection are associated with high economic costs to both the individual and society. In the early 1990s, the cost of treating an infected total joint replacement was

estimated to be between 50,000 and 60,000 dollars.[7] With an annual incidence of 3500 to 4000 infected total joint replacements, direct treatment costs at that time represented 150 to 200 million dollars per year,[7] and more than half of these costs were due to infected total knee replacements. A large proportion of the costs of treating these patients has fallen on academic and tertiary referral centers, with an estimated net loss from caring for each patient of approximately 15,000 to 30,000 dollars.[7, 36] Because many of these tertiary centers receive direct and indirect public funding, these costs are borne by state and federal tax payers.

TABLE 4. OUTCOMES OF TREATMENT OF INFECTED TOTAL KNEE ARTHROPLASTY

Treatment	Outcome
Antibiotic suppression	8.8% functional prosthesis[13]
Débridement and prosthesis retention	5 of 7 independent ambulators and 5 of 7 pain free, mean ROM 9–87 degrees if infection eradicated[4]
	100% good/excellent results and KSS 91 points if infection eradicated[41]
Resection arthroplasty	58–100% functional ambulators with gait aid[37,43]
	Mean ROM 39–52 degrees[37,43]
	68% satisfactory outcome[6]
Arthrodesis	
External fixation	80% persistent pain with nonunion[39]
	27% persistent pain with union[39]
	53% walk >6 blocks with union[39]
Intramedullary nail	14% persistent pain with union[33]
	100% functional ambulators with union[33]
Reimplantation	
One stage	11% ambulation limited by pain[33]
	Mean flexion 87 degree[44]
Two stage	Mean HSS 78 with 72% good/excellent results[8]
	Mean ROM 94 degrees[8]
	Mean KSS 77 degrees[9]
	Mean ROM 92 degrees[9]
Articulating spacer	Mean HSS 80 points[11]
	Mean ROM 5–91 degrees[11]
Amputation	30% daily ambulators and 52% confined to wheelchair[47]

HSS, Hospital for Special Surgery knee rating scale; KSS, Knee Society clinical rating score; ROM, range of motion.

REFERENCES

1. Insall JN, Thompson FM, Brause BD: Two-stage reimplantation for the salvage of infected total knee arthroplasty. J Bone Joint Surg Am 1983; 65:1087.
2. Arden GP, Tinning RN: Total replacement of the knee. J Bone Joint Surg Br 1975; 57:119.
3. Brodersen MP, Fitzgerald RH, Peterson LFA, et al: Arthrodesis of the knee fol-

lowing failed total knee arthroplasty. J Bone Joint Surg Am 1979; 61:181.
4. Schoifet SD, Morrey BF: Treatment of infection after total knee arthroplasty by debridement with retention of the components. J Bone Joint Surg Am 1990; 72:1383.
5. Rand JA, Bryan RS: Reimplantation for the salvage of an infected total knee ar-

throplasty. J Bone Joint Surg Am 1983; 65:1081.
6. Rand JA: Alternatives to reimplantation for salvage of the total knee arthroplasty complicated by infection. J Bone Joint Surg Am 1993; 75:282.
7. Sculco TP: The Economic Impact of Infected Total Joint Arthroplasty. American Academy of Orthopaedic Surgeons, In-

structional Course Lectures. 1993; 42: 349.

8. Goldman RT, Scuderi GR, Insall JN: 2-stage reimplantation for infected total knee replacement. Clin Orthop 1996; 331:118.

9. Hanssen AD, Rand JA, Osmon DR: Treatment of the infected total knee arthroplasty with insertion of another prosthesis: The effect of antibiotic-impregnated bone cement. Clin Orthop 1994; 309:44.

10. Hofmann AA, Kane KR, Tkach TK, et al: Treatment of infected total knee arthroplasty using an articulating spacer. Clin Orthop 1995; 321:45.

11. Masri BA, Kendall RW, Duncan CP, et al: Two-stage exchange arthroplasty using a functional antibiotic-loaded spacer in the treatment of the infected knee replacement: The Vancouver experience. Semin Arthroplasty 1994; 5(3):122.

12. Hanssen AD, Osmon DR, Nelson CL: Prevention of deep periprosthetic joint infection. An Instructional Course Lecture, The American Academy of Orthopaedic Surgeons. J Bone Joint Surg Am 1996; 78: 458.

13. Bengtson S, Knutson K: The infected knee arthroplasty: A 6-year follow-up of 357 cases. Acta Orthop Scand 1991; 62(4):301.

14. Wilson MG, Kelley K, Thornhill TS: Infection as a complication of total knee-replacement arthroplasty: Risk factors and treatment in sixty-seven cases. J Bone Joint Surg Am 1990; 72:878.

15. Greene KA, Wilde AH, Stulberg BN: Preoperative nutritional status of total joint patients: Relationship to postoperative wound complications. J Arthroplasty 1991; 6(4):321.

16. England SP, Stern SH, Insall JN, et al: Total knee arthroplasty in diabetes mellitus. Clin Orthop 1990; 260:130.

17. Gherini S, Vaughn BK, Lombardi AV Jr, et al: Delayed wound healing and nutritional deficiencies after total hip arthroplasty. Clin Orthop 1993; 293:188.

18. Maderazo EG, Judson S, Pasternak H: Late infections of total joint prostheses: A review and recommendations for prevention. Clin Orthop 1988; 229:131.

19. American Dental Association and American Academy of Orthopaedic Surgeons Expert Panel: Antibiotic prophylaxis for dental patients with total joint replacements. Am Acad Orthop Assoc Bull 1997; 45(3):1.

20. Salvati EA, Robinson RP, Zeno SM, et al: Infection rates after 3175 total hip and total knee replacements performed with and without a horizontal unidirectional filtered air-flow system. J Bone Joint Surg Am 1982; 64:525.

21. Gold DA, Scott SC, Scott WN: Soft tissue expansion prior to arthroplasty in the multiply-operated knee. J Arthroplasty 1996; 11(5):512.

22. Petrie RS, Hanssen AD, Osmon DR, et al: Metal-backed patellar component failure in total knee arthroplasty: A possible risk for late infection. Am J Orthop 1998; 27(3): 172.

23. Weiss A-PC, Krackow KA: Persistent wound drainage after primary total knee arthroplasty. J Arthroplasty 1993; 8(3): 285.

24. Windsor RE, Bono JV: Infected total knee replacements. J Am Acad Orthop Surg 1994; 2:44.

25. Duff GP, Lachiewicz PF, Kelley SS: Aspiration of the knee joint before revision a' arthroplasty. Clin Orthop 1996; 331:132.

26. Barrack RL, Jennings RW, Wolfe, MW, et al: The Coventry Award: The value of preoperative aspiration before total knee revision. Clin Orthop 1997; 345:8.

27. Palestro CJ, Swyer AJ, Kim CK, et al: Infected knee prosthesis: Diagnosis with In-111 leukocyte, Tc-99^m sulfur colloid, and Tc-99^m MDP imaging. Radiology 1991; 179(3):645.

28. Lonner JH, Desai P, Dicesare PE, et al: The reliability of analysis of intraoperative frozen sections for identifying active infection during revision hip or knee arthroplasty. J Bone Joint Surg Am 1996; 78: 1553.

29. Mariani BD, Martin DS, Levine MJ, et al: The Coventry Award: Polymerase chain reaction detection of bacterial infection in total knee arthroplasty. Clin Orthop 1996; 331:11.

30. Gerwin M, Rothas KO, Windsor RE, et al: Gastrocnemius muscle flap coverage of exposed or infected knee prosthesis. Clin Orthop 1993; 286:64.

31. Younger ASE, Duncan CP, Masri BA: Surgical exposures in revision total knee arthroplasty. J Am Acad Orthop Surg 1998; 6:55.

32. Wasielewski RC, Barden RM, Rosenberg AG: Results of different surgical procedures on total knee arthroplasty infections. J Arthroplasty 1996; 11(8):931.

33. Ellingsen DE, Rand JA: Intramedullary arthrodesis of the knee after failed total knee arthroplasty. J Bone Joint Surg Am 1994; 76:870.

34. Booth RE Jr, Lotke PA: The results of spacer block technique in revision of infected total knee arthroplasty. Clin Orthop 1989; 248:57.

35. Whiteside LA: Treatment of infected knee arthroplasty. Clin Orthop 1994; 299: 169.

36. Hebert CK, Williams RE, Levy RS, et al: Cost of treating an infected total knee replacement. Clin Orthop 1996; 331:140.

37. Lettin AWF, Neil MJ, Citron ND, et al: Excision arthroplasty for infected constrained total knee replacements. J Bone Joint Surg Br 1990; 72:220.

38. Knutson K, Hovelius L, Lindstrand A, et al: Arthrodesis after failed knee arthroplasty: A nationwide multicenter investigation of 91 cases. Clin Orthop 1984; 191: 202.

39. Rand JA, Bryan RS, Chao EYS: Failed total knee arthroplasty treated by arthrodesis of the knee using the Ace-Fischer apparatus. J Bone Joint Surg Am 1987; 69: 39.

40. Teeny SM, Dorr L, Murata G, et al: Treatment of infected total knee arthroplasty: Irrigation and debridement versus two-stage reimplantation. J Arthroplasty 1990; 5(1):35.

41. Mont MA, Waldman B, Banerjee C, et al: Multiple irrigation, debridement, and retention of components in infected total knee arthroplasty. J Arthroplasty 1997; 12(4):426.

42. Borden LS, Gearen PF: Infected total knee arthroplasty: A protocol for management. J Arthroplasty 1987; 2(1):27.

43. Falahee MH, Matthews LS, Kaufer H: Resection arthroplasty as a salvage procedure for a knee with infection after a total arthroplasty. J Bone Joint Surg Am 1987; 69:1013.

44. Goksan SB, Freeman MAR: One-stage reimplantation for infected total knee arthroplasty. J Bone Joint Surg Br 1992; 74: 78.

45. Scott IR, Stockley I, Getty CJM: Exchange arthroplasty for infected knee replacements: A new two-stage method. J Bone Joint Surg Br 1993; 75:28.

46. Rosenberg AG, Haas B, Barden R, et al: Salvage of infected total knee arthroplasty. Clin Orthop 1988; 226:29.

47. Pring DJ, Marks L, Angel JC: Mobility after amputation for failed knee replacement. J Bone Joint Surg Br 1988; 70:770.

NECROTIZING FASCIITIS AND SOFT-TISSUE INFECTIONS

Allen T. Bishop and Steven B. Schnall

Summary

- Necrotizing fasciitis is a frequent cause of severe morbidity and death.
- Because laboratory (blood and urine) studies are of limited value, early diagnosis requires a high index of suspicion and astute clinical observation.
- Myonecrosis (gas gangrene) is a rare, often rapidly fatal necrotizing infection of muscle caused by both clostridial and nonclostridial organisms. It may occur after trauma or spontaneously.
- For both necrotizing fasciitis and myonecrosis, early diagnosis followed by prompt medical and surgical treatment markedly decreases the severity of morbidity and the frequency of death.
- Mycobacterial (acid-fast) musculoskeletal infection, both tuberculous and nontuberculous, is often difficult to diagnose and treat.
- Diagnosis requires bacteriological culture of tissue for tuberculosis, atypical mycobacteria, fungi, and both aerobic and anaerobic bacteria.
- Treatment requires antibiotic sensitivity studies because mycobacteria have widely varying resistance to chemotherapeutic agents.
- Musculoskeletal fungus infection can be superficial or deep. Diagnosis and treatment require specific fungus culture studies.

Necrotizing fascial infections are rapidly progressive, severe lesions with serious morbidity and relatively frequent mortality. Their dramatic presentation and the occurrence of clusters of cases in a single geographic area result in alarming articles about the condition in the media ("flesh-eating bacterial infections").[1] Necrotizing fasciitis is a severe, fulminant infection that spreads along fascial planes beneath seemingly normal skin. The relatively benign appearance of the extremity is misleading and the fascial necrosis beneath normal or cellulitic skin frequently unrecognized.[2] Unfortunately, delay in diagnosis may result in increased morbidity, including amputation or death. Immediate aggressive surgical débridement through extensile incisions or life-saving amputation in combination with broad-spectrum antibiotic therapy[2] and hemodynamic and nutritional support[3] may be necessary to control these limb- and life-threatening soft-tissue infections.[2]

The initial description of necrotizing fasciitis is attributed to Jones.[4] A Civil War surgeon, he coined the phrase "hospital gangrene" in a report to the U.S. Sanitary Commission in 1871. Necrotizing erysipelas,[5] hemolytic streptococcal gangrene,[6] Meleney's gangrene (or postoperative bacterial synergistic gangrene), idiopathic scrotal gangrene (Fournier's gangrene), monomicrobial necrotizing cellulitis,[7] and gram-negative synergistic necrotizing cellulitis[8] are

synonyms for the condition. Necrotizing fasciitis is now the preferred term, as suggested by Wilson.[9] Necrotizing fasciitis is distinct from clostridial myonecrosis or "gas gangrene": fascial rather than muscle necrosis is the primary disease. Myonecrosis may occur in a minority of patients.

Most patients present with a history of a break in the skin as a result of trauma, surgery, intravenous drug abuse,[10] or a dermatological condition.[11–13] Nevertheless, necrotizing infections have also occurred without a history of trauma,[14] termed primary or idiopathic necrotizing fasciitis.[11] Other risk factors include an immunocompromised state,[10, 15] debilitating disease,[2] atherosclerotic vascular disease,[3] diabetes mellitus,[10, 16] alcoholism,[14] pregnancy,[14] age, hypertension, malnutrition, and obesity.

The overall reported mortality of necrotizing soft-tissue infections is high, with a reported range from 4%[17] to as great as 76%.[14] Increased mortality has been associated with the presence of multiple risk factors,[12] age greater than 40, positive blood cultures,[13] delay in surgical débridement or amputation,[2] and the presence of hemodynamic instability (septic shock).

CLINICAL PRESENTATION

The presence of rapidly progressive cellulitis and painful swelling in an extremity, often developing in a matter of hours, requires consideration of necrotizing fasciitis as the diagnosis. The cellulitic area is tender to palpation, with edema of the extremity proximal to the erythema.[5, 18] When present, the edema is frequently impressive, later resulting in bullae and cutaneous discoloration (Fig. 1). Obvious clinical features such as subcutaneous gas, cutaneous bullae, and patchy cutaneous discoloration are usually absent at initial presentation and cannot be relied on in making a diagnosis of necrotizing fasciitis.[14] The relatively benign appearance of the extremity is frequently misleading, resulting in delay of diagnosis and increased morbidity or death.[18] In some cases, a traumatic or surgical wound, intravenous injection site, ulceration, or dermatological skin eruption is identifiable as the likely initial location of the infection. As the infection progresses, bacterial enzymes open soft-tissue planes, and the infection advances rapidly with concomitant soft-tissue necrosis.[16] The infection spreads rapidly along fascial planes, belied by minimal skin involvement. Systemic signs of sepsis, including elevated temperature, increased pulse, and hypotension (septic shock), may occur rapidly. Hemodynamic instability and multisystem organ failure similar to toxic shock syndrome is often present.[19] Again, skin bullae, crepitance, skin necrosis, and fever are frequently absent at presentation.

Evaluation of the patient at initial presentation may require an assessment of the fascial necrosis. When a wound

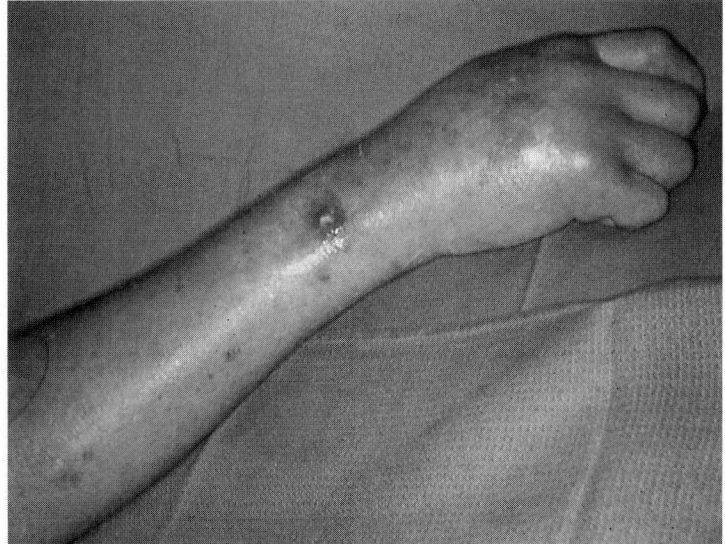

Fig. 1. Necrotizing fasciitis. Swelling of forearm and hand is prominent, with rapidly advancing cellulitis in an infection arising at an IV site.

is present, drainage of a brownish, watery exudate is suggestive. Fascial destruction results in a degloving phenomenon, allowing easy elevation of the skin from subcutaneous tissues. When an open wound cannot be examined, a small bedside incision will demonstrate the characteristic exudate and fascial destruction.[9] When found, immediate surgical treatment should be rendered. If rapidly available, a frozen-section biopsy of the subcutaneous tissue may confirm the diagnosis.[20]

Imaging studies may at times be helpful. Although subcutaneous gas is only occasionally seen in necrotizing fasciitis, it may be visualized when present on standard radiographs. Computed tomography[21, 22] and magnetic resonance imaging[23, 24] may be useful to demonstrate fascial changes. The urgent nature of the problem in many cases precludes the use of such studies. Surgical exploration and culture will provide the most certain diagnosis as well as needed therapeutic intervention.

BACTERIOLOGY

Meleney, in a classic article, described necrotizing fasciitis as "hemolytic streptococcal gangrene" based on the presence of group A β-hemolytic streptococci in all of his original group of patients.[6] Subsequently, however, it has become clear that a broad spectrum of bacteria may cause necrotizing fasciitis. For example, noncholera vibrios,[25] *Aeromonas hydrophila,*[26] other gram-negative aerobic bacilli,[27, 28] and anaerobes[29, 30] are frequently reported in such cases. Giuliano et al[31] described two types of necrotizing fasciitis on the basis of culture results. Type I consists of a combination of anaerobic bacteria and facultative anaerobic bacteria such as Enterobacteriaceae and streptococci other than group A. Type II consists of cases in which group A streptococci were isolated alone or in combination with *Staphylococcus aureus* or *Staphylococcus epidermidis.* In his series, most were type I, and only 19% were type II.[31] In another study, 52% of patients had a single organism.[18] Most commonly, particularly in the past decade, group A

β-hemolytic streptococci have been isolated from fasciitis wounds. Polymicrobial infections tend to have a longer incubation period than monomicrobial infections, making them more difficult to diagnose. No differences in survival have been observed attributable to bacteriology, however.[32] Because many of these infections are polymicrobial,[2] broad-spectrum antibiotics are mandatory pending final cultures.

TREATMENT

Once diagnosed, the most important intervention is aggressive surgical débridement.[2, 6, 9, 10, 17] The infectious process involves the fascia, which liquefies. At operation, necrotic fat weeps muddy brown serous fluid (Fig. 2), and thrombosis of subcutaneous vessels is usually present. Inspection of the underlying muscle is imperative because of the occasional presence of myositis and myonecrosis. Only extensive surgical débridement can control infection. Delayed or incomplete radical excision may lead to disseminated infection. All necrotic skin, fat, fascia, and muscle must be débrided and fasciotomy extended well beyond the area of cellulitis to contain the infection (Fig. 3). Amputation may be necessary in medically unstable patients and in limbs demonstrating progression of infection at reexploration. Early redébridement in 12 to 24 hours should be performed and repeated as necessary. Worsening medical condition dictates immediate reoperation, including consideration for amputation. Multiple débridements and ultimately skin grafts are required in most cases. Broad-spectrum antibiotic coverage should be started empirically, including penicillin, clindamycin, or metronidazole and an aminoglycoside. Hemodynamic monitoring with a Swan-Ganz catheter with fluid resuscitation and dopamine support is indicated, as is nutritional supplementation.[32] Nutritional needs are similar to those of a severely burned patient. Consideration of hyperalimentation for these patients is indicated.[33]

Enhanced fibrin deposition and vascular occlusions in the skin are the basis for most complications that occur in

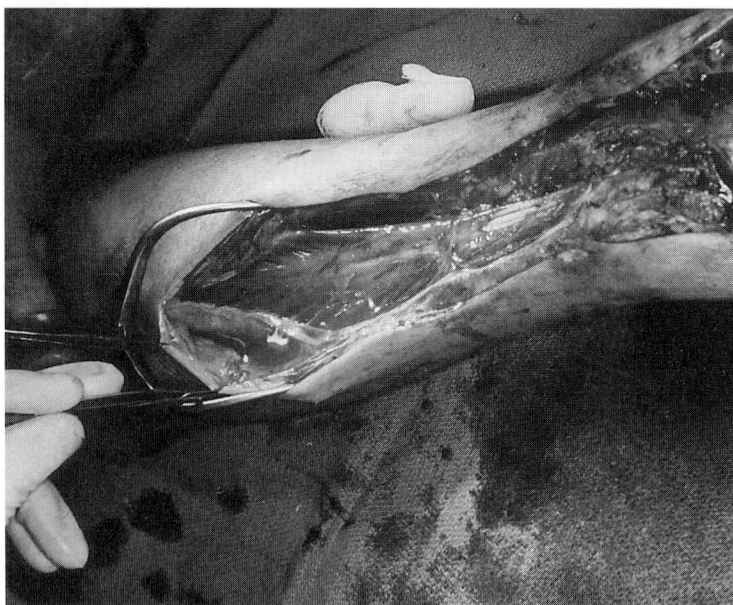

Fig. 2. Necrotizing fasciitis. At operation, necrotic fat weeps muddy brown serous fluid.

necrotizing fasciitis. A diminution in complications has been reported with the use of heparin 300 to 500 U/kg/day.[34] Hyperbaric oxygen has not been of substantial benefit,[35] unless anaerobic organisms are demonstrated.[36, 37]

GAS GANGRENE

Clostridial myonecrosis, or gas gangrene, is a rare but often rapidly fatal infection. Classically, gas gangrene is caused by *Clostridium perfringens,* occurring as a complication of trauma or surgery. It is a rare disorder, with an estimated 900 to 1000 cases per year.[38] Nontraumatic, or spontaneous, gas gangrene is less common. Infection in such cases is usually caused by *Clostridium septicum*; underlying malignancy is often present. Gas gangrene may also result from nonclostridial infection. Nonclostridial gangrene is most commonly seen in diabetic patients, usually caused by a mixture of aerobic, anaerobic, gram-positive,

and gram-negative species. Diagnosis of spontaneous myonecrosis, as in necrotizing fasciitis, is difficult because of its insidious onset and lack of an obvious predisposing event.

Clostridia are gram-positive, spore-forming, obligate anaerobic bacilli found in soil, the human gastrointestinal tract, and the female genital tract.[39] Culture requires an anaerobic environment supplemented with reducing agents. Pathological examination, including Gram stain, is important for early diagnosis.

Myonecrosis, or gas gangrene, occurs when there is both contamination of tissues with clostridia and a low oxygen tension environment, fostering production of toxins and further growth of the organism. Even though almost 90% of major wounds can be shown to be contaminated with clostridial organisms, gas gangrene develops in fewer than 2%, demonstrating the importance of host and wound factors.[40] Most cases of gas gangrene involve traumatic or postoperative wounds. Patients with diabetes mellitus, im-

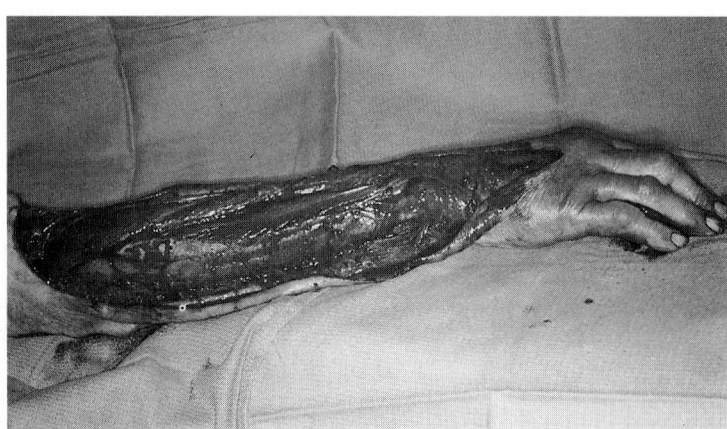

Fig. 3. Necrotizing fasciitis. All necrotic skin, fat, fascia, and muscle must be débrided and fasciotomy extended well beyond the area of cellulitis to contain the infection.

mune compromise, vascular insufficiency, or malignancy are at greater risk.

Symptoms include massive edema, discoloration of the overlying skin, and hemorrhagic bullae and blebs. Patients may have a low-grade fever, tachycardia, and severe local pain. Drainage when present has a foul odor. Rapid progression is the rule. Gas gangrene can advance as rapidly as 2 cm/hour, and it is universally fatal if not treated.

Gram stain of any fluid will identify clostridial organisms. The muscles become necrotic, and renal failure secondary to acute tubular necrosis can occur. Radiographs may show gas in the soft tissues, but lack of such findings should not dissuade the physician from the diagnosis, because rapid progression to septic shock and death can occur if the diagnosis is delayed.

Prevention should be the cornerstone of treatment, and appropriate débridement and incision and drainage of wounds with a potential for development of this disease should be recognized. Closure of any wound that might suggest the possibility for development of a gangrenous infection should be condemned.

TREATMENT

Prompt emergency surgical consultation for exploration and débridement is essential. Resuscitative measures before and after surgery should include oxygen, tetanus toxoid prophylaxis, and intravenous fluids as needed. Antibiotics are an essential adjunct to surgical débridement. It is best to begin triple-antibiotic treatment, such as penicillin, gentamicin, and clindamycin, to cover all possible gas-forming organisms. Once *Clostridium* is isolated, high-dose penicillin G is the drug of choice, but combinations with cephalosporins and aminoglycosides should be used inasmuch as the contaminated wound and necrotic muscle allow mixed flora to flourish.[39]

Hyperbaric oxygen therapy remains controversial.[41–44] Although no randomized, prospective studies in humans have been reported, animal data and clinical experience with hyperbaric oxygen therapy suggest that, when used in conjunction with an operation and antibiotics, hyperbaric oxygen therapy significantly reduces morbidity and mortality in cases of clostridial infection.[45, 46]

MYCOBACTERIAL INFECTIONS

MYCOBACTERIUM TUBERCULOSIS INFECTION

Tenosynovitis attributed to tuberculosis has been reported since 1777, and subsequent descriptions have been provided by Dupuytren, Virchow, and others. Now, however, tenosynovial tuberculosis is rare and seldom mentioned in standard medical or surgical texts.[47] Like other mycobacterial infections, tuberculosis in the hand is an indolent process resulting in gradually progressive diffuse digital swelling (dactylitis) and chronic tenosynovitis reminiscent of rheumatoid arthritis. Signs of acute inflammation such as warmth and pain are not prominent. Radiographs demonstrate only soft-tissue swelling. The Mantoux skin test is positive and the sedimentation rate elevated. Malnutrition,

advanced age, immunosuppression, ethanol abuse, and a history of pulmonary tuberculosis are risk factors for mycobacterial musculoskeletal infection. Treatment should include surgical tenosynovectomy for both diagnosis and treatment, with postoperative chemotherapy with isoniazid, rifampin, and pyrazinamide for several months.[47]

ATYPICAL MYCOBACTERIAL INFECTION

Atypical mycobacteria are widely distributed in nature and are only infrequently human pathogens. The mycobacteria are grouped by the Runyon classification according to pigmentation and growth characteristics (Table 1). Most have been implicated in infections, although *Mycobacterium marinum*, *Mycobacterium kansasii*, *Mycobacterium terrae*, and *Mycobacterium avium-intracellulare* are most common.[48, 49] Musculoskeletal manifestation of infection involves the wrist and hand in almost one-half of cases.[50]

M. marinum is endogenous to both fresh and salt-water fish and proliferates in fresh or salt-water enclosures, especially when not frequently replenished. All types of bathing places, aquariums, fish farms, and fish tanks qualify as potential sources of infection. Fish, shrimp, snails, and crabs may become infected and transfer the organism to humans.[51] *M. marinum* may cause infection varying from subcutaneous granulomas with sinus tracts to sporotrichoid-like nodules, tenosynovitis, bursitis, arthritis, and osteomyelitis.[52] There is usually a history of puncture wound or trauma within 6 months of symptoms onset that could have allowed the organism to pass the skin barrier. The patients are usually normal hosts having no underlying diseases. Flexor tenosynovitis involving a digit, the wrist, or both is common. Symptoms of carpal tunnel syndrome may be present. The typical swimming pool granuloma is a localized superficial granuloma involving little more than deep dermis and presenting as an ulcerated nodule. The patients are usually normal hosts having no underlying diseases.

TABLE 1. RUNYON CLASSIFICATION OF MYCOBACTERIA	
Runyon Type	**Characteristic**
Group I M. marinum M. kansasii	*Photochromogens* (cream-colored colonies turning yellow on exposure to light)
Group II M. gordonae M. szulgai	*Scotochromogens* (produce orange pigment independent of light)
Group III M. avium-intracellulare M. terrae	*Nonchromogens* (white colonies that do not develop pigment)
Group IV M. fortuitum M. chelonae M. ulcerans	*Rapid growers* (form cream-colored colonies in 1 week or less compared with the 10–28 days required by the other groups; are resistant to most antituberculosis drugs but often susceptible to amikacin, doxycycline, erythromycin, kanamycin)

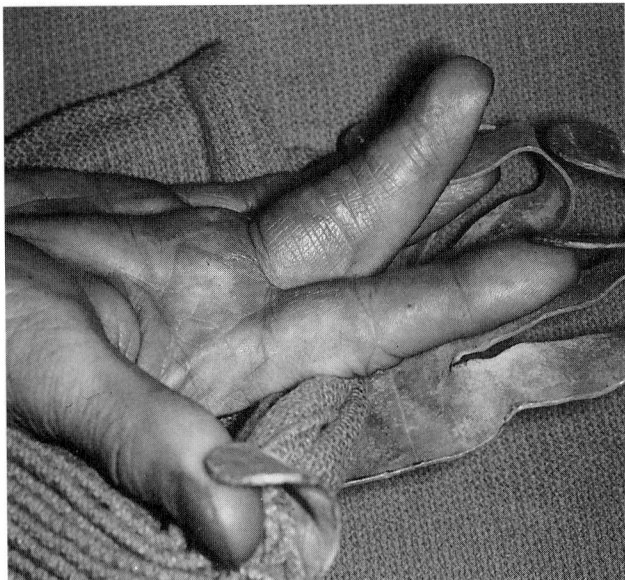

Fig. 4. Atypical mycobacterial infection. This shows mycobacterial flexor tenosynovitis with painless marked distention of the flexor sheath reminiscent of rheumatoid disease.

M. avium-intracellulare is an organism found in soil, water, and domestic poultry. In humans it may cause pulmonary disease, localized skin and subcutaneous infections, arthritis, osteomyelitis, and disseminated sepsis. Before 1982, disseminated sepsis was extremely rare. However, *M. avium-intracellulare* has become the most frequently isolated organism in patients terminally ill with AIDS.[50] Primary musculoskeletal disease remains rare, although multifocal osteomyelitis may occur in immunocompromised hosts and young children. Focal septic arthritis and osteomyelitis are even less common. History of a puncture wound, closed trauma, treatment with oral prednisolone or local steroid injections, and immunodeficiency are risk factors. The organism is difficult to eradicate because of mul-

tiple drug resistance and the immunocompromised nature of most of its hosts. No combination of chemotherapy appears particularly effective *in M. avium-intracellulare* infection, including the use of five or more agents.[53]

Other mycobacteria have been reported to cause hand infection, including *M. kansasii* and *M. terrae*.[48, 49, 54] Most cases have been pulmonary involvement, but hand infections caused by penetrating wounds from pins, fish fins, or wooden splinters or incurred while gardening have occurred. *Mycobacterium fortuitum* has been isolated from soil, house dust, milk, and saliva as well as fish, frogs, and cattle.[55] *M. fortuitum* infections have been associated with trauma and prosthetic devices and can infect an operative incision. Clinically, *M. fortuitum* infections may present in the hand as indolent subcutaneous masses, cold abscesses, tenosynovitis, or joint synovitis. Other species causing hand infections include *Mycobacterium malmoense, Mycobacterium chelonae,* and *Mycobacterium szulgai*.[56–58]

DIAGNOSIS

Because of the indolent nature of mycobacterial infection, lack of clinical suspicion, and special growth requirements, diagnosis is usually delayed. Indolent inflammation after a puncture wound or arising in an immunocompromised host should suggest the possibility of an atypical mycobacterial infection (Fig. 4). Tuberculin skin testing is not a reliable indicator of atypical mycobacterial disease.[48] Diagnosis in all instances requires an incisional biopsy of the involved tissue, with culture submission for tuberculosis, atypical mycobacteria, and fungi, as well as aerobic and anaerobic bacteria. Florid tenosynovial proliferation is generally seen, reminiscent of rheumatoid disease (Fig. 5). Request for sensitivities to antibiotics must be stressed because of widely varying resistance to chemotherapeutic agents. At biopsy, histological examination should be performed, although synovial lesions may not be diagnostic.[51, 59] Forms and components of the inflammatory reaction from *M. marinum*–infected tissue included diffuse granulomatous inflammation, focal granulomatous inflammation, fibrous

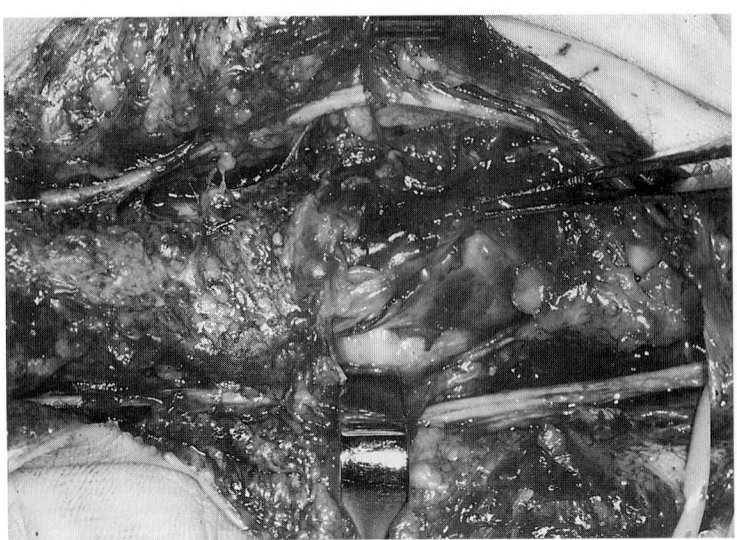

Fig. 5. Atypical mycobacterial infection. Florid tenosynovial proliferation is present at surgical exploration.

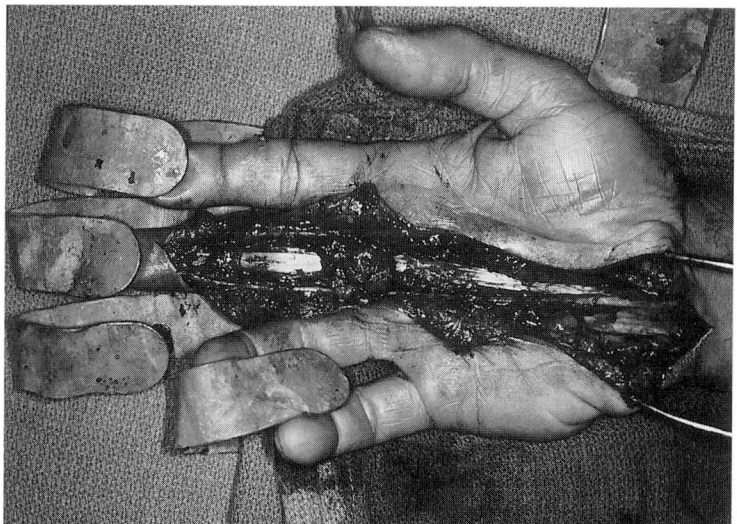

Fig. 6. Atypical mycobacterial infection. Flexor tenosynovitis requires wide sheath exposure and tenosynovectomy sparing all annular pulleys. Intraoperative cultures and histological samples confirm the diagnosis.

exudates and caseation, and acid-fast bacilli seen on Ziehl-Neelsen–stained sections.[51] Synovial lesions may resemble rheumatoid disease, although careful examination will often reveal the presence of small, well-formed granulomas consisting of nodular collections of epithelioid cells and multinucleated giant cells. In addition, poorly formed granulomas and several dense collections of plasma cells may be observed.

Growth in culture requires special culture media and temperatures. For example, *M. marinum* is a rapidly growing photochromogen, requiring 2 to 8 weeks in culture with best growth at 30°C to 32°C. Little or no growth occurs at 37°C.[52] *M. fortuitum* is distinguished in the laboratory by growth of nonpigmented colonies within 48 hours at 20°C on Lowenstein-Jensen medium. Isolation of mycobacteria from a hand should prompt a search for pulmonary foci by chest radiograph, because infection may occur by either hematogenous spread or direct inoculation.[49]

TREATMENT

Although spontaneous healing of cutaneous lesions has been mentioned in the literature, tenosynovitis has not.[52] Currently, treatment recommendations for most of these infections include both surgical débridement and postoperative pharmacological therapy. Abscesses require drainage, and synovectomy of involved joints and tendon sheaths is probably necessary (Fig. 6). Superficial (cutaneous) infections may be managed by débridement alone with satisfactory resolution. The length of postoperative chemotherapy depends in part on the antibiotic resistance of the organism, but it is commonly continued for several months.[48, 52, 55] Institution of drug therapy in most instances should begin immediately after surgery, although empiric treatment may need to be modified once sensitivities are obtained. The rapid growers (*M. fortuitum* and *M. chelonae)* are resistant to conventional mycobacterial agents but may be susceptible to amikacin and doxycycline.[60–62]

M. terrae is also resistant to drug therapy, and *M. avium-intracellulare* responds poorly in immunocompromised patients to regimens of even five or more agents.[53, 63, 64] Consultation with an infectious disease specialist is indicated for the postoperative management of mycobacterial infections.

FUNGAL INFECTIONS

Fungal infection of the extremities may broadly be divided into cutaneous, subcutaneous, and deep infections. The organisms involved may be true pathogens, capable of infecting normal hosts, or opportunists. These fungi cause infection in patients with immune compromise, such as diabetics, patients using steroids or immunosuppressives, and those with a myeloproliferative disorder or HIV infection. This section deals with subcutaneous and deep infections.

SUBCUTANEOUS FUNGAL INFECTIONS

Subcutaneous infection is most commonly caused by *Sporothrix schenckii*. The most common form of sporotrichosis is the lymphocutaneous variety. Most cases result from handling plants or soil, often with the recollection of a penetrating injury from a thorn, scratch, animal bite, or wood sliver.[65, 66] Sporotrichosis skin lesions begin with a papule at the site of inoculation, with subsequent development of metastatic lesions along lymphatic channels. These channels become indurated and cord-like, with the development of violaceous abscesses that drain seropurulent material.[67]

DEEP INFECTION

Deep fungal infections of the upper extremity have three common presentations: tenosynovial infections of the flexor or extensor compartments, septic arthritis, and osteomyelitis. Definitive diagnosis requires identification of the organism on specific fungal cultures. True pathogens causing deep infections include histoplasmosis, blastomycosis, coccidioidomycosis, and paracoccidioidomycosis. Opportunistic infections include aspergillosis, candidiasis, mucormycosis, and cryptococcosis.[67] Histoplasmosis is caused by *Histoplasma capsulatum* and is endemic as a subclinical primary pulmonary infection in the Mississippi-Ohio River Valley region. Cases of tenosynovial infection have been reported. Blastomycosis occurs in the same region of North America but at a much lower incidence. Cutaneous lesions may occur with systemic infection, including subcutaneous nodules, which may develop draining peripheral ulcerations. Septic arthritis and lytic epiphyseal lesions may also be commonly seen. Coccidioidomycosis is a rare fungal infection found in arid regions of the southwestern United States and northern Mexico. It is most commonly a self-limiting pulmonary infection; hematogenous spread to the upper extremity occurs in a minority of patients causing metaphyseal osteomyelitis or septic arthritis.[67] Treatment of deep infection, including opportunistic infections, should combine surgical débridement and intravenous antifungal agents such as amphotericin B.

REFERENCES

1. Fernandez Guerrero ML: Streptococcal gangrene and so-called "flesh-eating bacteria disease": A rare and devastating disease. Revista Clinica Española 1999; 199: 84.
2. Wang KC, Shih CH: Necrotizing fasciitis of the extremities. J Trauma-Injury Infect Crit Care 1992; 32:179.
3. Majeski JA, Alexander JW: Early diagnosis, nutritional support, and immediate extensive debridement improve survival in necrotizing fasciitis. Am J Surg 1983; 145: 784.
4. Jones NF, Conklin WT, Albo VC: Primary invasive aspergillosis of the hand. J Hand Surg Am 1986; 11:425.
5. Hammar H, Wanger L: Erysipelas and necrotizing fasciitis. Br J Dermatol 1977; 96:409.
6. Meleney FL: Hemolytic streptococcus gangrene. Arch Surg 1924; 9:317.
7. McHenry CR: Monomicrobial necrotizing fasciitis complicating pregnancy and puerperium. Obstet Gynecol 1996; 87:823.
8. Stone HH, Martin JD Jr: Synergistic necrotizing cellulitis. Ann Surg 1972; 175: 702.
9. Wilson B: Necrotizing fasciitis. Am J Surg 1952; 18:416.
10. Gonzalez MH: Necrotizing fasciitis of the upper extremity. J Hand Surg Am 1996; 21:689.
11. Gonzalez MH: Upper extremity infections in patients with diabetes mellitus. J Hand Surg Am 1999; 24:682.
12. Gonzalez-Ruiz A: Varicella gangrenosa with toxic shock-like syndrome due to group A streptococcus infection in an adult: Case report. Clin Infect Dis 1995; 20:1058; discussion, 1061.
13. Snider JM, McNabney WK, Pemberton LB: Necrotizing fasciitis secondary to discoid lupus erythematosus. Am Surg 1993; 59:164.
14. McHenry CR: Idiopathic necrotizing fasciitis: Recognition, incidence, and outcome of therapy. Am Surg 1994; 60:490.
15. Laursen MB, Dossing KV: Necrotizing fasciitis. Ugeskrift Laeger 1998; 160:6533.
16. Schecter W: Necrotizing fasciitis of the upper extremity. J Hand Surg Am 1982; 7:15.
17. Bessman AN, Wagner W: Nonclostridial gas gangrene: Report of 48 cases and review of the literature. JAMA 1975; 233: 958.
18. Gonzalez MH: Necrotizing fasciitis and gangrene of the upper extremity. Hand Clin 1998; 14:635.
19. Erstad BL, Witte CL, Talkington DF: Toxic shock-like syndrome. Pharmacotherapy 1992; 12:23.
20. Stamenkovic I, Lew PD: Early recognition of potentially fatal necrotizing fasciitis: The use of frozen-section biopsy. N Engl J Med 1984; 310:1689.
21. Wysoki MG: Necrotizing fasciitis: CT characteristics. Radiology 1997; 203:859.
22. Rogers JM: Usefulness of computerized tomography in evaluating necrotizing fasciitis. South Med J 1984; 77:782.
23. Brothers TE: Magnetic resonance imaging differentiates between necrotizing and nonnecrotizing fasciitis of the lower extremity. J Am Coll Surg 1998; 187:416.
24. Revelon G: Acute swelling of the limbs: Magnetic resonance pictorial review of fascial and muscle signal changes. Eur J Radiol 1999; 30:11.
25. Howard RJ: Necrotizing soft-tissue infections caused by marine vibrios. Surgery 1985; 98:126.
26. Furusu A: *Aeromonas hydrophila* necrotizing fasciitis and gas gangrene in a diabetic patient on haemodialysis. Nephrol Dial Transplant 1997; 12:1730.
27. Freeman HP: Necrotizing fasciitis. Am J Surg 1981; 142:377.
28. Mentec H: Necrotizing fasciitis, caused by *Neisseria meningitidis,* simultaneously involving an arm and a leg. Ann Dermatol Venereol 1993; 120:889.
29. Jacobson JM, Hirschman SZ: Necrotizing fasciitis complicating intravenous drug abuse. Arch Intern Med 1982; 142:634.
30. Rein JM, Cosman B: *Bacteroides* necrotizing fasciitis of the upper extremity: Case report. Plast Reconstr Surg 1971; 48:592.
31. Giuliano A: Bacteriology of necrotizing fasciitis. Am J Surg 1977; 143:52.
32. Sudarsky LA: Improved results from a standardized approach in treating patients with necrotizing fasciitis. Ann Surg 1987; 206:661.
33. Al-Sogair SM, Moawad MK, Al HYM: Fungal infection as a cause of skin disease in the eastern province of Saudi Arabia: Tinea pedis and tinea manuum. Mycoses 1991; 34:339.
34. Hammar H: Coagulation and fibrinolytic systems during the course of erysipelas and necrotizing fasciitis and the effect of heparin. Acta Dermatol Venereol 1985; 65:495.
35. Barzilai A, Zaaroor M, Toledano C: Necrotizing fasciitis: Early awareness and principles of treatment. Isr J Med Sci 1985; 21:127.
36. Monestersky J, Myers R: Hyperbaric oxygen treatment of necrotizing fasciitis. Am J Surg 1995; 169:187.
37. Brown DR: A multicenter review of the treatment of major truncal necrotizing infections with and without hyperbaric oxygen therapy. Am J Surg 1994; 167:485.
38. Cline KA, Turnbull TL: Clostridial myonecrosis. Ann Emerg Med 1985; 14:459.
39. Valentine EG: Nontraumatic gas gangrene. Ann Emerg Med 1997; 30:109.
40. Altemeier WA, Furste WL: Gas gangrene. Surg Gynecol Obstet 1947; 84:507.
41. Hennessy MJ: *Aeromonas hydrophila* gas gangrene: A case report of management with surgery and hyperbaric oxygenation. Orthopedics 1988; 11:289.
42. Cohn GH: Hyperbaric oxygen therapy: Promoting healing in difficult cases. Postgrad Med 1986; 79:89.
43. Gaietta T: Considerations on collateral treatments used with hyperbaric oxygenation in the therapy of gas gangrene. Minerva Med 1982; 73:2959.
44. Alvis HJ: What hyperbaric medicine has to offer the industrial physician. J Occup Med 1967; 9:304.
45. Gibson A, Davis FM: Hyperbaric oxygen therapy in the management of *Clostridium perfringens* infections. N Z Med J 1986; 99:617.
46. Stemens MB: Gas gangrene: Potential for hyperbaric oxygen therapy. Postgrad Med J 1996; 99:217.
47. Jackson RH, King JW: Tenosynovitis of the hand: A forgotten manifestation of tuberculosis. Rev Infect Dis 1989; 11:616.
48. Love GL, Melchior E: *Mycobacterium terrae* tenosynovitis. J Hand Surg Am 1985; 10:730.
49. Love GL, Melchior E: Synovial hand infection from *Mycobacterium terrae.* J Hand Surg Br 1988; 13:335.
50. Rolfe B, Sowa DT: Mixed gonococcal and mycobacterial sepsis of the wrist. Clin Orthop 1990; 257:100.
51. Collins RJ: Synovial involvement by *Mycobacterium marinum:* A histopathological study of 25 culture-proven cases. Pathology 1988; 20:340.
52. Lacy JN: Mycobacterium marinum flexor tenosynovitis. Clin Orthop 1989; 238:288.
53. Rosenzweig DY: Pulmonary mycobacterial

infections due to *Mycobacterium intracellulare-avium* complex: Clinical features and outcome in 100 consecutive cases. Chest 1979; 75:115.

54. Halla JT, Gould JS, Hardin JG: Chronic tenosynovial hand infection from *Mycobacterium terrae*. Arthritis Rheum 1979; 22:1386.

55. Maher DP: *Mycobacterium fortuitum* infection following treatment of a ganglion cyst: Case report and literature review. Orthop Rev 1989; 18:1193.

56. Prince H, Ispahani P, Baker M: A *Mycobacterium malmoense* infection of the hand presenting as carpal tunnel syndrome. J Hand Surg Br 1988; 13:328.

57. Stratton CW, Phelps DB, Reller LB: Tuberculoid tenosynovitis and carpal tunnel

syndrome caused by *Mycobacterium szulgai.* Am J Med 1978; 65:349.

58. Stern PJ, Gula DC: *Mycobacterium chelonei* tenosynovitis of the hand: A case report. J Hand Surg Am 1986; 11:596.

59. Travis WD: The histopathologic spectrum in *Mycobacterium marinum* infection. Arch Pathol Lab Med 1985; 109:1109.

60. Dalovisio JR, Pankey GA: Activity of amikacin, erythromycin and doxycycline against *Mycobacterium chelonei* and *Mycobacterium fortuitum.* Tubercle 1978; 59:277.

61. Dalovisio JR, Pankey GA: In vitro susceptibility of *Mycobacterium fortuitum* and *Mycobacterium chelonei* to amikacin. J Infect Dis 1978; 137:318.

62. Wallace RJ Jr, Dalovisio JR, Pankey GA:

Disk diffusion testing of susceptibility of *Mycobacterium fortuitum* and *Mycobacterium chelonei* to antibacterial agents. Antimicrob Agents Chemother 1979; 16:611.

63. Deenstra W: Tenosynovitis of the hand caused by *Mycobacterium terrae.* Eur J Clin Microbiol Infect Dis 1989; 8:722.

64. Petrini B: *Mycobacterium terrae* tenosynovitis. Pathology 1990; 22:106.

65. Rowe JG, Amadio PC, Edson RS: Sporotrichosis. Orthopedics 1989; 12:981.

66. Hay EL, Collawn SS, Middleton FG: *Sporothrix schenckii* tenosynovitis: A case report. J Hand Surg Am 1986; 11:431.

67. Hitchcock TF, Amadio PC: Fungal infections. Hand Clin 1989; 5:599.

section 5 chapter 10

ORTHOPAEDIC SURGERY IN THE IMMUNOCOMPROMISED HOST

James V. Luck, Jr, and Colby Young

Summary

- Although AIDS and HIV infection attract significant attention, more common causes of immune impairment include drug complications (among them consequences of chronic corticosteroid use), diabetes mellitus, malnutrition, chronic liver disease, and aging.
- Treatment of HIV-positive patients presents real but acceptable risks to health care workers; all clinicians should adhere closely to published guidelines regarding precautions.
- Symptomatic HIV patients seem to be at increased risk for late prosthetic joint infections; infection risk for asymptomatic patients is approximately the same as that for HIV-negative patients.
- Patients with alcoholism present multiple medical and orthopaedic challenges in addition to reduced immune function.

Were it not for an awesomely complex and adaptive system of host immunity, the ongoing battle between microbe and human would be lost on the initial assault. However, each of the many facets of this complex system may be subject to impairment from a wide variety of sources. The magnitude and consequences of these impairments are highly varied depending on the extent and location of the defects. These defects may be especially consequential in musculoskeletal trauma and reconstructive patients requiring the extensive implantation of hardware or devitalized bone graft materials.

Although much attention has been focused over the last decade on immune impairment as a consequence of infection with immunodeficiency virus, other causes of immunodeficiency affect a greater proportion of our patients. Some of the more common causes include complications of pharmacological agents, metabolic diseases like diabetes mellitus, malnutrition, chronic liver disease, and aging. In less severe instances, the patients appear clinically healthy and basic lab tests are often normal. However, if undetected, most immune impairments will progress, eventually resulting in a series of infections, many of which have musculoskeletal significance. In many instances, the affects can be lessened or even corrected with proper management. Awareness of these impairments and their medical management will assist the surgeon in facilitating patients' recovery and lessening the risk of both early and late postoperative infection. With proper preoperative evaluation and management, most patients with immune system impairment remain potential candidates for elective surgery.

IMMUNE SYSTEM REVIEW AND DEFINITION OF TERMS

The immune system is mediated by two categories of cells, phagocytes and lymphocytes, as well as secreted proteins and peptides, including cytokines, antibodies, and complement. The phagocytes, including polymorphonuclear leukocytes, monocytes, and macrophages, are part of the innate system that identifies, engulfs, and destroys microorganisms such as bacteria and foreign materials. The adaptive system, or acquired immunity, involves a "learned" response, which is highly antigen specific and is principally mediated by the lymphocyte lineage. Lymphocytes are generally divided into thymus-derived, or T, lymphocytes and bone marrow–derived, or B, lymphocytes. T cells that have not had an initial encounter with a specific antigen are called naïve lymphocytes. The process in which a naïve lymphocyte has an initial encounter with a specific antigen is termed "priming." Once priming occurs, the naïve lymphocytes then proliferate, allowing large numbers of these

TABLE 1. AIDS CASES AND ANNUAL RATES PER 100,000 POPULATION, BY AREA AND AGE GROUP, REPORTED THROUGH JUNE 1999, UNITED STATES

| Area of Residence | July 1997–June 1998 | | July 1998–June 1999 | | Cumulative Totals | | |
	No.	Rate	No.	Rate	Adults/ Adolescents	Children < 13 Years Old	Total
Alabama	604	14.0	467	10.7	5,508	67	5,575
Alaska	41	6.7	30	4.9	448	5	453
Arizona	546	12.0	738	15.8	6,501	27	6,528
Arkansas	227	9.0	189	7.4	2,644	38	2,682
California	6,283	19.5	5,737	17.6	112,444	581	113,025
Colorado	316	8.1	339	8.5	6,586	28	6,614
Connecticut	892	27.3	622	19.0	10,518	173	10,691
Delaware	161	21.9	177	23.8	2,238	21	2,259
District of Columbia	941	177.6	750	143.4	11,468	166	11,634
Florida	5,410	36.9	5,683	38.1	71,815	1,353	73,168
Georgia	1,368	18.3	1,635	21.4	20,789	194	20,983
Hawaii	128	10.7	140	11.7	2,280	15	2,295
Idaho	39	3.2	29	2.4	459	2	461
Illinois	1,765	14.7	1,285	10.7	22,102	246	22,348
Indiana	484	8.3	353	6.0	5,573	37	5,610
Iowa	97	3.4	73	2.6	1,185	9	1,194
Kansas	145	5.6	146	5.6	2,165	11	2,176
Kentucky	310	7.9	306	7.8	2,988	23	3,011
Louisiana	1,058	24.3	904	20.7	11,466	118	11,584
Maine	41	3.3	42	3.4	856	9	865
Maryland	1,628	32.0	1,634	31.8	19,136	293	19,429
Massachusetts	763	12.5	1,250	20.3	14,281	202	14,483
Michigan	802	8.2	714	7.3	10,161	106	10,267
Minnesota	176	3.8	206	4.4	3,450	22	3,472
Mississippi	359	13.1	432	15.7	3,783	53	3,836
Missouri	545	10.1	492	9.0	8,451	56	8,507
Montana	34	3.9	18	2.0	298	3	301
Nebraska	75	4.5	74	4.5	981	9	990
Nevada	466	27.8	257	14.7	3,968	27	3,995
New Hampshire	53	4.5	47	4.0	820	9	829
New Jersey	2,484	30.8	2,061	25.4	38,614	730	39,344
New Mexico	220	12.8	125	7.2	1,858	8	1,866
New York	11,273	62.1	7,655	42.1	129,882	2,204	132,086
North Carolina	812	10.9	789	10.5	9,226	113	9,339
North Dakota	10	1.6	6	0.9	100	—	100
Ohio	792	7.1	585	5.2	10,373	119	10,492
Oklahoma	298	9.0	185	5.5	3,338	26	3,364
Oregon	236	7.3	198	6.0	4,438	16	4,454
Pennsylvania	1,891	15.7	1,806	15.0	21,757	300	22,057
Rhode Island	134	13.6	120	12.1	1,890	20	1,910
South Carolina	772	20.4	984	25.7	8,275	77	8,352
South Dakota	17	2.3	17	2.3	151	4	155
Tennessee	690	12.8	769	14.2	7,335	48	7,383
Texas	4,456	23.0	3,715	18.8	49,795	363	50,158
Utah	150	7.3	154	7.3	1,731	21	1,752
Vermont	21	3.6	16	2.7	350	4	354
Virginia	998	14.8	912	13.4	11,442	161	11,603
Washington	523	9.3	393	6.9	8,798	33	8,831
West Virginia	122	6.7	64	3.5	968	9	977
Wisconsin	222	4.3	183	3.5	3,283	27	3,310
Wyoming	4	0.8	8	1.7	159	2	161
Subtotal	**51,882**	**19.4**	**45,514**	**16.8**	**679,125**	**8,188**	**687,313**
U.S. dependencies, possessions, and associated nations							
Guam	—	—	7	4.7	26	—	26
Pacific Islands, U.S.	—	—	—	—	4	—	4
Puerto Rico	2,012	52.6	1,448	37.5	22,640	387	23,027
Virgin Islands, U.S.	63	53.9	33	27.9	408	16	424
Total[1]	**54,140**	**19.9**	**47,083**	**17.1**	**702,748**	**8,596**	**711,344**

[1] U.S. totals presented in this report include data from the United States (50 states and the District of Columbia) and from U.S. dependencies, possessions, and independent nations in free association with the United States. Totals include 550 persons whose area of residence is unknown.
From Centers for Disease Control and Prevention: HIV/AIDS Surveillance Report 1999; 11:1.

"memory" T cells to be available to interact with a specific antigen in the future.

Lymphocytes and monocytes have a wide variety of surface receptors or markers that can be identified by binding specific monoclonal antibodies. These "cluster designations" have been given CD numbers such as CD4, which is a specific binding site for the HIV.

Antigens, wherever encountered, are taken up by antigen-presenting cells (APCs) and presented to lymphocytes. The antigens are bound on the surface of the APC with peptides termed major histocompatibility complex (MHC) molecules. Some APCs are migratory, such as Langerhans' cells, taking antigens from the skin and other epithelial surfaces to regional nodes and presenting them to T cells. Once in these tissues, a separate signal then directs the cells to the appropriate location for immune function. Others, like follicular dendritic cells located in B-cell areas of lymph nodes, are static and bind antigen using complement receptors. Circulating B cells are also capable of directly binding antigen. Antigen binding is followed by activation and differentiation. B-cell blasts progress to antibody-forming cells and ultimately to plasma cells. These processes are known as adaptive immunity. Adaptive immunity can be divided into two types: cell mediated and humoral. T cells are examples of cell-mediated immunity, whereas B cells are humoral through the production of antibody.

B-LYMPHOCYTE AND PLASMA CELL INDUCTION

It is well established that induction of antibody response and conversion from B cells to plasma cells is facilitated by primed helper CD4 cells. Once the antigens are bound to the antibody on the B-cell surface, the antigens are internalized, processed, and expressed on the B-cell surface with the MHC complex. This complex allows for recognition of helper CD4 cells. These responses are linked. Once this linked complex is expressed, lymphokines are then produced, allowing for amplification and clonal expansion. It is at this phase that differentiation into plasma cells occurs, which then excretes newly formed antibody.

CD8-MEDIATED IMMUNITY

Cytotoxic T cells function by inducing apoptosis (programmed cell death). These cells recognize antigen by MHC class I molecule-peptide interaction. Once activated, CD8 cells recognize target cells, induce the release of secretory granules from the T cells that are cytotoxic, and induce apoptosis. In addition, CD8 cells release cytokines, which allows for increased activity of theses CD8 cells and their cytotoxic effect.

Thus, humoral immunity may function in one of three ways. It may bind to bacteria and directly neutralize them. Antibody may coat bacteria, undergo opsonization, and facilitate phagocytosis. Alternatively, it may activate the complement cascade, which through opsonization facilitates phagocytosis or lysis.

ORTHOPAEDIC SURGERY ON THE HIV-POSITIVE PATIENT

HIV infection represents one of the most common causes of major immune system impairment. As of 1996, there were an estimated 21.8 million people living with HIV infection worldwide, 13 million of whom lived in sub-Saharan Africa.[1] According to the Centers for Disease Control (CDC), as of October 8, 1999, 711,344 cases of AIDS have been reported (Table 1).[2] Based on data from 1994 and 1995, AIDS was the most common cause of death among Americans 22 to 45 years of age.[1] The incidence of reported new cases of AIDS has declined since 1992, and death from AIDS has declined since 1995 (Fig. 1).[3]

The prevalence of HIV-positive individuals in the United States has been variously estimated from calculations based on AIDS prevalence and studies of different populations such as volunteer blood donors, job corps applicants, and sexually transmitted disease clinics. It is estimated that 0.2% to 0.5% of the U.S. population is HIV-positive.[1, 4] In high endemic areas, trauma centers report that up to 10.4% of their emergency trauma patients are HIV-positive.[5] In anonymous serosurveys conducted by the CDC at multiple institutions, 0.2% to 8.9% of emergency room patients and

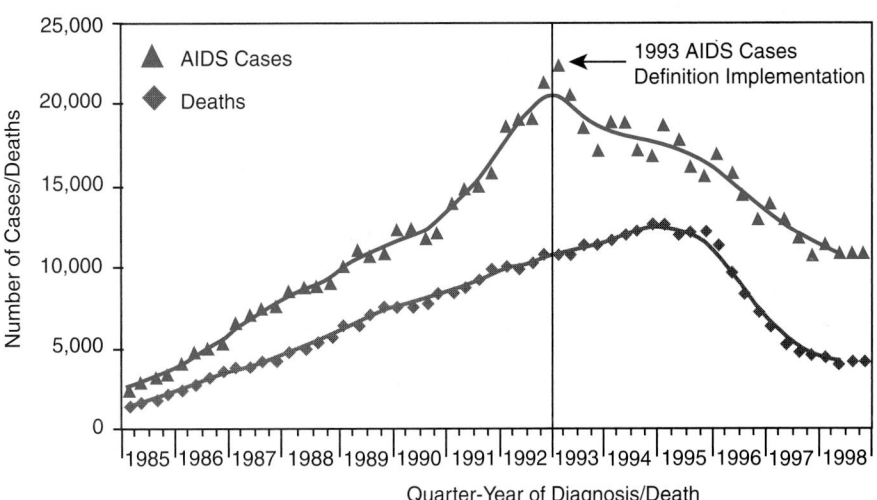

Fig. 1. Estimated incidence of AIDS. This is the estimated incidence of AIDS, by quarter year of diagnosis, and number of deaths, by quarter year of death, among adults* with AIDS† in the United States from 1985 to 1998. (From Centers for Disease Control: CDC guidelines for national human immunodeficiency virus case surveillance, including monitoring for human immunodeficiency virus infection and acquired immunodeficiency syndrome. (Persons aged ≥13 years. Adjusted for reporting delays. Data reported through June 1999.) (MMWR Mor Mortal Wkly Rep CDC Surveill Summ 1999; 48:3.)

0.1% to 7.8% of all hospital admissions were found to be HIV-positive.[5] Orthopaedic surgeons practicing in high endemic areas may anticipate that 3% to 10% of their acute trauma cases are HIV-positive. Elective surgical case rates are generally lower than emergency rates but highly variable.

Surgery on the HIV-positive patient, elective or emergent, involves some special risks, which may be divided into two categories: risk to the patient and risk to health care personnel. Because of concern about these issues, some orthopaedic surgeons may pursue nonoperative management of fractures usually treated surgically and are reluctant to recommend elective surgery in the HIV-positive patient. Such decisions cannot be condoned and may have legal implications.

There has been extensive study of the risks to health care personnel caring for HIV-positive patients. Recommendations of methodologies to reduce this risk in the practice of orthopaedics have been developed and published by the Task Force on AIDS of the American Academy of Orthopaedic Surgeons (AAOS) and also by the Occupational Safety and Health Administration (OSHA) and are mandated for hospital employees.[6, 7] To date, there have been 49 well-documented occupational seroconversions among health care workers. None has followed suture needle injuries, the most common being surgical percutaneous injury.[8] In a CDC report, zidovudine (ZVD) was shown to be effective in the prevention of seroconversion after percutaneous exposure to HIV-contaminated blood.[9, 10] If the AAOS/CDC/OSHA recommendations are closely followed, the risk to health care personnel, although real, can be reduced to an acceptable level. In a trauma setting, the patient's HIV status is often unknown, so adherence to these recommended universal precautions is essential.

Surgeons have expressed concern about the complications and outcome of operations on the HIV-infected patient because of immune system compromise. Early postoperative complications of greatest concern in the HIV-positive patient include sepsis and impaired wound healing. The late postoperative complication of primary concern in the HIV-positive orthopaedic patient is implant infection resulting from bacteremia, which some authors speculated is at increased risk.[11-13] The risk of early and late septic complications is theoretically increased because of impaired cellular and humoral immunity.

PATHOPHYSIOLOGY OF IMMUNITY IMPAIRMENT

The HIV is a member of the lentivirus subfamily of the Retroviridae family. Retroviruses are enveloped RNA viruses that are dependent on a DNA polymerase termed reverse transcriptase.[14] HIV is a single-strand RNA composed of 9300 nucleotide base units, genetic encoding segments, and a replication promoter region. Two major types have been identified. HIV-1 is prevalent. HIV-2 is still principally found in people from West Africa.[15] There are nine worldwide currently classified HIV-1 subtypes based on variations in the envelope gene (env), of which the largest portion (48%) are subtype B.[15] HIV mutates at an extremely rapid rate, creating "swarm" or "quasi-species" within the same individual host. The env gene mutates much more frequently than the gene responsible for encoding reverse transcriptase (pol), which accounts for the relative large number of patients responsive to reverse transcriptase inhibitor therapy. Mutation frequency and strain variation have additional significance on the validity of screening and confirmatory diagnostic tests for HIV.

Immunity impairment in HIV infection involves many components of host defenses, some of which are directly related to cellular invasion by the virus and others to secondary effects. The CD4+ T lymphocyte, which is responsible for cellular immunity, is the primary target cell in HIV infection. CD4 is a protein found on one subset of mature T lymphocytes and is essential for binding of HIV envelop glycoprotein. CD4 is also present in smaller amounts on macrophages and thymus cells. HIV is reproduced in both CD4+ T cells and macrophages. In addition to effects in cellular immunity, differentiation of the B lymphocyte, responsible for humoral immunity, is also impaired.[16] Studies have shown decreased humoral response to specific antigens, including strains of *Staphylococcus aureus.* Additional derangements occur in the monocyte/macrophage cell line and the production of gamma interferon and lymphokines, products of antigenically stimulated lymphocytes.[16]

As the disease progresses, the absolute polymorphonuclear leukocyte count drops to levels that impair phagocytosis.[17] This is believed to be the result of a direct HIV effect on stem cells but may be further reduced by marrow-suppressing drugs such as ZVD and other first- and second-generation reverse transcriptase inhibitors used to treat AIDS.[18] Malnutrition, which may be the consequence of both the disease process and therapeutic medications, causes hypoalbuminemia and lymphopenia, which may further impair host immunity.[19, 20]

In addition to their crucial role in the immune system, CD4 lymphocytes and lymphokines are important in wound healing. Lymphokines activate fibroblast proliferation and participate in their regulation.[21-23] Fishel and coinvestigators[22] documented the migration of CD lymphocyte subsets into healing wounds, which peaks at 7 days. Furthermore, experimental impairment of both cellular and humoral immunity by cyclosporin A was shown to reduce wound tensile strength to a significant degree at 10 days.[24]

Autoimmune dysfunction also occurs with AIDS. As a result of B-cell dysfunction, there are increased circulating immune complexes. One manifestation of this phenomenon is platelet deficiency, which, if uncorrected, can result in excessive bleeding at surgery. Immunodeficiency-associated thrombocytopenic purpura may be the result of an autoimmune globulin directed against platelet antigens similar to the immunoglobulin (Ig) G produced in idiopathic thrombocytopenic purpura.[25] It seems somewhat paradoxical that autoimmune afflictions should occur in individuals with reduced immunity, but such reactions are common among AIDS patients. This platelet deficiency is treated initially with steroids and, if persistent, with splenectomy. The former further reduces host resistance to infection, and the latter is associated with an increased risk of septicemia.[25, 26] Despite treatment, the platelet deficiency persists in 80% of those treated with steroids and in about 50% after splenectomy. Bleeding problems may be further compounded by the development of autoimmune inhibitors to clotting fac-

TABLE 2. THIRTY-DAY MORTALITY AFTER GENERAL SURGICAL PROCEDURES IN PATIENTS WITH AIDS			
Time Period	30-Day Mortality (%) After Elective Procedures	30-Day Mortality (%) After Emergent Procedures*	Type of Procedure
1982–1985	43% (24)	57% (7)	Thoracotomy, laparotomy, craniotomy
1984–1988	9% (22)	46% (13)	Abdominal

Values in parenthesis represent number of procedures.

*The authors believed that this very high postoperative mortality rate was the result of progression of opportunistic infection, Kaposi's sarcoma, or lymphoma as well as the fact that these patients were critically and chronically ill at the time of surgery during a period when our capacity to manage the complications of AIDS was very limited.

tors. These lupoid antibodies will result in a prolonged activated partial thromboplastin time but in most cases will not result in excessive bleeding at surgery. Allogeneic blood transfusion often required in AIDS patients because of anemia, related to both the disease and pharmacological agents, can be immunosuppressive. These adverse effects include decrease in helper/suppressor ratio, reduced natural killer cell function, impaired antigen presentation, suppressed lymphocyte blastogenesis, and impaired delayed hypersensitivity.[27]

Several groups studied neutrophil bactericidal capacity in HIV-positive patients. This capacity is dependent on chemotaxis, phagocytosis, and secretion of oxygen-dependent and oxygen-independent microbicides. Using cultures of *S. aureus* as the target organism, Murphy and coworkers compared 90-minute bacterial survival in washed neutrophils from 19 AIDS patients, who had no active infections and were on no drugs, with that in 17 healthy controls.[28] Bacterial survival in the AIDS patients was significantly higher: 32.5% compared with 13.8% in the controls. Reduced bacterial killing against *S. aureus* was also demonstrated by Ellis and associates[17] in patients with AIDS and Kaposi's sarcoma. These two studies suggest impairment of all three leukocyte bactericidal functions: chemotaxis, phagocytosis, and secretion of microbicides in patients with AIDS.

As a result of this complex and widespread immune system impairment, patients with advanced HIV infection have increased susceptibility to common pathogens as well as to opportunistic infections. Many of these pathogens include those commonly etiological in musculoskeletal infections. Ganesh and associates[29] showed that the carriage rate for *S. aureus* in nose, throat, and perineum was twice that for the asymptomatic HIV-positive individual (49%) compared with HIV-negative controls (27%). Krumholz et al[30] reported 44 episodes of community-acquired bacteremia in 38 AIDS patients at San Francisco General Hospital. The most common infecting organisms in order were *S. aureus, Streptococcus pneumoniae, and Escherichia coli*,

and presenting infections included pneumonia, central catheter phlebitis, cellulitis, and urinary tract infection. Typical for AIDS patients with a bacterial infection, these patients often present with minimal inflammatory response and appear deceptively benign: only 57% of these patients were febrile, including pyarthrosis and other orthopaedic infections.

SURGICAL COMPLICATIONS AND OUTCOME

Impaired defenses to common surgical pathogens and delayed would healing are causes for concern about the outcome of orthopaedic procedures on the HIV-positive patient. Robinson, Wilson, and coworkers[31, 32] reported a reduction in the elective mortality rate in surgical procedures on patients with AIDS, reflecting the improvement in management of opportunistic infections and preterminal AIDS. Unfortunately, the 30-day mortality rate remained unchanged between 1982 and 1986 (Table 2).

Diettrich et al[20] reported the 30-day mortality in HIV-positive patients without AIDS to be roughly comparable to that for the HIV-negative population after surgical intervention in 20 patients with a positive titer with or without AIDS (Table 3).

Greene and coworkers[33] reviewed 26 orthopaedic procedures on HIV-positive hemophiliacs performed between 1984 and 1988. There were no surgical site infections, but there was one intravenous site cellulitis. Five patients had a protracted postoperative fever but did not experience clinical infection. Investigations by Buehrer[33a] and Greene and their coworkers suggest that the outcome and functional result of orthopaedic procedures in hemophiliacs with or without a positive HIV titer were similar to those for patients treated before 1982 who were presumed HIV-negative (Table 4).

Hoekman[33b] and Paiement[33c] and their associates investigated the incidences of postoperative infections in trauma patients with and without a positive HIV titer. Hoekman et al studied 171 individuals treated without prophylactic admin-

TABLE 3. THIRTY-DAY MORTALITY IN HIV-POSITIVE PATIENTS WITH AND WITHOUT AIDS (1986–1990)		
Procedure	Patients HIV-Positive	Patients with AIDS (%)
Elective	0/40	1/26 (4)
Emergent	0/24	7/30 (3)

TABLE 4. SURGICAL WOUND INFECTIONS IN HEMOPHILIACS WITH AND WITHOUT A POSITIVE HIV TITER			
Study	HIV Negative	HIV Positive	AIDS
Buehrer et al[33a]	0%	1.4%	1.5%
Greene et al[33]	0%	0%	0%

istration of antimicrobial agents, whereas Paiement and associates treated 476 patients with prophylactic antimicrobial agents. The rate of infection is remarkably similar between the Hoekman and Paiement studies, with no increase in the asymptomatic HIV-positive groups compared with the HIV-negative groups but a significant increase in the HIV-positive patients (Table 5).

To date, there has been much speculation but few studies of the effect of HIV infection on the incidence of late prosthetic joint infection. Ragni and associates,[34] in a mail survey of 115 hemophilia centers, studied the rate of postoperative infection in orthopaedic procedures performed on 66 HIV-positive patients with CD4 counts below 200 at surgery. CD4 counts under 200 qualifies these patients for the diagnosis of AIDS. Sixty-six patients had 74 procedures resulting in 10 infections in the first 5 months postoperatively. Five of these patients had preoperative evidence of infection. The overall rate of infection was 10 of 66 (15.2%). The rate of infection for joint replacement was 9 of 34 (26.5%) compared with 1 of 40 (2.5%) for other procedures.

Our Hemophilia Treatment Center at Orthopaedic Hospital (Los Angeles) found the incidence of spontaneous hematogenous joint infections in hemophiliacs increased significantly after HIV-1 was introduced into the donor blood pool.[35] In the period between 1973 and 1980, there were three such infections in a stable population of 480 hemophiliacs that varied less than 6% per year. In the subsequent 7-year period from 1981 to 1988, there were 13. In the group of hemophiliacs with CD4 counts less than 200, which would currently qualify for the diagnosis of AIDS, the incidence of musculoskeletal infection was 11.0% compared with 1.1% in all other hemophiliacs at this center. Both of these differences were statistically significant. All of these infections involved either arthropathic or prosthetic joints. In the six prosthetic joints, the time from implantation to infection was 6 months to 15 years. As in the Krumholz study, infected joints in the HIV-positive patient with less than 200 CD4 cells appeared deceptively benign, and fever was usually low grade or absent. Other literature reports of hematogenous pyarthrosis in hemophiliacs have increased since the introduction of HIV. According to Gilbert,[36] there were four cases reported before 1982 and more than 20 since.

Because of the deceptively benign appearance of these infections in immunosuppressed patients, joint aspiration for culture is performed when there is any suspicion of infection based on a change in the clinical picture. These patients typically present with increased pain and difficulty with range of motion but may be afebrile, and the involved joint is usually not particularly swollen or erythematous. After aspiration, the joint is immobilized. If the clinical suspicion is high, broad-spectrum antibiotics may be started while awaiting culture results. If purulent material is aspirated or the Gram stain is positive, the joint is washed out, usually with arthroscopic lavage.

Gilbert[36] reported on a multicenter study on total knee replacements in hemophiliacs. The rate of infection in the 134 patients was 10.5%, with the earliest 6 months postoperatively. All patients were HIV-positive at the time of infection, with CD4 counts ranging from 66 to 449 (mean, 202). Gilbert stated that he "restricts joint arthroplasty to intelligent, cooperative patients who are aware of the risks and will rapidly treat any infection to prevent hematogenous spread to the replacement." Both Wiedel and Ragni indicated that their centers are reluctant to perform joint replacement on patients with CD4 counts below 200.[36]

Our Hemophilia Treatment Center studied the incidence of infection in 93 joint replacements performed in 62 hemophiliacs between 1968 and 1991.[28] At surgery, 25 patients were HIV-negative and 25 were HIV-positive. The status of the 12 patients who had surgeries performed between 1978 and 1985 was unknown. There were no early postoperative infections in any of these patients. The incidence of late postoperative infection in the HIV-negative group was 8%, which is similar to the average in other studies on HIV-negative hemophiliacs (10%).[37–39] This high incidence of late hematogenous prosthetic joint infection in hemophiliacs before HIV infection may be a consequence of bacteremia from frequent intravenous self-administration of clotting factor concentrate. The incidence of late prosthetic joint infection in the patients known to be HIV-positive at surgery was 18%. The earliest infection occurred 5 months postoperatively. Because of the small numbers in each group, this difference is not statistically significant but may represent a trend. It seems likely that the already high risk of infection in hemophiliacs is magnified by the immune system impairment caused by HIV infection. It is interesting to note that the incidence of late infection of knee replacements in HIV-positive hemophiliacs of 10.4% reported by Gilbert is essentially the same as that reported in multiple studies before the advent of HIV.

Unger and associates[40] reported on 26 total knee replacements in hemophiliacs between 1984 and 1991 with 1 to 9 years follow-up. Even though all patients were HIV-positive, no early or late infections were reported. The degree of symptomatology and CD4 levels were not reported for these patients.

TABLE 5. PERCENTAGE OF WOUND INFECTIONS			
		HIV Titer	
Study	No. Patients	Negative	Positive
Hoekman et al[33b]	171	5%	1% asymptomatic, 23% symptomatic
Paiement et al[33c]	476		
Clean and clean-contaminated		4%	0%
Open fractures		11%	56%

It is uncertain how applicable the data on late infection of prosthetic joints in hemophiliacs is to nonhemophiliac HIV-positive patients. Both logic and some data suggest that the risk of late infection increases as the immune system impairment worsens. In our study, the risk essentially doubled. However, the risk of late infection in HIV-negative hemophiliacs (10%) is much higher than that for the general HIV-negative population (<1%). In our study, the risk doubled in the HIV-positive group. If this were true for the HIV-positive nonhemophiliac population, the risk would be less than 2%, which would be far more acceptable than 18% as it is in hemophilia. The only study of which we are aware that attempts to deal with this question was by Lehman, Paiement, and coauthors,[41] presented at the annual meeting of the American Academy of Orthopaedic Surgeons in 1999. They performed a retrospective study of total joint replacements on 19 HIV-positive patients without hemophilia and 9 patients with a history of intravenous drug abuse with a median follow-up of 5 years. Four patients had a history of both. In the HIV-positive group without a history of intravenous drug abuse, the rate of infection was 21%. For the intravenous drug abuse group it was 21%, and for the group with both risk factors it was 50%. The results of this small population suggest that the risk of late infection of prosthetic joints in HIV-positive patients is similar in hemophiliac and non-hemophiliac populations.

Opportunistic infections, common in patients with AIDS, are very rarely causative of orthopaedic implant infection. Mycobacterial infections, including atypical strains, are common in patients with advanced HIV infection. Hawkins and associates[42] reported disseminated *Mycobacterium avium–intracellulare* (MAI) infection in 53% of patients dying of AIDS at Sloan Kettering Cancer Center. McLaughlin, Tierney, and Harris reported one patient in whom MAI infection developed in both prosthetic hips. Both sides demonstrated prosthetic loosening for many years.[43] The patient had clinical AIDS at the time of apparent *Mycobacterium* infection. Hawkins reported positive blood cultures in 98% and bone marrow aspirations in 100% of patients with MAI. The prostheses in this patient could have become infected either through hematogenous seeding or from the adjacent bone. Loosening with hyperemic interface membrane would predispose to this complication. Fungal infections are also common in HIV-positive patients, but to the best of our knowledge there have been no reports of fungal prosthetic joint infection related to HIV infection.

VIRAL HEPATITIS

Like HIV, hepatitis B and C viruses (HBV) and (HCV) have a significant effect on host immunity. Before describing the immune impairment mechanisms, it seems appropriate to review the prevalence and transmissibility of these viruses in the clinical setting. Today chronic viral hepatitis is more prevalent among hospitalized patients than HIV and represents a greater risk to health care personnel. Several studies reported a range of 0.5% to 5% HBV carriers among hospitalized patients.[44-46] Despite the availability of a safe, effective recombinant HBV vaccine, hepatitis B remains the most common occupationally acquired blood-

borne disease in the health care setting.[44] The risk of transmission from a needlestick contaminated with HBV-infected blood is estimated to be 30%, which is approximately 300 times that for HIV. In a study of surgeons, 17% were HBV-positive not from vaccine. Fourteen percent of those still susceptible to HBV had not received the vaccine.[44] The CDC estimated that 5100 U.S. health care workers acquired HBV occupationally in 1991 and that 125 of these would die from consequences of this disease.[44, 47]

HCV was identified in 1989[48] as the probable cause of most cases of non-A, non-B hepatitis. It is a small single-stranded RNA virus and part of the Flaviviridae family. HCV genomes are heterogeneous but closely related. A portion of the cloned genome has been used to develop an immunoassay to detect antibodies against HCV (anti-HCV) in the serum.

HCV is transmitted principally through the bloodborne route. It is estimated that 90% of recipients of blood from an HCV-positive donor will contract the disease. Transmission via transplanted organs and musculoskeletal allografts has been reported. Sexual transmission is much less likely than HIV but remains controversial and poorly defined. It is estimated that nearly 4 million Americans are infected with HCV, with a moderately increased prevalence in minorities: 3.2% of blacks, 2.1% of Hispanics, and 1.5% of non-Hispanic whites.[48-50] The incidence appears to be declining since 1989. In 1997 it was estimated that 30,000 new cases occurred annually.[48] Most infections are subclinical, but virtually all patients demonstrate liver cell damage, as evident from elevated serum aminotransferase levels.[48] Approximately 85% of infected individuals have chronically elevated liver enzymes and chronic active hepatitis.[48, 51] At least 20% will experience cirrhosis within two decades after exposure. The incidence of hepatocellular carcinoma is elevated and estimated to be 1% to 5% after 20 years of infection.[48] The incidence is highest in those with cirrhosis. HCV is responsible for 8000 to 10,000 deaths annually, which is estimated to triple over the next 10 to 20 years. Persistent infection with intermittent viremia appears to occur in all infected individuals.

Screening tests for HCV use enzyme immunoassays to detect anti-HCV. The assays contain core HCV antigens. Polymerase chain reaction (PCR) tests detect HCV RNA and are used as a reference standard. The second-generation enzyme immunoassay (EIA-2) is 92% to 95% sensitive, but specificity has yet to be precisely established.[48] Positive EIA-2 tests should be confirmed with a recombinant immunoblot assay (RIBA). Even with a positive RIBA test result, the specificity is only 70% to 75% in low-risk donors. Positive individuals may require PCR testing. However, a single negative PCR does not mean the patient is not infected and intermittently viremic. Viral load can be determined by quantitative PCR. Treatment for hepatitis C is limited. Interferon-α has been the primary form of therapy, with an end of treatment response rate of 40% to 50% and a sustained response rate of 15% to 20%.[48] Treatment is recommended for those with persistently elevated serum alanine aminotransferase, who are at increased risk for cirrhosis.

The risk of HCV transmission to health care personnel from percutaneous injury is less per incident than HBV, but the prevalence and susceptibility are higher, creating a worrisome situation. Serosurveys among health care personnel have demonstrated rates ranging from 0% to 1.7%. One such survey, performed at the annual meeting of the American Academy of Orthopaedic Surgeons in 1991, showed that 0.8% of surgeons tested were positive.[52] This compares with 0.09% to 0.36% among U.S. blood donors. The percentage of surgeons testing positive in this study correlated with age (years in practice): 30 to 39 years, 0.4% positive; 40 to 49 years, 0.8%; 50 to 59 years, 1.2%; and 60 years and older, 1.4%. In addition to parenteral transmission from patient to health care personnel in the health care setting, transmission from surgeon to patient has been described as well. The risk of seroconversion after a percutaneous injury contaminated with HCV-positive blood has been estimated from 2.7% using first-generation EIAs to 10% in a study using second-generation EIAs and PCR testing for HCV RNA.

Chronic HBV and HCV patients demonstrate a wide variety of immune system impairments. Lymphocytic response to hepatitis B surface antigen is impaired, and interleukin (IL)-2 synthesis is reduced.[53] T- and B-cell populations were reduced in studies of mice infected with mouse hepatitis virus type 3.[54] Neutralizing antiviral antibody responses are delayed in both HIV and hepatitis B infections.[55] Cirrhosis secondary to chronic active hepatitis B or C leads to reduced phagocytosis, which may be the result of secondary malnutrition, common in both alcoholism and viral liver disease.[56, 57] Viral hepatitis patients are also plagued with the development of autoantibodies, hyperglobulinemia, and increased circulating immune complexes similar to that seen in HIV-infected patients. This can result in immune-mediated thrombocytopenia and other autoimmune disorders.[58] Peripheral T cells are reduced, leading to abnormal B-cell activation, which may account for the increase in circulating immune complexes and autoantibodies.

ALCOHOLISM

Alcoholic patients are predisposed to several musculoskeletal problems, including infection related to immune system impairment, ischemic necrosis, and myopathy. Decreased bone mass combined with balance impairment and battering resulting in predisposition to fractures and delayed fracture healing are also problems facing the alcoholic patient.[59] In addition, postoperative management may be complicated by alcohol withdrawal, manifestations of chronic hepatic failure, immune system impairment, and cardiomyopathy.

Although millions of Americans consume alcoholic beverages to varying degrees, approximately 10% eventually are diagnosed as alcoholics.[67] Various studies have estimated a wide prevalence of alcoholism ranging from 5% to 77%.[60, 67] Different types of patients and diagnostic criteria accounted for this large disparity. These studies established both major and minor criteria. The major criteria for the diagnoses of alcoholism include presence of withdrawal syndrome, tolerance to the effects of alcohol, presence of alcoholic blackout periods, and continued drinking despite medical or social contraindication. Minor criteria include alcohol-related physiological disorders and altered behavioral patterns such as gulping drinks and alcohol-related

automobile accidents. In an analysis of a population of orthopaedic patients using the CAGE (concern, anger, guilt, eye-opener), alcoholism was diagnosed in 31%.[60]

Although many different organ systems can be affected by alcoholism, including the liver, central nervous system, pancreas, and hematopoietic systems, fatty changes of the liver are the most common. Unchecked, these changes will eventually manifest as cirrhosis. Immune system impairment in alcoholics is multifactorial, resulting in an increased risk of infection, first described in 1785 by Benjamin Rush.[61]

EFFECTS OF ALCOHOL ON LEUKOCYTES

Granulocytopenia has been found in 4% to 8% of hospitalized alcoholic patients.[62] This is of particular consequence in alcoholics undergoing surgery and those with infection.[63] The acute reduction in leukocytes may be mild and has been shown to normalize within a few days of abstinence.[64] Evaluation of the marrow in chronic alcoholics demonstrates a decrease in the number of mature granulocytes. MacGregor[64] demonstrated that endotoxin injection did not show an increase in circulating polymorphonuclear neutrophil numbers, suggesting that there is a decrease in marrow reserve as well as a decrease in production and response to stimulation.

MacGregor and Gluckman[65, 66] found that alcohol causes a dose-dependent fall in granulocyte adherence.[67] Alcohol ingestion has also been found to impair normal chemotaxis of polymorphonuclear leukocytes. This is believed to result from a depressed level of complement associated with a serum inhibitor.[67] When alcohol abusers progressed to cirrhosis, 70% to 90% acquired a serum inhibitor to chemotactic factor that dramatically inhibited the chemotaxis-stimulating ability of their own serum even when normal serum was added. All patients' antibody response to keyhold limpet hemocyanin (KLH) immunization was poor, and delayed hypersensitivity to KLH could not be established. Edmondson[67] concluded that chronic alcoholics exposed to infectious agents requiring cell-mediated immunity (i.e., tuberculosis) for the first time may fail to respond in an adequate manner. Alcohol also demonstrates an effect on cell-mediated immunity by depressing both the development and expression of lymphocytes. McFarland and Libre[63] demonstrated that alcoholics with infection had decreased numbers of lymphocytes. Tennenbaum et al[68] demonstrated a correlation between alcoholic fatty liver disease and delayed hypersensitivity against new antigen in rats. In animal studies they noted atrophy of the spleen and thymus, in which B and T cells are produced. Antibody response to primary immunization was delayed. Improved liver function associated with alcohol withdrawal correlated with improved response to anergy testing. Nonalcoholic volunteers who were acutely intoxicated had normal delayed hypersensitivity reactions. Inhibition of cell-mediated skin test sensitization in alcoholics appears to be related to the degree and type of secondary hepatic disease.[64]

Alcohol also adversely affects humoral immunity. Excessive alcohol ingestion has been shown to interfere with antibody response to new antigens.[64]

ALCOHOLIC MYOPATHY

Heavy drinking can produce an acute alcoholic myopathy characterized by painful swollen muscles, high levels of serum creatine phosphokinase, and occasionally myoglobinemia and myoglobinuria.[69]

Alcoholic myopathy frequently follows a period of heavy drinking and has been reported in up to 22% of alcoholics with fatty liver degeneration or cirrhosis.[67] Rapid muscle wasting occurs. Serum creatine phosphokinase remains elevated for 10 to 14 days.[70]

OSTEONECROSIS

Alcoholism is a well-established risk factor for osteonecrosis involving the hip, knee, and shoulder. In theory, altered lipid metabolism resulting from alcohol and liver dysfunction results in occlusion of small vessels in the subarticular bone and consequent necrosis. These events are subsequently followed by attempted replacement, resorption of the subarticular bone, and eventual collapse, setting the stage for progressive degenerative arthritis. The exact pathophysiology of osteonecrosis remains obscure. The first lesions identified with MRI[71] include vascular congestion and bone marrow edema in the marrow spaces.[72] Core decompression has been advocated for the early phases of osteonecrosis, although after many studies the indications remain controversial.

BATTERED ALCOHOLIC SYNDROME

The battered alcoholic syndrome has been defined as an alcoholic patient in whom there are three or more fractures of different ages. In 1977, Oppenheim[73] undertook a retrospective study evaluating 100 consecutive charts of patients at a county hospital who sustained fractures requiring hospital admission. In his review, he found that fully 26% of the patients admitted for fractures were diagnosed as alcoholic, 62% of the patients admitted for a third fracture were alcoholic, and 8% of the study population had three or more fractures at various stages of healing. Oppenheim coined the term "battered alcoholic syndrome" to describe these patients. The diagnosis was made radiographically and/or by history of previous fractures. This determination is important in the treatment of alcoholic patients.

ALCOHOL EFFECTS ON BONE MINERAL DENSITY

Alcohol alters serum calcium metabolism and induces a low-grade osteomalacia associated with an increased fracture risk, especially in a patient population predisposed to falling.[74] Alcohol has been found to affect the frequency in which femoral neck fractures occur in men.[74] This appears to be related to the decreased mineral content and increased bone fragility found in alcoholic patients.[75] Bone biopsy specimens obtained from the iliac crest in middle-aged alcoholic men were comparable in bone density to that of an average elderly female.[74, 76] Kalbfleisch et al[77] demonstrated that alcoholics have increased osteoclastic activity as well as a magnesium and calcium diuresis. Alcohol is known to increase the parathyroid hormone level rapidly in normal males and stimulates the adrenal cortex in rodents.[78] Decreased physical activity associated with alcohol also facilitates low bone mineral content. Widened osteoid seams were present only in those alcoholics who underwent gastric resection.[79] However, alcoholics who were not socially or nutritionally impaired had bone mineral content only 3.3% less than normal controls.[80]

RECOMMENDATIONS

Given such significant associated morbidity, certain precautions should be taken when operating on patients with possible alcoholism. For patients requiring elective surgical procedures, abstinence from alcohol for 1 month before the procedure will reduce immunity impairment and diminish the morbidity and complications compared with those who do not abstain.[81] Chronic alcoholics are in need of vitamin replacement. An intravenous solution containing 100 mg thiamine, 1.0 mg folate, 2.0 g magnesium sulfate, and one ampule of a multivitamin per liter can correct the most frequently depleted nutrients. Oral supplements may also be used. Dehydration greatly increases the intraoperative and postoperative morbidity. Adequate fluid replacement therapy, even to the degree of modest hyperhydration, is essential. Correction of protein-calorie malnutrition, common in alcoholics, is discussed in the next section. A medical consult for preoperative evaluation and assistance in managing comorbid disease is strongly recommended, especially in those patients undergoing major surgery and those with advanced alcoholic liver disease. Alcoholic patients with advanced liver disease often have coagulation defects involving both platelets and clotting factor production. Preoperative evaluation should include partial thromboplastin time, prothrombin time, platelet count, and bleeding time. Defects in these coagulation systems are usually correctable with vitamin K, fresh frozen plasma or specific clotting factors, and platelet transfusion. Abnormalities in any of these tests should be evaluated by a hematologist.

Finally, in all chronic alcoholics, consideration must be given to the effects of abstinence during hospitalization. The symptoms of withdrawal can be managed with appropriate sedatives such as chlordiazepoxide (Librium), 25 to 75 mg IV or IM every 4 to 6 hours, which usually provides adequate amelioration of symptoms if begun early. Delirium tremens or "rum fits" bears a 5% mortality, and appropriate precautions, including hydration, control of hypertension, and sedation, must be instituted at the onset of symptoms. These patients require close monitoring, usually in an intensive care unit, with multispecialty team management.

MALNUTRITION

Malnutrition has a substantial effect on immune system competence. When compromised by malnutrition, patients are at increased risk for local infection, septicemia, and poor wound healing.[82–84] Among hospitalized populations, up to 50% of patients have some form of malnutrition.[85–89] Socioeconomic factors such as poor nutrition and alcoholism limit adequate nutritional intake. Absorption of nutrients may be compromised by gastrointestinal dysfunction, excessive antacids or proton pump inhibitors, or enteric losses from vomiting or diarrhea.[90] Psychological factors include clinical depression, anorexia, or bulimia. Neuromuscular diseases such as cerebral palsy are often associated with malnutrition. Hypermetabolic states and malignancies with severe wasting represent malnutrition also.

Surgery, trauma, infection, and other physiological stressors increase the basal metabolic demands, and endogenous stores of glycogen can be depleted within 12 hours. With the addition of physiological stressors, basal energy requirements may increase by 30% to 55%.[91] Body fat is

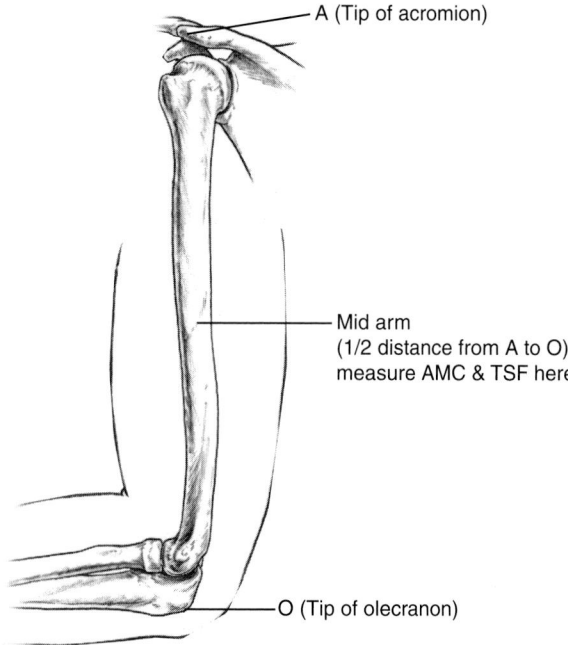

Arm muscle circumference (AMC) (cm) =
Arm circumference – [0.0314 x triceps skinfold (TSF) (mm)]

Fig. 2. Method of mid—upper arm circumference measurement. Muscle mass is estimated by subtracting 0.314 × the triceps skinfold measurement from the mid-upper arm circumference. (From Jensen JE: Nutrition in orthopaedic surgery. J Bone Joint Surg Am 1982; 64:1264.)

relatively unavailable as an energy substrate during times of stress, and muscle breakdown occurs to provide protein as the primary caloric source, resulting in negative nitrogen balance.[92] Negative nitrogen balance results in increased

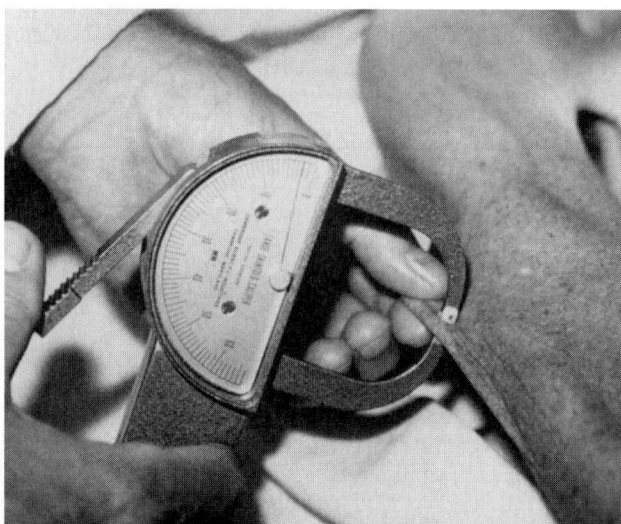

Fig. 3. Triceps skinfold measurement utilizing a skinfold caliper as designed by Lange, Harpenden, or Holtrain. (From Goodhart RS, Shills ME: Modern Nutrition in Health and Disease. Philadelphia, Lea & Febiger, 1980, p. 672; originally from Weinsier, Butterworth, Sahm: Handbook of Clinical Nutrition. Birmingham, University of Alabama Department of Nutrition Sciences, 1977.)

rate of impaired wound healing, infection, sepsis, and pneumonia.

Nutritional deficiencies may be documented with anthropometric evaluations including weight, height relationship, mid–upper arm circumference, and triceps skinfold measurement[93] (Figs. 2 and 3). Weight should be 90% or greater of ideal body weight for height. A mid–upper arm circumference of 19 cm or less for women and 24 cm or less for men and a triceps skinfold of 13 mm or less for women and 6 mm or less for men are indicative of malnutrition.[93] Ideally, all adult patients should have their weight and height measured and plotted on admission, and patients at risk should be monitored by daily weights, measurement of mid–upper arm circumference, and the triceps skinfold. There are many potential pitfalls, because moderately obese patients who appear well nourished may be in acute protein-calorie malnutrition. Local or generalized edema can also be misleading. Figure 4 presents an algorithm for evaluating elective surgical patients with possible malnutrition. Other clinical indications include supraclavicular, intercostal, or interosseous muscle wasting, a scaphoid abdomen, recent weight loss of more than 10 pounds, and

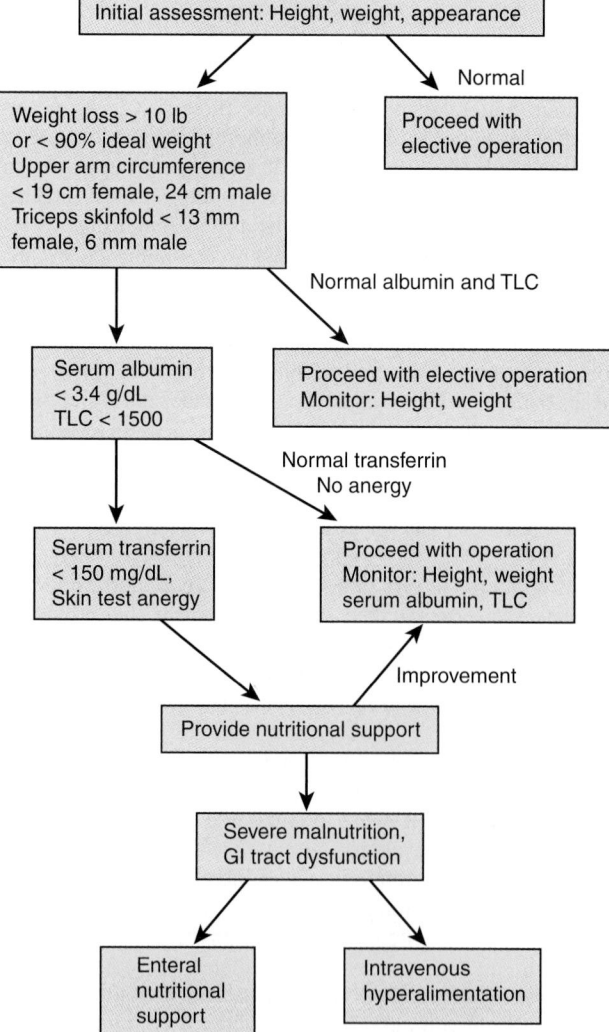

Fig. 4. Algorithm for evaluation of nutritional status and elective surgical decision-making. (Modified from Jensen JE: Nutrition in orthopaedic surgery. J Bone Joint Surg Am 1982; 64:1264.)

pitting edema.[91] Laboratory evaluation includes measurement of serum transferrin, serum albumin, and prealbumin.[94–96] Albumin is the most useful, and values below 3.5 g/dL are indicative of malnutrition. Total lymphocyte count (TLC) per cubic millimeter is also widely used, and normal anergy is returned after nutritional repletion.[97, 98] TLC levels should be above 1500 cells/mm³.[99] The albumin and TLC correlate inversely with mortality rate, prolonged hospital stays, and perioperative complications.[100] Serum transferrin is a more sensitive indicator of marginal protein depletion because of its relatively short half-life but is not readily obtainable in all hospital laboratories.

RECOMMENDATIONS

Given the potential risks imposed by malnutrition on the orthopaedic patient, nutritional parameters should be optimized before surgery. In addition to anthropometric measurements, preoperative laboratory testing of serum albumin and TLC should be performed on all patients at risk for malnutrition. The literature supports delaying elective cases in patients with decreased TLC (<1500 cells/mm³) and serum albumin (<3.5 g/dL) until adequate nutritional and metabolic status can be achieved.[83, 91, 101–103]

A multidisciplinary approach including the hospital dietitian should be used to reduce protein-calorie malnutrition. Oral versus enteral versus intravenous hyperalimentation should be evaluated, because trauma patients with associated abdominal disease and patients with full thickness burns, bowel obstruction, or prolonged ileus generally require total parenteral nutrition (TPN). Infection is the most frequent complication of TPN and is probably the result of more severe malnutrition and immune suppression combined with the risks of bacteremia associated with venous access ports, more critical illnesses, and more major surgical procedures. Cognizance of the patient's preoperative nutritional status using the physical examination parameters and laboratory tests described will help determine the patient's baseline metabolic status as well as the initial immunocompetence risk. Use of this basic regimen will help decrease the risk of complications in both elective and emergent surgical procedures.

MANAGEMENT OF THE POST-TRANSPLANT PATIENT

Transplant recipients are living longer, and in one study the 10 year post-transplant survival of patients receiving orthotopic heart transplantation was 80%.[104] There is an increased morbidity and mortality in post-transplant patients requiring subsequent surgical intervention.[104, 105] The majority of the complications, especially infection, occur as a consequence of immunosuppressive drug therapy. The risk of infection is determined by the intensity of the exposure to the pathogen and the net immunosuppressed state.[106–108] Figure 5 shows the timeline of specific opportunistic infections in relation to the immunosuppressive agent.[109] Since the early 1990s, a three-drug regimen consisting of azathioprine, cyclosporin A, and a glucocortico-

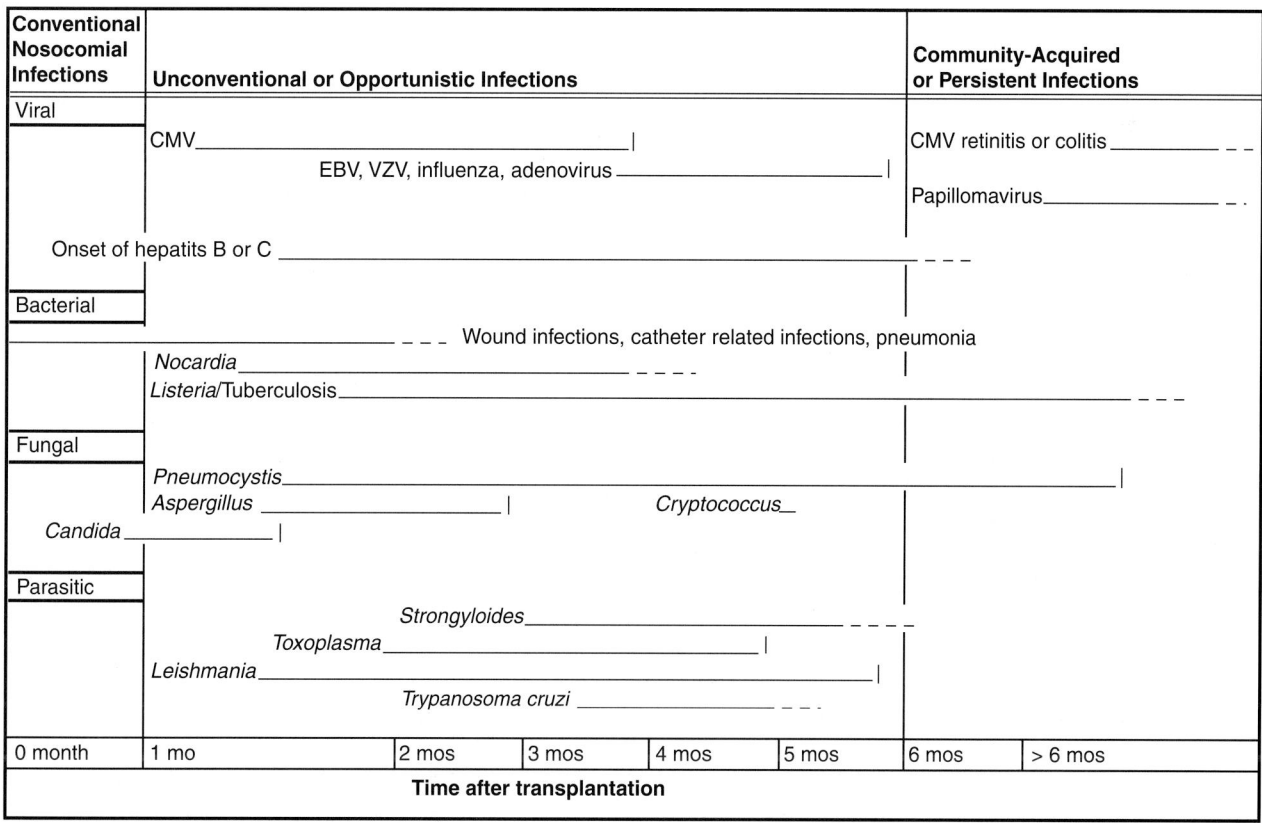

Fig. 5. Timeline of viral and opportunistic infections after major organ transplantation. (From Fishman JA, Rubin RH: Infection in organ transplant recipients. N Engl J Med 1998; 338:1741.)

steroid has been used[110, 111] for post-transplant immunosuppression. The risk of musculoskeletal infection in these patients is significantly increased.

Tannenbaum and coworkers[110] reported a 19% risk of infection in post-transplant patients receiving total joint replacements. Because immune suppression induces impairment of the inflammatory response and diminishes the signs and symptoms of infection, a high index of suspicion and a low threshold for intervention are warranted. If infection does occur, aggressive treatment should be implemented. Finally, in 10% of patients, there is chronic infection with HBV, HCV, cytomegalovirus, Epstein-Barr virus (EBV), or a variety of opportunistic agents. EBV has an increased risk of progressing to non-Hodgkin's lymphoma.[111–113] Included in the following section on pharmacological immune suppression is a description of some of the common drugs used in organ transplant patients.

PHARMACOLOGICAL IMMUNE SUPPRESSION

Pharmacological immune suppression is the most common form in most orthopaedic practices. Agents include corticosteroids, antibiotics, immunosuppressive drugs used to prevent rejection in organ transplant patients, and antivirals. Specific mechanisms of immune impairment and severity of risk are described for some of the more common agents.

Corticosteroids affect all leukocyte lines and inhibit neutrophil migration to inflammatory sites, decrease neutrophil adherence to vascular endothelium, and decrease the phagocytic and bactericidal activity of neutrophils.[114] This results in a decrease of neutrophils at sites of inflammation.[114, 115] An increased number of neutrophils in the immature form is highly suggestive of a superimposed infectious process.[115] Thrombocytosis can also occur and may increase the risk of thromboembolic complications after lower extremity surgery. Lymphocyte impairment results in T-cell activation inhibition and CD4 cell destruction. In high doses, steroids may also inhibit immunoglobulin production.[116] In addition to reduction of chemotaxis and bactericidal activity, steroids impair monocyte cytokine production (i.e., IL-1).[116–118]

Cyclosporin A blocks the transmission of the antigen-mediated signal of T cells through inhibition of the production of IL-2, a cytokine necessary for the induction of cytotoxic T lymphocytes,[119] and also inhibits production of IL-2, -3, and -4 and interferon-γ.[120] It is this step that allows increased risk of infection. Antibiotics, even those that are not normally nephrotoxic, cannot be assumed to be benign to the transplant recipient. Trimethoprim/sulfamethoxazole has been shown to exhibit a synergistic renal toxicity with cyclosporin A. Erythromycin, frequently given in penicillin-allergic patients, is contraindicated because both cyclosporin and erythromycin are metabolized by the cytochrome P-450 system. Erythromycin competitively inhibits cyclosporin A metabolism with subsequent increase in the serum cyclosporin A level and consequent renal toxicity.[121, 122]

Azathioprine is a cytotoxic agent used for immunosuppression, which in large doses suppresses both antibody production and cell-mediated immunity.[117, 123, 124] Leukopenia is the most common side effect that predisposes the patient to opportunistic infection. As with all immunosuppressive agents, drug levels and their effects should be closely monitored. If the peripheral absolute polymorphonuclear count drops below 1000, the patient is at significant risk for septicemia, which may result in hematogenous seeding of prosthetic joints or other devitalized reconstructive materials, including large skeletal allografts used for limb salvage reconstruction. Septicemia may also target pathological tissue such as an arthritic joint or fracture. Most chemotherapy patients require an implanted venous access port (VAP). Externalized VAPs carry a much greater risk of infection than subcutaneous ports and are a common source of septicemia in immunocompromised hosts.

THE ELDERLY PATIENT

The U.S. population is living longer. Over the last century, the population older than 65 years increased from 4% to 12% but is projected to nearly double in the next 30 years.[125, 126] It has been estimated that, because of the increase in the aging population, hip fractures are expected to increase by 80% between 1990 and 2030.[127] The elderly patient has also been subdivided into two main groups: younger and older elderly.[128] The older elderly, older than 75 years, have more medical comorbidities as well as increased psychosocial issues. It has been well documented in the general medical and orthopaedic literature that elderly patients as a group are immunocompromised.[125, 126, 129–132] Alterations in both humoral and cell-mediated immunity render the elderly patient more susceptible to infectious disease. Infection is the fourth most common cause of death among the elderly.[129]

Aging affects both humoral and cell-mediated branches of the immune system. Deficiency in humoral immunity increases the risk of bacterial and viral infections, whereas cell-mediated immunity, which is the more severely affected, is associated with infectious diseases such as pathogenic opportunistic organisms (fungi, parasites, mycobacteria).[133, 134] The immune system regulatory mechanisms also decrease with age. Many factors that modulate T-cell function are produced in the thymus, where a dramatic decrease in activity occurs in patients older than 40 years. In patients older than 65 years, the factors responsible for cell maturation and differentiation are virtually undetectable. Elderly-onset impaired immunity is related more to qualitative than quantitative changes in the T cells. A terminal differentiation antigen, the "senescent cell antigen," appears on aging cells, and naïve T-cell function is reduced.[129]

Humoral immunity is not as significantly diminished as cell-mediated immunity. Studies demonstrated a decrease in serum IgA as well as IgG.[133] These humoral changes suggest that there may be impairment in the ability of B cells to mount an appropriate antibody response to an antigenic challenge. Neutrophil counts are usually within normal limits but show decreased migratory ability.[135] Phagocytosis remains intact, but the magnitude of the metabolic burst associated with its ability to consume debris is limited.

Other factors associated with aging may contribute to the immunocompromised state. One study demonstrated nutritional advice, and dietary supplements given for 8 weeks resulted in improved skin testing, increased T-cell numbers, and increased lymphocyte proliferation with associated improvement in albumin, prealbumin, transferrin, retinol-binding protein, zinc, and iron.[136] Dietary supplementation, including zinc, given to patients older than 70 years for 1 month increased the number of circulating T cells. Vitamin C (500 mg/day) for 1 month enhanced lymphocyte proliferation. Exercise has also been shown to improve the immune status of the elderly.[135] A multidisciplinary approach to the elderly patient, including a thorough medical evaluation, exercise program, nutritional supplementation, and counseling, will improve their immune competence and reduce the risk of infection after trauma and elective surgery.

OTHER DISEASES ASSOCIATED WITH IMMUNE IMPAIRMENT

Sickle cell disease (SCD) patients have a well-established high incidence of osteomyelitis and septic arthritis principally with *Salmonella* and *S. aureus*. The risk of prosthetic joint infection in this patient population is estimated at 20% based on multiple studies. The mechanisms of immune impairment include reduced serum opsonic activity and antibiotic response as well as functional asplenia, which eliminates one of the important defenses against bacteremia.[137–140]

Congenital hypogammaglobulinemia is a genetic disorder of B-cell maturation that impairs IgG production. A milder form of this condition referred to as common variable hypogammaglobulinemia is seen in adults. These patients are especially prone to *Mycoplasma* infections.[138, 141]

Diabetes mellitus patients have reduced resistance to infection, which is the result of hyperglycemia, peripheral vascular disease, and a variety of immune system impairments. Leukocytes have reduced glycolysis. Chemotaxis is reduced, phagocytosis is impaired, and intracellular killing is decreased.[142–146] All of these defects are lessened with prevention of hyperglycemia. Antibody production is normal, but there is evidence that cell-mediated immunity is reduced.[147, 148] In addition, local hypoxemia from small vessel disease reduces oxygen-dependent bactericidal activity and results in skin breakdown and delayed healing with secondary colonization and risk of local infection and bacteremia. The incidence of postoperative infection in the diabetic patient population is increased in some orthopaedic procedures. Simpson and coworkers[149] reviewed lumbar spine decompressions in 62 diabetics and 62 age- and sex-matched nondiabetic controls. Twenty-four percent of the diabetics had delayed wound healing and drainage. Ten percent had infection with positive cultures. There were no wound problems or infections in the control group.

Collagen vascular disease processes are a consequence of immune system regulatory aberrations. Immune suppression in these patients is a consequence of both the disease and its medical management. Rheumatoid arthritis and collagen vascular disease are associated with an increased incidence of septic arthritis and other postoperative infections. This may be the consequence of chronic joint inflammation with hyperemia and frequent subclinical bleeding. Some studies identified a reduction in phagocytosis in rheumatoid patients.[150] Systemic corticosteroids and antimetabolites further predispose these patients to infection. To date, no studies documented an increased risk of late infection of prosthetic joints in this patient population.

SURGICAL MANAGEMENT

THE HIV-POSITIVE PATIENT
Screening Tests
Based on current basic and clinical knowledge, a general philosophy or guideline may be developed for elective and emergent surgery in the HIV-positive patient in various stages of disease. All patients with risk factors for HIV infection should be tested on a voluntary basis, and in our experience no patient has refused to be tested on a confidential basis. Highly sensitive screening tests for HIV, available since 1985, are based on antibody to the virus. The principal screening test is the enzyme-linked immunosorbent assay (ELISA). If the initial ELISA is positive, it is repeated. If both are positive the result is confirmed with an immunoelectrophoresis or immunoblot procedure such as Western blot or immunofluorescence assay. Sensitivity and specificity for the ELISA alone are greater than 98% for HIV-1. Combining the ELISA and the Western blot, the false-positive rate is no more than 0.00006%.[151] Home collection kits for highly confidential testing are now available.[152] There is a window of infectivity between exposure and seroconversion that may extend for several months. Some investigators attempted to determine the applicability of PCR as a screening test to detect HIV during this period.[153] The PCR amplifies proviral DNA to make it detectable. However, the specificity of the HIV PCR is not high due to cross-reaction with other DNA contaminating the specimen. One study reported an average sensitivity of 99% but a specificity of 94.7%.[157] The CD4 lymphocyte count, although somewhat variable within the same individual, is an accepted method of determining the degree of immune system impairment.

Surgical Decision-Making
Most clinical studies available do not demonstrate an increased incidence of early postoperative complications in asymptomatic HIV-positive compared with HIV-negative patients. Furthermore, most of the orthopaedic studies and the more recent general surgery studies do not show an increased incidence of early complications in symptomatic HIV-positive patients with CD4 counts above 200 undergoing elective procedures. The risk of complications after emergent surgery is consistently higher in patients with AIDS but has improved dramatically with better antiretroviral therapy. As the disease progresses and these impairments increase, the hazard of early complications increases. The risk of late prosthetic implant infection, although not yet completely quantified, may be increased, especially in hemophiliacs and patients with advanced immune impairment. Implant infection with opportunistic organisms, although rare, has been reported. In view of all of these factors, special management of the HIV-positive patient undergoing surgery seems warranted.

Our Hemophilia Treatment Center uses a protocol that serves as the basis for the following recommendations. These recommendations will be useful only in patients who are aware of their HIV status. Patients living in high endemic areas, especially those with risk factors identified in their medical history or physical findings suggestive of HIV infection, should be encouraged to have an ELISA screen with appropriate consent.

If the procedure is elective, decision-making about the advisability of surgery is crucial. As a result of improved reverse transcriptase agents and protease inhibitors, high viral loads are treatable to undectable levels, often resulting in CD4 count elevation. The prognosis and life expectancy for patients with AIDS have improved, making reconstructive surgery in these patients a serious consideration (see Fig. 2). After a thorough assessment of the patient's medical status, a thoughtful discussion of the risk-benefit ratio should ensue. In patients with more advanced disease, quality of life issues are often a principal consideration, especially in the patient's view. This must be balanced against the risk of early and late complications. The spectrum of disease in HIV infection is a continuum, and no single clinical factor is a reliable predictor of longevity or risk of surgery. Several components should be combined in determining a prognosis and assigning risk. The factors that seem to correlate best with surgical outcome in published studies are history of opportunistic infection, CD4 cell level less than 200, serum albumin less than 2.5 g/dL, and cutaneous anergy. Viral load combined with CD4 counts has been shown to be the best prognostic indicator and is especially valuable in elective surgery risk-benefit analysis. Several hemophilia centers have used a CD4 count of 200 as a cutoff point for joint replacement.[34, 41, 154] Jury trials have tended to render plaintiff decisions in these instances. In high-risk situations in which the patient persists in wishing elective surgery, consultation should be obtained with the infectious disease or hematology service as well as with another orthopaedic surgeon, and an open dialogue should be maintained with the patient. In emergent situations, such as open tibial fractures, early wound débridement and thorough irrigation are highly desirable, but decisions regarding definitive internal fixation might best await medical evaluation and stabilization. In most cases, the patient's HIV status is unknown at the time of the emergent procedure.

Preparation for Surgery

Once a decision is made to proceed with surgery, several steps to further reduce the risk are applicable to an emergent situation, whereas others are only feasible in elective surgery. The absolute polymorphonuclear leukocyte count should exceed 1000 and the platelet count 30,000. Granulocyte-stimulating factor may be used to elevate an unacceptably low white blood cell count, and platelet transfusions may be used when needed but must be given immediately before or during surgery. All patients with advanced disease should be carefully screened for opportunistic infections and brought under control before elective procedures are performed.

Several drugs used to suppress HIV, such as ZVD, didanosine (DDI), and zalcitabine (DDC) cause various degrees of marrow suppression. However, reverse transcriptase inhibitors such as lamivudine (3TC) and stavudine (D4T) are less likely to do this. Many symptomatic HIV-positive patients are chronically anemic and require transfusion before surgery. When clinically appropriate, marrow-suppressing drugs should be stopped a few days preoperatively and

resumed after the first postoperative week. Prophylactic antibiotics are indicated. Some investigators suggested continuation of prophylactic antibiotics longer than normal in patients with advanced HIV infection, but there are no data to demonstrate efficacy of this practice.

Intraoperative and Postoperative Management

Attention to the usual antisepsis precautions during surgery is essential, because hematomas and wound necrosis in the immunocompromised patient are more likely to result in wound breakdown and infection than in the general population. The HIV-positive patient with a prosthetic implant may be at increased risk of late hematogenous implant infection as host defenses diminish. Regular medical attention, prophylactic antibiotics before dental work and any invasive procedures, and early evaluation and treatment of possible infections are especially important. Many patients will require long-term venous access. Subcutaneous ports are less likely to become infected than those with external, percutaneous catheters. Wastell and associates[155] reported a rate of infection with Hickman catheters of 0.65/100 days. Tanner and associates[156] found a rate of infection in Hickman catheters of 50% compared with 5% for implanted subcutaneous ports placed in the upper extremity. These should be avoided whenever possible in joint replacement patients. Hemophilia patients and others who self-administer intravenous medicines should be carefully instructed to use meticulous antisepsis precautions. Some clinicians have raised the issue of using chronic prophylactic antibiotics in symptomatic HIV-positive patients with a joint replacement. To date, no studies have demonstrated a reduction in the rate of late infection with chronic prophylactic antibiotics in symptomatic HIV-positive patients with a joint replacement. Long-term use of trimethoprim-sulfamethoxazole as prophylaxis against pneumocystis pneumonia may offer some protection against *S. aureus* infection of prosthetic joints.

SURGICAL MANAGEMENT OF OTHER IMMUNE DISORDERS

Patients with a medical history and physical findings indicative of any immune impairment require special preoperative evaluation. In emergency settings, this may be limited to the physical assessment of nutrition and peripheral blood analysis of leukocyte and platelet counts. If indicated, additional evaluation can be accomplished postoperatively. For the elective surgical candidate, further testing and medical consultation are appropriate and are, in part, specific to the cause of immune compromise. A careful search for possible sources of infection is essential preoperatively in the elective patient and postoperatively for emergencies. This includes dental, dermatologic, pulmonary, genitourinary, and gastrointestinal screening. Whenever possible, identified infections should be resolved before elective procedures.

Other key elements are patient education and patient reliability. Regular medical check-ups and prescribed medical regimens will often improve host immunity and reduce the risk of late hematogenous infection. Immunocompromised patients who are unreliable are poor candidates for elective joint replacement and other procedures requiring significant implanted hardware. Intraoperative measures to reduce the risk of infection in the immunocompromised host are simply an extension of usual methods. The risk of these complications may be reduced through extra care and attention to detail. Incisions should be carefully planned to avoid margin necrosis, because the skin of many immunocompromised patients is frail. All tissues should be handled very gently by avoiding the use of crushing instruments and excessive thermal injury from electrocautery. Elimination of dead space with closure and placement of drains

helps prevent hematomas and seromas, which may be a focus for hematogenous bacterial seeding and eventual enzymatic wound breakdown. Wound closure should be secure. Suture removal should be later than normal because healing is delayed in these patients. The surgical site should be protected and not subjected to early range of motion or vigorous physical therapy until the wound appears stable without excessive swelling, hematoma, or necrosis. The postoperative follow-up should be at closer intervals, especially for the patient with prosthetic joints or large amounts of implanted hardware.

REFERENCES

Human Immunodeficiency Virus

1. Ward WW, Drotman DP: Epidemiology of HIV and AIDS. In Wormser (ed): AIDS and Other Manifestations of HIV Infection. New York, JB Lippincott, 1997, p 1.
2. Centers for Disease Control and Prevention. HIV/AIDS surveillance report. 1999; 11:1.
3. Centers for Disease Control and Prevention: Guidelines for national immunodeficiency virus surveillance. MMWR Mor Mortal Wkly Rep CDC Surveill Summ 1999; 48:1.
4. Karon JM, Buehler JW, Byers RH, et al: Projections of the number of persons diagnosed with AIDS and the number of immunosuppressed HIV-infected persons-United States, 1992–1994. MMWR Mor Mortal Wkly Rep CDC Surveill Summ 1992; 41:1.
5. Ward JW, Janssen RS, Jaffe HW: Recommendations for HIV testing services for inpatients. MMWR Mor Mortal Wkly Rep CDC Surveill Summ 1993; 42:1.
6. AAOS Task Force on AIDS and Orthopaedic Surgery: Recommendations for the Prevention of Human Immunodeficiency Virus (HIV) Transmission in the Practice of Orthopaedic Surgery. Rosemont, IL, American Academy of Orthopaedic Surgeons, 1989.
7. Department of Labor Safety and Health Administration: Occupational exposure to bloodborne pathogens: Final rule. Fed Register 1991; 56:64004.
8. Centers for Disease Control and Prevention: HIV/AIDS Surveill Rep 1995; 7:21.
9. Centers for Disease Control and Prevention: Case-control study of HIV seroconversion in health-care workers after percutaneous exposure to HIV infected blood—France, United Kingdom, and United States, January 1988–August 1994. MMWR Mor Mortal Wkly Rep CDC Surveill Summ 1995; 44:929.
10. Chang HJ, Luck JV, Bell DM, et al: Transmission of human immunodeficiency virus infection in the surgical setting. J Am Acad Orthop Surg 1996; 4: 279.
11. Kjaersgaard-Andersen P, Christiansen SE, Ingerslev J, et al: Total knee arthroplasty in classic hemophilia. Clin Orthop 1990; 256:137.
12. Esterhai J: Threats to health-care workers from human immunodeficiency virus and

hepatitis B. In Frymoyer J (ed): Orthopaedic Knowledge Update 4. Rosemont, IL, American Academy of Orthopaedic Surgeons 1993, p 164.
13. Jellis JE: Orthopaedic surgery and HIV disease in Africa. Int Orthop 1996; 20: 253.
14. McGrath MS: HIV: Overview and general description. In Cohen PT, Sande MA, Volberding PA (eds): The AIDS Knowledge Base. Waltham, MA, Massachusetts Medical Society, 1990, p 1.
15. Hu DJ, Dondero TJ, Rayfield MA, et al: The emerging genetic diversity of HIV: The importance of global surveillance for diagnostics, research, and prevention. JAMA 1996; 275:210.
16. Grant IH, Armstrong D: Management of infectious complications in acquired immunodeficiency syndrome. Am J Med 1986; 81:59.
17. Ellis M, Gupta S, Galant S, et al: Impaired neutrophil function in patients with AIDS or AIDS-related complex: A comprehensive evaluation. J Infect Dis 1988; 158:1268.
18. Hambleton J: Hematologic complications of HIV infection. In Sande MA, Volberding PA (eds): The Medical Management of AIDS. Philadelphia, WB Saunders, 1997, p 239.
19. Burack JH, Mandel MS, Bizer LS: Emergency abdominal operations in the patient with acquired immunodeficiency syndrome. Arch Surg 1989; 124:285.
20. Diettrich NA, Cacioppo JC, et al: A growing spectrum of surgical disease in patients with human immunodeficiency virus/acquired immunodeficiency syndrome experience with 120 major cases. Arch Surg 1991; 126:860.
21. Barbul A, Damewood RB, Wasserkrug BA, et al: Fluid and mononuclear cells from healing wounds inhibit thymocyte immune responsiveness. J Surg Res 1983; 34:505.
22. Fishel RS, Barbul A, Beschorner WE, et al: Lymphocyte participation in wound healing. Morphologic assessment using monoclonal antibodies. Ann Surg 1987; 206:25.
23. Neilson EG, Phillips SM, Jimenez S: Lymphokine modulation of fibroblast proliferation. J Immunol 1982; 128:1484.
24. Fishel R, Barbul A, Wasserkrug HL, et al: Cyclosporine A impairs wound healing in rats. J Surg Res 1983; 34:572.
25. Schneider PA, Abrams DI, Rayner

AA, et al: Immunodeficiency associated thrombocytopenic purpura (IDTP) response to splenectomy. Arch Surg 1987; 122:1175.
26. Ravikumar TS, Allen JD, Bothe A Jr, et al: Splenectomy: The treatment of choice for human immunodeficiency virus related immune thrombocytopenia? Arch Surg 1989; 125:625.
27. Bordin JO, Blajchman MA: Immunosuppressive effects of allogeneic blood transfusions: Implications for the patient with a malignancy. Hematol Oncol Clin North Am 1995; 9:205.
28. Murphy PM, Lane HC, Fauci AS: Concise communications. J Infect Dis 1988; 158:627.
29. Ganesh R, Castle D, McGibbon D, et al: Staphylococcal carriage and HIV infection. Lancet 1989; 2:558.
30. Krumholtz HM, Sande MA, Lo B: Community-acquired bacteremia in patients with acquired immunodeficiency syndrome. Am J Med 1989; 86:776.
31. Wilson SE, Robinson G, Williams RA, et al: Acquired immune deficiency syndrome (AIDS) indications for abdominal surgery, pathology, and outcome. Ann Surg 1989; 210:428.
32. Robinson G, Wilson SE, Williams RA: Surgery in patients with acquired immunodeficiency syndrome. Arch Surg 1987; 122:170.
33. Greene WB, DeGnore LT, White GC: Orthopaedic procedures and prognosis in hemophilic patients who are seropositive for human immunodeficiency virus. J Bone Joint Surg Am 1990; 72:2.
33a. Buehrer JL, Weber RJ, Meyer AA, et al: Wound infection rates after invasive procedures in HIV-1 seropositive versus HIV-1 seronegative hemophiliacs. Ann Surg 1990; 211:492.
33b. Hoekman P, VandePerre P, Nelissen J, Kwisanga B, et al: Increased frequency of infection after open reduction of fractures in patients who are seropositive for human immunodeficiency virus. J Bone Joint Surg Am 1991; 73:675.
33c. Paiement GD, Hymes RA, LaDouceur MS, et al: Postoperative infections in asymptomatic HIV-seropositive orthopaedic trauma patients. J Trauma 1994; 37: 545.
34. Ragni MV, Crossett LS, Herndon JH: Postoperative infection following orthopaedic surgery in human immunodeficiency virus-infected hemophiliacs with

CD4 counts 200/mm³. J Arthroplasty 1995; 10:716.

35. Teeny S, Luck JV Jr, Sanders N, et al: Musculoskeletal sepsis in HIV positive hemophiliacs. Conference on Musculoskeletal Problems in Hemophiliacs, Nat'l Hemophilia Foundation, New York, NY, March 10, 1989.

36. Gilbert MS: Hemophilia: The role of the orthopedic surgeon in the era of HIV infection. Southeast Asian J Trop Med Public Health 1993; 24:30.

37. Goldberg VM, Heiple KG, Ratnoff OD, et al: Total knee arthroplasty in classic hemophilia. J Bone Joint Surg Am 1981; 63:695.

38. McCullough NC, Ennis JE, Lovitt J, et al: Synovectomy or total replacement of the knee in hemophilia. J Bone Joint Surg Am 1979; 61:69.

39. Luck JV, Kasper CK: Surgical management of advanced hemophilic arthropathy. Clin Orthop 1989; 242:60.

40. Unger AS, Kessler CM, Lewis RJ: Total knee arthroplasty in human immunodeficiency virus-infected hemophiliacs. J Arthroplasty 1995; 10:448.

41. Lehman C, Paiement GD: Infection after total joint arthroplasty in patients with human immunodeficiency virus or intravenous drug abuse. Presented at the annual meeting of the American Association of Orthopaedic Surgeons, Anaheim, CA, 1999.

42. Hawkins CC, Gold JW, Whimby E, et al: *Mycobacterium avium* complex infections in patients with the acquired immunodeficiency syndrome. Ann Intern Med 1985; 105:184.

43. McLaughlin JR, Tierney M, Harris WH: *Mycobacterium avium intracellulare* infection of hip arthroplasties in an AIDS patient. J Bone Joint Surg 1994; 76:498.

Hepatitis

44. Panlilio AL, Shapiro CN, Schable CA, et al: Serosurvey of human immunodeficiency virus, hepatitis B virus, and hepatitis C virus infection among hospital-based surgeons. J Am College Surg 1995; 180:16.

45. Maynard JE: Nosocomial viral hepatitis. Am J Med 1981; 70:439.

46. Kelen GD, Green GB, Purcell RH, et al: Hepatitis B and hepatitis C in emergency department patients. N Engl J Med 1992; 326:1399.

47. Bell DM, Shapiro CN, Culver DH, et al: Risk of hepatitis B and human immunodeficiency virus transmission to a patient from an infected surgeon due to percutaneous injury during an invasive procedure. Infect Agents Dis 1992; 1:263.

48. NIH Consensus Statement: National Institutes of Health Consensus Development Conference Panel Statement: Management of hepatitis C. Hepatology 1997; 26:2S.

49. Alter MJ: Epidemiology of hepatitis C. Hepatology 1997; 26:62S.

50. McQuillan G, Alter MJ, Moyer L, et al: A population based serologic study of hepatitis C virus infection in the United States [abstract]. Presented at the IX International Symposium on Viral Hepatitis and Liver Disease, Rome, 1996, p 8A.

51. Seeff LB: Natural history of hepatitis C. Hepatology 1997; 26:21S.

52. Tokars JI, Chamberland ME, Schable CA, et al: A survey of occupational blood content and HIV infection among orthopaedic surgeons. JAMA 1992; 268:489.

53. Nagaraju K, Naik SR, Naik S: Chronic hepatitis B carriers have low lymphoproliferative responses to HbsAg and reduced interleukin-2 synthesis. Indian J Gastroenterol 1998; 17:83.

54. Jolicoeur P, Lamontagne L: Impaired T and B cell subpopulations involved in a chronic disease induced by mouse hepatitis virus type 3. J Immunol 1994; 153:1318.

55. Battegay M, Moskophidis D, Waldner H, et al: Impairment and delay of neutralizing antiviral antibody responses by virus-specific cytotoxic T cells. J Immunol 1994; 152:1635.

56. Abdel F, Abdel K, El-Shawarby L, et al: Some immunological aspects of chronic liver disease in Egyptian children. J Egypt Soc Parasitol 1991; 21:343.

57. Caregaro L, Alberino F, Amodid P, et al: Malnutrition in alcoholic and virus-related cirrhosis. Am J Clin Nutr 1996; 63:602.

58. De Noronha R, Taylor BA, Wild G, et al: Inter-relationships between platelet count, platelet IgG, serum IgG, immune complexes and severity of liver disease. Clin Lab Hematol 1991; 13:127.

Alcoholism

59. Elvy GA, Gillespie WJ: Problem drinking in orthopaedic patients. J Bone Joint Surg Br 1985; 67:478.

60. Beresford T, Low D, Adduci R, et al: Alcoholism assessment on an orthopaedic surgery service. J Bone Joint Surg Am 1982; 64:730.

61. Rush B: An inquiry into the effects of ardent spirits upon the human body and mind with an account of the means of preventing and of the remedies for curing them. Q J Stud Alcohol 1943; 4:321.

62. Liu YK: Effects of alcohol on granulocytes and lymphocytes. Semin Hematol 1980; 17:130.

63. McFarland W, Libre EP: Abnormal leukocyte response in alcoholism. Ann Intern Med 1963; 59:865.

64. MacGregor RR: Alcohol and immune defense. JAMA 1986; 256:1474.

65. MacGregor RR, Gluckman SG, Senior JR: Granulocyte function and levels of immunoglobulins and complement in patients admitted for withdrawal from alcohol. J Infect Dis 1978; 138:747.

66. MacGregor RR, Gluckman SG: Effect of acute alcohol intoxication on granulocyte mobilization and kinetics. Blood 1979; 52:551.

67. Edmondson HA: Pathology of alcoholism. Am J Clin Pathol 1980; 74:725.

68. Tennenbaum JI, Leevy CM, St. Pierre RL, et al: The effects of chronic alcohol administration on the immune responsiveness of rats. J Allergy 1969; 44:272.

69. Perkoff GT: Alcoholic myopathy. Ann Rev Med 1971; 22:125.

70. DiSilvio TV: Alcoholic myopathy and changes in serum enzyme activity. Clin Chem 1978; 24:1653.

71. Mitchell DG, Steinber ME, Dalinka MK, et al: Magnetic resonance imaging of the ischemic hip. Alterations within the osteonecrotic, viable, and reactive zones. Clin Orthop 1989; 244:60.

72. Henrigou P, Beaujean F: Abnormalities in the bone marrow of the iliac crest in patients who have osteonecrosis secondary to corticosteroid therapy or alcohol abuse. J Bone Joint Surg Am 1997; 79:1047.

73. Oppenheim WL: The "battered alcoholic syndrome." J Trauma 1977; 17:850.

74. Nilsson BE, Westlin NE: Changes in bone mass in alcoholics. Clin Orthop 1973; 90:229.

75. Alffram PA: An epidemiologic study of cervical and trochanteric fractures of the femur in an urban population. Acta Orthop Scand 1964; 65:9.

76. Saville PD: Changes in bone mass with age and alcoholism. J Bone Joint Surg 1967; 37:492.

77. Kalbfleisch JM, Lindeman RD, Ginn HE, et al: Effect of ethanol administration on urinary excretion of magnesium and other electrolytes in alcoholic and normal subjects. J Clin Invest 1963; 42:1471.

78. Santisteban GA, Swiniard CA: The effect of ethyl-alcohol on adrenal cortex activity in mice. Endocrinology 1956; 59:391.

79. Johnell O, Nilsson BE, Wiklund PE: Bone morphometry in alcoholics. Clin Orthop 1982; 165:253.

80. Dalen N, Feldreich AL: Osteopenia in alcoholism. Clin Orthop 1974; 99:201.

81. Tonnesen H, Rosenberg J, Nielsen HJ, et al: Effect of preoperative abstinence on poor postoperative outcome in alcohol misusers: Randomised controlled trial. Bone Miner J 1999; 318:1311.

Malnutrition

82. Hu SS, Fontaine F, Kelly B, et al: Nutritional depletion in staged spinal reconstructive surgery. Spine 1998; 23:1401.

83. Dickhaut SC, DeLee JC, Page CP: Nutritional status: Importance in predicting wound-healing after amputation. J Bone Joint Surg Am 1984; 66:71.

84. Hill GL, Pickford I, Blackett RL, et al: Malnutrition in surgical patients: An unrecognised problem. Lancet 1977; 1:689.

85. Bistrian BR, Blackburn GL, Hallowell E, et al: Protein status of general surgical patients. JAMA 1974; 230:858.

86. Bollet AJ, Owens S: Evaluation of nutritional status of selected hospitalized patients. Am J Clin Nutr 1973; 26:931.

87. Dudrick SJ, Duke JH: Nutritional complications in the surgical patient. In Artz CP, Hardy JD (eds): Management of Surgical Complications. Philadelphia, WB Saunders, 1975, 3rd ed, p 243.

88. Hill GL, Blackett RL, Pickford I, et al:

Malnutrition in surgical patients. An unrecognised problem. Lancet 1977; 1: 689.

89. Willard GD, Gilsdorf RB, Price TA: Protein-calorie malnutrition in a community hospital. JAMA 1980; 243:1720.

90. Dudrick SJ, Jensen TG, Rowlands BJ: Nutritional support: Assessment and indications. In Deitel M (ed): Nutrition in Clinical Surgery. Baltimore, Williams & Wilkins, 1980.

91. Jensen JE, Jensen TG, Smith TK, et al: Nutrition and orthopaedic surgery. J Bone Joint Surg Am 1982; 64:1263.

92. Kinney JM: Energy requirements of the surgical patients. In Ballinger WF, Collins JA, Drucker WR, et al (eds): Manual of Surgical Nutrition. Philadelphia, WB Saunders, 1975, p 223.

93. Dreblow DM, Anderson CF, Moxness K: Nutritional assessment of orthopedic patients. Mayo Clin Proc 1981; 56:51.

94. Shetty PS, Jung RT, Watrasiewicz KE, et al: Rapid turnover transport proteins: An index of subclinical protein energy malnutrition. Lancet 1979; 2:230.

95. Bistrian BR, Blackburn GL, Hallowell E, et al: Protein status of general surgical patients. JAMA 1974; 230:858.

96. Bistrian BR, Blackburn GL, Vitale J, et al: Prevalence of malnutrition in general medical patients. JAMA 1976; 235: 1567.

97. Copeland EM, MacFadyen BV, Dudrick SJ: Effect of intravenous hyperalimentation on established delayed hypersensitivity in the cancer patient. Ann Surg 1976; 184:60.

98. Law DK, Dudrick SJ, Abdou NI: The effects of protein calorie malnutrition on immune competence of the surgical patient. Surg Gynecol Obstet 1974; 139: 257.

99. Blackburn GL, Bistrian BR, Maini BS, et al: Nutritional and metabolic assessment of the hospitalized patient. J Parent Enteral Nutr 1977; 1:11.

100. Koval KJ, Maurer SG, Su ET, et al: The effects of nutritional status on outcome after hip fracture. J Orthop Trauma 1999; 13:164.

101. Mandelbaum BR, Tolo VT, McAfee PC, et al: Nutritional deficiencies after staged anterior and posterior spinal reconstructive surgery. Clin Orthop Res 1987; 234: 5.

102. Kay SP, Moreland JR, Schmitter E: Nutritional status and wound healing in lower extremity amputations. Clin Orthop 1987; 217:253.

103. Puskarich CL, Nelson CL, Nusbickel FR, et al: The use of two nutritional indicators in identifying long bone fracture patients who do and do not develop infection. J Orthop Res 1990; 8:799.

The Post-Transplant Patient

104. Bhatia DS, Bowen JC, Money SR, et al: The incidence, morbidity, and mortality of surgical procedures after orthotopic heart transplantation. Ann Surg 1997; 225:686.

105. Elmstedt E, Svahn T: Skeletal complica-

tions following renal transplantation. Acta Orthop Scand 1981; 52:279.

106. Rubin RH: Infection in the organ transplant recipient. In Rubin RH, Young LS (eds): Clinical Approach to Infection in the Compromised Host. New York, Plenum, 1994, 3rd ed, p 629.

107. Winston DJ, Emmanouilides C, Busuttil RW: Infections in liver transplant recipients. Clin Infect Dis 1995; 21:1077.

108. Rubin RH: Infectious disease complications of renal transplantation. Kidney Int 1993; 44:221.

109. Fishman JA, Rubin RH: Infection in organ transplant recipients. N Engl J Med 1998; 338:1741.

110. Tannenbaum TA, Matthews LS, Grady-Benson JC: Infection around joint replacements in patients who have a renal or liver transplantation. J Bone Joint Surg Am 1997; 79:36.

111. Hunt SA: Current status of cardiac transplantation. JAMA 1998; 280:1692.

112. Stein JP, Skinner EC, Freeman JA, et al: Radical cystectomy and lower urinary tract reconstruction after cardiac allograft transplantation. J Urol 1995; 153:415.

113. Cianio G, Antun RA, Norberg DG, et al: Prostate cancer after heart transplantation. J Urol 1995; 153:158.

Pharmacological Immune Suppression

114. Bowen DL, Fauci AS: Adrenal corticosteroids. In Gallin JI, Goldstein I, Snyerman R (eds): Inflammation: Basic Principles and Clinical Correlates. New York, Raven Press, 1988, p 877.

115. Dale DC, Fauci AS, Guerry D, et al: Comparison of agents producing a neutrophilic leukocytosis in man. Hydrocortisone, prednisone, endotoxin, and etiocholanolone. J Clin Invest 1975; 56:808.

116. Butler WT, Rossen RD: Effects of corticosteroids on immunity in man: I. Decreased serum IgG concentration caused by 3–5 days of high doses of methylprednisolone. J Clin Invest 1973; 52: 2629.

117. Atkinson JP, Frank MM: Complement-independent clearance of IgG-sensitized erythrocytes: Inhibition by cortisone. Blood 1974; 44:629.

118. Fauci AS: Alternate-day corticosteroid therapy. Am J Med 1978; 64:729.

119. Tannenbaum DA, Matthews LS, Grady-Benson JC: Infection around joint replacements in patients who have a renal or liver transplantation. J Bone Joint Surg Am 1997; 79:36.

120. Segal BH, Sneller MC: Infectious complications of immunosuppressive therapy in patients with rheumatic diseases. Rheum Dis Clin North Am 1997; 23:219.

121. Myers BD, Ross J, Newton L, et al: Cyclosporin-associated chronic nephropathy. N Engl J Med 1984; 311:699.

122. Amacher DE, Schomaker SJ, Retsema JA: Comparison of the effects of the new azalide antibiotic, azithromycin, and erythromycin estolate on rat liver cytochrome P-450. Antimicrob Agents Chemother 1991; 36:1186.

123. Schumacher HR (ed): Primer on the Rheumatic Diseases. Atlanta, GA, Arthritis Foundation, 1988, 9th ed, p 288.

124. Austin HA, Klippel JH, Balow JE, et al: Therapy of lupus nephritis: Controlled trial of prednisone and cytotoxic drugs. N Engl J Med 1986; 314:614.

The Elderly Patient

125. Ershler WB, Longo DL: The Biology of Aging: The Current Research Agenda. Cancer 1997; 80:1284.

126. Gilbert RS, Strauss E, Gilbert MS: Infection in the aged: Septic arthritis. Arch Am Assoc Orthop Surg 1998; 2:74.

127. Perron VD, Robinson BE: The aging process and functional assessment. Archives Am Assoc Orthop Surg 1998; 2:74.

128. Levy RN, Rowe JW: Editorial. Clin Orthop 1995; 316:2.

129. Chandra RK: The relation between immunology, nutrition and disease in elderly people. Age Aging 1990; 19:25.

130. Norman DC, Toledo SD: Infections in elderly persons: An altered clinical presentation. Clin Geriatr Med 1992; 8:713.

131. Yoshikawa TT: Approach to the diagnosis and treatment of the infected older adult. In Hazzard WR, Bierman EL, Blass JP, et al (eds): Principles of Geriatric Medicine and Gerontology. New York, McGraw-Hill, 1994, 3rd ed, p 1157.

132. Fox RA (ed): Immunology and Infection in the Elderly. Edinburgh, Churchill Livingstone, 1984, p 289.

133. Chandra RK (ed): Nutrition, Immunity, and Illness in the Elderly. New York, Pergamon, 1985.

134. Banks DA, Fossel M: Telomeres, cancer, and aging: Altering the human life span. Cancer Aging 1997; 278:1345.

135. Burr ML, Milbank JE, Gibbs D: The nutritional status of the elderly. Age Aging 1982; 11:89.

136. Patterson BM, Cornell CN, Carbone B, et al: Protein depletion and metabolic stress in elderly patients who have a fracture of the hip. J Bone Joint Surg Am 1992; 74: 251.

Other Diseases

137. Ebong WW: Septic arthritis in patients with sickle-cell disease. Br J Rheumatol 1987; 26:99.

138. Brennan PJ, Pia DeGirolamo M: Musculoskeletal infections in immunocompromised hosts. Orthop Clin North Am 1991; 22:389.

139. Acurio MT, Friedman RJ: Hip arthroplasty in patients with sickle-cell hemoglobinopathy. J Bone Joint Surg Br 1992; 74:367.

140. Hanker GJ, Amstutz HC: Osteonecrosis of the hip in the sickle-cell diseases. J Bone Joint Surg Am 1988; 70:499.

141. Johnston CLW, Webster ADB, Taylor-Robinson D, et al: Primary late onset hypogammaglobulinemia associated with inflammatory polyarthritis and septic arthritis due to *Mycoplasma pneumoniae*. Ann Rheum Dis 1983; 42:108.

142. Rayfield EJ, Ault MJ, Keusch GT, et al: Infection and diabetes: The case for glucose control. Am J Med 1982; 72:439.

143. Sbarra AJ, Karnovsky ML: The biochemical basis of phagocytosis: 1. Metabolic changes during the ingestion of particles by polymorphonuclear leukocytes. J Biol Chem 1959; 234:1355.

144. Perille PE, Nolan JP, Finch SC: Studies of the resistance to infection in diabetes mellitus: Local exudative cellular response. J Lab Clin Med 1962; 59:1008.

145. Brayton RG, Stokes PE, Schwartz MS: Effect of alcohol and various diseases on leukocyte mobilization phagocytosis and intracellular bacterial killing. N Engl J Med 1970; 282:123.

146. Bagdade JD, Root RK, Bulger RJ: Impaired leukocyte function in patients with poorly controlled diabetes. Diabetes 1974; 23:9.

147. MacCuish AC, Urbaniac SJ, Campbell CJ: Phytohemagglutinin transformation and circulating lymphocyte subpopulation in insulin-dependent diabetic patients. Diabetes 1974; 23:708.

148. Casey JI, Heeter BJ, Klyahevich KA: Impaired response of lymphocytes of diabetic subjects to antigen of *Staphylococcus aureus.* J Infect Dis 1977; 136:495.

149. Simpson JM, Silveri CP, Balderston RA, et al: The results of operations on the lumbar spine in patients who have diabetes mellitus. J Bone Joint Surg Am 1993; 75:1823.

150. Brennan PJ, De Girolamo MP: Musculoskeletal infections in immunocompromised hosts. Orthop Clin North Am 1991; 22:389.

Surgical Management

151. Wilber JC: HIV antibody testing: Methodology. In Cohen PT, Sande MA, Volberding PA (eds): The AIDS Knowledge Base. Waltham, MA, Massachusetts Medical Society, 1990, p 1.

152. Tao G, Kassler WJ, Branson BM, et al: Home collection kits for HIV testing: Evaluation of three strategies for dealing with insufficient dried blood specimens. J Acquired Immune Defic Syndr 1997; 15: 312.

153. Essary LR, Kinard SJ, Butcher A, et al: Screening potential corneal donors for HIV-1 by polymerase chain reaction and a colorimetric microwell hybridization assay. Am J Ophthalmol 1996; 122:526.

154. Luck JV, Hansjaj KK, Dorey FJ, et al: Risk factors for late infection in hemophiliacs with total hip and knee arthroplasties. Presented at the meeting of the American Academy of Orthopaedic Surgeons, New Orleans, 1994.

155. Wastell C, Corless D, Keeling N: Surgery and human immunodeficiency virus-1 infection. Am J Surg 1996; 172:89.

156. Tanner AG, Skinner CJ, McBride MO: A prospective comparative study between externally sited (Hickman), chest implanted (Port-O-Cath), and arm implanted (PASport) for long term venous access in AIDS patients. Int Conf AIDS 1994;10: 219.

157. Kenten JH, Casadei J, Link J, et al: Rapid electrochemiluminescence assays of polymerase chain reaction products. Clin Chem 1991; 37:1626.

ARTHRITIDES
ARTHROPATHIES

RAJ K. SINHA AND HARRY E. RUBASH

OVERVIEW OF ARTHRITIS

Michael H. Huo and Omer A. Ilahi

Summary
- The care of arthritic conditions costs more than $65 billion annually.
- A multispecialty team approach is required to treat arthritis patients effectively pre- and postoperatively.
- Inflammatory arthritides present special challenges to the orthopaedic surgeon.

Rheumatic and arthritic diseases have been recognized as clinically relevant entities since ancient Greece. Gout was first described in the 1600s in the medical literature. Major advances in diagnosing various rheumatic diseases occurred in the 19th century, with publications describing rheumatoid arthritis (RA), osteoarthritis (OA), juvenile chronic polyarthritis, ankylosing spondylitis, lupus erythematosus, and many others.

Treatment of these arthritic conditions has evolved over the past century. Currently, clinicians and researchers continue to investigate and institute exciting medical, rehabilitative, and surgical treatment protocols in the management of these conditions. This chapter serves as an introduction to the following chapters in this section of the textbook. We focus on several general issues in arthritis and address social and economic impact, rehabilitation, and surgical principles.

SOCIAL AND ECONOMIC IMPACT

Arthritic diseases are characterized by chronic pain, deformity, and progressive physical and psychological disability. These issues affect not only the patients but also the families and society at large. Clinicians must understand some of these issues to best manage the patient's overall needs.

These disease entities generally cause physical dysfunction, possibly leading to social dysfunction. Physical impairments can easily affect functions of daily living, such as mobility, ambulation, stair climbing, dressing, hygiene care, cooking, eating, and so on. In addition, decreased physical capabilities will result in decreased productivity at work and increased loss of work time. Moreover, the impact of these physical impairments can result in psychological distress such as depression. Clinicians often overlook the potential impact of arthritis on the rest of the family. The caregivers may have to alter their own lifestyle and work schedule to provide care. Marriages can be faced with significant challenges in regard to financial burden, sexual problems, and care of children. Adjustment to some of these challenges is even more difficult for children with chronic arthritis conditions.

The economic impact of any disease entity can be divided into two broad components: direct costs and indirect costs. Direct costs include those dollars spent to treat the disease, whereas indirect costs represent the financial impact secondary to loss of productivity and wages. It has been estimated that the overall total costs of all musculoskeletal conditions, excluding fracture care, approximated $65 billion in 1992. Direct costs accounted for only 25% of the total, whereas indirect costs accounted for 75%. Additionally, the costs for osteoporosis and related fracture care totaled more than $10 billion.[1]

Surgical procedures for musculoskeletal conditions accounted for nearly 10% of the 37 million operations performed in the United States in 1985. It was estimated that more than 250,000 hip and knee replacement surgeries were performed that year for arthritic conditions and for fractures in selected cases. The direct costs of joint replacement surgeries were more than $4 billion and approached nearly 25% of the overall direct costs for all musculoskeletal conditions.[2]

The most significant factor contributing to the large indirect costs of care for arthritic conditions is work disability. One of the conditions that have been extensively studied is RA. It has been reported that fewer than 50% of the patients with RA remain gainfully employed 10 years after diagnosis.[3] Both functional status and clinical disease severity have been demonstrated to be reliable predictors of work disability.[4] It is prudent for the clinician to be aware of the patient's clinical, psychological, and functional parameters early in the disease course to be best able to advise the patient on how to remain productive most effectively.

In addition to the staggering overall costs of caring for arthritic conditions, financial impact directly on the patients themselves has been calculated and reported for some specific disease entities. It has been reported that the mean direct costs per capita for an OA patient was $2043 compared with $1591 for the nonarthritic cohort. The difference was considerably more when the indirect costs were included. On average, 10% of OA patients reduced work hours and 14% retired early. This was in contrast to 1.7% and 3.4% of nonarthritic patients, respectively.[5] In another study, RA patients experienced a 50% decrease in earnings over a 9-year period. Additionally, the contribution to overall family income from their earnings decreased from 69% to 32% in this period, thus placing increased hardship on the family and spouses.[6] The disability and deteriorating earning potential for the majority of these patients continue to escalate with prolonged duration and progression of the disease process.

REHABILITATION

Rehabilitation of arthritic conditions should be functionally oriented rather than disease oriented for rheumatology care. There are four key elements in arthritis rehabilitation: (1) realistic goals should be defined based on measurable functional deficits and potential for improvement; (2) realistic patient expectations should be outlined based on pa-

807

tient education; (3) preventive measures should be instituted to maintain maximal functional capacity and minimize deterioration with disease progression; (4) enhancement and supplementation become necessary when prevention has failed. The most critical element is patient education, which would allow the patients themselves to achieve voluntary adaptation of behaviors and beliefs conducive to improved health and functional status. The spectrum of patient education should focus on medical knowledge, communication abilities, psychosocial adjustments, vocational and recreational adaptations, and financial counseling.

Rehabilitation of arthritic patients must take the form of an interdisciplinary approach that enhances communication, cooperation, and coordination of all patient needs. The team generally consists of a rehabilitation physician, clinical nurse coordinator, physical and occupational therapists, recreational therapist, social worker, vocational counselor, and psychiatric counselor. The contributing role of each member should be clearly defined. Team case management meetings must be held regularly. The designed program must be modified as patient needs change over time.

A variety of psychosocial factors may influence the health status of arthritis patients. The clinician must be aware of these issues to formulate the best therapeutic program both medically and rehabilitatively for these patients. Depression in particular is common. It has been reported that the frequency of depression was as high as 33% for patients with OA of the hips and knees, 37% for RA patients, and nearly 50% for those with fibromyalgia.[7] The relationship between depression and perception of pain, disability, and loss of valued activities is independent of disease activity itself. Given the relationship between health status and psychosocial factors, great effort has been devoted to testing psychosocial interventions that may improve patients' pain, emotional states, and function. It is hoped that these improvements will be reflected in reduced health care utilization and costs.

SURGICAL MANAGEMENT

The end results of various entities of arthritis are relatively similar in regard to joint destruction. They lead to pain and loss of function. Surgery may be indicated to reconstruct the joint and surrounding structures to relieve pain and improve function. In some selected situations, surgery may be indicated to prevent these consequences.

Two important principles must be observed and followed by the surgeon who treats patients with arthritic conditions, especially those with multiple joint involvement such as in RA. First, the surgeon should be familiar with the different disease entities, anatomic alterations, and associated technical challenges, which are different for patients with OA. Second, the surgeon should be part of a multispecialty team, including rheumatologists, nurses, therapists, social workers, and, most importantly, the patient. The patient must be involved as a part of the surgical planning, sequence of reconstructive surgeries, and rehabilitation protocols. This involvement generally allows the patient to be educated, to feel a sense of control and participation, and, most importantly, to have realistic expectations regarding surgery outcome.

PREOPERATIVE PLANNING

Nonsurgical treatments should be optimized before considering surgical options. Bracing, walking aids, therapy, injections, and maximizing pharmacological therapies should all be implemented. If these measures have failed and the patient's functional parameters deteriorate, arthroplasty or arthrodesis is then indicated. General medical issues such as cardiopulmonary status, carious teeth, urinary tract infection or incontinence, prostatic hypertrophy, and airway problems should be evaluated. One factor that is difficult to evaluate objectively before surgery is the patient's motivation and ability to participate sufficiently in the rehabilitation program after surgery. Patient education and involvement with the multispecialty team are invaluable.

Patients with systemic inflammatory arthritis are susceptible to infection. The dose of medications that may adversely affect the immune system, such as corticosteroids and methotrexate, should be kept to a minimum. Skin lesions in psoriatic arthritis patients should be cleared up as much as possible before surgery. Many patients are also chronically anemic, which makes preoperative autologous blood donation difficult. Selective use of erythropoietin may be indicated in certain clinical settings.

In addition to the systemic problems presented by patients with inflammatory arthritis, the involvement of multiple joints requires special considerations. The ability to use crutches or a walker must be assessed before surgery. On occasion, it may even be necessary to perform reconstructive surgery such as shoulder or elbow arthroplasty or wrist arthrodesis to fulfill the prerequisites that the patient be able to use walking aids to assist with the rehabilitation program after surgery of the lower extremities. Painful foot deformities may require orthoses or surgical correction before arthroplasty of the hips and knees. Associated problems of the lumbosacral spine should be identified and addressed with therapy, medications, or surgery. The cervical spine is significantly involved in 30% to 40% of the patients with RA.[8] Preoperative evaluation with flexion-extension radiographs is standard protocol because the majority of these patients are asymptomatic.

PERIOPERATIVE AND POSTOPERATIVE CARE

The bone quality and soft-tissue integrity may be compromised in patients with inflammatory arthritis. These changes may pose technical challenges to the surgeon. Selection of implants and choice of fixation must be based on the same principles as for patients with OA: fit of prostheses, stability of fixation, restoration of anatomic offset, balance of ligaments, equalization of leg lengths, and preservation of bone stock. Cementless fixation can be as durable as cemented fixation in performing hip arthroplasty in patients with inflammatory arthritis. It is not routinely necessary to use more constrained implants in knee arthroplasty to balance the ligaments. Resurfacing of the patella, however, is generally recommended in patients with inflammatory arthritis.[9]

Rehabilitation after surgery is of critical importance. The duration of supervised therapy should be determined by the patient's progress in reaching rehabilitation goals. It may be necessary to use orthotic devices in patients with multiple joint involvement resulting from inflammatory arthritis.

Proper patient education is critical to ensure complete understanding of the limitations and exercise routines after arthroplasty as well as active participation in the rehabilitation program. It is necessary to educate the patient not only to protect and use the operated joint properly but also to protect the unoperated joints. Finally, routine follow-up is necessary for the surgeon to determine the progress of improvements after surgery, to obtain objective measures of outcome and, most importantly, to recognize both early and late complications.

ANESTHETIC CONSIDERATIONS

Patients with severe rheumatic diseases may pose special, important challenges for anesthetic management during surgery. The patients often have severe deformities, chronic illness, poor nutrition, associated alterations of the airway anatomy or pulmonary functions, and comorbid conditions.[10] There are generally four areas of difficulties:

1. Airway and oral cavity deformities may prevent intubation by orotracheal or nasotracheal techniques.
2. On occasion, even bronchoscopy-assisted techniques may be difficult.
3. Manipulation of the cervical spine may risk neurological deficit in patients with an unstable cervical spine or cervical myelopathy from the primary disease process.
4. Laryngeal edema may increase the risk of airway obstruction after extubation.

It is, therefore, appropriate to use regional anesthesia when possible. Regional techniques are practical for the majority of extremity surgeries. However, general anesthesia is necessary for most spinal procedures. All patients should undergo evaluation of potential airway difficulties before surgery regardless of whether regional or general technique is planned.

Spinal or epidural anesthesia may not be practical in patients with ankylosing spondylitis because of fusion of the spinal column. Interscalene block may be applied for upper extremity surgeries, although it may compromise inspiratory function because the block may result in unilateral temporary paralysis of the diaphragm. Thus, intubation using bronchoscopy-assisted technique with the patient awake is preferred.

Postoperative analgesia management should be no different from that for patients without inflammatory arthritis. It is, however, necessary to have a heightened awareness of potential adverse effects on the pulmonary function of these patients, because access to the airway is generally difficult.

CONCLUSION

Care for patients with arthritis is a major part of the clinical practice of all orthopaedic surgeons. It is necessary for the surgeon to appreciate not only the medical and surgical issues but also the psychological and financial implications in the care of these patients. The surgical care of these patients will undoubtedly continue to improve with newer implants and techniques. A successful outcome is not dependent exclusively on the surgery. The surgeon must work closely with a multispecialty team to address all patient needs before and after reconstructive surgery.

REFERENCES

1. Yelin E, Callaghan LE: The economic cost and social and psychological impact of musculoskeletal conditions. Arthritis Rheum 1995; 38:1351.
2. Felts W, Yelin E: The economic impact of the rheumatic diseases in the United States. J Rheumatol 1989; 16:867.
3. Pincus T, Callaghan LF: What is the natural history of rheumatoid arthritis? Rheum Dis Clin North Am 1993; 119:123.
4. Reisine S, McQuillan J, Fifield J: Predictors of work disability in rheumatoid arthritis patients. Arthritis Rheum 1995; 38:1630.
5. Gabriel SE, Crowson CS, O'Fallon WM: Cost of osteoarthritis: Estimates from a geographically defined population. J Rheumatol 1995; 22:23.
6. Meenan RF, Yelin EG, Nevitt M, et al: The impact of chronic disease. Arthritis Rheum 1981; 24:544.
7. Hawley DJ, Wolfe F: Depression is not more common in rheumatoid arthritis: A 10-year longitudinal study of 6,153 patients with rheumatic disease. J Rheumatol 1993; 20:2025.
8. Boden SD, Dodge LD, Bohlman HH, et al: Rheumatoid arthritis of the cervical spine: A long-term analysis with predictors of paralysis and recovery. J Bone Joint Surg Am 1993; 75:1282.
9. Boyd AD Jr, Ewald FC, Thomas WH, et al: Long-term complications after total knee arthroplasty with or without resurfacing of the patella. J Bone Joint Surg Am 1993; 75:674.
10. Sharrock NE: Anesthetic considerations. In Kelley WN, Harris Jr ED, Ruddy S, et al (eds): Textbook of Rheumatology, 5th ed, Philadelphia, WB Saunders, p 1640.

OSTEOARTHRITIS

P. John Kumar and Gerald Levy

Summary
- Osteoarthritis is the second leading cause of disability in the United States.
- The estimated cost to treat arthritis in the United States is over 60 billion dollars per year.
- The incidence increases with increasing age.
- The natural history of the disease is variable.
- Treatment is based on the location of the disease, severity of symptoms, and degree of disability.

DEFINITION

Osteoarthritis (OA) is a disease entity characterized by pain, stiffness, and swelling of the joints. The etiology is multifactorial and poorly understood. It is the most common form of arthritis and can usually be distinguished from inflammatory arthritides based on the clinical and radiological pattern of appearance, negative results of serological testing, and the absence of involvement of other organ systems. Other terms previously used to describe osteoarthritis include degenerative arthritis and hypertrophic arthritis.

HISTORICAL REVIEW

1899: Aspirin first used for treatment.
1900: Distinguished from inflammatory arthritis based on radiographs.
1960s: Charnley total hip developed and used successfully.
1970s: Use of ibuprofen for treatment.
1973: Total condylar knee replacement developed and used successfully.
1980s: Arthroscopy used to diagnose and treat early cases.

EPIDEMIOLOGY

The prevalence of symptomatic OA is estimated to be 12% of the U.S. population or approximately 20 million people.[1, 2] It is second to chronic heart disease in adults requiring Social Security disability payments. Although OA has been demonstrated in individuals in their second decade, the prevalence increases with age and increases exponentially after the age of 50. Reported radiographic prevalence rates are 20% for the knee in women older than 65 years of age and 70% for the hand in patients older than 65 years of age.[3, 4] The best study of incidence rates was the Framingham study. The incidence rate of symptomatic knee arthritis was 1% per year in patients older than 60 years with no prior history of disease, with a progression to symptomatic OA in patients with baseline radiographic OA of 4% per year.[5] The sex distribution of OA varies by

anatomic location. OA of the hip shows an equal distribution by gender. Disease in the knees or hands is more commonly seen in women.[3-5] Women have a greater tendency to form Heberden's and Bouchard's nodes.[6] There is evidence to suggest that OA may have a hereditary component. One manifestation of this hereditary influence is the familial tendency toward developmental dysplasia of the hip (DDH).

PATHOGENESIS

ETIOLOGY

The causes of OA are multifactorial and not fully understood. If an underlying cause can be identified, the patient is considered to have secondary OA. In patients in whom the cause is unknown, the OA is classified as idiopathic. Factors leading to OA include the following:

1. An excess load on the joint leading to tissue failure, such as occurs with trauma or repetitive impact sports. A loss of the normal protective reflexes can lead to severe changes, such as seen in the Charcot joint.
2. Altered bone or cartilage physiology or biochemistry, leading to failure, such as occurs with aging or in many disorders with secondary OA, such as Ehlers-Danlos syndrome, calcium pyrophosphate deposition disease (CPPD), or the mucopolysaccharidoses. Table 1 gives a classification of OA.[7]

PATHOLOGY

In the initial phase of the disease process, the cartilage layer is thicker than normal. Increased water content is found, which leads to increased proteoglycan synthesis. This results in increased proteoglycan concentration. As the disease progresses, the cartilage surface thins unevenly. The surface will usually thin most in the areas of maximum load, whereas other areas may appear normal (Fig. 1). The proteoglycan content decreases, surface integrity is lost, vertical clefts appear, and subchondral bone is exposed. Initially, the chondrocytes replicate in OA, increasing the cellularity of the cartilage. Later on, the tissue becomes hypocellular. The bony response to disease progression includes appositional bone growth in the subchondral region (sclerosis), the appearance of bony cysts due to microfractures, and peripheral osteophyte formation with subsequent synovial thickening and inflammation.[8, 9] These changes lead to the common complaints of decreased motion, stiffness, and pain.

BIOCHEMICAL AND MOLECULAR CHANGES

In the early phase of OA, the synthesis of cartilage constituents—proteoglycans, collagen, and hyaluronic acid—is increased. Cartilage loss occurs due to lysosomal proteases and collagenase. Production of collagenase is increased

TABLE 1. CLASSIFICATION OF OSTEOARTHRITIS

I. *Idiopathic*
  A. Localized
    1. Hands: e.g., Heberden's and Bouchard's nodes (nodal), erosive interphalangeal arthritis (nonnodal), carpal-1st metacarpal
    2. Feet: e.g., hallux valgus, hallux rigidus, contracted toes (hammer/cockup toes), talonavicular
    3. Knee:
      a. Medial compartment
      b. Lateral compartment
      c. Patellofemoral compartment
    4. Hip:
      a. Eccentric (superior)
      b. Concentric (axial, medial)
      c. Diffuse (coxae senilis)
    5. Spine:
      a. Apophyseal joints
      b. Invertebral joints (disc)
      c. Spondylosis (osteophytes)
      d. Ligamentous (hyperostosis, Forestier's disease, DISH)
    6. Other single sites: e.g., glenohumoral, acromioclavicular, tibiotalar, sacroiliac, temporomandibular
  B. Generalized (GOA) includes three or more areas above (Kellgren-Moore)
II. *Secondary*
  A. Trauma
    1. Acute
    2. Chronic (occupational, sports)
  B. Congenital or developmental
    1. Localized diseases: e.g., Legg-Calve-Perthes, congenital hip dislocation, slipped epiphysis
    2. Mechanical factors: e.g., unequal lower extremity length, valgus/varus deformity, hypermobility syndromes
    3. Bone dysplasias: e.g., epiphyseal dysplasia, spondylo-apophyseal dysplasia, osteonychondystrophy
  C. Metabolic
    1. Ochronosis (alkaptonuria)
    2. Hemochromatosis
    3. Wilson's disease
    4. Gaucher's disease
  D. Endocrine
    1. Acromegaly
    2. Hyperparathyroidism
    3. Diabetes mellitus
    4. Obesity
    5. Hypothyroidism
  E. Calcium deposition diseases
    1. Calcium pyrophosphate dihydrate deposition
    2. Apatite arthropathy
  F. Other bone and joint diseases
    1. Localized: e.g., fracture, avascular necrosis, infection, gout
    2. Diffuse: rheumatoid (inflammatory) arthritis, Paget's disease, osteopetrosis, osteochondritis
  G. Neuropathic (Charcot joints)
  H. Endemic
    1. Kashin-Beck
    2. Mseleni
  I. Miscellaneous
    1. Frostbite
    2. Caisson's disease
    3. Hemoglobinopathies

From Mankin M, Brandt K, Shulman L: Workshop on etiopathogenesis of osteoarthritis. J Rheumatol 1986; 13:1134.

with increased severity of the disease. Hyaluronan content decreases because of these enzymes even though the synthesis of hyaluronan has increased. Alteration occurs in the size and orientation of cartilage fibers, with a disruption of the cartilage network. This results in increased stress on the chondrocytes. Increased chondrocyte replication and metabolism follow, leading to the increase in cartilage constituents seen early in the disease (Figs. 2 and 3). As cartilage loss progresses, the aggrecan content decreases, which leads to loss of compressive stiffness, loss of elasticity, and increased hydraulic permeability.[8, 9]

Interleukin-1 (IL-1) may play a role in mediating cartilage degradation in OA by stimulating synthesis and secretion of the proteinases. IL-1 is produced in the synovium and in mononuclear cells and is present in higher concentrations in the chondrocytes in OA than in normal cartilage. However, IL-1 is also found in high concentrations in the joints of patients with rheumatoid arthritis. Also, IL-1 stimulates production of the proteases in their latent form; activation of these enzymes must still occur to result in joint destruction. It may simply be that IL-1 is involved in the process of joint destruction, independent of the underlying disease state.[9, 10]

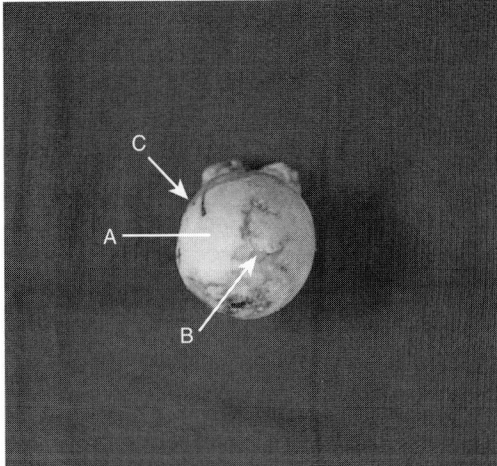

Fig. 1. Osteoarthritic femoral head. This femoral head was resected in a patient undergoing total hip arthroplasty. The cartilage is unevenly worn, with normal areas. *(A),* adjacent to areas with complete loss of cartilage down to bone *(B).* A surgical mark is noted *(C).*

GENETIC FEATURES

Genetic predisposition may play a role in the development of OA.[11–13] The most conclusive evidence of this comes from a twin study comparing 130 identical twins with 120 fraternal twins. The study was performed in women and evaluated radiographic changes in the hands and knees. Identical twins showed a concordance rate that was twice that of nonidentical twins at all sites.[11]

Other reports indicate increased familial incidence of OA in sites such as the distal interphalangeal joint of the hands in women,[12] and the familial defect detected in the complementary DNA of type II collagen on chromosome 12 in

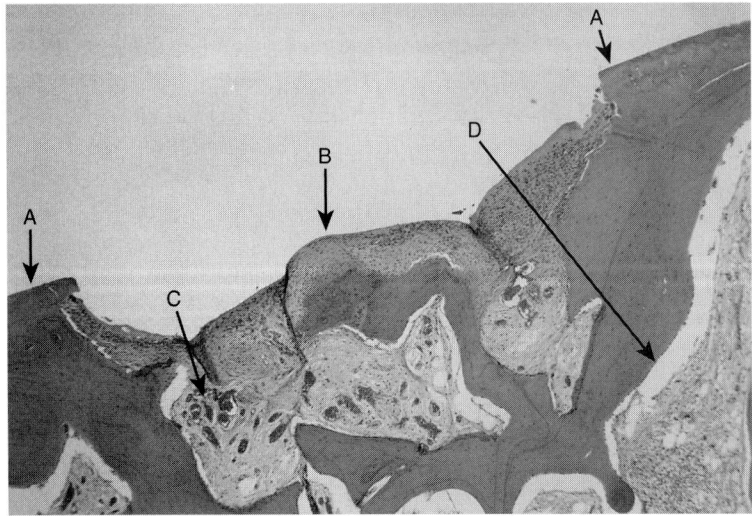

Fig. 2. Low-power H&E micrograph of section from femoral head. Areas of articular cartilage *(A)* are separated by an area of granulation *(B)*. The cartilage is thinner than normal. The area of granulation shows increased vascularity *(C)* with complete loss of cartilage. Osteoblastic rimming is also seen, indicating an attempt to support this deficient area. (Courtesy of Dr. Richard Miller and Dr. April Ewton, Southern California Permanente Medical Group.)

two families from Finland.[13] A familial tendency has also been noted for disorders leading to secondary OA such as occurs in DDH, CPPD, and the chondrodysplasias.

CLINICAL FEATURES

The symptoms and complaints of patients with OA are variable. The most common complaint is pain, often described as aching, burning, or stabbing. Pain is usually localized to the affected joint but can radiate to the joint above or below. It often includes the surrounding muscles, most likely from fatigue. The severity of pain perception is multifactorial and may correlate poorly with the physical examination's findings and radiographic appearance.

Less common is joint swelling, which may be due to either an effusion or bony enlargement from osteophytes. It is rarely caused by synovitis, which is a hallmark of inflammatory arthritis. The swelling caused by an effusion will usually vary with activity or trauma. As a result, the affected joint may be larger than its unaffected counterpart.

Another symptom is stiffness or loss of range of motion. Stiffness is usually of short duration (<10 min), present in the morning and after periods of rest, such as after getting up from a chair or out of a car after a period of time. Patients also complain of inability to perform activities that require dexterity or power such as manipulating small objects, opening jars, or kneeling. The chronic loss of motion can lead to contractures.

Crepitus is very common and may lead to undue concern by patients who fear that something dangerous is occurring when they hear sound emanating from within their joint.

Patients also complain of deformity such as Heberden's and Bouchard's nodes in the fingers, or bowing of the knees (Fig. 4).

Lower extremity involvement can produce complaints of a limp. This may be due to muscle weakness such as is seen in the Trendelenburg gait of hip arthritis or pain as seen in the antalgic gait of knee arthritis. Other manifestations of weakness include loss of grip strength, difficulty

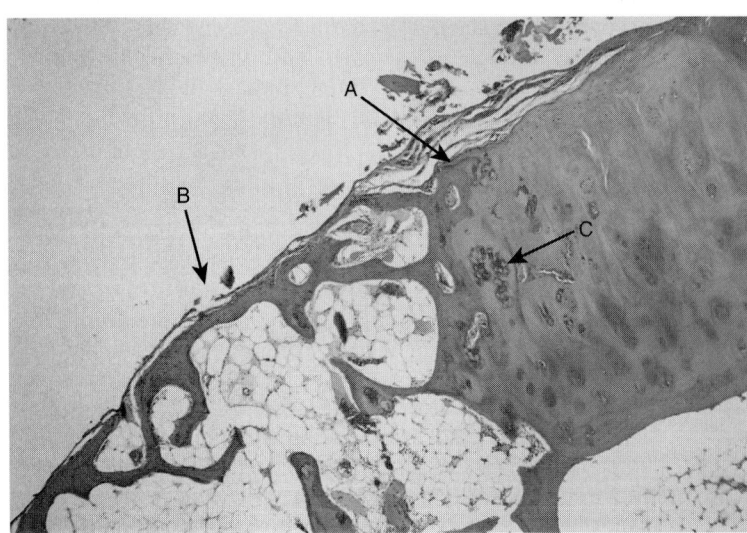

Fig. 3. High-power H&E micrograph of section from femoral head. An area of cartilage *(A)* is adjacent to an area of erosion to the level of subchondral bone *(B)*. Chondrocyte cloning *(C)* indicating increased synthesis of cartilage constituents is seen. (Courtesy of Dr. Richard Miller and Dr. April Ewton, Southern California Permanente Medical Group.)

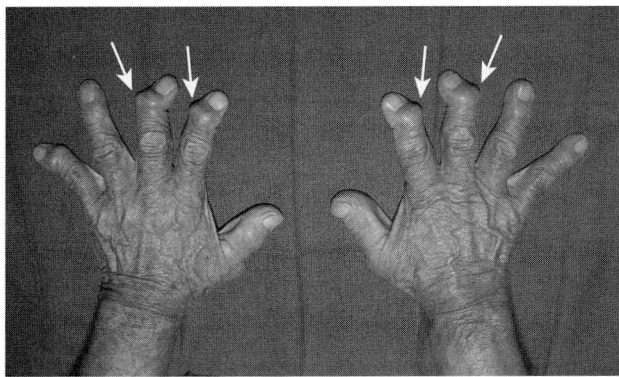

Fig. 4. Hands of a patient with OA. Severe deformity involving the distal interphalangeal joints of all of the fingers is noted. Deformity of the metacarpophalangeal joints of the thumbs is also demonstrated.

with ascending or descending stairs, and loss of endurance. The weakness is due to a combination of reflex inhibition due to pain and actual atrophy from disuse.

EVALUATION

Pertinent medical history that will affect the treatment offered to the patient should be obtained. The presence of underlying conditions leading to secondary OA, such as gout, Wilson's disease, CPPD, and so on, should be noted. If these conditions are not adequately treated, the patient will be symptomatic. A history of peptic ulcer, hepatic, or renal disease will affect pharmacological treatment options. Concurrent immunodeficiency disorders, severe peripheral vascular disease, and diabetes increase the risk of infection or other complications. Patients with a history of cardiac, pulmonary, cerebrovascular, hepatic, or renal disease may have a higher anesthetic risk profile, which possibly will affect the outcome of surgery. Patients with hematopoietic disorders require additional vigilance because of hypercoagulability leading to deep venous thrombosis or pulmonary embolism, or increased hemorrhage due to coagulation disorders.

The history should include handedness, occupation, hobbies and activities, use of ambulatory aids, and limitations brought on by the disease. Treatment will vary based on this information. The activities the patient performs, such as the nature of his or her job and leisure activities, will affect the type of treatment offered. Limitations in activities of daily living such as difficulty with stairs, transfers, ambulation, dressing, and hygiene guide the clinician to therapies appropriate for each patient.

Family history should also include a search for secondary causes of OA, such as DDH, bone dysplasias, Gaucher's disease, and so on. A history of other arthritic disorders, such as rheumatoid arthritis, systemic lupus erythematosus, ankylosing spondylitis, psoriatic arthritis, or Reiter's syndrome, should also be sought.

PHYSICAL EXAMINATION

Findings on examination include joint enlargement or effusion, crepitus, decreased range of motion, contracture, tenderness to palpation, angulatory or rotational deformity, and limp. Range of motion, contracture, and deformities should be carefully noted. Comparison should always be made to the contralateral side. The joints of the entire limb should be examined. For example, in a patient with knee arthritis, the ipsilateral hip and ankle as well as the contralateral knee should all be examined for range of motion, contracture, ligamentous stability, and muscle strength. The pinch and grip strength should be noted for the hand. Muscle strength and the presence of gait abnormalities should also be noted. Special attention should be paid to the most commonly involved joints of the cervical and lumbar spine, hip, knee, distal interphalangeal joints of the hands, carpometacarpal joint of the thumb, and the joints of the foot. The shoulder, elbow, wrist, sacroiliac joint, and ankle are less frequently involved unless there is a history of overuse or trauma. Neurological status, including sensation and reflexes, should be documented. A vascular examination, including pulses and the presence of decubiti or stasis changes of the skin, should also be noted.

INVESTIGATIONS

The diagnosis of OA is usually made clinically, with radiographic confirmation. The pathognomonic findings of osteoarthritis on plain radiographs include subchondral sclerosis, cystic change, marginal osteophytes, and asymmetric narrowing of the joint (Figs. 5 to 7). These findings may also be seen in end-stage avascular necrosis or ankylosing spondylitis. In avascular necrosis, the findings are usually limited to one half of the joint (femoral head), whereas in patients with ankylosing spondylitis the disease is generally bilateral, with characteristic changes in the spine and sacro-

Fig. 5. AP radiograph of the pelvis. Marginal osteophytes *(A)*, subchondral sclerosis *(B)*, and a cyst *(C)* are apparent. The joint space is asymmetrically narrowed, with a larger space at the periphery than in the center of the joint.

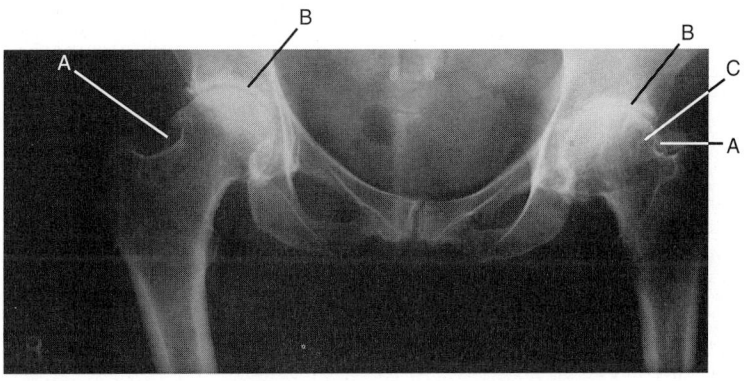

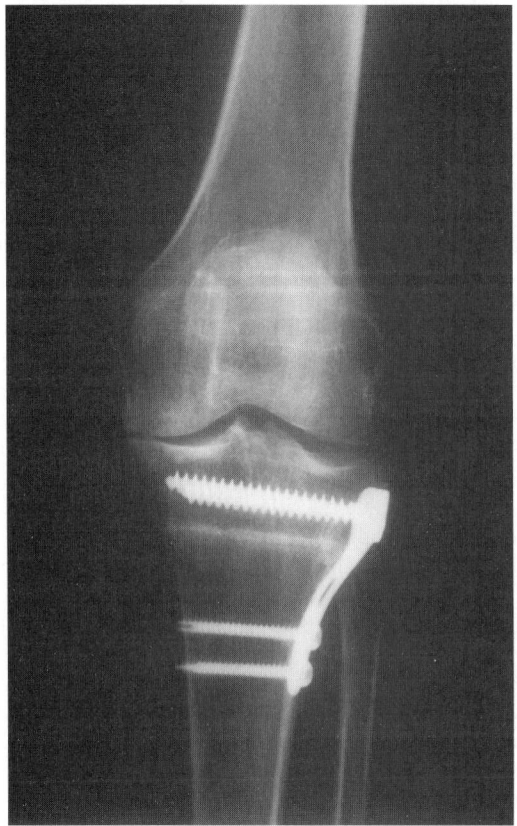

Fig. 6. AP radiograph of the knee. This view is of a 47-year-old man after a successful high tibial osteotomy. Medical compartment narrowing with flattening of the condyles and marginal osteophytes are apparent.

iliac joints. In contrast, inflammatory arthritis demonstrates symmetric joint space narrowing, with periarticular osteopenia and a paucity of osteophytes.

Imaging studies such as computed tomography or magnetic resonance imaging may be indicated to define the extent of disease in specialized cases. Examples include evaluation of neural compression in the spine, or to assess avascular necrosis (magnetic resonance imaging is best for

this). These studies are usually not helpful in distinguishing osteoarthritis from other forms of arthritis. Physical examination and plain radiographs are generally sufficient for this. Whole body bone scan may be useful to determine all of the joints involved by the arthritic process. Radiological findings may correlate poorly with clinical symptoms and should not dictate treatment.

Serological testing is of no benefit in making the diagnosis of OA. All serological markers are negative in OA. Similarly, joint fluid analysis will not make the diagnosis of OA but may rule out other disorders such as inflammatory arthritis, septic arthritis, or crystalline arthritis. For further information on this see Chapters 6-1, 6-3, and 6-4.

In the future, serological markers of OA may be measurable; however, it remains to be seen whether the marker will define the presence or absence of disease in the preclinical state or characterize the rate of progression of the disease, the severity of the disease, or the state of cartilage metabolism. The difficulty in establishing a marker lies in the multiple causes of OA and in the lack of knowledge of whether the marker concentration varies by type of body fluid or with renal or hepatic function. No marker has been established to date that is reproducible, reliable, or cost-effective.[14–16]

DIFFERENTIAL DIAGNOSIS

Osteoarthritis must be distinguished from other arthritides, most commonly inflammatory arthritis and avascular necrosis. Patients with inflammatory arthritis often have pain at rest, in contrast to patients with OA, who usually have pain with activity. Start-up stiffness abates rapidly in patients with OA, generally within 10 minutes. The pattern of joint involvement can help distinguish OA from inflammatory arthritis. Hand involvement in OA is primarily in the distal interphalangeal joints or carpometacarpal joint, whereas in inflammatory arthritis the metacarpophalangeal and proximal interphalangeal joints are involved. Patients with inflammatory arthritis also have significant synovitis, which is rarely seen in OA. Patients with avascular necrosis typically present with one joint involved. Table 2 and Chapters 6-3 and 6-9 give further details.

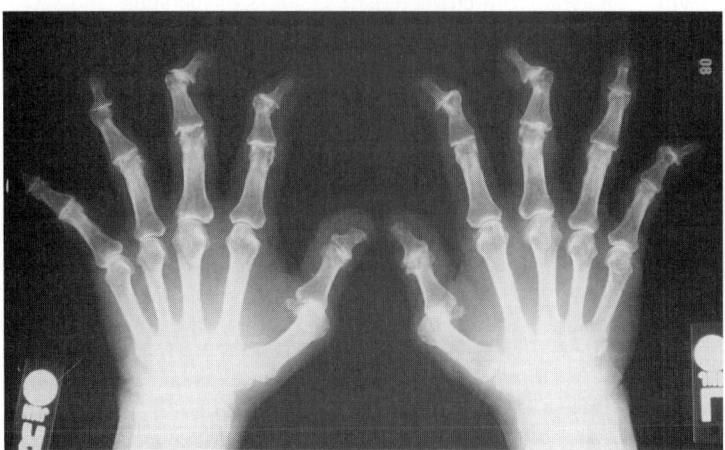

Fig. 7. AP radiograph of both hands from Figure 4. Marginal osteophytes with subluxation is demonstrated at the distal interphalangeal joints of the fingers as well as subluxation of the metacarpophalangeal joints of the thumbs.

TABLE 2. DIFFERENTIAL DIAGNOSIS OF OSTEOARTHRITIS (OA)

	Osteoarthritis	Rheumatoid Arthritis	Systemic Lupus Erythematosus	Ankylosing Spondylitis	Avascular Necrosis
Hand involvement	Distal interphalangeal joints, carpometacarpal joint of thumb Heberden's nodes	Metacarpophalangeal and proximal interphalangeal joints involved	Metacarpophalangeal and proximal interphalangeal joints involved	Nonspecific	Not involved
Radiographic appearance	Osteophytes, subchondral cysts and sclerosis, asymmetric joint space narrowing	Osteopenia, symmetric joint space narrowing, rare osteophytes	Osteopenia, symmetric joint space narrowing, rare osteophytes	Similar to OA; hallmarks are bamboo spine and fused sacroiliac joints	Collapse of involved bone, cysts; may appear like advanced OA in late stages
MRI	Not indicated	Not indicated	Not indicated	Not indicated	Signal loss in areas of avascularity
Laboratory tests					
Rheumatoid factor	Negative	Highly positive	Negative	Negative	Negative
Antinuclear antibody	Negative	Negative	Highly positive	Negative	Negative
HLA-B27	Negative	Negative	Negative	Highly positive	Negative
Synovial fluid volume	Normal to increased	Normal to increased	Normal to increased	Normal to increased	Normal to slightly increased
Clarity*	Clear	Clear to cloudy	Clear to cloudy	Clear	Clear
Cell count†	<2000	2000–80,000	2000–80,000	2000–80,000	<2000
%PMNs†	<25%	>50% but <85%	>50% but <85%	>50% but <85%	<25%

* The presence or absence of crystals should be noted. Negatively birefringent crystals indicate gout, positively birefringent crystals indicate calcium pyrophosphate deposition disease.
  † A cell count >80,000 with >85% PMNs indicates septic arthritis.
  PMN, polymorphonuclear neutrophil leukocyte.

MANAGEMENT

The overriding principle of treatment is pain control and improvement in function. Consideration must be given to the patient's functional demands, degree of impairment, age, and underlying medical conditions and past success or failure with other treatment modalities. The spectrum of the treatment options available for these disorders vary by the location to be treated and encompass all forms of orthopaedic management. Treatment must also be directed toward the underlying cause in secondary OA—gout, CPPD, and so on—to mitigate further damage.

The first line of treatment includes physical and occupational therapy. Emphasis should be placed on maintaining range of motion and strength. Exercises and modalities that focus on maintaining function and diminishing symptoms, without overloading the joint, are the mainstays of this treatment. The lower extremity requires closed chain exercises that avoid repetitive pounding as in jogging, tennis, or basketball. Examples of appropriate exercises are walking, bicycling, and swimming. The use of heavy weights should be avoided; weight training should emphasize maintaining range of motion with multiple repetitions. Warm soaks, hot baths, and ice packs are all beneficial, especially for involvement of the hand. Studies have shown improvement in function in patients with OA on a regular exercise program, although preoperative exercise has not been shown to have an impact on the outcome of patients undergoing total knee arthroplasty.[17, 18]

Pharmacological treatment options in OA are varied. One must consider the underlying medical condition and comorbidities of the patient prior to prescribing medication. The most commonly used medications include the analgesics such as acetaminophen and the nonsteroidal anti-inflammatory drugs (NSAIDs). These medications are commonly used in conjunction with physical therapy and are very effective in the treatment of OA.[19–22] Patient response to an individual NSAID may be variable; two to three different NSAIDs should be tried for more than 4 weeks each before this class of drugs can be considered a failure. The main risk with acetaminophen is liver toxicity. Risks with the NSAIDs include gastrointestinal upset or ulceration, nephrotoxicity, and increased blood pressure. The NSAIDs may have significant drug interactions that can lead to gastrointestinal ulceration if given with corticosteroids or hemorrhage if given with anticoagulants. Newer NSAIDs (cyclooxygenase-2–specific inhibitors) are less likely to cause gastrointestinal bleeding and renal problems but are significantly more expensive than the older NSAIDs.[22] These agents are generally reserved for those patients with previous history or a high risk of gastrointestinal bleeding from the older NSAIDs. The newer cyclooxygenase-2–specific agents are usually tolerated well by patients on warfarin, but careful monitoring of the INR is required. In this age of rising health-care costs, the practitioner must be cognizant of the costs of the pharmacological modes of treatment and carefully select the appropriate medication for the patient.

Other pharmacological treatment options in OA include glucosamine and chondroitin. There are limited studies on these medications to support their use in treatment of OA. Most studies show a decrease in pain with improvement in symptoms after 6 weeks of use.[23–25] However, the studies were of short duration and without long-term follow-up. The known side effect profile of these medications is minimal. Further investigation of these medications is warranted. There is no information to suggest that these medications alter the disease process or the course of the disease.

Narcotics should be reserved for short-term use in exacerbations of pain and for perioperative pain management. They may also be beneficial in patients with end-stage arthritis who are poor surgical risks.

Intra-articular medications include corticosteroids and newer cartilage derivatives. Corticosteroids should be used sparingly because of the detrimental effect of multiple injections into a single joint. It is our practice to inject a patient younger than 50 years of age only once unless there is an underlying condition or end-stage arthritis in the affected joint. In patients over 50 years of age with arthritis of the hip or knee, injections can be given as often as every 4 months for symptomatic relief. Corticosteroid injections in the lumbar spine can be very beneficial and even eliminate the need for surgery. Systemic corticosteroids are not indicated for routine treatment in OA, but they may be used in cases of spinal stenosis. See Chapter 8-5 for more details on spinal stenosis.

Other treatments include intra-articular injections using the cartilage derivatives, hylan GF-20 or sodium hyaluronate.[26, 27] These may offer symptomatic pain relief in a select population of patients. They are believed to work by providing a "cushion" in the joint. There are no long-term studies that demonstrate significant sustained improvement in symptoms. There is a risk of side effects, including short-term exacerbation of symptoms similar to a gout flare. At present, the cost of a course of these injections is considerable, approximately one fourth the cost of the implants used in total joint arthroplasty. There is no evidence to suggest that these injections alter the course of the disease. These injections should be used in patients with arthritis who have failed pharmacological intervention, do not desire surgery, or are poor surgical candidates.

SURGICAL TREATMENT

To understand the treatment options for OA in all locations is to understand orthopaedic surgery in its entirety. Inappropriate treatment of trauma or other conditions can lead to OA. For specific surgical treatment options, the reader is referred to the appropriate chapter based on the anatomic location of the disease. The success rate of surgical treatment varies by the age of the patient, the location of the disease, the activity level of the patient, patient compliance, the surgical skill employed, and, in the case of total joint arthroplasty, the components used. There are four basic types of surgery for OA: débridement and lavage, osteotomy, arthrodesis, and arthroplasty. Table 3 gives a treatment algorithm and Chapters 6-6, 6-7, and 11-2 describe surgical options in the shoulder, elbow, and ankle, respectively.

Débridement and lavage is useful in early stages of the disease in easily accessible joints such as the knee. It should be considered a temporizing measure. Several studies have shown the benefit of arthroscopic lavage in reducing pain in patients with OA. It is unclear whether this benefit is due to simply removing the inflammatory mediators present in the knee or to removing mechanical irrita-

---

TABLE 3. TREATMENT ALGORITHM FOR OSTEOARTHRITIS

Stage	Modality	Specific Modality	Notes
Initial presentation and mild radiographic appearance	Mechanical modifications Therapy Analgesics	Braces, canes/walker, weight loss Stretching, conditioning, range of motion, modalities (US/ice/heat/TENS) Acetaminophen 650 mg PO q4–6 hours, topical ointments	
Failure of above or initial presentation with moderate radiographic changes	NSAIDs and above modalities as effective Note: 2–3 different NSAIDs should be tried for 4 weeks each before this class of drugs can be considered a failure.	Ibuprofen 400–800 mg PO tid–qid Naproxen 250 mg tid–500 mg PO bid Indomethacin 25–50 mg PO tid Piroxicam 20 mg PO qd Diclofenac 50–75 mg PO bid ASA 650 mg PO q4–6 hours, etc.	Many other NSAIDs are available; consult a pharmacist for more information
Failure of above or intolerance to NSAIDs	Cartilage constituents	Glucosamine 1200 mg qd Chondroitin	These may supplant NSAIDs in the future
Failure of above or acute inflammation	Intra-articular corticosteroids		
Failure of above and mild to moderate radiographic changes	Intra-articular cartilage supplements	Hyalgan/Synvisc	
Failure of above	Surgery Mild radiographic changes Knee in patient <50 years old Moderate to severe radiographic changes Young physiological age <50 years old	Arthroscopic lavage Consider mosaicplasty or cartilage transplant Arthrodesis/arthroplasty depending on anatomic site Consider osteotomy or arthrodesis for knee or hip	

NSAIDs, nonsteroidal anti-inflammatory drugs; TENS, transcutaneous electrical nerve stimulation; US, ultrasonography.

tion from loose cartilage (or a torn meniscus), or if some other mechanism plays a role.[28, 29] Care should be taken to avoid aggressive débridement, which usually results in worsening of symptoms. Patients should be warned that they might feel worse after surgery or require further surgery as the disease progresses.

Osteotomy is useful in joints with malalignment from disease progression or prior injury that results in mechanical overload of a portion of the joint and sparing of another portion of the joint.[28] The surgical premise is to restore alignment and redistribute the mechanical forces to more normal areas of the joint. This is commonly performed in the knee and less often in the hip. These procedures are technically demanding and require extensive preoperative planning. Full details of these procedures can be obtained in Chapters 6-10 and 6-15.

Arthrodesis, or joint fusion, has a large role in the treatment of OA. It is commonly used in the hand, spine, ankle, and foot, and less commonly in the hip or knee.[28] It can be an excellent salvage procedure in these areas. It provides excellent pain relief but results in loss of motion and overload of the surrounding joints. It is also quite useful in the hip or knee of the young patient or manual laborer with isolated OA who is a poor candidate for total joint arthroplasty. See Chapters 6-10, 8-10, 11-2, 11-8, 12-12, and 12-15 for more details on arthrodesis.

Arthroplasty, or joint resurfacing, is available in several subtypes. Interposition arthroplasty involves placing a tissue graft, such as a tendon or fascia lata, into the joint. This is commonly used in the small bones, such as the carpometacarpal joint of the thumb. Resection arthroplasty[28] involves excision of the joint surfaces and supporting bone, with secondary filling of the space by scar tissue. This technique is often used in the salvage of infected total hip arthroplasty (see Chapters 6-18 and 12-12).

Resurfacing arthroplasty involves using foreign materials, most commonly cobalt chrome and ultra-high molecular weight polyethylene, as a new bearing surface. The limitation of this procedure, in the past, has been the limited durability of the polyethylene. However, newer cross-linked polyethylene is now available, as are metal-on-metal articulations with the promise of greater durability. Ceramic-on-ceramic prostheses are also under study. It remains to be seen whether the newer cross-linked polyethylene, metal-on-metal, or ceramic-on-ceramic materials will be more durable than the current polyethylene, as there are no long-term (>15 years) data on these new articulations.

Resurfacing arthroplasty is most commonly performed in the hips and knees; recent advances in technology are now allowing this to be used more in the shoulders, elbows, and ankles. A newer variation on resurfacing arthroplasty involves autologous cartilage in the form of grafts (mosaicplasty) or cultured chondrocytes[30] to fill cartilaginous defects in arthritis. There are no long-term studies on these two techniques (see Chapter 4-14).

TABLE 4. RESULTS OF NONOPERATIVE TREATMENT IN OSTEOARTHRITIS	
Treatment Modality	**Results**
Exercise[18]	Improvement in ambulation time and pain score for patients following an aerobic exercise or strengthening program compared with those going to a health education class without exercise in patients with knee osteoarthritis.
Acetaminophen[19]	Improvement in pain score following 4 weeks of therapy at 4000 mg/day
Ibuprofen[19]	Improvement in pain score following 4 weeks of therapy with either 1200 mg/day (analgesic dose) or 2400 mg/day (anti-inflammatory dose). No difference in improvement from acetaminophen.
Piroxicam[20]	Improvement in pain score, function, and effusion with either a 14- or 28-day course of piroxicam 20 mg/day. Continued benefit was seen in the 28-day group of patients.
Glucosamine/chondroitin[23]	Improvement in pain score, and physical examination score in U.S. naval personnel after 8 weeks treatment with glucosamine 1500 mg and chondroitin 1200 mg.
Glucosamine[24]	Improvement in pain scores in patients receiving 1 week of 400 mg/day intramuscular glucosamine followed by 2 weeks of oral glucosamine 1500 mg/day, compared with a control group receiving 1 week IM piperazine/chlorbutanol followed by 2 weeks placebo.
Glucosamine vs. ibuprofen[25]	Faster improvement in pain scores at 2 weeks in patients receiving 1200 mg/day ibuprofen than those receiving 1500 mg/day glucosamine. At 8 weeks, pain scores were significantly lower in the glucosamine group, although both groups had a significant decrease in pain scores from baseline.
Hylan G-F 20 vs. NSAID[26]	Three groups created; NSAID only, Hylan G-F 20 only, and NSAID + Hylan G-F 20. No difference seen between the groups at 12 weeks after therapy, but all three groups showed significant improvement from baseline. At 26 weeks, the NSAID + Hylan G-F 20 group showed the most improvement.
Sodium hyaluronate vs. naproxen[27]	Comparison of sodium hyaluronate, naproxen 500 mg bid, and placebo. At 26 weeks, the hyaluronate group had better performance on a 50-foot walk test with respect to pain than the placebo group.
Joint lavage vs. intra-articular corticosteroid injection[29]	Four groups studied: placebo, intra-articular corticosteroid alone, joint lavage with intra-articular placebo, and joint lavage with intra-articular steroid. Significant decrease in pain was seen for intra-articular steroid up to 4 weeks after injection, with a trend for decreased pain at 12 weeks. Joint lavage showed a significant decrease in pain for up to 24 weeks. The combination therapy showed additive effects.

NSAID, nonsteroidal anti-inflammatory drug.

COMPLICATIONS

Complications in patients with untreated osteoarthritis are limited to those caused by disease progression: loss of motion, pain, swelling, and decreased function. Complications from pharmacological intervention include side effects of the medication and end-organ toxicity (most commonly liver or kidney). Surgical complications include infection, hemorrhage, neurological injury, contracture, thrombosis (deep vein thrombosis or pulmonary embolism), and failure of the implants used. See Chapter 6-18 for the complications of total joint arthroplasty (which would include most complications of surgical treatment), and the appropriate section for other complications specific to the anatomic location or type of surgery.

RESULTS

The results of nonoperative treatment vary because there is no cure for OA. As the disease progresses, nonoperative treatments fail. The rate of progression is highly variable. The literature conflicts on the various nonoperative treatments because of this variability. It is for this reason that the clinician must be vigilant and carefully individualize the treatment for each patient. Some patients will respond to one form of treatment, whereas others with the same level of disease will not. Surgical intervention should not be performed cavalierly, but only when all other options have been exhausted. Table 4 gives data on nonoperative treatment. For data on operative treatment, refer to the appropriate chapter.

REFERENCES

1. Yellin E, Callahan L: The economic cost and social and psychological impact of musculoskeletal conditions. Arthritis Rheum 1995; 38:1351.
2. Lubeck D: The economic impact of arthritis. Arthritis Care Res 1995; 8:304.
3. Lawrence R, Helmick C, Arnett F, et al: Estimates of the prevalence of arthritis and selected musculoskeletal disorders in the United States. Arthritis Rheum 1998; 41:778.
4. Oliveria S, Felson D, Reed J, et al: Incidence of symptomatic hand, hip and knee osteoarthritis among patients in a Health Maintenance Organization. Arthritis Rheum 1995; 38:1134.
5. Felson D, Zhang Y, Hannan M, et al: The incidence and natural history of knee osteoarthritis in the elderly: The Framingham Osteoarthritis Study. Arthritis Rheum 1995; 38:1500.
6. Swanson A, Swanson G: Osteoarthritis in the hand. J Hand Surg 1983; 5:669.
7. Mankin H, Brandt K, Shulman L: Workshop on etiopathogenesis of osteoarthritis. J Rheum 1986; 13:1130.
8. Buckwalter J, Mankin H: Articular cartilage: Degeneration and osteoarthritis, repair, regeneration, and transplantation. In Cannon W (ed): Instructional Course Lectures. Rosemont, IL, American Academy of Orthopaedic Surgeons, 1998, p 487.
9. Brandt K, Mankin H: Pathogenesis of osteoarthritis. In Sledge C, Ruddy S, Harris E, et al (eds): Arthritis Surgery. Philadelphia, WB Saunders, 1994, p 450.
10. van den Berg W, van der Kraan P, van Beuningen H: Synovial mediators of cartilage damage and repair in OA. In Brandt K, Doherty M, Lohmander L (eds): Osteoarthritis. Oxford, Oxford University Press, 1998, p 157.
11. Spector T, Cicuttini F, Baker J, et al: Genetic influences on osteoarthritis in women: A twin study. BMF 1996; 312:940.
12. Cicuttini F, Spector T: What is the evidence that osteoarthritis is genetically de-

termined? Ballieres Clin Rheumatol 1997; 11:657.
13. Palotie A, Ott J, Vaisanen P, et al: Predisposition to familial osteoarthritis linked to type II collagen gene. Lancet 1989; 1:924.
14. Lohmander L, Felson D: Defining and validating the clinical role of molecular markers in osteoarthritis. In Brandt K, Doherty M, Lohmander L (eds): Osteoarthritis. Oxford, Oxford University Press, 1998, p 519.
15. Myers S: Synovial fluid markers in osteoarthritis. Rheum Dis Clin North Am 1999; 25:433.
16. Wollheim F: Serum markers of articular damage and repair. Rheum Dis Clin North Am 1999; 25:417.
17. D'Lima D, Colwell C, Morris B, et al: The effect of preoperative exercise on total knee replacement outcomes. Clin Orthop 1996; 326:174.
18. Ettinger W, Burns R, Messier S, et al: A randomized trial comparing aerobic exercise and resistance exercise with a health education program in older adults with knee osteoarthritis. JAMA 1997; 277:25.
19. Bradley J, Brandt K, Katz B, et al: Comparison of an antiinflammatory dose of ibuprofen, an analgesic dose of ibuprofen, and acetaminophen in the treatment of patients with osteoarthritis of the knee. N Engl J Med 1991; 325:87.
20. Ravaud P, Auleley G, Ayral X, et al: Piroxicam therapy: A double blind, randomized, multicenter study comparing 2 versus 4 week treatment in patients with painful knee osteoarthritis with effusion. J Rheum 1998; 25:2425.
21. Zhao S, Dedhiya S, Bocanegra T, et al: Health related quality-of-life effects of oxaprazosin and nabumetone in patients with osteoarthritis of the knee. Clin Ther 1999; 21:205.
22. Fung H, Kirschenbaum H: Selective cyclooxygenase-2 inhibitors for the treatment of arthritis. Clin Ther 1999; 21:1131.
23. Philippi A, Leffler C, Leffler S, et al: Glu-

cosamine, chondroitin, and manganese ascorbate for degenerative joint disease of the knee or low back: A randomized, double-blind, placebo-controlled pilot study. Military Med 1999; 164:85.
24. Crolle G, D'Este E: Glucosamine sulphate for the management of arthrosis: A controlled clinical investigation. Curr Med Res Opin 1980; 7:104.
25. Vaz A: Double-blind clinical evaluation of the relative efficacy of ibuprofen and glucosamine sulphate in the management of osteoarthritis of the knee in out-patients. Curr Med Res Opin 1982; 8:145.
26. Adams M, Atkinson M, Lussier A, et al: The role of visco supplementation with hylan G-F 20 in the treatment of osteoarthritis of the knee: A Canadian multicenter trial comparing hylan G-F 20 alone, hylan G-F 20 with non-steroidal anti-inflammatory drugs and non-steroidal anti-inflammatory drugs alone. Osteoarthritis Cartilage 1995; 3:213.
27. Altman R, Moskowitz R: Intraarticular sodium hyaluronate in the treatment of patients with osteoarthritis of the knee: A randomized clinical trial. J Rheum 1998; 25:2203.
28. Buckwalter J, Lohmander L: Surgical treatment of osteoarthritis. In Kuettner K, Goldberg V (eds): Osteoarthritic Disorders. American Academy of Orthopaedic Surgeons, Rosemont, IL, 1994, p 379.
29. Ravaud P, Moulinier L, Giraudeau B, et al: Effects of joint lavage and steroid injection in patients with osteoarthritis of the knee: Results of a multicenter, randomized, controlled trial. Arthritis Rheum 1999; 42:475.
30. Menche D, Vangsness C, Pitman M, et al: The treatment of isolated articular cartilage lesions in the young individual. In Cannon W (ed): Instructional Course Lectures. Rosemont, IL, American Academy of Orthopaedic Surgeons, 1998, p 505.

section 6 chapter 3
INFLAMMATORY ARTHRITIS

Timothy M. Wright and Aldo Vincent Londino

Summary

- The inflammatory arthritides comprise a varied group of illnesses with articular and systemic features.
- Most forms of inflammatory arthritis have a genetic predisposition, although the mechanism responsible for triggering inflammatory arthritis is poorly understood.
- The diagnosis of inflammatory arthritis is dependent on a careful history and physical examination and is based primarily on the pattern of articular involvement and associated nonarticular manifestations.
- Laboratory and radiographic studies aid in the diagnosis of inflammatory arthritis, but in themselves are not usually diagnostic.
- Approaches to treatment are directed toward the preservation of function, reduction of inflammation, and management of pain.
- In spite of advances in medical management, many patients progress to severe joint destruction necessitating surgical intervention.

In this chapter, we review the classification, pathogenesis, diagnostic approach, and management of inflammatory arthritis, a group of illnesses whose common features include inflammation of joints and periarticular structures of unknown cause, extra-articular disease manifestations, and a potentially chronic progressive course. The inflammatory arthritides can be divided broadly into three main categories, as listed in Table 1.

Rheumatoid arthritis (RA) is a systemic inflammatory disease in which joint inflammation and destruction predominates. It is characterized by a symmetric chronic polyarthritis involving the diarthrodial joints with prominent involvement of the small joints of the hands and feet. One of the first descriptions of findings consistent with RA was by Sydenham in the 17th century, although the term "rheumatoid arthritis" was not used until 1859 in a treatise by Garrod on "Gout and Rheumatic Gout."[1, 2] RA affects women two to three times more often than men and has a

TABLE 1. INFLAMMATORY ARTHRITIDES

Rheumatoid arthritis
Spondyloarthropathies
  Ankylosing spondylitis
  Psoriatic arthritis
  Reactive arthritis/Reiter's syndrome
  Inflammatory bowel disease–associated arthritis
Inflammatory arthritis associated with connective tissue diseases

peak incidence in the 4th to 5th decades, with a steadily rising prevalence with age.[3] The prevalence of RA varies throughout the world but generally ranges from 0.5% to 1% in most populations. Approximately 80% of RA patients test positive for rheumatoid factor, an autoantibody specific for the Fc portion of the immunoglobulin (Ig) G molecule.

The spondyloarthropathies are related diseases that are distinguished by inflammation of entheses, the sites of tendon and ligament attachments to bone with frequent involvement of the spine. Ankylosing spondylitis (AS), the prototypic spondyloarthropathy, usually begins in the second or third decade and has a male to female ratio of approximately 5:1. The development of AS is highly associated with the major histocompatibility complex (MHC) class I allele HLA-B27, which is present in over 90% of white people with this illness. The prevalence of AS varies among populations, in part related to the frequency of HLA-B27, and is generally 0.1% to 0.5% in white populations and rare in black populations.[4]

The related spondyloarthropathies are less common than AS, and together their prevalence rate approaches 0.1%. Reactive arthritis (or Reiter's syndrome), like AS, has a male predilection, and 50% to 75% of patients are HLA-B27–positive. Psoriatic arthritis and arthritis associated with inflammatory bowel disease (ulcerative colitis and Crohn's disease) occur equally among males and females. The HLA-B27 association is weaker and is seen primarily in a subset of these patients with spondylitis.

Inflammatory arthritis is also a common component of other systemic inflammatory diseases, including the autoimmune connective diseases (e.g., systemic lupus erythematosus, Sjögren's syndrome, systemic sclerosis, and polymyositis/dermatomyositis), polymyalgia rheumatica, and sarcoidosis. The inflammatory arthritides are to be distinguished from septic arthritis, which is in most cases acute and responds to appropriate antibiotic therapy and drainage. Two chronic inflammatory conditions that mimic the idiopathic inflammatory arthritides, however, are now known to be infectious in origin. These are Whipple's disease, which is caused by the actinomycete *Tropheryma whippelii*, and Lyme disease, which is caused by the spirochete *Borrelia burgdorferi*. Interestingly, the arthritis associated with these infections may persist long after the treatment with antibiotics, raising the possibility that the microorganisms can serve as a trigger for a chronic polyarthritis in susceptible individuals.

PATHOGENESIS

The pathogenesis of the inflammatory arthritides involves a complex interplay of cellular interactions and soluble inflammatory mediators that results in joint and periarticular tissue destruction and remodeling. It is now well recognized that genetic background plays an important role in the development of the inflammatory arthritides. Studies in the genetics of RA have defined the strong relationship between predisposition for disease and an amino acid sequence found on HLA-DR4 and HLA-DR1 molecules. The reason for the association between RA and these two MHC class II molecules is unclear but may be related to the ability to present certain peptides by the MHC molecules, thereby shaping the helper T-cell repertoire.

As noted earlier, RA is an inflammatory disease involving primarily diarthrodial joints. The proliferative synovium of RA is referred to as pannus. The pannus is characterized by proliferation of fibroblast-like synovial lining cells (pannocytes), neovascularization, and infiltration by a mixture of inflammatory cells (predominantly T cells, B cells, and macrophages). The pannus is a rich source of cytokines and matrix metalloproteinases (MMPs). The cytokines of the pannus include tumor necrosis factor-α, interleukin (IL)-1, IL-6, IL-8, and IL-15. Some of these (tumor necrosis factor-α, IL-1, IL-6) contribute to the proliferation of the pannocytes, inhibit chondrocyte matrix production, and act as autocrine and paracrine factors to stimulate MMP production. Others, such as IL-8, a polymorphonuclear chemoattractant, and IL-15, a T-cell chemoattractant and activator, are involved in perpetuating the inflammatory response.[5, 6]

The MMPs include collagenase, gelatinase, and stromelysin, which are capable of degrading the matrix components of cartilage and bone. As the inflammatory pannus extends to the capsular margin, there is invasion of the adjacent cartilage and bone, resulting in the typical "marginal erosion" of RA observed radiographically. There is also thinning of the articular cartilage across the joint and demineralization of subchondral bone, possibly due to the effect of cytokines and other soluble inflammatory mediators such as nitric oxide and prostaglandins.[7]

The spondyloarthropathies also have a well-defined genetic predisposition. The association, which is strongest for AS (>90%) and reactive arthritis (50% to 75%), is with the MHC class I allele HLA-B27. This association crosses all racial and ethnic groups and raises the possibility that a peptide, perhaps derived from an intracellular pathogen presented through the MHC class I pathway, may be responsible for the chronic inflammatory responses seen in these diseases. In support of this hypothesis is the fact that reactive arthritis is known to follow acute enteritis with one of several organisms (*Yersinia, Salmonella, Shigella, Campylobacter*) or venereal infection with *Chlamydia,* and recent evidence supports persistence of the organisms or their antigens in joint and skin lesions.[8] The importance of the HLA-B27 molecule in the pathogenesis of spondyloarthropathies is further supported by the spontaneous development of enthesitis with ankylosis in transgenic animals (rats and mice) expressing the human HLA-B27 gene.[9]

Synovial inflammation also occurs in the spondyloarthropathies. Histologically, it is similar to RA and can progress to joint erosions. What distinguishes this group of diseases is the inflammation of entheses. The reason for targeting entheses with a chronic inflammatory response in spondyloarthropathies is not known, and the biochemical and molecular aspects of this inflammation are not well characterized. The enthesitis of spondyloarthropathies is a distinguishing feature because it is accompanied by proliferative new bone formation that often results over time in bony ankylosis.

The arthritides associated with systemic inflammatory diseases (with the exception of adult Still's disease) are relatively mild chronic synovitis and/or tenosynovitis and do not generally result in erosive joint destruction.

CLINICAL FEATURES

The most important element in the assessment of patients with inflammatory arthritis is a detailed history and physical examination. When approaching a patient with articular pain, one of the key determinations to be made is whether the pain is mechanical or inflammatory in origin. Mechanical pain is typically associated with minimal stiffness (lasting less than 30 minutes), worsening with activity, and improvement with rest of the joint or joints involved. Inflammatory pain, in contrast, is usually associated with significant stiffness (usually lasting more than 1 hour) that is worse in the morning or after prolonged rest. Inflammatory arthritis is also generally improved with activity and often persists during periods of rest or inactivity. The location (peripheral, axial, large, small joints), extent (number of involved joints), pattern (symmetrical versus asymmetrical), and chronicity of joint complaints provide clues to the type of inflammatory arthritis.

RA results in synovitis of diarthrodial joints with a characteristic symmetrical pattern of joint involvement. RA is associated with significant morning stiffness that may last for hours. A prominent clinical feature is the striking degree of muscle atrophy that accompanies the arthritis, often out of proportion to the degree of inflammation present on examination. This presumably is the result of disuse atrophy because of the severity of the joint pain. RA typically affects the small joints of hands and feet (metacarpophalangeals, proximal interphalangeals, and metatarsophalangeals with sparing of distal interphalangeals) and commonly involves the wrists, elbows, shoulders, knees, and ankles. The hips and sacroiliac joints are less commonly affected and spine involvement is usually limited to the cervical spine. Synovitis in the apophyseal joints of the cervical spine can result in subluxation of cervical vertebrae, erosion of the odontoid, and superior migration of the odontoid encroaching on the foramen magnum. All of these can progress to neurological emergencies, threatening paralysis or death from compromise of the cervical spinal cord.

The chronic inflammation extending beyond the joint capsule into surrounding tissues results in loosening and/or detachment of tendons from pericapsular structures. Coupled with the invasion of cartilage and bone by pannus with subsequent loss of cartilage, this leads to the deformities commonly seen in RA patients. Typically, there is ulnar deviation of hands, ligamentous and capsular laxity at the metacarpophalangeal joints and proximal interphalangeal joints, resulting in swan neck and boutonniere deformities of the fingers. Subluxation occurs commonly with advanced disease at the metacarpophalangeal joints, wrist, and metatarsophalangeal joints.

As mentioned earlier, RA is a systemic illness, and patients may complain of constitutional symptoms of low-

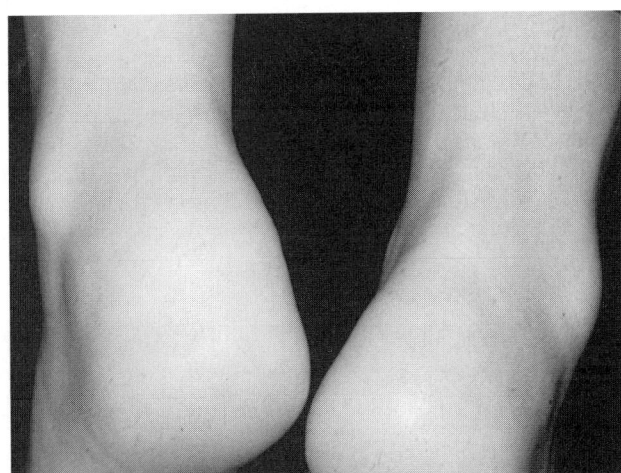

Fig. 1. Achilles enthesitis. This photograph shows a patient with ankylosing spondylitis.

grade fever, fatigue, and weakness. Extra-articular features include rheumatoid nodules, vasculitis, ocular inflammation (scleritis and episcleritis), pleuropericarditis, and pulmonary fibrosis. Rheumatoid nodules are firm, movable, soft-tissue masses seen in approximately 25% of RA patients. They occur on the extensor surfaces of the elbows, hands, knees, buttocks, Achilles tendons, and internal organs, including the lungs and heart. Felty's syndrome is a severe systemic variant occurring uncommonly in long-standing RA characterized by fever, splenomegaly, neutropenia, chronic leg ulcers, and recurrent bacterial infections.

The spondyloarthropathies are also systemic diseases with more variable constitutional symptoms. Stiffness of the affected joints is common and often lasts an hour or more. The hallmark of the spondyloarthropathies is enthesitis, the inflammation of ligaments, tendons, and joint capsules where they insert to bone. The common target of inflammation in AS is the axial skeleton with involvement of synovial joints and entheses. This process usually begins in the lumbar region and progresses in an ascending fashion. In cases of spondylitis, the spine becomes rigid over

time owing to the ankylosis that follows the enthesitis. Fusion of the spine may yield severe thoracic kyphosis and limited cervical spine mobility such that the patient may have difficulty visualizing his or her path ahead when walking. Involvement of the hips may result in bony ankylosis as well.

Sacroiliitis is common and is most often bilateral in AS, but often unilateral in the other spondyloarthropathies. Peripheral joints are less frequently affected in AS but are commonly involved in psoriatic arthritis, reactive arthritis, and inflammatory bowel-associated arthritis. The weight-bearing joints are more often affected than those of the upper extremity, and the pattern of involvement is asymmetric and oligoarticular. In the extremities, enthesitis is also a prominent feature of the spondyloarthropathies, with frequent involvement of the plantar fascia and Achilles insertion (Fig. 1). Dactylitis of the hands and/or feet may result in the appearance of characteristic "sausage digits," which contrasts with the fusiform articular swelling observed in RA.

Psoriatic arthritis, which occurs in about 6% of psoriasis patients, has five recognized patterns of joint involvement.[10] A common pattern is asymmetric, scattered, large and small joint, oligoarticular involvement, often with sausage digits—the pattern most often observed in reactive arthritis and inflammatory bowel disease associated arthritis. Psoriatic arthritis can also present with a pattern of hand involvement indistinguishable from RA. A third pattern, characteristic of psoriatic arthritis, is an asymmetric arthritis involving the distal interphalangeal joints of the hands and feet in association with psoriatic nail changes. A severe form of hand arthritis, arthritis mutilans, results from asymmetric proximal interphalangeal and distal interphalangeal joint involvement (Fig. 2). Finally, psoriatic arthritis patients may develop spondylitis that is indistinguishable from AS, in the presence or absence of peripheral arthritis. The skin disease usually antedates the joint involvement, but the converse may occur in as many as 10% of cases.

An extra-articular feature common to all spondyloarthropathies is anterior uveitis, which is linked to the HLA-B27 allele. Other extra-articular manifestations vary with

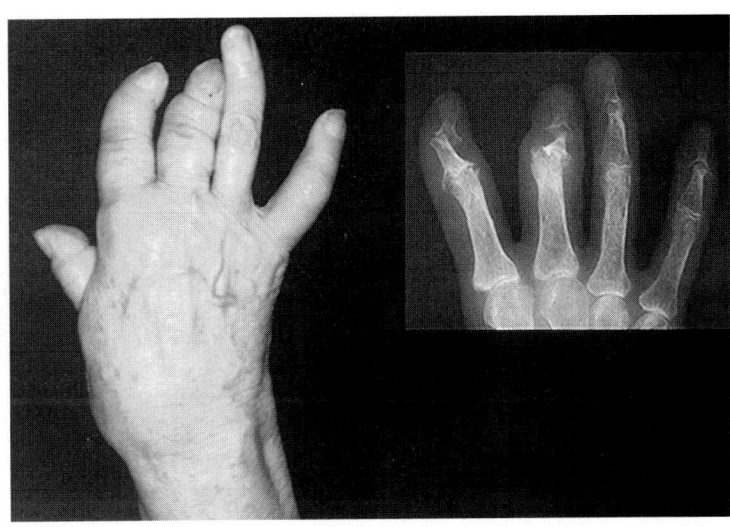

Fig. 2. Hand and corresponding radiograph. A patient with psoriatic arthritis demonstrates arthritis mutilans.

the specific form of arthritis. AS may be rarely complicated by aortitis, fibrotic valvular disease, and cardiac conduction defects. Mucocutaneous lesions are common extra-articular manifestations of reactive arthritis and include keratoderma blennorrhagicum (indistinguishable from pustular psoriasis), aphthous ulcers, urethritis, cervicitis, conjunctivitis, and circinate balanitis. Nail pitting is often observed in psoriasis patients with arthritis. Inflammatory bowel disease associated arthritis may also be associated with skin lesions (erythema nodosum and pyoderma gangrenosum).

INVESTIGATION

In general, laboratory test results should be considered as supportive, not diagnostic or specific, for the diagnosis of inflammatory arthritis. The erythrocyte sedimentation rate and C-reactive protein, two general measures of inflammation, can be helpful in differentiating inflammatory versus mechanical joint processes. Serial measurements can be used as markers to evaluate responses to therapy. However, they may not be useful in all patients.

Rheumatoid factor is an autoantibody with specificity for the FC portion of the IgG molecule. The IgM isotype is the most commonly assayed, but all isotypes of rheumatoid factor have been described. Seropositivity for rheumatoid factor in RA is correlated with the presence of nodules, more severe erosive disease, and HLA-DR4 positivity. In fact, rheumatoid factor negative RA is considered by many to represent a distinct disease entity with fewer erosions, more frequent remissions, and minimal extra-articular features. Rheumatoid factor is not, however, specific for RA and may be found in the sera of patients with a number of other systemic inflammatory diseases including autoimmune connective tissue diseases (systemic lupus erythematosus, Sjögren's syndrome, and overlap syndromes) and chronic infections (subacute bacterial endocarditis, tuberculosis, hepatitis). It is also important to note that the frequency of rheumatoid factor positivity (usually low titer) without an identifiable underlying illness increases with age.

Testing for HLA-DR4 and DR1 alleles in RA has not gained wide application in clinical practice, but it is useful in defining specific patient populations for research studies. It may prove useful as a marker for RA susceptibility in relatives of RA patients who present with inflammatory articular symptoms. It may also prove useful in identifying RA patients at the highest risk of severe disease, since this group more frequently has two doses of RA susceptibility alleles.[5]

There are no specific serological tests for the spondyloarthropathies. Determination of HLA-B27 status is not necessary when history, physical examination, and radiographic findings are consistent with spondyloarthropathy. In certain situations, testing for HLA-B27 can prove useful in supporting a diagnosis. These situations include the evaluation of juvenile spondylitis, recent-onset inflammatory low back pain without radiographic changes of sacroiliitis, inflammatory back or neck pain in middle-aged females, incomplete Reiter's syndrome, and limited (i.e., nonspondylitic) manifestations of AS.[11] However, the frequency of

HLA-B27 in the population must be kept in mind; it is 8% in the U.S. white population.

The radiographic changes of inflammatory arthritides often lag behind the articular symptoms by a period of months to years. Therefore, radiographs are not generally helpful in establishing a diagnosis in a patient with recent disease onset. Radiographs are useful in assessing the degree of joint damage and in following disease progression

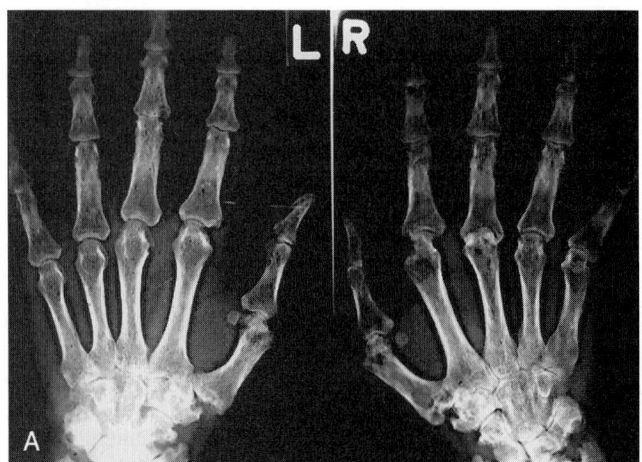

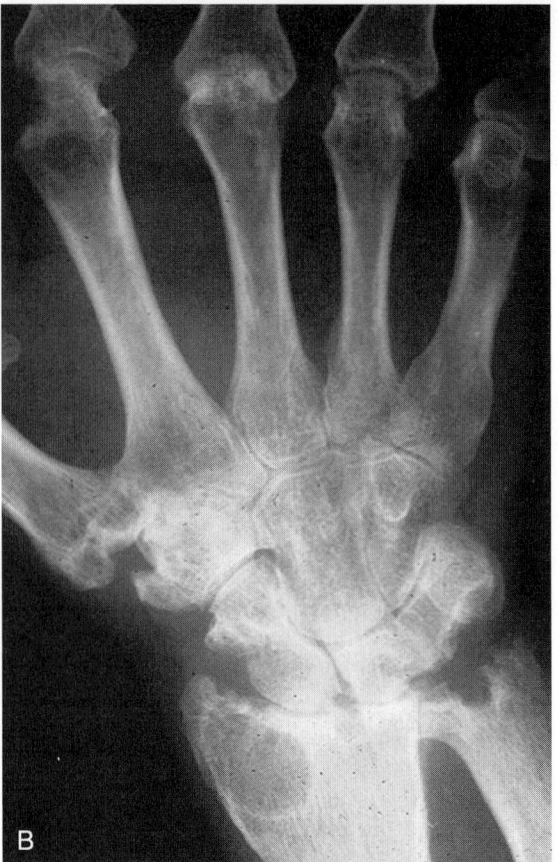

Fig. 3. Radiograph of the hands of a patient with long-standing (27 years) RA. *A,* Note the juxta-articular osteoporosis; joint space narrowing at the MCP, PIP and carpal joints; and extensive marginal erosions. *B,* The ulnar styloid erosion (enlarged view of the right hand) is characteristic of RA. (Courtesy of Dr. T. Benedek.)

as a function of therapy. The radiographic features of RA include juxta-articular osteoporosis (a relatively early finding), marginal erosions, and joint space narrowing (Fig. 3). Late in the course of RA subluxations and deformities may be observed and changes of secondary osteoarthritis may be present when the synovitis has "burned out."

In the spondyloarthropathies, radiographic sacroiliitis may be a relatively early finding and when present is strongly supportive of the diagnosis. Enthesitis of the spine is followed (after variable intervals) by syndesmophyte formation and subsequent bony ankylosis of the spine (bamboo spine). Enthesitis involving peripheral locations is frequently associated with periosteal new bone formation adjacent to the site of inflammation. Radiographs of peripheral joints in spondyloarthropathy patients may demonstrate pericapsular erosions, usually in conjunction with new bone formation, which distinguishes these from the marginal erosions of RA. When the erosions are pronounced, as may occur in psoriatic arthritis, they may lead to a "pencil in cup deformity," as shown in Figure 2.

DIFFERENTIAL DIAGNOSIS

The differential diagnosis of inflammatory arthritis is shown in Table 2. Early in the course of inflammatory arthritis, when the full extent or the pattern of joint in-

volvement is not yet evident, it may be difficult or impossible to establish an accurate diagnosis. Although at times frustrating for the patient and the physician, it is often better to allow a "tincture of time" to assist with defining the disease course and ultimate diagnosis, rather than to mislabel the patient. When extra-articular manifestations are present, they are often useful in narrowing the differential diagnosis.

In patients with established inflammatory arthritis, laboratory and radiographic studies can serve as important adjuncts to the history and physical examination in making a specific diagnosis. Evaluation of synovial fluid for crystals and infection is also essential when the clinical presentation raises suspicion of gout, pseudogout, or chronic infectious arthritis.

MANAGEMENT

The general approach is similar for all inflammatory arthritides: reduce inflammation, control pain, and preserve or restore function. A summary of the agents useful in the management of inflammatory arthritis is presented in Table 3. The cornerstone of medical management for inflammatory arthritis is the use of the nonsteroidal anti-inflammatory drugs (NSAIDs). The role of these agents is to suppress inflammation and to provide analgesia. The response to NSAIDs by patients is highly variable, and it is important to encourage at least a 6-week trial at a maximal tolerated dose before declaring the medication ineffective. Chronic administration of NSAIDs is not without hazard, however, and it is important to monitor patients closely for signs and symptoms of gastrointestinal side effects, impairment of renal function, and liver toxicity. Guidelines for the monitoring of toxicity of NSAIDs and other antirheumatic drugs are well-established.[12] Most of the experience with disease-modifying antirheumatic drugs has been in RA, although sulfasalazine, methotrexate, and cyclosporin A have been used in the spondyloarthropathies with some success.

In addition to medications to control pain and suppress inflammation, it is essential to include three other components in the management of patients with inflammatory arthritis: patient education, exercise, and assistive devices to facilitate activities of daily living. The process of patient education includes providing information regarding joint protection, compliance, medication toxicities, disease manifestations, and outcome. Often information can be provided in the way of detailed patient-oriented materials from the Arthritis Foundation or other support groups. Exercise, in particular stretching, posture, and nonimpact exercise programs (especially aquatics), are helpful for maintaining range of motion and improving strength. This is essential because deconditioning often increases stress on already inflamed or damaged joints and can lead to a downward spiral in function and mobility. It is beneficial to begin with a formal physical therapy program and have the patient receive training for a maintenance exercise program. Evaluation by the occupational therapist can often identify difficulties in routine aspects of daily life that can be improved by modifications of appliances or assistive devices.

TABLE 2. DIFFERENTIAL DIAGNOSIS OF INFLAMMATORY ARTHRITIS

Rheumatoid arthritis (RA)
  Seropositive RA
  Seronegative RA
Spondyloarthropathies
  Ankylosing spondylitis
  Reactive arthritis/Reiter's syndrome
  Psoriatic arthritis
  Inflammatory bowel disease–associated arthritis
Juvenile chronic arthritis (pediatric age group, see Chapter 9-8)
Other systemic inflammatory diseases associated with arthritis
  Systemic lupus erythematosus
  Sjögren's syndrome
  Systemic sclerosis (scleroderma)
  Polymyositis/dermatomyositis
  Mixed connective tissue disease ("overlap syndrome")
  Adult Still's disease
  Systemic vasculitis (e.g., Wegener's granulomatosis, polyarteritis nodosa)
  Polymyalgia rheumatica
  Sarcoidosis
Chronic infections associated with arthritis
  Whipple's disease
  Lyme disease
  Tuberculosis
  Fungal
  Viral (e.g., parvovirus)
  Subacute bacterial endocarditis
  Acute rheumatic fever
Crystalline arthropathies
  Calcium pyrophosphate dehydrate (CPPD) deposition disease (pseudogout, CPPD arthropathy)
  Gout
Amyloidosis

TABLE 3. MANAGEMENT OF INFLAMMATORY ARTHRITIS

Agent	Use	Special Considerations
Nonsteroidal anti-inflammatory drugs (NSAIDs)	Titrate to maximal tolerated dose or as necessary for control of pain, stiffness, and inflammation	Increased risk of gastrointestinal complications in patients with RA and in elderly. Consider using cyclooxygenase-2 selective NSAIDs or combined use of the prostaglandin E_1 analogue misoprostol or proton pump antagonist (omeprazole or lansoprazole) to reduce risk of gastric ulcers and bleeding; note the use of other agents (H2 blockers, sucralfate, antacids) to reduce gastrointestinal symptoms of NSAIDs should be avoided as they may mask symptoms and result in more severe complications (bleeding and perforation).
Narcotic analgesics	May need opioid analgesics for pain management and in particular for sleep	Preferable to avoid or limit the use of narcotics whenever possible, since patients with inflammatory arthritis are likely to have chronic pain that may be life-long.
Corticosteroids	Low-dose daily corticosteroids (prednisone 5–10 mg qd) are particularly helpful in reducing morning stiffness • Intra-articular corticosteroids are useful in flare of one or few joints and in the treatment of popliteal cyst • High-dose pulse steroids (methylprednisone 100–1000 mg IV qd × 3 days) can help control severe polyarticular flare of rheumatoid arthritis while beginning slow-acting DMARD[13]	Important to administer vitamin D 400 U/d and calcium supplement 1000–1500 mg qd in divided doses to help prevent bone loss; consider antiresorptive therapy (bisphosphonates, calcitonin) in patients found to be osteoporotic (e.g., by DEXA) or in high-risk groups
Disease-modifying antirheumatic drugs (DMARDs) Hydroxychloroquine Sulfasalazine Methotrexate Leflunamide Cyclosporin A Azathioprine Etanercept Infliximab		Recent studies have shown combination therapy to be superior to single agents.[14] Methotrexate is currently the current gold standard of DMARD monotherapy. Other agents (auranofin, intramuscular gold, D-penicillamine) are also effective, but long-term efficacy and tolerance due to side effects are poor. The DMARDs require regular monitoring for toxicity.[12]

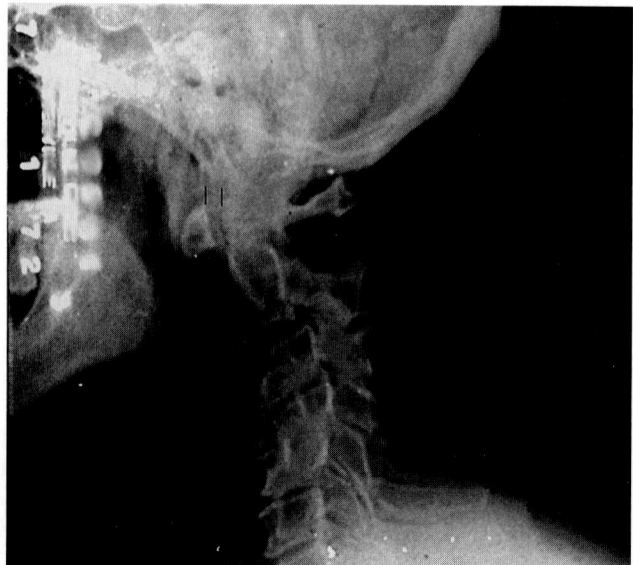

Fig. 4. Radiograph of the cervical spine of a 54-year-old patient with a 9-year history of RA. There is widening of the space between the odontoid process and the axial arch and severe malalignment and spondylosis of C2-C6. (Courtesy of Dr. T. Benedek.)

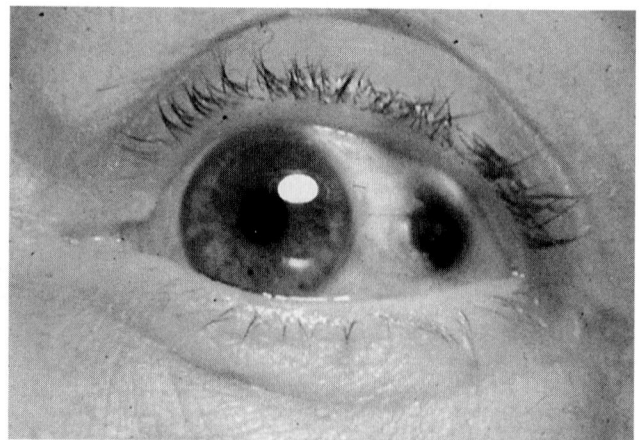

Fig. 5. Scleritis has resulted in scleromalacia perforans in this patient with RA. (Courtesy of Dr. T. Benedek.)

COMPLICATIONS

In spite of aggressive medical management, many patients with RA progress to severe joint destruction requiring total joint arthroplasty, most frequently of the knees. Hand deformities may require surgical intervention for cosmetic and functional improvement. Foot deformities frequently lead to difficulty with ambulation and pressure sores and may necessitate metatarsal resection or fusion. A severe complication of long-standing RA is cervical spine instability with C1-C2 subluxation (Fig. 4). This is particularly important to consider in the RA patient who is undergoing general anesthesia or has developed new occipital pain or neurological signs consistent with cervical cord compression. Persistent rheumatoid scleritis may result in scleromalacia perforans, an uncommon but serious ocular complication (Fig. 5).

Chronic inflammation of the hip joints in patients with AS and other spondyloarthropathies commonly leads to joint destruction, necessitating total hip arthroplasty. It is important to note that the rigid cervical spine in patients with AS (and others with spondylitis) may present difficulty in intubation, and there is a risk of fracturing the fused spine with manipulation. Cauda equina syndrome can occur in AS patients years after active inflammation has subsided.[15]

REFERENCES

1. Short CL: The antiquity of rheumatoid arthritis. Arth Rheum 1974; 17:193.
2. Frazer KJ: Anglo-French contributions to the recognition of rheumatoid arthritis. Ann Rheum Dis 1982; 41:335.
3. Lawrence RC, Helmick CG, Arnett FC, et al: Estimates of the prevalence of arthritis and selected musculoskeletal disorders in the United States. Arth Rheum 1998; 41: 778.
4. Lau CS, Burgos-Vargas R, Louthrenoo W, et al: Features of spondyloarthritis around the world. Rheum Dis Clin North Am 1998; 24:753.
5. Weyand CM, Goronzy JJ: The molecular basis of rheumatoid arthritis. J Mol Med 1997; 75:772.
6. Brennan FM, Zachariae CO, Chantry D, et al: Detection of interleukin-8 biological activity in synovial fluids from patients with rheumatoid arthritis and production of interleukin-8 mRNA by isolated synovial cells. Eur J Immunol 1990; 20:2141.
7. Muller-Ladner U, Gay RE, Gay S: Cellular pathways of joint destruction. Curr Opin Rheum 1997; 9:213.
8. Shumaker HR Jr: Reactive arthritis. Rheum Dis Clin North Am. 1998; 24:261.
9. Khare SD, Luthra HS, David CS: Animal models of human leukocyte antigen B27-linked arthritides. Rheum Dis Clin North Am 1998; 24:883.
10. Moll JM, Wright V: Psoriatic arthritis. Semin Arthritis Rheum 1973; 3:55.
11. Arnett FC: Histocompatibility typing in the rheumatic diseases: Diagnostic and prognostic implications. Rheum Dis Clin North Am 1994; 20:371.
12. Borigini MJ, Paulus HE: Rheumatoid arthritis. In: Weisman MH, Weinblatt ME (eds): Treatment of Rheumatic Diseases. Philadelphia: W.B. Saunders, 1995, p 31.
13. Iglehart IW III, Sutton JD, Bender JC, et al: Intravenous pulsed steroids in rheumatoid arthritis: A comparative dose study. J Rheum 1990; 17:159.
14. O'Dell JR: Triple therapy with methotrexate, sulfasalazine, and hydroxychloroquine in patients with rheumatoid arthritis. Rheum Dis Clin North Am 1998; 24:465.
15. Larner AJ, Pall HS, Hockley AD: Arrested progression of the cauda equina syndrome of ankylosing spondylitis after lumboperitoneal shunting J Neurol Neurosurg Psych 1996; 61:115.

section 6 chapter 4 CRYSTALLINE ARTHROPATHIES

Mary Chester M. Wasko and Timothy M. Wright

Summary
- Crystalline arthropathies are common causes of acute monoarthritis.
- Chronic forms of crystalline arthropathies may be confused with rheumatoid arthritis and osteoarthritis.
- The evaluation and treatment of crystalline arthropathies are different from those of other types of arthritis; therefore, establishing the correct diagnosis is mandatory for proper management.
- Arthrocentesis with polarized microscopic examination of synovial fluid is essential for accurate diagnosis.
- Acute and chronic treatment varies with the type of crystal deposition and the patient's other medical problems.

Gout and calcium pyrophosphate dihydrate (CPPD) deposition disease account for most cases of crystal-induced arthritis. The classic presentation of acute monoarthritis raises the suspicion of an underlying crystal-induced arthritis, but the clinical manifestations of chronic forms of these illnesses are far more protean and can be confused with rheumatoid arthritis and osteoarthritis. The crystalline arthropathies affect adults almost exclusively. However, they affect distinct patient subsets, produce different patterns of chronic joint disease with associated radiographic findings, and are managed somewhat differently. An understanding of these distinct clinical characteristics, coupled with appropriate synovial fluid examination and laboratory tests, will enable the clinician to establish the correct diagnosis and institute appropriate acute and long-term treatment.

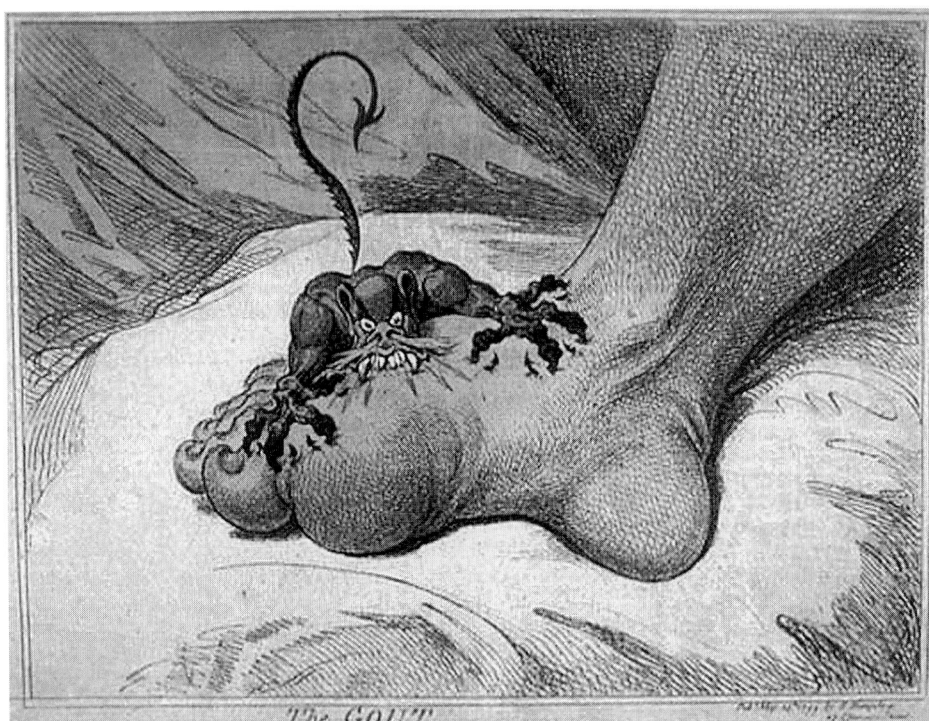

Fig. 1. Drawing by Gillray capturing the pain of "the gout."

Gout, the extremely painful acute joint inflammation (Fig. 1), due to the deposition of monosodium urate monohydrate (MSUM), has long been known as the "disease of kings." In fact, this arthritis historically has been attributed to an indulgent diet consisting of food and spirits high in purine content, afforded only by the wealthy. In modern times, gout has been recognized as a disease of middle-aged and older men and postmenopausal women, with men being affected at twice the rate of women (13.6/1000 men versus 6.4/1000 women).[1] Factors predisposing to hyperuricemia, such as renal insufficiency or the use of medications that alter uric acid metabolism and clearance, may result in high serum uric acid levels and clinical manifestations of gout. Although such factors can be modified to normalize the serum uric acid level in some cases, most cases of symptomatic hyperuricemia are idiopathic and require lifelong therapy.

In contrast to gout, CPPD deposition disease affects men and women equally, with a prevalence of clinical symptoms roughly half that of gout. In radiographic surveys, chondrocalcinosis, the radiographic correlate of CPPD deposition, is seen in 50% of individuals in the ninth decade of life.[2] Clinical features of CPPD deposition disease are more varied than in gout, and the CPPD crystals are more difficult to identify in synovial fluid, making the diagnosis more challenging to establish. Only about 25% of patients have a recognized condition predisposing to CPPD disease. In those with an underlying metabolic disease, such as hyperparathyroidism or hypomagnesemia, the condition may be easily corrected, but those with a familial predisposition can only be treated symptomatically.

PATHOGENESIS

The pathogenesis of crystal-induced arthritis can be divided into two parts. First, the mechanisms of crystal deposition, and second, the mechanisms underlying crystal-induced inflammation and joint damage. Uric acid is a normal by-product of purine metabolism. Hyperuricemia due to overproduction of uric acid may result from inherited metabolic defects (e.g., hypoxanthine-guanine phosphoribosyltransferase deficiency), excessive dietary intake of purine-rich foods, and states of increased cell turnover (psoriasis, hematological malignancies, cancer chemotherapy). The most common cause of hyperuricemia is underexcretion of uric acid. This may be due to an inherited defect in renal clearance or factors that reduce uric acid excretion such as renal insufficiency, lead toxicity, or medications (e.g., thiazide diuretics, furosemide, low-dose aspirin, cyclosporin A, and tacrolimus).

The accumulation of uric acid in tissues is dependent on sustained elevated serum uric acid levels that occur usually over the course of many years. High serum levels of uric acid lead to supersaturation of the extracellular fluids, leading to deposition of MSUM crystals in tissues when uric acid concentrations are in excess of 7 mg/dL, the aqueous solubility point of MSUM at 37°C. Although MSUM deposits (tophi) have been reported in many tissues, the most common sites are skin, synovial joints, and periarticular structures. It is important to note that asymptomatic hyperuricemia is common, and many patients with elevated uric acid levels never develop gout. Also, in the setting of acute gout, the serum uric acid level may be elevated, normal, or decreased. It is generally accepted that flux in uric acid levels (up or down) may precipitate an attack, and it is hypothesized that this is due to rapid expansion or fragmentation of MSUM crystals that induce an inflammatory response.

Deposition of CPPD results from the accumulation of another cellular metabolite of nucleic acid (nucleoside triphosphate) metabolism, namely pyrophosphate (PP_i). Normally, the production of PP_i is followed by its conversion to inorganic phosphate by pyrophosphatases. This is an enzyme- and magnesium-dependent process that can be inhibited by certain ions (Fe, Cu). The precise reasons for accumulation of PP_i and complexing with calcium ion in CPPD deposition disease are not clear. However, recent studies suggest that alterations in PP_i metabolic enzymes occur in older individuals.[3] In support of the role of altered pyrophosphatase enzyme activity in the pathogenesis of CPPD deposition disease are the associations with Wilson's disease, hemochromatosis, and hypomagnesemia. The accumulation of CPPD crystals generally occurs in hyaline cartilage (seen radiographically as chondrocalcinosis), tendons, bursae, synovium, and ligaments.

The pathogenesis of crystal-induced inflammation is believed to be similar regardless of the type of crystal. The accumulation of crystalline material (e.g., MSUM, CPPD) in the joint or periarticular tissues is asymptomatic and in most cases occurs over the course of many years. It is proposed that the inflammatory response is induced by the shedding of crystals into synovial fluid, the rapid expansion and dissolution of crystals in periarticular tissues, or changes in the protein coating of the crystals. The latter mechanism may involve coating crystals with immunoglobulin G, thereby promoting F_c receptor–mediated phagocytosis of crystals by polymorphonuclear neutrophil leukocytes (PMNs) and monocytes with the subsequent release of inflammatory mediators. Although the initial sequence of events is not clear, a recent study of MSUM crystal–induced inflammation in a rabbit model demonstrated that intra-articular injection of MSUM crystals resulted in the rapid production of interleukin-8 (IL-8, a potent PMN che-

moattractant) by synovial lining cells that preceded PMN accumulation.[4] Neutralization of IL-8 activity in their model using anti-IL-8 antibody resulted in reduced joint swelling and reduced PMN infiltration in response to MSUM crystals.

Other crystals are also associated with joint pathology. These include calcium oxalate crystals seen in renal failure patients, and calcium hydroxyapatite (basic calcium phosphate) crystals associated with a syndrome of calcific periarthritis, tendinitis, and destructive arthritis ("Milwaukee shoulder").[5, 6] These entities are relatively uncommon and are not discussed further in this chapter but are comprehensively reviewed elsewhere.

CLINICAL FEATURES

The clinical manifestations of gout follow a prolonged period, usually at least a decade, of asymptomatic hyperuricemia. The onset of acute gouty arthritis depends on the degree and duration of hyperuricemia. Often a discrete precipitating event, such as excess ethanol consumption, hospitalization for an acute illness, surgery, or trauma antedates an attack. The initial attack of gout usually occurs in a single lower extremity joint. The first metatarsophalangeal (MTP) joint is most commonly affected during the first bout. Acute gout at this site is known as podagra. Subsequent attacks may affect up to two or three joints, and rarely more. The shoulders, spine, and hips are virtually spared, perhaps owing to the warmer temperature of the joints near the torso. Polyarticular gout is relatively uncommon. It is most often associated with a chronic course of untreated tophaceous gout or with marked elevations of serum uric acid accompanying chronic renal insufficiency or immunosuppressive therapy with cyclosporin A or tacrolimus.

The pain in an acutely inflamed gouty joint is exquisite. It develops over a few hours, escalating to the point that the weight of a bedsheet is unbearable. The joint rapidly becomes swollen, red, and hot, often followed by desquamation of overlying skin as the attack remits (Fig. 2).

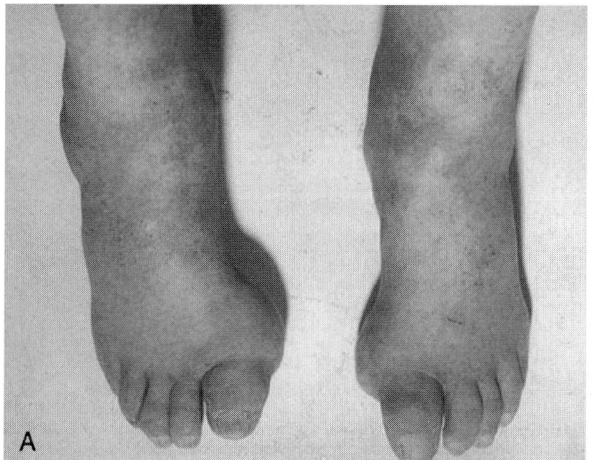
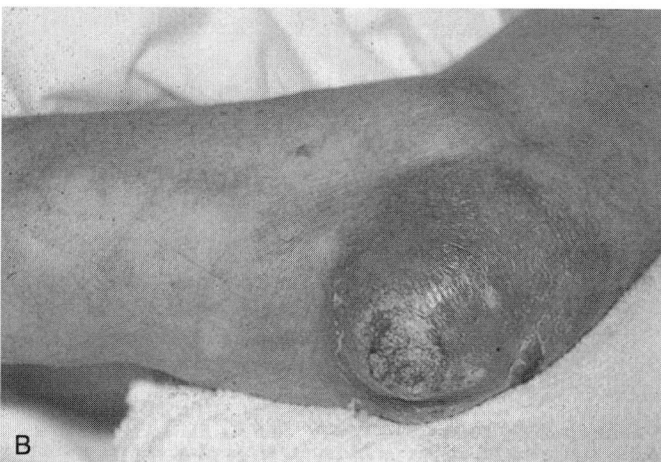

Fig. 2. Acute gout. This involves the MTP joints bilaterally *(A)* and the olecranon bursa *(B)*. Note the tophaceous material visible subcutaneously in the olecranon bursa and the intense erythema with desquamation. (Courtesy of Dr. T. Benedek.)

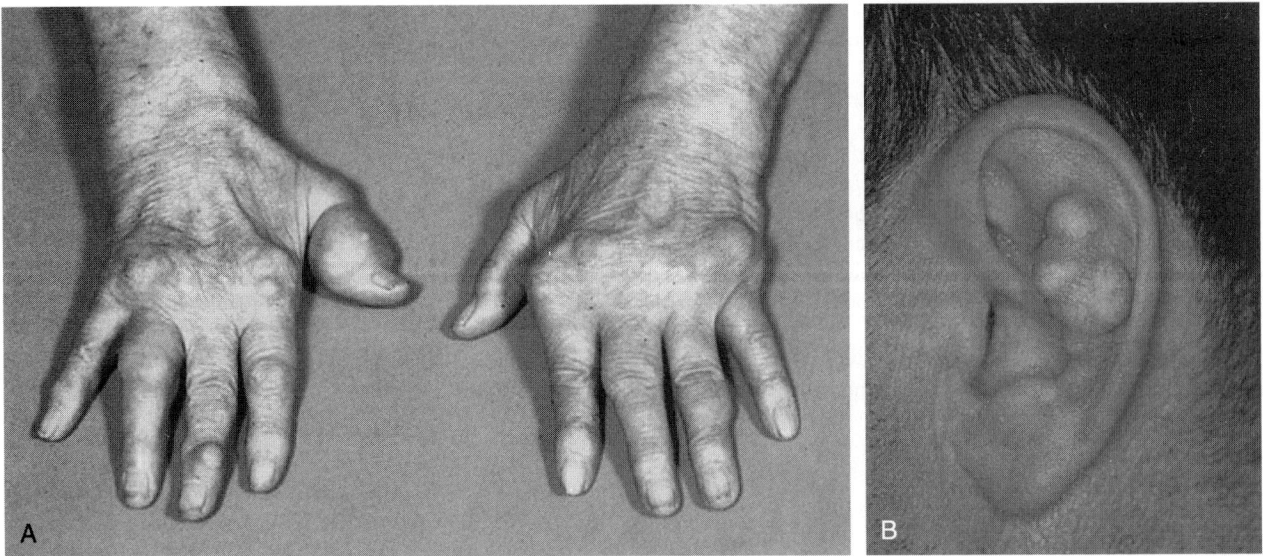

Fig. 3. Tophi. These are on the extensor surfaces of both hands *(A)* and antihelix of the auricle *(B)*. (Courtesy of Dr. T. Benedek.)

Fever and chills may accompany the joint symptoms. If untreated, most attacks will spontaneously subside within 3 to 14 days. Following a variable period of quiescence, often lasting over a year, acute gout recurs in over 90% of those affected. In subsequent attacks, the same joint or others may be involved, though again the joints near core body temperature are usually spared.

Tophaceous gout follows many years of sustained hyperuricemia. The presence of tophi on examination reflects total body stores of MSUM in excess of 30 times the normal amount. They occur over olecranon bursae, extensor surfaces of the finger joints, Achilles tendons, and first MTPs most frequently (Fig. 3). While usually asymptomatic, tophi may spontaneously drain chalky paste as they erode through skin. Examination of a simple touch preparation of this material (or a needle aspirate of a non-draining tophus) reveals sheets of MSUM crystals.

The renal manifestations of hyperuricemia include uric acid renal calculi, chronic interstitial nephritis, and acute renal failure seen in tumor lysis syndrome. The history of a prior kidney stone or chronic renal insufficiency in conjunction with episodic gouty arthritis warrants further search for underlying renal disease, as those patients should be managed long-term with a xanthine oxidase inhibitor to block uric acid production rather than a uricosuric, which might precipitate stone formation or worsening renal function (see later discussion).

The CPPD deposition disease may manifest as chondro-

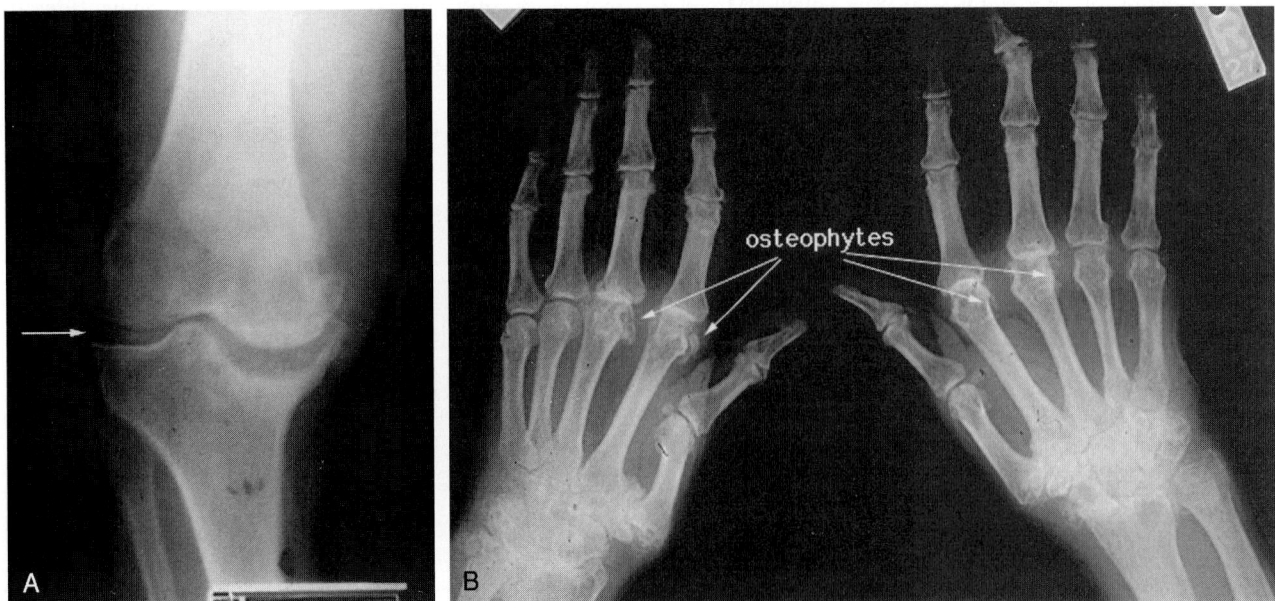

Fig. 4. Radiographs of CPPD deposition disease. Shown are chondrocalcinosis of the meniscal cartilage *(A)* and a radiograph of the hands demonstrating marked osteoarthritic changes at the wrist and the second and third MCP joints bilaterally *(B)*.

calcinosis, acute pseudogout, chronic arthropathy, or a combination of these. Chondrocalcinosis is defined as radiographically apparent CPPD deposition in hyaline or fibrocartilage, most commonly the knee menisci (Fig. 4A), symphysis pubis, and triangular fibrocartilage of the wrist. Acute pseudogout, as the name implies, clinically mimics attacks of acute gout, with abrupt onset of pain, swelling, and erythema of the affected joint or bursa. However, the attacks less frequently affect the first MTP and more often involve the knee or wrist. Synovial fluid examination is necessary to establish the correct diagnosis and rule out infection. Similar to gout, the attacks of pseudogout usually remit over the course of 1 to 2 weeks and often recur.

Chronic CPPD arthropathy shares features of osteoarthritis (OA) and rheumatoid arthritis (RA), both clinically and radiographically. Persistent, usually low-grade, stiffness, pain, and swelling occur in joints of a distribution seen in RA—the wrists, metacarpophalangeals (MCPs), and proximal interphalangeals. However, in contrast to RA, palpation of the joints reveals not only soft tissue and synovial hypertrophy, but also bony enlargement typical of OA. Radiographs demonstrate characteristic changes of OA in the MCP and wrist joints (Fig. 4B), which are not sites of primary osteoarthritis.

INVESTIGATION

Synovial fluid analysis is essential to establish the diagnosis of crystal-induced arthritis. An attack of acute gout or pseudogout is confirmed only by identification of MSUM or CPPD crystals within PMNs. Joint aspiration also is indicated to rule out infection. As septic arthritis may occur simultaneously with acute crystal-induced arthritis, joint fluid should always be sent for cell count with differential, glucose, Gram stain, and culture. Even a small amount of fluid in the hub of the aspirating needle can be adequate for crystal analysis and culture. Numerous other conditions may be confused with acute gout or pseudogout, including peripheral arthritis associated with rheumatoid arthritis, spondyloarthropathy, and acute sarcoidosis. See Differential Diagnosis section.

Using a microscope equipped with polarizing filters and a first-order red compensator to examine synovial fluid, the physician can promptly and definitively establish the diagnosis of acute gout or pseudogout. Both MSUM and CPPD crystals have a characteristic shape and are birefringent when viewed under polarized light. MSUM crystals are needle-shaped and appear yellow when parallel to the axis of the red compensator in polarized light, and blue when perpendicular (an easy pneumonic: YUP = yellow, urate, parallel). The CPPD crystals of pseudogout, by contrast, are rhomboid, rod-shaped, or square and appear blue when parallel to the axis of the red compensator in polarized light (the opposite of MSUM). It is important to note that surgical specimens to be examined for crystals should not be placed in formalin fixative, which will dissolve MSUM crystals.[8]

Radiographs may be helpful during the first attack of crystalline arthritis, although this is more often the case with pseudogout than with gout. The radiographic findings of gout result from pressure of soft tissue or articular tophi on adjacent bony structures, leading to pressure erosions in

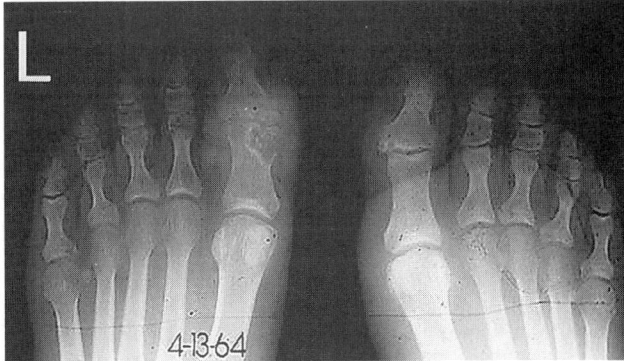

Fig. 5. Radiograph of tophaceous gout. This demonstrates partial destruction of the interphalangeal joint of the great toe on the left foot with overhanging edges surrounding the eroded area (left panel) and a small erosion with sclerotic margins at the interphalangeal joint of the great toe on the right foot. (Courtesy of Dr. T. Benedek.)

bone with a characteristic overhanging edge (Fig. 5). These have been described as resembling a rat bite taken out of bone. Tophi do not usually calcify and simply appear as a soft tissue mass on radiograph. However, because tophi do not develop until years following the first attack of acute gout, radiographs are seldom useful in establishing the diagnosis.

In contrast, the finding of chondrocalcinosis may be asymptomatic and antedate the onset of acute pseudogout. In the setting of an acutely inflamed joint, chondrocalcinosis found on the radiograph should alert the physician to the possible diagnosis of pseudogout. Radiographs in chronic CPPD arthropathy demonstrate osteoarthritic changes in atypical locations, in the absence of preceding trauma. Joint space narrowing, sclerosis, and osteophyte formation in the wrists, MCPs, and proximal interphalangeals typify hand radiographs in chronic CPPD arthropathy (see Fig. 4). These findings distinguish CPPD arthropathy radiographically from RA (characterized by osteopenia and periarticular erosions) with which it may be confused clinically. Other findings suggestive of CPPD arthropathy include scapholunate dissociation with scapholunate advanced collapse deformity in the wrist, and preferential patellofemoral narrowing and osteophytes with relative sparing of the medial and lateral compartments of the knee.

DIFFERENTIAL DIAGNOSIS

The differential diagnosis of acute gout and pseudogout is that of acute monoarthritis.[7] It is important to keep in mind this differential when approaching a patient with no prior history of arthritis as well as patients who have had prior episodes of crystal-induced arthritis (Table 1). In particular, it is important to evaluate the possibility of infection, and hence the need in most cases for immediate joint aspiration. Although strongly supportive of sepsis if extraordinarily high (over 100,000/mm³), cell counts in the synovial fluid can be misleading since there is overlap between elevated cell counts seen in septic and crystal-induced arthritis, and the cell type is predominantly PMNs in both cases. It is prudent, therefore, to send all monoarthritis

TABLE 1. DIFFERENTIAL DIAGNOSIS OF ACUTE GOUT AND PSEUDOGOUT

Septic arthritis
Septic bursitis
Cellulitis
Trauma
Hemarthrosis (hemophilia, anticoagulation therapy, subchondral fracture)
New-onset inflammatory arthritis
    Rheumatoid arthritis (presenting as monarthritis or oligoarthritis)
    Spondyloarthropathy (especially reactive arthritis or Reiter's syndrome)
    Sarcoid (acute periarthritis)

strate the classic periarticular "punched out" lesions with overhanging edges indicative of MSUM deposits. CPPD arthropathy often appears clinically as an inflammatory form of OA with a pattern of joint involvement typical of RA. The diagnosis of CPPD arthropathy is supported by the findings of radiographs demonstrating chondrocalcinosis and/or osteoarthritic changes in the MCPs and wrist (and the absence of marginal erosions), absence of extra-articular manifestations, and CPPD crystals in synovial fluid.

MANAGEMENT

Treatment for an acute attack of crystal-induced arthritis focuses on control of inflammation and pain management. Nonsteroidal anti-inflammatory drugs (NSAIDs) are effective and readily tolerated therapy in the otherwise healthy patient. Usually these medications promptly and effectively control pain and inflammation. Table 2 gives dosing guidelines and other treatment options.

In the absence of tophi or other indications for therapy to reduce uric acid (uric acid nephropathy or nephrolithiasis, chronic renal insufficiency, ongoing chemotherapy for malignancy), patients with a single attack of gout do not warrant further treatment for hyperuricemia. Correcting underlying factors that predispose to hyperuricemia should be made. These include elimination of drugs producing hyperuricemia, such as low-dose salicylates, thiazide diuretics, and cyclosporin, whenever possible, and avoidance of foods and beverages with high purine content. Infrequent

synovial fluid samples for polarized microscopy, Gram stain, and culture.

In the case of chronic forms of crystal-induced arthritis, the differential diagnosis is more limited and includes rheumatoid arthritis (and other inflammatory arthritides), osteoarthritis, and neuropathic joint disease (Charcot's joints). In the case of gout, the distinction is made based on the pattern of joint involvement (sparing axial and proximal joints), hyperuricemia, synovial fluid crystals, and, when present, uric acid nephrolithiasis or tophi. Radiographs, although not usually helpful in early acute gout, may demon-

TABLE 2. MANAGEMENT OF ACUTE GOUT AND PSEUDOGOUT

Agent	Use	Special Considerations
Nonsteroidal anti-inflammatory drugs (NSAIDs)	Maximal dose (e.g., indomethacin 50 mg three times a day) for 3 days, then taper gradually over 10 days	Adjust doses downward for geriatric patients and those at higher risk for NSAID complications. Traditional NSAIDs are contraindicated in patients with renal insufficiency, liver disease, coagulopathy, or peptic ulcer disease. The newer cyclooxygenase-2 specific inhibitors may be useful in the latter two situations.
Corticosteroids	Prednisone 40 mg qd for 3 days, then tapered off over 10 days Intravenous solumedrol 8–12 mg every 8 hours, tapered off over 10 days	Intra-articular corticosteroids are effective for monoarticular involvement with minimal systemic effects compared with oral and parenteral drugs. Patients with glucose intolerance should be monitored carefully for hyperglycemia following corticosteroid administration. Hypertension and fluid retention may accompany corticosteroid therapy. Those with known psychiatric disease or mood lability from prior steroid use should be cautioned and observed for steroid-induced exacerbations.
Adrenocorticotropic hormone (ACTH)	ACTH 40 to 80 U IM or IV every 8 hours for 2–3 days	ACTH may work via stimulation of endogenous cortisol production.[9] However, in patients on chronic corticosteroid therapy, such as in the organ transplant population, ACTH is effective in treating acute gout, suggesting other mechanisms of action.
Colchicine	Colchicine 0.6 mg orally every 1–2 hours (up to 8 mg total) until the attack subsides or gastrointestinal toxicity (nausea, vomiting, abdominal pain, or diarrhea) occurs	Colchicine's efficacy is greater for acute gout than pseudogout, and for those attacks of less than 24 hours' duration. Because it is likely to induce diarrhea and ambulation is difficult with acute attacks affecting the lower extremities, other treatment options are preferable. Dosage should be reduced in patients with hepatic or renal insufficiency and in the elderly. Intravenous colchicine therapy is **not recommended** because of the narrow therapeutic window and the risk of fatal complications.

recurrent attacks of gout can be managed acutely and may be effectively suppressed with daily low-dose colchicine (0.6 mg qd or bid) or NSAIDs.

If the patient has recurrent disabling attacks of gout (three to four per year) or other indications for uric acid lowering therapy (see earlier), further evaluation is necessary to determine appropriate long-term management of hyperuricemia. Options vary, depending on whether a patient is a uric acid underexcretor (<600 to 1000 mg uric acid/24 hour urine collection) or overproducer. Underexcretors with creatinine clearance greater than 50 mL/min may be managed with a uricosuric agent such as probenecid as long as compliance with increased fluid intake to prevent stone formation can be assured. The presence of tophi, uric acid renal calculi, chronic renal insufficiency, or uric acid overproduction are indications for use of the xanthine oxidase inhibitor allopurinol. In either case, the goal is to maintain the serum uric acid level at approximately 5 mg/dL. Uric acid lowering therapy should not be instituted during the course of an acute attack and should be delayed until after the attack has completely resolved (usually 4 to 6 weeks). It should be instituted in conjunction with low-dose NSAID or colchicine prophylaxis. Continued anti-inflammatory therapy (low-dose NSAID or colchicine) is necessary for several months after the target reduction of serum uric acid is achieved to prevent precipitating an acute gouty attack. If the serum uric acid level is lowered effectively, tophaceous deposits will resorb over the course of months to years.

Chronic management of patients with CPPD deposition disease is less satisfactory, in that only 25% have an identifiable metabolic disorder linked to their joint disease. Daily low-dose colchicine (0.6 mg qd or bid) may aid in preventing acute attacks, although this is not as effective as in gout. No specific treatment to modify calcium, pyrophosphate, and cartilage metabolism has been effective. For patients with chronic CPPD arthropathy, NSAIDs and low-dose corticosteroids may suppress synovitis. In otherwise healthy patients over the age of 50 with CPPD deposition disease, the only cost-effective screening is a serum calcium and parathyroid hormone level in search of occult hyperparathyroidism.

REFERENCES

1. Lawrence RC, Hochberg MC, Kelsey JL, et al: Estimates of the prevalence of selected arthritic and musculoskeletal diseases in the United States. J Rheumatol 1989; 16:427.
2. Ryan LM, McCarty DJ: Calcium pyrophosphate crystal deposition disease: Pseudogout, articular chondrocalcinosis. In McCarty DJ, Koopman WJ (eds): Arthritis and Allied Conditions: A Textbook of Rheumatology, 12th ed. Philadelphia, Lea & Febiger, 1993, p 1835.
3. Rosenthal AK: Calcium crystal-associated arthritides. Curr Opin Rheum 1998; 10: 273.
4. Nishimura A, Akahoshi T, Takahashi M, et al: Attenuation of monosodium urate crystal-induced arthritis in rabbits by a neutralizing antibody against interleukin-8. J Leukocyte Biol 1997; 62:444.
5. Schumaker HR Jr: Other crystals. In Klippel JH, Dieppe PA (eds): Rheumatology. London, Mosby-Year Book, 1994, p 17.5.1.
6. Uri DS, Dalinka MK: Crystal disease. Radiol Clin North Am 1966; 34:359.
7. Sack K: Monarthritis: Differential diagnosis. Am J Med 1997; 102:30S.
8. Simkin PA, Bassett JE, Lee QP: Not water, but formalin, dissolves urate crystals in tophaceous tissue samples. J Rheumatol 1994; 21:2320.
9. Ritter J, Kerr LD, Valeriano-Marcet J, et al: ACTH revisited: Effective treatment for acute crystal induced synovitis in patients with multiple medical problems. J Rheumatol 1994; 21:696.

section **6** chapter **5**

NEUROPATHIC ARTHROPATHIES

John S. Kirchner

Summary

- Charcot's arthropathy is a painless destructive disorder of the joints. After the etiology of the neuropathic condition can be established, treatment should be initiated. Treatment begins with control of the joint to prevent further destruction. After the reaction has subsided, treatment focuses on patient education and correction of deformities to prevent subsequent injury and deformities. With proper management, patient function can be optimized.

INTRODUCTION

Neuropathic arthropathies, known also as Charcot's arthropathies, were named after Jean Martin Charcot in 1868 after his description of a patient who had contracted tabes dorsalis.[1] Neuropathic arthropathies, when unrecognized and untreated, can result in joint destruction, loss of joint congruity, and altered overall bony architecture because of lack of protective sensation. This alteration of the bony architecture can lead to significant deformities that not only can cause high-contact pressure areas but also can affect

TABLE 1. OTHER ETIOLOGIES OF PERIPHERAL NEUROPATHIES
1. Tabes dorsalis
2. Leprosy
3. Syringomelia
4. Spina bifida
5. Meningomyelocele
6. Congenital insensitivity to pain
7. Chronic alcoholism
8. Spinal cord injury or compression
9. Peripheral nerve injuries

the patient's ability to ambulate and to perform normal activities of daily living. Although this condition is most commonly found in patients with diabetes mellitus (both insulin dependent and non–insulin dependent), other etiologies do exist. These etiologies are based on the presence of peripheral neuropathy and are listed in Table 1.[2] A common characteristic of all these disorders is the absence of or decrease in pain or protective sensation. This allows continued microtrauma to occur to the joints. This causes microfractures, subluxations, and dislocations that lead to progressive deformity. Evaluation and treatment are directed to prevention of injury or prevention of progression of the patient's deformities.[3] Progressive deformities can lead to areas of high-contact pressure, breakdown ulcers, subsequent infection, and osteomyelitis. These infections can lead to extended hospital stays and can necessitate partial or radical amputations. If infections continue to progress, sepsis and loss of life can occur.

PATHOGENESIS

Most modern literature centers around diabetic neuropathic arthropathies. Since the advent of treatment for syphilis, diabetes has become the most common and documented cause of neuropathic arthropathy.[4] Neurological dysfunction with diabetes involves both vascular and metabolic alterations.[5] Thought originally to be only a microvascular disease, diabetes has been found to also be a macrovascular entity. Atherosclerosis is more common and more severe in diabetic patients than in nondiabetic patients. Atherosclerosis occurs earlier, progresses at an increased rate, and is more often bilateral. Atherosclerosis in diabetic arteries is diffusely distributed along the vessel length, leading to a "lead pipe" appearance on radiographs.[6] The increased rate of atherosclerosis increases the tendencies for both clotting and thrombosis. This compromise in blood supply can lead to ischemia and subsequent cell death.

Along with the compromise in blood supply to the nerves that leads to cell death, alterations in the metabolic pathways are found in diabetics. The metabolic alterations are due to an alternative pathway through which glucose must be metabolized because there is a lack of insulin. Within the nerves themselves, there is a buildup of sorbitol and fructose and a decrease in the quantity of *myo*-inositol and sodium potassium–adenosine triphosphatase (ATPase).

The buildup of sorbitol and fructose, with the lack of sodium potassium–ATPase, leads to destruction of the sodium pump, which leads to depolarization, demyelination, nerve injuries, and subsequent nerve death.[7, 8] These alterations occur within both the small and the large myelinated fibers. This loss of small and large fibers causes progression in the losses of proprioception, light touch, and pain. As a result of the loss of pain and protective sensation, the patient will continue to cause increased stresses across the foot, leading to microfractures, cartilage degeneration, loss of normal joint congruity, subluxations, dislocations, and subsequent deformities.

Along with the loss of myelinated fibers, the patient will begin to have an autonomic neuropathy, leading to the inability to thermoregulate the extremity. This can lead to periods of flushing followed by periods of vasoconstriction. The autonomic neuropathy can cause anhidrosis that leads to drying of the skin, increased callus formation, and subsequent fissuring and cracking. This results in avenues for infection and ulceration.[9] With the loss of autonomic regulation, patients will develop periods of hyperemia that cause increased blood flow to the foot, which can lead to increased reabsorption of the mineral matrix.[10] This loss of mineral matrix can cause progressive weakening of the microstructure, leading to an increased chance for microfractures and deformities to occur.

CLINICAL PRESENTATION

During early stages of neuropathy the patient presents with occasional radiating paresthesia, hypersensitivity, and a "pins and needles" feeling within a nerve distribution. These symptoms continue to evolve, and the patient will start to complain of a more global paresthesia similar to the frequently documented "stocking glove" distribution. However, the proximal border is not usually complete.[11] As continuing cell death proceeds, the patient will begin to lose protective sensation. Loss of protective sensation is confirmed when the patient is unable to feel a 5.07 Semmes-Weinstein monofilament.[12] Along with the loss of small myelinated fibers, large myelinated fibers become ischemic, causing the patient to lose some muscle mass and therefore lose balance control, leading to an ataxic gait.[13] This ataxia can cause increased microtraumatic events as well as macrotraumatic events, leading to increased stresses and subsequent injuries to the involved joints.

The patient will present with a warm, swollen, potentially tender foot or ankle, depending on the severity of the neuropathy. The patient may or may not be able to recount a traumatic or inciting event. The patient may also have a history of previous infections, chronic fissures, hyperkeratotic lesions, nonhealing ulcers, and wounds. Many patients will have seen two or three other physicians before presentation in your office. Not infrequently, a history of hospital admission for intravenous antibiotics and elevation with resolution of symptoms will be present. The patient will also state that the appearance of the foot has been changing. Most patients with advanced neuropathy will usually complain of no pain or of an occasional burning or paresthesia. Some patients who have not progressed to profound

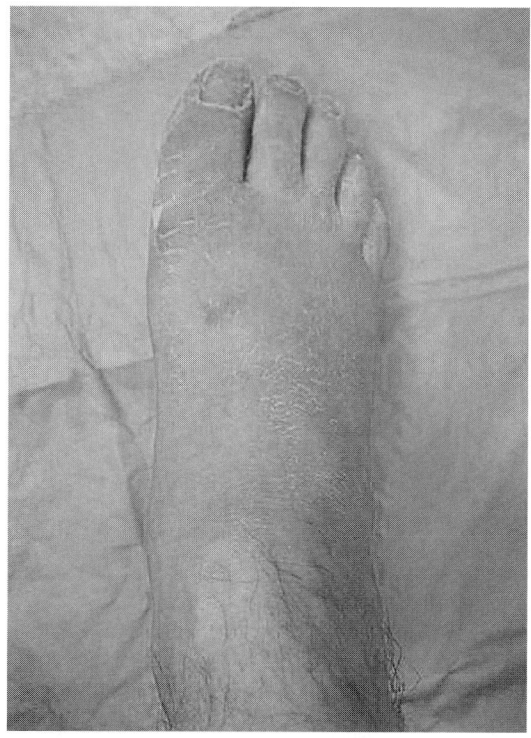

Fig. 1. Typical presentation of Charcot's joint. The joint is warm, edematous, and erythematous. Note the dry, tight appearance with lack of follicular growth.

neuropathy will complain of mild to moderate pain and discomfort.

On physical examination, most patients have some degree of obesity. Physical examination of the foot usually reveals a swollen and erythematous foot that is warm to the touch (Fig. 1).[14] The morphology of the foot varies with the stage, the pattern, and the previous Charcot's reactions. Frequently there are calluses and hyperkeratotic lesions located over the toes as well as on the plantar aspect of the foot. The patient's sensation varies with the degree of neuropathy present and can range from a slight loss of sensation to hypersensitivity to a dense neuropathy preventing adequate protective plantar sensation. The latter presentation is most likely if the patient has true Charcot's neuropathic arthropathy. Because artherosclerosis is extremely common within the diabetic population, pulses can occasionally be elicited in the noncompressible vessels. The skin will usually be shiny, tight, and dry, and follicular growth is usually not present on the patient's foot or lower extremity. The vasculopathy does not usually correlate well with the arthropathy itself, and palpable pulses are frequently present, along with significant alterations in sensation.[15]

INVESTIGATIONS

Laboratory work-up should consist of complete blood count, erythrocyte sedimentation rate, and glycosylated hemoglobin level. Good glucose control that decreases meta-

bolic by-products may assist in decreasing the rate of progression of the neuropathy itself.[16] However, no good clinical trials substantiate this hypothesis.[17]

Standing anteroposterior and lateral radiographs with a non-weightbearing oblique should be obtained and will closely correlate with the stage, pattern, and degree of neuropathic arthropathy. Early findings frequently include joint widening and stress fractures. Later changes include loss of joint space with sclerosis and fragmentation. As Charcot's neuropathy progresses, subsequent subluxation, dislocation, and alteration of the morphology of the foot are frequently found. Because of the increased sympathetic tone, osteoporosis is frequently present.[18]

A vascular work-up should be performed, especially if any invasive intervention to the foot is debated. This should include ankle brachial as well as toe brachial indices and patterns. Although these can be initially reliable, as further atherosclerosis of the patient's vessels continues, they can become misleading. Therefore, segmental pressures and waveforms can be very useful in the initial work-up. Transcutaneous partial oxygen pressure (tcPO$_2$) has frequently been used to evaluate the viability of the soft tissues. A tcPO$_2$ of around 20 is equivocal for wound healing. Therefore, a tcPO$_2$ of 30 or greater is a good indication that the soft tissues are viable and are capable of healing.[19, 20]

CLASSIFICATION

The disease process can be divided into three radiographically distinct stages as described by Eichenholtz[21] (Table 2). The first stage is the stage of development and fragmentation. This represents the acute destructive phase and is distinguishable by joint effusions, soft-tissue swelling, cartilage debris, intra-articular fractures, and fragmentation of the bone. These are usually initiated by a minimal traumatic event with continued ambulation and joint stresses on the extremity. Continued trauma causes further microfractures and stresses to propagate greater destruction. The second stage, the stage of coalescence, follows with lessening edema, healing of the fractures, and absorption of small debris. The final stage, the stage of consolidation or remodeling, demonstrates continuing repair or remodeling of the bone into its new morphology.

Charcot joints can be classified into basic anatomic regions that direct the treatment plan (Fig. 2).[22] Type 1 involves the midfoot regions (i.e., the metatarsal cuneiform and the metatarsal cuboid), as well as the navicular cuneiform joints. Type 1 is the most common and represents approximately 60% of all Charcot's feet. Type 1 Charcot's joints are typified by development of symptomatic bony prominences, occurrence of rocker-bottom

TABLE 2. EICHENHOLTZ STAGES
Stage 1: Development and fragmentation
Stage 2: Coalescence
Stage 3: Consolidation

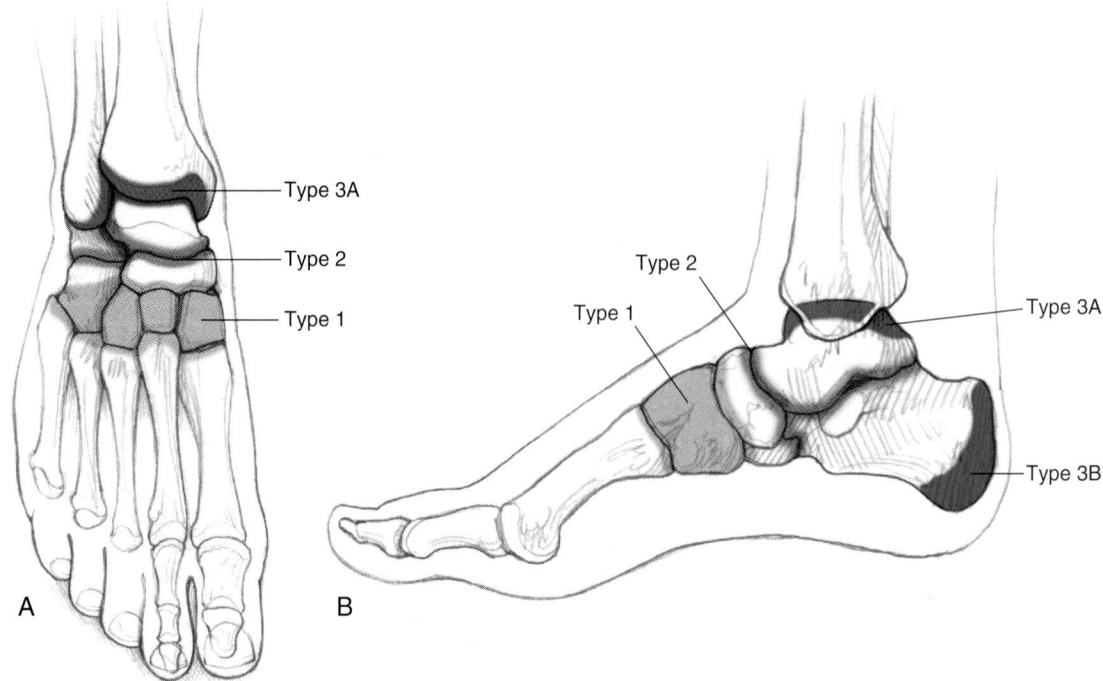

Fig. 2. Classification of Charcot's joints of the foot and ankle by anatomic region. (From Coughlin MJ, Mann RA: Surgery of the Foot and Ankle, 7th ed. Mosby, St. Louis, 1999, p 949.)

feet, or severe midfoot valgus deformities (Figs. 3 and 4). These bony prominences produce increased pressure leading to persistent ulceration on the plantar surface at the level of the midfoot (Fig. 5). These patients usually have a

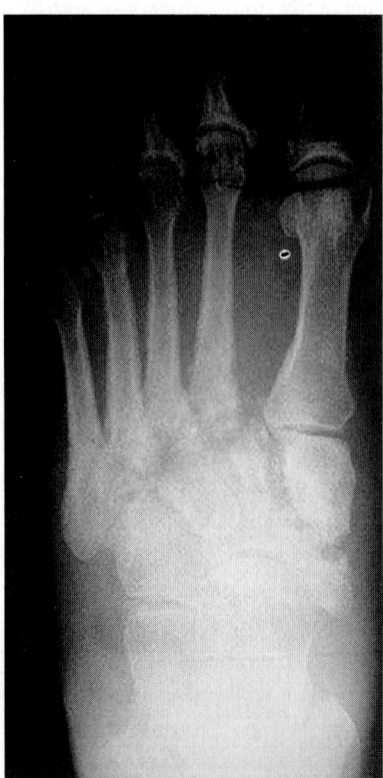

Fig. 3. Anteroposterior radiograph of type I Charcot's joint. Note the involvement of the tarsometatarsal and navicular cuneiform joints.

shorter period of immobilization necessary for bone healing and a lower likelihood of the necessity for long-term immobilization. They also have a higher proportion of hypertrophic bony changes and a lower incidence of erosive changes.

Type 2 Charcot's joints involve the hindfoot (i.e., the subtalar, talonavicular, and calcaneocuboid joints) (Figs. 6 and 7). These account for approximately 30% to 35% of Charcot's joints. These patients usually present with chronic, persistent skeletal instability. Although the ulcerations can occur on occasion from symptomatic bony prominences, many of these patients will not develop ulcerations. These patients tend to require longer periods of immobilization until Eichenholtz stage 2 or 3 has been noted. The subsequent deformity that occurs is usually beyond what can be easily contained in normal footwear and will usually displace off the normal weightbearing axis, causing the patient to have progressive deformities.

Type 3 Charcot's joints are split into two subgroups, type 3A and type 3B. Type 3A is associated with the tibiotalar joint. Type 3B is associated with the os calcis, with a pathological fracture of the tuberosity and subsequent pes planus deformity. Both type 3A and type 3B deformities are less common but are associated with a more discrete traumatic event. Type 3A deformities will present with chronic swelling and instability that require immobilization for approximately 1 year. These patients tend to drift into varus or valgus deformities, leading to increased pressures and subsequent ulceration over the malleoli. Unlike the previous two types, type 3 does not involve the joint specifically, but rather a pathological fracture that progresses. Attention should be paid to subsequent secondary changes that occur after consolidation has been completed.

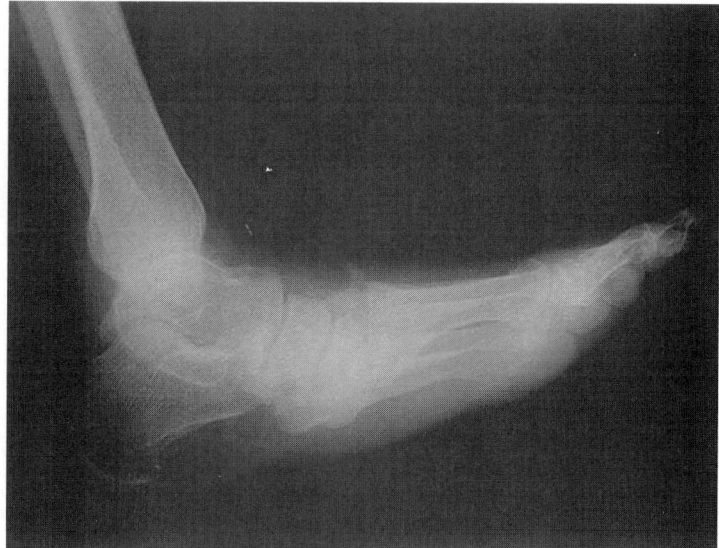

Fig. 4. Lateral radiograph of type I Charcot's joint.

TREATMENT

The main objectives in treatment of the Charcot foot are to achieve bony healing, to minimize soft-tissue breakdown and ulcerations, and to keep the patient at maximum ambulatory capacity (Fig. 8).[23] It is also important to emphasize to the patient that Charcot's arthropathy is a slow and lingering process and that at times it is necessary to be patient to maximize the objectives. The majority of Char-

cot's arthropathies can be treated conservatively. However, occasional surgical indications do arise.

Treatment depends on the stage of arthropathy, the pattern of arthropathy, the tissue viability, and the subsequent deformities. Initial treatment depends first on good patient education. This includes discussion of basic pathophysiology, use of well-chosen footwear, proper foot care, and importance of good glucose management. A team approach is prudent and should include the patient's orthopaedist,

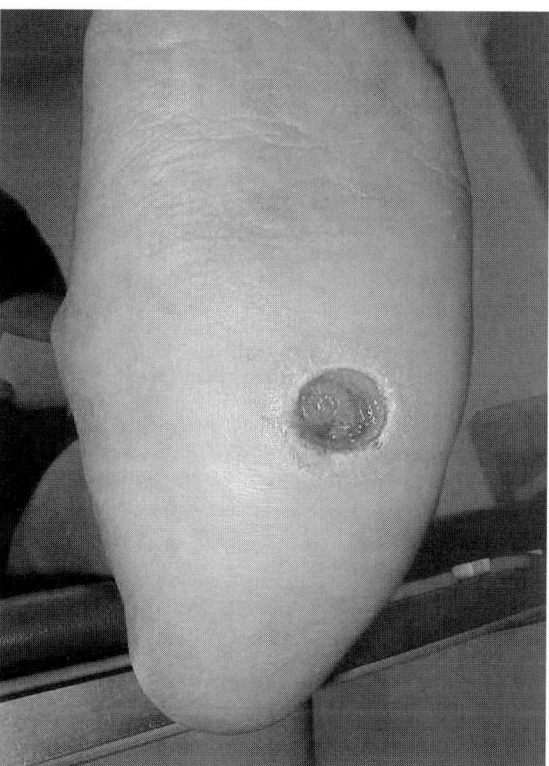

Fig. 5. Plantar ulceration caused by increased plantar pressure from underlying bony deformities.

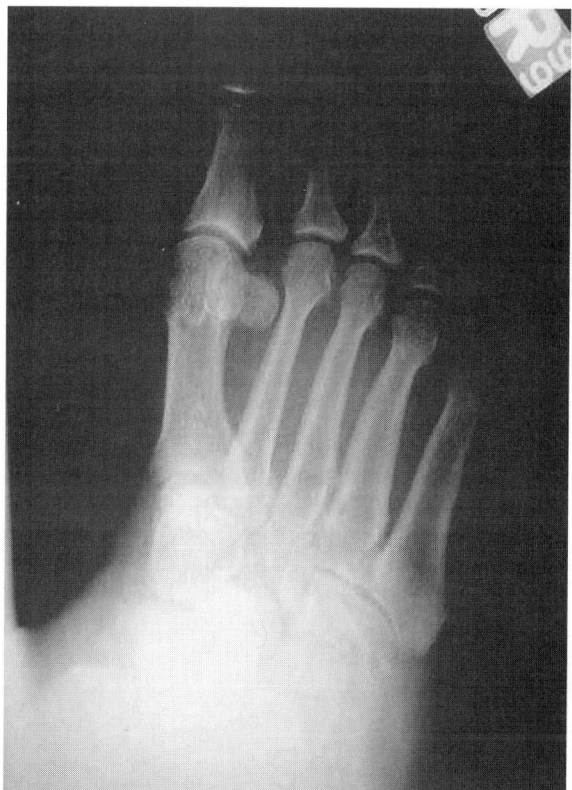

Fig. 6. Oblique radiograph of type II Charcot's joint. Note the involvement of the subtalar, talonavicular, and calcaneocuboid joints.

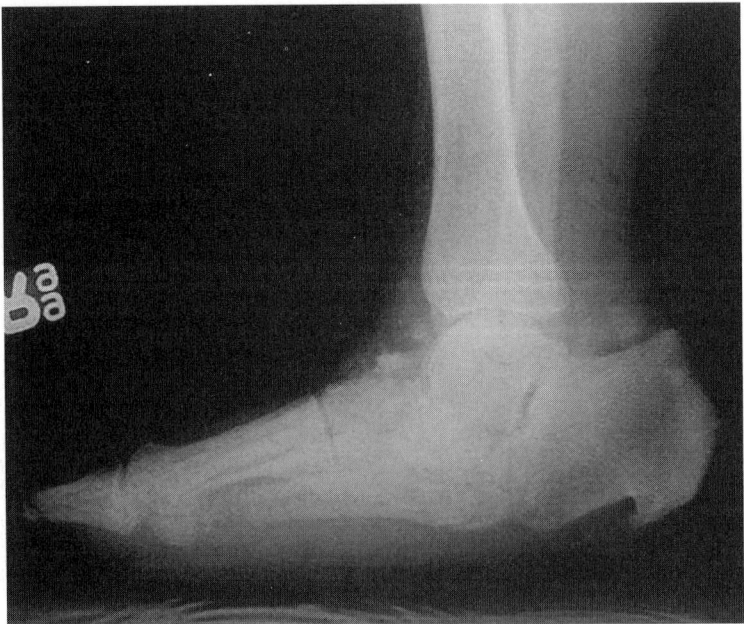

Fig. 7. Lateral radiograph of type II Charcot's joint.

internist, endocrinologist, and a vascular surgeon.[24] A well-educated pedorthist is an asset to the team. A pedorthist can advise the patient on the use of orthotics and proper footwear and on proper shoe fit. Important to the care of the patient with neuropathic arthropathy is a set of general guidelines that should be discussed with the patient. These are listed in Table 3.

After the patient has had initiation of Charcot's reaction, the first stage of treatment involves rest and elevation to diminish the swelling and to protect the foot. Protection can be either a pneumatic compressive boot or a total-contact cast. Cast changes should be frequent because swelling and edema can be decreased quickly, thereby

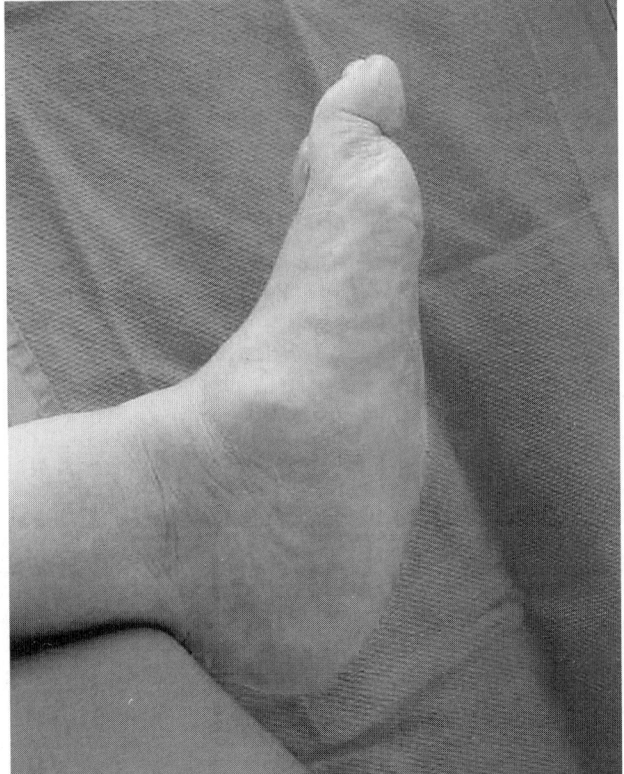

Fig. 8. Clinical picture of type I Charcot's joint with a rocker-bottom deformity.

TABLE 3. GENERAL PATIENT GUIDELINES

1. Cessation of smoking
2. Frequent inspection of the foot for fissures, cracks, ulcerations, and infections
3. Use of a parabolic mirror, especially in patients who have progressing retinopathy
4. Assistance of another person for routine foot inspections
5. Daily cleansing with a mild soap followed by thorough drying and use of a moisturizing, but not perfumed, lotion on all areas except for web spaces (an antifungal powder should be used in web spaces)
6. Avoidance of extremes in temperature, especially with bathing
7. Avoidance of hot-water bottles and ice packs
8. Proper shoe fit and shoe choice
9. Frequent inspections of the shoes, especially before putting them on
10. Use of cotton socks without a seam to absorb moisture as well as to provide increased protection
11. Avoidance of constrictive garments
12. Instruction to wear shoes at all times to prevent injury to the feet
13. Instruction to never go barefoot
14. Proper care and hygiene of the toenails
15. Instruction to not remove any corns or calluses unless the patient has adequate protective sensation
16. Frequent physician visits
17. Instruction that the patient should remove the shoes for all physician visits so an inspection can be performed

causing the cast to loosen. As the cast begins to loosen, there is an increased propensity for blisters and ulcerations to develop.[25] Prefabricated pneumatic walkers are innocuous in that they allow the patient the ability to increase pneumatic bladders as swelling decreases. A disadvantage of pneumatic walkers is that they are sometimes unable to accommodate the bony prominences and deformities associated with severe arthropathy. The pneumatic walker also relies on the patient to be compliant and to follow the physician's guidelines.

As Eichenholtz stage 1 resolves and progresses into stage 2, advancement to a more permanent immobilization device is necessary. Knowing when stage 1 has resolved and when advancement into stage 2 has occurred is a matter of clinical judgment. This can be assessed by the use of the water displacement test, which is preferably done at approximately the same time of day at each examination; this can eliminate the daily fluctuance of edema. Other techniques include use of an infrared thermometer. However, this can be quite expensive.[26] Once stage 2 has been reached, a more permanent mobilization device is used. This can be a Charcot restraint orthotic walker[27, 28] or a patellar tendon–bearing, double upright brace attached to the shoe, with an accommodative insert within the shoe.[29–31] This is usually continued until Eichenholtz stage 3 has been reached and bony consolidation has been noted. Eichenholtz stage 3 is then treated with a full-length, tri-layer, total-contact insert within accommodative footwear, taking into account bony prominences and soft-tissue ade-

quacy. This insert should be made by a properly trained pedorthist. At this point, the patient-physician relationship should advance to the prevention of recurrence of the disease and the prevention of skin or soft-tissue breakdown. It is within this stage that soft-tissue evaluation and treatment of residual deformities should be addressed and coupled with regular, well-spaced reevaluations.

CONCLUSION

The patient with Charcot's arthropathy can be managed using a team approach, with a well-educated orthopaedist as the director. If the patient presents to your office with a warm, swollen, painless joint, and infection can be ruled out, neuropathic arthropathy should be considered, especially if the patient's medical conditions or afflictions increase your suspicions. If the patient is not diabetic, or if diabetes can be ruled out, then other sources of neuropathic arthropathies should be investigated. The basic treatment for other neuropathic arthropathies should follow the same general guidelines as those for treatment of diabetic neuropathic arthropathies. Early treatments should involve immobilization and control of edema and protection from further destruction or deformity. Later stages are then directed toward correcting specific joint imbalances to prevent further injury to the surrounding soft tissue and bone. The last stage should be the prevention of further injury, ulceration, and infection and the maximization of patient function.

REFERENCES

1. Charcot JM: Sur quelques arthropathies quai paraissant dependre d'une lesion cerveau ou de la moelle epinere. Arch Physiol Norm Pathol 1868; 1:161.
2. Sanders LJ, Frykberg RG: Charcot foot. In Levin ME, O'Neal LW, Bowker JH (eds): The Diabetic Foot. St Louis, Mosby–Year Book, 1993, 5th ed, p 150.
3. Calhoun JH: Neuropathic arthropathy. In Sammarco GJ (ed): Foot and Ankle Manual. Malvern, Lea & Febiger, 1991, p 177.
4. Brodsky JW: The diabetic foot. In Coughlin MJ, Mann RA (eds): Surgery of the Foot and Ankle. St Louis, Mosby, 1999, 7th ed, p 940.
5. Greene DA, Feldman EL, Stevens M: Neuropathy in the diabetic foot: New concepts in etiology and treatment. In Levin ME, O'Neal LW, Bowker JH (eds): The Diabetic Foot. St Louis, Mosby–Year Book, 1993, 5th ed, p 144.
6. Brodsky JW: The diabetic foot. In Coughlin MJ, Mann RA (eds): Surgery of the Foot and Ankle. St Louis, Mosby, 1999, 7th ed, p 900.
7. Greene DA, Lattimer SA, Sima AAF: Sorbitol, phosphoinositides, and sodium-potassium-ATPase in the pathogenesis of diabetic complications. N Engl J Med 1987; 316:599.
8. Greene DA, Sima AAF, Albers J, et al: Diabetic neuropathy. In Rifkin H, Porte D (eds): Diabetes Mellitus: Theory and Prac-

tice. St Louis, Mosby–Year Book, 1990, 4th ed, p 721.
9. Brodsky JW: The diabetic foot. In Coughlin MJ, Mann RA (eds): Surgery of the Foot and Ankle. St Louis, Mosby, 1999, 7th ed, p 900.
10. Sanders LJ, Frykberg RG: Charcot foot. In Levin ME, O'Neal LW, Bowker JH (eds): The Diabetic Foot. St Louis, Mosby–Year Book, 1993, 5th ed, p 154.
11. Calhoun JH: Neuropathic arthropathy. In Sammarco GJ (ed): Foot and Ankle Manual. Malvern, Lea & Febiger, 1991, p 177.
12. Birke JA, Sims D: Plantar sensory threshold in the ulcerative foot. Lepr Rev 1986; 57:261.
13. Calhoun JH: Neuropathic arthropathy. In Sammarco GJ (ed): Foot and Ankle Manual. Malvern, Lea & Febiger, 1991, p 177.
14. Brodsky JW: The diabetic foot. In Coughlin MJ, Mann RA (eds): Surgery of the Foot and Ankle. St Louis, Mosby, 1999, 7th ed, p 945.
15. Calhoun JH: Neuropathic arthropathy. In Sammarco GJ (ed): Foot and Ankle Manual. Malvern, Lea & Febiger, 1991, p 179.
16. Calhoun JH: Neuropathic arthropathy. In Sammarco GJ (ed): Foot and Ankle Manual. Malvern, Lea & Febiger, 1991, p 183.
17. Greene DA: Glycemic control. In Dyck PJ, Thomas PK, Asbury AK, et al (eds): Diabetic Neuropathy. Philadelphia, WB Saunders, 1987, p 186.

18. Brower A, Allman R: Neuropathic osteoarthropathy. Orthop Rev 1985; 14:81.
19. Wyss CR, Harrington RM, Burgess EM, et al: Transcutaneous oxygen tension as a predictor of success after amputation. J Bone Joint Surg Am 1988; 70:203.
20. Early JS: Surgical intervention in diabetic neuropathy of the foot. Foot Ankle Clin 1997; 2:23.
21. Eichenholtz S: Charcot Joints. Charles C. Thomas, Springfield, IL, 1966.
22. Brodsky JW: The diabetic foot. In Coughlin MJ, Mann RA (eds): Surgery of the Foot and Ankle. St Louis, Mosby, 1999, 7th ed, p 948.
23. Brodsky JW: The diabetic foot. In Coughlin MJ, Mann RA (eds): Surgery of the Foot and Ankle. St Louis, Mosby, 1999, 7th ed, p 952.
24. Calhoun JH: Neuropathic arthropathy. In Sammarco GJ (ed): Foot and Ankle Manual. Malvern, Lea & Febiger, 1991, p 184.
25. Dhawan S, Conti SF: Use of total contact casting in the diabetic foot. Foot Ankle Clin 1997; 2:115.
26. Brodsky JW: The diabetic foot. In Coughlin MJ, Mann RA (eds): Surgery of the Foot and Ankle. St Louis, Mosby, 1999, 7th ed, p 953.
27. Boninger ML, Leonard JA, Jr: Use of bivalved ankle-foot orthosis in neuropathic foot and ankle lesions. J Rehabil 1996; 33: 16.

28. Morgan JM, Biehl WC, Wagner FW Jr: Management of neuropathic arthropathy with the Charcot restraint orthotic walker. Clin Orthop 1993; 296:58.

29. Gristina AG, Thompson WA, Kester N, et al: Treatment of neuropathic conditions of the foot and ankle with a patellar-tendon-bearing brace. Arch Phys Med Rehabil 1973; 54:562.

30. Guse ST, Alvine FG: Treatment of diabetic foot ulcers and Charcot neuroarthropathy using the patellar tendon-bearing brace. Foot Ankle Int 1997; 18:675.

31. Saltzman CL, Johnson KA, Goldstein RH, et al: The patellar tendon-bearing brace as treatment for neurotrophic arthropathy: A dynamic force monitoring study. Foot Ankle 1984; 13:14.

section 6 chapter 6

GLENOHUMERAL ARTHRITIS

Rick Placide and Gerald R. Williams, Jr

Summary

- Glenohumeral arthritis is not as common as arthritis that affects the lower extremities. It is seen in younger patients with potentially higher activity levels.
- Multiple types of glenohumeral arthritis exist; the most common are osteoarthritis, rheumatoid arthritis, post-traumatic arthritis, and cuff tear arthropathy.
- Nonoperative treatment is often successful and includes anti-inflammatory medications and other pharmacological agents, physiotherapy, and activity modification.
- The most commonly performed operative procedure for end-stage glenohumeral arthritis is shoulder replacement.
- Total shoulder replacement is preferred for patients older than 50 years who have an intact and functional rotator cuff and adequate glenoid bond stock for accepting a glenoid component.
- The problems of glenoid component wear and aseptic loosening will take longer-term follow-up to fully characterize.

Glenohumeral (GH) arthritis is not uncommon, although less so than hip and knee arthritis. Generally, arthritis of the GH joint can be defined as aseptic destruction of the GH articular surfaces, resulting in pain and progressive loss of GH motion and function.

There are many causes of GH arthritis; in some types, the cause is unclear (Table 1). GH arthritis can be broadly categorized as osteoarthritis (OA), inflammatory arthritis, and other arthritides.

OA can be divided into primary and secondary types. Primary OA does not have an identifiable cause. Causes of secondary OA include post-traumatic arthritis, such as arthritis of instability and intra-articular fracture. Inflammatory arthritides include rheumatoid arthritis (RA), inflammatory bowel disease, ankylosing spondylitis, and psoriatic arthritis. Crystalline arthropathies include gout and pseudogout. Rotator cuff arthropathy is a unique form of arthritis with a well-known pathoanatomy and a poorly understood cause. Additional types of GH arthritis include arthritis associated with acromegaly, GH dysplasia, atraumatic osteonecrosis secondary to corticosteroid use, alcoholism,

Gaucher's disease, sickle cell disease and irradiation, neuropathic arthropathy, and septic arthropathy. Figure 1 presents a breakdown in terms of causes leading to shoulder arthroplasty.

HISTORICAL REVIEW

The history of GH arthritis associated with rotator cuff deficiency begins in the middle 1800s when Robert Adams, a professor of surgery at the University of Dublin, presented what was probably the earliest description of GH degenerative joint disease associated with rotator cuff rup-

TABLE 1. TYPES OF GLENOHUMERAL ARTHRITIS
Osteoarthritis
Primary
Secondary
Post-traumatic
Instability
Inflammatory Arthritis
Rheumatoid arthritis
Ankylosing spondylitis
Psoriatic arthritis
Inflammatory bowel disease
Cuff Tear Arthropathy
Crystalline Arthropathy
Gout
Pseudogout
Osteonecrosis
Idiopathic
Corticosteroid induced
Alcoholism
Post-traumatic
Gaucher's disease
Post-irradiation necrosis
Hemaglobinopathies
Sickle cell disease
Hemophilia
Hemachromatosis
Neuropathic Arthropathy
Syringomyelia
Peripheral neuropathy
Septic Arthritis
Lyme Arthritis
Arthritis Associated with Acromegaly
Congenital
Glenohumeral dysplasia

DIAGNOSES LEADING TO SHOULDER ARTHROPLASTY

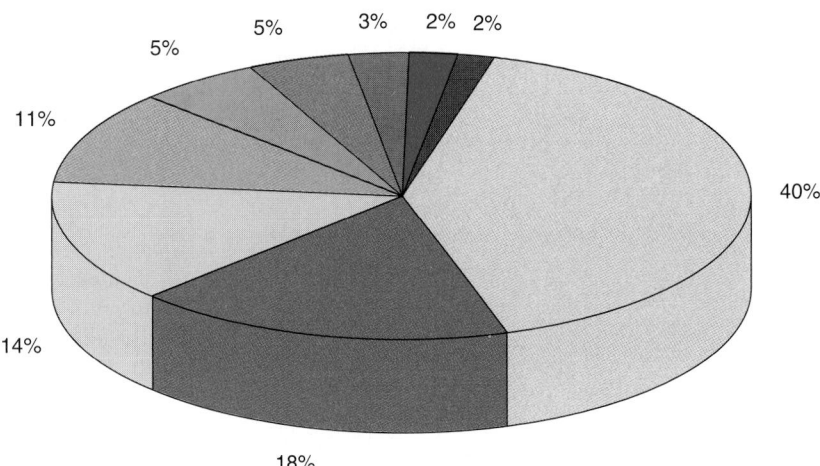

□ OA ■ TrA □ RCTc ■ RA □ AVN ■ MU/NU ■ I/D ■ FX ■ SA

Fig. 1. Shoulder arthroplasty. University of Pennsylvania Shoulder and Elbow Service (1992–1998) by diagnosis. OA: osteoarthritis; TrA: traumatic arthritis; RCTc: complete rotator cuff tear; RA: rheumatoid arthritis; AVN: avascular necrosis; MU/NU: malunion/nonunion; I/D: instability/dislocation; FX: fracture; SA: septic arthritis.

ture.[1, 2] He noted localized and generalized types of "chronic rheumatoid arthritis." The generalized type probably represented RA, and the localized type displayed characteristics consistent with what is now termed rotator cuff tear arthropathy. The characteristics of the localized type included rotator cuff tear, ruptured long head of the biceps, joint effusion, loss of articular cartilage, and marginal osteophytes.

In 1934 E. A. Codman[3] described a condition that he called hygroma of the subacromial bursa in a patient with GH degenerative joint disease and complete absence of the rotator cuff. In 1981 McCarty et al[4, 5] introduced the term "Milwaukee shoulder" to describe several patients with GH degenerative joint disease, recurring effusions, and large rotator cuff tears. Their analysis of the synovial fluid from these arthritic joints demonstrated active collagenases, proteases, and hydroxyapatite crystals, all thought to play a role in the joint destruction.

The term "cuff tear arthropathy" was first presented by Neer in 1977.[6] In 1983 Neer, Craig, and Fukuda[7] described GH joint arthritis associated with rotator cuff deficiency. They provided detailed gross pathological and histological findings as well as their thoughts on how nutritional and mechanical alterations may play a role in joint destruction. The term cuff tear arthropathy continues to be used to describe GH degenerative joint changes that are associated with a rotator cuff tear.

SHOULDER ARTHROPLASTY

The shoulder joint was the first large joint in humans to be replaced by an artificial prosthesis. The first successful shoulder replacement was performed in 1892 by the French surgeon Jules Emile Pean.[8] Prior to this, there had been unsuccessful attempts to replace joints in humans with animal bones and ivory. These substances proved too weak. However, in 1892, using a humeral prosthesis made of platinum and rubber, Pean replaced the proximal humerus

of a young man suffering from tuberculosis of the humerus and shoulder joint. The implant consisted of an iridescent platinum tube serving as the humeral shaft with several holes for soft-tissue attachments. A hardened rubber ball represented the humeral head. Metal anchors fixed the ball to the platinum tube at one end and to the scapula at the other end. The device remained in place for about 2 years; it had to be removed secondary to a chronic draining sinus and sepsis.

In the 1950s, an acrylic prosthesis was tried as a replacement for a proximal humerus, but it was soon abandoned because of implant failures and poor wear characteristics. At this time, many implants appeared that were of a constrained design. One of the more common constrained devices was the Michael Reese prosthesis. Early failure of the prosthesis itself or the anchoring points of the prosthesis to bone complicated this implant, like all other constrained implants.[9]

In 1950 Frederick Krueger used cadaver humeri to mold acrylic reproductions, then had a laboratory make prosthetic molds out of Vitallium.[10, 11] This was probably the first attempt at a nonconstrained implant based on human anatomy and made of a biomaterial superior to others of that time. In 1953 Charles S. Neer ushered in the modern era of shoulder arthroplasty when he presented a review of proximal humeral fractures associated with GH dislocation that were treated with a metallic humeral prosthesis.[12] According to Neer, the value of prosthetic replacement in GH reconstruction would be to reestablish a fulcrum for movement about the shoulder joint.

In 1955 Neer presented early results of articular replacement of the humeral head.[12–14] He stated that treatment of shoulder fracture/dislocations by reduction, arthrodesis, or excision of the head yielded unsatisfactory results. Treatment by reduction resulted in avascular necrosis of the humeral head secondary to soft-tissue damage; failure of treatment by arthrodesis was related to tuberosity displace-

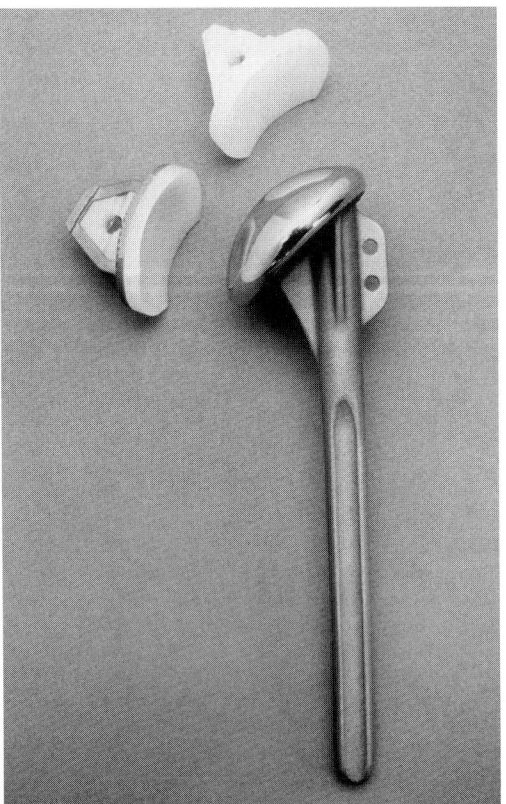

Fig. 2. The Neer prosthesis. It became the prototype for modern-day nonconstrained implant designs.

ment; and treatment by humeral head excision resulted in a flail joint without a fulcrum for motion. Neer went on to say that prosthetic replacement would be a logical solution.[13, 14] The Neer prosthetic design became the prototype for modern shoulder replacement (Fig. 2).

In 1974 Neer expanded his indications for GH replacement to include OA; a glenoid component was added around 1977.[6, 15] Since Neer's original total shoulder implant, a number of other implants have been designed. Second-generation implants offered the convenience of humeral head modularity and, in some cases, less conforming articular surfaces than the original Neer prosthesis had (Fig. 3). Third-generation implants have been designed to emphasize anatomic recreation of the humeral articular surface through the use of prosthetic humeral heads that have a variable inclination (i.e., neck-shaft angle) and that are offset with respect to the humeral head and shaft. Many of the principles of shoulder arthroplasty described by Neer in the 1950s are still important. The one-piece Neer component continues to have the longest follow-up and remains the gold standard by which to compare all other nonconstrained implants.

EPIDEMIOLOGY

Primary OA of the GH joint is not as common as in the weight-bearing joints, such as the hip or knee. In general, patients with OA of the shoulder joint are younger and more active than are patients with lower extremity arthritis.

This is particularly true for certain types of arthritis, such as secondary to instability or related to intra-articular fractures. Although there is much information regarding the epidemiology of OA in general, very little relates specifically to the GH joint.

RA can affect any synovial joint, including the GH, acromioclavicular (AC), and sternoclavicular (SC) joints. When the shoulder joint is involved, it tends to be in the setting of polyarticular involvement. The GH joint is most commonly involved without symptomatic involvement of the AC or SC joints.

Neer introduced the term "rotator cuff tear arthropathy" in 1977.[6] The incidence rate of rotator cuff tears is much higher than that of arthropathy associated with rotator cuff tears. Several cadaveric studies have been undertaken; the incidence rate of rotator cuff tears ranges from 5% to 10% for full-thickness tears to 30% when partial-thickness tears are included.[2, 7] Rotator cuff defects have also been shown to increase with age.[2] Hamada et al[16] concluded that massive rotator cuff tears would lead to arthropathy and would be accompanied by characteristic radiographic changes. In contrast, Rockwood et al[17] presented a group of patients with large rotator cuff tears who were treated with acromioplasty and cuff débridement. They concluded that these patients did not show radiographic progression of degenerative joint disease. It seems that rotator cuff tears do not necessarily lead to arthropathy; Neer et al[7] had estimated that about 4% of patients with complete rotator cuff tear would develop cuff tear arthropathy.

PATHOGENESIS

PRIMARY OA

Primary OA of the shoulder is likely to have a similar cause and pathogenesis as other joints in the body. Although the shoulder is not typically a weight-bearing joint, the muscles about the shoulder can generate significant forces within the joint. In contrast to rotator cuff arthropathy, the majority of patients with primary OA have an intact rotator cuff.[15, 18] Therefore, rotator cuff tears are not thought to be involved in the pathogenesis or perpetuation of primary GH OA. One feature often seen in GH OA is asymmetrical wear of the posterior glenoid. It is almost always present in conjunction with progressive contracture of the anterior capsule and, in severe cases, contracture of the subscapularis. It is not clear whether the anterior soft-tissue contracture is the primary pathogenic factor in the development of posterior glenoid wear or simply a result of joint deterioration. At the very least, it is a mitigating factor in the pathogenesis of asymmetric glenoid wear commonly seen in GH OA. One last factor worth mentioning is congenital hypoplasia of the glenoid. The influence of congenital glenoid hypoplasia on the development of OA is not known. However, there is some suggestion that patients with hypoplastic glenoids have a higher prevalence rate of GH OA than do patients without glenoid hypoplasia.[19, 20]

In RA, the immune-mediated events leading to joint destruction occur in conjunction with GH joint pathoanatomy. Some of the earlier changes that are observed in a joint affected by RA are damage to the microvasculature, synovial edema, and proliferation of synovial lining cells. The

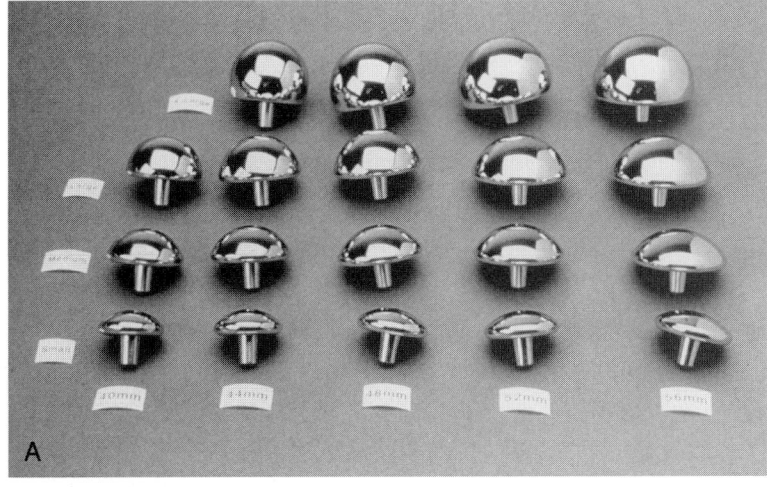

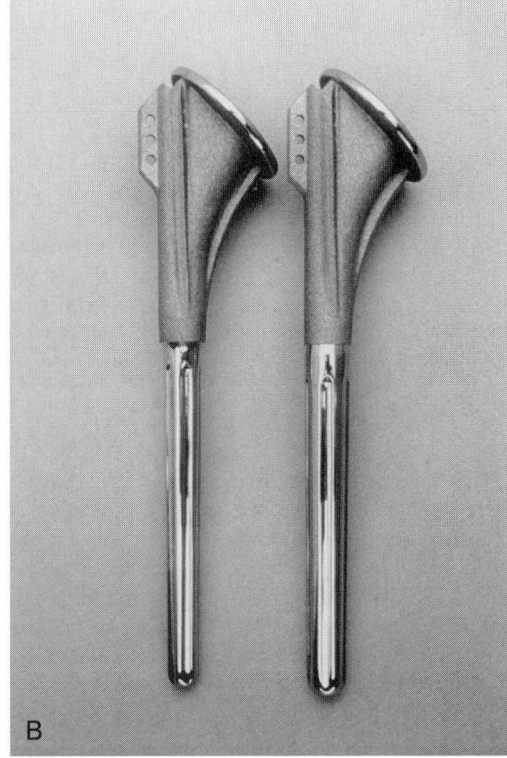

Fig. 3. Newer prostheses. *A* and *B,* These employ a modular head design and less conforming articular surfaces.

proliferating pannus destroys the articular cartilage and bone beginning at the synovial reflection at the anatomic neck of the humerus and extends onto the articular surfaces and through to the subchondral bone (Fig. 4).[21, 22] Two major pathoanatomical characteristics associated with the progression of RA in the shoulder are bone destruction (i.e., erosion) and rotator cuff insufficiency.

The precise cause of rotator cuff arthropathy is not known. When Codman[3] described what he called hygroma of the subacromial bursa in 1934, he thought this was a result of neglected rotator cuff tear. Neer et al[7] postulated that gross instability of the humeral head and proximal

migration of the humerus with subacromial impingement would occur following a massive rotator cuff tear. Subsequent inactivity and disuse about the joint would lead to a loss of a closed joint space and leaking of synovial fluid. These factors would then lead to disuse osteopenia and atrophy of the humeral head and glenoid as well as insufficient diffusion for articular cartilage nutrition. The combination of instability, inactivity and disuse, proximal humeral migration, and poor nutrition led to the ultimate finding of humeral head collapse.

Another theory to explain cuff tear arthropathy is the crystal-induced or crystal deposition theory.[4, 5, 23] In 1981,

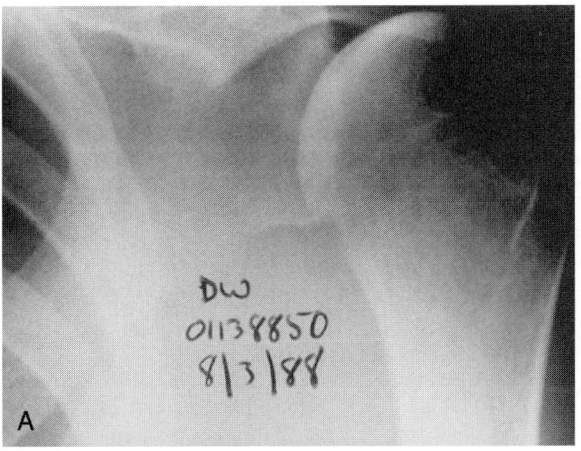

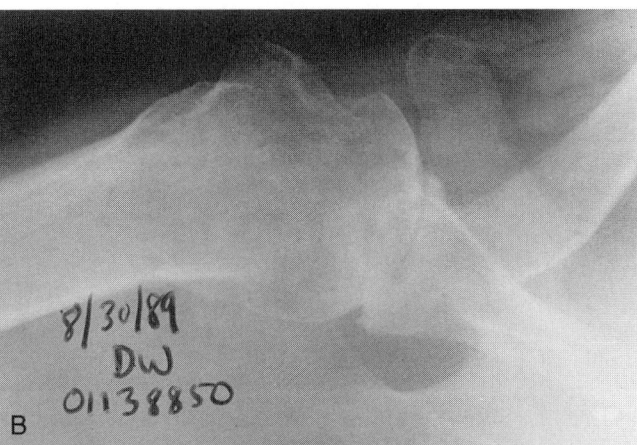

Fig. 4. Rheumatoid arthritis. Juxta-articular erosions begin at the anatomic neck of the humerus. Anteroposterior and axillary radiographs may demonstrate these erosive changes in addition to symmetrical joint space narrowing (*A* and *B*).

McCarty et al[4, 5] introduced the term "Milwaukee shoulder." They described a group of patients with GH degenerative joint disease, rotator cuff defects, and previously undescribed microscopic and biochemical findings. Scanning electron microscopy of the synovial fluid exhibited microspheroids containing hydroxyapatite and calcium phosphate crystals. Chemical analyses revealed active collagenase and neutral protease. In contrast to McCarty et al, Dieppe et al[23, 24] were unable to document the presence of active collagenase or neutral protease in synovial fluid in patients with Milwaukee shoulder and reported that 30% to 50% of all osteoarthritic joints contained hydroxyapatite and calcium phosphate crystals.

CLINICAL FEATURES

The general clinical features of GH arthritis are pain, decreased range of motion, poor function, and decreased quality of life. The specific clinical features seen in an individual patient depend on the type of arthritis present (Table 2). When examining a patient complaining of shoulder pain, a large differential diagnosis must be considered. In addition to arthritic conditions presenting with shoulder pain, other sources of shoulder pain include cervical spine/neck, cardiac, pulmonary, abdominal (diaphragmatic irritation), neoplastic, and traumatic.

OA of the GH joint has similar clinical features to OA at other joints such as the knee and hip. OA in its early stages may be asymptomatic. When signs and symptoms do present, they tend to be localized. The earliest chief complaint is likely to be pain that occurs with joint use and that is relieved by rest. With disease progression, the pain can be brought on by minimal amounts of activity and may even progress to resting or night pain. The patient's description of the pain is that it is usually vague and diffuse about the shoulder region in general. Other complaints include decreased range of motion, decreased function, and crepitus.

Physical examination reveals decreased motion and crepitus. There is a symmetrical restriction of both active and passive motions. However, there is a greater loss of external rotation compared with internal rotation secondary to anterior capsular and/or subscapularis contracture (Fig. 5). There may be a slight prominence of the coracoid process and loss of normal shoulder contour from a posteriorly subluxated humerus in the setting of posterior glenoid wear. Localized posterior joint line tenderness is also a common physical finding.

Generalized atrophy about the shoulder may be another finding, likely related to disuse and contracture. Specific spinati atrophy is absent, except in the unusual circumstance of concomitant rotator cuff rupture. Rotator cuff strength is usually good, even though the patient may be limited in ability to cooperate with the examination because of pain and fixed restrictions. Additional findings include joint enlargement secondary to synovitis and proliferative changes in bone and cartilage.

RA is characteristically an inflammatory disease of joints. However, it is a systemic disease with potentially significant extra-articular manifestations. Joint involvement is typically symmetrical and polyarticular and includes involvement of periarticular soft tissues as well as joint surfaces. It is unlikely for the patient with RA to present initially with monoarticular involvement of the shoulder.

The presenting complaints and physical findings can vary widely in severity from patient to patient. The patient will complain of pain, morning stiffness, swelling, and decreased function. RA is diagnosed primarily on clinical grounds, but radiographs and laboratory testing are useful. Published diagnostic criteria exist for RA and are based on physical examinations, laboratory tests, radiographs, synovial fluid analyses, and biopsy samples of rheumatoid nodules.[25]

Examination of a painful shoulder in a patient with RA must be done in the context of other joint involvement. Patients with RA frequently have involvement of the cervical spine. Therefore, radiculopathy and myelopathy must be considered. These patients may also have elbow involvement as another source of referred pain. Pinpointing the source of pain may prove difficult because multiple structures about the shoulder may be involved, including the GH joint, rotator cuff, various bursae, acromioclavicular joint, and muscles of the thorax. Examination is likely to reveal a boggy synovitis, generalized atrophy, and a

---

TABLE 2. COMPARISON OF SOME FEATURES OF OSTEOARTHRITIS, RHEUMATOID ARTHRITIS, AND ROTATOR CUFF TEAR ARTHROPATHY

	Osteoarthritis	Rheumatoid Arthritis	Rotator Cuff Tear Arthropathy
Physical Exam	• Pain • Decreased motion; ER loss > IR loss • Crepitus • Strength generally good	• Pain • Decreased strength • Morning stiffness • Swelling/synovitis	• Pain • Loss of active motion • Weakness • Effusion • Deltoid dysfunction
Radiographs	• Asymmetric joint space narrowing • Osteophytes • Subchondral sclerosis and cysts	• Osteopenia • Symmetric joint space narrowing • Juxta-articular erosions	• Superior humeral migration • Acromial erosion • Humeral head collapse
Additional Imaging	• CT most useful, especially to evaluate posterior glenoid erosion	• MRI most useful to evaluate the status of the rotator cuff • CT useful to evaluate glenoid bone stock	• MRI and CT useful for same reasons as osteoarthritis and rheumatoid arthritis

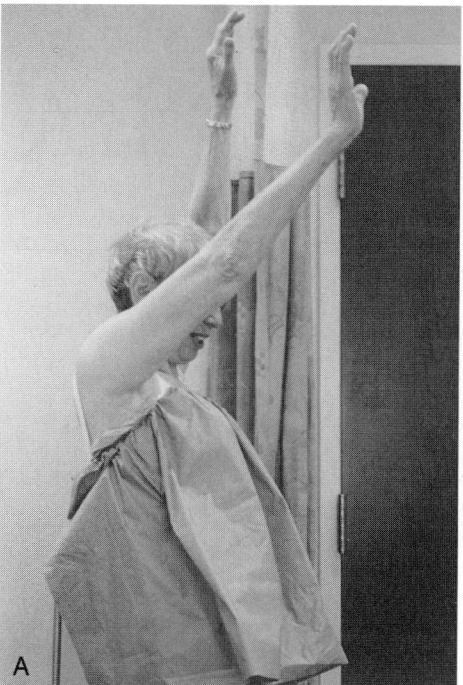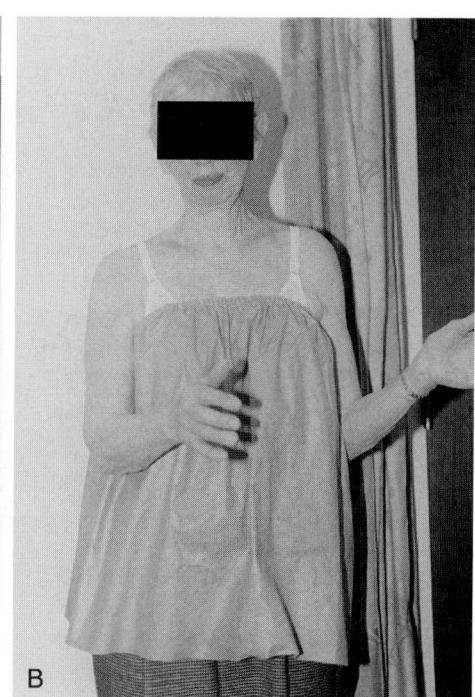

Fig. 5. Physical examination. This patient with primary glenohumeral osteoarthritis has symmetrical decrease in active and passive motion *(A)*, which is particularly evident with external rotation *(B)*.

decreased active and passive range of motion. In contrast to primary OA, the loss of active motion in RA is often greater than the loss of passive motion.

There is a higher incidence rate of dysfunctional or torn rotator cuffs in RA as compared with OA. Consequently, there may also be an element of weakness. Ennevaara[26] presented a series of 200 patients with RA, whose shoulders were studied by arthrography. He found that 21% had rotator cuff tears and that an additional 24% had evidence of tendon fraying. Kelly et al[27] reported on 42 shoulders in 37 patients with RA treated with Neer's total shoulder replacement. Rotator cuff disease was present in 34 shoulders, and cuff tears were present in 13 shoulders. This difference in rotator cuff integrity between primary OA and RA becomes important in surgical and nonsurgical treatment strategies.

The main complaints of patients with GH arthritis and massive rotator cuff tear are pain and loss of active range of motion. The pain typically interferes with sleep and is exacerbated with activity. The loss of motion is related to the rotator cuff defect, the GH incongruity, and the integrity of the coracoacromial arch. The role of the coracoacromial arch as a static humeral head containment mechanism is much more significant in the case of a large rotator cuff tear.[28] Coracoacromial arch insufficiency, when coupled with a massive rotator cuff tear, leads to marked decrease in active range of motion and function.[29] These complaints of pain and loss of motion will tend to be long-standing and progressive.

The severity of signs and symptoms will depend on rotator cuff tear size and chronicity. Smaller cuff tears leave enough residual cuff tissue so that the remaining, intact rotator cuff musculotendinous units may compensate for the loss. This is particularly true if the cuff defect has occurred gradually over many years without significant

trauma. In these partially compensated cuff tears, the (AP) rotator force couple remains relatively balanced, and overhead motion and function are often quite good (Fig. 6).[30, 31] Patients with larger tears may have insufficient cuff tissue intact to maintain a balanced force couple; consequently, they lose overhead motion and function.

Another finding during physical examination is recurrent swelling about the shoulder, reminiscent of Codman's description of hygroma of the subacromial bursa. Codman called this swelling the "fluid sign," thought to result from a communication between the GH joint space and the subacromial bursa.[3] Neer et al[7] reported that the majority of patients with rotator cuff tear arthropathy had significant recurrent swelling. Williams and Rockwood[32] reported in their series that a minority of patients had recurrent swelling, which may indicate a difference in patient population.

One final aspect of the clinical features is deltoid integrity. Patients with cuff tear arthropathy will often have had prior surgical attempts at rotator cuff repair. In addition to iatrogenic coracoacromial arch insufficiency, these prior surgical procedures might result in deltoid detachment or denervation. The resultant scenario of a large rotator cuff tear and deltoid dysfunction with or without coracoacromial arch insufficiency leads to an essentially functionless shoulder.[29]

INVESTIGATION

ROUTINE RADIOGRAPHS

The majority of patients presenting with GH arthritis can be diagnosed and given a treatment plan based on history, physical examination, and plain radiographs. The basic minimum radiographs taken in the evaluation of GH arthritis include an AP view in the scapular plane in internal and external rotation and an axillary view.

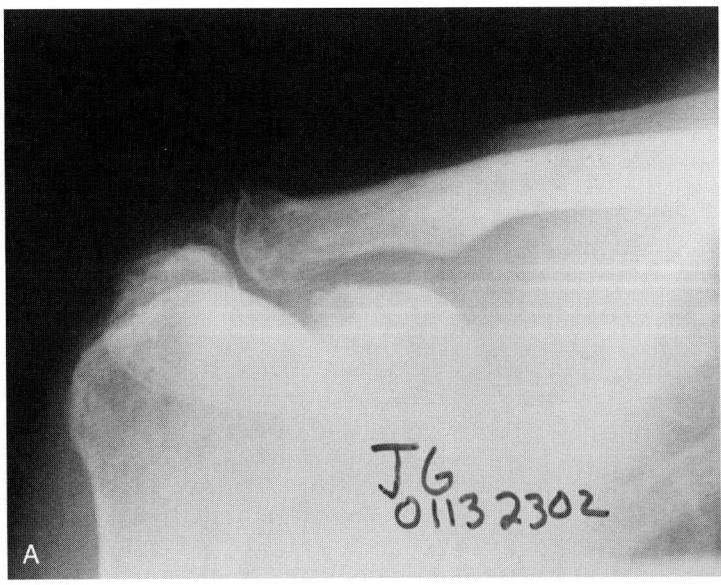

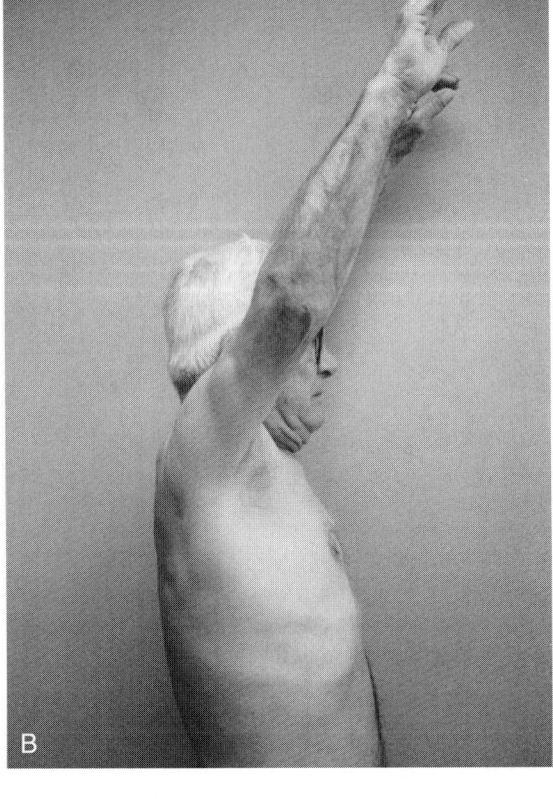

Fig. 6. Patients with cuff tear arthropathy may have surprisingly good function. This is demonstrated by this patient with relatively balanced anterior and posterior rotator cuff force couples remaining (*A* and *B*).

The cardinal radiographic features of GH OA are asymmetric joint space narrowing, subchondral sclerosis, subchondral cyst formation, and osteophyte formation. Osteophyte formation is especially common on the inferior aspect of the humeral neck. On the AP view, the glenoid side of the joint line should lie within 5 mm of the base of the coracoid process.[33] The axillary view is better than the AP view for evaluating GH joint space narrowing. This view can show humeral head flattening not appreciated on AP views. When glenoid erosion is present, the axillary view can give a rough estimate of posterior glenoid wear and posterior humeral head subluxation (Fig. 7).

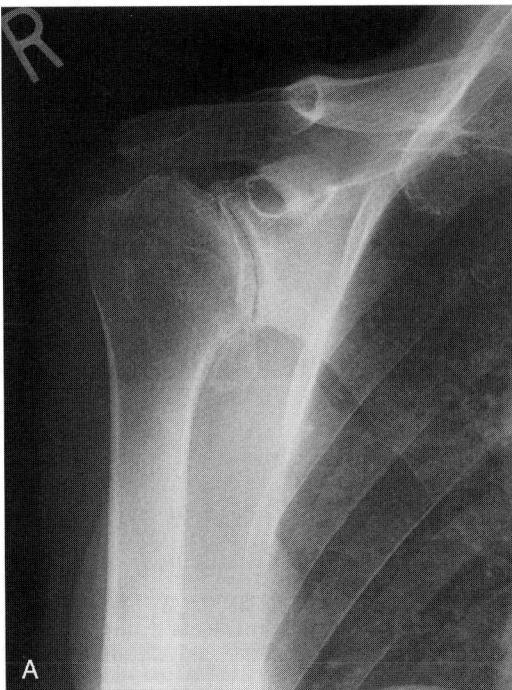

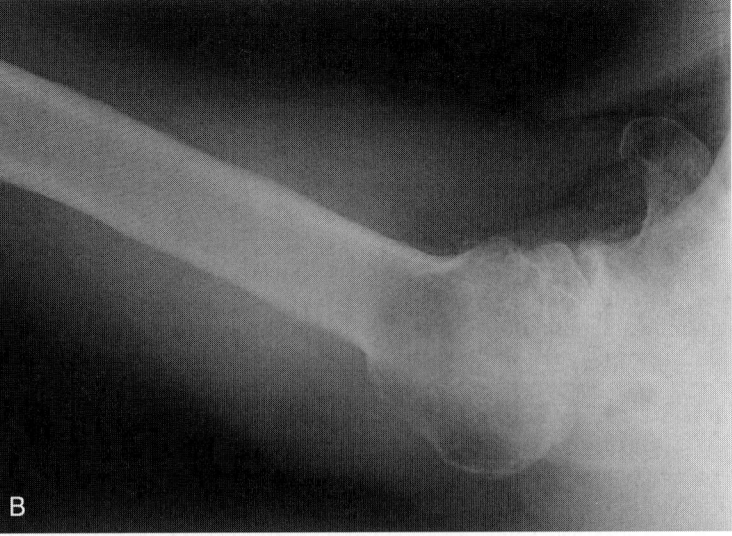

Fig. 7. Radiographs. This anteroposterior radiograph *(A)* of a patient with glenohumeral osteoarthritis reveals subchondral sclerosis, joint space narrowing, and a large inferior humeral osteophyte. The axillary view *(B)* reveals asymmetric posterior glenoid erosion and posterior humeral subluxation.

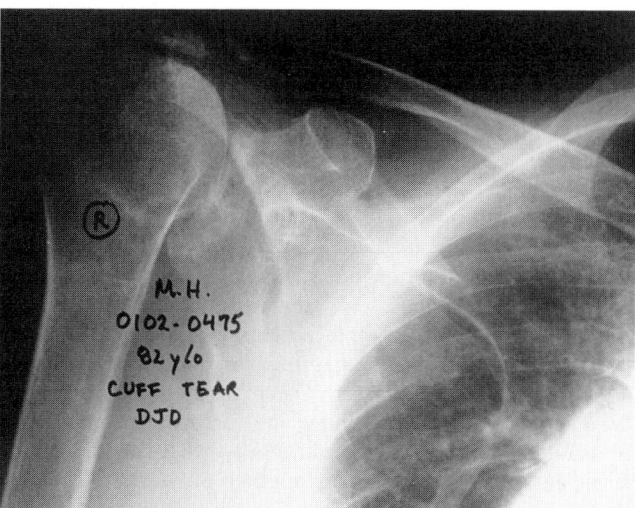

Fig. 8. Radiograph. Radiographic findings of cuff tear arthropathy include proximal humeral migration and scant osteophyte formation. Proximal humeral head collapse is a late radiographic finding that confirms the diagnosis.

The radiographic features of RA in the shoulder parallel those of any joint affected by RA. Cardinal features include regional osteopenia, symmetrical joint space narrowing, and juxta-articular erosions. These erosions are best seen at the synovial reflection on the superior aspect of the humeral head. Osteophytes are not a prominent feature but may be present. The AP view can also demonstrate central glenoid erosion. This is seen as medial migration of the glenoid joint surface as far medial as the base of the coracoid process and beyond. Additionally, in the case of rotator cuff insufficiency, the AP view will help determine superior migration of the humerus, contributing to superior glenoid erosion. The axillary view helps estimate joint space narrowing as well as medial erosion of the glenoid surface with respect to the coracoid process. The extent of humeral head deformity associated with juxta-articular erosions is best evaluated with the axillary view (see Fig. 4).

The radiographic findings in cuff tear arthropathy depend somewhat on the size and chronicity of the tear. The characteristic radiographic findings include proximal humeral migration with subsequent acromion erosion. This erosion can progress to involve the AC joint and lateral clavicle. Additional radiographic findings include superior humeral head collapse and a relative lack of osteophytes (Fig. 8). Again, the axillary view is most useful for evaluating glenoid erosion and medial migration.

The major use of a computed tomography scan in glenohumeral arthritis is for quantitating posterior glenoid erosion,[34] most often in cases of primary OA or post-traumatic arthritis. A computed tomography scan is obtained when the axillary plain film suggests a posterior glenoid deficiency or when external rotation is less than −20 degrees, even if the plain films are not suggestive of posterior glenoid deficiencies (Fig. 9). Computed tomography scan can also assist in evaluating glenoid bone stock, central glenoid erosion, and glenoid position (i.e., anteversion/retroversion).

Imaging of the rotator cuff can be performed using magnetic resonance imaging, arthrography, and sonography. Presently, magnetic resonance is the preferred method of imaging the rotator cuff in the setting of arthritis. It is accurate and noninvasive and may provide additional information regarding intra-articular disorder. Moreover, magnetic resonance imaging is helpful in quantifying cuff tear size, retraction, muscle atrophy, and fatty degeneration.[35]

Indications for obtaining a magnetic resonance image include inflammatory arthritis without fixed proximal humeral migration and early cuff tear arthropathy. If a patient with inflammatory arthritis has an intact or reparable cuff, especially if there is minimal fatty degeneration of the

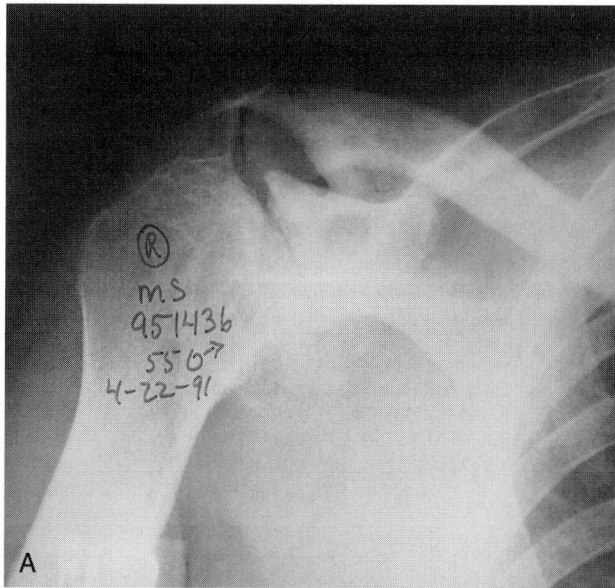
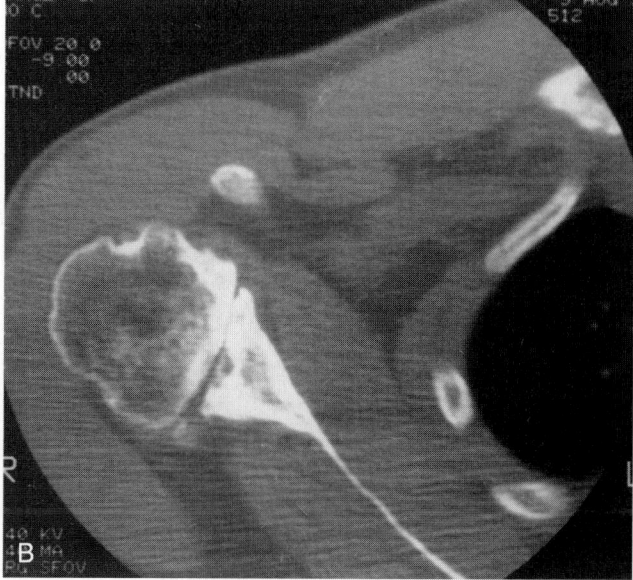

Fig. 9. Posterior erosion in patients with glenohumeral osteoarthritis. May be suspected on plain radiographs (A). Computed tomography scan confirms its presence (B).

muscle bellies, placement of a glenoid component would be more appropriate. Similarly, placement of a glenoid component in cuff tear arthropathy is made more likely if there is no fixed proximal humeral migration and a reparable cuff defect. A fixed proximal migration of the humerus or a large irreparable cuff tear is thought to cause eccentric loading of the humeral head on the glenoid and contribute to early loosening of the glenoid component.

MANAGEMENT

NONOPERATIVE
All patients with GH arthritis should exhaust nonoperative management strategies before considering surgery. These strategies include activity modification, individualized physical therapy, nonsteroidal anti-inflammatory drugs, disease-modifying antirheumatic drugs (for inflammatory arthropathies), and intra-articular corticosteroid injections. Additionally, new pharmacological oral and intra-articular therapies that target different aspects of the destructive pathways will likely soon be available. One caveat is that patients with inflammatory arthritis may need surgery sooner to avoid joint destruction so severe that the joint cannot be salvaged surgically.

OPERATIVE
Osteoarthritis
Operative management of GH OA is indicated when nonoperative measures have failed and symptoms are severe enough to justify further treatment. In general, surgical options for shoulder arthritis include (1) arthroscopic joint débridement, (2) arthroscopic contracture release with joint débridement, (3) osteotomy, (4) arthrodesis, (5) interpositional arthroplasty, and (6) shoulder arthroplasty (although shoulder arthroplasty may be the best treatment option for advanced degenerative GH arthritis, there are patients whose disease is less severe or whose age or activity level is not compatible with prosthetic replacement).

In the patient younger than 40 years who does not have severe radiographic deformity, arthroscopic joint débridement can be useful. Arthroscopy is an excellent diagnostic tool. Capsular release, performed arthroscopically or open, can be successful in the management of tight anterior soft tissues, particularly in postcapsulorrhaphy arthropathy when degeneration is mild. Arthrodesis has a limited role in the treatment of GH OA. Indications include cases of OA where there has been loss of rotator cuff and deltoid function, after multiple failed reconstructive attempts including failed shoulder arthroplasty, in patients who perform heavy manual labor, and in the treatment of joint destruction resulting from infection.

Burkhead and Hutton presented the results of soft-tissue interposition combined with hemiarthroplasty as an alternative to total shoulder replacement.[36] This procedure was performed in two different groups of patients: for young active patients with primary OA to spare revision surgery for eventual glenoid loosening and for patients undergoing revision of total shoulder arthroplasty where there was insufficient glenoid to support another prosthesis. They reported favorable results.

The use of hemiarthroplasty in the treatment of GH OA, as opposed to a total shoulder replacement, is controversial. Hemiarthroplasty for OA is indicated in the presence of irreparable rotator cuff tear and proximal humeral migration. The use of a glenoid component in these circumstances has been associated with premature glenoid loosening (Fig. 10).[37] For the majority of patients with GH OA, the procedure of choice is total shoulder arthroplasty, provided there is an intact or reparable rotator cuff and adequate bone for placement of a glenoid component.

Rheumatoid Arthritis (RA)
Several surgical options exist for the rheumatoid shoulder, depending on the severity of the destruction. Synovectomy, bursectomy, and contracture release, whether performed arthroscopically or open, are indicated only early in the disease process, prior to severe articular involvement and while joint surfaces are still congruent. Arthrodesis has a very limited role in managing RA about the shoulder because the other shoulder is likely to be involved. Arthrodesis may become an option, however, in certain revision situations characterized by unreconstructable bone deficiency, rotator cuff insufficiency, or anterosuperior humeral dislocation.

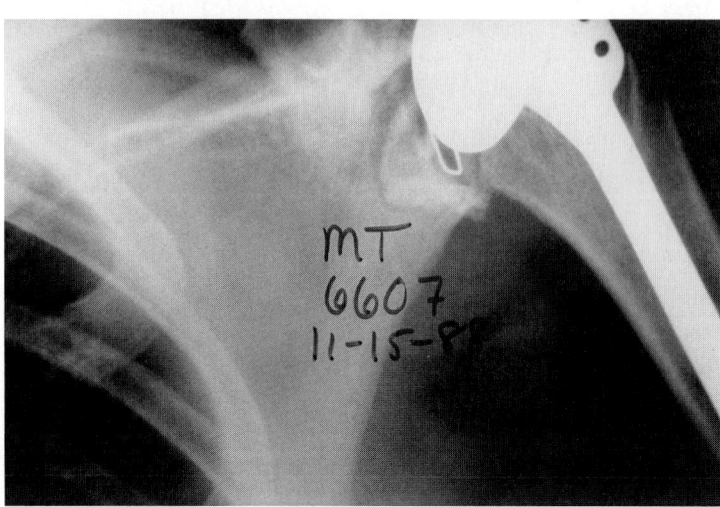

Fig. 10. Radiograph. Total shoulder arthroplasty in patients with fixed proximal humeral migration may lead to asymmetric superior loading of the glenoid component and early glenoid loosening.

Hemiarthroplasty is more commonly indicated in RA than in OA. In RA, hemiarthroplasty is performed for those patients without significant glenoid involvement as compared with humeral involvement, with an irreparable rotator cuff deficiency, with insufficient joint volume to accept a glenoid component, or with inadequate glenoid bone stock to support a prosthetic component (Fig. 11). Total shoulder arthroplasty may offer the best surgical option for those patients with RA of the shoulder. However, prerequisites for total shoulder arthroplasty in RA include an intact or reparable rotator cuff, adequate glenoid bone stock to accept a prosthesis, sufficient joint capsule space for a glenoid component, and no fixed proximal humeral migration (Fig. 12).

Rotator Cuff Tear Arthropathy

Several surgical procedures for rotator cuff tear arthropathy have been tried; some are no longer considered viable options. Although the idea of constrained and semiconstrained total shoulder arthroplasty would seem a reasonable way to manage cuff tear arthropathy, they both have met with unacceptably high rates of prosthetic loosening and implant failure. Unconstrained total shoulder arthroplasty has been reported for cuff tear arthropathy. However, the high-riding humeral head causes eccentric loading on the cemented glenoid component and ultimately may result in glenoid loosening. For that reason, some have recommended hemiarthroplasty for treatment of cuff tear arthropathy.[32, 38] Partial or complete rotator cuff repair may

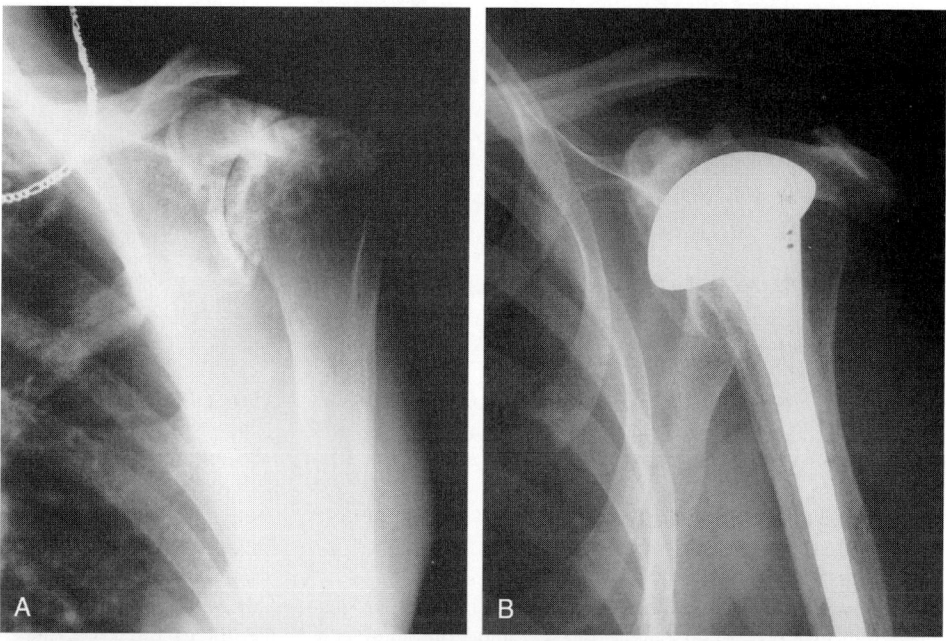

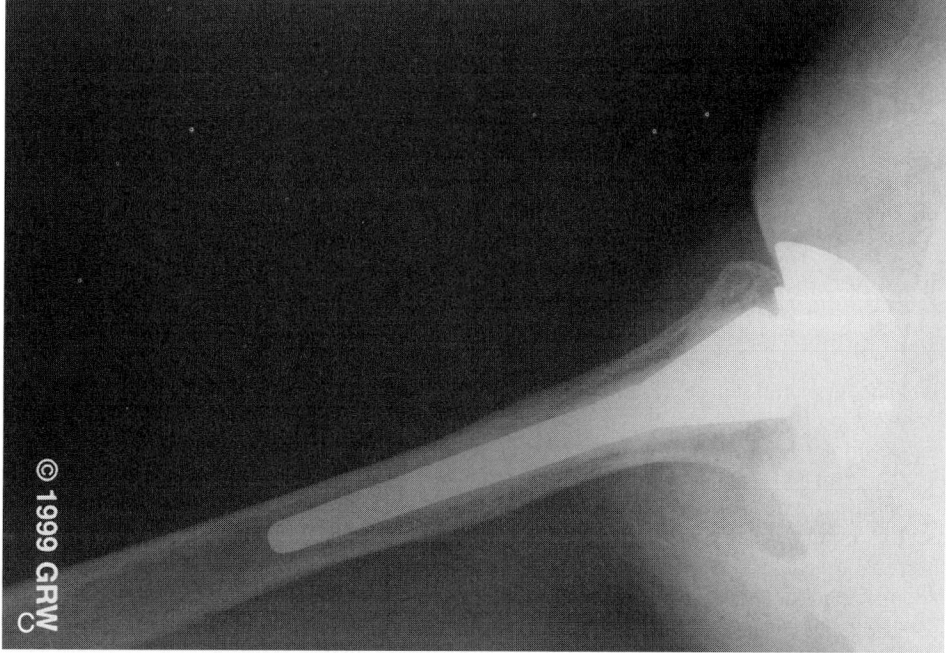

Fig. 11. Radiographs. This patient with rheumatoid arthritis exhibits fixed proximal humeral migration and severe glenoid erosion. Therefore, hemiarthroplasty was performed instead of total shoulder arthroplasty (*A* to *C*).

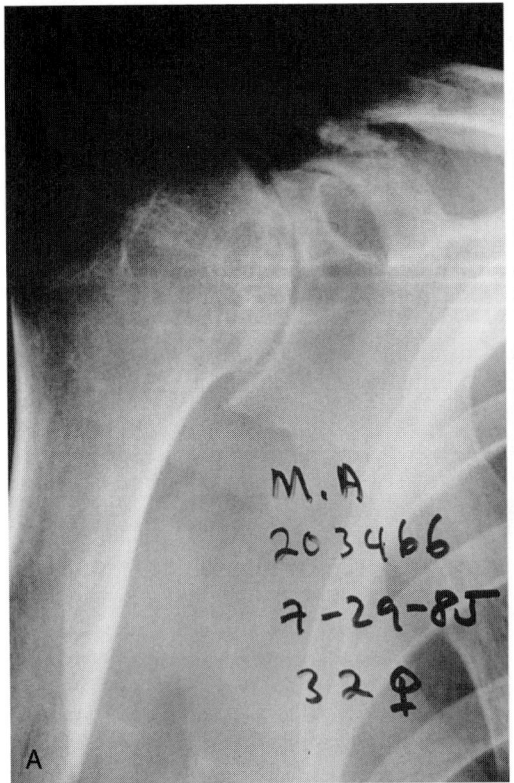

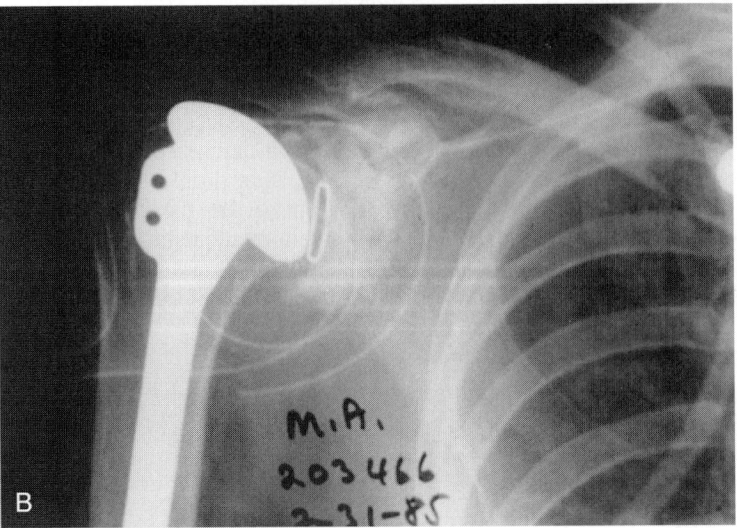

Fig. 12. Radiographs. Total shoulder arthroplasty in rheumatoid arthritis is reserved for patients with no fixed proximal humeral migration, an intact or reparable rotator cuff, and adequate glenoid bone for accepting a glenoid component (A and B).

be possible at the time of hemiarthroplasty. However, an intact coracoacromial arch and functioning deltoid are prerequisites.

Surgical Techniques for Total Shoulder Arthroplasty
Anesthesia and Patient Positioning

Anesthetic choices for shoulder arthroplasty include general, regional (i.e., interscalene block), and combined general and regional techniques. Interscalene block, when performed with a long-acting anesthetic, offers the advantage of prolonged postoperative pain control, decreased amount of postoperative pain, and decreased need for analgesics. The reported experience with interscalene block during shoulder surgery has been safe and reliable, although occasionally the block may be incomplete. The experience of surgery may make some patients extremely anxious and cause them to change position frequently or talk with the surgical team. Consequently, a combined general anesthetic and interscalene block are frequently used.

The most important principle of patient positioning is to provide adequate access to the humeral shaft during reaming and humeral stem insertion. This requires that the patient be positioned laterally on the operating table so the entire humerus and GH joint are unsupported by the table. The arm may then be maximally adducted, extended, and externally rotated to provide unobstructed instrumentation of the intramedullary canal. The patient's head and neck are cushioned and secured to the operating table; a horseshoe-shaped headrest may be used to allow unobstructed access to the top of the shoulder. A laterally placed pad or bolster against the patient's thorax helps to prevent inad-

vertent movement of the patient off the edge of the table during surgical manipulation. A mechanical shoulder positioner may be used to facilitate exposure and instrumentation of the shoulder (Fig. 13).

Deltopectoral Exposure

Shoulder arthroplasty is performed by an extended deltopectoral approach. The skin incision begins superior and medial to the coracoid process and extends inferolaterally toward the deltoid tuberosity. The deltopectoral interval is identified and dissected superiorly to the clavicle and inferiorly to the inferior margin of the pectoralis major tendon. The cephalic vein is preserved and may be taken laterally with the deltoid or medially with the pectoralis major. The upper 1 to 1.5 cm of the pectoralis major tendon may be released from the humerus for added exposure and correction of severe internal rotation contractures.

The conjoined tendon of the coracobrachialis and short head of the biceps brachii is identified deep to the deltopectoral groove. The claviopectoral fascia is incised laterally to the conjoined tendon. This incision is extended proximally to the coracoacromial ligament. The rotator cuff is inspected; if a full-thickness rotator cuff tear is identified, reparability is assessed. If there is any question whether the tendon can be repaired, the coracoacromial ligament is preserved. Otherwise, the coracoacromial ligament is incised to improve exposure. In most cases of primary or post-traumatic OA, the cuff is intact or reparable. In all cases of cuff tear arthropathy and many cases of RA, rotator cuff integrity cannot be restored adequately. Therefore, coracoacromial arch integrity must be maintained. The subscapularis tendon is exposed by retracting the conjoined tendon

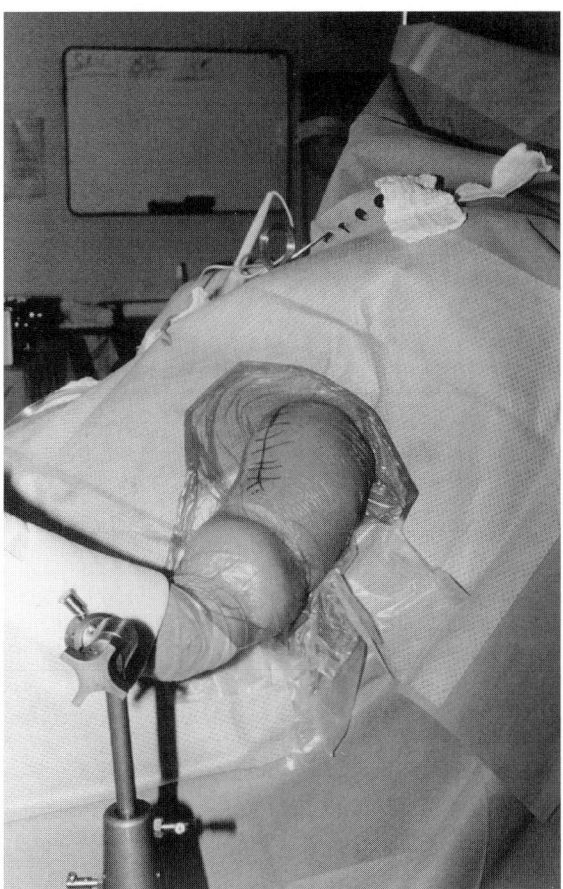

Fig. 13. View. Patients are positioned for shoulder arthroplasty in the semirecumbent or beach-chair position. The use of a mechanical shoulder holder assists in arm manipulation during surgery.

medially. The anterior humeral circumflex vessels are clamped and coagulated, and the axillary nerve is identified and protected throughout the remainder of the procedure.

Subscapularis Incision

The method of subscapularis incision depends on the extent of subscapularis and anterior capsular contracture. If preoperative passive external rotation with the arm at the side is greater than 10 degrees, the subscapularis is incised 1.5 to 2 cm medial to its insertion on the lesser tuberosity. After appropriate capsular release, the subscapularis may be repaired anatomically. Preoperative passive external rotation of −10 to +10 degrees indicates the need for added subscapularis length. In these circumstances, the subscapularis is released directly from its lesser tuberosity insertion to ensure maximal length. At the time of closure, the subscapularis is reinserted medial to the lesser tuberosity at the level of the humeral osteotomy site. Every centimeter of medial advancement yields approximately 20 to 30 degrees of external rotation. Severe internal rotation contractures (i.e., passive external rotation of less than −10 degrees) may require subscapularis Z-lengthening. This is most easily accomplished by direct release of the subscapularis from the lesser tuberosity, separation of the subscapularis from the underlying anterior capsule, and release of the

anterior capsule from the glenoid. This creates a medially-based subscapularis flap and a laterally-based capsular flap that can be used to lengthen the subscapularis (Fig. 14).

Humeral Preparation

After the subscapularis has been reflected medially and the capsule has been released, the humerus is dislocated by simultaneously adducting, extending, and externally rotating the arm. Humeral osteophytes are removed in order to define the region of the humeral anatomic neck. The humeral osteotomy can be made in one of two ways. In the first method, the osteotomy can be performed without a mechanical cutting guide by following the boundary of the humeral anatomic neck. The second method employs a mechanical cutting guide that enforces a predetermined "average" neck-shaft angle. This guide can be intramedullary or extramedullary. Retroversion can be determined using the known "average" relationship between the distal humeral epicondylar axis and the plane of the articular surface (e.g., 30 degrees). The goal of either osteotomy method is to place the humeral osteotomy in a location that permits anatomic placement of the prosthetic articular surface. Either method can be used successfully, and both have advantages and disadvantages.

Once the humeral osteotomy has been performed and the humeral head excised, the humeral canal is reamed with sequentially larger reamers. An appropriately-sized broach is then used to prepare the proximal metaphysis. The broach is left in place to protect the humeral metaphysis during posterior retraction of the humeral head required for glenoid exposure.

Glenoid Preparation

A humeral head retractor is placed between the humerus and the glenoid to displace the humeral metaphysis posteriorly. The glenoid is inspected, and a decision is made with regard to glenoid resurfacing. If adequate bone is available, the rotator cuff is intact and functional, and the patient's age and activity level are appropriate, glenoid resurfacing is preferred. The glenoid labrum is identified and circumferentially excised, starting anterior to the biceps anchor and extending to the posterior aspect of the biceps anchor. The biceps anchor itself is left attached to the superior glenoid.

A large number of glenoid components and reamer systems exist; each has advantages and disadvantages. However, important underlying principles of reaming are common to all systems. The surface contour of the reamed glenoid should match the contour of the glenoid component. In addition, the glenoid version should be corrected as much as possible so that the angular relationship between the implanted glenoid component and the plane of the scapula is nearly perpendicular. After reaming has been completed, the glenoid component is fixed to the native glenoid using either cemented or cementless techniques (Fig. 15).

Soft-Tissue Balancing

Appropriate tension in the capsule and rotator cuff insures maximal range of motion and stability. Soft-tissue tension is assessed by placing a trial humeral head on the broach or the trial humeral implant. A humeral head is selected

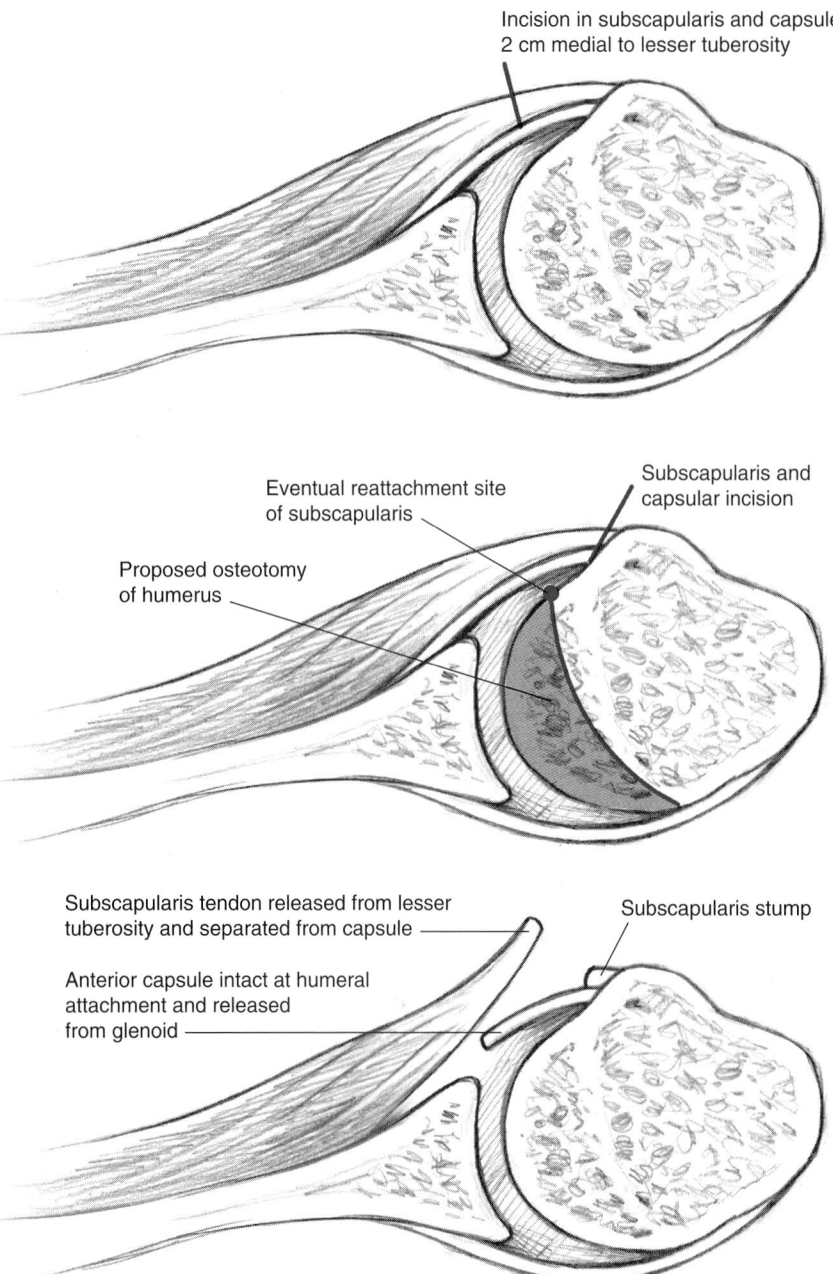

Incision in subscapularis and capsule
2 cm medial to lesser tuberosity

Eventual reattachment site
of subscapularis

Proposed osteotomy
of humerus

Subscapularis and
capsular incision

Subscapularis tendon released from lesser
tuberosity and separated from capsule

Anterior capsule intact at humeral
attachment and released
from glenoid

Subscapularis stump

Fig. 14. Diagram. The subscapularis may be incised 1.5 to 2.0 cm medial to its lesser tuberosity attachment and repaired anatomically in patients with more than 10 degrees of external rotation *(A)*. In patients with more than minus 10 degrees but less than plus 10 degrees of external rotation, the subscapularis is released directly from the lesser tuberosity with maximum length. It is advanced to the edge of the humeral osteotomy at the time of closure *(B)*. Subscapularis Z-lengthening is reserved for patients with less than −10 degrees of external rotation *(C)*. The subscapularis is released from the lesser tuberosity, and the capsule is released from the glenoid.

that approximates the size of the resected humeral head. With the trial implant reduced, the humeral head is translated posteriorly. The humeral head should subluxate approximately 50 percent of its diameter. In addition, the subscapularis should reach the proposed repair site with enough laxity to allow a minimum of 30 to 40 degrees of external rotation. This may require circumferential release of the subscapularis and excision of the anterior capsule. If the posterior capsule is too lax, a larger humeral head can be placed. However, if this larger head compromises subscapularis length, the smaller head size should be used in combination with a posterior capsular shift. This can be accomplished from the anterior approach "through the joint" with the prosthetic humeral head removed. Once a

humeral head size has been selected, the trial implant is removed. The final humeral component can be fixed to the humerus using either cemented or cementless techniques.

Closure

The technique of subscapularis repair depends on the method of subscapularis incision (see Fig. 14). If the tendon was incised medial to its insertion in anticipation of anatomic, tendon-to-tendon repair and subscapularis length is sufficient, anatomic repair of the subscapularis tendon is performed. If the tendon was released directly from the lesser tuberosity with maximum length because of loss of external rotation, two choices for repair exist. The decision is made by temporarily fixing the tendon to the humerus at

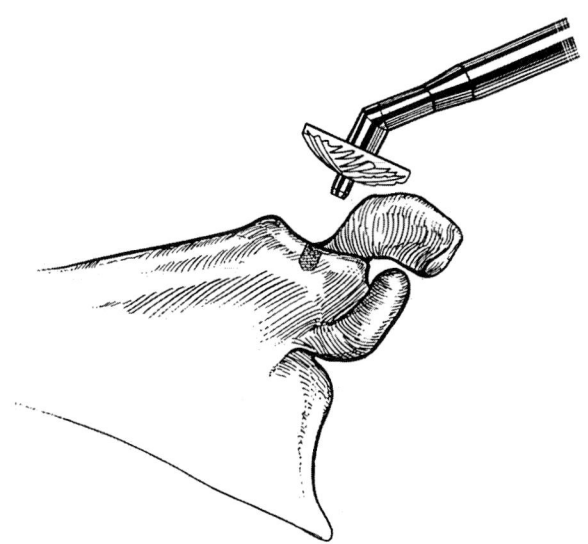

Fig. 15. Diagram. One of the most important concepts of glenoid component fixation is reaming the surface of the native glenoid to match the contour of the back of the glenoid component.

the level of the osteotomy. If the humerus externally rotates 30 to 40 degrees or more, the tendon is reattached through drill holes at the osteotomy site. If the subscapularis is too tight, the laterally based capsular flap is used to lengthen the tendon. The subcutaneous tissue and skin are closed in standard fashion over a closed-suction drainage system.

Postoperative Rehabilitation

The safe range of motion for rehabilitation is determined in the operating room after subscapularis closure. Passive mobilization within these safe limits commences on the first postoperative morning. An overhead pulley is added in 2 to 4 weeks, depending on the status of the subscapularis and rotator cuff. The patient is encouraged to use the arm as a helping hand during daily activities within the first or second postoperative week. Strengthening exercises for the rotator cuff, deltoid, and scapular stabilizers are added approximately 6 weeks postoperatively. Complete rehabilitation requires approximately 1 year.

RESULTS
General

The results of unconstrained total shoulder arthroplasty and hemiarthroplasty are generally favorable.[15, 39, 40] Most of these results, however, are short- to mid-term follow-up, and need to be viewed with caution until larger, long-term survival rates become available. Short-term and mid-term (up to approximately five years) follow-up demonstrate up to 90% good and excellent results of total shoulder arthroplasty.[41, 42] The results of constrained shoulder arthroplasty, on the other hand, have been fraught with complications and a relatively high reoperation rate. Complications include aseptic loosening, implant failure, and instability.[43] Presently, constrained implants are not approved for use in the United States. However, in Europe, more recent designs have met with reasonable success in selected patients as a salvage procedure.[44]

Osteoarthritis

Total shoulder arthroplasty in GH OA has been successful in relieving pain, increasing range of motion, and improving activities of daily living. Pain relief is more predictable in total shoulder arthroplasty than in hemiarthroplasty. Hemiarthroplasty, however, provides acceptable results in patients with concentric, rather than eccentric, glenoid wear patterns.[45] When deciding whether to use a glenoid component in OA, one must individualize each case and weigh the risks and benefits of possible improved pain relief versus early glenoid loosening. Pain relief and improved function can be expected in approximately 90% of patients with a survivorship of approximately 90% at 5 years.[15, 39, 40]

Rheumatoid Arthritis

As in OA, shoulder arthroplasty in RA reliably achieves relief of pain. Improved function, however, is dependent on the preoperative status of the rotator cuff, deltoid, and other periarticular soft tissues. Hemiarthroplasty is often indicated because of significant bone loss or proximal humeral migration associated with rotator cuff dysfunction. However, when glenoid bone stock is adequate and the head can be centered on the glenoid by virtue of an intact or reparable cuff, total shoulder arthroplasty provides superior pain relief. Boyd et al reported the results of total shoulder arthroplasty and hemiarthroplasty with the intent of more clearly outlining the indications for glenoid resurfacing.[46] They concluded that total shoulder arthroplasty and hemiarthroplasty demonstrated similar functional improvements. However, in the patients with rheumatoid arthritis, pain relief, range of motion, and patient satisfaction were greater in those receiving a total shoulder arthroplasty versus a hemiarthroplasty. Therefore, they recommended total shoulder arthroplasty for patients with inflammatory arthropathy.[46]

In 1997, Stewart and Kelly reported on total shoulder arthroplasty in rheumatoid arthritis.[47] There were 37 patients with a 7 to 13 year follow-up. Of the 37, 29 had no pain or slight pain and 4 had moderate or severe pain. Range of motion on average improved for elevation and external rotation. Most studies report good success with total shoulder arthroplasty in rheumatoid arthritis.[48–51] Good to excellent pain relief is achieved in 88% to 100% of patients in almost all follow-up studies. Most have improvement in their activities of daily living even though their active range of motion may remain limited. Hemiarthroplasty is indicated in the presence of fixed proximal humeral migration, irreparable rotator cuff insufficiency, or inadequate glenoid bone stock.

Rotator Cuff Tear Arthropathy

Presently, hemiarthroplasty is the treatment of choice for cuff tear arthropathy.[32, 38] Higher rates of glenoid loosening following total shoulder arthroplasty for cuff tear arthropathy have been reported because of superiorly eccentric loading of the glenoid component associated with proximal humeral migration. The results of follow-up studies are mixed because of the variations in the status of the rotator cuff, the condition of the humerus and the glenoid, and whether there was a previous attempt at a cuff repair. As with arthroplasty for OA and RA, pain relief is generally achieved with arthroplasty for cuff tear arthropathy.

Improvements in strength and function are less predictable because of persistent rotator cuff insufficiency. If the coracoacromial arch has been preserved and the deltoid is intact, satisfactory results can be expected in 80% to 85% of patients.

COMPLICATIONS

Potential complications include periprosthetic fracture, GH instability, infection, implant loosening, rotator cuff tear, and nerve injury. The complications encountered may be related to the underlying etiology leading to the replacement and whether it is early or late in the postoperative period.[41, 42]

Intraoperative periprosthetic fractures may be the result of technical error such as excessive reaming or careless manipulation of the extremity, and are more common in cases of revision arthroplasty or poor bone quality. There is a reported 3% prevalence rate of periprosthetic fractures.[42] Most are intraoperative and involve the humerus.[42] Management of intraoperative humeral fractures typically involves using rigid internal fixation and/or a long stem prosthesis at the time of surgery. Postoperative periprosthetic fractures, on the other hand, have reportedly been managed with operative and nonoperative measures. Some authors advocate aggressive treatment of these injuries because of the risk of nonunion.[52] Surgical options include open reduction with rigid internal fixation, long-stem prosthesis, plates, cerclage wires, cortical bone struts, and autologous bone grafting. Others feel that stable fractures can be managed nonoperatively.[53] Patients with rheumatoid arthritis may be at greater risk for intraoperative fracture because their bone is soft with thin cortices. These patients may also be at greater risk of nonunion.

One additional early complication that may occur at the time of surgery is nerve injury, usually involving the axillary nerve. Nerve injuries occur in less than 1% of cases; most are neuropraxias resulting from traction or contusion; and most resolve without operative intervention. However, blunt injury to neural structures other than the axillary nerve as well as nerve lacerations have been reported.[42, 54]

GH instability is often related to improper positioning of the components or inadequate balancing of the soft tissues.[55] Anterior instability is related to decreased retroversion of the humeral component and subscapularis dysfunction or disruption. Posterior instability is associated with increased retroversion of the humeral component and unrecognized or undercorrected posterior glenoid erosion resulting in increased glenoid component retroversion. Superior instability is associated with a torn or poorly functioning rotator cuff that may not provide sufficient force coupling to counter the superior pull of the deltoid. Patients with RA are especially at risk because their capsule and rotator cuff are affected by their disease. For patients without a functioning rotator cuff, maintaining an intact coracoacromial arch and a well-functioning deltoid is critical to help minimize this problem.

Infection is a complication that can present early (acute) or late (chronic). Acute infections tend to be wound-related. Chronic infections, on the other hand, tend to be from hematogenous spread from a site other than the shoulder. The most common infecting organisms, are *Staphylococcus aureus* and *Staphyloccus epidermidis*.[54]

Due to an excellent blood supply about the shoulder, this complication is rarely seen, with a reported incidence of 0.34 to 2.9%.[54] Presently, the literature is deficient in management (i.e. primary versus secondary exchange, resection arthroplasty, etc.), and in outcomes for infected shoulder arthroplasty compared to infected hip and knee arthroplasty. However, the patient with inflammatory arthropathy may be at increased risk due to poor healing ability and immunosuppression secondary to their systemic disease process and medications.

Implant loosening has been widely discussed, especially that of the glenoid component. Radiolucencies about the glenoid component are common and have been reported to occur in 30% to 100% of cases.[42] However, the clinical relevance of glenoid lucent lines is unclear. Glenoid loosening is much less common than glenoid radiolucency. Cofield and Edgerton found an overall glenoid loosening rate of 4.7%.[54] A variety of reasons have been proposed for glenoid component loosening, including glenoid replacement in the face of an irreparable rotator cuff tear, inadequate fixation, and various technical limitations (see Fig. 9). Rodosky and Bigliani reviewed the literature and found a glenoid revision rate from 0% to 12.5% in a variety of cases and follow-up time from surgery.[56] In 1997, Torchia, Cofield, and Settergren[51] reported on total shoulder arthroplasty performed with the Neer prosthesis. These patients had a diagnosis of OA, RA, or traumatic arthritis, and 79 patients with 89 implants were available for follow-up from 5 to 17 years postoperatively. Seventy-five (84%) glenoid components developed bone-cement radiolucencies. Thirty-nine (44%) showed radiographic evidence of loosening and this glenoid loosening was associated with pain.[59] Early results with tissue ingrowth glenoid components revealed that less radiographic evidence of loosening had occurred than in the cemented glenoid components.[13] Clearly, longer follow-up and further study are necessary to accurately characterize the survivorship of the cemented glenoid components and to determine the role of cementless glenoids.

Humeral component radiolucencies and loosening are much less common when compared to glenoid components. Loosening of the humeral component has been reported at 0.4% with a range of 0% to 6.9%.[64, 65] However, cementless fixation may be more commonly associated with subsidence and loosening than with cemented fixation. The absence of a radiodense cement mantle complicates the diagnosis, which requires a high index of suspicion.

Postoperative rotator cuff tear has a reported prevalence of about 2%.[22, 54] These can be managed operatively or nonoperatively, depending on the individual circumstances. Operative management carries the risk of re-rupture. However, surgical indications are similar to the nonprosthetic shoulder. Patients with inflammatory arthropathy may be at greater risk of postoperative cuff rupture and less likely to benefit from surgical repair. Certainly, each case must be individualized.

SUMMARY

GH arthritis is not as common as arthritis affecting the lower extremities, but it is encountered in younger patients with potentially higher activity levels. Although multiple types of GH arthritis exist, the most common are OA, RA, post-traumatic arthritis, and cuff tear arthropathy. The pathogenesis of all types of GH arthritis is poorly understood. The clinical presentation, prognosis, and recommended treatment are largely dependent on the arthritis type. Nonoperative treatment is often successful and includes anti-inflammatory medications and other pharmacologic agents, physiotherapy, and activity modification. When nonoperative measures fail, surgical management includes several options. However, the most commonly performed procedure for end-stage GH arthritis is shoulder replacement. The indications for total shoulder replacement versus humeral hemiarthroplasty continue to be refined. Presently, total shoulder replacement is preferred in patients older than 50 years with an intact and functional rotator cuff and adequate glenoid bone stock to accept a glenoid component. Short- to mid-term results are encouraging, with survivorship of approximately 95% at 5 years. The problems of glenoid component wear and aseptic loosening will take longer-term follow-up to fully characterize.

REFERENCES

1. McCarty DJ: Robert Adams' rheumatic arthritis of the shoulder: "Milwaukee shoulder: Revisited." J Rheumatol 1989; 16: 668.

2. Williams G, Rockwood C: Massive rotator cuff defects and glenohumeral arthritis. *In* Friedman RJ (ed): Arthroplasty of the Shoulder. New York, Thieme Medical Publishers, Inc., 1994, p 204.

3. Codman EA: Rupture of the Supraspinatus Tendon and Other Lesions In or About the Subacromial Bursa. Boston, Thomas Todd, 1934.

4. Halverson PB, Cheung HS, McCarty DJ, et al: "Milwaukee shoulder"—association of microspheroids containing hydroxyapatite crystals, active collagenase, and neutral protease with rotator cuff defects II: Synovial fluid studies. Arthritis Rheum 1981; 24:474.

5. McCarty DJ, Halverson PB, Carrera GF, et al: "Milwaukee shoulder"—association of microspheroids containing hydroxyapatite crystals, active collagenase, and neutral protease with rotator cuff defects I: Clinical aspects. Arthritis Rheum 1981; 24:464.

6. Neer CS: Total shoulder replacement: A preliminary report. Orthop Trans 1977; 1: 244.

7. Neer CS, Craig EV, Fukuda H: Cuff-tear arthropathy. J Bone Joint Surg Am, 1983; 65:1232.

8. Lugli T: Artificial shoulder joint by Pean (1893): The facts of an exceptional intervention and the prosthetic method. Clin Orthop 1978; 133:215.

9. Post M, Jablon M: Constrained total shoulder arthroplasty. Clin Orthop Rel Res 1983; 173:109.

10. Burkhead W: History and development of shoulder arthroplasty. *In* Friedman RJ (ed): Arthroplasty of the Shoulder. New York, Thieme Medical Publishers, Inc., 1994, p 1.

11. Krueger FJ: A vitallium replica arthroplasty on the shoulder. Surgery 1951; 30: 1005.

12. Neer CS, Brown THJ, McLaughlin HL: Fracture of the neck of the humerus with dislocation of the head fragment. Am J Surg 1953; 85:252.

13. Neer CS: Articular replacement for the humeral head. J Bone Joint Surg Am 1955; 37:215.

14. Neer CS: Indications for replacement of the proximal humeral articulation. Am J Surg 1955; 89:901.

15. Neer CS: Replacement arthroplasty for glenohumeral osteoarthritis. J Bone Joint Surg Am 1974; 56:1.

16. Hamada K, Fukuda H, Mikasa M, et al: Roentgenographic findings in massive rotator cuff tears: A long-term observation. Clin Orthop Rel Res 1990; 254:92.

17. Rockwood CA Jr, Williams GR Jr, Burkhead WZ Jr: Debridement of degenerative, irreparable lesions of the rotator cuff. J Bone Joint Surg Am 1995; 77:857.

18. Fenlin JM Jr, Frieman BG: Indications, technique, and results of total shoulder arthroplasty in osteoarthritis. Orthop Clin North Am 1998; 29:423.

19. Edelson JG: Localized glenoid hypoplasia: An anatomic variation of possible clinical significance. Clin Orthop Rel Res 1995; 321:189.

20. Wirth MA, Lyons FR, Rockwood CA Jr: Hypoplasia of the glenoid: A review of sixteen patients. J Bone Joint Surg Am 1993; 75:1175.

21. Cuomo F, Greller MJ, Zuckerman JD: The rheumatoid shoulder. Rheum Dis Clin North Am 1998; 24:67.

22. Rodnan G, Schumacher H, Zvaifler N: Rheumatoid arthritis. *In* Rodnan GP, Schumacher H, Zvaifler N (eds): Primer on the Rheumatic Diseases. Atlanta, Arthritis Foundation, 1983, 8th ed, p 38.

23. Dieppe P, Watt I: Crystal deposition in osteoarthritis: An opportunistic event? Clin Rheum Dis 1985; 11:367.

24. Dieppe PA, Cawston T, Mercer E, et al: Synovial fluid collagenase in patients with destructive arthritis of the shoulder joint. Arthritis Rheum 1988; 31:882.

25. Arnett FC: The American Rheumatism Association 1987 revised criteria for the classification of rheumatoid arthritis. Arthritis Rheum 1988; 31:315.

26. Ennevaara K: Painful shoulder joint in rheumatoid arthritis: A clinical and radiological study of 200 cases, with special reference to arthrography of the glenohumeral joint. Acta Rheumatol Scand Suppl 1967; 11:1.

27. Kelly IG, Foster RS, Fisher WD: Neer total shoulder replacement in rheumatoid arthritis. J Bone Joint Surg Br 1987; 69:723.

28. Flatow E, Weinstein D, Duralde X, et al:

Coracoacromial ligament preservation in rotator cuff surgery. J Shoulder Elbow Surg 1994; 3:73.

29. Wiley AM: Superior humeral dislocation: A complication following decompression and debridement for rotator cuff tears. Clin Orthop 1991; 263:135.

30. Burkhart SS: Fluoroscopic comparison of kinematic patterns in massive rotator cuff tears: A suspension bridge model. Clin Orthop 1992; 284:144.

31. Burkhart SS: Reconciling the paradox of rotator cuff repair versus debridement: A unified biomechanical rationale for the treatment of rotator cuff tears. Arthroscopy 1994; 10:4.

32. Williams GR Jr, Rockwood CA Jr: Hemiarthroplasty in rotator cuff-deficient shoulders. J Shoulder Elbow Surg 1996; 5:362.

33. Iannotti JP, Gabriel JP, Schneck SL, et al: The normal glenohumeral relationships: An anatomical study of one hundred and forty shoulders. J Bone Joint Surg Am 1992; 74:491.

34. Badet R, Boileau P, Noel E, et al: Arthrography and computed arthrotomography study of seventy patients with primary glenohumeral osteoarthritis. Rev Rhumatisme, English edition, 1995; 62:555.

35. Iannotti JP, Zlatkin MB, Esterhai JL, et al: Magnetic resonance imaging of the shoulder: Sensitivity, specificity and predictive value. J Bone Joint Surg Am 1991; 73:17.

36. Burkhead WZ Jr, Hutton KS: Biologic resurfacing of the glenoid with hemiarthroplasty of the shoulder. J Shoulder Elbow Surg 1995; 4:263.

37. Franklin JL, Barrett WP, Jackins SE, et al: Glenoid loosening in total shoulder arthroplasty. J Arthroplasty 1988; 3:39.

38. Pollock RG, Deliz ED, McIlveen SJ, et al: Prosthetic replacement in rotator cuff–deficient shoulders. J Shoulder Elbow Surg 1992; 1:173.

39. Cofield RH: Total shoulder arthroplasty with the Neer prosthesis. J Bone Joint Surg Am 1984; 66:899.

40. Neer CS, Watson KC, Stanton FJ: Recent experience in total shoulder replacement. J Bone Joint Surg Am 1982; 64:319.

41. Wirth MA, Rockwood CA Jr: Complications of shoulder arthroplasty. Clin Orthop Rel Res 1994; 307:47.

42. Wirth MA, Rockwood CA Jr: Complications of total shoulder replacement arthro-

plasty. J Bone Joint Surg Am 1996; 78: 603.

43. Post M: Constrained arthroplasty of the shoulder. Orthop Clin North Am 1987; 18: 455.

44. Grammont PM, Baulot E: Delta shoulder prosthesis for rotator cuff rupture. Orthopedics 1993; 16:65.

45. Levine WN, Djurasovic M, Glasson JM, et al: Hemiarthroplasty for glenohumeral osteoarthritis: Results correlated to degree of glenoid wear. J Shoulder Elbow Surg 1997; 6: 449.

46. Boyd AD Jr, Thomas WH, Scott RD, et al: Total shoulder arthroplasty versus hemiarthroplasty: Indications for glenoid resurfacing. J Arthroplasty 1990; 5:329.

47. Stewart MP, Kelly IG: Total shoulder replacement in rheumatoid disease: 7- to 13-year follow-up of 37 joints. J Bone Joint Surg Br 1997; 79:68.

48. Barrett WP, Thornhill TS, Thomas WH, et al: Nonconstrained total shoulder arthroplasty in patients with polyarticular rheumatoid arthritis. J Arthroplasty 1989; 4:91.

49. Friedman RJ, Ewald FC: Arthroplasty of the ipsilateral shoulder and elbow in patients who have rheumatoid arthritis. J Bone Joint Surg Am 1987; 69:661.

50. Kelly IG: Unconstrained shoulder arthroplasty in rheumatoid arthritis. Clin Orthop Rel Res 1994; 307:94.

51. Torchia ME, Cofield RH, Settergren CR: Total shoulder arthroplasty with the Neer prosthesis: Long-term results. J Shoulder Elbow Surg 1997; 6:495.

52. Bonutti PM, Hawkins RJ: Fracture of the humeral shaft associated with total replacement arthroplasty of the shoulder: A case report. J Bone Joint Surg Am 1992; 74:617.

53. Groh G, Heckman MM, Curtis RJ, et al: Treatment of fractures adjacent to humeral prosthesis. Orthop Trans 1994; 18:1072.

54. Cofield RH. Edgerton BC: Total shoulder arthroplasty: Complications and revision surgery. Instr Course Lect 1990; 39:449.

55. Moeckel BH, Altchek D, Warren RF, et al: Instability of the shoulder after arthroplasty. J Bone Joint Surg Am 1993; 75: 492.

56. Rodosky MW, Bigliani LU: Indications for glenoid resurfacing in shoulder arthroplasty. J Shoulder Elbow Surg 1996; 5: 231.

57. Cofield RH: Uncemented total shoulder arthroplasty: A review. Clin Orthop 1994; 307:86.

ARTHRITIS OF THE ELBOW

John A. King, James H. Herndon, and Matthew M. Tomaino

Summary

- Arthritis of the elbow requires treatment less frequently than arthritis of other major joints.
- The type of treatment is dictated by the type of arthritis present.
- Motion-preserving procedures are the treatment of choice.
- Surgical treatment of rheumatoid arthritis is stage-dependent and consists primarily of elbow synovectomy or total elbow arthroplasty.
- Treatment of post-traumatic arthritis is aimed at restoring motion and eliminating extrinsic and intrinsic disorders causing decreased motion and contributing to pain.
- Osteoarthritis is seen relatively infrequently, and the ulnohumeral articulation is usually preserved.

Arthritis affects the elbow less frequently than other major joints of the body. Rheumatoid and post-traumatic arthritis are the most common types of elbow arthritis requiring treatment. Osteoarthritis is seen less frequently. A careful history and physical examination to assess the clinical presentation are crucial to determine the cause of arthritis and the appropriate treatment.

The most common complaint causing patients to seek medical advice is pain. Instability in rheumatoid arthritis and stiffness in post-traumatic arthritis and osteoarthritis are also common. Less frequent are swelling, weakness, locking, neuritis, and deformity. Physical examination should include assessment of extra-articular manifestations of the arthritis such as skin quality, olecranon bursitis, or extensor surface nodules. Joint examination should include evaluation of both passive and active range of motion,

assessment for effusion or instability, and maneuvers that reproduce painful symptoms and measure strength. Assessment of the other joints of the ipsilateral and contralateral upper extremity and of the lower extremities must be included, as the order of treatment of the various joints may be altered. Radiographic features, laboratory evaluation, and synovial fluid analysis will frequently assist with the diagnosis. Treatment should be dictated by the type of arthritis. These treatments are discussed in later sections.

ANATOMY AND BIOMECHANICS

The elbow joint is composed of the complex articulations of the humerus, radius, and ulna. The ulnotrochlear and radiocapitellar joints provide motion through the arc of flexion and extension, but do not act as a true hinge, as there is a valgus/varus laxity of 3 to 4 degrees.[1] In addition, the proximal radioulnar and the distal radioulnar joints of the wrist provide rotation.

The normal elbow has a 165 to 170 degree arc of flexion and extension, 75 to 80 degrees of pronation, and 85 to 90 degrees of supination.[2] As shown by Morrey et al,[3] an arc of flexion and extension of 30 to 130 degrees and an arc of rotation of 50 degrees each for pronation and supination are required for most activities of daily living. Many patients affected with elbow arthritis can function adequately with less motion, especially if other joints are not affected. When considering options for surgical intervention, an attempt at restoring functional motion in addition to relieving pain is justified.

The center of the flexion-extension arc coincides with the center of the arc of curvature of the distal humerus and is bisected, in the lateral view, by a line drawn distally along the anterior cortex of the humeral shaft. In the anteroposterior plane, the axis of motion lies parallel to the distal articular surfaces of the trochlea and capitellum.[4] Failure to restore the center of motion with reconstruction may lead to instability, insufficient motion, or early failure of the procedure.

Maintaining joint stability is of paramount importance in providing a functional elbow. In extension, the bony articulation provides approximately 50% of the stability of the elbow, with the other 50% being provided by the soft tissues.[5] Ligamentous stability is provided by the lateral collateral ligament complex in varus stress and by the medial collateral ligament complex in valgus stress. In flexion, the articular surface provides approximately 75% of the resistance to varus stress but is less important when a valgus stress is applied. The anterior portion of the medial collateral ligament is the major restraint against a valgus force.[5, 6] The radial head is a secondary stabilizer and provides resistance to valgus load only if the medial collateral ligament is incompetent.[7]

Forces to which the patient will subject the elbow must also be considered when determining the best treatment option. Dynamic forces, such as those that occur when using the upper extremity to push up from sitting, when using an ambulatory aid, or lifting, can produce loads of more than six times body weight.[8] Joint reaction forces are in a posterior direction with flexion and anteriorly with extension.[9] Significant forces about the elbow must be considered, therefore, when designing reconstructive procedures and prosthetic implants.

RHEUMATOID ARTHRITIS

The prevalence of rheumatoid arthritis has been reported to be between 1% and 2% of the adult population. The incidence rate increases as the population ages, with 0.3% of adults younger than 35 years of age affected compared with 10% of those older than 65 years of age.[10] Between 20 and 50% of patients with rheumatoid arthritis will have some involvement of the elbow, but only 66% will complain of symptoms.[11] The majority of patients with elbow symptoms will also have involvement of the hand and wrist as well as the shoulder. Only 5% of rheumatoid patients experience isolated involvement of the elbow.[12] Therefore, treatment is dictated on many occasions by the status of other joint involvement.

PATHOGENESIS
As the disease progresses, the articular cartilage is replaced by pannus, and the supporting ligaments become incompetent. Severe loss of bone stock with subluxation or frank dislocation may occur.

CLINICAL FEATURES
Classification
The pattern of bony destruction has been classified by the American Rheumatism Association (ARA) into radiographic stages[13] and has been modified by several authors.[11, 14–16] In stage I, synovitis is prominent clinically. Osteoporosis is present on radiographs. With stage II, slight cartilage and bony destruction begins and joint space narrowing is present (greater than 1 mm of joint space remains). Mild or moderate degrees of erosive changes with small bone cysts also may develop (Fig. 1). In stage III, the bony architecture is altered. Less than 1 mm of the joint space remains and cystic formation is more common. Because bony destruction is more significant, slight instability in the coronal plane may be evident. Ferlic et al[14] further divided stage III into stage IIIA, some degree of joint space maintained, and stage IIIB, total loss of joint space in one radiographic view. Stage IV represents end-stage disease with gross destruction of the bony architecture. Radiographically, the joint space is lost in two views. Ankylosis or subluxation/dislocation may be present (Fig. 2).

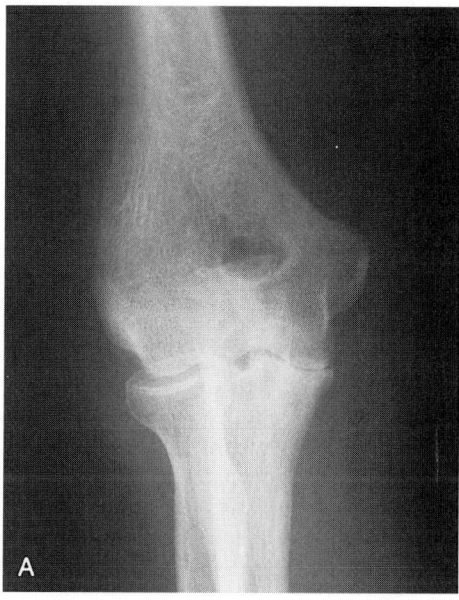
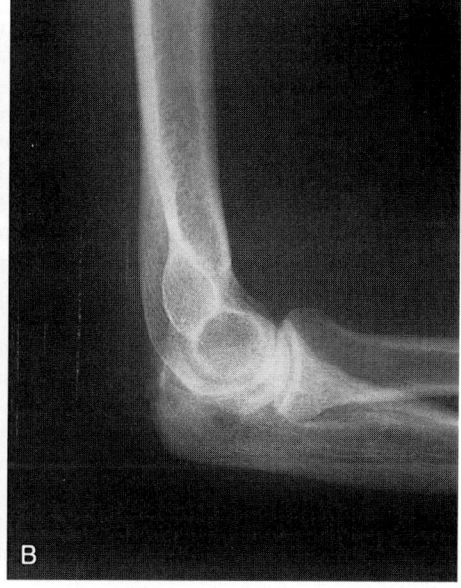

Fig. 1. Stage II rheumatoid arthritis. *A*, Anteroposterior view: joint space narrowing of the ulnohumeral joint. *B*, Lateral view: small bone cyst of the ulna.

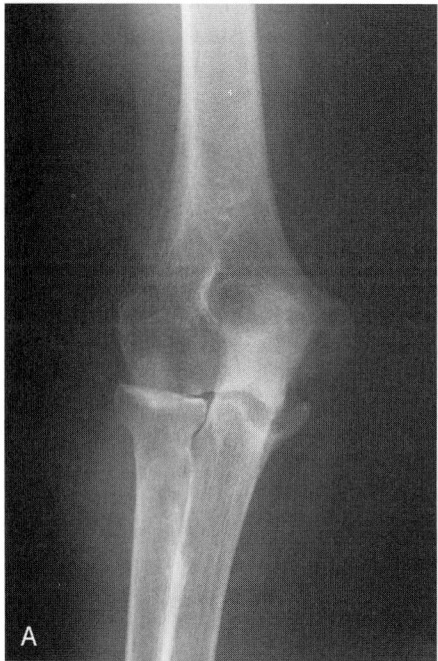 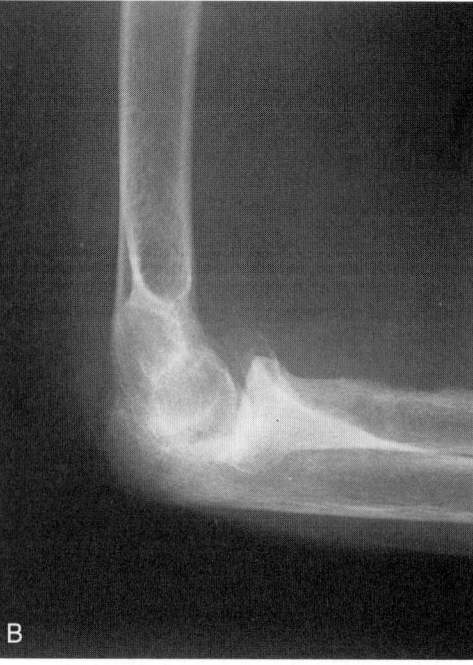

Fig. 2. Stage IV rheumatoid arthritis. *A* and *B*, Joint space is lost on both radiographic views.

Extra-Articular Manifestations

Rheumatoid arthritis at times can be difficult to differentiate from other inflammatory arthritides. The rheumatoid elbow is associated with many extra-articular manifestations that can aid in the diagnosis. Many of these features are associated with the intra-articular disorder secondary to synovitis. Olecranon bursitis is a frequent finding. Aspiration and injection of a corticosteroid may be beneficial. Excision should be entertained cautiously because it is followed by a high recurrence rate.

Synovitis of the elbow joint may also lead to nerve entrapment syndromes. Diagnosis is made with arthrography or magnetic resonance imaging. Injection may diminish synovitis and relieve pressure on the nerve, but surgical decompression is usually indicated.[17]

Ulnar nerve impingement may also be encountered secondary to medial synovitis or articular destruction or instability. Simultaneous ulnar nerve decompression and transposition should be considered when treating the symptomatic elbow with any reconstructive procedure. Rheumatoid nodules are a frequent finding and are more commonly found on the extensor surface of the elbow. No treatment is needed unless a nonhealing ulceration develops or the patient requests excision because of pain or cosmetic concerns. A high recurrence rate is noted with removal.

MANAGEMENT
Nonoperative Treatment

It should be recognized that rheumatoid arthritis is a systemic disease. As with most orthopaedic maladies, initial treatment should be nonoperative (Fig. 3). The nonoperative treatment is aimed at relieving pain, slowing the progression of the disease, and maintaining function of the involved limb. The patient must be monitored closely so that loss of motion, instability, and deformity of the elbow do not become so severe as to make surgical treatment

more difficult or lessen its effectiveness. The clinical course of the rheumatoid patient is variable and unpredictable.[18]

Although medication does not cure the disease, progression may be curtailed. There are currently three classes of medications being used in treatment of rheumatoid arthritis.[19] Salicylates and nonsteroidal anti-inflammatory drugs are the first line of treatment. The second-line drugs are the disease-modifying antirheumatic drugs. Gold, penicillamine, sulfasalazine, hydroxychloroquine, and methotrexate are examples. Typically this class of drugs improves symptoms for several months to years. Cytotoxic and immunoregulatory therapy are the third class of medication. This class includes glucocorticoids, azathioprine, cyclophosphamide, and cyclosporine. Glucocorticoids are given orally or intra-articularly. Use of corticosteroids orally should be limited and injection into the joint should not exceed three to four occasions per year. Other nonoperative measures include therapy to maintain motion and strength and to assist with activities of daily living. Rest and splints are helpful in periods of exacerbation, but care should be taken so that long-term or constant use of a splint does not lead to restricted motion.

Surgical Treatment

Surgical intervention of the rheumatoid elbow should be considered when nonoperative measures fail to halt the symptoms or progression of the disease process. Pain is the most common indication for surgery. In later stages of the disease, instability or bony destruction may be an indication. When ankylosis is present or the elbow has significant loss of motion, reconstruction may be needed to improve or maintain function.

The order of treatment of an ipsilateral shoulder and elbow pathological condition is controversial. The most disabling or painful joint should probably be addressed first. The surgeon should consider reconstruction of the elbow before that of the shoulder if both joints are involved equally. The shoulder reconstruction should be performed initially if significant loss of shoulder rotation is noted, because excessive loads in valgus, varus, or rotation may lead to early failure of the elbow reconstruction.[20]

The primary reconstructive options for the rheumatoid elbow include synovectomy with or without radial head excision, interposition arthroplasty, and total elbow arthroplasty (see Fig. 3). Several variables must be assessed to

determine which procedure is best suited for a particular patient. Age, health status, skin quality, bone stock, presence of instability, and range of motion determine which reconstructive option is most appropriate.

Elbow Synovectomy

The ideal candidate for elbow synovectomy is a rheumatoid patient with pain, persistent synovitis, crepitation with rotation, and slightly limited motion. Synovectomy is usually performed with open or arthroscopic techniques. Ra-

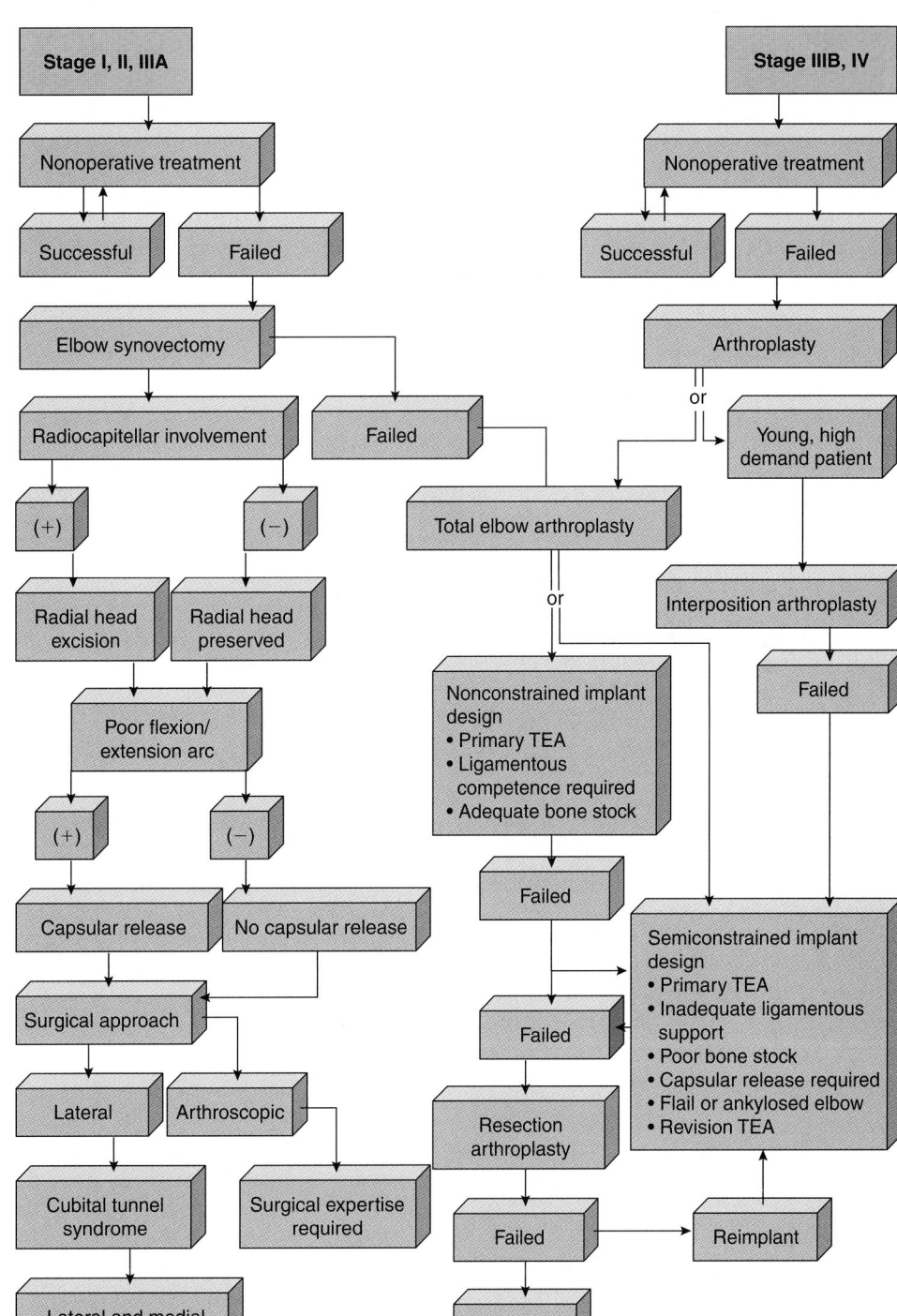

Fig. 3. Rheumatoid arthritis. This is a management algorithm. TEA = total elbow arthroplasty.

dioisotope injection remains experimental. Debate exists over the stage of the disease for which the procedure is indicated, whether the radial head should be excised or retained, and which approach is best.

The radiographic ARA stage of the disease for which synovectomy is indicated is controversial. Most authors feel that it is best reserved for early-stage disease (ARA stage I, II, and IIIA).[12, 14, 21–23] However, some studies claim adequate results in the later stages of the disease (ARA stage III and IV).[11, 16, 24–26] With articular destruction and ligamentous laxity beginning in stage III disease, some degree of instability is present in most elbows with this degree of involvement. Tulp and Winia[16] cited no statistical difference comparing the results in the treatment of stage I/II versus stage III/IV. Contrary to this claim, they found instability to be a predictor of failure, as have others.[27, 28]

Schemitsch et al[29] compared rheumatoid patients having primary unconstrained total elbow arthroplasty and those having total elbow arthroplasty following a failed elbow synovectomy and radial head excision. The primary arthroplasty group was more satisfied with regard to pain and functional status. More patients in the revision group required additional surgery and had symptoms of instability. It would appear, therefore, that elbow synovectomy should be reserved for the earlier stages of the disease before the occurrence of instability.[12]

Another controversial point regarding elbow synovectomy is whether to excise or retain the radial head. Most authors recommend excision because it is felt to contribute to pain relief. Better access to the joint is also provided when the radial head is excised.[28] However, late valgus instability may be a problem after its excision, leading to a poor outcome.[16, 23] If cartilage is present on the radial head and the articular surface is congruous with the capitellum, excision should be avoided. Results have been comparable with those of excision and may improve the longevity of the procedure, especially by preventing instability.[16, 25] The use of a Silastic radial head implant after head excision has been largely abandoned.

Several surgical approaches to the elbow have been used for synovectomy. Inglis et al[26] described a transolecranon approach. Most authors favor a lateral approach.[11, 14, 22, 25, 28] Some advocate a combined medial and a lateral approach.[14, 16] Rymaszewski et al[28] reported that cases in which the results deteriorated over time tended to have recurrence of medial-sided pain. Additionally, ulnar neuropathy, if not addressed, is a predictor of failure.[27] In that light, if significant medial pain or ulnar neuritis is present preoperatively, a medial exposure should be used so that ulnar nerve decompression and transposition can be performed at the same time as synovectomy.

Patient satisfaction after elbow synovectomy ranges from 70% to 90%.[12, 14, 16, 23, 27, 28, 30, 31] Some studies have shown no progression of the disease,[11, 25] whereas others show a gradual deterioration.[14, 27, 28] After synovectomy, the pronation-supination arc improves most reliably.[11, 14, 22, 27] The flexion-extension arc typically improves in 50% of patients with 25% unchanged and 25% worsened.[26] The strongest predictor of satisfaction with the procedure seems to be a low arc of rotation.[27]

Because gains in extension and flexion may be moderate at best, Lonner and Stuchin[11] performed an anterior capsular release in addition to synovectomy and radial head excision. They acknowledged that synovectomy and radial head excision address the intrinsic causes of lost motion but do not address secondary extrinsic contracture. In their series, the flexion contracture and flexion-extension arc improved more than in previous studies.

Patients with juvenile rheumatoid arthritis have a strong predilection to elbow stiffness, and because the preoperative flexion-extension arc of motion is limited, the results of synovectomy in this population are poor in as many as 50% of patients.[14]

In addition to elbow instability, persistent ulnar neuropathy, and poor preoperative motion in the sagittal plane, duration of symptoms longer than 5 years, recurrent synovitis, poor upper limb function, and poor general health status have all led to poor results.[27] In spite of these findings, open elbow synovectomy is a reliable procedure if the candidates are appropriately chosen.

Arthroscopic synovectomy results in excellent short-term outcome. Lee and Morrey[32] achieved 93% excellent to good results with the procedure. Unfortunately, by 42 months the favorable results had deteriorated to 57%. Radioactive synovectomy has also produced fairly good results in clinical trials, but the long-term benefit is uncertain.

Interposition Arthroplasty

Interposition arthroplasty has been reported for the rheumatoid elbow. The indications are the same as those for total elbow arthroplasty, but adequate stability must be present. Ljung et al[33] reported on 35 rheumatoid elbows that underwent interposition arthroplasty. At an average follow-up of 6 years, results were inferior to those of total elbow arthroplasty with one half progressing to a higher radiographic stage. A significant number developed bone loss, which occasionally made further reconstruction more difficult. The authors felt that total elbow arthroplasty was a better choice in late-stage disease. Interposition arthroplasty may still be a viable option in the younger patient with high demand.

Total Elbow Arthroplasty
Historical Development

The developmental history of total elbow arthroplasty has been divided into four periods by Coonrad.[34] Resection or interposition arthroplasty was the only option in the first period. In the late 1940s, custom hemiarthroplasties were used, but this second period was characterized by high rates of complications. In the third period, constrained metal-on-metal hinged prostheses produced good results initially, but a loosening rate of 27% to 41% developed because of high stresses transmitted to the bone-cement interface.[35–37] The fourth period signaled a change in prosthetic design that allowed the soft-tissue structures of the elbow to absorb a great deal of the forces. Nonconstrained and semiconstrained prostheses became more widely used and results improved. Increasing knowledge of biomechanics, triceps-sparing approaches, and improved cementing techniques all contributed to increased implant longevity. Additional design changes in the 1980s resulted in many of the current implants available. Changes in the articular surface and stem lengths of nonconstrained implants allowed greater stability. Changes to semiconstrained components were also designed to decrease the incidence rate of dislocation of the snap-fit designs. An anterior flange was added to the Coonrad-Morrey implant to decrease the rate of loosening. As a result, the rate of complications following total elbow arthroplasty is approaching that of other joint replacements.

Indications

The most common reason for elbow replacement is elbow pain with stage III or IV disease. Motion loss alone does not mandate total elbow arthroplasty unless the function of the joints in the ipsilateral upper extremity is poor, the elbow is ankylosed in a position that compromises function, or both elbows are ankylosed. Stiffness and ankylosis are, however, frequent indications for surgery in patients with juvenile rheumatoid arthritis. Instability secondary to poor ligamentous support and loss of bone stock are also indications for replacement and usually require a semiconstrained implant. Elbow arthroplasty is also useful when synovectomy or interposition arthroplasty fails.

Contraindications to elbow arthroplasty are active infection of the joint or adjacent soft tissues, neurological abnormalities such as a flaccid limb or increased tone from spasticity, and a neuropathic joint. Relative contraindications include a previous infection or osteomyelitis and skin or wound problems. Infection must be ruled out before proceeding with reconstruction and if wound problems exist, they must be addressed before surgery.

Implant Designs

The two categories of elbow replacement arthroplasty currently in use are resurfacing nonconstrained and semiconstrained implants (Fig. 4). Nonconstrained implants resurface the distal humerus and the proximal ulna. Adequate

bone stock and ligament competence are required because stability of the device is obtained by the soft-tissue supporting structures. Kudo and Iwano[38] found that 70% of the humeral implants used without stems had various degrees of subsidence. The loosening in these components followed a predictable pattern. Humeral components tended to rotate posteriorly with gross displacement requiring revision in 14% of cases. The addition of stems has significantly diminished this problem.[38, 39]

Semiconstrained implants evolved from fully constrained devices. The articulation of the humeral and ulnar components was altered to allow motion in an attempt to lessen the high rate of loosening seen with earlier constrained implants. Morrey modified the Coonrad elbow arthroplasty in 1978 to allow 8 degrees of varus-valgus laxity and 8 degrees of internal-external laxity within the device. In 1981, an anterior flange was also added to the humeral component to resist the posteriorly directed forces seen with elbow flexion.[15] The stresses were no longer directed only to the bone-cement interface, but were absorbed by the soft tissues that normally stabilize the elbow. The problem of loosening seen in early designs is no longer a major problem because of the addition of longer stems and the change in the articulation of semiconstrained components.[15, 21]

The indications for the two designs are similar. Semiconstrained implants should be used when there is poor bone stock or inadequate ligamentous support and when capsular or bony release is needed to achieve functional motion such as in ankylosis or juvenile rheumatoid arthritis. Capsular releases should never be performed when using nonconstrained devices.

Results

A review of the literature suggests that the outcome following total elbow arthroplasty is satisfactory in the majority of patients, with approximately 90% reporting little or no pain.[23] Cumulative survivorship analysis in recent studies ranges between 85 and 95% at 5 years, with most failures occurring within the first 2 years.[2, 15, 30, 40, 41] Range of motion typically increases to within the functional range with gains of 16 to 32 degrees in the flexion-extension arc and 26 to 34 degrees in the pronation-supination arc.[15, 21, 37, 41–45] Semiconstrained implants allow more improvement in extension because of the ability to perform an anterior capsular release.[23] In addition, Morrey et al described increased flexion strength of 92%, with gains in pronation and supination of 63% and 69%, respectively.[46] Extension strength did not improve, presumably because of triceps mobilization.

Complications

The results of total elbow arthroplasty are now approaching those of total knee and hip replacement, but complications remain relatively high. Gschwend et al,[43] in a review of the literature from 1986 to 1992, found a complication rate of 43% and a revision rate of 18%. In Morrey's experience, these complications have decreased from a reported 48% in 1981 to 22% in 1992.[15, 45] Common complications include instability, infection, triceps insufficiency, neuropraxia, delayed wound healing, and both intraoperative and postoper-

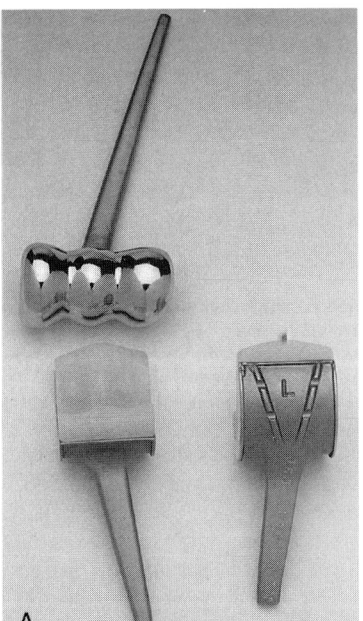
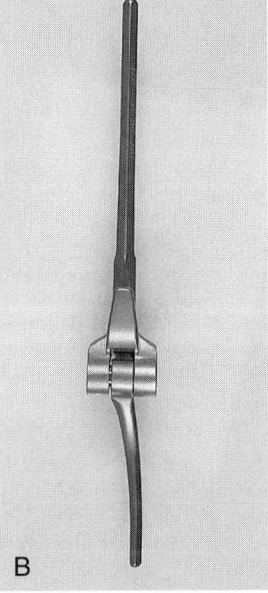

Fig. 4. Total elbow implant designs. *A*, Capitellocondylar nonconstrained implant of Ewald (Depuy, Warsaw, ID). *B*, Coonrad-Morrey semiconstrained implant (Zimmer, Warsaw, ID).

ative fracture.[34] Aseptic loosening has greatly diminished because of implant design modifications. Although most authors report radiolucencies in as many as 20% of arthroplasties,[21, 38–41, 43–45, 48, 49] only 2% to 6% are clinically relevant,[21, 46] and recent reports cite no evidence of significant clinical loosening.[15] The final outcome of these radiolucencies is uncertain at this time.

Instability has been a problem in the past with snap-fit semiconstrained prostheses such as the Pritchard-Walker implant,[34, 37] but design modifications have virtually eliminated those problems. Dislocation and subluxation are currently problems with nonconstrained designs. Since there is no linking mechanism between the humeral and ulnar components, adequate bone stock and soft-tissue support are required to provide stability. The incidence rate of instability varies between 3 and 21%, with most reports noting subluxation or dislocation in less than 9%.[21, 23, 37, 39, 41, 42, 44, 48]

Triceps insufficiency was a problem in the past with posterior approaches that detached the triceps insertion. Triceps weakness was noted in 29% of cases. Newer surgical approaches that reflect the triceps in continuity with the soft tissues distally, such as the extended Kocher approach and the Bryan-Morrey approach, have alleviated this problem.[15, 21, 43, 50]

Intraoperative fractures occur in approximately 2% to 5% of cases.[21, 39] These include cortical perforation and epicondyle fractures. Of course, the occurrence is more frequent in revision cases. Cortical perforations should be bypassed by longer stems. Epicondylar fractures may not heal, and if painful, excision may be necessary.[15] Postoperative fractures usually occur with injury. However, loosening of a prosthesis can lead to cortical thinning and fracture with only minimal trauma. Most of these fractures will heal with immobilization. If the component is loose, revision is required. If comminution is severe, the revision may need to be accomplished in stages, beginning with removal of the prostheses until the fracture heals.[50]

Permanent ulnar nerve complications following total elbow arthropolasty occur in 1% to 3% of cases.[12] Temporary problems are much more frequent and may take several months to resolve. The incidence rate ranges between 3% and 31%.[15, 21, 37, 41] Neuropraxia may occur even with decompression and transposition as described in the Bryan-Morrey approach[15] or the transtricepital approach of Gschwend.[43] The lateral Kocher approach may offer protection to the nerve.[21, 37] Ewald et al[21] showed a decrease in incidence rate of ulnar nerve complications with the Kocher approach compared to the posterior approach of Campbell. In addition to decompression of the ulnar nerve before dislocation, frequent reduction of the elbow during the procedure has been recommended.[51] Morrey and Bryan[50] also recommend that the ulnar nerve be explored and decompressed if motor weakness is present more than 12 hours after the procedure.

Infection continues to be a cause for early removal (Fig. 5). The incidence rate of deep infection is between 3 and 9%. Superficial wound problems occur more frequently.[15, 37, 40–43, 45, 49, 52, 53] Infection is more common after total elbow arthroplasty than replacement of other joints. Because the elbow is such a subcutaneous joint, it may be infected after local trauma or erosion of the overlying skin. It may also be caused by hematogenous seeding as seen with other joint replacements. Operative approach has not been associated with the onset of infection unless the skin is compromised from previous surgery.[53] Other factors associated with an increased rate of infection include pre-

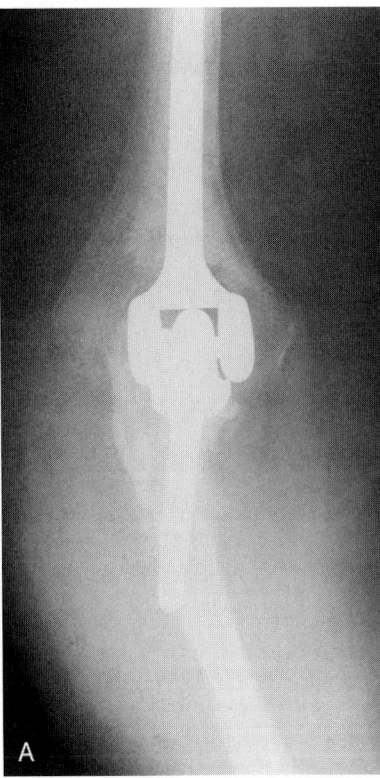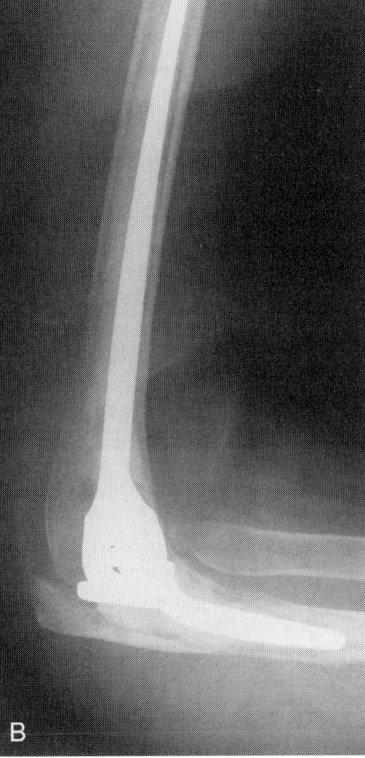

Fig. 5. Total elbow arthroplasty with infection and component loosening. *A* and *B*, A 65-year-old patient presented with a draining olecranon bursa and required removal of the components.

vious operation, previous infection in the region of the elbow, psychiatric illness, class IV rheumatoid arthritis, drainage from the wound after surgery, spontaneous drainage after 10 days, and reoperation for any reason.

Morrey and coworkers have found that certain methods of surgical technique and postoperative care lower the incidence rate of infection.[15, 50] The skin incision should, if possible, include old incisions and be straight and not directly over the olecranon tip. The triceps mechanism should be reflected in continuity with the ulnar periosteum and distal soft tissues. The tourniquet should be deflated before closure and the wound drained. If any skin problems are present preoperatively or develop postoperatively, they should be addressed aggressively. The elbow should be splinted in extension for a few days. Ljung et al[54] found fewer wound problems and no compromise in motion when the elbow was immobilized in a splint for 12 days postoperatively.

The most important step in preventing infection has probably been the addition of antibiotics into the polymethylmethacrylate used for fixation. Several authors have discovered that the use of antibiotic-impregnated cement has significantly diminished or eliminated this complication.[15, 21, 40]

Treatment of infection usually requires removal of the implant. Salvage of the components may be attempted but is usually successful only if the infection is diagnosed early and treated aggressively with débridement and parenteral antibiotics.[45, 53] Attempt at salvage is contraindicated in the older patient who may not tolerate the multiple surgical procedures and prolonged treatment course that may be needed.[53] If salvage attempts fail or if the patient is not a candidate, the components should be removed.

Revision

Most patients with an infected total elbow arthroplasty are best treated by resection arthroplasty. The surgical procedure should begin with débridement of all infected tissues including open wounds and bone. The triceps and muscular attachments to the epicondyles are spared so that these structures may assist in the stability of the resected joint. All foreign materials should be removed, taking great care not to create a fracture. An external fixator should be applied, possibly using a hinged fixator to improve postoperative motion. The proximal ulna should be contained within the humeral epicondyles to increase stability.[55] Figgie et al[56] obtained satisfactory results in seven of eight patients undergoing resection arthroplasty in which the ulna was contained. These patients exhibited no pain and had a range of motion of 85 degrees. The remaining patients in whom containment was not obtained developed significant instability that required arthrodesis for salvage. Arthrodesis in the rheumatoid elbow is probably only indicated in this type of situation.

Reimplantation is rarely indicated after removal of an infected implant. Indications include a compliant patient able to withstand the prolonged treatment, no fracture or significant bone loss at the time of removal of the components, and a sensitive organism able to be eradicated with 6 weeks of parenteral antibiotics. Wound problems should be resolved and antibiotics should be placed in the cement.[53, 57]

In revision total elbow arthroplasty, the rate of complications and reoperations is high. In a review of 33 revision arthroplasties, 60% had at least one complication.[55] Fracture with implant removal or severe bone stock loss may hamper the reconstruction options. In the same study, 24% sustained a cortical penetration. The goals of the revision are to restore the function of the upper extremity with minimal pain and adequate motion. With new implant designs, the rate of success has risen significantly.

POST-TRAUMATIC ARTHRITIS

Arthritis and sequelae secondary to injury are seen more frequently in the elbow than in other types of arthritis. Injuries to the elbow can cause intra-articular pathological lesions predisposing the joint to later degeneration. Compression or shearing injuries to the articular surface can cause chondral damage even if no fracture or dislocation is evident. Injury from dislocation, fracture, or both is more obvious. The most common fracture types leading to post-traumatic pathological conditions involve the distal humerus or radial head. With damage to supporting soft-tissue structures and bony architecture of the joint, secondary changes are not infrequent, despite adequate treatment of the acute injury.

PATHOGENESIS AND CLINICAL FEATURES

The primary clinical feature of post-traumatic arthritis is loss of motion. Pain, crepitation, and swelling may be present, especially if degenerative changes have begun. Complaints of locking or clicking are typically signs of chondral damage, loose bodies, or intra-articular incongruity. Instability is usually not present unless ligaments are incompetent or the bony structures are distorted from malunion or nonunion.

Stiffness stems from elbow contracture with loss of motion in all planes. Causes of contractures are classified as intrinsic or extrinsic. Intrinsic causes include loose bodies, intra-articular incongruity from articular cartilage irregularity or bony malunion, degenerative joint changes such as osteophytes, and fibrous or bony ankylosis. Extrinsic causes result from soft-tissue damage at the time of injury or secondary changes from periods of decreased motion such as protective immobilization post-injury. Extrinsic causes include ligamentous or capsular contracture, scarring of musculotendinous structures, and heterotopic ossification (Fig. 6).[58]

INVESTIGATIONS

The history of the patient is important in identifying factors that may lead to the development of pathology after elbow trauma. The time and type of injury and previous treatment rendered may assist in treatment decisions. Knowledge of prior treatment should include that of nonoperative as well as operative management. Information concerning periods of immobilization is particularly useful. The adequacy of previous operative intervention may be an issue as well. However, even when previous treatment was appropriate, post-traumatic arthritis or related problems may develop.

Physical examination should include evaluation of both active and passive range of motion and the quality of that motion. If passive motion is greater than active motion,

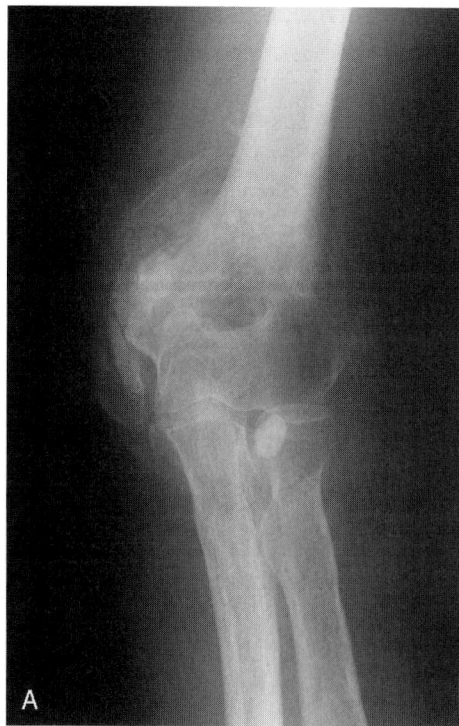

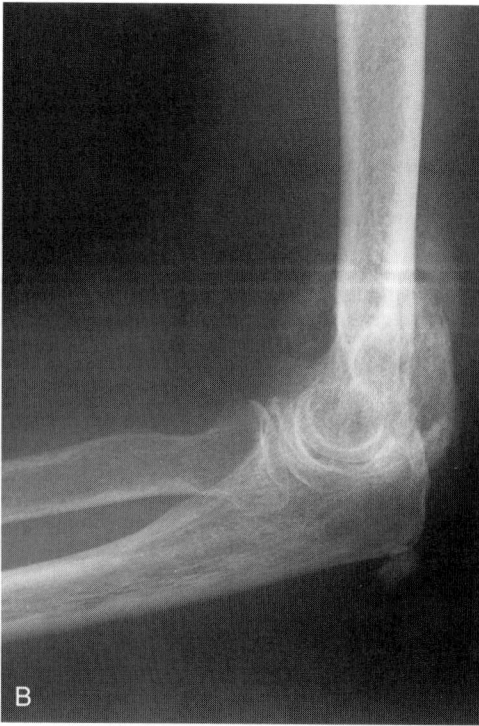

Fig. 6. Post-traumatic arthritis with class II heterotopic ossification (A, B).

and a soft end point is detected on examination, nonoperative treatment may be indicated to stretch contracted soft tissues. With a hard bony end point, nonoperative measures are less likely to be effective, as bony impingement may limit the arc of motion.

Examination should include evaluation of old scars, especially when planning surgical intervention. The presence of instability may stem from incompetent ligamentous structures or bony malunion. Strength assessment should be made. If weakness is present, it should be determined whether this is secondary to disuse or represents a neurological deficit. A flail elbow may be secondary to neurological injury or perhaps a supracondylar humerus nonunion.

Radiographic evaluation is useful in detecting possible intrinsic pathological lesions such as intra-articular incongruity, osteophytes, and loose bodies. If radiographs reveal no intrinsic pathological condition, the elbow can be evaluated by arthrography, trispiral tomography, or computed tomography. In cases of normal findings by radiographs and arthrography, loss of motion may be secondary to extrinsic factors alone. Heterotopic ossification, if present, can be classified by plain radiographs, but computed tomography is frequently needed to identify the exact location. Injury radiographs, if available, may assist in determining the etiology of the symptoms and signs. Magnetic resonance imaging is typically less helpful in the elbow with post-traumatic arthritis.

MANAGEMENT
Nonoperative Treatment
Nonoperative treatment is dictated primarily by symptoms. Pain is treated with nonsteroidal anti-inflammatory drugs and possibly intra-articular injection of corticosteroid. In-

stability may be improved with functional bracing. Contractures may show improvement with physical therapy, which may also improve symptoms of pain and instability and loss of motion. If the contracture has been present for more than 6 months, no improvement is noted with therapy, or a bony hard end point of motion is present, nonoperative treatment will most likely be ineffective. Surgical intervention should then be considered.

Surgical Treatment
In considering surgical treatment options, several factors must be addressed (Fig. 7). Improvement in range of motion is a surgical priority, since stiffness is the most common complaint. Treatment alternatives should address extrinsic and intrinsic causes of contracture including heterotopic ossification if present. Contracture may be addressed by open or arthroscopic techniques. Articular cartilage abnormalities will need to be addressed if significant. Options will be directed by the amount of cartilage wear and the age and functional level of the patient. These options include interposition arthroplasty with or without distraction, allograft arthroplasty, and total elbow arthroplasty. Significant instability and presence of infection may also alter treatment alternatives. Arthrodesis of the elbow with post-traumatic arthritis is indicated only if all other options are contraindicated.

Contracture Release
Post-traumatic contracture release is indicated when motion of the elbow is not functional. Typically if the elbow exhibits a flexion contracture of greater than 30 degrees or cannot flex greater than 110 degrees, and the patient is unsatisfied with the motion, release is warranted. The only contraindication is the inability of the patient to comply

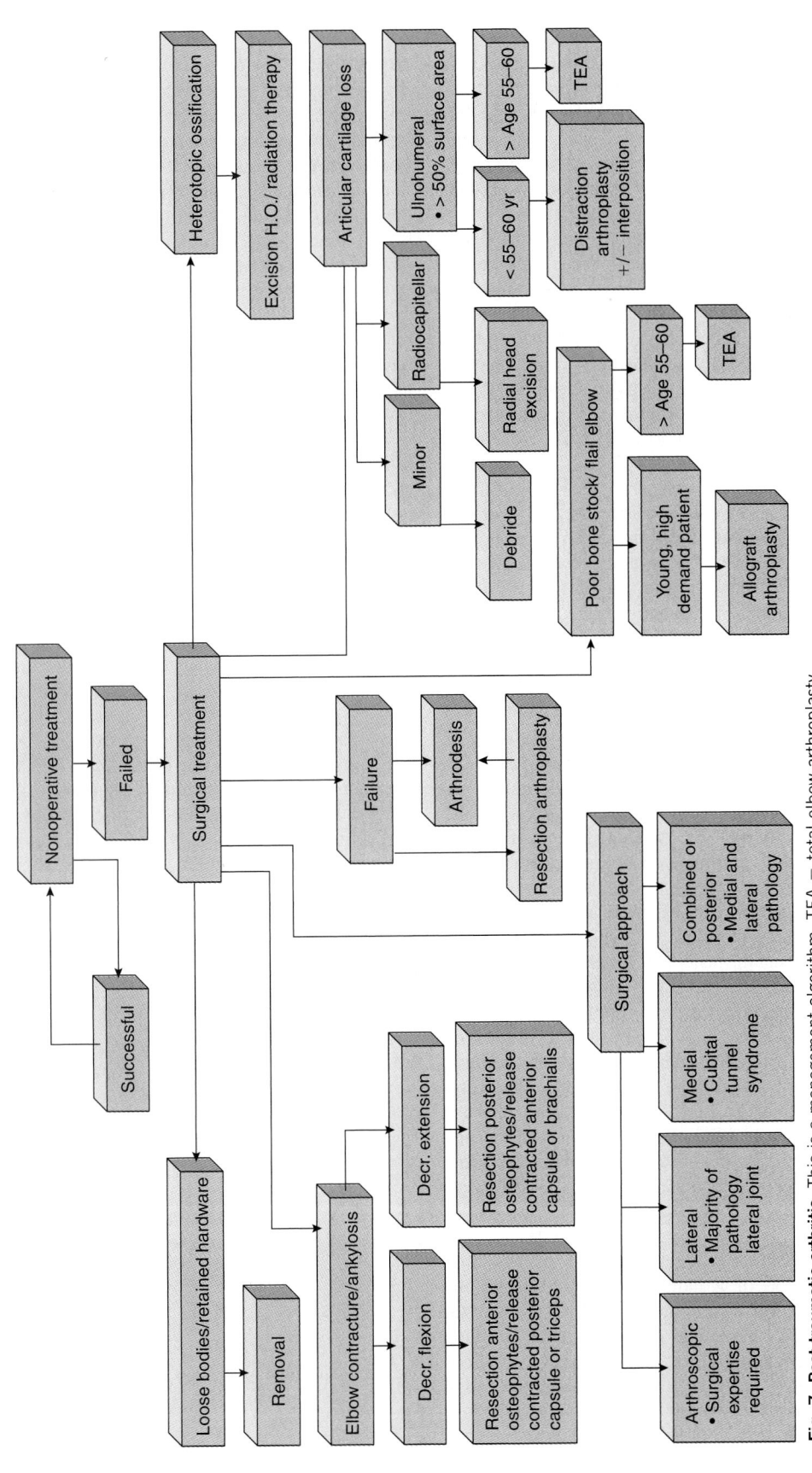

Fig. 7. Post-traumatic arthritis. This is a management algorithm. TEA = total elbow arthroplasty.

with the postoperative regimen.[59] An additional procedure may be needed, in addition to the contracture release, if significant degeneration of articular cartilage or severe instability is noted preoperatively or intraoperatively after contracture release. An extended Kocher approach or medial approach is used for the procedure.[59–61] We routinely use the lateral approach, especially if the proximal radioulnar joint or radiocapitellar joint is involved. If no significant lateral pathological lesion is noted preoperatively and ulnar neuritis is present, a medial approach is preferred.[61] If a pathological lesion is present laterally and ulnar neuritis is present, a combined approach is used, although in some cases, a long midline posterior incision might be chosen. All loose bodies should be removed and intra-articular fibrosis débrided and lysed. All involved structures must be addressed at the time of surgery. The motion regained with contracture release is significant and averages between 45 and 65 degrees.[59–61] However, if both intrinsic and extrinsic causes are present, results may not be as satisfactory.[58]

If heterotopic ossification is present and is a limiting factor, excision should be performed. The surgical approach may be dictated by its location. Posteromedial ossification may involve the ulnar nerve and anterolateral ossification may involve the posterior interosseous nerve, requiring decompression. Traditionally it has been recommended that excision of heterotopic bone be delayed until the bone has "matured" at 12 to 18 months. However, results have not been diminished with excision performed as early as 3 months after injury.[62, 63] McAuliffe and Wolfson[63] achieved greater than 100 degrees of motion with excision of heterotopic ossification performed early in elbows with severe limitation of motion or complete ankylosis. Radiation therapy is used postoperatively, with 1000 cGy divided into four or five fractions or a single dose of 700 or 800 cGy administered within 72 hours postoperatively.[62, 63]

Arthroscopic techniques can be used to address post-traumatic pathological conditions in the elbow. Capsular contractures as well as intrinsic abnormalities can be addressed arthroscopically. Results are comparable to those achieved with open techniques, with significant improvement in motion and decrease of pain.[64, 65] Arthroscopy on an elbow with post-traumatic changes may be difficult, however, because of intra-articular fibrosis. The skill level of the arthroscopist must be high and the surgeon must be prepared to discontinue the arthroscopic procedure and convert to open techniques. Ulnar nerve pathology and heterotopic ossification cannot be addressed arthroscopically and would require an open technique.[66]

Radial Head Excision

Intra-articular malunion of a radial head fracture, chronic subluxation or dislocation of the radial head, or a capitellar fracture may lead to degenerative changes of the proximal radioulnar or radiocapitellar joint. If intra-articular incongruity exists and causes pain or loss of motion, the radial head may be excised. Radial head replacement is not indicated in this setting. After fracture, pain relief is good in most patients. Broberg and Morrey found 90% patient satisfaction with excision.[67] The time interval from injury to excision had no bearing on the result. Excision of the chronically subluxated or dislocated radial head also is reli-

able in relieving pain if present, but does not reliably improve motion.[68]

Interposition Arthroplasty

Significant loss of articular cartilage within the ulnohumeral joint may necessitate additional procedures. Some type of resurfacing arthroplasty may be required. In patients older than 60 years of age, total elbow arthroplasty may be indicated. However, because of the higher incidence of complications in this population undergoing elbow replacement, a biological resurfacing should be employed in those younger than 55 to 60 years.[69]

Interposition or fascial arthroplasty is indicated when greater than 50% of the articular cartilage of the ulnohumeral joint is involved or when significant intra-articular malunion is present that would require recontouring.[58] Other indications include pain, ankylosis, and loss of motion.

The principles of contracture release are followed in addition to the procedure of interposition arthroplasty. If ligamentous instability exists preoperatively or is present following contracture release, a hinged external fixator may be needed (Fig. 8). The hinge allows the patient to regain motion while maintaining stability.[12, 58]

Contraindications to the procedure include sepsis, severe bone loss, significant instability, muscular weakness, and evidence of a neuropathic joint.[70, 71] Relative contraindications include an elbow that will be used in heavy labor or with ambulatory aids. Interposition arthroplasty has been less effective when osteoporosis is present or when the elbow is ankylosed in a good position.[71]

Knight and Van Zandt found that 78% of patients were satisfied with the procedure at long-term follow-up.[70] No distraction device was used in their series. Morrey used a distraction device when significant articular cartilage destruction or intra-articular adhesions were present. Satisfac-

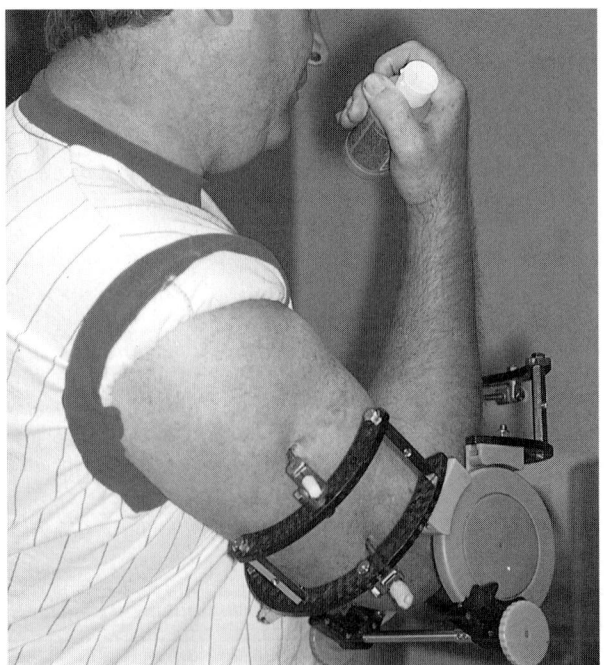

Fig. 8. Distraction arthroplasty.

tion was 96% at a shorter follow-up period. A gain in motion of approximately 60 degrees was achieved.[58]

Complications tend to be high because of the complex nature of the procedure.[58] Most patients requiring interposition/distraction arthroplasty have had previous surgeries and may have had multiple incisions. Skin slough may develop and lead to infection if a good soft-tissue envelope is not present.[70] Infection should be treated aggressively with appropriate skin coverage. The fascial implant, if used in the initial procedure, should be removed. If bone débridement is required, all attempts should be made to retain the epicondyles. A resection arthroplasty without capture of the ulna by the humeral epicondyles universally leads to a poor result.

As with any revision surgery about the elbow, nerves such as the ulnar and posterior interosseous nerves are at risk. Ulnar nerve decompression and anterior transposition should be considered. The nerve is not only at risk during débridement of the joint, but it may also be kinked during elbow dislocation during placement of the resurfacing membrane. Therefore, the elbow should be frequently reduced during this portion of the procedure. The posterior interosseous nerve is also at risk with anterolateral débridement of extrinsic pathology. Decompression of this nerve should be considered when surgery approaches its location. Tardy ulnar nerve palsy may occur with the development of late valgus instability.

Instability may occur from ligamentous incompetence or bony resection at the time of surgery. Too much bony resection may lead to resorption, especially of the distal humerus. Knight and Van Zandt noted that 13 of 45 patients exhibited some degree of subluxation.[70] Triceps avulsion may occur even with use of a triceps-sparing approach.[58] Repair should be performed if this develops. Even with no evidence of triceps detachment, extensor weakness may be a problem secondary to shortening the musculotendinous length across the elbow.[70]

Total Elbow Arthroplasty

Total elbow arthroplasty is indicated in the post-traumatic elbow when the patient is older than 55 to 60 years of age.[69] In addition, joint replacement may be used for a flail elbow with severe ligamentous incompetence or bone loss and with nonunion of a distal humerus fracture. Nonconstrained implants require stability and good bone stock and do not allow significant capsular release. Therefore, most post-traumatic elbows undergoing prosthetic arthroplasty should have semiconstrained devices implanted. With this design, ligamentous stability is not an issue and extrinsic as well as intrinsic factors may be addressed at the time of surgery. Contraindications are the same as for total elbow replacement in the rheumatoid elbow.

Results of total elbow arthroplasty in the post-traumatic elbow have not been as good as those noted with the rheumatoid elbow. Complications are higher and the need for reoperation is greater.[12, 69, 72] Kraay et al[40] showed a cumulative survival rate for elbow replacement in this population of 73% at 3 years and 53% at 5 years. Ramsey et al evaluated 53 patients with total elbow arthroplasty for post-traumatic arthritis and noted a 38% complication rate.[73] The rate was decreased to 16% by using the Coonrad-Morrey implant and by limiting patient selection.

As in other reconstructive procedures, the complications

of elbow replacement in this population will remain significant. Results may be marginal because many patients have had previous operations, with avascular bone and fibrosis, and occult sepsis may be present.[40]

Allograft Arthroplasty

In patients younger than 55 to 60 years of age, elbow replacement with a prosthesis is usually not a viable alternative. Options include arthrodesis and allograft arthroplasty when severe bony deformities are present. Dean et al reviewed long-term results in 23 patients with allograft arthroplasties, 20 of which were post-traumatic.[74] Satisfactory results were achieved in 10 of 14 followed at least 7.5 years. However, complications were noted in 70% and included infection, nonunion, fracture, bone resorption, instability, and nerve palsy. Cartilage deterioration was noted in all, but the joints universally functioned better than would be predicted from radiographs. Use of the allograft did not preclude other later reconstructive procedures.

OSTEOARTHRITIS

Primary osteoarthritis of the elbow accounts for only 1 or 2% of all osteoarthritis seen clinically.[75] The cause of the condition is unknown but has been associated with heavy labor and repetitive use of the arm. There may also be a link between throwing athletes and osteochondritis dissecans and the development of osteoarthritis.[23, 76] Repetitious throwing may lead to lax medial constraints followed by posteromedial impingement and secondary osteophytes and loose bodies.

PATHOGENESIS AND CLINICAL FEATURES

The typical patient is a middle-aged male with loss of motion and impingement pain at end ranges of motion, especially in extension. Pain is not usually noted in the mid-range of motion until the later stages of the disease. Symptoms of catching or locking may be present, especially with articular incongruity or when loose bodies are present. Ulnar neuritis may be observed secondary to compressive osteophytes medially. Swelling may be evident but is not typical. Patients usually do not seek medical advice unless a loss of 30 to 40 degrees of extension is evident or locking is painful. Radiographs reveal enlargement of the olecranon and coronoid processes and obliteration of the corresponding fossae of the distal humerus (Fig. 9). The ulnohumeral joint is usually preserved at initial presentation. A cubital tunnel view may reveal osteophytes compressing the ulnar nerve. Computed tomographic arthrography may be helpful in identifying loose bodies not visible on plain radiographic films.

MANAGEMENT

Nonoperative treatment, including activity modification and rest, may be helpful. If weakness is present, the patient may be instructed in strengthening. Nonsteroidal anti-inflammatory medication may relieve pain in later stages but early in the disease process does not help impingement pain. Corticosteroid injection may improve symptoms, but its benefit is usually temporary.

Surgical intervention is indicated when symptoms are not improved with nonoperative treatment or the efficacy of treatments is questioned. Early in the disease, radio-

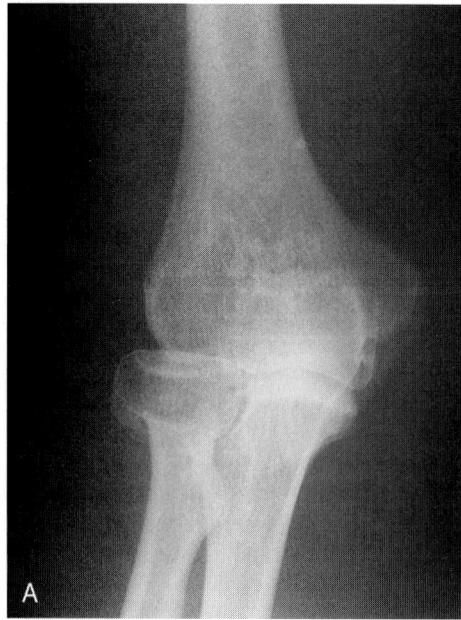 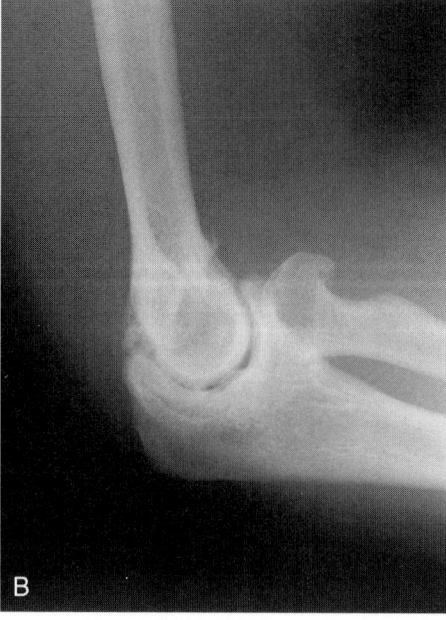

Fig. 9. Osteoarthritis. *A* and *B,* The ulnohumeral joint is preserved. Osteophytes of the coronoid and olecranon fossae and processes are typical.

graphs may be normal and symptoms of locking or pain may stem from loose bodies or chondral damage. The most common area of symptomatic chondromalacia is in the radiocapitellar joint followed by the posterior olecranon. Arthroscopy can be used to diagnose and treat chondral defects and loose bodies.[66, 77] As the disease progresses and osteophytes become more prominent, range of motion decreases and secondary capsular contracture may develop. Surgical correction should address the intrinsic and extrinsic causes of loss of motion as well as ulnar neuritis. Posteriorly, osteophytes should be débrided from the olecranon process and fossa and loose bodies removed. Occasionally, the posterior capsule requires release to regain full flexion. Anteriorly, the coronoid process and fossa should be débrided and loose bodies excised. The anterior capsule may need release if posterior débridement does not restore full extension. Ulnar nerve symptoms may require decompression and anterior transposition. The radial head may be débrided or resected if involved. Débridement and capsular release may be accomplished in the same manner as that described for post-traumatic arthritis. The approach used can be lateral, medial, or combined, depending on the pathological condition present, as in the post-traumatic elbow. The débridement and capsular releases may also be accomplished by arthroscopic techniques.

Tsuge and coworkers reported a 20-year experience with a posterolateral approach requiring sectioning of the lateral collateral ligament and reflection of the triceps off the olecranon. Ulnar neuritis was treated with decompression and medial epicondylectomy. The joint was débrided posteriorly and anteriorly with excision of the anterior capsule. The radial head was not routinely excised, but osteophytes were débrided. Both the collateral ligament and the triceps were repaired at completion of the procedure. Among 58 patients, results were satisfactory in 88% retaining over 70 degrees of motion.[78, 79]

A technique termed the ulnohumeral arthroplasty by Morrey offers a different approach (Fig. 10). A posterior approach is used, and the tip of the olecranon process is osteotomized. A fenestration with a trephine is made in the olecranon fossa into the anterior elbow joint, thus débriding the olecranon and coronoid fossae. The coronoid process may then be resected and loose bodies removed

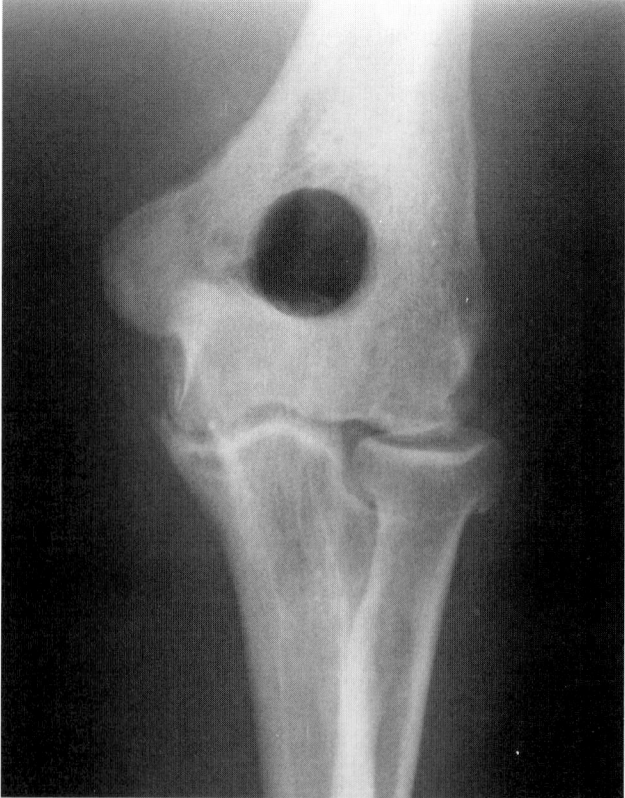

Fig. 10. Ulnohumeral arthroplasty. Fenestration of the olecranon fossa débrides the osteophytes of the olecranon and coronoid fossae.

through the fenestration with the elbow flexed. Release of the anterior capsule, if a flexion contracture still exists, may be accomplished but is difficult. Morrey[75] achieved satisfactory results in 87% of cases with this technique. The flexion-extension arc of motion improved 32 degrees. If the radiocapitellar joint is involved or anterior osteophytes extend significantly to the medial aspect of the joint, another approach should be considered.

Débridement of the osteoarthritic elbow can also be performed arthroscopically in a method similar to the ulnohumeral arthroplasty. If the ulnar nerve is involved or a large amount of bone will need to be resected, an open approach should be used.[66] Anterior pathological lesions are addressed initially, followed by posterior arthroscopy. Osteophytes and loose bodies are excised. The olecranon fossa

may be fenestrated with a drill in the center, followed by enlargement of the hole with a burr to greater than 1 cm.[80, 81] Relief of symptoms and range of motion also compare with results using open techniques.

Because osteoarthritis is a progressive disease, symptoms and pathological conditions may recur. The most common problem is recurrence of impingement pain and flexion contractures. Loose bodies and ulnar nerve symptoms do not commonly return.[12] If the pathological condition does worsen and involves significant amounts of articular cartilage, options include distraction arthroplasty for the younger patient and total elbow arthroplasty in patients older than 60 years of age. Results and complications are similar to those seen with reconstruction of the post-traumatic elbow.

REFERENCES

1. O'Driscoll SW, An K, Korinek S, et al: Kinematics of semiconstrained total elbow arthroplasty. J Bone Joint Surg Br 1992; 74:297.
2. Boone DC, Azen SP: Normal range of motion in the joint in male subjects. J Bone Joint Surg Am 1979; 61:756.
3. Morrey BF, Askew LJ, An KN, et al: A biomechanical study of normal functional elbow motion. J Bone Joint Surg Am 1981; 63:872.
4. Morrey BF, Chao EYS: Passive motion of the elbow joint: A biomechanical analysis. J Bone Joint Surg Am 1976; 58:501.
5. Morrey BF, An KN: Articular and ligamentous contributions to the stabilities of the elbow joint. Am J Sports Med 1983; 11:315.
6. Morrey BF, An KN: Functional anatomy of the ligaments of the elbow. Clin Orthop 1985; 201:84.
7. Morrey BF, Tanaka H, An KN: Valgus stability of the elbow: Definition of primary and secondary constraints. Clin Orthop 1991; 265:187.
8. Morrey BF, An KN: Biomechanics of the elbow. In Morrey BF (ed): The Elbow and Its Disorders, 2nd ed. Philadelphia, WB Saunders, 1993, p 53.
9. Pearson JR, McGinley DR, Butzel LM: A dynamic analysis of the upper extremity: Planar motion. Hum Factors 1963; 5:59.
10. Smyth CJ: Rheumatoid arthritis. A major rheumatic disease. In Clayton ML, Smyth CJ (eds): Surgery for Rheumatoid Arthritis: A Comprehensive Team Approach. New York, Churchill Livingstone, 1992, p 9.
11. Lonner JH, Stuchin SA: Synovectomy, radial head excision, and anterior capsular release in stage III inflammatory arthritis of the elbow. J Hand Surg Am 1997; 22:279.
12. Morrey BF, O'Driscoll SW: Elbow arthritis. In Norris TR (ed): Orthopaedic Knowledge Update: Shoulder and Elbow. Rosemont, IL, AAOS, 1997:379.
13. Steinbrocker O, Traeger CH, Batterman RC: Therapeutic criteria in rheumatoid arthritis. JAMA 1949; 140:659.
14. Ferlic DC, Patchett CE, Clayton ML, et al:

Elbow synovectomy in rheumatoid arthritis: Long-term results. Clin Orthop 1987; 220:119.
15. Morrey BF, Adams RA: Semiconstrained arthroplasty for the treatment of rheumatoid arthritis of the elbow. J Bone Joint Surg Am 1992;74: 479.
16. Tulp NJ, Winia WP: Synovectomy of the elbow in rheumatoid arthritis: Long-term results. J Bone Joint Surg Br 1989; 71: 664.
17. Ishikawa H, Hirohata K: Posterior interosseous nerve syndrome associated with rheumatoid synovial cysts of the elbow joint. Clin Orthop 1990; 254:134.
18. Smyth CJ: Clinical and laboratory features of rheumatoid arthritis. In Clayton ML, Smyth CJ (eds): Surgery for Rheumatoid Arthritis: A Comprehensive Team Approach. New York, Churchill Livingstone, 1992, p 23.
19. Smyth CJ: Medical aspects of management of rheumatoid arthritis. In Clayton ML, Smyth CJ (eds): Surgery for Rheumatoid Arthritis: A Comprehensive Team Approach. New York, Churchill Livingstone, 1992, p 39.
20. Goldberg VM, Figgie HE III, Inglis AE, et al: Current concepts review: Total elbow arthroplasty. J Bone Joint Surg Am 1988; 70:778.
21. Ewald FC, Simmons ED, Sullivan JA, et al: Capitellocondylar total elbow replacement in rheumatoid arthritis: Long-term results. J Bone Joint Surg Am 1993; 75: 498.
22. Herold N, Schrocler HA: Synovectomy and radial head excision in rheumatoid arthritis. Acta Orthop Scand 1995; 66:252.
23. O'Driscoll SW: Elbow arthritis: Treatment options. JAAOS 1993; 1:106.
24. Eichenblat M, Hass A, Kessler I: Synovectomy of the elbow in rheumatoid arthritis. J Bone Joint Surg Am 1982; 64: 1074.
25. Copeland SA, Taylor JG: Synovectomy of the elbow in rheumatoid arthritis: The place of excision of the head of the radius. J Bone Joint Surg Br 1979; 61:69.
26. Inglis AE, Ranawat CS, Straub LR: Synovectomy and debridement of the elbow in

rheumatoid arthritis. J Bone Joint Surg Am 1971; 53:652.
27. Gendi NS, Axon JMC, Carr AJ, et al: Synovectomy of the elbow and radial head excision in rheumatoid arthritis: Predictive factors and long-term outcome. J Bone Joint Surg Br 1997; 79:918.
28. Rymaszewski LA, Mackay I, Amis AA, et al: Long-term effects of excision of the radial head in rheumatoid arthritis. J Bone Joint Surg Br 1984; 66:109.
29. Schemitsch EH, Ewald FC, Thornhill TS: Results of total elbow arthroplasty after excision of the radial head and synovectomy in patients who had rheumatoid arthritis. J Bone Joint Surg Am 1996; 78: 1541.
30. Alexaide MM, Stanwyck TS, Figgie MD, et al: Minimum ten-year follow-up of elbow synovectomy for rheumatoid arthritis. Orthop Trans 1990; 14:255.
31. Brumfield RH, Resnick CT: Synovectomy of the elbow in rheumatoid arthritis. J Bone Joint Surg Am 1985; 67:16.
32. Lee BPH, Morrey BF: Arthroscopic synovectomy of the elbow for rheumatoid arthritis: A prospective study. J Bone Joint Surg Br 1997; 79:770.
33. Ljung P, Jonsson K, Larsson K, et al: Interposition arthroplasty of the elbow with rheumatoid arthritis. J Shoulder Elbow Surg 1996; 5:81.
34. Coonrad RW: Comments on the historical milestones in the development of elbow arthroplasty: Indications and complications. In Tullos HS (ed): Instructional Course Lectures, Vol XL. Park Ridge, IL: AAOS, 1991, p 51.
35. Dee R: Total replacement arthroplasty of the elbow for rheumatoid arthritis. J Bone Joint Surg Br 1972; 54:88.
36. Garrett JC, Ewald FC, Thomas WH, et al: Loosening associated with GSB hinge total elbow replacement in patients with rheumatoid arthritis. Clin Orthop 1977; 127: 170.
37. Weiland AJ, Weiss A-PC, Wills RP, et al: Capitellocondylar total elbow replacement. J Bone Joint Surg Am 1989; 71:217.
38. Kudo H, Iwano K: Total elbow arthroplasty with a non-constrained surface-re-

placement prosthesis in patients who have rheumatoid arthritis: A long-term follow-up study. J Bone Joint Surg Am 1990; 72: 355.

39. Sjoden GOJ, Lundberg A, Blomgren GA: Late results of the Souter-Strathclyde total elbow prosthesis in rheumatoid arthritis. Acta Orthop Scand 1995; 66:391.

40. Kraay MJ, Figgie MP, Inglis AE, et al: Primary semiconstrained total elbow arthroplasty. J Bone Joint Surg Br 1994; 76: 636.

41. Ruth JT, Wilde AH: Capitellocondylar total elbow replacement. J Bone Joint Surg Am 1992; 74:95.

42. Ewald FC, Scheinberg RD, Poss R, et al: Capitellocondylar total elbow arthroplasty: Two- to five-year follow-up in rheumatoid arthritis. J Bone Joint Surg Am 1980; 62: 1259.

43. Gschwend N, Simmen BR, Matejovsky Z: Late complications in elbow arthroplasty. J Shoulder Elbow Surg 1996; 5:86.

44. Lyall HA, Cohen B, Clatworthy M, et al: Results of the Souter-Strathclyde total elbow arthroplasty in patients with rheumatoid arthritis: A preliminary report. J Arthroplasty 1994; 9:279.

45. Morrey BF, Bryan RS, Dobyns JH, et al: Total elbow arthroplasty: A five-year experience at the Mayo Clinic. J Bone Joint Surg Am 1981; 63:1050.

46. Morrey BF, Askew LJ, An KN: Strength function after elbow arthroplasty. Clin Orthop 1988; 234:43.

47. Inglis AE, Pellicci PM: Total elbow replacement. J Bone Joint Surg Am 1980; 62:1252.

48. Poll RG, Rozing PM: Use of the Souter-Strathclyde total elbow prosthesis in patients who have rheumatoid arthritis. J Bone Joint Surg Am 1991; 73:1227.

49. Lo IKY, King GJW: Arthroscopic radial head excision. Arthroscopy 1994; 10:689.

50. Morrey BF, Bryan RS: Complications of total elbow arthroplasty. Clin Orthop 1982; 170:204.

51. Ljung P, Ahlmann S, Knutson K, et al: Intraoperative monitoring of ulnar nerve function during replacement of the rheumatoid elbow via the lateral approach. Acta Orthop Scand 1995; 66(2):132.

52. Morrey BF, Bryan RS: Infection after total elbow arthroplasty. J Bone Joint Surg Am 1983; l65:330.

53. Wolfe SW, Figgie MP, Inglis AE, et al: Management of infection about total el-

bow prostheses. J Bone Joint Surg Am 1990; 72:198.

54. Ljung P, Bornmyr S, Svensson H: Wound healing after total elbow replacement in rheumatoid arthritis: Wound complications in 50 cases and laser-doppler imaging of skin microcirculation. Acta Orthop Scand 1995; 66(1):59.

55. Morrey BF, Bryan RS: Revision total elbow arthroplasty. J Bone Joint Surg Am 1987; 69:523.

56. Figgie MP, Inglis AE, Mow CS, et al: Results of reconstruction for failed total elbow arthroplasty. Clin Orthop 1990; 253:123.

57. Figgie HE III, Inglis AE, Ranawat CS, Rosenberg GM: Results of total elbow arthroplasty as a salvage procedure for failed elbow reconstruction operations. Clin Orthop 1987; 219:185.

58. Morrey BF: Post-traumatic contracture of the elbow. J Bone Joint Surg Am 1990; 72:601.

59. Husband JB, Hastings H II: The lateral approach for operative release of post-traumatic contracture of the elbow. J Bone Joint Surg Am 1990; 72:1353.

60. Mansat P, Morrey BF: The column procedure: A limited lateral approach for extrinsic contracture of the elbow. J Bone Joint Surg Am 1998; 80:1603.

61. Weiss A-PC, Sachar K: Soft tissue contractures about the elbow. Hand Clin 1994; 10:439.

62. Hastings H, Graham TJ: The classification and treatment of heterotopic ossification about the elbow and forearm. Hand Clin 1994; 10(3):417.

63. McAuliffe JA, Wolfson AH: Early excision of heterotopic ossification about the elbow followed by radiation therapy. J Bone Joint Surg Am 1997; 79:749.

64. Jones GS, Savoie FH III: Arthroscopic capsular release of flexion contracture (arthrofibrosis) of the elbow. Arthroscopy 1993; 9:277.

65. Phillips BB, Strasburger S: Arthroscopic treatment of arthrofibrosis of the elbow joint. Arthroscopy 1998; 14:38.

66. Savoie FH, Field LD: Cartilage lesions, osteoarthritis, and contracture. In Green DP, Hotchkiss RN, Pederson WC (eds): Green's Operative Hand Surgery, 4th ed. New York, Churchill Livingstone, 1999, p 249.

67. Broberg MA, Morrey BF: Results of delayed excision of the radial head after

fracture. J Bone Joint Surg Am 1986; 68: 669.

68. Bell SN, Morrey BF, Bianco AJ: Chronic posterior subluxation and dislocation of the radial head. J Bone Joint Surg Am 1991; 73:392.

69. Morrey BF, Adams RA, Bryan RS: Total replacement for post-traumatic arthritis of the elbow. J Bone Joint Surg Br 1991; 73: 607.

70. Knight RA, Van Zandt IL: Arthroplasty of the elbow: An end result study. J Bone Joint Surg Am 1952; 34:610.

71. Wright PE, Froimson AI, Stewart MJ: Interposition arthroplasty of the elbow. In Morrey BF (ed): The Elbow and Its Disorders, 2nd ed. Philadelphia, WB Saunders, 1993, p 611.

72. Inglis AE, Inglis AE Jr, Figgie MD, et al: Total elbow arthroplasty for frail and unstable elbows. J Shoulder Elbow Surg 1997; 6:29.

73. Ramsey ML, Adams RA, Morrey BF: Instability of the elbow treated with semiconstrained total elbow arthroplasty. J Bone Joint Surg Am 1999; 81:38.

74. Dean GS, Holliger EH IV, Urbaniak JR: Elbow allograft for reconstruction of the elbow with massive bone loss. Clin Orthop 1997; 341:12.

75. Morrey BF: Primary degenerative arthritis of the elbow: Treatment by ulnohumeral arthroplasty. J Bone Joint Surg Br 1992; 74:409.

76. Esch JC, Baker CL: Valgus extension overload. In Surgical Arthroscopy: The Shoulder and Elbow. Philadelphia: JB Lippincott; 1993, p 287.

77. Ogilvie-Harris DJ, Schemitsch E: Arthroscopy of the elbow for removal of loose bodies. Arthroscopy 1993; 9:5.

78. Tsuge K, Mizuseki T: Debridement arthroplasty for advanced primary osteoarthritis of the elbow. J Bone Joint Surg Br 1994; 76:641.

79. Tsuge K, Murakami T, Yasunaga Y, et al: Arthroplasty of the elbow: Twenty years' experience of a new approach. J Bone Joint Surg Br 1987; 69:116.

80. Ogilvie-Harris DJ, Gordon R, MacKay M: Arthroscopic treatment for posterior impingement in degenerative arthritis of the elbow. Arthroscopy 1995; 11(4):437.

81. Redden JF, Stanley D: Arthroscopic fenestration of the olecranon fossa in the treatment of osteoarthritis of the elbow. Arthroscopy 1993; 9:14.

ARTHRITIS OF THE HIP

David L. Boardman and Jay R. Lieberman

section
6
chapter
8

Summary
- Arthritis of the hip affects up to 2% of adults.
- The causes of hip arthritis are degenerative, inflammatory, infectious, traumatic, and developmental.
- Pain is the primary symptom for which patients seek medical treatment.
- Nonoperative treatment includes nonsteroidal anti-inflammatory drugs (NSAIDs), weight reduction, activity modification, exercise, and use of external supports.
- End-stage degeneration often requires surgical treatment, most commonly hip replacement.

INTRODUCTION

The hip joint consists of a nearly spherical ball at the proximal end of the femur that articulates within the deep bony constraint of a pelvic socket. Formation of normal anatomy depends on the articular congruity and forces transmitted across the joint as it develops.[1] Other than a thickening of the anterior joint capsule, which acts as a check to extension, and a thin fibrocartilaginous labrum at the periphery of the acetabulum, soft tissues play little role in the stability of the hip. Smooth articular hyaline cartilage lubricated by synovial fluid provides a virtually frictionless bearing surface.

Strong juxta-articular muscles, primarily flexors, extensors, and abductors, power the joint through a functional range of motion: 120 degrees of flexion/extension, 70 degrees of abduction/adduction, and 80 degrees of internal/external rotation.[2] In the normal state, the hip provides a painless platform for activities ranging from the ordinary (e.g., sitting) to the very specialized (e.g., punting a football). Static equilibrium in the frontal plane during single-limb stance is afforded by pull of the abductors, which counteracts the moment of body mass (Fig. 1).[3] The resultant joint reaction force can vary from two to five times body weight, depending on the activity, with maximal forces measured during stair climbing (Table 1).

Unfortunately, the joint is sensitive to developmental abnormalities and is susceptible to mechanical and biochemical damage, all of which can precipitate arthritis. Symptomatic arthritis of the hip is common, affecting as many as 2% of adults.[4] The associated economic impact of this condition is enormous, amounting to a tremendous loss of productivity in the working and in the retired populations and to millions of dollars spent in medical care. Many causes of hip arthritis exhibit genetic inheritance patterns, but expression of disease is multifactorial, suggesting developmental and environmental factors in pathogenesis. Osteoarthritis is by far the most common of the diseases of the hip, with a slight preponderance in white males, and has a clear linear increase in prevalence with age. All other causes of hip arthritis combined do not approach the number of new cases of osteoarthritis diagnosed and treated per year.[5]

Though the possible causes are numerous, the end result of all causes of arthritis is the degradation of articular cartilage through a particular combination of inflammatory cellular mediators. Potential triggers for this cascade in the hip are biomechanical (e.g., developmental dysplasia, cumulative microtrauma, or catastrophic injury), biochemical (e.g., infection, autoimmune disease, or metabolic abnormality), or both (e.g., osteonecrosis). Determining a specific diagnosis is of most benefit early in the progression of disease, when treatment options have the potential to prevent or delay end-stage degeneration.

Most forms of arthritis were originally described and differentiated in the 19th century, although presumably people have always suffered from arthritis of the hip. Two major milestones in the treatment of hip arthritis have been the development of acetylsalicylic acid in the mid 1800s (with the subsequent derivation of potent nonsteroidal anti-inflammatory medications) and Sir John Charnley's advance of total hip arthroplasty in the early 1960s,[6] a procedure now widely held to be the most successful operation of the last 25 years.

PATHOGENESIS

The tissue types that comprise a joint include hyaline cartilage, bone, synovium, and ligament; all of these tissues are involved in the pathogenesis of arthritis. In response to an appropriate stimulus, the immune response will affect these tissues through a complex cascade of cellular and humoral mechanisms, initiated by cells of both lymphoid and myeloid lineage. Intercellular communication is achieved through production of interleukins and cytokines, which in turn launch the inflammatory response via release of arachidonic acid from cell membrane phospholipids. Oxidation of the arachidonic acid produces prostaglandins, leukotrienes, and thromboxanes, the mediators of inflammation.[7]

TABLE 1. ACTIVITY-SPECIFIC PEAK HIP FORCES	
Activity	**Approximate Peak Hip Force**
Walking normal speed	2.5–3.0 BW
Walking fast	3.5 BW
Arising from chair	3.5 BW
Stair climbing	4.0–7.5 BW

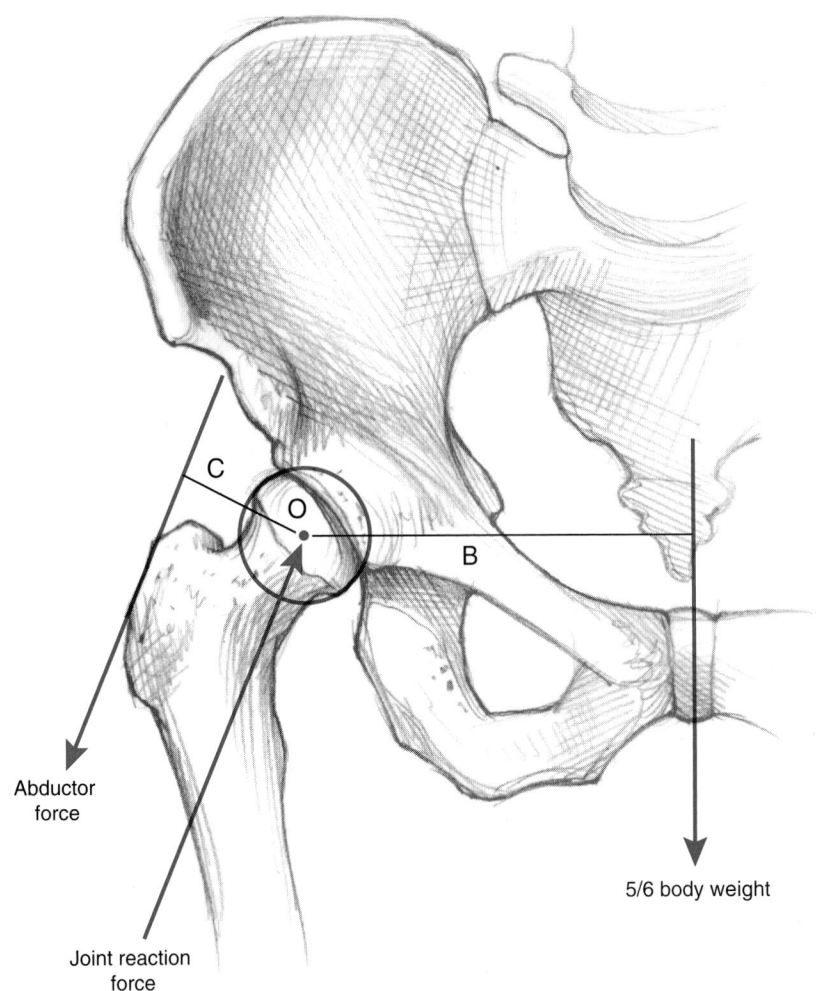

Abductor
force

Joint reaction
force

C

O

B

5/6 body weight

Fig. 1. Forces about the hip. The force of body weight acts through the hip center of rotation (O) at a distance (B), producing a given torque of body weight. In static equilibrium, the abductor force works at a distance (C) from the hip center to provide an equal and opposite torque. Because the moment arm (C) is considerably shorter than the moment arm (B), the abductor force can be two to three times the body weight force in single limb stance. The joint reaction force exerted on the hip is the sum of the force of body weight and the compensatory abductor force.

Osteoarthritis, although not a classic inflammatory condition, results from primary disease of articular cartilage. The condition occurs either when normal tissue succumbs to overwhelming or repetitive compressive mechanical forces or when more reasonable loads adversely affect abnormal cartilage. Many believe that nearly all cases of hip osteoarthritis can ultimately be linked to some degree of developmental abnormality or collagen mutation.[8] Cellular adaptations to articular injury lead to pathologic alterations in water content, collagen structure, and proteoglycan composition, with eventual degeneration of cartilage and focal loss of joint space.[9] In the hip, reactive changes in the other tissues typically include formation of a medial hypertrophic acetabular osteophyte, subchondral bony sclerosis, a cysts, synovitis, and external rotation ligamentous contracture.[4]

Rheumatoid arthritis, a more classic inflammatory condition, results from disease affecting primarily the synovial tissue. A faulty immune response to native antigens leads to proliferation of monocytes and leukocytes that infiltrate the synovium, causing edema and hypertrophy. This synovitis is associated with the release of local inflammatory mediators that cause pain and that can erode cartilage and bone and distort the soft-tissue support of a joint, rendering it unstable.[10] In the hip, the cartilage wears diffusely, and bony deterioration of the acetabulum leads to superior and medial protrusion of the hip into the pelvis.[11] The systemic nature of inflammatory arthritides can result in diffuse osteopenia and simultaneous involvement of many joints, both large and small.

Septic arthritis results from a severe inflammatory response mounted in reaction to local infection, typically bacterial. Immune response to organisms trapped in the synovium causes subsequent edema and increased production of synovial fluid, leading to elevated articular pressure and congested blood flow. Rupture of the synovial membrane and direct seeding of the joint disrupts the nutrient supply to the articular cartilage and permits immediate contact with destructive proteolytic enzymes.[12] In the hip, this entire reaction commonly interrupts the bony blood supply, leading to osteonecrosis of the femoral head. As with other causes of osteonecrosis, subsequent collapse and erosion of cartilage and subchondral bone lead to the loss of articular congruity and destruction of the joint.

CLINICAL FEATURES

A patient with osteoarthritis of the hip typically experiences insidious onset of groin and thigh pain of variable duration. Occasionally, the pain may also radiate into the buttocks. Associated features include a component of stiffness that limits sitting, standing, walking, and donning socks and shoes. These symptoms fluctuate in severity, often being worse early in the morning and exacerbated by weightbearing activity (Table 2). Patients are usually older than 55 years and may or may not relate a specific inciting injury, childhood hip disorders (such as developmental dysplasia of the hip, Legg-Calvé-Perthes disease, slipped capital femoral epiphysis, etc.), a history of heavy manual labor, other arthritic joints, or a positive family history. Unlike with the knee, osteoarthritis of the hip has no association with body weight.[5, 13]

A very common early physical finding associated with osteoarthritis of the hip is loss of internal rotation. The hip may be irritable to passive range of motion, particularly at the extreme of internal rotation, causing pain in the groin. As the disease progresses, the patient can develop flexion contracture of the affected hip, and subsequent pelvic obliquity can create effective and/or real leg-length inequality. Potential gait abnormalities include antalgia and an abductor lurch. Both patterns develop as a mechanism of reducing painful joint reaction forces with weightbearing, but an ipsilateral trunk lean might also be secondary to abductor weakness.[14]

Rheumatoid arthritis typically affects the small joints of the hands and feet before it affects the hip (Table 3).[15] Further, early involvement of the hip may be subtle because synovitis can be relatively asymptomatic, and the deep location within the pelvis hides the stigmata of swelling and deformity seen with superficial joints.[4] When synovitis progresses, symptoms of pain and stiffness similar to those seen with osteoarthritis occur.

Bilateral hip pain and stiffness in association with back stiffness, pain, and decreased thoracic respiratory excursion

---

TABLE 3. CLASSIFICATION CRITERIA FOR RHEUMATOID ARTHRITIS

Four of the following seven criteria are required for the diagnosis. Criteria 1 to 4 must have been present for at least 6 weeks.
1. Morning stiffness in and around the joints, lasting at least 1 hour before maximal improvement.
2. At least 3 of 14 joint areas simultaneously have had soft-tissue swelling or fluid (not bony overgrowth) observed by a physician. The 14 areas are right and left proximal interphalangeal joints, metacarpophalangeal joints, metatarsalphalangeal joints, wrist, elbow, knee, and ankle.
3. At least one area being the wrist, metacarpophalangeal joint, or proximal interphalangeal joint.
4. Simultaneous involvement of the same joint areas (as defined in 2) on both sides of the body (bilateral involvement of proximal interphalangeal joints, metacarpophalanageal joints, or metatarsalphalangeal joints) is acceptable without absolute asymmetry.
5. Subcutaneous nodules over bony prominences, extensor surfaces, or in juxta-articular regions observed by a physician.
6. Demonstration of abnormal amounts of serum rheumatoid factor.
7. Radiographic changes typical of rheumatoid arthritis, which must include erosions or unequivocal bony decalcification localized in or most marked adjacent to involved joints.

From American College of Rheumatology, 1987.

---

constitute a common presentation for ankylosing spondylitis, the most common seronegative spondyloarthropathy to involve the hip.[16] Reiter's syndrome and psoriatic arthritis rarely affect the hip.

Special mention should be made regarding hip pain in the young patient. Osteoarthritis is rare in this age group, barring significant precipitating trauma or severe developmental dysplasia. However, a young adult with pain should have a radiograph to rule out the presence of hip dysplasia, which can lead to severe osteoarthritis over time. Sustained polyarticular symptoms in the child, often in association with temperature spikes and diffuse lymphadenopathy, should trigger suspicion of juvenile rheumatoid arthritis, which frequently involves the hip.[4] Acute isolated pain in the hip with high fevers and inability to bear weight should be treated as septic arthritis until proved otherwise.[12] Spontaneous onset of hip pain in a young adult man with appropriate risk factors is a common presentation for osteonecrosis.[17] Although rare, unprecipitated hip pain in the older adult can indicate a hematogenously seeded septic joint or crystalline arthropathy such as gout or pseudogout.

INVESTIGATION

After the history and the physical examination, the benchmark for evaluating an arthritic hip is the radiograph. A standard weightbearing anteroposterior view of the pelvis is a cost-effective and reasonably safe means of determining the extent of involvement, allowing useful comparison of both hips and frequently giving clues to the underlying disease.[18] However, when the joint shows substantial destruction, as is often the case in the first radiograph of the older adult, further work-up for a specific diagnosis rarely

---

TABLE 2. CLASSIFICATION CRITERIA FOR OSTEOARTHRITIS OF THE HIP

Clinical Criteria

Hip pain and
• internal rotation less than 15 degrees and
• erythrocyte sedimentation rate less than 44 mm/h
or
Hip pain and
• internal rotation greater than 15 degrees and
• morning stiffness less than 60 minutes and
• age greater than 50 years and
• pain on internal rotation

Clinical and Radiographic Criteria

Hip pain and at least two of the following:
• erythrocyte sedimentation rate less than 20 mm/h
• radiographic osteophytes
• radiographic joint space narrowing

From American College of Rheumatology, 1987.

offers any clinical significance because treatment options decrease with advanced disease.

On radiograph, osteoarthritis typically appears hypertrophic, with marginal osteophyte formation, lateral displacement of the hip center, and focal joint space narrowing superiorly (Fig. 2). Conversely, inflammatory arthritis exhibits local osteopenia, diffuse joint space narrowing, lack of osteophytes, and medial or superior migration of the hip center (Fig. 3). Degenerative changes associated with irregularity of the femoral head and acetabulum, with or without superior displacement of the hip center, typically represent osteoarthritis secondary to a childhood hip disorder (Fig. 4). In contrast, sclerosis and collapse of a femoral head well contained by a round acetabulum is a common picture in osteonecrosis (Fig. 5). Progressive deterioration of the osteonecrotic hip can lead to joint space narrowing and degenerative arthritis.

Other imaging studies of potential use include lumbosacral spine radiographs for differentiating potentially confusing pain generators in the back and associated sacroiliac involvement. Magnetic resonance imaging has become the standard imaging modality for diagnosing patients with suspected early osteonecrosis[19] or for ruling out a stress fracture of the hip. Computed tomography has some role in evaluating patients with suspected osteochondral fractures or loose osteochondral fragments causing mechanical symptoms or patients with acetabular dysplasia out of plane from standard radiographs. Bone scintigraphy, although frequently nonspecific, can be useful for detecting localized abnormalities in the pelvis and femur.

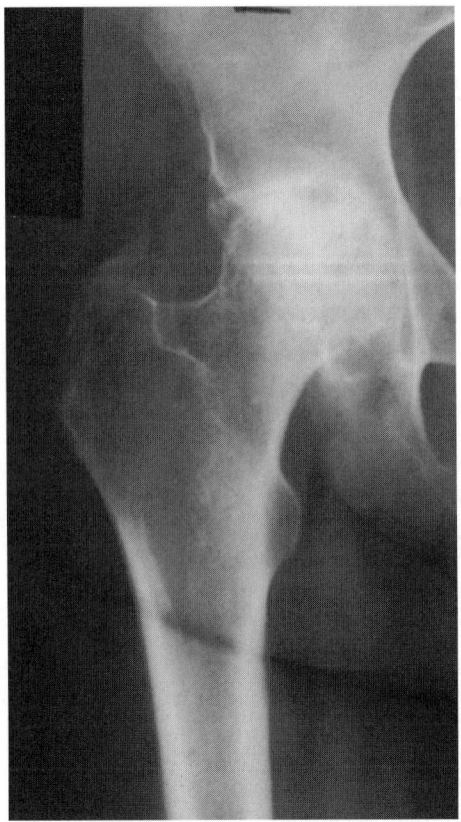

Fig. 3. Anteroposterior radiograph. This is a hip affected by rheumatoid arthritis.

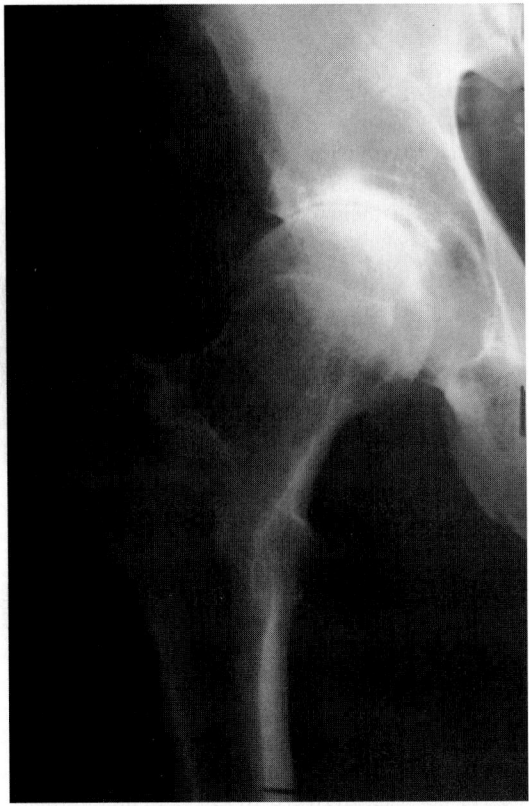

Fig. 2. Anteroposterior radiograph. This is a hip affected by osteoarthritis.

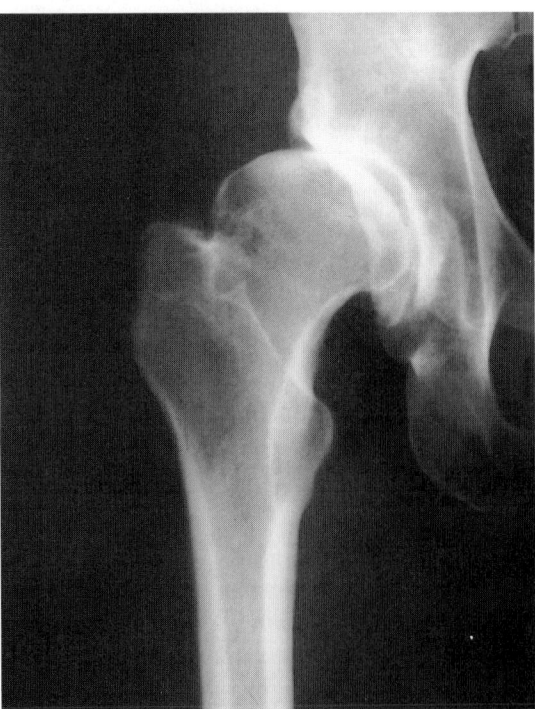

Fig. 4. Anteroposterior radiograph. This is a hip affected by dysplasia.

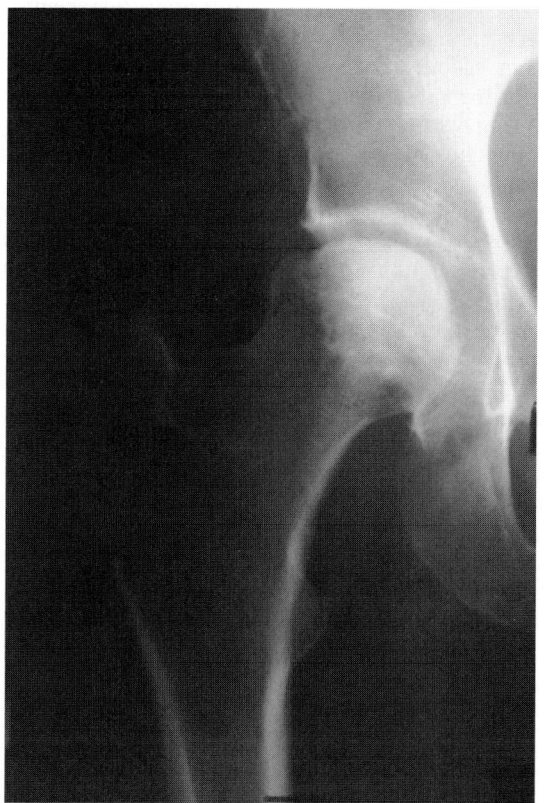

Fig. 5. Anteroposterior radiograph. This is a hip affected by osteonecrosis.

Arthrocentesis is necessary for diagnosis of septic arthritis. It often demonstrates frank pus, bacteria on Gram's stain, white blood cell counts greater than 50,000 cells per milliliter, predominantly polymorphonuclear neutrophils,

and a definitive organism on culture. Conclusive diagnosis of crystalline arthropathy also necessitates arthrocentesis, demonstrating the weakly negatively birefringent needle-shaped crystals seen with gout versus the positively birefringent rhomboid-shaped crystals seen with pseudogout. Synovial fluid analysis can also help differentiate inflammatory arthritis from osteoarthritis, with white blood cell counts in the former case reaching as high as 75,000 cells per milliliter (Table 4).

Certain serological laboratory tests can be of help. Rheumatoid factor is present in 70% to 80% of patients with rheumatoid arthritis. Antinuclear antibodies are frequently present in patients with either rheumatoid arthritis or systemic lupus erythematosus. Uric acid levels can be elevated in patients with gout, and multiple enzyme, hormone, or electrolyte-level abnormalities can give clues to any of the diverse causes of osteonecrosis. HLA-B27 is positive for as many as 90% of patients with ankylosing spondylitis[16] and can be present with other seronegative spondyloarthropathies such as Reiter's syndrome.

DIFFERENTIAL DIAGNOSIS

Conditions commonly confused with arthritis of the hip are listed in Table 5 along with useful clinical tests to help differentiate the true diagnosis. For a list of common adulthood causes of hip arthritis and a guide for clinical evaluation, see Table 6.

MANAGEMENT

The goals of managing a patient with arthritis of the hip are to reduce pain, increase range of motion, and optimize function. For the patient with mild to moderate disease, effective nonoperative treatment options include activity modification, low-impact exercise, anti-inflammatory medication, weight loss, and use of assistive walking devices.[4]

TABLE 4. ARTHROCENTESIS: SYNOVIAL FLUID TESTS		
Test	**Result**	**Clinical Suspicion**
Direct visualization	Straw-colored–translucent	Normal
	Turbid	Inflammation, infection
	Pus	Infection
	Blood	Hemarthrosis, sickle cell disease
	Fat	Intra-articular fracture
White blood cell count	<1000 wbc/mm³	Osteoarthritis, normal
	>1000 and <50,000	Infection (immunocompromised host)
		Tuberculosis, gonococcus
		Well-treated inflammatory arthritis
	>50,000 and <100,000	Infection
		Inflammatory arthritis
	>100,000	Infection
Neutrophil differential	<50%	Normal, noninflammatory arthritis
	>50% and <90%	Inflammatory arthritis
	>90%	Infection
Gram's stain	Positive	Bacterial infection
		Contaminant
Culture	Positive	Infection
	Negative	Treated or suppressed infection
Polarized microscopy	Negatively birefringent crystals	Gout
	Positively birefringent crystals	Pseudogout

Surgical treatment can include arthroscopy for the patients with persistent mechanical symptoms and mild disease, redirectional osteotomy of the pelvis and/or femur for the younger patient with focal disease, fusion for the younger patient with diffuse disease, and total hip arthroplasty for the older patient with diffuse disease.

Most patients, regardless of age and extent or severity of disease, warrant a trial of conservative treatment to avoid unnecessary risks of surgery. Limiting activities that necessitate high joint forces, such as running, hiking, and excessive stair-climbing, will theoretically improve symptoms. The use of a cane, one or two crutches, or even a walker to unload the hip with weightbearing is often beneficial. Weight loss very likely plays a role in hip symptomatology, and maintenance of functional range of motion through a supervised low-impact exercise regimen seems essential. None of these interventions has obvious complications; however, exercise is the only one of these modalities with documented results in treating patients with arthritis of the hip.[20]

Medical management of hip arthritis often begins with NSAIDs, although evidence shows that these medications offer an efficacy rate similar to that of acetominophen.[21] Aspirin, the prototypical NSAID, reduces inflammation by interfering with cyclooxygenase, an enzyme necessary for the production of such cellular mediators as prostaglandins, prostacyclins, and thromboxanes. Because of its short half-life and toxicity profile, aspirin has been largely replaced by the dozens of chemically related NSAIDs that allow lower doses and once or twice daily administration. Different NSAIDs have varying efficacy in different patients, warranting a trial-and-error approach with as many as four different preparations before abandoning this line of treatment.[22]

Attendant risks of NSAIDs include gastrointestinal irritation and bleeding as well as renal toxicity. Prostaglandins are known to have essential functions in the maintenance of the gastric mucosal lining, and prolonged use of these medications will predictably lead to erosions and possibly ulcerations of the stomach lining. A newer set of these medications, COX-2 inhibitors, specifically inhibits the subtype of cyclooxygenase that is present in periarticular tissues, sparing the gastric mucosa and theoretically decreasing intestinal bleeding complications.[23] All NSAIDs are excreted in the kidney and, as such, renal function should be periodically monitored in patients on long-term therapy.[22] Other potent medications used in the treatment of inflammatory arthritides, such as steroids, methotrexate, penicillamine, and gold, have complex profiles of drug interactions, adverse reactions, and side effects, making them most prudently managed by rheumatology consultants.

Hip arthroscopy has limited indications in the treatment of certain aspects of hip arthritis.[24] Early changes of osteoarthritis may include tearing of the acetabular labrum, osteochondritis dissecans, and formation of loose bodies, all of which can cause painful mechanical symptoms that have been successfully alleviated with hip arthroscopy. Synovectomy of the hip involved with inflammatory arthritis can be performed arthroscopically with less morbidity than when done open. Finally, there is guarded support in the literature that some cases of pyogenic arthritis of the hip can be adequately decompressed, diagnosed, and treated with the use of an arthroscopic washout in conjunction with parenteral antibiotics.[25, 26] However, open irrigation and débridement are still necessary for most patients. Complications of hip arthroscopy include iatrogenic injury to the articular surface, infection, neurovascular injury, and compression/traction palsies from distraction of the joint.

If the arthritis is limited and localized, redirectional osteotomy of either the proximal femur or the acetabulum may be indicated.[27] These procedures are also best performed on younger patients before the arthritis has progressed significantly. The goal of these procedures is to delay the progression of the arthritis in order to preserve the hip joint and avoid a total hip arthroplasty. Special radiographs and/or computed tomography scans should be taken preoperatively to evaluate the congruity of the joint and the articular space adjacent to the areas of focal involvement. Osteotomies about the femur can change any combination of the varus/valgus alignment, flexion, and axial rotation,

TABLE 5. CONDITIONS COMMONLY CONFUSED WITH ARTHRITIS OF THE HIP

Condition	Diagnostic Tests

Radicular low back pain	Physical examination
	   Nerve root tension signs
	   Neurologic deficit
	Lumbar spine radiographs
	MRI
	Local anesthetic injection of hip
	Epidural block

Trochanteric bursitis/
   abductor tendinitis
	Physical examination
	   Pain localized to trochanter
	   Pain with resisted abduction
	Local anesthetic injection of trochanter

Early osteonecrosis	Radiograph MRI
Femoral neck nonunion	History Radiograph CT scan
Acetabular nonunion	History CT scan

Intra-articular loose
   body
	Physical examination
	   Mechanical sensation with range
	      of motion
	MRI
	CT arthrography

Acetabular labral tear	Physical examination
	   Mechanical sensation with range
	      of motion
	MRI

Saroiliac arthritis	Physical examination
	   Pain with figure of four position
	      (FABER)
	Bone scan

Psoas tendinitis	Physical examination Pain with resisted hip flexion Bone scan Tendonography

Piriformis syndrome	Physical examination
	   Pain with resisted external rotation
	   Pain with palpation of piriformis

TABLE 6. DIFFERENTIAL DIAGNOSIS OF COMMON ADULTHOOD FORMS OF HIP ARTHRITIS

Condition	Presentation	Examination	Diagnostic Studies
Osteoarthritis	Age: typically >55 years Gender: slightly more men Onset: insidious Symptoms: groin pain, stiffness, limp Unilateral typically	Limited internal rotation Pain with extremes of motion Antalgia vs abductor lurch Flexion contracture, pelvic obliquity Variable leg-length discrepancy Abductor weakness/inhibition	Plain radiographs
Post-traumatic	Age: variable (can be young): 5 to 15 years after injury Gender: more common in men Onset: typically insidious Symptoms: same as those of osteoarthritis Unilateral nearly always	Similar to that for osteoarthritis Contracture more variable	Plain radiographs CT scan helpful if joint destruction is focal
Dysplasia	Age: typically <50 years Gender: more common in women Onset: typically insidious and chronic, limp during childhood Symptoms: waddling gait with leg-length discrepancy Bilateral not uncommon Previous surgery in childhood Family history commonly positive	Pain with extremes of motion Typically anteverted: intoed Contracture variable Leg-length discrepancy common Abductor weakness secondary to shortened moment arm	Plain radiographs Oblique radiographs/false profile CT scan for three-dimensional assessment
Osteonecrosis	Age: variable (depending on cause) Gender: traumatic more common in men Onset: typically acute Symptoms: groin pain Bilateral not uncommon	Acute pain with weightbearing Irritable range of motion Pain with internal rotation Antalgic gait True abductor weakness rare	Plain radiographs MRI
Sepsis	Age: Most common in childhood Gender: equal Onset: acute onset, typically with fever, chills, systemic illness Symptoms: inability to bear weight Unilateral typically	All hip motion irritable, held in flexed position	Plain radiographs CBC ESR Aspiration Ultrasonography
Rheumatoid	Age: usually >40 years (unless juvenile onset) Gender: more common in women Onset: insidious, starts in small joints Symptoms: early swelling and deformity before large joint pain Bilateral common	Deformity of feet and hands Thin skin, sequelae of immunosuppresion use Groin pain Hip irritability and limited range of motion	Plain radiographs Radiographs of hands and feet Serum rheumatoid factor, antinuclear antibody
Ankylosing spondylitis	Age: usually >40 years Gender: more common in men Onset: insidious Symptoms: groin pain, associated back and sacroiliac symptoms, decreased respiratory reserve Bilateral common	Decreased spine motion Sacroiliac joint irritability Decreased chest wall expansion Groin pain with considerable hip stiffness	Plain radiographs Serum HLA-B27 Pulmonary function tests
Crystalline arthropathy	Age: usually >50 years Gender: more common in men Onset: typically quite acute Symptoms: sharp groin pain, episodic, variable relationship to activity Unilateral typically	Irritable range of motion Groin pain Antalgic gait Hot joint	Plain radiographs Serum uric acid Arthrocentesis with crystal examination

with attendant risks of infection, nonunion, leg-length inequality, osteonecrosis, and failure to relieve symptoms. Similar risks accompany periacetabular osteotomies, which are complex three-dimensional procedures that can provide significant pain relief and slow the progression of the osteoarthritis.[28]

Hip arthrodesis can eliminate arthritis pain by eliminating motion at the joint.[29, 30] Changes in the modern work force and patient concerns regarding limitations in range of motion have decreased the popularity of hip fusion. However, the procedure is still ideally indicated for adults with incapacitating and severe arthritis who are younger than 40 years and who participate in heavy labor. The joint should be placed in 5 to 10 degrees of adduction, 10 degrees of external rotation, and 25 degrees of flexion to allow sitting. The procedure can be performed successfully with any one of a number of internal fixation options. Contraindications include patients with symptomatic arthritis of adjacent joints such as the spine, contralateral hip, and ipsilateral knee, which will be expected to compensate for lost range of motion. Complications include infection, nonunion, malposition, and development of degenerative changes in adjacent joints.

Septic arthritis of the hip, in any age category, is considered a surgical emergency, requiring operative lavage and intravenous antibiotics[12]; the specifics are discussed in the chapter about orthopaedic infections. Treatment of childhood hip dysplasia and the various stages of osteonecrosis can include surgery as well, and the reader is referred to the chapters dedicated to these subjects. Finally, total hip arthroplasty consistently offers drastic improvements in pain, stiffness, and quality of life for the older individual with end-stage arthritis of the hip. Total hip arthroplasty is not often performed in patients younger than 60 years. Although these patients receive excellent pain relief, there are concerns that these more active individuals will wear out the joint and require a number of revision procedures during their lifetime.

REFERENCES

1. Ganey TM, Ogden JA: Pre- and post-natal development of the hip. In Callaghan JJ, Rosenberg AG, Rubash HE (eds): The Adult Hip. Philadelphia, Lippincott-Raven, 1998, pp 39–55.
2. Magee DJ: Orthopaedic Physical Assessment. Philadelphia, WB Saunders, 1997, 3rd ed, pp 463–465.
3. Burstein AH, Wright TM: Fundamentals of Orthopaedic Biomechanics. Baltimore, Williams & Wilkins, 1994, pp 1–39.
4. Brown CR: Arthritis and allied conditions. In Callaghan JJ, Rosenberg AG, Rubash HE (eds): The Adult Hip. Philadelphia, Lippincott-Raven, 1998, pp 561–573.
5. Brandt KD, Slemenda CW: Osteoarthritis: Epidemiology, pathology and pathogenesis. In Schumacher HR, Klippel JH, Koopman WJ (eds): Primer on the Rheumatic Diseases. Atlanta, Arthritis Foundation, 1993, 10th ed, pp 184–188.
6. Charnley J: Low-Friction Arthroplasty of the Hip. New York, Springer-Verlag, 1970.
7. Springfield DS, Bolander ME, Friedlander GE, et al: Molecular and cellular biology of inflammation and neoplasia. In Simon SR (ed): Orthopaedic Basic Science. Rosemont, IL, American Academy of Orthopaedic Surgeons, 1994, pp 250–255.
8. Harris WH: Etiology of osteoarthritis of the hip. Clin Orthop 1986; 213:20.
9. Mankin HJ, Mow VC, Buckwalter JA, et al: Form and function of articular cartilage. In Simon SR (ed): Orthopaedic Basic Science. Rosemont, IL, American Academy of Orthopaedic Surgeons, 1994, pp 1–44.
10. Wilder RL: Rheumatoid arthritis: Epidemiology, pathology and pathogenesis. In Schumacher HR, Klippel JH, Koopman WJ (eds): Primer on the Rheumatic Diseases. Atlanta, Arthritis Foundation, 1993, 10th ed, pp 86–89.
11. Cracchiolo AC: Rheumatoid arthritis. In Amstutz HC (ed): Hip Arthroplasty. New York, Churchill Livingstone, 1991, pp 745–65.
12. Berman AT, Quartararo L: Septic arthritis. In Callaghan JJ, Rosenberg AG, Rubash HE (eds): The Adult Hip. Philadelphia, Lippincott-Raven, 1998, pp 575–591.
13. Felson DT, Anderson JJ, Naimark A, et al: Obesity and knee osteoarthritis: The Framingham study. Ann Intern Med 1988; 109:18.
14. Hoppenfeld S: Examination of gait. In Hoppenfeld S (ed): Physical Examination of the Spine and Extremities. New York, Appleton-Century-Crofts, 1976, pp 133–141.
15. Lachiewicz PF: Rheumatoid arthritis of the hip. J Am Acad Orthop Surg 1997; 5:332.
16. Khan MA: Ankylosing spondylitis. In Schumacher HR, Klippel JH, Koopman WJ (eds): Primer on the Rheumatic Diseases. Atlanta, Arthritis Foundation, 1993, 10th ed, pp 154–158.
17. Aaron RA: Osteonecrosis: Etiology, pathophysiology and diagnosis. In Callaghan JJ, Rosenberg AG, Rubash HE (eds): The Adult Hip. Philadelphia, Lippincott-Raven, 1998, pp 451–466.
18. Greenspan A: Orthopaedic Radiology: A Practical Approach. New York, Gower Medical Publishing, 1992, pp 11.1–14.14.
19. Hayes CW, Balkissoon AA: Magnetic resonance imaging of the musculoskeletal system II: The hip. Clin Orthop 1996; 322:297.
20. Minor MA, Hewett JE, Webel RR, et al: Efficacy of physical conditioning exercise in patients with rheumatoid arthritis and osteoarthritis. Arthritis Rheum 1989; 32:1396.
21. Bradley JD, Brandt KD, Katz BP, et al: Comparison of an anti-inflammatory dose of ibuprofen, an analgesic dose of ibuprofen, and acetaminophen in the treatment of patients with osteoarthritis of the knee. N Engl J Med 1991; 325.
22. Berger RG: Nonsteroidal anti-inflammatory drugs: Making the right choices. J Am Acad Orthop Surg 1994; 2:255.
23. Lane NE: Pain management in osteoarthritis: The role of COX-2 inhibitors. J Rheumatol 1997; 49:20.
24. McCarthy JC, Day B, Busconi B: Hip arthroscopy: Applications and technique. J Am Acad Orthop Surg 1995; 3:115.
25. Blitzer C: Arthroscopic management of septic arthritis of the hip. Arthroscopy 1993; 9:414.
26. Bould M, Edwards D, Villar R: Arthroscopic diagnosis and treatment of septic arthritis of the hip joint. Arthroscopy 1993; 9:707.
27. Brand RA: Hip osteotomies: a biomechanical consideration. J Am Acad Orthop Surg 1997; 5:282.
28. Trousdale RT, Ekkenkamp A, Ganz R, et al: Periacetabular and intertrochanteric osteotomy of osteoarthrosis in dysplastic hips. J Bone Joint Surg Am 1995; 1:73.
29. Callaghan JJ, McBeath AA: Arthodesis. In Callaghan JJ, Rosenberg AG, Rubash HE (eds): The Adult Hip. Philadelphia, Lippincott-Raven, 1998, pp 749–759.
30. Sponseller PD, McBeath AA, Perpich M: Hip arthrodesis in the young patient: A long-term follow-up study. J Bone Joint Surg Am 1984; 66:853.

section 6
chapter 9

OSTEONECROSIS

Nobuhiko Sugano

Summary
- Osteonecrosis has an enormous socioeconomic and public health impact because it often afflicts young males. It also often involves young females with collagen-vascular diseases that require corticosteroid treatment.
- Nonoperative treatment almost always fails, especially if the hip is involved.
- The natural history is influenced by the precise cause, site, and extent of the infarct.
- The early diagnosis can be extremely difficult.
- The treatment options are controversial.
- Treatment varies depending on the stage, location, and extent of the lesion.

DEFINITION AND TERMINOLOGY

Many terms have appeared in the literature for the name of the clinical syndrome osteonecrosis. Aseptic necrosis was initially used to distinguish the condition from sequestra due to bone infections. Avascular necrosis, ischemic necrosis, or infarction of bone presumed a uniform cause and pathogenesis. Ischemic necrosis and avascular necrosis generally are used for areas of epiphyseal or subarticular involvement, whereas bone infarction usually is reserved for metaphyseal or diaphyseal involvement. However, the pathogenesis is still unknown, and the causes of osteonecrosis are varied. Therefore, a term more neutral in its presumption of causation is preferable. In 1993, Association Research Circulation Osseous (ARCO) proposed the following definition and terminology. "Bone" is an organ that consists of mineralized tissues. Bone necrosis is a disease that causes death of bone and is called *osteonecrosis*.[1]

HISTORICAL REVIEW

The first publication dealing with necrosis of bone was "A Practical Essay on a Certain Disease of the Bones Termed Necrosis," by James Russell, published in 1874. In 1910, G. Axhausen described a clear distinction between septic and aseptic necrosis, and introduced decompression and bone graft into the femoral head for treatment. A classification system for osteonecrosis into stages with therapeutic and prognostic implications was first utilized in 1973. Each subsequent decade saw advances in the treatment of osteonecrosis. In the 1950s, prosthetic hemiarthroplasty was introduced. This evolved into the use of total hip replacement for end-stage disease in the 1960s. The following decade saw the introduction of rotational osteotomy, and during the 1980s the use of vascularized fibula grafts gained popularity. Today, all of these options are applied, depending on patient age and cause and stage of osteonecrosis.

EPIDEMIOLOGY

The number of patients with nontraumatic osteonecrosis of the femoral head is believed to have increased throughout the world. This is partly due to an improved awareness of the condition and development of diagnostic imaging techniques sensitive enough to detect it. However, a real increase in the disease burden is undeniable, especially after the mid-1970s, as seen by the yearly number of new patients with osteonecrosis by the author (Fig. 1). A tenfold increase in the incidence of osteonecrosis was noted from 1965 to 1985, probably due to the increase in corticosteroid usage. Osteonecrosis occurs in 5% to 25% of patients taking corticosteroids. The male-to-female ratio is approximately 1.6 : 1 and the prevalent age is in the third to fifth decade in idiopathic and alcohol-associated osteonecrosis.[2] Female preponderence in collagen-vascular disease or autoimmune disease resulted in the same trend as steroid-induced osteonecrosis. Both hips are often involved, with prevalences ranging from 42% to 72%, and development of osteonecrosis in bilateral hips has been suggested to be simultaneous or sequential.[3] Osteonecrosis accounts for 5% to 10% of total hip replacements performed in the United States.[4]

PATHOGENESIS

ETIOLOGY

Various clinical conditions are associated with the development of osteonecrosis. These are traumatic disruption of the blood supply (femoral head dislocation and femoral neck fracture), dysbaric disorders, exogenous corticosteroid therapy and Cushing's disease, alcoholism, hemoglobinopathies, Gaucher's disease, and irradiation.

Traumatic osteonecrosis usually develops after dislocation of the hip or subcapital fracture of the femoral neck. Osteonecrosis after intertrochanteric fracture of the femur

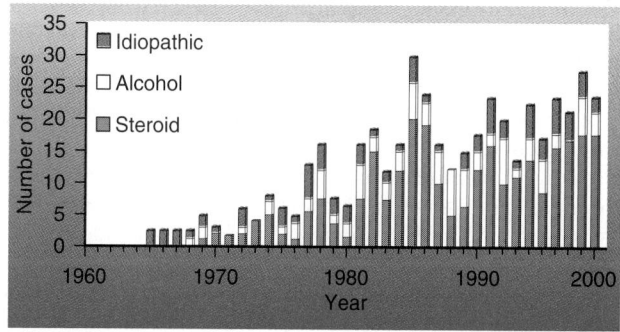

Fig. 1. New cases. Yearly number of new cases of osteonecrosis at the Osaka University Hospital, Japan.

or minor contusion of the hip is rare.[5, 6] The incidence of osteonecrosis after dislocation is reported to be 10% to 25%, depending on the severity of injury and associated femoral head or acetabular fractures.[7–9] Dislocation of the adult hip ruptures the ligamentum teres, disrupting the arterial supply to the femoral head. The superior retinacular artery also may be compromised. Reduction of the hip will not restore blood flow through the ligamentum teres but may relieve any vascular embarrassment that had occurred as a result of twisting or stretching of the retinacular vessels.[10, 11] Therefore, prompt reduction after injury (within 12 hours) may reduce the incidence of osteonecrosis.[12] In intracapsular femoral neck fractures, the sinusoidal vascular bed is interrupted and the subsynovial retinacular vessels, including the lateral epiphyseal, superior metaphyseal, and inferior metaphyseal vessels, also may be disrupted or damaged severely. The only remaining blood supply to the femoral head may come through the ligamentum teres, provided that it was functional before fracture.[13, 14] The prevalence of osteonecrosis after intracapsular fractures depends on the reestablishment of adequate blood flow from the remaining intact vasculature or revascularization. Therefore, it may be associated with the severity of displacement or rotation of the fractured fragments. It has been reported that osteonecrosis is seen in 11% to 16% of patients with a Garden stage I or stage II fracture and in 20% to 28% of patients with a Garden stage III or stage IV fracture.[15, 16] The incidence of osteonecrosis may be increased by use of magnetic resonance imaging (MRI), which can detect asymptomatic lesions in the early course of the disease.[17]

Dysbaric osteonecrosis occurs in tunnel workers use of compressed air (caisson disease) and deep-sea divers. Caisson disease was quite common in the early part of this century, but it is uncommon now as a consequence of U.S. Occupational Safety and Health Administration standards mandating safe working pressures and decompression schedules.[18] Osteonecrosis does not occur below atmospheric pressures of 17 psi. The risk of osteonecrosis in divers is related to the depth of the dive, number of dives, uncontrolled decompression, and low oxygen concentrations. Osteonecrosis is not believed to be a risk at depths of less than 30 m. Dysbaric osteonecrosis supposedly develops as a result of nitrogen gas embolization after rapid decompression. Both epiphyseal lesions and the metadiaphyseal lesions are commonly seen.

The increased prevalence of osteonecrosis in patients receiving corticosteroid therapy for collagen-vascular diseases, nephrosis, asthma, uveitis, or organ transplantation is well known. Steroid-associated osteonecrosis accounts for 10% to 30% of osteonecrosis cases, depending on the treatment center. It has been difficult to separate the effects of corticosteroids from those of underlying associated diseases, particularly in patients with vasculitis or renal failure. Osteonecrosis also occurs in patients with Cushing's disease and in patients receiving short-term high-dose corticosteroid treatment for cerebral edema or long-term softtissue corticosteroid infiltration.[19, 20] The threshold of corticosteroid use in determining the risk for development of osteonecrosis is still unclear. Many studies have suggested a correlation between osteonecrosis and the mean daily or peak dose, and have suggested that high doses, even for a short duration, present more significant risks than the cumulative dose. A maximum oral corticosteroid dose of 30 mg/day or greater is generally regarded as increasing the risk for osteonecrosis. The rash introduction of highdose and pulsed corticosteroid therapy proved to be associated with high rates of osteonecrosis.[21, 22]

Alcohol-associated osteonecrosis makes up 10% to 40% of cases, depending on the center.[23] Studies from Japan have determined the relative risks of developing osteonecrosis with varying doses of alcohol.[24, 25] The risk of developing femoral head osteonecrosis was estimated by adjusted relative odds obtained by a conditional logistic regression model. The elevated relative odds were observed for occasional drinkers (relative odds = 3.2; 95% confidence interval, 1.1 to 9.2) and regular drinkers (relative odds = 13.1; 95% confidence interval, 4.1 to 42.5) with a significant dose-response relationship ($p < .001$). For current drinkers, the relative odds were 2.8, 9.4, and 14.8 for less than 320, 320 to 799, and 800 g/wk or more of ethanol intake, respectively. A cumulative ill effect was found in more than 3200 g drink-year individuals, that is, in drinkers of more than 320 g/wk for 10 years.

Hemoglobinopathies, including most notably sickle cell disease (hemoglobin SS), hemoglobin SC disease, and sickle thalassemia are associated with localized areas of epiphyseal and metadiaphyseal osteonecrosis.[23] Sludging of sickled erythrocytes within the sinusoidal vascular bed results in functional occlusion. But in most cases, osteonecrosis occurrs in the epiphyseal and metadiaphyseal marrow cavities of the humerus, tibia, and femur.[26, 27] The incidence of osteonecrosis in hemoglobin SS disease is 4% to 12%. In hemoglobin SC disease, the incidence is 20% to 68%. There was a slight predominance in females (male-tofemale ratio, 1 : 1.6), and in individuals below the age of 25 years, especially in children between the ages of 6 and 15 years.[28]

Etiological associations are less well established for diverse conditions such as hyperlipidemia, pancreatitis, and hyperuricemia. The prevalence of chronic alcoholism in these patient populations may be a significant factor. Pregnancy has been reported to be an etiological factor, but the number of cases is small and a causal relationship has not been established.

The relatively high incidence rate of osteonecrosis in systemic lupus erythematosus is likely related to corticosteroid therapy. Vasculitis with interruption of the arterial blood supply has been suggested as a possible additional mechanism because some patients with collagen-vascular disorders not treated with steroids have been reported to develop osteonecrosis.[29, 30]

GENETIC FEATURES

There have been few known genetic features. Rare instances of multiple idiopathic osteonecrosis in several members of a family have been reported, suggesting a hereditary predisposition in some cases.[31] Hypofibrinolysis has been reported to be associated with familial osteonecrosis.[32] At my institution, one familial case of osteonecrosis of the femoral head was found in a male with a history of corticosteroid treatment for nephrosis and his son who was also treated with corticosteroids for systemic lupus erythematosus. Although an etiological factor such as thrombophilia, hypofibrinolysis, or corticosteroids may be related to the pathogenesis, some other genetic features, including vascular anatomy of the femoral head and endothelial cell behaviors, may exist. Analysis of the genetic aspects of the pathogenesis needs to be expanded.

PATHOPHYSIOLOGY

A uniform concept of the pathophysiology of osteonecrosis is vascular occlusion and ischemia of bone leading to bone death. The mechanical interruption of circulation to the femoral head after hip dislocations or femoral neck fractures is the most obvious pathological mechanism. Cellular or gas embolization in the sinusoids probably plays the central role of blood supply occlusion in Gaucher's disease, hemoglobinopathies, and dysbaric disorders. However, the pathogenesis of alcohol- or corticosteroid-associated osteonecrosis is not so clear. There have been several mechanisms proposed for the pathogenesis. Fat embolism from a fatty liver was proposed because the microscopic fat emboli in the end arteries of bone and other organs were found.[33] Marrow fat cell hypertrophy was suggested to contribute to the pathogenesis by compression of the sinusoidal vascular bed, which causes venous stasis and elevated intraosseous marrow pressure.[34] Because the marrow cavity is a compartment encased by a nonexpandable shell of bone, attention has been focused on elevated intraosseous pressure (IOP) as a pathogenic mechanism. An elevated IOP within the osteonecrotic femoral head and decreased venous drainage and stasis have been shown.[35, 36] IOP has also been shown to be elevated in the contralateral asymptomatic and preradiograph negative hips that develop biopsy-proven osteonecrosis. It has been described that in normal femoral heads, the resting IOP is about 15 mm Hg and a transient elevation of about 10 mm Hg occurs with a stress test injecting 5 mL of normal saline within the bone. In osteonecrosis, an abnormal resting IOP of above 30 mm Hg is recorded, and sustained elevations of greater than 10 mm Hg for more than 5 minutes are observed with the stress test. Other observers have not found IOP measurements to be reproducible, specific, or sensitive for the diagnosis of osteonecrosis.[37–40] An experimental study showed that increased IOP to 30 to 45 mm Hg increased endosteal, periosteal, and cancellous new bone formation but did not produce osteonecrosis.[41] Elevated IOP is observed not only in osteonecrosis but also in osteoarthritis and can also be related to elevations in intra-articular pressure and compressive loads.[42, 43] Thus, an elevated IOP does not seem to be causally related to the pathogenesis of osteonecrosis and is a nonspecific and secondary, but potentially contributory, factor.[23]

Alcohol and corticosteroids have been suggested to be directly cytotoxic to osteocytes. Steroid-induced osteoporosis with subsequent microfracture has also been proposed. Vascular occlusion secondary to vasculitis is also a possible cause. However, there is still little evidence for these putative mechanisms.

The final common pathway for nontraumatic osteonecrosis is intravascular coagulation with microcirculatory thrombotic occlusion.[44] Arteriolar and other intravascular thromboses have been reported in many studies. Microcirculatory thrombosis associated specifically with fat emboli have been described.[44] Elevated fibrinopeptides and fibrin degradation products, indicating the presence of dissemi-

nated intravascular coagulation (DIC), have been measured in some cases of osteonecrosis, providing indirect evidence of ongoing thrombosis. DIC, focal intravascular coagulation in the subchondral microcirculation, and osteonecrosis have been observed in human and animal examples of the Shwartzman and Arthus phenomena. Finally, hypofibrinolysis and thrombophilia have been demonstrated in many cases of osteonecrosis thought to be idiopathic.[32] Both hypofibrinolysis and thrombophilia are accompanied by an increased incidence of thrombotic events. Conditions capable of triggering intravascular coagulation include familial thrombophilia (resistance to activated protein C, decreased protein C, protein S, or antithrombin III), hyperlipemia and embolic lipid (alcoholism and hypercortisonism), hypersensitivity reactions (allograft organ rejection, immune complexes, and antiphospholipid antibodies), bacterial endotoxic (Shwartzman) reactions and various viral infections, proteolytic enzymes (pancreatitis), tissue factor release (inflammatory bowel disease, malignancies, neurotrauma, and pregnancy), and other prothrombotic and hypofibrinolytic conditions.[2]

PATHOLOGY

Although many staging systems have been proposed[35, 45–47] (Table 1), the latest version of ARCO staging is used in this chapter because it is simple and describes both the pathological features of osteonecrosis and its imaging findings.

Although various pathological mechanisms may be related to development of osteonecrosis with variable etiological factors, an ischemic event is still the origin. Six hours of complete anoxia generally is regarded as sufficient to result in death of the hematopoietic marrow. Osteocytes, osteoblasts, and osteoclasts may survive 6 to 48 hours of anoxia before irreversible cell damage and death occur. Little attention has been focused on the marrow fat cells' ability to survive anoxia. Their survivability after anoxia ranges from 2 to 5 days or more. Care must be taken in the diagnosis of cell death by light microscopy. Histological analysis can be complicated by improper preparation, fixation, decalcification, and staining of the specimen. Although functional cell death may have occurred, documentation of cell death is not possible until sufficient cytoplasmic (coagulation) or nuclear (pyknosis, karyorrhexis, and karyolysis) changes occur. It takes 48 to 72 hours before the degree of cell autolysis is sufficient to be recognized histologically. Because viable osteocytes within bony lacunae frequently appear pyknotic, pyknosis alone is not a reliable sign of cell death in osteonecrosis. The partial disappearance of trabecular cell nuclei alone is not considered as evidence of osteonecrosis because there is a normal attrition of osteocytes with age. Complete osteocyte autolysis may take 48 hours to 4 weeks or longer. However, complete absence of osteocytes within localized areas of trabecular bone is a reasonably reliable indicator of osteonecrosis, if artifactual loss can be excluded. The initial histological phase of osteonecrosis is a phase of cell death (stage 0). This histological phase can be obtained in femoral neck fractures because the ischemic event is quite clear. During this phase, the gross appearance of the femoral head is unchanged and sectioning of the femoral head shows no architectural changes of the bone and cartilage

TABLE 1. STAGING SYSTEMS OF OSTEONECROSIS

Staging System	Stage and Imaging Findings						
Marcus		1 Asymptomatic; radiograph: mottled density	2 Asymptomatic; radiograph: demarcated sclerosis	3 Onset of pain; radiograph: crescent sign	4 Pain with activity; radiograph: depression of femoral head	5 Pain with activity; radiograph: joint space narrowing	6 Pain at rest; radiograph: degenerative arthritis
Ficat	0 Asymptomatic; elevated IOP	1 Pain, limited movement; radiograph: normal; elevated IOP	2 Pain, limited movement; radiograph: diffuse porosis, sclerosis, or cysts; elevated IOP	Transition — Radiograph: flattening, crescent sign	3 Increased pain and limited movement; radiograph: collapse	4 Radiograph: decreased joint space, osteophytes	
Steinberg	0 Imaging: normal histology only	1 Radiograph: normal; MRI/bone scan positive	2 Radiography: cysts or sclerosis	3 Radiograph: crescent sign	4 Radiograph: flattening of femoral head	5 Radiograph: joint space narrowing	6 Radiograph: advanced degenerative changes
ARCO	0 Imaging: normal histology only	1 Radiograph: normal; MRI/bone scan: positive	2 Radiograph: mottled or demarcating sclerosis, cysts		3 Radiograph: crescent sign, flattening, collapse without degenerative changes	4 Radiograph: joint space narrowing, osteophytes	

IOP, intraosseous pressure; MRI, magnetic resonance imaging; ARCO, Association Research Circulation Osseous.

except for the fracture site. There is no obvious intervening zone between the central zone of cell death and the surrounding viable zone.

Bone death initiates an inflammatory response to the dead tissue. Between the necrotic zone and the viable zone, increased vascularity and perivascular inflammatory cell infiltration can be identified. Then a reactive interface with reparative fibrous tissue appears in the margin of the necrotic zone. Resorption of the necrotic bone and new bone formation are initially poor. During this phase (stage 1), radiographs do not reveal any density changes. This phase of osteonecrosis can be detected only by MRI. In osteonecrosis after femoral neck fracture (Fig. 2A), it takes 4 weeks or more after injury for the reactive interface to be detectable by MRI.[17] A marginal reparative reaction appears as a band of low signal intensity on T_1-weighted images and a band of high signal intensity on T_2-weighted images (Fig. 2B). Histologically, the band represents the reactive interface (Fig. 2C) and empty lacunae are seen in the necrotic bone within the band. During this phase of nontraumatic osteonecrosis, the three zones (necrotic, reparative, and viable zones) are also seen in specimens obtained by core biopsy specimens.[48] If the core specimen is obtained from the viable zone to the necrotic zone, it is possible to recognize these zones macroscopically (Fig.

3B). Although the nuclei of the cartilage cells are seen, the subchondral bone and marrow cells reveal complete disappearance of the nuclei (Fig. 3C). Arteriolar and sinusoidal thromboses are found in the necrotic zone close to the reactive interface (Fig. 3D).

With the further entry of blood vessels into the necrotic zone, a repair process consisting of bone resorption and formation produces the radiological appearance of lucency and sclerosis (stage 2). Toward the outer margin of the reactive interface, previously dead cancellous bone is partially invested by fiber or lamellar bone (Fig. 4A). This area is surrounded by a zone of reinforcing viable trabecular bone that represents a demarcating sclerosis on radiograph (Fig. 4B). This type of bone formation has classically been referred to as creeping substitution or creeping apposition. In this stage, there is no articular buckling or collapse of the femoral head.

The supporting bony architecture is weakened by continued resorption of trabecular bone. The stress of weightbearing can result in subchondral fracture with focal cartilage buckling and eventual collapse (stage 3) (Fig. 5A). Fragmentation and compaction of subchondral bony fracture debris lead to the development of a subchondral lucent area along the fracture line (crescent sign) (Fig. 5B). A crescent sign is usually seen on the lateral views of the femoral

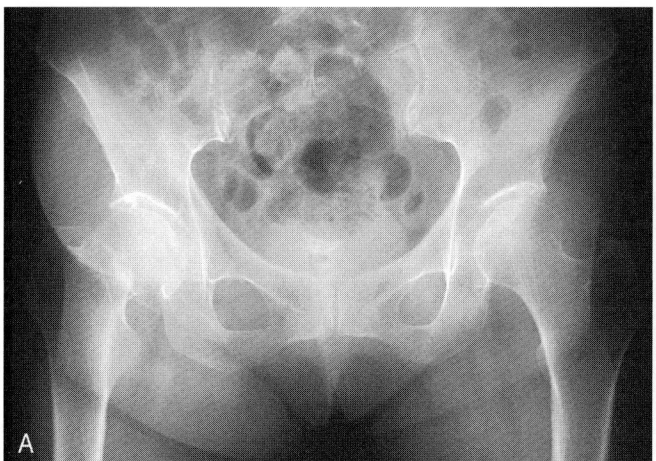

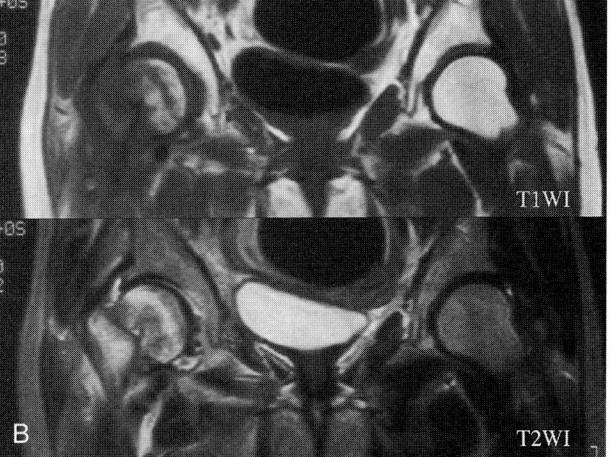

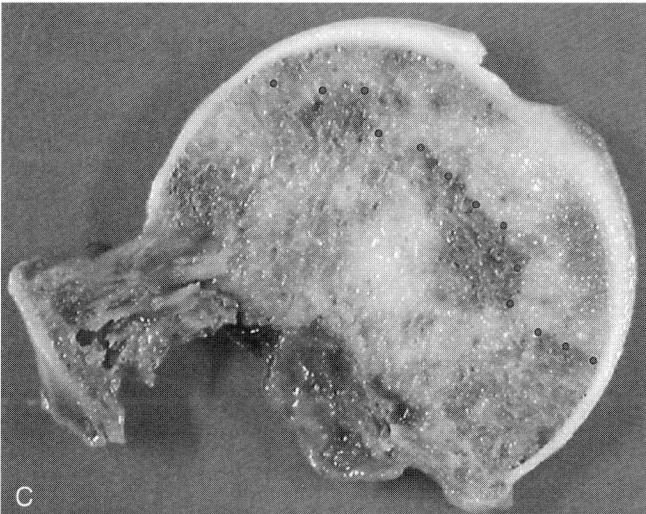

Fig. 2. **Views.** *A,* Intracapsular femoral neck fracture in the right hip in a 79-year-old woman. The patient underwent replacement arthroplasty 5 weeks after injury because of some medical complications. *B,* Preoperative magnetic resonance imaging (MRI) showed a low intensity band on T_1-weighted images and a high signal intensity band on T_2-weighted images in the subchondral area. *C,* A coronal section of the femoral head revealed a fibrous reactive interface in accordance with the band on MRI (*green dotted line*).

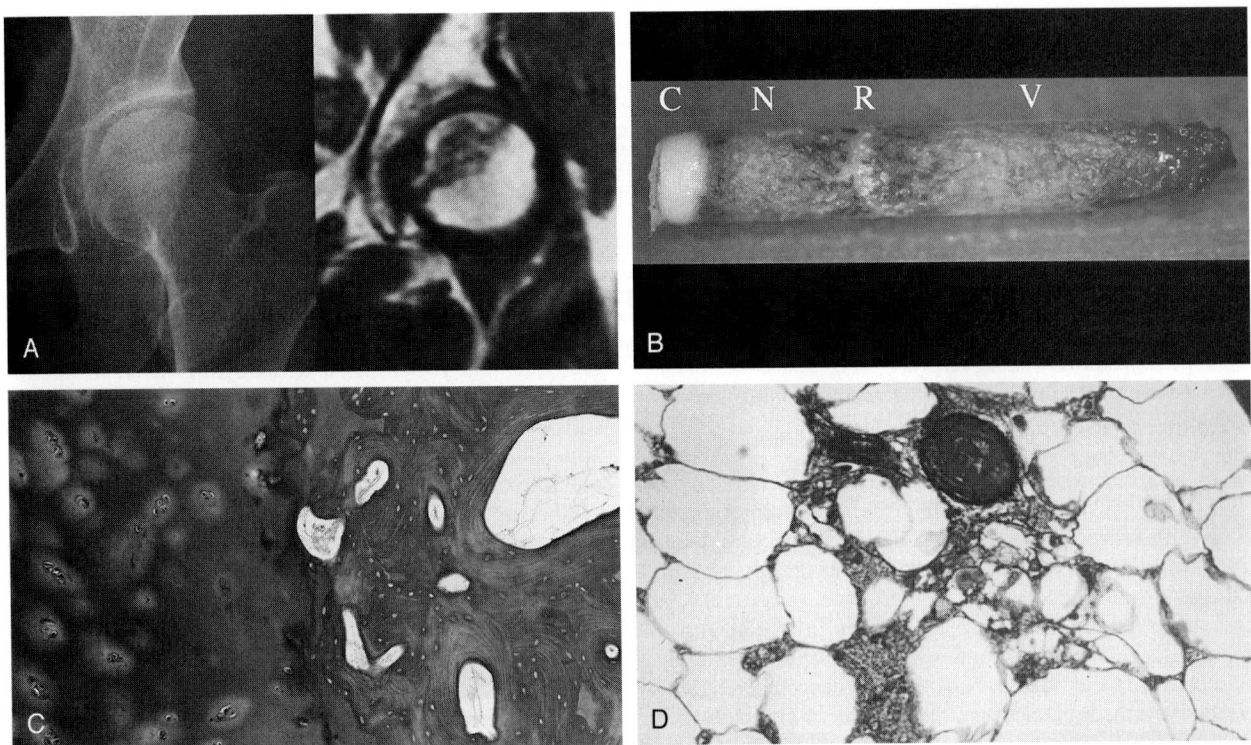

Fig. 3. Views. Steroid-induced osteonecrosis in a 40-year-old woman with Evans' syndrome. The right hip became symptomatic 2 years after the start of corticosteroid treatment but the left hip was asymptomatic. *A,* Radiograph showed no abnormality in the left hip (stage 1) and a low signal intensity band was detected on T1-weighted images. *B,* An 8-mm core biopsy specimen was obtained during a bone grafting procedure. A cartilage layer (C), a subchondral necrotic bone layer (N), a fibrous reactive layer (R), and a viable intact layer (V) are seen. *C,* The nuclei of the cartilage are intact and the subchondral bone and marrow cells reveal complete disappearance of the nuclei (×100, hematoxylin-eosin). *D,* Arteriolar and sinusoidal thromboses are found in the necrotic zone close to the reactive interface (×100, Masson).

head because it often is located in the anterior part of the femoral head. Resorption of bone also may cause fractures deep in the femoral head leading to segmental collapse.

The articular buckling and collapse cause an incongruent articular surface that eventually results in the degenerative arthritis of the joint (stage 4).

CLINICAL FEATURES

Pain is the usual initial presenting symptom. It is most often reported in the groin, but radiating pain to the ante-

rior thigh is common. It has been controversial whether the pain is more pronounced in the established or developing infarct (stage 0). Frequently, asymptomatic osteonecrosis (stage 1) is found as an incidental finding in the contralateral hip during MRI performed for symptomatic osteonecrosis. In MRI screening studies of high-risk patients with renal transplantation and systemic lupus erythematosus, stage 1 hips have usually been asymptomatic when osteonecrosis is detected.[49, 50] The most obvious cause of pain in osteonecrosis may be a microfracture of the cancellous bone due to reparative response to the dead bone. This

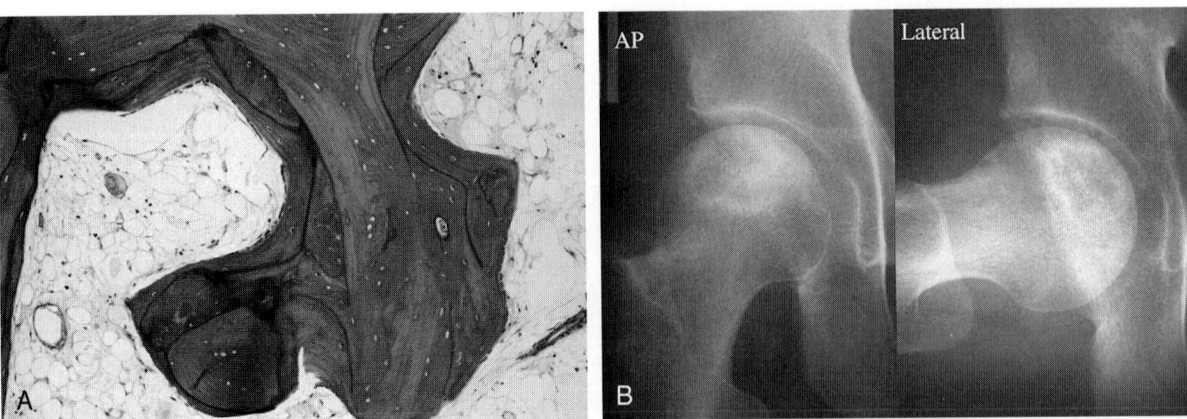

Fig. 4. Histology. Histology of stage 2 osteonecrosis. *A,* Bone formation on the dead core is observed with osteoblast lining (×100, hematoxylin-eosin). *B,* Radiograph shows demarcating sclerosis.

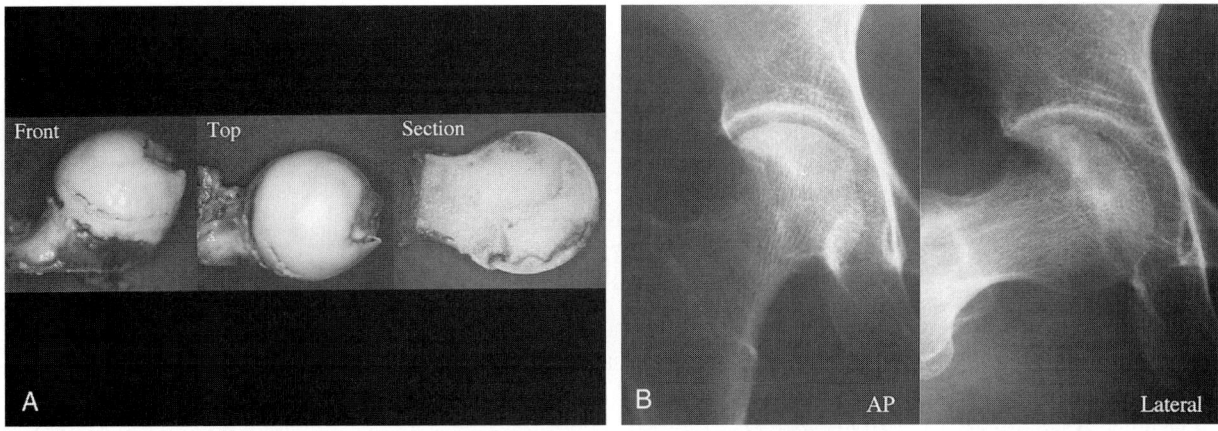

Fig. 5. Views. *A,* A femoral head of a 37-year-old man with idiopathic osteonecrosis shows a fold of the cartilage in the anterior part of the head. An axial section of the femoral head shows a subchondral fracture in the anterior part of the head. *B,* Radiograph showed crescent sign (a radiolucent zone) in the anterior part of the subchondral area on the lateral view.

may not manifest on radiograph or may show a crescent sign or slight flattening of the femoral head. Pain can be very intense and sudden in onset or it can be insidious and chronic. Pain is sometimes present even at rest and is worse with hip motion and weightbearing. Patients commonly exhibit an antalgic gait. On physical examination, a corresponding decrease in range of motion, particularly flexion and internal rotation, is observed.

INVESTIGATION

In the absence of specific causes (e.g., hemoglobinopathies), laboratory studies are normal. Blood counts, C-reactive protein, and rheumatoid factor are normal and these can rule out septic or rheumatoid arthritis. Hypofibrinolysis may be found in cases of osteonecrosis. Hypofibrinolysis is usually associated with low levels of stimulated tissue plasminogen activator, elevated levels of plasminogen activator inhibitor, and, often, high levels of lipoprotein A. Decreased levels of the antithrombotic proteins C or S and resistance to activated protein C decrease regulation of the prothrombotic factors V and VIII.

The finding of imaging studies such as radiography, MRI, and bone scan according to stage are summarized in Table 2. MRI or bone scan findings may not be clearly divided in each stage because the staging primarily refers to radiographic findings.

DIFFERENTIAL DIAGNOSIS

Although many different techniques have been used to diagnose osteonecrosis as early as possible using radiographs, venography, bone marrow pressure measurement, biopsy, computed tomography, bone scans, and MRI, no single modality has been shown to provide the ideal solution for accurate diagnosis. An alternative method is to use clinical diagnostic criteria. The Japanese multicenter study of osteonecrosis proposed diagnostic criteria for the standardized clinical definition of nontraumatic osteonecrosis of the femoral head.[48] The most effective and simple diagnostic criteria for osteonecrosis are chosen as follows: (1) collapse of the femoral head without joint space narrowing or acetabular abnormality on radiographs (including the crescent sign), (2) demarcating sclerosis in the femoral head without

			TABLE 2. FINDINGS OF IMAGING STUDIES IN EACH STAGE		
Imaging Study	**Stage**				
	0	**1**	**2**	**3**	**4**
Radiograph	Negative	Negative	Demarcating sclerosis; cystic radiolucency	Crescent sign Collapse	Degenerative changes (e.g., joint space narrowing, osteophytes)
Bone scan	Negative	Cold in hot or cold	Cold in hot	Cold in hot or hot	Hot or cold in hot
MRI	Negative	A low-intensity band on T_1WI; a double-line sign on T_2WI	A low intensity band on T_1WI; a double-line sign on T_2WI	A low signal intensity area within the band on T_1WI; an inhomogeneous signal intensity area within the band on T_2WI; bone marrow edema in the viable zone	A low-intensity band on T_1WI; a low or inhomogeneous intensity on T_2WI

MRI, magnetic resonance imaging; T_1WI, T_1 = weighted image; T_2WI, T_2 = weighted image.

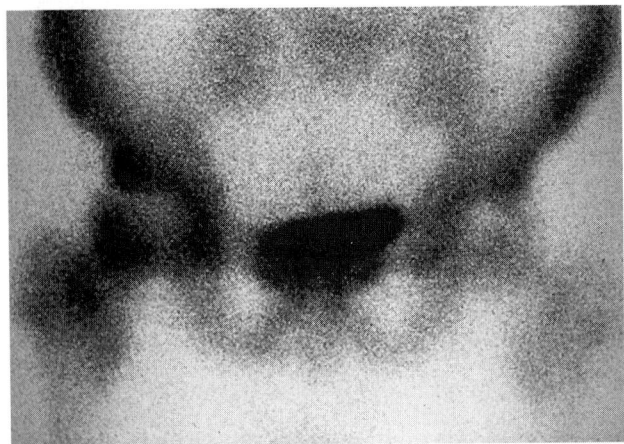

Fig. 6. Scan. Bone scan shows the "cold in hot" appearance in the bilateral hips.

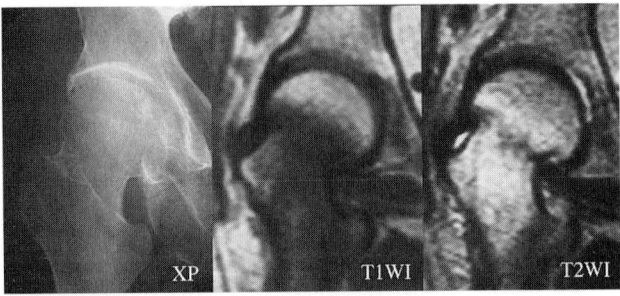

Fig. 7. Fracture. This shows an occult fracture of the femoral neck in the right hip of a 62-year-old man. The fracture line was still unclear on radiograph 1 week after injury. Magnetic resonance imaging shows low intensity area on T_1-weighted images and a low intensity line with surrounding high intensity area on T_2-weighted images.

joint space narrowing or acetabular abnormality, (3) "cold in hot" on bone scans (Fig. 6), (4) low-intensity band on T1-weighted images (band pattern) (see Fig. 3A), (5) trabecular and marrow necrosis on histology. With any sets of two positive criteria out of five, the sensitivity and specificity of diagnosis were 91% and 99%.

Differential diagnosis for stage 1 osteonecrosis may be fatigue fracture, inflammatory disease, nonspecific synovitis, and transient osteoporosis. MRI is useful to rule out these conditions. A low signal intensity line on T_1-weighted images and a high signal intensity area around the line on T_2-weighted images are seen in fatigue or occult fractures (Fig. 7). Normal intensity of the femoral head and some effusion or synovial swelling may be observed in synovitis. Most of the femoral head and sometimes the neck show diffuse low intensity on T_1-weighted images and high intensity on T_2-weighted images in transient osteoporosis (Fig. 8A). Osteonecrosis usually shows a low-intensity band on T_1-weighted images and a double-line sign that is characterized by an outer low-intensity and an inner high-intensity line on T_2-weighted images,[51] although bone marrow edema around the necrotic lesion may

be seen just after collapse has occurred.[49] Bone scan is useful to increase the diagnostic accuracy because it shows a pattern of cold in hot in osteonecrosis and a pattern of diffuse hot accumulation without a cold area in transient osteoporosis (Fig. 8B). Bone scan also may be useful to diagnose mulitple sites of osteonecrosis. For stage 2 or 3, the radiographs will establish the precise diagnosis in almost all cases. However, it is important to rule out bone tumors, which fulfills the diagnostic criteria (Fig. 9). For advanced stage 4 osteonecrosis, the underlying cause may be obscure. It is hard to differentiate it from degenerative osteoarthritis and post-traumatic arthritis.

MANAGEMENT

NONOPERATIVE TREATMENT

Nonoperative treatment that is limited to observation and/or protected weightbearing has not been effective in preventing progression.[52–54] No differences in disease progression were observed when patients were evaluated according to whether they used steroids, had excessive alcohol intake, or had idiopathic disease.[54, 55] The Japanese study of osteonecrosis proposed a radiographic classification[56] and later an MRI classification[51] (Fig. 10) based on the location of the lesion. Small lesions located medially or centrally such as

TABLE 3. INDICATIONS OF NONOPERATIVE AND OPERATIVE TREATMENTS ACCORDING TO STAGE. IOP, INTRAOSSEOUS PRESSURE					
Stage	0	1	2	3	4
Nonoperative treatment	Indicated for small lesions				
Core decompression	Indicated for high IOP				
Vascularized bone graft					
Angular or rotational osteotomy	Indicated for lesions which can be relocated to less weightbearing area				
Prosthetic arthroplasty					

Good indication
Limited indication
Contraindication

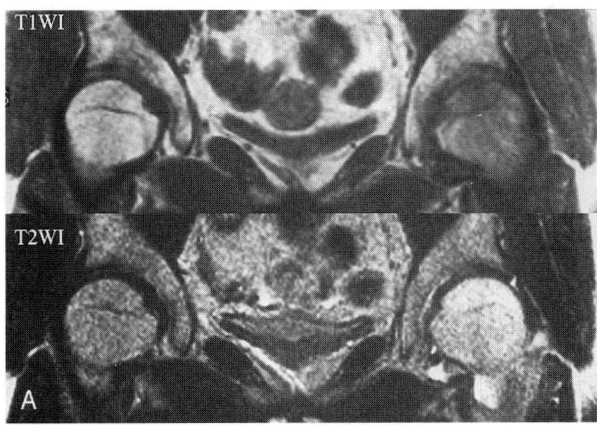
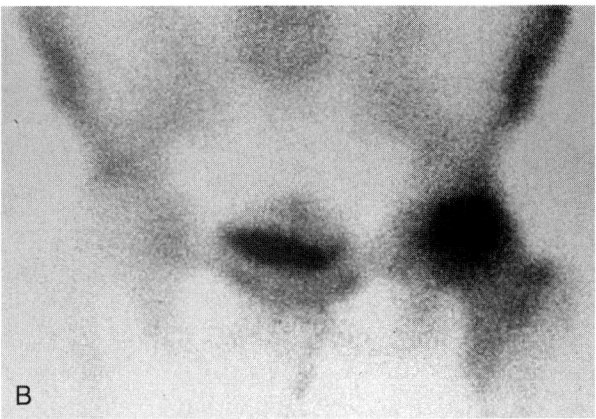

Fig. 8. Scans. This is from a 42-year-old male with transient osteoporosis in the left hip. *A,* Magnetic resonance imaging shows a low intensity area of the entire femoral head on T$_1$-weighted images and a high intensity area on T$_2$-weighted images. *B,* Bone scan shows a diffuse increased accumulation of the isotope.

type A or type B are much less likely to progress to collapse than the lesions occurring in most of the weight-bearing areas. In such cases, it may be reasonable to follow the patient's condition with watchful waiting, because osteonecrosis may heal without developing subchondral fracture and collapse. If progression of the infarct is seen, treatment should be instituted.

OPERATIVE TREATMENT

Prosthetic arthroplasty can relieve pain and restore hip function quickly. However, an effort should be made to avoid prosthetic arthroplasty if the stage is early and the femoral head reveals no collapse, because the patients are usually young and active. Arthrodesis is probably not a good option because of the high incidence of bilateral involvement. Several joint-preserving operations have been proposed for the treatment of early-stage disease and even some for treatment of later stages. They include core decompression, structural and nonstructural bone grafting, vascularized bone grafting, and femoral osteotomy (Table 3). The procedures of osteotomy and prosthetic arthroplasty are described elsewhere in this book.

Core decompression may be considered as a treatment option because the procedure prevents collapse, especially in Ficat stage.[1, 56] However, as described earlier under

Pathogenesis, elevated IOP is not causally related to the pathogenesis of osteonecrosis and intervention tends to be unsuccessful in stage 2 or later. Because fracture of the femur is a major postoperative risk, attention to surgical technique and weightbearing protection for 2 to 3 months are essential.

Several bone grafting procedures have been proposed. The use of a cancellous graft with core decompression seems to have about the same results as core decompression alone and to be associated with similar risks. Using a fibular strut graft, prevention of collapse can be achieved in up to 90% of patients. The procedure is not much more involved than core decompression alone, unless an autograft is used. The risks are the same as those for core decompression without grafting. If an allograft is used, however, transmission of blood-borne disease is possible. A vascularized fibular graft provides about the same outcome as core decompression with a nonvascularized fibular graft, but it is more complex and costly.

Because most of the lesions are located in the anterosuperior portion of the femoral head, various types of femo-

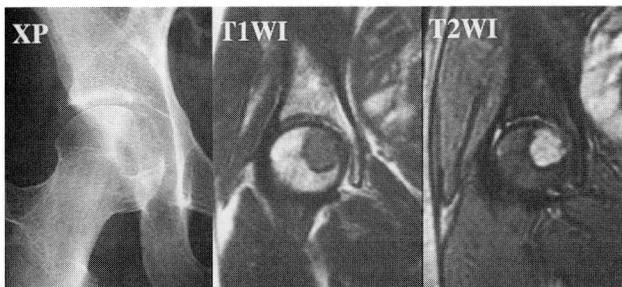

Fig. 9. Radiograph. This is from a 24-year-old female with chondroblastoma in the right hip. Radiograph showed a lucent area in the epiphysis of the femoral head with a marginal sclerosis and subchondral fracture. The lesion shows low intensity on T$_1$-weighted images and high intensity on T$_2$-weighted images.

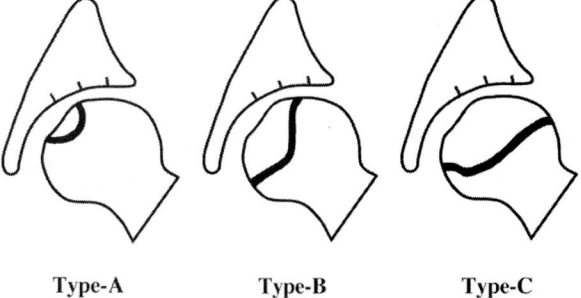

Type-A   **Type-B**   **Type-C**

Fig. 10. Classification. This is the Japanese Investigation Committee classification of osteonecrosis. The classification scheme consists of three types (A, B, and C) and is based on the central coronal section of the femoral head on T$_1$-weighted images. Type A lesions occupy the medial one-third or less of the weightbearing portion, type B, the medial two-thirds or less of the weightbearing portion, and type C, greater than two-thirds of the weightbearing portion.

TABLE 4. CLINICAL OUTCOME OF EACH OPERATIVE TREATMENT

Treatment Type	Success Rate in Each Stage				
	0	1	2	3	4
Core decompression	100%	25%–96%	14%–82%	0%–60%	
Vascularized bone graft			89%	57%–77%	68%
Angular osteotomy			47%–83%	47%–87%	
Rotational osteotomy			89%	73%	70%

ral osteotomies that move the necrotic lesion outside the weightbearing area have been proposed. They may reduce symptoms by reducing the stresses across the lesion and may let the lesion heal without further deformation of the femoral head. The procedures include angular osteotomy and rotational osteotomy. The major risk of angular osteotomy is nonunion. When preceded by angular osteotomy, prosthetic arthroplasty is probably more difficult if the procedure becomes necessary. Rotational osteotomy is highly demanding technically and is difficult even for the experienced hip surgeon to perform well. The risks are similar to those associated with angular osteotomy, although the proximal femur is less deformed, making subsequent prosthetic arthroplasty easier. Osteotomy, especially rotational osteotomy, may stabilize symptoms even in stage 3. Long-term benefit may be achieved in patients with smaller infarcts that can be completely rotated out of the weightbearing area.

Probably the most commonly performed procedure for advanced osteonecrosis of the femoral head is prosthetic arthroplasty, despite the concerns related to prosthetic failure in younger patients. The explanation is that few or no good alternatives are available, especially in cases of bilat-eral or potentially bilateral disease. Bipolar arthroplasty is an option, although total hip arthroplasty seems preferable because pain relief is more certain. Also, the complication rate is no higher than that associated with bipolar arthroplasty.

COMPLICATIONS

Complications of ostenecrosis are a progression to arthritis, subluxation or dislocation, fracture, and secondary infection. Arthritis is ususally secondary to subchondral fracture. Subluxation or dislocation occurs as the degree of collapse increases. Fracture may occur if the lesion is extensive to the whole femoral head. Secondary infection without operation is very unlikely in any stage. Osteochondromatosis and free bodies are sometimes developed after osteochondral fragmentaion in the knee but seldom in the hip.

RESULTS

Clinical outcomes of the operative procedures are listed in Table 4.

REFERENCES

1. Gardeniers JWM: The ARCO perspective for reaching one uniform staging system of osteonecrosis. In Schoutens A, Arlet J, Gardeniers JWM, et al (eds): Bone Circulation and Vascularization in Normal and Pathological Conditions. New York, London, Plenum Press, 1993, pp 375–380.
2. Collaborative Osteonecrosis Group: Symptomatic multifocal osteonecrosis: A multicenter study. Clin Orthop, 1999; 369:312.
3. Sugano N, Nishiii T, Shibuya T, et al: The contralateral hip in patients with unilateral non-traumatic osteonecrosis of the femoral head. Clin Orthop 1997; 334:85.
4. Mankin HJ: Nontraumatic necrosis of bone (osteonecrosis). N Engl J Med 1992; 326:1473.
5. Arlet J: Nontraumatic avascular necrosis of the femoral head: Past, present, and future. Clin Orthop 1992; 267:12.
6. Baixauli EJ, Baixauli F Jr, Baixauli F, et al: Avascular necrosis of the femoral head after intertrochanteric fractures. J Orthop Trauma 1999; 13:134.
7. Epstein HC: Traumatic dislocation of the hip. Clin Orthop 1973; 92:116.

8. Roeder LF Jr, DeLee JC: Femoral head fractures associated with posterior hip dislocations. Clin Orthop 1980; 147:121.
9. Upadhyay SS, Moultoj A, Srikrishnamurthy K: An analysis of the late effects of traumatic posterior dislocation of the hip without fractures. J Bone Joint Surg Br 1983; 65:150.
10. Sevitt S, Thompson RG: The distribution and anastomoses of arteries supplying the head and neck of the femur. J Bone Joint Surg Br 1965; 47:560.
11. Shin SS: Circulatory and vascular changes in the hip following traumatic hip dislocation. Clin Orthop 1979; 140:255.
12. Brav EA: Traumatic dislocation of the hip. J Bone Joint Surg Am 1962; 44:1115.
13. Cato M: A histological study of avascular necrosis of the femoral head after transcervical fracture. J Bone Joint Surg Br 1965; 47:749.
14. Sevitt S: Avascular necrosis and revascularization of the femoral head after intracapsular fracture: A combined arteriographic and histologic study. J Bone Joint Surg Br 1964; 46:270.

15. Banks HH: Factors influencing the results in fractures of the femoral neck. J Bone Joint Surg Am 1962; 44:931.
16. Barnes R, Brown JT, Garden RS, et al: Subcapital fractures of the femur. A prospective review. J Bone Joint Surg Br 1976; 58:2.
17. Sugano N, Masuhara K, Nakamura N, et al: MRI of early osteonecrosis of the femoral head after transcervical fracture.. J Bone Joint Surg 1996; 78:253.
18. Jones JP Jr, Behnke AR Jr: Prevention of dysbaric osteonecrosis in compressed-air workers. Clin Orthop 1978; 130:118.
19. Fast A, Alon M, Weiss S, et al: Avascular necrosis of bone following short-term dexamethasone therapy for brain edema. Case report. J Neurosurg 1984; 61:983.
20. Roseff R, Canoso JJ: Femoral osteonecrosis following soft tissue corticosteroid infiltration. Am J Med 1984; 77:1119.
21. Zizic TM, Marcoux C, Hungerford DS, et al: Corticosteroid therapy associated with ischemic necrosis of bone in systemic lupus erythematosus. Am J Med 1985; 79:596.

22. Ono K, Tohjima T, Komazawa T: Risk factors of avascular necrosis of the femoral head in patients with systemic lupus erythematosus under high-dose corticosteroid therapy. Clin Orthop 1992; 277:89.

23. Aaron RK: Osteonecrosis: Etiology, pathophysiology, and diagnosis. In Callaghan JJ, Rosenberg AG, Rubash HE (eds): The Adult Hip. Philadelphia, Lippincott-Raven 1998, pp 451–466.

24. Ono K, Sugioka Y: Epidemiology and risk factors in avascular necrosis of the femoral head. In Schoutens A, Arlet J, Gardeniers JWM et al (eds): Bone Circulation and Vascularization in Normal and Pathologic Conditions. New York, Plenun Press, 1993, pp 243–248.

25. Hirota Y, Hirohata T, Fukuda K, et al: Association of alcohol intake, cigarette smoking, and occupational status with the risk of idiopathic osteonecrosis of the femoral head. Am J Epidemiol 1993; 137: 530.

26. Diggs LW: Bone and joint lesions in sickle cell disease. Clin Orthop 1967; 52: 119.

27. Keely K, Buchanan GR: Acute infarction of long bones in children with sickle cell anemia. J Pediatr 1982; 101:170.

28. Iwegbu CG, Fleming AF: Avascular necrosis of the femoral head in sickle-cell disease. J Bone Joint Surg Br 1985; 67:29.

29. Siemsen JK, Brook J, Meister L: Lupus erythematosus and avascular bone necrosis. A clinical study of three cases and review of the literature. Arthritis Rheum 1962; 5:492.

30. Smith FE, Sweet DE, Brunner CM, et al: Avascular necrosis in SLE. An apparent predilection for young patients. Ann Rheum Dis 1976; 35:227.

31. Mitchell DG, Steinberg ME, Dalinka MK, et al: Magnetic resonance imaging of the ischemic hip. Alterations within the osteonecrotic, viable, and reactive zones. Clin Orthop 1989; 244:60.

32. Glueck CJ, Glueck HI, Welch M, et al: Familial idiopathic osteonecrosis mediated by familial hypofibrinolysis with high levels of plasminogen activator inhibitor. Thromb Haemost 1994; 71:195.

33. Jones JP, Sakovich L: Fat embolism of bone. A roentgenographic and histological investigation with use of intra-arterial Lipiodol in rabbits. J Bone Joint Surg Am 1966; 48:149.

34. Wang GJ, Sweet D, Reger SI, Thompson RC: Fat-cell changes as a mechanism of avascular necrosis of the femoral head in cortisone-treated rabbits. J Bone Joint Surg Am 1977; 59:729.

35. Ficat RP: Idiopathic bone necrosis of the femoral head: Early diagnosis and treatment. J Bone Joint Surg Br 1985; 67:3.

36. Hungerford DS, Lennox DW: The importance of increased intraosseous pressure in the development of osteonecrosis of the femoral head: Implications for treatment. Orthop Clin North Am 1985; 16:635.

37. Camp JF, Colwell CW: Core decompression of the femoral head for osteonecrosis. J Bone Joint Surg Am 1986; 68:1313.

38. Hauzeur JPH, Pasteels JL, Orloff S: Bilateral non-traumatic aseptic osteonecrosis in the femoral head. J Bone Joint Surg Am 1987; 69:1221.

39. Kiaer T, Pedersen NW, Kristensen K, et al: Intra-osseous pressure and oxygen tension in avascular necrosis and osteoarthritis of the hip. J Bone Joint Surg Br 1990; 72:1023.

40. Learmonth ID, Maloon S, Dall G: Core decompression for early atraumatic osteonecrosis of the femoral head. J Bone Joint Surg Br 1990; 72:387.

41. Welch RD, Johnston CE, Waldron MJ, et al: Bone changes associated with intraosseous hypertension in the caprine tibia. J Bone Joint Surg Am 1993; 75:53.

42. Downey DJ, Simkin PA, Taggart R: The effect of compressive loading on intraosseous pressure in the femoral head in vitro. J Bone Joint Surg Am 1988; 70:871.

43. Goddard NJ, Gosling PT: Intra-articular fluid pressure and pain in osteoarthritis of the hip. J Bone Joint Surg Br 1988; 70:52.

44. Jones JP Jr: Intravascular coagulation and osteonecrosis. Clin Orthop 1992; 277:41.

45. Stulburg BN. Editorial comment. Clin Orthop 1997; 334:2.

46. Marcus ND, Enneking WF, Massam RA: The silent hip in idiopathic aseptic necrosis. Treatment by bone grafting. J Bone Joint Surg Am 1973; 55:1351.

47. Steinberg ME, Hayken GD, Steinberg DR: A quantitative system for staging avascular necrosis. J Bone Joint Surg Br 1995; 77B:34.

48. Sugano N, Kubo T, Takaoka K, et al: Multicenter study of diagnostic criteria for nontraumatic osteonecrosis of the femoral head. J Bone Joint Surg Br 1999; 81:590.

49. Kubo T, Yamazoe S, Sugano N, et al: Initial MRI findings of non-traumatic osteonecrosis of the femoral head in renal allograft recepient. Magn Reson Imaging 1997; 15:1017.

50. Sugano N, Ohzono K, Masuhara K, et al: Prognostication of osteonecrosis of the femoral head in patients with systemic lupus erythematosus by magnetic resonance imaging. Clin Orthop 1994; 305:190.

51. Mitchell DG, Rao VM, Dalinka MK, et al: Femoral head avascular necrosis: Correlation of MR imaging, radiographic staging, radionuclide imaging, and clinical findings. Radiology 1987; 162:709.

52. Patterson RH, Bickel WH, Dahlin DC: Idiopathic avascular necrosis of the head of the femur: A study of fifty-two cases. J Bone Joint Surg Am 1964; 46:267.

53. D'Aubigne M, Postel M, Mazabraud A, et al: Idiopathic necrosis of the femoral head in adults. J Bone Joint Surg Br 1965; 47: 612.

54. Musso ES, Mitchell SN, Schink-Ascani M, et al: Results of conservative management of osteonecrosis of the femoral head. A retrospective review. Clin Orthop 1986; 207:209.

55. Sugano N, Takaoka K, Ohzono K, et al: Prognostication of nontraumatic avascular necrosis of the femoral head: Significance of location and size of the necrotic lesion. Clin Orthop 1994; 303:155.

56. Ohzono K, Saito M, Takaoka K, et al: Natural history of nontraumatic avascular necrosis of the femoral head. J Bone Joint Surg Br 1991; 73:68.

57. Fairbank AC, Bhatia D, Jinnah RH, et al: Long-term results of core decompression for ischaemic necrosis of the femoral head. J Bone Joint Surg Br 1995; 77:42.

OSTEOTOMY/ARTHRODESIS/RESECTION

Rajit Saluja

Summary

- Unilateral osteoarthritis of the hip in a young patient poses a difficult challenge for the treating physician.
- Extensive reviews showed that primary osteoarthritis is very rare and that in the majority of cases an underlying mechanical abnormality exists that predisposes the hip to early osteoarthritis.
- Studies of hip biomechanics showed that anatomic abnormalities either on the femoral or acetabular side can lead to elevated stress transmission across the hip joint.
- Femoral or acetabular osteotomies are generally performed to reduce the stress across the hip and subsequently either decrease the risk of osteoarthritis or slow the progression of early osteoarthritis.
- In a young patient who already has advanced osteoarthritis, salvage osteotomy may still be of some benefit. However, if the individual is involved in a heavy labor occupation or has restricted mobility in the hip joint, arthrodesis of the joint can provide durable pain-free results.
- Resection arthroplasty is usually not recommended as a primary treatment for osteoarthritis in the young patient. Rather, it is reserved for the treatment of infection after arthroplasty either as the first stage of a two-stage revision or as a definitive procedure in an individual unable to tolerate a major revision because of compromised medical status.
- Osteotomies have been shown to be successful at slowing down the development or the progression of osteoarthritis in a young patient with underlying anatomic abnormality.

INTRODUCTION

Unilateral osteoarthritis of the hip in the young patient is a difficult problem. Total hip arthroplasty has been shown to be a very successful procedure in the older patient and has established high levels of expectations. However, even with the current advancements in prosthetic design, bearing surfaces, and fixation techniques, joint replacement has not provided durable results in the young population. As a result, alternative surgical treatments need to be explored for young, active patients. The surgical options currently available for these patients with osteoarthritis include resection arthroplasty, arthrodesis, and osteotomy.

At this time, resection arthroplasty is generally not recommended as a reasonable form of primary surgical treatment for a young patient with osteoarthritis. It is men-

tioned here for historical interest only. Resection arthroplasty, also known as Girdlestone's arthroplasty, was first described in 1817 by Schmalz for the treatment of tuberculosis of the hips in children. In 1943, Girdlestone described this operation for the treatment of septic arthritis involving gunshot wounds secondarily infected with tubercle bacilli.[1,2] His operation included removal of the femoral head and greater trochanter along with a wide excision of the abductors[2] (Fig. 1). Currently, this procedure is generally reserved for the treatment of an infected total joint arthroplasty. The procedure has been modified such that the abductors and the greater trochanter are preserved. It is performed either as the first part of a two-stage revision that includes removal of the infected prosthesis and cement along with a thorough débridement of the bone and joint or as a definitive procedure in the multiply-operated hip joint with severe infection. The latter is generally performed in an elderly, low-demand patient who either has an infection with a resistant organism for whom revision surgery is not recommended or in a patient whose medical condition precludes a second operation. Studies showed that Girdlestone's arthroplasty has a 90% success rate in eradicating infection but generally leads to poor functional results. The patient is left with a leg length discrepancy greater than 2 inches along with a Trendelenburg gait and a need for ambulatory aids. Ambulation is often limited by the increased oxygen consumption, which has been measured as 264% of normal.[3]

Arthrodesis is also an available option for the treatment of unilateral osteoarthritis of the hip in the young active patient. This procedure is most commonly performed for post-traumatic or postinfectious arthritis or for the salvage of a failed total hip arthroplasty in a young patient. The usual techniques include extra-articular or intra-articular fusion or a combination of these two. With the current fixation techniques, fusion rates of greater than 90% can be achieved.[4–7] A popular technique is the AO technique, which uses a laterally placed cobra plate along with an anterior compression plate, supplemented with bone grafting[6] (Fig. 2). The optimal position for fusion has generally been accepted as 30 degrees of flexion, 0 to 5 degrees of adduction, and 10 to 15 degrees of external rotation.[8] Some surgeons also choose to use a hip spica cast to protect their fixation.

Once a successful fusion is attained, the patient can function at a very high level, including working at strenuous occupations involving manual labor. However, with a fused hip, added stress is placed on the other joints in the body, most commonly the lumbosacral spine, the contralateral hip, and the ipsilateral knee. Up to 60% of patients may experience low back pain, 45% to 57% may experience ipsilateral knee pain and 17% to 28% may experience contralateral hip pain.[9, 10] The nonunion rate is highest in

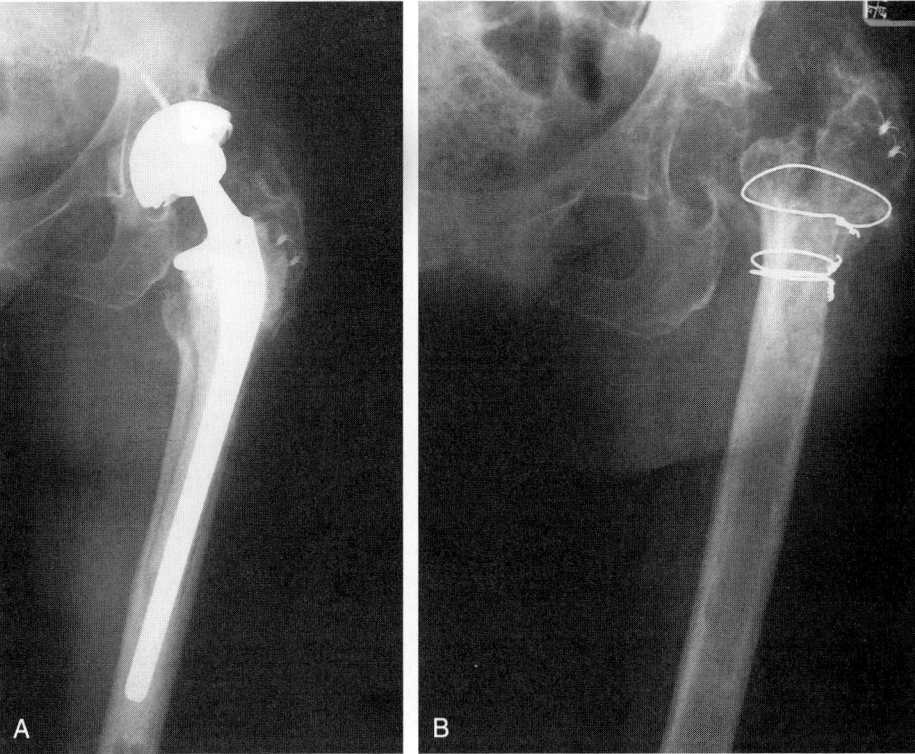

Fig. 1. Treatment of an infected total joint arthroplasty by Girdlestone's resection arthroplasty.

the avascular necrosis group.[5] If the secondary joint complaints become intolerable with age, the patient may choose to undergo a takedown of the arthrodesis with conversion to a total hip arthroplasty. Fusion takedown surgeries are technically more demanding and fraught with higher complication rates compared with routine primary total hip arthroplasty. These risks include a higher rate of infection, loosening, nerve palsy, heterotopic ossification, and weakness of abductors, which may even predispose to dislocation.[11, 12]

Whereas arthrodesis and Girdlestone's arthroplasty are procedures for treatment of advanced osteoarthritis of the hip, osteotomies are procedures directed at the treatment of a preosteoarthritic hip or a hip with very early osteoarthritis. Osteotomies are considered joint-preserving procedures with the underlying goal of halting the progression of preosteoarthritis or of early osteoarthritis to severe end-stage osteoarthritis. This is achieved by redirecting the functional articular cartilage on either the femoral or acetabular side or a combination of both sides of the hip joint.

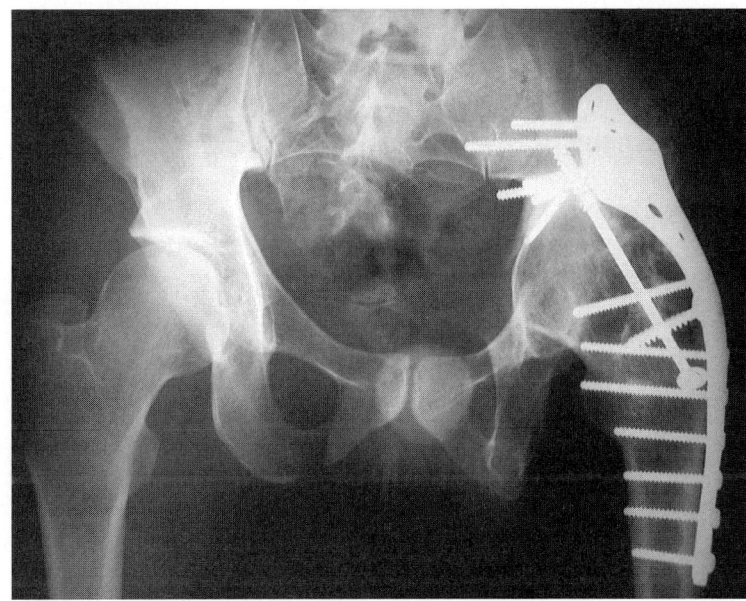

Fig. 2. Laterally placed cobra plate.

PATHOGENESIS

For a joint to function properly, a balance must exist between the stresses acting on the joint and the ability of the joint to withstand those stresses. However, if a preexisting anatomic deformity is present in the hip joint, a disproportionate increase in stress may develop and subsequently lead to osteoarthritis. This has been described as secondary osteoarthritis, whereas primary osteoarthritis or idiopathic osteoarthritis is considered to be a biological failure of articular cartilage in the absence of mechanical derangement or deformity and is very rare or nonexistent.[13, 14] In fact, reviews of large series of patients with osteoarthritis showed that more than 90% of patients had significant abnormalities in the hip joint, which predisposed them to osteoarthritis.[13] The underlying abnormalities included hip dysplasia, Legg-Calvé-Perthes disease, slipped capital femoral epiphysis, and various epiphyseal dysplasias. In the presence of anatomic abnormalities in a hip joint, the compressive stress of the hip joint (measured in kilograms per squared centimeter) is increased. This compressive stress is a function of the total force acting on the hip joint, the weightbearing surface area of the joint, and the point at which the total force (R) passes through the weightbearing surface and the distribution of forces on that surface.[15] Of all these factors, the area of the weightbearing surface is believed to be critical, and this is determined by the relative positions of the femoral head and acetabulum. Because the stress or the pressure on the hip is reflected by the total force divided by the area of the weightbearing surface, a uniform force applied over a smaller area will lead to higher stress or pressure. If the pressure exceeds the tolerance limit of the cartilage, degenerative changes will ensue with time (Fig. 3).[15]

Therefore, it is the goal of the treating surgeon to correct the underlying anatomic abnormality by performing corrective osteotomies, which will redirect the femoral or acetabular articular surfaces. This, in turn, will alter the magnitude of the combined force acting on the hip and the total area of the weightbearing surface over which this force is applied. The goal is to decrease the resultant stress or pressure across the hip joint and prevent the development or progression of osteoarthritis.[16] These osteotomy procedures are considered reconstructive if the joint surfaces are congruous and no signs of secondary osteoarthritis are present. However, even after early osteoarthritis develops, a salvage-type osteotomy can be performed with the same surgical goals as just mentioned to improve function and delay the need for total hip arthroplasty.[14]

CLINICAL FEATURES

Careful evaluation is required in the treatment of a young patient with hip disease. It is essential to first establish the underlying mechanical abnormality on radiographs and verify that the individual either has a hip at risk or has early osteoarthritis because of increased stress across the joint. Next, the patient's age, body habitus, and activity level are assessed, along with the functional limitations resulting from the hip disease. These limitations are generally due to symptoms of pain, limp, and extremity weakness. The pain may result from early arthritic changes in the joint or be secondary to fatigue of the abductor muscles and at the same time also manifest as a limp.[14]

A thorough physical examination is also undertaken to assess the specific cause of pain, type of gait, range of motion, and strength, particularly of the abductor muscles. Weakness of the hip abductors is generally exhibited as a

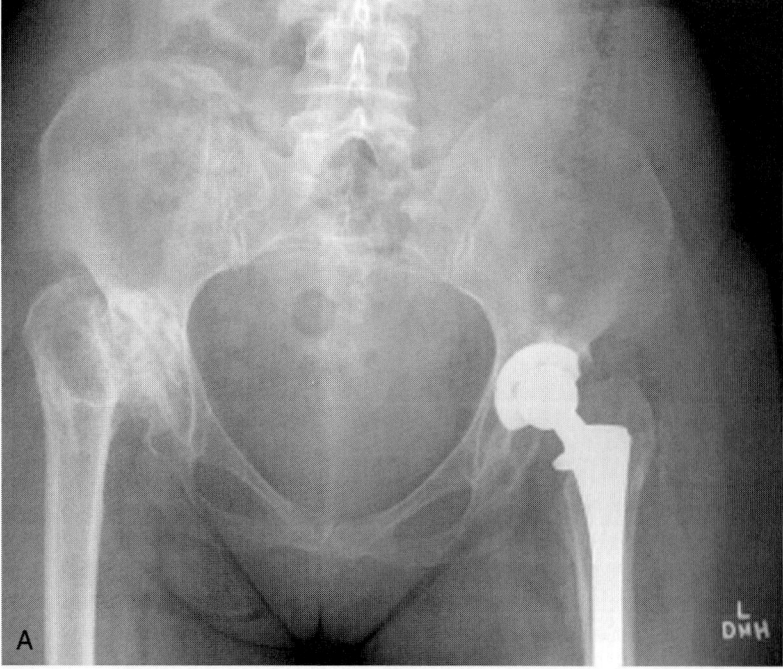
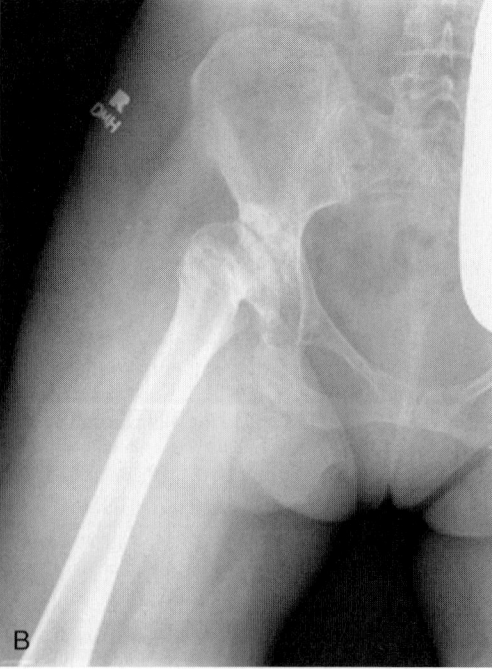

Fig. 3. Views. *A*, AP radiograph of developmental hip dysplasia with severe arthrosis of both hips. The left hip has undergone total hip arthroplasty. *B*, Lateral view of arthritic left hip.

positive Trendelenburg sign or gait, but in some cases it may not be immediately evident. In such cases, the weakness may be elicited by allowing an individual to perform a weightbearing exercise such as walking or running. With time, the muscles around a hip with underlying disease will fatigue, a limp may become more obvious, and pain may develop in the peritrochanteric region. This is analogous to the stress test a cardiologist administers to establish the underlying cardiac disease.

Furthermore, the range of motion may also be limited, especially if early osteoarthritis is present, and may often lead to flexion and adduction contractures. Osteotomy may improve the functional arc of motion and help resolve the contractures, but it will not increase the overall motion.[14]

INVESTIGATION

To define the mechanical abnormality on radiographs, an anteroposterior (AP) view of the pelvis along with lateral and false profile views of the hip are necessary. The AP view allows evaluation of the lateral coverage of the femoral head by the acetabulum and can be measured as the center edge angle (CEA) of Wiberg, in which a CEA of greater than 20 degrees is considered normal.[17] The false profile view is an oblique view taken at 65 degrees with the patient standing. It allows evaluation of the anterior coverage of the head by the acetabulum and is measured as the CEA of acetabular ventral inclination (VCA). VCA of greater than 20 degrees is considered normal[18] (Fig. 4). Once the lack of acetabular coverage of the femoral head is defined, signs of increased stress in the hip can be evaluated. The shape of the acetabular "sourcil" (eyebrow),

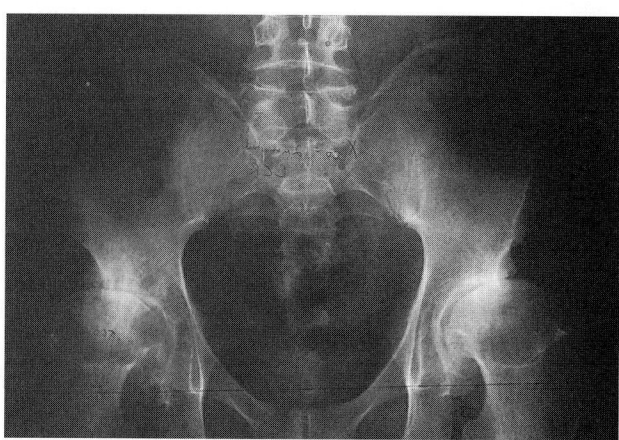

Fig. 5. Degenerative changes in a hip with elevated stress. (From Canale ST [ed]: Campbell's Operative Orthopaedics, 9th ed, vol 1, St. Louis, Mosby, 1998, p 1040.)

which is an area of subchondral bony condensation in the acetabular roof, represents the magnitude of the stress across the hip joint. In a hip with normal stress, the sourcil appears narrow and wide, but in an uncovered hip with increased stress, the sourcil becomes more triangular and lateralized.[15] With time, a hip with elevated stress will begin to demonstrate degenerative changes such as narrowing of the cartilage height, cystic changes, and eventually osteophytes (Fig. 5).

More recently, computed tomography (CT) evaluation of acetabular coverage was performed and showed some early use in both preoperative planning of surgeries and computer-assisted osteotomies. Once these techniques are optimized in the future, more widespread use can then be envisioned.[14, 19, 20]

GOALS, INDICATIONS, AND CONTRAINDICATIONS

The goals of osteotomy are to decrease the joint stress, improve the functional range of motion, and relieve pain. An osteotomy can be performed either through the pelvis or through the proximal femur, depending on where the primary deformity lies. In the majority of dysplasia cases, the primary deformity is in the acetabulum with a deficiency in the anterolateral coverage of the femoral head. These are best treated with a pelvic osteotomy. In the absence of osteoarthritis, reconstructive osteotomies, of which there are two groups, can be performed. These osteotomies redirect the acetabulum and increase the coverage of the femoral head with functional hyaline cartilage. The first group of osteotomies includes the single innominate osteotomy (Salter),[21, 22] which is typically performed in young children, and its most common variation, the triple innominate osteotomy (Steel),[23] which is performed in adolescents and young adults. The second group includes the spherical (Dial, Wagner)[14] and the Bernese (Ganz)[24] periacetabular osteotomies. In the presence of osteoarthritis, salvage osteotomies such as the Chiari[25] or the shelf, in which the redirected part of the pelvis increases the coverage of the femoral head with fibrocartilage instead of hyaline cartilage, can be performed.

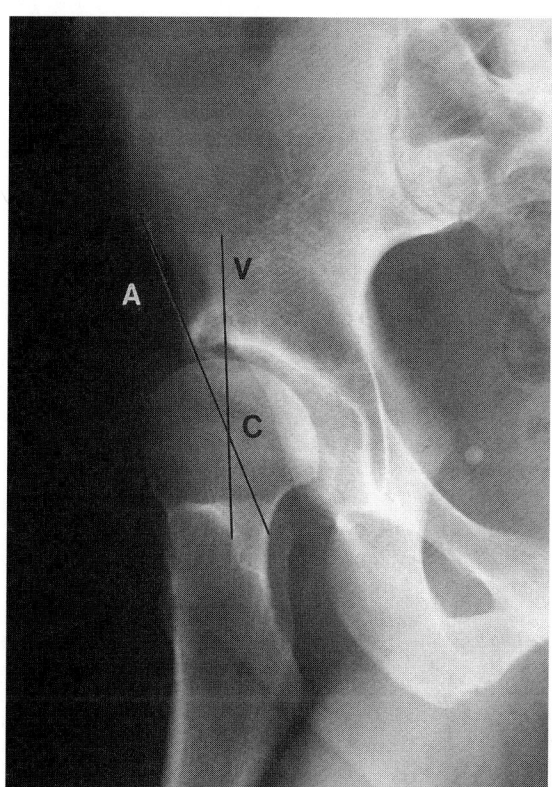

Fig. 4. Angle of acetabular ventral inclination (VCA).

In cases of hip disease secondary to osteonecrosis, slipped capital femoral epiphysis (SCFE), and dysplasia in which pelvic osteotomy has been performed but residual deformity remains in the proximal femur, treatment involves a proximal femoral osteotomy. A varus intertrochanteric osteotomy is performed for correction of residual coxa valga after a dysplastic hip has been previously treated with a pelvic osteotomy. In a dysplastic hip with evidence of advanced osteoarthritis in the form of a subcapital osteophyte and narrowing in the lateral cartilage height, a valgus extension intertrochanteric osteotomy can be performed. The severe extension deformity and the accompanying retroversion and varus seen in SCFE can be treated with a flexion derotation intertrochanteric osteotomy.

PROCEDURES

PREOPERATIVE PLANNING

Once the primary deformity has been identified and the location of the corrective osteotomy established, thorough preoperative planning is essential before proceeding with surgery. This planning begins with a review of the radiographs. The CEA and VCA are measured from the AP pelvis and false profile radiographs to establish the magnitude of deformity. Additional radiographs may be obtained with the hip in abduction and adduction to simulate the femoral head coverage obtained by performing a varus or valgus osteotomy, respectively, and may also be combined with flexion and extension to determine their effects on

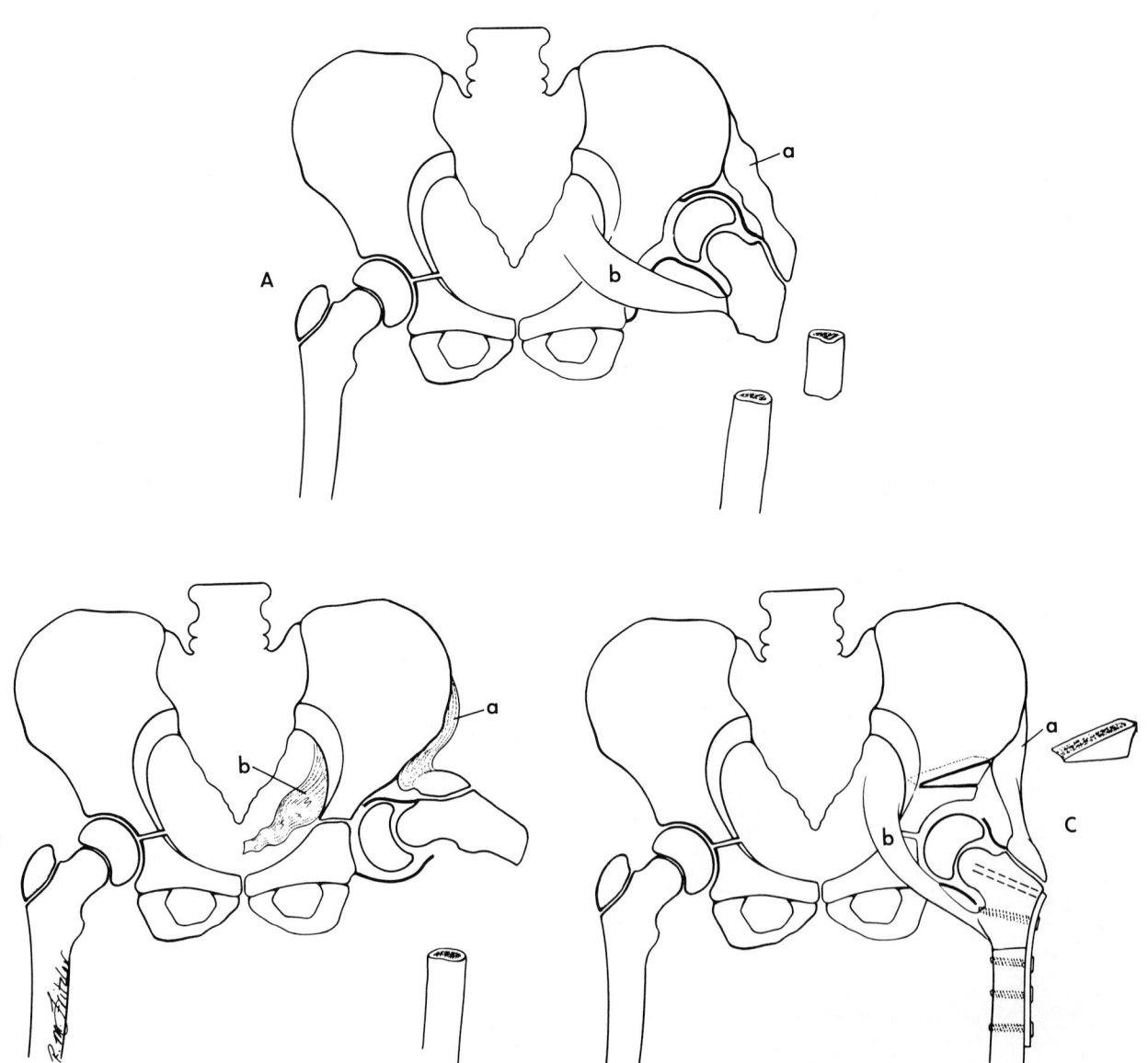

Fig. 6. Technique for open reduction, primary femoral shortening, and Salter osteotomy. *A,* The femoral head is dislocated. Gluteal muscles (a) are retracted and slightly shortened. The iliopsoas muscle (b) is intact. The capsule is interposed between the femoral head and the ilium. A segment of femur is resected. *B,* The proximal femur is abducted and the iliopsoas tendon (b) divided. The capsule is incised on the inferior surface parallel to the femoral neck. *C,* Operation is complete. Gluteal muscles (a) are tight. The iliopsoas muscle (b) is reattached. Salter osteotomy is complete with the graft in place. Femoral fragments are fixed with Campbell hip screw. (From Canale ST [ed]: Campbell's Operative Orthopaedics. St. Louis, CV Mosby, 1998, vol 1, 9th ed, p 1040.)

femoral head coverage. Fluoroscopy has also been used and may improve the accuracy over preoperative simulation radiographs, especially when biplanar corrections or corrections in which rotation is combined with angulation are required. Fluoroscopy is most useful when performed personally by the operating surgeon.[14] With all the information obtained from the radiographs, paper tracings and templates can be made to determine more precisely the magnitude and direction of correction. Furthermore, CT scans with three-dimensional reconstruction may also be used to simulate the effects of the osteotomy. They have enormous potential for use in the future with the anticipated improvements in preoperative planning software.

TECHNICAL DETAILS
Pelvic Osteotomies
Innominate Osteotomy

This osteotomy was first described by Salter and is typically used in young children and rarely in adolescents and young adults. The iliofemoral approach to the hip is used, and an opening wedge complete supra-acetabular osteotomy of the iliac bone just above the acetabulum is per-

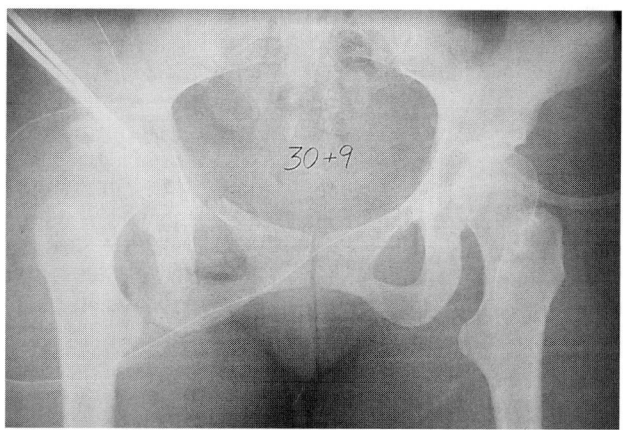

Fig. 8. Radiograph view of triple innominate osteotomy. (From Canale ST [ed]: Campbell's Operative Orthopaedics, 9th ed, vol 1, St. Louis, Mosby, 1998, p 826; originally from Ganz R, Klave K, Uinh TS, et al: A new periacetabular osteotomy for the treatment of hip dysplasias. Clin Orthop 1988; 232:26.)

formed. Anterior, outward, and downward displacement of the distal segment is then carried out, and the rotation of the acetabulum hinges across the symphysis pubis. The new position is maintained by a triangular-shaped bone graft taken from the proximal portion of the ilium and secured with internal fixation, which is either a threaded pin or cortical screw.[21, 22] Typically, the adductor and the iliopsoas tendons are released and the capsule is left intact. Because only limited correction is obtained in the adolescent and adult as a result of the stiffness of the pubic symphysis, this osteotomy is only an option for cases with mild dysplasia and a CEA greater than 15 degrees[14] (Fig. 6).

Triple Innominate Osteotomy

This procedure, first described by Steele, combines a standard innominate osteotomy with a high ischial osteotomy and a pubic osteotomy close to the acetabulum.[23] A posterior approach is used to perform the ischial cut, and then an iliofemoral approach is used to perform the innominate osteotomy. The pubic cut is made through the same approach. The osteotomy cuts are typically stabilized with cortical screws. This procedure is used more frequently in the adolescent and young adult because a larger correction can be obtained than that typically seen with the standard innominate osteotomy alone. However, because the ischial cut is typically some distance from the joint, any significant correction may create a noticeable deformity at the ischial osteotomy site and predispose this site to nonunion (Figs. 7 and 8).

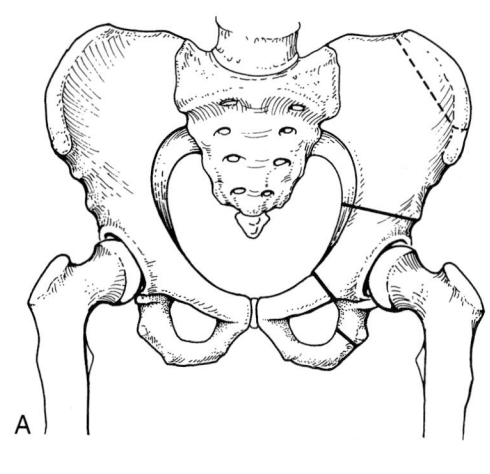

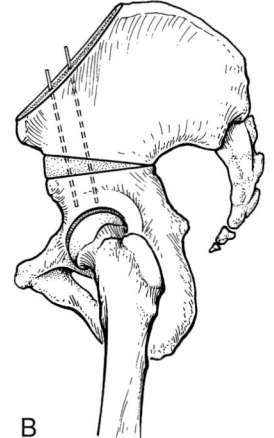

Fig. 7. Steel triple innominate osteotomy. *A,* Osteotomies to be performed in the iliac wing and superior and inferior pubic rami. Note the wedge of bone to be taken as a graft from the most superior portion of the ilium. *B,* Lateral view shows the graft in place and fixation with two Kirschner wires. (From Canale ST [ed]: Campbell's Operative Orthopaedics. St. Louis, CV Mosby, 1998, vol 1, 9th ed, p 1040.)

Periacetabular Osteotomy

Spherical Osteotomies (Dial, Wagner). An anterior Smith-Petersen approach is used, and the osteotomy requires the use of special curved gouges to perform a circumferential cut 15 mm from the articular surface of the acetabulum. The capsule is preserved to maintain the blood supply to the acetabulum. The acetabulum is then rotated over the femoral head, and significant correction can be obtained. The technique is demanding and at times difficult to reproduce and, therefore, not used as frequently.

Bernese's or Ganz's Osteotomy. First described by Ganz in 1983, this procedure addresses many of the problems encountered in the various other pelvic osteotomies. The technique uses an anterior Smith-Petersen approach and is a triplanar osteotomy of four cuts performed sequentially.[24] A special osteotome with a 15-mm blade bent at a 30-degree angle to the shaft is required. An intraoperative image intensifier is very helpful, with the patient positioned on a radiolucent table such that both an anterior view and a false profile view can be obtained intraoperatively to confirm the position of the cuts and the magnitude of correction.

1. The ischium is scored to a depth of 5 to 10 mm and basically serves as a barrier for the final cut to keep it from exiting into the ischial tuberosity.
2. The pubic ramus is then divided from the acetabulum, and a Gigli saw can simplify this cut after the obturator nerve and soft tissues are protected.
3. The supra-acetabular osteotomy is then performed with both an inside limb and an outside limb. The inside limb is above the anteroinferior iliac spine and is performed with an oscillating saw. The posterior cut forms a 120-degree angle with the anterior limb and is performed with an osteotome. Only the first 15 mm is osteotomized; the rest breaks spontaneously. A Schanz screw is placed into the supra-acetabular bone to lever it for the correction.
4. The fourth osteotomy is performed with an osteotome going 4 cm below the pelvic rim at a 50-degree angle relative to the quadrilateral surface. The acetabulum is then rotated around the center of the femoral head and the osteotomy is stabilized with two cortical screws[24] (Figs. 9 and 10).

This technique offers several advantages over others. A single approach is generally used, and large corrections in all directions can be obtained. The blood supply to the acetabulum is preserved, and the posterior column of the pelvis is left intact, which, in turn, requires minimal internal fixation for stability. The shape of the pelvis is minimally altered and allows for normal childbirth in females.[24]

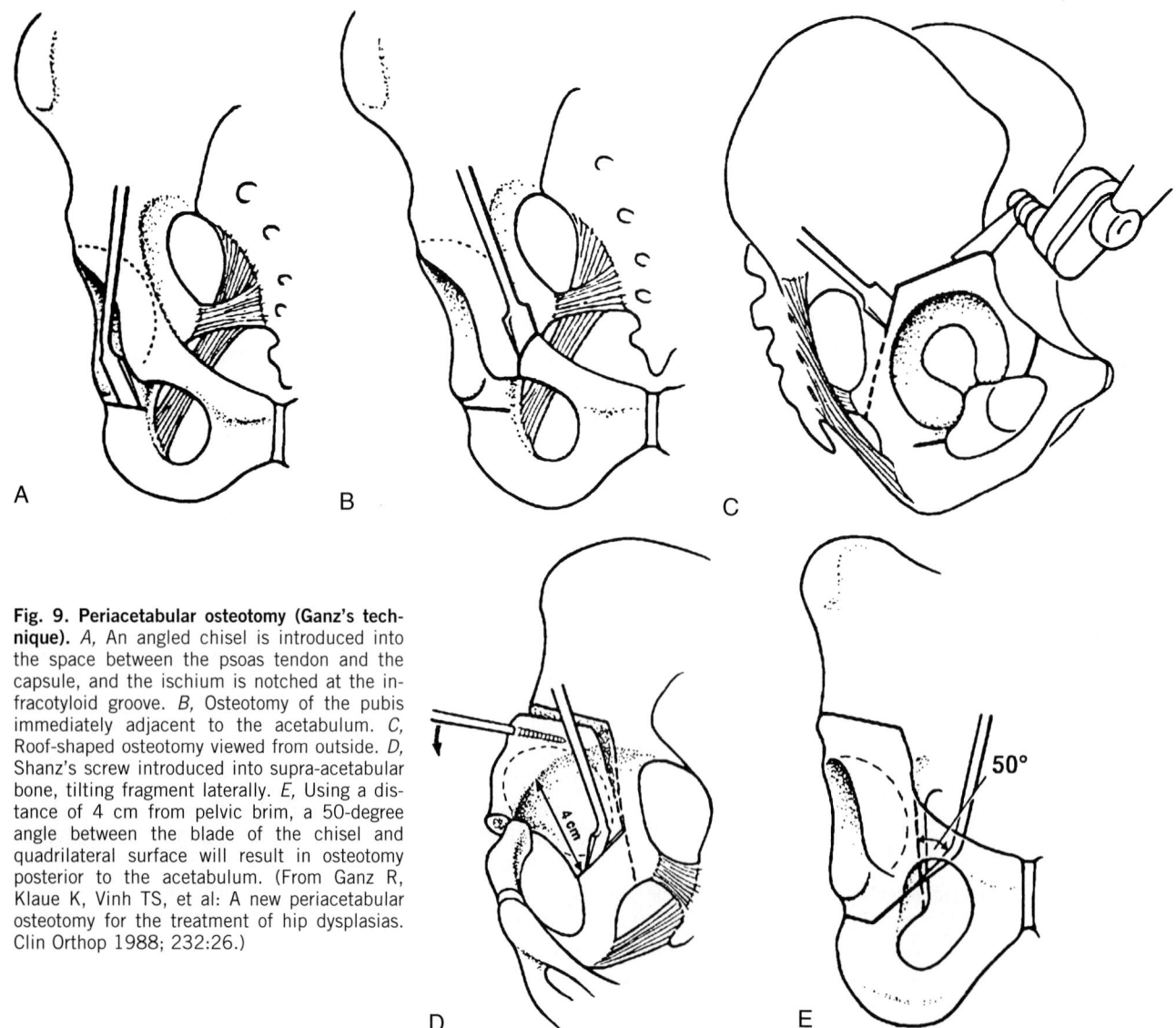

Fig. 9. Periacetabular osteotomy (Ganz's technique). *A,* An angled chisel is introduced into the space between the psoas tendon and the capsule, and the ischium is notched at the infracotyloid groove. *B,* Osteotomy of the pubis immediately adjacent to the acetabulum. *C,* Roof-shaped osteotomy viewed from outside. *D,* Shanz's screw introduced into supra-acetabular bone, tilting fragment laterally. *E,* Using a distance of 4 cm from pelvic brim, a 50-degree angle between the blade of the chisel and quadrilateral surface will result in osteotomy posterior to the acetabulum. (From Ganz R, Klaue K, Vinh TS, et al: A new periacetabular osteotomy for the treatment of hip dysplasias. Clin Orthop 1988; 232:26.)

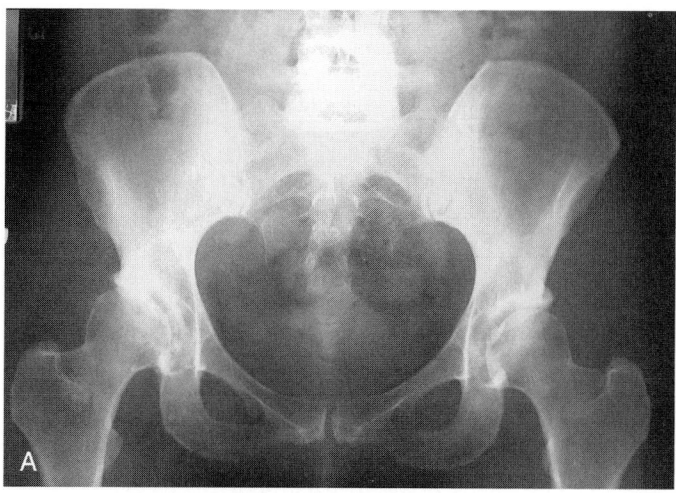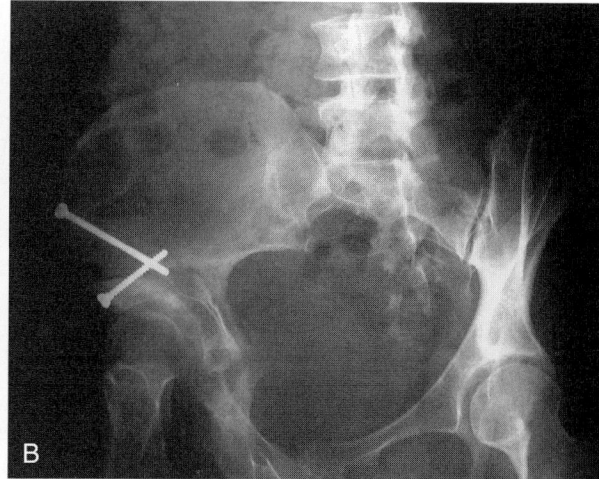

Fig. 10. Periacetabular osteotomy. The acetabulum is rotated around the center of the femoral head, and the osteotomy is stabilized with two cortical screws. (From Canale ST [ed]: Campbell's Operative Orthopaedics, 9th ed, vol 1, St. Louis, Mosby, 1998, p 1052.)

Salvage Osteotomy
Chiari's Osteotomy

This technique was first described by Chiari in 1953 and is now indicated in very dysplastic hips with moderate osteoarthritis.[14] An anterior approach to the hip is used with the patient in the supine position. The osteotomy is made at

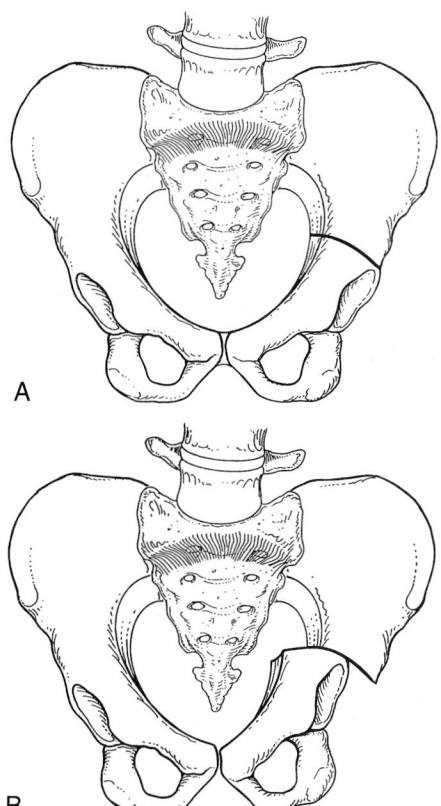

Fig. 11. Chiari's medial displacement osteotomy. *A,* A line of osteotomy extending from immediately superior to lip of acetabulum into sciatic notch. Osteotomy may be curved to facilitate femoral head coverage. *B,* A completed osteotomy with medial displacement of the distal fragment for interpositional capsular arthroplasty. (From Canale ST [ed]: Campbell's Operative Orthopaedics. St. Louis, CV Mosby, 1998, vol 1, 9th ed, p 1040.)

the superior margin of the joint capsule and is directed at a 10-degree angle toward the inner table of the ilium. The distal pelvic fragment is then displaced medially, thereby placing the femoral head beneath the cancellous bone of the ilium with the capsule of the hip joint interposed in between. The osteotomy is then stabilized with internal fixation screws. It is theorized that the interposed capsule subsequently undergoes metaplasia with eventual formation of fibrocartilage in response to weightbearing across the joint[14, 25, 26] (Figs. 11 and 12).

Femoral Osteotomy
Varus Intertrochanteric Osteotomy

This procedure is performed through a lateral approach on a fracture table. A lateral opening wedge osteotomy is the technique of choice because it avoids any shortening of the limb. A 90-degree AO angled blade plate is used to obtain rigid internal fixation. An intraoperative image intensifier is essential during the procedure. It helps in accurate placement of the blade and allows for control over the magnitude of correction. Typically, the femoral shaft must be displaced medially by approximately 10 to 15 mm to keep the knee centered under the femoral head[14, 27, 28] (Fig. 13).

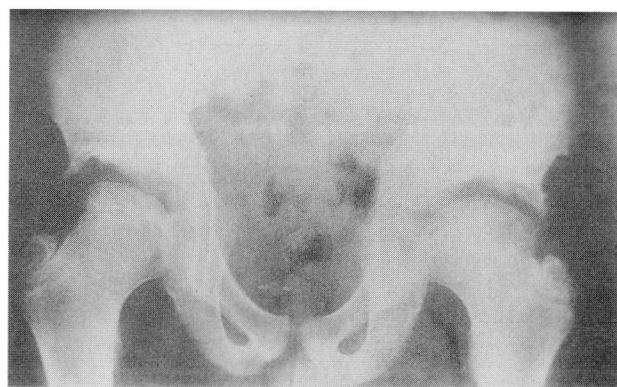

Fig. 12. Radiographic view of Chiari's osteotomy. (From Morrey BF [ed]: Reconstructive Surgery of the Joints, 2nd ed, vol 2, New York, Churchill Livingstone. Copyright Mayo Foundation 1996, p 1095–1096.)

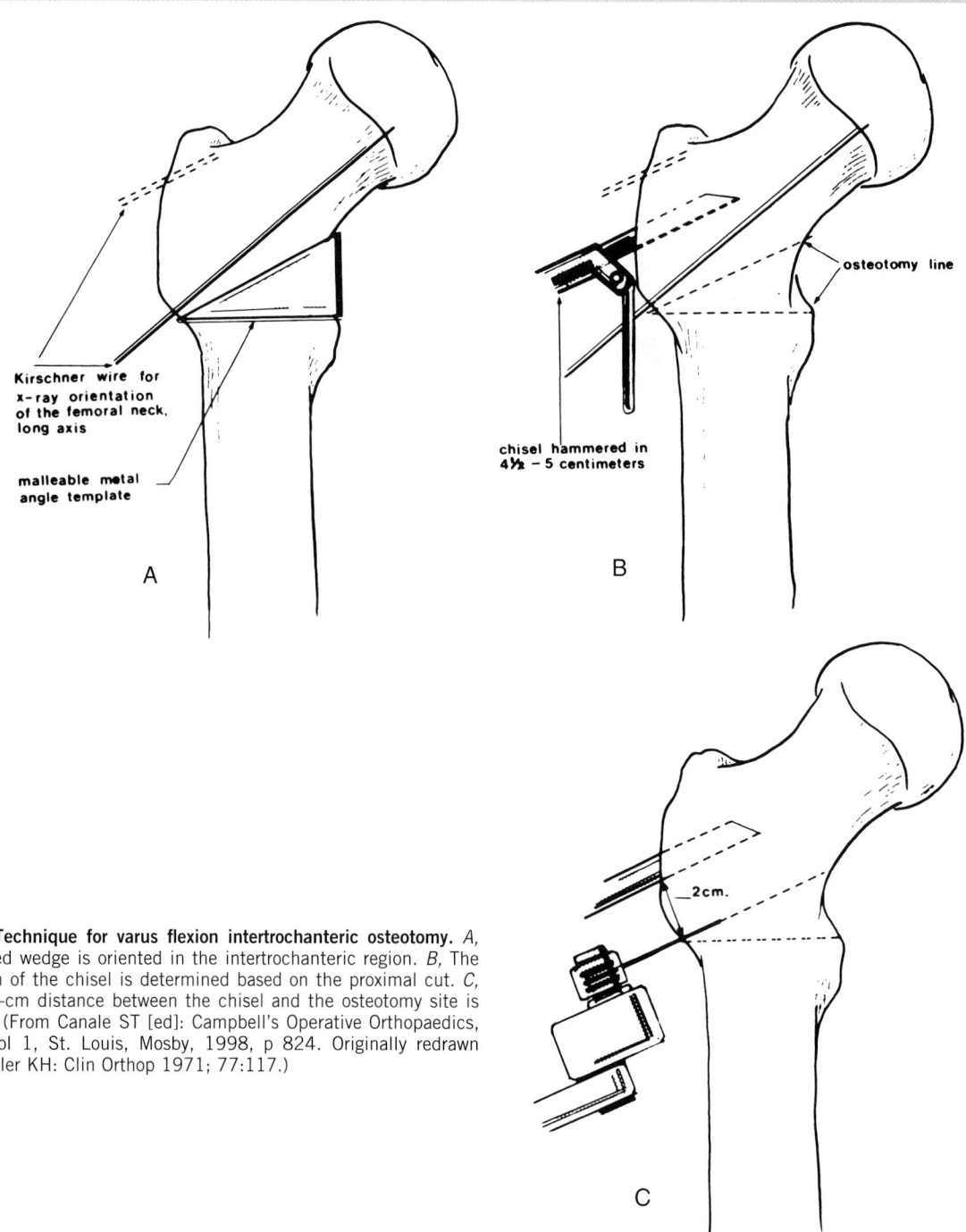

Fig. 13. Technique for varus flexion intertrochanteric osteotomy. *A,* The desired wedge is oriented in the intertrochanteric region. *B,* The orientation of the chisel is determined based on the proximal cut. *C,* At least 2-cm distance between the chisel and the osteotomy site is desirable. (From Canale ST [ed]: Campbell's Operative Orthopaedics, 9th ed, vol 1, St. Louis, Mosby, 1998, p 824. Originally redrawn from Mueller KH: Clin Orthop 1971; 77:117.)

Valgus Extension Osteotomy

A prerequisite for this procedure is a preoperative radiograph or fluoroscopic examination with the hip in adduction confirming the presence of signs of osteoarthritis along with the capital drop osteophyte articulating with acetabular floor osteophytes and opening up of the lateral joint space. The procedure is performed with the patient in the supine position using a lateral approach on a fracture table. The valgus angle of the osteotomy is determined by the angle formed by the axis of femoral shaft in the neutral position and in the adducted position, which ensured contact between the capital drop osteophyte and the acetabular floor osteophytes. The magnitude of extension is calculated by determining the flexion required to position the capital drop osteophyte in contact with the posterior part of the acetabulum on a lateral radiograph. An AO blade plate is used to obtain rigid internal fixation. The iliopsoas tendon is also released, and the shaft of the femur is lateralized to restore the mechanical axis[14, 28, 29] (Fig. 14).

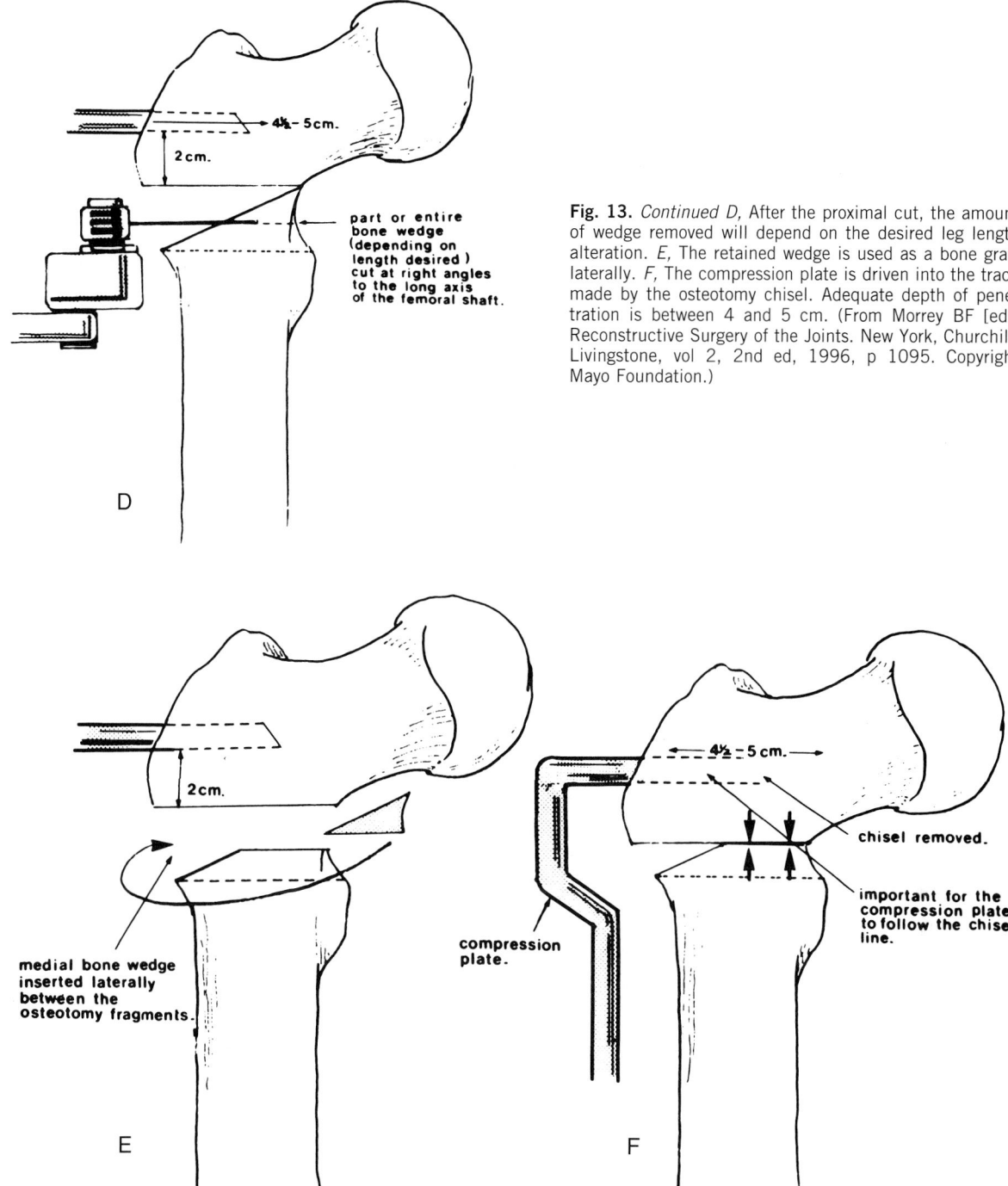

Fig. 13. *Continued D,* After the proximal cut, the amount of wedge removed will depend on the desired leg length alteration. *E,* The retained wedge is used as a bone graft laterally. *F,* The compression plate is driven into the track made by the osteotomy chisel. Adequate depth of penetration is between 4 and 5 cm. (From Morrey BF [ed]: Reconstructive Surgery of the Joints. New York, Churchill-Livingstone, vol 2, 2nd ed, 1996, p 1095. Copyright Mayo Foundation.)

POSTOPERATIVE MANAGEMENT

After pelvic osteotomies, indomethacin (Indocin) is generally recommended to decrease the risk of ectopic bone formation. Some form of thromboembolism prophylaxis must also be used postoperatively. The patient is gradually mobilized with crutches and remains partially weightbearing (20 pounds). Active movements, which could jeopardize the reinserted muscles, are avoided for a minimum of 6 weeks. Once bony healing is verified on radiographs, usually by 8 to 12 weeks, weightbearing is advanced. The use of a cane is recommended until the hip abductors are strong enough to maintain hip stability as evidenced by the disappearance of the Trendelenburg sign.[24] After a Chiari osteotomy, partial weightbearing is recommended for at least 3 months to allow adequate time for the interposed capsule to remodel.[14]

After a femoral osteotomy alone, the risk of heterotopic bone formation is not significant enough to require prophylaxis, but thromboembolism prophylaxis is recommended.

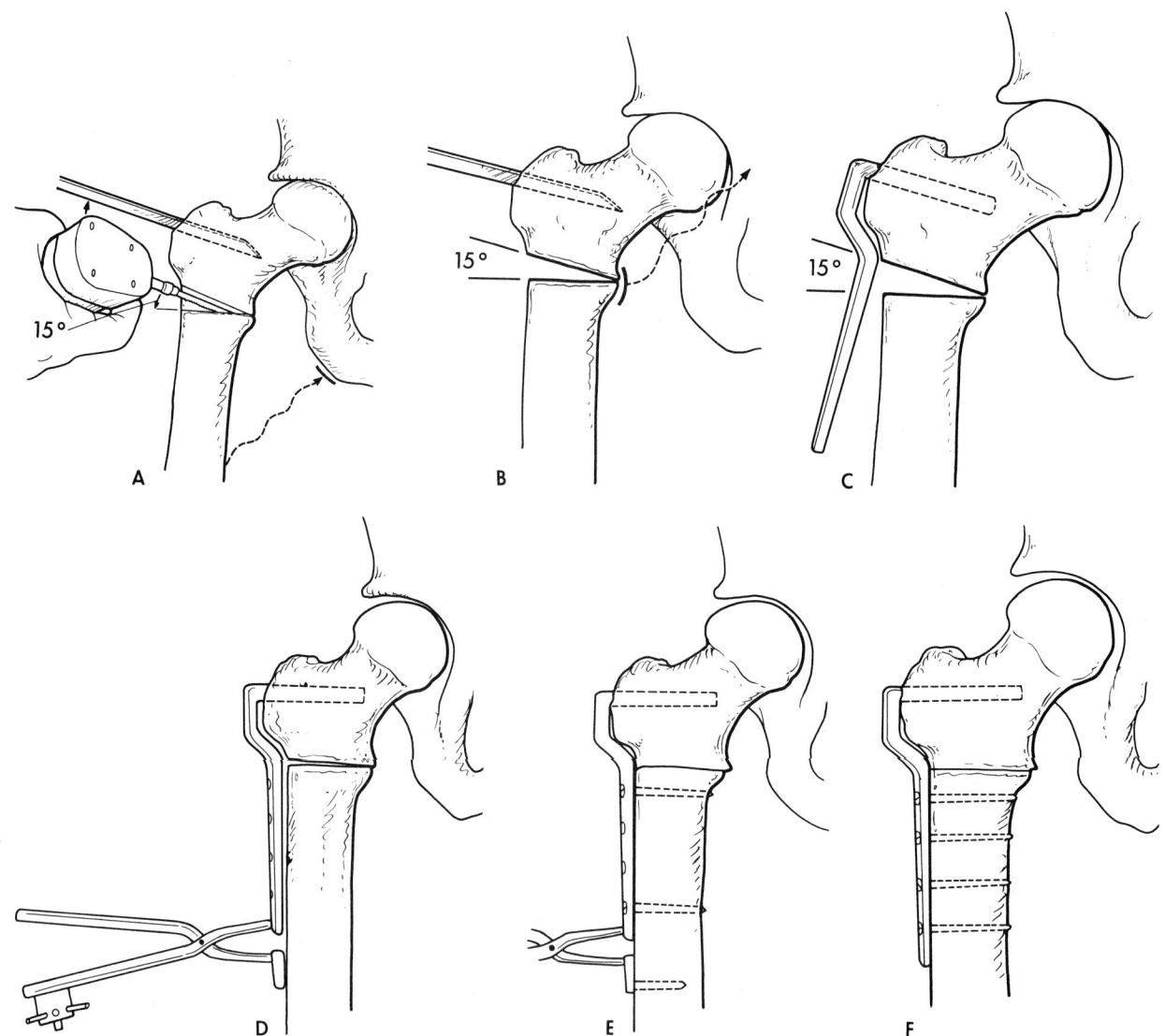

Fig. 14. Technique of valgus osteotomy with right-angled compression plate. *A,* A lateral wedge is cut to achieve 15-degree valgus correction. *B,* A wedge of bone removed. *C,* A right-angled compression plate is inserted into a prepared slot in the trochanteric area. *D,* Closure of the wedge and application of compression. *E* and *F,* Screws are inserted for fixation of compression plate. (From Mueller KH: Osteotomies of the hip. Clin Orthop 1971; 77:117.)

Crutch walking is begun postoperatively with protected weightbearing for 8 to 10 weeks. Once adequate bone healing is evident radiographically, weightbearing is advanced and a cane is subsequently used. There are typically no restrictions against active movements unless some muscle reattachment or trochanteric advancement has been carried out.

COMPLICATIONS

Complications are summarized in Table 1.

RESULTS

There are limited reports in the literature on the use of the single innominate osteotomy in the adult population. At a minimum follow-up of 2 years, Salter reported that 94% of patients experienced complete or significant relief of pain. An average 19-degree improvement in CEA was also reported.[21, 22]

There are several reports on the use of the triple innominate osteotomy in the adolescent and young adult population. According to Kleuver et al,[30] at a minimum follow-up of 8 years, 81% of patients had improvement in symptoms, and the average CEA improved by 19 degrees and the VCA by 26 degrees. Kleuver et al[31] also reported on a series of 11 patients with a minimum follow-up of 10 years. Significant improvements were noted in the hip score, range of motion, and limp, and the average CEA improved by 30 degrees. No clinical or radiographic deterioration was noted, even after 10 years, except in two individuals with underlying neuromuscular disease, and caution is advised in these patients.

Trousdale et al[18] reported on the results after the Bernese

		TABLE 1. OSTEOTOMY COMPLICATIONS	
Type of Osteotomy	**Complication**	**Type of Complication**	**Methods of Avoiding Complication**
Innominate	Infection 9%	Surgical débridement	Perioperative abx Meticulous surgical technique
Triple innominate	Nerve palsy <1% Nonunion of ischial cut	Transient and usually resolves Generally asymptomatic; if symptomatic, bone graft and ORIF	May need to expose nerve at risk Make cuts closer to acetabulum
	Heterotopic ossification 35% grade I	Asymptomatic in most cases; if symptomatic consider resection	Indocin
Periacetabular (Ganz)	Sciatic nerve palsy <1% Intra-articular osteotomy 1.5%	Transient and usually resolves Let heal; if symptomatic, will eventually need THA	May need to expose nerve at risk Intraoperative fluoroscopy
	Heterotopic ossification 33%	Most asymptomatic; excise if symptomatic	Indocin
	Pressure from screws over crest	Screw removal after osteotomy heals	Obtain good layer of soft tissue over screws
Chiari	Nonunion 6%	Bone graft and plating	Confirm good contact between osteotomy surfaces; use better internal fixation
Femoral osteotomy	Nerve palsy 3% Delayed union <1% Wound problems 4% Femoral neck fracture <1%	Transient and usually resolves Bone graft Débridement Additional fixation; screws across fracture site	May need to expose nerve at risk Rigid internal fixation Meticulous surgical technique Intraoperative fluoroscopy during osteotomy and blade plate insertion

ORIF = open reduction and internal fixation; THA = total hip arthroplasty; abx = antibiotics.

periacetabular osteotomy in 42 patients with a minimum follow-up of 2 years and an average follow-up of 4 years. The average Harris Hip Score improved by 62 points, and 96% of the patients had good or excellent results. The average VCA improved by 26 degrees and the average CEA by 28 degrees.[37]

Even after salvage procedures such as the Chiari osteotomy, fairly good results are obtained. Several large series with a follow-up of more than 10 years reported good or excellent results in greater than 90% of patients. The results are better if the osteotomy is performed before age 40 and in individuals with a lesser degree of arthrosis. Ninety percent of patients will not need a total hip arthroplasty for at least 10 to 15 years if the flexion/extension arc is at least 90 degrees at surgery.[14, 26]

In reviewing osteotomies of the proximal femur, Morscher[27] reported 90% good to excellent results in a series of 1819

patients who underwent varus intertrochanteric osteotomy. Some degree of leg shortening was encountered but was minimized by the use of an opening wedge instead of a closing wedge osteotomy.

Valgus extension osteotomy has also been shown to produce favorable results. Maistrelli et al[32] reported 67% good or excellent results with an 11- to 15-year follow-up. Better results were obtained in patients younger than 40 years with preoperative flexion greater than 60 degrees. Radiographic improvement was seen in 54% of hips at 5 years and in 39% at 11 to 15 years. Santore and Bombelli[33] reported that 75% of patients had satisfactory results at an average follow-up of 11 years. Gotoh et al[29] reported that if the capital drop osteophyte was greater than 3 mm in width and the roof osteophyte of the lateral edge of the acetabulum was greater than 5 mm in length, 75% of patients had good pain relief at 15 years.

REFERENCES

1. Berman AT, Mazur D: Conversion of resection arthroplasty to total hip replacement. Orthopedics 1994; 17:1155.
2. Girdlestone GR: Acute pyogenic arthritis of the hip. Lancet 1943; 1:419.
3. Kantor GS, Osterhamp JA, Dorr LD, et al: Resection arthroplasty following infected total hip replacement arthroplasty. J Arthroplasty 1986; 1:83.
4. Barmada R, Abraham E, Ray RD: Hip fusion utilizing the cobra head plate. J Bone Joint Surg Am 1976; 58:541.
5. Brien WW, Golz RJ, Kuschner SH, et al: Hip joint arthrodesis utilizing anterior compression plate fixation. J Arthroplasty 1994; 9:171.
6. Kostuik J, Alexander D: Arthrodesis for failed hip arthroplasty. Clin Orthop 1984; 188:173.
7. Schneider R: Hip arthrodesis with the cobra head plate and pelvic osteotomy. Reconstr Surg Traumatol 1974; 14:1.
8. Lindahl O: Hip-joint arthrodesis: To find the best position. Acta Orthop Scand 1966; 34:317.
9. Callaghan JJ, Brand RA, Pedersen DR: Hip arthrodesis. J Bone and Joint Surg Am 1985; 67:1328.
10. Sponseller PD, McBeath AA, Perpich M: Hip arthrodesis in young patients. J Bone Joint Surg Am 1984; 66:853.
11. Amstutz HC, Sakai DN: Total joint replacement for ankylosed hips. J Bone Joint Surg Am 1975; 57:619.
12. Kilgus DJ, Amstutz HA, Wolgin MA, et al: Joint replacement for ankylosed hips. J Bone Joint Surg Am 1990; 72:45.
13. Harris WH: Etiology of osteoarthritis of the hip. Clin Orthop 1986; 213:20.
14. Millis MB, Murphy SB, Poss R: Osteotomies about the hip for the prevention and treatment of osteoarthritis. Am Acad Or-

thop Surg Instruct Course Lect 1996; 46: 209.

15. Legal H: Introduction to the biomechanics of the hip. In Toennis D, Legal H, eds: Congenital Dysplasia and Dislocation of the Hip in Children and Adults. New York, Springer-Verlag, 1987, p 26.

16. Hsin J, Saluja R, Eilert RE, et al: Evaluation of the biomechanics of the hip following a triple innominate osteotomy of the innominate bone. J Bone Joint Surg Am 1996; 78:855.

17. Wiberg G: Studies on dysplastic acetabula and congenital subluxation of the hip joint with special reference to the complication of osteoarthritis. Acta Chir Scand Suppl 1939; 83:58.

18. Trousdale RT, Ekkernkamp A, Ganz R, et al: Periacetabular and intertrochanteric osteotomy for the treatment of osteoarthritis in dysplastic hips. J Bone Joint Surg Am 1995; 77:73.

19. Klaue K, Wallin A, Ganz R: CT evaluation of coverage and congruency of the hip prior to osteotomy. Clin Orthop 1988; 232:15.

20. Langlotz F, Bachler R, Berlemann U, et al: Computer assistance for pelvic osteotomies. Clin Orthop 1998; 354:92.

21. Salter RB: Innominate osteotomy in the treatment of congenital dislocation and subluxation of the hip. J Bone Joint Surg Br 1961; 43:518.

22. Salter RB, Hansson G, Thompson GH: Innominate osteotomy in the management of residual congenital subluxation of the hip in young adults. Clin Orthop 1984; 182:53.

23. Steel HH: Triple osteotomy of the innominate bone. J Bone Joint Surg Am 1973; 55:343.

24. Ganz R, Klaue K, Vinh TS, et al: A new periacetabular osteotomy for the treatment of hip dysplasias. Clin Orthop 1988; 232:26.

25. Chiari K: Medial displacement osteotomy of the pelvis. Clin Orthop 1974; 98:55.

26. Migaud H, Duquennoy A, Gougeon C, et al: Outcome of Chiari pelvic osteotomy in adults. Acta Orthop Scand 1995; 66:127.

27. Morscher EW: Intertrochanteric osteotomy in osteoarthritis of the hip. In Riley LH Jr (ed): The Hip: Proceedings of the Eight Open Scientific Meeting of The Hip Soci-

ety. St. Louis, MO, CV Mosby, 1980, p 24.

28. Mueller KH: Osteotomies of the hip. Clin Orthop 1971; 77:117.

29. Gotoh E, Inao S, Okamoto T, et al: Valgus-extension osteotomy for advanced osteoarthritis in dysplastic hips. J Bone Joint Surg Br 1997; 79:609.

30. Kleuver M, Huiskes R, Kauer JMG, et al: Three-dimensional displacement of the hip joint after triple pelvic osteotomy. Acta Orthop Scand 1990; 69:585.

31. Kleuver M, Kooijman MAP, Pavlov PW, et al: Triple osteotomy of the pelvis for acetabular dysplasia. J Bone Joint Surg Br 1997; 79:225.

32. Maistrelli GL, Gerundini M, Fusco U, et al: Valgus-extension osteotomy for osteoarthritis of the hip. J Bone Joint Surg Br 1990; 72:653.

33. Santore RF, Bombelli R: Long-term follow-up of the Bombelli experience with osteotomy for osteoarthritis: Results at 11 years: The hip. In Proceedings of the 11th Open Scientific Meeting of The Hip Society. St. Louis, MO, CV Mosby, 1983, p 106.

section **6** chapter **11**

PRIMARY TOTAL HIP ARTHROPLASTY

William B. Macaulay and Eduardo A. Salvati

Summary

- Approximately 150,000 primary total hip arthroplasty (THA) procedures are performed each year in the United States alone.
- The majority are performed for the treatment of osteoarthrosis.
- Primary THA will continue to be commonly performed throughout the world, because the population older than 65 years is expected to triple by the year 2050.
- The key objectives of primary THA are to relieve hip pain and to improve ambulation, range of motion, and function, thereby reversing the deficit caused by hip disorder.
- Despite better than 90% good to excellent long-term results, primary THA should be reserved for those individuals in whom conservative treatment has failed.

Primary THA is the most commonly performed hip reconstructive procedure today. Its effectiveness in relieving hip pain and reversing the functional loss caused by hip disease is unparalleled. More than half of the 150,000 primary THAs performed each year in the United States are performed for primary or secondary osteoarthritis. The remainder are performed to treat other hip disorders such as inflammatory arthritides (such as rheumatoid arthritis, an-

kylosing spondylitis, systemic lupus erythematosus, and psoriasis), post-traumatic arthritis, femoral neck fractures and its complications, tumor, vasculopathies (such as hemophilia, sickle cell disease, and osteonecrosis), and metabolic diseases (such as calcium pyrophosphate deposition disease, hemochromatosis, ochronosis, gout), among others.

HISTORICAL REVIEW

Sir John Charnley is generally regarded as the father of primary THA research. Many of his pioneering advances in the understanding of hip biomechanics, lubrication, biomaterials, prosthetic design, and operating theater environment remain unchallenged. He progressively incorporated these concepts into the practice of "low frictional torque arthroplasty" (LFA) at The Wrightington Centre for Hip Surgery at Wigan in England. Many technical improvements have been made during the last four decades, but many modifications to LFA have not withstood the test of time. The surgeon in training is encouraged to review Charnley's description of the evolution of LFA and the fundamentals, which serve as the scientific basis for the concepts we espouse today.[1]

Charnley's advances followed a number of attempts to reconstruct the arthritic hip. Biological interposition grafts at the hip (fascia lata and periarticular soft tissue) were being performed both in Europe and the United States at the outset of the 20th century. Smith-Petersen introduced the concept of mold arthroplasty[2] in 1923. This later gave rise to the "cup arthroplasty," which was perfected by Aufranc.[3] Charnley, however, was most influenced by the work of the Judet brothers in France. In the 1940s, they developed and implanted a heat-cured acrylic femoral head prosthesis[4] with catastrophic results because of loosening and breakage of the material. Thompson[5] and Moore[6] developed metallic femoral endoprostheses, but cartilage loss and bone lysis on the acetabular side highlighted the need for pelvic resurfacing. The concurrent metal-on-metal designs of McKee and Watson-Farrar[7] and Ring[8] resulted in high loosening rates and metallosis. Charnley's work would focus on overcoming the problems associated with these forerunning designs.[1]

LFA, as described by Charnley, was founded on the low-friction principle that emphasized the use of a small-diameter prosthetic head (22.225 mm) in combination with a large outer diameter socket with maximal plastic thickness (Fig. 1). Originally, Charnley used polytetrafluoroethylene (PTFE) (Teflon) sockets to articulate with smooth, monolithic stainless steel femoral components (both fixed with a methylmethacrylate grout). Teflon/steel provided one-fifth the friction of high molecular weight polyethylene/steel; however, its wear rate was later found to be 1000 times greater. This translated into clinical disaster for Charnley's first 300 LFAs performed. Polytetrafluoroethylene-wear debris-laden periprosthetic granulomas were the first dramatic example of primary THA–associated "particle disease"[9] as it is now known. Fortunately, Charnley persisted and switched to high molecular weight polyethylene sockets. When stainless steel femoral components began to demonstrate fatigue failure at an alarming rate, improved stem design and forging processes were used to solve the problem. Charnley's choice of methacrylate as a grout proved serendipitous (especially for femoral compo-

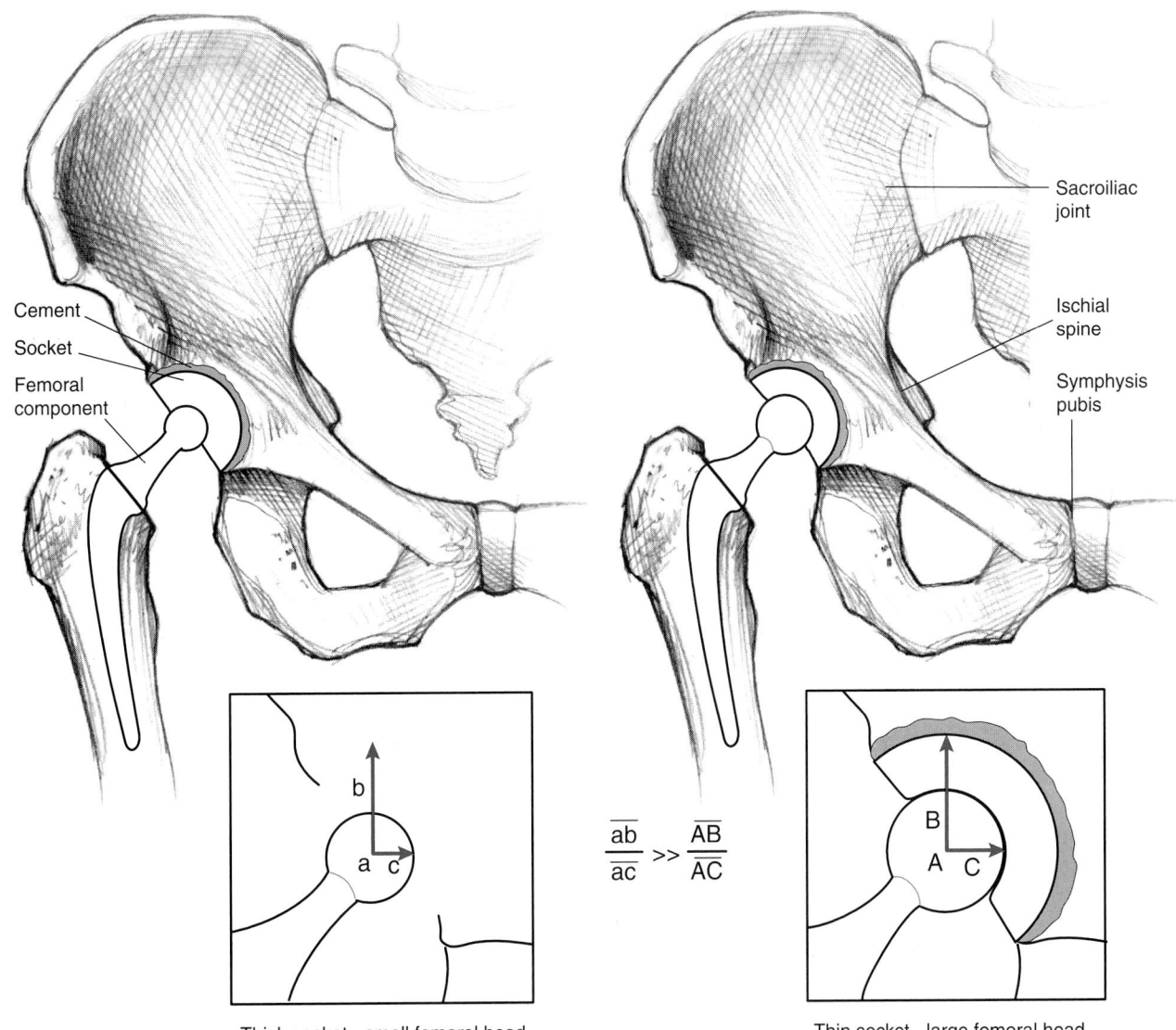

$$\frac{\overline{ab}}{\overline{ac}} \gg \frac{\overline{AB}}{\overline{AC}}$$

Thick socket - small femoral head

Thin socket - large femoral head

Fig. 1. Low frictional torque principle. The thick socket/small femoral head construct on the left favors the socket remaining stationary and fixed. Although the construct on the right provides greater range of motion and improved stability, the cup longevity is compromised.

nent fixation), and the material has yet to be significantly improved on, although the technique of application has been significantly refined.

Charnley's theory included techniques to minimize the joint reactive force at the hip (Fig. 2) by medializing the socket while lateralizing the abductor muscles insertion via trochanteric osteotomy. Charnley increased the stability of his LFA by advancing the greater trochanter and tensioning the abductors. Trochanteric migration, nonunion, wire breakage, and increased operative time have relegated the indication of trochanteric osteotomy to cases requiring more extensive hip reconstruction rather than replacement (i.e., developmental dysplasia of the hip). This transition was made possible with the advent of femoral head modularity and Morse tapers, which provided the ability to increase stability by changing the prosthetic neck length and offset. Other modifications in primary THA include press-fit porous-coated metal sockets with ultra-high molecular weight polyethylene inserts, cobalt-chrome alloy modular femoral heads, alternative bearing surfaces, and certain types of uncemented femoral components. Some of these so-called advances have encountered a higher rate of clinical failures, particularly in the early experience. The ultimate judgment on the relative success of these and other modifications of Charnley's LFA will rest on the 25-year and longer term clinical results.

CLINICAL FEATURES

When considering primary THA, the surgeon should explore several key aspects of the patient's history and physical examination. Failure to be thorough in this regard could predispose the patient to increased risk of complications such as infection, excessive bleeding, heterotopic ossification, intraoperative fracture, dislocation, early loosening, and leg length discrepancy.

Ensuring that the symptoms are referable to the hip joint is of paramount importance. The patient with the painful hip will generally point to the ipsilateral inguinal region anteriorly, describing a classic "groin pain" that is exacerbated with activity and weightbearing. Lumbosacral disease can commonly refer symptoms to the hip. Patients will often describe buttock pain posterior to the hip with or without concomitant low back and posterior thigh pain and radicular symptoms. Rarely, intrapelvic disorders (such as hernia, iliopsoas abscess or hematoma, vascular insufficiency, ovarian cyst, intrapelvic tumor, or prostatitis) can refer pain to the hip or cause hip activity-related pain. If other conditions coexist or if the source of the hip pain is unclear, confirmation can be obtained with an intra-articular injection of a local anesthetic that will provide immediate pain relief for the patient with isolated intra-articular hip disease.

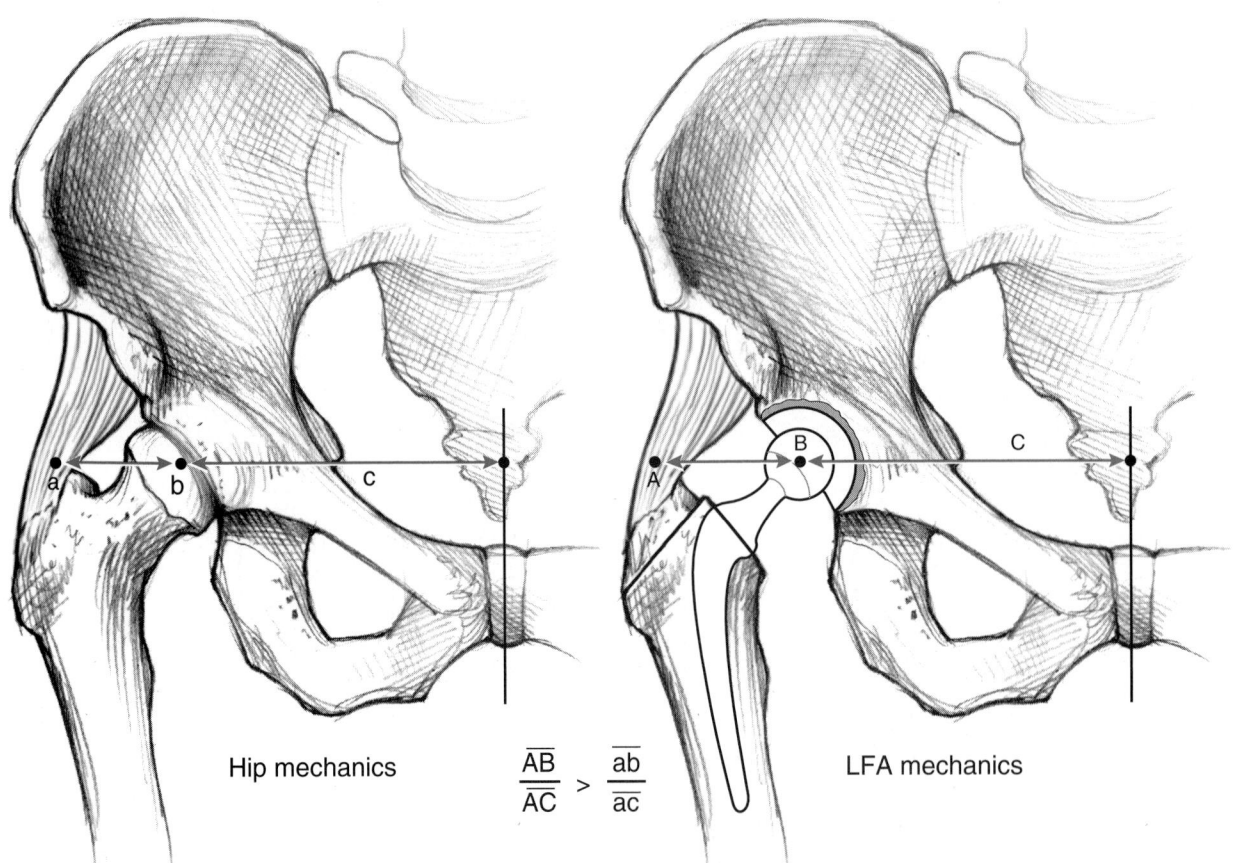

Hip mechanics $\qquad \dfrac{\overline{AB}}{\overline{AC}} > \dfrac{\overline{ab}}{\overline{ac}} \qquad$ LFA mechanics

Fig. 2. Biomechanics of low frictional torque arthroplasty (LFA). Charnley's LFA *(right)* optimized the lever arms acting at the hip by making AB/BC ≫ ab/bc, thereby decreasing the joint reactive force, which should decrease long-term wear. aA, bB, and cC represent the greater trochanteric insertion of the abductor musculature, center of hip rotation, and the body's center of gravity, respectively.

The hip reconstructive surgeon should conduct a thorough medical history. Many hip diseases of childhood (e.g., developmental dysplasia, sepsis, Perthes' disease, slipped capital femoral epiphysis, polio) could have a direct impact on the hip joint status in adulthood. Family history (i.e., sickle cell anemia) and social history (i.e., caisson working) can be illustrative with regard to diagnosis and prognosis. The patient's employment and recreational activity/proclivity are pertinent and should be explored. Obtaining a history of an immunocompromised state, bleeding dyscrasia, inflammatory arthropathy, osteomalacia, and previous trauma/irradiation can be critical to perioperative management and implant choice.

Information regarding the progression of the severity of hip pain and loss of function and ambulation can be a useful guide in choosing the appropriate timing of primary THA (Table 1). How severe is the hip pain? How far can the patient walk? Has the patient ever used or considered using an ambulatory aid such as a cane, crutch, or walker? How well can the patient negotiate stairs (with or without a banister), place socks, cut toenails, sit in a chair, get into a car, use public transportation, or engage in sexual activity? The timing of primary THA is a decision arrived at jointly by the patient and surgeon and can be influenced greatly by patient-related biases. What is the patient's pain tolerance? How comfortable is the patient with the prospect of surgery and making the time commitment necessary for rehabilitation? Is the patient willing to explore conservative management fully (i.e., activity concessions, ambulatory aids, weight loss, physiotherapy, systemic or local medications). Perhaps the most pertinent question is "Is your current hip situation acceptable?" The answer to this question can be enlightening and can help guide the course of the encounter with the patient. In the current environment of outcome studies and cost containment in health care, reliable health measurement indices such as the SF-36 Health Status Survey or Western Ontario and McMaster (WOMAC) Universities Osteoarthritis Index should be considered pre- and postoperatively. The Harris hip score is currently perhaps the most widely used hip pain/function instrument.[10]

TABLE 1. HIP PAIN QUESTIONNAIRE*

How severe is your hip pain?
Is the pain getting better or worse or staying the same?
How long has the hip been hurting?
How far can you walk?
Do you use a cane, crutch, walker, or wheelchair?
Is getting in and out of a car difficult?
Is your overall hip situation acceptable or unacceptable?
Occupation?
For recreation, what physical activity do you engage in?
With whom do you live?
Does the pain allow you to sit, lie down, or sleep comfortably?
Medications for hip pain?
Do they help?
Can you climb/descend stairs without a banister?
Can you climb/descend stairs one after the other?
Can you cut your toenails on the affected side?
Can you put your socks on the affected side?

* Answers to these questions allow an assessment of the patient's pain, prognosis, and functional limitations.

Physical examination of the hip patient begins without manipulation. The gowned patient's gait, without ambulatory aids, is observed for limp, coxalgia, pace, cadence, and lurch. A Trendelenburg gait (leaning toward the affected hip, while the pelvis tilts away at stance phase) can be indicative of a hip joint reaction force compensation with inadequate abductor muscle force. Patients are examined for discomfort as they rise from a chair, mount the examination table, and lie down. Lower extremity deformity, symmetry, atrophy, skin integrity and discoloration, hirsutism, and edema can be visually inspected. Leg length measurements, in the form of patient comfort in stance on blocks, are most helpful.

The balance of the examination, including vascular, neurological, and joint range of motion, requires manipulation. Palpation of the femoral, popliteal, posterior tibial, and dorsalis pedis should be documented and, if absent, should be identified with Doppler ultrasonography. Motor strength, sensation, reflexes, and balance are critical and may pinpoint concomitant lumbosacral disease. While the patient is supine (with the affected side away from the examination room wall), the hips should be examined for irritability at the extreme ranges of motion, passive "log roll," flexion contraction via the Thomas test, extent of flexion, abduction, adduction, and internal/external rotation (with the hip at 45 degrees and 90 degrees of flexion, respectively). If the patient has a pelvic tilt while standing, reassess if it persists while sitting to define hip contracture versus lumbosacral fixed deformity. Palpation of the greater trochanter and anterior hip joint capsule and use of the Patrick test or apprehension test can be helpful in selected patients.

INVESTIGATION

High-quality plain radiography remains the primary diagnostic tool for the hip under consideration for primary THA. For the evaluation of unilateral hip disease, anteroposterior (AP) orthopaedic pelvis and bilateral frog lateral hip radiographs comprise the minimal requirement. Our preference is that any patient who has decided to undergo primary THA should be further evaluated with a lumbosacral series and weightbearing AP and lateral radiographs of both knees. The information gathered with these radiographs (e.g., pelvic obliquity, relative anatomic distances, adjacent joint disease), in conjunction with the physical examination, usually is all that is necessary for comprehensive preoperative planning. At 6-week follow-up, a single AP radiograph of the operated hip with the beam centered over the socket (in addition to an orthopaedic AP pelvis and frog lateral view of the operated hip) is useful to determine the version of the acetabular prosthesis when compared with the AP pelvis radiograph.[11] For unusual deformities of the lower extremities that might affect mechanical alignment (e.g., previous long bone fracture, hemihypertrophy, multiple enchondromatosis, coxa vara, fibrous dysplasia), the surgeon should obtain long radiographs to determine the mechanical axis and the offset that should be built into the hip reconstruction. Computed tomography (CT) of the hip should be reserved for the rare instance of severe pelvic bony deficiency or profound deformity such as that observed in severe femoral dysplasia. Magnetic resonance imaging (MRI) is occasionally useful for diagnos-

TABLE 2. PREOPERATIVE THA TESTING*

Radiographic

Anteroposterior pelvis
Frog lateral both hips
Chest radiograph

Nonradiographic

Electrocardiogram
Urinalysis
Blood testing
  Complete blood count
  Basic serum chemistries (lytes, blood urea nitrogen, creatinine,
    glucose)
  Prothrombin time/partial thromboplastin time

*This list will vary depending on medical consultation, hospital/anesthesia policy, and regional tendencies. This list represents the minimum that will be done for patients older than 40 years at our hospitals.

ing early osteonecrosis of the hip, cartilage damage, or labral disease. Both CT and MRI can be used to assess heterotopic ossification in post-traumatic conditions and its anatomic relation to neurovascular structures. A *faux profil* (false profile) plain radiograph can be useful for the dysplastic acetabulum when a pelvic osteotomy is being contemplated.

Routine laboratory testing for patients who undergo primary THA is a controversial subject. The type of tests ordered preoperatively depends on the age and health of the patient, the policy of local regulatory agencies, the institution where the operation takes place, level of comfort of the physician performing the preoperative medical clearance, and the medicolegal atmosphere. It has become clear that too many tests are ordered and that a trend toward more selective testing should be promoted.[12] In general, preoperative THA patients undergo (1) electrocardiogram, (2) urinalysis, (3) chest radiography, and (4) blood tests, including complete blood count, basic serum chemistries, and coagulation studies (Table 2).

GOALS, INDICATIONS, AND CONTRAINDICATIONS

The primary goal of primary THA surgery is to relieve the pain and disability resulting from intra-articular hip joint disease. This should be severe enough to interfere significantly with the patient's ability to ambulate, perform activities of daily living, earn a livelihood, sleep without pain, drive a car, or engage in recreational and sexual activities. Ideally, the candidate for primary THA has failed conservative management. The patient's desire to ambulate without a cane or limp or without a leg length discrepancy or to have increased hip range of motion is generally not an indication to undergo primary THA if present as a single complaint. However, the association of several of these findings may justify its indication.

The decision process with regard to the performance and timing of primary THA is a complex subject in which the patient should be well educated and informed of the advan-

tages and disadvantages of continuing in a conservative approach or surgery. The patient would be underserved by following an absolute algorithm. Charnley stated that "to enunciate golden rules to guide the choice of patients for total hip replacement was an impossible task," nor should we try.[1] Nevertheless, the goals of pain relief and improved function should always provide the cornerstone for the decision. Patient-related biases are unavoidable, but the prudent hip surgeon will offer conservative treatment or more conservative surgical options to the patient who is young, active, and not in pain or disabled enough to justify primary THA. The risk-benefit ratio is of paramount importance, because complications such as deep infection or recurrent dislocation, although rare, are tragic for the patient who "was getting by" before primary THA surgery.

PREOPERATIVE PLANNING

Preoperative planning for primary THA is essential for minimizing complications and optimizing the construct. It is a simpler task than that for the revision surgery (refer to Chapters 6–12 and 6–13 on revision THA for details). Planning begins with a detailed medical history, focused physical examination, and a selective radiographic and laboratory work-up as previously described. The thorough medical history will define the severity of pain resulting from hip disease and rule out other sources of hip pain such as referred pain from the lumbosacral spine. The focused physical examination will yield vital information regarding true and apparent leg length, pelvic obliquity, neurovascular abnormality, and so on. A selective radiographic and laboratory work-up will save money by eliminating unnecessary tests and by decreasing complications (which are the most costly aspect of hip replacement surgery).

The preoperative planning is simpler in the virgin hip because there are no previous incisions, altered anatomy, or hardware with which to cope. Restoring proper hip mechanics can best be achieved through the careful preoperative templating of high-quality radiographs. Radiograph-related magnification should always be considered in patients with extreme body habitus. Although the radiographic magnification of the "average" patient approximates 15% to 20%, very thin patients have magnification of 12.5%, whereas very obese patients can have magnification of upward of 25%.[13] Restoring the center of hip rotation, offset, and leg length equality should be achieved while providing a construct with good range of motion that is stable and not prone to dislocation.

Primary hybrid (uncemented acetabular shell/cemented femoral stem) THA is currently considered state of the art,[14] and the templating of this most commonly used construct is discussed here. The principles are analogous when cemented cups and uncemented femoral components are used. However, uncemented femoral components require more precision on the AP and lateral radiographs because of the nature of the fixation. Templating for primary THA should begin proximally with the acetabular side. On the AP pelvis radiograph, we place a dot at the inferolateral border of the teardrop and another dot at the superolateral margin of the acetabulum. The convex side of the acetabular template is then juxtaposed to these dots at an abduction angle of approximately 40 degrees. The projected center of rotation is marked with a dot.

At this point, it is necessary to make a decision regarding leg length. The preoperative information gathered from the block test and clinical examination of leg length is essential and should coincide with the relative hip length on the AP pelvis radiograph. For example, one can draw the interteardrop line (a line connecting the nadirs of the teardrops) and place a dot at this level on both femora. Then the difference in height relative to the lesser trochanter is calculated. Usually the arthritic side is short, and this difference should be added by placing an X that same distance directly above the proposed center of rotation of the templated acetabulum. The surgeon will want the templated center of the prosthetic head to fall over this X as well. Careful thought must be given to lengthening more than 3 cm. Restoring equal leg lengths is not always desirable in patients with long-standing shortening because compensatory mechanisms may be established in the lumbosacral spine, knee, and ankle. They may perceive the reconstructed limb to be long when equalized and may be unhappy. The block test preoperatively is the best way to predict this. If in doubt, shortening is better tolerated than lengthening.

TECHNICAL DETAILS

ENVIRONMENT

Aseptic technique is important for all surgical procedures, but none more so than for primary THA. Because of bacteria's ability to shroud themselves in a glycocalix and the enormous suffering and economic impact associated with periprosthetic joint infections, the operative wound must be exposed to as low a bacterial load as possible. To this end, we use isolator suits, a clean air laminar flow enclosure, and perioperative antibiotics. Isolator suits control bacterial shedding by the members of the operative team within the enclosure.[1] There should be no extraneous individuals within the enclosure, and traffic within the operating room

outside the enclosure should be kept to a minimum. Clean air filters remove 99.9% of particles larger than 1 μm (thus all bacteria).[15] Laminar airflow shunts airborne particles (and bacteria) away from the wound and under the walls of the enclosure (Fig. 3). Anesthesia personnel and the patient's upper body remain outside the enclosure. For those bacteria that, nonetheless, do settle in the operative wound, frequent pulse lavage and intraoperative antibiotics can be helpful.[15]

THE OPERATIVE TEAM

The primary THA operative team consists of the surgeon, anesthesiologist, surgical assistants, scrub technician, and circulator. The team that works together most often will be the most efficient, with all members able to anticipate the next step of the procedure and avoid unnecessary delays. Decreasing operative time is an important step toward minimizing the incidence rate of serious postoperative complications such as infection and venous thromboembolism.

Although remaining outside the enclosure, the anesthesiologist and circulator are integral players on the operative team. The THA-efficient anesthesiologist helps keep patient preparation and room turnover time to a minimum. The anesthesiologist is proficient in regional anesthesia (epidural and spinal), which can be refined with deliberate intraoperative hypotension,[16] which will lower blood loss and avoid fluid overload. The efficient circulator will anticipate potential delays/problems and have equipment and supplies ready on request, thereby decreasing surgical time.

For the surgical technique (involving a posterolateral approach to the hip) outlined later, two or three surgical assistants are preferable. One surgical assistant is mandatory. The more familiar the assistant is with both human hip anatomy and the surgeon's technique, the simpler the procedure will be. In an academic setting, the assistants change on a rotational basis. The time for these rotational stints should be maximized for efficiency but not be so long as to compromise the assistant diversity of training.

Fig. 3. Clean air enclosure. The enclosure incorporates high-efficiency particulate air filters, laminar airflow, and isolator suits to keep the exposure of the surgical wound to airborne bacteria and particles as low as possible.

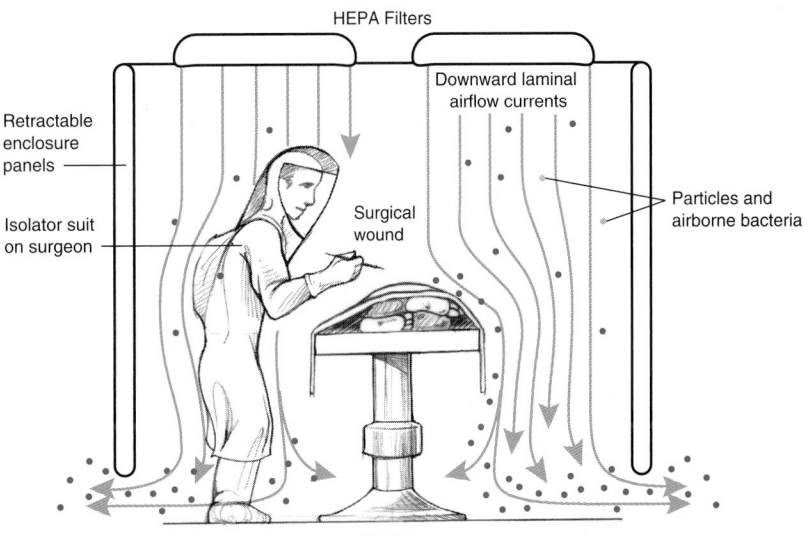

We prefer that the surgeon stand behind the laterally positioned patient, with the first assistant on the same side of the operating table toward the foot. The last assistant stands in front of the patient toward the foot and holds the leg when needed. The second assistant, if available, stands opposite the surgeon.

PATIENT POSITIONING

The operating table is placed in the center of the enclosure; the head of the patient protrudes through an opening in the enclosure toward the anesthesiologist. This table placement corresponds to an area directly beneath the lights, equidistant from the enclosure panels to the front and back of the patient. This also provides a maximal amount of space near the foot of the patient for instrument trays and equipment.

We prefer to position patients in the lateral decubitus position on a custom-designed hip table (Medrecon, Garwood, NJ). This table's main attractive feature for hip replacement surgery is a height-adjustable pelvic holder, which uses a vertical padded rest over the sacrum and a shorter concave padded rest over the pubis. This holder prevents forward/backward rolling of the pelvis. The height adjustment feature allows both pelves to be positioned neutrally, in line with the spine, avoiding tilting of the pelvis in the frontal plane. This neutral positioning of the pelvis in space reduces the guesswork in positioning of the acetabular component in the correct abduction and anteversion. The torso is supported with a posterior padded rest and with an inflatable axillary cushion, which relieves shoulder pressure. The down leg is well padded (including the area of the fibular head), and a cushioned pad is placed between the legs before draping. Determining leg length by comparing knee height or malleolar height is too imprecise and unreliable to justify access to the down leg.

SKIN PREPARATION AND DRAPING

We prefer a preliminary povidone scrub of the patient's hip and thigh area by the circulator (in addition to the scrub and shave done in the holding area) immediately before the final skin preparation with povidone by a scrubbed member of the operative team who has donned the isolator suit. Skin preparation includes the hip area from L4 to the umbilicus, down to below the knee circumferentially, around the thigh, and up to the groin. During this preparation, the leg is held aloft and abducted and in external rotation by unscrubbed personnel. With the leg aloft, a sterile bottom sheet is placed, followed by a top sheet, which is connected to a U-drape from below. A sterile folded half-sheet then encloses the unprepared distal part of the leg, which is covered with a stockinette. The skin is dried with towels, and marking lines are placed on the skin with a sterile pen to ensure precise skin closure. A sterile transparent plastic shower curtain separates the lower half of the patient from the anesthesia team. It is taped directly to the enclosure panels after placement of an extremity drape. All exposed skin is then covered with adhesive, povidone-laden Vi-Drape. After affixing the suction, pulse lavage, and use of an electrocautery, the patient is ready for the incision.

APPROACH AND SURGICAL TECHNIQUE

We use the posterolateral approach for all primary THA cases. Surgeons complain that this approach increases the rate of dislocation. However, if the components are positioned with proper version and the external rotators and posterior capsule are formally repaired, the rate of dislocation will be less than 1%. Protection of the skin edges (with moist lap pads) and peri-incisional tissues (with delicate retractor placement and avoidance of bulky Charnley self-retaining retractors) is of paramount importance during the approach. With the patient positioned and prepared as just described, bony landmarks and the intended incision are marked with a pen as shown in Figure 4. The superior margin of the greater trochanter is marked, as are the posterior and anterior margins of the greater trochanter of the femur. The insertion of the gluteal sling is estimated, as is the approximate location of the acetabulum relative to the superior margin of the greater trochanter based on the AP pelvis radiograph. The curvilinear skin incision should be centered over the neck of the femur where the bulk of the work is to be performed. The length of the incision will depend on the size of the patient and the depth of the surgical wound. It should be long enough to perform the operation with minimal trauma to the surrounding tissues. However, care should be taken not to make it unnecessarily long either proximally or distally. The lower part of the incision is linear from the top of the trochanter (in line with the femur) but centered slightly posteriorly. The upper part of the incision curves posteriorly at an angle of approximately 140 degrees relative to the inferior linear portion.

The incision is carried through the skin (and subcutaneous adipose tissue in line with the skin incision) with a large blade. A new no. 11 blade is used to incise the tensor and gluteal fascia in line with the skin incision. Hemostasis is achieved using electrocautery. This fascial incision should be made directly lateral to the greater trochanter; one should take care to avoid being too anterior or posterior. The appropriately centered fascial incision will be rewarded with the absence of tensor or gluteal musculature lateral to the greater trochanter. Superiorly, the gluteus maximus should be divided bluntly after the fascial incision is made. The sciatic nerve is identified posteriorly and deep within the wound. The gluteal sling is located inferiorly and posterior and divided using an electrocautery over its proximal half after being held under tension with a Hibbs retractor. Care is taken to stay superficial during this maneuver to avoid the first of the perforating vessels immediately beneath the gluteal sling.

After traversing the trochanteric bursa, the posterior border of the gluteus medius is identified and the piriformis tendon palpated with an index finger. A thin Hohmann retractor (bent midshaft at a right angle, thin-bent Hohmann) is placed over the piriformis tendon and under the posterior border of the gluteus minimus muscle, which has been separated from the capsule with a Cobb elevator. Next, an Aufranc retractor is swept from the piriformis tendon, along the posterior capsule, and under the femoral neck. With the appropriate amount of pressure, this maneuver clearly exposes the piriformis and conjoined tendons, which are divided at their insertion on the greater trochanter and separately tagged with "short" no. 2 braided nonabsorbable suture. These "short" external rotators are retracted posteriorly to protect the sciatic nerve further (Fig. 5), and the entire posterior capsule is thusly exposed. Next, a posterior capsular flap is created by incising the capsule at its insertion on the posterior intertrochanteric crest area

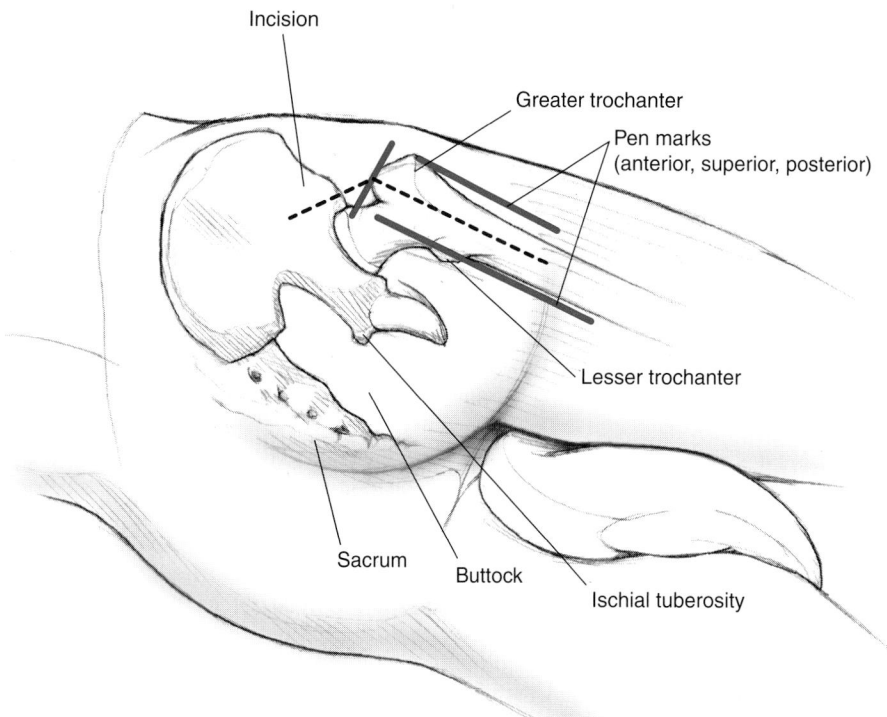

Fig. 4. Bony landmarks and proposed incision. This is a posterolateral view of the laterally positioned patient on the hip table. The bony pelvis and femur are shown with dotted lines (hidden). Superior is left, and inferior is right. The bony landmarks are displayed with straight lines. The curvilinear incision has a 140-degree angle at the superior aspect of the palpable greater trochanter.

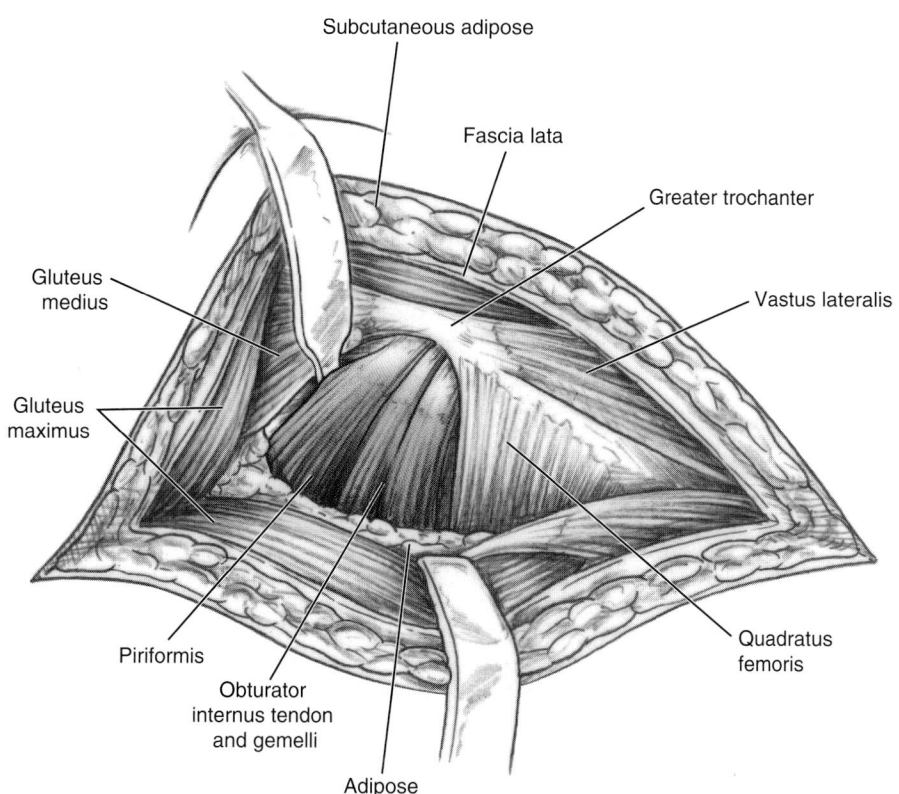

Fig. 5. External rotators and capsule exposed. This is a posterolateral view of the open incision with a clear view of the piriformis and conjoined tendons overlying the posterior hip joint capsule. This exposure is aided with a superior thin-bent Hohmann and inferior Aufranc retractor.

of the neck. For a right hip (see Fig. 5), for example, the capsule is incised posterosuperiorly toward the 10 to 11 o'clock position (along the inferior border of the gluteus minimus) back to the edge of the acetabulum, incising the labrum. A similar linear incision is made in the capsule from the lower posterior femoral neck, posteroinferiorly toward the 7 o'clock position, stopping near the tip of (but not touching) the Aufranc retractor. Particular attention is devoted to protecting the sciatic nerve. This posterior capsular flap is then tagged with two "long" no. 2 braided nonabsorbable sutures (spread by 1 to 1.5 cm) at its distal base and retracted posteriorly. The femoral head is gently dislocated by internal rotation and flexion of the hip, bringing the femoral head to be replaced superficially into the wound.

Two tagging sutures (no. 0 absorbable) are then placed proximally within the superior half of the quadratus femoris muscle, which is divided with electrocautery. Care is taken to cauterize the medial femoral circumflex artery before it is transected and the posterior femoral neck completely denuded of soft tissue. In this fashion, the proximal aspect of the lesser trochanter is visualized, and the femoral neck cut can be marked at an appropriate height above the lesser trochanter as templated preoperatively. We prefer the use of the reciprocating saw to perform the femoral neck osteotomy. The orientation of this osteotomy should avoid flexion and extension, which can be made easier by placing a folded drape below the knee so that the femur is parallel with the floor while the leg is kept vertical. The angle of the osteotomy relative to the long axis of the length of this osteotomy from the neck toward the greater trochanter is determined based on the proximal geometry of the implants and insertion devices. Care is taken to avoid overthinning the greater trochanter, which will predispose it to fracture. As soon as the osteotomy is made with the reciprocating saw, the wound is lavaged to remove bone debris (and its associated osteoblast and osteoinductive factors, i.e., bone morphogenetic proteins) to decrease the risk of postoperative heterotopic ossification. If significant subchondral cysts are found on the pelvic side, cancellous autograft bone is removed and prepared for later insertion into these defects. Attention is turned to the acetabulum while unsterile personnel tilt the hip table 20 degrees posteriorly.

Exposure of the acetabulum is obtained with the hip in extension. First, a C-retractor is placed over the anterior lip of the acetabulum, further moving the femur anteriorly. The remaining capsule and reflected head of the rectus femoris are divided at the 1 o'clock position on the acetabulum (relaxing the anterior capsule more and further improving anterior exposure), and a smooth Steinmann pin is placed into the pelvis 2 cm above the acetabulum, improving superior visualization by retraction of the gluteus minimus and medius. The Aufranc retractor is placed inferiorly adjacent and distal to the capsule enhancing inferior exposure. A "wide-bent" Hohmann retractor is then placed outside the labrum, but inside the capsule, and secured into the ischium with gentle taps with the mallet. Again, care is taken to avoid injuring the sciatic nerve during this maneuver.

The labrum and soft-tissue pulvinar within the acetabular notch can now be removed with a long-handled scalpel and a large curet, respectively. Hemispheric reaming is begun at a size 6 to 8 mm below the preoperatively templated size and aiming medially to the quadrilateral surface. Preoperative radiographs will help the surgeon anticipate how much medialization is necessary based on thickness of the teardrop. Often in cases of severe osteoarthritis the head of the femur is lateralized relative to the teardrop with interposition of large medial osteophytes. These osteophytes must not be confused with the medial wall. Once reaming medially has abutted the quadrilateral surface, reaming is performed at the desired version angles (40 degrees abduction and 20 degrees anteversion), preserving the medial wall. Reaming is continued with sequentially larger reamers (increasing by 2-mm increments). As the reamers increase in size, the entire surface of the acetabulum is reamed. Bleeding corticocancellous bone should comprise the entire hemisphere to receive the press-fit shell. When the reamer's diameter is approximately 2 mm smaller than the size that was preoperatively templated, a press-fit trial is tried. The preoperatively templated acetabular shell is then press-fit into the socket, which has been underreamed by 2 mm. We prefer to use hemispheric shells without holes if there are no significant bony defects. Contained cystic defects can be filled with the cancellous autograft from the native femoral head, as mentioned. If there is any doubt that excellent press-fit fixation will be obtained, we prefer the use of a cluster hole cup so that one or two screws can be inserted into the posterosuperior safe zone.[17] The desired polyethylene liner (chosen based on thickness, internal diameter, wear prognosis, and posterior elevation) is inserted under direct visualization without intervening soft tissue and impacted into place. Activation of the locking mechanism is verified, and any remaining anterior or posterior osteophyte is removed at this time with an osteotome. Retractors are removed, and attention is turned to the femoral side.

The leg is brought into 90 degrees of hip internal rotation, flexion, and adduction so that the surgeon can prepare the proximal femur. The surgeon should be aware that this position twists the proximal vasculature of the lower extremity; thus, time in this position should be limited to decrease the risk of postoperative deep venous thrombosis. Exposure is ensured with the use of a "jaws" (or Stirchfield) retractor anterior to the femoral neck and an Aufranc retractor medially adjacent to the jaws. A crown (or thinbent Hohmann) retractor protects the abductor musculature during broaching. Soft tissue is removed from the area of the neck and posterior greater trochanter. Anterior femoral osteophytes are removed at this time. The femoral neck osteotomy is revised with the reciprocating saw if necessary. A canal finder will identify the long axis of the femur. Femoral canal broaching is performed based on a prosthesis-specific protocol in the desired anteversion with sequentially larger broaches. Again, fatty exudate from the canal (with osteoinductive biological factors) is simultaneously suctioned to decrease the risk of postoperative heterotopic ossification. Enough space is created for a 2-mm minimum cement column. Trial reduction can be carried out with modular broaches and a head and neck assembly or with a separate trial prosthesis. The lesser trochanter to center of head distance should be measured and can be matched within 2 mm in the vast majority of cases. The trial reduction ensures that soft-tissue balance, range of motion, and hip joint stability have been achieved.

The trials are removed, and the cement restrictor is placed to the desired depth (1 to 2 cm distal to the tip of the prosthesis). The canal is thoroughly irrigated, cleaned of debris, and dried with vaginal packing as the cement is mixed. The canal is filled in retrograde fashion with a cement gun with polymethylmethacrylate (PMMA) cement of the appropriate consistency with pressurization. The femoral stem is inserted within the cement column (with associated distal or proximal centralizers) in the desired anteversion and neutral varus/valgus alignment. Excess cement is removed, and care is taken not to sink the prosthesis too deeply if it is of a collarless design. The cement is allowed to cure. We preheat the PMMA and the stem (to 40°C) to reduce the polymerization time, but this practice should only be undertaken with an experienced operative team. In addition, heated PMMA and stem reduce cement porosity and has a detrimental effect on the mechanical properties.[18] The templated modular femoral head is tapped into place on the Morse taper and the construct gently relocated under visualization. The posterior capsular flap and short external rotators are formally repaired by placing the "long" and "short" braided sutures through drill holes in the posterior greater trochanter with Keith needles and tying them separately (Fig. 6). The superior quadratus femoris is repaired with free needles passing the tagged No. 0 absorbable suture mentioned previously through the distal portion of the muscle and tying the two sutures. The wound is vigorously irrigated with antibiotic-laden saline to remove any remaining bone, soft tissue, or cement debris. The tensor fascia is repaired with interrupted No. 2 nonabsorbable suture beginning distally. As this closure approaches the trochanteric flare, two small tubes to a self-suction drain are placed under the tensor fascia anteroinferiorly, exiting 5 cm from the wound edge. The surgeon may opt to use figure-of-eight knots over the greater trochanter. As the closure of the tensor layer approaches thin fascia superiorly, absorbable no. 0 suture should be used. This same suture can be used for inverted deep subcutaneous knots, but 2-0 sutures should be used immediately subcutaneously. Staples are applied on the skin. We cover the wound with nonstick antibacterial dressing, gauze, and two abdominal pads. This dressing is

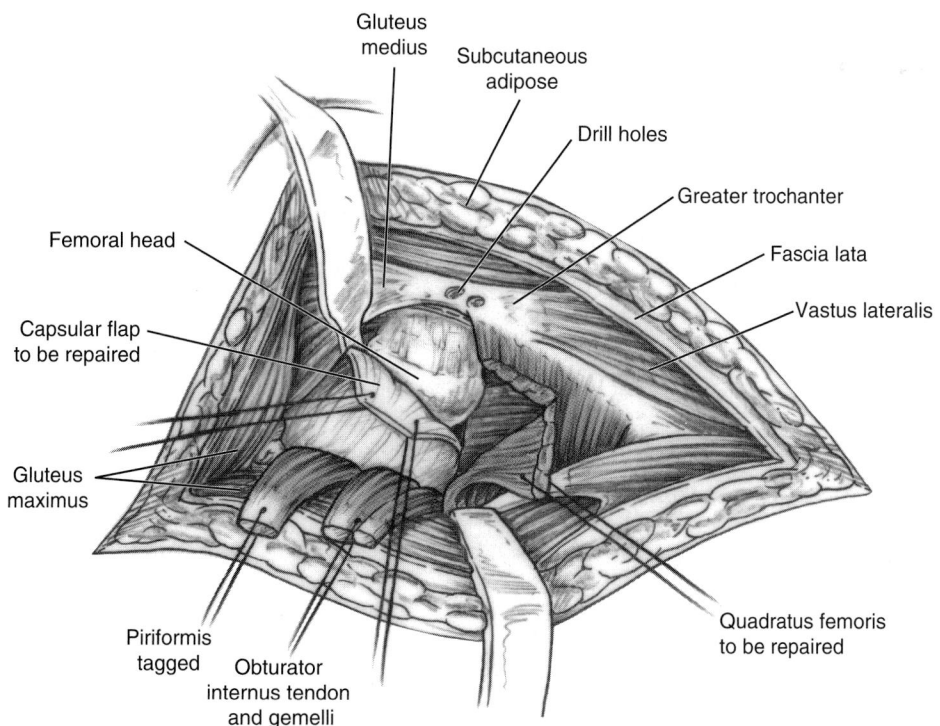

Fig. 6. Incision closure: formal repair of the capsule and external rotators. This is a posterolateral view of the open incision immediately before formal repair of the capsular flap and short external rotator tendons. The capsular flap tagged with a "long" suture and the tendons tagged with a "short" suture are seen in the center and posterior aspect of the wound, respectively. The quadratus femoris muscle (seen inferiorly) is tagged, and the superior defect in the muscle is repaired via free needle placement of the doubled sutures into the distal portion of the muscle near the femur.

covered loosely with wraps with minimal elastic capacity in a hip spica fashion. Placement of the hip spica is facilitated by the use of the hip table mentioned earlier.

COMPLICATIONS

A detailed discussion of the common complications after total hip arthroplasty, as well as their management, can be found in Chapter 6–18.

RESULTS

Hybrid total hip arthroplasty has had outstanding clinical results, particularly with the advances introduced in the 1980s and 1990s. Advances were made in component design, cement insertion technique, and manufacturing techniques, all of which contributed to the high success rates. In addition, the change from cementing both the acetabular and femoral components to hybrid fixation (i.e., cementless fixation of the acetabular cup with cemented fixation of the femoral stem) made a tremendous impact on the overall longevity of primary THA.

For example, Clohisy and Harris[19] showed that at 10-year follow-up 96% of 196 Harris-Galante cups were still implanted, and of the 4% that had been revised, all were well fixed at the time of revision. Similarly, other authors demonstrated outstanding results with press-fit porous-coated acetabular components.[20,21]

With regard to cemented femoral stems, Madey et al[22] reported on 356 Charnley stems inserted with second-generation cement techniques (plugging the femoral canal, pressure lavage of the canal, and retrograde injection of the cement with a cement gun) and found 3% overall loosening and 5% loosening after 15-year follow-up. Similarly, Mulroy et al[23] showed 2% loosening at an average 15-year follow-up. With third-generation cement techniques (i.e., the addition of PMMA precoated onto the proximal aspect of the femoral component), results have been similar in several series, although with shorter follow-up.[24–26] Continued observation will demonstrate the true longevity of the hybrid THA.

REFERENCES

1. Charnley J: Low Friction Arthroplasty: Theory and Practice. London, Churchill Livingstone, 1979.
2. Smith-Petersen MN: Evolution of mold arthroplasty of the hip. J Bone Joint Surg Br 1949; 30:59.
3. Aufranc OE: Constructive hip surgery with a vitallium mold: A report of 1000 cases of arthroplasty of the hip over a 15 year period. J Bone Joint Surg Am 1957; 39:237.
4. Judet R, Judet J: Essais de reconstruction prothetique de la hanche apres resection de la femorale. J Chir 1949; 65:17.
5. Thompson FR: Two and a half years experience with vitallium intramedullary prosthesis. J Bone Joint Surg Am 1954; 36:489.
6. Moore AT: The self locking metal hip prosthesis. J Bone Joint Surg Am 1957; 39:811.
7. McKee GK, Watson-Farrar J: Replacement of arthritic hips by the McKee-Farrar prosthesis. J Bone Joint Surg Br 1966; 48:245.
8. Ring PA: Complete replacement arthroplasty of the hip by the Ring prosthesis. J Bone Joint Surg Br 1968; 50:720.
9. Harris WH: Osteolysis and particle disease of the hip. Acta Orthop Scand 1994; 65(1):113.
10. Harris WH: Traumatic arthritis of the hip after dislocation and acetabular fractures: An end result study using a new method of result evaluation. J Bone Joint Surg Am 1969; 51:737.

11. McLaren RH: Prosthetic hip angulation. Radiology 1973; 107:705.
12. Callaghan JJ, Rosenberg AG, Rubash HE (eds): The Adult Hip. Philadelphia, Lippincott-Raven, 1998.
13. Clarke IC, Gruen T, Matos M, et al: Improved methods for quantitative radiographic evaluation with particular reference to total hip arthroplasty. Clin Orthop 1976; 121:83.
14. National Institutes of Health: Consensus statement on total hip replacement. 1994; 12:12.
15. Lidwell OA, Lowbury EJL, Whyte W, et al: Effect of ultraclean air in operating rooms on deep joint sepsis in the joint after total hip or knee replacement: A randomised study. BMJ 1982; 285:10.
16. Sharrock NE, Mineo R, Urquhart B: Hemodynamic response to low-dose epinephrine infusion during hypotensive epidural anesthesia for total hip replacement. Reg Anesth 1990; 15:295.
17. Wasielewski RC, Cooperstein LA, Kruger MP, et al: Acetabular anatomy and the transacetabular fixation of screws in total hip arthroplasty. J Bone Joint Surg Am 1990; 72:501.
18. Parks ML, Walsh HA, Salvati EA, et al: Effect of temperature on the polymerization rate and mechanical properties of four bone cements. Clin Orthop 1998; 355:238.
19. Clohisy JC, Harris WH: The Harris-Galante porous-coated acetabular component

with screw fixation. J Bone Joint Surg Am 1999; 81:66.
20. Latimer HA, Lachiewicz PF: Porous-coated acetabular components with screw fixation. J Bone Joint Surg Am 1996; 78:975.
21. Tompkins GS, Jacobs JJ, Kull LR, et al: Primary total hip arthroplasty with a porous-coated acetabular component. J Bone Joint Surg Am 1997; 79:169.
22. Madey SM, Callaghan JJ, Olejniczak JP, et al: Charnley total hip arthroplasty with use of improved techniques of cementing. J Bone Joint Surg Am 1997; 77:53.
23. Mulroy WF, Estok DM, Harris WH: Total hip arthroplasty with use of so-called second generation cementing techniques. J Bone Joint Surg Am 1995; 77:1845.
24. Berg RA, Kull LR, Rosenberg AG, et al: Hybrid total hip arthroplasty. Clin Orthop 1996; 333:134.
25. Oishi CS, Walker RH, Colwell CW Jr: The femoral component in total hip arthroplasty: Six to eight year follow-up of one hundred consecutive patients after use of a third generation cementing technique. J Bone Joint Surg Am 1994; 76:1130.
26. Clohisy JC, Harris WH: Primary hybrid total hip replacement performed with insertion of the acetabular component without cement and a precoat femoral component with cement. J Bone Joint Surg Am 1999; 81:247.

section
6
chapter
12

REVISION TOTAL HIP ARTHROPLASTY: THE FEMORAL SIDE

Arthur L. Malkani

Summary

- Problems that require revision of the femoral compartment are rapidly increasing, as the service life of the prosthesis is extended.
- Pain is the most common clinical symptom.
- Preoperative planning, including surgical approach, is critical. Removing the implant and addressing bone loss require a variety of instrumentation, prosthetic devices, and the availability of allograft bone.
- Compensating for bone loss is one of the major technical challenges.
- Complications after femoral revision total hip arthroplasty are increased, rehabilitation is slower, and the results are not as spectacular as with primary total hip arthroplasty.

Revision total hip arthroplasty is the procedure by which an existing (but failed) total hip prosthesis is removed and replaced by a new prosthesis. Failure of total hip arthroplasty, as a result of either loosening or sepsis, is not uncommon. However, the bone loss and compromised soft tissue that are encountered during revision present the surgeon with a number of challenges to provide a stable and durable arthroplasty, challenges that are not encountered in primary hip replacement. In aseptic loosening of a total hip arthroplasty, when the bone loss from the proximal femur is minimal and adequate cancellous bone is available for interdigitation of cement, revision total hip arthroplasty with a cemented femoral component is usually feasible and appropriate. For most patients who require a revision total hip arthroplasty, the situation—a smooth, sclerotic endosteal surface of the proximal femur deficient in both cancellous and cortical bone—makes the surgical procedure more complex. In such situations, an extensively coated stem, a modular femoral component, a calcar femoral replacement component, or an impaction grafting technique using morselized cancellous allograft may be a better treatment option. Thus, for an individual patient, the choice of the femoral component for implantation during revision

total hip arthroplasty is based on the extent of femoral bone loss, the quality of the soft tissue and bone, the experience of the treating surgeon, and the availability of different types of prostheses. Consequently, preoperative planning must be thorough and provide the surgeon with multiple options that can be selected on the basis of the intraoperative findings.

HISTORY AND EPIDEMIOLOGY

Revision total hip arthroplasty constitutes a major portion of the hip surgery performed at secondary and tertiary referral centers. The incidence of revision total hip arthroplasty continues to increase as patients who had an initially successful primary total hip arthroplasty experience aseptic loosening of the arthroplasty 10 to 20 years later. The early results of cemented femoral component revisions, in the 1980s, documented failure rates of 4% to 29% (Table 1), with radiographic evidence of probable femoral component loosening in as many as 44% of all revisions at 10-year follow-up.[1–7] More recent experiences have demonstrated a decrease in the incidence of aseptic loosening with the introduction of modern cementing techniques.[8–12]

PATHOGENESIS

Aseptic loosening is the most common cause of failure for which revision total hip arthroplasty is performed. Willert et al[13] identified large foreign body granulomas at the bone-cement interface; histiocytes and foreign body giant cells containing particles of polymethylmethacrylate (fragmented bone cement) were found in clinical material retrieved from surgical biopsies in patients who had aseptically loosened total hip arthroplasties. These granulomatous lesions consisted of well-organized tissue containing histiocytic-monocytic and fibroblastic reactive zones. Immunohistological evaluation has revealed the presence of multinucleated giant cells and C3 bireceptor-bearing monocyte-macrophages.[14] Explant cultures of the pseudomembrane and synovial tissue derived from osteoarthritic patients undergoing revision for cemented hip implant failure

TABLE 1. RESULTS OF FEMORAL COMPONENT REVISION IN THE 1980s				
Study	No. Hips	Average Follow-Up (Years)	Failed Revision That Required Further Revision (%)	Radiographically Loose (%)
Callaghan et al (1985)[6]	139	3.6	4.3	12
Kavanagh et al (1985)[2]	166	4.5	6	44
Pellicci et al (1982),[5] (1985)[4]	116	8.1	19	29

have been shown to produce interleukin (IL)-1, tumor necrosis factor, and prostaglandin E_2, which may implicate the cells of the prosthesis-associated pseudomembrane in the pathogenesis of aseptic loosening.[15]

Although the final common pathway at the cellular level has yet to be fully elucidated, particulate debris emanating from the prostheses' articulating surfaces, acetabular and femoral components' nonarticulating surfaces, and polymethylmethacrylate (if present) initiate the process.[16] Currently, it appears that the submicron particles stimulate circulating monocytes to produce cytokines, in particular IL-1, IL-2, and tumor necrosis factor, which recruit macrophages into the location of the particles. The failure of the macrophages to digest or dissolve the foreign particle causes cell death, with the elaboration of more cytokines and the recruitment of additional macrophages. During this process, bone erosion occurs, and there is radiographic evidence of bone lysis and resorption. Although metal, polyethylene, and polymethylmethacrylate particles have been identified in the reactive tissue obtained during revision total hip arthroplasty, histological analysis with electron microscopy has demonstrated that particles emanating from the high-density polyethylene acetabular component are encountered with the greatest frequency[17, 18] (Fig. 1). Particle size has been identified as an important factor in the biological response. Particles larger than 10 μm do not elicit a cytokine response. Submicron particles and those smaller than 10 μm do elicit a cytokine response.[17, 18]

Although aseptic loosening is multifactorial, Jasty et al,[16] on the basis of their postmortem studies of the hip in patients with well-functioning total hip arthroplasties, suggested that debonding of the cement-femoral component interface is the initial event that leads to loosening. This debonding contributes to fracture of the cement mantle with the release of polymethylmethacrylate particles. Others suggested that increased hoop stresses within the cement mantle cause longitudinal fractures of the polymethyl-

methacrylate, with the subsequent release of polymethylmethacrylate particles.

In cementless total hip arthroplasties, the initial event that leads to loosening is (1) lysis of bone adjacent to the prosthesis, associated with the biological response to wear-generated particles; (2) stress relief resorbtion of bone adjacent to the prosthesis resulting from the mismatch between stiffness of the prosthesis and stiffness of bone; or (3) the initial fixation having not been secure, so that the prosthesis simply became loose as a result of repetitive cyclic loading.

CLINICAL FEATURES

Pain is the most common clinical symptom in patients presenting with aseptic loosening of their total hip arthroplasty. On physical examination, findings that should raise the suspicion of a loose femoral component include painful range of hip motion, thigh atrophy, a positive Trendelenburg sign, and an antalgic gait. It may be difficult to differentiate between thigh pain of the type that occurs with a well-fixed cementless femoral component and that seen with a loose cementless component. However, there are usually radiographic changes indicative of an unstable femoral component (e.g., a circumferential radiolucent line about the femoral component, migration of the femoral component, and no evidence of "spot welding"). The differential diagnosis of a painful total hip includes infection and neurovascular entities such as spinal stenosis, lumbar disk herniation, and claudication.

INVESTIGATIONS

Radiographic findings in patients who have aseptic loosening of a femoral component are quite variable. In those who have a cemented total hip arthroplasty, radiolucent lines at the bone-cement interface as described by Gruen et

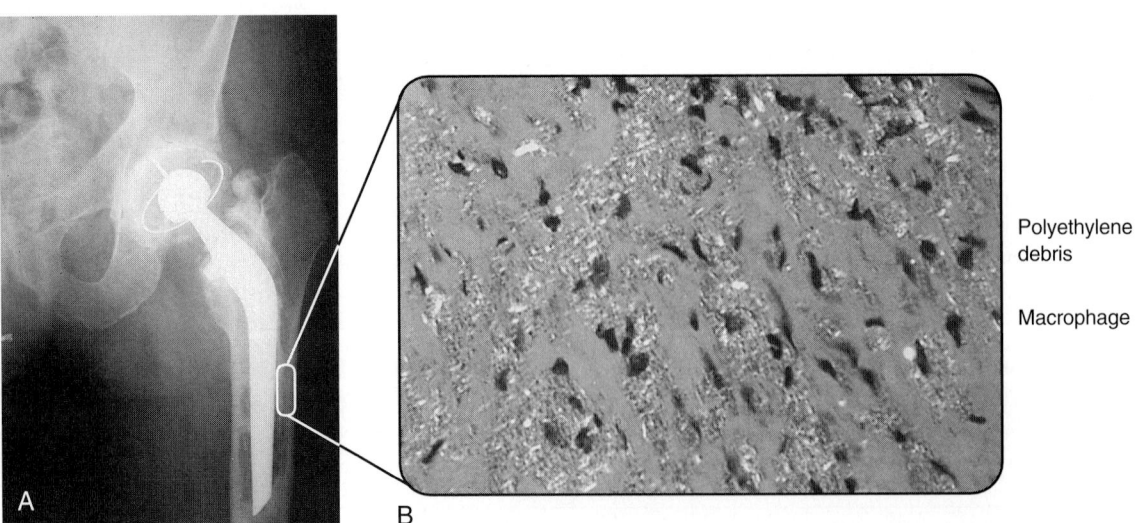

Polyethylene debris

Macrophage

Fig. 1. View. Pathogenesis of aseptic loosening of a cemented femoral component *(A). B,* Polarized light microscopy demonstrates macrophages and polyethylene wear debris at the bone-cement interface. The exact sequence of events is not fully known. (Courtesy Thomas Bauer, Cleveland Clinic.)

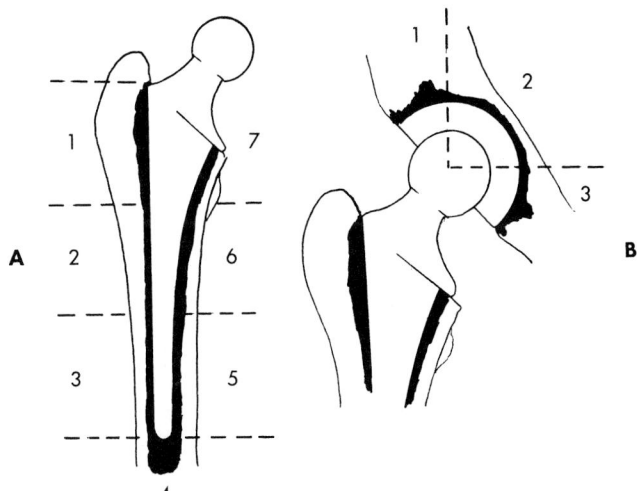

Fig. 2. Gruen's zones. Seven delineated sections around the femoral component for zonal evaluation of looseness and progressive loosening. (From Crenshaw et al: Campbell's Operative Orthopaedics, 8th ed, vol 1, Philadelphia, Mosby, 1992, p 559; redrawn from Amstutz HC, Smith RK: J Bone Joint Surg Am 1979; 61:1161.)

al[19] are usually a prominent feature (Fig. 2). Radiolucent lines 2 mm in width and a progressive increase in the width of a radiolucent line observed on serial radiographs are thought to be important and suggestive of loosening. A circumferential radiolucent line 2 mm or larger at the bone-cement interface is highly suggestive of loosening. Subsidence—sinking of the femoral component within the femoral canal—is a radiographic finding strongly suggestive of loosening. Radiographically evident fracture of the femoral component or cement mantle is also strongly suggestive of loosening.[20]

Radiographic findings in a patient who has aseptic loosening of a cementless femoral component are more subtle.[21] Subsidence of the femoral component and debonding of the porous coating are radiographic findings consistent with loosening of cementless femoral components. Radiolucent lines at the prosthesis-bone interface of cementless femoral components usually have a sclerotic edge adjacent to the osseous side of the interface and may or may not be significant. Radiolucent lines are significant if they are noted to become progressively wider with serial radiographs. Radiolucent lines adjacent to nonporous portions of a cementless femoral component are common and of no clinical significance. A sclerotic buildup of bone at the tip of the femoral component, referred to as a pedestal, is thought to be indicative of micromotion and thus may be a radiographic finding consistent with loosening.

Modifications of the surgical technique used to prepare and insert polymethylmethacrylate have reduced the incidence of aseptic loosening from as high as 40% to 3% at 10 or more years after surgery.[1–9] Although the diagnosis of aseptic loosening of a total hip arthroplasty is suspected from the patient's history, it is usually confirmed by physical examination and radiographic analysis. An arthrogram can also help to establish the diagnosis if contrast material is seen to extend into the interface between the bone and cement. Arthrography has proved to be less helpful in the

evaluation of a patient who has a cementless femoral component.[22] Although bone scans using technetium methylene diphosphonate have also been used to assist in the diagnosis of a painful total hip, they are rarely diagnostic and generally are of limited value.[23]

If the patient who has a painful total hip arthroplasty had a history of infection of the hip before total hip arthroplasty, or if wound drainage has continued beyond the first few days after total hip arthroplasty, the possibility of septic loosening must be considered. If radiographic changes occur within the first year after surgery, septic loosening is more likely than aseptic loosening. In such clinical situations, the erythrocyte sedimentation rate and a C-reactive protein determination may be helpful. If these are elevated in patients who do not have a collagen disease, they are suggestive of infection. If infection is suspected, then the hip should be aspirated and any fluid recovered from the joint submitted for cell counts and culture and sensitivity studies.[24] If the result of aspiration is not definitive, further information can be obtained by indium-labeled autologous leukocyte scanning, which accurately identifies sepsis in up to 93% of patients who have infected total hip arthroplasties.[22, 23]

GOALS, INDICATIONS, AND CONTRAINDICATIONS

GOALS

The surgical objectives of revision total hip arthroplasty are to do the following:

Alleviate pain.
Restore normal mechanics about the hip.
Provide adequate soft-tissue tension.
Achieve rigid fixation of the implant to host bone, resulting in a stable and durable implant and compensating for lost bone.

INDICATIONS

The indications for revising a total hip arthroplasty are summarized in Table 2. The primary indication for revision total hip arthroplasty is pain in the presence of objective evidence of a pain-producing abnormality such as loosening.[22] Total hip revision operations for unexplained pain rarely succeed in relieving pain. Invariably, the pain caused by loosening occurs with activities such as standing and walking. Most patients will indicate that they have experienced a dramatic reduction in their ability to walk without pain. Frequently, the patient will have resorted to the use

TABLE 2. INDICATIONS FOR REVISION TOTAL HIP ARTHROPLASTY
Pain
Loosening
Recurrent dislocation
Excessive heterotopic bone formation
Massive progressive osteolysis
Infection

of a cane or crutch when walking. Patients will describe pain that is severe during the first few steps with weight-bearing activities and then subsides after 10 or so steps only to recur while walking a variable distance. Putting on or removing socks and shoes, climbing stairs, and rising from a chair are usually painful for patients who have aseptic loosening of a total hip arthroplasty.

Occasionally, the lysis of bone associated with debris particles generated by a total hip arthroplasty prosthesis will create excessive destruction of the osseous tissue. This can be appreciated when repeat radiographs are performed on a regular basis. When progressive destruction of bone is appreciated from such radiographic analysis, a surgeon will sometimes suggest early surgical intervention even though the patient is not experiencing significant pain. Such advice is based on the premise that earlier surgical intervention will permit the revision total hip arthroplasty to be performed with a less drastic surgical procedure.

CONTRAINDICATIONS

Once it is established that a patient has a symptom-producing loosened femoral component, a frank discussion of the risks and benefits of surgery should take place. Patients who have significant associated medical conditions may find that the risk of surgery outweighs the potential for relief of pain that can be anticipated with revision surgery. Other patients may decide to postpone surgery if the pain they are experiencing is insufficient to warrant a major surgical procedure.

PROCEDURES

PREOPERATIVE PLANNING

The first step in preoperative planning is thorough assessment of the patient, including examination of the patient's surgical scars from previous incisions, the neurovascular status of the extremity, leg length discrepancy, and abductor function. Radiographs with a 100-mm marker should be performed to determine the extent of bone loss from the proximal femur and widening of the femur at the isthmus. The extent of bone loss influences implant selection. A sense of the quality of bone in the proximal femur can also be obtained from these radiographs.

It is prudent to have several options available because there are often unexpected intraoperative events, such as fracture or discovery of unanticipated extensive bone loss, which render the original plan for reconstruction of the femoral component inappropriate. Two important aspects to consider in planning are (1) how to remove the failed implant along with any polymethylmethacrylate and (2) the length of the revision stem that will be necessary to bypass areas of osteolysis or other defects that serve as stress risers that can contribute to postoperative femoral fracture. All these factors will have an impact on the choice of the optimal operative approach.

SURGICAL APPROACHES

A number of surgical approaches exist.[25-29] The one chosen for an individual patient will depend on several factors:

Previous approaches to the hip.
Overall surgical objectives.

Specific needs of the femur (the need to remove cement or a well-fixed implant with proximal or distal porous coating, extent and quality of trochanteric bone, existing soft-tissue tension).
Bone graft requirements.
The surgeon's experience.

No single approach can satisfy the requirements of all femoral component revisions, and each operation should be individualized on the basis of its specific objectives. Inadequate exposure at revision total hip arthroplasty can be frustrating and often leads to complications. In general, the patient should be positioned in a such a way as to allow extended exposure of the pelvis and femur without movement of the pelvis, which can lead to loss of orientation of acetabular anteversion during surgery. If possible, previous incisions should be used, but not at the cost of compromising the exposure for the revision operation.

The approach selected should allow for proximal extension on to the ilium and distally along the femoral shaft should the need arise. An extensile approach on to the pelvis may be required to minimize bone loss. Extension distally may be required to remove failed or broken femoral components, to remove polymethylmethacrylate, or to manage distal intraoperative femoral fractures. The best approach is the one that provides optimum exposure of the hip joint to facilitate removal of old implants and fulfills the other surgical objectives without compromising host bone or soft tissue.

The approaches for revision of total hip arthroplasty can be divided into three categories[29]:

1. Standard-anterolateral, posterolateral.
2. Trochanteric-transtrochanteric, trochanteric slide, extended trochanteric osteotomy.
3. Complex extensile.

For most patients, an anterolateral or a posterolateral approach will provide adequate exposure to meet the surgical objectives. More complicated and complex approaches may be necessary for patients who have distally fixed, extensively porous coated femoral components or securely fixed, distal polymethylmethacrylate. Standard approaches (e.g., anterolateral or posterolateral) are adequate for patients who have a loose femoral component that will be relatively easy to remove. The basic advantage of the posterolateral approach is that the abductor mechanism is not compromised. If necessary, the posterior approach can be converted intraoperatively to a transtrochanteric or extended trochanteric osteotomy.

The transtrochanteric approach (Fig. 3) is used for more difficult revisions. The traditional trochanteric osteotomy retains the gluteus medius and minimus attachments and requires that the osteotomized trochanteric fragment be reattached to the proximal femur. In patients who have considerable proximal femur bone loss or well-fixed, proximal, coated, porous femoral components, there is no trochanteric bed or proximal femur to which the trochanteric fragment can be attached. This leads to trochanteric nonunion and a postoperative limp with or without pain.[26] The trochanteric slide (Fig. 4) was developed to allow the gluteus medius and minimus attachments as well as the attachment of the vastus lateralis to remain in continuity, pre-

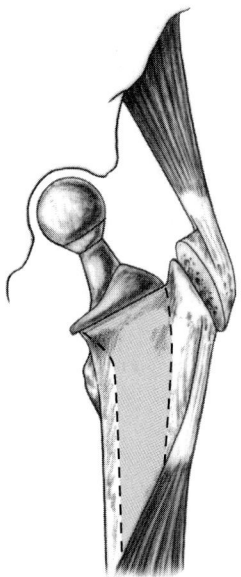

Fig. 3. Transtrochanteric osteotomy.

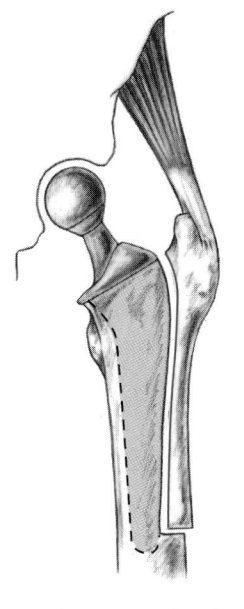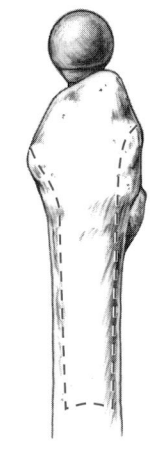

Anteroposterior view   Lateral view

Fig. 5. Extended trochanteric osteotomy. The length of the extended osteotomy varies based on the specific goals. This type of surgical exposure allows access to well-fixed long-stem femoral implant or a well-fixed distal cement mantle.

cluding proximal migration of the trochanteric fragment with the gluteus medius and the gluteus minimus attached.[28] The extended trochanteric osteotomy (Fig. 5) provides greater access to the femur and is especially helpful for removal of well-fixed implants or distal polymethylmethacrylate.[25] Because the extended trochanteric osteotomy creates a larger fragment, it allows for increased surface area of contact between the fragment and the proximal femur, decreasing the incidence of trochanteric nonunion. The trochanteric fragment created by an extended trochanteric osteotomy must be manipulated intraoperatively with great care to avoid a fracture of the trochanteric fragment.

Any transtrochanteric approach requires careful secure fixation of the osteotomized trochanter to the femur using multiple circumferential wires or cables. Initial secure fixation is essential to minimize the incidence of "trochanter problems," such as fragmentation, nonunion, proximal displacement, and abductor insufficiency. Special trochanter gripping devices may be of value.

IMPLANT REMOVAL

The loosened or fractured femoral component must be extracted from the femur with as little damage as possible to the femur and its soft tissues and minimal disruption of the vascular supply. Polymethylmethacrylate can be removed with osteotomes, high-speed cutting drills, or ultrasonic cutting instruments. Each has advantages and disadvantages, depending on the location of the polymethylmethacrylate and the degree of fixation to the femur. As mentioned, preoperative planning should take into account this portion of the operation to ensure that the proper instruments are available. For cemented components, a wide variety of equipment is necessary to remove the implant along with all residual polymethylmethacrylate. With the use of a flexible light source allowing visualization within the depths of the femoral canal, a pituitary rongeur (e.g., Ferris Smith) within a narrow femoral canal can help remove small pieces of polymethylmethacrylate and debris. If the cement mantle is well fixed, specialized cement removal equipment such as back-cutting osteotomes, high-speed burs, and ultrasonic cement cutting instruments are invaluable.[30] If the distal cement mantle is well fixed, a cortical window or an extended trochanteric osteotomy is useful to provide further exposure. However, an extended trochanteric osteotomy presumes that this possibility was planned preoperatively and was incorporated into the initial

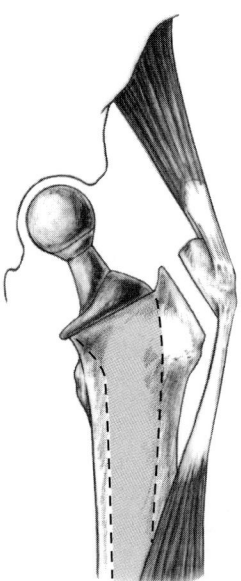

Fig. 4. Trochanteric slide osteotomy. The trochanter with attached musculature is displaced anteriorly or posteriorly to gain surgical exposure.

exposure, because it is not possible to convert most surgical exposures of the hip to an extended trochanteric osteotomy midway through the exposure.

Flexible osteotomes and powered instruments (greater than 2000 rpm) that have needle-tip cutting tools are useful for removal of well-fixed, proximal, porous coated femoral components. An extended trochanteric osteotomy is essential for the removal of extensively porous coated femoral components. Furthermore, it may be necessary to cut the femoral component into segments to minimize destruction of the femur during removal of a femoral component.

MANAGEMENT OPTIONS

After removal of the femoral component, residual polymethylmethacrylate, and debris, the next task is to restore the integrity of the femur. This may involve use of cancellous allograft chips to fill defects with structurally intact femoral cortices. Alternatively, femurs with large cortical defects that weaken the femur may require cortical strut allografts secured with wire, cables, or other fastening devices to restore the structural integrity and the biomechanical strength of the femur.

The optimum implant design and mode of fixation for revision total hip arthroplasty remain controversial. Treatment options should be individualized and largely depend on the following:

Quality of the host bone.
Activity level of the patient.
Resources available.
Experience of the treating surgeon.

The American Academy of Orthopaedic Surgeons (AAOS) Committee on the Hip has provided some general guidelines for treatment based on the classification of femoral bone loss[31, 32] (Table 3). Paprosky et al[33] also developed a very helpful classification scheme for femoral component revision (Table 4). The extent of bone loss noted on preoperative radiographs may not reflect the actual bone deficiency encountered intraoperatively during removal of the primary implant and polymethylmethacrylate. Thus, as

TABLE 4. CLASSIFICATION SCHEME FOR FEMORAL COMPONENT REVISION DEVELOPED BY PAPROSKY ET AL

Type	Description
1	Minimal metaphyseal and diaphyseal bone loss
2A	Absent calcar extending just below the intertrochanteric level
2B	Anterolateral metaphyseal bone loss
2C	Absent calcar with posteromedial metaphyseal bone loss
3A	2A plus diaphyseal bone loss
3B	2B plus diaphyseal bone loss
3C	2C plus diaphyseal bone loss

mentioned, it is important to have more than one plan available to address unforeseen circumstances that may be encountered during surgery (such as a femoral fracture). The component chosen for implantation during a revision total hip arthroplasty varies depending on the specific situation (Fig. 6). Choices include the following:

A standard cemented femoral component.
A cemented long-stem femoral component.
An extensively coated femoral component.
An impacted morselized cancellous graft followed by a cemented, tapered femoral component.
Structural allografts with a long-stem femoral component.
A calcar replacement femoral component.
A modular femoral component.
An allograft-prosthetic composite.
A segmental replacement (tumor-type) prosthesis.

TECHNICAL DETAILS

Reconstruction of the femur with a long-stem fully porous coated femoral component, after removal of the femoral component and residual polymethylmethacrylate, is composed of three stages:

1. Preparation of the proximal and distal femur.
2. Establishing the compatibility of the selected implant size and the femur as well as restoration of leg length equality through reduction with a trial femoral component.
3. Insertion of the final revision component.

Reconstruction of the femur is initiated with reaming of the isthmus of the femur to accommodate the stem portion of the femoral component. The isthmus of the femur is reamed to allow passage of the component without fracture of the femur. The proximal femur is broached to accept the selected size (based on the preoperative radiographs). If loss of the calcar femorale has occurred, a long-stem, fully porous coated femoral component with a calcar replacement can be used to compensate for the bone loss.

A trial femoral component of the length and size determined by the preoperative radiographs is inserted. It should pass smoothly without force. A trial reduction is performed with an appropriately sized trial femoral head to match the acetabular articular surface (22, 26, 28, or 32 mm). The neck length of the trial femoral head can be altered to

TABLE 3. AAOS CLASSIFICATION OF FEMORAL DEFECTS IN REVISION TOTAL HIP ARTHROPLASTY

Segmental
  Proximal
    Partial
      Complete
    Intercalary
    Greater trochanter
Segmental
  Cancellous
  Cortical
  Ectasia
Combined segmental and cavitary
  Malalignment
    Rotational
    Angular
  Stenosis
  Discontinuity

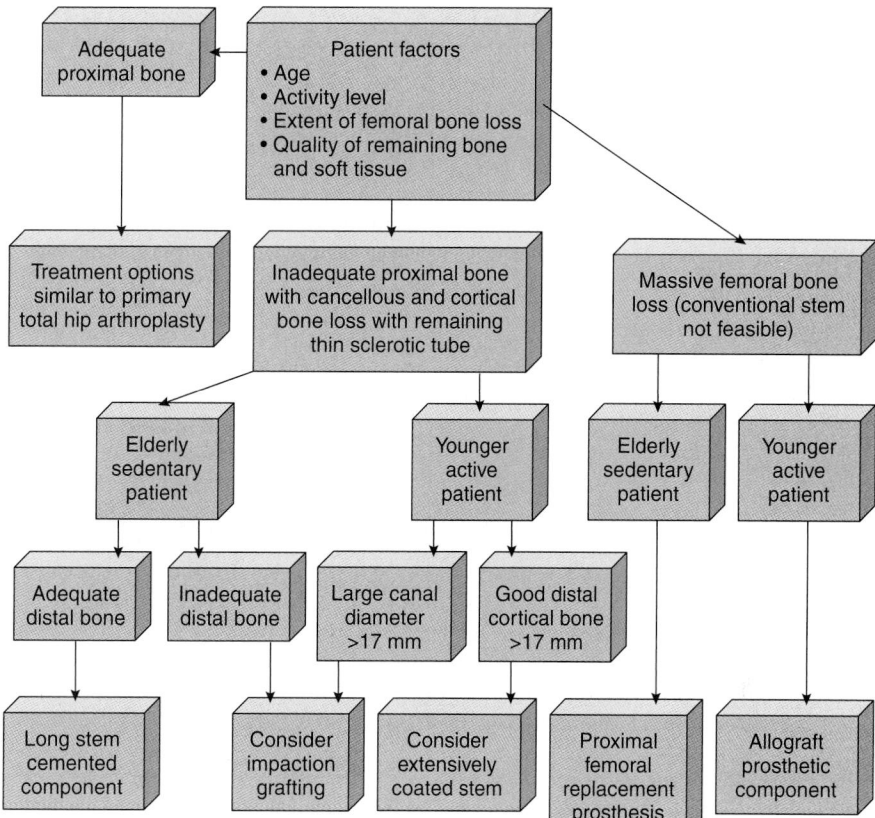

Fig. 6. Decision-making guidelines for choosing management options for femoral component revision.

correct leg length inequality as determined by the distance from a pin inserted in the supra-acetabular region (inserted before dislocation of the hip and removal of the loosened femoral component) and a fixed point on the proximal femur (a small score on the femur). If the extremity was 2 cm short, based on the preoperative examination, the femoral component and adjustment of the femoral head and neck should permit the leg to be lengthened 2 cm. If the hip is stable and leg length has been restored, the hip is dislocated and the trial components are removed.

The final revision long-stem, fully porous coated femoral component is then inserted. Because it is larger in diameter than the trial component, it will require blows with a mallet to insert. A second trial reduction with the trial femoral head and neck component is performed to ensure stability and restoration of correct leg length. Once the latter has been confirmed, the final revision femoral head and neck are applied to a cleaned Morse taper on the proximal aspect of the femoral component. The hip is reduced one final time, and stability is checked with flexion, adduction, and external rotation. The hip should also be checked in extension and external rotation. The trochanteric fragment is reattached using the technique previously described. The fascia, subcutaneous fat, and skin are closed in routine fashion with interrupted sutures.

POSTOPERATIVE MANAGEMENT

In general, postoperative management of a femoral revision hip arthroplasty is similar to that of a primary total hip arthroplasty. However, although the potential complications of femoral revision hip arthroplasty are similar to those of primary hip arthroplasty, these complications are, in general, much more frequent after a femoral revision operation. Management after a femoral revision hip arthroplasty should, therefore, differ from postoperative management of primary hip arthroplasty to minimize these complications.

If the femoral component hip revision operation consisted of cementing a conventional femoral component, assuming that secure fixation was achieved, the postoperative management need not differ from that of primary hip arthroplasty. However, if the femoral component revision included a trochanteric osteotomy, insertion of a cementless femoral component, or an intraoperative fracture of the femur, prolonged postoperative protected weightbearing is desirable. This will minimize the likelihood of trochanteric complications, improve the probability of tissue ingrowth that will secure the femoral component, and allow union of a femoral-shaft fracture, if present.

Because there is an increased incidence of infection after femoral revision hip arthroplasty, it may be wise to administer prophylactic antibiotics until the results of all of the surgical tissue specimens submitted to the microbiology laboratory are known. Heterotopic bone formation is generally more common and more marked in femoral revision hip arthroplasty than in primary hip arthroplasty; it is, therefore, wise to administer effective heterotopic bone formation prophylaxis, such as diphosphonates, nonsteroidal anti-inflammatory drugs, or low-dose local radiation therapy (800 to 2100 Gy) beginning within 5 days of the revision operation in high-risk patients.[34]

COMPLICATIONS AND RESULTS

COMPLICATIONS

Although complications associated with femoral component revision of a total hip arthroplasty are qualitatively the same as those with a primary hip arthroplasty, their frequency is generally greater after a femoral revision of a total hip arthroplasty than after primary hip arthroplasty.[34] Complications that can occur include the following:

Thromboembolism.
Heterotopic bone formation.
Abductor insufficiency limp.
Repeat loosening failure.
Intraoperative femur fracture.
Dislocation.
Infection.
Neurovascular injury.

Although infection and neurovascular complications are by far the least frequent complications, they are certainly the most devastating. The incidence of dislocation after revision total hip arthroplasty can be high. Meticulous attention to component position, soft-tissue tension, abductor mechanism repair, and avoidance of impingement should be considered to minimize the incidence of dislocation.

Periprosthetic Femoral Fractures

Periprosthetic femoral fractures after revision hip arthroplasty can occur intraoperatively at implant and cement mantle removal or during broaching or insertion of the final implant. At the Mayo Clinic, between 1989 and 1993, the second leading cause of revision total hip arthroplasty behind aseptic loosening was fracture.[35] The highest incidence of periprosthetic femoral fractures at revision hip

arthroplasty have been reported with the use of a proximally coated, large-diameter metaphyseal filling implant.[36, 37] Fractures can also occur around a loose implant secondary to the osteolytic process. Periprosthetic fractures about the femur have been classified by the location of the fracture with respect to the stem. According to the Vancouver classification system, type A fractures are proximal fractures around the trochanters, type B are fractures extending to the tip of the stem, and type C are fractures distal to the stem.[38] The classification is further subdivided into type B1 if the stem is stable, B2 if the stem is loose, and B3 in cases of significant bone loss. The management of periprosthetic femoral fractures in large part depends on the stability of the existing implant, location of the fracture, and quality of the host bone. In general, if the implant remains well fixed, then the fracture can be treated with internal fixation either with cerclage wires, cortical strut grafts, or with plate fixation. If the implant is loose, then the fracture should be bypassed with a long-stem implant. In these difficult cases, internal fixation is also usually necessary (Fig. 7).

RESULTS
Cemented Femoral Component Revision

The 7- to 10-year results of cemented femoral component revisions demonstrated failure rates of 9% to 29% and radiographic evidence of probable loosening as high as 44%.[1–7] Furthermore, the strength of the bone-cement interface is lower for revision than for a primary cemented hip replacement.[39] The most likely reason for the generally less than satisfactory results of cemented femoral component revision is the limited cancellous bone available for interdigitation. Despite this, it is still a viable alternative, especially in the elderly. Indeed, a 6.7% revision rate and a

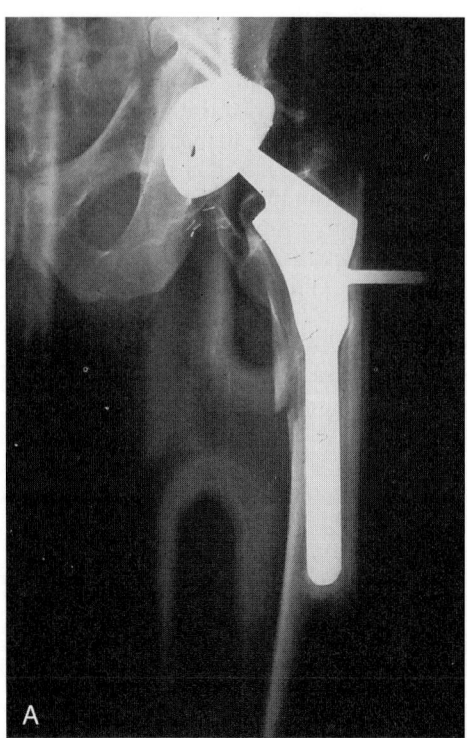
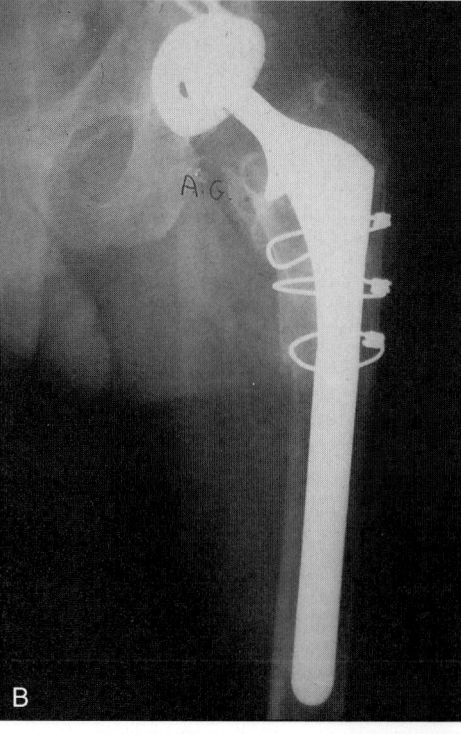

Fig. 7. Periprosthetic femoral fracture. Anteroposterior views of 62-year-old patient who had a periprosthetic fracture and loose femoral component *(A)* whose extensively coated revision implant was stable at 4-year follow-up *(B)*.

20% loosening rate have been reported in a group of elderly patients (60 hips, mean follow-up of 8.9 years).[3] Using improved cementing techniques, Katz et al[10] reviewed 47 hips at a minimum 10-year follow-up and reported a radiographic failure rate of 26%. At an average follow-up of 15 years, Mulroy and Harris[11] reported a 26% failure rate in 43 patients who underwent femoral component revision using second-generation cementing techniques.

Proximal Porous Coated Implants

Although they were developed in an attempt to improve on the results of cemented femoral component revisions, proximal porous coated femoral components have not achieved results that surpass those of cemented revisions. Failure rates as high as 20% have been reported at a relatively short-term follow-up.[36, 37, 40] Berry et al[36] reviewed the Mayo Clinic experience of 375 consecutive proximal coated femoral components and reported a failure rate of 20% (mean follow-up of 4.7 years) and an intraoperative fracture incidence of 26% (Table 5). Modular, proximally porous coated implants have been used in femoral component revisions with some success.[41, 42] Proximally porous coated femoral implants have been unsatisfactory at short-term follow-up because proximal ingrowth can be difficult and unpredictable in the compromised host proximal femur.[37] In general, proximal porous coated femoral components should be used only when there is adequate bone available in the proximal femur to provide implant stability and predictable ingrowth.

Extensively Coated Implants

A failure rate of 11% in 83 hips undergoing femoral component revision with an extensively coated stem has been reported (mean follow-up of 9 years).[43] The major concern with extensively coated stems is the potential for proximal stress shielding.[43–46] Extensively coated stems can also be extremely difficult to remove should the need arise. However, Paprosky's group[44] has reported excellent long-term results (see Table 5) using an extensively porous coated curved stem that achieves distal fixation. Moreland and Bernstein[45] reviewed 165 patients treated with an extensively coated stem with an average follow-up of 5 years and reported a 4% failure rate. They also expressed concern over the extent of severe stress shielding in certain patients and did not recommend this technique in patients with osteoporosis or large canal diameters. The results of extensively coated stems have been superior to those of cemented long stems and proximally coated uncemented stems in patients undergoing revision total hip arthroplasty. Extensively coated stems that provide distal fixation are also useful in cases of periprosthetic femoral fractures when a long-stem implant is needed to bypass the fracture line and when the proximal femoral bone is compromised and distal fixation is a more predictable option (see Fig. 7).

Impacted Morselized Cancellous Allograft

Gie et al[47] reported an alternative method to restore lost proximal bone by using impacted cancellous allograft and cement. Their technique of femoral component revision relies on rigid impaction of morselized allograft followed by cementing of a collarless, polished, tapered stem into the cancellous bed (Fig. 8). In Elting's[48] report on 60 patients treated with impaction grafting with a 2- to 5-year follow-up, 48% of patients experienced an average of 2 to 8 mm of femoral component subsidence. There were no cases of femoral component loosening. The overall revision rate was 10%; three cases of revision were due to fracture

| | | | Failed Revisions That |
Variable	No. Hips	Average Follow-Up (Years)	Required Further Revision (%)
Cemented Components			
Marti et al (1990)[3]	60	8.9	6.7
Pierson and Harris (1994)[9]	46	8.8	7.0
Smith and Harris (1997)[12]	52	10–13	2.0
Katz et al (1995)[10]	47	10	26
Mulroy and Harris (1996)[11]	43	15	26
Uncemented Components			
Proximal porous coated			
Malkani et al (1996)[37]	69	3	9.0
Cameron (1997)[41]	62	2.6	16.1
Woolson and Delaney (1995)[40]	25	5.5	20.0
Berry et al (1995)[36]	375	4.7	20.0
Extensively coated			
Lawrence et al (1993)[46]	174	5	4.6
Aribindi (1998)[44]	287	5–10	2.0
Moreland and Bernstein (1995)[45]	165	5	4.0
Impaction Grafting			
Gie et al (1993)[47]	56	2.5	4.0
Elting et al (1995)[48]	60	2–5	10.0

TABLE 5. RESULTS OF FEMORAL COMPONENT REVISION

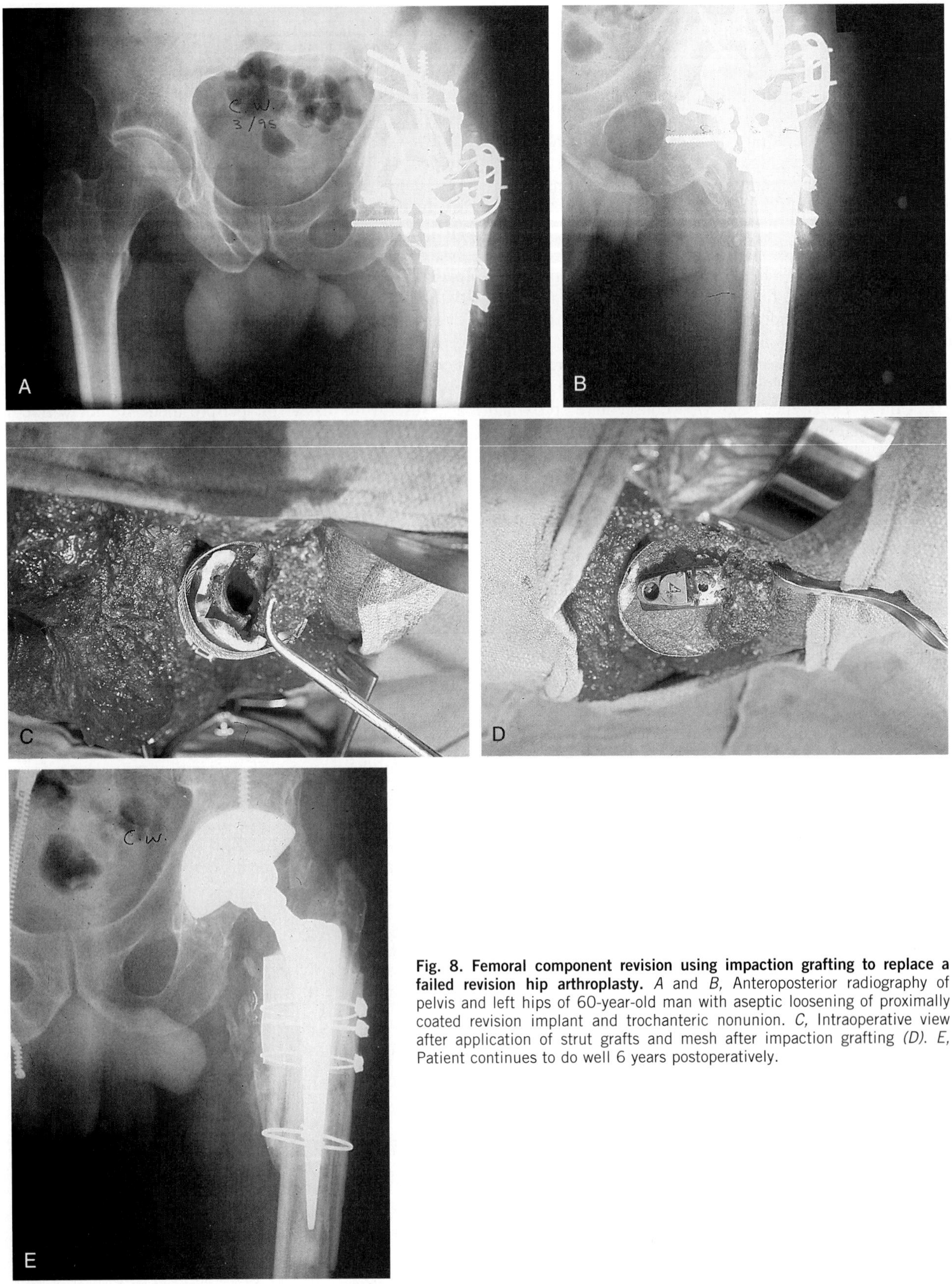

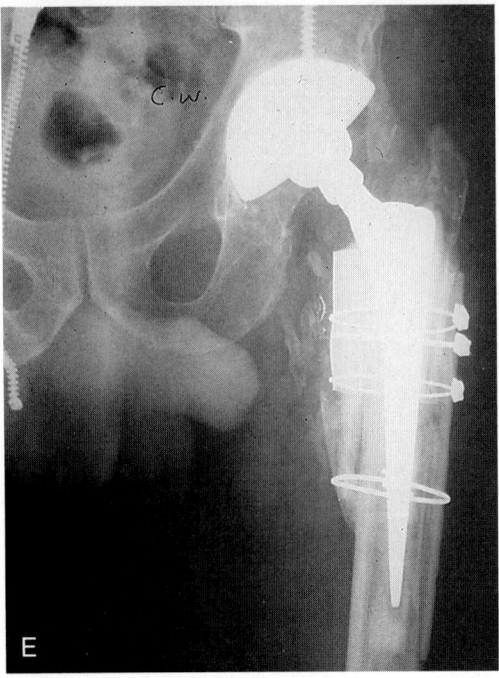

Fig. 8. Femoral component revision using impaction grafting to replace a failed revision hip arthroplasty. *A* and *B*, Anteroposterior radiography of pelvis and left hips of 60-year-old man with aseptic loosening of proximally coated revision implant and trochanteric nonunion. *C*, Intraoperative view after application of strut grafts and mesh after impaction grafting *(D)*. *E*, Patient continues to do well 6 years postoperatively.

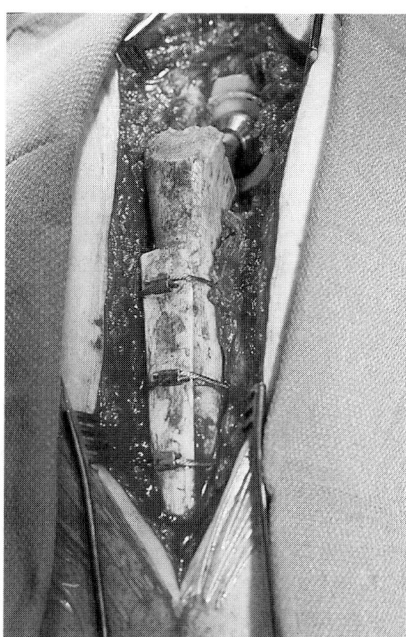

Fig. 9. Allograft prosthetic composite with cortical strut graft overlying allograft-host junction. This is an intraoperative view.

and three patients required acetabular revision (see Table 5). Knight and Helming[49] reviewed 31 consecutive patients undergoing femoral component revision using impaction revision with a collarless polished tapered stem. Their incidence of intraoperative fracture was 16% in this difficult patient population. Difficulty with the surgical technique was encountered in 94% of the patients and was associated with varus or valgus malalignment. The authors endorsed this type of reconstructive procedure and recommended improvement in the surgical technique of impaction grafting. Nelissen et al[50] obtained biopsy samples of four patients requiring secondary procedures after impaction grafting. They were able to demonstrate bone remodeling and partial restoration of bone stock. Masterson et al,[51] in their multicenter study, expressed concern over the variable and at times deficient cement mantle noted with this type of reconstruction technique.

In a cadaveric model, Malkani et al[52] reported similar rates of femoral component subsidence and torsion to failure when they compared a primary cemented implant with the same stem in a revision model using impacted morselized cancellous allograft. The indications for impaction grafting are still evolving. Controversy exists regarding the ideal implant design and the stem surface finish. There is a risk of intraoperative femoral fracture with impaction grafting, but this can be minimized with careful attention to surgical technique and, in certain cases, by using cortical strut grafts and cerclage wires to minimize hoop stress. Cortical strut grafts have been used with success to restore the integrity of the proximal femur at revision total hip arthroplasty.[53, 54] A 98% union rate has been reported using cortical strut grafts in 106 patients, with an average time to union of 7.3 months.[55]

Allograft Prosthetic Composites

In cases of massive proximal femoral bone loss that cannot be salvaged with standard prosthetic components, allograft prosthetic composites or bioimplants are alternatives (Fig. 9). These are essentially salvage procedures with high risks, mainly indicated when alternatives such as resection arthroplasty are not acceptable to the patient with massive proximal femoral bone loss. An 80% success rate has been reported in 186 patients who had a proximal femoral allograft (mean follow-up of 4 years).[56] The femoral implant is fixed to the allograft proximal femur with cement and, if possible, press fit into the host bone distally. The host-allograft junction can be secured with either plates or cortical strut grafts as needed. It is advisable to avoid placing screws in the allograft because this may contribute to fracture as the allograft resorbs. The complication rates for allograft prosthetic composites are high, especially those of dislocation, infection, and nonunion at the host-allograft junction.[56–58] Frequently, a hip spica cast or an abduction orthosis is necessary postoperatively to minimize the incidence of dislocation.

Segmental Femoral Replacement Prosthesis

The segmental femoral replacement prosthesis is of limited use in revision hip arthroplasty. Survival in patients after revision total hip arthroplasty has been reported to be 81% at 11 years.[59] The incidence of dislocation approaches 20%, similar to the rate for allograft prosthetic composites. Use of this procedure should be limited to elderly patients who have massive proximal femoral bone loss and a sedentary lifestyle and who prefer greater hip function than that achieved with resection arthroplasty, which has significant limitations. It is more commonly used after reconstruction following tumor surgery (Fig. 10).

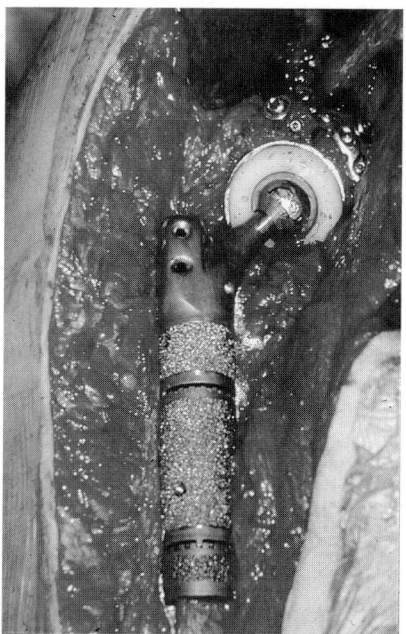

Fig. 10. Segmental replacement prosthesis (tumor-type implant) for massive proximal femoral bone loss in an elderly patient. This is an intraoperative view.

REFERENCES

1. Estok DM, Harris WH: Long-term results of cemented femoral revision surgery using second-generation techniques: An average 11.7 year follow-up evaluation. Clin Orthop 1994; 299:190.

2. Kavanagh BF, Ilstrup DM, Fitzgerald RH: Revision total hip arthroplasty. J Bone Joint Surg Am 1985; 67:517.

3. Marti RK, Schüller HM, Besselaar PP, et al: Results of revision hip arthroplasty with cement. J Bone Joint Surg Am 1990; 72:346.

4. Pellicci PM, Wilson PD Jr, Sledge CB, et al: Long-term results of revision total hip replacement. J Bone Joint Surg Am 1985; 67:513.

5. Pellicci PM, Wilson PD Jr, Sledge CB, et al: Revision total hip arthroplasty. Clin Orthop 1982; 170:34.

6. Callaghan JJ, Salvati EA, Pellicci PM, et al: Results of revision for mechanical failure after cemented total hip replacement. J Bone Joint Surg Am 1985; 67:1074.

7. Turner RH, Mattingly DA, Scheller A: Femoral revision total hip arthroplasty using a long-stem femoral component: Clinical and radiographic analysis. J Arthroplasty 1987; 2:247.

8. Rubash HE, Harris WH: Revision of nonseptic, loose, cemented femoral components using modern cementing techniques. J Arthroplasty 1988; 3:241.

9. Pierson JL, Harris WH: Cemented revision for femoral osteolysis in cemented arthroplasties: Results in 29 hips after a mean 8.5-year follow-up. J Bone Joint Surg Br 1994; 76:40.

10. Katz RP, Callaghan JJ, Sullivan PM, et al: Results of cemented femoral revision total hip arthroplasty using improved cementing techniques. Clin Orthop 1995; 319:178.

11. Mulroy WF, Harris WH: Revision total hip arthroplasty with use of so-called second-generation cementing techniques for aseptic loosening of the femoral component. A fifteen-year-average follow up study. J Bone Joint Surg Am 1996; 78:325.

12. Smith SE, Harris WH: Total hip arthroplasty performed with insertion of the component with cement and acetabular component without cement. J Bone Joint Surg Am 1997; 79:1827.

13. Willert HG, Bertram H, Buchhorn GH: Osteolysis in alloarthroplasty of the hip. The role of bone cement fragmentation. Clin Orthop 1990; 258:108.

14. Santavirta S, Konttinen YT, Bergroth V, et al: Aggressive granulomatous lesions associated with hip arthroplasty. Immunopathologic studies. J Bone Joint Surg Am 1990; 72:252.

15. Appel AM, Sowder WG, Siverhus SW, et al: Prosthesis-associated pseudomembrane-induced bone resorption. Br J Rheumatol 1990; 29:32.

16. Jasty M, Maloney WJ, Brogden CR, et al: The initiation of failure in cemented femoral components of hip arthroplasties. J Bone Joint Surg Br 1993; 73:551.

17. Goldring SR, Schiller AL, Roelke MS, et al: The synovial-like membrane at the bone-cement interface in loose total hip replacements and its purposed role in bone lysis. J Bone Joint Surg Am 1983; 65:575.

18. Jiranek WA, Machado M, Jasty M, et al: Production of cytokines around loosened cemented acetabular components: Analysis with immunohistological techniques and insight to hybridization. J Bone Joint Surg Am 1993; 75:863.

19. Gruen TA, McNeice GM, Amstutz HC: "Modes of failure" of cemented stem-type femoral components. A radiographic analysis of loosening. Clin Orthop 1979; 141:17.

20. Kavanagh B, Fitzgerald RH Jr: Clinical and roentgenographic assessment of total hip arthroplasty: A new hip score. Clin Orthop 1985; 193:133.

21. Engh CA, Massin P, Suthers KE: Roentgenographic assessment of the biologic fixation of porous-surfaced femoral components. Clin Orthop 1990; 257:107.

22. Evans BG, Cutler JM: Evaluation of the painful total hip arthroplasty. Orthop Clin North Am 1992; 23:303.

23. Lieberman JR, Huo MH, Schneider R, et al: Evaluation of painful hip arthroplasties: Are technetium bone scans necessary? J Bone Joint Surg Br 1993; 95:475.

24. Barrack RL, Harris WH: The value of aspiration of the hip joint before revision total hip arthroplasty. J Bone Joint Surg Am 1993; 75:66.

25. Younger TI, Bradford MS, Magnus RE, et al: Extended proximal femoral osteotomy: A new technique for femoral revision arthroplasty. J Arthroplasty 1995; 10:329.

26. Frankel A, Booth RE Jr, Balderston RA, et al: Complications of trochanteric osteotomy: Long-term implications. Clin Orthop 1993; 288:209.

27. Frndak PA, Mallory TH, Lombardy AV Jr: Translateral surgical approach to the hip: The abductor muscle split. Clin Orthop 1993; 295:135.

28. Glassman AH, Engh CA, Bobyn J: A technique of extensile exposure for total hip arthroplasty. J Arthroplasty 1987; 2:11.

29. McCrory BJ, Harris WH: Trochanteric osteotomy for total hip arthroplasty: Six variations and indications. J Am Acad Orthop Surg 1997; 4:248.

30. Klapper RC, Cailloutte JT, Callaghan JJ, et al: Ultrasonic technology in revision total joints. Clin Orthop 1992; 285:147.

31. D'Antonio JA: Classification and management of acetabular abnormalities in total hip arthroplasty. Clin Orthop 1989; 243:126.

32. D'Antonio JA, McCarthy JC, Bargar WL, et al: Classification of femoral abnormalities in total hip arthroplasty. Clin Orthop 1993; 296:133.

33. Paprosky WG, Lawrence WJ, Cameron H: Femoral defect classification: Clinical application. Orthop Rev Suppl 1990; 16:9.

34. Vaughn BK: Other complications of total hip arthroplasty. In Callahan JJ, Dennis DA, Paprosky WG, et al (eds): OKU Hip and Knee Reconstruction. Rosemont, IL, American Academy of Orthopaedic Surgeons.

35. Lewallen DG, Berry DJ: Periprosthetic fracture of the femur after total hip arthroplasty. J Bone Joint Surg Am 1997; 79:1881.

36. Berry DJ, Harmsen WS, Ilstrup D, et al: Survivorship of uncemented proximally porous coated femoral components in revision total hip arthroplasty. Clin Orthop 1995; 319:168.

37. Malkani AL, Lewallen DG, Cabanela ME, et al: Femoral component revision using an uncemented, proximally coated, long-stem prosthesis. J Arthroplasty 1996; 11:411.

38. Duncan CP, Masri BA: Fractures of the femur after hip replacement. In Instructional Course Lectures. Rosemont, IL, American Academy of Orthopaedic Surgeons, 1995, vol 44, p 293.

39. Dohmae Y, Bechtold JE, Sherman RE, et al: Reduction in cement-bone interface shear strength between primary and revision arthroplasty. Clin Orthop 1988; 236:214.

40. Woolson MD, Delaney TJ: Failure of a proximally porous-coated femoral prosthesis in revision total hip arthroplasty. J Arthroplasty 1995; 10(suppl):S22.

41. Cameron H: Experience with proximal ingrowth implantation in hip revision surgery. Acta Orthop Belg 1997; 63(suppl 1):66.

42. Chandler HP, Ayres DK, Tan RC, et al: Revision total hip replacement using the S-ROM femoral component. Clin Orthop 1995; 319:130.

43. Engh CA, Glassman AH, Griffin WL, et al: Results of cementless revision for failed cemented total hip arthroplasty. Clin Orthop 1988; 235:91.

44. Aribindi R, Barba M, Solomon MI, et al: Bypass fixation. Orthop Clin North Am 1998; 29:319.

45. Moreland JR, Bernstein ML: Femoral revision hip arthroplasty with uncemented, porous-coated stems. Clin Orthop 1995; 319:141.

46. Lawrence JM, Engh CA, Macalino GE: Revision total hip arthroplasty: Long-term results without cement. Orthop Clin North Am 1993; 24:635.

47. Gie GA, Linder L, Ling RSM, et al: Impacted cancellous allografts and cement for revision total hip arthroplasty. J Bone Joint Surg Br 1993; 75:14.

48. Elting JJ, Zicat BA, Mikhail WEM, et al: Impaction grafting: Preliminary report of a new method for exchange femoral arthroplasty. Orthopedics 1995; 18:107.

49. Knight JL, Helming C: Collarless polished tapered impaction grafting of the femur during revision total hip arthroplasty. J Arthroplasty 2000; 15:159.

50. Nelissen RGHH, Bauer TW, Weidenhielm DS, et al: Revision hip arthroplasty with the use of cement and impaction grafting. Histological analysis of four cases. J Bone Joint Surg Am 1995; 77:412.

51. Masterson EL, Masri BA, Duncan CP, et al: The cement mantle in femoral impaction allografting. J Bone Joint Surg Br 1997; 79:908.

52. Malkani AL, Voor MJ, Fee KA, et al: Femoral component revision using im-

pacted morselized cancellous graft: A bio-mechanical study of implant stability. J Bone Joint Surg Br 1996; 78:973.

53. Pak JH, Paprosky WG, Jablonsky WS, et al: Femoral strut allografts in cementless revision total hip arthroplasty. Clin Orthop 1993; 295:172.

54. Head WC, Wagner RA, Emerson RH, et al: Restoration of femoral bone stock in revision total hip arthroplasty. Orthop Clin North Am 1993; 24:697.

55. Emerson RH Jr, Malinin PI, Cuellar AD, et al: Cortical strut allograft in reconstruc-tion of the femur and revision total hip arthroplasty. Clin Orthop 1992; 285:35.

56. Allan DG, Lavoie GJ, McDonald S, et al: Proximal femoral allografts in revision hip arthroplasty. J Bone Joint Surg Br 1991; 73:235.

57. Gross AE, Allan DG, Lavoie GJ, et al: Revision arthroplasty of the proximal fe-mur using allograft bone. Orthop Clin North Am 1993; 24:7705.

58. Gross AE, Hutchison CR: Proximal femo-ral allografts for reconstruction of bone stock in revision arthroplasty of the hip. Orthop Clin North Am 1998; 29:313.

59. Malkani AL, Simm FH, Chao EY: Custom made segmental femoral replacement pros-theses in revision total hip arthroplasty. Orthop Clin North Am 1993; 24:727.

section 6 chapter 13

REVISION THA: ACETABULUM

Fares S. Haddad, Bassam A. Masri, Donald S. Garbuz, and Clive P. Duncan

Summary

- Revision of the failed acetabular component is a major undertaking that is complicated by loss of bone stock, by a sclerotic bony bed, and by soft tissue scarring and dysfunction. The principles of acetabular reconstruction are to restore the bio-mechanics of the hip, to restore acetabular integ-rity and continuity, to obtain prosthetic contain-ment and sound fixation, and to improve the bone stock.
- Acetabular revision surgery demands careful pre-operative evaluation and planning, a wide expo-sure, educated preoperative and intraoperative decision-making, the ability to assess and classify acetabular defects, and the availability of a range of reconstructive techniques.
- The challenge of reconstituting the acetabulum depends on the degree and type of bone loss.
- The principles of maximizing host bone-implant contact and implant stability have borne fruit with regard to cementless revision.

Despite the excellent results of total hip arthroplasty, an increasing number of hips require revision operations. In contrast to femoral fixation, changes in prosthetic design and improved cementing have not dramatically improved the longevity of acetabular fixation. Long-term studies of cemented total hip replacements uniformly reveal an earlier and higher acetabular failure rate.[1, 2] Acetabular loosening is also a concern with cementless cups, particularly if the components have been in situ for more than 10 years.[3, 4] Acetabular revision surgery is therefore likely to increas-ingly challenge the reconstructive surgeon.

Revision of the acetabular component presents a number of unique problems. These include difficulties with expo-sure and surgical access if the femoral component is sol-idly fixed, difficulties with the assessment and management of bone loss, and difficulties in achieving rigid fixation within a suboptimal bony surface.[5] The aims of acetabular revision include the creation of a stable acetabular bed, secure prosthetic fixation with freedom of orientation, bony

reconstitution, and the restoration of a normal hip center of rotation with acceptable biomechanics. In this chapter, we review the etiological factors, diagnosis, and management of the failed acetabular component, and the available re-constructive options.

PATHOGENESIS

INDICATIONS FOR ACETABULAR REVISION

Common indications for revision arthroplasty include asep-tic loosening of one or both components, periprosthetic infection, recurrent dislocation, polyethylene wear with or without osteolysis, periprosthetic fracture, and exchange at the time of femoral revision for a variety of indications, including malposition, excessive wear, or an excessively large internal diameter (Table 1). All but the first indica-tion may occur in the presence of solidly fixed implants.

Aseptic loosening is the most common cause of long-term failure for both cemented and cementless cups. Inter-vention should be planned before osteolysis and prosthetic movement result in irretrievable bone loss. Because acet-abular failure occurs more frequently than femoral loosening, there are occasions when the socket has to be revised in the presence of a solidly fixed cemented or ingrown femo-ral stem. The femoral component can generally be pre-served in these situations unless a nonmodular component

---

TABLE 1. INDICATIONS FOR ACETABULAR REVISION

Well-Fixed Component
Polyethylene wear
Osteolysis
Infection
Instability at the time of femoral revision
Loose Component
Aseptic loosening of one or both components
Polyethylene wear
Osteolysis
Infection
Instability at the time of femoral revision
Acetabular fracture

shows evidence of damage to the surface of the femoral head, or is malpositioned and requires revision to ensure stability of the hip joint (Fig. 1).

Sepsis may be treated with débridement and component retention if diagnosed in its earliest stages, but in most cases requires removal of the components with either a single-stage revision using antibiotic-loaded cement, or a two-stage reconstruction, particularly if the use of bone graft or cementless prostheses is desirable.[6]

Dislocation may occur secondary to component malposition, inadequate femoral offset, poor soft-tissue tension, poor patient compliance, and for unexplained reasons. Not all cases require revision of the components, and a change of liner, a different femoral head size, or tensioning of the abductors by advancing the greater trochanter may suffice. In some cases, however, the acetabular height or orientation must be changed, or, rarely, a constrained socket may be necessary.

Asymptomatic osteolysis may be seen with solidly ingrown cementless acetabular components.[3, 4, 7, 8] The path of least resistance for wear particles in these cases is through holes in the metal shell and through noningrown areas into the trabecular bone of the ilium, ischium, and pubis. Loosening and symptoms may not become apparent until extensive bony destruction has occurred. If osteolysis is seen in association with a loose cemented or cementless cup, that component should be revised before further bone loss ensues. If there is osteolysis in the presence of a well-fixed cemented cup, the polyethylene liner should be revised, if possible, or the entire cup should be revised if the component is nonmodular, or if the shell is of suboptimal design with a poor locking mechanism. When there is osteolysis around an uncemented cup, treatment will depend on the stability of the cup, its design, and on the degree of osteolysis and whether it is accessible without cup removal. If the socket is ingrown, stable, and of satisfactory design, the liner only may be changed, and any defects grafted at the same time, when technically feasible. If the socket is well fixed, but is nonmodular, or is damaged due to excessive wear or to a broken locking mechanism, it should be revised.

Acetabular fracture may occur intraoperatively during component insertion, postoperatively after trauma, or as a pathological fracture secondary to severe osteolysis. This usually leads to failure of the acetabular component, and requires reconstruction as in other cases of aseptic loosening. The configuration of the defect created by the fracture of these components should be considered. A large cementless component with screw augmentation may be used if there is adequate rim remaining to achieve component stability. Otherwise, a protrusion ring or cage with morselized allograft and fixation of the acetabular component with cement is an alternative. If there is a transverse acetabular fracture or posterior column fracture, fixation with a plate, packing of the fracture site with morselized bone graft, and insertion of a component without cement but with screws usually provides a satisfactory solution if there is otherwise sufficient bone stock. If in addition to the fracture the acetabular bone stock is also deficient, an acetabular reconstruction cage can be used to secure the superior aspect of the hemipelvis to the ischium with a morselized graft at the fracture site and cementing of the acetabular component, in addition to plating of the posterior column.

The revision of a well-fixed acetabular component may also be necessary *at the time of femoral revision.* This is indicated when polyethylene wear or damage is seen with a nonmodular component. It may also be necessary if the orientation of the cup is deemed unsatisfactory at the time of trial reduction, or if a femoral head of the appropriate size is not available.

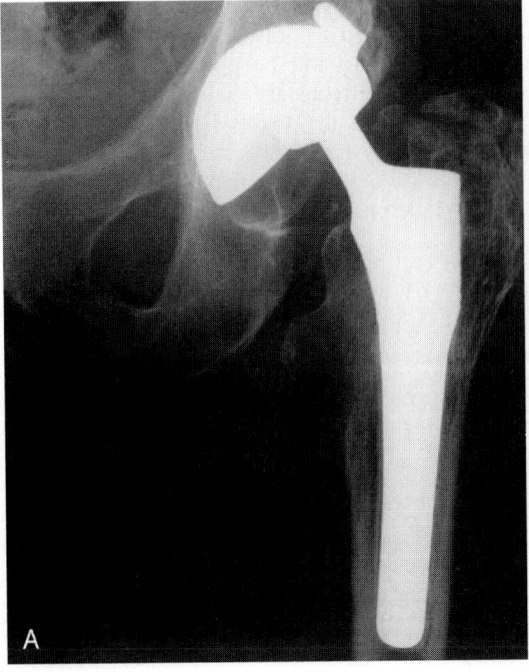
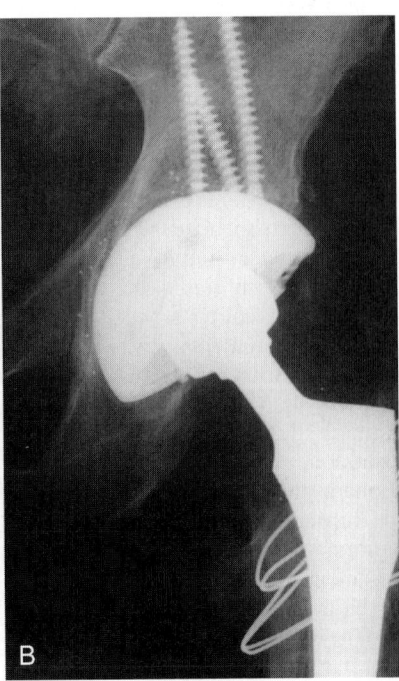

Fig. 1. Polyethylene wear. *A,* Severe polyethylene wear led to metal-on-metal contact, and damage to this well-fixed uncemented acetabular component. *B,* A trochanteric slide allowed wide access, and without revising the femoral stem the acetabular component was carefully removed, and replaced with a cementless hemispheric porouscoated shell. A 28-mm head was used to allow a greater polyethylene thickness in the revision acetabular liner.

INVESTIGATIONS

The diagnosis of acetabular component failure is usually made on the basis of the patient's history in association with a review of serial radiographs. The majority of acetabular revisions are adequately imaged preoperatively with plain radiographs, including anteroposterior, lateral, and Judet's oblique views. The initial radiographic assessment involves an assessment of the nature of existing components, the length and stability of the femoral component, and any migration of the acetabular component. It is often difficult to truly appreciate the type and extent of any bony deficit present on the acetubular side before surgery.

Careful study of the oblique radiographs usually demonstrates the acetabular anatomy sufficiently to characterize the bone deficiency and remaining support for the acetabulum. The posterior column and anterior rim are seen on the iliac oblique radiographs and the anterior column and posterior rim are seen on the obturator radiographs. Particular attention should be paid to the integrity of the acetabular roof, the posterior column, and the medial wall, as they are important contributors to the stability of the acetabulum and are common sites of bone deficiency. The acetabular roof is seen on the anteroposterior radiographs and the obturator oblique radiograph where the anterior and posterior columns converge. Posterior column deficiencies may be seen on the iliac oblique radiograph and by a deficiency of the ilioischial line on the anteroposterior radiograph. If there is a deficiency of the ilioischial line combined with a deficiency of the anterior column, pelvic discontinuity is likely (Fig. 2). Medial wall deficiencies should be suspected when there is a deficiency of the teardrop but may be obscured by an overlying metal-backed cup.

Migration from the original acetabular position indicates bone loss in the direction of failure. If the initial radiographs are unavailable for comparison, the next preferred reference is an anatomically normal contralateral hip. Superior migration from the original or ideal acetabular position is measured from the inferior border of the teardrop. If there is severe medial wall lysis with obliteration of the teardrop, the superomedial border of the obturator foramen is an alternative reference point. Medial or lateral migration is measured from the medial border of the teardrop, if present, or from the ilioischial line.

Additional imaging techniques are occasionally necessary. Computed tomography (CT) has been used to define the medial wall and it may have a particular application when the medial wall is obscured by a metal-backed cup. If a customized acetabular impant or double cup is being considered for reconstruction of a complex pelvic defect, a CT scan may be very useful to define the anatomy and occasionally to manufacture a preoperative foam model of the bone defect.[9, 10] CT can accurately characterize discrete periacetabular deficiencies such as isolated lytic lesions associated with screw holes and fixation screws.

PROCEDURES

THE SURGICAL ANATOMY OF THE ACETABULUM

The hemipelvis can be thought of as an inverted Y with the limbs of the letter Y representing the anterior and posterior columns of the acetabulum.[11] The acetabulum can be divided into four regions: the anterior column, the posterior column, the roof, and the medial wall.

The anterior column extends from the superior pubic ramus to the iliac wing. Radiographically, it is seen best on the obturator oblique view. The iliopectineal line delineates the anterior column on both anteroposterior and Judet's views of the pelvis. Disruption of this line indicates significant bone loss affecting the anterior column.

The posterior column extends from the ischium to the iliac wing. Radiographically, the ilioischial line (Köhler's line) demarcates the posterior column, and disruption of this line indicates significant bone loss affecting the posterior column. Discontinuity or a gap indicates separation of

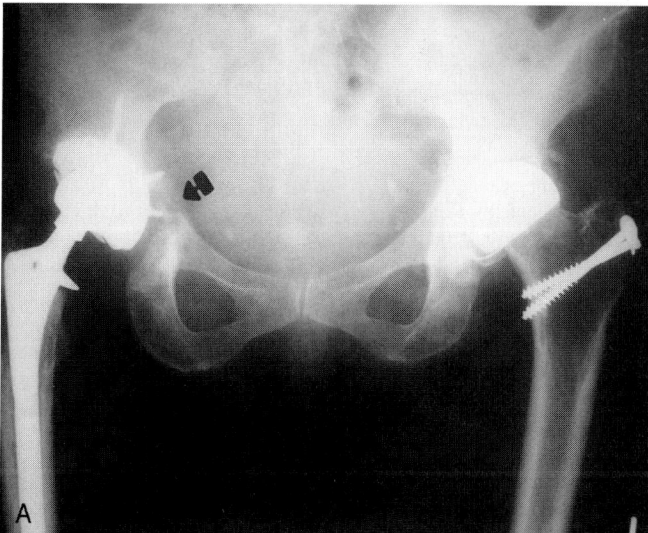
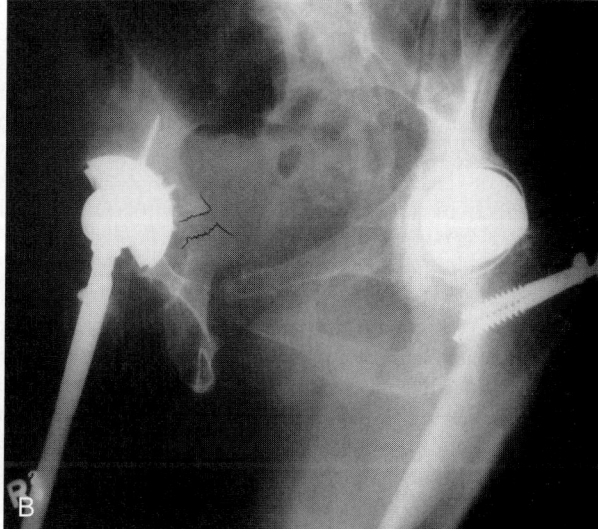

Fig. 2. Pelvic dissociation. Anteroposterior (A) and iliac oblique (B) radiographs demonstrate a pelvic dissociation.

TABLE 2. THE AMERICAN ACADEMY OF ORTHOPAEDIC SURGEONS CLASSIFICATION SYSTEM FOR ACETABULAR DEFICIENCIES IN TOTAL HIP ARTHROPLASTY

Type 1. Segmental deficiencies
      Peripheral
          Superior
          Anterior
          Posterior
      Central (medial wall absent)
Type 2. Cavitary deficiencies
      Peripheral
          Superior
          Anterior
          Posterior
      Central (medial wall intact)
Type 3. Combined deficiencies
Type 4. Pelvic discontinuity
Type 5. Arthrodesis

the upper and lower halves of the pelvis through the acetabulum, a condition known as pelvic discontinuity.

The junction between the anterior and posterior columns and the ilium is the roof, with its associated superior rim of the acetabulum. This is the important weightbearing surface of the acetabulum.

The medial wall of the acetabulum consists primarily of the quadrilateral plate, which separates the hip joint from the pelvic cavity. Radiographically, this is seen as the medial limb of the teardrop shadow.[12] The acetabular notch defines the inferior border of the acetabular cavity. It is defined radiologically by the inferior segment of the teardrop and the posterosuperior margin of the obturator foramen; it is defined surgically by the transverse acetabular ligament.

CLASSIFICATION OF BONE LOSS

The greatest difficulty in acetabular revision surgery is the evaluation and management of bone loss. This may be caused both by the failure process and at the time of implant removal, and is the major factor dictating the type of reconstruction and bone graft required. A number of authors have produced classification systems for bone loss about the hip.[13, 14] These have been devised to quantify the severity of acetabular bone loss, to explain the indications for particular revision arthroplasty techniques, and to assess the results of these interventions. The classification that is recommended by the American Academy of Orthopaedic Surgeons (AAOS) is that of D'Antonio and colleagues.[15, 16] The AAOS classification system is outlined in Table 2.

The AAOS system is based on the division of acetabular deficiencies into segmental (type 1), cavitary (type 2), combined segmental and cavitary (type 3), pelvic dissociation (type 4), and hip fusion (type 5). Segmental deficiency comprises bone loss in the supporting hemispheric structure of the acetabulum, whereas cavitary deficiency is defined as localized volumetric loss of bone without disruption of the acetabular rim. In this system, the acetabular rim includes the medial wall. Both segmental and cavitary defects may be peripheral or central, and peripheral deficiencies may be superior, anterior, or posterior. If the medial

wall is absent, in whole or in part, this is by definition a segmental central deficiency. On the other hand, if the medial wall is deficient, but still intact, this is a cavitary central deficiency. In cases of pelvic discontinuity, the bone loss extends from the anterior to the posterior column and separates the superior and inferior portions of the acetabulum. The fused hip is included in this system because of the technical difficulties that are encountered during reconstruction.

PREOPERATIVE PLANNING

A detailed preoperative plan should be made to ensure that all the required equipment, allograft bone, staff, and time are available (Table 3).

The assessment of any leg length discrepancy and the requirement for associated femoral component revision are essential to the preoperative planning of the acetabular reconstruction. If the femoral component also needs to be revised, the subsequent ability to change component head size, length, and offset will afford more freedom to the acetabular reconstruction. If there is no independent indication to revise the femoral component, additional consideration must be given to choosing a position, version, and height for acetabular revision that will minimize the risk of instability. Review of the initial operative reports is vital to ensure that the correct equipment is available at the time of surgery. Occasionally, it will be necessary to revise a well-fixed femoral component to achieve an acceptable reconstruction with satisfactory hip biomechanics and no instability. Templating determines the approximate component size and position and provides a guide to the entire procedure before the surgeon begins the operation. Templating should be performed in both the anteroposterior and lateral views on the basis of anatomic landmarks.

In the absence of a normal contralateral hip, the radiological anatomy can be used to determine the ideal acetabular position (and migration from this ideal position) even in the presence of previously abnormal anatomy, such as hip dysplasia, or the presence of severe bone lysis. The acetabular position is determined by Ranawat's method,

TABLE 3. PREOPERATIVE PLANNING FOR ACETABULAR REVISION

General patient factors
Hip factors
    Previous approach(es)
    Leg length discrepancy
    Mobility
    Stability
    Femoral component
Exclusion of sepsis
Estimation and classification of any bone loss and residual bone quality

Summary of reconstructive options
Planning the surgical approach
Templating the appropriate implants
Determining the need for bone graft—both type and quantity
Determining the plan of action if the femur also needs to be addressed at the time of surgery
Planning a fallback position in case a complication occurs and the planned operation is no longer possible

using the intersection of Shenton's line and the ilioischial line, and measuring the true pelvic height. Ranawat defined the inferomedial acetabulum by measuring 5 mm medial to the intersection of these two lines. The acetabular height is one-fifth of the height of the pelvis measured at this point.[17] These measures can be used to determine the true inferior and superior location of the acetabulum.

Usually, components of a slightly larger size than a primary arthroplasty are required, but it may be necessary to use a component of much larger size when a large defect is encountered. Overlying the radiographs with templates will approximate the component size required and indicate the need for nonstandard oversized components. It will also detemine the new center of rotation of the hip joint and alert the surgeon to inadvertent raising of the joint line. Due to the progressive nature of bone loss secondary to osteolysis or component migration, complete up-to-date imaging should be available to ensure that the plan devised in the clinic is still appropriate. Where there is massive bone loss, it is prudent to template for a number of options in order of preference, such that one or more fallback strategies are available. The precise templating technique will depend on the method of fixation chosen as the aims of cementing, bone ingrowth, reconstruction cage reconstruction, impaction grafting, and structural allograft reconstruction are different.

PROCEDURES

SURGICAL APPROACH

The surgical exposure will depend on the location and extent of any bone defects, the type of reconstruction planned, as well as the previous experience and training of the surgeon. Consideration should be given to an extensile approach. If there is any history of instability, the soft-tissue tethers that lend stability to the joint should be carefully considered. The direction of instability should be determined from the history, from radiographs, and from the records of any closed reduction of the components. This will help to determine whether preservation of the anterior or the posterior soft-tissue envelope is more important during exposure.

The particular design of the acetabular component will not usually influence the surgical approach as good circumferential visualization is required for the removal of any acetabular component. More extensive exposure of the outer table of the ilium is required if a reconstruction cage with a prominent flange is to be removed or inserted, or if allograft reconstruction of a superolateral or posterior column deficiency is necessary. When such access is necessary, an electrocautery can be used on the outer table of the ilium from the acetabular rim. The abductor musculature is then elevated superiorly and anteriorly, taking care not to dissect or strip posteriorly toward the sciatic notch as that would place the superior gluteal neurovascular bundle at risk. It is not necessary to completely clear the ilium, and the abductor muscles should only be lifted sufficiently to allow the cage or plate to be placed beneath them.

Whichever approach is chosen, a number of landmarks are useful for orientation, particularly when there are extensive bone defects. These include the superior pubic ramus, the obturator foramen, the ischium, and the level of the true floor of the acetabulum. It is not always necessary to directly visualize these structures, but their identification aids the safe placement of retractors and helps to define the ideal position for the reconstruction. The ischium may be required for the fixation of a cage or plate and serves as a reference point for the identification of the sciatic nerve, which must be protected. The cotyloid notch should be identified in all cases. It serves as the best guide to the anatomic position of the true acetabulum.

In general, anterolateral approaches to the hip, such as the Hardinge and the vastus slide, should be reserved for simple acetabular revisions.[18] Unlike posterolateral approaches, these approaches are not extensile proximally as they cannot be converted to a trochanteric osteotomy without compromising the blood supply of the trochanteric fragment. If a trochanteric osteotomy is likely to be necessary, it should be performed before the anterior one-third to two-thirds of the abductors have been unnecessarily detached. Furthermore, exposure of the ischium and the posterior column is more difficult with anterolateral approaches than with posterolateral approaches. For these reasons the posterior approach is certainly more versatile as it allows ready extension of the exposure to a classic trochanteric osteotomy, a trochanteric slide,[19] or an extended trochanteric osteotomy[20] if the exposure proves difficult. These specialized approaches have been designed to allow a safe and wide intraoperative exposure and decrease the risk of femoral fractures during exposure of the joint, or during implant positioning or removal.[18] A carefully planned approach will avoid excessive soft-tissue devitalization, uncontrolled bone avulsions, and excessive retraction and manipulation, which may lead to periprosthetic fractures or poor implant positioning and fixation. The length and exact location of any trochanteric osteotomy should be estimated preoperatively to allow sufficient access, and leave a fragment that remains well vascularized. To this end, it is vital not to excessively strip the trochanteric fragment during mobilization after trochanteric osteotomy.[18]

Of the commonly used surgical approaches, the widest exposure of the acetabulum is provided by a classic trochanteric osteotomy with proximal retraction of the trochanteric fragment and the attached abductor muscles. This is particularly appropriate when the femur has been medialized as a result of migration of the acetabular component into the pelvis. Particular attention should be paid to the sciatic nerve in these instances, as the medial migration of the femur can render it very superficial. Trochanteric osteotomy also provides the widest exposure of the superolateral rim of the acetabulum when this is required for the purpose of placing a reconstruction cage or a bulk allograft. Similar exposure can be achieved using the trochanteric slide.

We favor the trochanteric slide in most instances where a trochanteric osteotomy would be considered. This approach affords particularly good access to hips where there is close approximation of the proximal femur to the acetabulum such as severe protrusio, when there is marked preoperative stiffness, or when there is a history of joint instability. The comprehensive acetabular exposure is particularly helpful when total or superior acetabular allografts are required to allow fixation of acetabular cages or plating of the posterior column. Dynamizing the trochanteric fragment can be used to advantage when significant limb lengthening or shortening is anticipated. Cases in which dynamic instability may be a problem, such as isolated revision of the acetabular component when a solid monoblock femoral component does not require revision, also benefit from this approach. The abductors may be tensioned by advancing the trochanter distally to avoid postoperative dislocation. The attachment of the abductor mechanism to proximal femoral allografts is also facilitated by this approach.

A very extensive exposure of the acetabulum may be required for massive acetabular allografts and for the management of some cases of pelvic discontinuity. When very extensive access to both the anterior and posterior columns is needed, the choice lies between a triradiate approach and a two-incision approach (posterior and ilioinguinal or iliofemoral). The triradiate approach combines the posterior, transtrochanteric, and anterior exposures.[21] The anterior limb may be extended into an ilioinguinal approach. The incision can, however, cause problems with skin necrosis when scars from previous surgery are present and when the superior angle is not sufficiently large.

The removal of an intrapelvic acetabular component or infected intrapelvic cement via any of the conventional approaches to the hip is associated with a risk of serious injury to pelvic viscera. The sigmoid colon or cecum, rectum, bladder, and iliac vessels are the principal structures at risk in any penetration of the floor of the true acetabulum. The risk of injury to these structures by traction on the prosthesis or cement is made higher by the intense fibrous reaction that they can provoke. Preoperative assessment by arteriography of the iliac vessels is advisable when the protrusion is substantial and the possibility exists of the vessels lying interposed between the acetabular component and the pelvis. Eftekhar and Nercessian[22] reported four such cases in which the intrapelvic components were removed under direct vision using the lateral two windows of a modified ilioinguinal approach.

IMPLANT REMOVAL

Once the acetabulum has been exposed, the previous component, cement, foreign material, and any membrane present are removed. A combination of hand tools, power tools, and ultrasonic tools may be needed for implant and cement removal. Implant removal may be very straightforward if the previous component is loose, but requires a wide exposure, patience, and the appropriate tools if it is well fixed. The implant should not be levered out as this risks fracturing the acetabular rim or removing acetabular bone stock with the implant. Curved osteotomes and pneumatic-driven gauges can be used to break the bone-implant interface without loss of bone stock.

Solidly fixed cementless acetabular components are removed using sequential curved osteotomes with careful dissection between metal and bone to preserve bone stock. Great care has to be taken not to remove excessive amounts of bone. The screws are removed first. If they are stripped, their heads are cut off with metal cutting burs, the shell is removed, and the rest of the screw subsequently cored out with trephines. In some situations, it may be

TABLE 4. AVAILABLE OPTIONS FOR ACETABULAR REVISION
Liner exchange
Polyethylene wear and osteolysis
Acute infection
Cementless revision
Standard porous-coated hemispheric components
Jumbo cups
High hip center
Customized or eccentric sockets
Oblong cups
Threaded cups (now discouraged)
Constrained cups
Bipolar prostheses
Cemented revision
Alone
Constrained
With reconstruction rings or cages
With mesh
With large segmental grafts
Mesh reconstruction with impaction grafting
Reconstruction cages
Bone graft
Autograft
Allograft
Morselized with any of the other options
Bulk
Simple
Complex
Saddle prosthesis

necessary to transect the acetabular component to remove it without destroying further bone stock. This is usually performed using high-speed metal cutting burs.

Solidly fixed cemented components should be debonded from the cement. Controlled fractures can then be performed within the cement mantle, and the cement fragments can then be removed. Care has to be taken to remove the cement from within the keying holes. Alternatively, acetabular extractors are available where the polyethylene can be drilled and the extractor threaded through it. It is wise to always ensure that the cement prosthesis bond is already compromised, as the forceful extraction of the entire composite with keying holes may lead to the inadvertent removal of medial bone.

The remaining bony acetabulum is débrided with curets to remove any incompetent bone. Reamers may be required to achieve adequate débridement, but care has to be taken to not remove useful bone, or damage intrapelvic muscle or organs if there is a massive defect. After careful assessment of the acetabular bone stock, a decision is made as to the type and size of reconstruction required. It is important to assess any movement between the superior and inferior parts of the acetabulum. This suggests pelvic discontinuity and requires stabilization prior to reconstruction.

MANAGEMENT OPTIONS

The reconstruction options should be considered with reference to the available bone stock. The management of bone defects depends on their size, on their location, and on the existing center of rotation of the hip (Table 4). The factors that must be considered are the following:

- The percentage of host bone contact available.
- Whether the residual bone is biologically capable of ingrowth.
- The integrity of the acetabular columns and roof.
- The center of rotation and whether a high hip center is an acceptable alternative.
- The type and quantity of bone graft required.

Whatever option is chosen for reconstruction of the acetabulum, a stable construct is mandatory. At present, the most common reconstructive option in North America is a cementless porous-coated hemispheric cup. This can be a standard component placed in the anatomic position if the defects are small, or a high hip center where better residual bone may be available. Alternatively, a very large uncemented component—a jumbo cup—may be used to bridge a large defect. Other options based on biological ingrowth include some customized cups, eccentric cups, and oblong cups.

The decision-making is not always straightforward. For example, there are several reconstructive options available for a superior dome deficiency, including the high hip center, bulk allograft reconstruction, contained impaction allografting, and customized components such as oblong cups. The choice of reconstruction is controversial and all options require careful templating and measurement of the resulting hip center of rotation.

The choice of bone graft has a great influence on the reconstruction. Small segmental defects can be ignored if they are peripheral. If central or contained, they can be reconstructed with morselized bone graft. Uncontained defects may be converted into contained cavitary defects with mesh support, and then become suitable for reconstitution with a morselized allograft. Larger segmental and combined defects may require a bulk allograft. A femoral head allograft may be shaped appropriately and fixed to the pelvis to reconstruct a superior deficiency, while a larger defect may require a distal femoral allograft for reconstruction in a similar manner.[23, 24] Massive defects may require the use of a total acetabular allograft. Because the incorporation of a bone graft depends on the stability of the final reconstruction, a stable acetabular construct is mandatory. Furthermore, biological fixation by means of bone ingrowth requires a substantial amount of contact with host bone. If there is 70% host bone contact, a cementless component may be fixed without a structural graft. If there is 50% to 70% contact, structural grafting may be necessary. With less than 50% host bone contact a cementless component should not be used, and alternative methods of fixation must be considered. These include the use of a cemented acetabular component or the use of reconstruction rings or cages.

Inadequate columns represent the most severe bone deficiency and should be recognized preoperatively, as a complex reconstruction will be required. This deficiency is suspected when the acetabulum has migrated superiorly and laterally a considerable distance (over 3 cm). Close scrutiny of the posterior column on the iliac oblique radiograph and inspection of ischial lysis and the ilioischial line on the anteroposterior radiograph will suggest this deficiency. If there is pelvic discontinuity, specialized reconstruction plates and cages such as the Burch-Schneider cage (Sulzer,

Baar, Switzerland) or the GAP cup (Osteonics, Allendale, NJ) are required to stabilize the posterior column, along with a considerable volume of allograft bone.

TECHNICAL DETAILS
High Hip Center
The issue of a high hip center continues to be debated.[25] While the use of a small cup placed at a high center of rotation has been recommended,[26] this is not universally accepted. Although this method allows reconstruction with biological ingrowth, there are nevertheless concerns regarding the increased risk of impingement on both the ilium and ischium, which may lead to instability. In such circumstances, the femoral component often impinges on the anterior acetabular column in flexion and internal rotation, and on the ischium and posterior column in extension and external rotation. This can be avoided by increasing the offset of the femoral component. It may also be necessary to release the rectus femoris and/or resect the anterior inferior iliac spine or a portion of the ischium. The use of a small component often necessitates the use of a 22-mm head to ensure an adequate polyethylene thickness. Many modern modular femoral component designs do not allow the use of a 22-mm head, or provide a very limited head-neck ratio for these heads. This worsens the potential problem of impingement and dislocation that is seen with such reconstructions. Great caution is advised when inserting adjuvant screws at a high hip center. The peripheral half of the superior and inferior posterior quadrants provides the best fixation while minimizing the risk of vascular injury. The acceptance of a high hip center may also necessitate femoral revision in order to provide a stable reconstruction, and may require advancement of the greater trochanter to restore satisfactory soft tissue tension. While a superior position of the hip center alone does not increase the joint reaction, superolateral placement does.[27] This may contribute to high femoral loosening rates in association with high hip centers.[28] If a high hip center is accepted, it is recommended that the cup not be lateralized as well, because of the adverse biomechanical consequences and worse functional outcome.

Liner Change with or Without a Bone Graft
A liner change may be attempted for the management of polyethylene wear when the cementless component is well fixed, and of an acceptable design.[29] The acetabular component must be modular, must have a good locking mechanism for the liner, and new liners must be readily available. Because most of the acetabular liners that will undergo such an operation are of older designs and were most probably sterilized using gamma radiation in an oxygen environment, there is a risk of degradative oxidation, which worsens with time because these liners remain on the shelf for a long period of time. The surgeon should personally check the date of sterilization on the package prior to inserting such components, and a liner that has been on the shelf for more than 2 to 3 years should not be used.[30] If there is acetabular or trochanteric osteolysis, but the components are well fixed, the resulting defect may be grafted with an autograft and/or allograft. Liner exchange is also occasionally performed as part of the acute débridement that is performed for early postoperative or acute

hematogenous infection. If there is acetabular or trochanteric osteolysis, but the components are well fixed, the resulting defect may be grafted with an autograft and/or allograft.[29, 31]

Revision with a Cementless Hemispheric Acetabular Component

Revision to a cementless hemispheric porous-coated acetabular cup is the present North American standard. These implants can be used for most isolated cavitary or segmental defects and for many combined deficiencies (Fig. 3). The reconstruction relies on the ability to achieve biological fixation of the component to the underlying host bone. This requires intimate host bone contact and rigid implant stability. Cementless acetabular components should therefore not be used when the host biology does not allow for stability or for bone ingrowth. This includes the severely osteopenic pelvis, pelvic osteonecrosis after irradiation, tumors, metabolic bone disorders, and allograft reconstructions with less than 50% host bone contact. They should also not be used in the presence of pelvic discontinuity unless the structure of the pelvic ring has been restored with a plate.

Once the decision to attempt a cementless reconstruction is made, hemispheric reamers are used to prepare the acetabular cavity. Sequentially larger reamers are used until there is three-point contact with the ilium, ischium, and pubis. The reaming should be performed in the desired orientation of the final implant, with approximately 20 degrees of anteversion and 40 degrees of abduction. Reaming down to, but not through, the medial wall may improve coverage. Removing residual posterior column bone should be avoided. It is important to achieve host bone contact in a least part of the dome and posterior column. Either the reamer heads or trial cups can be used before choosing and

inserting the definitive implant. Acetabular component position and orientation are critical for postoperative stability. Relying on an elevated liner for stability is unwise because the liner may decrease the safe range of motion, and may lead to impingement, instability, and early loosening.[32]

Line-to-line reaming is often employed in the revision setting, and the fixation augmented with screws in almost all cases. Screw fixation is more frequently employed in the revision rather than the primary setting because bone loss makes press-fit less likely, and underreaming to press-fit the acetabular component increases the risk of intraoperative acetabular fractures. The screws should be directed towards the safe quadrants, and anterior screws should only be inserted with great caution.[33]

If there is more than 30% uncovering of the component, structural bone graft augmentation may be necessary. In addition, a morselized allograft is inserted and packed or reverse-reamed into any cavitary defects. This method can also be applied to medial wall uncontained defects by placing the graft onto the medial membrane or obturator internus muscle, and gently packing it down before inserting the cementless acetabular component. In such circumstances, it is important to ensure that the component is in contact with host bone over at least 50% of its surface.

On occasion, a large concentric deficiency necessitates the use of large hemispheric cementless acetabular components. These are the so-called jumbo cups. By definition, any acetabular component with an outside diameter greater than 70 mm is a jumbo cup. The principles of reconstruction with these cups are identical to those outlined for standard cementless components. The availability of such large components has expanded the role of porous-coated revisions to larger defects provided that there is a satisfactory rim fit and more than 50% host bone contact. Loss of

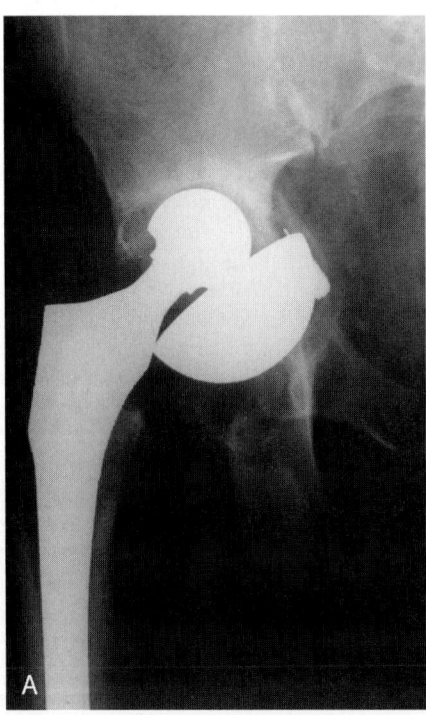
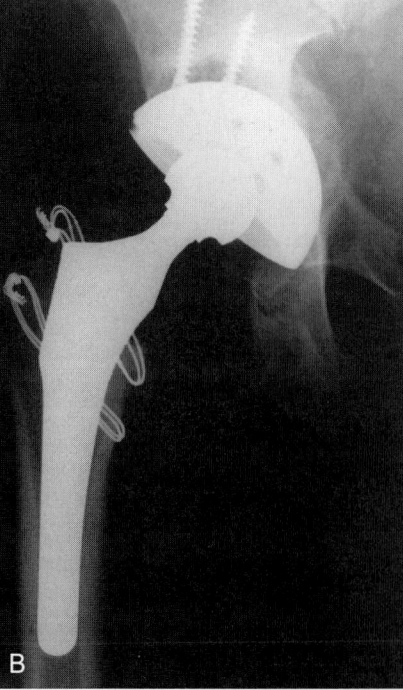

Fig. 3. Cementless reconstruction. *A,* A loose uncemented acetabular component that has migrated medially and eroded the acetabular bone stock. *B,* The acetabulum was exposed with a trochanteric slide. This allowed a circumferential exposure without removal of the well-fixed femoral component. A morselized allograft was used to reconstruct the resulting cavitary defect, and a cementless hemispheric porous-coated component with a stable rim support supplemented with screws.

the anterior column is not a contraindication to revision with a hemispheric porous-coated cup as adequate fixation can usually be obtained into the dome and posterior column. These are, however, contraindicated without supplementary techniques if there is pelvic discontinuity or severe loss of the dome.

Eccentric and Oblong Components

Customized sockets may also be used to manage protrusio defects. The preferred treatment is to fill the floor with morselized allograft and insert a cementless porous-coated cup with stable rim contact. If it is thought undesirable to graft, deep or eccentric cups are available. These lateralize the center of rotation while maintaining good host bone contact. The lateralization may be effected through eccentric metal shells, but also to a degree through the use of a lateralized polyethylene socket (up to 4 mm before the liner shell locking mechanism is overstressed).

When an acetabular implant loosens and migrates superiorly, it may create an oblong-shaped defect with a long craniocaudal dimension but a narrow anteroposterior diameter. This can be classified as a superior segmental defect, but is also not infrequently part of a combined defect in association with a medial cavitary defect. In most cases this defect can be converted to a hemispheric one for reconstruction with a large cementless porous-coated component. If the defect is large, however, this may lead to damage to the anterior or posterior column, or to both, and would threaten implant stability. The options are then restricted to the use of structural allografts, the acceptance of a high hip center, or the use of reconstruction rings. Oblong cups were designed as an alternative that combines the advantages of restoration of the hip center with biological ingrowth.[34] They resemble two overlapping hemispheres with a variety of diameters and inclinations. There are both central or dome screw options, and peripheral screw holes. The short-term results are promising but longer-term data are awaited.[35] These oblong cups are difficult to use because two diameters have to be controlled simultaneously, and errors in cup positioning are not infrequent. Furthermore, their failure leads to worsening bone loss, and we prefer structural allograft instead.

Cemented Reconstruction

Using cement for revision of the acetabular component has led to failure rates of between 10% and 20% at less than 10 years' follow-up.[36-40] Rarely, when there is a good cancellous bed, and the rim is preserved such that cement pressurization is possible, cemented revision may be successfully employed. The main indications for the use of cement in acetabular revision are the severely osteopenic patient in whom uncemented fixation is difficult and is associated with a high risk of fracture, in association with ring or cage reconstruction, and in association with structural or particulate allografting. Cement is also advocated for acetabular reconstruction in the face of abnormal bone such as that seen after irradiation or in metabolic bone disorders. In these situations, augmentation with a reinforcement cage is recommended.

Constrained Sockets

Constrained sockets essentially allow a snap fit of the femoral head into the plastic liner.[41] This gives partial constraint against dislocation (Fig. 4). They are available in both cemented and cementless designs. The secondary forces generated at the implant-bone interface are very high and demand sound primary fixation. Although these sockets reduce the dislocation rate after revision surgery, they also have a number of drawbacks. In order to capture the head, the liner has to cover more than a hemisphere; this reduces the range of motion of the hip and also increases the production of polyethylene wear particles. A larger femoral head (32 mm if possible) should therefore be used so that a reasonable range of motion can be obtained before impingement occurs, provided that an adequate polyethylene thickness is maintained.

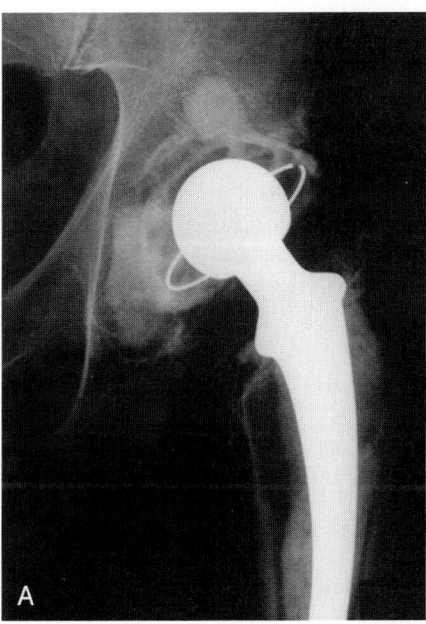 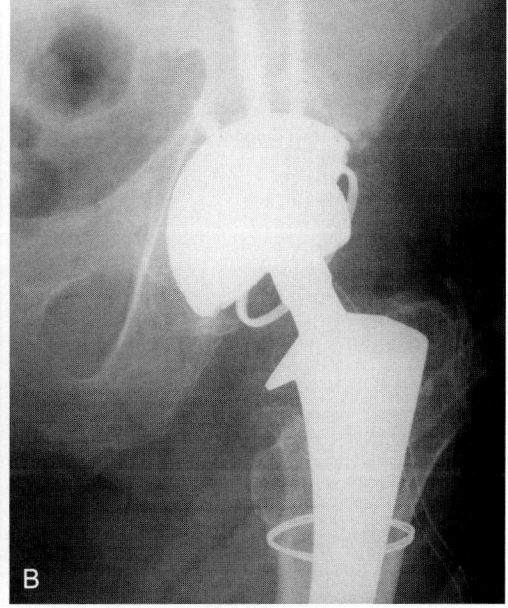

Fig. 4. Constrained socket. *A,* Loose femoral stem and recurrent dislocation in an uncooperative elderly man. *B,* An extended trochanteric osteotomy was used, and both components were revised. It was possible to obtain excellent fixation with a hemispheric porous-coated shell. A snap-fit constrained acetabular liner was used to enhance stability.

Reconstruction Cages

When large defects are present, a mechanically stable environment cannot be provided by routine acetabular fixation techniques alone. A more rigid construct is provided by reconstruction rings or cages that are secured to the surrounding pelvis (Fig. 5). The reconstruction helps to contain the graft, protects it from overload, and prevents motion between the allograft and the acetabular component. These cages also help to lateralize the hip center back to its anatomic position, to span or bridge a large defect such as a pelvic discontinuity, or to reinforce a deficient acetabular roof. Once the allograft is protected and supported by the reconstruction cage, the acetabular component of the arthroplasty can then be inserted independent of the bone graft or metal cage. This is usually in the form of an all-polyethylene cup, which is cemented inside the metal reconstruction cage.

These devices were initially used to manage protrusio defects but have now been employed to address more significant bone loss such as severe combined defects. They convert uncontained defects (segmental or combined) into contained defects and help to contain the particulate bone graft used to reconstruct the bony deficiency. They are also employed when the bone is so poor that it either cannot mechanically support a cementless component or does not have the biological potential for bone ingrowth.

When using any of these devices, it is critical that the ring or cage be secured to solid bone. If host bone is too distant for the device to span the defect, then a bulk allograft should be considered, to supplement host bone in returning the center of the hip back to its normal anatomic location. The flange of the cage should nevertheless rest on host bone, allowing host bone contact and protection of the underlying segmental allograft. Postoperative weightbearing has to be restricted for at least 3 months.

Allograft Reconstruction

The advantages of bone grafting in acetabular reconstruction include the ability to restore bone stock, to rebuild a normal hip center and hip biomechanics, and to increase bone stock for future revisions. Disadvantages include increased operative time, potentially increased morbidity, the possibility of graft failure, and disease transmission. Both morselized and structural allografts are commonly used in acetabular reconstruction. The defects addressed are usually too large to autograft, but an available autograft should either be mixed in with the morselized allograft or placed at the interfaces to take advantage of its osteoinductive properties. There is increasing interest in bioactive ceramics. Oonishi et al[42] described the successful use of hydroxyapatite granules as an alternative to morselized allograft bone to reconstruct acetabular defects. In such circumstances, the graft is not structural or weightbearing in function, and the precise type of graft used may therefore be of limited significance.

When there is a massive segmental or a large combined cavitary and segmental defect it may not be possible to obtain adequate bone-implant contact for cementless reconstruction. On occasion, the defect is so large that it cannot be spanned with a reconstruction cage. Such complex cases require the use of bulk allografts (Fig. 6). These include allograft femoral heads, distal femurs, or proximal tibias as figure-of-7 grafts, or whole acetabula. A very wide exposure is necessary for the insertion of such grafts. Chandler and Penenberg[43] recommend aligning the trabeculae of the graft to those of the host, although no data are available to

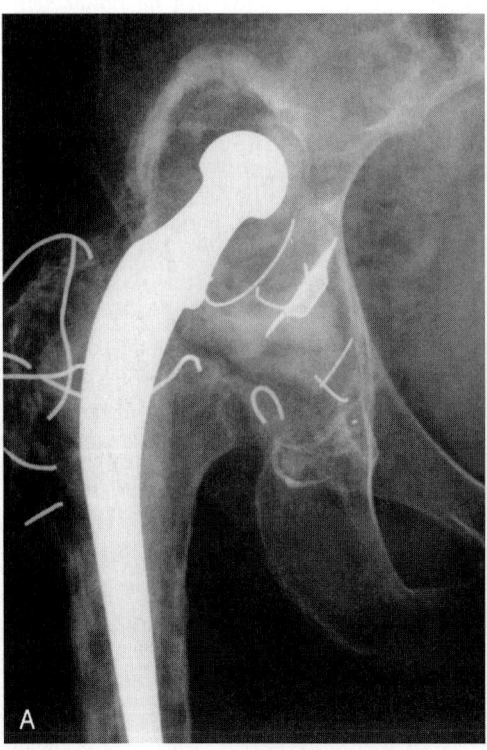
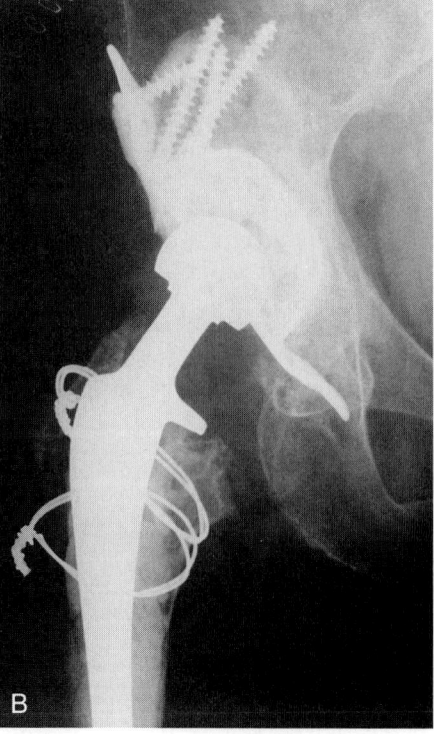

Fig. 5. Reconstruction cage. *A,* Severe combined cavitary and segmental bone loss following the aseptic failure of a cemented revision hip arthroplasty. *B,* A trochanteric slide gave satisfactory access. A morselized femoral head allograft was packed into the defect and a Burch-Schneider reconstruction cage was inserted to span the defect and protect the graft. A polyethylene acetabular component was cemented within the cage with freedom of orientation.

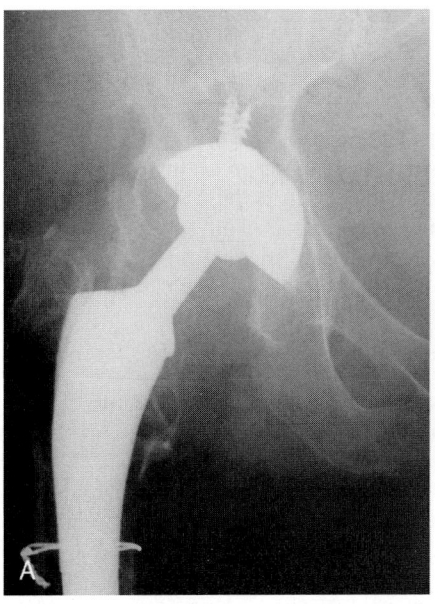
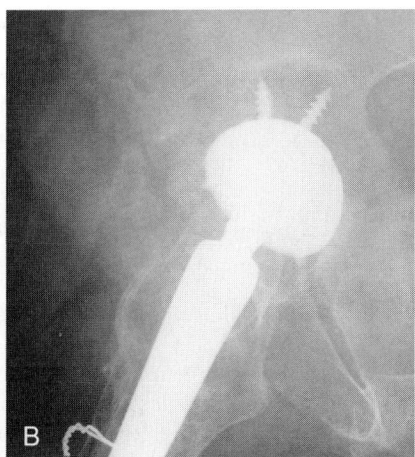
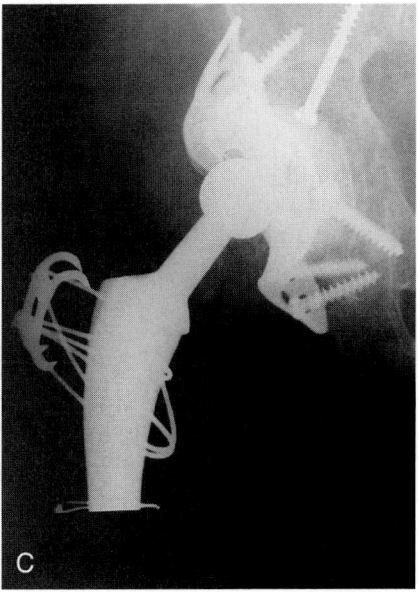

Fig. 6. Structural allograft. *A* and *B,* Polyethylene and titanium wear with massive osteolysis in an uncemented total hip arthroplasty. The femoral head articulates with the acetabular shell. The latter is still stable and ingrown anteriorly in spite of loss of most of the posterior column. *C,* Excellent access was achieved using a trochanteric slide. A structural acetabular allograft was trimmed to fit the defect and fixed with screws both superiorly and inferiorly. This was then protected with a reconstruction cage, and a cemented polyethylene socket was inserted.

support this. As a rule, the acetabular component should be cemented into the graft, as the allograft will not grow into a porous-coated implant.[44, 45] Certainly, if more than 50% of the structural support is provided by the allograft, the revision component should be cemented.

Bulk allografts, and whole acetabula in particular, are used in cases where until recently the only available treatment would have been resection arthroplasty. Graft union can usually be achieved and leads to an improvement in the net acetabular bone stock even if the revision component fails. The ultimate bone stock is greatly improved by avoiding graft lysis, fragmentation, and collapse. This is effected through stable primary graft fixation, and the avoidance of graft overload. There is also evidence for the use of structurally strong grafts (from young male donors), the avoidance of a freeze-dried allograft or multiple blocks of allograft, and for minimizing the exposure of cancellous allograft surfaces to the host. High clinical and radiological loosening rates have been reported but there are few if any reliable alternatives to the use of bulk allograft in these cases. Ultimately, direct comparisons of the long-term results of reconstruction with jumbo cups, reconstruction rings, morselized graft, and mesh and structural allograft may clarify the precise indications for each of these techniques.

Saddle Prostheses

Saddle prostheses are usually employed to bridge massive acetabular defects following the excision of pelvic tumors. They are also used in some centers for the salvage of failed acetabular reconstructions where the bone stock is insufficient for any of the previously detailed techniques. This implant allows load transmission between the residual iliac bone and the femur. A saddle-shaped cobalt-chrome surface bears directly on the upper part of the ilium proximally, and is cemented into the femur distally. A number of options for length and offset are available on the femoral side, and similar prostheses can be custom-designed to bridge specific defects.

POSTOPERATIVE PROCEDURE

The postoperative mobilization protocol will vary depending on the use of bone grafting, the security of the fixation, and any associated femoral reconstruction. We advocate 6 weeks of feather weightbearing followed by 6 weeks of 50% weightbearing with crutches or a walker in the straightforward cases, and more prolonged toe touching in the more complex cases.

RESULTS

CEMENTLESS REVISION

The early and midterm results of cementless acetabular revision have been universally successful.[46–51] Lachiewicz and Poon[48] followed 57 revision Harris-Galante porous-coated implants (Zimmer, Warsaw, IN) for a minimum of 5 years and a mean of 7 years. All the implants were well fixed with no radiological evidence of loosening.

In spite of the excellent reported results with hemispheric porous-coated cups, there are still concerns regarding late osteolysis, particularly where screws have been used, regarding the effects of modularity on the production of wear debris, and regarding the use of extended lip liners which may decrease the range of movement and promote dislocation through earlier impingement. Ongoing work to improve the wear characteristics of polyethylene, allied to improvements in hemispheric shell and liner locking mechanisms, and reduction in the number of screw holes may decrease the production of particulate debris and the resulting osteolysis.

JUMBO CUP

Jasty[52] has reviewed 19 acetabular reconstructions with a jumbo cup where there was at least a 4-cm defect in the medial wall and loss of the anterior column. The acetabulum was reamed up to the appropriate size while preserving the dome and posterior column. The medial wall was grafted with morselized allograft. At a mean follow-up of 10 years, the only failure had occurred in a patient with pelvic discontinuity. All the others had good graft incorporation and no evidence of implant loosening. There are concerns, however, about stress shielding in relation to these large implants, and regarding the sacrifice of posterior column bone in particular, as that is extremely difficult to graft if the jumbo cup fails.

CUSTOMIZED SOCKETS

Sutherland[50] used customized eccentric sockets in six patients with AAOS type III defects, but noted aseptic failure in three of them. These failures occurred, however, in first-generation implants that were used without appropriate reamers and with limited screw options.

RECONSTRUCTION RINGS AND CASES

Rosson and Schatzker[53] reviewed 66 acetabula that had been reconstructed with either the Müller ring (46 cases) or the Burch-Schneider antiprotrusio cage (20 cases) at a mean follow-up of 5 years. Five hips required rerevision, all after Müller ring insertion. The use of bone graft and cement instead of cement alone with the implants reduced the failure rate from 13% to 6%, and reduced the number of circumferential radiolucent lines at the bone-implant interface from 39% to 2%. The authors concluded that the Müller ring should be used for acetabula with isolated peripheral segmental defects or cavitary defects confined to one or two sectors. The Burch-Schneider antiprotrusio cage should be used for medial segmental defects, extensive cavitary defects, and combined deficiencies.

Berry and Müller[54] reported a series of 42 failed hip arthroplasties with massive acetabular bone deficiencies revised with the Burch-Schneider antiprotrusio cage, evaluated after 2 to 11 years. They had a 12% failure rate due to sepsis and a further 12% aseptic failure rate. The remaining 32 (76%) showed no evidence of acetabular component failure or loosening. The authors believe that because the cage acts as a bridge from host bone to host bone it protects the bone graft from resorption.

BONE GRAFT

The success of a bone grafting procedure is ultimately dependent on the surgeon's ability to provide a mechanically stable environment for graft incorporation. If movement or graft overload occurs it will lead to resorption or loosening. Whatever option is chosen for the reconstruction of the acetabular component, a stable construct is mandatory.

TECHNICAL DETAILS
Allograft Reconstruction

Animal experiments, primarily in a goat model, have shown rapid union of the graft to the host bone.[55] Morselized bone chips can be tightly packed to replace any bone loss, resulting in a complete layer with no gaps. During the revascularization phase, the open structure of this cancellous bone allows more rapid blood vessel invasion than the more solid cortical bone used in bulk or structural allografts. Moreover, apposition of new bone precedes osteoclastic function in the cancellous autograft. Thus, the bone is replaced without significant structural weakening as long as the graft has a stable fit and the host bed is well vascularized. The rate and extent of allograft incorporation remain unpredictable, however, and clinical success does not necessarily reflect the fate of the bone graft. Plain radiography does not necessarily prove the solidity of the reconstructed acetabulum, although bony consolidation does suggest satisfactory load bearing.

Garbuz et al[56, 57] distinguished contained from uncontained defects. They used a combination of techniques, including structural allografts, reinforcement rings and morselized graft. They recommended morselized allograft packing for contained defects followed by a cementless prosthesis for young patients and a reinforcement ring with a cemented cup in older patients. For uncontained defects, they favored the use of structural allografts.

Structural Femoral Head Grafts

There is still some controversy regarding the use of structural femoral head grafts. Morsi et al[58] reviewed 29 shelf acetabular allografts at an average follow-up of 7 years. Twenty-five (86%) were successful, both clinically and radiologically. The authors emphasized, however, that at least 50% of the cup must be supported by host bone. Harris's group has reported excellent short-term but poor medium-term results with the use of femoral head structural allografts to support acetabular reconstructions.[59] The failure rate increased with the percentage coverage of the component provided by the allograft.[52]

Saddle Prostheses

Nieder et al[60] reported the use of saddle prostheses for the salvage of gross loss of pelvic bone stock in 76 patients with failed hip arthroplasties. After early migration and settling of the prostheses, a useful and stable articulation was achieved in most cases, albeit with limited function and a restricted range of motion. The authors emphasize that this is a useful salvage alternative to excision arthroplasty or amputation, but that it cannot offer the durability or functional results of formal acetabular reconstruction.

ACKNOWLEDGMENTS

Fares S. Haddad was supported by the John Charnley and BOA/Wishbone trusts and by the Norman Capener Travelling Fellowship.

REFERENCES

1. Sutherland CJ, Wilde AH, Borden LS, et al: A ten-year follow-up of one hundred consecutive Müller curved-stem total hip replacement arthroplasties. J Bone Joint Surg Am 1982; 64:970.
2. Smith SW, Mankiletow A, Harris WH: Vastus-psoas release for acetabular exposure in revision hip surgery. J Arthroplasty 1997; 12:568.
3. Smith SE, Estok DM II, Harris WH: Average 12-year outcome of a chrome-cobalt, beaded, bony ingrowth acetabular component. J Arthroplasty 1998; 13:50.
4. Hastings DE, Tobin H, Sellenkowitsch M: Review of 10-year results of PCA hip arthroplasty. Can J Surg 1998; 41:48.
5. Hungerford DS, Jones LC: The rationale for the cementless revision cemented arthroplasty failures. Clin Orthop 1988; 235:12.
6. Masterson EL, Masri BA, Duncan CP: Treatment of infection at the site of total hip replacement. J Bone Joint Surg Am 1997; 79:1740.
7. Owen TD, Moran CG, Smith SR, et al: Results of uncemented porous-coated anatomic total hip replacement. J Bone Joint Surg Br 1994; 76:25.
8. Rorabeck CH, Bourne RB, Mulliken BD, et al: Acetabular osteolysis with cementless cups: A 5 to 7 year follow-up. Acta Orthop Belg 1997; 63:83.
9. John JF, Talbert RE, Taylor JK, et al: Use of acetabular models in planning complex acetabular reconstructions. J Arthroplasty 1995; 10:661.
10. Robertson DD, Sutherland CJ, Lopes T, et al: Preoperative description of severe acetabular defects caused by failed total hip replacement. J Comput Assist Tomogr 1998; 22:444.
11. Judet R, Judet J, Letournel E: Fractures of the acetabulum: Classification and surgical approaches for open reduction, preliminary report. J Bone Joint Surg Am 1964; 46:1615.
12. Bowerman JW, Sena JM, Chang R: The teardrop shadow of the pelvis: Anatomy and clinical significance. Radiology 1982; 143:659.
13. Masri BA, Masterson EL, Duncan CP: The classification and radiographic evaluation of bone loss in revision hip arthroplasty. Orthop Clin North Am 1998; 29:219.
14. Masri BA, Duncan CP: Classification of bone loss in total hip arthroplasty. Instr Course Lect 1996; 45:199.
15. D'Antonio JA, Capello WN, Borden LS, et al: Classification and management of acetabular abnormalities in total hip arthroplasty. Clin Orthop 1989; 243:126.
16. D'Antonio JA: Periprosthetic bone loss of the acetabulum. Orthop Clin North Am 1992; 23:279.
17. Crowe JF, Mani VJ, Ranawat CS: Total hip replacement in congenital dislocation and dysplasia of the hip. J Bone Joint Surg Am 1979; 61:15.
18. Glassman AH, Engh CA, Bobyn JD: A technique of extensile exposure for total hip arthroplasty. J Arthroplasty 1987; 2:11.

19. Masterson EL, Masri BA, Duncan CP: Surgical exposure in revision total hip arthroplasty. J Am Acad Orthop Surg 1988; 6:84.
20. Younger TI, Bradford MS, Magnus RE, et al: Extended proximal femoral osteotomy: A new technique for femoral revision arthroplasty. J Arthroplasty 1995; 10:329.
21. Stiehl JB, Harlow M, Hackbarth D: Extensile triradiate approach for complex acetabular reconstruction in total hip arthroplasty. Clin Orthop 1993; 294:162.
22. Eftekhar NS, Nercessian O: Intrapelvic migration of total hip prostheses. Operative treatment. J Bone Joint Surg Am 1989; 71:1480.
23. Paprosky AG, Magnus RE: Principles of bone grafting in revision total hip arthroplasty: Acetabular technique. Clin Orthop 1994; 298:147.
24. Penner M, Garbuz DS: Role and results of segmental allografts for acetabular segmental bone deficiency. Orthop Clin North Am 1998; 29:263.
25. Kelley SS: High hip center in revision arthroplasty. J Arthroplasty 1994; 9:503.
26. Harris WH: Reconstruction at a high hip center in acetabular revision surgery using a cementless acetabular component. Orthopaedics 1998; 21:991.
27. Doehring TC, Rubash HE, Shelly FJ, et al: The effect of superior and superolateral relocations of the hip-center on hip joint forces: An experimental and analytical analysis. J Arthroplasty 1996; 11:693.
28. Pagnano W, Hanssen AD, Lewallen DG, et al: The effect of superior placement of the acetabular component on the rate of loosening after total hip arthroplasty. J Bone Joint Surg Am 1996; 78:1004.
29. Maloney WJ, Herzwurm P, Paprosky W, et al: Treatment of pelvic osteolysis associated with a stable acetabular component inserted without cement as part of a total hip replacement. J Bone Joint Surg Am 1997; 79:1628.
30. Masri BA, Salvati EA, Duncan CP: Polyethylene properties and their role in osteolysis after total joint arthroplasty. In Tanaka S, Haminishi C (eds): Advances in Osteoarthritis. Tokyo, Springer-Verlag, 1998, pp 271.
31. Schmalzried TP, Fowble VA, Amstutz HC: The fate of pelvic osteolysis after reoperation. No recurrence with lesional treatment. Clin Orthop 1998; 350:128.
32. Murray DW: Impingement and loosening of the long posterior wall acetabular implant. J Bone Joint Surg Br 1992; 74:377.
33. Wasielewski RC, Cooperstein LA, Kruger MP, et al: Acetabular anatomy and the transacetabular fixation of screws in total hip arthroplasty. J Bone Joint Surg Am 1990; 72:501.
34. DeBoer DK, Christie MJ: Reconstruction of the deficient acetabulum with an oblong prosthesis: Three- to seven-year results. J Arthroplasty 1998; 13:674.
35. Cameron HU: Modified cups. Orthop Clin North Am 1998; 29:277.
36. Kavanagh BF, Fitzgerald RH: Multiple revisions for failed total hip arthroplasty not

associated with infection. J Bone Joint Surg Am 1987; 69:1144.
37. Kershaw CJ, Atkins RM, Dodd CAF, et al: Revision total hip arthroplasty for aseptic failure. J Bone Joint Surg Br 1991; 73:564.
38. Marti RK, Schuller HM, Besselaar PP, et al: Results of revision of hip arthroplasty with cement. J Bone Joint Surg Am 1990; 72:346.
39. Pellicci PM, Wilson PD Jr, Sledge CB, et al: Long-term results of revision total hip replacement. A follow-up report. J Bone Joint Surg Am 1985; 67:513.
40. Raut VV, Siney PD, Wroblewski BM: Cemented revision for aseptic acetabular loosening. J Bone Joint Surg Br 1995; 77:357.
41. Goetz DD, Capello WN, Callaghan JJ, et al: Salvage of a recurrently dislocating total hip prosthesis with use of a constrained acetabular component. J Bone Joint Surg Am 1998; 80:502.
42. Oonishi H, Iwaki K, Kin N, et al: Hydroxyapatite in revision of total hip replacements with massive acetabular defects. J Bone Joint Surg Br 1996; 79:87.
43. Chandler H, Penenberg BL: Bone Stock Deficiency in Total Hip Replacement. Classification and Management. Thorofare, NJ, Slack, 1989.
44. Hooten JP, Engh CA, Engh CA: Failure of structural acetabular allografts in cementless revision hip arthroplasty. J Bone Joint Surg Br 1994; 76:419.
45. Hooten JP, Engh CA, Heekin RD, et al: Structural bulk allografts in acetabular reconstruction. J Bone Joint Surg Br 1996; 78:270.
46. Hedley AK, Gruen TA, Ruoff DP: Revision of failed total hip arthroplasties with uncemented porous-coated anatomic components. Clin Orthop 1988; 235:75.
47. Padgett DE, Kull L, Rosenberg A, et al: Revision of the acetabular component without cement after total hip arthroplasty. J Bone Joint Surg Am 1993; 75:663.
48. Lachiewicz PF, Poon ED: Revision of a total hip arthroplasty with a Harris-Galante porous-coated acetabular component inserted without cement. J Bone Joint Surg Am 1998; 80:980.
49. Silverton CD, Rosenberg AG, Sheinkop MB, et al: Revision of the acetabular component without cement after THA. J Bone Joint Surg Am 1996; 78:1366.
50. Sutherland CJ: Treatment of type III acetabular deficiencies in revision total hip arthroplasty without structural bone graft. J Arthroplasty 1996; 11:91.
51. Tanzer M, Drucker D, Jasty M, et al: Revision of the acetabular component with an uncemented Harris-Galante porous coated prosthesis. J Bone Joint Surg Am 1992; 74:987.
52. Jasty M: Jumbo cups and morselized graft. Orthop Clin North Am 1998; 29:249.
53. Rosson J, Schatzker J: Use of reinforcement rings to reconstruct deficient acetabula. J Bone Joint Surg Br 1992; 74:716.
54. Berry DJ, Müller MR: Revision arthroplasty using an anti-protrusio cage for

massive acetabular bone deficiency. J Bone Joint Surg Br 1992; 74:711.

55. Slooff TJ, Van Horn J, Lemmens A, et al: Bone grafting for total hip replacement for acetabular protrusion. Acta Orthop Scand 1984; 55:593.

56. Garbuz D, Morsi E, Mohamed N, et al: Classification and reconstruction in revision acetabular arthroplasty with bone stock deficiency. Clin Orthop 1996; 324: 98.

57. Garbuz D, Morsi E, Gross AE: Revision of the acetabular component of a total hip arthroplasty with a massive structural allograft. Study with a minimum five-year follow-up. J Bone Joint Surg Am 1996; 78: 693.

58. Morsi E, Garbuz D, Gross AE: Revision total hip arthroplasty with shelf bulk allografts. J Arthroplasty 1996; 11:86.

59. Kwong LM, Jasty M, Harris WH: High failure rate of bulk femoral head allografts

in total hip acetabular reconstructions at 10 years. J Arthroplasty 1993; 8:341.

60. Nieder E, Elson RA, Engelbrecht E, et al: The saddle prosthesis for salvage of the destroyed acetabulum. J Bone Joint Surg Br 1990; 72:1014.

section
6
chapter
14

ARTHRITIS OF THE KNEE

Jonathan L. Schaffer, Peter J. Gard, and Daniel Solomon

Summary
- Arthritis of the knee affects a significant number of patients older than 40 years and is a leading cause of disability in the elderly.
- Osteoarthritis (OA) is more common than all forms of inflammatory arthritis combined.
- Accurate clinical evaluation facilitates treatment and selection of patients who warrant further investigation.
- The treatment course should be individualized for each patient based on lifestyle and general health considerations.
- Medical management of knee OA includes pharmaceuticals, weight loss, and regular exercise such as quadriceps strengthening, which are effective in the early stages of knee arthritis.
- Surgical interventions for knee OA are effective means of reducing pain and producing functional improvement.

INTRODUCTION

DEFINITION

The arthritides are a very broad group of diseases (see Chapter 6–1). Although the literal definition of arthritis implies joint inflammation, not all arthritides are inflammatory. A more appropriate term for the noninflammatory degenerative changes is osteoarthrosis. Loss of articular cartilage thickness is the final common pathway of all progressive forms of arthritis. In this chapter, arthritis of the knee is defined as cartilage loss or joint space narrowing severe enough to produce positive clinical or radiographic findings. OA is the most common form of knee arthritis and is more frequently observed than all other causes of degeneration in aggregate. Important inflammatory arthritides of the knee include rheumatoid, crystalline, septic, and spondylytic variants and posttraumatic cases. These arthritides are not discussed in detail here. OA of the knee is defined by the American College of Rheumatologists as (1) knee pain plus radiographic osteophytes or

(2) knee pain, age greater than 40 years, and morning stiffness less than 30 minutes in duration.

HISTORICAL REVIEW

Fossils found in the British Isles from the Roman and Saxon times show a high prevalence of arthritis.[1] Before the 20th century, arthritis of the knee most likely resulted from trauma or sepsis. Studies of skeletal remains from medieval times curiously suggest a much lower incidence of OA than is currently seen. Case reports of reactive arthritis (secondary to the venereal epidemics in large cities) and tuberculosis appear in hospital records of 19th-century London.[2] The earliest descriptions of inflammatory arthritis are from the 18th century, and rheumatoid arthritis (RA), such as suffered by the famous impressionist painter Pierre Auguste Renoir, was well described by the late 19th century.[3]

The incidence of degenerative OA has increased dramatically during the 20th century because the life expectancy of the population has increased. This trend is likely to increase further as the baby boomer generation ages. It is estimated that some form of arthritis will affect 60 million Americans by the year 2020 compared with 40 million in 1995.[4]

Early arthritis treatments consisted essentially of physical therapy, herbal potions, or plain quackery. Effective and widely available analgesic medications are a relatively recent advance. Aspirin was first mass produced and marketed in 1897 by Bayer, although ancient physicians, including Hippocrates, knew of the analgesic properties of the bark of the willow tree (which contains salicylate). In 1950, the Nobel Prize was awarded for the discovery of the anti-inflammatory effects of adrenocorticoid extract, resulting in successful treatment of inflammatory disorders with exogenous corticosteroids. The last years of the 20th century witnessed the development of cyclo-oxygenase selective nonsteroidal anti-inflammatory medications. The first surgically efficacious treatment for knee OA was tibial osteotomy, developed by Coventry around 1965.[5] Total joint and partial joint arthroplasty were first attempted around 1950 but not widely used until the 1970s.

EPIDEMIOLOGY

The American College of Rheumatology classifies OA as primary or secondary. An estimated 42 million Americans are affected by arthritis, and arthritis of the hip and knee are the leading cause of disability among adults. Each year, arthritis results in millions of physician visits and more than one-half million hospitalizations. Estimated medical costs for arthritis patients total billions of dollars annually. The single largest risk factor for arthritis of the knee is increasing age.[6] Other risk factors for OA of the knee include genetic predisposition, obesity, and female gender.[7] Among women, about 1% per year experience symptomatic knee arthritis.[8] Arthritis of the knee occurs more commonly in males with previous knee injuries. Abnormal joint anatomy or alignment, previous significant joint injury or surgery, joint instability, disturbances of joint or muscle innervation, or inadequate muscle strength may increase the risk of OA. Local biochemical factors also play a role.

Racial differences are difficult to assess and may prove to be negligible when confounding factors are adjusted for. Some studies suggest lower incidences among black populations from Jamaica, South Africa, Nigeria, and Liberia (1% to 4% with radiographic OA) compared with European populations. Another showed no difference between whites and blacks in North Carolina.[9] Rural populations may have higher rates of both hip and knee OA. Although OA is frequently defined by the presence of radiographic changes, the principal risk factors for radiographic knee arthritis may differ from those associated with the reporting of knee pain, which include psychosocial factors and general health status.

ANATOMY AND BIOMECHANICS

Motion of the knee that is coordinated, stable, adequate in range, and sufficiently powered is a prerequisite for good knee function. Undesirable motion causes eccentric loading, cartilage degeneration, and meniscal tears. OA commonly results from a primary mechanical problem, which causes loading of the articular cartilage beyond its limits.

The obvious and dominant motion of the knee is flexion. However, the knee has much more potential motion available. It has six degrees of freedom: three translations (anteroposterior, medial-lateral, and inferior-superior) and three rotations (flexion-extension, internal-external, and adduction-abduction). In the healthy knee, these six degrees of freedom are controlled by ligaments, the joint capsule, bony congruency, the menisci, and coordinated neuromuscular contractions. Deficiency in any part of this scheme will lead to abnormal motion, allowing for abnormal loading, often leading to degenerative arthritis. The absence of knee motion may also be detrimental because the knee articular surface must experience some loading and motion to circulate the nourishing synovial fluid and prevent ligament shortening and tissue atrophy.

The menisci play a significant role in load distribution. Experimentally, the load-bearing area of each condyle is reduced from 6 cm² to 2 cm² if the menisci are removed. This has implications for the underlying articular cartilage, which suffers irreparable damage if its critical load factor (36 kg/cm²) is consistently exceeded. Intact menisci also enhance knee stability, particularly in the sagittal plane and

rotationally. The medial meniscus is firmly attached at its outer rim to the capsule and medial collateral ligament and moves very little. The smaller lateral meniscus is more mobile and allows the lateral condyle to glide backward and forward. The lateral femoral condyle moves backward on the tibia with increasing flexion. In full extension, the tibia is maximally externally rotated in the "screw home" position. This is the position where the knee can support standing with the least muscular contraction.

Shape and size of the articular surfaces determine loading, stability, and range of motion. The femoral condyles are biconvex. The medial tibial condyle is biconcave in sagittal and frontal planes, whereas the lateral tibial condyle is concave in the frontal plane but convex in the sagittal plane. The intercondylar spines of the tibia resist lateral subluxation. Under load, the opposing surfaces of the knee achieve improved congruency that contributes to overall stability. Conversely, a variation in shape or relative size of articular surfaces can affect wear. For example, a congenitally small lateral femoral condyle contributes to lateral compartment arthritis by diminishing lateral compartment contact area and producing a valgus orientation of the leg, thus increasing the load on this compartment.

Ligaments function to stabilize the knee. The medial collateral ligament resists valgus angulation, whereas the lateral collateral ligament resists varus angulation. The anterior cruciate ligament (ACL) resists anterior displacement of the tibia (especially when the knee is flexed) and internal rotation. The posterior cruciate ligament (PCL) resists posterior displacement of the tibia and external rotation.

All muscles crossing the knee can contribute to dynamic stability of the knee by contracting at the appropriate phase of gait. One would instinctively think that increased muscle contraction across the joint will increase the joint load. However, the vector of muscle force can realign the knee, unloading a compartment under compression. Muscles can partly compensate for altered knee mechanics. For example, contraction of the quadriceps femoris muscle tends to pull the tibia anteriorly, an action normally resisted by the intact ACL. In the knee with a deficient ACL, the resulting unopposed anterior subluxation causes excessive load on articular surfaces. To avoid this, the body compensates by using a "quadriceps avoidance" gait. Building up the hamstring muscles also compensates for a deficient ACL by holding the tibia in a neutral position against forces (e.g., quadriceps) that would drive it forward.

PATHOGENESIS

Articular cartilage functions to absorb the stress of a mechanical load by its elasticity and ability to deform. It also provides a smooth surface to facilitate gliding motion of the joint. The histological appearance of articular cartilage is that of chondrocytes embedded in a matrix of collagen and proteoglycan. The collagen provides cartilage stability and is formed by the continuous process of synthesis and degradation. This process is dependent on the balance of growth factors and enzymes. Alterations in this balance, with increases in degradation or reduction in synthesis, will predispose the development of arthritis.

The initiating event of knee arthritis may be mechanical or inflammatory or may be due to inherent joint or cartilage deficiency. Local factors, mechanical loading, obesity, and repeated injury then propagate the degenerative process. Stiffening of subchondral bone makes it a less effective shock absorber, and radiological changes of subchondral sclerosis are common in OA. Although most often considered sequelae of arthritis, such changes may be initiating events. Alterations in subchondral bone are seen before changes in cartilage in one guinea pig model,[10] whereas in humans bone changes by scintigraphy have been shown to predict radiographic progression in the knee.[11]

As the disease process advances, articular cartilage is lost. After the loss of "shock-absorbing" articular cartilage, load is transferred onto a smaller area of subchondral bone, and, in keeping with Wolf's law, this bone hypertrophies, and subchondral sclerosis worsens. A rarer but illuminating mechanism of knee arthritis initiation is seen in Paget's disease, an idiopathic hypertrophy of cortical bone. If Paget's disease affects the periarticular bone, bone fails to conform as well, load is concentrated, and cartilage is destroyed. Interestingly, generalized reduction in bone mineral density, as in osteoporosis, is negatively correlated with knee OA.[12]

Osteophytes form by endochondral ossification into soft-tissue spaces and develop on the margins of articular cartilage. They typically occur in OA, in which peripheral articular cartilage persists, but are rarely seen in RA, in which articular cartilage is removed from the margins first and probably globally throughout the knee. Two specific injury types associated with OA of the knee are meniscal tears and cruciate ligament damage. OA of the knee is most common after meniscal tear and partial meniscectomy, especially when there is accompanying damage to the ACL.[13-15]

Instability may be the cause of some cases of knee OA, such as in an ACL-deficient knee, but it may result from the arthritic process. Instability resulting from knee OA comes from loss of articular cartilage and bone, occasionally from ligament stretching, and rarely if ever from ligament rupture. Exceptions include the ACL, which becomes abraded by osteophytes or degraded by local synovitis, or a collateral ligament, which becomes stretched on the convex side of a severely varus or valgus knee. Instability results in increased joint deformity and subluxation. The tibia frequently subluxates laterally in knee OA.

The forces on the knee are multiples of body weight (more than five times body weight per knee during vigorous activity). Body weight can, therefore, have significant influence on the forces across the knee, and overweight people are at higher risk for knee OA and may also be at increased risk for hand and hip OA.[16] Furthermore, being overweight accelerates disease progression in knee OA. This may be a purely mechanical effect, or it may be related to altered local proprioception and tissue factors in obese people.[17]

The nervous system has a large role in joint function, providing pain feedback, proprioception, and complex muscle coordination. A subtle variation in the quality of these functions may initiate or accelerate joint disease. Whether these potential mechanisms are clinically significant factors in the cause of OA remains uncertain.

CLINICAL FEATURES

PATIENT HISTORY

Pain, swelling, stiffness, deformity, and loss of function are salient historical features of knee arthritis (Table 1). Careful history taking will define arthritis of the knee as inflammatory or noninflammatory and mono- or polyarthritic. Conditions requiring urgent evaluation and management are suggested by the history of an acute hot, swollen joint and the presence of fever or constitutional symptoms. Septic

TABLE 1. CLINICAL, ROENTGENOGRAPHIC, LABORATORY, AND SYNOVIAL FLUID ALTERATIONS WITH VARIOUS TYPES OF KNEE ARTHRITIS

Diagnosis	Symptoms	Physical Examination	Characteristic Roentgenographic Alterations
Osteoarthritis	Brief morning stiffness Pain after activity (early disease stage) Pain with activity (progressive stages) Night pain (advanced stage)	Normal ROM (early stages) Decreased ROM (late stages) Minimal swelling or inflammation Deformity (late stages) Crepitation	Peripheral osteophyte formation Asymmetric joint space narrowing Subchondral sclerosis Subchondral cysts
Rheumatoid arthritis	Morning stiffness >60 min Usually polyarticular Swelling and inflammation	Pain with motion and weightbearing Decreased motion Swollen and inflamed Effusion	Osteopenia Periarticular erosions and cysts Symmetric joint space narrowing Effusion
Septic arthritis	Severe pain Decreased ROM	Significant swelling and inflammation Decreased ROM Pain with weightbearing	Normal except for soft-tissue swelling (early) Joint space narrowing (late) Soft-tissue swelling
Gout	Afflicts first MTP joint most commonly Severe pain Decreased ROM	Swollen and inflamed Decreased ROM	
Pseudogout	Commonly afflicts the knee joint Variable from mild to severe	Variable swelling and inflammation	Calcification of cartilaginous structures

TABLE 1. CLINICAL, ROENTGENOGRAPHIC, LABORATORY, AND SYNOVIAL FLUID ALTERATIONS WITH VARIOUS TYPES OF KNEE ARTHRITIS *(continued)*

Laboratory Abnormalities	Synovial Fluid Appearance	Fibrin Clot	Mucin Clot	WBC/mm³	PMN (%)	Sugar (% Blood Level)
None	Slightly turbid	Small	Good	<2000	<25	~100
Elevation of ESR and CRP, positive rheumatoid factor, alteration of serum complement	Turbid	Large	Fair to poor	5000–50,000	>65	75
Elevation of ESR and CRP	Very turbid or purulent	Large	Poor	50,000–100,000	>80	<50
Elevation of ESR and CRP	Turbid	Large	Fair to poor	5000–50,000	>75	90
Elevation of serum uric acid (variable)	Negative birefringent crystals with examination under UV light microscopy					
Elevation of ESR and CRP	Turbid	Large	Fair to poor	5000–50,000	>75	90
	Positive birefringement crystals with examination under UV light microscopy					

ROM = range of motion; MTP = metatarsophalangeal; WBC = white blood cell; PMN = polymorphonuclear leukocytes; ESR = erythrocyte sedimentation rate; CRP = C-reactive protein; UV = ultraviolet.

arthritis must be ruled out immediately in such a patient. The differential diagnosis of such a patient includes not only infection and systemic rheumatic disease but gout and pseudogout as well. In contrast, chronic progressive symptoms are usually those of OA.

A patient's pain should be evaluated in detail both for diagnosis and to appreciate its effect on the functional status of the patient. The time of onset, quality, radiation, and factors that relieve or aggravate the pain are important clues for diagnosis. Knee pain may be intermittent early in the course of degenerative arthritis. Importantly, not all knee pain is arthritic but may result from periarticular disorders, such as bursitis, or may be referred, especially from the hip.

Pain arising from articular surfaces is characteristically made worse by movement and better by rest. In the early stages, OA pain may be most noticeable when activity has ceased and the patient is relaxing. With disease progression, knee pain may occur earlier in activity. Pain occurring at rest or at night is a sign of advanced arthritis, although night pain is much more common in hip arthritis than knee arthritis. The pain may be localized or diffuse[5] and is frequently described as achy in nature. In general, pain will localize to the worst affected joint compartment. Diffuse knee pain may be associated with synovitis, effusion, and whole knee involvement or may represent pain referred from another site (e.g., the hip or lumbar radiculopathy). Pain from an arthritic knee rarely radiates elsewhere. A history of weakness or altered sensation suggests a neurological abnormality and is not a typical feature of arthritis.

In contrast, the pain of RA is characteristically episodic and associated with evidence of inflammation, such as redness, swelling, warmth, and constitutional symptoms. Morning stiffness lasting more than 1 hour is characteristic of systemic rheumatic disease, especially RA. Morning stiffness may also be a feature of OA but is generally no more than 30 minutes in duration. Knee pain from OA is typically worse at the end of the day.

Swelling around the knee from acute synovitis is characteristic of inflammatory arthritis. Synovial thickening and production of excess fluid (an effusion) cause swelling. Most osteoarthritic knees have little effusion, but occasionally an active synovitis is present and a large effusion may form. Rarely, an arthritic joint will spontaneously bleed into the synovial space, causing a painful, tense hemarthrosis. This is most common among patients with pseudogout or hemophilia and may also be seen in patients taking anticoagulant medications.

Deformity is a late manifestation of OA. Because of its insidious nature, deformity is often advanced before patients notice it. Loss of medial joint space results in a varus deformity and is the most common deformity associated with knee OA. Valgus deformity is more common in RA. Pain and stiffness may prohibit full knee flexion or extension and may eventually lead to the development of soft-tissue contractures and a fixed flexion deformity of the joint. A fixed flexion deformity in the knee produces an inefficient gait and contributes to reduced endurance.

The clinician must determine the effect of arthritis on the functional status of the individual patient. Loss of motion, joint pain, and contractures can interfere with dressing, toileting, bathing, stair climbing, getting out of a chair, and getting out of cars. The clinician should make the following inquiries: How far can you walk? Can you keep up with people your own age? Do you use a cane? Can you get up from a toilet? How many stairs can you climb with and without holding the rail? Do you use a cane? Can you get in and out of a car? How does this condition affect your daily life? A thorough review of systems is recorded. Constitutional symptoms such as fever, fatigue, and weight loss may suggest that arthritis is part of a systemic disorder. Additionally, symptoms in many joints warrant consideration of a systemic rheumatic disease. A history of trauma or surgery to the knee should be sought, and concomitant medical problems such as thyroid disease, psoriasis, inflammatory bowel disease, and chronic immunosuppression noted. Attention must be directed to eliciting a family history of arthritis, and the impact of arthritis on the life of the patient should be appreciated. The patient's occupation, leisure activities, and domestic situation should be noted. Does the patient have adequate support systems and access to appropriate resources? Has loss of function caused depression? Is the patient responsible for the care of others? Has the condition impacted on the patient's ability to earn an income? A complete list of the patient's medications should be noted, including the use of analgesics and their type, strength, frequency, and perceived efficacy. Previous drug interactions must be documented.

PHYSICAL EXAMINATION

After a detailed history, the physical examination will help distinguish between inflammatory versus mechanical disorders. Examination of the joint may be summarized as "look, feel, move, measure." Gait is usually the first observation as the patient enters the examination room. It may be antalgic, with a shortened stance phase on the affected leg, altered in speed or stride length. A "thrust" may be evident, with an increasing deformity (varus more common than valgus) during stance and push-off phase. The clinician should observe how well the patient rises from the chair and climbs on to the examination table. The entire limb must be exposed and, for comparison, the contralateral limb similarly displayed. Observe for scars and skin quality, muscle wasting (especially quadriceps femoris), deformity, and swelling around the knee or thigh. Palpation may elicit warmth, tenderness, or swelling. Synovial thickening or bogginess is typical of inflammatory arthritis. Signs of an effusion include a positive bulge sign and a patella tap. Local inflammation may be a feature of OA but is generally less marked.

Passive movement of the knee may be measured visually or more formally with a goniometer. The straight extended knee is at zero degrees, and any flexion beyond that is counted in degrees positive. Hyperextension, or motion in the negative direction, is rare in arthritis but not uncommon in neurological imbalance, in ligamentous laxity, and in youth. Active range of motion is tested and measured in the same way. Differences in active and passive range in extension, known as "quadriceps lag," should be recorded. Preservation of passive motion, but a reduced range of active motion, is typical of soft-tissue disorders or injury, whereas reduction of both active and passive ranges of motion is consistent with mechanical joint problems, synovitis, or soft-tissue contractures.

Joint stability can be tested by the application of physiological loads. Varus and valgus forces test collateral ligament stability. The clinician should note whether a varus or valgus deformity is correctable to neutral alignment. Neutral alignment in the disease-free knee is typically about 6 degrees of valgus from the femoral shaft to the tibial shaft ("anatomic" axis of the knee). Stability of the cruciate ligaments can be tested using the Lachman, drawer, and pivot shift tests. Rupture of the ACL will result in laxity of the knee, allowing for excess anterior movement of the tibia. The Lachman test is performed in 30 degrees of flexion, and the tibia is grasped and drawn forward. The degree that the tibia comes forward is estimated and compared with the other knee. The anterior drawer test is similar except the knee is at 90 degrees as the tibia is drawn forward. Placement of the examiner's thumb pulps on the femoral condyles and the heels of the hands on the tibia best differentiate movement as the tibia comes forward during the anterior drawer test. Some sense of the end point of the test is also useful. A softer end point is more indicative of ligament rupture. The pivot shift test is performed with the knee in extension, the tibia internally rotated, and a valgus stress applied while the knee is gradually flexed. In an ACL-deficient knee, this brings the subluxated tibia to a reduced position with a pivot or slight jumping sensation. It is uncomfortable if performed roughly but is a reliable sign, particularly if done under anesthetic.

Crepitus may be heard or palpated as a grinding sensation and may be patellofemoral, tibiofemoral or from soft tissue. It may result from abnormal articular surfaces or from synovitis but is a nonspecific sign and may also be found in otherwise normal knees. Neurovascular status examination of the lower limbs and a general medical assessment are prudent actions, particularly if surgery is contemplated. If a systemic rheumatic disease is being considered, extra-articular manifestations of arthritis, including tendon nodules, pericarditis, pleuritis, and hepatosplenomegaly, should be noted.

INVESTIGATION

The diagnosis of OA is essentially a clinical one that is confirmed by radiographs. It is critical to distinguish inflammatory arthritis from OA. Medical intervention for RA has progressed significantly, and many effective disease-modifying therapies are available. The use of laboratory tests is guided by the differential diagnosis formulated after the history and exam. However, no laboratory tests are required to diagnose OA.

LABORATORY TESTS

Inflammatory arthritis may produce elevations in erythrocyte sedimentation rate, C-reactive protein, and rheumatoid factor. These values also increase with age and are nonspecific. If there is clinical suspicion of RA, then the rheumatoid factor should be tested, remembering that this may be positive in other rheumatic diseases and may be negative in RA. The definitive diagnosis of gout depends on demonstration of monosodium urate crystals in synovial fluid. Serum levels of uric acid may be normal in the acute phase but may be elevated chronically and are most useful for monitoring treatment of hyperuricemia. Serum uric acid levels consistently greater than 10 mg/dL are associated with greater than 90% chance of an acute attack of gout. Aspiration of synovial fluid is critical when evaluating the patient with an acute febrile, monoarthritis to exclude infection. Fluid should be sent for Gram stain and culture and examined under polarized light for crystals. High leukocyte counts in synovial fluid suggest inflammation (such as rheumatoid or crystalline arthritis), although frankly purulent fluid ($>75,000 \times 10^9$/L), suggests septic arthritis. Synovial biopsy is useful only in rare circumstances when diagnosis cannot be confirmed with synovial fluid analysis and other standard diagnostic tests.

RADIOGRAPHIC IMAGING

Standard views include standing anteroposterior (AP), lateral, tunnel, and skyline (or Merchant's or Laurin's projections). The AP views are examined for soft-tissue abnormalities, bone quality, joint space width, osteophytes, and subchondral changes (cysts and sclerosis) (Fig. 1). The femoral condyle may appear squared after chronic medial meniscal resection with secondary arthritis. A square lateral condyle with increased joint space is suggestive of discoid lateral meniscus. The Schuss view (posteroanterior flexed weightbearing view) is suggested as the most accurate method for the evaluation of joint space width in early stages of femorotibial OA in routine clinical use. Calcification of the menisci is pathognomonic of chondrocalcinosis, a finding associated with pseudogout. The arthritis of the neuropathic knee is very characteristic with dramatic joint destruction, deformity, and soft-tissue bony debris (Fig. 2). The lateral view is examined for patella height relative to the joint line and condylar deformity. The cysts or erosion of RA are periarticular, whereas the cysts of OA are subchondral. Long films, including the hip, knee, and ankle, are taken to assess limb alignment and determine the correction required during an osteotomy or knee replacement. Bone scans are positive in early arthritis as well as reflex sympathetic dystrophy (RSD), stress fractures, and other conditions. Magnetic resonance imaging may be useful in the early stages of chondromalacia or osteonecrosis of the knee or to detect mechanical derangement of the knee, but it has little role in the diagnosis or management of OA. Radiographic staging schemes are used in clinical studies but are rarely used in routine orthopaedic practice.

DIFFERENTIAL DIAGNOSIS

Several conditions can mimic knee arthritis. Arthritis of the hip can produce anterior thigh and knee pain. All patients complaining of knee pain require a hip examination. One joint should be isolated while the other is tested to determine the likely site of disease. If a distinction between knee and referred pain is difficult, injection of the knee with local anesthetic will reduce local pain but not referred pain.

The third and fourth lumbar nerve roots supply sensation to the knee and its overlying skin. Irritation of nerve roots produces pain, which may mimic arthritis. This type of pain may have a burning quality, is exacerbated by nerve

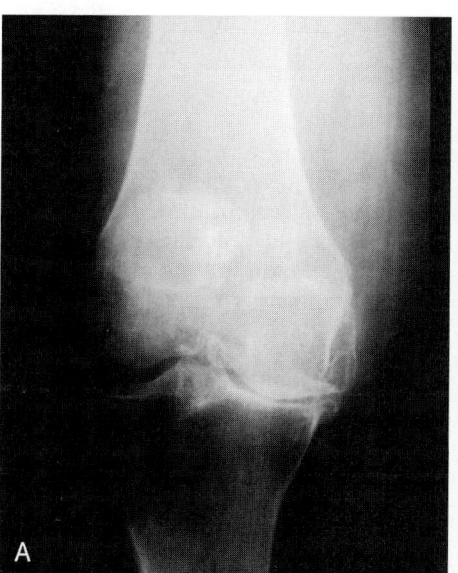
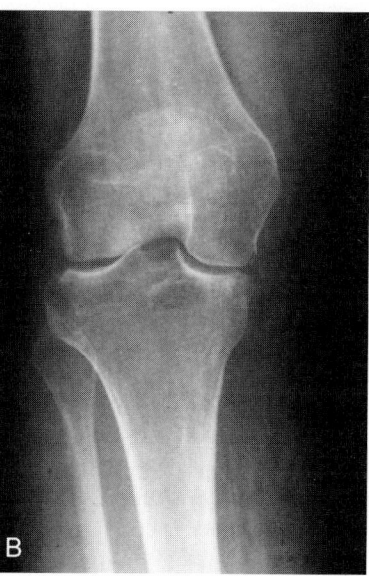
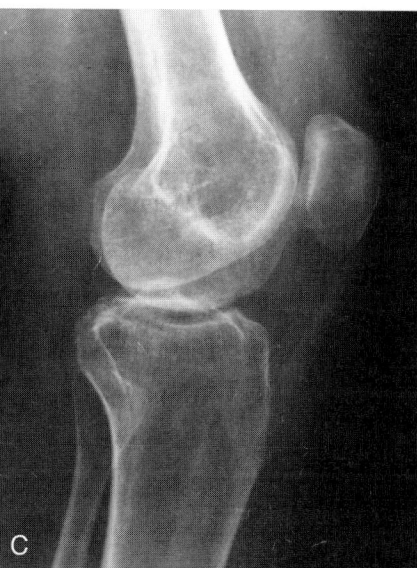
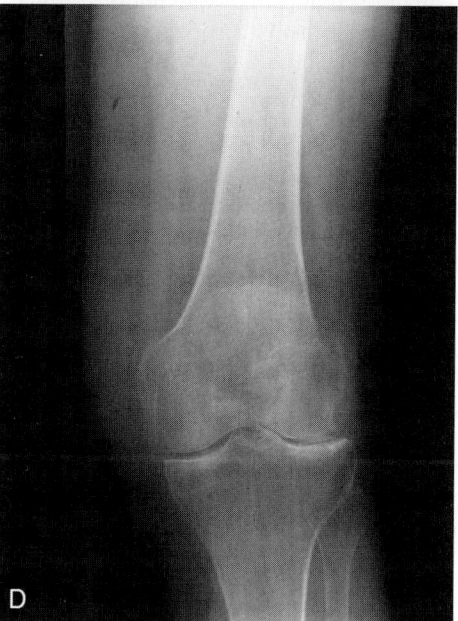

Fig. 1. Roentgenographic examination of patients with arthritic afflictions of the knee. *A,* Anteroposterior roentgenogram of the right knee in a retired 67-year-old teacher with osteoarthritis, primarily afflicting the medial compartment. There are peripheral osteophytes about the medial femoral condyle and the medial aspect of the tibial plateau with loss of the medial articular cartilage (joint space). Sclerosis of subchondral bone of both the medial femoral condyle and tibial plateau. *B* and *C,* Anteroposterior and lateral roentgenograms of the right knee in a 40-year-old woman with rheumatoid arthritis. There is osteopenia of the femur, tibia, and fibula. Erosions of the distal femur and tibia, both medially and laterally, can be seen in the area of the synovial reflections on the anteroposterior view. The articular cartilage thickness is reduced both medially and laterally. There are erosions of the medial subchondral bone, which are best seen on the lateral view. There is a large cyst of the proximal tibia, which is best seen on the anteroposterior view. *D,* Anteroposterior roentgenogram of the left knee in a 55-year-old with a 20-year history of rheumatoid arthritis. There are erosions of the distal femur in the area of the synovial reflections and osteopenia of the femur and tibia. The loss of articular cartilage (joint space) laterally with subchondral sclerosis is characteristic of secondary degenerative arthrosis. Excessive valgus angulation of the mechanical axis of the knee can be seen.

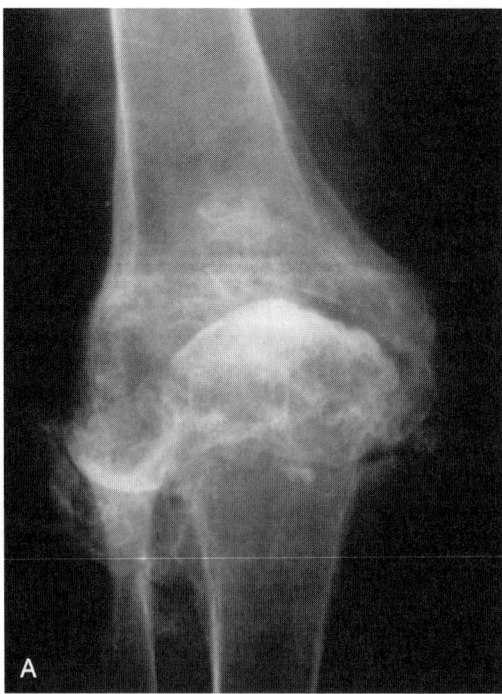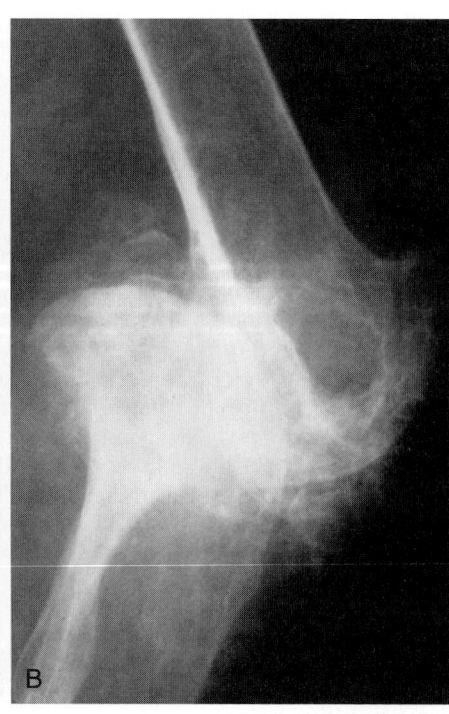

Fig. 2. Arthritis of the neuropathic knee. *A and B,* Anteroposterior and lateral roentgenograms of the right knee in a 64-year-old man with insulin-dependent diabetes mellitus and a Charcot joint. The knee is painless, but the patient complains of instability. The femorotibial articulation is dislocated with the tibial plateau subluxated proximally (best appreciated on the anteroposterior view) and posteriorly (best appreciated on the lateral view). The anatomy of the distal femur and proximal tibia has been completely distorted by the neuropathic process. Calcification of soft tissue, characteristic of the neuropathic process, can be visualized on both the anteroposterior and lateral views.

stretch tests, and may be accompanied by motor or reflex changes. Tendinitis or bursitis around the knee can produce pain, mimicking OA, but will have focal tenderness and occasional swelling and will generally be self-limiting. A meniscal tear will generally give some mechanical features of internal derangement such as catching, clicking, locking, or giving way. Meniscal tears and arthritis are often coexistent and can be differentiated by determining whether the pain emanates from the joint line or the chondral surfaces. Rare conditions like osteonecrosis of the femoral condyles or tumors causing knee pain can masquerade as OA. Features such as pain that is disproportionate to radiographic changes, unusual pain distribution or constant pain, or night pain unrelated to activity are not typical of knee arthritis.

MANAGEMENT

PREVENTION

Established arthritis of the knee with loss of articular cartilage is generally irreversible, so that prevention and slowing of progression of OA are vitally important in reducing the burden of disability in the community. Avoidance of obesity[9] and maintenance of activity with age should be encouraged.

For patients with inflammatory arthritis, disease should be controlled with disease-modifying drugs. (The issue of treatment of this disease is discussed in Chapter 6-3). Injury to the knee predisposes to OA. Sensitive MRI of the injured knee reveals "bone bruising," which previously went undetected. Apparently, benign knee injuries may result in long-term sequelae. The "knee-conscious" athlete may choose to reduce exposure to sports with the highest knee injury rates, such as football, downhill skiing, and others that require sudden changes in direction. Correction of limb malalignment (e.g., after fracture) is imperative for long-term integrity of the knee. After sporting injuries,

arthroscopic treatment of meniscal tears has largely replaced the older technique of open total meniscectomy, a procedure with a high rate of subsequent OA.[18] Preservation of menisci is paramount to reducing arthritis rates. ACL deficiency frequently leads to arthritis by subsequent meniscal and osteochondral injury and malalignment.[14, 15] Although not yet proven, reconstructing the ACL may lessen knee arthritis.[19]

NONPHARMACOLOGICAL TREATMENT

Weight reduction, physical therapy, and structured exercise programs are important management strategies for established arthritis. Therapeutic exercises decrease pain, increase muscle strength, and improve endurance and aerobic capacity.[20] Ideally, exercise should be daily and sustained and can involve simple activities like walking or cycling.[21] Water-based exercise may benefit those with advanced disease because it relieves weight and offers modest levels of resistance to motion. Identifying and eliminating provocative activities may reduce symptoms. Good lower limb strength may protect the knee from OA.[22, 23] Other means to reduce symptoms include stabilizing the joint, reducing impact forces, and distributing load. Therapeutic heat and cold, electrotherapy, ultrasonography, acupuncture, hydrotherapy, and spa treatments are widely used, although the effects and benefits have not been fully established. A cane can provide considerable weight relief in the affected knee and is a useful adjunct in nonoperative management. Shoe inserts for correction of angular deformities as well as knee braces may provide symptomatic relief.

PHARMACOLOGICAL TREATMENT

Acetaminophen is better than placebo and as effective as ibuprofen or naproxen for mild to moderate pain from OA. It is well tolerated and lacks the common complications associated with use of nonsteroidal anti-inflammatory agents (NSAIDs).[24] NSAIDS are frequently prescribed for all forms of arthritis and can be an effective analgesic for mild to moderate knee arthritis. They are more effective if taken continuously over days or weeks rather than intermittently. However, chronic use may increase the risk of adverse reactions, including gastric ulcerations, fluid retention, and renal impairment, especially in the elderly.

The Arthritis, Rheumatism, and Aging Medical Information System (ARAMIS) Post-Marketing Surveillance Program (PMS) prospectively monitored patient status and outcomes, drug side effects, and the economic impact of illness for more than 11,000 arthritis patients at eight participating institutions in the United States and Canada.[25] Analysis of these data indicated that patients with OA and RA are 2.5 to 5.5 times more likely than the general population to be hospitalized for NSAID-related gastrointestinal (GI) events. The absolute risk for serious NSAID-related GI toxicity remains constant, the cumulative risk increases over time, and there are no reliable warning signals. More than 80% of patients with serious GI complications had no prior GI symptoms. Independent risk factors for serious GI events are age, prednisone use, NSAID dose, disability level, and previous NSAID-induced GI symptoms. In addition, the clinical effectiveness of antacids, H_2 antagonists, in preventing NSAID-induced gastric ulcers is unclear. Currently, limiting nonselective NSAID use is the only way to decrease the risk of NSAID-related GI events. The anti-inflammatory actions of NSAIDs are mediated by the inhibition of COX-2, whereas the GI and renal toxicities are mediated by the inhibition of the constitutively expressed COX-1. Selective COX-2 inhibitors have now been approved for clinical use. Although their precise role in management of OA has not yet been defined, they are equally effective with less GI bleed risk. Tramadol may be useful for patients who do not receive adequate pain relief with acetaminophen and are at risk for NSAID-related toxicities.[26] Propoxyphene is no more effective than acetaminophen or ibuprofen and is not generally recommended.

Glucosamine sulfate, a nutritional supplement, has been anecdotally reported to provide symptomatic relief without serious adverse effects. A recent meta-analysis[26a] suggests it may be better than placebo for knee OA. However, no definitive clinical trials have provided convincing evidence of efficacy. Chondroitin sulphate is similarly a "nutraceutical" but again lacks scientific validation, and neither supplement is approved by the Food and Drug Administration for OA. Topical capsaicin acts selectively on a subpopulation of primary sensory neurons with a nociceptive function and can be effective local analgesia for knee pain.[27] Similarly, liniments and elastic bandages can provide symptomatic relief in mild cases.

Intra-articular steroid injections may also decrease knee pain, but the results are generally short term and are generally recommended no more than three or four times a year.[28] Best results are from use in acute flare-ups of inflammatory arthritis. However, if frequent injections are required, surgical intervention should be considered. "Visco-supplementation" with hyaluronic acid has been approved for use, and preliminary studies suggest a brief duration of benefit after injection into the knee.[29] Acute calcium pyrophosphate dihydrate arthritis has been reported after intra-articular hyaluronate injection.

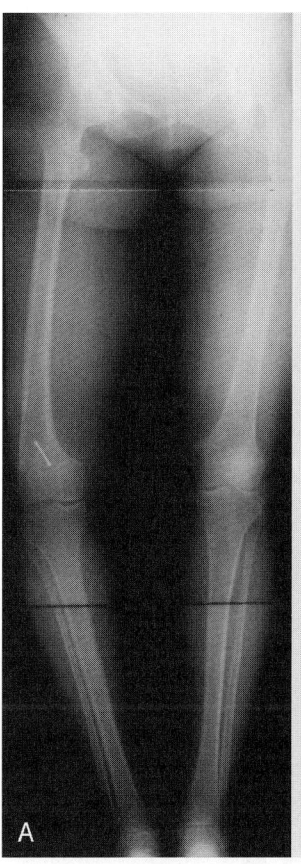
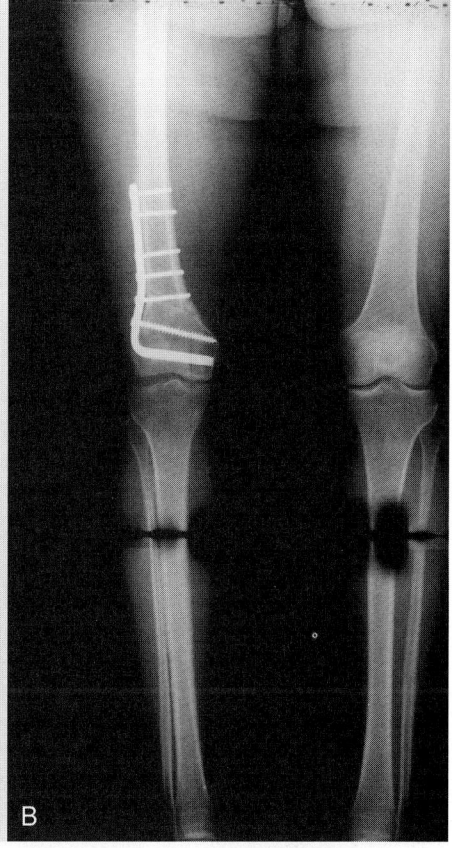

Fig. 3. Severe posttraumatic varus deformity treated with distal femoral valgus osteotomy. *A,* Full-length anteroposterior roentgenogram of both legs in a 32-year-old woman with right knee pain. She experienced a right femoral fracture as a child, which healed with a varus deformity. The mechanical axis falls outside (medial) to the knee. The varus deformity has also precipitated recurrent pretibial pain from stress fractures in the right leg. *B,* Full-length anteroposterior roentgenogram of both legs 1 year after a distal femoral valgus osteotomy. Fixation of the osteotomy was performed with a blade plate and screws. The mechanical axis falls through the medial aspect of the femorotibial articulation. She is asymptomatic and active as an emergency medical technician.

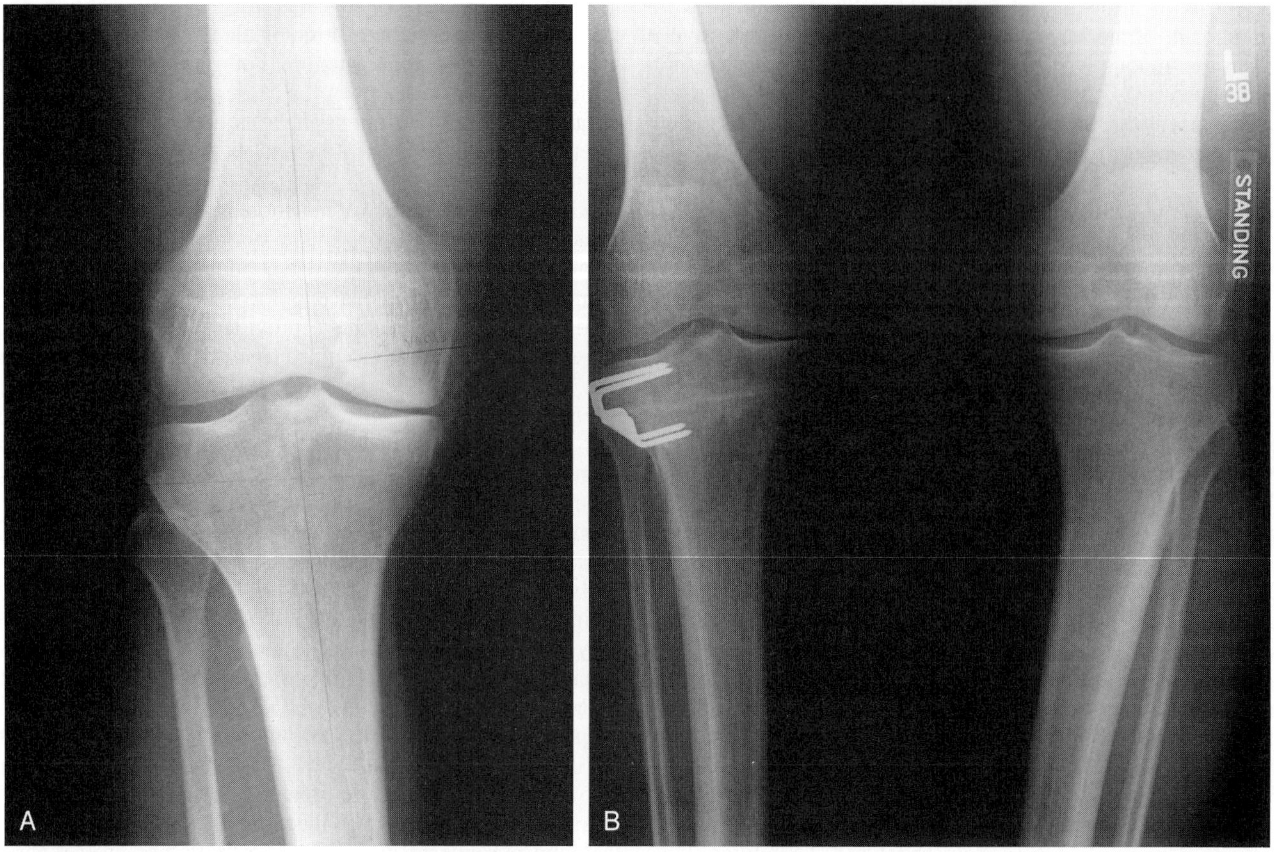

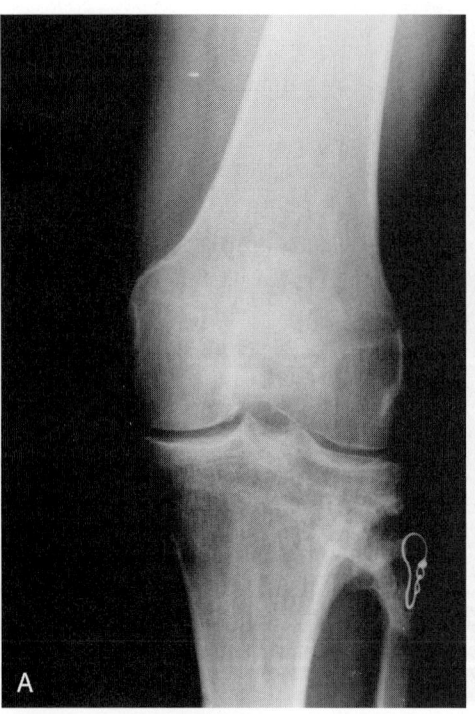

Fig. 4. **A painful right knee in a 57-year-old with a mild varus deformity treated with a proximal tibial valgus osteotomy.** *A*, Anteroposterior roentgenogram of the right knee with 3 degrees of varus deformity and narrowing of the medial joint space. *B*, Anteroposterior roentgenogram 15 months after a proximal tibial valgus osteotomy. Fixation of the osteotomy was performed with two Coventry stepped staples. The normal valgus mechanical alignment has been restored and slightly overcorrected. The patient is asymptomatic.

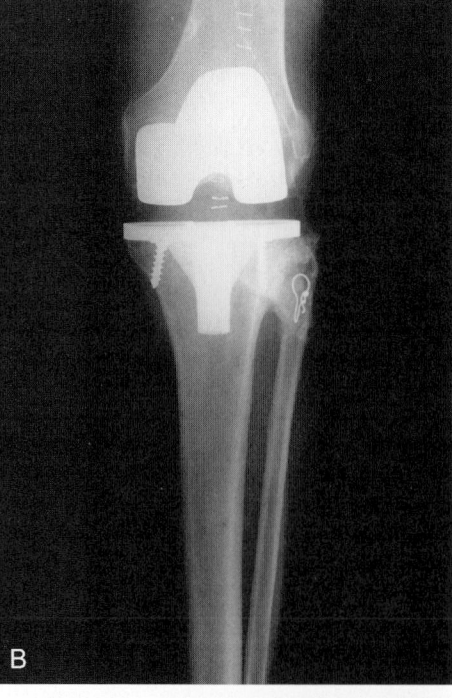

Fig. 5. **Severe pain of the right knee with osteoarthritis 8 years after a valgus proximal tibial osteotomy in a 65-year-old treated with a total knee arthroplasty.** *A*, Anteroposterior roentgenogram of the right knee with an 11-degree valgus deformity. Evidence of healing of an old valgus osteotomy is evident. The joint space is narrowed bilaterally, laterally greater than medially. *B*, Anteroposterior roentgenogram after a hybrid total-knee arthroplasty. The valgus alignment of the knee has been restored to a normal angulation of 7 degrees.

SURGICAL MANAGEMENT
Synovectomy
Synovectomy can be used to treat severe active RA of the knee that has not responded to medical management for at least 6 months. The method of synovectomy is open operation, arthroscopic, or by radioisotope. Pigmented villonodular synovitis, which has its highest incidence in the knee, may require similar treatment.

Arthroscopy
Arthroscopic lavage and débridement may provide relief of symptoms. It is well tolerated with minimal morbidity and rapid recovery and probably works by removing debris and degradative enzymes. Removal of unstable menisci and loose articular cartilage should also be achieved. Because some studies have shown no benefit or even worsening of symptoms in a proportion of patients with OA, one should be selective in offering arthroscopic treatment.[30] Patients with less knee deformity benefit more than patients with large angulations of the knee. Prior surgery, advanced disease, and the presence of rest pain predispose to poor results. However, many surgeons believe that arthroscopic débridement is a successful palliative, temporizing treatment for the osteoarthritic knee.[31]

Osteotomy
Osteotomy of the femur or the tibia is performed to restore the normal mechanical axis and the 5 to 7 degrees of valgus alignment of the femorotibial articulation in a patient with a painful knee and malalignment of the extremity. The compartment opposite the deformity must be normal for the corrective osteotomy to be successful. The patient must also have a stable knee (stability of the collateral and cruciate ligaments) and a near-normal range of motion. Assessment of the mechanical axis requires full-length AP roentgenograms demonstrating the hip, knee, and ankle joints on the film. Normally, the mechanical axis (a line from the center of the hip to the center of the ankle) falls through the center of the knee or just to the lateral aspect of the knee. Either a varus or valgus deformity of the knee can be treated with an osteotomy. A severe varus deformity (greater than 5 to 6 degrees) or a valgus deformity is best treated with a distal femoral osteotomy (Fig. 3). Careful preoperative planning to determine the exact degree of deformity and the degree of operative correction necessary is obligatory to restore alignment. A varus distal femoral osteotomy for a valgus deformity should not incorporate overcorrection. In contrast, a valgus osteotomy of either the distal femur or proximal tibia should incorporate 5 degrees of overcorrection. The mechanical forces after distal femoral osteotomy are of such magnitude that secure internal fixation is mandatory. In contrast, the large cancellous surfaces and the compressive forces of the quadriceps muscle after proximal tibial osteotomy permit less secure fixation, customarily with staples. A short period of immobilization with a cast brace or a cylinder cast permits early union of the large cancellous surfaces.

The typical clinical situation amenable to treatment is a mild varus deformity with medial joint space pain treated with a proximal tibial valgus osteotomy (Fig. 4). Prerequisites to a successful proximal tibial osteotomy require ligamentous stability and a near-normal range of motion with a

normal lateral compartment. Osteotomy is not recommended in the treatment of deformities associated with inflammatory arthritis because the underlying disease afflicts the articular cartilage of all three compartments of the knee.

Arthroplasty
Indications for knee arthroplasty are severe pain daily, rest pain several days per week, transfer pain either several days per week or daily pain, and destruction of most of the joint space as seen radiographically (Fig. 5). Younger age, comorbidity, technical difficulties, and lack of motivation generally sway the decision against surgery, whereas the desire to be independent and return to work sways the decision for surgery. The concept of 6 degrees of freedom is particularly important to the knee replacement surgeon, who has under his or her total control the positioning of the replacement components. Correct functioning of the prosthetic knee is dependent on correct placement of all the components in all six orientations. Failure in this regard is a frequent yet subtle cause of disappointing results in knee arthroplasty, leading to premature wear, component loosening, and diminished or painful motion (Fig. 6).

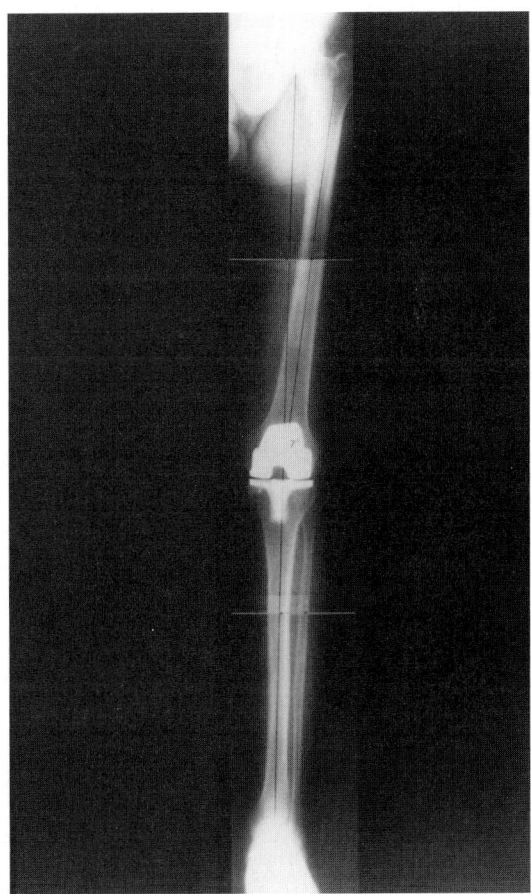

Fig. 6. Anteroposterior roentgenogram after a cemented total-knee arthroplasty. Correct placement of the components with restoration of the mechanical alignment of the extremity after total-knee arthroplasty is necessary for excellent long-term results. Full-length anteroposterior roentgenograms are required to document restoration of both the mechanical and anatomical axes. The anatomic (femorotibial) axis has been restored to 7 degrees of valgus alignment. The mechanical axis falls through the center of the knee.

Arthrodesis

This is the salvage procedure of choice for the multiply failed knee arthroplasty. Revision arthroplasty may not be an option because of infection, but arthrodesis may be necessary.

Excision Arthroplasty

This procedure is rarely undertaken and then only as a last resort after failed knee arthroplasty.

Experimental Surgical Methods

Meniscal allograft may be used in the early stages of knee OA secondary to meniscectomy. An entire meniscus is set into the place of the damaged meniscus and immediately begins load sharing. Definitive results are unavailable.[32] Osteochondral grafting has been attempted in young sufferers of focal OA. This might entail replacing an entire femoral or tibial condyle. Achieving a stable and congruent mechanical construct is technically challenging. Cartilage engineering is finding a role in focal defects of the knee. Chondrocyte cultures are placed beneath a periosteal membrane over the defect and proliferate and mature in situ. Techniques such as abrasion arthroplasty, drilling, and microfracture of subchondral bone expose marrow cells that are capable of differentiation. They produce only fibrocartilage, however, and thus do not offer a long-term cure.

REFERENCES

1. MacLennan WJ: History of arthritis and bone rarefaction: Evidence from paleopathology onwards. Scott Med J 1999; 44: 18.
2. Storey GO, Scott DL: Arthritis associated with venereal disease in nineteenth century London. Clin Rheumatol 1998; 17:500.
3. Boonen A, van de Rest J, Dequelcer J, et al: How Renoir coped with rheumatoid arthritis. BMJ 1997; 315:1704.
4. Lawrence RC, Helmick CG, et al: Estimates of the prevalence of arthritis and selected musculoskeletal disorders in the United States. Arthritis Rheum 1998; 41: 778.
5. Coventry MB: Osteotomy of the upper portion of the tibia for degenerative arthritis of the knee: A preliminary report. Clin Orthop 1989; 248:4.
6. Creamer P, Lethbridge-Cejku M, Hochberg MC: Where does it hurt? Pain localization in osteoarthritis of the knee. Osteoarthritis Cartilage 1998; 6:318.
7. Felson DT, Zhang Y, Hannan MT, et al: Risk factors for incident radiographic knee osteoarthritis in the elderly: The Framingham study. Arthritis Rheum 1997; 40:728.
8. Felson DT, Zhang Y, Hannan MT, et al: The incidence and natural history of knee osteoarthritis in the elderly: The Framingham Osteoarthritis Study. Arthritis Rheum 1995; 38:1500.
9. Jordan JM, Linder GF, Renner JB, et al: The impact of arthritis in rural populations. Arthritis Care Res 1995; 8:242.
10. Pastoreau PC, Chiomel AC, Bonnet J: Evidence of early subchondral bone changes in meniscectomized guinea pig: A densitometric study using dual energy X-ray absorptiometry subregional analysis. Osteoarthritis Cartilage 1999; 7:466.
11. Dieppe P, Cushnaghan J, Young P, et al: Prediction of the progression of joint space narrowing in osteoarthritis of the knee by bone scintigraphy. Ann Rheum Dis 1993; 52:557.
12. Hockberg MC, Altman RD, Brandt KD, et al: Guidelines for the medical management of osteoarthritis II: Osteoarthritis of the knee. Arthritis Rheum 1995; 38:1541.
13. Mikosz RP, Andriacchi TP: Anatomy and biomechanics of the knee. In Callaghan JJ, Dennis DA, Paprosky WG (eds): Hip and Knee Reconstruction. American Academy of Orthopaedic Surgeons, Rosemont, IL, 1995, p 227.
14. Jacobsen K: Osteoarthritis following insufficiency of the cruciate ligaments in man: A clinical study. Acta Orthop Scand 1977; 48:52.
15. Neyret P, Donell ST, Dejour H: Results of partial meniscectomy related to the state of the anterior cruciate ligament: Review of 20 to 35 years. J Bone Joint Surg Br 1993; 75:36.
16. Felson DT, Chaisson CE: Understanding the relationship between body weight and osteoarthritis. Baillieres Clin Rheumatol 1997; 11:671.
17. Felson DT, Zhang Y, Anthony JM, et al: Weight loss reduces the risk for symptomatic knee osteoarthritis in women: The Framingham study. Ann Intern Med 1992; 116:535.
18. Sommerlath K, Gillquist J: The long-term course of various meniscal treatments in anterior cruciate ligament deficient knees. Clin Orthop 1992; 283:207.
19. Clatworthy M, Amendola A: The anterior cruciate ligament and arthritis. Clin Sports Med 1999; 18:173.
20. Minor MA, Hewett JE, Webel RR, et al: Efficacy of physical condition and exercise in patients with rheumatoid arthritis and osteoarthritis. Arthritis Rheum 1989; 32: 1396.
21. Kovar PA, Allegrante JP, MacKenzie CR, et al: Supervised fitness walking in patients with osteoarthritis of the knee: A randomized, controlled trial. Ann Intern Med 1992; 116:529.
22. Slemenda C, Mazzuca S, Brandt K, et al: Lower extremity lean tissue mass and strength predict increases in pain and in functional impairment in knee osteoarthritis. Arthritis Rheum 1996; 39:S212.
23. Slemenda S, Heilman DK, Brandt KD, et al: Reduced quadriceps strength relative to body weight: A risk factor for knee osteoarthritis in women? Arthritis Rheum 1998; 41:1951.
24. Towheed TE, Hocherg MC: A systematic review of randomized controlled trials of pharmacological therapy in osteoarthritis of the knee, with an emphasis on trial methodology. Semin Arthritis Rheum 1997; 26:755.
25. Singh G, Rosen Ramey D: NSAID induced gastrointestinal complications: The ARAMIS perspective 1997. J Rheumatol 1998; 51:8.
26. Schnitzer TJ: Non-NSAID pharmacological treatment options for the management of chronic pain. Am J Med 1998; 105: 45S.
26a. McAlindon TE, LaValley MP, Gulin JP, et al: Glucosamine and chondroitin for treatment of osteoarthritis: A systematic quality assessment and meta-analysis. JAMA 2000; 283:1469.
27. Deal CL, Schnitzer TJ, Lipstein E, et al: Treatment of arthritis with topical capsaicin: A double-blind trial. Clin Ther 1991; 13:383.
28. Kirwan JR, Rankin E: Intra-articular therapy in osteoarthritis. Baillieres Clin Rheumatol 1997; 11:769.
29. Marshall KW: Viscosupplementation for osteoarthritis: Current status, unresolved issues and future directions. J Rheumatol 1998; 25:2056.
30. Harwin SF: Arthroscopic débridement for osteoarthritis of the knee: Predictors of patient satisfaction. Arthroscopy 1999; 15: 142.
31. McGinley BJ, Cushner FD, Scott WN: Débridement arthroscopy: 10 year followup. Clin Orthop 1999; 367:190.
32. Johnson DL, Bealle D: Meniscal allograft transplantation. Clin Sports Med 1999; 18: 93.

OSTEOTOMIES ABOUT THE KNEE

section 6 chapter 15

Stephen G. Manifold, Michael A. Kelly, Lars Richardson, and Thomas J. Gill

Summary

- Knee osteotomy in younger patients with osteoarthritic knees can delay the need for joint arthroplasty, therefore decreasing the risk of future revision arthroplasty. This is important because of the tremendous impact of revision surgery on the patient and its cost to society, which has been estimated to be nearly $230 million per year.
- The most important factor determining the success of an osteotomy is correction of the overall limb alignment.
- The osteotomy technique should include rigid fixation that will allow early range of knee motion.
- Preferred indications for osteotomy include age younger than 50 years, unicompartmental osteoarthritis, limb alignment deformity of less than 10 degrees, and a flexion arc of at least 90 degrees.
- Contraindications include inflammatory arthritides, knee flexion contracture of 10 degrees or more, and tibiofemoral subluxation greater than 1 cm.

Deviations from normal anatomic relationships can increase the forces across articular cartilage. Degenerative arthrosis of joints such as the knee may result from such malalignment. Abnormal tibiofemoral relationships also increase the stresses in the ligamentous structures around the knee, further advancing deformity.

Corrective osteotomies of the knee were originally introduced as an alternative to total knee arthroplasty in younger patients with degenerative joint disease. These patients were typically younger than 65 years old, and the durability of total joint implants in this patient population was uncertain at that time. The potential of an osteotomy to delay joint arthroplasty in these patients and therefore decrease the risk of undergoing future complex revision procedures made this an attractive alternative. However, improvements in technology and surgical techniques and the excellent clinical experience with knee arthroplasty have expanded the indications for joint replacement and decreased the role of osteotomies. Although the indications have become more limited, there is still a patient population for which this is an attractive surgical alternative. Additionally, with the advent of cartilage resurfacing procedures, osteotomies may become an integral component in the treatment of those patients with cartilage lesions and malalignment of the knee.

HISTORICAL REVIEW

Osteotomies of the long bones in the lower extremity were used initially to treat deformities resulting from trauma and developmental disorders. The first report of an osteotomy of the tibia was by Volkmann[1] in 1875, who performed the procedure to correct a deformity of the knee joint. Jackson and Waugh[2] were the first to describe osteotomy for the correction of varus or valgus malalignment of the knee secondary to degenerative osteoarthritis. Correction of the deformity was the primary goal of the procedure. These patients were also noted to have considerable relief of pain following the osteotomy. Coventry[3] reported on his extensive experience with proximal tibial valgus osteotomy in which a lateral approach was used and a wedge-shaped closing osteotomy was performed proximal to the level of the tibial tubercle. This has been the preferred osteotomy technique for the osteoarthritic varus knee for the past two decades.

High tibial osteotomy (HTO) has historically been a lateral closing wedge procedure performed for varus knees with medial compartment arthrosis. Techniques for medial opening wedge osteotomies have been developed that are successful and reproducible, with relatively low patient morbidity rates. Distal femoral osteotomy (DFO) remains the procedure of choice for valgus knees with lateral compartment arthrosis. Like HTOs, DFOs can be either closing wedge or opening wedge procedures.

Differences between the results of proximal tibial osteotomy for varus malalignment compared with those for valgus malalignment became evident and led to changes in the recommended procedure for patients with valgus knee deformities. Several authors noted the increased obliquity of the joint line following proximal tibial varus osteotomy[4] (Fig. 1). This is caused by the greater loss of bone from the lateral femoral condyle in a valgus deformity compared with a varus deformity. This obliquity was initially believed to be of little importance, but subsequent studies demonstrated that over time the joint obliquity resulted in medial subluxation of the femur on the tibia.[5–7] Consequently, proximal tibial osteotomy for valgus knee deformities greater than 10 to 12 degrees was abandoned and replaced with distal femoral varus osteotomy. This osteotomy not only corrects the malalignment but also restores the joint line parallel to the ground (Fig. 2).

This chapter reviews the current indications, contraindications, and surgical techniques for proximal tibial valgus and distal femoral varus knee osteotomies. The most common complications associated with these osteotomies and ways to avoid them are also discussed.

BASIC FEATURES

Alignment of the knee is assessed using the mechanical and anatomic axes of the limb (Fig. 3). The mechanical axis is defined by a straight line passing from the center of the hip joint through the center of the knee and continuing

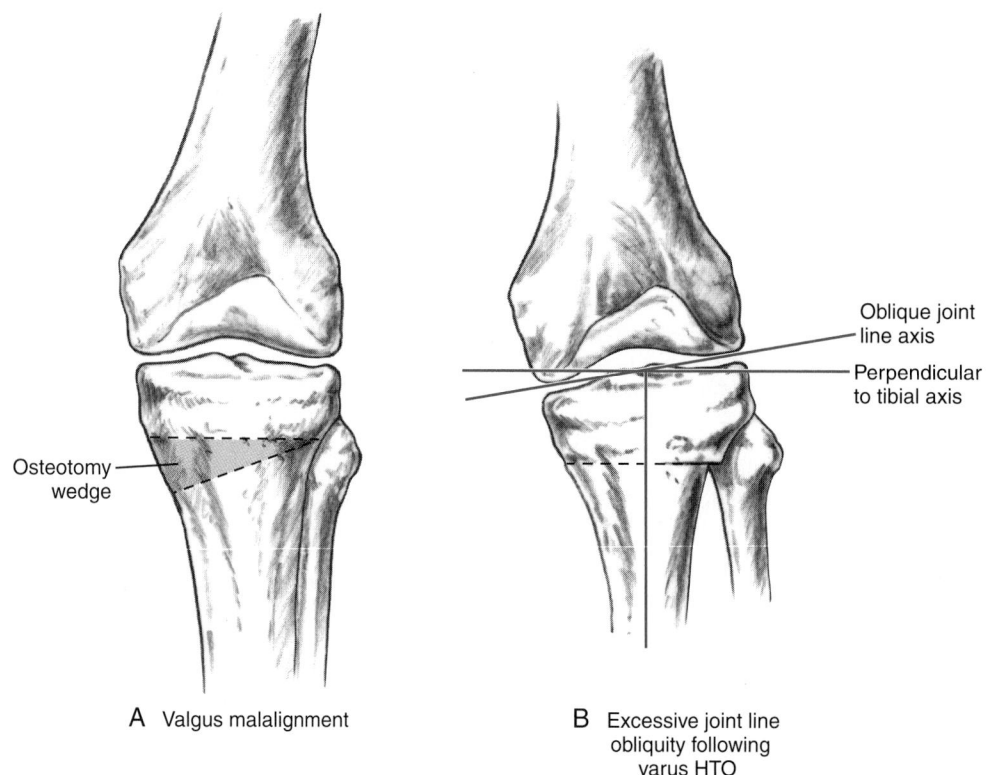

A Valgus malalignment

B Excessive joint line
obliquity following
varus HTO

Oblique joint
line axis

Perpendicular
to tibial axis

Osteotomy
wedge

Fig. 1. Joint line obliquity following varus HTO. *A,* Knee with significant valgus malalignment. *B,* Varus osteotomy of the proximal tibia has corrected the overall alignment but has created obliquity of the joint line.

through the center of the ankle mortise. The mechanical axis of the leg and the long axis of the tibia are colinear. The normal mechanical axis therefore is measured as 0 degrees. The anatomic axis is defined by the angle of intersection between a line drawn along the shaft of the femur and a line drawn along the shaft of the tibia. This angle is normally between 5 and 7 degrees of valgus. In a normally aligned knee, approximately 60% of the weight-

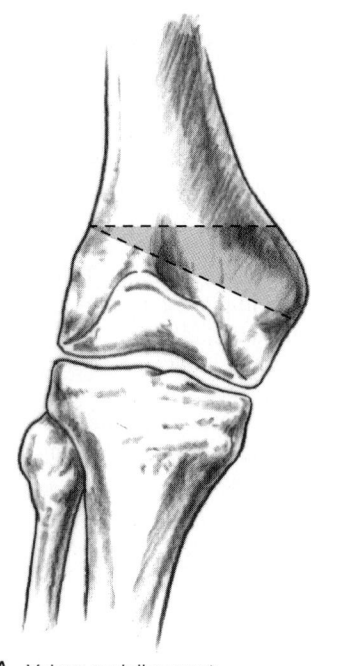

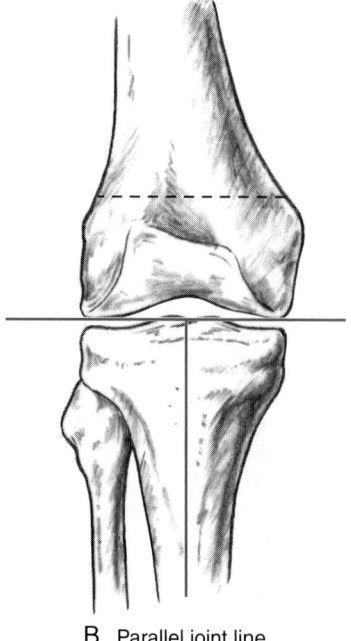

Perpendicular
to tibial axis

Fig. 2. Parallel joint line following DFO. *A,* Valgus knee with proposed osteotomy wedge from distal femur. *B,* After closure, joint line is parallel to floor.

A Valgus malalignment

B Parallel joint line
after DFO

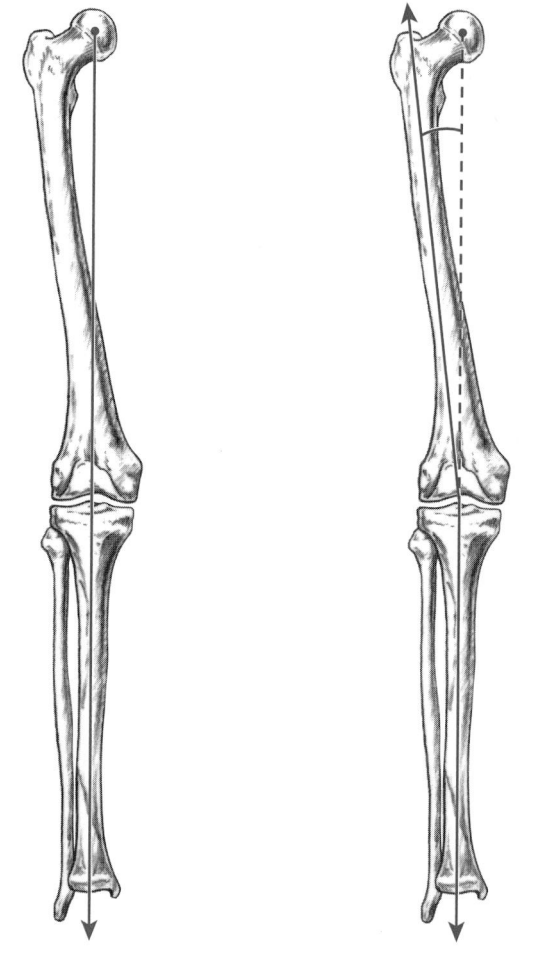

A Mechanical axis

B Anatomic (femorotibial) axis
normal 5-7° valgus

Fig. 3. Methods of assessing limb alignment. *A,* Mechanical axis passing from center of hip through center of knee and tibial plafond. Normal is 0 degrees. *B,* Anatomic (femorotibial) axis formed by intersection of femoral and tibial shaft axis lines. Normal is 5 to 7 degrees of valgus.

bearing force passes through the medial compartment and 40% through the lateral joint space.[8] In addition, the joint line of the knee is parallel to the ground.

The change in knee alignment that occurs in unicompartmental tibiofemoral osteoarthritis results in the mechanical axis passing either through the medial or lateral compartment of the knee rather than through the center. Consequently, there is a redistribution of the forces passing through the joint, with a greater percentage of the weight-bearing force passing through the medial compartment in a varus knee and through the lateral compartment in a valgus knee. Significant deviations from the mean can lead to abnormal articular contact pressures (see Fig. 1B). Medial compartment contact forces have been shown to increase with varus deformity.[9] This increased force causes further articular cartilage destruction, leading to worsening malalignment. A vicious cycle is established. Ultimately, full-thickness cartilage loss in the involved compartment ensues, followed by underlying bone loss if the malalignment is not corrected. This bone loss occurs primarily from the

medial plateau of the proximal tibia in a varus knee and from the lateral femoral condyle in a valgus knee.

CLINICAL FEATURES

Pain is the predominant symptom in osteoarthritis of any joint, including the knee. Typically, the patient reports a worsening of pain with activities, such as prolonged standing, walking, or running, in which the knee joint is subjected to increased loads. Pain is often improved during sedentary activities in which the load on the knee is reduced. The pain is usually well localized to the affected compartment in unicompartmental disease, with the unaffected compartment being relatively asymptomatic. Knee pain that is poorly localized may indicate more diffuse involvement of the other compartments with osteoarthritis. The onset of discomfort is most commonly insidious with a gradual progression of symptoms as the cartilage continues to deteriorate. A sudden onset of joint line pain may indicate other disorders, such as a degenerative meniscal tear or osteonecrosis. Additional complaints of intermittent swelling and stiffness may be reported.

Careful physical examination of patients with unicompartmental osteoarthritis and malalignment is important. The most obvious finding is the varus or valgus standing deformity of the limb. The clinical degree of deformity can be measured with a goniometer. The location and type of prior incisions associated with previous surgeries, such as a medial meniscectomy or open reduction of a lateral tibial plateau fracture, that may have predisposed to the development of the malalignment, should be noted. Joint line palpation should localize tenderness over the symptomatic compartment and verify that no tenderness exists over the other compartments, including the patellofemoral joint. In addition, the surrounding soft tissue of the knee should be palpated to eliminate other sources of pain, such as tendinitis of the patellar or pes anserine tendons. An assessment of the range of motion of the knee is mandatory. The presence and severity of any flexion contracture, extension lag, or lack of motion should also be documented. Finally, the status of the knee ligaments must be determined by testing for mediolateral and anteroposterior instability.

The clinician should perform a complete examination of the entire extremity. The hip should be examined for excessive femoral anteversion, which has been implicated in increased force transmission through the medial compartment of the knee. Similarly, increased internal tibial torsion or excessive supination of the foot can also overload the medial joint space. The possibility of referred knee pain from ipsilateral hip osteoarthritis must also be eliminated. Perhaps the most important factor is the magnitude of an adductor moment as noted on gait analysis.[10] Patients with low adduction moments at the knee compensate for the varus deformity by shortening the gait stride and toeing out. Conversely, patients with high adduction moments toe-in during ambulation and have a more normal stride. Wang et al[11] reported on the results of proximal tibial osteotomy at an average follow-up period of 5.9 years and found that 100% (14/14) of patients with a low adduction moment had excellent or good results compared with 64% (9/14) of patients with a high adduction moment. In addition, the recurrence rate of deformity was greater in the high-adduc-

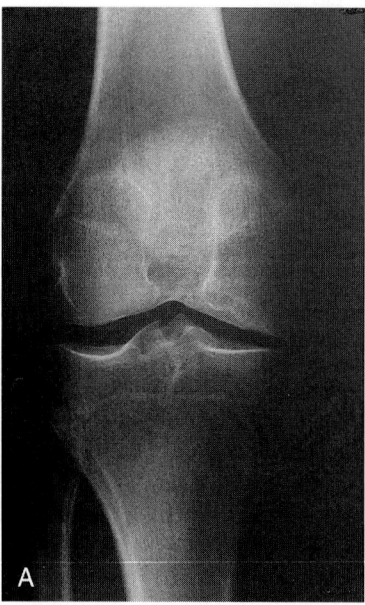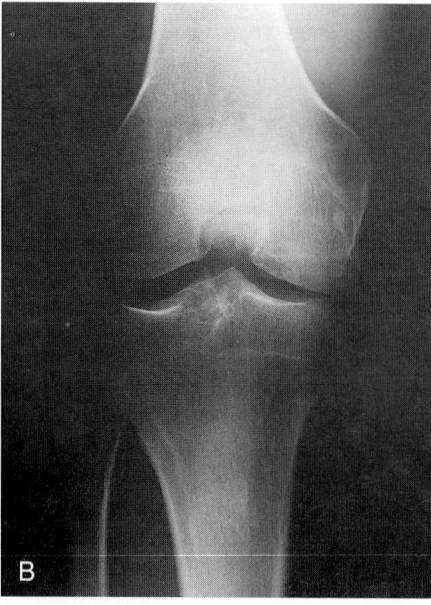

Fig. 4. Radiographic assessment of joint space narrowing. *A,* Standing anteroposterior radiograph showing mild medial joint space narrowing. *B,* 45-degree standing anteroposterior radiograph of the same knee demonstrating more severe narrowing of joint space.

tion-moment group than in the low-adduction-moment group (71% versus 21%), suggesting that the compensatory gait mechanisms may continue postoperatively.

INVESTIGATION

The information obtained from the history and physical examination is often sufficient to determine the potential benefit of a knee osteotomy. In some instances, more information concerning the condition of the compartments of the knee is required. In addition to routine knee radiographs, which include standing anteroposterior, lateral, and Merchant's views, a standing 45-degree anteroposterior radiograph should be obtained. This view more clearly demonstrates the extent of joint space narrowing compared with the regular standing anteroposterior view (Fig. 4). Full-length films with the three-joint standing view are also essential for preoperative planning (see below).

Preoperative stress views of the varus knee can demonstrate medial collateral ligament laxity. This laxity can be eliminated by a medial opening wedge osteotomy, which can restore anatomic tension to the medial soft tissues.[12]

Patients with unicompartmental osteoarthritis and malalignment may also have mechanical symptoms, such as locking or catching, which may indicate meniscal disorder. When mechanical symptoms exist, magnetic resonance imaging (MRI) is useful in identifying meniscal tears. Routine use of preoperative MRI in patients with malalignment is not indicated when these mechanical symptoms are absent. Degenerative tears are often ubiquitous in a malaligned osteoarthritic knee. If they are asymptomatic, they do not need to be addressed before the osteotomy. Patients with an osteoarthritic, malaligned knee and more diffuse pain throughout the knee require careful evaluation before an osteotomy. If radiographic evidence of degenerative changes, such as joint space narrowing or osteophytes, exists in the opposite joint space or in the patellofemoral joint, an osteotomy procedure can be expected to yield poor results. Evaluation becomes more difficult in those patients with diffuse

pain and radiographically normal opposite joint spaces. A technetium bone scan can be helpful in this situation by providing information concerning the condition of the opposite joint space.[13] Increased uptake on the scan is indicative of osteoarthritic involvement of the space and may discourage use of corrective osteotomy.

The role of knee arthroscopy prior to osteotomy has been examined. The rationale behind preosteotomy arthroscopy involves direct visualization and assessment of the articular cartilage of the opposite joint space. Significant alterations in the articular surface would seem to preclude osteotomy and the subsequent loading onto this abnormal surface. Accurate assessment of the thickness of the articular surface, however, is difficult.[14] Moreover, Keene et al[15] evaluated the results of high tibial osteotomy at a minimum 5-year follow-up in patients who underwent arthroscopy before osteotomy. The rate of good and excellent results was unrelated to the preosteotomy arthroscopic findings in the lateral and patellofemoral compartments. Consequently, routine use of arthroscopy before osteotomy is not recommended.

GOALS, INDICATIONS, AND CONTRAINDICATIONS

GOALS

The goal of osteotomy about the knee is to correct the abnormal mechanical axis of the knee and redistribute the weightbearing forces away from the osteoarthritic compartment onto the relatively unaffected cartilage. This serves to alleviate pain and potentially allows for cartilage regeneration in the narrowed joint space. Fujisawa et al[16] performed arthroscopy at yearly intervals on patients following HTO and noted the regeneration of normal-appearing articular cartilage by 2 years. The newly formed cartilage was found to have characteristics more typical of fibrocartilage than hyaline cartilage and was, therefore, more likely to undergo degeneration over time.[17] Consequently, the patient must understand that the purpose of an osteotomy is to correct malalignment and to relieve pain, not to create a "normal" knee.

In knees with medial compartment arthritis and varus deformity, the medial femoral and tibial condyles display significantly more osteosclerosis than the lateral condyles. When the sclerosis was quantitatively measured after HTO, the values normalized within 1 year.[18] Histological studies examining patients undergoing HTO have reported a quantitative comparison of pre- and postoperative synovial biopsy samples. At the time of hardware removal following HTO (mean 21 months), the amount of collagen fragments had decreased by nearly 90%, and CD68 lining cells typical of macrophages had decreased by 50%. It was concluded that the decrease in cartilage fragments postoperatively had alleviated the preoperative synovitis.[19]

The mechanism of pain relief has been debated. It is thought to occur primarily by removal of the abnormal force from the narrowed joint space, which allows healing of the subchondral bone microfractures associated with osteoarthritis and malalignment. In addition, some authors have ascribed pain relief to lowered intraosseous venous pressure following unloading of the joint space.[20] Regardless of the mechanism, the primary objective of the surgeon must be to obtain a balanced knee following osteotomy that allows for symmetric loading of the joint spaces. The exact amount of correction required to obtain this objective is not clearly defined. Vainionpaa et al[21] reviewed 5- to 10-year results of tibial osteotomy and determined that recurrence of varus deformity was minimized by obtaining postoperative anatomic valgus alignment of 7 to 10 degrees. Similarly, Insall et al[22] performed a long-term follow-up study of HTO and recommended that at least 10 degrees of postoperative valgus be achieved. Keene et al[15] noted that significantly better results were associated with those knees that had 7 to 13 degrees of valgus angulation compared with those with less than 7 degrees. The common conclusion of these and similar studies is that for a varus knee, the alignment must be corrected to at least the normal anatomic axis of 5 to 8 degrees of valgus and that, preferably, a small amount of overcorrection (approximately 5 degrees) should be achieved. The goal in realignment of a valgus knee is to achieve an anatomic axis of approximately 2 to 3 degrees of valgus while avoiding overcorrection into varus alignment.

INDICATIONS AND CONTRAINDICATIONS

One important factor that contributes to a satisfactory outcome following osteotomy is proper patient selection. Knee osteotomy outcomes depend not only on the overall angular deformity of the knee but also on patient age, range of motion, knee stability, and gait analysis. Patient expectations and cosmesis are additional factors that require consideration in choosing a candidate for osteotomy.

The angular deformity of the limb should not exceed 10 degrees of varus on the preoperative radiographs when considering an HTO.[23] Similarly, preoperative valgus deformity should not exceed 15 degrees in patients being considered for DFO. Deformities greater than these values are often associated with significant ligamentous laxity and tibiofemoral subluxation, both of which are contraindications to knee osteotomy (Table 1). The presence of laxity and/or

TABLE 1. KNEE OSTEOTOMY		
	Indications	Contraindications
Absolute	Unicompartmental osteoarthritis	Inflammatory arthritides
	Varus < 10 degrees	Tibiofemoral subluxation > 1 cm
	Valgus < 15 degrees	Flexion contracture > 10 degrees
	Flexion arc > 90 degrees	Severe ligamentous laxity
		Severe patellofemoral arthritis
Relative	Age < 50 years	Females (cosmesis)
	Increased activity level	High adductor moment
		Tibial plateau bone loss

subluxation results in asymmetric loading of the tibial plateaus, which persists following an osteotomy and therefore undermines the outcome. Insall et al[24] noted increased ligamentous laxity and subluxation in knees with varus deformity greater than 15 degrees, leading to poor results following osteotomy. The same authors stated that knee osteotomy in patients with deformity between 10 and 15 degrees may be suitable if there is no subluxation on the weightbearing radiographs.

An adequate knee range of motion is also a necessary prerequisite to osteotomy. The overall range of motion is usually not significantly improved following osteotomy and should not be considered a goal of the procedure by either the surgeon or the patient. A preoperative flexion arc of at least 70 to 90 degrees is recommended to avoid the postoperative complication of stiffness and decreased function. Healy et al[25] noted the close association between functional improvement and maintenance of the preoperative arc of motion of the knee in a follow-up study of 21 patients undergoing DFO for valgus malalignment. Restricted motion is often associated with a fixed flexion contracture of the knee[26] that, if greater than 10 to 15 degrees, is also a contraindication to osteotomy. Preoperative physical therapy emphasizing stretching and range-of-motion exercises may be employed. However, if the contractures are fixed, significant improvement is not likely, and osteotomy should be avoided.

Patients suffering from inflammatory arthritis have worse results from osteotomy than patients with osteoarthritis. In one study, 36 patients with rheumatoid arthritis had 39% poor results at short-term follow-up, and most good outcomes had deteriorated within 3 years.[27] Isolated patellofemoral compartment disease and tricompartmental arthrosis generally do not benefit from HTO. Poor preoperative range of motion does not improve with HTO. Varus deformity greater than 10 degrees is also associated with poor results.[28] As the deformity increases, there is a greater laxity in the lateral soft tissues as well as more advanced disease in the medial compartment.

There is a lack of universal agreement on the ideal age of patients undergoing osteotomy. This continues to change as the results of total knee arthroplasty (TKA) remain favorable over long-term follow-up periods. In addition, recent studies have examined the results of TKA in patients younger than 55 years and have noted estimated survival rates of 99% at 10 years[29] and 94% at 18 years.[30] Consideration of physiological age and activity level is often more important than the actual chronological age of the patient. Osteotomy is better suited for patients with increased activity levels involving heavy labor or high-demand sports because of the potential for increased wear and subsequent early failure of total joint arthroplasties in these patients.[31] The authors of this chapter generally reserve knee osteotomies for those patients younger than 50 years of age who are expected to continue with their high activity levels postoperatively.

The cosmesis of the limb must be taken into consideration during preoperative discussions with a patient who is a potential candidate for knee osteotomy. This is particularly true for female patients as overcorrection during an HTO may result in a limb that is in noticeable valgus. This outcome frequently results in patient dissatisfaction.

Distal femoral varus osteotomy is indicated for young, heavy, active patients with lateral compartment arthritis. Distal femoral osteotomy is recommended when the valgus deformity is greater than 12 degrees or if the postoperative tibial joint line will have more than 10 degrees of obliquity following HTO.[32] The goal of the procedure is to produce a tibiofemoral angle of zero degrees and a horizontal joint line.[33]

As with HTO, DFO is designed to treat unicompartmental arthrosis. Inflammatory arthritides are not amenable to DFO. The procedure is generally not successful in the setting of significant preoperative contractures.[34] A range of motion of 90 degrees combined with a flexion contracture of less than 20 degrees is recommended.

PROCEDURE

PREOPERATIVE PLANNING

Preoperative planning is a critical factor in the ultimate outcome of knee osteotomy. Correct intraoperative alignment of the knee is facilitated by accurate preoperative determination of the size of the bone wedge to be removed. This requires obtaining standing three-joint radiographs, which allow evaluation of the mechanical and anatomic axes of the lower limb. This determination of the wedge size is at best an estimate due to the magnification of the radiographs; as a result, the ultimate decision on limb alignment must be made intraoperatively.

The angle formed by the femoral and tibial anatomic axes is the simplest method of measuring limb alignment. This angle normally measures 5 to 8 degrees of valgus on a radiograph taken with the patient weightbearing on the affected limb. The overall alignment of a varus osteoarthritic knee not only should be corrected to this normal degree of valgus but should also include approximately 5 degrees of overcorrection such that the anatomic axis measures 10 to 13 degrees of valgus[35] (Fig. 5). The mechanical axis of the lower limb can also be used to determine the wedge size. This axis deviates from a normal value of 0 degrees in a varus or valgus malaligned knee (Fig. 6). The angle of this deviation can be measured to determine the appropriate wedge size to be removed. It is recommended that between 2 and 6 degrees of overcorrection be added

to this measurement to avoid recurrence of a varus knee.[35, 36]

The angle of required correction determined preoperatively is used to predict the thickness of the bone wedge to be removed. It is estimated that each degree of the angle correlates roughly with 1 mm of bone-wedge thickness.[4] Therefore, if a knee is malaligned in 10 degrees of varus, and overcorrection into 10 degrees of valgus is desired, a 20-mm bone wedge should be removed. This estimation, usually reliable in women, tends to be less predictable in men due to the larger bone size, which leads to undercorrection of the deformity. The surgeon must therefore be aware that these preoperative templates serve as useful guides but may not be exact in the dimensions necessary to achieve full correction of the deformity intraoperatively.

In the absence of careful planning there have been wide variations in correction reported. Miniaci et al[37] reported a method for calculating the desired degree of correction (see Fig. 6). Line 1 is drawn from the medial hinge to the center of the tibiotalar joint. Line 2 is drawn from the center of the femoral head through the junction of the middle and medial thirds of the lateral plateau and extends

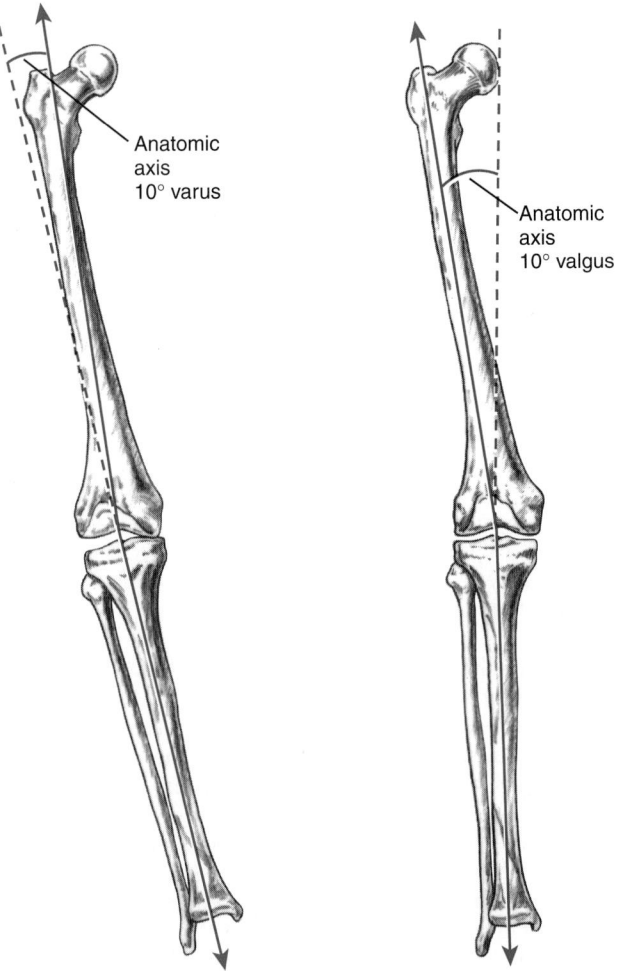

A Varus malalignment   B Desired overcorrection

Fig. 5. Desired overcorrection of malaligned limb. *A,* Knee with 10 degrees of varus malalignment. *B,* Desired alignment of limb with overcorrection of anatomic axis to 10 degrees of valgus.

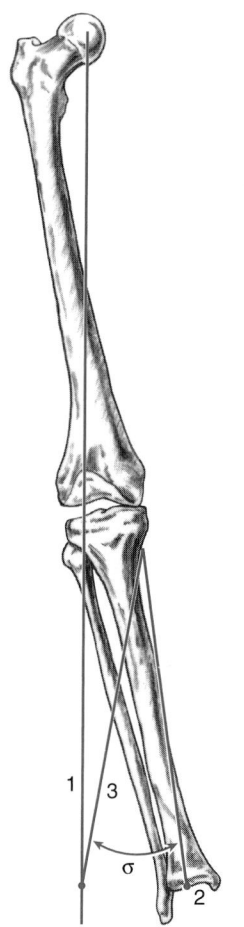

Fig. 6. View. This is the Miniaci method for preoperative planning of desired correction.

Intraoperative efficiency can be facilitated by determining the necessary instrumentation for the procedure. This should include a fluoroscopic image intensifier for intraoperative imaging and a radiolucent operating table. Variable-angle cutting guides or jigs are extremely useful in performing accurate osteotomy cuts and should be readily available in the operating room (Fig. 7). Sharp osteotomes and a sagittal saw are also basic requirements for the procedure.

Finally, the method of internal fixation must be determined and the necessary equipment made available. Coventry[3] described fixation with large staples, which continues to be the preferred method of fixation by many surgeons with or without additional cast immobilization. Fixation of the osteotomy site can also be achieved with the use of an L-shaped buttress plate or blade plate, which provides more rigid fixation but does require more extensive soft-tissue exposure. Our preferred fixation technique utilizes a low-profile, L-shaped buttress plate for an HTO and a 90-degree blade plate for a DFO.

HTO: LATERAL CLOSING WEDGE

Once proper patient selection and preoperative planning have been completed, the specific operative technique for the osteotomy must be chosen. Classically, a closing lateral wedge osteotomy is performed proximal to the tibial tubercle for a varus knee[38] and a closing medial wedge osteotomy for valgus deformity. Alternative techniques for HTO include dome osteotomy, opening medial wedge osteotomy, and distraction lengthening with an external fixator.[39] Opening wedge osteotomies have the potential advantage of decreasing the incidence of patella infera and improving medial collateral ligament laxity but the disadvantage of requiring iliac crest bone graft with associated donor site morbidity. Proponents of distraction lengthening emphasize

to the projected level of the ankle. Line 3 connects the medial hinge and the projected ankle point. The resultant angle defines the desired osteotomy. The use of a mechanical jig maximizes surgical precision.

Alternatively, a simple, accurate method for determining the amount of correction needed involves the use of 3-foot standing films, a tape measure, and tracing paper. Mark the center of the femoral head and the center of the tibiotalar joint on the radiograph. Tape the tracing paper to the tibia, and mark the outline of the tibia. Next, select the desired level for the osteotomy, which should be just proximal to the tibial tubercle at the metaphyseal flare, and cut the tracing paper at this level, leaving a lateral hinge. The distal end of the tibial tracing is then released from the radiograph. If a medial opening wedge osteotomy is planned, move the distal end of the tracing laterally until the mechanical axis passes through the lateral aspect of the lateral tibial spine, and then retape the paper to the radiograph. Measure the opening at the medial cortex of the tracing (typically 15 to 20 mm). This represents the amount of opening that must be achieved intraoperatively, taking radiographic magnification into account. At the time of osteotomy, this same distance can be measured from a fluoroscan machine or directly by using the known width of an osteotome placed into the osteotomy site.

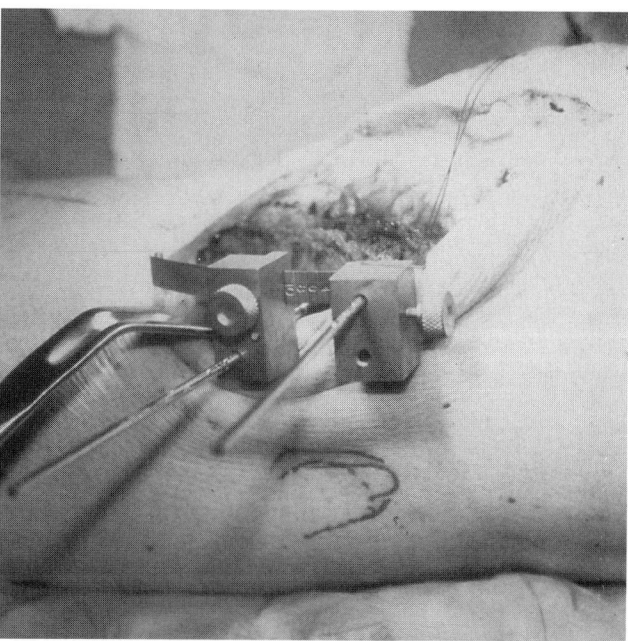

Fig. 7. Variable angle cutting guide. The guide allows placement of the distal pin at the desired angle of correction.

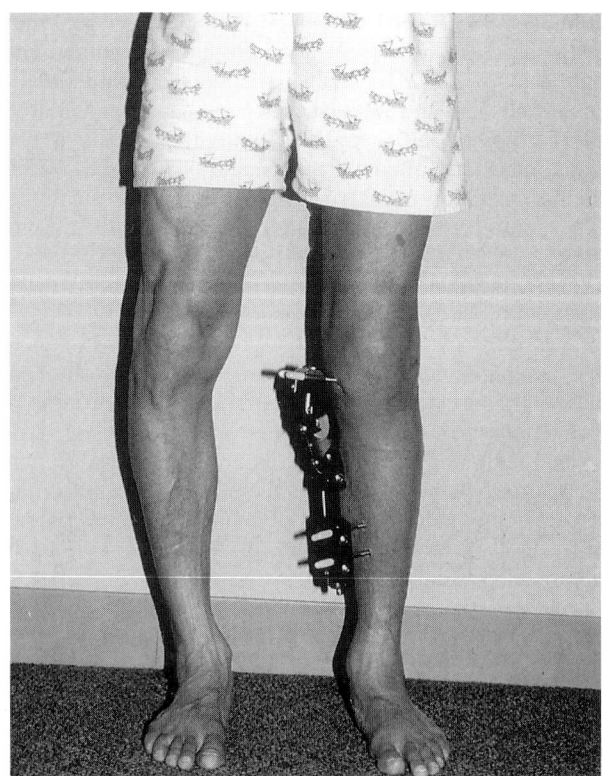

Fig. 8. View. This is the postoperative clinical correction with external fixator in place. (Courtesy William I. Sterett, M.D.)

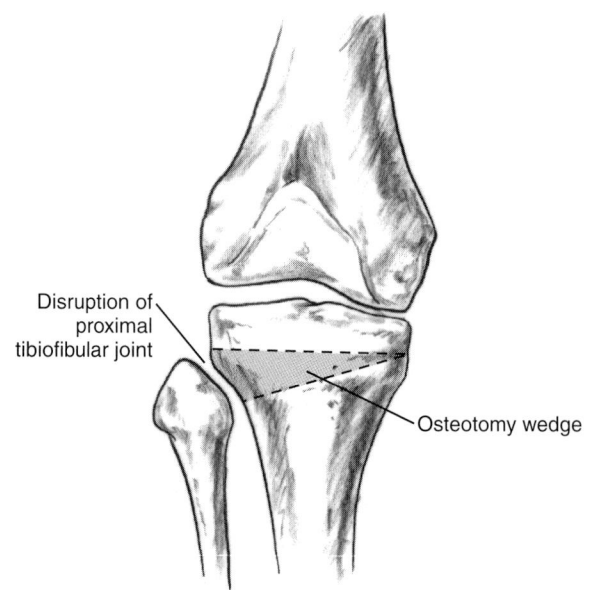

Fig. 9. Proximal tibiofibular joint disruption. The fibula should slide freely in a proximal direction during closure of the osteotomy site.

the ability to precisely titrate the desired degree of wedge opening as well as the lack of need for bone graft. However, the potential for pin tract infections with the use of external fixation in a knee that may ultimately require TKA is a concern (Fig. 8). We continue to use the closing lateral wedge technique for tibial osteotomies and the closing medial wedge for distal femoral osteotomies. The details of these techniques are described here.

The knee is first prepared and draped in the usual sterile fashion followed by inflation of the thigh tourniquet. We prefer a vertical midline skin incision over the anterior aspect of the knee. This incision can be utilized later for TKA without concern for potential problems with wound healing as can occur with horizontally oriented incisions. Care should be taken not to create excessively large skin flaps to minimize devascularization of the skin. In addition, the extensor mechanism and knee joint should not be violated during the dissection. After the overlying muscle and periosteum have been elevated from the lateral crest of the tibia during HTO, the proximal tibiofibular joint must be addressed. Closure of the tibial osteotomy site requires fibular osteotomy, fibular head resection, or tibiofibular joint dissociation. We prefer the latter technique for minimizing the risk of injury to the common peroneal nerve. A periosteal elevator is used to disrupt the joint to enable the fibular head to move freely on the tibia (Fig. 9). It is important to continue the soft-tissue dissection over the posterior aspect of the tibia to avoid inadvertent injury to the posterior neurovascular structures.

The site of the osteotomy is then outlined with methylene blue, based on the preoperative templating. This level should be 2 cm distal to the joint line of the knee for HTO. Placement of ⅛-inch Steinmann's pins is facilitated by the use of templates and cutting guides that incorporate the precise angle of desired correction (Fig. 10). The position of the pins should be checked with the C-arm image intensifier to verify that they are parallel to the joint line in both the anteroposterior and lateral planes to avoid rotational malalignment during osteotomy closure.

A sagittal saw is used to begin the HTO along the proximal limb of the wedge. Retractors are placed along the posterior surface of the proximal tibia to protect the posterior neurovascular structures from injury. Similarly, a retractor is also placed deep to the patellar tendon to prevent inadvertent sectioning of the tendon with the saw. A second osteotomy is then made along the distal limb of the wedge. These cuts should extend only three-quarters of the way across the tibia so as to prevent inadvertent division

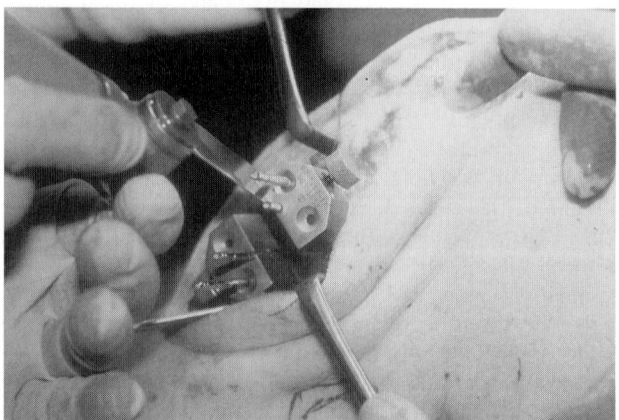

Fig. 10. Cutting guide template for HTO. The saw blade is maintained parallel to the cutting guide to remove the appropriate sized wedge.

of the medial tibial cortex, which can result in translation of the osteotomy fragments during closure. The wedge is removed, and several drill holes are made to perforate the medial cortex; however, the periosteal hinge is left intact. Closure of the osteotomy site is performed by applying a gentle valgus force to the tibia. Excessive force must be avoided in order to prevent inadvertent fracture of the proximal tibia (Fig. 11). If resistance is encountered, complete disruption of the tibiofibular joint should be verified. Once the osteotomy site is closed, overall alignment can be checked with a long alignment rod. Undercorrection of the deformity should be avoided as this will result in early recurrence of symptoms.

Fixation of the HTO is achieved with the use of a low-profile L-buttress plate applied to the lateral aspect of the proximal tibia. Care must be taken to avoid fixation of the osteotomy site in malrotation and to not allow penetration of the proximal screws into the knee joint. Gentle retraction of the lateral soft tissues should be performed to prevent injury to the common peroneal nerve during application and fixation of the buttress plate. Once alignment has been corrected and the fixation device applied, the tourniquet is deflated, and hemostasis is achieved. This is followed by thorough irrigation of the wound and layered closure over a suction drain. The fascia over the proximal tibia should not be closed following an HTO in order to prevent the formation of a compartment syndrome in the leg. We do not utilize cast immobilization following osteotomy; instead, we place a light compressive dressing on the wound.

HTO: MEDIAL OPENING WEDGE

An alternative method of treatment for genu varum is the medial opening wedge osteotomy (Fig. 12). The procedure can be performed using either internal fixation, such as a Puddu plate with associated tricortical iliac crest bone graft, or external fixation and hemicallostasis. External fix-

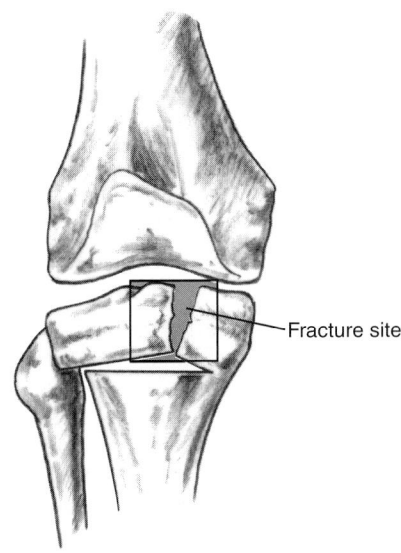

Fig. 11. Complication of proximal tibia fracture during HTO. Excessive force during closure and an incomplete osteotomy can create an intra-articular fracture of the proximal fragment.

Fracture site

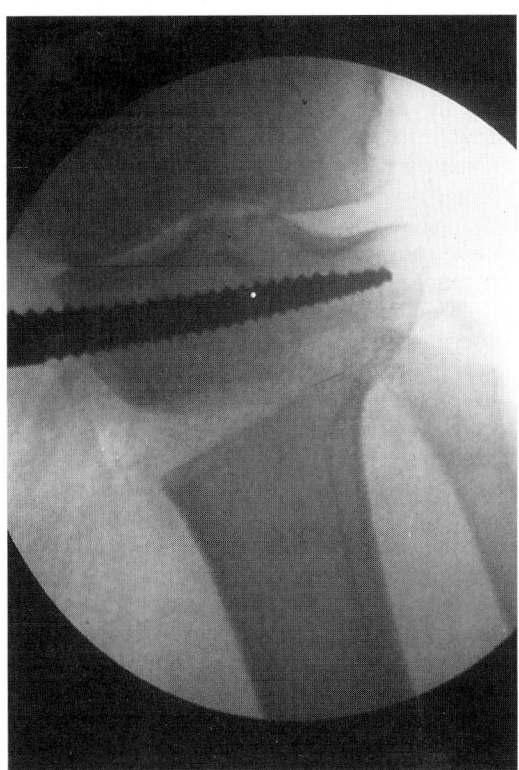

Fig. 12. Intraoperative radiograph. This measures degree of correction with opening wedge osteotomy.

ation and hemicallostasis have been reported to be easier, shorter, and less traumatic. They allow earlier rehabilitation and result in more accurate correction of the tibiofemoral axis than other forms of osteotomy[40] (see Fig. 3). One of the first to describe the technique was Magyar et al.[39] Although 20% of pin sites became infected, they noted improvement in the (Hospital for Special Surgery) knee score from 71 to 94.

When performing distraction osteogenesis, the proximal fixator pins must be placed in the subchondral bone. We recommend placement at least 14 mm distal to the articular surface to avoid intracapsular penetration by the pins and the theoretical risk of joint sepsis from a pin-tract infection. The distal pins are placed in the tibial diaphysis in bicortical fashion. A 2-cm incision is made on the anteromedial tibia at the level of the metaphyseal flare. A ¼-inch drill bit is used to make a corticotomy. Next, a ⅛-inch drill bit is placed through the corticotomy and, under fluoroscopic control, a series of corticotomies are made circumferentially in the proximal tibia. Care is taken to avoid penetrating the lateral cortex so that an intact lateral hinge is preserved. Once the corticotomies are complete, a ¼-inch osteotome is used to "connect the dots," finishing the osteotomy. Neither the medial collateral ligament nor the insertion of the patellar ligament is damaged using this technique.

An osteoclasis is performed, the fixator is attached, and the medial cortex is distracted to the desired amount of opening/correction. This distance is typically 2 cm. The distance on the distractor must be recorded because there is not a one-to-one correlation between distraction at the fixator and distraction at the osteotomy site. The fixator is then shortened, compressing the osteotomy site. For the next 3 to 5 days, the patient is allowed to be weightbearing as tolerated in the fixator, representing the rest phase for the osteotomy. Distraction is generally begun on day 5 at the rate of 1 mm per day at the osteotomy site. Once the desired degree of correction is obtained and documented on 3-foot standing radiographs, no further distraction is performed. The patient continues weightbearing as tolerated while the immature bone in the osteotomy site begins to take form. Generally, by week 10 to 12, the fixator is ready to be removed. We typically recommend the use of crutches, with partial weightbearing, for 2 weeks after removal of the fixator. Patients are usually ready to return to full sporting activities at 6 months.

The main advantage of this technique is the ability to "dial-a-correction." Regardless of the preoperative planning, adjustments can be made as many as 3 weeks postoperatively if more or less correction is desired. The use of 3-foot standing radiographs confirms that an appropriate correction has been accomplished. Because no bone is removed (in fact, bone is "added"), there is no limb-shortening or patella infera with this technique. Patients can be weightbearing immediately, lax collateral ligaments are generally corrected, and future TKAs are not compromised.

Patient selection is critical to the success of this technique. The patient must make frequent office visits to monitor the pin tracts and must be capable of performing meticulous pin care. Patients with low pain thresholds should also be forewarned; the process of distraction can cause discomfort. When a superficial pin-tract infection occurs, as it does in at least 65% of cases, a short course of antibiotics is almost universally successful when given early. There is seldom a need to remove or replace pins. There is a theoretical risk of osteomyelitis from a pin tract that could compromise a future TKA. To date, we are unaware of any increased risk of sepsis with subsequent TKA. Nonunion has not been a significant issue.

For patients who cannot tolerate an external fixator for 3 months, we use the Puddu plate with autogenous tricortical iliac crest bone graft (Fig. 13). The current plate is an H-shape with a metal block between the holes in sizes ranging from 5 to 17.5 mm. This technique has all the advantages of the distraction osteogenesis procedure with the added benefit of not needing an external fixator. Disadvantages of the technique include the need to restrict weightbearing for at least 8 weeks, increased risk of nonunion, and the need for autogenous bone graft. The use of bone substitutes such as demineralized bone paste has recently been introduced, although there are no short- or midterm results in the literature. Another disadvantage is that, like the closing wedge osteotomy, correction of deformity is a one-time opportunity. Thus, the risk for under- or overcorrection persists.

DISTAL FEMORAL OSTEOTOMY

When performing a DFO, the surgeon should also plan for a potential future TKA; a DFO does not compromise future reconstructive procedure. Results of osteotomies immobilized postoperatively have a high incidence rate of arthrofibrosis. Thus, rigid internal fixation should be used to allow

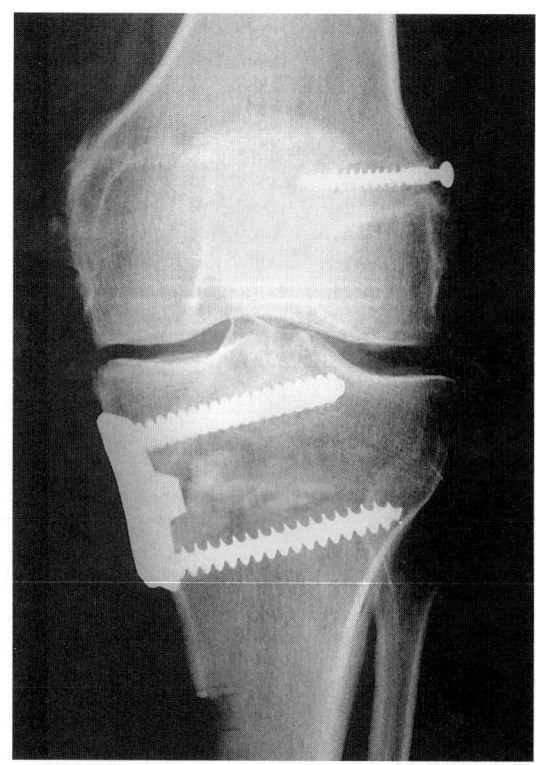

Fig. 13. Radiograph. This demonstrates internal fixation of opening wedge osteotomy. (Courtesy William I. Sterett, M.D.)

postoperative rehabilitation and prevent loss of correction. Staples are an unacceptable fixation method for DFOs. Fixed-angle devices, such as a 95-degree blade plate or dynamic compression screw, provide more consistent results.[41]

DFOs can be performed as a medial closing wedge or lateral opening wedge. When a closing wedge is chosen, we recommend rigid internal fixation with a blade plate due to the large forces experienced in the distal femur. As in the tibia, either an external fixator or internal fixation can be used to perform a lateral opening wedge osteotomy. Because a closing wedge DFO does not pose the same problems with a future TKA as those seen with HTO, the only real advantage of opening wedge procedures is the ease of operation and exposure from the lateral side. The risks of pin-tract infections, nonunion, and hardware failure are not insignificant when performing opening wedge DFOs.

The dissection during a DFO involves periosteal elevation from the anterior, posterior, and medial aspects of the distal femur, with special care taken not to injure the collateral ligaments at their insertion onto the epicondyles. During DFO, the distal arm of the wedge should be directed obliquely such that it is parallel to the joint line. The proximal arm of the wedge is directed perpendicular to the shaft of the distal femur at the desired angle of the wedge to be removed. Before making the actual osteotomy in a DFO, a 90-degree blade plate is inserted laterally at an angle that is complementary to that of the osteotomy until the plate impinges proximally against the lateral cortex (Fig. 14). We prefer not to place the plate on the medial

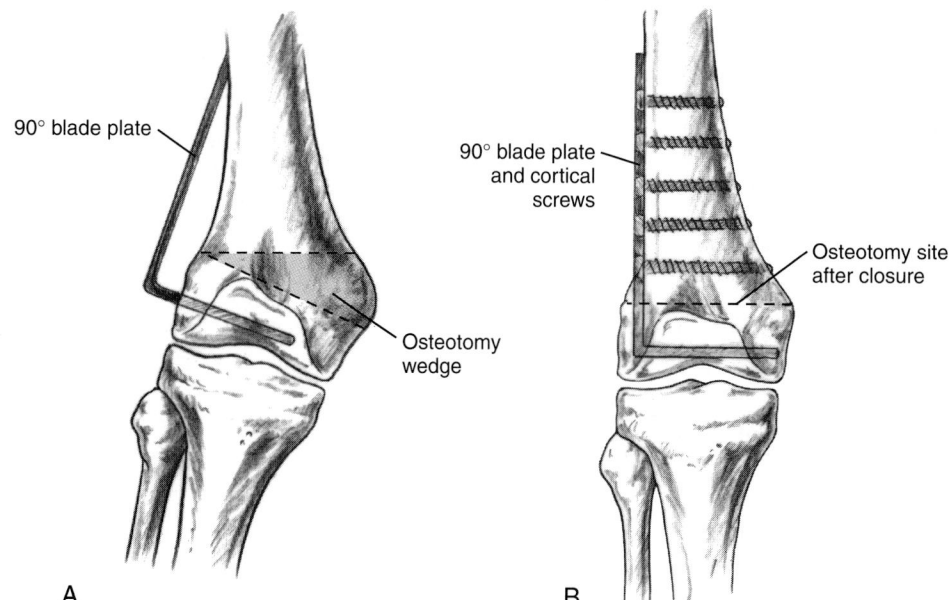

Fig. 14. Insertion of 90-degree blade plate in supracondylar femoral osteotomy. *A,* Before osteotomy, the blade plate is inserted until the proximal portion of the plate abuts against the lateral cortex of the distal femur. *B,* After closure of the osteotomy, the blade plate is fully seated against the lateral cortex.

90° blade plate

Osteotomy wedge

90° blade plate and cortical screws

Osteotomy site after closure

A

B

cortex so as to avoid potential encroachment on the vessels in Hunter's canal located on the proximal medial aspect of the distal femur. The osteotomy in a DFO is made from a medial to a lateral direction, with the knee in a flexed position to allow the posterior neurovascular structures to fall away from the bone. The cuts should not extend across the entire diameter of the bone so as to avoid violation of the lateral cortex. Gentle closure of the osteotomy is performed by applying a varus force to the distal fragment; alignment is checked to verify that the limb is in 2 to 3 degrees of valgus. For a DFO, the partially seated blade plate, which was inserted before the osteotomy, is fully seated following closure of the osteotomy. The appropriate-length screws secure the plate to the lateral aspect of the distal femur. Patellar tracking should be assessed at this point as maltracking of the patella may occur following correction of a valgus knee deformity. A lateral release and/or proximal realignment of the quadriceps can be performed as needed.

POSTOPERATIVE MANAGEMENT

The tenets of postoperative management following knee osteotomy include early restoration of motion and protected weightbearing until healing has occurred. The knee is placed in a continuous passive motion (CPM) machine in the recovery room with range-of-motion settings of 0 to 60 degrees. Initial pain control is achieved with patient-controlled analgesia administered intravenously or through an epidural catheter. The flexion limit on the CPM machine is advanced 10 degrees or more per day as tolerated by the patient, with the goal of achieving 90 degrees of flexion at the time of hospital discharge. Most patients are able to be discharged on the 2nd or 3rd postoperative day with a hinged brace applied to the affected leg, which permits range-of-motion exercises.

Crutches are used for toe-touch weightbearing ambulation for the first 6 to 8 weeks, during which time isometric strengthening exercises of the leg are also performed. After this time, progression to full weightbearing can begin if clinical and radiographic evidence of healing is present. Full-weightbearing ambulation without assistive devices is typically achieved by the 3rd or 4th postoperative month. Most patients are able to resume activities of daily living by 4 to 6 months following the procedure; return to full activity, including heavy labor and sports, can be anticipated by 6 months postoperatively.

COMPLICATIONS AND RESULTS

COMPLICATIONS

Complications following osteotomies about the knee are often directly related to poor surgical technique, including poor preoperative planning, inadequate handling of soft tissues, incorrect osteotomy technique, and inadequate fixation. In addition, prolonged immobilization or overaggressive rehabilitation can lead to postoperative complications. The incidence rate of specific complications has been reported to be relatively low (Table 2), and with continued improvements in technique and fixation these rates may be expected to decline further.

The most common complication following knee osteotomy is undercorrection of the deformity. The incidence rate has been reported to be approximately 10% to 15%[22, 35] and is directly related to surgical technique. Engel and Lippert[42] noted undercorrection of the deformity in 8 of 20 (40%) patients undergoing valgus tibial osteotomy. This rate decreased to 0% (0 of 13 patients) following the development of a comprehensive preoperative protocol emphasizing careful patient selection and accurate preoperative planning. Inadequate correction can lead to early recurrence of the deformity and a progression of symptoms requiring TKA. Hernigou et al[35] reported on proximal tibial osteotomy for varus deformity and found that only 19 of 68 knees that were corrected to a hip-knee-ankle angle of less than 183 degrees had a good result.

TABLE 2. COMPLICATIONS OF KNEE OSTEOTOMY

	Incidence	Prevention	Treatment
Undercorrection	10%–15%	Preoperative planning Intraoperative technique	TKA if becomes symptomatic
Delayed Union or Non-union	0%–4% for HTO	Osteotomy proximal to tubercle Rigid internal fixation	Bone grafting and rigid fixation
Infection	1%–2%	Minimize soft-tissue dissection Antibiotic prophylaxis	Wound incision and drainage (if deep) and antibiotics
Vascular injury	Rare (<0.5%)	Proper retractor placement Flex knee during osteotomy	Direct repair of vascular graft
Peroneal palsy	<1%	Careful soft-tissue retraction Avoid osteotomy of proximal third of fibula	Loosen compressive dressing Ankle-foot orthosis if prolonged Expectant management
Thromboembolic disease	3%–5%	Early range of motion Low-dose Coumadin	Heparinization and high-dose Coumadin
Intraoperative fracture	1%–2%	Avoid incomplete osteotomy Avoid forceful closure Complete dissociation of proximal tibular/fibular joint	Articular reduction and rigid internal fixation

The rate of delayed union or nonunion of the osteotomy site is slightly higher in DFOs (0% to 8%)[25] versus HTOs (0% to 4%).[43] The overall union rates for osteotomies about the knee are high generally because of the broad cancellous surface of the proximal tibia and distal femur. In addition, the use of internal fixation provides a more rigid construct and promotes healing, compared with simple cast immobilization in which there is greater potential for motion at the osteotomy site. The treatment of an osteotomy nonunion is similar to that of a fracture nonunion: it consists of removal of fibrous tissue from the nonunion site, generous packing of bone graft, and application of rigid internal fixation if not already present. The possibility of infection as the underlying cause of the nonunion should always be considered. The reported rates of infection following knee osteotomy are from 1% to 2%[14, 21] The majority of these infections are superficial and require only local wound care and a short course of oral antibiotics. Deep infections require more aggressive treatment consisting of wound débridement and intravenous antibiotics. Hardware may be left in place if the construct is stable. However, if implant breakage has occurred, all hardware should be removed. Temporary fixation with an external fixator may be utilized until the infection has been eradicated and bone grafting and stable internal fixation can be performed. The risk of infection can be reduced by gentle handling of the soft tissues and minimizing the size of the skin flaps.

Neurovascular injuries are rare and are best prevented by proper positioning and use of tissue retractors. Peroneal nerve palsies may occur in fewer than 1% of cases involving osteotomy of the proximal tibia.[14, 22] Careful dissection over the lateral aspect of the tibia as well as disruption of the proximal tibiofibular joint rather than an osteotomy of the proximal one-third of the fibular shaft minimizes this complication. Evidence of peroneal palsy in the recovery room should be treated initially by releasing the compressive bandage and flexing the knee. A prolonged palsy of the nerve may require the use of an ankle-foot orthosis. Injury to the popliteal artery is best prevented by complete periosteal stripping of the soft tissues over the posterior surface of the tibia and placement of retractors posteriorly. The knee should also be flexed during the osteotomy to relax the posterior neurovascular structures. Injury to the anterior tibial artery can also occur during lateral dissection and lead to a compartment syndrome in the anterior compartment of the leg. Thromboembolic disease has been reported in up to 5% of patients following HTO.[21, 23] Contributing factors to this complication may include traumatic handling and retraction of soft tissues during the procedure as well as prolonged postoperative cast immobilization. The use of stable internal fixation allows earlier range of motion and potentially reduces the risk of deep vein thrombosis. In addition, prophylactic anticoagulation with Coumadin or aspirin may be used for several weeks postoperatively.

Intraoperative fracture of the proximal tibia or distal femur may occur during forced closure of the osteotomy site. This is most often due to inadequate completion of the osteotomy across the far cortex. Attempted closure results in a fracture through the articular surface. This can be prevented by ensuring that the osteotomy is complete and, in HTO, that the proximal tibiofibular joint has been adequately disrupted. Treatment of this complication includes accurate reduction of the articular surface and rigid internal fixation.

Increased difficulty in performing a TKA can be considered a long-term complication of knee osteotomy. Exposure for the arthroplasty can be difficult in patients with previous HTO due to the formation of scar tissue over the proximal tibia and possible shortening of the patellar ligament (patella infera).[44] This can lead to possible avulsion of the patellar ligament from the tibial tubercle or to decreased vascularity of the wound, resulting in impaired healing and increased rates of deep infection.[45] Staeheli et al[46] reported on the results of TKA following failed proximal tibial osteotomy in 35 patients and noted results comparable to those of arthroplasty in knees that had not undergone prior osteotomy. Additionally, no increased rates of intraoperative or postoperative complications were noted. In contrast, Windsor et al[47] examined the results of 45 knee arthroplasties following HTO with a minimum follow-up of 2 years and noted excellent results in 51% and poor results in 16% of the knees. Difficulty with exposure was encountered in many of the cases due to patella infera and, in addition, the authors noted the potential for excess removal of bone from the posterior tibial plateau because of anterior tilting, which can occur following HTO. They concluded that arthroplasty following HTO yields results that are more similar to those of revision knee arthroplasty. Similar rates of excellent or good results were reported by Mont et al[48] in their review of 73 TKAs following HTO with an average follow-up of 73 months. Bergenudd et al[49] compared the results of knee arthroplasty in 14 patients with previous osteotomies to those of 99 patients without osteotomy. No differences were found in the postoperative knee scores, range of motion, or requirement for later revision between the two groups at an average follow-up of 6 years. However, there was a significantly greater rate of postoperative complications following arthroplasty in the osteotomy group (57%) compared with the non-osteotomy group (22%).

The reported experience with TKA following osteotomy of the distal femur, although limited, has yielded results similar to those following HTO.[50, 51] Beyer et al[50] reported the results of arthroplasty following failed DFO in 17 knees, with an average follow-up of 4.8 years. According to the Hospital for Special Surgery rating scale, there were 58% excellent and 42% good results, with no fair or poor results noted. The authors did note that the arthroplasties were technically demanding, with exposure difficulty due to extensive scarring being the most common problem (6 of 17 knees). The authors concluded that previous DFO does not preclude a satisfactory clinical outcome following TKA. It is likely that as techniques for performing knee osteotomies improve, regarding preservation of bone stock and reducing the incidence of patella infera,[52] the complication rates associated with conversion to TKA will be minimized.

The type of hardware used for fixation of the osteotomy site often determines whether a TKA is performed as a staged procedure. Staple fixation usually does not pose any problems with the arthroplasty technique and can often be ignored. If the staples are prominent or interfere with making the correct bony cuts, they can be easily removed at the time of the arthroplasty. Staged procedures are recommended for those patients with buttress plate fixation. The first stage includes removal of the hardware, followed by approximately 6 months to allow the bone holes to fill in so that no stress risers are present. The second stage consists of the TKA.

SHORT-TERM RESULTS AND OUTCOMES

Numerous studies have shown that, when performed correctly, knee osteotomy can yield satisfactory results.[5, 22, 35, 53–57] These results, however, tend to deteriorate over time as the osteoarthritic process progresses and TKA becomes

necessary. Stuart et al[58] monitored 113 knees treated with HTO for varus osteoarthritis for a minimum of 5 years and noted recurrence of varus deformity in only 18% of the knees. However, progression of the medial compartment arthritic process was observed in 83% of the knees. The study concluded that the long-term probability of arthritic progression is much higher following HTO than that of significant varus recurrence.

Coventry[5] reported good results in 88% of patients followed for 1 to 9 years after HTO for osteoarthritis. Insall et al[22] noted excellent or good results in 97% of patients at 2 years and 85% at 5 years following HTO. This rate decreased to 63% at a mean follow-up of 8.9 years, with only 37% of patients followed for more than 9 years having no pain. The authors concluded that the passage of time was the most important factor in determining the result and that knee arthroplasty was more suitable for those patients older than 60 years of age. Yasuda et al[55] reported similar long-term results, with a 63% satisfaction rate at post–10-year follow-up. These authors could not correlate patient age with deteriorating results but did note a relationship between achieving a femorotibial angle of 164 to 168 degrees at the time of bony union of the HTO and satisfactory 10-year results. Hernigou et al[35] reviewed the results of proximal tibial osteotomy with a mean follow-up of 11.5 years and noted even poorer long-term results, with only 45% of the knees having excellent or good results after 10 years. Healy and Riley[56] observed a smaller rate of deterioration following HTO, with 96% (24 of 25 patients) excellent or good results at 2 years compared with 80% (4 of 5 patients) at 9 years. The authors attributed the lower rate to their strict criteria for patient selection and precise surgical technique. The average preoperative femorotibial angle was 7 degrees varus, and patients with two- to three-compartment osteoarthritis were excluded. A study by Rinonapoli et al[57] reviewed the 10- to 12-year results of HTO and noted 55% of the knees with an excellent or good outcome. A higher percentage of fair and poor results was noted in those patients with follow-up greater than 15 years. The authors concluded that HTO provides a long period of pain relief and function with deterioration of these results occurring over time, particularly after 15 years. A subjective outcome study was performed by Nagel et al[59] on 37 knees following HTO and revealed that 82% of the patients were satisfied and would have the operation again. However, using the Tegner and Lysholm system to evaluate functional results, the authors found that the patients were not able to return fully to their preoperative level of function following the osteotomy (5.4 points preoperatively versus 4.8 points postoperatively). This study demonstrates the importance of establishing patient expectations prior to performing a knee osteotomy.

Reports on the results of DFO are fewer. However, similar to HTO, reliable short-term results can be achieved followed by deterioration over longer periods of time. Healy et al[25] reported on 23 patients who underwent a DFO for valgus deformity and noted 83% excellent or good results at an average follow-up of 4 years. However, of the 15 patients in the study with osteoarthritis, 93% (14 of 15) had excellent or good results. The authors concluded that DFO is a reliable procedure for the treatment of valgus deformity due to osteoarthritis. McDermott et al[60] studied the results of DFO in 24 patients with osteoarthritis at an average follow-up of 8.3 years. Using the Hospital for Special Surgery knee score, 71% of the patients had excellent or good results, with only 13% of the knees having been converted to a knee arthroplasty. Finkelstein et al[61] reported on the long-term follow-up of supracondylar femoral osteotomy in 21 knees with lateral compartment osteoarthritis. At an average of 133 months, 13 of 21 knees (62%) were still successful. Using the Kaplan-Meier survivorship analysis, the authors noted a 64% probability of survival at 10 years.

CONCLUSION

Knee osteotomy still has a place in the treatment of patients with osteoarthritis of the knee, although the indications for its use have become more limited as the indications for TKA have expanded. In addition, the techniques for performing HTO and supracondylar femoral osteotomy continue to evolve in an effort to minimize the postoperative complications associated with these procedures. It is likely that with the introduction of successful cartilage resurfacing procedures in younger, more active patients, orthopaedic surgeons will increase their utilization of osteotomies of the knee.

REFERENCES

1. Volkmann R: Osteotomy for knee joint deformity. Edinburgh Med J, translated from Berl Klin Wochenschr 794, 1875.
2. Jackson JP, Waugh W: Tibial osteotomy for osteoarthritis of the knee. J Bone Joint Surg Br 43:746, 1961.
3. Coventry MB: Osteotomy of the upper portion of the tibia for degenerative arthritis of the knee: A preliminary report. J Bone Joint Surg Am 47:984, 1965.
4. Bauer GCH, Insall J, Koshino T: Tibial osteotomy in gonarthrosis (osteoarthritis of the knee). J Bone Joint Surg Am 51:1545, 1969.
5. Coventry MB: Osteotomy about the knee for degenerative and rheumatoid arthritis: Indications, operative technique, and results. J Bone Joint Surg Am 55:23, 1973.
6. Shoji H, Insall J: High tibial osteotomy for osteoarthritis of the knee with valgus deformity. J Bone Joint Surg Am 55:963, 1973.
7. Harding ML: A fresh appraisal of tibial osteotomy for osteoarthritis of the knee. Clin Orthop 114:223, 1976.
8. Kettelkamp DB, Chao EY: A method for quantitative analysis of medial and lateral compression forces at the knee during standing. Clin Orthop 83:202, 1972.
9. Hsu RWW, Himeno S, Coventry MB, et al: Normal axial alignment of the lower extremity and load-bearing distribution at the knee. Clin Orthop 255:215, 1990.
10. Prodromos CC, Andriacchi TP, Galante JO: A relationship between gait and clinical changes following high tibial osteotomy. J Bone Joint Surg Am 67:1188, 1985.
11. Wang J-W, Kuo KN, Andriacchi TP, et al: The influence of walking mechanics and time on the results of proximal tibial osteotomy. J Bone Joint Surg Am 72:905, 1990.
12. Murphy SB: Tibial osteotomy for genu varum: Indications, preoperative planning, and technique. Orthop Clin North Am 25:477, 1994.
13. Coventry MB: Upper tibial osteotomy. Clin Orthop 182:46, 1984.
14. Coventry MB: Upper tibial osteotomy for osteoarthritis. J. Bone Joint Surg Am 67:1136, 1985.
15. Keene JS, Monson DK, Roberts JM, et al: Evaluation of patients for high tibial osteotomy. Clin Orthop 243:157, 1989.
16. Fujisawa Y, Masuhara K, Shiomi S: The effect of high tibial osteotomy on osteoarthritis of the knee: An arthroscopic study of 54 knee joints. Orthop Clin North Am 10:585, 1979.
17. Mankin HJ: The response of articular cartilage to mechanical injury. J Bone Joint Surg Am 64:460, 1982.
18. Akamatsu Y, Koshino T, Saito T, et al: Changes in osteosclerosis of the osteoarthritic knee after high tibial osteotomy. Clin Orthop 334:207, 1997.
19. Nakashima K, Koshino T, Saito T: Synovial immunohistochemical changes after high tibial osteotomy for osteoarthritis of the knee: Two-year prospective follow-up. Bull Hosp Jt Dis 57:187, 1998.
20. Arnoldi CC, Lemperg RK, Linderholm H: Intraosseous hypertension and pain in the knee. J Bone Joint Surg Br 57:360, 1975.
21. Vainionpaa S, Laiake E, Kirves P, et al: Tibial osteotomy for osteoarthritis of the knee: A five to ten year follow-up study. J Bone Joint Surg Am 63:938, 1981.
22. Insall JN, Joseph DM, Msika C: High tibial osteotomy for varus gonarthrosis: A long-term follow-up study. J Bone Joint Surg Am 66:1040, 1984.
23. Aglietti P, Rinonapoli E, Stringa G, et al: Tibial osteotomy for the varus osteoarthritic knee. Clin Orthop 176:239, 1983.
24. Insall J, Shoji H, Mayer V: High tibial osteotomy: A five-year evaluation. J Bone Joint Surg Am 56:1397, 1974.
25. Healy WL, Anglen JO, Wasilewski SA, et al: Distal femoral varus osteotomy. J Bone Joint Surg Am 70:102, 1988.
26. Insall JN: Osteotomy. In Insall JN, Windsor RE, Scott WN, et al (eds): Surgery of the Knee, 2nd ed. New York, Churchill Livingstone, 1993, pp 635–676.
27. Chan RN, Pollard JP: High tibial osteotomy for rheumatoid arthritis of the knee: A one to six year follow-up study. Acta Orthop Scand 49:78, 1978.
28. Surin V, Markhede G, Sundholm K: Factors influencing results of high tibial osteotomy in gonarthrosis. Acta Orthop Scand 46:996, 1975.
29. Duffy GP, Trousdale TR, Stuart MJ: Total knee arthroplasty in patients 55 years or younger: 10- to 17-year results. Clin Orthop 356:22, 1998.
30. Diduch DR, Insall JN, Scott WN, et al: Total knee replacement in young active patients. J Bone Joint Surg Am 79:575, 1997.
31. Holden DL, James SL, Larson RL, et al: Proximal tibial osteotomy in patients who are fifty years old or less: A long-term follow-up study. J Bone Joint Surg Am 70:977, 1988.
32. Coventry MB: Proximal tibial varus osteotomy for osteoarthritis of the lateral compartment of the knee. J Bone Joint Surg Am 69:32, 1987.
33. McDermott AG, Finkelstein JA, Farine I, et al: Distal femoral varus osteotomy for valgus deformity of the knee. J Bone Joint Surg Am 70:110, 1988.
34. Healy WL, Anglen JO, Wasilewski SA, et al: Distal femoral varus osteotomy. J Bone Joint Surg Am 70:102, 1988.
35. Hernigou PH, Medevielle D, Debeyre J, et al: Proximal tibial osteotomy for osteoarthritis with varus deformity. J Bone Joint Surg Am 69:332, 1987.
36. Maquet P: The treatment of choice in osteoarthritis of the knee. Clin Orthop 192:108, 1985.
37. Miniaci A, Ballmer FT, Ballmer PM, et al: Proximal tibial osteotomy: A new fixation device. Clin Orthop 246:250, 1989.
38. Gariepy R: Genu varum treated by high tibial osteotomy. In Proceedings of the Joint Meeting of the Orthopaedic Associations of the English-Speaking World. J Bone Joint Surg Br 46:783, 1964.
39. Magyar G, Toksvig-Larson S, Lindstrand A: Open wedge tibial osteotomy by callus distraction in gonarthrosis: Operative technique and early results in 36 patients. Acta Orthop Scand 69:147, 1998.
40. Calista F, Pegreffi P: High tibial osteotomy: Osteotomy imminus or hemocallostasis with monoxial external fixation? Chir Organi Mov 81:155, 1996.
41. Edgerton BC, Mariani EM, Morrey BF: Distal femoral varus osteotomy for painful genu varum: A five to 11 year follow-up study. Clin Orthop 288:263, 1993.
42. Engel GM, Lippert FG III: Valgus tibial osteotomy: Avoiding the pitfalls. Clin Orthop 160:137, 1981.
43. Tjornstrand B, Hagstedt B, Persson BM: Results of surgical treatment for nonunion after high tibial osteotomy in osteoarthritis of the knee. J Bone Joint Surg Am 60:973, 1978.

44. Gill T, Schemitsch EH, Brick GW, et al: Revision total knee arthroplasty after failed unicompartmental knee arthroplasty or high tibial osteotomy. Clin Orthop 321: 10, 1995.

45. Jackson M, Sarangi PP, Newman JH: Revision total knee arthroplasty: Comparison of outcome following primary proximal tibial osteotomy or unicompartmental arthroplasty. J Arthroplasty 9:539, 1994.

46. Staeheli JW, Cass JR, Morrey BF: Condylar total knee arthroplasty after failed proximal tibial osteotomy. J Bone Joint Surg Am 69:28, 1987.

47. Windsor RE, Insall JN, Vince KG: Technical considerations of total knee arthroplasty after proximal tibial osteotomy. J Bone Joint Surg Am 70:547, 1988.

48. Mont MA, Antonaides S, Krackow KA, et al: Total knee arthroplasty after failed high tibial osteotomy: A comparison with a matched group. Clin Orthop 299:125, 1994.

49. Bergenudd H, Sahlstrom A, Sanzen L: Total knee arthroplasty after failed proximal tibial valgus osteotomy. J Arthroplasty 12: 635, 1997.

50. Beyer CA, Lewallen DG, Hanssen AD: Total knee arthroplasty following prior osteotomy of the distal femur. Am J Knee Surg 7:25, 1994.

51. Cameron HU, Park YS: Total knee replacement after supracondylar femoral osteotomy. Am J Knee Surg 10:70, 1997.

52. Westrich GH, Peters LE, Haas SB, et al: Patella height after high tibial osteotomy with internal fixation and early motion. Clin Orthop 354:169, 1998.

53. Rudan JF, Simurda MA: Valgus high tibial osteotomy. A long-term follow-up study. Clin Orthop 268:157, 1991.

54. Ivarsson I, Mynerts R, Gillquist J: High tibial osteotomy for medial osteoarthritis of the knee: A 5 to 7 and 11 year follow-up. J Bone Joint Surg Br 72:238, 1990.

55. Yasuda K, Majima T, Tsuchida T, et al: A ten- to 15-year follow-up observation of high tibial osteotomy in medial compartment osteoarthrosis. Clin Orthop 282:186, 1992.

56. Healy WL, Riley LH Jr: High tibial valgus osteotomy: A clinical review. Clin Orthop 209:227, 1986.

57. Rinonapoli E, Mancini GB, Corvaglia A, et al: Tibial osteotomy for varus gonarthrosis: A 10- to 21-year follow-up study. Clin Orthop 353:185, 1998.

58. Stuart MJ, Grace JN, Ilstrup DM, et al: Late recurrence of varus deformity after proximal tibial osteotomy. Clin Orthop 260:61, 1990.

59. Nagel A, Insall JN, Scuderi GR: Proximal tibial osteotomy: A subjective outcome study. J Bone Joint Surg Am 78:1353, 1996.

60. McDermott AGP, Finkelstein JA, Boynton EL, et al: Distal femoral varus osteotomy for valgus deformity of the knee. J Bone Joint Surg Am 70:110, 1988.

61. Finkelstein JA, Gross AE, Davis A: Varus osteotomy of the distal part of the femur: A survivorship analysis. J Bone Joint Surg Am 78:1348, 1996.

section
6
chapter
16

KNEE ARTHROPLASTY

Yram J. Groff, Anton Y. Plakseychuk, and Lawrence S. Crossett

Summary
- Total knee arthroplasty (TKA) is currently the standard treatment for a variety of end-stage arthritic disorders of the knee and has consistently shown survival rates of 95% to 97% between 10 and 15 years.
- The primary goal of this intervention is to alleviate pain and to restore function to the knee.

Approximately 150,000 total knee replacements are performed every year in the United States. The long-term success of TKA has been well documented; several authors reported survival rates from 95% to 97% between 10 and 15 years.[1–5] These results are the best among those of any joint replacement, and at this point little evidence of a declining survivorship curve has been noted. The evolution of surgical technique and prosthetic design has produced consistently excellent results. Despite this apparent success, controversy continues regarding issues such as optimal method of fixation, retention versus substitution of the posterior cruciate ligament (PCL), and prevention of complications, especially those related to the patellofemoral articulation.

INDICATIONS

In general terms, the indication for prosthetic replacement of the knee is severe, unrelenting pain that is due to a global lack of intact articular cartilage and that is refractory to other modalities of treatment. A variety of different conditions can render the knee arthritic enough to be a candidate for replacement. The associated pain should be of a magnitude significant enough to warrant a major operative intervention. Before an operation is considered, nonoperative modalities should be exhausted. These traditionally have included activity modification, weight reduction, nonsteroidal anti-inflammatory drugs, the use of a cane in the contralateral hand, and possibly intra-articular injection of steroid. Newer investigational alternatives include viscosupplementation materials for intra-articular injection and articular cartilage constituents to be taken orally, such as glucosamine and chondroitin sulfate.

Contraindications to knee replacement are mostly related to the overall medical condition of the patient. Patients with severe medical problems may not be candidates for major elective surgery. Active infection in the knee is perhaps the only absolute contraindication to prosthetic implantation. Virtually all other conditions related to the knee can be accommodated with modern techniques and design implants.

Once it has been established that operative intervention is warranted and desired, the specific type of operation must be determined. This is influenced by the physiological age, functional demands, rehabilitation potential, and desires of the patient. Surgical options include arthroscopic débridement, osteotomy, and arthroplasty, be it uni-, bi-, or tricompartmental. Once the decision is made to proceed with TKA, further technical details must be considered, such as the design of the implant, PCL retention versus substitution, method of fixation to the skeleton (e.g., cemented versus noncemented), and specific components.

TECHNICAL CONSIDERATIONS
Posterior Cruciate Ligament

The role of the PCL in TKA is controversial. Since the introduction of the posteriorly stabilized design in 1978, few surgeons have advocated routine sacrifice of the PCL without prosthetic substitution, but the equally excellent long-term results of TKA performed with cruciate-retaining and cruciate-substituting implants ensures that this debate will continue. Early claims that retention of the PCL would allow better range of motion, better joint stability, more normal gait, and enhanced prosthetic longevity compared with PCL-substituting knee designs have not been supported by recent clinical and basic science research.[6, 7] The argument in favor of PCL preservation is that the joint line is maintained, the proprioceptive function of the ligament is retained, the contact point of the knee is centralized, and femoral rollback is promoted. However, PCL retention brings the following potential difficulties into TKA:

1. Functional retention of the PCL requires a flattened tibial articular surface to allow for rollback. The consequent mismatch of the bearing surfaces is thought to lead to increased polyethylene wear.[1] This is accentuated in the case of unrecognized PCL contracture. In addition, the suggestion that PCL retention improves femoral rollback has been challenged.[6]
2. Postoperative avulsion or intraoperative excessive recession of the PCL can increase the flexion gap, resulting in instability in flexion.[9]
3. Preserving the PCL in the face of flexion contracture or significant valgus deformity makes soft-tissue balancing very difficult. In addition, accounting for a diseased ligament makes balancing exceedingly difficult.
4. PCL retention makes a wide proximal tibial exposure difficult, and accurate placement of the tibial component may be jeopardized.

These reservations notwithstanding, the range of motion after TKA averages roughly 115 degrees with both cruciate-retaining and posteriorly stabilized designs. Gait analysis and isokinetic muscle-testing studies do not support a difference between the two systems in regard to temporospatial gait variables, knee range of motion during stair climbing, and isokinetic muscle strength.[6, 7] Nonetheless, PCL substitution may hold many advantages.

1. Resection of the PCL allows greater exposure and simplifies correction, because there is no need to balance a contracted or damaged PCL.
2. Resection of the PCL allows for removal of posterior osteophytes and loose bodies and simplifies gap balancing by facilitating the resection of additional bone.
3. The surgeon is not restricted to a particular depth of tibial resection, because there is no need to balance the PCL.
4. PCL substitution allows the implantation of a more conforming articular polyethylene surface and a consequent decrease in polyethylene wear, at least in theory.

Similar prosthetic longevity established for the posteriorly stabilized condylar implant (98% survivorship at 14 years)[10] and for the cruciate-retaining design (96% at 10 years)[3] will feed this discussion until longer follow-up results are published.

Cement Versus Cementless Fixation

The orthopaedic surgeon must choose between two forms of fixation: cement versus cementless. Cementless fixation of TKA was developed because of concern about the long-term durability of cemented component fixation. The idea was that the future of knee reconstructive surgery would be directed toward cementless fixation, which would be able to provide younger, more active patients with a more lasting cure for disabling arthritis. The early clinical results of cemented and cementless TKA in younger patients were similar, with no significant difference in knee score, at an average of 2.8 years after surgery.[11] Review of the same group of patients in the 10-year survival analysis revealed higher mechanical failure and revision rate for aseptic loosening in the cementless group.[12] Screw fixation appears to be the optimal method of securing an uncemented tibial tray, but osteolysis remains the main nemesis of cementless fixation. Meanwhile, clinical survival for cemented posterior stabilized knee prostheses at 15 years is reported at 94.6%,[10] and in many other studies 10-year survival is reported as greater than 96%. On the basis of these results and others like them, cementing has become the standard method of fixation for all three components in most knee replacements. Cementless fixation, particularly of the tibia, has proven to be problematic with several designs. Thus, despite early excitement over "biological fixation," this method has largely fallen out of favor.

Rotational Considerations

Although TKA has clearly established itself as one of the most successful surgeries in all of orthopaedics, of those knee replacements that need to be revised, roughly half are due to patellofemoral problems.[13] The intraoperative determination of appropriate component rotation is critical in this regard.[14] An area of intense investigation in TKA is the selection of accurate landmarks for rotational alignment of the components, particularly the femoral component. This issue is crucial because a lack of proper patellar tracking can lead to pain and crepitus, excessive component wear, and loosening. Patellofemoral malalignment is one of the more insidious pitfalls encountered in this operation, and it can be manifest as patellar subluxation, dislocation,[13, 15, 16] fracture[17, 18] or excessive patellar wear.[19]

Component positioning obviously is a large determinant of patellar tracking, but a variety of other factors must be taken into account. The most common problem is excessive lateral retinacular tightness with a relatively weak vastus medialis. A large Q angle in the valgus knee is also a contributing factor, as can be postoperative hemarthrosis and overly aggressive rehabilitation.

These other factors notwithstanding, component position is the most critical factor that the surgeon can control to avoid patellofemoral complications. Excessive internal rotation of the tibial tray causes the tibia to be externally rotated under the femur. This effectively lateralizes the tibial tubercle and increases the Q angle, resulting in patellar instability. The same effect is created if the tibial tray is translated medially on the tibial plateau. The corollary is true of the femoral component: internal rotation of the femoral component on the femur effectively medializes the trochlear groove and leaves the patella relatively lateralized, as does medial translation of the femoral component on the femur. Similar concerns apply to the position of the patellar component on the patella and, if anything, it should be medialized. The surgeon must be cognizant of all these issues as the components are implanted.

Determining rotational alignment is not always as straightforward as one might hope. Many different approaches have been tried to achieve reliably appropriate rotation of the femoral component. In the classic method, the external rotation of the femoral component is determined by creating a rectangular flexion gap. Other methods use anatomic landmarks as reference points, including the posterior femoral condyles, the transepicondylar axis, and the trochlear groove. All of these methods have their shortcomings, but it seems that the gap-balancing method is the most adept at accommodating individual variations in anatomy and pathoanatomy.

Intraoperative analysis of patellar tracking is essential. Ideally, no patient should leave the operating room with a patella that does not track down the middle of the trochlear groove. This assessment is best performed after the release of the tourniquet to remove the potential binding effect on the extensor mechanism. Once patellofemoral problems have been diagnosed in the postoperative period, a computed tomography scan may be necessary to evaluate the rotational alignment of the components.[20]

TECHNIQUE REVIEW

The patient is positioned in a supine position with a tourniquet placed high on the thigh. In general, an anterior approach is the preferred technique, although a lateral approach has been described for the valgus knee.[14] An anterior midline longitudinal skin incision is made, centered over the femur proximally and extending distally to a point just medial to the tibial tubercle. Previous surgical incisions should be used when feasible to maintain blood supply to the skin. A skin bridge of at least 6 cm should be maintained between parallel incisions, and old incisions should be traversed as close to 90 degrees as possible. It should be recalled that the lateral wound edge is more hypoxic than the medial edge of the incision. A medial parapatellar arthrotomy is then created, taking care to leave a cuff of tissue around the patella for eventual closure. The cruciates are resected (PCL resection depending on implant design, of course). The lateral meniscus is removed, taking care to avoid injury to the popliteal muscle. The medial meniscus is resected, leaving behind a thin rim of the tissue to ensure that the deep medial collateral ligament will not be compromised in any way. Osteophytes are resected for accurate sizing and balancing. Once the exposure is complete, ligament balancing and bone resections follow.

Philosophies differ regarding preparation of the femur and tibia to accept prostheses and the balancing of the soft-tissue envelope. The more common techniques are presented next. However, it should be kept in mind that bone resections are virtually never altered to accommodate soft-tissue contractures. Soft tissue must be released to restore

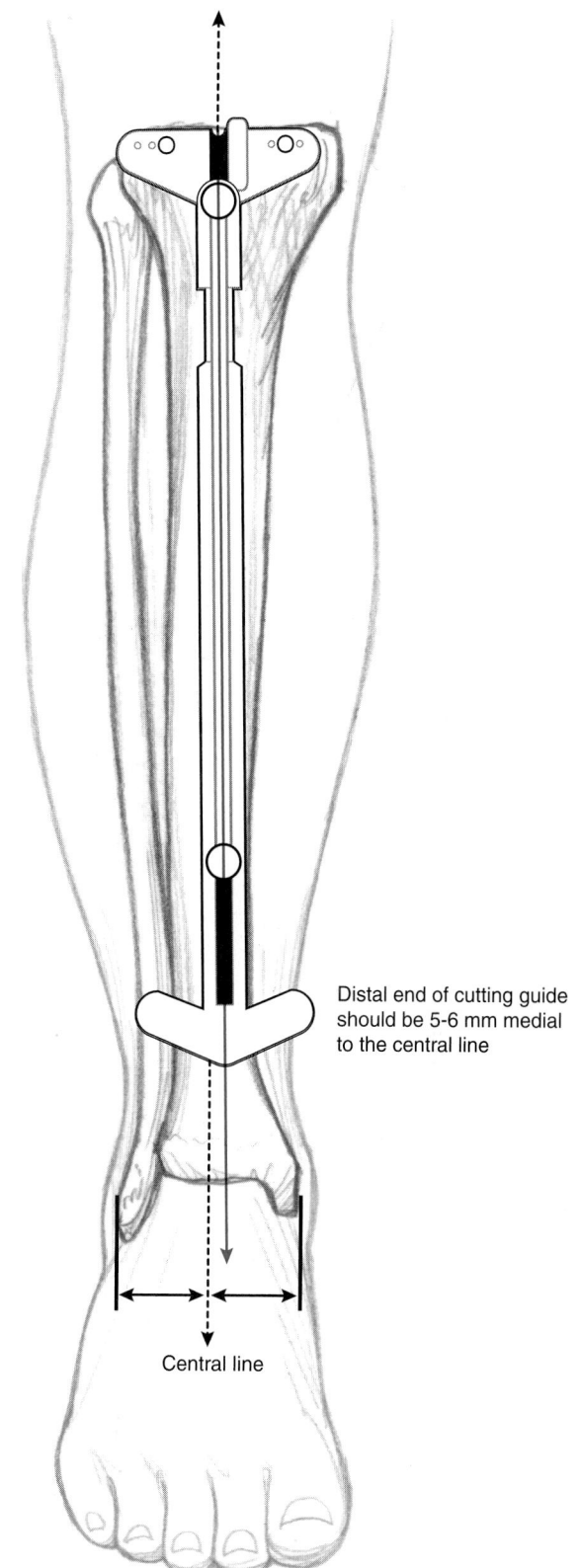

Distal end of cutting guide should be 5-6 mm medial to the central line

Central line

Fig. 1. The tibial cut with a minimum of 3 degrees posterior slope. The distal aspect of the cutting guide was moved 5 to 6 mm medially from center line, because the center of the ankle was not equidistant between the malleoli.

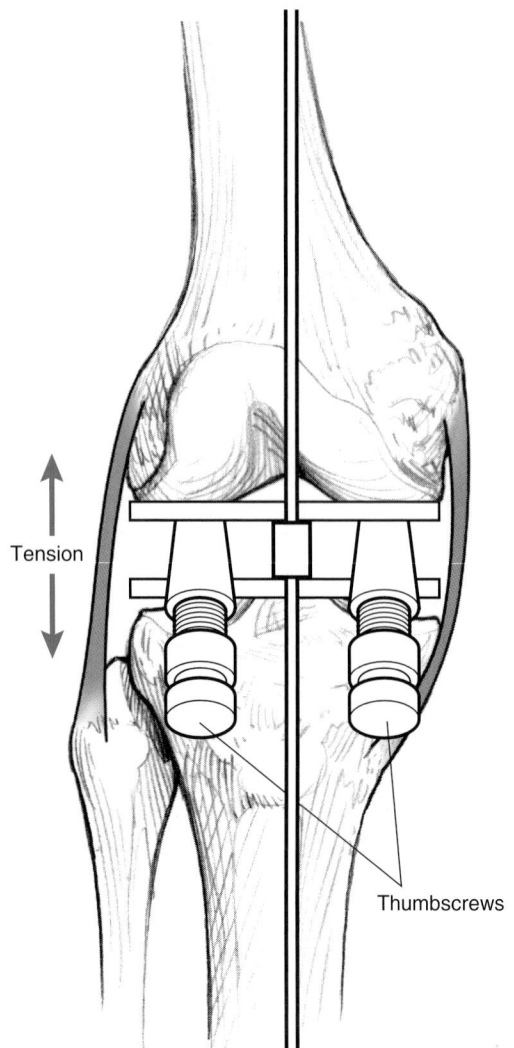

Fig. 2. Restoration of the limb axis with tensioning device. By adjusting the medial and lateral thumbscrews, the alignment rod is brought into the mechanical axis. If not, then further soft-tissue releases are necessary to restore the axis of the limb.

the overall limb alignment, and appropriate bone cuts are made to ensure proper component positioning.

FLEXION-EXTENSION GAP (CLASSIC) METHOD

With the classic technique, popularized by John Insall,[21] ligament balancing is performed before any bone resections (with the one exception of severe flexion contracture). This method is predicated on the fact that improper ligament balance can adversely influence the accuracy of bone cuts. Logistically, it is nearly impossible to perform any ligament releases without initially removing some bone, and so typically the tibial resection is done first. The tibia is cut perpendicular to the long axis of the tibia (Fig. 1). Then the ligaments are balanced such that overall alignment of the limb is restored. This is done in extension with the aid of a tension device (Fig. 2). Subsequently, the posterior femoral cut is made such that the flexion gap is a rectangle. A tension device is again useful at this juncture to

facilitate estimation of the symmetry of the gap to be created, based on the balance of the knee previously established. The rotation of the femoral component is automatically determined by rotating the femoral cutting block until a rectangle, and not a trapezoid, is created (Fig. 3). Next, the distal femur is resected to create an extension gap that is equal to the flexion gap in size and balance (Fig. 4). Insall popularized the use of different sized blocks to confirm the balance and symmetry in flexion and extension. In extension, the knee should come to full extension. If the knee does not come to full extension, posterior capsule should be released from the posterior femur until full extension is achieved (Fig. 5). Once the soft tissues have been balanced and the appropriate bone cuts made, the knee is prepared to accept a prosthesis.

No technique is flawless, and this one is no exception. Some concerns have been voiced regarding this methodology. First, the femoral cuts are dependent on the tibial cut, and any malalignment of the tibial cut will be magnified as the operation progresses. Second, knee stability in extension is due to ligamentous and capsular contributions. Flexion stability has no significant capsular component. Conse-

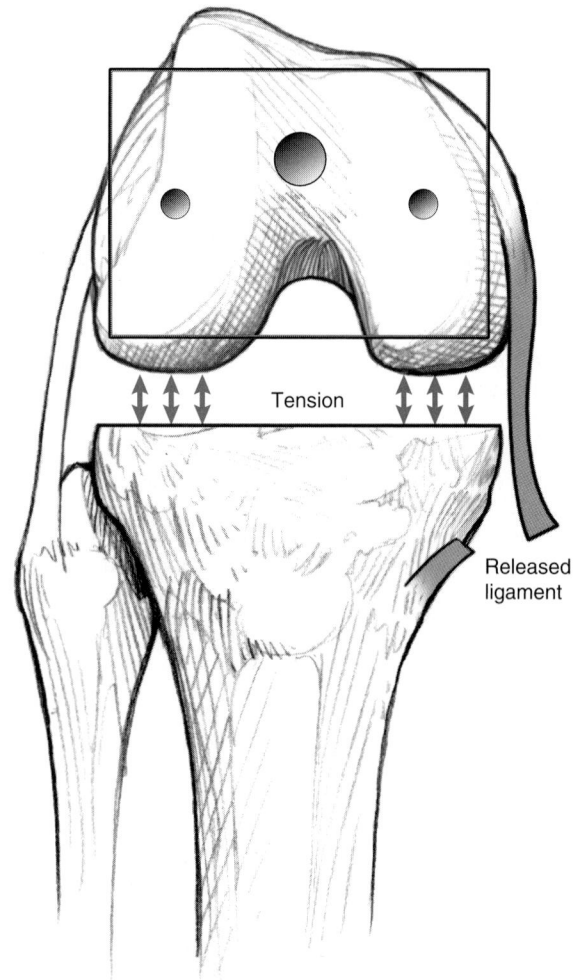

Fig. 3. The femoral cutting block. The tensor rests on the tibial surface, and two prongs are attached to the cutting block. Tensioning up to 25 pounds externally rotates the intramuscular alignment guide within the canal and creates a rectangular flexion space.

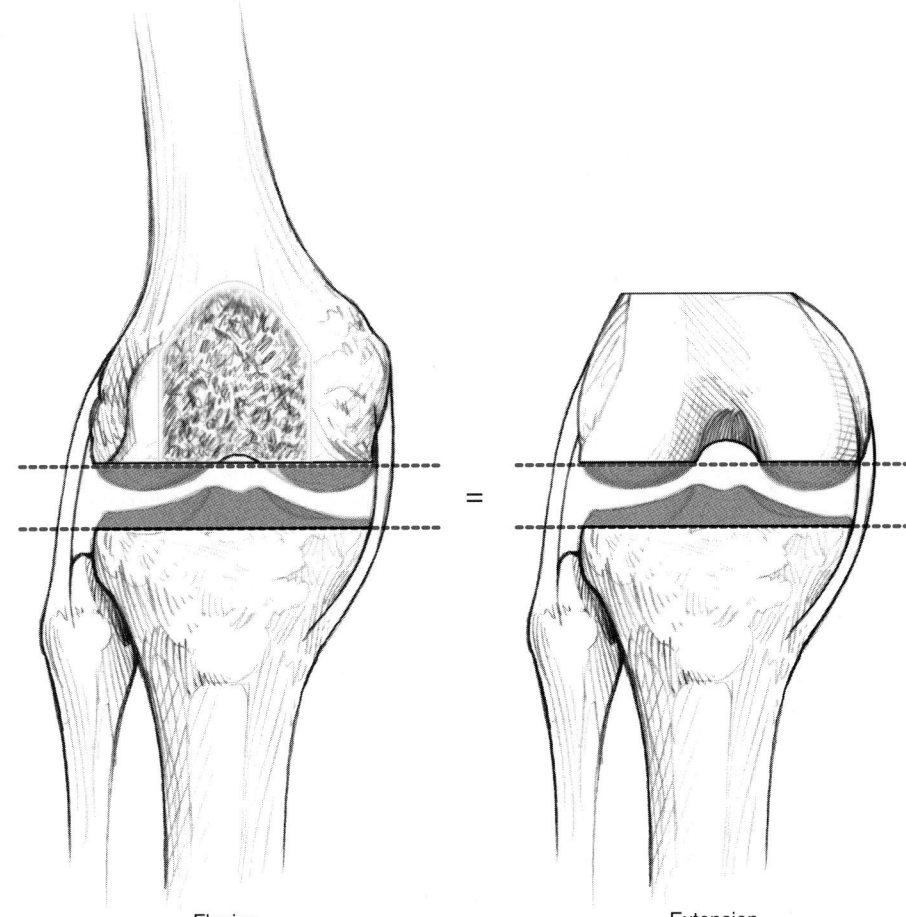

Fig. 4. Flexion-extension gaps. These are equal and rectangular.

Flexion

Extension

quently, ligament releases (or lack thereof) in extension may influence the rotation of the femur in flexion and may lead to patellofemoral problems if the rotational alignment of the femoral component is inaccurate. Another caveat is that posterior capsular contracture spuriously decreases the extension space and will cause an excessively large distal femoral resection if not corrected before the cut. If not accounted for beforehand, the ligaments will be loose; with no contribution from the posterior capsule, midflexion instability of the knee will result. Questions have also been raised as to the reproducibility of the soft-tissue tensioning device. Table 1 presents some common scenarios encoun-

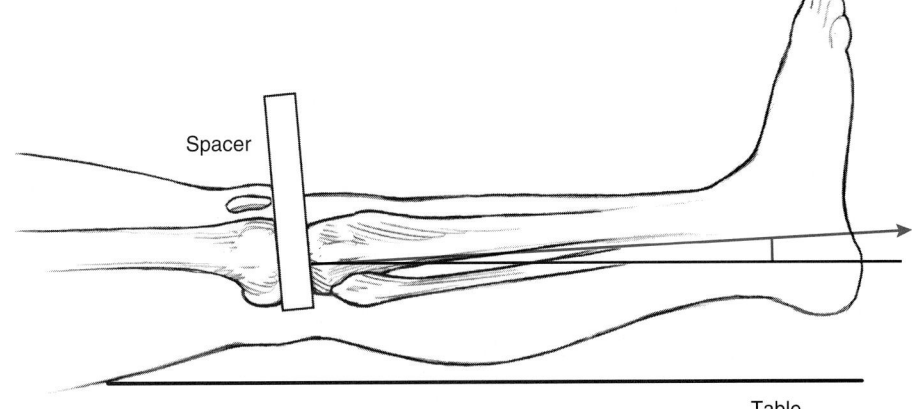

Fig. 5. Extension of the knee. In extension, the knee should come to full extension or slight recurvatum with a 10- or 12-mm spacer block.

Spacer

Table

tered in the classic method along with their causes and appropriate solutions.

MEASURED RESECTION

In the early 1980s, as intramedullary cutting guides were developed, the technique of measured resection, or the "anatomic" method, gained popularity. The goal of this method was to restore the normal anatomy of the knee more accurately. The measured resection technique is rooted in anatomic studies of the knee joint.[22] With this method, the tibia is cut parallel to the anatomic joint line (3 degrees of varus relative to the long axis of the tibia), and the distal femur is cut in 9 degrees of valgus, resulting in an overall joint alignment of 6 degrees of valgus. In addition, the posterior femoral cut is made parallel to the posterior femoral condyles, assuming no gross malalignment of the limb. As surgeons returned to cutting the tibia perpendicular to the long axis of the bone, an additional 3 degrees of external rotation of the posterior femoral cutting guide became necessary to avoid medialization of the trochlear groove of the implant and resultant patellofemoral complications. This has been confirmed in radiographic studies.[23] After all bone cuts are made and trial components have been inserted, attention is turned to balancing the soft tissues.

This philosophy is derived mainly from proponents of PCL-sparing implants, in which maintenance of the level of the joint line is critical to the function of the ligament. The philosophy has evolved to incorporate PCL-substituting designs, but its roots lie in PCL retention. According to this technique, the deformity dictates not only the amount of soft-tissue release needed for correction of limb alignment but also the thickness of the bone to be resected. Ligament balancing is performed after all bone cuts have been made and trials inserted. Results with this method rival those of the classic method. However, skeptics criticize it as "cookbook" surgery and believe that it neglects the central role of soft-tissue balancing in knee arthroplasty. In addition, although tension is reliably equalized between the medial and lateral compartments, there is often asymmetry between the flexion and the extension gaps, with consequent instability through at least part of the range of motion.

UNICOMPARTMENTAL ARTHROPLASTY

Unicompartmental arthroplasty (UA) is used to treat unicompartmental arthrosis by replacing only the arthritic compartment of the knee and preserving the contralateral and the patellofemoral articulations. Despite nearly 25 years of experience, the role of unicompartmental knee replacement continues to be debated. Proponents of UA point out that the procedure has several advantages over osteotomies[24] and tricompartmental knee replacement,[25] although careful patient selection is widely regarded as one of the most critical determinants of success. Compared with osteotomies, UA has a higher success rate and fewer early complications. It also allows for concomitant intra-articular intervention, if necessary, and has a shorter recovery time. Relative to total knee replacement, UA has the advantages of preserving both cruciate ligaments and, consequently, near-normal kinematics. It reliably yields excellent motion and is relatively conservative in terms of bone resection. Objectively, patients report that a unicondylar replacement feels more like a native knee.[25] Skeptics are quick to point out, however, that, despite its theoretical advantages, UA has proven to have a survivorship significantly inferior to that of TKA (10-year survivorship of 85%[26] versus more than 96%[10]). Furthermore, results of revision after UA seem to be no better than revision after TKA,[27] although this is contested in the literature.[28, 29]

These arguments notwithstanding, UA may play a role in the armamentarium against gonarthrosis when osteotomy is contraindicated and the patient is too young or too heavy to be a candidate for TKA. The ultimate decision to proceed with uni- versus bi- or tricompartmental replacement must be made at the time of arthrotomy after visual inspection of the entirety of the articular cartilage of the knee. Involvement of more than one compartment with more than Outerbridge grade III changes precludes UA. Absence of the anterior cruciate ligament is another contraindication

TABLE 1. FLEXION-EXTENSION BALANCING

Problem	Reason	Solution
Flexion gap is too small (FG < EG = 10 mm).	Underresection of proximal tibia (<7 mm removed from normal side).	Recut 2–4 mm from tibia.
	Oversizing of the femoral component.	Recut posterior femoral condyles, downsize femoral component.
Flexion gap is too large (FG > EG = 10 mm).	Overresection of the posterior.	1. Use a larger femoral component with posterior buildup. 2. Resect additional distal femur.
Flexion and extension gaps are too large (EG = FG > 10 mm).	Overresection of the tibia.	Use thicker tibial component or insert.
Flexion and extension gaps are too small (EG = FG < 10 mm).	Underresection of the tibia.	Recut 2–4 mm from tibia.
Extension gap is too small (EG < FG = 10 mm).	Underresection of the distal femur (flexion contracture with 10 mm block).	Resect additional distal femur.
Extension gap is too large (EG > FG = 10 mm).	1. Overresection of the distal femur. 2. Excessive ligamentous laxity.	Augments on the distal femur (requires stemmed femoral component).

FG, flexion gap; EG, extension gap.

for UA, because it reflects a level of ligamentous laxity that almost invariably leads to bicompartmental disease. Last, a significant inflammatory component to the arthrosis is a relative contraindication to UA, because the risk of contracompartmental involvement in subsequent years is high. With all these caveats in mind, however, UA may be an appropriate therapeutic option for the properly selected patient.

REFERENCES

1. Malkani AL, Rand JA, Bryan RS, et al: Total knee arthroplasty with the kinematic condylar prosthesis. J Bone Joint Surg Am 1995; 77:423.
2. Ranawat CS, Padgett DE, Ohasi Y: Total knee arthroplasty for patients younger than 55 years. Clin Orthop 1989; 248:27.
3. Ritter MA, Herbst SA, Keating EM, et al: Long-term survival analysis of a posterior cruciate retaining total condylar total knee arthroplasty. Clin Orthop 1994; 309:136.
4. Buechel FF: Cementless meniscal bearing knee arthroplasty: 7- to 12-year outcome analysis. Orthopaedics 1994; 17:833.
5. Whiteside LA: Cementless total knee replacement: Nine- to 11-year results and 10-year survivorship analysis. Clin Orthop 1994; 309:185.
6. Schlepkow P: Three-dimensional kinematics of total knee replacement systems. Arch Orthop Trauma Surg 1992; 111:204.
7. Stiehl JB, Komistek RD, Dennis DA, et al: Fluoroscopic analysis of kinematics after posterior-cruciate retaining knee arthroplasty. J Bone Joint Surg Br 1995; 74:884.
8. Maily T, Scott WN: Posterior stabilized knee arthroplasty. In Rand JA (ed): Total Knee Arthroplasty. New York, Raven Press, 1993.
9. Ochsner JL, McFarland G, Baffes GC, et al: Posterior cruciate avulsion in total knee arthroplasty. Orthop Rev 1993; 22:1121.
10. Ranawat CS, Flynn WF, Saddler S, et al: Long-term results of the total condylar knee arthroplasty: A 15-year survivorship study. Clin Orthop 1993; 286:94.
11. Rand JA: Cement or cementless fixation in total knee arthroplasty? Clin Orthop 1991; 273:52.

12. Rorabeck CH, Neil HL: Total knee replacement: Should it be cemented, cementless, or hybrid? Presented at annual meeting of the American Academy of Orthopaedic Surgeons, San Francisco, 1997.
13. Ranawat C: The patellofemoral joint in total condylar arthroplasty: Pros and cons based on 5- to 10-year follow-up observations. Clin Orthop 1986; 205:93.
14. Keblish PA: The lateral approach to the valgus knee. Surgical technique and analysis of 53 cases with over two year follow-up evaluation. Clin Orthop 1991; 271:52.
15. Merkow R, Soudry M, Insall J: Patellar dislocation following total knee replacement. J Bone Joint Surg Am 1985; 67:1321.
16. Briard J, Hungerford D: Patellofemoral instability following total knee replacement. J Arthroplasty 1989; 4:87.
17. Figgie M, Goldberg V, Figgie H: Salvage of the symptomatic patellofemoral joint following cruciate substituting total knee arthroplasty. Am J Knee Surg 1988; 1:48.
18. Figgie M, Goldberg V, Figgie H: The effects of alignment of the implant on fracture of the patella after total knee arthroplasty. J Bone Joint Surg Am 1989; 71:1031.
19. Berger RA, Seel MJ, Luttell L, et al: Component malrotation causing patellofemoral complication in total knee arthroplasty. Presented at the meeting of American Association of Orthopaedic Surgeons, New Orleans, 1994.
20. Berger RA, Crossett LS: Determining the rotation of the femoral and tibial components in total knee arthroplasty: A com-

puter tomography technique. Oper Tech Orthop 1998; 8:128.
21. Insall J: Surgery of the Knee. New York, Churchill Livingstone, 1984, p 620.
22. Krackow KA: Intraoperative alignment and instrumentation. In Krackow KA (ed): The Technique of Total Knee Arthroplasty. St. Louis, CV Mosby, 1990.
23. Crossett LS, Kugler J, Berger RA, et al: The Determination of Femoral Component Rotation in Total Knee Arthroplasty.
24. Broughton NS, Newman JH, Baily RA: Unicompartmental replacement and high tibial osteotomy for osteoarthritis of the knee: A comparative study after 5–10 years' follow-up. J Bone Joint Surg Br 1986; 66:447.
25. Laurencin CT, Zelicof SB, Scott R, et al: Unicompartmental versus total knee arthroplasty in the same patient: A comparative study. Clin Orthop 1991; 273:151.
26. Scott RD, Cobb AG, McQueary FG, et al: Unicompartmental knee arthroplasty: Eight to 12-year follow-up evaluation with survivorship analysis. Clin Orthop 1991; 271:96.
27. Lai CH, Rand JA: Revision of failed unicompartmental knee arthroplasty. Clin Orthop 1993; 287:193.
28. Levine WN, Ozuna RM, Scott RD, et al: Conversion of failed modern unicompartmental arthroplasty to total knee arthroplasty. J Arthroplasty 1996; 11:797.
29. Otte KS, Larsen H, Jensen TT, et al: Cementless AGC revision of unicompartmental knee arthroplasty. J Arthroplasty 1997; 12:55.

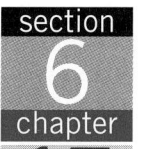

section **6** chapter **17**

REVISION TOTAL KNEE ARTHROPLASTY

Raj K. Sinha

Summary
- Despite the success of total knee arthroplasty (TKA), the number of revision procedures continues to increase.
- Prior to revision surgery, the exact cause of failure of the primary TKA must be determined.
- Adherence to principles of limb alignment and ligament balance provides the greatest chance for success in revision TKA.
- The results of revision TKA are inferior to those of primary TKA.

Total knee arthroplasty (TKA) is one of the most successful operations in medicine for resolving arthritis-related pain and deformity and restoring function. Despite success rates of primary TKA of over 95%[1] with a longevity of approximately 10 to 15 years, the number of revision procedures appears to be increasing. This is due in part to factors outside the control of surgeons, such as the increased number of primary TKAs currently performed, the increased lifespan of patients today, and the high activity level of younger patients who have received TKAs. However, several other factors contribute to TKA failures.

These include component design, surgical technique, the premature introduction of potential "advances" into the marketplace without proper study, the high percentage of arthroplasties performed by surgeons who perform very few annually,[2] and infection. As a result, the revision surgeon faces several technical issues, from bone loss to malalignment to poor soft tissue coverage. Subsequently, it is understandable that the results of revision TKA are inferior to those of primary TKA.

HISTORICAL REVIEW

Several different designs of knee arthroplasty have had fair results, including the University of California–Irvine, polycentric, Duocondylar, geometric, and Duopatellar designs, among many others. The first prosthesis designs to meet with widespread success were the total condylar[3] and the kinematic designs.[4] Despite success in achieving pain relief, these arthroplasties did not return the knee to near-normal kinematic function and were technically challenging for the surgeon. As such, there were concerns regarding longevity, early loosening, mode of component fixation, and technique for insertion.

To address these concerns, several "advances" were introduced, some of which met with widespread acceptance prematurely. One advance was the instrumentation used for the porous coated anatomic (PCA) component (Howmedica, Rutherford, NJ). Although the new instruments and improved surgical technique made it easier for surgeons to restore limb alignment, they failed to establish correct femoral component rotation or ligament balance. As a result, there were problems with patellar instability and early loosening.[5–7] The underlying problems were not recognized, however, and instead research focused on improving patellar component fixation and patellar alignment. Metal-backed patellar components were introduced, but the resulting polyethylene was too thin, leading to rapid early wear and failure with metal-on-metal articulation.[8] In addition, attention directed to patellar alignment led to the use of soft-tissue procedures and tibial tubercle osteotomies, both of which added additional surgeries, and complications.[9]

Similarly, with a lack of attention to ligament balancing, problems with femorotibial instability surfaced. With cruciate-retaining components, there is the potential for increased anteroposterior translation of the femur on the tibia. In addition to mechanical instability and pain, this sliding caused a higher rate of polyethylene wear.[10] Also, with the measured-resection technique introduced by the PCA group, there was a tendency to create small flexion and extension gaps, leading to the use of polyethylene inserts as thin as 2 mm in some portions.[5] Coupled with poor ligament balance and improper rotation, these articular inserts were subject to rapid wear and led to further instability, pain, osteolysis, and loosening.

To further compound problems with component design, there were several manufacturing processes that resulted in inferior inserts. Such flawed techniques included heat isostatic pressing,[11] carbon-reinforced polyethylene,[12] gamma-irradiation in air,[13, 14] machining of the polyethylene bearing surface,[14] and the use of uncemented and titanium femoral components.[15, 16] Thus, although surgeons widely claim that TKA is a reproducible and reliable procedure,

the orthopaedic literature has shown only a few prosthesis designs to be durable and reliable (LCS, IB-I/II, AGC, Kinematic, Total Condylar).[1, 3, 4, 17, 18]

Finally, the role of the surgeon's ability merits mention. Although most of the previously mentioned causes for failure have been corrected or eliminated, TKA remains a technically challenging procedure that requires a high degree of skill and experience.[2] Iatrogenic causes for failure are myriad and range from malalignment to infection. The successful completion of revision TKA procedures also requires a high degree of technical and cognitive ability.

PATHOGENESIS

Patients with failed TKAs usually present with pain. There are several causes for pain that necessitate revision TKA. These can be grouped into the following categories: loosening, polyethylene wear, instability, malalignment, malrotation, fracture, infection, poor range of motion (ROM), stiffness, reflex sympathetic dystrophy, unrecognized hip or spine osteoarthritis, and pain of unknown cause. Although malalignment and malrotation can be causes of pain themselves, these problems can also contribute to or exacerbate the other problems of wear, loosening, and instability. It is extremely important to identify the source of pain in the TKA prior to attempting surgical correction. Attempts to identify the cause for pain intraoperatively can be very frustrating for the patient and surgeon. It is likely that no particular source may be found and the revision surgery would fail to resolve the preoperative pain.[19]

The preoperative evaluation of the painful TKA begins with radiographs, including standing anteroposterior, lateral, flexion weight-bearing and Merchant views. Most problems can be identified on this series of radiographs. Radiolucencies at the prosthesis-cement, bone-cement, or bone-prosthesis interfaces, especially if progressive in width, are characteristic of loosening. Change of component position may be the result of loosening or fracture. Asymmetric femorotibial spaces suggest polyethylene wear. Subluxation of the tibia posteriorly relative to the femur in cruciate-retaining TKAs indicates instability due to posterior cruciate ligament insufficiency or rupture, or excessive polyethylene wear. In posterior stabilized TKAs, femorotibial subluxation may be the result of mismatched flexion and extension gaps, a fractured polyethylene post, or excessive wear. On the Merchant view, loosening, subluxation, dislocation, and bony impingement of the patella are readily identified. When infection is suspected, elevated erythrocyte sedimentation rate, C-reactive protein, or white blood cell count may support the diagnosis. The definitive test for infection is positive aspiration. Adjunctive tests for infection include radionuclide scans, which also may be used to confirm mechanical loosening. Finally, computed tomography can be used to assess component rotation.[20]

GOALS

The basic goals of revision TKA are to resolve pain and restore function. Thus, it is critical to identify the cause for failure so that this can be corrected surgically. Table 1 outlines the causes for failure and the appropriate surgical treatment.

TABLE 1. CAUSES FOR FAILED TOTAL KNEE ARTHROPLASTY

Diagnosis	Reason	Treatment
Loosening	Failure of cement mantle	Revise
	Fibrous ingrowth	Revise with cement
	Osteolysis	Bone graft, revision as needed
Polyethylene wear	Tibial insert too thin	Change insert
	Malalignment	Change insert, correct alignment
	Imbalance	Change insert, correct imbalance
	Metal-backed patella	Revise patella, revise femur if damaged
Instability	Ruptured posterior cruciate ligament	Revise to posterior stabilized TKA
	Polyethylene wear	Change tibial insert
	Fractured PS post	Change tibial insert
	Patellar	Check femoral/tibial component rotation, revise as needed
	Flexion/extension gap imbalance	Balance gaps as indicated
Fracture	Supracondylar	Intramedullary nail vs. femoral revision with intramedullary stem
	Tibial shaft	Revise tibial component with intramedullary stem
	Patella	Good bone stock—open reduction and internal fixation ± revision
		Poor bone stock—resect component, excise fragment, augmented tendon repair
Poor range of motion	Patella too thick	Recut patella and revise component
	Femoral component too big	Downsize femoral component
	Flexion/extension gap imbalance	Balance gaps
	Patella infera	Address joint line

PS = posterior stabilized.

Loosening. In the case of cementless components, loosening is usually the result of a lack of bony ingrowth. Revision to a cemented component is indicated. For cemented components, loosening may occur due to cement mantle fracture or osteolysis. Revision TKA is usually necessary, with particular attention to restoration of bone stock and the appropriate use of stems and wedges (see Technical Details section).

Polyethylene Wear. If the original articular insert was too thin, a thicker insert should be placed while maintaining flexion-extension gap balance (see Technical Details section). In the case of malalignment, the polyethylene insert should be revised along with the appropriate component revision to restore limb alignment. When wear occurs secondary to ligament imbalance, polyethylene insert exchange should be coupled with the appropriate component revision to resolve the imbalance.

Instability. In TKAs in which the posterior cruciate ligament (PCL) is retained, rupture of the PCL can result in femorotibial instability, which is easily addressed by converting to a posterior-stabilized TKA, provided that the flexion-extension gaps are balanced. Instability due to tibial articular polyethylene insert wear or post fracture can be resolved by exchanging the damaged insert. Patellar instability is almost always the result of femoral, tibial, or combined malrotation and thus can rarely be addressed by soft tissue procedures such as lateral release or tubercle osteotomy. Instead, revision of the malrotated components should be undertaken with appropriate revision of the patellar button if it is worn. Malrotation can also cause patellar impingement pain, especially if the patellar button is undersized. In this case, the button should be exchanged and the malrotation corrected. Occasionally, impingement can occur without malrotation, and in this case, patellar button revision or débridement of the offending osteophyte should suffice. Finally, instability may be the result of imbalanced flexion and extension gaps, which then should be corrected (see Technical Details section).

Fracture. Periprosthetic supracondylar fracture of the femur can be treated with a retrograde statically locked intramedullary nail or open reduction and internal fixation with a dynamic condylar screw plate. In the latter situation, bone graft should be used at the fracture site. Alternatively, a distal femoral fracture that extends under the component can be effectively treated by revising the femoral component and using a press-fit intramedullary stem to stabilize the fracture.[21] Fractures of the tibial shaft that are well distal to the component can be treated by open reduction and internal fixation. Those adjacent to the tibial stem are best treated with revision of the tibial component to one with a long press-fit stem that sufficiently bypasses the fracture. Fractures of the patella are especially challenging, as failed treatment results in severe extensor lag with extreme debility. If there is sufficient bone stock, then open reduction and internal fixation should be performed, and the component should be revised only if loose. If the bony fragments are thin or avascular, then excision followed by primary repair and augmentation should be performed.[22, 23]

Poor ROM. Limited extension usually results from an overly thick polyethylene insert that blocks full extension. Exchange to a smaller insert usually resolves this problem but may lead to flexion instability. In that case, proper balancing of the flexion and extension gaps is required (see Technical Details section). Poor flexion is usually the result of an "overstuffed anterior compartment." This means that the patella–patellar button construct is too thick or that the femoral component is too large and thus displaces the patella anteriorly. To correct this problem, revision of the patellar component to a smaller one, or revision of the femoral component, or both, may be necessary. Poor flexion may also result from an overly thick polyethylene insert. If that is the case, then proper balancing of the flexion and extension gaps is required to correct the problem. Finally, flexion may be limited by patella infra, especially after a previous lateral closing wedge high tibial osteotomy.[24] Correction of this problem is often frustrating. If the joint line had been elevated, then revision of the femoral component with distal augments to lower the joint line may be effective. Otherwise, restoration of balanced flexion and extension gaps has the greatest chance for success (see the Technical Details section). In addition, certain patients are prone to poor ROM after TKA for no apparent reason. Low pain threshold limiting the effectiveness of physical therapy, abnormal propensity for scar formation, obesity, and heavy musculature have all been implicated. Revision surgery is unlikely to resolve these issues.

INDICATIONS AND CONTRAINDICATIONS

Revision TKA is indicated when the source of the patient's pain is clearly identified, and the patient is a good candidate in terms of compliance, bone stock, and medical condition. Contraindications include poor medical condition, recurrent infected TKA, poor soft tissue coverage, ruptured extensor mechanism, and poor bone stock, among others.

PROCEDURE

PREOPERATIVE TEMPLATING

Before revision surgery, a preoperative template and surgical plan should be prepared. Good-quality anteroposterior, lateral, and Merchant's radiographs of the operative limb, as well as a lateral radiograph of the contralateral limb, are required. The contralateral knee lateral radiograph helps to establish the correct component size, especially if the knee has never been operated on. When malalignment is suspected, then full-length standing views of the limb are required.

Templates should be used to determine component size, the need for stems and augments, the need for various types of bone grafts, and the potential for specialized components such as hinged TKAs or tumor-type prostheses.

The primary indication for the use of a stem is the situation in which there is insufficient bone stock to support a conventional component. For example, after removal of an ingrown cementless femoral component, quite often the anterior femur is deficient (Fig. 1). In that case, a femoral stem bypasses the defect and stabilizes the prosthesis. Other relative indications include assistance with alignment, supplemental support when augments are used, and the use of constrained polyethylene inserts, in which case the stems theoretically decrease the shear stress at the component-cement interface.

For augments, the appropriate usage is in case of uncontained bone defects greater than 5 mm in depth. Additional applications would be to change the position of the joint line, to balance asymmetric bone loss, and to help balance the flexion and extension gaps. Nonstructural bone grafts such as cancellous bone are used only when the components are stable and have adjacent isolated osteolytic cavities. Structural allograft may be used in situations of extreme bone loss. In those conditions, the fixation of the

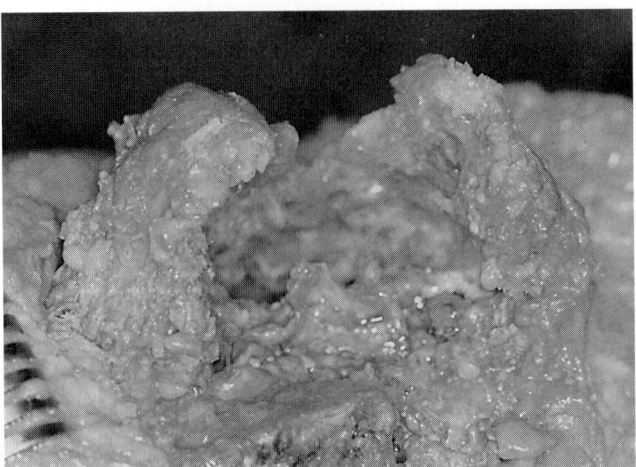

Fig. 1. Distal femur after removal of femoral component demonstrating significant anterior bone loss. Because there is insufficient bone in the anterior femur, a femoral stem is indicated to stabilize the component.

allograft to host bone is supplemented by long intramedullary stems affixed to the components. Typically, the stem and component are cemented to the allograft bone and press-fit into the host bone. Alternatively, in situations of extreme bone loss or when both the medial and lateral collateral ligaments are incompetent, a rotating hinged TKA may be utilized.

Constrained articular inserts may be used when a single collateral ligament is incompetent or when a larger post is necessary to confer stability. In cases of minor imbalances of the flexion-extension gaps, a constrained insert may be used, especially in elderly patients with osteoporotic bone in whom component revision may cause excessive bone loss. However, in severe flexion-extension mismatches, relying on a constrained insert to solve the problem is inviting further complications.

TECHNICAL DETAILS (FLEXION-EXTENSION GAP BALANCING)

The basic steps for performing a posterior-stabilized revision TKA are as follows:

Exposure. A standard midline incision followed by a medial parapatellar arthrotomy should be used, as this provides the greatest exposure. A total synovectomy should follow, primarily to release adhesions and to create space for the new components. If additional exposure is required after synovectomy, specialized techniques such as rectus snip or V-Y turndown[25] can be employed.

Removal of Components. Cemented components are easily removed by using flexible or curved osteotomes. The osteotome should be directed at the prosthesis-cement interface and the initial step is to disrupt the bond between the prosthesis and the cement (Fig. 2). Once this interface is disrupted circumferentially, the components can be disimpacted from the cement mantle. The remaining cement is removed piecemeal with osteotomes, rongeurs, and a bur to preserve bone stock. For cemented patellar components, I prefer to use an oscillating saw to carefully cut the fixation pegs. A bur is then used to remove the pegs and then to

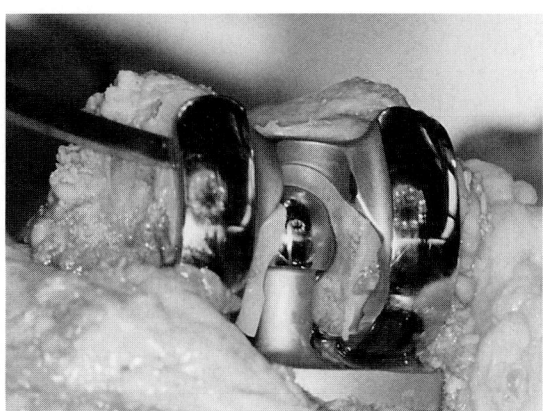

Fig. 2. Example of osteotome utilized to disrupt the prosthesis-cement interface. Note that the osteotome is directed with the curve pointing toward the prosthesis. This technique helps to minimize loss of bone during component removal.

remove cement. For bone-ingrowth prostheses, flexible osteotomes should be used to carefully disrupt the bone-prosthesis interface. Alternately, a Gigli saw can be used to disrupt the interface, particularly under the anterior flange of the femoral component.

Reestablish the Proximal Tibia. The proximal tibia is cut with an intramedullary or extramedullary guide. The cut should be perpendicular to the long axis of the tibia and alignment should be confirmed prior to continuing (Fig. 3). The recut tibia is then prepared for a new trial implant. If there is significant proximal metaphyseal bone loss, an intramedullary stem should be used for additional support. In addition, medial and lateral defects should be addressed with hemiblocks (Fig. 4). Hemiblocks are preferable over wedges and half-wedges, as the latter have poor resistance to shear stress.[26] Contained defects and those less than 5 mm in depth can be filled with cement. Proper rotation of the tibial component is set by placing it so that the midpoint of the tray lies adjacent to the medial third of the tubercle. The trial tibial component is then impacted into the tibia.

Restoring Limb Alignment. Once the tibial component is placed, the leg is brought into full extension. A lamina spreader is placed between the distal femur and proximal tibia. Leg alignment can be estimated by aligning a Bovie cord from a point 2 cm medial to the anterior superior iliac spine to the center of the ankle. The cord should pass through the center of the knee. If it does not, then the appropriate releases should be performed to restore alignment.

Determining the Flexion Gap. Estimate the size of the new femoral component from the preoperative template or lateral radiograph of the contralateral knee. If the anterior and posterior bone stock is sufficient, then an intramedullary stem is not required. In that case, a standard intramedullary cutting guide can be utilized. If bone loss is present and an intramedullary stem will be required, then this stem can be used to place the cutting guide and to set the flexion gap and rotation. Place the appropriate intramedullary cutting guide into the femur. With the knee flexed to 90 degrees, the knee is distracted. The femoral cutting guide is rotated to create a rectangular gap between the

bottom of the cutting guide and the tibial tray (Fig. 5). The guide is pinned, and the anterior and posterior cuts are made. Any posterior defects that would require augments are addressed at this time, and the cuts are freshened to accommodate the augments. The guide is removed, and a spacer block is placed to determine the size of the flexion gap.

Balancing the Flexion and Extension Gap. The distal femoral cut is freshened, with particular attention to defects that may require augmentation (Fig. 6). The leg is brought to full extension and the spacer blocks are used to determine the size of the extension gap. If the extension gap matches the flexion gap, then final component trials can be placed. If there is a mismatch, then additional bone resection or augments will be necessary. The various options are outlined in Table 2. The guiding principles are as follows. Resection or augmentation of the proximal tibia affects the flexion and extension gap equally. Resection or augmentation of the posterior femoral condyles affects the flexion gap only. Resection or augmentation of the distal femur affects the extension gap only.

Establishing the Joint Line. Once the gaps are balanced, the final trial components are placed, and the appropriately sized articular spacer (as determined by the spacer blocks during flexion-extension gap balancing) is placed. The articulation of the femoral component with the tibial

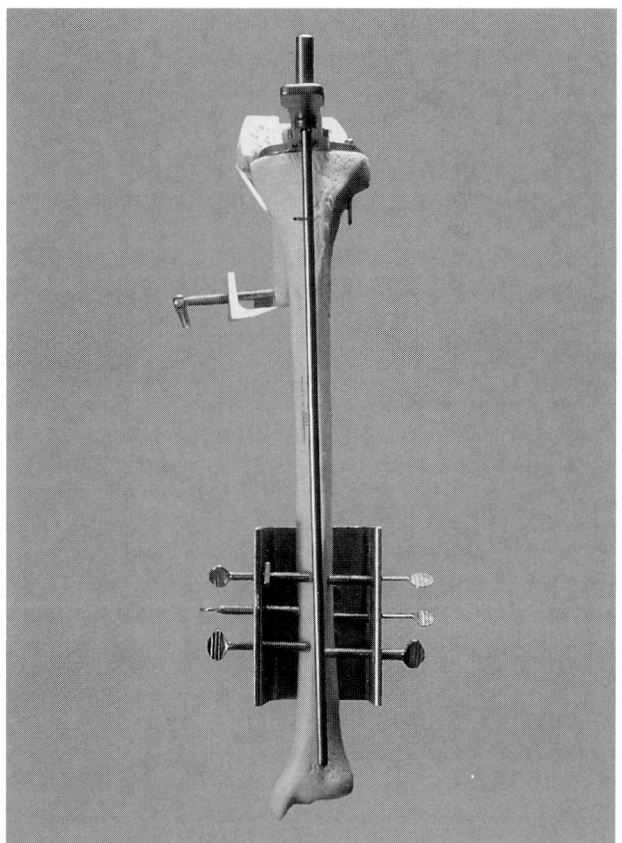

Fig. 3. Tibial alignment guide confirms that the proximal tibial cut is perpendicular to the long axis of the femur. The alignment rod should fall along the tibial crest or within the center of the mortise. The second metatarsal is an unreliable landmark for referencing the perpendicularity of the proximal tibial cut.

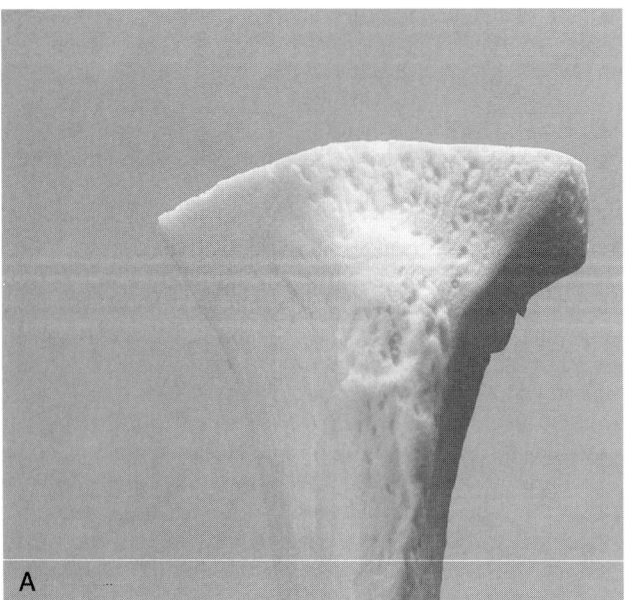
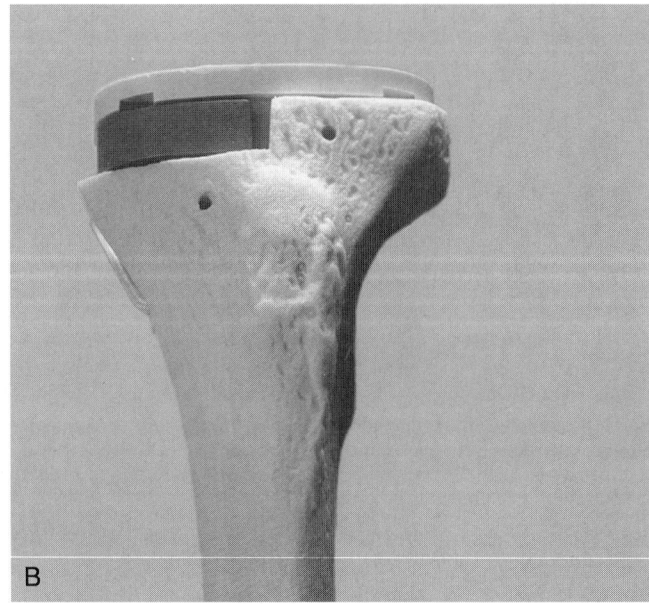

Fig. 4. Views. *A,* Example of a medial defect in the proximal tibia after component removal. Although a wedge may be used, a hemiblock is preferred because it loads the cement in compression rather than in shear. *B,* The tibial component with hemiblock used to correct the medial tibial defect.

component should be at the level of the native joint line, or no more than 8 mm proximal to that point.[27] The native joint line can be estimated by the position of the meniscal scar, as being 1.5 cm proximal to the top of the fibular head, or as being 1.5 cm distal to the distal pole of the patella. If the joint line has been brought too far proximally, then the distal femur should be augmented. This will decrease the extension gap, and therefore the posterior

femur will need to be increased in size to decrease the flexion gap as well. The situation of a lowered joint line very rarely occurs, but if it does, the only solution is to augment the proximal tibia, which then affects the flexion and extension gaps equally.

Determining the Need for Constrained Inserts. Once the final trial components are placed, the knee should be tested with a varus and valgus stress. If there is asymmet-

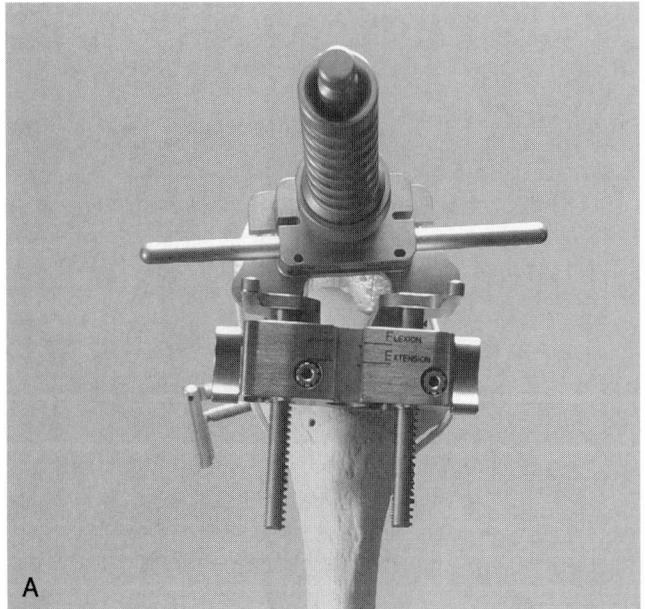
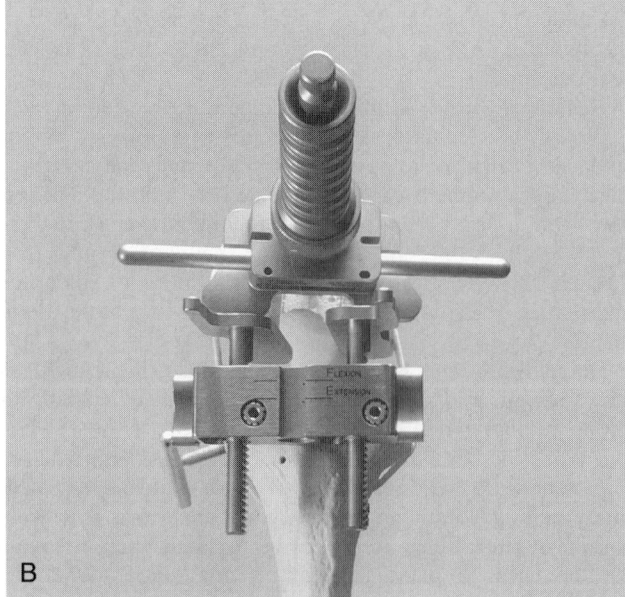

Fig. 5. Setting femoral component rotation. *A,* A tensor is placed between the corrected proximal tibia and posterior femur, with the knee at 90° of flexion, in order to distract the flexion space. The IM cutting guide for the femur has been placed. However, it is rotated internally, as demonstrated by the trapezoidal flexion space. *B,* The IM guide was rotated externally to create a rectangular flexion space. Now the correct femoral component rotation has been determined.

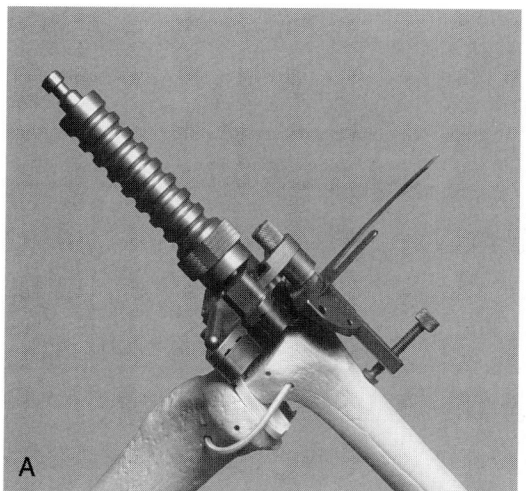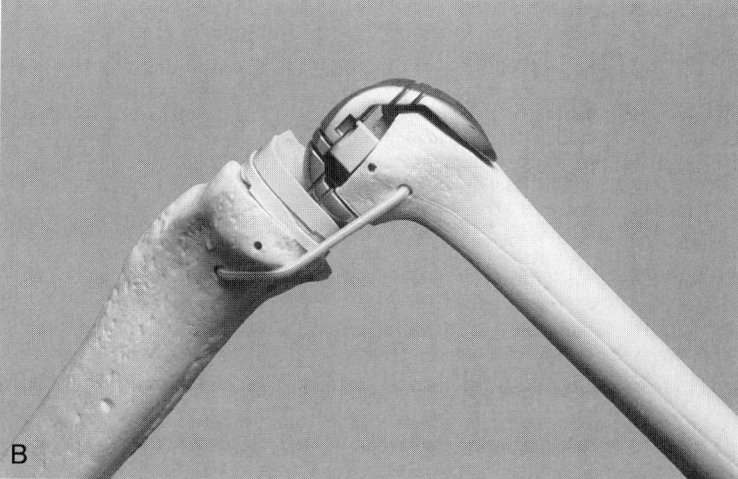

Fig. 6. Distal femoral cut. *A,* The distal femoral cut is freshened to help determine the extension gap. The batwing can be used to reference the level of the previous distal femoral cut. In this example, the batwing was placed at the level of the medial distal femoral cut. *B,* With the distal cut having been freshened, there was a residual lateral defect. An augment was used to correct the distal lateral femoral defect.

ric laxity, then a constrained implant may be required. Full extension and flexion past 90 degrees should be achieved. In addition, there should be no liftoff of the femoral component from the articular component at 90 degrees of flexion. If there is liftoff, the risk for femorotibial dislocation exists and a constrained insert should be used. The larger post of a constrained insert should prevent dislocation. If there is significant liftoff, then the gaps are grossly mismatched and should be rebalanced.

Patellar Resurfacing. If the patella is greater than 12 mm thick and does not appear avascular, it can be resurfaced with the appropriate implant. If it is too thin or appears avascular, a patelloplasty should be performed. In both situations, patellar tracking should be carefully inspected and the threshold for performing a lateral release should be low. Finally, with all the trial components in place, the soft tissues should be assessed to ensure that a tension-free closure can be accomplished.

POSTOPERATIVE REGIMEN

A bulky dressing with intra-articular drains and a knee immobilizer are used routinely. All are removed on the second postoperative day and flexion is begun in physical therapy. Isometric exercises and weightbearing as tolerated are usually allowed on the first postoperative day. When structural allograft is used, touchdown weightbearing is maintained for up to 3 months. Physical therapy focused on ROM, quadriceps strengthening, ambulation, and stair climbing is instituted for 6 weeks. Patients are allowed to progress to no ambulatory aids at their own pace.

RESULTS

The results after primary knee arthroplasty have been quite good. TKAs have been shown to be durable, with 94% survivorship after 10 years of follow-up.[1] In addition, they have improved the functional level in young patients as well as in elderly patients.[28] These are the primary reasons that TKA is one of the most rewarding operations in all of medicine.

Revision TKA has not been quite as successful, however. Functional scores are lower and durability has not been demonstrated. For example, Peters et al[29] reviewed 57 revision TKAs and found Hospital for Special Surgery scores to be only 82 (compared to greater than 92 in primary TKA[28]), and survivorship estimated to be 75% at 99-month follow-up. Similarly, Haas et al[30] showed Hospital for Special Surgery scores to be 76 after revision TKA. However, Gustilo et al[31] suggested that correct alignment and ligament balance would result in only slight deterioration of the results over time. Several factors correlate with diminishing results in revision TKA, including bone loss, the number of operations, valgus alignment, and history of infection.

CONCLUSION

Revision TKA is a complex and often difficult procedure. There are several possible problems with the failed TKA, and all must be addressed at the time of surgery for there to be any chance for success. Adherence to the principles of limb alignment and ligament balance help the surgeon address the technical problems at the time of surgery and provide the patient with a good outcome.

TABLE 2. MATCHING THE EXTENSION GAP TO FLEXION GAP	
Situation	**Solution**
Extension gap = flexion gap	None needed
Extension gap < flexion gap	Resect distal femur
	Augment posterior femur
Extension gap > flexion gap	Augment distal femur
Extension gap = flexion gap (but both larger than available insert sizes)	Augment proximal tibia

REFERENCES

1. Font Rodriguez DE, Scuderi GR, Insall JN: Survivorship of cemented total knee arthroplasty. Clin Orthop 1997; 345:79.
2. Lavernia CJ, Guzman JF: Relationship of surgical volume to short-term mortality, morbidity, and hospital charges in arthroplasty. J Arthroplasty 1995; 10:133.
3. Insall J, Scott WN, Ranawat CS: The total condylar knee prosthesis: A report of two hundred and twenty cases. J Bone Joint Surg Am 1979; 61:173.
4. Ewald FC, Jacobs MA, Miegel RE, et al: Kinematic total knee replacement. J Bone Joint Surg Am 1984; 66:1032.
5. Lindstrand A, Ryd L, Stenström A: Polyethylene failure in two total knees: Wear of thin, metal-backed PCA tibial components. Acta Orthop Scand 1990; 61:575.
6. Skinner HB, Mabey MF, Paganelli JV, et al: Failure analysis of PCA revision total knee replacement tibial component: A preliminary study using the finite element method. Orthopedics 1987; 10(4):581.
7. Maruyama M, Terayama K, Sunohara H, et al: Fracture of the tibial tray following PCA knee replacement: A report of two cases. Arch Orthop Trauma Surg 1994; 113:330.
8. Bayley JC, Scott RD, Ewald FC, et al: Failure of the metal-backed patellar component after total knee replacement. J Bone Joint Surg Am 1988; 70:668.
9. Merkow RL, Soudry M, Insall JN: Patellar dislocation following total knee replacement. J Bone Joint Surg Am 1985; 67:1321.
10. Blunn GW, Walker PS, Joshi A, et al: The dominance of cyclic sliding in producing wear in total knee replacements. Clin Orthop 1991; 273:253.
11. Bloebaum RD, Nelson K, Dorr LD, et al: Investigation of early surface delamination observed in retrieved heat-pressed tibial inserts. Clin Orthop 1991; 269:120.
12. Wright TM, Astion DJ, Bansal M, et al: Failure of carbon fiber-reinforced polyethylene total knee-replacement components: A report of two cases. J Bone Joint Surg 1988; 70:926.
13. Li S, Burstein AH: Ultra-high molecular weight polyethylene: The material and its use in total joint implants. J Bone Joint Surg Am 1994; 76:1080.
14. Schmalzried TP, Callaghan JJ: Wear in total hip and knee replacements. J Bone Joint Surg Am 1999; 81:115.
15. Nilsson KG, Kärrholm J, Linder L: Femoral component migration in total knee arthroplasty: Randomized study comparing cemented and uncemented fixation of the Miller-Galante I design. J Orthop Res 1995; 13:347.
16. Peters PC Jr, Engh GA, Dwyer KA, et al: Osteolysis after total knee arthroplasty without cement. J Bone Joint Surg Am 1992; 74:864.
17. Ritter MA, Worland R, Saliski J, et al: Flat-on-flat, nonconstrained, compression molded polyethylene total knee replacement. Clin Orthop 1995; 321:79.
18. Buechel FF, Pappas MJ: New Jersey low contact stress knee replacement system: Ten-year evaluation of meniscal bearings. Orthop Clin North Am 1989; 20:147.
19. Jacobs MA, Hungerford DS, Krackow KA, et al: Revision total knee arthroplasty for aseptic failure. Clin Orthop 1988; 226:78.
20. Berger RA, Crossett LS, Jacobs JJ, et al: Malrotation causing patellofemoral complications after total knee arthroplasty. Clin Orthop 1998; 356:144.
21. Peyton RS, Booth RE: Supracondylar femur fractures above an Insall-Burstein CCK Total Knee: A new method for intramedullary stem fixation. J Arthroplasty 1998; 13(4):473.
22. Emerson RH, Head WC, Malinin TI: Extensor mechanism reconstruction with an allograft after total knee arthroplasty. Clin Orthop 1994; 303:79.
23. Cadambi A, Engh GA: Use of a semitendinosus autogenous graft for rupture of the patellar ligament after total knee arthroplasty. J Bone Joint Surg Am 1992; 74:974.
24. Windsor RE, Insall JN, Vince KG: Technical considerations of total knee arthroplasty after proximal tibial osteotomy. J Bone Joint Surg Am 1988; 70:547.
25. Younger AS, Duncan CP, Masri BA: Surgical exposures in revision total knee arthroplasty. J Am Acad Orthop Surg 1998; 6:55.
26. Chen F, Krackow KA: Management of tibial defects in total knee arthroplasty. Clin Orthop 1994; 305:249.
27. Figgie HE, Goldberg VM, Heiple KG, et al: The influence of tibial-patellofemoral location on function of the knee in patients with the posterior stabilized condylar knee prosthesis. J Bone Joint Surg Am 1986; 68:1035.
28. Diduch DR, Insall JN, Scott WN, et al: Total knee replacement in young, active patients. Long term follow-up and functional outcome. J Bone Joint Surg Am 1997; 79:575.
29. Peters CL, Hennessey R, Barden RM, et al: Revision total knee arthroplasty with a cemented posterior-stabilized or constrained condylar prosthesis. J Arthrop 1997; 12:896.
30. Haas SB, Insall JN, Montgomery W III, et al: Revision total knee arthroplasty with use of modular stems inserted without cement. J Bone Joint Surg Am 1995; 77:1700.
31. Gustilo T, Comadoll JL, Gustilo RB: Long-term results of 56 revision total knee replacements. Orthopedics 1996; 19:99.

MANAGEMENT OF COMPLICATIONS AFTER JOINT ARTHROPLASTY

section 6 / chapter 18

Nicholas G. Sotereanos, Robert F. Hube, Sokratis E. Varitimidis, and Ulrich Schietsch

Summary
- Management of complications of joint arthroplasties is one of the most challenging problems in orthopaedic surgery.
- In the majority of the cases treatment of these complications is nonoperative.
- Pulmonary embolism, and sepsis secondary to joint infection can put the patient's life at risk.
- Early recognition and management of complications is crucial for an optimal result.
- Preoperative planning and teamwork are essential to overcome difficulties in the surgical treatment of complications in joint replacement.

Joint replacement has revolutionized the treatment of arthritic conditions of the hip and knee. In the United States over 300,000 patients undergo hip and knee replacements every year. After any major surgical procedure, complications can occur. Arthroplasty, mainly performed in patients older than 65 years, is complicated by high morbidity, which is often accepted as the norm. Comorbidity factors certainly contribute to general complications.

The goal in total joint arthroplasty is prevention of systemic and local complications and, if they occur, the diagnosis and adequate management of them. Careful preoperative preparation, suitable anesthesia, and efficient surgery will help decrease perioperative and postoperative complications and mortality.

GENERAL CONCERNS

MORTALITY

The cumulative postoperative mortality rate increases with age. In a study to investigate the mortality and cumulative postoperative survival rate of older Americans undergoing total hip arthroplasty (THA), total perioperative mortality was found to be 0.95% and increased with age.[1] Those 85 years of age or older had a mortality rate of 3.75%.[2-4] Intraoperative complications are rare, but postoperative complications account for a significant increase in morbidity and thus a poor outcome (Table 1).

DEEP VENOUS THROMBOSIS AND PULMONARY EMBOLISM

A number of secondary risk factors for thromboembolism have been identified, including increased age, previous venous thromboembolism, prolonged immobilization, varicose veins, obesity, and cardiac dysfunction. These factors are often present in patients who have undergone joint arthroplasty of the lower extremity. The development of a postoperative proximal deep vein thrombosis (DVT) or life-threatening pulmonary embolus cannot be predicted. Thus, the optimal defense in patients who undergo hip or knee arthroplasty is prevention. This routine use of prophylaxis is necessary; prophylaxis should be relatively free of adverse effects, easy to use, and cost-effective. There must be a commitment on the part of the surgeon to provide this regimen to all patients in whom a high-risk procedure is performed. Without prophylaxis, DVT occurs in 40% to 80% of patients undergoing hip or knee arthroplasty and is the most common cause of readmission to hospital after THA.[5]

Detection of vascular complications can be difficult. In a large percentage of these patients the involved extremity will be asymptomatic. Patients who have had a THA or total knee arthroplasty (TKA) have been shown to be at

risk for thromboembolic complications, and a simple and accurate method of early diagnosis of DVT has been sought for decades. Ascending venography has been the standard with which other methods of evaluation have been compared. Problems related to ascending venography, however, such as discomfort, renal impairment, and reaction to the contrast medium, have prompted the search for noninvasive tests. Plethysmography, radioactive fibrinogen uptake, and Doppler testing appeared to be useful for the evaluation of patients who are clinically suspected of having DVT.[6, 7]

However, because of the lack of accuracy, these modalities have limited use for the screening of patients who do not have clinical symptoms. Ultrasonography has been reported to be highly accurate in the detection of thrombi both in patients in whom there is a clinical suspicion of DVT and in high-risk patients.[8, 9] As with any diagnostic study, ultrasound has its limitations. The three most common causes of false-negative ultrasonograms are the location of the clot, the size of the clot, and inexperience on the part of the technician. Borris et al.[10] reported that only 2 of 11 thrombi less than 1 cm in length were detected with the compression test in 60 patients who had undergone a THA. Also, the adductor hiatus of the thigh has been described as a blind spot for examination with ultrasonography. Comerota et al[11, 12] recommended the use of adjunctive ultrasonography tests, such as Doppler flow studies, to examine the region of the adductor hiatus, but others have not found such studies to be useful. False-positive interpretations of ultrasounds are usually a result of echogenic areas being confused with clot material.

A lack of experience on the part of the technician is believed to be the most common cause of false-negative ultrasonograms. Acute clots are rarely visualized on real-time scans, which forces the technician to depend on the compression test. This examination may be technically difficult because acute clots are soft and partially compressible and may deceive an inexperienced technician.[13] The accuracy of the test increases with experience. Over a 4-year period, Woolson and Pottorff[14] were able to increase the sensitivity of the ultrasonography test from 67% to 83% when evaluating proximal veins after TKA. They concluded that there was a time-dependent learning curve for ultrasonography because they were able to detect the thrombi on a second ultrasound in two of the five extremities in which the ultrasonogram had initially been interpreted as negative. Garino et al[9] found similar results, citing lack of technical experience as a cause of false-negative findings.

The 1986 Consensus Conference of the National Institutes of Health on the management of thromboembolic disease strongly recommended the use of effective prophylaxis (dextran, adjusted-dose heparin, or low-dose warfarin) in high-risk patients. Even with the use of these prophylactic methods, the rate of DVTs (half of which occur in proximal veins) is still 15% to 30% by the time of discharge from the hospital. About 50% of fatal pulmonary emboli occur between 7 and 14 days after the operation, and 36% occur between days 14 and 90. Significant decreases in rates of DVT have been achieved with dose-adjusted heparin, warfarin sodium (Coumadin), low-molecular-weight heparin, and aspirin therapy. Adjuncts to these treatments include elastic hose and sequential compression

TABLE 1. MANAGEMENT OF GENERAL COMPLICATIONS AFTER HIP AND KNEE TOTAL JOINT ARTHROPLASTIES

Complication	Conservative Treatment	Operative Treatment
Deep venous thrombosis	Anticoagulant treatment	Surgical treatment for massive iliofemoral thrombi
Pulmonary embolism	Anticoagulant treatment (for microembolism)	Surgical treatment for massive pulmonary emboli
Infection, sepsis	None	Irrigation, débridement, and antibiotics for early infection; implant removal, antibiotics for 6 wks and reimplantation after eradication of infection

devices. The sequelae of thromboembolic events can be devastating, so that particular vigilance should be maintained in this high-risk group of patients. It is common in our practice to obtain noninvasive Doppler's ultrasound examinations on all high-risk patients even if asymptomatic.

POSTOPERATIVE INFECTION, SEPSIS

Deep wound infections cause significant numbers of failures in lower extremity joint replacement.[2] The most common pathogens in orthopaedic procedures are *Staphylococcus aureus* and *Staphylococcus epidermis.*

Certain prophylactic measures are effective in preventing postoperative infections. In malnourished patients, for instance, preoperative enteral feeding to improve nutrition can significantly change the rate of postoperative infections; parenteral feedings have not proved efficacious.[15] The use of ultra–clean air operating rooms and antibiotic prophylaxis is a well-established therapy that has been proved to decrease the postoperative infection rate. Usually a first- or second-generation cephalosporin is given just before surgery and every 8 hours for 2 days thereafter. Another method of providing prophylaxis is using antibiotic loaded cement or mixing 1.2 g of tobramycin with each 40 g of cement when performing cemented arthroplasties. With these measures, wound infection rates of 1.2% after THA have been obtained. A disadvantage of this procedure is weakening of the cement by loading with antibiotics.

Postoperative infections are manifested by a painful joint that cannot be related to other factors. The erythrocyte sedimentation rate and the C-reactive protein level are elevated. Scintigraphy is another reliable technique for differentiating infections from aseptic loosening, but cannot be used in an early infection because of poor specificity. The standard to diagnose an infected hip or knee is still an aspiration although the sensitivity has been reported to be 60% to 75%. It can be improved by repeated aspiration and should be performed under sterile conditions to prevent new infections. Aspiration can show false-negative results when performed while the patient is receiving antibiotics. Radiographic changes with lysis of periprosthetic bone and cyst formation are present in a septic joint.

The treatment of hip and knee infections after total joint replacement is operative. In cases of early infection, débridement with retention of the prosthesis can be effective. Polyethylene modular implants should be removed and replaced to allow for débridement of the covered surfaces. The failure rate correlates with the duration of the infection, and pathogenicity of the infecting organism. In late or chronic infections a one-stage or two-stage reimplantation is an option. The two-stage reimplantation contains insertion of a temporary antibiotic-loaded cement spacer for at least 6 weeks and antibiotic suppression (Figs. 1 and 2). Recurrent infections or failed reimplantations can be treated by arthrodesis. In cases of life-threatening sepsis secondary to an infected TKA, an above-knee amputation may be required.

WOUND PROBLEMS

Wound-healing problems can lead to deep infection and for this reason should be treated aggressively with surgical

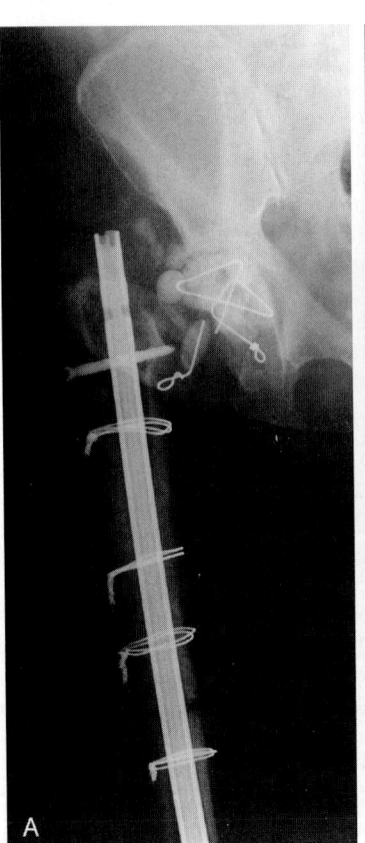
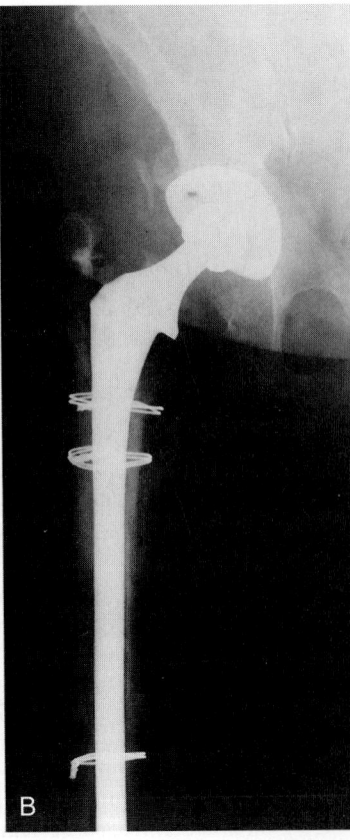

Fig. 1 Removal. *A,* Removal of implants after infection of total hip arthroplasty. Antibiotic-loaded cement beads were placed in the arthroplasty space. Temporary intramedullary nailing was performed due to an osteotomy of the femur that was done to facilitate removal of the femoral component. *B,* Six weeks after the removal of the prosthesis a new implant was inserted.

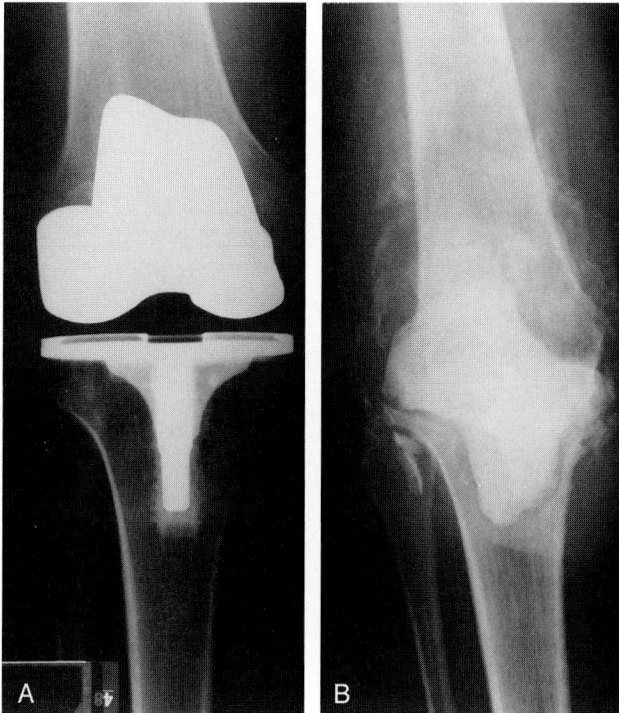

Fig. 2 Arthroplasty. *A,* Infected total knee arthroplasty. *B,* The prosthesis was removed and a cement spacer was placed. The patient needed three débridements before achieving negative cultures of the tissues in the knee joint.

débridement. A deep infection should be ruled out before administrating antibiotic suppression. To prevent wound problems, old incisions should be used and no parallel new incisions performed. This frequently leads to skin necrosis. In knee replacement, lateral skin flaps have to be avoided, because anastomoses of blood supply are rare in this region. For treatment of necrotic areas after TKA, the gastrocnemius and free flaps can be used.

HIP ARTHROPLASTY

PERIPROSTHETIC FRACTURES

Periprosthetic fractures are among the most devastating complications of primary and revision THA (Table 2). The incidence has been reported as 0.1% in primary THA and as 4.2% in revision THA.[16] These fractures can occur from a few days to a few years after surgery. The fracture rate increases with predisposing factors, such as loosening of the prosthesis, osteolysis of the femoral component, osteoporosis, and rheumatoid arthritis. The risk factors known to lead to increased falls in older patients also make them more susceptible to periprosthetic fractures.

Periprosthetic fractures after THA can occur as fracture of the acetabulum but are most commonly associated with fractures of the femur.[17-19] The classification system as described by Mallory et al[20] divides the fractures into three simple patterns:

Type 1: undisplaced fracture limited to the proximal aspect of the femoral component.

Type 2: fracture that spirals distally but does not extend beyond the tip of the implant.

Type 3: fracture at the distal aspect of the femoral component.

Late periprosthetic fractures may occur around loose cemented femoral components, usually as a consequence of osteolytic bone deficiency. The type of prosthesis and the presence of preexisting stressors play a role in determining where the fractures occur. The site of fracture and the prefracture interface influence treatment.

Optimal reconstruction may sometimes warrant the use of special implants such as cable plates and structural allografts. Techniques that achieve fracture healing as well as component stability are desirable. Treatment can consist of both operative and nonoperative therapies, depending on the location of the fracture. Fractures proximal to the tip of a fixed prosthesis, such as an avulsion fracture of the greater or lesser trochanter, can usually be treated nonoperatively or with limited internal fixation; fractures at the tip of the prosthesis usually require implant revision or the use of internal fixation (Fig. 3). Fractures below the prosthesis can be managed operatively if displaced or nonoperatively if nondisplaced. Individual evaluation is necessary in the determination of fracture care.

Periprosthetic acetabular fractures are relatively rare, but they are associated with a poor prognosis with regard to survival of the acetabular component. It is possible, however, to achieve union and to salvage a functional prosthesis in patients who have sustained a rare undisplaced fracture. Acetabular fractures are typically associated with high-energy trauma and usually require revision of the acetabular component, frequently requiring additional fixation and/or bone grafting if the supportive anterior or posterior columns of the acetabulum are displaced.

HETEROTOPIC OSSIFICATION

Heterotopic ossification after THA occurs in about 50% of primary hip arthroplasties.[21] It varies from fine islands of

TABLE 2. MANAGEMENT OF COMPLICATIONS AFTER TOTAL HIP ARTHROPLASTY

Complication	Conservative Treatment	Operative Treatment
Periprosthetic fractures	Traction, non-weightbearing	Open reduction and internal fixation; implant revision may be necessary
Heterotopic ossification	Prevention (indomethacin, diphosphonates, irradiation)	Removal of heterotopic bone.
Dislocation of the prosthesis	Closed reduction under anesthesia	Open reduction when closed reduction fails; revision of implants may be required
Neurovascular injuries	None	Repair of vessel or nerve (nerve injury is catastrophic)

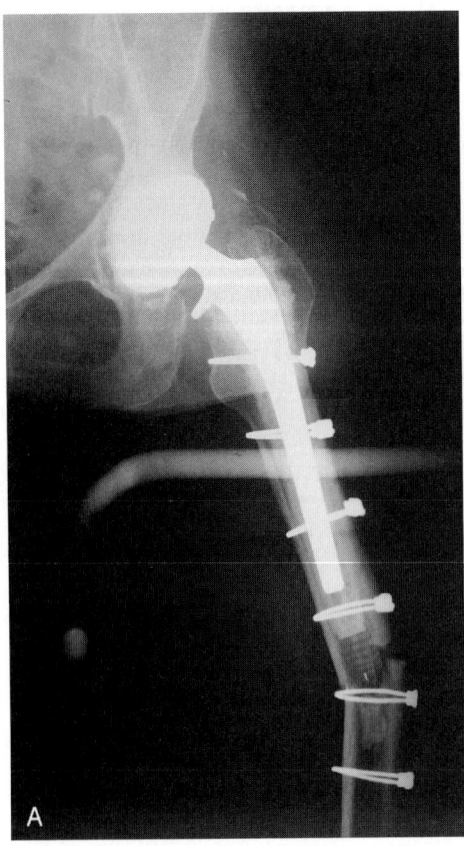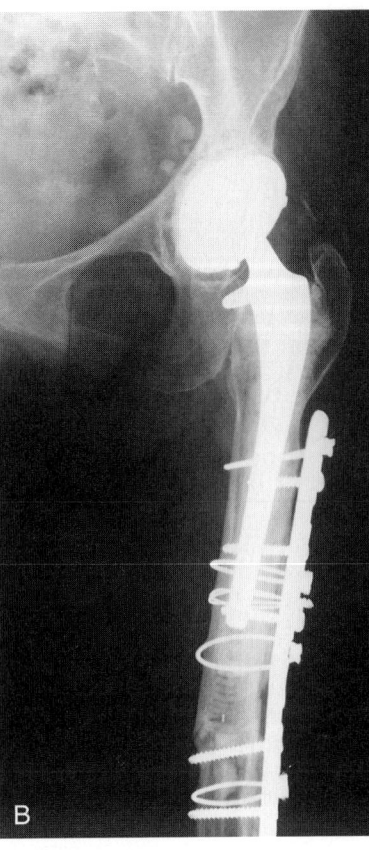

Fig. 3 Periprosthetic femoral fracture. *A,* Periprosthetic femoral fracture 3 cm below the tip of a femoral component of a total hip arthroplasty. *B,* Open reduction and plating with screws and wires was performed for fixation of the fracture.

bone within soft tissue to almost complete ankylosis. In 2% to 10% of patients it results in pain and decreased range of motion.[22] The cause is unknown although there appears to be a metaplasia of local fibroblasts into osteoblastic cells that produce bone.

Identified risk factors are patients who have developed heterotopic ossifications after previous surgery, patients with hypertrophic osteoarthritis, young male patients, and patients with ankylosing spondylitis. Technical factors include prolonged surgery and the surgical approach. It has been shown that the incidence is higher after a transtrochanteric, anterior, and lateral approach compared with the posterolateral approach.

Heterotopic ossification can be seen radiographically within the second or third week. The widely used grading system for heterotopic ossifications is the classification of Brooker et al.[23] It describes four grades:

Grade 1: islands of bone within the soft tissues about the hip.
Grade 2: bone spurs from the proximal femur or pelvis leaving at least 1 cm between opposing bone surfaces.
Grade 3: bone spurs from the proximal femur or pelvis with less than 1 cm between opposing bone surfaces.
Grade 4: ankylosis of the hip.

Several methods of prevention have been recommended. Treatment with nonsteroidal anti-inflammatory medications has been shown to be successful in preventing heterotopic bone formation after THA. Kjaersgaard-Admundson and Ritter[24] demonstrated that 25 mg of indomethacin 3 times a day for the first 2 weeks after surgery is sufficient to prevent severe grades of heterotopic ossification. Other authors recommend 4 to 6 weeks of treatment with indomethacin. Diphosphonates also have been advocated for prophylaxis of heterotopic bone formation.[25]

The other therapeutic limb of prophylaxis is low-dose radiation therapy. It may be indicated in high-risk patients as described above and has been administered successfully to this patient group and to patients who have undergone excision of massive heterotopic bone formation.[26] Different doses are reported. More recent studies showed improved results using a single dose of 700 cGy within 3 days of surgery.[27, 28] In cases with massive bone formation and associated pain and motion restriction, excision of heterotopic bone followed by low-dose irradiation has shown good results.

DISLOCATION AND EARLY INSTABILITY

Early instability is defined as dislocations within 3 months of surgery.[2, 16] It is the most common technical instability after THA (Fig. 4). Rates of dislocation for primary arthroplasties range from 1% to 4%; revision rates are much higher, with various studies reporting rates between 5% and 30%. Causes are multifactorial. The most significant is previous hip surgery. Other causes are a posterolateral approach, impingement of components and retained osteophytes, component design, inadequate soft tissue tension, weakness of the abductor mechanism, and patient noncompliance. Most dislocations are caused by component malposition, occurring more often in female patients. There is no

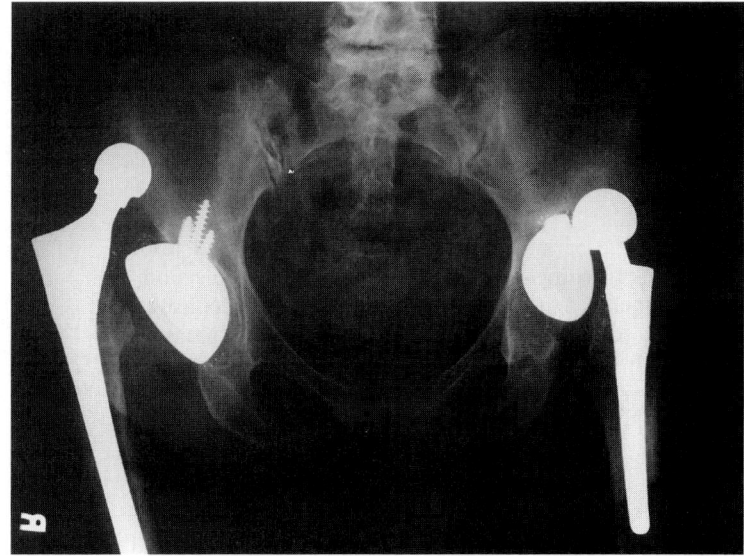

Fig. 4 Prostheses. This shows bilateral dislocation of hip prostheses. The left prosthesis dislocated secondary to aseptic loosening of the cup. The right prosthesis dislocated secondary to malposition of the acetabular component.

correlation with age, height, or weight for postoperative dislocations.

To avoid postoperative dislocations there are a few precautions. In the postoperative period, regardless of surgical approach, patients have a "safe zone" for hip motion. Motion beyond 60 degrees of flexion, less than 10 degrees of abduction, and any internal or external rotation should be avoided. A simple method for educating patients involves instructions to avoid reaching the palm of the hand beyond the knee (to avoid flexion), avoid reaching the palm across the contralateral shoulder (to avoid twisting), to keep a pillow between the knees for 6 weeks (to avoid adduction), and finally to keep the toes pointing straight (to avoid rotation). Arthroplasties usually dislocate within the first year after surgery, but late dislocations have been reported and result more often in patients with recurrent dislocations.

Dislocations are evaluated clinically, radiographically, and by history. Usually the patient gives a history of hip flexion followed by an audible and perceived "clunk" and severe pain at the hip. The leg is shortened and malrotated and the patient is unable to ambulate. The rotation of the femur is indicated by the position of the lesser trochanter and shows an anterior or posterior dislocation.

The initial management of dislocation is closed reduction. After the procedure a hip abduction brace is required for at least 6 weeks. Physical therapy and occupational therapy are needed to evaluate and reeducate the patient regarding hip precautions. In cases of soft-tissue interposition or recurrent dislocation an open reduction has to be performed. Often it requires repositioning of the acetabular component or trochanter advancement. In patients with recurrent dislocations a constrained acetabular component may be required.

Daly and Morrey[29] concluded that the results of operative treatment of an unstable THA can be optimized when a precise determination of the cause of the instability is made and appropriate measures are applied. Chronic dislocations warrant surgical intervention, but success in obtaining a stable construct is only 70%.

NEUROVASCULAR INJURIES

Although neurovascular injuries are uncommon in THA, the complications are devastating.[30-33] The most important factor in avoiding neurovascular injuries and their significant complications is a sound knowledge of hip anatomy.

Nerves can be damaged by direct trauma, traction, leg lengthening, or injury from heat of polymerization of polymethyl methacrylate during surgery. Postoperatively, the nerves can be damaged from compression by a hematoma, dislocation of the hip, or direct compression at the femoral head. Injuries to the sciatic nerve are most common. Other injuries are to the femoral and obturator nerves. The incidence of nerve palsy has been reported to range from 0% to 3.5% after primary hip arthroplasty and up to 7.6% after revision hip replacement.

The most common cause of nerve injury after THA is stretching due to leg lengthening or retraction. Overlengthening of the leg should be avoided. Edwards et al[30] reported that the amount of lengthening correlates with sciatic nerve damage. Injury to the peroneal branch occurred with lengthenings of 1.9 to 3.7 cm and complete sciatic nerve palsy with lengthenings of 4 cm and more. In revision surgery, somatosensory-evoked potentials have been used successfully to monitor sciatic nerve function. In difficult cases the sciatic nerve should be exposed and protected.

If nerve palsy occurs, an accurate diagnosis of the cause has to be established. Wound hematomas should be evacuated, bone cement in the area of the injured nerve removed, and after leg lengthening, the knee flexed to take tension off the sciatic nerve. The prognosis of partial nerve palsies is better than that of complete palsies. Patients who retain motor function after surgery have a better prognosis. The recovery of mild nerve injuries can take days to weeks. In severe cases recovery may not or just partially occur and can take 12 to 24 months.

The incidence of vascular injuries after THA is rare and has been reported in the range of 0.1% to 0.3%.[34] Most injuries occur in revision surgery. The causes are similar to those for nerve injuries. More common are vascular injuries after drilling of transacetabular screws for uncemented acetabular components. Screws should be placed only in the posterior quadrants of the acetabulum. If screws are placed in the anterior quadrants, injury to the external iliac vessels can occur. Other precautions are avoiding long and sharp retractors, and positioning refractors carefully and against bone.

The source of intraoperative bleeding must be identified. Excessive bleeding may require an additional incision or retroperitoneal exposure. If bleeding occurs uncontrollably from retroperitoneal sources at the sciatic notch, an arteriogram and embolization should be completed. Bleeding of the iliac vessels should be temporarily clamped to prevent additional blood loss and a vascular surgeon should be called.

LIMB LENGTH INEQUALITY

To remain or achieve equal limb length, accurate preoperative planning and templating are necessary. It is not always possible to equalize preexisting shortening in cases of hip dysplasia and revision arthroplasty. Overlengthening may result in neural injuries. This fact should be explained to the patient before surgery. In primary hip arthroplasty incorrect templating or positioning of the components and insufficient resection of bone from the femoral neck can result in lengthening of the leg. Patients are likely to be bothered by leg length inequality of more than 1 cm. This is one of the most common reasons for lawsuits against orthopaedic surgeons in the United States. This problem can be avoided by exact length measurements intraoperatively, utilizing a fixed point of reference at the iliac wing and marking the greater trochanter prior to the dislocation, then exactly measuring leg length differences before the components are implanted.

KNEE ARTHROPLASTY

PERIPROSTHETIC FRACTURES

Supracondylar fractures of the femur represent the most common type of periprosthetic fracture after TKA (Table 3). Hirsh et al[35] reported that an average of 3 to 4 years lapsed between the TKA and the fracture. Risk factors include osteopenia, neurological disorders, notching of the anterior femoral cortex at the time of surgery, rheumatoid arthritis, steroid therapy, and revision TKA. It has also been found that osteolysis, defined as inflammatory bone resorption caused by prosthetic wear debris, can lead to significant bone loss with subsequent fracture. Patients usually give a history of stumbling followed by hyperflexion of the knee. Severe pain, inability to ambulate, and obvious deformity of the femur are usually present. A complete radiographic series must be obtained, to include the entire length of the femur and tibia, to assess the length of the fracture and associated pathological changes.

These fractures present with an extremely wide range of fracture patterns. There is no standard classification currently reported in the orthopaedic literature. Treatment usually is based on the amount of comminution and the quality of bone adjacent to the implant. If the implant is loose at the bone-implant interface, immediate revision arthroplasty should be performed. Many treatment options are

TABLE 3. MANAGEMENT OF COMPLICATIONS AFTER TOTAL KNEE ARTHROPLASTIES

Complication	Conservative Treatment	Operative Treatment
Periprosthetic fracture	Traction, non-weight-bearing	Open reduction and internal fixation
Patellar mal-tracking	None	Revision total knee arthroplasty
Patellar instability	None	Revision total knee arthroplasty
Patellar clunk	None	Open or arthroscopic débridement of soft tissue around the patella

available, but closed treatment is usually reserved for minimally displaced fractures. Culp et al[17] discourage the use of closed methods because, in their study, treatment with traction and casts was followed by nonunion in 20%, malunion in 23%, and substantial decrease in range of motion.

Treatment innovations involve the insertion of intramedullary devices through the implant via a relatively small surgical incision while avoiding extensive periosteal stripping. Union rates, as well as postoperative function, have been improved with this technique. Intramedullary retrograde nails can be inserted through relatively small surgical incisions by splitting the patellar tendon and inserting the nail (Fig. 5B). One series of periprosthetic supracondylar femur fractures[36] treated with a titanium supracondylar retrograde nail showed promising results, with all cases going on to union with minimal deformity and loss of function. In this patient population, minimally invasive procedures are associated with less perioperative and intraoperative morbidity.

PATELLOFEMORAL COMPLICATIONS

Patellofemoral complications have been reported as the most common reason for revision knee arthroplasty and have accounted for up to 50% of reoperations.[37] They include patellofemoral maltracking and instability, patellar fracture, patellar clunk syndrome, tendon rupture, and patellar component failure.[38–44]

Patellofemoral maltracking may result in anterior knee pain, crepitus, excessive polyethylene wear, and patellar component failure. It is caused by several factors, including extensor mechanism imbalance[44] with a tight lateral retinaculum, a preexisting valgus angulation of the knee, malposition of the components (Fig. 6), and asymmetric patellar resection. Internal rotation of the tibial and femoral components and lateralization of the patellar component may lead to lateral subluxation of the patella. To avoid patellofemoral instability intraoperative evaluation of patellar tracking is essential. If the patella has the tendency to subluxate laterally with knee flexion, the component position should be carefully assessed to avoid internal rotation of the tibia and femur. Depending on the cause, in more severe cases a tibial tubercle transposition or an implant revision is considered.

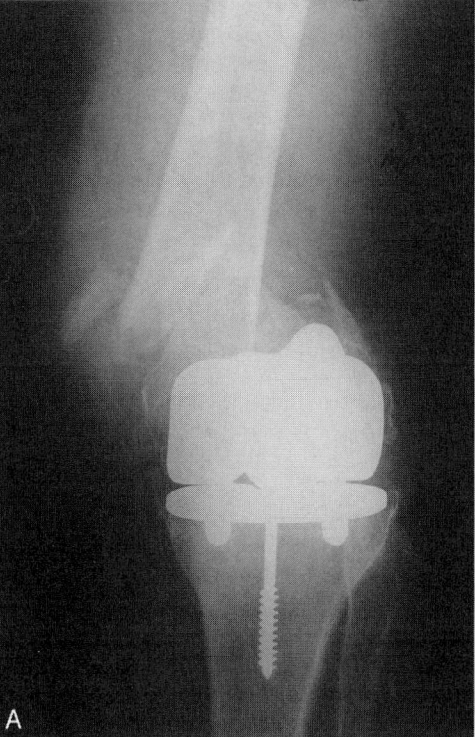
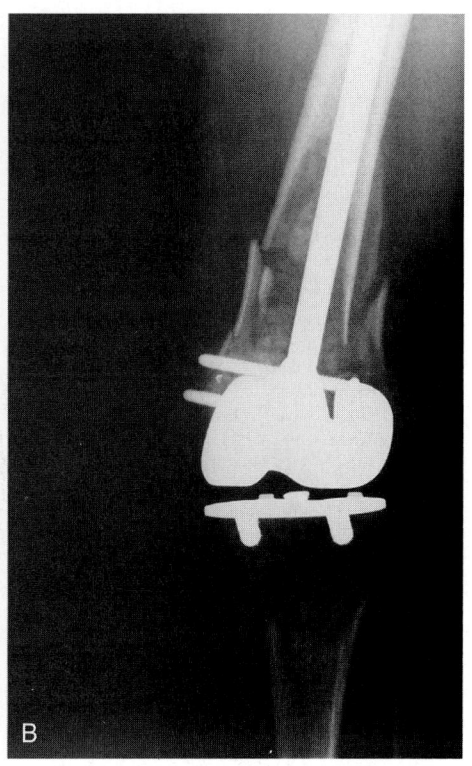

Fig. 5 Fracture. *A*, Periprosthetic femoral fracture above a left knee prosthesis. *B*, The fracture was managed with retrograde intramedullary nailing.

Patella fractures are not uncommon after TKA[41] and can be caused by a number of factors, including excessive resection of the patella, vascular compromise associated with lateral release, and patellar instability secondary to component malrotation. The surgeon should preserve as much of the blood supply to the patella as possible. If a lateral retinacular release is necessary, the superior lateral geniculate artery should be avoided. Poor results of surgical treatment of patellar fractures after TKA have been reported. In nondisplaced fractures conservative treatment is recommended. Displaced fractures may require patellectomy.

In patellar clunk syndrome,[38] a fibrous hypertrophic nodule develops at the posterior aspect of the quadriceps tendon just above the proximal pole of the patella. This nodule can become entrapped in the intercondylar notch of the femoral component. It causes a "clunk" at 30 to 45 degrees of flexion. The treatment is débridement of the fibrous nodule, which can be performed open or arthroscopically.

Rupture of the patellar or quadriceps tendon after TKA is a rare but severe complication. Quadriceps tendon rupture is often associated with a lateral retinacular release because of tendon weakening and devascularization. Patellar tendon ruptures occur often in knees that have undergone prior surgery. Several techniques of repair and augmentation and grafting are described but the results are poor. Often substantial extensor lags and limited knee motion occur. Most common techniques include hamstring augmentation and more recently bone-tendon allograft for augmentation of the extensor mechanism.

NEUROVASCULAR INJURIES

Peroneal nerve palsy is the only common nerve injury after TKA. It is caused by lateral retractors placed at the fibular head but more often by stretching of the nerve in cases with valgus deformity and flexion contracture. This appears in knees with rheumatoid arthritis and can be avoided by

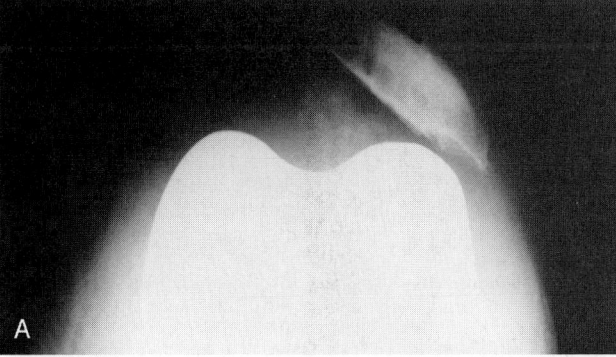
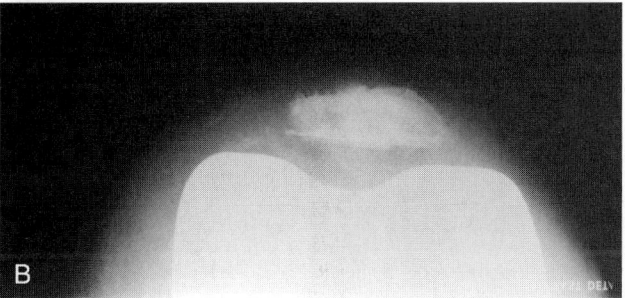

Fig. 6 Tibial component. *A*, Patellar instability secondary to malpositioned tibial component of a knee arthroplasty. *B*, Revision and correct placement of the tibial component restore patellar stability.

exploration of the nerve prior to the procedure. Incomplete peroneal nerve palsy recovers more often than complete peroneal nerve palsy. In cases where the palsy continues for more than 1 year, surgical exploration at the fibular head should be considered.

Arterial thromboembolism after TKA is rare and often associated with peripheral vascular disease. The complication is devastating and frequently results in amputation. In cases with peripheral vascular disease, use of a tourniquet should be avoided. Preoperative arterial Doppler testing and consultation with a vascular surgeon should be obtained.

REFERENCES

1. Eketund A, Rydell N, Nilsson OS: Total hip arthroplasty in patients 80 years of age and older. Clin Orthop 1992; 281:101.
2. Hube RF, Cohen PZ, Sotereanos NG, et al: Postoperative complications of lower extremity surgical procedures in older patients. TEM 1998; 20:55.
3. Seagroatt V, Tan HS, Goldacre M: Elective total hip replacement: Incidence, emergency readmission rate and postoperative mortality. BMJ 1991; 303:1431.
4. Zuckermann JD, Skovron ML, Koval KJ, et al: Postoperative complications and mortality associated with operative delay in older patients who have a fracture of the hip. J Bone Joint Surg Am 1995; 77: 1551.
5. McNally MA, Mollan RAB: Venous thromboembolism and orthopaedic surgery. J Bone Joint Surg Br 1993; 75:517.
6. Leutz DW, Stauffer ES: Color duplex Doppler ultrasound scanning for detection of deep venous thrombosis in total hip and knee arthroplasty patients. Incidence, location and accuracy compared with ascending venography. J Arthroplasty 1994; 9: 543.
7. Woolson ST, McCrory DW, Walter JF, et al: B-mode ultrasound scanning in the detection of proximal venous thrombosis after total hip replacement. J Bone Joint Surg Am 1990; 72:983.
8. Froehlich JA, Dorfman GS, Cronan JJ, et al: Comparison ultrasonography for the detection of deep venous thrombosis in patients who have a fracture of the hip. A prospective study. J Bone Joint Surg Am 1989; 71:249.
9. Garino JP, Lotke PA, Kitziger KJ, et al: Deep venous thrombosis after total joint arthroplasty. The role of compression ultrasonography and the importance of the experience of the technician. J Bone Joint Surg Am 1996; 78:1359.
10. Borris LC, Christiansen HM, Lassen MR, et al: Comparison of real-time B-mode ultrasonography and bilateral ascending phlebography for detection of postoperative deep venous thrombosis following elective hip surgery: Thromb Haemost 1989; 61:363.
11. Comerota AJ, Katz ML, Greenwald LL, et al: Venous duplex imaging: Should it replace hemodynamic tests for deep venous thrombosis? J Vasc Surg 1990; 11:53.
12. Comerota AJ, Katz ML, Grossi RJ: The comparative value of noninvasive testing for diagnosis and surveillance of deep vein thrombosis. J Vasc Surg 1988; 7:40.
13. Wright DJ, Shepard AD, McPharlin M, et al: Pitfalls in lower extremity venous duplex scanning. J Vasc Surg 1990; 11:675.
14. Woolson ST, Pottorff GT: Venous ultrasonography in the detection of proximal vein thrombosis after total knee arthroplasty. Orthop Trans 1992; 16:115.
15. Smith TK: Nutrition: Its relationship to orthopaedic infections. Orthop Clin North Am 1991; 23:373.
16. Sotereanos NG, Hube RF, Cohen PZ, et al: Hip dislocations and periprosthetic fractures. TEM 1998; 20:63.
17. Culp RW, Schmidt RG, Hanks G, et al: Supracondylar fracture of the femur following prosthetic knee arthroplasty. Clin Orthop 1987; 222:212.
18. Kavanagh BF: Femoral fractures associated with total hip arthroplasty. Orthop Clin North Am 1992; 23:249.
19. Mallory TH, Engh CA: Femoral fractures during noncemented total hip arthroplasty. J Bone Joint Surg Am 1989; 71:1135.
20. Mallory TH, Klaus TJ, Vaughn BK: Intraoperative femoral fractures associated with cementless total hip arthroplasty. Orthopedics 1989; 12:213.
21. Thomas BJ: Heterotopic bone formation after total hip arthroplasty. Orthop Clin North Am 1992; 23:347.
22. Maloney WJ, Kzushell RJ, Jasty M, et al: Incidence of heterotopic ossification after total hip replacement: Effect of the type of fixation of the femoral component. J Bone Joint Surg Am 1991; 73:191.
23. Brooker AF, Bowerman JW, Robinson RA, et al: Ectopic ossification following total hip arthroplasty. J Bone Joint Surg Am 1973; 55:1629.
24. Kjaersgaard-Amundson P, Ritter MA: Short-term treatment with nonsteroidal anti-inflammatory medications to prevent heterotopic bone formation after total hip arthroplasty: A preliminary report. Clin Orthop 1992; 279:157.
25. Thomas BJ, Amstutz HC: Results of the administration of diphosphonate for the prevention of heterotopic ossification after total hip arthroplasty. J Bone Joint Surg Am 1985; 67:400.
26. Warren SB, Brooker AF Jr: Excision of heterotopic bone followed by irradiation after total hip arthroplasty. J Bone Joint Surg Am 1992; 74:201.
27. Healy WL, Lo TCM, DeSimone AA, et al: Single-dose irradiation for prevention of heterotopic ossification after total hip arthroplasty. A comparison of doses of five hundred and seven hundred centigray. J Bone Joint Surg Am 1995; 77:590.
28. Hedley AK, Mead LP, Hencren DH: The prevention of heterotopic bone formation following total hip arthroplasty using 600 rad in a single dose. J Arthroplasty 1989; 4:319.
29. Daly PJ, Morrey BF: Incorporated operative correction of an unstable total hip arthroplasty. J Bone Joint Surg Am 1992; 74:1334.
30. Edwards BN, Tullos HS, Noble PC: Contributory factors and etiology of sciatic nerve palsy in total hip arthroplasty. Clin Orthop 1987; 218:136.
31. Johanson NA, Pellici PM, Tsairis P, et al: Nerve injury in total hip arthroplasty. Clin Orthop 1983; 175:214.
32. Schmalzried T, Amstutz HC, Dorey FJ: Nerve palsy associated with total hip replacement. J Bone Joint Surg Am 1991; 73:1074.
33. Wasielewski RC, Crosset LS, Rubash HE: Neural and vascular injury in total hip arthroplasty. Orthop Clin North Am 1992; 23:219.
34. Nachbur B, Meyer RP, Verkkala K, et al: The mechanism of severe arterial injury in surgery of the hip joint. Clin Orthop 1979; 141:122.
35. Hirsh DM, Bhalla S, Roffman M: Supracondylar fracture of the femur following total knee replacement: Report of four cases. J Bone Joint Surg Am 1981; 63: 162.
36. Hanks GA, Matthews HH, Routson GW, et al: Supracondylar fracture of the femur following total knee arthroplasty. J Arthroplasty 1989; 4:289.
37. Dennis DA: Patellofemoral complications in total knee arthroplasty: A literature review. Am J Knee Surg 1992; 5:156.
38. Beight JL, Yao B, Hozack WJ, et al: The patellar "clunk" syndrome after posterior stabilized total knee arthroplasty. Clin Orthop 1994; 299:139.
39. Boyd AD Jr, Ewald FC, Thomas WH, et al: Long-term complications after total knee arthroplasty with or without resurfacing of the patella. J Bone Joint Surg Am 1993; 75:674.
40. Brick GW, Scott RD: The patellofemoral component of total knee arthroplasty. Clin Orthop 1988; 231:160.
41. Hozak WJ, Goll SR, Lotke PA: The treatment of patellar fractures after total knee arthroplasty. Clin Orthop 1988; 236:123.
42. Kirk P, Rorabeck CH, Bourne RP: Management of recurrent dislocation of the patella following total knee arthroplasty. J Arthroplasty 1992; 7:229.
43. Leblanc J: Patella complications in total knee arthroplasty. Orthop Rev 1989; 3: 296.
44. Lynch AF, Rorabock CK, Bourne RB: Extensor mechanism complications following total knee arthroplasty. J Arthroplasty 1987; 2:135.

PARTICULATE DISEASE

Stuart B. Goodman

Summary
- All joint replacement implants generate wear debris.
- The wear particles stimulate a process that leads to osteoclast-mediated bone resorption, known as *osteolysis.*
- Osteolysis is often silent and requires frequent follow-up.
- Treatment usually requires thorough surgical débridement accompanied by revision of worn components and appropriate bone grafting.

DEFINITIONS

Particulate disease is a term that is used to describe the adverse clinical and radiographic manifestations of excessive wear debris from joint replacement arthroplasties.[1] Particulate disease is commonly associated with *periprosthetic osteolysis,* which is the pathological destruction of bone ascribed to the biologic reaction to wear debris (Fig. 1).[2-7]

HISTORICAL REVIEW

Particulate disease is not a recent phenomenon. Sir John Charnley[8] first noted rapid wearing of the plastic acetabular component that used bearing surfaces composed of polytetrafluoroethylene and stainless steel. Early loosening and progressive periprosthetic bone resorption, frequently after only a few years of use, lead to the abandonment of this coupling, and the use of polyethylene as one of the articulating materials. Willert and Semlitsch[9] underlined the importance of the foreign body and chronic inflammatory reaction to wear particles in the etiology of loosening and osteolysis, and postulated some of the early biological processes and cellular interactions. Numerous histological descriptions of retrieved periprosthetic tissue interfaces were forthcoming. For example, Goldring and associates[10] first likened the interface surrounding loose cemented implants to rheumatoid synovium ("pseudosynovium"). They employed the methods of cell biology to demonstrate greater production of prostanoids, cytokines, and metalloproteinases by the pseudomembrane and related these factors to periprosthetic bone resorption. In vivo, in vitro, and human retrieval studies have subsequently shown that particles of different materials activate a cascade of pro- and anti-inflammatory mediators that modulate a variety of cellular processes at the prosthetic interface.[11-25] What Jones and Hungerford[26] originally thought to be "cement disease" has now become known as *particulate disease,* in recognition that all types of wear particles may potentially participate in this adverse biological reaction.

EPIDEMIOLOGY

All implants used for joint replacement generate wear debris. Wear debris is formed at normally functioning total joint articulations (such as with the ball and socket of a hip replacement), at modular interfaces (such as at the junction of the femoral trunion and ball, or polyethylene insert and metallic backing), during third body wear (when bone particles or debris become interposed within the joint articulation), at areas of impingement (such as when the femoral neck impinges on the acetabular cup at extremes of motion), and at nonarticulating interfaces as a result of abrasion with the surrounding bone or debris.[27]

Prosthetic wear, particulate disease, and osteolysis are more common with cementless implants than cemented ones, and with modular rather than monoblock components.[1]

ETIOLOGY, PATHOGENESIS, AND PATHOLOGY

The following factors (list based on the work of Albrektsson and Albrektsson[28]) determine the interface surrounding a joint replacement:

- The design, material properties, topography, and other surface characteristics of the implant.
- The presence of voids and gaps.
- The initial implant stability and subsequent parameters of mechanical loading.
- Local biological stimuli, such as coatings and growth factors.
- The vascularity and viability of the prosthetic bed.
- Constitutional factors, including the general health and metabolic state of the host.

Surgical factors are of paramount importance in determining the interface characteristics and the eventual clinical outcome of the implant.

Mechanically loose implants are surrounded by a thick fibrous tissue layer. In some cases, a synovial-like layer is present at the bone-implant interface. As loosening progresses and larger prosthetic displacements occur, the fibrous membrane thickens. A thin bony encapsulation may surround the fibrous tissue layer. Motion at the articulating and nonarticulating surfaces produces wear debris, which accumulates locally within the tissues and especially within macrophages. This accumulation begins a series of events that results in osteolysis, the destruction of bone in the prosthetic bed.

Osteolysis results from increased local synthesis of bone-resorbing factors by activated macrophages, fibroblasts, osteoblasts, and other cells. Particles are phagocytosed but

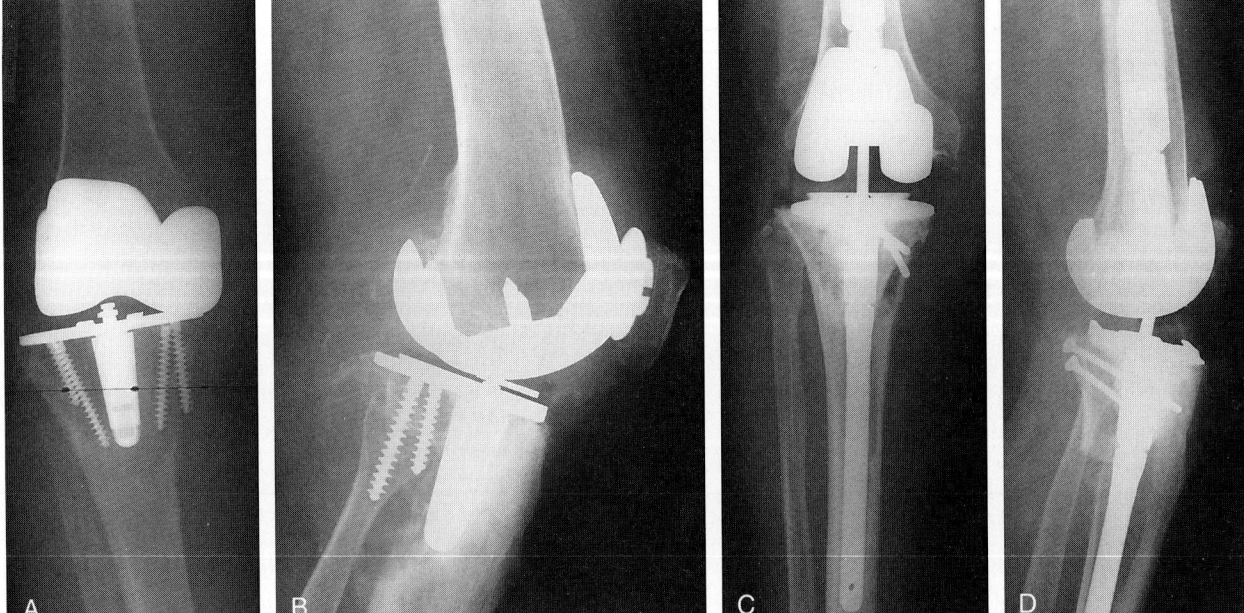

Fig. 1. Total knee replacement with severe osteolysis. *A,* Anteroposterior radiograph of a cementless total knee replacement demonstrating varus deformity with subluxation, and complete wear-through of the polyethylene liner with metal-on-metal articulation. Note the large area of osteolysis around the tibial component, especially around the stem and screws. *B,* Lateral radiograph of this cementless total knee replacement. The polyethylene of the metal-backed patellar component has worn. There is severe osteolysis, primarily involving the posterior half of the proximal tibia. The posterior metaphysis is severely eroded, and the posterior cortical outline is barely discernible. The tibial stem and screws have no supporting bone. A malignant tumor was suspected, and an initial biopsy of the tibia performed at another hospital showed a foreign body reaction to wear debris without malignant changes in the tissues. *C* and *D,* Postoperative anteroposterior (*C*) and lateral (*D*) radiographs of the revision total knee replacement. The knee has been revised with long-stem, cemented, more constrained tibial and femoral components (Zimmer-constrained Condylar Knee total knee replacement). The tibial foreign body granuloma has been excised, and the bony defect has been reconstructed with a cortical-cancellous tibial allograft, two cortical lag screws, and cancellous allograft bone impacted into the proximal tibial defect. The metaphyseal portions of each prosthesis are cemented in place, and the stems of the components are press-fit into the diaphysis. The patellar component has been excised; there was insufficient bone stock for a new patellar component.

are unable to be digested.[29] Through autocrine and paracrine signaling mechanisms, phagocytosed particles stimulate increased macrophage accumulation, proliferation, and the synthesis of bone-resorbing factors. In conjunction with osteoblasts, fibroblasts, osteoclasts, and other cells, bone-resorbing factors such as prostaglandin E_2, cytokines and growth factors such as interleukin-1, interleukin-6, tumor necrosis factor, and platelet-derived growth factor, metallo-proteinases, lysosomal enzymes, chemokines, and other factors are released locally into the interfacial tissues and synovial fluid interface.[11–25] These substances stimulate the differentiation, maturation, and activation of osteoclasts, producing localized bone resorption. Particles also interfere with osteoblast function, thus affecting both bone formation and degradation.[30–31]

The indigestible particles are eventually egested and recirculated. Particles migrate throughout the interface, through non-osseointegrated areas and gaps, and into the cancellous bone.[32] The normal gait cycle produces waxing and waning periods of greater intra-articular pressure, which may serve as a pumping mechanism for the movement of particles around the prosthesis into the effective joint space.[33] Increased local bone resorption and decreased bone formation undermine the bony support of the prosthesis.

The primary reaction to particulate debris is a nonspecific foreign body–type reaction, composed of sheets of macrophages, foreign body giant cells, and other cells containing phagocytosed particles in a fibrous tissue stroma (Fig. 2). In some patients, however, there may be an immune reaction to the particle-protein complex.[34] One study suggested that severe, progressive osteolysis may be due to an uncoupling of the events encompassing the foreign body response and reactive fibrosis, resulting in an aggressive granulomatous reaction due to activated fibroblasts and macrophages.[35]

CLINICAL INVESTIGATION

Osteolysis secondary to particle disease is usually associated with excessive prosthetic wear. If the diagnosis is obvious, the lesion should be defined radiographically, and treatment instituted. In this regard, simple radiographic evaluations, such as oblique radiographs and computed tomography, may be useful.

Further investigations may be necessary to rule out other specific diagnoses. These tests may include measurements of the erythrocyte sedimentation rate (ESR) and C-reactive protein (CRP), complete blood count, blood tests (measurements of calcium, phosphorus, and alkaline phosphatase; serum protein electrophoresis), white blood cell scan, and specific metabolic and rheumatological tests. Aspiration arthrogram (with or without dye injection and infusion of local anesthetic) may be useful in further defining pros-

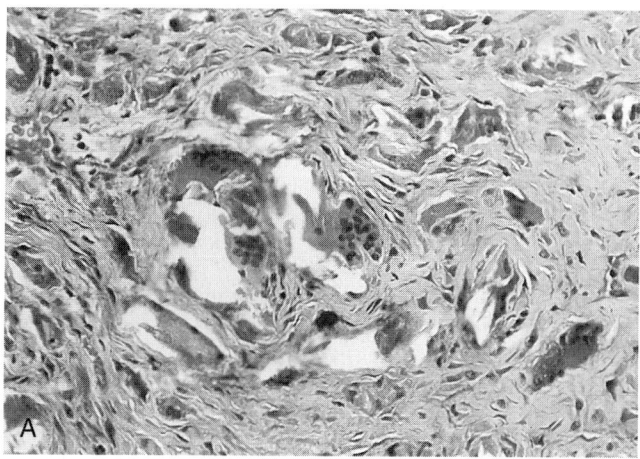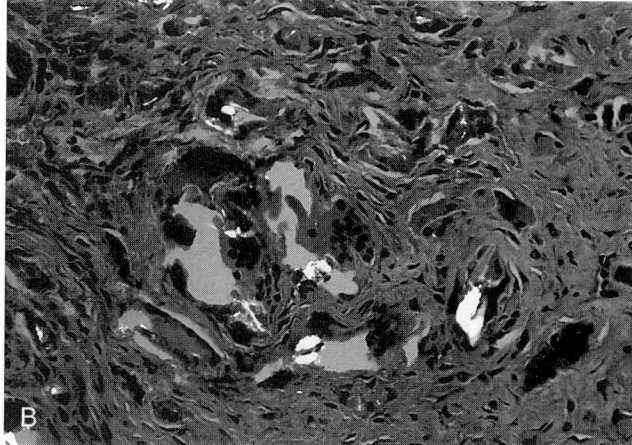

Fig. 2. Histology of tissue retrieval from a loose hip replacement. *A,* This tissue, harvested from a loose cemented hip replacement, demonstrates mono- and multinucleated foreign body cell and chronic inflammatory cells in a fibrovascular stroma. *B,* When polarized light is employed, birefringent polyethylene particles are seen adjacent to and within some of the foreign body cells.

thetic loosening and the joint as the pain generator, respectively. Culture of the joint fluid may reveal infection of the prosthesis. Biopsy and pathological examination of a suspicious lesion may also be necessary prior to definitive treatment.

DIFFERENTIAL DIAGNOSIS

The differential diagnosis of particle-induced osteolysis includes the following conditions:

- Mechanical loosening of the prosthesis.
- Polyethylene wear without component loosening.
- Periprosthetic radiographic changes associated with bone remodeling (e.g., "stress shielding").
- Prosthetic infection.
- Metabolic disorders, such as hyperparathyroidism.
- Bone resorption associated with a rheumatic disorder.
- Primary and metastatic bone and soft tissue tumors.

Simple mechanical loosening is usually associated with linear osteolysis, that is, slowly progressive, thin radiolucent lines of about 2 mm in thickness surrounding a loose prosthesis. The clinician searches for these radiolucent lines when assessing the stability of a total joint replacement. Particle disease is associated with progressive ballooning and scalloping in the bone surrounding a prosthesis. These areas are wider than 2 mm and balloon out from the prosthesis, eroding both cancellous and cortical bone. Significant wear of the components is usually apparent and may occur in the absence of mechanical loosening. In addition, progressive osteolysis may result in component loosening.

Bone remodeling changes, generally seen proximally around femoral stems, result in osteopenia and cortical rounding rather than scalloping of the calcar region and adjacent bone. Distal cortical thickening may also be present. Prosthesis wear is generally absent. Infection of a total joint replacement (TJR) is commonly painful with range of motion and may be associated with systemic

symptoms, abnormal laboratory as well as (ESR, CRP) radiographic (rapid osteolysis without prosthetic wear, periosteal new bone formation, abnormal white blood cell scan) findings. A positive bacterial culture after joint aspiration is diagnostic. Metabolic and rheumatological disorders, such as hyperparathyroidism, gout, and rheumatoid arthritis, are diagnosed from appropriate findings on history physical examination and laboratory evaluation. The diagnosis of a bone tumor around a joint prosthesis is extremely difficult but usually the tumor is not associated with prosthetic wear and must be confirmed by biopsy and histopathological examination.

MANAGEMENT

Management of particulate disease and osteolysis consists of (1) continued observation and conservative measures, (2) pharmacological therapy, and (3) surgical procedures.

OBSERVATION AND CONSERVATIVE MEASURES

Clinical observation and documentation of the radiographic progression of prosthetic loosening, wear, and osteolysis are the cornerstones of the early treatment of particulate disease. Clinical and radiographic observations should be stepped up from yearly follow-up to more frequent evaluations. Patients should be informed about the condition and appropriately counseled about weight loss, activity restriction, the use of walking aids, and the importance of continued, regular follow-up.

PHARMACOLOGICAL THERAPY

Pharmacological therapy for particulate disease is controversial. The use of analgesics and nonsteroidal anti-inflammatory drugs (NSAIDs) may be indicated to control pain and inflammation in the more advanced stages of loosening and osteolysis in patients who are not candidates for surgery. NSAIDs also have theoretical advantages in that they decrease synthesis of prostaglandin E_2 and proinflammatory cytokines. Animal studies involving the use of oral bis-phosphonates (which reduce osteoclast-mediated bone resorption) are encouraging, and clinical trials are ongoing.[36] Targeted pharmacological therapy, such as the use of specific cytokine inhibitors or receptor antagonists, is enticing; however, the plethora and redundancy of participating cytokines and factors in the proinflammatory cascade may make this approach extremely difficult.

SURGICAL PROCEDURES

- Débridement, synovectomy.
- Replacement of worn component(s).
- Replacement of entire prosthesis.
- Bone grafting of defects (autograft, allograft, synthetic bone substitutes).
- Special implants (e.g., eccentric acetabular cups, tibial and femoral wedges).
- Fixation of fractures.

Any surgical procedure for particulate disease should be accompanied by débridement of the soft tissues and bone, and a complete synovectomy should be performed. Bone ingrowth is impeded by residual particulate debris and granuloma. Therefore, eradication of the remnants of the foreign body and the chronic inflammatory reaction to particles is necessary to optimize the outcome of the new reconstruction.

Particulate disease is secondary to prosthetic wear. Worn components should be replaced, and predisposing factors, such as suboptimal implant materials, prosthetic design issues, and malalignment, should be addressed. This may entail replacement of some or all of the prosthetic components. Special or custom implants may be needed for reconstruction. Whether cemented or cementless components should be used is controversial and should be determined by the surgeon's preference and expertise. Pathological fractures secondary to osteolysis should be fixed (in addition to the previously described prosthesis issues), so that early motion and return to function can be instituted. Bone grafting is usually necessary, although small defects may be filled with polymethylmethacrylate when cemented implants are used. Autografts, allografts, and specialized techniques such as cancellous impaction grafting are employed to reconstitute larger bone defects. Contained defects are easier to reconstruct; very large, noncontained defects may require strut grafts or structural allografts.

COMPLICATIONS

Complications from particulate disease may be local or systemic.

LOCAL COMPLICATIONS

- Symptoms of chronic synovitis without bone destruction.
- Asymptomatic destruction of bone without evidence of prosthetic loosening.
- Symptomatic destruction of bone without prosthetic loosening.
- Destruction of bone with prosthetic loosening.
- Pathological fracture.

- Prosthetic fracture.
- Malignant degeneration of periprosthetic tissues (controversial).

Particulate disease is generally silent. In other words, while progressive wear of the components and bone destruction proceed, there are usually no clinical symptoms. Synovitis and pain may occur with more advanced component wear, and high-pitched "squeaky" sounds indicate complete wear-through of the polyethylene, resulting in metal-on-metal articulation. Progressive deformity, especially in the knee, may indicate eccentric polyethylene wear. If the prosthesis bed is sufficiently undermined, loosening of the component may ensue. Pathological bone fracture and prosthesis fracture are relatively uncommon and are usually accompanied by increasing pain. Whether malignant degeneration of the periprosthetic tissues can occur secondary to excessive wear and particulate disease is controversial.

SYSTEMIC COMPLICATIONS

- Increased levels of wear debris byproducts in body fluids and remote organs, without symptoms.
- Increased levels of wear debris byproducts in body fluids and remote organs, with symptoms.

Wear particles and byproducts are stored locally in the periarticular tissues and systematically, generally in the reticuloendothelial system. Some byproducts are excreted in the urine and elsewhere. Increased levels of some of metallic alloys and byproducts have been found in the blood, urine, and other organs, but the clinical significance of these findings is unknown. One of my patients with bilateral loose, cemented cobalt chrome alloy and polyethylene components had systemic signs, including fever of unknown origin and inguinal lymphadenopathy, which abated after bilateral cementless revision procedures were performed.

RESULTS

Despite the rising incidence rate of particulate disease, few reports on the outcome of revisions specifically for this phenomenon have been presented.[1, 2, 37–46] Indeed, such cases are usually grouped with revisions for mechanical loosening without osteolysis, thus confounding the data.

The results for revision cases associated with osteolysis depend on (1) the size and location of the bone defects and (2) the type of prosthesis currently in situ. Irrespective of whether hip or knee replacements are considered, the best results are obtained for cases that are diagnosed and treated early in the disease, when bone defects are small and easily replenished. Higher complication rates and poorer clinical outcomes are reported with extensive bone grafting procedures, especially the use of large bulk allografts, and larger, more constrained prostheses.

With the advent of newer, more wear-resistant materials, better prosthetic designs and instrumentation, improved surgical technique, and pharmacological manipulation of the prosthetic interface, it is hoped that revisions for particulate disease will decrease in number and extent.

REFERENCES

1. Wright TM, Goodman SB: Implant Wear: The Future of Total Joint Replacement. Rosemont, IL, American Academy of Orthopaedic Surgeons, 1996.

2. Anthony PP, Gie GA, Howie CR, et al: Localized endosteal bone lysis in relation to the femoral components of cemented total hip arthroplasties. J Bone Joint Surg Br 1990; 72:971.

3. Maloney WJ, Jasty M, Harris WH, et al: Endosteal erosion in association with stable uncemented femoral components. J Bone Joint Surg Am 1990; 72:1026.

4. Maloney WJ, Jasty M, Rosenberg A, et al: Bone lysis in well fixed cemented femoral components. J Bone Joint Surg Br 1990; 72:966.

5. Maloney WJ, Peters P, Engh CA, et al: Severe osteolysis of the pelvis in association with acetabular replacement without cement. J Bone Joint Surg Am 1993; 75:1627.

6. Maloney WJ, Smith RL: Periprosthetic osteolysis in total hip arthroplasty: The role of particulate wear debris. J Bone Joint Surg Am 1995; 75:1449.

7. Bell RS, Schatzker J, Fornasier VL, et al: Study of implant failure in the Wagner resurfacing arthroplasty. J Bone Joint Surg Am 1985; 67:1165.

8. Charnley J: Low Friction Arthroplasty of the Hip. New York, Springer-Verlag, 1979.

9. Willert HG, Semlitsch M: Reactions of the articular capsule to wear products of artificial joint prostheses. J Biomed Mater Res 1977; 11:157.

10. Goldring SR, Schiller AL, Roelke M, et al: The synovial-like membrane at the bone cement interface in loose total hip replacements and its proposed role in bone lysis. J Bone Joint Surg Am 1983; 65:575.

11. Chiba J, Rubash HE, Kim KJ, et al: The characterization of cytokines in the interface tissue from failed cementless total hip replacements with and without femoral osteolysis. Clin Orthop 1994; 300:304.

12. Glant TT, Jacobs JJ: Response to three murine macrophage populations to particulate debris: Bone resorption in organ cultures. J Orthop Res 1994; 12:720.

13. Goodman SH, Chin RC, Chiou SS, et al: A clinical-pathological-biochemical study of the membrane surrounding loosened and nonloosened joint arthroplasty. Clin Orthop 1989; 244:182.

14. Goodman SB, Huie P, Song Y, et al: Loosening and osteolysis of cemented joint arthroplasties: A biological spectrum. Clin Orthop 1997; 337:149.

15. Goodman SB, Huie P, Song Y, et al: Cellular profile and cytokine production at prosthetic interfaces. J Bone Joint Surg Br 1998; 80:531.

16. Goodman SB: The effects of micromotion and particulate materials on tissue differentiation: Bone chamber studies in rabbits. Acta Orthop Scand 1994; 65(Supp 258):1.

17. Jiranek WA, Machado M, Jasty M, et al: Production of cytokines around loosened cemented acetabular components: Analysis with immunohistochemical techniques and in situ hybridization. J Bone Joint Surg Am 1993; 75:863.

18. Kodaya Y, Revell PA, Al-Saffar N, et al: Bone formation and bone resorption in failed total joint replacements arthroplasties: Histomorphometric analysis with histochemical and immunohistochemical technique. J Orthop Res 1996; 14:473.

19. Murray DW, Rushton N: Macrophages stimulate bone resorption when they phagocytose particles. J Bone Joint Surg Br 1990; 72:988.

20. Pollice F, Silverton SF, Horowitz SM: Polymethytlmethacrylate-stimulated macrophages increase rat osteoclast precursor recruitment through their effect on osteoblasts in vitro. J Orthop Res 1995; 13:325.

21. Quinn J, Joyner C, Triffitt JT, et al: Polymethylmethacrylate-induced inflammatory macrophages resorb bone. J Bone Joint Surg Br 1992; 74:652.

22. Shanbhag AS, Jacobs JJ, Black J, et al: Macrophage/particle interactions: Effect of size, composition and surface area. J Biomed Mater Res 1994; 28:81.

23. Ohlin A, Johnell O, Lerner UH: The pathogenesis of loosening of total hip arthroplasties: The production of factors by periprosthetic tissues that stimulate in vitro bone resorption. Clin Orthop 1990; 253:287.

24. Shanbhag AS, Jacobs JJ, Black J, et al: Cellular mediators secreted by interfacial membranes obtained at revision total hip arthroplasty. J Arthroplasty 1995; 10:498.

25. Sabokbar A, Rushton N: Role of inflammatory mediators and adhesion molecules in the pathogenesis of aseptic loosening in total hip arthroplasties. J Arthroplasty 1995; 10:810.

26. Jones LC, Hungerford DS: Cement disease. Clin Orthop 1987; 225:193.

27. McKellop HA: Wear modes, mechanisms, damage, and debris: Separating cause from effect in the wear of total hip replacements. In Galante JO, Rosenberg AG, Callaghan JJ (eds): Total Hip Revision Surgery. New York, Raven Press, 1995, p 21.

28. Albrektsson T, Albrektsson B: Osseointegration of bone implants: A review of an alternative mode of fixation. Acta Orthop Scand 1987; 58:567.

29. Campbell P, Ma S, Yeom B, et al: Isolation of predominantly submicron-sized UHMWPE wear particles from periprosthetic tissues. J Biomed Mater Res 1995; 29:127.

30. Allen MJ, Myer BJ, Millet PJ, et al: The effects of particulate cobalt, chromium and cobalt-chromium alloy on human osteoblast-like cells in vitro. J Bone Joint Surg Br 1997; 79:475.

31. Yao J, Cs-Szabo G, Jacobs JJ, et al: Suppression of osteoblast function by titanium particles. J Bone Joint Surg Am 1997; 79:107.

32. Schmalzried TP, Kwong LM, Jasty M, et al: The mechanism of loosening of cemented acetabular components in total hip arthroplasty. Analysis of specimens retrieved at autopsy. Clin Orthop 1992; 274:60.

33. Schmalzried TP, Jasty M, Harris WH: Periprosthetic bone loss in total hip arthroplasty: Polyethylene wear debris and the concept of the effective joint space J Bone Joint Surg Am 1992; 74:849.

34. Hicks DG, Judkins AR, Sickel JZ, et al: Granular histiocytosis of pelvic lymph nodes following total hip arthroplasty: The presence of wear debris, cytokine production and immunologically activated macrophages. J Bone Joint Surg Am 1996; 78:482.

35. Santavirta S, Konttinen YT, Begroth V: Aggressive granulomatous lesions associated with hip arthroplasty: Immunopathological studies. J Bone Joint Surg Am 1990; 72:252.

36. Shanbhag AS, Hasselman CT, Rubash HE: Inhibition of wear debris mediated osteolysis in a canine total hip arthroplasty model. Clin Orthop 1998; 344:33.

37. Gie G, Linder L, Ling RSM, et al: Impaction cancellous allografts and cement for revision total hip arthroplasty. J Bone Joint Surg Br 1993; 75:14.

38. Knight JL, Gorai PA, Atwater RD, et al: Tibial polyethylene failure after primary porous-coated anatomic total knee arthroplasty. J Arthroplasty 1995; 10:748.

39. Peters PC Jr, Engh GA, Dwyer KA, et al: Osteolysis after total knee arthroplasty without cement. J Bone Joint Surg Am 1992; 74:864.

40. Kim Y-H, Oh J-H, Oh S-H: Osteolysis around cementless porous-coated anatomic knee prosthesis J Bone Joint Surg Br 1995; 77:236.

41. Cadambi A, Engh GA, Dwyer KA, et al: Osteolysis of the distal femur after total knee arthroplasty. J Arthroplasty 1994; 9:579.

42. Ezzet KA, Garcia R, Barrack RL: Effects of component fixation method on osteolysis in total knee arthroplasty. Clin Orthop 1995; 321:86.

43. Whiteside L: Effect of porous-coating configuration on tibial osteolysis after total knee arthroplasty. Clin Orthop 1995; 321:92.

44. Lewis PL, Rorabeck CH, Bourne RB: Screw osteolysis after cementless total knee replacement. Clin Orthop 1995; 321:173.

45. Robinson EJ, Mulliken BD, Bourne RB, et al: Catastrophic osteolysis in total knee replacement: A report of 17 cases. Clin Orthop 1995; 321:98.

46. Engh G, Parks NL, Ammeen DJ: Tibial osteolysis in cementless total knee arthroplasty: A review of 25 cases treated with and without tibial component revision. Clin Orthop 1994; 309:33.

MUSCULOSKELETAL TUMORS

DEMPSEY SPRINGFIELD

PATHOPHYSIOLOGY OF BONE TUMORS

Michael J. Klein

Summary
- The behavior of neoplasia of bone is reflected by its presentation.
- The patient's symptoms and the appearance of a lesion on a plain radiograph help the physician understand the tumor's behavior.
- An understanding of how to interpret these clues gives the physician a more thorough understanding of the patient's prognosis.
- The orthopaedic surgeon must work with the radiologist and pathologist to fully understand a neoplasia of bone.

The rarity of bone tumors and their location in sites that are externally invisible without imaging techniques present unique problems in their diagnosis and management. The incidence of primary malignant bone neoplasms (excluding myeloma) is approximately 1 case per 100,000 individuals per year.[1] True benign bone tumors occur at about half this frequency. Certain non-neoplastic space-occupying lesions of bone often grouped with neoplasms, such as nonossifying fibroma/fibrous cortical defect and osteochondroma, are much more common than bone tumors and are not included in these statistics. Because successful treatment of a disease depends on the collection of enough cases to demonstrate the response of that particular disorder to some standardized treatment, both the classification and treatment of bone tumors are still in the process of evolution.

CLASSIFYING TUMORS

Epithelial tumors (i.e., tumors of ectodermal or endodermal embryonic origin) are classified by deciding their site of origin and by observing their differentiation and growth characteristics. The type of extracellular connective tissue matrix produced by the neoplastic cells is also used to classify primary bone tumors (as it is in other tumors of mesodermal origin). In addition to its neoplastic cells, a tumor may form bone, cartilage, fibrous tissue, or other extracellular connective tissue elements, and there are benign and malignant variants of each type (Table 1). Certain types of primary bone tumors such as giant cell tumor and Ewing's sarcoma do not produce specific types of extracellular matrix and are of controversial origin. However, each of these tumor types is readily recognizable microscopically and therefore may be histologically classified.

Biologically, tumors are conventionally separated into benign and malignant types.

In the sense used in this chapter, a *benign* tumor is a space-occupying lesion that may cause morbidity in a patient, but if it is not located in a vital area, it will not ordinarily result in the death of the host if left untreated. Most tumors of bone classified as benign are indolent and quite self-limited. Other bone tumors considered benign may behave in a locally aggressive fashion. A *malignant* tumor is a space-occupying lesion that will almost invariably result in the death of the host if left untreated. Although the death of the host may result from local complications of a malignant tumor, death is more often a consequence of distant spread or *metastasis* of tumor cells to the lungs or to other vital organs.

TUMORS: BENIGN VERSUS MALIGNANT

Patients with bone tumors usually present with pain; however, they may present with a painful mass or even with a painless mass. The symptoms and signs depend on the indolence or aggressiveness of a tumor and its interaction with a given host. The most characteristic symptom associated with bone tumors is pain present at night. As this pain becomes more progressive, it is usually severe enough to wake patients from their sleep. In certain tumors, the onset and relief of pain is characteristic enough to make a specific diagnosis. For example, in osteoid osteoma, aspirin usually relieves the intense nocturnal pain associated with the tumor. This is believed to be related to the unique innervation of this lesion combined with its biosynthesis of prostaglandins.[2, 3]

Certain characteristics are so typically reproducible in benign and malignant tumors of bone that their identification enables physicians to infer their biological potential with great reproducibility. When a neoplasm grows within a bone, the tumor cells, the adjacent marrow, and the cancellous bone compete for the limited space that exists inside the surrounding compact bone envelope. Because this tissue is of limited compressibility, the intraosseous pressure may rise to a point where its vascular supply becomes compromised. Unless some intervening tissue is decompressed, osteonecrosis of the adjacent bone and necrosis of some of the tumor cells will be inevitable. The usual response by the adjoining normal bone associated with a benign tumor is increased host osteoclastic activity, which tends to remove the bone at its interface with the tumor; in these cases, spontaneous tumor necrosis and osteonecrosis are seldom a prominent feature. This will result in radiolucency if the area of bone resorption is sufficiently large. In rapidly growing malignant tumors, there is seldom control over the rate of intertrabecular spread of tumor; spontaneous tumor necrosis and irregular osteonecrosis are usual features, but there may be no discernible radiographic change. On the other hand, a tumor growing in bone may sometimes induce new bone at its periphery, causing radiodensity.

Differences in the response of the host bone to different kinds of tumor depend on the biology of the tumor and on the response idiosyncratic to the particular host. The overall pattern of host response can be used as a template to

TABLE 1. CLASSIFICATION OF BONE TUMORS

Tumors Forming Bone Matrix

Benign	Malignant	
Osteoid osteoma	Osteosarcoma (central)	Osteosarcoma (surface)
Osteoblastoma	Conventional	Parosteal
	Telangiectatic	Periosteal
	Small cell	Dedifferentiated
	Low grade	parosteal
	Gnathic	High-grade surface
	Secondary	

Tumors Forming Cartilage of Chondroid Matrix

Benign	Malignant
Osteochondroma	Chondrosarcoma
Enchondroma	Conventional
Periosteal Chondroma	Central
Chondroblastoma	Peripheral
Chondromyxoid Fibroma	Dedifferentiated
	Mesenchymal
	Clear cell

Tumors of Fibrous Origin

Benign	Malignant
Nonossifying fibroma	Fibrosarcoma
Desmoplastic fibroma	Malignant fibrous histiocytoma

Tumors of Marrow/Hematopoietic Origin

Benign	Malignant
	Lymphoma
	Plasma cell myeloma
	Granulocytic sarcoma

Tumors of Neural Elements

Benign	Malignant
Schwannoma	Malignant peripheral nerve sheath tumor
Neurofibroma	Primitive neuroectodermal tumor
	Metastatic neuroblastoma
	Ewing's sarcoma*

Tumors of Notochordal Elements

Benign	Malignant
Benign notochordal remnant	Chordoma

Vascular Tumors

Benign	Malignant
Hemangioma	Hemangioendothelioma
Epithelioid hemangioma	Epithelioid hemangioendothelioma
	Angiosarcoma
	Hemangiopericytoma

Epithelial Tumors

Benign	Malignant
	Adamantinoma
	Metastatic carcinoma

Muscle Tumors

Benign	Malignant
Leiomyoma	Leiomyosarcoma
Rhabdomyoma	Rhabdomyosarcoma

Adipose Tissue Tumors

Benign	Malignant
Lipoma	Liposarcoma

Tumors of Mixed Origin

Benign	Malignant
Benign mesenchymoma	Malignant mesenchymoma

Tumors of Unknown Origin

Benign	Malignant
Giant cell tumor	Malignant giant cell tumor

Tumor-Like Space-Occupying Lesions

Benign Bone	Benign Joint
Simple cyst	Pigmented villonodular synovitis
Aneurysmal bone cyst	Synovial chondromatosis

predict the biological behavior of any given tumor, but it must be kept in mind that characteristic radiographic findings are pictures that reflect statistical probabilities. Occasionally, a tumor that is radiologically benign proves to be malignant and vice versa. In the most slowly growing benign tumor, for example, the adjacent bone may actually wall off the tumor with a zone of reactive bone. This osseous shell, which is an attempt by the host bone to redistribute force, is best appreciated in weightbearing bones[4] both radiographically and histologically. This pattern of destruction is sometimes described as *marginated* (Fig. 1). In a faster-growing benign tumor, destruction of adjacent normal bone proceeds but without enough time or stimulus for reactive new bone formation. On a radiograph, the area between where the bone is radiographically normal and where it is obviously abnormal, or where the *transition zone* is narrow, and the lesion appears geographically circumscribed (Fig. 2A). A histological section corresponding to the edge of the lesion will reveal that it ends rather abruptly, with little or no extension into the marrow spaces between the normal osseous trabeculae surrounding the lesion (Fig. 2B).

Cytologically, the cells of a benign tumor are relatively uniform in comparison to one another, and the size and chromatin distribution of the tumor cell nuclei are similar

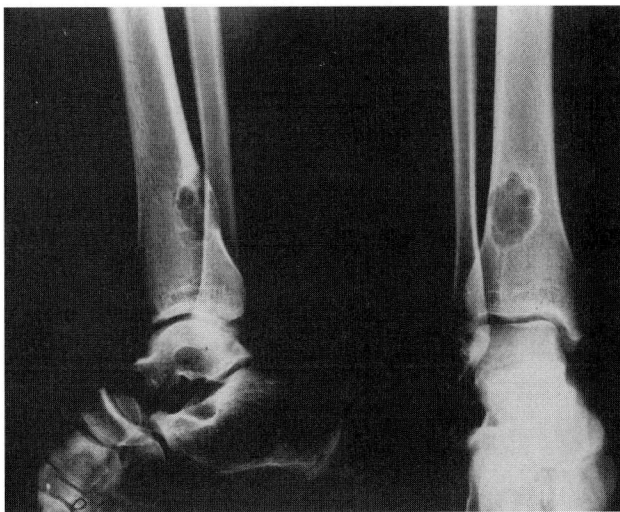

Fig. 1. Lesion. This shows a marginated, geographically circumscribed lesion in the metadiaphyseal region of the right tibia. Anteroposterior and lateral views of the right lower leg and foot of a 19-year-old male. Eccentric, intracortical, scalloped, sclerotic lesion is almost pathognomonic of nonossifying fibroma.

to those of normal-appearing cells in the same tissue. Mitotic divisions may be encountered in a benign tumor; however, the proliferation is orderly in that there is no significant degree of accompanying necrosis of tumor tissue, and the mitotic divisions are normal in configuration and usually low in absolute number.

In certain osseous tumors, the distinction between benign and malignant may be blurred. In giant cell tumor, for example, although the tumor is usually confined to one anatomic site and is considered benign, it is often locally aggressive. Even though the radiological transition zone may be relatively sharp, histological examination of the boundary between normal bone and tumor interface often demonstrates extension of tumor into the intertrabecular spaces of the adjacent osseous trabeculae (Fig. 3). Because these interosseous extensions are not always accessible to curettage, they may be responsible for the high frequency of local recurrence of giant cell tumor after simple curettage. Less frequently, a chondroblastoma may behave in a locally aggressive manner. Histologically, both giant cell tumor and chondroblastoma may show a significant degree of mitotic activity and, occasionally, atypical mitotic figures are identifiable in a benign giant cell tumor. Nuclear pleomorphism is not the norm in either tumor, and in the absence of fracture or matrix calcification, the degree of necrosis in both tumors is limited. Although considered benign, approximately 5% of giant cell tumors and 1% of chondroblastomas give rise to lung metastases. Which particular tumor will eventually metastasize is not predictable by studying the morphology of the primary neoplasm. When they do occur, these lung metastases are usually few in number, of limited growth potential, and do not usually result in the death of patients. For this reason, even when they metastasize, both tumors are regarded as benign. Even though frank vascular invasion may be seen in the soft tissues outside of a bone containing a giant cell tumor,

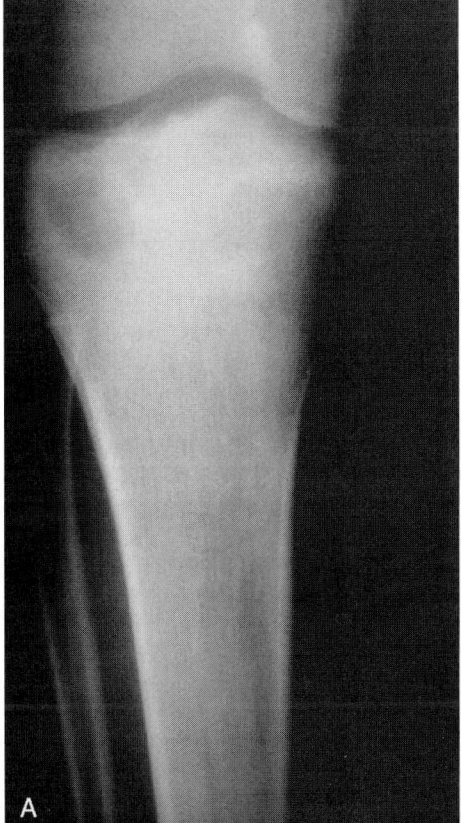

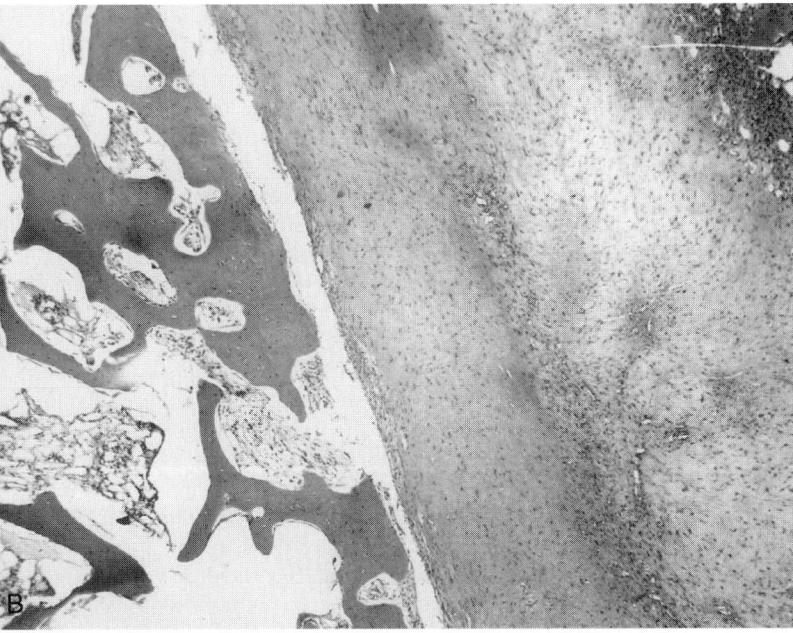

Fig. 2. Chondroblastoma. *A,* Geographically circumscribed osteolysis without marginal sclerosis in the epiphyseal end of the right tibia of an 18-year-old male. The findings are consistent with a benign tumor. *B,* Low-power histological section reveals a sharply circumscribed margin between the chondroid matrix (right) and bone without sclerosis (left) (magnification ×40).

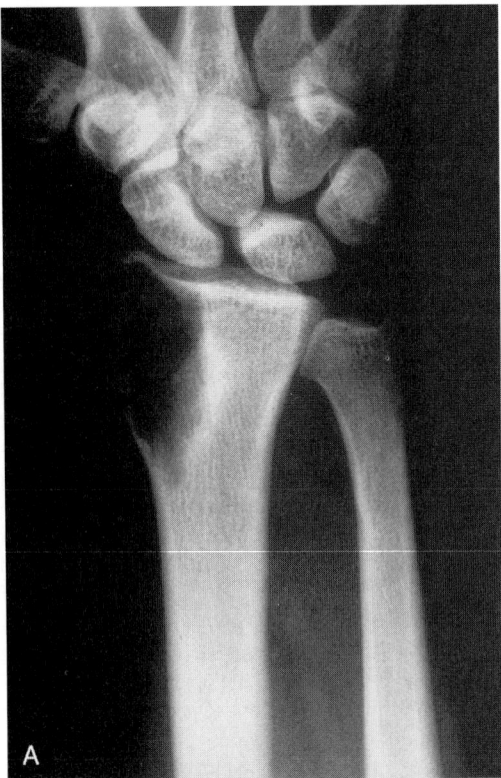

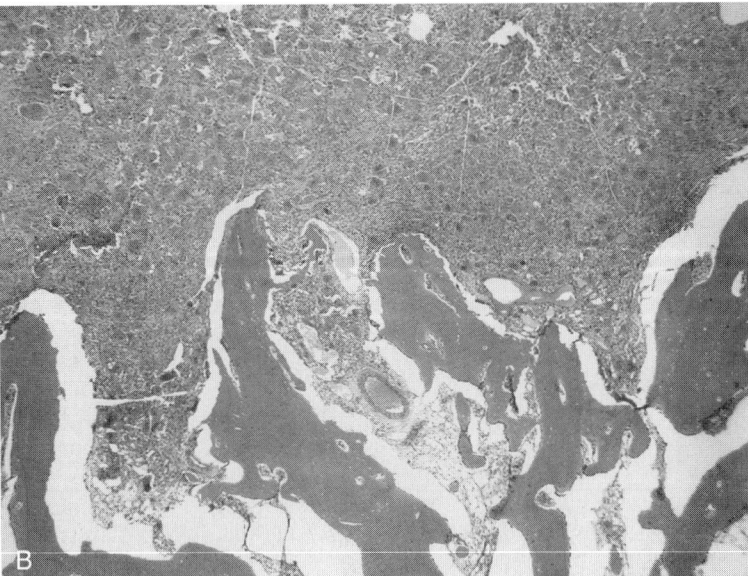

Fig. 3. Giant cell tumor. *A,* Radiograph of the right wrist of a 30-year-old female with swelling and wrist pain. Eccentric, radiolucent lesion of radius is seen extending to the articular end. There is fairly sharp circumscription medially and proximally and thinning of the medial distal cortex. *B,* Low-power view of the interface between giant cell tumor (top) and adjacent bone (bottom) reveals slight intertrabecular extension of the giant cell tumor despite the fairly circumscribed edge seen on the radiograph (magnification ×20).

there has been no positive correlation between this event and the subsequent development of pulmonary metastases.

GROWTH PATTERNS

Malignant bone tumors possess characteristic growth patterns that help to distinguish them from a benign tumor. In general, malignant tumors grow at a rate faster than that at which the surrounding host bone is reabsorbed. In addition, they usually display invasive local extension into the surrounding osseous and interosseous tissues. The consequence of this growth pattern is that malignant tumors are usually not well circumscribed radiographically. In some instances, the marrow or adipose tissue between normal intertrabecular spaces of cancellous bone or the haversian canals of the cortical bone are filled with tumor cells without any substantial structural alterations of the surrounding normal bone. This pattern of growth is sometimes referred to as *permeative* (Fig. 4).[4, 5] Despite the subtle changes often seen on plain radiographs, this growth pattern is clinically associated with the most malignant behavior. Very often, there is associated tumor extension into the adjacent soft tissues to produce an extraosseous tumor mass in the complete absence of demonstrable cortical destruction. This attests to the ability of malignant tumors to penetrate haversian and Volkmann's canals within the compact bone. In more slowly growing malignant tumors, often there are areas bordering the tumor in which osteoclast function is active enough to cause irregular bone destruction. In this type of destruction, sometimes referred to as *moth-eaten,*[5] some areas of the tumor interface with bone are indistinct, and some are obvious. This reflects differen-

tial growth and differential responses in various areas of the tumor (Fig. 5).

EFFECTS OF TUMORS

Because the most common primary bone tumors produce extracellular osseous or cartilaginous matrix, secondary mineralization or ossification may be superimposed on bone destruction. If the extracellular tumor matrix is osseous, it may be trabeculated or arranged in sheets. This, in turn, gives rise to rather coarse linear radiodensities or diffuse radiodensities resembling cotton or cumulus clouds (Fig. 6). If the tumor produces cartilage, its matrix grows in clonal nodules of varying sizes, analogous to a bag of marbles. These nodules are radiolucent, because cartilage is composed primarily of water. However, when these nodules reach sufficient size, they undergo calcification and endochondral ossification in the same way that cartilage is replaced by bone in normal development.[6] Calcification of cartilage appears flocculent or stippled on plain radiographs. Endochondral ossification, often taking place at the periphery of cartilage lobules, tends to be trabeculated and curved or even ring-like (Fig. 7). The rounded edges of these cartilage spherules exert pressure on the endosteal cortex. This causes slowly evolving endosteal scalloping as osteoclastic reabsorption remodels the inner cortex.

Regardless of their biological potential, bone tumors exert secondary effects on the host bone and on the periosteum, which contains osteoprogenitor cells in its innermost layer. If this inner layer of the periosteum is irritated or physically separated from the cortical surface, the osteoprogenitor cells differentiate into osteoblasts, and new bone

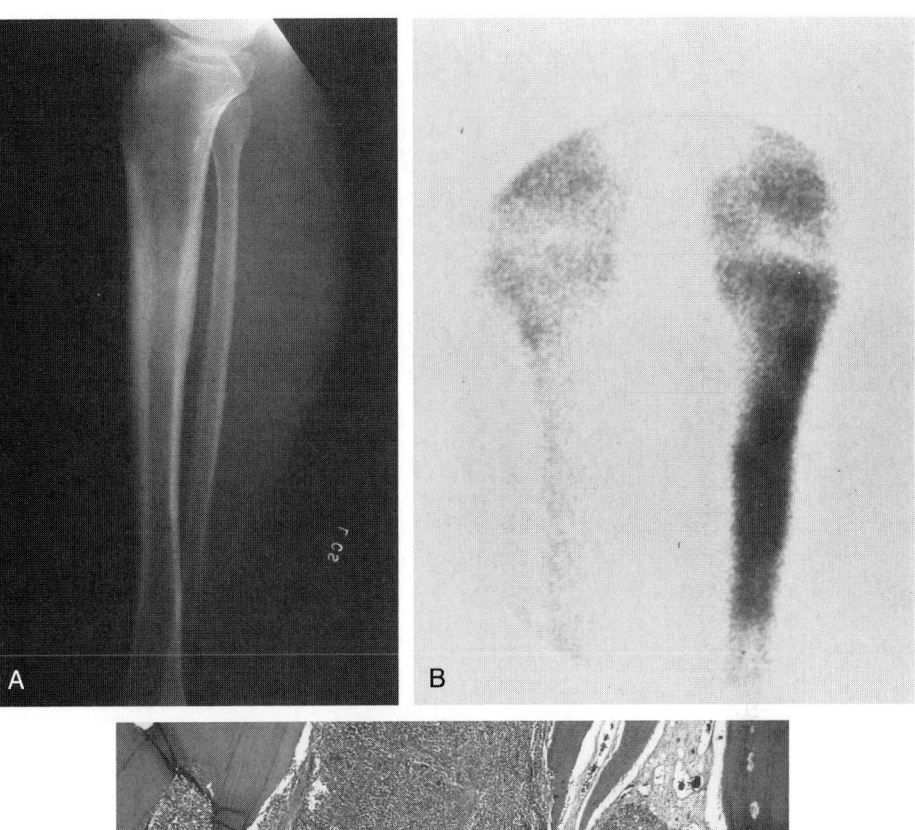

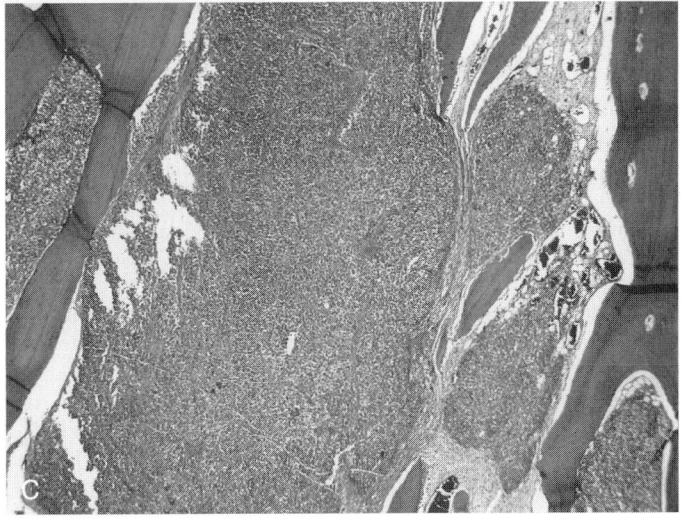

Fig. 4. Ewing's sarcoma. *A,* Lateral radiograph of an 18-year-old high school football player demonstrates slight thickening of the upper cortex of the left tibia with apparent slight density of the medullary cavity due to the circumferential thickening of the cortex. *B,* Technetium-99 bone scan reveals diffuse uptake of the radioisotope. Correlated with the plain radiograph, there is extensive permeation of the marrow spaces by tumor without corresponding radiographic evidence of bone destruction. *C,* Low-power biopsy sample of the corticomedullary junction demonstrates intact cortex and cancellous bone. There is total replacement by small round tumor cells of marrow fat and extension through haversian systems with very little osseous destruction (magnification ×40).

production is stimulated. Even if a tumor does not physically dissect the germinative layer of the periosteum from the bone surface, the elevated intraosseous pressure internally generated may cause secondary periosteal lifting, particularly in young individuals in whom the Sharpey fibers anchoring the periosteum to the cortex have laxity. New bone produced by the periosteum may be of sufficient radiodensity to detect on routine radiograph, and the pattern of this ossification may be somewhat indicative of the biological potential of the associated tumor. These reactions may also be associated with non-neoplastic diseases. In general, the more solidly formed the periosteal reaction, the slower is the evolution of periosteal elevation and the more indolent the behavior of the underlying lesion (Fig. 8). Disruption or discontinuity in periosteal new bone formation indicates a greater rate of associated tumor growth

and is highly correlated with malignant behavior.[7] The most familiar of these reactions is the discontinuous single periosteal new bone line open at one end, termed Codman's triangle (Fig. 9A). Both continuous and discontinuous periosteal reactions may be vertically arranged ("hair-on-end," see Fig. 9A to C), radially arranged ("sunburst"), or in layers ("onion-skin"; Fig. 10). Any soft-tissue mass appearing to be in continuity with an intraosseous lesion, particularly if the intervening cortex is intact, almost invariably means that an underlying bone tumor is malignant.

Bone tumors affect individuals of all ages, but in general, primary bone tumors have their greatest frequency in young individuals. The notable exceptions to this rule are chondrosarcoma, which is most frequently seen in the 5th to 7th decades, and plasma cell myeloma, which is unusual before the 5th decade. Metastatic carcinoma, although not a

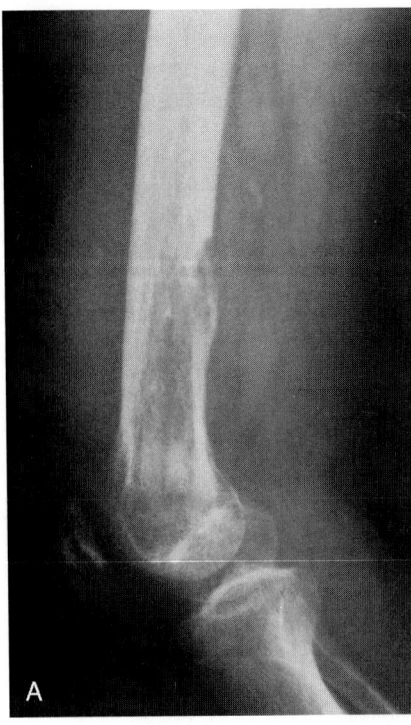

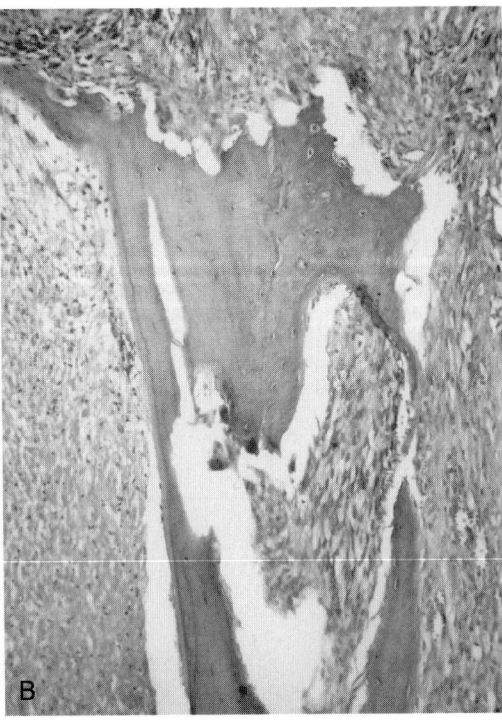

Fig. 5. Views. *A,* "Moth-eaten" osteolysis. Lateral radiograph of the distal femur of a 52-year-old male with fibrosarcoma. There are irregularly defined proximal borders for this radiolucent lesion. The posterior cortex is radiolucent with a large posterior soft-tissue mass. *B,* Medium power photograph of the femoral cortex of the patient in *A.* A cellular, spindle-cell lesion abuts a fragment of cortex with ragged, scalloped edges indicative of osteoclast activity. One haversian canal (bottom center) is expanded and filled with tumor. The superior border of this haversian canal contains several active osteoclasts (×100).

primary bone tumor, is very important in considerations of skeletal tumors because it is the most frequent malignant tumor to affect bones. The majority of individuals who die of widespread metastatic carcinoma harbor metastatic carcinoma in their skeleton even though they may not present with bone lesions clinically. Although carcinoma may spread to parenchymal organs via lymphatics, metastatic carcinoma to the skeleton is invariably bloodborne. Metastatic carcinoma usually affects more than one site in a single bone, and it often affects more than just one bone. Primary bone tumors of vascular origin and cartilage tumors associated with Ollier's disease are the only notable

primary tumors to present with some frequency as multiple discrete osseous lesions. Individuals with metastatic carcinoma are usually in their 5th decade or older. Occasionally, carcinoma may first manifest itself clinically as a skeletal metastasis from an occult primary tumor. When a pathologist is called upon to predict the site of the primary carcinoma in this circumstance, it may be difficult or impossible to do so from the morphological features alone of the metastases. The effects on host bone by metastatic carcinoma depend on events in the surrounding host bone. Usually, metastatic disease presents radiographically as radiolucent lesions. This is because the most frequent sec-

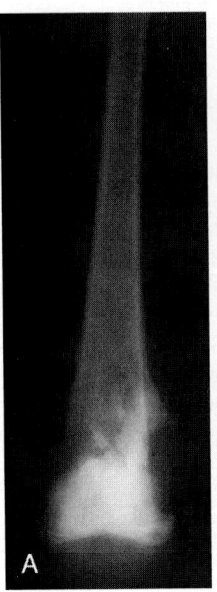

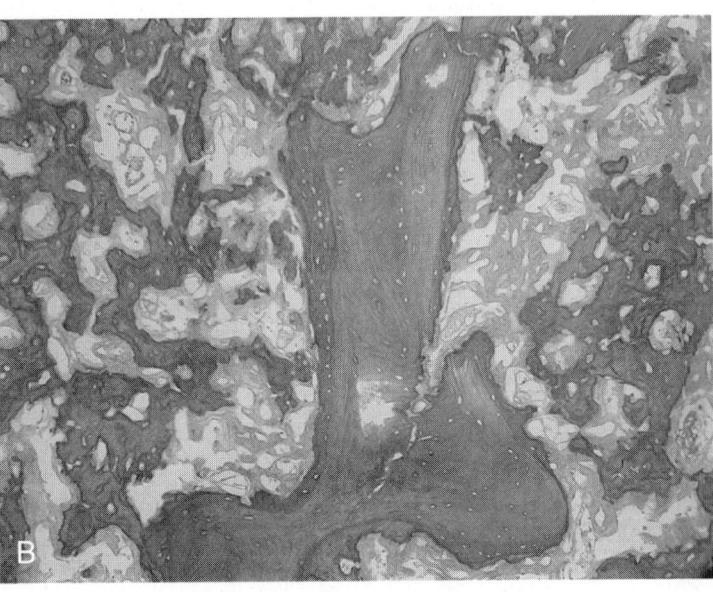

Fig. 6. Osteosarcoma. *A,* Distal left femur in a 10-year-old male. The tumor has diffuse "cumulus cloud–like" radiodensity and extends into the soft tissue to form an open periosteal "Codman's triangle" superolaterally. *B,* Low-power photograph of sclerosing osteosarcoma in *A* after chemotherapy and excision of the distal femur. Only the lamellar center of the trabecula, extending from the top to bottom in the middle of this photograph, is derived from the patient's own cancellous bone. The remaining marrow spaces are filled with immature bone produced by the tumor cells and replacing the normal fatty marrow. This bone is what produces the radiodensity seen in the plain radiograph (magnification ×40).

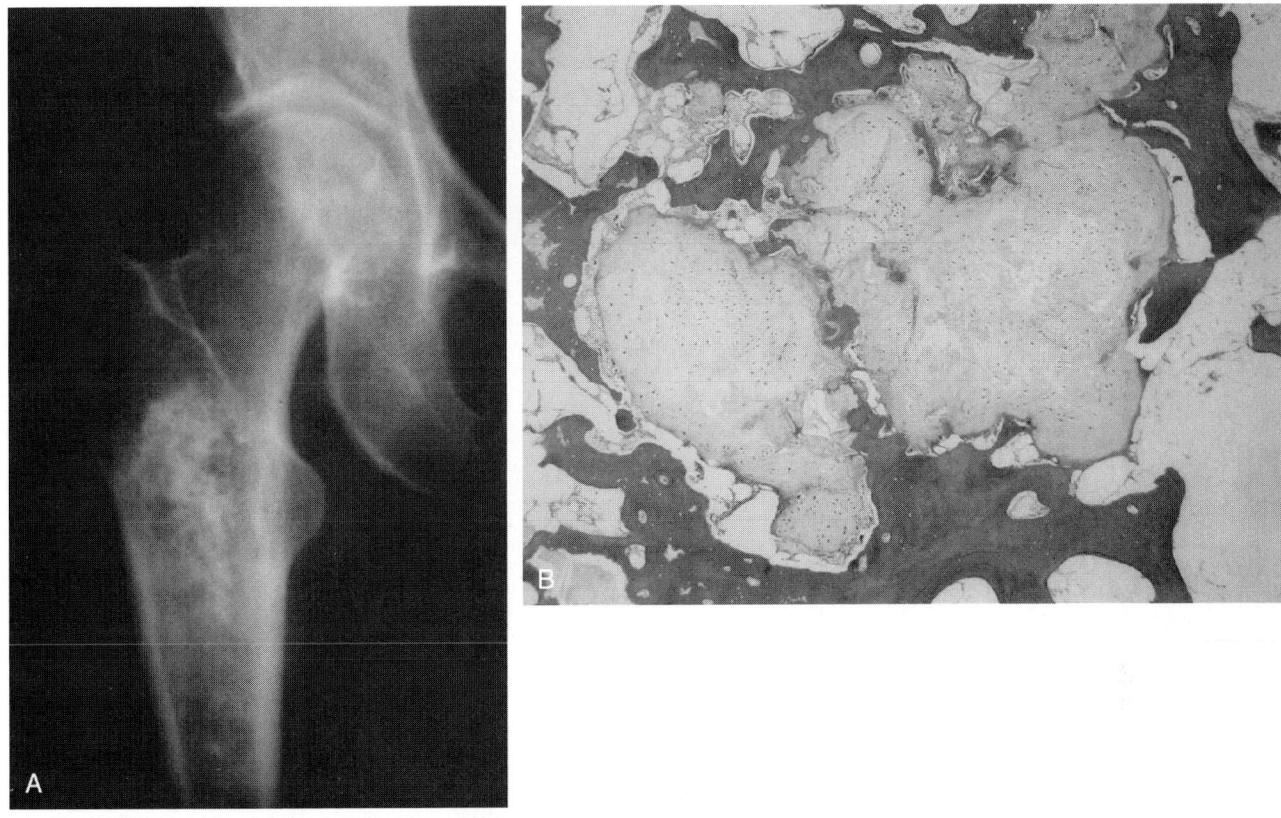

Fig. 7. Low-grade chondrosarcoma. *A,* Shown in a 53-year-old female. The lesion is ill-defined, radiolucent, and extends from the diaphysis to above the intertrochanteric line of the right femur. Note slight scalloping of the lateral and medial cortex and slight thickening of the medial cortex. There are aggregates of stippled "popcorn-like," curlicue, and rings of bone due to endochondral ossification. *B,* Low-power view. Lobules of hyaline cartilage with slightly myxoid cellular appearance demonstrate intertrabecular extension and endochondral ossification, resulting in the rings seen in the radiographs (magnification ×40).

Fig. 8. Osteoid osteoma. *A,* The lesion cannot be perceived due to diffuse periosteal reaction that has resulted in the continuous, fusiform expansion of the medial cortex. *B,* Outer femoral cortex derived from patient in *A.* Periosteal new bone is highly interconnected, contains new haversian systems, and is becoming compact (magnification ×20).

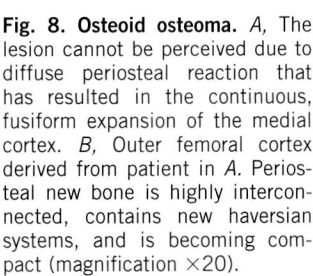

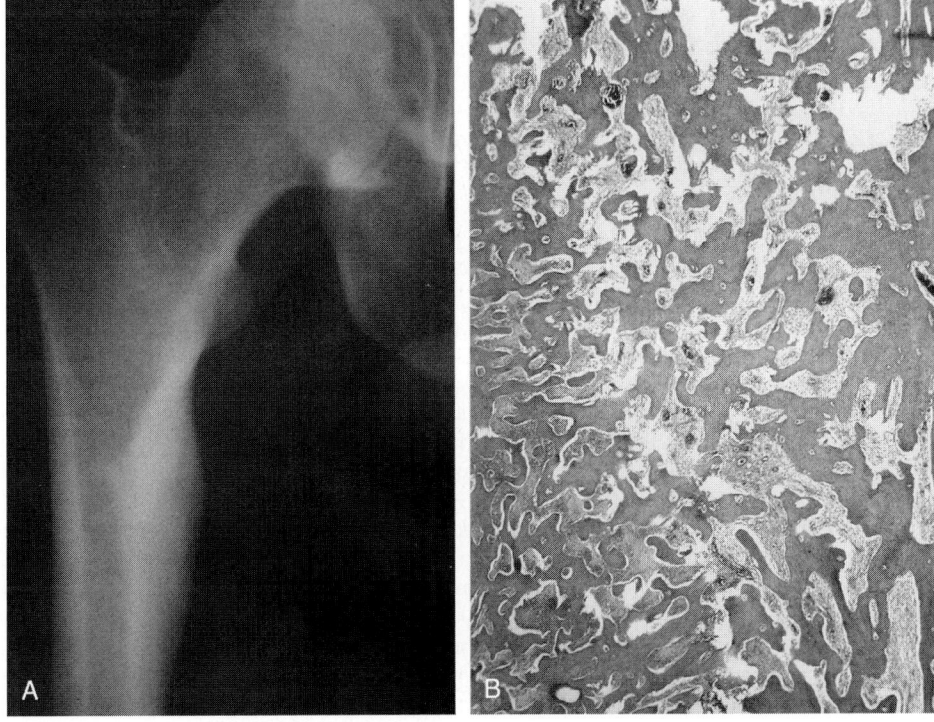

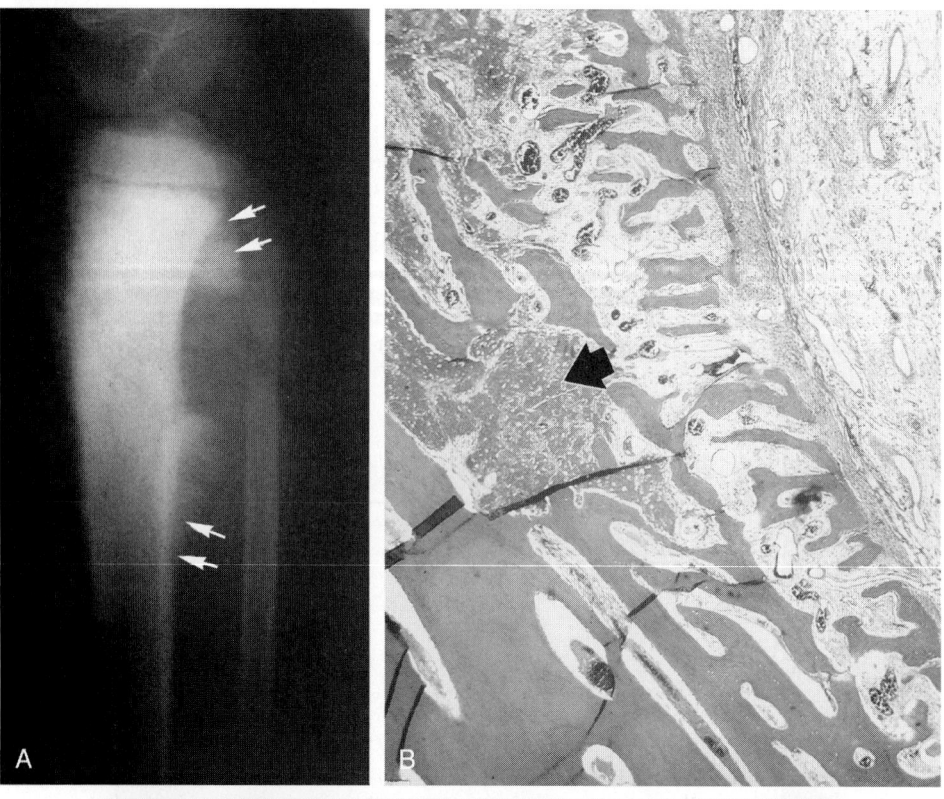

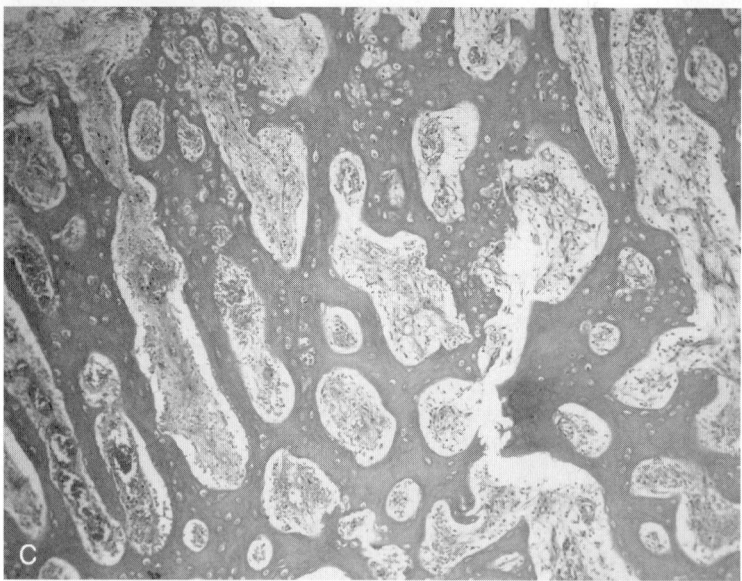

Fig. 9. Views. *A,* Osteosarcoma of the proximal tibia in a 12-year-old male. There is a discontinuous ossifying periosteal reaction that is open at its lower and upper edges, forming two Codman's triangles *(arrows).* The remaining periosteal reaction is delicately striate, interrupted, and perpendicular to the tibial shaft ("hair-on-end") *B,* Codman's triangle, low-power photograph. Delicate and interrupted periosteal reaction is hair-on-end toward the upper right and merges with the underlying cortex in the lower right corner. Tumor is not seen in the subperiosteal regions until the periosteum is widely lifted from the cortical surface (center left, *arrow*) (magnification ×20). *C,* Hair-on-end periosteal reaction demonstrates hypercellularity of the most superficial portions of the periosteal reaction (top), where the collagen structure of the new bone is most immature. In its more mature portions (bottom), there are haversian canals, less cellularity, and more trabecular connectivity connectivity (magnification ×40).

ondary effect is the activation of osteoclasts by cytokines produced by the tumor cells.[8] Less often, there is secondary activation of osteoblasts, and radiodense lesions are formed when new bone is produced.

While any portion of a bone may be affected by a bone tumor, certain neoplasms reproducibly affect particular areas of a bone. For example, osteosarcoma most frequently arises in the metaphyses of rapidly growing long bones. It is not surprising, then, that osteosarcoma is seen most often in the distal femur and proximal tibia of teenagers and that it has greater frequency in taller individuals than in shorter

ones. Occasionally, osteosarcoma arises in association with a preexisting bone lesion, such as Paget's disease, or in previously irradiated bone. In these circumstances, it occurs in middle-aged or elderly individuals rather than in adolescents. On the other hand, Ewing's sarcoma parallels the skeletal distribution of red marrow, so it tends to affect the axial skeleton in older individuals and the more distal appendicular skeleton in young children. Giant cell tumor almost always occurs after the growth plates have closed. It affects females at a younger age than males, who reach skeletal maturity at a later age. Chondroblastoma is usually

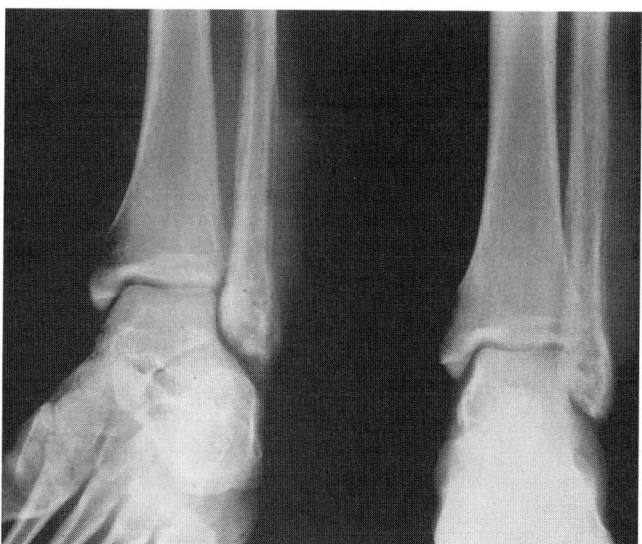

Fig. 10. Ewing's sarcoma of the fibula. Discontinuous "onionskin"-type periosteal reaction and soft-tissue mass are suggestive of a malignant tumor.

associated with a secondary ossification center, usually in skeletally immature individuals. Epiphyses, apophyses, and epiphysioid bones are the most frequently affected. Metastatic carcinoma usually affects the axial skeleton, and it rarely occurs distal to the femur or the humerus. It may affect the medullary cavity, the cortex, or both. Although it can extend into overlying soft tissue, it is distinctly rare for metastatic carcinoma to form a soft-tissue mass without having an underlying intraosseous component. As metastatic carcinoma usually has more than one discrete focus in the bone, there may be some clinical confusion with a primary bone tumor if a metastatic locus is solitary and the primary tumor is unknown. Renal cell carcinoma and thyroid carcinoma are notorious for this type of clinical presentation.

HOW TUMORS ARISE

In general, tumors are thought to arise as clonal genetic abnormalities of cells, resulting in limited growth in the case of most benign tumors. In the case of malignant tumors, these clonal abnormalities result in unrestricted local growth and metastatic potential. The clonal genetic abnormalities, or *oncogenes*, may act by either producing a faulty gene product that fails to prevent progression of the cell cycle (suppressor genes) or directly promoting tumor growth by creating a new gene product (transforming genes). The first description of a human tumor-suppressor gene alteration leading to the development of malignant bone tumors was that of the retinoblastoma gene.[9] Whereas the normal product of this gene suppresses the expression of cell cycle progression genes,[10] absence of both retinoblastoma alleles induces tumors.[11] Humans with a single retinoblastoma allele alteration have a risk for the development of retinoblastoma 36,000 times greater than the normal population. Their risk for the development of osteosarcoma is 2000 times normal.[10]

Transforming genes may arise as autosomal mutations leading to the unmasking of oncogenes. The most widely studied transforming gene arising from such mutations is the p53 gene. In its naturally occurring (wild) state, p53 acts as a tumor suppressor, with negative regulation of the cell cycle.[12] Mutations of the p53 gene eventuate in the initiation of the G1 phase of the cell cycle.[13, 14] Overexpression of p53 can be shown in about 30% of high-grade osteosarcomas[10] and is associated with highly aggressive variants.[15] Transforming genes may also arise as new gene products, which prevent the inhibition of cell division. The latter group includes fixed chromosomal translocations such as that found in the Ewing's sarcoma/primitive neuroectodermal tumor complex associated with a translocation of the short arms of chromosomes 11 and 22.[16, 17] Certain other bone tumors arise in the background of preexisting benign conditions with a heritable pattern (e.g., chondrosarcomas arising in multiple hereditary osteochondroma) or in syndromes from presumed gene mutations in which an inheritance pattern is not known (e.g., chondrosarcoma in Ollier's disease). Although rare, there are at least two inherited syndromes that predispose individuals to develop bone sarcomas: the Li-Fraumeni syndrome and the Rothmund-Thomson syndrome.[10] The Li-Fraumeni syndrome is characterized by inherited mutations of the p53 gene. The usual types of tumors in individuals with this syndrome are breast carcinoma and soft-tissue sarcomas; osteosarcomas of bone are also reported.[18, 19] The Rothmund-Thomson syndrome includes cutaneous lesions and skeletal dysplasia associated with adnexal tumors of the skin and an increased frequency of osteosarcoma.[22–22] The disorder is believed to originate from increased chromosomal fragility and deficiency in DNA repair.[23, 24] Certain high-grade malignant tumors may also arise as secondary clonal abnormalities engrafted on lower-grade malignant tumors that preceded them (e.g., dedifferentiated chondrosarcoma and dedifferentiated parosteal osteosarcomas).[25, 26]

CLINICAL MANAGEMENT

Clinical management of bone tumors is tailored to the individual type of lesion, its histological grade, and its local extent in the host. The process of making this assessment is termed staging. The standard tumor, lymph node, metastasis (TNM) classification (Table 2) originated by the American Joint Commission on Cancer[27] has limitations

TABLE 2. TNM CLASSIFICATION FOR BONE TUMORS				
Stage	**Grade**	**Tumor**	**Node**	**Metastasis**
Stage IA	$G_{1,2}$	T_1	No	Mo
Stage IB	$G_{1,2}$	T_2	No	Mo
Stage IIA	$G_{3,4}$	T_1	No	Mo
Stage IIB	$G_{3,4}$	T_2	No	Mo
Stage III	Not defined			
Stage IVA	Any G	Any T	N_1	Mo
Stage IVB	Any G	Any T	Any N	M_1

From Hermanek P, Sobin LH (eds): TNM Classification of Malignant Tumors. Berlin, Springer-Verlag, 1987, 4th ed.

TABLE 3. MUSCULOSKELETAL ONCOLOGY STAGING SYSTEM (AMERICAN JOINT COMMITTEE TASK FORCE ON BONE TUMORS)		
Stage	**Grade**	**Site**
Benign	G_0	
IA	G_1	T_1
IB	G_1	T_2
IIA	G_2	T_1
IIB	G_2	T_2
III	Metastases (any G)	Metastases (any T)

From Enneking WF: A system of staging musculoskeletal neoplasms. Clin Orthop 1986; 204:9.

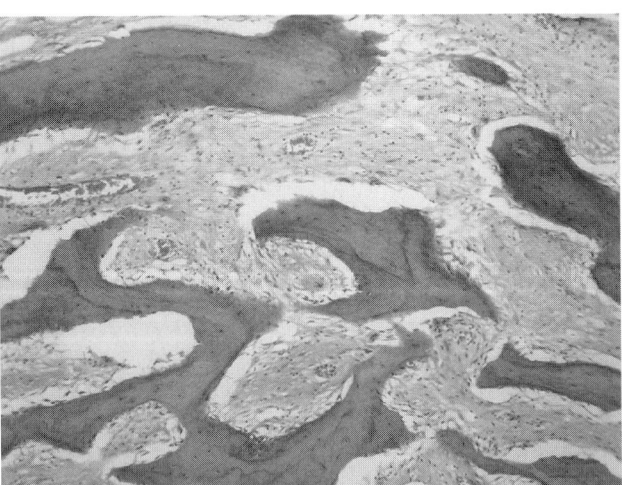

Fig. 11. Parosteal osteosarcoma, grade 1. The fibrous tissue between the trabeculae is not visibly hypercellular, and the spindle cells are bland. It is difficult, without radiographic correlation, to state that this lesion is a low-grade osteosarcoma (magnification ×200).

when applied to bone tumors. In this system T_1 refers to tumors that are intracortical, and T_2 refers to those that are extracortical, but tumors arising on the bone surfaces and not invading the interior of the bone cannot be properly classified. Whereas stage IV tumors are metastatic, there is no stage III defined for bone tumors. In addition, the presence of lymph nodes in this staging system is seldom relevant in bone sarcomas because they rarely metastasize to lymph nodes.

The Enneking Musculoskeletal Tumor Society staging system is based on both the tumor grade and the extent of disease (Table 3).[28] It is applicable to benign and malignant bone tumors (whether they arise within the bone or its surface) and is easily understood. There are only three stages in this system, designated by I, II, and III. In grades I and II, the suffix A or B is added, depending on whether the lesion is intracompartmental (T_1) or extracompartmental (T_2). Unless there is metastatic disease, the clinical stages are based primarily on the histological grading of the tumor. G_0 refers to benign tumors. G_1 refers to a tumor that is either locally aggressive or of low-grade malignancy with a relatively small likelihood of metastasis; unless it is extracompartmental, it is automatically designated stage I. G_2 refers to a high-grade malignant tumor and is designated stage II regardless of its local extent. Any tumor with metastases is automatically designated stage III.

The extent of local surgical treatment depends largely on the compartmentalization of the tumor. This is usually determined by preoperative imaging studies. Histological grading, on the other hand, is central to the Musculoskeletal Tumor Society staging system, because the decision to add adjunctive chemotherapy or radiation therapy depends entirely on the diagnosis and grade. The most important input required from the pathologist is whether the tumor is high- or low-grade. Because it should be obvious to any experienced pathologist whether a tumor is high- or low-grade, the system at first seems simple and reproducible (Figs. 11 and 12). Unfortunately, the histological grading of sarcomas has not been uniformly and objectively standardized. Broders and colleagues[29] created a four-tiered grading system for soft-tissue sarcomas, based on extent of cellularity, anaplasia, mitotic activity (number of mitoses and atypical mitoses), quantity of necrosis, and the extent of infiltrative growth. They further recognized that certain

soft-tissue sarcomas, regardless of their grade, always tend to behave as high-grade tumors.

There have been many attempts to regroup this grading system, sometimes adding criteria and sometimes changing the number of tiers to three or even two.[28, 30–32] A three-tiered system allows for the distinction of malignancies of intermediate grade, and it may be more suited to the prediction of survival and recurrence patterns.[33] Four-tiered grading systems, if grades I–II are considered low grade and III–IV high grade, become slightly and unnecessarily more complicated than two-tier systems, which do not attempt to segregate tumors of intermediate malignancy.[33] Whereas in soft-tissue tumors, the two most important parameters for the grading of sarcomas are probably a combination of mitotic counts and degree of necrosis,[33–35] in

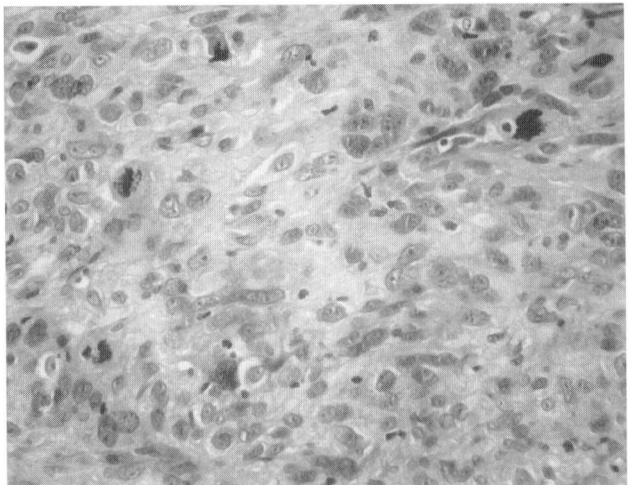

Fig. 12. Fibrosarcoma, grade 4. The spindle cells demonstrate enlarged nuclei with prominent nucleoli. Many of the nuclei are plump, although there is only moderate pleomorphism of the nuclei. There are four to five mitoses in this field (magnified ×400), and all are atypical.

bone tumors the method is somewhat less clear. One grading method, with good supporting data based on counting the number of mitoses per 10 high-power fields, has been suggested for differentiating grade II from grade III chondrosarcoma.[36] On the other hand, there have not been a large number of similar studies to objectively grade other types of bone sarcoma. The need for *biological* grading (*i.e.*, assigning a grade based on the anticipated behavior of a given tumor type)—hinted at by Broders—was strongly favored by Mirra because "histological grade (in terms of degree of anaplasia) and potential for metastasis are not always coupled. A 'sclerosing' variant of intramedullary osteosarcoma . . . usually exhibits histologic grade 1 anaplasia, yet is associated with a 40–50% metastatic rate within 2 years."[1] Similarly, Enzinger and Weiss[33] cited

studies using the histological type and tumor subtype as a "shortcut" to establish the grade of soft-tissue sarcomas.[31, 37] This is possible because some tumors that have a relatively low mitotic rate and lack significant pleomorphism are known to have a high rate of metastasis. Occasional tumors may escape histological or biological grading. Clear cell chondrosarcoma, which is usually considered an indolent tumor of low-grade malignancy in young adults, demonstrates widespread metastatic behavior not only to the lungs but also to many other bones in about 20% of cases. Why this unusual pattern of disease takes place only once in five times or which of the tumors is destined to behave in a malignant fashion have yet to be reproducibly predicted. This, in turn, precludes the precise staging that is required for treatment protocols.

REFERENCES

1. Mirra J: Bone Tumors: Clinical, Radiologic, and Pathologic Correlations. Philadelphia, Lea and Febiger, 1989.
2. O'Connell JX, Nanthakumar SS, Nielsen GP, et al: Osteoid osteoma: The uniquely innervated bone tumor. Mod Pathol 11: 175, 1998.
3. Wold LE, Pritchard DJ, Bergert J, et al: Prostaglandin synthesis by osteoid osteoma and osteoblastoma. Mod Pathol 1:129, 1988.
4. Madewell JE, Ragsdale BD, Sweet DE: Radiographic and pathologic analysis of solitary bone lesions I: Internal margins. Radiol Clin North Am 19:715, 1981.
5. Lodwick GS, Wilson AJ, Farrell C, et al: Determining growth rates of focal lesions of bone from radiographs. Radiology 134: 577, 1980.
6. Sweet DE, Madewell JE, Ragsdale BD: Radiographic and pathologic analysis of solitary bone lesions III: Matrix patterns. Radiol Clin North Am 19:785, 1981.
7. Ragsdale BD, Madewell JE, Sweet DE: Radiographic and pathologic analysis of solitary bone lesions II: Periosteal reactions. Radiol Clin North Am 19:749, 1981.
8. Mundy GR: Hypercalcemina of malignancy revisited. J Clin Invest 82:1, 1986.
9. Zhou Y, Li J, Xu K, et al: Further characterization of retinoblastoma gene-mediated cell growth and tumor suppression in human cancer cells. Proc Natl Acad Sci U S A 91:4165, 1994.
10. Dorfman HD, Czerniak B: Bone Tumors. Mosby, New York, 1998, p 66.
11. Reed JC, Zha H, Aime-Sempe C, et al: Structure-function analysis of bcl-2 family proteins: Regulators of programmed cell death. Adv Exp Med Biol 406:99, 1996.
12. Finlay C, Hinds PW, Levine AJ: The p53 proto-oncogene can act as a suppressor of transformation. Cell 57:1083, 1989.
13. El-Deiry WS, Tokino T, Velculescu VE, et al: WAF-1, a potential mediator of p53 tumor suppression. Cell 75:817, 1993.
14. Sheikh MS, Li XS, Chen JC, et al: Mechanisms of regulation of WAF-1/Cip-1 gene

expression in human brast carcinoma: Role of p53 dependent and independent signal transduction pathways. Oncogene 9: 3407, 1994.
15. Radig K, Schneider-Stock R, Oda Y, et al: Mutation spectrum of p53 gene in highly malignant human osteosarcomas. Gen Diagn Pathol 142:25, 1996.
16. Turc-Carel C, Aurias A, Mugneret F, et al: Chromosomes in Ewing's sarcoma I: An evaluation of 85 cases and remarkable consistency of t(11,22)(q24,;q12). Cancer Genet Cytogenet 32:229, 1988.
17. Whang-Peng J, Triche TJ, Knutsen T, et al: Cytogenetic characterization of selected round cell tumors of childhood. Cancer Genet Cytogenet 21:185, 1986.
18. Malkin D.: p53 and the Li-Fraumeni syndrome. Biochim Biophys Acta 1198:197, 1994.
19. Strong LC, Williams WR, Tainsky MA: The Li-Fraumeni syndrome: From clinical epidemiology to molecular genetics. Am J Epidemiol 135:190, 1992.
20. Cumin I, Cohen JY, David A, et al: Rothmund-Thomson syndrome and osteosarcoma. Med Pediatr Oncol 26:414, 1996.
21. Judge MR, Kilby A, Harper JI: Rothmund-Thomson syndrome and osteosarcoma. Br J Dermatol 129:723, 1993.
22. Sim FH, DeVries EM, Miser JS, et al: Osteoblastic osteosarcoma (grade 4) with Rothmund-Thomson syndrome. Skeletal Radiol 21:543, 1992.
23. Orstavic KH, McFadden N, Hagelsteen J, et al: Instability of lymphocyte chromosomes in a girl with Rothmund-Thomson syndrome. J Med Genet 31:570, 1994.
24. Shinya A, Nishigori C, Morikawi S, et al: A case of Rothmund-Thomson syndrome with reduced DNA repair capacity. Arch Dermatol 129:332, 1993.
25. Bridge JA, DeBoer J, Travis J, et al: Simultaneous interphase cytogenetic analysis and fluorescence immunophenotyping of dedifferentiated chondrosarcoma: Implications for histopathogenesis. Am J Pathol 144:215, 1994.
26. Johnson S, Tetu B, Ayala AG, et al: Chondrosarcoma with additional mesenchymal component (dedifferentiated chon-

drosarcoma) I: A clinicopathologic study of 26 cases. Cancer 58:278, 1986.
27. Hermanek P, Sobin LH (eds): TNM Classification of Malignant Tumors. Berlin, Springer-Verlag, 1987, 4th ed.
28. Enneking WF: A system of staging musculoskeletal neoplasms. Clin Orthop 204:9, 1986.
29. Broders AC, Hargrave R, Meyerding HW: Pathological features of soft tissue fibrosarcoma. Surg Gynecol Obstet 69:267, 1939.
30. Costa J, Wesley RA, Glatstein, E, et al: The grading of soft tissue sarcomas: Results of a clinicohistopathologic correlation in a series of 163 cases. Cancer 53:530, 1984.
31. Mandard AM, Chasley JC, Mandard JC, et al: The pathologist's role in a multidisciplinary apprach for soft part tissue sarcomas: A reappraisal (39 cases). J Surg Oncol 17:69, 1981.
32. Myhre-Jensen O, Kaae S, Madsen EH, et al: Histopathological grading in soft-tissue tumors: Relation to survival in 261 surgically treated patients. Acta Pathol Microbiol Immunol Scand 91:145, 1983.
33. Enzinger FM, Weiss SW: Soft Tissue Tumors. St. Louis, C.V. Mosby, 1995, 3rd ed.
34. Albus-Lutter CE, de Stefani E, van Unnik JAM: Clinicopathologic relations in soft tissue sarcomas. In Management of Soft Tissue and Bone Sarcomas. New York, Raven Press, 1986.
35. Enzinger FM: Clinicopathological correlation in soft tissue sarcomas. In Management of soft tissue and bone sarcomas. New York, Raven Press, 1986.
36. Evans HL, Ayala AG, Rohmsdahl MM: Prognostic factors in chondrosarcoma of bone: A clinicopathologic analysis with emphasis on histologic grading. Cancer 40:818, 1977.
37. Russell WO, Cohen J, Cutler S, et al: Staging system for soft tissue sarcoma. In American Joint Committee for Cancer Staging and End Results Reporting. Chicago, American College of Surgeons Task Force on Soft Tissue Sarcoma, Chicago, 1980.

BIOPSY

Mark T. Scarborough and Gerard Powell

Summary

- The biopsy is one of the most important steps in the management of a patient with a musculoskeletal tumor.
- Correctly performed, the biopsy can result in an accurate and timely diagnosis, with an excellent chance of limb salvage.
- Decisions regarding the type of biopsy, the location of the puncture or incision, and handling of the tissue require extensive thought and experience.
- Staging studies should be done before the biopsy to help develop a differential diagnosis, guide the location of the biopsy, and look for metastatic or multicentric disease.
- There are four main methods of biopsy: fine needle aspiration, needle (true cut), incisional, and excisional.
- Careful evaluation of a tumor with plain radiographs, bone scans, magnetic resonance imaging, computed tomography, angiography, and/or ultrasound facilitates accurate diagnosis.
- If the staging studies reveal a potentially malignant or aggressive tumor, then referral to a musculoskeletal oncologist is advised.

The biopsy is one of the most important steps in the management of a patient with a musculoskeletal tumor. As William F. Enneking said, "knowing the diagnosis is never a hindrance when planning treatment."[1] Correctly performed, the biopsy can result in an accurate and timely diagnosis, with an excellent chance of limb salvage. Conversely, a poorly planned and performed biopsy can make local control of the tumor difficult and sometimes result in an unnecessary amputation.[2, 3] Biopsies are not technically difficult procedures, but the decisions regarding the type of biopsy, the location of the puncture or incision, and handling of the tissue require extensive thought and experience. Thus, a musculoskeletal oncologist should perform the biopsy of bone and soft-tissue tumors to minimize complications and optimize the chances for limb salvage. In 1982 Mankin et al[2] reported the outcome of patients that had undergone biopsy of a musculoskeletal tumor in a referring institution compared with those that had the biopsy done in the tertiary care institution. The findings of this multicenter study revealed a high incidence of biopsy-associated complications (17.3%), major errors in diagnosis (18.2%), nonrepresentative tissue or technically poor biopsies (10.3%), and alterations in ultimate treatment (18.2%). Furthermore, avoidable amputations (4.5%) and adverse effects on prognosis (8.5%) were also common. In a follow-up study 10 years later, similar findings were noted.[3] The rate of diagnostic error was 17.8%; nonrepresentative biopsies, 8.4%; biopsy complications, 15.9%; alterations in treatment, 19.3%; and unnecessary amputation, 3%. In both studies complications were more common when the biopsy was done in the referring institution rather than in the

TABLE 1. BIOPSY PROBLEMS AND SOLUTIONS

Problem	Solution
Transverse incisions make soft-tissue coverage after resection difficult	Use longitudinal incisions
Hematomas can contaminate uninvolved tissues	Plug bone biopsy cavities with cement; use drains when needed; place drains in line of incision
Pathological fractures may occur at a biopsy site or through tumor	Plug bone biopsy cavities with cement; protect patient from weightbearing
Tumor tissue may be necrotic or heterogeneous	Obtain frozen section to ensure adequacy of specimen
The pathologist may need to do multiple special studies to make a diagnosis	Discuss case preoperatively with the pathologist, provide adequate tissue, obtain frozen section, and put tissue in appropriate media under guidance of pathologist
Assuming a bone lesion is metastatic disease and proceed with internal fixation (e.g., nail) without a biopsy	Obtain a careful history and physical examination; do preoperative staging studies; do a biopsy prior to prophylactic internal fixation; do not do prophylactic internal fixation of bones affected by sarcoma
Poorly planned or executed biopsy of sarcomas can make definitive treatment more difficult	Refer potential sarcomas to an orthopaedic oncologist before biopsy
Arthroscopic biopsy or biopsy through a joint can contaminate the joint (e.g., juxta-articular synovial sarcoma)	Avoid arthroscopic biopsy of juxta-articular get preoperative radiographs and staging studies
Assuming a soft-tissue lesion is a lipoma or ganglion cyst	If considering excision stage preoperatively, consider before excision
Assuming a deep soft-tissue lesion is a hematoma or Baker's cyst	Do preoperative staging studies; the mass is suspicious, refer for biopsy
Contaminating the neurovascular bundle	Careful staging and biopsy technique can avoid contamination of neurovascular bundle
Doing biopsy or an excision as a means of deciding who should be referred	Refer potential sarcomas to an orthopaedic oncologist prior to biopsy

tertiary care institution. These studies underscore the importance and complexity of performing the biopsy of musculoskeletal tumors. Careful planning will minimize the complications associated with biopsy of musculoskeletal tumors (Table 1).

GOALS, INDICATIONS, AND CONTRAINDICATIONS

There are four main methods of biopsy: fine needle aspiration (FNA), needle (true cut), incisional, and excisional (Table 2). The goal of each is to obtain sufficient tissue to make a diagnosis. For all malignant tumors it is important that a histological grade be assigned to the tumor. Grading usually requires more tissue, and only a few tumors can be graded based only on FNA. Biopsy is important when a tumor needs treatment or when there is a reasonable chance that it needs treatment. Those tumors of the musculoskeletal system that can be diagnosed from their presentation (e.g., nonossifying fibroma, enchondroma, exostosis) and that do not need treatment do not need to be biopsied. There are few contraindications to a biopsy when a specific diagnosis is needed.

PROCEDURES

PREOPERATION PLANNING

Careful planning of the biopsy is essential to ensure an accurate diagnosis.[1, 4–8] Staging studies should be done before the biopsy. The staging studies help develop a differential diagnosis, guide the location of the biopsy, and look for metastatic or multicentric disease. Sometimes the biopsy procedure can alter the staging studies, making evaluation of tumor extent difficult. Direct consultation with the pathologist should be done *before* the biopsy.

Advances in radiology have revolutionized the treatment of musculoskeletal tumors. Careful evaluation of a tumor with plain radiographs, bone scans, magnetic resonance imaging (MRI), computed tomography (CT) scans, angiography, and/or ultrasound facilitates making an accurate diagnosis. The radiographic information is complementary to the pathological information. The radiographic characteristics of a tumor are just as important as the histological features. The radiographic studies are the guide for determining where to perform a biopsy. In difficult anatomic settings (e.g., pelvis and spine), the biopsy can be done under CT guidance.

The pathological evaluation of musculoskeletal tumors is very difficult. Given the rarity of these tumors, there are few pathologists with extensive experience with mesenchymal tumors. The tumor tissue is often a heterogeneous collection of tumor cells and host reaction. For example, the fracture callus surrounding a pathological fracture of bone containing an aneurysmal bone cyst looks histologically similar to the malignant osteoid of an osteosarcoma. In such cases clinical, radiographic, and pathological coordination and biopsy selection remote from the fracture callus will facilitate an accurate diagnosis. To assist the pathological evaluation we recommend consultation with the radiologist and pathologist before biopsy. This allows the pathologist to develop a differential diagnosis to guide the selection of specialized tests such as immunohistochemistry panels, cytogenetics, molecular studies, and electron microscopy. The pathologist and radiologist can also help select the biopsy target.

	TABLE 2. TYPES OF BIOPSY				
Type	**Procedure**	**Sample Obtained**	**Indications**	**Pros**	**Cons**
FNA	Fine needle aspiration of tumor	Cells	Some round cell tumors, metastatic carcinomas, recurrent tumors, select primary tumors	Minimally invasive	Requires very experienced pathologist, small tumor sample, inadequate amount of tissue for extensive pathological study
Needle	Tissue removed with core needle	Small cores of tissue	Some round cell tumors, metastatic carcinomas, recurrent tumors, select primary tumors	Minimally invasive; avoids a surgical procedure	Small sample size; may not be enough tissue for the pathologist to do sophisticated tests
Incisional	Open surgical biopsy	Large sample	Tumors requiring extensive pathological evaluation	Allows frozen section to ensure adequacy of specimen; can proceed with excision if indicated	Requires a surgical procedure
Excisional	En bloc excision of tumor	Entire lesion and some normal tissue	Small subcutaneous lesions, cases with clear diagnosis radiographically, select malignant tumors	Allows for a single procedure	If the lesion is presumed benign, and turns out to be malignant, then more extensive surgery, adjuvant therapy, or even amputation may be necessary

TABLE 3. PRINCIPLES OF BIOPSY

1. Consult with the pathologist and radiologist before the biopsy.
2. Make sure the pathologist knows the differential diagnosis and all of the special studies that may be required to make a diagnosis.
3. Do staging studies before the biopsy.
4. Avoid transverse incisions.
5. Plan the exact path and method of the biopsy to avoid contaminating uninvolved tissues (especially the neurovascular bundle and joints).
6. Do a frozen section to assure the collection of adequate, representative tissue.
7. Avoid creating hematomas.
8. Prevent pathological fracture with protected weightbearing.
9. Place drains in line of and close to the incision.
10. Refer to an orthopaedic oncologist before the biopsy if all of the above steps cannot be performed or if uncomfortable performing the definitive treatment.

TECHNICAL DETAILS

True cut and FNA biopsies are typically done in the outpatient clinic or radiology suite, and open biopsies (incisional and excisional) are done in the operating room. FNA is done by placing a small-gauge needle in the tumor and then aspirating cells. The aspirate is placed on a glass slide and fixative is applied. The sample consists primarily of a small quantity of individual cells. FNA is a simple procedure that is done in the clinical setting. The sample is easy to obtain but the interpretation of the histological preparation is difficult.[9] FNA of musculoskeletal tumors is quite controversial.[10] In some select clinical situations FNA is very helpful. Because only cells are obtained, tumors that are homogeneous are easier to evaluate than those with a mixed cell population. Round cell tumors such as myeloma, lymphoma, and Ewing's sarcoma are examples. Diagnosis of a metastatic lesion in a patient with a known malignancy is sometimes feasible with FNA because a small sample may suffice. Also, some cases of metastatic carcinoma have characteristic cells and are readily identified. The paucity of material obtained by FNA limits extensive evaluation with sophisticated techniques such as cytogenetics, electron microscopy, and flow cytometry.

A needle (true cut) biopsy is the other minimally invasive technique of biopsy. This can be done percutaneously under guidance by palpation or with the assistance of ultrasound, fluoroscopy, CT, or operative MRI. The technique is usually done with local anesthesia and utilizes a needle that cuts a small sample of tissue. Several samples can be obtained. Careful placement and marking of the needle tract is important to allow later excision of the tract at the time of surgical resection. This decreases the risk of local recurrence along the biopsy tract. The needles are manually directed or mechanical with a firing mechanism. The samples obtained are cores of tissue that measure approximately 10 mm in length and 2 mm in width. The size of the sample allows for extensive pathological evaluation, including frozen sections, immunohistochemistry, flow cytometry, and electron microscopy. Indications for needle biopsy include accessible bone and soft-tissue tumors that are potentially diagnosed with a small tumor sample. Many pathologists are not experienced enough to make accurate diagnoses of musculoskeletal tumors biopsied with a needle.

An incisional biopsy is a surgical procedure. Large amounts of tissue are available for the pathologist. There are strict principles in doing an incisional biopsy (Table 3). Transverse incisions should *never* be done to biopsy lesions on the extremities. Transverse incisions are more difficult to excise than longitudinal incisions and may make it necessary to do more extensive reconstructive procedures at the time of surgical resection of the tumor. The approach taken for the biopsy should be carefully planned to avoid the neurovascular bundle and to minimize contamination of tissues. Incision placement is important to allow for excision of the scar at the time of tumor resection. The most direct route is taken from the skin to the tumor, taking into consideration the best place for the incision for the surgical resection. Placement of the incision requires considerable knowledge of approaches for surgical resection. Cut a 1-cm square block of tissue from the tumor. A frozen section analysis should be done to ensure that diagnostic tissue has been obtained. Cultures should be taken. Drains may be used if necessary but should be placed in line with the skin incision and should not be near the neurovascular bundle (Fig. 1). Strict hemostasis is important to avoid distant tumor implantation. Tourniquets may

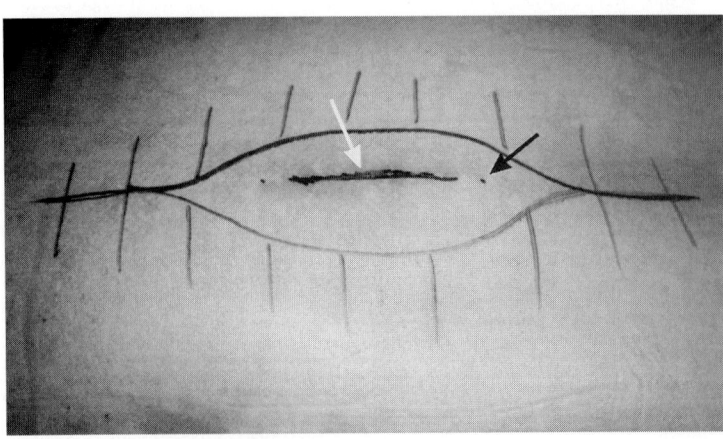

Fig. 1. Sarcoma. This patient had a high-grade soft-tissue sarcoma located within the subcutaneous tissue. He received preoperative radiation therapy following a generous incisional biopsy. Fortunately the drain was placed in line with the incision (*black arrow*), allowing easy excision of the drain tract. The incision was longitudinal, which facilitated primary closure without a flap (*white arrow*).

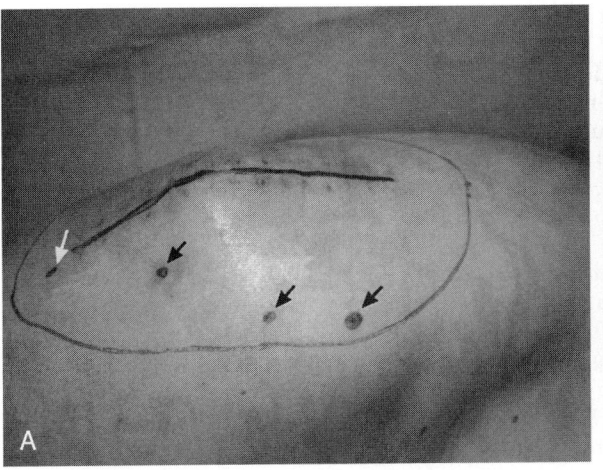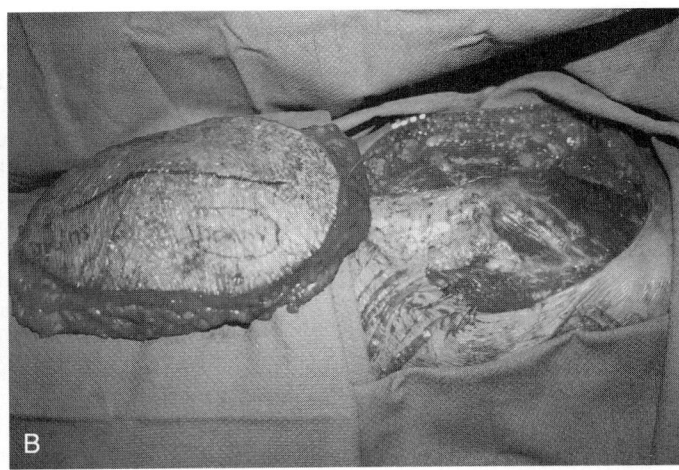

Fig. 2. Chondrosarcoma. This patient had a high-grade extraskeletal chondrosarcoma. The biopsy was performed through a longitudinal incision (*white arrow*) but the drains were placed several centimeters medial and not in line with the incision (*black arrows*). This poor placement necessitated excision of more soft tissue and required a flap for closure. Had the drainage tube been placed in line with the incision, primary closure would have been possible.

be used for biopsy, but the limb should not be exsanguinated (a maneuver that could cause tumor embolization). Arthroscopic biopsy of juxta-articular masses should not be done, to avoid joint contamination.

Excisional biopsies should be done only in well-selected cases. An excisional biopsy involves removal of the entire lesion. This type of biopsy is typically done with some classic benign lesions such as exostoses, lipomas, and ganglia. Orthopaedic oncologists occasionally do excisional biopsies of carefully selected malignant tumors given a classic radiographic appearance and appropriate clinical and radiographic setting.

COMPLICATIONS AND RESULTS

There are a number of significant complications from biopsies. The most significant is obtaining the wrong diagnosis. This occurs most often when there is limited communication between the surgeon and pathologist. Whenever the pathological diagnosis seems inconsistent with the clinical

setting it is vital that the surgeon confirm the diagnosis with the pathologist and assure that the pathologist is aware of the clinical situation. It is embarrassing to obtain no diagnosis but usually not dangerous. Doing a frozen section during the biopsy reduces the risk of this complication. Postoperative bleeding is a complication that can increase the tissue at risk and hemostasis is important. A postoperative infection is also a complication that can have significant adverse effects on the patient's care. Attention to detail is the single most important aspect of doing a biopsy to reduce complications and optimize patient care (Fig. 2).

The biopsy is an important part of the treatment of musculoskeletal tumors. Careful planning is essential to optimize chances for local control of the tumor and to facilitate limb salvage. Careful radiographic staging and consultation with both the pathologist and radiologist help create a plan for the type and route of biopsy. If the staging studies reveal a potentially malignant or aggressive tumor, then referral to a musculoskeletal oncologist is advised.

REFERENCES

1. Enneking W: Personal communication, 1999.
2. Mankin HJ, Lange TA, Spanier SS: The hazards of biopsy in patients with malignant primary bone and soft-tissue tumors. J Bone Joint Surg Am 1982; 64:1121.
3. Mankin HJ, Mankin CJ, Simon MA: The hazards of biopsy, revisited. J Bone Joint Surg Am 1996; 78:656.
4. Enneking WF, Spanier SS, Goodman MA: Current concepts review: The surgical staging of musculoskeletal sarcoma. J Bone Joint Surg Am 1980; 62:1027.
5. Heare TC, Enneking WF, Heare MM:

Staging techniques and biopsy of bone tumors. Orthop Clin North Am 1989; 20: 273.
6. Simon MA: Current concepts review: Biopsy of musculoskeletal tumors. J Bone Joint Surg Am 1982; 64:1253.
7. Springfield DS, Rosenberg A: Biopsy: Complicated and risky (editorial). J Bone Joint Surg Am 1996; 78:639.
8. Simon MA: Biopsy. In Simon MA, Springfield DS (eds): Surgery for Bone and Soft-Tissue Tumors. Philadelphia, Lippincott, 1988, pp. 55–65.
9. Kilpatrick SE, Geisinger KR: Soft tissue

sarcomas: The usefulness and limitations of fine-needle aspiration biopsy. Am J Clin Pathol 1998; 110:50.
10. Ryan M: Cytology and mesenchymal pathology: How far will we go? Am J Clin Pathol 1996; 106:561.
11. Joyce MJ, Mankin HJ: Caveat arthroscopes: Extra-articular lesions of bone simulating intra-articular pathology of the knee. J Bone Joint Surg Am 1983; 65:289.

IRRADIATION FOR MUSCULOSKELETAL TUMORS

Dempsey Springfield

Summary

- Irradiation of bone tumors, both primary and secondary, can be of value to patients. It is a local treatment not unlike surgery.
- Chemotherapy is systemic treatment.
- Irradiation can reduce the magnitude of the surgical resection, thus preserving function.
- It is important for orthopaedic surgeons to understand the basic principles of irradiation and to know when it can be used to the benefit of the patient.

Irradiation plays an important role in the management of musculoskeletal tumors. Irradiation is a local treatment similar to an operation often used in conjunction with surgery to help eradicate a primary tumor when an adequate surgical resection without adjuvant irradiation would lead to excessive morbidity. Irradiation is the definitive oncological treatment of some primary musculoskeletal tumors (i.e., myeloma and lymphoma of bone), and metastatic carcinoma to bone is usually best controlled by irradiation. During the past 20 years, irradiation's role in the management of musculoskeletal tumors has changed. Many advances have been made in the methods of administration.

ADMINISTRATION

The means of administering irradiation depends on the clinical situation. The goal of treatment is to administer the highest feasible dose to the tissue containing the tumor, with the least amount of irradiation to surrounding normal tissue. High-energy linear accelerators delivering 10 to 25 mv are used primarily. Their beams are capable of penetrating deeply enough to treat musculoskeletal tumors with a limited surface dose. They also have rapid fall-off of irradiation at the edge of the field, so normal tissues outside the field of treatment receive limited irradiation. This is called "conventional external beam" irradiation (Fig. 1). Modern equipment allows the patient and beam to be adjusted so numerous beam portals can be designed to optimize the patient's treatment. These instruments are combined with computer-assisted planning so that accuracy of treatment has increased dramatically over the past decade. Only plain radiographs used to be utilized for planning.

Brachytherapy is often used for administering irradiation to patients with musculoskeletal tumors[1-3] (Fig. 2). This technique was first used early in the last century but until recently was not used for musculoskeletal tumors. Brachytherapy is administered by placing hollow catheters in the bed of the tumor at the time of the operation after the tumor has been resected. The wound is closed, and the radioactive material is loaded later. Usually the radioactive material is placed within a week of the operation and is left in place from 24 to 72 hours. After the radioactive source is removed, the catheters are removed, usually at the bedside. Brachytherapy allows high doses of irradiation to be administered to a limited amount of tissue. It is more convenient than external-beam treatment because it is given over a day or two; external-beam treatment is given over a period of 5 to 6 weeks.

IRRADIATION SENSITIVITY

The effect of irradiation is not dependent on its method of administration. Irradiation acts on the DNA template.[4] Irradiation damages the DNA and leads to either the death of the cell or its inability to reproduce. A tumor cell's DNA is more sensitive to irradiation than is a normal cell's DNA. Therefore, the tumor is more affected by the irradiation than is normal tissue. The reasons tumor cells are more sensitive are thought to be a combination of the tumor's potential inherent radiosensitivity, the tumor cell's poor healing capacity, the tumor cell's lower oxygen tension and nutrients, and the tumor cell's increased cell cycle rate. By giving the irradiation in daily doses over weeks, the cumulative differential effects are magnified, and the therapeutic advantages are improved.

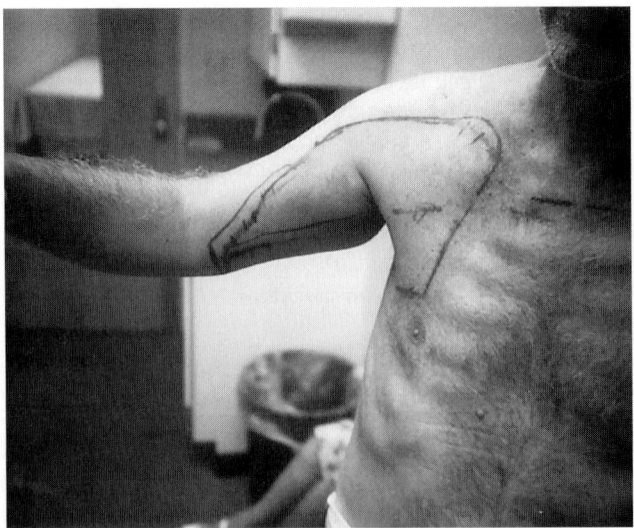

Fig. 1. Preoperative external beam irradiation. It is administered on an outpatient basis, usually once 5 days a week. The "field" of treatment is marked on the patient's skin so the tissue treated is kept constant. Often the size of the field is reduced after 30 cGy so that less normal tissue is exposed to the full irradiation dose. This is called "shrinking field treatment." This patient is approximately halfway through his preoperative irradiation for a soft-tissue sarcoma in his axilla.

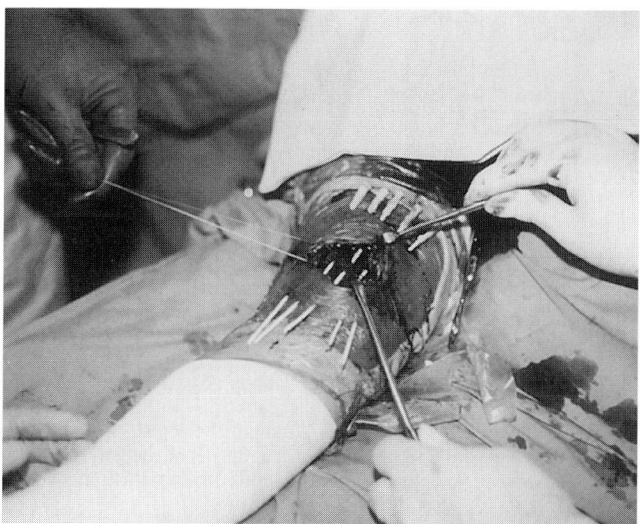

Fig. 2. Brachytherapy. It is used to shorten the time needed to administer the irradiation. As illustrated by this photograph, catheters are placed in the wound after the tumor has been resected. Careful measurements are needed at the time of catheter placement so all tissue can be treated afterward. The wound is closed, and radioactive beads are placed within the catheters. After the radioactive beads have been removed, the catheters are pulled from the wound.

Normal cells and tumor cells are capable of repairing the damage done by irradiation. Normal cells have greater healing capacity than do tumor cells; this allows the radiation oncologist to administer lethal doses of irradiation to the tumor without doing irreparable damage to the adjacent normal tissues. Spacing the treatments by a minimum of 6 hours and usually 24 hours optimizes the difference in healing potentials between tumor and normal cells. Another disadvantage tumor cells have that permits irradiation to do more damage to them than to normal cells is that tumor cells are more likely to be in a vulnerable part of their cell cycle. Cells are most resistant to irradiation during the S-phase, whereas those in the late G2 phase and undergoing mitosis are the most sensitive. Because tumor cells are generally more likely to be in late G2 or mitosis at any one time, more of the tumor cells will be damaged. Local factors affect the irradiation sensitivity of tissues. For example, increased oxygen tension increases the sensitivity of the cells to radiation, and hypoxia reduces a cell's sensitivity to radiation.

It is not understood why some tumors are inherently more sensitive to irradiation than others, but clinical experience has clearly demonstrated differences. Myeloma tumor cells, for instance, are exquisitely sensitive to irradiation, whereas the cells of a chondrosarcoma are much more resistant. All cells are affected by irradiation; if enough irradiation is given, all cells will be irreparably damaged, but the concepts of "resistance" and "sensitivity" refer to the relative effect of therapeutic doses of irradiation. Some tumors are thought to be resistant because they do not shrink with irradiation, but the cells are clinically sensitive. Their solid matrix prevents shrinkage. Osteosarcoma is an example. Although osteosarcoma cells are as sensitive to irradiation as breast cancer cells, the osteosarcoma usually does not reduce in size due to its solid matrix. (Neither

osteosarcoma nor breast cancer is cured with irradiation alone.) Additional experience and research are needed to more thoroughly explore sensitivity of specific cell types.

Musculoskeletal tumors that are considered sensitive to irradiation and that are often treated with irradiation alone are plasmacytoma/myeloma, lymphoma of bone, Ewing's sarcoma, giant cell tumor of bone, hemangioendothelioma, and Langerhans' cell histiocytosis.

Musculoskeletal tumors that are considered resistant to irradiation and that are rarely treated with irradiation, even as an adjuvant to surgery, are chondrosarcoma and osteosarcoma.

All other tumors of the musculoskeletal system are considered sensitive enough to irradiation that irradiation is often used as an adjuvant to surgery but not as the primary treatment.

The more irradiation given, the more tumor cells killed, but the higher the dose, the more the damage to normal tissues. Therefore, the dose administered needs to be selected to optimize the chance of curing the tumor while doing the least amount of damage to the normal tissues within the field of treatment. Figure 3 shows the relationship between dosage for cure and dosage for complications. The therapeutic range of treatment is the dose that achieves the highest point on the cure curve while keeping the risk of complications as low as possible.

ADJUVANT IRRADIATION

Adjuvant treatment with irradiation, in conjunction with surgery, can be given before the operation (preoperative), during the operation (intraoperative), after the operation (postoperative), or a combination of these.[5–10] The most common time when irradiation is given as adjuvant is after the operation (postoperative irradiation), but most radiation oncologists prefer to give the irradiation before the operation (preoperative irradiation). The single most important benefit of preoperative irradiation is the ability to tailor the treatment to the limits of the tumor rather than having to treat the entire operative field, which is considerably larger than the tumor. Preoperative irradiation doses can be lower than postoperative irradiation doses; theoretically, preoperative irradiation reduces the risk of releasing tumor cells into the blood stream from the mechanical pressure that occurs during surgical removal. Also, irradiated cells are less likely to be able to survive and metastasize, as compared with nonirradiated cells. The principal disadvantage of preoperative irradiation is the adverse effects of irradiation on wound healing. Operating on an irradiated extremity is associated with more postoperative wound complications as compared with operations done on nonirradiated tissue. The majority of wound complications are managed with minimal difficulty, but they do add to the patient's morbidity level. When preoperative irradiation is used, it is best to wait for at least 2 weeks before doing an operation.

Intraoperative irradiation is indicated when the operative bed needs adjuvant irradiation and there are adjacent normal structures that are in the way of conventional external beam irradiation. Usually, this is encountered with retroperitoneal tumors where the bowel lies between the source of irradiation and the tumor. The surgeon opens the abdomen and resects the tumor. Then the patient is given a

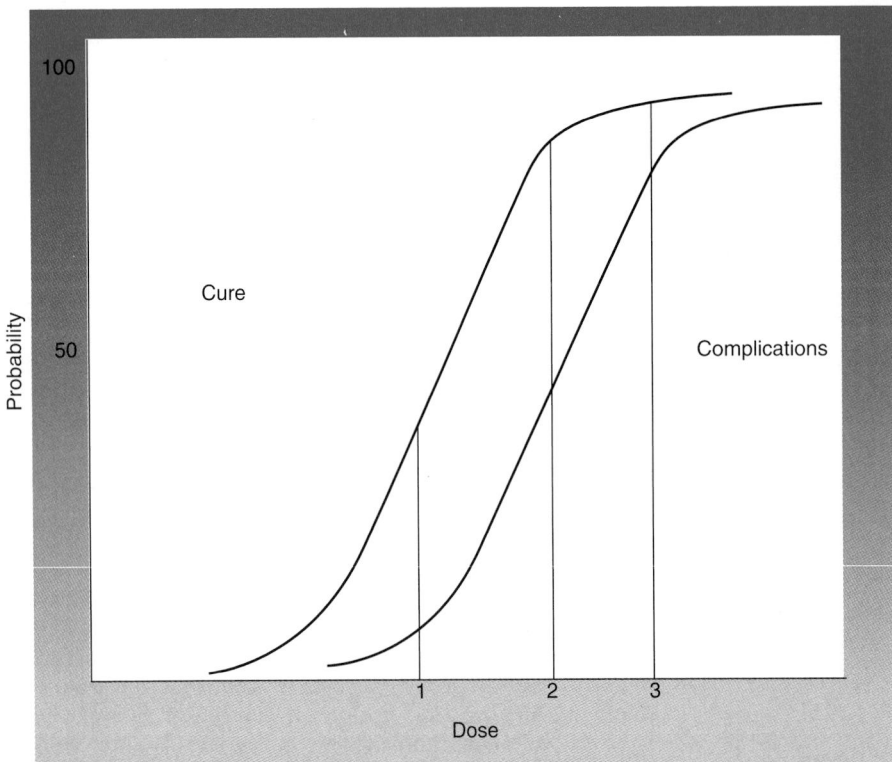

Fig. 3. These curves show the relationship between risk for cure and risk for complications. Higher doses are associated with higher cures and more complications. By selecting the optimum dose for a particular situation, the radiation oncologist can offer the patient the best chance for cure with the least risk. In this illustration, dose 2 is the best.

single large dose of irradiation with the bowels held out of the irradiation field. Additional conventional external beam irradiation is usually given either before the surgery or after the operation.[11]

IRRADIATION FOR SOFT-TISSUE SARCOMAS

Rhabdomyosarcoma, particularly of the head, neck, or genitourinary system, is often treated with irradiation and is considered sensitive to irradiation. As much of the tumor as possible is removed, and irradiation is used only for close, or positive, margins. Until the late 1960s, other soft-tissue sarcomas were considered resistant to irradiation. In the 1960s some radiation oncologists used irradiation as a means of controlling large inoperable soft-tissue sarcomas and found them to be sensitive to irradiation. These early results were encouraging and led to the use of adjuvant irradiation in conjunction with nonamputative surgery for soft-tissue sarcoma of the extremities. Adjuvant irradiation is now an accepted method of treating soft-tissue sarcoma and allows limb salvage in most patients with less than 5% prevalence of local recurrence.[8] Adjuvant irradiation for soft-tissue sarcoma can be given preoperatively or postoperatively. When given preoperatively, the dose is usually between 50 Gy and 55 Gy (Fig. 4). A higher preoperative dose leads to an unacceptable incidence and severity of complications. When irradiation is given postoperatively, the dosage given is at least 60 Gy and often 65 Gy.

External Beam Technique. The administration of irradiation to an extremity must be done carefully to reduce the risk of complications. Originally this was not appreciated, and circumferential irradiation was frequently used. This led to a high incidence of circumferential fibrosis and distal edema. Now a longitudinal strip of tissue along the extremity is spared from irradiation. This allows adequate lymphatic drainage and has effectively eliminated the incidence of circumferential fibrosis. Giving the irradiation from different directions while the beam concentrates on the tumor reduces the dose to uninvolved normal tissues while exposing the tumor to the full dose. Usually, approximately 180 cGy is given each day, 5 days a week. Accelerated courses can be given by administering treatment twice a

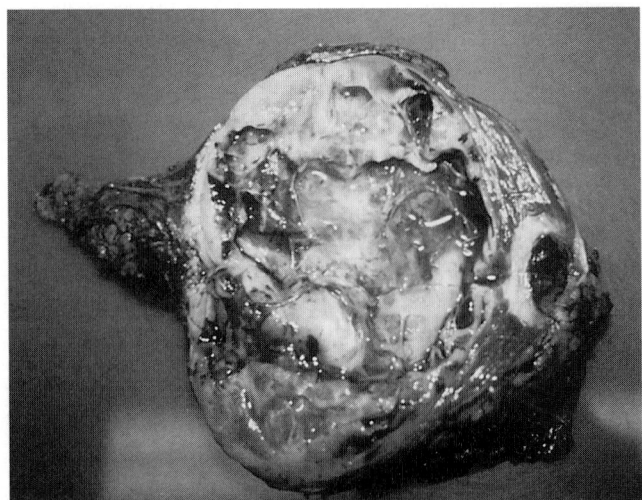

Fig. 4. Soft-tissue sarcoma. It was resected after preoperative irradiation. The majority of the tumor is necrotic. The periphery has thickened, and the adjacent muscles are less inflamed than before irradiation. The relatively close surgical margin is associated with less than 5% local recurrence when preoperative irradiation is used.

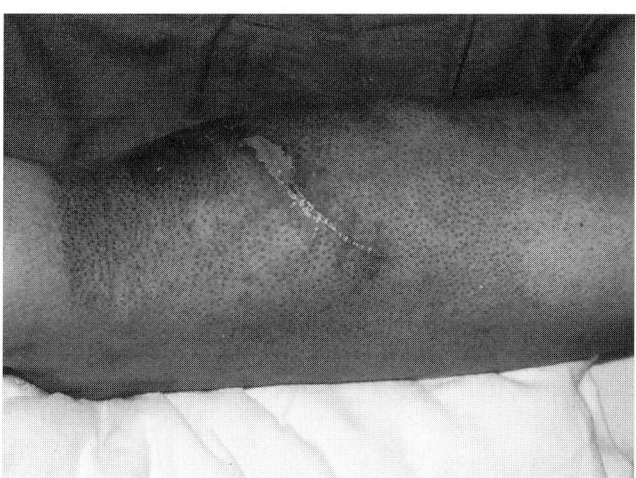

Fig. 5. This patient completed preoperative irradiation 2 weeks before this photograph. Immediately after treatment, there were blisters along his biopsy incision that cleared without specific treatment. The skin is still not completely recovered; in our experience, 2 to 3 weeks after preoperative irradiation is usually sufficient time for the tissue to recover enough to tolerate surgery.

day, separated by 6 to 8 hours. This is associated with more local inflammation during the treatment. Most patients notice mild generalized fatigue during the first week of treatment, but this passes spontaneously. After 4 or 5 weeks, some patients develop skin erythema and, occasionally, blistering, but this heals within 7 to 10 days after treatment is discontinued (Fig. 5). Unless blistering is severe, treatment is not suspended until the entire planned dose is given.

Extra-abdominal desmoid (aggressive fibromatosis) is also treated with irradiation, either primarily or in conjunction with operation.[12, 13] These locally aggressive but benign soft-tissue tumors are difficult to control. Irradiation

has been used as a primary treatment for inoperable lesions or as an adjuvant for lesions that have been only partially removed or for those that have recurred. Patients who have a resection with negative margins do not need adjuvant irradiation.

IRRADIATION FOR BONE TUMORS

Patients with eosinophilic granuloma can be treated with low doses (lower than 15 Gy) of irradiation and expect a high incidence rate of control. In general, irradiation is used only for patients with a recurrent eosinophilic granuloma, patients with cord compression from eosinophilic granuloma, or adults with resistant painful lesions caused by eosinophilic granuloma. Lymphoma and myeloma are malignant bone lesions that are treated with irradiation with or without chemotherapy. The recommended dosage is between 55 and 65 Gy. Irradiation was considered the treatment of choice for Ewing's sarcoma until adjuvant chemotherapy began to improve the overall survival rate of these patients. Ewing's sarcoma is considered a "radiosensitive" neoplasm and does respond by shrinking, but the risk of local recurrence is debated. Many retrospective reviews suggest that surgical resection is associated with a better overall survival rate.[14] Currently, operation is the treatment of choice for a primary Ewing sarcoma, but irradiation can be used for tumors that are not amenable to resection (e.g., spine). Other sarcomas of bone are considered "radio-resistant," but irradiation may be used as an adjuvant when a complete surgical resection is not possible or when the chance of morbidity of the resection is greater than the patient will accept.

Irradiation can be of significant benefit to a patient with a musculoskeletal tumor. Often, it allows limb salvage when an amputation would otherwise be necessary. Some tumors that occur in the skeleton can be treated with irradiation alone, saving the patient a major resective surgery. It is important that the orthopaedist understand the use of irradiation for musculoskeletal neoplasia.

REFERENCES

1. Delannes M, Thomas L, Martel P, et al: Low-dose-rate intraoperative brachytherapy combined with external beam irradiation in the conservative treatment of soft tissue sarcoma. Int J Radiat Oncol Biol Phys 2000; 47:165.
2. Habrand JL, Gerbaules A, Pejouvic MH, et al: Twenty years' experience of interstitial iridium brachytherapy in the management of soft tissue sarcomas. Int J Radiat Oncol Biol Phys 1991; 20:405.
3. Schray MRF, Gunderson LL, Sim FH, et al: Soft tissue sarcoma: Integration of brachytherapy, resection, and external irradiation. Cancer 1990; 66:451.
4. Spiro I, Suit H: Introduction to Radiation Therapy. In Simon M, Springfield D (eds): Surgery for Bone and Soft-Tissue Tumors. Philadelphia, Lippincott-Raven Publishers, 1998.
5. Cheng EY, Dusenbery KE, Winters MR,

et al: Soft tissue sarcomas: Preoperative versus postoperative radiotherapy. J Surg Oncol 1996; 61:90.
6. Mundt AJ, Awan A, Sibley GS, et al: Conservative surgery and adjuvant radiation therapy in the management of adult soft tissue sarcoma of the extremities: Clinical and radiobiological results. Int J Radiat Oncol Biol Phys 1995; 32:977.
7. Pao WJ, Pilepich MV: Postoperative radiotherapy in the treatment of extremity soft tissue sarcomas. Int J Radiat Oncol Biol Phys 1990; 19:907.
8. Sadoski C, Suit HD, Rosenberg A, et al: Preoperative radiation, surgical margins, and local control of extremity sarcomas of soft tissues. J Surg Oncol 1993; 52:223.
9. Tepper JE, Suit HD: Radiation therapy of soft tissue sarcomas. Cancer 1985; 22:73.
10. Wanebo HJ, Temple WJ, Popp MB, et al:

Preoperative regional therapy for extremity sarcoma: A tricenter update. Cancer 1995; 75:2299.
11. Alektiar KM, Hu K, Andderson L, et al: High-dose-rate intraoperative radiation therapy (HDR-IORT) for retroperitoneal sarcomas. Int J Radiat Oncol Biol Phys 2000; 47:157.
12. Ballo MT, Zagars GK, Pollack A, et al: Desmoid tumor: Prognostic factors and outcome after surgery, radiation therapy, or combined surgery and radiation therapy. J Clin Oncol 1999; 17:158.
13. Goy BW, Lee SP, Eilber F, et al: The role of adjuvant radiotherapy in the treatment of resectable desmoid tumors. In J Radiat Oncol Biol Phys 1997; 39:659.
14. O'Connor MI, Pritchard DJ: Ewing's sarcoma: Prognostic factors, disease control, and the reemerging role of surgical treatment. Clin Orthop 1991; 262:78.

CHEMOTHERAPY

Linda Granowetter

section 7 chapter 4

Summary
- Bone and soft-tissue sarcomas are a diverse group.
- Adequate biopsy sampling for histological, immunochemical, cytogenetic, and biological studies is essential for determining appropriate treatment regimens.
- Adjuvant chemotherapy is recommended for Ewing's sarcoma, high-grade sarcoma, and rhabdomyosarcoma.
- The role of chemotherapy for nonrhabdomyosarcoma soft-tissue sarcomas is less clear but may be appropriate for high-grade and/or advanced tumors.

Sarcomas of bone and soft tissue are relatively rare tumors, but they comprise nearly 15% of childhood cancers. Among adults, bone and soft-tissue sarcomas comprise only 1% of all malignancies. Osteosarcoma, Ewing's sarcoma, and rhabdomyosarcoma are most common in adolescents and young adults, whereas chondrosarcoma and the soft-tissue sarcomas, with the exception of rhabdomyosarcoma, are more common in adults. The relative infrequency of these tumors makes clinical research difficult. Nonetheless, through multicenter, randomized clinical trials, remarkable success in the treatment of many sarcomas using adjuvant and neoadjuvant chemotherapy is one of the more exciting advances in the treatment of cancer in the last quarter century. Multidisciplinary approaches to the treatment of these tumors have resulted in excellent cure rates. For example, in 1975 a young adult presenting with an osteosarcoma of the extremity without evidence of metastatic disease would most likely be treated with amputation and, despite radical surgery, would have a 60% to 80% chance of developing metastases and dying. With chemotherapy, 75% of patients with nonmetastatic osteosarcoma

are cured. The goal of this chapter is to discuss the role of chemotherapy in the treatment of bone and soft sarcomas and to summarize the expectations for cure.

METHOD OF TREATMENT

Multidisciplinary interaction is essential in the treatment of a patient with a sarcoma. It is imperative that the orthopaedist be in communication with the diagnostic radiologist, the oncologist, and the pathologist as soon as the diagnosis of sarcoma is entertained. In the absence of the correct pathological diagnosis, chemotherapy cannot be given. A biopsy sample provides the tissue for essential histology and immunohistochemical, cytogenetic, and/or molecular studies. Many sarcomas are now characterized by distinct cytogenetic aberrations (Table 1). These cytogenetic variations are not only helpful in diagnosis, but there is also a growing body of data suggesting that specific molecular variations among histological subtypes of sarcoma may be associated with different outcomes.[1, 2] Although specific chemotherapy is not yet based on the demonstration of molecular markers, it is imperative that we continue to expand our knowledge of molecular and cytogenetic variations among histologically similar tumors, and it is likely that in the very near future molecular phenotypes will guide the management of these patients.

Another reason for coordination of planning before biopsy sampling is that for some sarcomas, such as those comprising the Ewing's sarcoma family, complete staging requires bone marrow aspirates and biopsies. These studies can be performed at the time of the diagnostic biopsy. In some instances, imaging studies point so clearly to a sarcoma that will be treated with chemotherapy that it is possible to place indwelling central venous access at the time of the biopsy. In order to facilitate these procedures, the orthopaedic surgeon must work with the imaging specialist, the pathologist, and the oncologist.

TABLE 1. EXAMPLES OF CYTOGENETIC ABNORMALITIES IN BONE AND SOFT TISSUE SARCOMAS				
Tumor	Translocation	Fusion Gene	%	Possible Implications
ESFT[1]	t(11;22)(q24;q12)	EWS/FLI1	97	Most common, best prognosis
ESFT	t(21;22)(q22;q22)	EWS/ERG	2	Possibly poorer prognosis
ESFT	t(7;22)(p22;q12)	EWS/ETV-1 EWS/E1A-F	2	Possibly poorer prognosis
RMS[2]	t(2;13)(q35;q14)	PAX3-FKHR	95	Better prognosis
RMS	t(1;13)(p36;q14)	PAX7-FKHR	5	Poorer prognosis
Synovial Sarcoma	t(X;18)(p11.2;q11.2)	SYT-SSX	?	unknown

[1] ESFT = Ewing's sarcoma family of tumors
[2] RMS = Rhabdomyosarcoma

TABLE 2. EXAMPLES OF ESTABLISHED CHEMOTHERAPY REGIMENS FOR SARCOMAS

Sarcoma	Chemotherapy Agents	5-year Survival
Osteosarcoma non-metastatic	High-dose methotrexate Cisplatin Doxorubicin +/− Ifosfamide	75%
Ewing's sarcoma bone and soft tissue	Vincristine Doxorubicin Cyclophosphamide Ifosfamide Etoposide	60%–65%
Rhabdomyosarcoma nonmetastatic extremity	Vincristine Actinomycin-D Cyclophosphamide	65%

Not all sarcomas should be resected before chemotherapy. Ewing's sarcoma, osteosarcoma, and rhabdomyosarcoma have been shown to be particularly chemotherapy-sensitive; extensive resection before chemotherapy is often not indicated. Chemotherapy for osteosarcoma usually facilitates limb-sparing surgery and does not result in an increased risk of chemotherapy resistance. For Ewing's sarcoma, chemotherapy before surgical resection or irradiation of the primary lesion is the standard of care. The standard of care for rhabdomyosarcoma is total resection before chemotherapy when possible; however, in selected patients, chemotherapy and/or radiation therapy is appropriate before resection to avoid excessively morbid surgery, particularly an amputation.[3, 4]

ROLE OF CHEMOTHERAPY

Adjuvant chemotherapy is clearly established for osteosarcoma of bone, Ewing sarcoma of bone and soft tissue, and rhabdomyosarcoma. For the large group of nonrhabdomyosarcoma sarcomas of soft tissue, the indications for chemotherapy are less clear. In general, adjuvant chemotherapy is restricted to high-grade sarcomas with a propensity for metastasis, in which chemosensitivity has been documented. Table 2 lists the more common sarcomas and the role of chemotherapy for these sarcomas. Table 3 lists the chemotherapy agents most commonly used and the most common side effects associated with these agents. Following is a more detailed discussion of chemotherapy for the sarcomas in which chemotherapy is the standard of care.

OSTEOSARCOMA

The peak incidence of osteosarcoma occurs in the second decade of life. With the exception of radiation-induced osteosarcoma and osteosarcoma secondary to Paget's disease, the majority of osteosarcomas occur in adolescents. Patients with low-grade or parosteal osteosarcoma should be treated with surgery alone. However, the majority of osteosarcoma patients have high-grade osteosarcoma; they should be treated with chemotherapy. At presentation, approximately 85% of patients with osteosarcoma have no evidence of metastatic disease. When metastases occur, the most common site is lung, followed by bone. If patients with nonmetastatic osteosarcoma are treated with surgery alone, 50% will develop pulmonary metastases within 6 months of initial surgery, and as many as 80% will eventually succumb to pulmonary metastases. Irradiation is not used in the treatment of osteosarcoma.[5]

In the late 1970s osteosarcoma was demonstrated to be sensitive to chemotherapy. The history of the use of chemotherapy for osteosarcoma included an era of significant controversy. Some centers reported significant survival rates (20% to 40%) with surgery alone. Thus, in the early 1980s, some clinicians believed that chemotherapy should be reserved for patients who developed metastases, whereas others believed that chemotherapy should be used as adju-

TABLE 3. SOME COMMON TOXICITIES OF CHEMOTHERAPEUTIC AGENTS

Chemotherapeutic Agent	Common Early and Transient Effects	Late Effects
Vincristine	Constipation Numbness of fingers/toes Jaw pain Bone pain	
Doxorubicin	Myelosuppression Mucositis	Potential cardiomyopathy
Cyclophosphamide	Myelosuppression Syndrome of inappropriate antidiuretic hormone Hemorrhagic cystitis	Secondary leukemia (rare) Infertility
High-dose methotrexate	Mucositis Renal dysfunction Liver dysfunction	
Ifosfamide	Myelosuppression Fanconi's syndrome Hemorrhagic cystitis	Secondary leukemia (rare) Infertility
Etoposide	Myelosuppression Allergy-anaphylaxis	Secondary leukemia (rare)
Cisplatin	Renal dysfunction Tinnitus Neuropathy	Hearing loss Renal dysfunction Infertility (uncommon)

vant therapy after definitive surgery. At that time there was increasing interest in limb-sparing surgery, and neoadjuvant chemotherapy (chemotherapy given before resection) was introduced.

The Multi-Institution Osteosarcoma Trial was designed to compare treatment with chemotherapy after surgery with the same therapy given only at relapse. Patients without metastases at diagnosis were eligible for this trial after resection or amputation. This trial demonstrated that although many patients could be salvaged with aggressive surgery and chemotherapy after relapse, disease-free survival was dramatically improved in patients who received neoadjuvant chemotherapy.[6, 7]

Today, the standard of care for osteosarcoma patients is "induction" (neoadjuvant) chemotherapy, generally for 2 months, followed by surgical resection and then chemotherapy for 6 to 8 months. Although there is a variety of chemotherapy protocols, the agents included in virtually all regimens are high-dose methotrexate, cisplatin, and doxorubicin. Ifosfamide and ifosfamide with etoposide have also been shown to be useful in the treatment of osteosarcoma, but increased survival when these agents are used in initial therapy has not yet been documented. Current treatment programs in the United States and Europe for osteosarcoma are investigating these agents.

There is a direct correlation between the percent necrosis of an osteosarcoma and the survival of the patient. To date, no improvement in survival has been documented with alteration in the drugs or doses used postoperatively for patients whose osteosarcoma had limited necrosis, but current regimens are investigating the role of intensified chemotherapy for those patients who have demonstrated less than good histological response and are evaluating biological predictors of response.

Patients with metastatic osteosarcoma at diagnosis have a less sanguine prognosis; however, chemotherapy followed by aggressive resection of the primary tumor and metastases when possible may result in survival. Patients with fewer than five resected pulmonary nodules and no bone metastases have survival rates of close to 40%.

EWING'S SARCOMA

The Ewing sarcoma family of tumors consists of Ewing's sarcoma and primitive peripheral neuroectodermal tumors (PNET). These tumors occur mainly in bone but may occur in soft tissue. For many years, Ewing's sarcoma and PNET soft-tissue tumors were not treated with the same regimens as the more common bone tumors; however, with the recognition of the shared molecular characteristics[8] of these tumors and neuroectodermal derivation of these tumors, current treatment regimens are similar for bone and soft-tissue variants. The natural history of the Ewing sarcoma bone tumors is that less than 10% of patients who have no clinical evidence of metastasis at the time of diagnosis survive when treated with surgery and/or radiation, without chemotherapy. The most common sites of metastases are lung, bone, and bone marrow. Multiagent chemotherapy regimens produced dramatically improved survival, with 5-year disease-free survival rates of close to 60% by the early 1980s.[9] Regimens including vincristine, actinomycin D, doxorubicin, and cyclophosphamide were the most ef-

fective early protocols. More recently, ifosfamide and etoposide have been demonstrated to be superior to earlier regimens.[10] Current treatment regimens for Ewing sarcoma include vincristine, doxorubicin, and cyclophosphamide alternating with ifosfamide and etoposide for 9 to 12 weeks before definitive local control, which may be radiation therapy or surgery. This is followed by ongoing chemotherapy for 6 to 12 months.

Patients with metastases at the time of diagnosis have a worse prognosis; however, patients with pulmonary metastases alone may have survival rates as high as 40% when treated with radiation to the lungs, aggressive local control, and chemotherapy. Patients with bone metastases at diagnosis have a worse prognosis, but aggressive chemotherapy and local control will result in some survivors.[11]

RHABDOMYOSARCOMA

Rhabdomyosarcoma is a soft-tissue sarcoma of protean manifestations: one-third of patients have disease in the head and neck; one-third have it in the trunk (usually, the genitourinary system), and one-third have it in an extremity. As with all sarcomas, metastasis at presentation is a bad prognostic feature. The most common site of metastasis is lung. Patients with a primary rhabdomyosarcoma in an extremity not infrequently have regional lymph nodes. Specific histological subtypes are also prognostic variables. Patients with alveolar rhabdomyosarcoma have a relatively poor survival rate compared with those with embryonal rhabdomyosarcoma. Rhabdomyosarcoma of the extremity is most often alveolar and, thus, generally high-risk. All patients with rhabdomyosarcoma should be treated aggressively with surgery and chemotherapy. The agents shown to be most effective against rhabdomyosarcoma in the pediatric intergroup rhabdomyosarcoma studies are vincristine, cyclophosphamide, and actinomycin D. Although doxorubicin, cisplatin, ifosfamide, and ifosfamide plus etoposide regimens have all shown efficacy, they have not been shown to improve survival when compared with vincristine, cyclophosphamide, and actinomycin D in prospective randomized trials in pediatrics.[12] Regimens such as doxorubicin, ifosfamide, and DTIC have been demonstrated to be useful in the rare adult rhabdomyosarcoma.[13]

NONRHABDOMYOSARCOMA SOFT-TISSUE SARCOMAS

Biologically, the nonrhabdomyosarcoma soft-tissue sarcomas are a diverse group of tumors.[14, 15] However, due to the rarity of these tumors, chemotherapy trials do not distinguish among the varying kinds of tumors. Studies comparing the survival of patients treated with adjuvant chemotherapy with that of historical control patients for whom chemotherapy was not employed suggest a role for adjuvant chemotherapy. However, randomized trials have not consistently demonstrated overall survival benefits for patients treated with adjuvant chemotherapy. Patients with nonmetastatic, fully resected, small tumors (smaller than 5 cm) are generally not considered candidates for therapy. Adult patients with high-grade tumors that are not resectable or for whom radiation is considered inappropriate may be candidates for chemotherapy in the context of clinical trials. In pediatrics, patients with nonrhabdomyosarcoma tumors generally have a better outlook than their adult counterparts, with over 80% survival after 5 years.[16] Factors associated with lower event-free survival are tumor size smaller than 5 cm, high histological grade, intra-abdominal primary tumor, and microscopic disease after resection. The administration of adjuvant chemotherapy and the absence or presence of microscopic residual after surgery did not correlate with the occurrence of metastatic disease. In pediatric trials, patients with completely resected tumors have not been shown to benefit from chemotherapy. Those with microscopic residual may be treated with radiation therapy. If chemotherapy is shown to be useful for patients with metastatic disease or in the adjuvant setting, future clinical trials may include chemotherapy for patients at high risk of metastatic disease, such as those with high histological grade or large tumor size.

CONCLUSION

Successful chemotherapy regimens have been clearly established for osteosarcoma, the Ewing sarcoma family of tumors, and rhabdomyosarcoma. The role of chemotherapy in the treatment of adult and pediatric nonrhabdomyosarcoma soft-tissue sarcomas remains controversial. Clinical trials for patients with soft-tissue sarcoma are necessary to define the role of chemotherapy for patients with advanced, unresectable, or high-grade disease. Future chemotherapy regimens for these patients will incorporate information learned about the prognosis of these tumors based on molecular classifications and will allow better tailored chemotherapy regimens.[17] Ultimately, it is hoped that new avenues of treatment will be based on biological markers, such as molecular subtype of tumor.

REFERENCES

1. Kelly KM, Womer RB, Sorensen PH, et al: Common and variant gene fusions predict distinct clinical phenotypes in rhabdomyosarcoma. J Clin Oncol 15; 1831, 1997.

2. de Alava E, Kawai A, Healey JH, et al: EWS-FLI1 fusion transcript structure is an independent determinant of prognosis in Ewing's sarcoma. J Clin Oncol 16; 1248, 1998.

3. Baker LH, Bierman S: NCCN Practice Guidelines: Bone Cancers. NCCN Proceedings Oncol 1999:365.

4. Antman KH: Adjuvant therapy of sarcomas of soft tissue. Semin Oncol 24; 556, 1997.

5. Meyers PA, Gorlick R: Osteosarcoma. Pediatr Clin North Am 44; 973, 1997.

6. Link MP, Goorin AM, Miser AW, et al: The effect of adjuvant chemotherapy on relapse-free survival in patients with osteosarcoma of the extremity. N Engl J Med 314; 1601, 1986.

7. Link MP, Goorin AM, Horowitz M, et al: Adjuvant chemotherapy of relapse-free survival high-grade osteosarcoma of the extremity. Clin Orthop 270; 8, 1991.

8. Delattre O, Zucman J, Melot T, et al: The Ewing family of tumors: A subgroup of small-round-cell-tumors defined by specific chimeric transcripts. N Engl J Med 331; 294, 1994.

9. Granowetter L, West DC: The Ewing's sarcoma family of tumors: Ewing's sarcoma and peripheral primitive neuroectodermal tumor of bone and soft tissue. In Walterhouse DO, Cohn SL (eds): Diagnostic and Therapeutic Advances in Pediatric Oncology. Boston, Kluwer, 1997, p 254.

10. Grier H, Krailo M, Link M, et al: Improved outcome in nonmetastatic Ewing's sarcoma and PNET of bone with the addition of ifosfamide and etoposide to vincristine, adriamycin, cyclophosphamide, and actinomycin: A Children's Cancer Group and Pediatric Oncology Group report (abstract). Proc Am Soc Clin Oncol 13; 421, 1994.

11. Ladenstein R, Lasset C, Pinkerton R, et al: Impact of megatherapy (MGT) in children with high-risk Ewing's tumors in complete remission: A report from the EBMT solid tumor registry. Bone Marrow Transplant 15; 697, 1995.

12. Pappo AS, Shapiro DN: Rhabdomyosarcoma: Biology and therapy. In Walterhouse DO, Cohn SL (eds): Diagnostic and Therapeutic Advances in Pediatric Oncology. Boston, Kluwer, 1997, p 309.

13. Antman K, Crowley J, Balcerzak SP, et al: A Southwest Oncology Group and Cancer and Leukemia Group B phase II study of doxorubicin, dacarbazine, ifosfamide, and mesna in adults with advanced osteosarcoma, Ewing's sarcoma, and rhabdomyosarcoma. Cancer 82; 1288, 1998.

14. Hibshoosh H, Lattes R: Immunohistochemical and molecular genetic approaches to soft tissue tumor diagnosis: A review. Semin Oncol 24; 515, 1997.

15. Zahm SH, Fraumeni JF Jr: The epidemiology of soft tissue sarcoma. Semin Oncol 24; 504, 1997.

16. Spunt SL, Poquette CA, Hurt YS, et al: Prognostic factors for children and adolescents with surgically resected nonrhabdomyosarcoma soft tissue sarcoma: An analysis of 121 patients treated at St. Jude Children's Research hospital. J Clin Oncol 17; 3697, 1999.

17. Grier H: Soft tissue sarcoma: Apples, oranges, and passion fruit. J Clin Oncol 17; 3695, 1999.

CLINICAL PRESENTATION AND RECOMMENDED EVALUATION OF A PATIENT WITH A SUSPECTED BONE TUMOR

Terrance D. Peabody

Summary
- The history, physical examination, and plain radiographs are critical in making decisions about any bone lesion. From these data, a treatment plan or further evaluation can be developed.
- Often a specific diagnosis can be made without additional information.
- When a specific diagnosis cannot be made, additional radiographic tests are usually necessary before taking a biopsy sample.
- The biopsy is the last test to be done in most circumstances.

Within orthopaedic surgery, the variability of symptoms and physical findings in patients diagnosed with a "bone tumor" is matched only by the heterogeneous appearance, unclear cause, and unpredictable behavior of these lesions. Fortunately, true bone neoplasms are rare.[1] Most radiographic abnormalities are post-traumatic or inflammatory. Many are noted incidentally on imaging studies performed for an unrelated condition. In addition, many "bone tumors" may be considered by some surgeons to be more developmental (e.g., osteochondroma, nonossifying fibroma) or reparative (e.g., aneurysmal bone cyst) than neoplastic.

The problem is that the rarely encountered primary bone malignancy is both limb-threatening and requires aggressive systemic medical therapy and radical operative procedures for preservation of life. The challenge, then, is for the orthopaedic surgeon to be able, based on what is commonly a nonspecific patient interview, to recognize and identify a bone lesion. Based on physical examination and imaging studies, the surgeon must differentiate inflammatory or post-traumatic from neoplastic processes, benign from malignant lesions, and primary from secondary (metastatic) lesions. A consistent and organized approach, in addition to training, experience, and consultation, is necessary (Fig. 1).

PATIENT EVALUATION

In the evaluation of patients with bone tumors, the clinical history and physical examination are often nonspecific and contribute limited information to the development of a differential diagnosis.[2] The age of the patient is the single most important historical detail.[3]

As shown in Table 1,[4, 5] most neoplastic conditions have a predilection for certain age groups. Common benign neoplasms and developmental conditions, such as osteochondroma, unicameral bone cyst, chondroblastoma, histiocytosis, and osteoid osteoma, are seen in immature and growing bone. Malignant neoplasms that occur in the young skeleton include osteosarcoma, leukemia, Ewing's sarcoma, and metastatic neuroblastoma. Giant cell tumors and lymphoma are commonly diagnosed in young adults. In contrast, in patients more than 40 years of age, a malignant-appearing bone lesion is more likely to be metastatic carcinoma or myeloma than a primary bone sarcoma. Benign-appearing bone lesions noted in adults are commonly persistent neoplasms that originate in youth; e.g., enchondroma.

Patients with a bone tumor often have complaints that are nonspecific and variable. Although in most cases pain and swelling are the result of trauma or of a degenerative disorder, the surgeon must consider a neoplasm as a potential cause for these symptoms. The patient must be carefully queried about the onset of symptoms, a history of trauma, and any recent changes in activity level. The surgeon must ask about the character of the symptoms and whether there have been any changes in those symptoms over time. Aggravating factors, especially the relationship of symptoms to activities, should be noted. Anti-inflammatory medication may relieve pain from inflammatory conditions or benign conditions such as osteoid osteoma. The patient's use of high-dose narcotics should be a source of concern. Medications that alleviate the symptoms should be identified. Finally, taking a history of similar problems in the past, including documenting any previous imaging studies, is important. An imaging abnormality that is stable over time rarely needs intervention. As always, the treating surgeon must attempt to identify whether the symptoms are, in fact, referred from another part of the body. The purpose of obtaining this history is to help discern whether the underlying bone abnormality is responsible for the patient's symptoms.

It is common for a bone lesion to be noted incidentally in the course of evaluating a patient for a traumatic, degenerative, or inflammatory condition. The surgeon must attempt to sort out in detail the source of the patient's symptoms.[1] Are two conditions present? Rarely do asymptomatic lesions require operative intervention. Most of these can be observed with serial examination and imaging studies. Treatment should be directed at the underlying inflammatory or degenerative condition. In contrast, symptomatic bone lesions often require treatment. Strictly speaking, pain related to bone neoplasms is not activity-related. Pain due to neoplasms is often vague and may be severe at rest or at night. The underlying mechanism for pain is poorly understood but may be due to compromised structural integrity with eventual fracture, endosteal or periosteal expansion, prostaglandin production, or soft-tissue compression.

When pathological fracture has occurred, the patient or family should be asked whether pain or symptoms were present before the fracture. The lack of prior symptoms

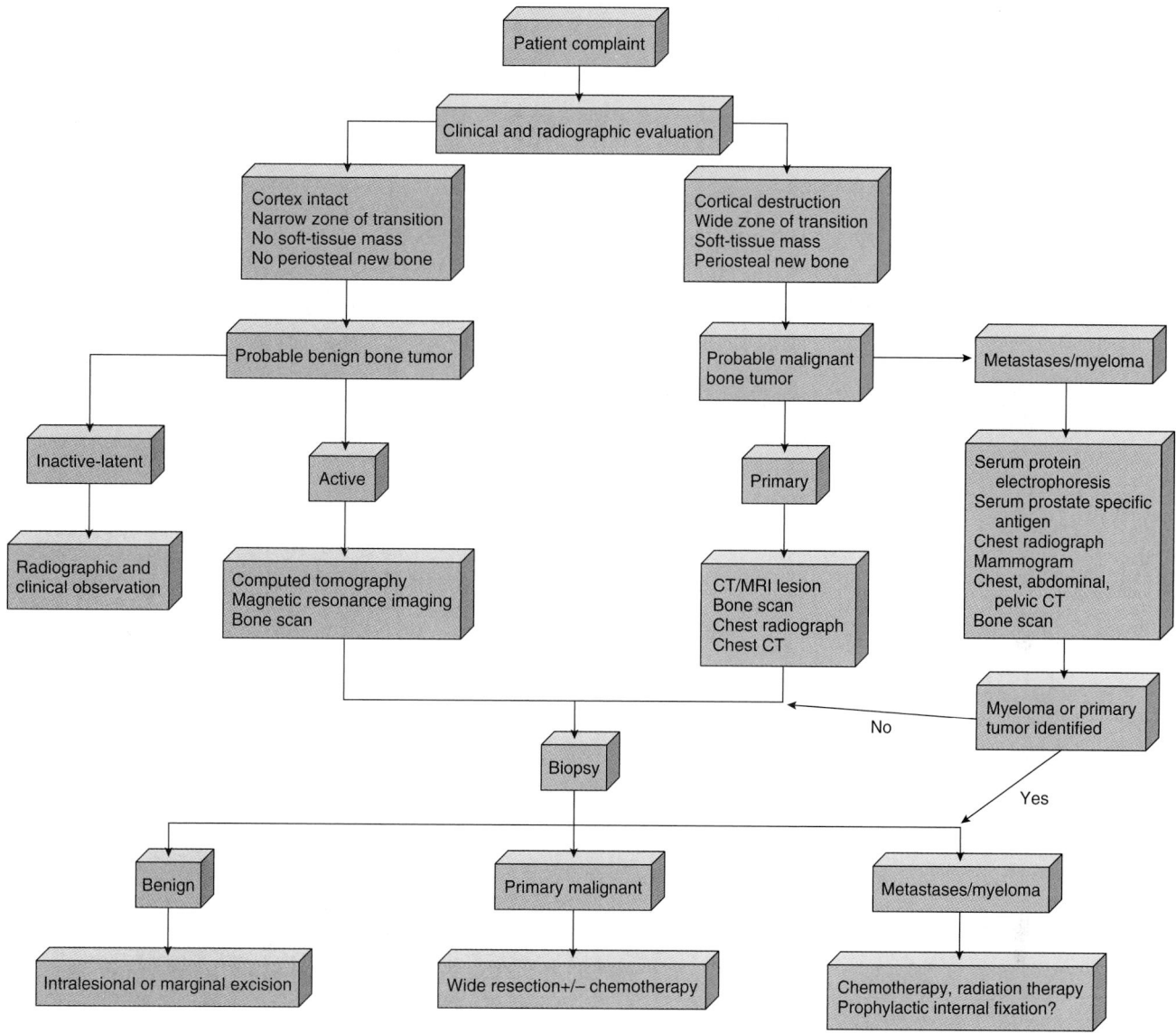

Fig. 1. Flow diagram. This is a recommended diagnostic strategy in the evaluation of a patient with a suspected bone neoplasm.

and a benign radiographic appearance will, in most instances, denote a benign cause, and it is likely that the lesion can be carefully observed and the fracture allowed to heal. A history of symptoms before fracture may indicate a more active benign or malignant process, and the surgeon may need to consider intervention in the form of a biopsy (Fig. 2).

Other systemic symptoms such as fever, weight loss, and anorexia are rarely associated with bone neoplasms and are nonspecific. They may occur in both inflammatory and neoplastic conditions but are most common in older individuals with metastatic carcinoma or advanced marrow cell tumors.

The patient's medical history is informative in cases of suspected metastatic disease or in conditions where multiple bones are involved; e.g., in multiple hereditary exostoses. Endocrine abnormalities may be seen in patients with polyostotic fibrous dysplasia (McCune-Albright syndrome) or histiocytosis (diabetes insipidus). Rarely, sarcomas are

the result of malignant degeneration of preexisting non-neoplastic disease such as Paget's disease or bone infarction. A patient's medical history and comorbidities are probably most important in assessment of the patient's ability to tolerate a particular treatment regimen. Specifically, cardiac disease and renal insufficiency will severely limit a patient's ability to tolerate chemotherapy. Severe peripheral vascular disease or uncontrolled diabetes mellitus may limit a patient's ability to tolerate the rigors of limb salvage procedures.

Because of the relative rarity of primary bone malignancies, little is known about the role of nutritional or environmental agents in the cause of this disease. One risk factor known to be associated with bone and soft-tissue sarcomas is exposure to high-dose radiation. In most cases, however, the cause of the bone neoplasm is unknown.

Few familial or heritable syndromes have been described in patients with bone tumors. Multiple hereditary exostosis

TABLE 1. BONE TUMOR CHARACTERISTICS

Histology	Age at Diagnosis (yrs)	History	Location	Radiographic Characteristics	Bone Scan	Computed Tomography	Magnetic Resonance Imaging	Clinical Syndrome	Malignant Potential
Osteochondroma	5–25	Painless, firm mass, skeletally immature inflammed bursa	Metaphyseal, long bone	Broad-based or pedunculated exostosis apex away from joint	Positive	Absence of cortical bone destruction	Marrow continuous with underlying bones	Multiple hereditary exostoses, autosomal dominant	Extremely rare in solitary disease, up to 10% in multiple disease, heralded by growth and pain in adulthood
Enchondroma	20–40	Common incidental radiographic finding	Metaphyseal, long bones or small bones of hands and feet	Radiolucency, narrow zone of transition, internal calcification (punctate), little endosteal scalloping except small bones	Positive	Punctate calcification, minimal endosteal scalloping	May contain low-signal areas, no soft-tissue mass	Dyschondroplasia (Ollier's disease) associated with hemangiomas (Maffucci's)	Rare, higher with multiple disease
Chondrosarcoma	40–60	Pain, swelling, mass	Axial skeleton	Radiolucency, punctate calcification, cortical bone destruction, wide zone of transition	Positive	Punctate calcification, minimal endosteal scalloping	May contain low-signal areas, no soft-tissue mass	Same as enchondroma	N/A
Chondroblastoma	10–30	Pain (joint)	Epiphyseal, humerus, distal femur, proximal tibia	Radiolucency, narrow zone of transition, punctate calcification may be seen	Positive	Punctate calcification	Nonspecific	None	None
Chondromyxoid Fibroma	10–30	Pain	Metaphyseal, long bones, pelvis	Radiolucency, eccentric	Positive	"Expanded" periosteum	Nonspecific	None	N/A
Giant Cell Tumor	25–45	Pain (joint or spine)	Epiphyseal, distal femur, proximal tibia, spine	Radiolucent, wide zone of transition, septated cortical destruction	Positive (halo)	Cortical bone destruction, abnormal marrow	Soft-tissue mass	Differentiate from hyperparathyroidism (Brown's tumor)	N/A
Aneurysmal Bone Cyst	10–30	Pain, swelling	Metaphysis, long bones	Radiolucency, expanded bone, narrow zone of transition, internal septation	Positive (halo)	Expanded rim of cortical bone	Fluid-fluid levels	May be secondary to other benign tumors	N/A
Unicameral Bone Cyst	5–25	Pathological fracture	Metaphysis, long bones	Radiolucency, central cortex expanded, fallen leaf sign, septated	Positive (halo)	Expanded rim of bone, septations	Signal changes consistent with fluid	N/A	N/A
Fibrous Dysplasia	15–35	Pain, deformity	Metadiaphyseal, may be polyostotic	Narrow zone of transition, radiolucent, ground-glass appearance, shepherd's crook deformity	Positive	Ground-glass appearance	Nonspecific, no soft-tissue mass	Endocrine abnormalities, café-au-lait spots (McCune-Albright syndrome)	Very low
Osteoid Osteoma	5–25	Night pain relieved with ASA, NSAID	Diaphyseal, long bone, posterior elements spine	Radiolucent nidus (small), surrounding cortical thickening	Positive	Central radiolucent nidus	Extensive inflammation	N/A	None

Tumor	Age	Symptoms	Location	Radiographic					
Osteoblastoma	10–30	Pain	Spine, posterior elements flat bones	Radiopaque, mature periosteum	Positive	Reactive bone formation	Nonspecific	N/A	Confused with osteoblastoma-like osteosarcoma
Osteosarcoma	10–30	Pain, limp, swelling, mass	Metaphyseal, long bones, pelvis	Radiopaque/radiolucent, wide zone of transition, cortical destruction, immature periosteal reaction	Positive	Cortical bone loss	Marrow and cortical bone replacement, soft-tissue mass	Li-Fraumeni, retinoblastoma, Paget's disease	N/A
Fibrosarcoma	20–40	Pain, swelling, mass	Metaphyseal, long bones	Radiolucency, immature periosteal new bone, wide zone of transition	Positive	Cortical and medullary bone replacement	Cortical and medullary bone replacement, soft-tissue mass	N/A	N/A
Malignant Fibrous Histiocytoma	40–60	Pain, swelling, mass	Metaphyseal, long bones	Radiolucency, wide zone of transition, immature periosteal reaction, may be underlying disease (bone infarction)	Positive	Cortical and medullary bone replacement	Cortical and medullary bone replacement, soft-tissue mass	Dedifferentiated tumors (infarcts)	N/A
Nonossifying Fibroma (Fibrous Cortical Defect)	5–25	Incidental finding, pathological fracture	Metaphysis, long bones	Cortical, eccentric lucency, narrow zone of transition	Variable	Cortical bone loss	Nonspecific	Jaffe-Campanacci disease (café-au-lait spots)	None
Chordoma	40–60	Pain (sacral or cervical)	Midline sacrum or upper cervical spine	Subtle radiolucency, sacrum or cervical spine	Positive	Cortical bone destruction	Cortical and medullary replacement with soft-tissue mass	N/A	N/A
Adamantinoma	20–40	Pain, swelling	Tibia	Mixed, patchy radiolucencies, cortical-based	Positive	Cortical and medullary bone resplacement	Marrow and cortical bone replacement	N/A	N/A
Langerhans' Cell Histiocytosis (Eosinophilic Granuloma)	Birth–20	Pain, limp, swelling	Diaphyseal, long bones, flat bones	Central radiolucency, narrow zone of transition, variable periosteal bone formation, vertebra plana	Positive or negative	Central radiolucency, surrounding periosteal new bone	Nonspecific marrow changes	Letterer-Siwe (infancy), Hand-Schüller-Christian (toddler), eosinophilic granuloma	None
Metastatic Neuroblastoma	Birth–10	Pain, limp, swelling	Diaphyseal, long bones, flat bones	Central radiolucency, variable zone of transition, often multiple	Positive or negative	Central radiolucency	Nonspecific marrow changes	N/A	N/A
Metastatic Carcinoma	40–70	Pain, history of carcinoma	Axial skeleton	Radiolucency, radiopacity, wide zone of transition, often multiple	Positive	Cortical and medullary destruction	Cortical and medullary bone loss, often soft-tissue mass	N/A	N/A
Lymphoma	30–50	Pain, swelling	Diaphysis, long bones, flat bones	Subtle radiolucency or radiopacity	Positive	Variable cortical and medullary replacement	Marrow and cortical bones loss, large soft-tissue mass	N/A	N/A
Myeloma	50–70	Pain, swelling	Axial skeleton	Radiolucency (punched-out), narrow zone of transition	Positive or negative	Medullary replacement, endosteal scalloping or destruction	Marrow and cortical replacement	N/A	N/A
Leukemia	Any	Pain, swelling	Variable	Variable	Positive or negative	Variable	Marrow, bone replacement	N/A	N/A

Data from Shajowicz F: In Tumors and Tumorlike Lesions of Bone. New York, Springer, 1994; and from Wold LE, McLeod RA, Sim FH, et al: In Atlas of Orthopaedic Pathology. Philadelphia, WB Saunders, 1990.

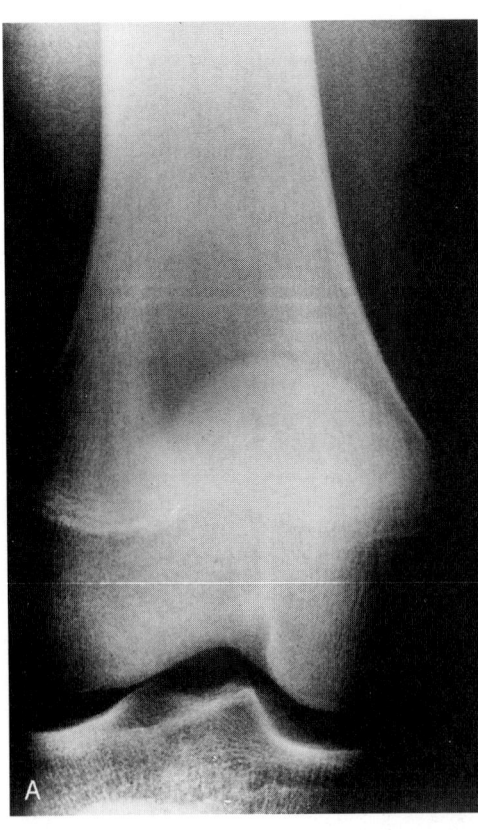
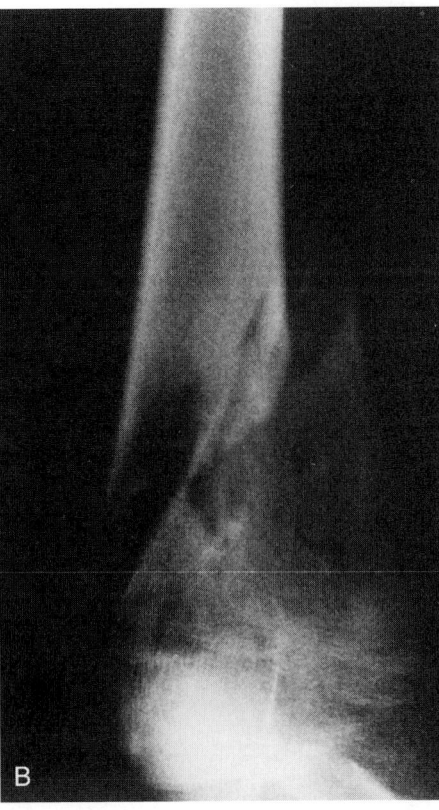

Fig 2. Pathological fracture secondary to osteosarcoma. *A,* Anteroposterior lateral radiograph of a 16-year-old boy who complained of knee pain. A subtle radiolucent lesion is noted in the distal femoral metaphysis, which appears to be entirely intramedullary. There is no associated cortical reaction. *B,* Films taken 2 months later, after an injury to the distal thigh. The patient sustained a pathological fracture of the distal femur. A history of pain prior to the fracture may indicate an underlying active benign or malignant process.

is a condition that appears to be inherited, in many patients as an autosomal dominant trait. Li-Fraumeni syndrome refers to a germline *TP53* mutation that has been associated with an increased incidence of breast, bone, and soft-tissue sarcomas.[6] It is estimated that approximately 30% of osteosarcomas examined contain a *TP53* mutation. An increased incidence of osteosarcoma is also seen in patients with a history of retinoblastoma.[7] Both the *TP53* and the *Rb* gene, in their wild form, are important in regulating the cell cycle, and mutations of the genes probably predispose these individuals to the development of malignant tumors.[8, 9]

PHYSICAL EXAMINATION

Examination of the involved body part, adjacent joint, and skin may provide additional information for formulating a differential diagnosis. Expansile lesions may be palpable in subcutaneous bones such as the tibia or ulna. A palpable mass of new onset in the distal thigh or pelvis is worrisome and may indicate an underlying aggressive benign or malignant process (Fig. 3). Restriction in the range of motion may be noted in patients with a bone tumor and may be associated with a soft-tissue mass or significant surrounding inflammation. Skin examination may reveal changes suggestive of other mesenchymal neoplasms, such as café-au-lait spots (neurofibromatosis or nonossifying fibroma) or hemangiomas that are occasionally associated with cartilage tumors (Maffucci's syndrome). In evaluating

for possible metastatic disease, physical examination of the breast and prostate may reveal a primary site.

As with the patient history, the patients must be fully evaluated for more common degenerative conditions such as arthritis, tendinopathy, and referred pain. These conditions may be responsible for the symptoms, as opposed to the underlying radiographic abnormality. The surgeon may wish to consider diagnostic injection of a joint, tendon, or bursa in an effort to determine whether an underlying inflammatory condition is responsible for the patient's symptoms rather than the underlying bone abnormality.

IMAGING STUDIES
Radiographs

For most patients, a bone tumor will be diagnosed on a plain radiograph of the involved extremity. This imaging study is the single most valuable of all available tests.[2, 3] In most cases, the radiographic appearance of the lesion, in combination with knowledge of the patient's age, allows the surgeon to determine whether a radiographically identified bone lesion is likely to be benign or malignant. In some cases, such as most instances of nonossifying fibroma, the radiograph will be diagnostic and will be the only necessary imaging study (Fig. 4).

Interpreting a radiograph requires an organized approach that includes assessing the location of the tumor, the reaction of the host bone to the tumor, the internal characteristics of the lesion, and any associated soft-tissue mass. Utilizing this assessment, the surgeon will, in almost all cases,

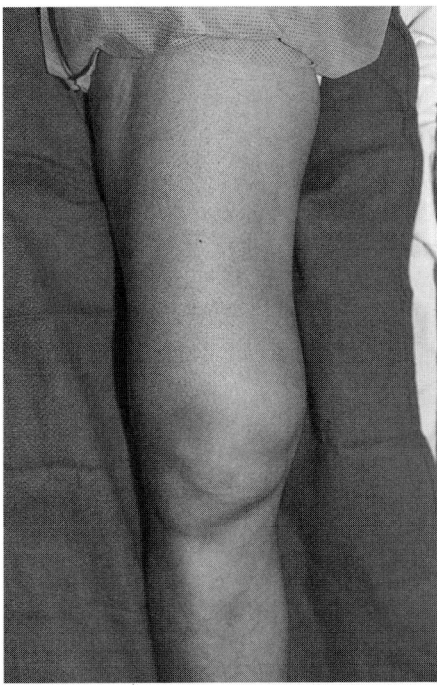

Fig. 3. Soft-tissue mass associated with lymphoma of bone. This is a photograph taken from an anterior perspective of a distal thigh mass in a 35-year-old woman. She was subsequently diagnosed as having lymphoma of bone.

be able to distinguish benign from malignant tumors and tumors that require operative intervention from those that can safely be observed.

Bone tumors of particular histological features occur most commonly in certain types of bones and in specific locations within bones, particularly long bones (see Table 1). Adamantinoma is most commonly located in the tibia or fibula. Chordoma is, in almost all cases, located in the axial skeleton in the cervical spine or sacrum. Marrow cell tumors (lymphoma, histiocytosis, and Ewing's sarcoma) are often diagnosed in the flat bones of the pelvis, spine, and scapula (Fig. 5). When these occur in a long bone, they tend to be located in the diaphysis. In contrast, tumors located in an epiphyseal location are usually one of two types. In the skeletally mature patient, an epiphyseal lesion is usually a giant cell tumor of bone; in the young patient, it is most commonly a chondroblastoma (Fig. 6). However, most tumors affecting long bones are found in the metaphyses. This is true for both malignant and benign tumors.

Evaluation of the host bone reaction to a tumor is essential when the differential diagnosis is formulated. Latent or slowly progressive lesions tend to be surrounded by dense sclerotic bone, resulting in a well-defined tumor with a narrow zone of transition to normal bone (Fig. 7). Malignant tumors, in contrast, often enlarge rapidly, overwhelming the host bone's ability to respond. These lesions tend to be radiolucent, with a permeative or "moth-eaten" appearance. The lesion may be poorly defined, and the transition from tumor to normal bone is vague. This is described as a wide zone of transition. With an increase in the rate of

growth, the cortical bone may be expanded, scalloped, or destroyed and, at times, a soft-tissue mass may be evident (Fig. 8).

In addition, the surgeon should carefully evaluate the nature and extent of periosteal new-bone formation. Immature periosteal new bone, perpendicular new-bone formation ("sunburst" appearance), and periosteal laminations of bone ("onion-skinning") are worrisome features that indicate an active process and very possibly an underlying malignancy (Fig. 9). In contrast, mature periosteal new bone is seen with stress fractures, subacute infection, and some benign bone tumors such as eosinophilic granuloma (Fig. 10).

Internal characteristics may reveal the underlying tumor type. Intralesional calcification in the form of punctate radiopacities is characteristic of cartilage tumors (Fig. 11). Ossification may appear immature (amorphous) or mature and well-defined and is seen in benign and malignant bone-forming lesions (osteoblastoma, osteosarcoma) (Fig. 12). Internal septations are less specific and may be seen in many histological types of bone tumors.

Tumors may be seen that appear to have developed on the surface of the bone. These surface lesions may be

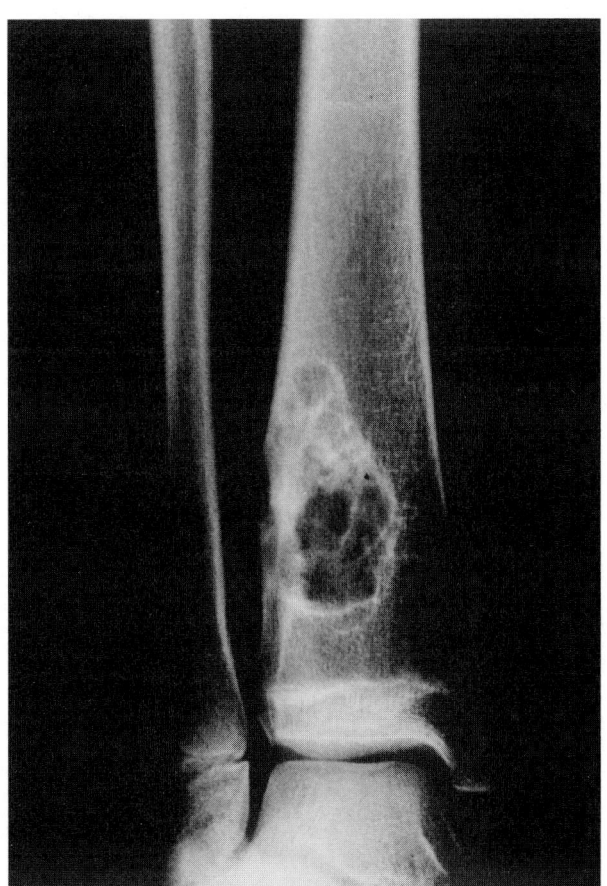

Fig. 4. Nonossifying fibroma. This is an anteroposterior radiograph of the ankle taken after a soft-tissue injury. Incidentally noted is an eccentric radiolucent lesion of the distal tibia with a narrow zone of transition. This radiograph is diagnostic of a nonossifying fibroma, and no additional imaging or biopsy sampling was necessary.

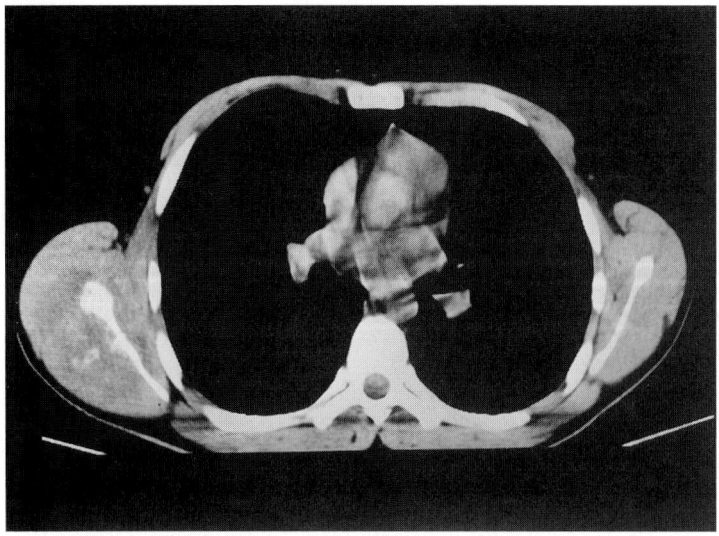

Fig. 5. Ewing's sarcoma of the scapula. A 14-year-old boy complained of pain in the shoulder. No radiographic abnormality was noted. A trans-scapular view demonstrated periosteal elevation and a soft-tissue mass associated with a probable lesion of the underlying scapula. A computed tomography image of the patient demonstrates a large soft-tissue mass associated with an underlying bone abnormality of the scapula, subsequently diagnosed as Ewing's sarcoma.

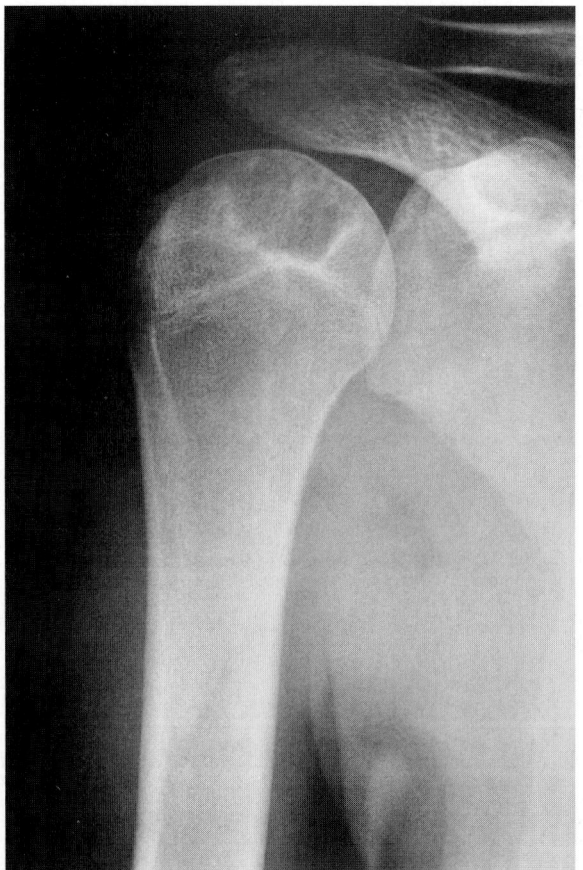

Fig. 6. Chondroblastoma of the proximal humerus. This is an external rotation radiograph of the proximal humerus of a 16-year-old girl, demonstrating a radiolucent lesion of the epiphysis of the proximal humerus with internal calcification. The patient had a biopsy; findings were consistent with chondroblastoma.

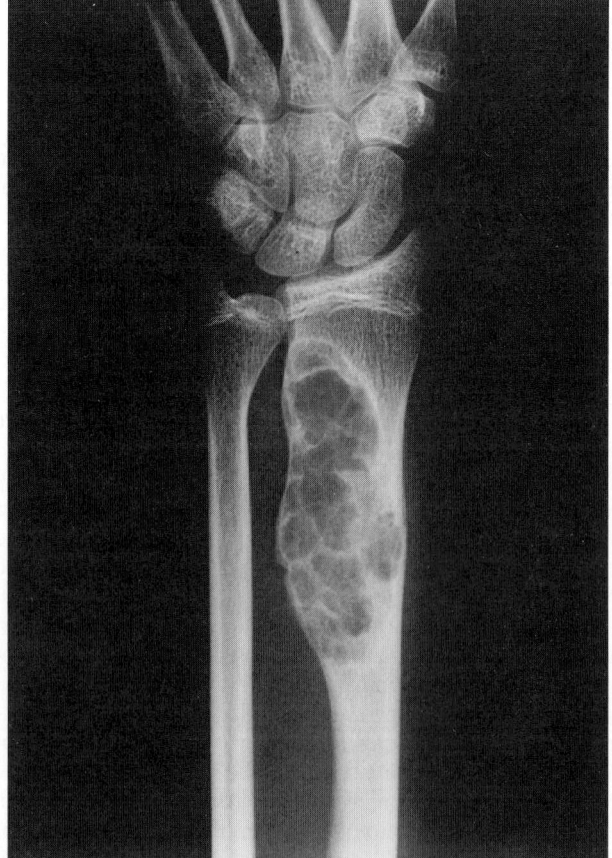

Fig. 7. Benign-appearing bone neoplasms. This is an anteroposterior radiograph of the distal forearm of a 14-year-old girl diagnosed with a nonossifying fibroma of the distal radius. The zone of transition is narrow between the lesion and the underlying bone. Dense sclerotic bone resulting in a well-defined tumor with a narrow zone of transition is characteristic of a benign bone neoplasm.

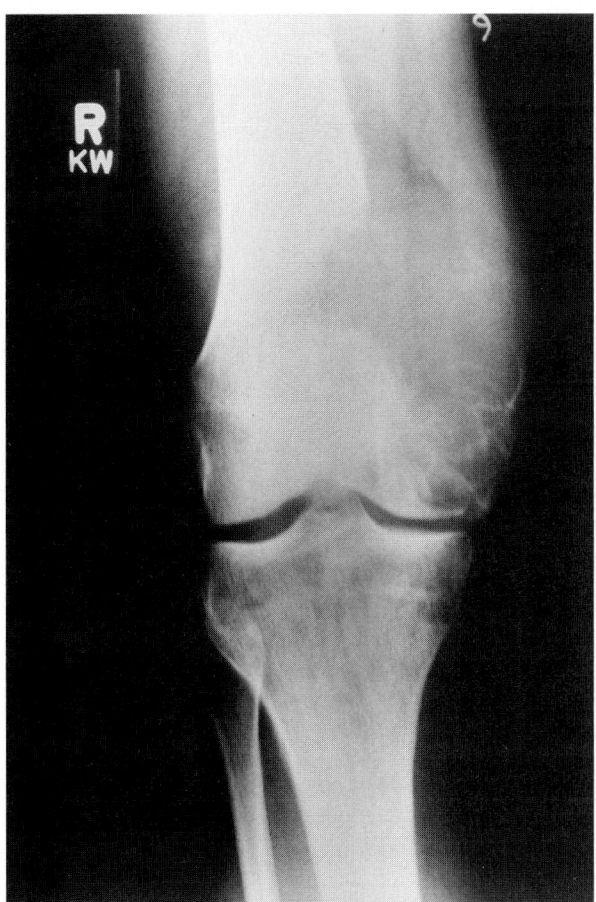

Fig. 8. Giant cell tumor of the distal femur. This is an anteroposterior radiograph of the distal femur of a 35-year-old woman complaining of knee pain. This bone lesion is associated with a wide zone of transition, cortical destruction, and a soft-tissue mass, all of which would indicate a rapid rate of growth in what subsequently proved to be a giant cell tumor of bone.

benign (for example, parosteal chondroma) or malignant (for example, parosteal osteosarcoma).

Multifocal bone disease may be seen in both benign and malignant conditions. Examples of polyostotic diseases include fibrous dysplasia, histiocytosis, metastatic disease, and myeloma.

Serial radiography in the initial evaluation of a bone lesion and subsequent follow-up is important in the evaluation and treatment of a patient with a bone tumor. If the patient has had a previous radiograph, it is most helpful to obtain that radiograph for direct comparison. If there has been no change in the size or nature of the lesion over time, it is likely that no intervention is required and that symptoms are probably referable to some other cause.

Technetium Bone Scanning

The value of bone scanning is for identifying patients with multifocal disease. Patients who have benign bone lesions known at times to be multifocal (e.g., fibrous dysplasia), metastatic disease from carcinoma, or a bone sarcoma (bone is the second most common metastatic site of dis-

ease) should have a whole-body bone scan (Fig. 13). Regardless of its cause or whether it is inflammatory, benign, or malignant, a radiographically apparent lesion is likely to show increased scintigraphic activity. Therefore, a bone scan is not specific. A few neoplasms may not show increased scintigraphic activity on the bone scan. At times, despite a normal bone scintigram, a skeletal survey will reveal multiple osseous sites of disease in cases of histiocytosis and multiple myeloma.

Computed Tomography

Computed tomography (CT) remains very useful in the evaluation of bone tumors. Cortical bone is better visualized with CT than with magnetic resonance imaging (MRI), and it allows precise identification of cortical destruction, fracture, and intralesional mineralization. CT images have an appearance that is virtually diagnostic of many cartilage tumors and hemangiomas of bone (Fig. 14). CT remains the test of choice in evaluating a patient for possible osteoid osteoma (Fig. 15). In many ways, it is equivalent to MRI of the spine and pelvis. CT is commonly used for directing the performance of needle biopsies, especially for lesions in these locations.

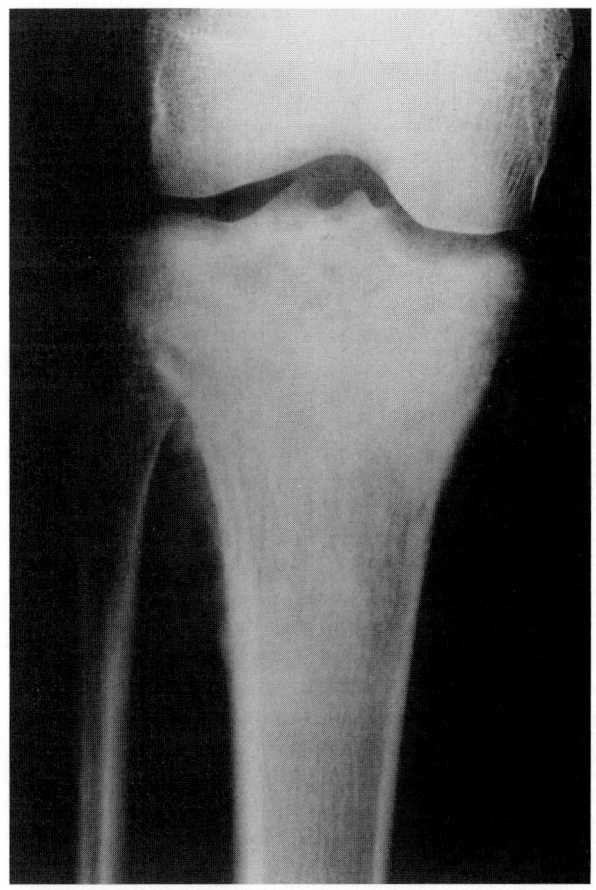

Fig. 9. Sunburst appearance of a malignant tumor. This is an anteroposterior radiograph of the proximal tibia of a 15-year-old girl diagnosed with an osteosarcoma. Of note is the perpendicular periosteal mineralization, or so-called sunburst appearance, suggesting a rapid rate of growth of the underlying malignancy.

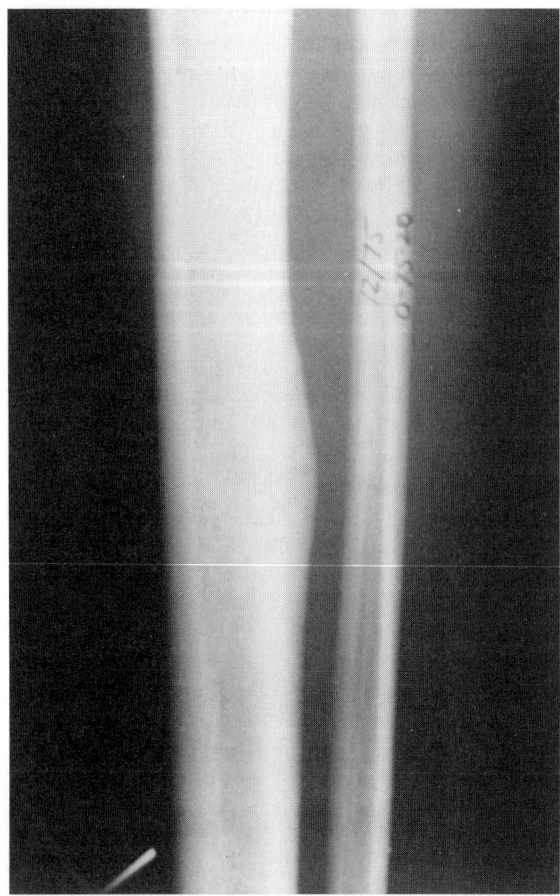

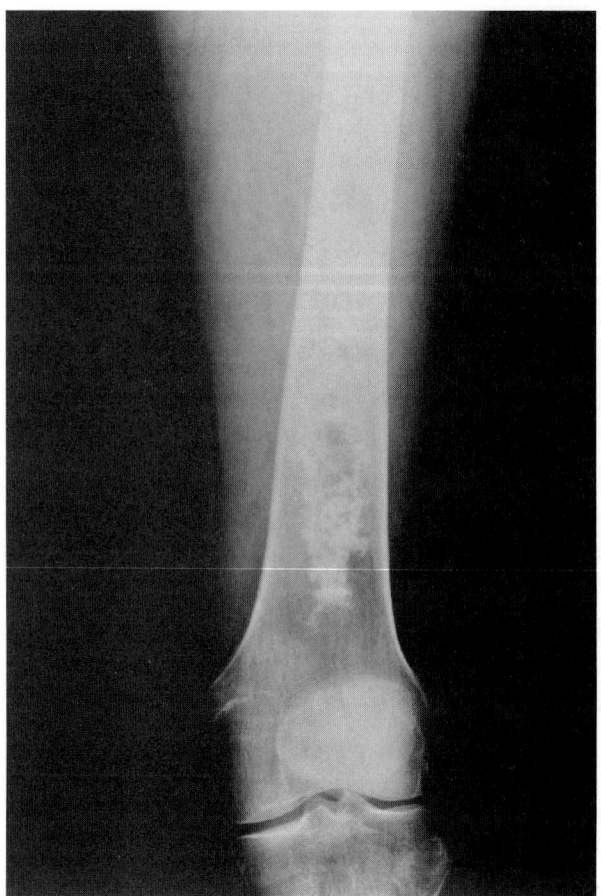

Fig. 10. Stress fracture with mature periosteal new bone. This is an anteroposterior radiograph of a child who sustained a stress fracture of the tibia, demonstrating mature periosteal new bone.

Fig. 11. Calcification associated with an enchondroma. This is an anteroposterior radiograph of a 60-year-old woman with an incidental finding of a lesion of the distal femur. The lesion has punctate calcifications within the intramedullary canal without any evident endosteal scalloping, cortical destruction, or soft-tissue mass. Radiographically, this lesion appears to be an enchondroma.

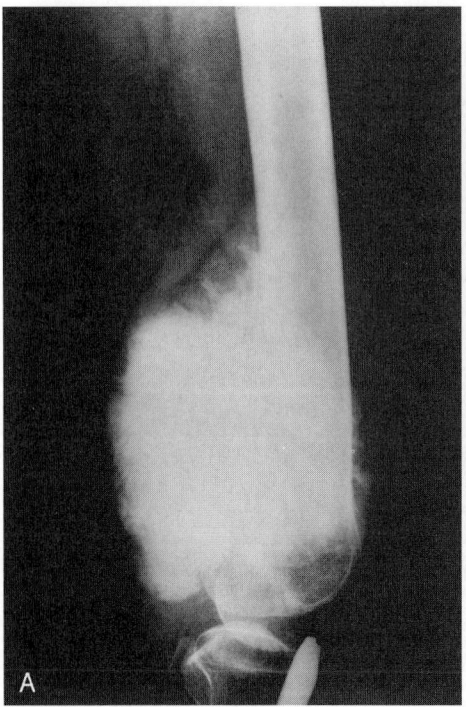

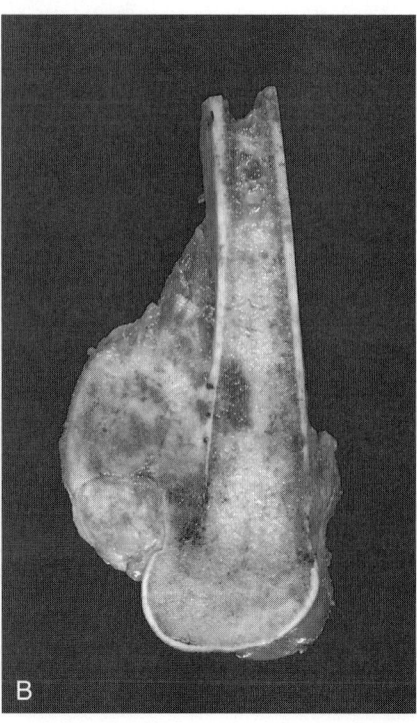

Fig. 12. Parosteal osteosarcoma. *A,* Lateral radiograph of a 35-year-old woman who underwent intramedullary rodding of her tibia for a fracture after a motor vehicle accident. A large radiodense lesion is noted on the posterior surface of the femur, with internal characteristics of ossification. *B,* Specimen photograph after resection of the distal femoral parosteal osteosarcoma, demonstrating a tumor arising from the surface of the bone.

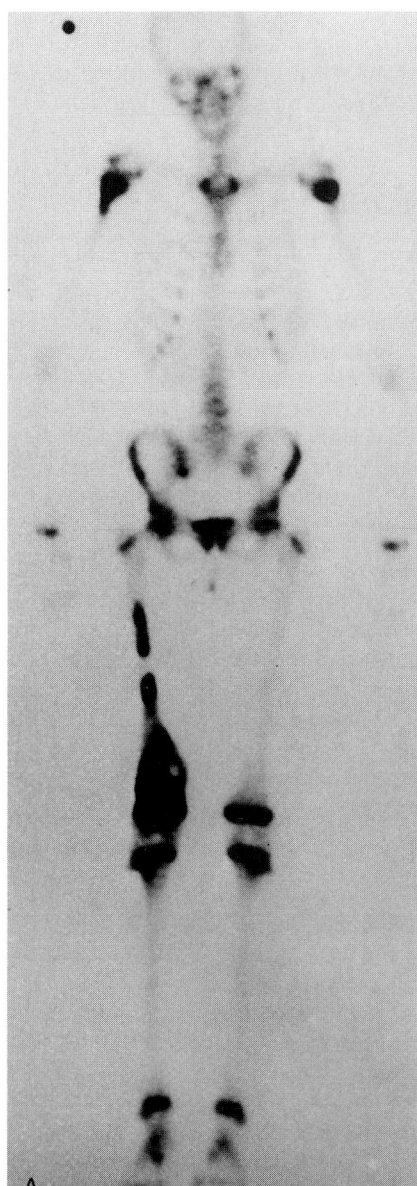

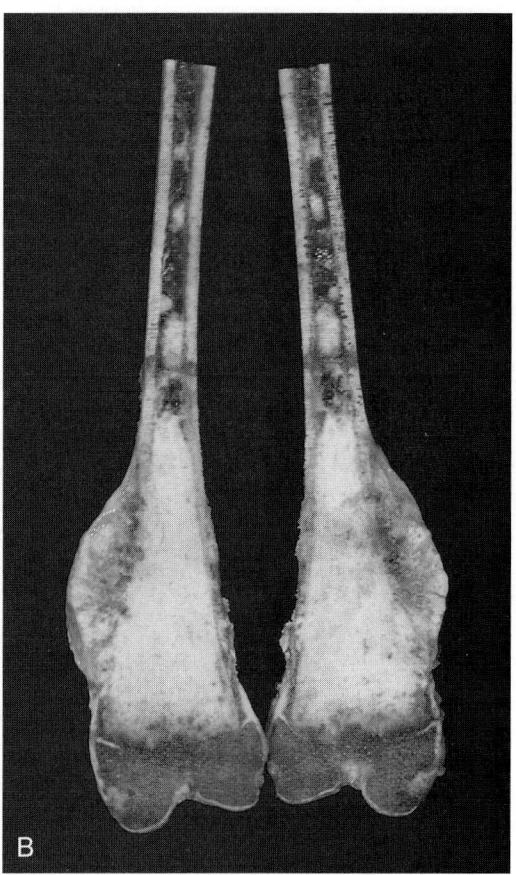

Fig. 13. Skip metastases. *A,* A technetium bone scan of an adolescent woman diagnosed with osteosarcoma of the distal femur, demonstrating two proximal areas of activity suggestive of skip metastases and, on careful examination, increased activity of the right proximal humeral metaphysis, which subsequently proved to be metastatic osteosarcoma. *B,* Photograph of the resected distal femur, demonstrating the multiple sites of osteosarcoma within the femur, consistent with skip metastases from the distal primary.

Fig. 14. Hemangioma. The computed tomographic image is characteristic of hemangioma with a "polka-dot" appearance.

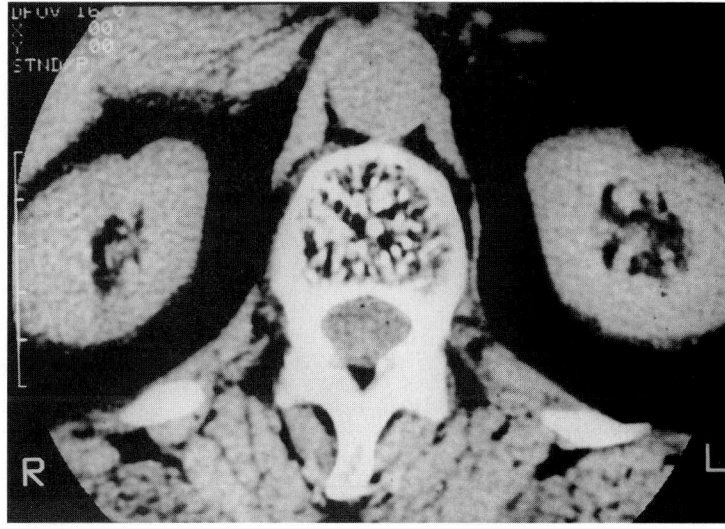

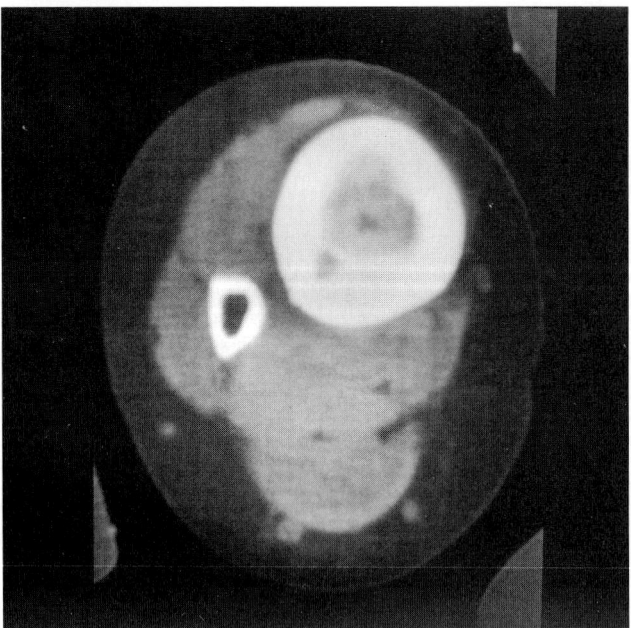

Fig. 15. Osteoid osteoma. This computed tomographic image demonstrates a small radiolucent nidus within the posterior cortex of the tibia, diagnostic of an osteoid osteoma.

CT of the chest, abdomen, and pelvis is also recommended in the evaluation of patients with suspected metastases of unknown origin; it should also be done as part of routine staging of a patient with a bone sarcoma for possible pulmonary metastases.

Magnetic Resonance Imaging

The value of MRI in assessing a bone tumor lies in defining the extent of the tumor within the bone marrow, including "skip metastases" and associated soft-tissue masses. Some tumors are noted to have a significant soft-tissue mass despite little in the way of radiographic change (as in lymphoma and other marrow cell tumors) (Fig. 16). For benign bone tumors, fluid-fluid levels are often seen in cases of aneurysmal bone cyst. MRI may also show an associated joint effusion and intra-articular tumor extension, and it delineates the association of bone tumors with surrounding neurovascular structures.

PET, Thallium Scanning

Newer imaging modalities such as positron emission tomography (PET) and thallium scanning are still investigational. PET may be useful in detecting nonpulmonary metastatic disease. Thallium scanning has been used in determining the response of malignant bone tumors to preoperative chemotherapy.

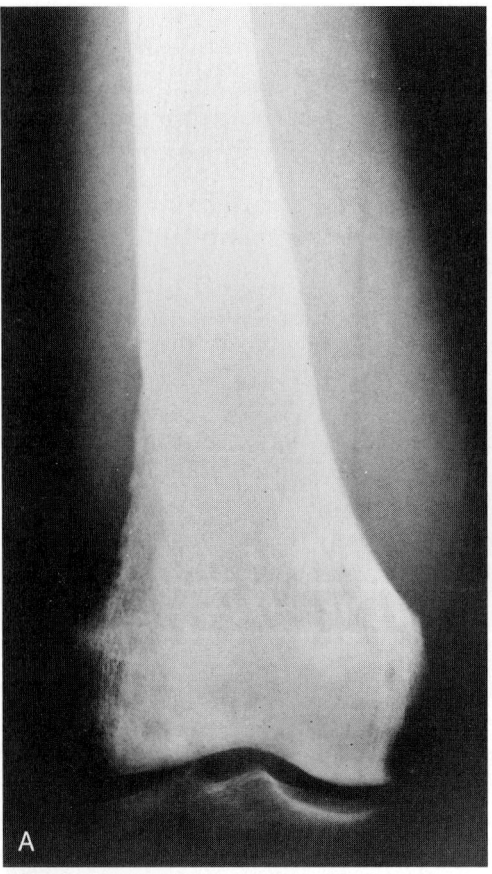

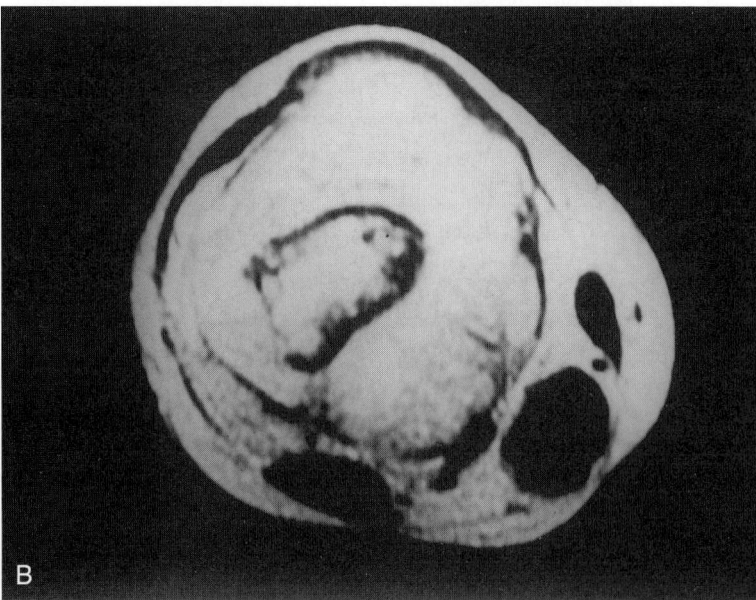

Fig. 16. Marrow cell tumors. *A,* Anteroposterior radiograph of the distal femur, demonstrating increased density of the distal femur but no significant cortical destruction. A very large soft-tissue mass is shown in *B,* a T_2-weighted image of the distal femur, indicating the soft-tissue mass to be out of proportion to the radiographic changes seen. This is characteristic of marrow cell tumors, in this case a large cell lymphoma.

EVALUATION OF A PATIENT FOR METASTASES OF UNKNOWN ORIGIN

For patients older than 40 years who have a malignant-appearing radiographic lesion, the most common underlying cause is metastatic carcinoma or myeloma. These lesions are commonly radiolucent but may be radiopaque. They may be multifocal or solitary. It is relatively common for complaints of skeletal pain leading to the diagnosis of metastatic disease to be the first sign of metastatic carcinoma. The most common primary tumors are breast, lung, prostate, kidney, and thyroid carcinoma. In patients suspected to have metastases who do not have a known primary lesion, a suggested evaluation, including serological and imaging studies, is recommended prior to biopsy. This is outlined in Figure 1.

FORMULATION OF A DIFFERENTIAL DIAGNOSIS

Based on the patient's history, physical examination, and the results of imaging studies, the surgeon can formulate a provisional differential diagnosis. In the most general terms, a surgeon must decide the growth and malignant (metastatic) potential of the neoplasm. This will dictate treatment, ranging from serial radiographic observation to biopsy to resection.

Latent bone tumors such as nonossifying fibroma or osteochondroma can safely be observed. Asymptomatic, benign-appearing cartilage tumors similarly may be observed. Serial radiographs at 3-, 6-, and 12-month intervals during the first year may be preferred. Disproportionate growth or radiographic change should prompt a biopsy. When the diagnosis is unclear, the decision is more difficult as to whether to observe or to proceed with a bone biopsy. That decision is based on the surgeon's perception of the underlying process and the natural history of that process. Is this lesion likely to grow and place the patient at risk for pathological fracture? More important, is the lesion malignant and likely to place not only the limb but also the patient's life in jeopardy? Does the lesion appear to be inflammatory, benign, or metastatic, or is it a primary bone malignancy?

Patients with lesions suspicious for primary bone sarcoma should be referred to a tertiary center that is likely to be responsible for the eventual treatment of the patient. Poorly performed biopsies or ill-advised exploratory operative procedures may compromise the ability of the subsequent surgeon not only to preserve the limb but also to save the patient's life.[10] If it is decided that tissue must be obtained for a diagnosis, a biopsy is performed. A biopsy has been described as a technically straightforward procedure but one that requires significant preparation and planning. It may also be associated with complications that, in case of malignancy, may limit the surgeon's ability to preserve the involved limb.

BIOPSY

A biopsy may be open or closed. A closed biopsy including the use of needles or trephine is associated with a more

TABLE 2. SYSTEM OF ENNEKING FOR THE STAGING OF BENIGN TUMORS OF BONE

Stage	Definition	Behavior
1	Latent	Remains static or heals spontaneously
2	Active	Progressive growth but limited by natural barriers
3	Locally invasive	Progressive growth not limited by natural barriers

Data from Enneking WF, Spanier SS, Goodman MA: A system for the surgical staging of musculoskeletal sarcomas. Clin Orthop Rel Res 1980; 153:106.

limited exposure; in the setting of a virtually diagnostic radiograph, a fine needle aspirate or needle biopsy may be diagnostic despite the limited amount of tissue obtained. These biopsies are often performed in the evaluation of spine and pelvic lesions in conjunction with axial imaging by CT.

More commonly, an open biopsy is performed for a bone lesion. In that situation, incisions must be longitudinal and oriented in such a way that they can later be resected en bloc with the underlying bone tumor. Knowledge of common flaps and approaches used in bone tumor surgery is important so that future limb salvage surgery is not precluded. Standard orthopaedic approaches in intramuscular or intravenous planes are not commonly used. Dissection is performed directly over the lesion through muscle, without creating flaps or contaminating additional compartments, and avoiding regional nerves and vascular structures. Whenever possible, tissue for analysis should be obtained from the soft-tissue component as opposed to bone. If a bone biopsy sample must be obtained, it is important to do this through a circular or elliptical opening in the bone to minimize any potential fracture risk. Postoperative hematomas must be avoided. Hemostasis may be obtained by use of cautery, bone wax, gel foam, or methylmethacrylate. Drains may be used and should be placed in line with and close to the incision. An intraoperative frozen section should be obtained for confirmation of the presence of diagnostic tissue. Cultures for bacteria, fungus, and acid-

TABLE 3. SYSTEM OF ENNEKING FOR THE STAGING OF BONE SARCOMAS

Stage	Grade*	Site ¥	Metastasis £
IA	G_1	T_1	M_0
IB	G_1	T_2	M_0
IIA	G_2	T_1	M_0
IIB	G_2	T_2	M_0
III	G_1 or G_2	T_1 or T_2	M_1

* G_1 = low-grade, G_2 = high-grade.
¥ T_1 = intracompartmental, T_2 = extracompartmental.
£ M_0 = no regional or distant metastases, M_1 = regional or distant metastases.
Data from Enneking WF, Spanier SS, Goodman MA: A system for the surgical staging of musculoskeletal sarcomas. Clin Orthop Rel Res 1980; 153:106.

			Metastases in Regional	
Stage	Grade*	Primary Tumor ¥	Lymph Nodes §	Distant Metastases £
IA	G_1 or G_2	T_1	N_0	M_0
IB	G_1 or G_2	T_2	N_0	M_0
IIA	G_3 or G_4	T_1	N_0	M_0
IIB	G_3 or G_4	T_2	N_0	M_0
III	Not defined			
IVA	Any G	Any T	N_1	M_0
IVB	Any G	Any T	Any N	M_1

TABLE 4. SYSTEM OF THE AMERICAN JOINT COMMITTEE ON CANCER FOR STAGING OF BONE SARCOMAS

* G_1 = well differentiated, G_2 = moderately differentiated, G_3 = poorly differentiated, G_4 = undifferentiated.
Note that Ewing's sarcoma and malignant lymphoma are defined as G_4.
¥ T_1 = tumor is confined within the cortex, T_2 = tumor expands beyond the cortex.
§ N_0 = no metastases within regional lymph nodes, N_1 = metastases in regional lymph nodes.
£ M_0 = no distant metastases, M_1 = distant metastases.
Data from American Joint Committee on Cancer. In Beaches OH, Myers MH (eds): Manual for Staging. Philadelphia, JB Lippincott, 1997, 5th ed, p 143.

fast bacilli should be obtained. In the case of benign tumors, definitive surgery may proceed immediately if the preoperative diagnosis, based on imaging studies, matches the intraoperative frozen section results.

STAGING OF BONE TUMORS

Benign bone tumors are classified into stages 1, 2, and 3 according to the staging system described by Enneking et al.[11] The system integrates clinical, histological, and imaging characteristics to rank the tumors in increasing stages of aggressiveness (Table 2). Benign-appearing lesions that are asymptomatic and are considered latent (stage 1) can usually be observed radiographically. Benign active (stage 2) or aggressive (stage 3) lesions often require additional studies with CT or MRI and are likely to require pathological confirmation and resection by means of curettage and bone graft or resection if they are in an expendable location.

Two staging systems are currently being used in the classification of malignant bone tumors. The Musculoskeletal Tumor Society system divides tumors according to grade, intracompartmental or extracompartmental location, and the presence or absence of metastases (Table 3). For bone sarcomas, intracompartmental tumors are defined as those that are intraosseous or, for surface tumors, those that are confined to a paraosseous location. The presence of soft-tissue extension or intraosseous or extrafascial extension, in the case of surface lesions, makes these lesions extracompartmental.

The American Joint Committee on Cancer (Table 4) has defined a staging system for sarcomas of bone.[12] It is very similar to that used by the Musculoskeletal Tumor Society. More in keeping with a four-stage system used for other tumors, the American Joint Committee puts tumors considered well-differentiated or moderately differentiated into a low-grade classification similar to that used by Enneking. Poorly differentiated or undifferentiated tumors are considered high-grade. The presence of metastases places the patient in stage IV, with stage III currently being undefined. A T_1 tumor (A) is defined as one that is confined to

the cortex, and a T_2 tumor is considered as extending beyond the cortex. Obviously, the American Joint Committee on Cancer and the Enneking systems are more similar than they are different.

These staging systems allow for an estimation of patient prognosis based on various factors. These factors include tumor grade and extent and the presence or absence of metastases. These factors are obviously based on relatively crude measurements of the result of the interaction between the tumor and the host. Research is currently under way on examining the role of various molecular-oncology markers in the determination of patient prognosis. It is likely that a staging system will be developed based on these molecular markers and that it will more accurately stratify patient information regarding relative risk categories so that specific treatment regimens involving surgery, chemotherapy, and radiation therapy may be more selectively administered and better evaluated.

SUMMARY

The clinical presentation of a patient with a bone tumor is highly variable. Nevertheless, a surgeon using an organized and consistent approach of eliciting the proper historical detail, medical history, and physical examination findings in conjunction with useful imaging studies can formulate a useful differential diagnosis. Based on the surgeon's perception of the underlying disease and its natural history, observation or operative intervention may be indicated. It is important to understand the patient's symptoms and their possible relationship to the underlying neoplasm, to interpret radiographic studies accurately, and to use other imaging studies efficiently in the evaluation of bone neoplasms. This careful approach is important in the optimal use of resources, including avoiding unnecessary operative intervention and imaging tests that are not particularly useful while guaranteeing that tumors that place the life and limb of the patient in danger are evaluated efficiently so that a timely and accurate diagnosis may be made and treatment initiated.

REFERENCES

1. Springfield DS: Evaluation of bone and soft tissue tumors. In Lewis M (ed): Musculoskeletal Oncology: A Multidisciplinary Approach. Philadelphia, WB Saunders, 1992, p 1.
2. Simon MA: Diagnostic strategies. In Simon MA, Springfield DS (eds): Surgery for Bone and Soft Tissue Tumors. Philadelphia, Lippincott-Raven, 1998, p 21.
3. Shives TS: The age of the patient: Clinical evaluation, biopsy, and staging of bone tumors. In Chapman M (ed): Operative Orthopaedics. Philadelphia, JB Lippincott, 1988, p 887.
4. Schajowicz F: Tumors and Tumorlike Lesions of Bone. New York, Springer, 1981.
5. Wold LE, McLeod RA, Sim FH, et al: In Atlas of Orthopaedic Pathology. Philadelphia, WB Saunders, 1990.
6. Li FP, Fraumeni JF: Soft-tissue sarcomas, breast cancer, and other neoplasms: A familial syndrome? Ann Intern Med 1969; 71:747.
7. Araki N, Uchida A, Kimura T, et al: Involvement of the retinoblastoma gene in primary osteosarcomas and other bone and soft-tissue tumors. Clin Orthop Rel Res 1991; 270:271.
8. Chen PL, Chen YM, Bookstein R, et al: Genetic mechanism of tumor suppression by the human p53 gene. Science 1990; 250:1576.
9. Lonbardo F, Veda T, Huvos AG, et al: p53 and MOM2 alterations in osteosarcomas: Correlations with clinicopathologic and proliferative rate. Cancer 1997; 79: 1541.
10. Mankin HJ, Mankin CJ, Simon MA: The hazards of biopsy revisited. J Bone Joint Surg Am 1996; 78:659.
11. Enneking WF, Spanier SS, Goodman MA: A system for the surgical staging of musculoskeletal sarcomas. Clin Orthop Rel Res 1980; 153:106.
12. American Joint Committee on Cancer: Bone. In Beahrs OH, Myers MH (eds): Manual for Staging. Philadelphia, JB Lippincott, 1997, 5th ed, p 143.

section
7
chapter
6

BENIGN BONE TUMORS

Theodore W. Parsons III

Summary
- Benign bone tumors are common. Some need no treatment, either remaining of no consequence to the patient or spontaneously resolving. Others should be simply curetted, and still others require extensive surgery and cannot only locally recur but metastasize.
- The patient's age, presenting symptoms, physical examination, and plain radiographs are usually all that are necessary to distinguish between the benign bone tumors and assure the patient that the lesion is benign. Sometimes a biopsy is necessary to be definitive.
- All benign lesions not sampled should be observed to ensure they behave as predicted. This chapter is a brief description of the common benign bone tumors.

Benign bone lesions are encountered by the practicing orthopaedist with some frequency; they are seen four or five times more often than malignant bone lesions. Many of these lesions are discovered by chance at the time of routine radiographs, often prompting orthopaedic referral. Appropriate treatment depends on recognition, and frequently observation and patient reassurance are all that is required.

Although there are more than two dozen recognized benign bone lesions, for simplicity the most commonly encountered lesions can be grouped into five categories: osseous, chondroid, fibrous, cystic, and giant-cell lesions (Table 1). The more common tumors are briefly discussed here in terms of their clinical, radiographic, and histologic presentation.

OSSEOUS TUMORS

OSTEOID OSTEOMA

Osteoid osteoma (OO) is a common benign lesion that is characterized by a well-demarcated, very vascular center (nidus) with a surrounding zone of reactive bone sclerosis. Typically, the nidus is less than 1 to 1.5 cm in diameter.

TABLE 1. COMMON BENIGN BONE TUMORS
Osseous Lesions:
Osteoid osteoma
Osteoblastoma
Chondroid Lesions:
Osteochondroma
Enchondroma
Chondroblastoma
Fibrous Lesions:
Nonossifying fibroma
Fibrous dysplasia
Cystic Lesions:
Solitary bone cyst
Aneurysmal bone cyst
Giant-Cell Lesions:
Giant-cell tumor

OO accounts for some 10% to 12% of all benign bone lesions, with a male/female ratio of nearly 3:1. The peak prevalence is in the second decade, with some 80% of patients presenting between age 5 and 25 years.

Nearly 50% of all cases of OO present in the long bones of the lower extremities, with the femoral neck being the single most frequent site.[1] In the upper extremities, OO is most commonly seen around the elbow. When presenting in long bones (70%), the lesion tends to appear near the end of the shaft. Presentation in the tubular bones of the hand and feet is also encountered. Although OO rarely occurs in the axial skeleton, it is likely to be found in the lumbar spine, almost exclusively in the posterior elements.

The most common clinical symptom is *pain of increasing severity that is relieved by aspirin* or other nonsteroidal anti-inflammatory agent. The pain is typically worse at night and is often referred to the nearest joint. Some 80% of patients demonstrate these clinical symptoms.[2] Reactive inflammation associated with these lesions may cause arthritic-like symptoms and even soft-tissue swelling. Lesions in the spine are often associated with a painful scoliosis and may present with neurological symptoms. The pain, reactive sclerosis, and inflammatory changes have been attributed to high levels of prostaglandin E_2 and prostacyclin in the nidus.[3]

Radiographically, the lesion classically demonstrates a well-demarcated *nidus* (radiolucent) surrounded by a sclerotic zone of reactive bone. When the lesion occurs in cancellous bone, or more particularly in lesions that are juxta-articular, the amount of surrounding sclerosis may be minimal, or even absent, often making the diagnosis difficult. Computed tomography (CT) or magnetic resonance imaging (MRI) is often necessary to adequately identify the nidus, especially in locations that are more difficult to visualize, such as the spine (Fig. 1).

Histologically, the nidus presents as a network of thin, woven trabecular bone in a background of loose, vascular connective tissue with prominent osteoblasts.

Radiographically, the differential diagnosis includes osteomyelitis, bone abscess, bone island, and even stress fracture. Although the lesions are known to spontaneously regress,[4] symptoms generally require treatment of some kind.

OSTEOBLASTOMA

Benign osteoblastoma, although rare, is mentioned here because it is histologically quite similar to OO. It is generally larger than 2 cm in size and used to be referred to as giant osteoid osteoma. It has a predilection for the spine. It generally lacks the typical pain pattern seen with OO (although it is also a painful lesion), and the surrounding sclerosis is minimal.

CHONDROID TUMORS

OSTEOCHONDROMA

Solitary osteochondroma (OCE) is a developmental abnormality that results in an exophytic outgrowth from the surface of the bone, which is covered by a cartilaginous cap. It is likely the most common benign lesion, accounting for some 35% of benign bone lesions. OCE has a male/female ratio of almost 2:1 and generally presents in the second or third decade. OCE most commonly appears in the appendicular skeleton in the metaphysis of the major long bones, but it is not uncommon on the scapula or ilium. Some 35% of OCE occurs around the knee.[5]

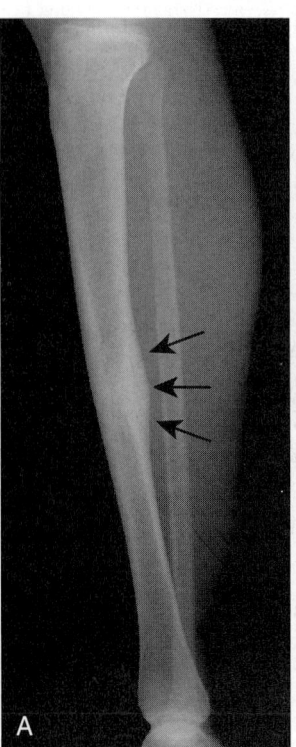
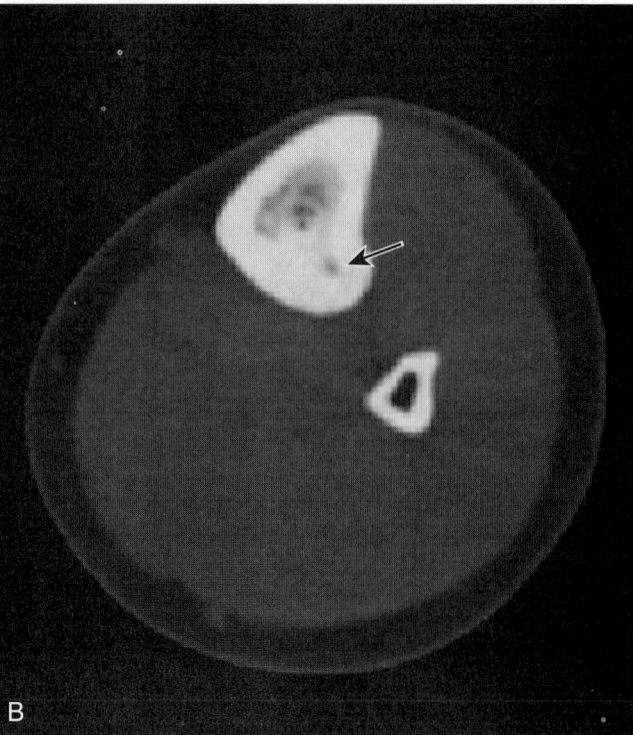

Fig. 1. Views. *A,* Lateral radiograph of tibia showing the classic appearance of an osteoid osteoma in the diaphyseal bone. Note the abundant reactive bone surrounding the nidus (*arrows*), which is not well visualized on plain film. *B,* CT scan of lesion seen in *A.* The radiolucent nidus is well visualized on axial imaging (*arrow*) and is surrounded by dense, reactive bone.

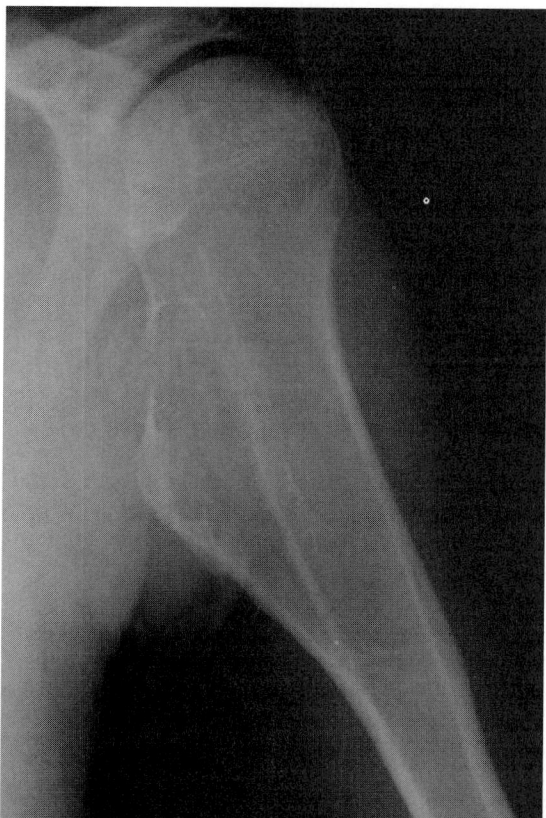

Fig. 2. View. Radiograph of the proximal humerus shows a large, sessile osteochondroma. Note that the lesion appears to be an extension of the natural cortex of the humerus. There is no mineralization of the cartilage cap. This lesion was symptomatic because of impingement on the neurovascular bundle.

Histologically, hyaline cartilage is noted overlying normal cancellous bone (with persistent primary trabeculae) and covered with a fibrous perichondrium.

Radiographically, the differential diagnosis includes parosteal osteosarcoma, juxtacortical myositis ossificans, and periosteal chondroma.

ENCHONDROMA

Enchondroma (ENCH) is a common lesion composed of mature cartilage that accounts for some 24% of all benign bone lesions. The lesion may present at any age and has no sex predilection. Approximately 60% of ENCH cases are found in the hands and feet. The femoral metaphysis ranks second (17%), followed by the proximal humerus (7%).[8]

ENCH is an asymptomatic lesion generally discovered by chance when imaging is performed for other reasons, although it occasionally presents as a pathological fracture. Any lesion presenting as painful, in the absence of fracture, should be evaluated for malignancy.

Radiographically, the lesion is centrally located and may show expansion of the bone and cortical thinning. In major long bones, the lesion is almost always metaphyseal in location. In small long bones, the lesion is often diaphyseal or may be epiphyseal in location. Mineralization is variable, and lesions may show areas of *stippled calcification* or *popcorn balls,* or there may be minimal mineralization seen only on CT or MRI (Fig. 3). CT and MRI can be helpful in delineating the extent of the lesion and in evaluating endosteal scalloping, which may signify malignant transformation. Focal lytic areas within an otherwise well-mineralized lesion should also arouse suspicion for malignancy.

Although often discovered by chance, patients may complain of a firm mass that has been present for years. Symptoms may result from fracture, bursal formation, impingement on surrounding structures, decreased joint motion from mass effect, or malignant transformation.

Radiographically, lesions may present as a sessile surface lesion (especially on flat bones) or as a pedunculated mass. The stalk of the lesion (which generally points away from the nearest joint) *shares the cortex of the adjacent bone,* and the intramedullary contents of the host bone flow into the lesion (Fig. 2). The OCE is covered with a lobulated *cartilage cap,* which may be mineralized. This cartilage cap is active in the immature skeleton and slowly grows via endochondral ossification (hence its warmth on bone scintigraphy).

If OCE growth continues after skeletal maturity, or if the cartilage cap exceeds 1–2 cm in thickness, then malignant transformation of the lesion must be considered. The risk of this transformation is likely less than 1% in the solitary lesion. CT or MRI is often helpful in delineating the details of the lesion and in assessing the size of the cartilage cap.

Osteochondromatosis (multiple hereditary exostosis) is an autosomal-dominant disorder resulting in multiple OCEs associated with bone deformities of the affected sites.[6] Malignant degeneration is reported to be as high as 25% of cases but is likely to be as low as 1% to 2%.[7]

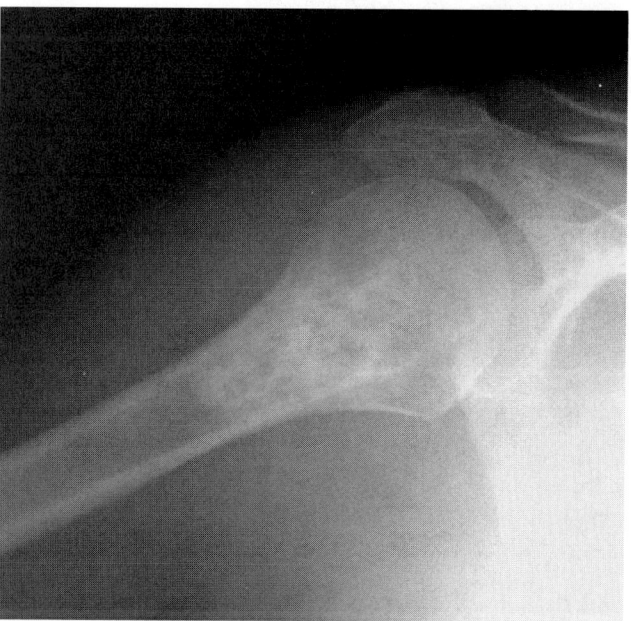

Fig. 3. View. Radiograph of the proximal humerus shows the common appearance of an enchondroma. Note the central location of this lesion and the presence of uniform calcification. This particular lesion lacks mild expansion, and the endosteal scalloping is very subtle. The appearance of these cartilage lesions can vary considerably.

Enchondromatosis (multiple enchondromas, presenting as Ollier's or Maffucci's syndrome) frequently presents with unilateral involvement of the appendicular skeleton. Often, bone deformity is severe as a result of the diffuse lesions. The prevalence of malignant transformation is approximately 25%.[9]

Histologically, the lesion is composed of mature cartilage of variable cellularity. These lobules of cartilage are incompletely separated by thin fibrovascular septae. The tremendous variation in cellularity of these lesions can make interpretation difficult for the pathologist, and the knowledge of clinical behavior and location is paramount in making the appropriate diagnosis.

Radiographically, the differential diagnosis includes low-grade chondrosarcoma, bone infarct, and fibrous dysplasia.

CHONDROBLASTOMA

Chondroblastoma (CBMA) is a benign lesion of immature cartilage cells that classically involves the epiphysis of major long bones in the immature skeleton. This lesion is relatively rare, accounting for less than 1% of bone lesions. CBMA generally presents in adolescents, with a male/female ratio of approximately 1.4:1.[10]

One-third of these lesions occur around the knee (distal femur/proximal tibia), followed by the proximal humerus and the proximal femur. Other typical locations include the periacetabular region and the calcaneus.[11]

The common presenting symptom is pain. Symptoms referred to the joint (stiffness, swelling, etc.) are frequently encountered as well.

Radiographically, CBMA typically presents as a well-demarcated, eccentrically located lytic lesion of the epiphysis with a sclerotic rim. These lesions are usually 4 cm or less in size. Some 25% to 30% of these tumors show sparse trabeculation or calcification, often best seen on CT scan. Larger lesions may expand or even break through the cortex[12] (Fig. 4).

Rare cases of multifocal lesions have been reported. CBMA may also behave in an aggressive fashion clinically, and pulmonary metastases are well documented.[13]

Histologically, closely packed chondroblasts (*cobblestone appearance*) with scattered multinucleated giant cells and areas of immature cartilaginous matrix are common. Fine, linear, calcified deposits (*chicken-wire calcification*) are typical.

Radiographically, the differential diagnosis includes giant-cell tumor, aneurysmal bone cyst, osteomyelitis, and clear-cell chondrosarcoma.

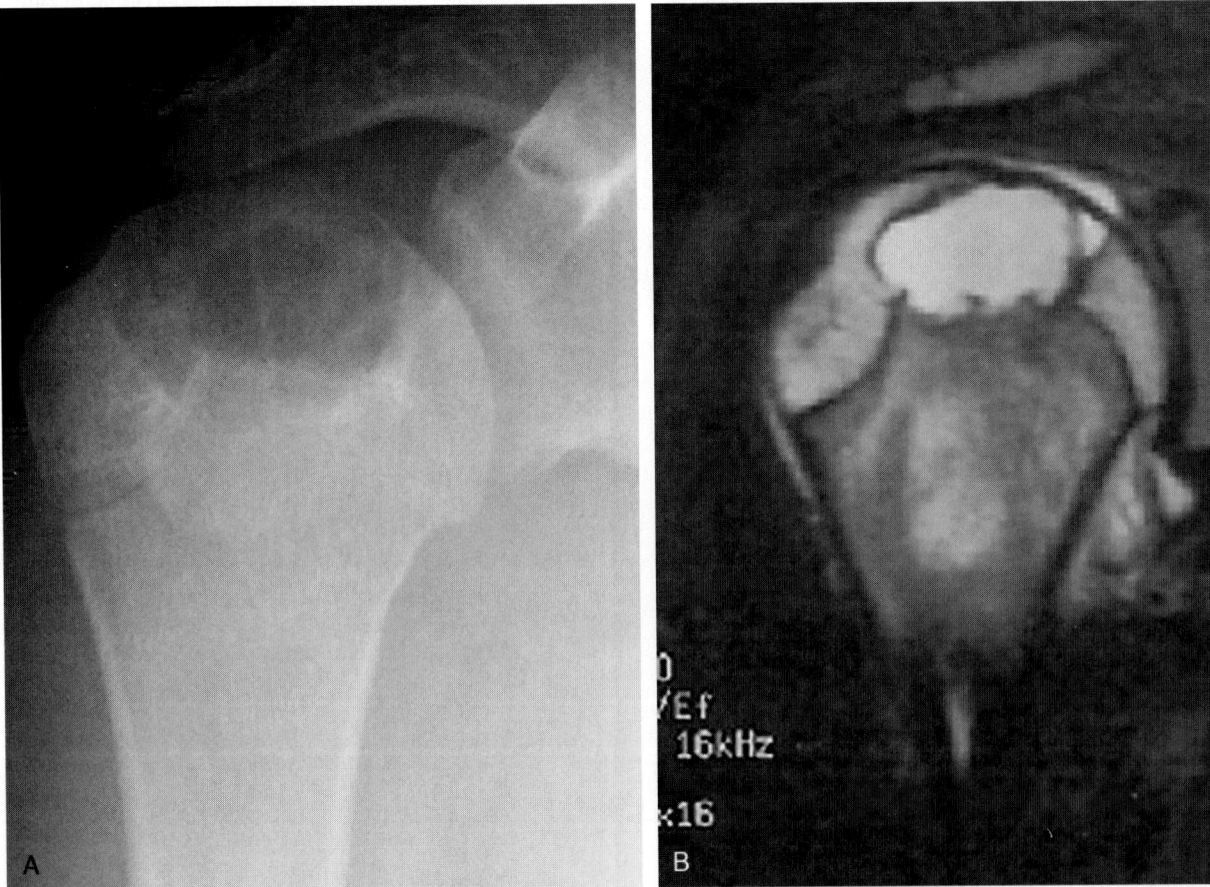

Fig. 4. Views. *A,* Radiograph of the proximal humerus showing a large chondroblastoma in the epiphysis. The size of this lesion has led to subchondral bone destruction and breakthrough into the joint. This particular lesion has neither mineralization nor a sclerotic margin. *B,* MRI (T$_2$-weighted, fat saturation coronal image) of lesion seen in *A.* Note the classic epiphyseal location with local bone destruction. There is little edema in the surrounding marrow signal. The complete destruction of the subchondral bone is clearly delineated.

FIBROUS TUMORS

NONOSSIFYING FIBROMA (FIBROUS CORTICAL DEFECT)

Nonossifying fibroma (NOF) is a metaphyseal fibrous lesion seen predominantly in skeletally immature individuals. These lesions are found in some 30% of individuals with open physes and may represent a developmental condition rather than a neoplasm per se. There is a slight male predominance, and most lesions are identified in the second decade. The distal femoral metaphysis is the most common site, followed by the proximal tibial and the distal tibial metaphyses. Lesions of the upper extremity are far less common.[14]

NOF is generally found by chance, as most lesions are asymptomatic. Larger lesions may cause mechanical pain, and pathological fractures through these lesions are not uncommon.[15]

Radiographically, NOF presents as an eccentrically located lytic metaphyseal tumor with distinct and frequently sclerotic margins. The overlying cortex is generally intact, but it may be thinned and is frequently expanded. Although matrix mineralization is absent, a "bubbly" or trabecular pattern at the periphery of the lesion is common (Fig. 5). These lesions may be multifocal and associated with other anomalies.[16] The natural history appears to be

spontaneous regression over time, often leaving an area of denser, benign-appearing bone.

Histologically, NOF is characterized by a dense population of spindle cells with a prominent storiform pattern. Multinucleated giant cells and xanthomatous foci are common.

Radiographically, the differential diagnosis includes fibrous dysplasia and desmoplastic fibroma.

FIBROUS DYSPLASIA

Fibrous dysplasia (FIBDYS) is a dysplastic condition of bone characterized by intramedullary fibrous proliferations in which scattered trabeculae of woven bone are present. The lesion may present in a monostotic form, which is far more common, or a polyostotic form, which is generally unilateral and involves only one extremity. The diagnosis is generally made in the first three decades of life, with a slight female predominance. The most common sites include the ribs, proximal femur, and the tibia.[17]

Monostotic lesions are usually asymptomatic and are discovered by chance. In those cases where the lesions are symptomatic, pain, swelling, deformity, or pathological fracture may be present.[18]

Polyostotic lesions may be associated with extraskeletal manifestations, such as café au lait spots or axillary freckling. Various endocrinopathies, such as Albright's syndrome (precocious puberty in females, polyostotic lesions, café au lait spots), hyperthyroidism, and Cushing's syndrome, are well documented.

Radiographically, FIBDYS appears as a geographic, intramedullary lesion with a *ground glass* appearance. The density of the lesions varies with the amount of immature bone produced. Cortical thinning and expansion of the bone contour is common (Fig. 6). Areas of punctate calcification may be seen. Extensive involvement of the bone can lead to significant deformities, such as *shepherd's crook* deformity of the proximal femur.[19]

Histologically, the lesion is characterized by whorls of spindle cells, with scattered trabeculae of woven bone (*Chinese C's and O's*) that lack rimming osteoblasts. The lack of osteoblastic rimming clearly distinguishes this as neoplastic rather than reactive bone formation.

Radiographically, the differential diagnosis is fairly broad, as FIBDYS can mimic many lesions. One should consider desmoplastic fibroma, osteofibrous dysplasia, nonossifying fibroma, and even chondroid lesions.

CYSTIC LESIONS

SOLITARY BONE CYST

Solitary bone cyst (SBC) is a common lesion of the immature skeleton, characterized by an intramedullary fluid-filled cavity that forms in the metaphysis, juxtaposed to or near the physis. The lesion generally presents between ages 3 and 14 years, with a male/female ratio of approximately 2:1. Some 80% of lesions are found in the proximal humerus and proximal femur, but other locations such as the calcaneus and ilium are also seen.[20]

Most lesions are asymptomatic, but patients may present with pain, swelling, and deformity following pathological fracture.

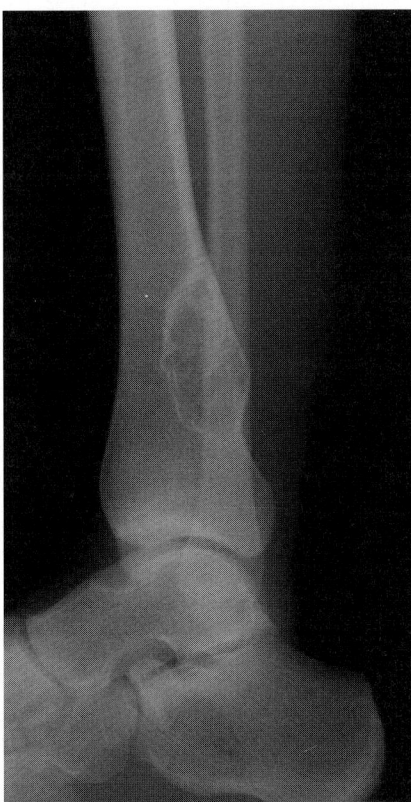

Fig. 5. View. Lateral radiograph of the tibia shows the classic appearance of nonossifying fibroma. Note the distinct margins of the lesion, which is eccentrically located and causes mild expansion of the cortex. The bubbly pattern seen is a common presentation as is the metaphyseal location.

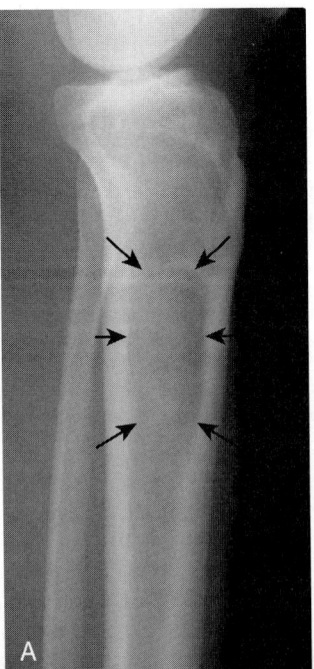

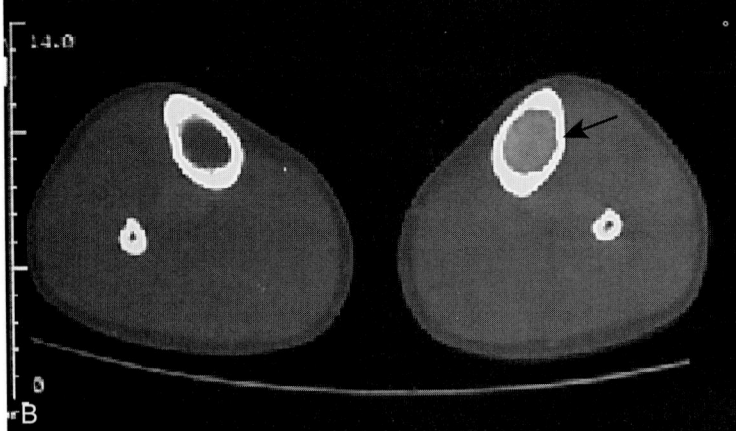

Fig. 6. Views. *A,* Lateral radiograph of the proximal tibia showing common "ground glass" appearance of fibrous dysplasia (*arrows*). Note the modest expansion of the cortical contour and the modest thinning of the cortex overlying the lesion. No calcification is seen. *B,* CT scan through lesion seen in *A.* Note the increased density of the intramedullary contents (*arrow*) compared with that of the contralateral tibia. This axial view also demonstrates the modest expansion of the bone and the cortical thinning.

Radiographically, the lesion presents as a geographic intramedullary lucency. The cortex is often markedly thinned and the bone contour frequently expanded (Fig. 7). Reactive periosteal changes are rarely seen, unless there has been a pathological fracture. Occasionally, a piece of fractured cortex may drop into the cyst, and the *fallen fragment sign* is noted on plain films. The lesion may abut or even cross the physis; this is generally seen in younger children and has been referred to as an *active cyst.* In older children, the lesion tends to be in a more metadiaphyseal or diaphyseal location and has been referred to as an *inactive cyst.* SBC regresses and heals following skeletal maturity.[21, 22]

Histologically, a scant layer of fibrous tissue (not a true lining) with scattered inflammatory and multinucleated giant cells is observed. Focal deposits of hemosiderin are common.

Radiographically, the differential diagnosis includes fibrous dysplasia and aneurysmal bone cyst.

ANEURYSMAL BONE CYST

Aneurysmal bone cyst (ABC) is a locally destructive, blood-filled, multilocular, cystic lesion of bone. ABC accounts for some 3% of primary bone lesions. Approximately 80% of lesions occur in patients younger than 20 years of age, with the peak incidence in the second decade. There is no clear sex predilection. Although any bone may be affected, the most common sites include the femur, tibia, and spine.[23]

Clinically, the lesion presents with pain and swelling, the duration of which can be highly variable. Lesions near joints may present with symptoms referred to the joint (swelling, stiffness, etc.), and lesions of the spine may cause neurological symptoms.

Radiographically, the classic appearance is that of a lytic lesion with a "blowout" or "ballooned" appearance to the cortex. A thin rim of bone surrounds the lesion. The multilocular pattern of ABC gives rise to the *soap-bubble* appearance of the lesion. Generally, ABC is eccentric in

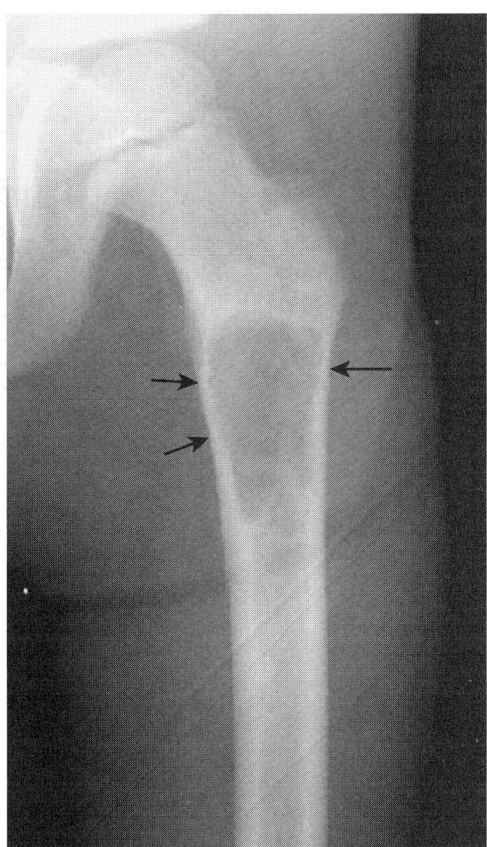

Fig. 7. View. Anteroposterior radiograph of the proximal femur demonstrates the common appearance of a simple bone cyst. The lesion is in the classic metaphyseal location and has thinned the overlying cortex (*arrows*). Marked cortical thinning and modest enlargement of the bone is common with SBC.

location and involves the metaphysis, but diaphyseal and even epiphyseal locations are seen. In the spine, ABC typically originates in the posterior elements. CT and MRI are useful in documenting the multilocular nature of the lesion (*fluid-fluid levels* are commonly seen) and in demonstrating the thin rim or bone that surrounds the lesion[24] (Fig. 8).

Histologically, the lesion is characterized by loose septae of fibrous tissue, inflammatory cells, and multinucleated giant cells, surrounding *lakes of blood*. Focal areas of reactive bone are commonly seen.

Secondary ABC superimposed on a preexisting lesion is common and often reflects features of both underlying processes.[25]

Radiographically, the differential diagnosis includes giant-cell tumor, fibrous dysplasia, telangiectatic osteosarcoma, and simple cyst.

GIANT-CELL LESIONS

GIANT-CELL TUMOR

Giant-cell tumor (GCT) is an aggressive, destructive epiphyseal lesion characterized by abundant multinucleated giant cells. GCT accounts for some 5% of primary bone lesions, with approximately 70% of lesions presenting in patients from the age of 20 to 40 years. It is very rare in patients younger than 20 years of age. There appears to be a slight female predominance. Nearly 50% of cases present around the knee (distal femur, proximal tibia), followed by the distal radius and the sacrum.[26]

Clinically, GCT presents with pain or symptoms referred to the joint (swelling, stiffness, etc.). A mass effect may be present from soft-tissue extension, and pathological fractures are not uncommon.

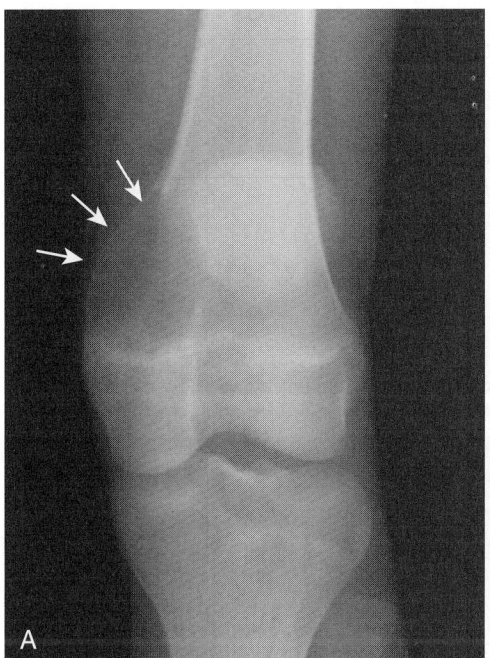
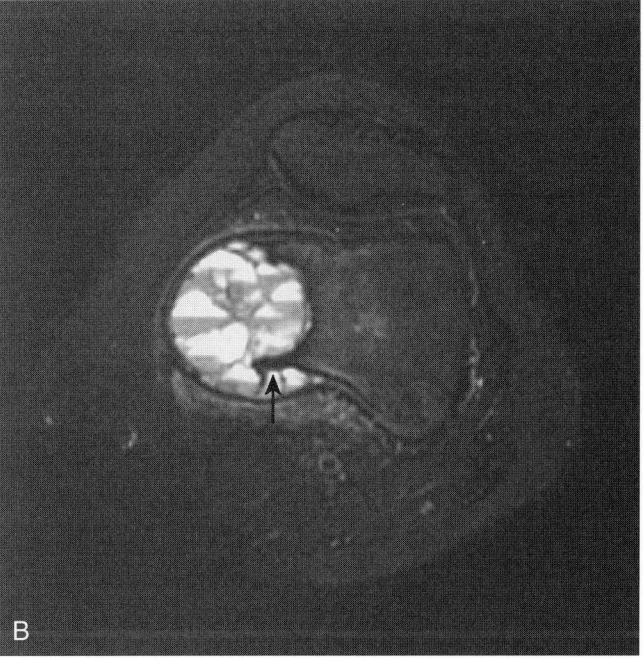

Fig. 8. Views. *A,* Anteroposterior radiograph of the distal femur showing an eccentric, metaphyseal, aneurysmal bone cyst. Note that the lesion is focally destructive, has caused a marked expansion or "blowout" of the cortex, and is covered with a thin rim of bone (*arrows*). *B,* MRI (T$_2$-weighted, fat saturation axial image) of the lesion seen in *A.* The extent of the local destruction is well visualized, and the appearance of the multiple cavities with fluid-fluid levels is classic for aneurysmal bone cyst. Note the original cortical margin extending into the lesion (*arrow*).

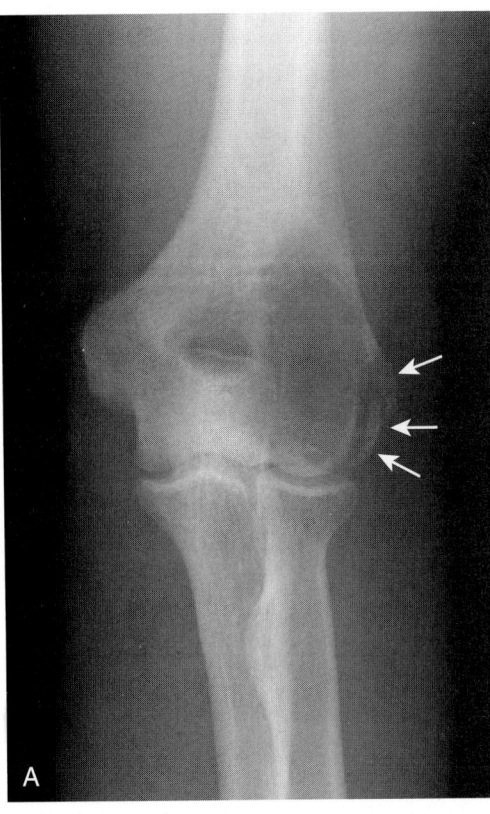
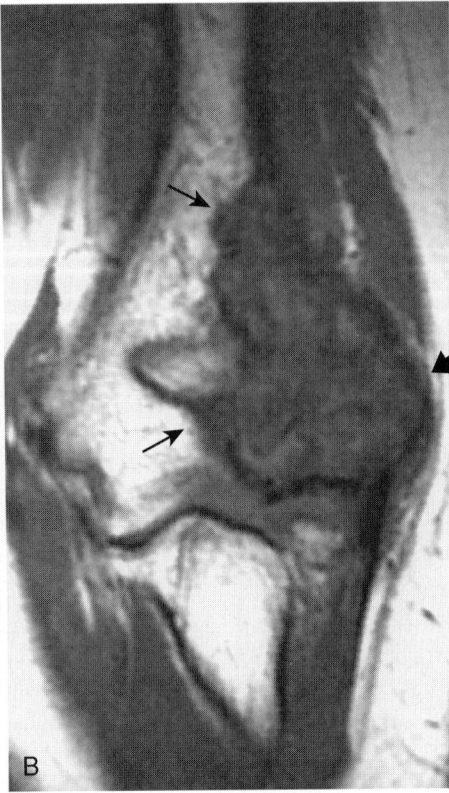

Fig. 9. Views. *A,* Anteroposterior radiograph of the distal humerus showing poorly marginated giant-cell tumor that involves the bone all the way to the subchondral articular surface. There is evidence of modest expansion of the bony contour, pathological fracture (*arrows*), and a paucity of any periosteal reaction. This lesion most commonly presents around the knee. *B,* MRI (T$_1$-weighted, coronal image) of the lesion seen in *A.* Note the extensive involvement of subchondral bone and the tumor expanding the lateral aspect of the bone (*large arrow*). The stark contrast (without edema) between normal marrow and the lesion on T$_1$ imaging is common in giant-cell tumor (*arrows*).

Radiographically, the tumor classically presents as a lytic, eccentric, subchondral lesion that involves the epiphyseal/metaphyseal region of bone. Tumor destruction that extends to the subchondral surface of the joint is common. The cortex is frequently thinned, often expanded, and may be completely destroyed in areas. Although a geographic lesion, its borders are usually not well defined, and trabeculation within the tumor is generally absent. Periosteal reaction, if at all present, is minimal[27] (Fig. 9).

GCT has been classified radiographically into three grades, based on its appearance and behavior.[28] However, the clinical behavior of the lesion and its appearance (both radiographic and histological) show no clear correlation,

and there appears to be no true prognostic value in grading this tumor. GCT is rarely multicentric; pulmonary metastases are well documented; and malignant transformations have been reported.[29] This tumor appears to have the ability to behave anywhere from locally aggressive to frankly malignant.

Histologically, the lesion consists of a stroma of plump mononuclear cells, with abundant multinucleated giant cells. The nuclei of both stromal and giant cells are similar in appearance.

Radiographically, the differential diagnosis includes aneurysmal bone cyst, chondroblastoma, clear-cell chondrosarcoma, and osteosarcoma.

REFERENCES

1. Dorfman HD, Czerniak B: Osteoid osteoma. In Bone Tumors. St. Louis, Mosby, 1998, p 85.
2. Healy JH, Ghelman B: Osteoid osteoma and osteoblastoma: Current concepts and recent advances. Clin Orthop 204; 76: 1986.
3. Greco F, Tamburrelli F, Ciabattoni G: Prostaglandins in osteoid osteoma. Int Orthop 15; 35:1991.
4. Jackson RP, Reckling FW, Mants FA: Osteoid osteoma and osteoblastoma: Similar histologic lesions with different natural histories. Clin Orthop 128; 303:1977.
5. Dorfman HD, Czerniak B: Osteochondroma. In Bone Tumors. St. Louis, Mosby, 1998, p 331.

6. Peterson HA: Multiple hereditary osteochondroma. Clin Orthop 239:222, 1989.
7. Schmale GA, Conrad EU, Raskinel WH: The natural history of hereditary multiple exostoses. J Bone Joint Surg Am 76; 986: 1994.
8. Dorfman HD, Czerniak B: Enchrondroma. In Bone Tumors. St. Louis, Mosby, 1998, p 253.
9. Schwartz HS, Zimmerman NB, Simion MA, et al: The malignant potential of enchondromatosis. J Bone Joint Surg Am 69; 269:1987.
10. Dorfman HD, Czerniak B: Chondroblastoma. In Bone Tumors. St. Louis, Mosby, 1998, p 296.

11. Bloem JL, Simon MA: Chondroblastoma: A clinical and radiological study of 104 cases. Skeletal Radiol 14; 1:1985.
12. Huvos AG, Marcove RC: Chondroblastoma of bone: A critical review. Clin Orthop 95; 300:1973.
13. Huvos AG, Higinbotham NL, Marcove RC, et al: Aggressive chondroblastoma: Review of the literature on aggressive behavior and metastases with a report of one new case. Clin Orthop 126; 266:1977.
14. Dorfman HD, Czerniak B: Nonossifying fibroma. In Bone Tumors. St. Louis, Mosby, 1998, p 492.
15. Arata MA, Peterson HA, Dahlin DC: Pathological fractures through nonossifying fibromas: Review of the Mayo Clinic

experience. J Bone Joint Surg Am 63; 980:1981.

16. Mirra JM, Gold RH, Rand F: Disseminated nonossifying fibromas in association with café-au-lait spots (Jaffe-Companacci syndrome). Clin Orthop 168; 192:1982.

17. Dorfman HD, Czerniak B: Fibrous dysplasia. In Bone Tumors. St Louis, Mosby, 1998, p 441.

18. Harris WH, Dudley HR Jr, Barry RJ: The natural history of fibrous dysplasia. J Bone Joint Surg Am 44; 207:1962.

19. Grabias SL, Campbell CJ: Fibrous Dysplasia. Orthop Clin North Am 8; 771:1977.

20. Dorfman HD, Czerniak B: Solitary bone cyst. In Bone Tumors. St. Louis, Mosby, 1998, p 879.

21. Neer CS, Francis KC, Marcove RC, et al:

A follow-up study of one hundred seventy-five cases: Treatment of unicameral bone cyst. J Bone Joint Surg Am 48; 731: 1966.

22. Cohen J: Unicameral bone cysts: A current synthesis of reported cases. Orthop Clin North Am 8; 715:1977.

23. Dorfman HD, Czerniak B: Aneurysmal bone cyst. In Bone Tumors. St Louis, Mosby, 1998, p 855.

24. Vergel De Dios AM, Bond JR, Shives TC, et al: Aneurysmal bone cyst: A clinicopathologic study of 238 cases. Cancer 69; 2921:1992.

25. Martinez V, Sissons HA: Aneurysmal bone cyst: A review of 123 cases including primary lesions and those secondary to

other bone pathology. Cancer 61; 2291: 1988.

26. Dorfman HD, Czerniak B. Conventional giant-cell tumor of bone. In Bone Tumors. St. Louis, Mosby, 1998, p 559.

27. Goldenberg RR, Campbell CJ, Bonfiglio M: Giant-cell tumor of bone: An analysis of two hundred and eighteen cases. J Bone Joint Surg Am 52; 619:1970.

28. Campanacci M, Baldini N, Boriani S: Giant-cell tumor of bone. J Bone Joint Surg Am 69; 106:1987.

29. Maloney WJ, Vaughan LM, Jones HH, et al: Benign metastasizing giant-cell tumor of bone: Report of three cases and review of the literature. Clin Orthop 234; 208: 1989.

section 7 chapter 7

MALIGNANT BONE TUMORS

Marco Manfrini

Summary

- Primary tumors of bone are rare, and they are less common than metastatic lesions, generally carcinomas.
- Bone tumors are defined by both histology (Schajowicz/WHO classification) and surgical staging (Enneking).
- Osteosarcoma is a malignant tumor composed of mesenchymal cells that produce osteoid and immature bone.
- Ewing's sarcoma is a malignant tumor composed of poorly differentiated small round cells. The genotypic lesion is precisely the same as in peripheral neuroectodermal tumor and Askin's tumor.
- Chondrosarcoma is a malignant tumor composed of chondrocytes that fill the medullary canal and invade cancellous bone.
- Malignant fibrous histiocytoma is an intramedullary, high-grade sarcoma, most commonly localized in the long bones.

Primary bone malignancies are rare. Much more frequently, a skeletal lesion is secondary spread of a tumor (usually carcinoma) that has arisen in another organ. Nevertheless, in the last 20 years, a progressive increase in interest in sarcoma of bone has been displayed all over the world. In this period, in fact, significant advances have been made in classification, diagnostic management, molecular genetics, and, over all, the treatment of these diseases.

CLASSIFICATION AND STAGING

A reliable classification of bone tumors should distinguish between neoplasms that show well-defined features, not only in their histological appearance but also in their clinical, imaging, treatment, and prognostic characteristics and, increasingly, in their genetic background. However, it is practical and traditional to group tumors according to their histogenesis. The still more used, histological classification is one proposed by Schajowicz in 1972 and then adopted by the World Health Organization (WHO) (Table 1). Bone tumors are also defined as low-grade when their histological grade is 1 or 2 according to Broder's grading. Their growth is slow but more progressive than that of benign lesions, and some may indolently grow to huge sizes. Grade 1 or 2 tumors may manifest progression in malignancy over time, transforming to high-grade neoplasms. High-grade malignant tumors (Broder's grade 3 and 4) generally grow rapidly and invade adjacent structures. Cell differentiation and function are decreased and anomalous. Growth is invasive and infiltrative; thus, the tumor lacks well-defined limits.

Histological classification (type and grade) is not sufficient to describe a tumor's behavior. It is also necessary to stage the malignant bone tumor in each patient. The goals of a staging system are to group patients with similar risks of death and to use this classification as a guide to treatment. There are numerous staging systems, but the one in widespread use for malignant primary tumors of bone was devised in 1980 by Enneking.[1] This staging system was devised to be simple to use and is employed primarily as a surgical staging system.

This system is based on the concept of compartments separated by a natural barrier to tumor spread. Natural barriers are cortical bone, fascia and fascial septa, articular cartilage, joint capsule, and tendons. Fat and interstitial tissue, such as the tissue around neurovascular bundles, are extracompartmental. Any natural barrier, such as cortical bone, fascia, and even articular cartilage, can be breached by an aggressive tumor. Other thin barriers are the perios-

TABLE 1. HISTOLOGICAL CLASSIFICATION OF BONE TUMORS			
Differentiation or Histogenesis	**Benign**	**Low-Grade Malignant**	**High-Grade Malignant**
Fibrous and histiocytic	Histiocytic fibroma Giant cell tumor Desmoid fibroma	Grade 1 and 2 fibrosar-coma	Grade 3 and 4 fibrosarcoma *Malignant* fibrous histiocytoma (MFH)
Cartilaginous	Exostosis Chondroma Chondroblastoma Chondromyxoid fibroma	*Central CS (grade 1, 2)* *Peripheral CS* *Periosteal CS* *Clear cell CS*	*Central CS (grade 3)* *Dedifferentiated CS* *Mesenchymal CS*
Osseous	Osteoid osteoma Osteoblastoma	*Parosteal OS* *Periosteal OS* Low-grade central OS	*Classic OS* *Telangiectatic OS* *Small cell OS* Osteosarcomatosis
Hemopoietic			Lymphoma Plasmacytoma
Vascular	Hemangioma Lymphangioma	Hemangioendothelioma Hemangiopericytoma	Angiosarcoma Hemangiopericytoma
Nervous	Neurinoma Neurofibroma		*Ewing's sarcoma* *Peripheral neuroectodermic tumor*
Epithelial	Osteofibrous dysplasia	Adamantinoma	
Notochordal		Chordoma	

CS = chondrosarcoma; OS = osteosarcoma.

teum, the synovial membrane, and the sheaths of the major nerves. Where the joint capsule, the ligaments and the tendons insert into an epiphysis or metaphysis, the only barrier is a thin cortex with vascular perforations through which the tumor may easily extend from the cancellous bone into adjacent structures.

The surgical staging system (Enneking's) employs the following three parameters (Table 2):

- G indicates histological grade.
- T signifies local anatomic extension.
- M indicates metastases.

Sarcomas of bone are staged as I (low-grade malignancy—G1, M0), II (high-grade malignancy—G2, M0), or III (with metastases—any G, M1). Different stages are subdivided into A and B according to whether the tumor is intracompartmental (T1) or extracompartmental (T2).

Primary tumors of bone are rare. Among malignant tumors, the most frequently observed is plasmacytoma, but it is more a systemic malignancy of bone marrow than a true primary tumor of bone. The major primary sarcomas of bone are therefore osteosarcoma, Ewing's sarcoma, and chondrosarcoma. These three neoplasms and their main subvarieties are described in this chapter. Only the principal features of other, less common tumors (malignant fibrous histiocytoma, chordoma and adamantinoma) are considered.

OSTEOSARCOMA

Osteosarcoma is a malignant tumor composed of mesenchymal cells producing osteoid and immature bone.[2] Most are intramedullary, but they may originate on the bone's surface. The types are classic high-grade, periosteal, parosteal, radiation-associated, and low-grade intramedullary osteosarcomas.

CLASSIC OSTEOSARCOMA
Epidemiology and Clinical Features

Osteosarcoma represents only 0.2% of all malignancies, with an incidence rate estimated as two to three new cases per million people per year. Most of the new cases occur in the second decade of life, but this tumor may present at any age. In the older adult, it is usually secondary to radiation, Paget's disease, or another preexisting lesion. Males are more commonly affected than females in a ratio of 1.5:1 to 1.7:1. Seventy percent of osteosarcomas occur in the distal femur, proximal tibia, or proximal humerus, suggesting a relationship to rapid bone growth sites; however, osteosarcoma may arise anywhere in the skeleton. They usually grow in the metaphysis or metadiaphysis but tend to invade the epiphysis even when the growth plate is still open.

Pain is usually the first symptom, but most patients relate the pain to trauma. Later, a mass develops, often in association with decreased motion in the adjacent joint. A patient with an osteosarcoma only rarely has systemic symptoms. Pathological fracture may occur, mainly in os-

TABLE 2. ENNEKING (MUSCULOSKELETAL TUMOR SOCIETY) STAGING SYSTEM FOR BONE TUMORS

Low-grade I
    Intracompartmental IA
    Extracompartmental IB
High-grade II
    Intracompartmental IIA
    Extracompartmental IIB
Metastatic III
    Intracompartmental IIIA
    Extracompartmental IIIB

teolytic forms. An elevation of serum alkaline phosphatase value is more common than elevation of serum lactate dehydrogenase (LDH), although both have been related to an adverse prognosis. Other laboratory values are normal.

At presentation, 80% of osteosarcomas are stage IIB lesions, only 5% are stage IIA, and about 15% are stage III lesions. Without the use of chemotherapy, 80% to 90% of patients with osteosarcoma die of metastases, notwithstanding surgical ablation of the primary tumor; therefore, 80% to 90% of patients have subclinical micrometastases at presentation.

In most patients with osteosarcoma, no predisposing factor is identified. Exposure to radiotherapy in infancy may explain the rare cases of radiation-induced osteosarcoma in very young patients, whereas a genetic predisposition to osteosarcoma has been demonstrated in the survivors of heritable retinoblastoma.

No characteristic cytogenetic abnormality has been found. A wide spectrum of highly complex chromosomal changes have been observed (e.g., germline mutations of the tumor suppressor gene p53, overexpression of oncogenic *fos*, alteration of gene CDK4 or SAS).

Imaging

Conventional radiography is usually diagnostic. Typically, osteosarcoma starts within the medulla but breaches the cortex and expands into the soft tissues. It is usually a mix of poorly defined radiolucencies and radiodensities but it may manifest as an entirely dense or lucent lesion (Fig. 1). The pure osteolytic form is typical of the telangiectatic variety. Soft-tissue extension is evident in 90% of cases and appears as irregular, cloud-like radiodensities or, rarely, perpendicular stripes of density (sun-ray image). Along the cortex, a triangular buttress of immature bone (Codman's triangle) produced by the periosteum is frequently recognized.

Commonly, isotopic (technetium 99m deposition) bone scan is intensely hot, even beyond what is seen on a plain radiograph. This activity on the bone scan indicates the extent of bone reaction to the tumor. Computed tomography (CT) demonstrates the intraosseous and extraosseous extension of the tumor and the intratumoral radiodensities, but magnetic resonance imaging (MRI) is the best way to determine the medullary tumor borders, epiphyseal invasion, and borders of the soft-tissue mass. A CT scan of the lungs is routinely performed. Metastases to the lung appear as radiodense round nodules.

Histopathology and Differential Diagnosis

Microscopically, osteosarcoma has a wide range of histological presentations, but the characteristic feature is high-grade sarcomatous cells producing osteoid and woven bone. The cells are large, with striking pleomorphism, hyperchromia, prominent nucleoli, and frequent atypical mitoses. The tumor matrix varies from slender seams of osteoid to islands or sheets of woven bone (Fig. 2).

The most relevant diagnostic feature is invasion of the marrow spaces, which traps the host trabecular bone. The cortex is also permeated and usually breached with invasion of surrounding soft tissues. Endosteal and periosteal production of reactive bone occurs. Rarely, osteosarcoma plugs are found in the adjacent veins. Skip metastases,

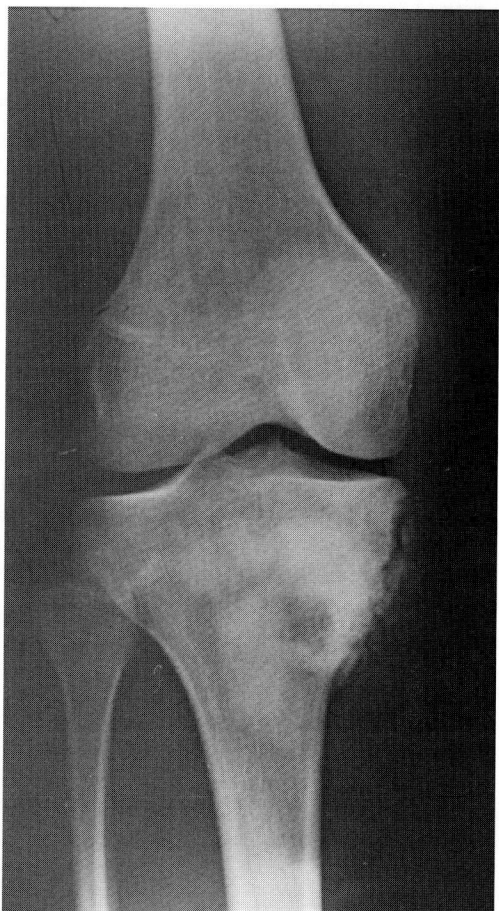

Fig. 1. Conventional osteosarcoma of proximal tibia. A poorly defined mixed radiolytic and radiodense lesion is associated with a periosteal reaction. (From McCarthy EF, Frassica FJ: Pathology of Bone and Joint Disorders. Philadelphia, WB Saunders, 1998, p 208; originally from Frassica FJ, McCarthy EF: Orthopaedic pathology. In Miller MD [ed]: Review of Orthopaedics. Philadelphia, WB Saunders, 1996, 2nd ed, p 303.)

usually in the same but also in the adjacent cross-joint bone, have been reported in a variable percentage of cases (from 2% to 20%). Radiographic diagnosis of osteosarcoma may be easy, but imaging alone is occasionally misleading. Osteolytic osteosarcoma can mimic malignant fibrous histiocytoma, fibrosarcoma, aneurysmal bone cyst, or even giant cell tumor. Diaphyseal osteosarcoma may resemble Ewing's sarcoma or lymphoma. Rarely, a small sclerotic osteosarcoma may resemble a bony island.

Course and Prognosis

Modern treatment of a classic high-grade osteosarcoma consists of surgical resection preceded and followed by multidrug systemic chemotherapy. Before chemotherapy, the 5-year disease-free survival rate was around 15% to 20%. Current neoadjuvant chemotherapy for stage II osteosarcoma has a 65% to 70% 5-year disease-free survival rate.[3] Metastases (mainly to the lung) usually occur in the first 2 to 3 years. There are, however, rare cases of metastases occurring 5 to 10 years after treatment.

PERIOSTEAL OSTEOSARCOMA

Periosteal osteosarcoma is a rare variant of osteosarcoma (about 2% to 3% of all cases), predominantly chondroblastic and originating from the periosteum, usually in a long bone diaphysis. Preferred locations are tibial and femoral diaphyses. Such tumors are less common in the humerus and are rare in other long bones.

Periosteal osteosarcoma generally grows more slowly than classic high-grade osteosarcoma. Metastases, usually to lung, have been observed in only 15% of cases. Surgical resection without chemotherapy is the standard treatment.

PAROSTEAL OSTEOSARCOMA

Parosteal osteosarcoma is a variant of osteosarcoma (6% of all osteosarcomas). It originates at the surface of a long-bone metaphysis, with abundant production of dense bone and low-grade anaplasia. It displays a slight preference for females and usually appears in patients aged between 20 and 50 years. The most typical site is the posterior aspect of the distal femur (60% of the cases). The patient usually only complains of loss of motion in the adjacent joint. Radiographic diagnosis is usually easy; the tumor appears as a lobulated mass of intense radiodensity fused to the cortex with a broad base that tends to wrap around the bone (Fig. 3).

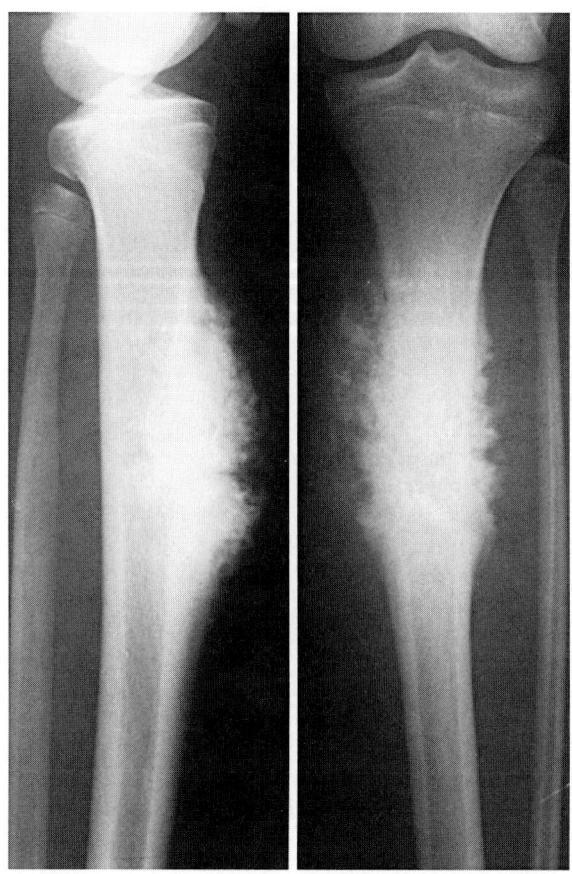

Fig. 3. Views. Lateral (*left*) and anteroposterior (*right*) radiographs of parosteal osteosarcoma of the tibia. A well-defined surface mass contains stippled and linear radiodensities. (From McCarthy EF, Frassica FJ: Pathology of Bone and Joint Disorders. Philadelphia, WB Saunders, 1998, p 213.)

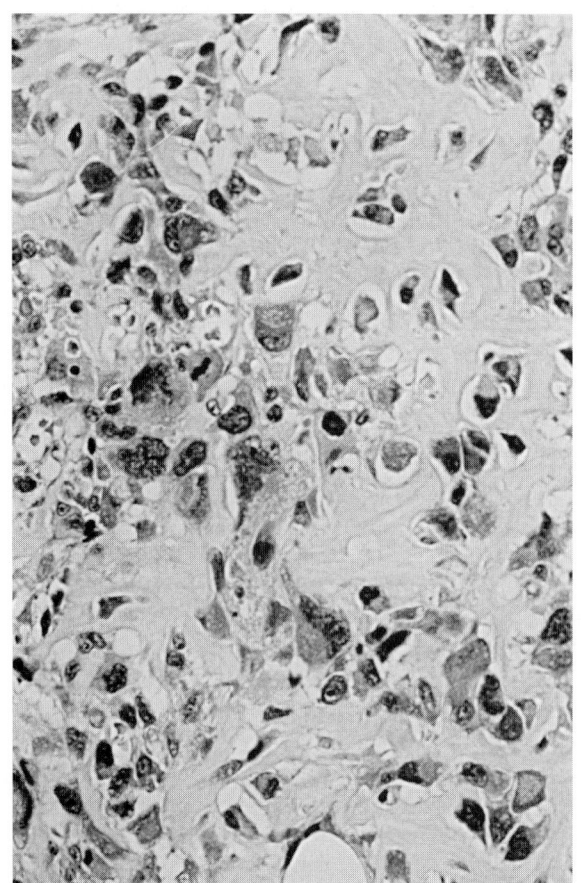

Fig. 2. Photomicrograph of conventional osteosarcoma. Bizarre pleomorphic cells are present in an osteoid matrix. (From McCarthy EF, Frassica FJ: Pathology of Bone and Joint Disorders. Philadelphia, WB Saunders, 1998, p 209.)

Parosteal osteosarcoma grows slowly but relentlessly. A complete surgical resection is curative in 90% of patients.

EWING'S SARCOMA AND PERIPHERAL NEUROECTODERMAL TUMOR

Ewing's sarcoma is a malignant tumor composed of poorly differentiated small round cells. The discovery of Ewing's sarcoma–associated cytogenic translocation t(11;22) (q24-12), found in Ewing's sarcoma, peripheral neuroectodermal tumor (PNET), and Askin's tumor, established that these lesions are different phenotypic presentations of the same genotypic disorder.

Ewing's sarcoma usually displays an aggressive growth. There are, however, cases in which sarcoma remains intraosseous from 1 to several years. Metastases, usually multiple, appear most frequently in the lungs, followed by skeleton and lymph nodes.

Before the use of chemotherapy, long-term survival was less than 10%. Presently, with multimodal treatment, it is around 60% to 70%. A more favorable prognosis can be expected for younger patients, in distal appendicular locations, and in cases of small tumor volume.

Ewing's sarcoma is three times less common than osteosarcoma. It is more common in males than in females, at a

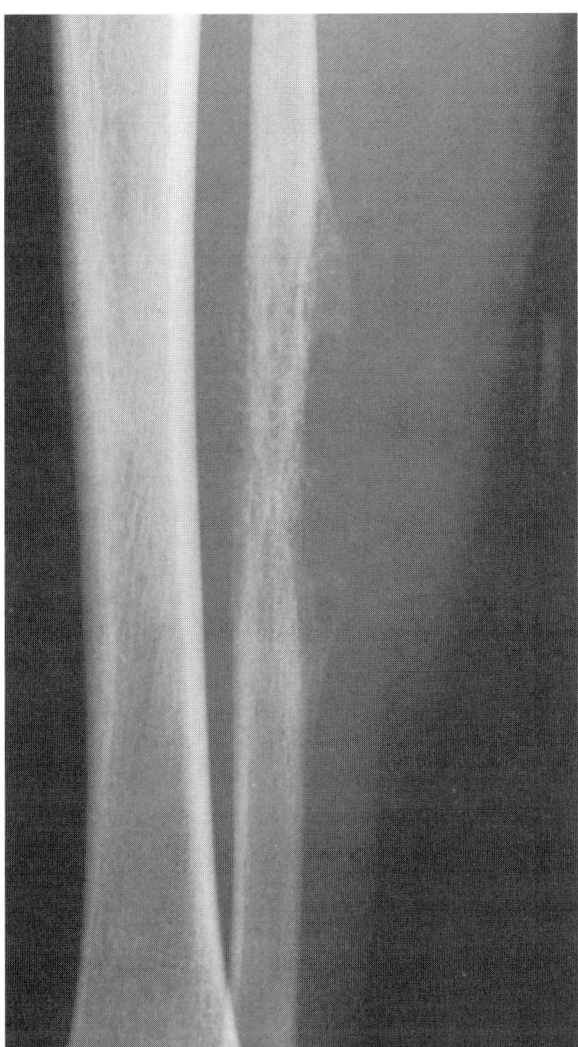

Fig. 4. Radiograph of a Ewing's sarcoma. It shows the characteristic lytic appearance of such tumors. A diaphyseal location, as in this case involving the fibula, is most common. The periosteum is generally elevated in such cases, resulting in Codman's triangle and an associated soft-tissue mass. (From Wold LE, McLeod RA, Sim FH, et al: Atlas of Orthopedic Pathology. Philadelphia, WB Saunders, 1990, p 212.)

ratio of 1.5:1. Ninety percent of the cases occur in patients aged 5 to 25 years, with a peak incidence between 10 and 20 years. Ewing's sarcoma occurs as frequently in flat and short bones as in long bones. Within the appendicular skeleton, the most common localization is the femur, followed by the tibia, humerus, fibula, and forearm bones. In the trunk, the most common location is the pelvis, followed by the vertebrae and sacrum, scapula, ribs, and clavicle. In long bones, the tumor is common in the midshaft but may involve a larger portion or even the entire bone.

Pain is the earliest symptom. Swelling is also a common and early sign. Occasionally, however, no soft-tissue mass is appreciated, even for a long time. Low-grade fever is not infrequent.

The typical radiographic appearance of Ewing's sarcoma is permeative osteolysis with a laminated periosteal reac-

tion (Fig. 4). The majority of patients have an extraosseous component. Usually, the extent of Ewing's sarcoma, shown by MRI, CT, and isotope scan, is greater than what appears on plain radiographs.

Ewing's sarcoma is composed of small, round, closely packed cells without any matrix. The cells have a homogenous appearance. Their cytoplasm is scarce and pale with poorly defined limits. The nuclei are round to oval, with a distinct nuclear membrane and one or more tiny nucleoli. Mitotic figures are rare (Fig. 5). The cytoplasm contains glycogen. Intracellular glycogen can be detected by electron microscopic examination and is stained by PAS. The cells are stained by vimentin. When immunohistochemical analysis shows positive reactions to S 100 and NSE and electron microscopy shows dendritic processes, neurotubes, and dense-core neurosecretory granules, the tumor is labeled a PNET.

Many lesions must be considered in differential diagnosis: Ewing's sarcoma may mimic osteomyelitis, histiocytosis, lymphoma, or metastatic neuroblastoma. In difficult cases, the chromosomal abnormality t(11;22) (q24-12) may be detected by means of reverse transcriptase polymerase chain reaction.

Patients with Ewing's sarcoma should be treated with multidrug systemic chemotherapy before having the primary tumor treated specifically.[4] Once they have received two to four courses of chemotherapy, the primary tumor is re-evaluated, and a decision is made whether to do a surgical resection or irradiation. There remains some controversy as to which is better; the treatment of the primary tumor is individualized.

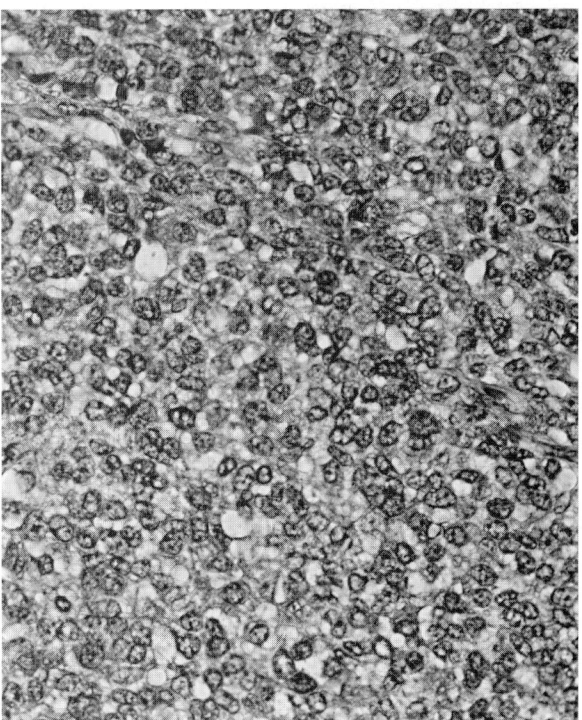

Fig. 5. Photomicrograph of Ewing's sarcoma. Sheets of small round blue cells are present. (From McCarthy EF, Frassica FJ: Pathology of Bone and Joint Disorders. Philadelphia, WB Saunders, 1998, p 260.)

CHONDROSARCOMA

Chondrosarcoma is a mesenchymal tumor producing cartilage. It is subdivided into several types. They are classified according to their site of origin as follows:

- Central chondrosarcomas arise within the medullary canal.
- Peripheral chondrosarcomas arise on the surface of the bone (usually in association with a previous osteochondroma).
- Extraosseous chondrosarcomas occur in the soft tissues.

CENTRAL CHONDROSARCOMA
Epidemiology and Clinical Features
Among the primary sarcomas of the skeleton, central chondrosarcoma is third in frequency, after osteosarcoma and Ewing's sarcoma. The male-to-female ratio ranges from 1.5:1 to 2:1. The tumor occurs predominantly in adults, with a peak incidence between 30 and 70 years of age; its occurrence is uncommon before 30 years and exceptional before puberty. The most frequent sites are the proximal femur and the pelvis, followed by the proximal humerus and the scapula. Pain is the most common presenting symptom in patients with central chondrosarcoma.

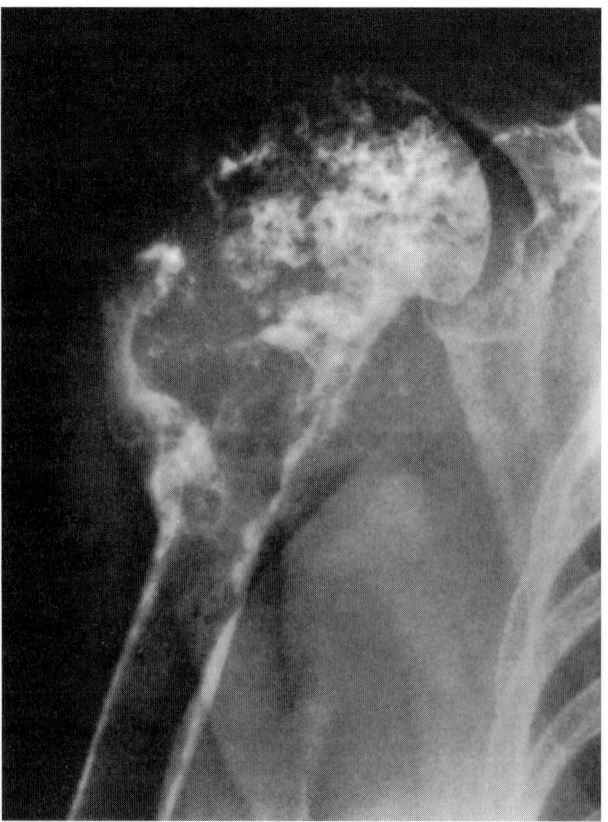

Fig. 6. Radiograph showing a destructive lesion in the proximal humerus in an adult patient. The lesion is partially calcified, showing multiple areas of ring-like calcification. These features are indicative of a hyaline cartilage tumor. The extensive cortical destruction and associated soft-tissue extension of the tumor support a malignant diagnosis. (From Wold LE, McLeod RA, Sim FH, et al: Atlas of Orthopedic Pathology. Philadelphia, WB Saunders, 1990, p 88.)

Imaging
The radiographic appearance of a central chondrosarcoma is that of irregularly distributed calcification with endosteal resorption (Fig. 6). Periosteal reaction is common and may induce a chronic enlargement of the affected segment. An extraosseous component is not uncommon and is best seen on CT or MRI.

Histopathology
The histological diagnosis of chondrosarcoma can be particularly difficult, especially for the lower histological grades. Clinical correlation is critical.

Chondrosarcoma may display a progression of malignancy (transformation); in the same individual tumor, it is possible to find two or more histological grades, even combined with a benign enchondroma.

Low-grade chondrosarcoma is composed of chondrocytes filling the medullary canal with invasion of the cancellous bone. Chondrosarcoma of higher grade is more cellular and less well-differentiated, and contains mitotic figures.

Course and Prognosis
Distant metastases are very rare in low-grade central chondrosarcomas (0 to 10%), uncommon in medium-grade tumors (20% to 30%), and common in high-grade tumors (50% to 60%). Metastases can occur many years (even 20) after the onset of symptoms, nearly exclusively to lung. The treatment of chondrosarcoma is surgical resection.[5] Chemotherapy is used only for patients with established metastases.

PERIPHERAL CHONDROSARCOMA
Epidemiology and Clinical Features
Peripheral chondrosarcomas arise from preexisting osteocartilaginous exostoses. They are more common in patients with multiple heritable exostoses. The male-to-female ratio is 2:1, and the tumors usually occur in patients between 20 and 50 years of age. The pelvis and proximal femur are the most common sites. The principal complaint is an enlarging mass.

Imaging
On a radiograph, peripheral chondrosarcoma has a large, irregularly ossified and calcified cartilaginous cap. CT or MRI best enables determination of the size and extent of the lesion.

Histopathology
The earliest evidence of malignancy in peripheral chondrosarcoma is thickening of the cartilaginous cap to more than 2 cm, although few tumors metastasize. As the lesions progress, cytological changes consistent with chondrosarcoma occur in the cap.

Course and Prognosis
Complete surgical resection almost always results in cure. Local recurrence is usually due to disruption of the cartilage cap at the time of excision. Metastatic disease is rare.

MALIGNANT FIBROUS HISTIOCYTOMA

Malignant fibrous histiocytoma is an intramedullary high-grade sarcoma less common than osteosarcoma and seen in all age groups except children. It is most commonly localized in the metaphysis of a long bone—femur, tibia, or humerus.

Pain and swelling are usually of short duration, and pathological fracture is common. Malignant fibrous histiocytoma is a purely osteolytic tumor. The osteolysis may be uniform, with ill-defined borders; sometimes, scattered or confluent radiolucent areas give a moth-eaten appearance. The cortex is usually permeated or destroyed. Atypical mitoses are common. Malignant fibrous histiocytoma of bone is often associated with abnormal bone (infarcts, old chondroma and chondrosarcoma, radiated bone, Paget's disease, or osteomyelitis). Treatment of malignant fibrous histiocytoma is identical to that of osteosarcoma.

CHORDOMA

Chordoma is a low-grade malignancy originating from remnants of the notochord.[6] These remnants have been found at the base of the skull, in the sacrococcyx, and, more rarely, in the vertebral bodies. The chordoma arises from these remnants.

Although rare, chordoma is the most common neoplasm of the sacrum. They arise caudally in the midline. The male-to-female ratio ranges from 2:1 to 3:1. This tumor is seen in adults, with a maximum incidence rate after 50 years of age. Owing to the slow growth, symptoms of a sacral chordoma are mild and of long duration. The tumor tends to bulge anteriorly, and a rectal examination provides its earliest clinical evidence. Surgical resection is the treatment.

ADAMANTINOMA

Adamantinoma is a rare, low-grade malignant tumor whose epithelium-like component is reminiscent of the ameloblastoma of the jaw bones.[7] Adamantinoma may affect patients at any age but is more common between 20 and 40 years. Always located in the diaphysis, adamantinoma affects the tibia in 80% of cases. Most patients complain of mild pain. On a radiograph, one or multiple, usually eccentric, osteolytic lesions can be seen involving the anterior cortex of the tibia. Anterior bowing of the tibia is a common finding. Adamantinoma is composed of epithelium-like cell aggregates, surrounded by a fibro-osseous stroma. Complete surgical resection is the treatment of choice.

REFERENCES

1. Enneking WF, Spanier SS, Goodman MA: A system for the surgical staging of musculoskeletal sarcoma. Clin Orthop 1980; 153: 106.
2. Philip T, Blay JY, Brunat-Mentigny M, et al: Osteosarcoma. Br J Cancer 2001; 84:78.
3. Stiller CA, Craft AW, Corazziani I: Survival of children with bone sarcoma in Europe since 1978: Results from the EUROCARE study. Pediatr Radiol 2001; 37:760.
4. Paulussen M, Ahrens S, Dunst J, et al: Localized Ewing's tumor of bone: Final results of the cooperative Ewing's Sarcoma Study CESS 86. J Clin Oncol 2001; 19: 1818.
5. Bjornsson J, McLeod RA, Unni KK, et al: Primary chondrosarcoma of long bones and limb girdles. Cancer 1998; 83:2105.
6. McMaster ML, Joldstein AM, Brimley CM, et al: Chordoma: Incidence and survival pattern in the United States, 1973–1995. Cancer Cause Control 2001; 12:1.
7. Qureshi AA, Shott S, Mallini BA, et al: Current trends in the management of adamantinoma of long bones: An international study. J Bone Surg Am 2000; 82:1122.

section
7
chapter
8

MANAGEMENT/SURGERY

F. W. Marsden

Summary

- Bone tumors display a wide spectrum of biological behavior. This ranges from benign latent neoplasms such as osteomas to highly malignant and aggressive tumors, such as Ewing's sarcoma and osteogenic sarcoma. Management decisions are best when they are made with knowledge of the tumor—its nature and biological activity—and its location.
- Significant advances in the management of malignant bone tumors have been made over the last two decades. This has been due to the advent of effective chemotherapy, with the prospect of survival from diseases that were previously almost universally fatal. Improved imaging has led to better definition of tumor sites and, as a result, less radical surgery.
- Before the availability of effective chemotherapy, the development of resection surgery, and reconstructive methods, amputation was the most commonly used procedure for malignant tumors and many aggressive benign lesions.
- Most patients with a nonmetastatic sarcoma of bone will survive. If surgery is performed, the majority of these operations are limb-sparing procedures.
- The goals of management of bone tumors are as follows:
    Removal of the tumor with avoidance of local recurrence.
    Restoration of limb function by either reconstructive surgery or a prosthesis, with successful rehabilitation.
    Local control of sarcomas of bone has to be achieved along with systemic treatment intended to prevent metastatic disease. This overrides all other considerations. Survival is possible only if effective local control is achieved by complete removal of the primary tumor mass.

HISTORICAL REVIEW

Until recently, surgery for malignant and locally aggressive bone tumors was dominated by amputation. Amputations for tumors were often performed without recognition of the biological activity of the tumor and were notable for their radical nature. The most common operation for tumors in the proximal part of the lower limb was a hindquarter amputation.[1] Although some limb-sparing surgery was done using prosthetic implants, surgery for bone sarcoma followed the principles expressed by Cade,[2] who, from 1931, advocated preoperative radiotherapy followed by amputation.

"Ablation of the limb was always done at or above the joint proximal to the affected bone; in the case of the femur, disarticulation of the hip; and in tumors of the humerus, disarticulation at the shoulder. No amputation through the affected bone was done and so local recurrence at stump level was avoided." Jaffe's[3] presentation of results of survival after treatment with high-dose methotrexate for osteosarcoma encouraged a more optimistic outlook not only for survival but also for less radical surgery. Although amputation initially remained the most common procedure, the level of selection was extended distally. It was realized that it was no longer necessary to interpose a joint between the level of section and the tumor.

Massive endoprosthetic systems began to be developed at centers in both Europe and North America. In 1981, the Mayo Clinic convened an international conference to discuss "tumor prostheses for bone and joint reconstruction."[4] This symposium has reconvened every 2 years since then as the International Symposium on Limb Salvage. Cautious evaluation of limb salvage procedures was undertaken by many centers as well as public health bodies.[5] The indications for limb salvage surgery have now been more clearly defined to the degree that the majority of operations being performed for aggressive as well as malignant tumors of bone are limb-sparing procedures.

It has also become recognized that surgery alone has no role in the management of sarcomas of bone. Multimodality treatment involving chemotherapy combined with an operation is now standard practice. Apart from gaining enhanced survival, it has been recognized that chemotherapy can facilitate the operation by "down-staging" the tumor, allowing for less radical resections and, as the result, enhanced preservation of function.

THE SURGICAL DECISIONS

BENIGN TUMORS

Staging studies must define the biological activity of benign tumors to predict the likelihood of local recurrence. This, in turn, determines the nature of the surgical procedure. Latent tumors as well as active tumors that are unlikely to recur locally are treated by local excision or by intralesional curettage. Should the integrity of the bone be threatened by the removal of the tumor, bone grafting, with or without internal fixation, is used. However, some active lesions and all aggressive lesions require more than simple excision. Adjuvant treatments, then, are as appropriate in the management of benign but aggressive tumors as they are in the management of malignant bone tumors (Table 1).

TABLE 1. SUMMARY OF TREATMENT OPTIONS FOR BENIGN TUMORS				
Tumor Type	Induction Treatment	Adjuvant	Surgery-Excision	Surgery-Reconstruction
Giant cell tumor	Embolization (for control of surgical blood loss)	Alcohol Phenol Liquid nitrogen	Lesional "soft" curettage + lavage, bur	Autograft Allograft Bone substitute Cement
			Wide	Autograft Allograft
			En bloc	Anatomic allograft Endoprosthesis Resection-arthrodesis
Aneurysmal bone cyst	Embolization (for regression and for control of surgical blood loss)	Liquid nitrogen	Lesional excision ± lavage, bur	Autograft Allograft Bone substitute Cement
Simple bone cyst	Steroid injection Osteoinduction Bone marrow Bone substitutes		None Lesional excision Curettage	Autograft Allograft Bone substitute Cement
Eosinophilic granuloma	Steroid injection		None Local excision (rarely)	None Autograft (very rarely)
Osteochondroma			Local excision	None Autograft ± internal fixation
Enchondroma			Lesional excision	Autograft Allograft Bone substitute Cement
Osteoid osteoma			Excision of nidus: open, en bloc percutaneous (computed tomography control)	
Osteoblastoma (giant osteoid osteoma)			En bloc excision	Autograft, allograft, ± internal fixation

The management of a giant cell tumor, which has a high rate of local recurrence, is an example. Most of these tumors occur at the ends of long bones and, provided there is sufficient ability to preserve joint function, can be treated by curettage as well as appropriate adjuvant agents. Principles appropriate to the surgical management of an aggressive giant cell tumor are as follows:

Access must be gained to all areas occupied by the tumor. The tumor should be approached through a sufficiently wide window to ensure that this access is gained.

Care must be taken during the removal of tumor material so as not to contaminate surrounding tissues. Wet packs should be used to exclude the surrounding tissue space.

All material must be removed from the cavity within the bone, but aggressive curettage must be avoided at this stage. Otherwise, tumor cells will be driven deeply into the marginal bone, thus extending rather than limiting the tumor compartment. Piecemeal removal with sponge-holding forceps and "soft" curettage is appropriate. Pulse lavage systems are useful once all adherent macroscopic tumor tissue is removed.

It is then appropriate to apply more aggressive methods to deal with residual fossae that may contain residual tu-

mor. A high-speed bur, coupled with copious irrigation, can be used at this stage. Chemical treatment of the cavity using phenol or alcohol is also advocated. Cryotherapy, using liquid nitrogen, has proved most effective in avoiding local recurrence.[6] Its potential for complications, such as damage to surrounding skin and to soft tissue and late fracture, demands caution in use.

RECONSTRUCTION AFTER LESIONAL EXCISION

Lesional excision as described leaves a large cavity that must be reconstituted. It is usually not possible to fill this solely with autologous bone. Morselized allograft bone is an ideal supplement (Fig. 1C). Bone substitutes are also available for this purpose and are best used mixed with autologous bone. These substances are osteoconductive (coralline derivatives and other hydroxyapatite products) or osteoinductive ("bioactive" ceramics and carriers for biological materials such as bone marrow and bone morphogenic proteins).[7]

The use of bone cement is also popular. The heat generated with the curing of the polymethylmethacrylate has an adjuvant effect. The depth of necrosis is only 1 to 2 mm, so it is not clear whether polymethylmethacrylate is a true adjuvant. The major advantage of this method of treatment

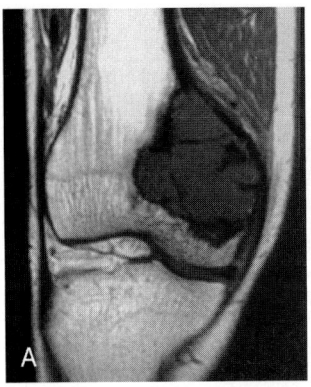
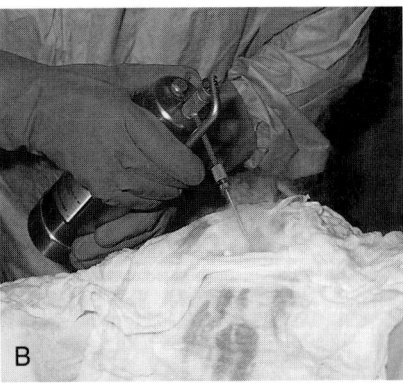
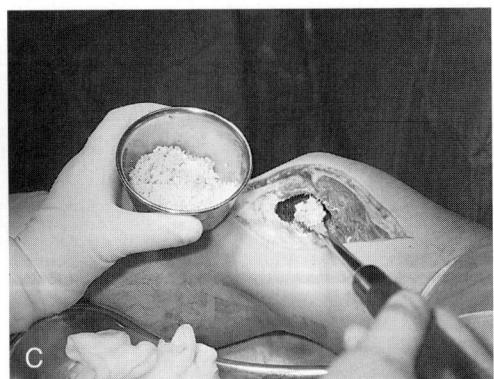

Fig. 1. Giant cell tumor. *A,* Tumor involves the metaphysis of the femur. *B,* Cryotherapy using liquid nitrogen. The more conventional technique is to pour the fluid. Three "freeze-thaw" cycles are used. Alternatively, spray delivery, as seen here, gives controlled delivery and access to the cavity after tumor evacuation. *C,* The cavity is filled and packed with morcellized allograft bone. Autologous bone is preferred for the final layer.

is that it provides immediate structural support for sub-chondral bone and articular cartilage.

EN BLOC EXCISION

When a locally aggressive benign tumor has destroyed or threatened the integrity of the joint surface to such a degree that reconstruction is not practical, an en bloc excision of the tumor, with a margin of unaffected bone, is appropriate. In these circumstances, it becomes necessary to consider an endoprosthetic reconstruction using a tumor prosthesis or an allograft, techniques more commonly used in the management of malignant tumors.

OTHER BENIGN TUMORS

ANEURYSMAL BONE CYST

Aneurysmal bone cysts are probably not true neoplastic lesions; they may represent a reactive phenomenon rather than a true neoplastic process of an overgrowth of a single cell type. They exhibit grades of behavior[8] and can be destructive, difficult to control, and prone to local recurrence. Angiography with selective embolization of identified feeder vessels is a useful induction treatment for these tumors. There are occasions when this can be effective as a sole treatment modality for tumors in inaccessible locations.

Most of these cases, however, require curettage with the same careful technique as described for giant cell tumors. The resultant bone defect requires reconstruction using similar grafting techniques.

SIMPLE BONE CYST

The discovery of a simple bone cyst often follows a pathological fracture. Spontaneous healing can follow, although this is not as common as might be hoped. It is preferable to allow the fracture to heal before considering further treatment. Initially, especially in patients younger than 10 years, these lesions always extend to the physis. As the bone grows, the cyst migrates distally, so intervention surgery is best delayed as long as possible. Recurrent fractures will force the decision to operate in some cases. Thus,

there is interest in and some success with aspiration and steroid injection or installation of bone marrow and other osteoinductive materials. Reported success with these methods, however, is variable.[9]

EOSINOPHILIC GRANULOMA (LANGERHANS' CELL HISTIOCYTOSIS)

This lesion is seen predominantly in the pediatric age group and may mimic a high-grade malignant tumor or osteomyelitis. Imaging studies often continue to compound the confusion and concern; therefore, biopsy sampling is usually required. Fortunately, most of these lesions are self-limiting and heal spontaneously without further intervention. The injection of steroids often aborts the process and appears to stimulate healing.[10]

OSTEOID OSTEOMA

Osteoid osteoma is a painful lesion that may be successfully treated with aspirin or nonsteroidal anti-inflammatory drugs. Successful surgery requires complete removal of the nidus of osteoid tissue. Complete removal may be accomplished with either a resection of a block of bone containing the nidus or a direct curettage. Computed tomography scan localization and percutaneous radiofrequency ablation are also used.

The management of benign tumors is summarized in Table 1.

MALIGNANT TUMORS OF BONE

Other chapters cover the important issues of staging studies, particularly biopsy technique. It is necessary, however, that management plans be firmly in the mind of the surgeon at an early stage of evaluation of these tumors. These plans can be frustrated by such events as poorly placed biopsy scars and the complications of induction treatment.

The role of surgery for a malignant tumor is to achieve local control. The role of chemotherapy is to gain systemic control at an early stage. Survival from the disease process is dependent on effective chemotherapy. However successful chemotherapy may be, all is lost if the surgery is such that there is local recurrence. This then must be the overriding principle in surgical management.

PRINCIPLES OF SURGERY FOR MALIGNANT BONE TUMORS

RESECTION MARGINS

A safe margin of resection[11] implies that when the tumor is removed, no single cell is left behind. Because it is beyond our physical capacities to know exactly where this single cell might be, a safe margin of normal tissue must exist around the resected specimen. Involvement of vital structures with the tumor, such as the major blood vessels and major nerves of the limb, usually precludes successful limb salvage.

LIMB SALVAGE OR AMPUTATION?

With staging studies complete, the diagnosis, the biological activity, and the anatomy of the tumor determine whether limb salvage is appropriate. Those tumors known to be responsive to chemotherapy are treated with induction (alternatively called neoadjuvant) therapy. Effective chemotherapy can have the affect of "down-staging" a tumor such that a situation that initially appeared treatable only by amputation can be converted into one treatable by a salvage procedure.[12]

To decide whether limb salvage surgery is appropriate, one must ask whether, after total removal of all tumor tissue, the subsequent reconstructive surgery will result in a limb that is less acceptable to the patient than an amputation and prosthesis.

The more distally placed the tumor is in the limb, the more likely the answer will be "no" and that an amputation will be done. The converse, however, is also true.

THE ROLE OF CHEMOTHERAPY

The primary role of chemotherapy has, historically, been that of control of systemic disease, as covered in Chapter 7-4. The local effect on the tumor is important in the surgical management. The route of administration of the chemotherapy[13] and the relative abilities of regional (intra-arterial) compared with systemic chemotherapy to gain enhanced local control is a point of contention. Whatever type of chemotherapy is used as induction treatment, its local effect is of significance to the surgeon. Hardening of the tumor, its encapsulation, and the extent of necrosis can make the definition of the tumor mass more readily appreciated by the surgeon, making tumor resection and subsequent reconstruction easier and thus safer. The local response is also significant in surgery for Ewing's sarcoma, in which effective chemotherapy can totally eliminate the extraosseous soft-tissue mass. Uncertainty can exist about whether the planned resection is based on where the tumor has been brought to by chemotherapy or where it was before the commencement of chemotherapy. In balance, it seems reasonable practice to base the subsequent resection on the staging of the tumor at surgery rather than at presentation.

Tumor bulk and involvement with major vessels and especially major nerves are the two major factors in determining whether a limb is salvageable. Pathological fracture,

TABLE 2. INDICATIONS AND CONTRAINDICATIONS FOR LIMB SALVAGE SURGERY

Contraindications	Indications
Safe resection not possible	Tumor resectable with wide margin (5 cm bone, 1.0 cm soft tissue)
Arterial reconstruction not possible	Skeletal reconstruction possible
Involvement of major nerve(s) (e.g., sciatic)	Soft-tissue reconstruction possible
Late-stage disease*	Resulting function should be better than an amputation
Pathological fracture*	Result must be cosmetically and emotionally acceptable

* These are relative, but not absolute, contraindications.

if the extent of tumor spill is limited, is not necessarily a contraindication for limb salvage surgery.[14] However, pathological fracture in the face of a massive soft-tissue component invariably indicates the need for amputation. The indications and contraindications for limb salvage are outlined in Table 2.

LIMB SALVAGE SURGERY: PRINCIPLES

Any limb salvage operation has three distinct phases:

1. Tumor resection.
2. Skeletal reconstruction.
3. Soft-tissue reconstruction and cover (Fig. 2).

RESECTION

A safe resection margin for any malignant tumor must include the entire tumor compartment. Skin incisions must be planned to include the biopsy track. The tumor must be regarded as occupying the surgical space created by the biopsy as well as its original location. The "footprint" of the biopsy has to go as well as the tumor.

A safe margin is achieved only when the last tumor cell is included in the resection. Skip lesions and the reactive zone, as detected by preoperative imaging, provide an appropriate guide, but for safety a margin of uninvolved tissue is appropriately included with the tumor. The tumor must not be seen during the resection procedure. During resection, and particularly as the mass is being mobilized for removal, muscles can slide away from around the tumor capsule, creating a "retraction" effect, thereby exposing the tumor. If this is to be anticipated, it should be prevented by a limited number of anchoring sutures within the surrounding muscle cuff.

The recommended 1 cm of soft-tissue cover may have to be compromised in situations of close proximity to the neurovascular bundle. This compromise is safer in the presence of a good chemotherapy response but represents a risky variation if there has been little alteration in the tumor or poor physical definition of the tumor mass. The use of frozen section is a helpful guide throughout the resection phase of the operation. Confirmation of the margin can be obtained by submitting a specimen of bone marrow at the level of bone transection. The specimen should be taken from the tumor side of the line rather than

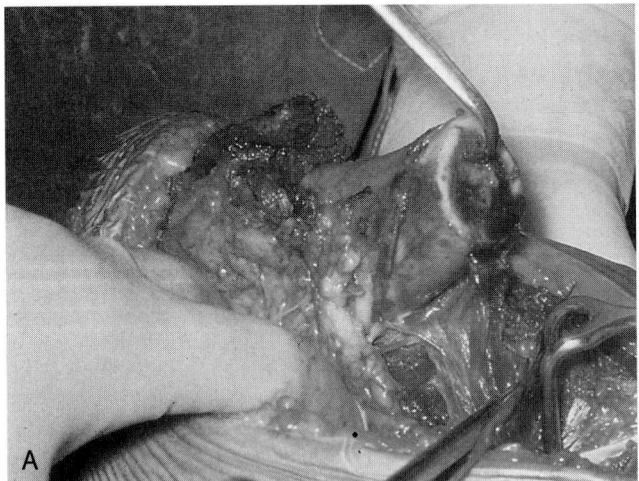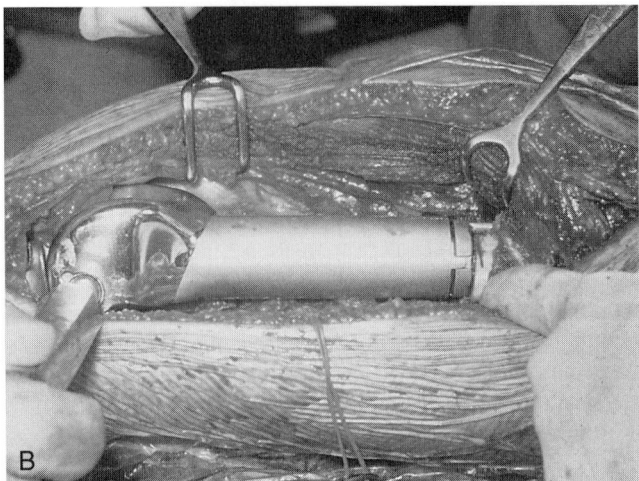

Fig. 2. Resection of an osteosarcoma of the distal femur. *A,* The tumor is removed and enveloped in a cuff of surrounding soft tissue. The tumor must not be exposed. *B,* Endoprosthetic reconstruction follows.

from the bone destined to remain. Furthermore, soft-tissue margins can be similarly checked. This can become of particular relevance in deciding the nature of tissue change from chemotherapy effect. This can produce staining and physical changes, seen as local tissue abnormalities during the procedure.

Preoperative staging must include evaluation of intra-articular spread, which in turn determines whether the joint resection can be intra-articular or extra-articular, in which the joint with its intact surrounding capsule is included in the resection.

SKELETAL RECONSTRUCTION

Opportunities for local excision and grafting for malignant tumors are rare. Skeletal reconstruction after cavity excision is possible in some low-grade tumors such as a metaphyseal stage 1A chondrosarcoma. The use of local adjuvant agents, such as liquid nitrogen, may have a role in this situation.

Intercalary Reconstruction

Tumors limited to the diaphysis of a long bone and with a clear margin of separation of either joint are managed by intercalary resection. Allograft reconstruction is most practical under these circumstances. An allograft replacement never fully incorporates. Creeping substitution occurs at the junctional zones. To enhance this, local supplementary autologous grafting is recommended. Supplementary fixation must always be used to secure lasting stability. This can be in the form of an intramedullary device or with the use of plates and screws. I favor plating with complete screw fixation throughout the length of the graft (Fig. 3A and B).

Supplementary use of cement throughout the medullary cavity of the allograft further enhances the fixation. Such fixation must remain in place permanently.

Vascularized autologous grafting, most commonly with the ipsilateral fibula, can also be used in diaphyseal reconstructions. This has the advantage of establishing a permanent biological solution. The limitations are those of mechanical instability and strength throughout the healing phase.

RESECTION INVOLVING MAJOR JOINTS

Endoprosthetic replacement, or allograft reconstruction, is necessary when there is need to remove a joint adjacent to or involved in the tumor.

THE ROLE OF ALLOGRAFTS

The versatility of allograft[15, 16] reconstruction allows its use in a wide range of anatomic situations.

Soft-tissue attachment, through retained ligaments, or directly to the graft is a distinct advantage.

Failure of transplanted joint surfaces, however, has led to the use of composite reconstructions using allograft bone with conventional endoprosthetic joint replacement components.

ENDOPROSTHETIC SYSTEMS

There are two major groups of systems in use for reconstruction after tumor resection: customized[17] and modular.[18] The customized device is manufactured as a special match for a particular patient and a particular tumor resection. This calls for appropriate preoperative planning and the fabrication of a device matched specifically for the planned procedure. The modular prosthesis is built up from a range of individual components at the time of the operation. A particular feature of such devices is that individual components, rather than the whole prosthesis, can be revised should the need arise.

Both systems have their unique advantages and disadvantages (Table 3). Consequently, both systems have their own individual enthusiasts and detractors.

Other variations in prosthetic design are in the type of joint and the method of stem fixation. Constrained, or hinged, joints are favored for those reconstructions necessary when significant soft-tissue resection has occurred. In these circumstances, the mechanics of the joint, particularly of the knee, can be so altered that a mechanical match is less important than it would be in conventional knee replacement. A rotating hinge relieves a significant amount of mechanical stress, particularly at the anchor points of the prosthetic reconstruction.

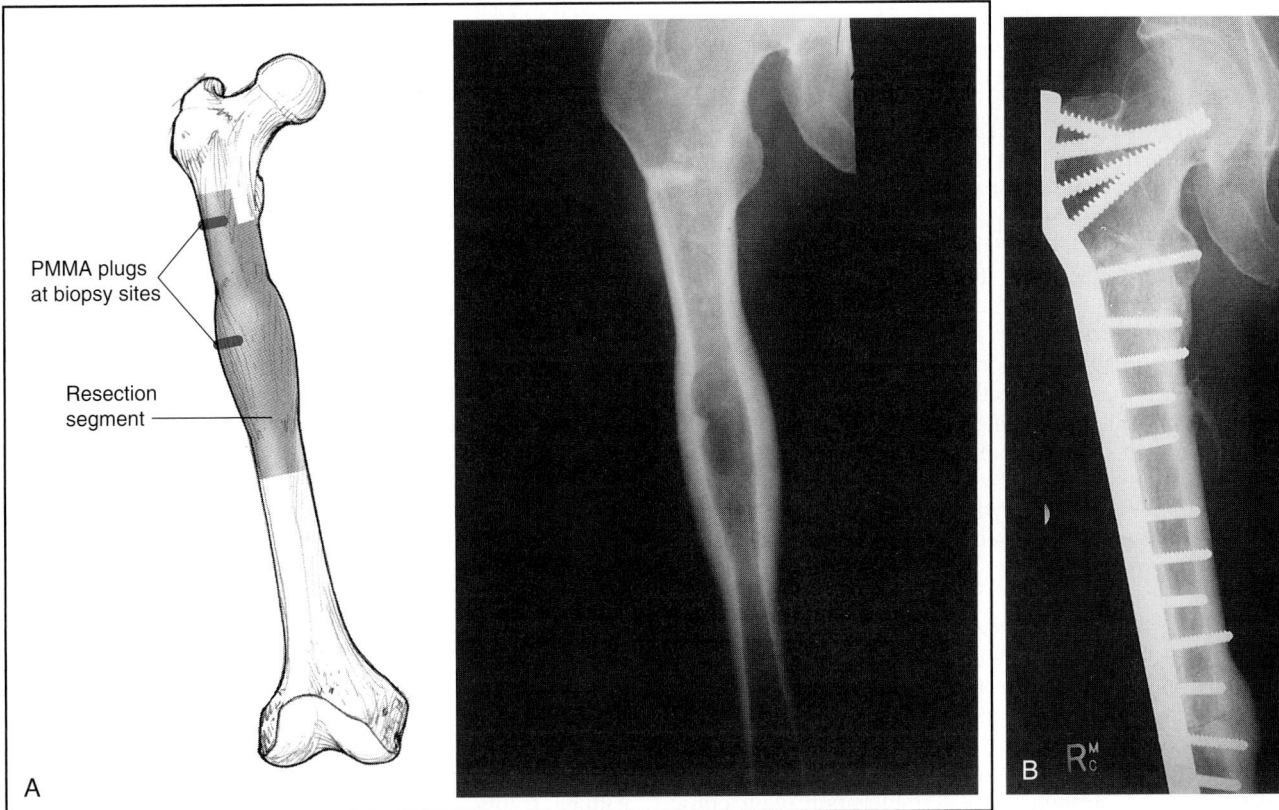

Fig. 3. Chondrosarcoma in the diaphysis of the femur. *A,* Two biopsy sites have been sealed by plugs of bone cement. This is a useful guide for the subsequent resection. *B,* Intercalary allograft reconstruction has been performed. The junctional zones have healed and incorporated with the allograft.

There is also variation in fixation with the use of either cemented stem fixation, which produces early rigidity and mechanical security to the system, or fixation without cement. In the latter case, stability is obtained from cross-screw fixation and later stability from bone ingrowth. Stems are rendered osteoconductive with a porous metal surface or with a hydroxyapatite coating.

SOFT-TISSUE RECONSTRUCTION

The reconstruction, prosthetic or biological, must be covered by healthy and adequate soft tissue. Skin closure must be without tension. Primary wound healing must be achieved, even at the expense of function. There are special considerations and circumstances in different regions.

Hip and Proximal Femur

An effective method of soft-tissue ingrowth allowing for lasting attachment of soft tissue to metallic implants has yet to be achieved. It is difficult to retain abductor function around a metal implant. Allografts have a distinct advantage at this level in providing soft-tissue anchorage.

Distal Femur and Knee

The problems here usually relate to the adequacy of soft-tissue cover. The sharing of muscle groups and the technique of spreading of residual muscles are necessary to gain appropriate cover of the implant. This is especially so when a wide resection of soft tissue is necessary to gain a safe margin. A constrained knee hinge may be preferred in this circumstance.

TABLE 3. COMPARATIVE MERITS OF MODULAR AND CUSTOMIZED ENDOPROSTHESES	
Modular	**Customized**

Availability
  Access and proximity to an appropriate manufacturer are not necessary.
  Time delays waiting fabrication avoided.
Adaptability
  The modularity of these systems allows for late change at the time of surgery should new circumstances arise.
  Selective revision possible; not all of the component needs to be removed should there be a focal failure of the system.
	Anatomic match
	  A more accurate anatomic match for the patient is possible.
	Design variations possible
	  Mechanical, as well as anatomic, variations can be customized.
	Preoperative planning
	  The use of a customized system demands careful and detailed evaluation of the tumor and planning of the surgical procedure.

Knee and Proximal Tibia

The difficulty associated with achieving anchorage of the patellar tendon is a limiting factor on the functional outcome of resection surgery and reconstruction of tumors of the proximal tibia. If an endoprosthetic system is used, soft-tissue techniques such as the use of gastrocnemius flaps and the relocation of the fibula are used to provide a site for attachment of the patellar tendon. An allograft, in association with conventional knee replacement components, is often preferable in this situation.

Resection Arthrodesis

This is an alternative to endoprosthetic reconstruction, particularly when massive resection, with associated soft-tissue loss, is such that poor function resulting from instability can be foreseen. The choice lies between the turn-up/turn-down procedure described by Enneking and Shirley[19] or an allograft segment together with a long intramedullary nail. These can provide rugged reconstructions but with the sacrifice of knee motion.

Shoulder and Proximal Humerus

In the normal individual, shoulder joint function relies significantly on the integrity of the enclosing muscular and capsular envelope. Tumors about the shoulder needing significant soft-tissue resection are associated with loss of function of the shoulder joint. Reconstructions to restore this are limited. Scapulohumeral stabilization, with consequent retention and ability to transmit scapular movement to the humerus, should be attempted. The shoulder joint does not need to be arthrodesed unless the patient needs a stronger shoulder girdle. It must be remembered, however, that preservation of hand function is the primary goal of limb salvage procedures about the shoulder. Consequently, replacement of the proximal humerus may, in most cases, serve to occupy space and provide scapular stability rather than replacing glenohumeral movement. Resection of the shoulder joint and scapula without endoprosthetic recon-

struction (Tikhoff-Lindberg procedure[20]), or its modification as described by Capanna et al,[21] preserves hand and forearm function in a similar manner.

Pelvis

The anatomic location of pelvic tumors determines the options for reconstruction.[22]

Resection of lesions involving the sacroiliac joint often requires graft reconstruction of the pelvis-sacral ring, but satisfactory function can be achieved without necessarily performing this reconstruction. Similarly, lesions involving the iliac wing usually do not require restoration of pelvic ring integrity.

Prostheses available after acetabular and para-acetabular resections include the saddle prosthesis and also customized components. These resections are also managed by a range of other methods, including the following:

Allograft reconstruction in association with endoprosthetic replacement.
Pelvis-femoral arthrodesis, with or without allograft reconstruction.
Iliofemoral arthrodesis with internal fixation and autologous grafting.
On occasion, no reconstruction.

Tumors restricted to the ischium or ischiopubic area of the pelvis are more likely to be treatable by resection without reconstruction, provided integrity of the hip joint can be maintained. Without this, allograft reconstruction, iliofemoral arthrodesis, or no reconstruction are options appropriate to particular circumstances (Fig. 4).

LIMB SALVAGE IN EARLY CHILDHOOD

Conventional reconstruction after limb-sparing surgery in the growing child is limited by the inevitable limb length discrepancy that follows if the physis is included in the resection.

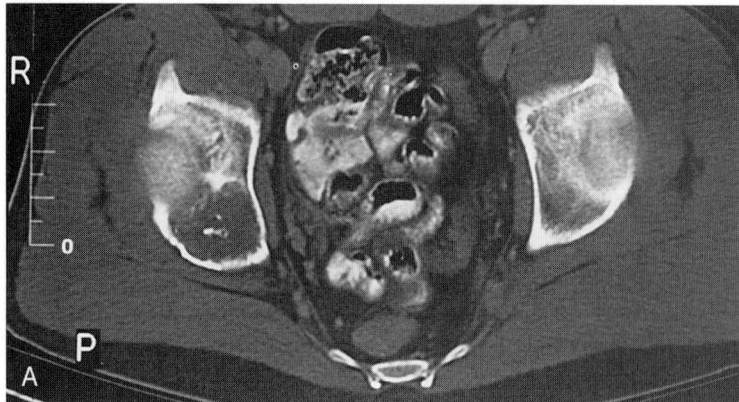
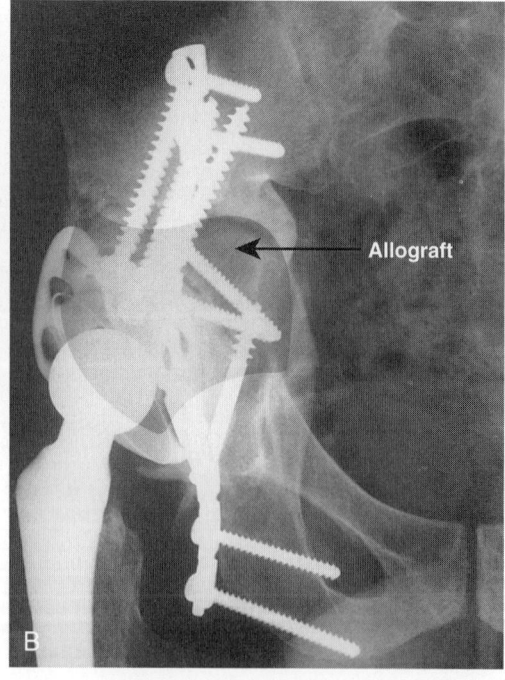

Fig. 4. Clear cell chondrosarcoma. *A,* The tumor involves the acetabulum. *B,* Resection has been followed by a reconstruction using an anatomically matched allograft with plate and screw fixation and a total hip replacement with an acetabular reinforcement ring.

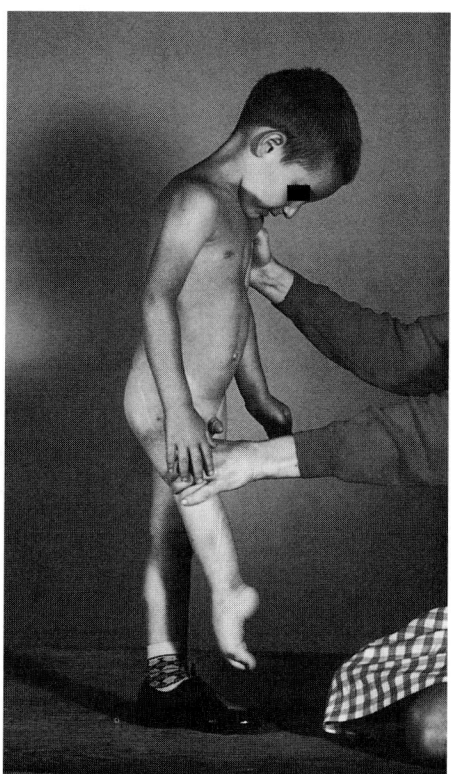

Fig. 5. Rotationplasty. The ankle now functions like a knee joint. A modified below-knee prosthesis is fitted. (Courtesy Dr. Robert Gillespie, Buffalo, NY.)

GROWING (EXPANDABLE) PROSTHESES

Expandable endoprostheses[23, 24] have been developed with the capability to expand the device at intervals by repeat operations. Care needs to be exercised in their use. A child

amputee has significant limitations, but those limitations are clearly defined and can be constantly challenged.

ROTATIONPLASTY

This procedure was first developed for proximal femoral focal deficiencies.[25] The limb is turned through 180 degrees, usually at the knee, so that the posture of the foot and ankle is reversed. This has the effect of extending the level of amputation distally such that the ankle and foot function as for a below-knee amputee. This principle was developed and applied to tumor surgery.[26, 27] The tumor and surrounding limb segment are excised with preservation of the major neurovascular structures. The distal limb is turned through 180 degrees, and continuity is reestablished with the foot and ankle reversed (Fig. 5).

The indications, limitations, and complications of these reconstructive procedures are summarized in Table 4.

AMPUTATION

UPPER LIMB

The outcomes after proximal amputation of the upper limb are so devastating that operations such as forequarter amputation and, to a lesser extent, shoulder disarticulation can only be considered in view of a total lack of any reconstructive option or brachial plexus involvement. The importance of hand function is such that indications for high proximal upper limb amputations resemble a threat to life rather than a threat to the limb.

LOWER LIMB

The high level of function of the below-knee amputee, particularly in fit young individuals, is such that there is little place for limb preservation procedures for tumors in the distal parts of the lower limb. This being said, there are means of doing limb salvage surgery for malignant tumors

---

TABLE 4. INDICATIONS, LIMITATIONS, AND COMPLICATIONS OF RECONSTRUCTIVE PROCEDURES

Procedure	Indications	Limitations/Complications
Local resection	Low grade, intracompartmental (Ia) Minimal diaphyseal, metaphyseal involvement	Limited indications
Intercalary resection/reconstruction	Diaphyseal involvement	Limited indications
Allograft	Any location: joint surfaces need prosthetic replacement	Infection (local + potential for transmitted disease) Late degradation and mechanical failure of internal fixation Fracture
Endoprosthetic reconstruction	Joint and adjacent long bone	Local infection Mechanical failure Loss of host bone by Osteolysis Stress shielding Loss of growth potential Local metallosis Distant metal ion accumulation
"Growing prosthesis"	Skeletal immaturity	Need for repeated surgery Activity restriction
Vascularized transfer	Diaphyseal; low mechanical demand	Early mechanical failure Limitation of early rehabilitation
Rotationplasty	Knee joint (or hip) in early childhood	Emotional and social acceptance
Bone transport	Diaphyseal; low mechanical demand	Limited indications prolonged delay to rehabilitation

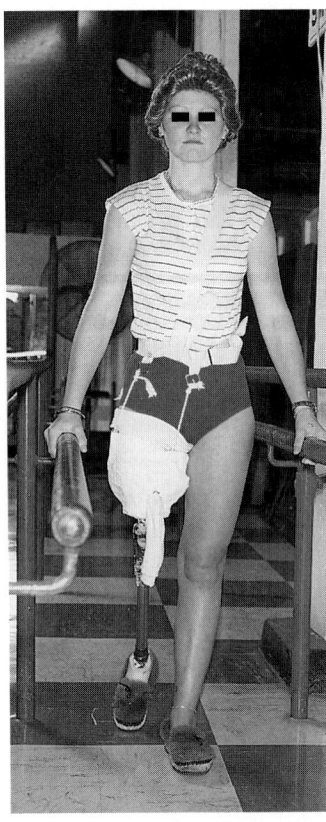

Fig. 6. Postoperative prosthetic fitting after an above-knee amputation for a distal femoral osteosarcoma. Early resumption of gait and establishment of the rehabilitation program are essential after amputations for tumors.

of the foot and lower leg. The situation changes dramatically above the knee. Surgical principles involved in amputations for tumors are not substantially different from those appropriate for any young patient. Maximum preservation of stump length and the use of "reconstructive techniques"

such as myoplasty and myodesis are of particular importance.[28] Unfortunately, most amputations performed in the lower limb for tumors of the femur must be at a higher level than might be desired. To be of functional use, an amputation stump in the leg must extend below the level of the buttock fold. The level of bone section necessary to achieve this must extend well distal to the lesser trochanter. An amputation stump shorter than this has no ability to drive a conventional above-knee prosthesis. For this reason, there is no gain to the patient in compromising or risking tumor clearance to achieve such a short femoral stump. The type of prosthesis necessarily fitted at this level has to emulate a hip disarticulation (tilting table) prosthesis.

Above the level of the hip joint, however, it is appropriate to aim to preserve as much of the pelvic ring as possible without compromising tumor clearance. This may mean significant modification of placement or development of skin and soft-tissue flaps. There are many opportunities to enhance function even if hemipelvectomy (or hindquarter) amputation seems necessary. Preservation of much of the iliac wing and of the ischium is important subsequently for dressing, seating, and prosthetic fitting.

The use of continuous regional anesthesia and rigid cast dressing techniques is important in the control of postamputation pain. Postoperative prosthetic fitting, as originally developed by Burgess and Romano,[29] continues to have special benefit, even for high-level amputees (Fig. 6).

QUALITY OF LIFE

Although the advantages of limb salvage surgery are obvious, differences in quality of life as perceived by the patients who have had amputations and those who have had successful limb salvage can be to a surprisingly lesser degree than might be expected. Patient selection, preoperative counseling, and continuing support are of major concern to the surgeon in the management of bone tumors.[30] Ultimate quality of life for each individual must then be reckoned with in deciding between amputation and limb salvage.

REFERENCES

1. Gordon-Taylor G, Munro R: Technique and management of hindquarter amputation. Br J Surg 1952; 39:536.
2. Cade S: Bone sarcoma. Ann R Coll Surg Edin 1967; 12:83.
3. Jaffe N: Osteogenic sarcoma: State of the art with high-dose methotrexate treatment. Clin Orthop 1976; 120:95.
4. Chao EY-S, Ivins JC (eds): Tumor Prostheses for Bone and Joint Reconstruction. New York, Thieme-Stratton, 1983.
5. National Institutes of Health: Limb-sparing treatment of adult soft-tissue sarcomas and osteosarcomas: Consensus Development Conference Statement 1984.
6. Marcove RC: A 17-year review of cryosurgery in the treatment of bone tumors. Clin Orthop 1982; 163:231.
7. Lane JM, Bostrom MP: Bone grafting and new composite biosynthetic graft materials. Instr Course Lect 1998; 47:525.

8. Campanacci M, Capanna R, Picci P: Unicameral and aneurysmal bone cysts. Clin Orthop 1986; 204:25.
9. Hashemi-Nejad A, Cole WG: Incomplete healing of simple bone cysts after steroid injections. J Bone Joint Surg Br 1997; 79:727.
10. Yasko AW, Fanning CV, Ayala AG, et al: Percutaneous techniques for the diagnosis and treatment of localized Langerhans cell histiocytosis (eosinophilic granuloma of bone). J Bone Joint Surg Am 1998; 80:219.
11. Malawer M, Buch R, Reaman G, et al: Impact of two cycles of preoperative chemotherapy with intra-arterial cisplatin and intravenous doxorubicin on the choice of surgical procedure for high-grade bone sarcomas of the extremities. Clin Orthop 1991; 270:214.
12. Enneking WF: A system of staging musculoskeletal neoplasms. Clin Orthop 1986; 204:9.

13. Winkler K, Bielack S, Delling G, et al: Effect of intra-arterial versus intravenous cisplatin in addition to systemic doxorubicin, high-dose methotrexate, and ifosfamide on histologic tumor response in osteosarcoma. Cancer 1990; 66:1703.
14. Jaffe N, Spears R, Eftekhari F, et al: Pathologic fracture in osteosarcoma: Impact of chemotherapy on primary tumor and survival. Cancer 1987; 59:701.
15. Mankin HJ, Springfield DS, Gebhardt MC, et al: Current status of allografting for bone tumors. Orthopedics 1992; 15:1147.
16. Sim FH, Frassica FJ: Use of allografts following resection of tumors of the musculoskeletal system. Instr Course Lect 1993; 42:405.
17. Unwin PS, Cobb JP, Walker PS: Distal femoral arthroplasty using custom-made

prostheses: The first 218 cases. J Arthroplasty 1993; 8:259.

18. Capanna R, Morris HG, Campanacci D, et al: Modular uncemented prosthetic reconstruction after resection of tumors of the distal femur. J Bone Joint Surg Br 1994; 76:178.

19. Enneking WF, Shirley PD: Resection-arthrodesis for malignant and potentially malignant lesions about the knee using an intramedullary rod and local bone grafts. J Bone Joint Surg Am 1977; 59:223.

20. Marcove RC, Lewis MM, Huvos AG: En bloc upper humeral interscapulo-thoracic resection: The Tikhoff-Lindberg procedure. Clin Orthop 1977; 124:219.

21. Capanna R, van Horn JR, Biagini R, et al: The Tikhoff-Lindberg procedure for bone tumors of the proximal humerus: The clas-

sical "extensive" technique versus a modified "transglenoid" resection. Arch Orthop Trauma Surg 1990; 109:63.

22. Enneking WF, Dunham WK: Resection and reconstruction for primary neoplasms involving the innominate bone. J Bone Joint Surg Am 1978; 60:731.

23. Lewis MM: The use of an expandable and adjustable prosthesis in the treatment of childhood malignant bone tumors of the extremity. Cancer 1986; 57:499.

24. Unwin PS, Walker PS: Extendible endoprostheses for the skeletally immature. Clin Orthop 1996; 322:179.

25. Torode IP, Gillespie R: Rotationplasty of the lower limb for congenital defects of the femur. J Bone Joint Surg Br 1983; 65: 569.

26. Winkelmann WW: Rotationplasty. Orthop Clin North Am 1996; 27:503

27. Merkel KD, Gebhardt M, Springfield DS: Rotationplasty as a reconstructive operation after tumor resection. Clin Orthop 1991; 270:231.

28. Marsden FW: Amputation: Surgical technique and postoperative management. Aust N Z J Surg 1977; 47:384.

29. Burgess EM, Romano RL: The management of lower extremity amputees using immediate postsurgical prostheses. Clin Orthop 1968; 57:137.

30. Tomeno B, Antract P, Ouakine M: Psychological management, prevention and treatment of phantom pain after amputation for tumors. Int Orthop 1998; 22: 205.

SOFT-TISSUE TUMORS

section 7 chapter 9

PRESENTATION AND EVALUATION

William G. Ward, Sr

Summary
- Large deep-seated masses are usually malignant; small innocuous-appearing superficial nodules are usually benign but may be malignant.
- Most soft-tissue sarcomas present as asymptomatic masses in otherwise healthy individuals.
- Magnetic resonance imaging is the imaging modality of choice for soft-tissue tumors.
- Sarcoma metastases are most commonly pulmonary; chest radiographs and chest computed tomography scan are the studies of choice for metastatic surveillance.
- Accurate diagnosis requires histological examination.
- The biopsy should not compromise the ability to perform a subsequent complete resection of all tumor-contaminated tissues.

A soft-tissue tumor can be broadly defined as any abnormal mass arising in soft tissues. By convention, tumors of solid organs or reticuloendothelial tissues are excluded. Soft-tissue tumors are classified by histogenic origin and identified histologically by their extracellular matrix. Both benign and malignant processes arise within each histogenic type. Benign tumors vastly outnumber malignant tumors. A primary malignant tumor of soft tissue is termed a sarcoma. Although metastases to soft tissue and extension of primary bone sarcoma are not primary soft-tissue tumors, they should be considered in the differential diagnosis of soft-tissue masses. The larger the tumor, the worse the prognosis; hence the importance of an early diagnosis.[1, 2]

During the past 2 decades our understanding and management of soft-tissue sarcomas has dramatically changed. Amputation gave way to limb salvage surgery.[3, 4] Adjuvant irradiation and systemic chemotherapy now play significant roles in management.[4, 5] Diagnostic studies to evaluate the tumor's extent have been developed (computed tomography [CT] and magnetic resonance imaging [MRI]) and the understanding of the genetic basis of tumors should lead to a means of curing a patient.[6–10]

EPIDEMIOLOGY

The average annual incidence rate of malignant soft-tissue tumors is estimated at 2 per 100,000 population, compared with an incidence rate of 300 benign soft-tissue neoplasms per 100,000 population.[11–14] There are approximately 5500 new soft-tissue sarcomas diagnosed annually in the United States.[12] Approximately 15% of soft-tissue sarcomas occur in patients younger than 15 years old, 45% occur in patients 15 to 55 years old, and 40% occur in patients older than 55 years.[15] Approximately 40% of soft-tissue sarcomas occur in the lower extremity, 20% in the upper extremity, 10% in the head and neck, and 30% in the trunk.[15]

CLINICAL FEATURES AND PRESENTATION

Most soft-tissue tumors present as an asymptomatic mass, rarely causing symptoms until it has achieved considerable

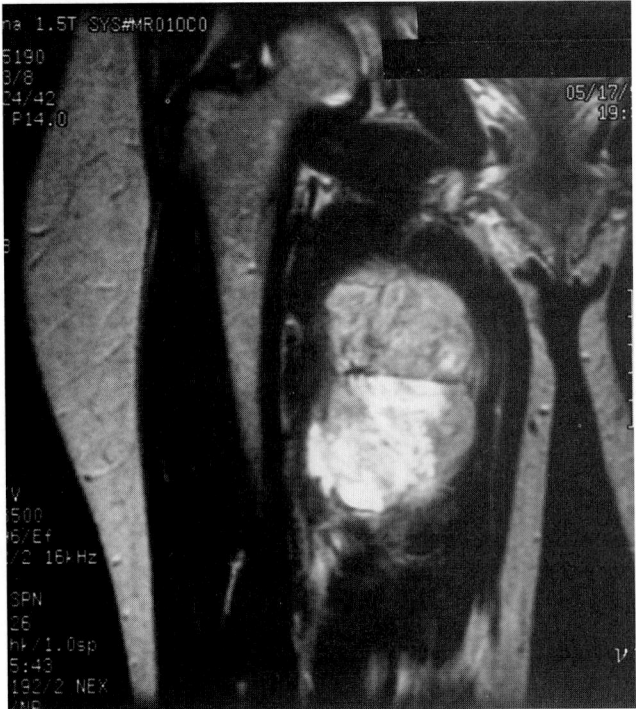

Fig. 1. MRI. This frontal plane (MRI) scan reveals a large inhomogeneous groin mass in a 39-year-old woman. Her initial physician attributed this mass to a "pulled muscle." The patient, being fully aware that she had not sustained any trauma to account for a pulled muscle, refused to accept this diagnosis and insisted on an MRI. Biopsy revealed extraosseous Ewing's sarcoma.

nificant skin changes that the majority of soft-tissue tumors cause is stretching of skin over the mass (Fig. 3).

Most true neoplasias continually increase in size. Whereas some benign processes may stabilize or become latent, few true neoplasms shrink. Individual tumor masses that vary in size are most often benign. Hemangiomas can develop intermittent clotting of tortuous vessels causing intermittent localized swelling and edema. Ganglions also frequently fluctuate in size.

STAGING AND CLASSIFICATION OF SOFT-TISSUE TUMORS

Tumor staging systems or classifications are based on histological grade and aggressiveness of the lesion and on the anatomic extent, both locally and distant. The staging system devised by Enneking and adopted by the Musculoskeletal Tumor Society is the one most familiar to orthopaedic surgeons[16, 17] (Table 1). The higher the assigned stage, the worse the prognosis and the greater the margins required to achieve a cure. Malignant tumors are divided into two stages (high and low) based on histological grade. Two subdivisions of each stage reflect whether or not the tumor has extended beyond the local tissue compartment (defined as an anatomic space bounded by fascia, bone, periosteum, or other tissue border). The third or highest malignant stage is metastatic. The American Joint Committee on Cancer (AJCC) staging of soft-tissue sarcomas is similar[2] (Table 2). It is based on size, grade, depth, and extent, including the presence or absence of metastases. This system is more cumbersome and difficult to use in managing individ-

size. Patients and occasionally physicians may minimize the significance of the mass. Most lesions deep to the fascia and over 5 cm in any dimension are malignant (Fig. 1), especially if they are firm and fixed to the surrounding bone or soft tissues. Most superficial masses, particularly those smaller than 5 cm, are benign, but superficial benign nodules often feel no different from superficial malignant nodules to either the patient or the examining physician (Fig. 2). Because of this difficulty in establishing an accurate diagnosis on clinical grounds alone, a fine needle aspiration biopsy (FNAB), an open biopsy, or an excisional biopsy of a superficial lesion is appropriate when there is any question of the diagnosis.

Pain in a soft-tissue lesion should raise the level of suspicion that the mass is malignant. Pain can be caused by rapid growth. Internal hemorrhage or internal edema will cause capsular or pseudocapsular stretching and pain. With extensive necrosis and secondary inflammation, the surrounding skin may become erythematous and warm. Occasionally, if there is a significant or exuberant inflammatory reaction around the tumor, the skin may be edematous or have a peau d'orange appearance (resembling the skin of an unpeeled orange). Traumatically induced hematomas, as from contusions or muscle ruptures, extend along the fascial planes and are observable as ecchymosis in the dependent portion of the body in the subcutaneous tissues. With internal tumor hemorrhage, however, the hematoma is contained within the tumor's pseudocapsule. The hemorrhage does not migrate along fascial planes and there will be no subcutaneous ecchymosis or bruising. The only sig-

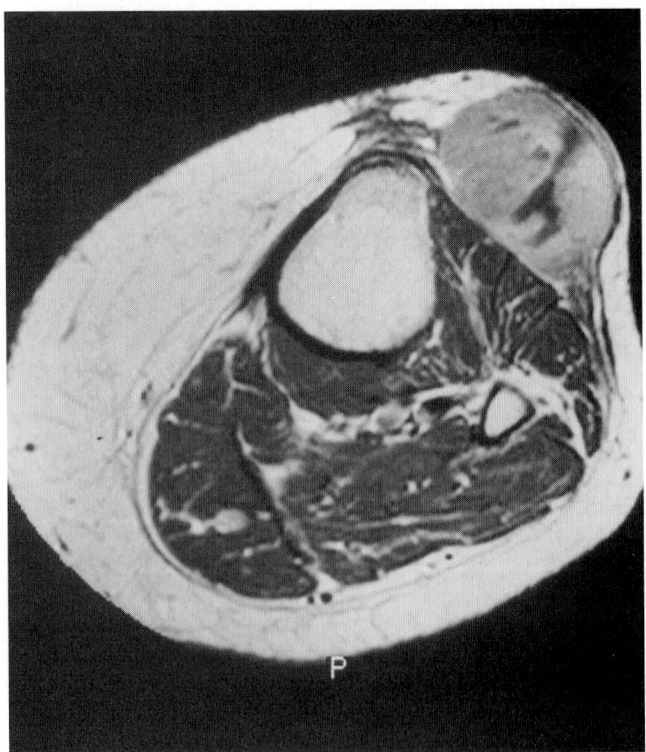

Fig. 2. MRI. This is an axial plane MRI scan of a 4-cm high-grade malignant fibrous histiocytoma in the anterolateral calf of a 50-year-old woman. Note the relatively sharp demarcation between normal tissue and the tumor.

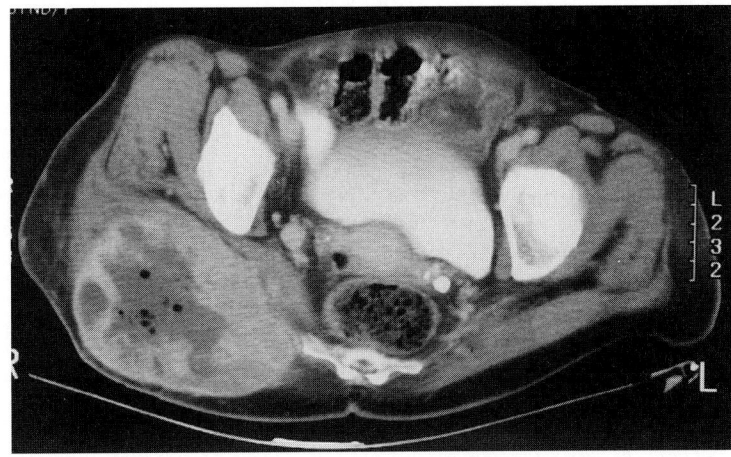

Fig. 3. Computed tomography. This cross-sectional CT scan reveals a large buttock sarcoma with internal hemorrhage, first noted after a fall on stairs. Despite the lack of subcutaneous bruising, it was diagnosed as a simple hematoma and aspirated twice by her family physician. Her general surgeon then performed a formal incision and drainage on two separate occasions. Only after a wound dehiscence with extruding tumor did the surgeon consider the diagnosis of a malignancy. Despite radical buttockectomy and chemotherapy, the patient died 1 year later of pulmonary metastases.

ual patients, but may allow a better categorization of patients for comparison of results from different series and different treatment modalities. The interested reader should consult the latest edition of the *AJCC Cancer Staging Manual* for specific details.

INVESTIGATION

The first investigational step is obtaining a complete history. Questioning should include how long the mass has been present; changes in size; its growth rate; the presence, type, and character of pain; pain-aggravating and -relieving factors; history of prior cancers; and a thorough review of systems for other systemic diseases. Eliciting a history of trauma may be helpful but can be misleading. Post-traumatic hematoma should not be diagnosed on the basis of history alone.

The physical examination should be complete. The mass itself should be palpated to determine its size (measured in centimeter), depth, contour, texture, and mobility and to determine if it is solid, cystic, or multiloculated. Examination should determine if it is warm, tender, erythematous, or pulsatile (Table 3). Auscultation can detect bruits. The distal neurovascular status, including edema, should be determined. Aneurysms and pseudoaneurysms are pulsatile and have a bruit. A lesion that is firm, solid, and fixed to the surrounding structures is more likely malignant or aggressive than one that is soft, cystic, and mobile. A lesion that is hot, erythematous, and exquisitely tender is most likely an abscess, not a tumor.

Radiographic evaluation begins with plain radiographs of the lesion. Soft-tissue calcifications noted on the radiograph of the lesion vary with the underlying cause. In myositis ossificans, a mature ossification rim surrounds immature calcifications. Hemangiomas may contain multiple calcified phleboliths appearing as smooth rounded calcifications. Malignant neoplasms such as synovial cell sarcoma may have dysplastic, irregular-appearing calcifications in approximately one-fourth of cases. Regional bones may manifest erosive changes from an adjacent tumor. If malignancy is suspected, then a chest radiograph for metastases is indicated. If malignancy is confirmed, a chest CT scan is indicated owing to its additional approximate 15% sensitivity.[18]

MRI is the imaging study of choice for soft-tissue lesions. MRI reveals the extent of the tumor, its tissue homogeneity or inhomogeneity, the nature of its margin, the tumor's anatomic relationship to surrounding structures, surrounding edema, inherent vascularity and it will demonstrate involvement of key anatomic structures such as neurovascular bundles (Fig. 4). Gadolinium enhancement reflects the vascularity of lesions. Internal signal inhomogeneity is usually a characteristic of malignancy. MRI usually cannot provide a histologically accurate diagnosis except in classic cases of lipomas, cysts, and hemangiomas. A lesion with a multitude of MRI-demonstrated tortuous vessels in combination with phleboliths on plain radiographs can be conclusively diagnosed as a hemangioma. A lipoma has the same imaging characteristics as the surrounding subcutaneous fat and should be free of internal signal inhomogeneity. Inhomogeneity may reflect a lipoma-like liposarcoma. Ganglion cysts should present a homogeneous signal characteristic of fluid, that is, dark on T_1-weighted and bright

TABLE 1. SOFT-TISSUE TUMOR STAGING AND SURGICAL MARGIN	
Stage	**Margin Recommended**
Benign	
1. Latent	Marginal
2. Active	Wide; if marginal, consider adding adjuvant*
3. Aggressive	Wide or marginal + adjuvant*
Malignant	
I. Low grade	Wide
a. Intercompartmental	
b. Extracompartmental	
II. High grade	Radical or wide ± adjuvant**
a. Intracompartmental	
b. Extracompartmental	
III. Metastatic	Radical or wide + systemic adjuvant therapy*

* Adjuvants used for benign aggressive lesions treated with a marginal margin include phenol, freeze/thaw, and cauterization.
** Adjuvant therapy possibilities include radiation therapy (local treatment) and chemotherapy (systemic treatment).
Based on data from Enneking WF, Spanier SS, Goodman MA: A system for the surgical staging of musculoskeletal sarcoma. Clin Orthop 1980; 153: 106–120.

TABLE 2. AMERICAN JOINT COMMITTEE ON CANCER SOFT-TISSUE SARCOMA STAGING

Primary Tumor (T)

TX	Primary tumor cannot be assessed
TO	No evidence of primary tumor
T1	Tumor $\leq$ 5 cm in greatest dimension
T1a	Superficial tumor
T1b	Deep tumor
T2	Tumor > 5 cm in greatest dimension
T2a	Superficial tumor
T2b	Deep tumor

Superficial tumor is located exclusively above the superficial fascia without invasion of the fascia; deep tumor is located either exclusively beneath the superficial fascia, or superficial to the fascia with invasion of or through the fascia, or superficial and beneath the fascia. Retroperitoneal, mediastinal, and pelvic sarcomas are classified as deep tumors.

Regional Lymph Nodes (N)

NX	Regional lymph nodes cannot be assessed
N0	No regional lymph node metastasis
N1	Regional lymph node metastasis

Distant Metastasis (M)

MX	Distant metastasis cannot be assessed
M0	No distant metastasis
M1	Distant metastasis

Histopathologic Grade (G)

GX	Grade cannot be assessed
G1	Well differentiated
G2	Moderately differentiated
G3	Poorly differentiated
G4	Undifferentiated

Stage Grouping

Stage I		
A	(Low grade, small, superficial and deep)	G1–2, T1a–1b, N0, M0
B	(Low grade, large, superficial)	G1–2, T2a, N0, M0
Stage II		
A	(Low grade, large, deep)	G1–2, T2b, N0, M0
B	(High grade, small, superficial, or deep)	G3–4, T1a–1b, N0, M0
C	(High grade, large, superficial)	G3–4, T2a, N0, M0
Stage III		
	(High grade, large, deep)	G3–4, T2b, N0, M0
Stage IV		Any G, any T, N1, M0
	(Any metastasis)	Any G, any T, N0, M1

Modified from American Joint Committee on Cancer: Soft tissues. The original source for this material is Fleming ID, Cooper JS, Henson DE, et al (eds): AJCC Cancer Staging Manual, 5th ed. Philadelphia, Lippincott-Raven, 1997, pp 149–156. Used with the permission of the American Joint Committee on Cancer, Chicago, IL.

TABLE 3. DIFFERENTIAL DIAGNOSIS OF SOFT-TISSUE MASSES

Symptoms/Findings	Likely Diagnosis
Large, firm, or fixed	Sarcoma
Warm, erythematous, tender	Abscess
Ecchymosis	Hemorrhage, trauma
Variable size	Ganglion, hemangioma
Pulsatile	Pseudoaneurysm; metastasis or extension of renal or thyroid carcinoma or myeloma
Transilluminates	Ganglion
Paresthesias/percussion sign	Neural tumor or tumor compressing a nerve

community general radiologist with little experience interpreting the MRIs of musculoskeletal neoplasms. Referral to an experienced musculoskeletal oncologist may avoid disasters from MRI misinterpretations.

When MRI is unobtainable (e.g., patient refusal due to severe claustrophobia, intraocular metallic debris, etc.), then CT scan with contrast is the next best imaging study for soft-tissue tumors. CT is the best study for demonstrating bony architecture, including heterotopic ossifications such as myositis ossificans. It is also excellent for CT-guided biopsies, as is discussed below.

Biopsy provides the definitive histological diagnosis. Open biopsy performed through a longitudinal incision with dissection directly through soft tissues and muscles, avoiding intermuscular planes, is the gold standard. Neurovascular bundles should be avoided to minimize tumor contamination of vital structures as all tumor-contaminated tissues will ultimately require resection. A frozen section pathological analysis of biopsy material should always be

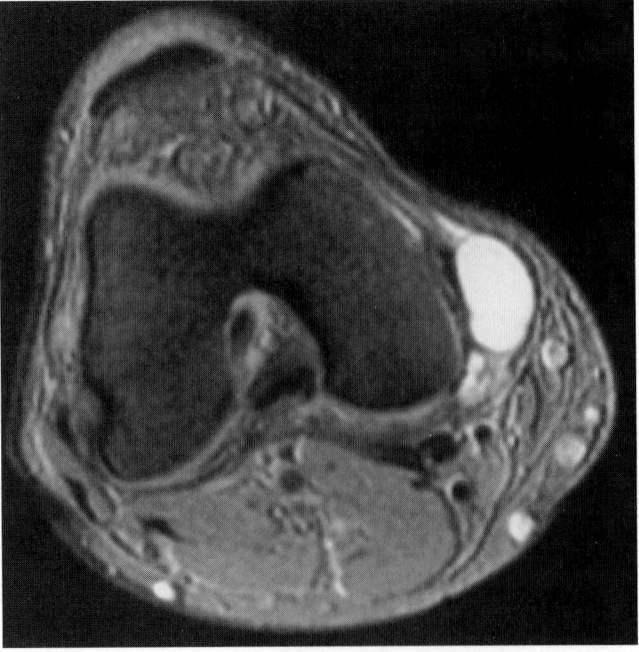

Fig. 4. MRI. This T_2-weighted MRI scan reveals a ganglion on the medial aspect of the knee. The mass had been present for 6 months and spontaneously resolved 1 week after the MRI was done.

on T_2-weighted imaging and should be in characteristic locations for ganglion cysts. Whenever lesions are inhomogeneous in signal or located in aberrant locations, beware of myxoid sarcomas masquerading as a ganglion.

Soft-tissue sarcomas create a pseudocapsule of compressed surrounding tissue. Thus, on MRI scans, they often appear encapsulated and sharply marginated. Inexperienced radiologists may interpret such lesions as benign (see Fig. 2). Conversely, some benign soft-tissue tumors can be infiltrative neoplasms. Thus, rarely from an MRI can the physician reliably separate benign from malignant tumors, or vice versa. The orthopaedist should personally inspect all studies, especially when the MRI has been interpreted by a

obtained to verify adequacy of tissue sampling, including an adequate amount of tissue for special stains or analyses such as flow cytometry.

Core needle biopsy can be performed in the office under local anesthesia. It is cost-effective and usually affords adequate tissue for accurate diagnosis. An FNAB is another option.[19, 20] It is nearly painless and can be performed without local anesthesia in the office.[19, 20] (See Chapter 7-2 for a more thorough discussion of biopsy.)

MANAGEMENT OVERVIEW

The mainstay of soft-tissue tumor management is complete surgical resection of all but asymptomatic, inactive, benign lesions. Locally aggressive and malignant lesions require a wide surgical margin. Ganglion cysts, lipomas, and a number of other nonmalignant, nonaggressive localized lesions can be "shelled-out," properly referred to as a marginal excision. A soft-tissue sarcoma should always be excised with a circumferential cuff of normal tissue. Except for small lesions (generally less than 3 to 5 cm) that can be resected as excisional biopsies, resection is best performed after appropriate staging and anatomic mapping of the lesion. It is inappropriate to perform a "debulking biopsy," as this spreads tumor throughout the soft tissues and predisposes the patient to multiple local recurrences, metastases, and death.

The proper management sequence consists of an initial history and physical examination, followed by appropriate imaging, and then a biopsy. The biopsy should not compromise the ability to ultimately resect all contaminated tissues. Use of preoperative chemotherapy in sarcoma management is gaining popularity. Adjuvant chemotherapy in high-grade soft-tissue sarcomas adds an approximately 10%

to 12% likelihood of survival.[5] Chemotherapeutic response varies widely by patient and by sarcoma, and therefore treatment must be individualized. Further management discussions follow in subsequent chapters.

COMPLICATIONS

The most serious and frequently encountered complications arise from misdiagnosis and consequent mismanagement. Misdiagnosing a soft-tissue sarcoma as a ganglion, hematoma, pulled muscle, or isolated muscle hypertrophy will delay diagnosis and increase the risk of tumor progression and metastasis. Improper biopsy may create local tumor spread, converting a limb-salvageable lesion to one requiring amputation. Whereas complications and functional deficits may occur following tumor resection, chemotherapy, and radiation treatment, none are as troubling to the patient and the involved physicians as a loss of life, limb, or function that results from a delayed or missed diagnosis. Tumor recurrence is best avoided by appropriate staging with appropriate imaging, proper planning, adequate resection, and appropriate adjuvant therapy. All these steps require an initial index of suspicion of the nature of the lesion.

TREATMENT RESULTS

The functional results of soft-tissue tumor treatment depend on four primary factors: (1) histologic type and aggressiveness of the lesion, (2) anatomic extent, (3) adequacy of resection, and (4) tissue sacrifice required for resection. Discussion of the results for the specific entities are covered elsewhere in this book and in standard textbooks of soft-tissue tumors and in multiple journal articles.

REFERENCES

1. Brennan MS, Casper ES, Harrison LB: Soft tissue sarcoma. In Devita VT Jr, Hellman S, Rosenberg SA (eds): Cancer: Principles and Practice of Oncology, 5th ed. Philadelphia, Lippincott-Raven, 1997, pp 1739–1788.
2. American Joint Committee on Cancer: Soft tissues. In Fleming ID, Cooper JS, Henson DE, et al (eds): AJCC Cancer Staging Manual, 5th ed. Philadelphia, Lippincott-Raven, 1997, pp 149–156.
3. Enneking WF: In Simon MA, Springfield D (eds). Surgery for Bone and Soft Tissue Tumors. Philadelphia, Lippincott-Raven, 1998, pp xv–xvi.
4. Yang JC, Chang AE, Baker AR, et al: Randomized prospective study of the benefit of adjuvant radiation therapy in the treatment of soft tissue sarcomas of the extremity. J Clin Oncol 1998; 16:197.
5. Tierney JF, Mosseri V, Stewart LA, et al: Adjuvant chemotherapy for soft-tissue sarcoma: Review and meta-analysis of the published results of randomised clinical trials. Br J Cancer 1995; 72:469.
6. Hurwitz Mr: Diagnostic and prognostic molecular markers in cancer. Am J Surg 1992; 164:299.
7. Kamagai SG, McGuire MH: Cellular and Molecular Biology. In Simon MA, Springfield D (eds): Bones and Soft Tissues. Philadelphia, Lippincott-Raven, 1998, pp 9–20.
8. Li FP, Fraumeni JF Jr: Soft-tissue sarcomas, breast cancer, and other neoplasms, a familial syndrome? Ann Intern Med 1969; 71:747.
9. Culotta E, Koshland DD Jr: Molecule of the year: p53 sweeps through cancer research. Science 1993; 261:1958.
10. Malkin D, Li FP, Strong LC, et al: Germ line p53 mutations in a familial syndrome of breast cancer, sarcomas, and other neoplasms. Science 1990; 250:1233.
11. Cutler SJ, Young IL: Third National Cancer Survey. Incidence data. Natl Cancer Inst Monogr 41, 1975.
12. Parker SL, Tong T, Bolden S, et al: Cancer Statistics, 1997. Ca Cancer J Clin 1998; 47:5.
13. Rantakko V, Ekfors TO: Sarcomas of the soft tissues in the extremities and limb girdles. Analysis of 240 cases diagnosed in Finland in 1960–1969. Acta Chir Scand 1979; 145:384.
14. Rydholm A, Berg N: Size, site and clinical incidence of lipoma. Acta Orthop Scand 1983; 54:929.
15. Enzinger FM, Weiss SW. Soft Tissue Tumors. St Louis, Mosby–Year Book, 1988.
16. Enneking WF, Spanier SS, Goodman MA: A system for the surgical staging of musculoskeletal sarcoma. Clin Orthop 1980; 153:106.
17. Enneking WF: Staging musculoskeletal tumors. In Enneking WF (ed): Musculoskeletal Tumor Surgery. New York, Churchill Livingstone 1983, pp 88–89.
18. Chalmers N, Best JJK: The significant of pulmonary nodules detected by CT but not by chest radiography in tumour staging. Clin Radiol 1991; 44:410.
19. Kilpatrick SE, Ward WG, Chauvenet AR, et al: The role of fine-needle aspiration biopsy in the initial diagnosis of pediatric bone and soft tissue tumors: An institutional experience. Mod Pathol 1998; 11:923.
20. The Papanicolaou Society: Guidelines of the Papanicolaou Society of Cytopathology for fine-needle aspiration procedure and reporting. Mod Pathol 1997; 10:739.

BENIGN SOFT-TISSUE TUMORS

Lawrence R. Menendez, Larissa B. Isterabadi, and Alexander Fedenko

Summary
- Benign soft-tissue tumors in the extremities are common. Most are subcutaneous and need no treatment or a simple excision.
- Lipoma, schwannoma, and hemangioma account for the majority of these neoplasia.
- There are numerous others, some that can be mistaken for malignant tumors and some that need more than simple excision. A brief description of each is provided.

BENIGN FIBROUS TISSUE TUMORS

Benign tumors, such as nodular fasciitis and proliferative myositis, grow rapidly, reaching their final size within 2 weeks. They are highly cellular due to proliferations of fibroblasts. These types of tumors rarely recur and never metastasize. Other less cellular tumors, such as elastofibroma, have marked amounts of collagen and elastic fibers. Tumors of this kind are slow-growing and rare.

NODULAR FASCIITIS (PSEUDOSARCOMATOUS FASCIITIS)

Incidence Rate. Nodular fasciitis was not recognized until first reported in 1955 by Konwaler et al.[1] It occurs frequently and is the most common fibroblastic-type tumor seen in the soft tissues.

Sex. There is no predilection for one sex.

Age. This tumor occurs most frequently in adults from 20 to 40 years of age. It occurs infrequently in children and rarely in the elderly.

Localization. The upper extremity is the most common site, particularly the volar aspect of the forearm. Other less common sites are the thoracic wall and back. Tumors of the head and neck occur more frequently in children. The tumors are found in deep subcutaneous tissue, usually near the deep fascia or occasionally within striated muscle.

Gross Pathology. The lesion is a small, fixed nodule with whitish-gray appearance. The nodule may be firm, soft, or gelatinous, depending on the amount of mucus-filled cystic cavities or collagen within it. The cut surface displays a poorly encapsulated and well vascularized nodule. The nodule may have a stellate appearance due to the extension of the tumor into the surrounding subcutaneous tissue and muscle fibers.

Histological Findings. Large, immature fibroblasts of consistent size and shape are seen with large, pale, staining nuclei. Mitotic figures are common. The fibroblasts are arranged as intertwining bundles with an abundant reticular network surrounding them. There are increased amounts of ground substance and varying amounts of collagen. The fibroblasts and proliferation of capillaries resemble granulation tissue. Inflammatory cells are abundant, especially lymphocytes and macrophages. Giant cells and erythrocytes are also common (Fig. 1).

ELASTOFIBROMA (ELASTOFIBROMA DORSI)

Incidence Rate. This pseudotumoral lesion is rare and self-limited.

Sex. This tumor occurs more often in women.

Age. It is typically seen in patients older than 55 years. It is rare in young adults, adolescents, or children.

Localization. The tumor is found exclusively in the subscapular area, beneath the latissimus dorsi and rhomboideus muscles. It adheres to the ligaments and fascia of the thoracic wall at the level of the seventh and eighth ribs. Only a few isolated cases have documented the tumor found in other locations, such as greater trochanter, deltoid region, and foot. Unilateral presentation is typical in 90% of patients.[2]

Gross Pathology. The cut surface is gray-white and glistening, with a fibrous appearance. Fatty lobules and hyperemia may be seen on the surface. The lesions are firm and fairly large, with a diameter up to 10 cm. Margins are poorly defined.

Histological Findings. There is decreased cellularity, with sparse numbers of mature fibrocytes. Thick, irregular, swollen fibrous bands are seen. These intertwining bands are composed of equal amounts of collagen and elastic fibers.

PROLIFERATIVE MYOSITIS

This type of tumor is analogous to nodular fasciitis in clinical and anatomic presentation, except that it occurs in deep or intramuscular areas. However, the pathological findings are unique.

Histological Findings. Proliferation of fibroblastic cells occurs in stroma of skeletal muscle tissue. Clusters of peculiar giant cells near sarcolemma of adjacent skeletal muscle fibers are seen. These giant cells are basophilic and resemble rhabdomyoblasts or ganglion cells. However, they appear to be modified fibroblasts.[3]

FIBROMATOSES

Fibromatoses vary in their presentation; some are characteristic of benign lesions and others of fibrosarcoma, with a more infiltrative growth. However, neither type of fibromatosis metastasizes. There are superficial, fascial fibromatoses (palmar fibrosis) and deep, musculoaponeurotic fibromatoses (extra-abdominal desmoid tumor). Nodules of palmar fibrosis begin as highly cellular and then progress to hypocellular and collagenized. These nodules are pain-

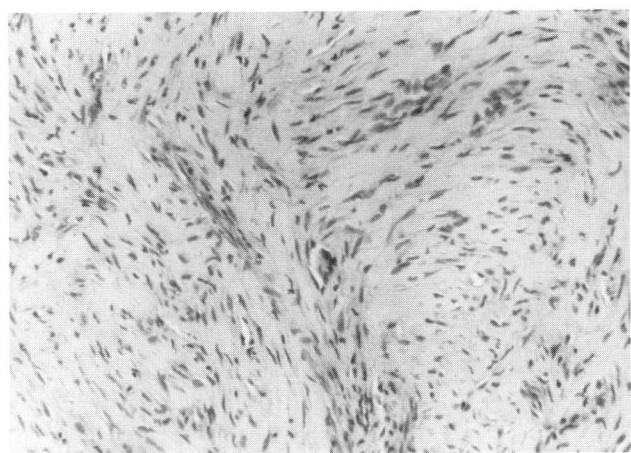

Fig. 1. Nodular fasciitis. Interlacing bundles of plump fibroblasts are demonstrated (×160).

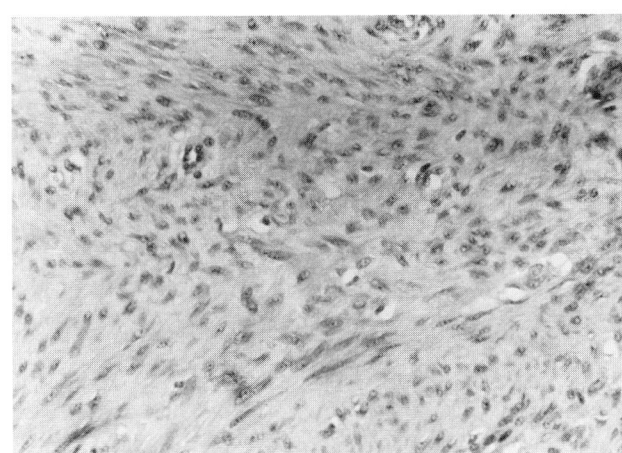

Fig. 3. Extra-abdominal desmoid. There is uniform fibroblast proliferation, separated by bands of collagen (×160).

less and may resolve without treatment. Many cases are also associated with plantar fibromatosis or penile fibromatosis. Desmoid tumors are more aggressive and are often labeled as nonmetastasizing fibrosarcoma. Recurrence rates are high for these types of deep fibromatosis.

EXTRA-ABDOMINAL DESMOID TUMOR (AGGRESSIVE FIBROMATOSIS, MUSCULOAPONEUROTIC FIBROMATOSIS)

Incidence Rate. This is not a rare type of tumor. Three to four cases per million are recorded in the United States annually.[4]

Sex. There is a slight predilection for women. This type of tumor is often seen in the abdominal wall of recently pregnant women. However, studies have shown varying statistics on predilection for one sex.[5]

Age. The age of presentation varies from childhood to 40 years old, with the most common age from 25 to 35 years old. Desmoid tumors are rare in infants and the elderly.

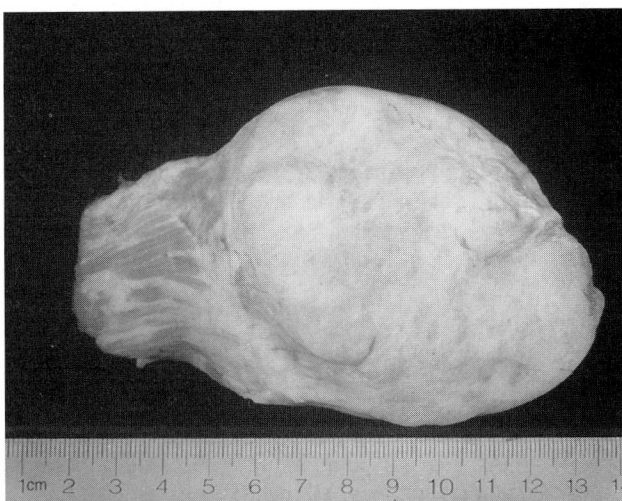

Fig. 2. Extra-abdominal desmoid tumor. This is a desmoid tumor of the thigh, showing involvement of the skeletal muscle.

Localization. Tumors are either deep within musculature or in the superficial fascial plane. The most frequent site is in the proximal extremities: shoulder, axilla, buttock, and groin. Another common location is the trunk. Tumors often arise on or within the abdominal wall. Rarely are they seen in the hand or foot.

Gross Pathology. Margins are poorly defined, with the tumor invading the musculature. Tumor size is 5 to 10 cm in diameter typically. It is firm and hard. The cut surface of the tumor displays a glistening white, scarlike appearance (Fig. 2).

Histological Findings. Fibroblasts, fibrocytes, and collagen predominate. The fibroblasts are spindle-shaped, with plump nuclei. However, mitotic activity is rare. The fibroblasts are arranged in intertwining bundles, separated by large bands of collagen. Overall, the tumor is very hypocellular. There is little vascularization, and yet no tissue necrosis. Multinucleate giant cells may be present, resembling malignancy (Fig. 3).

PALMAR FIBROSIS (DUPUYTREN'S DISEASE, DUPUYTREN'S CONTRACTURE)

Incidence Rate. This disease occurs frequently. It is the most common type of fibromatosis. In the elderly age 65 years and older, 20% will be afflicted.[6]

Sex. It is common in both men and women, with a slight predilection for men.

Age. The disease is rare in children and adolescents. It is most frequent in middle-aged and elderly persons.

Localization. Nodules are seen on the ulnar aspect of the palm on the hand. The nodules are located just beneath the skin. It is rare for any other parts of the hand or wrist to be affected.

Gross Pathology. Single or multiple lesions are firm and usually less than 1 cm in diameter. There is a thin, poorly defined capsule. The cut surface of the fibrous lesion is gray-white or gray-yellow, depending on the stage of development and collagenization. The nodules blend with the palmar aponeurosis and superficial fascia.

Histological Findings. Many plump, spindle-shaped fibroblasts arranged in whirls are seen within this highly

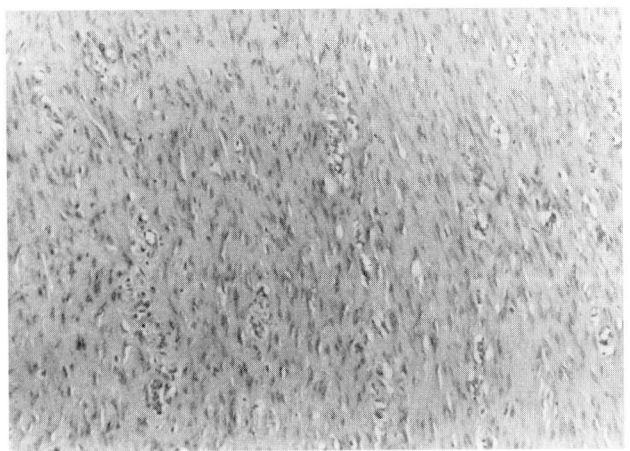

Fig. 4. Palmar fibromatosis. The lesion is composed of parallel fascicles of fibroblasts, separated by collagen (×100).

cellular tumor. Mitotic figures are not uncommon. Also seen are giant cells, hemosiderin, chronic inflammatory cells, and microhemorrhages. Moderate amounts of collagen are interspersed between fibroblasts. Fibrocollagenous cords resemble tendons. In the later stages of development, the lesions appear scar-like and disorganized. Nodules become hypocellular with increasing amounts of collagen (Fig. 4).

FIBROUS TUMORS OF INFANCY AND CHILDHOOD

MYOFIBROMATOSIS (CONGENITAL GENERALIZED FIBROMATOSIS)

Fibrous tumor of infancy and childhood may be either equivalent to those seen in adults or unique to infants and children and therefore vastly different in their prognosis and course of treatment. Myofibromatosis is a type of smooth-muscle tumor with multiple lesions. This multiple form is almost always fatal, especially during the first days or weeks of life. Myofibroma is the solitary form of the disease, which is often misdiagnosed for other tumors, such as fibrosarcoma. Patients present with a swelling or mass in the dermis or subcutaneous area.

Incidence Rate. This is a rare type of tumor, which almost exclusively affects infants.

Sex. It is almost twice as common in men as in women.

Age. This disease is present at birth or during the first few months. It is seen occasionally in adults.

Localization. Solitary lesions are found in the subcutaneous and muscular planes. The most common sites are head and neck region, craniofacial bones, and shoulder girdle. Less commonly, they are found in the extremities. Multiple lesions are seen in the same locations as well as in the viscera.

Gross Pathology. They occur as multiple or single tumors several centimeters in diameter, which may have peripheral satellite lesions. The nodules are firm, with a white-gray or pink color. They are poorly encapsulated and difficult to discern from surrounding tissue.

Histological Findings. Within highly cellular areas, fibroblasts and myofibroblasts are arranged as bundles or nodules. These eosinophilic cells have large ovoid nuclei

with many mitotic figures. The surrounding stroma is rich in collagen and highly vascularized. There are often areas of extensive necrosis and weak radiodensity due to minute calcification.[7] Margins are difficult to delineate, with the tumor blending into surrounding tissues. Immunostaining is positive for vimentin and actin but not desmin or S-100 protein.[8]

BENIGN FIBROHISTIOCYTIC TUMORS

Benign fibrohistiocytic tumors share similar histological features but differ in their nature of growth. Fibrous histiocytomas have good growth potential but are not metastatic. The recurrence rate for these tumors may be as high as 50%.[9] Xanthomas are relatively painless and slow-growing. They are not true tumors but "pseudotumors," composed of collections of lipid within histiocytes. Xanthomas usually arise in response to a disturbance in serum lipids and may be associated with the five subtypes of essential[10] or secondary hyperlipidemia disease states.

FIBROUS HISTIOCYTOMA (DERMATOFIBROMA, HISTIOCYTOMA CUTIS, SCLEROSING ANGIOMA)

Incidence Rate. This is a frequently occurring tumor. They are more common in the cutaneous tissue than in the deeper tissues.

Sex. There does not appear to be a predilection for one sex.

Age. Adults from the age of 20 to 40 years are most commonly affected.

Localization. Both cutaneous and deeply situated fibrous histiocytomas occur frequently in the extremities. Skin lesions may be referred to as sclerosing hemangiomas.[11]

Gross Pathology. Cutaneous lesions are often protrusive or pedunculated. They appear red-brown or blue-black due to hemosiderin deposits. Cutaneous nodules are typically less than 3 cm in diameter, whereas the deeply situated ones are greater than 5 cm. Lesions are yellow-white in color and may contain isolated areas of hemorrhage. Margins are well defined. Often, multiple lesions are present.

Histological Findings. Short, intertwining fascicles, composed of spindle-shaped fibroblastic cells, are the predominant finding. There is a storiform or whorled appearance. Occasional histiocytes and giant cells are seen with phagocytosed lipid and hemosiderin. Lymphocytes and xanthoma cells may also be present. Cells are well differentiated, with little mitotic activity. In some cases, there may be increased hyalinization of stroma and vessels, thus leading to the incorrect term sclerosing angioma. In the deeply situated lesions, a more storiform pattern is evident (Fig. 5).

XANTHOMA

Incidence Rate. Xanthomas occur quite frequently.

Sex. There is no sex predilection.

Age. Xanthomas may present at any age.

Localization. Depending on the different clinical subtype, xanthomas occur in particular sites. Most common locations include buttocks, elbows, knees, fingers, eyelids, and palmar skin creases. Sites of frequent trauma, such as tendons of hands and feet, are common locations. The Achilles tendon is particularly affected.

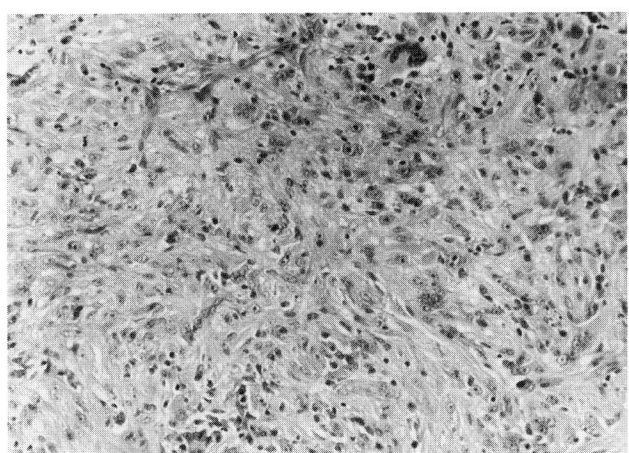

Fig. 5. Benign fibrous histiocytoma. Histiocytes and giant cells are seen in fibroblastic collagenized stroma (×160).

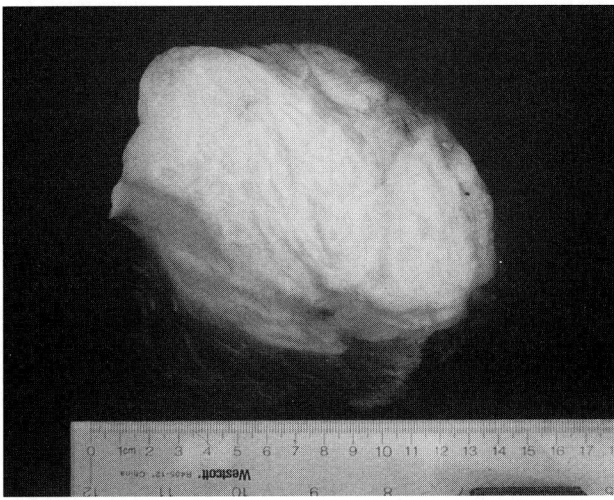

Fig. 6. Lipoma. Lipoma involving the thigh with a distinct multilobular pattern is seen.

Gross Pathology. Average size of the lesions is a few centimeters in diameter. The cut surface may be white, yellow, or brown. This depends on the amounts of fibrous tissue, lipids, or hemorrhage present. Multiple lesions are common. They are firmly attached to tendons.

Histological Findings. There are sheets of foamy and nonfoamy histiocytes, with small amounts of inflammatory cells. There may be fibrosis and hemosiderin granules. Extracellular cholesterol is seen. The common identifying features are multiple, clear vacuoles within xanthoma cells, which are filled with cholesterol.

BENIGN LIPOMATOUS TUMORS

Lipomas are usually asymptomatic and not recognized until they have reached large sizes. Lipomas are frequently seen in obese people and increase in size during rapid weight gain. However, the mass does not decrease in size with weight loss. Therefore, the mature lipocytes of a lipoma do not participate in normal fat metabolism. Lipomas gradually enlarge over time, and they may remain unchanged for years. There is great size diversity in these lesions. The clinical presentation of angiolipomas is that of intense, intermittent pain that decreases as the tumor reaches its final size. The pain is not associated with any type of trauma to the area but is triggered by light touch or palpation. The tumor is usually not palpable. Tumors are more often found in deep than superficial tissues. Multiple lesions are more common than solitary ones.[12]

LIPOMA

Incidence Rate. Lipomas are the most common type of mesenchymal neoplasm. Because of the fact that most remain unreported, the incidence rate of lipomas is unknown.

Sex. There is no true sex predilection reported in the literature. It is commonly believed that the superficial type of tumor occurs more frequently in women, whereas the deeper, multiple forms are more common in male patients.[13]

Age. Lipomas present in individuals age 40 to 60 years. It is at this age when fat begins to accumulate in the body in greater amounts. Lipomas are very rare in individuals 20 years and younger.

Localization. Solitary lipomas of the subcutaneous or superficial type are most commonly found in the upper back, neck, shoulder, and abdomen. Less frequently, these lipomas are found in the buttocks and axilla. Deeper, less commonly occurring lipomas are usually detected at a later stage because they do not bother the patient until they reach a large size. These types of lipomas are seen in the hands, feet, periosteum, forehead, scalp, thorax, and pelvis.

Gross Pathology. Lesions are typically soft, lobular-shaped, and encapsulated by a thin membrane. The surface varies from yellow to orange. A common feature of lipomas is a greasy surface. Deep lipomas have a thin, more prominent capsule and increased variance in shape (Fig. 6).

Histological Findings. Microscopically, lipomas do not differ much from the fat that surrounds them. They are composed of mature lipocytes, which tend to be larger in size. The typical lipoma contains decreased amounts of stroma and is well vascularized. Fibrous connective tissue and mucoid substances are also seen in the stroma (Fig. 7).

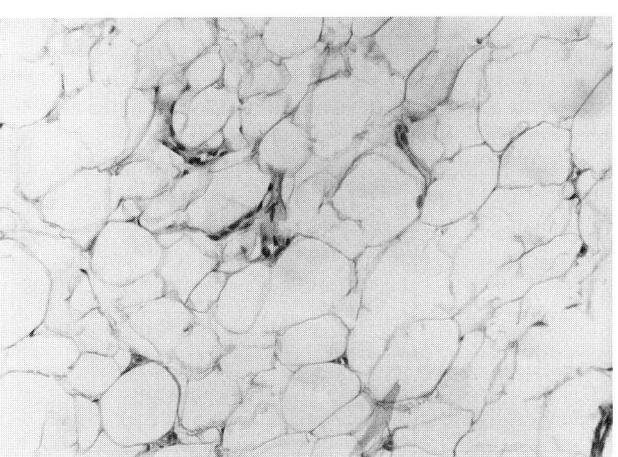

Fig. 7. Lipoma. Lipoma consisting of mature fat cells shows slight variation in cellular size and shape (×160).

ANGIOLIPOMA

Incidence Rate. Angiolipomas are relatively rare tumors.

Sex. Males are more commonly affected.

Age. Tumors occur in young adults from 15 to 20 years of age. Rarely are they seen in children or the elderly.

Localization. Typical presentation is in the forearm. Other less frequent sites are trunk and upper arm.

Gross Pathology. Lesions have a thin capsule. There is an irregular, indistinct border between the tumor and adjacent tissue. Tumors are small, less than 2 cm in diameter. Yellow fat lobules predominate, with interspersed red areas of vascularity. The tumors are typically firmer than lipomas.

Histological Findings. Mature lipocytes are interspersed within a vascular network of capillaries. This vascular network is more prominent in the subcapsular region of the tumor. Perivascular or interstitial fibrosis may be present. Unlike lipomas, fibrin microthrombi are often seen occluding the vessels.[14] The vascular component of the tumor is more prominent than the adipose component.

BENIGN TUMORS OF SMOOTH MUSCLE

On average, leiomyomas of deep soft tissues tend to be much larger than those found in the skin. This is best explained by the fact that leiomyomas of soft tissue show few symptoms and thus are detected at a much later stage. Because of the fact that many leiomyomas may undergo calcification at the periphery, radiography proves to be an effective means of detection. The high vascularization of leiomyomas may suggest the incorrect diagnosis of a malignancy.[15]

LEIOMYOMA (FIBROMYOMA, VASCULAR LEIOMYOMA, LEIOMYOMA OF DEEP SOFT TISSUE)

Incidence Rate. Leiomyomas are rare, compared with other benign tumors of the soft tissues.

Sex. Both sexes are affected equally.

Age. Middle-aged individuals from 35 to 50 years are commonly affected. Leiomyomas are rare in children.

Localization. Most leiomyomas are located in the deep musculature of the extremities. Other common locations are the abdominal cavity and retroperitoneum.

Gross Pathology. Leiomyomas are well-encapsulated and circumscribed lesions. Under light, they are slightly grayish or white. Lesions undergo significant myxoid change and may appear gelatinous.

Histological Findings. Deeply seated lesions usually undergo regressive changes. The well-patterned order of their intersecting follicles with stubby-ended nuclei makes them easily recognizable as smooth muscle tumors. In some cases, nuclear palisading or perinuclear vacuolization can be seen in the lesions.[16] Leiomyomas may also be recognized by the large amounts of myxoid substance that accumulate between cells.

BENIGN TUMORS AND TUMOR-LIKE LESIONS OF BLOOD VESSELS

Hemangiomas are benign vascular neoplasms. They are thought to be hamartomatous malformations of blood vascular tissue.[17] Capillary hemangiomas are composed of

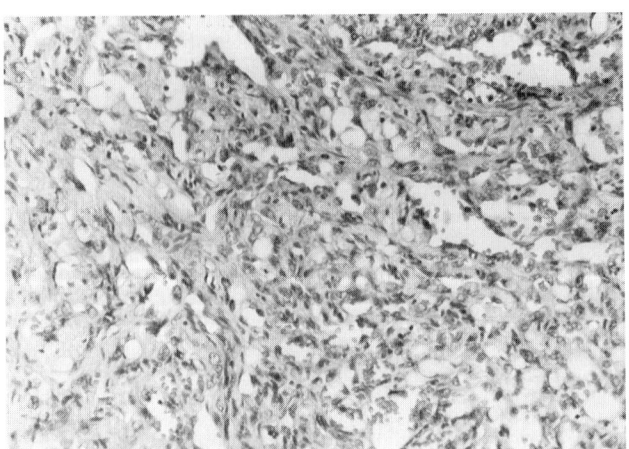

Fig. 8. Capillary hemangioma. The tumor consists of small vessels lined by flattened endothelium (×160).

large numbers of intersecting capillaries, which are highly anastomosing with the systemic circulation. There is no order to their arrangement. The capillaries of the tumor in cavernous hemangiomas are tortuous, with large dilations and few anastomoses. Cavernous hemangiomas vary in size over time and are painful during clotting episodes. On the other hand, capillary hemangiomas remain stable in size and are relatively painless.

HEMANGIOMA (CAPILLARY HEMANGIOMA, CAVERNOUS HEMANGIOMA, ANGIOMA, VASCULAR NEVUS)

Incidence Rate. Hemangiomas are very common soft-tissue tumors and comprise 7% of all benign tumors.[18]

Sex. Capillary and cavernous hemangiomas affect females more often than males.

Age. These lesions most often occur in children and adolescents.

Localization. They are most frequently found in the subcutaneous tissue and skin, especially in the face and oral cavity. Deeper-seated lesions are found in the fascia, musculature, and internal organs, such as the liver.

Gross Pathology. Lesions are soft, compressible, and highly vascular. Capillary hemangiomas are red, whereas the cavernous hemangiomas are bluish when viewed from the skin surface. A thin, poorly defined capsule may be present. The defining characteristic of hemangiomas is the massive, vascular network comprising the lesion and extending outward.

Histological Findings. Margins are difficult to identify because of the extensive infiltration into surrounding normal tissue. Vascular networks are composed of bundles of capillaries or wide, dilated vascular channels. These vascular proliferations intertwine among the previously normal tissue. Capillaries and channels are lined by a flattened, mature, single layer of endothelium. Collagenous thickening of the vessel walls may be seen. Dystrophic calcification may be seen in cavernous hemangiomas (Fig. 8).

TUMORS OF LYMPH VESSELS

The majority of these tumors arise during a developmental abnormality in early life. Less frequently, they may be due to obstruction from surgery or infection.[19] It is unclear if these tumors are true neoplasms. They are composed of overgrowth of lymphatic vessels that have collections of fluid within them.

LYMPHANGIOMA (CAVERNOUS LYMPHANGIOMA, CYSTIC LYMPHANGIOMA, HYGROMA CYSTICUM COLLI)

Incidence Rate. These tumors are relatively rare.

Sex. No predilection for one sex is found.

Age. Lymphangiomas are usually present at birth as a congenital abnormality. However, they may not appear clinically until the first few years of life.

Localization. The most common locations are those that are rich in lymphatics, such as the head, neck, and axilla. Other less common sites include omentum, mesentery, fingers, spleen, liver, gastrointestinal tract, and bone.

Gross Pathology. The tumors are sponge-like and easy to compress. Tumors may be composed of one large cystic cavity, as in cystic lymphangioma. When multiple microscopic cysts are present, it is termed cavernous lymphangioma. Multiple tumors are occasionally present. Proliferation of blood vessels may also occur within the tumor.

Histological Findings. Cystic cavities are lined by an attenuated endothelium. Within these lacunae may be proteinaceous fluid with lymphocytes and few erythrocytes. Surrounding these lacunae are collagen and smooth muscle cells.

BENIGN PERIVASCULAR TUMORS

First described in 1924 by Masson, glomus tumors were previously thought to be forms of angiosarcomas.[20] Glomus tumors are unique benign, vascular types of tumors that are derived from the glomus body. They frequently occur in the nail bed of the fingers. The clinical presentation of this tumor is sharp, stabbing pain that radiates out from the lesion. This pain may be brought on by sudden changes in temperature or minor trauma to the lesion.

GLOMUS TUMOR (GLOMANGIOMA)

Incidence Rate. Glomus tumors are relatively uncommon.

Sex. There is an equal division between men and women. However, in the common subungual region, they occur mainly in women (3:1).[21]

Age. They occur during early adult life, usually from the ages of 20 to 40 years. Rarely do they occur in childhood.

Localization. Nail beds of fingers and toes as well as upper extremities are affected. In the trunk region, it is only found in the stomach.

Gross Pathology. Nodules are small, usually less than 1 cm in diameter. Often, they are difficult to visualize when located in the nail bed. Lesions are pink or bluish-red due to dilated vessels within it. A thin, fibrous capsule is present.

Histological Findings. Tumors are composed of a fine network of vascular channels. Surrounding these channels are rims of epithelioid, glomus cells. The glomus cells are round with ample cytoplasm filled with fine granules. Spindle-shaped glomus cells resemble smooth muscle cells.

Nonmyelinated nerve fibers are located between the thick-walled vessels. Surrounding collagen stroma may be myxoid in appearance.

BENIGN TUMORS OF PERIPHERAL NERVES

Morton's neuroma occurs on the digital plantar nerve, between the heads of the third and fourth metatarsals. Pain is triggered by traumatic compression of the nerve between the two heads of the metatarsals. Morton's neuroma is not true neoplasm; it is fibrosing of tissue adjacent to the nerve affected. Granular cell tumors are also benign tumors of neural origin. There is no pain reported with these tumors, and they occur predominantly in black people. Neurilemomas and neurifibromas are both composed of cells that resemble Schwann's cells. Neurilemoma presents with pain on compression or with light trauma to the area. It is typically a palpable mass. The growth of these tumors is usually limited to small sizes. Patients with neurofibromas often have café au lait skin spots, especially in the axilla, due to increased melanin production. Neurofibromas are generally slow-growing tumors, except during puberty and pregnancy.

NEURILEMOMA (BENIGN SCHWANNOMA, NEURINOMA, PERINEURAL FIBROBLASTOMA)

Incidence Rate. It is an unusual type of tumor.

Sex. Both sexes are equally affected.

Age. The tumor may present at any age, although it occurs most commonly in middle-aged adults (20 to 50 years).

Localization. Tumors are frequently localized in spinal nerve roots as they exit the spinal canal through the intervertebral foramen. Nerves to the mediastinum, retroperitoneum, or peripheral nerves may be involved.

Gross Pathology. Nodules are fusiform in shape and extend along the direction of nerve. The tumor is well encapsulated in the nerve sheath. The cut surface is firm and shiny. They may be pink, white, or yellow. The diameter is usually less than 5 cm.

Histological Findings. Histologically, there are two alternating components: Antoni A and B. Antoni A is composed of intersecting bundles of spindle-shaped cells. Nuclei are palisading around eosinophilic areas (Verocay's bodies). Cells create a whorling appearance around central hyaline areas. Antoni B areas are distinguished by decreased cellularity and loosely organized cells. Mitotic figures are infrequent. S-100 protein is associated,[22] especially in Antoni A areas (Fig. 9).

NEUROFIBROMA (SOLITARY NEUROFIBROMA, NEUROFIBROMATOSIS, VON RECKLINGHAUSEN'S DISEASE)

Incidence Rate. This is an unusual type of tumor. The incidence rate is 1 in every 2500 to 3000 live births.[23]

Sex. The solitary form of neurofibroma has no predilection for one sex. However, the multiple form associated with von Recklinghausen's disease occurs typically in boys.

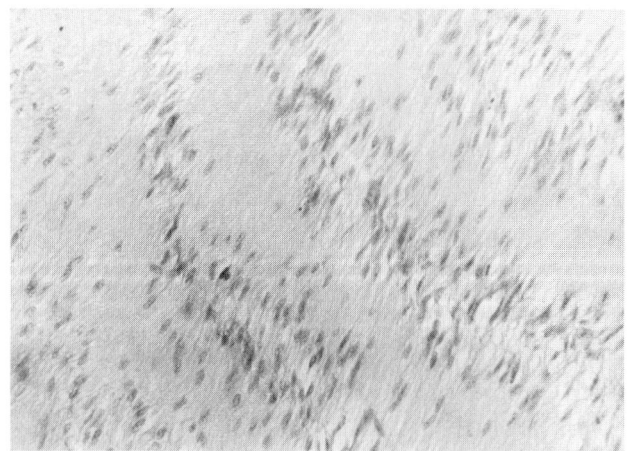

Fig. 9. Schwannoma. Prominent nuclear palisading and formation of Verocay bodies are seen (×160).

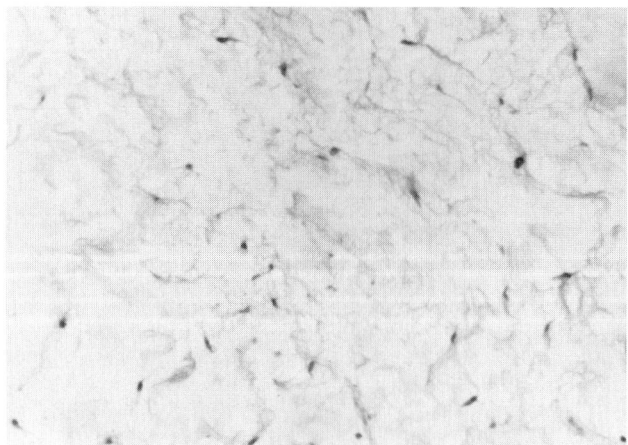

Fig. 11. Myxoma. The tissue is characterized by a paucity of cells in mucoid matrix. Note almost complete absence of vessels (×160).

Age. Solitary neurofibroma occurs in young adults from the ages of 20 to 40 years, and multiple form occurs in young children.

Localization. The solitary form is localized to the subcutaneous and dermal tissues, and the multiple form may occur in any organ or part of the body. Occasionally, the tumors are limited to one area (segmental neurofibromatosis).[23]

Gross Pathology. Tumors have a firm consistency with a thin, translucent capsule. They may be obviously associated with a nerve or have only microscopic associations with small unmyelinated nerve fibers. The cut surface is gray and pink.

Histological Findings. Loose intersecting bundles of spindle cells are seen, creating an undulating pattern. There are varying amounts of collagen and mucoid material in the surrounding stroma. Mitotic figures and necrosis are rare (Fig. 10).

BENIGN SOFT-TISSUE TUMORS OF UNCERTAIN TYPE

Myxomas are benign soft-tissue tumors that do not metastasize, rarely recur, and are successfully treated by local

excision. Many cases have been reported in the last 30 years. Myxomas are typically solitary lesions. Multiple intramuscular myxomas are often associated with fibrous dysplasia of bone. The presentation is that of a relatively painless mass that is mobile. Lesions grow slowly to their large sizes.

MYXOMA (INTRAMUSCULAR MYXOMA)

Incidence Rate. This is a relatively rare type of tumor.

Sex. Myxomas are seen equally in both men and women.

Age. Tumors may occur at any age. Adults are most commonly affected after 40 years of age. They are rare in children.

Localization. Most frequently, tumors are seen in the large musculature of the limbs. Locations include thigh, shoulder, buttocks, and arm.[24]

Gross Pathology. Lesions are globose or ovoid. Average diameter is 5 to 10 cm but may reach up to 21 cm. A thin pseudocapsule is present. The tumor may infiltrate within the musculature or be attached below the muscle to the fascia. The surface has a gray-white, glistening, translucid appearance. The cut surface is soft, slimy, and mucoid.

Histological Findings. The tumor is hypocellular. There is abundant mucoid material that is chiefly mucopolysaccharide and hyaluronidase-sensitive. The matrix is composed of a loose network of reticulin fibers and varying amounts of mature collagen fibers. Sparse spindle-shaped cells have small, pyknotic nuclei with dense chromatin. There is a decreased amount of vessels. Small cystic cavities are occasionally present (Fig. 11).

BENIGN TUMORS OF SYNOVIAL TISSUE

Giant cell tumors are typically slow-growing and self-limited in size to small lesions. Classic presentation is that of soft, nontender, nonmobile nodules. When located in tendinous sheaths, they do not change shape or position with movement of the tendon. Giant cell tumors may present in a localized or nodular form or as a diffuse villous or villonodular form. The localized form of the giant cell tumor was initially described in 1852 by Chas-

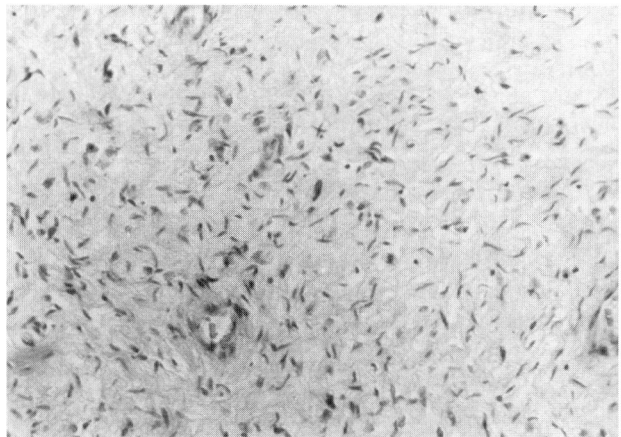

Fig. 10. Neurofibroma. This lesion consists of Schwann's cells associated with collagen fibrils and myxoid stroma (×160).

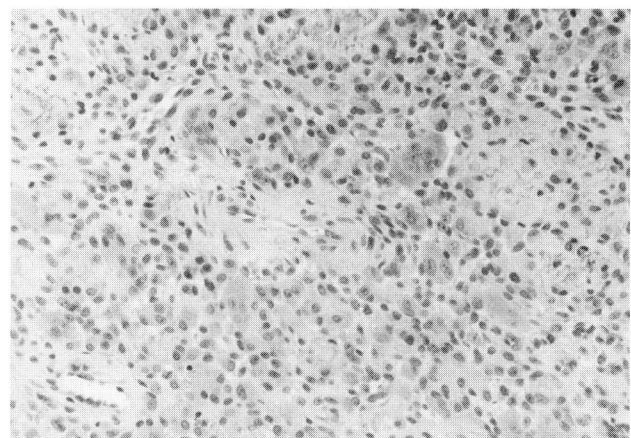

Fig. 12. Tenosynovial giant cell tumor. The tumor is composed of round synovial-like cells, multinucleated giant cells, and scattered inflammatory cells (×250).

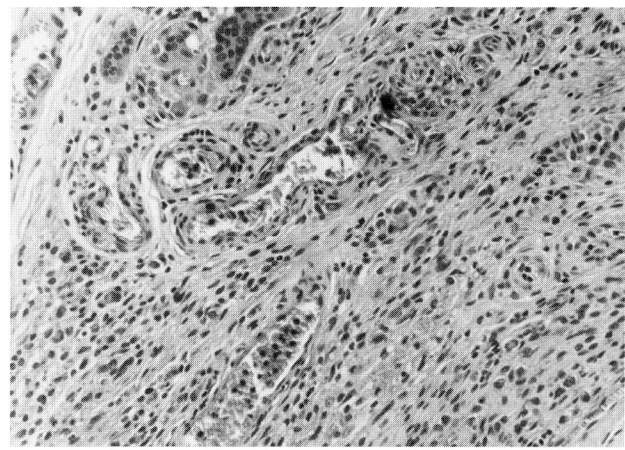

Fig. 13. Pigmented villonodular synovitis. This is a diffuse type of tenosynovial giant cell tumor. Mixed round and spindle cells with pseudoglandular spaces are demonstrated (×250).

saignac as "cancer of tendon sheath."[25] Lesions typically appear in the synovial lining of tendons or joints.

TENOSYNOVIAL GIANT CELL TUMOR: LOCALIZED TYPE (NODULAR TENOSYNOVITIS, LOCALIZED VILLONODULAR TENOSYNOVITIS)

Incidence Rate. These tumors are relatively rare.

Sex. There is a predilection for females.

Age. Adults from the ages of 30 to 50 years are most commonly affected. However, it is possible to see giant cell tumors in any age group.

Localization. These lesions are found in the tendinous sheaths and peritendinous tissue. Tumors are observed most frequently in the hands and are the most common type of neoplasm here.[26] Less frequent locations include feet, ankles, and knees.

Gross Pathology. Well-circumscribed lesions are lobular. They are typically small, less than 4 cm in diameter. The cut surface may have areas of white, yellow, gray, and brown, depending on the presence of fat and hemosiderin. In early stages, the tumor is soft and elastic and does not adhere to surrounding tissue, tendon, or bone. In later stages of fibrous scarring, tumors are hard and adhere to surrounding tissues.

Histological Findings. A dense, collagenous capsule is present. Fibrous scarring maturation is typically seen by the time of excision. Tumors are composed of multinucleated giant cells, mononuclear cells, and xanthoma cells in varying numbers. Histiofibroblastic hyperplasia is noted. Small, cystic spaces may be present. Shallow grooves created by the underlying tendon may be seen in the lesion.[27] No villi are evident. Decreased amounts of hemosiderin are present, compared with the diffuse type of giant cell tumor (Fig. 12).

TENOSYNOVIAL GIANT CELL TUMOR: DIFFUSE TYPE (PIGMENTED VILLONODULAR SYNOVITIS, PROLIFERATIVE SYNOVITIS)

Incidence Rate. The diffuse type of giant cell tumor is relatively uncommon.

Sex. There is a slight predilection for females.

Age. Tumors may occur anywhere from the ages of 10 to 75 years. However, 20 to 40 years is the most frequent age of presentation.[28]

Localization. Unlike the localized form, the diffuse form is found most commonly in the knee and foot. Less frequently, it is seen in the wrist and fingers.

Gross Pathology. The tumors commonly present as multiple, soft, spongy lesions. They are brown, yellow, or rustlike, depending on amounts of hemosiderin present. There does not appear to be a clearly defined collagenous capsule to this diffuse type of giant cell tumor. Commonly, the lesion is secondary, arising from a primary intra-articular tumor.

Histological Findings. Varying amounts of hemosiderin are seen within histiocytes. Villous hyperplasia of synovial membrane and capillary hyperplasia are well demonstrated. Sheets of polymorphic, rounded cells grow in an expansile manner into surrounding tissue. Cystic clefts are typically seen. Cells resemble those of the localized form of the tumor: chronic inflammatory cells and multinucleated giant cells. However, there are decreased numbers of giant cells in the diffuse type. Collagen is present in varying proportions throughout the stroma, and the tumor may at times appear hyalinized (Fig. 13).

CARTILAGINOUS SOFT-TISSUE TUMORS

Chondromas are benign soft-tissue tumors of mature, hyalinized cartilaginous nodules. The lesions are slow-growing, painless, and present during the middle decades of a patient's life. Tumors are not detected radiographically, unless calcification of cartilaginous nodules is present. Computed tomography scan and magnetic resonance imaging are the optimal choices in visualizing the exact location and extent of the tumor.[29]

CHONDROMA OF SOFT PARTS (EXTRASKELETAL CHONDROMA, SYNOVIAL CHONDROMATOSIS)

Incidence Rate. Extraskeletal chondromas are relatively rare.

Sex. Tumors are more frequently seen in males.

Age. Chondromas present from the ages of 30 to 60 years.

Localization. Lesions grow within the synovial membrane, tendinous sheath, or bursae, unlike periosteal chondromas.[30] Common locations in the distal extremities include fingers, hands, toes, and feet.

Gross Pathology. Lesions are round, smooth, and easily dissectable through a surrounding plane of areolar tissue. The appearance of the lesion is white, shiny, and smooth, resembling mature cartilage. Nodules are rarely larger than 3 cm in diameter and are typically attached to tendons or tendon sheaths.

Histological Findings. The tissue is composed of mature hyaline cartilage arranged in well-defined lobules. Cells are large and arranged in bundles. The pleomorphism of large nuclei may lead to the incorrect diagnosis of chondrosarcoma. Ossification, fibrosis, myxoid change, or hemorrhage may be present within the lesion. Calcification is often associated with focal cellular necrosis (Fig. 14).

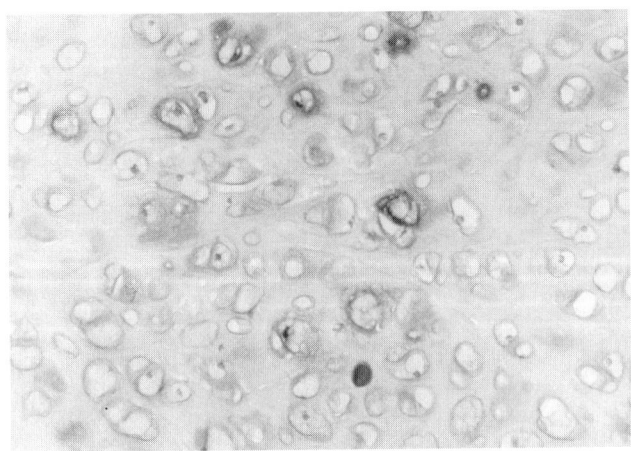

Fig. 14. Chondroma. This chondroma of soft parts consists of mature hyaline cartilage (×250).

REFERENCES

1. Konwaler BE, Keasbey L, Kaplan L: Subcutaneous pseudosarcomatous fibromatosis (fasciitis): Report of 8 cases. Am J Clin Pathol 25; 241:1955.
2. Jarvi OH, Saxen E: Elastofibroma dorsi. Acta Pathol Microbiol Scand 51; 83:1961.
3. El-Jabbour JN, Bennet MH, Burke MM, et al: Proliferative myositis: An immunohistochemical and ultrastructural study. Am J Surg Pathol 15; 654:1991.
4. Reitamo JJ, Hayry P, Nykuri E, et al: The desmoid tumor: Incidence, sex, age and anatomical distribution in the Finnish population. Am J Clin Pathol 77; 665:1982.
5. Brodsky JT, Gordon MS, Hajdu SI, et al: Desmoid tumors of the chest wall: A locally recurrent problem. J Thorac Cardiovasc Surg 104; 900:1992.
6. Enzinger F, Weiss S: Soft Tissue Tumors. St. Louis, Mosby-Year Book, 1995, p 201.
7. Baer JW, Radkowski MA: Congenital multiple fibromatosis: Case report with review of the world literature. Am J Roentgenol 118; 200:1973.
8. Bracko M, Cindro L, Golouh R: Familial occurrence of infantile myofibromatosis. Cancer 69; 1294:1992.
9. Franquemont DW, Cooper PH, Shmookler BM, et al: Benign fibrous histiocytoma of the skin with potential for local recurrence: A tumor to be distinguished from dermatofibroma. Mod Pathol 3; 58:1990.
10. Fredrickson DS, Lees RS: A system for phenotyping hyperlipoproteinemia. Circulation 31; 321:1965.
11. Carstens PHB, Schrodt GR: Ultrastructure of sclerosing hemangioma. Am J Pathol 77; 377:1974.
12. Enjoji M, Tsuneyoshi M, Hashimoto H: Subcutaneous angiolipoma: A clinicopathologic observation. Fukuoka Acta Medica 67; 82:1976.
13. Solvonuk PF, Taylor GP, Hancock R, et al: Correlation of morphologic and biochemical observations in human lipomas. Lab Invest 51; 469:1984.
14. Sandberg AA, Turc-Carel C: The cytogenetics of solid tumor: Relation to diagnosis, classification and pathology. Cancer 59; 387:1987.
15. Herrin K, Willen H, Rydholm A: Deep-seated soft tissue leiomyomas: A report of four cases. Skeletal Radiol 19; 363:1990.
16. Enzinger F, Weiss S: Soft Tissue Tumors. St. Louis, Mosby-Year Book, 1995, p 470.
17. Enneking W: Musculoskeletal Tumor Surgery. New York, Churchill Livingstone, 1983, p 1175.
18. Watson WL, McCarthy WD: Blood and lymph vessel tumors. Surg Gynecol Obstet 71; 569:1940.
19. Flanagan BP, Helwig EB: Cutaneous lymphangioma. Arch Dermatol 113; 24:1977.
20. Masson P: Le glomus neuromyoarterieal des regions tactiles et ses tumeurs. Lyon Chir 21; 257:1924.
21. Shugart RR, Soule EH, Johnson EW: Glomus tumor. Surg Gynecol Obstet 117; 334:1963.
22. Weiss SW, Langloss JM, Enzinger FM: The role of the S-100 protein in the diagnosis of soft tissue tumors with particular reference to benign and malignant Schwann cell tumors. Lab Invest 49; 299:1983.
23. Lowman RM, LiVolsi VA: Pigmented (melanotic) schwannomas of the spinal canal. Cancer 46; 391:1980.
24. Hashimoto H, Tsuneyoshi M, Daimaru Y, et al: Intramuscular myxoma: A clinicopathologic, immunohistochemical, and electron microscopic study. Cancer 58; 740:1986.
25. Chassaignac CME: Cancer de la gaine des tendons. Gaz Hosp Civ Milit 47; 185:1852.
26. Jones FE, Soule EH, Coventry MB: Fibrous histiocytoma of synovium (giant cell tumor of tendon sheath, pigmented nodular synovitis). J Bone Joint Surg Am 51; 76:1969.
27. Wright CJE: Benign giant cell synovioma. Br J Surg 38; 257:1951.
28. Campanacci M: Bone and Soft Tissue Tumors. New York, Springer-Verlag, 1990, p 1102.
29. Wong L, Dellon AL: Soft tissue chondroma presenting as a painful finger: Diagnosis by magnetic resonance imaging. Ann Plast Surg 28; 304:1992.
30. DelSignore JL, Torre BA, Miller RJ: Extraskeletal chondroma of the hand: Case report and review of the literature. Clin Orthop 254; 147:1990.

MALIGNANT SOFT-TISSUE TUMORS

H. Thomas Temple

Summary
- Soft-tissue tumors are rare and diverse.
- Radiographs and magnetic resonance imaging (MRI) are the most widely used studies for evaluating and characterizing soft-tissue tumors.
- Either needle or open biopsy may be the optimal choice to obtain tissue samples.
- Biopsies should be performed by the surgeon who will perform the definitive procedure.
- Tumor grade and size are the most important factors in predicting patient survival.

Soft-tissue sarcomas are a rare[1] and diverse group of neoplasms that vary clinically, radiographically, and microscopically.

History and physical examination, appropriate imaging studies, and staging are necessary in the initial management of patients with malignant soft-tissue tumors. After this, prompt referral to centers with individuals experienced in sarcoma treatment is necessary when the biopsy and definitive care are performed.

Because soft-tissue sarcomas are rare and heterogeneous, the diagnosis is often missed or delayed, and many patients undergo inappropriate biopsy and unplanned resection before referral.[2, 3] Poorly placed incisions may contaminate normal adjacent tissues, including nerves, vessels, and joints, so that limb salvage and survival can be compromised.[4]

HISTORY AND PHYSICAL EXAMINATION

Soft-tissue sarcomas occur in patients of all ages, and males are more often affected than females.[1] The peak incidence of sarcoma is between the third and eighth decades of life and, in general, increases with advancing age.[5]

The chief complaint is usually an expanding, often painless mass. Although malignant tumors generally grow more rapidly than benign lesions, occasionally benign tumors such as lipomas, traumatized hemangiomas, and even posttraumatic pseudotumors can grow very rapidly. Conversely, some sarcomas, such as synovial sarcoma, can grow insidiously over many months and even years.[6]

In those patients complaining of pain, symptoms are frequently worse at night. These symptoms are inconsistently relieved by aspirin or nonsteroidal anti-inflammatory medicines. Occasionally, the chief complaint is radiating pain, exacerbated by certain positions or activities, and suggests tumor impingement or encasement of nerves. Vascular claudication is rare, even in patients with neglected tumors surrounding the vessels.

Certain soft-tissue tumors tend to occur in specific anatomic sites. Epithelioid sarcoma, for example, is common in the hand and upper extremity, whereas synovial sarcoma is the most common deep-seated malignancy of the foot.[6]

Some patients with malignant tumors of soft parts complain of fevers, sweats, and chills that mimic infection. This, unfortunately, may result in the administration of antibiotics for a presumed abscess and, in some cases, incision and drainage. The erroneous clinical diagnosis of infection may be reinforced when a biopsy sample of a tumor composed of small, round, blue-staining cells is misinterpreted as acute or chronic infection on needle biopsy specimens. One of the principles of tumor surgery is to perform a biopsy in every infection and to culture every tumor. This simple maxim can avoid terrible mistakes in diagnosis.

Weight loss and anorexia, a nonproductive cough, and diffuse skeletal pain can be symptoms of disseminated disease.

A medical history of previous malignancy, radiation therapy, or administration of alkylating agents is important. For example, soft-tissue sarcomas are not uncommon[7] in patients surviving retinoblastoma, and secondary sarcomas are reported in postirradiated tissues.[8, 9]

On physical examination, tumor size and its relationship to adjacent structures (i.e., superficial to the fascia and mobile or deep and fixed to underlying muscle, periosteum, or bone) or to vascular structures and nerves should be noted. A thrill or bruit may be detected in patients with highly vascular tumors. Dysesthesias on percussion can be elicited in patients with tumors arising within or around nerves. Neurological deficits are uncommon in patients with appendicular tumors but are occasionally seen in patients with pelvic sarcomas.

Skin changes may be observed in patients with vascular tumors and in patients with neglected tumors that fungate. Café au lait spots are associated with neurofibromatosis, and neurofibrosarcoma occurs in 5% of patients with neurofibromatosis.[10–12] Dermatofibrosarcoma protuberans is a superficial dermis-based lesion that frequently ulcerates the skin. It is important to determine whether the mass involves overlying dermis, because wide margins of skin must then be excised along with the mass, necessitating muscle flaps and split-thickness skin grafts for wound closure.

Although nodal metastases are uncommon, the regional lymph nodes should be palpated in all patients with soft-tissue masses.[13] Certain tumors like epithelioid sarcoma have a higher rate of lymphatic spread, especially in the upper extremity, and some surgeons routinely sample lymph nodes in these patients at resection.[14] However, because nodal spread is infrequent, routine node sampling is not recommended for most soft-tissue sarcomas.[13]

LABORATORY DATA

Laboratory data are rarely helpful in establishing a diagnosis but are important in excluding other causes of a mass such as infection. In extraordinary cases, soft-tissue sarcomas produce parathyroid hormone analogues with serum and urine abnormalities of calcium and phosphorus. Patients with diffuse metastatic disease may be anemic and exhibit a mild leukocytosis.

IMAGING

Biplanar radiographs should be obtained before any other imaging study in all patients who present with a soft-tissue mass. Plain radiographs demonstrate internal tumor matrix, bone invasion, periosteal reaction, and, on close inspection, intralesional fat.

Technetium-labeled bone scans are most useful for detecting osseous metastases and for determining whether adjacent bone is secondarily involved, but they are not routinely used in evaluating soft-tissue masses. Soft-tissue sarcomas often have scintigraphic uptake, but there is no correlation between blood flow, histological type or grade, and intensity of uptake on routine bone scan.[15]

Computed tomography (CT) is the study of choice in evaluating pulmonary metastases, because the lungs are the most common metastatic site of soft-tissue sarcomas. This should be part of the initial evaluation in all patients with known or suspected malignancies of soft parts. If osseous involvement is suspected on the initial radiographic evaluation, CT is useful for delineating the extent of cortical destruction.

After radiographs, MRI is the most widely used study for evaluating and characterizing soft-tissue tumors. The MRI should always include images with IV contrast (gadolinium). Although sonography is also beneficial for delineating tumor size and character (cystic or solid), it is not as effective as MRI for surgical planning. Heterogeneity is common in many sarcomas and is caused by differences in cellularity within the tumor, areas of necrosis, and varying degrees of collagenous matrix, mineralization, and hemosiderin deposition. This feature is well demonstrated on MRI and can thus serve as a guide for needle placement at biopsy to avoid areas of hemorrhage and necrosis and lead to viable tissue for diagnosis.

Gadolinium-enhanced MRI is useful in the initial evaluation of soft-tissue tumors and demonstrates overall tumor vascularity; it is also useful in differentiating tumor recurrence from postoperative tissue changes such as edema, fluid collections, and inflammation. T_1-weighted images with and without contrast are compared to determine vascularity.

For surgical planning, MRI is critical for assessing the exact location of the tumor, its size and depth, and its relationship to adjacent bones, joints, and neurovascular structures. Usually, when a tumor effaces a neurovascular bundle, a subtle fat plane separates the tumor from nerve or vessel, an important observation in anticipation of tumor resection (Fig. 1).

Soft-tissue sarcomas arising within joints are rare, as is intra-articular tumor extension.[16] Tumors arising adjacent to

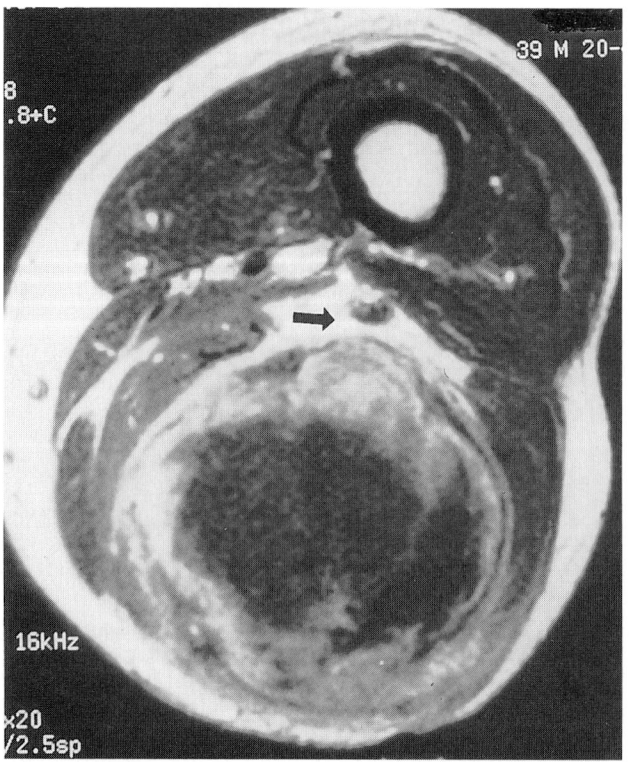

Fig. 1. Neurofibrosarcoma. Note the fat plane between the tumor mass and the sciatic nerve *(arrow)* in this 39-year-old man with a large neurofibrosarcoma of the posterior thigh.

joints often appear to extend into the joint directly. They are, however, usually covered by a synovial reflection that is demonstrated on MRI on close inspection. Synovial tissue is an effective barrier to tumor spread; thus, tumors contained by synovial tissue can be resected, preserving the joint without compromising tumor-free margins. An exception to this is a lesion that arises in the popliteal fossa that closely adheres to or involves bone and capsule. These tumors can extend along the cruciate ligaments, and extra-articular resection is necessary to achieve tumor-free margins. In the rare instance when the joint is violated by tumor, joint resection and reconstruction are necessary. These procedures are technically more difficult. Diminished postoperative function follows, especially if the extensor mechanism is compromised.

ANATOMIC COMPARTMENTS

Sarcomas grow centripetally along the path of least resistance. Fascia, periosteum, and articular cartilage are generally effective barriers to tumor growth in contrast to muscle and fat, which are poor obstacles to tumor infiltration. For this reason, sarcomas tend to infiltrate muscle and fat but are generally confined to single compartments or muscle groups by investing fascia. Sarcomas are surrounded by a pseudocapsule, a rind of reactive tissue. Tumor cells penetrate this pseudocapsule, and the presence of microscopic disease beyond the tumor mass demands wide excisions or resection of entire compartments to achieve tumor-free margins.

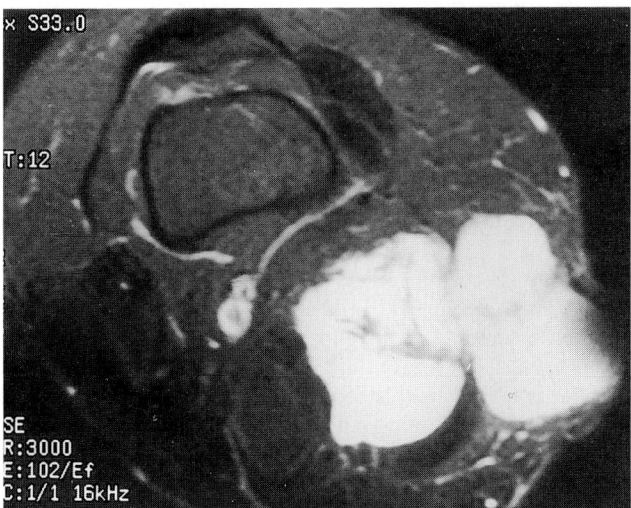

Fig. 2. Myxoid liposarcoma. This large myxoid liposarcoma arises in the posterior muscles of the thigh but extends between muscle groups and involves more than one compartment.

Disease-free margins are more difficult to obtain when tumors exceed well-delineated boundaries and thus become extracompartmental. Some subcutaneous tumors, for example, tend to infiltrate extensively into fat and overlying dermis and along fascial planes, making wide excision difficult and sometimes impossible. Sarcomas arising between muscle groups may involve more than one compartment, requiring extensive resection and often uncertain tumor margins (Fig. 2). The distinction between intracompartmental and extracompartmental tumors then is important for the radiologist, pathologist, and especially the surgeon for the purpose of biopsy, pathological interpretation, and resection, respectively.

BIOPSY

At biopsy, only one compartment should be violated, because sarcomas are easily implanted in normal adjacent tissue. Contamination of more than one compartment requires extended surgical excision with increased risk of local disease recurrence, larger radiation fields, and diminished postoperative function. In the appendicular skeleton, open biopsies should be longitudinal with minimal exposure of normal adjacent tissue (Fig. 3). Hemostasis must be obtained before wound closure, and drains should be used liberally and brought out in line with the biopsy track. Needle biopsies are more prevalent in diagnosing soft-tissue sarcomas, and practical knowledge of compartments and limb salvage principles is essential to avoid inappropriate needle placement. Biopsy is generally guided by CT, and needle placement should be directly over the tumor in line with the anticipated surgical incision and through only one compartment.

The needle should be inserted into areas of viable tumor only, and multiple passes through the same skin puncture should be obtained. Because of tumor heterogeneity, limited or misdirected core specimens may underestimate tumor grade and, hence, metastatic potential. Treatment options vary according to grade and tumor extent, and errors

in biopsy will, therefore, result in inappropriate management of these patients.

Needle biopsy is a relatively inexpensive procedure with a low risk of hemorrhage and infection.[17] The diagnostic accuracy of fine-needle aspiration varies between 64% and 96%.[18, 19] The fundamental problem with fine-needle biopsy and even core-needle biopsy is one's confidence in the diagnostic interpretation and accuracy, given the small amount of tissue available to analyze. Histological heterogeneity and areas of necrosis and hemorrhage within the tumor conspire to make pathological interpretation difficult. Finally, a number of studies highlight the diagnostic challenge of differentiating benign from malignant soft-tissue tumors; intraobserver variability ranges from 16% to 39%.[20–23]

The advantage of open biopsy is that adequate tissue is usually obtained for all diagnostic procedures as well as research activities. At surgery frozen sections are obtained to prove that adequate tissue has been procured. An experienced pathologist can usually make a definitive diagnosis so that the surgical resection can be performed immediately for some tumors, thus avoiding a second operation. The disadvantages are that, although sufficient tissue is obtained for diagnosis, further processing and special staining are needed for final pathological interpretation. Thus, the cost

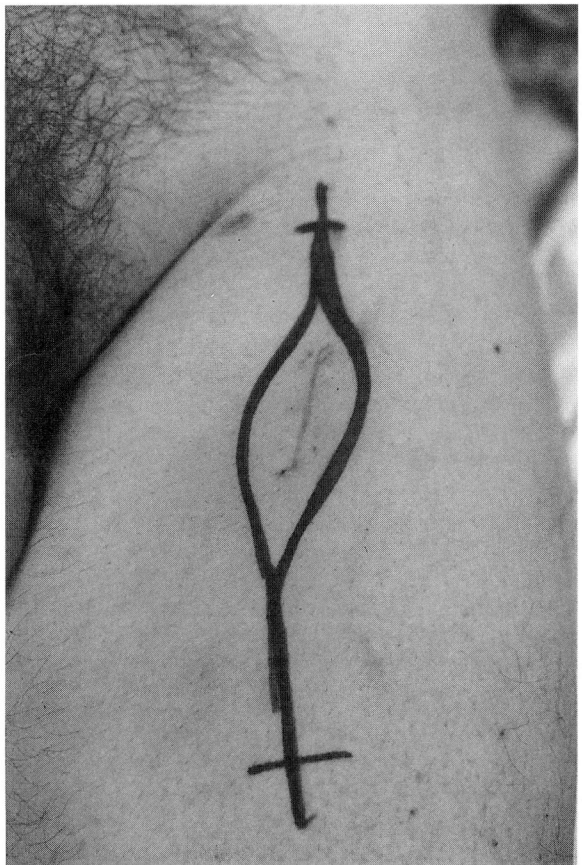

Fig. 3. Malignant fibrous histiocytoma. This patient had a malignant fibrous histiocytoma of the thigh and underwent open biopsy. The incision and the drain site must be ellipsed with the underlying tumor. Biopsies should be performed through longitudinal incisions in the appendicular skeleton.

of open biopsy is significantly higher than needle biopsy alone, and the risks of hematoma, contamination of adjacent tissues, and wound infection are greater.[24]

The hazards of biopsies are well known.[4, 24] In one series, 17.8% of musculoskeletal tumors were misdiagnosed and the overall outcome was altered in 16.6% of patients.[4] Unnecessary amputations were performed in 3% of patients as a result of poorly performed biopsies.[4] From 1982 to 1996, the incidence of biopsy-related problems has remained unchanged.[4, 24] Biopsy-related complications, however, were 2 to 12 times greater in community hospitals than in referral hospitals. Thus, the biopsy should be performed by the surgeon who will perform the definitive procedure in an institution familiar with the care of patients with soft-tissue sarcomas.[4]

STAGING

Staging includes a careful history and physical examination, appropriate imaging studies, and biopsy. In defining tumor type and disease extent, staging helps to guide treatment and predict survival. Tumor staging classifications stratify patients into groups based on prognostic factors such as tumor size, grade, depth, and distant spread. The Musculoskeletal Tumor Society classification[25] is a surgical classification based on histological grade, location, intra- or extracompartmental location, and the presence or absence of metastasis (Table 1). Hadju[26] proposed a classification that considers tumor size (greater or less than 5 cm), grade (high or low), and depth (prefascial or subfascial). The TMN classification relies on tumor size, grade (low, intermediate, and high), presence or absence of distant metastases, and presence or absence of nodal disease.[27] Grade and size are the most important factors in predicting survival in patients with soft-tissue sarcomas, because large high-grade tumors present the greatest risk for metastases.[28–30]

ADJUNCT THERAPY

Surgical excision with negative tumor margins combined with radiotherapy is highly effective in controlling local disease.[31–35] Tumor cells often penetrate beyond the tumor mass and its investing pseudocapsule, so-called satellite lesions. Radiation therapy effectively extends the margins obtained with surgery by eliminating microscopic disease at the tumor periphery.

TABLE 1. HISTOLOGY		
Anatomic Extent	**Low-Grade Histology**	**High-Grade Histology**
Limited to compartment of origin	IA	IIA
Extension beyond compartment of origin	IB	IIB
Distant metastasis	III	III

Metastases, either lymphatic or hematogenous, regardless of histological grade or limitation to the anatomic compartment of origin, are stage III.

I = low grade; II = high grade; A = within the anatomic compartment in which the tumor originated; B = extension beyond the anatomic compartment in which the tumor originated.

Radiotherapy can be used preoperatively, postoperatively, or both. The advantages of preoperative radiation are the use of less radiation over a potentially smaller field,[36–38] the greater tumoricidal effects in better oxygenated (nonoperated) tissue, tumor volume reduction before resection, and a lower risk of transplanting tumor cells at resection. Preoperatively, patients receive approximately 50 Gy of radiation followed by tumor resection 2 to 3 weeks later when the erythema and tissue induration resolve. For close margins, a postoperative boost using either brachytherapy or external beam radiation over a smaller field can be administered. The advantages of preoperative radiation are mitigated, in part, by significant wound morbidity.[39]

Patients are often referred to sarcoma centers because of unplanned surgical intervention.[2] These patients are particularly difficult to treat because of inadequate staging (frequently no imaging studies are performed before resection), surgical violation of tissue planes, and presence of residual tumor, either gross or microscopic. In a group of 65 patients referred to an oncology unit after unplanned resection, sarcoma was identified histologically in only 35% of patients after tumor bed excision.[2] Not surprisingly, 22% of patients had a local recurrence, a rate much higher than that observed for patients initially treated at this center.[2] Because residual tumor is often present in tumor beds in patients with unplanned excisions, it is best managed by tumor bed excision and radiation.

The use of chemotherapy in nonmetastatic soft-tissue sarcomas is controversial. Chemotherapy is reserved for patients with large (greater than 5 cm) high-grade tumors because they are at greatest risk for having a metastasis. Chemotherapeutic trials initially compared single-agent doxorubicin with no treatment[40–42] and, later, combined therapy with no treatment.[43, 44] A meta-analysis[45] of 13 randomized trials of adjuvant chemotherapy versus no chemotherapy for patients with soft-tissue sarcoma demonstrated an overall survival benefit, because fewer local recurrences and distant metastases were observed in chemotherapy-treated patients. Furthermore, there was a trend favoring combined therapy over single-agent therapy. The literature is difficult to interpret because these studies include a variety of high-grade soft-tissue sarcomas that are histologically, biologically, and clinically diverse. In addition, study protocols use different inclusion criteria and diverse drug regimens, and they report end results differently.

Patients presenting with metastatic disease should have preoperative chemotherapy, if their medical condition permits; standard local disease control with radiation and surgery; and pulmonary resection of lung metastases. The 5-year survival in patients with advanced sarcoma with resectable lung metastases ranges from 31% to 40%.[46–48] Patients with unresectable pulmonary metastases or extrapulmonary disease have a dismal prognosis and are best treated with systemic chemotherapy alone.[49]

SURGICAL EXCISION

The goal of surgery is to achieve tumor-free margins and to preserve the limb when possible but not at the expense of achieving tumor-free margins or optimal function. Optimal function does not always follow limb salvage surgery, and sometimes a patient is better served by an amputation. Although amputations for soft-tissue sarcoma are uncommon,[50, 51] relative contraindications to limb salvage include diffuse pulmonary or extrapulmonary metastases at presentation, neurovascular involvement, particularly nerve bundles, associated osseous involvement with pathological fracture or joint extension, and large tumors in distal sites, particularly the foot, where resection results in an insensate and functionally useless extremity.

Exposures are extensile, with large skin flaps preserving major vessels and nerves and as much normal muscle as possible. Because sarcomas are highly implantable, the biopsy track, even core-needle tracks, should be excised with the underlying tumor. Large soft-tissue defects are covered with either rotational or free flaps and split-thickness skin grafts. Meticulous hemostasis is critical, and large closed suction drains are used postoperatively to avoid hematoma and seroma formation, which may compromise flap viability. To optimize postoperative surveillance for tumor recurrence, the use of vascular clips is limited to delineating the margins of the tumor bed for the purpose of planning postoperative radiotherapy. Wound dehiscence is more commonly seen early postoperatively but may occur 3 to 4 weeks after surgery, especially in patients who received preoperative irradiation. Aggressive wound débridement and antibiotic administration are necessary for wound dehiscence and deep infection.

FOLLOW-UP OF SOFT-TISSUE SARCOMAS

Clinical examination augmented with MRI, particularly gadolinium-enhanced MRI, is used to monitor patients postoperatively for tumor recurrence. Postoperative surveillance is performed every 4 months for 2 years. Because the lungs are the most common site of metastatic disease spread, CT scans and posteroanterior and lateral chest radiographs are alternated every 4 months. Repeat bone scans are obtained if patients complain of bone pain to exclude osseous metastases. During the second through fifth postoperative years, MRIs are obtained every 6 months along with alternating chest radiographs and CT scans. After the fifth postoperative year, the patient is monitored annually by clinical examination and chest radiographs.

Postoperative imaging is difficult because of distorted anatomy after resection and the use of rotational or free flaps for soft-tissue coverage, which, to the unsuspecting observer, can be confused with recurrent tumor. Metal clip artifacts along vessels distort MRIs. The use of allografts fixed with plates or metal prostheses in patients requiring bone resection and skeletal reconstruction cause such distortion that MRI for local recurrence is uninterpretable. When metal artifact obscures MRI and clinically local recurrence is a concern, ultrasound-directed biopsy is indicated.

SUMMARY

Soft-tissue sarcomas present diagnostic and therapeutic challenges. For this reason, tumor staging and biopsy are best performed in the treating institution by individuals experienced in sarcoma management. Errors in biopsy are frequent and can compromise both life and limb.

Surgery remains the mainstay of local disease control and, when augmented by radiotherapy, results in few local tumor recurrences. The role of chemotherapy is evolving in patients with large high-grade sarcomas, although this is still controversial. Finally, long-term surveillance is necessary to monitor local and distant tumor relapse.

REFERENCES

1. Parker SL, Tong T, Bolden S, et al: Cancer statistics 1997. CA Cancer J Clin 1997; 46:9.
2. Noria S, Davis A, Kandel R, et al: Residual disease following unplanned excision of a soft tissue sarcoma of an extremity. J Bone Joint Surg Am 1996; 78:650.
3. Giuliano AE, Eilber FR: The rationale for planned reoperation after unplanned total excision of soft tissue sarcomas. J Clin Oncol 1985; 3:1344.
4. Mankin HJ, Mankin CJ, Simon MA: The hazards of biopsy revisited. J Bone Joint Surg Am 1996; 78:656.
5. Enzinger FM, Weiss SW: General considerations. In Soft Tissue Tumors, 3rd ed. St. Louis, Mosby–Year Book, 1995, p 1.
6. Scully SP, Temple HT, Harrelson JM: Synovial sarcoma of the foot and ankle. Presented at the meeting of the American Orthopaedic Foot and Ankle Society meeting, Boston, 1998.
7. Mall AC, Imhof SM, Bouter LM, et al: Secondary primary tumors in patients with retinoblastoma: A review of the literature. Ophthal Genet 1997; 18:27.
8. Cahan WG, Woodward HQ, Higinbothan

NL, et al: Sarcoma arising in irradiated bone: Report of eleven cases. Cancer 1948; 1:3.
9. Huvos AG, Woodward HQ, Cahan WG, et al: Postradiation osteogenic sarcoma of bone and soft tissue: A clinicopathologic study of 66 patients. Cancer 1985; 55: 1244.
10. Hope DG, Mulville JJ: Malignancy in neurofibromatosis. Adv Neurol 1981; 29: 33.
11. Knight WA III, Murphy WK, Gottleib JA: Neurofibromatosis associated with malignant neurofibromas. Arch Dermatol 1973; 107:747.
12. D'Agostino AN, Soule EH, Miller RH: Sarcomas of the peripheral nerves and somatic soft tissues associated with multiple neurofibromatosis (von Recklinghausen's disease). Cancer 1963; 16:1015.
13. Weingrad DN, Rosenberg SA: Early lymphatic spread of osteogenic and soft-tissue sarcomas. Surgery 1978; 84:231.
14. Steinberg BD, Gelberman RH, Mankin HJ, et al: Epithelioid sarcoma in the upper extremity. J Bone Joint Surg 1992; 74:28.

15. Sinnett HD, Rowell NP, McCready VR, et al: Demonstration of blood flow patterns in human soft tissue sarcomas using 99m Tc-labeled hexamethyl propyleneamineoxime. Br J Surg 1990; 77:454.
16. Enzinger FM, Weiss S: Synovial Sarcoma in Soft Tissue Tumors. St. Louis, Mosby–Year Book, 1988, 2nd ed, p 661.
17. Skrzynski MC, Biermann JS, Montag A, et al: Diagnostic accuracy and charge-savings of outpatient core needle biopsy compared with open biopsy of musculoskeletal tumors. J Bone Joint Surg Am 1996; 78: 644.
18. Akerman M, Rydholm A, Persson BM: Aspiration cytology of soft tissue tumors: The 10 year experience at an orthopedic oncology center. Acta Orthop Scand 1985; 56:407.
19. Barth AB, Merino MJ, Solomon D, et al: A prospective study on the value of core needle biopsy and fine needle aspiration in the diagnosis of soft tissue masses. Surgery 1992; 112:536.
20. Presant CA, Russell WO, Alexander RW, et al: Soft tissue and bone sarcoma histopathology peer review: The frequency of

disagreement in diagnosis and the need for second pathology opinions. The South Eastern Cancer Study Group experience. J Clin Oncol 1986; 4:1658.

21. Skiraki M, Enterline HT, Brooks JJ, et al: Pathologic analysis of advanced adult soft tissue sarcomas, bone sarcomas and mesotheliomas. The Eastern Cooperative Oncology Group experience. Cancer 1989; 64:484.

22. Alvegard TA, Berg NO: Histopathology peer review of high-grade soft tissue sarcoma: The Scandinavian Sarcoma Group experience. J Clin Oncol 1989; 7:1845.

23. Harris M, Hartley AL, Blair V, et al: Sarcomas in North West England: Histopathology peer review. Br J Cancer 1991; 64:315.

24. Mankin HJ, Lange TA, Spanier SS: The hazards of biopsy in patients with malignant primary bone and soft tissue tumors. J Bone Joint Surg Am 1982; 64:1121.

25. Enneking WF, Spanier SS, Goodman MA: A system for the surgical staging of musculoskeletal sarcoma. Clin Orthop 1980; 153:106.

26. Hadju SI: History and classification of soft tissue tumors. In Pathology of Soft Tissue Tumors. Philadelphia, Lea & Febiger, 1979, p 5.

27. American Joint Committee for Cancer Staging and End-Result Reporting: Manual for Staging of Cancer. Lippincott, Chicago, 1988.

28. Coindre JM, Terrier O, Bui NB, et al: Prognostic factors in adult patients with locally controlled soft tissue sarcoma. A study of 546 patients from the French Federation of Cancer Centers Sarcoma Group. J Clin Oncol 1996; 14:869.

29. Pisters PW, Leung DH, Woodruff J, et al: Analysis of prognostic factors in 1,041 patients with localized soft tissue sarcomas of the extremities. J Clin Oncol 1996; 14:1679.

30. Nakanishi H, Tomita Y, Ohsawa M, et al: Tumor size as a prognostic indicator of histologic grade of soft tissue sarcoma. J Surg Oncol 1997; 65:183.

31. Wilson AN, Davis A, Bell RS, et al: Local control of soft tissue sarcomas of the extremity: The experience of a multidisciplinary sarcoma group with definitive surgery and radiotherapy. Eur J Cancer 1994; 30A:746.

32. Barkley HT, Marin RG, Romsdahl MM, et al: Treatment of soft tissue sarcomas by pre-operative irradiation and conservative surgical resection. Int J Radiat Oncol Biol Phys 1988; 14:693.

33. Abbatucci JS, Boulder N, DeRanier J, et al: Local control and survival in soft tissue sarcomas of the limbs, trunk walls and head and neck: A study of 113 cases. Int J Radiat Oncol Biol Phys 1986; 12:579.

34. Bell RS, O'Sullivan B, Liu FF, et al: The surgical margin in soft tissue sarcoma. J Bone Joint Surg Am 1989; 71:370.

35. Berlin O, Stener B, Angervall L, et al: Surgery for soft tissue sarcoma in the extremities. Acta Orthop Scand 1990; 61:475.

36. Nielsen OS, Cummings B, O'Sullivan B, et al: Preoperative and postoperative irradiation of soft tissue sarcomas: Effect of radiation field size. Int J Radiat Oncol Biol Phys 1991; 21:1595.

37. Suit HD, Mankin HJ, Wood WC, et al: Preoperative, intraoperative, and postoperative radiation in the treatment of primary soft tissue sarcoma. Cancer 1985; 55:2659.

38. Suit HD, Mankin HJ, Wood WC, et al: Treatment of the patient with stage M0 sarcoma of soft tissue. J Clin Oncol 1988; 6:854.

39. Bujko K, Suit HD, Springfield DS, et al: Wound healing after preoperative radiation for sarcoma of soft tissues. Surg Gynecol Obstet 1993; 176:124.

40. Antman K, Ryan L, Borden E, et al: Pooled results from three randomized adjuvant studies of doxorubicin versus observation in soft tissue sarcoma: 10 year results and review of literature. In Salmon SE (ed): Adjuvant Therapy of Cancer VI. Philadelphia, WB Saunders, 1990, p 529.

41. Wilson RE, Wood WC, Lerner HL, et al: Doxorubicin chemotherapy in the treatment of soft tissue sarcoma: Combined results of two randomized trials. Arch Surg 1986; 121:1354.

42. Gherlinzoni F, Bacci G, Picci P, et al: A randomized trial for the treatment of high grade soft tissue sarcomas of the extremities: Preliminary observations. J Clin Oncol 1986; 4:552.

43. Ravaud A, Bui NB, Coindre JM, et al: Adjuvant chemotherapy with CyVADIC in high risk soft tissue sarcoma: A randomized prospective trial. In Salmon SE (ed): Adjuvant Therapy of Cancer VI. Philadelphia, WB Saunders, 1990, p 556.

44. Bramell V, Rousse J, Steward W, et al: Adjuvant CYVADIC chemotherapy for adult soft tissue sarcoma—Reduced local recurrence but no improvement in survival: A study of the European Organization for Research and Treatment of Cancer Soft Tissue and Bone Sarcoma Group. J Clin Oncol 1994; 12:1137.

45. Jones GW, Chouinard E, Patel M: Adjuvant Adriamycin (doxorubicin) in adult patients with soft-tissue sarcomas: A systematic overview and quantitative meta-analysis. Clin Invest Med 1991; 14:A772.

46. Girard P, Spaggiari L, Baldeyrou P, et al: Should the number of pulmonary metastases influence the surgical decision? Eur J Cardiothorac Surg 1997; 12:385.

47. Van Geel AN, Pastorino U, Jauch KW, et al: Surgical treatment of lung metastases: The European Organization for Research and Treatment of Cancer, Soft Tissue, and Bone Sarcoma Group study of 255 patients. Cancer 1996; 77:675.

48. Choong PF, Pritchard DJ, Rock MG, et al: Survival after pulmonary metastasectomy in soft tissue sarcoma: Prognostic factors in 214 patients. Acta Orthop Scand 1995; 66:561.

49. Lewis JJ, Brennan MF: Soft tissue sarcomas. Curr Probl Surg 1996; 33:817.

50. Barr LC, Thomas JM: Major amputation for soft tissue sarcoma of the extremities. Eur J Cancer 1991; 27:S162.

51. Karakousis CP, Emrich LJ, Rao U, et al: Feasibility of limb salvage and survival in soft tissue sarcomas. Cancer 1986; 57:486.

MANAGEMENT AND SURGERY

Rodolfo Capanna and Domenico A. Campanacci

A soft-tissue mass is a quite common clinical finding in medical practice and it may be the expression of a nontumoral condition (e.g., myositis, hematoma) or of a benign or malignant soft tissue tumor. Usually, the evaluation of the history, the physical examination, and the imaging studies allow the distinction between tumoral and nontumoral conditions. When the distinction is not clear, and

especially when a soft-tissue tumor is suspected, a biopsy is mandatory.

The treatment of soft-tissue tumors is based on surgical removal, which should achieve different surgical margins according to the histological type (benign or malignant) and the extent of the tumor.

Radiation therapy is commonly employed as adjuvant

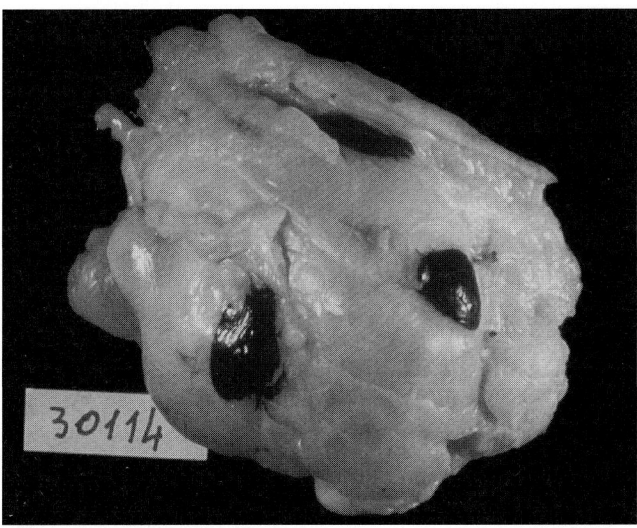

Fig. 1. The surgical specimen is marked with black ink by the surgeon in the areas at risk for contamination.

treatment in malignant soft tissue sarcomas to improve local control of the disease.

Several different chemotherapeutic protocols have been used, including intravenous preoperative and postoperative regimens for local and systemic control of high-grade sar-

comas. Isolated local hyperthermic perfusion of the limb is recommended for unresectable tumors of the extremities.

BIOPSY

The biopsy is the last step in the diagnostic procedure and the first step in the management of a soft-tissue tumor. It is a surgical procedure, and it must be carried out with care because an inappropriately done biopsy may jeopardize the possibility of performing conservative surgery later on. The biopsy may be excisional, incisional, core needle, or fine needle aspirate (FNA). Refer to Chapter 7-2 for a thorough discussion of biopsy.

SURGERY

MARGINS

After tumor excison, the areas of the surgical specimen considered at risk for contamination are marked with black ink by the surgeon (Fig. 1). This technique allows the pathologist a better histological evaluation of margins (Fig. 2). Surgical excision is the treatment of choice for soft-tissue tumors, and in the case of either conservative or ablative surgery, the resection margins are evaluated following the Musculoskeletal Tumor Society criteria, which classify the margins as radical, wide, marginal, or intralesional (Fig. 3).

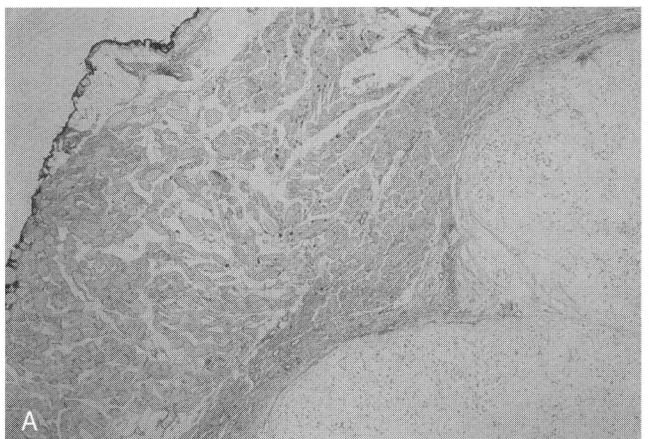

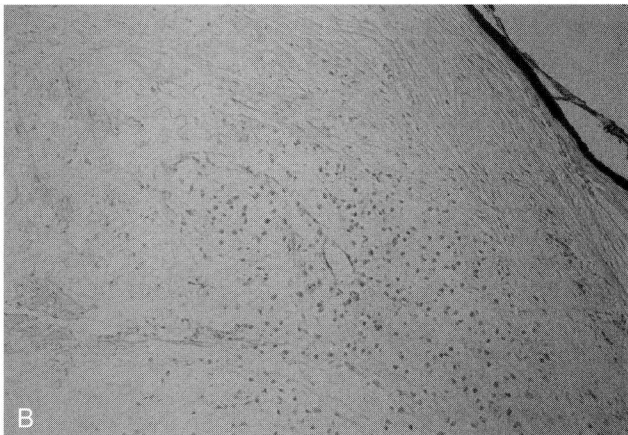

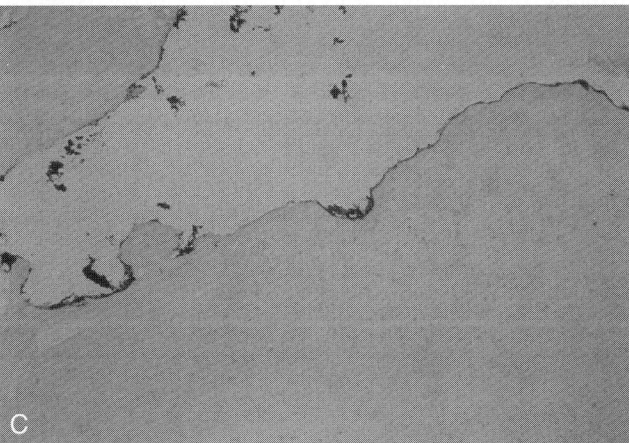

Fig. 2. Views. *A*, **Wide margin:** the tumor is covered by a cuff of healthy tissue. *B*, **Marginal margin:** the tumor is covered by the reactive pseudocapsule. *C*, **Intralesional margin:** the dissection plane passes through the tumoral tissue.

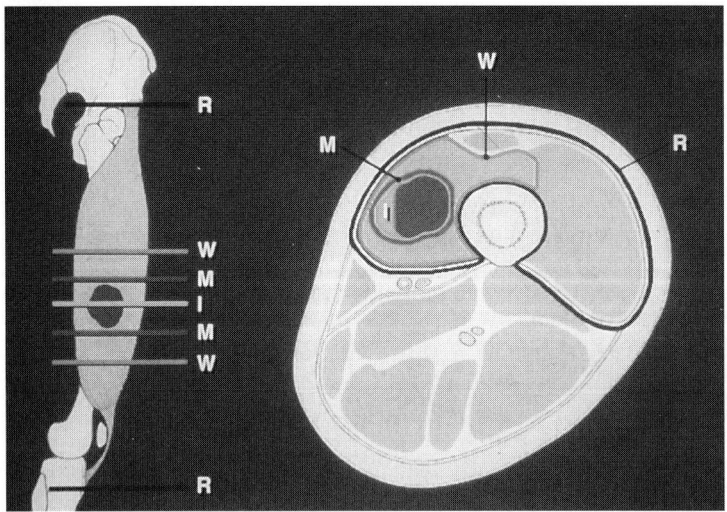

Fig. 3. Classification of surgical margins of Musculoskeletal Tumor Society. I, intralesional, **M,** marginal; **W,** wide; **R,** radical.

Intralesional

In an intralesional margin, the pseudocapsule of the tumor is violated by the surgeon and the dissection is carried out passing through the tumoral mass. This kind of margin is unacceptable in malignant soft-tissue tumors because it exposes the patient to a very high risk of local recurrence, reduced to 60% in the case of association with postoperative radiation therapy. An intralesional margin may be accepted in the case of benign tumors (lipoma) or locally aggressive lesions (desmoid tumor) when they extend around important anatomic structures such as vessels or nerves. In these benign conditions, conservative surgery with intralesional margins is justified and postoperative radiation therapy can be considered to decrease the risk of local recurrence of desmoid tumor.

Marginal

With a marginal excision, the tumor is excised following a dissection plane represented by the pseudocapsule of the tumor.

A marginal excision is an adequate treatment for most benign soft-tissue tumors, and local recurrence is infrequent if the tumors are excised completely. Some benign conditions, such as desmoid tumor and neurofibroma, have locally aggressive behavior, and they are not delimited by a real capsule. The neurofibroma should be carefully dissected from the nerve of origin with marginal margins using magnifying visual equipment. The desmoid tumor should be excised, covered by a cuff of healthy tissue (wide margins); in the case of marginal excision, owing to the contiguity with nerves or vessels, postoperative radiation therapy is recommended.

The pseudocapsule of a malignant soft-tissue sarcoma is an area of reactive tissue potentially contaminated by tumoral cells, and tumoral skip lesions may be present around this area. For this reason, a marginal excision is not an adequate treatment for soft tissue sarcomas, exposing the patient to a high risk of local recurrence (40% to 60%).[1, 2] Only in selected cases of low-grade soft-tissue sarcoma may restricted areas of marginal margin be accepted to preserve nerves and vessels and to avoid amputation. In these cases, the dissection must include the vascu-

lar adventitia and the perineurium. Postoperative radiation therapy is often recommended.

Wide

For wide margins, the tumoral mass is resected en bloc with a cuff of surrounding healthy tissue. The wide excision may leave in site tumoral skip lesions, especially in high-grade soft-tissue sarcomas, and the local recurrence rate ranges between 15% and 30%.

Radical

For radical margins, the entire anatomic compartment containing the tumor is removed (e.g., whole quadriceps excision for a tumor of the anterior thigh). The local recurrence rate after this procedure is extremely low (2%) and usually no further adjuvant treatment to improve local control is required.

RECONSTRUCTIVE PROCEDURES

In most cases, the surgical excision of soft-tissue tumors does not require any reconstructive procedure. In other cases, radical or wide margins can be achieved only with the sacrifice of important anatomic structures, requiring reconstruction.

When the tumor is in contact with the bone but is clinically mobile and the bone scan results are negative, removal of the tumor with periosteal stripping is recommended (Fig. 4A). An increased uptake on the bone scan is indicative of a periosteal reaction at that level with involvement of the periosteum in the pseudocapsule; in this case, a tangential resection of the cortex en bloc with the tumor must be performed and reconstruction by autografts or allografts is required (Fig. 4B). If adjuvant radiation therapy must be employed, autogenous grafts are preferred and a preventative osteosynthesis by a plate or intramedullary rod is recommended. If the bone scan finding is positive and CT scan or magnetic resonance imaging (MRI) shows erosion of the cortex, circumferential en bloc removal of the entire bony segment adjacent to the tumor and consequent reconstruction are mandatory (Fig. 4C).

The relationship of the tumor with vessels must be evaluated. Angiography may be needed but usually MRI is

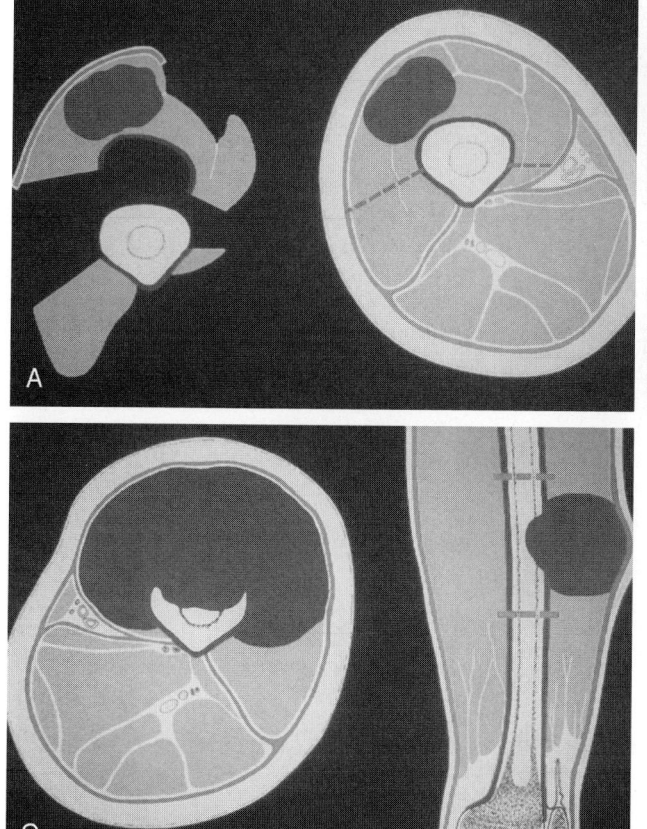

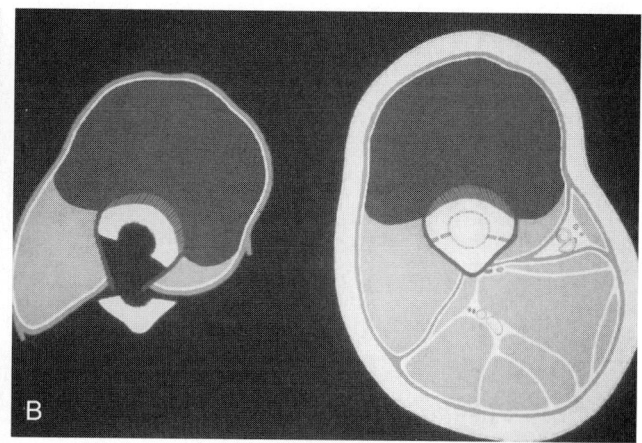

Fig. 4. Views. *A,* When the tumor is adjacent to the cortical bone and the bone scan results are negative, a periosteal stripping should be performed. *B,* If there is an increased uptake on the bone scan, a tangential cortical resection is recommended. *C,* When CT or MRI shows the erosion and tumoral extension into the bone, a segmental resection has to be performed.

sufficient. If the vessels immediately adjacent can be dissected free without opening the tumor, removing just the adventitial membrane, and achieving marginal margins, adjuvant radiation therapy should be employed to decrease the risk of local relapse. When the vessels are contained within the mass, a vessel resection en bloc with the tumor must be performed. In this case, a vessel bypass is required, using a synthetic prosthesis, which is more compatible with radiation therapy than an autogenous vein graft (Fig. 5). Nevertheless, irradiation of a vascular prosthesis produces a risk for infective complications.

In case of tumoral contiguity with a primary nerve trunk, marginal margins with dissection of the perineurium and postoperative radiation therapy may be considered. If the nerve trunk is contained within the tumoral mass and sacrifice of the nerve is required, a microsurgical reconstruction with nerve grafts may be performed. This technique is not indicated in old patients with low reparative potential, in defects of the common sciatic nerve, in long defects (>10 cm), and when postoperative radiation therapy has to be delivered. In these cases, alternative procedures such as muscular transpositions or stabilizing arthrodeses may be considered.

A soft-tissue sarcoma may occasionally extend into a joint cavity or, rarely, it may arise within a joint. When preoperative MRI demonstrates joint cavity involvement, an extrarticular resection of the joint en bloc with the tumor should be performed. The skeletal defect may be

reconstructed by an arthrodesis or an arthroplasty using autografts, allografts, or prostheses.

In soft-tissue sarcomas with superficial locations, ulcerated lesions, recurrences with multiple skin incisions, and especially when they arise in distal extremities (hand and foot), a wide skin excision is often required. In these cases, a rotational or a free microsurgical fasciocutaneous or muscular flap can be used for reconstruction.

When radical surgery is performed and an entire muscle is removed, if the muscle is necessary for functional recovery, in selected patients a motor unit transplantation can be performed. The deltoid may be replaced by a latissimus dorsi innervated rotational flap (Itoh technique).[3] The reconstruction of the quadriceps and sural triceps can be achieved by a free latissimus dorsi flap with microsurgical anastomosis of the vessels and of the motor nerve with a branch of the femoral nerve (thigh) and of the posterior tibialis (leg).[4] In the same way, the en bloc removal of the flexor or extensor muscles of the forearm can be replaced by a free gracilis flap with microsurgical suture of the vessels and motor nerve.

AMPUTATION

Limb salvage surgery is feasible in more than 90% of cases of soft tissue sarcomas. The advances observed in surgical reconstruction and the possibility of repairing vessel resections and nerve defects and replacing wide skin

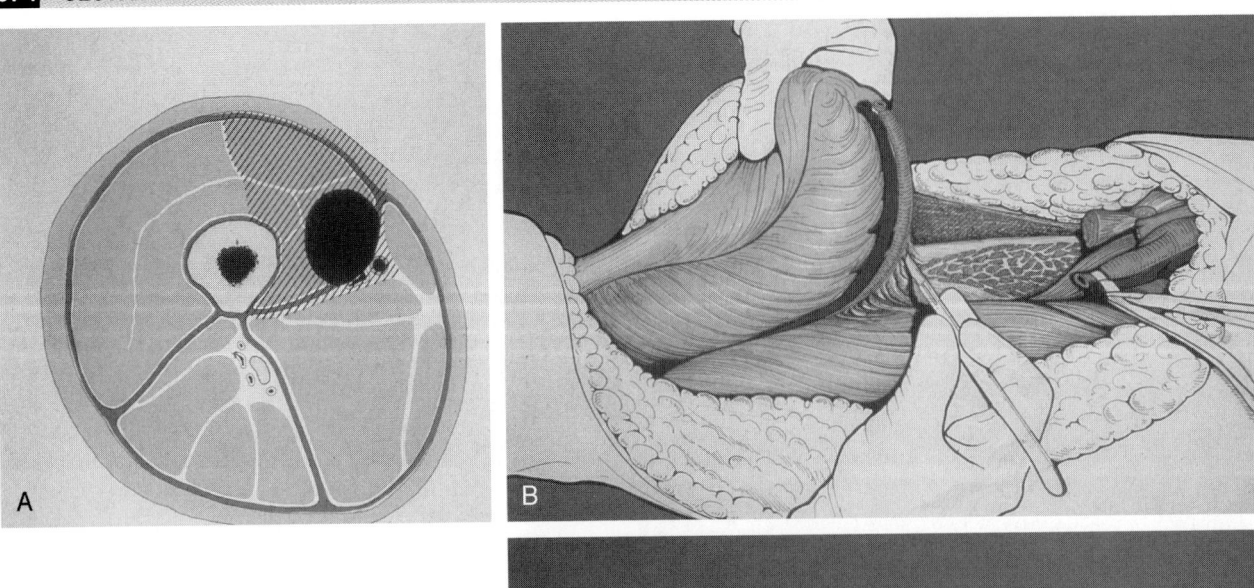

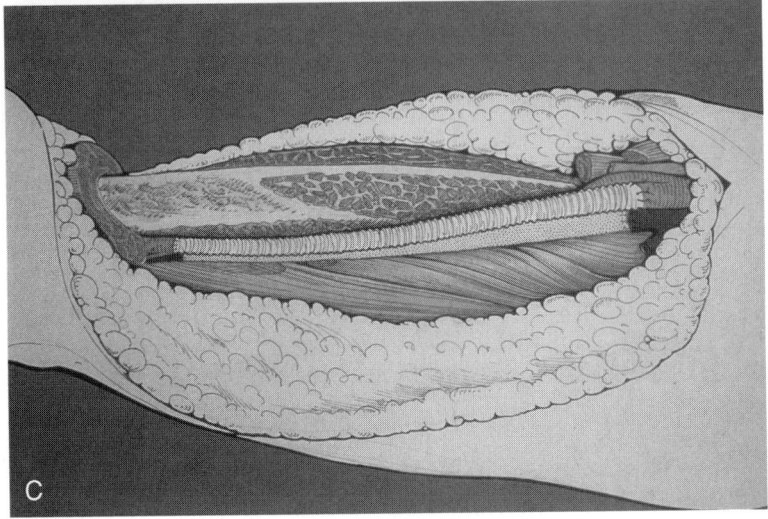

Fig. 5. Views. These show when the vessels are contained or infiltrated by the tumor. *A*, Wide margins may be achieved by resecting the vessels en bloc with the tumor. *B*, A reconstructive bypass with synthetic graft is used for reconstruction *(C)*.

loss with microsurgical techniques have expanded the indications for conservative surgery.[5]

At present, an amputation is rarely required. The basic indications for ablative surgery are the following:

- Patients with a compromised general status, in whom demanding reconstructive procedures, prolonged surgical time, and possible blood loss would be hazardous to their life.
- Simultaneous extensive involvement of vessels and nerves, when function of the limb cannot be restored after resection and reconstructive techniques. In these cases, the function achievable with an external prosthesis has to be preferred to an unfunctional limb.
- Soft tissue sarcomas with multiple skip lesions or local recurrences along the limb. In these situations, besides the lesions detectable with preoperative imaging, there may be a microdissemination of the tumor and conservative surgery would not guarantee an adequate local control.

SURGICAL RE-EXCISION

There are patients without evident local recurrence who have been inadequately treated with an intralesional or marginal excision (Fig. 6). These patients should have a complete re-excision of the operative site to achieve a wide

margin. Radiation should also be considered. The persistence of microscopic and macroscopic tumoral areas has been demonstrated in 35 to 59% of cases.[6–8] When the histology was positive for viable tumor, the recurrence risk was higher by 1.5 to 3 times as compared with patients with negative histology. Nevertheless, no influence on overall survival was demonstrated.[9]

RADIATION THERAPY

The treatment of soft tissue sarcomas with high-dose radiation therapy alone (≥6000 cGy) was associated with inadequate local control, resulting in a recurrence in two thirds of cases, and a very high incidence of radiation-induced complications was observed.[10] Nevertheless, when used as an adjuvant to surgical excision, radiation therapy was shown to be successful in improving local control of the disease.[11] Randomized trials demonstrated the efficacy of radiation therapy when either marginal or wide margins had been achieved.[1, 2] Therefore, radiation therapy may allow sterilization of the residual tumoral cells along the reactive pseudocapsule and of the skip lesions at the tumor periphery. However, the indications for adjuvant radiation therapy are still controversial, and some surgical oncolo-

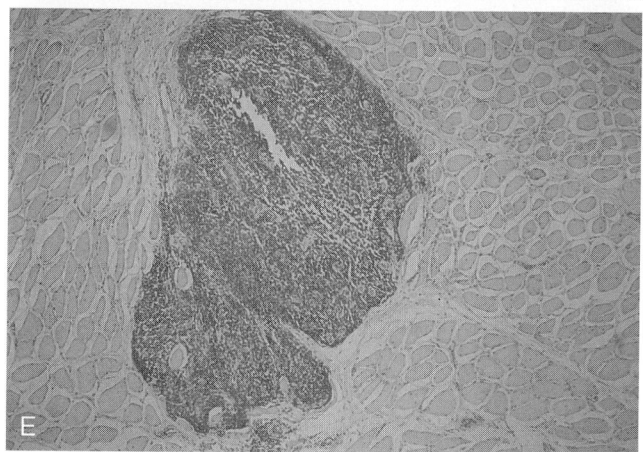

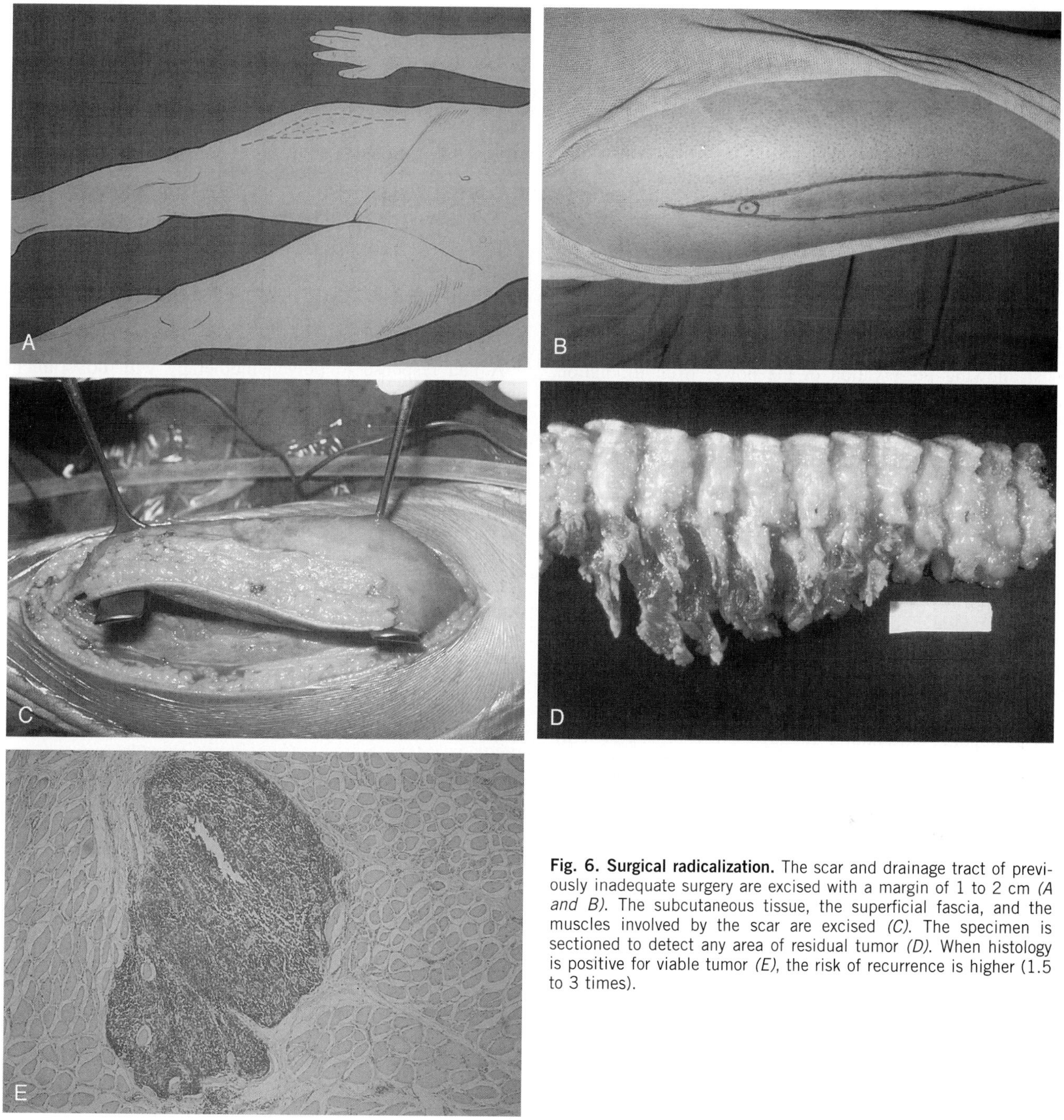

Fig. 6. Surgical radicalization. The scar and drainage tract of previously inadequate surgery are excised with a margin of 1 to 2 cm *(A and B)*. The subcutaneous tissue, the superficial fascia, and the muscles involved by the scar are excised *(C)*. The specimen is sectioned to detect any area of residual tumor *(D)*. When histology is positive for viable tumor *(E)*, the risk of recurrence is higher (1.5 to 3 times).

gists are concerned about radiation-induced complications and recommend irradiation only in cases of high-grade lesions or when the surgical margins are contaminated by tumor.[1, 2]

Radiation therapy can be delivered preoperatively, intraoperatively, or postoperatively.

PREOPERATIVE RADIATION THERAPY

The advantages of preoperative radiation therapy are the following:

1. The exact limits and volume of the tumor are defined by accurate imaging techniques (MRI) and irradiation of healthy tissue is limited.

2. Irradiation is more effective if the tumoral mass is well vascularized (the effects of surgical excision may decrease the oxygenation of the residual tumoral cells).

3. The target volume may be smaller, allowing preservation of the contiguous joints.

4. The tumoral necrosis and the pseudocapsule thickening may help prevent dissemination during surgical excision.

The disadvantages are the following:

1. The tumor remains in situ for a long time and it may be at risk, especially in bad responders.

2. This technique was associated with a high rate of postoperative radiation-induced complications.[13, 14]

The average dose employed is 5000 to 5400 cGy on the initial target volume (180 to 200 cGy/day in 28 to 30 fractions) followed by a boost (1000 to 1600 cGy), which may be delivered with conventional postoperative irradiation, with postoperative brachytherapy, or with intraoperative radiation therapy.

INTRAOPERATIVE RADIATION THERAPY

Irradiation of the surgical bed after tumor removal is performed with a dose of 1000 to 2000 cGy followed by postoperative external radiation therapy (3500 to 4000 cGy). This technique is indicated in retroperitoneal sarcomas, allowing preservation of the bowel from irradiation, and in other sites when is not possible to implant catheters for brachytherapy for anatomic reasons.[15]

POSTOPERATIVE RADIATION THERAPY

Postoperative radiation therapy can be delivered by external beam irradiation, by interstitial brachytherapy, or with a combination of both techniques.

External beam irradiation is given with a total dose of 6000 to 7000 cGy with fractions of 180 to 200 cGy/day. Circumferential irradiation of the limb and of long bones should be avoided to prevent distal lymphedema and pathological fractures. The local control is reported to range between 78% and 92% and local complications account for 6 to 16% of cases. No differences between preoperative and postoperative radiation therapy were observed in terms of overall survival and local control of the disease, although preoperative radiation therapy was associated with a higher rate of complications.[16] The current trend is to hyperfraction the dose up to three fractions per day to decrease the damage to healthy tissue and to increase the total dose.

Interstitial curietherapy (brachytherapy) can be employed alone with high doses (4000 to 4500 cGy in 90 to 110 hours) or in association with external beam irradiation therapy.[17] The combined treatment consists of low-dose brachytherapy (1500 to 3500 cGy in 45 to 50 hours) delivered 1 week after surgery followed by a dose of 3500 to 4500 cGy of external beam irradiation after 1 month. After tumor excision, plastic catheters are positioned in the surgical bed, and, after 5 to 7 days, they are filled with radioactive sources ([192]I). This technique allows focal irradiation of the surgical bed, preserving the surrounding healthy tissue.

High-dose brachytherapy alone was associated with a high rate of complications (35%) and local recurrence at the margins of the field of treatment (30%) owing to the rapid fall-off of dose around the implant.[18] The combined treatment (brachytherapy plus external radiation therapy) allows an increase in the total dose with a lower risk of complications and a decrease in the local recurrence rate at the periphery of the implant. In our experience on 145 patients treated with limb salvage for a soft-tissue sarcoma, local recurrences occurred in 2.5% of cases when combined treatment was performed (brachytherapy plus external radiation therapy), in 12.5% of cases when preoperative or postoperative radiation therapy was delivered, and in

23% of cases treated with surgery alone. The high dose of irradiation delivered with combined treatment determined the increase of postoperative complications (26% versus 13%), which required surgical revision in 85% of cases.[5]

CHEMOTHERAPY

NEOADJUVANT CHEMOTHERAPY WITH OR WITHOUT RADIATION THERAPY

Several different protocols have been proposed for locally advanced soft-tissue sarcomas to reduce the tumor mass. These protocols are used in an attempt to convert a tumor from one requiring an amputation to one that can be safely resected while saving the limb.

A bad response to polychemotherapy with doxorubicin and dacarbazine with or without cyclophosphamide was reported by Pisters et al in 1997.[19] More encouraging results were observed with doxorubicin monochemotherapy associated with radiation therapy. Unresectable tumors became resectable in 40% of cases, and no differences were observed in terms of necrosis, limb salvage, local recurrence, and complications between intra-arterial and endovenous delivery of doxorubicin.[20, 21] At present, a polychemotherapy protocol is under trial, consisting of three preoperative cycles of mesna, doxorubicin, ifosfamide, and dacarbazine (MAID). Postoperative radiation therapy is associated when inadequate surgical margins are obtained.

ISOLATED LOCAL PERFUSION WITH RECOMBINANT TUMOR NECROSIS FACTOR

Recombinant tumor necrosis factor alpha (rTNF-α) presents a powerful antineoplastic activity by selective destruction of tumoral vessels, but, owing to the high toxicity in humans, the drug must be delivered by perfusion of limb in isolated circulation. The rTNF-α activity is synergic with melphalan, doxorubicin, and interferon and it is improved by hyperthermia.

The hyperthermic perfusion with rTNF-α, interferon-γ, and melphalan allowed a complete response in 35% of cases and a partial response in 50 to 60%. Moreover, after perfusion, limb salvage became feasible in 85 to 90% of patients with an unresectable tumor with a recurrence rate of 13%.[22, 23] The association of rTNF-α with doxorubicin in hyperthermic perfusion determined a good response in 60% of cases and a fair response in 28% of cases, and limb salvage surgery was performed in 75% of cases.[24]

Although rTNF-α is delivered in isolated perfusion, cardiovascular and lung toxicity and renal failure due to rhabdomyolysis may be observed. For this reason, this technique is indicated in selected cases with locally advanced soft-tissue sarcomas to avoid an amputation.

ADJUVANT CHEMOTHERAPY

The efficacy of adjuvant chemotherapy in improving the systemic control of soft tissue sarcomas is controversial. Several trials of monochemotherapy with doxorubicin or polychemotherapy including doxorubicin have been proposed. When a significant difference in disease-free survival was demonstrated, the studies were criticized for the small number of patients or for the modality of randomization.

A meta-analysis of data reported in the literature (1546 cases) showed an improvement of survival at 2 and 5 years in patients treated with adjuvant chemotherapy.[25] Recently, a randomized study with a polychemotherapeutic protocol with epirubicin and high-dose ifosfamide showed such a significant difference in both disease-free survival and overall survival that the randomization was interrupted.[26] Adjuvant chemotherapy should be considered for a patient who can safely tolerate the drugs and who has a high-grade soft-tissue sarcoma greater than 5 cm in diameter.

REFERENCES

1. Gustafson P: Soft tissue sarcoma, epidemiology and prognosis in 508 patients. Acta Orthop Scand 1994; 65:2.
2. Stotter AT, A'Hern RP, Fischer C, et al: The influence of local recurrence of extremity soft tissue sarcoma on metastasis and survival. Cancer 1990; 65:1119.
3. Itoh Y, Sasaki T, Ishiguro T, et al: Transfer of latissimus dorsi to replace a paralyzed anterior deltoid. J Bone Joint Surg Br 1987; 69:647.
4. Ihara K, Shigetami M, Kawai S, et al: Functioning muscle transplantation after wide excision of sarcomas in the extremities. Clin Orthop 1999; 358:140.
5. Capanna R: Le traitement des sarcomes des tissus mous: Cahiers d'enseignement de la SOFCOT. Conferences d'Enseignement, 1998; p 175.
6. Goodlad JR, Fletcher CD, Smith MA: Surgical resection of primary soft tissue sarcoma. Incidence of residual tumor in 95 patients needing re-excision after local resection. J Bone Joint Surg Br 1996; 78:658.
7. Noria S, Davis A, Kandel R, et al: Residual disease following unplanned excision of soft tissue sarcoma of an extremity. J Bone Joint Surg Am 1996; 78,5:650.
8. Zormig C, Peiper M, Schroder S: Reexcision of soft tissue sarcoma after inadequate initial operation. Br J Surg 1995; 82:278.
9. Lewis JJ, Leung D, Woodruff JM, Brennan MF: Extremity soft tissue sarcoma: Are two operations better than one? International Society of Limb Salvage, IX Symposium, New York, 1997.
10. Tepper JE, Smit HD: Radiation therapy alone for sarcomas of soft tissue. Cancer 1985; 56:475.
11. Pisters PW, Harrison LB, Leung DH, et al: Long term results of a prospective randomized trial of adjuvant brachytherapy in soft tissue sarcoma. J Clin Oncol 1996; 14:859.
12. Rydholm A: Surgery without radiotherapy in soft tissue sarcoma. Acta Orthop Scand 1997; 273:117.
13. Bujko K, Suit MD, Springfield DS, Convery K: Wound healing after preoperative radiation for sarcomas of tissue. Surg Gynecol Obstet 1993; 176:124.
14. Eilber FR, Eckardt JJ, Rosen G, et al: Preoperative therapy for soft tissue sarcoma. Hematol Oncol Clin North Am 1995; 9:817.
15. Willet CG, Suit MD, Topper JE: Intraoperative electron beam radiation therapy for retroperitoneal soft tissue sarcoma. Cancer 1991; 68:278.
16. Cheng EY, Dusembery KE, Winters MR, Thompson RC: Soft tissue sarcoma: Preoperative vs postoperative radiotherapy. J Surg Oncol 1996; 61:90.
17. Alekhteyar KM, Leung DM, Brennan MF, Harrison LB: The effect of combined external beam radiotherapy and brachytherapy on local control and wound complications in patients with high grade soft tissue sarcoma of the extremities with positive microscopic margins. Int J Radiat Oncol Biol Phys 1996; 36:321.
18. Habrand JL, Gerbaulet A, Pejonic MH: Twenty years experience of interstitial iridium brachytherapy in the management of soft tissue sarcomas. Int J Radiat Oncol Biol Phys 1991; 20:405.
19. Pisters PW, Patel SR Varma DGK, et al: Pathologic complete response following preoperative multimodality therapy for stage IIIB extremity soft tissue sarcoma. Proc ASCO 1997; 16:499.
20. Badellino F, Canavese G, Palumbo R, et al: Surgery after concomitant radiochemotherapy treatment in advanced soft tissue sarcomas (STS): Feasibility and activity of a multimodality limb sparing protocol. International Society of Limb Salvage, IXth Symposium, New York, 1997.
21. Eilber FR, Eckardt JJ, Rosen G, et al: Neoadjuvant chemotherapy and radiotherapy in the multidisciplinary management of soft tissue sarcoma of the extremities. Surg Oncol Clin North Am 1993; 2:611.
22. Eggermont AM, Schraffordt Koeps M, Lienard D, et al: Isolated limb perfusion with high dose tumor necrosis factor alpha in combination with interferon-gamma and melphalan for non resectable extremity soft tissue sarcomas: A multicentric trial. J Clin Oncol 1996; 14;10:2653.
23. Meller I, Gutman M, Schlush L, et al: Hyperthermic isolated limb perfusion with high dose necrosis factor alpha and melphalan as a limb preserving modality in patients with extensive soft tissue sarcomas. International Society of Limb Salvage, IX Symposyum, New York, 1997.
24. Di Filippo F, Lise M, Rossi CR, et al: Hyperthermic autoblastic perfusion with a TNF and doxorubicin for the treatment of soft tissue limb sarcoma in candidates for amputation: Results of phase 1 study. Proc ASCO 1997; 16:501.
25. Tierney JF, Mosseri V, Stewart LA, et al: Adjuvant chemotherapy for soft tissue sarcoma: Review and meta-analysis of the published results of randomized clinical trials. Br J Cancer 1995; 72:469.
26. Frustaci S, Gherlinzoni F, De Paoli A, et al: Preliminary results of an adjuvant randomized trial on high risk extremity soft tissue sarcomas. Proc ASCO 1997; 16:468.

METASTATIC SKELETAL DISEASE

Denis R. Clohisy

Summary
- The most common bone cancers that orthopaedists treat are skeletal metastases.
- Bone destruction at sites of metastatic bone tumors is performed by osteoclasts.
- Bone formation at sites of metastatic bone tumors is performed by osteoblasts.
- Treatments that inhibit osteoclast formation can decrease skeletal complications of osteolytic metastatic bone tumors.
- The most useful test to evaluate for the presence of metastatic bone disease is a bone scan.
- The most useful test for searching for an unknown primary tumor in a patient with a suspected skeletal metastasis is a computed tomography (CT) scan of the chest and abdomen.

The term *metastatic bone disease* generally refers to skeletal disease manifested as cancer that has spread from a distant site to one or more bones. This definition, however, is not completely accurate, in that most general discussions of metastatic bone disease include reference to multiple myeloma, a malignancy that actually arises from within bone. Because the general concept that defines the clinical presentation, pathophysiology, and treatment of both truly metastatic bone cancers and myeloma bone tumors are similar, these tumors are discussed together in this chapter.

Tumors that are considered metastatic bone disease include both solid and hematological malignancies. By far the majority of patients with metastatic bone disease have solid tumors. The solid tumors that have clear predisposition for spreading to the skeleton include cancers arising from the breast, prostate, lung, kidney, and thyroid. In the majority of patients with skeletal metastases from solid tumors, either breast or prostate is the primary cancer site. This fact reflects both the high incidence of these two cancers and the high frequency with which these cancers metastasize to bone. In fact, up to 80% of women who die from breast cancer and more than 90% of men who die from prostate cancer have skeletal metastases. The hematological malignancy that most commonly causes skeletal disease is multiple myeloma.

Cancer can have devastating localized or systemic effects on the skeleton. Systemic effects are mediated by circulating tumor-secreted cytokines, involve only bone resorption, and do not require the presence of bone-residing tumors. This systemic effect of cancer on the skeleton, called *humoral hypercalcemia of malignancy,* is encountered only rarely in general orthopaedic practice. Localized effects of bone-residing metastases occur only at sites of metastatic tumor deposits in bone, and they can result in bone destruction, bone formation or both. Localized effects of cancer on the skeleton can cause skeletal pain, immobility, and, ultimately, fracture. Complications of localized effects of cancer on the skeleton are commonly seen in general orthopaedic practice.

After cancer cells become established in bone, they can influence bone cells locally at sites of tumor deposit to make bone, destroy bone, or both. Understanding the pathophysiology of the interaction between bone metastases and bone cells is of value to the practicing orthopaedic surgeon, because the cell biology of this interaction provides the basis for various treatments and imaging modalities.

PATHOGENESIS

PATHOLOGY
All metastatic tumor sites show histological evidence of the primary tumor and also of a cellular reaction of normal host cells to the tumor. The type of cellular response to tumors varies somewhat among tumor types and may even vary within the confines of an individual tumor. The cellular response of bone to tumors results in bone formation, bone destruction, or both. Metastatic tumors that predominantly destroy bone are myeloma and metastases from primary tumors in the kidney, thyroid, and lung. Skeletal metastases from the prostate primarily form bone, and skeletal metastases from the breast generally have areas of significant bone formation and bone destruction. The mechanism for tumor-induced bone resorption is tumor stimulation of osteoclastic bone destruction, and that for tumor-induced bone formation is tumor stimulation of osteoblastic bone production (Fig. 1).

Understanding the cell biology of the effects of skeletal metastases on bone requires a general understanding of the two cell populations that normally reside in bone. They are cells of hematopoietic origin and cells of mesenchymal origin. The most important cells of hematopoietic origin are cells of the monocyte/macrophage lineage and their precursor cells. These cells are important because they form osteoclasts. The cells of mesenchymal origin, which are most important for understanding the cell biology of the effects of skeletal metastases on bone, are bone marrow stromal cells and osteoblasts. Bone marrow stromal cells are critical for regulating skeletal homeostasis. They are contained in the bone marrow microenvironment, and they play a role in both bone resorption and bone formation. Osteoblasts are important because they make bone.

PHYSIOLOGICAL BONE RESORPTION
Osteoclasts, the body's principal bone-resorbing cells, are influenced either directly or indirectly by virtually all bone metastases. Osteoclast-mediated skeletal resorption is accomplished in two steps. The first step requires osteoclast-

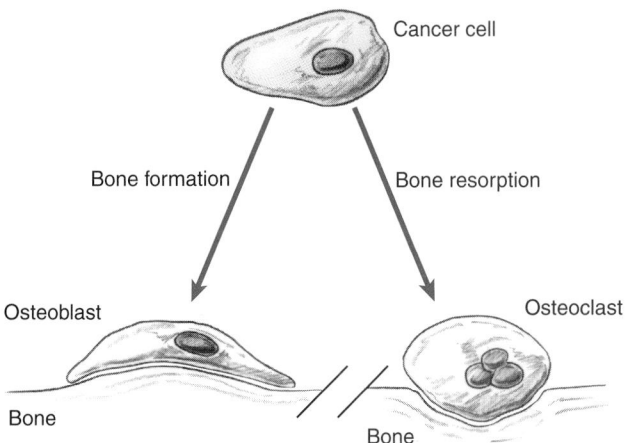

Fig. 1. Tumor-induced bone resorption and tumor-induced bone formation. Bone-residing cancer cells initiate a series of steps that ultimately result in osteoblastic bone formation, osteoclastic bone resorption, or both.

dependent acidification of bone surfaces, which causes demineralization of bone. The second step requires bone matrix destruction by osteoclast-secreted lysosomal-type enzymes, such as cathepsin K.

Changes in bone resorption can reflect changes in osteoclast number, which may be due to alterations in either survival or formation of osteoclasts. Changes in osteoclast survival would reflect a change in the frequency of programmed death (apoptosis) of osteoclasts. Bisphosphonates are proposed to accelerate osteoclast apoptosis; colony-stimulating factor-1 (CSF-1) or macrophage colony-stimulating factor (M-CSF) is proposed to inhibit osteoclast apoptosis. Osteoclast formation is regulated by tightly controlled interactions between specific hematopoietic osteoclast precursor cells and cells of mesenchymal origin, either bone marrow stromal cells or osteoblast lineage cells. Hematopoietic osteoclast precursor cells that are uniquely capable of differentiating into osteoclasts are cells of monocyte/macrophage lineage, which have been shown to express cell surface receptors for both M-CSF and the osteoclast-differentiating protein called osteoprotegrin ligand (OPGL),[1] also termed osteoclast differentiation factor (ODF) and TRANCE/RANK ligand (Fig. 2).[2] A variety of secreted and cell-associated cytokines or cytokine receptors have been postulated as affecting osteoclast formation in vivo. The agents required for osteoclast formation to occur in vivo are osteoprotegrin (OPG),[3] CSF-1, and OPGL. Cytokines or hormone may also directly stimulate osteoclasts to resorb bone in vivo. Molecules that have been proposed to perform this function in vivo include OPGL, CSF-1, and proteins from the transforming growth factor (TGF) family.

Changes in bone resorption can reflect changes in the bone-resorbing activity of existing osteoclasts. Osteoclast size in vivo is a recognized measure of the level of osteoclastic bone resorption, with an increase in size representing an increase in bone resorption. Bisphosphonates have been shown to decrease the bone-resorbing capabilities of osteoclasts and parathyroid hormone (PTH), PTH-related protein (PTH-rP), and OPGL have been shown to increase the bone-resorbing capabilities of osteoclasts.

TUMOR-INDUCED BONE RESORPTION

The most devastating effect that a skeletal metastasis can have on bone is to stimulate bone resorption. Examples of metastatic bone tumors that usually induce bone destruction are multiple myeloma and metastatic cancer from the lung, thyroid, kidney, or breast. Tumor-induced bone resorption (tumor osteolysis) causes skeletal pain and may ultimately cause skeletal fracture.

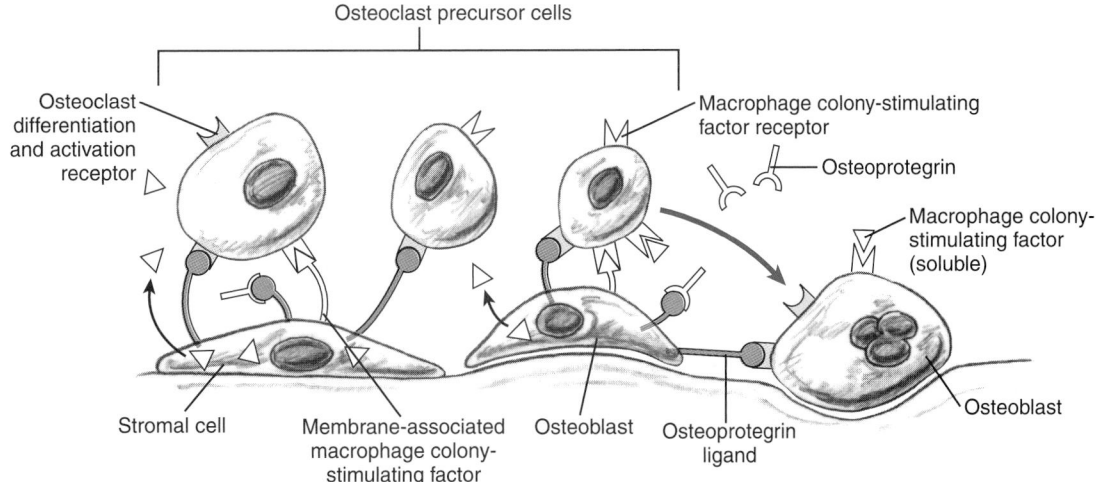

Fig. 2. Regulation of osteoclast formation and osteoclast activation by macrophage colony-stimulating factor (M-CSF) and the osteoprotegrin/ osteoprotegrin-ligand system. Osteoclast formation requires interaction of osteoclast precursor cells with both M-CSF and osteoprotegrin ligand (OPGL). M-CSF exerts its influence by binding to the M-CSF receptor on osteoclast precursor cells and mature osteoclasts. It stimulates both formation and activation of osteoclasts and can act in either a soluble or membrane-associated form. OPGL is a cell surface protein on osteoblasts and bone marrow stromal cells. It stimulates formation and activation of osteoclasts by binding to the osteoclast differentiation and activation receptor (ODAR). ODAR is found on osteoclast precursor cells and on mature osteoclasts. Osteoprotegrin (OPG) is a secreted protein that acts as an antagonist to the OPGL/ODAR pathway and is therefore a negative regulator of osteoclast formation and activation.[1, 3] Each of the molecules presented in this figure has an alternative name; these are provided by Yasuda and colleagues.[2]

Investigations into the mechanisms by which tumors destroy bone have revealed the consistent finding, in both humans and animals, that tumors destroy bone by stimulating osteoclasts. An increase in osteoclast-mediated bone resorption at sites of tumor reflects increases in both the number of osteoclasts and the amount of bone resorption per osteoclast.[4-6]

Several tumor-secreted products have been proposed as being responsible for these influences on osteoclasts and their precursor cells, including PTH-rP and M-CSF.[4, 7] A feedback loop that involves PTH-rP and the bone microenvironment at sites of osteolytic breast cancer tumors has been characterized.[8] In this loop, tumor-secreted PTH-rP induces stromal cells to stimulate osteoclast-mediated bone resorption (Fig. 3).

The fact that metastatic bone tumors promote their own growth and development by inducing osteoclast formation has been used to develop new therapies to prevent or treat patients with skeletal metastases. Because bisphosphonates are suspected to both induce osteoclast apoptosis and decrease osteoclastic bone resorption, these agents have been used to determine whether inhibition of osteoclast activity would reduce skeletal complications of metastatic bone cancer or decrease the frequency of skeletal metastasis in patients at risk for such tumors. The bisphosphonate pamidronate has been shown to decrease both pain and the frequency of skeletal complications in patients with metastatic breast cancer and multiple myeloma.[9-11] The bisphosphonate clodronate has been demonstrated to reduce the incidence and the number of new bony and visceral metastases in women with breast cancer who are at risk for distant metastases.[12] The exact mechanism by which inhibition of osteoclast-mediated bone resorption decreases bone tumor growth and spread can only be speculated.

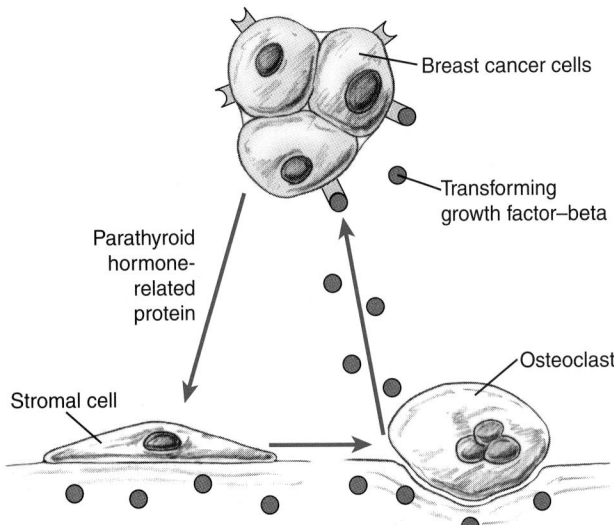

Fig. 3. Proposed parathyroid hormone–related protein (PTH-rP) and bone-residing transforming growth factor-β (TGF-β) feedback loop directed by breast cancer metastases in bone. Breast cancer tumor–secreted PTH-rp induces bone marrow stromal cell to stimulate osteoclast-mediated bone resorption. This localized bone resorption releases TGF-β from the bone matrix. The TGF-β interacts with adjacent breast cancer cells and stimulates them to increase their production of PTH-rP. Tumor-secreted PTH-rP then initiates the cycle again.[7, 8]

PHYSIOLOGICAL BONE FORMATION

Understanding how cells of mesenchymal origin influence both bone formation and bone resorption permits one to comprehend the influence of tumor metastases on the skeleton. Bone formation is initiated when there is increased OPGL gene expression in stromal/osteoblast cells.[2] Increased expression of OPGL on the surface of such cells causes osteoclast formation by cell-cell contact that is communicated from membrane-associated OPGL to osteoclast precursor cells bearing the osteoclast differentiation and activation receptor (ODAR) (see Fig. 2).[13]

Osteoblasts are derived from mesenchymal precursor cells, which are uniquely capable of forming bone. Bone formation occurs in two steps. The first step is osteoblast production of osteoid, that is, type I collagen and noncollagenous proteins. The second step is a passive biochemical reaction that involves mineralization of the osteoid matrix with calcium and phosphorous. Signals to osteoblasts that stimulate osteoid production can be received by the osteoblasts during the process of adhesion or direct contact with the bone matrix or through interaction of either soluble or membrane-associated, osteoblast-targeted cytokines and hormones. Examples of agents that stimulate osteoblast production of bone matrix are transforming growth factor-β (TGF-β), fibroblast growth factor, and the bone morphogenetic proteins.[14]

TUMOR-INDUCED BONE FORMATION

Bone formation at sites of tumor metastases is very common. Examples of metastatic bone tumors that typically produce radiographic evidence of bone formation are cancers that spread from the prostate or breast. Bone formation at these sites requires production of osteoblast matrix and then mineralization of that matrix. Osteoblasts produce the osteoid matrix, and mineralization of the matrix is a passive biochemical event that requires calcium and phosphate. It is believed, however, that even in the case of "purely" bone-forming metastases, tumor-induced osteolysis precedes tumor-induced bone formation; as a result, the tumor-induced bone resorption at these sites is suspected to cause the skeletal pain.

Tumor-induced bone formation is performed by osteoblasts that have been directed by tumors to divide, to produce bone, or both. Several tumor-secreted bone growth factors have been proposed as potential mediators of this process. They include TGF-β, fibroblast growth factor, and the bone morphogenetic proteins. In addition, an interesting new scenario for tumor-induced bone formation has been proposed. This scenario is based on studies of prostate cancer–secreted urinary plasminogen activator (uPA). It has been shown that the amino-terminal fragment of uPA is secreted by prostate cancer cells, that the fragment contains an epidermal growth factor–like domain, and that it acts as a growth factor for osteoblasts (Fig. 4).[15]

Means of identifying and treating metastatic tumor deposits that are stimulating bone production have exploited the fact that radioactive calcium analogues are incorporated, through a passive biochemical reaction with phosphorus, into the osteoid matrix present at sites of tumor. Two such radioactive analogues are technetium 99m and strontium 89. Technetium 99m is used when a bone scan is performed. This radionuclide is incorporated into the

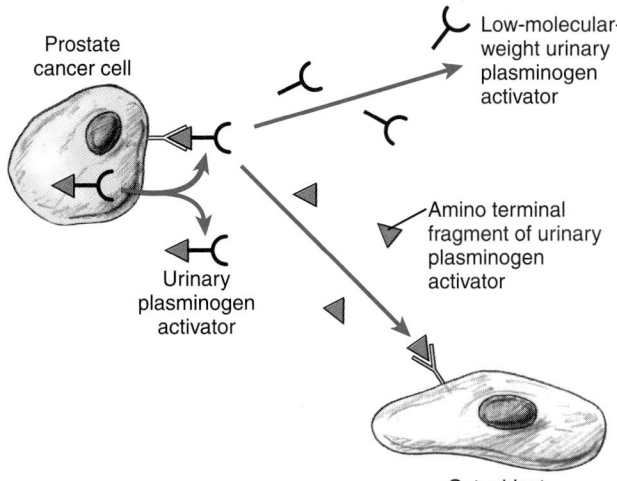

Fig. 4. Proposed mechanism of prostate cancer cell stimulation of osteoblasts. Prostate cancer–secreted urinary plasminogen activator (uPA) binds to the prostate cancer cell uPA receptor and is then enzymatically cleaved into a low-molecular-weight uPA and an amino-terminal fragment of uPA (ATF). ATF contains an epidermal growth factor–like domain that binds to osteoblasts and acts as an osteoblast growth factor.[14]

osteoid matrix at sites of tumor through a passive biochemical reaction with phosphorus, enabling extremely sensitive identification of bone-forming metastases. Strontium 89 is a radioactive calcium analogue that provides an energetic beta particle for radiation therapy of osteoblastic metastases. Like technetium 99m, strontium 89 is deposited at sites of osteoid mineralization, where tumor cells have induced osteoblasts to produce bone collagen matrix, and the isotope kills tumor cells at these sites. Treatment with agents such as strontium 89 can be a very effective and palliative therapy for painful osteoblastic metastases.[16]

ADHERENCE OF NORMAL CELLS TO THE BONE MARROW MICROENVIRONMENT

Knowledge about the adherence of cells to the bone marrow microenvironment is important in that it provides a background upon for discussion of the adherence of tumor cells. The bone marrow microenvironment is a complex milieu of a wide variety of cells, cytokines, and extracellular matrix. Adhesive interactions between cells within this environment and the extracellular matrix permit selected cells to be retained within the bone and most likely direct the growth and survival of selected populations of cells. These interactions are mediated via cell surface adhesion receptors.[17]

ADHERENCE OF CANCER CELLS TO THE BONE MARROW MICROENVIRONMENT

After cancer cells have moved into the blood stream, they must adhere to elements within the bone marrow microenvironment to form a skeletal metastasis. Adherence within the bone marrow microenvironment localizes tumor cells to skeletal sites and may potentiate tumor cell growth. Stimulation of tumor cell growth may occur because (1) adherence of tumor cells allows interaction of these cells with extracellular matrix proteins and normal bone marrow cells

and (2) adherence exposes tumor cells to the cytokine-rich environment of the bone marrow microenvironment. Both integrins and cell adhesion molecules appear to be critical for the attachment of tumor cells to the extracellular matrix of bone. Breast cancer cells use the integrin $\alpha_v\beta_3$ to attach to bone and the integrin $\alpha_4\beta_1$ as an important molecule for attachment of other metastatic cancer cells to bone. They also use both vascular cell adhesion molecules (VCAMs) and intercellular cell adhesion molecules (ICAMs) to attach to bone. Future advances in the treatment and prevention of skeletal metastases will likely involve novel therapeutic agents designed to block the adhesive interactions between cancer cells and the extracellular matrix.

CLINICAL FEATURES AND INITIAL EVALUATION

Diagnosis of patients with metastatic bone disease is typically established in one of two possible clinical settings. In the first and most common setting, the patient is known to have a primary tumor, and skeletal metastases are suspected either because of positive findings on routine cancer screening protocols or from an evaluation of musculoskeletal symptoms. In the second setting, the patient presents without a history of cancer and is evaluated for musculoskeletal symptoms.

The patient whose presentation with musculoskeletal symptoms results in a first-time diagnosis of skeletal metastases usually is being evaluated for complaints of bone pain. Typically, the pain is described as being constant, being present without activity and at night, and increasing over time. Finally, patients with advanced skeletal destruction may complain of severe activity-related pain or may present with a pathological skeletal fracture through a site of tumor. Symptoms that follow any of these patterns must be further evaluated in all patients to exclude the possibility of malignancy-related pain.

Evaluation of patients in whom malignancy-related pain is suspected should be initiated with a detailed medical history, review of symptoms, and physical examination. The objective of this initial portion of the evaluation is to thoroughly evaluate the region of symptoms and, in a patient who does not have a history of metastatic cancer, to identify a primary malignancy. Information particularly important to evaluate in the medical history includes:

- Assessment of previous cancers and their treatment.
- Tobacco use.
- Date of last mammogram (women).
- Date of last serum prostate-specific antigen test (men).

The review of systems should be comprehensive and must include questions that evaluate the following aspects:

- Details of the presenting symptoms.
- Changes in weight or appetite.
- Presence of a cough or hemoptysis.
- Breast mass, breast skin retraction, or nipple discharge.
- Fever, chills, or night sweats.
- Hematuria.

Physical examination should be comprehensive. It should focus on identifying potential sites of primary tumor and must include a detailed examination of the symptomatic site. Specific components of the physical examination that may provide clues to a primary tumor and that define the site of symptoms are as follows:

- Inspection for adenopathy, bruising, and skin lesions.
- Chest auscultation.
- Palpation for abdominal organ enlargement or tenderness.
- Palpation of "asymptomatic" bones to detect sites of additional skeletal metastases.
- Palpation of the symptomatic region to search for a mass.
- Complete neurological examination of the region that contains the symptomatic site.
- Examination of the arterial supply to the symptomatic region.

If the examining physician still suspects that skeletal pain is malignancy-related after completion of the initial clinical evaluation, radiographs of symptomatic sites should be obtained. Radiographs should be biplanar and should provide sufficient bony detail to ascertain whether a skeletal neoplasm is present. Although the appearance of metastatic bone tumors can vary significantly according to the site of primary tumor and the severity of disease, certain general features are evident with all malignant tumors. Radiographs of metastatic tumors characteristically reveal a process that is destructive and is not well marginated. Hematological malignancies, such as myeloma and lym-

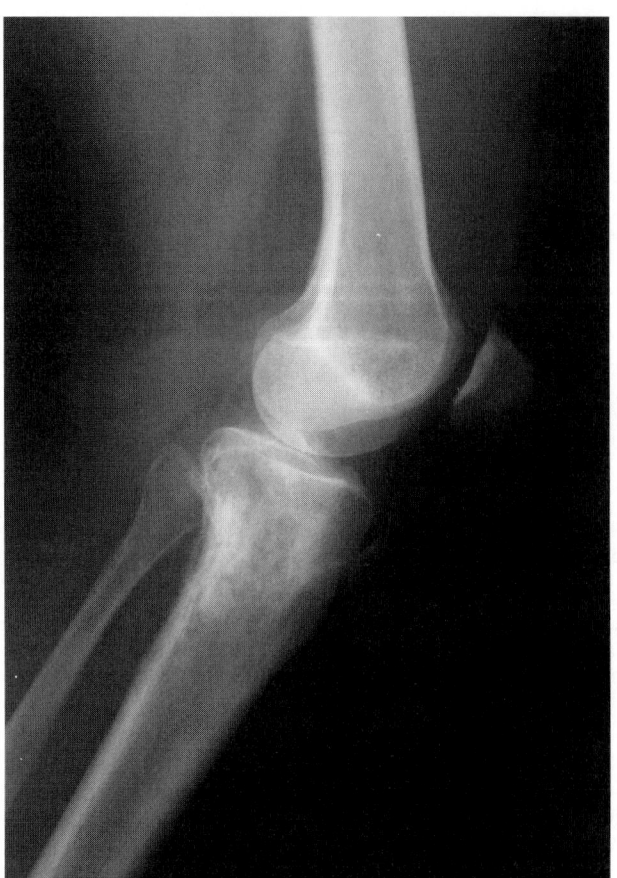

Fig. 6. Radiograph of osteoblastic bone metastasis from prostate cancer.

phoma, as well as metastases from solid tumors in the lung, kidney, and thyroid have a purely destructive effect on the bone, and they are permeative at their margins (Fig. 5). In contrast, radiographs of a bone metastasis from prostate cancer is often purely bone-forming (Fig. 6), and radiographs of a bone metastasis from breast cancer are mixed (Fig. 7), that is, they both destroy bone and form bone.

When a bone lesion seen on radiographs is suspected of being malignant, the findings from the patients medical history, review of symptoms, and physical examination should be combined to determine the nature of the lesion as well as, potentially, the site of primary tumor. In most patients who have symptomatic skeletal metastases and no previous history of cancer, however, the site of primary tumor has not been identified after completion of this initial evaluation.[18] Evaluation of these patients must move to investigations that can further add to identification of the primary tumor and, in selected cases, staging of either the entire skeleton or the site of symptomatic tumor.

INVESTIGATIONS

The majority of patients who present with skeletal pain and in whom a suspicious bone lesion is detected on radiographs need further investigation to determine the site of primary tumor. This investigation should initially involve

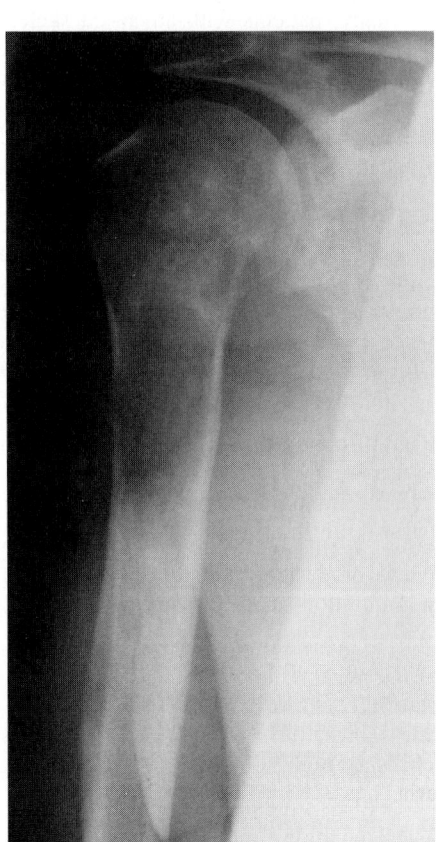

Fig. 5. Radiograph of osteolytic bone metastasis from renal cell carcinoma.

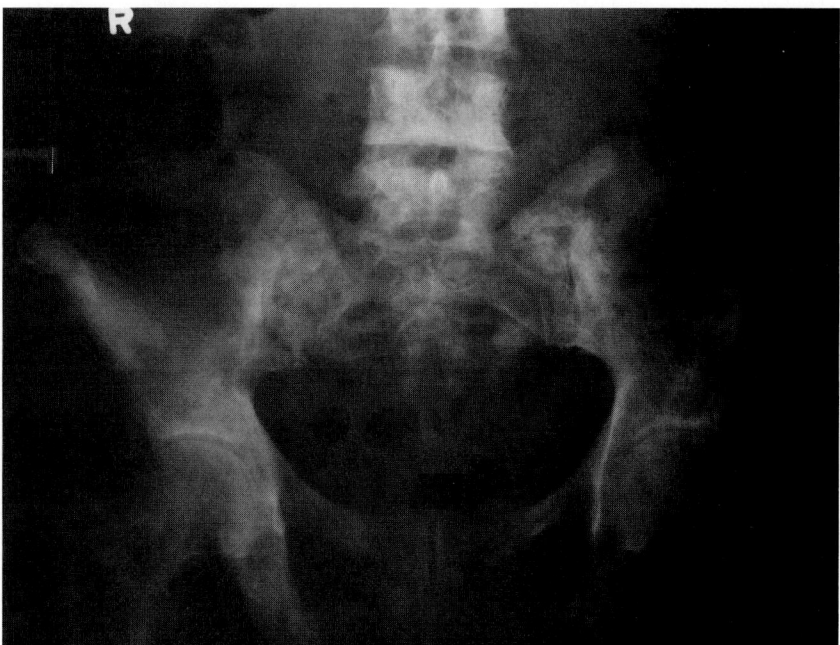

Fig. 7. Radiograph of mixed osteoblastic and osteolytic bone metastases from breast cancer.

diagnostic laboratory studies and usually requires additional imaging. Laboratory studies should include a complete blood count in all cases. In selected cases, additional laboratory tests should be performed; for example, serum immunoelectrophoresis for suspicion of myeloma, erythrocyte sedimentation rate and C-reactive protein measurements for suspicion of infection, and prostatic-specific antigen measurement for suspicion of prostate cancer. Serum calcium and phosphorus measurements should be obtained in all patients with myeloma and in patients in whom either multiple sites of skeletal metastases or humoral hypercalcemia of malignancy is suspected.

Imaging studies beyond routine radiographs are needed to evaluate all patients in whom the site of primary tumor has not been established by information obtained in the medical history, review of systems, and physical examination. In patients who do not have a known primary site of tumor, the most efficient means of obtaining a diagnosis is to perform a computed tomography (CT) scan of the chest, abdomen, and pelvis. This method of evaluation has been shown to establish the diagnosis in 28% of patients with tumors of unknown origin that are not established by initial clinical evaluation, serological analysis, and chest radiographs.[18] As one might expect, primary tumors diagnosed in this fashion are those located at sites inaccessible to physical examination, that is, cancers of the kidney and lung (Fig. 8).

Imaging studies in addition to those that focus on detecting the site of primary tumor may be needed to further evaluate specific sites of skeletal tumor. CT or magnetic resonance imaging (MRI) should be considered when additional information about a specific site of skeletal tumor is needed. The objectives of additional imaging with either modality can be two fold: (1) to establish the precise extent of bone destruction at a metastatic site and (2) to determine the local stage of a skeletal tumor. Establishing the precise

extent of skeletal destruction is necessary when radiographs do not provide sufficient information to direct the surgeon's decision about the role of prophylactic surgical stabilization. This information is best obtained and easiest to interpret from CT scans (Fig. 9).

Determining the local stage of a skeletal tumor is necessary when the lesion may represent a primary bone malignancy, such as osteosarcoma. Also, it is important to determine the precise extent of intramedullary tumor when one is planning surgical stabilization of a metastasis. An example of the latter circumstance is a skeletal metastasis that must be treated with surgical stabilization, could be stabilized with any of several methods of internal fixation, and has ill-defined margins on radiographs. In such a case, if the method of surgical stabilization depends on the intramedullary extent of the tumor, MRI can be used to precisely define the intramedullary extent of tumor.

Other imaging studies may be needed to accurately stage the extent of disease beyond the known skeletal site. Some diseases that produce skeletal tumors require specific staging studies, and others require more general staging studies. An example of a disease that requires a specific study for staging is myeloma, for which a skeletal survey is needed. Evaluation with a skeletal survey involves radiographs of the skull and the entire axial and appendicular skeleton. The number of skeletal sites identified with tumor in part determine the extent of disease and contribute to estimation of the prognosis for survival.

Most patients with skeletal metastasis, however, have not myeloma but, rather, metastases from malignancies arising from the breast, prostate, kidney, or lung. In these patients, a bone scan should be used to determine the extent of skeletal involvement. A bone scan of the entire skeleton should be reviewed in all patients who have skeletal metastases from solid tumors. Such scans are performed with the bone-seeking isotope technetium 99m. This radiopharma-

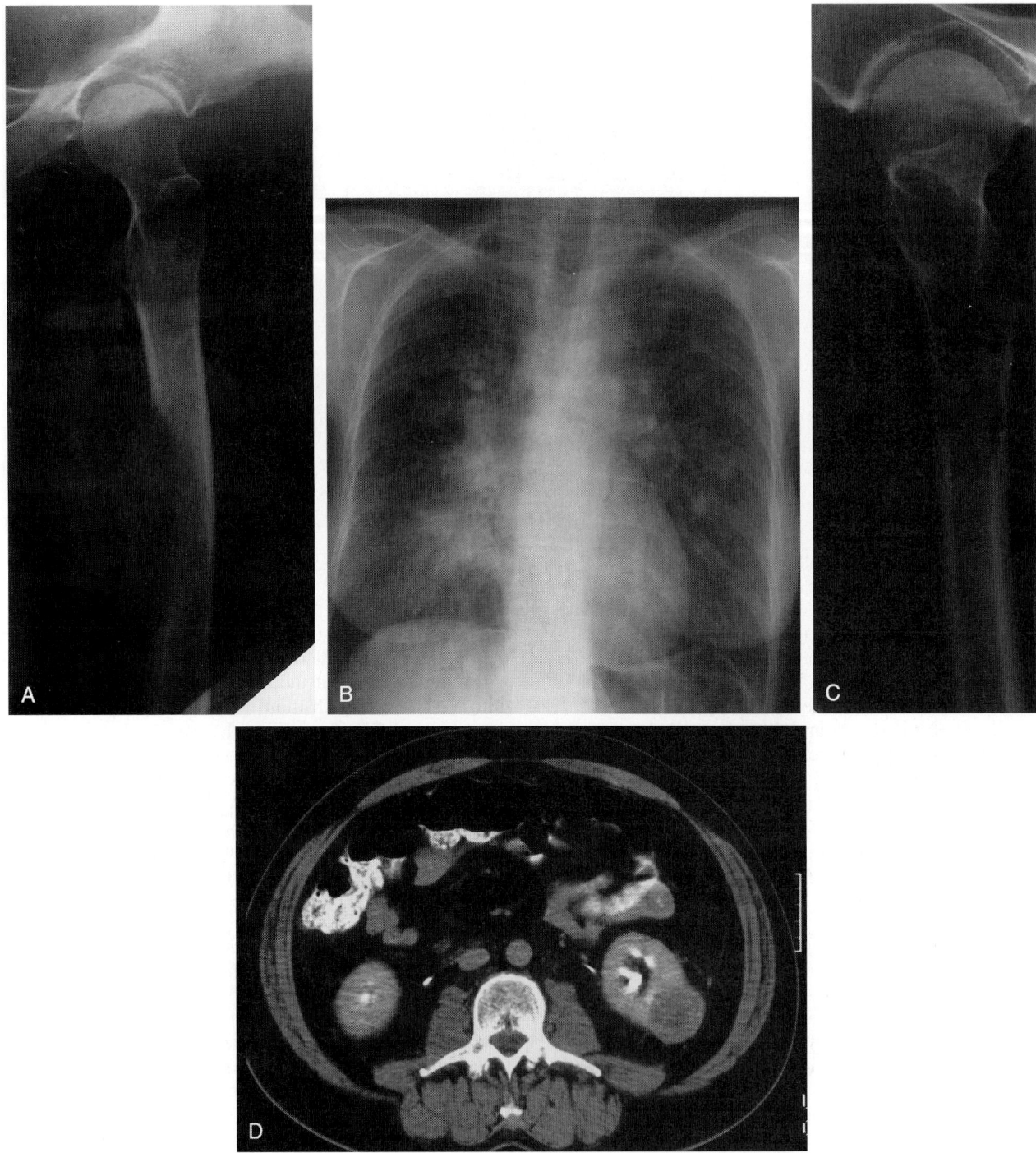

Fig. 8. Primary (extraosseous) cancers diagnosed in patients with destructive bone lesions. *A* and *B,* A 54-year-old woman with a history of tobacco use presented with continuous thigh pain at night and with any movement. Radiograph of the femur (*A*) reveals an osteolytic lesion, and chest radiograph (*B*) shows a right-sided lung cancer. *C* and *D,* A 62-year-old man presented with thigh discomfort when standing up from a chair and when bearing weight. Radiograph of the hip (*C*) shows a subtle osteolytic lesion in the proximal femur, and an abdominal CT scan (*D*) reveals a left renal mass that was determined to be a carcinoma.

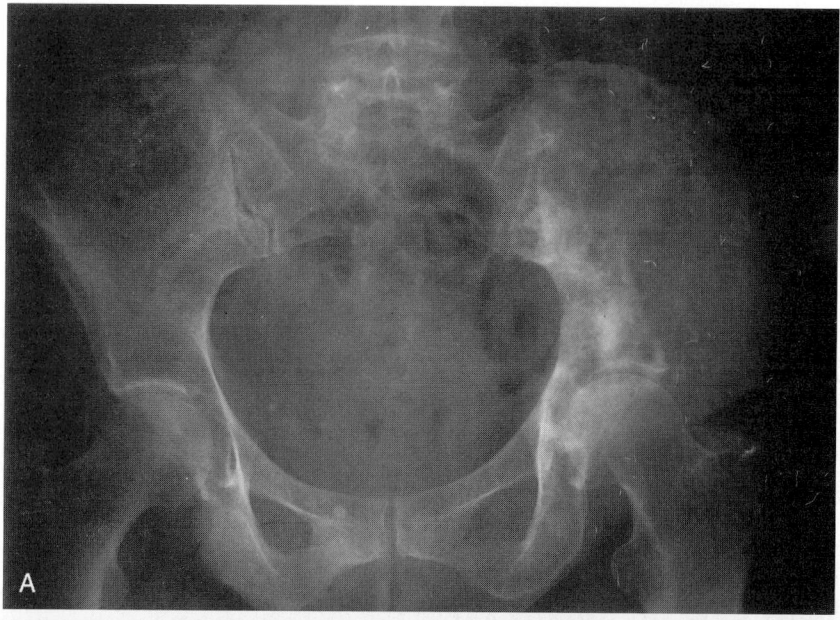

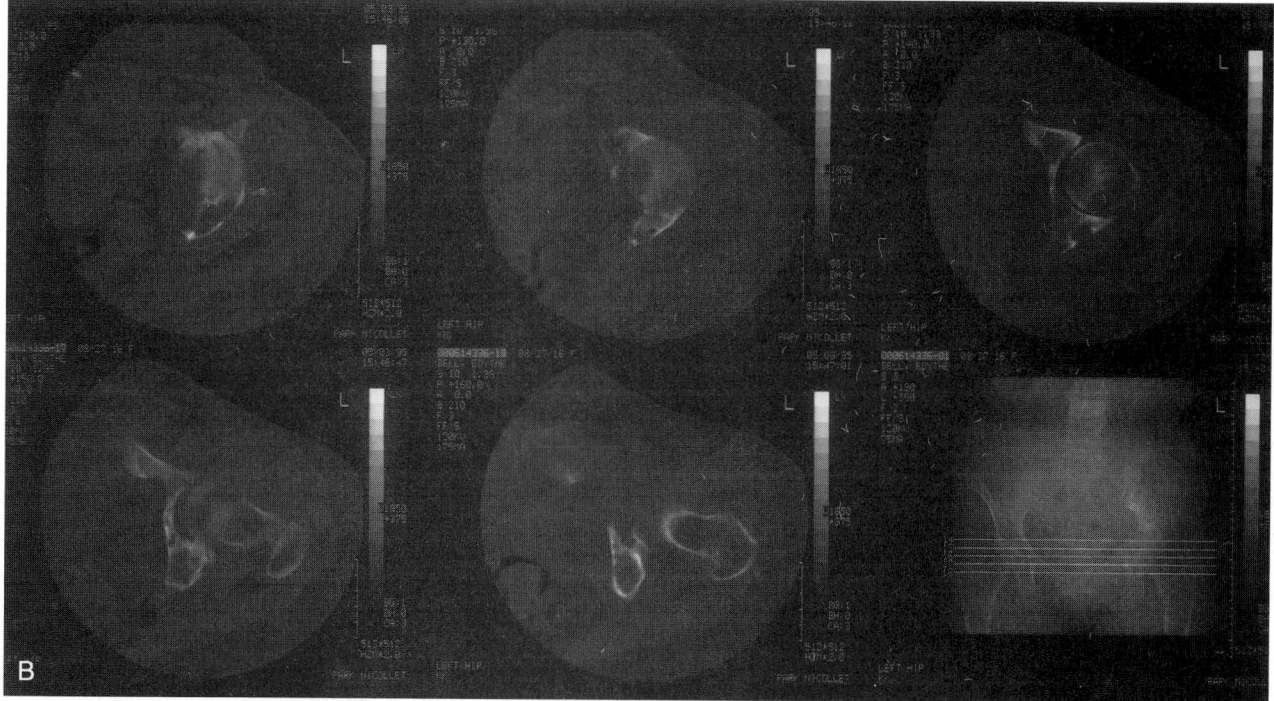

Fig. 9. Axial imaging with computed axial tomography to determine the precise extent of skeletal destruction. Radiograph of a breast cancer metastasis to the hemipelvis (*A*) does not reveal the full extent of skeletal destruction in the periacetabular region, which is appreciated on a CT scan of the same region (*B*).

ceutical is deposited at sites of bone metastasis that are stimulating the production of new bone. The bone scan is very sensitive for bone-forming metastases, but is not necessarily specific for them. As a result, it is often necessary to evaluate sites of metastases identified by bone scan with biplanar radiographs (Fig. 10). This is particularly applicable in the patient in whom there was no previous evidence of skeletal metastases before bone scanning.

PREOPERATIVE EVALUATION

Patients with metastatic skeletal disease who are judged candidates for surgical treatment must undergo a comprehensive evaluation to establish each patient's ability to tolerate anesthesia, and to maintain hemostasis as well as the risk of fracture in skeletal sites that will not be treated with the first procedure. As a minimum, the evaluation should include the following:

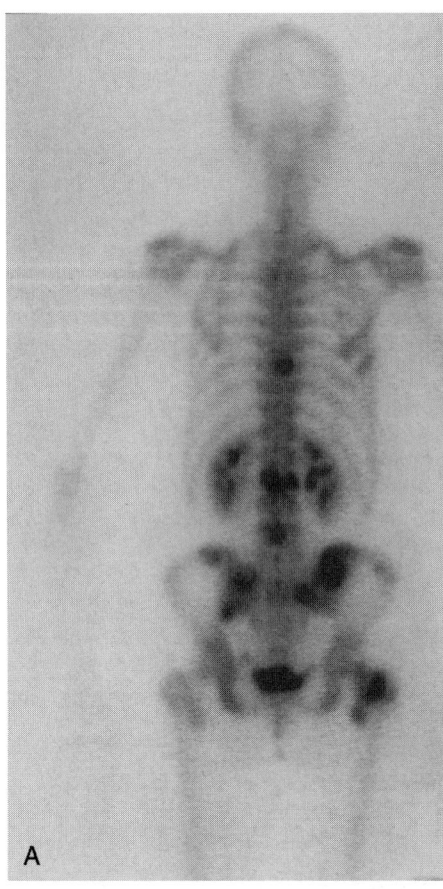
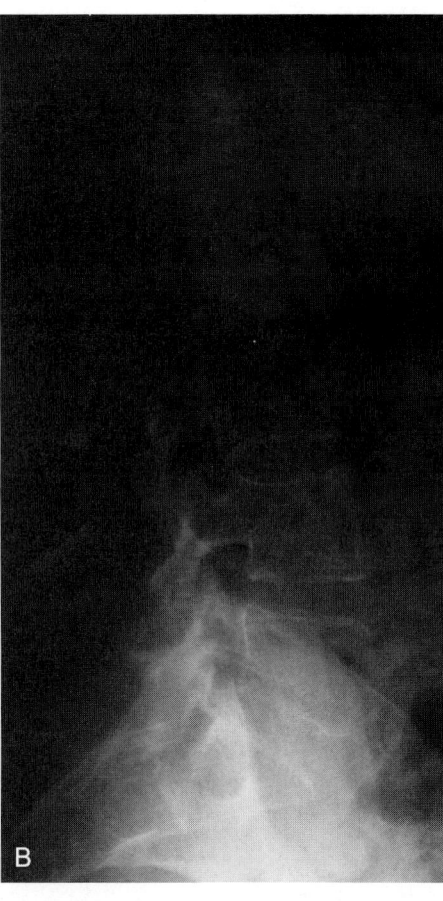

Fig. 10. Bone scan identifies skeletal metastases. *A,* Bone scan of the entire skeleton in a patient with lung cancer that is known to have spread to the proximal femur reveals additional skeletal lesions. *B,* Radiograph of the lumbar spine further characterizes metastatic lesions that involve the twelfth thoracic and second lumbar vertebrae.

- Assessment of fluid status.
- Assessment of the ability to tolerate a fluid challenge.
- Hemoglobin measurement.
- Electrocardiogram.
- Serum potassium determination.
- Chest radiograph.
- Careful history to identify recent or past bleeding episodes.
- Review of recent medications, including anticoagulants and agents that inhibit platelet function.
- Platelet count.
- Serum coagulation studies.

The vascularity of tumor metastases at sites that will be treated with surgery should be assessed in patients who have metastatic tumor types that are characteristically vascular and are in anatomic sites at which excessive bleeding could not be controlled by a tourniquet. Skeletal metastases from renal and thyroid carcinomas are characteristically vascular, and tumor locations at which bleeding could not be controlled by a tourniquet include the spine, scapula, pelvis, proximal humerus, and proximal femur. In patients who have skeletal metastases from primary malignancies of the kidney and the thyroid and who need surgical treatment in the spine, scapula, pelvis, proximal humerous, or proximal femur, tumor vascularity should be evaluated by an arteriogram. If the arteriogram shows feeder arterial vessels that provide substantial blood flow to the tumor, emboliza-

tion of the feeder vessels should be performed on the day of surgery, and the effectiveness of the embolization should be confirmed prior to surgery (Fig. 11). If the arteriogram indicates that there is no significant blood flow to the tumor, surgery can be performed without embolization.

Patients who have multiple sites of skeletal metastases must be identified before any single site is treated with surgery, because they may benefit from surgery at more than one site or from modification of standard postoperative rehabilitation. For example, a patient who has a pathological fracture through a metastasis in the proximal femur, which should be treated with surgery, may also have metastases in one or both humeri or may have a second metastasis in the ipsilateral distal femur. If a metastasis were present in one or both humeri, a pathological fracture of the humerus might occur during postoperative rehabilitation, when the patient is relying on crutches or a walker for pivots, transfers, and walking. Addressing any humeral lesion in advance, with either radiation or surgical stabilization, and modifying the patient's use of ambulatory aids (i.e., platform crutches) are obviously preferred to dealing with a pathological fracture shortly after the first surgical procedure. If the patient had a metastatic lesion in the ipsilateral distal femur, a different method might be chosen for surgical stabilization; an intramedullary rod may be preferred to a hip screw and side plate, because the former would span the second lesion, providing prophylactic treatment for it.

Assessment for the presence of skeletal metastases at

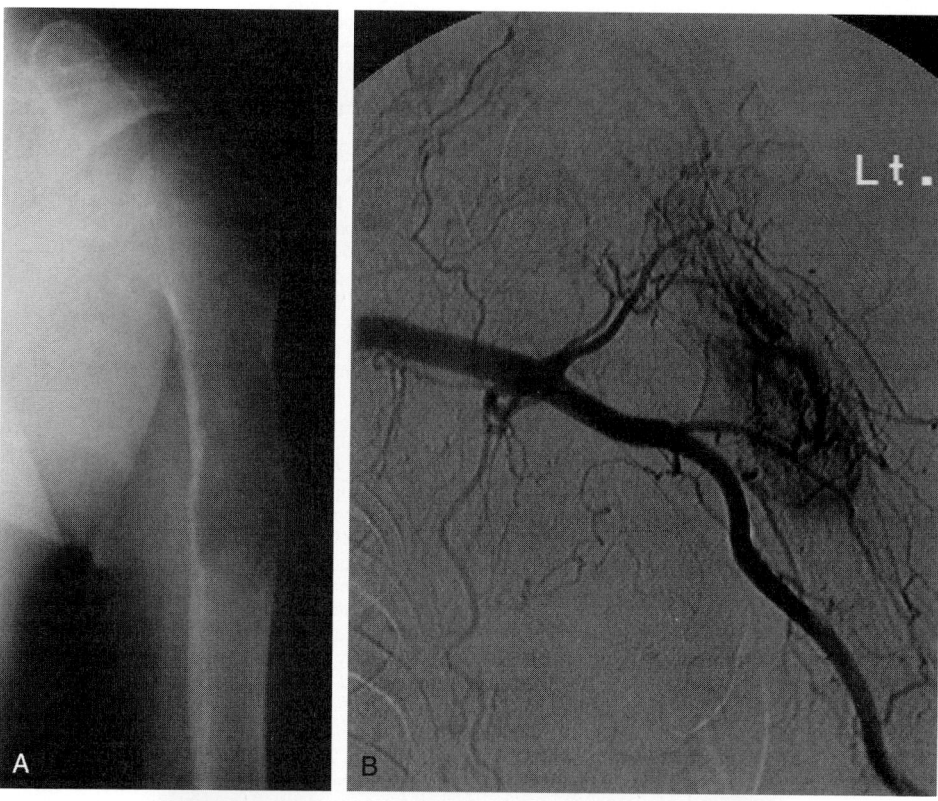

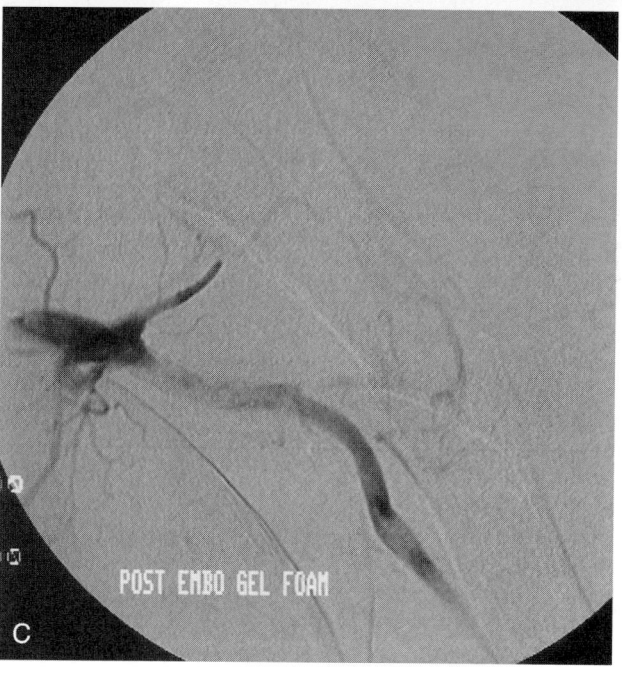

Fig. 11. Preoperative embolization of a metastatic renal cell cancer in a skeletal location that is not accessible to a tourniquet. An osteolytic renal cell metastasis involving the proximal humerus (*A*) is evaluated by arteriogram (*B*) and then is embolized (*C*) prior to surgical treatment.

locations other than the site for which surgery is planned should, at a minimum, involve a careful history and physical examination that focus on identifying other such sites. The history should determine whether the patient has skeletal pain at other sites during inactivity or while rising from a sitting position, walking, or lifting. Physical examination should include forceful palpation or percussion of the spine and appendicular skeleton. Evaluation for the presence of skeletal metastases at occult sites with bone scanning is suggested in patients who are poor historians, have diffuse complaints of skeletal pain, or are difficult to examine. Anatomic sites that are suspicious for skeletal metastases on the basis of history, physical examination, or bone scan should be evaluated with biplanar radiographs to determine whether a tumor is present and, if so, whether surgical stabilization is indicated.

REFERENCES

1. Simonet WS, Lacey DL, Dunstan CR, et al: Osteoprotegerin: A novel secreted protein involved in the regulation of bone density. Cell 1997; 89:309.
2. Yasuda H, Shima N, Nakagawa N, et al: Osteoclast differentiation factor is a ligand for osteoprotegerin/osteoclastogenesis-inhibitory factor and is identical to TRANCE/RANKL. Proc Natl Acad Sci U S A 1998; 95:3597.
3. Lacey DL, Timms E, Tan H-L, et al: Osteoprotegrin ligand is a cytokine that regulates osteoclast differentiation and activation. Cell 1998; 93:165.
4. Clohisy DR, Ogilvie CM, Ramnaraine MLR: Tumor osteolysis in osteopetrotic mice. J Orthop Res 1995; 13:892.
5. Clohisy DR, Palkert, D, Pekurovsky I, et al: Human breast cancer induces osteoclast activation and increases the number of osteoclasts at sites of tumor osteolysis. J Orthop Res 1996; 14:396.
6. Clohisy DR, Ramnaraine MLR: Osteoclasts are required for bone tumors to grow and destroy bone. J Orthop Res 1998; 16:660.

7. Guise TA, Yin JJ, Taylor SD, et al: Evidence for a causal role of parathyroid hormone-related protein in the pathogenesis of human breast cancer-mediated osteolysis. J Clin Invest 1996; 98:1544.
8. Guise TA: Parathyroid hormone-related protein and bone metastases. Cancer 1997; 80(Suppl):1572.
9. Adami S: Bisphosphonates in prostate cancer. Cancer 1997; 80(Suppl):1664.
10. Berenson JR, Lichtenstein A, Porter L, et al: Efficacy of pamidronate in reducing skeletal events in patients with advanced multiple myeloma. N Engl J Med 1996; 334:488.
11. Hortobagyi GN, Theriault RL, Porter L, et al: Efficacy of pamidronate in reducing skeletal complications in patients with breast cancer and lytic bone metastases. N Engl J Med 1996; 335:1785.
12. Diel IJ, Solomayer EF, Costa SD, et al: Reduction in new metastases in breast cancer with adjuvant clodronate treatment. N Engl J Med 1998; 339:357.
13. Hsu H, Lacey DL, Dunstan CR, et al: The TNFR-related protein RANK is the osteo-

clast differentiation and activation receptor (ODAR) for OPG ligand. Presented at the American Society of Bone and Mineral Research Second Joint Meeting, 1–6 December 1998, San Francisco, CA.
14. Goltzman D: Mechanisms of the development of osteoblastic metastases. Cancer 1997; 80(Suppl):1581.
15. Rabbani SA, Gladu J, Mazar AP, et al: Induction in human osteoblastic cells (SaOS2) of the early response genes fos, jun, and myc by the amino terminal fragment (ATF) of urokinase. J Cell Physiol 1997; 172:137.
16. Robinson RG: Strontium-89–precursor targeted therapy for pain relief of blastic metastatic disease. Cancer 1993; 72:3433.
17. Rougraff BT, Kneisl JS, Simon MA: Skeletal metastases of unknown origin: A prospective study of a diagnostic strategy. J Bone Joint Surg Am 1993; 75:1276.
18. Verfaillie CM: Adhesion receptors as regulators of the hematopoietic process. Blood 1998; 92:2609.

section 7
chapter 14

NONSURGICAL MANAGEMENT OF BONE METASTASES

Peter Kirkbride

Summary
- Radiotherapy is a mainstay of palliative treatment for painful bone metastases.
- Local radiotherapy is effective in relieving pain in up to 80% of patents, but the optimal treatment schedule is not defined.
- Wide-field radiotherapy may be of value in selected patients.
- There is increasing evidence for the value of systemic agents, especially bisphosphonates.
- One should not overlook the importance of appropriate analgesia for patients who have pain from bone metastases.

Bone metastases are a common complication of many cancers, especially those of breast, lung, prostate, thyroid, and kidney, and are the most common cause of intractable pain in patients with cancer.[1] Estimates vary, but between 30% and 70% of patients with cancer are thought likely to develop bone pain at some time. In the absence of impending or actual fracture, surgery is rarely used, but many other treatments are available to the patient with bone metastases. The intent of treatment is usually pain relief, although benefits such as improved mobility and prevention of fracture may also ensue.

Local radiotherapy has long been known to be effective in relieving bony pain. In 1948, Paterson, from the Christie Hospital in Manchester, United Kingdom, first proposed treatment schedules aimed at palliating symptoms rather than curing tumors. The first randomized trial comparing different radiation schedules for treating bone metastases was performed by the Radiation Therapy Oncology Group (RTOG) in the 1970s. The results of this trial were published twice, with conflicting conclusions[2, 3]; accordingly, there has been debate about the optimal treatment regimen ever since. Most randomized trials published since 1986 suggest that a single treatment or fraction is as efficacious as a longer course, although controversy exists about the appropriate end points that should be used to evaluate radiotherapy in this situation.

Endocrine therapy has long been used to treat patients with bone metastases from breast and prostate cancer, but until the 1990s, other systemic therapies were rarely used. There is now evidence that both chemotherapy and bisphosphonates can be valuable in selected patients.

CLINICAL FEATURES

Metastases to bone can be asymptomatic, in which case there may not be any indication for palliative treatment. Most cause moderate to severe pain that is usually unrelenting and is often exacerbated by motion or weightbearing. It can be very difficult for a patient to accurately localize the site of the pain, but a bone that is tender on palpation is probably the site of a painful metastasis, and this finding is often used by radiation oncologists to assist treatment planning. Plain radiographs may show lytic or sclerotic lesions, often with associated bone destruction, although a technetium 99m bone scan is a more sensitive method of detecting bone metastases. Patients with bone metastases may have a raised serum calcium level, and it is estimated that 40% to 50% of patients with breast cancer have hypercalcemia at some point. Because hypercalcemia may be initially asymptomatic but can insidiously progress to become life-threatening, serum calcium should usually be determined when bone metastases are suspected.

RADIOTHERAPY

The radiation used in radiotherapy consists of high-energy "photons" that are generated following a complex series of interactions in a linear accelerator (x-rays), or directly from the nucleus of a radioactive isotope, such as cobalt 60 (gamma-rays). The rays used for therapy are similar to those used in diagnostic imaging but are more powerful and penetrating and can cause damage and death of both normal and tumor cells.

Exactly how radiotherapy relieves the pain caused by bone metastases is not well understood, but there is wide acceptance that it is a highly effective tool in this situation. However, there has been less agreement about (1) the optimal way in which radiotherapy should be used and (2) whether a short course of large doses or "fractions" of radiotherapy, as used in the United Kingdom, is as effective as the more prolonged course favored in the United States. In addition, there is debate about whether further benefits can be obtained by widening the target of the radiotherapy, such as by employing half-body irradiation (HBI) or intravenous injection of radioisotopes such as strontium 89, which can be thought of as "systemic radiation."

Radiotherapy is also commonly used in the treatment of impending or actual pathological fractures, often in conjunction with surgical fixation. As with bone metastases, the optimal scheduling and dosing of radiotherapy for pathological fractures are unknown.

PRINCIPLES OF PALLIATIVE RADIOTHERAPY

A large proportion of radiation treatment is delivered with palliative intent, accounting for more than 50% of the workload in some radiotherapy centers. The decision-making process associated with the administration of palliative radiotherapy can be quite complex; interested readers are referred to "Rules for the Practice of Palliative Radiotherapy" as proposed by Mackillop.[4] Because palliative radiotherapy is given with the intent of preventing or relieving symptoms, complete elimination of the tumor is not necessary, and radical doses are not usually employed. Thus, it is common to use much shorter treatment times than the 6 to 7 weeks used for curative treatment, but the optimal scheduling is not well defined in many situations. It should be noted that radiotherapy can provide rapid and durable

pain relief often in the absence of any radiographic evidence of response, so patient-reported symptoms are used to evaluate its effect. Such end points can be difficult to obtain reliably and consistently, however. Accordingly, it is difficult to derive good estimates of the efficacy of palliative radiotherapy from much of the published literature.

The exact area or field treated with radiation, of course, varies with each case. In general, the field includes the bone deemed to be the source of the patient's symptoms, with a margin to allow for movement and day-to-day variation. It is usual to keep the field as small as is practical and to shield out as much normal tissue, especially bowel, as possible to minimize side effects. A typical field is shown in Figure 1.

LOCAL RADIOTHERAPY

Paterson[5] first recognized that palliation could be achieved with "at least one-half but better still, two-thirds of a tumour lethal dose," and that palliative radiotherapy could be given over short periods, such as 1, 4, or 8 days. His recommendations set the standards in the United Kingdom, whereas in North America, Fletcher[6] advised doses such as 30 Gy in 10 fractions over 2 weeks and 20 Gy in 5 fractions over 1 week, depending on the location of the treatment. Neither researcher could provide any data to substantiate the recommendations, but current palliative radiotherapy practices appear to be derived from them. Many

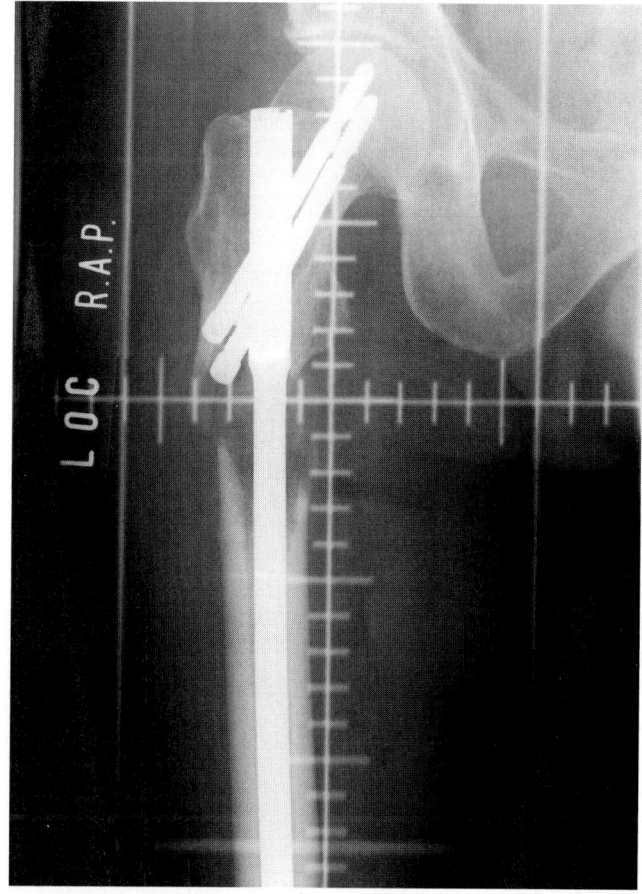

Fig. 1. Simulator radiograph. It shows a treatment field for a patient with painful metastases in his lumbar spine.

different radiotherapy treatment regimens have been used, and there is a lack of good clinical trial data to allow us to judge their relative merits.

One review summarized retrospective studies evaluating more than 100 patients and published since 1969, in which reported response rates varied from 65% to 100%.[7] Noteworthy were the uses of single fractions in doses as high as 18 Gy and of more radical-type fractionation schemes, such as 50 Gy in 5 weeks. Response criteria used in these reports were highly variable and included subjective interpretations of patients' charts. No consistent definitions of the terms "complete relief" or "partial relief" of pain in the context of radiotherapy for bone metastases currently exist. However, in randomized studies, the reported response rates are lower, probably because of the use of more stringent response criteria. A 2000 analysis of 12 published randomized controlled trials suggested that pain relief rates vary between 30% and 60%.

The RTOG trial, first published in 1982, randomly assigned more than 1000 patients to receive a 15- or a 5-fraction regimen (for solitary metastases) or a 10- or a 5-fraction regimen (for multiple metastases). In this study, the primary end point was pain relief; the results were prospectively collected but physician-assessed, and there were no measures of toxicity. The results of this trial were published twice and caused confusion. In the first analysis in 1982, it was concluded that the low-dose short-course schedules were as effective as the high-dose protracted programs,[2] but the subsequent reanalysis published in 1985 arrived at the completely reverse opinion.[3] In retrospect, the design of this study was flawed, and the contradictory results of the two analyses make any interpretation extremely difficult.

Since then, more studies have been performed and published. Price and colleagues[9] randomly assigned 288 patients with a life expectancy of more than 6 weeks to receive either 8 Gy as a single fraction or 30 Gy over 2 weeks. Pain was evaluated with patient self-assessment using a validated tool, and the analgesic requirement was also recorded and taken into account. End points used were "partial response," defined as an improvement in pain score with some or reduced analgesic requirement, and "complete response," defined as no pain, no analgesic requirement. In this trial, there was no difference in total pain relief, in rate of pain relief, or in duration of response in the patients whose pain responded to treatment. Although toxicity was not specifically reported, there was no difference in acute side effects. Other published trials also support the hypoth-

esis that single-fraction radiotherapy is as effective as a multifraction regimen in this situation,[10, 11] although a Canadian study has produced a contradictory conclusion.[12] Survival times in all the groups of patients are very similar.

With at least some evidence that single fraction radiotherapy is as effective as more prolonged treatment, why is this modality not more commonly used? An unpublished, informal survey of Canadian radiation oncologists showed that although 60% of responding physicians in Canada prefer single-fraction radiotherapy because of convenience and greater or similar efficacy, there were still concerns about the duration of response, acute complications, and patient tolerance. In health care systems in which the physician is remunerated on the basis of the number of fractions of treatment delivered, there may even be a financial incentive to prolong treatment times.

WIDE-FIELD RADIOTHERAPY

"Wide-field" or "systemic" radiation therapy uses either HBI or radioactive isotopes, such as strontium 89. The response rates and duration of response are comparable to those achieved with local radiation, although one study suggests superior results for fractionated HBI in terms of duration and need for re-treatments.[13]

At present, the efficacy of strontium, used either alone or in conjunction with local irradiation, is confined to the treatment of bone metastases from prostatic cancer, because this agent has an affinity for osteoblastic lesions. There is evidence that this approach is beneficial in both the treatment of known painful metastases and the prevention of future lesions. Further research is proceeding, in particular with the use of newer isotopes, such as rhenium 186 and samarium 153.

Side effects of radiation treatment vary according to the area of the body being treated. Unfortunately, most investigators do not report toxicity. Nevertheless, Table 1 lists the toxicities that have been reported from local and wide-field irradiation. Most trials were carried out before 5-hydroxytryptamine ($5HT_3$) antagonists were available. It would appear, from studies utilizing these agents, that the incidence of acute side effects, especially nausea and vomiting, are similar for both single-fraction and multifraction treatment regimens. In the HBI trials, the toxicity rates tend to increase with dose, ranging from 30% to 60% for gastrointestinal toxicity, and from 20% to 40% for hematological toxicity, with occasional pulmonary toxicity. In the strontium trials, there was no significant gastrointestinal toxicity,

TABLE 1. RATES OF TOXICITIES FROM LOCAL AND WIDE-FIELD RADIATION THERAPY (RT)				
Toxicity	Single-Fraction RT	Multiple-Fraction RT	Half-Body Irradiation	Strontium Therapy
Gastrointestinal (nausea, vomiting, diarrhea)	30–75%	25–35%	30–60%	10%
Neurological (paraparesis)	<1%	<1%	NR	NR
Hematological (leukopenia, thrombocytopenia)	NR	<10%	20–40%	30–40%
Pathological fracture	8%	5–18%	NR	NR

NR = not reported.

and hematological effects, although not uncommon, were usually mild. There are no late toxicity data in any of these trials, although in an as-yet-unpublished British trial, there were no differences in numbers of fractures after treatment or the rate of paraplegia developing from a treated area.[13a]

RE-IRRADIATION

Once radiotherapy has been used to treat a bone metastasis, can it be used again? The physician who believes that re-irradiation is not often possible may not refer patients who might benefit from further radiotherapy back to the radiation oncologist. Bone is comparatively tolerant of the effects of radiation, and in radical treatments, doses of 60 to 70 Gy can be used. Although the biological effects of the more rapidly given 20- to 30-Gy irradiation regimens used in palliation are greater than those of the same doses used as part of a radical treatment, there is usually scope for at least one re-treatment without any risk of complication. The therapeutic effect of the second course may not be as great as that of the initial treatment, however, so if the first course achieved only minimal pain relief, other options may be more appropriate.

PATHOLOGICAL FRACTURES

One of the complications of bone metastases is the development of a pathological fracture through an affected area of bone, especially the long bones of the arm and leg. The indications for surgical intervention to prevent fracture in an at-risk limb are described elsewhere in this book (see Chapters 7-16 and 7-18), but radiotherapy has also been used to prevent pathological fractures. In addition, after surgical correction, most patients should receive postoperative radiotherapy to the involved bone. Although the benefit of radiotherapy in relieving bone pain is well established, the effectiveness of this treatment in preserving structural integrity and preventing or delaying fractures through at-risk lesions is less clear. For example, two studies of metastatic breast cancer in the femur noted that although radiotherapy to lytic bone metastases gave rates of pain relief of 70% to 81%, the radiographic reossification rates were only 17% to 31%.[14, 15] One of these studies, however, noted that of 59 patients who presented with nonfractured lesions in the humerus, only 4 had a subsequent pathological fracture. Two fractures occurred during the time of radiation, and those were the only fractures in a group of 39 patients who were classified as being at high risk for fracture according to the criteria of Beals et al.[16] The authors of this study concluded that radiotherapy is effective initial management of patients with long-bone metastases from breast cancer and that surgical prophylaxis is usually not warranted.[15] Nevertheless, it would seem prudent for both a radiation oncologist and an orthopaedic surgeon to assess patients thought to be at risk for pathological fracture.

Customarily, after surgical fixation, patients receive "adjuvant" radiation (Fig. 2). Although this practice seems intuitively sensible, its value has never been demonstrated. In addition, a wide range of different fractionation regimens are employed, usually derived from the treatment prescriptions more commonly used for pain. Whether short

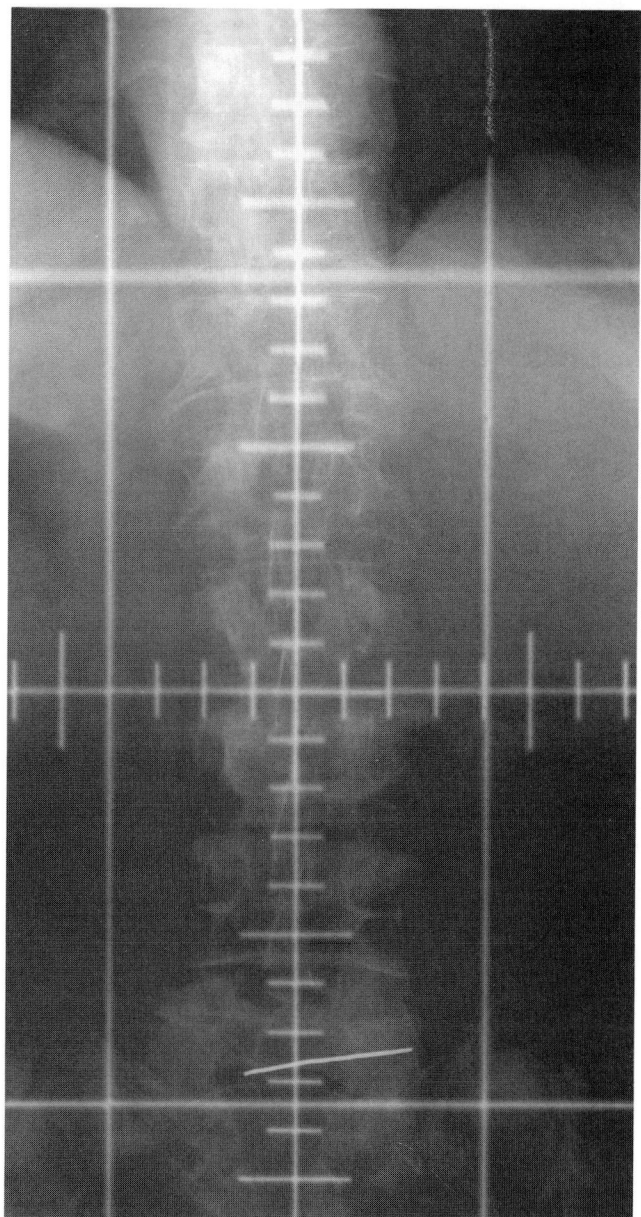

Fig. 2. Simulator radiograph. It shows a treatment field for radiation therapy following surgical fixation of a pathological fracture of the femur.

one- or two-fraction treatment regimens are as effective as longer courses in producing reossification is currently unknown. It is also quite possible that there may be a subset of patients, perhaps those who are completely ambulatory and pain free after surgery, who may not require additional radiation, especially if they have a poor prognosis from the underlying malignancy (e.g., lung cancer).

SYSTEMIC THERAPY

Traditionally, bone metastases have been thought to respond poorly to systemic anticancer therapies, although this belief probably reflects the insensitivity of response assess-

TABLE 2. UNION INTERNATIONALE CENTRE DE CANCER (UICC) CRITERIA FOR ASSESSMENT OF RESPONSE IN BONE METASTASES	
Complete response	Complete disappearance of all lesions on radiograph for at least 4 weeks.
Partial response	Partial decrease in size of lytic lesions, recalcification of lytic lesions, or decreased density in blastic lesions. No new lesions appearing.
No change	No change in number or size of lesions for at least 8 weeks.
Progressive disease	Increase in the size of existing lesions or appearance of new lesions.

ment more than true resistance to treatment. The Union Internationale Centre de Cancer (UICC) criteria rely on radiographic responses (Table 2), yet patients report significant symptom improvement without any demonstrable radiographic changes. In hormonally influenced diseases, such as prostate and breast cancers, the response to endocrine therapy can be significant. In other situations, chemotherapy can be of value, whereas bisphosphonates, although not having known specific anticancer actions, have been shown to significantly benefit patients with myeloma and breast cancer by delaying the onset of skeletally related events, such as pathological fractures, hypercalcemia, and radiation treatments.[17]

ANTINEOPLASTIC THERAPY
Endocrine Therapy

In the patient with breast cancer whose original tumor demonstrated the presence of receptors for estrogen, progesterone, or both, there is a good chance that metastases will respond to hormonal manipulations, particularly if the patient has had a long disease-free interval and the metastatic disease is predominantly skeletal rather than visceral. Tamoxifen, an antiestrogen, is usually the first choice, but patients who experience relapse after their disease responds to first-line therapy can have significant responses to second- or third-line treatment, such as with an aromatase inhibitor (anastrozole) or a progestagen (megestrol acetate). Response rates of up to 70% have been reported,[18] but in practice, the levels of symptomatic benefit may be greater (see earlier).

Prostate cancer is also a hormonally sensitive tumor, and up to 80% of patients experience some response to endocrine therapy.[18a] Orchiectomy has long been the preferred first-line treatment, but the introduction of luteinizing hormone–releasing hormone antagonists such as leuprolide has led many patients to opt for this therapy rather than undergo surgical castration. However, unlike breast cancer, prostate tumors relapsing after first-line hormonal therapy respond poorly to subsequent endocrine therapy.

Chemotherapy

Chemotherapy does not result in radiographic improvement in bone metastases in the vast majority of cases, response rates being as low as 0.[20] Research has therefore concen-

trated on assessing its value in producing symptomatic benefit. There is now evidence that if the appropriate end points are used (pain relief, consumption of analgesics, quality of life), chemotherapy may be beneficial to some patients. The preponderance of evidence comes from studies of patients with breast cancer, but perhaps the best-designed trial was that conducted in Toronto in patients with hormone-resistant prostate cancer, and skeletal metastases, traditionally a group of patients who are not thought to benefit from systemic therapy. The study showed that 29% of patients treated with a combination of mitoxantrone and prednisone had responses in terms of a decrease in pain without an increase in analgesic requirement, with a median duration of effect of 43 weeks.[19] However, in other solid tumors, such as non–small cell lung cancer and bowel cancers, chemotherapy appears to be of limited value in the treatment of bone metastases.

Bisphosphonates

Bisphosphonates, such as clodronate and pamidronate, are potent inhibitors of osteoclastic bone resorption and have been standard therapy for the treatment of malignant hypercalcemia for many years. Studies have now focused on their potential benefit in preventing skeletal complications of malignant disease. These agents appear to be most effective in lytic rather than sclerotic bone disease. Randomized trials have accordingly demonstrated these agents to have benefit in patients with myelomatosis and metastatic breast cancer,[17, 21] through reducing the proportion of and delaying time to the development of skeletal events. Further research is going on to evaluate their effectiveness in bone metastases from other primary tumors, especially prostate cancer, for which early results are promising despite the fact that bone metastases from prostate cancer are usually sclerotic.[22] Currently, both clodronate and pamidronate are administered intravenously (the oral clodronate form, although available, is unpredictably absorbed). As newer, more potent, and better-absorbed agents of this type are being developed, it is likely that these drugs will be increasingly used in the management of skeletal metastases.

ANALGESIA

Bone metastases are often but not invariably painful. In many cases, the pain is only mild and can be effectively controlled with oral analgesics. In particular nonsteroidal anti-inflammatory drugs (NSAIDs) can be very effective, probably owing to their antiprostaglandin action. If bone pain cannot be controlled by NSAIDs alone, the additional use of opioids, together with a referral for radiation therapy, is recommended. If pain relief from radiotherapy is only partial, or if the radiotherapy is not possible, long-term opioid therapy may be needed. The initial use of long-acting analgesics, such as slow-release morphine (usually 30 mg orally q12h), initially is preferred, with shorter-acting agents (e.g., morphine sulfate, hydromorphone) used for "breakthrough" pain, as required. NSAIDs may still be useful for patients taking opioids, but for patients with difficult pain problems, such as the neuropathic pain often seen with nerve root involvement, other coanalgesics, such as corticosteroids and antidepressants, can be beneficial.

REFERENCES

1. Foley KM: Analgesic management of bone pain. In Weiss (ed): Bone Metastasis. Boston, Hall, 1981, p 348.
2. Tong D, Gillick L, Hendrickson F: The palliation of symptomatic osseous metastases: Final results of the study by the radiation oncology group. Cancer 1982; 50:893.
3. Blitzer P: Reanalysis of the RTOG study of the palliation of symptomatic osseous metastasis. Cancer 1985; 55:1468.
4. Mackillop WJ: The principles of palliative radiotherapy: A radiation oncologist's perspective. Can J Oncol 1996; 6:5.
5. Paterson R: The Treatment of Malignant Disease by Radium and X-Rays. London, Edward Arnold, 1948.
6. Fletcher G: A Textbook of Radiotherapy. Philadelphia, Lea & Febiger, 1966.
7. Kirkbride P, Mackillop WJ, Priestman TJ, et al: The role of palliative radiotherapy for bone metastases. Can J Oncol 1996; 6: 33.
8. Kirkbride P, Warde P, Panzarella A, et al: A randomised trial comparing the efficacy and safety of single fraction radiation therapy plus ondansetron with fractionated radiation therapy in the palliation of skeletal metastases. Int J Radiat Oncol Biol Phys 2000; 48:147.
9. Price P, Hoskin P, Easton D, et al: Prospective randomised trial of single and multifraction radiotherapy schedules in the treatment of painful bony metastases. Radiother Oncol 1986; 6:247.
10. Niewald M, Tkocz H-J, Abel U, et al: Rapid course radiation therapy vs. more standard treatment: A randomized trial for bone metastases. Int J Radiat Oncol Biol Phys 1996; 36:1085.
11. Nielsen OS, Bentzen SM, Sandberg E, et al: Randomized trial of single dose versus fractionated palliative radiotherapy of bone metastases. Radiother Oncol 1998; 47:233.
12. Ratanatharathorn V, Powers WE, Moss WT, et al: Bone metastasis: Review and critical analysis of random allocation trials of local field treatment. Int J Radiat Oncol Biol Phys 1999; 44:1.
13. Zelefsky MJ, Scher HI, Forman JD, et al: Palliative hemiskeletal irradiation for widespread metastatic prostate cancer: A comparison of single dose and fractionated regimens. Int J Radiat Oncol Biol Phys 1989; 17:1281.
13a. Peat I, Spooner D, Hardwick M, et al: The Birmingham-Leicester Pain Study. Clin Oncol 2000; 12:328.
14. Keene JS, Sellinger DS, McBeath AA, et al: Metastatic breast cancer in the femur: A search for the lesion at risk of fracture. Clin Orthop 1986; 203:282.
15. Cheng DS, Seitz CB, Eyre HJ: Nonoperative management of femoral, humeral, and acetabular metastases in patients with breast carcinoma. Cancer 1980; 45:1533.
16. Beals RK, Lawton GD, Snell WE: Prophylactic internal fixation of the femur in metastatic breast cancer. Cancer 1971; 28: 1350.
17. Hortobagyi GN, Theriault RL, Lipton A, et al: Long-term prevention of skeletal complications of metastatic breast cancer with pamidronate: Protocol 19 Aredia Breast Cancer Study Group. J Clin Oncol 1998; 16:2038.
18. Muss HB: Endocrine therapy for advanced breast cancer: A review. Breast Cancer Res Treat 1992; 21:15.
18a. Huggins C, Stevens R, Hodges C: Studies on prostatic cancer: The effects of castration on advanced carcinoma of the prostate gland. Arch Surg 1941; 43:209.
19. Tannock IF, Osoba D, Stockler MR, et al: Chemotherapy with mitoxantrone plus prednisone or prednisone alone for symptomatic hormone-resistant prostate cancer: A Canadian randomized trial with palliative end points. J Clin Oncol 1996; 14: 1756.
20. Whitehouse J: Site-dependent response to chemotherapy for carcinoma of the breast. J R Soc Med 1985; 78:18.
21. Berenson JR, Lichtenstein A, Porter L, et al: Long-term pamidronate treatment of advanced multiple myeloma patients reduces skeletal events: Myeloma Aredia Study Group. J Clin Oncol 1998; 16:593.
22. Papopoulos SE, Handy NA, van der Plujim G: Bisphosphonates in the management of prostate carcinoma metastatic to the skeleton. Cancer 2000; 88:3047.

section
7
chapter
15

SURGICAL MANAGEMENT OF THE SPINE

J. Dominic Femino and James D. Bruckner

Summary
- Symptomatic metastatic disease of the spine occurs in approximately 5% of patients with cancer, or 18,000 patients annually in the United States.[1]
- Most patients with metastatic spine disease do not require surgical intervention and are best managed with nonoperative modalities, including chemotherapy, hormonal therapy, radiation therapy, and steroids.
- The goals of surgical treatment are to control pain, prevent or improve neurologic deficits, allow mobility, and maintain the highest possible quality of life.
- Indications for surgery include spinal instability, progressive neurologic deficit, failure of radiotherapy, need for a tissue diagnosis, and intractable pain.
- Contraindications for surgery include short life expectancy (generally less than 3 to 6 months), generally poor medical status (with special attention to immunologic and nutritional states), multiple areas of epidural compression, and inadequate bone stock.
- The surgical approach and reconstruction depend on several variables, including the location and nature of the tumor in the individual patient as well as the surgeon's experience and familiarity with various instrumentation systems and techniques.

The spine is the most frequent site of skeletal metastases.[2, 3] In the United States, symptomatic spinal metastases occur in 5% of patients with a malignancy, or approximately 18,000 patients per year.[1] If asymptomatic spinal metastases are included, the incidence is several times higher. An overall spinal metastatic rate of 36% was found in autopsy cases of 832 patients dying from neoplastic disease.[4] Twenty-six percent of the lesions were not detectable radiographically but were confirmed histologically.

A variety of primary malignancies can metastasize to the spine. Among those most likely are carcinoma of the breast, lung, prostate or kidney, and myeloma or lymphoma. In a review of 10 published studies comprising 1477 patients with spinal epidural metastases, Brihaye et al[5] found the following occurrence for primary tumors: breast, 16.5% of patients; lung, 15.5%; prostate, 9.2%; kidney, 6.5%; gastrointestinal, 4.6%; thyroid, 3.6%; hematosarcoma, 10.8%; miscellaneous, 20.5%; and unknown, 12.5%. In women, breast carcinoma has been reported to account for up to 54% of symptomatic spinal metastases.[6]

On the basis of autopsy studies, spinal metastasis is most frequent in the lumbar spine and least frequent in the cervical spine.[7] However, symptomatic vertebral metastases are much more common in the thoracic and thoracolumbar spine. In a review of 1585 cases of symptomatic metastatic spinal tumors, Brihaye et al[5] found that 70.3% localized to the thoracic and thoracolumbar spine, 21.6% to the lumbar and sacral spine, and 8.1% to the cervical spine. Metastases in the thoracic spine may become symptomatic earlier because of epidural compression and the relatively small space available to the cord. The normally kyphotic thoracic spine may make pathological fracture more likely than in the lordotic lumbar and cervical spine.[8]

Advances in medical management of metastatic cancer have lengthened patient survival, making surgical intervention for spinal metastases more useful as a means of preserving quality of life. Historically, palliative posterior decompression has yielded no better results than radiation alone for neurological compromise. With advances in radiological imaging, surgical technique, and spinal instrumentation, spinal metastases can be resected en bloc and spinal stability reliably restored. However, there remains a lack of uniformity in surgical approach, resection and reconstruction technique, and indications for surgical intervention in these complex patients.

Despite advances in the surgical treatment of metastatic disease of the spine, the surgeon should keep in mind that most patients do not require surgical intervention. A multidisciplinary approach should be used in the treatment of these patients, with participation of a medical oncologist, radiation oncologist, neurosurgeon, and orthopaedic surgeon. Most patients can be treated with a combination of radiation therapy, chemotherapy, hormonal therapy, and steroids. Successful operative treatment requires good clinical judgment and appropriate patient selection.

PATHOGENESIS

A detailed account of the pathogenesis of skeletal metastases is described in Chapter 7–13. However, some special considerations regarding the spine should be emphasized. The vertebral bodies are particularly susceptible to metastatic deposits because of the epidural venous plexus of Batson.[9] The plexus is a collection of valveless vessels that allow bidirectional flow. Batson suggested that increased intra-abdominal or intrathoracic pressure diverts venous flow into the epidural space from the pelvic or azygous systems and into the vertebral trabecular system. Thus, metastatic emboli are deposited anteriorly in the vertebral bodies.

Spinal deformity and neural compromise are preceded by replacement of marrow elements and bony trabeculae of the vertebral body with neoplastic tissue. If there is enough trabecular destruction, the vertebral end plates collapse. At end-stage collapse, the posterior wall of the vertebral body is retropulsed, compromising the spinal canal. Asdourian et al[10] classified patterns of vertebral body collapse, finding localized kyphotic deformities in the thoracic spine and symmetric vertebral body collapse in the cervical and lumbar spine. Direct extension of the neoplasm from the vertebral body into the spinal canal also may cause neurological compromise. Neurological symptoms may develop acutely or over many weeks.

CLINICAL FEATURES

Spinal metastases may present with various clinical signs and symptoms. Pain is by far the predominant symptom, occurring in up to 96% of symptomatic patients.[11] It is usually well localized and unremitting. It may be progressive and may occur at night. There may not be a clear association with activities, as is characteristic of mechanical back pain. In one study, radicular symptoms were noted in 65%, and motor weakness was a presenting symptom in 76% of patients, including 17% who were paraplegic. Half of the patients reported numbness or paresthesias. No patients reported bowel and bladder dysfunction as an initial symptom, but 57% were found to have this symptom on initial evaluation.[11] Constans et al[6] found isolated bowel and bladder dysfunction as a presenting complaint in only 2% of 600 patients.

Three predominant patterns of symptom progression have been described.[6] In 30% of patients, symptoms occur acutely with rapid progression to maximal neurological deficit within 48 hours. Sixty percent show subacute neurological deterioration over 7 to 10 days. Symptoms develop insidiously over a 4- to 6-month period in 10% of patients.

Clinical features may vary depending on the level of spine involvement. Encroachment on cervical nerve roots produces radicular symptoms in the upper extremity. Focal weakness and hyporeflexia in the arms represent damage to the anterior horn cells and peripheral roots in the cervical region. Lower extremity signs may be insidious and include spasticity, hyperreflexia, and a positive Babinski's sign. These signs and symptoms may also be present in the patient with degenerative disease and stenosis of the cervical spine.

Thoracic metastases may present with localized pain that progresses to radicular pain with perithoracic or periabdominal dysesthesias or hypoesthesia. Localized sensory loss may progress to sensory loss below the level of the lesion, with spasticity and hyperreflexia in the legs. Later, weakness develops in the lower extremities, with hyperreflexia and dorsiflexion of the toes (Babinski's sign) completing the clinical picture. Bladder and bowel involvement occurs in association with paraplegia.

Metastatic lesions involving the lumbosacral vertebrae may cause epidural compression of the cauda equina, resulting in saddle anesthesia and loss of bowel and bladder control.

Examination should include a thorough history and a detailed neurological examination. Localized tenderness should be assessed by palpation and percussion at all levels. Complete motor and sensory testing should be performed. Spasticity, clonus, and hyperreflexia indicate a lesion above the level of the conus medullaris. A rectal examination should be performed on all patients suspected

of having metastatic disease of the spine, and a postvoiding residual urine volume should be measured in those suspected of having bladder dysfunction.

INVESTIGATION

Preoperative imaging studies should begin with plain radiographs in anteroposterior and lateral views. Any lytic lesion visualized on plain radiographs should raise the suspicion of metastatic disease. Blastic lesions should raise the suspicion of metastatic breast or prostate carcinoma. Finally, patients with vertebral body collapse, particularly at multiple levels, should be suspected of having metastatic disease; however, up to 70% of a vertebral body may be destroyed before bony metastases are visible on plain radiographs.[12]

Total body technetium 99m bone scans are a useful screening tool to determine the presence or absence of multiple bony lesions in the spine and remainder of the skeleton. They are used frequently as a staging study in patients to rule out the presence of metastatic carcinoma.[13] The shortcoming of bone scans is that they are nonspecific and will yield positive results for a multitude of benign pathological processes. They also poorly demonstrate specific anatomic details.

Myelography is useful in detecting epidural spinal metastases. Computed tomographic (CT) myelography is useful in detecting central and foraminal sites of compression. The disadvantages of myelography are that it is an invasive procedure and carries the risks of dural puncture, local bleeding complications, acute neurological deterioration, and contrast toxicity. However, in the patient with previous spinal surgery, myelography is an extremely valuable modality because images are not degraded by artifact from preexisting hardware.

Magnetic resonance imaging (MRI) is the most valuable imaging modality in evaluating spinal metastases. MRI most reliably shows the anatomic location and extent of tumor involvement. MRI is superior in defining the soft-tissue extent of tumor and in visualizing compression around the spinal cord and nerve roots. It is also valuable in detecting metastatic abnormalities in the bone marrow of the vertebral bodies. Anatomy and tumor location can be assessed more effectively with direct axial, coronal, and sagittal images. We recommend MRI scans for all patients suspected of having metastatic spinal disease. A limited sagittal screening MRI of the entire spine can be obtained quickly and is relatively inexpensive. More detailed studies can then be carried out at abnormal sites as indicated.

Blood studies are useful as both diagnostic tests to determine the primary site of a metastatic tumor and as an adjunct to assess the patient's acceptability as a surgical candidate. Diagnostic blood studies should include prostate-specific antigen for prostate carcinoma, carcinoembryonic antigen for colon, pancreas, breast, lung, and ovarian cancer, and serum protein electrophoresis for multiple myeloma. Other studies include a complete blood count, calcium, phosphorus, alkaline phosphatase, blood urea nitrogen, serum creatinine, total protein, albumin, and transferrin.

Patients with extensive bone marrow replacement from skeletal metastases or with myelosuppression from chemotherapy or radiation therapy may have pancytopenia. Hypercalcemia or hypocalcemia may be present in patients with metastatic cancer and should be corrected preoperatively. A patient's general nutritional status should be optimized before surgery. Serum albumin and transferrin are good indicators of nutritional status and should be checked preoperatively and monitored closely after any major operation.

GOALS, INDICATIONS, AND CONTRAINDICATIONS

The goals of surgical management of metastatic disease of the spine are to (1) control pain that cannot be successfully managed by nonoperative means, (2) prevent neurological deficits or improve an existing neurological deficit, (3) stabilize the spine and allow mobility, and (4) allow the patient to enjoy the highest possible quality of remaining life. With these goals in mind, one must consider indications and contraindications to surgical intervention very carefully. The patient's overall medical status must be considered carefully when deciding whether surgery is an appropriate means of management. The risks of surgery and length of recovery should be weighed against the patient's general health, quality of life, and expected survival. Generally, patients with an expected survival less than 3 months are more appropriately managed by medical means.[14] Patient age is another factor to be considered. Elderly patients are generally less likely to tolerate large surgical procedures well. Patients with four or more separate levels of tumor involvement are generally less likely to benefit from surgical intervention and are probably better treated by medical means.[15] Bone density is a consideration because patients with severe osteopenia may be unable to support internal fixation for spinal stabilization. Finally, the degree of mechanical and neurological instability should be estimated. This is often difficult to assess. Several classification schemes may assist in making this determination.

The most widely used classification system was developed by Harrington.[16] Harrington's system classifies patients based on their neurological stability and mechanical stability as predictors of the need for surgical intervention. Harrington's five classes are as follows: I, no significant neurological involvement; II, bony involvement by tumor without collapse or bony instability; III, neurological involvement without bony involvement; IV, painful bony collapse without significant neurological compromise; V, bony collapse and associated significant neurological compromise. Harrington recommended that class I, II, and III patients be treated by nonoperative means and that class IV and V patients are more appropriately treated with an operation.

Kostuik and Weinstein[17] devised a system to predict mechanical instability by dividing the vertebral body into six zones of potential tumor involvement. Each vertebra is divided into anterior, middle, and posterior columns and left and right sides. Lesions involving three or more zones may result in mechanical instability and are suitable for surgical intervention. Lesions involving five or six zones are considered to be severely unstable.

Tokuhashi et al[18] proposed a scoring system using six categories to help determine whether a patient is a good candidate for surgery: general condition, number of vertebral metastases, metastases to internal organs, extraspinal bone metastases, primary site, and severity of neurological compromise. Each category carries a score of 0, 1, or 2, with a maximum possible score of 12. They propose that patients with a score less than 5 are more appropriate for palliative surgery and that patients with a score of 9 to 12 are more appropriate for excisional surgery.

Although authors vary in their indications for an operation, principles that are widely accepted[19] as surgical indications for metastatic disease of the spine are as follows:

1. Intractable pain unresponsive to nonoperative measures such as bracing and radiotherapy.
2. Progressive neurological changes during or after radiotherapy.
3. The presence of a radioresistant tumor.
4. The need for a specimen to make a histological diagnosis.
5. Decompression of the neural elements with debulking of the tumor mass.
6. Spinal instability or major destruction of vertebral bone architecture.

PROCEDURES

Advances in surgical techniques for stabilizing the spine and improved survival with various therapies have made more aggressive surgical intervention possible. We believe that a wide margin of resection should be the goal of surgical tumor resection, even for metastatic disease, because this often affords the best relief of pain and leaves "normal" bone for anchoring hardware, implants, and bone graft. The proximity of neural and vascular structures may not allow true wide margins, but a true wide margin is ideal.

Usually, metastatic disease is located in the vertebral bodies. Surgical resection should, therefore, be done anteriorly to provide complete decompression. Posterior laminectomy alone may not provide adequate decompression and may result in increased instability. Combined anterior and posterior procedures may be necessary if anterior decompression is not satisfactory or if posterior stabilization is needed as an adjunct to anterior resection and stabilization. In a review of patients treated with anterior or posterior decompression, Weinstein and McLain[23] found that patients treated with anterior decompression had a 78% mean neurological improvement rate and those treated with posterior decompression had a 33% neurological improvement rate.

BIOPSY

The need for diagnostic tissue to confirm the presence of metastatic disease or as the initial diagnostic procedure for a bony spinal lesion with an unknown primary tumor is, in itself, an indication for surgical intervention. Biopsy may also assist the medical oncologist by obtaining tissue for hormonal receptor evaluation. There are two primary means by which tissue can be obtained: percutaneous needle biopsy and open biopsy.

Percutaneous needle biopsy has been advanced by the use of CT scans to guide the placement of the biopsy needle. A large-bore needle should be used whenever possible to obtain a core of tissue. Alternatively, a fine needle may be used to aspirate malignant cells. All levels of the spine may be reached, although needle placement is more difficult in the cervical and thoracic spine. The overall accuracy rate in obtaining diagnostic tissue varies in the literature from 75%[20] to 95%.[21] In a large review of more than 9500 percutaneous biopsy procedures, Murphy and Gilula[22] reported an overall complication rate of 0.2%. There were two deaths, and four patients had permanent neurological damage. Overall, the use of percutaneous biopsy is becoming increasingly effective and is more easily tolerated by the patient compared with open biopsy.

Open biopsy is used when a tissue diagnosis cannot be obtained percutaneously. The selection of the surgical approach should be that of a potential future definitive operation. A posterior approach is used for lesions in the posterior spinal elements. Open biopsy of lesions in the vertebral bodies can be done through a transpedicular approach or through a costotransversectomy. Biopsies can be safely taken from cervical body lesions through an anterior approach. When there is a significant soft-tissue component to the lesion, this tissue should be obtained as the primary specimen. If this is not diagnostic, a trephine may be used to take bony specimens. Intraoperative frozen sections should be obtained to ensure that the tissue is diagnostic, and the surgeon should confirm with the pathologist that there is an adequate amount of tissue to perform the necessary stains and immunocytochemical studies. All biopsy lesions also should be cultured for aerobic, anaerobic, and fungal and acid-fast bacilli.

CERVICAL SPINE

The cervical spine is the least common region of the spine for metastatic disease, but several approaches to cervical resection have been described. In the past, transoral and submandibular approaches were popular. However, the transoral approach introduces the risk of infection. More useful alternative extraoral approaches include the prevascular extraoral, retrovascular extraoral, far lateral, transclival transcervical, anterior retropharyngeal, and anterolateral approaches. We prefer an extensile modification of these approaches that potentially allows access to the ventral spine from the clivus to C7.

The procedure is performed supine with continuous somatosensory evoked potential monitoring. While the patient is awake, Gardner-Wells tongs are applied with 10 pounds of traction. The neck is then extended as far as possible as determined by the patient's symptoms and changes in cortical evoked potentials.

Fiberoptic nasotracheal intubation is performed with the patient awake. General anesthesia then is administered. If only the submandibular portion of the incision is to be used, it may be made on the right side if the surgeon is right-handed. If the inferior extension of the incision is to be used, the incision is best made on the left side to avoid injury to the recurrent laryngeal nerve. A transverse submandibular incision is made, extended posterior to the angle of the mandible, and then directed in a gentle curve lateral to the posterior border of the sternocleidomastoid (Fig. 1). From there, the incision extends distally to approximately the midcervical spine and then curves anteri-

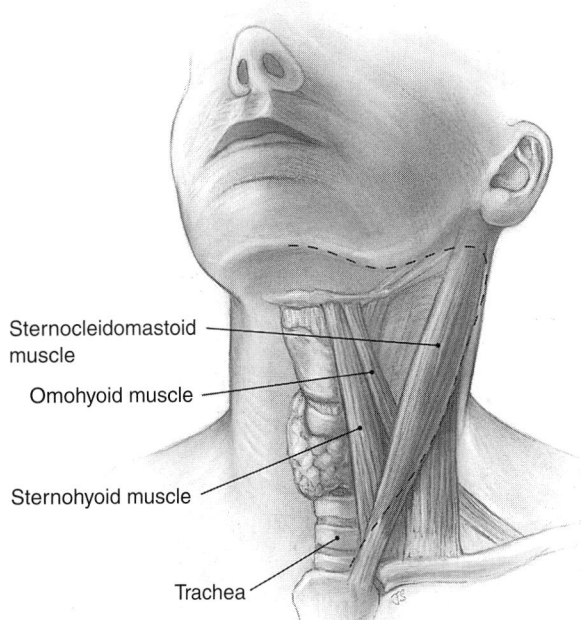

Fig. 1. Skin incision and anatomic landmarks for an extensile approach to the anterior cervical spine. In general, the submandibular portion of the incision is reserved for exposure of the clivus and first cervical vertebra. (From Simon MA, Springfield D: Surgery for Bone and Soft-Tissue Tumors. Philadelphia, Lippincott-Raven, 1998, p 437.)

orly, crossing the clavicle and ending in the suprasternal notch. Large medial and lateral flaps of skin and platysma are created, exposing the sternocleidomastoid and strap muscles as well as the pharynx, thyroid gland, edge of mandible, and submaxillary fossa. The anterior border of the sternocleidomastoid muscle is mobilized throughout its length. The omohyoid muscle is identified deep to the sternocleidomastoid muscle and transected. The mandibular branch of the facial nerve is identified and protected. The middle layer of cervical fascia is then identified and incised medial to the carotid sheath. This enables visualization of the trachea and the thyroid gland.

The hypoglossal nerve is identified, using a nerve stimulator if necessary, and completely mobilized. Once this nerve is identified, the stylohyoid and digastric muscles can be divided safely and reflected. The superior laryngeal neurovascular bundle can then be identified. The dissection then proceeds superiorly above the level of C3. At this point, the various branches of the internal carotid artery (superior thyroid, lingual, ascending pharyngeal, and facial) with their accompanying veins need to be ligated to allow progressive mobilization of the carotid sheath laterally. The superior laryngeal nerve is fully mobilized and protected. Superior retraction in the submaxillary triangle places the facial nerve at risk and should be controlled carefully. If superior visualization is inadequate, the temporomandibular joint may be dislocated anteriorly (Fig. 2).

The prevertebral fascia is incised, exposing the longus colli muscles. These may be reflected laterally to expose the transverse processes and the vertebral artery. The exposure must enable visualization of the upper, lower, and

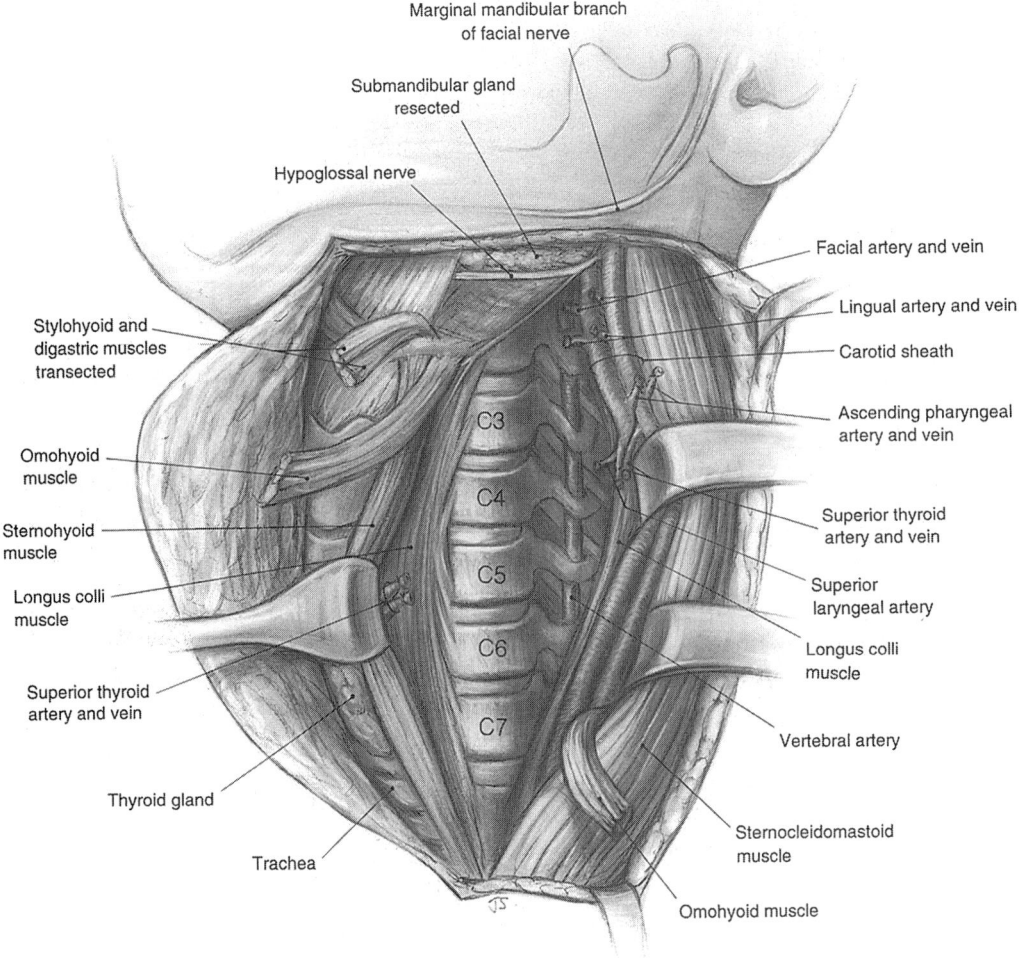

Fig. 2. Exposure of the anterior cervical spine after mobilization of the sternocleidomastoid and strap muscles, and the pharynx and thyroid gland. If wider exposure of the first two cervical vertebrae is desired, then the submaxillary gland may be resected and the mandible subluxed anteriorly. (From Simon MA, Springfield D: Surgery for Bone and Soft-Tissue Tumors. Philadelphia, Lippincott-Raven, 1998, p 438.)

lateral extents of the tumor mass. Vertebral resection is accomplished by diskectomy at levels above and below the lesion, followed by careful dissection through the transverse processes or vertebral body using a power bur or curet and Kerrison's rongeurs. Injury to the vertebral arteries in the transverse foramen must be avoided. If the tumor involves a vertebral artery, preoperative arteriography and a vertebral occlusion test to assess cerebral collateral circulation should be performed. If collateral circulation is adequate, unilateral vertebral artery embolization and sacrifice may allow more complete tumor resection. Reconstruction is typically performed with structural autograft or allograft recessed into normal vertebral bone above and below (Fig. 3). It may be augmented with rigid internal fixation using a low-profile anterior cervical spine plate. Interbody titanium cages, filled with allograft or autograft, also may be used in the reconstruction of anterior segmental defects. Polymethylmethacrylate may be used as an augmentation to bone grafting if the bone quality is poor.

If additional stabilization is required, posterior cervical fusion with instrumentation may be performed. In the

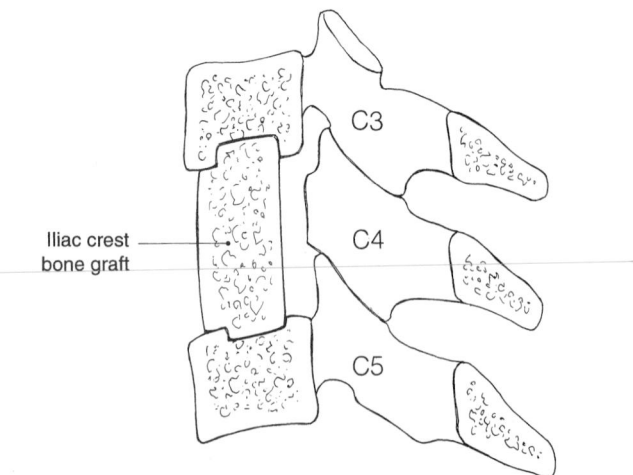

Fig. 3. A tricortical autograft iliac crest graft or an appropriately sized allograft used to reconstruct the vertebral defect. Care is taken to inset the graft slightly into the normal vertebral end plate above and below the resection. (From Simon MA, Springfield D: Surgery for Bone and Soft-Tissue Tumors. Philadelphia, Lippincott-Raven, 1998, p 439.)

prone position, a standard posterior midline incision is used to expose the posterior elements at the appropriate levels. A high-speed bur is used to decorticate the bone, and bone graft is applied. Stabilization is performed with lateral mass plates and screws or with wiring techniques.

Rigid stabilization is one of the goals of surgical intervention so that the patient may be mobilized as quickly as possible. Usually, we protect the patient in a rigid cervical collar for 6 to 12 weeks and monitor the fusion radiographically.[24]

THORACIC SPINE

Posterior decompression and stabilization alone for metastatic disease of the thoracic spine have limited utility. Anterior decompression and stabilization provide superior access to the vertebral bodies, facilitating removal of the diseased segment. The anterior approach generally is a superior means of accessing the thoracic spine for purposes of vertebral body resection and reconstruction.

The patient is secured in a lateral decubitus position with an axillary roll. We use somatosensory evoked potential monitoring throughout the procedure. An oblique incision is used over the rib of the involved vertebral body. The serratus anterior and latissimus dorsi are mobilized or split to access the rib. The periosteum over the rib is divided, and the rib resected to facilitate access to the vertebral body. Sometimes more than one rib needs to be resected. The lung is deflated or retracted to visualize the vertebral bodies and adjacent vessels. The parietal pleura is divided longitudinally, and the intercostal vessels are dissected and ligated at the levels of planned resection. The disk spaces superior and inferior to the involved vertebral body are identified with the assistance of radiography. These disks are excised. A corpectomy is performed with the use of rongeurs, curets, and a high-speed bur. Extreme care should be taken to protect the spinal cord posteriorly. Epidural bleeding is controlled with bipolar cautery and thrombin-soaked pledgets. Every effort should be made to achieve a complete resection of the metastatic tumor (Fig. 4), keeping in mind that the proximity of neural and vascular structures makes a truly wide resection impossible.

Reconstruction is achieved with structural autograft, allograft, interbody titanium cages, or methylmethacrylate. Structural allograft and autograft should be notched or doweled into holes created with a burr in the superior and inferior normal vertebral bodies. Titanium cages packed with allograft or autograft are secured into position, with the irregular metallic mesh at each end impacted into the normal vertebral bodies. Methylmethacrylate can be used around Steinmann's pins or metal rods doweled into holes in the superior and inferior normal vertebral bodies. Anterior instrumentation has been improved to provide additional stabilization if needed. Vertebral body screws and longitudinal rod systems can provide rigid fixation if bone stock is adequate. Anterior instrumentation may preclude the use of posterior instrumentation and fusion.

However, posterior instrumentation may be used as an adjunct to the anterior procedure. In the prone position, a standard midline approach is used to visualize the posterior elements, including the costotransverse processes. Posterior instrumentation with one of a number of rod systems with pedicle and laminar hooks can be used to stabilize the

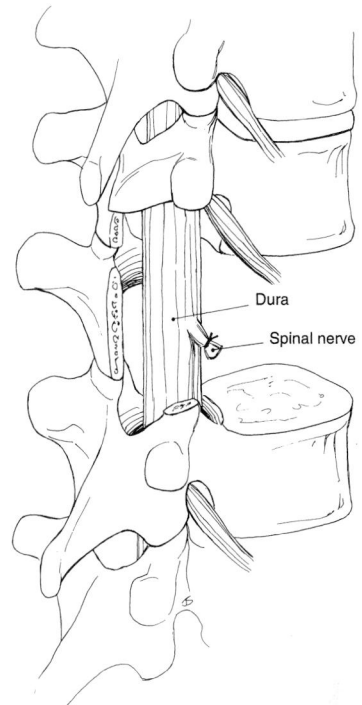

Fig. 4. Completed tumor resection. Reconstruction can now proceed. (From Simon MA, Springfield D: Surgery for Bone and Soft-Tissue Tumors. Philadelphia, Lippincott-Raven, 1998, p 443.)

spine posteriorly. Decortication is performed with a high-speed bur and allograft, or autograft is used to encourage fusion.

In almost all cases, we have been able to obtain rigid fixation with anterior, posterior, or combined procedures. Rigid stabilization allows immediate mobilization of the patient without the use of an external orthotic device.

LUMBAR SPINE

Metastatic lesions in the lumbar spine are usually approached by a retroperitoneal dissection from the left side, which avoids the liver. The patient is placed in a lateral position on the operating table. An oblique incision between the iliac crest and the 12th rib is made from the rectus abdominis anteriorly and may be extended posteriorly as far as the midline if necessary. The external oblique, internal oblique, and transversus abdominis muscles are split in line with the incision. This exposes the peritoneal fascia, which, with its contents, is elevated anteriorly by blunt dissection. Blunt dissection is extended medially until the great vessels and lumbar fascia are exposed. The femoral nerve, the genitofemoral nerve, and sympathetic chain should be identified and protected. The lumbar fascia is divided longitudinally, and the segmental vessels are ligated at the necessary levels.

When exposure is needed as low as the L5 and S1 bodies, a midline transperitoneal approach may be easier. In the supine position with the table flexed, a midline incision is made from the umbilicus to the symphysis pubis. The rectus abdominis and peritoneal fascia are divided

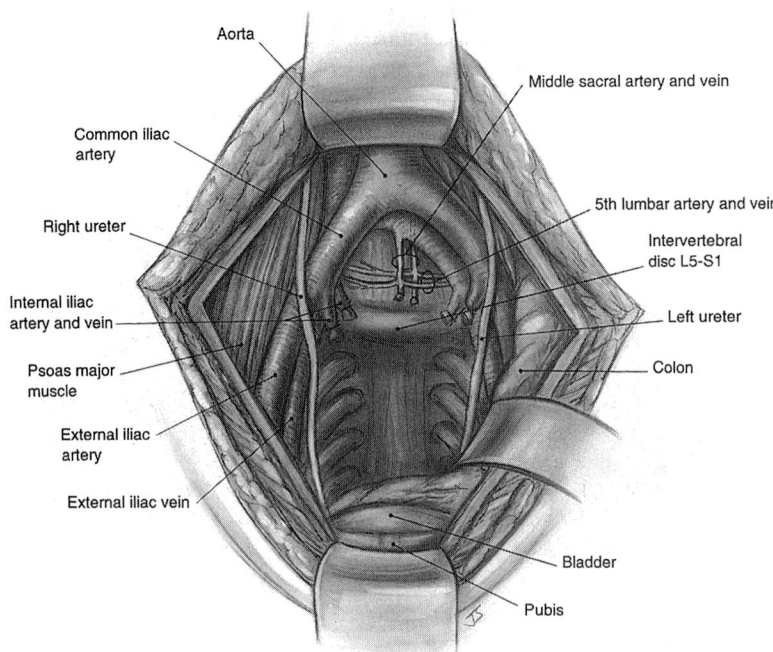

Aorta

Middle sacral artery and vein

Common iliac artery

5th lumbar artery and vein

Right ureter

Intervertebral disc L5-S1

Internal iliac artery and vein

Left ureter

Psoas major muscle

Colon

External iliac artery

External iliac vein

Bladder

Pubis

Fig. 5. Release of the abdominal wall muscles, including the rectus abdominis, from the pelvis, exposing the retroperitoneal space. Pelvic viscera are mobilized and retracted to one side or the other as the great vessels and ureters are identified. The extent of the anterior soft-tissue tumor mass determines which pelvic vessels are ligated. (From Simon MA, Springfield D: Surgery for Bone and Soft-Tissue Tumors. Philadelphia, Lippincott-Raven, 1998, p 446.)

longitudinally in the midline. The abdominal contents are retracted superiorly, and the bifurcation of the aorta and the common iliac veins are identified. The iliac vessels are mobilized and retracted laterally, creating direct access to the lower lumbar and upper sacral vertebral bodies and disks (Fig. 5).

After adequate exposure, diskectomies and a complete corpectomy can be performed as described previously. Reconstruction and stabilization can be accomplished with structural allograft, autograft, titanium cage, or methylmethacrylate. Anterior vertebral body screw and rod systems may provide rigid fixation. When lower lumbar corpectomy is performed and stabilization is needed to the pelvis or sacrum, posterior instrumentation is a good option. Posterior constructs such as the Galveston technique[25] or iliac or sacral screw systems can provide rigid pelvic fixation. Rods then extend to the lumbar spine and are secured with hooks or pedicle screws.

COMPLICATIONS AND RESULTS

Studies of surgical treatment for metastatic spine disease show promising results in improving neurological compromise, increasing mobility, and decreasing pain. Survival times are limited and range from 9.5 to 35.8 months postoperatively in this patient population.[26, 27] Thus, the primary objective of all treatment should focus on maintaining the best possible quality of remaining life.

Results of anterior decompression versus posterior decompression consistently support anterior decompression as superior in improving neurological function. Anatomically, the source of spinal cord compression is usually from the anterior vertebral body metastasis, so anterior decompres-

sion addresses the site of disease more directly. In their review, McLain and Weinstein[31] compared the neurological recovery of patients treated with anterior decompression versus posterior decompression. They reviewed 14 published studies comprising 1173 patients and found that 73% to 84% of patients in the anterior decompression group experienced neurological improvement, whereas 13% to 45% of patients in the posterior decompression group had neurological improvement. A satisfactory outcome was achieved in 73% to 89% of anterior decompressions and in 29% to 48% of posterior decompressions.

In 1985, Sundaresan et al[28] reported the results of anterior corpectomy and stabilization with methylmethacrylate and Steinmann pins in 101 patients. Only 15% of the patients were ambulatory before surgery. After surgery, 78% of patients were ambulatory. There was no neurological deterioration as a result of the operation. The complication rate was 10%, and there was a 30-day mortality rate of 8%.

Harrington[29] found that 82% of patients with neurological compromise secondary to vertebral malignancy improved at least one functional grade after decompression and stabilization, and 88% experienced good to excellent relief of spinal pain with restoration of walking ability. In another review by Harrington,[30] 77 patients underwent anterior decompression and stabilization as a treatment for vertebral collapse and spinal cord compression from metastatic malignancy. Preoperatively, all patients had pain; postoperatively, 94% had significant pain relief or no pain at all. Sixty-two patients (81%) were nonambulatory preoperatively, and 66% of these were ambulatory postoperatively. Of 15 patients (19%) who were paraplegic or quadriplegic preoperatively, 4 (27%) had complete recovery, 5

(33%) improved, and 6 (40%) remained unchanged. There was a 10% surgical morbidity rate and a 10% mortality rate at 6 weeks postoperatively.

Miller et al[26] reported on 27 patients with metastatic disease of the cervical and upper thoracic spine treated with anterior resection and coaxial double-lumen methylmethacrylate reconstruction. At 1 month postoperatively, there were significant improvements in spinal axial pain, radiculopathy, gait, and Frankel grade. Twenty-one patients (77%) experienced no complications. Two patients (7%) experienced complications related to instrumentation failure. There were no neurological complications or infections. They concluded that their methylmethacrylate reconstruction technique provided excellent results.

In 1999, Wise et al[32] reviewed 80 patients undergoing surgical treatment for metastatic disease of the spine to determine the surgical complication and survival rates and risk factors for complications. They found a mean survival time after diagnosis of 26.0 months (range, 1-107.25 months). Mean survival postoperatively was 15.9 months (range, 0.25–55.5 months). Six patients showed no change in Frankel grade, 19 improved one Frankel grade, and 1 deteriorated one Frankel grade; 1 patient had paraplegia. Thirty-five complications occurred in 20 patients (25%). Sixty patients (75%) had no complications. There were no intraoperative deaths. Complications were statistically more likely to occur in patients with significant neurological deficits and those who had preoperative radiation therapy.

In another 1999 study of 76 patients undergoing anterior surgical procedures, Weigel et al[33] found neurological improvement in 58%. Ninety-three percent were able to ambulate postoperatively. Pain relief was noted in 89%, and 80% were satisfied with their surgical intervention. There were complications from 19% of the operations and local tumor recurrence in 22% of the patients, with paraplegia ultimately developing in 18%.

Although these overall results are encouraging, controversies in the surgical treatment of metastatic spine disease remain. Improvements in resection and reconstruction techniques will be made. Careful patient selection remains the most important factor in determining a beneficial outcome for the patient and maintenance of optimum quality of remaining life.

REFERENCES

1. Black P: Spinal metastasis: Current status and recommended guidelines for management. Neurosurgery 1979; 5:726.
2. Harrington KD: Metastatic disease of the spine. J Bone Joint Surg Am 1986; 68:1110.
3. Berrettoni BA, Carter JR: Mechanisms of cancer metastasis to bone. J Bone Joint Surg Am 1986; 68:308.
4. Wong DA, Fornasier VL, MacNab I: Spinal metastases: The obvious, the occult and the imposters. Spine 1990; 15:1.
5. Brihaye J, Ectors P, Lemort M, et al: The management of spinal epidural metastases. Adv Tech Stand Neurosurg 1988; 16:121.
6. Constans J, de Divitiis E, Donzelli R, et al: Spinal metastases with neurological manifestations: Review of 600 cases. J Neurosurg 1983; 59:111.
7. Suen KC, Lau LL, Yermakov V: Cancer and old age: An autopsy study of 3,535 patients over 65 years old. Cancer 1974; 33:1164.
8. Nottebaert M, von Hochstetter AR, Exner GU, et al: Metastatic carcinoma of the spine: A study of 92 cases. Int Orthop 1987; 11:345.
9. Batson OV: The role of the vertebral veins in the metastatic process. Ann Intern Med 1942; 16:38.
10. Asdourian PL, Mardjetko S, Rauschning W, et al: An evaluation of spinal deformity in metastatic breast cancer. J Spinal Disord 1990; 3:119.
11. Gilbert RW, Kim JH, Posner JB: Epidural spinal cord compression from metastatic tumor: Diagnosis and treatment. Ann Neurol 1978; 3:40.
12. Edelstyn GA, Gillespie PJ, Grebbell FS: The radiological demonstration of osseous metastases: Experimental observation. Clin Radiol 1967; 18:158.
13. Galasko CS: Skeletal metastases. Clin Orthop 1986; 210:18.
14. O'Connor MI, Currier BL: Metastatic bone disease. Orthopaedics 1992; 15:611.
15. Siegal T, Tiqva P, Siegal T: Vertebral body resection for epidural compression by malignant tumors: Result of forty-seven consecutive operative procedures. J Bone Joint Surg Am 1985; 67:375.
16. Harrington KD: Anterior cord decompression and spinal stabilization for patients with metastatic lesions of the spine. J Neurosurg 1984; 61:107.
17. Kostuik JP, Weinstein J: Differential diagnosis and surgical treatment of metastatic spine tumors. In Frymoyer J (ed): The Adult Spine: Principles and Practice. New York, Raven Press, 1991, p 861.
18. Tokuhashi Y, Matsuzaki H, Teviyama S, et al: Scoring system for the preoperative evaluation of metastatic spine tumor prognosis. Spine 1990; 15:1110.
19. Asdourian PL: Metastatic disease of the spine. In Budwell KH, DeWald RL (eds): The Textbook of Spinal Surgery. Philadelphia, Lippincott-Raven, 1997, 2nd ed, p 2007.
20. Tehranzadeh J, Freiberger RH, Ghelman B: Closed skeletal needle biopsy: Review of 120 cases. AJR Am J Roentgenol 1983; 140:113.
21. Mink J: Percutaneous bone biopsy in the patient with known or suspected osseous metastases. Radiology 1986; 161:191.
22. Murphy WA, Destouet JM, Gilula LA: Percutaneous skeletal biopsy 1981: A procedure for radiologists—results, review and recommendations. Radiology 1981; 139:545.
23. Weinstein JN, McLain RF: Tumors of the spine. In Rothman RA, Simone FA (eds): The Spine. Philadelphia, WB Saunders, 1992, 3rd ed, p 1279.
24. Bruckner JD, Conrad EU III: Spine. In Simon MA, Springfield D (eds): Surgery for Bone and Soft Tissue Tumors. Philadelphia, Lippincott-Raven, 1988, p 435.
25. Allen BL Jr, Ferguson RL: The Galveston technique for L rod instrumentation of the scoliotic spine. Spine 1982; 7:276.
26. Miller DJ, Lang FF, Walsh GL, et al: Coaxial double-lumen methylmethacrylate reconstruction in the anterior cervical and upper thoracic spine after tumor resection. J Neurosurg 2000; 92:181.
27. Caspar W, Pitzen T, Papavero L, et al: Anterior cervical plating for the treatment of neoplasms in the cervical vertebrae. J Neurosurg 1999; 90:27.
28. Sundaresan N, Galicich JH, Lane JM, et al: Treatment of neoplastic epidural cord compression by vertebral body resection and stabilization. J Neurosurg 1985; 63:676.

29. Harrington KD: Orthopedic surgical management of skeletal complications of malignancy. Cancer 1997; 80:1614.

30. Harrington KD: Anterior decompression and stabilization of the spine as a treatment for vertebral collapse and spinal cord compression from metastatic malignancy. Clin Orthop 1988; 233:177.

31. McLain RF, Weinstein JN: Tumors of the spine. Semin Spine Surg 1990; 2:157.

32. Wise JJ, Fischgrund JS, Herkowitz HN, et al: Complication, survival rates, and risk factors of surgery for metastatic disease of the spine. Spine 1999; 24:1943.

33. Weigel B, Maghsudi M, Neumann C, et al: Surgical management of symptomatic spinal metastases: Postoperative outcome and quality of life. Spine 1999; 24:2240.

section 7 chapter 16

METASTATIC DISEASE OF THE UPPER EXTREMITY

H. Thomas Temple

Summary

- Twenty percent of all skeletal metastases occur in the upper extremity, most often the humerus.
- Upper extremity skeletal metastases distal to the elbow are very uncommon.
- In general, fracture through an upper extremity skeletal metastasis produces much less disability than a pathological fracture through a lower extremity metastasis. Therefore, the indication for prophylactic internal fixation of an upper extremity skeletal metastasis is less clear.
- Staging and biopsy of upper extremity skeletal metastases are necessary to exclude the possibility of a primary bone tumor or a second primary carcinoma.
- Physical therapy and occupational therapy are important to maximize the functional outcome after operative therapy for an upper extremity skeletal metastasis or a pathological fracture.
- Preoperative embolization of feeding vessels to highly vascular tumors can substantially reduce operative blood loss.
- Symptomatic and functional results are improved by postoperative radiation therapy.
- Amputation is indicated for uncontrolled metastasis growth with recurrent pathological fractures, sepsis, or hemorrhage.

The frequency of skeletal metastases in patients with cancer is variable, ranging from 12% and 85% in autopsy studies.[1, 2] Approximately 20% of skeletal metastases occur in the collective bones of the upper extremity.[2] Of these, the humerus is the most common site of cases.[1] Although the clavicle and scapula are commonly involved, metastatic disease of the humerus presents the greatest challenge to orthopaedic surgeons in an effort to relieve pain and restore function. Metastases below the elbow, particularly the hand, represent less than 1% of all metastases.[3]

The morbidity of pathological fracture of the bones in the upper extremity is not as significant as that in the lower extremity. Partly for this reason, the indications for prophylactic internal fixation of impending pathological fractures in the upper extremity, especially the humerus, are not as clearly defined as those for fractures in the peritrochanteric region of the hip.

For pathological fractures of the humerus and forearm, internal fixation often supplemented with polymethylmethacrylate (PMMA) and radiotherapy is usually necessary. Prosthetics are reserved for patients with large, destructive periarticular lesions about the proximal or distal humerus. Fractures or impending pathological fractures through solitary lesions in patients with known and unknown primary cancers require tumor staging and biopsy to exclude the possibility of a primary bone tumor.

After surgery, physical and occupational therapy are important adjuncts to surgical treatment in maintaining joint motion and restoring strength.

HISTORY

Generally, patients with metastatic bone lesions have a history of a primary cancer for which they have been diagnosed and treated. The most common malignancies disseminating to bone arise in breast, lung, prostate, thyroid, and kidney. Therefore, the history should focus on a review of systems specific to these organs. Myeloma is the most common primary tumor arising within bone, but, because its management is similar, it can be included in the general category of metastatic disease.

A history of a mass in the breast, the date and results of the last mammogram, and a family history of breast cancer are important details in a woman presenting with an aggressive lesion or lesions of bone. For women previously undergoing treatment for breast cancer, the initial date of presentation, tumor type and grade, treatment rendered, and number of lymph nodes positive for cancer are important prognostic factors. Estrogen receptor status of the tumor cells is important for treatment purposes. Patients with lung carcinoma present with a nonproductive cough and weight loss; a history of tobacco use is frequent. Metastases in patients with prostate cancer usually occur late in the disease course, and these men will often have a history of transurethral resection or radical prostatectomy. Renal cell carcinoma is frequently asymptomatic, although these patients may complain of hematuria. Patients with multiple myeloma may complain of diffuse skeletal pain and fatigue. Occasionally, patients present with more than one primary cancer, and discovery of this condition starts with a thorough history.

Patients with metastatic disease involving the upper extremity often complain of pain. The pain is usually insidious and described as a diffuse ache. Initially, symptoms are present with activity but later are associated with rest as well, particularly at night. The pain is inconsistently relieved by anti-inflammatory medicines and other nonnarcotic analgesics. Interestingly, there is no direct relationship between pain and the extent of skeletal involvement in patients with metastatic disease.[4] Furthermore, pain often precedes the radiographic appearance of bone metastases by several weeks or months. Occasionally, patients with known primary tumors are completely asymptomatic and referred for solitary or multiple abnormalities on surveillance bone scans.

Patients with pathological fractures present with sudden pain and deformity that occurs spontaneously or with minor trauma. Pathological fracture also can occur during or immediately after radiotherapy for known bone metastases.

PHYSICAL EXAMINATION

A general and complete physical examination is important in all patients with suspected metastases. Examination of the affected extremities includes a basic musculoskeletal examination to assess any deformity or swelling, skin discoloration, or fixed contractures. Assessment of joint range of motion, palpation of the involved extremity and regional lymph nodes, and neurovascular assessment are necessary.

RADIOLOGICAL STUDIES

Plain radiographs are essential in the initial evaluation of patients with suspected metastatic disease of bone and should include the entire involved bone, including the joint above and below the lesion, because metastatic deposits may be multiple in a single long bone. This is important to assess because internal fixation must bypass all defects to avoid fractures above and below the fixation devices.

Technetium 99 pyrophosphate scintigraphy is useful in detecting other sites of tumor involvement in the skeleton. Focal areas of uptake should be imaged with biplanar radiographs to assess the size of the lesion and the extent of cortical disruption. Bone scintigraphy is inconsistent in demonstrating sites of skeletal involvement in patients with myeloma. Woolfenden et al[5] studied 562 sites in patients with myeloma using radiographs and bone scintigraphy. It was found that bone scintigraphy underestimated or failed to show radiographically evident disease in 27% of patients.[5] For this reason, a general skeletal survey should be part of the initial work-up for patients with this myeloma.

Computed tomography (CT) is an excellent study to assess the degree of cortical destruction and has been used to make quantitative measurements of bone destruction to predict the risk of fracture in patients with metastatic disease of bone.[6] For routine screening and metastatic surveillance, CT has limited application.

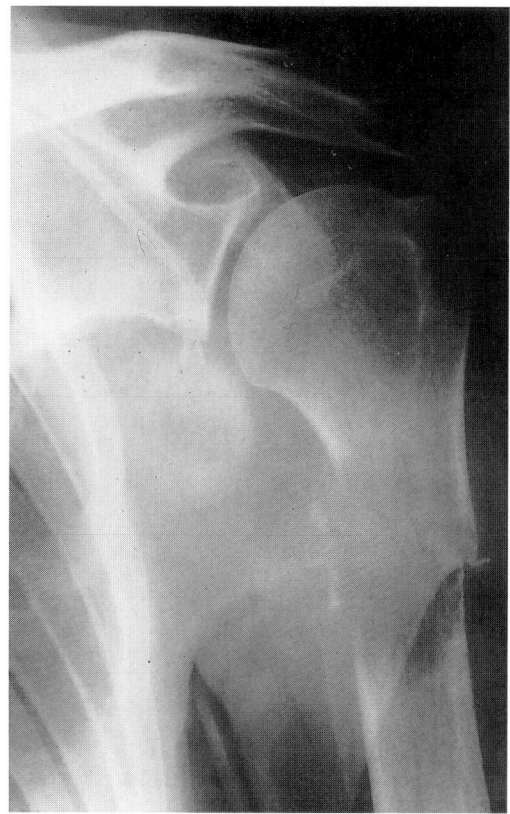

Fig. 1. Metastatic disease in the proximal humerus. A 45-year-old man with a history of renal cell carcinoma and an aggressive radiolucent abnormality in the proximal humerus consistent with metastatic disease. There is an associated pathological fracture.

Magnetic resonance imaging (MRI) is the best study for assessing the degree of intra- and extraosseous tumor extension, but it has a limited role in the diagnosis and treatment of patients with metastatic disease. It can be used to evaluate periarticular sites of tumor involvement and to assess accurately the extent of tumor in bone in patients with infiltrative bone lesions above or below the primary lesion in whom internal fixation is planned.

Angiography is useful in evaluating hypervascular metastases such as renal cell carcinoma in patients in whom internal fixation or tumor resection is planned. Before resection, embolization of the feeding vessels can significantly limit intraoperative blood loss[7, 8] (Figs. 1 to 3).

IMPENDING PATHOLOGICAL FRACTURE

No definitive criteria exist for prophylactic internal fixation in patients with metastatic disease in the upper extremity. Most data pertain to the risk of pathological fracture in patients with proximal femoral disease, because this is a very common site of metastatic disease spread and fractures in this area are associated with significant morbidity.

Beals et al[9] recommended internal fixation for femoral metastatic lesions 2.5 cm or greater. This guideline was based on retrospective data of patients with femoral defects and has not been tested in other skeletal sites. Others found geometric measurement of tumor size to be unreliable in

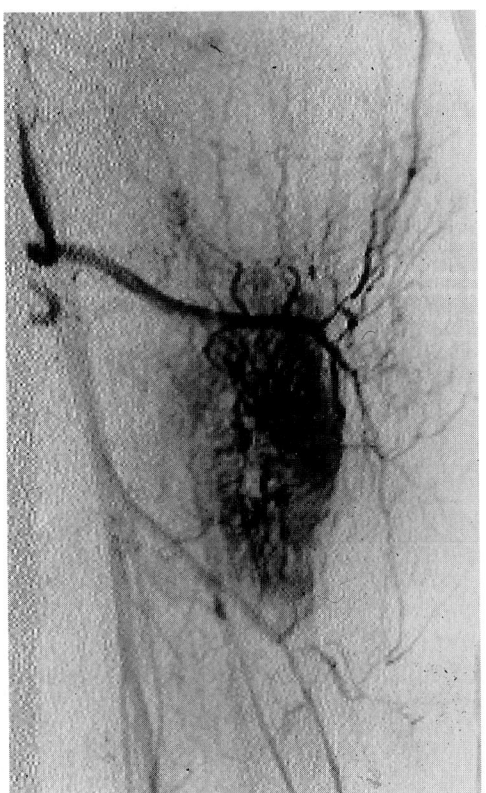

Fig. 2. Angiogram demonstrating a significant tumor blush and a prominent feeding vessel.

Hipp et al[6] applied engineering principles using CT to assess the risk of pathological fracture in bone. They evaluated the load-bearing properties of bone after making careful measurements of bone lost as a result of tumor destruction, the modulus of remaining bone, the location of the defect with regard to applied loads, and the types of loads applied. Fundamentally, this approach quantitatively analyzed the defect with regard to size and location within a bone as well as predicting load to failure from anticipated forces, taking into consideration premorbid functional levels. Although this study assessed risk for metastatic tumors in the spine only, it is a compelling model for assessing pathological fracture risk in patients with lesions in other sites as well.

The problem of predicting pathological fracture risk is the reliance on plain radiographs, specifically size (greater than 2.5 cm) and extent of cortical involvement (more than 50%) in predicting risk of fracture. Metastatic lesions, especially lytic or permeative abnormalities, are difficult to assess accurately by plain radiography and even conventional CT.[10] Premonitory symptoms such as pain and dysfunction can be absent in patients with impending pathological fractures and are not reliable in assessing pathological fracture risk. Premorbid function in patients with metastatic disease is very important and should be assessed in all patients with impending pathological fractures. For example, a lesion in the nondominant upper extremity certainly poses less potential morbidity than a

assessing pathological fracture risk in patients with metastatic disease of bone.[10, 11]

Fidler[12] retrospectively studied 66 patients with metastatic bone disease and assessed the degree of bone destruction from plain radiographs. He concluded that lesions occupying less than 50% of the cortex of bone were at minimal risk of fracture (2.3%) compared with those occupying 50% to 75%, in which the risk was 60%, and even more of the cortex, in which the risk was higher still. Unfortunately, this study did not stratify risk based on tumor location or type of bone destruction, whether lytic, blastic, or mixed.

Mirrels[13] attempted to calculate the relative risk of pathological fracture in all long bones by analyzing 78 metastatic lesions that had been irradiated without prophylactic surgical intervention. He identified 51 patients without fracture in 6 months subsequent to radiation and 27 fractures in patients who sustained a fracture 6 months after radiation. Risk was analyzed based on site, associated pain, radiographic appearance of the lesion (lytic, blastic, or mixed), and size of the metastatic deposit. Based on these criteria, points were assigned and tallied. Patients with total scores less than 7 were not at significant risk of pathological fracture, whereas those with scores greater than 7 were at substantial risk to warrant prophylactic internal fixation. In this series, patients with lesions in the upper extremity with only mild pain and radiographic involvement less than one-third of the diameter of bone were at minimal risk for a pathological fracture.

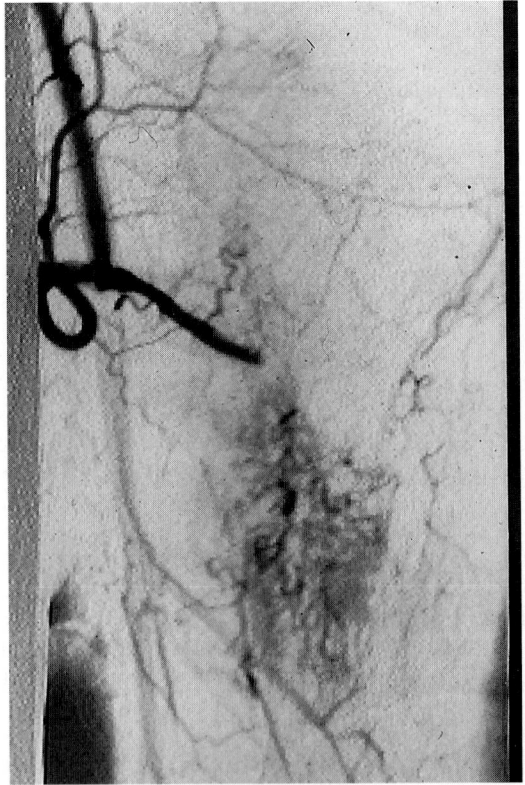

Fig. 3. Embolization of feeding vessel. The feeding vessel was embolized with Gelfoam angiographically, resulting in significant diminution of tumor vascularity.

lesion in the lower extremity or even the dominant upper extremity in a young, active patient. Finally, the patient's comorbid conditions should be considered before prophylactic internal fixation. Patients with extensive visceral metastases or hepatic insufficiency rarely survive long and are at significant risk for intra- and perioperative complications, which may preclude any benefit from internal fixation, even in patients with pathological fractures. Other conditions that place a patient at significant perioperative risk are hypercalcemia, malnutrition, anemia, and myelosuppression resulting from extensive radiation or chemotherapy.

Many patients with impending pathological fractures of the humerus can be managed by radiation alone and a functional brace.[14–17] Decisions to intervene in patients with metastases to the upper extremities involve a careful assessment of the patient's overall medical condition, the size and location of the defect, and the patient's preoperative functional status. The goal of intervention should be to prevent pathological fracture, relieve pain, and restore useful function. If intervention is undertaken, care must be exercised in positioning and preparing the patient on the operating table, because pathological fracture can easily occur and thus alter the surgical plan and render stabilization more difficult.

TREATMENT

Before surgical treatment, attention to the patient's overall medical status is important. Nutritional deficits and metabolic abnormalities should be treated before surgical intervention.

Before undertaking operative intervention, especially open intralesional surgery, angiographic evaluation and therapeutic embolization are prudent in patients with highly vascular tumors such as hypernephroma, myeloma, and occasionally thyroid carcinoma. Embolization substantially reduces intraoperative blood loss if surgery follows embolization within 24 to 48 hours.[7, 8]

All patients with symptomatic and radiographically measurable disease in the upper extremity should undergo radiation therapy. Whereas many patients with impending pathological fractures of the humerus can be treated with radiation alone, surgical stabilization is more reliable in relieving pain and restoring function in patients with pathological fractures of the humerus.[16, 18, 19] Townsend et al[20] studied 64 surgical interventions in 60 consecutive patients with impending or pathological fracture, 35 of whom were treated with postoperative radiotherapy and 29 were not. They found that radiation therapy and prefunctional status were the only significant predictors of normal postoperative function. They also demonstrated that postoperative pain relief was less reliable in the patients treated by surgery alone and that second-site surgery was more likely in patients who were not treated with adjunct radiotherapy.

CLAVICLE

Metastatic lesions in the clavicle rarely require surgical intervention. Resection is appropriate for tumors in the distal one-third of the clavicle that are symptomatic after radiation. Symptomatic middle one-third lesions of the clavicle, especially those that are significantly displaced and compromising the overlying skin, can be stabilized with 3.5-mm compression plates and screws and augmented with PMMA.

SCAPULA

Patients with lesions of the scapula are generally treated with radiotherapy, gentle range of motion, and anti-inflammatory or narcotic analgesics for pain control. For extensive, destructive lesions, especially those involving the glenohumeral joint, scapulectomy may be necessary. Suspending the humerus from the chest wall or the residual clavicle, a variation of the Tikhoff-Lindberg procedure,[21] is recommended.

HUMERUS

Patients with large, destructive lesions of the humeral head are best treated with proximal humeral resection and standard hemiarthroplasty or proximal humeral replacement followed by radiotherapy. Replacement of the glenoid is unnecessary. An intact rotator cuff and preservation of the axillary nerve result in optimal postoperative function in these patients. In those in whom the rotator cuff is insufficient, proximal migration of the humerus can occur and cause painful impingement on attempted abduction.

A variety of internal fixation devices are available to stabilize the humerus in patients with metastatic bone lesions. For tumors in the surgical neck or diaphysis, interlocking nails[22] or Rush's rods and cement[18] can be used to stabilize the bone and restore function. Anterograde nail placement can result in rotator cuff problems if the cuff tear is not repaired or in impingement if the nail is prominent. Also the axillary nerve can be injured during the approach, resulting in loss of deltoid function. Rush's rods or Ender's nails should always be supplemented with PMMA because these devices do not have sufficient rigidity to resist bending or rotation and can even result in distraction of the fractured bone ends.

Interlocked nails can be placed either retrograde through a posterior triceps splitting incision or anterograde through a deltoid splitting incision. These devices are rigid enough to resist bending, and the static locking screws proximally and distally prevent rotation. The advantages of interlocking nails include immediate stability, limited surgical exposure, and low morbidity.[22] Adjunctive cementation may be necessary for large, destructive cavitary lesions.

Plates and screws supplemented with cement are effective in patients with solitary destructive tumors in the distal metadiaphysis and diaphysis as well. Tumor curettage followed by cementation results in better local tumor control, and the addition of 4.5-mm compression plates and screws results in a stable construct. The exothermic effects of the PMMA in conjunction with postoperative radiotherapy limits or prevents further tumor growth. The surgeon, however, must be certain that tumor does not extend proximal or distal to the plate and screw construct, because this can result in a fracture above or below the plate (Figs. 4 and 5). For this reason, if plates and screws are contemplated, a limited MRI evaluation with either sagittal or coronal views using fast spin echo inversion recovery sequences is useful to evaluate the extent of tumor involvement within bone.

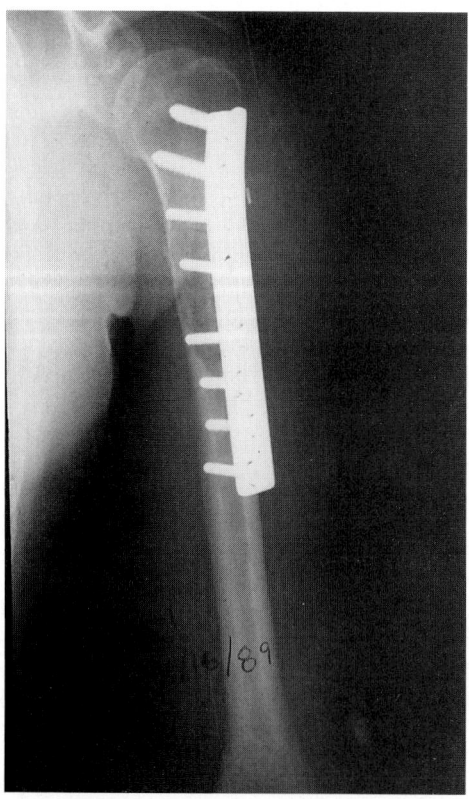

Fig. 4. Large, destructive lesion in the humerus. A 75-year-old patient with myeloma and a large radiolucent abnormality in the proximal humeral metaphysis who underwent stabilization without cementation.

For destructive middiaphyseal tumors between 2.5[23] and 4 cm,[3] resection and shortening of the humerus followed by plate fixation is a reasonable alternative procedure.

Lesions in the distal humerus and around the elbow are more difficult to treat and generally require an extensile exposure by splitting the triceps in a V fashion and reflecting it proximally. Olecranon osteotomy should be avoided because postoperative radiation therapy may interfere with subsequent healing, resulting in a nonunion. Plates and screws (either 4.5-mm compression plates or pelvic reconstruction plates) placed in both the medial and lateral columns of the distal humerus supplemented with PMMA is effective in stabilizing these defects. In one study, the use of double plates was found to be biomechanically superior to the use of a single plate or intramedullary fixation with Rush's rods.[24] Occasionally, for highly destructive tumors near the elbow, total elbow arthroplasty and distal humeral replacement are needed.

Another alternative for treating distal humeral lesions is crossed Ender's nails with insertion sites in the medial and lateral epicondyles of the distal humerus. This construct should be augmented by PMMA.

Rarely, wide local resection and segmental reconstruction are performed in patients with solitary metastatic disease secondary to renal cell carcinoma and only after careful staging rules out other sites of metastases and if the primary tumor is resectable.

FOREARM

Metastatic lesions below the elbow are unusual.[25] For destructive and painful tumors in the proximal radius, radial head excision is appropriate and effective in relieving pain with minimal loss of function. Tumors in the shafts of the ulna or radius can be stabilized with 3.5-mm compression plates and screws supplemented with PMMA. Alternatively, Rush's pins can be placed through the radius styloid distally or through the ulna proximally. A third option for large, destructive lesions is diaphyseal resection and conversion to a one-bone forearm.

HAND

Metastases to the hand are very rare.[26, 27] Metastatic tumors of the hand generally arise from lung or renal primary sites.[28–30] Radiotherapy alone is usually sufficient to control local disease, decrease pain, and restore function. Transarticular amputation is appropriate for metastases in the middle or distal phalanges. For highly destructive lesions of the proximal phalanges or metacarpals, ray resection is indicated.

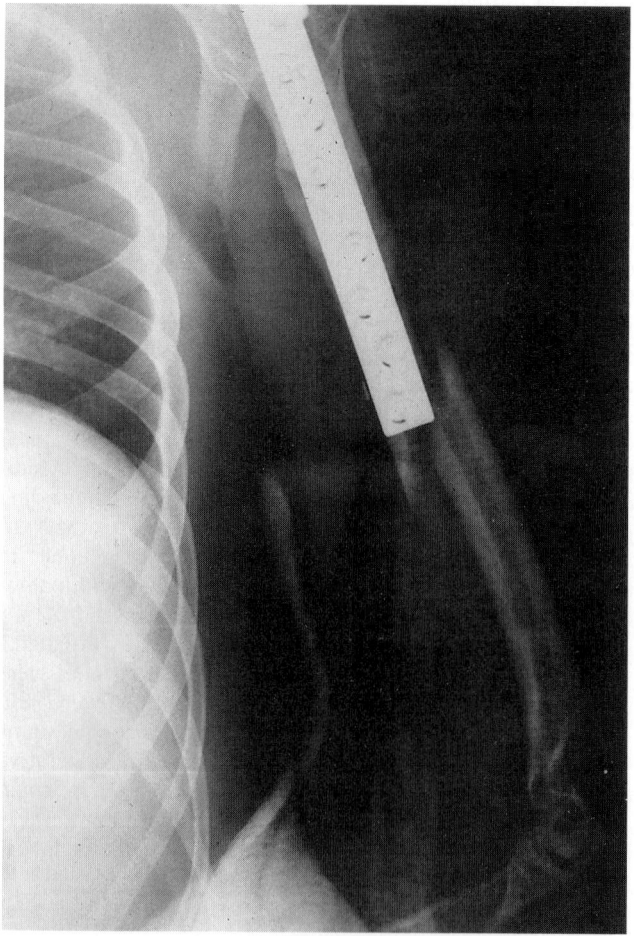

Fig. 5. Fracture in the humerus. The humerus fractured below the plate as a result of tumor extending distally beyond the plate and screw construct. A magnetic resonance image may have been helpful in the preoperative evaluation of this patient to assess tumor extension.

POSTOPERATIVE MANAGEMENT

Rehabilitation is an important component of postoperative care. In patients with upper extremity metastases, efforts to improve joint motion and muscle strength facilitate improvements in patient self-reliance and independence. This, in turn, results in a measurable improvement in quality of life. During rehabilitation and thereafter, however, the risk of pathological fracture is still present in patients with disseminated disease. Bunting et al,[31] in a prospective study of 54 patients with metastatic bone disease, reported 16 fractures in 12 patients during the course of rehabilitation. Patients at greatest risk were younger and female with advanced disease and lytic metastases; 5 of 16 fractures occurred in the humerus.

SOLITARY LESIONS

Solitary destructive tumors in patients with known or unknown primary tumors require clinical staging and biopsy before definitive treatment to rule out the possibility of a primary bone tumor. Primary tumors of bone, in particular chondrosarcoma and occasionally fibrosarcoma, malignant fibrous histiocytoma, and even osteosarcoma, can mimic metastatic tumors. The treatment of primary bone tumors, of course, is different from that for metastatic tumors of bone and involves wide local resection and chemotherapy. Intralesional surgery for presumed metastatic tumors of bone contaminates normal adjacent tissue and joints and compromises limb salvage and potential survival.[32]

UNKNOWN PRIMARY TUMORS

When patients in their fifth and sixth decades and beyond present with pain and radiographic abnormalities of bone in multiple sites, this usually represents either metastases or myeloma. A vigilant search for the primary tumor of origin must be undertaken and is usually initiated by the orthopaedic surgeon. This begins with a thorough history and physical examination to include radiographs of the area in question as well as a bone scan or skeletal survey to demonstrate other sites of tumor. Posteroanterior and lateral chest radiographs, CT of the chest, abdomen, and pelvis, and directed laboratory studies are needed before biopsy. The majority of primary tumor sites are identified on history and physical examination and radiographic studies.[33] If the preoperative evaluation does not identify the primary tumor, the biopsy will ultimately lead to the underlying primary in only 35% of cases.[33]

MAJOR PALLIATIVE AMPUTATION

Occasionally, amputation is required for pain relief in patients with large fungating tumors in whom attempts at local disease control have failed.[34, 35] Indications for palliative amputation are uncontrolled tumor growth with recurrent pathological fracture, sepsis, and hemorrhage.[34] This can lead to satisfactory results and improvement in quality of life in terminally ill patients.

SUMMARY

Upper extremity bone metastases are not uncommon and may result in significant morbidity if untreated. The humerus is the most commonly affected bone, and for many metastatic tumors in this location, radiation and functional bracing are adequate. For predominately lytic lesions that occupy more than 50% of the cortex and in patients with concomitant disease in their lower extremities who must rely on their upper extremities to ambulate, prophylactic internal fixation and radiation are indicated. The type of fixation depends on the size and location of the defect. Occasionally, joint arthroplasty is necessary in patients with large, destructive periarticular tumors. These patients require aggressive preoperative medical management and postoperative rehabilitation to fully realize the goals of surgery, specifically pain relief and restoration of function. Solitary lesions must be staged to assess the local and distant extent of disease and tumor type. The orthopaedic surgeon, in concert with medical and radiation oncologists, is pivotal in the overall management of the patient with upper extremity metastases.

REFERENCES

1. Clain A: Secondary malignant disease of bone. Br J Cancer 1965; 19:15.
2. Jaffe HK: Tumors and Tumorous Conditions of the Bones and Joints. Philadelphia, Lea & Febiger, 1958.
3. Rock MG: Metastatic lesions of the humerus and upper extremity. In Eilert RE (ed): Instructional Course Lectures XLI. Rosemont, IL, American Academy of Orthopaedic Surgeons, 1992, p 329.
4. Galasko CSB: Pathologic fractures secondary to metastatic cancer J R Coll Surg Edinb 1974; 19:351.
5. Woolfenden JM, Pitt MJ, Durie BGM, et al: Comparison of bone scintigraphy and radiology in multiple myeloma. Radiology 1980; 134:723.
6. Hipp JA, Springfield DS, Wilson HC: Predicting pathologic fracture risk in the management of metastatic bone defects. Clin Orthop 1995; 312:120.
7. Bowers TA, Murray JA, Charnsangavej C, et al: Bone metastases from renal carcinoma: The preoperative use of transcatheter arterial occlusion. J Bone Joint Surg Am 1982; 64:749.
8. Carpenter PR, Ewing JW, Cook AJ, et al: Angiographic assessment and control of potential operative hemorrhage with pathologic fractures secondary to metastases. Clin Orthop 1977; 123:6.
9. Beals RK, Lawton GD, Snell WE: Prophylactic internal fixation of the femur in metastatic breast cancer. Cancer 1971; 28: 1350.
10. Keene JS, Sellinger DS, McBeath AA, et al: Metastatic breast cancer in the femur: A search for the lesion at risk of fracture. Clin Orthop 1986; 203:282.
11. Zickel RE, Mouradian WH: Intramedullary fixation of pathological fractures and lesions of the subtrochanteric region of the femur. J Bone Joint Surg Am 1976; 58: 1061.
12. Fidler M: Prophylactic internal fixation of secondary neoplastic deposits in long bones. BMJ 1973; 849:341.
13. Mirrels H: Metastatic disease in long bones: A proposed scoring system for diagnosing impending pathologic fractures. Clin Orthop 1989; 249:256.
14. Albright JA, Gillespie TE, Butuad TR: Treatment of bone metastases. Semin Oncol 1980; 7:418.

15. Cheng DS, Seits CB, Eyre HJ: Nonoperative management of femoral, humeral and acetabular metastasis in patients with breast cancer. Cancer 1980; 45:1533.

16. Flemming JE, Beals RK: Pathologic fracture of the humerus. Clin Orthop 1986; 203:258.

17. Schocker JD, Brady LW: Radiation therapy for bone metastasis. Clin Orthop 1982; 169:38.

18. Lewallen RP, Pritchard DJ, Sim FH: Treatment of pathologic fractures or impending fractures of the humerus with Rush rods and methylmethacrylate: Experience with 55 cases in 54 patients, 1968–1977. Clin Orthop 1982; 166:193.

19. Sim FH, Pritchard DJ: Metastatic disease in the upper extremity. Clin Orthop 1982; 169:83.

20. Townsend PW, Rosenthal HG, Smalley SR, et al: Impact of postoperative therapy and other perioperative factors on outcome after orthopaedic stabilization of impending or pathologic fractures due to metastatic disease. J Clin Oncol 1994; 12:2345.

21. Malawer MM, Sugarbaker PH, Lampert M, et al: The Tikhoff-Lindberg procedure: Report of ten patients and presentation of a modified technique for tumors of the proximal humerus. Surgery 1985; 97:518.

22. Redmond BJ, Biermann JS, Blasier RB: Interlocking intramedullary nailing of pathologic fractures of the shaft of the humerus. J Bone Joint Surg Am 1996; 78:891.

23. Peabody TD, Finn HA: Humerus. In Simon MA, Springfield D (eds): Surgery for Bone and Soft Tissue Tumors. Philadelphia, Lippincott-Raven, 1998, p 713.

24. Damron TA, Heiner JP, Freund EMN, et al: Biomechanical analysis of prophylactic fixation for pathologic fractures of the distal third of the humerus. J Bone Joint Surg Am 1994; 76:839.

25. Leeson MC, Makley JT, Carter JR: Metastatic skeletal disease distal to the elbow and knee. Clin Orthop 1986; 206:94.

26. Kerin R: Metastatic tumors of the hand. J Bone Joint Surg Am 1983; 40:263.

27. Wu KK, Guise ER: Metastatic tumors of the hand. A report of six cases. J Hand Surg 1978; 3:271.

28. Branson FW, Eschner EG, Sanes S, et al: Secondary carcinoma of the phalanges. Radiology 1951; 57:864.

29. Colson GM, Willcox A: Phalangeal metastases in bronchogenic carcinoma. Lancet 1948; 1:100.

30. Hicks MC, Kalmon EH, Glasser SM: Metastatic malignancy to phalanges. South Med J 1964; 57:85.

31. Bunting R, Lamont-Havers W, Schweon D, et al: Pathologic fracture risk in rehabilitation of patients with bony metastases. Clin Orthop 1985; 192:222.

32. Mankin, HJ, Mankin CJ, Simon MA: The hazards of biopsy revisited. J Bone Joint Surg Am 1996; 78:656.

33. Rougraff BT, Kneisl JS, Simon MA: Skeletal metastases of unknown origin: A prospective study of a diagnostic strategy. J Bone Joint Surg Am 1993; 75:1276.

34. Malawer MM, Buch RG, Thompson WE, et al: Major amputations done with palliative intent in the treatment of local bony complications associated with advanced cancer. J Surg Oncol 1991; 47:121.

35. Pack GT, Ehrlich HE, Gentil FD: Radical amputations of the extremities in the treatment of cancer. Surg Gynecol Obstet 1947; 84:1105.

section
7

chapter
17

SURGICAL MANAGEMENT OF METASTATIC DISEASE OF THE PELVIS*

Mary I. O'Connor

Summary

- The pelvis is the third most frequent site of metastatic bone disease. Associated bone destruction results in pain and compromised ambulation and necessitates medical evaluation and treatment. With increased longevity of patients with metastatic bone disease, management of pelvic metastases has become more problematic and challenging.

- The key objective of medical and surgical management is relief of pain and prompt restoration of function, specifically ambulation.

- Patient selection for surgical treatment is critical. Surgical treatment is considered only in patients with significant bone metastases who have a satisfactory prognosis for survival.

- Periacetabular metastases are extremely challenging, and reconstructive techniques are designed to transmit weightbearing stress from diseased to intact bone. Protrusio devices are frequently incorporated into the acetabular construct.

- Complications include bleeding and postoperative hip arthroplasty dislocation. The risk of complications may be decreased by careful attention to surgical technique and component positioning, consideration of preoperative embolization, and selective use of constrained acetabular liners.

Advances in treatment have increased the life expectancy of patients with metastatic bone disease. As these patients live longer, orthopaedic issues of bone destruction with impending or actual fracture become more problematic, particularly in the pelvis. After the spine and ribs, the pelvis is the third most frequent site of bony metastases. Metastatic disease involving the pelvis often results in significant pain and functional disability. Management of these lesions is extremely challenging, and surgical treatment is reserved for selected patients who have a reasonable life expectancy.

HISTORICAL REVIEW

In the past, management of pelvic metastases was typically nonoperative. Radiotherapy, chemotherapy, analgesics, and restriction of ambulation were the mainstays of palliative care. As advances in chemotherapy resulted in improved survival, restricting these patients to nonambulatory status became undesirable. Surgeons began to apply to pelvic metastases the knowledge that had been gained in successful pelvic limb salvage procedures for sarcoma and complex acetabular arthroplasty revisions. This evolution in the treatment of patients with pelvic metastases is ongoing, as treatment guidelines and reconstructive techniques continue to be refined.

CLINICAL FEATURES

Patients with pelvic metastases typically present to an orthopaedic surgeon for evaluation of pain or are referred for evaluation of a destructive bone lesion. Because bone metastases are the presenting symptom in approximately 23% of patients,[1] orthopaedic surgeons will evaluate patients with bone metastases in whom the diagnosis of carcinoma has not yet been established. Subsequent referral of the patient to a medical oncologist is appropriate for further diagnostic studies, delineation of systemic treatment options, estimation of remaining life expectancy, and general medical evaluation, including assessment of metabolic, hematological, and nutritional status.

Pain from pelvic metastases is common in the region of the lesion. Discomfort may be worse at night and not be relieved by rest. Pain that is exacerbated with weightbearing is worrisome for impending or pathological fracture. Patients may also present with referred pain to the knee from a hip lesion or radicular symptoms from impingement of a pelvic tumor on local nerves or nerve roots, or they may have pain referred to the pelvis from spinal metastases. It must be noted, however, that in some patients the metastases may be asymptomatic until pathological fracture occurs, particularly in the periacetabular region.

Physical examination should emphasize the spine, pelvis, and lower extremities. Range of motion, motor strength testing, and neurovascular status should be assessed, and palpation is necessary to detect any local tenderness or soft tissue masses. The upper extremities should also be reviewed, as metastases or other clinical disorders may involve these areas and affect postoperative rehabilitation.

Once identified, pelvic metastases can be classified by anatomic location. Lesions may involve one or more of the three major anatomic regions of the pelvis: (1) the iliosacral, (2) the periacetabular, and (3) the ischiopubic. Frequently, patients have multiple metastases with one large, more symptomatic lesion.

INVESTIGATION

Pelvic metastases may result in lytic, sclerotic, or mixed bone lesions. Some pelvic metastases may be difficult to appreciate on routine radiographs, as metastases are typically within cancellous bone with minimal periosteal reaction. Osteopenia may further hinder identification of osteolytic lesions. Bone scintigraphy, computed tomography (CT), and magnetic resonance imaging (MRI) may be necessary to identify pelvic metastases. Surgical decision making is dependent on the extent of bone and soft tissue involvement. In some patients, both MRI and CT scans are obtained to better define the lesion and the degree of compromised bone.

The surgeon should be confident of the diagnosis of pelvic metastatic disease before performing an operative procedure. This is especially important in the patient with a solitary bone lesion. Periacetabular chondrosarcomas occur in older patients and should not be mistaken for metastatic disease. Patients may also have more than one primary tumor. Needle biopsy is often used to establish a diagnosis of metastatic disease. If the clinical setting is consistent with metastases from a patient's known primary tumor and

a preoperative biopsy has not been performed, the diagnosis should be confirmed by intraoperative frozen section.

TREATMENT GOALS, INDICATIONS, AND CONTRAINDICATIONS

GOALS

The goals of treatment of patients with pelvic metastases are to relieve pain, restore function in the shortest possible time, prevent pathological fracture, and avoid treatment-related complications.

INDICATIONS

Consideration of operative treatment is influenced by the degree of clinical symptoms, the location and extent of metastatic destruction, and the life expectancy and activity status of the patient. The importance of careful patient selection cannot be overstated.[2] Although significant medical complications accompany immobilization (pneumonia, decubitus ulcers, difficulty with nursing care), operative reconstruction of the periacetabular region is a complex undertaking associated with operative morbidity. A life expectancy of at least 4 months, and perhaps 6 months, is necessary for patients to benefit from such surgery.

Osteolytic metastatic lesions that compromise weight-transmitting areas, namely the periacetabular region, should be considered for operative stabilization in patients with pain and functional compromise. Pathological fracture of the periacetabular region is an appropriate indication for considering operative intervention. Radiation is ineffective for relief of pain that is related to biomechanical weakness, intra-articular destruction, or fracture. Surgical treatment should also be considered for asymptomatic periacetabular lesions that are large and are at clear risk of fracture. Resection of the femoral head and neck (Girdlestone's procedure)[3] can be considered in patients with acetabular disease and actual or impending intrapelvic displacement of the femoral head for whom other reconstructive options are not appropriate.

Wide en bloc resection for attempted cure is rarely appropriate for metastatic disease. However, in patients with late unifocal metastasis from a thyroid carcinoma or a hypernephroma, such a procedure can be considered. The author has had clinical experience with extended survival in such patients with hypernephroma, but analysis of patients with unifocal bone metastasis diagnosed at least 6 months after nephrectomy failed to show improved survival compared with patients who had a solitary metastasis to bone at the time the primary carcinoma was diagnosed (Trousdale R, Rock MG, unpublished data). Thus, radical curative excision should be considered very cautiously in such patients.

A new invasive, but nonoperative, technique for treatment of acetabular metastasis is percutaneous osteoplasty—that is, injection of acrylic bone cement into the metastatic lesion under fluoroscopic guidance.[4] Indications for percutaneous osteoplasty (or percutaneous acetabuloplasty)[5] have not been well defined. Cotten et al[4] first described this technique and their early experience with it in 1993, noting that it was still an experimental palliative procedure that should be "offered only to patients who cannot undergo surgery" and "must be performed in combination with radiation therapy." Weill et al[5] have added a second small series to the literature. With further experience with this technique, indications and efficacy can be better assessed.

CONTRAINDICATIONS

Sclerotic metastases are typically treated with nonoperative modalities, as they pose less risk of fracture. Also, some minimally displaced pathological fractures will heal with nonoperative treatment. Fractures due to prostate or breast metastases may progress to union because of the amount of reactive bone in the lesion and the longer survival of the patient. Primarily lytic and destructive metastases such as lung and renal lesions, however, usually do not heal.[6]

Operative intervention is generally not considered in patients with osteolytic metastatic lesions in non-weight-transmitting regions of the pelvis, namely the ischiopubic and iliac wing, even if fracture occurs. These lesions are generally treated with radiation therapy and protected ambulation. Infrequently, operative intervention can be considered if the non-weightbearing lesion is relatively radioresistant and if local progression of the metastasis would subsequently compromise the periacetabular region.

When the goals of pain improvement and preservation or restoration of function cannot be realistically achieved, operative intervention is not indicated. Patients who would still have significant pain and functional compromise related to extensive nonpelvic metastases are not good surgical candidates. In patients with extensive bone destruction involving most of the ilium, insufficient bone remains for adequate reconstruction. Although hemipelvic allograft and total hip arthroplasty reconstruction in such a situation would be considered after sarcoma resection, such a complex procedure is not recommended for metastatic disease.[2]

Specific treatment options are detailed in Table 1, including brief notations on indications, contraindications, and typical outcomes of each method. Systemic therapy refers to the use of chemotherapeutic, hormonal, radionuclide, or biphosphonate agents.[7] Systemic therapy and radiotherapy are typically used in patients with bone metastases. Embolization may be performed preoperatively or as a specific treatment.

PROCEDURES

PREOPERATIVE PLANNING

Operative strategy is determined by the location and extent of bone compromise. Bone compromise occurs as a result of tumor destruction, radiation osteolysis, or fracture. Soft tissue involvement, particularly tumor extension into the sciatic notch, also influences surgical planning.

Adequate imaging of the pelvis is critical to defining the degree of metastatic compromise. Appropriate radiographic studies include plain radiography, MRI, and CT. Extent of the disease is best determined by MRI, but CT provides superior imaging of cortical bone and the integrity of cancellous bone. Areas of cancellous bone may show marrow signal abnormality on the MRI scan but still be of sufficient strength for periacetabular reconstruction as determined by CT. Actual bone compromise may be more extensive, however, and should be anticipated. This is particularly true in patients who were previously irradiated, as

hyperemia of the adjacent bone results in weakening and increased risk of reconstructive compromise.

Use of a classification scheme can aid in preoperative planning. Harrington[8, 9] divided metastatic destruction of the periacetabular region into four classes. In class I, the periacetabular bone is sufficiently intact for conventional hip arthroplasty with a cemented polyethylene acetabular component. Such patients have a structurally intact rim, dome, and medial wall.

Class II patients have loss of the medial wall but a structurally intact dome and rim. Use of a protrusio device and a cemented polyethylene acetabular component is sufficient to transfer stress from the deficient medial bone to the intact rim (see Technical Details).

Class III patients have destruction of not only the medial wall but also the acetabular roof and rim. Unfortunately, most patients present with these challenging class III lesions. Weightbearing stress must be transferred to the intact ilium and sacrum via Steinmann's pin or screw placement combined with cementation of the acetabular defect, a protrusio device, and hip arthroplasty. Allan et al[2] have reported on the use of bulk bone grafts as a substitute for cementation of the tumor defect combined with reinforcement rings.

Class IV patients have a solitary metastasis and a reasonable chance of cure with wide en bloc resection of the metastatic lesion. Surgical planning includes adequate resection to obtain negative bone and soft-tissue margins. Reconstructive options, which are the same as those for pelvic limb salvage procedures,[10] are beyond the scope of this chapter.

Other authors suggest alternative classification schemes.[11, 12] Regardless of the system employed, the surgeon must identify the areas of both bone destruction and relatively intact bone to plan the reconstructive procedure.

Because selection of the femoral component used in hip arthroplasty reconstruction is influenced by the location and extent of disease in the femur, preoperative planning must also include imaging the entire femur for potential metastatic involvement. Plain radiographs and bone scintigraphy are appropriate, and typically a portion of the proximal femur is included in the CT and MRI scanning of the pelvis. Use of a cemented long-stem femoral component is appropriate in many patients with metastatic disease, with the necessary caution regarding the potential for fat and methacrylate monomer emboli.

Preoperative embolization should be considered in metastatic lesions with significant vascularity (e.g., renal cell carcinoma, myeloma). Even with embolization, severe blood loss can occur, and this potential should be discussed with the anesthesiologist.

Specific instrumentation needs are dependent on the type of reconstruction selected, as discussed in the following section.

TECHNICAL DETAILS

The reconstructive goal of the procedure is to provide the patient with a pelvis that will last for his or her anticipated lifespan. The reconstruction should noticeably reduce the patient's pain and provide adequate hip range of motion, leg length, hip stability, and durability of the reconstruction.[8]

TABLE 1. TREATMENT OPTIONS FOR METASTATIC DISEASE OF THE PELVIS

Treatment Type	Indications	Specific Treatment	Contraindications	Outcome
Nonoperative	Asymptomatic metastases, especially sclerotic with little fracture risk Symptomatic metastases with low risk of fracture	Systemic therapy and radiotherapy only	Large lytic metastasis in weightbearing acetabulum	Clinical improvement Strengthening of bone may occur but is not immediate Continued radiographic follow-up appropriate
Nonoperative	Large vascular lytic periacetabular metastases in patient at high risk of operative complications	Embolization of vascular supply to metastasis	Patient with extended life expectancy	Potential improvement in symptoms and delay in tumor progression, often temporary Embolization can be repeated
Nonoperative	Lytic metastasis involving acetabular dome	Percutaneous osteoplasty (methylmethacrylate injection under fluoroscopic control)	Metastasis with fracture into hip joint, destruction of subchondral bone, and destruction of posterior acetabulum	Diminished pain and improved weightbearing
Resection of femoral head and neck (Girdlestone procedure)	Impending or actual pathological acetabular fracture with intrapelvic displacement of femoral head in patient in whom other reconstructive options are not appropriate	Excision of femoral head and neck	Other reconstructive options suitable	Variable pain relief, limb shortened, ambulatory aids required[3]
En bloc resection of metastasis	Isolated metastasis with potential for cure	Wide en block resection of metastasis No skeletal reconstruction following resection of portion of ilium or ischiopubic region Consideration of skeletal reconstruction following extensive iliac or periacetabular resection with pelvic limb salvage techniques	Multiple metastases	Potential for cure of disease in selected patients
Intralesional excision of periacetabular metastasis without THA[13]	Metastasis localized to superior acetabular dome with articular surface preserved	Curettage of lesion, reconstruction of defect with custom polyethylene device, methacrylate, and Steinmann pins to support articular surface	More extensive acetabular involvement	Abstract presentation of new technique reports improved function No published data to date
Intralesional excision of periacetabular metastasis with THA	Treatment or prevention of pathological fracture of proximal femur with minor periacetabular involvement	Acetabular curettage/reaming and use of cemented THA	Significant periacetabular involvement (requires more extensive acetabular reconstruction)	Good improvement in pain and satisfactory function
Intralesional excision of periacetabular metastasis with specialized pelvic reconstruction and THA	Significant periacetabular lesion at risk of fracture in patient with adequate life expectancy (more than 4–6 months)	Debulking of periacetabular metastasis Reconstruction of defect with methylmethacrylate reinforced with screws/pins (or bulk allograft) combined with protrusio acetabular device and cemented THA	Inappropriate surgical candidate	Generally good improvement in pain and function Complex procedure with associated morbidity

THA, total hip arthroplasty.

The reconstructive construct should be anchored to remaining bone of sufficient mechanical strength and should permit transfer of weightbearing stress from diseased to intact bone. Optimally, the weightbearing stress is transmitted along a line 15 degrees medial to the vertical line, as this is the normal weightbearing stress across the pelvis.[9]

Such a reconstruction should not migrate medially. Fixation of the reconstruction should be secure.

For most extensive metastases, the technique of tumor curettage and acetabular reconstruction with methylmethacrylate reinforced with Steinmann's pins or a protrusio device and screws, or both, is utilized. Methacrylate alone in large bone defects is limited in its ability to resist tensile and shear stresses. The classic Harrington technique[8] involves using threaded Steinmann's pins to create a "cage" in the periacetabular region to support a reinforcement shell and a cemented polyethylene acetabular component (Fig. 1). Pins are drilled from the deficient acetabular dome into the intact proximal and medial ilium or sacroiliac region to transfer stress to this region. Note that pins may exit the medial ilium and then reenter the more posterior ilium and thereby place nearby neurovascular structures at risk. Palpation of the medial ilium via finger placement through the sciatic notch or deficient acetabulum will guide the surgeon in proper pin placement. Additional pins are placed from the anterior iliac crest inferiorly into the deficient socket to improve rotational stability. If necessary, mesh can be placed medially to prevent extrusion of cement. A polyethylene acetabular component is then cemented in place.

A modification of the classic Harrington technique is the use of cancellous screws inserted into the ilium extending proximal to the defect, with cementation into the defect and placement of a protrusio (or reinforcement) ring or cage with a cemented polyethylene acetabular component (Fig. 2).[2, 12] Screws for fixation of the protrusio ring are also placed. Care is taken to ensure that the polyethylene acetabular component is properly positioned. As the protrusio device is seated against the pelvis in a somewhat vertical fashion, the acetabular component must be positioned so that it is independent of the ring.

Selection of the most appropriate protrusio device is dependent on the degree of bone loss. The surgeon should be familiar with each device that may be considered. De-

vices vary in overall size, size options, shape, flange location, and size and acetabular depth. The author prefers to have several devices available at the time of surgery, as bone loss may be more extensive than predicted and individual patient anatomy at times favors one design over another.

There are three basic designs of protrusio devices, and for the purpose of discussion they can be classified as shells, rings, and cages. Reinforcement shells have a small peripheral rim that rests against the acetabular rim, most notably in the iliac region (e.g., Müller's ring, Oh-Harris protrusio shell). Such devices are designed to protect the deficient medial acetabular region by transmitting stress to the intact acetabular rim. Some designs permit screw fixation through the shell. Although such devices can be used for Harrington class II lesions with isolated deficiency of the medial wall, the author prefers to use reinforcement rings or cages.

Reinforcement rings have a short superior rim for oblique screw fixation into the ilium, multiple internal screw holes for placement of superior screws into the ilium, and an inferior hook that captures the inferior medial acetabulum, the condyloid notch (e.g., Ganz's ring). Longer, somewhat flexible flanges for more proximal transverse screw fixation into the ilium are featured in one device (Osteonics Restoration GAP II acetabular cup). In patients with an intact condyloid notch, the author favors the Ganz ring for medial defects and combined medial and partial superior defects. Manipulation of the hook to slightly decrease its contour will facilitate insertion of the hook around the condyloid notch. Although the acetabular profile of the GAP cup is deeper, the anterior and posterior

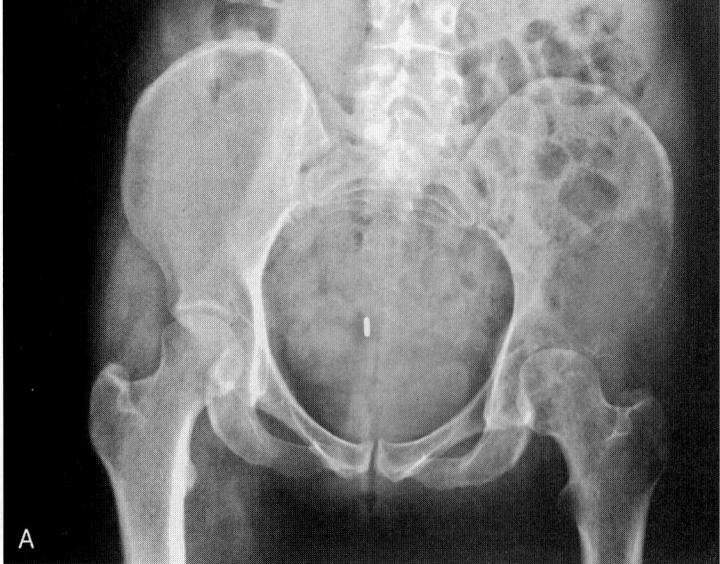
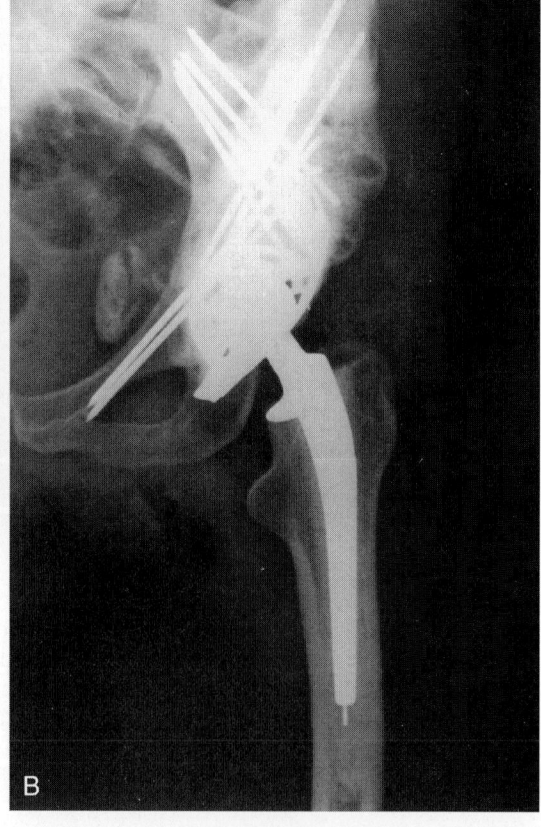

Fig. 1. The classic Harrington reconstructive technique for class III periacetabular metastases. *A,* Extensive destruction of the left ilium and periacetabular region secondary to breast carcinoma in a 33-year-old woman. *B,* After surgical tumor debulking, reconstruction was performed with methylmethacrylate reinforced with threaded Steinmann's pins, a protrusio cage, and a cemented polyethylene acetabular component and arthroplasty.

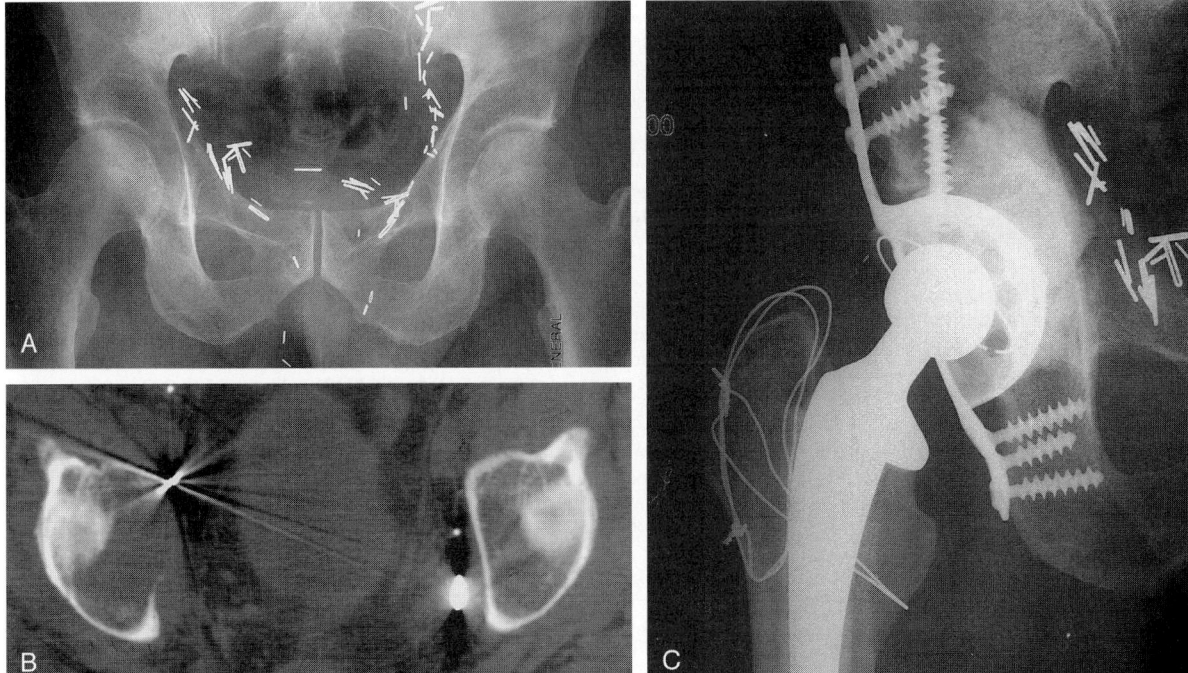

Fig. 2. Periacetabular reconstruction with protrusio cage and methylmethacrylate augmentation. This is a case of impending pathological fracture due to metastatic prostate carcinoma in a 62-year-old man. *A,* Bone loss in the right superior and medial acetabulum with lucent change and loss of the ilioischial and iliopectineal lines. *B,* Computed tomography better demonstrates medial bone loss. *C,* Postoperative radiograph following curettage, cement augmentation, and placement of a protrusio cage, cemented polyethylene acetabular component and cemented femoral component. Note the trochanteric osteotomy.

aspects of the Ganz ring can be slightly bent to deepen its outline. With use of the GAP cup, more extensive dissection of the abductors off the wing to the ilium is necessary to utilize the superior flanges. These flanges can easily be cut with a large bolt cutter at surgery to shorten them.

Protrusio cages have a large superior flange for transverse screw fixation into the ilium, multiple internal screw holes, and an inferior flange for ischial fixation (e.g., Burch-Schneider cage, DePuy's protrusio cage, Smith and Nephew contour reconstruction cage). The inferior flange of most cages is fixed to the surface of the ischium with screws, although the Burch-Schneider cage can also be slotted into the ischium. Cages are used in patients with more global acetabular bone loss (e.g., Harrington class III lesions) to transfer stress from deficient to intact bone of the superior ilium and inferior ischium. Sufficient bone must be present for fixation of the cage. In cases of extreme bone loss, techniques can be combined.

Implantation of cages requires more dissection of the abductors off the ilium for seating the iliac flange. Although it is generally preferable to avoid trochanteric osteotomy in patients with metastatic pelvic disease, such an osteotomy is often needed for surgical exposure. In such cases, the trochanteric region should be shielded from postoperative radiotherapy.

Several technical points merit emphasis. The author typically curets the tumor cavity and, if necessary, contours the protrusio device so that it is well seated against host bone. With flanged devices, one screw is drilled and measured for each flange and the device is removed. The tumor cavity is then cemented and the protrusio device placed against the doughy cement. The two initial flange screws are quickly replaced to provide preliminary fixation to the cage. Dome screws are promptly drilled and placed before the cement hardens. Additional rim or flange screws can then be placed.

The polyethylene acetabular component should have an adequate cement mantle. It is acceptable to downsize the component to achieve a better mantle of cement, particularly as polyethylene wear is not a concern in patients who have a limited lifespan. The author uses an acetabular liner instead of an acetabular component in small patients. Constrained liners can also be used to minimize the risk of dislocation and avoid the use of a postoperative brace. Finally, the length and offset of the femoral neck must be sufficient to avoid impingement against the protrusio device.

The author does not have any experience with the more limited surgical technique of tumor curettage and cavity reconstruction with a polyethylene acetabular reconstructive device, cement, and Steinmann's pins without hip arthroplasty, as recently presented by Rupert et al.[13] Such a technique is attractive for patients with a dome lesion and an intact articular surface. Further clinical experience with this technique is needed.

POSTOPERATIVE MANAGEMENT

Postoperative functional rehabilitation is individualized and is determined by the extent of surgery, the integrity of residual pelvic bone, and the overall medical status of the patient. Weightbearing is protected in the postoperative period and is gradually increased. Patients who have under-

TABLE 2. COMPLICATIONS OF PELVIC SURGERY

Complication	Frequency	Avoidance	Treatment
Infection/wound healing problems	1 in 26,[2] 2 in 58,[8] 0 in 58,[11] 1 in 12,[12] 3 in 17[15]	Perioperative antibiotics Meticulous surgical technique Avoidance of postoperative seroma or hematoma	Surgical débridement, antibiotics Possible rotational muscle flap for adequate soft tissue coverage of reconstruction
Dislocation of total hip arthroplasty or saddle prosthesis	2 in 26,[2] 0 in 58,[8] 1 in 58,[11] 5 in 12,[12] 2 in 17[15]	Appropriate placement of acetabular component (independent of protrusio device) Adequate neck length of femoral component to avoid impingement Avoidance of 22 mm femoral head component Use of constrained acetabular linear	Closed reduction and hip abduction brace Chronic dislocation may require revision to constrained linear
Reconstructive mechanical failures	1 in 26,[2] 5 in 58,[8] 1 in 12,[12] 2 in 17[15]	Thorough curettage to remove tumor and minimize postoperative tumor progression Postoperative radiotherapy and chemotherapy	Activity restriction Excisional arthroplasty can be considered
Extensive intraoperative blood loss (>8 L)	1 in 26,[2] 1 in 58[8]	Preoperative angiography and consideration of embolization	Rapid curettage of tumor Placement of methylmethacrylate to cauterize bone
Pulmonary embolism	3 in 26,[2] 1 in 58[8]	Early patient mobilization Prophylactic low-dose anticoagulation	Consultation with pulmonary medicine Anticoagulation
Operative deaths	1 in 26,[2] 2 in 58[8]	Control of intraoperative hemorrhage Avoidance of pulmonary embolism	
Neurovascular injury	1 in 58,[8] 1 in 17[15]	Careful placement of hardware and protection of sciatic and femoral nerve	Neurosurgical consultation for nerve laceration

gone extensive reconstruction are instructed to use a cane or crutch for the remainder of their lives. The author avoids early postoperative hip range-of-motion exercises by a physical therapist because of the need for soft tissue healing of the more extensive soft tissue dissection and to minimize the risk of dislocation. For extensive operations, a hip abduction brace is used for 6 weeks unless a constrained liner was implanted.

Prophylactic antibiotics are administered in the perioperative period. In many patients, low-dose prophylactic anticoagulation is cautiously administered to decrease the risk of deep vein thrombosis.

COMPLICATIONS AND RESULTS

COMPLICATIONS

Complications are, unfortunately, common after extensive pelvic surgery. The risk of a specific complication is related to the extent of surgery and the method of reconstruction. Table 2 lists the most common complications, their frequency in the larger published series of surgical management of metastatic pelvic disease, and strategies to minimize and treat such complications. Note that most mechanical failures of reconstruction are related to local tumor progression, often despite postoperative radiotherapy.

TABLE 3. OUTCOMES: PAIN RELIEF AND AMBULATION FOR SURGICAL TREATMENT OF ACETABULAR METASTASES

Clinical Series, Year	Surgical Technique	Postoperative Pain	Postoperative Ambulatory Status
Harrington,[8] 1981	THA with cement/protrusio ring/Steinmann pins	Minimal in 37 patients; moderate in 10; severe in 4 (total 51 patients at 6 months postoperative)	No aids in 20 patients; cane in 19; crutches in 6; nonambulatory in 6 (51 patients at 6 months postoperative)
Allan et al,[2] 1995	THA with protrusio device and bulk allograft or cement	Minimal in 14 of 16 patients (3 months postoperative)	"Only 55% of the patients regained complete independence after surgery. Twenty-five percent required partial assistance and 31% required total care."
Stark and Bauer,[12] 1996	THA with protrusio device	Minimal in 11 of 12 patients	Surviving patients "fully ambulatory without crutches" (3 of 12 patients)
Aboulafia et al,[15] 1995	Saddle prosthesis	Minimal in 5 of 9 patients	Cane in 5 patients; nonambulatory in 4

THA, total hip arthroplasty.

SHORT-TERM RESULTS AND OUTCOMES

Several factors influence the results of surgical treatment. Patient survival is principally determined by the histological features of the primary tumor. In Harrington's study,[8] patients with metastatic breast cancer had a mean length of survival of 29 months, compared with 13 months for the remaining patients with other types of tumors. However, patient death within several months of surgery was common in some series. Allan et al[2] noted that only 50% of their patients were alive 6 months after surgery. Stark and Bauer[12] reported that 4 of their 12 patients with acetabular metastases died less than 4 months after surgery. Giurea et al[14] reported that 33 of 43 patients who underwent surgical treatment of a pelvic metastasis, with or without skeletal reconstruction, died after a median of 12 months. These results underscore, again, the importance of patient selection for operative intervention.

Differing survival of patients, variation in extent of disease, differences in surgical technique, and disease progression at other anatomic sites limit analysis of clinical series regarding outcome. In general, relief of pain and maintenance or restoration of ambulation are achieved (Table 3).[3, 11, 12, 15] The literature does not identify one surgical technique as being superior to another for acetabular reconstruction. Allan et al[2] found no difference in outcome after use of their modified Harrington technique compared with use of a bulk graft to the acetabulum combined with a protrusio device. Whether larger numbers of patients with increased survival would better define differences in outcome with various techniques is unknown. Continued efforts to improve surgical techniques and patient outcomes are warranted.

REFERENCES

1. Conroy T, Malissard L, Dartois D, et al: Natural history and development of bone metastasis: Apropos of 429 cases [in French]. Bull Cancer 1988; 75:845.
2. Allan DG, Bell RS, Davis A, Langer F: Complex acetabular reconstruction for metastatic tumor. J Arthroplasty 1995; 10: 301.
3. Kantor GS, Osterkamp JA, Dorr LD, et al: Resection arthroplasty following infected total hip replacement arthroplasty. J Arthroplasty 1986; 1:83.
4. Cotten A, Deprez X, Migaud H, et al: Malignant acetabular osteolyses: Percutaneous injection of acrylic bone cement. Radiology 1995; 197:307.
5. Weill A, Kobaiter H, Chiras J: Acetabulum malignancies: Technique and impact on pain of percutaneous injection of acrylic surgical cement. Eur Radiol 1998; 8:123.
6. Enneking WP: Musculoskeletal Tumor Surgery, Vols 1 and 2. New York, Churchill Livingstone, 1983.
7. Aaron AD: Treatment of metastatic adenocarcinoma of the pelvis and the extremities. J Bone Joint Surg Am 1997; 79:917.
8. Harrington KD: The management of acetabular insufficiency secondary to metastatic malignant disease. J Bone Joint Surg Am 1981; 63:653.
9. Harrington KD: Orthopedic surgical management of skeletal complications of malignancy. Cancer 1997; 80:1614.
10. O'Connor MI: Malignant pelvic tumors: Limb-sparing resection and reconstruction. Semin Surg Oncol 1997; 13:49.
11. Levy RN, Sherry HS, Siffert RS: Surgical management of metastatic disease of bone at the hip. Clin Orthop 1982; 169:62.
12. Stark A, Bauer HC: Reconstruction in metastatic destruction of the acetabulum: Support rings and arthroplasty in 12 patients. Acta Orthop Scand 1996; 67:435.
13. Rupert C, Kollender Y, Malawer M: New approaches and surgical strategies in the management of metastatic malignant periacetabular tumors. Presented at the 4th Combined Meeting of the American and European Musculoskeletal Tumor Societies, May 6–10, 1998, Washington, DC.
14. Giurea A, Ritschl P, Windhager R, et al: The benefits of surgery in the treatment of pelvic metastases. Int Orthop 1997; 21: 343.
15. Aboulafia AJ, Buch R, Mathews J, et al: Reconstruction using the saddle prosthesis following excision of primary and metastatic periacetabular tumors. Clin Orthop 1995; 314:203.

LOWER EXTREMITY METASTASES

Frank J. Frassica, Steven A. Lietman, and Deborah Anne Frassica

Summary

- Lower extremity metastases are common in cancer patients and often involve the proximal femur, the subtrochanteric region, and the femoral diaphysis.
- Clinical problems in patients with lower extremity metastases include pain, inability to ambulate, and fractures.
- Activity-related pain is common and is an important warning sign of impending fracture.
- The indications for prophylactic surgery of the femur include 50% cortical bone destruction and long lytic lesions in high-stress regions such as the subtrochanteric region of the femur and the femoral diaphysis.
- Preoperative arterial embolization is used for highly vascular lesions, such as renal cell carcinoma.
- Interlocking intramedullary rods are used for diaphyseal lesions in the femur and tibia; in general, the surgery is performed without exposing the metastatic lesion.
- Prosthetic devices are used when rigid internal fixation is not feasible or the articular surfaces have been damaged.
- In patients with progressive lesions despite maximum radiation, wide resection and prosthetic arthroplasty are performed.
- External beam irradiation is used after surgery to minimize disease progression.

Metastases to the skeleton of the lower extremity are common in cancer patients.[1, 2] Frequent sites of involvement in the lower extremity include the pelvis, hip, subtrochanteric region of the femur, and the diaphysis of the femur. Clinical problems in patients with lower extremity metastases include pain, inability to ambulate, and fracture. The location and pattern of bone metastases are important in planning a course of treatment. The goal of treatment for the patient is to control pain, maintain ambulatory ability, and improve the quality of remaining life.

Operative treatment is recommended for patients with impending or complete fractures who are medically fit and have a reasonable life expectancy. Unfortunately, there are no absolute criteria to predict life expectancy. We generally recommend surgery if we expect the patient to live more than 6 to 8 weeks.

HISTORICAL REVIEW

In the past, many patients with metastatic cancer were treated with a very futile and pessimistic approach. Before the development of internal fixation and prosthetic devices, there was little that could be done from a surgical perspective. Patients with untreated lower extremity fractures often lost their will to live and died in severe pain.

The development of intramedullary rods and plates enabled surgeons to stabilize pathological fractures. Achieving rigid internal fixation was difficult as there was often substantial bone destruction. In addition, fatigue failure of the implant and pullout of the device from the compromised bone were major problems. In 1976, Sim and Harrington reported the use of polymethylmethacrylate (PMMA) to supplement the internal fixation of pathological fractures.[3] The PMMA may serve two important functions. First, it can improve the pullout strength of screws in plate fixation; the surgeon can lock an intramedullary rod in the medullary cavity by first placing PMMA into the canal and then advancing the rod into the PMMA-filled canal. Second, the PMMA can be used to fill large defects, which reduces the deformation of the implant during loading. The PMMA facilitates rigid fixation so that the patient can bear full weight on the lower extremity immediately following surgery.

Intramedullary rods play an important role in stabilizing lesions of the femur. The original intramedullary devices, such as the Kuntscher nail and AO nail (first-generation nails), were unlocked. When these devices were used to treat pathological lesions, it was often necessary to supplement the fixation with cement by opening the fracture site and filling the proximal and distal canals with methylmethacrylate. With the development of interlocking nails, rigid fixation is achieved by locking the rod proximally and distally with the interlocking screws.

The development and refinement of prosthetic devices was also an important advance. In the early era there were only a few stems for the femoral neck lesions (Austin Moore and Muller unipolar stems). Currently, there are stems for the proximal femur that are specifically designed to address the degree of bone destruction. When the bone destruction is so extensive that internal fixation is not feasible, the diseased bone can be resected and the defect reconstructed with a custom or modular prosthesis.[4]

CLINICAL FEATURES

Patients with lower extremity metastases usually present with pain or a pathological fracture. A smaller percentage of patients may present with asymptomatic lesions. Cancer patients with lower extremity pain should be questioned closely about their symptoms. Patients often describe a dull aching pain that is made worse on ambulation. Patients often describe difficulty walking secondary to a combination of pain and weakness. Night pain is a common feature.

INVESTIGATION

A careful evaluation should be performed before surgery.[1] High-quality plain radiographs in two planes are the first step. Cone-down views (such as an anteroposterior view of the proximal third of the femur) are useful for detecting subtle bone destruction. Patients are asked where their pain is located, and radiographs are taken of the appropriate site. When planning for surgery, it is important to have an anteroposterior view of the entire bone to prevent placing the end of an internal fixation device or a prosthesis at the level of a second lesion.

A technetium bone scan is a useful test for determining if the patient has more than one lesion. It is also useful for looking for other lesions and for serving as a baseline. The bone scan is sensitive in detecting metastatic foci. False negatives can occur in patients with myeloma and melanoma and in large destructive lytic lesions where there is virtually no remaining bone.

Before undertaking lower extremity surgery, it is important to know if there are any destructive lesions in the upper extremity or cervical spine. This assessment can be made from either a recent technetium bone scan or plain radiographs of the humeri. One must be careful in regard to placing a patient on a walker or crutches if he or she has upper extremity lesions; they may fracture. Cervical spine bone destruction or instability is an important consideration for the anesthesiologist in preventing neurological injury.

GOALS, INDICATIONS, AND CONTRAINDICATIONS

GOALS

The goal of surgery is to attain rigid internal fixation so that the patient can ambulate without pain and avoid postoperative complications.

INDICATIONS

The indications for prophylactic internal fixation vary with each patient. There are many different grading schemes and recommendations in the literature.[4–8] The general guidelines that the authors use in the lower extremity are the following:

- Cortical bone destruction in the diaphysis or diametaphyseal greater than 50% (the amount of cortical destruction on anteroposterior and lateral radiographs is measured).
- Purely lytic lesions in high-stress regions with weight-bearing pain (femoral neck, subtrochanteric femoral region, femoral diaphysis).
- Femoral neck lesions with greater than 25% to 50% bone destruction.
- Metaphyseal lesions with 50% to 75% bone destruction.

These guidelines must be used with a measure of common sense. If a patient has a purely lytic destructive lesion with only 25% to 50% bone destruction and marked weightbearing pain, then we recommend prophylactic internal fixation.

CONTRAINDICATIONS

The contraindications to surgery are relative. In the following scenarios, we do not recommend surgery:

- The terminal patient is a poor candidate. If we believe that the patient will not survive the surgery or the postoperative recovery we discourage surgery. It is very difficult to predict survival, and we generally recommend surgery only if we believe that the patient's survival will be at least 4 to 6 weeks.
- Patients who are severely immunocompromised with an absolute white blood cell count below 500 to 1000/mm³, who have an active infection, or who have fevers of unknown origin are at high risk for postoperative infection.
- Patients with platelet counts below 50,000/mm³ or who have a prolonged prothrombin are at risk for both intra- and postoperative bleeding. In cases of severe thrombocytopenia, we transfuse the patients with platelets on the morning of surgery. If the prothrombin time is prolonged, we treat a patient with intramuscular vitamin K and fresh-frozen plasma to correct the prothrombin time to normal.

ROLE OF EMBOLIZATION

Several of the metastatic carcinomas to bone can be extremely vascular. Their vascularity can be so prominent that biopsy sampling alone can result in severe hemorrhage. The metastatic lesions that are particularly vascular include metastatic renal cell cancer, some thyroid carcinomas, multiple myeloma, and metastatic hemangiopericytoma. Severe bleeding can occur in three scenarios: (1) during intramedullary reaming of the femoral or tibial shaft, (2) during curettage of a lesion, and (3) during the resection of a lesion that has destroyed the cortex and extended into the soft tissues. The bleeding may be so extensive that the surgeon must abandon the procedure. These lesions are best treated with embolization before surgery. With modern techniques, the lesion can be embolized up to a week before surgery. A longer time between embolization and surgery allows peripheral vessels to hypertrophy.

OPERATIVE TREATMENT

The surgical treatment of lower extremity metastases is accomplished with intramedullary rods, plates, and screws and prosthetic devices, depending on the anatomic locations and the pattern of bone destruction.

FEMORAL NECK AND INTERTROCHANTERIC REGIONS

Femoral neck lesions are usually treated with bipolar prosthetic arthroplasty[4, 9–13] (Fig. 1). If the destructive process is confined to the femoral neck, with excellent bone stock remaining in the femoral head, one should consider stabilizing the femoral neck with 7.0- or 7.3-mm cannulated screws, just as for a conventional nondisplaced femoral neck fracture. The authors do this occasionally for the young, active patient who does not want prosthetic arthroplasty.

Bipolar hemiarthroplasty may be performed through either the anterior or posterior approach. We prefer the anterior Hardinge approach because it allows more extensile exposure of the femur. The exposure of the femur is easily

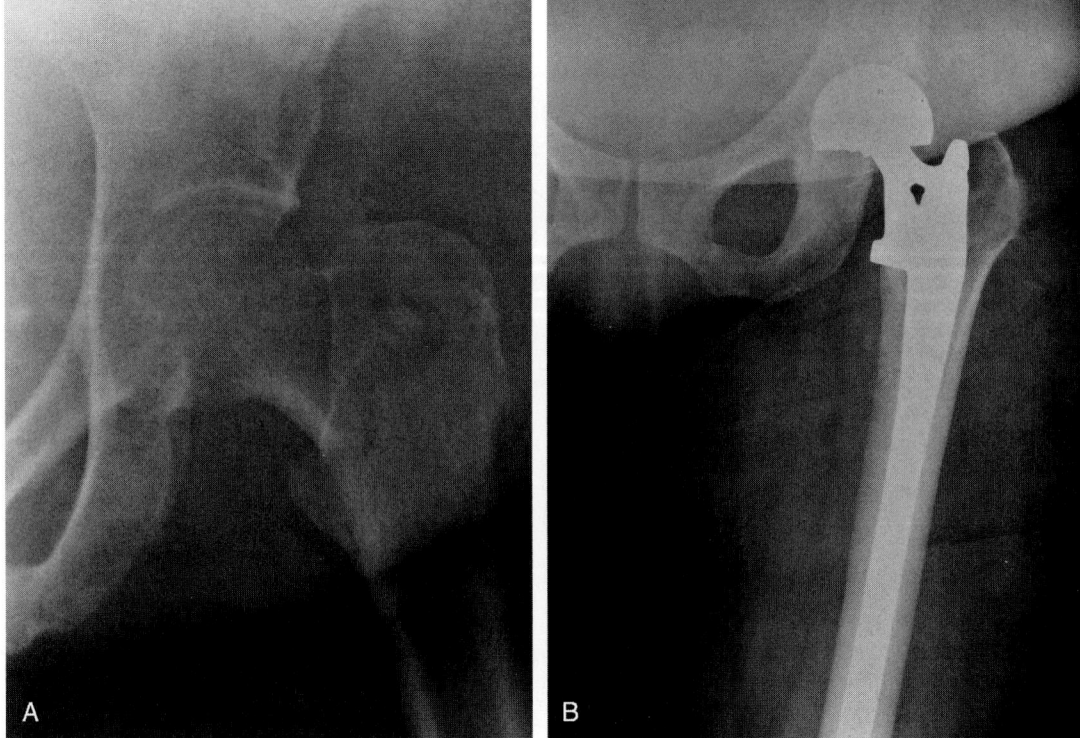

Fig. 1. Views. *A,* Anteroposterior radiograph demonstrating a pathologic fracture through the base of the femoral neck in a patient with metastatic melanoma. A preoperative magnetic resonance imaging scan had shown extensive disease in the femoral diaphysis. Because of loss of the entire femoral neck following resection and involvement of the intertrochanteric region, a long-stem head and neck prosthesis was chosen. *B,* Anteroposterior radiograph following reconstruction with a long-stem cemented bipolar head and neck prosthesis.

extended by further splitting the vastus lateralis and developing flaps by elevating the vastus lateralis subperiosteally. The extended exposure can be used to curettage the tumor so that the gaps can be filled with PMMA as necessary.

The acetabulum is palpated and, if there are no defects, the bipolar device is used. If there are defects in the articular cartilage, the acetabulum is reamed, and an acetabular component is placed.

The femoral component is selected based on the following amount of bone destruction:

- Femoral neck involvement alone: a standard femoral component is cemented into place.
- Femoral neck and intertrochanteric: a head and neck prosthesis that allows matching the head and neck replacement with the size of the defect.
- Extensive femoral neck and intertrochanteric involvement: a custom or modular proximal femoral replacement

SUBTROCHANTERIC LESIONS

Subtrochanteric lesions are prone to fracture secondary to the high local stresses. If the intertrochanteric region is intact, the authors prefer to stabilize subtrochanteric lesions with a reconstruction nail (Fig. 2). If there is substantial destruction of the greater trochanter, it may be difficult to use the reconstruction nail. The nail must be centered in the trochanter to guide the interlocking screws up the neck into the femoral head. With extensive destruction in the

trochanter, the nail will tend to drift laterally, making proximal interlocking impossible. If there is substantial destruction, a dynamic hip screw with PMMA augmentation can be used. If rigid fixation cannot be achieved with this technique, the proximal femur should be resected and reconstructed with a custom or modular proximal femoral replacement (Fig. 3).

Patients are placed supine on the fracture table in the same manner as for standard femoral nailing. It is crucial to make sure that one can visualize the femoral head well on both the anteroposterior and lateral fluoroscopic views. The only major difference from standard femoral nailing is the starting point in the piriformis fossa. One must be careful not to place the starting hole too posteriorly. The starting hole should be just in the midline or slightly anterior to it. Posterior nail placement may preclude targeting of the interlocking screws into the head.

FEMORAL SHAFT LESIONS

Femoral shaft lesions are treated with standard interlocking nails.[14] If any of the cortical bone is intact, we generally perform the nailing in a closed fashion and do not supplement the fixation with PMMA. With larger nails, there is little or no room for cement in the medullary cavity. The nail is always locked proximally and distally. Modern nails are quite rigid, and we counsel the patient that a femur with a large lesion may fracture during placement of the nail. To avoid fracture, we often over-ream the canal to a diameter 1.5 to 2.0 mm larger than the diameter of the nail.

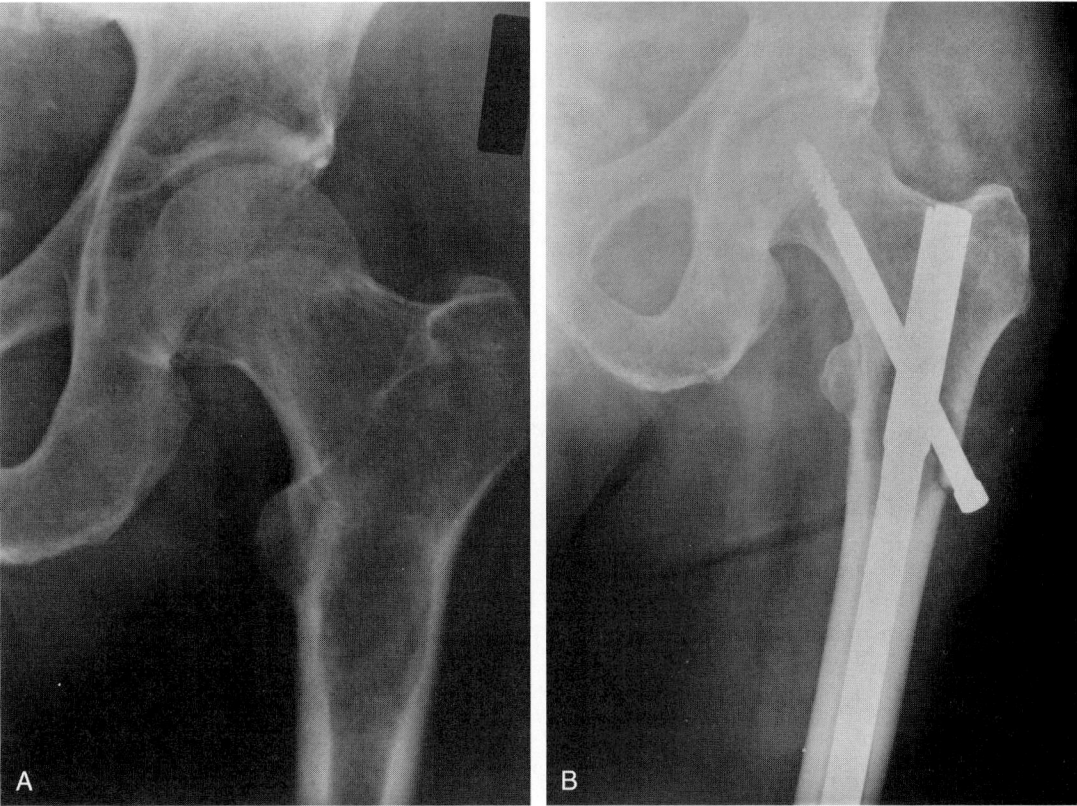

Fig. 2. Views. *A,* Anteroposterior radiograph demonstrating a lytic destruction lesion in the subtrochanteric region of the femur in a patient with metastatic breast cancer. In addition to the lytic diaphyseal lesion, there was diffuse involvement of the trochanteric region. *B,* Anteroposterior radiograph following stabilization with a reconstruction nail and treatment with external beam irradiation.

FEMORAL METAPHYSEAL LESIONS

Metaphyseal lesions can be treated with either standard intramedullary nails or plate fixation. The more distal the lesion, the greater the difficulty of achieving fixation with an intramedullary device. If the bone destruction occurs at the level of the supracondylar region, we prefer plate fixation with PMMA augmentation. Plate options include a 90-degree blade plate, femoral buttress plate, or a dynamic condylar screw. We prefer the dynamic condylar screw because of the ease of insertion and the excellent purchase with the screw in the medial femoral condyle. The PMMA can be placed through existing cortical defects, through a small window, or through the screw holes.

A lateral approach to the femur is used. Patients are placed supine on a fluoroscopic table, and the limb is prepared from the toes to hip. A sterile tourniquet is used. Depending on the amount of exposure necessary, the sterile tourniquet can be used for the entire procedure or the distal exposure. The vastus lateralis is elevated from posterior to anterior, and Bennett's retractors are placed. If there is substantial bone destruction in the femur, we prefer to place the dynamic condylar screw before curetting the tumor. This is important because, if the curettage is done first and the femur is extremely weak, the femur may fracture when the internal fixation device is placed. If the femur does not fracture, the patient can bear full weight immediately postoperatively. With fracture, the fixation de-

vice must be protected with partial weightbearing until the fracture heals.

The distal compression screw is placed first, and the plate chosen is laid into position. At this point, all the screws can be placed to achieve fixation and then the intramedullary cavity can be augmented, depending on the amount of bone destruction. If there is mild bone destruction (less than 25% cortical involvement), one can use the internal fixation device alone. Augmenting the fixation with PMMA for bone destruction greater than 25 percent is recommended. If the cortices are intact, we place the PMMA through the screw holes. The PMMA is mixed and placed into 5 mL–syringes while it is wet (if one waits for the doughy stage it will be very difficult to inject the PMMA). The PMMA can be placed in stages by removing three or four screws and placing the syringe firmly into the screw and injecting the cement. Alternatively, if there is an area of major bone destruction (greater than 75% cortical bone destruction), one can remove this cortex and inject the PMMA through the defect.

TIBIAL METAPHYSEAL LESIONS

Destructive lesions of the tibial metaphysis are less common than lesions in the femur. We prefer plate fixation with PMMA augmentation. A medial or lateral approach is chosen based on the side of the greatest bone destruction. For lateral lesions, we use lateral tibial plateau plates. The

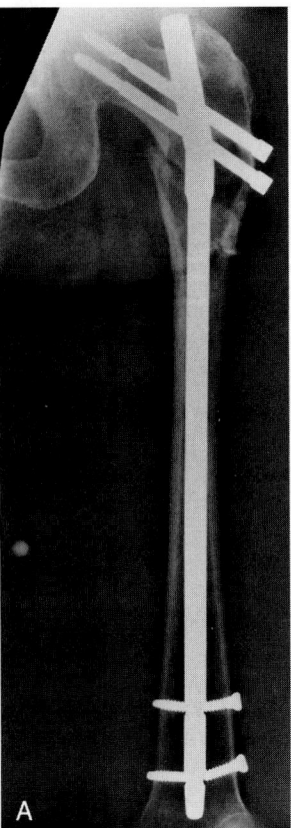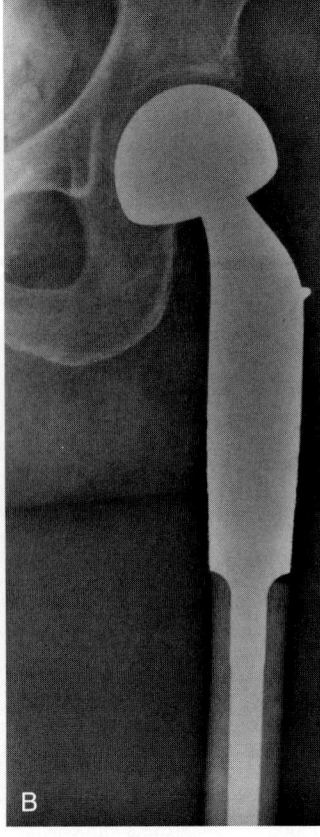

Fig. 3. Views. *A,* Anteroposterior radiograph of the femur in a patient with solitary myeloma of bone who underwent stabilization with a reconstruction nail. Note that the patient had progressive disease with fatigue failure of the proximal portion of the nail. The patient had been treated with 4500 cGy of external beam irradiation. *B,* Anteroposterior radiograph following wide resection and reconstruction with a cemented custom proximal femoral replacement. The patient, who went on to develop multiple myeloma and was treated with a bone marrow transplant, is now free of disease 6 years following resection and reconstruction.

plates come in different lengths (5, 7, and 9 holes), and a plate is chosen that extends at least three screws below the level of the cortical bone destructions. On the medial side, medial buttress plates are used.

The patient is placed supine on the fracture table, and a tourniquet is used. Carefully raise the fasciocutaneous flaps and expose the tibia subperiosteal. The most compromised cortex is opened, and the lesion is curetted. The plate is then chosen and contoured. The PMMA can be placed with one of three techniques. One, the PMMA can be placed and allowed to harden. Then the plate and screws are applied by drilling through the PMMA. Two, the plate can be placed, and then the PMMA can be placed through the cortical defect and through the screw holes. Three—the easiest technique—fix the plate to the tibia, and then remove the screws, keeping them in order so that they can be replaced quickly. The PMMA is then mixed and placed into the defect. The plate is applied, and the screws are inserted. The PMMA monomer can be cooled in the refrigerator to allow greater working time.

TIBIAL DIAPHYSIS

Metastatic lesions of the tibial diaphysis are uncommon. When they do occur, they can be fixed rigidly with an intramedullary nail locked both proximally and distally. PMMA augmentation is usually not used in the diaphysis because there is little room for the cement when the nail fills the intramedullary cavity. At the proximal and distal diametaphyseal regions it may be necessary to fill defects with PMMA.

The patient is placed supine on a fluoroscopic table, and the standard tibial nailing technique is used. The procedure is performed closed unless there are large diametaphyseal lesions. With large lesions, the nail is placed closed, and then the proximal or distal area is exposed as necessary. The nail is withdrawn, and the PMMA is placed into the defect. With fluoroscopic guidance, the nail is advanced across the site of the defect to its distal location. The PMMA is allowed to harden, and the interlocking screws are placed.

FOOT AND ANKLE LESIONS

Foot and ankle lesions are uncommon. Carcinomas of the lung and kidney and melanomas are the most likely cancer to metastasize to the foot and ankle.[15, 16] Most lesions can be treated with external beam irradiation alone. When necessary, the most common surgery that is necessary is curettage and cement augmentation. If the joint surfaces have been destroyed, a resection, arthrodesis, and then irradiation can be performed.

SOLITARY LESION AND EXCELLENT PROGNOSIS

A patient with a solitary metastatic lesion and an excellent prognosis may be a candidate for resection of the lesion.[17] In most cases a cure cannot be expected with resection; however, excellent local control of the metastatic lesion can be achieved. The reason to consider a resection of a metastatic deposit in bone is that intralesional surgery and irradiation will not provide permanent local control. A certain percentage of patients will have progressive local disease despite treatment. Failures occur more frequently in patients who survive longer than 2 to 3 years. In patients who survive up to 5 years, the failure of reconstructions of the femur can be as high as 30% to 40%.[18] Therefore, the patient with a solitary lesion and an expected survival of more than 3 to 5 years should be considered a candidate for a primary resection and reconstruction. We rarely treat patients with primary resection. A young patient with a solitary metastatic focus of renal cell carcinoma is the best candidate for resection and reconstruction.

PROGRESSIVE LOCAL DISEASE DESPITE IRRADIATION

Local control of metastatic lesions can be achieved in approximately 70% to 80% of patients.[19, 20] Most patients will succumb to their disease before progression becomes apparent. Patients with an expected prolonged survival (those with breast, prostate, and thyroid carcinoma) may have progression for 2 or 3 years after successful treatment. When progression occurs, there are two options: a second course of external beam irradiation or resection and reconstruction. If the patient has only a single site of disease, we favor resection and reconstruction. If the patient has multiple bone lesions or visceral disease with progression, we recommend a second course of irradiation.

Patients who have had maximum irradiation and progression are treated with resection and reconstruction if they have a reasonable life expectancy (more than 3 months) and are medically fit. For these situations, we try to achieve a wide surgical margin; there is not an option for further external beam irradiation.

DESTRUCTION OF THE JOINT SURFACES

When the articular surfaces have been destroyed, some form of arthroplasty is necessary. When only the subchondral bone is involved, standard resurfacing arthroplasties can be performed. If there has been major destruction of the proximal femur, distal femur, or proximal tibia, custom or modular arthroplasty is usually necessary.

SEVERE BONE DESTRUCTION

Rigid internal fixation or arthroplasty is an absolute requirement for the patient with metastatic disease. Patients must be allowed to bear full weight after surgery with a minimum risk for fixation failure. If the bone destruction is so severe that rigid fixation is not feasible, then resection and reconstruction should be performed.

Failed internal fixation devices are difficult to salvage with a second internal fixation device. The quality and quantity of the bone are poor. In this scenario, we tend to resect the diseased bone and internal fixation device together and reconstruct with a custom prosthesis (see Fig. 3).

POSTOPERATIVE CARE

Infections are common in the cancer patient, and a specific program should be followed to avoid them. Patients are treated with a first-generation cephalosporin intravenously for 48 hours or until all the drains are removed. Gentamicin is added for patients who are immunocompromised. Patients who have undergone lower extremity surgery are treated with low-dose Coumadin for 4 weeks after surgery.

Patients are mobilized out of bed on the first postoperative day. If rigid fixation has been achieved, patients are allowed to bear full weight immediately. Two crutches or a walker is recommended for 6 weeks to reduce the risk of falling.

RADIATION THERAPY

External beam radiotherapy is the prime modality for treatment of painful lower extremity metastases that are not at high risk for a pathological fracture.[19] The lesion is treated with a generous margin (3 to 5 cm) to prevent marginal recurrences. In treating the proximal femur, fields encompassing the supraacetabular region and the pubis are generally used to facilitate matching should additional treatment be needed for pelvic metastases in the future. The most commonly used dose-fractionation pattern is 3000 cGy in 10 fractions over 2 weeks. This is very well tolerated by the majority of patients and will result in pain relief in approximately 80% of patients. If patients are debilitated or have transportation difficulties, shorter courses of treatment may be more convenient. Options for more rapid treatment include 2000 cGy in five fractions or a single fraction of 800 cGy.

PAIN CONTROL

Control of pain is important for maintaining each patient's quality of life. The clinician should devise a regimen that controls pain and minimizes sedation. Long-acting slow-release narcotic agents are the mainstays of treatment.[20] The patient should also be treated with stool softeners and laxatives to prevent constipation and impaction.

REFERENCES

1. Frassica FJ, Gitelis S, Sim FH: Metastatic bone disease: General principles, pathophysiology, evaluation, and biopsy. In Eilert RE (ed): Instructional Course Lectures, XLI. Rosemont, IL, American Academy of Orthopedic Surgeons, 1992, pp 293–300.
2. Habermann ET, Lopez RA: Metastatic disease of bone and treatment of pathologic fractures. Orthop Clin North Am 1989; 20: 469.
3. Harrington KD, Sim FH, Enis JE, et al: Methylmethacrylate as an adjunct in internal fixation of pathologic fractures: Experience with 375 cases. J Bone Joint Surg Am 1976; 58:1047.
4. Sim FH: Metastatic bone disease of the pelvis and femur. In Eilert RE (ed): Instructional Course Lectures, XLI. Rosemont, IL, American Academy of Orthopedic Surgeons, 1992, pp 317–327.
5. Hipp JA, Springfield DS, Hayes WC: Predicting pathologic fracture risk in the management of metastatic bone defects. Clin Orthop 1995; 312:120.
6. Mirels H: Metastatic disease in long bones: A proposed scoring system for diagnosing impending pathologic fractures. Clin Orthop 1989; 249:256.
7. Beals RK, Lawton GD, Snell WE: Prophylactic internal fixation of the femur in metastatic breast cancer. Cancer 1971; 28: 1350.
8. Fidler M: Prophylactic internal fixation of secondary neoplastic deposits in long bones. Br Med J 1973; 1:341.
9. Levy RN, Sherry HS, Siffert RS: Surgical management of metastatic disease of bone at the hip. Clin Orthop 1982; 169:62.
10. Borel Rinkes IH, Wiggers T, Bouma WH, et al: Treatment of manifest and impending pathologic fractures of the femoral neck by cemented hemiarthroplasty. Clin Orthop 1990; 260:220.
11. Finn HA: Hip and proximal femur. In Simon MA, Springfield D (eds): Surgery for Bone and Soft-Tissue Tumors. Philadelphia, Lippincott-Raven, 1998, pp 683–703.
12. Behr JT, Dobozi WR, Badrinath K: The treatment of pathologic and impending fractures of the proximal femur in the elderly. Clin Orthop 1985; 198:173.
13. Lane M, Sculco TP, Zolan S: Treatment of pathological fractures of the hip by endoprosthetic replacement. J Bone Joint Surg Am 1980; 62:954.
14. Peabody TD, Finn HA: Femoral diaphysis and distal femur. In Simon MA, Springfield D (eds): Surgery for Bone and Soft-Tissue Tumors. Philadelphia, Lippincott-Raven, 1998; p 705.
15. Hattrup S, Amadio PC, Sim FH, et al: Metastatic tumors of the foot and ankle. Foot Ankle 1988; 8:243.
16. Healey JH, Turnbull AD, Miedema B, et

al: Acrometastases: A study of 29 patients with osseous involvement of the hands and feet. J Bone Joint Surg Am 1986; 68: 743.

17. Sim FH, Frassica FJ, Chao EYS: Orthopaedic management using new devices and prostheses. Clin Orthop 1995; 312:160.

18. Yazawa Y, Frassica FJ, Chao EYS, et al: Metastatic bone disease: A study of the surgical treatment of 166 pathologic humeral and femoral fractures. Clin Orthop 1990; 251:213.

19. Frassica DA, Frassica FJ: Nonoperative management. In Simon MA, Springfield D (eds): Surgery for Bone and Soft-Tissue Tumors. Philadelphia, Lippincott-Raven, 1998, p 663.

20. Frassica DA, Frassica FJ, Sim FH: Supportive measures for patients. In Simon MA, Springfield D (eds): Surgery for Bone and Soft-Tissue Tumors. Philadelphia, Lippincott-Raven, 1998, p 625.

SPINE

STEVEN R. GARFIN

section 8 chapter 1

MECHANISMS OF DISK AND MUSCULOSKELETAL BACK PAIN

Robert F. McLain and Gordon R. Bell

Summary

- Localized, persistent back pain may be caused by a variety of structures and a variety of pathological processes.
- Pain may be generated by bone tissue in response to physical distortion, inflammation, intraosseous disorder, or periosteal injury.
- Muscle pain and spasm may result from direct injury, resulting in either damage to the muscle tissue or swelling and pressure. Muscle pain may occasionally result from compartment syndromes and can be severe and unremitting until the pressure is released.
- Pain in facet joints, as with other synovial joints, may result from articular degeneration, fracture of the subchondral bone, ligament damage, strain of the surrounding muscles, and distention of the joint capsule itself.
- Although there is some controversy, evidence indicates that the intradiskal disorder itself can produce pain directly.
- Mechanical distortion or disruption of fibers of the posterior longitudinal ligament is a likely source of pain in disk protrusion or rupture and in other spinal disorders.
- Injuries to the dorsal root ganglion produce numbness, weakness, local pain, and radicular pain.
- Back pain in degenerative disk disease represents a combination of mechanisms.
- Back pain should be managed via a judicious combination of medical management, physical therapy, and occasional surgical intervention.

Back pain can result from a wide variety of musculoskeletal disorders. Destructive lesions expand the bony cortex and produce fractures or impending fractures in the weakened bone. Soft-tissue expansion caused by tumor or infection may elevate the periosteum away from the bone, producing local pressure and disrupting pain-sensitive nerve endings. Vascular compression may produce ischemia or venous congestion; and neural compression may cause pain, paresthesias, or paralysis. Some neoplastic lesions, such as osteoid osteoma and osteoblastoma, may exacerbate factors that produce pain directly, and the degenerating disk itself may produce factors or peptides that produce or magnify pain sensations.

Localized, persistent pain is the symptom that most often prompts the patient to seek medical treatment, but it is nonspecific and, by itself, provides little insight into the nature of the pain generator. The spine may be affected by a variety of pathological disorders—traumatic, neoplastic, inflammatory, metabolic, or degenerative—and the mechanisms by which these disorders produce pain are diverse. The physician must identify the anatomical source and

physiological cause of the pain, if possible, while excluding systemic or malignant processes that could threaten the patient's life. Irrespective of cause, the objective of treatment is to improve function and reduce pain, and the physician may use a variety of modalities to accomplish that goal.

POTENTIAL PAIN GENERATORS

The musculoskeletal system consists of the bones and articulations of the skeleton, and the ligaments, muscles, and tendons that connect and manipulate them are diverse tissues with radically different characteristics. Diagnosing the cause of pain based on the character and intensity of the symptoms is difficult. Severe, localized low back pain can be caused by a wide variety of disorders, ranging from the most benign to the most malignant. Conversely, a specific pathological process can produce a spectrum of very different symptoms depending on the situation and the patient. As the intervertebral disk degenerates, for example, it may stimulate local nerve endings mechanically or chemically, producing either localized, focal pain or diffuse, poorly localized back pain. Alternatively, the same degenerative disk may directly compress or chemically irritate the nerve roots or dorsal root ganglion, causing radicular pain symptoms. Injuries or disorders may directly affect any of the spinal column's component tissues or may indirectly affect the overlying integument, musculature, or neural elements associated with or contained within the skeletal framework. Many of these tissues are richly innervated.

BONE AND PERIOSTEUM

Bone is a composite tissue involved in a variety of physiological processes and capable of mounting a dynamic biological response to injury or stress. Fine nerve endings containing substance P and calcitonin gene-related peptide (CGRP) have been found in the marrow, periosteum, and cortex of long bones as well as in the associated muscles and ligaments.[2, 3] There is a higher density of substance P–immunoreactive and CGRP-immunoreactive fibers in epiphyseal rather than diaphyseal marrow, and fibers from the abundantly innervated periosteum are known to pass through the cortex into the marrow space by way of the Volkmann's canals. These two neuropeptides have been associated with a variety of actions. Both play a role in nociception, and both have been shown to accelerate and aggravate experimental arthritis after local infusion.[4, 5] Vasoactive intestinal peptide (VIP) and a number of other pain-related neuropeptides have also been localized to fine nerve fibers found in cancellous bone of the epiphysis and in the periosteum.[3] VIP is a vasodilator,[6] whereas neuropeptide Y is a powerful vasoconstrictor.[7] Fibers containing these neuropeptides aggregate at the osteochondral junction of the epiphyseal plate; VIP fibers run in the marrow spaces, whereas neuropeptide Y fibers follow the small vessels nourishing the epiphysis. The primary role of these peptides is probably to regulate growth, but these or similar peptides may also play a role in bone pain, possibly by triggering intraosseous hypertension or ischemia.

Bone is capable of responding to physical distortion, inflammation, intraosseous disorder, and periosteal injury by transmitting pain signals proximally. Primary bone pain may be generated by microfracture and subsidence in osteoarthritis, by periosteal elevation and distortion in infection or tumor, by vascular congestion and infarction in sickle cell crisis, and by mechanical distortion in fractures. In vertebral fractures, pain is initially produced when intramedullary nerve fibers and receptors in the broken bone and torn periosteum are stretched or disrupted and when injury results in pressure on receptors in the muscle and soft tissue overlying the fracture (Fig. 1). Hematoma accumulates rapidly, expanding until the pressure within the compartment is significantly elevated. The expanding hematoma triggers further pain receptors as it distends the fascia and soft tissue around the fracture. It may generate ischemic pain as pressure within the fracture obstructs blood flow to the adjacent tissues. Damaged tissues release bradykinin, histamine, potassium, and neurotransmitters, which sensitize nociceptive nerve endings, alter vascular permeability, and stimulate the influx of inflammatory cells. Edema, inflammation, and irritation of the injured muscle ensue, triggering muscle spasms and involuntary muscular contractions. These gross muscular contractions further displace the fracture fragments, causing further tissue damage and increased deformity and producing uncontrolled pain. In a patient with multiple extremity fractures, this cascade may lead to life-threatening hemorrhage and systemic shock.[8]

The tough, fibrous periosteal sheath that adheres to the outer cortex of the vertebral body is highly vascular and copiously supplied with both free and encapsulated nerve endings. The complex of free nerve endings is thought to generate painful discharges, whereas the encapsulated endings are thought to be sensitive to pressure.[9, 10] Periosteal nerve endings are immunoreactive for a wide variety of pain-related and vasoactive neuropeptides.[11] There is an extensive ramification of substance P–reactive nerve fibers in both the superficial and deep layers of the periosteal sheath,[12] and some encapsulated, glomerular-type receptors from the same tissue have also demonstrated substance P immunoreactivity. Encapsulated substance P–reactive nerve endings have been reported in the posterior longitudinal ligament of the spine, implicating that structure as a source of low back pain as well.[13]

PARASPINOUS MUSCLES AND TENDONS

Muscular pain and spasm are common components of low back pain. Muscular pain may result from direct injury, such as a blow or laceration, which damages muscle tissue and the intrafascicular nerve fibers that supply it, or from the swelling and pressure produced by the hematoma and the edema that subsequently forms. Pain may result from indirect injuries, such as athletic injuries, in which muscle is torn or ruptured as it strains against an excessive resistance force. Pain may also occur when overuse, inflammation, or ischemia causes the muscle to swell within its compartment, raising the intramuscular pressure and producing further ischemia. In major musculoskeletal injuries, persistent muscle spasm may result in severe pain as well as further trauma to the muscle and other tissues of the soft-tissue envelope. Persistent spasm may also be seen in more benign disorders, such as facet arthropathy or segmental instability.

Muscular pain receptors may be either chemonociceptive or mechanonociceptive and may respond to stimuli as either specific or polymodal receptors. Chemonociceptive endings may respond to metabolites that accumulate during

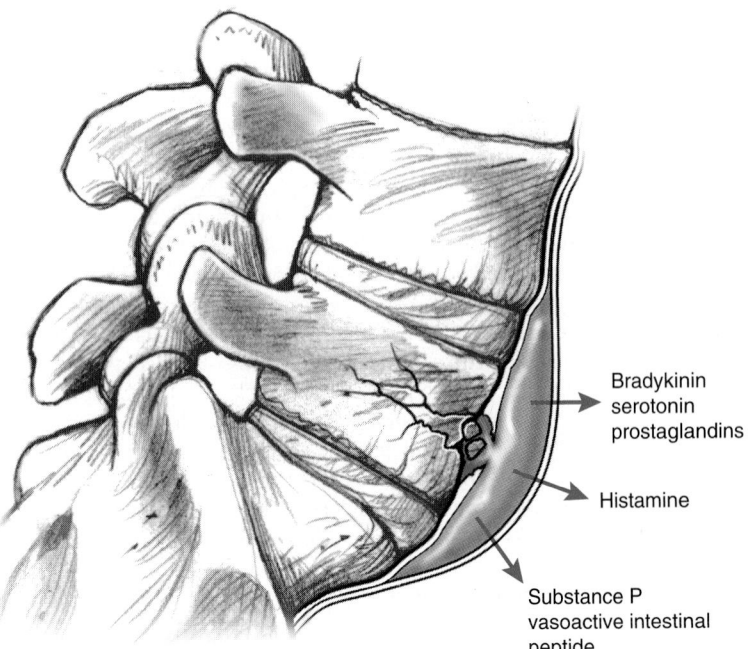

Bradykinin
serotonin
prostaglandins

Histamine

Substance P
vasoactive intestinal
peptide

Fig. 1. Pain in the bone and periosteum. Trauma initiates a series of mechanical and inflammatory reactions that may generate focal or radicular pain. After a vertebral fracture, disrupted nerve endings in the damaged muscle, fascia, periosteum, and bone will generate acute pain directly. Fracture hematoma, edema, and soft-tissue swelling will expand and distort tissues, stimulating pressure- and stretch-sensitive mechanoreceptors and nociceptors. Hematoma can generate enough pressure to compromise the nerve roots or cauda equina. Even after the injury is stabilized, inflammatory mediators and pain-related neuropeptides continue to seep into the surrounding tissues, stimulating and sensitizing receptors in the surrounding soft tissues.

anaerobic metabolism, the products of cell injury produced by injury or ischemia, or to chemical irritants such as bradykinin, serotonin, and potassium. Mechanonociceptive units may respond to stretch, pressure, or disruption. Some receptors may also respond to thermal stimuli.[14, 15] The primary nociceptive endings in muscle are unencapsulated free nerve endings similar to those seen in periarticular tissues, which transmit their impulses centrally by way of type III and IV afferent fibers. Intramuscular mechanoreceptors may also produce pain impulses when exposed to noxious stimuli.

Experimental studies demonstrated that intramuscular injection of CGRP in combination with either substance P or neurokinin A elicits a significant pain sensation, although none of the neuropeptides produces muscular pain when injected alone.[16, 17] It is thought that the neurogenic inflammatory response produced by CGRP, which results in persistent vasodilatation, erythema, and edema formation, may also serve to sensitize nociceptors to the presence of other pain-related neuropeptides.[18, 19] This type of receptor sensitization, combined with increases in intramuscular blood flow and interstitial edema, may be a primary cause of muscular pain.

A more ominous type of muscle pain occurs when excessive pressure in or around the muscle results in ischemia. Compartment syndromes occur in patients with bleeding disorders, vascular injuries, musculoskeletal trauma, systemic infections, and constrictive dressings or casts. Compartment syndromes can occur in virtually any muscle group and have even been reported in the paraspinous muscular compartments.[20] Pain is severe, unremitting, and disproportional to any injury the patient may have sustained. The clinical condition mimics the symptoms produced by experimental tourniquet pain, and it is likely that the pathophysiology of the two conditions is similar.[21, 22] Like tourniquet pain, compartment syndrome pain is progressive in intensity and rapidly resolves when pressure is released, either by removing the constricting dressing or by performing a surgical release of the compartmental fascia.[23, 24]

FACET JOINTS

These joints are specialized to meet specific demands of function: articular cartilage absorbs and distributes loads, and subchondral bone resists deformation. The blood supply coursing through the subchondral trabeculae supports and nourishes the cartilage; ligaments maintain alignment and constrain joint excursion; and musculotendinous units flex, extend, and stabilize the joint. Derangement or subluxation of the joint may accelerate articular degeneration or cause fracture of the subchondral bone, attenuation or disruption of the ligaments, and excessive strains and injury to the muscles. Nerve endings in these tissues may signal actual or impending tissue damage, producing the sensation of pain.

Synovial joints have a dual pattern of innervation. Primary articular nerves are independent branches from larger peripheral nerves, which specifically supply the joint capsule and ligaments. Accessory auricular nerves reach the joint after passing through muscular or cutaneous tissues to which they provide primary innervation.[25–27] Both primary and accessory articular nerves are mixed afferents, containing both proprioceptive and nociceptive nerve fibers. Freeman and Wyke[28] described four basic types of afferent nerve endings in articular tissues and documented the presence of those endings in a variety of joints. Although the type IV receptors (free nerve endings) are the only ones thought to be exclusively nociceptive, it is known that the proprioceptive endings of types I to III are capable of responding to excessive joint excursion as a noxious stimulus, and these types have an important role in mediating protective muscular reflexes that maintain joint stability.[29, 30] Deandrade[31] and Kennedy[32] and their colleagues demonstrated that the presence of a joint effusion, a common finding in patients with inflammatory, traumatic, or degenerative joint disease, can produce significant reflex inhibition of the quadriceps mechanism. Histological studies have demonstrated receptors in ligaments,[26, 33, 34] capsule[28, 35] and meniscal tissues,[36] as well as fat and muscle.[28, 37] Giles and Harvey[38] demonstrated nociceptive free nerve endings in capsular tissue from human lumbar facets and reported similar endings in the apophyseal synovium. Others identified free nerve endings and encapsulated mechanoreceptors in human cervical facets and synovium.[39] These nociceptive free nerve endings are supplied by small myelinated type III nerve fibers and small unmyelinated type IV fibers. These periarticular receptors respond to either mechanical (capsular distention, ligamentous instability, direct trauma) or chemical stimuli.[40]

It was previously thought that the synovium was a relatively insensitive tissue[41] and that the pain of synovitis was produced by capsular distortion and release of inflammatory mediators. Using antisera against specific neuronal markers, investigators re-examining synovial tissue found greater numbers of small-diameter nerve fibers than were previously reported using standard histological methods.[42, 43] Nearly all of these fibers have been immunoreactive for vasoactive and pain-related neuropeptides. Substance P, a neuropeptide strongly associated with pain perception and transmission, has been shown to accumulate in synovial fluid after intra-articular capsaicin injection and is known to trigger plasma extravasation and vasodilatation in surrounding tissues.[44–46] Substance P levels are higher in arthritic joints, and infusion of the neuropeptide into joints with mild disease appears to accelerate the degenerative process.[5] CGRP has also been implicated as a mediator in the early stages of arthritis.[47, 48] Whether these peptides directly stimulate pain receptors or simply make them more sensitive to noxious stimuli is not known. It is clear that sensitization has a primary role in pain production, and that several mechanisms of sensitization exist. Induction of experimental arthritis results in sensitization of free nerve endings in the joint capsule.[49] Intra-articular infusion of prostaglandins or bradykinin produces a similar effect,[50, 51] suggesting that local sensitization of free nerve endings is at least partly responsible for the pain of arthritic and inflamed joints.

In conditions of inflammation, hemarthrosis, and pyarthrosis of the larger peripheral joints, pain is produced by the distention of the joint capsule. Acute inflammation liberates chemical pain mediators that directly stimulate chemonociceptors and sensitize receptors in the fat pads and joint capsule.[52, 53] Synovial irritation results in edema, synovial hypertrophy, and effusion, which stretch and distort the capsule. Any subsequent motion of the joint increases the tension within the capsule, increasing pain. Joint motion may also cause the release of noxious neuropeptides, kinins, and inflammatory agents, which act on receptors in the capsule and periosteum. Inflammation results in the appearance of, or increase in, spontaneous activity in fine joint afferents and in an increase in sensitivity to movement.[54] By immobilizing the patient in a brace, these mechanisms are attenuated.

Whether all these same reactions occur within the spinal facet joints is unclear, but these are synovial joints and most likely respond in a way similar to the larger extremity articulations.

INTERVERTEBRAL DISK

Considerable controversy exists as to whether and how the intervertebral disk may generate focal back pain. The confusion arises, at least in part, from difficulties in separating disk tissues from peridiskal tissues, such as the periosteum and posterior longitudinal ligament, and from frank differences of opinion as to the presence and extent of innervation within the disk itself. Some authors failed to find any nerve fibers in the annulus fibrosus, contending that endings reported by others were actually residing in adherent portions of the posterior longitudinal ligament.[55–57] Other authors reported finding nerve endings within the layers of the outer annulus but only in limited areas.[58] More recent studies, however, consistently demonstrated fine nerve endings in the outer one-third of the annulus.[59, 60] Using histochemical techniques, Weinstein et al[61] demonstrated fine nerve fibers in the annulus fibrosus of the rat disk, which were immunoreactive for a variety of pain-related neuropeptides: substance P, CGRP, and vasoactive intestinal peptide. The presence of free nerve endings in the outer annulus and in the adjacent longitudinal ligaments suggests that intradiskal disorder can produce pain directly (Fig. 2).

The intervertebral disk receives its innervation from the sinuvertebral nerve, which supplies the posterior longitudinal ligament, ventral dura, and posterior and posterolateral annuli, and from the gray ramus communicans, which innervates the lateral and anterior aspects of the disk.[62] Branches of the gray rami also innervate the periosteum of the lumbar vertebral bodies and may provide some fibers to the posterolateral annulus in addition to those of the sinuvertebral nerve. These fine nerves primarily terminate in free nerve endings within the outer laminae of the annulus. Encapsulated receptors have also been located in the superficial layers of the disk.[60, 63] Ascending and descending nerve fibers provide considerable overlap of innervation within the spinal canal, with branches of a given sinuvertebral trunk supplying tissues one or two spinal levels higher. Pain resulting from disk degeneration may be referred to adjacent levels by this overlap, making it difficult to localize the pain generator clearly.

The close proximity of the intervertebral disk to the dorsal root ganglion, a structure uniquely sensitive to irritation, provides an additional way for intradiskal disorder to produce pain. Irritating neuropeptides and prostaglandins may sensitize or directly stimulate the dorsal root ganglion neurons.

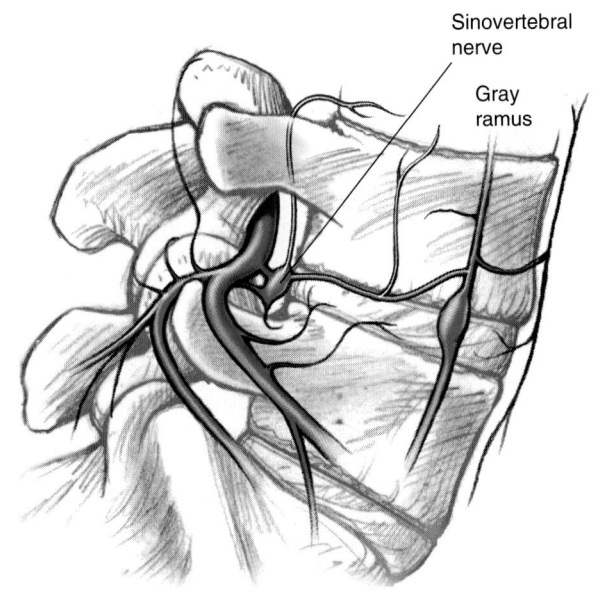

Fig. 2. Pain in the intervertebral disk. Innervation of the vertebral motion segment comes from two primary sources. The gray ramus communicans provides fine branches anteriorly that supply the outer layers of the anterior and lateral annulus and periosteum. The recurrent sinuvertebral nerve leaves the root and returns through the intervertebral foramen to innervate the posterior longitudinal ligament, posterior annulus, root sheath, and dura. These branches ramify with each other and with branches from adjacent levels of the spine, providing considerable segmental overlap. (From McLain RF: Neural mechanisms of musculoskeletal back pain. Pain Digest 1993; 3:82.)

POSTERIOR LONGITUDINAL LIGAMENT

The posterior longitudinal ligament is the most richly innervated of the spinal ligaments. The posterior longitudinal ligament contains a variety of endings thought to be sensitive to pressure, distortion, or chemical irritation. These nerve endings, supplied by ramifying branches of the sinuvertebral nerves, may be particularly important to the production of back pain because of the intimate relationship of the posterior longitudinal ligament and the posterior layers of the annulus fibrosus. The interdigitation of annular fibers and the posterior longitudinal ligament has resulted in some controversy as to whether nerve endings identified histologically actually resided in the disk or the ligament. Nerve endings may be found in both structures, but they are more numerous and varied in the posterior longitudinal ligament.

Numerous free nerve endings and a number of encapsulated nerve endings may be found in normal human posterior longitudinal ligaments. Both encapsulated endings and free nerve endings are immunoreactive for substance P, implicating the posterior longitudinal ligaments as a source of low back pain.[13, 48, 64]

These intraligamentous free nerve endings, because of their intimate proximity to the outer layers of the annulus fibrosus, are prime suspects for the production of localized back pain in patients with disk degeneration or herniation. Mechanical distortion or disruption of fibers overlying the posterolateral aspect of the intervertebral disk is a likely source of pain in disk protrusion or rupture as well as in cases of segmental instability, in which disk mechanics are significantly altered. Chemical irritation by herniated nuclear material, prostaglandins, or neuropeptides eluted from the degenerating disk stimulates nociceptive endings in these tissues as well.

DORSAL ROOT GANGLION

Compression and injury of spinal nerves and the dorsal root ganglion produce numbness, weakness, and local or radicular pain. Lindblom and Rexed[65] first implicated the dorsal root ganglion as a source of back pain in 1948. They noted that dorsolateral disk herniations sometimes resulted in dramatic compression and interstitial damage to the dorsal root ganglia of cadavers they examined. Since their work, the importance of the dorsal root ganglion in disorders of the spine has become widely appreciated.

The dorsal root ganglion is exquisitely sensitive to direct pressure, generating prolonged neural discharges after a brief compression. The nerve root itself responds to this same stimulus only after it has become inflamed and sensitized.[66–68]

Irritation of the dorsal root ganglion and nerve root often results from herniation of the intervertebral disk. In the absence of direct compression, pain may still be generated through chemical mediators. Noxious substances elaborated by the disk into the tissues and fluids immediately adjacent to the ganglion sensitize the afferent pathways and may even generate pain directly. A number of neuropeptides,

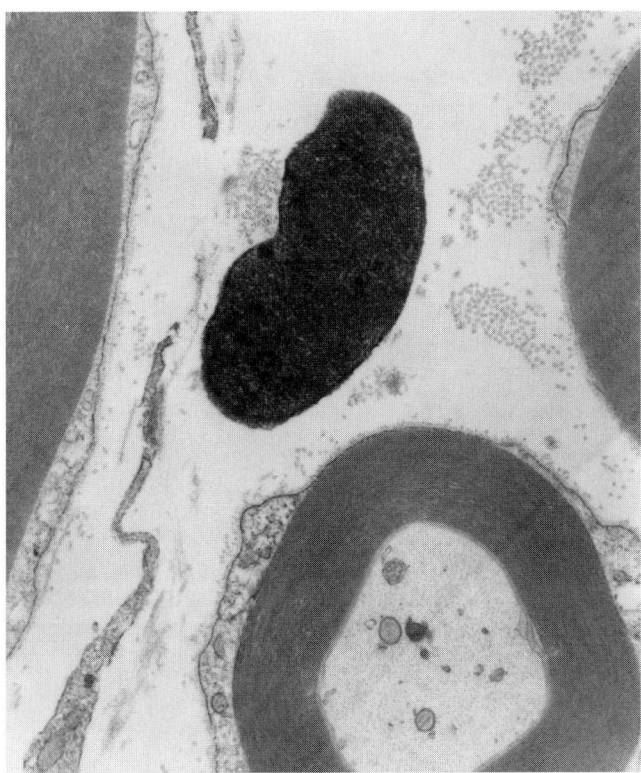

Fig. 3. Pain from the dorsal root ganglion. Electron micrograph shows afferent neurons passing through the dorsal root ganglion of an adult rabbit exposed to low-frequency whole-body vibration. Tissue was immunohistochemically stained using an avidin-biotin process, demonstrating marked immunoreactivity to substance P in a small number of specific, unmyelinated nerves. (From McLain RF: Neural mechanisms of musculoskeletal back pain. Pain Digest 1993; 3:82.)

prostaglandins, and inflammatory enzymes have been proposed as possible sources of dorsal root ganglion irritation (Fig. 3). Whole body vibration has been shown through a number of epidemiological studies to be a prime contributor to early degenerative disease and chronic back pain.[69, 70] Using a physiologically appropriate whole-body vibration stimulus, Weinstein and others first demonstrated that vibration was transmitted to the spinal column and, then, that short-term vibration exposure resulted in marked changes in dorsal root ganglion neuropeptide profiles.[71–73] The localized decrease in substance P and increase in VIP seen after low-frequency vibration exposure reflects the same changes seen after peripheral nerve injury and suggests a mechanism by which low-intensity physiological stimuli may produce back and leg pain. Subsequent studies using the same model found subtle but consistent changes in the cellular structure of dorsal root ganglion neurons exposed to low-frequency whole-body vibration.[74, 75] These changes are similar to those seen after direct nerve injury, with increased neuronal nuclear clefts, nuclear porosity, and mitochondrial and lysosomal volumes. These findings confirm the ability of indirect stimuli to produce neuropeptide and ultrastructural changes in dorsal root ganglion neurons, changes that may explain how whole-body vibration can generate clinically significant back pain and degeneration.

BACK PAIN IN DEGENERATIVE DISK DISEASE

The pathological conditions associated with disk degeneration present several possible pathways of pain production. As the disk ages, the proteoglycan matrix native to the healthy disk changes in composition and character. The nuclear matrix holds less water, and the disk loses some of its resilience and turgor. As the disk desiccates, horizontal and vertical clefts and tears form in the annulus. As a result, the mechanical stability of the vertebral segment is compromised, the disk loses height and begins to bulge, and the facet joints begin to override each other. Throughout the process, the deteriorating disk spills inflammatory mediators into the local soft tissues and the perineural spaces.

In phase 1 of this degenerative cascade, loss of mechanical stability results in abnormal motion and pain despite a relatively benign-appearing radiographic picture. Micromotion appears to precede actual spondylosis or listhesis, but even small sagittal or translational excursions can precipitate spasm and pain. Disk clefts and fissures may disrupt free nerve endings in the outer annulus or may serve as an avenue for neural in-growth from the surrounding tissues.[60] This phase may represent the clinical condition of internal disk disruption. During this process plain radiographs, myelogram, and computed tomography scan may be normal, and magnetic resonance imaging studies may show only desiccation and occasional clefts. The neurological examination will also be normal in most cases. In these patients, diskography is often the only positive objective study.

As segmental instability increases, excessive sagittal flexion or extension may inflame or injure the facet joints, triggering pain production from a secondary generator.

Whether stimulated directly by diskogenic pain or by the secondary facet arthropathy, patients frequently experience paraspinous muscle spasm as a result of muscular splinting and protective contractions. The pain from muscle spasm can be intense and may persist after the underlying generator has calmed down. The vicious cycle of spasm-pain-disability-weakness-activity-spasm is often the last part of the pain puzzle to be solved.

Over time, more overt signs of disk damage or degeneration develop. Disk space narrowing, osteophyte formation, sagittal malalignment, and/or spondylolisthesis herald phase 2 of the natural progression of disk degeneration. The clinical syndrome of degenerative disk disease may now be recognizable: mechanical back pain, restricted range of motion, and intermittent leg pain, all of which are associated with clearly recognizable radiographic changes. Radiographs show end-plate sclerosis, osteophyte formation, disk space narrowing, sagittal collapse, and early signs of instability: translation or excessive motion on flexion and extension films. Later, severe disk changes may be evident: vacuum disk phenomena and end-plate erosions and cysts, which are usually accompanied by complete collapse of the intervertebral space. There is considerable overlap between the condition of degenerative disk disease, as defined here, and more advanced conditions of segmental instability, degenerative scoliosis, and spinal stenosis. Patients with severe disk degeneration can present with diskogenic back pain, segmental instability, spinal stenosis, and pseudoclaudication.

Phase 3 represents the successful, natural conclusion to this process that we all hope for: consolidation of the disk/osteophyte complex, with reestablished stability and resolution of pain. When this end is met in a timely fashion, conservative therapy will have been successful. If the patient cannot function and cope sufficiently to achieve this end, then surgery may have to be considered.

SUMMARY

The rational treatment of any musculoskeletal problem requires that treatment options be applied in the order of ascending risk and potential injury. Understanding the nature of the patient's pain problem will lead the physician to make the most prudent therapeutic choices. The goal of the proper treatment plan is to keep the patient functioning at the highest possible level throughout his or her life, with an acceptable level of pain; such a patient has the opportunity to be an asset to, rather than a burden on, the community. The majority of patients will be well cared for with a judicious combination of medical management, physical therapy, and an occasional surgical intervention, well timed and tailored to the patient's needs.

REFERENCES

1. Marsh BW, Bonfiglio M, Brady LP, et al: Benign osteoblastoma: Range of manifestations. J Bone Joint Surg Am 1975; 57:l.
2. Bjurholm A, Kreicbergs A, Brodin E, et al: Substance P and CGRP immunoreactive nerves in bone. Peptides 1988; 9:165.
3. Bjurholm A, Kreicbergs A, Terenius L, et al: Neuropeptide Y–, tyrosine hydroxylase–, and vasoactive intestinal peptide–immunoreactive nerves in bone and surrounding tissues. J Auton Nerv Sys 1988; 25:119.
4. Colpaert FC, Donnerer J, Lembeck F: Effects of capsaicin on inflammation and on the substance P content of nervous tissues in rats with adjuvant arthritis. Life Sci 1989; 32:1827.
5. Levine JD, Clark R, Devor M, et al: Interneuronal substance P contributes to the severity of experimental arthritis. Science 1984; 226:547.
6. Said SI, Mutt V: Polypeptide with broad biological activity: Isolation from small intestine. Science 1970; 169:1217.
7. Lundberg JM, Terenius L, Hokfelt T, et al: Neuropeptide Y (NPY)–like immunoreactivity in peripheral noradrenergic neurons and effects of NPY on sympathetic function. Acta Physiol Scand 1982; 116:477.
8. Chapman MW: Orthopaedic management of the multiply injured patient. In Evarts CM (ed): Surgery of the Musculoskeletal System. New York, Churchill-Livingstone, 1989, 2nd ed, p 19.
9. Cooper RR: Nerves in cortical bone. Science 1968; 160:327.
10. Ralston HJ, Miller MR, Kasahara M: Nerve endings in human fasciae, tendons, ligaments, periosteum, and joint synovial membrane. Anat Rec 1960; 136:137.
11. Hill EL, Elde R: Distribution of CGRP-, VIP-, DH-, SP-, and NPY-immunoreactive nerves in the periosteum of the rat. Cell Tissue Res 1991; 264:469.
12. Gronblad M, Liesi P, Korkala O, et al: Innervation of human bone periosteum by peptidergic nerves. Anat Rec 1984; 209:297.
13. Liesi P, Gronblad M, Korkala O, et al: Substance P: A neuropeptide involved in low back pain? Lancet 1983; i:1328.
14. Kumazawa T, Mizumura K: Thin fiber receptors responding to mechanical, chemical and thermal stimulation in the skeletal muscle of the doe. J Physiol 1977; 273:179.
15. Mense S, Schmidt RF: Muscle pain: Which receptors are responsible for the transmission of noxious stimuli? In Rose CF (ed): Physiological Aspects of Clinical Neurology. Oxford, England, Blackwell Scientific, 1977, p 265.
16. Pedersen-Bjergaard U, Nielsen LB, Jensen K, et al: Algesia and local responses induced by neurokinin A and substance P in human skin and temporal muscle. Peptides 1989; 10:1147.
17. Pedersen-Bjergaard U, Nielsen LB, Jensen K, et al: Calcitonin gene-related peptide, neurokinin A, and substance P: Effect on nociception and neurogenic inflammation in human skin and temporal muscle. Peptides 1991; 12:333.
18. Fuller RW, Conradson TB, Dixon CMS, et al: Sensory neuropeptide effects in human skin. Br J Pharmacol 1987; 92:781.
19. Piotrowski W, Foreman JC: Some effects of calcitonin gene-related peptide in human skin and on histamine release. Br J Dermatol 1986; 114:37.
20. Carr D, Gilbertson L, Frymoyer J: Lumbar paraspinal compartment syndrome: A case report with physiologic and anatomic studies. Spine 1985; 10:816.
21. Smith GM, Egbert LD, Markowitz RA, et al: An experimental pain method sensitive to morphine in man: The submaximal effort tourniquet technique. J Pharmacol Exp Ther 1966; 154:324.
22. Sternbach RA, Murphy RW, Zimmermans G, et al: Measuring the severity of clinical pain. In Bonica JJ (ed): Advances in Neurology. New York, Raven Press, 1974, vol 4.
23. Matsen FA: Compartment syndrome: A unifying concept. Clin Orthop 1975; 113:8.
24. Mubarak SJ, Owen CA: Double incision fasciotomy of the leg for decompression of compartment syndromes. J Bone Joint Surg Am 1977; 59:184.
25. Gardner E: The distribution and termination of nerves in the knee joint of the cat. J Comp Neurol 1944; 80:11.
26. Gardner E: The innervation of the knee joint. Anat Rec 1948; 101:109.
27. Wyke B: Articular neurology: A review. Physiotherapy 1972; 58:94.
28. Freeman MAR, Wyke BD: The innervation of the knee joint: An anatomical and histological study in the cat. J Anat 1967; 101:505.
29. Eckholm J, Eklund G, Skoglund S: On the reflex effects from the knee joint of the cat. Acta Physiol Scand 1960; 50:167.
30. Palmer I: Pathophysiology of the medial

ligament of the knee joint. Acta Chir Scand 1958; 115:312.

31. Deandrade JR, Grant C, Dixon A: Joint distention and reflex muscle inhibition in the knee. J Bone Joint Surg Am 1967; 47: 313.

32. Kennedy JC, Alexander IJ, Hayes KC: Nerve supply of the human knee and its functional importance. Am J Sports Med 1982; 10:329.

33. DeAvila GA, O'Connor BL, Visco DM, et al: The mechanoreceptor innervation of the human fibular collateral ligament. J Anat 1989; 162:1.

34. O'Connor BL, Gonzales J: Mechanoreceptors of the medial collateral ligament of the cat knee joint. J Anat 1979; 129:719.

35. Grigg P, Hoffman AH, Fogarty KE: Properties of Golgi-Mazzoni afferents in cat knee joint capsule as revealed by mechanical studies in isolated joint capsule. J Neurophysiol 1982; 47:31.

36. O'Connor BL, McConnaughey JS: The structure and innervation of the cat knee menisci, and their relation to a sensory hypothesis of meniscal function. Am J Anat 1978; 153:432.

37. Dee RM: The innervation of joints. In Sokoloff L (ed): The Joints and Synovial Fluid. New York, Academic Press, 1978, vol 1, p 177.

38. Giles LGF, Harvey AR: Immunohistochemical demonstration of nociceptors in the capsule and synovial folds of human zygapophyseal joints. Br J Rheumatol 1987; 26:362.

39. McLain RF: Mechanoreceptor endings in human cervical facet joints. Spine 1994; 19:495.

40. Wyke B: The neurology of joints: A review of general principles. Clin Rheum Dis 1981; 7:233.

41. Kellgren JH, Samuel EP: Sensitivity and innervation of the articular cartilage. J Bone Joint Surg Br 1950; 32:84.

42. Gronblad M, Konttinen Y, Korkala O, et al: Neuropeptides in synovium of patients with rheumatoid arthritis and osteoarthritis. J Rheumatol 1988; 15:1807.

43. Kidd BL, Mapp PI, Blake DR, et al: Neurogenic influences in arthritis. Ann Rheum Dis 1990; 49:649.

44. Lam FY, Ferrell WR: Inhibition of carrageenan induced inflammation in the rat knee joint. Ann Rheum Dis 1989; 48:928.

45. Lam FY, Ferrell WR: Neurogenic component of different models of acute inflammation in the rat knee model. Ann Rheum Dis 1991; 50:747.

46. Yaksh TL: Substance P release from knee joint afferent terminals: Modulation by opioids. Brain Res 1988; 458:319.

47. Konttinen Y, Rees R, Hukkanen M, et al: Nerves in inflammatory synovium: Immunohistochemical observations on the adjuvant arthritic rat model. J Rheumatol 1990; 17:1586.

48. Konttinen Y, Gronblad M, Antti-Poika I, et al: Neuroimmunohistochemical analysis of peridiscal nociceptive neural elements. Spine 1990; 15:383.

49. Grigg P, Schaible HG, Schmidt RF: Mechanical sensitivity of group III and IV afferents from posterior articular nerve in normal and inflamed cat knee. J Neurophysiol 1986; 55:635.

50. Neugebauer V, Schaible HG, Schmidt RF: Sensitization of articular afferents to mechanical stimuli by bradykinin. Pflugers Arch 1989; 415:330.

51. Schaible HG, Schmidt RF, Willis WD: Spinal mechanisms in arthritis pain. In Schaible HG, Schmidt RF, Vahle-Hinz C (eds): Fine Afferent Nerve Fibers and Pain. Weinheim, Germany, Wiley-VCH Publishers, 1987, p 399.

52. Heppelmann B, Schaible HG, Schmidt RF: Effects of prostaglandin El and E2 on the mechanosensitivity of group III afferents from normal and inflamed cat knee joints. In Fields HL, Dubner R, Cerverof F (eds): Advances in Pain Research and Therapy. New York, Raven Press, 1985, p 91.

53. Heppelmann B, Pfeffer A, Schaible HG, et al: Effects of acetylsalicylic acid and indomethacin on single group III and IV sensory units from acutely inflamed joints. Pain 1986; 26:337.

54. Schaible HG, Schmidt RF: Effects of an experimental arthritis on the sensory properties of fine articular afferent nerves. J Physiol 1985; 54:1109.

55. Parke WW: The innervation of connective tissues of the spinal motion segment. Presented at the International Symposium on Percutaneous Lumbar Discectomy, Philadelphia, 1987.

56. Pedersen HE, Blunk CFJ, Gardner E: The anatomy of the lumbosacral posterior rami and meningeal branches of spinal nerves (sinu-vertebral nerves). J Bone Joint Surg Am 1956; 38:377.

57. Stillwell DL: The nerve supply of the vertebral column and its associated structures in the monkey. Anat Rec 1956; 12(5):139.

58. Hirsch C: Studies on the mechanism of low back pain. Acta Orthop Scand 1951; 20:261.

59. Bogduk N, Tynan W, Wilson AS: The innervation of the human lumbar intervertebral discs. J Anat 1981; 132:39.

60. Yoshizawa H, O'Brien JP, Smith WT: Neuropathology of the intervertebral disc removed for low back pain. J Pathol 1980; 132:95.

61. Weinstein JN, Pope M, Schmidt R, et al: Neuropharmacologic effects of vibration on the dorsal root ganglion: An animal model. Spine 1988; 13:521.

62. Bogduk N: The innervation of the lumbar spine. Spine 1983; 8:286.

63. Malinsky J: The ontogenetic development of nerve terminations in the intervertebral discs of man. Acta Anat 1959; 38:96.

64. Korkala O, Gronblad M, Liesi P, et al: Immunohistochemical demonstration of nociceptors in the ligamentous structures of the lumbar spine. Spine 1984; 9:156.

65. Lindblom K, Rexed B: Spinal nerve injury in dorsolateral protrusions of the lumbar disks. J Neurosurg 1948; 5:413.

66. Howe JF, Loeser JD, Calvin WH: Mechanosensitivity of dorsal root ganglia and chronically injured axons: A physiologic basis for the radicular pain of nerve root compression. Pain 1977; 3:25.

67. Howe JF: A neurophysiological basis for the radicular pain of nerve root compression. In Bonica JJ (ed): Advances in Pain Research and Therapy. New York, Raven Press, 1979, vol 3, p 647.

68. Wall PD, Devor M: Sensory afferent impulses originate from dorsal root ganglia as well as from the periphery in normal and nerve injured rats. Pain 1983; 17:321.

69. Frymoyer JW, Pope MH, Costanza MC, et al: Epidemiologic studies of low back pain. Spine 1980; 5:419.

70. Kelsey JL, Hardy RJ: Driving of motor vehicles as a risk factor for acute herniated lumbar intervertebral disc. Am J Epidemiol 1975; 102:63.

71. Weinstein JN: Mechanisms of spinal pain: The dorsal root ganglion and its role as a mediator of low back pain. Spine 1986; 11:999.

72. Weinstein J, Pope M, Schmidt R, et al: Neuropharmacologic effects of vibration on the dorsal root ganglion: An animal model. Spine 1988; 13:521.

73. Weinstein JN, Claverie W, Gibson S: The pain of discography. Spine 1988; 13:1344.

74. McLain RF, Weinstein JN: Ultrastructural changes in dorsal root ganglion neurons associated with whole body vibration. J Spinal Dis 1991; 4:142.

75. McLain RF, Weinstein JN: Nuclear clefting in dorsal root ganglion neurons: A response to whole body vibration. J Comp Neurol 1992; 322:538.

ADULT SCOLIOSIS

Glenn M. Amundson and Marc A. Asher

Summary

- The prevalence of scoliosis in adults increases with age and is said to be 15% for people older than 60 years; the prevalence appears to be higher in females.
- Scoliosis continues to progress in the majority of patients who presented with it as adolescents.
- Reduction in pulmonary function seems to be largely a product of age, smoking status, and co-existing pulmonary disease.
- Pain unrelieved by conservative measures is the most common indication for surgical intervention.
- Determination of fusion levels, method of spinal fixation, and surgical approaches should be individualized, based on the characteristics of the scoliotic curvature.
- Major complications are much more frequent in adult than in adolescent patients.

The management of adult scoliosis patients includes assessment, nonsurgical and surgical treatment, and postoperative care. It is much more difficult in the adult than in the adolescent patient. The complication rate of surgery is significantly higher in the adult. The age-related issues of osteopenia, smoking history, disk degeneration with secondary arthritis, spinal stiffness, and other medical illnesses are much more significant factors in the treatment of the adult.

Adult patients are defined as individuals older than 18 years of age who are physiologically and skeletally mature and who have a Cobb angle scoliosis greater than 10 degrees in the coronal plane. There are four major categories of adult scoliosis patients: (1) young adults without spinal degenerative changes who have a history of adolescent idiopathic scoliosis, (2) older adult patients with a history of adolescent scoliosis and extensive degenerative change, (3) those who develop scoliosis de novo after adulthood, most commonly in the degenerative lumbar spine, and (4) adult scoliosis associated with neuromuscular conditions, including post-traumatic paraplegia. Osteoporosis, rapid decompensating disk degeneration, and extensive surgical decompressions for spinal stenosis facilitate the development and progression of adult scoliosis. Degenerative curves have several typical characteristics, including a decrease in lumbar lordosis, short reciprocating curves without significant scoliosis above the lumbar levels, a rotatory subluxation most commonly at L3 or L4 or lateral listhesis of one vertebral body on another, and spinal stenosis.[1]

EPIDEMIOLOGY

The prevalence of adult scoliosis shares a positive correlation with the age range of the study population and has

been reported as 1.4% to 9%.[1-5] Kostuik and Bentivoglio[2] found that the prevalence of curves involving the adult thoracolumbar and lumbar spine was 3.9% in a review of 5000 intravenous pyelograms. Carter and Haynes[3] examined 6594 thoracic radiographs and found a 4.7% prevalence of thoracic curves greater than 10 degrees in patients age 25 to 75 years old. Perennou and associates[4] defined the frequency and characteristics of degenerative lumbar scoliosis in the adult low back population. The prevalence was 7.5%, and it increased with age: 2% before age 45 years, 15% after 60 years. Of patients who initially presented with low back pain, 86% were subsequently discovered to have scoliosis. Radicular pain was more related to unstable deformities and was more common in women, particularly at the L3-4 level. Perennou et al concluded that most degenerative cases of scoliosis seem to originate from minor childhood scoliosis and evolve due to disk degeneration. The male-to-female ratio varies from 1:1 to 1:2.[1]

NATURAL HISTORY

Curve progression in the adult patient with an idiopathic curve pattern has been well defined.[6, 7] Weinstein and Ponseti,[7] in a classic study with an average follow-up period of 40 years, found that 68% of adolescent idiopathic curves progressed after skeletal maturity. Thoracic curves progressed the most, with those measuring 50 degrees to 75 degrees progressing almost 1 degree per year and 30 degrees over the 40-year follow-up period. Thoracolumbar curves increased an average of 22.3 degrees during the same period, approximately 0.5 degree per year on average. Lumbar curves progressed an average of 0.24 degree per year. Progression was greatest when there was a lumbar curve, the fifth vertebra was not well seated, and the apical rotation exceeded 33%. The adolescent patient with the worst prognosis for later difficulty as an adult is one who presents with an unbalanced lumbar or thoracolumbar curve, the fifth lumbar vertebra not parallel to the sacrum, and the curve emanating from the lumbosacral junction. Curves less than 30 degrees at skeletal maturity tended not to progress, regardless of location.

Progression in degenerative lumbar curves has been reported to occur at 1 degree to 6 degrees per year, with an average of 3.3 degrees per year.[1, 3] Curves with a poorer prognosis include those with a pattern where the apex falls at L2-3 or L3-4, those with a grade III rotation, those that are imbalanced, and those with a secondary compensatory curve that is sharp and angular at L4-5 and L5-S1.[8] Patients with degenerative scoliosis who are also osteoporotic do appear to be at higher risk for progression.[9] Curve progression may not occur at a constant rate. Young adult curves may progress slowly or be stable. Middle-aged and older adult curves undergoing increased degenerative changes in the disks, facets, and ligaments may progress at an accelerated rate.

CLINICAL FEATURES

PAIN

Pain is often the chief complaint of patients who present to the spinal surgeon for treatment. Multiple pain generators exist in patients with adult scoliosis. Pain can be secondary to muscle fatigue, trunk imbalance, loss of lumbar lordosis, facet arthropathy, osteoporosis, or spinal stenosis. In a review of adult patients with idiopathic lumbar and thoracolumbar scoliosis, Kostuik and Bentivoglio[2] found that 60% complained of pain. This was similar to the prevalence in 100 age-matched patients without curvature. In fact, if all adult patients with scoliosis are considered, numerous studies suggest that the overall prevalence of pain averages 60% to 80% and is no greater than in control subjects.[1] It is unclear whether a correlation exists between the presence or severity of back pain and the magnitude of the curve. One long-term follow-up study showed no correlation.[10] Another study, however, found that in curves exceeding 45 degrees, the prevalence and severity of pain complaints increased significantly.[2] Jackson et al[11] found the incidence of back pain in adults with scoliosis and in a comparable group of adults without spinal deformity to be the same. Severity of pain, however, was greater in scoliotic patients. The clinical course of back pain in adults without spinal deformity and in scoliotic patients was different: 64% improvement in adults without scoliosis versus 83% persistence and progression in adults with scoliosis. Of the scoliotic patients, 51% had significant pain. Pain increased with age and degree of scoliotic curvature.

There appears to be a correlation between pain and curve location. All studies seem to agree that thoracic curves are rarely a source of pain. In general, patients with curves involving the lumbar spine more commonly complain of back pain. Compensatory lumbosacral fractional curves are the most painful and disabling. Pain appears to peak from the ages of 40 to 60 years, particularly in patients with thoracolumbar and lumbar curves greater than 45 degrees with apical degeneration, rotation, and coronal imbalance.[1] Most series show a higher prevalence of radiculopathy in patients with degenerative lumbar curves. Radicular leg pain may occur in conjunction with spinal stenosis, foraminal stenosis, or rotatory subluxation. Grubb et al[12] reported a 100% prevalence of stenotic symptoms in patients with degenerative curves, compared with 14.2% in those with preexisting adolescent idiopathic curves.

Precise evaluation of pain is made difficult because pain in adults is often multifactorial and may be totally unrelated to the deformity. The importance to the patient of cosmesis and underlying psychosocial factors such as depression, job dissatisfaction, and substance abuse are difficult to determine objectively.

EVALUATION

HISTORY AND PHYSICAL EXAMINATION

Adult scoliosis patients usually seek medical treatment because of the magnitude of their deformity, a complaint of or documented progression, back and/or radicular pain, or a combination of the above. Evaluating adults with scoliosis is much more difficult than evaluating adolescents because the usual criteria for operative treatment are often difficult to interpret or missing in adults. A history of curve progression is important. Curve progression is implicated from changes in clothes fit, increase in rib hump, loss of height, or altered waist line. Documentation of curve progression by serial radiographs is ideal but frequently unavailable.

Pulmonary compromise is difficult to attribute to scoliosis in the setting of chronic smoking or other pulmonary disease. The literature presents conflicting data on the incidence of cardiopulmonary complications secondary to scoliosis. Kostuik[8] found that functionally important respiratory dysfunction was not observed, even in curves of 100 degrees or more. However, ventilation was often decreased by up to 25% of normal predicted values. Exceptions to this overall favorable picture are patients with idiopathic scoliosis associated with marked thoracic lordosis. In a 20-year follow-up study on the natural history of untreated adult idiopathic scoliosis, Pehrsson and colleagues[13] showed a decline in pulmonary function equal to that predicted on the basis of aging alone. Unlike other causes of scoliosis, adolescent idiopathic scoliosis was not associated with an increase in mortality rate. Vital capacity was the strongest predictor of the development of respiratory failure, followed by the scoliotic angle. Respiratory failure occurred only in patients with a vital capacity of less than 45% predicted and angle greater than 110 degrees. Smokers and patients with underlying pulmonary disorders appear to be more susceptible to the detrimental pulmonary effects of curve progression.[1] Patients who have pulmonary symptoms or who are being considered for thoracoplasty or anterior procedures should have pulmonary function tests before surgery. Any extensive thoracotomy, thoracoabdominal approach, or thoracoplasty can be anticipated to disrupt the rib cage and result in at least short-term reduction in pulmonary function. Following a thoracoplasty, pulmonary functions recover more slowly in adult patients than in adolescent patients, if at all (Fig. 1).

The physical examination is comparable to the evaluation of all patients with spinal disorders. For any patient older than 40 years of age, a preoperative chest radiograph and electrocardiogram are advisable as well as a thorough evaluation by an internist.

Imaging Studies

The initial radiographic analysis includes 36-inch standing, posteroanterior, and lateral films as well as supine side-bending films. A long-cassette supine hyperextension film with the patient lying over a bump will assess flexibility in the sagittal plane. Magnetic resonance imaging or computed tomography myelograms are useful in evaluating patients with stenotic or radicular symptoms. Discography and facet and nerve blocks have proved helpful in localizing pain generators and can result in the extension of fusion levels.[12]

TREATMENT

NONSURGICAL TREATMENT

The basic approach to nonoperative care is similar to the treatment for all chronic, painful spinal disorders. It in-

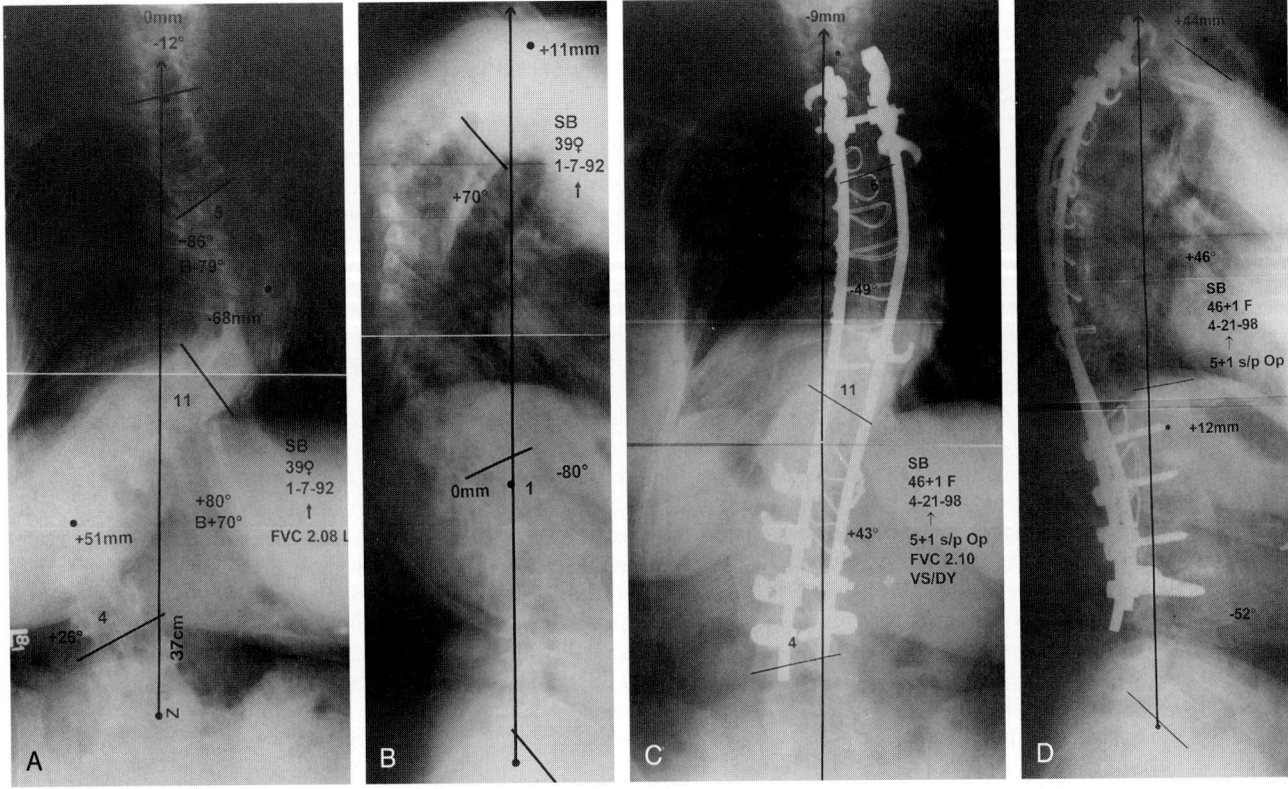

Fig. 1. Standing 36-inch posteroanterior and lateral radiographs. *A* and *B,* A 39-year-old female with previously untreated idiopathic scoliosis presents with shortness of breath and back pain. Treatment consisted of left-side transthoracic and retroperitoneal exposure with thorough diskectomies and arthrodesis, T10-11 through L3-4 motion segments. Following a period of halo-gravity traction, posterior segmental spinal instrumentation and fusion was performed. *C* and *D,* Standing 36-inch posteroanterior and lateral radiographs 5 years, 1 month postoperative show satisfactory alignment of her spine. Her pulmonary function, although not improved, has not deteriorated, and she is very satisfied with the outcome at this point.

cludes physical therapy, nonsteroidal anti-inflammatory medications, a low-impact or aqua-aerobics exercise program, and nerve root or facet blocks. None of these measures has ever been shown to affect the natural history of the adult's spinal deformity; they are instituted only to reduce symptoms. Other measures, including estrogen and calcium, are important for preventing postmenopausal osteoporosis. Patients who are not operative candidates but who have persistent pain despite maximal nonoperative treatment may obtain some relief by bracing, although there is no evidence to suggest that they prevent curve progression in the adult. To be effective, orthotics must be stiff and fitted carefully to the patient's deformity; however, they are poorly tolerated.

SURGICAL TREATMENT
Cessation of smoking and nutritional evaluation promote healing and limit postoperative infections and are of particular importance for the operative candidate.[1] The candidate's preoperative total serum lymphocyte count, serum albumin level, and prealbumin level should be well within the normal range before an elective spinal reconstructive procedure is performed. Some form of perioperative enteral or parenteral hyperalimentation may be advisable for the older patient who has medical problems and reduced protein stores.

Indications
The indications for surgery in adult patients with scoliosis include structurally significant curves with documented progression, back pain in the area of spinal curvature unresponsive to nonoperative care, thoracic curves greater than 60 degrees with loss of pulmonary function in whom progression is thought probable without history of concomitant respiratory disorder, progressive loss of neurological function and muscle fatigue due to increasing decompensation in the coronal or sagittal plane, significant curves (greater than 50 degrees) with associated deformity that is unacceptable to the patient and that the physician believes has a high probability of continued progression.[1, 2, 14]

Pain, the most common indication, accounts for about 85% of surgical cases.[2] Patients with significant axial pain in the area of their scoliosis and who have a curvature greater than 50 degrees to 60 degrees may be assisted by spinal stabilization. In these patients, there is a 69% to 95% reduction in the severity of pain, but the patient must be cautioned that there is a 15% to 20% chance that the pain will be no better after fusion surgery.[1] The frequency of pain may be unchanged.

Significant thoracic curves that have more than 10 degrees of documented progression are considered for stabilization.[14] Young adults (less than 35 years) with progressive thoracolumbar or lumbar curves of 45 degrees or more deserve consideration for stabilization.[2] A younger patient with truncal imbalance of 4 cm or more and whose major curve of 40 degrees or more extends to L3 or L4 and is accompanied by a compensatory curve at L4, L5, or the sacrum is a fusion candidate. Kostuik[2] has found that the primary curve may be reduced significantly by rebalancing only the lower compensatory curve. This approach should be used only if the lower curve is painful.

Fusion Levels

Determining fusion levels in the young adult who does not have significant degenerative change is similar to that for the adolescent patient. Sagittal plane considerations are equally as crucial in the adult as in the adolescent patient. The end vertebrae should be stable and neutral, and the sagittal plane profile should be corrected to as near physiological as possible. "Stable" means that the top and bottom of the fusion should be intersected by a line through the center of the sacrum (the center sacral line). "Neutral" means that there is no segmental rotation at the top or bottom of the fusion area. In most cases, it is preferable for the top and bottom of the fusion to be parallel to the shoulders and the sacrum at the completion of treatment. The fusion should not stop at or near the apex of a scoliotic deformity. Stopping a fusion at the apex of a sagittal kyphosis commonly results in a progressive junctional kyphosis. In the adult patient, the cephalad and caudad ends of the fusion should extend into areas of lordosis. Correction of an adult's deformity is more difficult to achieve than in the adolescent because of the increased rigidity of the curves and averages 30% to 40%. A factor that hinders achievement of coronal plane balance is the ability of the lower lumbar fractional curve to compensate for curve correction above it. Segments that should be included in the fusion include those with rotatory subluxation, spinal stenosis, and posterior column deficiencies as a result of a previous laminectomy or bilateral spondylolysis. However, in general, segments in the lumbar spine with only mild degenerative changes do not need to be included in a fusion if there is no underlying degenerative deformity or central, lateral recess, or foraminal stenosis. Unlike the adolescent patient, it is unusual for an adult patient to tolerate a primary distractive force extending to the L4 or L5 level. Distraction as a primary corrective force in the lumbar spine is contraindicated in the adult patient as it results in loss of normal lordosis. Preservation of segmental lumbar lordosis is critical; loss of the segmental lumbar lordosis predisposes to accelerated degeneration in remaining spinal segments. Thus with thoracic correction, primary distraction can be used safely to the L1 or L2 level, but by the L3 level a compression force is indicated.

Spinal Fixation

In general, the planned operation should provide enough immediate postoperative stability to allow for early ambulation. This requires the use of stiff, segmental fixation in the adult with scoliosis. Multilevel segmental instrumentation is useful in lowering stress concentrations and preventing fractures at the bone-metal interface. Osteoporosis is a potential problem when instrumenting the older adult spine, and the posteriorly overgrown facet joints are likely to be an obstacle to correction. Therefore, for most adults who are middle-aged and older, anterior segmental spinal instrumentation is not helpful. In this population, it is generally better to combine anterior structural bone graft with posterior instrumentation. With long fusions to the sacrum, it is preferable to have four points of fixation in the sacrum. Alternatives include two sacral screws with two intrasacral rods, bilateral S1 pedicle screws combined with a Galveston-type technique in the ilium, or bilateral S1 pedicle screws combined with long iliac screws. Constructs utilizing four sacral screws have also been described but are not favored by the senior author of this chapter. With long fusions to the sacrum, it is also important to segmentally fix L3-4 and L4-5 to capture the midlumbar spine in the construct. Structural anterior interbody grafts from L3 to the sacrum reduces the pull-out forces on the distal fixation points.

Surgical Approaches

The adult scoliotic patient's curve magnitude, location, flexibility, and sagittal plane balance determine whether a posterior, anterior, or circumferential fusion is needed. Lumbar curves, severe rotational subluxations, and laminectomized and kyphotic segments are more apt to benefit from anterior release, realignment, and structural grafting procedures. Anterior surgery helps increase the likelihood of obtaining a solid fusion and the amount of correction. Patients with severe, out-of-balance, highly inflexible curves may benefit from either triplane osteotomies or vertebral column resection procedures. In most cases, if anterior and posterior surgeries are contemplated, the anterior surgery is performed before the posterior surgery. With respect to staging of anterior and posterior procedures, Jeffrey and colleagues[15] compared 11 multiply-staged patients to 13 single-staged patients. Infection rates were less, and costs were 30% lower in the single-stage deformity-correction group.

Thoracic Curves

Generally, patients with thoracic scoliosis that requires surgery have a posterior operation only for scoliosis less than 70 degrees and kyphosis less than 60 degrees. If a patient has either kyphosis greater than 60 degrees or scoliosis greater than 70 degrees to 75 degrees, particularly if associated with ankylosis and coronal imbalance, an anterior release and fusion is added to the surgical regimen of posterior fusion and stabilization. The first stage consists of anterior diskectomies, osteotomies as necessary, and bone grafting using the harvested rib. The second stage is done posteriorly, with complete facetectomies and osteotomies as necessary, followed by curve correction with instrumentation, thoracoplasties as necessary, and bone grafting. With curves of this magnitude and rigidity, a substantial amount of mobility can be gained by resecting the ribs that have autofused to the ankylosed vertebral segments.

Thoracoplasties may be considered whenever a rib prominence of more than 3 cm exists.[1] The primary indications for thoracoplasty in patients with significant prominence include improved cosmetic result, increased spinal correction, diminished pain at the site of prominence, and added fusion mass. The complications of thoracoplasty in adult scoliosis are few. Thoracoplasty results are poorer in very angular deformities; if too much rib is resected, the rib cage can be destabilized. The most common complication of thoracoplasty is a pneumothorax.

Thoracolumbar/Lumbar Curves

Mobile curves less than 75 degrees that maintain lumbar lordosis without lumbosacral involvement can be managed by a single-stage anterior fusion with instrumentation. Segmental instrumentation systems, spanning the entire curve in the adult, are indicated; they preserve distal motion segments best. If there is significant osteoporosis, methylmethacrylate is used to augment the construct. Autogenous bone graft is used, usually consisting of excised ribs. A 0% pseudoarthrosis rate can be achieved, although most series report a small number of pseudarthroses.[2] Some loss of lordosis is common with anterior systems, but the amount can be decreased by using a stiffer rod, placing the screws as posteriorly as possible in the vertebral body, and using anterior interbody bone blocks to maintain a lordotic posture. Kostuik and colleagues[16] reported correction in the frontal plane for patients younger than 50 years as 72% and 60% for those older than 50 years. Trammell and colleagues[17] reported an average correction of 63% in their patients instrumented with the Zielke device. They believed that high-risk groups consisted of patients with a curve greater than 60 degrees and those older than 50 years with rigid deformity. This technique can be used from T9 or T10 to L5. Further extension above this level is rarely of value because the disk spaces are so narrow that little additional correction is gained in the adult.

If a fixed, oblique lumbosacral take-off exists, fusion must be extended across the lumbosacral junction. Failure to do so can lead to pelvic obliquity if the lumbar curve is corrected alone. In these situations requiring fusion to the sacrum, a combined approach is preferred. A posterior fusion alone can lead to loss of lumbar lordosis and a high rate of pseudarthrosis. The anterior stage includes placement of wedged femoral allografts in the L4-5 and L5-S1 disk spaces to maintain lordosis. The marrow cavity of the allograft is packed with autogenous bone graft. The posterior stage includes segmental instrumentation that incorporates the intrasacral rod or the Luque-Galveston transiliac or the sacroiliac screw pelvic fixation techniques. The specific treatment of thoracolumbar and lumbar curves depends on the locality of pain, presence of lumbosacral involvement on discography, extent of flexibility, and the presence or absence of an associated lumbar kyphosis secondary to degenerative changes. If the L5-S1 disk is part of the pain complex, then fusion to the sacrum is necessary and requires both anterior and posterior surgery. If the curve is flexible and the L5-S1 disk is part of the pain complex, then fusion to the sacrum is necessary and requires both anterior and posterior surgery. If the curve is flexible and the L5-S1 disk was not a source of pain, then a single-stage posterior segmental instrumentation and fusion is performed. If a kyphosis is present, an anterior release is added to facilitate curve correction. The anterior release is followed by posterior segmental instrumentation to derotate the spine and restore lordosis. Utilizing the classification and treatment techniques, 86% of 92 patients with disabling pain before surgery had pain relief. The pseudoarthrosis rate was 5%. Complications were greater in patients older than 50 years.[2]

The most common indications for surgery in adult onset scoliosis are nerve root symptoms and spinal stenosis. Decompression alone has been advocated for patients with severe stenosis, no coronal or sagittal imbalance, no rotatory subluxations, and stabilizing anterior osteophytes.[18] Also advocated is single-root decompression when preservation of facets is possible. However, if greater decompression is necessary or if the facets are sacrificed, there is a high potential for progressive deformity. If the curve associated with stenosis is relatively less severe (less than 70 degrees) with only mild subluxations of the vertebral bodies (less than 5 mm), reasonable coronal and sagittal balance, and flexibility, then a single-stage posterior decompression, instrumentation, and fusion can be performed (Fig. 2). If, however, the curve is larger, has subluxations greater than 5 mm, has imbalance in either plane, and is stiff, then a combined anterior and posterior procedure is required.[18] Grubb and associates[12] reported on their treatment of adult degenerative cases as resulting in a 70% reduction in pain and 33% pseudarthrosis rate. All pseudoarthrosis was in patients fused to the sacrum with posterior procedures alone. Preoperative assessment included the use of discography. Performing anterior diskectomies with structural outer body femoral ring allografts restores disk space height, lumbar lordosis, and foramina height resulting in an indirect decompression.

Double Thoracic and Lumbar Curves

In less severe (less than 60 degrees) and balanced double thoracic and lumbar curves, a single-stage posterior fusion with segmental instrumentation is adequate. If the curve is more severe (less than 70 degrees) or imbalanced, then a two-stage approach is required. The more rigid, unbalanced curve is released and fused anteriorly during the first stage. Both curves are then fused posteriorly with segmental instrumentation.[1]

COMPLICATIONS IN ADULT SCOLIOSIS

Complications in the surgical treatment of adult scoliosis are based on numerous factors. Major complications are much more frequent than in adolescents and depend on approach, spinal level of deformity, and the patient's age. Major complications include pseudarthrosis (0% to 33%), residual pain (5% to 15%), thromboembolism (1% to 20%), neurological injury (1% to 5%), mortality (1% to 5%), and infection (0.5% to 5%).[1, 19, 20] Complications are more likely to occur in older patients, those who are osteoporotic, those with significant comorbidities, and those with long fusions to the sacrum.

The transition syndrome complication is caused by breakdown adjacent to a fusion and involves a combination of increasing deformity and/or canal compromise that is symptomatic to the patient. Proximal and distal transition syndromes are more likely to occur in the adult population than the pediatric group. The usual causes of distal transition syndrome include fusing the spine in a position of hypolordosis or stopping at a segment with degenerative deformity. The most common causes of proximal junctional transition syndrome are stopping the fusion too close to the sagittal apex or destabilizing the proximal junction by ligamentous disruption. In a general review of complications

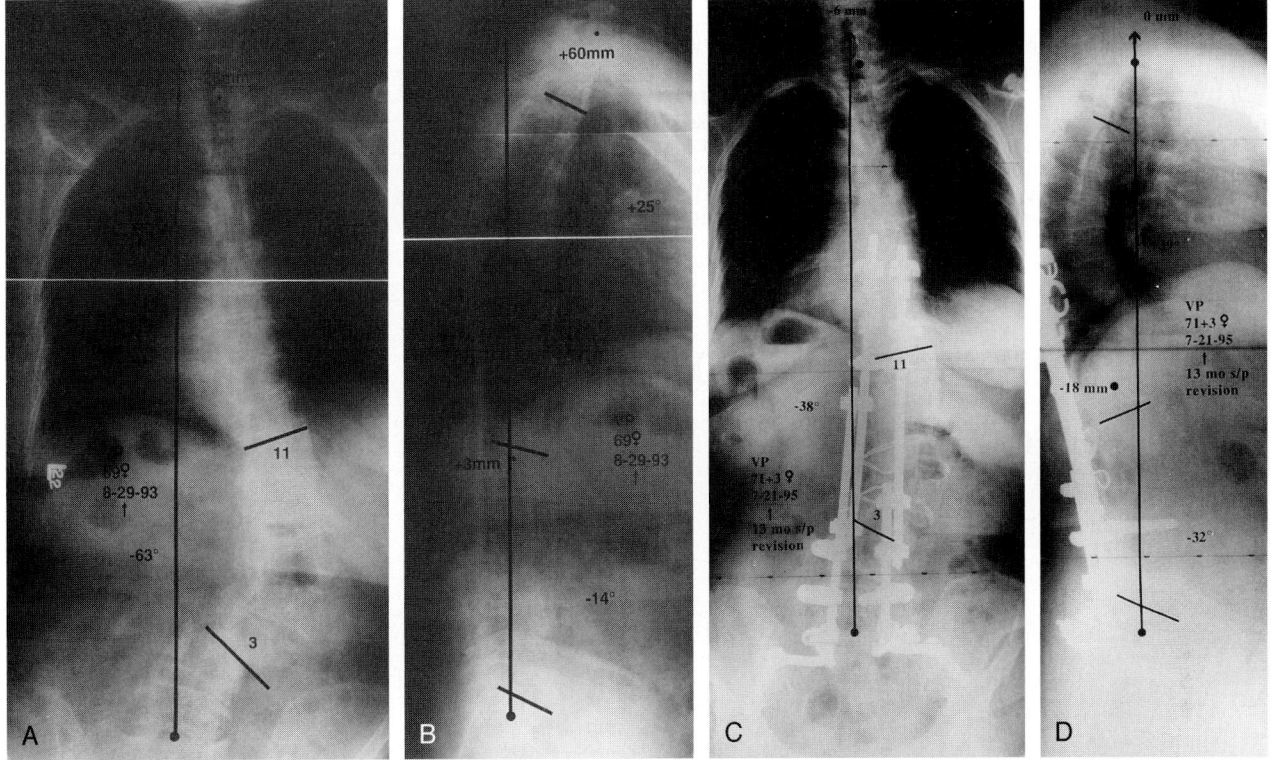

Fig. 2. Standing 36-inch posteroanterior and lateral radiographs. *A* and *B*, A 69-year-old female with degenerative scoliosis, back pain, central stenosis, and foraminal stenosis. Posterior decompression and instrumented arthrodesis was done with good relief of symptoms. However, she developed a pseudarthrosis at L5-S1, requiring revision. *C* and *D*, Thirteen months later she had a satisfactory clinical outcome; radiographs show satisfactory spinal alignment.

of adult reconstructive spinal surgery for deformity, Nelson and Trammell[20] noted 80% of patients had at least one complication, 67% minor and 33% major.

SUMMARY

Adult scoliosis affects a diverse patient population. The scoliosis may develop before or after skeletal maturity. Pain is the most common presenting complaint, but neurological symptoms, curve progression, and cosmetics may necessitate surgical intervention, particularly when multimodality, nonoperative treatment has failed. Coronal and sagittal plane spinal balance must be maintained or restored to maximize symptom relief and a lasting result. Although controversial, in addition to the standard imaging modalities, investigation of the adult with painful spinal deformity may be facilitated by discography and diagnostic facet and nerve blocks. When indicated, fusion across the lumbosacral junction is optimized by an anteroposterior procedure augmented by instrumentation extended to the pelvis. Surgical treatment of adult scoliosis provides satisfactory relief of pain and halts progression of deformity, although the complication rate is significantly higher than in the adolescent counterpart.

REFERENCES

1. Rhee JM, Deckey JE, Bradford DS: Surgical management of adult scoliosis. Semin Spine Surg 1998; 10:339.
2. Kostuik JP, Bentivoglio J: The incidence of low-back pain in adult scoliosis. Spine 1981; 6:268.
3. Carter OD, Haynes SG: Prevalence rates for scoliosis in US adults: Results from the first National Health and Nutrition Examination Survey. Int J Epidemiol 1987; 16:537.
4. Perennou D, Marcelli C, Herisson C, et al: Adult lumbar scoliosis: Epidemiologic aspects in a low-back pain population. Spine 1994; 19:123.

5. Witt I, Vestergaard A, Rosenklint A: A comparative analysis of x-ray findings of the lumbar spine in patients with and without lumbar pain. Spine 1984; 9:298.
6. Ascani E, Bartolozzi P, Logroscino CA, et al: Natural history of untreated idiopathic scoliosis after skeletal maturity. Spine 1986; 11:784.
7. Weinstein SL, Ponseti IV: Curve progression in idiopathic scoliosis. J Bone Joint Surg Am 1983; 65:447.
8. Kostuik JP: Adult scoliosis: The lumbar spine. In Bridwell KH, DeWald RL (eds): The Textbook of Spinal Surgery. Philadelphia, Lippincott-Raven, 1997, p 733.

9. Velis KP, Healey JH, Schneider R: Osteoporosis in unstable adult scoliosis. Clin Orthop 1988; 237:132.
10. Nachemson A: Adult scoliosis and back pain. Spine 1979; 4:513.
11. Jackson RP, Simmons EH, Stripinis D: Incidence and severity of back pain in adult idiopathic scoliosis. Spine 1983; 8:749.
12. Grubb SA, Lipscomb HJ, Suh PB: Results of surgical treatment of painful adult scoliosis. Spine 1994; 19:1619.
13. Pehrsson K, Bake B, Larsson S, et al: Lung function in adult idiopathic scoliosis: A 20-year follow-up. Thorax 1991; 46:474.

14. Balderston RA: Adult scoliosis: The thoracic spine. In Bridwell KH, Dewald RL (eds): The Textbook of Spinal Surgery. Philadelphia, Lippincott-Raven, 1997, p 715.

15. Jeffrey D, Boachie-Adjei O, Wilson M: One-stage versus two-stage anterior and posterior spinal reconstruction in adults: Comparison of outcomes including nutritional status, complication rates, hospital costs, and other factors. Spine 1992; 17: 310.

16. Kostuik JP, Carl A, Ferron S: Anterior Zielke instrumentation for spinal deformity in adults. J Bone Joint Surg Am 1989; 72: 898.

17. Trammell TR, Benedict F, Reid D: Anterior spine fusion using Zielke instrumentation for adult thoracolumbar and lumbar scoliosis. Spine 1991; 16:307.

18. Bridwell KH: Degenerative scoliosis. In Bridwell KH, Dewald RL (eds): The Textbook of Spinal Surgery. Philadelphia, Lippincott-Raven, 1997, p 777.

19. Bradford DS: Adult scoliosis. In Lonstein JE, Winter RB, Bradford DS, et al (eds): Moe's Textbook of Scoliosis and Other Spinal Deformities. Philadelphia, WB Saunders, 1994, p 369.

20. Nelson LM, Trammell TR: Complications and outcome of adult reconstructive spinal surgery. Presented at the annual meeting of the Scoliosis Research Society, Dublin, 1993.

section 8 chapter 3 — LUMBAR SPONDYLOLISTHESIS

Louis G. Jenis and Howard S. An

Summary
- Lumbar spondylolisthesis is a spinal disorder that presents in pediatric, adolescent, and adult populations.
- There is a range of clinical symptoms and nerve root entrapment syndromes.
- Diagnostic modalities include radiography, magnetic resonance imaging, computed tomography, and epidural and nerve root injections.
- Management can include nonoperative and operative techniques, depending on type and degree of spondylolisthesis, presence of nerve root symptoms, and extent of axial pain.

Lumbar spondylolisthesis is defined as a spinal condition in which slippage of the entire or part of the vertebral segment occurs on adjacent levels. Several types of spondylolisthesis exist in pediatric, adolescent, and adult patients and differ by etiology.

HISTORICAL REVIEW

The initial description of spondylolisthesis was by Herbiniaux in 1782 and was related to difficulty with childbirth in patients with high-grade slippage due to narrowing of the birth canal. The first attempt at classification of spondylolisthesis was by Neugebauer in 1882 based on facet joint dysplasia. This was followed by Capener in 1932 who classified slippage based on the presence or absence of a pars interarticularis defect. Newman and Stone developed a more contemporary classification by subdividing types by etiology.[1] Wiltse et al[2] expanded the classification into five categories in 1976, and their classification has become the most popular method of defining spondylolisthesis (Table 1).

EPIDEMIOLOGY

The natural history of spondylolisthesis has been extensively studied but remains inconclusive because of the various causes and degrees of slippage known to occur. Dysplastic spondylolisthesis is an uncommon form of slippage and is found more often in females.[2] Symptoms usually present earlier in life than other forms of spondylolisthesis, and when slippage is greater than 25% significant neural compression is often found.[3] Requirements for surgical stabilization are also more common in this deformity.[4, 5]

The incidence of spondylolysis with or without isthmic spondylolisthesis in childhood is 4.4% and in adulthood is 6%, with a 2:1 male to female ratio.[6] Prevalence is increased in certain ethnic groups, such as Yukon Eskimos, in whom incidence estimates of 50% have been reported.[7] Slippage may occur following the development of pars defects, usually during the adolescent growth spurt, but is unlikely to progress in adulthood.

Several authors have described risk factors for the development of clinical symptoms and radiographic progression of slippage.[8–11] No one risk factor allows prediction of progression, and several factors must always be considered (Tables 2 and 3).

PATHOGENESIS

Studies have evaluated the anatomy and biomechanical responses of the lumbar and lumbosacral spine to external

TABLE 1. WILTSE CLASSIFICATION OF SPONDYLOLISTHESIS	
Class	**Description**
I: Congenital	Congenital anomaly of the lumbosacral junction
II: Isthmic	Stress fracture or healed intact but elongated pars interarticularis
III: Degenerative	Secondary to intersegmental instability
IV: Traumatic	Acute fractures in area other than pars interarticularis
V: Pathological	Due to intrinsic bone disease leading to fracture and slippage

TABLE 2. RISK FACTORS FOR PROGRESSION OF SPONDYLOLISTHESIS
Clinical
Age—earlier onset carries increased risk
greatest risk during adolescent growth spurt
uncommon after skeletal maturity
Sex—possible increase risk in females
Symptoms—children with repeated episodes of back pain
Deformity—postural deformity/gait abnormality
Radiographic
Slip type—dysplastic spondylolisthesis increased risk
Degree of slippage—grade 2 or greater carries increased risk
Slip angle

forces.[12] Under normal conditions, the anterior column of the lumbar spine experiences 80% of the total axial load, whereas the posterior column undergoes the remaining 20% in the erect position.[13] The biomechanical loads at the lumbosacral disk include those arising from gravity and muscle contraction with a resulting combined force vector directed anteriorly and inferiorly. The resulting force leads to compression at the disk perpendicular to the vertebral end plates. In addition, an anteriorly directed shear force exists along the intervertebral disk, which is held in check by intact annulus fibrosus and posterior structures including the pars interarticularis, facet capsules, and ligaments. Therefore, a normal spinal functional unit (cranial and caudad vertebrae and intervertebral disk) converts the forces acting in the lumbar region to intervertebral compression, creating a load-bearing and force-dispersing situation.[13] This tension-band principle depends on an intact passive (disk) anterior column and active (musculature) posterior column.[14]

Isthmic spondylolisthesis leads to a condition in which the posterior constraints are no longer capable of altering the shear component of forces. The pars interarticularis is the supporting high-stress cortical area at the junction of the superior and inferior articular processes. In flexion, the anterior region of the pars is subjected to compression while the posterior region experiences traction force. The converse is present in extension, resulting in significant localized dynamic forces applied in all positions of motion. Spondylolysis or pars disruption may be unilateral or bilateral. Bilateral pars defects may allow forward slippage to occur, since the posterior elements no longer are attached to the vertebral body (Fig. 1). Steffee and Sitkowski[15] have described three structures believed to be responsible for maintaining the L5 vertebra in normal position, including the pars interarticularis, annulus fibrosis, and posterior longitudinal ligament and the iliolumbar ligaments. When

TABLE 3. RISK FACTORS FOR LOW BACK PAIN IN ADULT SPONDYLOLISTHESIS
Slip > 10 mm
Disk degeneration at level of slippage
Low lumbar index
Increased lumbar lordosis
Defect in pars at L4

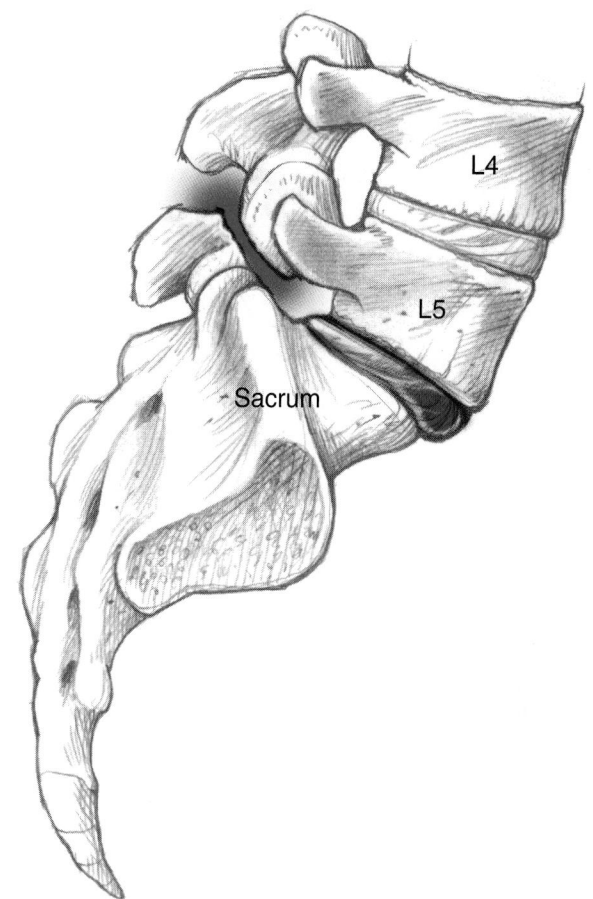

Fig. 1. Lateral schematic representation. This shows L5 spondylolysis with spondylolisthesis of L5 on S1. Note the pars interarticularis defect.

these structures become incompetent, forward slippage may occur. As the spondylolisthesis increases, the lever arm of inferiorly directed forces also magnifies, leading to greater instability. The biomechanics of isthmic spondylolisthesis must be considered when surgical intervention is warranted.

Degenerative spondylolisthesis is found most commonly at the L4-5 level and may be related to disk degeneration and facet joint orientation. In the lumbosacral region, facet joint orientation assumes a coronal alignment as compared with the more sagittal configuration of the upper lumbar spine.[16] In addition, the lower lumbar facet joints have been described as having a combined coronal and sagittal alignment, providing a J-shaped joint. Disk degeneration and height loss may lead to ligamentous and facet capsular laxity. Those individuals with a more sagittal orientation at the L4-5 facet articulation may be prone to the development of subluxation associated with the degenerative process (Fig. 2).[16]

CLINICAL FEATURES

Patients with spondylolisthesis may be asymptomatic, present with altered posture, or experience significant symptoms. In the pediatric patient, symptoms usually

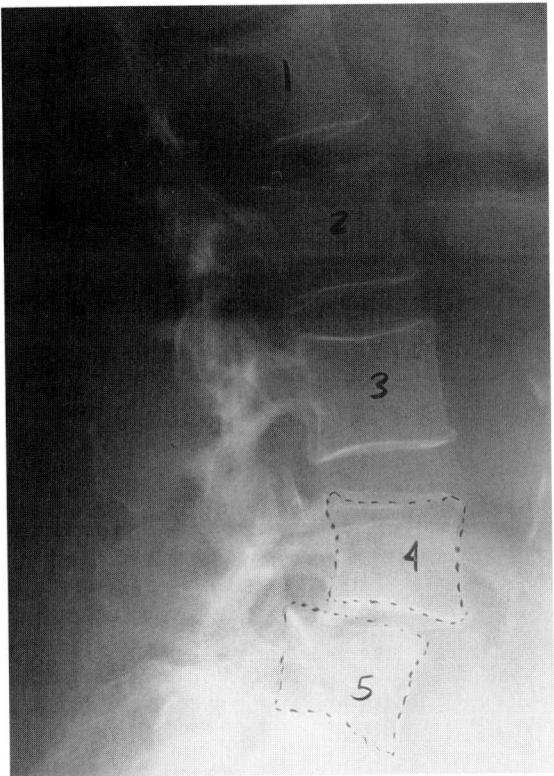

Fig. 2. Lateral radiograph. This shows a patient with degenerative spondylolisthesis of L4 on L5. Note the disk height loss at the L4-5 level.

present during the adolescent growth spurt, despite the slip's initiating several years previously. Often a traumatic event will be related to the onset of symptoms. Varying degrees of low back pain may develop and relate to repetitive mechanical activities such as sporting or lifting. Hyperextension maneuvers as seen in football linemen and gymnasts may exacerbate or initiate symptoms. Pain may be relieved with rest and activity modification. Radicular symptoms may develop from disk herniation or foraminal stenosis related to the listhetic segment. A high-degree slip with an intact posterior arch (dysplastic spondylolisthesis) may rarely present with a cauda equina syndrome and significant bowel or bladder dysfunction.

Physical examination may reveal tight hamstring muscles with limited hip and knee extension leading to a crouched-gait position. Theories proposed on the causes of the knees-bent and hip-flexed standing position (Phalen-Dickson sign) include verticality of the sacrum and nerve root irritation from instability or compression leading to the tight hamstrings.[17] The patient will often ambulate with a short, waddling gait, which may be more evident with high-degree listhesis. Other findings may include a short trunk with a transverse abdominal groove and flattening of the lumbosacral spine with progressive pelvic flexion or a palpable step-off of the spinous processes at the listhetic level.

Adults with isthmic spondylolisthesis may also present with varying degrees of low back and leg pain. Acute episodes of low back pain may occur and not be related to

the slippage but rather to self-limited muscle strain. Chronic low back pain is often mechanical in nature and may relate to disk degeneration at or above the listhetic level, segmental instability, or irritation of the dorsal root ganglion of the exiting nerve root near the foramen. Spondylolisthesis at the L5-S1 level may cause L5 radiculopathy from nerve compression due to a hypertrophied pars defect in the lateral spinal canal or in the neuroforamen from annular bulging or traction. Pain in the L5 root distribution, weakness of the extensor hallucis longus, and diminished sensation on the dorsum of the foot and great toe are common features.

Adult patients with degenerative spondylolisthesis may present with similar intermittent mechanical low back pain related to disk degeneration but also with symptoms of lower extremity claudication. Activity-related leg pain, weakness, or numbness might substantially incapacitate the patient. Exacerbating conditions often include walking variable distances or prolonged standing requiring leaning forward or sitting for symptom relief. The upright or extended lumbar spine leads to diminution of the spinal canal due to disk bulging and hypertrophied ligamentum flavum buckling with thecal sac compression. The canal dimensions are increased, with lumbar flexion providing neurological decompression. Differentiation of neurogenic claudication from vascular sources is important in the evaluation of the patient with activity-related leg pain.

The most common classification of spondylolisthesis is that of Wiltse et al (see Table 1).[1-3] This classification provides several types and causes of spondylolisthesis but lacks in description of the severity of the deformity.

Dysplastic or congenital spondylolisthesis is due to abnormalities at the lumbosacral junction, including the neural arch of L5 and the upper dome of the sacrum with varying degrees of listhesis. The posterior elements migrate anteriorly as they remain attached to the vertebral body, which results in compression of the cauda equina.

Isthmic spondylolisthesis occurs from a lesion within the pars interarticularis (spondylolysis) and is the most common form of listhesis in children and adults. Spondylolysis is most common at L5 (87%) followed by L4 (10%) and L3 (3%).[18]

Subtypes of isthmic spondylolisthesis include actual separation of the pars from a stress reaction or acute fracture and elongation of the pars without disruption, representing a continuum of healed stress fractures. The vertebral body slips anteriorly, leaving the posterior elements in place and preventing thecal sac compression.

Degenerative spondylolisthesis occurs in adults as wear of the disk and facet joint leads to segmental instability. Although degenerative spondylolisthesis may occur at any level of the lumbar spine, it is more common at the L4-5 level.

Traumatic spondylolisthesis develops from an acute fracture of the vertebra other than the pars region, allowing secondary slippage to occur. Fractures may involve the pedicle or posterior elements and listhesis may progress over a prolonged period.

Pathological spondylolisthesis results from a systemic or local inherent bone disorder, causing weakening and possibly fracture of the supporting pars, pedicle, and other aspects of the vertebrae and causing slippage.

TABLE 4. MARCHETTI AND BARTOLOZZI CLASSIFICATION OF SPONDYLOLISTHESIS

I. Developmental
    High dysplastic
    Low dysplastic
II. Acquired
        Traumatic
            Acute fracture
            Stress fracture
        Postsurgery
        Pathological
        Degenerative

Postsurgical spondylolisthesis occurs following lumbar decompressive procedures in which iatrogenic instability emerges due to excessive removal of supporting structures.

A more recent classification has been proposed by Marchetti and Bartolozzi[19] that further categorizes spondylolisthesis into developmental types, including high- or low-grade dysplasia and acquired forms, with further grouping according to cause (Table 4).

INVESTIGATION

Plain radiographic evaluation is indicated in the pediatric or adolescent patient with new-onset low back or radicular pain and in the adult patient with prolonged mechanical back or leg pain. Initial evaluation should include standing anteroposterior and lateral radiographs to accentuate any minor spondylolisthesis that may be present and reducible in the supine position. Oblique images may identify spondylolysis in the pars either unilaterally or bilaterally, as evidenced by a bony defect with or without sclerotic margins. The classic "Scotty-dog" sign is often seen on these images.

The lateral standing view is most helpful in diagnosing spondylolisthesis, allowing several descriptive and quantitative measurements to be made from this image. The degree of slippage or translation of the vertebra can be measured by the technique of Meyerding (Fig. 3).[20] The anteroposterior surface of the superior surface of the caudad vertebra is divided into fourths, and the posterior border of the cranial vertebra (listhetic segment) is calculated to fall into one of these quarters—that is, grade I is 0% to 25% slippage, grade II is 25% to 50%, grade III is 50% to 75%, and grade IV is greater than 75%. Taillard's[21] method of measuring translation is more specific in that the distance of the posterior cortex of the cranial vertebra is related to the posterior cortex of the caudad vertebra and expressed as a percentage displacement. Owing to remodeling changes that may take place over time along the posterior cortex of each vertebra, measurement errors are possible. Boxall et al recommend measuring the percentage translation relative to the cranial vertebra (opposite of Taillard's method), since bony erosion and hypertrophy are not as evident as on the caudad vertebra.[8]

The lateral standing radiograph may also be used to assess the angle of deformity at the listhetic level (Fig. 4). The slip angle may be determined by the intersection of a line parallel to the superior border of the cranial vertebra and, if at the L5-S1 level, a line drawn perpendicular to the posterior cortex of the sacrum.[8] As an alternative, the angle can be measured from the intersection of a line from the anterior cortex of L5 and posterior cortex of the sacrum.[22]

Sacral inclination is also measured from the standing lateral radiograph and is a determination of the degree of compensatory pelvic rotation in response to kyphosis at the lumbosacral junction (Fig. 5). The angle of inclination is calculated by the intersection of a vertical line and a line on the posterior aspect of the sacrum. Normal sacral inclination is slightly forward in the standing position. This angle increases with a greater degree of spondylolisthesis as the sacrum assumes a more vertical position.

In the event of equivocal findings on radiographs, the use of radioactive technetium bone scanning may elicit areas of increased bone turnover suggestive of an acute or subacute pars stress fracture. However, chronic spondylolytic defects often do not possess significant bone turnover and lack the "hot" appearance on scans. Single photon

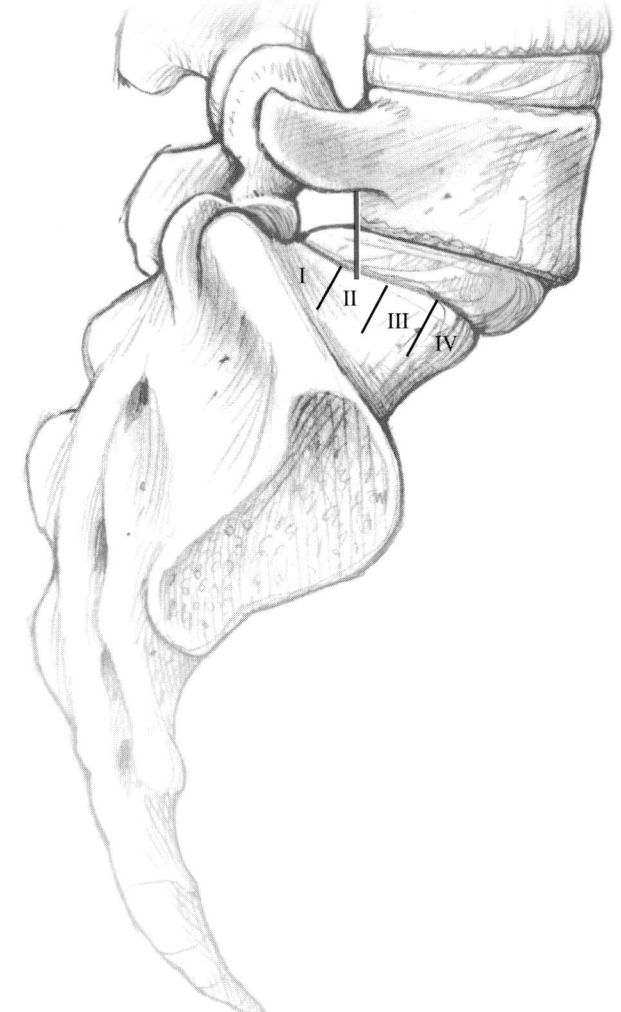

Fig. 3. Lateral schematic view. The lumbosacral junction depicts Meyerding's technique of quantifying translation of spondylolisthesis.

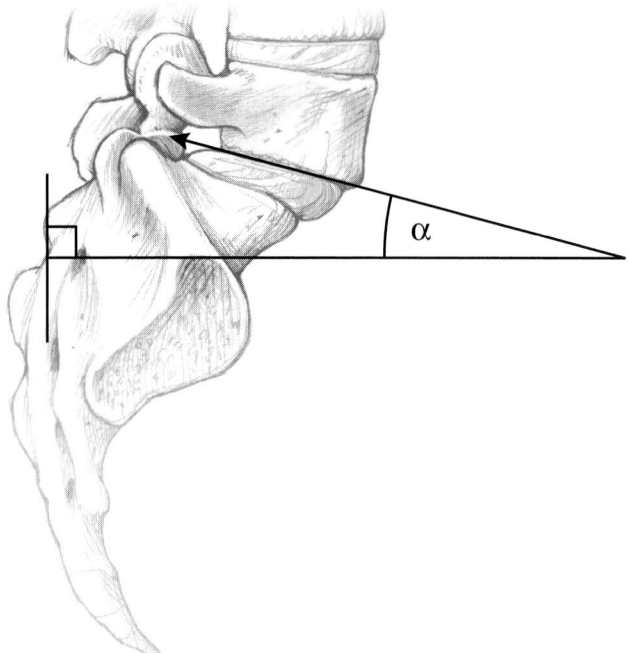

Fig. 4. Lateral schematic view. The lumbosacral junction depicts the technique of defining the slip angle.

lolysis are able to resume their normal activities following resolution of symptoms without any specific restrictions placed. If slippage is between 25% and 50%, then activities should be restricted, including avoidance of hyperextension and repetitive trauma, until skeletal maturation.

Adult patients with spondylolysis or spondylolisthesis should be treated according to their presenting symptoms. Mechanical low back pain is treated with an aggressive physical therapy and pain control program. Symptoms of nerve root compression may similarly be treated with an exercise regimen and anti-inflammatory drugs. Selective nerve root and epidural steroid injections are adjuvant treatments for leg pain.

OPERATIVE MANAGEMENT

ADOLESCENT PATIENT
The indications for surgical intervention in the adolescent patient with spondylolysis or spondylolisthesis include intractable low back pain not responsive to conservative treatment, presence of neurological signs, significant gait

emission computed tomography bone scanning provides more detail of the posterior elements and may be a more sensitive diagnostic tool.[23, 24]

Further diagnostic tests available for the evaluation of spondylolisthesis include computed tomography and magnetic resonance imaging (MRI). Computed tomography can be used to assess the degree of slippage and also define bony anatomy that is suspected to cause nerve root or thecal sac compression. The indications for myelography are limited by the availability of MRI. Radiculopathy or symptoms of neurogenic claudication are best evaluated with an MRI scan, which allows definition of the spinal canal and its structures throughout the lumbar spine. In degenerative or isthmic spondylolisthesis, nerve root impingement may occur in the central canal, lateral recess, or neuroforamina[25] and this can be adequately assessed with this modality.

NONOPERATIVE MANAGEMENT

Adolescent patients with spondylolysis or low-grade spondylolisthesis are initially managed with a conservative program of short-term rest and restriction of aggravating activities. Anti-inflammatory and non-narcotic pain medications may be used on a limited basis. Strengthening exercises may be initiated following resolution of the acute symptoms and gradual return to routine activities and sports participation. Patients with an acute pars fracture or those who do not respond to an exercise program of lumbar and abdominal stabilization are candidates for brace immobilization. An antilordotic brace worn full time for 3 to 6 months with gradual weaning can be associated with beneficial results.[26]

Patients with grade I or less spondylolisthesis or spondy-

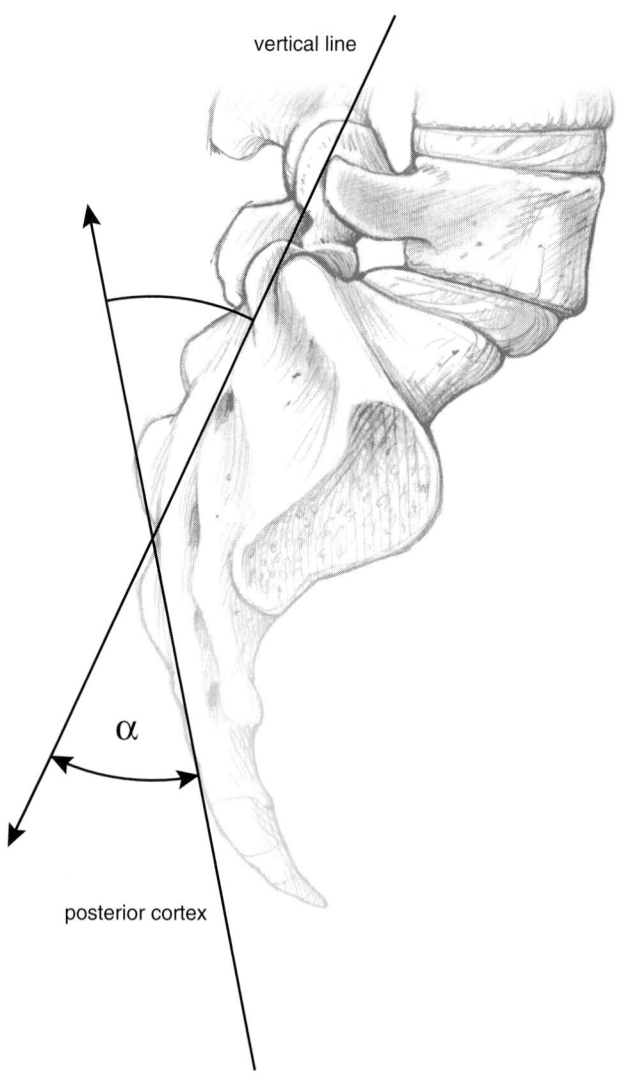

Fig. 5. Lateral schematic view. The lumbosacral junction depicts sacral inclination.

TABLE 5. OPERATIVE TREATMENT OPTIONS FOR ADOLESCENT SPONDYLOLYSIS

Segmental fusion—posterior/posterolateral
Direct repair of pars defect
    Screw fixation (Buck's)
    Wiring procedures—around transverse process or pedicle screw

abnormalities, radiographic progression of slippage, or spondylolisthesis greater than 50% translation.[4, 27]

The operative treatment of spondylolysis is seldom necessary. However, several options are available for dealing with recalcitrant pain (Table 5). Repair of the pars defect is an option for treatment of L1 to L4 disorders in patients younger than 25 years of age and with no evidence of significant intervertebral disk or facet joint degeneration.[28] This may be accomplished by transverse process–spinous process wiring or screw fixation along with débridement of the nonunion site.[28] Defects at the L5 level are not as amenable to direct repair and likely should be treated with a posterolateral intertransverse process in situ arthrodesis.

Surgical treatment of adolescent spondylolisthesis is varied and differs by the technique of fusion utilized, use of instrumentation, and performance of reduction maneuvers (Table 6). Progression of spondylolisthesis of less than 50% or intractable back pain is best managed by posterolateral in situ arthrodesis.[29] This can be performed through a midline incision and bilateral fascial and muscle-splitting approach to the intertransverse process area. The fascial incision is placed approximately two fingerbreadths off the midline. The facet joint capsules are removed and the joints denuded of articular cartilage, and copious amounts of autogenous bone graft are harvested from the iliac crest and packed into the joints and the surrounding decorticated region. Postoperatively, a rigid thoracolumbosacral orthosis may be used for immobilization until early graft consolidation occurs.

The presence of neurological compromise often indicates that a decompressive procedure should be considered. Removal of the loose posterior elements at L5, including the fibrocartilagenous pars region (Gill's procedure) may accomplish neural decompression, but has been associated with progression of the slippage if not accompanied by arthrodesis.[30] Foraminotomy may also be performed when indicated. Other investigators have found that arthrodesis without direct decompression may diminish symptoms of neurological compromise. However, the time frame for recovery is variable and not predictable.[3, 4, 31]

TABLE 6. OPERATIVE TREATMENT OPTIONS FOR ADOLESCENT SPONDYLOLISTHESIS

Posterior spinal fusion in situ
Posterolateral spinal fusion with Gill's laminectomy
Posterior lumbar interbody fusion
Anterior lumbar interbody fusion
Anterior or posterior dowel graft fusion (spondyloptosis)

Note: reduction of high-grade spondylolisthesis may be performed concomitant with fusion

Adolescent spondylolisthesis of greater than 50% is an indication for fusion, which can be accomplished with a posterior in situ technique (Fig. 6). The fusion may need to be extended up to the L4 level (L5 spondylolisthesis) due to the anteriorly migrated position of the L5 transverse process and subsequent diminished surface area available for fusion incorporation. Postoperative immobilization should include a pantaloon brace or cast. Other techniques of in situ fusion for high-grade slippage include anterior lumbar and posterior dowel interbody arthrodesis. In high-grade slips in which posterior fusion alone is thought not to be successful, then anterior fusion can be considered without reduction. The procedure can be performed by transperitoneal or retroperitoneal exposure and with varied bone grafts. Anterior exposure at the lumbosacral junction carries a risk of retrograde ejaculation due to potential injury to the lumbosacral plexus and must be considered carefully prior to recommending this surgery to the adolescent patient. Posterior decompression and interbody fusion

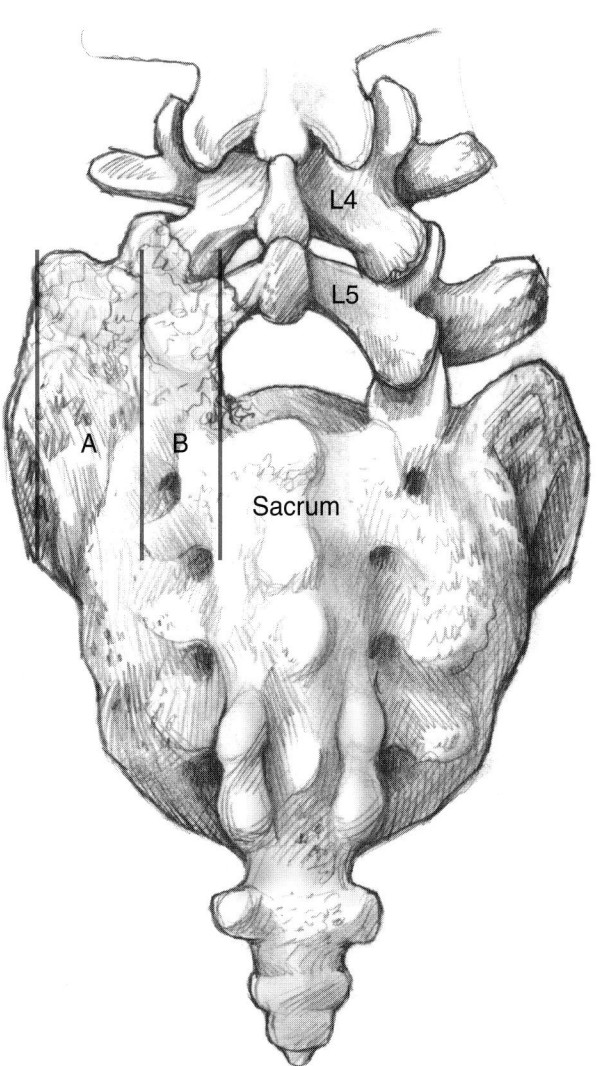

Fig. 6. Posterior view. The lumbosacral spine depicts in situ fusion on the left. *A*, Intertransverse process bone graft. *B*, Midline posterior bone graft.

TABLE 7. OPERATIVE TREATMENT OPTIONS FOR ADULT ISTHMIC SPONDYLOLISTHESIS
Posterior spinal fusion in situ
Posterolateral spinal fusion with nerve root decompression
Posterior lumbar interbody fusion combined with posterolateral fusion
Anterior lumbar interbody fusion with or without posterior fusion
Anterior or posterior dowel graft fusion (spondyloptosis)
Note: arthrodesis technique may be augmented with the use of internal fixation

may be used for very large slips or spondyloptosis.[32] Autograft fibula may be inserted through the posterior aspect of the sacrum through the displaced vertebral body of L5 up to the anterior cortex to accomplish fusion.

The role of reduction in the operative treatment of spondylolisthesis is controversial. The advantages of reduction include restoration of lumbar mechanics, increased surface area for fusion incorporation, and improved spinal alignment and cosmetic appearance.[33–35] The indications for reduction have been proposed and include the presence of neurological deficit (cauda equina syndrome) due to progressive deformity, slip progression greater than 50%, cosmetic deformity related to the compensatory hyperlordosis of the middle and upper lumbar spine resulting in the classic waddling gait appearance, and chronic disabling back pain.[34]

Options for reduction and arthrodesis include noninstrumented and instrumented techniques. Traction with serial extension casting and posterolateral fusion can be applied to flexible deformities in the younger patient in whom the role of instrumentation is limited. Reduction may also be accomplished by posterior decompression and manually levering the L5 vertebral body onto the sacrum, followed by interbody fusion.[15] Posterior instrumentation is used to hold the reduction while fusion occurs. The technique of gradual instrumented reduction accomplishes restoration of anatomic alignment by corrective forces and stress relaxation of the viscoelastic properties of the spine.[34] This is achieved with application of corrective forces, including distraction, posterior translation, and lumbosacral extension. Finally, others have recommended L5 vertebrectomy with anterior and posterior fusion of L4 onto S1 (Gaines' procedure).[36]

Although theoretical advantages of spondylolisthesis reduction exist, long-term follow-up studies comparing this technique with in situ fusion are lacking. This remains a high-risk procedure and not well defined in terms of absolute indications.

ADULT PATIENT

Operative management of the adult patient with spondylolysis or isthmic spondylolisthesis remains varied (Table 7). The most common indication for surgery is back pain refractory to nonoperative treatment. Chronic low back pain is a common finding in the adult population, and the identification of the "pain generator" remains a challenge. Degenerative changes at the level of the slippage or at adjacent levels may be the source of symptoms, and detailed

analysis is needed. Provocative discography, although controversial, allows for subjective analysis of the degenerated disk as a possible pain source and may assist in surgical planning. Patients with single-level degeneration with low-grade spondylolisthesis may be managed with in situ posterolateral intertransverse fusion. Whether to apply instrumentation such as pedicle screw fixation remains disputed. Improved fusion rate and greater initial postoperative stability are accepted by proponents of pedicle screw fixation as advantages in their use.[37, 38] Other investigators have not identified the advantage of instrumentation in the management of degenerative lumbar disorders.[39, 40]

Some investigators have advocated interbody fusion to restore lumbosacral biomechanics and increase surface area for fusion in isthmic spondylolisthesis.[41] Anterior lumbar interbody fusion can be achieved by various techniques and combined with posterolateral fusion. Newer threaded cage devices have been used as an anterior lumbar interbody fusion procedure for low-grade slips (less than grade 1). Posterior lumbar interbody fusion can be used to accomplish direct nerve root decompression while also providing the advantage of interbody arthrodesis. The role of interbody fusion is based on surgeon preference and has several advantages in the management of large-degree slips (greater than grade 1) (Fig. 7).

Lumbar radiculopathy associated with spondylolisthesis may also be an indication for surgical intervention. Lumbosacral spondylolisthesis may contribute to an L5 radiculopathy from stenosis in the lateral spinal canal from the hypertrophied pars fibrocartilagenous defect or in the neuroforamen from disk bulging and collapse. Decompression

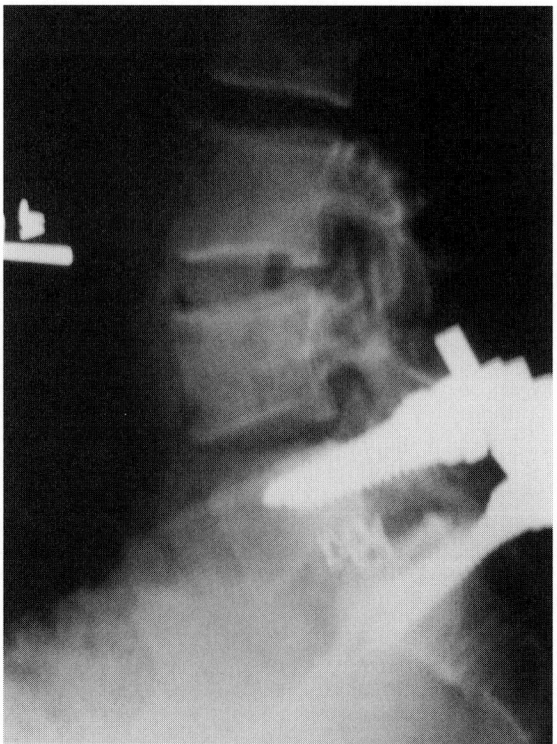

Fig. 7. Lateral radiograph. This shows L5-S1 grade II spondylolisthesis treated with instrumented posterolateral fusion and interbody fusion with mesh cages.

alone in these situations may be considered in the absence of associated back pain. However, the typical adult patient with isthmic spondylolisthesis has a high incidence of back pain and needs to be evaluated for possible arthrodesis.

The indications for surgical management in the adult patient with degenerative spondylolisthesis are intractable leg pain from neurogenic claudication or radiculopathy and/or back pain due to segmental instability. The treatment of degenerative spondylolisthesis usually involves posterior decompression accompanied by arthrodesis. Herkowitz and Kurz[42] performed a randomized, prospective study comparing patients undergoing decompression alone and those with concomitant fusion. They reported that 96% of patients who had a concomitant bilateral posterolateral fusion experienced good to excellent results, whereas patients treated with decompression alone had 46% good to excellent results. This study, while not using instrumentation, did detail the benefit of fusion in this condition. Several studies have since shown that instrumentation can increase the fusion rate in degenerative spondylolisthesis. The effects of various transpedicular,[38, 43–47] Luque rectangle,[48] and combined distraction and compression rod instrumentation[49] have been documented.

The presence of L4-L5 degenerative spondylolisthesis without obvious motion on dynamic preoperative flexion-extension lateral radiographs and essentially no remaining disk space (end plate to end plate contact) is a relative indication for an noninstrumented posterolateral fusion following decompression. However, when instability is documented or in the presence of a "wide" disk space, the addition of instrumentation is an option to prevent further postoperative listhesis secondary to the destabilization effects of the decompressive laminectomy.[50] An isolated L4-L5 instrumented fusion, or "floating fusion," is an effective means of treating this problem. Another indication for adding instrumentation to fusion is for significant slippage and subsequent kyphotic deformity for which correction is deemed necessary.

CONCLUSION

Many types of lumbar spondylolisthesis present in the adolescent and adult patient. The clinical spectrum of such abnormalities may vary widely, contributing to the diagnostic and management challenge when treating patients with this condition. Management consists of nonoperative and operative treatment protocols, and a sound understanding of the pathoanatomy and biomechanics is essential to providing relief of symptoms.

REFERENCES

1. Newman P: The etiology of spondylolisthesis. J Bone Joint Surg Br 1963; 45:39.
2. Wiltse L, Rothman S: Spondylolisthesis: Classification, diagnosis, and natural history. In Wiesel S (ed): Seminars in Spine Surgery. Philadelphia, W.B. Saunders, 1993, p 264.
3. Wiltse L, Hutchinson R: Surgical treatment of spondylolisthesis. Clin Orthop Rel Res 1964; 35:116.
4. Hensinger R, Lang J, MacEwen G: Surgical management of spondylolisthesis in children and adolescents. Spine 1976; 1: 207.
5. Newman P: A clinical syndrome associated with severe lumbo-sacral subluxation. J Bone Joint Surg Br 1965; 47:72.
6. Fredrickson B, Baker D, McHolick W, et al: The natural history of spondylolysis and spondylolisthesis. J Bone Joint Surg Am 1984; 66:699.
7. Stewart T: The age incidence of neural arch defects in Alaskan natives, considered from the standpoint of etiology. J Bone Joint Surg 1953; 35:937.
8. Boxall D, Bradford D, Winter R, Moe J: Management of severe spondylolisthesis in children and adolescents. J Bone Joint Surg Am 1979; 61:479.
9. Saraste H, Brostrom L, Asparisis T: Prognostic radiographic aspects of spondylolisthesis. Acta Radiol 1984; 25:427.
10. Saraste H: Long term clinical and radiological follow-up of spondylolysis and spondylolisthesis. J Pediatric Orthop 1987; 7:631.
11. Virta L, Osterman K: Radiographic correlations in adult symptomatic spondylolisthesis: A long term follow-up study. J Spinal Disord 1994; 7:41.

12. Schlegel K, Pon A: The biomechanics of posterior lumbar interbody fusion in spondylolisthesis. Clin Orthop Rel Res 1985; 193:115.
13. Lowery G, Harms J: Principles of load sharing. In Bridwell K, DeWald R (eds): The Textbook of Spinal Surgery. Philadelphia, Lippincott-Raven, 1997.
14. Bridwell K: Load sharing principles: The role and use of anterior structural support in adult deformity. Instruct Course Lect AAOS 1996; 45:109.
15. Steffee A, Sitkowski D: Reduction and stabilization of grade IV spondylolisthesis. Clin Orthop Rel Res 1988; 227:82.
16. Grobler L, Robertson P, Novotny J, Ahern J: Decompression for degenerative spondylolisthesis and spinal stenosis at L4-5: The effects of facet joint morphology. Spine 1993; 18:1475.
17. Phalen G, Dickson J: Spondylolisthesis and tight hamstrings. J Bone Joint Surg Am 1961; 43:505.
18. Rowe G, Roache M: Etiology of the separate neural arch. J Bone Joint Surg Am 1953; 35:102.
19. Marchetti P, Bartolozzi P: Classification of spondylolisthesis as a guideline for treatment. In: Bridwell K (ed): The Textbook of Spinal Surgery. Philadelphia, Lippincott-Raven, 1997, p 1211.
20. Meyerding H: Spondylolisthesis: Surgical treatment and results. Surg Gynecol Obstet 1932; 54:371.
21. Taillard W: Etiology of spondylolisthesis. Clin Orthop Rel Res 1976; 117:30.
22. Wiltse L, Winter R: Terminology and measurement in spondylolisthesis. J Bone Joint Surg Am 1983; 65:768.
23. Bellah R, Summerville D, Treves S, Micheli L: Low back pain in adolescent athletes: Detection of stress injury to the pars interarticularis with SPECT. Radiology 1991; 180:509.
24. Collier B, Johnson R, Carrera G, et al: Painful spondylolysis or spondylolisthesis studied by radiography and single-photon emission computed tomography. Radiology 1985; 154:207.
25. Jinkins J, Rauch A: Magnetic resonance imaging of entrapment of lumbar nerve roots in spondylolytic spondylolisthesis. J Bone Joint Surg Am 1994; 76:1643.
26. Bell D, Ehrlich M, Zaleske D: Brace treatment for symptomatic spondylolisthesis. Clin Orthop Rel Res 1988; 236:192.
27. Harris I, Weinstein S: Long term follow-up of patients with grade III and IV spondylolisthesis. J Bone Joint Surg Am 1987; 69:960.
28. Bradford D, Iza J: Repair of the defect in spondylolysis or minimal degrees of spondylolisthesis by segmental wire fixation and bone grafting. Spine 1985; 10:673.
29. Burkus J, Lonstein J, Winter R, et al: Long-term evaluation of adolescents treated operatively for spondylolisthesis: A comparison of in-situ arthrodesis only with in-situ arthrodesis and reduction followed by immobilization in a cast. J Bone Joint Surg Am 1992; 74:693.
30. Amuso S, Neff R, Coulson D, Laing P: The surgical treatment of spondylolisthesis by posterior element resection. J Bone Joint Surg Am 1970; 52:529.
31. Johnson L, Nasca R, Dunham W: Surgical management of isthmic spondylolisthesis. Spine 1988; 13:93.
32. Bohlman H, Cook S: One stage decompression and posterolateral and interbody

fusion for lumbosacral spondyloptosis through a posterior approach. J Bone Joint Surg Am 1982; 64:415.

33. Amundson G: The advantages of reduction in spondylolisthesis. Semin Spine Surg 1994; 6:46.

34. Edwards C, Curcin A: Instrumented reduction of high-grade spondylolisthesis. In: Wiesel S (ed): Seminars in Spine Surgery. Philadelphia, W.B. Saunders, 1994, p 34.

35. Heller J, Schimandle J, Garfin S: The operative reduction of spondylolisthesis: Indications, results and complications. In Wiesel S (ed): Seminars in Spine Surgery. Philadelphia, W.B. Saunders, 1994, p 22.

36. Gaines R, Nichols W: Treatment of spondyloptosis by two stage L5 vertebrectomy and reduction of L4 onto S1. Spine 1985; 10:680.

37. Chang P, Seow K, Tan S: Comparison of the results of spinal fusion for spondylolisthesis in patients who are instrumented with patients who are not. Singapore Med J 1993; 34:511.

38. Zdeblick T: A prospective, randomized study of lumbar fusion: Preliminary results. Spine 1993; 18:983.

39. Bernhardt M, Swartz D, Clothiaux P, et al: Posterolateral lumbar and lumbosacral fusion with and without pedicle screw internal fixation. Clin Orthop Rel Res 1992; 284:109.

40. McGuire R, Amundson G: The use of primary internal fixation in spondylolisthesis. Spine 1993; 18:1662.

41. Steffee A, Sitkowski D: Posterior lumbar interbody fusion and plates. Clin Orthop Rel Res 1988; 227:99.

42. Herkowitz H, Kurz L: Degenerative lumbar spondylolisthesis with spinal stenosis. J Bone Joint Surg Am 1991; 73:802.

43. Bridwell K, Sedgewick T, O'Brien M, et al: The role of fusion and instrumentation in the treatment of degenerative spondylolisthesis with spinal stenosis. J Spinal Dis 1993; 6:461.

44. Chen J, Chen W, Huang T, Shih O: Posterior transpedicular Zielke instrumentation in spondylolisthesis. Orthop Rev 1992; 21:75.

45. Kabins M, Weinstein J, Spratt K, et al: Isolated L4-L5 floating fusion using the variable screw placement system: Unilateral vs. bilateral. J Spinal Dis 1992; 5:39.

46. Mardjetko S, Connolly P, Shott S: Degenerative lumbar spondylolisthesis: A meta-analysis of literature 1970–1993. Spine 1994; 20:2256S.

47. Yuan H, Garfin S, Dickman C, Mardjetko S: A historical cohort study of pedicle screw fixation in thoracic, lumbar and sacral spinal fusions. Spine 1994; 19:2279S.

48. Knox B, Harvell J, Nelson P, et al: Decompression and Luque rectangle fusion for degenerative spondylolisthesis. J Spinal Disord 1989; 2:223.

49. Fujiya M, Saita M, Kaneda K, et al: Clinical study on stability of combined distraction and compression rod instrumentation with posterolateral fusion for unstable degenerative spondylolisthesis. Spine 1990; 15:1216.

50. Bridwell K: Acquired degenerative spondylolisthesis without lysis. In: Bridwell K ed: The Textbook of Spinal Surgery, 2nd ed. Philadelphia, Lippincott-Raven, 1997.

section 8 chapter 4

CERVICAL DISK DISEASE

Jeffrey S. Fischgrund and Harry N. Herkowitz

Summary

- Cervical degenerative disk disease occurs as part of the normal aging process and is often asymptomatic.
- Commonly occurring symptoms include neck pain, radiculopathy, and myelopathy.
- Neck pain and radiculopathy usually resolve with nonoperative modalities.
- Operative treatment is most successful when radiological findings correlate with both subjective complaints and objective patient findings.

Cervical disk degeneration occurs in the majority of the population and, although often symptomatic, can lead to neck pain, radiculopathy, and myelopathy. Axial neck pain is usually treated nonoperatively, whereas treatment options for cervical radiculopathy include nonsurgical management as well as various surgical procedures. A thorough understanding of the anatomy, pathophysiology, as well as natural history of cervical degenerative disk disease must be understood before the clinician can embark on a treatment protocol.

PATHOGENESIS

The cervical spine is made up of seven cervical vertebrae, of which C3, C4, C5, and C6 are considered typical verte-

brae, in that they are nearly identical in anatomic configuration. Although the body height is typically greater posteriorly than anteriorly, the typical cervical lordosis is caused by an increased thickness of the intervertebral disk anteriorly compared with posteriorly.[1] The upper surface of each cervical vertebral body is concave, and this concavity is accentuated by a bony shelf that projects upward from the posterolateral aspect of each side of the body. This bony shelf is known as the uncinate process. Along the inferior border of each typical vertebral body, there is a posterolateral ridge of bone that opposes or articulates with the uncinate process of the inferior vertebral body, thus forming the neurocentral joint (joint of Luschka).

Cervical nerve roots exit the spinal canal through the neural foramina in an anterolateral and inferior direction. The boundaries of the neural foramen are formed by the inferior and superior surfaces of the adjacent pedicles posterolaterally, the medial aspect of the facet joint and the adjacent part of the articular column anterolaterally, the posterolateral aspect of the uncus, the intervertebral disk, and the inferior part of the superior adjacent vertebrae.[2]

Degenerative changes in the cervical spine are frequently seen on plain radiographs and have been noted to increase with age. Friedenberg and Miller noted that in an asymptomatic group 25% of the patients in the 5th decade of life exhibited degenerative changes in one or more intervertebral disks, and this number increased to 75% by the 7th decade.[3] This degenerative process is characterized by a gradual decrease in the water content of the disk. As the disk hydration decreases, the strain increases on the annulus, which eventually fibrillates and weakens. Soft-disk ruptures occur when a sequestered amount of nuclear material herniates through a tear in the posterior annulus. Continued degeneration of the disk eventually causes loss of structural integrity, thus leading to annular weakening and protrusion. This protrusion, as well as osteophyte formation, leads to hard disk ruptures. The combination of osteophyte formation and disk rupture results in a decrease in the cross-sectional area of the neural foramina, thus leading to nerve root compression.

The pathomechanic cause of symptoms in cervical radiculopathy may be direct mechanical compression of the affected nerve root.[1] Additionally, stretching of the nerve root over either an osteophyte or soft-disk herniation can exacerbate the symptoms. Resultant muscle weakness, sensory disturbances, as well as pain may be due to the production of neuropeptides and/or other pain-producing chemicals. Cell bodies of the primary afferent neurons contained in the dorsal root ganglion produce various neuropeptides that are transported to central and peripheral terminals.[4] Substance P causes vasodilation and release of histamine, leading to the inflammatory cascade and pain.[5] Calcitonin gene-related peptide is found in the primary sensory neurons and has been implicated in mediating sensory modalities such as nocioception and mechanical reception.[6] Other pain-producing chemicals released during tissue damage that sensitize pain fibers include bradykinin, serotonin, histamine, potassium ions, and prostaglandins.[5]

CLINICAL FEATURES

Complaints of neck pain are common and frequently occur without radicular pain or neurological deficit. The pain is usually referred cranially toward the occiput and may be associated with headaches as well as bilateral and unilateral shoulder pain. Studies to locate the "pain generator" may include provocative injections in either the facet joints or the cervical disk. Unfortunately, there has been little, if any, evaluation of these procedures in a controlled or randomized study. Relief of neck pain after cervical fusion is usually within the expected improvement rate of the natural history of the disease process. Therefore, surgical intervention for neck pain alone is discouraged until a more accurate diagnostic method is developed.

The first through seventh cervical nerve roots exit above the correspondingly numbered cervical vertebrae, whereas the eighth cervical nerve exists between C7 and T1. Nerve root compression at a specific level in the spine may cause the classic symptoms of motor, sensory, and reflex deficits. However, because there is a fairly high degree of functional overlap among the spinal nerve roots, the classic findings described in numerous textbooks are often not seen (Table 1).

Patients with cervical radiculopathy will often have a positive Spurling sign. This test is performed by having the patient rotate and laterally bend the head toward the affected side, while applying a vertical compressive force to the top of the head. A positive test causes exacerbation of radicular symptoms. Head and neck extension can also recreate radicular symptoms. The shoulder abduction relief sign is performed by placing the painful extremity in the abducted position with the palm of the hand resting on the top of the head. This maneuver will frequently reduce radicular pain, presumably by decreasing nerve root tension.

Cervical myelopathy can be precipitated by either a large central disk herniation or more commonly by severe spondylitic changes. Symptoms vary widely but include a deterioration in gait and manual dexterity, generalized weakness, and/or urinary urgency or frequency. The most common complaint is lower extremity weakness, with further progression leading to loss of proprioception. The combination of these two problems leads to the characteristic wide-based myelopathic gait. Long tract findings of spasticity and hyperreflexia in the arms are usually accompanied by lower motor neuron findings, which result in muscle wasting and fasciculations. Generally, the lower extremities are hyperreflexic, whereas upper extremity reflexes may be either hypo- or hyperreflexic, depending on the level of the lesion in the cervical spine. A positive Hoffmann's sign is indicative of upper motor neuron disease and is found by flicking the nail of the middle finger and observing the abnormal reflexive contraction of either the thumb or index finger. An inverted brachioradialis reflex is demonstrated by tapping the brachioradialis tendon and noting an abnormal reflex contraction of the spastic

TABLE 1. NEUROLOGICAL TESTING OF THE UPPER EXTREMITY

Nerve Root	Reflex	Sensation	Muscle
C4	None	Back of neck Scapula	None
C5	Biceps	Lateral arm	Deltoid Biceps
C6	Brachioradialis	Lateral forearm Thumb, index finger	Wrist extensors Biceps
C7	Triceps	Middle finger	Triceps Wrist flexors Finger extensors
C8	None	Ring, little finger	Finger flexors Intrinsics
T1	None	Medial arm, forearm	Intrinsics

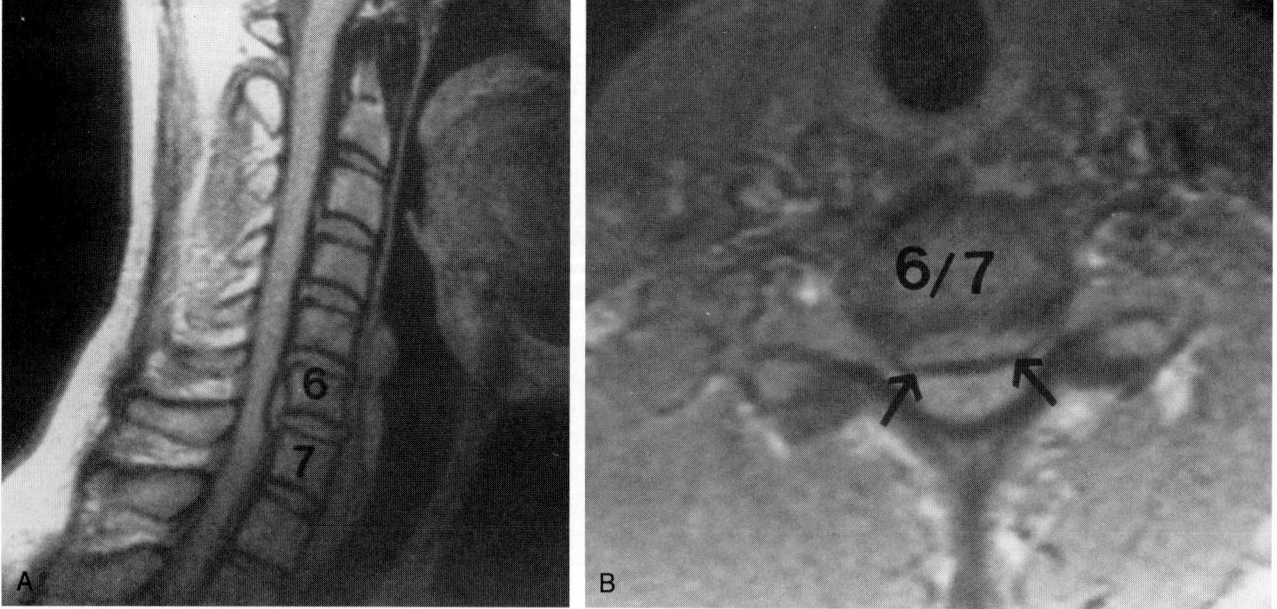

Fig. 1. Disk herniation. *A* and *B*, Sagittal and axial magnetic resonance imaging demonstrating a disk herniation at C6-7.

finger flexors.[7] Assessment of the jaw jerk reflex is important in those patients who have global hyperreflexia. This reflex is a stretch reflex involving both the masseter and temporalis muscles, and it is innervated by the fifth cranial nerve (trigeminal). An absent or diminished reflex is indicative of disease along the course of the nerve. A normal jaw jerk reflex will exclude disease above the foramen magnum, whereas hyperreflexic reflex is indicative of intracranial disease or systemic disease.

INVESTIGATION

The standard radiographic technique for evaluation of the cervical spine includes obtaining lateral, anteroposterior (AP), and oblique views. Degenerative changes that can be seen on these films include intervertebral disk space narrowing, osteoarthritis of the apophyseal joints, and uncovertebral arthrosis. Flexion-extension view of the cervical spine may also be obtained if subluxation is clinically suspected.

Because radiographs do not directly visualize the neural elements, further imaging tests are necessary to assess neural compression. The use of water soluble, nonionic myelographic agents can provide visualization of the entire spinal canal. A major disadvantage is that it is relatively invasive and somewhat nonspecific. Accuracy rates for myelography are similar to those for computed tomography (CT) scans and range from 70% to 90%.[8] However, numerous studies showed that myelography, as well as CT scans and magnetic resonance imaging (MRI) scans, have a relatively high incidence of radiographic abnormalities in patients who are asymptomatic.[9] Therefore, it is extremely important to correlate the patient's symptoms with the abnormal findings on the radiological test and then make the appropriate treatment recommendations.

MRI of the cervical spine is noninvasive, involves no radiation exposure, and provides excellent resolution of the cervical disk as well as the neural elements (Fig. 1). This test must be interpreted with caution because there is a fairly high prevalence of false-positive findings. Boden et al[9] found that 19% of 63 asymptomatic patients had major abnormalities on cervical spine MRI.

GOALS, INDICATIONS, AND CONTRAINDICATIONS

Before discussing the treatment of cervical radiculopathy and myelopathy, one must understand the natural history of the disease process. The results of surgical intervention should be compared with the natural history of the disease before definitive treatment is recommended.

Lees and Turner[10] reported on 95 patients with cervical spondylosis. Fifty-one patients presented with symptoms of a cervical radiculopathy without evidence of myelopathy. During long-term follow-up (2 to 19 years), no patient experienced myelopathy if it was absent at initial presentation. Forty-five percent of the study group with radicular pain had only a single episode without recurrence, whereas 30% continued to have mild symptoms and 25% had persistent or worsening symptoms. The authors concluded that wearing a collar often relieved symptoms but that any or no treatment will often give the same final result.

Forty-four of Lees and Turner's patients had radiological and objective evidence of a cervical myelopathy. All patients recorded at 10-year follow-up had exacerbation of symptoms for at least 1 year followed by either a static period or mild improvement. Those patients with mild disability at initial presentation had the best prognosis, with no significant progression during the study period. Of the 15 patients who initially had severe disability secondary to myelopathy, 14 remained moderately or severely disabled after 10 to 20 years of follow-up. It was concluded that the course of cervical spondylitic myelopathy may be prolonged and that long periods of nonprogressive disability are the rule with rare instances of progressive deterioration.

Numerous treatment options are available for patients who present with either neck pain or cervical radiculopathy. Rarely is surgical treatment considered initially unless a severe fixed neurological deficit is present or a rapidly progressive neurological deficit is evolving. The majority of patients will respond well to either various medications or physical therapy programs. The most common medications used are nonsteroidal anti-inflammatory drugs (NSAIDs). Because mechanical compression of nerve roots can lead to an inflammatory response, NSAIDs, by decreasing the inflammation, will usually cause the patient's pain to subside.

Other nonsurgical management modalities include physical therapy. Therapy programs should include both an active exercise program and passive program for pain modulation.

Current indications for surgery in cervical radiculopathy are as follows[11]: (1) persistent or recurrent arm pain not responsive to a trial of conservative treatment (3 months), (2) progressive neurological deficit, (3) static neurological deficit associated with radicular pain, (4) confirmatory imaging study consistent with clinical findings (CT myelogram and/or MRI).

ANTERIOR SURGICAL PROCEDURES

ANTERIOR DISKECTOMY AND FUSION

After the induction of general anesthesia, the patient is positioned supine on the operating room table. A small rolled towel should be placed between the scapulae to slightly extend the neck. Generally, a left-sided approach is preferable to decrease the risk to the recurrent laryngeal nerve. On the left, the nerve enters the thorax within the carotid sheath. It then loops under the aortic arch and ascends into the neck beside the trachea and esophagus. On the right side, however, it may leave the carotid sheath at a high level and cross anteriorly behind the thyroid, thus leaving itself more susceptible to injury with a right-sided incision.

The incision may be transverse or longitudinal, following the anterior border of the sternocleidomastoid muscle. Knowledge of anatomic landmarks is helpful in placement of the skin incision. Generally, the hyoid bone is at the level of C3, the thyroid cartilage is at C4-5, and the cricoid cartilage lies at the level of C6. A transverse incision is preferred for a one- or two-level fusion, whereas the longitudinal approach is best suited for three or more levels. Once through the skin and platysma muscles, the approach proceeds medial to the sternocleidomastoid muscle. The carotid sheath is retracted laterally and the esophagus and trachea medially, using hand-held blunt retractors. The vertebral bodies and disks can then be identified by palpation in the midline. Once the prevertebral fascia and longus colli muscles have been dissected away from the vertebral bodies, a spinal needle should be inserted in the appropriate disk space and lateral radiographs obtained to identify the surgical level accurately[12] (Fig. 2).

A flap of the anterior longitudinal ligament is then raised by sharp dissection and through this opening, the intervertebral disk is removed. After disk removal with pituitary rongeurs and curets, the cartilaginous end plates are also

removed. The posterior longitudinal ligament should be visualized but not incised if the ligament is intact. If a tear is seen in the ligament or a sequestered fragment is suspected, then resection of the ligament is performed. After complete ligament resection, a micro nerve hook can be used to probe the posterior border of the superior and inferior adjacent vertebrae for sequestered disk fragments. Removal of posterior osteophytes is not routinely recommended unless a significant motor deficit is present preoperatively because resorption of the osteophytes often occurs after a solid fusion.[13, 14]

Autologous bone graft is usually harvested from the iliac crest at least 2 cm behind the anterosuperior iliac spine. Two vertical cuts are made approximately 10 to 15 mm apart at the top of the crest. After appropriate trimming, the graft is horseshoe shaped and consists of cancellous bone surrounded by cortical bone on three sides (tricortical).[15]

The prepared disk space is then distracted after holes are made in the end plates with either a curet or power bur. Distraction can be accomplished either by the addition of weights to a previously placed head-hold or tong traction or manually by the anesthesiologist. The bone graft should be tamped into position and countersunk approximately 1 to 2 mm in relation to the anterior cortical edges of the adjacent bodies (Fig. 3). Postoperatively, the patient is usually placed in a rigid cervical collar for approximately 6 weeks.

CERVICAL CORPECTOMY

The technique of anterior cervical diskectomy and fusion becomes increasingly difficult over multiple levels, and the rate of successful fusion decreases as the number of attempted fusion levels increase, Therefore, it is recommended that partial corpectomies be performed for patients with multiple-level spondylotic myelopathy or myeloradiculopathy.[16–18]

The standard anterior cervical approach is used, and diskectomy should be completed at the appropriate levels. Small rongeurs as well as high-speed burs are used to create a trough in the center of the vertebral body. Bone and disk should be removed until the posterior longitudinal ligament is completely visualized. Posterior osteophytes are then removed with small rongeurs after deepening the trough. Fusion may be attempted with either an autologous or allograft fibular strut or iliac crest graft. The graft should be notched at both ends with a high-speed bur. After distraction on the neck, the graft should be placed into notches made in the center of the remaining superior and inferior vertebral bodies. Using this technique, it is important to preserve the anterior portion of the vertebral bodies to serve as an effective barrier against graft dislodgement.

ANTERIOR DISKECTOMY WITHOUT FUSION

Anterior diskectomy without fusion has developed as an alternative to cervical fusion based on the premise that if successful results of anterior fusions occur with pseudarthrosis, then diskectomy alone can be performed. Most authors who advocate this procedure reported good early results; the majority of the patients experienced a spontaneous fusion at the surgical level as well as some degree of postoperative kyphosis. Unfortunately, many of these stud-

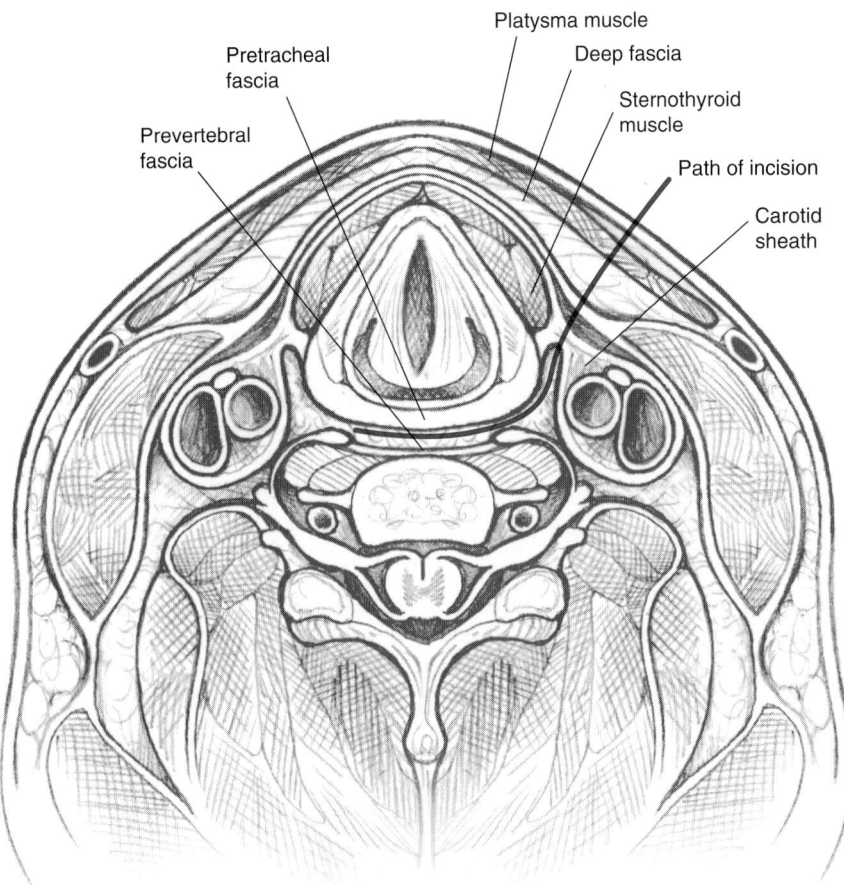

Pretracheal fascia

Prevertebral fascia

Platysma muscle

Deep fascia

Sternothyroid muscle

Path of incision

Carotid sheath

Fig. 2. Approach for anterior cervical diskectomy and fusion. The dissection proceeds through the platysma muscles and then medial to the carotid sheath and lateral to the trachea and esophagus.

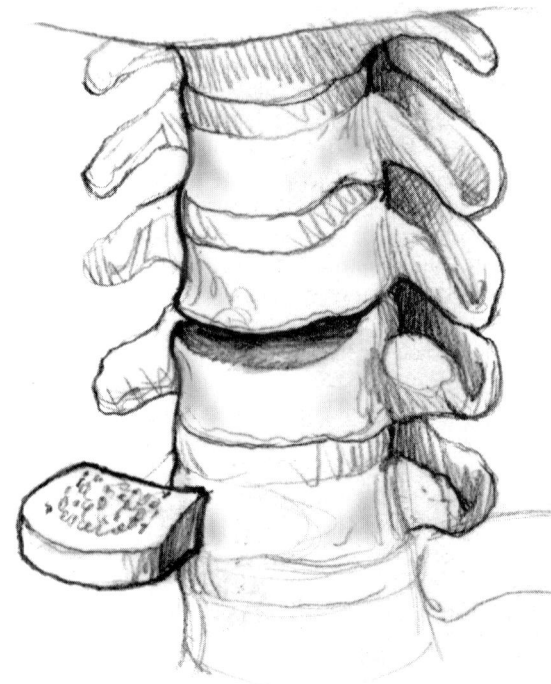

Fig. 3. Insertion of a tricortical iliac crest graft. This graft was placed after diskectomy at the C5-6 interspace.

ies examine only the neurological recovery rate and fail to highlight the significant problem with postoperative neck pain. Most longer term studies of anterior cervical diskectomy without fusion noted postoperative cervical and/or interscapular pain in up to 50% of the patients.[19]

AUTOGRAFT VERSUS ALLOGRAFT

In an attempt to eliminate donor site problems while maintaining acceptable fusion rates, many surgeons have substituted allograft for autologous bone in anterior cervical fusions. Allograft eliminates the need for a second surgery to obtain the bone graft, thereby decreasing the operative time, morbidity, and pain at the donor site. For one-level procedures, the clinical outcome is comparable for allograft and autograft fusions. However, for multilevel anterior cervical procedures, the nonunion rate using allograft bone has been found to be significantly higher and frequently is associated with collapse of the grafts and narrowing of the interspace.[20]

ANTERIOR CERVICAL INSTRUMENTATION

To increase the fusion rate of anterior cervical fusion and improve the clinical outcome, several authors advocated the use of anterior cervical instrumentation. The anterior cervical plate provides increased stability postoperatively after anterior cervical decompression. Additionally, the plate can act as a buttress to prevent graft extrusion in the immediate postoperative phase before fusion occurs. However, the anterior cervical plate adds additional time and expense to the surgical procedure. Improper use of the plate can lead to postoperative dislodgement with subsequent esophageal irritation and perforation. In the case of multiple-level cervical fusion in which the fusion rate is known to be lower or after a multiple-level cervical corpectomy in which cervical stability is in question, the use of a plate may increase the chance of a successful fusion and decrease the need for postoperative immobilization in a halo brace.

POSTERIOR SURGICAL PROCEDURES

The decision to perform either anterior or posterior surgery for cervical radiculopathy or myelopathy remains controversial. Simeone[21] recommended the posterior approach for (1) unilateral radiculopathy at one or more levels (posterior foraminotomy), (2) cervical myelopathy with spinal cord compression at three or more levels (laminectomy or laminoplasty), and (3) spinal cord compression secondary to congenital spinal stenosis or acquired stenosis from posterior compression.

The most common posterior cervical procedures performed for radiculopathy and myelopathy are laminotomy with foraminotomy, laminectomy, and laminoplasty. These procedures vary in the amount of decompression of neural elements that is achieved.[22]

FORAMINOTOMY

Laminotomy and foraminotomy require that only a minimal amount of lamina be removed to expose the lateral edge of the dura. Resection of the medial aspect of the facet joint will allow visualization of the exiting nerve root in its foramen. This technique is adequate for relieving nerve root compression within the foramen from either disk material or uncovertebral or facet spurs. It does not decompress the spinal cord and has minimal effect on cervical spine stability.

Limited surgical exposure is used to visualize the lamina and facet joint subperiosteally. The lamina immediately adjacent to the interspace is then thinned with a bur and removed to allow visualization of the lateral edge of the dura. The laminotomy should be directly over the junction of the nerve root and the dura (Fig. 4). If the patient was noted preoperatively to have a soft-disk herniation, the root can be gently retracted and the annulus incised. Fine pituitary rongeurs can then be used for removal of disk fragments.

LAMINECTOMY

Laminectomy may be considered in patients with myelopathy caused by multiple-level cervical spondylitic changes. Laminectomies are contraindicated in patients with preexisting cervical kyphosis or fractures and in children unless a fusion is performed at the same time. A significant concern regarding this procedure is the development of postoperative cervical kyphosis or instability. This kyphosis is directly related to the amount of facet joint resection. Raynor et al[23] showed that a 50% facetectomy allows visualization of 3 to 5 mm of the nerve root, whereas a 70% resection allows visualization of 8 to 10 mm. These authors concluded that resection of greater than 50% of the facet joint significantly compromises facet strength. Zdeblick et al[24] noted that segmental hypermobility of the cervical spine results if a foraminotomy involves resection of more than 50% of the facet.

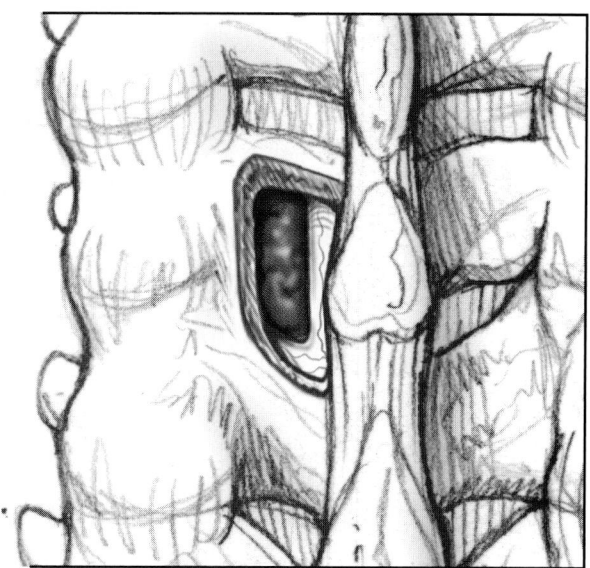

Fig. 4. Laminotomy. This procedure should expose the lateral edge of the dura and the margin of the exiting nerve root.

Positioning the patient for a laminectomy is similar to the positioning for a laminotomy or foraminotomy. However, extension of the spine should be avoided because this markedly decreases the space available for the cord. After adequate exposure of the cervical spine, a high-speed fine bur is used to create longitudinal troughs at the junctions of the facet and lamina. The bur drilling should continue until the troughs have been thinned down to the remaining anterior cortex. At this point, a fine 1-mm Kerrison rongeur can be used to complete the cutting of the longitudinal troughs through the anterior cortex of the lamina. With this technique, there is no need to place any instruments between the cord and the lamina, thereby preventing iatrogenic cord injury. After completion of the troughs, the lamina can be lifted off en bloc. The remaining ligamentum flavum may be released with either a knife or curet.

LAMINOPLASTY

Cervical laminoplasty evolved in Japan in response to the high incidence of postlaminectomy deformity seen after extensive cervical laminectomy. The advantage of the laminoplasty procedure is that it does not violate the facet joints while maintaining additional stability on the "hinged side" of the procedure. After positioning in the prone position, a subperiosteal dissection of the lamina from C2 to C7 is generally performed. Two bony gutters are then made with high-speed burs from the upper to the lower most involved vertebrae. The gutters should be made just medial to the facet joint and pedicle. These gutters are continued bilaterally until the inner cortex is reached. On the side exhibiting the greatest narrowing or the side with the most significant radiculopathy, the bur should go through the inner cortex and break through at one segment. Next, a 1-mm Kerrison rongeur is used to remove the inner cortex from proximal to distal on the side from which the lamina is to be elevated. At this point, nonabsorbable heavy sutures should be passed through the base of each spinous process at each segment to be elevated. The surgeon should now gently put pressure along the spinous

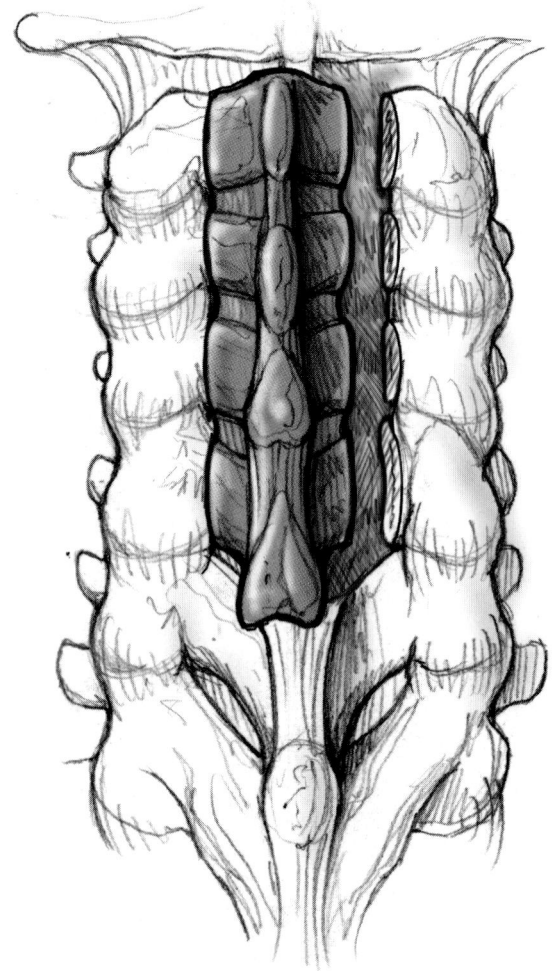

Fig. 5. Laminoplasty. This is a schematic illustration.

processes to open up the lamina on the side where the trough has been completed through both cortices. It is very important that adhesions are not present between the dural sac and undersurface of the lamina. If the laminae are elevated with significant dural adhesions present, there is a significant risk of tethering of nerve roots on the hinged side, causing a postoperative radiculopathy.[25] The previously placed sutures are then down to the facet capsules on the hinge side, thereby preventing hinge closure (Fig. 5).

COMPLICATIONS AND RESULTS

Complications of surgery for cervical disk disease can be divided with those occurring at the graft site and those occurring in the neck. Donor site pain is the most common patient complaint after spinal arthrodesis with autologous bone grafting. The ilium is the most common area from which bone graft is harvested, and the list of reported complications is extensive.[26] These include prolonged pain, cosmetic deformity, infection, hematoma, gait disturbance, ilium fracture, peritoneal perforation, hernia, and injuries to the lateral femoral cutaneous, superior cluneal, and ilioinguinal nerve. To minimize complications, the approach to the posterior ilium should be within 8 cm of the posterior

superior iliac spine to avoid cluneal nerves. When approaching the anterior ilium, the incision should end at least 2 cm lateral to the anterosuperior iliac spine to avoid injury to the lateral femoral cutaneous nerve.

The most common problem seen postoperatively in the neck after cervical surgery is a transient sore throat or difficulty swallowing. The risk of injury to the trachea and esophagus can be decreased by proper placement of blunt retractors. Although perforating injuries of the esophagus are rare, when they do occur they can be life threatening.[27] The most common neurological complication seen after anterior cervical surgery is temporary unilateral paralysis of the vocal cords. As mentioned, the risk to the recurrent laryngeal nerve can be decreased by using a left-sided approach.

Flynn[28] compiled the replies of 704 neurosurgeons describing more than 35,000 anterior cervical interbody fusions. In this large series, there were 100 cases of significant permanent myelopathy or myeloradiculopathy. Seventy-five percent of these patients had an immediate deficit postoperatively, whereas 25% of the patients experienced a deficit in the postoperative recovery phase. Analysis of the data led Flynn to conclude that, regardless of the cause of the myelopathy, reoperation had little effect on the ultimate status of the neurological deficit. In addition, most surgeons were unable to determine the cause of the neurological deterioration.

RESULTS

Robinson reported on the first large series of patients treated with anterior interbody fusion for cervical disk disease in 1962.[14] Overall, 73% of patients had either an excellent or good result. He noted that patients who had multiple-level fusions had worse results than those who had single-level disease. DePalma et al[29] noted that after a mean follow-up of 6 years 63% of the patients were considered to have satisfactory results. Pseudarthrosis was noted in 12% of the patients; however, this did not statistically affect the result. The lack of correlation between a successful fusion and patient outcome can be explained by the fact that even though bone union does not occur, a stable fibrous union does. In addition, removal of the degenerative disk can alleviate some of the mechanical pressure on the nerve root while distraction of the disk space and neural foramina occurs, although much of the initial height of the interspace gained by the bone graft may be lost.[30]

Neurological recovery after surgery for cervical myelopathy depends on the degree of spinal cord compression. Fujiwara[31] noted that surgical results generally are poor in most patients who have less than 30 mm^2 of spinal cord area before surgery. Okada[32] also noted that atrophy of the spinal cord was predictive of an unsatisfactory result.

Emery et al[33] reviewed the results of 108 patients with cervical spondylitic myelopathy treated with either anterior diskectomy or partial or subtotal corpectomy. At final follow-up, 87% of the patients had improvement of their gait and 92% had recovery of a motor deficit. Generally, those patients with better preoperative neurological function were associated with a better neurological outcome.

Unlike the surgical management of lumbar disk herniations, the surgical approach to cervical soft-disk herniations has remained controversial. Excellent results have been reported by using either the posterior or anterior approach. Henderson et al[34] reported on 736 patients who had a posterior foraminotomy for cervical radiculopathy and noted an overall excellent or good result in 91% of the cases. However, recurrent signs of radiculopathy were present in 20% of the cases, and 14% of the patients required a second posterior surgical procedure. Herkowitz et al,[35] in their prospective study, compared the results of anterior cervical diskectomy and fusion versus laminotomy/foraminotomy in patients with the diagnosis of cervical disk herniation. Overall, after a follow-up of 4 years, the patients who had an anterior procedure performed had an excellent or good rate of 94%, whereas those patients who had a posterior procedure performed had an excellent or good rate of 75%. On the basis of this study, it was concluded that anterior cervical diskectomy and fusion had the best long-term results in the surgical management of posterolateral soft-disk herniation. Posterior laminectomy and foraminotomy may be considered when there are technical limitations of the anterior approach and when prior anterior cervical surgery has restricted access to the level.

Currently, no prospective, randomized studies are available that compare surgical approaches in results of cervical myelopathy. Many available studies are retrospective reviews of different procedures that have been performed at the same institution. In general, for two- or three-level decompressions, the results of corpectomies are significantly better than those for anterior diskectomies and fusions. In addition, two- or three-level anterior decompressions generally have a more favorable neurological recovery rate compared with laminectomies.

REFERENCES

1. Lestini WF, Wiesel SW: The pathogenesis of cervical spondylolisthesis. Clin Orthop 1989; 239:69.
2. Payne EE, Spillane JD: The cervical spine. An anatomico-pathological study of 70 specimens. Brain 1957; 80:571.
3. Friedenberg ZB, Miller WT: Degenerative disc disease of the cervical spine. J Bone Joint Surg Am 1963; 55:1171.
4. Chatani K, Kawakami M, Wainstein J, et al: Characterization of thermal hyperalgesia, C-fold expression, and alterations in neuropeptides after mechanical irritation of the dorsal root ganglion. Spine 1995; 20:277.
5. Cavanaugh J: Neural mechanisms of lumbar pain. Spine 1995; 20:1804.
6. Ahmed M, Bjurholm A, Kreicbergs A, et al: SP and CGRR-immunoreactive nerve fibers in the rat lumbar spine. Neuro-Orthopedics 1991; 12:19.
7. Montgomery D, Brower R: Cervical spondylotic myelopathy. Clinical syndrome and natural history. Orthop Clin North Am 1992; 23:487.
8. Bell GR, Ross JS: Diagnosis of nerve root compression. Orthop Clin North Am 1992; 22:405.
9. Boden SD, McCowin PR, Davis DO, et al: Abnormal magnetic resonance scans of the cervical spine in asymptomatic subjects. J Bone Joint Surg Am 1990; 72:1178.
10. Lees F, Turner J: Natural history and prognosis of cervical spondylolisthesis. BMJ 1963; 2:1607.
11. Fischgrund J, Herkowitz H: Cervical degenerative disease. In Garfin S, Vaccaro A (eds): Spine Knowledge Update. Rosemont, Ill, American Academy of Orthopaedic Surgeons, 1997; p 75.
12. Herkowitz H: Anterior cervical surgery in cervical spondylolisthesis. Presented at the meeting of the American Academy of Orthopaedic Surgeons, Washington, DC, 1992.
13. Connolly E, Seymour R, Adams J: Clinical evaluation of anterior cervical fusion for degenerative cervical disc disease. J Neurosurg 1965; 23:431.
14. Robinson R, Walker A, Ferlic D: The results of anterior interbody fusion of the cervical spine. J Bone Joint Surg Am 1962; 44:1569.
15. Jones AA, Dougherty PJ, Sharkey NA, et al: Iliac crest bone graft. Osteotome versus saw. Spine 1993; 18:2048.
16. Bernard T, Whitecloud T: Cervical spondylotic myelopathy and myeloradiculopathy. Anterior decompression and stabilization with autogenous fibula strut graft. Clin Orthop 1987; 221:149.
17. Boni M, Cherubino P, Benazzo F: Multiple subtotal somatectomy: Technique and evaluation of a series of 39 cases. Spine 1984; 9:358.
18. Hanai K, Fujiyoshi F, Kamei K: Subtotal vertebrectomy and spinal fusion for cervical spondylotic myelopathy. Spine 1986; 11:310.
19. Yamamoto I, Ikeda A, Shibuya N, et al: Clinical long-term results of anterior discectomy without interbody fusion for cervical disc disease. Spine 1991; 16:272.
20. Zdeblick T, Ducker T: The use of freeze-dried allograft bone for anterior cervical fusions. Spine 1991; 16:726.
21. Simeone F: Surgical management of cervical disc disease: Posterior approach. Semin Spine Surg 1989; 1:239.
22. Fischgrund J, Herkowitz H, Brower R: Posterior cervical laminectomy and laminoplasty. Operative Tech Orthop 1993; 3:187.
23. Raynor R, Pugh J, Shapiro I: Cervical facetectomy and its effect on spine strength. J Neurosurg 1985; 63:278.
24. Zdeblick TA, Zou D, Warden KE, et al: Cervical stability after foraminotomy. J Bone Joint Surg Am 1992; 74:22.
25. Kimura I, Oh-Hama M, Shingo H: Cervical myelopathy treated by canal-expansive laminaplasty. J Bone Joint Surg 1984; 66:914.
26. Fischgrund J, Kurz L, Herkowitz H: Techniques of bone graft harvesting for cervical fusions. Semin Spine Surg 1995; 7:27.
27. Newhouse K, et al: Esophageal perforation following anterior cervical spine surgery. Spine 1989; 14:1051.
28. Flynn T: Neurologic complications of anterior cervical interbody fusion. Spine 1982; 7:536.
29. DePalma A, Rothman R, Lewinnek G, et al: Anterior interbody fusion for severe cervical disc degeneration. Surg Gynecol Obstet 1972; 134:755.
30. Fischgrund J, Herkowitz H: Anterior surgical procedure for cervical disc disease. In An H (ed): Surgery of the Cervical Spine. London, UK, Martin-Dunitz, 1994, p 195.
31. Fujiwara K, Yonenobu K, Ebara S, et al: The prognosis of surgery for cervical compression myelopathy. J Bone Joint Surg Br 1989; 71:393.
32. Okada K, Shirasaki N, Hayashi H, et al: Treatment of cervical spondylotic myelopathy by enlargement of the spinal canal anteriorly followed by arthrodesis. J Bone Joint Surg Am 1991; 73:352.
33. Emery S, Bohlman H, Bolesta M, et al: Anterior cervical decompression and arthrodesis for the treatment of cervical spondylotic myelopathy. J Bone Joint Surg Am 1998; 80:941.
34. Henderson C, Hennessy H, Shuey H, et al: Posterior-lateral foraminotomy as an exclusive operative technique for cervical radiculopathy. A review of 846 consecutively operated cases. Neurosurgery 1983; 13:504.
35. Herkowitz H, Kurz L. Overholt D: Surgical management of cervical soft disc herniation. A comparison between the anterior and posterior approach. Spine 1990; 15:1026.

section
8
chapter
5

THORACIC DISK HERNIATIONS

Srdjan Mirkovic

Summary

- Thoracic disk herniations are a difficult diagnostic entity because of limited clinical findings and uncommon presentation.
- Although magnetic resonance imaging facilitates diagnosis, the high incidence of asymptomatic disk herniations must be considered.
- Overdiagnosis and overaggressive treatment should be avoided.
- Conservative treatment in the absence of neurological findings is best.
- Surgery should take into account disk consistency, disk location, level of disk herniation, and the surgeon's experience.

INTRODUCTION

Thoracic disk herniation (TDH) is a difficult diagnostic entity because of atypical clinical presentation and its rarity. A high level of suspicion must be maintained, and consideration should be given to the differential diagnosis in order to avoid delaying treatment. Magnetic resonance imaging (MRI) is the diagnostic modality of choice. Overtreatment, particularly in the presence of asymptomatic lesions, should be avoided.

The true prevalence of trauma causing TDH is controversial. Some have reported up to 50% prevalence of traumatically induced TDH. Computed tomography (CT) in conjunction with autopsy studies suggests an 11% prevalence. In addition, a 14.5% prevalence of TDH was found in a group of patients with neoplastic involvement of the thoracic spine. Objective neurological findings are rare, with an incidence of 1:1,000,000 per year. Thoracic diskectomies represent only 0.2% to 2.0% of all operations for clinically significant TDHs.

Scheuermann's disease, with myelopathy secondary to thoracic disk calcification, has been reported in younger patients. Twisting and torsional movements and heavy lifting have also been described as precipitating factors. Thoracic spondylosis in the elderly with disk calcification, posterior degenerative facet changes, and ligamentum flavum hypertrophy, may be a contributing cause to thoracic myelopathy and stenosis. Degenerative changes are considered the major predisposing factor.

Unlike cervical and lumbar disk herniations, TDH tends to undergo calcification, which can be a helpful radiographic feature. The anatomic narrowing of the spinal canal diameter and the proximity of the spinal cord to the posterior margin of the vertebral bodies may lead to thoracic myelopathy secondary to cord compression in the presence of TDH.

Conservative management is recommended in the absence of neurological involvement. In the presence of progressive neurological compromise and thoracic myelopathy as well as intractable radiculopathy, surgical intervention is indicated. Disk consistency, level of herniation, disk location, and the surgeon's experience determine the optimal surgical approach.

HISTORY

The first TDH leading to spinal cord injury was reported in 1838. A traumatic TDH at the T12-L1 level caused by lifting, with ensuing paraplegia and subsequent death, was described at the beginning of the 20th century. The first surgical approach in the treatment of TDH appears to have been performed in 1922. Two additional surgical cases were reported during the next 10 years.

CLINICAL ASPECTS

Due to the extreme variation in the clinical presentation of TDH, the disorder remains a difficult diagnostic entity. A third of patients present in their fifth decade, and 80% of TDHs occur in the fourth to sixth decade. The male-to-female ratio has been reported as 1.5:1.

The most frequent initial symptom is pain (Table 1). The pain may be intermittent, dull, sharp, constant, or shooting. The pain distribution depends on the disk location and may be axial, unilateral, or bilateral. Circumferential pain radiating around the chest wall is frequently reported. Atypical pain can occur at times, simulating renal disease or degenerative hip disease in the presence of T11 disk herniations. A unilateral lower extremity distribution can mimic lumbar disk herniations. T1 or T2 TDH can be confused with degenerative cervical disease in patients who present with upper extremity pain, Horner's syndrome, and neck pain. Symptoms are often aggravated by sneezing, coughing, and an increase in activities. The symptoms are improved with rest.

Sensory changes are the second most common presentation. This may involve dysesthesias, paresthesias, and numbness. Sensory changes in the absence of pain may be the only initial presentation. Infrequently, motor weakness and bladder dysfunction present before pain and sensory changes. Sensory and motor dysfunction are the primary findings in 60% of symptomatic patients (Table 2). Given the generally long delay in diagnosis at the time of presentation, 30% of patients may exhibit bladder abnormalities, and 18% may have both bowel and bladder disturbances. A chronic history of symptoms is frequent. Delay in diagnosis and misdiagnosis are common due to the varied and nonspecific clinical presentation.

TABLE 1. INITIAL SYMPTOMS OF TDH	
Initial Symptoms	**Occurrence**
Pain	57%
Sensory	24%
Motor	17%
Bladder	2%

Data from Arce CA, Dohrmann GJ: Herniated thoracic disks. Neurol Clin 1985; 3:383.

TABLE 2. SYMPTOMS ON TDH PRESENTATION		
	Occurrence	
Symptoms	**Arce & Dohrmann**	**Stillerman & Weiss (n = 51)**
Motor and sensory	61%	
Motor only	6%	
Sensory only	15%	39%
Weakness		59%
Bladder/sphincter	30%	
Bowel and bladder		18%
Radicular pain only	9%	16%

Based on data from Arce CA, Dohrmann GJ: Herniated thoracic disks. Neurol Clin 1985; 3:383 and Stillerman CB, Weiss MH: Management of thoracic disk disease. Clin Neurosurg 1992; 38:325.

Other neurological disorders should also be considered in rendering treatment. Physical examination early in the course of TDH is unremarkable. Sensory changes with diminished light touch and pinprick may be present as the only finding. In cases of significant spinal cord compression secondary to TDH, upper motor neuron signs may develop with onset of weakness, spasticity, hyperreflexia, decreased sensation to pinprick and light touch, gait disturbances, and a positive Babinski sign. Occasionally, a large centrolateral disk herniation may cause a Brown-Séquard syndrome.

The natural history of TDH is variable. In younger patients, more acute progression from thoracic pain to progressive myelopathy may be seen. More frequently, predominantly in the middle-aged population, disk degenerative changes lead to gradual onset of symptoms secondary to spinal cord compression. The commonly accepted perception of symptom progression from pain to sensory disturbances and on to weakness and neurological demise is, instead, the exception.

INVESTIGATION

MRI is the imaging modality of choice for suspected TDH. MRI allows both axial and sagittal (Fig. 1) imaging with highly specific and sensitive anatomic definition. The MRI sensitivity in imaging of the thoracic spine has increased the frequency of TDH diagnoses, allowing follow-up of smaller cases. Specifically, sagittal MRI of the thoracic spine allows visualization of thoracic disk degeneration,

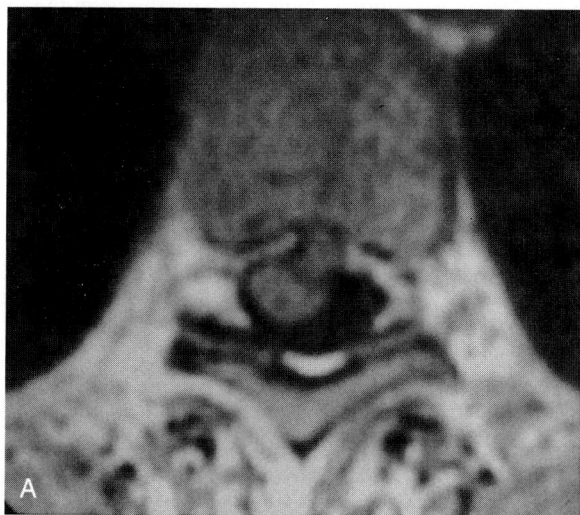
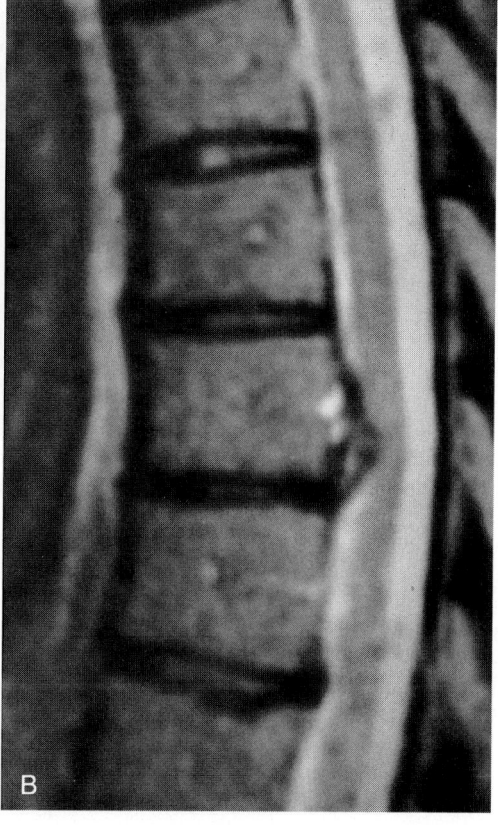

Fig. 1. MRI. *A,* Sagittal MRI of a T8-9 TDH. *B,* Axial MRI of a T9-10 centrolateral TDH.

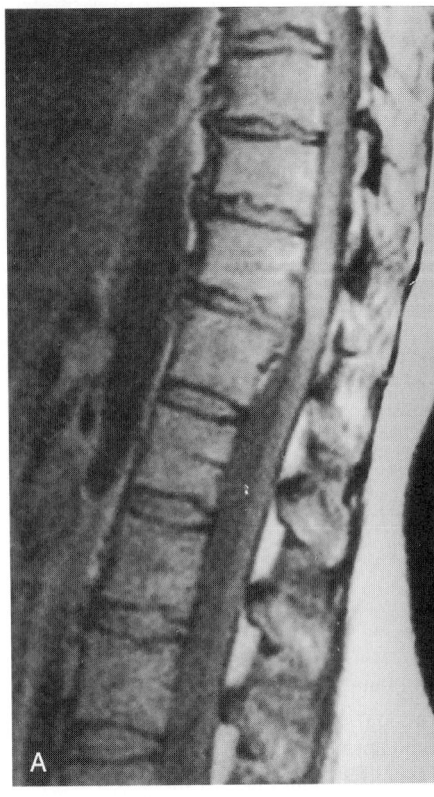 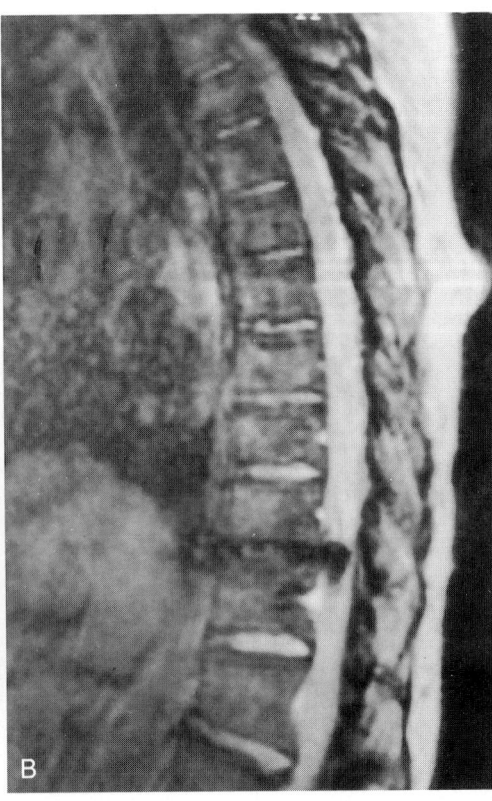

Fig. 2. MRI. *A*, T$_1$-weighted sagittal MRI of isointense T11-12 TDH. *B*, T$_2$-weighted sagittal MRI of a T10-11 TDH.

which is superior to other radiographic techniques. One should exercise caution in correlating MRI studies with clinical presentation due to the high prevalence of asymptomatic TDHs.

Herniated disk material is isointense or slightly hypointense on T$_1$-weighted images relative to adjacent disk levels (Fig. 2). On the T$_2$-weighted images, disk herniations appear hypointense. The myelogram effect produced by T$_2$-weighted images, with the cerebrospinal fluid appearing brighter than the spinal cord, allows better contrast between the spinal cord and low-intensity disks or osteophytes (Fig. 2). Calcified disk herniations can be distinguished from soft-disk herniations due to their hypointense presentation on both T$_1$- and T$_2$-weighted sequences. T$_2$-weighted or gradient echo sequences allow the best assessment of disk degeneration.

In addition, MRI has the advantage of identifying multiple disk herniations on sagittal sequences without the need for multilevel axial imaging required with CT myelography. MRI allows better differentiation between disk herniations and neurogenic tumors. Volume averaging, pulsatile cerebrospinal fluid motion, scoliosis, and motion artifact may compromise imaging quality.

CT myelography allows better identification of disk calcifications than does MRI (Fig. 3). It also can clearly demonstrate encroachment on the spinal cord in the presence of lateral herniations (Fig. 4). The sensitivity and specificity of CT myelography is equal to that of MRI. The main disadvantage of CT myelography, in addition to being more invasive, is the need to perform axial cuts at multiple levels.

Myelograms are particularly useful in determining the correct operative level by comparing them to intraoperative anteroposterior and lateral radiographs. The correct level is

determined intraoperatively by counting ribs from the most inferior rib superiorly on the anteroposterior radiographs or counting vertebrae from the fifth lumbar vertebra superiorly on the lateral radiographs.

Plain radiographs have low specificity in the diagnosis of TDH. Osteophyte formation, segmental kyphosis, and disc narrowing are commonly seen in the degenerative process, with or without TDH. Disk calcifications can be seen radiographically in 70% of patients, with TDH in 4% to 6% of patients without herniations.

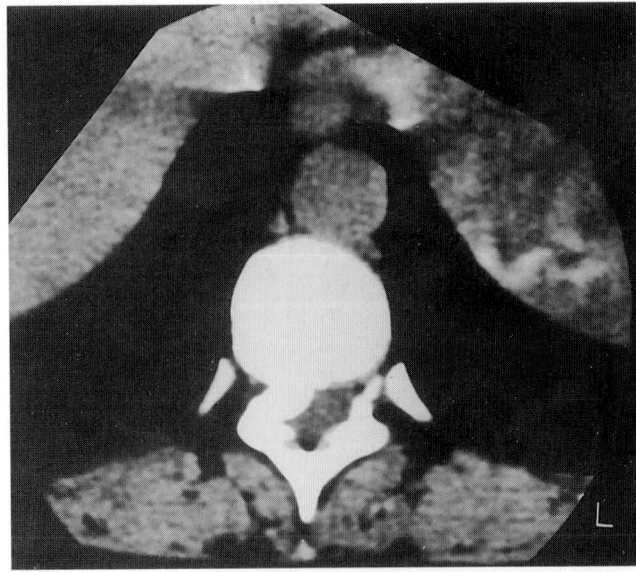

Fig. 3. Computed tomography scan. This is a lateral calcified TDH.

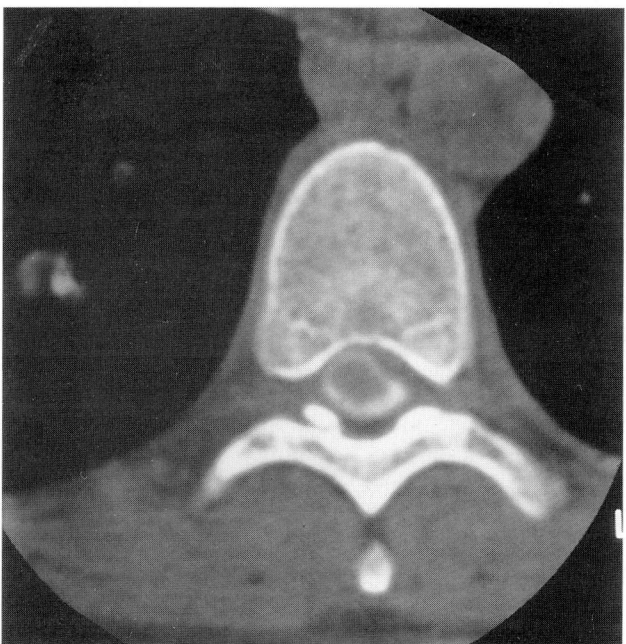

Fig. 4. Computed tomography myelogram. Soft T8-9 TDH eneroaching on the spinal canal.

Extension of disk material and indentation of the spinal cord beyond the posterior margin of the adjacent vertebral bodies is a key feature of TDH. Classification of TDH according to location and level is helpful in determining the surgical approach. Location may be central, lateral, centrolateral, or intradural. Clinically, patients with central herniations may present with symptoms consistent with myelopathy, whereas lateral protrusions can elicit radicular symptoms. Rarely, intradural herniations are seen. Overall, 26% of cases occur at the T11-12 level, while 75% occur between T8-12. Seventy percent of TDH cases are either central or centrolateral. The increased frequency of thoracolumbar disc herniations may be attributed to increased motion at this level and early disk degeneration.

The surgical approach is influenced by the disk herniation and consistency. Differentiation between soft- and hard-disk herniations should be made on MRI and CT myelography. The goals of treatment are pain reduction and reversal of neurological deterioration.

INDICATIONS AND CONTRAINDICATION

The absolute indication for surgical intervention is the patient who presents with myelopathy. Patients with chronic unrelenting pain unresponsive to nonsurgical management constitute relative surgical indications. Surgery is contraindicated in patients with ongoing medical conditions predisposing them to increased surgical risk.

PROCEDURE

The appropriate surgical approach is based on the location of the disk herniation relative to the spinal cord (Table 3), disk consistency, the level of herniation, and the surgeon's familiarity with the different approaches. The patient's

medical condition and age must be taken into consideration before surgery.

Surgical approaches are either anterior or posterior. Anterior approaches are transthoracic, trans-sternal, and thoracoscopic. Posterior approaches are lateral extracavitary, costotransversectomy, and transpedicular.

Anterior approaches are performed with the patient in the lateral decubitus position. A double lumen and a tracheal tube are used to allow unilateral lung ventilation. Somatosensory and motor potential spinal monitoring is instituted for both anterior and posterior procedures. Patients are approached from the left side, unless the herniation is on the right side, in which cases a right transthoracic approach can be used. Patients are secured to the operating table with Stulberg's hip positioners, avoiding the use of bean bags, which may interfere with the operative field. Hips and knees are flexed, and all extremities are carefully padded. An axillary roll is used under the arm. The head is secured in a neutral position with pillows or blankets. The iliac crest is included in the operative field when iliac crest bone harvesting is necessary.

Posterior approaches are performed with the patient in the standard prone position.

The correct surgical level is determined by identifying the rib leading to the corresponding level of the disorder. Ribs attach to the transverse processes and to the superior aspect of the vertebra at the level of the pedicle. The T11-12 thoracic disk, for example, can be located on anteroposterior radiographs by following the twelfth rib to its costovertebral attachment located at the superior aspect of the twelfth thoracic vertebra and thus the inferior border of the T11-12 disk. The correct surgical level can also be identified by counting vertebra from either L5-S1 or T12 proximally on the lateral intraoperative radiograph. The presence of a transitional lumbar vertebra should be ruled out on the anteroposterior and lateral radiographs.

In high TDHs, the surgical level is ascertained by obtaining an intraoperative swimmer's view and counting distally from C1-2.

TABLE 3. SURGICAL APPROACHES		
Levels	**Disk Herniation**	**Approaches**
Soft Disks		
T1-4	Central, centrolateral	Trans-sternal
	Central, centrolateral	Medial clavisectomy
	Centrolateral, lateral	Costotransversectomy
T4-12	Central, centrolateral, lateral	Transthoracic
	Central, centrolateral, lateral	Thoracoscopy
	Centrolateral, lateral	Lateral
	Central, centrolateral, lateral	Costotransversectomy
	Lateral	Transpedicular
Calcified Disks		
T1-4	Central, centrolateral	Trans-sternal
	Central, centrolateral	Medial clavisectomy
	Lateral	Costotransversectomy
T4-12	Central, centrolateral, lateral	Transthoracic
	Lateral	Lateral
	Lateral, centrolateral	Costotransversectomy

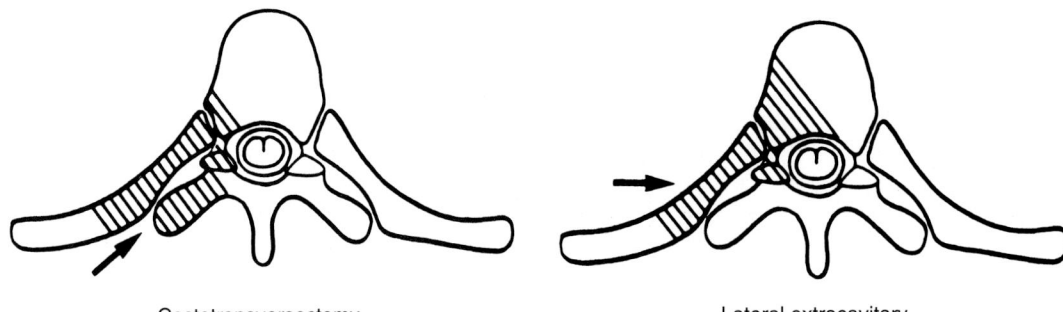

Costotransversectomy   Lateral extracavitary

Fig. 5. View. This shows the extent of bony resection *(crosshatch)* and angle or approach *(arrows)* to disk space with costotransversectomy (left) and lateral extracavitary (right) procedures. (From Orthopaedic Knowledge Update: Spine, AAOS, Rosemont, IL, 1997, p 92; originally from Cybulski G: Thoracic disk herniations: Surgical technique. Contemp Neurosurg 1992; 14:1.)

POSTERIOR APPROACHES

Lateral (Extracavitary) (Fig. 5). This is an extrapleural exposure, facilitating thoracolumbar junction visualization without the need to elevate the diaphragm. An attempt should be made to close any violations of the pleura. If this is not possible, a chest tube is placed. The lateral (extracavitary) approach is applicable for any level of TDH and is particularly indicated for centrolateral and lateral soft disks (Fig. 6) as well as lateral calcified disk herniations. The procedure entails excision of portions of the costotransverse joint, rib, facet, and pedicle. By extending the rib resection laterally, additional visualization of the spinal cord, nerve root, and disk space can be obtained without retraction of the cord. Segmental vessels can be dissected in the trough of the vertebral bodies and are clipped or ligated, and the intercostal nerves generally need not be sacrificed. Multiple levels can be exposed, including the thoracolumbar junction. Anterolateral fusions with either rib or strut graft can be performed through this approach. The procedure can entail significant paraspinal muscle disruption and bone removal, which can increase operative time as well as blood loss. Any ventral dural tears can be difficult to repair. If segmental nerves are sacrificed at multiple levels, significant chest wall numbness can ensue. The numbness can be bothersome if it involves a significant amount of the breast in the female patient.

Costotransversectomy. Costotransversectomy (see Fig. 5) allows access to central, centrolateral, as well as lateral thoracic disk herniations. A curved paramedial incision is made with its apex 2 cm from midline. The paraspinal muscles are retracted medially or split transversely. The posteromedial portion of the rib transverse process articulation and the superior aspect of the vertebral body inferior to the disk herniation are resected. The pleura is mobilized and reflected anterolaterally. This allows exposure of the underlying transverse process and the pedicle inferiorly, allowing lateral exposure to the underlying disk herniation. A cavity into which the herniated fragments are pushed is created by removing the posterosuperior and posteroinferior vertebral bodies bordering the disk herniation.

The main advantage of costotransversectomy is enhanced visualization of centrolateral and lateral disk herniations without the need to enter the pulmonary cavity. Central disk herniations in patients in whom a thoracotomy is contraindicated can also benefit from this approach. This approach is contraindicated for large central calcified disk herniations and in the presence of large osteophytes. The approach also has the disadvantage of requiring some disruption of paraspinal muscles as well as more aggressive bone resection.

Transpedicular (Fig. 7). This is a midline approach entailing resection of the facet joint and the medial portion of the pedicle ipsilateral and caudal to the herniated disk. For excision of the pedicle, usually a bur is used, flush with the vertebral body. In the presence of hard-disk herniations, a trough is created with a high-speed bur, into which the hard disk can be pushed and removed with pituitaries. This minimizes manipulation of the neural structures. The approach is indicated for soft lateral disk herniations in medically compromised individuals.

The main disadvantage is limited visualization, which hinders management of central and centrolateral disk fragments as well as of calcified disks and osteophytes. Segmental instability may ensue following facet, pedicle, and

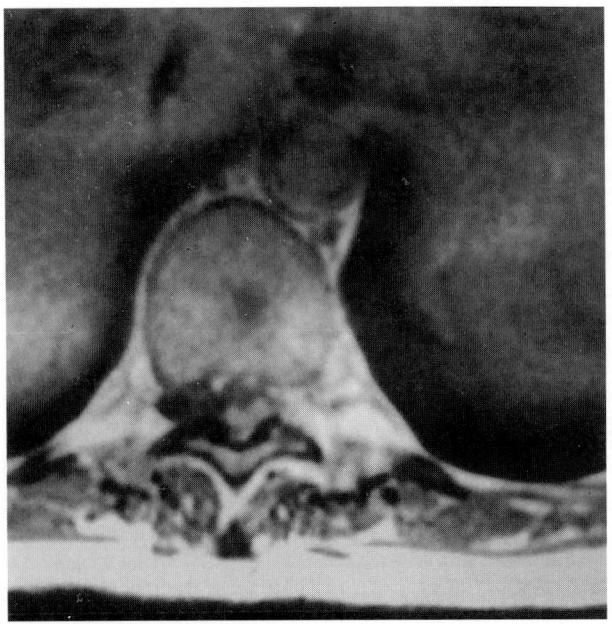

Fig. 6. MRI. Axial MRI of a foraminal T7-8 TDH herniation.

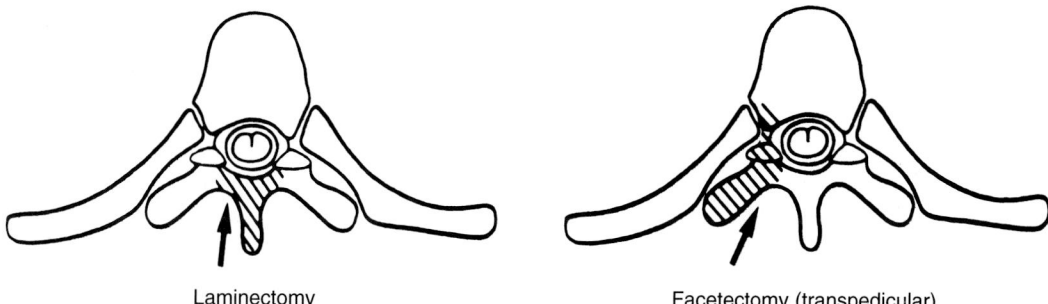

Laminectomy   Facetectomy (transpedicular)

Fig. 7. View. This shows the extent of bony resection *(crosshatch)* and angle of approach *(arrows)* to disk space with laminectomy (left) and facetectomy/pediculectomy (right) procedures. (From Orthopaedic Knowledge Update: Spine, AAOS, Rosemont, IL, 1997, p 93; originally from Cybulski G: Thoracic disk herniation: Surgical technique. Contemp Neurosurg 1992; 14:1.)

diskectomy. Because of limited visualization, access to dural tears or any intradural disorder is compromised.

The advantage of the approach is that it involves limited disk dissection with diminished operative time as well as bleeding, thus minimizing complications.

Laminectomy. In the majority of cases, this approach for thoracic disk herniations should be avoided because of the high prevalence of poor results in more than 50% of patients, including high rates of paraplegia. The complications associated with laminectomy stem from inadequate exposure, which compromises the anterolateral access to the herniated disc. Because of the tethering effect of the intradural dentate ligaments, only limited retraction of the thoracic spinal cord is possible.

ANTERIOR APPROACHES

Transthoracic. This transpleural approach (Fig. 8) is the most adaptable, allowing excellent central and centrolateral visualization from T4 to the thoracolumbar junction. A left-sided chest approach is preferable in the middle and lower thoracic spine, which avoids manipulation of the inferior vena cava and the liver. For TDHs in the upper thoracic spine, a right-sided approach, avoiding the heart, carotid, and subclavian vessels, is preferred. The appropriate rib to resect is the rib caudal to the level of the disk herniation, articulating with the corresponding inferior vertebral body. Ligation of the segmental vessel may not always be necessary. The rib is excised at its base at the

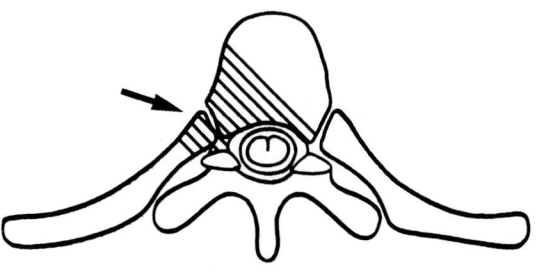

Anterolateral (transthoracic)

Fig. 8. View. This shows the extent of bony resection *(crosshatch)* and angle of approach *(arrow)* to disk space with transthoracic approach. (From Orthopaedic Knowledge Update: Spine, AAOS, Rosemont, IL, 1997, p 93; originally from Cybulski G: Thoracic disk herniation: Surgical technique. Contemp Neurosurg 1992; 14:1.)

point of articulation with the vertebral body. The superior aspect of the inferior pedicle is either partially or completely removed, and the disk space is incised. Partial diskectomy using curets and pituitaries is then performed. If the disk is calcified, a bur can be used to create a trough by resecting the posterolateral portion of each vertebral body. The calcified disk can then be pulled into the trough, minimizing the manipulation of the cord and nerve root. If extensive vertebrectomy is performed, the rib can be used for fusion.

The advantage of the transthoracic approach is excellent visualization anteriorly and anterolaterally, allowing safe decompression and dural manipulation under direct visualization. The approach is particularly recommended for calcified disks with large osteophytes and midline thoracic disk herniations extending behind the vertebral body. The extent of bone removal is limited, diminishing the possibility of destabilization and optimizing anterior interbody graft placement. The intercostal nerves need not be disturbed, decreasing the likelihood of neuralgia and chest sensory changes.

The main disadvantage relates to thoracotomy, requiring chest tube placement and possible pulmonary complications. Disk herniations located at the thoracolumbar level may require resection of the diaphragm.

Trans-sternal/Medial Clavisectomy. Access to the upper thoracic spine (T2-4) can often be difficult, using the previously discussed approaches. An alternative is to use an anterior trans-sternal splitting approach or a medial clavisectomy approach extending distally from a cervical Smith-Robinson exposure, leaving the sternum intact. This approach is recommended in the presence of central and centrolateral disk herniations. The plane of dissection is between the left, common carotid artery and the esophagus, trachea, innominate artery, and the thyroid gland.

The disadvantages entail splitting the sternum and questionable shoulder instability in the younger, active individual. The thoracic duct can be injured in this approach, leading to a chylous leak.

Thoracoscopy (Fig. 9). The surgical positioning is the same as that for the anterior transthoracic approach. Accurate cannula placement, depending on the location of the TDH, is paramount in optimizing visualization. The assistance of a thoracic surgeon experienced in thoracoscopy can be useful.

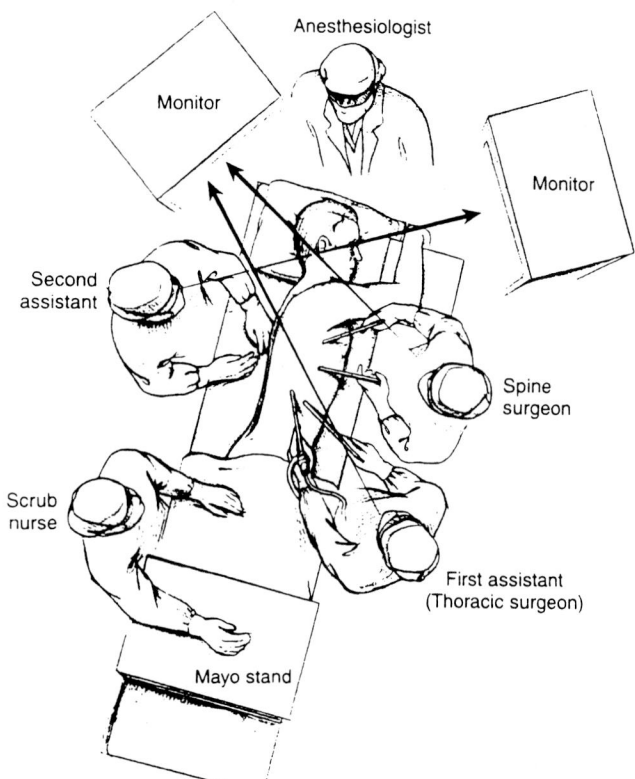

Fig. 9. Thoracoscopy. This shows surgical approach, instrumentation, and personnel positioning. (From Regan JJ, McAfee PC, Mack MJ: Atlas of Endoscopic Spine Surgery. St. Louis, Quality Medical Publishing, Inc., 1995.)

The surgeon and first assistant stand anterior to the patient. The surgeon holds working instruments and suction irrigation, and the first assistant has a fan retractor and the camera. If the surgeon needs to use both hands for sharp instrument manipulation, a second assistant is needed to hold the suction irrigation. The second assistant is placed on the opposite side of the patient, facing a second monitor. This assistant must adjust to the mirror imaging that occurs when facing the spine from the back. Optimal visualization must be maintained at all times, allowing clear distinction between the dura and disk material. Instrumentation is similar to that of open procedures; however, instruments are 8 to 10 inches long, requiring some practice in their use.

Thoracoscopic diskectomy is particularly indicated in the treatment of TDH located in the midthoracic spine, typically at the T5-8 levels. Approaching the spine on the side of the disk herniation is preferable, with soft-disk herniations being more amenable to thoracoscopic diskectomies.

Advantages include decreased post-thoracotomy complications, earlier rehabilitation, diminished surgical trauma, and decreased cost.

Intercostal neuralgia is the most common postoperative complication. Disadvantages include injury to the lung parenchyma and hemidiaphragm as well as injury to the great vessels. Neurological injury, including paraplegia, remains the most catastrophic complication.

Important surgical principles include avoiding instrumentation crowding and ensuing fencing by spacing the portals;

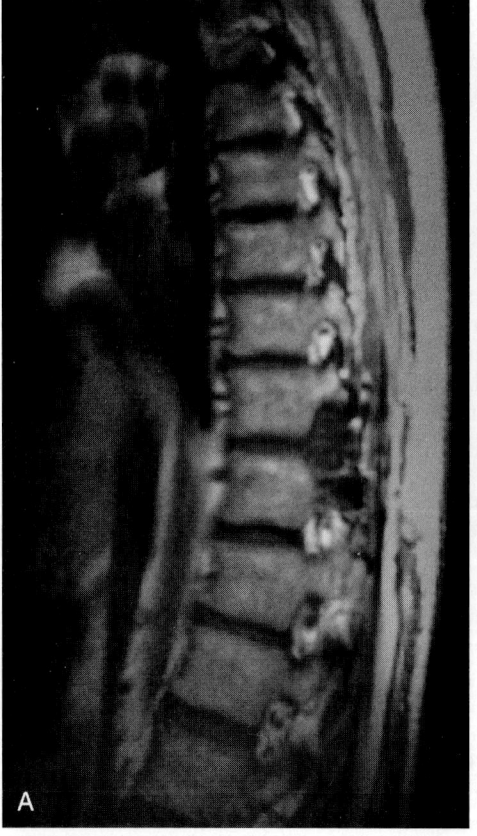

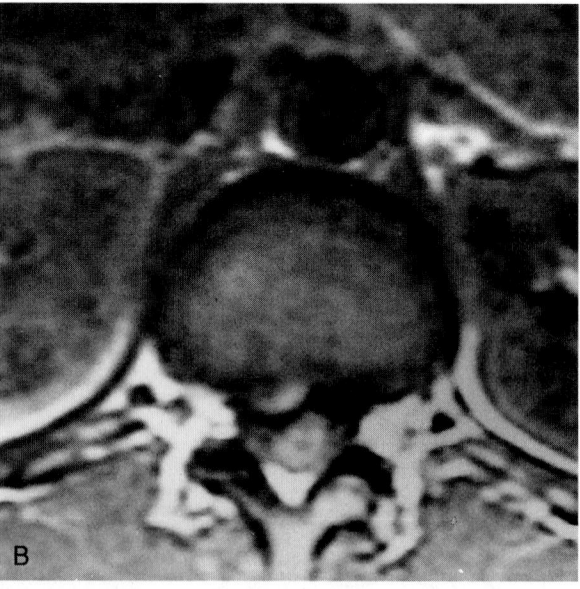

Fig. 10. MRI. *A,* Sagittal MRI of a far lateral TDH. *B,* Axial MRI of a soft TDH.

placement of the camera and instrumentation at a 180-degree arc in the same direction; and moving one instrument at a time, avoiding simultaneous movement of instruments and camera.

Practice in a laboratory setting prior to surgery allows familiarization with thoracoscopic orientation and development of tactile sensation when working with long instruments at a significant distance from the disorder. Thoracoscopy may be best suited for far lateral disk and soft-disk herniations (Fig. 10). Dural tears are not amenable to ar-throscopic repair. Smaller tears can be tamponaded; larger tears necessitate an open thoracotomy. Difficulty can arise using straight instruments while working through a fixed hole; however, the development of angled instruments may obviate some of these difficulties. Thoracoscopy is absolutely contraindicated in patients with pleural adhesions and patients with pulmonary disorders who may not be able to tolerate single lung ventilation. Thoracoscopy is relatively contraindicated in patients with a history of previous thoracotomy and/or thoracostomy.

REFERENCES

Albrand OW, Corkill G: Thoracic disk herniation: Treatment and prognosis. Spine 1979; 4:41.

Arce CA, Dohrmann GJ: Herniated thoracic disks. Neurol Clin 1985; 3:383.

Awwad EE, Martin DS, Smith KR Jr, et al: Asymptomatic versus symptomatic thoracic disks: Their frequency and characteristics as detected by computed tomography after myelography. Neurosurgery 1991; 28:180.

Benson MKD, Byrnes DP: The clinical syndromes and surgical treatment of thoracic intervertebral disk prolapse. J Bone Joint Surg Br 1975; 57:471.

Bohlmann HH, Zdeblick TA: Anterior excision of herniated disks. J Bone Joint Surg Am 1988; 70:1039.

Brown CW, Deffer PA Jr, Akmakjian J, et al: The natural history of thoracic disk herniations. Spine 1992; 17:S97.

Carson J, Gumbert J, Jefferson A: Diagnosis and treatment of thoracic disk protrusions. J Neurol Neurosurg Psychiatry 1971; 34: 68.

Currier BL, Eismont FJ, Green BA: Transthoracic disk excision and fusion for herniated thoracic disks. Spine 1994; 19:323.

Cybulski G: Thoracic disk herniation: Surgical technique. Contemp Neurosurg 1992; 14:1.

el-Kalliny M, Tew JM Jr, van Loveren H, et al: Surgical approaches to thoracic disk herniations. Acta Neurochir (Wien) 1991; 111:22.

Hulme A: The surgical approach to thoracic intervertebral disk protrusions. J Neurol Neurosurg Psychiatry 1960; 23:133.

Jefferson A: The treatment of thoracic intervertebral disk protrusions. Clin Neurol Neurosurg 1975; 1:1.

Kurz LT, Pursel SE, Herkowitz HN: Modified anterior approach to the cervicothoracic junction. Spine 1991; 16:S542.

Le Roux PD, Haglund MM, Harris AB: Thoracic disk disease: Experience with the transpedicular approach in twenty consecutive patients. Neurosurgery 1993; 33:58.

Lesoin F, Rousseaux M, Autricque A, et al: Thoracic disk herniations: Evolution in the approach and indications. Acta Neurochir (Wien) 1986; 80:30.

Love JG, Schorn VG: Thoracic disk protrusions. JAMA 1965; 191:627.

Maiman DJ, Larson SJ, Luck E, et al: Lateral extracavitary approach to the spine for thoracic disk herniation: Report of 23 cases. Neurosurgery 1984; 14:178.

Marinacci AA, Courville CB: Radicular syndromes simulating intra-abdominal surgical conditions. Amer Surg 1962; 28:59.

O'Leary PF, Camins MB, Polifroni NV, et al: Thoracic disk disease: Clinical manifestations and surgical treatment. Bull Hosp Joint Dis Orthop Inst 1984; 44:27.

Otani K, Shunichi M, Shibasaki K, et al: The surgical treatment of thoracic and thoracolumbar disk lesions using the anterior approach. Spine 1977; 2:266.

Patterson RH Jr, Arbit E: A surgical approach through the pedicle to protruded thoracic disks. J Neurosurg 1978; 48:768.

Perot PL Jr, Munro DD: Transthoracic removal of midline thoracic disk protrusions causing spinal cord compression. J Neurosurg 1969; 31:452.

Ravichandran G, Frankel HL: Paraplegia due to intervertebral disc lesions: A review of 57 operated cases. Paraplegia 1981; 19: 133.

Rosenthal D, Rosenthal R, de Simone A: Removal of a protruded thoracic disk using microsurgical endoscopy: A new technique. Spine 1994; 19:1087.

Ross JS, Perez-Reyes N, Masaryk TJ, et al: Thoracic disk herniation: MR imaging. Radiology 1987; 165:511.

Simmons EH, Evans DC, Bailey SI: Thoracic disk disease. J Bone Joint Surg Am 1975; 57:475.

Simpson JM, Silveri CP, Simeone FA, et al: Thoracic disk herniation: Re-evaluation of the posterior approach using a modified costotransversectomy. Spine 1993; 18: 1872.

Singounas EG, Kypriades EM, Kellerman AJ, et al: Thoracic disc herniation: Analysis of 14 cases and review of the literature. Acta Neurochir (Wien) 1992; 116:49.

Stillerman CB, Weiss MH: Management of thoracic disk disease. Clin Neurosurg 1992; 38:325.

Williams MP, Cherryman GR, Husband JE: Significance of thoracic disc herniation demonstrated by MR imaging. J Comput Assist Tomogr 1989; 13:211.

Wood KB, Garvey TA, Gundry C, et al: Magnetic resonance imaging of the thoracic spine: Evaluation of asymptomatic individuals. J Bone Joint Surg Am 1995; 77:1631.

LOW BACK PAIN AND SCIATICA

Todd J. Albert and Kush Singh

Summary

- Low back pain and sciatica are widespread disorders. Although low back pain can be very debilitating, its natural history is commonly favorable.
- Other potentially dangerous diagnoses such as tumor or infection must be ruled out before arriving at a diagnosis of sciatica. A thorough understanding of the neuroanatomy of the lumbar spine aids in the proper treatment and understanding of the cause of this common occurrence.
- Unless there is progressive neurological deficit and/or cauda equina syndrome, once the diagnosis of sciatica has been made, the appropriate conservative treatment should be started, and the patient should be allowed to heal.

DEFINITION

Sciatica and low back pain (LBP) are unique entities. Sciatica is one of the most clearly defined categories of common and painful back disorders. Sciatica is a symptom; leg pain associated with back pain is not always caused by lumbar disk herniation. On the other hand, lumbar disk degeneration is recognized as probably the most common cause of LBP.

HISTORICAL REVIEW

Descriptions of sciatica date back to 400 BC when Hippocrates described pain associated with the sciatic nerve. More than 2000 years later, Italian physician Domenico Contugno[1] in 1874 recognized the relationship between sciatic nerve disorder and leg pain. In 1911 Joel Goldthwait[2] suggested that a herniated disk causes sciatica. In 1934 Mixter and Barr[3] confirmed the association of sciatica and a "ruptured intervertebral disk" by surgically removing a herniated disk. Since then, causes and treatments of sciatica have been explored further.

EPIDEMIOLOGY

The Arthritis and Rheumatism Council of the United Kingdom[4] conducted a study on LBP and sciatica in the 1950s. In the study, 40% of men and 33% of women 35 years and older gave a history of LBP and leg pain. Pain was present in 11% of males and 19% of females. The study defined sciatica as pain radiating from the back down one or both legs. This pain was secondary to radiculopathy or mechanical pressure and inflammation of the L5 and S1 nerve roots. The origin of the mechanical pressure was in soft tissue (herniated disk), bone, or a combination of the two. Sciatica, suggestive of a herniated disk, was found in 3.1%

of men and 1.3% of women. The highest prevalence was in 55- to 64-year-old men, with 9.6% experiencing sciatica; the peak prevalence in women was 5%, occurring after the age of 64 years. In a similar study conducted in Sweden, the lifetime history of sciatica was 3.6% in those younger than 25 years and 22.4% among those 45 to 54 years old.

Schmorl and Junghanns[5] found diffuse degeneration of intervertebral disks in 100% of autopsies in persons older than 90 years of age. Hirsch and Schajowicz and others confirmed these findings. Thus, although LBP is not universal, disk degeneration is present in most, if not all, segments of the population after a certain age.

In an incidence study conducted in southeastern London, Dillane et al[6] recorded 605 attacks of LBP during 24,977 person-years. The incidence rates of herniated nucleus pulposus (HNP) were 2.0 and 1.2 per 1000 person-years for men and women, respectively. In Copenhagen, Gyntelberg[7] conducted a study on the incidence of sciatica in a sample of 4753 men age 40 to 59 years. Eleven percent of the men reported sciatic pain during 1 year of observation.

RISK FACTORS

Similar risk factors are associated with LBP and sciatica. These factors can be characterized into two categories: occupational and individual (Table 1).

OCCUPATIONAL FACTORS

It is difficult to control the number of confounding factors when comparing occupations. For example, workers with LBP may change to a less strenuous job. The result is a shift from heavy to light jobs in prevalence of back pain. Furthermore, another problem arises in defining a heavy versus a light job. Consequently, there is no general consensus as to all occupational risk factors for LBP and sciatica.

Several studies have shown that heavy physical labor correlates with a higher incidence of LBP as well as sciatica. Klein et al[8] found the highest rates of back sprain/strains among workers in physically heavy industries and with physically heavy occupations. Over 10 years, Lenino et al[9] found that LBP was more common among Finnish blue-collar workers than among white-collar workers. Similarly, Wickstrom et al[10] found a higher prevalence of sciatica in concrete reinforcement workers than in computer technicians.

There is considerable disagreement whether static posture—in particular, prolonged sitting and bent-over working postures—increases risk of back pain. Magora[11] found that those with static work postures, i.e., those who either sat or stood during most of the work day, had an increased risk of LBP. However, frequent changes in posture were

TABLE 1. RISK FACTORS FOR LOW BACK PAIN AND SCIATICA	
Occupational	**Individual**
1. Heavy physical work	1. Age and sex
2. Static work postures	2. Posture
3. Frequent bending and twisting	3. Anthropometry
4. Lifting, pushing, and pulling	4. Muscle strength
5. Repetitive work	5. Physical fitness
6. Vibrations	6. Spine mobility
	7. Smoking (?)

also found to increase the risk of back pain. Thus, no conclusions were made.

It is difficult to evaluate bending and twisting as causes of LBP and sciatica because these movements are most commonly associated with lifting. However, a large number of studies report an association between these two movements. Troup et al[12] found the combination of movements to be the most frequent cause of back injuries in England. Kelsey et al[13] found that twisting or holding a load far away from the body increased the relative risk 12 times for reporting LBP and 4 times for reporting sciatica.

Several studies have established that back pain can be triggered by lifting, but the frequency at which back pain occurs after lifting varies from 15% to 64% in these same studies.[14] Magora[11] found that sudden unexpected maximal efforts were particularly harmful.

The National Institute of Occupational Safety and Health[15] estimated in 1981 that one-third of the U.S. work force lifted in excess of what was considered acceptable and that lifting was a major cause of LBP. Likewise, in a retrospective study of a general practice population, Frymoyer et al[16] found LBP to be associated with repetitive heavy lifting, pushing, and pulling.

In general, repetitive work increases the incidence of LBP. The effects of this risk factor are particularly striking in assembly line industries, where there is a higher incidence of LBP among manual workers than among office employees.[17]

Several studies suggest that LBP occurs at an earlier age in subjects exposed to vibration. In these studies, there is an increasing risk of LBP in drivers of tractors and trucks and pilots of airplanes. Kelsey and Hardy[18] found that truck driving increased the risk of disk herniation by a factor of four and that tractor driving and car commuting (20 miles more per day) increased the risk by a factor of two. Several authors report an association between automobile use and LBP.

INDIVIDUAL FACTORS

Individual factors also influence the incidence of LBP. LBP usually begins early in life, with the frequency of symptoms usually peaking between the ages of 35 and 55 years. Biering-Sørensen[19] reported a difference in age pattern between women and men affected by sciatica. Women have a large increase in prevalence and incidence from 50 to 60 years; men have a prevalence maximal at age 40 years. The discrepancy between male and female is likely due to the earlier development of osteoporosis in females.

However, Svensson et al[20] did not find a significant difference between age groups in their study of women in Goteborg, Sweden, whereas Hult[21] and Horal[22] reported increasing prevalence up to age 50 years but not thereafter.

Age is a major factor influencing the prevalence of sciatica and operations for herniated disk. The majority of operations for disk herniation causing sciatica are in patients 35 to 50 years old, although older individuals have more symptoms. In this older population, sciatica is often the result of spinal stenosis. The leg pain is more frequent when walking and standing, whereas in the younger population with disk hernias, the pain is provoked more frequently with sitting.

Gender appears to be of less importance than age with respect to low back symptoms. Sciatica seems to be equally distributed between sexes. Most cross-sectional surveys indicate the incidence and prevalence of sciatica are similar in males and females.[23]

In general, postural deformities, such as scoliosis, kyphosis, lordosis, and leg length discrepancy do not seem to increase risk of LBP. The only evidence for true association of LBP occurs in scoliosis with curves of 80 degrees or more.[24]

According to anthropometric data, no strong correlation exists between height, weight, and body build and LBP. Westrin[25] studied several anthropometric factors in addition to height and weight, including length of tibia and femur and width of femoral condyles and malleoli, but was unable to correlate these factors to LBP. However, Gyntleburg[7] and other authors found increased height to be associated with a higher than average risk of back pain. Also, it appears that LBP and sciatica occur more frequently in very obese patients.[26]

Some investigators have found poor strength in abdominal and back muscles in patients with back pain, whereas others have found no difference or differences only in selected types of strength activities. Whether a weakness is primary or secondary to back pain is still unknown. Chaffin and Park[27] evaluated isometric lifting strength in relation to job demands in 411 workers in 103 different jobs. A follow-up conducted a year later showed the incidence rate of LBP to be three times higher in those individuals who did not have strength equal to or above that required by the job. The study was later expanded by Chaffin et al[28] in order to reach statistical significance.

Physical fitness appears to reduce the risk of chronic LBP and increase the rate of recovery after a back pain episode. Cady et al[29] found that, among 1652 firefighters in the Los Angeles area, the fittest firefighters had fewer injuries. In the study, several fitness factors were used to obtain an "overall fitness score" in order to compare fitness levels between firefighters. Still, the role of physical exercise in the prevalence of LBP is difficult to determine. Svensson et al[20] found LBP to be more common in men who were less physically active during their free time; Videman et al[30] found the opposite in nurses.

Most patients with back pain have reduced spinal mobility. Pain is associated with all movements, particularly at the end of the range of motion, although it is unlikely that spine mobility is a factor in the causation of back pain. Biering-Sørensen[19] found that increased risk of recurrence was associated with reduced spine motion in subjects with previous LBP. Contrarily, increased risk for future LBP was associated with less spine mobility in previously healthy subjects. Troup et al[31] found that flexibility was a poor predictor of future back pain, whereas subjects with ongoing back pain experienced poor sagittal flexibility.

It is unclear whether smoking is a risk factor or only a confounding factor. Kelsey,[32] Frymoyer et al,[16] and others have found an association between smoking, HNP, and LBP. Other studies have not confirmed this association.

PATHOGENESIS

HNP is the most common cause of sciatica, although other causes are prevalent. LBP, on the other hand, is most commonly caused by lumbar disk degeneration. As the intervertebral disk ages, the nucleus pulposus and annulus receive less nutrients via diffusion. Collagen and proteoglycan synthesis is disrupted and, as a result, there is loss of water content from the intervertebral disk.

At this point, there is a relative increase in collagen, accompanied by broader fiber bundles and a disappearance of ground substance in the nucleus. As its nutritional requirements are not met, the nucleus solidifies, and cracks appear because of the decline in efficiency in distributing stresses from vertical and torsional loads.

Due to the hydrostatic nature of the intervertebral disk, it absorbs and dissipates movement forces applied to the axial skeleton. The fluid nature of the nuclear gel absorbs forces as well as intimately contacts the elastic coil structure of the annulus. The remaining support for this force transmission is provided by the various ligaments and muscles attached to processes, body, and posterior arch of the vertebral segment.

Abnormal nuclear movement or disk failure can occur in one of three ways:

1. Herniation of nuclear material through the end plate.
2. Alteration of nuclear-annular integrity from within, resulting in a progressive outward disruption of annular integrity.
3. Alteration of annular integrity from the outside of the annulus, caused by forces applied to the motion segment that exceed normal annular resistance. This cleaves the outer fibers and can extend inward, eventually communicating with the nucleus and creating a path for nuclear migration.

The spine can withstand several different types of forces, three of which—compression, torsion, and bending—can cause an HNP (Figs. 1 to 4).

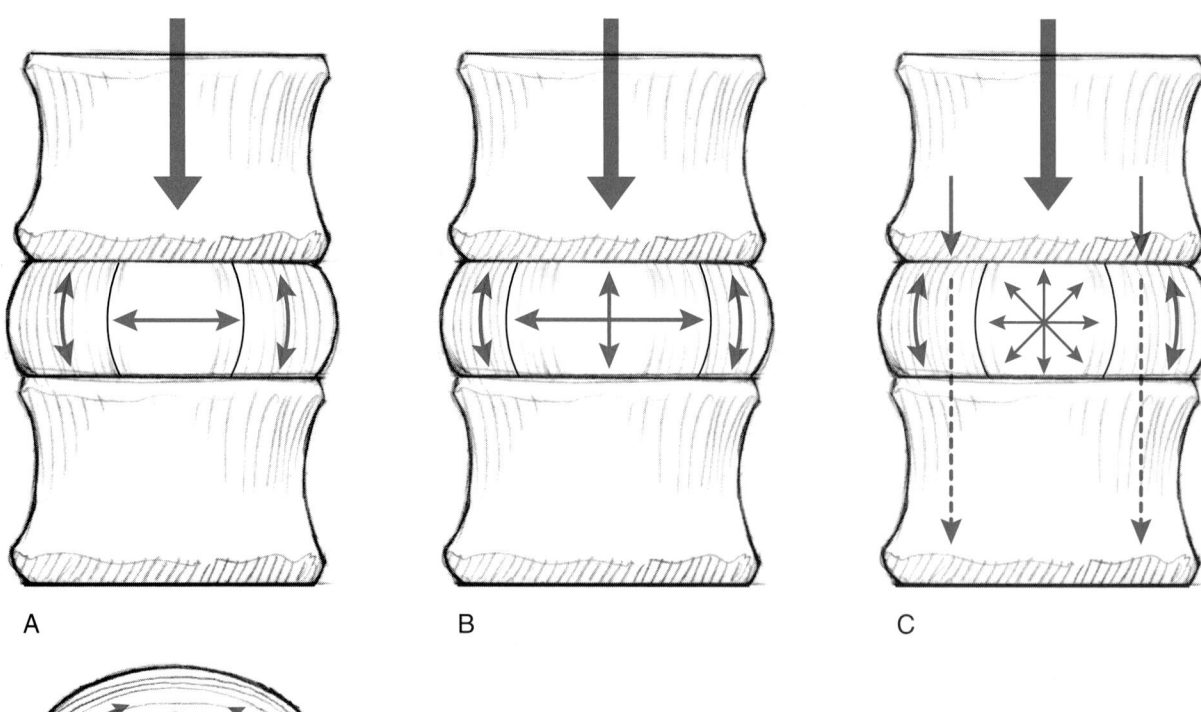

A   B   C

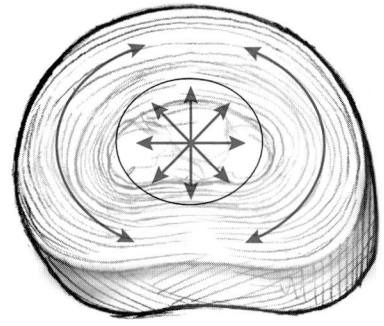

Fig. 1. Distribution of forces in the annulus fibrosus. This shows weight transmission in an intervertebral disk. *A,* Increasing pressure in the nucleus pulposus due to compression. Annular tension rises as the pressure is exerted radially onto the annulus fibrosus. *B,* The annulus does not expand radially because the tension in the annulus is exerted on the nucleus. Nuclear pressure is then exerted on the vertebral end plates. *C,* Both the nucleus pulposus and the annulus fibrosus bear the weight. The radial pressure in the nucleus braces the annulus, and the pressure on the end plates transmits the load from one vertebra to the next.

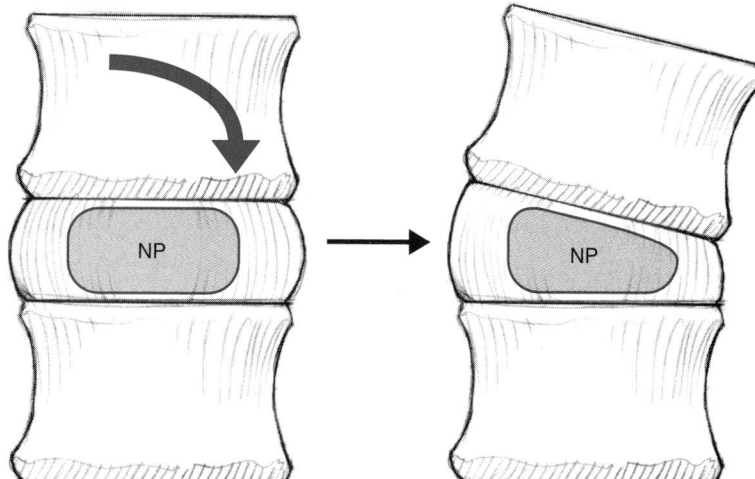

Fig. 2. Distribution of forces in the annulus fibrosus. As a rocking motion occurs, the annulus is stretched opposite the direction of movement and compressed in the direction of movement.

COMPRESSION

Compressive loads place a great deal of pressure on the nucleus, causing a decrease in size because of the loss of a small amount of water (5%) and bulging of the annulus, which absorbs the rest of the compressive load. Normally, the annular fibers increase tension, increasing angulation in the collagen lamellar pattern. Herniation occurs when compression increases the nuclear pressure and annular tension until end-plate fracture (1500 to 2000 pounds), at which point the end plate fails. The appearance on radiograph of the HNP with subsequent bone-healing is similar to that of a Schmorl node, caused by the vertical prolapse of the intervertebral disk.

The nucleus-annulus junction changes as it ages, with repeated compressive loads causing annular fissures from within the disk and localized bulging of the nuclear material partway through but still enclosed by the annulus. This bulging may compromise an adjacent nerve root.

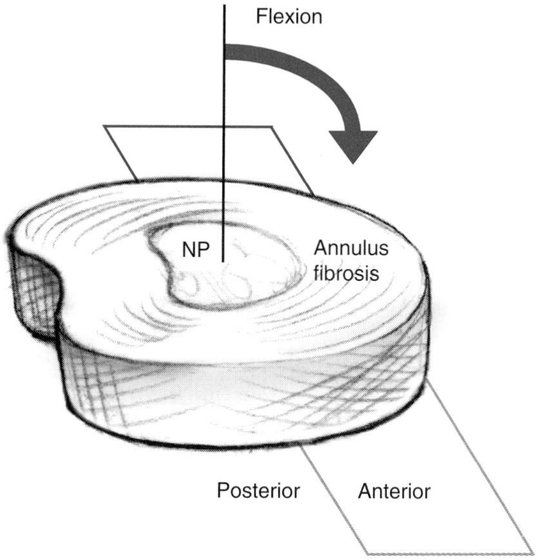

TORSION

Tensile and shear stresses in the annulus may result from the application of torsion (twisting or rotating on the long axis). Peripheral annular fibers are affected most, and forces decrease considerably toward the center of the disk at the nucleus. If forces are large enough, facet joints may become damaged and vertebral segments permanently rotated. Possibly, the nerve root may be compressed by the medial migration of the pedicle, with the resulting myelographic defect mimicking a disk herniation.

End plates are usually not damaged in a forced rotational injury because the force is greatest on the outer annular

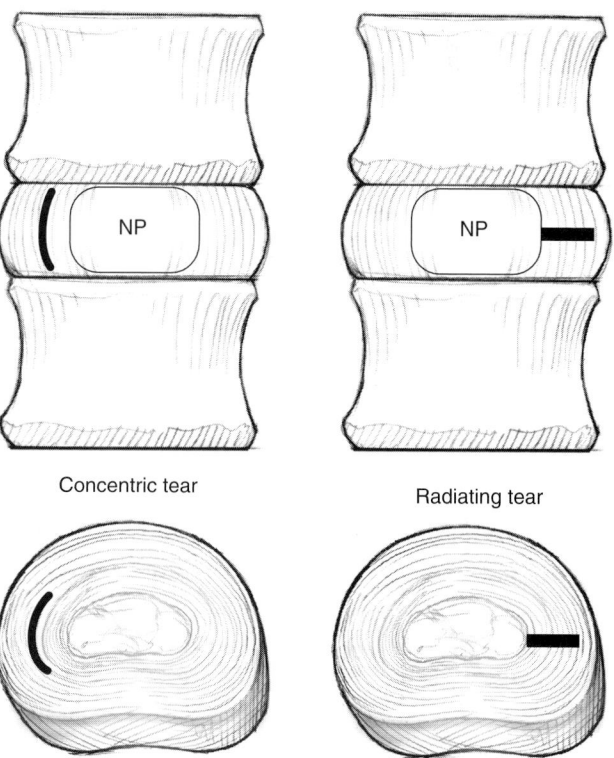

Concentric tear

Radiating tear

Fig. 4. Annular tears.

Fig. 3. Distribution of forces in the annulus fibrosus. Concave disks have an increased amount of annulus fibrosus to resist the posterior stretch that occurs with flexion.

fibers. As a result of initial and subsequent strains, the first radial fissures start here and move inward to the nuclear cavity, forming a pathway through which the nuclear material can extrude.

Torsional stress is maximal in the posterolateral portions of the annulus because they are thinner and weaker than the rest of the annulus. As the shape of the posterior vertebral border to which the annulus is attached is more "round" (L5 to S1), the closer the stress riser is to the midline. As the shape becomes more "flat" (L4 to L5), stress risers and resulting annular damage occur more laterally.

BENDING

Bending occurs when the upper surface of a disk tilts with respect to its lower surface. Unlike in torsional stresses, nuclear pressure remains fairly constant, and no end-plate failure occurs. However, posterior annular fibers may fail as tension is increased with forward bending. Unlike compression and torsion, in which forces distribute evenly around the cross-section of a disk, forward bending localizes forces to the posterior collagenous fibers and may cause failure of the annulus in this area. This bending disrupts the posterior annulus, cleaving the annulus or separating the annular fibers from the end plate or vertebral body and may extend to the nuclear territory, creating a pathway for nuclear herniation, much as in torsional injury.

Nuclear migration through the annulus is the result of a variety of stresses on the spinal cord. Aging, with molecular alteration of the nucleus pulposus and annulus fibrosus, and repeated mechanical stresses to the motion segment contribute to the herniation of the nucleus pulposus.[33]

CLINICAL FEATURES

SYMPTOMS

Sciatica is pain radiating down the posterior aspect of the leg in the distribution of the sciatic nerve and it may be associated with symptoms of paresthesia or weakness. Symptoms of sciatica are usually divided into two categories: pain and nerve dysfunction.

The pain can be further divided into two types: radicular and referred. Radicular pain is sharp and typically radiates in the distribution of a specific nerve root that commonly extends to the calf or foot. Referred pain is duller and does not relate to a specific nerve root. A reduction in the axonal traffic of a particular root may cause nerve dysfunction if the sciatic pain is the result of excessive axonal traffic. Currently, it is believed that pain may be induced by both mechanical and chemically mediated factors. In those patients with obvious symptoms of radiculopathy but no visible herniation on radiological examination or surgery, it appears that intradiscal space and epidural space communication is sufficient for inducing effects on the nerve roots. Thus, annular disruption with a discrete leakage of nucleus pulposus material in the spinal canal, with no visible herniation, could be sufficient to induce symptoms of sciatica.[34]

Sciatic pain is induced by mechanical or biological factors either by direct stimulation of axons or by neuroischemia. Vascular impairment can be induced by both mechanical and biological factors, resulting in a nutritional deficit of the nerve tissue and subsequent ischemia of the nerve.

Several theories have been developed to describe the mechanism of pain in sciatica. The nucleus pulposus material was primarily in contact with the surrounding meninges rather than the axons in studies where pain was thought to be caused by direct stimulation of nerve roots.[35, 36] On the same lines, the spinal dura mater contains nerve endings that may be responsible for sciatic pain.[37]

Nerve dysfunction may be present in motor and sensory nerves and usually coincides with pain, although the two are assumed to be opposites. However, pain and dysfunction are considered separately because they usually result from different pathophysiological events. Both mechanical deformation and the irritation of nuclear components may cause nerve dysfunction. Mechanical deformation, which includes compression and tension, at higher pressures (greater than 400 mm Hg) may separate the nodes of Ranvier, thus directly affecting normal nerve conduction. At much lower pressures, mechanical deformation may indirectly affect nerve conduction by impairing vascular supply.[38-40] Nucleus pulposus–induced nerve dysfunction may be the result of direct neurotoxic effects, the action of inflammatory agents, or vascular impairment.

Symptoms of sciatica are variable but are associated with five areas of the body: back, buttock, thigh, calf, and foot. They may occur in all five areas or only a few.

The midline lumbosacral area, the sacroiliac joint region, the posterosuperior iliac spine, the high iliac crest area, and the low midline sacrococcygeal region are all included in the back. Commonly, pain is originally felt in the lumbosacral region and may refer to the other areas, often as a mechanical sharp pain that leaves the back with a fragile, unstable sensation. Any sudden and severe movement increases the pain to the point where the legs may buckle or the back will "give."

The proximal extent of the leg defines the area of the buttock. Symptoms of sciatica in the proximal leg, which include a deep and cramp-like pain, should be separated from pain in the middle of the buttock, which is indicative of root interference caused by root tension, root irritation, or root compression.

Pain in the posterior thigh tends to be the sharpest component of sciatica and may be described as having an associated superficial "burning-sensitive" feeling. Unless the patient has a very sensitive bowstring sign, no pain is felt in the popliteal fossa region.

Calf symptomatology is mixed. Pain is usually felt in the belly of the gastrocsoleus or peroneal muscles and is usually cramp- and vise-like. In addition, paresthesia may occur in the lateral calf (fifth root) or posterior calf (first root). Most patients have pain below the knee when their sciatica is due to an HNP.

The most common symptom in the foot is paresthesia involving the lateral border or undersurface of the foot (S1 root) and the dorsum of the foot (L5 root). Pain in the belly of the extensor brevis muscle is uncommon.

L4, L5, and S1 nerve root syndromes are typical in sciatica.[41] Compression of nerve roots cranial to L4 is uncommon, and compression of lower sacral nerve roots produces pain unlike that of sciatica (Table 2). Pain from a herniated disk is greater after being exacerbated by an

TABLE 2. NERVE ROOT SYNDROMES		
	L4 Syndrome	**L5 Syndrome**	**S1 Syndrome**
Pain Originates	Laterally in upper gluteal region	Most lateral part of gluteal region and in muscle tensor fasciae latae	Maximus gluteal muscle laterally of its central region
Radiates	Anterior and medial side of thigh below groin and down to the knee	Down posterolateral side of thigh and lateral side of calf down to region of lateral malleolus	Down into posterolateral side of the thigh and leg into heel (often further along lateral edge of foot into little toe)
Diminished Reflexes	Knee jerk	None	Ankle jerk (decreased or absent)
Characteristic Tenderness	Adductor muscles of thigh and upper lateral part of the gluteal muscles	Most lateral part of the gluteal region, the peroneus nerve where it crosses the fibula, and leg extensor musculature	Spread out in posterolateral part of thigh and leg
Decreased Dermal Sensitivity	L4 (anterior surface of leg)	L5 (distally in medial part of foot and big toe)	Lateral, distal part of foot and little toe
Paresis	Quadriceps and adductor muscles (rarely severe)	Brevis and longus extensor muscles of big toe	Plantar flexion muscles of foot (if severe, suspect coexisting S2 syndrome)

increase in intra-abdominal pressure, sitting, and so on. Pain from stenosis is worsened with standing and walking.

L4 Syndrome

Pain originates laterally in the upper gluteal region and radiates to the anterior and medial side of the thigh down to the knee (Fig. 5). Occasionally the pain extends further down the anterior side of the leg, but it never reaches the foot. The knee jerk reflex is diminished and is occasionally absent. In addition, the adductor muscles of the thigh, especially their proximal attachments, as well as the upper lateral part of the gluteal muscles (gluteus medius and minimus) are characteristically tender. Dermal sensitivity is decreased in the L4 distribution area and is most obvious on the anterior surface of the leg. Paresis of the adductor and quadriceps muscles is rarely severe because L2 and L3 also innervate them.

L5 Syndrome

Pain originates in the most lateral part of the gluteal region and in the muscular tensor fasciae latae, just cranial to the greater trochanter. It radiates down to the region of the lateral malleolus along the posterolateral side of the thigh and lateral side of the calf. From here, pain radiates distally to the medial foot and into the big toe as a band on the dorsum of the foot. The most lateral part of the gluteal region, the peroneal nerve where it crosses over the fibula, and the extensor musculature of the leg are all typically tender to palpation.

Dermal sensitivity is often decreased in the L5 distribution area, most obvious distally in the medial part of the foot and on the big toe.

Characteristic of the L5 syndrome is a paresis of the brevis and longus extensor muscles of the big toe. In severe cases of L5 syndrome, the power of extension in all toes and the whole foot is reduced considerably. Bilateral and simultaneous comparison of the power of extension in the big toes is useful in examining the extensor muscles. If only slight, the paresis can be observed by exhausting the muscles with repeated testing at short intervals. Early evidence of motor paresis is apparent in the brevis extensor muscle of the big toe of L5 and can be recorded by electromyography.

S1 Syndrome

Pain originates slightly lateral to the central region of the gluteus maximus muscle and radiates downward into the lateral posterior side of the thigh and leg into the heel and often continues along the lateral edge of the foot to the little toe. Areas of maximal tenderness to palpation are spread out in the lateral posterior part of the thigh and leg.

The ankle jerk reflex, which is conducted mainly via S1 and only to a minor degree via S2, is decreased or absent. S1 dermal sensitivity is decreased most reliably in the lateral distal part of the foot and the little toe.

Slight muscular atrophy of the plantar flexor muscles of the foot may occur in severe S1 syndromes, but paresis of the plantar flexor muscles of the foot is seldom enough to noticeably affect normal gait because they are also innervated by S2. Severe paresis of the plantar flexion of the foot indicate a coexisting S2 syndrome.

NEUROANATOMY

There is a progressive obliquity of the dorsal and ventral nerve roots due to the inequality of lengths of the adult spinal cord and vertebral column (Fig. 6). This is especially apparent in the lumbar spine. Distal to the L2 vertebra, the bundle of nerve roots forms the cauda equina. Each of these nerve roots must travel distally before exiting under their respective pedicle (L3 nerve root under L3 pedicle, etc.). The nerve roots do so in a specific orientation, with the more proximal nerve roots traveling laterally and the L5 nerve root traveling paracentrally (S1 to S4 are located closest to the spine). As a result, each nerve tra-

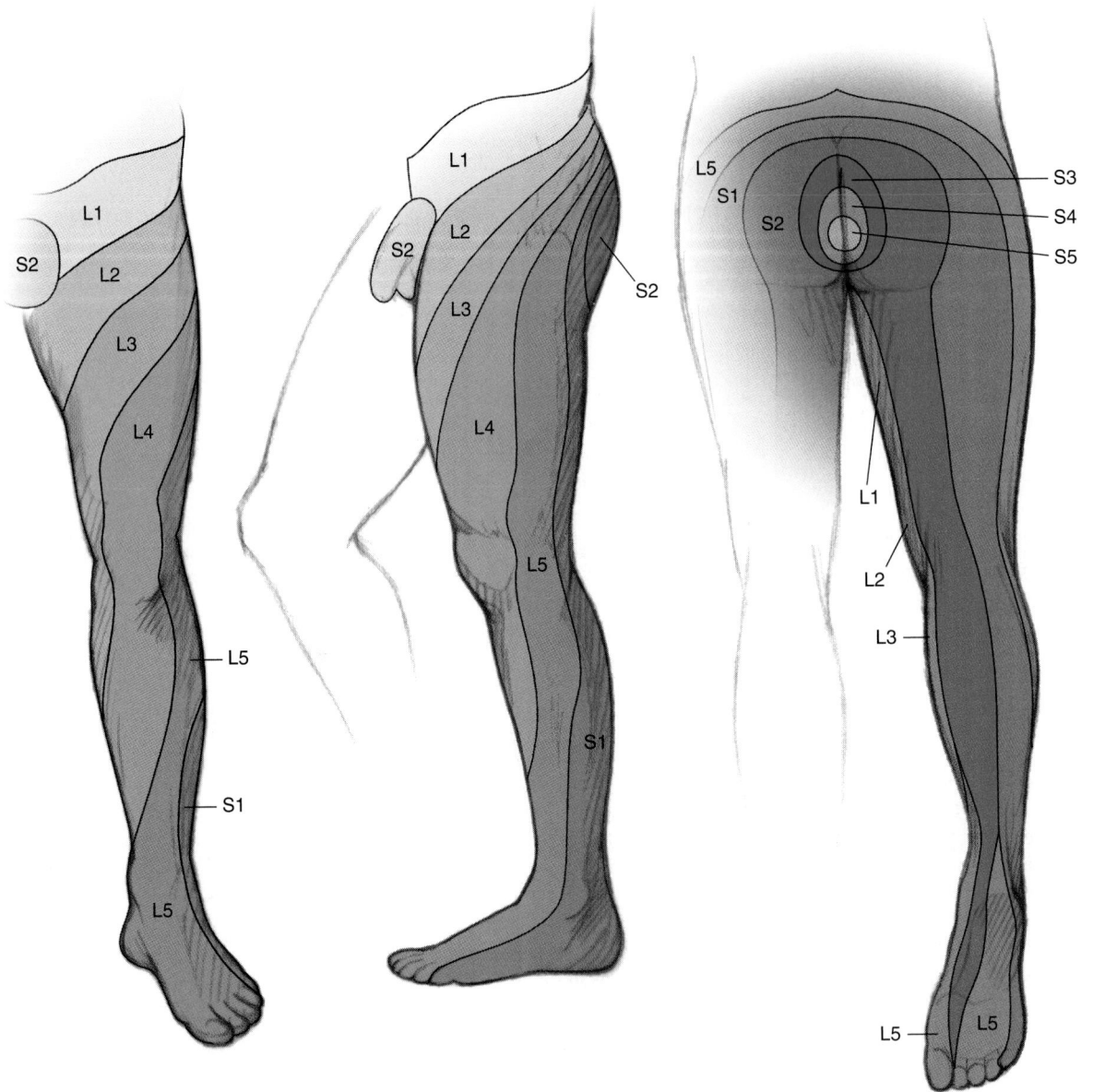

Fig. 5. Lumbosacral dermatomes. This shows gluteal distribution of lumbosacral dermatomes of the lower extremity.

verses its superior disk space (L4 traverses L3-4 disk space, etc.).

PHYSICAL EXAMINATION

The straight leg raising test (Fig. 7), first described by J.J. Forst in the late 1800s, is the classic test of sciatic nerve (L4, L5, S1) irritation. Its purpose is to stretch the dura. The test involves raising the leg with the knee extended while the patient lies supine on the examining table.

The patient will feel pain along the anatomic course of the sciatic nerve to the lower leg, ankle, and foot when the leg is stretched and its nerve roots and corresponding dural attachment are inflamed. Symptoms should not be produced in the lower leg until the leg is raised past 30 to 35 degrees because there is no dural involvement until the leg is raised. As the angle is increased between 30 and 60 to 70 degrees, tension is applied to the dura and nerve roots

and the rate of deformation of the roots diminishes. At elevations above 70 degrees, symptoms produced may also be related to mechanical LBP secondary to muscle strain or joint disease. Only when the patient's radicular symptomatology is reproduced (not just back pain) is the test considered positive. Some patients experience limitation of motion and posterior thigh pain secondary to hamstring muscle tightness. The extent of tightness is determined by raising the nonpainful side first, quantifying the amount of painless motion.

Another common test of sciatica is the Lasègue test. Although frequently mistaken as a straight leg test, the Lasègue test involves the supine patient, with hip flexed to 90 degrees, slowly extending the knee until sciatic pain is elicited. The test is difficult to interpret because of multiple joint involvement; as a result, the test is less valuable than the straight leg raising test.

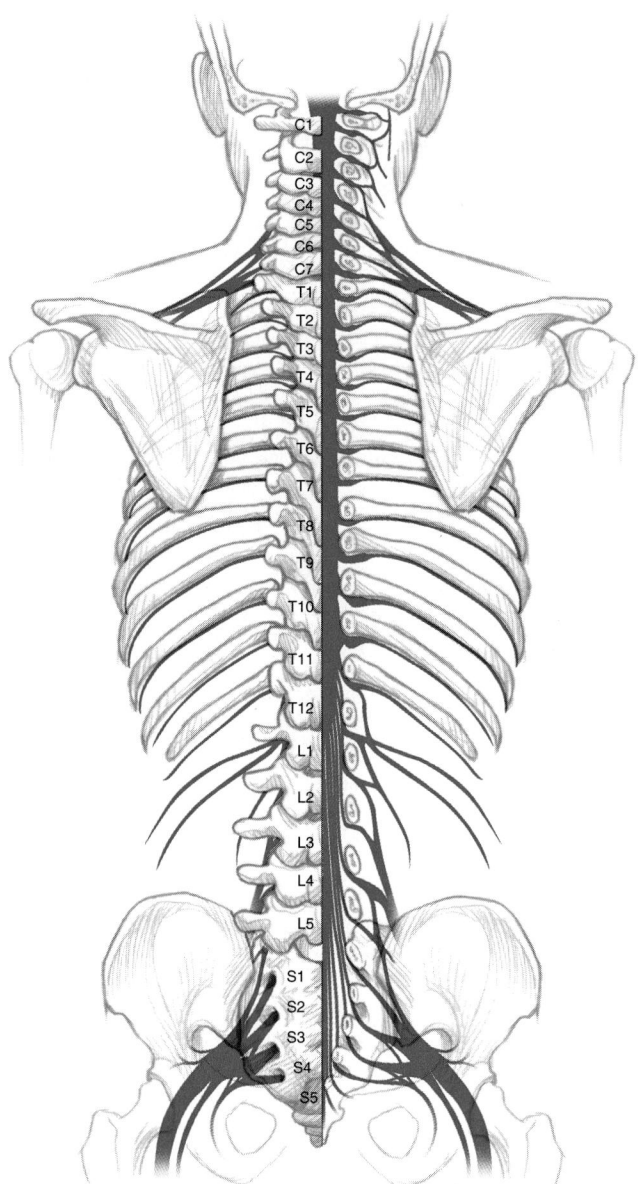

Fig. 6. Distribution of the nerve roots of the spinal cord.

prevalent condition, especially when the natural history of LBP and sciatica is so favorable (80% resolution in 2 to 6 weeks).

Plain radiographs are only useful after 4 to 6 weeks of symptoms unless, when indicated, to rule out tumor and infection and to define instability. Magnetic resonance imaging (MRI) is the preferred technique for initial imaging studies because it allows better visualization of soft-tissue structures (intervertebral disks) and offers adequate imaging of bony structures. Several investigators have assessed the accuracy of MRI in the diagnosis of posterolateral disk herniation with sciatica. In a prospective evaluation of surface coil MRI, computed tomography (CT), and myelography for lumbar disk herniation and canal stenosis, comparisons were made between diagnostic imaging and surgical findings. There was an 82.6% agreement between surgical findings with MRI regarding the type and location of disease, 83% agreement with CT, and 71% with myelography, whereas combined MRI and CT findings produced a 92.5% agreement.[42]

MRI is the best diagnostic technique for the diagnosis of disk prolapses associated with sciatica. The noncontained extruded disk can often be defined separately from the contained protrusion. A globular mass of intermediate-signal-intensity nuclear material without a low-signal-intensity outline around the whole outer margin can be seen on T_1-weighted images. This is more apparent on T_2-weighted images when the nuclear content (higher signal intensity) passes through the posterior longitudinal ligament–annulus fibrosus complex (low signal). The sequestered disk prolapse where the nuclear material has passed through the annulus and is no longer in communication with the parent nucleus is also seen.

Boden et al[43] performed MRI studies on 67 individuals who had never had LBP, sciatica, or neurogenic claudica-

The patient with positive results from the straight leg raising test has pain that radiates to the lower leg. To confirm the presence of nerve irritability, a Bragard test should be conducted. During the straight leg raising test, the raised leg should be lowered until the pain is relieved. The foot is dorsiflexed at that position, stretching the posterior tibial branch of the sciatic nerve and causing a recurrence of pain, commonly referred to as a positive Lasègue sign.

INVESTIGATION

IMAGING

The physician should allow at least 6 weeks before conducting an imaging study on a patient unless symptoms clearly require that one be ordered. It is both costly and inefficient to conduct an imaging study hastily on such a

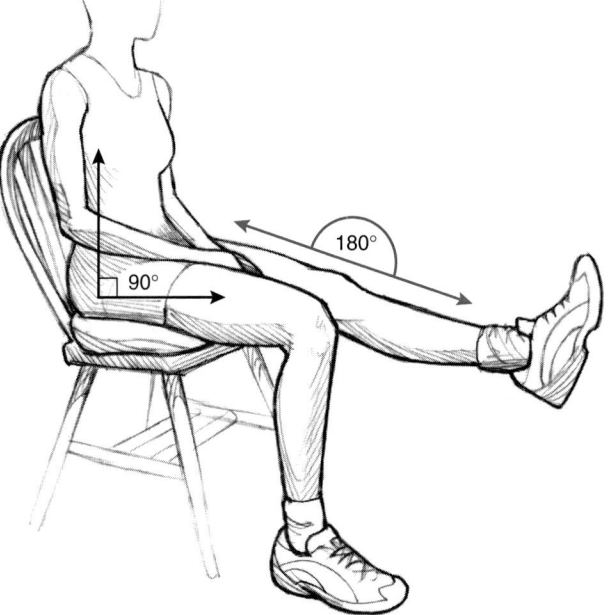

Fig. 7. Straight leg raising test.

tion. About one-third of the subjects were found to have a substantial abnormality. The authors concluded that, in view of these findings in asymptomatic subjects, abnormalities on magnetic resonance images must be strictly correlated with age and any clinical signs and symptoms before operative treatment is contemplated.

Although both lumbar CT and myelography are helpful tools in the diagnosis of the causation of sciatica, the sensitivity and specificity of both tests are questionable. The prevalence of positive findings in the asymptomatic population causes a problem with both of these imaging methods. Structural evidence of a herniated disk is fairly prevalent (10% to 25%) among healthy young individuals.

Bell et al[44] conducted a study of their own on 122 patients. Although myelography was accurate only 83% of the time, it was better than CT for both disk hernias and stenosis.

When using CT for a definitive diagnosis of disk herniation, specific criteria include: (1) focal and asymmetric disk protrusion, dorsolateral in position, directly underlying the nerve root traversing that disk; (2) demonstrable nerve root compression and/or displacement; and (3) postimpingement swelling of the affected nerve root caudal to the herniation with enlargement of the nerve and an indistinct margin due to edema, inflammatory exudate, or prominence of adjacent epidural veins. MRI also has positive findings on asymptomatic individuals as described by Boden et al[43] (up to 30% of disk degeneration, bulges, and hernias in asymptomatic young people).

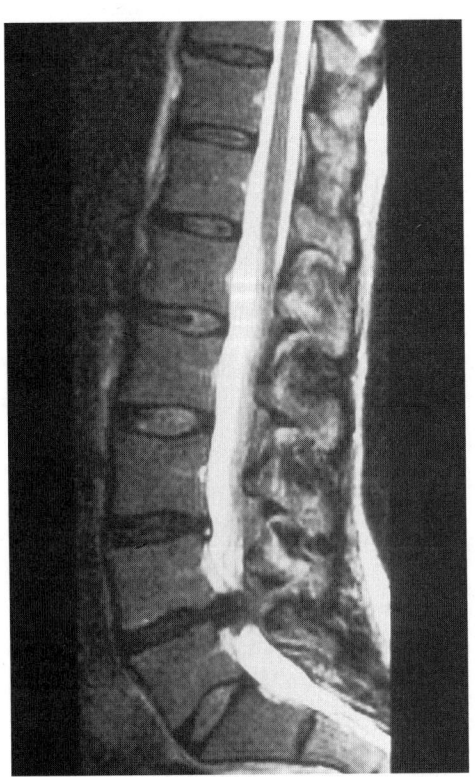

Fig. 8. MRI of an L4-5 disk protrusion.

DIFFERENTIAL DIAGNOSIS

Leg pain mimicking sciatica, also known as sciatic pain, may arise from several sources, the most common of which is radicular pain from nerve root tension, irritation, and/or compression from disk material or osseous encroachment on the canal or lateral recess. Root compression or irritation may also be derived from benign or malignant extradural or intrathecal tumors. Moreover, peripheral vascular disease, which may mimic stenotic radicular pain in a sciatic distribution, may cause intermittent claudication.

Diagnostic modalities for sciatica due to disk hernia include CT, myelography, MRI, and CT-diskography. In order to rule out other possibilities in a differential diagnosis, several other diagnostic tools may be used. Radiograph studies and laboratory tests are ideal for identifying tumors, infections, and rheumatic diseases. These should be employed earlier at 6 weeks if tumor or infection is suspected. CT can be used for measurements of dural sac area in order to rule out spinal stenosis. Although diskography can be used to diagnose discogenic back pain, for the diagnosis of disk herniation it has proved unreliable with a specificity of only 35%.[43, 44]

The differential diagnosis of a herniated disk with radiculopathy includes other conditions such as intradural tumors or cysts, meningiomas, neurofibromas, and ependymomas. Perhaps the most common cause of radiculopathy other than herniated disks is spinal stenosis. Extensions increase the pain if spinal stenosis with neurogenic claudication is present. On the other hand, flexion increases the pain when an HNP is the underlying cause (Figs. 8 and 9).

The physical examination is used to identify patients who have a true radiculopathy. A consistent history and physical findings can be used to determine if a true radiculopathy (often including pain, reflex loss, sensory changes, and weakness) is the underlying cause. It should be stressed that imaging tests are usually not necessary until a minimum of 4 to 6 weeks have passed because of the favorable natural history of LBP and sciatica.

DIFFERENTIAL DIAGNOSIS OF SCIATICA
The differential diagnosis of sciatica is outlined in Table 3.

MANAGEMENT/TREATMENT

Treatment for sciatica and LBP can be either surgical or nonsurgical. The various treatment methods have specific goals. The Quebec Task Force on Spinal Disorders[45] listed them as increase rest, diminish spasm, diminish inflammation, reduce pain, increase strength, increase range of motion, increase endurance, alter joint tissue, alter nerve tissue, increase function, modify work environment, modify social environment, and modify psychological states.

NONSURGICAL
The natural history of sciatica is predominantly that of spontaneous improvement. Hakelius[46] conducted a study of patients with sciatica treated with a corset and rest. Within 1 month, 38% of the patients had improved; by 2 months 52% had improved, and by 3 months 73% had improved. The Quebec Task Force on Spinal Disorders[45] studied the available literature on low back conditions and evaluated

TABLE 3. DIFFERENTIAL DIAGNOSIS OF SCIATICA
I. Intraspinal Causes 　A. Causes Proximal to Disk 　　Conus and cauda equina lesions (e.g., neurofibroma, epen- 　　dymoma, and intraspinal metastasis) 　B. Disk Level 　　Herniated disk 　　Stenosis (canal or recess) 　　Infection—osteomyelitis or diskitis (with nerve root pres- 　　sure) 　　Inflammation—arachnoiditis 　　Neoplasm—benign or malignant with nerve root pressure II. Extraspinal Causes 　A. Pelvis 　　Cardiovascular condition (e.g., peripheral vascular disease) 　　Gynecological conditions 　　Orthopaedic conditions (e.g., osteoarthritis of hip) 　　Sacroiliac joint disease 　　Neoplasms (invading or compressing lumbosacral plexus) 　B. Peripheral Nerve Lesions 　　Neuropathy (resulting from diabetes, tumor, or alcohol) 　　Local sciatic nerve conditions (trauma, tumor) 　　Inflammation (herpes zoster)

11 diagnostic areas and 13 treatment categories for LBP and lumbar disk disease. In this analysis, the only effective mode of treatment was brief bedrest and back school information programs. Also, nonrandomized control studies showed that nonsteroidal anti-inflammatory medication was effective. In a nonrandomized retrospective study, Saal and Saal[47] reported that more than 90% of patients with disk extrusions and radiculopathy had a successful outcome with nonsurgical treatment.

A variety of nonsurgical treatments are available, including braces, heat, ice, biofeedback, traction, manipulation, steroids (orally or injected epidurally), massage, and acupuncture. No definitive proof exists, however, as to the efficacy of these treatments on improvement beyond that of the natural history of herniated lumbar disks. Bedrest remains the treatment of choice; based on clinical and biological research, the duration of treatment should be restricted. For patients with sciatica, the information is less certain, but 24 to 48 hours appears optimal. If the sciatica is not relieved by bedrest, additional efficacious treatment includes exercise, although aerobic programs appear more appropriate than flexion exercises when the underlying disorder is a lumbar disk herniation.

SURGICAL
Indications
There is no indication for surgery earlier than 6 weeks to 3 months unless there is a progressive neurological deficit or a cauda equina syndrome.

The cauda equina consists of all the nerve roots from L1 distally. Paralysis of all these roots results in the loss, variably depending on the degree of nerve impingement, of motor and sensory function of the pelvic viscera, the pelvic floor, and both lower extremities. The cauda equina syndrome has been described as a complex of symptoms and signs consisting of LBP, unilateral sciatica, motor weakness of the lower extremities, sensory disturbance, and loss of

visceral function (i.e., bowel and bladder function), together with saddle anesthesia. Cauda equina syndrome is caused by compression of all or a portion of the nerves of the cauda equina. The lesions that may produce cauda equina compression include fracture, tumor, infection, spinal stenosis, and diskal hernia.

Before any type of surgical intervention, it is essential to clinically diagnose the cause of the sciatica, determine the anatomic level of the lesion, and support these impressions by an appropriate imaging study. If there is not a confluence of the patient's clinical presentation, the anatomic level, and the structural lesion as demonstrated by myelography, CT scanning, or MRI scanning, the potential for a poor result increases dramatically.

Contraindications
Disabilities with major nonorganic components are usually a relative contraindication to surgical intervention. Because of its systemic effects and known association with neuropathy, diabetes mellitus negatively influences the outcome of lumbar spine surgery. Other contraindications include a misdiagnosis (e.g., another pathological process causing leg symptoms), incorrect level, painless disk herniation (operation should not be done if no pain is present), and those patients with a poor potential for recovery.

Techniques for Sciatica
In most instances, surgery is performed to relieve sciatic pain, the effectiveness of the procedure depending on the identification and relief of pressure. Ideally, a mechanical nerve root compression will be found whenever an operation is done to relieve sciatica. The most common techniques used in the treatment of sciatica include open (conventional) diskectomy, microsurgical diskectomy, and percutaneous diskectomy.

Open (Conventional) Diskectomy. In those patients with a herniated disk who do not respond well to conservative treatment, open diskectomy has proved to be safe and effective. Conventional diskectomy can be expected initially to provide good to excellent results in 90% to 95% of cases with proper patient selection, although the long-term success rate may decrease to 70% in these patients over the subsequent decade due to recurrence or scarring. Conventional diskectomy has a low mortality rate, estimated to be 0.03%, as well as a low prevalence of neurological complications (less than 0.5%) and minor complications (4.7% of cases).[50]

Microsurgical Diskectomy. Microsurgical diskectomy involves the use of a small incision (2.5 to 3 cm), the operating microscope for high magnification, and intense illumination of the operative field. Theoretical technical advantages include improved visualization of microanatomy, preservation of epidural fat, meticulous hemostasis, minimal nerve root trauma, and minimal dissection of paravertebral muscles.[51]

There are several benefits to the use of microsurgical diskectomy, including apparent economic advantages over conventional diskectomy because of the decreased hospital stay, although overall postoperative time is similar.[52] Most reports claim at least a 90% success rate at relieving leg pain, although there is somewhat less success at relieving back pain.[53, 54]

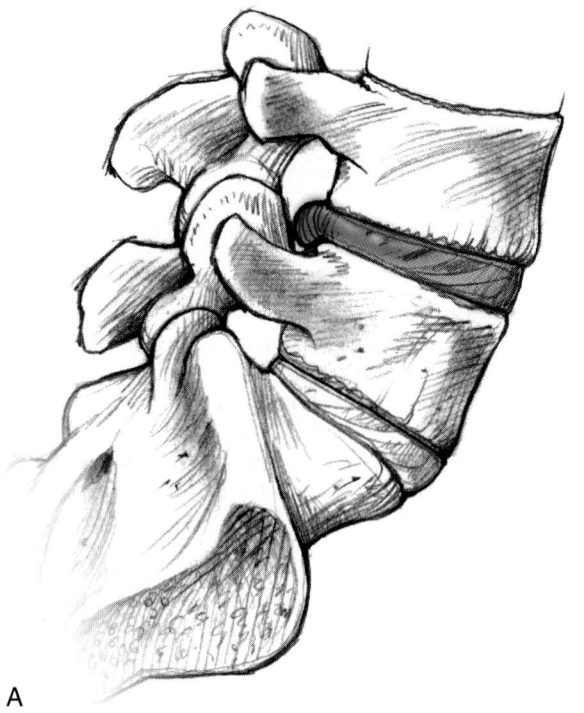

A

Fig. 9. Views. *A,* Herniated nucleus pulposus. *B,* Nuclear protrusion. A nuclear bulge weakens the intact annulus fibrosus. *C,* Nuclear prolapse. The posterior vertebral canal is occupied by a free fragment passing through a completely torn annulus fibrosus.

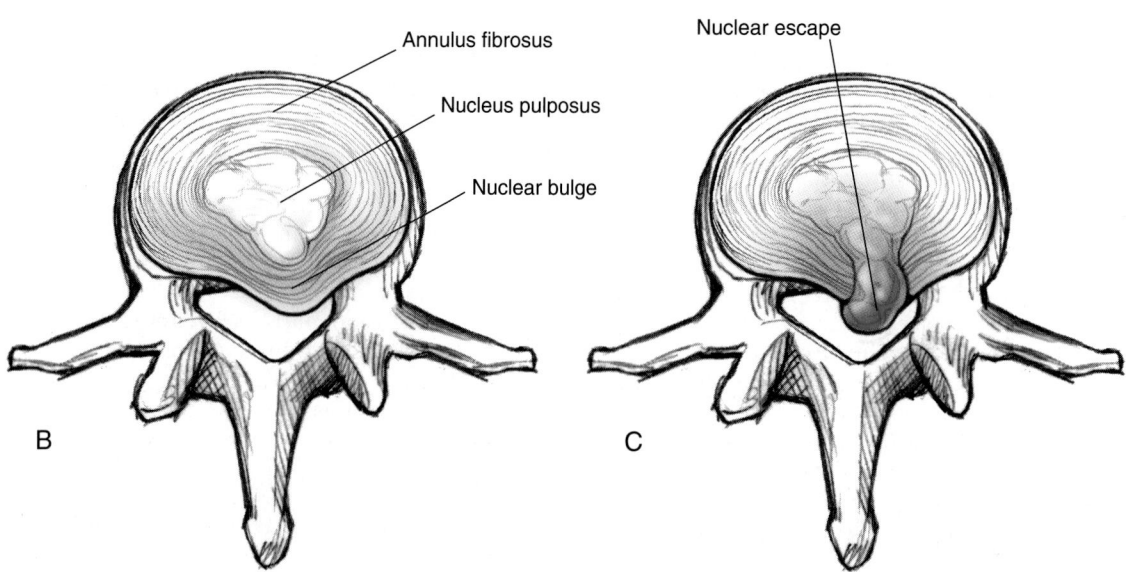

Annulus fibrosus

Nucleus pulposus

Nuclear bulge

Nuclear escape

B

C

Percutaneous Diskectomy. The newest technical method of removing a disk, percutaneous diskectomy, functions by mechanically decompressing the disk. Various approaches have been reported, including both posterolateral and lateral approaches, usually with manual removal of disk material with forceps after confirmation of location with fluoroscopy. Early trials indicate that this treatment was effective in 65% to 75% of patients.[55, 56]

COMPLICATIONS
Nonsurgical
After an initial successful course of conservative treatment, some individuals have recurrent sciatica that becomes inca-

pacitating. Symptoms may be completely absent between episodes as low-grade pain may become increasingly severe. Continued conservative management is indicated if the intensity of symptoms is within the patient's tolerance and if the recurrent episodes are not too disabling. However, if the frequency and intensity of attacks are severe enough, surgery should be seriously considered.

Surgical
Low back surgery should be undertaken only for the proper indications. The most frequent problem during operation is injury of the neural elements, which can involve an isolated nerve root or the cauda equina. Injury of the major vascular visceral structures can also occur, usually during

removal of the disk when an instrument violates the anterior longitudinal ligament.

Postoperative complications include wound infection, cauda equina syndrome, and urinary retention. These patients should be observed for the first 48 hours.

Concerns with microsurgical diskectomy include the relatively high recurrence rate,[57] missed pathological processes (extruded fragments, recess stenosis), an excessive number of dural tears,[58] and disk space infection. There has also been reported a case of bowel perforation following the procedure.[59] However, the success rate of microsurgical diskectomy appears to be superior to that of chemonucleolysis,[60, 61] and comparable to that of conventional diskectomy.[58, 62]

Complications associated with percutaneous diskectomy include leg dysesthesia and paraspinal muscle spasm. Early trials indicate that this treatment was effective in 65% to 75% of patients.[55, 56]

RESULTS/RECOVERY

As is the case with LBP, recovery from sciatica is thought to be favorable. Probably the most important proof of this assertion is Weber's[62] prospective study in which the outcomes of surgically and nonsurgically treated patients with unequivocal sciatica due to lumbar disk herniations were identical 4 and 10 years after the intervention. In the study, all 280 patients were treated with 14 days of bedrest, after which 87 patients (31%) had improved and surgery was

not a consideration. Surgery was elected for 67 (25%) candidates because of major neurological symptoms, fixed scoliosis, or severe pain, unmanageable for them and their treating physician. Of the 126 remaining patients who were divided randomly, 60 received operative therapy, and at the end of 1 year 65% of these surgically treated patients were rated as having a good result. Of the other 66 patients randomized to nonoperative treatment, 17 (26%) required an operation during the first year, and 49 (74%) continued with conservative therapy. However, only 24% were rated as having good health.

Similar outcomes between the two groups were seen only after 4 years. Weber's study does not prove that conservative treatment is as effective as operative intervention; however, most patients can resume function, and pain can be adequately managed with nonoperative treatment. In that study, the immediate surgery patients were not compared with nonoperative patients.

The conclusion reached by the Weber and other studies is that surgical intervention reduces the period of symptoms of disability in those patients. The key element for success is patient selection, which must be analyzed as to the condition being treated, the operation chosen, and the patient characteristics, the most important of which are psychosocial function and workers' compensation. In short, the natural history of a disease should be the standard by which surgical success is judged. Only when we know that we can improve on the natural history can we be certain of our surgical indications.

REFERENCES

1. Contugno D: De Ischiade Nervosa: Commentarios. Napoli, Apud Frat, Simonios, 1874.
2. Goldthwait J: The lumbo-sacral articulation: An explanation of many cases of "lumbago," "sciatica," and paraplegia. Boston Med Surg J 1911; 164:365.
3. Mixter WJ, Barr JS: Rupture of the intervertebral disc with involvement of the spinal canal. N Engl J Med 1934; 211: 210.
4. Hirsch C, Jonsson B, Lewin T: Low back symptoms in a Swedish female population. Clin Orthop 1969; 63:171.
5. Schmorl G, Junghanns H: The human spine in health and disease. New York, Grune and Stratton, 1971.
6. Dillane JB, Fry J, Kalton G: Acute back syndrome: A study from general practice. Br Med 1966; 2:82.
7. Gyntlenburg F: One year incidence of low back pain among male residents of Copenhagen aged 40–59. Dan Med Bull 1974; 21:30.
8. Klein BP, Jensen RC, Sanderson LM: Assessment of workers' compensation claims for back strains/sprains. J Occup Med 1984; 26:443.
9. Lenino P, Aro S, Hasan J: Trunk muscle function and low back disorders: A ten-year follow-up study. J Chronic Dis 1987; 40:289.
10. Wickstrom G, Hanninen K, Lehtinen M, et al: Previous back syndromes and present back symptoms in concrete reinforcement

workers. Scand J Work Environ Health 1978; 4:47.
11. Magora A: Investigation of the relation between low back pain and occupation—physical requirements: Sitting, standing and weight lifting. Ind Med Surg 1972; 41:5.
12. Troup JDG, Roantree WB, Archibald RM: Survey of cases of lumbar spinal disability: A methodological study. National Coal Board, 1970.
13. Kelsey JL, Golden AL, Mundt DJ: Low back pain/prolapsed lumbar intervertebral disc. Rheum Dis Clin North Am 1990; 16(3):699–716.
14. Brinckmann P: Injury of the annulus fibrosus and disc protrusions: An in vitro investigation of human lumbar discs. Spine 1986; 11:149.
15. NIOSH: Work practices guide for manual lifting. Washington, DC, DHHS (NIOSH) Publication No 81–122, 1981.
16. Frymoyer JW, Pope MH, Clements JH, et al: Risk factors in low back pain: An epidemiological survey. J Bone Joint Surg Am 1983; 65:213.
17. Bergquist-Ullman M, Larsson U: Acute low back pain in industry: A controlled prospective study with special reference to therapy and confounding factors. Acta Orthop Scand 1977; 170:1.
18. Kelsey JL, Hardy RJ: Driving of motor vehicles as a risk factor for acute herniated lumbar intervertebral disc. Am J Epidemiol 1975; 102:63.

19. Biering-Sørenson F: A prospective study of low back pain in a general population: Occurrence, recurrence, and aetiology. Scand J Rehabil Med 1983; 15:71.
20. Svensson HO, Andersson GBJ, Johansson S, et al: A retrospective study of low back pain in 38- to 64-year old women: Frequency and occurrence and impact on medical services. Spine 1988; 13:548.
21. Hult L: The Munkfors investigation. Acta Orthop Scand 1954; 16:1.
22. Horal J: The clinical appearance of low back disorders in the city of Gothenburg Sweden. Acta Orthop Scand 1969; 118:1.
23. Heliovaara M: Epidemiology of Sciatica and Herniated Lumbar Intervertebral Disc. Helsinki, The Research Institute for Social Security, 1988, p 1.
24. Collis DK, Ponseti IV: Long-term follow-up of patients with idiopathic scoliosis not treated surgically. J Bone Joint Surg Am 1969; 51:424.
25. Westrin C-G: Low back sick-listing: A nosological medical insurance investigation. Scand J Soc Med 1973; 7:1.
26. Ikata T: Statistical and dynamic studies of lesions due to overloading on the spine. Shikoku Acta Med 1965; 40:262.
27. Chaffin DB, Park KS: A longitudinal study of low back pain as associated with occupational weightlifting factors. Am Ind Hyg Assoc J 1973; 34:513.
28. Chaffin DB, Herrin GD, Keyserling WM: Preemployment strength testing: An updated position. J Occup Med 1978; 20:403.

29. Cady LD, Bischoff DP, O'Connell ER, et al: Strength and fitness and subsequent back injuries in fire fighters. J Occup Med 1979; 21:269.

30. Videman T, Numminen T, Tola S, et al: Low back pain in nurses and some loading factors of work. Spine 1984; 9:400.

31. Troup JDG, Foreman TK, Baxter CE, et al: The perception of back pain and the role of psychophysical tests of lifting capacity. Spine 1987; 12:645.

32. Kelsey JL: An epidemiological study of the relationship between occupations and acute herniated lumbar intervertebral discs. Int J Epidemiol 1975; 4:197.

33. McCulloch JA, Macnab I: Sciatica and Chymopapain. Baltimore, Williams and Wilkins, 1983, p 24.

34. Olmarker K: Mechanical and biochemical injury of spinal nerve roots: An experimental perspective. In Weinstein JN, Gordon SL, eds: Low Back Pain: A Scientific and Clinical Overview. Rosemont, IL, American Academy of Orthopaedic Surgeons, 1996, p 215.

35. Cavanaugh JM, Ozaktay AC, Vaidyanathan S: Mechano- and chemosensitivity of lumbar dorsal roots and dorsal root ganglia: An in vitro study. Trans Orthop Res Soc 1994; 19:109.

36. Kawakami M, Weinstein JN, Hashizume H, et al: Pathomechanisms of pain-related behaviour produced by intervertebral disc in the rat. Helsinki, Finland, Trans Int Soc Studies Lumbar Spine, 1995, p 53.

37. El-Mahdi MA, Abdel Latif FY, Janko M: The spinal nerve root "innervation" and a new concept of the clinicopathological interrelations in back pain and sciatica. Neurochirurgie 1981; 24:137.

38. Olmarker K, Rydevik B, Holm S, et al: Effects of experimental graded compression on blood flow in spinal nerve roots: A vital microscopic study on the porcine cauda equina. J Orthop Res 1989; 7:817.

39. Rydevik B, Lundborg G, Bagge U: Effects of graded compression on intraneural blood flow: An in vivo study on rabbit tibial nerve. J Hand Surg Am 1981; 6:3.

40. Rydevik B, Nordborg C: Changes in nerve function and nerve fibre structure induced by acute, graded compression. J Neurol Neurosurg Psychiatry 1980; 43:1070.

41. Herlin L: Sciatic and Pelvic Pain Due to Lumbosacral Nerve Root Compression. Springfield, MA, Charles C Thomas, 1966, p 11.

42. Modic MT, Masaryk T, Boumphrey F, et al: Lumbar herniated disc disease and canal stenosis. AJNR Am J Neuroradiol 1986; 7:709.

43. Boden SD, Davis DO, Dina TS, et al: Abnormal magnetic-resonance scans of the lumbar spine in asymptomatic subjects. J Bone Joint Surg Am 1990; 72:403.

44. Bell GR, Rothman RH, Booth RE, et al: A study of computer assisted tomography: Comparison of metrizamide myelography and computed tomography in the diagnosis of herniated lumbar disc and spinal stenosis. Spine 1984; 9:552.

45. Nachemson A, Spitzer WO, LeBlanc FE, et al: Scientific approach to the assessment and management of activity-related spinal disorders: A monograph for clinicians: Report of the Quebec Task Force on Spinal Disorders. Spine 1987; 12:S1.

46. Hakelius A: Prognosis in sciatica: A clinical follow-up of surgical and nonsurgical treatment. Acta Orthop Scand 1970; 129:1.

47. Saal JA, Saal JS: Nonoperative treatment of herniated lumbar intervertebral disc with radiculopathy: An outcome study. Spine 1989; 14:431.

48. Frymoyer JW: Back pain and sciatica. N Engl J Med 1988; 318:291.

49. Hill GM, Ellis EA: Chemonucleolysis as an alternative to laminectomy for the herniated lumbar disc: Experience with patients in a private orthopedic practice. Clin Orthop 1987; 225:229.

50. Maroon JC, Abla A: Microlumbar discectomy. Clin Neurosurg 1986; 33:407.

51. Kahanovitz N, Viola K, Mculloch J: Limited surgical discectomy and microdiscectomy: A clinical comparison. Spine 1989; 14:79.

52. Mixter WJ, Barr JS: Rupture of the intervertebral disc with involvement of the spinal canal. N Engl J Med 1934; 211:210.

53. Thomas AM, Afshar F: The microsurgical treatment of lumbar disc protrusion. J Bone Joint Surg Br 1987; 69:696.

54. Davis GW, Onik G: Clinical experience with automated percutaneous lumbar discectomy. Clin Orthop 1989; 238:98.

55. Friedman WA: Percutaneous discectomy: An alternative to chemonucleolysis? Neurosurgery 1983; 13:542.

56. Rogers LA: Experience with limited versus extensive disc removal in patients undergoing microsurgical operations for ruptured lumbar discs. Neurosurgery 1988; 22:82.

57. Schwartz AM, Brodkey JS: Bowel perforation following microsurgical lumbar discectomy: A case report. Spine 1988; 13: 104.

58. Maroon JC, Abla A: Microdiscectomy versus chemonucleolysis. Neurosurgery 1985; 16:644.

59. Zieger HE: Comparison of chemonucleolysis and microsurgical discectomy for the treatment of herniated lumbar disc. Spine 1987; 12:796.

60. Nystrom B: Experience of microsurgical compared with conventional technique in lumbar disc operations. Acta Neurol Scand 1987; 76:129.

61. Sachdev VF: Microsurgical lumbar discectomy: A personal series of 300 patients with at least 1-year of follow-up. Microsurgery 1986; 7:55.

62. Weber H: 1982 Volvo award in clinical science: Lumbar disc herniation: A controlled, prospective study with ten years of observation. Spine 1983; 8:131.

section 8 chapter 7

SPINAL STENOSIS

Alexander R. Vaccaro and Dan A. Zlotolow

Summary
- Spinal stenosis consists of narrowing of the spinal canal, resulting in compromise of the neural elements.
- Clinical features of spinal stenosis include neurogenic intermittent claudication, with discomfort and weakness in the buttock, thigh, or lower leg aggravated by walking and by extension of the spine.
- Another clinical feature is cauda equina syndrome, with saddle anesthesia and bowel and bladder dysfunction.

ANATOMY

The size of the central vertebral canal varies widely not only from individual to individual but also among racial groups and along the course of the spine.[1-3] At the level of the pedicles, the central canal is defined anteriorly by the posterior vertebral body, laterally by the two pedicles, and posteriorly by the superior aspect of the lamina and the medial aspect of the superior apophyseal joints. The cross-sectional area in this axial plane decreases from L1 to L4 and widens again at L5. In the midsagittal plane, the canal is indented anteriorly by the intervertebral disk and the

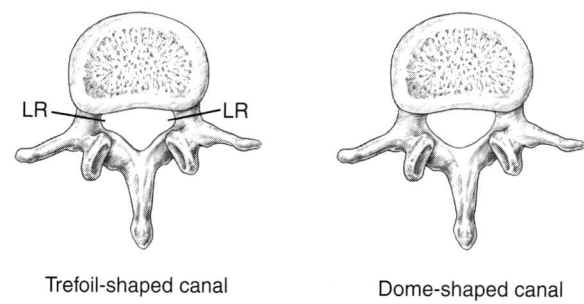

Trefoil-shaped canal

Dome-shaped canal

Fig. 1. Axial canal shape.

posterior longitudinal ligament and posteriorly by the superior aspect of the lamina and the ligamentum flavum. The midsagittal diameter is widest at L1, reducing in size down to L4, and widening again at L5. In the coronal plane, the narrowest diameter exists across the pedicles; L1-3 is roughly equal and then L4 and L5 become sequentially wider.[4] The adult canal size has been shown to correlate directly with placental size; the majority of development is completed by late infancy.[5] Specifically, the midsagittal diameter is primarily determined by early growth, whereas the interpedicular distance continues to widen until puberty. Eventual canal size may be decreased in preterm deliveries; the L3 vertebral level is the most affected by antenatal factors.[6] Repressed early growth followed by normal or accelerated growth, along with development of the normal lordotic curvature of the lumbar spine, has been theorized to result in a trefoil-shaped lumbar canal.[4] Trefoil-shaped canals contain paired lateral recesses that are not seen in dome-shaped canals (Fig. 1). The lumbar root must first pass through this lateral recess along the medial pedicle before exiting through the intervertebral foramen. This effectively decreases the capacity of the canal even though the cross-sectional area may be within normal limits.

Canal capacity is also affected by posture and fluctuates with activity. In extension, the intervertebral disk bulges posteriorly, whereas the ligamentum flavum and the superior aspect of the lamina protrude anteriorly. In addition, the facet joints sublux anteriorly, further reducing the dimensions of the central canal (Fig. 2). Ambulation results

in cyclical compression and expansion of the spinal canal in a set pattern; compression occurs during the double-supporting phase of each gait cycle. Not surprisingly, maximum backward tilt of the pelvis occurs at this stage of the gait cycle.[7]

Nutrition to the spinal nerve roots is provided equally by the arterial system and the cerebrospinal fluid (CSF).[8] Arterial blood flows in an ascending manner in the extradural or peripheral nerve root and in a descending pathway in the intradural or cauda equinal portion of the nerve root. A watershed area, or area where descending and ascending blood flows converge, often exists in the area of the dorsal root ganglion (Fig. 3A).[9, 10] The relatively hypervascular dorsal root ganglion has separate arterial supply and a blood-brain barrier that is not as impenetrable as those found in peripheral nerves.[9] The venous system in the lumbar spine is valveless with generous anastomoses.[10] The venous system is poorly developed in the nerve roots themselves; multiple arteriovenous anastomoses are present.[11]

PATHOPHYSIOLOGY

Any process or condition that narrows the spinal canal results in spinal stenosis. Spinal stenosis may be classified as congenital, which includes idiopathic and achondroplastic, or acquired, which includes degenerative, combined, spondylolisthetic, iatrogenic, posttraumatic, or any combination of these. Once the level of narrowing crosses a certain threshold, neurogenic intermittent claudication may develop. If the stenosis is severe, the patient may manifest symptoms consistent with a cauda equina syndrome, including perineal saddle anesthesia and urinary dysfunction. However, several studies have shown that 20% to 25% of people older than 40 have marked narrowing of the lumbar spinal canal yet remain asymptomatic.[12–14]

Spinal stenosis can result from either bony or soft-tissue encroachment into the spinal canal. Skeletal disease leading to canal narrowing may include degenerative changes at the apophyseal joints, osteophyte formation at the cranial edge of the lamina, and vertebral translation or spondylolisthesis. Degenerative spondylolisthesis is seen in 50% of men with bilateral claudication.[15] Soft-tissue disease contributing to spinal stenosis may include thickening of the

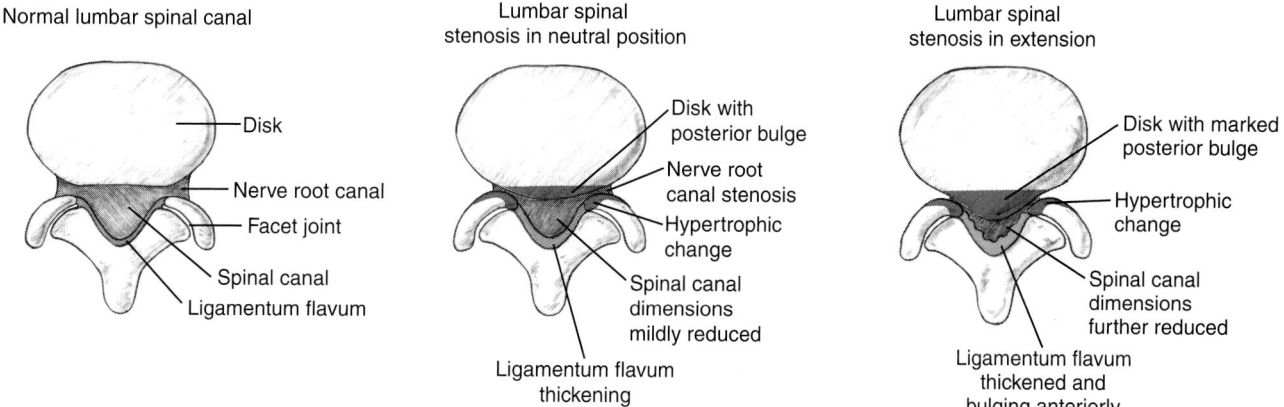

Fig. 2. Lumbar spinal canal in health and disease. (Redrawn from Klippel JH, Dieppe PA [eds]: Rheumatology. St. Louis, Mosby, 1994, Section 5, p 6.5, figure 6.7.)

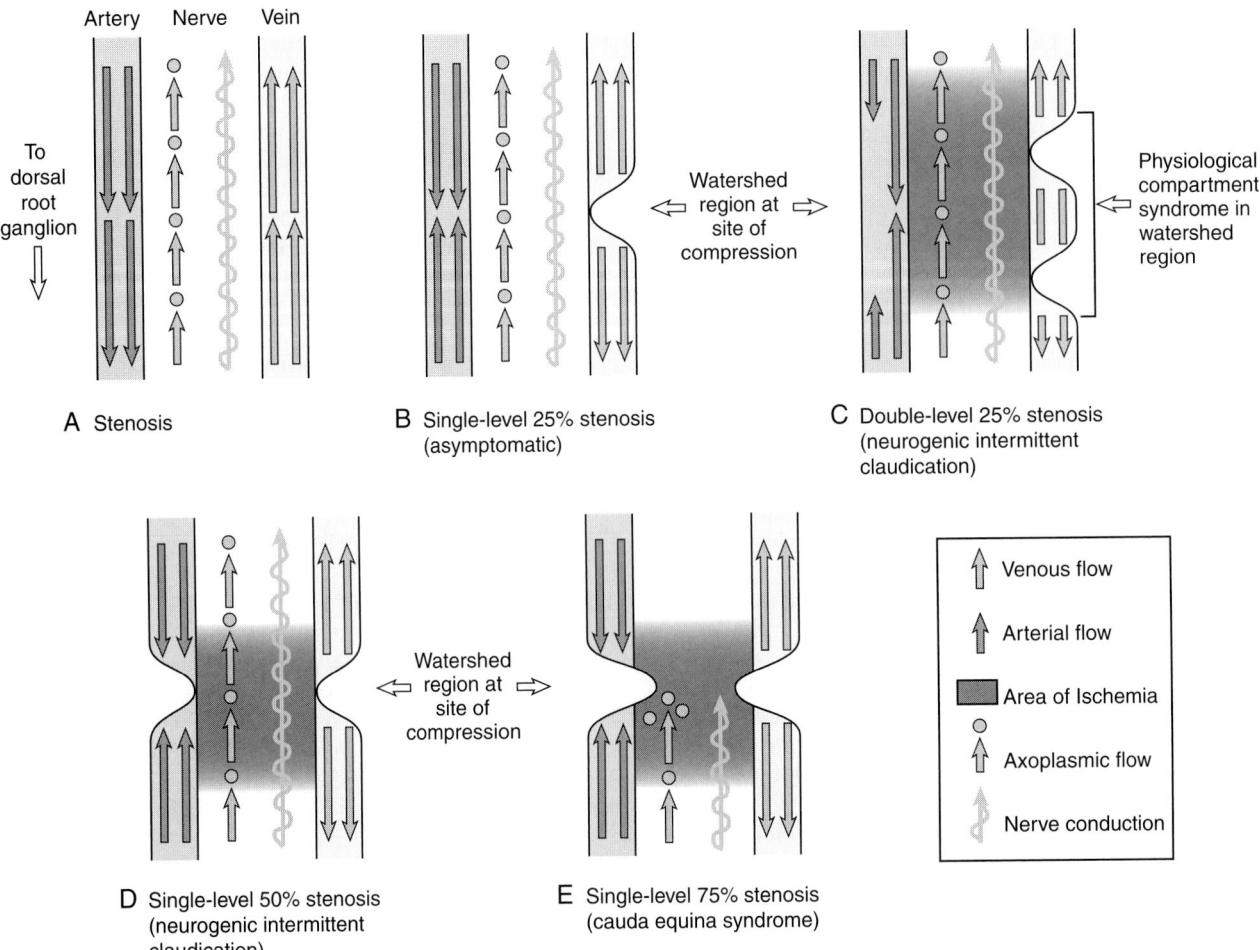

Fig. 3. Pathophysiology. These are models of spinal stenosis *(A–E)*.

ligamentum flavum, posterior longitudinal ligament hypertrophy, or a bulging or herniated intervertebral disk.[4] In patients with symptomatic degenerative disease, the ligamentum flavum has been shown to hypertrophy in response to mechanical stress, the degree correlating with the age of the patient.[16] This response was not found in patients without degenerative changes and, therefore, is not a pure age-related phenomenon.

The critical canal dimensions at which spinal stenosis becomes symptomatic are unclear. In the midsagittal plane, a diameter of less than 12 mm has been proposed as being probably pathological and less than 10 mm as being unequivocally pathological.[17] Animal studies seem to agree that 50% relative stenosis or greater leads to clinical symptoms and signs.[18–20] Schönström et al[21] compared the transverse areas of the dural sac at the L2-3 level between theoretical, experimental, and clinical examples of stenosis against normal controls. The average control transverse canal area was 178 mm² versus 90, 70, and 42 mm² for clinical, experimental, and theoretical stenosis, respectively.

The emergence of claudication symptoms during ambulation may be due to cyclical compression of an already narrowed canal in combination with greater metabolic activity of the spinal nerves without the concomitant ability to increase nutrient delivery to those nerves. Multiple studies showed that the normal vasodilation that occurs in the spinal nerves in response to exercise is inhibited by compression of the nerves.[22, 23] Furthermore, the normal pulsatile flow of CSF may be reduced in the stenotic segments.[9] A decrease in the vascular and CSF flow may cause toxic compounds and proteolytic enzymes to leak from leukocytes, resulting in increased vascular permeability and local inflammation.[24] Whether the vascular insufficiency is the result of arterial compromise, venous congestion, or capillary bed stasis is unknown. Regardless, it appears that regional tissue ischemia may play a role in causing claudication symptoms. The degree to which compression of the neural elements directly causes dysfunction is also unknown.

Some patients with radiographically stenotic canals remain asymptomatic, suggesting that compression of the neural elements may be only one of multiple factors leading to disease. When one considers that patients tend to be in an age group in which arteriosclerosis is common and vascular claudication often coexists, it is easy to hypothesize that neural ischemia may be worsened in some cases by arterial disease. Disease of the arteries of the lower limb has been found more frequently in spinal stenosis patients than in controls.[15]

There is much evidence for neural ischemia in stenotic canals.[9, 11, 19, 20, 22, 25–27] Jespersen et al[22] demonstrated that nerve root blood flow in a porcine model of spinal stenosis was lower than in the control pigs and decreased further during exercise. Slight hyperemia in the white matter at the level of stenosis was also noted after exercise, indicating a nutritional deficit. Hyperemia of the spinal nerves during the first 10 minutes after decompression has also been described.[27] Dilatation of the vessels was most prominent in the venules. Other studies showed that raising systemic blood pressure[28] and administering vasodilating drugs[29, 30] can serve to protect against or treat claudication. Even angiography has been shown to have a therapeutic effect.[31]

With slow nerve compression, compromise of the venules has been shown to occur at 50 to 60 mm Hg, capillaries at 20 to 50 mm Hg, and arterioles at 100 to 170 mm Hg in animals with a mean arterial pressure (MAP) of 150 mm Hg.[27] Others reported electrophysiological changes with compression pressures near MAP in normotensive, hypotensive, and hypertensive animals.[32, 33] These results indicate that in single-level stenosis models arteriolar compromise may lead to ischemia and subsequent neural dysfunction (see Fig. 3D).

The venous pathways in the cauda equina are valveless and contain a series of arteriovenous anastomoses. These may function to drive venous return in a retrograde fashion distal to the compressive lesion. Exercise has been shown to increase arterialization of veins, resulting in venous hypertension. Venous hypertension, in turn, causes engorgement of the venules in an already compromised spinal canal.[11] The result may be similar to a small-scale compartment syndrome, eventually causing retrograde stasis and arteriolar compromise (see Fig. 3C).[27] Cadaveric examinations of patients with lumbosacral spinal stenosis has revealed preservation of the major radicular arteries, albeit very convergent and straightened, but collapse, congestion, and decrease in the number of the venules.[34] Moreover, local arterial flow has been shown to compensate for single-level disease by shifting the watershed region from the normal location at the dorsal root ganglion to the area of stenosis (see Fig. 3B).[9]

Two-level stenosis has been found to cause nerve dysfunction at lower compression pressures than are necessary in single-level stenosis.[15, 23, 24] Baker et al[23] described a 75% reduction in blood flow in a two-level model compared with no change in a single-level model at the same low compression pressure. Two-site disease appeared to be necessary for venous congestion, which led to loss of vasodilation during exercise. Arteriolar compromise may play a larger role in single-level stenosis, accounting for the necessary high compression pressures experienced in single-level symptomatic models compared with multiple-level symptomatic models. Among 49 random patients with neurogenic claudication, 46 were found to have two-level stenosis,[15] suggesting that two-level pathology may be common in this patient population. This explains the discrepancy in clinical versus theoretical levels of significant stenosis as described by Schönström et al[21] as well as Watanabe and Parke[34] in cadaveric examinations.

Direct neural compromise independent of ischemia has been proposed by Verbiest[35] as a significant causative factor in symptomatic spinal stenosis. Jespersen et al[19] showed that, for reasons that are unclear, nerve conduction impairment occurred before a decrease in regional blood flow in pigs subjected to both 50% and 75% acute-onset stenosis. Shear forces generated as a result of compression have been theorized to cause neural damage, affecting nutrient uptake ability and leading to edema, which may then cause local vascular insufficiency.[36] This may be true for acute compression as seen with herniation of the nucleus pulposus but seems unlikely in the slowly progressive stenosis that results in claudication. In a later study, the same principal author concluded that axonal disruption from compression was not likely in gradual compression, because impairment of nerve conduction progressively increased over the first 2 hours of compression.[37]

Using a gradual compression model with ameroid constrictors, Cornefjörd et al[38] showed that, between 1 and 2 weeks of gradually increasing compression, a threshold was reached whereby axoplasmic flow of substance P was impeded. Ameroid constrictors are made up of a rigid circumferential shell enclosing a slowly expansile (approximately 2 weeks) material that is wrapped around the nerve root between the spinal cord and the dorsal root ganglion. Substance P is produced in the dorsal root ganglion in response to noxious stimuli and is involved in pain transmission. At 1 week after constriction, substance P levels were high in the nerve root cranial to the constrictor but low in the dorsal root ganglion located just caudal to the constrictor. This indicated increased production in response to constriction as well as adequate transport within the axons. By the second week, the dorsal root ganglion exhibited high levels of substance P, whereas levels in the proximal nerve root declined, illustrating that a specific threshold was reached whereby proximal flow of substance P was inhibited. Kawakami et al[39] found an increase not only of substance P but also of calcitonin gene-related peptide and vasoactive intestinal peptide (VIP) in the dorsal root ganglion in a similar model using suture constrictors. There was no concurrent increase proximal to the site of stenosis. They concluded that not only was axonal transport of these molecules impeded but that the significant increase of substance P and VIP in the dorsal root ganglion was due principally to increased production in response to nerve irritation.

A blockage of axoplasmic flow has been associated with cauda equina-like symptoms in an animal model. Delamarter et al[20] found that with greater than 55% to 60% stenosis in a dog model, the cortical evoked potential waveform flattened and paralysis of the tail with urinary incontinence developed. After 3 months of constriction, complete loss of axons was seen at the constriction site, with wallerian degeneration noted in the motor nerve fibers caudad and sensory nerve fibers cephalad to the level of constriction. There was also histological evidence of the interruption of axoplasmic flow at the level of the stenosis. Direct neural compromise may, therefore, be a greater factor in cauda equina syndrome pathogenesis than in neurogenic claudication (see Fig. 3E).

In summary, neurogenic claudication is likely due to compression of the cauda equina with ambulation. The nerve fibers in this setting become ischemic, with temporary dysfunction resulting from the inability of the nerves to keep up with increased metabolic requirements. Direct neural damage results as a consequence of exposure to deleterious metabolites and oxygen free radicals as well as shear forces. Diabetes, atherosclerosis, and other factors such as multilevel stenosis may lower the threshold level for symptomatic stenosis. Severe compression leading to axonal loss and blockade of axoplasmic flow, however, may be linked to a cauda equina syndrome presentation. The differences in histopathology between these two manifestations of essentially the same disease entity may help explain their different prognoses and rationales for treatment.

CLINICAL FEATURES

Symptomatic spinal stenosis is a relatively common disease affecting predominantly men older than 50 years, many of whom have a history of heavy manual labor. Acute symptomatic spinal stenosis from a herniated nucleus pulposus more often leads to the clinical entity known as sciatica. The symptoms associated with neurogenic intermittent claudication are caused by chronic slowly progressive or stable stenosis. Patients typically present with discomfort with walking, usually in the thighs, calves, and feet. They may complain of tired or heavy feeling legs. Forty percent of patients will exhibit these symptoms bilaterally.[40] The distance walked until symptoms begin is referred to as the threshold distance, and the maximum distance that the patient can walk without stopping is referred to as the tolerance distance. For each patient, these distances will vary from day to day and even during the same walk. Patients generally report gradually stooping over and slowing down. Once still, many have to continue leaning forward to relieve their symptoms. Flexion of the lumbar spinal canal increases the geometric area available for the neural elements. Many patients adopt a "simian stance," with the hips and knees slightly flexed to maintain spinal flexion. Similarly, patients may not experience symptoms while going up hills or stairs or while riding a bicycle, activities performed in a flexed posture. However, walking down hills or extending the spine often results in worsening of symptoms. Most patients with spinal stenosis also have concomitant back pain (65%) and standing discomfort (94%) in addition to their radicular symptomatology.[41] Because of its gradually progressive course, some patients may first present months to years after the initial onset of symptoms. The symptoms and onset may vary considerably between individuals.

The physical examination is often remarkable for its lack of objective abnormalities. Findings may be limited to a decrease or lack of lumbar extension and tenderness to palpation over several segments of the lumbar spine. Overall, neurological signs such as straight leg raising, reflexes, and strength are normal. Some researchers advocated the use of a treadmill to record objective threshold and tolerance distances as well as to observe the speed and posture changes that occur with the onset of symptoms. More precise localization of patient discomfort is also possible in this controlled setting. The comparison of treadmill tolerances over time can serve as a means to monitor the progression of the disease.[4, 42]

DIFFERENTIAL DIAGNOSIS

INTERMITTENT CLAUDICATION FROM VASCULAR INSUFFICIENCY

Patients with vascular insufficiency often present with a history of leg pain and weakness brought on by walking. They also report having to take short breaks to relieve symptoms before resuming their activities. Moreover, these patients tend to have identical historical profiles and symptom patterns as those with spinal stenosis. Differentiating between the two is often difficult, particularly because these two diseases often coexist. Unlike spinal stenosis, however, patients with vascular insufficiency often have a stable tolerance distance from day to day. Their symptoms are not affected by posture and, in fact, may report having more pain going up stairs. A typical patient with vascular insufficiency cannot tolerate walking or cycling and usually has greater symptoms in one leg than the other. On examination, the presence of a femoral bruit or a lack of peripheral pulses is often encountered. In complex cases, particularly mixed claudication, Doppler scans or other vascular studies as well as vascular surgical consultation may be necessary.[43]

SCIATIC CLAUDICATION

Insufficiency of the inferior gluteal artery can result in referred pain in a root or radicular distribution. The spinal examination and imaging studies are usually normal in this clinical situation.[4] Diagnostic confusion arises when what would otherwise be an incidental finding of spinal stenosis on the imaging studies is mistakenly interpreted as the source of the symptoms. Such cases may require angiography or vascular surgical consultation if the diagnosis of spinal stenosis is suspect.

REFERRED PAIN

Lower lumbar spondylosis may cause referred pain in the buttocks, thighs, and upper calves as well as mechanical low back pain aggravated by walking. However, other activities not specific for spinal stenosis may also induce symptoms, with pain occurring in a more proximal distribution.

SPACE-OCCUPYING LESIONS

Spinal tumors and synovial cysts can decrease the space available for the neural elements, producing a clinical picture identical to neurogenic intermittent claudication. Imaging studies are, therefore, critical in differentiating these from other causes of spinal stenosis. Back pain accompanied by night pain, fevers, or weight loss indicates the need for a more extensive work-up.

HERNIATED NUCLEUS PULPOSUS

A large, central herniation can compress the cauda equina and present with a clinical picture identical to neurogenic intermittent claudication. However, unlike the latter, the onset of symptoms is usually abrupt.

PERIPHERAL NERVE ENTRAPMENT

Although some entrapment syndromes may mimic spinal stenosis, these can be differentiated with the use of imag-

TABLE 1. DIFFERENTIAL DIAGNOSIS	
Condition	Distinguishing Feature
Vascular intermittent claudication	Not affected by posture
Sciatic claudication	Angiography
Referred pain	More proximal distribution
Space-occupying lesions	Imaging studies
Herniated nucleus pulposus	Abrupt symptoms
Peripheral nerve entrapment	Electromyography
Distress	Inconsistent symptoms

ing techniques and more importantly electromyography and nerve conduction velocities.[44] They can also occur concurrently and further complicate the treatment and prognosis.

DISTRESS

Inconsistent or fluctuating clinical symptoms as well as exaggerated or inappropriate signs may raise suspicion of a functional component to the pain. Litigation and psychological factors can confuse the diagnosis, even when symptomatic spinal stenosis is present, and pose the greatest diagnostic and treatment challenge (Table 1).

INVESTIGATIONAL MODALITIES

PLAIN FILMS

A normal plain radiograph nearly excludes spinal stenosis as the source of symptoms. Plain films can demonstrate changes associated with canal compromise such as narrowing of the disk spaces, apophyseal joint osteoarthritis, structural lumbar scoliosis, and degenerative spondylolisthesis (Fig. 4).[40, 45] However, because degenerative changes in this age group are so common, an "abnormal" film is not diagnostic.

MAGNETIC RESONANCE IMAGING

At any one spinal segment, magnetic resonance imaging (MRI) and computed tomography (CT) with contrast have been found to be comparable at demonstrating spinal stenosis.[46] Yet MRI, unlike CT scans with contrast, is noninvasive and allows multiplanar visualization especially useful in multilevel stenosis. A good quality MRI will clearly depict the spinal cord, cauda equina, subarachnoid space, epidural fat, intervertebral disks, and vertebral ligaments (Fig. 5). On T_1-weighted images, stenosis is marked by a loss of the epidural fat pad, whereas T_2-weighted images will reveal loss of the CSF surrounding the dural sac. Other signs may be hypertrophy of the ligamentum flavum and degeneration of the intervertebral disk.[47]

COMPUTED TOMOGRAPHY

CT is a second-line imaging test. A CT scan allows measurement of the cross-sectional area of the central canal, degree of lateral recess stenosis, articular facet hypertrophy, enlargement of laminae, hyperplasia and ossification of the ligamentum flavum, and degree of disk prolapse. The classic shape of a pathologically narrowed canal (i.e., trefoil) can be clearly visualized on CT (Fig. 6). Although the

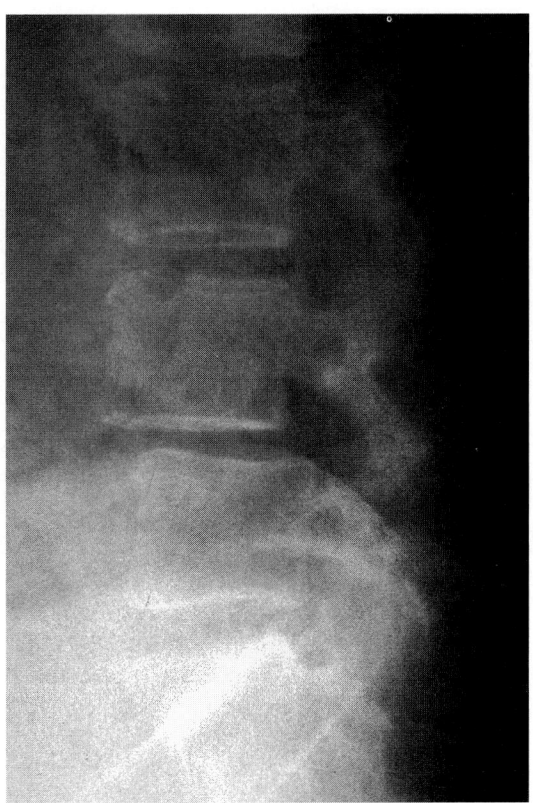

Fig. 4. Degenerative listhesis. This lateral radiograph is of a patient with neurogenic intermittent claudication.

trefoil shape usually indicates severe stenosis, this shape can also be seen in asymptomatic patients.

Most standard CT protocols inaccurately determine the degree or extent of spinal stenosis (10% of cases) as a result of not including lumbar segments above the L3 level.[40] Willen et al[47] demonstrated that conventional CT scanning did not reveal a significant number of stenotic lesions, and they advocated the use of axially loaded CT

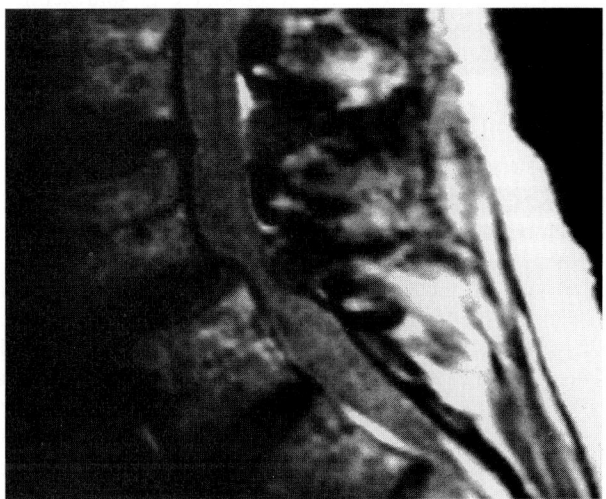

Fig. 5. Degenerative spondylolisthesis. This MRI is of a patient with spinal stenosis.

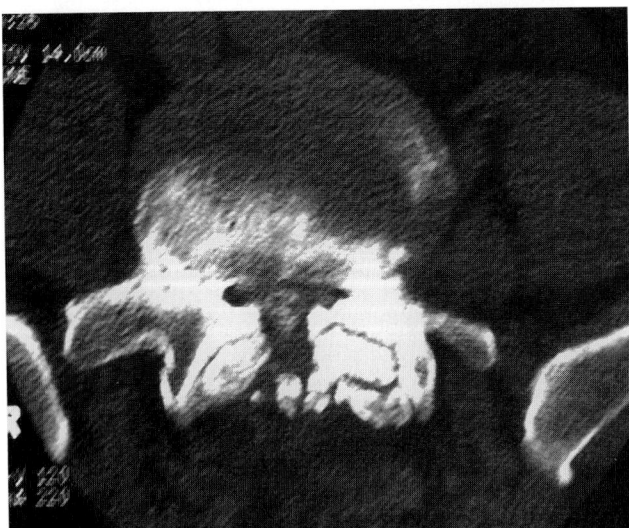

Fig. 6. Spinal stenosis. This CT scan shows the classic trefoil shape and degenerative changes.

myelography or MRI when the cross-sectional area of the dural sac on conventional CT scanning is below 130 mm^2 or when there is suspicion of a narrowed lateral recess.

MYELOGRAPHY

Although often overlooked for CT and MRI, myelography continues to be useful, particularly in visualizing multiple-level disease. One advantage of myelography is its ability to demonstrate posturally dependent stenosis of the central canal. Used in combination with CT, myelography can reveal disease not visible with either modality alone (Fig. 7).[48]

ELECTROMYELOGRAPHY

If used selectively, electromyelography and nerve conduction velocities are useful for ruling out peripheral neuropathies and peripheral nerve entrapment.[44] Many patients with spinal stenosis, however, may have abnormalities on electromyography.[40, 49] Therefore, judicious use of this modality, reserved for patients for whom there is some clinical suspicion of peripheral nerve disease, will avoid diagnostic confusion.

MANAGEMENT

The prevailing opinion, in general, is that the natural course of lumbar spinal stenosis is one of progressive worsening, although the course is variable and can be slow and the pain tolerable. Although the pathoanatomy does not improve, and in fact progresses over time, the pain need not. The Maine Lumbar Spine Study (Part III) found that, at 1 year follow up, only 28% of nonoperatively treated patients reported no changes or gradual improvement in symptoms.[50] If symptoms of stenosis are of relatively recent onset and are well tolerated by the patient, reassurance that this spinal disorder is not life threatening, accompanied by an appropriate conditioning program and regular follow up, is frequently all that is needed. Patients will generally benefit from a clear explanation of the pathophysiology of the normal aging process related to the

spine and how this at times manifests as low back pain, leg pain, and weakness. Fortunately, the vast majority of patients respond to a brief duration of activity restriction, an exercise protocol, and mild medication usage, obviating the need for surgical intervention.[51] Surgical treatment should, therefore, be reserved for cases refractory to medical management and for patients in whom neurological deficits are either poorly tolerated or who are unlikely to recover without it.

NONSURGICAL TREATMENT

The goals of treatment of symptomatic lumbar spinal stenosis are primarily to improve the patient's level of function while decreasing lower extremity discomfort.

Activities Restriction/Physical Therapy

A brief duration of bedrest or activity restriction is often beneficial during an acute exacerbation of low back or leg pain resulting from spinal stenosis. This assists in alleviating the discomfort of paravertebral muscle spasms so that the patient may begin early mobilization techniques. These may involve postural training, appropriate lifting techniques, and a graded exercise program. Although researchers extensively evaluated the benefits of flexion versus extension exercises, no one technique has been proven significantly superior in the long run.[52, 53] Evidence suggests that the combination of bedrest and controlled physical activity is the most effective nonoperative treatment for low back pain associated with various lumbar degenerative disorders, including spinal stenosis.[54]

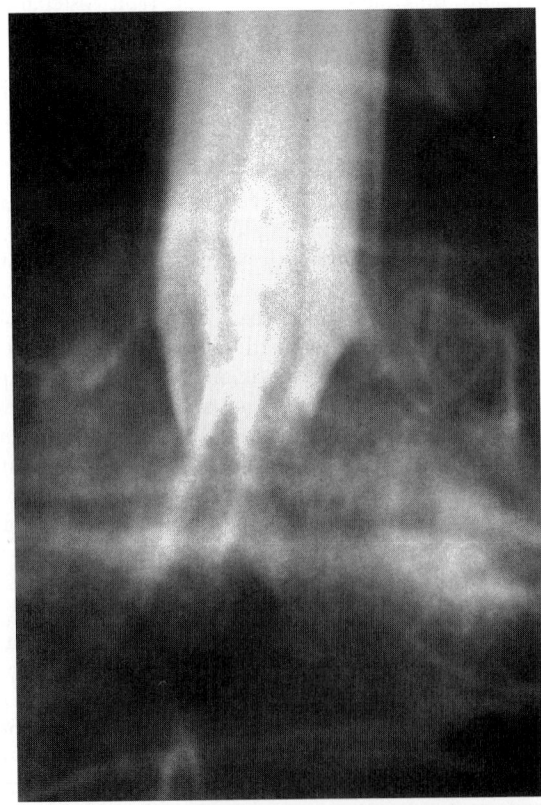

Fig. 7. Myelogram. This is a view of a complete block of contrast flow.

Drugs

Medications often used in the management of spinal stenosis include nonsteroidal anti-inflammatory drugs (NSAIDs),[55–57] analgesics, muscle relaxants, and antidepressants. Generally, the majority of studies demonstrated the superiority of NSAIDs over placebo treatment. NSAIDs mediate their effect by decreasing nociceptive impulses resulting from local inflammation as a result of mechanical neural irritation. The side effects of gastrointestinal irritation and renal toxicity often restrict their use. When specific NSAIDs are compared directly, their efficacy appears to be roughly equivalent.[58–60]

Some patients may require the addition of mild narcotics for symptomatic relief, particularly during acute exacerbations. The role of narcotics in the treatment of spinal stenosis is uncertain. The potential for addiction, sedation, and constipation in the elderly population often restricts their use as a long-term treatment strategy.

Acute exacerbations may benefit from epidural steroid injections. Retrospective reviews found that approximately 60% to 80% of spinal stenosis patients obtained some relief from four or five epidural injections (up to three to four injections over time in a series). Up to 25% of these patients reported excellent long-term relief.[61, 62] Most clinical trials are split between showing positive and neutral results from epidural steroid use.[63–73]

Many other drugs have been considered in the treatment of spinal stenosis, although their efficacy remains unproven. Systemic corticosteroid use has been evaluated in a small number of clinical trials, but results have been inconclusive.[74, 75] Muscle relaxants can be habituating, offer little if any additive relief in combination with NSAIDs,[75] and often cause more sedation than muscle relaxation. Antidepressants, used in multiple chronic pain syndromes, have been studied but show no clear efficacy in improving radicular symptoms in patients with spinal stenosis.[56, 57, 60, 76–78] Calcitonin, because of its use in spinal stenosis secondary to Paget's disease, has been tried on patients without Paget's disease, although results in this population have not been as impressive.[79] Various injection therapies are also in use. Trigger point injections of local anesthetics and selective nerve root injections may offer some relief of symptoms, whereas facet joint injections with corticosteroids have been demonstrated to have negative results in a small number of randomized trials.[68]

Miscellaneous

The beneficial use of traction,[80] spinal manipulation,[81] and braces and corsets[82] has not been proven. Spinal manipulation, in addition, may place patients with osteoporosis or metabolic bone disease at risk for iatrogenic vertebral compression fractures.[83, 84]

Future Therapy

Because the cause of neurogenic intermittent claudication may be neural ischemia, patients may benefit from vasodilating drugs. One study evaluated the benefit of intravenous administration of lipoprostaglandin E_1 in 40 patients with symptomatic intermittent neurogenic claudication. After 10 days of injections, 31 patients reported a favorable response in walking ability and leg numbness at an average follow-up of 2.5 months. However, patients with advanced disease and radicular pain did not show any noticeable improvement.[30] Successful treatment of neurogenic intermittent claudication has been reported using beraprost sodium, an orally effective prostaglandin I_2 analogue. The patient's symptoms, although mild, completely resolved 1 month after initiation of therapy.[29]

SURGICAL TREATMENT

The basic principles of surgical management of spinal stenosis are to provide sufficient neural decompression to relieve symptoms while preserving the mechanical stability of the spine (Table 2). If the spinal decompression is not adequate, neurogenic intermittent claudication may persist. Alternatively, if the decompression is overzealous, the stability of the spine may be compromised, perhaps leading to back pain or deformity (spondylolisthesis).

Surgical decompression is absolutely indicated in the patient with a rapidly progressive neurological deficit with demonstrable thecal sac compression on advanced imaging studies. However, the presence of a cauda equina syndrome resulting from a space-occupying lesion such as a large central disk herniation is seen in less than 5% of patients with spinal stenosis.[85] The clinical presentation of this syndrome includes bowel or bladder dysfunction, saddle anesthesia, and variable loss of motor or sensory function. Consensus has been reached that urgent surgical intervention is beneficial in this setting and in progressive neurologic deterioration, yet objective evidence determining the optimal timing of surgery is sparse. Animal studies showed faster recovery of neurological function after immediate decompression versus decompression that was delayed for 1 to 6 hours.[86] However, other studies indicated that surgical intervention within 6 hours may be unnecessary.[87, 88] It should, however, be treated urgently but not necessarily emergently.

In general, surgery is often beneficial on an elective basis in a patient with persistent, incapacitating neurogenic claudication despite an aggressive trial of nonoperative management. The clinical success of surgical intervention is predicated on the preoperative correlation of the available imaging studies with the patient's symptomatology and physical examination. If the predominant symptom is back pain and not lower extremity claudication, a decompressive procedure is usually not helpful. In fact, surgery in this setting may lead to worsening of the patient's axial back complaints. There are, however, a small group of patients with stenosis who have mainly back pain and who otherwise provide a history exactly the same as the neurogenic claudicant. This small group is helped by decompression but are difficult to diagnose. The duration or chronic-

---

TABLE 2. SURGICAL PRINCIPLES

Back pain is not an indication for surgery.
Patient factors greatly affect surgical outcome.
The surgical procedure should provide sufficient decompression of the neural elements.
Mechanical stability should be preserved.
Mechanical stability should be restored if compromised by a thorough decompression.
Instrumentation is used for correction of angular deformities, fusion of multiple levels, and revision of prior spinal surgeries.
Fusion success may not correlate with clinical outcome.

ity of symptoms has also been correlated with outcome after a surgical decompression. A duration of claudicatory symptoms more than 4 years has been associated with a poorer prognosis.[89]

The extent of decompression should be designed to adequately relieve pressure on the symptomatic neural elements while maximally preserving spinal stability. Some researchers advocated "prophylactic" decompression of asymptomatic stenotic segments during an index procedure to avoid the potential for future symptomatology.[90] However, the importance of treating all levels of a multilevel stenosis has been questioned.[91] In general, however, this multilevel disorder is best treated by decompressing all involved levels.

Patient characteristics have been shown to impact surgical outcome significantly. Certain patients may experience a poor prognosis after surgical decompression despite having appropriate indications for surgery. Factors associated with a poor outcome are history of cigarette smoking, young age, diabetes, hip joint arthrosis, a preoperative lumbar spine fracture, previous surgery, obesity, and female gender.[92, 93]

Proper patient selection may have a greater impact on the success of the decompression than the type of procedure that is performed.[92–96] There is some controversy regarding laminotomy versus laminectomy; the latter is a more extensive decompression and subsequently carries a higher theoretical risk of iatrogenic instability. Studies have found no significant difference between laminotomy and laminectomy in either relief of symptoms or postoperative listhesis.[95] However, the general recommendation is a multiple-level laminectomy for degenerative stenosis, because many patients may require disk or anterior canal osteophyte excision as well.[90] Also, laminotomy per se does not address the central involvement, unless wide, bilateral laminotomies extending to the midline are performed.

Care in preserving the integrity of the spinal facet joints and pars interarticularis is imperative during the decompression procedure in a spine without evidence of deformity. The removal of a complete facet joint or greater than 50% of both facets has been shown to result in instability, whereas removal of greater than one third of the pars interarticularis bilaterally may result in a symptomatic pars fracture with late slippage.[97] The degree of postoperative spondylolisthesis or vertebral slippage has been found to correlate inversely with ambulatory ability and has been reported in up to 20% of patients. Slippage in the postoperative setting is often associated with the extent of the decompression, trauma to the facet joints, size of the disk space, and preoperative presence of spondylolisthesis or scoliosis.[96] If mechanical instability is identified, a fusion is often required to avoid symptomatic progression of a spinal deformity. A decompression followed by an arthrodesis has been shown to have a better clinical outcome than decompression alone in patients with symptomatic degenerative spondylolisthesis or with a long duration of symptoms.[94, 98–100]

Currently, there is controversy as to the efficacy of instrumented (Fig. 8) versus noninstrumented fusions in the treatment of specific spinal deformities in the setting of spinal stenosis. In a meta-analysis of the literature from 1975 to 1995, instrumented fusions after decompression for

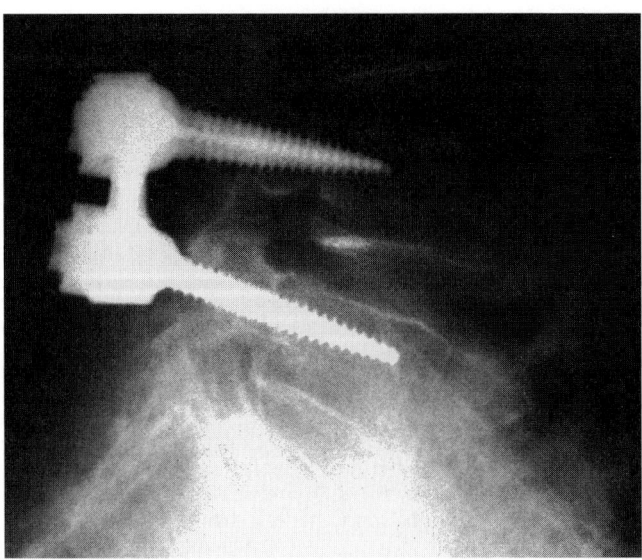

Fig. 8. Posterior lumbar fusion with pedicle screws. A lateral view on radiograph is shown here.

degenerative spondylolisthesis were shown to provide a better outcome, particularly in patients with long-standing symptoms.[94] Noninstrumented fusions, however, are less invasive and less expensive and provide comparable or superior results to instrumented fusions in certain stenotic patient subgroups.[101] Studies have demonstrated superior fusion success rate in instrumented versus noninstrumented fusions in patients treated surgically for degenerative spondylolisthesis. However, the presence of a solid fusion does not necessarily correlate with eventual patient outcome.[102] In general, the use of instrumentation may be beneficial in the correction of angular deformities, fusion of multiple motion segments, and revision procedures, particularly in the setting of a spinal deformity or in recurrent spinal stenosis with translational or angular instability.[103] Currently, no well-designed multicenter randomized, prospective studies exist evaluating the efficacy of instrumentation and fusion in the management of various forms of spinal stenosis.

In a meta-analysis of the literature[104] reviewing 74 journal articles on surgical treatment of lumbar spinal stenosis, 64% of patients were found to have a good or excellent result at follow-up. In general, the success rate for surgical correction of spinal stenosis decreases because patients are monitored over a longer time period. A 90% success rate at 1 year slowly declines to a 67% at 5 years.[105] The reoperation rate for failed spinal stenosis surgery has been reported to be between 5% and 23%.[106] Revision surgery is not as effective on average, with reported success rates between 25% and 80%.[107, 108] Failure of operative treatment of spinal stenosis may be attributed to poor patient selection, inadequate decompression, resultant instability, patient comorbidities, or postoperative complications. Immediate failure of decompression surgery may be the result of an incorrect diagnosis, inadequate decompression technique, and concomitant psychosocial issues such as litigation, low education, and psychiatric disease.[109] Late recurrence is understandable, considering the degenerative process continues, unless a fusion is performed.

REFERENCES

1. Eisenstein S: The morphometry and pathological anatomy of the lumbar spine in South African negroes and caucasoids with specific reference to spinal stenosis. J Bone Joint Surg Br 1977; 59:173.
2. Porter RW, Hibbert C, Wellman P: Backache and the lumbar spinal canal. Spine 1980; 5:99.
3. Postacchini F, Ripani M, Carpano S: Morphometry of the lumbar vertebrae. An anatomic study in two caucasoid ethnic groups. Clin Orthop 1983; 172: 296.
4. Porter RW: Spinal stenosis of the central and root canal. In Jayson MIV (ed): The Lumbar Spine and Back Pain. New York, Churchill Livingstone, 1992, p 313.
5. Porter RW, Pavitt D: The vertebral canal: I. Nutrition and development, an archaeological study. Spine 1987; 12:901.
6. Papp T, Porter RW, Craig CE, et al: Significant antenatal factors in the development of lumbar spinal stenosis. Spine 1997; 22:1805.
7. Takahashi K, Kagechika K, Takino T, et al: Changes in epidural pressure during walking in patients with lumbar spinal stenosis. Spine 1995; 20:2746.
8. Rydevik B, Holm S, Brours MD: Nutrition of the spinal nerve roots: The role of diffusion from the cerebrospinal fluid. Transactions of the 30th Annual Meeting of the Orthopedic Research Society, Atlanta, 1994, p 276.
9. Yoshizawa H, Kobayashi S, Hachiya Y: Blood supply of the nerve roots and dorsal root ganglia. Orthop Clin North Am 1991; 22:195.
10. Garfin SR, Rydevik B, Lind B, et al: Spinal nerve root compression. Spine 1995; 20:1810.
11. Parke WW: The significance of venous return impairment in ischemic radiculopathy and myelopathy. Orthop Clin North Am 1991; 22:213.
12. Hitselberger WE, Witten RM: Abnormal myelograms in asymptomatic patients. J Neurosurg 1968; 28:204.
13. Weisel SW, Tsourmas N, Feffer HL, et al: A study of computer-assisted tomography: I. The incidence of positive CAT scans in an asymptomatic group of patients. Spine 1984; 9:549.
14. Boden SD, Davis DO, Dina TS, et al: Abnormal magnetic-resonance scans of the lumbar spine in asymptomatic subjects. J Bone Joint Surg Am 1990; 72: 403.
15. Porter RW, Ward D: Cauda equina dysfunction. The significance of two-level pathology. Spine 1992; 17:9.
16. Fukuyama S, Nakamura T, Ikeda T, et al: The effect of mechanical stress on hypertrophy of the lumbar ligamentum flavum. J Spine Disord 1995; 8:126.
17. Resnick D, Niwayama G: Degenerative disease of the spine. In Resnick D (ed): Bone and Joint Imaging. Philadelphia, WB Saunders, 1989, p 413.
18. Kim NH, Yang IH, Song IK: Electrodiagnostic and histologic changes of graded caudal compression on cauda equina in dog. Spine 1994; 19:1054.

19. Jespersen SM, Christensen K, Svenstrup L, et al: Spinal cord and nerve root blood flow in acute double level spinal stenosis. Spine 1997; 22:290.
20. Delamarter RB, Bohlman HH, Dodge LD, et al: Experimental lumbar spinal stenosis. Analysis of the cortical evoked potentials, microvasculature, and histopathology. J Bone Joint Surg Am 1990; 72: 110.
21. Schönström N, Bolender NF, Spengler DM, et al: Pressure changes within the cauda equina following constriction of the dural sac. Spine 1984; 9:604.
22. Jespersen SM, Hansen ES, Hoy K, et al: Two-level spinal stenosis in minipigs. Hemodynamic effects of exercise. Spine 1995; 20:2765.
23. Baker AR, Collins TA, Porter RW, et al: Laser Doppler study of porcine cauda equina blood flow. The effect of electrical stimulation of the rootlets during single and double site, low pressure compression of the cauda equina. Spine 1995; 20:660.
24. Olmarker K, Rydevik B: Single- versus double-level nerve root compression. An experimental study on the porcine cauda equina with analyses of nerve impulse conduction properties. Clin Orthop 1992; 279:35.
25. Cornefjörd M, Takahashi K, Matsui H: Impairment of nutritional transport at double level cauda equina compression. Neuro-Orthop 1992; 13:107.
26. Evans JG: Neurogenic intermittent claudication. BMJ 1964; 2:985.
27. Olmarker K, Rydevik B, Holm S, et al: Effects of experimental graded compression on blood flow in spinal nerve roots. A vital microscopic study on the porcine cauda equina. J Orthop Res 1989; 7:817.
28. Lind B, Massie JB, Lincoln T, et al: The effect of induced hypertension and acute graded compression on impulse propagation in the spinal nerve roots of the pig. Spine 1993; 18:1550.
29. Kato H, Emura S, Ngashima K, et al: Successful treatment of intermittent claudication due to spinal canal stenosis using beraprost sodium, a stable prostaglandin I2 analogue. Angiology 1997; 48: 457.
30. Murakami M, Takahashi K, Sekikawa T, et al: Effects of intravenous lipoprostaglandin E1 on neurogenic intermittent claudication. J Spinal Disord 1997; 10: 499.
31. Kikuchi S, Watanabe E, Hasue M: Spinal intermittent claudication due to cervical and thoracic degenerative spine disease. Spine 1996; 21:313.
32. Garfin SR, Cohen MS, Massie JB, et al: Nerve-roots of the cauda equina. The effect of hypotension and acute graded compression on function. J Bone Joint Surg Am 1990; 72:1185.
33. Lind B, Massie JB, Lincoln T, et al: The effects of induced hypertension and acute graded compression on impulse propagation in the spinal nerve roots of the pig. Spine 1993; 18:1550.

34. Watanabe R, Parke WW: Vascular and neural pathology of lumbosacral spinal stenosis. J Neurosurg 1986; 64:64.
35. Verbiest H: A radicular syndrome from developmental narrowing of the lumbar vertebral canal. J Bone Joint Surg Br 1954; 36:230.
36. Olmarker K, Rydevik B, Hansson T, et al: Compression-induced changes in the nutritional supply to the porcine cauda equina. J Spine Disord 1990; 3:25.
37. Olmarker K, Holm S, Rydevik B: Importance of compression onset rate for the degree of impairment of impulse propagation in experimental compression injury of the porcine cauda equina. Spine 1990; 15:416.
38. Cornefjörd M, Olmarker K, Farley DB, et al: Neuropeptide changes in compressed spinal nerve roots. Spine 1995; 20:670.
39. Kawakami M, Weinstein JN, Spratt KF, et al: Experimental lumbar radiculopathy. Immunohistochemical and quantitative demonstrations of pain induced by lumbar nerve root irritation of the rat. Spine 1994; 19:1780.
40. Hall S, Bartleson JD, Onofrio BM, et al: Lumbar spinal stenosis: Clinical features, diagnostic procedures and results of treatment in 68 patients. Ann Intern Med 1985; 103:271.
41. Dillin W, Watkins R: Natural history of lumbar spinal stenosis, clinical features. Semin Spine Surg 1994;6:84.
42. Deen HG Jr, Zimmerman RS, Lyons MK, et al: Measurement of exercise tolerance on a treadmill in patients with symptomatic lumbar spinal stenosis: A useful indicator of functional status and surgical outcome. J Neurosurg 1995; 83: 27.
43. Dodge LD, Bohlman HH, Rhodes RS: Concurrent lumbar spinal stenosis and peripheral vascular disease. Clin Orthop 1988; 230:141.
44. Saal JA, Dillingham MF, Gamburd RS, et al: The pseudoradicular syndrome. Lower extremity peripheral nerve entrapment masquerading as lumbar radiculopathy. Spine 1988; 13:926.
45. Porter RW: Spinal stenosis and neurogenic claudication. Spine 1996; 21: 2046.
46. Deen HG, Zimmerman RS, Swanson SK, et al: Assessment of bladder function after lumbar decompressive surgery for spinal stenosis: A prospective study. J Neurosurg 1994; 80:971.
47. Willen J, Danielson B, Gaulitz A, et al: Dynamic effects on the lumbar spinal canal. Axially loaded CT-myelography and MRI in patients with sciatica and/or neurogenic claudication. Spine 1997; 22: 2968.
48. Griffiths HJ: Imaging of the lumbar spine. Gaithersburg, MD, Aspen, 1991, p 68.
49. Seppalainem AM, Alaranta H, Soini J: Electromyography in the diagnosis of lumbar spinal stenosis. Electromyogr Clin Neurophysiol 1981; 21:55.
50. Atlas JS, Richard A, Deyo RB, et al: The

Maine lumbar spine study: Part III. Spine 1996; 21:1787.

51. Wiesel SW, Cuckler JM, Deluca F, et al: Acute low back pain: An objective analysis of conservative therapy. Spine 1980; 5:324.

52. Hemborg B, Moritz U, Hamberg J: Intra-abdominal pressure in trunk muscle activity during lifting: II. Effects of abdominal muscle training in chronic low back patients. Scand J Rehab Med 1985; 17:15.

53. Jackson CP, Brown MD: Analysis of current approaches and a practical guide to prescription of exercise. Clin Orthop 1983; 179:46.

54. Nelson MA: Lumbar spinal stenosis. J Bone Joint Surg Br 1973; 555:506.

55. Hickey RFJ: Chronic low back pain: A comparison of diflunisal with paracetamol. N Z Med J 1982; 95:312.

56. Amile E, Weber H, Holme I: Treatment of acute low back pain with piroxicam: Results of double blind placebo controlled trial. Spine 1987; 12:473.

57. Berry H, Bloom B, Hamilton EB, et al: Naproxen sodium, diflunisal, and placebo in the treatment of chronic back pain. Ann Rheum Dis 1982; 41:129.

58. Videman T, Osterman K: Double-blind parallel study of piroxicam versus indomethacin in the treatment of low back pain. Ann Clin Res 1984; 16:156.

59. Vignon G: Comparative study of intravenous ketoprofen versus aspirin. Rheum Rehabil 1976; 15:83.

60. Ward N, Bokan JA, Philips M, et al: Antidepressants in concomitant chronic back pain and depression: Doxepin and desipramine compared. J Clin Psychiatry 1984; 45:54.

61. Liebergall M, Fast A, Olshwanger D, et al: The role of epidural steroid injections in the management of lumbar radiculopathy due to disk disease or spinal stenosis. Pain Clin 1986; 1:35.

62. Rosen CD, Kahanovitz N, Bernstein R: A retrospective analysis of the efficacy of epidural steroid injections. Clin Orthop 1988; 228:270.

63. Mathews JA, Mills SB, Jenkins VM, et al: Back pain and sciatica: Controlled trials of manipulation, traction, sclerosant, and epidural injections. Br J Rheumatol 1987; 26:416.

64. Snock W, Webner H, Jorgensen B: Double blind evaluation of extradural methyl prednisolone for herniated lumbar discs. Acta Orthop Scand 1977; 48:635.

65. Yates DW: A comparison of the types of epidural injection commonly used in the treatment of low back pain and sciatica. Rheumatol Rehab 1978; 17:181.

66. Beliveau P: A comparison between epidural anesthesia with and without corticosteroid in the treatment of sciatica. Rheumatol Phys Med 1971; 11:40.

67. Bush K, Hillier S: A controlled study of caudal epidural injections of triamcinolone plus procaine for the management of intractable sciatica. Spine 1991; 16: 572.

68. Cuckler JM, Bernini PA, Wiesel SW, et al: The use of epidural steroids in the treatment of lumbar radicular pain: A

69. Brevik H, Hesla PE, Molnar I, et al: Treatment of chronic low back pain and sciatica: Comparison of caudal epidural injections of bupivacaine and methylprednisolone with bupivacaine followed by saline. In Bonica JJ, Albe-Fessard DG, (eds): Advances in Pain Research and Therapy. New York, Raven Press, 1976, vol 1, p 927.

70. Dilke TFW, Burry HC, Grahame R: Extradural corticosteroid injection in the management of lumbar nerve root compression. BMJ 1973; 2:635.

71. Goodkin K, Gullion CM, Agras WS: A randomised, double-blind, placebo-controlled trial of trazodone hydrochloride in chronic low back pain syndrome. J Clin Psychopharmacol 1990; 10:269.

72. Green LN: Dexamethasone in the management of symptoms due to herniated lumbar disk. J Neurol Neurosurg Psychiatry 1975; 38:1211.

73. Haimovich IC, Beresford HR: Dexamethasone is not superior to placebo for treating lumbosacral radicular pain. Neurology 1986; 36:1593.

74. GutKnecht DR: Chemical meningitis following epidural injections of corticosteroids. Am J Med 1987; 82:570.

75. Basmajian JV: Acute back pain and spasm. A controlled multi-center trial of combined analgesics and anti-spasm agents. Spine 1989; 14:438.

76. Berry H, Hutchinson DR: Tizadinide and ibuprofen in acute low-back pain: Results of a double-blind multicenter study in general practice. J Int Med Res 1988; 16: 83.

77. Alcoff J, Jones E, Rust P, et al: Controlled trial of imipramine for chronic low back pain. J Fam Pract 1982; 13: 841.

78. Jenkins DG, Ebbutt AF, Evans CD: Tofranil in the treatment of low back pain. J Int Med Res 1976; 4:28.

79. Porter W, Miller CG: Neurogenic claudication and root claudication treated with calcitonin. A double-blind trial. Spine 1988; 13:1061.

80. Weber H: Traction therapy in sciatica due to disk prolapse. J Oslo City Hosp 1973; 23:167.

81. Curtis P: Spinal manipulation: Does it work? Occup Med 1988; 3:31.

82. Morris JM: Low back bracing. Clin Orthop 1974; 103:120.

83. Gallinaro P, Cartesegna M: Three cases of lumbar disc rupture and one of cauda equina associated with spinal manipulation (chiroprosis). Lancet 1983; 1:411.

84. Dan NG, Saccasan PA: Serious complications of lumbar spinal manipulation. Med J Aust 1983; 2:672.

85. Shapiro S: Cauda equina syndrome secondary to lumbar disk herniation. Neurosurgery 1993; 32:743.

86. Delamarter RB, Sherman JE, Carr JB: Cauda equina: Evoked potentials, somatosensory (physiology) nerve compression syndromes. Spine 1991; 16:1022.

87. Shapiro S: Cauda equina syndrome secondary to lumbar disk herniation. Neurosurgery 1993; 32:743.

88. Kostuit JP, Harrington I, Alexander D, et al: Cauda-equina syndrome and lumbar disk herniation. J Bone Joint Surg 1986; 68:386.

89. Jonsson B, Annertz M, Sjoberg C, et al: A prospective and consecutive study of surgically treated lumbar spinal stenosis. Part II: Five year follow-up by an independent observer. Spine 1997; 22:2938.

90. Postacchini F: Management of lumbar spinal stenosis. J Bone Joint Surg Br 1986; 78:154.

91. Grob D, Humke T, Dvorak J: Degenerative lumbar spinal stenosis. Decompression with and without arthrodesis. J Bone Joint Surg Am 1995; 77:1036.

92. Airaksinen O, Herno A, Turunen V, et al: Surgical outcome of 438 patients treated surgically for lumbar spine stenosis. Spine 1997; 22:2278.

93. Lehto MU, Honkkanen P: Factors influencing the outcome of operative treatment for lumbar spinal stenosis. Acta Neurochir 1995; 137:25.

94. Niggemeyer O, Strauss JM, Schulitz KP: Comparison of surgical procedures for degenerative lumbar spinal stenosis: a meta-analysis of the literature from 1975 to 1995. Eur Spine J 1997; 6:423.

95. Thomas NW, Rea GL, Pikul BK, et al: Quantitative outcome and radiographic comparisons between laminectomy and laminotomy in the treatment of acquired lumbar stenosis. Neurosurgery 1997; 41: 567.

96. Johnsson K-E, Willner S, Johnsson K: Postoperative instability after decompression for lumbar spinal stenosis. Spine 1986; 11:107.

97. Abumi K, Panjabi MM, Kramer KM, et al: Biomechanical evaluation of lumbar spinal stability after graded facetectomies. Spine 1990; 15:1142.

98. Vaccaro AR, Garfin SR: Degenerative lumbar spondylolisthesis with spinal stenosis: A prospective study comparing decompression with decompression and intertransverse process arthrodesis: A critical analysis. Spine 1997; 22:368.

99. Tile M, McNeil SR, Zarins RK, et al: Spinal stenosis. Results of treatment. Clin Orthop 1976; 115:104.

100. Herkowitz HN, Kurz LT: Degenerative lumbar spondylolisthesis with spinal stenosis. A prospective study comparing decompression with decompression and intertransverse process arthrodesis. J Bone Joint Surg Am 1991; 73:802.

101. Katz JN, Lipson SJ, Lew RA, et al: Lumbar laminectomy alone or with instrumented or noninstrumented arthrodesis in degenerative lumbar spinal stenosis. Patient selection, costs, and surgical outcomes. Spine 1997; 22:1123.

102. Fischgrund JS, Mackay M, Herkowitz HN, et al: 1997 Volvo Award winner in clinical studies. Degenerative lumbar spondylolisthesis with spinal stenosis: A prospective, randomized study comparing decompressive laminectomy and arthrodesis with and without spinal instrumentation. Spine 1997; 22:2807.

103. Herkowitz HN: Management of syndromes related to spinal stenosis. In Weinstein JN, Rydevik BL, Sonntag

VKH (eds): Essentials of the Spine. New York, Raven Press, 1995, p 177.

104. Turner JA, Ersek M, Herron L, et al: Surgery for lumbar spinal stenosis. Attempted meta-analysis of the literature. Spine 1992; 17:1.

105. Whiffen JR, Neuwirth MG: Spinal stenosis. In Bridwell KH, DeWald RL (eds): The Textbook of Spinal Surgery. Lippincott, Philadelphia, 1997, 2nd ed, p 1561.

106. Tuite GF, Stern JD, Doran SE, et al: Outcome after laminectomy for lumbar spinal stenosis. J Neurosurg 1994; 81: 699.

107. Jonsson B, Stromqvist B: Repeat decompression of lumbar nerve roots. J Bone Joint Surg Br 1993; 75:894.

108. Herno A, Airaksinen O, Saari T: Long-term results of surgical treatment of lumbar spinal stenosis. Spine 1993; 18:1471.

109. Gill K, Frymoyer JW: The management of treatment failures after decompressive surgery. Surgical alternatives and results. In Frymoyer JW (ed): The Adult Spine: Principles and Practice. Lippincott-Raven, New York, 1991, 1st ed, p 1849.

section 8 chapter 8

WHIPLASH

Jack E. Zigler, Marion McGregor, and John J. Triano

Summary
- More than 1.5 million Americans suffer whiplash injuries in motor vehicle accidents each year.
- 25% of patients with whiplash-associated disorders will develop chronic pain.
- Patients disabled longer than 6 months account for 46% of total costs.
- Special diagnostic testing may be appropriate in a small percentage of patients with chronic complaints despite adequate conservative care.

DEMOGRAPHICS

Neck pain is a frequent occurrence following vehicular trauma. Although classically considered a hyperextension/hyperflexion soft-tissue strain phenomenon, the term "whiplash" has been expanded to more generally include perceived neck pain after inertial loads are applied to the head in a motor vehicle accident.[1] The average patient is in his or her third or fourth decade. National Highway Traffic Safety Administration data in 1995 indicate that there were 2,900,000 motor vehicle accidents in the United States during that year, 53% of which included whiplash complaints. The financial impact of whiplash is huge. More than $29 billion is spent annually on whiplash injuries and associated litigation in the United States alone.[2]

Low-speed accidents appear to be more significant in producing whiplash injuries than high-speed trauma. Foret-Bruno et al[3] reported that the whiplash injury rate was 36% at velocity changes below 9.3 mph, whereas it was only 20% at velocity changes above 9.3 mph. Olsson et al[4] found that 78% of whiplash injuries occurred at less than 12.5 mph. Approximately 20% of individuals involved in rear-end collisions will develop symptoms. Symptom onset is usually within 24 hours of the accident. Hildingsson and Toolanen[5] reported on 93 patients, finding that 65 were symptomatic within 1 hour, 77 were symptomatic at 5 hours, and 85 were symptomatic within 15 hours.

Twenty-five percent of those injured will develop chronic pain, and 10% will complain of severe pain. The Quebec Task Force cohort study demonstrated that more than one-fifth (22.1%) recovered within 1 week of injury, 50% of the whiplash subjects recovered at 30 days, and 64% recovered by 60 days.[6] Several other studies have shown persistent symptoms at greater than one year in variable numbers of patients (3%, 15%, 27%, 40%, and 43%).[6-10] This demonstrates the difficulty in interpreting data from retrospective studies that use different methodologies in collecting information from medical or insurance records.

Radanov et al[11] reported prospectively on 117 patients referred from primary care physicians. Injury-related symptoms persisted in 44% after three months, 30% after 6 months, 24% after 12 months, and 18% at 24 months postinjury. In comparing patients who had persisting symptoms with those who had recovered, the authors noted that the symptomatic patients were older, had rotated or inclined head positions at the moment of impact, reported a greater variety of subjective complaints at the time of initial evaluation, and were initially more concerned with the possibility of long-term symptoms or disability.

Many patients have persisting symptoms. Chronic symptoms most commonly include neck ache, headache, and stiffness. In Hohl's study,[8] follow-up neck radiographs taken an average of seven years post injury in patients with no preexisting degenerative changes showed that 39% had developed degenerative disk disease. This was compared with an expected prevalence of only 6% in age-matched controls. Interestingly, however, the development of degenerative changes had no correlation with the presence or absence of persisting symptoms.

A recent study of the late sequelae of whiplash in Lithuania, where there were no medicolegal implications to the injury, retrospectively reviewed 200 individuals 1 to 3 years after their motor vehicle accident.[12] Their incidence of neck pain, headache, subjective cognitive dysfunction, psychological disorders, and low back pain was compared with a sex- and age-matched geographic cohort group. No significant differences were found. In logistic regression analysis, only a family history of neck pain was an important risk factor for ongoing symptoms.

EPIDEMIOLOGY

Modern epidemiology involves both the estimation of disease/disorder rates and the evaluation of relationships between attributes that may be involved in the disease/disorder process. In the case of the whiplash injury, as pointed out by Bogduk[6] in his editorial regarding the Quebec Task Force findings: "there is no decent epidemiology . . ." This is to be expected, given that the term "whiplash" describes an event rather than a syndrome or disease. The event has been described as "an acceleration-deceleration mechanism of energy transferred to the neck"[6] and is commonly associated with soft-tissue and occasionally bony injuries. The diversity of symptoms associated with this event is seemingly endless. Included are headaches, temporomandibular disorders,[13] zygapophysial joint pain[14] and/or neck sprain,[15] vertebral artery injury,[16] cognitive deficits,[17] and even disturbance of eye movements.[18] Controversy exists as to whether one should distinguish between a separate disorder called "whiplash" and other elements of post hyperflexion-hyperextension injury such as concussion. The epidemiologist is faced with the difficult task of determining exactly what to count.

The Quebec Task Force resolved the "event versus syndrome" issue by referring to "whiplash-associated disorders" (WAD)[6] rather than to the term "whiplash." They attempted to restrict their evaluation to soft-tissue injury related to motor-vehicle collisions, a cohort study conducted in Quebec, and only the small number of articles deemed scientifically worthy of review. Although understandable, this tact has been criticized[2] and does not address the epidemiological problem of which numbers are most appropriate to count.

Given the limitations, few attempts have been made to provide the clinical community with estimates of the magnitude of the "whiplash-associated disorder" problem. Evans[19] estimated in 1992 that neck injuries associated with motor vehicle accidents occur in approximately one million people in the United States each year. This translates to approximately 3.9 per thousand in the U.S. population and agrees with Barnsley's estimate of 3.8 per thousand.[1] Interestingly, Galasko's[15] estimate of the incidence in the United Kingdom at 250,000 per annum agrees with both Barnsley and Evans, working out to about 4.5 per thousand per year. Galasko's estimate is based on an evaluation of both police records and hospital records. The above three very consistent estimates differ greatly from those reported by the Quebec Task Force.

The Quebec Task Force chose to tally only the *compensated* whiplash injury rates. Although a number of breakdowns of their data are available, an overall incidence rate in their terms is reported as 70 per 100,000. This translates to 0.7 per thousand, and as expected, is substantially lower than the reports above. The rate of *compensated* WADs varies tremendously, from a reported low in Australia of 0.4 per thousand[20] to a high of 7 per thousand in the province of Saskatchewan in Canada.[6] Saskatchewan's rate is double that of Galasko's estimate, which appears to include uncompensated injuries, and is therefore especially surprising.

In light of the estimates provided, it is reasonable to suggest that the incidence of the nebulous entity described as "whiplash-associated disorder" is between 1 and 10 per thousand. Variability can be attributed to discrepancies in diagnosis, counts that may or may not consider claims, as well as elements of lifestyle, such as numbers of cars on the roads, and the potential impact of seatbelt legislation.

Discrepancies in diagnosis reflect two important issues. The first is the diversity of clinical symptomatology reviewed earlier, which may or may not be attributed to the disorder. The second is the controversy regarding psychological factors and secondary gain. This controversy is significant, ranging from the belief that whiplash soft-tissue type injuries do not exist to complete models regarding their pathogenesis. A rational perspective is provided by Mayou and Radanov.[21] They propose that, as with other physical disorders, the *interaction* between the predisposing event, psychological variables, and social consequences (litigation, work-time-income loss, etc.) is key in determining the level of amplification, should it exist.

Unfortunately, at this time, so little is understood regarding this area that the prevalence of symptom amplification cannot be clearly described from the perspective of epidemiology. The authors have found, in an initial evaluation of 73 patients being seen for neck pain at a large multidisciplinary setting, physicians suspected 11 (15%) of symptom amplification. This was confirmed in a second data set with a rate of 14%, where the somatization scale on the SCL90 psychological test was used for cross-validation. If Mayou and Radanov are correct, and syndromes resulting from whiplash should be expected to have the same rates of amplification that are seen in other physical disorders, then a prevalence rate of 14% to 15% amplification in neck pain patients may be realistic.

PATHOGENESIS

BIOMECHANICS

More people claim injury from car accidents of low energy impact than from incidents where the damage requires towing the vehicle from the scene.[22] Since it is counterintuitive, this fact has motivated much controversy on causation of complaints associated with WAD and their relation to the mechanism of injury. Most judgments of injury are based on the circumstances observed in the most common type of collision, where an unsuspecting occupant of a stationary vehicle is struck from behind. The vehicle absorbs some of the impact energy with the remainder causing a forward acceleration. The inertia of the resting occupant results in the head and neck being forced into extension as the seat back pushes the torso forward. As the vehicle comes to rest, the head and torso continue to move forward until arrested by the seat constraints, resulting in a rapid deceleration and elastic recoil—the "whiplash" action from which the injury gets its common name.

The biomechanical effects of injury are influenced significantly by several factors (Table 1). A good history will include questions about these details as means to assess causation and prognosis. It is the balance of competing factors that yield the basis for the acute, nociceptive pain generation.

Early models of WAD mechanisms portrayed the head as being tethered to the body by a flexible, segmented rod. When exposed to a sudden acceleration or deceleration, the neck would smoothly bend, causing compression loading of one side and tension on the other. We now know that this is too simplistic. Unfortunately, there is little information describing neck motions in response to the low accelerations claimed to cause many whiplash injuries.[6] Tissue damage appears to be a related function of both the head/neck displacements and the forces and moments that overload the tissues. The primary mechanism of injury is the local bending moment at any given vertebral segment. The further the separation of the head from the headrest, the higher the torque created from head impact.[23] Volunteers tested for impacts creating lateral bending and hyperextension motions have reported minor strain symptoms at 60 to 70 degrees and 70 to 90 degrees respectively under torques of approximately 200 in-lb.[24]

Impact forces are rapid and create head/torso accelerations faster than the spinal muscles can respond. The reflex reactions that follow create a second set of loads to the spinal structures. As a result there are two opportunities for injury. The first is from the unguarded impact response and the second is from the reaction phase of muscle response. In fact, muscle guarding in anticipation may have significant preventive effects.[25] Figure 1 shows the bracing capacity of the neck muscles to protect against injury from low and moderate velocity collision. At the same time, the static maximum loads of Figure 1 represent the injury potential from marked startle response within the neck muscles.

At higher impact velocities, intersegmental motions exceed the physiological range. Within the first 50 to 75 milliseconds, complex S-shaped neck configurations are achieved causing focal bending stresses that may occur anywhere in the spine depending on the direction of the

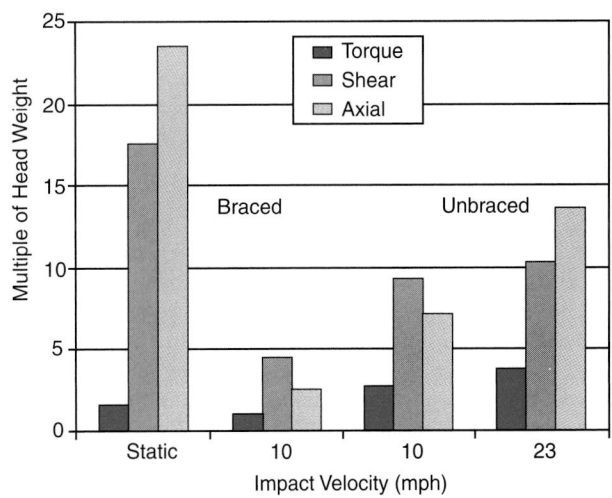

Fig. 1. Neck muscle bracing. The effect of neck muscle bracing in volunteers compared with that in cadavers (unbraced) under impact velocities of 10 and 23 miles per hour. The "static" impact represents the maximum loads achieved before overcoming volunteer muscle resistance to head movement. (Adapted from Gadd CW, Culver CC, Nahum AM, et al: A study of responses and tolerances of the neck. In Backaitis SH [ed]: Biomechanics of Impact Injury and Injury Tolerances of the Head-Neck Complex. Warrendale, PA, Society of Automotive Engineers, 1993, pp 73–85.)

impact force.[26] During the whipping motions of the spine, pressure gradients develop across the spinal cord and intervertebral foramina.[27] The result may be any combination of damage to the anterior or posterior soft-tissues, disk, facet joints, and neural tissues. Injury to the temporomandibular joint may arise from extreme neck extension while the mouth is open, followed by strong anterior neck compartment muscle contraction.

Because the spine tolerates shear and axial stresses better than bending moments, the direction of loading can make the difference between severe and mild or no injury for a specific accident. High energy rear-end collisions that break the seat backs actually reduce the risk for cervical whiplash. At the same time, they increase the incidence of low back injury as the passenger, falling backward with the broken seat, shifts the bending moment from the cervical to the lumbar spine. Similarly, impacts from other directions or with the passenger in altered postures at the moment of impact will have complex bending stresses at different spinal locations. Front-end collisions may also transfer stress through the legs or arms that are often braced against the floorboard or steering wheel.

CLINICAL FEATURES

PATIENT EVALUATION

Neck pain and stiffness are the most common neck complaints following motor vehicle accidents. One cannot overemphasize the importance of a clear and accurate history in evaluation of the postaccident patient. Preexisting medical conditions, preexisting neck pain and/or headache, and prior treatments for those conditions must be documented and addressed. Similarly, any history of prior neurological signs or symptoms must be ascertained by the physician

TABLE 1. FACTORS TENDING TO ENHANCE OR REDUCE MECHANISMS OF INJURY DURING A MOTOR VEHICLE COLLISION

Factor	Prognostics
Occupant age	Not important
Occupant sex	Female (70%); Men 1.5 times risk of severe injury
Occupant position	Front > rear; passenger > driver
Occupant posture	Asymmetric > symmetric
Occupant anticipation	Relaxed > braced
Impact direction	Side/oblique (neck or low back) > front (neck or low back) > rear (neck)
Impact energy	High > low (hard tissue/disc); low > high (soft tissue)
Head rest use	Shoulder height > occipital height
Air bag deployment	Reduced mortality; increased injury to head, face, chest
Seat/shoulder belt use	Reduced mortality; increased injury to chest, thorax
Seat integrity	Intact—increased neck injury. Broken—increased low back injury (rear-end collision only)

Adapted from Borenstein DG, Wiesel SW, Boden SD: Neck Pain: Medical Diagnosis and Comprehensive Management. Philadelphia, WB Saunders, 1996, p 28.

doing the initial evaluation. Early and accurate documentation of these preexisting conditions will be of immeasurable help later in the course of treatment, when it may be necessary from both medical and medicolegal perspectives to dissect out those areas of continuing disability that are the result of the index trauma.

Position of the head at the moment of impact, location within the involved vehicle, seat belt usage, seat back breakage, head or facial injuries, loss of consciousness, and any transient paresis must all be discussed with the patient and incorporated into the medical record. Types of vehicles and relative rates of speed may also be helpful to the treating physician in estimating the forces and vectors involved, helping to focus the assessment, and suggesting other areas of potential injury.

Physical examination should include observation of the neck for the patient's resting posture, as well as neck motion as the patient follows the physician's movements when entering the examination room. Palpation for tenderness and muscle spasm, attempting to localize the involved tissues, is often helpful in focusing on the more involved areas. Global tenderness from the occiput to the interscapular regions is commonly found for the first few days after injury. Palpation of the cervical spine anteriorly through the neck may locate discrete tenderness that may be an indication of anterior column injury in response to cervical hyperextension.

A neurological screening examination should be performed to rule out radiculopathy or myelopathy. Any suggestion of post-traumatic objective upper or lower motor neuron involvement after vehicular trauma should immediately trigger a more thorough evaluation. The cervical spine should be immobilized and an initial lateral cervical spine radiograph should be scrutinized for any suggestion of prevertebral soft-tissue swelling, fracture, or soft-tissue ligamentous disruption. Other views should be carefully evaluated. With clinical evidence of acute myelopathy, a magnetic resonance imaging (MRI) scan should be obtained to screen for extrinsic or intrinsic cord injury. A computed tomography (CT) scan may be necessary to diagnose occult bony injury, or to better evaluate skeletal trauma.

In the majority of patients, however, no objective neurological abnormalities will be found. The typical findings of cervical muscle tenderness and spasm with restricted range of motion should be followed by review of routine neck radiographs. Anteroposterior, lateral, and open-mouth views should be utilized in general screening of these patients. Any suspicious or positive finding would trigger additional views or studies. Flexion-extension lateral views are usually of little value in acute-phase diagnosis, since protective muscle spasm may mask underlying instability. They may be more useful after initial conservative treatment has reduced the protective muscle spasm.

INVESTIGATION

INJECTION THERAPIES

Selective nerve root blocks may add clinical information to the cause of ongoing post-whiplash pain. These blocks can occasionally be therapeutic as well, with small amounts of corticosteroids administered along with the local anesthetic agents. There are surprisingly few data to scientifically demonstrate the efficacy of these blocks, however.

Nerve blocks are typically done under fluoroscopic image intensification, and the operator must have an excellent knowledge of cervical anatomy. Placement of the needle tip at the exit foramen of the nerve root in question and the achievement of hypoalgesia in the sensory distribution of that root are necessary for a successful block. Temporary relief of pain may indicate a favorable result with surgical decompression and/or stabilization.

The proximal cervical roots have been referred to as "the forgotten roots." Symptoms of pain, numbness, or dysesthesias over the back of the scalp, the side of the face, or the top of the shoulder may suggest involvement of the C2, C3, or C4 roots respectively. Blocks may be therapeutic as well as diagnostic, but surgical decompression or neurectomies may occasionally be required.

The role of trigger point injections is unclear. Although they are a commonly used modality in the treatment of chronic soft-tissue pain, more recent randomized studies have failed to establish efficacy over acupuncture or vapocoolant-accupressure in low back pain.[28]

Cervical facet blocks are occasionally used for both diagnostic and therapeutic reasons. Cervical facet sclerotomes have been mapped in healthy subjects.[29] Long-term results of facet injections with depot corticosteroids have been disappointing, with no longer-lasting pain relief than injection with local anesthetic alone.[30]

CERVICAL DISCOGRAPHY

CT and MRI revolutionized the diagnostic imaging of the cervical spine. Despite their advantages, correlation of symptoms with imaging data is not always possible.[31, 32] Abnormal imaging findings are found in up to 28% of asymptomatic individuals.[33] Conversely, Schellhas[32] demonstrated that symptomatic and significant annular tears may be present in disks that appear normal on MRI. Provocative or analgesic diskography offers a dynamic test of a potentially symptomatic disk, which can furnish additional information to the patient's database.

The role of cervical diskography as a diagnostic screening tool continues to be controversial despite increasing amounts of scientific evidence to validate its use. Older articles tended to deride diskography as poorly sensitive,[34, 35] painful, expensive, and without diagnostic value.[36] Some proponents argued against the conclusions of these researchers.[8, 37, 38] In the early 1980s, proponents of diskography became more numerous, and although significant polarization in the medical community regarding the usefulness of this modality still exists, advocates of diskography are becoming more numerous as the scientific evidence for its utility mounts.

Cervical diskogenic syndrome as a separate clinical entity, initially termed internal disk disruption, was popularized by Crock,[39] who described disk lesions unassociated with rupture or other easily defined anatomic disorder. He postulated an internal biochemical basis for the frequently described symptoms of deep-seated, dull aching neck pain, commonly associated with generalized nondermatomal limb pain, headache, and constitutional symptoms.

Several authors have reported that using cervical diskography as a surgical screening tool leads to good-to-excellent postoperative results in 93%, 70%, and 73% of patients.[40–42] Complication rates are generally reported as quite low in centers where diskography is done routinely. Guyer[43] noted an inverse relationship between complication rate and number of procedures done per month. In his series, Guyer reported 1.49% complications based on the number of disks injected. Connor and Darden[44] reported complications in 4/31 (13%) of their patients, while in a much larger series of 4400 disk injections in 1357 patients performed by an experienced radiologist, Zeidman et al[45] reported significant complications occurring in less than 0.6% of the patients and 0.16% of the cervical disks.

At present, cervical diskography is a highly specialized diagnostic procedure best performed by an individual with special expertise and experience. A positive result requires both an abnormal anatomic lesion as well as concordant pain reproduction with provocative diskography, and/or specific pain relief with analgesic disk injection. Results of diskography should not serve alone as a surgical indication, but should be incorporated into the gestalt of the individual patient's clinical situation.

INSTANTANEOUS HELICAL AXIS TESTING

Several studies have shown that the frequency of WADs has increased over time.[15, 21, 46] This increased frequency is associated with higher costs at a time when cost-benefit issues are paramount in the health care industry. Publication of the Quebec Task Force report[6] has resulted in greater interest in the quality investigation of this phenomenon. Such investigations must create clearer definitions of WADs. It is very likely that WADs cannot be studied as a whole, but rather that individual disorders within this group must be evaluated with respect to guidelines for appropriate treatment.

Continuing to confound this area of clinical study is the controversy surrounding the degree of symptom amplification that may be associated with hyperflexion-hyperextension injuries, especially in light of the litigation that frequently accompanies motor vehicle accidents where injury is suspected. Attempts have been made to distinguish between "malingering," post-trauma cognitive disorders,[47] and psychological stresses that would be expected due to post-traumatic chronic pain complaints.[21]

New technologies are constantly created with the hope of clarifying some of these concerns. With the onset of MRI, improved imaging of soft-tissue damage has led to greater appreciation of the whiplash patient whose lesion had no possibility of being viewed before. Unfortunately, the MRI does not provide motion analysis of the patient. As such, those victims of WAD whose biomechanical lesion is best viewed dynamically, while in motion, continue to be misdiagnosed.

A promising new technology involves the evaluation of instantaneous helical axis motion. The instantaneous helical axis (IHA) is a mathematical description of three-dimensional movement. In the case of the cervical spine, the movement of the head is calculated relative to the trunk. Characteristics of the IHA have been assembled to describe differences between a pool of patients seeking treatment for neck-related complaints and a pool of normal individuals. Patients under care for their neck complaints were divided into those suspected of amplifying their symptoms and those reporting their complaints accurately. Eighty-four percent correct classification was achieved using this model. The results of the study were confirmed in a second data set.[48]

In addition to identifying symptom amplifiers, there is the potential to evaluate relationships between patterns of motion, clinical status, and clinical outcome. In a small population of whiplash-injured patients and other mechanical neck pain patients, it was observed that the average intersection of the IHA (piercing point) in the sagittal plane during flexion and extension was different for those with upper versus lower cervical spine pain.[49] In addition, no differences were found between patients experiencing mechanical spine pain versus those with WAD.

Initial work has been completed looking at patterns of cervical motion in postfusion patients. Differences in the behavior of the IHA have been observed between symptomatically resolved post–neck fusion cases and those with residual and/or recurrent problems.[50] Fusion cases were studied in this initial investigation, because they provide the most dramatic circumstances for alteration in IHA movement that can be expected to occur clinically. With further research, insights should be available for the evaluation of pattern distortions in mechanical neck pain patients such as those with WAD. Treatment protocols tailored more specifically to the biomechanical idiosyncrasies of individual patients may provide greater clinical success.

MANAGEMENT

MEDICAL TREATMENT

Early mobilization following whiplash trauma is preferable to the traditional recommendations of rest and a cervical collar. Three-quarters of these patients will improve within a few months. Although early aggressive interventional therapy is empirically attractive, there is no scientific evidence proving its efficacy.

Collars for immobilization should have very limited usage, and should be reserved for those instances where severe spasm or radicular pain with neck motion is present. If necessary, collars should be removed several times a day, and discontinued after 5 to 10 days. There is no place for chronic use of a cervical collar in the management of post-whiplash neck pain.

Initial medical therapy has traditionally included prescriptions of nonsteroidal anti-inflammatory drugs (NSAIDs), muscle relaxants, and non-narcotic analgesics. Some practitioners have advocated treatment of acute whiplash with intramuscular or oral corticosteroids, but no scientific evidence exists for use of these medications.

In a prospective study of whiplash patients, no benefit of outpatient physical therapy could be identified when compared with a home rehabilitation program. Most of the therapeutic modalities that are commonly prescribed have not been scientifically validated. Although facet joint pain has been found in over half of chronic whiplash pain patients, intra-articular steroid injections were not found to be effective for long-term pain relief.

The Quebec Task Force has suggested that treatment for whiplash be based on the degree of injury, as determined by the presenting signs and symptoms. For a grade I injury (pain, stiffness, or tenderness without any physical signs) work restrictions are not generally necessary. Non-narcotic analgesics and NSAIDs are appropriate in grade II injuries, where there are musculoskeletal signs. Neurological signs (decreased or absent deep tendon reflexes, motor weakness, sensory deficit) may require narcotic medications, as well as appropriate work restrictions.

Patients remaining symptomatic after two months of treatment fall into a subacute group with a poorer overall prognosis. The financial burden of whiplash injury results mainly from the 15% to 30% that become chronic. Patients with disabilities lasting between 2 and 6 months account for 38% of the total costs, and those disabled longer than 6 months account for 46% of the total cost to society.

Surgical treatment for injuries resulting from whiplash is very infrequent. Instability, mechanical pain, and neurological compression are all rare sequelae of whiplash. Acute instability, such as in unrecognized facet dislocation following hyperflexion, should generally be diagnosed from the initial postinjury radiographs. A dislocation that spontaneously reduces may remain undiagnosed for 1 to 2 weeks, until protective cervical muscle spasm subsides and allows the instability to be visualized on flexion-extension lateral films. Focal interspinous tenderness, interspinous widening on lateral radiograph, or evidence of soft-tissue disruption on MRI scan may also be helpful in making this diagnosis. Posterior cervical fusion is indicated for soft-tissue capsular and ligamentous injuries, with generally excellent results. Unilateral facet fractures may be treated with immobilization, but late pain from post-traumatic facet arthritis may require later fusion. Diagnostic facet joint blocks, or interspinous ligament blocks are occasionally useful in diagnosis when soft-tissue strains without mechanical disruption are suspected.

Cervical myelopathy or radiculopathy rarely result from whiplash trauma. Central cord syndromes or episodes of transient quadriparesis may rarely follow whiplash in individuals with preexisting canal stenosis. Those cases must be addressed on an individual basis. Nerve root irritation secondary to disk herniation or foraminal compression occurs in a very small number of patients. Only a history clearly negative for any preexisting neck and arm pain in an individual symptomatic immediately following vehicular trauma should make one suspicious of whiplash-related injury as the causative factor.

Other than progressive myelopathy, these neurological injuries should all be treated conservatively, with the expectation that the majority will improve. Only after failure of nonoperative treatment, persistent radicular irritability, and a correlative anatomic lesion, should surgical intervention be considered. Although a pure nerve root irritation caused by a posterolateral soft-disk herniation or foraminal stenosis can be addressed by a posterior laminoforamenotomy, the presence of axial neck pain should suggest mechanical disruption of the disk as well. If diskogenic pain is contributing to the patient's pain and disability, then anterior cervical diskectomy and fusion is the procedure of choice. This procedure has an excellent track record for technical fusion and satisfactory patient outcome.

ADDITIONAL TREATMENT: THE ROLE OF MANIPULATION

Increased function is promoted by the appropriate and limited use of chiropractic manipulation, mobilization, massage, and exercises. Manipulation provides pain relief and increased motion.[51-53] Flexibility exercises that emphasize self-stretching, bilaterally symmetrical activity (e.g., walking, swimming), and low-intensity resistive efforts can be initiated early, generally within the first 2 weeks. Exercise should be goal-directed and focus on those activities that support return to preinjury status and function.[54]

Manipulation has earned scientific and clinical recognition. Its use in general practice is growing but deserves cautionary comment. As emphasized by the Quebec Task Force, these procedures should only be attempted by clinicians skilled and experienced in their use. Manipulation applies controlled loading of the spine that must alter motion segment behavior without interfering with tissue healing. The skills to perform these procedures are complex and do not transfer from one manual process (e.g., surgical tool handling or physical therapy soft-tissue work) to another.[55-57]

Patients with activity intolerance that persists beyond 12 weeks should undergo multidisciplinary reassessment.[6] If significant life style interruption, family disruption, or work dissatisfaction is involved, a psychological consultation may be useful to quantify and address psychosocial factors that may hinder further recovery. A focused, goal-directed rehabilitation program should be initiated while passive treatments, like manipulation and physical therapy modalities, should be limited. Nociceptive pain generators may require a return to passive treatment as an adjunctive method to sustain continued patient activation.[58, 59] Rehabilitation objectives should address postural and ergonomic faults, proper spinal biomechanics, improved range of motion, strengthening, and endurance. Aquatherapy in neck-deep water can provide a smooth transition to more aggressive patient activation. Intensity of the exercise is controlled by depth of the water, speed of movement, and resistance boards or aqua gloves.[60] As the patient progresses to land-based exercise, special attention should be given to the muscular balance for the thorax and shoulder girdle as a foundation for neck function.[61] Typical cervical muscle imbalances found in WAD syndrome patients include weakness of the deep neck flexors and hypertonicity of the suboccipital extensors.[62] Overactivity of the scalenes, sternomastoid, pectoral muscles, and upper trapezius are also commonly present. The patient should be trained in appropriate relaxation techniques complementing progressive resistance exercises to restore muscular balance and function.

DISCUSSION

Practice guidelines regarding the diagnosis and treatment of whiplash should incorporate the current knowledge base discussed in this chapter. Patients should be mobilized as soon as possible after injury. Earlier identification of those individuals who will remain refractory to treatment, possibly utilizing techniques like IHA testing, may allow for better allocation of health care resources.

REFERENCES

1. Barnsley L, Lord S, Bogduk N: Whiplash injury. Pain 1994; 58:283.
2. Freeman MD, Croft AC, Rossignol AM: "Whiplash associated disorders: redefining whiplash and its management" by the Quebec Task Force. A critical evaluation. Spine 1998; 23:1043.
3. Foret-Bruno J, Dauvilliers F, Tamere C: Influence of the seat and headrest stiffness on the risk of cervical injuries. 13th International Technical Conference on Experimental Safety Vehicles, Scottsdale, AZ, 1991.
4. Olsson J, Bunketop O, Carlsson G, et al: An indepth study of neck injuries in rear end collisions. International IRCBI Conference: September 12–14, 1990.
5. Hildingsson C, Toolanen G: Outcome after soft-tissue injury of the cervical spine. A prospective study of 93 car-accident victims. Acta Orthop Scand 1990; 61:357.
6. Spitzer WO, Skovron ML, Salmi LR, et al: Scientific monograph of the Quebec Task Force on Whiplash-Associated Disorders: Redefining "whiplash" and its management. Spine 1995; 20:1S.
7. Dvorak J, Valach L, Schmid S: Injuries of the cervical spine in Switzerland. Orthopade 1987; 16:2.
8. Hohl M: Soft-tissue injuries of the neck in automobile accidents. Factors influencing prognosis. J Bone Joint Surg Am 1974; 56:1675.
9. Pearce JM: Whiplash injury: a reappraisal. J Neurol Neurosurg Psychiatry 1989; 52:1329.
10. Gargan MF, Bannister GC: Long-term prognosis of soft-tissue injuries of the neck. J Bone Joint Surg Br 1990; 72:901.
11. Radanov BP, Sturzenegger M, Di Stefano G: Long-term outcome after whiplash injury. A 2-year follow-up considering features of injury mechanism and somatic, radiologic, and psychosocial findings. Medicine (Baltimore) 1995; 74:281.
12. Schrader H, Obelieniene D, Bovim G, et al: Natural evolution of late whiplash syndrome outside the medicolegal context. Lancet 1996; 347:1207.
13. Kolbinson DA, Epstein JB, Burgess JA: Temporomandibular disorders, headaches, and neck pain following motor vehicle accidents and the effect of litigation: Review of the literature. J Orofac Pain 1996; 10:101.
14. Lord SM, Barnsley L, Wallis BJ, et al: Chronic cervical zygapophysial joint pain after whiplash. A placebo-controlled prevalence study. Spine 1996; 21:1737.
15. Galasko CS, Murray PM, Pitcher M, et al: Neck sprains after road traffic accidents: A modern epidemic. Injury 1993; 24:155.
16. Friedman D, Flanders A, Thomas C, et al: Vertebral artery injury after acute cervical spine trauma: Rate of occurrence as detected by MR angiography and assessment of clinical consequences. AJR Am J Roentgenol 1995; 164:443.
17. Lorenz J, Kunze K, Bromm B: Differentiation of conversive sensory loss and malingering by P300 in a modified oddball task. Neuroreport 1998; 9:187.
18. Gimse R, Bjorgen IA, Straume A: Driving skills after whiplash. Scand J Psychol 1997; 38:165.
19. Evans RW: Some observations on whiplash injuries. Neurol Clin 1992; 10:975.
20. Mills H, Horne G: Whiplash—manmade disease? N Z Med J 1986; 99:373.
21. Mayou R, Radanov BP: Whiplash neck injury. J Psychosom Res 1996; 40:461.
22. Partyka S: Whiplash and other inertial force neck injuries in traffic accidents. Paper from Mathematical Analysis Division, National Center for Statistics and Analysis, Atlanta, GA, 1981.
23. Mertz H Jr, Patrick LM: Investigation of the kinematics and kinetics of whiplash. In Backaitis SH (ed): Biomechanics of Impact Injury and Injury Tolerances of the Head-Neck Complex. Warrendale, PA, Society of Automotive Engineers, 1993, p 43.
24. Gadd CW, Culver CC, Nahum AM: A study of responses and tolerances of the neck. In Backaitis SH (ed): Biomechanics of Impact Injury and Injury Tolerances of the Head-Neck Complex. Warrendale, PA, Society of Automotive Engineers, 1993, p 73.
25. Pope MH, Aleksiev A, Hasselquist L, et al: Neurophysiologic mechanisms of low-velocity non-head-contact cervical acceleration. In Gunzburg R, Szpalski M (eds): Whiplash Injuries: Current Concepts in Prevention, Diagnosis, and Treatment of the Cervical Whiplash Syndrome. Philadelphia, Lippincott-Raven, 1997, p 89.
26. Panjabi MH, Gauer JN, Cholewicki J, et al: Whiplash trauma injury mechanism: A biomechanical viewpoint. In Gunzburg R, Szpalski M (eds): Whiplash Injuries: Current Concepts in Prevention, Diagnosis, and Treatment of the Cervical Whiplash Syndrome. Philadelphia, Lippincott-Raven, 1997, p 79.
27. Svensson MY: Injury biomechanics. In Gunzburg R, Szpalski M (eds): Whiplash Injuries: Current Concepts in Prevention, Diagnosis, and Treatment of the Cervical Whiplash Syndrome. Philadelphia, Lippincott-Raven, 1997, p 69.
28. Garvey TA, Marks MR, Wiesel SW: A prospective, randomized, double-blind evaluation of trigger-point injection therapy for low-back pain. Spine 1989; 14:962.
29. Dwyer A, Aprill C, Bogduk N: Cervical zygapophyseal joint pain patterns I: A study in normal volunteers. Spine 1990; 15:453.
30. Barnsley L, Lord SM, Wallis BJ, et al: Lack of effect of intraarticular corticosteroids for chronic pain in the cervical zygapophyseal joints. N Engl J Med 1994; 330:1047.
31. Parfenchuck TA, Janssen ME: A correlation of cervical magnetic resonance imaging and diskography/computed tomographic disograms. Spine 1994; 19:2819.
32. Schellhas KP, Smith MD, Gundry CR, et al: Cervical diskogenic pain. Prospective correlation of magnetic resonance imaging and diskography in asymptomatic subjects and pain sufferers. Spine 1996; 21:300.
33. Boden SD, McCowin PR, Davis DO, et al: Abnormal magnetic-resonance scans of the cervical spine in asymptomatic subjects. A prospective investigation. J Bone Joint Surg Am 1990; 72:1178.
34. Lindblom K: Diagnostic puncture of intervertebral disk in sciatica. Acta Orthop Scand 1948; 17:131.
35. Scoville W, Whitcomb B, McLaurin R: The cervical ruptured disk: Report of 115 operative cases. Trans Am Neurol Assoc 1951; 76.
36. Holt EP: Fallacy of cervical diskography. JAMA 1964; 188:799.
37. Cloward RB: Cervical diskography defended. JAMA 1975; 233:862.
38. Cloward RB: Cervical diskography: Technique, indications and use in diagnosis of ruptured cervical disk. AJR Am J Roentgenol 1958; 79:563.
39. Crock HV, Bedbrook GM: Practice of Spinal Surgery. New York, Springer-Verlag, 1983, p 319.
40. Roth DA: Cervical analgesic diskography. A new test for the definitive diagnosis of the painful-disk syndrome. JAMA 1976; 235:1713.
41. Whitecloud TSI, Seago RA: Cervical diskogenic syndrome. Results of operative intervention in patients with positive diskography. Spine 1987; 12:313.
42. Siebenrock KA, Aebi M: Cervical diskography in diskogenic pain syndrome and its predictive value for cervical fusion. Arch Orthop Trauma Surg 1994; 113:199.
43. Guyer RD, Ohnmeiss DD, Mason SL, et al: Complications of cervical diskography: Findings in a large series. J Spinal Disord 1997; 10:95.
44. Connor PM, Darden BV: Cervical diskography complications and clinical efficacy. Spine 1993; 18:2035.
45. Zeidman SM, Thompson K, Ducker TB: Complications of cervical diskography: Analysis of 4400 diagnostic disk injections. Neurosurgery 1995; 37:414.
46. Versteegen GJ, Kingma J, Meijler WJ, et al: Neck sprain in patients injured in car accidents: A retrospective study covering the period 1970–1994. Eur Spine J 1998; 7:195.
47. Schmand B, Lindeboom J, Schagen S, et al: Cognitive complaints in patients after whiplash injury: The impact of malingering. J Neurol Neurosurg Psychiatry 1998; 64:339.
48. McGregor M, Block AR, Blumenthal SL, et al: Symptom amplification and neck pain patients: An objective test. Presented at the North American Spine Society and American Spine Society Meeting, April 26–29, 1998, Charleston, SC.
49. McGregor M, Triano JJ, Kohlbeck FJ: Instantaneous helical axis location for upper versus lower neck pain. ACC Convention, March 18–20, 1999, Orlando, FL.
50. Triano JJ, McGregor M, Zigler J: An objective model for discriminating neck pain using instantaneous kinematic parameters. Presented at the Seventeenth Annual Houston Conference on Biomedical Engineering Research, February 11, 1999, Houston, TX.

51. Triano JJ, McGregor M, Hondras MA, et al: Manipulative therapy versus education programs in chronic low back pain. Spine 1995; 20:948.

52. Cassidy JD, Lopes AA, Yong-Hing K: The immediate effect of manipulation versus mobilization on pain and range of motion in the cervical spine: A randomized controlled trial [see comments]. J Manipulative Physiol Ther 1992; 15:570.

53. Hurwitz EL, Aker PD, Adams AH, et al: Manipulation and mobilization of the cervical spine. A systematic review of the literature. Spine 1996; 21:1746; discussion 1759.

54. Borenstein DG, Wiesel SW, Boden SD: Neck Pain: Medical Diagnosis and Comprehensive Management. Philadelphia, WB Saunders, 1996.

55. Cohen E, Triano JJ, McGregor M, et al: Biomechanical performance of spinal manipulation therapy by newly trained vs. practicing providers: Does experience transfer to unfamiliar procedures? J Manipulative Physiol Ther 1995; 18:347.

56. Triano JJ, McGregor M, Skogsbergh D, et al: Rating of skill in lumbar spinal manipulative therapy. Proceedings of the International Conference on Spinal Manipulation, 1994, Palm Springs, CA.

57. Triano JJ, Skogsbergh D, McGregor M, et al: Biomechanical parameters of skill in lumbar spinal manipulative therapy. Proceedings of the International Conference on Spinal Manipulation, 1994, Palm Springs, CA.

58. Triano JJ, McGregor M, Skogsbergh DR: Use of chiropractic manipulation in lum-

bar rehabilitation. J Rehabil Res Dev 1997; 34:394.

59. Lewit K: Role of manipulation in spinal rehabilitation. In Leibenson C (ed): Rehabilitation of the Spine: A Practitioner's Manual. Baltimore: Williams & Wilkins, 1996, p 195.

60. Ruoti RG, Morris DM, Cole AJ: Aquatic Therapy. Philadelphia, Lippincott, 1997, p 85.

61. Leibenson C: Active rehabilitation protocols. In Leibenson C (ed): Rehabilitation of the Spine: A Practitioner's Manual. Baltimore, Williams & Wilkins, 1996, p 355.

62. Treleaven J, Jull G, Atkinson L: Cervical musculoskeletal dysfunction in post-concussional headache. Cephalalgia 1994; 14: 273.

CHRONIC LOW BACK PAIN

section 8
chapter 9

Tom G. Mayer, Robert J. Gatchel, and Trent H. Evans

Summary

- All too often, the patient with chronic low back pain (CLBP) is either over- or undertreated. In some cases, the chronic patient simply becomes an annuity for a health provider, who provides unrelenting high-cost palliative care of no durable value either to the patient or society; in other cases, the patient is simply ignored and as a result becomes nonproductive.
- CLBP represents the highest cost of ongoing welfare benefits under the Social Security Disability Income program for workers younger than 45 years.
- The average age for workers to fall under Social Security Disability Income for CLBP is 35 to 40 years; they continue to receive benefits for being nonproductive for a far longer time than patients with other common disabilities (cardiovascular, arthritis, or even psychiatric illnesses).
- Developing programs that are effective in helping patients become productive at work, at recreation, and at home remains a vital goal for those involved in treating CLBP.
- Functional restoration has been demonstrated empirically to be a very effective treatment method for CLBP.

DEFINITION

In more than 90% of cases, back pain is a brief, time-limited condition for which the treatment chosen often appears irrelevant to the outcome.[1] From the onset of symptoms, about 50% of patients with acute low back pain are no longer disabled within 2 weeks, 70% recover in 1 month, and about 90% recover within 3 to 4 months.[2] Of those whose symptoms persist for more than 3 to 4 months, the majority will continue to be disabled and unable to work at the end of 1 year, and the greatest number of these individuals will continue to be disabled after 2 years. These patients often have extensive medical treatment, compensation costs, and settlement awards that make their contribution to the problem disproportionate to that of the entire group suffering CLBP. Most studies demonstrate that the mean cost of low back pain care is more than 10 times greater than the median cost, implying that the relatively small number of chronic cases encompass the majority share of social and financial losses. The most disabled 5% of workers with occupational low back pain account for 85% of costs over 15 years in the United States.[3]

Even in situations of CLBP, it has been estimated that a structural diagnosis is made only 60% of the time. When a physical diagnosis is made in these cases, it may be irrelevant to the primary causes of persistent pain and disability.[2] The severity of low back pain, particularly in the workers' compensation setting, is much more dependent on the chronicity of the condition and the disability created than on the inciting event (in contrast to other events with orthopaedic trauma). The majority of worker injuries to the low back involves the soft tissues with an initial diagnosis of sprains and strains of musculoligamentous tissues. In most cases, soft-tissue injuries have a relatively brief healing period. Imperfect healing may result in biomechanical dysfunction and *permanent impairment* of important supporting elements. Degenerative disk arthritis, chronic pain, and disability may follow. In this case, socioeconomic cost in terms of loss of human productivity, medical cost, and disability-related indemnity benefits escalate dramatically.

Because a structural diagnosis is often not made in CLBP patients, or even when made may not be materially

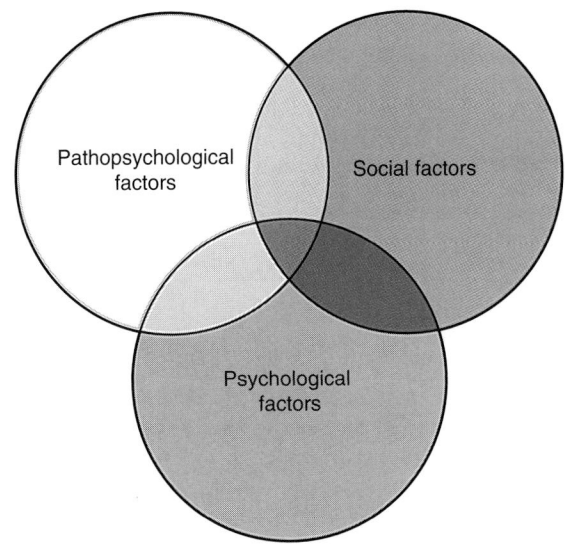

Fig. 1. Model. This is the biopsychosocial model of chronic pain.

related to ongoing pain and disability, patients suffering from CLBP have commonly been categorized as having a psychogenic or nonorganic problem. This view stems from the conventional medical perspective that classifies the nature of pain as either organic or psychogenic. This simplistic perspective falls short of adequately elucidating the chronic pain phenomenon. A strong amount of evidence suggests high comorbidity between psychological disturbances and physical disorders for medical patients in general, and more significantly for chronic pain patients.[4–8] There has been little allowance for these comorbid conditions in the unidimensional traditional medical model. The more recent biopsychosocial model of pain (Fig. 1) addresses these comorbid conditions, which are highlighted in the next section.

HISTORICAL REVIEW

New terms and concepts have emerged in the scientific literature in an attempt to conceptualize pain more adequately. Engel[9] coined the term "psychogenic pain," which evolved into the "pain-prone disorder." Melzack and Wall[10] developed the "gate-control theory of pain," attempting to explain the various psychophysiological aspects that interplay in pain perception. This model asserts that the dorsal horns of the spinal cord serve a gate-like capacity, regulating the transmission and intensity of nerve signals from peripheral fibers to the central nervous system. According to this model, psychological processing plays a significant role in the resulting pain experience. Consequently, pain is viewed not as a result of a specific biological stimulus but as the result of an interaction between psychological and physiological reactions. Before the gate-control theory, psychological correlates of pain were conceptualized as mere epiphenomena.[11] In addition to physiological and psychological factors, sociocultural variables have also been noted to have an important impact in the onset and maintenance of pain.[12] Mechanic[13, 14] noted the manner in which a patient responds to symptoms may be conceptualized as an

operation of the social implications of that behavior. Some examples of this include evasion of unwanted work and responsibilities, special attention from others, and financial compensation. Other behavioral concomitants of symptom expression include how individuals observe their bodies, define and interpret their symptoms, take therapeutic action, and implement available sources of help.[15]

As a result of these developments, the biopsychosocial model of pain emerged as a comprehensive means of assessing, conceptualizing, and treating low back pain. This multidimensional model takes into account a patient's physiological, biological, cognitive, affective, behavioral, and social factors in attempting to understand the reported pain. Further, these factors are viewed as interdependent. For example, biological conditions may initiate and perpetuate a physiological disturbance. Psychological factors impact the patient's perception and assessment of the physical stimuli. Social factors impact the individual's behavior in reaction to the pain experience. Turk[11] identified three hallmarks of the biopsychosocial model of pain: integrated action, reciprocal determinism, and evolution. He notes that "no single factor in isolation—pathophysiological, psychological, or social—will adequately explain chronic pain status." It has been asserted that it is important to conceptualize low back pain and other chronic illnesses as an ongoing, long-term, fluid condition with reciprocal interplay among the patient's biological, psychological, and social factors.[16] The dynamic nature of these factors, along with variations in illness duration, explains the diversity with which low back pain is manifested among patients or within the same individual throughout the course of illness.

EPIDEMIOLOGY

Low back pain disability is the most expensive benign medical condition in industrialized countries and is the number one cause of disability in people younger than 45 years. For those older than 45 years, it is the third leading cause of disability, becoming progressively less of a factor during later years when function and productivity become of less concern than survival.[3] It has been estimated that in any one year, about 3% to 4% of the population in all industrialized countries has temporarily disabling low back pain and that more than 1% of the working-age population is "totally and permanently disabled" by this problem.[17] Low back pain has an estimated lifetime prevalence rate of 60% to 80%; 40% of these patients later experience recurrences, with 10% developing CLBP.[18] From a financial point of view, data from 1960 to 1975 revealed the medical bill for low back pain care to be $16 billion annually, slightly more than 50% of which was expended for surgical treatment.[19] Although there are no firm statistics available, it has been estimated that the cost of all aspects of low back pain care, including medical, compensation, legal, vocational, retraining, occupational modifications, and lost industrial productivity, may be in the range of 40 to 50 billion dollars annually.[2] A more startling trend is the disproportionate increase in low back pain disability as measured against population growth. It has been reported that low back pain disability increased at a rate 14 times the population growth from 1957 to 1976.[20]

PATHOGENESIS

Loss of the capacity to perform physical tasks may be associated both with structural lesions and decrements in physical capacity. An example of the first factor is a tibial fracture; an example of the second is the joint stiffness and muscle atrophy attendant on prolonged immobilization and pain-induced neural inhibiting influences that may, in some cases, go on to chronic pain and dysfunction. This example delineates general principles of behavior of the human organism following musculoskeletal injury. Soon after injury, effects of the trauma on structural factors predominate. Inflammation leads to repair of the tissue with the original mesothelial elements or, in the case of large defects, replacement with collagenous scar equivalents. In more significant trauma, the period of immobilization/inactivity may be prolonged and lead to dysfunctional behaviors, abetted by a variety of psychosocial and cultural factors. These dysfunctional behaviors may be succeeded by loss of physical capacity, measured by deterioration of a variety of basic elements of performance such as motion, strength, endurance, and agility.[22, 23] The longer the period of inactivity, the greater the opportunity for disuse to create physical capacity deficits, leading to decreased human performance. Ultimately, these changes lead to a variety of psychosocial and affective concomitants such as depression, medication abuse, and disability habituation. Pain may be a parallel factor, but its direct relationship to changes in muscles or other mesothelial structures remains a conundrum. Although pain may be a potent distractor of attention and inhibitor of function through a variety of fear-mediated mechanisms, its very subjectivity may create a simultaneous excuse for a patient to avoid recovery.

Passage of time is the critical factor. Physical capacity deficits are rarely a factor in human performance in the acute post-traumatic stages, but they become a gradually increasing factor accompanying inactivity and disuse. As time passes, functional deficits become the dominant physical impairment disabling the more chronic patient. Strength testing during the early post-traumatic time is hampered by invalid measurements because of pain-induced neuromuscular inhibition. There is also some limited concern that overaggressive attempts at achieving performance might actually exacerbate the injury during acute phases of occupational injury. Given usual soft-tissue healing periods, such concerns should no longer be necessary 1 to 2 months post-trauma. Although testing may be feasible from that point forward, deconditioning produced by inactivity is likely to make its appearance only after that acute period. Epidemiologically, the majority of occupational musculoskeletal cases will have resolved spontaneously by then. However, even as the healing process approaches a plateau, the cascade of progressive joint immobility, muscle inhibition/atrophy, decreased cardiovascular conditioning, and musculotendinous contracture will routinely follow disuse associated with occupational musculoskeletal injury if not actively dealt with. Many patients will recognize the problem and respond to gentle encouragement. Others will require consistent supervision and coaching on a group or individual basis.

Does atrophy or contracture represent the whole problem? The term "deconditioning syndrome" has been applied to the cumulative disuse changes produced in the chronically disabled patient suffering from spinal and other musculoskeletal chronic dysfunction. The syndrome is produced initially by the immobilization and inactivity attendant on injury, supplemented by disruption of spinal soft tissues and scarring resulting from degenerative change, surgical approaches, or repetitive microtrauma. As pain perception is enhanced, learned protective mechanisms lead to a *dynamic* vicious cycle of inactivity and disuse. As physical capacity decreases, the likelihood increases of fresh sprains/strains to unprotected joints, muscles, ligaments, and disks. The disruption of soft-tissue homeostasis accelerates pain, and dysfunction is typically perceived by the patient as a "recurrence" or "reinjury," but it is really secondary to a cycle of healing contracture and deconditioning. The concept of joint and muscle *inhibition* must be introduced to account for much of the measured loss of human performance. In normal subjects, there is generally a level of activity that is tolerated without overuse symptoms that is specific to that individual. The point at which overuse pain is produced is related to age, gender, body size, and current status of physical capacity. The degree to which the *overuse threshold* is exceeded determines the degree of injury. In deconditioning, there is a progressive shift of the activity/symptom curve to the left so that less and less activity is tolerated before overuse pain appears. This pain is perceived as reinjury by an already inhibited patient. Activity is further suppressed, and the level of physical capacity declines concomitantly. The relationship of activity and symptoms continues to shift until a steady state of relative inactivity and functional decline comes into balance. In certain individuals, such disability may simply involve eliminating a few home or recreational activities. In others, particularly those with heavier job demands and fewer transferable skills, the deconditioning may have devastating consequences, including total disability from work.

CLINICAL FEATURES

As early chronicity of impairment and disability lead to greater stress, fear of injury, and disuse of the injured body part, there is a tendency to develop a "weak link" in the injured musculoskeletal functional unit. The low back, which used to serve the patient so well, now breaks down after 1 hour of weeding in the garden. For those individuals developing such a problem, simple whole-person reconditioning is insufficient. Only by identifying the more specific elements of human performance primarily responsible for the weak link, such as rigidity of facet joints in the low back, can an effective therapeutic plan be developed.

The recognition of deconditioning associated with knee meniscal injuries and surgery in World War II and popularized by highly visible football players two decades later led to a therapeutic revolution in combined surgical and rehabilitation treatment of the knee that goes on today. Although facilitated by easy visual access, the concepts translate nicely to spinal and upper extremity disorders. Inactivity leads to loss of general body functional performance ability, well recognized by any athlete, with uniform loss of *functional capacity*. On the other hand, the injured area sustains more profound loss of para-articular soft-tissue function, becoming progressively greater as the period of disuse and immobilization increases. These changes create a weak link in the localized extremity joint or spinal region, whose *physical capacity* must be measured separately. What are the elements of performance that are of value in characterizing extremity physiological "functional units"? Such factors as range of motion, strength, neurological status, endurance combined with whole body aerobic capacity, and activities of daily living measurements are some of the major factors traditionally assessed.

INVESTIGATION

Evaluation of extremity neurological function (straight leg raising, lower extremity strength, sensation and reflexes in dermatomal/myotomal patterns) is still viewed by the majority of clinicians as the ideal objective spine functional evaluation, but these neurological characteristics may be irrelevant for several reasons. First, they are a measure of acute change when noted in relation to surgical pathology. In the chronic situation, persistence of neurological changes generally reflects epidural fibrosis or other permanent, noncorrectable anatomic abnormalities. In addition, the neurological deficits, although emanating from spinal structures, are perceived by the patient as *extremity abnormalities* producing pain, sensory changes, and weakness of arms/legs. In sum, what the clinician currently views as standard "objective" functional tests may provide no useful information to overcome spinal deconditioning.

When dealing with musculoskeletal disability, the various psychosocial and socioeconomic components associated with the physical symptoms are likely to make self-report of pain symptoms an unreliable gauge of treatment progression. For this reason, indirect, objective assessment of function is necessary. In fact, such quantitative measures are necessary for deriving any objective information about the spine, as compared with extremity rehabilitation, for which functional tests may be an adjunct luxury only. Objective, quantitative measurements of function provide the clinician with a definition of patient physical capacity; succeeding tests document changes in performance with treatment. Suboptimal effort demonstrates the degree to which barriers to recovery impede physical performance and lead to changes in psychosocial treatment interventions. Finally, at *maximum medical recovery,* the quantitative tests outline the patient's work capacity and the functional elements often required as part of impairment/disability evaluation.

MANAGEMENT

Pain clinics have proliferated over the past 35 years in response to the recognition that surgical correction of structural deficits could address spinal pain perception in only a small percentage of chronic patients and, in some cases, was associated with prolongation of disability (as in the "failed back surgery syndrome").[24–27] Poor surgical results in compensation patients associated with psychosocioeconomic disincentives have been documented from several quarters.[2, 20, 28–30] However, successful outcome studies using objective criteria from the large number of pain clinics actively treating chronically disabled back (and other) pain patients have failed to materialize. Rather, patient subjective reports of level of pain, use of medication, and levels of stress have appeared as criteria of improvement in the

pain literature. The originators of pain management made brilliant diagnostic contributions to the field by recognizing the importance of psychosocial factors to the CLBP problem.

The major problems arose not in diagnosis but in treatment. Behavioral modification principles were translated from simple animal models to complex human contingencies. Generally, passive physical therapy approaches and unquantified reactivation programs do not address the physical inhibition and deconditioning components of chronic pain. Pain, a subjective verbalized perception refractory to external measurement, remains the major focus of both the treatment process and outcome goals. Increased pain all too often results in return to primary or palliative care level passive modalities, sympathetic attention, inactivity, and avoidance behavior. Disability and its modification were most often ignored.

FUNCTIONAL RESTORATION

In response to the traditionally poor outcomes provided by pain clinics, *functional restoration* was developed and demonstrated to be therapeutically effective.[2, 31] Functional restoration, as a subset of chronic pain management, is a type of tertiary care that utilizes physical/functional capacity measurements and psychosocial assessments to organize a physician-directed, interdisciplinary-team treatment approach to restore patients to productivity. Multiple disciplines are required on site, with all patients having the benefit of access to each specialized group of health providers in an intensive program individualized to the initial assessments. An additional feature of these programs is the attention to outcome monitoring for all patients, with structured clinical interviews at 1 year. These interviews focus on specific objective factors related to cost and disability (such as return to work, health care utilization, injury recurrence, etc.).

The physical/functional capacity measurements are a vital aspect of developing an effective treatment program for disabling spinal disorders. These measures allow a quantitatively directed and individualized training progression approach to treatment. These quantified approaches address the great difficulty in assessing lumbar spine functioning caused by the lack of visual feedback to the deep, well-camouflaged spinal structures. This problem, combined with the absence of a comparison, contralateral side, makes it impossible to use the usual visual and semiquantitative physical capacity testing that assesses deficits and documents progress in extremity rehabilitation. This issue has not been generally recognized by clinicians, who often continue to rely on subjective self-reports or physical measures that are either inaccurate or irrelevant. More accurate methods are necessary for objective quantification.[31–34]

Following the initial physical/functional capacity and psychosocial assessment, a preprogram phase of treatment is initiated, whose duration and frequency are determined by degree of physical inhibition and psychosocial barriers that interfere with participation in the tertiary care team approach. In this phase, the physical and occupational therapists are involved primarily in patient confidence-building so as to overcome inhibition and fear of injury limiting physical performance, including mobilization and stretching designed to prepare the patient for the intensive muscle training portion of tertiary care. Psychologists and disability managers should be available to deal with early psychological (e.g., depression, substance use, psychosis, etc.) and social (e.g., financial, transportation, child care needs, etc.) barriers to program participation.

After physical and emotional stabilization, the patient enters an intensive phase of tertiary care. Program duration, education, and counseling are tailored to individual requirements. The program takes advantage of the *environment of function,* which is critical to the rehabilitation experience. Physical progress occurs through a quantitatively directed exercise program, supplemented by periodic objective human performance testing to document progress.[31, 35–40] If necessary, a postintensive phase of optional *work transition* may be added for those individuals lacking jobs to return to, requiring work simulation for particularly strenuous jobs, or possibly having to shift directly into a focused vocational rehabilitation placement or retraining option.

The reconditioning and work simulation aspects of the program involve therapists using active therapeutic exercise. Very little passive care (manipulation, injections, etc.) is used as these procedures provide an excuse for the patient to slip back into dependency.[41] If independence is to be achieved, the patient's own personal responsibility for accomplishing increasing physical tasks, with therapists as coaches, is essential. Terms such as "use it or lose it" and "no pain, no gain" are often used to motivate patients. Obviously, occasional pain control techniques, through use of nonhabituating anti-inflammatory medications or thermal modalities, is reasonable and can be used with minimal interference to the active therapeutic approach. Injections, if used sparingly and focused on *function* rather than *pain,* may also be helpful. For example, using intra- or para-articular cortisone injections may provide a potent localized anti-inflammatory to facilitate joint mobilization. Once accomplished, such mobilization may facilitate other aspects of the reconditioning process. Once diarthrodial joints are moving again, pain distraction from rigid arthritic joint capsules and surfaces declines, permitting stretching of spastic muscles after mild overuse and the training of muscles through a more physiological range. Quantification is necessary to optimally achieve these aspects of the program. The indirect assessments confirm functional deficits and psychosocial barriers to effort, leading to a combination of education and exercise training to resolve the deconditioning syndrome. Initial treatment is directed toward mobilizing and strengthening the injured weak links in the biomechanical chain, while whole body work simulation integrates the performance of this link with other parts of the body deconditioned by inactivity.

The cognitive-behavioral multimodal disability management program is based on diagnosis of psychosocioeconomic barriers to functional recovery for the individual. Specific treatments are designed for identified barriers. Initial treatment may be pharmacological, involving detoxification from habituating opiate and tranquilizer medications, use of antidepressants and anti-inflammatory medications, occasionally including antipsychotics.[42] Remaining treatments include a cognitive-behaviorally based program of education and counseling, including stress management, that is time-limited and aggressively oriented toward sequential goal-setting. Vocational planning, pain control skills, health education, and legal/administrative awareness components are provided. Failure to meet mutually prearranged goals could result in dismissal from the program.

COMPLICATIONS

The patient's ultimate socioeconomic outcomes depend on the maintenance of treatment goals. Under treatment supervision, patients generally achieve a much higher level of physical and functional capacities, which must be continued in a fitness maintenance program. The patient must be educated on an individualized program, based on the training level he or she has achieved. Repeated objective physical quantification leads to feedback to the patient on maintenance of physical capacity, which can be correlated with job demands. Relevant pieces of durable medical equipment or memberships in appropriately equipped fitness centers need to be suggested. The repeated physical testing, usually performed at 3- and 6-month postintensive intervals on a voluntary basis, comprises objective human performance tests and self-report tests of pain, disability, depression, and treatment satisfaction as one aspect of outcome monitoring.

RESULTS

The above functional restoration approach to the treatment of low back pain disability has received increasing attention in recent years because of its documented clinical efficacy.[2] Research has shown that the functional restoration program, when fully implemented, is associated with substantive improvement in various important societal outcome measures (e.g., return to work and resolution of outstanding legal and medical issues) in chronically disabled patients with spinal disorders in 1-year follow-up studies,[34, 39, 43–46] and a 2-year follow-up study.[31] For example, in the 2-year follow-up study by Mayer et al,[43] 87% of the functional restoration treatment group was actively working at 2 years as compared with only 41% of a nontreatment comparison group. Moreover, about twice as many of the nontreatment group of patients had additional spine surgery and unsettled workers' compensation litigation relative to the treatment group. The nontreatment group continued with an approximately five-times higher rate of patient visits to health professionals and higher rates of recurrence or reinjury. Thus, the results demonstrate the striking impact that a functional restoration program can have on these important outcome measures in a chronic group consisting primarily of workers' compensation cases (traditionally the most difficult cases to treat successfully).

Finally, it should be noted that the original functional restoration program was independently replicated by Hazard et al[34] in this country as well as by Bendix and Bendix[44] and Bendix et al[45] in Denmark; Hildebrandt et al[46] in Germany; and Corey et al[47] in Canada. The fact that different clinical treatment teams, functioning in different states (Texas and Vermont) and countries, with markedly different economic/social conditions and workers' compensation systems, produced comparable outcome results speaks highly for the robustness of the research findings and utility as well as the fidelity of this functional restoration approach. Hazard[33] has also reviewed the overall effectiveness of functional restoration.

REFERENCES

1. Deyo R: Conservative therapy for low back pain: Distinguishing useful from useless therapy. JAMA 1983; 250:1057.
2. Mayer TG, Gatchel RJ: Functional Restoration for Spinal Disorders: The Sports Medicine Approach. Philadelphia, Lea & Febiger, 1988.
3. Frymoyer JW: Epidemiology of spinal diseases. In Mayer TG, Mooney V, Gatchel RJ (eds): Contemporary Conservative Care for Painful Spinal Disorders. Philadelphia, Lea & Febiger, 1991.
4. Gatchel RJ: Psychological disorders and chronic pain: Cause-and-effect relationships. In Gatchel RJ, Turk DC (eds): Psychological Approaches to Pain Management: A Practitioner's Handbook. New York, Guilford, 1996.
5. Katon W, Sullivan MD: Depression and chronic mental illness. J Clin Psychiatry 1990; 51:3.
6. Kinney RK, Gatchel RJ, Ellis E, et al: Major psychological disorders in chronic TMD patients: Implications for successful management. J Am Dent Assoc 1992; 123:49.
7. Kinney RK, Gatchel RJ, Polatin PB, et al: Prevalence of psychopathology in acute and chronic low back pain patients. J Occup Rehabil 1993; 3:95.
8. Polatin PB, Kinney RK, Gatchel RJ, et al: Psychiatric illness and chronic low back pain. Spine 1993; 18:66.
9. Engel GL: Psychogenic pain and the pain-prone patient. Am J Med 1959; 26:900.
10. Melzack R, Wall PD: Pain mechanisms: A new theory. Science 1965; 150:971.
11. Turk DC: Biopsychosocial perspective on chronic pain. In Mayer TG, Mooney V, Gatchel RJ (eds): Contemporary Conservative Care for Painful Spinal Disorders. Philadelphia, Lea & Febiger, 1996.
12. Dworkin SF: Illness behavior and dysfunction: Review of concepts and application to chronic pain. Can J Physiol Pharmacol 1990; 69:662.
13. Mechanic D: Response factors in illness: The study of illness behavior. Social Psychiatry 1966; 1:11.
14. Mechanic D: Social psychological factors affecting the presentation of bodily complaints. New Engl J Med 1972; 286:1132.
15. Mechanic D: Illness behavior: An overview. In McHugh S, Vallis T (eds): Illness Behavior: A Multidisciplinary Model. New York, Plenum, 1985.
16. Dworkin SF, Von Korff MR, LeResche L: Multiple pains and psychiatric disturbance: An epidemiological investigation. Arch Gen Psychiatry 1990; 47:239.
17. Gatchel RJ, Polatin, PB, Mayer TG: The dominant role of psychosocial risk factors in the development of chronic low back pain disability. Spine 1995; 20:2702.
18. Anderrson GBJ, Pope MH, Frymoyer JW, et al: Epidemiology and cost. In Pope MH, Anderrson GBJ, Frymoyer JW, et al (eds): Occupational Low Back Pain: Assessment, Treatment, and Prevention. St. Louis, Mosby-Year Book, 1991.
19. Holbrook T, Grazier K, Kelsey J, et al (eds): The Frequency of Occurrence, Impact, and Cost of Musculoskeletal Conditions in the United States. Chicago, American Academy of Orthopedic Surgeons, 1984.
20. Fordyce W: Back pain, compensation, and public policy. In Rosen J, Solomon L (eds): Prevention in Health Psychology. Hanover, VT, University Press of New England, 1985.
21. Mayer TG, Kondraske G, Beals SB, et al: Spinal range of motion: Accuracy and sources of error with inclinometric measurement. Spine 1997; 22:1976.
22. Kondraske G.: Towards a standard clinical measure of postural stability. In Kondraske G, Robinson C (eds): Proceedings of the Eighth Annual Conference of the IEEE Engineering in Medicine and Biology Society 1986; 3:1579.
23. Kondraske G: Human performance: Measurement, science, concepts and computerized methodology. Neurology (in press).
24. Turner J, Ersek M, Herron L, et al: Patient outcomes after lumbar spinal fusions. JAMA 1992; 268:907.
25. van Tulder M, Koes B, Bouter L: Conservative treatment of acute and chronic nonspecific low back pain: A systematic review of randomized controlled trials of the most common interventions. Spine 1997; 22:2128.
26. Faas A, Van Eijk J, Chavannes A, et al: A randomized trial of exercise therapy in patients with acute low back pain. Spine 1995; 20:941.
27. Stuckey S, Jacobs A, Goldfarb J: EMG biofeedback training, relaxation training, and placebo for the relief of chronic back pain. Percept Motor Skills 1986; 63:1023.
28. Beals R: Compensation and recovery from injury. West J Med 1984; 104:233.
29. Dzioba R, Doxey N: A prospective investigation into the orthopaedic and psychologic predictors of outcome of first lumbar surgery following industrial injury. Spine 1984; 9:614.
30. Jackson R, Boston D, Edge A: Lateral mass fusion: A prospective study of a consecutive series with long-term follow-up. Spine 1983; 10:828.
31. Mayer T, Gatchel R, Mayer H, et al: A prospective two-year study of functional restoration in industrial low back injury: An objective assessment procedure. JAMA 1987; 258:1763.
32. Gatchel R, Mayer T, Hazard R, et al: Functional restoration: Pitfalls in evaluating efficacy. Spine 1992; 17:988.
33. Hazard R: Spine update: Functional restoration. Spine 1995; 20:2345.
34. Hazard R, Fenwick J, Kalish S, et al: Functional restoration with behavioral support: A one-year prospective study of chronic low back pain patients. Spine 1989; 14:157.
35. Mayer T, Pope P, Tabor J, et al: Physical progress and residual impairment quantification after functional restoration: Lumbar mobility. Spine 1994; 19:389.
36. Brady S, Mayer T, Gatchel R: Physical progress and residual impairment quantification after functional restoration: Isokinetic trunk strength. Spine 1994; 18:395.
37. Spengler D, Bigos S, Martin N, et al: Back injuries in industry: A retrospective study: Overview and cost analysis. Spine 1986; 11:241.
38. Kohles S, Barnes D, Gatchel R: Improved physical performance outcomes following functional restoration treatment in patient with chronic low back pain: Early versus recent training results. Spine 1990; 15: 1321.
39. Mayer T, Gatchel R, Kishino N: Objective assessment of spine function following industrial injury: A prospective study with comparison group and one-year follow-up. Spine 1985; 10:482.
40. Hazard R, Sobel J, Hartigan C: The effect of compensation involvement on the reporting of pain and disability by patients referred for rehabilitation of chronic low back pain. Spine 1997; 22:2016.
41. Mooney V, Robertson J: The facet syndrome. Clin Orthop 1976; 115:149.
42. Ward N: Tricyclic antidepressants for chronic low back pain: Mechanisms of action and predictors of response. Spine 1986; 11:661.
43. Mayer TG, Gatchel RJ, Kishino N, et al: A prospective short-term study of chronic low back pain patients utilizing novel objective functional measurement. Pain 1986; 25:53.
44. Bendix T, Bendix A: Different training programs for chronic low back pain: A randomized blinded one-year follow-up study. Seattle, WA, International Society for the Study of the Lumbar Spine, 1994.
45. Bendix AF, Bendix T, Vaegter K, et al: Multidisciplinary intensive treatment for chronic low back pain: A randomized, prospective study. Cleveland Clin J Med 1996; 63:62.
46. Hildebrandt J, Pfingsten M, Saur P, et al: Prediction of success from a multidisciplinary treatment program for chronic low back pain. 1997; Spine 22:990.
47. Corey DT, Koepfler LE, Etlin D, et al: A limited fuinctional restoration program for injured workers: A randomized trial. J Occup Rehabil 1996; 6:239.

COMPLICATIONS OF SPINAL SURGERY

S. Tim Yoon and Serena S. Hu

Summary
- Complications of spinal surgery can be minimized by careful identification of spinal pathology and by evaluating coexisting medical, social, and psychological issues.
- Intraoperative complications include bleeding, dural tears, instrumentation-related problems, intrathoracic injury, and neurological injury.
- Major types of postoperative complications include infection, deformity, and pain.
- Clinicians should be vigilant in preventing, identifying, and promptly treating any complications.

Although the benefits of spinal surgery can be great to the patient, surgical complications can occur, sometimes with devastating results. The spinal surgeon must guard against complications during all stages of surgery: preoperative, operative, and postoperative. The reported complications are varied, complex, and dependent on the type of spinal surgery involved. A detailed discussion of all spinal complications is beyond the scope of this chapter, but the important and more common complications are discussed within the framework of the surgical stage at which they become prominent. The methods used to prevent or manage these complications are discussed.

PREOPERATIVE

Prevention of surgical complications begins with careful preoperative assessment and planning. The first step is to avoid an incorrect diagnosis. At times, this may not be a simple task. A wide array of spinal and non-spinal diagnoses must be considered. Even when a spinal pathological lesion is diagnosed, there may well be another pathological lesion that is the real cause of the patient's morbidity. For example, a patient with low back pain and radiographic evidence of degenerative lumbar spine may have a dissecting aortic aneurysm, metastatic tumor, or sacroiliitis that may be the true cause of the back pain. As with most fields of medicine, arriving at the proper diagnosis begins with a careful history. Knowledge of the epidemiology of spinal disorders is helpful in diagnosis. For example, children with back pain, unlike adults, have been reported to have as high as 86% likelihood of having a defined spinal pathological conditon.[1, 2] The surgeon should perform a thorough spinal and orthopedic examination and, when appropriate, a more general physical examination. Imaging or electrophysiologic studies should be used in a selective manner.

After the proper diagnosis has been made, an individualized treatment plan can be formulated. The patient may have significant medical, social, and psychological issues that must be carefully addressed before a surgical course of action is recommended. Evaluations by anesthesiologists, internists, or other surgeons may be critical in assessing operative risk and to bring the patient to his or her optimal condition prior to surgery. Family members as well as the patient should be educated in the nature of the surgery, its expected results, its usual postoperative course, and its potential complications. Good preoperative planning can be a vital part of preventing surgical complications and promoting a satisfying experience for the patient and family.

OPERATIVE

EXCESSIVE BLOOD LOSS

Excessive blood loss can generally be managed by aggressive blood replacement by the alert anesthesiologist; however, it can still cause significant morbidity. Recognizing the causes and risk factors for excessive blood loss, using meticulous surgical technique, and using appropriate ancillary support measures can minimize the possibility of complications.

Morbidities related to large blood loss are systemic in nature. Large blood loss leads to sudden or extended loss of intravascular volume and reduced oxygen delivery. This leads to complications related to systemic hypotension and hypoperfusion, which can lead to renal failure, adult respiratory distress syndrome, cardiac ischemia, and central nervous system ischemia. Large blood loss may require random donor blood transfusion, which incurs the risk of transfusion reaction (1 in 25,000 per unit)[3] and infectious disease transmission. Although the risk of infectious disease transmission has been reduced significantly with better screening methods, there is still a small degree of risk with each transfused unit of blood product (1 in 190,000 units for human immunodeficiency virus, 1 in 63,000 units for hepatitis B virus, 1 in 125,000 for hepatitis C virus).[4–6] Rapid transfusion and volume replacement entails the risk of over-resuscitation, causing cardiac decompensation due to excessively high central venous pressures. This in turn can lead to pulmonary edema, hypoxia, hypotension, and cardiac arrest.

Risk factors for excessive hemorrhage fall into patient-related and procedure-related categories. The patient may have an intrinsic or an acquired coagulopathy. Intrinsic coagulation deficiencies more commonly involve deficiencies in factor VIII, factor IX, or von Willebrand factor.[7] Major surgery can be performed safely in these patients by replacing the missing factor, unless circulating inhibitors to factors are present. Acquired coagulopathy can be caused by the use of nonsteroidal anti-inflammatory drugs, malnutrition, cirrhosis, hypothermia, and intraoperative disseminated intravascular coagulation. The surgeon should be alert for signs of coagulopathy during the surgery by taking note of the level of oozing and clot formation. When heavy bleeding is encountered, coagulation profiles and platelet count should be measured and abnormalities corrected with fresh whole blood, fresh frozen plasma, cryoprecipitate, or platelet transfusion. We do this routinely and regularly during lengthy procedures, so that these problems can be addressed early in their course.

Some procedures are more likely to cause excessive blood loss. Patients with paralytic spinal deformity, large stiff spinal deformity, or osteoporotic bone are more likely to have heavy bleeding. High blood loss is more common in surgery for major deformity, in which extensive surgical exposure is necessary. General oozing from a wide exposure combined with lengthy surgical times are the major factors. Decancellation procedures or corrective osteotomy can lead to heavy bleeding from exposed cancellous bone. Procoagulant materials such as thrombin-soaked Gelfoam, and collagen matrix are useful adjuvants that should be used in liberal quantities to control bleeding.

Major vessel injury is rare but is life-threatening. During the anterior approach to the spine, the vena cava, aorta, large segmental vessels, and iliac vessels are encountered. A left-sided anterior approach in the lumbar spine decreases risk to the vena cava, which is significantly more fragile and more difficult to repair than the aorta. The risks to the large vessels are significantly greater if there has been previous abdominal or retroperitoneal surgery due to the adhesions and distortion of normal anatomy. Retractors should be placed with great care to protect the large vessels. A tear in the vena cava or aorta is life threatening and the assistance of a vascular surgeon may be necessary to repair the tear. A significant decrease in vessel diameter can lead to chronic venous return problems or extremity claudication symptoms. Although the major vessel injury is rare with posterior spinal surgery, aortic or vena caval injury has also been reported with posterior diskectomies by the surgeon's inadvertently pushing an instrument through the anterior annulus.[8]

During autologous bone graft procurement, other arteries are at risk. When approaching the posterior iliac crest, the superior gluteal artery is at risk as it exits the pelvis through the greater sciatic notch. Injury to the superior gluteal artery can cause massive hemorrhage that can be very hard to control. When lacerated, the artery has a tendency to retract into the pelvis, and it may not be possible to safely control the bleeding from the posterior approach. In this case, the patient should be turned to the supine position and the artery ligated using a retroperitoneal approach. When approaching the anterior iliac crest, the vessels at risk include the fourth lumbar, the iliolumbar, and the deep iliac circumflex arteries. Injuries to these arteries occur when the abdominal wall or iliac muscle is perforated with a sharp instrument.[9]

Precautions can be taken to minimize the bleeding and mitigate its effects. Predonated autologous blood should be an option when there is a likelihood of the patient's needing blood transfusion. Perioperative blood salvage should be used intraoperatively whenever more than 20% blood volume loss is predicted.[10–12] Acute normovolemic hemodilution immediately preoperatively dilutes the concentration of red blood cells, reducing the number of red blood cells lost per unit volume of blood loss. The phlebotomized

blood can be transfused as needed, reducing the nonautologous blood transfusion and providing fresh coagulation factors.[13] Hypotensive anesthesia is a commonly used technique that reduces arterial blood loss by lowering arterial blood pressure. However, this technique may not be applicable in patients with chronic or poorly controlled hypertension, coronary artery disease, or other cardiovascular disease.[14, 15]

DURAL TEAR

The dura can be lacerated during surgery, causing leakage of cerebrospinal fluid and severe headache. The dura is at risk whenever the operation occurs in close proximity to it. Dural tears have been reported during laminectomy, foraminotomy, diskectomy, facet excision, decortication, and instrumentation. The dura is especially at risk during a posterior decompression of spinal stenosis in which the dura may be scarred to the surrounding tissue. Dural tears are the most common complication following a repeat laminectomy.[16] Meticulous care must be used to separate the dura from the ligamentum flavum using an instrument such as the Penfield elevator prior to decompression. Revision surgery with the presence of scar may make separation of dura from adjacent structures difficult, if not impossible. Often, a sharper instrument, such as a small curette, is needed to create a plane between scarred dura and bone. In general, intimate knowledge of the anatomy and meticulous surgical technique are the best methods to guard against this all too common complication.

When a dural tear occurs, it must be repaired if possible. Unfortunately, this may not be a simple task. Adequate exposure is important. Soft tissue and bony tissue must be removed to allow proper inspection of the full length of the tear. The neural elements within the dural tear should be inspected for damage. A fine nonabsorbable suture is used to close the tear and Gelfoam placed over the repair. If there is large loss or attenuation of dural tissue and a simple repair is not possible, interpositional fascial or fat graft may be needed. Fibrin glue can be used to augment the repair. During the repair, great care should be taken to avoid any further damage to neural elements, such as with the repair stitch or direct suctioning on the nerve roots. Occasionally, if adequate closure is not possible, a drain may be placed in the lumbar area to decompress the tear until sufficient healing has occurred.[17] Postoperatively, the patient should be supine for at least 48 hours to reduce cerebrospinal fluid pressure and spinal headache.[16] Patients with persistent headaches and/or fluid collection after surgery may need a magnetic resonance imaging (MRI) scan or myelogram to determine whether they have a persistent cerebrospinal fluid leak (Fig. 1).

INSTRUMENTATION

Instrumentation-related complications include sagittal or coronal decompensation, neurological injury, or failure of fixation. The more commonly described instrumentation-related complications are described in this section.

Loss of lumbar lordosis, which leads to flatback syndrome, is a significant complication that is related to certain types of instrumentation. When first introduced, the Harrington rod was a significant advance in instrumentation, but it is now well recognized that when this instru-

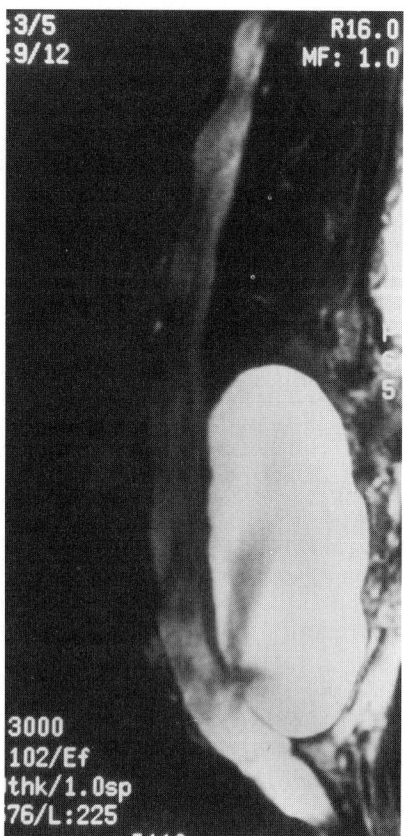

Fig. 1. MRI of patient with persistent headache and back swelling after revision decompression of lumbar spine. MRI demonstrates pseudomeningocele with flow artifact corresponding to the actual dural leak. The patient was re-explored, with primary repair of a small durotomy, without further recurrence of symptoms.

ment is used in distraction mode in the lumbar spine, significant loss of lordosis can develop.[18, 19] Anterior instrumentation systems have the potential for producing loss of lordosis because they compress through the anterior spine. The loss of lordosis following instrumentation with Dwyer's and Zielke's systems is well documented.[20, 21] Even when using the modern solid rod constructs for anterior surgery, the surgeon must be careful to maintain anterior disk heights with structural grafts or implants to maintain the lumbar lordosis.

Posterior instrumentation systems may use a solid rod with wires, hooks, or pedicle screws. The use of segmental sublaminar wires are favored in situations in which the bone is of poor quality, especially in patients with neuromuscular scoliosis. A rigid construct with excellent sagittal contour control can be obtained with segmental wires.[22] However, because the sublaminar wire enters the spinal canal, there is a risk of injuring the neural elements. Injuries to the dura, nerve root, and spinal cord have been reported.[23, 24] The wire should be shaped into the largest possible radius of curvature to cause the least intrusion into the spinal canal, and meticulous surgical technique must be used.[25] To avoid the risks of sublaminar wires, some surgeons have used the spinous process wires.[26] Even with this, dural tear and intradural injury have been reported.[27]

Furthermore, because spinous process fixation is biomechanically not as strong as sublaminar wires, its use is limited to smaller, more flexible curves in the pediatric population.

Unlike fixation with sublaminar wires, instrumentation with hooks on the posterior bony elements (lamina, pedicle, and transverse process) allow application of both distractive and compressive corrective forces.[28, 29] Because of the ability to rotate the rod, selectively distract, and compress, hook fixation may save segments in comparison to sublaminar wires alone.[30] As with sublaminar wires, sublaminar hooks enter the spinal canal and can cause neurological complications. However, they are safer than sublaminar wires. Instrumenting with hooks alone usually entails fewer points of fixation as compared with segmental wires. Therefore, the corrective forces are concentrated on a smaller number of segments, making hooks more likely to cut through bone if too much force is applied or if the bone is soft. Hook dislodgment can be a problem, especially if the rod is not sufficiently well contoured (Fig. 2). It should be addressed as soon as it is identified, especially if it occurs at the end of the instrumentation.

Pedicle screws provide superior biomechanical fixation, making them a very valuable tool in spinal surgery. Experience is needed to use them safely, however. The pedicle itself may be damaged by a screw that is too large in diameter or by improper insertion.[31] If the pedicle wall is penetrated, neurological injury may result by impingement by the displaced pedicle bone or by the screw itself. An error in the inferior medial direction is more likely to injure the nerve root as it exits the neural foramen. A gross error may injure any neurological structure in the vicinity, including the spinal cord, conus medullaris, or nerve roots (Fig. 3). The incidence of neurological injury is 3.2% according to a self-reported database system by the Scoliosis Research Society.[32] In another study, the rates of transient nerve root injury and permanent neurological injury were reported to be 2.4% and 2.3%, respectively.[31] Fluoroscopic imaging, especially in the thoracic region, can assist pedicle screw placement. A small laminotomy can also be used to help identify the pedicle anatomy. In the lumbar region, if the anatomy is not too distorted, an experienced surgeon can safely place pedicle screws using just anatomic landmarks.[33] After hardware placement, radiographs should be taken to confirm proper positioning.

INTRATHORACIC

Among the different intrathoracic complications, pneumothorax is the more common problem and can sometimes occur insidiously. Central line placement, barotrauma, ruptured pulmonary bleb, and direct surgical injury are potential causes of pneumothorax.[34, 35] A postoperative chest radiograph should be obtained routinely, especially when a thoracoplasty has been performed or a central venous line has been placed. For a significant pneumothorax, a chest tube should be placed.

Less common intrathoracic complications are pulmonary contusion, hemothorax, and chylothorax. Pulmonary contusion can result from excessively vigorous retraction during anterior surgery. The pulmonary parenchymal damage that results may manifest itself as hypoxia in the operating

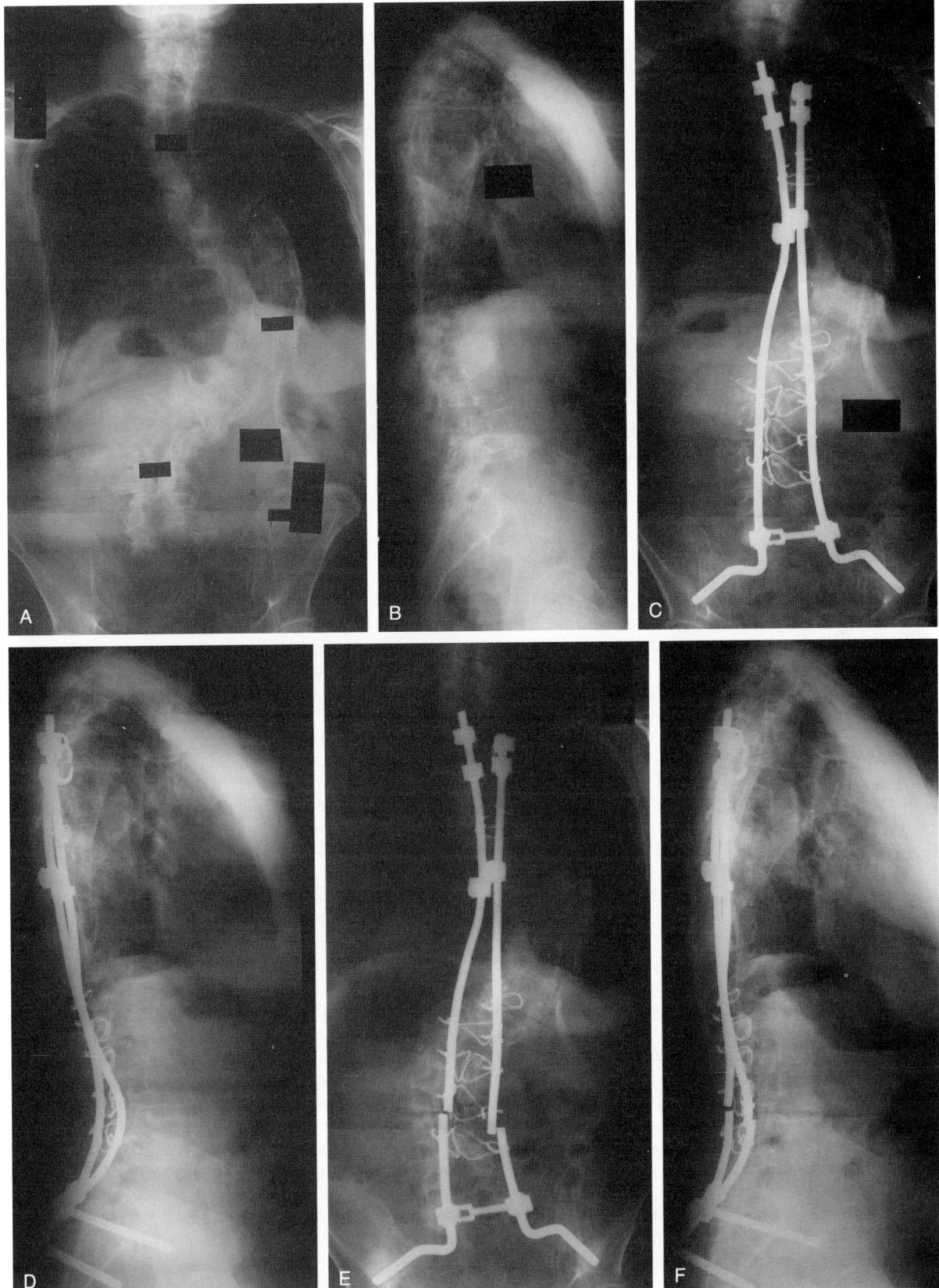

Fig. 2. Patient views. This patient noted a "pop" in her back about 2 years after combined anterior/posterior fusion for adult scoliosis. *A* and *B*, Preoperative radiographs. *C* and *D*, Postoperative radiographs. About 2 years postoperatively, the first rod was noted to be broken; the second rod was broken a few months later. *E* and *F*, Note obvious radiolucency in the fusion mass, through the L3-4 disk space, consistent with pseudarthrosis. Patient has declined revision surgery for now.

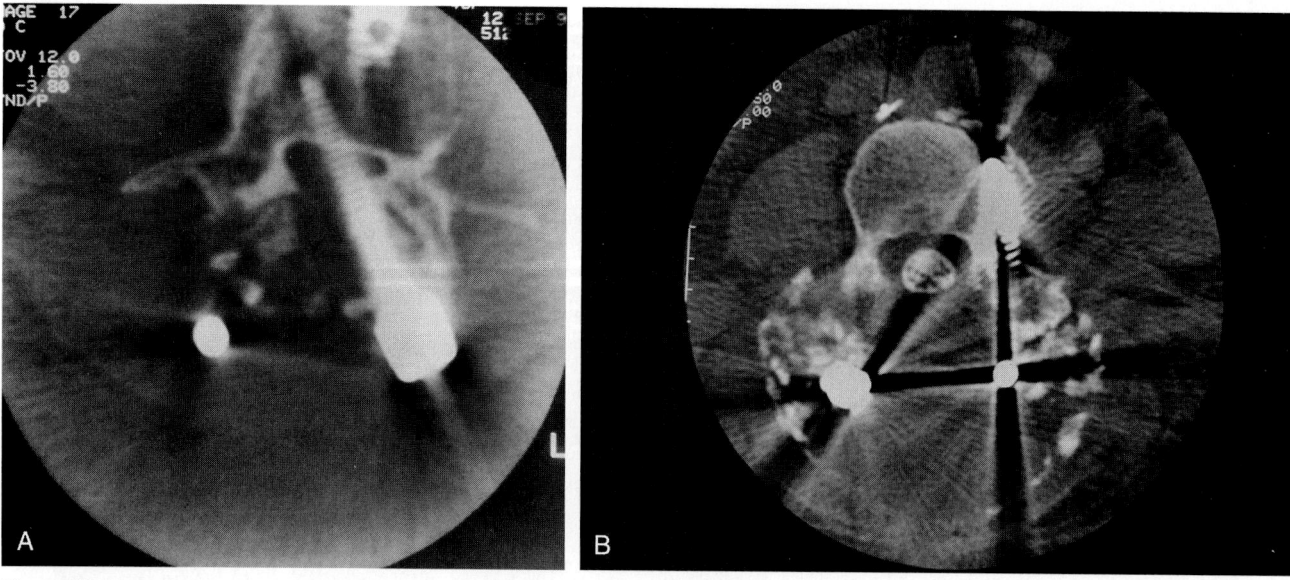

Fig. 3. CT scans. *A*, CT scan of patient who was referred for leg pain, weakness, and back pain after lumbar fusion. She underwent surgery for revision of lumbar fusion with removal of the offending screw. The leg pain and neurological deficit partially improved. *B*, This patient was noted to have quadriceps weakness after revision lumbar fusion surgery for flatback deformity. CT scan demonstrates lateral penetration of screw with impingement of L3 nerve root. The fusion was revised with removal of the screw, with partial improvement of weakness.

room or perhaps a day after the surgery. Supportive therapy with supplemental oxygen or continued intubation is the usual treatment. Hemothorax can result from damage to an intercostal vessel during rib resection or bleeding from segmental vessels around the vertebral body after an anterior spinal surgery. It may manifest itself as excessive bloody chest tube output and may necessitate a return to the operating room for exploration and ligation of the offending vessel. Chylothorax can result from accidental injury to the thoracic duct during anterior spinal approach.[36] If the duct laceration is noted during surgery, the duct should be repaired. If the duct laceration is not identified until the postoperative time period, institution of a nonfat diet is generally sufficient to stop the chyle leak.[37]

NEUROLOGICAL INJURY

Although the rate of neurological injury is relatively low, it can be a particularly serious complication. These complications range from transient radicular sensory dysfunction to permanent radicular motor loss or paraplegia from spinal cord injury. Direct surgical trauma or traction during deformity correction is the main cause of these complications. The rate of neurological injury varies with the type of procedure being performed. Procedures that involve surgical maneuvers close to neurological elements (especially the spinal cord) or those procedures that involve translation of the spine or correction of kyphosis have a significantly higher risk of neurological complication.

In scoliosis surgery, the type of instrumentation used affects the rate of neurological complications. Interestingly, neurological injury was nonexistent in the days of cast immobilization after surgery. With the advent of instrumented fusion, the neurological complication rates have increased. This is due to two major factors. First, instrumented fusions entail hardware that can potentially damage neural elements through direct physical contact. Second,

modern instrumentation systems used for significant deformity correction can cause cord or root damage by stretch or compression.

Rigid deformities, both coronal and sagittal, particularly when congenital, are associated with a higher risk of neurological injury. Distraction instrumentation, osteotomies, or curve correction beyond preoperative flexibility are associated with significantly higher risk.[38] Associated intracanal aberrations such as tethered cord, diastematomyelia, and syrinx can all lead to cord injury if curve correction is performed in their presence. A preoperative MRI scan of the spine is useful to identify these abnormalities[39] and is recommended in patients with congenital scoliosis or rapidly progressive scoliosis. In rare instances, paraplegia can occur even when instrumentation is not used. This is more common in congenital kyphosis. Achondroplastic dwarfs have a high rate of cord injury with posterior instrumented fusions owing to their very narrow spinal canal.[40] Every effort must be taken to use the least intrusive instrumentation in these patients.

With anterior spinal surgery, both mechanical and vascular injury to neurological elements can occur. Accidental intrusion into the spinal canal can occur during anterior diskectomy or vertebrectomy. Cord damage can occur during screw placement in the vertebral body. The risk of injury is higher with scoliosis surgery, in which the rotation of the spine can distort the anatomy. During the anterior approach, the sympathetic lumbar chain can be divided. The sympathectomy will manifest itself as ipsilateral leg warmth due to hypoperfusion and will often resolve within 6 months. Injury of the hypogastric plexus or presacral nerves can lead to impotence or retrograde ejaculation. Ischemic injury to the spinal cord can occur when segmental vessels are divided, especially in the watershed region between the fifth and ninth thoracic vertebrae. Fortunately, this complication rarely occurs if only unilateral division of the segmental vessel is performed. Some authors advocate the temporary occlusion of the segmental vessels in combination with electrophysiological monitoring before permanent ligation.

The risk of neurological injury for treatment of spondylolisthesis is dependent on the type of surgery. When laminectomy and foraminotomy are performed, there is a potential for injuring a nerve root or the cauda equina. In situ lumbar fusion without decompression has a very low incidence of neurological complication; however, cauda equina syndrome or foot drop can occur even after in situ fusion of high-grade spondylolisthesis.[41] Deliberate significant surgical reduction is rarely indicated and is associated with a high rate of neurological complication. Although cauda equina syndrome is the more feared complication, the L5 nerve root is the most commonly injured structure during reduction.[42] Reduction of spondylolisthesis produces tension on the nerve roots as the proximal spine is translated superiorly and posteriorly. The risk of excessive tension can be decreased if an anatomic reduction is not the goal and a slow controlled reduction is performed with full visualization of the nerve root.[43]

Whenever significant risk for neurological injury is anticipated, spinal monitoring in the form of electrophysiological monitoring and/or the wakeup test should be used. Somatosensory evoked potential (SEP) and motor evoked potential (MEP) monitor two parallel but independent electrophysiological monitoring systems. With SEP, peripheral nerves are stimulated with electrodes and the resultant cortical electrical signals are extracted and monitored. SEP, however, does not monitor the motor pathways. With MEP, the motor cortex or the rostral spinal cord is stimulated with an electrical or magnetic stimulus and the response distally in the muscle or large peripheral nerve is recorded. The combination of SEP and MEP are theoretically better than either alone.[44, 45] Anesthetic agents modulate the electrophysiological signal so that the anesthesiologist and the electrophysiologist must coordinate their technique to get the best readings. The wakeup test consists of lightening the anesthesia and asking the patient to move his or her feet and demonstrating full ankle plantarflexion and dorsiflexion.[46] It is a more definitive test of the integrity of the spinal cord motor pathway. However, care is necessary during this test. The patient may become physically agitated and become extubated.[47] Spontaneous respiration can generate negative pressures in the open veins in the surgical field and cause venous air emboli. Despite the potential problems, wakeup tests are cheap and effective and can be performed safely by an experienced anesthesiologist. The use of transient bilateral ankle clonus, which is normally present while patients are recovering from general anesthesia, to monitor spinal cord integrity, has been reported to have a 100% sensitivity and 99.7% specificity.[48] On the occasion that a spinal cord injury is noted by monitoring, the cause must be sought and rectified. Improper instrumentation or overly aggressive curve correction may be the offending cause, and if so, the hardware should be removed or the amount of correction reduced. Hypotension or anemia may also cause cord ischemia, which can be associated with heavy surgical blood loss. Careful monitoring to prevent such volume loss combined with aggressive resuscitation with intravenous fluids and blood products are important countermeasures.

OTHER

Malignant hyperthermia is an infrequent complication triggered by certain anesthetic agents, especially succinylcholine and halogenated inhalants. Cellular hypermetabolic activity causes elevated temperature, respiratory acidosis, muscle rigidity, tachycardia, and/or arrhythmias. Patients with Duchenne's muscular dystrophy, arthrogryposis, and osteogenesis imperfecta are especially at risk. Prompt administration of dantrolene as well as supportive measures are necessary to treat this potentially fatal complication.[49]

Ophthalmological complications, while rare, can cause significant disturbance in vision. These perioperative ophthalmic complications include posterior optic nerve ischemia, occipital lobe infarcts, and central retinal vein thrombosis.[50] Avoiding excessive hypotension and prolonged dependent position of the head may help prevent this complication.

POSTOPERATIVE

INFECTION

Surgical wound infections occur with different frequency, depending largely on the type of surgery. A review of 7769 spinal cases from 1950 to 1982 showed an overall rate of wound infection at 2.5%.[51] The infection rate for posterior surgery was significantly higher than that for anterior surgery (2.6% vs 0.9%). Patients undergoing revision surgery and adult populations were at higher risk. Patients with myelodysplasia had an especially high risk of infection (7.9%). The use of instrumentation and longer time of surgery were also relative risk factors. The use of allograft did not increase the infection rate. Prophylactic antibiotics has become a standard part of spinal surgery since the 1970s, dramatically reducing infection rates. Surgery for idiopathic scoliosis had an infection rate drop from 2.3% to 0.1% after institution of prophylactic antibiotics.[35]

Clinical judgment is important in early diagnosis of wound infection. Although an elevated temperature and white blood cell count can suggest an infection, these measures are nonspecific. Erythema or wound drainage raises the index of suspicion. If necessary, the wound can be aspirated and cultured. However, the diagnosis is often clear before any culture results are available. As soon as the diagnosis has been established or strongly suspected, the wound should be incised, pulse lavaged, and closed over drains. It is not uncommon after revision spine surgery for the wound to drain for short periods of time postoperatively. However, for patients with persistent drainage that is not decreasing (particularly if hardware is present), a more aggressive approach with incision and drainage is preferred. Appropriate antibiotics should be instituted after consultation with infectious disease specialists. In the majority of cases, prompt surgical incision and débridement will allow the hardware to be retained.

POSTOPERATIVE DEFORMITY

Despite the best efforts during surgery, significant spinal imbalance in the coronal or sagittal plane can be noted postoperatively. Coronal imbalance occurs when curves are overcorrected relative to the compensatory curve or vice versa. If the imbalance is mild, it may be treated with bracing; however, it may progress and require surgical intervention. Shoulder height discrepancy can occur in patients with double thoracic spinal curves who have only the lower curve included in the fusion. Special care should be taken to assess the magnitude and flexibility of the upper curve to decide whether to include that curve in the fusion. Significant loss of lumbar lordosis can cause severe back pain or early fatigability. The patient may have a forward lean, and standing radiographs will show significant sagittal plane decompensation. As discussed in the instrumentation section, the choice of instrumentation or improper application of distraction over the lumbar spine can contribute to this complication. Improper patient positioning prior to surgery (with lumbar spine in flexion) may also be a contributing factor. If the deformity is severe and painful, corrective surgery may be needed.[52, 53]

The crankshaft phenomenon is a late complication of posterior fusion in children with significant growth potential remaining. The posterior fusion mass acts as a tether preventing growth in the posterior column while the anterior column of the spine continues to grow and spins around the posterior. This can lead to significant and progressive rotatory scoliosis, as can be measured by increasing rib-vertebral angle difference. Crankshaft can be avoided by delaying spinal fusion until the child is more skeletally mature or by performing a combined posterior and anterior spinal fusion.[54] Risk factors for the development of crankshaft include curve greater than 50 degrees, open triradiate cartilage, Risser stage 0 to 1, female gender and age less than 11 years, and male gender and age less than 13 years.[54,55]

Curve lengthening, or "adding on," is an extension of the curve to levels that were not part of the original curve. This can result from improper selection of fusion levels. Sometimes this can occur despite proper level selection, more commonly when the child's spine is fused before his or her adolescent growth spurt. If prolonged brace wear does not control curve progression, an extension of the fusion should be performed.

POSTOPERATIVE PAIN

Pseudarthrosis can be a cause of late postoperative pain. It can be seen with progression of deformity, spinal imbalance, or hardware failure. Development of these problems should be assumed to be secondary to pseudarthrosis until proven otherwise. Pseudarthrosis is more likely to occur with fusion in the lumbosacral levels or the thoracolumbar levels. Adults, smokers, and patients with neuromuscular curves have an increased risk of pseudarthrosis.[56] Posterior fusion alone of adult patients with thoracic kyphosis not correctable to less than 50 degrees is associated with a higher reported incidence of pseudarthrosis.[57] Older flexible anterior systems are also known to be associated with a higher incidence of pseudarthrosis in adults and of instrumentation failure.[58]

Pseudarthrosis may be difficult to diagnose on plain radiographs (68% sensitive). Other imaging methods used to help make the diagnosis include motion radiography, tomography, computed tomography, bone scan, and MRI. Even with these sophisticated methods, their predictive value either has been disappointing or has not been established. Failure of modern instrumentation most often indicates persistent micromotion through a pseudarthrosis. If the deformity is progressive or the pain is significant and other causes of pain have been ruled out, surgical exploration, reinstrumentation, and further bone grafting of the pseudarthrosis is indicated. Anterior fusion may be necessary to increase the rate of fusion in the presence of failed posterior fusion.

Adjacent segment degeneration refers to degeneration of motion segments adjacent to the fused levels of the spine. The most common abnormalities are adjacent segment facet joint arthrosis, spinal stenosis, disk degeneration, and degenerative spondylolisthesis.[59] More often, the lower adjacent level to a long fusion is involved, although adjacent segments above can also be involved. The proper selection of the fusion levels, especially the lower level, is important. Fusion to L4 or below increases the likelihood of developing low back pain.[60]

Other causes of postoperative pain include arachnoiditis, nerve root adhesions, and prominent hardware. Arachnoiditis is inflammation of the pia arachnoid membrane surrounding the spinal cord or cauda equina. Any intrusion into the dural space can cause arachnoiditis. Extradural scar may also form and impinge on the involved nerve root, causing a radiculopathy. Prominent hardware can cause bursitis or skin erosion. Thin, small patients are more likely to have this complication. If desired, after the fusion mass is sufficiently mature, the hardware can be removed.

CONCLUSION

As mentioned at the beginning of this chapter, careful preoperative evaluation and diagnosis are key to successful spinal surgery. Certainly some diagnoses (scoliosis, spondylolisthesis, spinal stenosis) are more likely to have a successful patient outcome and significant pain relief than others (degenerative disk disease, failed back surgery). Spinal surgery is very complex, and a wide range of potential complications can occur during and after surgery. All spine surgeons should be aware of these complications and maintain a highly vigilant stance in preventing, identifying, and promptly treating any complications.

REFERENCES

1. Hensinger RN: Back pain in children. In Bradford D, Hensinger R: The Pediatric Spine. New York: Thieme, 1985, p 41.
2. Thompson G: Back pain in children. J Bone Joint Surg Am 1993; 6:928.
3. Haller GS, Shulman BJ, Taylor PD: Anesthesia for surgery of the spine. In Lonstein J (ed): Moe's Textbook of Scoliosis and Other Spinal Deformities. Philadelphia, W.B. Saunders, 1995, p 595.
4. Remis RS, Delage G, Palmer RW: Risk of HIV Infection from Blood Transfusion in Montreal. CMAJ 1997; 157(4):375.
5. Whyte GS, Savoia HF: The risk of transmitting HCV, HBV or HIV by blood transfusion in Victoria. Med J Austral 1997; 166(11):584.
6. Gresens CJ, Holland PV: Current risks of viral hepatitis from blood transfusions. J Gastroenterol Hepatol 1998, 13(4):443.
7. Donaldson WR, Levine WN: Coagulation

and thromboembolism in orthopedics. In Kasser J (ed): Orthopedic Knowledge Update 5. Rosemont, IL, American Academy of Orthopaedic Surgeons, 1996, p 53.

8. Anda S: Anterior perforations in lumbar discectomies: A report of four cases and a CT study of the prevertebral lumbar anatomy. Spine 1991; 16:54.

9. Fowler BL, Dall BE, Rowe DE: Complications associated with harvesting autogenous iliac bone graft. Am J Orthop 1995; 24(12):895.

10. American Association of Blood Banks: Guidelines for Blood Salvage and Reinfusion in Surgery and Trauma. Arlington, VA: American Association of Blood Banks, 1990.

11. Kruger LM, Colbert JM: Intraoperative autologous transfusion in children undergoing spinal surgery. J Ped Orthoped 1985; 5(3):330.

12. Bovill DF: The efficacy of intraoperative autologous transfusion in major orthopedic surgery: a regression analysis. Orthopedics 1986; 9(10):1403.

13. Laks H: Acute hemodilution: its effect on hemodynamics and oxygen transport in anesthetised man. Ann Surg 1974; 180: 103.

14. Malcolm-Smith NA, McMaster MJ: The use of induced hypotension to control bleeding during posterior spinal fusion for scoliosis. J Bone Joint Surg Br 1983; 65(3):255.

15. Grundy BL, Nash CL Jr, Brown RH: Deliberate hypotension for spinal fusion: prospective randomized study with evoked potential monitoring. Can Anaesth Soc J 1982; 29(5):452.

16. Wiesel SW: The multiply operated lumbar spine. Instructional Course Lectures 1985; 34:68.

17. Kitchel SH, Eismont FJ, Green BA: Closed subarachnoid drainage for management of cerebrospinal fluid leakage after an operation on the spine. J Bone Joint Surg Am 1989; 71(7):984.

18. Aaro S, Ohlen G: The effect of Harrington instrumentation on the sagittal configuration and mobility of the spine in scoliosis. Spine 1983; 8(6):570.

19. Lagrone MO: Treatment of symptomatic flatback after spinal fusion. J Bone Joint Surg Am 1988; 70(4):569.

20. Dwyer AF: Experience of anterior correction of scoliosis. Clin Orthop Rel Res 1973; 93:191.

21. Moe JH, Purcell GA, Bradford DS: Zielke instrumentation (VDS) for the correction of spinal curvature. Analysis of results in 66 patients. Clin Orthop Rel Res 1983; 180:133.

22. Luque ER: Segmental spinal instrumentation for correction of scoliosis. Clin Orthop Rel Res 1982; 163:192.

23. Johnston CED: Delayed paraplegia complicating sublaminar segmental spinal instrumentation. J Bone Joint Surg Am 1986; 68(4):556.

24. Wilber RG: Postoperative neurological deficits in segmental spinal instrumentation. A study using spinal cord monitoring. J Bone Joint Surg Am 1984; 66(8):178.

25. Goll SR: Depth of intraspinal wire penetration during passage of sublaminar wires. Spine 1988; 13(5):503.

26. Drummond D: Interspinous process segmental spinal instrumentation. J Pediatr Orthoped 1984; 4(4):397.

27. Liebergall M: Dural penetration by interspinous process segmental spine instrumentation: case report. J Spinal Disord 1989; 2(1):56.

28. Bradford DS: Adult scoliosis. Current concepts of treatment. Clin Orthop Rel Res 1988; 229:70.

29. Bridwell KH: Spinal instrumentation in the management of adolescent scoliosis. Clin Orthoped Rel Res 1997; 335:64.

30. Lenke LG: Ability of Cotrel-Dubousset instrumentation to preserve distal lumbar motion segments in adolescent idiopathic scoliosis. J Spinal Disord 1993; 6(4):339.

31. Esses SI, Sachs BL, Dreyzin V: Complications associated with the technique of pedicle screw fixation. A selected survey of ABS members. Spine 1993; 18(15):2231; discussion, 2238.

32. Scoliosis Research Society: Morbidity and Mortality Committee Report. Rosemont, IL, SRS, 1987.

33. Bradford RCT Jr: The spine. In Master Techniques in Orthopaedic Surgery. Philadelphia: Lippincott-Raven, 1997.

34. Anderson PR: Postoperative respiratory complications in non-idiopathic scoliosis. Acta Anaesthesiol Scand 1985; 29(2): 186.

35. Transfeldt EE: Complications of treatment. In: Lonstien JE, et al (eds): Moe's Textbook of Scoliosis and Other Spinal Deformities. Philadelphia: WB Saunders; 1995: 460.

36. Colletta AJ, Mayer PJ: Chylothorax: An unusual complication of anterior thoracic interbody spinal fusion. Spine 1982; 7(1): 46.

37. DeHart MM, et al: Management of retroperitoneal chylous leakage. Spine 1994; 19(6):716.

38. MacEwen GD, Bunnell WP, Sriram K: Acute neurological complications in the treatment of scoliosis. A report of the Scoliosis Research Society. J Bone Joint Surg Am 1975; 57(3):404.

39. Bradford DS, Heithoff KB, Cohen M: Intraspinal abnormalities and congenital spine deformities: a radiographic and MRI study. J Pediatr Orthoped 1991; 11(1):36.

40. Lutter LD: Anatomy of the achondroplastic lumbar canal. Clin Orthop Rel Res 1977; 126:139.

41. Maurice HD, Morley TR: Cauda equina lesions following fusion in situ and decompressive laminectomy for severe spondylolisthesis: Four case reports. Spine 1989; 14(2):214.

42. An HS, Glover JM: Complications and revision surgery in adult spinal deformity. In Bridwell KH, DeWald RI (eds): The textbook of spinal surgery. Philadephia: Lippincott-Raven; 1997:797.

43. Bradford DS, Boachie-Adjei O: Treatment of severe spondylolisthesis by anterior and posterior reduction and stabilization. A

long-term follow-up study. J Bone Joint Surg Am 1990; 72(7):1060.

44. Balzer JR, et al: Simultaneous somatosensory evoked potential and electromyographic recordings during lumbosacral decompression and instrumentation. Neurosurgery 1998; 42(6):1318.

45. Stephen JP: Cotrel-Dubousset instrumentation in children using simultaneous motor and somatosensory evoked potential monitoring. Spine 1996; 21(21):2450.

46. Vauzelle C, Stagnara P, Jouvinroux P: Functional monitoring of spinal cord activity during spinal surgery. Clin Orthop Rel Res 1973; 93:173.

47. Engler GL: Somatosensory evoked potentials during Harrington instrumentation for scoliosis. J Bone Joint Surg Am 1978; 60(4):528.

48. Hoppenfeld S: The ankle clonus test for assessment of the integrity of the spinal cord during operations for scoliosis. J Bone Joint Surg Am 1997; 79(2):208.

49. Madi-Jebara S: [Intraoperative malignant hyperthermia: apropos of a case]. J Med Libanais 1997; 45(1):36.

50. Stevens WR: Ophthalmic complications after spinal surgery. Spine 1997; 22(12): 1319.

51. Transfeldt EE, Lonstein JE, Winter RB: Wound infections in reconstructive spinal surgery. Orthop Trans 1985; 9:128.

52. Bradford DS, Tribus CB: Current concepts and management of patients with fixed decompensated spinal deformity. Clin Orthop Rel Res 1994; 306:64.

53. Farcy JP, Schwab FJ: Management of flatback and related kyphotic decompensation syndromes. Spine 1997; 22(20):2452.

54. Lee CS, Nachemson AL: The crankshaft phenomenon after posterior Harrington fusion in skeletally immature patients with thoracic or thoracolumbar idiopathic scoliosis followed to maturity. Spine 1997; 22(1):58.

55. Lapinsky AS, Richards BS: Preventing the crankshaft phenomenon by combining anterior fusion with posterior instrumentation. Does it work? Spine 1995; 20(12): 1392.

56. Larsen JM, Capen DA: Pseudarthrosis of the lumbar spine. J Am Acad Orthop Surg 1997; 5(3):153.

57. Winter RB, Moe JH, Wang JF: Congenital kyphosis. Its natural history and treatment as observed in a study of one hundred and thirty patients. J Bone Joint Surg Am 1973; 55(2): 223.

58. Trammell TR, Benedict F, Reed D: Anterior spine fusion using Zielke instrumentation for adult thoracolumbar and lumbar scoliosis. Spine 1991; 16(3):307.

59. Lee CK: Accelerated degeneration of the segment adjacent to a lumbar fusion. Spine 1988; 13(3):375.

60. Cochran T, Irstam L, Nachemson A: Long-term anatomic and functional changes in patients with adolescent idiopathic scoliosis treated by Harrington rod fusion. Spine 1983; 8(6):576.

section 8 chapter 11

SPINAL BIOMECHANICS

Geoffrey M. McCullen, Nathaniel Ordway, and Hansen A. Yuan

Summary

- Vertebral articulations have six "degrees of freedom" with translation and rotation about three orthogonal axes.
- The intervertebral disk is a composite structure with the nucleus pulposus gelatinous core surrounded by the circumferential, multilayered fibers of the anulus fibrosis and the framing end plates.
- The load at the L3-4 disk ranges from 30 kg while lying flat to more than 300 kg while lifting.
- Facet joints provide resistance against intervertebral torsion and shear forces and carry only a small proportion of compressive spinal loads.
- A "junctional" segment occurs at a transition point within a structure where two dissimilar mechanical zones meet. Within the spine, there are four "junctional" segments: (1) occipitocervical, (2) cervicothoracic, (3) thoracolumbar, and (4) lumbosacral.
- Anatomic structures with similar mechanical functions have been grouped into "columns" (Holdsworth, Denis).

Clinical Summary

- Injury force vectors include compression, distraction, flexion, extension, rotation, and shear. Each results in a recognized fracture pattern.
- Torsional stiffness decreases dramatically when more than 50% of a cervical facet joint is resected.
- In the lumbar spine, a total of one facet joint can be excised if the supraspinous and interspinous ligaments are competent.
- Rigid spinal implants augment spinal fusion success. However, as the rigidity of a construct is increased, device-related vertebral osteoporosis (stress shielding) becomes apparent.

The spine serves two distinct roles by providing the body's central, mobile axis and protecting the neural elements. The proper blending of flexibility and stability is required to simultaneously fulfill these functions. This is accomplished by a linked structure containing 24 mobile vertebrae connected at 74 stable articulations that allow motion. As such, the spine is a true masterpiece of evolution.

Adjacent vertebrae meet at three articulations known as the "triple joint complex," a tripod-shaped array with the discovertebral joint anteriorly and paired facet joints posteriorly. Compressive loads are transmitted primarily through the vertebral bodies and disks. Posterior ligaments serve as a countering tension band. Thus, these loads are effectively

"balanced" in both the coronal and sagittal plane for optimal load bearing and efficient energy utilization.

"Instability" occurs when the bony and ligamentous elements are compromised and a spinal segment demonstrates a greater than normal range of motion under physiological loads, which may cause pain, deformity, or neurological compromise.

In this chapter we review (1) the laboratory and analytic methods used to study spine biomechanics; (2) the biomechanical properties of the bony and ligamentous elements that contribute to spinal stability; (3) the clinically useful structural paradigms by which stability is assessed; (4) the effects of traumatic, degenerative, and pathological conditions on the maintenance of spinal stability; and (5) some of the clinically relevant biomechanical changes occurring after surgical intervention.

METHODS OF SPINAL MECHANICAL ASSESSMENT

Vertebral articulations have six "degrees of freedom" with translation and rotation about three orthogonal axes (Fig. 1). Because the spinal column is a linked system, the application of a single force or torque does not produce a single corresponding translation or rotation. Rather, forces on the spine result in combinations of motion encompassing all of the six degrees of freedom. Certain spinal motions always occur in combinations and are referred to as "coupling." For example, in the lumbar spine, lateral bending is coupled to axial rotation. The converse is also true. In the cervical spine, coupling is a function of intact facet joints with intact vertebral rings.[1]

Because in vivo spine biomechanical testing is prohibitive, knowledge of spinal function has most often used cadaveric specimens tested under a variety of loading sequences (loading rate, direction, and magnitude) within a materials testing machine to produce load-deformation plots. A functional spinal unit (FSU), consisting of two vertebral bodies (dissected free of muscle), the intervertebral disk, and ligamentous attachments, is the most frequently studied spine preparation (Fig. 2). After first assessing the response of the intact specimen to a given load, the effect of alterations (through progressive excision/release of a selected spinal component) is then analyzed.

Unfortunately, human cadaveric spine specimens demonstrate great specimen-to-specimen variability in regard to age, size, shape, extent of degenerative change, and bone mineral quality. To avoid these study variations, the calf spine, with controlled age and size, has been effectively used.[2]

Information gathered through anatomic dissections and cadaveric and animal spine mechanical testing has been

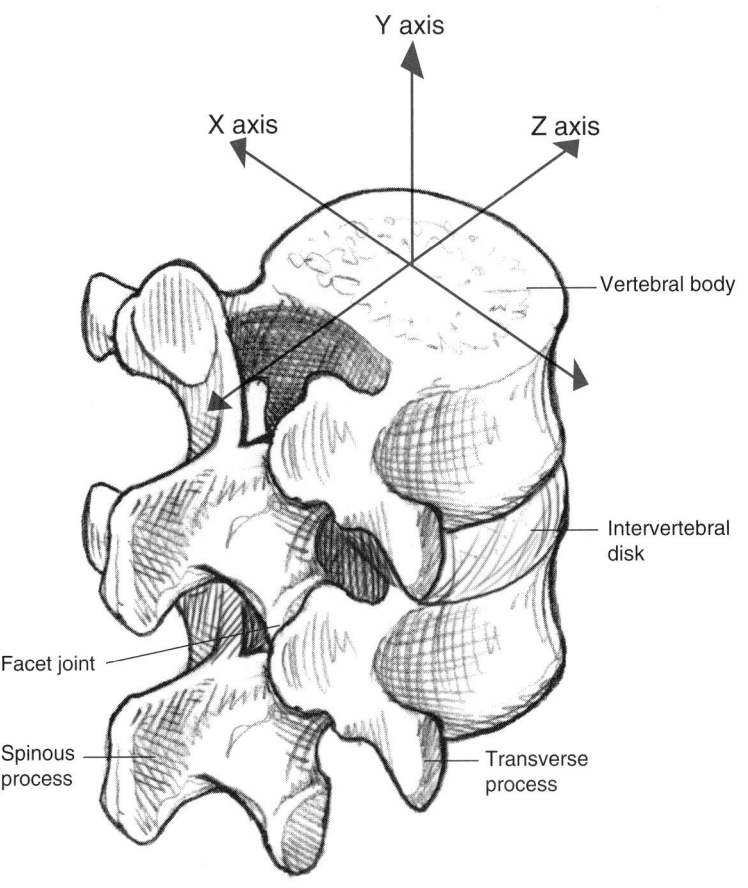

Y axis

X axis

Z axis

Vertebral body

Intervertebral disk

Facet joint

Spinous process

Transverse process

Fig. 1. Coordinate system. A coordinate system (represented by the *x*, *y*, and *z* axes) is placed in the center of the vertebra. Vertebrae have six "degrees of freedom" by translating along and rotating around each of these three axes.

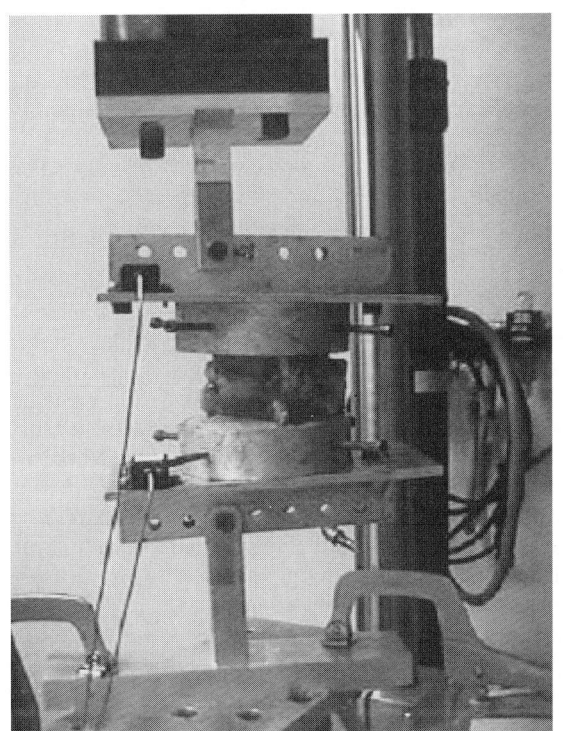

Fig. 2. Function spinal unit within a material testing machine. Generally used for determining material properties, such machines are used to study spinal biomechanics.

extended into mathematical models through finite element analysis (FEA). Detailed "mesh" figures, each line replicating one aspect of the complex spinal anatomy, are assigned specific material property values. Such a model allows absolute repeatability. However, creating such a model requires making numerous assumptions and simplifications that must be validated.

STRUCTURAL PROPERTIES OF SPINAL COMPONENTS

VERTEBRAL BODY

Compressive load is transmitted from the superior to the inferior vertebral end plate through the vertebral body's cortical shell and cancellous core. The shell accounts for only 10% of vertebral strength, whereas the trabecular centrum provides the dominant compressive strength.[3, 4] The allowable load before failure depends on bone mineral density (BMD)[3, 5] and the stress-responsive cancellous trabecular architecture.[6] The portion of the vertebral body overlying a normal nucleus pulposus is stronger than the surrounding bone.[7] When the disk degenerates, the strength of the bone adjacent to the nucleus decreases.[7]

INTERVERTEBRAL DISK

The intervertebral disk is a composite structure with the nucleus pulposus gelatinous core surrounded by the circumferential, multilayered fibers of the annulus fibrosis and the framing end plates (Fig. 3). The ability of the disk to function relies on a well-hydrated nucleus pulposus serving as the pressurized core. The nucleus is composed of a hydrophilic proteoglycan gel with a loosely bound network of collagen fibers (predominantly type II).[8] The hydrophilic proteoglycan maintains a very high water content, approximately 90% at birth and decreasing with age.[9, 10] The chondrocytes, producers of the extracellular matrix, are responsive to the mechanical environment. Increased cellular activity has been observed in response increases in compressive loading.[11]

The annulus is composed of collagen fibers (type I) in 15 to 25 distinct concentric laminated bands, approximately 1 mm thick, called lamellae.[12] The fibers of the lamellae are alternately oriented at an angle of 60 degrees with respect to the vertebral axis. The inner lamellae are connected to the end plates, whereas outer layers attach directly to the vertebral body through Sharpey fibers. This structural array makes the anulus capable of contributing greatly to torsional rigidity.[13]

The end plates are thin (average thickness, 0.6 mm) layers of hyaline cartilage.[14] The outer portion, toward the vertebral body, has a high collagen content. Progressing toward the nucleus the proteoglycan content of the end plate increases.

With prolonged loading, the disk exhibits "creep" (the deformation of a structure as a function of time after introduction of a maintained load) as water is forced across adjacent end plates.[15–17] This fluid flux results in a 20% loss of water content and a 13% to 36% reduction of hydrostatic pressure within the nucleus.[15, 16] With cyclic loading and unloading, fluid shifts across the disk and end plates and creates a metabolite transport system delivering nutrients and removing products of metabolism from the avascular disk.[18] Calcification of the end plate may create an impermeable barrier to solute transport.[14]

To study the mechanisms that lead to a herniated disk, studies have hyperflexed, laterally bent, and then compressed (to 8000 N) cadaveric lumbar intervertebral joints to replicate the forces generated when lifting a heavy object.[19] Nearly half of the tested disks failed with posterior disk prolapse after such a loading sequence. The most susceptible disks are those of the lower lumbar spine, especially those demonstrating a greater degree of degenerative change. Nuclear extrusion is almost always posterior and central or on the side away from a component of a lateral bending stress.

FACET JOINTS

Facet joints provide resistance against intervertebral torsion and shear forces and carry only a small proportion of compressive spinal loads. In the lumbar spine, the facet joints absorb one-third of an intervertebral shear force while the disk resists the remainder.[4] Facets function to protect the disk from torsion[13] and, in lordotic postures, transmit one-sixth of the compressive loads.[20, 21] When asymmetrically aligned (referred to as tropism), paired facets will unequally resist these shear forces with a tendency to rotate toward the more obliquely aligned facet.

The facet joint capsule plays a dominant role in resisting flexion, providing 39% of the joint's resistance.[22, 23] Oriented in a direction perpendicular to the plane of the facet joint, capsular fibers have optimal orientation to provide this support. In the lumbar spine, the outer layer of the capsule is made up of dense connective tissue with parallel bundles of collagenous fibers running from medial to lateral across the joint. The inner layer is composed of elastic fibers.[23] The capsule is innervated.

LIGAMENTS

The spinal ligaments work in concert with the intervertebral disk and the capsular ligaments to limit joint motion. This ability is dependent on the location, orientation, physical properties, resting tension of the ligament, and type of loading. Ligaments are most effective at carrying tensile loads along the axis of their fibers. In compression, ligaments tend to buckle.

The anterior longitudinal ligament (ALL) arises from the anterior aspect of the basioccipital region of the skull and travels caudally with a firm attachment to the anterior vertebral bodies, but no connection to the anulus, before terminating at the sacrum.[24] The deep layer spans between one intervertebral articulation, whereas the intermediate and superficial layers extend across two to five segments. The ALL is strongest in the upper cervical, lower thoracic, and lumbar regions with the ability to tolerate a load of 680 N before failure.[25, 26] In flexion, the ALL is relaxed, and all other spinal ligaments are under tension. In extension, the ALL is under maximal strain.[22]

The posterior longitudinal ligament (PLL), like the ALL, begins at the basiocciput but completes its course caudally at the coccyx. The PLL widens at each disk level, and its fibers are firmly attached to the anulus. It is richly innervated with small, unmyelinated C-type nerves, which may transmit painful stimuli.

The supraspinous and interspinous ligaments provide 19% of the intervertebral joint's resistance to flexion.[20] In flexion, these ligaments are under the highest strains.[22] The

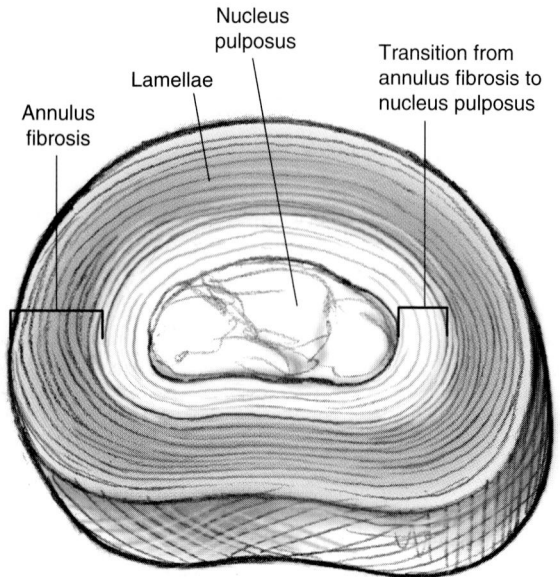

Fig. 3. Intervertebral disk. The intervertebral disk is a composite structure. The annulus fibrosis is a tough, multilayered fibrous mesh that confines the gelatinous, high-pressured nucleus pulposus.

Annulus fibrosis

Lamellae

Nucleus pulposus

Transition from annulus fibrosis to nucleus pulposus

supraspinous ligament in the lumbar spine has demonstrated a load-to-failure of 750 N.[26] Interactions between collagen fibers of these ligaments allow forces to be transmitted along alternative pathways after a partial transection.[27] In addition, these ligaments are well innervated and may form the basis of a proprioceptive feedback mechanism for protection of the spine.[28]

The ligamentum flavum, composed almost entirely of elastic fibers, connects adjacent laminae and provides 13% of the spine's resistance to flexion.[20] It is strongest in the lower thoracic spine and weakest in the midcervical region.[26] These ligaments, in a resting position in vivo, are pretensioned to prevent redundant fibers from buckling into the neural canal during spine extension. Posterior spinal instrumentation and fusion leads to stress shielding of the posterior ligaments, including the ligamentum flavum, with diminished tensile properties and histological changes.[29]

The occipitoatlantoaxial region of the spine does not have intervertebral disks and relies on a strong ligamentous network to maintain stability while allowing significant motion. The apical ligament connects the apex of the odontoid to the occiput and is able to tolerate a load of 125 N to 420 N before failure.[26] Stronger alar ligaments (200 N load to failure) span from the superolateral aspect of the odontoid to the occiput and restrain rotation.[30]

Half of the available cervical rotation arises from the atlantoaxial articulation.[31] The transverse ligament, with an in vitro strength of 350 N, forms a sling around the posterior portion of the odontoid.[30] This ligament is essential to securing the rotatory pivot point at the odontoid and in restricting flexion and anterior displacement of the atlas relative to the axis.

PARASPINAL MUSCULATURE

Paraspinal muscles are responsive to load and, therefore, are "active" spine stabilizers. As the spine faces increasing loads, progressive muscle recruitment through a specialized activation pattern has been predicted using FEA and confirmed by electromyography.[32] At high loads and with a more flexed posture, muscles play a crucial role in stabilizing the spine compared with the passive ligamentous restraints. Trunk twisting does not load the trunk muscles very much.[33] In the upright posture, the lumbar back muscles exert a net posterior shear force on the L1-4 segments and an anterior shear force on L5.[34] Muscle dysfunction reduces the role of facet joints in transmitting load and shift loads to the disks and ligaments.[35]

REGIONAL STRUCTURAL VARIATIONS

CERVICAL

In addition to the triple-joint complex, the subaxial cervical spine has two additional articulations between vertebrae. The "uncovertebral joints" consist of an uncinate process, which projects upward from the lateral surface of the lower vertebral body, and its corresponding recess located on the inferolateral surface of the upper vertebral body. The major biomechanical function of uncovertebral joints includes the regulation of extension and lateral bending motion followed by torsion, which is mainly provided by the posterior uncovertebral joint.[36]

The cervical facet joints, aligned within the coronal plane, are similar to overlapping shingles on a roof. When isolated in the lab, the average allowable cervical facet motions are 19 degrees of flexion, 14 degrees of extension, 28 degrees of lateral bending, and 17 degrees of rotation.[1] However, when constrained within an intact spine, the range of motion is much less. An intact vertebral ring with competent facet joints is necessary to provide axial rotational and lateral bending stability but accounts for little flexion-extension stability.[1]

THORACIC

The thoracic portion of the spine is morphologically unique for several reasons[37]: the resting sagittal plane alignment is kyphotic[38]; the facet joints, similar to those of the cervical spine, lie in the frontal plane; and the ribs,[19] through attachments at the costotransverse junctions, limit motion and provide additional stability to lateral bending and axial rotation.[39] A discontinuity of the chest, as with removal of the sternum, completely negates the stiffening effect of the rib cage.

LUMBAR

The lumbar spine demonstrates great flexibility and transmits loads up to four times body weight.[40] The sagittal alignment is lordotic. Facet joints adopt a more curved appearance with a greater surface within the coronal plane. The thick, firm iliolumbar ligaments travel to the transverse processes of L5. In the upright lordotic posture, the pars interarticularis at L5 (and occasionally L4) faces greater stress, occasionally resulting in fatigue fractures (spondylolysis).

JUNCTIONAL

A junctional segment occurs at a transition point within a structure in which two dissimilar mechanical zones (with differing physical dimensions or material properties) meet. Within the spine, there are four such junctional segments[37]: occipitocervical,[28] cervicothoracic,[19] thoracolumbar, and lumbosacral.[20] Each of these regions face unique loads and focal stresses.

CLINICAL PARADIGMS TO ASSESS SPINAL STABILITY

COLUMNAR CONCEPTS AND LOAD SHARING

To define spinal stability, anatomic structures with similar mechanical functions have been grouped into columns (Fig. 4). Holdsworth described two spinal columns.[41, 42] The anterior column, transmitting compressive load, consists of the vertebral body and intervertebral disk, the ALL, and the PLL. The posterior column, carrying tensile stress, includes the paired facet joints, the neural arch, and the interspinous ligaments. Disruption of more than one column defines an "unstable" injury. Holdsworth emphasized the importance of the posterior ligaments, functioning as a tension band to effectively balance the load that travels through the anterior column.

Denis later added to the work of Holdsworth with the development of the three-column classification.[43] The anterior column consists of the anterior two-thirds of the verte-

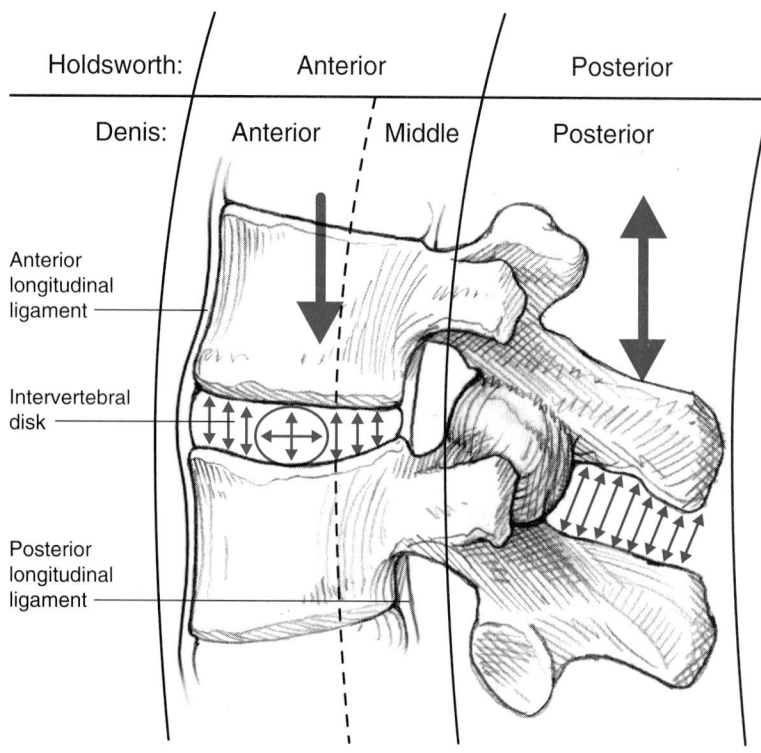

Holdsworth: Anterior | Posterior

Denis: Anterior | Middle | Posterior

Anterior longitudinal ligament

Intervertebral disk

Posterior longitudinal ligament

Fig. 4. Holdsworth two-column and Denis three-column concepts. A compressive load is transmitted through the anterior column. A healthy nucleus pulposus underload causes tensile forces to be developed within the annulus. Tensile forces within the posterior column ligaments effectively balance the spinal segment in the sagittal plane.

bral body/disk and the ALL. The middle column includes the posterior third of the vertebral body and disk with the PLL. The posterior column incorporates everything posterior to the PLL. Using this paradigm, disruption of more than two columns indicates instability. However, not all columns contribute equally to spinal stability. Actually, the middle column is not of great importance in regard to biomechanical stability compared with the contributing elements within the anterior or posterior columns.[44]

Sagittal plane balance requires functional anterior and posterior columns. The concept of "load sharing" in the spine refers to the ability of the anterior or posterior columns to carry a large portion of their required physiological loads. Severe, anteroposterior column disruption is unlikely to be stabilized by reconstructive efforts that support only one column unless the remaining column is capable of contributing.[45] Posterior fixation has very little effect on the magnitude of the compressive loads transmitted across the vertebral bodies and disks.[46]

SPINAL MECHANICAL DISORDERS

TRAUMA

The specific spinal injury that occurs is a function of the rate, magnitude, and direction of the applied load as well as the specific structural properties of the segment facing the load. Possible injury vectors include compression, distraction, flexion, extension, rotation, and shear.[8, 47]

When a compression load is applied to the spine, the highest stresses concentrate in the middle of the end plate in the cancellous bone under the nucleus and in the middle of the posterior wall cortex. With increasing load, the vertebral body fails, resulting in a compression fracture of the

superior or inferior end plate. If the load continues, the body "bursts," the pedicles are driven apart, and the middle column retropulses posteriorly, obstructing a portion of the neural canal. A "stable burst" implies the posterior ligamentous "tension band" is intact, allowing minimal kyphosis. Cervical and mid- and lower lumbar "burst" fractures are typically caused by an axial compressive load.[42]

A flexion-compression moment is the cause of nearly half of thoracolumbar junctional injuries.[48] The anterior column is compressed while the posterior ligamentous complex is placed under tension. The anterior vertebral body fails followed by middle column bony retropulsion and posterior ligament disruption. The ALL remains intact. The PLL may be stretched depending on the severity of the posterior tensile forces. "Unstable" burst fractures occur with disruption of the posterior ligaments.[41] With the loss of the posterior "tension band," early or late progressive kyphosis at the injured zone is possible.

Flexion-distraction forces occur less frequently than flexion-compression forces. Tensile failure can occur through ligament or bone or through a variable path that includes both.[49] Chance[50] first described three cases involving the thoracolumbar spine in 1948. He observed a fracture line through the spinous process, lamina, transverse processes, and pedicle and exiting on the superior surface of the vertebral body just anterior to the neural foramen. When the axis of rotation in a flexion-distraction injury is located within the anterior vertebral body, the result is a compression fracture of the anterior vertebral body and posterior ligament disruption with unilateral or bilateral facet joint disruption-dislocation. Alternatively, when the center of rotation is brought anterior to the vertebral column, an effective distraction force is applied to all three columns. In a thoracolumbar "seat belt" injury, the fulcrum is located at the anterior abdominal wall. Posterior and middle columns disrupt in tension on an intact ALL hinge.

Extension is a rare mechanism in the thoracic and lumbar spine but is more frequently seen in the cervical region. The ALL is inevitably torn with variable injury to the anterior anulus fibrosis. The posterior compressive forces generated may fracture the lamina, with posterior ligaments remaining in continuity. The presence of posterior segmental translation greater than 3 mm in the cervical spine and 5 mm in the thoracic and lumbar spine usually indicates a significant shear component and a three-column ligamentous injury.

The facet joint, in concert with the anulus, is a primary structure opposing *rotation*. When such forces are applied one facet joint may fracture and dislocate anteriorly, whereas its counterpart fails in tension with disruption of the joint capsule. When occurring within the thoracolumbar spine, these fractures traverse multiple ribs and transverse processes. A Holdsworth "slice" fracture of the thoracolumbar spine, the result of a rotational force, proceeds anteriorly through the superior vertebral body after facet joint failure.[41]

The most destabilizing of all injury mechanisms is that of a shear force. There is failure of all three columns representing the highest risk for concurrent neurological compromise.[51] A fracture-dislocation resulting from a shear mechanism frequently affects the facet joints, allowing the vertebral body to translate with failure of the ALL, PLL, and anulus fibrosis. Surgical exploration often demonstrates complete ligament discontinuity. Multiple fractures may occur at the transverse processes and ribs. These are three-column injuries.

DEGENERATIVE CASCADE

The internal pressures developing with a disk, in vivo, with a given load and posture have been determined.[40] The load at the L3-4 disk ranges from 30 kg while lying flat to more than 300 kg while lifting a 20-kg weight with the back bent and knees straight. Disk degeneration is an inevitable result of the metabolic alterations that result directly from aging and the immense mechanical loads.

The disk nucleus is 80% water in youth and desiccates progressively after 30 years of age.[9] Proteoglycan synthesis in adults is five times less than within an immature disk and even lower within a spondylolisthetic disk.[17, 52–54] There is no systematic change in collagen content.[54] In the degenerative disk, lactic acid accumulates and the pH drops. Below a pH of 6.8, the proteoglycan synthesis markedly decreases.[17]

A disk without a well-hydrated nucleus is unable to function properly. Stress concentrations occur as the load is transferred from the nucleus to the anulus.[15, 55] The altered tensile properties of the anulus with age lead to lower energy to failure and tears of the fibers.[38] Such structural changes further adversely affect chondrocyte metabolism. The healing capacity of the nucleus and anulus is poor. The facets are forced to take on an increased proportion of the axial loads, up to 70%,[20] ultimately resulting in facet joint arthropathy. Increased motion between vertebra is then allowed. End plates are subjected to stress concentra-

tion sites along the periphery.[15] Calcification of the articular cartilage of the end plate and age-related end-arteriole vascular changes restrict the exchange of water and nutrients to the chondrocyte, and the products of metabolism accumulate.

To maintain mechanical stability with aging, the components of the spine, including ligament, bone, and facet joint, thicken and hypertrophy.[56] The result is a stiffening of the motion segment and a narrowing of the neural canal (spinal stenosis).

PATHOLOGICAL PROCESSES

In cases of recognized tumor or infectious infiltration of a vertebra, it is advantageous for the clinician to diagnose impending vertebral collapse accurately. The association between vertebral body collapse and the size and location of the metastatic lesions has been studied clinically.[57] For the thoracic region, tumor size and costovertebral joint destruction are predictive of impending collapse (50% to 60% involvement of the vertebral body and no destruction of other structures or 25% to 30% vertebral body involvement with costovertebral joint destruction). For the thoracolumbar and lumbar spine, tumor size and pedicle destruction are predictive of collapse (35% to 40% of the vertebral body alone or 20% to 25% involvement with posterior element destruction).

Several studies attempted to simulate pathological destruction in the laboratory by drilling the vertebral body centrum.[58, 59] No threshold defect size has been noted beyond which failure consistently occurs. Vertebral strength is predicted by the product of bone mineral density and the remaining intact vertebral body cross-sectional area (the vertebral strength index).[58]

MECHANICAL CHANGES RESULTING FROM SURGERY

POSTERIOR CERVICAL DECOMPRESSION

A cadaveric study has been used to analyze the biomechanical alterations after sequential facet resections to replicate decompressive procedures.[60] Study groups included the intact specimen; after C5 laminectomy; and after 25%, 50%, 75%, and 100% bilateral facetectomies. Torsional stiffness decreased dramatically when more than 50% of the facets were resected. In a subsequent study, the stabilizing role of the facet capsule was examined after resection of the cervical facet joint capsule alone without bone disruption.[61] In torsion, the displacement increased 19% after a 50% capsular resection. Great care should be made to avoid greater than 50% facet resection.

ANTERIOR CERVICAL FUSION

After an anterior decompression (diskectomy or corpectomy), anterior reconstruction with a structural load-bearing graft for fusion is required. Proper sizing and contouring of the graft to obtain physiological cervical lordosis are essential. Placement of too large an anterior graft in the cervical spine leads to overdistraction, unloading of the facets, and increased compressive forces on the bone graft.[62] This would potentiate the risk of collapse and pseudarthrosis.

LUMBAR DISKECTOMY

Surgical injury to the anulus and removal of the nucleus adversely affect the mechanical properties of the segment and even alter coupled motions within adjacent segments.[63-65] In one study using the whole lumbar spine, the level above the diskectomy showed an increased anteroposterior translation in flexion and increased lateral translation with lateral bending irrespective of the amount of disk removed.[63] Sagittal plane symmetry is disrupted, leading to asymmetric facet joint movements. Subtotal diskectomy, inducing significantly less abnormal motion than total diskectomy in all loading modes, is favored.[63-65]

LUMBAR LAMINECTOMY/FACETECTOMY

Biomechanical studies have been performed to assess the effect of posterior lumbar surgical decompression, including laminectomy and facetectomy.[21, 37, 66] One study used fresh human lumbar functional spinal units and a sequential injury pattern beginning with transection of the supraspinous and interspinous ligaments followed by progressive facet excisions.[37] Unilateral or bilateral partial medial facetectomies did not affect lumbar spine stability. In another study examining three motion segments, progressive alterations of the lumbar facet joints were stable under physiological compression-flexion loads unless the supraspinous and interspinous ligaments are violated.[66] Therefore, at any one motion segment, a total of one facet joint can be excised if the supraspinous and interspinous ligaments are competent.

LUMBAR FUSION

Rigid spinal implants augment spinal fusion success. However, as the rigidity of a construct is increased, device-related vertebral osteoporosis (stress-shielding) becomes apparent.[67] The increased fusion mass resulting from the use of rigid instrumentation more than compensates for the loss of compressive, torsional, or flexural rigidity resulting from osteopenia.[67]

Arthrodesis significantly alters the biomechanics of the spine, requiring an increased compensatory motion and mechanical loading in the adjacent free segments, particularly within the facet joints.[68-72] Posterior fusions produce the largest amount of stress, whereas lateral fusion, constructed at a point closer to the center of spinal rotation, cause the least.[73] Such change in the adjacent segment motion pattern becomes more pronounced as the fixation range extends and as the rigidity of the construct increases.[68, 71, 74]

In a 1996 retrospective review, juxtafusion degeneration was estimated in approximately 35% of patients; the occurrence was associated with advanced patient age and with the use of an interbody fusion.[75] In a study using single-photon emission computed tomography to evaluate patients with back pain 4 years after lumbar fusion, 62% demonstrated lesions in the vertebral bodies and apophyseal joints in the free motion segment adjacent to the fused segment.[61]

Semirigid devices have been developed on the premise that the undesirable effects of rigid devices (juxtafusion degeneration, device-related vertebral osteoporosis, stress shielding of the fusion mass) will be decreased. Polymer washers, which dissolve with time, decrease rigidity and diminish the effects of stress shielding.[76]

CONCLUSION

A detailed understanding of spine biomechanics is essential to the surgeon who is examining a patient with back pain or performing complex spinal decompressive and reconstructive procedures. This is accomplished through an appreciation of the complex bony, articular, and ligamentous spinal components; their material properties; allowable motions; and transmitted loads. Trauma, tumors, infections, degenerative processes, and surgical interventions alter spinal mechanics at both the involved and the adjacent levels.

REFERENCES

1. Onan OA, Heggeness MH, Hipp JA: A motion analysis of the cervical facet joint. Spine 1998; 23:430.
2. Wilke HJ, Krischak ST, Wenger KH, et al: Load-displacement of the thoracolumbar calf spine: Experimental results and comparison to known human data. Eur Spine J 1997; 6:129.
3. Bell GH, Dunbar O, Beck JS, et al: Variation in strength of vertebrae with age and their relation on osteoporosis. Calcif Tissue Res 1967; 1:75.
4. Silva MJ, Keaveny TM, Hayes WC: Load sharing between the shell and centrum in the lumbar vertebral body. Spine 1997; 22:140.
5. Hansson TH, Keller TS, Panjabi MM: A study of the compressive properties of lumbar vertebral trabeculae: Effects of tissue characteristics. Spine 1987; 12:56.
6. Smit TH, Odgaard A, Schneider E: Structure and function of vertebral trabecular bone. Spine 1997; 22:2823.
7. Keller TS, Hansson TH, Abram AC, et al: Regional variations in the compressive properties of lumbar vertebral trabeculae: Effects of disc degeneration. Spine 1989; 14:1012.
8. Ferguson RL, Allen BL: A mechanistic classification of thoracolumbar spine fractures. Clin Orthop Rel Res 1984; 189:77.
9. Eyre DR: Biochemistry of the intervertebral disc. Int Rev Connect Tissue Res 1979; 8:227.
10. Urban JPG, McMullin JF: Swelling pressure of the intervertebral disc: Influence of proteoglycan and collagen contents. Biorheology 1986; 22:145.
11. Brickley-Parsons D, Glimcher M: Is the chemistry of collagen in the intervertebral disc an expression of Wolff's law? A study of the human lumbar spine. Spine 1984; 9:148.
12. Marchand F, Ahmed AM: Investigation of the laminate structure of the lumbar anulus fibrosis. Spine 1990; 15:402.
13. Krismer M, Haid C, Rabi W: The contribution of anulus fibers to torque resistance. Spine 1996; 21:2551.
14. Roberts S, Menage J, Urban JPG: Biochemical and structural properties of the cartilage end-plate and its relation to the intervertebral disc. Spine 1989; 14:166.
15. Adams MA, McMillan DW, Green TP, et al: Sustained loading generates stress concentrations in lumbar intervertebral discs. Spine 1996; 21:434.
16. McMillan DW, Garbutt G, Adams MA: Effect of sustained loading on the water content of intervertebral discs: Implications for disc metabolism. Ann Rheum Dis 1996; 55:880.
17. Ohshima H, Urban JPG: The effect of lactate concentrations and pH on matrix synthesis rates in the intervertebral disc. Spine 1992; 17:1079.
18. Magnusson ML, Aleksiev AR, Spratt KF, et al: Hyperextension and spine height changes. Spine 1996; 21:2670.
19. Adams MA, Hutton WC: Prolapsed intervertebral disc: A hyperflexion injury. Spine 1982; 7:184.
20. Adams MA, Hutton WC: The mechanical function of the lumbar apophyseal joints. Spine 1983; 8:327.

21. Lorenz M, Patwardhan A, Vanderby R: Load bearing characteristics of lumbar facets in normal and surgically altered spinal segments. Spine 1983; 8:122.

22. Panjabi MM, Goel V, Takata K: Physiological strains in lumbar ligaments. Spine 1982; 7:192.

23. Yamashita T, Minaki Y, Ozaktay AC, et al: A morphological study of the fibrous capsule of the human lumbar facet joint. Spine 1996; 21:538.

24. Przybylski GJ, Patel PR, Carlin GJ, et al: Quantitative anthropometry of the subatlantal cervical longitudinal ligaments. Spine 1998; 23:893.

25. Chazal J, Tanguy A, Bourges M, et al: Biomechanical properties of spinal ligaments and a histological study of the supraspinal ligament in traction. J Biomech 1985; 18:167.

26. Myklebust JB, Pintar F, Yoganandan N, et al: Tensile strength of spinal ligaments. Spine 1988; 13:526.

27. Dickey JP, Bednar DA, Dumas GA: New insight into the mechanics of the lumbar interspinous ligament. Spine 1996; 21:2720.

28. Jiang H, Russell G, Raso VJ, et al: The nature and distribution of the innervation of human supraspinal and interspinal ligaments. Spine 1995; 20:869.

29. Kotani Y, Cunningham BW, Capuccino A, et al: The effects of spinal fixation and destabilization on the biomechanical and histologic properties of spinal ligaments: An in vivo study. Spine 1998; 23:672.

30. Dvorak J, Schneider E, Saldinger P, et al: Biomechanics of the craniocervical region: The alar and transverse ligaments. J Orthop Res 1988; 6:452.

31. Penning L, Wilmink JT: Rotation of the cervical spine: A CT study in normal subjects. Spine 1987; 12:732.

32. Ladin Z, Murthy KR, DeLuca CJ: Mechanical recruitment of low back muscles. Spine 1989; 14:927.

33. Schultz A, Andersson G, Haderspeck K, et al: Analysis and measurement of lumbar trunk loads in tasks involving bends and twists. J Biomech 1982; 15:669.

34. Bogduk N, Macintosh JE, Pearcy MJ: A universal model of the lumbar back muscles in the upright position. Spine 1992; 17:897.

35. Kong WZ, Goel VK, Gilbertson LG, et al: Effects of muscle dysfunction on lumbar spine mechanics: A finite element study based on a two-motion segment model. Spine 1996; 21:2197.

36. Kotani Y, McNulty PS, Abumi K, et al: The role of anteromedial foraminotomy and uncovertebral joints in the stability of the cervical spine. Spine 1998; 23:1559.

37. Abumi K, Panjabi M, Kramer KM, et al: Biomechanical evaluation of lumbar spinal stability after graded facetectomies. Spine 1990; 15:1142.

38. Acaroglu ER, Iatridis JC, Setton LA, et al: Degeneration and aging affect the tensile behavior of human anulus fibrosis. Spine 1995; 20:2690.

39. Oda I, Abumi K, Lu D, et al: Biomechanical role of the posterior elements, costovertebral joints, and rib cage in the stability of the thoracic spine. Spine 1996; 21:1423.

40. Nachemson A, Morris JM: In vivo measurements of intradiscal pressure. J Bone Joint Surg Am 1964; 46:1077.

41. Holdsworth FW: Fractures, dislocations, and fracture-dislocations of the spine. J Bone Joint Surg Am 1970; 52:1534.

42. Holdsworth FW, Hardy A: Early treatment of paraplegia from fractures of the thoracolumbar spine. J Bone Joint Surg Br 1953; 35:540.

43. Denis F: The three-column spine and its significance in the classification of acute thoracolumbar spinal injuries. Spine 1983; 8:817.

44. James KS, Wenger KH, Schlegel JA, et al: Biomechanical evaluation of the stability of thoracolumbar burst fractures. Spine 1994; 19:1731.

45. McCormack T, Karaikovic E, Gaines RW: The load sharing classification of spine fractures. Spine 1994; 19:1741.

46. Edwards AG, McNally DS, Mulholland RC, et al: The effects of posterior fixation on internal intervertebral disc mechanics. J Bone Joint Surg Br 1997; 79:154.

47. Allen BL, Ferguson RL, Lehmann TR, et al: A mechanistic classification of closed, indirect fractures and dislocations of the lower cervical spine. Spine 1982; 7:1.

48. Cotler, JM, Vernace JV, Michalski JA: The use of Harrington rods in thoracolumbar fractures. Orthop Clin North Am 1986; 17:87.

49. Gertzbein SD, Court-Brown CM: Flexion-distraction injuries of the lumbar spine. Clin Orthop 1988; 227:52.

50. Chance GQ: Note on a type of flexion fracture of the spine. Br J Radiol 1948; 21:452.

51. Gertzbein SD: Neurologic deterioration in patients with thoracic and lumbar fractures after admission to the hospital. Spine 1994; 19:1723.

52. Bayliss MT, Johnstone B, O'Brien JP: Proteoglycan synthesis in the human intervertebral disc: Variation with age, region and pathology. Spine 1988; 13:972.

53. Ohshima H, Tsuji H, Hirano N, et al: Water diffusion pathway, swelling pressure and biomechanical properties of the intervertebral disc during compressive loading. Spine 1991; 14:1234.

54. Urban JPG, McMullin JF: Swelling pressure of lumbar intervertebral discs: Influence of age, spinal level, composition and degeneration. Spine 1988; 13:179.

55. McNally DS, Shackleford IM, Goodship AE, et al: In vivo stress measurement can predict pain on discography. Spine 1996; 21:2580.

56. Fukuyama S, Nakamura T, Ikeda T, et al: The effect of mechanical stress on hypertrophy of the lumbar ligamentum flavum. J Spinal Disord 1995; 8:126.

57. Taneichi H, Kaneda K, Takeda N, et al: Risk factors and probability of vertebral body collapse in metastases of the thoracic and lumbar spine. Spine 1997; 22:239.

58. Dimar JR, Voor MJ, Zhang YM, et al: A human cadaver model for determination of pathologic fracture threshold resulting from tumorous destruction of the vertebral body. Spine 1998; 23:1209.

59. McGowan DP, Hipp JA, Takeuchi T, et al: Strength reductions from trabecular destruction within thoracic vertebrae. J Spinal Disord 1993; 6:130.

60. Zdeblick TA, Zou D, Warden KE, et al: Cervical stability after foraminotomy. J Bone Joint Surg Am 1992; 74:22.

61. Zdeblick TA, Abitbol JJ, Kunz DN, et al: Cervical stability after sequential capsule resection. Spine 1993; 18:2005.

62. Olsewski JM, Garvery TA, Schendel MJ: Biomechanical analysis of facet and graft loading in a Smith-Robinson–type cervical spine model. Spine 1994; 19:2540.

63. Goel VK, Goyal S, Clark C, et al: Kinematics of the whole lumbar spine: Effect of discectomy. Spine 1985; 10:543.

64. Goel VK, Nishiyama K, Weinstein JN, et al: Mechanical properties of lumbar spinal motion segments as affected by partial disc removal. Spine 1986; 11:1008.

65. Panjabi MM, Krag MH, Chung TQ: Effects of disc injury on the mechanical behavior of the human spine. Spine 1984; 9:707.

66. Cusick JF, Yoganandan N, Pintar FA, et al: Biomechanics of sequential posterior lumbar surgery. J Neurosurg 1992; 76:805.

67. McAfee PC, Farey ID, Sutterlin CE, et al: Device-related osteoporosis with spinal instrumentation. Spine 1989; 14:919.

68. Chow DHK, Luk KD, Evans JH, et al: Effects of short anterior lumbar interbody fusion on biomechanics of neighboring unfused segments. Spine 1996; 21:549.

69. Dekutoski MB, Schendel MJ, Ogilvie JW, et al: Comparison of in vivo and in vitro adjacent segment motion after lumbar fusion. Spine 1994; 19:1745.

70. Lee CK: Accelerated degeneration of the segment adjacent to a lumbar fusion. Spine 1988; 13:375.

71. Nagata H, Schendel MJ, Transfeldt EE, et al: The effects of immobilization of long segments of the spine on the adjacent and distal facet force and lumbosacral motion. Spine 1993; 18:2471.

72. Quinnel RC, Stockdale HR: Some experimental observations of the influence of a simple lumbar floating fusion on the remaining lumbar spine. Spine 1981; 6:263.

73. Lee CK, Langrana NA: Lumbosacral spinal fusion: A biomechanical study. Spine 1984; 9:574.

74. Shono Y, Kaneda K, Abumi K, et al: Stability of posterior spinal instrumentation and its effects on adjacent motion segments in the lumbosacral spine. Spine 1988; 23:1550.

75. Rahm MD, Hall BB: Adjacent-segment degeneration after lumbar fusion with instrumentation: A retrospective study. J Spinal Disord 1996; 9:392.

76. Even-Sapir E, Martin RH, Mitchell MJ, et al: Assessment of painful late effects of lumbar spinal fusion with SPECT. J Nucl Med 1994; 35:416.

77. Goel VK, Lim TH, Gwon J, et al: Effects of rigidity of an internal fixation device: A comprehensive biomechanical investigation. Spine 1991; 16:S155.

section
8
chapter
12

SPINE FUSION: BIOLOGICAL AND MECHANICAL CONSIDERATIONS

Geoffrey M. McCullen, Navin Kilambi, and Steven R. Garfin

Summary

- Structural grafts are used to reconstruct the anterior column of the spine to transmit compressive loads and maintain physiological sagittal plane alignment.
- Nonstructural cancellous autograft is preferred for posterior fusion techniques.
- Revascularization of dense cortical structural graft first requires osteoclastic bone resorption, resulting in weakening of the structural properties of the graft for 6 weeks to 6 months after implantation.
- To obtain a solid fusion, attention to both biological and biomechanical principles is required.
- Host systemic factors known to affect spinal fusion include use of corticosteroid and nonsteroidal anti-inflammatory drugs, smoking, poor nutrition, and metabolic disorders.
- Local factors that may adversely affect the soft-tissue bed and diminish graft healing capacity include infection, tumor, radiation therapy, previous surgery, and vertebral instability.

Clinical Summary

- Alternatives to autologous bone graft for spinal fusions include allograft, ceramics (hydroxyapatite [HA], calcium phosphate, coralline products, composites), demineralized bone matrix (DBM), and bone morphogenic protein (BMP).
- Fresh frozen and freeze-dried structural allografts (fibula and iliac crest) have been successfully used for single-level anterior cervical interbody fusions.
- Freeze-dried cancellous allograft, when used for posterior thoracolumbar spinal fusion in skeletally immature patients, has demonstrated a low pseudarthrosis rate. However, poor results have been obtained when used for posterior cervical fusion in children and for posterior fusions in adults.
- Application of ceramics in spinal fusion has been slow to evolve secondary to the brittle nature of the materials and often incomplete incorporation.
- DBM is best used to extend autologous or allograft bone in posterior spinal fusions.
- BMP also appears to be successful when used alone without autograft.

Spinal fusions are used primarily in four clinical scenarios: (1) reconstruction of a vertebral element left incapacitated by tumor, infection, or surgical decompression; (2) correction or prevention of deformity; (3) intersegmental instability developing from traumatic or degenerative changes; and (4) reduction of pain originating from a definable degenerative site.

In the early 1900s, Albee[1] and Hibbs[2] independently described techniques for posterior spinal fusion for prevention of progressive deformity in patients with Pott's disease. Since that time, great progress has been made in fusion techniques. This is reflected in the variety of fusion methods (anterior interbody, posterior interbody, posterior intertransverse process, and combined), choices of grafting materials (autograft, allograft, bone substitutes), and the concomitant use of instrumentation.

For optimal healing capacity in spinal fusions, autograft is the best material possessing three critical properties: (1) osteogenesis, the ability to directly produce bone; (2) osteoinduction, the release of factors capable of stimulating osteoprogenitor cells to differentiate; and (3) osteoconduction, a structural lattice onto which new bone can grow and develop.

The biological incorporation of autograft into a solid fusion follows the sequence observed in fracture healing: induction, inflammation, soft callus, hard callus, and remodeling.[3] These processes may occur simultaneously within different segments of the graft. Disruption of a particular step may lead to pseudarthrosis.

GRAFT REQUIREMENTS

Interbody and strut grafts are used to reconstruct the anterior column of the spine to transmit compressive loads and maintain physiological sagittal plane alignment. In vivo, lumbar intradiscal pressures have been shown to support physiological loads between 2400 and 3300 N.[4] To withstand these compressive loads, structural grafts must include a substantial cortical component. Grafts currently used include tricortical iliac crest, fibula, and allograft diaphyseal (femur, humerus) "ring" segments (Table 1).

Autologous tricortical iliac crest is an optimal structural graft. Because of their compressive strength, 7-mm autologous sections taken from the anterosuperior iliac spine is able to bear significantly higher axial loads (3200 N) than comparable sections taken from the posterior crest (1400 N).[5] The cancellous density within these tricortical segments is the most significant factor in the prediction of load to failure. An autologous fibula graft is stronger than iliac crest in compression (12600 N load to failure) but has a smaller cross-sectional area and less cancellous bone.[5]

Nonstructural cancellous autograft is preferred for posterior fusion techniques (Table 2). Posterior interlaminar grafts are now infrequently used in isolation. Dorsal to the axis of rotation, such grafts experience tensile forces, which promote fibroblast formation and limit the healing capacity.[6] Alternatively, by virtue of more ventral positioning closer to the spine axis of rotation, intertransverse process (posterolateral) lumbar fusions face less disruptive ten-

TABLE 1. STRUCTURAL GRAFT MATERIALS IN SPINAL FUSIONS

Type	Properties			Effectiveness in Spine	
	Osteogenic	Inductive	Conductive	Animal	Clinical
Autograft tricortical	+	+	+	+	+ (Gold standard)
Allograft cortical "ring"	−	−	+	+	+ (Slow, incomplete incorporation)
Ceramics					
HA/TCP	−	−	+	+/−	+ (Cervical spine interbody with plate fixation)
Coralline HA					

HA, hydroxyapatite; TCP, tricalcium phosphate.

sile forces. The vascular supply to intertransverse process graft appears to come primarily from the decorticated transverse processes but may also receive contributions from the overlying muscle.[7, 8]

Revascularization of dense cortical graft first requires osteoclastic bone resorption. Thus, when compared with porous cancellous bone, the process is much slower and results in weakening of the structural properties of the graft for 6 weeks to 6 months after implantation.[9] Newer cage devices, designed to be packed with cancellous bone, substitute a durable and biocompatible synthetic material (titanium, carbon fiber) for the cortical structural component that does not weaken with revascularization.[10] Ultimately, the rate and extent of incorporation of autograft in a spinal fusion are dependent on the size and type of graft as well as the host systemic and local environments.

SYSTEMIC FACTORS

Several host systemic factors known to affect spinal fusion include corticosteroid and nonsteroidal anti-inflammatory drugs (NSAIDs), smoking, poor nutrition, and metabolic disorders.

NSAIDs are known to affect the inflammatory phase of bone osteogenesis adversely. An animal model studying the effect of indomethacin on posterior spinal fusion demonstrated a 10% fusion rate compared with 45% in the control group.[11] Histologically, the indomethacin group showed bone graft involution, predominant fibrous tissue, and scant periosteal reaction at the decorticated laminar surface. Similarly, in a human clinical study of lumbar spine fusion, a 4% nonunion rate was seen in the control group compared with 17% in those who had received perioperative ketorolac.[12] Therefore, NSAIDs are best avoided during the induction and inflammatory phases of graft incorporation (for 1 week preoperatively to approximately 6 weeks postoperatively).

Smoking adversely affects spine bone graft incorporation, presumably through hypoxemia and nicotine effects. The average partial pressure of oxygen in smokers is 78% versus 93% in nonsmokers.[13] Nicotine is likely to play an inhibitory role in the neovascularization of the bone graft.[14–16] Smokers are three times more likely than nonsmokers to develop nonunion in posterior lumbar fusions.[12, 13]

Clinical parameters commonly used to assess nutritional status of surgical patients are the serum albumin level (an index of visceral protein mass) and the total lymphocyte count (an indicator of immune competence). Serum albumin less than 3.5 g/dL and a total lymphocyte count less than 1500 cells/mm^3 are consistent with malnutrition. In one study, up to 25% of patients (42% when older than 60 years) undergoing elective spinal fusion were considered malnourished by these criteria.[18] For malnourished patients, the risk for postoperative infection was more than 15 times greater than for the adequately nourished group.

TABLE 2. NONSTRUCTURAL GRAFT MATERIALS IN SPINAL FUSIONS

Type	Properties			Effectiveness in Spine	
	Osteogenic	Inductive	Conductive	Animal	Clinical
Autograft cancellous	+	+	+	+	+ (Gold standard)
Allograft cancellous	−	−	+	+	+ (Only in TL spine, skeletally immature)
Ceramics					
HA/TCP	−	−	+	+	+ (Only as autograft expander)
Calcium sulfate					
Coralline HA					
DBM	−	+	−	+	+ (Only as autograft expander)
BMP	−	++	−	++	Not studied
Composites					
Collagraft/Healos	−	−	+	+	Not studied (used with bone marrow aspirate)

HA, hydroxyapatite; TCP, tricalcium phosphate; DBM, demineralized bone matrix; BMP, bone morphogenic protein; TL, thoracolumbar.

LOCAL FACTORS

Local factors may adversely affect the soft-tissue bed and diminish graft healing capacity. Infection, tumor, radiation therapy (XRT), previous surgery, and vertebral instability create scar, diminish the intrinsic vascular supply, alter local immune responsiveness, and jeopardize the optimal mechanical environment.

The biological and biomechanical effects of XRT on posterior bone graft healing in the spine have been studied in animal models.[19, 20] Bone healing is influenced by the timing of the radiation dose. Specimens receiving immediate postoperative irradiation demonstrate marked fibrous tissue formation and are less stiff compared with controls and those receiving delayed postoperative dosing. Preoperative XRT also affects the histological score, graft maturation, and mechanical strength but to a lesser degree than in the group treated immediately postoperatively. If adjuvant radiation therapy is required after a posterior fusion, it should be delayed for 3 to 6 weeks postoperatively.

At surgery, careful preparation of the fusion site is important. Trauma to the soft-tissue envolope should be minimized. Decortication exposes local bone marrow to the fusion site and provides a source of osteoinductive proteins. Primary technical requirements for interbody fusions include complete removal of the disk and cartilage; preservation of the end plate; proper graft sizing and contouring for load-bearing distribution; and restoration of intervertebral height and sagittal contour. The interbody graft area should include 30% of the total end-plate area, at a minimum, to prevent end-plate fracture and graft subsidence.

CONSTRUCT RIGIDITY AND GRAFT IMPLICATIONS

The optimal rigidity of a spinal construct necessary to increase the likelihood of arthrodesis while avoiding device-related stress shielding and osteoporosis has yet to be determined. Animal, clinical, and biomechanical studies sought to address these issues. Animal models showed that, as the rigidity of the instrumentation is increased, the rigidity of the resultant fusion mass is increased at the cost of creating vertebral osteoporosis.[22–24] After implant removal, a rebound in the bone mineral density within the vertebra is seen.[22]

Several human clinical studies attempted to analyze the relationship between construct rigidity and graft healing. Atrophic pseudarthroses have been associated with intact facet joints or retained hardware, which are believed to contribute to stress shielding and graft atrophy.[25, 26] The addition of an anterior interbody fusion leads to a higher rate of resorption of the lateral intertransverse process fusion mass, although the overall fusion success rate across the motion segment may improve.[27]

Alternatively, a prospective, randomized clinical trial comparing posterolateral constructs using constructs of varying stiffness found that the best results were obtained with the use of rigid pedicle screw instrumentation.[12] Histologically, instrumented fusion bone closely resembles cortical bone. Noninstrumented fusions cover a signifi-cantly wider area, effectively increasing the moment of inertia, but are less dense.[28]

BIOLOGICAL AUGMENTATION OF SPINAL FUSIONS

Mechanical loading of a crystalline structure causes a deformity and the creation of an electrical dipole or charge differential across the material. "Streaming potentials" occur when an extracellular electrolyte solution flows past the fixed crystalline structure. The cellular elements of bone are able to respond to these electrical signals. Compressive loading induces electronegative charge and the formation of osteoblasts, whereas a tensile zone is electropositive and promotes fibroblast proliferation.[6]

Implanted, direct current stimulators and externally applied pulsed electromagnetic fields (PEMF) may enhance cellular responsiveness in spinal fusions. A direct current electrical stimulator was first used clinically in posterolateral lumbar spine fusions in 1974 and was found to promote an earlier, immature fusion.[29] In 1988, a prospective, randomized study on direct current stimulation in posterolateral fusion demonstrated a 54% fusion rate in the control group compared with an 81% success rate in the stimulated group.[30]

Several clinical studies examined the effectiveness of PEMF in lumbar interbody fusions. Eleven of 13 patients with a failed posterior lumbar interbody fusion experienced a definite increase in fusion mass after PEMF application.[31] In a prospective, randomized, double-blind study of 98 patients undergoing lumbar interbody fusion, successful arthrodesis was obtained in 92% of those receiving PEMF versus 65% of the control group.[32]

Ultrasound stimulation has been introduced to improve fusion success with hypothesized beneficial effect on protein synthesis, vascularization, and matrix calcification. In a rabbit posterolateral fusion model, low-intensity ultrasound, begun on postoperative day 3 and used for 20 minutes daily for 6 weeks, caused a significant increase in the fusion rate, stiffness, and load to failure of the fusion mass.[33]

AUTOGRAFT DISADVANTAGES

Increased operative morbidity and limitations of supply remain the significant disadvantages of autograft use. Major complications have occurred in 9%, including wound infection (2.5%), hematoma requiring intervention (3%), sensory loss (1%), and osteomyelitis (1%). Minor complications have been frequent (21%) and include superficial infection, wound healing problems, slowly resolving pain, and temporary sensory loss.[34] Residual pain at the site of harvest is, unfortunately, a common problem.[34–36] Up to 50% of patients described postoperative harvest site pain.[36] Pain lasting more than 3 months has been reported in 15%.[35] Permanent nerve injuries can occur.[34–36] The most frequently injured nerve is the lateral femoral cutaneous nerve, at risk during anterior iliac harvesting. Proximal anterior thigh numbness or dysesthetic meralgia paresthetica has been reported in as many as 10%.[35] Transection of

TABLE 3. COSTS OF SELECTED AUTOGRAFT SUBSTITUTES/EXPANDERS

Type	Cost
Allograft (freeze dried)	
Femoral diaphyseal segment (6–10 cm)	$410–$530
Fibular diaphyseal segment (5–10 cm)	$235–$300
Iliac crest	
Tricortical (1–2.2 cm)	$435–$775
Bicortical	$225–$375
Morcelized bone graft (freeze dried)	
Cancellous	
1- to 15-mm chips	40 cc = $375
Finely crushed	30 cc = $575
Corticocancellous (add 10% for fresh frozen)	40 cc = $345
Ceramics	
Pro-osteon	30 cc = $550
Osteoset	100 pellets = $270
Demineralized bone matrix (DBM)	
Grafton	
Gel	1 cc = $118; 5 cc = $481; 10 cc = $754 25 cc = $1340
Putty	10 cc = $798
Composites	
Collagraft	Three strips = $545 Six strips (10.3 mm) = $995

the cluneal nerves during harvest of the posterior iliac may cause bothersome buttock numbness.

To avoid these significant complications, a number of alternatives to autologous bone graft for spinal fusions have been developed, among them allograft, ceramics (HA, calcium phosphate, coralline products, composites), DBM and BMP (Tables 1–3).

ALLOGRAFTS

In 1880 the Scottish surgeon Macewen performed the first allograft surgery when he successfully transplanted the tibia of a child into the infected humerus of another child.[37] Currently, more than 150,000 musculoskeletal allograft procedures are performed annually.[38] The use of allografts has increased secondary to advances in sterile procurement, storage, and the desire to avoid donor site morbidity. The physical properties of an allograft are determined by many factors, including the specific site from which the graft was taken; age, sex, and physical characteristics of the donor; and preparation/sterilization method used.

There are disadvantages arising with the use of allograft bone, including antigenicity, slow and incomplete incorporation, biological and mechanical changes occurring with preparation, and potential for infectious disease transmission (HIV, hepatitis B and C) depending on the processing technique.

Histological analysis has shown that at 8 months after implantation revascularization into an allograft is less pronounced than a 1-month post-transplant autograft.[9, 39] Fresh and fresh frozen allograft evoke a detectable humoral and cell-mediated immunity.[40] During graft remodeling, mono-

nuclear cells are present in greater number, indicating that some degree of graft "rejection" is occurring.[9]

The risk of receiving a bone or soft-tissue allograft that is infected with HIV is extremely low. Statistically, if well screened (social history, HIV antibody and antigen status, risk groups, serologies [Venereal Disease Research Laboratories], lymph node biopsy, and analysis of other grafts from the same donor), the risk of HIV infection in allograft bone procedures is 1 in 1.67 million.[41] Since instituting improved screening and preparation techniques in 1985, no cases of HIV transmission have been reported in allograft bone implantations.[42]

Allograft bone for use in spinal fusion is preserved by either deep freezing or freeze drying with benefits of reducing antigenicity[39] and increasing storage time. For fresh frozen graft preparation constant temperatures between $-20°C$ and $-70°C$ are required. The biomechanical properties of the bone are preserved.[43–45] Shelf life is approximately 5 years at $-70°C$ and decreases to 6 months at $-20°C$.[15]

Freeze drying or "lyophilization" involves dehydration of the bone by sublimation (i.e., from solid state to gas state). After sterile procurement, the graft is rinsed, lavaged with saline and alcohol, and frozen. The frozen water molecules are then removed under vacuum, and the bone is stored in vacuum packaging at room temperature with an indefinite shelf life. "Rehydration" of the graft with normal saline is required at least 1 hour before use.[45] Freeze-dried cortical allograft does not provoke an immunological response and is the least antigenic.[40] However, there is a sacrifice in strength in compression[10, 44, 45] and torsion[44] when preserved in this fashion.

Currently, ethylene oxide (ETO) and gamma radiation are the two most prevalent allograft sterilization methods. ETO is best used for sterilizing small grafts because it must thoroughly diffuse into the material and be completely removed. Gamma radiation requires large doses (2–3 Mrad) to achieve sterilization. The osteogenic, osteoinductive, and biomechanical properties are adversely affected by both of these sterilization techniques. There is almost complete loss of osteogenic potential after ETO application.[47, 48] After 2.5-Mrad gamma radiation, a 50% loss of osteogenic potential is experienced[48] without affecting mechanical properties.[49] A significant decrease in tension, compression, and torsional strength occurs after a 6-Mrad exposure.[50]

There are two accepted indications for the use of either fresh frozen or freeze-dried allograft bone in spine surgery: (1) when autograft quantity is insufficient and (2) when a structural element is needed (either as an anterior interbody or strut graft spanning several segments).

Fresh frozen and freeze-dried structural allografts (fibula and iliac crest) have been successfully used for single-level anterior cervical interbody fusions.[51, 52] A 5% nonunion rate has been reported for both autograft and allograft when used at a single level. However, with two-level cervical interbody fusion, the rates of nonunion rise to 17% for autograft and 63% for allograft.[52] Anterior cervical strut grafts after corpectomy for spondylosis have demonstrated a 41% pseudarthrosis rate with allograft compared with 27% with autograft.[53]

Femoral ring segments have been used successfully for lumbar interbody fusions.[54] Morcellized autograft bone, packed within the medullary canal of the ring, is recommended. Posterior instrumentation and fusion may augment stability and improve the anterior allograft fusion rate.[47, 54]

Freeze-dried cancellous allograft, when used for posterior thoracolumbar spinal fusion in skeletally immature patients, has been highly effective with a very low pseudarthrosis rate.[55–58] However, poor results have been obtained when used for posterior cervical fusion in children.[59] An unacceptably high pseudarthrosis rate also occurs when allograft is used in posterior fusions in adults.[47, 60, 61] Allograft alone should not be used for intertransverse process fusions in adults.[61]

BONE SUBSTITUTES

Ceramics constitute a family of synthetic, biodegradable materials and include HA, tricalcium phosphate (TCP), and coral-based products. Unlike allografts, there is no risk of antigenicity or infectious disease transmission. Applications in spinal surgery have been slow to evolve secondary to the brittle nature of the materials and often incomplete incorporation.

HA and TCP are created by a high-temperature (>1100°C) process called sintering whereby calcium phosphate crystals are fused into a polycrystalline ceramic. They are available as porous or dense intact implants (as cancellous or cortical analogues) or granular particles. The density directly determines the mechanical stability and the rate of resorption/incorporation. Dense ceramics implanted in the spine tend to become surrounded by fibrous tissue.[62] Porous ceramics demonstrate good host cellular ingrowth but are more brittle and may fracture.[62, 63] HA resorbs very slowly (if at all), whereas TCP usually is completely resorbed by 6 weeks. Mixing of HA and TCP into a "biphasic" ceramic combines the advantages of each material. Internal fixation may improve the revascularization of the ceramic and diminish the crumbling of the brittle edges.[64]

Norian SRS (Norian Corp, Cupertino, CA) is an osteoconductive bone substitute made of a specific combination of monocalcium phosphate, TCP, and calcium carbonate. The brittle nature of the material currently limits spine applications, which require a structural component. In a cadaveric study, Norian successfully augmented pedicle screw pull-out strength by 68%.[65] Future applications may be realized in minimally invasive spinal fusion techniques.

Natural coral is a calcium carbonate crystalline exostructure made by invertebrates through extraction of calcium and phosphorus from the sea. Structurally, coral is very similar to cancellous bone. The genus of the coral determines the ultimate pore size: Goniopora produces large pores (500–600 μm), and Porite creates smaller pores (200–250 μm). Biocoral (Inoteb, St. Gonnery, France) appears not to provoke an acute or chronic inflammatory reaction.

The coral-based ceramics are created by a thermodynamic process that replaces the original calcium carbonate of the coral with HA (Pro-Osteon, Interpore, Irvine CA). Bone ingrowth into such implants in the spine appears to occur rapidly and consistently for both block and granular forms.[60, 66]

Composite substitutes, combining materials of different properties, have been commercially developed. Collagraft (Zimmer, Warsaw, IN), a combination of calcium phosphate ceramic (65 HA:35 TCP) and bovine type I dermal collagen, is provided in strips or as a paste. Healos (Orquest Inc, Mountainview, CA) is cross-linked bovine type 1 collagen coated with crystalline HA. The collagen serves as a conductive matrix and improves the bony interface between the ceramic and the spin.[68] To add osteoinductive capabilities, autologous bone marrow obtained from an iliac crest aspiration can be mixed with these materials. A collagen-biphasic calcium phosphate composite mixed with autologous bone (3:1) compared favorably with autologous bone alone in a canine model.[69] However, in another study, the addition of Collagraft significantly decreased the effectiveness of the autograft.[70] Antibodies to bovine collagen have been found in 7% of those receiving Collagraft.[71] However, this immunological response was found not to be associated with significant adverse sequelae.

DEMINERALIZED BONE MATRIX

DBM is formed by acid extraction of cortical and corticocancellous allograft bone. This process leaves osteoinductive noncollagenous proteins, bone growth factors, and collage, which lack intrinsic structural capabilities. It is available freeze dried as a powder/granules or delivered within a gel or putty carrier. The human bone is sterilized without the use of radiation or ETO processing to preserve the osteoinductive proteins (Grafton, Osteotech Inc, Shrewsbury, NJ).

DBM is best used to extend autologous or allograft bone in posterior spinal fusions. When DBM is added to autograft, less graft is needed to induce a similar amount of new bone formation.[72, 73] Rabbits implanted with DBM have demonstrated a more mature fusion mass as evidenced by greater trabecular bone formation on radiographs and by histological analysis.[78]

However, when an ample amount of bone graft is available, adding DBM does not increase the probability of obtaining a successful fusion.[73] In fact, one study suggested a possible inhibitory effect of DBM in this setting.[68] When used alone, DBM produces osteoid but may be unable ultimately to create a solid fusion.[72]

BONE MORPHOGENIC PROTEINS

In 1978, Urist isolated a low-molecular-weight osteoinductive protein from bone matrix gelatin.[74] He termed this product "bone morphogenic protein." Nine BMPs have since been identified.[75] Representing less than 0.001% of the wet weight of marrow-free compact bone, BMP is not accessible until the bone matrix is demineralized.[74]

BMP induces formation of cartilage and bone in vivo and stimulates a cascade of activity that is similar to fracture repair, including the differentiation of perivascular mesenchymal cells into cartilage and bone.[76] BMP, analyzed extensively within animal studies of the posterior lumbar spine, appears able to augment the healing capacity of autograft through induction of additional bone-forming cell.[68, 77–79] BMP, when added to autograft in a canine model, demonstrated two to three times greater bone formation, a larger fusion mass, and higher fusion rates than autograft alone.[78]

BMP also appears to be successful when used alone without autograft.[75, 80–82] In a rabbit lumbar intertransverse process fusion model, a higher proportion of animals attained a solid fusion when a bovine bone–derived osteoinductive protein (BMP) extract was used than when autologous bone graft was used.[80] Using the same model, with recombinant BMP-2 (rhBMP-2), all of the rhBMP-2 rabbits fused compared with 42% of the autograft group.[75] The rhBMP-2 fusions were biomechanically stronger and stiffer.

Human BMP extract is not currently commercially available for use in the spine. BMP created by recombinant DNA technology may improve future accessibility, but the current high costs are restrictive.

FUTURE DIRECTIONS

In 1992, a meta-analysis of the clinical lumbar spine fusion literature was attempted.[83] Only 47 published reports met inclusion criteria. Among these articles, success was variably reported because of the divergent outcome assessment protocols that had been used. Overall, it appeared that 68% of patients had a satisfactory outcome after fusion. Pseud-

arthrosis was recognized in 14%. Chronic pain at the bone graft donor site occurred in 9%.

To improve patient outcomes, methods have been sought to decrease the rate of pseudarthrosis and reduce the complications of autologous bone harvest. In addition, standardized patient outcome measures have been developed to improve the ability to assess and compare newer forms of treatment.

To obtain a solid fusion, attention to both biological and biomechanical principles is required. Recombinant and extracted osteoinductive bone proteins (BMPs), which have markedly improved fusion rates in animal spinal models, hold the most promise. Current and future studies will emphasize development of the ideal delivery system for BMP. Human clinical trials to validate safety and efficacy must be completed before general clinical use. Further, advances in "structural" devices that provide an osteoconductive matrix capable of withstanding physiological loads while serving as a carrier of osteoinductive BMPs are likely.

Operative techniques in spine surgery will continue to evolve toward the minimally invasive route. Decreasing the surgical disruption to the soft-tissue bed will result in less scar formation, improved vascularization of the graft, and improved healing rates. Such improvements in technology are likely to positively influence the patient outcomes of the future.

BIBLIOGRAPHY

1. Albee FH: Transplantation of a portion of the tibia into the spine for Pott's Disease. JAMA 1911; 57:885.
2. Hibbs RA: An operation for progressive spinal deformities. N Y Med J 1911; 93: 1013.
3. McKibbon B: The biology of fracture healing in long bones. J Bone Joint Surg Br 1978; 60:150.
4. Nachemson A, Morris JM: In vivo measurements of intradiscal pressure. J Bone Joint Surg Am 1964; 46:1077.
5. Smith MD, Cody DD: Load-bearing capacity of corticocancellous bone grafts in the spine. J Bone Joint Surg Am 1993; 75: 1206.
6. Bassett AL: Current concepts of bone formation. J Bone Joint Surg Am 1962; 44: 1217.
7. MacNab I, Dall D: The blood supply of the lumbar spine and its application to the technique of intertransverse lumbar fusion. J Bone Joint Surg Br 1971; 53:628.
8. Toribatake Y, Hutton WC, Tomita K, et al: Vascularization of the fusion mass in a posterolateral intertransverse process fusion. Spine 1998; 23:1149.
9. Goldberg VM, Stevenson S: Natural history of autografts and allografts. Clin Orthop 1987; 225:7.
10. Brantigan JW, Steffee AD, Geiger JM: A carbon fiber implant to aid interbody lumbar fusion—A biomechanical analysis. Spine 1991; 16(suppl):270.
11. Dimar JR, Ante W, Zhang YP, et al: The effects of nonsteroidal anti-inflammatory drugs on posterior spinal fusions in the rat. Spine 1996; 21:1870.

12. Glassman SD, Rose SM, Dimar JR, et al: The effect of postoperative nonsteroidal anti-inflammatory drug administration on spinal fusion. Spine 1998; 23:834.
13. Brown CW, Orme TJ, Richardson HD: The rate of pseudarthrosis in patients who are smokers and patients who are nonsmokers. Spine 1986; 11:942.
14. Daftari TK, Whitesides TE, Heller JG, et al: Nicotine on the revascularization of bone graft: An experimental study in rabbits. Spine 1994; 19:904.
15. Riebel GD, Boden SD, Whitesides TE, et al: The effect of nicotine on incorporation of cancellous bone graft in an animal model. Spine 1995; 20:2198.
16. Silcox DX, Daftari T, Boden SD, et al: The effect of nicotine on spinal fusion. Spine 1995; 20:1549.
17. Zdeblick TA: A prospective, randomized study of lumbar fusion. Spine 1993; 18(8): 983.
18. Klein JD, Hey LA, Yu CS, et al: Perioperative nutrition and postoperative complications in patients undergoing spinal surgery. Spine 1996; 21:2676.
19. Bouchard JA, Koka A, Bensusan JS, et al: Effects of irradiation on posterior spinal fusion. Spine 1994; 19:1836.
20. Emery SE, Brazinski MS, Koka A, et al: The biological and biomechanical effects of irradiation on anterior spinal bone grafts in a canine model. J Bone Joint Surg Am 1994; 76:540.
21. Closkey RF, Parsons JR, Lee CK, et al: Mechanics of interbody spinal fusion. Spine 1993; 18(8):1011.
22. Craven TG, Carson WL, Asher MA, et al.

The effects of implant stiffness on the bypassed bone mineral density and facet fusion stiffness in the canine spine. Spine 1994; 19(15):1664.
23. McAfee PC, Farey ID, Sutterlin CE: Device-related osteoporosis with spinal instrumentation. Spine 1989; 14:919.
24. McAfee PC, Farey ID, Sutterlin CE: The effect of spinal implant rigidity on vertebral bone density. A canine model. Spine 1991; 16(suppl):190.
25. Heggeness MH, Esses SI: Classification of pseudarthrosis of the lumbar spine. Spine 1991; 168(suppl):S449.
26. Heggeness MH, Esses SI, Mody DR: A histologic study of lumbar pseudarthrosis. Spine 1993; 18(8):1016.
27. Gill K, O'Brien M: Observations of resorption of the posterior lateral bone graft in combined anterior and posterior lumbar fusion. Spine 1993; 18(13):1885.
28. Kleiner JB, Odom JA, Moore MR, et al: The effect of instrumentation on human spinal fusion mass. Spine 1995; 20(1):90.
29. Dwyer AF, Wickham GG: Direct current stimulation in spinal fusion. Med J Aust 1974; 1:73.
30. Kane WJ: Direct current electrical bone growth stimulation for spinal fusion. Spine 1988; 13:363.
31. Simmons JW: Treatment of failed posterior lumbar interbody fusion (PLIF) of the spine with pulsing electromagnetic fields. Clin Orthop 1985; 193:127.
32. Mooney V: A randomized double-blind prospective study of the efficacy of pulsed electromagnetic fields for interbody lumbar fusions. Spine 1990; 15:708.

33. Glazer PA, Heilmann MS, Lotz JC, et al: Use of ultrasound in spinal arthrodesis. Spine 1998; 23:1142.

34. Younger EM, Chapman MW: Morbidity of bone graft donor sites. J Orthop Trauma 1989; 3:192.

35. Kurz LT, Garfin SR, Booth RE: Harvesting autologous iliac bone grafts. Spine 1989; 14:1324.

36. Summers BN: Donor site pain from the ilium. J Bone Joint Surg Br 1989; 71:677.

37. Macewen W: Observations concerning transplantation on bone. Proc R Soc Lond 1881; 32:232.

38. Mowe J: Annual questionnaire of accredited tissue banks. American Association of Tissue Banks, McLean, VA, 1992.

39. Heiple KG, Chase SW, Herndon CH: Comparative study of the healing process following different types of bone transplantation. J Bone Joint Surg Am 1963; 45:1593.

40. Frielaender GE, Strong DM, Sell KW: Studies on the antigenicity of bone. I: Freeze-dried and deep frozen allograft in rabbits. J Bone Joint Surg Am 1976; 58:854.

41. Buck BE: Bone transplantation and HIV. Clin Orthop 1989; 240:129.

42. Tomford WW: Transmission of disease through transplantation of musculoskeletal allografts. J Bone Joint Surg Am 1995; 77:1742.

43. Brantigan JW, Cunningham BW, Warden K, et al: Compression strength of donor bone for posterior lumbar interbody fusion. Spine 1993; 18:1213.

44. Pelker RR: Effects of freezing and freeze drying on biomechanical properties of rat bone. J Orthop Res 1984; 4:405.

45. Wolfinbarger I, Zhang Y, Adam BT, et al: A comprehensive study of physical parameters, biomechanical properties, and statistical correlations of iliac crest bone wedges used in spinal fusion surgery: Mechanical properties and correlation with physical parameters. Spine 1994; 19:304.

46. Czitrom AA: Principles and techniques of tissue banking. Instr Course Lect 1993; 42:359.

47. Herron LD, Newman MD: The failure of ethylene oxide gas-sterilized freeze dried bone graft for thoracic and lumbar fusion Spine 1989; 14:496.

48. Munting E, Wilmart J, Wijne A, et al: Effect of sterilization on osteoinduction: Comparison of five methods in demineralized rat bone. Acta Orthop Scand 1988; 59:34.

49. Zhang Y, Homsi D, Gates K, et al: A comprehensive study of physical parameters, biomechanical properties, and statistical correlations of iliac crest bone wedges used in spinal fusion surgery: Effect of gamma irradiation on mechanical and material properties. Spine 1994; 19:304.

50. Komender A: Influence of preservative on some mechanical properties of human haversian bone. Mater Med Pol 1976; 8:13.

51. Young WF, Rosenwasser RH: An early comparative analysis of the use of fibular allograft versus autologous iliac crest graft for interbody fusion after anterior cervical discectomy. Spine 1993; 18:1123.

52. Zdeblick TA, Ducker TB: The use of freeze-dried allograft bone for anterior cervical fusions. Spine 1991; 16:726.

53. Fernyhough JC, White JI, LaRocca H: Fusion rates in multi-level cervical spondylosis comparing allograft fibula with autograft in 126 patients. Spine 1991; 16(Suppl):S563.

54. Butterman GR, Glazer PA, Bradford DS: The use of bone allografts in the spine. Clin Orthop 1996; 324:75.

55. Blanco JS, Sears CJ: Allograft bone use during instrumentation and fusion in the treatment of adolescent idiopathic scoliosis. Spine 1997; 22:1338.

56. Knapp D, Jones ET: Use of cortical cancellous allograft for posterior spinal fusion. Clin Orthop 1988; 229:99.

57. McCarty RE, Peek RD, Morrissy RT, et al: Allograft bone in spinal fusion for paralytic scoliosis. J Bone Joint Surg Am 1986; 68:370.

58. Yazici M, Asher MA: Freeze-dried allograft for posterior spinal fusion in patients with neuromuscular spinal deformities. Spine 1997; 22:1467.

59. Stabler CL, Eismont FJ, Brown MD, et al: Failure of posterior cervical fusions using cadaveric bone graft in children. J Bone Joint Surg Am 1985; 67:370.

60. An HS, Lynch K, Toth J: Prospective comparison of autograft vs allograft for adult posterolateral lumbar spine fusion: Differences among freeze-dried, frozen and mixed grafts. J Spinal Disord 1995; 8:131.

61. Jorgenson SS, Lowe TG, France J, et al: A prospective analysis of autograft versus allograft in posterolateral lumbar fusion in the same patient. Spine 1994; 19:2048.

62. Toth JM, An HS, Lim TH, et al: Evaluation of porous biphasic calcium phosphate ceramics for anterior cervical interbody fusion in a caprine model. Spine 1995; 20:2203.

63. Emery S, Fuller DA, Stevenson S: Ceramic anterior spinal fusion. Spine 1996; 21:2713.

64. Fuller DA, Stevenson S, Emery SE. The effects of internal fixation on calcium carbonate. Spine 1996; 21:2131.

65. Lotz JC, Hu SS, Chiu DFM, et al: Carbonated apatite cement augmentation of pedicle screw fixation in the lumbar spine. Spine 1997; 22:2716.

66. Holmes R, Mooney V, Bucholz R, et al: A coralline hydroxyapatite bone graft substitute. Clin Orthop 1984; 188:252.

67. Martin RB, Chapman MW, Holmes RE, et al: Effects of bone ingrowth on the strength and non-invasive assessment of coralline hydroxyapatite material. Biomaterials 1989; 10:481.

68. Helm GA, Sheehan JM, Sheehan JP, et al: Utilization of type I collagen gel, demineralized bone matrix, and bone morphogenetic protein-2 to enhance autologous bone lumbar spinal fusion. J Neurosurg 1997; 86:93.

69. Zerwekh JE, Kourosh S, Scheinberg R: Fibrillar collagen-biphasic calcium phosphate composite as a bone graft substitute for spinal fusion. J Orthop Res 1992; 10:562.

70. Muschler GF, Negami S, Hyodo A, et al: Evaluation of collagen ceramic composite graft materials in a spinal fusion model. Clin Orthop 1996; 328:250.

71. Delustro F, Dasch J, Keefe J, et al: Immune responses to allogeneic and xenogeneic implants of collagen and collagen derivatives. Clin Orthop Rel Res 1990; 260:263.

72. Frenkel SR, Moskovich R, Spivak J, et al: Demineralized bone matrix: Enhancement of spinal fusion. Spine 1993; 18:1634.

73. Morone MA, Boden SD: Experimental posterolateral lumbar spinal fusion with demineralized bone matrix gel. Spine 1998; 23:159.

74. Urist MR: Solubilized and unsolubilized bone morphogenetic protein. Proc Natl Acad Sci USA 1978; 78:1828.

75. Schimandle JH, Boden SD, Hutton WC: Experimental spinal fusion with recombinant human bone morphogenetic protein-2. Spine 1995; 20:1326.

76. Urist MR, Lietze A, Mizutani H, et al: A bovine low molecular weight bone morphogenic protein (BMP) fraction. Clin Orthop Rel Res 1982; 162:219.

77. Fischgrund JS, James SB, Chabot MC, et al: Augmentation of autograft using rhBMP-2 and different carrier media in the canine spinal fusion model. J Spinal Disord 1997; 10:467.

78. Lovell T, Dawson EG, Nilsson OS, et al: Bone morphogenic protein augmentation of experimental spinal fusion. Clin Orthop 1986; 243:266.

79. Sheehan JP, Kallmes DF, Sheehan JM, et al: Molecular methods of enhancing lumbar spine fusion. Neurosurgery 1996; 39:548.

80. Boden SD, Schimandle JH, Hutton WC: Lumbar intertransverse-process spinal arthrodesis with use of a bovine bone-derived osteoinductive protein. J Bone Joint Surg Am 1995; 77:1404.

81. Boden SD, Schimandle JH, Hutton WC, et al: In vivo evaluation of a resorbable osteoinductive composite as a graft substitute for lumbar spinal fusion. J Spinal Disord 1997; 10:1.

82. Sandhu HS, Kanim LEA, Toth JM, et al: Experimental spinal fusion with recombinant human bone morphogenetic protein-2 without decortication of osseous elements. Spine 1997; 22:1171.

83. Turner JA, Ersek M, Herron L, et al: Patient outcomes after lumbar spinal fusions. JAMA 1992; 268:907.

PEDIATRIC ORTHOPAEDICS

**JAMES C. DRENNAN AND
KENNETH GUIDERA**

FAILURE OF FORMATION OF THE LIMBS

R. M. Bernstein and H. G. Watts

Summary

- Children with limb deficiencies and amputations differ considerably from adult amputees and are best served by treatment in a specialized pediatric center.
- Approximately 30% of children with congenital limb deficiencies have multiple limb involvement.
- Upper extremity congenital limb deficiencies outnumber lower extremity congenital limb deficiencies by a ratio of 3:1.
- In congenital limb deficiencies, length discrepancies remain proportional throughout growth.
- Molecular genetics is rapidly increasing the understanding of the causes of limb deficiencies.

Children with limb deficiencies present complex diagnostic and therapeutic issues for the treating physician. The presence of one congenital abnormality may signal the presence of congenital anomalies in other organ systems. Thus, the physician must be familiar with these associations and carefully evaluate the entire child. Many of these deformities may require multiple surgeries or ablative procedures. Because these deformities often produce feelings of helplessness and anxiety for the parents, expert psychological and social support is also required. Thus, it is desirable that the child be evaluated and treated in a center that specializes in congenital limb deficiencies.

Children with amputations differ considerably from adult amputees. For instance, amputation in childhood is more often the result of congenital defects, and childhood amputees more often have upper extremity involvement as well as multiple limb involvement. In addition, children are more agile and easier to train to use devices, are already dependent on other persons, and seldom have associated chronic diseases to complicate their care. Because children are constantly growing in length and girth and are more likely to abuse their prosthesis, they require more frequent adjustments and repairs than adults. Their skin may be more tolerant of prosthetic wear, and they rarely develop neuromas or phantom pain. However, they are more likely to require surgical modifications of their stumps. Finally, they often have more special needs in prosthetic components than their adult counterparts. Because of these differences, adolescent amputees should not be considered small adults.

DEFINITIONS AND NOMENCLATURE

Several systems of terminology have been and are still in use throughout the world. Hemimelia, ectromelia, peromelia, and dysmelia, among other terms, may mean different things to different people (Table 1).

In 1973 a committee of the International Society for Prosthetics and Orthotics produced an international terminology accepted by the World Health Organization and the International Standards Organization.[1]

The basics of the International Terminology are simple:

Name the side (L, R, or B).

Decide whether the deficiency is longitudinal or transverse. Transverse deficiency resembles a surgical amputation, with no remaining distal part. (Small remnants of rudimentary fingers or toes, or "nubbins," do not count as remaining distal parts). Longitudinal deficiency encompasses everything else.

If transverse, name the level of loss (e.g., "left transverse forearm deficiency, proximal third").

If longitudinal, name the missing bones (as nouns), modified by "partial" or "total" (absence), from proximal to distal (e.g., "right longitudinal deficiency, radius, total; rays 1 and 2"). ("Ray" refers to a metacarpal or metatarsal and all of its associated phalanges.)

Further embellishments such as "hypoplastic" or "fused" may be used.

EPIDEMIOLOGY

The overall incidence of congenital limb deficiencies ranges from 5 to 9.7 per 10,000 live births[2, 3] (Table 2). There is a 3:1 ratio of upper extremity to lower extremity deficiencies. In addition, there is a high rate of extraskeletal involvement in patients with limb deficiencies. Up to 80% with heritable limb deficiencies have associated nonmusculoskeletal abnormalities compared with 53% of birth registry patients with limb deficiencies. Upper limb deficiencies are more likely to have associated anomalies than lower limb deficiencies. Thus, an assessment of the craniofacial, cardiovascular, gastrointestinal, genitourinary, and central nervous systems should be performed in any child with a congenital limb deficiency.

PATHOGENESIS

MOLECULAR GENETICS

Limb development begins in the 4th week of gestation and is complete by the eighth week. A complex interaction of cell groups, genes, growth factors, and programmed cell death results in a complete limb. Under- or overexpression of these factors can result in limb deficiencies or duplications.

The apical ectodermal ridge (AER), a group of cells at the tip of the limb bud, affects proximal-distal growth of the limb. Fibroblast growth factors are active in this area, and removal of the AER will result in truncation of the limb in a temporal fashion. The zone of polarizing activity (ZPA) is a group of cells on the posterior portion of the limb bud adjacent to the AER. The ZPA affects anteroposterior development of the limb apparently through the protein product of the sonic hedgehog gene (shh). Transferring

TABLE 1. SYNONYMS USED IN PAST LITERATURE

Synonyms for limb deficiencies
  Melia: Greek root word for "limb"
  Amelia: "a" meaning absence; "melia" meaning limb
  Phocomelia: literally meaning a limb like a seal (i.e., the marine animal); used for a hand or foot attached directly to the trunk
  Hemimelia: literally meaning half a limb; in practice, a longitudinal deficiency
  Meromelia: "partial limb"; synonym for hemimelia
  Intercalary: a part missing from the middle (e.g., absent radius with five-rayed hand)
  Terminal: a longitudinal deficiency with a long bone and its related distal part missing totally (e.g., absent fibula and missing fourth and fifth rays)
Terms more commonly used in the European literature
  Peromelia: peros meaning maimed (Greek)
  Ectromelia: ectro meaning miscarriage (Greek); a combining form signifying the congenital absence of a part
  Dysmelia: Greek root word; a combining form signifying difficult, painful, bad, disordered, abnormal

the ZPA to the anterior side of the limb bud results in mirror-image duplication of the digits. The dorsal ectoderm patterns the dorsal-ventral axis through the protein product of the *wnt7a* gene. Lack of this ectoderm (or gene product) results in ventral structures forming on the dorsal side of the limb. Finally, homeobox *(HOX)* genes occur in all species and apparently act as transcription factors. Various *HOX* genes play roles in anteroposterior and proximal-distal patterning as well as digit identity.[4]

These areas and proteins form a complex web of interaction, producing a normally aligned and developed limb. Given that these genes interact in a variety of ways, it is not surprising that the loss of a variety of these gene products will result in similar limb deformities.

VASCULAR

Although definitive evidence is lacking, there is some suggestion that some limb deficiencies may have a vascular cause. These may be secondary to constriction or thrombosis of the vascular supply to the affected part. For instance, amniotic band syndrome (previously called Streeter's dysplasia) often results in terminal amputations. Presumably, the fibrotic bands from the amnion wrap around the digit or limb. While the part grows, the amniotic band does not. Thus, a circumferential vascular constriction occurs, resulting in amputation. Another example is Poland's syndrome

TABLE 2. INCIDENCE OF LIMB DEFICIENCIES PER 10,000 LIVE BIRTHS

Variable	Incidence
Overall	5–9.7
Fibular deficiency	1.07
Tibial deficiency	0.01–0.2
Proximal femoral focal deficiency	0.05–0.2
Congenital constriction band syndrome	0.66–11.4

(unilateral absence of the sternocostal head of the pectoralis major associated with ipsilateral breast hypoplasia and terminal transverse limb defects), which may result from a disruption of the embryonic subclavian arterial system.[5]

TOXINS AND VITAMINS

A number of known teratogens affecting limb bud development exist, the most famous of which is thalidomide (an angiogenesis inhibitor). The affect of vitamins on limb bud development has been investigated. Retinoic acid may have some affect on normal limb bud development. In addition, Yang et al[6] reported that periconceptional multivitamin use reduced the risk of transverse limb deficiency.

CONGENITALLY "ACQUIRED" LIMB DEFICIENCY

The most common congenitally "acquired" deficiency is associated with congenital constriction band syndrome, a sporadically occurring condition. Although considered a focal germplasm defect by Streeter, most believe that this results from constriction of the circulation in the limbs of the fetus as a result of entanglement after rupture of the amnion. Thus, the resulting limb deficiencies may be better thought of as having a vascular occlusive cause. These constriction bands may also result in growth abnormalities of the limbs or intrauterine amputations. Associated deformities include syndactyly, craniofacial defects, visceral anomalies, and clubfoot.[7, 8]

CLINICAL FEATURES

GENERAL
Physical Examination

The physical examination for any child with a limb deficiency involves a thorough evaluation of the entire child. The presence of one congenital anomaly should spur the search for others. A prime example is the VATER association of *v*ertebral anomalies, imperforate *a*nus, *t*racheoesophageal abnormalities, and *r*enal or radial abnormalities (Table 3).

Additionally, a deficiency is usually not focal. Thus, in so-called proximal femoral focal deficiency (PFFD), there

TABLE 3. DIFFERENTIAL DIAGNOSIS (MORE COMMON DISEASES)

Upper Extremity Deficiencies
Holt-Oram syndrome (AD)
(Thrombocytopenia–absent radius) syndrome (AR)
Radial clubhand (S)
Fanconi's anemia (AR)
VATER association (S)

Lower Extremity Deficiencies
Isolated tibial deficiency (S)
Cleft hand, absent tibia syndrome (AD)
Fibular deficiency (S)
Proximal femoral focal deficiency (S)

AD = autosomal dominant; AR = autosomal recessive; S = sporadic.

is usually hypoplasia of the lateral femoral condyle, absence of the anterior cruciate ligament, and often fibular deficiency as well as deletion of one or more of the lateral rays of the foot. In fibular deficiency, associated ankle instability and tarsal coalitions are often present.

Each portion of the limb must be examined and the range of motion of the joints, stability of the joints, motor examination, and alignment of the limb recorded. Functional limb length discrepancies should be assessed. In upper limb deficiencies, an occupational therapist may assist in the evaluation to determine how the child performs certain tasks.

Investigation

Radiographs of all suspicious bones or joints should be obtained. Scanograms of the lower extremities should be performed to determine the anticipated limb length discrepancy at skeletal maturity. If a knee or hip flexion contracture is present, a lateral scanogram should be taken to avoid mistaking the apparent shortening for true shortening.

An additional investigation that may be useful in later years is an arthrogram to evaluate the location and depth of reduction of the femoral head in the hip joint in patients with PFFD. An unossified proximal tibial anlage in tibial deficiency or an unossified femoral head in PFFD may be identifiable by ultrasonography or magnetic resonance imaging (MRI). An MRI may help demonstrate the presence of a quadriceps tendon insertion in children with tibial deficiency. In patients with congenital scoliosis (e.g., VATER association), an MRI of the spinal cord should be obtained before surgical correction and stabilization of the spine.

Renal ultrasonography should be obtained in any patient with evidence of congenital scoliosis or cardiac involvement to investigate the presence of renal anomalies.

Because thrombocytopenia may accompany a radial deficiency (i.e., thrombocytopenia–absent radius [TAR] syndrome) a complete blood count, including a platelet count, should be obtained in these patients.

Tibial and fibular deficiencies are usually distinguishable on physical examination. In tibial deficiencies, the foot is unstable and in equinovarus at the end of a short, functionless limb. In fibular deficiencies, the foot is usually in equinovalgus and articulates with a variably shortened and anteriorly bowed tibia.

CLINICAL FEATURES OF SPECIFIC ENTITIES
Congenital Deficiency of the Femur (Congenital Short Femur and PFFD)

Congenital deficiencies of the femur form a continuum from simple hypoplasia to total absence. The deficiencies may be diffuse or limited to the upper or lower portions and are often associated with other limb deficits or indeed other organ anomalies. Treatment can range from acceptance to amputation and fitting with a prosthesis. A standardized approach is not easy. Subtleties of hip, knee, or ankle strength and motion, along with the aesthetic wishes of the family, may play a pivotal role in the final plan, and no one treatment will ever be correct for every child.

Classification systems can be used to organize clinical material for presentation in the medical literature or to help the orthopaedic surgeon make clinical decisions for an individual child; sometimes they serve both functions. Aitken's[9] classification of PFFD is an example of the former. It focuses entirely on the radiograph appearance of the bones of the upper end of the femur and the pelvis. This plays a moderately small role in the overall decision-making. Similarly, the classifications of Pappas,[10] Fixsen and Lloyd-Roberts,[11] and Amstutz[12] are primarily radiographic "groupings." By contrast, the classification by Gillespie and Torode[13] is concise, practical, and useful. This classification has been modified[14] and separates longitudinal deficiencies of the femur into three types (Fig. 1).

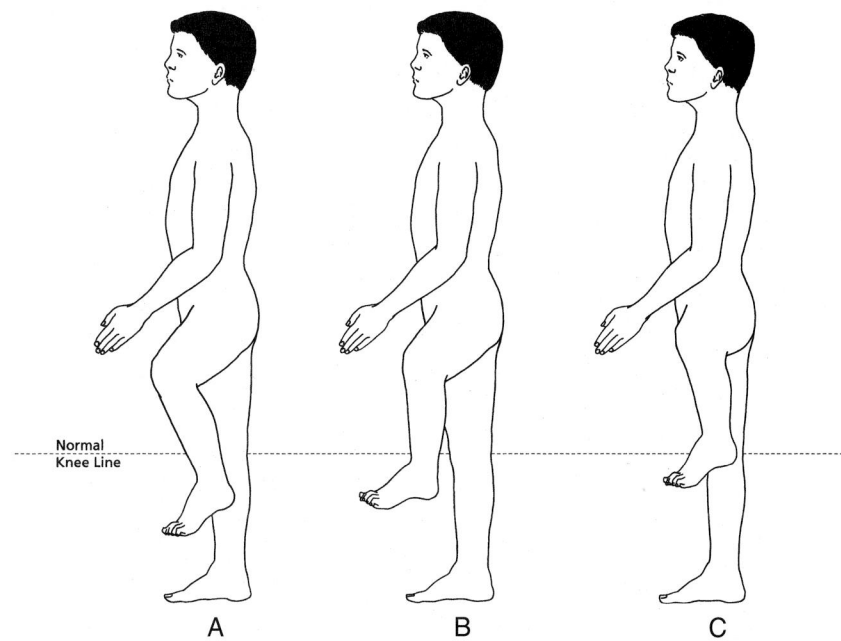

Fig. 1. Modified Gillespie and Torode classification of proximal femoral focal deficiency. (Redrawn from Gillespie R: Classification of congenital abnormalities of the femur. In Herring J, Birch J [eds]: The Child with a Limb Deficiency. Rosemont, IL, American Academy of Orthopaedic Surgeons, 1998.)

Normal
Knee Line

A   B   C

1. Type A: congenital short femur. In extension, the foot lies opposite the midpoint of the contralateral tibia. The overall length discrepancy is 20% or less. This type is best treated by leg equalization procedures (epiphyseodesis, lengthening, or a combination).
2. Type B: the thigh is very short, and there is external rotation of the hip and flexion contracture of the hip and knee. Overall length discrepancy is about 40%. This type is best treated with a prosthesis. However, fitting may be difficult because of the hip and knee flexion contractures. Van Nes rotationplasty or knee fusion and foot ablation are options.
3. Type C: the thigh is extremely short and pistoning of the hip is apparent. There is almost no femur radiographically. The overall length discrepancy is more than 50%. There is dysplasia of the hemipelvis and no acetabular development. This is easier to fit with a prosthesis than type B.

Congenital Short Femur. For children with congenital shortness of the femur who have a stable hip and knee (or when a stable knee and hip is the result of surgical intervention), limb lengthening may be indicated.

The current guideline for the amount of leg equalization to be gained by epiphyseodesis is usually given as 5 cm. This is not based on any scientific evidence but on opinion. The parents need to decide between the disadvantages of being an extra inch shorter in height (e.g., 7½ cm versus 5 cm epiphyseodesis) versus the need to gain those extra centimeters with a lengthening that may result in significant added complications.

Children whose limbs are predicted to have a discrepancy at maturity in the range of 5 to 15 cm can be considered for lengthening. We prefer to lengthen using Ilizarov's biology (i.e., lengthening of a healing callus) while using a unilateral apparatus (such as Wagner's) for its safety and convenience.

For discrepancies predicted to be in excess of 20 cm, serious consideration should be given to amputation and prosthetic fitting. Keep in mind that the need to equalize the extremities does not have to be accomplished by a single technique. A difference of 20 cm could, for example, be made up with an acceptance of a 2-cm difference, the addition of a 1-cm lift inside the shoe, an epiphyseodesis of 7 cm, and a final lengthening of 10 cm. A lengthening of 10 cm is within reason, whereas a lengthening of 20 cm is beyond the margin of current practice.

PFFD. The management of children with PFFD has been confused by an array of classification systems that have focused on the radiograph appearance of the hip. The major decisions in caring for the child with a PFFD involves treatment of the large limb shortening and depends very little on the anatomy of the hip.

Making Up for the Marked Leg Length Difference. Amstutz[12] made a significant contribution by pointing out that the length of a congenitally short bone remains proportional throughout growth compared with the normal limb. This allows the orthopaedic surgeon to predict the ultimate limb length difference at the end of growth while the child is still an infant.

A leg length difference that is anticipated to be greater than 40% to 50% of the normal length at maturity will require heroic efforts and is not likely to leave the child with a well-functioning extremity if lengthened.

If lengthening is not realistic, the options for making up for the limb length difference are to (1) remove the foot and fit the child as a below-knee (B-K) amputee, accepting the huge difference in knee heights; (2) remove the foot and shorten the limb so that the child can be fitted as an above-knee (A-K) amputee; (3) perform a van Nes rotationplasty.

To fit the child as a BK amputee, the foot is removed by a Syme or Boyd amputation and an extra-long BK prosthesis is used. This is a simple solution but is cosmetically unappealing because of the great difference in knee heights, which is especially obvious when the child is sitting.

To shorten and fit at the AK level, the limb is shortened sufficiently so that the child will be able to function well as an AK amputee. To do that, the foot needs to be removed. This can be done either as a Syme or Boyd amputation (Fig. 2). Many surgeons favor a Syme amputa-

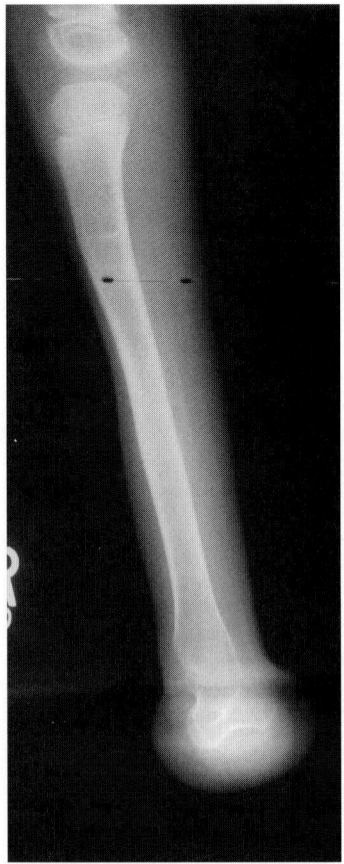

Fig. 2. Lateral radiograph of a Boyd amputation. Note the fusion of the calcaneus to the distal tibia and the bulbous stump, again allowing the use of a self-suspending socket. Unlike in this example, we prefer to shorten the tibia so that the stump comes to lie at the level of the opposite calf at skeletal maturity. This allows the patient to be fitted with a more cosmetic prosthesis.

tion because of its simplicity. However, Syme's amputations done in infancy have a tendency toward "pencil-point thinning" of the distal tibia compared with a Boyd amputation. The issue of heel-pad migration is probably overblown, because children's skin will modify to the pressures applied, as witnessed by children with untreated clubfeet who are able to walk on the dorsum of their feet without skin breakdown. However, good scientific evidence to help one choose between these two procedures is not available, and the choice tends to involve the surgeon's personal preference. A transdiaphyseal amputation is ill advised because children younger than 12 years who undergo such amputations have a high likelihood of experiencing "terminal overgrowth" spikes of bone, which complicate prosthetic fitting and may require one or more stump revisions.[15]

Ultimately, the end of the stump on the deficient side should be sufficiently short to allow room for a standard mechanical knee joint in the prosthesis to be at the level of the opposite, normal knee. Although orthopaedic surgeons have often focused on the end of the bony stump as seen on a scanogram, it must be remembered that almost 3 cm of room is needed for the soft tissues, the socket padding, and the thickness of the socket itself. To this must be added 7 cm for the knee joint. An ideal aim is to have the end of the bone of the stump 10 cm proximal to the knee joint on the opposite side.

The van Nes rotationplasty is an alternative to the fitting as an AK amputee. The leg is rotated 180 degrees so that the ankle can be used as a substitute for the knee.[16] A prosthesis is applied to the foot to behave similarly to a BK prosthesis (although the socket commonly includes a thigh support attached with outside hinges). For this to be successful, there are three requirements: the length must be appropriate, the ankle must be sufficiently normal to function as a substitute knee, and the psychological acceptance of the procedure is within the bounds of the patient, the family, and the medical personnel caring for the child.

At maturity, the reversed ankle should be at approximately the level of the opposite knee joint. Plantar flexion and dorsiflexion of the foot are composite of the motion at the ankle and the subtalar joints. The axis of rotation for the purposes of the prosthesis is taken to be at the tip of the lateral malleolus. The limb can be shortened an appropriate amount at the time of rotation or knee fusion (see later discussion).

The ankle needs to have an appropriate range of motion and sufficient strength to power a prosthesis. A foot with all five rays is more likely than one with fewer rays to have these requirements but not invariably.

There has been concern that children who have the operation at a young age will experience derotation. This has led some to advocate waiting until the child is older than 10 years.[17] Torode and Gillespie[16] as well as Krajbich[18] showed that, if the rotation is done through the knee fusion with appropriate shortening and muscle releases, later derotation is not a problem.

The psychological issues are important. Concerns may vary among age groups and cultures. In those medical centers where the van Nes procedure is frequently selected, there are usually other children who can act as models for a potential patient and their parents. The psychology of the medical staff cannot be ignored. If the medical personnel feel that such procedures are bizarre, it is clear that they will not be offered or that, if offered, they will be presented in such a manner that no patient would accept the choice. As a consequence, one sees centers in the United States where they have a moderately large group of children who have had the procedure and those that have no children who have had the procedure.

Additionally, prosthetic facilities must be considered. The prosthesis that is required to fit a child after a van Nes procedure is difficult to fit. If good prosthetic facilities are not available, this operation should be avoided.

Enhancement of Prosthetic Function. Most children with PFFD live with the anatomic knee held in flexion. They will often sit on the thigh section of their prosthesis. This gives decreased control and power over the prosthesis and aligns the vertical axis of the prosthesis more laterally to the center of gravity, requiring a child to lurch laterally in stance. Function is greatly enhanced if the femur is fused to the tibia. When this is done, the fusion must be done with the knee in full extension. In the past, this procedure was not as frequently performed but is now considered routine.

As discussed, most children who have had conversion of their PFFD extremity to that of an AK level end up with a stump that is too long. At the time of knee fusion, the distal femoral or proximal tibial physis (or both) should be considered for excision. Proper application of growth data using the Anderson-Messner-Green[19, 20] charts can alleviate that fear. Moseley's[21] straight line graph does not differentiate between the growth contributed by the femur compared with the tibia, so it does not provide the answer for this calculation.

Before Definitive Surgery. Regardless of what the decision is for ultimate management, there is a period when the difference in leg lengths can be considerable yet it is too early to do anything definitive surgically. Lifts greater than 5 cm in height tend to lead to ankle sprains. Ankle-foot orthoses can be used to decrease this likelihood. However, when the difference gets to 8 cm or 9 cm, an extension prosthesis can be made that has a hole in the front of the prosthesis distally through which the forefoot extends. If tried at too young an age when the length difference is less than 5 cm, there is not enough room below the socket to fit a foot on the end of such a prosthesis.

Reconstruction of the Hip Joint. In the past, a great deal of focus was placed on the radiograph of the upper end of the femur. The radiographic appearance of the bone is often the focus, and the cartilage and soft tissues are forgotten. If there is absolutely no acetabulum, this does not alter the discussion of the management (given previously) as to length decisions. If, alternatively, the acetabulum is satisfactorily formed and there is some element of secondary center of the femur in the acetabulum and some segment of upper femur that are not joined, surgery may be considered. One should wait until there is sufficient ossification of the two fragments so that they can be fused together. There is certainly no rush to do this, and more complications occur from proceeding too soon before there is adequate bone stock.

Fusion of the Distal Femur to the Pelvis. The distal femur can be fused to the pelvis in order to use the knee joint as a replacement for the hip joint.[22] This can be done at the time of rotation rather than excision of the knee. This gives the theoretical advantage of having a stable hip. However, the knee joint does not allow reasonable rotation. In addition, once it is fused to the pelvis, the distal femur has some capacity to grow and the hip joint will (depending on the orientation of the distal femur at the time of fusion to the pelvis) grow to a point that is a mechanical disadvantage. Although there have been a small number of reports of such cases, most surgeons believe that this is not a useful procedure and have avoided it.

TAR SYNDROME

DEFINITION

TAR syndrome was initially reported as a variable deficiency of the radius associated with thrombocytopenia.[23] Schoenecker et al[24] later recognized its association with variable deficiencies of knee formation together with internal tibial torsion. These authors suggested the name TARK syndrome, adding the K for the knees, but this term did not catch on. In patients with the most severe form characterized by phocomelia (in which the hands virtually articulate with the scapulae) and stiff knees, walking is precarious and function is markedly inhibited as a result of the lack of knee motion.

PHYSICAL EXAMINATION AND DIFFERENTIAL DIAGNOSIS

The usual distinction between those children with simple radial deficiencies and those with the added thrombocytopenia is that the latter usually have five rays in their hands, which should prompt a close look at the child's platelet count.

In the mildest manifestation, the forearm shortening may be slight and there are no lower extremity deformities. However, such children may have severe platelet deficiency and have been known to die from exsanguination because physician suspicion was not raised.

Those with lower extremity involvement may have only medial lateral instability or severe knee formation deficiencies to the extent of having total lack of segmentation at the knee joint (Fig. 3), together with severe knee flexion deformities of 45 to 90 degrees. The feet point medially, usually about 45 degrees because of a combination of medial tibial torsion and medial spin through the subtalar joint. When examining these children, one should look for functional rather than anatomic losses.

Other conditions associated with radial deficiencies are Holt-Oram syndrome, Fanconi's anemia, VATER association, and simple congenital radial clubhand.

GENETICS

Although the inheritance of the condition is considered to be autosomal recessive,[23] Hedberg and Lipton[25] indicated that the exact mode of inheritance is not fully clear.

CLASSIFICATION AND INCIDENCE

The literature groups all TAR patients together, which is confusing. We have developed our own classification system, as follows (Fig. 4):

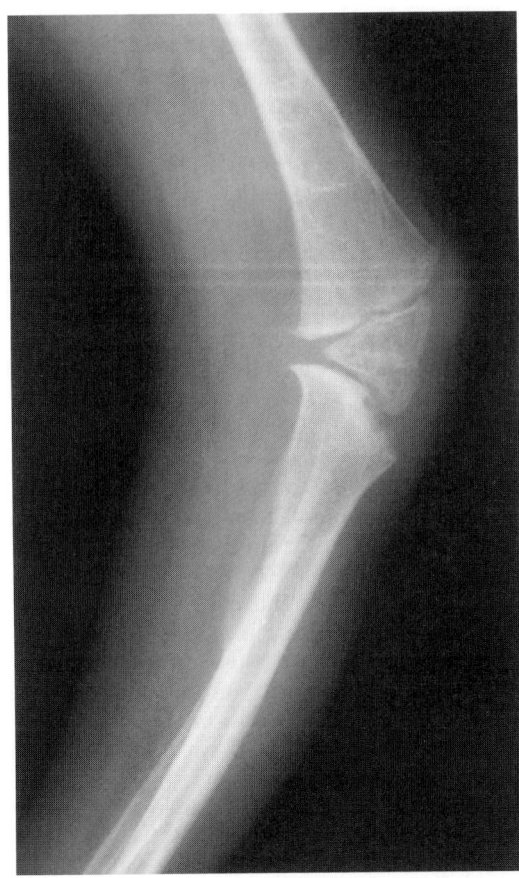

Fig. 3. Thrombocytopenia–absent radius (TAR) syndrome. Lateral radiograph of a 3-year-old boy with TAR syndrome shows lack of segmentation between the distal femoral and proximal tibial epiphyses.

Group A: children with upper extremity involvement only.

Group B: children with upper extremity involvement with additional limited knee involvement, allowing a range of motion of 60 degrees or more. (These children usually have knee ligament instability and mildly internally rotated feet and their arms usually have some humerus.)

Group C: children with phocomelic upper extremities (usually no humerus) and with absent or limited knee motion, allowing less than 60 degrees range of motion. Radiographs of the knees frequently show distal femoral flattening or femoral-tibial synchondrosis. The feet may be internally rotated 45 to 80 degrees.

The percentage of individuals in the three groups is not known. The numbers that are reported will depend on the source of information. Information from orthopaedic departments will describe a high proportion of group B and group C patients, because children with lower extremity problems are usually referred to the orthopaedic surgeon. Hand surgeons will report a higher proportion of group A patients, because those patients would ordinarily be referred to hand surgeons. Such children may not be recognized as having TAR syndrome but rather diagnosed as having simple deficiency of the radius. This is especially true of older children who have gone beyond the period of

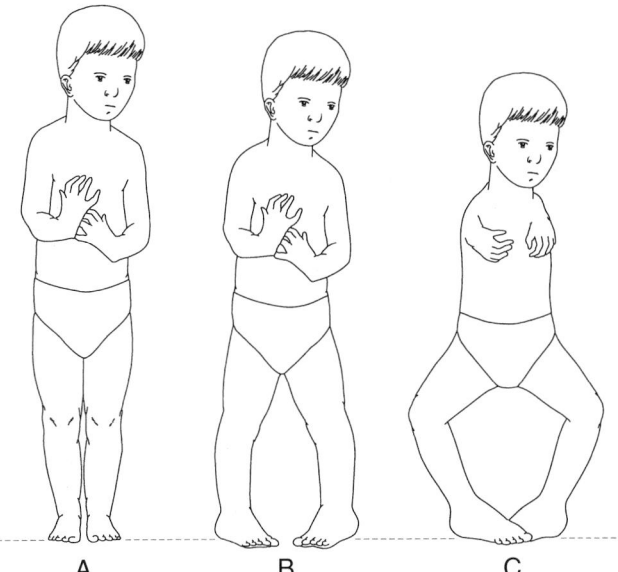

Fig. 4. Classification of thrombocytopenia–absent radius syndrome patients. *A,* Radial clubhands with five digits. Note the normal height and normal lower extremities. *B,* Radial clubhands with five digits, slightly shorter stature, unstable knee ligaments; flexion/extension arc of the knees 60 degrees or more; internal rotation of the tibias. *C,* Patients have very short arms, often with no humerus, and short stature; hips are externally rotated; tibias are internally rotated; feet are further internally rotated; flexion/extension arc of the knees is less than 60 degrees.

low platelet counts. Hematologists will probably report a lower proportion of group A patients.

MANAGEMENT
Thrombocytopenia

Thrombocytopenia is evident from birth and gradually improves, so that by age 1 to 3 years the platelet counts may be sufficiently high to allow operation. However, surgery may precipitate a sudden drop in the platelet count. Appropriate blood transfusions need to be available.

Upper Extremities

Group A patients: the upper extremities of these children can be managed similarly to those of children with congenital clubhands (see Chapter 12–20).

Group B patients: these children may have very short arms with limited elbow motion, and the arms are usually better left untreated.

Group C patients: these children are phocomelic. Their upper extremity function is better than most doctors recognize. They are able to transfer objects from one hand to the other using their mouths as an intermediate transfer. All of our children have become good computers users, managing well with their fingers (or occasionally with a mouth stick). Toileting in public facilities is a major problem as is independent dressing. Successful independence has come from occupational therapy help and the provision of long-handled tools. Surgery has not helped.

Lower Extremities

Group A patients: these children have no lower extremity problems.

Group B patients: these children usually require soft-tissue surgery to stabilize their knees and may need osteotomies to improve alignment of their tibias.

Group C patients: these children present some of the most difficult challenges in orthopaedics. In our experience, all of these children walked independently during childhood. How many will end up in wheelchairs as adults is not known.

Should the feet be left alone so they can be used as upper extremity substitutes? None of the children we have seen have successfully used their feet for prehension, because limited knee motion prevented their ability to reach their mouths with their feet. Consequently, we have operated on the feet to correct the internal rotation by a combination of surgery at the subtalar joint and the tibia.

Should the legs be straightened out at the knees? Easy walking requires knees that are straight. Getting into or out of a chair (especially without the use of one's arms) requires the knees to be bent in order to get the feet under the center of gravity of the body. The major difficulty these children suffer is their inability to sit down from standing and to get up from a chair once they are seated, because their arms are too short to use for assistance. If they should fall down, getting on their feet becomes a Herculean feat. Several of the children have devised ways to manage this with the aid of a "helper dog." The most successful compromise has been to straighten one knee and leave the other flexed.

The use of surgery to straighten the knees by lengthening tendons and ligaments or by gradual straightening at the knee joint using any number of different apparatus (such as Ilizarov's gradual soft-tissue distraction) has not been successful because the knees rapidly return to their preoperative positions. Furthermore, these operations do not increase the total amount of motion in the knee joint but only change the position of the arc of knee motion. Creating a joint by cutting through the block of cartilage in fused knees has been performed in two children. Although this has provided some motion, it has not converted a group C child into a group B child.

It is the consensus of individuals in group C that the upper extremity shortness is not the major source of interference to their quality of life. Rather, it is the limitation of motion at the knees that is the factor determining functional outcome. There are currently no obvious or easy solutions.

CONCLUSION

While caring for a child with a limb deficiency can be very gratifying, the physician must have a thorough knowledge of the associated anomalies and the available resources for psychological support and prosthetic production. Children with limb deficiencies are not small adults. Thus, these children are best treated in clinics specializing in child amputees.

REFERENCES

1. Day H: The ISO/ISPO classification of congenital limb deficiency. In Bowker J, Michael J (eds): Atlas of Limb Prosthetics: Surgical, Prosthetic, and Rehabilitation Principles. St. Louis, MO, Mosby–Year Book, 1992.

2. Banister P: Congenital malformations: Preliminary report of an investigation of reduction deformities of the limbs, triggered by a pilot surveillance system. Can Med Assoc J 1970; 103:466.

3. Froster-Iskenius UG, Baird PA: Limb reduction defects in over one million consecutive live births. Teratology 1989; 39:127.

4. Johnson RL, Tabin CJ: Molecular models for vertebrate limb development. Cell 1997; 90:979.

5. Weaver D: Vascular etiology of limb defects: The subclavian artery supply disruption sequence. In Herring J, Birch J (eds): The Child With a Limb Deficiency. Rosemont, IL, American Academy of Orthopaedic Surgeons, 1998.

6. Yang Q, Khoury MJ, Olney RS, et al: Does periconceptional multivitamin use reduce the risk for limb deficiency in offspring? Epidemiology 1997; 8:157.

7. Higginbottom M, Jones K, Hall B, et al: The amniotic band disruption complex: Timing of amniotic rupture and variable spectra of consequent defects. J Pediatr 1979; 95:544.

8. Foulkes G, Reinker K: Congenital constriction band syndrome: A seventy-year experience. J Pediatr Orthop 1994; 14:242.

9. Aitken G: Proximal femoral focal deficiency: Definition, classification and management. In Aitken G (ed): Proximal Femoral Focal Deficiency: A Congenital Anomaly. Washington, DC, National Academy of Sciences, 1969.

10. Pappas A: Congenital abnormalities of the femur and related lower extremity malformations: Classification and treatment. J Pediatr Orthop 1983; 3:45.

11. Fixsen J, Lloyd-Roberts G: The natural history and early treatment of proximal femoral dysplasia. J Bone Joint Surg Br 1974; 56:86.

12. Amstutz H: The morphology, natural history, and treatment of proximal femoral focal deficiency. In Aitken G (ed): Proximal Femoral Focal Deficiency: A Congenital Anomaly. Washington, DC, National Academy of Science, 1969.

13. Gillespie R, Torode I: Classification and management of congenital abnormalities of the femur. J Bone Joint Surg Br 1983; 65:557.

14. Gillespie R: Classification of congenital abnormalities of the femur. In Herring J, Birch J (eds): The Child with a Limb Deficiency. Rosemont, IL, American Academy of Orthopaedic Surgeons, 1998.

15. Pellicore R, Sciora J, Lambert C, et al: Incidence of bone overgrowth in the juvenile amputee population. Inter-Clin Inform Bull 1974; 8:1.

16. Torode I, Gillespie R: Rotationplasty of the lower limb for congenital defects of the femur. J Bone Joint Surg Br 1983; 65:569.

17. Kostuik J, Gillespie R, Hall J, et al: Van Nes rotational osteotomy for treatment of proximal femoral focal deficiency and congenital short femur. J Bone Joint Surg Am 1975; 57:1039.

18. Krajbich I: Rotationplasty in the management of proximal femoral focal deficiency. In Herring J, Birch J (eds): The Child with a Limb Deficiency. Rosemont, IL, American Academy of Orthopaedic Surgeons, 1998.

19. Anderson M, Messner M, Green W: Distribution of lengths of the normal femur and tibia in children from one to eighteen years of age. J Bone Joint Surg Am 1964; 46:1197.

20. Anderson M, Green W, Messner M: Growth and predictions of growth in the lower extremities. J Bone Joint Surg Am 1963; 45:1.

21. Moseley C: A straight line graph for leg length discrepancies. J Bone Joint Surg Am 1977; 59:174.

22. Steel H, Lin P, Betz R, et al: Iliofemoral fusion for proximal femoral focal deficiency. J Bone Joint Surg Am 1987; 69:837.

23. Hall J, Levin J, Kuhn J, et al: Thrombocytopenia with absent radius (TAR). Medicine 1969; 48:411.

24. Schoenecker P, Cohn A, Sedgwick W, et al: Dysplasia of the knee associated with the syndrome of thrombocytopenia and absent radius. J Bone Joint Surg Am 1984; 66:421.

25. Hedberg VA, Lipton JM: Thrombocytopenia with absent radii: A review of 100 cases. Am J Pediatr Hematol Oncol 1988; 10:51.

section 9 chapter 2 — CONGENITAL ABSENCE OF THE FIBULAE

James A. Harder

Summary

- The most common long-bone absence in the body, 1:10,000 live births.[1]
- Has no genetic inheritance pattern.
- Treatment plans must restore normal lifestyle without undue physical, psychological, or mental anguish.
- Important associated abnormalities involve the tibia, the knee, and the femur.
- Other associated anomalies most often involve the cardiovascular or genitourinary systems.

Congenital absence of the fibula is a deficiency present at birth in which the fibula is either completely or partially absent, the foot is normal or abnormal, and there is a degree of associated leg length discrepancy (LLD) (Fig. 1).

The knee may also be unstable with absent cruciate ligaments. There may be valgus of the knee, which is dynamic and secondary to a lax medial collateral ligament and/or fixed, owing to a secondary hypoplastic lateral femoral condyle.

HISTORICAL REVIEW

Congenital absence of the fibula is a partial or complete deficiency of the lower extremity in which there may be associated anomalies of the foot and knee, with some degree of leg length inequality. Terminology to describe the deficiency is, according to Franz and O'Rahilly,[2] fibular hemimelia, or according to the International Society for Prosthetics and Orthotics (ISPO),[3] congenitally absent fibula, partial or complete. The longitudinal deficiency sometimes extends into the foot. It is useful to include a description of the deficiencies of the foot and the foot's position and range of motion, e.g., absent fourth and fifth rays, with foot in fixed equinus and valgus (Franz and O'Rahilly) or absent fourth and fifth metatarsals and phalanges, with the foot in fixed equinus and valgus (ISPO). The tibia may also be shortened and bowed anterolaterally as compared with the normal side.

Further classification is described by Achterman and Kalamchi[4] as type IA and IB, in which the fibula is partially absent, and type II, in which the fibula is entirely absent. The most recent classification was developed by Birch et al,[5] in which the classification tries to help the physician and the family with decision-making. The emphasis is on the presence or absence of a functional foot and, secondly, on the amount of shortening. This classification helps with the decision to choose a treatment pathway of ablating the foot by amputation or maintaining a functional foot and considering a program of limb equalization. A functional foot needs to have three or more metatarsals and be plantigrade or be able to be made plantigrade by the correction of contractures. No mention is made of the foot being mobile either passively or actively. The classification then goes on to quantitate and group the leg length inequality by expressing the LLD as a percentage of that of the opposite normal side. Type IA has a discrepancy of 5% or less; type IB has a discrepancy of 6% to 10%; type IC has a discrepancy of 10% to 30%; and type ID has a discrepancy of greater than 30%. Type IIA patients have a nonfunctional foot and have upper extremity function that precludes the use of their feet for prehension. Type IIB

TABLE 1. CLASSIFICATION OF FIBULAR DEFICIENCY	
Type	**Management**
Type IA	Shortening 5% or less	No treatment? Shoe lift?
Type IB	Shortening 6% to 10%	Equalization by epiphyseodesis or by one lengthening
Type IC	Shortening of 10% to 30%	Minimum of two staged lengthenings +/− epiphyseodesis
Type ID	Shortening of 30% or more	Requires "heroic" reconstruction; amputation is a viable option
Type IIA	Nonfunctional foot with functional uppers	Early amputation
Type IIB	Nonfunctional foot with abnormal uppers that may require the feet for prehension	Defer decision for amputation until functional patterns are established

From Birch JG, Lincoln TL, Mack PW: Functional classification of fibular deficiency. In Herring JA, Birch JG (eds): The Child With a Limb Deficiency. AAOS, 1997, p 161.

patients may need their feet for prehension activities due to associated upper limb abnormalities. A classification of fibular deficiency (Birch et al) is provided in Table 1.

EPIDEMIOLOGY

Fibular deficiency is said to be the most frequent long-bone absence.[1] The reported incidence rate is said to be about 1 in 10,000 live births.[6] There is no evidence of genetic transmission of the defect. Males and females are affected almost equally (1.6:1.0). About one-third of fibular deficiencies are bilateral. Associated genetic disorders are primarily syndromic, and associated anomalies most often involve the cardiac and genitourinary systems.

PATHOGENESIS

The pathogenesis of fibular deficiency is not clear. The deficiency may be complete or partial and be associated with a LLD, anterolateral bowing of the tibia, a dimple at the apex of the tibial bow, tarsal coalition, or absence of tarsals, metatarsals, or phalanges. The femur may have some degree of shortening and demonstrate a hypoplastic lateral condyle. The hypoplastic lateral femoral condyle will result in valgus angulation of the residual tibia. The knee may have absent cruciate ligaments and a lax medial collateral ligament. There may be significant femoral retroversion, which persists with growth and results in an obvious medial heel whip during the swing phase of gait.[7]

INVESTIGATION

When a child is born with a musculoskeletal abnormality such as a congenitally deficient fibula, it must be assumed that other abnormalities may be present, and a thorough search must be undertaken. This search must involve a complete history and physical examination. Dysmorphic features should lead to a genetic consultation. Careful as-

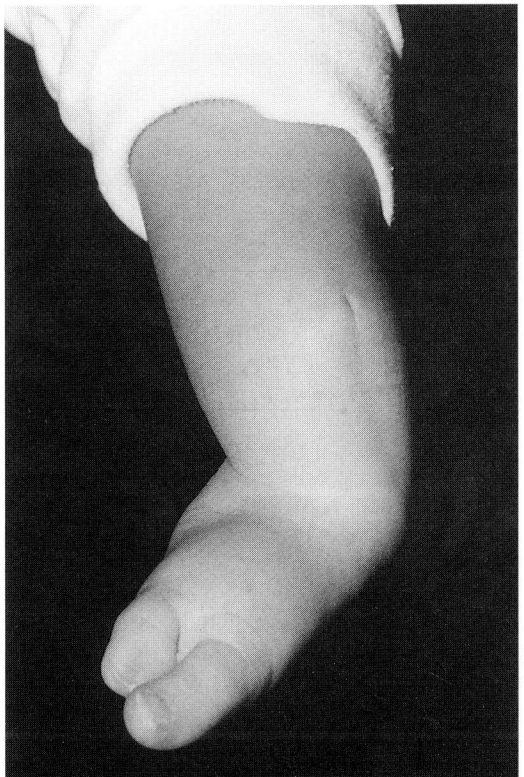

Fig. 1. Anteroposterior photograph. Lower leg with a congenitally absent fibula and absent fourth and fifth metatarsals and phalanges complete.

sessment of the cardiac and genitourinary systems is necessary, as these most often have associated anomalies. A chest radiograph and a cardiology consult with or without an echocardiogram may be helpful in assessing the cardiovascular system. A urinalysis, routine and microscopic; abdominal ultrasonography; and perhaps a consultation with a pediatric urologist investigates the genitourinary system. Radiographs of the spine, pelvis, and lower limbs will help to rule out vertebral anomalies as well as detect the often associated anomalies of acetabular dysplasia, proximal femoral focal deficiency, congenitally short femur, and lateral femoral condylar hypoplasia. Radiographs with anteroposterior and lateral views of the affected extremity will also delineate the deficiencies of the affected lower limb.

MANAGEMENT

Management of the child with a fibular deficiency is divided into the following:

1. The foot deformity.
2. The LLD.
3. The valgus deformity.
4. The unstable knee.
5. The prosthetic fitting.

FOOT DEFORMITY

The foot must at least be plantigrade in order for it to function during gait. Valgus and equinus contractures, therefore, must be released in order to maintain a plantigrade position. The foot must have three or more rays or metatarsals in order for it to function as an effective weightbearing surface in the adult. It is a bonus if the foot is powered by dorsiflexors and plantarflexors. These improve the efficiency of gait by adding energy to the stance phase. If the foot meets these requirements for salvage, posterior and lateral releases should be performed as necessary to provide a plantigrade foot. Sensation of the foot will be normal. However, range of motion of the foot will be variable and depend on joint contractures and the functional muscle groups present. Further weakness of the existing muscle groups and loss of strength can be expected after soft-tissue release or bone lengthening.

If the foot is of less than three rays and is fixed in equinus and valgus, there is likely an associated tarsal coalition. The likelihood of successfully transforming the foot into a stable plantigrade walker is doubtful. This type of foot is best amputated in order to provide the patient with the best functional result. The Syme or Boyd type of amputation is the most successful in providing a long-term excellent functional result.

Syme's Amputation

The Syme amputation was originally designed as a salvage procedure and provides direct full end-bearing on the heel pad. When performing this procedure on the congenitally abnormal foot, modifications to the classic Syme procedure are necessary. The surgery is performed by excising the talus, calcaneus, and forefoot. The heel/sole pad is folded and sutured anteriorly, with the excess pad trimmed to fit (Fig. 2).

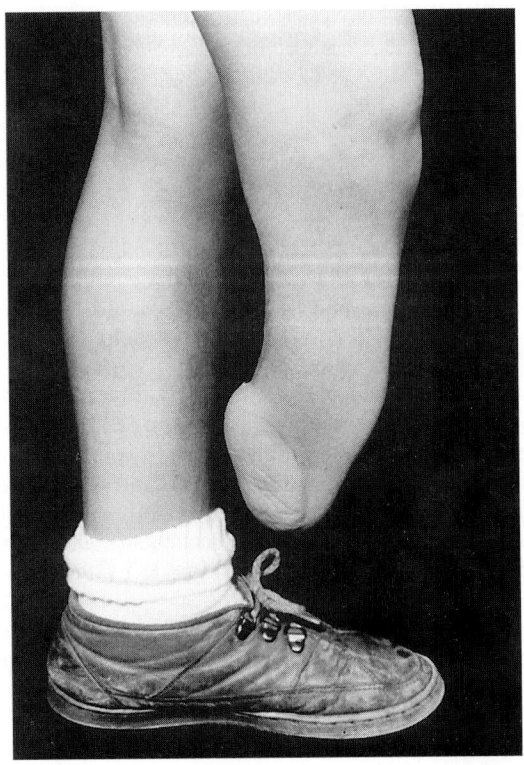

Fig. 2. Lateral view. Completed Syme's amputation shows the preservation of the entire sole of the foot, which is necessary as part of the flap. The heel is often fixed in equinus, and therefore extra flap length is necessary. The heel pad is behind the end of the stump rather than on the end of it.

The incision is made beginning anterior to the medial and lateral malleoli and carried dorsally over the top of the foot over the neck of the talus. As it is difficult to judge the length of the anterior flap in the congenitally abnormal foot, the second incision is carried along the lateral and medial sides of the foot at the junction of the sole and dorsum of foot skin. This distal incision crosses the dorsum of the foot at the base of the toes. The incision is deepened, and the toes, metatarsals, talus, and calcaneus are removed, leaving the sole of the foot with its soft tissues intact and undisturbed. Dissection must always be extraperiosteal to prevent formation of bone by remnants from the remaining periosteum. When removing the talus and calcaneus, care must be taken to protect the neurovascular bundle on the medial side of the foot near the medial malleolus. Care must also be taken to remove the calcaneus extraperiosteally but not to damage the delicate weightbearing structure of the heel pad. The cartilaginous calcaneal apophysis must be completely removed; portions of the calcaneal apophysis left behind will develop into bone fragments, which could be painful on weightbearing. The tourniquet is released, hemostasis is obtained, and the flap trim line is made to allow for a relaxed fit with no tension on the suture line. The Achilles tendon is identified and released with the excision of the calcaneus. A Penrose drain is inserted at the base of the flap and protrudes through the apices of the incision at the medial and lateral malleoli as the flap is brought up and sutured into position. The tibialis anterior and the long extensors are left sufficiently long so as to allow suturing into the deep layers of the posterior flap. The long extensors sutured into the anterior deep tissues of the flap will resist the pull of the triceps surae posteriorly, as the Achilles tendon will reattach itself to the soft tissues of the posterior heel pad. The wound is closed in layers with *interrupted sutures* to allow for best fit. Any excess skin is eased into position with the sutures; "dog ears" are not trimmed but left to contract. *Trimming dog ears at the apex of the incision will compromise the blood supply of the distal flap.* The heel pad may be stabilized with a vertical pin into the tibia or simply dressed so that the heel pad remains in the neutral position. If the foot was in significant fixed equinus, the actual heel pad will remain posterior to the distal tibia. This is due to the contracted soft tissues posteriorly. *The distal end of the tibia is not shortened or disturbed.* Ring sequestrum and overgrowth spikes are thereby avoided.

Care must be taken to keep the heel and sole pad in the neutral position during healing as it will serve as an excellent weightbearing surface. The patient will be able to walk without prosthesis by end-weightbearing directly on the pad. This feature is particularly useful when going to the bathroom at night or taking a shower. The heel pad is somewhat bulbous and, therefore, the Syme prosthesis is usually self-suspending (Fig. 3).

Boyd Amputation

The Boyd amputation gives an additional measure of length to the residual limb and stabilizes the heel pad by fusing a small portion of the calcaneus directly to the epiphysis of the distal tibia (Fig. 4). The Achilles tendon

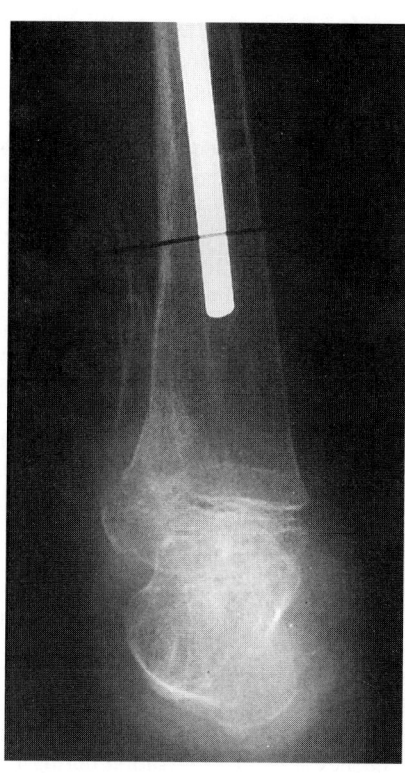

Fig. 4. Anteroposterior radiograph. This shows the lower leg after a Boyd amputation. The calcaneus has been placed on the end of the tibial epiphysis. Transverse osteotomies have been performed across the epiphysis of the tibia and across the calcaneus.

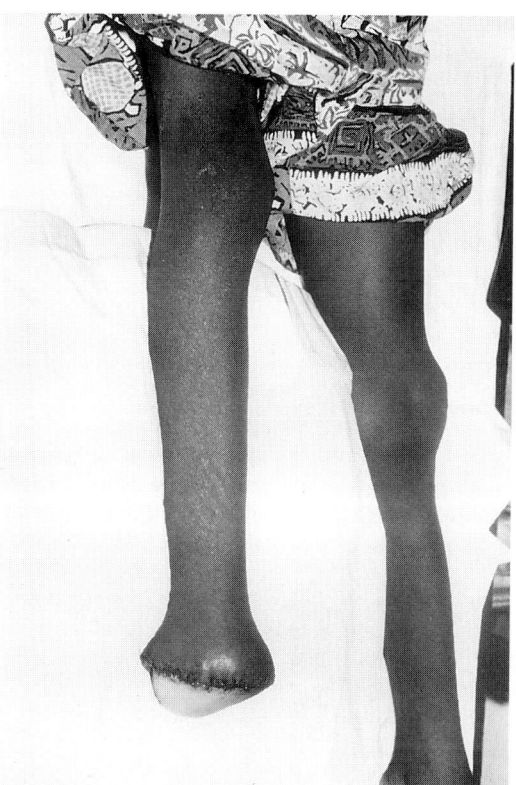

Fig. 3. Anteroposterior photograph. This shows the lower leg after a Syme amputation. Notice the bulbous end of the residual limb. This bulbous architecture is useful for suspending the prosthesis.

remains attached to the remnant of calcaneus. The extensor tendons are sutured into the deep tissues of the posterior flap. The patient must be old enough to have sufficient cancellous bone in the distal tibial epiphysis to allow for fusion. The calcaneus must be ossified enough to allow a transverse osteotomy through cancellous bone. In the 6- to 12-month-old child, there is not enough cancellous bone in the distal tibial epiphysis and the calcaneus to accomplish a successful fusion. The Boyd amputation also requires a longer flap. Special care must be taken to dissect out all of the heel and sole pad as shown in Figure 2 and to trim the flap to size after the remnant of calcaneus has been fixed to the exposed cancellous bone of the tibial epiphysis with a vertically oriented pin. Note that the terminal bone end of the residual limb (the calcaneal apophysis) is undisturbed and, therefore, development of a ring sequestrum or a bony overgrowth spike is avoided. *Leaving the terminal bone end undisturbed in pediatric amputations is very important to avoid distal end complications.*

LEG LENGTH DISCREPANCY

LLD is quantified by calculating the shortening as a percentage of the opposite normal tibial length. The discrepancy is then divided into categories (see Table 1).

If the discrepancy is less than 5%, it may require no treatment, a shoe lift, or perhaps at most an epiphyseodesis of the opposite distal tibial physis. Timing of the distal tibial epiphyseodesis is important and based on the growth rate of the physis. Growth at the distal tibial physis will be 4 to 6 mm/year in a normal tibia.

If the discrepancy is 6% to 10%, then appropriately timed epiphyseodesis of the distal and/or the proximal opposite tibia or one lengthening of the shortened tibia will be the treatment of choice.

If the shortening is between 10% and 30%, a minimum of two lengthenings of the shortened tibia will be required, and epiphyseodesis of the opposite side may have to be added to accomplish leg equalization. A Symes or Boyd amputation is certainly a consideration as the LLD reaches 30%, even if the foot is functionally satisfactory. Two to three lengthenings will be accompanied by a significant morbidity. The lengthenings require the highest level of expertise as well as a multidisciplinary team approach to be successful. Each lengthening will take about 12 months, and protection of the lengthened bone with an orthosis will be necessary thereafter to prevent tibial fracture. Participation in recreational sports will be limited while the lengthened tibia is gaining strength. Sometimes an orthosis is necessary for an indefinite period to protect the lengthened tibia from fracture. After repeated lengthenings, the function of the foot declines as the muscle groups will be weakened. The foot must be kept plantigrade during the lengthenings. At the completion of lengthening, the ankle joint may be rigid.

Careful attention needs to be given to the knee, as there may be a tendency toward subluxation during the lengthening process. If the Ilizarov technique of lengthening is used, it may be necessary to extend the Ilizarov construct above the knee to prevent knee joint subluxation or dislocation and to include the foot in the construct to prevent equinus contracture. Tibial bowing will be corrected during the lengthening. Valgus deformity due to lateral condyle hypoplasia will be corrected by performing a distal femoral varus osteotomy and by extending the Ilizarov frame above the knee. If there is a significant portion of fibula remaining proximally, it can be transported distally to offer better lateral ankle joint stability.

Tibial Bowing

The tibia is bowed anterolaterally and is most severely affected when the fibula is completely absent. There will be a dimple at the apex of the bow (Fig. 5). The bowing can be accommodated within the prosthesis during the early years of walking. As subcutaneous fat is lost and the tibia grows longer, the deformity becomes more obvious and more difficult to accommodate into the socket. In order to help decide whether tibial osteotomy is indicated, it is useful to look at the end of the tibia in relation to the weightbearing line in the anteroposterior and lateral planes. When the end of the tibia falls lateral to the lateral femoral condyle in the anteroposterior plane and is posterior to the weightbearing line in the lateral plane, an osteotomy is indicated. As there is sometimes a persistent flexion contracture at the knee, this will contribute to the position of the end of the tibia in the lateral view and should be considered when correcting the valgus deformity with an osteotomy. There is minimal increased risk of pseudoarthrosis after osteotomy as the osteotomy is in the proximal one-third of the tibia.

The technique preferred by the author is the oblique osteotomy through the proximal tibia by approaching from the anterolateral side, as described by Harder[8] and Rab.[9] This technique allows the osteotomy to be performed at the site of most deformity and avoids the tibial tubercle. The anterior compartment muscles are reflected laterally, and the tibia is exposed subperiosteally. The site and the plane

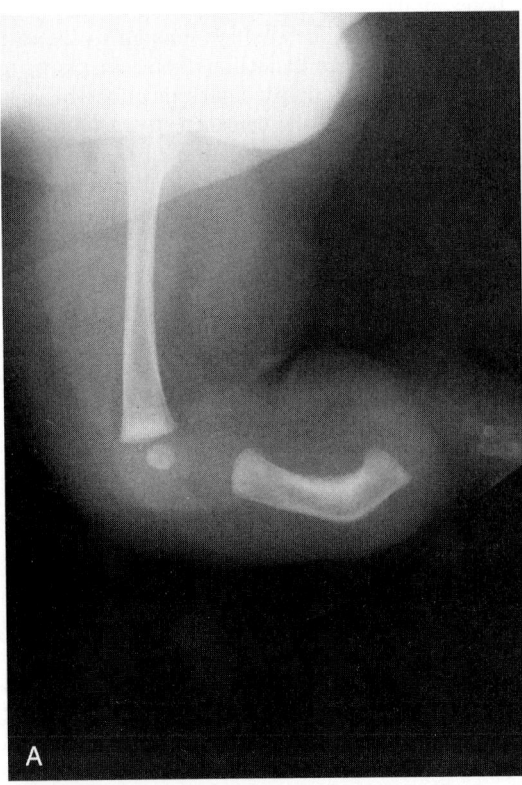 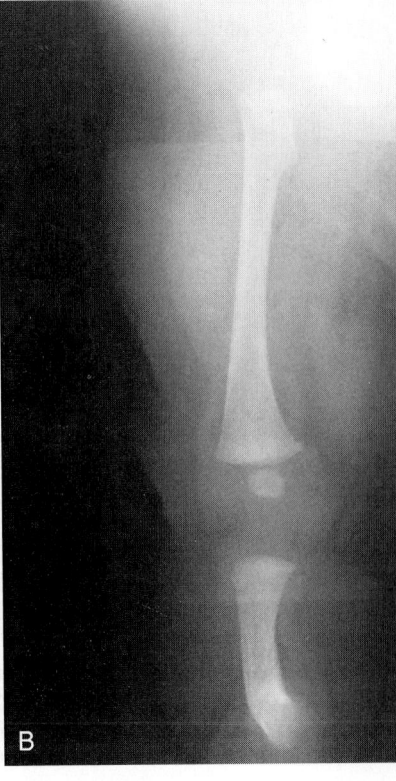

Fig. 5. Radiographs. These are anteroposterior *(A)* and lateral *(B)* radiographs of lower leg of a child who has complete absence of the fibula. Notice the anterior and lateral tibial bowing.

of the osteotomy is selected (Fig. 6C and D). The osteotomy is performed with a sagittal saw and osteotomes, being careful to protect the neurovascular bundle posteriorly and to exit the tibia posteriorly and proximally, well clear of the proximal tibial physis. The plane of the osteotomy must be parallel to the operating table in order not to introduce internal or external rotation. A threaded Steinmann pin is placed in the center of the osteotomy perpendicular to the plane of the osteotomy and used to stabilize the bone as the valgus correction is dialed to neutral. The end of the tibia should be in line with the anterosuperior iliac spine and the center of the knee joint. Another threaded Steinmann pin is added to maintain the corrected

relationship. A blood-clotting agent, such as Surgicel or Tisseel, can be spread over the open osteotomy before apposing the surfaces. This decreases bleeding and tension within the compartments postoperatively. The wound is irrigated and closed over the pins. A long leg cast is applied to help stabilize the osteotomy and to reduce postoperative discomfort. The cast is bivalved to allow for soft-tissue swelling. The cast and the pins are removed after there is sufficient evidence of healing seen on radiograph. The Syme prosthesis can be refitted after pin removal with end-weightbearing as tolerated. The prosthesis will maintain alignment and protect the healing osteotomy. Weightbearing will promote continued healing of the osteotomy.

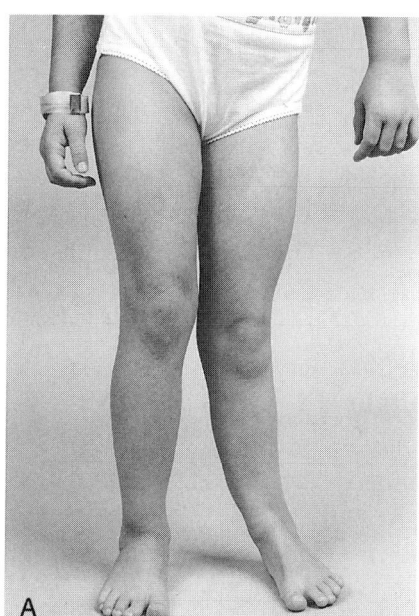

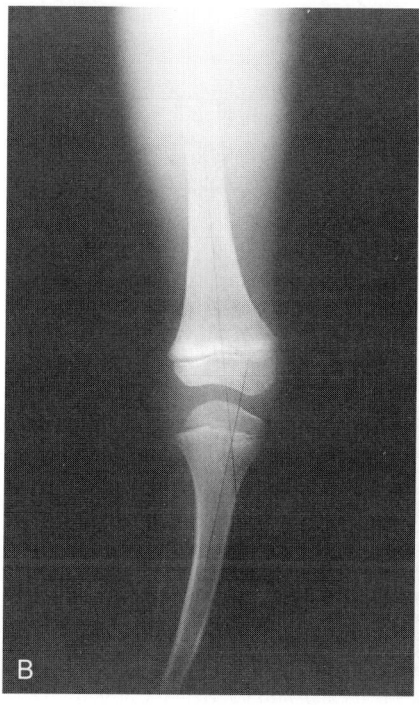

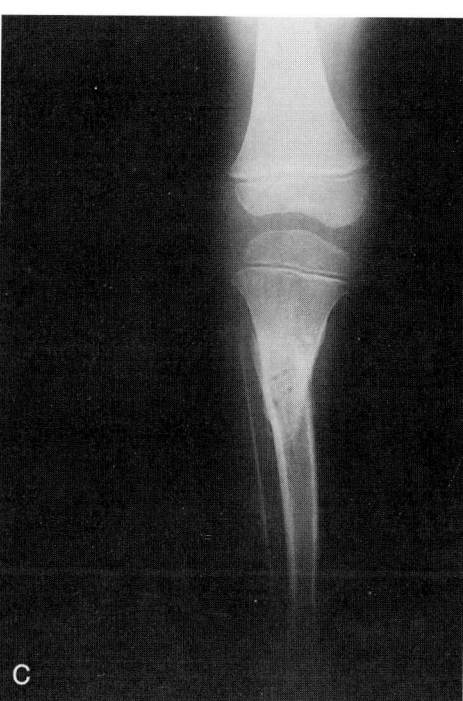

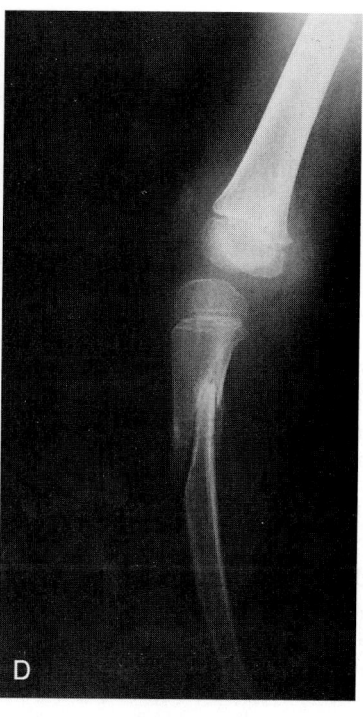

Fig. 6. Photographs and radiographs. *A,* Photograph of child with fibular hemimelia. Note the valgus deformity at the knee, resulting from a combination of medial collateral ligament laxity of the knee and lateral condylar hypoplasia of the femur. *B,* Anteroposterior radiograph of the child in *A,* showing the valgus deformity at the knee. Notice the hypoplastic lateral femoral condyle and the valgus deviation of the tibia. *C,* Anteroposterior radiograph of the patient with fibular hemimelia who has had a corrective proximal tibial osteotomy for valgus deformity of the tibia. The weightbearing line will now fall within the plane of the knee joint. *D,* Lateral radiograph of a patient with fibular hemimelia who has had a proximal tibial osteotomy for correction of valgus deformity of the tibia. Notice that the osteotomy exits the posterior tibia well clear of the proximal tibia growth plate. Retractors must be placed to protect the neurovascular bundle posteriorly.

VALGUS DEFORMITY

Valgus deformity of the knee can result from hypoplasia of the lateral femoral condyle of the femur. The diagnosis is easily made by taking an anteroposterior and lateral radiograph of the distal femur and noticing the smaller lateral femoral condyle (see Fig. 6B). The valgus deformity is structural and does not improve over time. If the deformity, as measured on a long standing radiograph, results in the weightbearing line passing medial to the ankle joint or the distal end of the tibia, the deformity should be corrected. This may be done by medial closing or lateral opening wedge osteotomy of the distal femur above the physis. Centralize the distal condyles (lateralize or medialize the distal fragment), and restore the alignment along the mechanical axis of the limb. The type of fixation used depends on the age of the patient. Care must be taken not to damage the distal femoral physis while performing the osteotomy. This can be accomplished by imaging by means of intraoperative fluoroscopy and by placing a smooth K-wire about 1 cm parallel and proximal to the physis. The K-wire will protect the physis while the osteotomy is being made at a more proximal level.

THE UNSTABLE KNEE

Congenital absence of the fibula may result in an unstable knee secondary to a lax medial collateral ligament of the knee, secondary to absent cruciate ligaments, or both. The instability pattern may be in one plane only or may be multidirectional. Valgus instability is successfully managed conservatively. The prosthesis is brought above the femoral condyles (patellar tendon socket [PTS] or patellar tendon–bearing with supracondylar extension). If rotatory stability is a significant problem, it can be managed by using a silicone rubber sleeve extending from the prosthesis to the thigh or by using outside knee hinges and attaching a thigh corset to the below-knee prosthesis.

THE PROSTHETIC FITTING

The prosthesis used for a patient with a congenital absence of the fibula consists of a socket and a terminal device. The socket consists of a rigid outer shell made of a polyester resin and a flexible inner shell made of pelite or silicone. If the residual limb is bulbous enough, the suspension will be from the bulbous end of the distal tibia. The inner shell of pelite, which is shaped to the residual limb, will be narrow above the bulbous end to give the necessary suspension. Putting on the flexible shell is made possible by cutting slits into the narrowed section so that the bulbous end can expand the pelite as it is passed through the narrowed segment. The pelite liner is then pushed into the rigid outer prosthesis and stays on by friction fit. The pelite liner is usually separated from the skin of the residual limb by a nylon or woolen stocking. The fit must be intimate, as "pistoning" of the prosthesis on the residual limb causes excess perspiration and skin irritation. The type of terminal device, which is attached to the end of the rigid socket, depends on the LLD. The Syme foot–type of terminal device takes up the least amount of space and is designed to be used when the LLD is 1 to 2 cm or less. As the space for the terminal device increases (i.e., there is more of a LLD), the choice of terminal devices is increased and includes devices with multiaxis ankle motion as well as devices with energy-storing features.

CONGENITAL ABSENCE OF THE TIBIA

1. A very rare anomaly, 1:1,000,000[10] (Fig. 7).
2. Usually associated with congenital abnormalities of the upper thigh, hip, foot, upper limb, and sometimes spine.
3. Can be bilateral (most commonly associated with complete absence or type Ia)
4. Distinguish between type Ia and Ib with an anteroposterior radiograph of the knee. Type Ia demonstrates the presence of femoral condyle hypoplasia. If the physician is uncertain, obtain an arthrogram or a magnetic resonance image (MRI) of the knee.
5. Brown's procedure (centralization of the fibula) has very strict prerequisites for only a small chance of success in type Ia.

Congenital abnormality of the tibia is a longitudinal deficiency of the tibia that will be complete or incomplete. The fibular head will be palpable proximal to the knee joint line. The fibula is usually foreshortened and angulated medially. It is high-riding (the head of the fibula is above the knee joint line) and prominently palpable along the lateral side of the knee. The foot may demonstrate polydactyly and be fixed in equinus and varus. The knee joint may be unstable, and there may be a flexion contracture present at birth (see Fig. 7).

There may be associated anomalies of the leg and hip joint as well as abnormalities of the upper limbs and sometimes the spine (Fig. 8A).

HISTORICAL REVIEW

Congenital absence of the tibia is a rare abnormality that results in severe deformity and diminished function of the

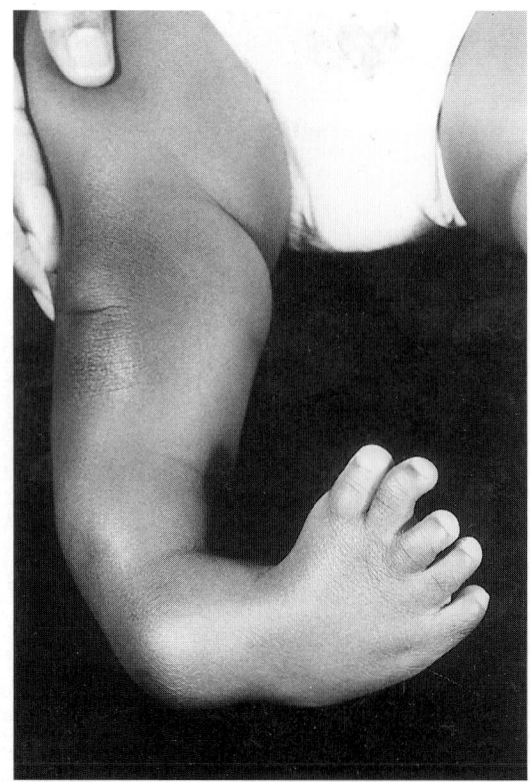

Fig. 7. Photograph. This is a child with congenitally absent tibia type Ia. Polydactyly is frequently present.

knee joint and the lower leg. There is an associated wide range of abnormalities that usually accompany this deformity as described by Schoenecker.[11] Varied deformities of the hip have been recorded; they include hip dislocation, congenital coxa vara, congenital short femur, and proximal femoral focal deficiency (see Fig. 8A). The hands may show deficiencies, be hypoplastic, or have syndactyly. Ab-

normalities of the spine may be failures of formation of the vertebral segments or partial failure of formation (hemivertebrae).

Two autosomal-dominant inheritance patterns were described by Clark[12] and Lenz.[13] Cases may also occur sporadically.

Schoenecker et al[14] as well as Jones and Lloyd-Roberts[15]

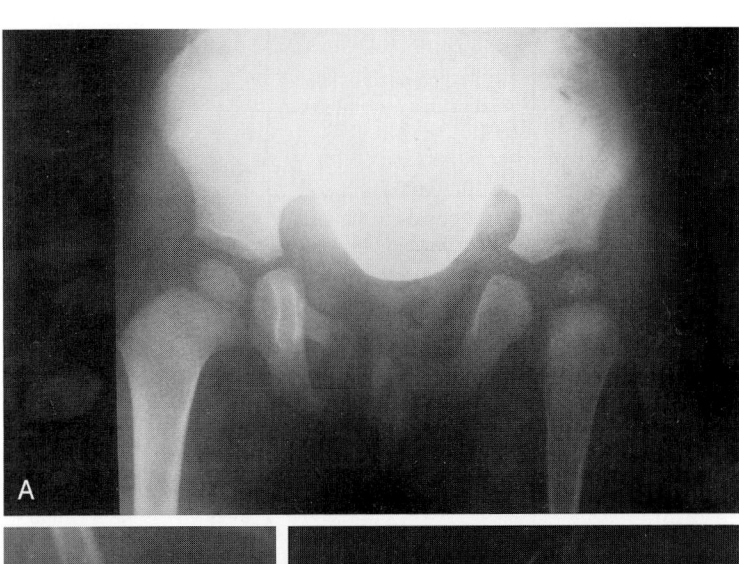

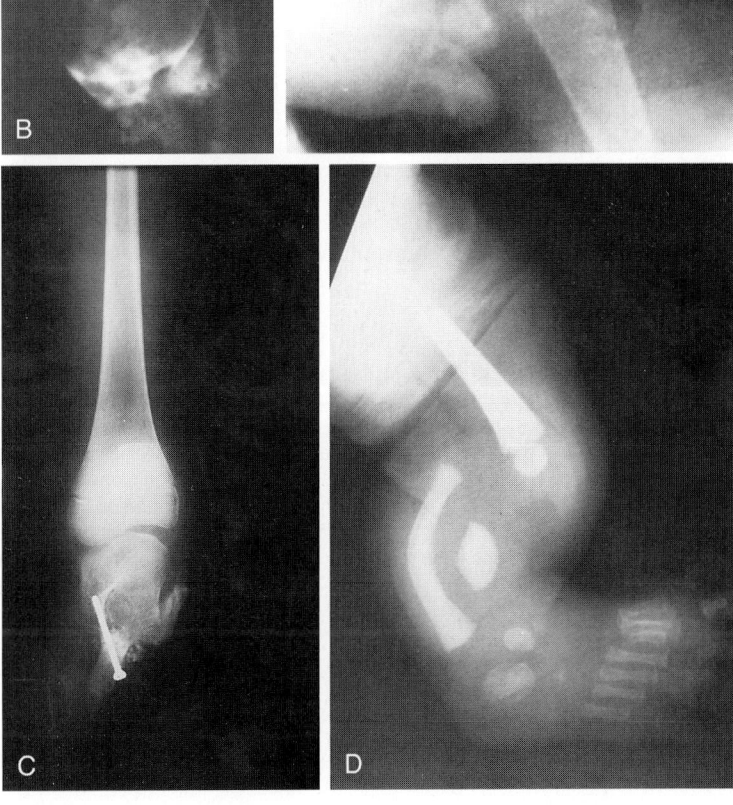

Fig. 8. Radiographs. *A,* Anteroposterior radiograph of the pelvis of a patient with congenital absence of the tibia. Notice the hypoplastic hemipelvis and abnormal proximal femur. There is also an associated congenitally shortened femur on the affected side. *B,* Anteroposterior and lateral radiograph of an arthrogram of the knee of a patient with type Ia congenital absence of the tibia. On the anteroposterior and lateral views, notice the hypoplastic rounded cartilaginous end of the femur outlined by the contrast. The intercondylar notch is absent. The tibia plateau is not outlined. The tibia is completely absent. *C,* Anteroposterior radiograph of a child's leg with type II congenital absence of the tibia. The proximal tibia is present, and the lateral condyle of the femur is hypoplastic. The child has had the distal fibula transferred into the remnant of the proximal tibia in order to gain tibial length. The calcaneus was also preserved at the time of the foot amputation to add length. *D,* Radiograph of a child with type III congenital absence of the tibia. A central portion of the tibia is present. The proximal tibia and the distal tibia are absent. The distal femur will be hypoplastic.

have developed a classification that is very useful in clinical decision-making. The classification has four types of congenitally absent tibia (Fig. 9).

Type I is the most common form of congenital absence of the tibia and may be bilateral. Females are affected twice as often as males.[16] Type I is divided into subgroups Ia and Ib. Type Ia demonstrates a completely absent tibia. This may be difficult to determine at birth as the proximal tibial remnant is sometimes present and completely cartilaginous. A clue, which hints at complete absence, can be

Type	Description	Treatment
Type Ia 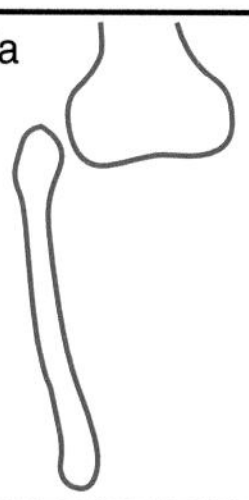	• Complete absence of the tibia • Hypoplastic distal femoral condyles • High-riding head of fibulae • Absent tibia confirmed on MRI	• Knee disarticulation at a convenient time before independent standing is anticipated (8 months)
Type Ib 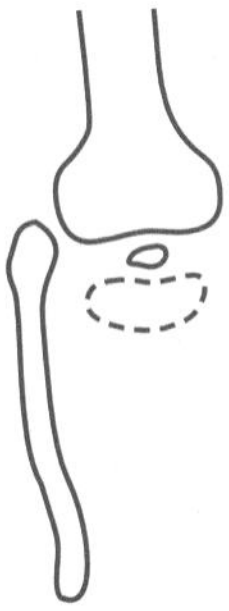	• Small portion of the distal tibia is present but not visible on radiograph • Distal femoral condyle and joint line appear relatively normal on radiograph • Arthrogram or MRI will demonstrate the cartilaginous proximal tibia	• Maintain ROM • Treat in a long-leg prosthesis until the proximal tibia ossifies • Osteotomize and move the fibulae into the tibia and ablate the deformed foot into a streamlined residual limb (modified Brown's procedure) • Move head of fibulae into alignment along proximal tibia • Length must be preserved, and a good end-weightbearing surface must be obtained. Ablate through joints rather than across bone. • Fit with B/K prosthesis, outside hinges, and a thigh lacer if necessary for knee joint stability
Type 2 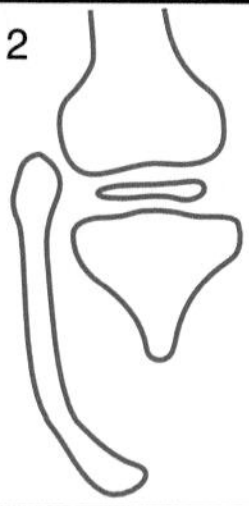	• Proximal tibia is visible on radiograph • Joint line appears normal • Distal femoral condyles are normal	• Treatment as for Type Ib
Type 3 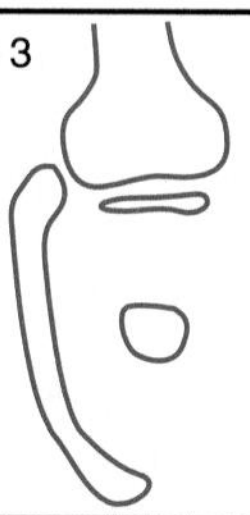	• Rudimentary midsection of the tibia is present	• Chopart's or Syme's amputation of the foot to maintain length and give a good end-bearing residual limb • Proximal one-third of the fibulae may need to be resected to allow for good socket fit and knee joint motion • Outside hinges and a thigh lacer may be necessary to gain knee stability
Type 4 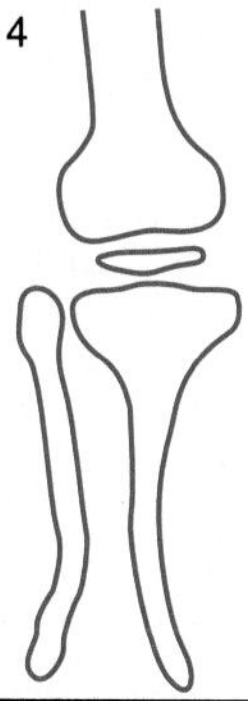	• The proximal section and midsection of the tibia are present • There is no ankle joint • The distal tibial and fibular bones diverge	• Ankle joint development is usually suboptimal and may compromise ultimate function • Leg length inequality is significant • Syme's amputation is the most functional form of treatment • The foot and ankle articulation may be salvaged in some circumstances. In these instances the lower leg must be lengthened.

Fig. 9. Classification of congenitally absent tibia.

provided by a radiograph of the knee showing hypoplastic distal femoral condyles on the affected side (see Fig. 8B and C). If the distal femur is poorly ossified, and the joint outline cannot be delineated on the anteroposterior radiograph, an arthrogram can be helpful in outlining the distal hypoplastic femur (see Fig. 7A and B). In type Ib, there is a cartilaginous portion of the proximal tibia that allows the knee joint to develop more normally in utero. An anteroposterior radiograph and an arthrogram of the knee will demonstrate a tibial plateau and a small cartilaginous fragment of the proximal tibia. An MRI will also demonstrate the cartilaginous anlage of the tibia and outline the tibial plateau.

In type II (see Fig. 8C), a portion of the proximal tibia is ossified at birth and is visible on a radiograph. The anteroposterior radiograph of the knee will show a normal relationship between the tibia and fibula, and there will be no evidence of femoral condylar hypoplasia.

Type III (see Fig. 8D) is very rare and is characterized by the central portion of the tibia being visible on radiograph and the proximal plateau region as well as the distal ankle joint being absent. The foot may be present and deformed.

Type IV is characterized by the proximal portions and midportions of the tibia being present and the ankle joint being absent as the tibia and fibula splay at the distal end. The foot may show a variety of anomalies ranging from deficiencies to polydactyly and syndactyly.

PATHOGENESIS

The pathogenesis of congenitally absent tibia is obscure. There have been reports of autosomal-dominant inheritance patterns and increased incidence rates when a family member is born with a tibial deficiency.[11, 16] The most common type of deficiency is type I, complete absence of the tibia. It is clear from Loder's work[16] that there is a 2:1 female-to-male ratio in type I. The ratio of the type Ia to Ib is 6:1 (Ia is also more often bilateral).

INVESTIGATION

Investigation of the child born with a congenitally absent tibia consists of a thorough history and physical examination to assess the other associated congenital abnormalities in other systems as well as the musculoskeletal system. The anomalies should be documented by photograph and radiograph. The knee should be assessed for stability and the presence of a prominent high-riding fibular head. Palpation may detect the presence of a remnant of proximal tibia.

Anteroposterior and lateral radiographs of the affected areas of the musculoskeletal system should be taken. The radiographs help to classify the type of congenital absence of the tibia and document and characterize other associated anomalies, such as hypoplasias, duplications, hemivertebrae, abnormal hip, and congenitally short femur. In type Ia, there is an associated hypoplasia of the femoral condyles evident on the anteroposterior radiograph of the knee. If the distinction between type Ia and Ib is not made by physical examination and radiograph of the knee, further imaging studies should be done. The best and least invasive test is an MRI of the knee. If an MRI is not available,

an arthrogram of the knee should be performed (see Fig. 8B and C). The arthrogram will outline the knee joint and the contour of the tibial plateau as well as the contour of the femoral condyles. The presence of normal femoral contours indicates proximal tibial cartilaginous anlage. Type III may also require an MRI or an arthrogram to prove presence or absence of a cartilaginous proximal tibia. Type IV will require an anteroposterior and lateral radiograph of the lower leg and will show splaying of the tibia and fibula with an abnormal articulation at the ankle joint and an abnormal foot.

MANAGEMENT

Type Ia is best treated by disarticulation amputation through the knee. The Brown procedure has a slim chance of success and usually ends in a knee disarticulation amputation because of uncontrollable knee flexion contracture. Loder[16] reviewed the world literature on the Brown procedure and concluded that patients must be chosen very carefully in order to have a successful result. Criteria for a successful result include (1) strong quadriceps function, (2) active knee motion from 10 degrees to 80 degrees, and (3) varus or valgus laxity of less than 5 degrees.

If these criteria are not met, knee disarticulation amputation is the procedure of choice. The quadriceps mechanism with the patellae is sutured to the posterior hamstrings. The end of the femur is left undisturbed. When the child pulls to standing, the child is fitted with a straight-leg-above-knee prosthesis or a prosthesis with a four-bar linkage knee that has been set into considerable stability. In the first 24 months of walking, many children do well with the straight-leg prosthesis, which does not have a knee joint. When the prosthesis is aligned and a knee joint is present, the weightbearing line will pass anterior to the knee joint on the lateral view, giving the leg significant inherent stability. The knee does not collapse with standing but bends with crawling and when sitting in a chair. This stable configuration in the early phases of walking allows the patient to trust the prosthesis. After the patient increases in strength and gains some experience with the stable prosthesis, the stability of the knee joint can be decreased. Suspension of the socket needs to be adequate to allow for crawling. The author of this chapter has found that a belt made of foam rubber that goes around the waist and is incorporated into the proximal thigh socket works very well. The belt is attached to the socket by laminating it into the upper rim and forming a flexible waist belt. The belt is usually held with Velcro. The prosthesis remains in place with crawling and is rotationally stable with walking.

Type Ib and type II should be treated with ablative surgery to the abnormal foot. *Preservation of residual limb length is of utmost importance for functioning in type Ib.* Sometimes, leaving the calcaneus or the talus in place allows added length to be preserved (see Fig. 8C). At a later stage when the proximal tibia has ossified, the fibular head can be osteotomized distally, brought down, and fused to the tibial plateau below the physis. The remaining distal fibula is then brought distally and medially to be set into the distal tibial remnant. The reconstruction is stabilized with screws and held postoperatively in an above-knee cast. Prosthetic fitting includes giving added stability to the knee by extending the prosthesis proximally, by using a Silastic sleeve, or by adding side hinges and a thigh corset to the PTS prosthesis.

Type III (see Fig. 8D) has a small residual remnant of tibia distally and a deformed foot.[11] After a Syme or Chopart type of amputation, the leg can be fitted with a prosthesis. The knee is stabilized by extending the prosthesis proximally with a PTS socket, by using a Silastic sleeve, or by using side hinges and a thigh corset.

Type IV has an abnormal ankle joint articulation with a deformed and malpositioned foot.[11, 16] The best and most functional treatment is the Syme amputation and prosthetic fitting. Consideration can also be given to correcting the foot malposition, followed by leg lengthening. Function, however, is influenced by the strength of the lengthened tibia and the motion and strength at the ankle and foot. An orthosis will be necessary to protect the tibia and maintain position of the foot.

REFERENCES

1. Kruger LM: Fibula deficiencies. In Herring JA, Birch JG (eds): The Child With a Limb Deficiency. AAOS, 1997, p 151.
2. Franz CH, O'Rahilly R: Congenital skeletal limb deficiencies and duplications. Am J Anat 1951; 89,135.
3. Kay HW, Day HJ, Henkel HL, et al: The proposed international terminology for the classification of congenital limb deficiencies. Dev Med Child Neurol 1975; 34,1.
4. Achterman C, Kalamchi A: Congenital deficiency of the fibula. J Bone Joint Surg Am 1979; 61,133.
5. Birch JG, Lincoln TL, Mack PW: Functional classification of fibular deficiency. In Herring JA, Birch JG (eds): The Child With a Limb Deficiency. AAOS, 1997, p 161.
6. Froster UG, Baird PA: Congenital defects of lower limbs and associated malformations: A population based study. Am J Med Genet 1993; 45,60.
7. Harder JA: Gait analysis of the child with a lower limb deficiency. In Herring JA, Birch JG (eds): The Child With a Limb Deficiency. AAOS, 1997, p 331.
8. Harder JA: Fractures and Dislocations of the Proximal Tibia and Fibula. In Letts RM (ed): Management of Pediatric Fractures. New York, Churchill Livingstone, 1994, p 611.
9. Rab GT: Oblique tibial osteotomy for Blount's disease (tibia vara). J Pediatr Orthop 1988; 8,715.
10. Fernandez-Palazzi F, Bendahan J, Rivas S: Congenital deficiency of the tibia: A report on 22 cases. J Pediatr Orthop 1998; 7,298.
11. Schoenecker PL: Tibial deficiency. In Herring JA, Birch JG (eds): The Child With a Limb Deficiency. AAOS, 1997, p 209.
12. Clark MW: Autosomal dominant inheritance of tibial meromelia: Report of a kindred. J Bone Joint Surg Am 1975; 57,262.
13. Lenz W: Genetics and limb deficiencies. Clin Orthop 1980; 148,9.
14. Schoenecker PL, Capelli AM, Millar EA, et al: Congenital longitudinal deficiency of the tibia. J Bone Joint Surg Am 1989; 71,278.
15. Jones D, Barnes J, Lloyd-Roberts GC: Congenital aplasia and dysplasia of the tibia with intact fibula: Classification and management. J Bone Joint Surg Br 1978; 60,31.
16. Loder RT: Fibula transfer for congenital absence of the tibia (Brown procedure). In Herring JA, Birch JG (eds): The Child With a Limb Deficiency. AAOS, 1997, p 223.

ACQUIRED AMPUTATIONS IN CHILDREN

Yoshio Setoguchi and Dawn Marie Ickes

Summary

- In the pediatric amputee population, approximately 35% to 40% of patients have acquired amputations.
- Treatment of child amputees works best with specialized centers with multidisciplinary teams.
- Acquired amputations are due to trauma or diseases such as infections, vascular disorders, and congenital anomalies.
- Prosthetic prescriptions should consider not only the physical factors but also the developmental and psychosocial needs of the child and family.
- Children are not miniature adults; therefore, treatment should be geared toward their developmental and growth needs.

Acquired amputations in children are secondary to trauma or disease. Past surveys indicated that in most specialized child amputee clinics acquired amputations account for approximately 35% to 40% of cases. However, this statistic varies according to the geographic areas from which the clinic receives its patients.

Acquired amputations can be classified into two basic subcategories: traumatic amputations and acquired amputations secondary to various diseases such as infections, vascular disorders, tumors, and congenital anomalies, not including limb reduction deformities.

HISTORY OF CHILD AMPUTEE CLINICS

Before the management of acquired amputations in children can be discussed, it is necessary to have some knowledge of the history of the establishment of child amputee clinics, especially in the United States. The field of prosthetics and management of amputees dates back to before the 1900s. There are published reports of prostheses made out of metals, and some that resembled crutches. A major focus on prosthetic rehabilitation and the emphasis on research into prosthetic fabrication techniques, new designs in prosthetic components, and concepts of a team approach to the care of these patients did not begin until after World War II. With the advancement of military medicine, more and more soldiers were returning from the war with amputations.

In 1946, the Michigan Children's Commission noted that, although the emphasis was on rehabilitation of adults, primarily the injured soldiers, a number of child amputees were being seen in orthopaedic clinics and fitted with prostheses. However, the results were poor, and most of the children rejected their prostheses because they were inadequate for their needs and uncomfortable. The prostheses were designed and developed for adults and did not take into consideration the particular needs for children. That year, Aitken and Frantz at the Mary Free Bed Hospital in Grand Rapids, Michigan, organized the first Juvenile Amputee Program in this country. Using the concept of a multidisciplinary team approach, the clinic emphasized not only fitting of the child with the best prosthetic devices available modifying them to meet specific needs, but instructing and training the child in its use, a model idea at that time. As many other clinics soon learned, the prosthetic needs of children differed from age to age, especially in the early formative years, and the child was not a miniature adult to whom adult prosthetic principles and modes of fitting could be applied.

In 1955 funds were made available from the Children's Bureau of the U.S. Department of Health, Education, and Welfare to establish a national pilot program for child amputee clinics. Following Grand Rapids, the University of California at Los Angeles (UCLA) and New York University were funded.

Soon after the funding of these clinics, funding was made available from the National Institutes of Health programs to establish research centers where the emphasis of prosthetic research was dedicated to the particular needs of children. Unfortunately, the initial period of strong funding (15 to 20 years) for research died down, and only recently have new funds been made available.

The concept and effectiveness of prosthetic clinics specifically for children have continued to be viable. Currently, approximately 70 centers exist throughout the United States and Canada. Many such clinics are available in Asia and Europe. In the United States and Canada, communications and exchange of technologies and training methods are made possible through an organization, whose concept was established in 1959, now called the Association of Children's Prosthetics and Orthotics Clinics (ACPOC).

To develop an effective program for the care and management of acquired amputations, as the early clinics learned, it is important to have a clinic devoted to the care of children. General growth and development, and the psychosocial issues of the amputations on the patients and also on the family are very important areas of focus in the treatment assessment.

ETIOLOGY

Before treatment is begun, one needs to know the cause of the amputations (Table 1). Trauma continues to be a major cause of morbidity and mortality in children. The causes differ slightly according to the age of the child and where the family lives. (This is especially true in third world countries.) In young, preschool-age children, the most common causes are power tools such as lawn mowers, meat or food grinders, and powered farm equipment. In the preado-

TABLE 1. CAUSES OF TRAUMATIC AMPUTATIONS
Young Children
Power tools
Lawn mowers
Meat grinders
Farm equipment
Preadolescents
Power tools
Vehicular accidents
Burns, including electrical
Gunshot and explosion
Adolescents
Vehicular accidents
Gunshot and explosions
Power tools

lescent period, power tool and machinery accidents are most frequent, followed by vehicular accidents, electrical injuries, gunshot and explosions wounds, and railroad accidents. In the adolescent years, vehicular accidents, both automobile and motorcycles, gunshot wounds, and power tool injuries are the leading causes.

In metropolitan areas, the majority of amputations are caused by motor vehicular accidents, burns, and commercial machinery injuries. In rural areas, farm equipment accidents, such as large lawn mowers, and hunting accidents are more common. In the third world countries, other causes include train accidents, electrical and flame burns, and war-related injuries, such as gunshot and land mine explosions.

Diseases that might lead to amputations can be classified into tumors, infections, vascular malformations, neurological disorders, and other miscellaneous disorders. Up until the development of limb salvage techniques and improved survival from chemotherapy, the most frequent acquired amputations were in children, especially during the second decade of life, were bone malignancies (i.e., osteogenic sarcomas).

TREATMENT

The treatment of accident-related injuries starts with a discussion of prevention. A thorough understanding of the factors involved in the accidents will lead to effective safety programs such as education, legislation, regulations, and research and development of safety features for both equipment and motor vehicles.

The decrease in the use of amputations as a treatment option in limb malignancies has been a result of the improved survival rate resulting from chemotherapy and, more importantly, of the development of new limb salvage procedures.

As for amputations secondary to infections, early recognition and treatment are the only means of prevention. Many of the cases are due to very sudden and rapid onset of disseminated coagulopathy as is seen in meningococcemia. Even with early and appropriate medical treatment, the limb gangrenes are difficult to prevent.

GENERAL TREATMENT CONSIDERATIONS

It is important for those involved in the prosthetic and rehabilitation management to understand the complexities of some of the problems encountered in children with acquired amputations. Some factors that need to be considered at the time of amputation or in the immediate postoperative period that will have long-term effects on the prosthetic program are as follows:

1. Length of residual limb. In the past, the minimal length of stump needed for utilization of the most proximal joint determined the level of the amputation. However, more recently, with the advent of stump lengthening, the recommendation now is to save any joint possible, even with a very short, nonfunctioning stump, with the understanding that stump lengthening in the future might make the patient more functional. Therefore, the current concept is that if the joint is functional, one should save as much of the distal stump as possible. However, one should not save length with skin grafts, as they do not respond well to lengthening.
2. Condition of the skin coverage of the amputation stump. Scar tissue is not a good medium for weightbearing or absorption of friction and skin forces. Yet, if it means providing additional length to the stump, grafts should be considered. However, this may lead to longer rehabilitation as well as more frequent prosthetic problems.
3. Function of most proximal joint. If one is uncertain of function, it is best to save the joint. However, if adequate function is not anticipated, then a disarticulation may be the treatment of choice.
4. Associated injuries. The type and duration of treatment of other injuries should be considered in the treatment of the amputation. This is especially true for patients with malignancies who are undergoing chemotherapy. The morbidity and debilitation caused by the therapy will affect prosthetic training and, ultimately, function.

ASSESSMENT

Prosthetic prescription should be a team decision involving the medical staff and the patient and family (Fig. 1). The role of the team is to provide a comprehensive evaluation of the amputation, the physical status of the patient, the amputation site, including the proximal joint(s), the factors surrounding the amputation, and the reactions of the patient and family to the injury and resultant disabilities.

Initial evaluation should include a comprehensive psychosocial assessment by a social worker or psychologist with experience in pediatric issues and rehabilitation needs. Several issues are important to the team in developing a treatment plan (Table 2).

1. Family's ability to handle stress. It is important to know how the parents and the patient handled the emotional impact of the accident and the news of the amputation. The social worker needs to assess the family's ability to work through grief and loss and their readiness to comply with the rehabilitation program. Families that are still in the grief stages often find it difficult to proceed

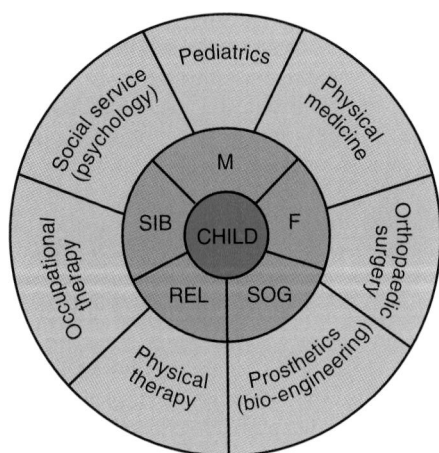

Fig. 1. Team approach to the treatment of the limb-deficient child. Inner circle: treatment to include, in addition to the patient, mother (M), father (F), siblings (SIB), relatives (REL), and grandparents (SOG). Outer circle: treatment team.

with the prosthetic fitting and training program. They may express their grief by reacting negatively to the function and appearance of the prostheses.
2. Blame and guilt issues related to the accident. It is important for the team to understand the factors surrounding the trauma and amputations. Often when the injury is secondary to an accident, there is the question of whether there was someone to blame. When disease processes led to the amputations, parents often wonder whether amputation could have been prevented if they had recognized the problems sooner. Failure of the team to assess, recognize, and treat these issues may have a negative effect on the treatment program. At times, the team becomes the object of the family/patient's anger and resentment.
3. Family's ability to handle rehabilitation issues. These issues must be dealt with if the patient is to progress through a positive prosthetic program. In addition, the ability of the family to understand that they have a major role in the treatment is vital to a successful program. The family's commitment to a full-time wearing pattern, appropriate training program, and a well-fitting and functional prosthesis is essential.
4. Future well-being and financial issues. The rehabilitation program is a very expensive process. The team must help the family learn of the resources available to them and how to maximize them for the patient's benefit. In addition, parents must be made aware of the child's future needs, the availability of high-technology devices and their impact on the child's function, the activities

---

TABLE 2. PREPROSTHETIC ASSESSMENTS: FACTORS TO CONSIDER

Family's ability to handle stress
Blame and guilt issues related to the accident
Family's ability to handle rehabilitation issues
Future well-being and financial issues
Support groups

that the child is expected to participate in both in school and at home, and the future educational and vocational potentials and, in rare instances, limitations.

5. Support groups. Many clinics provide support groups for the new amputees and their families. These groups provide tremendous support to many families. In some cases, simply a one-to-one contact with one family with a child with similar circumstances may be more helpful.

PHYSICAL THERAPY

Preprosthetic assessment begins with the status of the amputated limb (Table 3). The condition of the patient's skin has a direct bearing on the course of treatment. Adequate skin coverage is imperative for success with prosthetic fitting. Damaged tissues do not tolerate compression, shear, or torsional forces as well as normal tissues. This can mean sacrificing some length to provide good skin coverage over the distal portion of the stump.

The physical therapist assesses the amputation scar location with respect to the level of amputation and the prosthetic options as they relate to the weightbearing surfaces of the residual limb. Scar tissue mobility is of equal importance and any areas of adherence to underlying bone, fascia, or soft tissues need to be addressed to provide appropriate treatments.

The control of edema and swelling after amputation surgery is necessary to ensure suitable fitting with a prosthesis. Proper positioning of the amputated limb and postoperative exercises can help control edema. Shrinker socks, residual limb wrapping with elastic bandage, and semirigid or rigid postoperative dressings assist with edema control and shaping of the limb. Inadequate postoperative care can lead to a poorly shaped residual limb, which can lead to difficulties with the prosthetic fitting.

Joint stability has an effect on the decisions made with regard to the type of prosthesis selected for a particular amputation level. Differences in joint stability and ligamentous laxity are taken into consideration when prosthetic decisions are made. Additionally, residual limb muscle strength is assessed and has an impact on the type of prosthesis that is ultimately prescribed for the patient. Lack of proximal stability or irreparable muscular weakness will necessitate a more stable prosthesis, which may be less desirable for the patient.

In many cases, improvements in muscle strength are plausible. A strengthening program can be initiated as soon as the sutures are removed and muscular contractions will not create adverse stretching of the scar. Active exercise can help control edema, improve residual limb circulation, and decrease the chances of scar tissue adhesion. Postural and balance reeducation exercises are also begun as soon

as possible after amputation surgery in the seated and standing positions. For the lower extremity amputee, good standing balance is very important because many activities of daily living will be done without a prosthesis.

It is very important that new amputees begin practicing good hygiene habits immediately. Checking the skin regularly and noting any areas of discoloration, adverse reddening, breakdown, or rash must become a part of the lifestyle early on, because the need for this will span the rest of their lives. Untreated skin problems can become extremely problematic for prosthetic use.

The sensory assessment provides information regarding areas of decreased sensation or hypersensitivity, both of which can create problems with prosthetic fitting and training. Increased sensitivity is very common after amputation surgery. Stump desensitization programs are more effective when they are initiated as soon as possible after the surgery. The patient is taught gentle self-massage three times per day for 5 to 10 minutes; the amount of pressure and the duration of the massage are increased as tolerated. The program is modified with younger patients, for whom the parents perform the massage and encourage the child's involvement. Transverse friction massage across the scar site is also taught to patients to decrease hypersensitivity and prepare the scar for contact with the prosthesis. Areas of decreased sensation are mapped and the information is relayed to the physician and the prosthetist.

Measurement of the available range of motion in any involved and/or proximal joints is necessary for the identification of joint contractures. Flexion contractures are the most common after amputation surgery, and prevention is the best treatment. Teaching proper postoperative positioning and stretching exercises to both patients and their parents will undoubtedly benefit patients if they are compliant with the program. Active and passive stretching, coupled with positioning the susceptible joints into extension while the patient is resting, can assist with the prevention and treatment of flexion contractures.

The treatment of an existing contracture can be done by using the same techniques used for prevention with the additional use of modalities such as ultrasound waves or heat, which relaxes the patients and the muscles that are contracted. Counterbalance force with weights in prone or supine position can also be used to help treat contractures.

Functional limitations without a prosthesis are dependent on the level of the amputation. The therapist ensures that the patient knows how to transfer to and from the floor, into and out of chairs, cars, and bathtubs and how to dress without the prosthesis. It is important to identify any difficulties the patient may have with such activities and make recommendations or provide special training to assist the patient.

Determining the type of prosthetic device to prescribe is dependent on the patient's developmental age and cognitive capabilities, functional need for the device, lower extremity stability, and parental attitudes. An understanding of the amputee's capabilities and functional needs, at different stages of development, guides the prosthetist in selecting components and fabricating a prosthesis. The age of the patient affects decisions made regarding the stability that the prosthesis provides and the complexity of the components used.

TABLE 3. PREPROSTHETIC ASSESSMENT
Evaluate:
Skin condition (presence of scar)
Range of motion and strength of proximal joints
Edema and swelling
Developmental status

PROSTHETIC ORIENTATION

Some basic issues that the prosthetic team must address and assess before developing a prescription and treatment program are discussed below.

1. Developmental age. A developmental age of at least 1 year should be reached prior to prosthetic fitting. Fitting should be performed as soon as the wound and the stump have healed sufficiently to tolerate it.
2. Cognitive function. Cognitive abilities must be carefully assessed in designing the prosthetic program. It is important not to overwhelm the patient with large numbers of components. Simple devices with simple control sources make it easier for the patient to learn to operate and use the prosthesis. One example for upper extremity amputees is when there is more than one function to control with a single cable, such as terminal device operation and elbow lock control operation. The general rule is to start with active terminal device operation with passive elbow lock control. Later, when the patient has a good understanding of the terminal device operation, one can activate the elbow lock system. In the lower extremity, it generally is not necessary to prescribe an energy-stored foot for children younger than 5 years who have not yet developed the normal adult heel-toe pattern of gait and would not maximize the functions of these high-energy active feet. In addition, the knee joint for the above-knee (A/K) and hip disarticulation (H/D) prostheses before the age of approximately 3 years is not necessary and actually may be hazardous. The patients are not aware of the function of the knee joint and, therefore, will likely not lock it (extend the knee fully) before putting weight on the prosthesis.
3. Functional versus cosmetic. Many upper extremity amputees and their families come to the clinic expecting a true replacement of the lost arm, particularly the lost hand. They are appalled at the sight of a terminal device that does not resemble a normal hand. Careful orientation by the team, especially the occupational therapist, in describing the benefits and limitations of the various terminal devices is important. Often, the initial training begins with the most functional device, and then the more cosmetic device is added. However, the patient and families make the ultimate decision. In the lower extremity, the prescription of an endoskeletal or exoskeletal prosthesis relates to cosmesis. The cosmesis is provided by a custom-shaped foam mold with a cosmetic hose. For the very young child, this system is not very durable.

UPPER EXTREMITIES

Successful upper extremity prosthetic fitting starts with a strong and consistent commitment by the parents and child. The parents must understand that most children with one or both upper extremity amputations can usually function quite well without prosthetic fittings. They can learn to become extremely functional with the one remaining limb, the use of the residual (amputated side) limb, or the use of their feet. Children can be very adaptable and will develop excellent functional abilities with what they have. There-fore, if a prosthesis is to become a functional part of the child's upper extremities, the child must develop a full-time wearing pattern and learn to integrate the prosthesis into a spontaneous, effective use pattern in bimanual activities. In addition, the family has to commit their resources to ongoing prosthetic training, usually starting twice weekly and continuing at least once a week or once every other week during the first 6 months. The commitment must be made to ensure that the prosthesis continues to fit and function well. This entails frequent adjustments by the prosthetist as the child grows, and repairs must be made as soon as breakage or poor function is noted.

In order for upper extremity prosthetic fitting to be successful, the prosthesis should be as simple as possible in operation, have a minimal number of components, be lightweight, and have good suspension and good stability of socket fit. The more complex the prosthetic prescription, the more likely it is that the child will reject the prosthesis.

LOWER EXTREMITIES

General factors to consider in prescribing lower extremity prostheses for children include the need for stability, easy control, good fit, and function. Child amputees will not wear a prosthesis that is not stable. If the foot is not flat on the floor during weightbearing, the child will feel insecure and will not want to stand on it. In infant amputees, one must be aware of their base of support and position of the lower extremities during weightbearing and ambulation. Prosthetists must align the prosthesis with a wide base of support with the hips and knees flexed (normal side) to lower the center of gravity. As the child narrows the base of support, the alignment can be changed to a more normal adult type.

In the young A/K or bilateral A/K amputee, the initial fitting without a knee joint may provide the necessary stability to ensure rapid weightbearing and ambulation. Knee joints are usually added between 3 and 4 years of age.

SOCKET FIT AND SUSPENSION

The key to successful wearing in child amputees is comfort. The skin may not demonstrate any irritation. The only clue that the patient is uncomfortable may be in the gait pattern. A classic example of this is in the very young below-knee (B/K) amputee, who presents with excessive knee flexion and a tendency to walk on the prosthetic toe, the problem could be one of alignment, but it is more likely to be pressure of the socket over the anterior distal end of the stump. Appropriate socket adjustment usually will correct the problem. Good suspension in the A/K patient often will minimize circumduction and subsequent poor gait pattern.

Other sources of suspension such as sleeves, silicone sockets, and modified suction sockets may help but may also cause problems such as skin irritation, increased perspiration, and the necessity of frequent replacements.

ALIGNMENT PROBLEMS

Flexion contractures, deformities at the knee, and functional limitations of the ankle lead to problems in alignment and providing the patient with a cosmetically-functionally acceptable prosthesis. One example of this is in the

B/K amputee with a valgus deformity at the knee. To obtain the best alignment with the typical slight lateral thrust of the knee at midstance, the foot needs to have sufficient inset to achieve weightbearing over the foot. This may cause a bowing effect on the final shape of the prosthesis.

PROSTHETIC PRESCRIPTIONS

As pediatric patients age, their prosthetic prescriptions become more similar to those of adult amputees. However, as in the congenital amputees/limb deficiencies, some fitting principles apply to the young acquired amputee.

In the child amputee, before the age of 12 months, the standard approach to an upper extremity unilateral fitting is to perform the fitting when the child has developed good sitting balance. This is usually at 6 to 8 months of age. The first fitting is usually a passive type in which the child does not actively open the terminal device. The terminal device is usually activated with appropriate harness fitting at 15 to 18 months of age. As noted, the elbow lock control system is not activated until 3 to 3½ years of age.

In the lower extremity, the age of the child affects the timing of initial fitting and the prescription of various mechanical joints. In the infant amputee, prosthetic fitting is instituted when the child starts to pull to stand. This is generally at 8 to 12 months of age but may be later in high-level amputees and bilateral amputees.

Knee joints are usually not added until the patient has developed an effective, safe gait on the pylon/extension type prosthesis. Although knee joint introduction is delayed, the hip joint is added with the first fitting of the H/D prosthesis to allow sitting.

The prescription for the bilateral acquired amputee depends to a great degree on the level of the amputation. Bilateral B/K amputees are fitted just as unilateral amputees, that is, when the child has developed abilities to pull up to stand.

When the bilateral amputations are asymmetric, with one side being below the knee and the other above the knee, usually the length of the B/K side determines the ultimate length of the prostheses. The younger child especially is fitted with a pylon extension type on the A/K side until balance and endurance are obtained. Some older children, if their balance and coordination are not good, are fitted in a similar manner.

The bilateral A/K amputees (both A/K and through-knee levels) are usually fitted at our clinic with bilateral stubbies without knee joints until good stability and comfort are obtained. The prostheses are then gradually lengthened until the appropriate height is reached. Then knee joints are added. Usually at this point, patients will require assistive devices such as canes or crutches.

Bilateral H/D amputees generally do not become good prosthetic users. In the young child, sitting balance is very important. If stability is a problem, he or she is fitted with a bucket or bilateral H/D socket attached to a square piece of wood to provide a good base of support. Prosthetic fitting can be attempted, but the success rate is low. Devices such as sway walker and reciprocal gait systems have been tried with limited success. These children usually find that a wheelchair is more efficient energy-wise and provides much faster mobility. Careful and thorough discussion by the team with the parents and, when appropriate, with the patient is essential for successful function.

CONCLUSION

The child amputee with an acquired amputation is not a miniature adult. His or her needs are different, and the prosthetic management must be tailored to developmental as well as functional needs. In addition, the special needs secondary to the cause of the amputation must be taken into account in planning the prosthetic prescription and subsequent training. An experienced, well-coordinated team is essential for maximum success in the rehabilitation.

REFERENCES

1. Academy of Orthopedic Surgeons: Atlas of Limb Prosthetics. St. Louis, MO, CV Mosby, 1987.
2. Aitken G: The child with an acquired amputation. Inter-Clinic Inform Bull 1968; 7(8).
3. Blank JE, Dormans JP, Davidson RS: Perinatal limb ischemia: Orthopedic implications. J Pediatr Orthop 1996; 16:90.
4. Burke JF, Quinby WC Jr, Bondoc C, et al: Patterns of high tension electrical injury in children and adolescents and their management. J Hand Surg 1977; 133:492.
5. Dormans JP, Azzoni M, Davidson RS, et al: Major lower extremity lawn mower injuries in children. J Pediatr Orthop 1995; 15:78.
6. Edholm CD: A history of ACPOC. ACPOC News 1998; 43:1.
7. Kon M: Firework injuries to the hand. Ann Chir Main Memb Super 1991; 10: 443.
8. Letts M, Davidson D: Epidemiology and prevention of traumatic amputations in children. In Herring J, Birch J (eds): The Child With a Limb Deficiency. Rosemont, IL, American Academy of Orthopedic Surgeons, 1998, p 235.
9. Letts RM: Farm machinery accidents in children. In Dosman JA, Cockcroft DW (eds): Principles of Health and Safety in Agriculture. Boca Raton, FL, CRC Press, 1986, p 357.
10. Nixon J, Corcoran A, Fielding L, et al: Fatal and nonfatal accidents on the railways: A study of injuries to individuals, with particular reference to children and to nonfatal trauma. Accid Anal Prev 1985; 17:217.
11. Pyper JA, Black GB: Orthopaedic injuries in children associated with the use of off-road vehicles. J Bone Joint Surg Am 1988; 70:275.
12. Setoguchi Y, Rosenfelder R: The Limb Deficient Child. Springfield, IL, Charles C Thomas, 1982.
13. Shapiro MJ, Luchtefeld WB, Durham RM, et al: Traumatic train injuries. Am J Emerg Med 1994; 12:92.
14. Slauterbeck JR, Britton C, Moneim MS, et al: Mangled extremity severity score: An accurate guide to treatment of the severely injured upper extremity. J Orthop Trauma 1994; 8:282.
15. Stucky W, Loder RT: Extremity gunshot wounds in children. J Pediatr Orthop 1991; 11:64.
16. Tooms RE: The amputee. In Morrissy RT (ed): Lovell and Winter's Pediatric Orthopaedics. Philadelphia, PA, JB Lippincott, 1990, 3rd ed, vol 2, p 1023.
17. Tooms RE: Acquired amputations in children. In Atlas of Limb Prosthetics. St. Louis, MO, CV Mosby, 1987, p 553.
18. Trautwein LC, Smith DG, Rivara FF: Pediatric amputation injuries: Etiology, cost, and outcome. J Trauma 1996; 41:831.

section
9
chapter
4

GENETICS I

Benjamin A. Alman and Michael J. Goldberg

Summary
- The genetic cause of many musculoskeletal disorders is now known.
- Data from the human genome project and new advances in gene searching techniques will likely identify the genes involved in most common disorders treated by orthopaedists.
- New ways in which genes can be inherited (parental effect and unstable DNA mutations) explain the inheritance pattern in some disorders that do not follow classic mendelian inheritance.

Many of the musculoskeletal conditions treated by orthopaedists have a genetic component to their cause. A basic knowledge of genetics is, therefore, necessary to give patients appropriate information about their disorders and to know when to refer them for a comprehensive genetic evaluation.

Research into the genetics of human disease is progressing at a staggering pace. Advances in research technique and knowledge from the human genome project are helping to make the identification of genes responsible for inherited disorders a common occurrence. Gene defects that predispose to common diseases, such as some cancers, have been identified, and novel ways in which genes can be inherited have been discovered. The knowledge from this research produced new diagnostic tests, improved our ability to provide genetic and prenatal counseling, and led to a better understanding of the pathophysiology of many disease processes. It is likely that genes will be identified that are responsible for, or predispose to, many musculoskeletal conditions, such as clubfoot, scoliosis, Dupuytren's contracture, and osteoarthritis. In fact, some familial forms of osteoarthritis are already known to be related to mutations in the type II collagen gene. Although gene therapy is not yet a reality, the knowledge of cellular pathways altered by gene defects can suggest novel treatments for some conditions.

Because the information about genetic disorders is increasing at such a rapid pace, the most up-to-date information is rarely available in a traditional textbook. The Internet has become an excellent source for obtaining up-to-date detailed information on specific inherited disorders and genes. One good site for this is the on-line mendelian inheritance in humans at http//www.ncbi.nlm.nih.gov/Omim, which can be searched by disease name, responsible gene, or clinical findings.

HISTORICAL REVIEW

1866 Gregor Mendel proposes basic rules of inheritance.
1910 Thomas Hunt Morgan determines that some genetic traits are sex linked.

1944 Oswald Avery, Colin MacLeod, and Maclyn McCarty show that DNA is responsible for inherited traits.
1953 James Watson and Francis Crick discover the double-helix structure of DNA.
1964 Charles Yanofsky shows that DNA sequences correspond to protein sequences.
1978 The human insulin gene is cloned.
1980 Human gene is successfully introduced and expressed by bacteria and the first transgenic mouse is reported.
1990 Human genome project begins, as does the first use of gene therapy (on a patient with severe immunodeficiency).

HOW ARE DISEASES INHERITED?

There are estimated to be about 3 billion base pairs of DNA, making up about 70,000 genes, which are located on 23 chromosomes in the nucleus of human cells. DNA is composed of pairs of nucleic acids. There are four nucleic acids: guanine, cytosine, adenosine, and thymine (abbreviated G, C, A, and T). The DNA in chromosomes is arranged into genes, which are preceded by a segment of DNA responsible for controlling the gene. The DNA in a gene is transcribed into messenger RNA (mRNA), which leaves the nucleus and is translated into a protein product in the cytoplasm. Three nucleic acids in a row encode for one protein residue, and some nucleic acid sequences give information about where to start or stop transcription and translation. These genes are responsible for the behavior of every cell in the body and encode information for structural genes (e.g., collagen), enzymes (e.g., lysosomal enzymes), and cell-regulating genes (e.g., growth factors).[1]

Mutations are a permanent change in the DNA sequence. When a mutation is present in the zygote (the fertilized oocyte), it will be found in all the cells in the body and is termed a germline mutation. When a mutation occurs in only one cell, either during or after development, it will be present in only a subset of the cells in the mature individual and is termed a somatic mutation. Some genes have many alternative forms and are called polymorphic. Such polymorphic genes are used in forensic medicine to determine the origin of a DNA sample. Many polymorphic variants and mutations do not have deleterious effects and are part of the normal process of genetic heterogeneity that makes each individual unique. However, others predispose to or cause disease.

Mutations in DNA can range from a change in a single nucleic acid to complete chromosome rearrangement. Mutations of a single nucleic acid are termed point mutations and may change a protein's function by altering its structure. Such mutations tend to occur in hot spots in DNA, such as at a CG dinucleotide. Larger scale mutations can occur, causing deletions of portions of a gene, duplications of a gene, or a rearrangement of a gene. These may cause complete lack of a gene or an abnormal protein structure or may alter the normal relationship between the control portion of the DNA and the portion coding for the protein product (e.g., may produce too much of a gene product).

New mutations may occur by a chance mistake made when a cell reproduces and needs to copy its DNA (replication). One can imagine that with 3 billion base pairs, a mistake in one pair is not that unlikely. New point mutations occur in the DNA in sperm, with a higher frequency with advanced paternal age. Thus, there is an increased incidence of some disorders (e.g., achondroplasia) in the children of older fathers. Environmental factors, such as radiation, can also cause mutations during cell replication. Disorders that are inherited can, therefore, also occur because of a new mutation in a child whose parents are unaffected and do not carry the mutation.

MENDELIAN INHERITANCE

In the last half of the 1800s, Gregor Mendel formulated laws that explained the inheritance of diseases. Advances in molecular genetics, however, have shown many ways in which diseases can be inherited without following these laws. Despite this, Mendel's laws still explain the inheritance patterns of most genetic disorders. Mendelian inheritance is based on the fact that in the normal situation 22 of the 23 chromosomes exist as pairs, one maternally and one paternally derived. These paired chromosomes are called autosomes. The remaining chromosome pair is the sex chromosomes that exist as a pair of X chromosomes in females and a single X chromosome and a single Y chromosome in males. During reproduction, each parent normally contributes one copy of each of the chromosomes to the child. Thus, all of the genes located on the autosomes exist in duplicate copies, one of maternal origin and one of paternal origin. Each copy of the gene is termed an allele. When a gene mutation is present on one allele, it is called a heterozygous mutation. When present on both alleles, it is termed homozygous.

Autosomal-dominant disorders (Fig. 1) are caused by genes in which only one of the two alleles needs to be affected to cause the disorder (heterozygous). When one

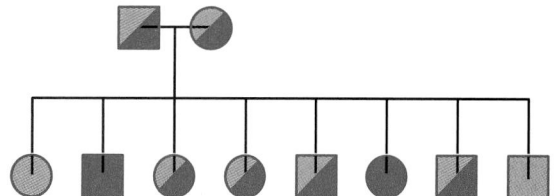

Fig. 2. Pedigree of an autosomal recessive disorder. A half-blackened square or circle means the causative gene is present in one allele, and a completely blackened square or circle means the causative gene is present in both alleles. Because the disease requires both alleles to be affected, only individuals with completely blackened squares or circles are affected, but individuals with half-blackened squares or circles are carriers.

parent has one copy of the mutant gene, he or she will have the disease and will pass it on to one-half of the children, who will also be affected by the disease. Males and females are equally affected. Some of the musculoskeletal disorders inherited in this manner are many types of Charcot-Marie-Tooth disease, neurofibromatosis, osteogenesis imperfecta, and achondroplasia.

Autosomal-recessive disorders (Fig. 2) are caused by genes in which both alleles need to be affected to cause the disease. Thus, if both parents carry the gene mutation on one allele, neither will have the disease, but one-fourth of their children will inherit both copies of the mutant gene and have the disease, whereas one-half of the children will carry the mutation in one allele to pass it on the next generation. Sometimes the carriers manifest mild manifestations of the disease. Mutations disturbing enzyme function are often inherited in an autosomal-recessive manner, such as the mucopolysaccharidoses.

X-linked disorders are caused by genes located on the X chromosome. Mutations in genes on the X chromosome, like those in genes on the autosomes, can cause disease in a dominant (heterozygous mutation) or recessive (homozygous mutation) fashion. Because males carry only one X chromosome, both dominant and recessive disorders produce the disease. In the dominant type, the disease from an affected father is transmitted to all of the daughters but none of the sons. In general, the males exhibit more severe clinical manifestations of the disease than do females. For example, Rett's syndrome is an X-linked dominant disorder that gives a picture similar to cerebral palsy in females but is lethal in males. X-linked recessive diseases are transmitted from a mother who carries the gene mutation but exhibits mild or no clinical manifestations, to one-half of the sons, who have the disease. One-half of the daughters are carriers. Duchenne's muscular dystrophy is an example of an X-linked recessive disorder.

NONMENDELIAN WAYS TO INHERIT GENES

Some diseases were known to be inherited but did not fit well into the mendelian modes of inheritance. Some of these disorders may be multifactorial, in that a variety of genes and environmental factors may be important. Others may exhibit variable penetrance in which other factors modulate the severity of the disease. Other novel ways in

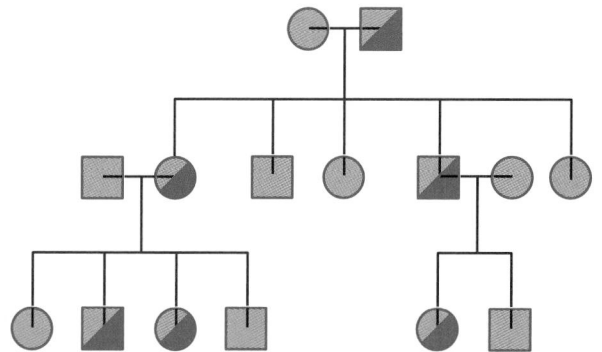

Fig. 1. Pedigree of an autosomal dominant disorder. Males are represented as squares and females as circles. A blackened half of a square or circle means that a gene causing a disorder is present in one of the two alleles. Because only one allele causes the disease, all of the individuals that are half blackened are affected.

which genes can be inherited were identified that do not fit into mendelian laws.

PARENTAL EFFECTS

Mendelian inheritance assumes genes of paternal and maternal origin to be equally weighted in terms of effect. However, this has turned out not to be the case in some disorders. One mechanism for this is termed imprinting. Because there are double copies of each gene, one of the copies is inactivated. This occurs by a process called methylation, which usually turns off either the maternal gene or the paternal gene in a random manner. When a gene is imprinted, the copy from one of the parents is always turned off. This is the case in Prader-Willi syndrome, in which gene mutation is inherited from the father, but the normal maternal copy is always turned off.[2]

The process of chromosome division normally produces 23 pairs of chromosomes. It was thought that any error in the division of chromosomes resulted in a trisomy (an extra copy of one chromosome). Surprisingly, it was found that an embryo can self-correct for the extra chromosome by removing it. Thus, when there is an error causing an extra chromosome (e.g., two from the mother and one from the father), the cell will remove one of the extra chromosomes. However, it removes the extra chromosome in a random fashion so that there is a one-third chance that the embryo will be left with two chromosomes of maternal origin. This phenomenon is called uniparental disomy (Fig. 3). The implications of uniparental disomy are just beginning to be explored. However, it is known that some cases of Prader-Willi syndrome are caused by uniparental disomy.[2]

UNSTABLE DNA MUTATIONS

There are regions along DNA where a series of three nucleotides are repeated for a variable number of times. The purpose of the repeats is not known, but their length usually remains the same through successive generations. However, in some families, the length of the repeats increases over successive generations and is termed unstable. The increasing length can cause the disease when it reaches a threshold size or can predispose the segment of DNA to divide abnormally during cell division, producing a secondary gene abnormality (Fig. 4). The fragile X syndrome and myotonic dystrophy are two musculoskeletal diseases caused by unstable DNA mutations.[3]

GENETIC CAUSES OF MUSCULOSKELETAL DISEASE

A wide variety of musculoskeletal disorders are caused by gene defects, and it is beyond the scope of this text to cover them all. Because we now know the types of genes that cause many of the disorders, it is helpful to group them by the type of responsible gene. These diseases can be broadly grouped into those caused by mutation in a structural protein gene (such as osteogenesis imperfecta caused by a collagen mutation); genes important in normal development (such as achondroplasia caused by a mutation in fibroblast growth receptor type III); or a gene coding for an enzyme (such as a lysosomal enzyme causing a mucopolysaccharidosis). Knowing the causative gene often makes it easier to understand the various clinical manifestations of a disorder. For instance, spondyloepiphyseal dysplasia is caused by a mutation in type II collagen, which

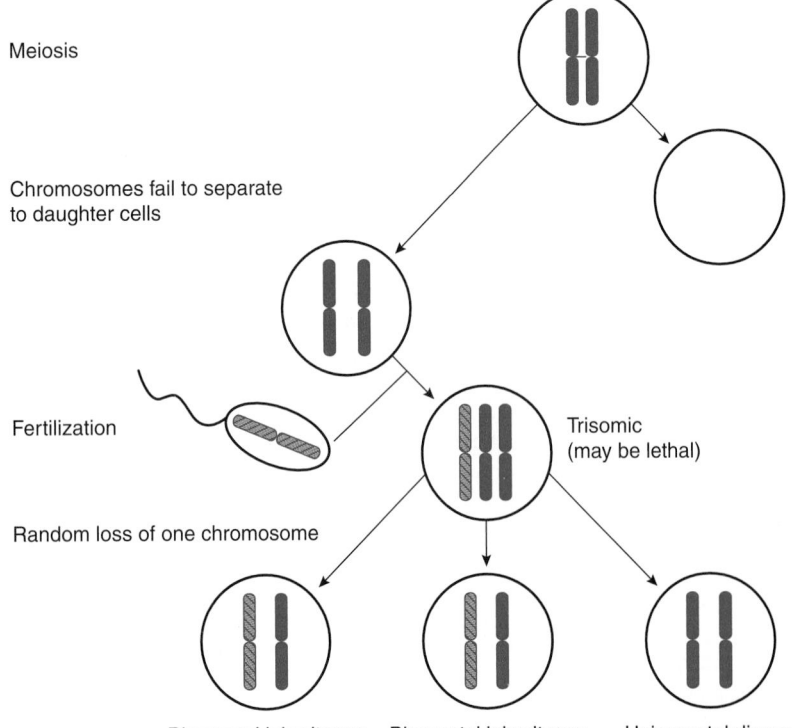

Meiosis

Chromosomes fail to separate
to daughter cells

Fertilization

Random loss of one chromosome

Trisomic
(may be lethal)

Biparental inheritance   Biparental inheritance   Uniparental disomy

Fig. 3. A diagrammatic representation of uniparental disomy. This shows how an error in replication producing a trisomy can be corrected, giving two chromosomes from a single parent.

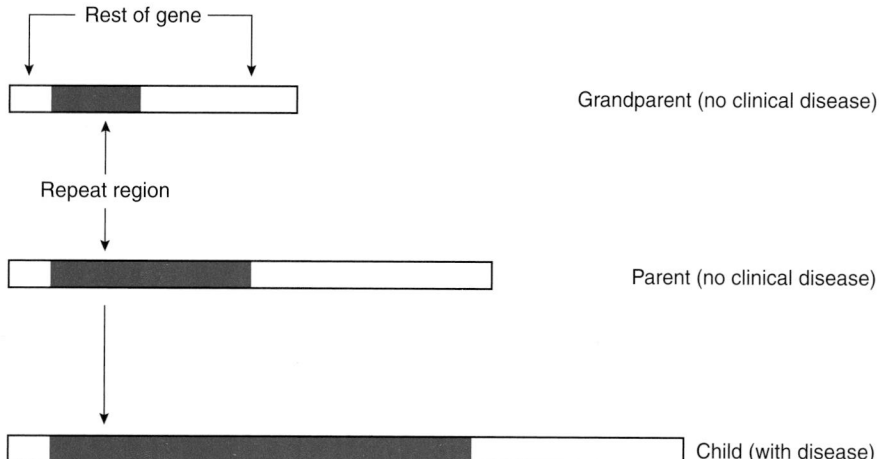

Fig. 4. A diagrammatic representation of an unstable trinucleotide DNA repair. This shows how the region becomes larger in successive generations, causing disease when it reaches a threshold length.

plays a role in cartilage and in the eye. Affected individuals, therefore, have abnormalities of the growth plates, articular cartilage, and eyes. Currently, the area of developmental genes is one of intense research. Developmental biologists are making substantial progress in understanding the sequence of gene expression in normal development. Abnormalities in these pathways lead to a variety of musculoskeletal disorders.

Some disorders are caused by a large chromosomal abnormality (e.g., trisomy 21, causing Down's syndrome). Others are due to the environmental effect on DNA replication in the embryo and fetus (e.g., fetal alcohol syndrome), and in many cases we do not yet know the underlying responsible gene. For the remainder of this chapter, disorders caused by structural genes are discussed. The next chapter deals with disorders caused by genes important in developmental regulation, genes encoding for enzymes, chromosome abnormalities, and genes that are not yet identified. Many genetic disorders are covered in separate chapters in this text, such as many of the neuromuscular disorders.

STRUCTURAL GENES

Four representative disorders that are caused by mutations in structural genes are now discussed.

OSTEOGENESIS IMPERFECTA

- Osteogenesis imperfecta (OI) is the most common inherited disorder causing increased fracture susceptibility in children.
- It is associated with a wide variation in severity.
- Treatments depend on severity of disease. Biphosphonate therapy and intramedullary fixation are used in the more severe cases.

DEFINITION AND EPIDEMIOLOGY

OI is characterized by osteopenic bones that fracture with minimal trauma. The disease varies greatly in the severity of bone involvement and in the occurrence of other findings, such as blue sclera, deafness, ligamentous laxity, and cardiovascular defects. Silence classified the disorder into four types based on clinical findings and inheritance pattern (Table 1); however, patients do not always fall neatly into these four categories. Other investigators classify patients by severity, commonly dividing patients into more and less severely affected categories, termed congenita and tarda. The more severe type, congenita, presents with fractures early in life, whereas the less severe type, tarda, does not present with fractures until children are several years old. The disorder is estimated to occur in about 20 individuals per 100,000 population.

PATHOGENESIS

OI is caused by a gene defect in type I collagen. Most types are inherited in an autosomal-dominant manner, but other modes of inheritance can occur. There are a variety of defects that cause a variable clinical picture ranging from milder forms, in which the collagen structure is normal but there is a decreased amount of collagen, to more severe forms, in which there is a mutation causing a structural abnormality in collagen. The structural defect in collagen interferes with the ability of bone to act like a fiber-reinforced material, allowing the bone to deform more with smaller loads applied and to fracture with a smaller than normal force. Thus, although OI is often called a "brittle"

TABLE 1. SILLENCE CLASSIFICATION OF OSTEOGENESIS IMPERFECTA				
Type	Inheritance	Biochemistry	Severity	Sclera
I	Autosomal dominant	Half normal amount type I collagen	Mild	Blue
II	Autosomal dominant	Mutation in type I collagen	Usually fatal	Blue
III	Autosomal recessive	Mutation in type I collagen	Severe	Blue
IV	Autosomal dominant	Mutation resulting in short pro-α-I chains	Mild	Normal

bone disease, its biomechanical behavior is actually more like "taffy" than like a true brittle material such as glass.[4, 5]

INVESTIGATION

The cardinal feature of OI is fractures occurring with less trauma than would be expected. However, a variety of other features are associated with the collagen abnormality or occur because of the bone weakness. Blue sclera occurs in some individuals; however, the specificity of this finding is low, because many normal newborns also have blue sclera.[6] Hearing loss can occur either from a conductive or a sensorineural cause.[7] Dental involvement may be present, and its presence is used to subclassify the Sillence types. Some individuals have thin skin, cardiac abnormalities (mild valvular disease), hernias, or hyperextensible joints.[8] The fragile bones lead to bowing of the limbs, short stature, scoliosis, and kyphosis.

Radiographs show different degrees of abnormality depending on the severity of involvement. Mild cases show only osteopenia. Bones may be thin and gracile. However, in the more severe cases, they are deformed with a thin cortex and have radiographic evidence of multiple fractures (Fig. 5). A displaced fracture of the apophysis of the olecranon suggests this diagnosis.[9]

DIFFERENTIAL DIAGNOSIS

The most severe forms present soon after birth and are easy to diagnose based on clinical and radiographic findings. Cases that are inherited in an autosomal-dominant

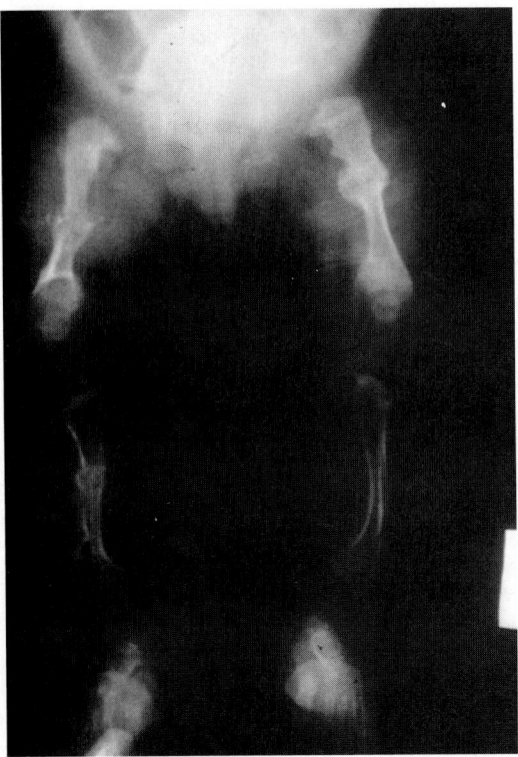

Fig. 5. Radiographic appearance of severe OI. Bones are osteopenic with a thin cortex. There are multiple fractures, resulting in bowing of the bones.

manner are also easy to diagnose based on the family history. However, in the remainder of cases, one needs to consider a metabolic, dietary, or drug-induced cause; idiopathic juvenile osteoporosis; and child abuse. Often the metabolic causes of osteopenia and fracture susceptibility will show some abnormality of the growth plate on radiographs to aid in the diagnosis. The history will aid in diagnosing a dietary or drug cause. Idiopathic juvenile osteoporosis is a diagnosis of exclusion but usually presents in a slightly older child (8 to 14 years) than does OI. It can be hard to distinguish child abuse from a mild form of OI. Looking for nonorthopaedic manifestations of child abuse or OI may help. The fracture pattern alone will not help in this differential diagnosis. Rarely, a child with OI will also be abused. This is a difficult diagnostic situation. When in doubt, it is best to contact the child abuse services involved with the case to help with the diagnosis.[10, 11]

MANAGEMENT

Traditional orthopaedic management focuses on treating fractures and straightening deformed bones. Because the bones are already osteopenic, it is best to avoid prolonged immobilization. However, one still needs to treat fractures appropriately or nonunion will result.[12] At some centers special orthotic devices such as vacuum pants are used to try and mobilize these individuals.[13, 14] When the bones frequently fracture and cause deformity interfering with function, intramedullary fixation is often used. Multiple osteotomies are necessary to straighten the bone for this fixation.[14] The initial recommendations for removing deformed segments of bone from the periosteal sleeve, performing multiple longitudinal osteotomies of the removed segment, and then replacing the segments onto an intramuscular (IM) device in "shish kebob" manner have been abandoned in favor of in situ osteotomies in most centers (Fig. 6). Sometimes these can be performed percutaneously.[15] The IM devices can be an expanding or nonexpanding type. The expanding devices have the advantage of "growing" with the child and may not need to be replaced as often but have a higher hardware failure rate. Comparative series have not shown a clear advantage of one type of device over another. Spinal deformity can occur from the osteopenic bones.[16] The presence of six biconcave-shaped vertebra predicts the occurrence of progressive scoliosis. Bracing is ineffective.[17] Spinal instrumentation and fusion can stabilize the deformity in the less severe types of OI; however, in more severe cases the bone is not strong enough to hold instrumentation, and the fusion mass deforms, making surgical treatment results unpredictable.[18, 19] Basilar invagination is an uncommon but potentially fatal deformity that can be treated with posterior fossa decompression and occipitocervical fusion. However, like surgical treatment for scoliosis, the results of occipitocervical fusion are also unpredictable in severe types of OI.[20, 21] Individuals can experience painful arthritis in adulthood, and this can be treated with total joint replacement.[22]

Previous attempts to increase bone mass in these patients failed. However, series using intravenous pamidronate show promising results for improving bone density.[23] Well-designed trials to determine whether this treatment im-

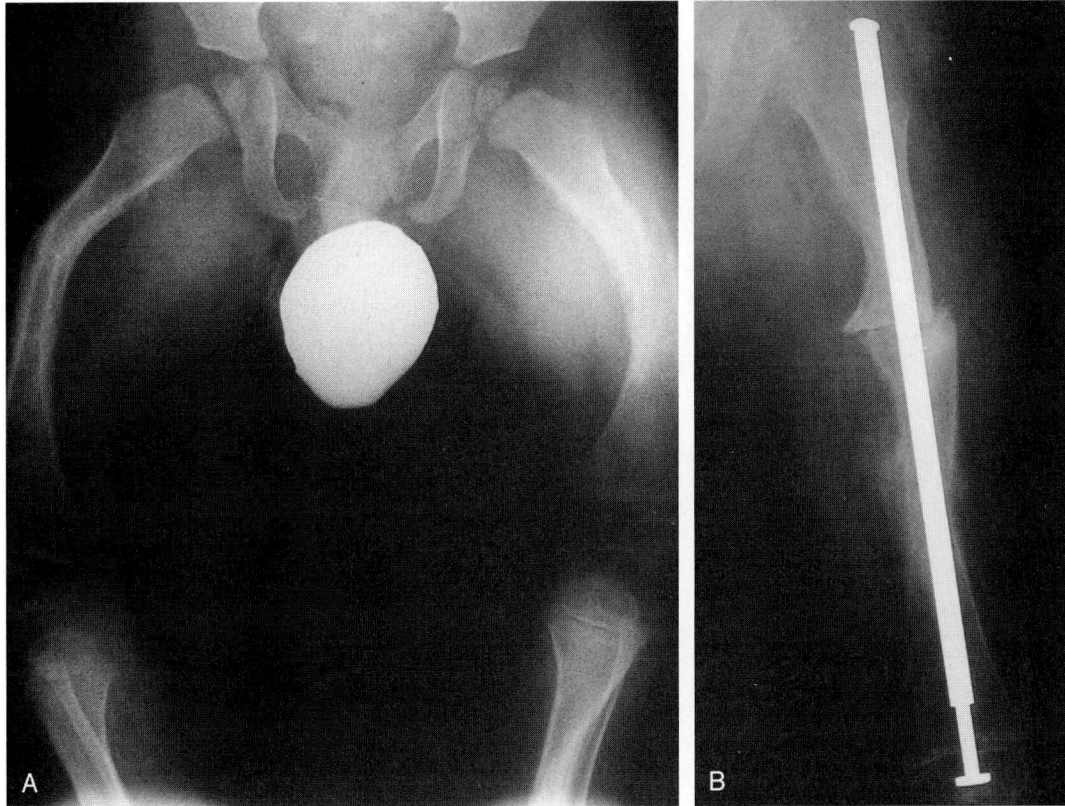

Fig. 6. Views. *(A)* A bowed femur treated with multiple osteotomies and *(B)* placement of an elongating IM rod in a patient with osteogenesis imperfecta.

proves the children's function, decreases fracture incidence, or interferes with growth are still needed, but this therapy is probably warranted in the more severe cases. Study of the use of an oral biphosphonate would also be helpful.

COMPLICATIONS

With age the fracture incidence decreases in these children.[24] Whether this is due to increased bone strength resulting from maturity or to the individuals becoming more careful is unclear. Nonunion from inadequate fracture treatment needs to be managed with appropriate therapy. Some reports suggested that OI predisposes to osteosarcoma,[25] although this has not been substantiated. Although hyperthermia with anesthesia has been reported, patients with OI are probably not at increased risk for true malignant hyperthermia.[26]

SPONDYLOEPIPHYSEAL AND MULTIPLE EPIPHYSEAL DYSPLASIA

- These are skeletal dysplasias that result in short stature, early arthritis, and, in some cases, spinal deformity.
- They are associated with a wide variation in severity.
- Treatments are individualized and include osteotomies, total joint replacement, and spinal surgery.
- Cervical instability may occur.

SPONDYLOEPIPHYSEAL DYSPLASIA
Definition and Pathogenesis

Spondyloepiphyseal dysplasia is a short-trunk dwarfism with abnormalities of the physes and spine. The term is used for a variety of disorders that can broadly be classified into congenita and tarda.[27] The congenital forms present at birth are caused by mutations in type II collagen and are inherited in an autosomal-dominant manner.[28] The tarda form is milder; most patients experience manifestations by about 4 years of age, although some symptoms do not present until adolescence. The tarda form is an X-linked condition due to a mutation in the SELDIN gene, although the cellular mechanism by which this causes the disease is unknown.[29]

Investigation

Affected individuals have short limbs and trunk. The congenita forms are associated with coxa vara, valgus alignment at the knees, scoliosis, kyphosis, and increased lumbar lordosis (Fig. 7). The hands are normal. Severe myopia, retinal detachments, and sensorineural hearing loss can be present. The skeletal deformities may give affected individuals a waddling gait pattern with increased lumbar lordosis and a protuberant abdomen. The tarda form presents with hip pain or stiffness (generally in the second decade of life), flattened vertebrae (platyspondylisis), and, in many cases, scoliosis.

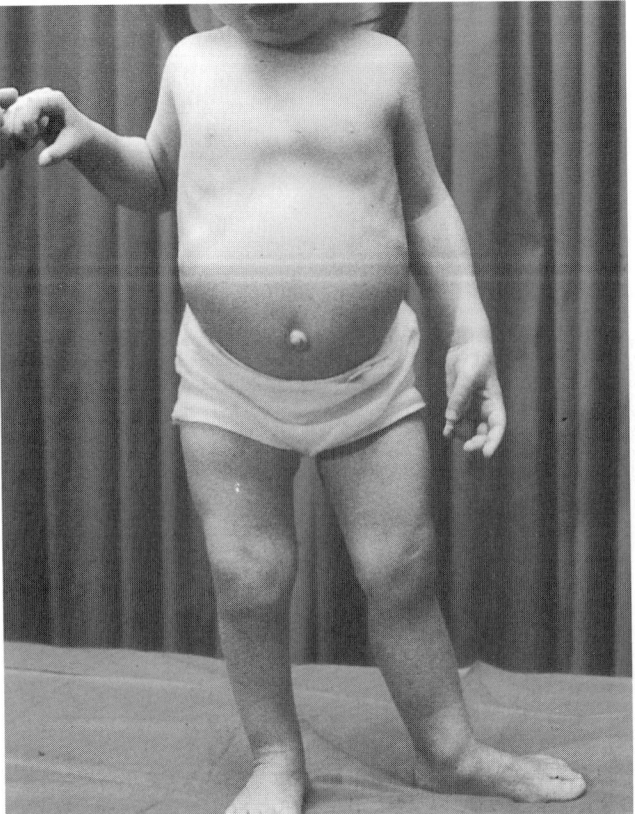

Fig. 7. Typical appearance of an individual with spondyloepiphyseal dysplasia.

The vertebrae are flattened (platyspondylisis), and there is failure or delay of ossification of the proximal femoral epiphysis, os pubis, distal femoral epiphysis, talus, and calcaneus. The hips show coxa vara (Fig. 8). In the tarda form, the involvement is less severe. The hips show radiographic changes similar to Perthes' disease, and the spine shows platyspondyly.[27, 30]

Differential Diagnosis

A variety of other skeletal dysplasias can have a similar appearance clinically, including multiple epiphyseal dysplasia and pseudoachondroplasia. However, the constellation of clinical and radiographic findings usually gives the correct diagnosis.

Management

Odontoid hypoplasia (Fig. 9) can predispose to upper cervical instability and can cause myelopathy.[31] This should be evaluated with flexion extension views of the cervical spine before the patient undergoes anesthesia. More severely involved individuals are at higher risk for cervical instability. Lower extremity malalignment may be treated with osteotomies. The delay in proximal femoral ossification should not be mistaken for dislocation of the hips.[32] Pain resulting from degeneration of the articular cartilage of the hips can be treated with osteotomies but may well require total joint replacement. Depending on the degree of deformity, a custom prosthesis may be necessary.[33] Scoliosis and kyphosis are treated using the usual treatment principles for these spinal deformities.

Complications

Because the disorder is related to a structural abnormality in type II collagen, deformity can recur after osteotomies in skeletally immature individuals, and osteotomies to change joint loading for pain may not do as well as in other conditions.[34] Although most individuals with lower extremity deformity will not require surgery, if it is contemplated, it is probably best to realign the entire lower extremity rather than concentrate on a single joint.[35]

MULTIPLE EPIPHYSEAL DYSPLASIA
Definition

This disorder causes short stature and premature arthritis as a result of a defect in the epiphyses of bones. There is some similarity in presentation to the tarda form of spondyloepiphyseal dysplasia, but there is minimal spinal involvement, if any. There is variability in severity of the

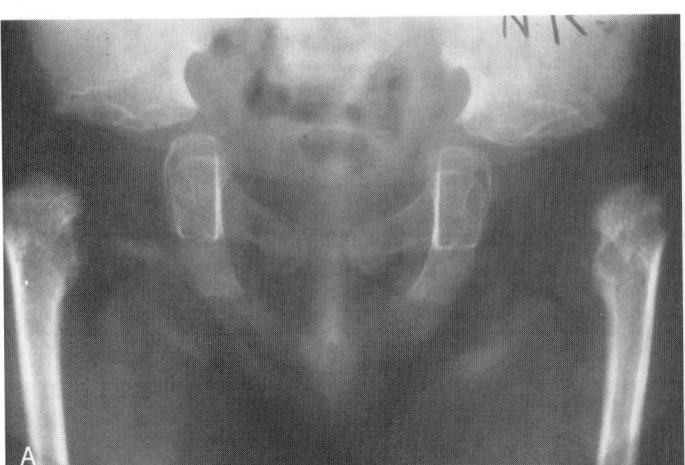
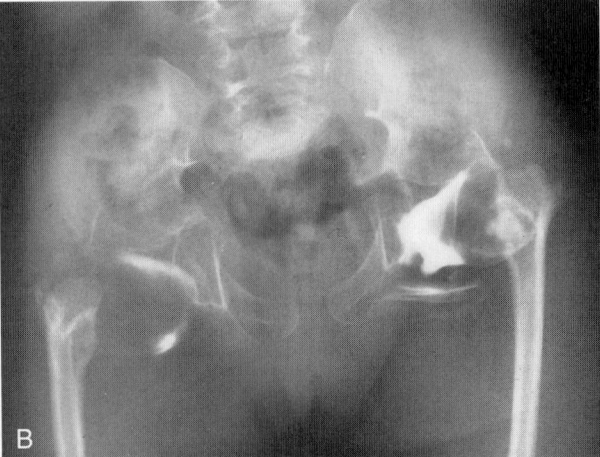

Fig. 8. Pelvic radiograph (*A* and *B*). This is from an individual with spondyloepiphyseal dysplasia. Although it appears that the femoral heads are absent, arthrograms reveal their presence and severe varus alignment.

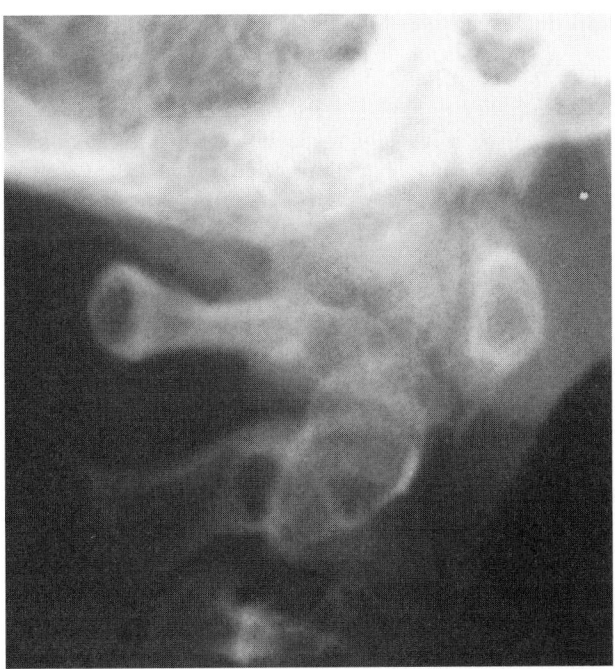

Fig. 9. Odontoid hypoplasia in a patient with spondyloepiphyseal dysplasia.

disorder, and there can also be variability of severity within a single family.[36] Multiple epiphyseal dysplasia may be caused by a mutation in cartilage oligomeric protein[37] (whose function in cartilage is not yet completely understood) or by a mutation in type IX collagen.[38] Interestingly, mutations in these genes are also responsible for pseudoachondroplasia.

Pathogenesis

Although the precise mechanism by which the mutations cause this disorder is not yet known, chondrocytes are known to contain cytoplasmic inclusion bodies in which there is a large quantity of proteoglycans. This results in abnormal growth plate function, leading to short stature, and abnormal articular cartilage function, leading to early degenerative arthritis. Occasionally, there is avascular ne-

crosis of an epiphysis, most commonly at the proximal femur.[39] It is inherited in an autosomal-dominant manner.

Investigation and Differential Diagnosis

The hips are often most severely involved, and the proximal femoral epiphyses are late in appearance, irregular in shape, and fragmented (Fig. 10). This appearance is quite similar to that seen in Legg-Perthes disease, although here multiple sites are involved, which all have a similar radiographic appearance. The hips do not go through the changes in radiographic appearance with time, typical of the stages of Legg-Perthes disease.[36, 39–41]

Management

Most patients present with hip symptoms. More severe involvement early in life predicts a worse outcome.[36] In younger patients (younger than 8 years), containment of the femoral head within the acetabulum is advocated, although femoral osteotomy is usually not performed because of underlying coxa vara. There are no comparative studies that show an advantage to containment.[39] Older patients may have hinge abduction or incongruity of the lateral portion of the femoral head, which may be improved by osteotomy of the proximal femur. Knee deformity may be treated with osteotomy, although malalignment in younger individuals may recur with growth.[35] Osteochondritis dissecans can occur and is treated using the usual treatment principles.[42] Because there is an intrinsic abnormality of the articular cartilage, osteotomies are at best temporizing procedures, and many individuals ultimately undergo total joint arthroplasty. Involvement of other joints, such as the shoulder, can occur. Treatment for these is individualized and may require total joint replacement in adulthood.[43]

MARFAN'S SYNDROME

- This is a disorder of connective tissue resulting in a tall, thin body habitus with lax joints and scoliosis.
- Patients have variable skeletal involvement; scoliosis is common. Cardiovascular abnormalities need appropriate therapy.
- Scoliosis does not respond as well to brace treatment as in idiopathic scoliosis. Meningoceles may be present.

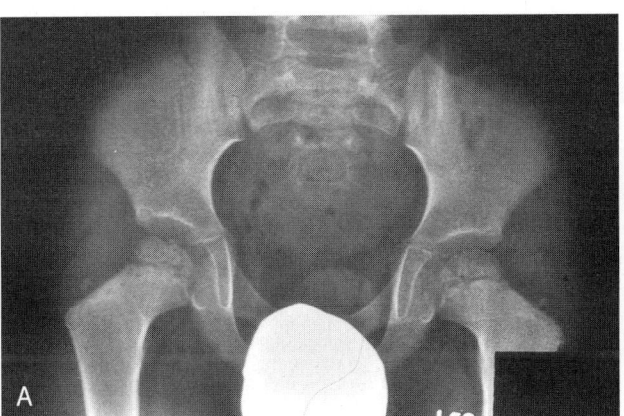
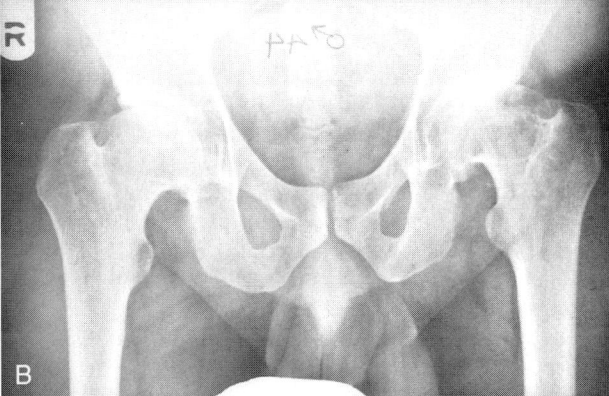

Fig. 10. Typical radiographic appearance of hips in multiple epiphyseal dysplasia.

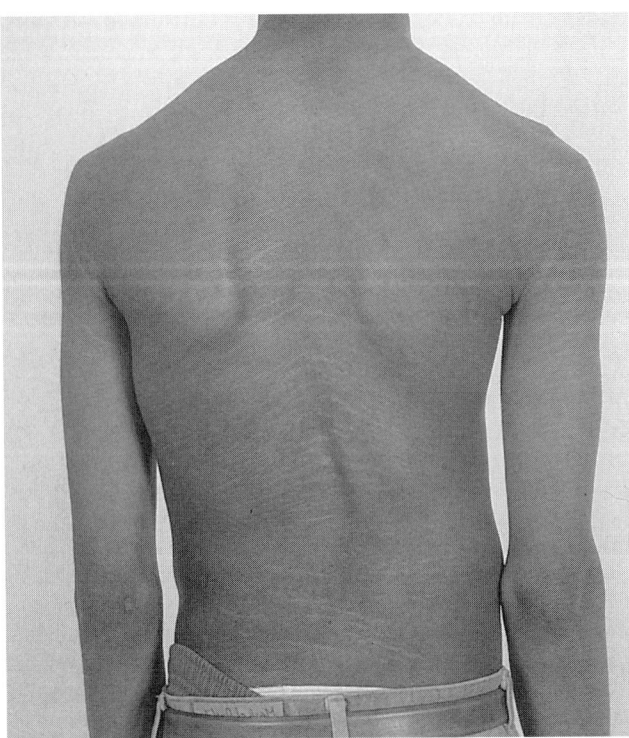

Fig. 11. Physical appearance of the back of a patient with Marfan's syndrome. Note the scoliosis and striae in the skin.

DEFINITION

Marfan's syndrome is a disorder characterized by tall stature with long limbs and digits. It is caused by a mutation in the fibrillin gene.

PATHOGENESIS

The fibrillin gene plays a structural role in the connective tissues, and the defects in patients with Marfan's syndrome lead to abnormalities in the skeletal, cardiovascular, and ocular systems. The cardiovascular anomalies may be life threatening. It is inherited in an autosomal-dominant manner, although about one-fourth of cases are thought to be due to new mutations. The fibrillin gene is located on two chromosomes, 5 and 15. Interestingly, the gene on the 15th chromosome gives Marfan's syndrome, whereas the gene on the 5th chromosome gives contractual arachnodactyly.[44–46]

DIAGNOSTIC FEATURES

Patients have a tall and thin body habitus, may have ectopia lentis, or other eye abnormalities, have crowded teeth, and exhibit a variety of cardiovascular problems (including aortic root dilatation, aortic or mitral regurgitation, and congestive heart failure).[47] There can be scoliosis and possibly spinal arachnoid cysts, joints are lax, digits are long (arachnodactyly), and striae are present on the skin (Fig. 11). Occasionally, there are painful hips as a result of protrusio acetabuli.[48]

Radiographs show a widened lumbosacral canal (often demonstrated only with a computed tomography scan) and an increased length-width ratio of the metacarpals (a ratio averaging digits two through four greater than 8.8 in males and 9.4 in females is abnormal).

DIFFERENTIAL DIAGNOSIS

The diagnosis is usually made based on clinical findings, including involvement of the skeleton, and at least on extraskeletal manifestation (ectopia lentis, aortic dilatation or dissection, or dural ectasia). The use of "span greater than height" to make the diagnosis does not work well, because at least one-half of normal adult males have an arm span greater than their height.

MANAGEMENT

Progressive scoliosis requires operative intervention. Bracing does not work as well as in idiopathic scoliosis and should be reserved for curves less than 40 degrees.[49] Surgery in children younger than 5 years has a worse result with a high complication rate, and operative intervention should be delayed beyond this age if possible.[50] Meningoceles may be present (particularly in the anterior sacral region) and can be treated with surgical patching of the communication from the dural sac.[51, 52] Protrusio acetabuli occurs in some individuals (Fig. 12). Surgery to arrest the triradiate cartilage is reported to arrest the protrusio.[48]

COMPLICATIONS

Cardiac complications are the main cause of mortality. The use of β-blockers and surgery to reconstruct the cardiovascular dilatation significantly extends life expectancy.[53, 54] One should always evaluate an affected individual's cardiac function before contemplating operative intervention.

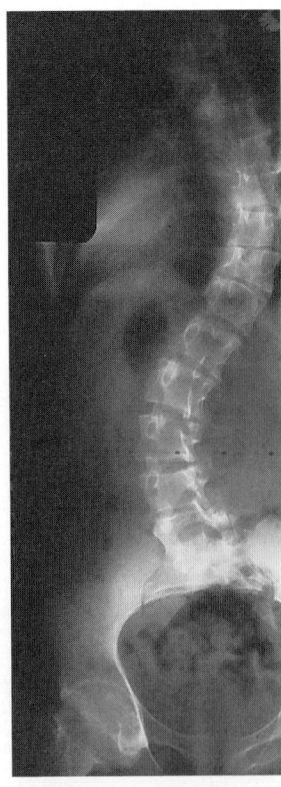

Fig. 12. Spine radiographs. This is from a patient with Marfan's syndrome, showing scoliosis and protrusio acetabula.

REFERENCES

1. Jaffurs D, Evans CH: The human genome project: Implications for the treatment of musculoskeletal disease. J Am Acad Orthop Surg 1998; 6:1.

2. Nichollo RD, Saitok S, Horsthemke B: Imprinting in Prader-Willi and Angelman syndromes. Trends Genet 1998; 14:194.

3. Shapiro LR: The fragile X syndrome. A peculiar pattern of inheritance. N Engl J Med 1991; 325:1736.

4. Cole WG: Etiology and pathogenesis of heritable connective tissue diseases. J Pediatr Orthop 1993; 13(3):392.

5. Alman B, Frasca P: Fracture failure mechanisms in patients with osteogenesis imperfecta. J Orthop Res 1987; 5(1):139.

6. Sillence D, Butler B, Latham M, et al: Natural history of blue sclerae in osteogenesis imperfecta. Am J Med Genet 1993; 45(2):183.

7. Stewart EJ, O'Reilly BF: A clinical and audiological investigation of osteogenesis imperfecta. Clin Otolaryngol 1989; 14(6):509.

8. Vetter U, Maierhofer B, Muller M, et al: Osteogenesis imperfecta in childhood: Cardiac and renal manifestations. Eur J Pediatr 1989; 149(3):184.

9. Stott NS, Zionts LE: Displaced fractures of the apophysis of the olecranon in children who have osteogenesis imperfecta. J Bone Joint Surg Am 1993; 75(7):1026.

10. Augarten A, Laufer J, Szeinberg A, et al: Child abuse, osteogenesis imperfecta and the grey zone between them. J Med 1993; 24:171.

11. Dent JA, Paterson CR: Fractures in early childhood: Osteogenesis imperfecta or child abuse? J Pediatr Orthop 1991; 11(2):184.

12. Gamble JG, Rinsky LA, Strudwick J, et al: Non-union of fractures in children who have osteogenesis imperfecta. J Bone Joint Surg Am 1988; 70(3):439.

13. Letts M, Monson R, Weber K: The prevention of recurrent fractures of the lower extremities in severe osteogenesis imperfecta using vacuum pants: A preliminary report in four patients. J Pediatr Orthop 1988; 8(4):454.

14. Wilkinson JM, Scott BW, Clarke AM, et al: Surgical stabilisation of the lower limb in osteogenesis imperfecta using the Sheffield telescopic intramedullary rod system. J Bone Joint Surg Br 1998; 80(6):999.

15. McHale KA, Tenuta JJ, Tosi LL, et al: Percutaneous intramedullary fixation of long bone deformity in severe osteogenesis imperfecta. Clin Orthop 1994; 305:242.

16. Porat S, Heller E, Seidman DS, et al: Functional results of operation in osteogenesis imperfecta: Elongating and nonelongating rods. J Pediatr Orthop 1991; 11(2):200.

17. Ishikawa S, Kumar SJ, Takahashi HE, et al: Vertebral body shape as a predictor of spinal deformity in osteogenesis imperfecta. J Bone Joint Surg Am 1996; 78(2):212.

18. Hanscom DA, Winter RB, Lutter L, et al: Osteogenesis imperfecta. Radiographic classification, natural history, and treatment of spinal deformities. J Bone Joint Surg Am 1992; 74(4):598.

19. Engelbert RH, Gerver WJ, Breslau-Siderius LJ, et al: Spinal complications in osteogenesis imperfecta: 47 patients 1–16 years of age. Acta Orthop Scand 1998; 69(3):283.

20. McAllion SJ, Paterson CR: Causes of death in osteogenesis imperfecta. J Clin Pathol 19XX; 49(8):627.

21. Sawin PD, Menezes AH: Basilar invagination in osteogenesis imperfecta and related osteochondrodysplasias: Medical and surgical management. J Neurosurg 1997; 86(6):950.

22. Papagelopoulos PJ, Morrey BF: Hip and knee replacement in osteogenesis imperfecta. J Bone Joint Surg Am 1993; 75(4):572.

23. Glorieux FH, Bishop NJ, Plotkin H, et al: Cyclic administration of pamidronate in children with severe osteogenesis imperfecta. N Engl J Med 1998; 339(14):947.

24. Daly K, Wisbeach A, Sanpera I Jr, et al: The prognosis for walking in osteogenesis imperfecta. J Bone Joint Surg Br 1996; 78(3):477.

25. Gagliardi JA, Evans EM, Chandnani VP, et al: Osteogenesis imperfecta complicated by osteosarcoma. Skeletal Radiol 1995; 24(4):308.

26. Porsborg P, Astrup G, Bendixen D, et al: Osteogenesis imperfecta and malignant hyperthermia. Is there a relationship? Anaesthesia 1996; 51(9):863.

27. Spranger JW, Langer LO Jr: Spondyloepiphyseal dysplasia congenita. Radiology 1970; 94(2):313.

28. Lee B, Vissing H, Ramirez F, et al: Identification of the molecular defect in a family with spondyloepiphyseal dysplasia. Science 1989; 244(4907):978.

29. MacKenzie JJ, Fitzpatrick J, Babyn P, et al: X linked spondyloepiphyseal dysplasia: A clinical, radiological, and molecular study of a large kindred. J Med Genet 1996; 33(10):823.

30. MacDermot KD, Roth SC, Hall C, et al: Epiphyseal dysplasia of the femoral head, mild vertebral abnormality, myopia, and sensorineural deafness: Report of a pedigree with autosomal dominant inheritance. J Med Genet 1987; 24(10):602.

31. Nakamura K, Miyoshi K, Haga N, et al: Risk factors of myelopathy at the atlantoaxial level in spondyloepiphyseal dysplasia congenita. Arch Orthop Trauma Surg 1998; 117(8):468.

32. Crossan JF, Wynne-Davies R, Fulford GE: Bilateral failure of the capital femoral epiphysis: Bilateral Perthes disease, multiple epiphyseal dysplasia, pseudoachondroplasia, and spondyloepiphyseal dysplasia congenita and tarda. J Pediatr Orthop 1983; 3(3):297.

33. Huo MH, Salvati EA, Lieberman JR, et al: Custom-designed femoral prostheses in total hip arthroplasty done with cement for severe dysplasia of the hip. J Bone Joint Surg Am 1993; 75(10):1497.

34. Stanescu R, Stanescu V, Bordat C, et al: Pathologic features of the femoral heads in a patient aged 14½ years with spondyloepiphyseal dysplasia with osteoarthritis. J Rheumatol 1987; 14(5):1061.

35. Ferrone JD Jr: Congenital deformities about the knee. Orthop Clin North Am 1976; 7(2):323.

36. Treble NJ, Jensen FO, Bankier A, et al: Development of the hip in multiple epiphyseal dysplasia. Natural history and susceptibility to premature osteoarthritis. J Bone Joint Surg Br 1990; 72(6):1061.

37. Briggs MD, Hoffman SM, King LM, et al: Pseudoachondroplasia and multiple epiphyseal dysplasia due to mutations in the cartilage oligomeric matrix protein gene. Nat Genet 1995; 10(3):330.

38. Muragaki Y, Mariman EC, van Beersum SE, et al: A mutation in the gene encoding the alpha 2 chain of the fibril-associated collagen IX, COL9A2, causes multiple epiphyseal dysplasia (EDM2). Nat Genet 1996; 12(1):103.

39. Mackenzie WG, Bassett GS, Mandell GA, et al: Avascular necrosis of the hip in multiple epiphyseal dysplasia. J Pediatr Orthop 1989; 9(6):666.

40. Mandell GA, MacKenzie WG, Scott CI Jr, et al: Identification of avascular necrosis in the dysplastic proximal femoral epiphysis. Skeletal Radiol 1989; 18(4):273.

41. Andersen PE Jr, Schantz K, Bollerslev J, et al: Bilateral femoral head dysplasia and osteochondritis. Multiple epiphyseal dysplasia tarda, spondylo-epiphyseal dysplasia tarda, and bilateral Legg-Perthes disease. Acta Radiol 1988; 29(6):705.

42. Versteylen RJ, Zwemmer A, Lorie CA, et al: Multiple epiphyseal dysplasia complicated by severe osteochondritis dissecans of the knee. Incidence in two families. Skeletal Radiol 1988; 17(6):407.

43. Ingram RR: The shoulder in multiple epiphyseal dysplasia. J Bone Joint Surg Br 1991; 73(2):277.

44. Tsipouras P, Del Mastro R, Sarfarazi M, et al: Genetic linkage of the Marfan syndrome, ectopia lentis, and congenital contractural arachnodactyly to the fibrillin genes on chromosomes 15 and 5. The International Marfan Syndrome Collaborative Study. N Engl J Med 1992; 326(14):905.

45. Francke U, Furthmayr H: Marfan's syndrome and other disorders of fibrillin. N Engl J Med 1994; 330(19):1384.

46. Ramirez F: Fibrillin mutations in Marfan syndrome and related phenotypes. Curr Opin Genet Dev 1996; 6(3):309.

47. Dervanian P, Mace L, Folliguet TA, et al: Surgical treatment of aortic root aneurysm related to Marfan syndrome in early childhood. Pediatr Cardiol 1998; 19(4):369.

48. Steel HH: Protrusio acetabuli: Its occurrence in the completely expressed Marfan syndrome and its musculoskeletal component and a procedure to arrest the course of protrusion in the growing pelvis. J Pediatr Orthop 1996; 16(6):704.

49. Joseph KN, Kane HA, Milner RS, et al: Orthopedic aspects of the Marfan phenotype. Clin Orthop 1992; 277:251.

50. Sponseller PD, Sethi N, Cameron DE, et al: Infantile scoliosis in Marfan syndrome. Spine 1997; 22(5):509.
51. Raftopoulos C, Delecluse F, Braude P, et al: Anterior sacral meningocele and Marfan syndrome: A review. Acta Chir Belg 1993; 93(1):1.
52. Smith MD: Large sacral dural defect in Marfan syndrome. A case report. J Bone Joint Surg Am 1993; 75(7):1067.
53. Salim MA, Alpert BS, Ward JC, et al: Effect of beta-adrenergic blockade on aortic root rate of dilation in the Marfan syndrome. Am J Cardiol 1994; 74(6):629.
54. Gray JR, Bridges AB, West RR, et al: Life expectancy in British Marfan syndrome populations. Clin Genet 1998; 54(2):124.

section 9 chapter 5

GENETICS II: GENETIC SYNDROMES WITH ORTHOPAEDIC MANIFESTATIONS

Keith R. Gabriel

Summary
- Autosomal dominant is the most common pattern of inheritance among these conditions.
- In addition to musculoskeletal manifestations, other organ systems are almost always involved.
- Orthopaedic intervention is usually, but not always, indicated for treatment of these conditions.
- A multidisciplinary approach will usually optimize diagnosis and treatment.

ACHONDROPLASIA

- Achondroplasia is the most common form of short-limb disproportionate dwarfism.
- Inheritance is autosomal dominant; genetic defect is on chromosome 4.
- Abnormalities at the foramen magnum and occipitocervical region may lead to death in infancy.
- Thoracolumbar kyphosis generally resolves spontaneously; spinal stenosis may require surgical intervention.
- Limb lengthening and growth hormone treatment remain controversial.

DEFINITION

Achondroplasia, the most common form of dwarfism, is recognizable by the rhizomelic, disproportionate shortening and unique facial features.

HISTORICAL REVIEW

The term "achondroplasia," first used by Parrot[1] in 1878, is technically incorrect because cartilage formation is not truly absent. The responsible gene was localized in 1994.[2]

EPIDEMIOLOGY

The incidence rate of achondroplasia is on the order of 1 in 20,000 to 1 in 50,000 live births. The inheritance is autosomal dominant with essentially complete penetrance. New mutations are responsible for 80% to 87% of cases. There is an increased incidence rate of achondroplasia associated with increased paternal age. Germ-line mosaicism (spermatogonial mutation) may account for occasional affected children from normal parents. Homozygous forms present with extremely severe and often lethal manifestations.

Achondroplasia results from missense mutations at residue 380 of 4p16.3, the gene for fibroblast growth factor receptor 3 (FGFR3).[2] The resulting deficiency of endochondral bone formation suggests a gene-dosage effect. Histopathological studies show shortening of epiphyseal and physeal cartilage plates, more pronounced in homozygous than in heterozygous patients. Biopsy information regarding cellular organization of the physis is conflicting, but immunostaining reveals a normal distribution of major matrix constituents.[3] Appositional growth areas and periosteal bone growth appear normal. Regional differences, which produce the rhizomelic pattern of shortening, remain unexplained.

CLINICAL FEATURES

Many features of the achondroplastic phenotype are explained by the mismatch of normal periosteal and appositional bone growth in the presence of slowed endochondral ossification. Normal development of the surrounding soft-tissue envelope contributes to the appearance.

Individuals are recognizable even at birth by the enlarged neurocranium with frontal bossing, flattening of the nasal bridge, midface hypoplasia, and prominence of the mandible. True megalencephaly occurs, with disproportion between the base of the skull and the brain. Most patients have an arrested hydrocephalus, which does not require shunting. Underdevelopment of the midface occasionally leads to dental malocclusion, and otitis media is frequent.[4] The foramen magnum is small throughout life.

Intelligence is normal; however, motor milestones are frequently delayed by 3 to 6 months.[5] These delays have generally been attributed to mechanical issues such as the ligamentous laxity and disproportionate stature, but neurological factors must also be considered.

The abdomen is protuberant, and the lower ribs flare outward. The trunk is of nearly normal length, but with narrow circumference and flattening of the anteroposterior dimension. Respiratory difficulties may be due to the narrow chest wall diameter, but upper airway obstruction and brain-stem compression at the level of the foramen magnum may also be contributing factors.[6]

Most affected infants will have an angular kyphosis centered at the thoracolumbar junction, which resolves spontaneously with walking ambulation. An increased lumbar lor-

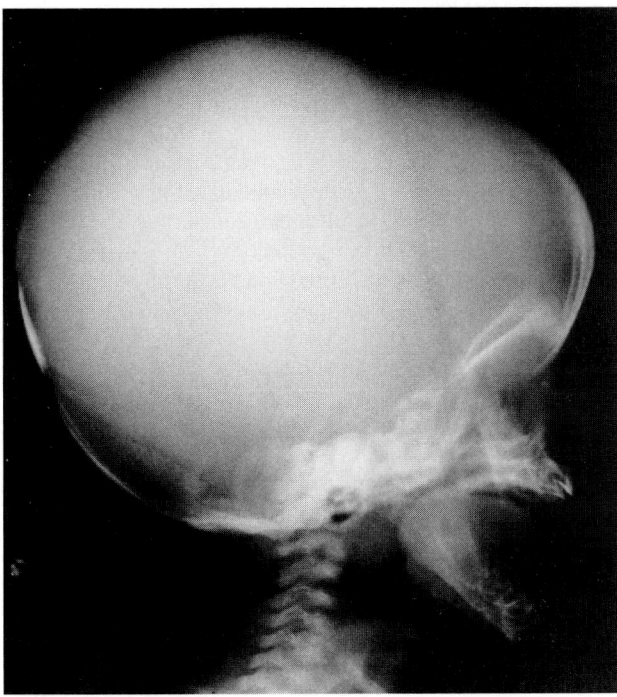

Fig. 1. Achondroplasia. This is a lateral skull radiograph of an affected infant. Typical findings include the enlarged calvarium and midface hypoplasia.

Normal development of the membranous portion of the clavicle leads to a broad-shouldered appearance. Abnormalities of the elbow joint include a moderate loss of extension and frequent dislocation of the radial head. The hands are short and broad. The middle finger is especially short, so that all the digits are approximately of the same length ("starfish hand"). With attempted approximation of the fingers in extension, a persistent space is seen between the long and ring fingers ("trident hand").

INVESTIGATION

Radiographs show characteristic abnormalities, even in infancy. Findings on the lateral skull film include midface hypoplasia, an enlarged calvarium with frontal prominence, and shortening of the base of the skull (Fig. 1). The small, funnel-shaped foramen magnum is best demonstrated by computed tomography (CT).

The anteroposteror (AP) spine radiograph demonstrates progressive narrowing of the interpedicular distances in the lumbar spine. Shortened pedicles and short vertebral bodies with mild posterior scalloping are seen on the lateral spine film. Before walking age, variable degrees of thoracolumbar kyphosis are expected, with anterior wedging of T-12 or L-1 (Fig. 2). Beyond walking age, the kyphosis generally resolves, and the lateral spinal radiograph will show an exaggerated lumbar lordosis with horizontal sacrum.

The pelvis appears short and broad in the AP radiograph (Fig. 3). Appositional and intramembranous growth of the

dosis then develops, accompanied by hip flexion contracture. Some degree of kyphosis with wedging of the apical vertebra persists in about 15% of cases.

Developmental spinal stenosis, especially in the lumbar segments, is extremely common.[4] Anatomic factors include narrowing of the interpedicular distance, thickening of the laminae and inferior facets, and shortening and thickening of the pedicles. The onset of symptoms is generally in the third decade but may be even in early childhood. Patients having persistent thoracolumbar kyphosis seem to have a higher incidence rate of symptomatic stenosis.

Some degree of scoliosis, including true kyphoscoliosis, is common in achondroplasia. The curves tend to be mild and not progressive.

Hip flexion contracture is nearly universal and is intimately related to anterior pelvic tilt and increased lumbar lordosis. As appositional cartilage growth continues normally, some overgrowth of the greater trochanter is expected. Epiphyseal deformity and articular cartilage abnormalities are not features of achondroplasia. Developmental dysplasia of the hip, coxa vara, and premature osteoarthritis of the hip are distinctly uncommon.

Moderate genu recurvatum is common in infancy. Angular deformities of the lower extremity, most often tibial bowing with genu varum and lesser degrees of ankle varus, develop in at least half of patients after walking age.[4] Normal appositional growth produces a relative overgrowth of the fibula, but whether this actually accounts for the genu varum remains unproven. Other mechanical factors, such as ligament laxity and obesity, may also contribute. An occasional patient will experience genu valgum, despite the relative overgrowth of the fibula.

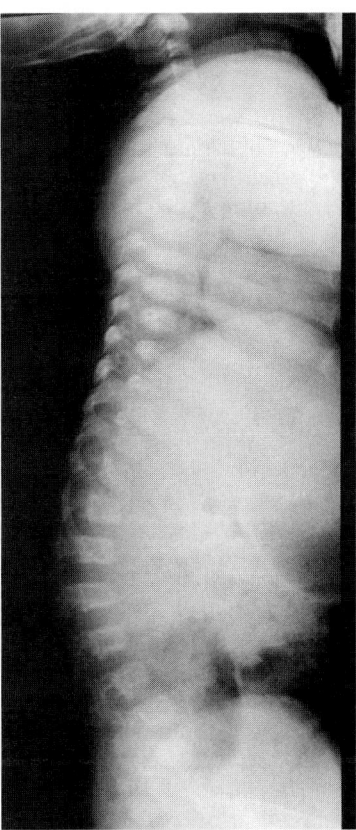

Fig. 2. Achondroplasia. This is a lateral radiograph of the spine of an affected infant. Thoracolumbar kyphosis is evident.

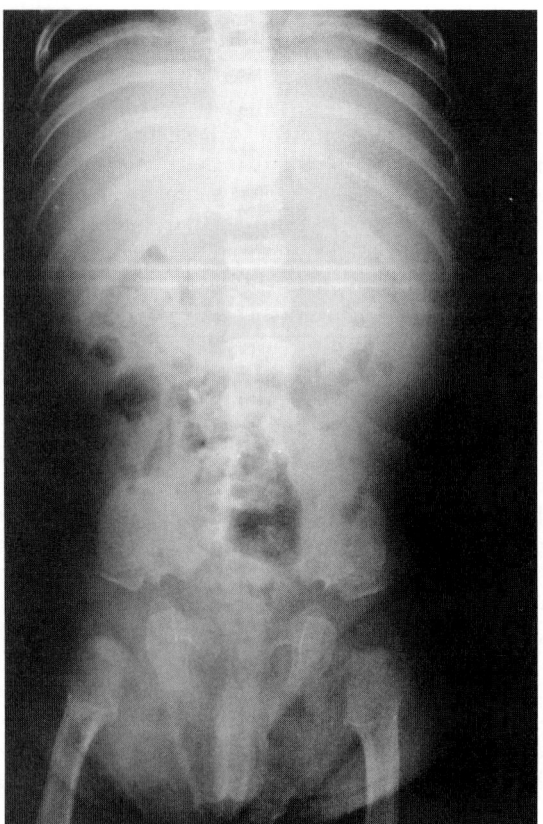

Fig. 3. Achondroplasia. This is an anteroposterior radiograph of the lumbar spine and pelvis of an affected infant. There is narrowing of the interpedicular distance distally in the lumbar spine. The "champagne glass" appearance of the pelvis is obvious.

ilia are unaffected, but there is poor growth at the base. The sacrosciatic notch is short. The acetabular roof is horizontal. The width of the pelvic inlet exceeds its depth, producing the "champagne glass" appearance.

Because of normal periosteal bone growth, the diaphyseal shaft diameter of the long bones is normal or somewhat enlarged. Bowing may occur, and sites of muscle attachment produce marked cortical thickening. During infancy, there may be areas of oval radiolucency in the proximal metaphyses of the femur and humerus. Metaphyseal flaring is seen, and the growth plates have a central V- or U-shaped depression (Fig. 4). The epiphyses are typically normal.

DIFFERENTIAL DIAGNOSIS

The diagnosis of achondroplasia is usually straightforward, based on the typical physical appearance and the characteristic radiographic findings of the skull, spine, and pelvis. At birth, there may be initial confusion with conditions such as severe osteogenesis imperfecta or achondrogenesis. In childhood, other possibilities include rickets, cretinism, and the mucopolysaccharidoses. The differentiation from severe hypochondroplasia, an allelic variant, may be arbitrary. Screening of at-risk pregnancies for homozygous achondroplastic fetuses is possible.[2]

MANAGEMENT

Large head size, structural abnormalities at the base of the skull and brain, and generalized hypotonia place affected infants at risk for neck extension injuries.[7] Parents should be cautioned about the need to support the infant's head during handling and positioning. Careful neurological examinations are especially important. Baseline magnetic resonance imaging (MRI) and somatosensory evoked potentials should be considered.

Initial management of thoracolumbar kyphosis in infants is simple observation. Early prohibition of unsupported upright sitting and selected extension bracing may help prevent persistent kyphosis after independent walking.[8] Surgical stabilization, including anterior and posterior fusion, is recommended for patients who do have marked continued kyphosis. If neurological symptoms are present, anterior decompression and fusion, combined with posterior fusion, should be considered. Posterior laminectomy is contraindicated. Because of small canal size, any form of posterior instrumentation extending into the canal is hazardous.

Nonoperative treatment for symptoms of the developmental spinal stenosis has had only mixed results. Adequate surgical treatment includes wide multilevel decompressive laminectomy, extending proximally three levels cephalad to the compression seen on myelogram or MRI and distally to the second sacral level. Less extensive de-

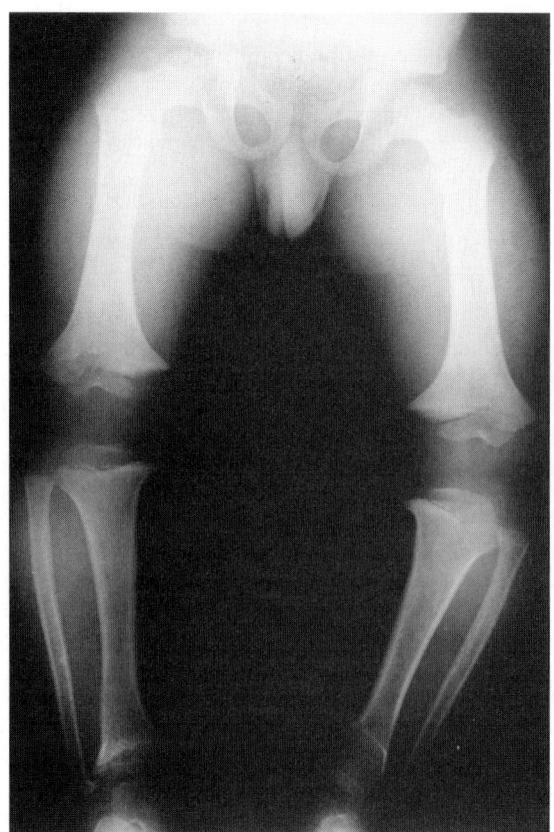

Fig. 4. Achondroplasia. This is an anteroposterior radiograph of the lower extremities of a 5-year-old boy. Genu varum with relative fibular overgrowth is evident. The metaphyses are flared, and the epiphyses are located within V-shaped depressions.

compression leads to the development of symptoms from compression adjacent to the level of surgery. Unless there is preexisting kyphosis, instability after even these extensive laminectomies is unusual; however, if instability does result, an anterior spinal fusion may be necessary. The transverse processes in achondroplasia are relatively small, so that the posterior fusion can be problematic. Primary treatment for scoliosis is seldom indicated.

Brace treatment is not effective in controlling genu varum. The joint surfaces of the knee are generally well preserved, and prophylactic realignment osteotomy is unnecessary. Those patients who have progressive knee laxity and pain may require osteotomy. Upper extremity anomalies rarely require treatment.

Surgical lengthening of the upper and lower extremities is technically feasible.[9] Recommended techniques and sequences for lengthening are quite variable. Advocacy groups such as the Little People of America and the Dwarf Athletic Association of America have been generally opposed to the lengthening performed only to increase stature.

Growth hormone therapy remains controversial. There is no evidence that affected individuals are actually growth hormone deficient, and the contribution of hormone administration to ultimate height is still under study.[10]

RESULTS/COMPLICATIONS

Standardized growth curves are available for patients with achondroplasia. Because trunk length is preserved, the sitting height of affected adults is normal. However, average standing height is below the third percentile. Expected adult standing height is 132 cm for males and 125 cm for females. Weight control is a lifelong concern for these individuals.[11]

Affected individuals have reduced reproductive fitness. The excess risk of death in achondroplastic infants is approximately 7.5% largely because of abnormalities at the craniocervical junction. Mortality rates are increased for all age groups; central nervous system and respiratory abnormalities are the predominant causes through childhood and early adult life.

HYPOCHONDROPLASIA

- This disorder encompasses a spectrum of dwarfism, from mild shortening to an appearance indistinguishable from achondroplasia.
- Inheritance is autosomal dominant.
- Hypochondroplasia and achondroplasia are allelic.
- Skeletal abnormalities are generally mild; surgery is infrequent.

DEFINITION

Hypochondroplasia is a variable form of short-limbed dwarfism. There is no characteristic facial appearance.

HISTORICAL REVIEW

Ravenna recognized this disorder and coined the term "hypochondroplasia" in 1913.[12] A description in the English language was provided in 1969 by Beals.[13] The genetic defect responsible for the majority of cases was defined in 1995.[14]

EPIDEMIOLOGY

The incidence and prevalence of hypochondroplasia are unknown. Transmission is autosomal dominant, and most cases represent new sporadic mutations. The majority of cases are due to a transversion at nucleotide 1620 of the gene for FGFR3.[14] This is the same gene locus (4p16.3) responsible for achondroplasia, but the mutation is different; hence, the disorders are allelic. Some patients, particularly those with milder forms, do not have this precise mutation.[15]

CLINICAL FEATURES

The facial appearance is generally normal, except perhaps for some mild frontal bossing. Trident hand and early thoracolumbar kyphosis are not features of hypochondroplasia.

Diminished height is recognized by early childhood. Trunk height is preserved; the shortening is primarily in the limbs. The pattern is not generally rhizomelic; rather, the shortening is distributed more proportionately in the segments of each limb. Mild joint laxity is common, but severe genu varum is unusual. Lumbar lordosis is less pronounced, and scoliosis is less frequent compared with achondroplasia. Symptomatic spinal stenosis eventually develops in about one-third of patients; however, neurological deficits are not common.[16]

INVESTIGATION

Radiograph findings are variable, according to the severity of each individual case. In general, the appearances are similar to those of achondroplasia but much less pronounced. Primary and secondary diagnostic criteria[17] are indicated in the accompanying table (Table 1).

DIFFERENTIAL DIAGNOSIS

There is wide variation in the severity of hypochondroplasia, and many mild cases are presumably unrecognized. More severe forms of hypochondroplasia are difficult to distinguish from mild forms of achondroplasia.

MANAGEMENT

Most of the skeletal manifestations of hypochondroplasia are mild, and orthopaedic treatment is usually not required.

TABLE 1. DIAGNOSTIC CRITERIA FOR HYPOCHONDROPLASIA	
Primary Criteria	**Secondary Criteria**
Narrowed lumbar interpedicular distance	Shortening of lumbar pedicles
Short, square iliac crests	Concavity of posterior vertebral bodies
Short, broad femoral necks	Elongation of distal fibula
Mild metaphyseal flaring	Shortening of distal ulna
Shortening of long tubular bones	Elongation of the ulnar styloid
Mild brachydactyly	

Occasionally, corrective osteotomy of the tibia may be indicated for symptomatic genu varum. Symptoms of spinal stenosis may be managed nonoperatively unless there are signs of neurological deficit.

RESULTS/COMPLICATIONS

Adult height in hypochondroplasia is between 127 cm and 152 cm. About 10% of patients will have mild mental retardation. Disabling symptoms are unusual, and life expectancy is normal.

DIASTROPHIC DYSPLASIA (DIASTROPHIC DWARFISM)

- This disorder is characterized by extreme short-limb dwarfism.
- The genetic defect maps to chromosome 5; there are several allelic disorders.
- Peculiar deformities include hitchhiker thumbs, cauliflower ears, and clubfeet.
- Severe spinal deformities and joint contractures develop in most patients.

DEFINITION

This is a rare dysplasia, characterized by extreme short-limb dwarfism and the almost universal combination of thumb, ear, and foot deformities.

HISTORICAL REVIEW

"Diastrophic" is based on a geologic term for bending and twisting of the earth's crust. Lamy and Maroteaux described the syndrome in 1960.[18] The responsible genetic defect was mapped to 5q32-q33.1 in 1996.[19]

EPIDEMIOLOGY

The syndrome is transmitted as an autosomal-recessive trait. The gene (5q32-q33.1) encodes a novel sulfate transporter, impaired function of which leads to undersulfation of proteoglycans in cartilage matrix.[20] Atypical features of affected cartilage include decreased numbers of chondrocytes, fibrotic foci, and abnormally large collagen fibrils in the intercellular matrix. There are several allelic variants of this dysplasia.[21]

CLINICAL FEATURES

Diastrophic dysplasia is recognizable at birth. Although the cranium is normocephalic, the face is long with a square jaw, narrow nasal bridge, and flared nostrils. Cleft palate is very common. Swelling of the pinnae of the ears develops by about 3 weeks of age and remains for several weeks. As the swelling resolves, the cartilage calcifies, and the pinnae deform into the typical cauliflower ear shape. Hearing remains normal. Patients have a characteristic soft, hoarse voice.

Abnormalities of the hands and feet are nearly universal and assist in establishing the diagnosis. The hands are broad and short. The characteristic hitchhiker thumb consists of disproportionate shortening of the first metacarpal, with thumb abduction and hypermobility. Rigid, resistant bilateral equinovarus foot deformities are expected. The deformity is centered in the midfoot, without the subtalar displacement seen in idiopathic clubfoot.

Shortening of the extremity is exacerbated by severe flexion contractures. Accentuated lumbar lordosis develops secondarily and becomes fixed. Symptoms of lumbar spinal stenosis are unusual. Severe, progressive spinal deformities include scoliosis and cervical kyphosis. Cervical kyphosis develops during the first 2 years of life and frequently progresses to cause myelopathy.

INVESTIGATION

Radiographs of the skull show the overlying calcifications of the pinnae. Occasionally, there are also intracranial calcifications.

Cervical kyphosis is centered in the mid-segments. The apical vertebrae are typically hypoplastic and wedged, and spina bifida occulta is seen in the mid- to lower cervical segments. Atlantoaxial instability is unusual, but flexion and extension lateral radiographs are necessary to evaluate for instability at the apex of the kyphosis. Flexion and extension MRI studies may be needed to assess the cord itself.

The ribs are short, with premature ossification of the costal cartilages. Severe and progressive kyphosis, scoliosis, or kyphoscoliosis of the thoracic or lumbar spine occurs in more than 80% of patients.[22] Although radiographs may show narrowing of the interpedicular distance in the distal lumbar spine, symptomatic spinal stenosis is unusual.

Radiographs of the pelvis show mild flaring of the iliac wings, accompanied by an unusual notch above the acetabulum. Femoral head ossification is delayed, with a central depression or unossified area. The resulting broad, flattened femoral head is poorly contained by the acetabulum, and hip dislocation or premature osteoarthritis is frequent.[23]

Radiographs of the long bones show rhizomelic shortening and metaphyseal flaring. Ossification of the epiphyses is delayed, and the eventual epiphyseal contours are irregular and flattened. The ulna and fibula are disproportionately short (Figs. 5 and 6). Genu valgum is common at the knee, but a corresponding valgus deformity of the ankles is rare. The wrist is deviated toward the ulna. The metacarpals are especially short, and the thumb metacarpophalangeal joint may be subluxed or dislocated in association with the hitchhiker deformity.

DIFFERENTIAL DIAGNOSIS

Multiple contractures and joint deformities sometimes lead to confusion with arthrogryposis syndromes. However, the hand and foot deformities of diastrophic dysplasia are relatively specific.

MANAGEMENT

Stable cervical kyphosis without neurological compromise may be observed. Posterior cervical fusion is recommended for instability or progression of the deformity when there are no neurological deficits. If there is any neurological compromise, anterior decompression and fusion should be combined with posterior fusion.

Deformities of the thoracolumbar spine have the dysplastic characteristics of rigidity, sharp angulation, and marked rotation. Many of these deformities will progress despite bracing, and surgical management may be indicated even in the very young patient. For patients who have not completed their spinal growth and when kyphosis is greater

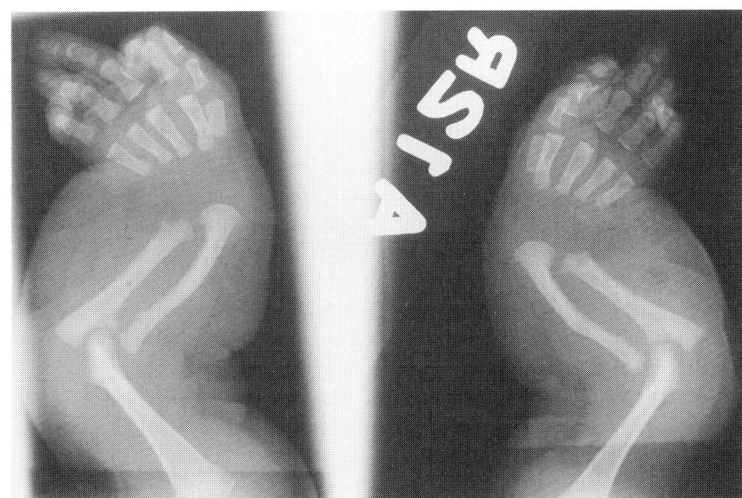

Fig. 5. Diastrophic dysplasia. These are radiographs of the upper extremities of an affected infant. Disproportionate shortening of the ulna, with ulnar deviation of the wrists, is evident even at birth.

than 50 degrees, anterior fusion combined with posterior fusion should be considered. Attempted correction of large kyphoscoliotic deformities with posterior instrumentation has been associated with neurological compromise. Fusion in situ should be strongly considered.

The equinovarus foot deformities tend to be rigid and do not respond to manipulation and casting. Complete correction is seldom achieved with standard soft-tissue surgery, and primary talectomy is often the best option.

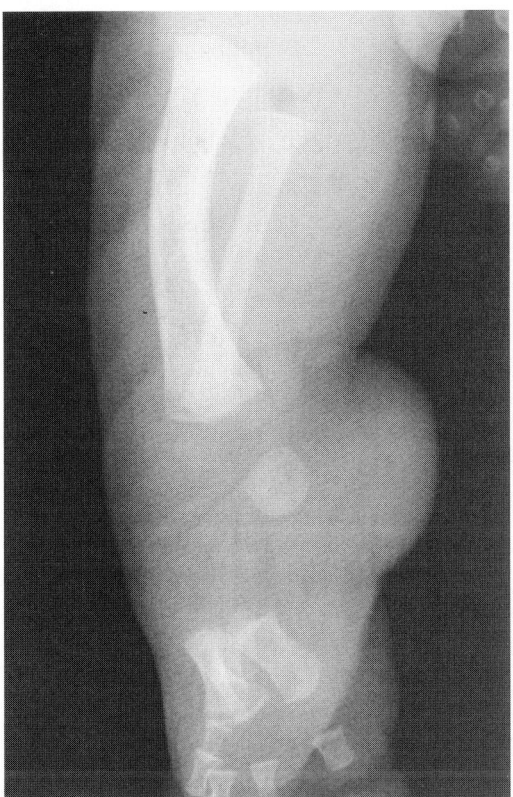

Fig. 6. Diastrophic dysplasia. This is a lateral radiograph of the leg and foot of an affected infant. This film suggests the severe, rigid foot deformity even though most of the midfoot and hindfoot structures remain unossified.

Conventional treatment for progressive hip dysplasia in these patients is hindered by concomitant knee flexion contractures and genu valgum. Attention should be directed toward maintaining functional range of motion of the lower extremity joints. Limitations are due to both extra-articular contractures and primary intra-articular deformity. Soft-tissue releases alone are frequently inadequate, and repositioning osteotomies may be needed. Total joint arthroplasty may be the best alternative for adult patients with premature osteoarthritis.

RESULTS/COMPLICATIONS

Some affected infants die of respiratory insufficiency, compounded by cleft palate with feeding abnormalities and possible aspiration. However, most patients have a normal life span. Intelligence is normal.

PRADER-WILLI AND ANGELMAN'S SYNDROMES

- These syndromes illustrate genetic imprinting; both result from absence of an identical part of chromosome 15.
- Prader-Willi syndrome results when the father's contribution is absent; Angelman's syndrome results when the mother's contribution is absent.
- Early-onset scoliosis is common in Prader-Willi syndrome; surgical stabilization is often indicated.
- Scoliosis occurs later in Angelman's syndrome.

DEFINITION

Prader-Willi and Angelman's syndromes have radically different phenotypes, although the genetic defect is similar. Prader-Willi syndrome includes hyperphagia, hypomentation, hypotonia, hypogonadism, and small hands. Angelman's syndrome includes small stature, severe mental retardation, seizures, athetosis, and characteristic facial features.

HISTORICAL REVIEW

The original report by Prader et al[24] in 1956 described the full clinical expression of the Prader-Willi syndrome.

Angelman reported three "puppet children" in 1965.[25] Subsequent authors objected to the possibly derisive label and supported the use of the eponym Angelman's syndrome.

EPIDEMIOLOGY

The incidence of Prader-Willi syndrome is on the order of 1 in 5000 live births, with a population prevalence of 1 in 20,000. The frequency of Angelman's syndrome is less well defined. Absence of a critical portion of chromosome 15, the 15q11.2-q13 segment, is responsible for the development of both syndromes.[26] If for any reason the child does not receive the male copy of 15q11.2-q13, Prader-Willi syndrome will result. This can occur if the father contributes a defective chromosome or if the father's chromosome is totally lacking and there are two copies of the maternal chromosome (uniparental maternal disomy). Deletions cause nearly 80% of Prader-Willi syndrome cases. If a defective chromosome is donated by the mother or if the father contributes both copies of chromosome 15 (uniparental paternal disomy), the child will have Angelman's syndrome.

CLINICAL FEATURES

Infants who have Prader-Willi syndrome begin life with hypotonia, a peculiar cry, poor feeding, cryptorchidism, and delayed milestones. The hypotonia is so characteristic that some authors recommend genetic testing for Prader-Willi syndrome based on that finding alone.[27] A recognizable facial appearance, which classically includes a narrow bifrontal diameter, strabismus, and upward-slanting, almond-shaped eyes, develops over the first 2 years (Fig. 7A). An insatiable appetite becomes apparent at about that same time, and central obesity develops. The feet and hands are disproportionately small, with somewhat delicate, tapering fingers. Patients have short stature, generally below the 10th percentile. There is no adolescent growth spurt. Many patients have relative hypopigmentation compared with their parents. Mental retardation is of variable severity.

A majority of Prader-Willi syndrome patients, 50% to 90%, will experience severe and progressive early-onset scoliosis. Lower extremity malalignments, especially genu valgum and pes planus, are common but seldom symptomatic.

The characteristic facies in Angelman's syndrome includes a large mandible and an open-mouthed expression. Patients have a great facility for protruding the tongue, which is large. Most have a happy disposition and are given to outbursts of excessive laughter. These patients have difficulty walking and usually have a jerky, ataxic, "puppet-like" gait. They are small. Mental retardation, absence of speech, hypotonia, and seizures are typical findings.

Patients with the Angelman's syndrome experience scoliosis in adolescence and adulthood.[28]

INVESTIGATION

The scoliosis of Prader-Willi syndrome is difficult to detect clinically because of truncal obesity (Fig. 7B). A high index of suspicion must be maintained, and periodic radiographs of the spine may be necessary.

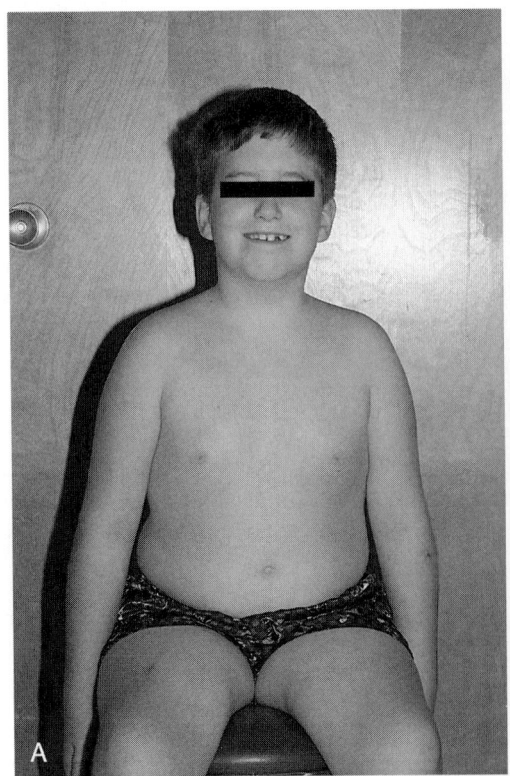
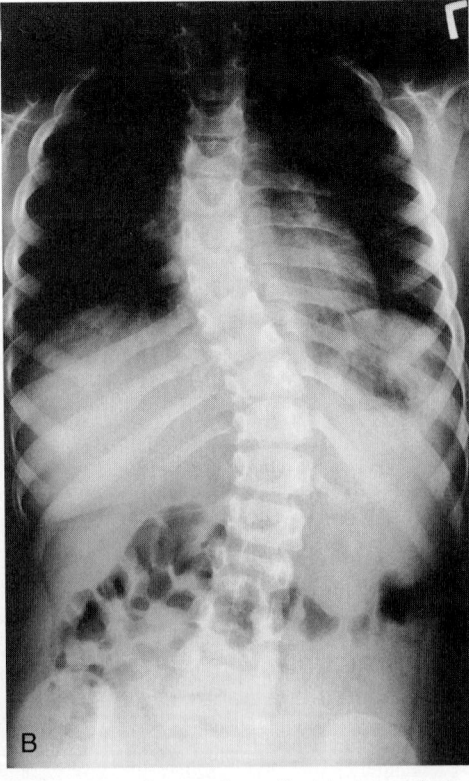

Fig. 7. Prader-Willi syndrome. *A,* Typical appearance of an affected boy. *B,* Even at age 6 years, the patient had a scoliosis of greater than 30 degrees. Despite the pelvic obliquity seen on this radiograph, lower extremity lengths were actually equal.

DIFFERENTIAL DIAGNOSIS

Prader-Willi syndrome is frequently diagnosed in early childhood, when the hyperphagia is manifested. Angelman's syndrome may be confused with cerebral palsy and, in females, Rett's syndrome.

MANAGEMENT

Current medical management of Prader-Willi syndrome frequently includes administration of growth hormone. Weight control through complex behavioral modification programs may be effective, but straightforward attempts at food restriction often result in intolerable psychological disturbance and outbursts of angry, defiant behavior.

Scoliosis in these patients is difficult to control by bracing because of obesity. Many patients require surgical spinal stabilization.[29] Lower extremity malalignments in the Prader-Willi syndrome seldom require treatment.

RESULTS/COMPLICATIONS

Historically, most patients with Prader-Willi syndrome did not live beyond the third decade because of complications of obesity. With optimal weight control, survival is improved. Any possible effect of growth hormone administration on longevity remains investigational. Patients with Angelman's syndrome have a normal life span.[26, 28]

BECKWITH-WIEDEMANN SYNDROME

- Several modes of inheritance have been documented for this syndrome.
- The gene abnormality is duplication of a specific band in chromosome 11.
- Omphalocele is common, as is severe hypoglycemia in the neonate.
- Orthopaedic features suggest a combination of spastic cerebral palsy and hemihypertrophy.
- Patients require repeated routine screening for Wilms' tumor.

DEFINITION

Infants with Beckwith-Wiedemann syndrome present with the triad of exomphalos (omphalocele or other umbilical abnormalities), macroglossia, and gigantism, which led to it being earlier known as EMG syndrome.

HISTORICAL REVIEW

The syndrome was first suggested by Wiedemann in 1964[30] and described in English by Beckwith in 1969.[31] An association with chromosome 11 was established in 1983.[32]

EPIDEMIOLOGY

The incidence of Beckwith-Wiedemann syndrome is 1 in 14,000. The inheritance pattern is anomalous, probably a result of at least partial imprinting.[33] The syndrome is associated with duplication of the p15.5 band of chromosome 11, the gene for insulin-like growth factor type I. This locus is near the Wilms' tumor gene (11p13), which may account in part for the high association with that and other tumors.

CLINICAL FEATURES

Tongue size is excessively large at birth and tends to regress with growth. Unusual linear indentations of the ear lobe are one of the diagnostic features, and posterior helical ear pits have also been described.

Omphalocele or other umbilical abnormalities are common. Visceromegaly is an important feature. In the pancreas, this is primarily due to islet cell hyperplasia. Neonatal hypoglycemia and seizures, resulting from overproduction of insulin in the first few days of life, have been implicated in the subsequent development of cerebral palsy. However, the spasticity seen most frequently is hemiplegia, which is not totally consistent with that cause.

Infants with this syndrome are large, usually in the 97th percentile by age 1 year. Children reach an average height of 2.5 standard deviations above the mean at or shortly after puberty.

From an orthopaedic standpoint, children with this syndrome seem to have the combination of hemihypertrophy and spastic cerebral palsy. Asymmetric growth affects about 20% of these patients. Scoliosis is common and is usually of an idiopathic pattern. Other less common findings include cavus feet, dislocated radial heads, and polydactyly.

INVESTIGATION

Increased placental size and excessive umbilical cord length, seen on prenatal ultrasonogram, may lead to the suspicion of Beckwith-Wiedemann syndrome even before birth.

These patients are at increased risk for tumor development, especially Wilms' tumor in those who have hemihypertrophy.[34] Periodic renal ultrasonographic screening is indicated at least through age 6 years. Investigation of the various orthopaedic manifestations is routine.

DIFFERENTIAL DIAGNOSIS

About 15% of all infants born with omphalocele will be found to have Beckwith-Wiedemann syndrome, and the syndrome should be considered in all infants born with abdominal defects. Beckwith-Wiedemann syndrome may be suspected in any overly large child with spastic cerebral palsy and is an important part of the differential for any child having hemihypertrophy.

MANAGEMENT

The scoliosis, limb length inequality, and cerebral palsy in these patients is managed according to the usual orthopaedic algorithms.

RESULTS/COMPLICATIONS

Complications in Beckwith-Wiedemann syndrome are primarily related to the initial omphalocele, the severe hypoglycemia, which develops shortly after birth, and the increased frequency of tumors later in childhood.

MULTIPLE HEREDITARY EXOSTOSES

- In this disorder, a similar phenotype may arise from three different genotypes; the abnormality may be on any one of the chromosomes 8, 11, or 19.
- In each case, the inheritance is autosomal dominant.
- Multiple osteochondromas may be located anywhere on the endochondral skeleton.
- Shortening of involved bones is common; problems are

magnified in the two-bone systems of the forearm and leg.
- Late transformation to chondrosarcoma may occur.

DEFINITION

This syndrome is characterized by the occurrence of multiple cartilaginous and bony exostoses, located on any bone formed by endochondral ossification. There is no involvement of any other organ system.

HISTORICAL REVIEW

The condition was described in a series of lectures delivered in 1786 and 1787 by John Hunter.[35] Eponymous credit is sometimes given to Ehrenfried,[36] who published a description of this syndrome in English in 1915. The preferred nomenclature, "hereditary multiple exostoses," was established by Jaffe in 1943.[37] Although many investigators noted the autosomal-dominant transmission of the disorder, it was not until 1993 that the several gene defects began to be defined.

EPIDEMIOLOGY

The condition is inherited as an autosomal-dominant trait with incomplete penetrance. Roughly one-third of cases represent new mutations. An unequal sex ratio with a preponderance of males is reported.

Currently, there are three separate gene loci known to be associated with hereditary multiple exostoses: *EXT1*, on 8q24.11-q24.13; *EXT2*, on 11p12-p11; and *EXT3*, on 19p. Each of these three genes has a tumor-suppressor function, which is lost with mutation at any one of the sites.[38] Multiple allelic variants have been identified.

Although *EXT* proteins are expressed in many tissues, the only known effect is specific to actively growing endochondral bone. Intramembranous bones such as the calvarium are spared. Individually, each mass resembles a solitary osteochondroma, both grossly and microscopically.

There have been proposals to subclassify this disorder. Carroll et al[39] showed relationships between the specific gene types and the predominant form (sessile or pedunculated) and location of the osteochondromas.

Additional genes, *EXTL1*, *EXTL2*, and *EXTL3*, have been identified that show high degrees of sequence homology with the three sites detailed previously. However, these "exostoses-like" genes are not actually associated with the clinical syndrome.

CLINICAL FEATURES

Diagnosis is usually made in childhood, typically between the ages of 2 and 12 years. Most patients present either because of known family involvement or because the parents discover a mass on their child. Subjective complaints are few, although some patients do experience local symptoms at prominent masses. Loss of joint mobility is common. There is shortening of involved bones. Patients are usually shorter than average but not below the normal range.

The two-bone systems of the forearm and leg warrant special considerations. Relative growth discrepancy and the local mass effects of exostoses can create incongruity and deformity at the wrist (Fig. 8) and ankle.

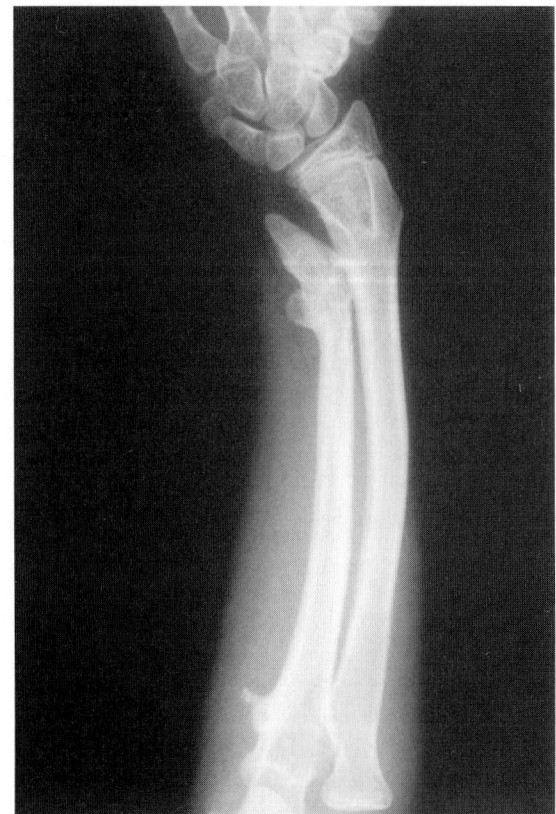

Fig. 8. Multiple hereditary exostoses. This is an anteroposterior radiograph of the forearm of a 12-year-old girl. Shortening of the ulna and resulting wrist deformity are evident.

INVESTIGATION

Radiographs of symptomatic areas or palpable masses are usually sufficient, and a full "skeletal survey" is seldom necessary. The exostoses each share the radiographic features of a solitary osteochondroma: metaphyseal location, directed away from the physis, medullary canal continuous with the subjacent bone, and a cartilage cap with variable calcification.

The appearance of the femoral neck, broad and short with multiple exostoses, is so characteristic as to be nearly diagnostic (Fig. 9). In the pelvis, exostoses may form at apophyseal areas of the ilium or at the ischiopubic synchondrosis. Scapular masses develop at the epiphysis of coracoid and acromion and along the growth areas of the body. Exostoses of the ribs tend to be near the anterior cartilaginous ends.

DIFFERENTIAL DIAGNOSIS

Multiple osteochondromas are one feature of the Langer-Giedion syndrome. Metachondromatosis is a disorder that includes both multiple exostoses and multiple enchondromas. Osteochondromas of the proximal medial tibia are seen in Turner's syndrome and in the very rare fibrodysplasia ossificans progressiva.

MANAGEMENT

The presence of an exostosis is not an indication for its removal. Patients should be advised to have routine, peri-

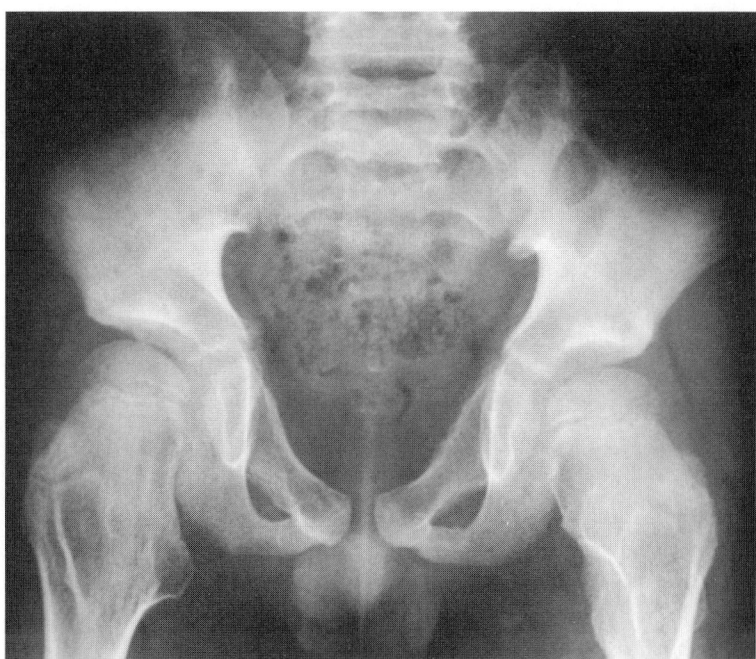

Fig. 9. Multiple hereditary exostoses. This is an antero-posterior radiograph of the pelvis of a 7-year-old boy. The appearance of the proximal femurs is nearly diagnostic.

odic examinations. Radiographs are requested selectively. It is especially important to monitor the wrist and ankle for differential growth or disruption of the joints. "Baseline" and periodic radiographs of the pelvis and spine are important because masses in those areas may be asymptomatic and yet have the greatest risk of undergoing later malignant degeneration.

Symptomatic lesions should be removed, as should those that create progressive deformity with growth. Lesions that continue to grow beyond skeletal maturity should be suspected of secondary chondrosarcoma and should be removed accordingly.

RESULTS/COMPLICATIONS

Life expectancy is normal, as is reproductive ability. Symptoms and disability related to the exostoses are unpredictable because of the wide variation in severity.

Malignant degeneration of the cartilage cap of an exostosis to secondary chondrosarcoma occurs in about 1% of patients.[40] This transformation is exceedingly rare in the pediatric age group and is of concern chiefly after the age of 30 years. Enlargement of an osteochondroma after skeletal maturity or spontaneous resting pain in a lesion is an indication for excisional biopsy.

FAMILIAL DYSAUTONOMIA (RILEY-DAY SYNDROME)

- It has a unique ethnic distribution among Ashkenazic Jews.
- Inheritance is autosomal recessive and maps to gene defect at 9q31-33.
- Nearly all patients experience scoliosis.
- Many orthopaedic aspects are secondary to pain insensitivity.

DEFINITION

The features of the Riley-Day syndrome are autonomic dysfunction and insensitivity to pain.

HISTORICAL REVIEW

The syndrome was first described by Riley et al in 1949.[41] The responsible genetic defect was localized in 1993.[42]

EPIDEMIOLOGY

The disorder is almost completely limited to persons of Ashkenazic Jewish heritage. Within that ethnic group, the incidence is about 1 in 3600 live births, and the gene carrier frequency is 1 in 30 persons. The inheritance is autosomal recessive. The responsible gene locus is 9q31-33. Specific biochemical defects are not yet defined.

CLINICAL FEATURES

Affected infants have poor suck responses and difficulty swallowing, resulting in frequent aspiration pneumonia. The absence of tears is noted even in infancy.

In childhood, manifestations of the dysautonomia include increased perspiration, blotchy skin coloration, wide swings in blood pressure and body temperature, and cyclic episodes of vomiting. Many patients have severe ataxia. Insensitivity to pain and temperature becomes more apparent with growth, and these children frequently sustain unrecognized fractures. Avascular disorders that mimic Perthes' disease at the hip and severe osteochondritis dissecans at the knee are common. These abnormalities may progress to frankly Charcot's syndrome joints. Scoliosis is nearly universal, and kyphosis occurs in about one-half of patients. The onset of spinal deformity is early, and progression is rapid.

In adulthood there is worsening of orthostatic hypotension, supine hypertension, and occasional bradyarrhythmias.

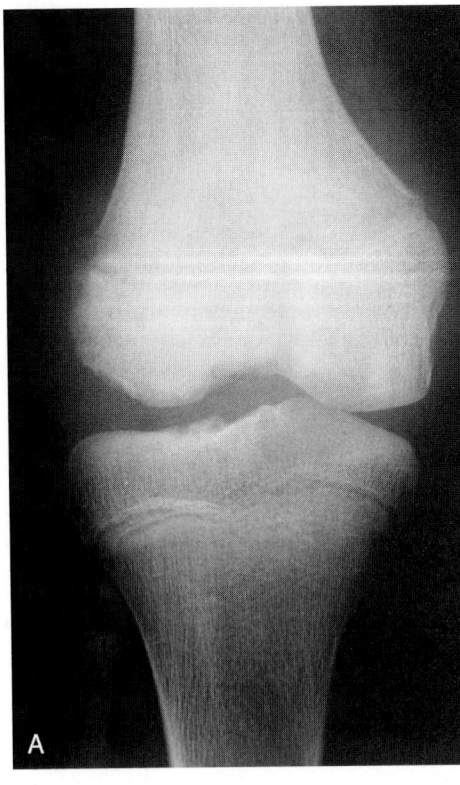 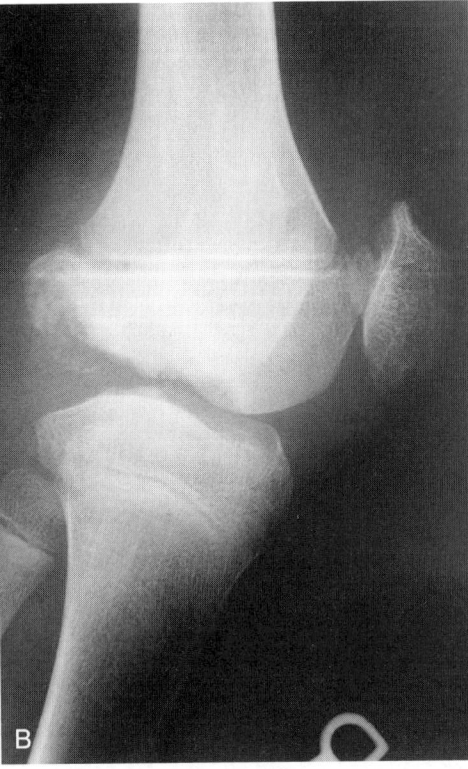

Fig. 10. Familial dysautonomia. Anteroposterior (*A*) and (*B*) lateral radiograph of the knee of a 10-year-old girl with Riley-Day syndrome. These Charcot syndrome–like changes in a patient with normal motor function should raise suspicion of an insensitivity syndrome.

Patients report poor balance, unsteady gait, and difficulty concentrating.[43]

INVESTIGATION

A family history will almost invariably include Ashkenazic Jewish heritage. The clinical diagnosis is based on five observations: diminished tear production, absence of fungiform papillae on the tongue, decreased deep tendon reflexes, miosis of the pupil after conjunctival instillation of methacholine chloride, and lack of an axon flare after intradermal histamine injection. Although individual radiographic findings are not diagnostic for this syndrome, the combination of occult fracture and avascular necrosis of weightbearing joints is highly suggestive (Fig. 10A and B), especially if there is also scoliosis. Diagnosis by genetic linkage studies, including prenatal diagnosis, is possible.[44]

DIFFERENTIAL DIAGNOSIS

The Biemond syndrome of congenital and familial analgesia and congenital sensory neuropathy with anhidrosis must be differentiated from Riley-Day syndrome. Neuropathological findings on sural nerve biopsy may be the best diagnostic criterion to differentiate familial dysautonomia from other forms of congenital sensory neuropathy.[45]

MANAGEMENT

Early gastrostomy and fundoplication may be needed to control vomiting and ensure adequate nutrition. Symptoms of orthostatic hypotension improve with the wearing of elastic stockings. The problem with fracture management is usually that of recognition rather than treatment because the fractures themselves heal well.

Brace management of the scoliosis is not practical for most patients because of cutaneous insensitivity, intolerance to external compression of the abdomen, ineffective body temperature control, and respiratory difficulty. Surgical stabilization is best offered as soon as curve progression is documented. Because patients do not have normal homeostatic responses, anesthesia is problematic. The surgical goal should be expeditious stabilization, not maximum correction.[46]

RESULTS/COMPLICATIONS

The mortality rate in infancy is high because of aspiration pneumonia. The inability of the body to respond to stress or hypoxia contributes to high death rates in childhood and adolescence. Homeostatic instability makes anesthesia hazardous for all age groups. Few patients survive beyond the fourth decade.

DOWN'S SYNDROME

- This disorder results from extra copies of chromosome 21.
- Incidence increases with increasing maternal age.
- Mental retardation is a characteristic feature.
- Ligament laxity and joint hypermobility are problematic.
- Occipitocervical and atlantoaxial instability may require surgical fusion.
- Scoliosis is common.

DEFINITION

Down's syndrome is the most frequent form of mental retardation. Patients are usually recognizable by the characteristic facial appearance and physical features.

HISTORICAL REVIEW

Down described this syndrome in 1866.[47] The chromosomal aberration causing the syndrome was first defined by Lejeune et al[48] in 1959.

EPIDEMIOLOGY

Down's syndrome is a chromosomal disorder caused by a triplicate state of all or a critical portion of chromosome 21, identified as 21q22.3.[49] The overall risk is 1 per 660 live births, and the relationship to advanced maternal age is well documented.

The extra dose of chromosomal material may come via several mechanisms. A true trisomy, resulting from meiotic nondisjunction of the chromosome 21 pair, is responsible in about 95% of patients.

Translocation of a significant portion of 21q to another chromosome is responsible for Down's syndrome in about 4% of patients. These robertsonian translocations are usually to the long arm of chromosome 14 or 22. Translocation of the long arm of one chromosome 21 to the other 21 is also possible. Translocation forms of Down's syndrome are not related to maternal age but do represent a very high recurrence risk.

About 1% to 2% of Down's syndrome cases are mosaic for a trisomic and a normal cell line. The variable proportions of trisomic and normal cells is probably responsible for the wide phenotypic variability in patients having mosaicism.

CLINICAL FEATURES

Facial features include round contours, slanted eyes with prominent epicanthal folds, and a short nose with flattening of the nasal bridge. Nearly all patients will have significant conductive hearing loss. About half will have congenital heart disorders, usually septal defects. Gastrointestinal tract anomalies may include duodenal atresia, imperforate anus, and Hirschsprung's disease. Mental retardation is a constant feature, but the degree of retardation is quite variable. Motor milestones are delayed; independent walking is usually achieved by age 2 years. Patients with Down's syndrome age prematurely and manifest the hallmarks of Alzheimer's disease at a much earlier age than do unaffected individuals.

Many of the orthopaedic manifestations of Down's syndrome are related to generalized hypotonia and ligament laxity. In the upper cervical spine, increased translational motion or frank instability may be seen at the occipitocervical and atlantoaxial articulations (Fig. 11).[50] Ten percent to 20% of affected persons have increased motion at one or both of these levels. Other abnormalities such as odontoid dysplasia and laminar defects of C-1 are quite frequent. A case of C2-3 instability has been identified.[51] Spondylolisthesis and precocious arthritis may be seen in the mid- to lower cervical spine.

Scoliosis is common in Down's syndrome, occurring in about one-half of patients. The curves usually follow an idiopathic pattern. In the lumbar spine, spondylolisthesis may occur in 5% to 6% of patients.

True congenital dislocation of the hips is unusual in Down's syndrome. However, spontaneous or habitual dislocation of the hip occurs in 4% to 5% of patients. The dysplasia is attributed to capsular laxity and generally be-

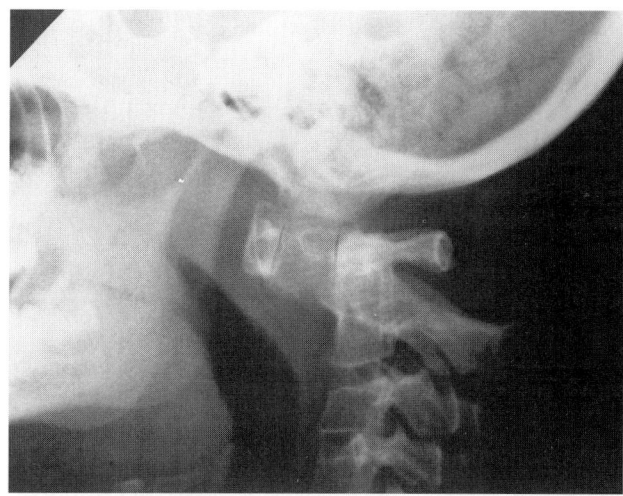

Fig. 11. Down's syndrome. Severely increased ADI is demonstrated on the lateral spine film of a 7-year-old.

comes manifest in later childhood or even after maturity. For unknown reasons, there is an increased risk of slipped capital femoral epiphysis compared with the general population.

Overall stature is short but proportional. The typical gait is broadly based and waddling, with noticeable out-toeing. The characteristic lower extremity alignment includes genu valgum and patellofemoral instability. Many patients are asymptomatic, even with frank recurrent patellar dislocation.

Most children with Down's syndrome have extremely flexible flat feet, with increased spacing between the great and second toes. Patients typically experience hallux valgus during adolescence.

The hands in Down's syndrome tend to be short, broad, and flat, with short fingers. Clinodactyly of the small finger and the transverse, or "simian," palmar crease are characteristic but not universal. All joints, especially the metacarpophalangeal joints, are hyperextensible.

Perhaps as many as 10% of patients with Down's syndrome will experience a polyarticular arthropathy, characteristically involving the feet. The cause and natural history of this arthropathy are not fully defined.

INVESTIGATION

Plain radiographs of the pelvis are practically diagnostic (Fig. 12). The iliac wings are broad and flared, an appearance likened to an elephant ear. The acetabular roof is nearly horizontal, with a resultant decrease in the acetabular index. These changes are so suggestive that analysis of the fetal pelvis by ultrasonogram may provide prenatal diagnosis.[52]

Good-quality radiographs of the cervical spine are mandatory. Lateral flexion and lateral extension plain films should be reviewed to assess upper cervical and occipitocervical stability. Questionable or "borderline" cases deserve flexion and extension MRI studies to evaluate possible cord changes. It may be necessary to obtain CT studies to define abnormalities of bone structure at the craniocervical junction.

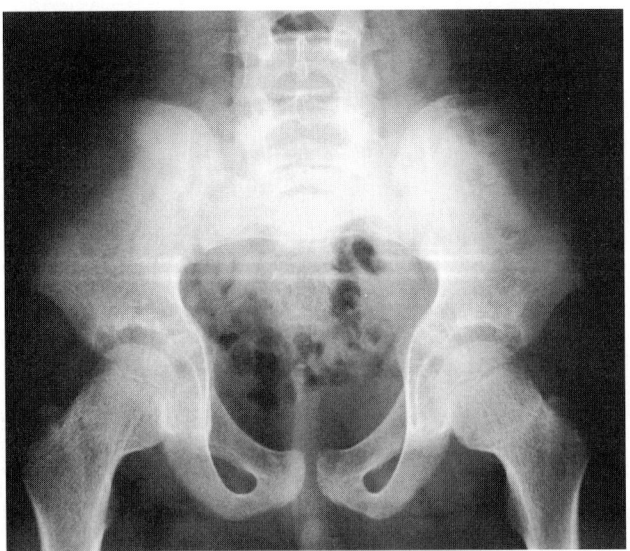

Fig. 12. Down's syndrome. This is an anteroposterior radiograph of the pelvis of an 11-year-old boy demonstrating broad ilial wings and horizontal superior acetabulum.

DIFFERENTIAL DIAGNOSIS

The diagnosis of Down's syndrome may be confirmed by cytogenetic techniques. This information is vital to genetic counseling because the risk of recurrence with subsequent pregnancy varies among the nondisjunction, translocation, and mosaic forms.

MANAGEMENT

The upper cervical spine presents significant management controversy. Screening radiographs are generally obtained before athletic participation or at about 3 to 4 years of age. Although screening may be required by sports organizations, the previous guidelines produced by the American Academy of Pediatrics have been retired.[53] Symptomatic patients and those whose atlanto-dens interval (ADI) exceeds 10 mm warrant surgical stabilization. A great many asymptomatic patients will have radiographic ADI measurement in the "gray zone" between 4.5 mm and 10 mm, for whom serial examinations are appropriate. Individual behavior and severity of mental retardation are risk factors that argue for or against operative stabilization, and flexion-extension MRI may help determine the risk of neural encroachment or cord compression.

No guidelines exist regarding the frequency of screening for occipitocervical instability or indications for occipitocervical fusion except for the symptomatic child. Recommended radiographic techniques differ among authors, and the "normal" excursions for Down's syndrome patients are still not adequately defined.[54, 55]

Scoliosis in Down's syndrome generally follows an idiopathic pattern, and treatment algorithms are routine. Similarly, management of lower lumbar spondylolysis and spondylolisthesis follows routine recommendations.

Nonoperative measures have usually been ineffective for control of habitual hip subluxation or dislocation. Operative capsulorrhaphy, combined with femoral and acetabular bony procedures, is generally required for symptomatic cases.

Genu valgum, with or without patellar instability, is frequently asymptomatic. Success of nonoperative interventions such as quadriceps strengthening and bracing for patellar instability is limited by underlying laxity and structural anomalies. Surgical reconstruction should be reserved for those with actual functional impairment.

Orthotic support does not seem to alter the natural history of severe flat feet and progressive hallux valgus in Down's syndrome. Once again, surgery should be reserved for those who experience functional impairment. Soft-tissue realignment is unreliable because of the generalized laxity. Bony reconstruction, including arthrodesis of the great toe metatarsophalangeal joint, should be considered.

Upper extremity abnormalities do not cause functional impairment for most patients; treatment interventions are seldom indicated.

RESULTS/COMPLICATIONS

The relative risk of leukemia and leukemoid reactions in Down's syndrome ranges from 10 to 20 times higher than the general population. Endocrinopathies, especially hypothyroidism, are also increased. Infections are more frequent and of greater severity than in unaffected individuals. Aggressive medical management of these issues, along with effective early surgical correction of congenital heart defects, has contributed to an improved longevity for Down's syndrome patients. Survival into the 60s is now common.

TURNER'S AND NOONAN'S SYNDROMES

- The phenotype in these syndromes is nearly identical.
- Turner's syndrome affects females; it is a chromosomal abnormality, lacking one of the X chromosomes.
- Noonan's syndrome affects males and females; it is a gene defect, located on chromosome 12.
- Scoliosis is common in both syndromes.
- Growth retardation and osteoporosis in Turner's syndrome are attributed to endocrine abnormalities.
- Noonan's syndrome must be distinguished from King-Denborough syndrome; malignant hyperthermia is part of King-Denborough syndrome.

DEFINITION

Turner's syndrome patients are female but do not have a full complement of two X chromosomes. The appearance includes short stature, webbed neck, cubitus valgus, and sexual infantilism.

Noonan's syndrome patients may be male or female and have normal karyotypes. The genetic defect maps to 12q24. The appearance is very similar to Turner's syndrome.

HISTORICAL REVIEW

Turner's syndrome was actually described first by Ullrich in 1930.[56] The 45,XO chromosomal aberration was demonstrated by Ford et al[57] in 1959.

Noonan's syndrome was first described in 1968.[58] Alternative names include "male Turner's syndrome" and "female pseudo-Turner's syndrome." In 1997, Brady et al[59] localized the responsible gene defect to 12q24.

EPIDEMIOLOGY

Turner's syndrome is associated with a single X chromosome. In about two-thirds of cases, this represents a straightforward 45,XO karyotype, with the mother contributing the single X chromosome. Approximately one-third of cases are XX/XO mosaic. A very small number of patients, 1% or fewer, represent deletion of only a portion of the X chromosome. The mechanisms that produce the phenotype remain unknown. Although intrauterine lethality is estimated in 95%, the syndrome is fairly common, affecting perhaps 1 in 2500 live births.

Although the location, 12q24, of the gene defect responsible for Noonan's syndrome is known, the mechanisms that produce the phenotype are not. The inheritance is autosomal dominant, with an incidence of about 1 in 1000.

CLINICAL FEATURES

The Turner's syndrome phenotype is female. At birth, features include webbed neck, widely spaced nipples, and edema of the hands and feet, which may persist for months. The low-set hairline, cubitus valgus, and short stature become more apparent in childhood. Osteoporosis may be evident even in childhood, resulting from both low estrogen and altered renal vitamin D metabolism.[60] In adolescence there is no puberty, and patients remain without secondary sexual characteristics unless exogenous hormone replacement is provided. A majority of patients, perhaps 80%, have cubitus valgus. Shortening of the small and ring finger metacarpals is characteristic. Genu valgum is frequent but usually requires no treatment. Some patients have a unique bony protuberance or actual osteochondroma at the proximal medial tibia. Idiopathic scoliosis is common in Turner's syndrome. Curve progression may be exacerbated by the administration of growth hormone.

Although males and females may have Noonan's syndrome, the phenotype is otherwise extremely similar to that of Turner's syndrome. Clinically, Noonan's syndrome is distinguished by the normal gonads, a high incidence of mental retardation, and congenital heart defects. Scoliosis is more frequent and more severe in Noonan's syndrome. Osteopenia may be seen in patients of either sex.[61] Significant bleeding diathesis and multiple coagulation abnormalities have also been described.[62]

INVESTIGATION

Orthopaedic aspects of both of these syndromes are investigated by usual radiographic methods.

DIFFERENTIAL DIAGNOSIS

There is no single physical feature diagnostic for either syndrome. Particular characteristics in each age group should arouse suspicion of Turner's syndrome. These include edema of hands and feet in the neonate, short stature in the child, and sexual infantilism in the adolescent. The short stature, with metacarpal and metatarsal shortening, is reminiscent of pseudohypoparathyroidism and pseudopseudohypoparathyroidism. Noonan's syndrome must be distinguished from King-Denborough syndrome because malignant hyperthermia is common in the latter.

MANAGEMENT

In Turner's syndrome, growth hormone administration through adolescence results in increases both in growth velocity and ultimate height. Growth hormone administration during childhood seems to improve the bone density. Cyclic sex hormones are usually provided from adolescence through adulthood. These hormonal replacements also help control osteoporosis. Relative timing of hormonal treatments will affect ultimate height.[63] Ovum transplantation supported by hormonal supplementation can result in successful pregnancy.

The neck webbing is a typical cutaneous feature, without underlying cervical abnormality. The cubitus valgum and genu valgum seldom cause any functional disability and do not require treatment interventions. Orthopaedic management of scoliosis in both of these syndromes follows standard algorithms.

RESULTS/COMPLICATIONS

Short stature is universal, with an adult height near 140 cm. Although there is a high incidence of learning disabilities, the general intelligence is normal. Overall medical status is excellent.

REFERENCES

Achondroplasia

1. Parrot JM: Sur les malformations achondroplastiques et le Dieu Ptah. Bull Soc Antropol 1878; 1:296.
2. Shiang R, Thompson LM, Zhu Y-Z, et al: Mutations in the transmembrane domain of FGFR3 cause the most common genetic form of dwarfism, achondroplasia. Cell 1994; 78:335.
3. Stanescu R, Stanescu V, Maroteaux P: Homozygous achondroplasia: Morphologic and biochemical study of cartilage. Am J Med Genet 1990; 37:412.
4. Hunter AGW, Bankier A, Rogers JG, et al: Medical complications of achondroplasia: A multicentre patient review. J Med Genet 1998; 35:705.
5. Hecht JT, Thompson NM, Weir T, et al: Cognitive and motor skills in achondroplastic infants: Neurologic and respiratory correlates. Am J Med Genet 1991; 41:208.
6. Tasker RC, Dundas I, Laverty A, et al: Distinct patterns of respiratory difficulty in young children with achondroplasia: A clinical, sleep, and lung function study. Arch Dis Child 1998; 79(2):99.
7. Pauli RM, Horton VK, Glinski LP, et al: Prospective assessment of risks for cervicomedullary-junction compression in infants with achondroplasia. Am J Hum Genet 1995; 56:732.
8. Pauli RM, Breed A, Horton VK, et al: Prevention of fixed, angular kyphosis in achondroplasia. J Pediatr Orthop 1997; 17(6):726.
9. Yasui N, Kawabata H, Kojimoto H, et al: Lengthening of the lower limbs in patients with achondroplasia and hypochondroplasia. Clin Orthop 1997; 344:298.
10. Tanaka H, Kubo T, Yamate T, et al: Effect of growth hormone therapy in children with achondroplasia: Growth pattern, hypothalamic-pituitary function, and genotype. Eur J Endocrinol 1998; 138(3):275.
11. Hunter AGW, Hecht JT, Scott CI Jr: Standard weight for height curves in achondroplasia. Am J Med Genet 1996; 62:255.

Hypochondroplasia

12. Ravenna R: Achondroplasie et chondrohypoplasie. Contribution clinique. Nouv Iconogr Salpet 1913; 26:157.
13. Beals RK: Hypochondroplasia. A report of five kindreds. J Bone Joint Surg Am 1969; 51:728.
14. Bellus GA, McIntosh I, Smith EA, et al: A recurrent mutation in the tyrosine kinase domain of fibroblast growth factor recep-

tor 3 causes hypochondroplasia. Nat Genet 1995; 10:357.

15. Ramaswami U, Rumsby G, Hindmarsh PC, et al: Genotype and phenotype in hypochondroplasia. J Pediatr 1998; 133(1): 99.

16. Wynne-Davies R, Walsh WK, Gormley J: Achondroplasia and hypochondroplasia. Clinical variation and spinal stenosis. J Bone Joint Surg Br 1991; 63(4):508.

17. Hall BD, Spranger J: Hypochondroplasia: Clinical and radiological aspects in 39 cases. Radiology 1979; 133:95.

Diastrophic Dysplasia

18. Lamy M, Maroteaux P: Le nanisme diastrophique. Presse Med 1960; 68:1977.

19. Treacher Collins Syndrome Collaborative Group: Positional cloning of a gene involved in the pathogenesis of Treacher Collins syndrome. Nat Genet 1996; 12: 130.

20. Satoh H, Susaki M, Shukunami C, et al: Functional analysis of diastrophic dysplasia sulfate transporter. Its involvement in growth regulation of chondrocytes mediated by sulfated proteoglycans. J Biol Chem 1998; 273(20):12307.

21. Hastbacka J, Superit-Furga A, Wilcox WR, et al: Atelosteogenesis type II is caused by mutations in the diastrophic dysplasia sulfate-transporter gene (DTDST): Evidence for a phenotypic series involving three chondrodysplasias. Am J Hum Genet 1996; 58:255.

22. Poussa M, Merikanto J, Ryoppy S, et al: The spine in diastrophic dysplasia. Spine 1991; 16:881.

23. Vaara P, Peltonen J, Poussa M, et al: Development of the hip in diastrophic dysplasia. J Bone Joint Surg Br 1998; 80(2): 315.

Prader-Willi and Angelman's Syndromes

24. Prader A, Labhart A, Willi H: Ein Syndrom von Adipositas, Kleinwuchs, Kryptorchismus und Oligophrenie nach Myatonieartigem Zustand im Neugeborenenalter. Schweiz Med Wochenschr 1956; 86:1260.

25. Angelman H: "Puppet children:" A report of three cases. Dev Med Child Neurol 1965; 7:681.

26. Cassidy SB, Schwartz S: Prader-Willi and Angelman syndromes. Disorders of genomic imprinting. Medicine (Baltimore) 1998; 77(2):140.

27. Miller SP, Riley P, Shevell MI: The neonatal presentation of Prader-Willi syndrome revisited. J Pediatr 1999; 134(2): 226.

28. Laan LAEM, den Boer AT, Hennekam RCM, et al: Angelman syndrome in adulthood. Am J Med Genet 1996; 66:356.

29. Rees D, Jones MW, Owen R, et al: Scoliosis surgery in the Prader-Willi syndrome. J Bone Joint Surg Br 1989; 71(4):685.

Beckwith-Wiedemann Syndrome

30. Wiedemann HR: Complexe malformatif familial avec hernie ombilicale et macro-glossie—un 'syndrome nouveau'?. J Genet Hum 1964; 13:223.

31. Beckwith JB: Macroglossia, omphalocele, adrenal cytomegaly, gigantism, and hyperplastic visceromegaly. Birth Defects Orig Art Ser 1969; V(2):188.

32. Waziri M, Patil SR, Hanson JW, et al: Abnormality of chromosome 11 in patients with features of Beckwith-Wiedemann syndrome. J Pediatr 1983; 102:873.

33. Weksberg R, Squire JA: Molecular biology of Beckwith-Wiedemann syndrome. Med Pediatr Oncol 1996; 27(5):462.

34. DeBaun MR, Tucker MA: Risk of cancer during the first four years of life in children from the Beckwith-Wiedemann Syndrome Registry. J Pediatr 1998; 132(3, Pt 1):398.

Multiple Hereditary Exostoses

35. Hunter J: The Works of John Hunter, F.R.S. With Notes by J. F. Palmer. Vol. I. London, Longman, Rees, Orme, Brown, Green and Longman, 1835.

36. Ehrenfried A: Multiple cartilaginous exostoses-hereditary deforming chondrodysplasia. A brief report on a little known disease. JAMA 1915; 64:1642.

37. Jaffe HL: Hereditary multiple exostoses. Ann Pathol 1943; 36:335.

38. Wuyts W, Van Hul W, De Boulle K, et al: Mutations in the EXT 1 and EXT 2 genes in hereditary multiple exostoses. Am J Hum Genet 1998; 62(2):346.

39. Carroll KL, Yandow SM, Ward K, et al: Clinical correlation to genetic variations of hereditary multiple exostosis. J Pediatr Orthop 1999; 19(6):785.

40. Schmale GA, Conrad EU III, Raskind WH: The natural history of hereditary multiple exostoses. J Bone Joint Surg Am 1994; 76:986.

Familial Dysautonomia (Riley-Day Syndrome)

41. Riley CM, Day RL, Greeley DM, et al: Central autonomic dysfunction with defective lacrimation: Report of five cases. Pediatrics 1949; 3:468.

42. Blumenfeld A, Slaugenhaupt SA, Axelrod FB, et al: Localization of the gene for familial dysautonomia on chromosome 9 and definition of DNA markers for genetic diagnosis. Nat Genet 1993; 4:160.

43. Axelrod FB: Familial dysautonomia: A 47-year perspective. How technology confirms clinical acumen. J Pediatr 1998; 132: S2.

44. Blumenfeld A, Slaugenhaupt SA, Liebert CB, et al: Precise genetic mapping and haplotype analysis of the familial dysautonomia gene on human chromosome 9q31. Am J Hum Genet 1999; 64(4):1110.

45. Axelrod FB, Pearson J, Tepperberg J, et al: Congenital sensory neuropathy with skeletal dysplasia. J Pediatr 1983; 102: 727.

46. Kaplan L, Margulies JY, Kadari A, et al: Aspects of spinal deformity in familial dysautonomia (Riley-Day syndrome). Eur Spine J 1997; 6(1):33.

Down Syndrome

47. Down JLH: Observations on an ethnic classification of idiots. London Hosp Clin Lect Rep 1866; 3:259.

48. Lejeune J, Gautier M, Turpin R: Etude des chromosomes somatiques de neuf enfants mongoliens. Coll R Acad Sci 1959; 248: 1721.

49. Delabar JM, Theophile D, Rahmani Z, et al: Molecular mapping of twenty-four features of Down syndrome on chromosome 21. Eur J Hum Genet 1993; 1:114.

50. Uno K, Kataoka O, Shiba R: Occipitoatlantal and occipitoaxial hypermobility in Down syndrome. Spine 1996; 21(12): 1430.

51. Citow JS, Munshi I, Chang-Stroman T, et al: C2/3 instability in a child with Down's syndrome. Case report and discussion. Pediatr Neurosurg 1998; 28(3):143.

52. Freed KS, Kliewer MA, Hertzberg BS, et al: Pelvic CT morphometry in Down syndrome: Implications for prenatal US evaluation—preliminary results. Radiology 2000; 214(1):205.

53. Committee on Sports Medicine and Fitness of the American Academy of Pediatrics. Atlantoaxial instability in Down syndrome: Subject review (RE9528). Pediatrics 1995; 96:151.

54. Karol LA, Sheffield EG, Crawford K, et al: Reproducibility in the measurement of atlanto-occipital instability in children with Down syndrome. Spine 1996; 21(21): 2463; discussion, 2468.

55. Wellborn CC, Sturm PF, Hatch RS, et al: Intraobserver reproducibility and interobserver reliability of cervical spine measurements. J Pediatr Orthop 2000; 20(1):66.

Turner's and Noonan's Syndromes

56. Ullrich O: Uber typische Kombinationsbilder multipler Abartungen. Z Kinderhilk 1930; 49:271.

57. Ford DE, Miller OJ, Polani PE, et al: A sex-chromosome anomaly in a case of gonadal dysgenesis (Turner's syndrome). Lancet 1959; 1:711.

58. Noonan JA: Hypertelorism with Turner phenotype. A new syndrome with associated congenital heart disease. Am J Dis Child 1968; 116:373.

59. Brady AF, Jamieson CR, van der Burgt I, et al: Further delineation of the critical region for Noonan syndrome on the long arm of chromosome 12. Eur J Hum Genet 1997; 5:336.

60. Rubin K: Turner syndrome and osteoporosis: Mechanisms and prognosis. Pediatrics 1998; 102 (2, Pt 3):481.

61. Takagi M, Miyashita Y, Koga M, et al: Estrogen deficiency is a potential cause for osteopenia in adult male patients with Noonan's syndrome. Calcif Tissue Int 2000; 66(3):200.

62. Sharland M, Patton MA, Talbot S, et al: Coagulation-factor deficiencies and abnormal bleeding in Noonan's syndrome. Lancet 1992; 339:19.

63. Chernausek SD, Attie KM: Role of oestrogen therapy in the management of short stature in Turner syndrome. Acta Paediatr Suppl 1999; 88(433):130.

METABOLIC CONDITIONS

Dennis P. Grogan and Harry K. W. Kim

section 9 chapter 6

Summary

- Hypophosphatemic vitamin D–resistant rickets is an X-linked dominant condition that presents with short stature, bowing of the legs, and hypophosphatemia.
- Metabolic bone disease associated with prematurity and total parenteral nutrition (TPN): be aware that TPN preparations may be deficient in calcium and phosphorus and that premature infants may retain the aluminum.
- Hereditary hypophosphatasia is associated with a decrease in the level of the liver-bone-kidney isoform of alkaline phosphatase.
- Renal osteodystrophy is a metabolic bone disease resulting from the abnormalities of mineral metabolism associated with chronic renal failure.
- Pseudohypoparathyroidism is a syndrome of hypoparathyroidism, hypocalcemia, increased parathyroid hormone (PTH), and unresponsiveness at the bone and kidney level to PTH. It may include characteristics of Albright's hereditary osteodystrophy.
- Caffey's disease (infantile cortical hyperostosis) is a self-limited condition that typically occurs in children younger than 6 months. Presenting symptoms include fever, irritability, soft-tissue swelling, and tenderness. Radiographs reveal layering of periosteal new bone formation.

HYPOPHOSPHATEMIC VITAMIN D–RESISTANT RICKETS

CLINICAL FEATURES

Hypophosphatemic vitamin D–resistant rickets (HPDR) is an X-linked dominant condition, with the mutant gene located in the distal part of the short arm of the X chromosome (Xp22.1–p22.2).[1] Clinically, these children present with short stature, bowing deformities of the lower extremities (anterior and lateral femoral bowing, genu varum or valgum), reduced growth rate, and hypophosphatemia (Fig. 1). Although the hypophosphatemia is evident shortly after birth, the decreased growth rate and bowed legs become apparent in early childhood and are usually the cause of parental concern.

PATHOGENESIS

The hypophosphatemia is the result of a primary inborn error of phosphate transport in the proximal nephron, with a resultant abnormality in the synthesis of 1,25-dihydroxyvitamin D. The exact pathogenesis of this condition remains the subject of intense research efforts.[2]

INVESTIGATION

Laboratory investigations should include serum phosphorus, calcium, and alkaline phosphatase. The serum phosphorus will always be low. The serum calcium will usually be normal because of the many homeostatic mechanisms present to maintain this mineral at normal levels; however, it may in fact be either low or high depending on the clinical situation and underlying metabolic condition. The alkaline phosphatase will usually be elevated, indicating increased bone metabolic activity.

Radiographic examinations should concentrate on the clinically involved areas, usually the lower extremities. There is often a bowing deformity that may include either the femur or the tibia or both. The appearance of the bones is also characteristic; the ends of the most rapidly growing bones demonstrate the most severe changes (i.e., the knee and wrist). The long bones are relatively shorter and wider; the shaft appears rarefied because of the lack of mineralization. The cortex can be thin and coarse. Transverse radiolucent bands or looser zones may be seen in more involved long bones. The growth plates are widened. The metaphyses are broader, concave, and flared, cupping over the edges of the growth plate at the most extreme (Fig. 2).

MANAGEMENT

Oral phosphate replacement (1 to 3 g of elemental phosphate per day in four to five doses) is recommended to replace the renal phosphate wasting. Large doses of vitamin D (20,000 to 75,000 IU per day) must be given to offset the hypocalcemic effect of the phosphate supplementation. On this treatment regimen, growth rate and radiological changes have been shown to improve.[2] A gene-dose effect has been observed in patients with HPDR; heterozygous girls respond better to medical treatment than hemizygous boys. To obtain improvement in the osteomalacia component, 1,25-dihydroxyvitamin D_3 must be substituted to obtain healing of the mineralization defect on the trabecular surfaces. There also exists a primary osteoblast defect in which the osteoblast is unable to produce an adequate amount of mineralized matrix, creating the characteristic hypomineralized periosteocytic lesions seen on histological exam.

Orthopaedic management of the bowing deformities of the lower extremities will depend on the severity of the deformity and must be combined with medical management. The objective of surgical treatment is to maintain joint alignment to minimize the risk for future degenerative disease. Femoral and tibial osteotomies are effective in the correction of the associated angular and torsional bony abnormalities. Rohmiller et al[3] showed that those children treated with medication plus surgical treatment had a significant improvement in the degree of bowing compared with children treated with medication only but did have a significant decrease in height. Also, obesity at presentation was

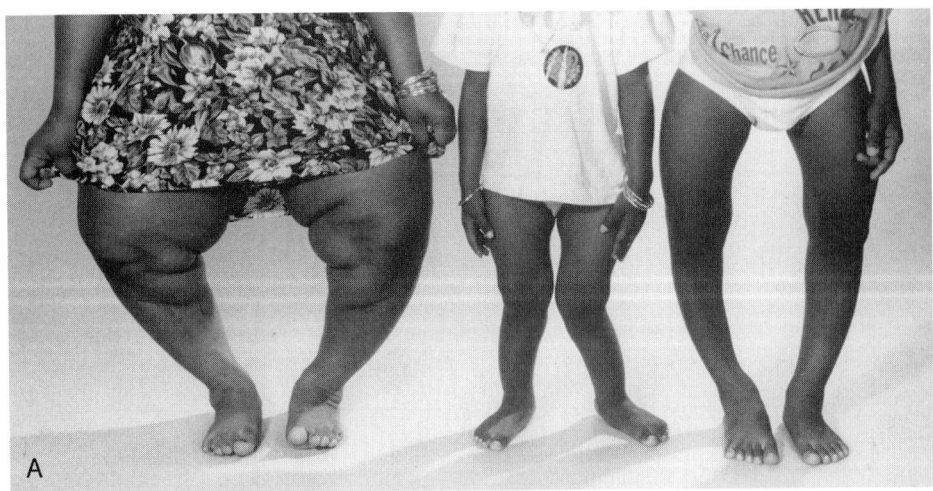

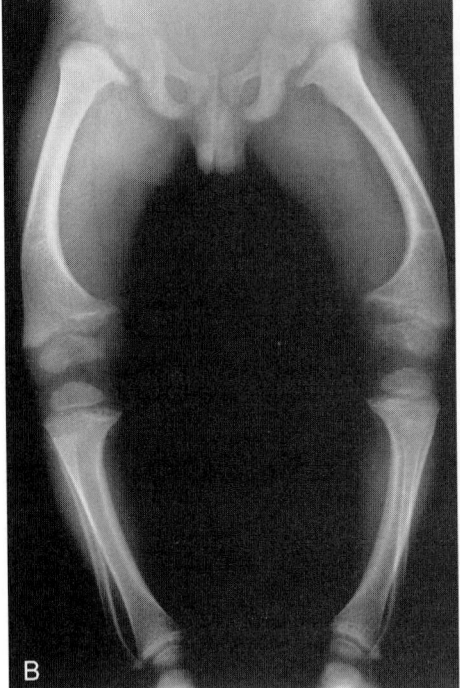

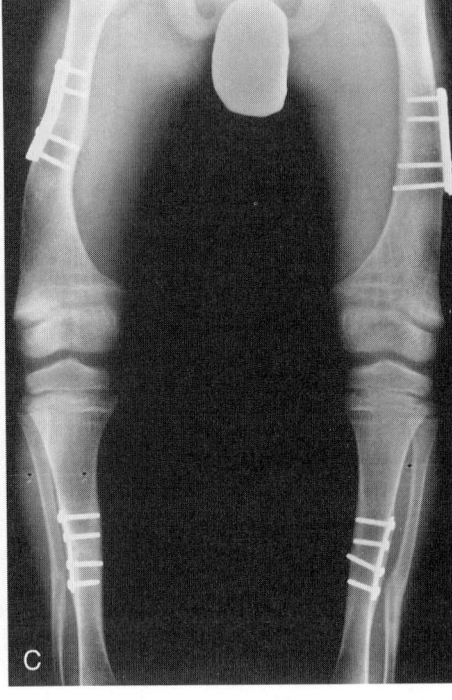

Fig. 1. Hypophosphatemic vitamin D–resistant rickets (HPDR). *A,* A mother and two daughters with HPDR. The mother underwent tibial osteotomies 20 years ago with recurrence of the varus deformity. The younger daughter has had tibial osteotomies with slight overcorrection into valgus. The older daughter has not yet undergone corrective osteotomies. *B,* A 3-year-old boy with HPDR. Deformity is noted in both the femurs and tibias. *C,* Patient in Fig. 1B 6 years later after bilateral femoral and tibial osteotomies with correction of deformity.

found to be a key indicator of future need for surgical management, even more significant than the bowing angle of either the femur or tibia at presentation.

DIFFERENTIAL DIAGNOSIS
The clinical, radiographic, and laboratory findings will differentiate rickets from other skeletal dysplasias, particularly metaphyseal chondrodysplasia. Familial short stature with physiological varus may require laboratory investigation to exclude rickets from consideration.

Metabolic Bone Disease Associated with Prematurity and TPN
Premature infants treated with long-term TPN are at risk for rickets or osteopenia. Factors associated with this condition are the lack of calcium and phosphorus in the TPN preparations and aluminum loading.[4, 5] Significant quantities of aluminum may be found in TPN preparations in the form of calcium and phosphate salts, heparin, and albumin. Because renal function in premature infants is developmentally reduced, the risk of aluminum retention is significantly increased. The aluminum has been noted to accumulate in bone, blood, and urine.[5]

Management and Prevention
Premature infants receiving TPN should be provided with as much calcium and phosphorus as permitted by the TPN preparations. Monitoring of these infants for evidence of metabolic bone disease, including hyperparathyroidism and vitamin D deficiency, should be done with periodic radiographic examination as well as serum calcium, phosphorus, PTH, 25-hydroxyvitamin D, and 1,25-dihydroxyvitamin D levels.

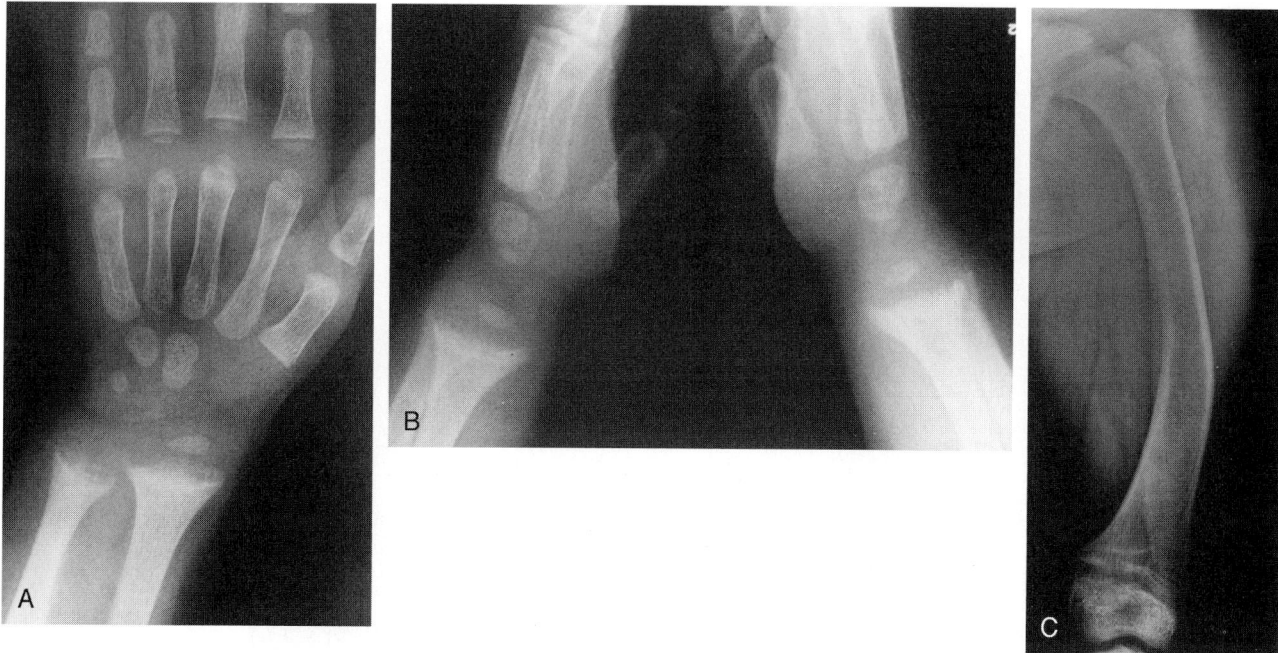

Fig. 2. Hypophosphatemic vitamin D–resistant rickets (HPDR). *A* and *B*, Anteroposterior and lateral radiographs of the left wrist of a 5-year-old girl with untreated HPDR. Note the broad metaphyses with flaring and cupping, widened growth plates, and coarse trabeculae. *C*, Anteroposterior radiograph of the femur of a 12-year-old girl with HPDR. Note the short broad bone with coarse trabeculae, varus deformity, and widening of the proximal and distal growth plates.

HEREDITARY HYPOPHOSPHATASIA

Hereditary hypophosphatasia is actually a group of rare hereditary diseases that are characterized biochemically by a decrease in the level of the liver-bone-kidney isoform of alkaline phosphatase. In the bone this enzyme is expressed by the osteoblasts, and it is required for normal mineralization of osteoid. Patients with a deficiency of this enzyme thus present with rachitic-like changes because of the abnormality of mineralization of bone and cartilage. The deficiency of alkaline phosphatase can also affect the normal processes of dentition.[6]

CLINICAL FEATURES

The spectrum of the disease is very broad depending on the age of onset and the severity of enzyme activity reduction. Because the disease tends to be more severe with a younger age of onset, a classification according to the age of onset (perinatal, infantile, childhood, and adult) is commonly used and has prognostic implications.[7] The perinatal type can be lethal in utero. The perinatal and infantile forms are transmitted in an autosomal-recessive fashion; the transmission of the other forms is less clear. Clinical presentation of the earlier-onset forms may include poor feeding, failure to thrive, irritability, hypotonia, and seizures. The childhood form can present with premature loss of primary teeth, long bone angular deformities, short stature, and delayed walking, with a clinical appearance similar to that of rickets.

INVESTIGATION

The level of tissue-nonspecific alkaline phosphatase activity (the liver-bone-kidney isoform) is reduced. This is the cir-

culating form of the enzyme. The substrates of the enzyme, including phosphoethanolamine, inorganic pyrophosphate and pyridoxal-5-phosphate, are elevated. Hypercalcemia and hypercalciuria are frequently observed in the younger age forms because of the lack of incorporation of serum calcium into bone.[6] Serum phosphate levels are also elevated in many patients. Vitamin D and PTH levels are normal. Radiographic findings are consistent with rickets. Severe hypomineralization of bone with rachitic changes may be seen in the younger age forms. Characteristic radiolucent areas can be seen extending from the growth plate into the metaphyseal bone. These are thought to represent areas of uncalcified bone matrix (Fig. 3).[8]

DIFFERENTIAL DIAGNOSIS

The differential diagnosis includes rickets.

MANAGEMENT

No specific treatment is available. Unlike individuals with rickets, these patients do not respond to vitamin D administration because their calcium level is normal or elevated. For this reason, administration of calcium and vitamin D, as in rickets, should be avoided. Hypercalcemia will respond to medical therapy. Bone healing after fracture and osteotomy may be delayed. Whenever possible, an intramedullary fixation device is preferred over plating if surgical intervention is required.

HEREDITARY HYPERPHOSPHATASIA (JUVENILE PAGET'S DISEASE)

Hereditary hyperphosphatasia is a rare hereditary disease with some clinical and biochemical features similar to

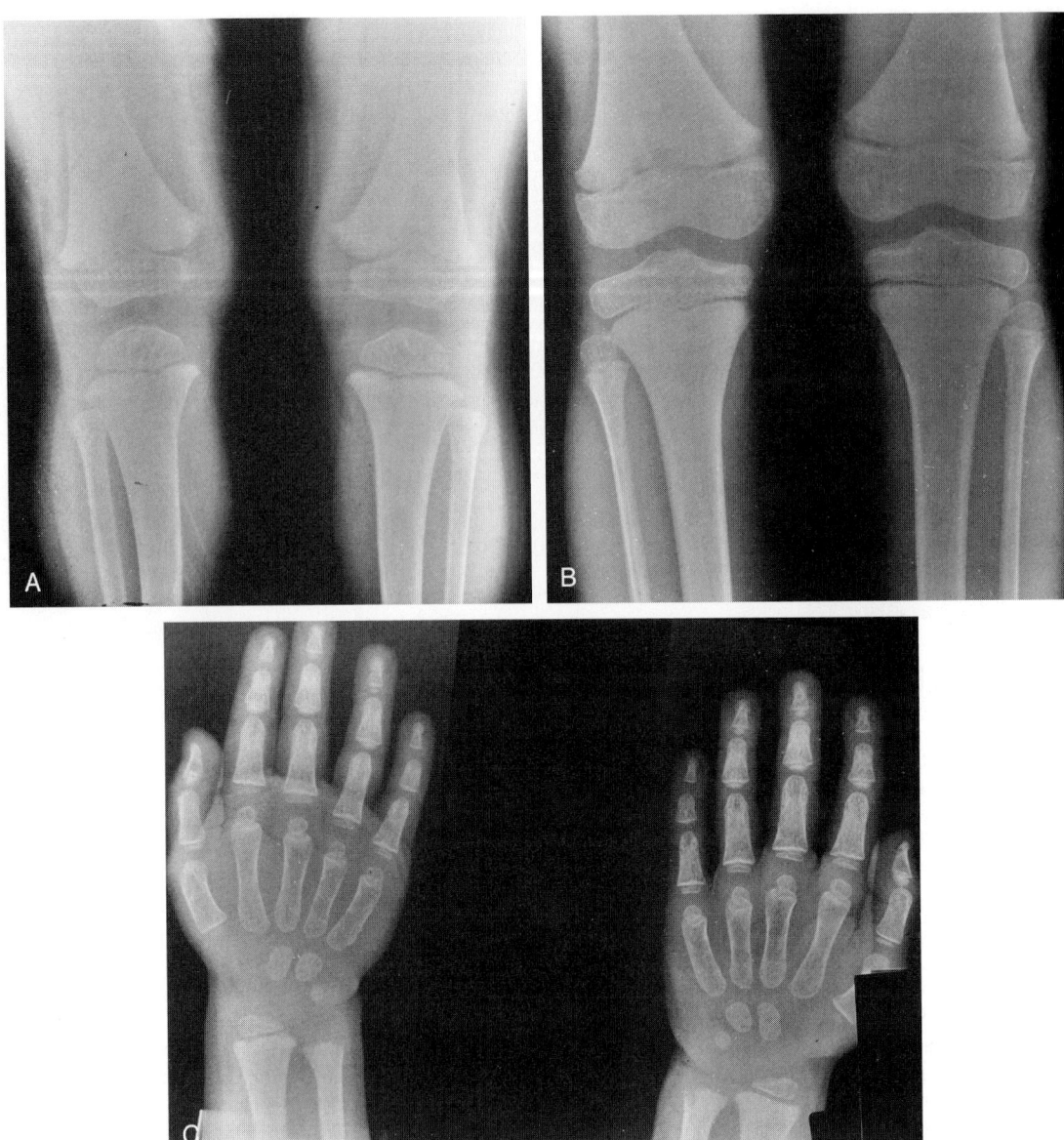

Fig. 3. Hereditary hypophosphatasia. *A,* A 6-year-old boy with hereditary hypophosphatasia. Note the central lucent areas extending from the growth plate of the distal femurs into the metaphysis bilaterally. *B,* Five years later these areas are improved. *C,* Anteroposterior radiographs of both wrists at age 6 demonstrate a similar lucent area extending from the distal growth plate of the ulna. These also resolved with growth.

those seen in adults with Paget's disease (increased bone remodeling, bone deformities, fractures, and elevated alkaline phosphatase activity). Early onset, diffuse skeletal involvement, and histomorphometric characteristics differentiate the disease from Paget's disease in adults.[9]

CLINICAL FEATURES

Patients with hereditary hyperphosphatasia present with bone pain, bony deformities, fractures, and decreased mobility. Unlike the adult form of Paget's disease, which tends to be localized and asymmetric, symmetric involvement of all bones is observed in the juvenile form.[7]

INVESTIGATION

Markedly elevated levels of serum alkaline phosphatase activity and hydroxyprolinuria are observed, indicating an increase in bone turnover. Serum calcium, phosphorus, vitamin D, and PTH levels are normal. Diffuse, symmetric bowing of the long bones and generalized osteopenia are observed radiographically.[9]

MANAGEMENT

Calcitonin and diphosphonates may improve the bone pain and radiographic parameters. Long-term use of calcitonin injection is limited by the development of antibodies against the calcitonin. Long-term effects of diphosphonates in children are not well defined and require further investigation before this form of treatment can be widely promoted.

RENAL OSTEODYSTROPHY

Renal osteodystrophy refers to a group of metabolic bone diseases that results from an alteration of mineral metabolism secondary to chronic renal failure. Five types of bone disease can occur based on their histological features: osteitis fibrosa cystica; rickets/osteomalacia; mixed, mild, and adynamic disease.[10] Various degrees of each of these disease processes may be present in an individual with renal failure.

PATHOGENESIS

The kidney is a key organ in the maintenance of mineral homeostasis and is crucial to normal bone metabolism. Loss of renal function affects not only calcium, phosphorus, and magnesium levels but also the ability to convert inactive vitamin D to a more active form (1,25-hydroxyvitamin D). The kidney is also a target organ for PTH and serves an important role in the degradation and excretion of the hormone. Generally, an alteration of renal function and mineral homeostasis can lead to either increased bone metabolism, as seen in osteitis fibrosa cystica, or decreased bone metabolism, as seen in renal rickets/osteomalacia.[11] Secondary hyperparathyroidism underlies the pathological processes associated with the increased bone metabolism seen in osteitis fibrosa cystica. Aluminum intoxication underlies the pathological processes associated with the decreased bone metabolism seen in osteomalacia. When the glomerular filtration rate falls below 25%, phosphate retention and hyperphosphatemia are observed. Hyperphosphatemia increases PTH secretion directly and by decreasing the level of serum ionized calcium also leads to secondary hyperparathyroidism over time. Phosphate retention may also stimulate PTH secretion through reduction of vitamin D_3 synthesis. Aluminum toxicity is frequently seen in patients undergoing hemodialysis with water contaminated with aluminum and in those patients receiving aluminum hydroxide as a phosphate-binding agent to lower the phosphate level. Normally, aluminum is excreted by the kidneys. In uremic patients the aluminum load is increased for the reasons mentioned, and its renal excretion is decreased. The excess aluminum becomes deposited at the interface between the osteoid and mineralized bone, further leading to reduction of bone mineralization and formation.

CLINICAL FEATURES

Manifestation of renal osteodystrophy in adult and pediatric patients differs considerably. Growth retardation, slipped epiphysis (epiphysiolysis), and angular deformities of the lower extremities are unique to pediatric patients, whereas bone pain, muscle weakness, and stress fractures are observed in both adult and pediatric patients (Fig. 4). Metastatic calcification, tendon rupture, and bursitis are uncommonly seen in pediatric patients. Unlike the idiopathic epiphysiolysis seen in adolescence that is limited to the capital femoral epiphysis (slipped capital femoral epiphysis), epiphysiolysis in uremic patients occurs at a much earlier age and can affect a variety of growth plates. The proximal and distal epiphyses of the femur, the distal epiphysis of the tibia, fibula, radius or ulna, and the proximal epiphysis of the humerus can be involved. These patients are also smaller in height and weight in comparison to the typically obese patients seen with idiopathic epiphysiolysis. Pediatric patients with chronic renal failure invariably have growth inhibition with one-third of the patients falling below the third percentile for height at the end stage of renal disease.[12] Uncontrolled uremia, secondary hyperparathyroidism, and early onset of uremia are associated with a greater incidence of epiphysiolysis. In a review of 31 children with renal osteodystrophy, all patients had secondary hyperparathyroidism at the time of diagnosis of slipped capital femoral epiphysis.[13] This study also showed a 95% prevalence of bilaterality. Angular deformities also tend to be more common in the patients with an earlier onset of uremia. Genu valgum is the most common angular deformity observed.[14] Bowing of the long bones in the lower extremities, ankle valgus, and scoliosis are also commonly seen in these patients. Mild degrees of slippage of the epiphysis and asymmetric growth disturbances of the physis are thought to contribute to these angular deformities (Fig. 5A).

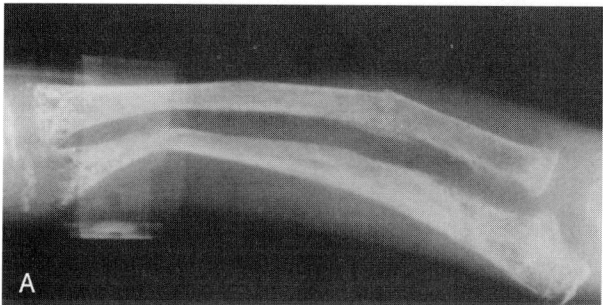
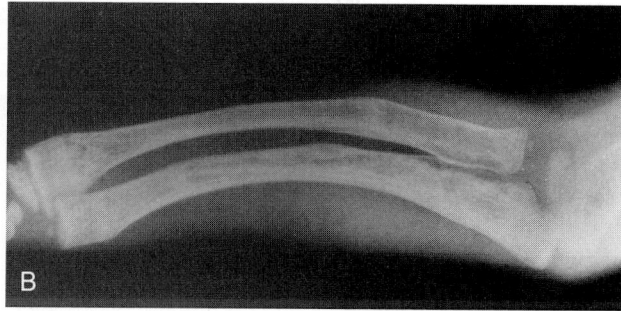

Fig. 4. Renal osteodystrophy. *A,* Anteroposterior radiograph of the forearm of a 6-year-old girl with renal failure. Note the widened growth plates and diffuse radiolucent areas throughout the radius and ulna. Both bones have sustained fractures after minimal trauma. *B,* After treatment of the child's renal disease, the appearance of the bones has significantly improved. The bowing deformity remains.

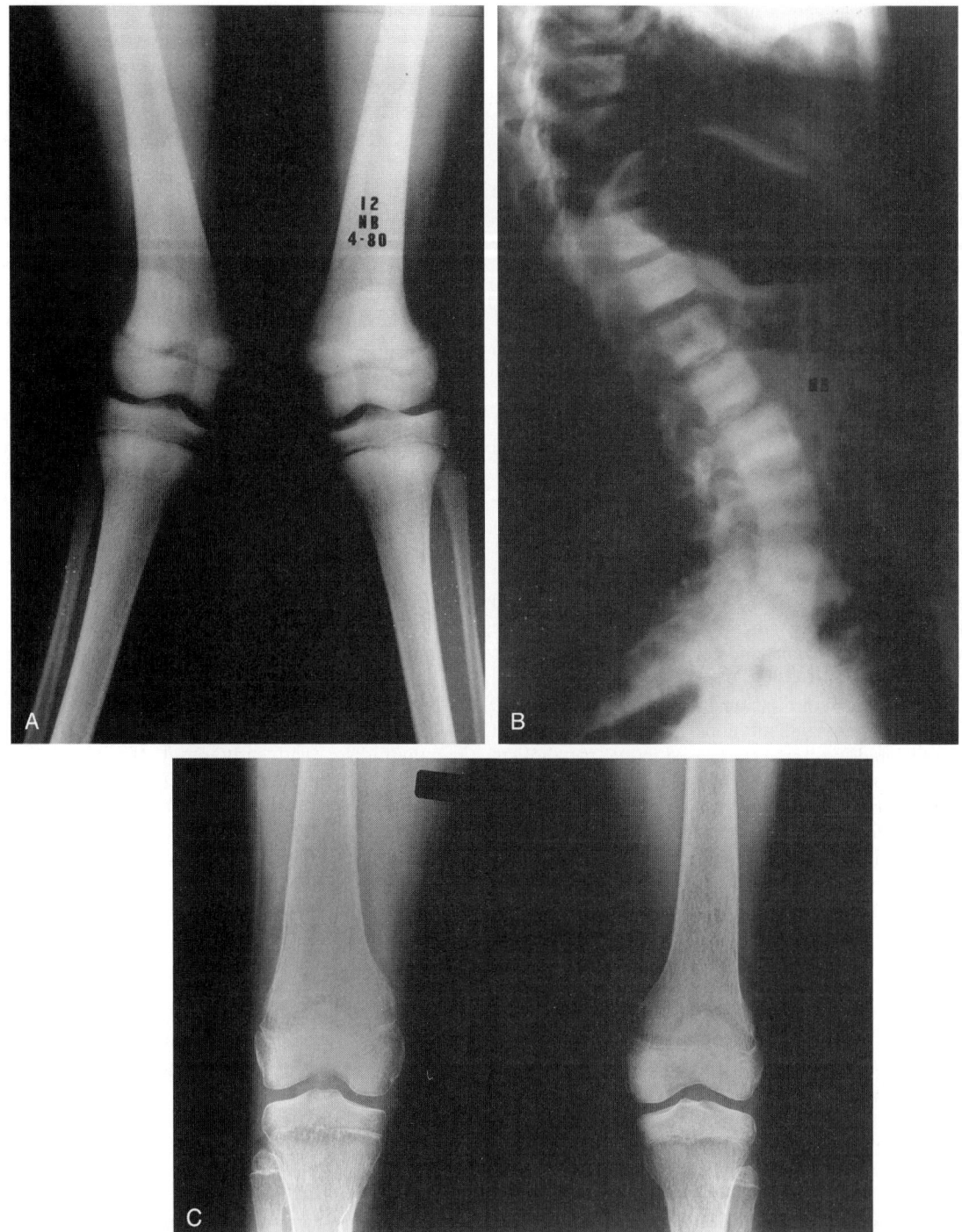

Fig. 5. Renal osteodystrophy. *A*, Anteroposterior radiograph of the lower extremities of a 12-year-old girl with chronic renal disease. Significant genu valgum, widening of the growth plates, and coarse trabeculation can be seen. *B*, Lateral view of the thoracolumbar spine of the same girl in Fig. 5A demonstrates the changes of alternating radiolucency with areas of osteosclerosis that is termed the "rugger-jersey spine." *C*, Anteroposterior radiograph of the knees of a 16-year-old boy with chronic renal disease demonstrating the osteosclerosis of the distal femurs and proximal tibias.

INVESTIGATION

Hyperphosphatemia, hypocalcemia, and hypermagnesemia are observed in undialyzed patients. With hemodialysis, serum calcium returns to normal. Serum PTH levels are elevated in most patients with end-stage renal disease. Patients with osteitis fibrosa tend to have higher levels of PTH than those with rickets/osteomalacia. Serum and plasma alkaline phosphatase levels are also elevated, especially in patients with severe secondary hyperparathyroidism. The serum alkaline phosphatase level falls with vitamin D therapy, and the enzyme level can be used to monitor the response to therapy. Radiographic features of renal osteodystrophy vary depending on the predominant disease process involved in the patient. Characteristic radiographic changes of all types include the "rugger-jersey spine" and osteosclerosis (Fig. 5B and C). Subperiosteal erosions, growth zone lesions in the metaphysis, brown tumors, and slipped epiphyses are typical of osteitis fibrosa. Rachitic changes are seen in patients with decreased bone metabolism and aluminum toxicity. In some patients, bone biopsy is useful to differentiate between different types of renal osteodystrophy and to determine the rate of bone formation (by dynamic tetracycline labeling). Bone biopsy can also confirm the presence of aluminum accumulation in the mineralization front.

MANAGEMENT

Management of renal osteodystrophy involves a multidisciplinary approach: achieving mineral homeostasis, controlling secondary hyperparathyroidism, preventing aluminum toxicity, treating skeletal deformities that are associated with decrease in function, and preventing complications such as avascular necrosis. Along with dialysis and renal transplantation, dietary manipulation, phosphate-binding agents, calcium supplementation, and vitamin D therapy have a role in maintaining normal levels of calcium and phosphorus and controlling the secondary hyperparathyroidism.[11] Parathyroidectomy may be beneficial for patients who do not respond to the conservative medical management. Aluminum toxicity is best managed by preventive measures such as decreasing the level of aluminum in the dialysate solution, using calcium carbonate instead of aluminum hydroxide, and decreasing dietary phosphate. In patients with aluminum toxicity, a chelating agent such as deferoxamine can be used to remove the aluminum. Orthopaedic problems, such as slipped capital femoral epiphysis and angular deformity of the lower extremities, should be managed initially by controlling the secondary hyperparathyroidism and the metabolic condition. Medical treatment alone can halt the progression of the slipped epiphysis.[13] When control of secondary hyperparathyroidism cannot be achieved within 2 months, surgical stabilization is warranted to prevent progression.[13] Unlike with idiopathic slipped capital femoral epiphysis of adolescence, single-screw fixation of capital femoral epiphysis in situ may not be adequate to prevent further slippage in uremic patients, who tend to be much younger at the time of the slip.[14] Concomitant medical therapy to control the metabolic disease is important to arrest progression of the slip after in situ pinning. In this situation, given the high prevalence of bilaterality, one should consider prophylactic pinning of the contralateral side. Whenever internal fixation is contemplated for fracture or osteotomy fixation, load-sharing devices such as intramedullary fixation should be used.

PSEUDOHYPOPARATHYROIDISM

CLINICAL FEATURES

The term pseudohypoparathyroidism (PHP) describes a heterogeneous syndrome characterized by hypoparathyroidism (hypocalcemia, hyperphosphatemia), increased plasma levels of PTH, and peripheral unresponsiveness to the biological actions of PTH.[15] These patients fail to show either a calcemic or a phosphaturic response to infused PTH. Two types of PHP have been described based on the patient's exact response to PTH. Among humans, PHP was actually the first disorder to be described that is characterized by diminished responsiveness to a hormone by otherwise normal target organs.

Some patients with PHP will also display resistance to multiple hormones that activate adenylate cyclase and express additional abnormalities such as hypothyroidism, hypogonadism, mental retardation, impaired olfaction, and a complex of characteristics referred to as Albright's hereditary osteodystrophy, including subcutaneous ossifications, brachydactyly, obesity, round facies, and short stature (Fig. 6).[15, 16] These multiple defects are believed to represent a generalized abnormality that impairs production of cyclic adenosine monophosphate (AMP) in all tissues (PHP type Ia).

PATHOGENESIS

The fact that cyclic AMP mediates many of the actions of PTH on kidney and bone led researchers to show that the unresponsiveness of these patients to infused PTH was due to a defect in the plasma membrane–bound adenylate cyclase complex that produces cyclic AMP in renal tubule cells.

INVESTIGATION

The PTH infusion test is the definitive diagnostic test for PHP. It enables the clinician to differentiate between the several variants of the syndrome. This test demonstrates the failure of the target organs (bone and kidney) to respond to PTH. The presence of Albright's hereditary osteodystrophy offers further evidence for the diagnosis.

MANAGEMENT

The pediatric endocrinologist will manage the diagnosis and treatment of this condition with the goal of maintaining a low- to mid-normal serum calcium concentration while avoiding hypercalciuria. Other hormonal dysfunctions should be searched for and addressed concurrently.

DIFFERENTIAL DIAGNOSIS

The clinical presentation of the child with type Ia PHP and Albright's hereditary osteodystrophy may be confused with the appearance of several genetic or neuromuscular conditions. The laboratory abnormalities (hypocalcemia and hyperphosphatemia) should lead to further investigations and referral to an endocrinologist.

IDIOPATHIC JUVENILE OSTEOPOROSIS

Idiopathic juvenile osteoporosis (IJO) is a rare disease affecting previously healthy prepubertal children. It presents between 8 and 14 years of age. A generalized decrease in bone mass (osteopenia) is observed in the absence of any known causes. Secondary forms of juvenile osteoporosis can result from prolonged anticonvulsant and glucocorticoid therapies, malabsorptive syndromes, endocrinopathies, inborn errors of metabolism (e.g., homocystinuria), and prolonged immobilization.

CLINICAL FEATURES

Previously healthy, prepubertal patients present with bone pain, low back pain, pain in the joints of the lower extrem-

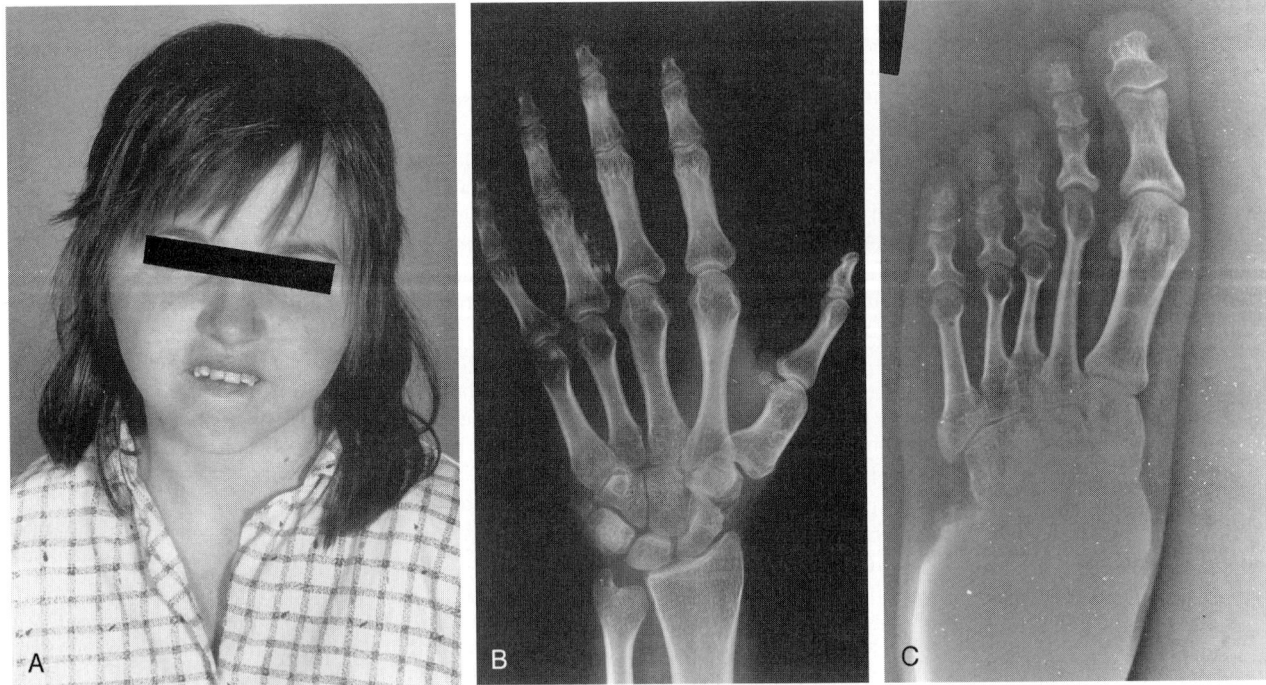

Fig. 6. Pseudohypoparathyroidism. This is a case of a 16-year-old girl with pseudohypoparathyroidism and Albright's hereditary osteodystrophy. *A*, Characteristic round facies. *B*, Anteroposterior radiograph of the left hand with shortening of the fourth and fifth metacarpals and three areas of subcutaneous ossification. *C*, Anteroposterior radiograph of the left foot demonstrating the shortening of the third and fourth metatarsals.

ity, feet pain, fractures after minimal trauma, or difficulty walking.[17] It affects more boys than girls (3 : 1), and family history is negative.[18] On physical examination, an increase in the thoracolumbar kyphosis, chest wall deformity, or angular deformities of the lower extremities may be found. The disease is usually self-limited, with spontaneous resolution at onset of puberty. The cause and the pathogenesis are unknown.

INVESTIGATION

Laboratory findings are variable. Serum calcium, phosphorus, and alkaline phosphatase levels are usually normal, but hypercalcemia, hypercalciuria, and elevated alkaline phosphatase activity have been reported in isolated cases. A negative calcium balance with increased fecal calcium level have also been reported. Vitamin D and calcitonin levels can be low to normal. Radiographic changes are characterized by severe osteopenia, increased thoracic kyphosis with biconcave vertebral bodies, and more involvement of the metaphysis than the diaphysis (Fig. 7).

DIFFERENTIAL DIAGNOSIS

The differential diagnosis includes osteogenesis imperfecta, secondary causes of osteoporosis, and Scheuermann's kyphosis.

MANAGEMENT

Given the self-limited course in most of the cases, a conservative treatment approach should be taken. Physical therapy and avoidance of prolonged immobilization after fractures are important components of any treatment plan. If specific biochemical abnormalities are found in the

work-up (e.g., low serum vitamin D or calcium malabsorption), calcium and vitamin D supplementation may be beneficial.[17] Correction of angular deformities may be indicated in those few patients in whom progressive deformities develop.

CAFFEY'S DISEASE (INFANTILE CORTICAL HYPEROSTOSIS)

CLINICAL FEATURES

Caffey's disease is an uncommon disorder with characteristic radiographic and clinical findings; it has been estimated to occur in 3 per 1000 patients younger than 6 months but seems to be decreasing in frequency. The typical child is younger than 6 months and presents with irritability, fever, and soft-tissue swelling and tenderness over the involved bones. Exacerbations and remissions can occur throughout the course of the disease. It is thought to be a self-limited condition that most often resolves without sequelae. Late recurrence and bony deformity have, however, been reported.[19]

PATHOGENESIS

The cause of Caffey's cortical hyperostosis remains unknown. Possible causes include infection (bacterial, viral, or fungal), inflammatory, metabolic, and genetic. Some studies have reported on families with several involved members.[19, 20] The theory that Caffey's disease represents the expression of a latent infectious agent promoted by another environmental factor[20] has similarities to a possible cause for Paget's disease of bone, which has been shown

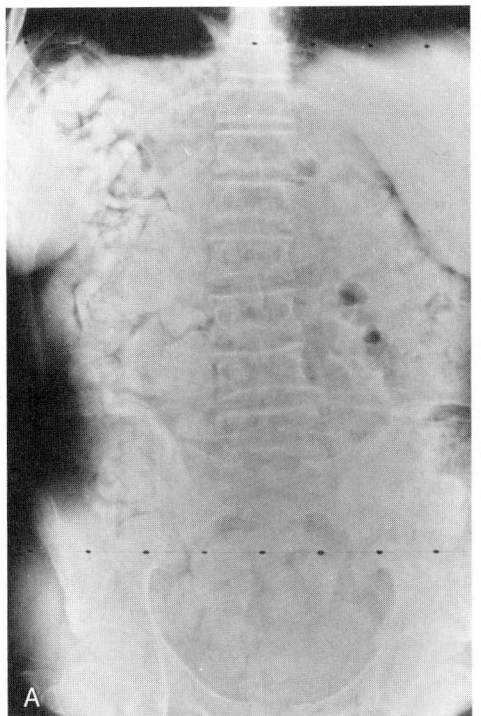
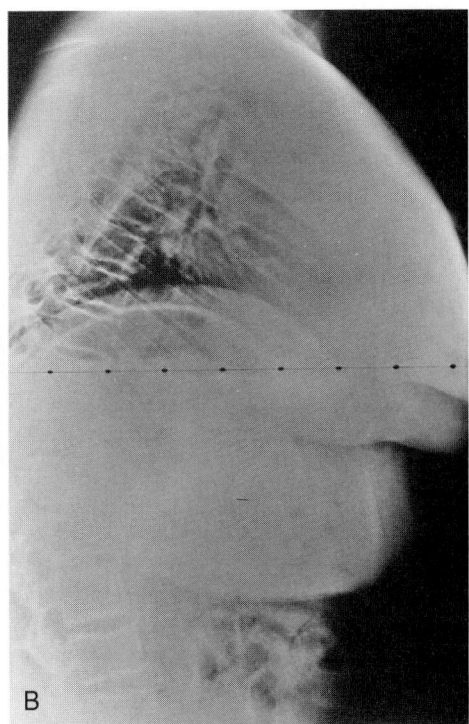

Fig. 7. Idiopathic juvenile osteoporosis. *A* and *B*, Radiographs of a 15-year-old boy with idiopathic juvenile osteoporosis of the thoracolumbar spine demonstrate flattening of the vertebral bodies with a biconcave appearance and increased kyphosis.

to have a strong familial occurrence and evidence for a viral cause (see Chapter 2–9).[22, 23]

INVESTIGATION

Laboratory findings include leukocytosis, anemia, elevated erythrocyte sedimentation rate, and elevated alkaline phosphatase. Radiographs reveal layers of periosteal new bone formation with cortical thickening of long bones (most commonly the humerus and ulna), the clavicles, and the mandible[24] (Fig. 8). Pleural effusions have been seen in children with lesions of the ribs.[19, 24]

DIFFERENTIAL DIAGNOSIS

The differential diagnosis includes trauma, osteomyelitis (particularly of the mandible), hypervitaminosis A, hyperphosphatemia, scurvy, infection (including syphilis), and

administration of prostaglandin E_1 and E_2 may resemble Caffey's disease radiographically. All of these conditions stimulate periosteal new bone formation.

MANAGEMENT

Treatment is supportive. Corticosteroids can be helpful in severe cases or during periods of exacerbation.[25]

SCURVY

Scurvy is caused by a deficiency of vitamin C (ascorbic acid), which is an essential factor for proper synthesis of collagen. This condition is now uncommon because of improved nutrition and vitamin C supplementation. It may be seen in infants who are fed heated cow's milk for a prolonged period without taking any juices or other products containing vitamin C. Heating can destroy vitamin C in the milk.

CLINICAL FEATURE

Nonspecific symptoms such as loss of appetite, irritability, and failure to thrive may be the earliest manifestation of scurvy. Gingival and subperiosteal hemorrhages can present later and are more indicative of scurvy. Patients with subperiosteal hemorrhage present with tender, swollen, and edematous extremities. Bone pain, tenderness, and fractures can be seen. Delayed wound healing and anemia are also observed.[26]

INVESTIGATION

Generalized osteoporosis and cortical thinning are seen on the radiographs. More specific radiographic manifestations of scurvy are subperiosteal elevation with new bone forma-

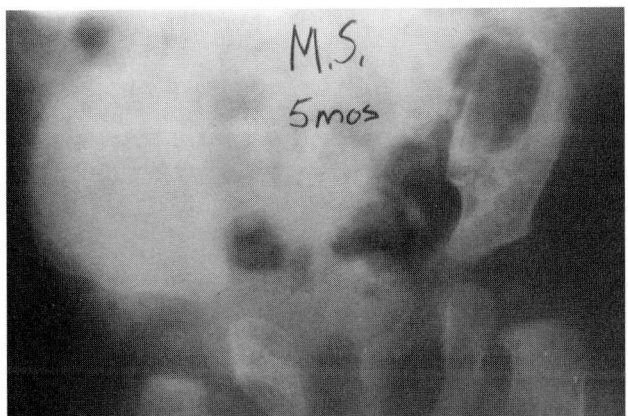

Fig. 8. Caffey's disease. This is an anteroposterior radiograph of the pelvis of a 5-month-old child with Caffey's disease involving the right iliac crest. Several other bones were involved simultaneously.

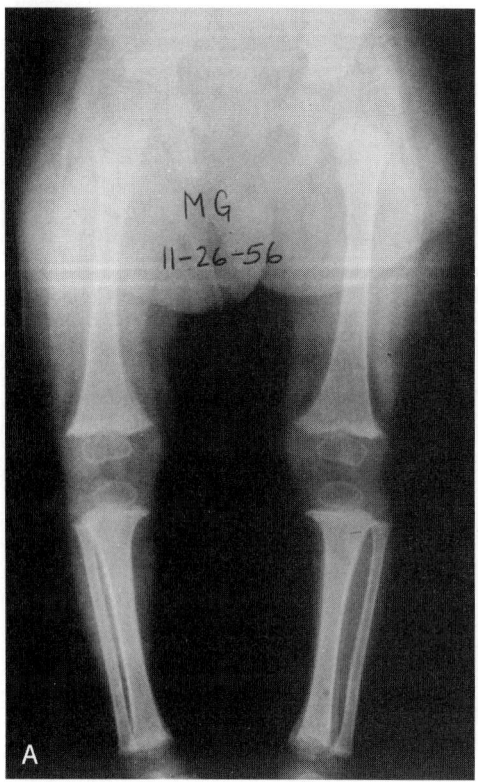
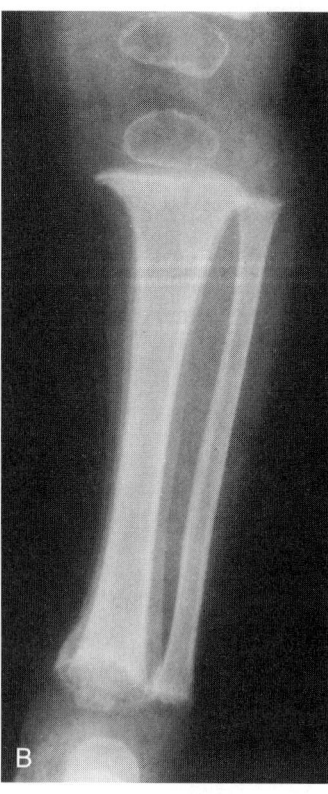

Fig. 9. Scurvy. *A,* Anteroposterior radiograph of the lower extremities of a 4-year-old child with scurvy. Note the lucent appearance of the epiphyses and the subperiosteal new bone formation along the left tibia. *B,* Close-up view of the left tibia with better detail of the periosteal elevation and new bone formation.

tion secondary to subperiosteal hematoma, epiphyseal separation, transverse metaphyseal lines ("scurvy line"), and a metaphyseal cleft at the peripheral junction of the metaphysis and physis ("corner sign") (Fig. 9A and B).[26]

MANAGEMENT

Patients recover rapidly with vitamin C administration.

ACKNOWLEDGMENTS

The authors would like to thank Claire Kenneally, MS, Nancy Pisciotto, RN, Janet Barber, Noelle Vallet, Susan Ellis, and the Media Resources Department of the Shriners Hospital for Children for their assistance with the preparation of this chapter.

REFERENCES

1. Thakker RV, Read AP, Davies KE, et al: Bridging markers defining the map position of X-linked hypophosphatemic rickets. J Med Genet 1987; 24:756.
2. Glorieux FH: Hypophosphatemic vitamin D resistant rickets. In Favus MJ (ed): Primer on the Metabolic Bone Diseases and Disorders of Mineral Metabolism. Kelseyville, CA, American Society for Bone and Mineral Research, 1990, p 182.
3. Rohmiller MT, Tylkowski C, Kriss VM, et al: The effect of osteotomy on bowing and height in children with X-linked hypophosphatemia. J Pediatr Orthop 1999; 19: 114.
4. Klein GL: Metabolic bone disease of total parenteral nutrition. In Favus MJ (ed): Primer on the Metabolic Bone Diseases and Disorders of Mineral Metabolism. Kelseyville, CA, American Society for Bone and Mineral Research, 1990, p 197.
5. Sedman AB, Klein GL, Merritt RJ, et al: Evidence of aluminum loading in infants receiving intravenous therapy. N Engl J Med 1985; 312:1337.

6. Ramage IJ, Howatson AJ, Beattie TJ: Hypophosphatasia. J Clin Pathol 1996; 49: 682.
7. Silve C: Hereditary hypophosphatasia and hyperphosphatasia. Curr Opin Rheumatol 1994; 6:336.
8. Pitt MJ: Rickets and osteomalacia. In Resnick D, Niwayama G (eds): Diagnosis of Bone and Joint Disorders. Philadelphia, WB Saunders, 1988, 2nd ed, p 2114.
9. Singer F, Siris E, Shane E, et al: Hereditary hyperphosphatasia: 20 year follow-up and response to disodium etidronate. J Bone Miner Res 1994; 9:733.
10. Hruska KA, Teitelbaum SL: Renal osteodystrophy. N Engl J Med 1995; 333:166.
11. Goodman WG, Coburn JW, Slatopolsky E, et al: Renal osteodystrophy in adults and children. In Favus MJ (ed): Primer on the Metabolic Bone Diseases and Disorders of Mineral Metabolism, first ed. Kelseyville, CA, American Society for Bone and Mineral Research, 1990, p 200.
12. Oppenheim WL, Salusky IB, Kaplan D, et al: Renal osteodystrophy in children. In

Castells S, Finberg L (eds): Metabolic Bone Disease in Children. New York, Marcel Dekker, 1990, p 197.
13. Loder RT, Hensinger RN: Slipped capital femoral epiphysis associated with renal failure osteodystrophy. J Pediatr Orthop 1997; 17:205.
14. Barrett IR, Papadimitriou DG: Skeletal disorders in children with renal failure. J Pediatr Orthop 1996; 16:264.
15. Levine MA: Parathyroid hormone resistance syndromes. In Favus MJ (ed): Primer on the Metabolic Bone Diseases and Disorders of Mineral Metabolism. Kelseyville, CA, American Society for Bone and Mineral Research, 1990, p 131.
16. Albright F, Burnett CH, Smith PH, et al: Pseudohypoparathyroidism: An example of the "Seabright-Bantam syndrome." Endocrinology 1942; 30:922.
17. Villaverde V, De Inocencio J, Merino R, et al: Difficulty walking. A presentation of idiopathic juvenile osteoporosis. J Rheumatol 1998; 25:173.
18. Castells S: Osteoporosis. In Castells S,

Finberg L (eds): Metabolic Bone Disease in Children. New York, Marcel Dekker, 1990, p 303.

19. Blank E: Recurrent Caffey's cortical hyperostosis and persistent deformity. Pediatrics 1975;55:856.

20. Bernstein RM, Zaleske DJ: Familial aspects of Caffey's disease. Am J Orthop 1995; 24:777.

21. Saul RA, Lee WH, Stevenson RE: Caffey's disease revisited. Further evidence for autosomal dominant inheritance with incomplete penetrance. Am J Dis Child 1982; 136:56.

22. Bataille R, Klein B: Etiology of Paget's disease of bone: A new perspective. Calcif Tissue Int 1992; 50:293.

23. Mills BG, Singer FR: Critical evaluation of viral antigen data in Paget's disease of bone. Clin Orthop 1987; 217:16.

24. Caffey J: Infantile cortical hyperostosis. J Pediatr 1946; 29:541.

25. Burg FD, Ingelfinger JR, Wald ER, et al (eds): Gellis and Kagan's Current Pediatric Therapy. Philadelphia, WB Saunders, 1996, p 223.

26. Tachdjian MO: Scurvy. In Pediatric Orthopedics. Philadelphia, WB Saunders, 1990, vol 2, p 918.

section 9 chapter 7

HEMATOPOIETIC CONDITIONS

Laurie O. Hughes and James Aronson

Summary

- Serious hematopoietic conditions may present initially to the orthopaedist with nonspecific musculoskeletal complaints.
- Radiographic changes are subtle.
- Collectively, these conditions may affect significant numbers of children each year.
- Marrow infiltration with abnormal cells or vascular compromise is the common pathway for this group of diseases.
- A high index of suspicion and knowledge of the appropriate work-up are keys to early referral and the judicious use of orthopaedic intervention.

LEUKEMIA

INTRODUCTION

Definition

Leukemia is a malignancy of the myeloproliferative system in which normal myeloproliferative cells are replaced by neoplastic hematopoietic tissue. Because of the location of the hematopoietic system within bone, bone pain is a common presenting complaint. Clinical and radiographic manifestations of leukemia in childhood may mimic a variety of orthopaedic disorders; therefore, leukemia must be considered in the differential diagnosis of any child with musculoskeletal pain or radiograph findings not fully explained by the clinical history and physical examination.

The acute forms of leukemia (acute lymphoblastic leukemia [ALL] and acute myelogenous leukemia [AML]) make up 98% of all childhood leukemias, as opposed to chronic myelogenous leukemia (CML), which is responsible for 2%.[1] Therefore, in this chapter we address the orthopaedic manifestations of the acute pediatric leukemias.

Historical Review

Heschl gave the first description of a leukemic skeletal lesion in 1854. Von Jaksch published the first radiographs of bone findings in acute leukemia (sclerosis and periosteal new bone formation) in 1901.[1] The so-called classic leukemic line, a linear metaphyseal lucency, was originally described by Baty and Vogt in 1935.[2] Radiographic evidence of leukemic bone involvement in pediatric patients at presentation has since been described by multiple authors, with a frequency ranging from 41% to 75%.[1]

Chemotherapy was introduced for the treatment of acute pediatric leukemia in the late 1960s, increasing the 5-year survival rate from approximately 4% to approximately 8%. By 1975, the 5-year survival rate of children with ALL had increased to 50%. At present the 5-year survival rate is 71%.[3]

Epidemiology

Leukemia is the most common form of childhood cancer, with an annual incidence of 40 per million. ALL represents 80% of pediatric leukemia cases; AML, 18%; and CML, 2%. The ratio of males to females is 1.44 to 1, and the ratio of whites to nonwhites is 2 to 1. The peak incidence of leukemia in children occurs at 4 years of age; those diagnosed at younger than 2 years or older than 10 years have a poorer prognosis.[1, 3]

PATHOGENESIS

Leukemia is the manifestation of cancerous proliferation of one of several different cell types (T cell, B cell). Mixed or undifferentiated types may rarely be seen. The T-cell type historically had the worst prognosis, although with newer chemotherapy regimens this is no longer the case. As the leukemic cells proliferate within the hematopoietic marrow, the child's small marrow reserve is quickly replaced by leukemic tissue. Bone pain results from massive proliferation of leukemic cells in the marrow and into the periosteum. Joint pain is the manifestation of referred pain from the metaphyseal periosteal lesion rather than from true joint disease (Fig. 1).

The hallmark of acute leukemia is the blast form, a relatively undifferentiated cell with diffusely distributed nuclear chromatin, one or more nucleoli, and basophilic cytoplasm. Under normal conditions, blast forms constitute fewer than 5% of the nucleated cells of the bone marrow; however, they predominate on bone marrow smears in leukemia (Fig. 2). They may usually be distinguished as lymphoid or myeloid blasts based on their morphology under

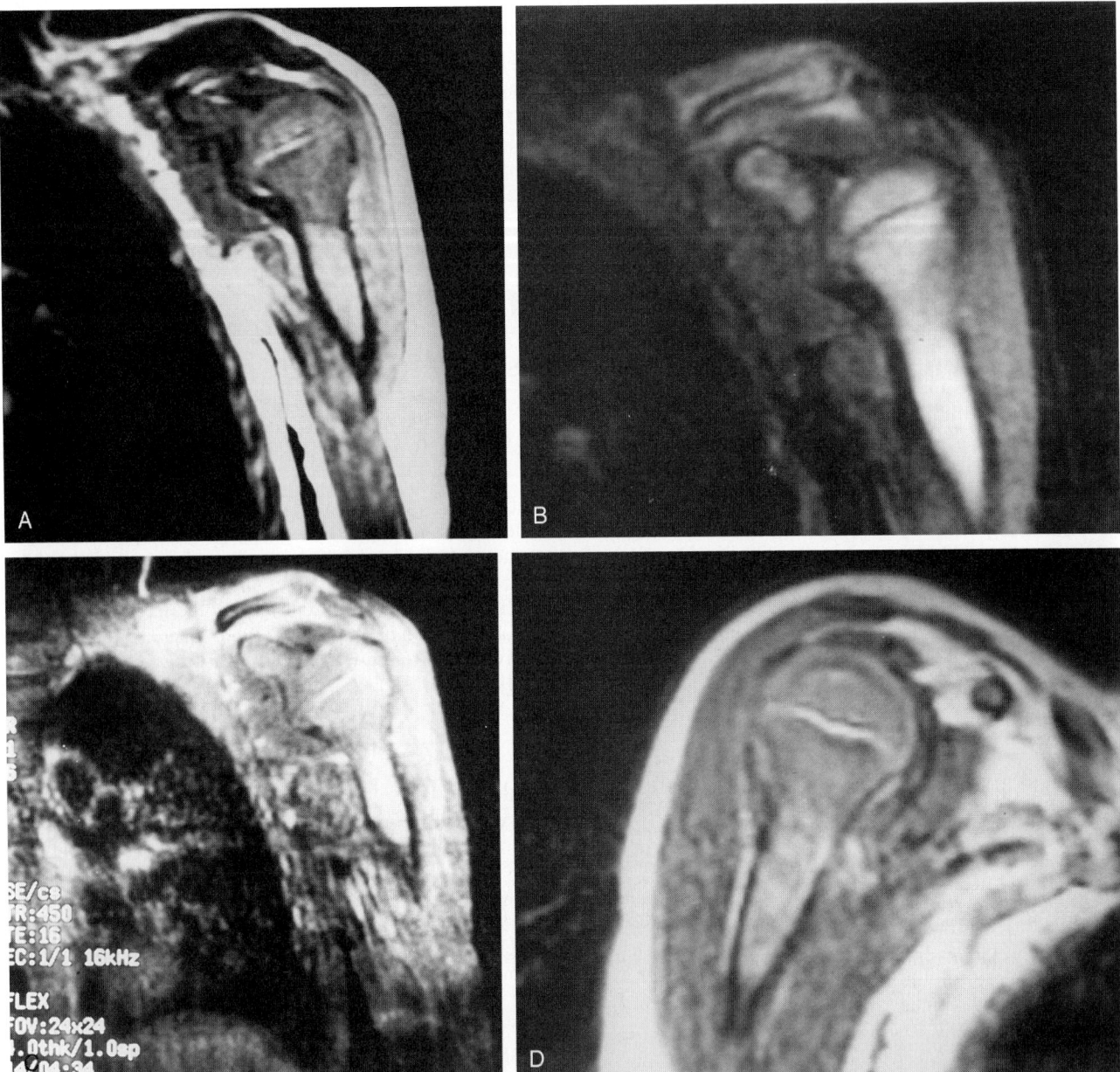

Fig. 1. Magnetic resonance imaging (MRI): leukemia. This is a case of a 5-year-old girl with left shoulder pain and decreased range of motion. MRI suggested a diffuse marrow abnormality and associated soft-tissue lesion before the diagnosis of leukemia. *A,* Coronal T_1-weighted image shows decrease of marrow signal throughout the left clavicle and proximal left humeral epiphysis and metaphysis. *B,* Coronal STIR image shows abnormal high signal intensity throughout the left clavicle and proximal left humerus. Associated high signal intensity in the soft tissues surrounding the left clavicle is seen compatible with aggressive cortical breakthrough. *C,* Postgadolinium fat-suppressed T_1-weighted image shows enhancement of the soft-tissue lesion surrounding the left clavicle. *D,* Coronal T_1-weighted image of the asymptomatic right shoulder shows abnormal low signal intensity of the proximal right humeral epiphyseal and metaphyseal marrow compatible with generalized marrow infiltration.

light microscopy. Wright/Giemsa–stained lymphoblasts typically have smooth, homogeneous nuclear material with indistinct nucleoli and only a small rim of light blue-staining cytoplasm, usually without granules. Myeloblasts have a lower nuclear/cytoplasmic ratio, more finely developed nuclear chromatin, and more distinct "punched-out" nucleoli. Cytoplasmic granules are more common and cytoplasmic inclusions (Auer's rods) are pathognomonic for AML. Cytochemical studies can further differentiate these leukemias into their various subtypes.[4]

CLINICAL FEATURES

Signs and symptoms include lethargy, pallor, purpura, fever, hepatosplenomegaly, lymphadenopathy, and bleeding tendencies. Bone pain is present in 21% to 59% of cases and is described as intermittent, localized, sharp, severe, and sudden in onset. It may be the only complaint at presentation in 20% to 33% of patients.[2] Night pain is common. Joint pain is manifested by arthralgia (which may be migratory) with or without arthritis. Sympathetic effusion may be present. Low back pain may be present

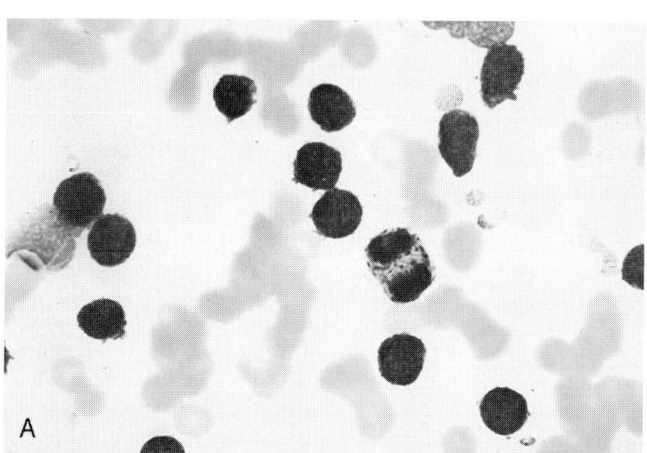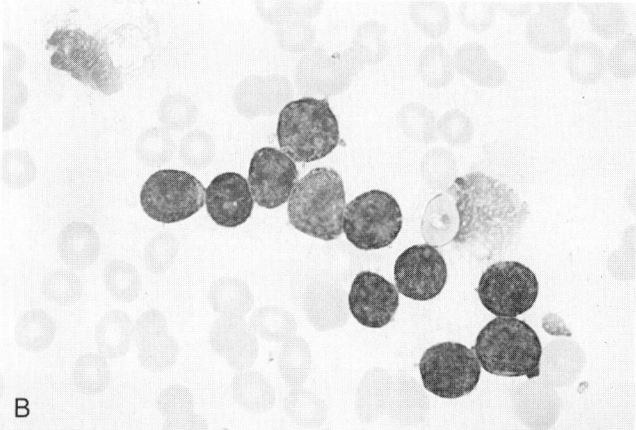

Fig. 2. Acute lymphoblastic leukemia (ALL). *A,* Hematoxylin and eosin (H&E) stain (×100) of bone marrow biopsy showing abundant uniform blue cells (lymphoblasts) predominating in the field, typical for ALL. A mitotic figure is present. *B,* Note homogeneous nuclei with finely dispersed chromatin, a small rim of blue cytoplasm and inconspicuous nucleoli.

secondary to osteoporosis and collapse of one or more vertebrae. Bone pain does not necessarily correlate with radiographic abnormalities. Each may be present in the absence of the other.[1]

INVESTIGATION

Roentgenographic findings at presentation have been reported to range from 41% to 75%.[1, 3] Bone changes eventually occur in 75% of patients during the course of this disease.[1-3] Typical radiographic findings in leukemia include osteopenia, lytic lesions, metaphyseal bands ("leukemic lines"), periosteal elevation, and sclerotic lesions. Pathological fractures occur, particularly in spine lesions. Aseptic necrosis is uncommon.

Osteopenia is the most common radiographic finding, occurring in up to 41% of cases. It is caused by infiltration of the normal bone marrow by leukemic cells and by altered bone metabolism resulting from chronic disease. Insufficiency fractures may result, particularly in vertebrae. Vertebral collapse indicates immediate neurological evaluation and intervention if necessary. Lytic lesions may be either geographic or permeative, occurring in up to 39% of patients. They occur more commonly in the metaphyses of long bones than in the flat bones. Their appearance in the small bones of the hands and feet should raise the possibility of leukemia as a diagnosis, because this seems to be fairly specific. These lesions are also potential sites of pathological fracture.[1] The presence of permeative changes may indicate a poor prognosis (Fig. 3).[3]

Metaphyseal bands were originally described in leukemia; however, they are found in a number of other chronic childhood diseases. They are more specific for leukemia after the age of 2 years. The band is a transverse area of decreased radiographic density adjacent to the physis (Fig. 4). A dense sclerotic band representing a growth arrest line occasionally occurs adjacent to the lucent band. These areas represent disruption of the normal growth process occurring at the physeal plates in the form of a generalized metabolic dysfunction. Periosteal elevation is seen in up to 50% of children with acute leukemia.[1, 3] It results from elevation of the periosteum by leukemic cells (see Fig. 3).

Sclerotic lesions are the most infrequent of the typical skeletal findings in acute leukemia, and pure osteosclerosis has been reported in 6% of patients,[2] whereas mixed sclerotic and lytic lesions have been identified in 18%. These lesions are usually metaphyseal and may be the result of simultaneous osteoblastic and osteoclastic activity in patchy areas within the bone.[1]

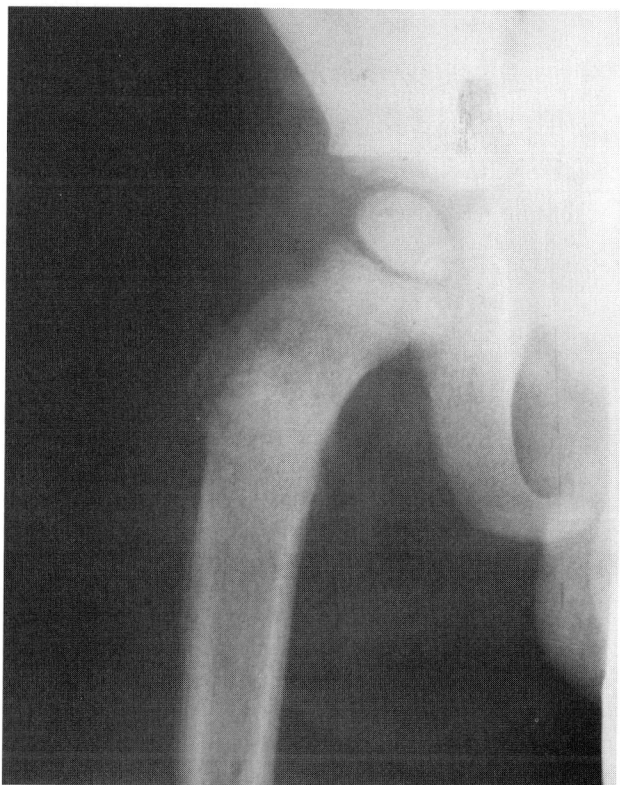

Fig. 3. Leukemic infiltration of bone. This is a case of a 5-year-old boy with right hip pain. Note the permeative pattern of lysis surrounding the greater trochanter and femoral neck. There is periosteal elevation along the lateral cortex. (Courtesy Joanna Seibert, MD.)

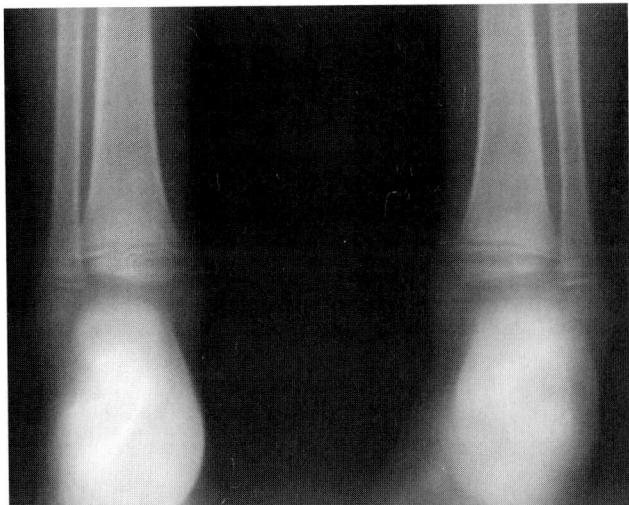

Fig. 4. Leukemic lines. These are leukemic lines proximal to distal tibial physis in a 3-year-old boy with acute lymphoblastic leukemia. Note the diffuse osteopenia throughout the distal tibias. (Courtesy Joanna Seibert, MD.)

Whether bone changes in acute leukemia signify a poor prognosis is controversial. Several authors independently concluded that no correlation exists between skeletal findings and survival rates, whereas others indicated that major skeletal involvement correlated with a better outcome. Heinrich, in a landmark study, reviewed 83 children with acute leukemia and found that children with one to four bone lesions have an "indolent" form of the disease and, therefore, have the highest survival rate (100% in his studies). Children without radiographic manifestations have a survival rate of 82%. They are thought to have a more aggressive form of the disease. Children with five or more skeletal lesions were also thought to have a more aggressive form of the disease (survival rate of 72%).[3]

On the basis of this information, a full skeletal survey is indicated in any child with a new diagnosis of acute leukemia. Baseline chest radiography is also indicated. Bone scanning does not correlate with symptoms or with prognosis.[5] Lesions may be "hot" or "cold" and do not differentiate the diagnosis from osteomyelitis or other malignancy. In one study, however, the presence of lesions was noted to help differentiate between the diagnosis of leukemia and rheumatoid arthritis.[5, 6] It may be helpful in directing attention to a specific site in the limping child.[7]

Laboratory work-up should include complete blood count (CBC) with peripheral smear and erythrocyte sedimentation rate (ESR). Bone marrow aspiration confirms the diagnosis. If the diagnosis is confirmed, chromosomal analysis should be performed to determine cell type. Spinal tap should be considered if central nervous system (CNS) involvement is suspected based on neurological examination. Anemia is present in most patients. Thrombocytopenia or thrombocytosis may be present. ESR is elevated in almost all cases. Peripheral white blood cell (WBC) count may be decreased, normal, or increased, although in ALL lymphocytosis predominates. Poor prognostic factors include WBC counts greater than 25×10^9/L, unfavorable phenotype,

age greater than 10 or less than 2 years, and more than five or fewer than one bony lesions on skeletal survey.[1, 3, 7]

DIFFERENTIAL DIAGNOSIS

Because the constitutional symptoms, laboratory findings (other than bone marrow analysis) and radiographic findings are generally nonspecific, the diagnosis of acute leukemia must be based on a high index of suspicion and the recognition of a clinical pattern that would be atypical for another disease. For example, the combination of fever, bone pain, increased ESR, and lytic lesions on plain radiograph is typical for osteomyelitis and demands aspiration of bone for confirmation of the diagnosis. A negative culture of the aspirate or a positive culture with subsequent failure of clinical response to antibiotics should raise suspicion of leukemia. Likewise, if septic arthritis is suspected based on arthralgia, fever, ESR, and effusion, lack of evidence of joint sepsis on aspiration or arthrotomy should also cause one to consider the diagnosis of acute leukemia. Fever, lymphadenopathy, hepatosplenomegaly, increased ESR, thrombocytopenia, anemia, decreased neutrophils, increased lymphocytes, blast cells on the peripheral blood smear, and an inconsistency between bone scan findings and clinical symptoms are important tip-offs in differentiating leukemia from sepsis.[2, 7]

The typical radiographic findings of leukemia may also be seen in Ewing's sarcoma, eosinophilic granuloma, metastatic neuroblastoma (or other metastatic childhood malignancy), primary lymphoma of bone, congenital hypoplastic anemia, and chronic granulomatous disease. The migratory nature of arthralgias and bone pain may confuse the diagnosis with that of juvenile rheumatoid arthritis or rheumatic fever. Bone scanning and radiographs may be helpful in this situation.

MANAGEMENT

Combination chemotherapy is the mainstay of treatment for acute pediatric leukemia. Current regimens for inducing remission consist of three or more chemotherapeutic agents, most often L-asparaginase and anthracyclines plus vincristine and prednisone. Methotrexate with or without cytarabine and hydrocortisone may be administered intrathecally for CNS involvement. Cranial irradiation may be used but is controversial. Further treatment phases after initial remission include intensification and continuation phases for a duration of at least 2 years. Bone marrow transplantation (BMT) is recommended for children who experience early relapse. Five-year event-free survival rates for ALL patients undergoing allogeneic transplantation are 30% to 50%. Patients with late relapse may respond to a second course of chemotherapy alone and are generally not considered candidates for transplantation. Autologous stem cell transplantation is currently being investigated. It carries the advantage of the absence of graft-versus-host disease (GVHD), but the risk of transplanting residual leukemic cells with the autograft.[4]

Musculoskeletal pain does not respond to salicylate treatment; however, the resolution of pain after chemotherapy or radiotherapy is a strong indicator of the effectiveness of treatment. Recurrence of bone pain at previous sites may be an indication of relapse. Bone lesions, particularly osteopenia and metaphyseal lucent lines, regress during peri-

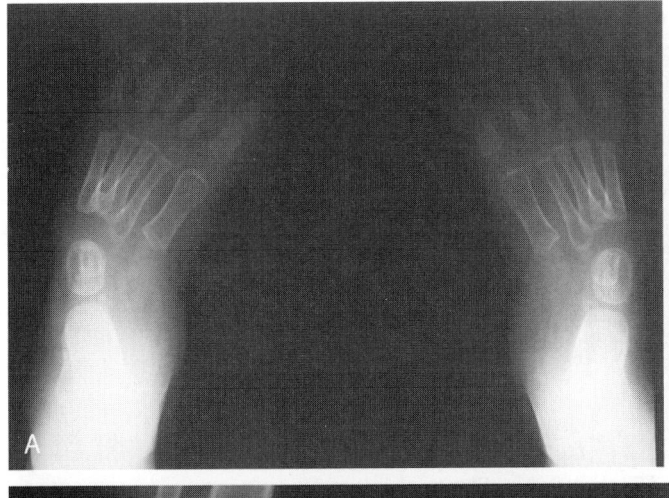

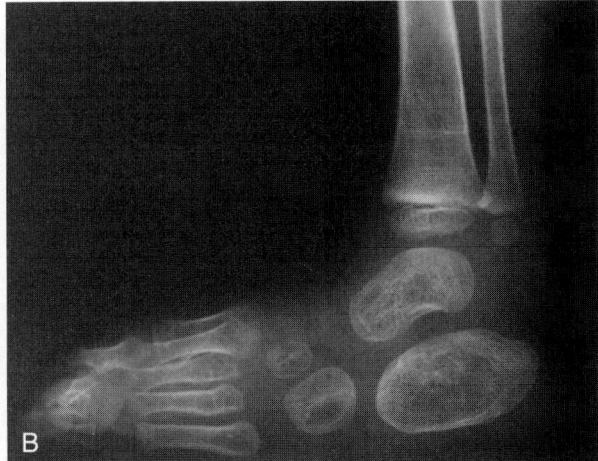

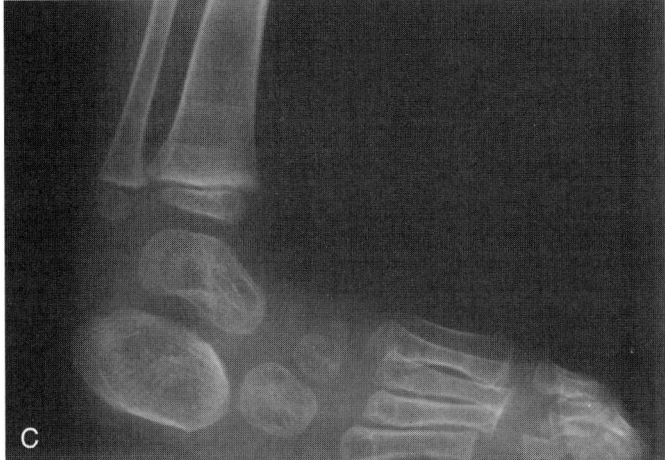

Fig. 5. Neurological complication of leukemia. *A*, Weight-bearing. Anteroposterior roentgenograms of both feet of a 3-year-old boy with acquired clubfoot deformity after vincristine-induced peroneal neuropathy. *B*, Weightbearing lateral of left foot. *C*, Weightbearing lateral of right foot. Note diffuse osteopenia and multiple "growth arrest" lines.

ods of remission. Pathological fractures should be treated using standard treatment methods.

COMPLICATIONS

Avascular necrosis may occur as a complication of chemotherapy and steroid treatment. Intrathecal leukemic infiltrates and the use of intrathecal methotrexate or other chemotherapeutic agents can produce a paraparesis with subsequent acquired musculoskeletal deformity. CNS involvement may also result in stroke with a subsequent hemi- or diplegic pattern. Vincristine is neurotoxic and may cause peripheral nerve paralysis, most commonly peroneal nerve palsy. Paresis should be treated with appropriate physical therapy and splinting and may be expected to resolve in some cases. Surgery should be considered for fixed deformity (Fig. 5).

RESULTS

The current 5-year survival rate for ALL is 86% and for AML is 24%.[3] Survival rate also appears to be related to the duration of symptoms before the initiation of treatment. As mentioned, bone pain regresses in response to treatment, as do most bone lesions seen on radiographs. Pathological fractures may be expected to respond to standard treatment within the expected time frame.

LANGERHANS' CELL HISTIOCYTOSIS

INTRODUCTION
Definition

Langerhans' cell histiocytosis (LCH) is a general term covering a spectrum of diseases that are manifestations of a nonneoplastic infiltration of normal tissue by cells of histiocytic origin. Although the disease may present in any form along the spectrum, there are three classic forms. Eosinophilic granuloma (EG) is a localized infiltration of bone by histiocytic cells. There may be single or multiple bony lesions, but there is no systemic involvement and the prognosis is generally good. Hand-Schüller-Christian disease involves children aged 3 years and older and includes bone lesions with or without soft-tissue extension and systemic involvement. Although many forms exist, the most classic triad for this disease is cranial bone defects, exophthalmos, and diabetes insipidus. It most commonly follows a chronic course. Letterer-Siwe disease is a fulminant form of the disease affecting children younger than 3 years. It is characterized by an acute course with multiple-organ involvement and an often grave prognosis. In any given patient, the possibility of conversion from one form to another exists.

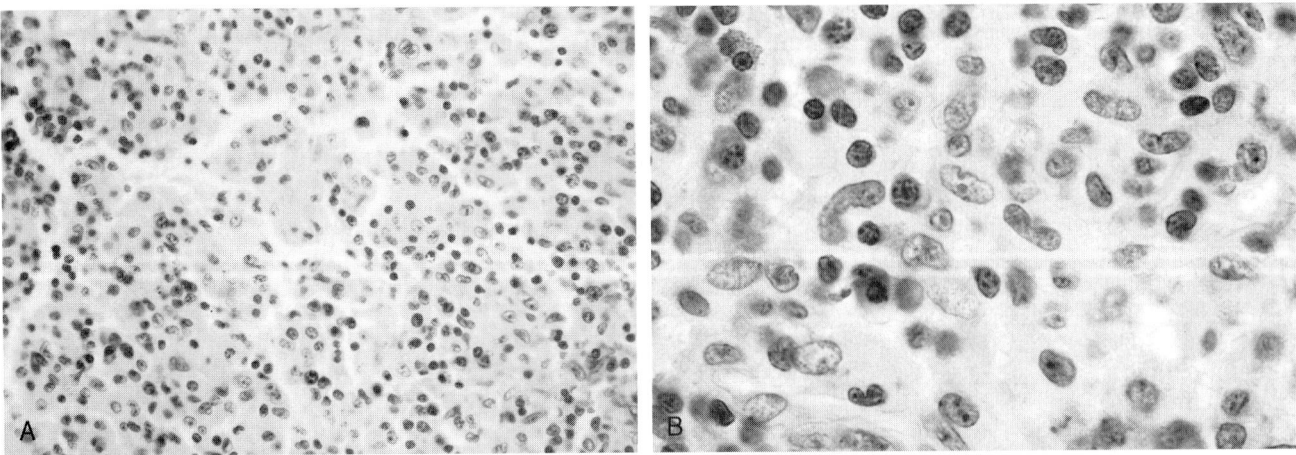

Fig. 6. Langerhans' cell histiocytosis. *A,* Hematoxylin and eosin (H&E) stain (×40). Sheets of histiocytes with large, clear, pink staining cytoplasm, giant cells, polymorphonuclear leukocytes (PMNs) and eosinophils are also seen. *B,* H&E stain (×100). Nuclear detail seen at this magnification includes oval shapes with characteristic nuclear grooves, finely dispersed chromatin, and distinct nucleoli. Cytoplasm is indistinct. Several giant cells and PMNs are present. An eosinophil is in the upper left corner.

Historical Review

LCH was first described as histiocytosis X by Lichtenstein in 1953. He recognized the three diseases as having a single histological appearance. In 1985, the term "Langerhans' cell histiocytosis" was recommended by the Histiocyte Society to replace the term "histiocytosis X."[8]

Epidemiology

LCH is a relatively uncommon condition with no obvious documented ethnic predilections. The frequency of disease has been estimated at two to five cases per million children per year.[9] Boys are slightly more commonly affected than girls.[10-12] Seventy to 90% of patients present with osseous lesions. The average age at presentation is about 6 to 7 years.[11, 12] Younger patients tend to have systemic involvement with a poorer prognosis.

PATHOGENESIS

Histiocytes are derived from bone marrow cells of the macrocyte/monocyte lineage. They come in many morphological forms, including foam cells, phagocytic macrophages, multinucleated giant cells, osteoclasts, and the typical Langerhans' cell.[13] Histologically, the lesion is distinguished by increased numbers of histiocytes with poorly defined cytoplasmic borders and an oval or indented nucleus. A central nuclear groove is characteristic. The chromatin is usually finely dispersed, and the nucleus may contain a small nucleolus. Some cells may show pleomorphism and hyperchromatism. Mitotic figures may be present, and a varying number of eosinophils, lymphocytes, or neutrophils may be seen. Occasionally, giant cells are present (Fig. 6).[9]

Pathological diagnosis of LCH is made by identification of specific inclusion bodies in the cytoplasm of these cells on electron microscopy and by positive immunostaining for S-100 protein and OKT6 antigen.[12] The trigger for proliferation of normal histiocytic cells into bony lesions is poorly understood. The disease may be an aberration of the immune system, resulting in poor regulation of histiocyte activation in response to some stimulus, possibly a virus.

Favara speculated that the activator, or cells that are subject to activation, are sequestered, most often in skin and bone, and that multisystem disease is a reflection of more extensive activation or loss of control of activation.[13]

CLINICAL FEATURES

The most common presentation of LCH is that of the solitary (or multiple) EG of bone. In this type, the patient typically presents with pain in a vertebral lesion, localized swelling in a flat bone (particularly the skull), or muscle wasting and limp because of a lesion in the pelvis or lower extremity. Pathological fracture may also be the presenting feature (Fig. 7). A simple EG may also present as an incidental finding on a radiological study done for another reason. Bone lesions are most commonly found in the skull, followed by the spine, ribs, lower extremities, pelvis, and upper extremities.

Systemic disease may be manifested as fever, rash, exophthalmos, respiratory disease, lymphadenopathy, anemia, hepatosplenomegaly, gingivostomatitis, or chronic otitis (with mastoid lesion). These may occur singularly or in association with each other or with a bony lesion. Diabetes insipidus is an important hallmark of systemic disease and may be the presenting complaint or may develop secondarily.[12]

INVESTIGATION

Hematological findings are highly variable. ESR may be moderately elevated. Anemia is common. Pancytopenia is rarer but should be considered evidence of hematological dysfunction and is a grave prognostic indicator. Radiographs show a rapidly destructive lytic lesion in the bone, most often in the skull, spine, or ribs (Figs. 8 and 9). There is generally no increased density in the peripheral bone. Satellite lesions may be present. In the flat bones and ribs, lesions may have a punched-out appearance. In the long bones, the metaphysis or diaphysis is most commonly affected. Epiphyseal lesions may rarely occur.[11] The osteolytic lesion may be surrounded by cortical scalloping and a moderate periosteal reaction. Vertebral lesions generally

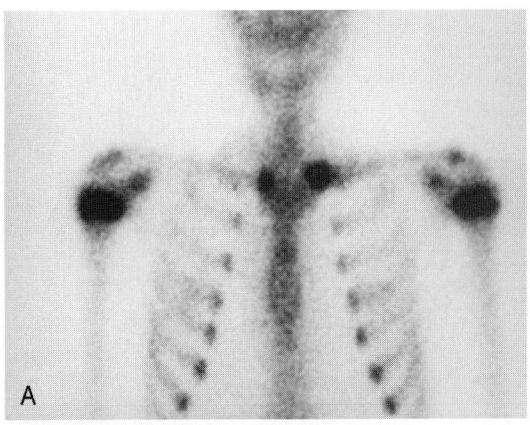

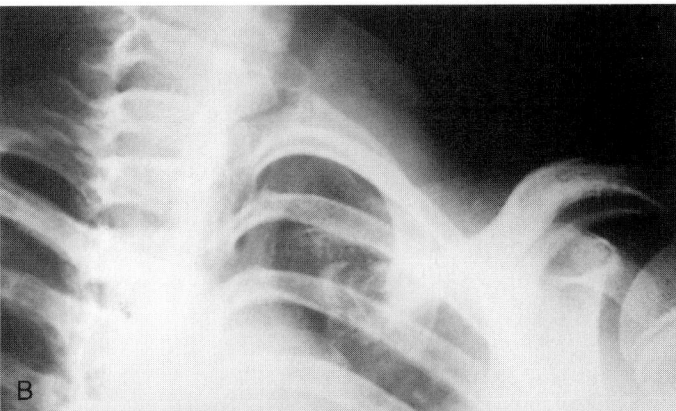

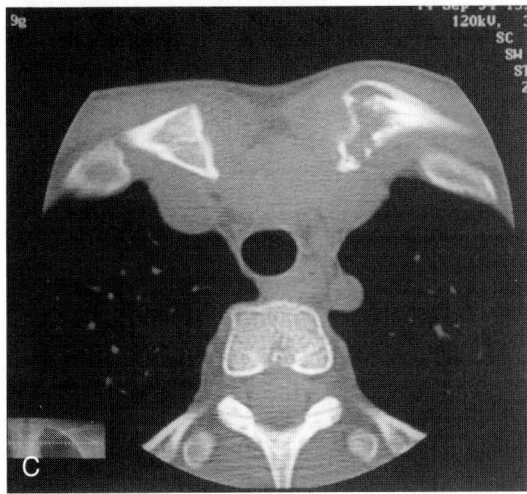

Fig. 7. Pathological fracture through eosinophilic granuloma (EG). *A,* Increased uptake on bone scan in the medial clavicle in this 11-year-old girl who experienced sudden chest wall pain while swimming. *B,* Oblique view of medial clavicle shows lytic lesion of the medial clavicle with pathological fracture. *C,* Preoperative computed tomography scan confirms bony destruction with cortical perforation in the medial clavicle. No adjacent soft-tissue mass was seen. EG was suspected in this otherwise healthy child. Biopsy confirmed the diagnosis.

spare the end plates and the perivertebral soft tissues, resulting in the presence of a typical vertebra plana (Fig. 10). Neural arches are involved less commonly. Sparing of the end plates portends a good prognosis for vertebral reexpansion.[11, 12, 14]

The diagnosis of LCH should be suspected based on the presence of a lytic lesion of the bone, particularly the skull or spine, with or without constitutional signs and symptoms described previously. Definite diagnosis can only be made histologically through biopsy of the lesion. Histological criteria include the proliferation of eosinophilic histiocytes on light microscopy, the presence of X bodies by electron microscopy, and positive OKT6 and S-100 protein immunology. At least two of these criteria must be present for diagnosis.[12] If multiple lesions are present, only biopsy of the most accessible lesion must be done. In the presence of typical vertebra plana with no other evidence of involvement, the diagnosis may be made presumptively and biopsy may be avoided, thus avoiding damage to the cartilaginous end plates.[11, 12] Lesions of the neural arch, however, require biopsy.

Once the diagnosis is established via biopsy, an investigation should be performed to detect the presence of other osseous lesions or systemic involvement. Complete ophthalmological, skin, gastrointestinal, and respiratory clinical exams should be performed. Work-up should also include CBC and ESR, ultrasound scan of the liver and the spleen, thoracic radiography, and examination of the urine for specific gravity. A careful neurological examination should be

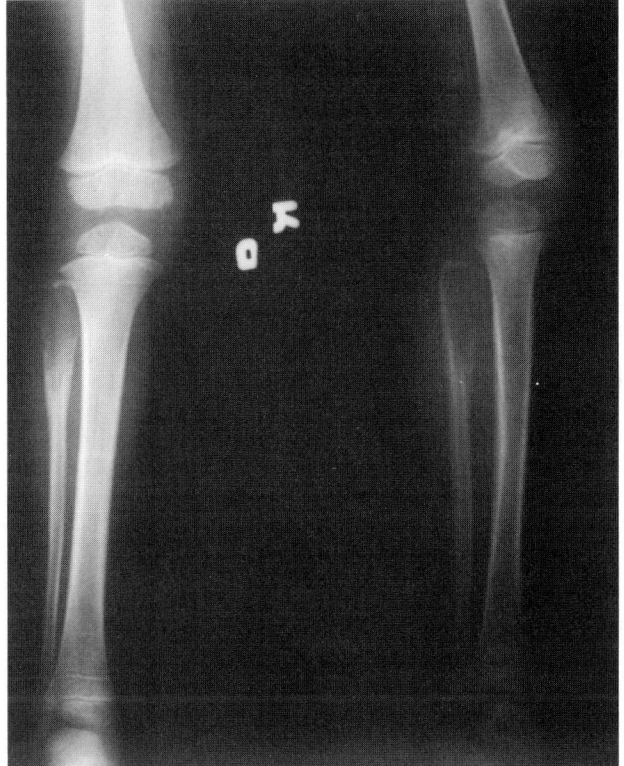

Fig. 8. Eosinophilic granuloma (EG). This moderately expansile lytic lesion in the proximal fibular metaphysis of a child is typical for EG/Langerhans' cell histiocytosis. (Courtesy Joanna Seibert, MD.)

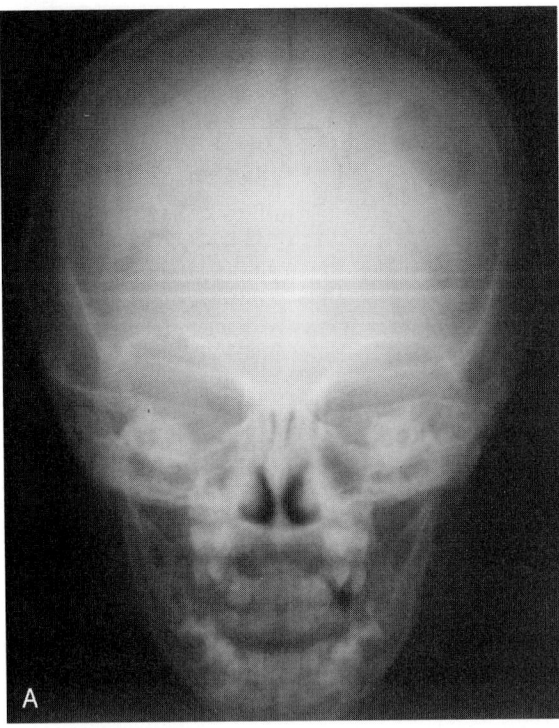
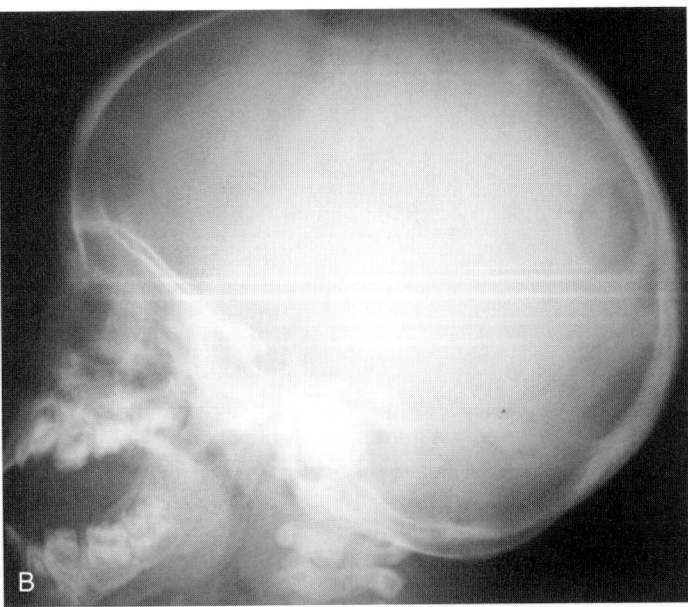

Fig. 9. Skull lesion in Langerhans' cell histiocytosis (LCH). *A,* Anteroposterior view of skull in a 1-year-old child. *B,* Lateral view of skull in the same child. There is a large lytic lesion typical for LCH. (Courtesy Joanna Seibert, MD.)

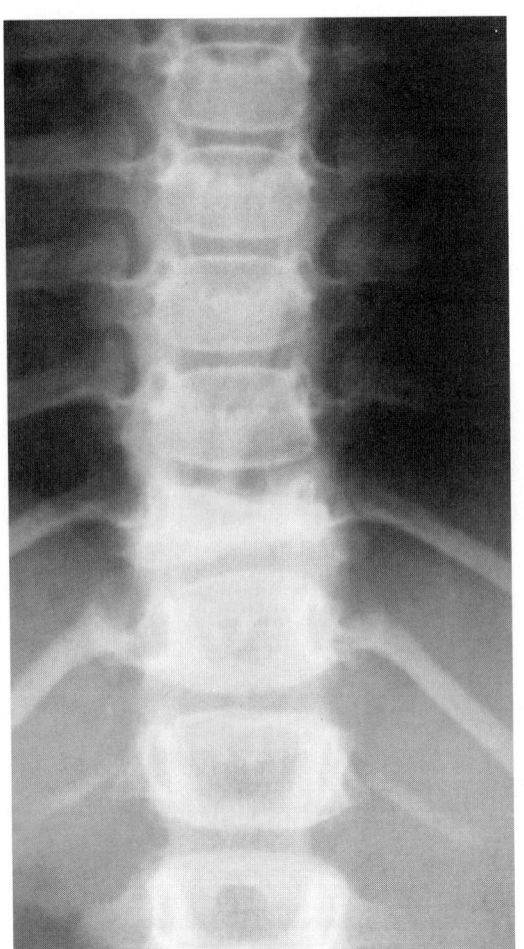

Fig. 10. Vertebra plana. Vertebra plana of T-10 resulting from Langerhans' cell histiocytosis. (Courtesy Joanna Seibert, MD.)

performed, particularly in the presence of skull or vertebral lesions.

Total skeletal radiography is indicated to search for the presence of other lesions. The use of technetium 99m (^{99m}Tc-methylene diphosphonate [MDP]) bone scintigraphy is controversial. Bone scanning is highly unreliable. Bollini reported five false-negative results (based on skeletal radiography); however, he noted finding seven lesions not present on radiograph in his series of 40 patients.[11] Sessa recommended skeletal survey only in the presence of negative findings on bone scan. In his series, however, 2 of 33 patients had positive findings on bone scan in the absence of a lesion on plain films and 4 of 33 patients had negative bone scans even though lesions were visible radiographically.[12] It appears, therefore, that the combined use of ^{99m}Tc-MDP bone scanning and skeletal radiography gives the most sensitivity for detection of multiple lesions. Computed tomography (CT) and magnetic resonance imaging (MRI) may be used to monitor lesions adjacent to critical structures (such as spine or skull lesions) for soft-tissue extension.

DIFFERENTIAL DIAGNOSIS

EG has been called the "great imitator" because, although it is technically a nonneoplastic process, its radiographic appearance is nonspecific and variable and mimics acute or subacute osteomyelitis, Ewing's sarcoma, leukemia, lymphoma of bone, or other malignant process. Nevertheless, there are a few clinical scenarios that are typical. Localization of lytic lesions in the skull should suggest the diagnosis of LCH, particularly in combination with diabetes insipidus (DI). Vertebra plana is another typical finding. The classic triad of exophthalmos, skull lesions, and DI is rarer but is typical for Hand-Schüller-Christian disease. In a child younger than 3 years, presentation may include primarily systemic symptoms with or without bony lesions. Osteomyelitis and leukemia should be high on the differential in this age group.

MANAGEMENT

Management of LCH is based on the clinical form and extent of the disease and its prognosis (Fig. 11). In the EG form, the prognosis is generally good. Bone lesions without systemic involvement tend to heal spontaneously, without any intervention at all. Asymptomatic isolated or multiple lesions should be treated with "watchful waiting." In lesions that are not easily accessible by an operation, such as vertebral lesions, or are progressive or recurrent after curettage, local injection of corticosteroids may be considered.[10, 12] Vertebral lesions should be treated with cast or brace immobilization until radiographically healed, even in the presence of neurological signs.[12, 14] Mammano et al[14] recommended at least 2 months of bedrest at the beginning of the immobilization period to avoid axial loading of the lesion.

In painful lesions, curettage and bone grafting may be indicated to facilitate rapid healing. Internal fixation with curettage and bone grafting may also be indicated in cases of pathological fracture or impending pathological fracture.

Although EG has an excellent prognosis, a small percentage of cases convert to the systemic form of the disease. Bollini, in his series and a review of the literature, reported a 7% transformation rate of solitary lesions to multiple ones and a 1% transformation rate of bone lesions to the generalized visceral form.[11] Because the likelihood of conversion decreases after the first year after diagnosis, a skeletal survey every 6 months for 2 years (possibly longer in younger patients) is recommended.[8] The prognosis for patients with systemic involvement is generally thought to be poorer than for those with bone lesions only. Lahey, in his series of 83 patients, reported mortality of greater than 50% in those who had organ dysfunction. Patient age is also an important prognostic factor. Patients younger than 3 years with the Letterer-Siwe form of the disease tend to have the most acute, fulminant course. Other poor prognostic factors include the presence of pulmonary lesions and hematopoietic dysfunction (pancytopenia). Both are more common in the Letterer-Siwe form of the disease. Thus, patients with extraosseous manifestations of any type should be more aggressively treated.

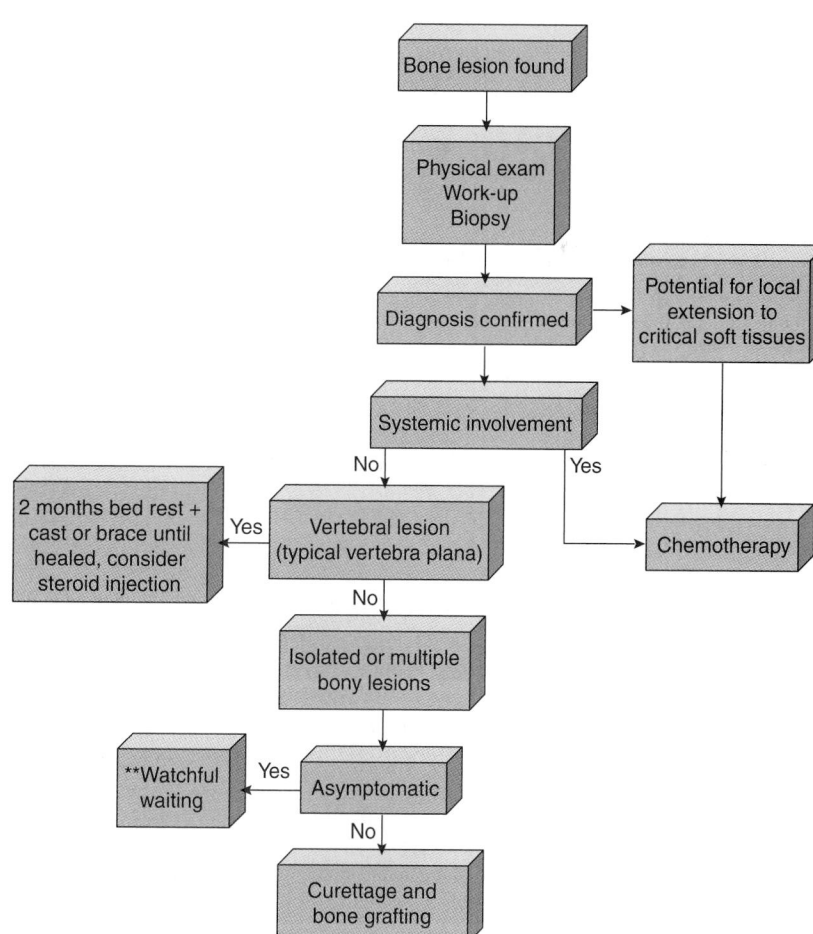

Fig. 11. Algorithm. This is an algorithm for management of Langerhans' cell histiocytosis.

** Internal fixation may be considered in cases of pathologic or impending fracture

Radiotherapy has been used in the past for patients with multifocal lesions; however, there is a risk of secondary malignant neoplasm. Additionally, some investigators reported no difference in the rapidity of healing of osseous lesions after radiotherapy.[11, 15] Radiotherapy is currently indicated for bone lesions only when the risk of curettage seems to be greater than the risk of radiotherapy. Chemotherapy is the mainstay of treatment for systemic involvement or, rarely, for an osseous lesion, which has a potential for rapid local extension to critical soft tissues, such as craniofacial or spinal sites. Prednisone and vinblastine have classically been used in the treatment of LCH, although other agents have been investigated.[12] Immunotherapeutic treatment has also been used with variable results.

COMPLICATIONS

Complications include the significant mortality rate already reported in patients with organ dysfunction. There is a strong association of DI with skull lesions. Neurological complications, although rare, have been reported as a result of direct compression of the spinal cord or nerve roots from extension of an adjacent osseous lesion, particularly in the cervical or upper thoracic spine. Epiphyseal lesions may extend across the growth plate but generally regress without damage to the physis. Curettage, however, may result in epiphysiodesis.[11] The rate of secondary malignant neoplasm after radiotherapy to bone lesions has been reported as 5%.[12] Theoretically, radiotherapy could also result in local destruction of growth plates in the zone of therapy.[12, 14] Chemotherapy and high-dose corticosteroids have the obvious complications of osteonecrosis (ON), neutropenia, infection, and death from overwhelming sepsis.

RESULTS

Overall, a benign outcome may be expected in 80% to 90% of patients with LCH.[12] Patients with solitary or multiple bone lesions are not at high risk for disease progression; thus, their prognosis is excellent. The prognosis for patients with systemic involvement is mentioned previously. Survival rate for Letterer-Siwe disease has improved from 30% to 63% with the use of modern chemotherapy.

SICKLE CELL DISEASE

INTRODUCTION
Definition
Sickle cell disease (SCD) is a general term that includes various forms of hereditary hemoglobinopathies characterized by the presence of the abnormal hemoglobin (Hgb) S. Sickle cell trait describes the heterozygous form in which both the Hgb A and Hgb S are present. It is largely asymptomatic. Sickle cell anemia refers to the homozygous state of Hgb S and generally results in the severest form of the disease, which is manifested as a chronic hemolytic anemia. SCD refers to several heterozygous forms of hemoglobinopathy in which Hgb S is present along with another abnormal gene for the structure of hemoglobin (Hgb C, β-thalassemia, or Hgb D).

Historical Review
SCD was first described by Herrick in 1910, who published his findings of sickled cells in a 20-year-old black man. In 1925 *Salmonella* osteomyelitis was reported in a patient with SCD by Carrington and Davison. The association of the two was recognized by Hodges and Holt in 1951.[16] In 1960, Sir John Dacie wrote that SCD was a disease of childhood and that few patients ever reached adult life. In a 1994 study of 3764 patients, Platt et al[17] documented a median age at death of 42 years for men and 48 years for women with sickle cell anemia and 60 years for men and 68 years for women with SCD.[17] Thus, as medical care has improved over the last 30 years, life expectancy has increased, and the population of patients experiencing orthopaedic complications of SCD has increased as well.

Epidemiology
The Hgb S gene is found predominantly in the black race, although it may less commonly be found in persons of Mediterranean descent. The incidence of the mutant allele for Hgb S in the black population of the United States is 8%; however, only about 1 in 40 has the homozygous state. Sickle cell anemia occurs in approximately 1 in 500 black children in this country.[18]

PATHOGENESIS
The abnormal Hgb S is characterized by substitution of glutamic acid by valine at the sixth position of the β globin chain. The substitution results in polymerization of Hgb under conditions of low oxygenation. As the Hgb polymerizes, RBCs assume an abnormal "sickle" shape, resulting in thromboembolic infarcts in the microcirculation of bone. This phenomenon is more likely in areas of the bone where the circulation is terminal and oxygen concentration is low. Stasis, hypoxia, and necrosis are the result. Perivascular fibrosis has also been noted in the bone marrow of patients with sickle cell anemia, and its presence increases with age. The contribution of this perivascular fibrosis to necrosis and infarction is unknown.[19, 20] A chronic hemolytic anemia is the result of destruction of the sickled red cells. As a response to this, erythoblastic activity increases with consequent expansion of the bone marrow cavity.[21]

Fetal Hgb (HbAF) is gradually replaced by sickle cell Hgb (HbSS) within the first year of life. The important contribution of retained HbAF in the adult circulation is discussed later.

CLINICAL FEATURES
Pain is the most common manifestation of SCD and is the result of underlying marrow ischemia or necrosis. Patients experience sudden, unrelenting pain in the affected bone. Fever, local tenderness, pain with range of motion, and occasionally swelling may be present. Pain crises are more frequent after the age of 3 years. After skeletal maturity, the frequency of symptoms decreases. Patients with Hb SS have much more frequent pain crises than do those with other variants. Precipitating factors include air travel, high altitude, stress, infection, and physical exertion. The common denominator for all of these is an increase in oxygen requirement.

Children with SCD are often well below the mean for height and weight, and skeletal maturity is delayed. Many, however, eventually have a normal growth spurt and are able to obtain at least average height. The mechanism for the delay in skeletal maturity is not understood.

Dactylitis, also known as hand and foot syndrome, may be the earliest manifestation of SCD. It occurs in 30% to 60% of patients and presents between the ages of 6 months and 4 years with painful, tender swelling of the hands or feet. Episodes are significantly more common during the colder months of the year. It is caused by infarction of the marrow of the small bones of the hands and feet. The hands are affected principally, with bilaterality in 50%. Fever is present in 55%.[22] Leukocytosis and elevation of the ESR are common. Dactylitis has not been reported after the age of 6 years, coinciding with the disappearance of hematopoietic marrow in the hands and feet. Radiographs may show some periosteal elevation after several days. Although dactylitis complicated by osteomyelitis is rare, high temperature, extreme tenderness, warmth and redness, or failure to resolve after hydration, analgesia, and warm compresses should suggest the possibility of osteomyelitis.[20, 23, 24]

Leg ulcers may present in late adolescence or early adulthood. They typically appear on the distal medial aspect of the tibia or posterior to the medial malleolus and begin as a small depression with central necrosis. If neglected, they can widen to encircle the entire lower leg. They are thought to be due to increased venous pressure caused by the expanded blood volume in the hypertrophied bone marrow. Poor tissue perfusion probably also plays a role.

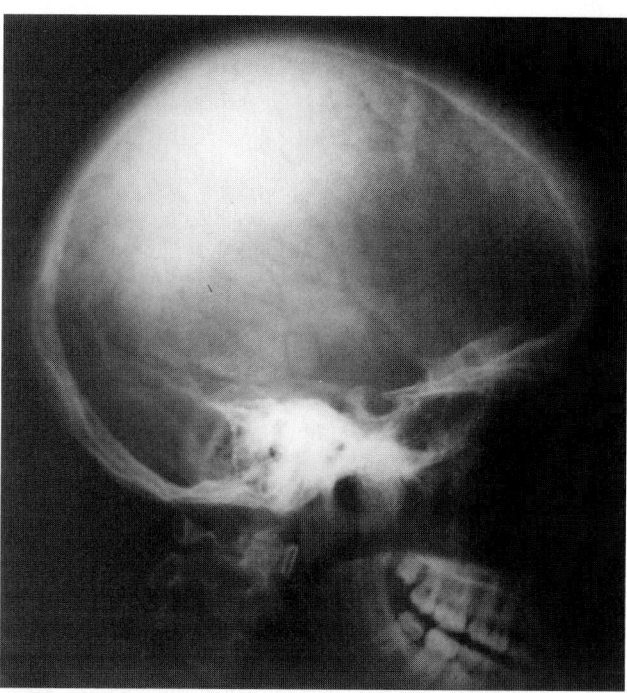

Fig. 12. "Hair-on-end" phenomenon. This is a lateral skull film showing "hair-on-end" phenomenon, a result of increased hematopoiesis in the skull causing peripheral radiation of the bony trabeculae. This finding is also typical for thalassemia. (Courtesy Joanna Seibert, MD.)

INVESTIGATION

Plain radiographic changes consist of two types: those related to marrow hyperplasia and those related to infarction and avascular necrosis.

Marrow hyperplasia results in increased size of the medullary spaces, thinning of the cortices, and osteoporosis. The calvarium demonstrates widening of the diploic space and may show a "hair-on-end" appearance as a result of peripheral radiation of bony trabeculae (Fig. 12). The effect of acute infarct cannot be seen on immediate plain radiographs; however, if severe, it may appear 7 to 14 days after the initial episode. Evidence of infarction includes lytic lesions, periosteal elevation, osteosclerosis, and necrosis of the epiphyseal region such as femoral and humeral heads.[25] The appearance of a lytic lesion with periosteal elevation suggests infarction but may be difficult to differentiate from acute osteomyelitis. Radiographic findings in dactylitis appear at about 14 days, much later than the subsidence of clinical findings with appropriate treatment. They include osteoporosis, periosteal elevation, coarsening of the trabeculae, and thinning of the cortex. These findings typically resolve 3 months to 1 year after onset.[21]

Characteristic changes in the vertebrae on plain film include osteoporosis and coarse trabeculation. A characteristic feature is flattening of the vertebral body with depression of the end plates so that a typical "fish vertebra" is produced.

Bone scanning has been suggested in differentiating acute infarct from osteomyelitis.[21] ^{99m}Tc-MDP scanning should show increased uptake in areas of osteomyelitis, although it is less consistently positive in areas of bone infarction.[26] Certainly, the presence of a "cold" bone scan

does not rule out infection but may indicate diaphyseal necrosis from an encircling, subperiosteal abscess. Keeley and Buchanan emphasized that because the efficiency of radionuclide scans has not been proved and because they are inconvenient and expensive and involve exposure to radioisotopes, their routine use is not justified for the diagnosis of osteomyelitis in patients who have SCD. Epps et al,[23] however, noted the usefulness of technetium or gallium scanning in the localization of multiple sites when osteomyelitis is suspected.

MRI has been used experimentally to document the appearance of the bone marrow in patients with SCD, and it may be used clinically in the detection of early ON of the femoral or humeral heads when there is pain in the absence of radiographic collapse (Fig. 13). Further clinical use of MRI, however, is not helpful.

Laboratory values in SCD are frequently abnormal. Anemia is common, and frequent transfusions may be required. A mild leukocytosis and elevation of the ESR may be present in acute infarct, particularly in dactylitis, even in the absence of osteomyelitis. Blood cultures should always be drawn in the event of a painful crisis if osteomyelitis is suspected.

DIFFERENTIAL DIAGNOSIS

Now that newborn screening of cord blood is performed in many areas, the condition of SCD is commonly known at birth. The first clinical manifestation is dactylitis, or less often, acute bony infarct. In this situation, the differentiation between infarct and osteomyelitis can present a difficult diagnostic dilemma.

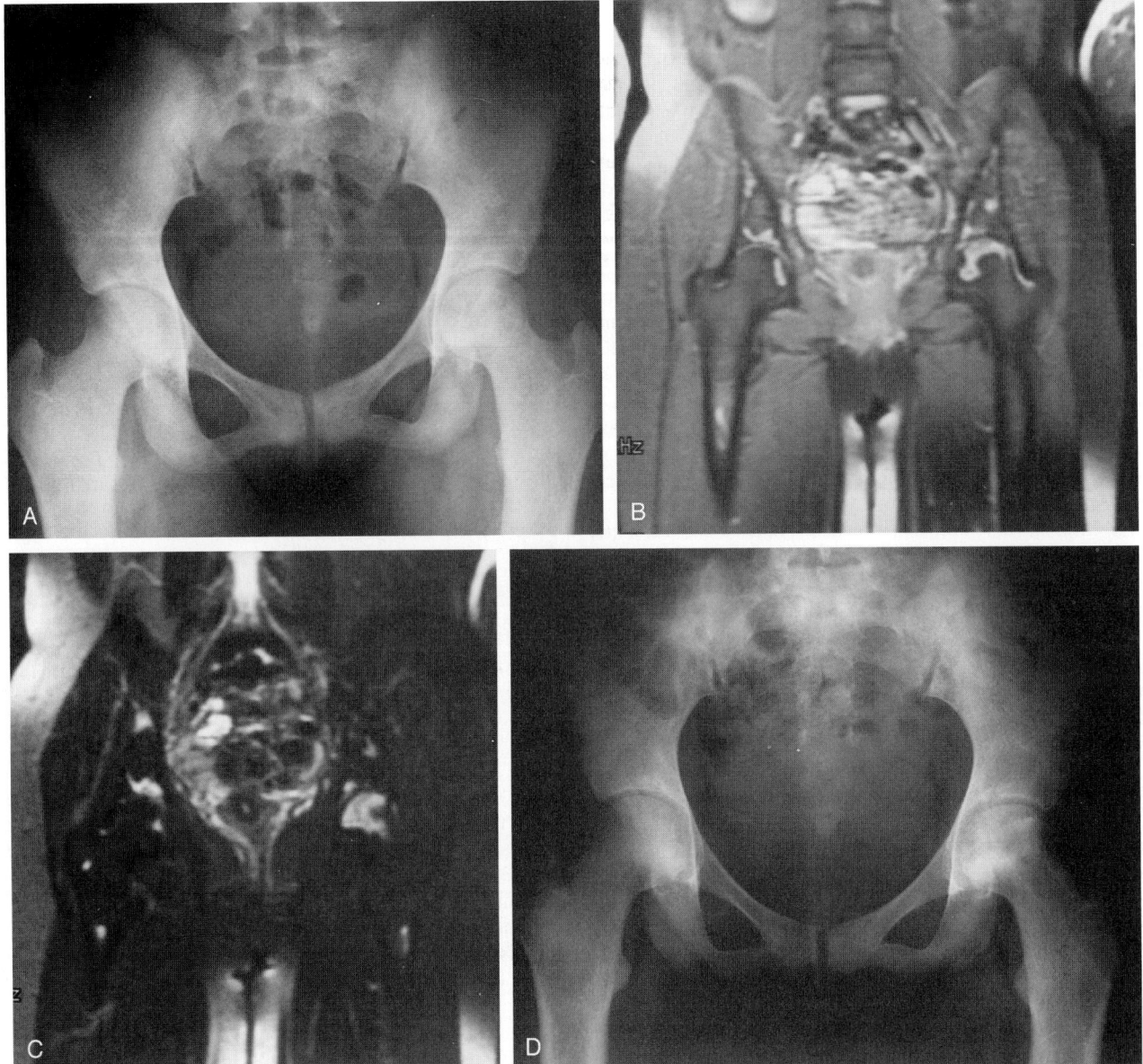

Fig. 13. Osteonecrosis (ON) of the hip in sickle cell disease. *A,* Plain anteroposterior pelvis of stage I ON in an 18-year-old woman with sickle cell anemia. There was no obvious evidence of ON on radiograph film; however, the patient complained of left hip pain. *B,* Coronal fast-spin echo proton density image with fat suppression shows extensive irregular high signal intensity throughout the proximal left femoral epiphysis. More localized signal abnormality within the medial portion of the proximal right femoral epiphysis is seen adjacent to the fovea. These changes are compatible with bilateral asymmetric osteonecrosis. Note additional high signal intensity lesion in the proximal right femoral diaphyseal marrow probably relating to the site of bone infarct. *C,* Coronal fast-spin echo T$_2$-weighted image with fat suppression shows more striking abnormal signal intensity throughout most of the proximal left femoral epiphysis compared with lower signal intensity of the adjacent metaphysis. *D,* Collapse of femoral head several months after core biopsy for stage I ON.

Osteomyelitis complicating SCD is primarily a disease of childhood. Most studies report a prevalence of *Salmonella* as the most common infecting organism (74% to 87% of cases)[16, 27] although in Epps' series *Staphylococcus* was most common.[23] *Klebsiella, Proteus,* and *Pseudomonas* have also been reported.[28] The prevalence of osteomyelitis complicating SCD in the United States is low, between 0.2% and 5.4%.[26] Nevertheless, osteoarticular infection can result in dire complications in this patient population, and its presence must always be suspected. Several tip-offs may

be helpful in differentiating osteoarticular infection from acute vaso-occlusive crisis.

1. Uncomplicated sickle cell crises with musculoskeletal pain should resolve in 3 to 7 days with hydration and anti-inflammatory medication. Failure of resolution of the crisis should suggest a diagnosis of infection.[26]
2. Generally, patients with osteomyelitis have a more pronounced clinical appearance of having a systemic infection and seem to be sicker than those having an acute bony infarction.[23]

3. Although leukocyte count and ESR can be elevated in both uncomplicated pain crises and osteomyelitis, osteomyelitis should cause a higher temperature and leukocyte count than pain crisis. ESR is unreliable in making the diagnosis but, in the case of osteomyelitis, can be monitored for response to treatment.[23, 24]

4. Blood cultures should be performed on every patient with severe enough acute pain crisis to warrant admission. A positive culture combined with bone pain establishes the diagnosis of osteomyelitis.

5. Cultures of stool for *Salmonella* species should be done.[23, 24]

6. Plain roentgenograms should be made of all bones thought to be involved and should be repeated at 10 to 14 days. Films will be negative in the first 7 to 14 days in both pain crisis and osteomyelitis. Lytic lesions and periosteal elevations that appear later in vaso-occlusive crisis may mimic osteomyelitis, but their presence at this stage in the face of continued symptoms should precipitate aspiration of the bone. A sequestrum seen on plain films is an obvious marker for osteomyelitis (Fig. 14). The presence of vertebral collapse beyond the usual fish mouth deformity on plain films should suggest the possibility of osteomyelitis, LCH, or even metastatic cancer.[20]

7. As discussed previously, the use of technetium and gallium scanning is controversial and may not help in the differentiation of osteomyelitis from bone infarction. In Epps'[23] series, however, they were helpful in localizing multiple sites of osteomyelitis, especially in the pelvis and spine.

8. Although sympathetic joint effusions may occur if bone infarcts involve the epiphyses of bone, aspiration should be performed to rule out septic arthritis (including gonococcal), inflammatory arthritis, gout, and Lyme disease.[20]

ON secondary to sickle cell anemia is ordinarily not confused with Legg-Calvé-Perthes disease (LCPD). LCPD tends to occur in children between 3 and 10 years of age, whereas ON secondary to SCD occurs in children older than 10 years. LCPD is more common in white children than in blacks and in boys than in girls, whereas ON of hemoglobinopathy is more common in blacks, with an even sex distribution. LCPD typically involves a large amount of the epiphysis and some of the metaphysis,

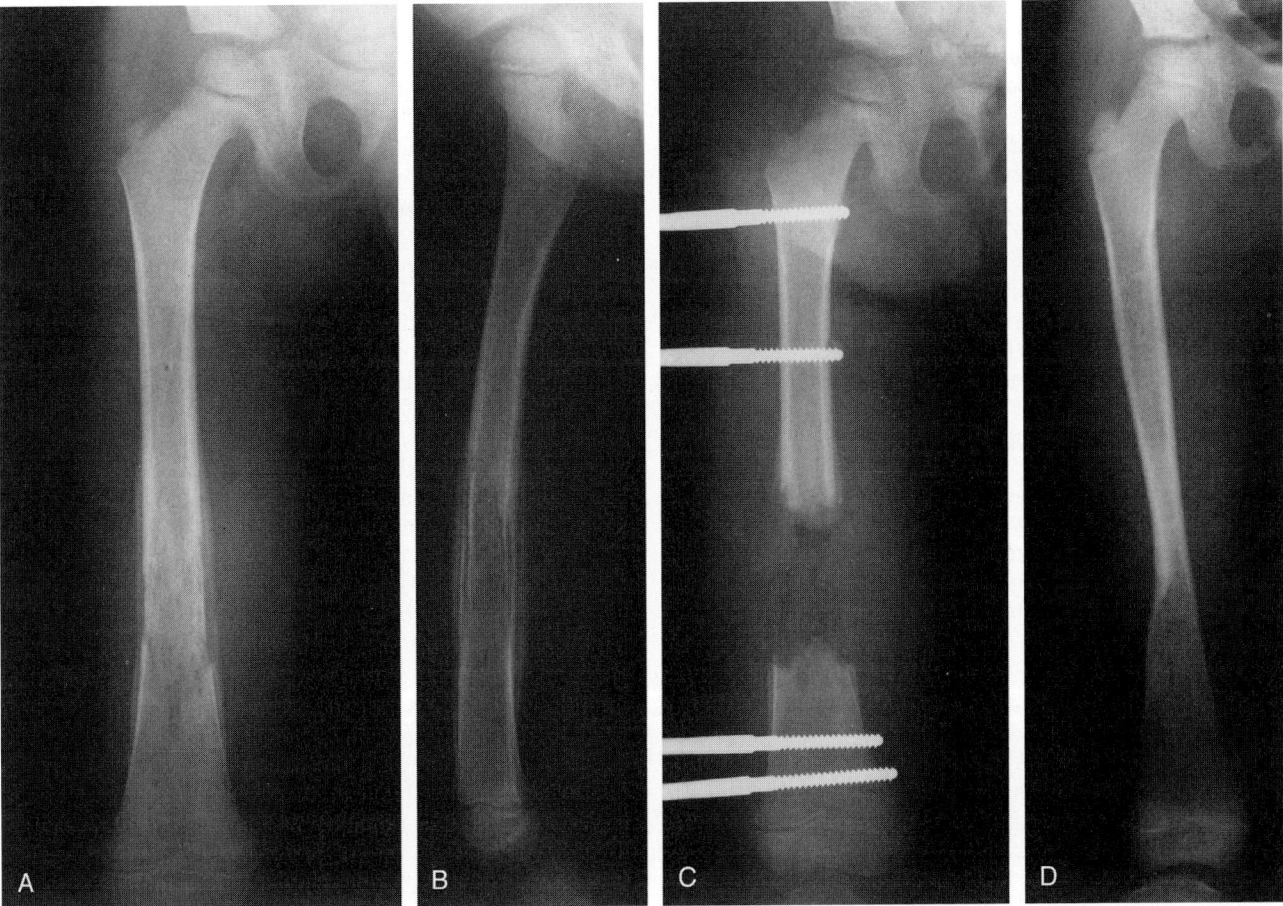

Fig. 14. Osteomyelitis in sickle cell disease (SCD). *A* and *B*, Anteroposterior and lateral roentgenograms of the femur in a 3-year-old girl with sickle cell anemia. This patient was treated for 3 weeks for pain crisis before referral for failure of symptoms to resolve. Note the diaphyseal location of the lesion, more typical for osteomyelitis in SCD than for acute hematogenous osteomyelitis in a normal child. The presence of the sequestrum surrounded by periosteal new bone (involucrum) results in a "bone-within-a-bone" appearance. *C*, This child was treated with external fixation and diaphysectomy in addition to long-term intravenous antibiotics. Cultures grew *Salmonella*. *D*, The patient eventually experienced reconstitution of the missing portion of her femur.

whereas ON of SCD usually involves a limited portion of the epiphysis and spares the metaphysis.

MANAGEMENT

Acute musculoskeletal pain crises should be treated with rest, hydration, oxygen therapy, nonsteroidal anti-inflammatory medications, and judicious use of narcotic analgesia. Warm compresses may be helpful. If the joint is involved, it should be splinted for a short time in the functional position and then gradually mobilized as symptoms subside. Most patients may be treated on an outpatient basis; however, occasionally admission for intravenous hydration is required. Fetal hemoglobin appears to have an inhibitory effect on Hgb S polymerization. Platt et al[29] found a correlation between low fetal hemoglobin levels and high pain rates. They also identified low fetal hemoglobin levels as a risk factor for early mortality.[17] The use of hydroxyurea to stimulate production of fetal hemoglobin is currently being investigated.[17, 29]

BMT has been used with modest success in Europe for young, symptomatic patients with SCD who have a human leukocyte antigen–compatible relative. GVHD is a serious potential complication of this procedure.[30]

Osteomyelitis should be managed with prompt operative decompression of the involved area. Antibiotic treatment should be withheld until Gram's stain and culture of the purulent material have been obtained. Initial empiric antibiotic treatment should include ampicillin or chloramphenicol combined with cefazolin or nafcillin until culture and sensitivity are determined. Consultation from a hematologist and an infectious disease specialist is recommended. Parenteral therapy should be continued for 6 to 8 weeks (see Fig. 14).

Special attention should be paid to the preparation of the SCD patient for surgery (Table 1). If an uncomplicated elective case is contemplated, the patient should receive preoperative transfusion with enough normal blood to raise the level of Hgb A to 60%. Fluids should be given during the preoperative period of fasting at 1½ to 2 times the usual hourly maintenance rate.[23] Hypothermia should be avoided. Close monitoring of oxygen tension and pH is mandatory perioperatively and intraoperatively. Partial pressure of oxygen (PO_2) should be kept at 95 mm Hg or above, and pulse oximetry should exceed 97%. Hematocrit level should ideally be kept to between 28% and 34%.[31] Hydration and oxygenation should be continued for at least 24 hours postoperatively to prevent sludging of sickle cells

in the glomeruli with resultant acute renal failure. Preoperative hematology and anesthesia consultations are recommended.

Tourniquets should be used with caution in these patients, because the local ischemia and vascular stasis they produce may precipitate sickling. In the absence of infection, the extremities should be completely exsanguinated before inflation of the tourniquet. Tourniquets should not be used in any operation for infection. Otherwise, preoperative preparation for the drainage of abscess is the same as for elective surgery. Leg ulcers should be treated with elevation and local wound treatment. Débridement may be necessary for large areas of necrosis. Protection of the ulcer with a soft sponge-rubber doughnut and a low-pressure elastic bandage may be beneficial. If ulcers persist despite aggressive local wound care, transfusion therapy and split-thickness skin grafting may be necessary. Oral zinc sulfate may also be beneficial. If facilities are available, consideration should be given to hyperbaric oxygen treatments to increase local tissue oxygenation.[18] The management of ON is described later.

COMPLICATIONS

Complications of SCD, besides acute pain crises and bone infarcts, include acute chest syndrome and pathological fracture, anemia, pyomyositis, and ON. The two primary orthopaedic complications of SCD are osteomyelitis (discussed previously) and ON.

ON affects primarily the femoral and humeral heads. As the RBCs sickle in the femoral capillaries, vaso-occlusion, anoxia, osteocyte death, and necrosis result. Intramedullary pressure may be increased by subsequent repair processing, leading to further bone resorption and collapse.[32]

The prevalence of ON of the femoral heads varies according to age and genotype. Among those with the HgSS genotype, the prevalence is 9% to 21% depending on the presence of the α-thalassemia gene. Those homozygous for α-thalassemia have a higher risk. Patients in the older age groups with SCD or sickle–β-thalassemia disease are at high risk for ON (older than 45 years). High hematocrit level, low fetal hemoglobin level, and frequent vaso-occlusive crises are also risk factors for the development of ON. The disease is bilateral in 54% of patients.[32] Although ON is uncommon among children younger than 15 years, patients having ON in childhood are likely to experience coxa magna, coxa plana, coxa breva, osteochondritis dissecans, and acetabular dysplasia.[33]

TABLE 1. PERIOPERATIVE CONSIDERATIONS IN SICKLE CELL PATIENTS		
Preoperative	**Intraoperative**	**Postoperative**
Hematology consultation	Avoiding hypothermia	IV at 1½ to 2 times maintenance
Anesthesia consultation	$PO_2 \geq 95$ mm Hg	Maintain oxygenation 24–48 hours
Transfuse until Hgb A = 60%	O_2 sat $\geq 97\%$	
Preop IV at 1½ to 2 times	Hct 28–34%	
Maintenance	Maintain neutral pH	
Broad-spectrum perioperative antibiotics (single dose)	Avoid tourniquet if possible	

Hgb, hemoglobin; PO_2, partial pressure of oxygen; O_2, oxygen; Hct, hematocrit; IV, intravenous.

Treatment of early ON includes rest, protected weight-bearing, and pain control with nonnarcotic pain medicines. Narcotic pain medicines should be used judiciously. Core decompression of Ficat stage I and early stage II disease has been proposed,[32] although only one study reported the results of this procedure in patients with SCD, and all three of their patients failed, requiring arthroplasty within 1 year.[31] Osteotomy may be an option in patients with a limited area of collapse (Fig. 15). Hernigou et al,[34] in 1993, reported injection of bone cement into the femoral head of 10 painful hips with early collapse. There were only two failures requiring revision at 5 years, and perioperative complications were minimal. Fusion is to be condemned because of the potential for bilaterality. Hemiarthroplasty is prone to failure because of soft acetabular bone.[31] Total hip replacement is considered to be the most reliable method of treatment of femoral head ON in carefully selected patients with severe disabling pain. Although results are favorable overall in terms of pain relief [35, 36] the high early and late complication rates are well reported.[33, 35–40]

ON of the humeral head in SCD is also age and genotype dependent. The prevalence is 2.7% in patients younger than 25 years, increasing to 20% in patients older than 35 years. Patients with Hgb SS and Hgb S–β-thalassemia are at highest risk. The presence of α-thalassemia is also a risk factor. Interestingly, about 79% of patients are asymptomatic at diagnosis. The disease is bilateral in 67% of patients, and there is a strong association of ON of the humeral head with ON of the hip. Treatment is symptomatic. Shoulder arthroplasty may be required for severe disabling pain, although Milner et al[41] reported only one shoulder arthroplasty in his series of 149 patients with ON of the humeral head.

Pathological fracture has been reported as a complication of long bone osteomyelitis in SCD. The incidence is higher in gram-negative infection. Ebong[28] reported treatment of the fractures conservatively, with casting or traction, plus treatment of the underlying osteomyelitis in the usual manner. Pyomyositis has also been reported as a complication of SCD, possibly secondary to infection complicating myonecrosis resulting from vascular occlusion.[42]

RESULTS

The overall failure rate of total hip arthroplasty in patients with SCD has ranged from 31% to 63%.[31, 35, 37, 38, 40] Hanker and Amstutz[40] reported that a failure rate of 50% could be expected by 5.4 years postoperatively. Nevertheless, five of their eight patients had significant pain relief. Bishop et al[35] reported good results in eight of 11 patients despite a high infection rate. "Good results" were based on improvement in the Harris Hip Score, including marked pain relief. Their revision rate was 33% at 7 years. Hickman and Lachiewicz[36] reported 13 primary and revision cementless arthroplasties. Nine had excellent or good clinical results at a mean follow-up of 6 years (revision rate of 33%). Clarke et al[31] reported a 59% revision rate at a mean follow-up of 6 years; mean hip scores improved from 11.5 of a possible 40 to 24.6. They called their results "mediocre."

The most common cause of failure is aseptic loosening. This may be due primarily to intraoperative difficulty in achieving optimal fixation. Areas of previous infarct may be sclerosed, causing eccentric reaming or even obliteration of the medullary canal. Adjacent nonsclerosed areas tend to be soft and of poor quality secondary to underlying bone marrow hyperplasia; thus, the risk of perforation and femoral fracture is high. The disease is ongoing, so even a well-fitted component is subject to loosening as a result of changes in the periprosthetic bone. The advantage of cementless over cemented implants is currently a matter of debate. In Hickman and Lachiewicz's[36] series of cementless arthroplasties, there were no early or late infections at a mean follow-up of 6 years, but a high rate of osteolysis (31%) was noted. Clarke et al,[31] Moran,[38] and Acurio and Friedman[37] also noted a lower incidence of femoral component loosening in cementless implants. Follow-up on such techniques is still short. The early and late infection rates are significant. Late hematogenous infection seems to be a particular problem because these patients have an already compromised immune system and frequent bacteremia secondary to chronic skin ulcers, sloughing of the intestinal mucosa, functional asplenia and frequent intravenous needlesticks. The relatively high incidence of gram-negative infections suggests the need for a gram-negative periopera-

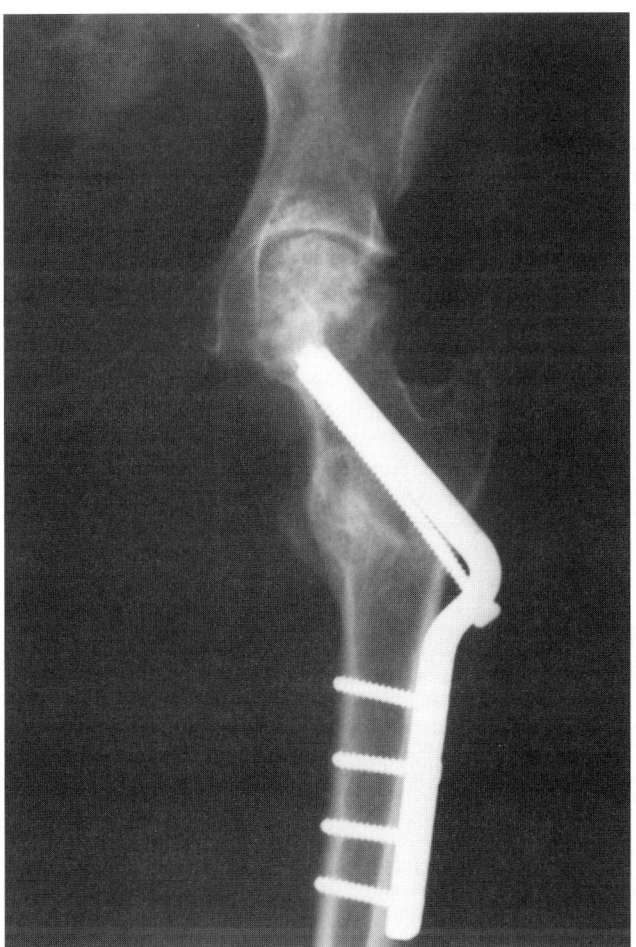

Fig. 15. Valgus osteotomy for osteonecrosis (ON). This is a case of a 20-year-old woman with sickle cell anemia and advanced ON of the femoral head treated with valgus osteotomy.

tive antibiotic prophalaxis.[38] Perioperative complications such as excessive blood loss, hematoma formation, vaso-occlusive crises, aplastic anemia crises, transfusion reactions, congestive heart failure, pneumonia, and urinary tract infections are also frequent. Principles of preoperative preparation described previously should be strictly followed, and preoperative hematology and anesthesia consultations should be obtained.

THALASSEMIA

INTRODUCTION
Definition
The predominant adult Hgb molecule is Hgb A, consisting of two α and two β globin chains. Two minor hemoglobins, $HgbA_2$ and HbF, consisting of two α chains and two chains that are similar in structure but not identical to the β chain, also exist. Thalassemia is a genetic defect in the production of one or more of these chains. The two major variants, β-thalassemia and α-thalassemia, are named in reference to the globin chain that is affected in that form of the disease. Thalassemia major (Cooley's anemia) refers to the homozygous form of β-thalassemia, whereas thalassemia minor refers to the heterozygous form. Thalassemia intermedia has a clinical expression intermediate between thalassemia major and minor and can either be homozygous with attenuated expression or a heterozygous variant.[43] Thalassemia minor is clinically manifested as a mild anemia, perhaps with some splenomegaly. It is often asymptomatic. Thalassemia major and its intermedia variants, alternatively, have significant orthopaedic implications.

Historical Review
Thalassemia was first described by Cooley in 1927. Up until the 1960s "Cooley's anemia" was an invariably fatal disease in the first 2 years of life. In the 1960s transfusion therapy was used to correct the hypoxia; however, iron overload became a significant cause of morbidity and mortality. In the 1970s, chelation therapy contributed significantly to the lifespan of patients receiving transfusion therapy by reducing iron overload. In the late 1980s, BMT resulted in cures for the disease in a select group of patients. The hope for the 21st century is gene therapy using the patient's own bone marrow. This technology is currently being investigated.[44]

Epidemiology
Thalassemia is most common in persons of Italian and Greek descent, hence the term "Mediterranean anemia." Prenatal diagnosis of thalassemia has reduced the birth rate of infants with the disease by about 90% in developed countries of Europe; however, it remains a significant problem in third world countries where prenatal screening and transfusion and chelation therapy are not widely available.

PATHOGENESIS
In β-thalassemia, there is a decrease in or absence of β globin chain production, resulting in precipitation of the excess α chains within the cell. Ineffectiveness of the aberrant Hgb molecule leads to intramedullary hemolysis, ineffective erythropoiesis, and marrow expansion.[45, 46] Ex-tramedullary hematopoiesis (EH) and hepatosplenomegaly may result.

Hemochromatosis from transfusion therapy can cause impaired pituitary function. Protein and vitamin D metabolism also appear to be impaired in this disease, although the exact pathogenesis is unclear. Endocrine and metabolic deficiencies thus contribute to impaired ossification and bony abnormalities.[47]

CLINICAL FEATURES
Untreated patients who have significant endogenous erythropoiesis undergo tremendous bone marrow expansion, particularly in the flat bones of the skull, resulting in the typical "Cooley's face" deformity (Table 2), including frontal bossing and maxillary prominence. If bone marrow suppression treatment is begun early in life, however, the physical appearance is normal.

Even in treated patients, frequent fractures may occur secondary to osteoporosis and cortical thinning. Of 62 patients with β-thalassemia, Exarchou et al[48] noted that one in three had sustained a fracture and in one in five they were multiple. Fractures most frequently involve the forearm, femur, and tibia. The most significant orthopaedic sequela of thalassemia is premature physeal fusion (PEF). This phenomenon has been reported to have an incidence of 14% to 50%[43, 48] in patients with the major and intermedia variants. It occurs in patients older than 10 years and is manifested by progressive shortening and angulation of involved limbs. The most frequently affected physes are the distal tibial and fibular, the proximal humeral, the distal femoral, the proximal fibular, and the proximal tibial, in that order. Colavita speculated that PEF is due to perforation of the cortex by the proliferating marrow and expansion beneath the periosteum across the peripheral physis. For instance, in the proximal humerus, the physis is almost completely covered by musculotendinous attachments except medially, where the arrest typically occurs. He also observed a greater incidence of EH and PEF in patients with the intermedia form, who typically do not undergo early and aggressive bone marrow suppression therapy.[43]

EH may result in hepatosplenomegaly, lymphadenopathy, or mass lesions from hypertrophied marrow extruding through the bone cortex. This is particularly significant in the spine where perivertebral masses can cause enlargement

---

TABLE 2. CLINICAL FEATURES OF THALASSEMIA MAJOR

Cooley's face
  Frontal bossing
    Maxillary prominence (untreated patients only)
Frequent fractures
Premature physeal fusion
Hepatosplenomegaly
Lymphadenomegaly
Soft-tissue masses
Spinal cord compression
Short stature
Delayed puberty
Leg ulcerations

of the posterior mediastinum,[43] and extradural hematopoietic tissue can result in spinal cord compromise.[49]

Children affected by thalassemia generally exhibit a mild form of growth retardation.[50] These children may have an underlying abnormality in vitamin D metabolism and endocrine function secondary to hemosiderosis. These abnormalities delay the onset of the adolescent growth spurt and contribute to osteoporosis.[48, 50]

In adolescents and young adults, leg ulcerations are common, ranging from trophic skin changes over the anteromedial distal tibia to 3 × 4 cm² ulcers with mild inflammatory changes surrounding them. The ulcers appear to be unrelated to the severity of the anemia or to the transfusion requirements and are precipitated or worsened by conditions of stasis, such as pregnancy, during which they are virtually untreatable. Ulcer development is probably related to impaired blood flow through capillary beds plugged with rigid thalassemic red cells. Impaired tissue oxygenation by these cells may also play a role in their pathogenesis.[51]

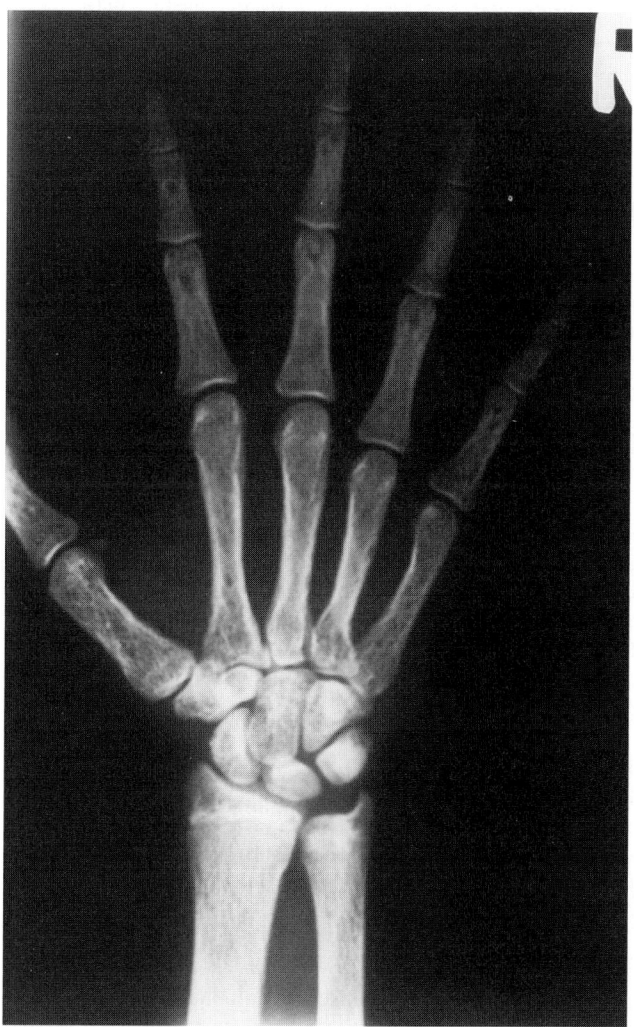

Fig. 16. Skeletal lesions in thalassemia. This is an anteroposterior radiograph of the hand of a 21-year-old white woman with thalassemia showing diffuse osteoporosis and cortical thinning, poor tubulation of the metaphyses, and multiple lytic lesions, primarily of the phalanges. (Courtesy Joanna Seibert, MD.)

INVESTIGATION

Roentgenographic findings are related to the marrow hyperplasia and include primarily osteoporosis and cortical thinning. Punched-out lytic lesions may also be seen (Fig. 16). In the skull, radial orientation of the bony trabeculae gives the characteristic "hair-on-end" appearance (see Fig. 12). Long bones may lack normal tubulation at their distal ends (Erlenmeyer's flask deformity). Vertebrae appear osteoporotic and may show some protrusion of disk material into the vertebral body (Schmorl's nodes). Physes affected by premature epiphyseal fusion show angular deformity and shortening. Laboratory findings in the untransfused patient include severe microcytic, hypochromic anemia with low reticulocyte count. Hgb electrophoresis should establish the diagnosis.

DIFFERENTIAL DIAGNOSIS

The differential diagnosis of thalassemia major is limited because patients are most often diagnosed at between 6 months and 2 years of life when the normal physiological anemia of the neonate fails to improve. Nevertheless, typical roentgenographic findings in thalassemia major strongly resemble those of metabolic bone disease (vitamin D–resistant rickets), leukemia, metastatic cancer (neuroblastoma, rhabdomyosarcoma), lymphoma, osteomyelitis, and, in the case of PEF, previous trauma or infection.

MANAGEMENT

Patients with thalassemia major require transfusion at 2- to 3-week intervals with enough leukocyte-poor RBCs to keep the baseline Hgb at least 10 to 10.5 g/dL. This transfusion regimen amounts to 25 to 30 units of blood per year, enough to cause significant enough iron overload to cause death from cardiac failure in the second decade of life. Chelation therapy with desferroxamine is required and should be begun after the age of 3 years. Desferroxamine must be administered by prolonged administration, usually via a subcutaneous pump. Oral chelation drugs are currently being investigated but are not yet available for clinical use.[44] Patients with thalassemia intermedia do not typically require transfusions to survive, at least until the third decade, when symptoms may become severe and chronic transfusion may be required.

Splenectomy is required in cases of massive splenomegaly with hypersplenism causing leukopenia, thrombocytopenia and an increasing transfusion requirement. The development of splenomegaly is delayed in patients maintained on a high transfusion regimen.[45]

BMT was introduced as a successful cure for thalassemia in 1982. Since then, the largest experience with BMT has been reported by Giardini et al in Pesaro, Italy, who had a 98% survival rate, 94% disease-free survival rate, and a 4% rejection rate in patients who met stringent clinical criteria. These criteria included age below 16 years, absence of hepatosplenomegaly or portal fibrosis, regular chelation prior to transplantation, and an HLA-identical donor. Mortality was, however, 20% in patients having either hepatosplenomegaly or portal fibrosis and 39% in those having both.[52] Thus, BMT is not an option in those patients not meeting strict criteria.

Roentgenographic abnormalities of bones regress with strictly managed transfusion therapy. Decompressive laminectomy or radiation therapy can result in recovery of patients with spinal cord compression due to periosteal extension of hematopoietic tissue into the spinal canal.[49]

Fractures in thalassemia are generally treated by conservative methods. Healing time is prolonged in these patients, fractures requiring long periods of immobilization. Refractures are common after cast removal. Despite the need for prolonged immobilization, early weightbearing with the use of walking casts or cast braces should be used whenever possible.[47] In the past, operative treatment was avoided in these patients as a result of their anemia and cardiac compromise. With the advent of chelation therapy, however, patients are living longer, more normal lives without the complications of hemochromatosis, making orthopaedic complications more frequent and significant and making operative treatment safer. Osteotomy may, therefore, be considered for significant angular deformity resulting from PES, and internal fixation of fractures may be considered when necessary (i.e., hip fractures). Careful preoperative evaluation of the patient's hematological and cardiac status is requested.

Leg ulcers are difficult to treat by conservative methods. If elevation, rest, and dressing changes fail, split-thickness skin grafting, often multiple times, may be required. Hyperbaric oxygen treatment should be considered, if available, because an increase in local tissue oxygenation should speed healing.[51]

COMPLICATIONS

Complications of poor compliance with transfusion therapy include worsening of the typical bony changes characteristic of marrow hyperplasia. (Conversely, stringent adherence to a transfusion/chelation protocol can cause regression of bony changes.) Poor compliance with chelation therapy almost certainly results in eventual cardiac failure from iron deposition in the myocardium. Endocrine abnormalities may also result from secondary hemosiderosis in glandular tissues. Toxicity of desferroxamine is rare except in very young children, in whom abnormalities of growth, vision, and hearing have been observed. Dose reduction can lead to clinical amelioration of these side effects.[44] Arthralgias are another complication of thalassemia and probably are related to underlying marrow proliferation, microfractures about the joints, and hemosiderin deposition in the tissues.

Leg ulcers and fractures are discussed previously.

Neurological complications may result from compression of the spinal cord by extramedullary hematopoietic tissue in poorly controlled disease. Patients with thalassemia intermedia are particularly at risk.

RESULTS

Well-managed patients now survive into the third and fourth decades of life. BMT is curative, but results are highly dependent on patient selection. Careful fracture management with attention to prolonged immobilization and early weightbearing if possible can have good results long term. One should be cognizant of the high risk of refracture in these patients.

FANCONI'S ANEMIA

INTRODUCTION
Definition
Fanconi's anemia is a severe childhood aplastic anemia and pancytopenia associated with multiple congenital abnormalities, including brownish pigmentation of the skin and skeletal abnormalities, primarily radial upper extremity deficiencies. It is not to be confused with Fanconi's syndrome, which is renal tubular insufficiency with cystinosis and secondary rickets.

Historical Perspective
In 1919 Smith reported aplastic anemia in a 6-year-old boy associated with nuchal, genital, umbilical, and areolar skin pigmentation. Fanconi, in 1927, described a similar syndrome in three brothers between the ages of 5 and 7 years. All had the marked skin pigmentation, mental retardation, and short stature. Two had hypogonadism. In 1921 Uehlinger reported on a patient with pigmentation and testicular hypoplasia associated with multiple renal and skeletal abnormalities and pancytopenia.[53] In the early 1980s, diagnosis with the chromosome breakage test became more specific, making early diagnoses before the onset of hematological abnormalities possible.[54] Fanconi's anemia is still a rare disease; only about 800 cases are reported in literature.

Epidemiology
Fanconi's anemia is inherited as an autosomal-recessive disorder with a low degree of penetrance. Male-female occurrences are about 2:1. The hematological disorder usually strikes patients aged 6 to 8 years, although this can vary from the second year to the fifth decade of life.[53]

PATHOGENESIS
The underlying hematological disorder is progressive bone marrow hypoplasia or aplasia of all elements and increasing infiltration of fat into the marrow. The chromosomes of patients with Fanconi's anemia have increased susceptibility to breakage when exposed to a DNA cross-linking agent such as diepoxybutane. Identification of this DNA fragility is required for diagnosis of the disease.[54] Fanconi's anemia is genetically characterized as a DNA repair disorder. The underlying defect may be a direct defect in the removal of DNA cross-links versus a defect in the ability of cells to respond to oxidative stress resulting from the interaction with cross-linking agents.[55] Chromosomal fragility is probably the underlying cause of these patients' high risk for leukemia or solid tumors and may explain the frequent presence of congenital anomalies, although the true pathogenesis is not completely understood.

CLINICAL FEATURES
Skeletal anomalies are present in about 40% of patients with Fanconi's anemia (Table 3). They primarily involve the radial side of the upper extremities and range from thumb hypoplasia or supernumerary thumb to radial hypoplasia or complete aplasia (radial clubhand) (Fig. 17). Other associated upper-extremity anomalies include ra-

TABLE 3. CLINICAL FEATURES OF FANCONI'S ANEMIA

Skeletal Anomalies	Nonskeletal Anomalies	Signs and Symptoms
Upper extremity anomalies (radial clubhand and its variants) Developmental dysplasia of the hips Clubfeet Lesser toe anomalies Sprengel's deformity Klippel-Feil syndrome Flatfeet	Skin pigmentation Growth retardation Hypogonadism Microcephaly Renal anomalies Micro-ophthalmia Strabismus Spasticity Undescended testis, other Hypospadias Deafness Inguinal hernia Obesity Gynecomastia	Pallor Fatigability Bleeding tendencies Acute febrile illness

dioulnar synostosis, congenital dislocation of the radial head, and thenar atrophy. Developmental dysplasia of the hips (DDH), clubfeet, and lesser toe abnormalities, Sprengel's deformity, Klippel-Feil syndrome, and flatfeet have also been described, although much less frequently.[53]

Abnormal brownish skin pigmentation occurs in 74% of patients, primarily in the intertrigenous regions such as the neck, axilla, and groin. Also frequently associated with Fanconi's anemia are (in descending order of frequency) genitourinary anomalies (primarily hypogonadism), growth retardation, microcephaly, micro-ophthalmia and strabismus, spasticity, cardiovascular anomalies, deafness, inguinal hernia, and gynecomastia.[53]

The onset of the hematological disturbance is usually delayed until the age of 6 to 8 years. The initial symptoms are anemia with pallor and fatigability. Symptoms related to thrombocytopenia, such as bleeding tendencies, may also be the presenting complaint. Initial onset may be associated with an acute febrile illness. The disease progresses slowly as the bone marrow evolves from hypoplasia to aplasia of all cellular elements. Untreated, most patients die within 5 years of onset.

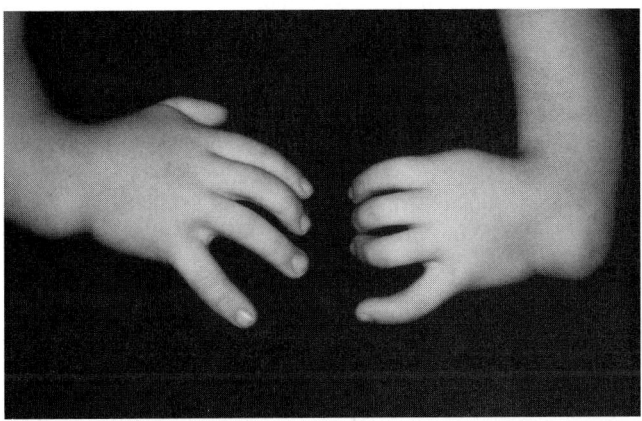

Fig. 17. Radial clubhand. This is an infant with radial clubhand deformity typical of Fanconi's anemia.

INVESTIGATION

CBC in the full-blown syndrome reveals macrocytic, hyperchromic anemia, leukopenia characterized by granulocytopenia with relative lymphocytosis, and thrombocytopenia. Early in the disease, one or two of these may be present. Bone marrow biopsy reveals hypoplasia or aplasia of all cellular elements. The degree of hypoplasia depends on the stage of the disease.[53]

Definitive diagnosis is made by exposure of lymphocytes to DNA cross-linking agents such as diepoxybutane. Increased chromosomal fragility in the presence of such agents is diagnostic of the disease. Investigation of skeletal anomalies should include radiographs of any positive findings on physical examination. Physical exam should also include plotting of height, weight, and head circumference on a growth chart, examination for nonskeletal congenital abnormalities, cardiac and renal ultrasonograms, and appropriate referral to hematology and genetics services.

DIFFERENTIAL DIAGNOSIS

There is considerable phenotypic variability and cross-over between Fanconi's anemia and the other congenital hypoplastic anemias. The hematological disorder alone, in the absence of congenital anomalies, has been noted in relatives of patients with full-blown Fanconi's anemia. Likewise, congenital malformations in the absence of the hematological disorder may be present.[53] In some families, DNA testing may be positive in the absence of any clinical manifestations of the disease.[54]

Fanconi's anemia must be differentiated from the other congenital hypoplastic anemias. About 40% of patients with congenital hypoplastic anemia have physical anomalies, primarily involving the thumbs. Triphalangeal thumbs, duplication, subluxation, and flattening of the thenar eminence have been noted. Other skeletal abnormalities include short stature, webbed neck, cleft palate and lip, abnormal eyes or ears, and renal abnormalities.[56] Among this group of patients are those with Diamond-Blackfan syndrome and thrombocytopenia-absent radius syndrome. Diamond-Blackfan syndrome is a slowly progressive, normocytic, normochromic red cell anemia affecting only the erythroid cell line. It is associated with the same skeletal anomalies as Fanconi's anemia; however, they seem to be less frequent and less marked. Its course is much milder, and remission after steroid treatment and BMT and even spontaneous remissions have been reported.[53] Thrombocytopenia-absent radius syndrome is discussed elsewhere in this chapter.

VATER syndrome includes vertebral defects, anal atresia, tracheoesophageal fistula, renal defects, and radial limb defects and must be considered in the differential diagnosis.

An important point is that the onset of the hematological disorder in Fanconi's anemia is delayed for several years after birth, whereas congenital anomalies are apparent at birth. Therefore, many patients may come to surgery before the bone marrow failure syndrome is diagnosed. Microcytosis and slowly progressive anemia are important clues to early diagnosis. Bone marrow failure should be considered and CBC performed in any patient with upper extremity anomalies, particularly those presenting for surgical treatment. Testing for sensitivity to diepoxybutane should be performed if there is any suspicion of Fanconi's anemia in a patient with these congenital anomalies.

MANAGEMENT

Nonoperative treatment of radial clubhand and other upper extremity abnormalities should be the first choice of treatment in patients with Fanconi's anemia. Patients requiring surgery should be operated on before the development of the hematological disorder, usually before age 6 years. Other congenital abnormalities, such as DDH and clubfeet, may be treated in the standard fashion.

Once the patients experience marrow failure, a prolonged period of preaplasia ensues, during which observation and periodic blood counts are needed. About 90% of patients ultimately experience full-blown aplastic anemia.[54] Androgen and corticosteroid therapy is the mainstay of treatment. Oxymetholone alternating with prednisone is most commonly used. The response rate is 50% to 75%, and remission is dose dependent. Dosing is limited, however, by the anabolic side effects of these agents. Androgen treatment has extended the lifespan of these patients by an average of 4 years. Most patients eventually fail androgens (although this may not happen until up to 20 years of treatment).[54]

BMT and cord blood transplantation have been successful in curing patients with human leukocyte antigen (HLA)–matched donors. Treatment of patients with HLA-mismatched donors is being investigated.[57, 58] Current work with certain hematopoietic growth factors, which stimulate hematopoietic progenitors in vitro, may promise new therapy in the future.[56, 59, 60]

COMPLICATIONS

The primary complication of Fanconi's anemia itself is the development of malignancies. There is a 10% to 15% risk of leukemia or solid tumors in this patient population. Complications of treatment by BMT include GVHD,[57, 58] transient decrease in linear growth,[61] toxicity from cyclophosphamide and other pre-BMT conditioning agents,[54, 57] and pneumonia. Perioperative complications can be avoided by early surgery, before the development of pancytopenia, and careful perioperative evaluation of hematological studies.

RESULTS

Overall, the results of surgical intervention in these patients are consistent with those with isolated congenital anomalies. BMT in HLA-matched donors has resulted in 2-year survival rates of 66% to 75% of those treated. The 2-year probability of survival in alternative donor transplant is only 29%.[57] Not every patient has a poor prognosis, and many have lived to have families of their own after androgen and corticosteroid treatment.[54]

THROMBOCYTOPENIA-ABSENT RADIUS SYNDROME

INTRODUCTION

The syndrome of thrombocytopenia and absent radius (TAR syndrome) is an autosomal-recessive genetic disorder characterized by hypomegakaryocytic thrombocytopenia and bilateral complete absence of the radii with presence of all five digits. TAR as a distinct clinical entity was first described by Hall et al[62] in 1969. Epidemiological studies have not been performed; however, Schoenecker et al[63] reported 21 cases culled from a pool of 50,000 children presenting for orthopaedic complaints over a period of 48 years (an approximate incidence of 1 in 2500 in this setting). TAR is two or three times as common as Fanconi's anemia. There is no ethnic predominance, although Hall[64] reported a slight preponderance of females. The condition is autosomal-recessive, with a 25% risk in subsequent offspring for the parents of an affected child. However, the extent of involvement and severity of abnormalities may be quite variable, even in the same family.

PATHOGENESIS

Although the mechanism for the embryogenesis of this condition is not completely understood, the predominant defect seems to be in the amebakaryocytic (white cell) precursors. Thrombocytopenia results from the decreased production of megakaryocytes. Hall[64] postulated that the primordial megakaryocyte plays a role in blood vessel formation, specifically in the normal vascular bifurcation of the developing limb during embryogenesis as well as in the formation of the heart and normal closure of the septum. A defect in megakaryocyte function would, therefore, explain the limb abnormalities and the frequent association of cardiac abnormalities in this syndrome.

CLINICAL FEATURES

The hematological manifestations of TAR present within the first few months of life and consist of episodic severe thrombocytopenia with platelet counts of 10×10^9/L or below (Table 4). Episodes of thrombocytopenia may be precipitated by stress, infections, or surgery. Petechiae, melena, or intracranial bleeding may occur. Between episodes, platelet counts generally range from 15×10^9/L to 30×10^9/L. After the first year of life, platelet counts increase spontaneously to almost normal by adulthood.[63, 64]

The skeletal abnormality in TAR is characterized by complete absence of the radius with the presence of four fingers and a thumb (Fig. 18). The condition is almost always bilateral. Clinodactyly of the small finger was present in 20 of 21 patients of Schoenecker et al.[63] Selective hypoplasia of the middle phalanx of the fifth finger

TABLE 4. CLINICAL FEATURES OF THROMBOCYTOPENIA-ABSENT RADIUS SYNDROME
Episodic bleeding tendencies (severe, first year of life; present in all)
Petechiae
Melena
Intracranial bleeding
Skeletal anomalies
Radial aplasia with presence of thumb (present in all)
Clinodactyly
Hypoplasia of P-2 fifth finger
Altered palmar contours
Humeral/ulnar anomalies
Knee deformities
Hip dislocation
Foot deformities
Clinical spine anomalies
Nonskeletal anomalies
Cardiac abnormalities (30%)
Cow's milk allergy

and altered palmar contours are characteristic findings.[65] The humerus and ulna may be normal or hypoplastic, and the overall upper extremity deformity can range from isolated absent radii to true phocomelia.[65]

Knee deformities are common but are not as consistently present as are the upper extremity deformities. Genu varum is the most common finding, usually in association with internal tibial torsion. Other findings include abnormal laxity of the joint, stiffness (less commonly), dislocation of the knee and hypoplasia, and absence or dislocation of the patella. Varying degrees of intra-articular bony and ligamentous abnormalities have been described.[63, 66] Hip dislocation and foot deformities may also be present. Upper limb involvement is generally more severe than lower limb involvement. Overall, the lower extremities are involved in 46% to 86% of patients, depending on the series.[63, 65] Cervical spine and craniofacial abnormalities may also be present. Cardiac abnormalities, primarily tetralogy of Fallot and atrial septal defects, are present in about 30% of cases. Cow's milk allergy is common and may precipitate episodes of thrombocytopenia and gastrointestinal bleeding, which, if untreated, can be fatal.

INVESTIGATION

Laboratory abnormalities include thrombocytopenia, described previously. Platelet aggregation and survival times are also reduced. Leukemoid reactions may occur, accompanying the episodes of thrombocytopenia. (WBC counts can rise to greater than 35×10^9/L with a left shift.) Eosinophilia is seen in 50% of patients, especially with exposure to cow's milk in those with cow's milk allergy. Anemia is common and is thought to be a result of bleeding. Long bone survey will detail the extent of skeletal involvement. Ultrasonography of the hips may be considered if clinical exam raises the suspicion of hip dislocation or subluxation. MRI of the knee may be helpful in preoperative planning to evaluate intra-articular ligamentous disease. Diagnosis of TAR may be made prenatally by ultrasonography. Chromosome analysis is normal.

DIFFERENTIAL DIAGNOSIS

TAR is a relative distinctive condition because of the consistent combination of complete radial aplasia, presence of a thumb, and thrombocytopenia. Roberts' syndrome is the only other condition in which complete bilateral radial aplasia and the presence of thumbs have been described. If thumbs are absent, other diagnoses, such as Fanconi's anemia, VATER syndrome, Diamond-Blackfan syndrome, trisomy 18, Holt-Oram syndrome, and isolated congenital radial clubhand, must be considered. In considering these diagnoses, careful evaluation of hematological abnormalities will be helpful in their differentiation.

MANAGEMENT

Platelet transfusion may be necessary during symptomatic episodes of thrombocytopenia during the first year of life. Leukocyte-poor or, if possible, single-donor platelets should be given to avoid the development of antibodies. The antifibrinolytic agent ϵ-aminocaproic acid (EACA) may be useful in decreasing bleeding and reducing platelet transfusion requirement, especially in nasopharyngeal and gingival bleed-

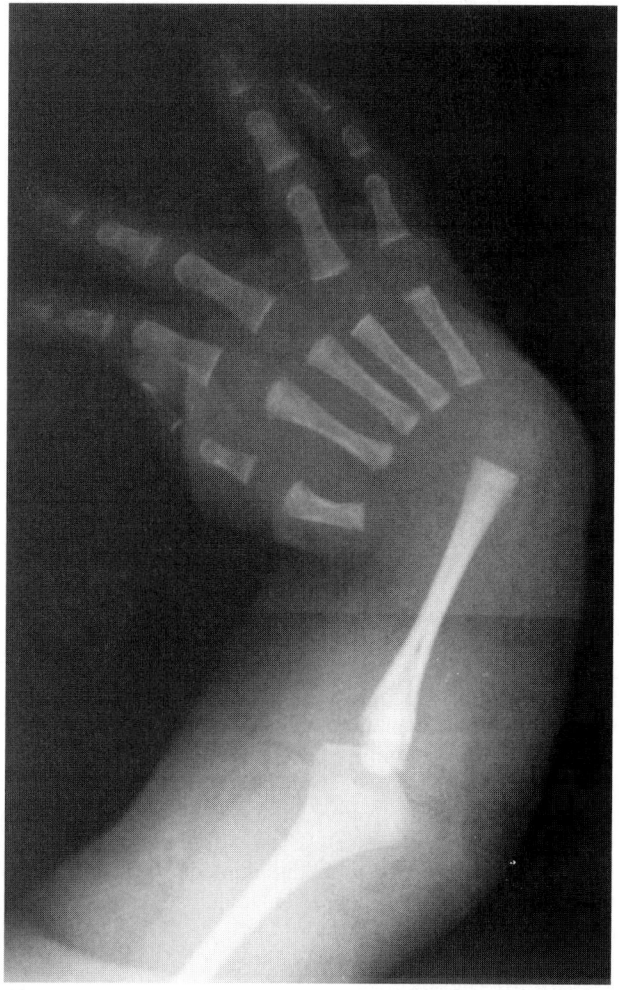

Fig. 18. Thrombocytopenia-absent radius syndrome (TAR) in a newborn. This is an anteroposterior roentgenogram of the forearm and hand in a newborn with TAR. Note the complete absence of the radius, presence of four fingers and thumb, and hypoplasia of the middle phalanx of the fifth finger.

ing.[65] Early in life, cardiac surgery may be necessary and is managed with perioperative platelet transfusion.

Initial treatment of orthopaedic conditions should be nonoperative until hematological abnormalities normalize. Splinting of the wrist is necessary to prevent progressive radial deviation. Bracing of knee deformities may be undertaken if possible, but experience with bracing has not been described. In Schoenecker's series of 21 patients, only one was braced, and knee deformities were so variable that no definite conclusions could be made regarding guidelines for timing and location of osteotomies. Schoenecker et al did note a high rate of recurrence of knee deformities after osteotomies before the onset of skeletal maturity. Patients appear to be out of danger of significant progression after skeletal maturity. Nevertheless, correction of knee deformities should be timed to coincide, if possible, with the onset of walking age.[63] Infants who are diagnosed prenatally should be delivered by cesarean section to minimize the risk of bleeding.

COMPLICATIONS

Bleeding episodes in the first year of life may lead to intracranial hemorrhage (with subsequent manifestations of mental retardation and cerebral palsy), glaucoma (from intraocular bleeding), bloody diarrhea, and even death. Obviously, hematological abnormalities should be carefully monitored perioperatively to prevent excessive intraoperative and postoperative bleeding. Schoenecker et al reported 3 patients of 14 (45 operations) who had delay in healing, which he attributed to thrombocytopenia.[63] As stated, recurrence of knee deformities after osteotomy is to be expected in the skeletally immature patient.

RESULTS

Overall, the prognosis for TAR patients surviving the first year of life is good. In the five patients Schoenecker et al[63] monitored to adulthood, all walked without braces and have adapted well to their functional limitations. The life span of these individuals, after the first 2 years of life, is comparable to that of the general population.

LYMPHOMA

INTRODUCTION
Definition

Primary non-Hodgkin's lymphoma of bone (PLB) is a rare extranodal form of lymphoma formerly known as reticulum cell sarcoma. Although non-Hodgkin's lymphoma may secondarily involve bone in up to 10% of patients, PLB is considered a separate clinical entity based on the presentation of initial symptoms of bone pain with single or multiple radiological bone lesions and with or without local or regional nodal involvement. Classically, the diagnosis of PLB excludes patients with dissemination of the disease within the first 6 months after diagnosis, although one study differs from this criterion.[67]

Historical Review

Lymphoma of the bone was first described by Oberling in 1928. In 1939 Parker and Jackson described 17 cases of "primary reticulum cell sarcoma of bone." Since then, more than 300 cases have been reported in the literature.[67–72]

Epidemiology

Primary lymphoma of bone is rare, constituting only about 3% of all primary malignant bone tumors and 5% of all extranodal lymphomas.[70, 71, 73] PLB comprises only 2.8% to 9% of childhood non-Hodgkin's lymphoma (NHL).[69] The average age of patients with PLB is about 40 years, with a wide range (first to seventh decade of life).[67, 70–72] In the pediatric population, the mean age for PLB is 13 years.[67] There is a slight male predominance,[71, 72] although this has not been found in the few series of PLB in childhood.[67, 69]

PATHOGENESIS

Lymphoma is considered a small round cell bone tumor arising from marrow elements. Most PLBs are B cell in origin, and the most common histological type is diffuse histiocytic lymphoma. The cells appear in sheets and are larger than a small lymphocyte. There is a moderate amount of cytoplasm with vesicular nuclei. Nucleoli are central, and nuclear indentation or multilobulation are frequent (Fig. 19). Reticulin fibers surround the cells.[67–70] Collagen fibers, sometimes dense, may be found.[73, 74] Undifferentiated or poorly differentiated types are also seen.

CLINICAL FEATURES

Bone pain is the most common initial symptom, occasionally accompanied by a palpable mass. PLB affects the lower half of the body most frequently, especially the long bones, but it can involve the short and flat bones. Constitutional symptoms such as anorexia, fever, weight loss, and general malaise may or may not be present. In children, locomotor disability may be the presenting complaint. Local or regional lymphadenopathy may be present on physical exam. Pathological fracture has been reported.[70]

INVESTIGATION

Physical examination should include palpation for bone pain and mass and for local, regional, and remote lymphadenopathy. A thorough neurological exam should be

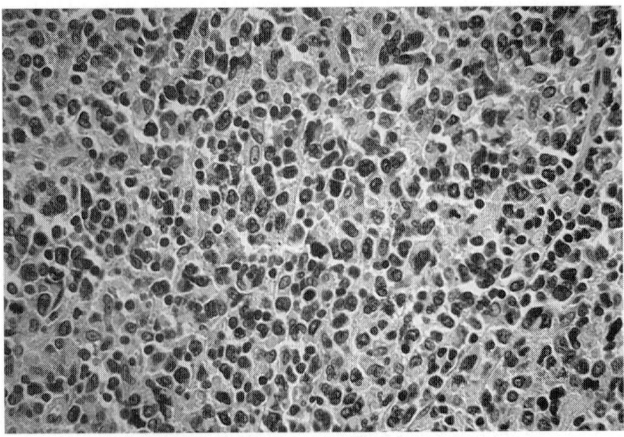

Fig. 19. Histopathology of primary non-Hodgkin's lymphoma of bone. This is the general appearance of a malignant round cell tumor of bone, but with more pleomorphism and more distinct cytoplasmic outlines than other round cell tumors such as Ewing's sarcoma. Nuclei stain relatively darkly with hematoxylin. Absence of intracellular glycogens on periodic acid–Schiff and positive stain for reticulin fibers would establish the diagnosis (hematoxylin and eosin ×100).

performed to rule out CNS involvement. Radiographs of PLB reveal diffuse lytic lesions in the diaphysis, metaphysis, and epiphysis. The joint may be involved in epiphyseal lesions.[74] Occasionally, lesions will be osteosclerotic or mixed lytic and osteosclerotic. There may be cortical erosion and destruction. Periosteal reaction is less frequent but occasionally present (Fig. 20).

CBC, ESR, chemistry profile, chest radiographs, CT scan of the chest and abdomen should be performed if malignancy is suspected. Routine laboratory evaluations will usually show no specific abnormalities other than a mildly elevated ESR. Hypercalcemia, when present, is a poor prognostic factor.[69]

Bone scintigraphy (^{99m}Tc-MDP) will detect 84% to 95% of lymphomatous bone lesions[75, 76] and should be performed to help rule out multifocal involvement.

Skeletal surveys with plain radiographs probably underestimate bone involvement.[76] Gallium 67 scintigraphy is not useful as a diagnostic test of bone involvement, because some lymphomas are not ^{67}gallium avid; however, it has been recommended for the evaluation of response to treatment.[75]

Lymphomas appear as heterogeneous hypointense lesions on both T_1- and T_2-weighted MRI images. This is in contrast to other small cell primary bone tumors, which tend to show marked hyperintensity on T_2-weighted images. This is thought to be secondary to the high reticulin fiber and collagen content in these tumors.[73, 74] Melamed et al[76] noted that MRI detected larger areas of marrow disease in his series of eight patients with primary multifocal osseous lymphoma than were evident on bone scan, particularly in the pelvis, hips, and lower lumbar spine.

Definitive diagnosis must be made by biopsy. Because the presentation of primary lymphoma of bone mimics that

of sarcoma, the diagnosis of lymphoma is often not considered at biopsy. Appropriate handling of the specimen is critical. If an extraosseous soft-tissue mass is present, a sample of it should be obtained with a sharp scalpel rather than a curet. This avoids creation of a cortical window and subsequent risk of pathological fracture. If soft-tissue mass is absent and the cortex must be opened, material should be removed with a knife or periosteal elevator, rather than a curet, to avoid crushing artifact on the slides. Incisional biopsy is far superior to needle biopsy to confirm the diagnosis of lymphoma. Frozen section will confirm adequacy of the material taken at biopsy. The pathologist should be alerted to the possibility of a diagnosis of lymphoma so that immunohistochemistry, electron microscopy, and flow cytometry may be performed to differentiate from other small round cell tumors.[72]

The average time from presentation to diagnosis is about 6 months,[67, 69] and often more than one biopsy is required to establish the diagnosis, especially if the prior steps are not followed.[72] This reflects the need to consider lymphoma in a differential diagnosis of any primary bone tumor.

DIFFERENTIAL DIAGNOSIS

Primary lymphoma of bone mimics bone sarcoma at presentation because of the clinical history of bone pain with or without mass and the radiographic appearance of diffuse lysis with minimal reactive bone formation. Therefore, the differential diagnosis is lengthy and should include other primary bone malignancies of the small round cell type, including Ewing's sarcoma, myeloma, and small cell osteosarcoma. Metastatic disease, especially metastatic neuroblastoma, clear cell carcinoma of the kidney, rhabdomyosarcoma, hepatoblastoma, and retinoblastoma in children and small cell lung carcinoma and melanoma in adults should be considered. The presence of pleomorphic and multilobulated nuclei and a reticulin-rich pattern and a lack of necrosis, hemorrhage, or intracellular glycogen favor diagnosis of lymphoma over Ewing's sarcoma. Absence of plasma cells rules out myeloma. Metastatic neuroblastoma should show pear- or carrot-shaped cells, true rosettes, and dense nuclear chromatin. Metastatic carcinoma should display abundant cytoplasm, large pleomorphic nuclei, and mucin positivity. Absence of such features suggests the diagnosis of lymphoma.[70]

Immunohistochemical markers specific for mesenchymal cell leukocytes, melanin, and neurodifferentiation can also help distinguish these tumors at biopsy.[72] The possibility of osteomyelitis should always be considered, and biopsy specimens should be sent for culture. The ESR should be much more elevated in osteomyelitis than in lymphoma, and clinical history and radiograph findings should also help make the distinction.

Hodgkin's disease may also present as a primary bone lesion. Although 9% to 35% of patients with known Hodgkin's disease experience extranodal skeletal disease, primary bone involvement is exceedingly rare.[77] Clinical presentation is identical to that of PLB, as is roentgenographic presentation (Fig. 21). Histology often shows a mixture of eosinophils, lymphocytes, plasma cells, histiocytes, and endothelial cells. Reed-Sternberg cells may be seen infrequently.[78] Misdiagnosis as Paget's disease, metastatic tu-

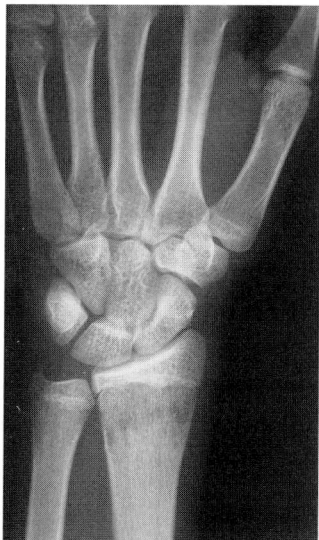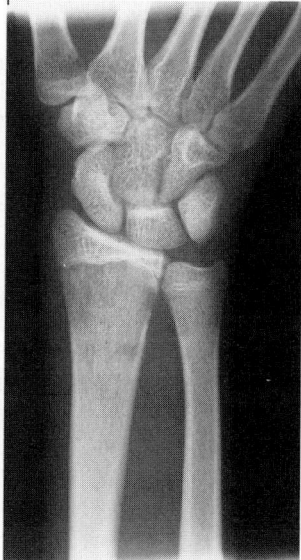

Fig. 20. Radiographic features of primary non-Hodgkin's lymphoma of bone. This 14-year-old girl presented with bilateral wrist pain. Anteroposterior views of bilateral wrists show permeative pattern of bone destruction in the metaphysis with minimal local reaction. Cortical destruction is evident in both wrists. Diagnosis was multifocal primary lymphoma of bone. (Courtesy Joanna Seibert, MD.)

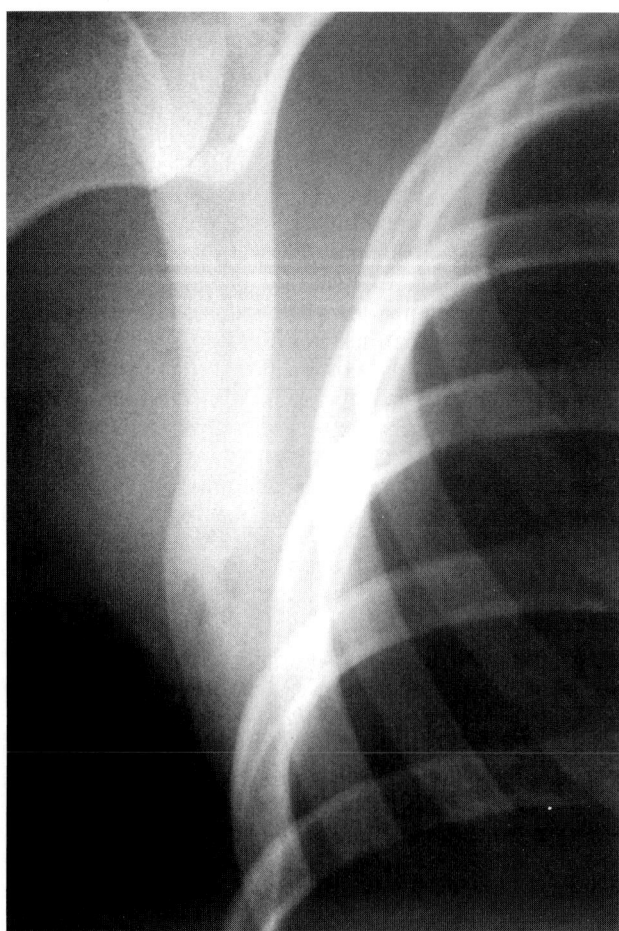

Fig. 21. Hodgkin's disease. This is a rare presentation of Hodgkin's disease as a primary bone lesion in the scapula of this 17-year-old boy. Note lytic lesions in distal lateral margin of scapula.

mor, chronic osteomyelitis, eosinophilic granuloma, and primary sarcoma of bone has been reported.[77] Fewer than 20 cases of primary Hodgkin's disease of the bone have been reported in the English literature.[77-79] Nevertheless, these reports emphasize the delay in diagnosis of these patients and the resulting poor survival rate. Therefore, primary Hodgkin's disease of the bone should also be considered on pathological examination of biopsy specimen.

MANAGEMENT

PLB is managed with multidrug chemotherapy with or without local radiotherapy to the primary site. Although the role of chemotherapy is well established, the role of radiation therapy has become less clear in recent years. Development of a second malignancy in the irradiated field has been documented in several studies,[67, 69] as have growth discrepancies of the extremities, local atrophy, and fibrosis.[67] Although a large, comparative study has not been done, several small studies suggested that the addition of radiotherapy to chemotherapy does not improve long-term survival.[67, 69] Radiation therapy is suggested by Wollner et al[67] only for lesions with demonstrated progression within the first few months of treatment. Radiation therapy alone

is to be condemned because it has a 50% recurrence rate.[68] Chemotherapy is the mainstay of treatment for lymphoma.

Surgery is reserved for diagnosis of lymphoma via open biopsy and management of complications such as pathological fracture and biopsy of the local site for persistent symptoms after treatment. Biopsy technique was discussed previously.

COMPLICATIONS

Pathological fracture may occur secondary to extensive bone lysis or to the creation of a cortical window during biopsy. Radiotherapy may impede normal remodeling of such fractures. Prophylactic fixation is not recommended for impending fractures, because good response to chemotherapy will result in resolution of radiographic findings. Also the possibility of Ewing's sarcoma and small cell osteosarcoma must be clearly ruled out before surgery other than a careful open biopsy is considered on such a lesion. Patients at risk for fracture should have protected weightbearing until after completion of medical treatment. The lesion can be stabilized, if necessary, after the diagnosis has been established and nonsurgical treatment completed.

Persistence of symptoms suggests recurrence or failure of the tumor to respond, which may necessitate repeat biopsy. Mechanical instability, infection, and ON should be considered as well in cases of persistent pain. As mentioned, the development of secondary malignancies after local radiation therapy has been reported.

RESULTS

The prognosis for PLB is better overall than in other forms of non-Hodgkin's lymphoma, primarily because in the classic definition of PLB more advanced stages of disease are excluded. Also the most common histological subtype in PLB is diffuse histiocytic lymphoma, which generally shows a good response to treatment.[70] Overall disease-free survival averages 70% to 90% at 5 years, depending on the treatment protocol used.[67-69] Radiograph findings generally resolve slowly in response to chemotherapy. Repeat plain radiography and possibly gallium scanning or MRI may be used to monitor response to treatment.

GAUCHER'S DISEASE

INTRODUCTION
Definition
Gaucher's disease is a genetic lipid storage disorder characterized by the accumulation of glucocerebroside in the reticuloendothelial (RE) system. It is caused by a deficiency of the enzyme glucocerebroside hydrolase. There are three forms of the disease. Type I is the most common and is characterized by the slow accumulation of glucocerebroside in the spleen, liver, and bones with sparing of the CNS. Type II, the acute neuropathic form, has its onset in infancy and is characterized by severe neural abnormalities. Most patients die within the first year of life. Type III, the subacute neuropathic form, has its onset in childhood and combines the features of type I with slowly progressive neural dysfunction. Type I is discussed specifically in this chapter because it is by far the most common and tends to be the most clinically significant for orthopaedic surgeons.

Historical Review

Gaucher's disease was first described by Phillippe Charles Earnest Gaucher in 1882.[80, 81] Amstutz described the orthopaedic manifestations in detail in 1966 in his classic paper.[82] In 1965 the specific enzyme deficit was discovered. In 1971, the autosomal-recessive mode of genetic transmission was proven.[80] Since then, several important studies described the nature and extent of the lipid storage in the marrow and spleen and the characteristic bone findings, including the natural history of ON in Gaucher's disease.[80, 83] In the 1990s, enzyme replacement therapy was successfully introduced and has been shown to reverse the bone marrow manifestations of Gaucher's disease.[84–86]

Epidemiology

Type I Gaucher's disease is an autosomal-recessive inborn error of metabolism that most often affects Jews of Ashkenazi (eastern European) origin. Types II and III are independent of ethnic origin.

PATHOGENESIS

Glucocerebroside hydrolase (β-glucosidase) is a lysosomal enzyme responsible for breaking the glycoside bond fixing a glucose to a ceramide (sphingosine plus a fatty acid), a material released from cell membranes on the death of a cell. In the absence of the enzyme, the glucosylceramide (glucocerebroside), which cannot itself be excreted by the body, is stored in macrophages of the RE system.[80] These lipid-laden macrophages, called Gaucher's cells, range from 20 to 80 μm and have one to several nuclei. Their cytoplasm is wrinkled appearing and contains striated rod-shaped inclusion bodies, giving it a crumpled-silk appearance. Gaucher's cells stain pale pink with hematoxylin and eosin and stain only slightly with oil-red-O and Sudan black B. The inclusions are autofluorescent and periodic acid–Schiff positive.[82, 87] The slow accumulation of these cells in the RE system results in visceromegaly. Thrombocytopenia, anemia, and structural changes in the bones develop secondary to marrow infiltration by the abnormal cells.

DNA studies and mutation analysis have been performed, and multiple genotypes have been identified. Four major genotypes exist, which tend to correlate with disease severity. Mutations associated with Jewish and non-Jewish ancestry have also been identified.[81]

CLINICAL FEATURES

Age at onset may range from 8 months to 70 years. The average age at symptom onset is 25 years. The younger the age at presentation, the more severe the disease seems to be.[81] Patients may present initially with one of two symptom complexes: bleeding manifestations or bone pain. In Zimran's[81] series of 53 patients, the most common presenting symptoms were epistaxis, easy bruising, or prolonged bleeding after superficial wounds. Postoperative, postpartum, and gastrointestinal bleeding also occurred (23 of 53 patients). Only seven patients presented with skeletal complaints. Amstutz and Carey,[82] however, reported that in 12 of their 20 patients the presenting symptoms were related to the skeletal system. They noted that skeletal manifestations became more prominent with the advancing age. Other presenting complaints may include abdominal protuberance from massive splenomegaly or fatigue secondary to anemia. History and physical examination may reveal brownish pigmentation of the exposed skin, pingueculae, cholecystitis, and poor dentition.[82]

There are three distinct clinical patterns of bone pain. Nonspecific dull pain, severe pain resulting from bone crisis, and pain caused by a complication such as osteomyelitis or pathological fracture. The most common pattern is that of a nonspecific dull ache, which lasts for a few days and is relieved by rest and symptomatic treatment. This type of pain tends toward chronicity, periodicity, and in some cases progressive joint degeneration. The most frequently involved sites are the hips, knees, shoulder, and spine.[82, 88, 89]

Bone crises are thus named because of their clinical (and etiological) similarities to sickle cell crises. They are thought to result from acute infarction of the bone and are marked by severe pain, local swelling, tenderness, and fever. The femur is more frequently involved, particularly the femoral head, and there is a relationship between frequent bone crisis and subsequent development of ON.[83] Crises tend to last from several days to 2 to 3 weeks, resolving with rest, hydration, and narcotics. The differential diagnosis of crisis versus osteomyelitis is difficult and is discussed later. Back pain also tends to follow one of the three typical patterns: mild, self-limited pain; acute bone crisis; and progressive pain caused by vertebral collapse. Subsequent fracture, kyphosis, and cord compression are rare but have been reported.[89] The lower extremities and spine tend to be more commonly involved than the upper extremities.

INVESTIGATION

Plain radiographs of affected long bones reveal areas of demineralization, either circumscribed or diffuse. There may be a moth-eaten, coarsely reticulated lattice-like appearance of the shaft. The cortex may be eroded, scalloped, or expanded (Fig. 22). Typically, the metaphysis, particularly the distal end of the femur, shows the Erlenmeyer flask deformity (Fig. 23). Osteosclerosis may also be seen. Periosteal reaction may become evident at approximately 6 weeks after a severe crisis.[82] Some patients have no radiographic evidence of bone involvement at all, whereas others have advanced radiographic changes. Radiographic findings generally correlate with the severity of the disease. The epiphyses are generally spared, except late in the course, and involvement is manifested as ON, particularly of the femoral and humeral heads.

Radiographs of the spine in the presence of gradually progressive back pain may reveal vertebral collapse. Three distinct patterns have been noted: rectangular collapse, central vertebral collapse, and anterior wedge collapse. Usually two or three vertebrae are involved without a characteristic site.[89]

Bone scan with ^{99m}Tc-MDP is typically normal in cases of mild pain without local tenderness and swelling. In acute bone crisis, however, delayed images showed decreased uptake consistent with bone infarcts. Bone scanning at 6 weeks and 6 months shows increased uptake and normal uptake, respectively (in the absence of pathological fracture). Interestingly, on the 6-week bone scan, a ring of increased uptake may be noted surrounding a photopenic

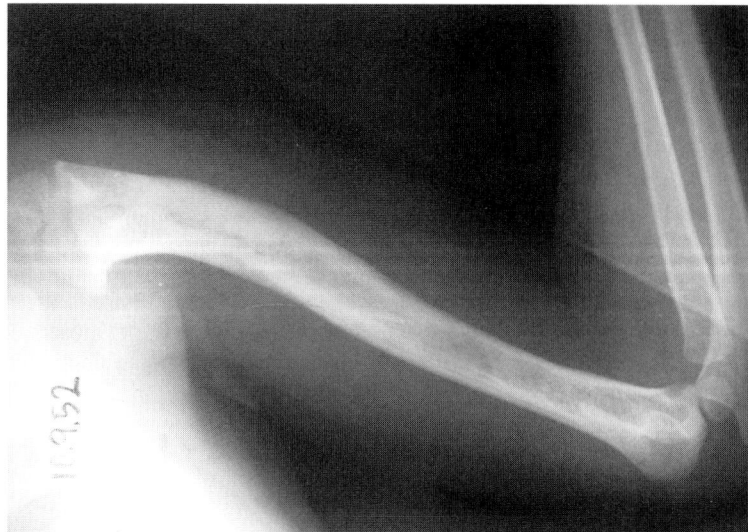

Fig. 22. Gaucher's disease. This is a lateral veiw of the humerus in a 5-year-old boy with Gaucher's disease. Diffuse lytic areas are mixed with some osteosclerosis and cortical expansion and bone proximally. Subtle endosteal scalloping is evident in the distal one-third of the shaft. (Courtesy Joanna Seibert, MD.)

area. This is possibly the result of an increase in the blood supply to the outer cortex during healing. The sensitivity of bone scan in crisis is 0.92.[88]

MRI of affected long bones reveals diffuse reduction of the marrow signals in both T_1- and T_2-weighted protocols. In acute crisis, however, intramedullary and subperiosteal hematoma has been identified by recognition of high signals on T_1- and T_2-weighted or on the proton density protocol.[90] MRI has also been used to monitor the response to treatment with enzyme replacement therapy (Fig. 24). After prolonged administration of replacement enzyme, marrow signals on T_1 and T_2 approach normal.[86]

Laboratory findings include thrombocytopenia, mild anemia, and occasionally pancytopenia. Thrombocytopenia tends to be more prominent in nonsplenectomized patients, whereas anemia is more common after splenectomy. Ab-

normal liver function tests, particularly prolonged prothrombin and partial thromboplastin times, are common. Most patients also have elevated serum acid phosphatase activities, serum ferritin levels, and angiotensin-converting enzyme activities. Low enzymatic activity of β-glucosidase is diagnostic of the disease. Cytopenia and liver function tests reflect the degree of organ involvement, whereas the serum chemistry findings listed previously do not correlate with the clinical severity of the disease.[81]

WBC count and ESR, although not typically elevated in patients with the milder form of skeletal complaints, are elevated in bone crisis. Typical WBC count in bone crisis may range from 13×10^9/L to 20×10^9/L. ESR in this situation ranges from 40 to 120 mm per hour.[88]

Diagnosis of Gaucher's disease has historically been established by identification of the typical Gaucher's cells in the bone marrow, liver, or spleen. Bone marrow biopsy is the traditional method of diagnosis. Enzymatic assay of the leukocyte acid β-glucosidase is, however, a less invasive method of diagnosis, making bone marrow biopsy necessary only when other hematological disorders, such as multiple myeloma, leukemia, or lymphoma are being considered. Mutation analysis may become more widely available in the future for diagnosis of Gaucher's disease.[81]

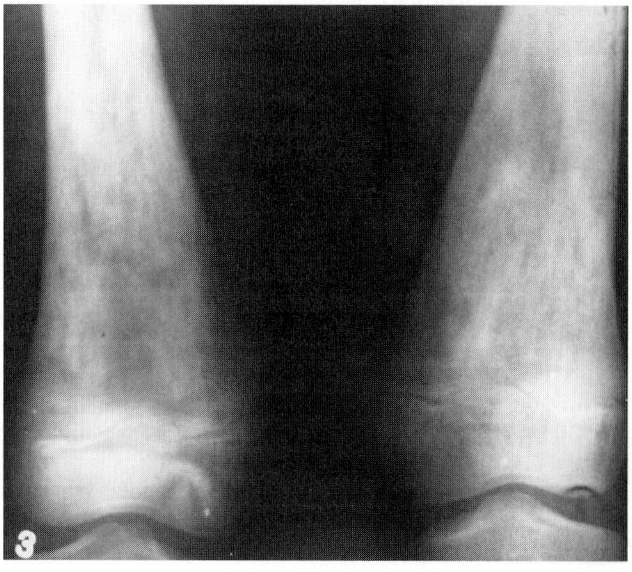

DIFFERENTIAL DIAGNOSIS

The initial diagnosis of Gaucher's disease should be considered in a patient presenting with bone pain of unknown cause, particularly in the presence of typical radiograph findings, bilateral ON of the femoral heads, positive family history, or Ashkenazi Jewish ancestry. A history of bleeding tendencies is also a tip-off to the diagnosis. Visceromegaly on physical exam and thrombocytopenia on CBC will usually be seen as signs of the disease. Thus, history and clinical exam should help establish the diagnosis. Because the bone findings may be typical of other marrow replacement conditions, multiple myeloma (in adults), lymphoma, leukemia, eosinophilic granuloma, and other storage diseases of the RE system should be considered in the differential.

Fig. 23. Erlenmeyer's flask deformities of distal femora. Mixed lytic and sclerotic lesions are present.

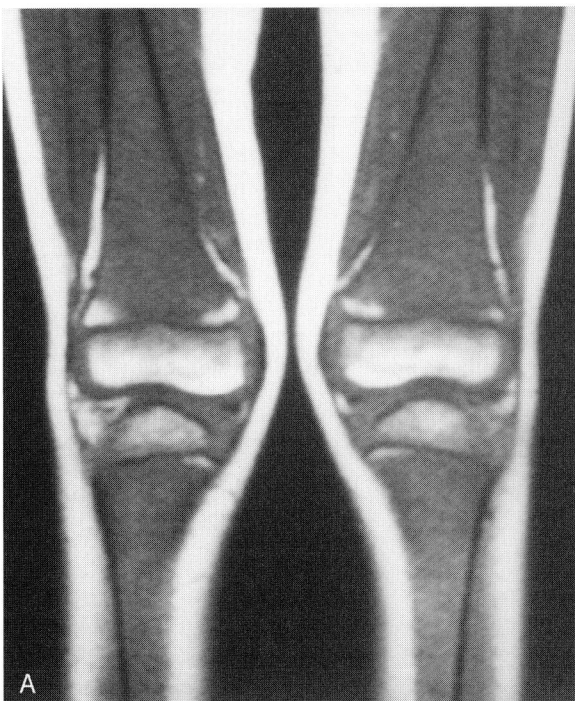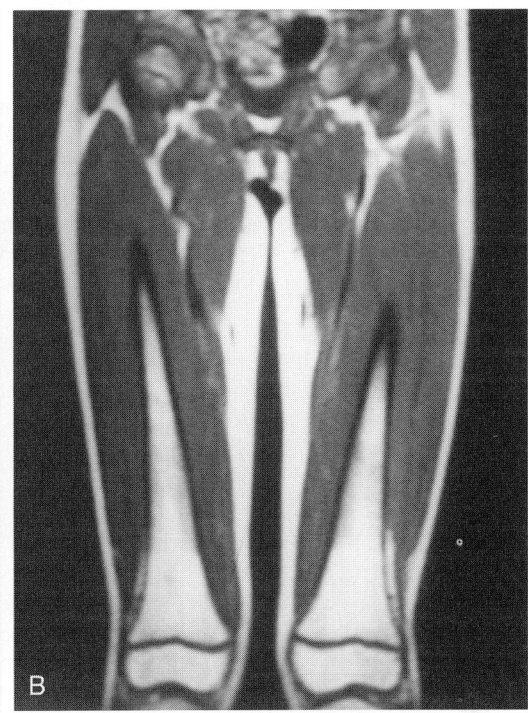

Fig. 24. Magnetic resonance imaging (MRI): Gaucher's disease. This is a 3-year-old child with Gaucher's disease type I before and after enzyme replacement therapy. *A*, Coronal T_1-weighted MRI of the knees shows marked decreased medullary signal intensity throughout the metaphyses and diaphyses of the distal femurs and proximal tibias. Less extensive marrow signal loss of the epiphyses is also seen. *B*, Coronal T_1-weighted image of the femurs after several years of alglucerase (Ceredase) enzyme therapy shows normalization of marrow signal intensity with return of high signal intensity fatty marrow throughout the diaphyses, metaphyses, and epiphyses. (From Allison JW, James CA, Arnold GL, et al: Reconversion of bone marrow in Gaucher disease treated with enzyme therapy documented by MR Pediatr Radiol 1998; 28:237.)

The most difficult diagnostic dilemma presenting to the orthopaedist is the differentiation of bone crisis from acute osteomyelitis. The clinical presentations of the two diseases are essentially the same, with acute severe bone pain, chills, fever, diaphoresis, tachycardia, leukocytosis, and elevated ESR. Radiographic changes in chronic Gaucher's disease include destructive and sclerotic lesions as well as periosteal reactions and may be confused with osteomyelitis. Additionally, invasive procedures such as bone aspiration, open biopsy, and débridement carry a significant risk of secondary infection of sterile but infarcted bone.[82, 91] Crisis is fairly common, occurring in up to 50% of patients with type I disease. Osteomyelitis is fairly uncommon, but its recognition is important if major disability is to be avoided. Patients presenting with acute signs and symptoms of a crisis should undergo a work-up in the following manner:

1. Multiple blood cultures should be obtained.
2. Bone scans should be performed immediately and at weekly intervals. Although decreased uptake on the initial bone scan does not rule out osteomyelitis, this finding is much more typical of acute bone crisis than acute infection. Sequential gallium scanning may also be considered.
3. CT scan of the affected part should be performed to rule out soft-tissue abscess.[91, 92]
4. MRI may be helpful because the finding of hemorrhage has been shown to be typical of bone crisis.[90]

If results of these studies are suspicious for infection or are inconclusive, needle biopsy of the affected area should be performed in the operating room under strict aseptic conditions. Needle biopsy is preferable to open biopsy to prevent wound breakdown. Preoperative consultation with an infectious disease specialist is recommended. Patients with Gaucher's disease tend to become infected with unusual organisms (*Bacteroides*, α-hemolytic *Streptococcus*, and *Proteus mirabilis* in Bell's series), and this should be taken into consideration in the submission of material for culture and in the planning of antibiotic coverage.[91]

Finally, preoperative planning should include a work-up for bleeding tendencies, as discussed in detail later.

MANAGEMENT

Currently, management of Gaucher's disease is based on the relatively recent development of a modified version of the deficient enzyme, which is recognized and taken up by the macrophage plasma membrane. Patients treated with this enzyme (alglucerase) at two weekly intervals for a year or more have shown elevation of their platelet counts and hematocrits, decreases in acid phosphatase levels, splenic and hepatic volumes, and resolution of the marrow changes by MRI and histological examinations.[80, 84, 86] This treatment is prohibitively expensive, however, for some patients, and modification of the treatment regimen to decrease expense has been the target of research.[80, 85] Gene therapy is the ultimate possible cure for Gaucher's disease and other inborn errors of metabolism and may be possible in the near future, because the gene locus for the deficient enzyme has been identified and the error in the nucleotide sequence defined.[80, 81]

The mainstay of treatment of the systemic manifestations of Gaucher's disease has been splenectomy when necessary for severe visceromegaly and thrombocytopenia. This measure is palliative only but can alleviate the hemorrhagic tendency. There is controversy as to whether splenectomy precipitates more severe skeletal involvement. There has been no conclusive evidence that splenectomy influences the onset or progression of skeletal disease.[81, 82] However, Katz et al[93] observed that pathological fractures are more common after splenectomy. Orthopaedic treatment of Gaucher's disease is limited to the treatment of the complications of the disease such as bone crisis, pathological fractures, ON, and osteomyelitis.

COMPLICATIONS

Bone crisis is a fairly common complication of Gaucher's disease, occurring in 10% to 32% of patients.[92] They should be treated much as a sickle cell crisis is treated, with supportive therapy such as bedrest, hydration, oxygenation, and narcotic pain medicine. Osteomyelitis should be ruled out, as discussed previously. If osteomyelitis is suspected based on the work-up and cultures have been taken, empirical broad-spectrum antibiotic treatment should be initiated. Crisis in the absence of infection should be expected to resolve within a few days to 2 to 3 weeks with supportive treatment.

There is a definite relationship between bone crisis and the subsequent development of pathological fracture. Katz et al[93] reported a series of 46 patients with type I disease who had a total of 23 fractures. Almost all occurred in splenectomized patients, and most occurred 2 months to 1 year after an acute crisis. Prolonged immobilization was also noted to be a risk factor for pathological fracture.[93]

Symptoms of pathological fracture include pain, swelling, and tenderness over the involved bone. Symptoms may be mild, however, and a history of trauma may be absent. Patients may continue to walk with a limp even in the presence of a fracture of the lower extremity. The typical site of fracture is in the metaphysis. Spine fractures may also present with mild but gradually progressive pain. Even a mild backache should be investigated to rule out vertebral fracture.[89]

Pathological fractures in Gaucher's disease require prolonged treatment times because formation of callus is exceedingly slow. Although evidence of callus may be seen on radiograph at 6 to 8 weeks, complete healing may take as long as 8 months. The initiation of weightbearing at 4 to 8 weeks is associated with gradual angulation and progression of the deformity at the fracture site. Femoral neck fractures treated nonoperatively tend to heal with varus deformity. The approach to pathological fracture, therefore, should include a high index of suspicion for fracture in a painful limb or back, early mobilization without weightbearing, prolonged protection of the fracture, and judicious use of surgical intervention when indicated, as in the case of femoral neck fractures. Weightbearing should not be allowed until good evidence of internal callus is seen.[93]

Pathological fractures of the spine usually heal without deformity. In the absence of progressive deformity or cord compromise, symptomatic treatment with or without bracing can be considered. Katz et al[93] recommended treatment of vertebral collapse and cord compromise with anterior decompression, strut grafting, and posterior instrumentation, keeping in mind that osteoporosis in these patients may compromise the stability of the instrumentation.[89]

ON is the most classically recognized orthopaedic complication of Gaucher's disease. Amstutz and Carey[82] reported ON of the femoral head in 75% of their patients. Bone crisis localized to the hip is usually the earliest sign of ON of the femoral head. Clinical presentation, laboratory values, and MRI findings are typical for bone crisis as described previously. Periosteal elevation is commonly seen along the femoral neck 6 weeks after the onset of the first crisis and is the earliest radiographic manifestation of ON. Several months later, classic signs of ON in the capital femoral epiphysis appear (Fig. 25). ON is bilateral in most cases, but onset is usually separated by 1 to 3 years. The average age of onset in Katz's series was 10 years. Treatment should consist of bedrest for 2 to 3 weeks followed by 1 to 3 weeks of non-weightbearing on the involved limb. Patients may discontinue the crutches when it is comfortable to do so. It does not appear that prolonged non-weightbearing treatment alters the natural history of ON in Gaucher's disease.[83] Total hip arthroplasty is the mainstay of treatment in adults with symptomatic ON of the femoral head resulting from Gaucher's disease. These individuals have a higher risk of intraoperative bleeding and aseptic loosening than do patients with idiopathic ON.

Humeral head ON is also common, although the need for total shoulder arthroplasty is rare because of the lack of weightbearing of this joint.[82]

Careful preparation of these patients for surgery is essential to avoid complications of hemorrhage and infection. Platelet counts, prothrombin time, partial thromboplastin time, liver enzymes, bleeding times, and platelet aggregation should be done preoperatively. Excessive bleeding may occur even when these tests are normal. Platelets, packed RBCs, and fresh frozen plasma should be available during the procedure, and the anesthesiologist should be made aware of the hemorrhagic tendency in these patients. Strict aseptic techniques should be followed. Immediate preoperative administration of broad-spectrum antibiotics in a one-time prophylactic dose should be given.

RESULTS

Results of enzyme treatment in Gaucher's disease are promising. Patients feel better, and histological and MRI findings suggest that the marrow normalizes after 1 to 2 years of therapy. Whether this form of treatment decreases the long-term morbidity of the skeletal system remains to be seen.

Splenectomy may significantly reduce hemorrhagic tendencies caused by thrombocytopenia, but the long-term effects of splenectomy on the skeletal system may be detrimental, as discussed previously.

Bone crisis tends to be self-limited when not associated with infection or pathological fracture; however, frequent bone crisis, particularly in the hip or shoulder, may herald subsequent radiographic evidence of ON. In most cases of pathological fracture, bone crisis has preceded fracture by about 6 weeks.

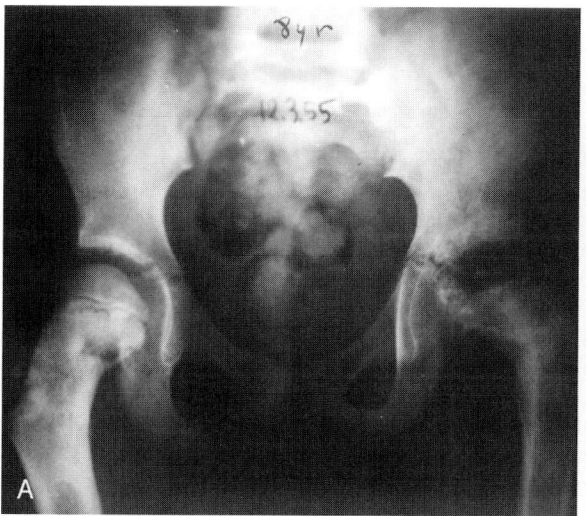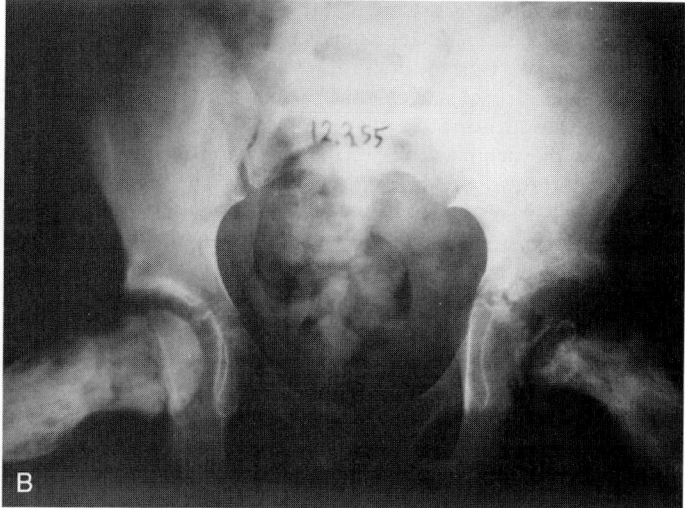

Fig. 25. Gaucher's disease. *A* and *B*, Anteroposterior and frog pelvis of 8-year-old boy with Gaucher's disease. Right hip shows mixed lytic and sclerotic lesions in the proximal femur without evidence of osteonecrosis (ON). Left hip shows primarily lytic lesions with severe ON of the femoral head. Disuse osteoporosis on the left is evident.

Pathological fracture is difficult to treat, and there is a high incidence of late deformity as a result of early weight-bearing and prolonged healing time. Although the results of only one hip fracture treated with internal fixation are reported in the literature,[93] internal fixation is recommended in femoral neck fractures, because nonoperative treatment invariably results in varus deformity.

The long-term outcome of osteomyelitis in Gaucher's disease has not been discussed in the literature. However, delay in diagnosis in three of Bell's patients led to unsatisfactory outcomes. Full recovery was evident within 1 year in the two patients in whom the infection was diagnosed early.[91]

The natural history of ON of the femoral head appears to be more benign than previously thought. Of the eight patients (13 hips) in Katz's[83] series, none required total hip arthroplasty at an average follow-up of 12 years. Total hip arthroplasty is the treatment of choice for disabling ON of the hips in the adult, and encouraging long-term results have been reported, although these patients do have a high risk of intraoperative bleeding and early aseptic loosening.[92]

GORHAM'S DISEASE

INTRODUCTION
Gorham's disease, also known as disappearing or vanishing bone disease, phantom bone, progressive osteolysis, massive osteolysis, and acute spontaneous absorption of bone, is a rare and unusual disorder of bone with uncertain cause, unpredictable prognosis, and unproven treatment.[94–97]

Definition
This acquired, insidious, and progressive resorption of a single bone can extend across joints and soft tissues to contiguous bones. Bone is replaced by nonmalignant angiomatosis that may spontaneously regress, stabilize with residual and permanent bone loss, or progress to death from local invasion of vital structures.

Historical Review
Jackson (1838) is credited with the first description of a "boneless" arm. One hundred years later several independent reports appeared between 1936 and 1937.[98] Gorham and Stout (1955) collected 24 cases (two of their own) with enough histological material to categorize the disease as a form of angiomatosis.[94] Torg and Steel (1969) attempted to elucidate radiographic stages.[99] Choma et al (1987) collected 97 cases to better describe the skeletal distribution and natural history.[100] On the basis of their own 11 cases treated at Mayo Clinic, Shives et al (1993) provided some hope for treatment.[101]

Epidemiology
With nearly 150 cases now documented, the disease is known to affect all ages from 4 weeks to 75 years, but with a definite predilection for adolescents and young adults. Males (64%) slightly outnumber females. Little more than half of the patients had documented trauma preceding the onset. The upper arm and shoulder girdle account for 26% of cases, whereas the mandible and femur comprise 15% and 11%, respectively. However, any bone can be affected, including the spine, metacarpals, and pelvis. Extension to contiguous bones is seen in 76%. The disease is fatal in 16% (10% secondary to chest wall invasion, 3% a result of spinal cord invasion, 2% from sepsis, 1% from aspiration), whereas only 5% are reported to regenerate the affected bones.

PATHOGENESIS
Without predilection to a location within a bone (epi-, meta-, or diaphysis) or to a type of bone (flat or long, cortical, or trabecular), an entire region of a bone gradually disappears radiographically. If preceded by a pathological fracture, the patient presents with pain, and the fracture does not heal. Rather, the ends of the fracture become thinned and may completely resorb over months or years, resulting in a swollen, painless nonunion. Biopsy samples routinely show large, thin-walled vascular sinusoids that

later result in a fibrous anlage of the original bone. Histology has not been pathognomonic. Hemangiomatosis and lymphangiomatosis have both been implicated, although cellular atypia are clearly absent. Occasionally, the bone will regenerate to a near-normal appearance. If the disease presents in the shoulder girdle, the clinical course is frequently disastrous with refractory chylothorax, erosion of the chest wall, cachexia, and death. If the disease occurs in a vertebra, structural instability and myelopathy also lead to high morbidity.[102]

INVESTIGATION

Routine laboratory is unremarkable except for sporadic reports of eosinophilia. Plain radiographs may show intramedullary and subcortical radiolucent foci followed by concentric shrinkage. Arteriography may show a "blush" within the affected area, and lymphangiography has also been shown to fill the lesion with dye. Technetium scintigraphy usually shows a relatively cold area surrounded by increased uptake in the delayed phase. CT scans merely delineate the structural bone loss, and to date MRI has not been diagnostic. When spinal or limb reconstructions are considered, CT and MRI can be helpful for preoperative planning.

DIFFERENTIAL DIAGNOSIS

Three distinct diseases may simulate the initial radiographic appearance. "Idiopathic hereditary osteolysis" is an autosomal-dominant condition affecting carpal or tarsal bones during childhood. "Idiopathic osteolyis with nephropathy" also affects carpal or tarsal bones, but renal involvement with azotemia and hypertension usually culminates in death by early adulthood. "Congenital hemangiomatosis" affects skin, subcutaneous tissues, muscle, and bone in an entire limb.

MANAGEMENT

Suspicious radiographic bone loss with prolonged limb swelling should lead to an early biopsy for a diagnosis. Although most authors reported poor results with autografting and internal fixation, occasional success follows structural allograft bridging.[103] In adults, limb salvage using metallic endoprostheses has been successful. Spinal stabilization by anterior and posterior fixation with allograft can protect the cord. Chylothorax seems refractory to simple chest tube drainage (one patient lost more than 50 L of chylous exudate over 40 days), so that more aggressive measures such as ligation of the thoracic duct and pleurodesis may be warranted. Medical treatments, including antibiotics, hormonal supplement (estrogens and androgens), calcium fluoride, vitamin D, vitamin B_{12}, and growth hormone have all been tried without success.[104]

Radiation therapy had been sporadically successful until Shives et al[101] published the Mayo Clinic experience in 11 patients. Whereas eight of nine autografts failed to obtain any union, six of eight patients receiving 30 Gy of radiation therapy experienced arrest of the disease.

COMPLICATIONS

Chylothorax from shoulder girdle involvement and paraplegia from spinal involvement both lead to death from decubiti, infection, and generalized cachexia. Even the more benign, self-limited involvement leads to bony nonunion, malunion, and limb dysfunction.

OSTEOPETROSIS

INTRODUCTION

Osteopetrosis, also known as Albers-Schönberg disease and marble bone disease, comprises a group of disorders characterized by increased bone radiopacity and defective bone resorption and remodeling. It was first described by the German radiologist Albers-Schönberg in 1904 and again by Kashner in 1922.[105] Traditionally, it has been classified into two phenotypic forms: the infantile-malignant autosomal-recessive form and the benign autosomal-dominant form. Within these two groups are a total of nine clinically heterogeneous subsets, including several autosomal-recessive intermediate groups that have a slightly later onset and generally milder clinical features than the infantile autosomal-recessive form. Another distinct intermediate autosomal-recessive subset is characterized by carbonic anhydrase II (CAII) deficiency. The incidence of osteopetrosis ranges between $1:100,000$ and $1:500,000$ people, although a single county in Denmark has reported an incidence of $5.5:100,000$ people.[106, 107] It is much more frequently seen in societies where inbreeding is common, although ethnicity and gender are not factors.

Pathogenesis

Osteopetrosis in all its forms results from a defect in osteoclast function. Osteoclasts are numerically normal, morphologically normal or abnormal, and functionally abnormal.[108] Whether the defect is in the maturation of osteoclasts from precursors or is a metabolic defect is not known. Bone marrow biopsy shows persistence of large amounts of calcified cartilage and primitive bone in the intramedullary spaces. Medullary cavities are very narrow. Hypocellularity, fibrosis, and spindle cell stroma may also be seen. Marrow spaces become obliterated, leading to pancytopenia and its complications. Quantitative CT scanning has shown that the increased radiopacity results from an increase in the amount of bone, not from an increase in density or mineral content.[109] Paradoxically, osteopetrotic bones are structurally weaker than normal bones because of the persistent accumulations of poorly organized mature bone and calcified cartilage.

Biochemical and genetic studies showed defects in macrophage and lymphocyte function in these patients, including defects in superoxide production.[110] Osteoblast dysfunction has also been implicated.[111] CAII deficiency is the only form that has been clearly identified biochemically. Deficiency of CAII prevents acid release, which is essential for bone mineral dissolution.[111]

CLINICAL FEATURES

Patients who suffer from the infantile-malignant autosomal-recessive type present within a few months of birth with failure to thrive, anemia and thrombocytopenia, hepatosplenomegaly, lymphadenopathy, bleeding tendencies, and fractures. Because of the lack of remodeling of the facial bones, the neural foramina become progressively smaller, leading to optic atrophy, deafness, oculomotor and facial palsies, and nasal obstruction. Obstructive sleep apnea may precipitate the need for tracheotomy.[107] Poor dentition and even osteomyelitis of the mandible are common. These patients have an increased susceptibility to infection and poor wound healing. Untreated, they rarely live beyond the age of 5 years.

Patients with the more benign, autosomal-dominant type have a normal life expectancy. They may have mild anemia, deafness, and facial palsies. Fractures are more common than in normal persons. An increased incidence of spondylolysis has been reported in these patients.[106] Within the autosomal-dominant group are two subsets: type I and type II. Autosomal-dominant type I is characterized by pronounced sclerosis of the cranial vault, whereas type II is characterized by alternating bands of increased and decreased radiopacity in the vertebrae (the so-called rugger jersey spine), pelvic endobones (a bone within a bone appearance), and marked osteosclerosis at the base of the skull. This type is associated with an especially increased risk of fractures and delayed fracture healing.[106]

INVESTIGATION

On radiograph, the bones are very dense and white (Fig. 26). The metaphyseal regions exhibit a flask-shaped deformity resulting from a lack of remodeling. Involvement may be nonhomogeneous, with some variability in radiodensity. The rugger jersey spine is an example of this phenomenon.

Laboratory findings in the patient with the infantile malignant forms include severe macrocytic anemia, reticulocytosis, teardrop red cells, circulating erythroblasts, and leukocytosis with immature myeloid elements. Thrombocytopenia, leukopenia, and hemolytic anemia eventually result from hypersplenism. Those with the autosomal-dominant forms exhibit a milder form of anemia without the other signs of stress erythropoiesis.

Bone marrow aspiration shows the characteristic histopathology mentioned previously. However, this technique is difficult in the sclerotic bone. Needle breakage is a significant risk.

Bone scanning with ^{99m}Tc-MDP shows widening of the metaphysis with increased tracer activity particularly in the metaphyses of the distal femur and proximal tibia.[105] This characteristic distribution may be used in the diagnosis of otherwise asymptomatic patients; however, radiographs are usually sufficient in establishing the diagnosis. Bone marrow immunoscintigraphy with ^{99m}Tc-Anti-NCA-95 shows a paucity of antibody accumulation in affected patients corresponding to the absence of hematopoietic marrow. The same study after successful BMT, however, shows a normal distribution of hematopoietic marrow. This study may be useful in monitoring response to treatment.[112]

DIFFERENTIAL DIAGNOSIS

Various other sclerosing bone diseases exist, including melorheostosis, X-linked hypophosphatemia with osteosclerosis, juvenile Paget's disease, craniometaphyseal dysplasia, fibrodysplasia (myositis) ossificans progressiva, osteopathia striata, Kenny-Caffey syndrome, hepatitis C–associated osteosclerosis, and idiopathic osteosclerosis. Most, like melorheostosis and Paget's disease, can be distinguished by their own characteristic radiographic features. Others have characteristic laboratory or phenotypic findings. Creatine kinase (CK) isoenzyme BB-CK is predominantly found in brain and is not normally detected in blood. However, it has been identified in the serum of patients with all types

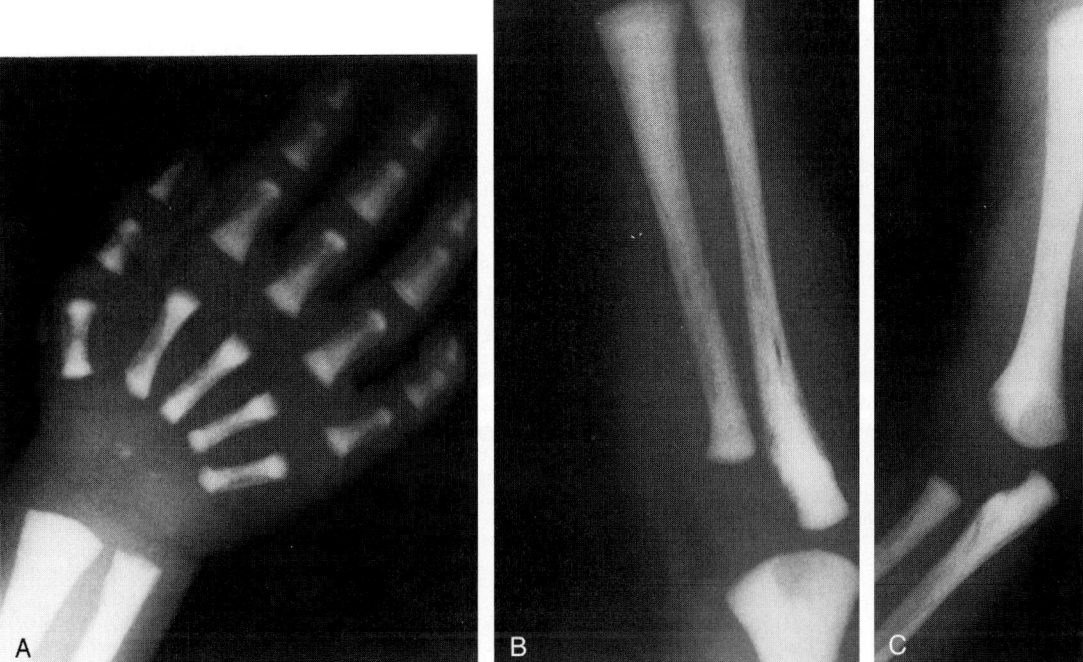

Fig. 26. Osteopetrosis. *A,* Anteroposterior (AP) radiograph of the right hand in a newborn with infantile malignant osteopetrosis. Marked but nonhomogeneous radiopacity is evident. *B,* AP forearm radiograph in the same patient. *C,* Oblique radiograph of elbow and humerus. Note the irregular pattern of sclerosis and apparent obliteration of medullary spaces.

of osteopetrosis, with the exception of the adult type I form. Its presence in the serum helps distinguish osteopetrosis from the other sclerosing bone disorders. Assay of cord blood in an affected newborn establishes the early diagnosis of malignant infantile osteopetrosis.[113]

MANAGEMENT

The treatment of choice for patients with infantile malignant osteopetrosis is BMT. The successful introduction of normal donor osteoclasts and hematopoietic cells results in restoration of normal hematopoiesis and improvement of radiographic findings.[108] Successful cord blood transplantation from an unrelated HLA-matched donor has also been reported.[114]

In milder disease or in the absence of a suitable donor, recombinant human interferon gamma, monocyte-macrophage colony-stimulating factor, and high-dose calcitriol have all been used, with varying success.[107]

Anemia and thrombocytopenia are treated symptomatically with transfusion of red cells and platelets. Erythropoietin and corticosteroid therapy may be of some benefit. Splenectomy is indicated for severe hypersplenism.[108]

Spondylolysis responds well to nonoperative treatment with the use of a lumbosacral corset or thoracolumbosacral orthosis. Several years of such treatment may be required before symptoms resolve and healing occurs.[106]

Fractures may be treated by conventional methods; however, healing times are generally prolonged. Sclerotic bone may be difficult to drill.

COMPLICATIONS

The primary complication of BMT is GVHD. Cord blood transplantation may present a slightly lower risk. Death from adult respiratory distress syndrome has been reported in two children who had previously been treated with recombinant interferon gamma and macrophage colony-stimulating factor. An autoimmune phenomenon has been implicated.[115] These patients have an abnormal immune system and are prone to wound healing problems and infection, particularly after surgery.

RESULTS

BMT results in a 5-year survival rate of at least 80% of patients with an HLA-identical donor. Experience with cord blood transplantation is limited but promising. Early transplantation offers the only hope for cure.

REFERENCES

Leukemia

1. Gallager DJ, Phillips DJ, Heinrich SD: Orthopedic manifestations of acute pediatric leukemia. Orthop Clin North Am 1996; 27:635.
2. Rogalsky RJ, Black GB, Reed MH: Orthopaedic manifestations of leukemia in children. J Bone Joint Surg Am 1986; 68:494.
3. Heinrich SD, Gallagher D, Warrior R, et al: The prognostic significance of the skeletal manifestations of acute lymphoblastic leukemia of childhood. J Pediatr Orthop 1994; 14:105.
4. Niemeyer CM, Sallan SE: Acute lymphocytic leukemia. In Nathan DG, Orkin SH (eds): Nathan & Oski's Hematology of Infancy and Childhood. Philadelphia, WB Saunders, 1998, 5th ed, vol 2, p 1245.
5. Clausen N, Gotze H, Pedersen A, et al: Skeletal scintigraphy and radiography at onset of acute lymphocytic leukemia in children. Med Pediatr Oncol 1983; 11:291.
6. Ostrov BE, Goldsmith DP, Athreya BH: Differentiation of systemic juvenile rheumatoid arthritis from acute leukemia near the onset of disease. J Pediatr 1993; 122:595.
7. Tuten HR, Gabos PG, Kumar SJ, et al: The limping child: A manifestation of acute leukemia. J Pediatr Orthop 1998; 18:625.

Langerhans' Cell Histiocytosis

8. Dimentberg RA, Brown KLB: Diagnostic evaluation of patients with histiocytosis X. J Pediatr Orthop 1990; 10:733.

9. Sullivan JL, Woda BA: Langerhans' cell histiocytosis. In Nathan DG, Orkin SH (eds): Nathan & Oski's Hematology of Infancy and Childhood. Philadelphia, WB Saunders, 1998, 5th ed, vol 2, p 1371.
10. Raney RB Jr, D'Angio GJ: Langerhans' cell histiocytosis (histiocytosis X): Experience at the Children's Hospital of Philadelphia, 1970–1984. Med Pediatr Oncol 1989; 17:20.
11. Bollini MD, Jouve JL, Gentet JC, et al: Bone lesions in histiocytosis X. J Pediatr Orthop 1991; 11:469.
12. Sessa S, Sommelet D, Lascombes P, et al: Treatment of Langerhans-cell histiocytosis in children. J Bone Joint Surg Am 1994; 76:1513.
13. Favara BE: Langerhans' cell histiocytosis pathobiology and pathogenesis. Semin Oncol 1991; 18:3.
14. Mammano S, Candiotto S, Balsano M: Cast and brace treatment of eosinophilic granuloma of the spine: Long-term follow-up. J Pediatr Orthop 1997; 17:821.
15. Cheyne C: Histiocytosis X. J Bone Joint Surg Br 1971; 53:366.

Sickle Cell Disease

16. Piehl FC, Davis RJ, Prugh SI: Osteomyelitis in sickle cell disease. J Pediatr Orthop 1993; 13:225.
17. Platt OS, Brambilla DJ, Rosse WF, et al: Mortality in sickle cell disease. N Engl J Med 1994; 330:1639.
18. Dover GJ, Platt OS: The sickle hemoglobinopathies. In Nathan DG, Orkin SH (eds): Nathan & Oski's Hematology of Infancy and Childhood. Philadelphia, WB Saunders, 1998, 5th ed, vol 1, p 762.
19. Mankad VN, Williams JP, Harpen MD,

et al: Magnetic resonance imaging of bone marrow in sickle cell disease: Clinical, hematologic and pathologic correlations. Blood 1990; 75:274.
20. Smith JA: Bone disorders in sickle cell disease. Hematol Oncol Clin North Am 1996; 10:1345.
21. Onuba O: Bone disorders in sickle cell disease. Int Orthop 1993; 17:397.
22. Stevens MC, Padwick M, Serjeant GR: Observations on the natural history of dactylitis in homozygous sickle cell disease. Clin Pediatr 1981; 20:311.
23. Epps CH Jr, Bryant DD, Coles MJM, Castro O: Osteomyelitis in patients who have sickle cell disease. J Bone Joint Surg Am 1991; 73:1281.
24. Greene WB, McMillan CW: *Salmonella* osteomyelitis and hand-foot syndrome in a child with sickle cell anemia. J Pediatr Orthop 1987; 7:716.
25. Omojola MF, Annobil S, Adzaku F: Bone changes in sickle cell anaemia. East Afr Med J 1993; 70:154.
26. Dalton GP, Drummond DS, Davidson RS, et al: Bone infarction versus infection in sickle cell disease in children. J Pediatr Orthop 1996; 16:540.
27. Givner LB, Luddy RE, Schwartz AD: Etiology of osteomyelitis in patients with major sickle hemoglobinopathies. J Pediatr 1981; 99:411.
28. Ebong WW: Pathological fracture complicating long bone osteomyelitis in patients with sickle cell disease. J Pediatr Orthop 1986; 6:177.
29. Platt OS, Thorington BD, Brambilla DJ, et al: Pain in sickle cell disease. N Engl J Med 1991; 325:11.
30. Vermylen C, Cornu G: Bone marrow transplantation for sickle cell disease. Am J Pediatr Hematol Oncol 1994; 16:18.

31. Clarke HJ, Jinnah RH, Brooker AF, et al: Total replacement of the hip for avascular necrosis in sickle cell disease. J Bone Joint Surg Br 1989; 71:465.

32. Milner PF, Kraus AP, Sebes JI, et al: Sickle cell disease as a cause of ON of the femoral head. N Engl J Med 1991; 325:1476.

33. Hernigou P, Galacteros F, Bachir D, et al: Deformities of the hip in adults who have sickle-cell disease and had avascular necrosis in childhood. J Bone Joint Surg Am 1991; 73:81.

34. Hernigou P, Bachir D, Galacteros F: Avascular necrosis of the femoral head in sickle-cell disease: Treatment of collapse by the injection of acrylic cement. J Bone Joint Surg Br 1993; 75:875.

35. Bishop AR, Roberson JR, Eckman JR, et al: Total hip arthroplasty in patients who have sickle-cell hemoglobinopathy. J Bone Joint Surg Am 1988; 70:853.

36. Hickman JM, Lachiewicz PF: Results and complications of total hip arthroplasties in patients with sickle-cell hemoglobinopathies. J Arthroplasty 1997; 12:420.

37. Acurio MT, Friedman RJ: Hip arthroplasty in patients with sickle-cell hemoglobinopathy. J Bone Joint Surg Br 1992; 74:367.

38. Moran MC: Osteonecrosis of the hip in sickle cell hemoglobinopathy. Ann Orthop 1995; 24:18.

39. Garden MS, Grant RE, Jebraili S: Perioperative complications in patients with sickle cell disease. Am J Orthop 1996; 25:353.

40. Hanker GJ, Amstutz HC: Osteonecrosis of the hip in the sickle-cell diseases. J Bone Joint Surg Am 1988; 70:499.

41. Milner PF, Kraus AP, Sebes JZ, et al: Osteonecrosis of the humeral head in sickle cell disease. Clin Orthop 1993; 289:136.

42. Smid WM, Breukelman F, Konings JG, et al: Pyomyositis in sickle cell disease: An unexpected diagnosis. Ann Hematol 1995; 70:277.

Thalassemia

43. Colavita N, Orazi C, Danza SM, et al: Premature epiphyseal fusion and extramedullary hematopoiesis in thalassemia. Skeletal Radiol 1987; 16:533.

44. Piomelli S, Loew T: Management of thalassemia major (Cooley's anemia). Hematol Oncol Clin North Am 1991; 5:557.

45. Orkin SH, Nathan DG: The thalassemias. In Nathan DG, Orkin SH (eds): Nathan & Oski's Hematology of Infancy and Childhood. Philadelphia, WB Saunders, 1998, 5th ed, vol 1, p 829.

46. Levin TL, Sheth SS, Ruzal-Shapiro C, et al: MRI marrow observations in thalassemia: The effects of the primary disease, transfusional therapy, and chelation. Pediatr Radiol 1995; 25:607.

47. Dines DM, Canale VC, Arnold WD: Fractures in thalassemia. J Bone Joint Surg Am 1976; 58:662.

48. Exarchou E, Politou C, Vretou E, et al: Fractures and epiphyseal deformities in beta-thalassemia. Clin Orthop 1984; 189:229.

49. Papavasiliou C: Clinical expressions of the expansion of the bone marrow in the chronic anemias: The role of radiotherapy. Int J Radiat Oncol Biol Phys 1994; 28:605.

50. Lapatsanis P, Divoli A, Georgaki H, et al: Bone growth in thalassaemic children. Arch Dis Child 1978; 53:963.

51. Gimmon Goldschmidt Z, Wexler MR, Rachmilewitz EA: Juvenile leg ulceration in beta-thalassemia major and intermedia. Plast Reconstr Surg 1982; 69:320.

52. Giardini C, Angelucci E, Lucarelli G, et al: Bone marrow transplantation for thalassemia: Experience in Pesaro, Italy. Am J Pediatr Hematol Oncol 1994; 16:6.

Fanconi's Anemia

53. Minagi H, Steinbach HL: Roentgen appearance of anomalies associated with hypoplastic anemias of childhood: Fanconi's anemia and congenital hypoplastic anemia (erythrogenesis imperfecta). AJR Am J Roentgenol 1966; 97:100.

54. Alter BP: Fanconi's anemia, current concepts. Am J Pediatr Hematol Oncol 1992; 14:170.

55. Strathdee CA, Buchwald M: Molecular and cellular biology of Fanconi anemia. Am J Pediatr Hematol Oncol 1992; 14:177.

56. Alter BP: Thumbs and anemia. Pediatrics 1978; 62:613.

57. Gluckman E, Auerbach AD, Horowitz MM, et al: Bone marrow transplantation for Fanconi anemia. Blood 1995; 86:2856.

58. Davies SM, Khan S, Wagner JE, et al: Unrelated donor bone marrow transplantation for Fanconi anemia. Bone Marrow Transplant 1996; 17:43.

59. Bagnara GP, Strippoli P, Bonsi L, et al: Effect of stem cell factor on colony growth from acquired and constitutional (Fanconi) aplastic anemia. Blood 1992; 80:382.

60. Guinan EC, Lopez KD, Huhn RD, et al: Evaluation of granulocyte-macrophage colony-stimulating factor for treatment of pancytopenia in children with Fanconi anemia. J Pediatr 1994; 124:144.

61. Sinohara O, Kato S, Yabe H, et al: Growth after bone marrow transplantation in children. Am J Pediatr Hematol Oncol 1991; 13:263.

Thrombocytopenia-Absent Radius Syndrome

62. Hall JG, Levin J, Kuhn J, et al: Thrombocytopenia with absent radius (TAR). Medicine 1969; 48:411.

63. Schoenecker PL, Cohn AK, Sedgwick W, et al: Dysplasia of the knee associated with the syndrome of thrombocytopenia with absent radius. J Bone Joint Surg Am 1984; 66:421.

64. Hall JG: Thrombocytopenia and absent radius (TAR) syndrome. J Med Genet 1987; 24:79.

65. Hedberg VA, Lipton JM: Thrombocytopenia with absent radii: A review of 100 cases. Am J Pediatr Hematol Oncol 1988; 10:51.

66. Tolo VT: Congenital absence of the menisci and cruciate ligaments of the knee. J Bone Joint Surg Am 1981; 63:1022.

Lymphoma

67. Wollner N, Lane JM, Marcove RC, et al: Primary skeletal non-Hodgkin's lymphoma in the pediatric age group. Med Pediatr Oncol 1992; 20:506.

68. Baar J, Burkes RL, Bell R, et al: Primary non-Hodgkin's lymphoma of bone. Cancer 1994; 73:1194.

69. Coppes MJ, Patte C, Couanet D, et al: Childhood malignant lymphoma of bone. Med Pediatr Oncol 1991; 19:22.

70. Desai S, Jamhekar NA, Soman CS, et al: Primary lymphoma of bone: A clinicopathologic study of 25 cases reported over 10 years. J Surg Oncol 1991; 46:265.

71. Dubey P, Ha CS, Besa PC, et al: Localized primary malignant lymphoma of bone. Int J Radiat Oncol Biol Phys 1997; 37:1087.

72. Lewis SJ, Bell RS, Fernandes BJ, et al: Malignant lymphoma of bone. Can J Surg 1994; 37:43.

73. Hermann G, Klein MJ, Abdelwahab IF, et al: MRI appearance of primary non-Hodgkin's lymphoma of bone. Skeletal Radiol 1997; 26:629.

74. Stiglbauer R, Augustin I, Kramer J, et al: MRI in the diagnosis of primary lymphoma of bone: Correlation with histopathology. Comput Assist Tomogr 1992; 16:248.

75. Bar-Shalom R, Israel O, Epelbaum R, et al: Gallium-67 scintigraphy in lymphoma with bone involvement. J Nucl Med 1995; 36:446.

76. Melamed JW, Martinez S, Hoffman CJ: Imaging of primary multifocal osseous lymphoma. Skeletal Radiol 1997; 26:35.

77. Chan K, Miller DR, Rosen G, et al: Hodgkin's disease in adolescents presenting as a primary bone lesion. Am J Pediatr Hematol Oncol 1982; 4:11.

78. Gross SB, Robertson WW, Lange BJ, et al: Primary Hodgkin's disease of bone. Clin Orthop 1992; 283:276.

79. Appell RG, Oppermann HC, Brandeis WE: Skeletal lesions in Hodgkin's disease. Pediatr Radiol 1981; 11:61.

Gaucher's Disease

80. Mankin HJ: Gaucher's disease: A novel treatment and an important breakthrough. J Bone Joint Surg Br 1993; 75:2.

81. Zimran A, Kay A, Gelbart T, et al: Gaucher disease. Clinical, laboratory, radiologic and genetic features of 53 patients. Medicine 1992; 71:337.

82. Amstutz HC, Carey EJ: Skeletal manifestations and treatment of Gaucher's disease. J Bone Joint Surg Am 1966; 48:670.

83. Katz K, Horev G, Grunebaum M, et al: The natural history of osteonecrosis of the femoral head in children and adoles-

cents who have Gaucher disease. J Bone Joint Surg Am 1996; 78:14.

84. Barton NW, Brady RO, D'ambrosia JM, et al: Replacement therapy for inherited enzyme deficiency-macrophage-targeted glucocerebrosidase for Gaucher's disease. N Engl J Med 1991; 324:1464.

85. Figueroa ML, Rosenbloom BE, Kay AC, et al: A less costly regimen of alglucerase to treat Gaucher's disease. N Engl J Med 1992; 327:1632.

86. Allison JW, James CA, Arnold GL, et al: Reconversion of bone marrow in Gaucher disease treated with enzyme therapy documented by MR. Pediatr Radiol 1998; 28:237.

87. Kolodny EH, Lebron D: Gaucher's disease. In Nathan DG, Orkin SH (eds): Nathan & Oski's Hematology of Infancy and Childhood. Philadelphia, WB Saunders, 1998, 5th ed, vol 2, p 1474.

88. Katz K, Mechlis-Frish S, Cohen IJ, et al: Bone scans in the diagnosis of bone crisis in patients who have Gaucher's disease. J Bone Joint Surg Am 1991; 73: 513.

89. Katz K, Sabato S, Horev G, et al: Spinal involvement in children and adolescents with Gaucher disease. Spine 1993; 18: 332.

90. Horev G, Kornreich L, Hadar H, et al: Hemorrhage associated with "bone crisis" in Gaucher's disease identified by magnetic resonance imaging. Skeletal Radiol 1991; 20:479.

91. Bell RS, Mankin HJ, Doppelt SH: Osteomyelitis in Gaucher disease. J Bone Joint Surg Am 1986; 68:1380.

92. Tauber C, Tauber T: Gaucher disease—The orthopaedic aspect. Arch Orthop Trauma Surg 1995; 114:179.

93. Katz K, Cohen IJ, Ziv N, et al: Fractures in children who have Gaucher disease. J Bone Joint Surg Am 1987; 69:1361.

Gorham's Disease

94. Gorham LW, Stout AP: Massive osteolysis (acute spontaneous absorption of bone, phantom bone, disappearing bone): Its relation to hemangiomatosis. J Bone Joint Surg Am 1955; 37:985.

95. Jones GB, Midgley RL, Smith GS: Massive osteolysis—Disappearing bones. J Bone Joint Surg Br 1958; 40:494.

96. Joseph J, Bartal E: Disappearing bone disease: A case report and review of the literature. J Pediatr Orthop 1987; 7:584.

97. Sage MR, Allen PW: Massive osteolysis: A report of a case. J Bone Joint Surg Br 1974; 56:130.

98. Jackson JBS: A boneless arm. Boston Med Surg J 1838; 18:368.

99. Torg JS, Steel HH: Sequential roentgenographic changes occurring in massive osteolysis. J Bone Joint Surg Am 1969; 51: 1649.

100. Choma ND, Biscotti CV, Bauer TW, et al: Gorham's syndrome: A case report and review of the literature. Am J Med 1987; 83:1151.

101. Shives TC, Beabout JW, Uuni KK: Massive osteolysis. Clin Orthop 1993; 294: 267.

102. Dewry GR, Sutterlin CE III, Martinez CR, et al: Gorham disease of the spine. Spine 1994; 19:2213.

103. Butler RW, McCance RA, Barrett AM: Unexplained destruction of the shaft of the femur in a child. J Bone Joint Surg Br 1958; 40:487.

104. Branco F, Horta JDS: Notes on a rare case of essential osteolysis. J Bone Joint Surg Br 1958; 40:519.

Osteopetrosis

105. el-Desouki M, al Herbish A, al Rasheed S, et al: Bone scintigraphy and densitometry in children with osteopetrosis. Clin Nucl Med 1995; 20:1061.

106. Martin RP, Deane RH, Collett V: Spondylolysis in children who have osteopetrosis. J Bone Joint Surg Am 1997; 79: 1685.

107. Stocks RMS, Wang MD, Thompson MD: Malignant infantile osteopetrosis. Arch Otolaryngol 1998; 124:689.

108. Alter BP, Young NS: The bone marrow failure syndrome. In Nathan DG, Orkin SH (eds): Nathan & Oski's Hematology of Infancy and Childhood. Philadelphia, WB Saunders, 1998, 5th ed, vol 1, p 310.

109. Kovanlikaya A, Loro ML, Gilsanz V: Pathogenesis of osteosclerosis in autosomal dominant osteopetrosis. AJR Am J Roentgen 1997; 168:929.

110. Yamamoto N, Naraparaju VR, Orchard PJ: Defective lymphocyte glycosidases in the macrophage activation cascade of juvenile osteopetrosis. Blood 1996; 88: 1473.

111. Lajeunesse D, Busque L, Menard P, et al: Demonstration of an osteoblast defect in two cases of human malignant osteopetrosis. J Clin Invest 1996; 98:1835.

112. Thelen MH, Eschmann SM, Moll-Kotowski M, et al: Bone marrow scintigraphy with technetium-99m anti-NCA-95 to monitor therapy in malignant osteopetrosis. J Nucl Med 1998; 39:1033.

113. Whyte MP, Chines A, Silva DP Jr, et al: Creatine kinase brain isoenzyme (BB-CK) presence in serum distinguishes osteopetrosis among the sclerosing bone disorders. J Bone Miner Res 1996; 11: 1438.

114. Locatelli F, Belluffi G, Giorgiani G, et al: Transplantation of cord blood progenitor cells can promote bone resorption in autosomal recessive osteopetrosis. Bone Marrow Transplant 1997; 20:701.

115. Madyastha PR, Jeter EK, Key LL: Cytophilic immunoglobulin G binding on neutrophils from a child with malignant osteopetrosis who developed fatal acute respiratory distress mimicking transfusion-related acute lung injury. Am J Hematol 1996; 53:196.

INFLAMMATORY ARTHRITIDES: JUVENILE RHEUMATOID ARTHRITIS, SERONEGATIVE SPONDYLOARTHROPATHIES, TRANSIENT SYNOVITIS, HEMOPHILIC ARTHROPATHY

Timothy P. Carey

Summary
- Rheumatic diseases of childhood encompass a broad spectrum of conditions that must be considered in the differential diagnosis of the child presenting with a painful or swollen joint.
- Juvenile rheumatoid arthritis (JRA) is the most common rheumatic disease of childhood and affects more than 200,000 children in North America.
- JRA is classified by the pattern of clinical involvement into three main groups: pauciarticular, polyarticular, and systemic onset.
- Seronegative spondyloarthropathies present with both spinal and peripheral arthritis symptoms; in childhood, the latter may predominate, and the condition may be confused with JRA.
- The majority of children affected with rheumatic disease have a good prognosis, but a significant percentage develop chronic disease with long-term complications.

DEFINITION

Childhood arthritis is a clinical entity that frequently presents to the orthopaedic surgeon for a first assessment. The multifaceted nature of inflammatory arthritides makes exact definition and classification challenging. Several subgroups of chronic inflammatory arthritis are recognized in children. The definition of juvenile arthritis, according to the American Rheumatology Association, consists of (1) chronic synovial inflammation of unknown cause; (2) onset younger than 16 years of age; (3) objective evidence of arthritis (swelling of a joint or limitation of motion with heat, pain, or tenderness) present in one or more joints for 6 consecutive weeks; and (4) exclusion of other diseases.[1]

Alternatively, the European League Against Rheumatism requires evidence of disease for 3 months and includes the seronegative spondyloarthropathies under the umbrella term "juvenile chronic arthritis."[2]

Seronegative spondyloarthropathies are defined as arthritis associated with sacroiliitis, spinal arthritis, and enthesitis. Seronegative arthritides refer to the absence of immunological markers such as rheumatoid factor or antinuclear antibodies (ANA) in the sera of affected patients. Clinical examples include ankylosing spondylitis or reactive arthritis such as Reiter's syndrome and arthritis associated with inflammatory bowel disease or psoriasis (Fig. 1).

Many other examples of "nonrheumatological" inflammatory arthritis involving children can present with similar clinical pictures. Chronic inflammatory arthritis can be seen in hemophilia, the result of recurrent hemarthroses. Tran-sient synovitis, an idiopathic condition, is often related to an antecedent respiratory infection and produces an acute inflammation of the hip joint that is self-limited.

HISTORY

In 1896 chronic joint disease was reported in the United States by Koplick. In 1897 George F. Still described chronic joint disease in children.[3] Pediatric rheumatology was developed as a subspecialty during the 1960s and 1970s.

EPIDEMIOLOGY

The incidence of rheumatic diseases in the United States is estimated as affecting approximately 200,000 children. A Mayo Clinic survey suggested an incidence of 13.9 per 100,000 children and a prevalence of 113 per 100,000. The multiple subtypes and protean manifestations of the disease undoubtedly lead to an underestimation of the true incidence.[4]

Typical ages of onset are characteristic for a number of rheumatic diseases and can be helpful in formulating differential diagnoses. Most rheumatic diseases are more common in females, with the exception of systemic onset JRA and the seronegative spondyloarthropathies.

Localized inflammatory arthritides are a very common cause of symptoms in children. Transient synovitis has been demonstrated to be the most common diagnosis in children who present with decreased range of motion of a joint or a limp or with hip pain.[5] Recurrent hemarthroses with resultant inflammatory arthropathy occur in hemophilia, an x-linked recessive deficiency of clotting factor VIII (hemophilia A) or IX (hemophilia B) affecting approximately 1.25/10,000 male births.[6]

PATHOGENESIS

The inflammatory response is the unifying element in all the entities. In certain inflammatory arthropathies, such as hemophilia, the cause is obviously due to recurrent hemarthroses, but the cause of the chronic inflammatory and immune responses in the rheumatic diseases of childhood is still unclear. The multiple factors that interact to create a chronic inflammatory response in these conditions are what set this response apart from the normal inflammation seen as a process of normal injury and repair throughout the human body. The inflammation appears to be antigenically stimulated, but whether the source of the antigen is environmental (e.g., infectious) or truly an autoimmune phenomenon continues to be explored.

The pathological features of inflammation involving diar-

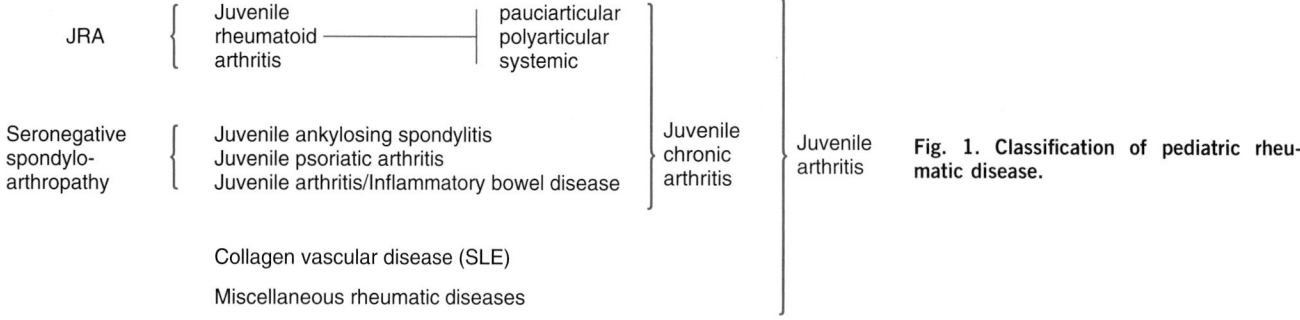

Fig. 1. Classification of pediatric rheumatic disease.

throdial joints is well known. An initial vascular response leads to increased capillary permeability and transudation of protein-rich sera into the extracellular space, followed by the exudative phase of inflammation, with migration of leukocytes to the site in response to chemotactic factors. Phagocytic cellular activity leads to the release of lysosomal hydrolytic enzymes, and fibroblastic and angioblastic activity occurs as part of an attempted healing phase.[7]

Histological examination of an involved joint reveals hypertrophic synovial villi with lymphocytic (predominantly T-cell) infiltration. In advanced cases, hypertrophy and hyperplasia of the synovium lead to formation of pannus (a granulation tissue composed of proliferating fibroblasts, blood vessels, and inflammatory cells), which advances over the cartilaginous surface. The action on articular cartilage leads to thinning and destruction of the cartilage and eventual exposure of subchondral bone. In the early stages, the pannus preferentially attacks the "bare" areas of the joint that are intra-articular but not covered by articular cartilage. This leads to the clinical manifestation of marginal erosions.

Additional clinical manifestation of rheumatic disease are due to the effects of inflammation on the periarticular tissues such as joint capsule ligaments and tendons. Capsular thickening and inflammation of surrounding muscles and tendons lead to contractures and decreased range of motion at joints. Extensive involvement of periarticular tissues can affect joint integrity and lead to joint subluxations. Chronic inflammation also leads to osteopenia.

A unique effect of chronic inflammation in the growing skeleton is growth stimulation of open physes. This can lead to limb-length discrepancy, although this depends predominantly on the amount of growth potential remaining at the onset of disease. In younger children, chronic inflammation can lead to growth stimulation. In the older child closer to skeletal maturity, the hyperemia can lead to premature physeal arrest.[8]

In hemophilic arthropathy, chronic inflammation of the synovium of the joint is incited by recurrent hemorrhage and deposition of iron in the joint. The iron deposits are phagocytosed by the synovial cells, leading to cell breakdown and release of enzymes, resulting in a hypertrophic synovitis with villous hypertrophy, increased vascularity, and chronic inflammatory cell infiltrates. The hypertrophic synovial villi are more friable and, in the presence of the clotting disorder, tend to bleed more easily, leading to recurrent hemarthrosis and setting up a cycle of chronic inflammation in the joint. This results in a rapidly progressive arthropathy.[9]

Transient synovitis presents with acute joint swelling owing to inflammation in the joint. The postulated process is likely similar to a reactive arthritis, perhaps an immune complex–mediated inflammation; tends to be short-lived; and does not truly fit into a chronic inflammatory picture.

CLINICAL FEATURES

Inflammatory arthritis must be considered in the child who presents with joint pain or limitation in range of motion. Patient age, distribution of the joints involved, and associ-

TABLE 1. CLINICAL FEATURES OF JUVENILE ARTHRITIS

	Pauciarticular	Polyarticular	Systemic
Frequency of Cases	50%	40%	10%
Number of joints	<5m	5 or greater	Variable
Age of onset	Early childhood; peak 1–2 yrs	Throughout childhood; peak at 1–3 yrs	Throughout childhood; no peak
Sex ratio (F:M)	5:1	3:1	1:1
Systemic involvement	Not present	Moderate	Prominent
Occurrence of chronic uveitis	20%	5%	Rare
Frequency of seropositivity			
Rheumatoid factors	Rare	10% (increases with age)	Rare
Antinuclear antibodies	75%–85%*	40%–50%	10%
Prognosis	Excellent except for eyesight	Guarded to moderately good	Moderate to poor

* Females with uveitis.
From Cassidy JT, Petty RE: Textbook of Pediatric Rheumatology. Philadelphia, WB Saunders, 1995, 3rd ed, p 146.

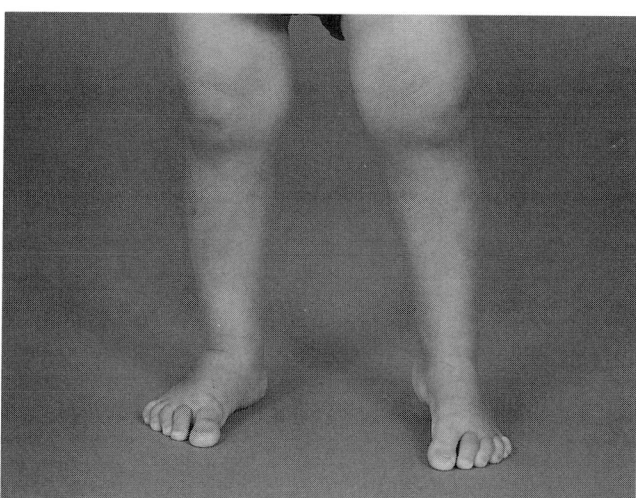

Fig. 2. Clinical photograph. This demonstrates bilateral knee effusions in an 18-month-old female with pauciarticular JRA.

TABLE 2. GUIDELINES FOR OPHTHALMOLOGICAL EXAMINATIONS IN CHILDREN WITH JRA

A. **No history of uveitis**
Pauciarticular disease—At initial diagnosis, then every 3 months for 2 years, then every 6 months for 7 years, then yearly.
Polyarticular disease—at initial diagnosis, then every 4–6 months for 5 years, then yearly.
Systemic onset disease—at initial diagnosis, then yearly.
B. **History of uveitis**
Inactive ocular disease—every 3 months.
Active ocular disease—as indicated by therapy.

ated systemic symptoms can all be useful in identifying the various types of inflammatory arthritides. JRA is usually divided into three subgroups: pauciarticular, polyarticular, and systemic onset disease (Table 1).[10]

Pauciarticular JRA is the most common subtype that is likely to present to the orthopaedic surgeon without previous diagnosis. The classic clinical presentation is that of a female toddler presenting with involvement of a knee or ankle (Fig. 2). The presentation is frequently that of a limp or decreased range of motion with fairly mild symptoms and often no significant pain except at range-of-motion extremes. Objective evidence of inflammation is present with swelling, increased warmth, decreased range of motion, and discomfort with motion, although patients can be pain-free. The condition most frequently involves the knee and the ankle; it is less likely to be seen with involvement of fingers, elbows, or wrists. Rarely is the hip or shoulder involved, and by definition fewer than five joints are affected. Systemic symptoms are rarely, if ever, seen. However, there can frequently be asymptomatic involvement of the anterior uveal tract of the eyeball with a chronic uveitis (iridocyclitis). This is often silent with respect to symptoms but can lead to permanent visual impairment. Up to 20% of patients with pauciarticular JRA have evidence of chronic uveitis. The majority of these (up to 90%) show evidence of ANA on serological testing. Guidelines for ophthalmological assessment in JRA are shown in Table 2).[11]

Polyarticular juvenile arthritis is less common and typically affects the slightly older age groups, although females are still preferentially affected. Presentation is with an insidious onset of symmetric arthritis involving the knees, wrists, and elbows, with five or more joints being involved within the first 6 months of the disease. An important subset of patients is that of females with the onset of disease in late childhood or adolescence and associated with a positive rheumatoid factor. This subgroup is at higher risk for a more chronic disease picture similar to adult rheumatoid arthritis. Systemic symptoms are variable but not usually severe. Uveitis occurs in only 5% of patients, in contrast to the pauciarticular patient population.

Systemic onset juvenile arthritis is the least common form. Systemic symptoms can precede the onset of arthritis. A classic clinical sign is a high-spiking daily fever, often occurring in the late afternoon or early evening, that can be associated with an evanescent (salmon-pink) erythematous macular rash with central clearing. Visceral disease is frequently seen with hepatosplenomegaly, lymphadenopathy, and pericarditis.

Seronegative spondyloarthropathies are, by definition, conditions that involve arthritis associated with sacroiliitis, spinal arthritis, and enthesitis (inflammation at sites of ligament or tendon attachment to bone). The clinical features vary somewhat with the subtype (Table 3). Males are more frequently affected than females in a ratio of four to one. The classic example of the condition is ankylosing spondylitis. Onset in childhood usually occurs in boys older than 8 years, with the development of asymmetric arthritis predominantly involving hips, knees, ankles, and toes. These symptoms can precede the onset of back pain and stiffness, although a more typical adult form with back symptoms predominating also occurs.[12]

An important subpopulation is a group of patients with so-called "SEA syndrome." This syndrome of seropositive enthesopathy and arthropathy (SEA) is in fact the most common type of spondyloarthropathy seen in pediatric patients. These patients have enthesitis and either arthritis or arthralgia. They are seronegative but do not fulfill a diagnostic criterion for any specific spondyloarthropathy. The significance of identifying SEA syndrome lies in the fact that it implies a high likelihood of evolution to a definitive spondyloarthropathy in time.[13]

TABLE 3. CLASSIFICATION OF SPONDYLOARTHROPATHY

Inflammatory spinal pain
or
Synovitis (asymmetric or predominantly lower limbs)
Plus one or more of the following:
    Positive family history.
    Psoriasis.
    Inflammatory bowel disease.
    Urethritis, cervicitis, or acute diarrhea within 1 month before arthritis.
    Buttock pain alternating in site.
    Enthesopathy.
    Sacroiliitis.

Other spondyloarthropathies seen include reactive arthritis following gastrointestinal or genitourinary infections and reactive arthritis associated with other diseases such as inflammatory bowel disease or psoriasis. The constellation of arthritis, conjunctivitis, and urethritis is known as Reiter's syndrome. This reactive arthritis is usually a postdysenteric infection in children as opposed to a sexually transmitted infection in adults. Typical organisms involved are *Salmonella*, *Shigella*, *Yersinia*, and *Campylobacter* species.

Inflammatory joint disease occurs in 7.5% to 20% of patients with inflammatory bowel disease. Peripheral arthritis is seen more commonly, involves predominantly the large joints, and is rarely destructive. It occurs slightly more frequently in girls and is not associated with HLA-B27, whereas axial skeletal involvement and sacroiliitis are associated with male predominance (4:1 male/female) and the presence of HLA-B27.

Juvenile psoriatic arthritis is another condition in which the diagnosis can be clouded by the delay in the appearance of the typical features of psoriasis. The most common clinical picture is more similar to that of JRA than to that of spondyloarthropathies with asymmetric arthritis of the large and small joints and increased incidence in females and an onset in early childhood. These patients can be ANA–positive and rheumatoid factor–negative. One of the features distinctive from JRA is that a dactylitis with small joint involvement occurs more often.[14]

Transient synovitis of the hip has a specific clinical course that is rarely mistaken for JRA and more often is a challenge to distinguish from septic arthritis of the hip. Monoarticular arthritis involving the hip is an unusual presentation for rheumatic disease in childhood. Typically, the patient with transient synovitis presents with a relatively sudden onset of symptoms related to the hip, including pain, muscle spasm, and restriction of motion, particularly internal rotation and extension. Often, patients have relatively mild symptoms one evening and awaken the following morning unable to bear weight. There can occasionally be a low-grade temperature, but an absence of signs of systemic toxicity is a useful feature distinguishing from septic arthritis. A history of a prodromal upper respiratory tract infection is often found.[15]

INVESTIGATION

There is no one test that definitively makes the diagnosis of juvenile arthritis or other arthropathies. The diagnosis is generally determined on the basis of history and physical examination, but distinguishing among the various subtypes and excluding other diseases are often aided by laboratory investigations.

HEMATOLOGY

A complete blood count may show anemia consistent with chronic disease in JRA and helps to rule out hemoglobinopathies, neoplasia, and collagen vascular disease. A leukocytosis occurs frequently in rheumatic disease that is active, and white blood cell counts can be quite high (30,000 to 50,000 per mm³) in systemic disease. A significant leukocytosis suggests septic processes as the major differential diagnosis.

The erythrocyte sedimentation rate and C-reactive protein are indices of inflammation but are nonspecific. The erythrocyte sedimentation rate is a simple test that reflects the presence of acute-phase reactants in the sera. It can be used to monitor disease activity, although it does not correlate with the articular response to medications. C-reactive protein is a specific acute-phase protein that is measured quantitatively; it is a more rapidly responsive monitor of inflammation.

SEROLOGY

Rheumatoid factor is an immunoglobulin M anti-immunoglobulin G antibody present in 15% to 20% of patients with JRA. It is not useful as a diagnostic aid, but it does assist with prognosis. The presence of rheumatoid factor tends to be associated with older age at onset and is rare under the age of 7. It is more commonly seen in polyarticular disease and long-standing disease.

Antinuclear antibodies are usually immunoglobulin G antibodies directed against nuclear antigens. The presence of ANA is higher in young girls with JRA. It is correlated highly with the presence of uveitis and, as such, it is an important test for identifying children with JRA at risk for this complication.

The HLA-B27 histocompatibility antigen is a normal finding in up to 8% of the population. However, there is a significantly increased prevalence in juvenile ankylosing spondylitis, being present in up to 92% of cases.

RADIOGRAPHIC ASSESSMENT

There can be limited findings early in the course of inflammatory arthropathy. The changes that may be present include soft-tissue swelling and osteopenia. The primary role for radiographs early in the course of the disease is to rule out other causes of inflammation of the joint and also to provide a base line for later changes.[16]

A magnetic resonance imaging scan is most likely to show early changes prior to radiographic changes. Signs of edema and joint effusions as well as early bone changes can be seen with this scan. This is not standard practice as it is not usually necessary for the diagnosis.

SYNOVIAL FLUID ANALYSIS

Joint aspiration and synovial biopsy are rarely indicated for purely diagnostic measures. They are most frequently indicated when septic arthritis is a serious consideration of differential diagnosis. Typically, inflammatory fluid in rheumatoid disease shows a leukocytosis ranging up to $50,000 \times 10^6$/L cell counts. Biopsy is indicated in situations in which the diagnosis is not clear so as to rule out other conditions of synovial involvement, such as tuberculosis, granulomatous involvement, or pigmented villonodular synovitis.

DIFFERENTIAL DIAGNOSIS

A broad spectrum of diagnoses presents to the orthopaedic surgeon as painful, stiff, or swollen joints. The challenge to the clinician is to have a differential diagnosis that is both broad enough to encompass the range of possibilities and focused enough to allow timely identification of disease processes, especially those that require immediate intervention.

Most of the inflammatory arthritides are diagnoses of exclusion. There is no single physical finding or laboratory investigation that can immediately identify patients with juvenile arthritis.

As indicated in the preceding section on clinical features, significant differences in age, sex, and distribution of the affected joints characterize the common subgroups of juvenile arthritis; thus, historical features are critical in narrowing the differential diagnosis.

A useful approach to the child with arthritic symptoms is to distinguish conditions with systemic symptoms from those with symptoms isolated to the musculoskeletal system. These groups can also be subdivided on the basis of the degree of acuity of the symptoms (i.e., acute versus insidious onset) (Table 4).

Obtaining a history of the nature of onset and duration of symptoms, combined with an assessment of the child's systemic health, age, and sex, should rapidly narrow the diagnostic possibilities.

The number and location of joints involved is also a critical piece of information. Monoarticular involvement is less commonly seen in childhood rheumatic diseases, and common hip pathologies, such as septic arthritis, Legg-Calvé-Perthes disease, and slipped capital femoral epiphysis, must be ruled out. Likewise, common knee problems such as patellofemoral syndrome should be easily diagnosed by appropriate history and physical examination.

MANAGEMENT

Early and appropriate diagnosis of the cause of inflammatory arthropathies will guide management. Self-limited problems such as transient synovitis are simply treated symptomatically, once urgent conditions such as septic arthritis have been ruled out. Recurrent hemarthrosis and inflammatory arthritis secondary to hemophilia is best managed by an aggressive treatment of the underlying bleeding disorder with clotting factor replacement. The incidence of long-term degenerative arthropathy due to recurrent hemorrhages has been decreased owing to an aggressive approach to management. Minor hemarthroses are treated by rest, ice, analgesics, and early factor replacement. Major hemarthroses, in addition to factor replacement and splinting, should have aspiration to decrease the amount of iron deposition in the synovium and decrease risk of chronic synovitis and subsequent recurrent bleeding. Recurrent hemarthroses (so-called "target joints") necessitate a more aggressive treatment. Prophylactic transfusions for 6 to 12 weeks have been recommended to treat these joints with some success. Synovectomy of these joints has also been shown to decrease the rate of hemarthrosis, although whether the progression of the hemophilic arthropathy is arrested is not clear. Synovectomy can be performed by arthroscopic or open techniques or by using radioactive agents such as yttrium.[17]

The management of rheumatic diseases is predominantly medical. The immediate objective of treatment is to provide pain relief and preserve joint function. Prevention of the development of deformities is critical to the latter goal. In the pediatric population, one must strive to promote normal growth and development as much as possible. The treatment team in chronic diseases like JRA includes the child and the family and usually a pediatric rheumatologist. Other team members include occupational therapists, physical therapists, social workers, and subspecialists such as psychologists, ophthalmologists, and orthopaedic surgeons.

Traditional treatment is begun with the simplest and the safest method, usually nonsteroidal anti-inflammatory drugs such as aspirin, Naprosyn, or ibuprofen, which are used as first-line treatment. The addition of other pharmacological agents depends on the response to the first-line drugs. With use of disease-modifying agents, such as antimalarials, gold compounds, and penicillin, may come the associated increased risks of greater toxicity. The traditional therapeutic pyramid of treatment is currently undergoing some revision. Recent changes in the management of these patients include early use of intra-articular steroid injections in cases of limited joint disease and the use of low-dose methotrexate in polyarticular disease.[18]

The orthopaedic surgeon may be involved in the joint injection stage. Occasionally, small children require sedation or even general anesthesia for the surgeon to accurately perform intra-articular injections. Accuracy of placement is an area of possible failure; the use of contrast

TABLE 4. DIFFERENTIAL DIAGNOSIS OF CHILDHOOD ARTHRALGIA AND ARTHRITIS

Acute Onset	Insidious Onset
Toxic Child	
Systemic JRA	Systemic JRA
Infection (bacterial, viral)	Infection (TB, fungal)
Leukemia	Sarcoidosis
Systemic lupus erythematosus	Neuroblastoma
Reiter's syndrome	
Reactive arthritis	Other neoplasia
Sickle cell disease	
Serum sickness	
Acute rheumatic fever	
Vasculitides	
Inflammatory bowel disease	
Well Child	
Trauma	Pauciarticular JRA
Transient synovitis	Polyarticular JRA
Reflex sympathetic dystrophy	Seronegative spondyloarthropathies
Hemophilia	Osteochondroses (Legg-Calvé-Perthes)
SCFE (acute)	SCFE (chronic)
Pigmented villonodular synovitis	Lyme disease
	Mechanical
	Discitis
	Osteoid osteoma
	Foreign body synovitis
	Hypermobility
	Patellofemoral syndrome

From Sherry D, Mosca V: Juvenile rheumatoid arthritis and seronegative spondyloarthropathies. In Morrissy RT, Weinstein SL (eds): Lovell and Winter's Pediatric Orthopaedics. Philadelphia, Lippincott-Raven, 1996, p 402.

material to confirm needle placement in some cases may be helpful. Indications for the use of intra-articular steroids during the management of pauciarticular JRA include disease that has not responded to appropriate nonsteroidal anti-inflammatory treatment and as an aid to therapy and bracing of a contracted joint. Triamcinolone hexacetonide is the agent most commonly used for intra-articular injections in a dose of 0.5 mg to 1.0 mg/kg. This is a relatively insoluble steroid preparation and can cause subcutaneous atrophy and hypopigmentation if injected too superficially. A beneficial effect is shown by most patients, and up to 60% of patients have a lasting effect for up to 6 months, 45% up to 1 year.[19, 20]

Physical measures to relieve pain and maintain joint function with the use of splints, exercise, and organized physical activity is a key component to ongoing treatment.

Surgical interventions are limited to older children with long-term sequelae such as joint contractures, dislocations, and end-stage arthritis. In any surgical intervention on JRA patients, a thorough preoperative evaluation of general medical status is necessary. JRA patients tend to have a greater propensity to bleed, often exacerbated by their medications. The osteopenia often seen with the disease can affect surgical planning in terms of implants used; as well, the small stature seen in patients with chronic rheumatic disease will sometimes necessitate custom implants for joint replacement surgery. A thorough assessment of the cervical spine for evidence of disease involvement is mandatory prior to any consideration regarding general anesthesia with endotracheal intubation.

Surgical interventions range from synovectomy to soft-tissue releases to joint replacement. Synovectomy does not seem to alter the long-term outcome of JRA and is therefore only indicated for assistance of the management of joint swelling and pain. Range of motion does not improve after synovectomy. Both arthroscopic and open techniques have been advocated but, regardless of technique, early and aggressive rehabilitation is essential for maintaining range of motion.

Soft-tissue releases are performed to release contractures for a functional joint position, to increase joint range of motion for function and possibly to improve articular cartilage nutrition, and to provide symptomatic relief. Encouraging results have been reported, particularly around the hip.[21]

Occasionally, realignment osteotomies about the knee are indicated for improvement of mechanical alignment in situations where altered growth or joint involvement has resulted in malalignment in either the coronal or sagittal planes.

Total joint replacement surgery is a mainstay of treatment in the adult population. An attempt is made to delay the procedures as long as possible to try to decrease the need for revision surgery in the future. Good short-term results have been reported in this patient population. Special attention must be paid to the technical difficulties associated with joint replacements in JRA and, as mentioned, frequently special implants are required.[22]

Occasionally, limb length equalization procedures are required in patients with JRA who have a significant degree of discrepancy. An epiphysiodesis on the longer limb is usually performed in a standard fashion once the accurate projections of ultimate discrepancy have been arrived at.

Seronegative spondyloarthropathy patients tend to require little input from the orthopaedic surgeon until much later. Those who go on to an adult form of the disease with typical findings of ankylosing spondylitis may require consideration for joint replacement surgery around the hips or even spinal realignment surgery, with osteotomies at a later date.

COMPLICATIONS

Transient synovitis appears to be a benign condition with no significant long-term sequelae, although long-term studies suggest a slightly increased incidence of radiological abnormalities involving the affected hip, predominantly the coxa magna. These studies did not confirm any increase in symptoms or degenerative disease. An association with Legg-Calvé-Perthes disease has been suggested, but there is no evidence of a direct causal relationship.

The major orthopaedic complication of hemophilia is hemophilic arthropathy occurring as a result of recurrent intra-articular bleeding and chronic synovitis. It is thought that an aggressive approach to the management of the bleeding disorder with prophylactic transfusion will result in a decrease in the incidence and severity of this problem. Other complications that may come to the attention of the orthopaedic surgeon are acute soft-tissue hematoma formations, which can result in an acute compartment syndrome in areas such as the forearm. Immediate surgical decompression is required, preceded by appropriate normalization of coagulation parameters to at least 50% of normal.[23]

Articular complications as a result of disease progression are the hallmark of chronic arthritis and were discussed previously. Leg length discrepancy as a result of growth disturbance may also require treatment.

Extra-articular complications can occur, especially with the systemic variety, but the one the orthopaedic surgeon should be most aware of is chronic uveitis, which can be asymptomatic and can lead to permanent visual deficits. One must also be aware of the complications of treatment, as many of the medications used have significant side effects.

OUTCOMES

As in any disease process with multiple subtypes, it is difficult to make generalizations regarding outcomes. Indeed, the tools used to measure outcomes significantly influence the results.

The global functioning scale of the American College of Rheumatology is one standard grading method, although it has not been specifically validated for children.

In general the overall prognosis for children with JRA is quite good; 70% to 90% have no serious disability carried into adulthood. Approximately 10% have serious functional disabilities that persist into adult life. A study of functional evaluation of patients with JRA at 15-year follow-up demonstrated remission rates of 70% for pauciarticular disease, 60% for polyarticular disease, and 80% for systemic onset disease. All of pauciarticular patients were functional class I or II versus 79% of polyarticular patients and 85% of systemic onset patients.[24]

In terms of specific subtypes, polyarticular disease with late age of onset and long duration of symptoms, associated with a positive rheumatoid factor, has a poorer prognosis. Hip joint involvement is a poor prognostic sign; if progressive, it can lead to significant disability.

Pauciarticular JRA patients tend to do very well from an arthritic viewpoint, but uveitis can cause continued problems. Systemic onset JRA has a variable prognosis, with approximately 50% recovering completely and the other 50% developing progressively more joint involvement and mild-to-moderate disability.

The disease-associated death rate, mainly due to infection and renal failure, has decreased with better management and is estimated at less than 1%.

REFERENCES

1. Brower EJ, Bass J, Baum J, et al: Current proposed revision of JRA criteria. Arthritis Rheum 1997; 20:195.
2. Ansell BM: Chronic arthritis in childhood. Ann Rheum Dis 1978; 37:107.
3. Still GF: On a form of chronic joint disease in children. Clin Orthop 1990; 259:4.
4. Towner SR, Michet CJ Jr, O'Fallon WM, et al: The epidemiology of juvenile rheumatoid arthritis in Rochester, Minnesota. Arthritis Rheum 1983; 26:1208.
5. Royle SG, Galasko C: The irritable hip: Scintography in 192 children. Acta Orthop Scand 1992; 63:25.
6. Greene WB, McMillan CW, Warren MW: Prophylactic transfusion for hypertrophic synovitis in children with hemophilia. Clin Orthop Rel Res 1997; 343:19.
7. Springfield DS, Bolander ME, Friedlander G: Molecular and genetic biology of inflammation and neoplasia. In Simon S (ed): Orthopaedic Basic Science, Chicago, American Academy of Orthopaedic Surgeons, 1994, p 219.
8. Simons S, Wiffen J, Shapiro F: Leg length discrepancies in monoarticular and pauciarticular juvenile rheumatoid arthritis. J Bone Joint Surg Am 1981; 63:209.
9. Arnold WD, Hilgartner MW: Hemophilic arthropathy: Current concepts of pathogenesis and management. J Bone Joint Surg Am 1977; 59:287.
10. Cassidy JT, Petty RE: Juvenile rheumatoid arthritis. In Textbook of Pediatric Rheumatology. Philadelphia, WB Saunders, 1995, 3rd ed, p 133.
11. Petty RE: Ocular complications of rheumatic diseases of childhood. Clin Orthop 1990; 259:51.
12. Burgos-Vargas R, Vazquez-Mellado J: The early clinical recognition of juvenile-onset ankylosing spondylitis and its differentiation from juvenile rheumatoid arthritis. Arthritis Rheum 1995; 38:835.
13. Cabral DA, Malleson PN, Petty RE: Spondyloarthropathies of childhood. Pediatr Clin North Am 1995; 42:1051.
14. Cassidy JT, Petty RE: Spondyloarthropathies. In Textbook of Pediatric Rheumatology. Philadelphia, WB Saunders, 1995, 3rd ed, p 224.
15. Del Beccaro MA, Champoux AN: Septic arthritis in transient synovitis of the hip: The value of screening lab tests. Am Emerg Med 1992; 21:1418.
16. Reed MH, Wilmot DM: The radiology of juvenile rheumatoid arthritis: A review of the English language literature. J Rheum 1991; 18:2.
17. Gilbert MS, Radomisli TE: Therapeutic options in the management of hemophilic synovitis. Clin Orthop Rel Res 1997; 343:88.
18. Giannini EH, Cawkwell GD: Drug treatment in children with juvenile rheumatoid arthritis: Past, present, and future. Pediatr Clin North Am 1995; 42:109.
19. Allen RC, Gross KR, Laxer RM, et al: Intraarticular triamcinolone hexacetonide in the management of chronic arthritis in children. Arthritis Rheum 1986; 29:997.
20. Sparling M, Malleson P, Wood B, et al: Radiographic follow-up of joints injected with triamcinolone hexacetonide for the management of childhood arthritis. Arthritis Rheum 1990; 33:821.
21. Moreno-Alvarez MJ, Espada G, Maldonado-Cocco JA, et al: Long-term follow-up of hip and knee soft-tissue release in juvenile chronic arthritis. J Rheum 1992; 19:1608.
22. Chmell MJ, Scott RD, Thomas WH, et al: Total hip arthroplasty with cement for juvenile rheumatoid arthritis: Results at a minimum of ten years in patients less than thirty years old. J Bone Joint Surg Am 1997; 79:44.
23. Greene WB: Disorders of hemostasis. In Morrissy RT, Weinstein SL (eds): Lovell and Winter's Pediatric Orthopaedics. Philadelphia, Lippincott-Raven, 1996, 4th ed, p 371.
24. Calabro JJ, Burnstein SL, Staley HL, et al: Prognosis in juvenile rheumatoid arthritis: A fifteen-year follow-up of 100 patients. Arthritis Rheum 1997; 20:285.

UPPER EXTREMITY (ACQUIRED ERB'S)

M. Mark Hoffer

Summary

- Most of these palsies resolve spontaneously. Palsies in shoulders with residual weakness are shoulder (Erb's), hand (Klumpke's), posterior cord, and mixed.
- Early management involves therapy for motion and monitoring for joint stability in the shoulder and elbow.
- Plexus exploration with repair in the first 6 months has been suggested by some investigators but is controversial for the neonatal palsies.
- Tendon transfers after return of muscle function reaches a plateau at 4 years, and earlier for patients with unstable joints, are the commonly accepted surgical procedures.

Neonatal brachial plexus palsies are noted at birth, with weakness involving all or part of the upper extremity. Occasionally, such palsies are bilateral.

HISTORICAL REVIEW

- Erb, in 1874, first described brachial palsy of the C5 and C6 roots that is due to shoulder dystocia.
- Klumpke, in 1885, described palsy of the lower portion of the plexus that is frequently seen in breech deliveries and occasionally is bilateral.

EPIDEMIOLOGY AND PATHOGENESIS

The incidence rate of birth palsies has been reported as varying from 0.4 to 2.5 per 1000 live births.[1] The shoulder palsy first described by Erb is most commonly a sequela of shoulder dystocia in the birthing of a large child. The hand palsy described by Klumpke most commonly results from the hyperextended shoulder due to a breech delivery and, as a consequence, is occasionally bilateral. Those palsies are occasionally seen with difficult deliveries that result in cesarean sections. Palsies of the upper extremities are also rarely seen in neonates who have undergone no birth trauma whatsoever. In that case, they are frequently bilateral, and they represent agenesis of anterior horn cells.

In the past, most birth palsies resulted in significant residuals.[2] Currently, with new obstetrical techniques, most of these palsies are transient, and 70% to 80% completely resolve.[1] The resolution may occur over time, with a return of motor function lasting up to 4 years. Some observers believe that if there is no significant return of muscle function in the key elbow flexors by 3 to 6 months, permanent residual effects will probably occur, justifying surgical exploration.[3, 4] It is unclear, however, whether the prognosis can be judged merely from this clinical evaluation.

Electromyograms of the muscles in such young children are difficult to obtain, and their validity to a prognostic judgment is not yet established.

Initial examination frequently shows a total palsy. Examination should be performed every month for the first year and every 3 months thereafter, until the muscle and sensory changes reach a plateau.

The residual deformities that occur then can be classified in four general types. The first and most common are the Erb's C5 to C6 palsies, which occasionally also involve the seventh root. There is residual weakness of the deltoid, biceps, external rotators of the shoulder and, when the seventh root is involved, of the wrist and elbow extensors. Posterior dislocations of the shoulder[5, 6] and of the radial head may be seen. Figure 1 is a photograph of a child with a typical Erb's palsy, demonstrating shoulder adduction, internal rotation, elbow extension, and wrist flexion, due to paralysis of the muscles innervated by C5-7 nerve roots.

The second type, Klumpke's palsy, involves C8 and T1 nerves. It results in residual weakness and some sensory loss in the muscles about the hand, especially on the flexor side.

Palsy due to damage to the posterior cord, the third type, does occur, although its pathogenesis is difficult to explain. There is paralysis of the muscles innervated by the axillary and radial nerves, and thus, weakness of shoulder abduction as well as of elbow, finger, and wrist extension. Anterior dislocation of the radial head may also occur.

Finally, some children have mixed palsies that cannot be fitted into the first three types. It is common, in adults with traumatic palsies, to observe complete loss of function that persists. This finding is extremely uncommon in birth palsies, however, especially with current obstetrical techniques.

INVESTIGATION

Radiographs of the shoulder and clavicle should be taken initially to rule out the more common clavicle fracture and proximal humeral fracture that can cause pseudoparalysis. Subsequent radiographs should be taken of any joints that have limited motion. Dislocation is best seen on the axillary view (Fig. 2). Some investigators have suggested that this is a difficult view to obtain, and they perform either magnetic resonance imaging (MRI)[7] or computed tomography (CT)[8] to verify the position of the contracted glenohumeral joint. Others have suggested that an arthrogram might be necessary when there is difficulty demonstrating the dislocation; also, they have found that many children with limited shoulder motion have deformed glenohumeral joints.[9] Performing MRI, CT, and arthrograms in such young patients often requires sedation or even, in some cases, general anesthesia. Usually, the axillary view is adequate.

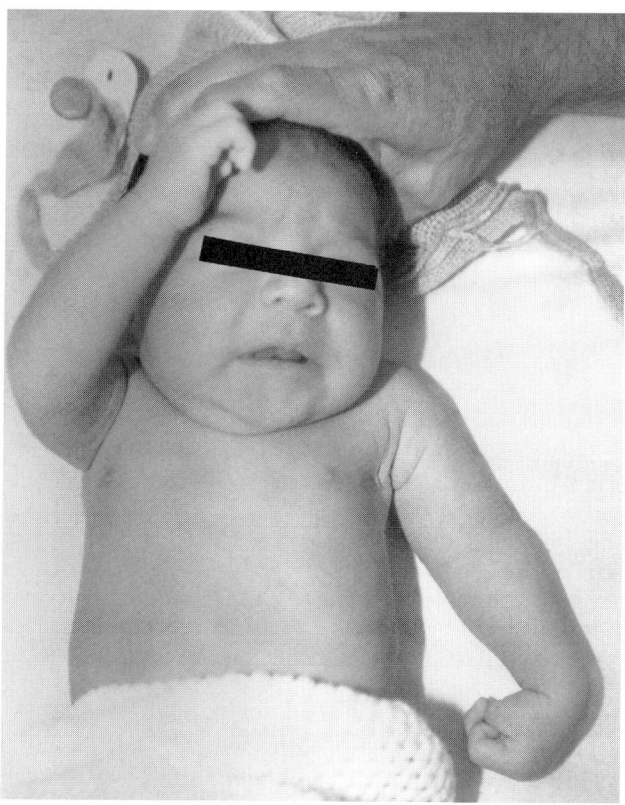

Fig. 1. Typical posture of brachial palsy. This is with shoulder adduction, internal rotation, and wrist flexion.

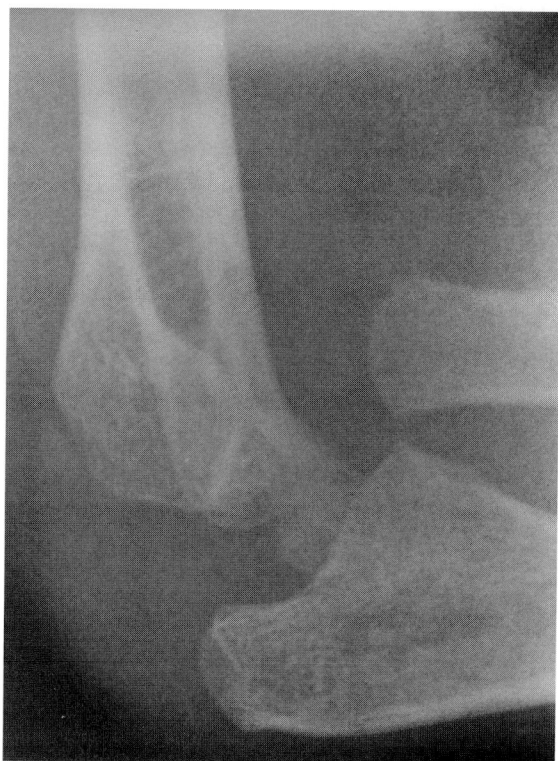

Fig. 3. Anterior dislocation of the radial head in a posterior cord palsy.

When supination contractures occur, radiographs of the elbow should be taken to rule out the anterior dislocation of the elbow frequently seen in posterior cord syndromes (Fig. 3). Also, posterolateral dislocation of the elbow due to persistent weakness of supination and pronation flexion contractures is frequently seen in patients with Erb's palsy (Fig. 4). A rarer total dislocation is seen in children with mixed palsies.

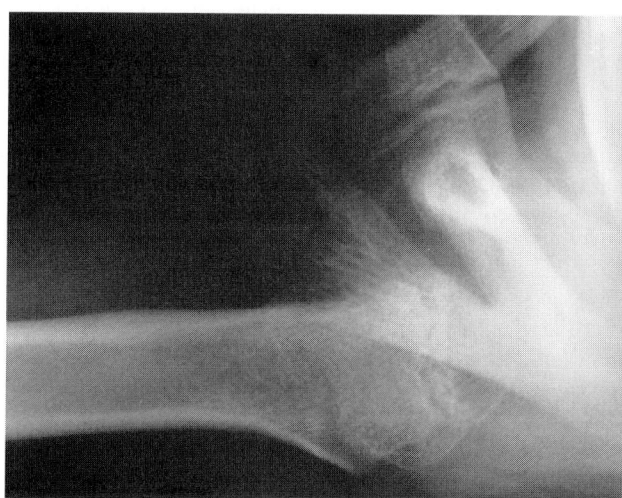

Fig. 2. Posterior dislocation of the glenohumeral joint. This is best seen on axillary view.

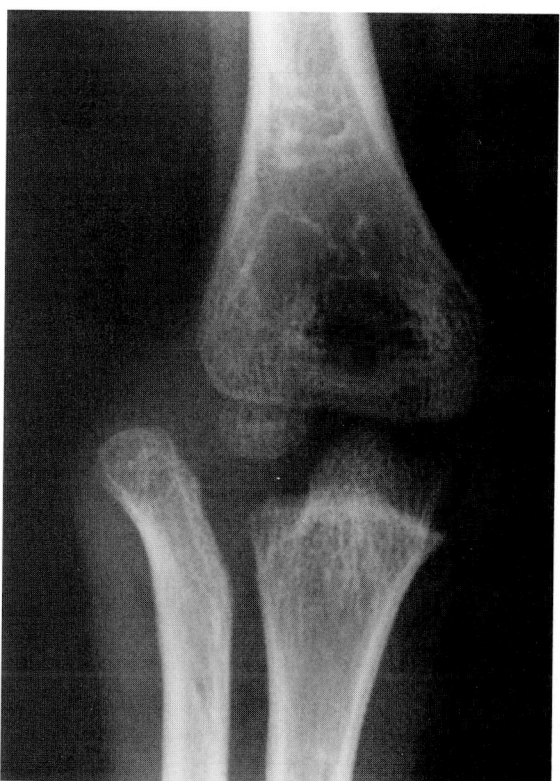

Fig. 4. Posterolateral dislocation of radial head in Erb's palsy.

TABLE 1. MANAGEMENT ALGORITHM FOR UPPER EXTREMITY PALSY				
0–4 years	Motor sensory examinations at 3 months abnormal	→	Range of motion Stretching	? Explore plexus
4 years +	Erb's palsy	→	Shoulder reconstruction* Elbow flexorplasty	
	Posterior cord syndrome	→	Biceps turnabout† Hand extensorplasties	

* Glenohumeral dislocation even before age 4 required reduction during shoulder reconstruction.
† Anterior dislocation of radial head requires biceps to ulna transfer.

Electromyograms are not helpful in a child with birth palsy. They require the use of sedation and are frequently difficult to obtain in such young patients. In the older child with acquired palsy, electromyograms are very helpful in the decision whether or when to explore the brachial plexus; in the adult with acquired palsy, they are traditional aids in the same decision-making process.

DIFFERENTIAL DIAGNOSIS

Differential diagnosis is usually not a problem in birth palsies, aside from the transient pseudoparalysis occurring from fracture. Determine whether the patient has torticollis, which may then represent a compression by a "compartment-like syndrome" about the plexus in the neck. It is also helpful to stimulate the startle reflex, which will demonstrate spontaneous motion in the upper extremity in newborns, in whom voluntary motion is difficult to obtain.

MANAGEMENT

The initial management of a patients with any of these palsies should consist of physical examination that includes motor, sensory, and range-of-motion evaluations. The child should then be seen at least every 3 months for the next 4 years, or until palsy has resolved. Therapists should be teaching the child's family stretching exercises to keep the range of motion that has been achieved. The range-of-motion exercise for external rotation should be performed with the elbow at the side. In the range-of-motion exercise for shoulder abduction, the therapist or other operator should restrain the child's scapula with one hand and elevate the humerus with the other (Table 1).

If there are persistent abnormal findings at 4 years of age, when muscle function changes have reached a plateau, one should be able to classify the patient's palsy as Erb's, Klumpke's, posterior cord, or mixed. At that point, appropriate tendon transfers should be performed. If, however, there is loss of motion, especially in the shoulder and elbow, before the child is 4 years old, it is extremely important to obtain appropriate radiographs to define the position of the joints. The surgical procedures are usually performed after the child is 4 years old. In the patient who has fixed contractures or dislocations prior to that age, earlier surgical procedures are advised.

In the patient with Erb's palsy, there are weak external rotators and some weakness of the deltoid and biceps, but an essentially normal hand. A release of the contracted pectoralis major and a transfer of the latissimus dorsi and teres major to the rotator cuff increase both the active external rotation and abduction in the shoulder. A simultaneous closed reduction of the posteriorly dislocated head may be required. A second procedure that may be necessary in the patient with Erb's palsy is an elbow flexorplasty to substitute for the weak biceps. In this procedure, the triceps may be utilized, a Steindler flexorplasty may be carried out, or a pectoralis major transfer may be utilized. In the case of a posterior dislocation of the radial head in the patient with Erb's palsy and weak biceps, the forearm is positioned in pronation and flexion, which is an advantage rather than a disadvantage; no effort should be made to relocate the radial head. If the radial head becomes prominent and bothersome when the child is an adult, it can be excised.

In the patient with posterior cord palsy with residual weakness in the entire shoulder abduction mechanism, an eventual glenohumeral fusion can be carried out; this procedure should rarely be performed before the child has completed growth, however, because the position varies with growth even in a solid fusion. In these patients, the supinator function of the biceps is unopposed by any function in the triceps, and supination contractures are noted early. When such contractures occur, a turnabout procedure, as described by Zancolli,[10] can improve the patient's ability to pronate (a more appropriate posture for a paralytic hand) while keeping the elbow joint stable. If the biceps has already dislocated anteriorly, elbow flexion will be locked, and marked improvement can be achieved with transfer of the biceps to the ulna. Finally, in posterior cord palsy, there is often weakness of finger and wrist extensors. A transfer of the flexor carpi ulnaris to the finger extensors, and even a transfer of the pronator teres to the central wrist extensor, which is a classic procedure for radial nerve palsy, are helpful.

Patients with residual effects of mixed or Klumpke's palsy occasionally need surgical procedures. Some may need the shoulder and elbow procedures mentioned previously. Some may require tendon transfers in the hand tailored to their specific weaknesses. Others may need humeral or forearm derotation osteotomies to accommodate deformities that have occurred secondary to muscle imbalance.

The following sections of the chapter describe the orthopaedic procedures commonly performed for neonatal palsies.

PROCEDURES AT THE SHOULDER

TENDON TRANSFERS FOR EXTERNAL ROTATION
Indications
Indications for tendon transfers are (1) internal rotation with weak but present deltoid and normal hand and (2) grade 4 to 5 strength pectoralis major, latissimus dorsi, and teres major muscle strength.

Procedure[11, 12]
A transverse incision is made in the axilla, the pectoralis major is released, and the tendons of the teres major and latissimus dorsi are released at their insertions, with careful attention given to the quadrangular space and the brachial plexus itself (Fig. 5). The combined tendons of the latissimus and teres major[13] are then transferred into the rotator cuff; sutures are used up into the area of the infraspinatus junction. A preformed shoulder spica case is then applied and is kept in place for 6 to 8 weeks. A therapy program with gradual active external rotation and gradual adduction is then permitted.

GLENOHUMERAL FUSION
Indications
This procedure is indicated in the patient to achieve a normally functioning hand and elbow after whatever tendon transfers are performed for posterior cord palsy. This surgery is performed upon completion of growth.

Procedure
A transverse incision is made over the shoulder just an inch distal to the acromion and is carried through the paralytic deltoid. The humeral head is denuded of cartilage, as is the glenoid. The acromion is tucked into the humeral head. A bone graft from the iliac crest may be necessary. Fixation is accomplished either with multiple compression screws and a shoulder spica cast or a reconstruction plate that is bent to fit about the acromion and humerus.

It is important to realize that the hardware alone may not hold these chronically osteoporotic paralytic bones and that the temporary shoulder spica, which is formed preoperatively, may need to remain in place postoperatively for at least 6 weeks. The humerus should be abducted far enough to permit 30 degrees of angulation between it and the vertebral line. The humerus should be slightly forward-flexed and slightly internally rotated. After the fusion is solid, gradual abduction exercises should be carried out.

PROCEDURES AT THE ELBOW

ELBOW FLEXORPLASTY
Indications
Indication for this procedure is weak elbow flexors with a normal hand. Four sets of procedures are available.

Procedure I: Steindler's Flexorplasty
A longitudinal incision is made along the medial border of the lateral forearm and humerus. The origin of the elbow flexors is located. The ulnar nerve and median nerve are

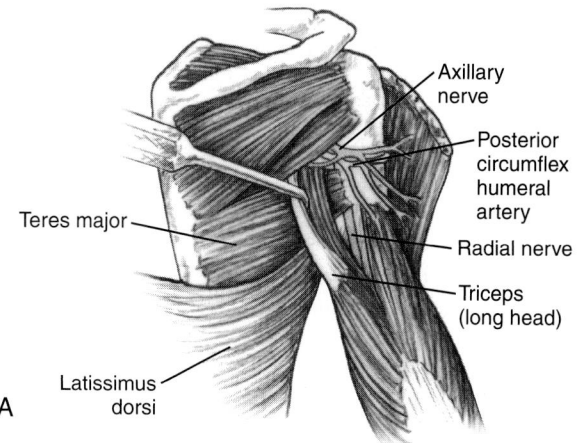

A

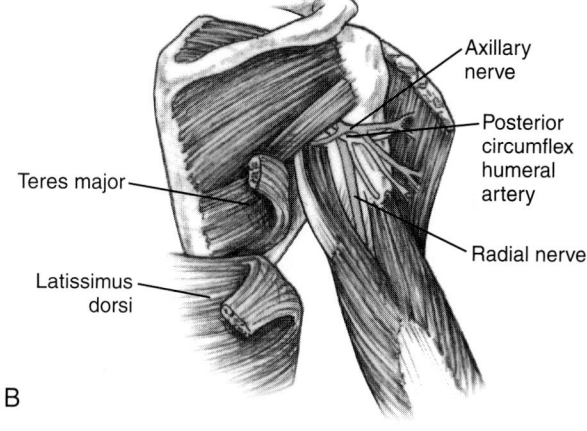

B

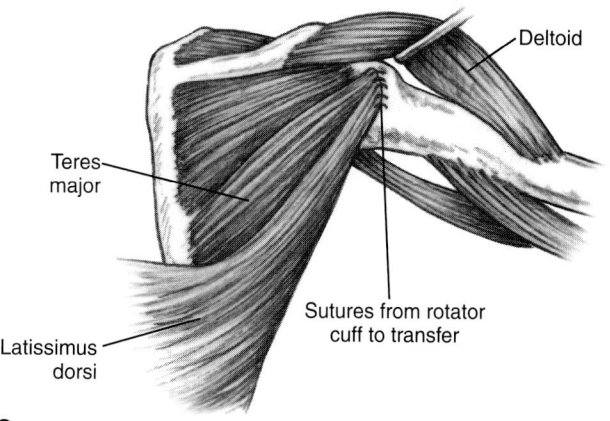

C

Fig. 5. Transfer of latissimus and teres major to posterior rotator cuff. (From Hoffer MM, Wickenden R, Roper S: Brachial plexus birth palsies. J Bone Joint Surg Am 1978; 60:692.)

located and protected. The origin is then brought to the junction of the middle and distal thirds of the humerus along with a chip of epicondyle. The chip of epicondyle should then be screwed in place with a compression screw in the anterior cortex. A long-arm cast is utilized for 6 to 8 weeks, after which active elbow flexion is begun and a brace is used to prohibit extension past 90 degrees for the next 2 to 3 months.

Procedure II: Pectoralis Major to Biceps

In this flexorplasty, the origin of the biceps is not released, because such a procedure is very disfiguring. A transverse incision is made in the axilla. The insertion of the pectoralis major is released from the humerus. Fascia lata is obtained from the thigh, sutured to this released pectoralis major, and carried subcutaneously to a second incision anterior to the elbow, where the biceps tendon is located. The fascia is then sutured into the biceps tendon so that the elbow is held at 90 degrees of flexion. A long-arm cast is utilized with sling for 6 to 8 weeks, after which active flexion is allowed, but a brace is used for the next few months to prohibit extension of the elbow past 90 degrees.

Procedure III: Triceps to Biceps

Indications. This procedure is performed for the patient with normal triceps and weak biceps.

Procedure. A longitudinal incision is made posteriorly in the distal two-thirds of the humerus. The triceps is located, and the radial nerve is located and protected. The triceps is then transferred anteriorly and laterally into the biceps tendon. A long-arm cast is applied for 6 to 8 weeks, after which a brace prohibiting flexion no more than 90 degrees is used for a few months.

Procedure IV: Biceps to Ulna

Indications. Dislocated radial head with supination contracture is the indication for a biceps to ulna flexorplasty.

Procedure. A zigzag incision is made in the antecubital fossa. The point of the zigzag incision is the lateral aspect of the elbow, with the proximal limb and distal limb and separated one from the other by approximately a 60-degree angle. The biceps is located and freed from its insertion. The neurovascular bundle is protected, and a suture of 1-0 self-absorbing material is placed in the biceps. Holes are drilled in the ulna, and the suture is driven through the drilled holes and tied to a piece of felt or cotton outside the skin. For 6 weeks, a long-arm cast holding the elbow at 90 degrees is used. Then the cast is removed, and the felt or cotton pad and suture are cut. The cast is reapplied and used for 2 weeks longer, after which active flexion is begun with a protective brace at 90 degrees of flexion for the next few months.

BICEPS TURNABOUT

Indications

The indication for a biceps turnabout procedure is supination contracture in a child without dislocation of the radial head.

Procedure

A zigzag incision is made in the elbow as noted previously in biceps to ulna. The biceps tendon is located, and a Z incision is made in the biceps tendon from the musculotendinous junction to its insertion so that the length of the central cut will permit the biceps to be flipped around and sutured to itself. The biceps is then carried about the radial head and neck as high as possible to avoid the posterior

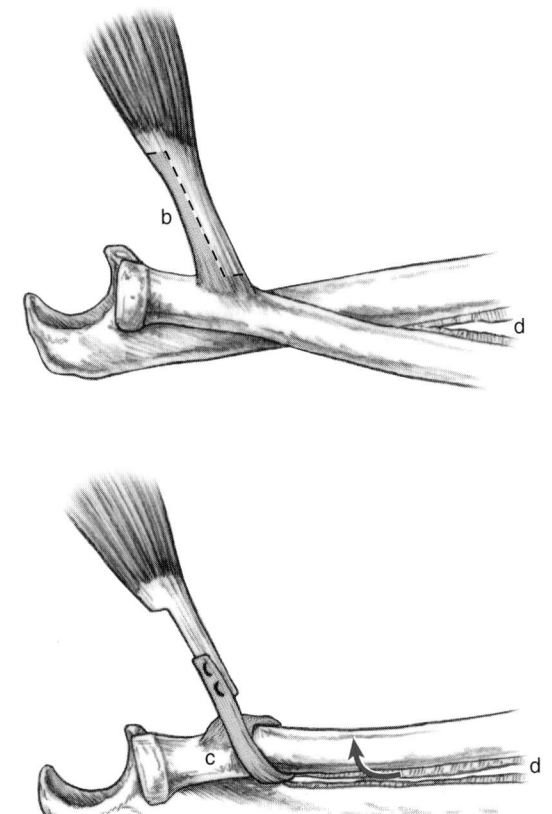

Fig. 6. Zancolli's turnabout biceps procedure. (From Zancolli E: Paralytic supination contracture of the forearm. J Bone Joint Surg Am 1967; 49:1276.)

interosseous nerve (Fig. 6). It is then sutured to itself to allow pronation and flexion. A long-arm cast is applied and kept in place for 6 to 8 weeks, after which flexion is permitted in a restrictive brace as described previously.

FINGER AND WRIST EXTENSORPLASTIES

INDICATIONS

The patient with posterior cord palsy who has normal wrist and finger flexors and normal pronator teres but weak wrist and finger extensors should undergo this procedure. The transfer of the finger flexors to the finger extensors that is frequently performed for radial palsies is not carried out in such a patient. Most children with posterior cord palsy have some residual weakness of these muscles, so the superficialis muscle group is not expendable.

PROCEDURE

An incision is made over the middle third of the forearm. The pronator teres is located and is transferred under tension to the extensor carpi radialis brevis. A separate incision is made over the volar distal third of the forearm, where the flexor carpi ulnaris is located and dissected into the distal two-thirds. The flexor carpi ulnaris is transferred subcutaneously to a third incision on the dorsum of the wrist into the combined finger extensors, with the wrist and fingers extended so that when the wrist is in neutral, the fingers are fully extended by the transfer. If a palmaris longus is present, it is also transferred, but subcutaneously along the radial border into the thumb extensor, which is taken out of its groove and Lister's tubercle to act as an abductor and extensor of the thumb. A long-arm cast is placed for 6 to 8 weeks, after which a splint is utilized with the wrist extended, and therapy to extend finger and thumb extensors is begun.

COMPLICATIONS

The complications for the procedures just described include the possible problems with anesthesia in young children, especially those who have had a challenge to the phrenic nerve. Therefore, preoperative radiographs of the chest are important for each patient.

Blood loss and nerve damage are concerns in relation to any surgery of the child's shoulder. In addition, because of the possibility of blood loss during glenohumeral fusion, blood transfusion may be needed. The patient's blood is usually typed and crossmatched before surgery, even for the tendon transfer procedures.

In the procedures about the elbow, a posterior interosseous nerve palsy is possible. It can be difficult to negotiate around the nerve because the radial head may be dislocated, and the position of the nerve may, therefore, be different from that noted in textbooks. Furthermore, the space between the elbow joint itself and the posterior interosseous nerve is limited by the size of the child and the supination contracture.

In the procedures in the hand and forearm, the biggest complaint has been the extensive scars that are necessary to perform the transfers.

RESULTS

The tendon transfers described in this chapter are standard procedures that have used for years in patients with polio or brachial plexus palsy. The cited articles attest to the relatively consistent good results that can be obtained with these procedures. When the procedures are performed in older patients whose joints have had significant loss of motion for many years, however, the results are not as predictable. Therefore, in patients with brachial plexus palsy, in whom procedures were previously delayed until after age 7, the age for surgery has crept down to 4 years and younger.

A bigger problem in terms of evaluation is the value of nerve repair in the neonate with brachial plexus palsy. There is no question that this is an important procedure in the palsies for which nerve repair is indicated; but the place of the procedure in the neonate, although it may be really important, is still difficult to establish.

REFERENCES

1. Jackson ST, Hoffer MM, Parrish N: Brachial palsy in the newborn. J Bone Joint Surg Am 1988; 70:1217.
2. Wickstrom J, Haslan ET, Hutchinson RH: Surgical management of residual deformities of the shoulder following birth injuries of brachial plexus. J Bone Joint Surg Am 1955; 37:27.
3. Birch R: Surgery for brachial plexus injuries. J Bone Joint Surg Br 1993; 75:346.
4. Gilbert A, Brokman R, Carlloz H: Surgical treatment of brachial plexus birth palsy. Clin Orthop 1991; 264:39.
5. Liebolt FL, Furey JG: Obstetrical paralysis and dislocation of the shoulder. J Bone Joint Surg Am 1953; 35:227.
6. Troum S, Floyd WE, Waters PM: Posterior dislocation of the humeral head in infancy associated with obstetrical paralysis. J Bone Joint Surg Am 1993; 75:1370.
7. Waters PM, Smith GR, Jaramillo D: Glenohumeral deformity secondary to brachial plexus birth palsy. J Bone Joint Surg Am 1998; 80:668.
8. Hernandez RJ, Dias L: CT evaluation of the shoulder in children with Erb's palsy. Pediatr Radiol 1988; 18:333.
9. Pearl ML, Edgerton B: Glenoid deformity secondary to brachial plexus birth palsy. J Bone Joint Surg Am 1998; 80:659.
10. Zancolli E: Paralytic supination contracture of the forearm. J Bone Joint Surg Am 1967; 49:1275.
11. Hoffer MM, Wickenden R, Roper S: Brachial plexus birth palsies. J Bone Joint Surg Am 1978; 60:691.
12. Phipps GJ, Hoffer MM: Latissimus dorsi and teres major transfer to rotator cuff for Erb's palsy. J Shoulder Elbow Surg 1995; 4:124.
13. Beck PA, Hoffer MM: Latissimus dorsi and teres major: Separate or conjoint tendons. J Pediatr Orthop 1989; 9:308.

section 9 chapter 10

THE CONGENITAL HAND

George E. Omer, Jr and Miguel A. Pirela-Cruz

Summary
- This chapter discusses malformations of the hand, including cleft hand, called central deficiency; ulnar club hand, called ulnar longitudinal arrest; curved or bent fingers, termed camptodactyly or clinodactyly; extra fingers or polydactyly; large digits or macrodactyly; short and stiff fingers termed brachydactyly; and constriction rings or bands.
- The clinical outcome of these difficult conditions is unpredictable and is related to unknown growth potential, individual anatomical abnormalities, and cooperation by the patient (and the family) for rehabilitation. These factors are as important as the timing and selection of the surgical procedures.

In the human embryo, the upper limbs first appear as small buds on the ventrolateral aspect of the body wall approximately 4 weeks after fertilization. At that time, the upper limb comprises an ectodermal sac filled with mesenchymal tissue. The mesenchyme has the ability to differentiate into the various connective tissue cells. Most bones appear as condensations of the mesenchymal cells to form a longitudinal core called the blastema. The apical ectodermal ridge on the limb bud is responsible for inducing the longitudinal growth and development of the limb mesenchyme.[1] Digits in the upper limb become distinguishable at 41 to 43 days and are fully separated approximately 10 days later.[2] One in approximately 555 to 626 newborns has a congenital malformation of the upper limb.[3, 4]

Pattern formation is the term used to describe spatial biological organization during development. Mechanisms involved in the control of pattern formation include cell-to-cell communication, control of cell growth, and tissue differentiation. These interactions lead to growth of the limb in proximal-to-distal, dorsal-and-ventral, and posterior-to-anterior (ulnar to radial digits) planes.[2, 5] Dysmorphogenesis of the limb, like other biological processes, has a fundamentally genetic basis.

Clinical geneticists recognize four major mechanisms of dysmorphogenesis: malformation, deformation, disruption, and dysplasia. Malformation refers to an interruption of normal morphogenesis, and the prognosis for normalization of malformation is limited. Examples are syndactyly, in which programmed cell death is interrupted, and split hand (ectrodactyly), in which mesenchyme is maldistributed. Surgical intervention is usually required. Deformation represents an alternation in shape of a part that has differentiated normally. Most deformations of the upper extremity involve large joints. Surgery is indicated in about 10% of cases. A disruption is a structural defect that results from destruction of a part that has differentiated normally. An example would be previously normal digits encircled by rings of amniotic membrane leading to tethering and embarrassment of blood flow, resulting in congenital constriction rings. Dysplasia refers to abnormal growth or differentiation of a part; for example, a hematoma. Prognosis for normalization of form is guarded because of discrepant growth and poor tissue differentiation of structure.

Current classifications of congenital hand malformations are based on descriptions of morphologic features or osseous anatomy[6] and provide a basis for practical clinical management of the patient. There is no "standard malformation," and there are no "routine" surgical techniques for these anomalies.

CLEFT HAND (CENTRAL DEFICIENCY)

Terms used to describe the cleft hand have included central hypoplasia, split hand, lobster claw, ectrodactyly, and oligodactyly.[7] The cleft hand occurs once in 90,000 live births, or from 4% to 6% of hand anomalies.[8, 9] Flatt[8] states that the cleft hand is a functional triumph and a social disaster. The variety of hands with this congenital deformity has led to discussion for appropriate classification. There is agreement that two general clinical types can be differentiated, usually termed typical and atypical.[8, 9] The typical type is usually bilateral and is characterized by a cleft between the index and ring fingers. A cross transverse bone is often found at the base of the cleft. The metacarpals show many abnormalities, such as two metacarpals supporting one digit, thickened metacarpals, or digital fusions.[7] The two remaining digits in each component may be webbed, with ring-small syndactyly somewhat more common. If true syndactyly of the thumb and index is present, it is the rule to find marked adduction contracture of the thumb. Typical or true cleft hand is often familial and is frequently associated with syndactyly and foot deformities, plus a significant number of other anomalies.[8]

The atypical type affects the index, long, and ring fingers, leaving the small fingers, which may be hypoplastic.[7–9] Little stumps of the three central fingers are usually present with rudimentary nails. In severe cases, only the thumb is present. The atypical type usually involves only one hand, and the feet are normal. Syndactyly is uncommon.[8]

Surgical treatment of the typical cleft hand depends on the degree of deformity. Several procedures to be considered include: (1) separation of syndactyly, (2) removal of a blocking transverse bone, (3) rotation or wedge osteotomies when indicated for correction of functional motion patterns, such as axial deviations, (4) correction of severe flexion contractures in the interphalangeal joints, (5) narrowing of the soft-tissue cleft, (6) widening the first interdigital (thumb-index) space, including transposition of the index finger when indicated[8, 9] (Fig. 1).

If there is syndactyly of the ring and little fingers, surgical release is done as the first procedure and allowed to heal before further surgery. After recovery, thumb mobility is assessed, and a decision is made either to simply close the central cleft or at the same time to increase the mobility of the thumb. If only the central cleft is closed, there must be good apposition of the distal ends of the metacarpals. Any transverse bony blocks should be excised, and the distal ends of the metacarpals must be approximated. The transverse intermetacarpal ligament should be reconstructed without forcing the metacarpals into a flat transverse plane that results in loss of grip with crossed fingers. A soft-tissue diamond-shaped skin flap is used to produce a more distant commissure as the cleft is reconstructed.[10]

If there is marked thumb adduction, most surgical procedures are based on the operation devised by Snow and Littler.[7–9, 11] A simpler technique was reported by Miura and Komada.[7, 12] An incision is made at the level of the metacarpal heads on the radial side of the base of the ring finger and runs across the fold of the cleft space to the ulnar side of the base of the index finger. A curved inci-

sion is added around the palmar base of the index finger at the level desired for the new thumb web space. A second dorsal incision is made to expose the bases of the thumb and index metacarpals. The fibrous band between the thumb and index metacarpal is released. The fascia of the adductor pollicis and first dorsal interosseous muscles is released. The index metacarpal is detached at its base, with the first dorsal interosseous muscle, and placed in the position of the third metacarpal and fixed with Kirschner's wires or a plate with screws. The rotation of the metacarpal should be checked by passively flexing the fingers into the palm to check for overlapping. The transverse metacarpal ligament is reconstructed between the index and ring fingers. The flap for the thumb index web is designed from the skin radial to the curved incision along the original cleft. Surgical treatment of the atypical cleft hand is designed to provide maximal function for the border digits so that they close across the central deficit for grasp. If the thumb and small finger cannot grasp, then it is useful to deepen the cleft with a Z-plasty.[8] Osteotomies near the base of the metacarpals may be needed to provide a maximal grasping position as well as tendon transfers for active motion. Infrequently, there are nubbins in the central part

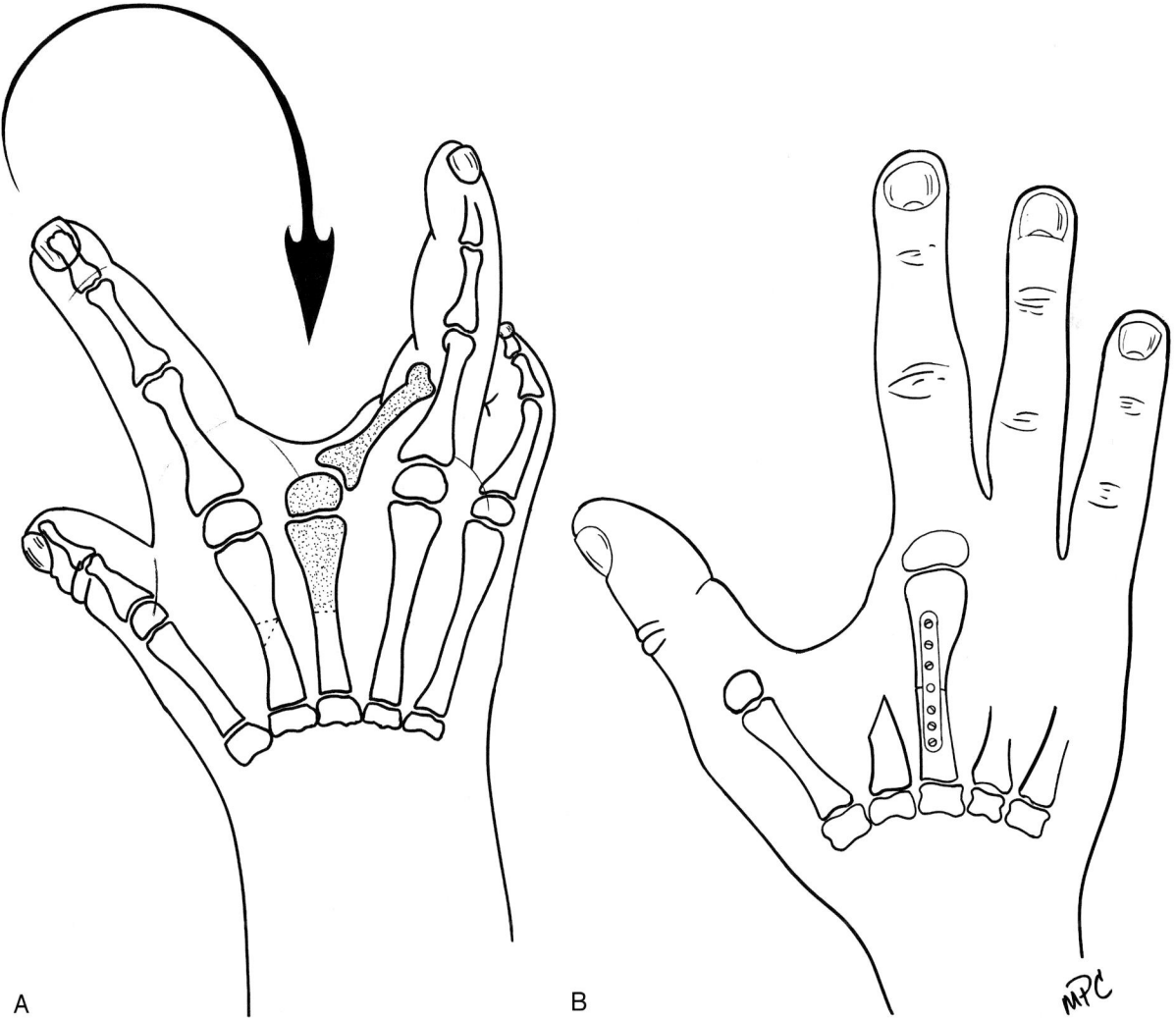

A   B

Fig. 1. Typical cleft hand deformity. *A* and *B,* Removal of the transverse blocking bone and transposition of the index ray to close the cleft.

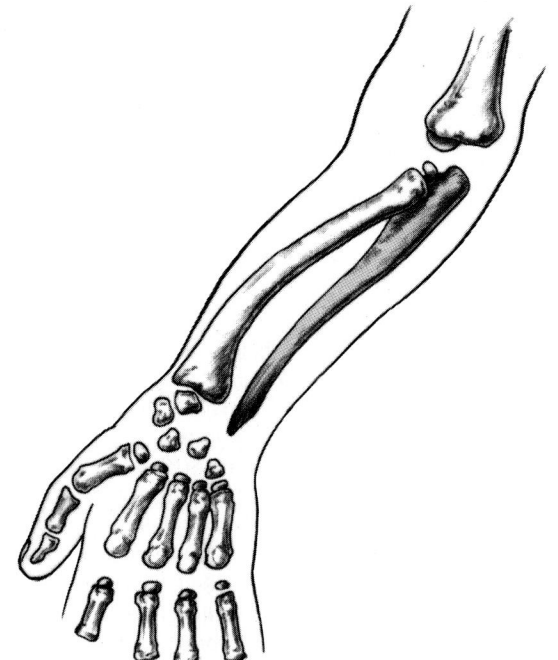

Fig. 2. Typical ulnar hemimelia.

of the hand, which should be removed. We have not done toe transfers in these cases, but toe transfers with microsurgical reconstruction have been reported.[13]

ULNAR CLUB HAND (ULNAR LONGITUDINAL ARREST)

Terms used to describe congenital ulnar ray deficiency include ulnar club hand, ulnar dysmelia, and para-axial ulnar hemimelia[7, 8, 14] (Fig. 2). Cases involve males at a ratio of 3:2, and left-side involvement is slightly more common. There is a 45% prevalence of anomalies in the contralateral

upper extremity. Clinical manifestations vary more widely in this deficiency than in any other longitudinal ray deficiency and include ectrodactyly, carpal hypoplasia, ulnar deviation of the hand, forearm shortening and bowing, defective elbow congruity with loss of motion, and hypoplasia of the proximal part of the extremity.[8, 14, 15] Ectrodactyly is the most common hand anomaly, and metacarpals are usually absent proximal to missing digits. Simple or complex syndactyly is the second most common hand anomaly. The extent of hand anomalies does not correlate with the extent of ulnar deficiency or with wrist or elbow deformities (Fig. 3). However, the hand anomalies determine, to a large extent, the patient's function.[14, 15]

Ulnar deviation of the wrist is a traditional concern. In our series, 7 of 15 wrists had ulnar deviation, but only 3 had more than 20 degrees.[14] Broudy and Smith[16] found ulnar deviation of the wrist in 8 of their 26 cases. Only three were greater than 20 degrees, and none were progressive. Combined data indicate that in the 30% of patients with ulnar deviation of the wrist, it is mild (20 degrees or less) in 57%, moderate (21 to 30 degrees) in 14%, and severe (more than 30 degrees) in 28% of cases. If ulnar deviation at the wrist is greater than 30 degrees for more than 6 months, resection of the ulnar anlage can be considered. Even then, resection may not be indicated. Our 2 patients with more than 30 degrees of ulnar deviation at the wrist have the same function—as evaluated by total active motion, grip, pinch, and activities of daily living—as those patients with neutral or less deviated wrists. It is appropriate to use serial ulnar gutter splints to maintain the wrist in neutral alignment. In early infancy, this should be done 24 hours a day. When the child is 1 year of age and is using the upper extremities to explore the environment, the splints should be worn only at night.

Present classifications[16–18] of ulnar longitudinal arrest do not prognosticate progression of the deformity or related function. The natural history in our series[14, 15] and the literature[16, 19] suggests that there is little progression of deformity. Surgical treatment is cautious and is utilized after conservative management of ulnar deviation of the

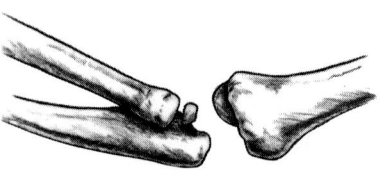

Normal relationship

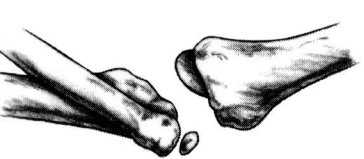

After dislocation of radial head

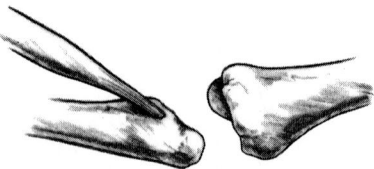

Unstable elbow with hypoplastic proximal radius

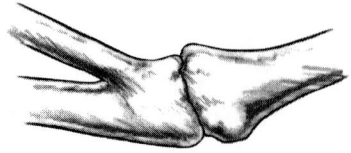

Ankylosed elbow

Fig. 3. Elbow deformities. These are deformities associated with ulnar deficiency syndrome.

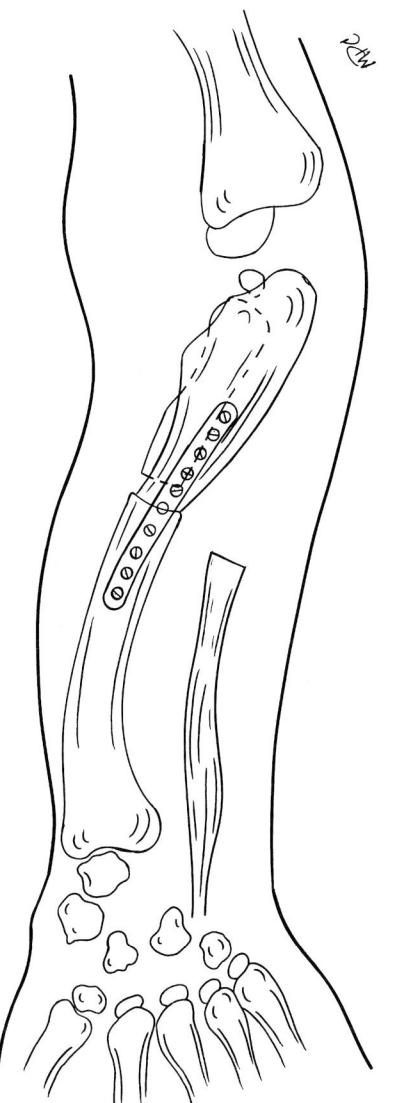

Fig. 4. View. This is a technique to obtain a "single-bone" forearm for stability.

wrist, radial head dislocation, and preservation of forearm pronation and supination. Standard techniques for syndactyly release, web space deepening, and metacarpal rotational osteotomy all provide measurable improvement in function. Resection of the distal ulnar fibrocartilaginous anlage is not indicated as frequently as indicated in the literature.[8] Creation of a one-bone forearm will increase elbow flexion and extension and will result in loss of forearm pronation and supination (Fig. 4). The procedure is indicated only when severe forearm instability or a marked decrease in motion prevents function.[16, 17]

CAMPTODACTYLY (CAMPYLODACTYLY, PALMAR CURVED OR BENT FINGERS, HAMMER FINGERS)

Camptodactyly usually occurs at the proximal interphalangeal (PIP) joint of the small finger. The extent of PIP joint flexion varies up to 90 degrees. About two-thirds of all patients have bilateral involvement, although the right hand is usually involved in unilateral cases. Other fingers may be involved, but the incidence decreases toward the radial side of the hand. There are two periods for clinical onset: the majority (84%) of cases appears during the first year of life and equally affects males and females; the second group (13%) of cases appears in adolescent females aged 10 years or older.[7] If untreated, the natural history is no improvement or gradual progressive worsening of the flexion contracture in more than 80% of cases through growth, then no progression after the age of 18 to 20 years.[7, 8] The prevalence is less than 1% of the population.[7, 8] The pathogenesis of the condition is unknown,[20, 21] but camptodactyly is commonly associated with many skeletal dysplasias and malformation syndromes.[23, 24] Isolated camptodactyly may be associated with a multitude of factors. Almost every structure at the base of the involved finger has been implicated as a deforming factor, including the lumbrical muscle, the flexor digitorum superficialis tendon, the dorsal extensor apparatus, the collateral ligaments, and the PIP volar plate. Dynamic muscular imbalance is the primary cause, and there is no single successful treatment because there is no single cause of the condition.

Treatment should begin with static and dynamic splinting. Splinting is particularly indicated when there are no obvious bony changes on lateral radiographs of the PIP joint. Dynamic splinting is useful with contractures of 40 to 60 degrees. The splint is centered dorsally over the PIP joint, with the palmar points over the proximal and middle phalanges. Ideally, the PIP joint should be passively fully extended before surgery is utilized, but when the contracture is more than 60 degrees, preoperative dynamic splinting is usually unproductive.[7, 8] In addition, constant splinting for a considerable period is necessary to maintain correction following surgery.

In the younger patient, soft-tissue operations are useful for PIP joint contractures of 40 degrees or more without obvious changes in lateral radiographs of the joint. The flexor digitorum superficialis tendon can be released in the palm or wrist if the involved joint can be corrected actively and passively. A transverse incision along the distal palmar crease at the base of the involved finger can be continued distally along the ulnar midlateral line[7] (Fig. 5). Tight or abnormal fascial structures are released, including the flexor tendon sheath, palmar plate, and portions of the accessory collateral ligaments; abnormal muscles and tendons are released.[20] The best operation in an adolescent is transferring the flexor digitorum superficialis through the lumbrical canal to either the lateral band or the central slip of the extensor apparatus[7, 8] (Fig. 6). Wood[7] prefers not to operate on adults with joints that cannot be passively corrected.

For fingers with severe flexion contractures and obvious bony changes, the common operation for postural improvement is an angulation osteotomy of the neck of the proximal phalanx (Fig. 7).[22] This is a closing dorsal wedge that is maintained with fine Kirschner's wires that are left in place up to 6 weeks. The motion is now in a different arc, and some tightening of the ulnar grasp is lost. An alternative procedure is joint arthrodesis.

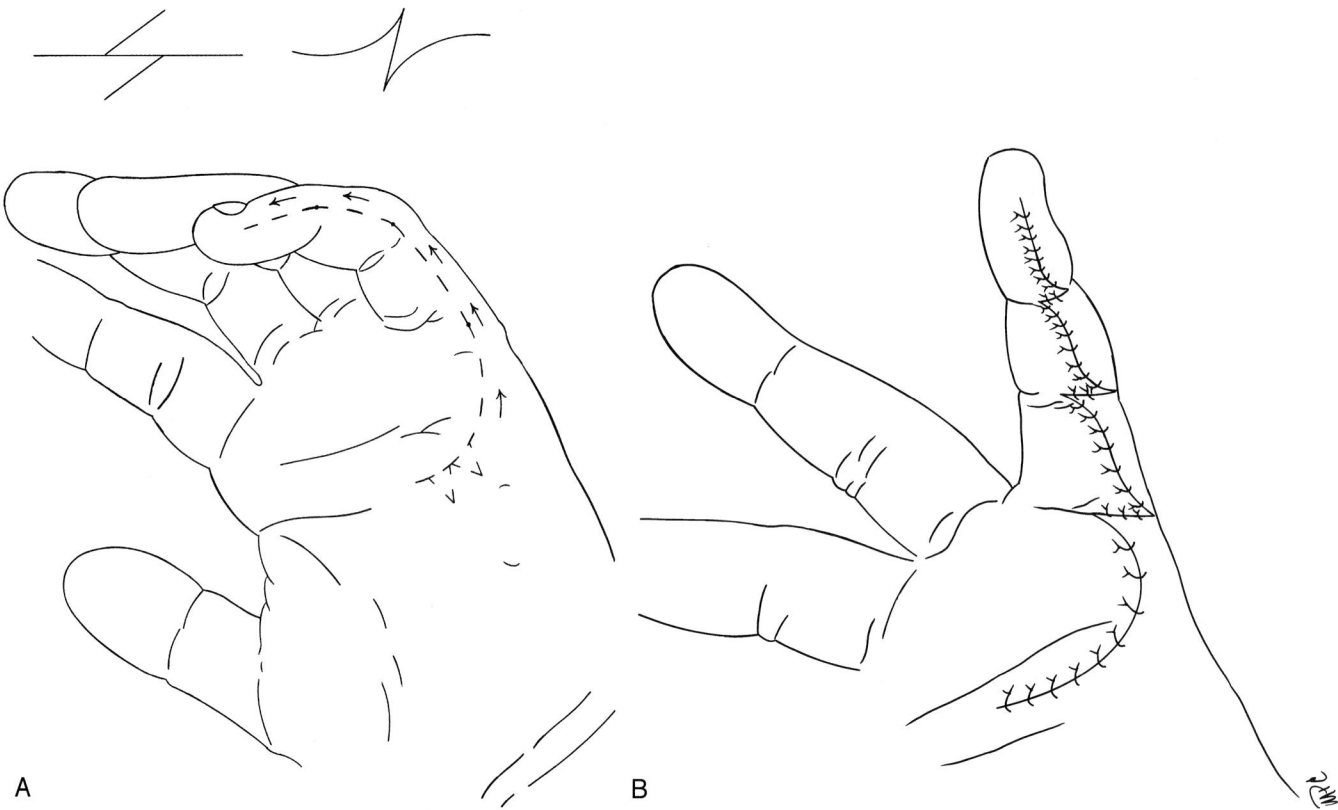

Fig. 5. Soft-tissue release for camptodactyly. *A* and *B*, Multiple Z-plasties may be required.

CLINODACTYLY (FINGER CURVATURE IN RADIAL/ULNAR PLANE)

Clinodactyly can occur in any finger, but it is most common as a radial deviation of the small finger at the distal interphalangeal joint. The usual cause is a delta phalanx, most often the middle phalanx. True shortening of the middle phalanx, termed brachymesophalangia, can occur.[8] An angulation of 10 degrees or less at the distal interphalangeal joint is commonly regarded as the upper limit of

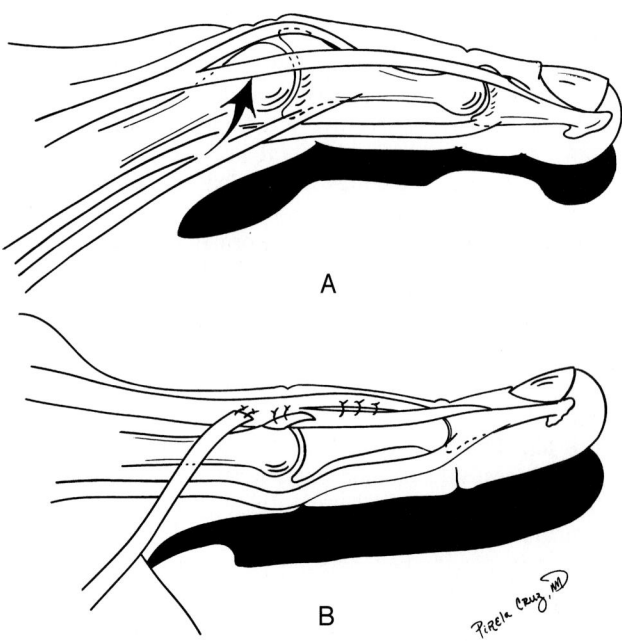

Fig. 6. View. *A* and *B*, Flexor digitorum superficialis transfer to correct camptodactyly.

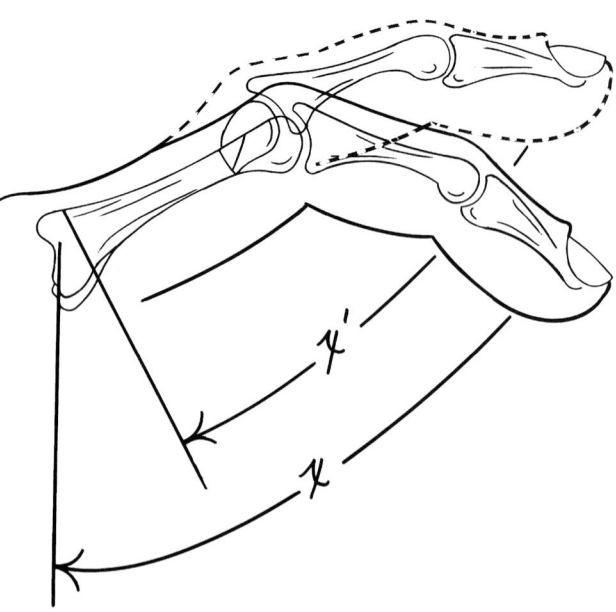

Fig. 7. View. This is a dorsal closing wedge osteotomy to correct camptodactyly.

normal.[23] Clinodactyly is usually bilateral and is more common in males. Prevalence is reported in 1% to 19.5% in normal children.[7, 8] Marked clinodactyly is important because it often indicates mental retardation, and it has been recorded in 35% to 79% of individuals with Down's syndrome.[23] It has been associated with more than 60 syndromes,[8] and clinical management of the condition should always include identifying any associated diseases.

Cooney[25] classified clinodactyly into four types: (1) simple, with bone deformity of the middle phalanx less than 45 degrees; (2) simple complicated, with bone deformity of the middle phalanx more than 45 degrees; (3) complex, with bone and soft tissue deformity less than 45 degrees, with syndactyly; (4) complex complicated, with 45 to 60 degrees of angulation with syndactyly, polydactyly, or gigantism. The complex cases usually demonstrate rotational as well as angulation deformity. Clinically, the finger deformity is cosmetic in the majority of cases, and surgical procedures are not always indicated. Barsky[26] believes that surgery should be postponed in simple syndactylies until the patient is at least 6 years of age. However, Flatt[8] recommends a closing wedge osteotomy in a simple, uncomplicated clinodactyly of 45 to 50 degrees (Fig. 8). The osteotomy is on the convex, usually ulnar, border of the finger. An opening wedge osteotomy with or without bone graft can also be performed. The surgical site is immobilized with Kirschner's wire fixation for 6 weeks. The wires should be placed from the ulnar side of the finger in a horizontal plane so that they do not penetrate the dorsal extensor mechanism.

In many complex clinodactylies, the cause of the significant angulation is a delta phalanx. If the angulation is sufficient to cause overlapping of fingers with functional impairment, then surgical correction is indicated. The longitudinal epiphysis of the delta phalanx must be interrupted and destroyed. This is usually done as a wedge osteotomy using bone cutters rather than an electrical saw. The phalanx may need lengthening, which can be done by two techniques: an opening wedge osteotomy can be done and bone packed into the space,[20] or a wedge osteotomy is based on the longer side of the phalanx and creates a wedge that is reversed and inserted from the shorter side of the phalanx.[27]

Additional soft-tissue procedures are needed to obtain correction and may include release of contractures, tightening of collateral ligaments, relocation of extrinsic tendons, and skin Z-plasties or flaps.[8] An alternative procedure in the young patient is a limited excision of the longitudinal epiphysis and filling the gap with a free fat graft.[28]

POLYDACTYLY (EXTRA FINGERS, MIRROR HAND)

Light[29] notes that upper limb polydactyly has an incidence of one per 1000 live births, with 80% of cases being ulnar polydactyly. Although each of the five digits can be duplicated, the small finger is the most common extra digit in African-Americans; the thumb is the most common extra digit in whites and Asian-Americans.[8, 29] More than 40 abnormalities and syndromes have been reported as associated with polydactyly, and the most common adjacent associated abnormality is syndactyly.[7, 8] The newborn patient with polydactyly should be carefully examined and evaluated for other associated abnormalities. Potential syndromes associated with polydactyly involve the eyes, orofacial abnormalities, the skin, bone dysplasia, trisomies 13 and 18, and mental retardation.[7, 8, 29]

Experimental studies suggest that polydactyly is a disorder of the balance between ectodermal and mesodermal cell growth and death in the developing hand.[30] There are several detailed classifications of polysyndactyly,[22, 31] but the usual designation for polysyndactyly is radial (thumb or

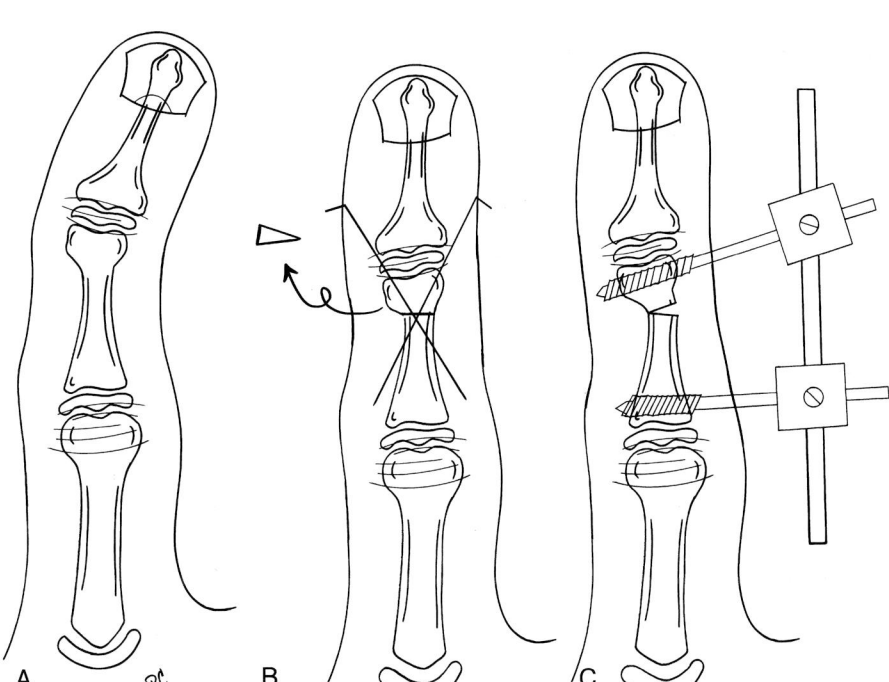

Fig. 8. View. *A, B,* and *C,* Closing and opening wedge osteotomies to correct clinodactyly of the finger.

A   B   C

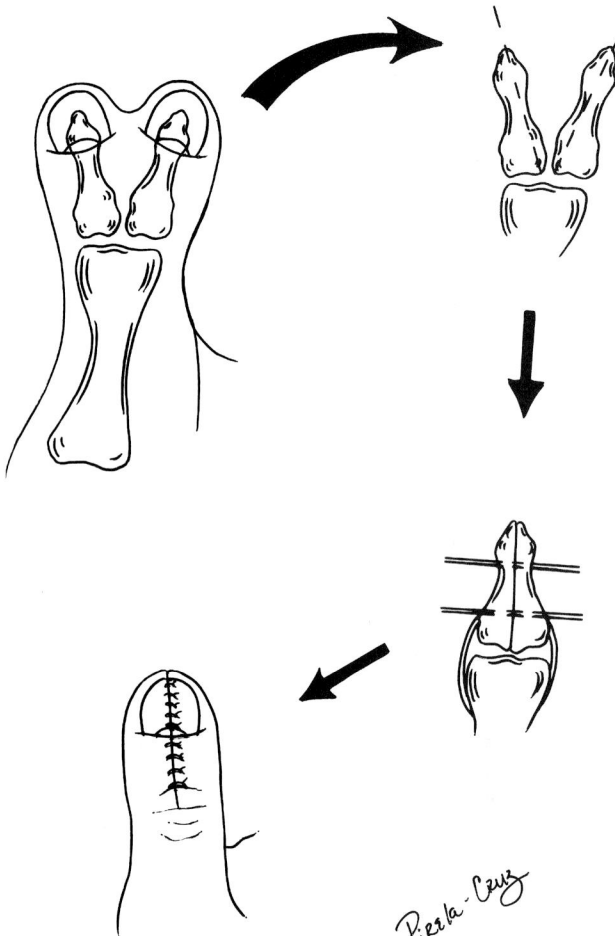

Fig. 9. View. This is the Bilhout-Cloquet procedure.

the metacarpal at the metacarpophalangeal joint. Kirschner's wires are used to stabilize osteotomies and ligament repairs. The insertion of extrinsic flexor or extensor tendons may be imbalanced, usually too radial on the distal phalanx of the retained thumb. When bifurcation occurs at the metacarpophalangeal joint level, the abductor pollicis brevis muscle tendon of insertion needs redirection from the deleted radial thumb to the ulnar thumb. If the longitudinal axis of motion is not restored or eccentric tendon forces are not adequately redirected, then residual angulation and late Z-collapse configuration is predictable.

The Bilhout-Cloquet procedure is a surgical technique in which the two component thumbs are merged by removing a composite central wedge of nail, bone, and soft tissue. The two halves are then joined at the midline.[7, 8, 29, 33] The procedure makes an attractive diagram but usually develops complications over the long term. Light[29] states that the Bilhout-Cloquet procedure should be reserved for cases of distal duplication in which the component elements are small and symmetrical (Fig. 9). Magnification should be used in matching the nail matrix after the central excision. The contralateral nail should be measured to determine the amount of nail to remove, and the radial paronychium is advanced to the border of the retained ulnar nail.

The technique of utilizing radial and ulnar soft-tissue sleeves is extended to include selective retention of proximal and distal portions of the double digits, the "on-top plasty." This procedure is indicated when neither skeletal unit is satisfactory. Transposition of skeletal segments is achieved through corresponding osteotomies in each digit, with excision of unused segments (Figs. 10 and 11).[7, 34]

Secondary deformity is often noted after surgical treatment of thumb polydactyly. Most common is a zig-zag collapse deformity that results from ineffective radial collateral ligament reconstruction at the metacarpophalangeal joint. The proximal thumb angles ulnarward, and the distal thumb angles radialward. Reconstruction requires stabilization of the metacarpophalangeal joint with arthrodesis. An alternative procedure includes metacarpal wedge osteotomy and collateral ligament reconstruction. With either procedure, the flexor and extensor tendons should be reinserted centrally on the distal phalanx.

Index polydactyly is unusual. It usually appears as duplication of the entire index ray. If the more ulnar index ray appears normal, simple resection of the more radial index ray is the procedure of choice.

Central polydactyly, involving the middle or ring fingers, is often associated with syndactyly. Excision of the skeletal units identified with one digit may result in instability in the residual digit. In addition, angular deformity and instability often requires secondary osteotomy and interphalangeal joint arthrodesis.[7] Two metacarpals may contribute to the support of a single proximal phalanx, or a single metacarpal will provide support to two proximal phalanges. Wood[7] has used the term *superdigit* for these cases of incomplete osseous syndactyly. The involved digits should be carefully evaluated to determine if surgery will result in instability. In some cases, excision of the entire dysplastic central polydactylous mass is the appropriate procedure.[7, 8, 29, 33]

Ulnar polydactyly involves the small finger. The condition may be classified as type A or B. Type A has bony continuity to the other skeletal elements; type B is a small

index), central (middle or ring), ulnar (little) or mirror hand. Radial polydactyly involves the thumb or the index finger. Thumb polydactyly is frequent, but index polydactyly is unusual. Several classifications have been developed to identify varied forms of thumb polydactyly, but the Wassel classification is used most often to distinguish six levels of bifurcation, plus a seventh group in which one thumb component is triphalangeal.[32]

Bilateral thumb duplication usually occurs at two different levels. Because the more ulnar of the two digits is typically more developed and of greater bulk, it is usually retained. The reconstructive plan must determine the skeletal elements to be retained and those to be excised. When duplication occurs at the interphalangeal or metacarpophalangeal joint level, the joint should be directly inspected for skeletal alignment and joint stability. The proximal surface of the interphalangeal or metacarpophalangeal joint may be incongruous to the digital axis. The articular surface might be shaved in the young patient, or osteotomies may be necessary. Because the retained digit is usually approached from its radial aspect, metacarpal osteotomies are usually closing wedge, and proximal phalangeal osteotomies are usually opening wedge.[29] An indicated bone graft for an opening wedge osteotomy can be fashioned from a deleted part. Reconstruction includes repositioning of the collateral ligaments and longitudinal narrowing of

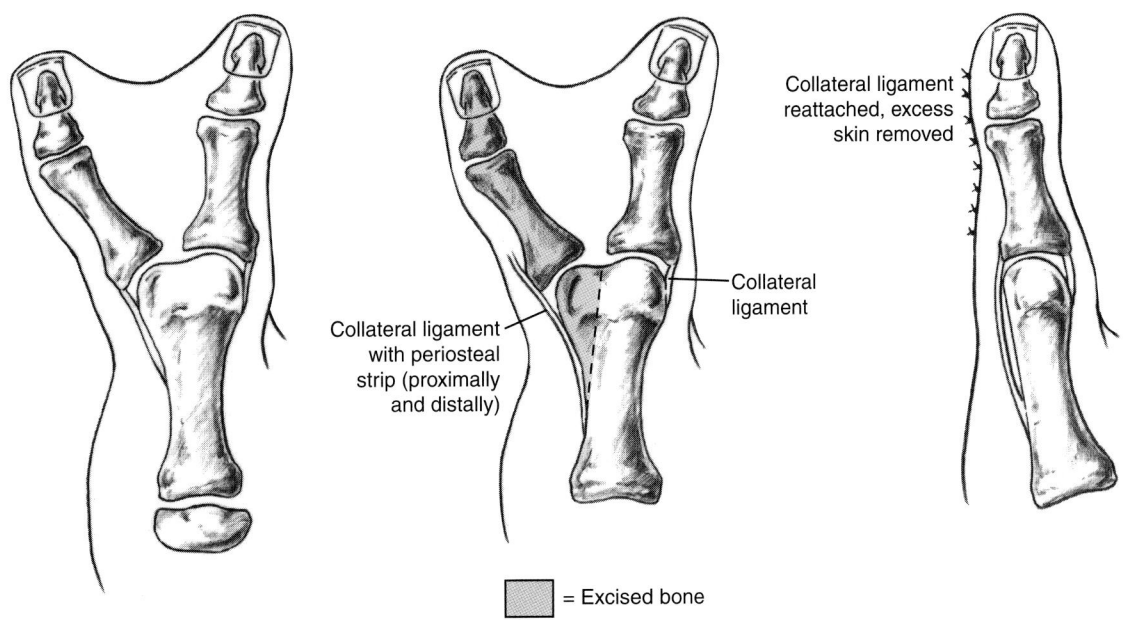

Collateral ligament
reattached, excess
skin removed

Collateral
ligament

Collateral ligament
with periosteal
strip (proximally
and distally)

☐ = Excised bone

Fig. 10. On-top plasty. *A* and *B,* Resection of a portion of the metacarpal head.

digit without bony continuity. Type B should be excised through an elliptical incision that allows identification and ligation of the neurovascular pedicle to the digit. Type A should be treated similar to thumb polydactyly.[7] Coaptation of soft tissue from both small finger components is helpful to provide contour and bulk.[29]

The mirror hand, or ulnar dimelia, involves the forearm, wrist, and hand. It is usually unilateral. There may be bilateral absence of the tibia as well as the radius.[7] The forearm consists of two ulnae without a radius, and the hand includes seven or eight fingers without a thumb. The wrist includes numerous carpal bones and frequently demonstrates carpal coalitions. Usually the wrist is flexed and

deviated to the side, usually radialward. The condition represents an excessive presentation of structures that normally arise from the medial epicondyle, resulting in strong and multiple wrist and finger flexors. In contrast, the wrist and finger extensors, which normally originate from the lateral epicondyle, are dysplastic and underdeveloped. As a result, the wrist is often fixed in a flexed position, and the elbow is stiff. Forearm rotation is limited or absent.[7, 29] The two olecranons are oriented about 60 to 120 degrees to one another.

Treatment begins at the elbow, and motion is enhanced by a combination of resecting the proximal 2 to 5 cm of the more lateral ulna and recontouring the distal humeral surface that abuts against this lateral ulna. Wrist position may be improved by tendon transfers to augment extension, but Wood[7] believes that a wrist arthrodesis is usually necessary. The number of digits is reduced from seven or eight digits to four fingers and a pollicized digit (Fig. 12). A nonfunctional most medial (ulnar) digit is removed, and the four most medial (ulnar) functional digits are retained. Pollicization consists of rotating and recessing the most normal or mobile of the three or four lateral (radial) digits and removing the other digits while salvaging their intrinsic muscles and extrinsic tendons. Shifts of tendon insertion positions of redundant wrist and finger flexors to wrist and finger extensors may improve finger balance.

MACRODACTYLY (MEGALODACTYLY, DIGITAL GIGANTISM, LARGE FINGERS)

Flatt[8] found a prevalence of macrodactyly in less than 1% of all congenital anomalies. The upper limb is affected more often than the lower limb.[35–37] The deformity is unilateral in 90% of patients, and there is an equal sex distribution. Syndactyly occurs in a small percentage of patients, as well as carpal tunnel syndrome. Multiple digits are involved two to three times as often as single digits.[35] The condition occurs most commonly in the index finger

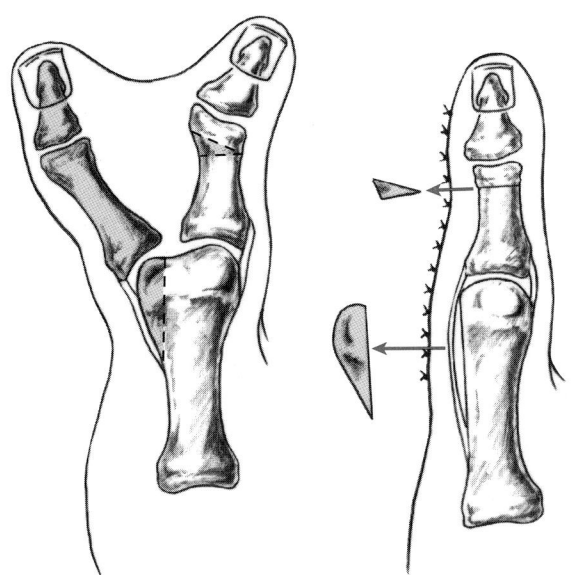

Fig. 11. On-top plasty. *A* and *B,* Resection of part of the metacarpal head and an osteotomy of the proximal phalanx to obtain a perpendicular interphalangeal joint surface.

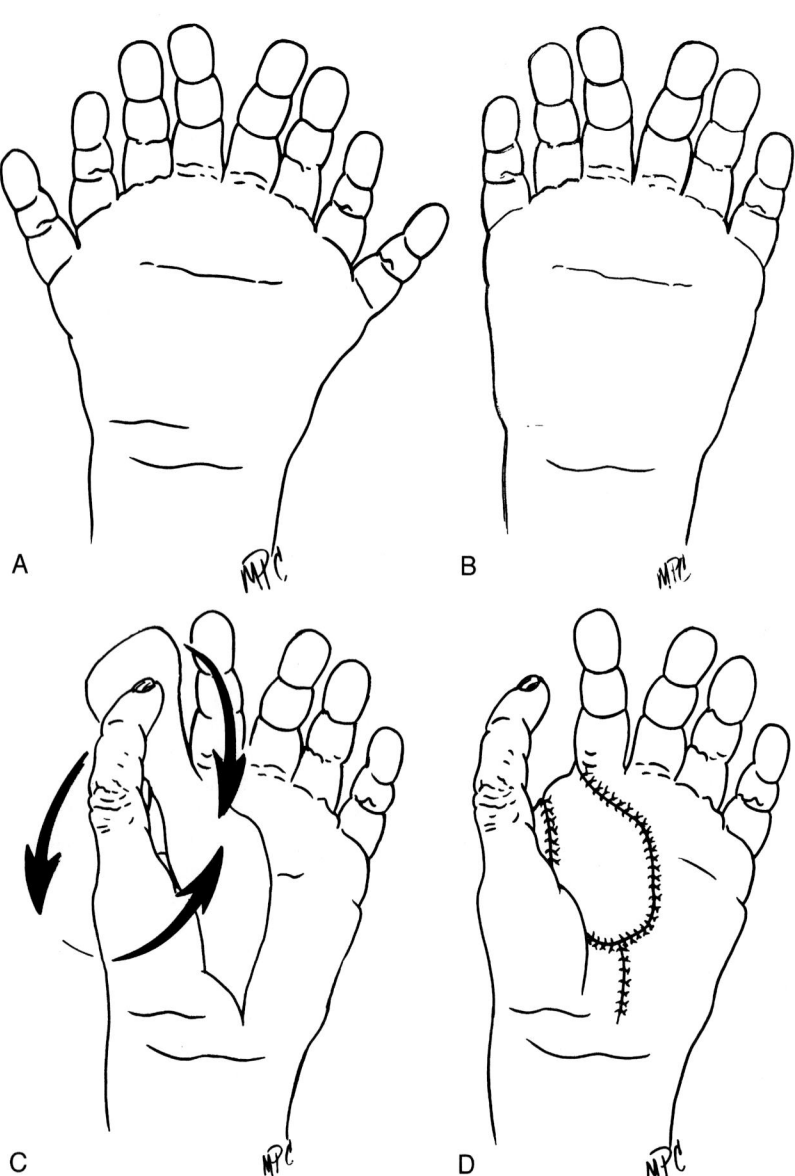

A

B

Fig. 12. View. *A* and *B*, Mirror hand. C, Fillet flap to reconstruct the first web space. *D*, Pollicization of a radial digit.

C

D

(Fig. 13), and then the long, thumb, ring, and little digits in descending frequency.[7] The most common two-digit combinations are thumb and index, then index and long. Syndactyly occurs in about 10% of cases.[8] Flatt[8] identifies the following four clinical forms of the condition.

TYPE I: GIGANTISM AND LIPOFIBROMATOSIS

This is the most common form of macrodactyly. It is usually unilateral and exhibits a "nerve territory oriented" distribution.[36] Median nerve distribution accounts for 85% of cases and ulnar nerve distribution for 15% of cases.[7] Type I is not inherited and does not show signs of neurofibromatosis. The affected peripheral nerve is usually normal to the level of the lower third of the forearm. The phalangeal medullary canals are always widened, but the metacarpals are not always involved. Blood vessels and tendons with their sheaths are not usually affected. The overgrowth is usually asymmetrical, and with growth the finger gradu-

ally begins to lose motion. There are two types of digital gigantism that are dependent on growth characteristics.[37] One type is present at birth, with further growth proportionate to the remaining uninvolved digits. The second type has disproportionate growth so that the involved digit increases in size at a faster rate than could be attributed to normal growth pattern. The second type is more frequently complicated by palmar overgrowth of soft tissues and metacarpal involvement. In both types, longitudinal and circumferential bone growth ceases at the time of epiphyseal closure.[38]

TYPE II: GIGANTISM AND NEUROFIBROMATOSIS

This condition is inherited as an autosomal dominant trait and demonstrates clinical characteristics: six or more café au lait spots, multiple neurofibromas on peripheral nerves, and pedunculated cutaneous tumors. The median nerve is involved most often. Osteochondral masses arising from the epiphyses can occur in both the phalanges and the

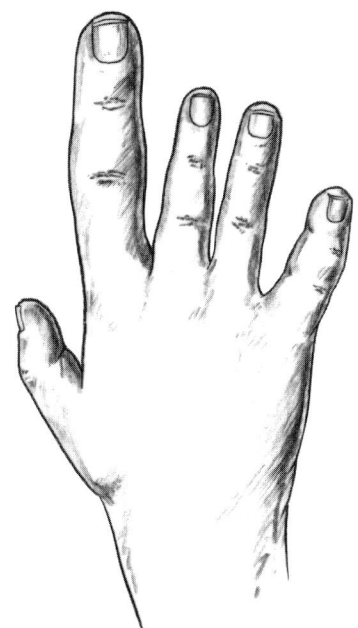

Fig. 13. Macrodactyly of the index finger.

metacarpals. These may involve the palmar plate and block flexion or displace tendons.

TYPE III: GIGANTISM AND DIGITAL HYPEROSTOSIS

Osteochondral masses arising from phalangeal or metacarpal epiphyses are the major problem. Peripheral nerves are not involved and are not enlarged. The digits rapidly become stiff because the osteochondral masses occurring in the palmar plates of the digital joints block motion. The digits are usually misshapen and stiff.

TYPE IV: GIGANTISM AND HEMIHYPERTROPHY

Gigantism is not always limited to a digit, hand, or extremity. Examination usually demonstrates that half of the body is involved. Massive hypertrophy of the thenar and hypothenar muscles is common, and similar muscular enlargement occurs in the forearm and arm. The hand is severely affected functionally, with ulnar drift of the fingers and thumb adduction during infancy and flexion contractures during adolescence. Surgical release is necessary.[8]

Deformity is the reason for treatment, and surgical ablation is the only treatment available. The parents of these patients must be told of the potential number of operations necessary and informed that function and appearance will still be abnormal. Surgery should be undertaken at an early date and must be aggressive.[7, 8, 37]

The procedure required most often is reduction of the diameter of the enlarged fingers.[7] This is done in two stages at least 3 months apart. First, the convex side is reduced. The neurovascular bundle is identified, and visible fat is removed from half of the digit. Tsuge[39] and Kelikian[36] proposed that the most effective technique would be to excise the very hypertrophic and tortuous digital nerve together with the surrounding adipose tissue, because it was noted that excision of the nerve results in only mini-

mal neurological impairment in young children. That result is not entirely predictable. In addition to soft-tissue removal, the phalanges of the older child or adult should be narrowed by removing up to one-fourth of each side of the phalanx. The thickened periosteum is removed. The bone is removed with a high-speed bur, primarily from the diaphysis. The epiphyseal plate is left intact unless growth arrest is done at the same time. The epiphyseal plate is removed with a high-speed drill and curettage across the entire plate. The remaining skin edges or flaps are now too large and may have inadequate blood supply. If the flaps are trimmed and closed without tension after cauterizing the bone and bleeding vessels and inserting a drain, the skin usually heals.

The finger may need shortening as a second stage of reconstruction. The simplest method is amputation through the distal joint, but that results in the loss of the nail. Tsuge[39] excises the end of the digit and reduces the size of the nail. Barsky[26] and Flatt[8] impaled a shortened distal phalanx on a sharpened middle phalanx. Tsuge[39] compresses the dorsal portion of the distal phalanx over the volar portion of the middle phalanx. This procedure often has a precarious blood supply through the dorsal flap.[38] If more shortening is indicated, the base of the proximal phalanx is excised. For lateral deviation, a lateral closing wedge is made at the point of greatest angulation. When indicated, the carpal tunnel is released using a standard volar incision that releases the entire transverse carpal ligament. Osteotomies are stabilized with Kirschner's wires, and 6 to 9 weeks of immobilization are usually required for bony union and soft-tissue homeostasis.

BRACHYDACTYLY (HYPOPLASTIC DIGITS, SHORT FINGERS, STUBBY FINGERS)

Brachydactyly is the term for a short digit in which the normal number of bones is present, but there is a size problem.[8] Ectrodactyly describes a digit with complete absence of one or more phalanges or the metacarpal. Symphalangia describes absence of the proximal interphalangeal joint with complete bony continuity of the proximal phalanx with the middle phalanx. The most commonly hypoplastic single bony segment is the middle phalanx, but any of the axial bones of the hand may be involved.[7, 8] Brachydactyly is a frequent autosomal-dominant malformation; predicting the occurrence or frequency of this condition is not a surgeon's expertise, and a genetic consultation is appropriate. It is equally important that parents realize that short fingers may never develop to the length and size of normal digits. Finger nubbins that have no skeletal support are not functional and are better removed for cosmesis. Flatt[8] believes that a single flail hypoplastic digit is probably not worth retaining because it will diminish coordinated hand function. Dobyns et al[7] advocate reconstruction of most hypoplastic digits when at least one-third the size of a normal digit is present (usual ratio is about 1:1 for digit and hand). Several techniques have been utilized: (1) syndactyly release or web deepening, (2) insert bone to increase length, (3) lengthening by distraction apparatus, (4) augmentation of another digit with the hypoplastic digit, and (5) toe-to-hand or hand-to-hand transfers, including whole digits.

The short digits in brachydactyly often have webbing of the fingers. Some of the cases have complex syndactyly. The skeleton must be separated early to encourage longitudinal growth. Procedures commonly used for syndactyly release can be used, but the surgeon should plan to deepen the web space considerably.[8] An example is Poland's syndrome, with absence of a portion of the pectoralis major muscle, hypoplasia of the ipsilateral hand, and syndactyly of the ipsilateral hand.[40]

Inserting bone into the finger cylinder will gain length and stability but may result in loss of circulation in the tip of the digit. The graft of choice is the proximal phalanx from either the third or fourth toes. Phalanges are transferred with their periosteum intact, and the capsule and palmar plate can also be moved with the phalanx to provide better stability and potential flexion.[41] The recipient finger is opened through a dorsal zig-zag approach that does not encroach on the end of the digit. The transferred phalanx is held in position with a small-diameter Kirschner wire for longitudinal fixation. If flexor or extensor tendons are present, they should be attached to the distal end of the transferred phalanx. Flatt[8] notes that the tourniquet should be deflatted and the end of the recipient finger observed for circulation. If blanching of the skin tip occurs and does not improve over several minutes, the transferred phalanx graft must be shortened until the tip is pink and remains pink around the shaft of the protruding Kirschner wire. The Kirschner wire is left in place for 6 to 9 weeks. Longitudinal growth of the transferred phalanx is usually poor; Carroll and Green[41] found no growth, but Snowdy and Omer[42] recorded growth over 8 years in one patient, and Flatt[8] states that growth is certainly unpredictable.

Distraction techniques are intended to retain circulation and sensibility for the involved digit. Flatt[8] recommends age 2 years as the earliest practical time to start distraction, which can be completed before school is begun. However, the bone to be lengthened must be at least 3 cm in length to accommodate two transverse Kirschner's wires on each side of the osteotomy site. The usual technique is to divide both periosteum and bone and to insert a bone graft when the desired length has been reached.[43] Pin penetration sites need meticulous toilet to prevent infections. A major problem is joint contracture distal to the osteotomy and is caused by stretched longitudinal musculotendinous units. The treatment is a slower rate of distraction. The daily lengthening should be done by the parents, who receive instructions and then must watch for complications while the surgeon performs frequent check-ups and assumes responsibility.

"On-top plasty," or intercalated transposition techniques, enhance the length of affected digits. These procedures are indicated for the skeletal components of the first or fourth web space and are performed with neurovascular pedicles or a skin subcutaneous neurovascular flap.[44] For example, if the index and long fingers are short, a transfer of the index finger onto the end of the long finger creates a wider first web space and a longer ulnar component of grasp.[7, 8] Extensive dissection and mobilization of the neurovascular bundles in the palm must be done because the fundamental problem with these techniques is the maintenance of good circulation. Extensive release of the fascial tissues is necessary, and even tendon lengthening may be required to avoid flexion contractures of the recipient digit.

Toe-to-hand transplantation can be done in children older than 1 year. Children younger than 18 months of age have not established patterns of hand use and tend to incorporate reconstructed digits better than older children. In hands that have no fingers, the goal of reconstruction is to provide sensation with two-finger pinch. The great or second toe from one foot can be transferred for use as the thumb to pinch against one or two minor toes from the opposite side.[45, 46] The vessels in symbrachydactyly and true transverse arrest are unpredictable. It is important to dissect the hand before doing the toe dissection to ensure that adequate recipient vessels are present. The advantage of toe transplantation over other techniques is the inclusion of a viable growth plate, which enables an 85% rate of growth as compared with the opposite digit.[46]

CONGENITAL RING SYNDROME (CONSTRICTION BANDS)

The incidence of these cases is about 1 in 15,000 births, and there is no evidence of an inherited defect.[47] The majority occur in the hand, and associated anomalies in other areas occur in approximately 50% of cases. Acrosyndactyly is a term describing terminal interconnection of syndactylized digits. Acrosyndactyly in congenital ring syndrome is associated with tiny clefts that pass from dorsal to palmar and appear to be remnants of web spaces. Swelling distal to the congenital ring ranges from none to massive swelling that is without function. Angulations, flexion contractures, and stiff joints are also complications. Neurological lesions are not uncommon in deep constriction rings. The critical criteria are identification of a compression band (hand, extremity, or even face or trunk) and relative anatomical normality of the part proximal to the band.[8] Patterson[47] noted four criteria for this syndrome, which may appear individually or in combination: (1) simple constriction rings, (2) constriction rings associated with deformity of the distal part with or without lymphedema, (3) constriction rings associated with soft-tissue merging fusions of distal parts, ranging from mild to gross acrosyndactyly, and (4) intrauterine amputations.

Simple constriction rings are treated with staged excision of the ring and Z-plasty of the defect. The Z-plasty flaps should be as large as possible and have an angle of about 60 degrees. Usually no more than one-half of the circumference of a digit is done at one operation. It is important to excise rather than incise the constricted ring; the depth of the excision should be performed meticulously to spare neurovascular structures in the depth of the constriction ring.

The common distal involvement is lymphedema. The distal subcutaneous tissues often have gross fatty tissue, and the excess fat can be trimmed from the skin flaps before closing. The distal swelling will begin to recede even when only half of the circumference has been released. The proper digital nerves and vessels can usually be found very closely adherent to the undersurface of the constriction ring, but it is more difficult to identify small nerves and vessels on the dorsum of the digit. The second operation can be scheduled approximately 3 months after the release of half of the constriction ring circumference. It is wise to inform parents that there will always be some cosmetic deformity.

The surgical challenge in children with constriction rings and acrosyndactyly is often the proper separation of the digits. The deformity is bilateral in half the cases, but the hands are not symmetrically involved. The distal tips of the fingers are drawn together, and it is often very difficult to allocate the appropriate tip to each finger. The tip of the long finger is usually the most palmar.[8] The fingers must be released early to encourage parallel longitudinal growth. That surgical decision may have to be combined with a decision regarding the salvage of three or four fingers. Surgical release often requires split-thickness skin grafts as well as appropriate Z-plasty flaps. Subsequently, a standard syndactyly release is indicated. Flatt[8] believes that severe cases must have release in the first 6 months of life and be completed by 1 year of age. A significant finding in Flatt's long-term study[8] is that there is loss of finger flexion, in both proximal and distal interphalangeal joints, in these patients.

REFERENCES

1. Upton J, Sinclair TM: Congenital anomalies: Shoulder region. In Peimer CA (ed): Surgery of the Hand and Upper Extremity. New York, McGraw-Hill, 1996, p 2001.
2. Zguricas J, Bakker WF, Heus H, et al: Genetics of limb development and congenital hand malformations. Plast Reconstr Surg 101:1126, 1998.
3. Conway H, Bowe J: Congenital deformities of the hands. Plast Reconstr Surg 18:286, 1956.
4. Lamb DW, Wynne-Davies F, Soto L: An estimate of the population frequency of congenital malformations of the upper limb. J Hand Surg 7:557, 1982.
5. Robinson LK: Genetics and dysmorphology: Approach to diagnosis of the child with a limb anomaly. In Peimer CA (ed): Surgery of the Hand and Upper Extremity. New York, McGraw-Hill, 1996, p 1993.
6. Swanson AB, Swanson G de G, Tada K: A classification for congenital limb malformation. J Hand Surg 8:693, 1983.
7. Dobyns JH, Wood VE, Bayne LG: Congenital hand deformities. In Green DP (ed): Operative Hand Surgery. New York, Churchill Livingstone, 1993, 3rd ed, p 251.
8. Flatt AE: The Care of Congenital Hand Anolamies. St. Louis, Quality Medical Publishing, 1994, 2nd ed.
9. Buck-Gramcko D: Cleft hands: Classification and treatment. Hand Clin 1:467, 1985.
10. Barsky AJ: Cleft hand: Classification, incidence, and treatment. J Bone Joint Surg Am 46:1707, 1964.
11. Snow JW, Littler JW: Surgical Treatment for Cleft Hand. Transactions of the International Society of Plastic and Reconstructive Surgery, Rome, Italy.
12. Miura T, Komada T: Simple method for reconstruction of the cleft hand with an adducted thumb. Plast Reconstr Surg 64:65, 1979.
13. Vilkki SK: Advances in microsurgical reconstruction of the congenitally adactylous hand. Clin Orthop Rel Res 314:45, 1995.
14. Johnson J, Omer GE Jr: Congenital ulnar deficiency: Natural history and therapeutic implications. Hand Clin 1:499, 1985.
15. Marcus NA, Omer GE Jr: Carpal deviation in congenital ulnar deficiency. J Bone Joint Surg Am 66:1003, 1984.
16. Broudy AS, Smith RJ: Deformities of the hand and wrist with ulna deficiency. J Hand Surg 4:304, 1979.
17. Ogden JA, Watson HK, Bohne W: Ulnar dysmelia. J Bone Joint Surg Am 58:467, 1976.
18. Swanson AB, Tada K, Yonenobu K: Ulnar ray deficiency: Its various manifestations. J Hand Surg Am 9:658, 1984.
19. Blair WF, Shurr DG, Buckwalter JA: Functional status in ulnar deficiency. J Pediatr Orthop 3:37, 1983.
20. Smith RJ, Kaplan EB: Camptodactyly and similar atraumatic flexion deformities of the proximal interphalangeal joints of the fingers. J Bone Joint Surg Am 50:1187, 1968.
21. Temtamy SA, McKusick VA: The Genetics of Hand Malformations, New York, Alan R. Liss, Inc., 1978, p 441.
22. Oldfield MC: Camptodactyly: Flexor contracture of the fingers in young girls. Br J Plast Surg 8:312, 1956.
23. Wynne-Davies R: Heritable Disorders in Orthopaedic Practice. London, Blackwell Scientific Publications, 1973, p 155.
24. Dudding BA, Gorlin RJ, Langer LO Jr: Oto-palato-digital syndrome: A new symptom-complex consisting of deafness, dwarfism, cleft palate, characteristic facies, and a generalized bone dysplasia. Am J Dis Child 113:214, 1967.
25. Cooney WP: Camptodactyly and clinodactyly. In Carter P (ed): Reconstruction of the Child's Hand. Philadelphia, Lea & Febiger, 1991.
26. Barsky AJ: Congenital Anomalies of the Hand and Their Surgical Treatment. Springfield, IL, Charles C Thomas, 1958.
27. Carstam N, Theander G: Surgical treatment of clinodactyly caused by longitudinally bracketed diaphysis. Scand J Plast Reconstr Surg 9:199, 1975.
28. Vickers D: Clinodactyly of the little finger: A simple operative technique for reversal of the growth abnormality. J Hand Surg Br 12:335, 1987.
29. Light TR: Congenital anomalies: Syndactyly, polydactyly, and cleft hand. In Peimer CA⁻ (ed): Surgery of the Hand and Upper Extremity. New York, McGraw-Hill, 1996, p 2111.
30. Nogami H, Ohira A: Experimental study on the pathogenesis of polydactyly of the thumb. J Hand Surg 5:443, 1980.
31. Light TR, Buck-Gramcko D: Polydactyly. In Buck-Gramcko D (ed): Congenital Malformations of the Hand and Forearm. Edinburgh, Churchill Livingstone, 1995.
32. Wassel HD: The results of surgery for polydactyly of the thumb. Clin Orthop Rel Res 64:175, 1969.
33. Simmons BP: Polydactyly. Hand Clin 1:545, 1985.
34. Light TR: Treatment of preaxial polydactyly. Hand Clin 8:161, 1992.
35. Barsky AJ: Macrodactyly. J Bone Joint Surg Am 49:1255, 1967.
36. Kelikian H: Congenital Deformitis of the Hand and Forearm, Philadelphia, WB Saunders, 1974, p 610.
37. Kalen V, Burwell DS, Omer GE Jr: Macrodactyly of the hands and feet. J Pediatr Orthop 8:311, 1988.
38. Dell PC: Macrodactyly. Hand Clin 1:511, 1985.
39. Tsuge K: Treatment of macrodactyly. Plast Reconstr Surg 39:590, 1967.
40. Ireland DCR, Takayama N, Flatt AE: Poland's syndrome: A review of 43 cases. J Bone Joint Surg Am 58:52, 1976.
41. Carroll RE, Green DP: Reconstruction of the hypoplastic digits using toe phalanges. J Bone Joint Surg Am 57:727, 1975.
42. Snowdy HA, Omer GE Jr, Sherman FC: Longitudinal growth of a free toe phalanx transplant to a finger. J Hand Surg 5:71, 1980.
43. Kessler I, Baruch A, Hecht O: Experience with distraction lengthening of digital rays in congenital anomalies. J Hand Surg 2:394, 1977.
44. Dobyns JH: Segmental digital transposition in congenital hand deformities. Hand Clin 1:475, 1985.
45. Gordon L: Toe-to-thumb transplantation. In Green DP: Operative Hand Surgery. New York, Churchill Livingstone, 1993, 3rd ed, p 1253.
46. Gilbert A: Congenital absence of the thumb and digits. J Hand Surg Br 14:6, 1989.
47. Patterson TJS: Congenital ring-constrictions. Br J Plast Surg 14:1, 1961.

section
9
chapter
11

IDIOPATHIC SCOLIOSIS

Mary E. Hurley and Vincent J. Devlin

Summary

- The estimated cost of screening and resultant treatment of idiopathic scoliosis exceeds $220 million dollars per year in the United States.
- The natural history of idiopathic scoliosis is determined by the degree of the curve at diagnosis, age at diagnosis, growth potential, and sex.
- Positive risk factors for progression are degree of curve at time of diagnosis, chronological age, Risser's sign, and growth potential.
- Negative risk factors for progression are family history, thoracic kyphosis, lumbar lordosis, lumbosacral transitional anomalies, and trunk balance.
- Staging is determined by radiographic Cobb's angle. Classification has traditionally been according to the King-Moe pattern. Classification systems are evolving with changes in surgical technique.
- Diagnosis relies on accurate screening and radiographic confirmation.
- Treatment is determined based on curve magnitude, curve location, and patient characteristics.
- Treatment options include observation, bracing, and surgical fusion.

DEFINITION

The term scoliosis derives from the Greek word for curvature. Scoliosis has been defined as the presence of a lateral curvature of the spine that exceeds 10 degrees as measured by the Cobb method. Curves below 10 degrees are referred to as spinal asymmetry. Idiopathic scoliosis is defined as the presence of scoliosis in the absence of all other spinal abnormalities such as congenital vertebral abnormalities, tumor, infection, trauma, postsurgical, and intraspinal disorder.

Idiopathic scoliosis occurs as a three-dimensional deformity that involves coronal, sagittal, and rotational components. All three components must be considered in the evaluation and treatment of scoliosis.

HISTORICAL REVIEW

Hippocrates first described the variation of etiology, relationship to pulmonary disease, and difficulty of treatment for certain curves in "De Articulation" of the Corpus Hippocraticum.[1]

Galen added the nomenclature of scoliosis, lordosis, and kyphosis.

Pare (1510–1590) introduced the steel corset made by armorers for correction of scoliosis as well as describing congenital scoliosis and cord compression as a cause of paralysis.

During the 19th century exercise and bracing remained the mainstay of treatment. Distraction on horizontal or vertical frames and plaster casting were developed.

The 20th century has seen the development and refinement of indications and techniques for surgical intervention:

- Successful spinal arthrodesis without the need for body casts.
- Refinement of anterior and posterior spinal surgical technique.
- Thoracoplasty.
- Harrington instrumentation.
- Segmental instrumentation.
- Intraoperative neurophysiological monitoring.
- Thoracoscopic and endoscopic spinal procedures.
- Bone graft substitutes and allograft bone graft.

EPIDEMIOLOGY

INFANTILE IDIOPATHIC SCOLIOSIS

Infantile idiopathic scoliosis affects children before the age of three. This type of scoliosis is much more prevalent in Europe and rarely reported in the United States. This type of scoliosis is more common in males.[2] Infantile curves may be progressive (15%) or resolving (85%). Infantile scoliosis is associated with plagiocephaly, mental retardation (13%), congenital dislocation of the hip (3.5%), and congenital heart disease (2.5%).[2]

Assessment of the radiographic relationships between the rib head and vertebral body as described by Mehta[3] continues to be the preferred method for differentiating progressive and resolving curves. The first relationship is the rib-vertebral angle difference (RVAD) (Fig. 1) and the second is described as the phase. An RVAD greater than 20 degrees combined with transition from phase I to phase II predicts progression in 80% of curves.

JUVENILE IDIOPATHIC SCOLIOSIS

Juvenile idiopathic scoliosis presents between age 4 years and adolescence. Juvenile scoliosis comprises 12% to 16% of all patients with idiopathic scoliosis. There is an increased prevalence in females reported by several authors.[4, 5] Curve progression is assessed by close clinical and radiographic follow-up especially during times of increased growth.

ADOLESCENT IDIOPATHIC SCOLIOSIS

Adolescent idiopathic scoliosis is responsible for the majority of curves that present for evaluation. These curves are most often noted around the time of the pubertal growth spurt. The prevalence of adolescent idiopathic scoliosis depends on the diagnostic criteria applied. When the threshold for the diagnosis of scoliosis is set at 10 degrees, the incidence is 25 per 1000 patients. If the threshold for diagnosis is increased to 20 degrees, the incidence drops to

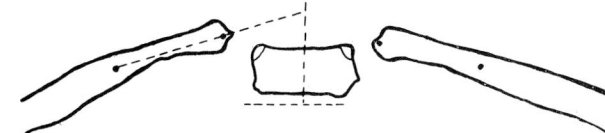

Fig. 1. Measurement of the rib-vertebral (RVA) angle. (From Mehta MH: The rib-vertebra angle in the early diagnosis between resolving and progressive infantile scoliosis. J Bone Joint Surg Br 1972; 54: 230.)

3 to 5 per 1000 patients. For curves greater than 30 degrees, prevalence is 1 to 3 per 1000 patients. If the threshold is extended to 40 degrees, the incidence drops to less than 1 per 1000. These rates of incidence are relatively constant across all populations.

Increasing curve magnitude is correlated with female sex. The female-to-male ratio for curves 10 degrees and greater is 1.4–2:1. For curves greater than 20 degrees, the ratio icreases to 5.4:1. For curves greater than 30 degrees, the female:male ratio increases to 10:1.

PATHOGENESIS

The cause and pathogenesis of idiopathic scoliosis are the focus of ongoing research. The importance of genotype is evident by the detection of hereditary patterns in mono- and dizygotic twins. However, no mode of inheritance has been confirmed.

Other areas of investigation regarding the causes of scoliosis are the following:

- Growth patterns.
- Hormonal influence.
- Abnormalities of connective tissue.
- Brain stem function.
- Postural reflexes.

- Equilibrium dysfunction.
- Chemical influences such as melatonin.

CLINICAL FEATURES

Idiopathic scoliosis may be brought to attention by many sources: school screening programs, primary care physicians, patients, or family members. Typical findings include postural abnormality as well as shoulder, rib, or pelvic asymmetry. Patients presenting with the primary complaint of pain must be evaluated with great caution as idiopathic scoliosis is not associated with pain in most cases. A thorough history and physical examination are mandatory.

The primary care physician should examine all children for asymmetry of the shoulders, trunk, and pelvis in the standing positon. Thoracic and lumbar prominences are best detected on the forward bend test. Every orthopaedic examination should include routine screening for scoliosis. All examinations are carried out with the child barefoot and undressed. Females may wear a sports bra or swimsuit. Hair is pulled away from the back so that a thorough examination can be carried out.

After an examination of the rest of the systems, the musculoskeletal examination starts with an inspection of the patient's anterior chest and thorax looking for asymmetry or rotation. The patient is examined from the side for abnormal kyphosis or lordosis. The back examination begins with the patient standing straight with both arms resting at the side. The position of the head over the sacrum is observed and any deviation from normal alignment measured with a plumb line and recorded. Asymmetry of the shoulders, scapula, or pelvis is noted. The skin is observed for sacral dimples, nevi, café au lait spots, or hairy patches giving clues to possible underlying intraspinal disorder. The posterior spinous processes are palpated for asymmetry, step-off, or tenderness (Fig. 2).

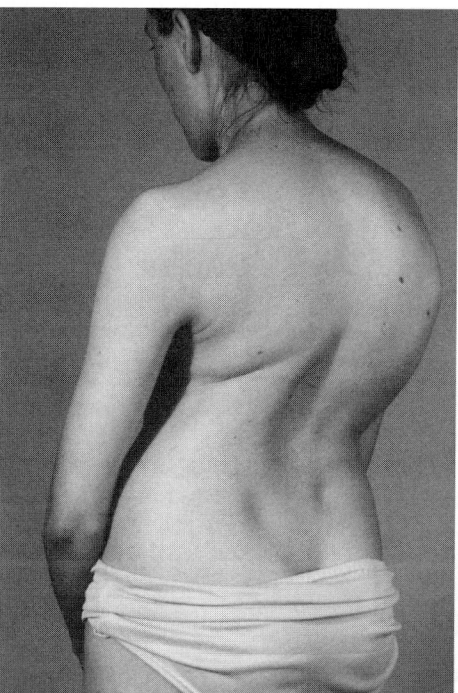
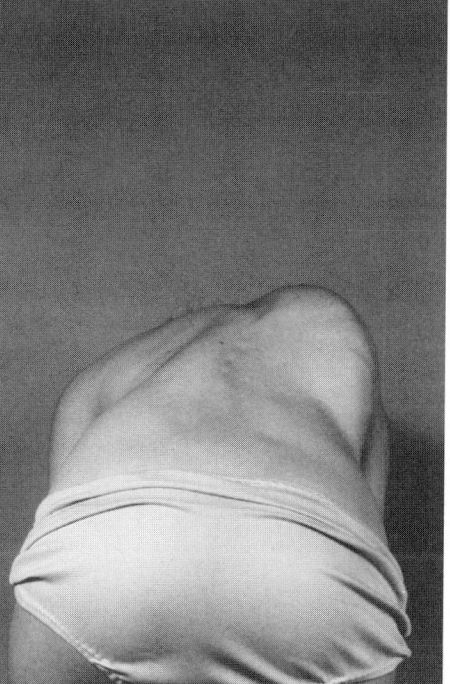

Fig. 2. This is an examination of the patient with thoracic prominence on forward bend.

After manual and visual examination in stance, the patient is asked to bend forward with the knees straight and the arms hanging freely. The spine is then inspected from posterior to assess for thoracic or lumbar prominence. A scoliometer may be used to measure the degree of prominence.

The upper and lower extremities are examined for full symmetric range of motion. Leg lengths are measured for asymmetry. Muscle tone is evaluated. A careful examination of the lower extremities for hamstring or tendo-Achilles tightness is carried out. Next, a neurovascular examination is undertaken, noting motor strength, deep tendon reflexes, sensation, and pulses. The abdominal reflex should be checked as well.[6] The patient's gait is evaluated.

INVESTIGATION

Radiographic evaluation of the patient is carried out with both standing posteroanterior and lateral 36-inch spine films. The use of 17-inch films pieced together is inadequate for evaluation and measurement. Lateral bending films are not needed for routine evaluation and are generally obtained only for preoperative planning. Oblique films, spot laterals, and other views may be indicated for specific problems.

The properly positioned and exposed films are assessed for degree of curve, type of curve, rotation, and skeletal age. The curve angle is measured by the Cobb-Lippman[7] technique. The top and bottom vertebrae that tilt maximally into the concavity of the curve being measured are identified as the *end vertebrae*. The end vertebra between two curves is the lower end vertebra of the top curve and the upper end vertebra of the bottom curve. Once the cephalad end vertebra is identified, the superior end plate, or pedicles if more clearly defined, is clearly marked with a line. A right angle to this line is then established. The caudal end vertebra is identified and a line drawn parallel to the end plate or pedicles. A right angle to this line is drawn to intersect with the previous right angle. The angle between these two lines measures the magnitude of the curve (Fig. 3). Careful identification of the end vertebra is

essential as this measurement will determine the baseline for all future measurements. Bending films are measured in the same manner utilizing the previously identified end vertebra.

The lateral film is measured for thoracic kyphosis and lordosis. The Cobb method is applied assigning kyphosis a positive value and lordosis a negative value. The normal thoracic kyphosis measures 20 to 40 degrees (T4-12) and normal lumbar lordosis 50 to 70 degrees (L1-S1).

The rotational component of the curve is measured by either the Nash and Moe[8] or Pedriolle[9] method. The Nash system is most commonly utilized. In this system the rotation is graded from zero to IV. Grade zero is when the pedicles of the apical vertebra are symmetric and equidistant from the sides of the vertebral body. Grade I rotation occurs when the pedicle on the convex side rotates away from the side of the vertebral body toward midline. In grade II the pedicle shadow aligns between the edge of the vertebra and the midline; in grade III the pedicle shadow is in the middle of the vertebra. Grade IV rotation brings the convex pedicle shadow across the midline to the concavity of the curve (Fig. 4).

Skeletal age can be determined from the iliac crests, vertebral bodies, or left wrist and hand film. The anteroposterior view of the hand is compared with standards found in the Greulich and Pyle Atlas.[10] The vertebral ring epiphyses fuse at skeletal maturity and can be most clearly identified on the lateral view. Risser[11] described the ossification of the iliac epiphysis in stages zero to 5 which correlate with skeletal maturity (Fig. 5). Complete excursion and cessation of spinal growth, Risser stage 5, denote fusion to the ilium and signal the end of height increase. Recent research has focused on growth velocity and other more accurate methods of predicting skeletal age.

The lifetime exposure to ionizing radiation in idiopathic scoliosis is not insignificant. Hoffman et al[12] reported on long-term risk for breast cancer and concluded that excess risk increased with time since exposure, increased number of radiographs, and with increased radiation dose to the breast. The overall lifetime risk has been projected at 1% to 2% among women followed for adolescent idiopathic scoliosis with serial radiographs.[13] Replacing the anteroposterior view with the posteroanterior view achieves a three- to sevenfold reduction in cumulative doses to the thyroid gland and breast tissue. This translates to a three- to fourfold reduction in the lifetime risk of breast cancer and half the lifetime risk of thyroid cancer.[14] Additional methods to minimize cumulative radiation include appropriate breast and gonadal shielding, beam collimation, tube filters, and high-speed film screen combinations.

Magnetic resonance imaging (MRI) evaluation may be indicated in certain clinical situations including patients with early onset of scoliosis (<11 years of age),[15] very rapidly developing scoliosis, certain left thoracic curves, abnormal neurological examination,[16] and curves associated with syndromes or congenital abnormalities. Bone scan, computed tomography, MRI, and laboratory work-up may be indicated in the patient with painful scoliosis.

DIFFERENTIAL DIAGNOSIS

Prior history of surgery (such as thoracotomy), tumor, infection, and radiation must be sought. The presence of

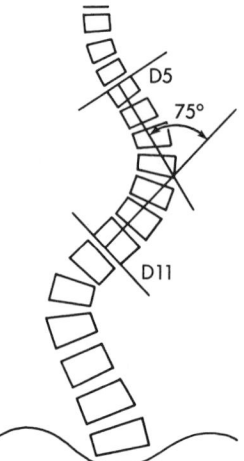

Fig. 3. Cobb's method for measuring the angle of a scoliotic curve. (Adapted from Cobb JR: Outline for the study of scoliosis. In Instr Course Lect, Ann Arbor, MI, American Academy of Orthopaedic Surgeons Instr Course Lect 1948; 5:261.)

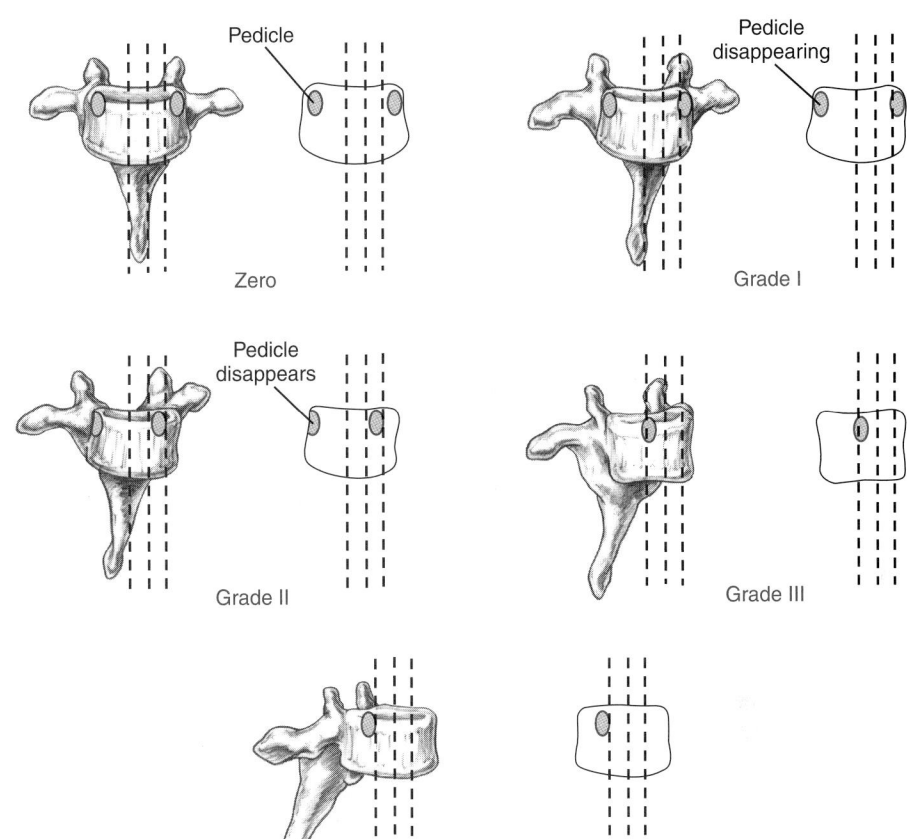

Fig. 4. Nash's method for measuring the rotational component of the curve. (Adapted from Nash C, Moe J: A study of vertebral rotation. J Bone Joint Surg Am 1963; 51:223.)

syndromes or congenital abnormality may be considered insignificant by the patient and family and must be carefully elicited. Family history is reviewed for scoliosis or other musculoskeletal abnormalities.

Painful scoliosis is evaluated for an underlying cause such as infection, tumor, or intraspinal lesions. In a retrospective study of 2442 patients with idiopathic scoliosis, the prevalence of back pain was found to be 23% (560/2442) at time of presentation with an additional 9% reporting back pain during the period of observation. Of the 560 patients presenting with back pain, 9% (n: 48) were found

to have an underlying pathological condition. The authors found a painful left curve or an abnormal neurological examination most predictive of an underlying pathological condition.[17]

Congenital scoliosis is identified radiographically. The presence of vertebral abnormalities differentiates congenital from idiopathic scoliosis. (See Chapter 9–12.)

Hysterical scoliosis has been reported and can be a difficult diagnosis. Diagnosis may need to be made under anesthesia. Evaluation by a psychiatrist is indicated when hysterial scoliosis is suspected.

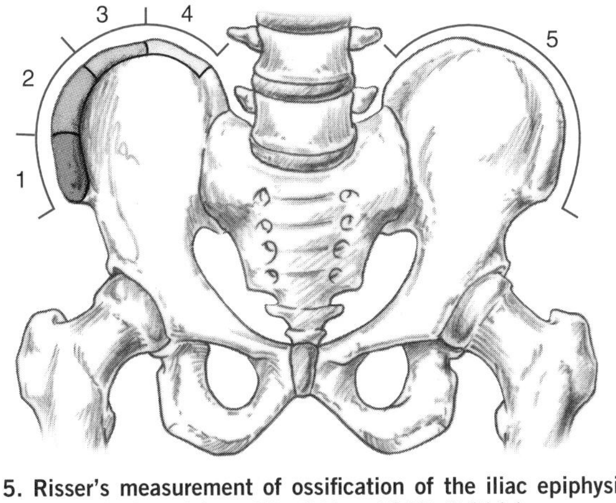

MANAGEMENT

Nonsurgical management of scoliosis requires diligent care on the part of the family and orthopaedic surgeon. The age of the patient, magnitude and type of curve, and curve progression over time must be carefully evaluated. For the very young skeletally immature patient (Risser 0–1), follow-up is needed at 4-month intervals until evidence of either curve progression or stability is established. For the older patient with less risk of progression, 6-month interval follow-up is indicated. For stable curves without evidence of progression, 9-month to 1-year follow-up may suffice.

Many methods of treating the scoliotic spine have been attempted. There is no evidence that exercise programs or electric stimulation regimens have altered the natural history of idiopathic scoliosis. While there is a great deal of interest in altered dietary intake, chiropractic adjustment,

Fig. 5. Risser's measurement of ossification of the iliac epiphysis in stages 0 to 5. (Adapted from Clin Orthop 1958; 2:111.)

acupuncture, and other nontraditional treatment methods, none have shown evidence of efficacy. However, the overall health of the patient with regard to adequate diet, exercise, and cardiovascular fitness should not be ignored.

Currently, bracing is the only non-operative management that has been shown to be effective in carefully selected patients.[18, 19] The goal of brace treatment is to prevent curve progression with the minimum of distress to the patient. There is no evidence that bracing will correct existing curves over the long term, and families should be made aware of this fact. Patient selection combined with diligent brace management is essential for successful outcome.

There is rarely an indication for bracing curves below 20 degrees. Patients who are Risser 0–1 and premenarchal with curves 20 to 29 degrees are candidates for bracing. In the Risser 2–4 patient with a curve 20 to 29 degrees, progression of 5 degrees should be documented before bracing is begun. A patient presenting with a curve of 30 or more degrees should be braced without waiting for evidence of progression. Patients who are Risser 4–5 are poor candidates for bracing as there is minimal growth remaining.

There are several types of braces and the appropriate one must be designed to fit the specific needs of the patient (Fig. 6). In general, if the curve apex is at T8 or below, an underarm brace can be utilized. For curves with an apex above T8 a Milwaukee style brace will be necessary. The Charleston nighttime bending brace has been advocated as

an alternative to a full-time brace regimen.[20] The Charleston brace passively corrects the spine in the opposite direction of the curve and is worn only during sleeping hours.

Brace wear has been prescribed as both a part-time (16 hours per day) and full-time (23 hours per day) regimen. Studies have shown that actual wearing time is much less than prescribed time in all groups. Recent studies demonstrate a dose-response in brace wear indicating that full-time wear is more effective in controlling progression of the curve.[21] Bracing is continued until skeletal maturity (Risser 4 or 5) and then weaned over the next year.

Relative contraindication to brace wear include curves greater than 45 degrees, patients unable to cope emotionally with bracing, severe thoracic hypokyphosis or lordosis, and high thoracic and cervicothoracic curves. Complications resulting from bracing include pressure sores, nerve compression with resultant neuralgia, stretch marks, esophageal reflux, decreased glomerular filtration rate, thoracic cage compression, increase in compensatory curves, psychological disturbances,[22–24] noncompliance, and curve progression despite a well-fitted brace.[25]

SURGICAL TREATMENT

The patient's age (chronological and skeletal), curve type, curve history, and the predicted long-term consequences of surgical versus nonsurgical treatment are all relevant factors in deciding whether or not to consider surgical treatment for a specific patient. The patient and family may be

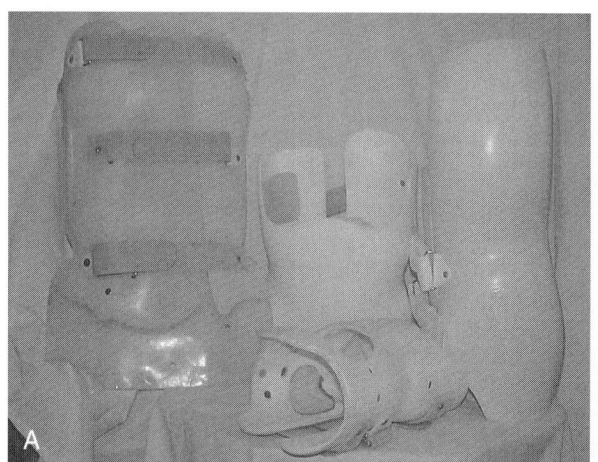
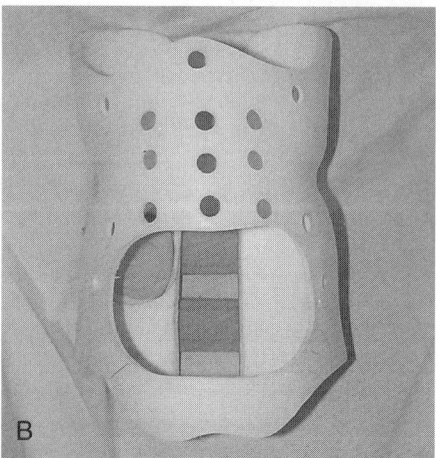
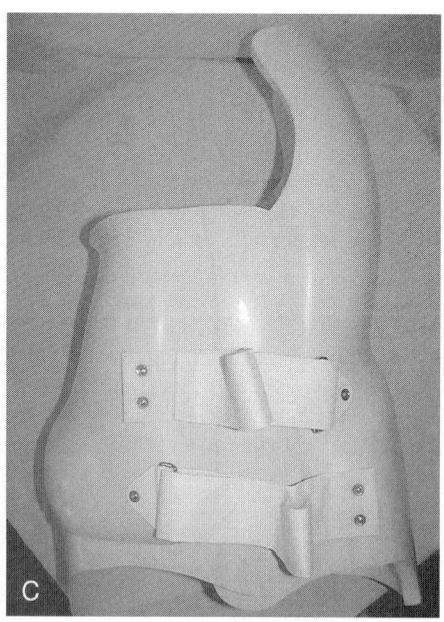

Fig. 6. Different types of braces.

most concerned with either the functional, cosmetic, or social outcome of treatment. Cosmetic and social concerns are more difficult to quantify and vary from patient to patient but are essential parts of preoperative discussion with the patient and family.

General surgical indications for fusion include a skeletally immature patient with a curve exceeding 40 to 50 degrees at presentation or one who progresses despite appropriate brace wear. Some curve patterns such as thoracolumbar or lumbar curves greater than 30 degrees with marked apical rotation, double major curves greater than 50 degrees, or significant coronal or sagittal imbalance are indications for surgical fusion even in the mature patient.

Preoperative planning ideally involves the patient and family through preoperative nursing education, hospital ward tours, child life specialist counseling, and peer support groups. A sufficient number of visits with the operative surgeon are required to thoroughly answer all questions.

A thorough history and physical examination including all major organ systems are required. If a significant cardiac history is elicited, appropriate work-up and clearance by the patient's cardiologist are obtained. Potential pulmonary complications can be identified with a careful history and physical exam. Patients with previous pulmonary disease, cardiothoracic surgeries, dyspnea with exertion, nocturnal dyspnea, hypokyphosis, or rigid thoracic curves may need preoperative pulmonary function tests. It is not necessary to obtain routine preoperative pulmonary function tests for mild to moderate idiopathic scoliosis.[26]

Careful neurological examination may reveal abnormalities warranting evaluation of the entire spinal axis with MRI. Abnormal curves such as left thoracic, rigid curves, painful curves, and rapidly progressive curves may also alert the surgeon to a potential underlying spinal disorder requiring clarification before surgical fusion. Arnold-Chiari malformations, syrinx, diastomatomyelia, and tumors warrant evaluation by a neurosurgeon.

Autologous or donor-directed blood donation should be considered and discussed with the family and informed consent obtained.[27] Erthyropoietin has been utilized to increase preoperative donation as well as postoperative hemoglobin levels. Close cooperation with the anesthesiologist utilizing intraoperative blood salvage, hypotensive anesthesia, and appropriate hemodilution techniques can reduce the need for transfusion. Special consideration should be undertaken with the patient who has specific religious tenets regarding blood products and transfusion.[28] Referral to institutions specializing in this type of care may be indicated.

Attention must be paid to the patient's menstrual history and the possibility of pregnancy. Sexual activity may be under-reported in the adolescent patient. Careful history taking with documentation of last menstrual cycle is needed. Some centers employ routine immediate preoperative serum pregnancy testing to avoid potential medical complications.

Patients who are underweight for height are evaluated for nutritional adequacy. The possibility of anorexia nervosa should be entertained and appropriate referral and treatment integrated with care of the surgical patient. Nutritional counseling for the obese patient may be helpful

though no studies have been published looking at these parameters and the impact on surgical fusion.

SURGICAL TREATMENT OF IDIOPATHIC SCOLIOSIS
Preoperative Evaluation
Deformity Analysis and Preoperative Planning

Standing 36-inch posteroanterior and lateral radiographs and supine right and left side bending radiographs are obtained before surgery.[29] Additional specialized radiographs including anteroposterior traction radiographs (best for thoracic curves exceeding 60 degrees), push-prone radiographs, and fulcrum apex bending radiographs have been described to assist with preoperative planning. Surgical decision-making involves selection of the spinal levels requiring arthrodesis, determination of the surgical approach (posterior, anterior, or combined), and selection of the type of spinal instrumentation.

Initially, experience with posterior Harrington's instrumentation led to the development of the concept of the stable zone as a guide to proper placement of posterior spinal instrumentation. This zone was defined by two vertical lines beginning at the lumbosacral facets and drawn perpendicular to a line across the iliac crest. It was recommended that Harrington's hooks be inserted in this zone to achieve a spinal fusion which was balanced over the sacrum.

Idiopathic thoracic scoliosis curve patterns were classified by King and colleagues. This classification does not take into account the sagittal profile of the spine. The five specific thoracic curve types are:

Type I

Double thoracic and lumbar curves
Thoracic and lumbar prominences
Both curves cross the midline
Lumbar curve may be larger than thoracic curve
Both curves are structural, with nearly equal flexibility
True double major curve

Type II

Thoracic and lumbar curves
Minimal lumbar prominence
Both thoracic and lumbar curves cross the midline
Lumbar curve is more flexible on side bending
False double major curve pattern

Type III

Thoracic curve
Minimal or no decompensation
Lumbar curve does not cross the midline

Type IV

Long thoracic curve
Marked decompensation
Curve reaches the midline at L4 which tilts into the curve

Type V

Double thoracic curve
Positive tilt of T1, with prominent left neckline
High left and right thoracic prominences
Upper left curve structural on side bending

The classification of thoracic curves described by King and colleagues combined with the exisiting classification of thoracolumbar and lumbar curves provides the most widely used classification for idiopathic scoliosis (Fig. 7).

Curve classification is used to determine appropriate fusion levels. Based on the King-Moe classification system, principles have evolved to guide selection of the spinal levels requiring posterior fusion and include the following:

- Fusion of all vertebrae in the measured major curve or curves.
- Fusion of major curves from a neutrally rotated cephalad vertebra to a neutrally rotated caudal vertebra.
- Fusion to the stable vertebra defined as the vertebra bisected by the midsacral reference line.

Type I curves generally require treatment by fusion of both curves. Traditionally, fusion is extended to L4 distally. Anterior surgery or use of posterior pedicular implants may permit the fusion to stop at L3. In type II curve patterns, where the lumbar curve is flexible and exists as a compensatory curve, selective fusion of only the thoracic curve may be performed. When the fusion is stopped at the stable vertebra, the fusion is balanced over the sacrum. The compensatory lumbar curve tends to correct spontaneously. This preserves valuable lumbar motion segments. In curve types III, IV, and V, fusion extends distally to the stable vertebra.

The above principles for determination of fusion levels were developed based on experience with posterior Harrington's instrumentation. As new posterior segmental spinal instrumentation systems (Cotrel-Dubousset, TSRH, Isola Moss-Miami) were introduced, additional principles evolved to guide selection of the fusion area. Experience with the CD system popularized additional criteria for fusion level selection when posterior segmental spinal instrumentation was utilized:

- The disc space below the lower instrumented vertebrae must open on both right and left side bending films.
- The lower surface of the lower instrumented vertebrae should become parallel or nearly parallel with the iliac crests on side bending films.

- The lower instrumented vertebrae should centralize over the sacrum and be intersected by the center sacral line.
- The lower instrumented vertebrae should derotate to a substantial degree.
- The above criteria are for use with hooks. In certain cases, the fusion may be stopped one level proximal to the level determined according to the above criteria if pedicle screws are utilized for fixation at the distal vertebral levels.

Based on experience gained with posterior segmental spinal instrumentation and improved understanding of the three-dimensional nature of idiopathic scoliosis, additional criteria to guide selection of fusion levels when using posterior spinal instrumentation have evolved. Asher developed the torsional concept of scoliosis and developed specific implants and instrumentation sequences which specifically address the correction of spinal deformity in three dimensions with emphasis on correction of the transverse plane deformity.[30, 31]

Various criteria exist for guiding selection of fusion levels when anterior fusion and instrumentation are utilized. Curve location, curve magnitude, and type of instrumentation utilized are factors which must be considered in decision-making. Since the pioneering work of Dwyer and Zeilke, the theoretical advantages of an anterior approach have been recognized. However, difficulty in obtaining and maintaining sagittal plane alignment has limited widespread acceptance of the anterior approach until recently. Various techniques have been developed to address this issue, including stiff rod constructs, structural bone grafting, use of anterior intervertebral spacers, and dual rod constructs. Recently, anterior fusion and instrumentation have been advocated for correction of select thoracic curve patterns. Currently, anterior instrumentation and fusion are the treatments of choice for certain thoracolumbar and lumbar curves. The criteria of Hall have been popularized.[32] These include that the patient be an adolescent or young adult with a lumbar or thoracolumbar curve 60 degrees or less. If there is a compensatory thoracic curve, it should correct

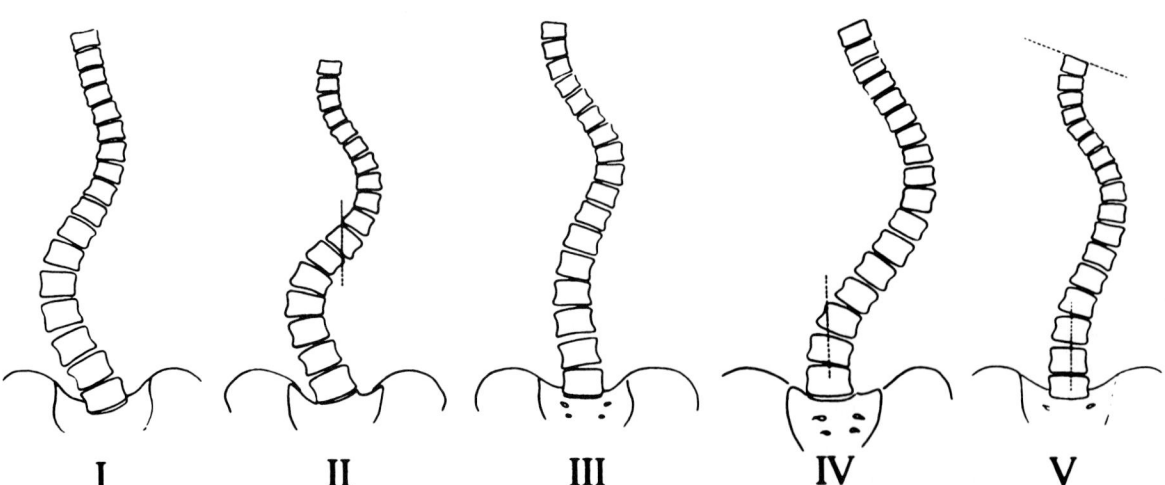

Fig. 7. King-Moe classification of idiopathic scoliosis. (From King HA, Moe JH, Bradford DS, et al: The selection of fusion in thoracic idiopathic scoliosis. J Bone Joint Surg Am 1983; 65:1202.)

to 20 degrees or less on the bend film, and there should be no abnormal kyphosis above the planned upper instrumentation level. Fusion levels are selected on the basis of a standing radiograph and a supine bend film toward the convexity as follows:

- On the standing film, if the regional horizontal apex is a disc space, two levels above and below should be fused.
- On the standing film, if the regional horizontal apex is a vertebral body, one vertebra above and one below should be fused.
- In addition, the instrumentation should extend to the vertebra above the first disc space that opens on the bending film toward the convexity.

As decision-making for scoliosis surgery has become more complex, alternative classification systems for idiopathic scoliosis have been proposed. A new comprehensive classification system for idiopathic scoliosis by Lenke and colleagues has been developed in order to facilitate comparison of various surgical treatments and appropriate analysis of outcome data. Six specific curve types are identified:

1. Primary thoracic.
2. Double thoracic.
3. Double major.
4. Triple major.
5. Primary thoracolumbar or lumbar.
6. Primary thoracolumbar or lumbar with a secondary thoracic curve.

These six curve types are further subclassified as A,B, C according to the relationship of the center sacral vertical line (CSVL) to the lumbar spine. This type of classification permits operative treatment of idiopathic scoliosis to be described in an algorithmic form (Fig. 8).

Surgical Approaches
Posterior Spinal Procedures
The posterior approach for fusion is commonly used for patients with idiopathic scoliosis. During the surgical procedure, the posterior spinal elements are exposed in a subperiosteal fashion and the facet joints are excised and

---

Curve Type

Type	Proximal Thoracic	Main Thoracic	Thoracolumbar/ Lumbar	Curve Type
1	Non-Structural	Structural (major*)	Non-Structural	Main Thoracic (MT)
2	Structural	Structural (major*)	Non-Structural	Double Thoracic (DT)
3	Non-Structural	Structural (major*)	Structural	Double Major (DM)
4	Structural	Structural (major*)	Structural	Triple Major (TM)
5	Non-Structural	Non-Structural	Structural (major*)	Thoracolumbar/Lumbar (TL/L)
6	Non-Structural	Structural	Structural (major*)	Thoracolumbar/Lumbar-Main Thoracic (TL/L - MT) Lumbar Curve>Thoracic by ≥5°

STRUCTURAL CRITERIA
(Minor Curves)

Proximal Thoracic: - Side Bending Cobb ≥ 25°
- T2 - T5 Kyphosis ≥ +20°

Main Thoracic: - Side Bending Cobb ≥ 25°
- T10 - L2 Kyphosis ≥ 20°

Thoracolumbar/Lumbar: - Side Bending Cobb ≥ 25°
- T10 - L2 Kyphosis ≥ +20°

*Major = Largest Cobb Measurement, always structural
Minor = All other curves with structural criteria applied

LOCATION OF APEX
(SRS definition)

CURVE	APEX
THORACIC	T2 - T11-12 DISC
THORACOLUMBAR	T12 - L1
LUMBAR	L1-2 DISC - L4

Modifiers

Lumbar Spine Modifier	CSVL to Lumbar Apex
A	CSVL Between Pedicles
B	CSVL Touches Apical Body(ies)
C	CSVL Completely Medial

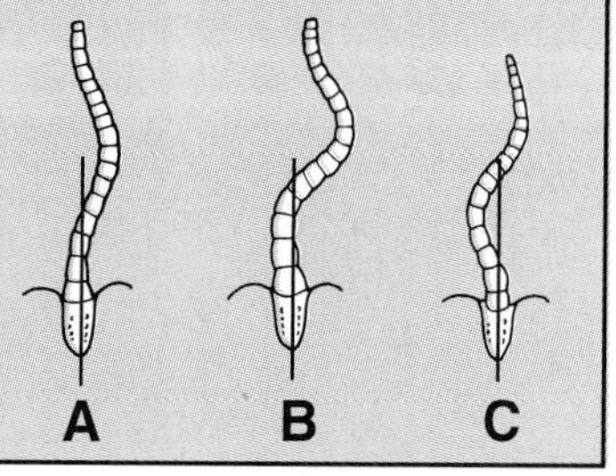

A   B   C

Thoracic Sagittal Profile T5 - T12		
-	(Hypo)	< 10°
N	(Normal)	10° - 40°
+	(Hyper)	> 40°

Curve Types (1-8) + Lumbar Spine Modifier (A, B, or C) + Thoracic Sagittal Modifier (-, N, or +)
Classification (e.g. 1B+):_____

Fig. 8. **Lenke's system of classification for idiopathic scoliosis.** (Courtesy of Dr. Lawrence Lenke.)

packed with autogenous iliac bone graft. Posterior spinal instrumentation is placed and the spinal curvature is partially corrected. Spinal implants used to achieve fixation to the posterior spinal elements may be hooks, wires (cables), and/or pedicular screws.[33, 34] The typical instrumentation construct consists of two parallel rods attached to the spine at multiple sites and connected at its cephalad and caudad aspect by a cross-linkage device thereby creating a rigid rectangular fixation construct. Various corrective forces may be applied to the posterior spinal elements to provide for deformity correction depending upon the implant system utilized. These include distraction, compression, translation, cantilever bending, and torsion-countertorsion (Fig. 9).

Anterior Spinal Procedures

Anterior spinal instrumentation and fusion have been most commonly indicated for patients with idiopathic thoracolumbar and lumbar curves. Recently, there has been interest in the use of anterior spinal instrumentation for thoracic deformities. Progress in minimally invasive surgical techniques has stimulated the development of thoracoscopic approaches to anterior spinal fusion and instrumentation.

For a typical thoracolumbar or lumbar curve, surgical exposure is achieved through a thoracoabdominal approach from the convex side of the curvature. Rib resection is generally performed two vertebral levels above the upper vertebrae requiring instrumentation. Exposure of the spine may be achieved through either the retropleural or trans-pleural route and requires release of the diaphragm from the chest wall. The disc, cartilaginous end-plates, and annulus are thoroughly excised. Vertebral body screws are placed across the mid-aspect of the vertebral body in the coronal plane. Currently, solid rods are the preferred linkage for connecting the vertebral body screws. After rod placement and correction of the curvature, the disc spaces are distracted and packed with rib graft and frequently with a structural spacer as well. This structural spacer may be a cortical ring allograft (femur or humerus) or a prosthetic cage. Compression forces are applied to the anterior spinal column. Wound closure is performed in the standard manner (Fig. 10).

Combined Anterior and Posterior Spinal Procedures

In certain cases of idiopathic scoliosis, both anterior and posterior procedures are indicated. When combined procedures are indicated, the anterior procedure consists of multilevel discectomy and fusion with non-structural grafting of the disc spaces. More recently, this has been performed through a minimally invasive thoracoscopic approach.[35] Anterior surgery is generally followed by posterior segmental spinal fixation to achieve correction of the spinal deformity (Fig. 11). Indications for combined approaches include the following:

- Large stiff curves (greater than 75 to 90 degrees).
- To prevent crankshaft (Risser 0, open triradiate cartilage, and before peak height velocity).[36]

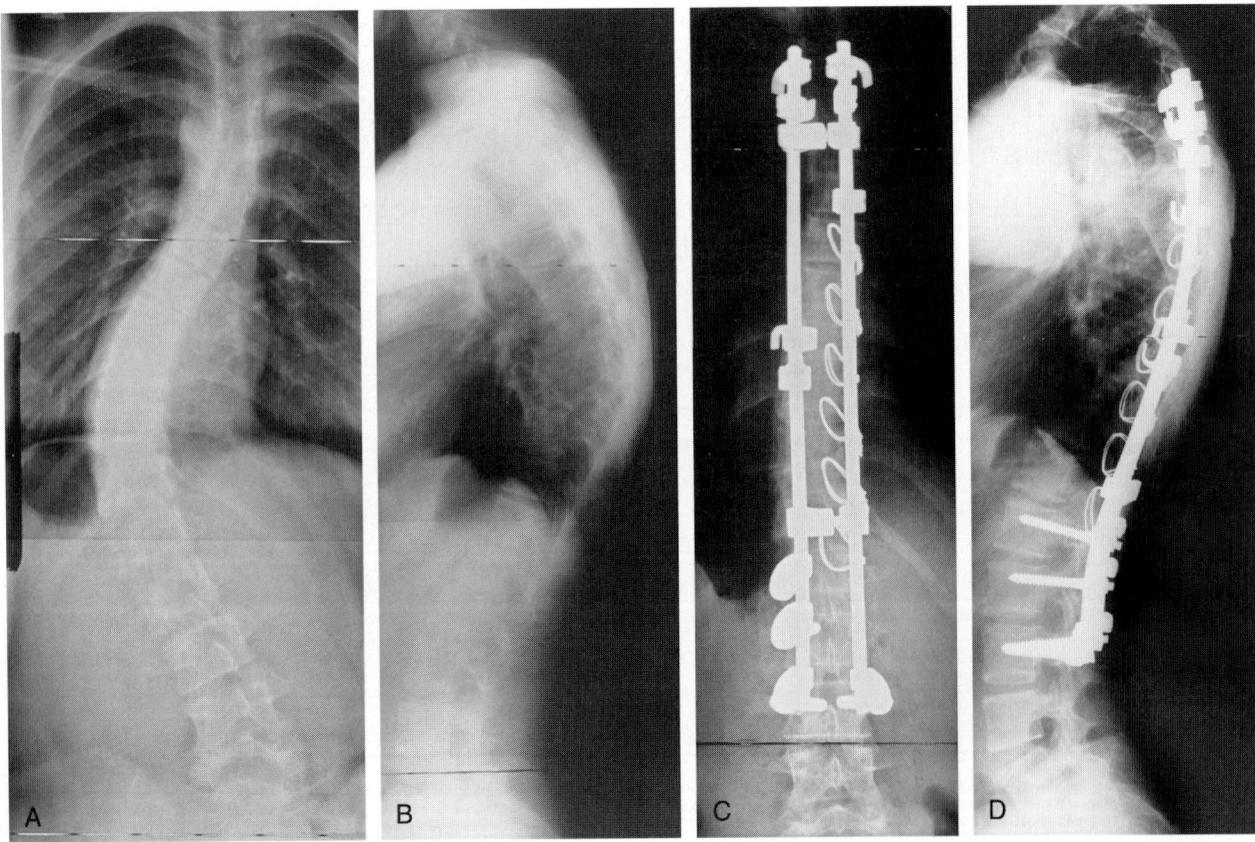

Fig. 9. Images. These are preoperative *(A, B)* and postoperative *(C, D)* images of posterior spinal fusion.

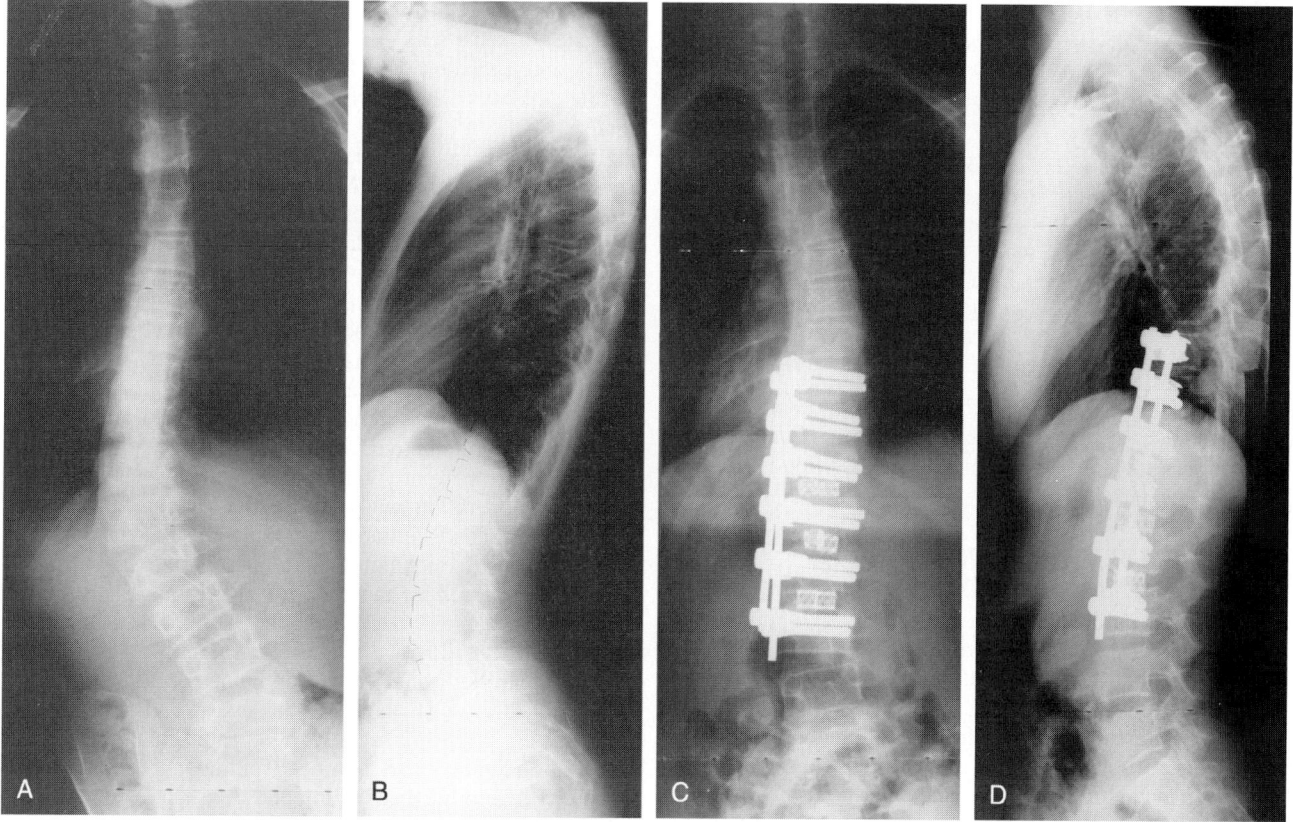

Fig. 10. Images. These are preoperative *(A, B)* and postoperative *(C, D)* images of anterior spinal fusion.

Fig. 11. Images. These are preoperative *(A, B)* and postoperative *(C, D)* images of combined anterior and posterior spinal procedure.

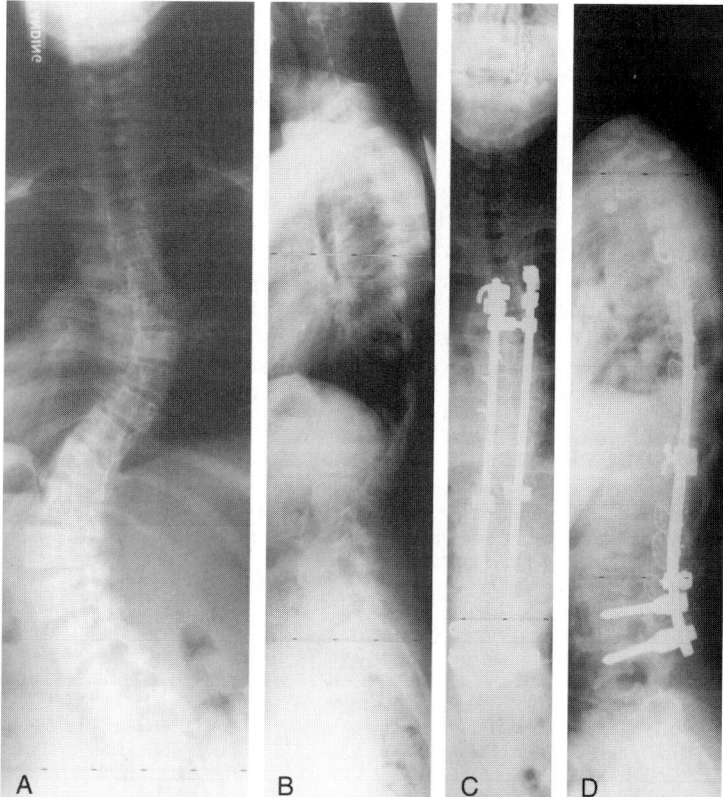

- To address coexistent sagittal plane abnormalities (thoracic lordoscoliois or excessive kyphosis).

ADJUNCTIVE PROCEDURES
Thoracoplasty

Thoracoplasty is used as an adjunct to spinal reconstructive procedures in order to decrease the magnitude of the thoracic rib prominence. It may be performed via an anterior or posterior approach. Thoracoplasty via the anterior approach may be performed as an open procedure or as a minimally invasive thorascopic procedure.[37]

Concave Rib Osteotomy

Sectioning of the concave ribs has been described as a useful method of achieving correction in stiff curves. This procedure is generally performed after insertion of the spinal instrumentation.

PERIOPERATIVE COMPLICATIONS OF SPINAL FUSION PROCEDURES

The risks of perioperative complications in spinal fusion have diminished with modern techniques of anesthesia, improved spinal instrumentation systems, intraoperative neurophysiological monitoring, and postoperative intensive care.[38, 39] Parents must be informed of the most common complications, including but not limited to hemorrhage, infection, pneumothorax, instrumentation failure, pseudarthrosis, trunk imbalance, neurological injury, and possible need for future surgery.

Intraoperative Considerations

Careful preoperative planning decreases the risks of intraoperative complications. Close communication with the anesthesiologist to determine the type and placement of intraoperative lines will facilitate proper positioning. The surgeon, before sterile preparation and draping of the patient, confirms adequate padding of all dependent body parts.

Avoidance of intraoperative neurological injury is of primary concern in the surgical treatment of scoliosis. The gold standard has been the Stagnara[40] wake-up test in which the patient is awakened intraoperatively in order to demonstrate motor competency. The introduction of somatosensory monitoring has decreased use of this method by allowing accurate monitoring of the dorsal spinal column function. The introduction of combined motor-evoked potential monitoring with somatosensory monitoring has demonstrated a sensitivity of 98.6% in predicting neurological status and specificity of 100% of normal data predicting normal findings when performed by an experienced monitor.[41]

The ultimate goal of surgery is a successful fusion of the selected spinal segments. Meticulous preparation of the fusion bed including facetectomies and decortication is critical. Application of abundant amounts of autologous bone harvested from the iliac crest supplemented with local bone graft and bone obtained from resected ribs has been the gold standard. Recent reports of dependable results utilizing freeze-dried or fresh-frozen allograft bone[42–44] have been encouraging and may possibly allow for decreased blood loss, operative time, and surgical morbidity. New synthetic osteoinductive and osteoconductive bone graft substitutes are currently being explored.

Close cooperation with the anesthesiologist utilizing intrathecal opioids,[45] intraoperative blood salvage, hypotensive anesthestic technique, and appropriate hemodilution techniques can reduce the need for blood transfusion.[46]

Postoperative Care

Patient-controlled analgesia, continuous epidural analgesia,[47] and the use of pain teams to assess and treat postoperative pain have enhanced patient comfort and recovery. Early mobilization and improved pulmonary toilet can be achieved due to adequate pain control.

Early and aggressive nutritional suport with total parenteral nutrition for nutritionally at-risk patients improves recovery time and wound healing. Removal of nasogastric tubes, Foley catheters, and invasive lines as soon as possible decreases the risk of postoperative sepsis. Peri-operative antibiotic coverage is maintained for 24 to 48 hours.

Postoperative bracing is infrequently required due to the rigidity of modern spinal instrumentation systems. Relative indications for bracing include an unfused minor curve in the skeletally immature patient, a noncompliant patient, and select anterior instrumentation and fusion procedures. Progressive prescribed activity following surgery will facilitate the patient's return to normal activities without risking hardware failure.

Late complications of trunk imbalance (sagittal and/or coronal), pseudarthrosis, hardware failure, curve progression, crankshaft phenomenon, and late infection should be recognized during follow-up and prompt management undertaken.

REFERENCES

1. Bradford DS, Lonstein JE, Ogilvie RB, Winter JW: Moe's Textbook of Scoliois and Other Spinal Deformities. Philadelphia, WB Saunders, 1987.
2. Wynne-Davies R: Familial (idiopathic) scoliosis: Causative factors, particularly in the first six months of life. J Bone Joint Surg Br 1975; 57:138.
3. Mehta MH: The rib-vertebra angle in the early diagnosis between resolving and progressive infantile scoliosis. J Bone Joint Surg Br 1972; 54:230.
4. Figueiredo UM, James JIP: Juvenile idiopathic scoliosis. J Bone Joint Surg Br 1981, 63:61.
5. Tolo VT, Giollespie R: The characteristics of juvenile idiopathic scoliosis and results of its treatment. J Bone Joint Surg Br 1978; 60:181.
6. Yngve D: Abdominal reflexes. J Pediatr Orthop 1997; 17(1):105.
7. Cobb J: Outline for the study of scoliosis. In Instructional Course Lectures. The American Academy of Orthopaedic Surgeons, vol 5. Ann Arbor, MI, JW Edwards Co., 1948.
8. Nash C, Moe J: A study of vertebral rotation. J Bone Jonit Surg Am 1969; 51: 2323.
9. Pedriolle R: La Scoliose. Paris, Maloine, 1979.
10. Greulich W, Pyle S: Radiographic Atlas of Skeletal Development of the Hand and Wrist, 2nd ed. Stanford, CA, Stanford University Press, 1959.
11. Risser J: The iliac apophysis: An invalu-

able sign in the management of scoliosis. Clin Orthop 1958; 11:111.

12. Hoffma DA, Lonstein JE, Morin MM, et al: Breast cancer in women with scoliosis exposed to multiple diagnostic x-rays. J Natl Cancer Inst 1989; 81:1307.

13. Levy AR, Goldberg MS, Hanley JA, et al: Projecting the lifetime risk of cancer from exposure to diagnostic ionizing radiation for adolescent idiopathic scoliosis. Health Phys 1994; 66:621.

14. Levy AR, Goldberg MS, Mayo NE, et al: Reducing the lifetime risk of cancer from spinal radiographs among people with adolescent idiopathic scoliosis. Spine 1996; 21:1540.

15. Lewonowski K, King JD, Nelson MD: Routine use of magnetic resonance imaging in idiopathic scoliosis patients less than eleven years of age. Spine 1992; 17:S109.

16. Schwend RM, Hennrikus W, Hall JE, et al: Childhood scoliosis: clinical indications for magnetic resonance imaging. J Bone Joint Surg Am 1995; 77:46.

17. Ramirez N, Johnston CE, Browne RH: The prevalence of back pain in children who have idiopathic scoliosis. J Bone Joint Surg Am 1997; 79:364.

18. Nachemson AL, Peterson LE, and members of the Brace Study Group of the Scoliosis Research Society: Effectiveness of treatment with a brace in girls who have adolescent idiopathic scoliosis. J Bone Joint Surg Am 1995, 77:815.

19. Rowe DE, Bernstein S, Riddick M, et al: A meta-analysis of the efficacy of non-operative treatments for idiopathic scoliosis. J Bone Joint Surg Am 1997; 79:664.

20. Price CT, Scott DS, Reed FR, et al: Nighttime bracing for adolescent idiopathic scoliosis with the Charleston Bending Brace: Long term follow-up. J Pediatr Orthop 1997; 17:703.

21. Rowe DE, Bernstein SM, Riddick MF, et al: A meta-analysis of the efficacy of non-operative treatments for idiopathic scoliosis. J Bone Joint Surg 1997; 79:664.

22. Fallstrom K, Nachemson A, Chochran T: Psychologic effects of treatment for adolescent idiopathic scoliosis. Orthop Trans 1984; 8:150.

23. Gratz R, Papalia-Finlay D: Psychosocial adaptation to wearing the Milwaukee brace for scoliosis. J Adolesc Health Care 1984; 5:237.

24. Myers B, Friedman S, Winer I: Coping with a chronic disability: Psychosocial observations of girl with scoliosis treated with a Milwaukee brace. Am J Dis Child 1970; 120:175.

25. Tachdjian M: Pediatric Orthopedics. Philadelphia, WB Saunders, 1990.

26. Vedantam R, Crawford AH: The role of preoperative pulmonary function tests in patients with adolescent idiopathic scoliosis undergoing posterior spinal fusion. Spine 1997; 22:2731.

27. Moran MM, Kroon D, Tredwell SJ, et al: The role of autologous blood transfusion in adolescents undergoing spinal surgery. Spine 1995; 20:532.

28. Safwat AM, Reitan JA, Benson D: Management of Jehovah's Witness patients for scoliosis surgery: The use of platelet and plasmapheresis. J Clin Anesth 1997; 9: 510.

29. Vaughan JJ, Winter RB, Lonstein JE: Comparison of the use of supine bending and traction radiographs in the selection of the fusion area in adolescent idiopathic scoliosis. Spine 1996; 21:2469.

30. Asher MA, Burton DC: A concept of idiopathic scoliosis deeformities as imperfect torsions. Clin Orthop Rel Res 1999; 364:11.

31. Asher MA: Isola instrumentation system for scoliosis. In Bridwell KH, DeWald RL (eds): The Textbook of Spinal Surgery, 2nd ed. Philadelphia, Lippincott-Raven, 1997, p 569.

32. Hall JE: Anterior surgery in the treatment of idiopathic scoliosis. J Bone Joint Surg Br 1994; 76:3.

33. Hamill CL, Lenke LG, Bridwell KH, et al: The use of pedicle screw fixation to improve correction in the lumbar spine of patients with idiopathic scoliosis: Is it warranted. Spine 1996; 21:1241.

34. Barr SJ, Schuette AM, Emans JB: Lumbar pedicle screws versus hooks. Results in double major curves in adolescent idiopathic scopiosis. Spine 1997; 22:1369.

35. Rothenberg S, Erickson M, Eilert R, et al: Thoracoscopic anterior spinal procedures in children. J Pediatr Surg 1998; 33:1168.

36. Roberto RF, Lonstein JE, Winter RB, et al: Curve progression in Risser stage 0 or 1 patients after posterior spinal fusion for idiopathic scoliosis. J Pediatr Orthop 1997; 17:718.

37. Mehlman CR, Crawford AH, Wolf RK: Video-assisted thoracoscopic surgery (VATS). Endoscopic thoracoplasty technique. Spine 1997; 222:2178.

38. Weis JC, Betz RR, Clements DG, Balsara RK: Prevalence of perioperative complications after anterior spinal fusion for patients with idiopathic scoliosis. J Spinal Disord 1997; 10:371.

39. McDonnell MF, Glassman SD, Dimar JR, et al: Perioperative complications of anterior procedures on the spine. J Bone Joint Surg Am 1996; 78:839.

40. Vauzelle C, Stangara P, Jouvinrou P: Functional monitoring of spinal cord activity during spinal surgery. J Bone Joint Surg Am 1973; 55:441.

41. Padberg AM, Wilson-Hoden TJ, Lenke LG, et al: Somatosensory- and motor-evoked potential monitoring without a wake-up test during idiopathic scoliosis surgery: An accepted standard of care. Spine 1998; 23:1392.

42. Stricker SJ, Sher JS: Freeze-dried cortical allograft in posterior spinal arthrodesis: Use with segmental intrumentation for idiopathic adolescent scoliosis. Orthopedics 1997; 20:1039.

43. Bridwell KH, O'Brien MF, Lenke LG, et al: Posterior spinal fusion supplemented with only allograft bone in paralytic scoliosis. Does it work? Spine 1994; 19:2658.

44. Blance JS, Sears CJ: Allograft bone use during instrumentation and fusion in the treatment of adolescent idiopathic scoliosis. Spine 1997; 22:1338.

45. Goodarzi M: The advantages of intrathecal opioids for spinal fusion in children. Paediatr Anaesth 1998; 8:131.

46. Burbi L, Gregoretti C, Borghi B, et al: Predeposit, intentional perioperative haemodilution and erythropoietin level in major orthopaedic surgery. Anaesthsia 1998; 53:27.

47. Shaw BA, Watson TC, Merzel DI, et al: The safety of continuous epidural infusion for postoperative analgesia in pediatric spine surgery. J Pediatr Orthop 1996; 16: 374.

SCOLIOSIS: CONGENITAL AND NEUROMUSCULAR

Thomas S. Renshaw

Summary

- Scoliosis, both the congenital and neuromuscular types, is frequently progressive and can lead to severe spinal deformity and poor quality of life.
- Neither congenital nor neuromuscular scoliosis has the natural history of, or responds to treatment like, idiopathic scoliosis.
- Both should be monitored periodically by clinical evaluation and radiographs.
- Orthotics are not effective in the treatment of either condition, and progressive curves must be surgically treated.
- In some instances, surgery is directly indicated without waiting for documentation of curve progression.

CONGENITAL SCOLIOSIS

Congenital scoliosis results from aberrant embryonic development of the spine, either by failure of formation in part or all of one or more vertebrae or partial or complete failure of segmentation of two or more vertebrae. Both types can occur in the same spine. It is the third most prevalent type of scoliosis after idiopathic scoliosis and deformity associated with neuromuscular diseases.[1] A brief review of the embryonic development of the spine is helpful for a better understanding.

FAILURE OF FORMATION

Complete bilateral failure of formation is rare. This results in the total absence of a vertebra and usually does not produce any deformity or asymmetry. The total or partial failure of midline fusion of the paired somites results in a butterfly vertebra but no curvature.

Most often, failure of formation involves one side of the vertebra. If incomplete or hypoplastic, a trapezoidal or wedge-shaped vertebra results. This usually results in a small curve, which may, but usually does not, progress or require treatment. If complete unilateral absence occurs, a hemivertebra exists on the opposite side. Several variations are possible. All or some of a vertebral body, pedicle, or posterior elements may be missing or hypoplastic. It is common for a hemivertebra to be more deficient anteriorly than posteriorly, and this often produces kyphoscoliosis.

The hemivertebra is considered incarcerated when its pedicle and vertebral edge align with those parts of the adjacent cranial and caudal vertebra. A hemivertebra with the involved vertebra displaced laterally (nonincarcerated) is more likely to develop progressive deformity. About 90% of hemivertebrae are nonincarcerated. Multiple hemivertebrae may occur sequentially or be separated by normal

or abnormal intervening vertebrae. They may occur on the same or on opposite sides of the spine.

The number of growth plates also has implications for the natural history. Hemivertebra is termed nonsegmented when there is no disk material or growth plate between the hemivertebra and its adjacent normal vertebra and is the least likely form to progress. The prognosis remains good when only one end is segmented, because each side of the spine has the same number of growth plates. The semisegmented type occurs in about 20% of cases. The fully segmented hemivertebra has two extra growth plates and is very likely to produce a continuously progressive curve. This situation is the most common, occurring in about two-thirds of hemivertebrae.

There are other factors in the natural course of congenital scoliosis caused by failure of formation. The more hemivertebrae that occur on the same side of the spine, the more likely it is that the curve will progress. Thoracolumbar and lower thoracic curves have a worse prognosis than do lumbar and high thoracic curves. Lumbosacral hemivertebrae may produce spinal decompensation and require treatment, despite a low numerical curve magnitude (Fig. 1).

FAILURE OF SEGMENTATION

This situation can be symmetrical or asymmetrical. Bilateral failure of segmentation results in two block vertebrae. This rarely induces a curve, and when a small curve is present, progression is not likely. Block vertebrae at multiple levels can shorten the length of the spine. Physiological consequences for the heart and lung do not occur unless nearly all the thoracic region is included (e.g., spondylothoracic dysplasia). Anterior symmetrical failure of segmentation produces congenital kyphosis. The rare posterior symmetrical failures result in progressive lordosis.

Unilateral failure of segmentation is more common, resulting in an unsegmented bar (Fig. 2). The bar acts as a tether on the concave side of the spine and causes a relentlessly progressive curve when growth potential remains on the opposite side. Occasionally, the convex side will have poor potential for growth, so the curve will progress more slowly.

MIXED ANOMALIES

Mixed anomalies do occur and occasionally are so complex that they are very difficult to classify, even with sophisticated three-dimensional imaging techniques. An unsegmented bar contralateral to a hemivertebra or, worse, to multiple hemivertebrae is virtually always progressive and needs prompt surgical stabilization without waiting for documentation of progression. At the opposite end of the spectrum, multiple variations on both sides of the spine may produce curves that vary from nonprogressive to rapidly

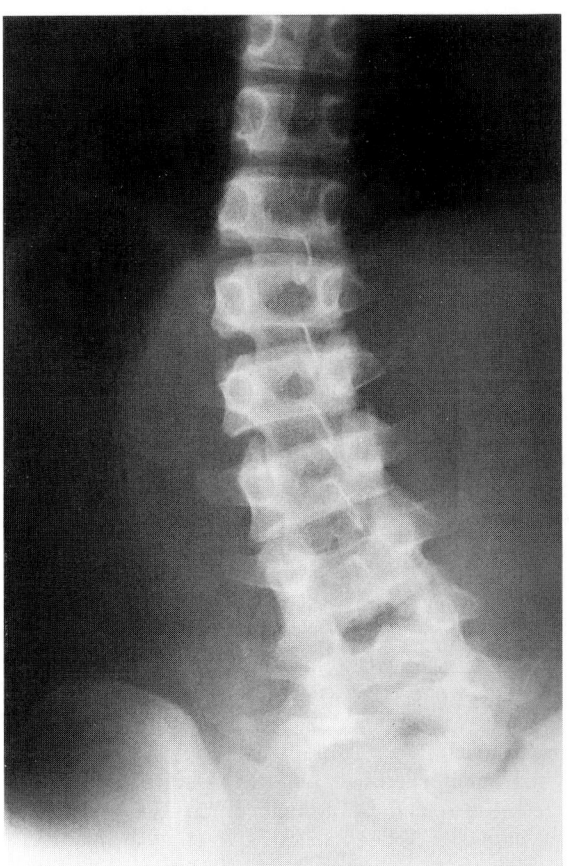

Fig. 1. Congenital scoliosis. Right hemivertebra at S1 produces right lumbosacral curve with compensatory left thoracolumbar curve and spinal decompensation. (From White AH: Spine Care. Mosby, 1995, p 1561.)

increasing. For optimal treatment to be provided, it is critical to monitor patients with congenital spine anomalies with standardized radiographs at appropriate intervals.

PATHOGENESIS

The specific causes of the disordered embryonic spinal anatomy are not known, but the problem likely occurs during the first 5 weeks of development. Teratogenic agents have been suspected as at least one cause of congenital spine abnormalities. Genetic studies have not been consistent in identifying risks of occurrence and patterns of anomalies.[2, 3]

Deformities evolve from asymmetrical growth of the spine: scoliosis from lateral imbalance, kyphosis from anterior anomalies, and the exceptionally rare congenital lordosis from posterior tethering. Fifty percent of congenital curves will progress to the point at which surgery will be needed. Thirty-five percent to 40% will progress to some degree but will not require surgery. Ten percent to 15% will be nonprogressive. Patient age and growth velocity are important factors in progressive curves. The younger the patient, the more potential there is for curve progression.[4] Progression usually accelerates during the rapid growth in the first 2 years of life and in the adolescent growth spurt.[5, 6]

It is important to document progression of both the structural anomaly and also the longer curve where the anomaly may be found at its apex. Any compensatory curves above and below the congenital curve and any sagittal plane deformity must also be monitored.[7]

OTHER ANOMALIES

Because all body systems develop simultaneously, it is not surprising that anomalies in other organ systems are encountered in 30% to 60% of patients with congenital scoliosis.[8] The most common are probably rib variants such as fusion or absence of ribs, but prevalence data are lacking. Anomalies are often found in the urinary tract (18% to 37%) and include unilateral renal agenesis, renal duplication, renal ectopia, and horseshoe kidney.[9] Spinal malformations are associated in 10% to 20% of congenital spinal deformities. Myriad anomalies, including myelodysplasia, Klippel-Feil syndrome, Arnold-Chiari malformation, and intraspinal defects (tethered cord, syringomyelia, diastematomyelia, lipomas, cysts, and others), are seen.[10, 11] Associated cardiac anomalies (5% to 10%) are generally seen with spinal variants in the thoracic region. Pulmonary hypoplasia, gastrointestinal problems, and other musculoskeletal defects such as limb deficiencies, Sprengel's deformity, cavovarus feet, clubfeet, and hip dysplasia can occur. Constellations of anomalies, such as the VATER syndrome and its variants, Holt-Oram syndrome, Aarskog syndrome, multiple pterygium syndrome, and Goldenhar's syndrome, also may include congenital spinal anomalies.

INVESTIGATION

Most cases of congenital scoliosis are detected by observing a clinically visible spinal deformity or during the evaluation of a cutaneous abnormality over the neural axis, such as a mass, hypertrichosis, vascular anomaly, or a sinus tract.

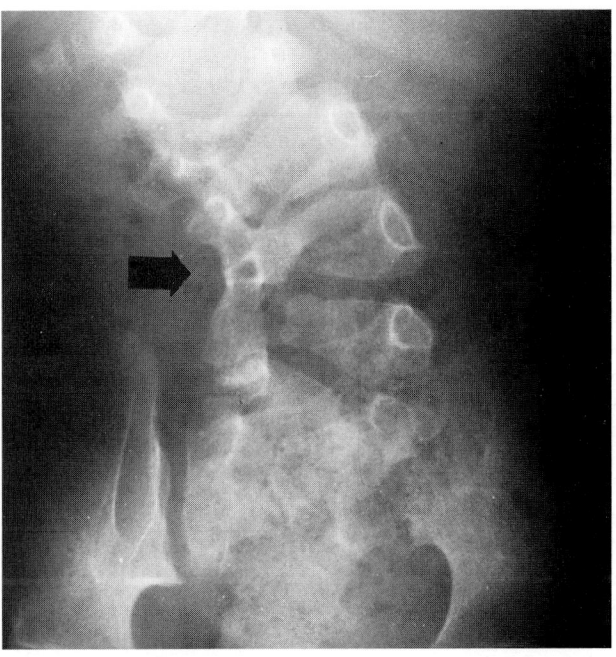

Fig. 2. Failure of segmentation. Left unilateral unsegmented bar at L3-5 produces right lumbar curve.

The diagnosis may be made during the evaluation of a radiograph taken for another reason such as a pulmonary problem. The physical examination will assess the entire musculoskeletal system and must include careful neurological evaluation and a search for abnormalities in other tissues or systems.

Imaging Studies

It is essential that high-quality radiographs of the entire spine in the frontal and sagittal projections be obtained as a baseline. These are routinely taken in the upright position. If the specific anomaly is not clear, an anteroposterior (AP) supine film may show much better bone detail. A chest radiograph in the newborn may afford the best assessment of the anomaly, but a unilateral bar may be cartilaginous and not seen until it ossifies. In older children, in whom it may be difficult to define the pathology, magnetic resonance imaging (MRI) or computed tomography (CT) scanning with three-dimensional reconstructions can be definitive.[12, 13] An ultrasound study of the urinary tract is always part of the initial work-up.

An MRI study is not necessary for every patient with congenital scoliosis, but it is indicated when (1) neurological deficit is present, (2) there is other evidence of intraspinal disorder, (3) there is rapid progression of the curve, and (4) surgical correction of the deformity is planned.

Radiographs at follow-up visits are necessary to document progression or lack thereof. It is not uncommon for physicians to disagree that real curve progression has occurred, because both inter- and intraobserver error in the radiographic measurement of congenital scoliosis is about 10 degrees.[14]

Management

The goals of management of congenital scoliosis are to stop the progression of increasing curves, maximize beneficial spinal growth, and obtain a balanced spine over a level pelvis. Management choices are observation, an orthosis, or an operation. When considering surgery at young ages, it must be remembered that a short and curved spine is better than a shorter and more curved one. This means that an early fusion may result in less deformity than ineffective nonsurgical management in an attempt to allow further growth of a deformed spine.[15]

Observation

Observation is appropriate for curves that are small (less than 30 degrees) and those that are nonprogressive, unless a stable curve is of severe magnitude or producing spinal imbalance. Evaluation should be repeated at intervals until skeletal maturity, because stable curves can increase in magnitude, especially during the adolescent growth spurt. Radiographic documentation is usually required at each visit.

Orthotics

Orthotic treatment will never control a progressing, structurally anomalous curve.[16] It is, therefore, appropriate only for flexible compensatory curves (either pre- or postoperatively) or to buy growth time in slowing the progression of a long flexible curve in which the anomalous segment is

the apex. With this latter situation, it may be necessary first to surgically stabilize the progressing defective area.

Surgery

The specifics of surgical treatment are beyond the scope of this chapter. Only principles and indications are presented. There are three types of procedures: those that stop progressive curves in situ, those that directly achieve some correction, and those that rely on future growth for some correction. Urgent surgery is needed for proven progressive curves, for those that are virtually certain to relentlessly increase regardless of the patient's age, and for those curves of severe magnitude or with major decompensation, even if these latter curves are not proven to be progressing. Awaiting further spinal growth in the face of a progressive congenital spinal deformity will only require a more complicated, riskier, less corrective procedure later.

In Situ Fusion. This is a prophylactic procedure that safely and effectively prevents the progression of small, short-segment curves.[17] Posterior in situ fusion is most commonly used to treat short unsegmented bars or hemivertebrae that have little anterior spinal growth potential. In spines with significant remaining anterior growth potential or more than one level of involvement, anterior and posterior in situ fusion should be performed. Otherwise, a posterior-only fusion may bend with time and plasticity. Unchecked anterior growth opposite a solid posterior fusion can result in relentless further rotation and curving, the so-called crankshaft phenomenon.[18] To prevent this, the addition of an anterior fusion should be considered in children younger than 10 years.

Convex Unilateral Anterior and Posterior Growth Arrest. This technique will stabilize a progressive curve and may enable continued growth from the concave side elements, thereby producing some correction.[19] It is best for the younger child with a small curve caused by a single or adjoining hemivertebra (Fig. 3). It is not appropriate if there is no concave growth potential.[20] The surgical approach may be through separate anterior and posterior incisions (with or without endoscopy) or via a posterior transpedicular approach.[21]

Hemivertebral Excision. This direct approach should produce substantial correction and a limited length of fusion.[22, 23] The major concern with this procedure is the risk of neurological injury either from direct trauma to the nerve roots or spinal cord or from vascular compromise. The procedure is particularly effective with lumbosacral hemivertebrae or curves at any level associated with large spinal imbalance.[24] The neurological risk is higher in the thoracic spine. Usually a short anterior and posterior fusion from the level above to the level below the excised segment will suffice. Short-segment posterior convex compression instrumentation adds stability.

Long Posterior Corrective Instrumentation and Fusion of the Entire Curve. This is appropriate for older children (more than 10 years) with flexible curves. It provides definitive treatment for the entire curve, not just the anomalous rigid segment; correction occurs in the nonstructural regions. Before correction, it is necessary to rule out intraspinal disease by obtaining an MRI. Intraoperative spinal cord monitoring is also suggested.

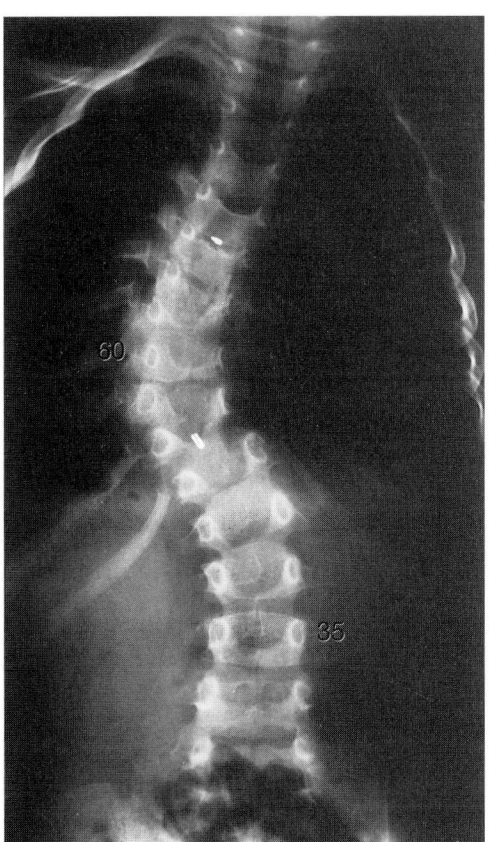

Fig. 3. Hemivertebrae causing small curve. In this view, two left low thoracic hemivertebrae result in a 60-degree left thoracic curve. The curve has been treated by a left anterior hemiepiphyseodesis and left posterior hemiarthrodesis.

Osteotomy or Vertebrectomy with Correction and Fusion. Large, rigid unbalanced curves can be corrected only by this complex, higher risk method. Much thought and planning and a thorough discussion of the neurological risk with the family are prerequisites. The anterior spine is approached and either osteotomies of a bar or a vertebrectomy is performed. Then, either staged or, more frequently, during the same anesthetic, osteotomies or excision of the posterior elements is accomplished, completely destabilizing the spine. Internal fixation compresses the convex side either anteriorly or posteriorly and shortens and translates the vertebral column while minimizing the risk to the spinal cord and nerve roots. Concave instrumentation is necessary to augment the fixation. This surgery should be performed only by very experienced spine surgeons.

Problems and Complications. These include death, paralysis, infection, instrumentation failure, failure of fusion, and syndrome of inappropriate antidiuretic hormone (SIADH), among many others. Mortality may occur from postoperative respiratory insufficiency resulting from severe thoracic deformity. Mechanical overdistraction of the spinal cord, vascular compromise of the cord, and direct impingement on the cord from translational instability may cause paraplegia, particularly with a concomitant intraspinal lesion. Preoperative MRI assessment, intraoperative spinal cord monitoring by evoked potentials, and gradual correc-

tion should help decrease the risk of neurological injury. Pseudarthrosis is avoided by rigid internal fixation and adequate bone grafting. Until more is known about allograft and bone graft substitutes in congenital spine deformities, autologous bone is probably the best choice for graft. It is wise to use a large volume of bone graft, because a large fusion mass is necessary to counteract the unbalanced forces of growth. To minimize the effects of SIADH, fluid loss should be replaced with blood or colloid, with limited crystalloid.

SACRAL AGENESIS

Sacral agenesis describes a rare spectrum of anomalous development of the caudal spine and neurological structures. The defect can range from unilateral hypoplasia of a portion of the sacrum to complete absence of the lower thoracic, lumbar, and sacral spine. Intercalary defects are rarely encountered. A useful classification system, based on the missing vertebral components and the spinopelvic articulation, has been developed (Figs. 4 to 7).[25] Associated anomalies can also be present in the more cephalad parts of the spine, most commonly congenital scoliosis. People with sacral agenesis usually have a motor nerve deficit similar in level to the skeletal defect or within one segment above or below. Sensory function is usually intact for several segments caudally.

The most important clinical significance of sacral agenesis is the loss of motor function. This parallels the absence

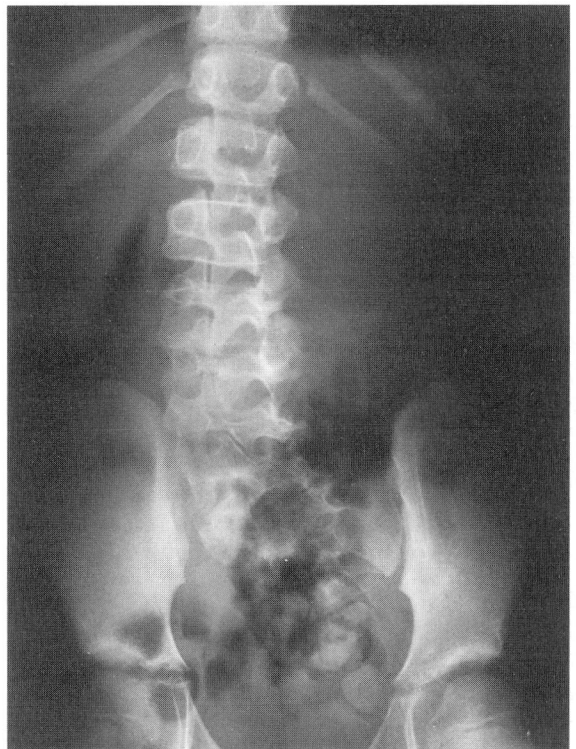

Fig. 4. Type I sacral agenesis. This is an anteroposterior radiograph showing absence of the right hemisacrum. (From Renshaw TS: Sacral agenesis: A classification and review of 23 cases. J Bone Joint Surg Am 1978; 60:373.)

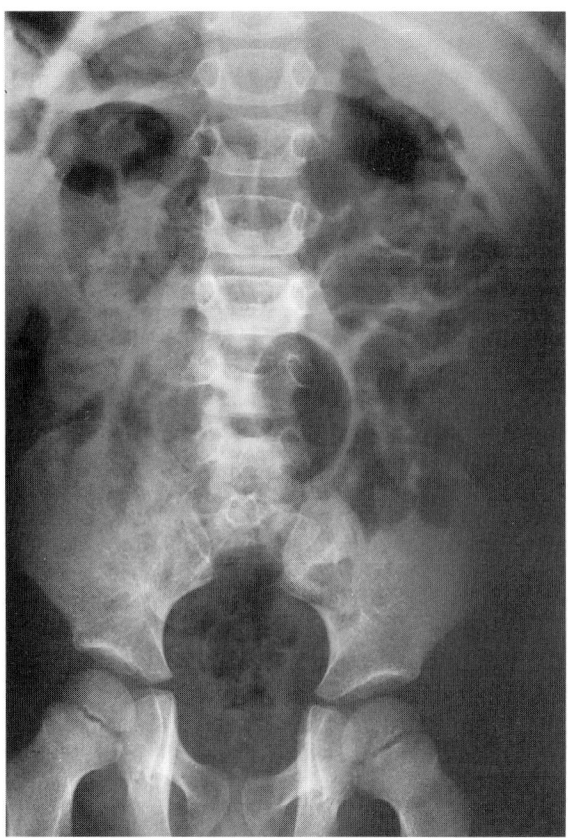

Fig. 5. Type II sacral agenesis. The sacrum is bilaterally absent caudal to a hypoplastic S1. (From Renshaw TS: Sacral agenesis: A classification and review of 23 cases. J Bone Joint Surg Am 1978; 60:373.)

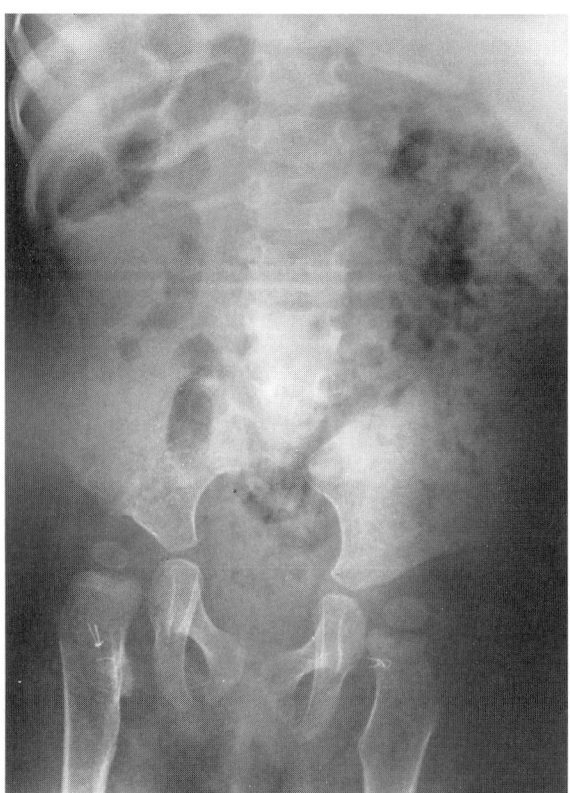

Fig. 6. Type III sacral agenesis. L4, L5, and the entire sacrum are absent. The ilia articulate with the sides of L3. (From Renshaw TS: Sacral agenesis: A classification and review of 23 cases. J Bone Joint Surg Am 1978; 60:373.)

of the spinal segments and ranges from minor weakness to completely functionless lower extremities. Regardless of the lumbar level, because the sacral neural elements are involved, bladder and bowel function is almost always affected.

Anomalies in other organ systems, especially the genitourinary tract, are common. Neurogenic bladder is present in all but the mildest cases, and unilateral renal agenesis and cryptorchidism are not infrequently encountered. Gastrointestinal tract anomalies also are common. Neurogenic bowel is the rule, and imperforate anus, rectovaginal fistula, and persistent cloacae also occur. Congenital cardiac malformations, myelomeningocele, and intraspinal neurological conditions must be ruled out. Studies such as ultrasonography, MRI, and CT imaging are helpful to define associated disease precisely.

PATHOGENESIS
Sacral agenesis occurs once in about 25,000 live births. The cause of the defect is not known, but in some instances it has been inherited.[26] An association with maternal diabetes has been reported in about 20% of cases.

CLINICAL FEATURES
The diagnosis is usually made at birth with radiographic confirmation of clinical findings. These findings vary depending on the severity of the defect and range from no

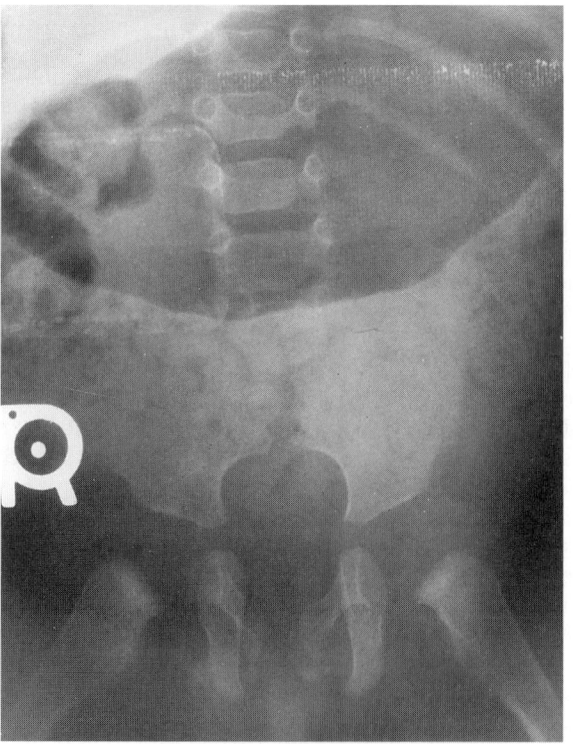

Fig. 7. Type IV sacral agenesis. L4, L5, and the entire sacrum are absent. L3 rests above an iliac amphiarthrosis. (From Renshaw TS: Sacral agenesis: A classification and review of 23 cases. J Bone Joint Surg Am 1978; 60:373.)

detectable deformity to severe deformation of the spine, pelvis, and lower extremities. Patients with sacral motor involvement only may only show urinary incontinence and dribbling. In contrast, the most severe "Buddha"-like involvement consists of a narrow, hypoplastic pelvis; marked atrophy of the buttocks with dimpling and a short intergluteal fold; tapered, hypoplastic lower extremities with hips flexed, abducted, and externally rotated; knee flexion contractures, often with popliteal pterygia; and foot deformities, usually either clubfeet or calcaneovalgus contractures. Severely affected individuals usually retain protective sensation in their feet.

INVESTIGATION

Plain radiographs usually suffice in defining the bony deficiencies and enable classification of the defective development. Supine radiographs show better detail than upright radiographs. Anomalies often occur in other systems and must be ruled in or ruled out.

MANAGEMENT
Neurological Deficit

This is a congenital absence problem and is not amenable to surgical improvement. Only if neurological deficit is progressive and shown to be caused by an associated, treatable intraspinal lesion is surgery likely to be of any benefit.

Spine

The entire spine must be assessed to rule out other problems, such as congenital scoliosis or kyphosis, that may require treatment. The major issue involves the method by which spinopelvic instability should be treated. Proponents of surgical stabilization for the unstable spinopelvic junction cite the need to free the upper limbs from trunk support, to protect internal organs from compression, to stabilize the spinopelvic junction so that hip and knee contractures can be corrected, and to prevent the development of a progressive rigid lumbopelvic kyphosis. Many cases of successful surgical fusion of the spine to the pelvis have been reported.[27]

The alternative to fusing an unstable spinopelvic junction is to leave it alone. Adults with such instability seldom actually have to use their arms to maintain adequate sitting balance. Reports of visceral compression are rare. Most patients with such severe involvement that they have spinopelvic instability do not have adequate lower extremity muscle power to functionally walk as adolescents and adults and will become wheelchair ambulators. In fact, in some cases, a mobile spinopelvic junction can help a young patient compensate for hip flexion contractures and thereby facilitate walking. It is recommended that spinopelvic fusion not be routinely performed, but that every patient's treatment be monitored and individualized.

Hips

Hip flexion contractures are almost inevitable in nonambulatory people with sacral agenesis, but they do not usually require treatment. Contractures are not common in those who walk. Whether subluxated and dislocated hips should be treated is dictated by the patient's actual or potential ambulatory status and whether the problem is bilateral or unilateral. Unilateral displacement in an ambulatory person should be treated to prevent painful mechanical arthritis and increased energy consumption during gait. Bilateral and perhaps even unilateral displacements in those who do not walk rarely benefit from treatment. Any pelvic osteotomy for acetabular dysplasia should be planned with utmost consideration of the status of spinopelvic stability and of the acetabular version.

Knees

Flexion contractures of considerable magnitude are probably best accepted, and the person will not have functional walking ability. The literature is rife with failed attempts at maintaining correction achieved by any means, including the latest gradual or sudden corrective methods. In some situations, bilateral knee disarticulation and prosthetic fitting will permit ambulation, especially if hip flexion contractures are not severe. However, in this situation, the walking is almost never continued into adulthood. If spinopelvic fusion is a possibility later on, the tibia and fibula from knee disarticulations should be frozen for use as autograft.

Feet

The presence of sensation in the feet of almost all people with sacral agenesis allows manipulation and casting and the safe use of orthoses. Clubfeet are extremely common in the more severe types, occurring in more than half of patients. Treatment by the standard methods of manipulation and casting or surgery is usually successful. Congenital vertical talus is often seen in the more involved cases and also responds well to surgical correction. Less commonly encountered deformities are calcaneovalgus and calcaneocavus. These, as well as congenital vertical talus, may not require treatment if the person is not able to walk.

RESULTS

Almost every child who has a stable spine, absence of contractures, and intact motor and sensory function below the hips will be able to walk if there are no severe associated anomalies.[28] Community ambulation is a rule when intact motor function extends to the fourth lumbar nerve root level. Even if the motor function in the lower extremities of a patient is limited, intact tactile sensation and proprioception allow standing or walking with orthotic support. Higher levels of motor involvement and knee disarticulation or a more proximal amputation level may be compatible with some degree of exercise ambulation in childhood, but usually not with functional ambulation as an adult.

NEUROMUSCULAR SCOLIOSIS

Scoliosis is common in children with neuromuscular disorders and differs from idiopathic scoliosis in several important aspects.[29] Besides neuromuscular involvement, scoliosis does the following:

- Develops earlier.
- Is less likely to be balanced by compensatory curves.
- Is more likely to be progressive.
- Will more likely progress throughout adulthood.
- Is much less responsive to orthotic treatment.

TABLE 1. THE PREVALENCE OF SCOLIOSIS IN VARIOUS NEUROMUSCULAR DISORDERS	
Disorders	**%**
Cerebral palsy	25
Myelomeningocele	60
Duchenne's muscular dystrophy	90
Spinal muscular atrophy (types I, II, III)	95
Infantile quadriplegia	100
Preadolescent quadriplegia	90
Friedreich's ataxia	95

- Is often accompanied by pelvic obliquity and lower extremity joint contractures.
- Will more often need surgery.[30]

Patients with comorbid factors, including a seizure disorder, hydrocephalus, malnutrition, gastroesophageal reflux, cardiac involvement, pulmonary problems, urinary tract dysfunction, and psychological issues, may have more perioperative problems and complications. Nevertheless, modern surgical techniques have made surgical correction and fusion of neuromuscular scoliosis a safe and effective means of preserving or improving quality of life. Each neuromuscular disease process is unique and requires an individualized approach to management.[31]

The most important priorities for a person with a neuromuscular disorder include communication, attending to

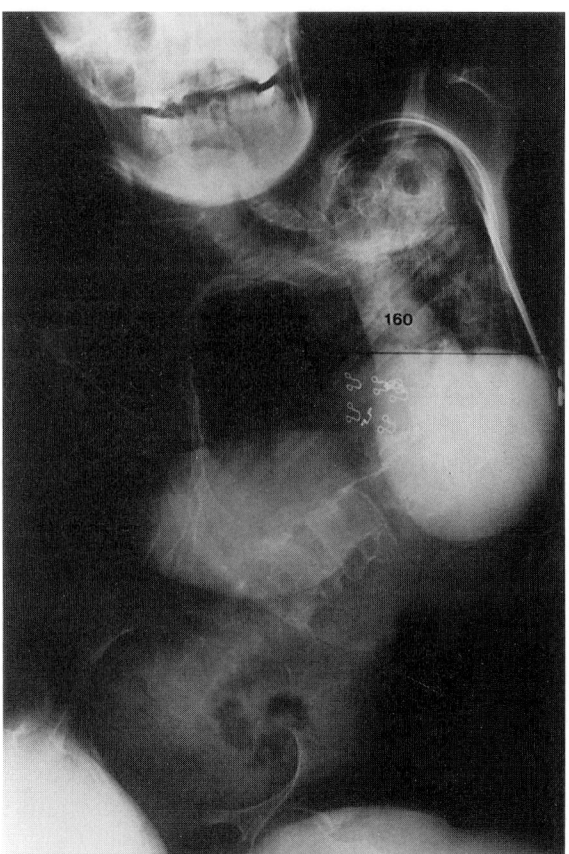

Fig. 9. Progression of untreated neuromuscular scoliosis. This view shows the same patient as in Figure 8 but 12 years later at age 29 years. She has had no treatment for her curve, which has progressed to 160 degrees.

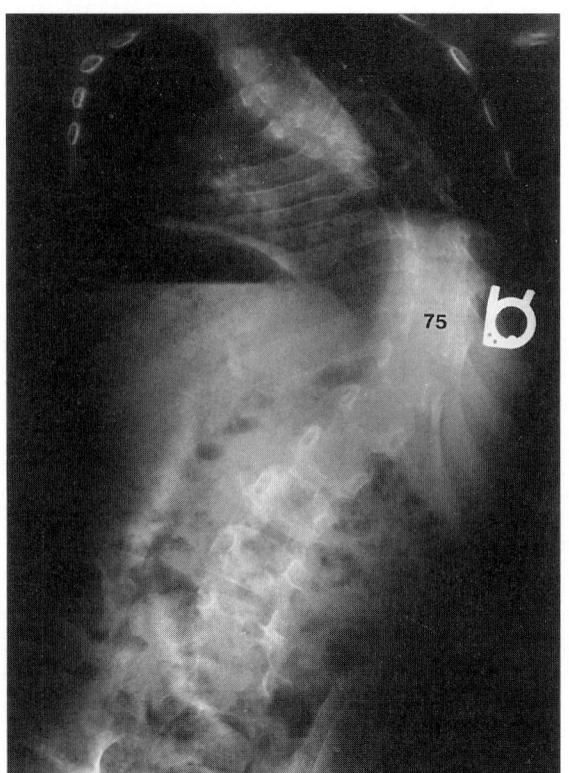

Fig. 8. Scoliosis in neuromuscular disorders. This view shows a 75-degree right thoracic curve in a 17-year-old girl with cerebral palsy.

one's own activities of daily living, achieving independent mobility in the environment, and walking. A balanced spine and a level pelvis are prerequisites for these critically important activities.

PATHOGENESIS

The prevalence of scoliosis in various neuromuscular disorders is listed in Table 1. Even though neuromuscular scoliosis is common, biomechanical causes and reasons for its progression are unknown. Trunk muscle weakness, muscle imbalance, osteopenia, pelvic obliquity, and central nervous system malfunction have all been hypothesized as having some causative role. More often than not, the natural history of untreated neuromuscular scoliosis is progression (Figs. 8 and 9). The onset and rate of progression vary with the condition, but progression throughout adulthood commonly occurs.

INVESTIGATION

The diagnosis is usually made by clinical examination of the back and confirmed by plain radiographs. Upright frontal and lateral plane studies are necessary to evaluate the scoliosis and sagittal alignment of the spine. For patients who cannot stand, sitting or supine radiographs may be necessary. Radiographs are used to confirm the diagnosis, determine curve magnitude, assess spinal balance, document progression, and plan and evaluate the results of surgical treatment. Other imaging studies may be needed to assess complex deformities and evaluate for associated pathological conditions.

In complex deformities, a CT scan with or without myelography or three-dimensional reconstruction will give excellent information. If intraspinal disease is suspected or other soft-tissue structures need to be evaluated, an MRI study is the imaging modality of choice. For surgical planning, supine maximum-bending AP radiographs or AP traction studies are often useful in selecting the fusion levels or deciding whether an anterior procedure will be needed to increase correctability.

MANAGEMENT

Regardless of the diagnosis, there are three options for managing neuromuscular scoliosis: observation, orthotic treatment, and surgical correction and fusion.

Observation

Observation is appropriate for those patients whose curves are small (less than 30 degrees) and do not require active treatment. It is also indicated for severely mentally handicapped patients in whom large spine deformity causes no discomfort or loss of function. It may be very difficult, however, to determine whether such patients have or are likely to have back pain from the severe deformity. A third indication is in the patient whose surgical risk precludes a procedure of the considerable magnitude of an extensive spinal fusion.

Orthotic Treatment

Orthotic treatment is more difficult in neuromuscular scoliosis. Reasons include poor muscle control, impaired sensation, pulmonary compromise, obesity, poor cooperation, and osteopenia of the ribs. In the majority of patients, regardless of the neuromuscular disease, orthotic treatment of scoliosis will not stop curve progression. It may, however, slow progression and allow for some beneficial growth of the spine in very young children until definitive fusion becomes unavoidable. In the occasional patient in whom orthotic treatment seems to have permanently halted curve progression, it is impossible to determine whether or not this represents the natural history of that individual's curve.

In young patients with very severe curves, it may be necessary to insert a corrective rod without performing a fusion and then provide external support for the rod with a custom-fitted orthosis. This allows for continued growth of the spine but requires periodic lengthening of the rod and a final definitive fusion procedure. Problems and complications are commonly seen with this treatment strategy.

Seating systems may be considered a form of orthotic treatment.[32] These are either custom-fabricated or commercially available modular equipment inserted into a wheelchair. The latter types are more adjustable for growth but usually do not support the spine as well. Seating systems are essential for those with compromised sitting balance. They begin with lateral pelvic support and a lap belt to hold the pelvis against the back of the chair. Lateral thoracic pads and a chest harness or thoracic vest support the trunk, and head supports and restraints may also be needed. In may be necessary to tilt the system back to enlist gravity into the support system. None of these wheelchair back modifications can be expected to prevent curve progression.

Surgery

Surgery is the definitive treatment for neuromuscular scoliosis. Its objectives are to stop curve progression, obtain safe correction, produce a solid arthrodesis of the curve, level an oblique pelvis, and balance the spine in the frontal and sagittal planes. This requires a long fusion, usually from the upper thoracic spine to the pelvis or occasionally to L5, with strong corrective internal fixation and a substantial mass of bone graft (Figs. 10 and 11).[33] Operative treatment should be considered when progressive curves reach 30 or 40 degrees or are substantially decompensated. One should not wait for skeletal maturity before considering a fusion. This may lead only to further progression of a rigid curve, so that correction will be less and the overall surgical risk may be higher. There is no absolute minimum age for spinal fusion surgery.[34]

Preoperative Considerations

All patients should have a general medical assessment, with particular attention to specific areas. The pulmonary evaluation may include respiratory function tests, if possi-

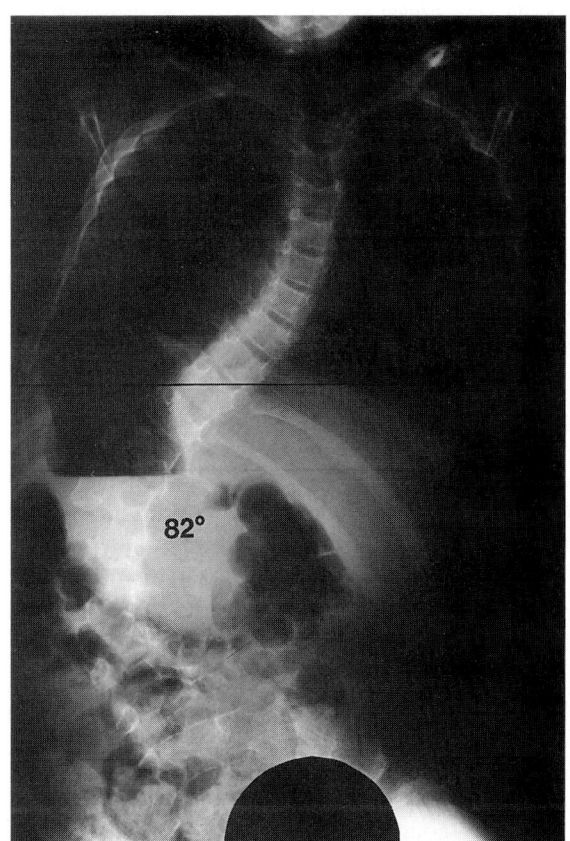

Fig. 10. Scoliosis in neuromuscular disorders. This view shows an 82-degree curve in a 14-year-old boy with cerebral palsy.

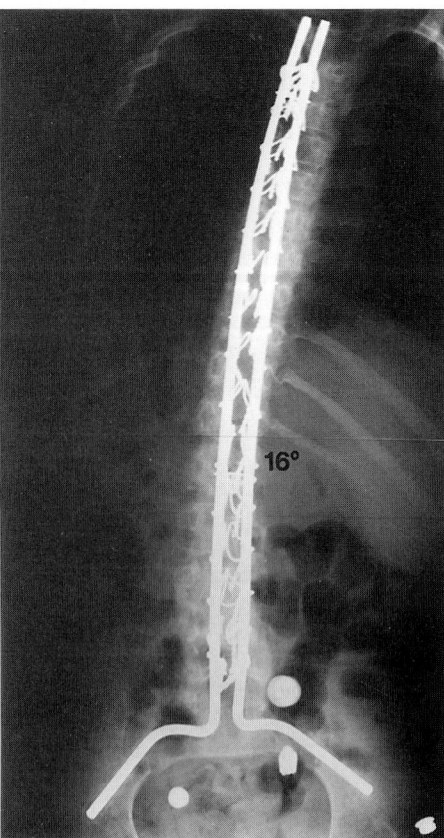

Fig. 11. Surgical management of neuromuscular scoliosis. This view shows the same patient as in Figure 10 1 year after corrective surgery. Note that the curve, which was very flexible, has been reduced to 16 degrees and the pelvic obliquity corrected.

ble, and blood gas analysis. Preoperative respiratory therapy may be beneficial. Cardiac involvement is common in many types of neuromuscular diseases and is usually asymptomatic. A chest radiograph and electrocardiogram comprise the initial evaluation studies. Coagulation studies are important to rule out coagulopathies. Of great importance is the assessment of the patient's nutritional state. Maximizing nutrition may take 6 weeks but will decrease the risks of postoperative infection, poor wound healing, and decubitus ulcers. Gastrointestinal problems such as gastroesophageal reflux and chronic constipation should be corrected before spinal surgery is performed. Neurological function should be documented, including intracranial pressure in those with hydrocephalus. If the patient is at risk for an allergy to latex, preoperative testing should be considered.

The patient's ambulatory status must be assessed. A marginal walker with a progressive disease may not walk postoperatively, and everyone must understand this before surgery. A posterior fusion with instrumentation is the most commonly performed procedure. Consideration should be given to a possible anterior release and fusion when necessary. Anterior surgery is indicated for enhancing correction in large rigid curves, in balancing severely decompensated spines,[35] to prevent the crankshaft phenomenon,[36]

and when posterior spinal elements are deficient or missing. Other preoperative considerations include the following:

- The type of segmental internal fixation.
- The means of achieving correction.
- The source and amount of the bone graft material.
- Techniques to minimize and replace blood loss.
- Thorough discussion of the indications, alternative treatment options, benefits, risks, complications, and problems associated with the procedure to secure informed consent; this discussion must be documented in the medical record.

Operative Considerations

Corrective spine surgery for neuromuscular scoliosis is a challenge for the surgeon and the anesthesiologist alike. Anesthesia issues include patient positioning, monitoring ventilatory status, depth of anesthesia, cardiac status, arterial blood pressure and gases, central venous pressure, core temperature, gastric status, urine output, coagulability, and blood loss.[13] Blood loss should be considered as percentage of blood volume, and both the suction collection and the weighed sponges should be totaled. Spinal cord monitoring of somatosensory and motor-evoked potentials is controversial in neuromuscular scoliosis,[37, 38] but may be valuable for patients who have functional lower extremities. Many patients will not be able to respond to the Stagnara wake-up test. Patients with myopathies are at increased risk for malignant hyperthermia, and halogenated agents may be contraindicated in these conditions.

Anterior surgery, if necessary, may be done either through an open incision or by endoscopic techniques. The anterior longitudinal ligament, annulus, and disk material are removed to mobilize the anterior column of the spine, and the vertebral end plates are exposed or removed and bone graft is applied to the disk spaces. Internal fixation may be used anteriorly and usually consists of rods attached to vertebral body screws.

Posterior fusion surgery involves clearing of the soft tissues from the posterior elements of the spine, including all ligaments and facet capsules that might interfere with the consolidation of the fusion mass. The corrective internal fixation is applied either before or after excision of the cartilage from the facet joints if one is performing a facet fusion. Finally, a large amount of local and homologous bone graft is applied to generate the fusion mass.

Postoperative Considerations

The patient's respiratory status is a major issue in the early postoperative period. As a rule of thumb, if the preoperative vital capacity was less that 50% of predicted, intubation and ventilatory assistance will be necessary for a few days. If the vital capacity was less than 30%, tracheostomy and ventilatory support may be needed for months or may even be permanent. An anterior thoracoabdominal approach may decrease vital capacity by about 25%.[39] During the postoperative period, it is essential that the patient receive continued monitoring of vital signs, cardiac status, hemodynamics, and fluid balance; assessment of hemoglobin and hematocrit and electrolytes if indicated; pain management;

antibiotic prophylaxis; positioning in bed with chest as vertical as possible; and any other specific needs. Once stabilized, the patient should be mobilized as soon as safety permits.

Complications

Problems and complications with spinal surgery range from death and paralysis to an asymptomatic pseudarthrosis that has no effect on the outcome.[40] Mortality in or after surgery may result from anesthetic problems, exsanguination, latex allergy, or, more commonly, postoperative pulmonary deterioration.

Paralysis could occur from spinal cord thrombosis or ischemia or a direct inadvertent traumatic event. Neurological complications are more likely when scoliotic curves exceed 90 degrees. Large kyphotic curves are at greatest risk, and methods to avoid lengthening the spine during correction should be considered. Although spinal cord monitoring techniques such as evoked potentials and the wake-up test detect injury after it has occurred, the more

rapid the detection and treatment, the better the chance for neurological recovery.

The development of a deep infection is always a risk. This is especially true in nutritionally compromised patients and those with more severe involvement with their diseases. It is very wise to assess the nutritional status of all patients at least 6 to 8 weeks preoperatively to detect and correct nutritional deficiencies. Myelomeningocele and cerebral palsy patients are particularly susceptible to infection.

Failure of instrumentation is usually a late finding, occurring as late as several years postoperatively. It most often signals a pseudarthrosis in the fusion mass. Supine radiographs provide the best bony detail, but still pseudarthroses often are not identified until rod fracture has occurred. Pseudarthroses are seen most often in people with myelomeningocele. A nonpainful pseudarthrosis with no loss of correction will not require treatment. However, if discomfort or significant loss of correction has occurred, reinstrumentation and repair of the fusion are necessary.

REFERENCES

1. Karlin LI: Congenital scoliosis. Spine 1998; 12:1.
2. McMaster MJ: Congenital scoliosis. In Weinstein SL (ed): The Pediatric Spine: Principles and Practice. New York, Raven Press, 1994, p 227.
3. Wynne-Davies R: Congenital vertebral anomalies: Etiology and relationship to spina bifida cystica. J Med Genet 1975; 12:280.
4. Renshaw TS: Congenital spinal deformity. In White AH (ed): Spine Care. St. Louis, MO, CV Mosby, 1995, p 1554.
5. McMaster MJ, Ohtsuka K: The natural history of congenital scoliosis: A study of two hundred and fifty-one patients. J Bone Joint Surg Am 1982; 64:1128.
6. Winter RB, Moe JH, Eilers VE: Congenital scoliosis: A study of 234 patients treated and untreated. I: Natural history and II: Treatment. J Bone Joint Surg Am 1968; 50:1.
7. Lonstein JE: Scoliosis. In Morrissy RT, Weinstein SL (eds): Lovell and Winter's Pediatric Orthopaedics. Philadelphia, Lippincott-Raven, 1996, 4th ed, p 625.
8. Beals RK, Robbins JR, Rolfe B: Anomalies associated with vertebral malformations. Spine 1993; 18:1329.
9. Drvaric DM, Ruderman RJ, Conrad RW, et al: Congenital scoliosis and urinary tract abnormalities: Are intravenous pyelograms necessary? J Pediatr Orthop 1987; 7:441.
10. McMaster MJ: Occult intraspinal anomalies and congenital scoliosis. J Bone Joint Surg Am 1984; 66:588.
11. Winter R, Lonstein J, Denis F, et al: Presence of spinal canal or cord abnormalities in idiopathic, congenital and neuromuscular scoliosis. Orthop Trans 1992; 16:135.
12. Barnes PD, Brody JD, Jaramillo D, et al: Atypical idiopathic scoliosis: MR imaging evaluation. Radiology 1993; 186:247.
13. Devlin VJ, Narvaez JC: Imaging strategies

for spinal deformities. Spine: State of the Art Rev 1998; 12:147.
14. Loder RT, Urquhart A, Steen H, et al: Variability in Cobb angle measurements in children with congenital scoliosis. J Bone Joint Surg Br 1995; 77:768.
15. Winter RB: Congenital scoliosis: Approach and treatment. Semin Spine Surg 1997; 9:80.
16. Winter RB, Moe JH, MacEwen GD, et al: The Milwaukee brace in the nonoperative treatment of congenital scoliosis. Spine 1976; 1:85.
17. Winter RB, Moe JH, Lonstein JE: Posterior spinal arthrodesis for congenital scoliosis: An analysis of the cases of two hundred ninety patients, five to nineteen years old. J Bone Joint Surg Am 1984; 66:1188.
18. Terek RM, Wehner J, Lubicky JP: Crankshaft phenomenon in congenital scoliosis: A preliminary report. J Pediatr Orthop 1991; 11:527.
19. Winter RB: Convex anterior and posterior hemiarthrodesis and hemiepiphyseodesis in young children with progressive congenital scoliosis. J Pediatr Orthop 1981; 1:361.
20. Winter RB, Lonstein JE, Denis F, et al: Convex growth arrest for progressive congenital scoliosis due to hemivertebrae. J Pediatr Orthop 1988; 8:633.
21. King AG, MacEwen GD, Bose WJ: Transpedicular convex anterior hemiepiphysiodesis and posterior arthrodesis for progressive congenital scoliosis. Spine 1992; 17:S291.
22. Bradford DS, Boachie-Adjei O: One-stage anterior and posterior hemivertebral resection and arthrodesis for congenital scoliosis. J Bone Joint Surg Am 1990; 72:536.
23. Callahan BE, Georgopoulos G, Eilert RE: Hemivertebral excision for congenital scoliosis. J Pediatr Orthop 1997; 17:96.
24. Holt DC, Winter RB, Lonstein JE, et al: Excision of hemivertebrae and wedge re-

section in the treatment of congenital scoliosis. J Bone Joint Surg Am 1995; 77:159.
25. Renshaw TS: Sacral agenesis: A classification and review of twenty-three cases. J Bone Joint Surg Am 1978; 60:373.
26. Phillips WA: Sacral agenesis. In Weinstein SL (ed): The Pediatric Spine: Principles and Practice. New York, Raven Press, 1994, p 259.
27. Winter RB: Congenital absence of the lumbar spine and sacrum: One-stage reconstruction with subsequent two-stage spine lengthening. J Pediatr Orthop 1991; 11:666.
28. Van Buskirk CS, Ritterbusch JF: Natural history of distal spinal agenesis. J Pediatr Orthop B 1997; 6:146.
29. Lonstein JE, Renshaw TS: Neuromuscular spine deformities. Instr Course Lect 1987; 36:285.
30. Renshaw TS, Drennan JC: Neuromuscular diseases. In Harris NH, Birch R (eds): Postgraduate Textbook of Clinical Orthopaedics. Oxford, England, Blackwell Science, 1995, p 49.
31. Dubowitz V: Muscle Disorders in Childhood. London, WB Saunders, 1995, 2nd ed.
32. Letts M, Rang M, Tredwell S: Seating the disabled. In The Atlas of Orthotics. St Louis, MO, CV Mosby, 1985, 2nd ed.
33. Broom MJ, Banta JV, Renshaw TS: Spinal fusion augmented by Luque rod segmental instrumentation for neuromuscular scoliosis. J Bone Joint Surg Am 1989; 71:32.
34. Dubousset J, Zeller RD: Therapeutic strategies in neuromuscular spinal deformities. Spine: State of the Art Rev 1998; 12:12.
35. Pascal-Moussellare H, Schwab FJ, Farcy J-PC: Fixed pelvic obliquity: A treatment approach. Spine: State of the Art Rev 1998; 12:41.
36. Dubousset J, Herring JA, Shufflebarger H:

The crankshaft phenomenon. J Pediatr Orthop 1989; 9:541.

37. Ashkenaze D, Mudiyam R, Boachie-Adjei O, et al: Efficacy of spinal cord monitoring in neuromuscular scoliosis. Spine 1993; 18:1627.

38. Schwartz DM, Drummond DS, Ecker ML, Neurophysiological monitoring during scoliosis surgery: A multimodality approach. Semin Spine Surg 1997; 9:97.

39. Gaudiche O, Dubousset AM, Pouliquen M: Anesthesiology for patients with neuromuscular diseases requiring spinal fusion surgery. Spine: State of the Art Rev 1998; 12:177.

40. Drummond DS, Ferguson RL, Banta JV: Advances in the treatment for neuromuscular scoliosis. Semin Spine Surg 1997; 9: 181.

section 9 chapter 13 CERVICAL: KLIPPEL-FEIL, TORTICOLLIS

Peter D. Pizzutillo

Summary
- Klippel-Feil syndrome (KFS) is clinically important because of its many associated conditions.
- KFS must be monitored to detect neurological impairment.
- Torticollis is most common in the newborn and resolves with stretching.
- Late-onset torticollis may be first sign of intraspinal tumor.

KFS was first described by Klippel and Feil in 1912 in a young man who appeared to have no neck and who died of nephritis. Autopsy revealed apparent massive fusion of all cervical vertebrae. Since that time, the term Klippel-Feil syndrome has been applied to individuals who may demonstrate nothing more than isolated congenital fusion of two cervical vertebrae. KFS is sporadic in nature, and only those with single-level fusions have been associated with a positive family history of similar cervical fusions. The incidence appears to be less than 1% of the population.

Although infants with KFS usually appear to be normal, they may present with torticollis. Congenital cervical anomalies that appear as torticollis must be distinguished from the more common congenital muscular torticollis in which the cervical spine is normal.

PATHOGENESIS

Hereditary transmission of KFS is rare and has only been reported in individuals with single-level cervical fusion. The majority occur sporadically. Embryologically, a failure of segmentation occurs when the cervical spinal column is still in its cartilage stage of development. No specific inciting cause has yet been discovered, but experimental research with early exposure to teratogens or to maternal hypotension in animal models has produced changes that mirror KFS. Early insult to the developing fetus is supported by the concomitant host of associated congenital anomalies.

Congenital muscular torticollis is thought to be the result of compartment syndrome involving the sternocleidomastoid compartment as a result of in utero head and neck position.

CLINICAL FEATURES

Patients with KFS may present for specific evaluation of neck cosmesis, or more commonly the cervical anomalies are detected incidentally in the work-up of other associated problems. The majority of individuals with KFS appear to be normal without the "classic triad" of short neck, low posterior hairline, and limited neck motion. Although most affected individuals will demonstrate normal flexion-extension and lateral rotation of the cervical spine, they will exhibit significant decrease in lateral side bending of the neck. Neurological examination is normal except in those with coexisting anencephaly or upper cervical intersegmental instability.

Additional evaluation will reveal other conditions such as scoliosis (60%), Sprengel's deformity (20%), renal anomalies (30%), hearing impairment (35%), synkinesis or mirror motions of the hands (15%), anomalies of the thumb and thenar eminence (26%), and cardiac anomalies (20%) (Table 1).

INVESTIGATION

Radiographs of the cervical spine should include lateral flexion-extension views, which will detect instability and more clearly delineate congenital segments in the young patient with little ossification of the cervical elements. The most common pattern of cervical involvement is fusion of C2-3, which is also most commonly associated with the development of neurological impairment. When occipitalization of C-1 coexists with congenital fusion of C2-3, the majority of individuals will progressively experience instability at C1-2.

Standing posteroanterior and lateral radiographs of the thoracic and lumbar spine will document the existence and magnitude of scoliosis and congenital anomalies. In addition, when Sprengel's deformity is present, these studies will document the position and orientation of the scapula and the existence of an omovertebral connection. When radiographs of the spine show widening of the interpedicular distance, magnetic resonance imaging (MRI) evaluation of the spinal cord will rule out the coexistence of diastematomyelia or syrinx.

TABLE 1. CONDITIONS ASSOCIATED WITH KLIPPEL-FEIL SYNDROME	
Associated Conditions	**Percentage**
Scoliosis	60
Hearing deficits	35
Renal anomalies	30
Hand anomalies	26
Sprengel's deformity	20
Cardiac anomalies	20
Synkinesis	15

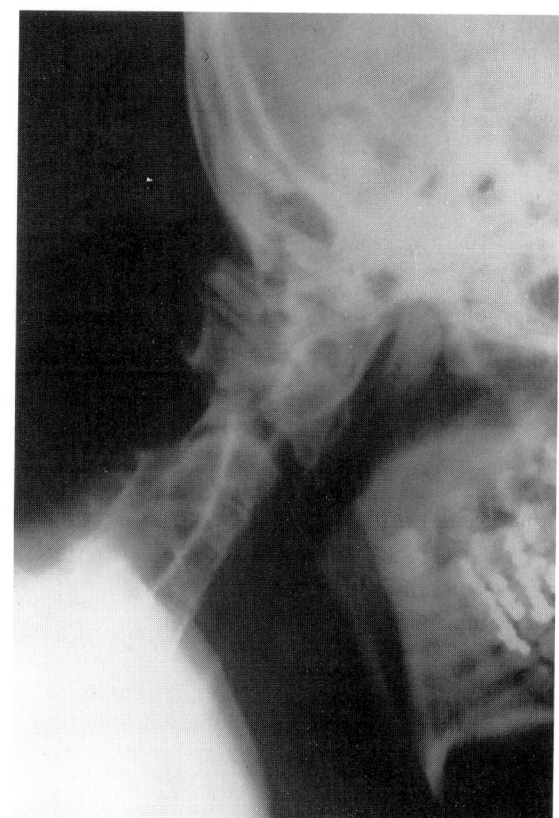

Fig. 1. Radiograph of Klippel-Feil syndrome.

Renal ultrasonography is performed to rule out renal anomalies, the most common of which is complete absence of one renal system. Other findings include ectopic kidney, horseshoe kidney, pelvic kidney, and hydronephrosis, which may be clinically silent.

Audiometry is routinely recommended in this population to detect the presence of hearing impairment, which may be conductive or sensorineural in nature. Early detection may avoid later problems in education and socialization.

When an infant presents with torticollis, radiographs of the cervical spine are needed to rule out the presence of congenital anomalies. Radiographs of the hips and pelvis are also recommended to rule out hip dysplasia, which may be clinically undetectable. Hip dysplasia occurs in 20% of infants with congenital muscular torticollis. In addition, ophthalmological evaluation may be indicated in those in whom visual disturbances are suspected as the cause of torticollis.

DIFFERENTIAL DIAGNOSIS

Radiographs of the cervical spine, including lateral flexion-extension views, are usually sufficient to confirm or rule out the presence of KFS or lesions of the cervical spinal column. In infants and children who have a high cartilage-bone ratio of the spinal column and in those with torticollis in whom neutral radiographs of the cervical spine may be difficult to obtain, other studies are indicated (Fig. 1).

Computed tomography (CT) scan and MRI are helpful in delineating confusing cervical anatomy, especially of the upper cervical spine and the occipitocervical junction. These studies may demonstrate "congenital scoliosis" of the cervical spine with hemivertebra, wedged vertebra, and miscellaneous changes that differ from the failure of segmentation seen in KFS. Congenital anomalies of the occipital condyles or of the lateral mass of C-1 are revealed and will influence decision making in treatment.

When torticollis is detected in the older child and is intermittent or fixed, MRI of the brainstem and cervical cord are indicated to rule out lesions such as syrinx or astrocytoma. When these studies are normal, CT scan is helpful in demonstrating the presence of rotary subluxation of C-1 and C-2, which frequently accompanies upper respiratory tract infection and posterior pharyngitis.

Occasionally, radiographs, CT scan, and MRI will not be able to identify instability problems clearly. When clinically suspected, cineradiography of the cervical spine will not only define pathological anatomy but also will demonstrate instability, which may be difficult to determine at the upper cervical spine or at the occipitocervical junction.

MANAGEMENT

Although the majority of patients with the KFS remain healthy and neurologically intact, there is sufficient concern regarding cervical instability and degenerative spine changes that serial follow-up is recommended. In childhood, asymptomatic patients may be clinically examined annually and be evaluated radiographically every 3 years as long as radiographic stability of the spine is documented. When hypermobility exists at the occipitocervical or upper cervical spine, there is a higher risk of neurological problems. These patients must be monitored closely and counseled against involvement in high-impact loading activities, such as football, wrestling, ice hockey, rugby and high diving, which may endanger the neck. When congenital fusion involves the cervical spine below C-2, degenerative disk changes and arthritis may develop with aging, but neurological problems are uncommon. These individuals may participate in most activities. Symptomatic treatment of pain resulting from degeneration may be needed, but surgical intervention has primarily been reserved to stabilize the cervical spine when instability has been documented.

The majority of KFS patients with scoliosis will require surgical intervention for progressive scoliosis. Those with Sprengel's deformity may require surgical intervention when severe limitation of shoulder motion exists.

Infants with torticollis from congenital anomalies of the cervical spine may obtain relief of their deformity by the application of customized orthoses or may require surgical realignment and stabilization later. Infants with torticollis and normal cervical spine are successfully treated by gentle stretching of the neck musculature. Only few individuals with congenital muscular torticollis will require surgical intervention.

Torticollis that develops in the older child secondary to rotary subluxation of C-1 and C-2 is successfully resolved with traction and bracing within 4 weeks of symptoms. When children present with fixed subluxation of C-1 and C-2, traction is usually successful in reducing the subluxation, but posterior C1-2 fusion is necessary to maintain the reduction. Open reduction of fixed rotary subluxation of C-1 and C-2 is dangerous and is not indicated. Acceptable cosmetic results in these patients may be obtained by posterior fusion from occiput to C-2 with maintenance of good alignment in a halo vest or cast.

The child with torticollis in whom an intraspinal lesion is detected requires immediate referral to a neurosurgeon.

COMPLICATIONS

Patients with KFS may experience complications when associated anomalies remain undiagnosed involving the cardiovascular system, renal system, and hearing deficits. Early detection is critical for good clinical results. In addition, problems of the spine such as undetected progressive scoliosis and occult low-grade instability of the cervical spine create their own problelms. The most serious of these is the development of myelopathy or the occurrence of a catastrophic neurological event in the unsuspecting patient.

Patients with congenital muscular torticollis may demonstrate persistent torticollis with marked limitation of cervical spine motion and progressive deformity of the facial bones and skull that eventually become irreversible. Reluctance to formally evaluate the hips may result in progressive hip dysplasia that will become symptomatic in the early years of the second decade. The profound dysplasia will then require complicated surgical interventions that may not be able to restore normal anatomy and stability.

RESULTS

The majority of individuals with KFS lead a normal life.

<table>
<tr><td>section
9
chapter
14</td><td># KYPHOSIS</td></tr>
</table>

Laurel C. Blakemore and George H. Thompson

Summary
- Kyphotic deformity in children and adolescents may be due to a variety of causes; postural kyphosis and Scheuermann's disease are the most common.
- Scheuermann's disease can be successfully managed by nonoperative means in skeletally immature children, but there are indications for surgical intervention.
- Congenital kyphosis, like congenital scoliosis, can cause severe deformity at an early age and, when progressive, is treated surgically.
- Kyphosis resulting from myelodysplasia is a challenging surgical problem, and treatment is associated with significant complications.
- Other causes of kyphosis in the pediatric population include infections such as tuberculosis, especially in developing countries, and iatrogenic causes.

Kyphotic deformities are characterized by an increased dorsal curvature in the sagittal plane of spinal alignment (Table 1). Postural round back and Scheuermann's disease are the most common causes of kyphosis. Other common causes include lumbar Scheuermann's disease, congenital kyphosis, myelodysplasia, and infectious and iatrogenic disorders.

The accepted range of normal thoracic kyphosis for a child or adolescent is 20 degrees to 40 degrees.[1] In the lumbar spine or thoracolumbar junction, any degree of kyphosis is considered abnormal. The mean thoracic kyphosis measurements in children younger than 10 years are 21 degrees and 24 degrees for males and females, respectively, increasing to 25 degrees and 26 degrees in adolescence.

POSTURAL ROUND BACK

Postural round back is the term used to describe an adolescent kyphotic deformity that can be voluntarily corrected both in the standing and prone positions. On forward bending, the kyphosis of postural round back is a smooth accentuation of normal kyphosis without abrupt angulation. Radiographs show a mild kyphosis without vertebral body wedging, disk space narrowing, or end-plate abnormalities. Schmorl's nodes are not typically seen. Postural round back may be improved with an exercise program emphasizing thoracic extension, although compliance may be diffi-

TABLE 1. CONDITIONS CAUSING KYPHOSIS

Postural kyphosis	Skeletal dysplasias
Scheuermann's disease	Achondroplasia
Lumbar Scheuermann's disease	Spondyloepiphyseal dysplasia
Congenital kyphosis	congenita
Neuromuscular disorders	Mucopolysaccharidosis
Myelodysplasia	Collagen disorders
Cerebral palsy	Marfan's syndrome
Rett's syndrome	Marie-Strümpell disease
Iatrogenic	Neurofibromatosis
Postlaminectomy	Metabolic disorders
Postirradiation	Juvenile osteoporosis
Incorrect fusion levels	Cystic fibrosis
Pseudarthrosis	Neoplastic
Infectious	Nutritional deficiencies
Tuberculosis	Vitamin A deficiency
Poliomyelitis	Nontropical sprue
Other bacterial/fungal infections	
Posttraumatic	
Fracture	
Spinal cord injury	

cult to achieve. This is a nonprogressive disorder, and orthotic management is rarely indicated.

Juvenile kyphosis was first distinguished from postural round back in 1920, when Holger Scheuermann[2] described the clinical and radiographic findings of a fixed dorsal kyphosis associated with end plate irregularities and anterior vertebral body wedging. In 1964 Sorensen[3] modified Scheuermann's definition of the radiographic findings, proposing that the wedging should involve three adjacent vertebrae and be at least 5 degrees in magnitude. Schmorl described disk protrusions through the end plate of the vertebrae, and suggested that this phenomenon was instrumental in producing the kyphosis seen in Scheuermann's disease.[4] However, Schmorl's nodes are also seen in areas of the spine not involved in the kyphotic deformity as well as in individuals with no evidence of Scheuermann's disease. Consequently, this theory has never gained wide acceptance. Most now consider the major radiographic criteria of Scheuermann's disease to include (1) kyphosis greater than 40 degrees, (2) wedging of one or more apical vertebrae of at least 5 degrees, (3) irregular vertebral end plates, and (4) narrowing of the intervertebral disk spaces in the kyphotic region.[5]

PREVALENCE

Estimates of the prevalence rate of Scheuermann's disease vary from 0.5% to 8% of the population.[3] Some authors described a higher prevalence rate in males or females, but generally there is not a clear gender predilection.[4, 6, 7] Radiographic findings of Scheuermann's disease are not seen before the onset of puberty, so the true age of onset of the disease is difficult to establish. Adolescent females typically demonstrate radiographic evidence at a younger age than do males, corresponding to their earlier onset of puberty.

PATHOGENESIS

In his initial description, Scheuermann postulated that the kyphosis was caused by avascular necrosis of the anterior

vertebral ring apophysis, leading to asymmetric growth and wedging of the vertebra. Later studies indicated that ring apophysis does not contribute to longitudinal growth of the spine and that ring apophysis was normal histologically. The matrix of the vertebral end plate in Scheuermann's disease demonstrates a lower collagen-proteoglycan ratio than normal, which may lead to abnormal end plate ossification and longitudinal growth.[1] Scoles et al[8] reported on histological alterations in biopsy specimens from two patients surgically treated for Scheuermann's disease. The disorganized enchondral ossification seen was virtually identical to the epiphyseal changes seen in tibia vara, or Blount disease, and slipped capital femoral epiphysis. They also reported anterior extension of the thoracic vertebral bodies in 94% of cadaver specimens meeting the radiographic criteria for Scheuermann's disease, postulating that this was analogous to the medial metaphyseal "beak" seen in Blount disease. This supports the hypothesis that Scheuermann's disease results from increased pressure on the anterior aspect of the vertebral body. The positive role of bracing in Scheuermann's disease also implicates a mechanical cause.

Bradford et al[9] postulated that early transient osteoporosis may be a causative factor and may precede radiographic changes. However, other studies using quantitative computed tomography failed to demonstrate osteoporosis.[10] There is a hereditary tendency, but an exact mode of genetic transmission has not been established. Other factors such as dietary deficiency and endocrine abnormalities have been found in association with Scheuermann's disease, but their role in the cause is unclear.[5]

CLINICAL CHARACTERISTICS

Scheuermann's disease presents in late childhood or early adolescence as a kyphotic deformity of the thoracic or thoracolumbar spine. Typically, the child's family or teacher has prompted the consultation because of his or her appearance. Pain is common, particularly in curves involving the thoracolumbar region, and is localized over the apex of the deformity. In fact, Scheuermann's disease is the most frequent cause of thoracic back pain in adolescents. Lumbar pain may be concurrent in the presence of marked compensatory lumbar lordosis.[10] Pain may be aggravated by standing, sitting, or physical activity and may subside at skeletal maturity, although the natural history of Scheuermann's disease includes back pain at a higher intensity than that seen in the general population.[7, 10] A family history of similar deformity may be present.

The kyphotic deformity is best visualized by observing the patient from the side in a forward-bend position (Fig. 1). The kyphosis is typically well circumscribed, with an apex in the mid- to lower thoracic region. The cervical and lumbar spine demonstrates varying degrees of compensatory lordosis, and the shoulder girdles tend to rotate anteriorly. In distinction from postural round back, the deformity in Scheuermann's disease does not completely correct on prone or standing hyperextension. Associated scoliosis is seen in approximately 30% of patients and is usually of mild to moderate severity. Many patients demonstrate associated tightness of the pectoral muscles, hip flexors, and hamstrings. Neurological abnormalities are rare and may indicate an associated extradural cyst or thoracic disk her-

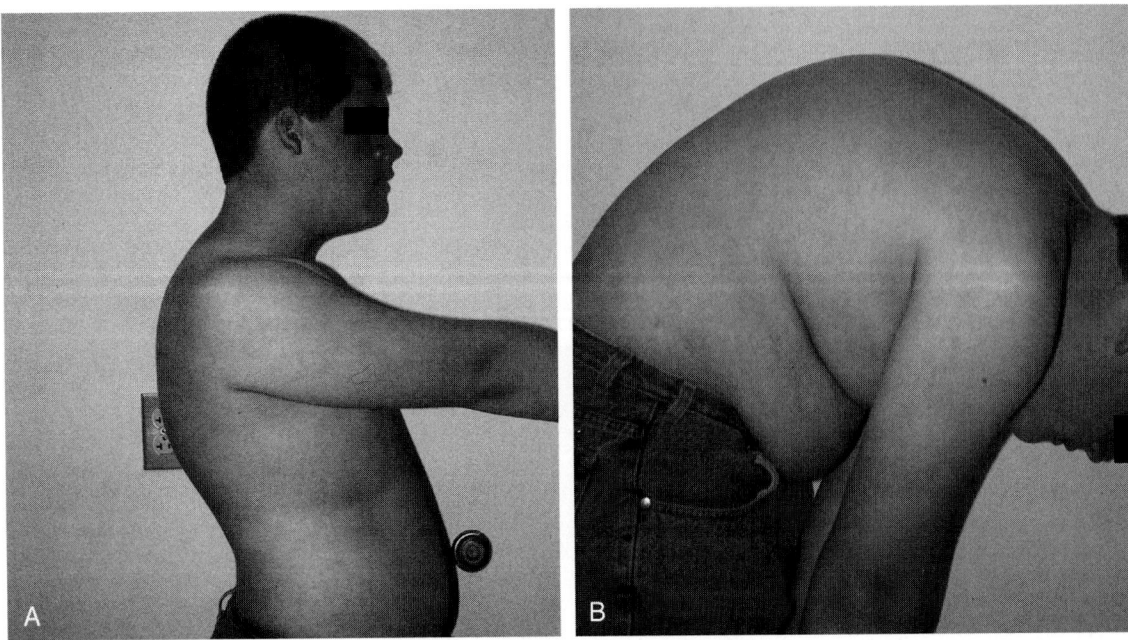

Fig. 1. Scheuermann's kyphosis. *A,* Observe the compensatory hyperlordosis in the cervical and lumbar spine of this 15-year-old boy. *B,* On forward bending, there is sharply angulated kyphotic deformity in the thoracic spine. Note reversal of the lumbar lordosis.

niation. Acute spinal cord compression at the apex of the kyphosis has also been reported in Scheuermann's disease, and the associated deformity is not always severe.[1, 11]

RADIOGRAPHIC ASSESSMENT

When evaluating a kyphotic deformity, standing posteroanterior (PA) and lateral radiographs of the entire spine should be obtained on long cassettes. An extension lateral radiograph over a radiolucent wedge is useful to assess the flexibility of the deformity.[6] The Cobb technique is used to measure the kyphosis between the superior end plate of the upper vertebral body and inferior end plate of the lower vertebral body most tilted into the kyphotic deformity. Angles of greater than 45 degrees are considered abnormal. Wedging is assessed by measuring the angle formed by the end plates of individual vertebral bodies (Fig. 2). Other radiographic findings include anterior detachment of the ring apophyses, anterior extensions of the vertebral bodies, and Schmorl's nodes (see Fig. 2). Associated scoliosis, spondylolysis, and spondylolisthesis are relatively common and should also be addressed.[6, 7]

DIFFERENTIAL DIAGNOSIS

Scheuermann's disease is often mistaken for postural round back, which is characterized by a smoother, more flexible kyphosis without the radiographic findings seen in Scheuermann's disease. Other causes of kyphotic deformity, such as congenital kyphosis resulting from an anterior failure of segmentation, can occasionally be difficult to distinguish from Scheuermann's disease.

TREATMENT

Treatment for Scheuermann's disease is based on the severity of the deformity, patient age, and presence of associated symptoms.

Observation

For deformities measuring less than 50 degrees in skeletally immature adolescents, observation is appropriate. If pain is present and other causes such as spondylolysis or disk herniation have been ruled out, nonsteroidal medications and physical therapy may be useful for short-term pain relief.

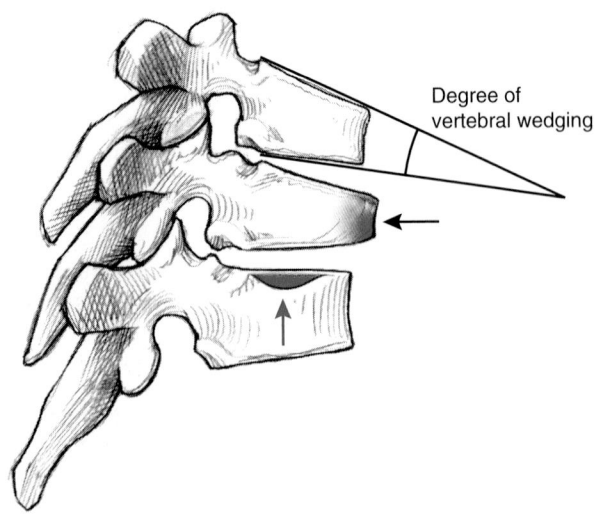

Degree of vertebral wedging

Fig. 2. Vertebral body wedging. The degree of vertebral body wedging is assessed by measuring the angle formed by the end plates of an individual vertebra. Schmorl's nodes *(lower arrow)* may be seen in the kyphotic section and anterior vertebral body extensions *(upper arrow)* in the area of the ring apophysis.

Exercises

Although exercise has not been proved to decrease kyphotic deformity in Scheuermann's disease, it may help relieve pain, decrease lumbar lordosis, and prevent progression. Thoracic extension and abdominal strengthening as well as hamstring stretching exercises added to an aerobic exercise program will usually improve symptoms.

Orthotic Treatment

The indications for orthotic treatment include progressive deformity in a skeletally immature adolescent or painful deformity, typically measuring 65 degrees or greater. Sachs et al,[12] in their report on the long-term results of Milwaukee brace treatment, included 45 degrees as the lower threshold for orthotic treatment. Most institutions use a low-profile Milwaukee brace, a cervical-thoracic-lumbar spinal orthosis with padded posterior uprights, which apply pressure over the apex of the deformity and act as a fulcrum for the three-point bending effect exerted by the brace. A standing lateral radiograph in the orthosis is obtained at fitting and at 4- to 6-month intervals thereafter. Physical therapy is initiated to reduce hamstring tightness and improve lumbar lordosis. In rigid curves, application of one or more Risser hyperextension casts can be beneficial to gain mobility before bracing. Partial reversal of vertebral body wedging is often seen after 12 to 18 months of full-time bracing.[10] Montgomery and Erwin[13] reported an average of 21 degrees of correction in 39 patients who completed a mean of 18 months of orthotic treatment. Those monitored more than 18 months showed an average loss of correction of 15 degrees. They recommended at least 18 months of full-time brace wear and indicated that correction of wedging to less than 5 degrees correlated with maintenance of correction. Sachs et al[12] monitored 120 patients for at least 5 years after brace treatment, which consisted of full-time wear for a mean of 14 months followed by a mean of 18 months of part-time wear. Their results showed that 69% maintained some correction and 22% had no improvement. An initial kyphosis of greater than 74 degrees was associated with progression of deformity. Most authors recommend continuing part-time brace wear until skeletal maturity is reached. Bradford et al[14] reported partial correction in skeletally mature patients as well.

Surgical Treatment

Murray et al[7] reported on the natural history of Scheuermann's disease in 67 patients with a mean kyphosis of 71 degrees who were monitored for a mean of 32 years. Although patients with Scheuermann's disease rated their back pain as more intense and differently localized than age-matched controls, they did not report increased use of medication for back pain or interference with their work or recreational activities. They also reported no increase in self-consciousness or preoccupation with their physical appearance. Restrictive lung disease was seen only when the kyphotic deformity exceeded 100 degrees. On the basis of these findings, the authors called for a review of the indications for operative treatment.

Most authors concur that operative indications for patients with Scheuermann's disease include the presence of a kyphotic deformity of 75 degrees or more that has not responded to bracing.[1, 10, 15] Disabling refractory back pain associated with a curve of at least 60 degrees in a skeletally mature patient may also be an indication for surgery. Neurological compromise secondary to the kyphotic deformity is an indication for surgical decompression. The goals of surgery are to halt progression, relieve symptoms, improve the deformity, and obtain a solid arthrodesis. Currently, a combined anterior and posterior spinal fusion is advocated, using posterior segmental spinal instrumentation.[16] Anterior release and arthrodesis enhance maximum safe correction and improve fusion rates. Most surgeons perform both the anterior and posterior procedures on the same day, although they may be staged a week apart. The anterior procedure can be performed either open, taking the rib corresponding to the most cephalad level to be fused, or thorascopically. Fusion can be performed using morselized or structural rib graft. The posterior instrumentation must include the entire deformity and, depending on the location of the apex, the upper lumbar spine to prevent junctional thoracolumbar kyphosis postoperatively. Postoperative immobilization is not generally required. Correction should not exceed 50% of the deformity or reduce the kyphosis to less than 40 degrees, because overcorrection can lead to junctional thoracolumbar kyphosis or worsened sagittal balance (Fig. 3).[1] Posterior instrumentation alone only provides stability on the tension side of the kyphotic deformity and is associated with a higher rate of pseudarthrosis. Lowe[10] postulated that posterior instrumentation alone may have a role in flexible curves that correct to 50 degrees or less on hyperextension. However, this is not the current recommendation for operative intervention. More recently, Ferreira-Alves et al[17] performed posterior-only instrumentation and fusion on 38 patients using a dynamic dual-rod technique followed by 9 months of postoperative immobilization in a hyperextension plaster jacket. Mean kyphosis was corrected from 68 degrees to 43 degrees at 5-year follow-up, with only one case of pseudarthrosis. The mean loss of correction was only 4 degrees. Their results question the need for anterior diskectomy and fusion with every case.

COMPLICATIONS

Many authors reported major complications associated with operative treatment for Scheuermann's disease.[10, 15, 17] Perioperative complications have included death, spinal cord injury, vertebral fracture, pulmonary embolus, wound hematoma, wound infection, pulmonary embolus, pericardial effusion, pneumothorax, and gastrointestinal obstruction. Delayed complications included pseudarthrosis, hardware failure, loss of correction, persistent pain, and worsened pulmonary function.

LUMBAR SCHEUERMANN'S DISEASE

Patients presenting with low back pain may demonstrate findings consistent with lumbar Scheuermann's disease. In the lumbar spine, radiographs demonstrate end plate irregularities, disk space narrowing, and Schmorl's nodes but no noticeable deformity or wedging of adjacent vertebrae. These adolescents tend to be athletic and often present with pain or scoliosis. Lumbar Scheuermann's disease is not

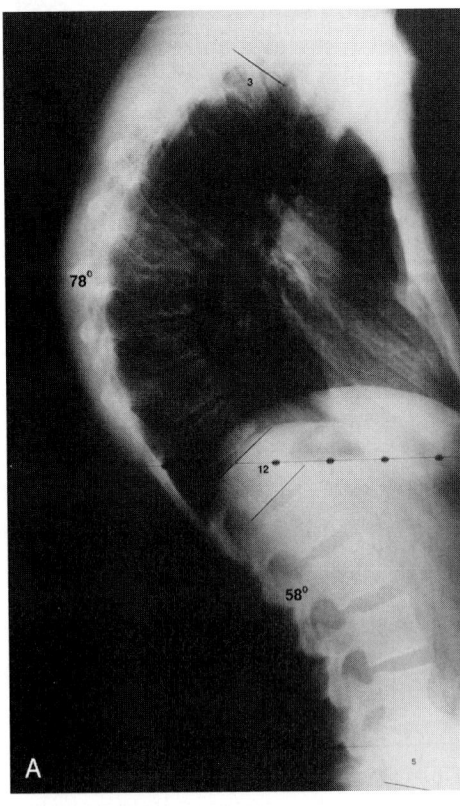
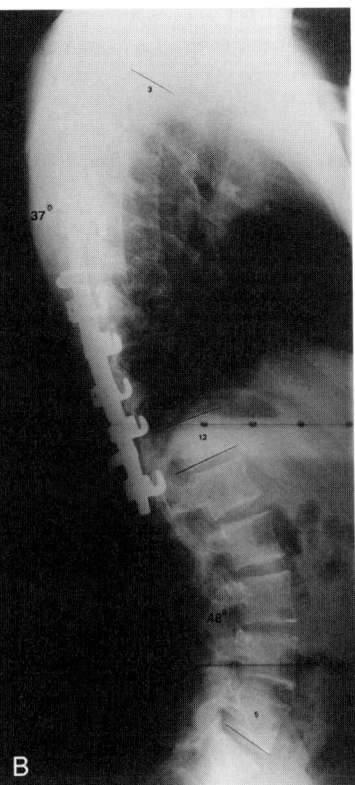

Fig. 3. Kyphosis resulting from Scheuermann's disease. *A,* Kyphosis in this 15-year-old boy was symptomatic and progressive despite bracing; preoperative kyphotic angle measures 78 degrees. The compensatory lumbar lordosis measured 58 degrees. Observe the vertebral body wedging at T7-10. *B,* Two years after anterior and posterior spinal fusion and Cortel-Dubousset instrumentation. The postoperative lateral radiograph shows reduction of the kyphotic angle to 37 degrees and of the compensatory lumbar lordosis to 48 degrees.

associated with progression or pain in adulthood. Treatment is symptomatic.

CONGENITAL KYPHOSIS

Congenital spinal deformities are caused by the abnormal formation and development of the vertebral elements. Spinal anomalies are postulated to develop from the 5th to 8th weeks of gestation, but the exact cause is unknown. Von Rokitansky is credited with the first description of this condition; in 1844 he described a thoracolumbar congenital kyphosis.[18] Congenital spinal deformity may be seen in isolation as well as in association with VACTERL syndrome, Jarcho-Levin syndrome, and Klippel-Feil anomaly. The most frequently associated condition is spinal dysraphism.[19] Other extraspinal anomalies seen with congenital spinal deformity include genitourinary, cardiac, and overlying cutaneous abnormalities. Congenital scoliosis is addressed in detail in Chapter 9-12.

When the congenital spinal malformation occurs in a primarily anterior or posterior position, kyphosis or lordosis will result. In 1973 Winter et al[18] classified congenital kyphosis according to the type of vertebral malformation; failure of formation (type I), failure of segmentation (type II), or mixed (type III) (Fig. 4). Failure of formation has the worst prognosis and is the most common cause of paraplegia resulting from spinal deformity. Failure of segmentation anteriorly may involve two to eight levels. Posterior defects of formation of the vertebral body, with intact posterior elements, typically involve one or several levels.

CLINICAL CHARACTERISTICS

Congenital kyphosis may be recognized at birth and progress rapidly, or it may not be identified until the adolescent growth spurt. Children typically demonstrate a sharp, angulated, rigid kyphosis. Kyphosis resulting from a defect of segmentation produces a more rounded deformity, which progresses less rapidly than kyphosis caused by failure of formation. A careful neurological examination is essential. Anomalies associated with congenital spinal deformity should be sought. Congenital kyphosis may be associated with back pain, often resulting from compensatory lumbar hyperlordosis.

RADIOGRAPHIC ASSESSMENT

Radiographic evaluation of a child with congenital kyphosis begins with standing posteroanterior and lateral radiographs of the entire spine. Flexibility of the deformity can be assessed by a supine lateral radiograph over an apical radiolucent wedge. Magnetic resonance imaging (MRI) scanning should also be performed on all children because of the high incidence rate of spinal cord abnormalities and compression (Fig. 5). Computed tomography (CT) myelography and tomograms are now used less frequently.

TREATMENT

Congenital kyphosis is nearly always progressive. Those curves that are nonprogressive may be monitored with close observation if there are no neurological deficits. Progressive kyphosis requires surgical intervention. The risk of paraplegia with progressive deformity has been recognized since 1955, when James[20] recommended early surgical in-

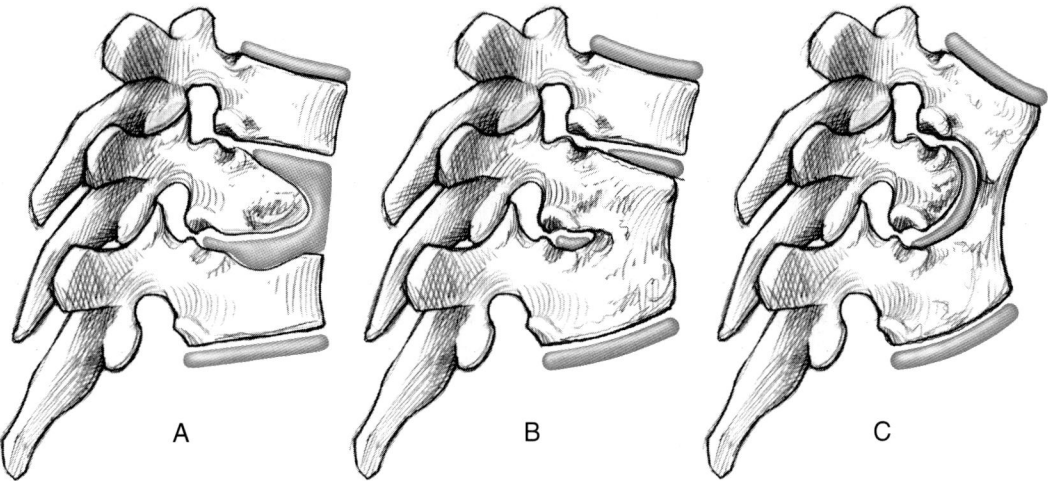

Fig. 4. Classification of Winter et al[18] of congenital kyphosis. *A,* Failure of formation. *B,* Failure of segmentation. *C,* Mixed (both).

tervention. Hodgson[21] first applied his technique for anterior osteotomy and fusion, which he used in the treatment of tuberculosis of the spine, to a patient with congenital kyphosis. Selection of the appropriate procedure depends on the patient's age, severity of the deformity, structural abnormality (i.e., failure of segmentation versus failure of formation), and neurological status. In children younger than 5 years with mild kyphosis (55 degrees or less) and no neurological compromise, limited posterior fusion is performed from the normal vertebral levels above and below the kyphosis. Postoperative immobilization in a Risser cast provides stability while the fusion heals; 6 months of immobilization and fusion augmentation is often required.

For more severe deformities or in older children and adolescents, combined anterior and posterior arthrodesis is necessary. Complete anterior diskectomy and excision of the anterior longitudinal ligament is followed by bone grafting. In cases caused by failure of segmentation, osteotomy of the anterior bony bar may be needed. If a neurological deficit is present, formal spinal cord decompression must be performed. If the neurological findings are limited to hyperreflexia without motor deficits, anterior and posterior fusion alone may allow neurological recovery.[22] The posterior procedure is usually completed on the same day, and segmental spinal instrumentation is used for stabilization rather than correction. Winter et al[22] reported on 94 patients 5 years of age or older who were treated surgically. Pseudarthrosis developed in 41% of patients who underwent posterior fusion alone compared with only 8% of those treated with combined anterior and posterior fusion.[22] Only those patients who were young and who had mild deformity showed good results with posterior fusion alone. Two patients in this series who were placed in halofemoral traction became paraplegic postoperatively; traction is, therefore, not recommended. Patients with a concomitant spinal cord anomaly should undergo neurosurgical evaluation and appropriate treatment, if indicated, before deformity correction. In addition, avoidance of traction and distraction instrumentation lessens the risk of neurological compromise.

LUMBAR KYPHOSIS CAUSED BY MYELODYSPLASIA

Lumbar kyphosis in patients with myelodysplasia presents the orthopaedic surgeon with a variety of difficult clinical problems. The reported incidence rate of lumbar kyphosis in myelodysplasia varies from 1% to 46%.[23] Three different types of kyphosis have been described: sharp angled, paralytic, and congenital. The terminology used to discuss

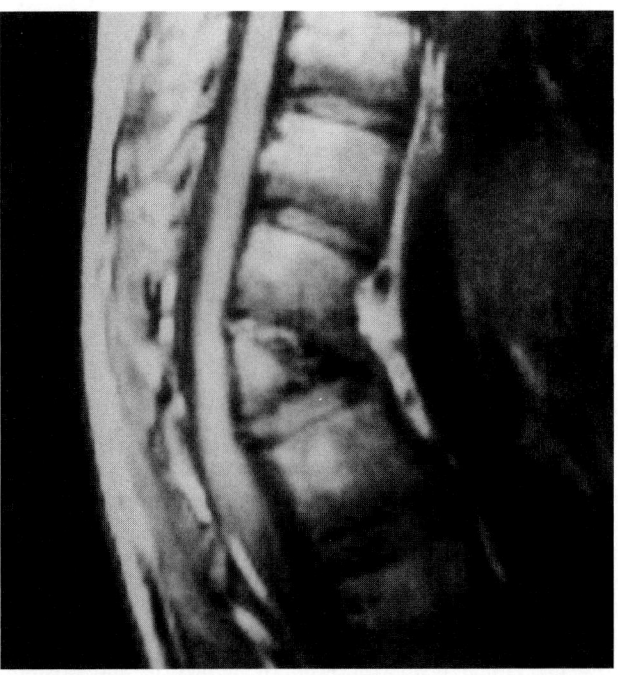

Fig. 5. Progressive kyphotic deformity. Based on magnetic resonance imaging (MRI) of the thoracolumbar junction in this 13-year-old boy, the deformity measured 55 degrees from T10 to L1. MRI reveals a type I congenital kyphosis with failure of anterior formation at the T12 vertebral level. Observe the mild impingement of the spinal cord at the T12 level.

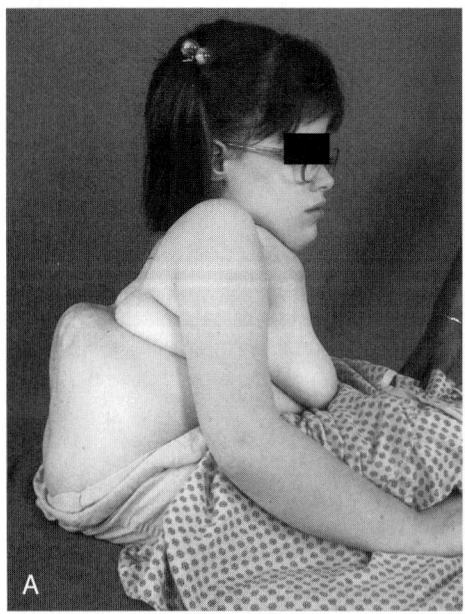 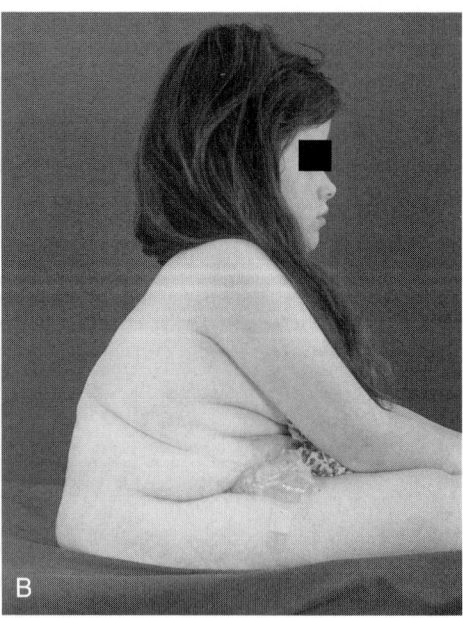

Fig. 6. T10-level myelodysplasia, severe rigid congenital kyphosis, and compensatory thoracic lordosis. *A,* This 16-year-old girl has shortness of breath from crowding of her abdominal contents. *B,* Postoperative view after complete vertebrectomy, posterior fusion, and Luque rod instrumentation. Sitting balance and cosmetic appearance are improved. Note the improved sitting height and spinal alignment.

kyphotic deformity in myelodysplasia can be confusing, because many authors refer to the sharp-angled curvature as congenital lumbar kyphosis. The sharp-angled or S-shaped type of kyphotic deformity is usually centered in the upper lumbar spine and lies distal to a rigid, lordotic lower thoracic segment. This curve typically measures 80 degrees or more at birth and is rapidly progressive, frequently at a rate of 8 degrees a year or more. Paralytic kyphosis associated with myelodysplasia is C shaped and less rigid; this pattern is caused by weakness of the trunk musculature, and it may progress rapidly or slowly.[24] The congenital type of curvature can occur anywhere along the spine and is usually due to an anterior defect of segmentation. In the remainder of this section, we address sharp-angled kyphotic deformity, which is unique to children with myelodysplasia.

Kyphotic deformity in children with myelodysplasia is associated with significant health and functional problems, including difficulty sitting upright, ulceration over the apex of the deformity, and respiratory compromise because of upward pressure from the abdominal contents. In addition, reduced abdominal capacity can cause poor nutrition and failure to thrive.[25] Because kyphosis is progressive in the majority of cases and surgical correctability is often limited, surgical treatment should be performed early.

The goals of treatment are to minimize the kyphotic deformity, halt further progression, and increase abdominal height. Moving the patient's center of gravity posteriorly also improves sitting balance (Fig. 6). Bracing is ineffective; most children with sharp-angled kyphosis will require surgical correction. Significant kyphosis present at birth can be managed at the time of sac closure by transpedicular decancellation and collapse of the vertebrae above and below the apical level, followed by reduction and posterior fixation using nonabsorbable sutures. Postoperative immobilization in a posterior plaster shell followed by an orthosis is continued for 1 year after surgery. Rigid kyphosis requires correction of the kyphotic segment as well as the

proximal rigid lordosis; excision of the apical vertebral body alone is associated with recurrent deformity.[25] Resection of the proximal vertebrae, between the lordotic and kyphotic apices, and reduction of the remaining vertebral bodies are followed by stabilization, depending on the age of the patient. Collapsing, flexible kyphosis may not require fusion until the child is nearing skeletal maturity, and it typically progresses only about 3 degrees a year.[24]

TREATMENT

Kyphosis correction in patients with myelodysplasia is complicated by the fact that the anterior structures, including the aorta and vena cava, are relatively shorter than the spine and limit the amount of correction that can be achieved. Posterior fusion in the immature child may fail because of tension forces in the fusion mass. Combined anteroposterior fusion in a young child results in insufficient trunk height to accommodate abdominal and pulmonary growth.[25] One method that addresses these problems involves removal of the ossific nuclei and posterior elements of the vertebrae one level above and below the apical segment. The apical vertebra is then translated forward, and tension band wiring is performed across these three levels, thus allowing continued growth in the vertebral bodies and gradual correction of the kyphosis.[25] In children older than 1 year of age, Luque's rod instrumentation is added without fusion. Alternatively, Lowe and Menelaus[26] described excision of the apical vertebrae, correction of the kyphosis and rigid compensatory curves, and internal fixation with threaded wires. Seven of their 11 patients experienced fusion, but two patients died in the postoperative period. Dunn[27] described a procedure involving complete excision of the intervertebral disks in the area of the kyphosis as well as posterior release, including the posterior longitudinal ligament in the proximal kyphotic section, followed by posterior instrumentation using a modified Luque's rod system. This technique can only be used in patients with thoracic-level neurological involvement, because the segmental nerves and vessels as well as the nonfunctioning spinal cord are sacrificed. Warner and Facker[28] compared a modification of the Dunn technique to Harrington rod fixation in 33 patients; they reported better correction and a lower incidence rate of complications with the modified Luque instrumentation. Banta[29] also reported successful results in six children with myelodysplasia and flexible collapsing kyphotic deformity with a mean of 95 degrees treated with anterior and posterior fusion using Luque's rod instrumentation. Of those with more rigid congenital kyphoses with a mean of 120 degrees, nine of 10 underwent posterior cordectomy, kyphectomy, and arthrodesis using Luque-Galveston instrumentation. One child died, and one experienced an asymptomatic pseudarthrosis; the remaining patients went on to apparently solid arthrodesis. Other authors recommended a variety of instrumentation methods, including tension band wire fixation, AO plates, Dwyer's cables, and pedicle screws.[30–32]

COMPLICATIONS

Spinal deformity surgery in myelodysplasia is associated with much higher complication frequencies than in other conditions. Excessive blood loss, infection, skin breakdown, recurrent deformity, and death are well-documented complications. Early kyphectomy is associated with an increased risk of late progression. Reported rates of pseudarthrosis have varied from 46% for posterior arthrodesis alone to 4% for combined anterior and posterior instrumentation and fusion.[29]

TUBERCULOSIS OF THE SPINE

Spinal tuberculosis, or Pott's disease, remains a significant problem in developing countries and continues to affect children and cause paraplegia in areas where it is common. *Mycobacterium tuberculosis* is the pathogen, and spinal infection is usually secondary to another source. Kyphotic deformity occurs as a result of collapse of the anterior spinal elements and can result in neurological compromise. Direct dural invasion or pressure from abscesses or bony sequestra can also lead to neurological deficit, which has been reported in as many of 61% of patients with spinal tuberculosis.[33]

The most common presenting complaint is pain, which may be accompanied by fever, malaise, and weight loss. Complete physical and neurological examination are essential. Radiographs may demonstrate disk space narrowing, vertebra plana, or kyphotic deformity. Loss of one vertebral body can result in as much as 35 degrees of kyphosis, most commonly in the thoracic spine.[34] MRI is the most useful imaging modality, and CT-guided biopsy is essential for definitive diagnosis. Differential diagnosis includes other pyogenic or fungal infections, sarcoidosis, and metastatic disease.

TREATMENT

Treatment is based on the neurological findings and degree of kyphotic deformity. Boachie-Adjei and Squillante[33] recommended that patients with Frankel grade C or D neurological deficits may be treated with chemotherapy and closely monitored for progression; significant neurological lesions (Frankel grade A or B), instability, or marked kyphosis should undergo immediate decompression anteriorly or posterolaterally depending on the anatomic location. In cases of circumferential involvement, anterior autologous iliac crest or fibular strut grafting may be followed by posterior fusion and instrumentation.

IATROGENIC KYPHOSIS

Children treated for intraspinal tumors are at risk for postlaminectomy or postirradiation kyphosis. The reported incidence rate of kyphotic deformity in this group is 26% and may be recognized as late as 6 years after treatment.[35] Younger age at treatment and more cephalad lesions increase the risk of kyphosis. There does not appear to be a correlation with the number of laminectomies performed.

TREATMENT

Prevention of postlaminectomy and postirradiation kyphosis includes exclusion of the spine from the radiation field, immediate fusion at the time of laminectomy, en bloc laminectomy followed by replacement of the posterior element block, and laminoplasty with posterolateral fusion. Some authors recommended early brace treatment to prevent progression of kyphosis, but more recently Otsuka et al[35] found no benefit from bracing and advocated surgical intervention. Flexible curves of mild to moderate severity may be adequately treated with posterior fusion and instrumentation alone, but larger, stiffer kyphotic deformities require anterior and posterior fusion.

REFERENCES

1. Tribus CB: Scheuermann's kyphosis in adolescence and adults: Diagnosis and management. J Am Acad Orthop Surg 1998; 6:36.
2. Scheuermann H: Kyfosis dorsalis juvenilis. Ugeskr laeger 1920; 82:385.
3. Sorensen KH: Scheuermann's Juvenile Kyphosis: Clinical Appearances, Radiography, Aetiology, and Prognosis. Copenhagen, Munksgaard, 1964.
4. Schmorl G: Die pathogenese der juvenilen kyphose. Fortschr geb. Röntgen 1930; 41: 359.
5. Bradford DS: Juvenile kyphosis. Clin Orthop 1977; 128:45.
6. Ascani E, LaRosa G: Scheuermann's kyphosis. In Weinstein SL (ed): The Pediatric Spine: Principles and Practice. New York, Raven Press, 1994, vol 1, p 557.
7. Murray PM, Weinstein SL, Sprat KF: The natural history and long term follow-up of Scheuermann's kyphosis. J Bone Joint Surg Am 1993; 75:236.
8. Scoles PV, Latimer BM, DiGiovanni BF, et al: Vertebral alterations in Scheuermann's kyphosis. Spine 1991; 16:509.
9. Bradford DS, Brown DM, Mose JH, et al: Scheuermann's kyphosis: A form of osteoporosis? Clin Orthop 1976; 118:10.
10. Lowe TG: Current concepts review: Scheuermann disease. J Bone Joint Surg Am 1990; 72:940.
11. Ryan MD, Taylor TKF: Acute spinal cord compression in Scheuermann's disease. J Bone Joint Surg Br 1982; 64:409.
12. Sachs B, Bradford D, Winter R, et al: Scheuermann's kyphosis: Follow-up of Milwaukee brace treatment. J Bone Joint Surg Am 1987; 69:50.

13. Montgomery SP, Erwin WE: Scheuermann's kyphosis: Long-term results of Milwaukee brace treatment. Spine 1981; 6: 5.

14. Bradford DS, Moe JH, Montalvo FJ, et al: Scheuermann's kyphosis and round back deformity: Results of Milwaukee brace treatment. J Bone Joint Surg Am 1974; 56:740.

15. Bradford DS, Moe JH, Montalvo FJ, et al: Scheuermann's kyphosis: Results of surgical treatment by posterior spine arthrodesis in twenty-two patients. J Bone Joint Surg Am 1975; 57:439.

16. Herndon WA, Emonds JB, Macaley LJ, et al: Combined anterior and posterior fusion for Scheuermann's kyphosis. Spine 1981; 6:125.

17. Ferreira-Alves A, Ressina J, Palma-Rodrigues R: Scheuermann's kyphosis: The Portuguese technique of surgical treatment. J Bone Joint Surg Br 1995; 77:943.

18. Winter RB, Moe JH, Wang JF: Congenital kyphosis: Its natural history and treatment as observed in the study of 130 patients. J Bone Joint Surg Am 1973; 55:223.

19. Winter RB, Lonstein JE, Boachie-Adjei O: Congenital spinal deformity. Am Acad Orthop Surg 1996; 45:117.

20. James JIP: Kyphoscoliosis. J Bone Joint Surg Br 1955; 37:414.

21. Hodgson AR: Correction of fixed spinal curves: A preliminary communication. J Bone Joint Surg Am 1965; 47:1221.

22. Winter RB, Moe JH, Lonstein JE: The surgical treatment of congenital kyphosis: A review of 94 patients age 5 years or older, with 2 years or more follow-up in 77 patients. Spine 1985; 10:224.

23. Carstens C, Koch H, Brocai DRC, et al: Development of pathological lumbar kyphosis in myelomeningocele. J Bone Joint Surg Br 1996; 78:945.

24. Banta JV, Hamanda JS: Natural history of the kyphotic deformity in myelomeningocele. J Bone Joint Surg Am 1976; 58:279.

25. Lindseth RE: Myelomeningocele spine. In Weinstein SL (ed): The Pediatric Spine: Principles and Practice. New York, Raven Press, 1994, p 1043.

26. Lowe GP, Menelaus MB: The surgical management of kyphosis in older children with myelomeningocele. J Bone Joint Surg Br 1978; 60:40.

27. Dunn HK: Kyphosis of myelodysplasia: Operative treatment based on pathophysiology. Orthop Trans 1983; 7:19.

28. Warner WC, Facker CD: Comparison of two instrumentation techniques in treatment of lumbar kyphosis in myelodysplasia. J Pediatr Orthop 1993; 13:704.

29. Banta JV: Combined anterior and posterior fusion for spinal deformity in myelomeningocele. Spine 1990; 15:946.

30. Martin JR, Kumar SJ, Gurlle JT, et al: Congenital kyphosis in myelomeningocele: Results following operative and nonoperative treatment. J Pediatr Orthop 1994; 14: 323.

31. McMaster MJ: The long-term results of kyphectomy and spinal stabilization in children with myelomeningocele. Spine 1988; 13:417.

32. Rodgers WB, Williams MS, Schwend RM, et al: Spinal deformity in myelodysplasia: Correction with posterior pedicle screw instrumentation. Spine 1997; 22:2435.

33. Boachie-Adjei O, Squillante RG: Tuberculosis of the spine. Orthop Clin North Am 1996; 27:95.

34. Rajasekaran S, Shanmugasundarum TK: Prediction of gibbus deformity in tuberculosis of the spine. J Bone Joint Surg Am 1987; 69:503.

35. Otsuka NY, Hey L, Hall JE: Postlaminectomy and postirradiation kyphosis in children and adolescents. Clin Orthop 1998; 354:189.

EMBRYOLOGY AND ANATOMY

Timothy M. Ganey and John A. Ogden

Summary

- Limb morphogenetic fields arise as a localized differentiation of the lateral plate mesoderm after the somites are defined.
- Interaction between the apical ectodermal ridge (AER) and the underlying mesoderm is responsible for establishment of the hip anlage and extension of the limb bud.
- Hox genes determine the primary and secondary axes of the developing embryo. They control associations such as proximal femur, lateral condyle, and fibula (thus, the concomitance of PFFD and fibular hemimelia).
- Limb development is specified by anteroposterior, dorsoventral, and proximodistal axes.
- Bone forms by both intramembranous and endochondral ossification.
- The large amount of epiphyseal cartilage, especially before secondary (epiphyseal) ossification develops, permits plastic deformation over time.
- Early departure from normal development carries a greater potential for complication.

Clinical Relevance

- Both congenital and environmental factors contribute to misguided development and morphological alteration.
- Longitudinal deficiencies may result from either genetic or environmental perturbation.
- Developmental hip dysplasia may occur in utero and lead to progressive postnatal morphological changes.
- Developmental hip dysplasia may occur postnatally in a mechanically unstable but morphologically normal hip at birth.
- The earlier that a hip abnormality is diagnosed, especially one with a major plastic deformation basis, the more likely it is that the process may be reversed and the less likely it is that major surgical intervention will be necessary.

The development of the hip joint will be used as an example of normal and abnormal embryologic processes in the immature skeletal system. The adult hip emerges over the course of coaptive development as an articulation between the head of the femur and the acetabulum, embodying individual responses to intrinsic demands initiated in the embryo and adapted to during progressive skeletal maturation. Developmental changes in either component affect the responsive growth of its companion, and balance between the two extends a mechanically stable range of motion through a course of skeletal maturation. A broad understanding of normal embryology establishes a framework for not only interpreting aberrance and inadequacies of skeletal development but for comprehending more specific mechanisms of bone biology as well.

CLINICAL RELEVANCE

When considering the development of the hip, it is important to remember the significance of changing anatomic differences between a child and an adult, particularly with respect to potential complications. Areas of major importance include (1) the complex cartilaginous components of the acetabulum; (2) the progressive development of the proximal femur from the functionally separate lesser trochanter, greater trochanter, and capital femoral epiphyses; and (3) the susceptibilities to vascular compromise that are associated with age and anatomy.

HISTORICAL REVIEW

The conceptual basis for embryology is the emergence of new identity from the context of previous order. Based on external and internal morphological criteria, Streeter[1] divided the human embryonic period into 23 stages termed *horizons.* Over the course of 8 weeks in humans, virtually all of the major differentiation processes affecting the forming skeleton are completed. The remainder of the 40-week gestation period is characterized by elaboration of the differentiated skeletal components. Congenital defects may result from either primary aberration in differentiation, from developmental abnormalities associated with growth, or from both.

Genetically controlled determinants propel development and initiate epigenetic, or cell-cell, interactions. Contact confers identifying features to individual cell condensations until they achieve a position along time and space coordinates appropriate for expression. Implicit in the notion of developmental specification is the concept of evolving potential, which for many tissues eliminates the perpetual capacity to differentiate. Thus, although an embryonic mesodermal cell may initially be endowed with an option to emerge as cartilage, bone, or even muscle, modifications imposed by location and adhesiveness, specifications imparted by extracellular matrix, and loss of cell mobility to a great extent restrict further adaptation. The chief characteristic of development is cumulative, progressive change to the extent invested by genetic option.

DEVELOPMENT OF THE HIP JOINT

Successful development of the vertebrate limb requires a complex set of interactions between the ectoderm and the underlying mesoderm.[2-4] The onset of limb development, initiated by mesodermal condensation in the lateral plate mesoderm, is dependent on inductive influences of both adjacent somite tissue[5] and the mesonephros.[6] Four weeks after fertilization, the lower limb buds are evident on the anterior lateral body wall at the level of the lumbar and first sacral somites.[7] Once the initial bud has formed, the epithelium at the leading margin of the bud thickens and assumes a pseudostratified appearance known as the AER. Further limb bud elongation occurs rapidly under the influence of the AER, and within a few days differentiation of an intricate pattern of cartilage, bone, muscles, and other support tissues occurs.

The remarkable degree of homology between different species of vertebrates has led to several insights into pattern imprinting.[8–10] From the available literature, a few basic tenets have evolved, perhaps the foremost being that the basic components of limb outgrowth are specified from most proximal to distal. This suggests that as cells divide in response to positional disparities, certain cells progressively adopt a more distal identity.[11] As the femur and the acetabulum emerge from this mesenchymal blastema as the most proximal aspect of the limb buds, they constitute the basis for further differentiation of more distal limb structures. Groups of cells become "committed" to certain zones or regions, whereas other groups continue to migrate and "commit" more distally. During the migration process, animal cells release traces of material in the matrix as footprints of their locomotion and adhesion.[12, 13] Although the phenomenon is poorly understood, traces of integrin proteins as well as other components of focal contacts in the tracks suggest that deposition and interactive recognition may extrude a patterned scaffold during the elaboration of the anlage.[14]

Separate studies support a genetic basis for simultaneous segmentation of the anteroposterior axis. Based on Lewis'[15] 1978 work in *Drosophila,* the vertebrate *Hox* genes have been elicited as candidates for pattern formation during development.[16, 17] In the context of the hip articulation, the proximal extent of the fibular developmental field involves the pubic portion of the pelvis and the proximal femur, whereas ischial and iliac portions of the hip bones and the distal femur are associated with the tibial developmental field.[18] It is important to realize that ontogenetic separateness extends to not only the skeleton but to the synovia, the ligaments of the joint, the muscles, and their intermuscular septa and tendons. These field patterns explain interrelationships of deficiency syndromes such as the association of fibular deficiency or absence with a hypoplastic femur or proximal femoral focal deficiency.[19]

EMBRYOPATHY VERSUS FETOPATHY

One of the challenges in evaluating hip disease is distinguishing changes that are genetically inherent from those engendered by development. Embryopathies, such as proximal femoral focal deficiencies and hypoplasia, require a different deliberation than do fetopathic conditions such as acetabular or femoral dysplasia, which usually responds well to closed reduction, bracing, casting, and, in some cases, open reduction. Recognizing the difference is key to implementing a corrective treatment strategy. Of the many characteristics of the immature skeleton, perhaps of foremost importance is developmental plasticity, or its ability to respond to mechanical, metabolic, and endocrine stimuli.

Development of bone through a cartilaginous anlage endows a capacity for joint articulation, growth in balance with muscle forces, and measured directional development.

Unfortunately, this modeling capacity also makes the developing hip susceptible to deforming external influences such as girding from uterine pressures, oligohydramnios, and breech presentation that confine or distort progressive fetal growth. Despite normal tissue differentiation of the acetabulum and the proximal femur, in some cases overriding deforming forces are able to modify the morphology of the hip joint. Understanding the natural history of the deforming forces allows the same biological plasticity to be exploited in corrective regimen. During the rapid postnatal expansion of the cartilaginous anlage, restoring direction and limiting aberrant forces can be used to guide the progressive force and to integrate the mechanical articulation of the hips to the loading dynamics of the child.

ACETABULUM

The acetabulum marks the convergence of three primary ossification centers: ischium, pubis, and ilium. The acetabulum is first apparent in the 14- to 15-mm embryo as a cellular depression proximal to the developing femur.[7] Essentially a skeletal blastema, further differentiation of the cartilaginous anlagen of the hipbone lags behind the shaft and the femoral head at all stages. Chondrification radiates from the conjunction of the three primordia, establishing an antecedent for the triradiate cartilage, which subsequently serves as a composite epiphysis for the acetabulum. In a manner inherent to all growth cartilage, enlargement of the acetabulum occurs by appositional and interstitial cell multiplication and through matrix elaboration.

Primary ossification centers for the three anlagen of the hip joint appear in the ileum at 38 to 39 mm, in the ischium variably between 105 to 124 mm, and in the pubis at 161 mm.[20] Each of the three ossification centers expands centrally, converging within the acetabulum until separated only by the triradiate cartilage (Fig. 1). The triradiate cartilage represents a composite epiphysis of the three contributing centers of the hipbone, integrating growth of the acetabulum proportionate to spherical growth of the capital femur.

The lateral cup-shaped articular cartilage forms the articular surface with the head of the femur, whereas the medial triradiate component forms a continuous buttress that separates the ileum, ischium, and pubis in the region of the acetabulum.[21] The triradiate cartilage assumes a Y shape: an anterior, slightly superiorly slanted component divides the ileum and the pubis; a posterior horizontal strip of cartilage separates the ileum and the ischium; and an inferior, nearly vertical component is located between the ischium and the pubis.

Within the triradiate cartilage, the physis is bipolar. The germinal zone runs along the center of each arm. Extending from the central germinal zone toward each metaphysis are the dividing and the hypertrophic zones. These zones are not as wide as in longitudinal bones, reflecting less rapid rates of endochondral ossification.[22]

Bone adjacent to each physis corresponds to a metaphysis and, accordingly, is capable of considerable remodeling. However, because this metaphyseal bone does not elaborate a subchondral plate until late in development, interstitial expansion of the physis and epiphysis may continue unimpeded. The interrelationship among the acetabular, articu-

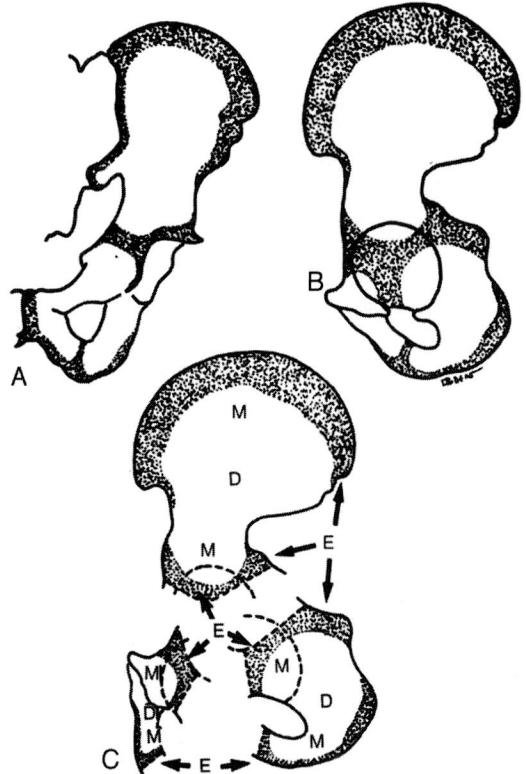

Fig. 1. The separate osseous entities from which the hip bone is composed. *A,* An anterior view does not permit a full appreciation of the acetabulum. *B,* In a true lateral view, a better grasp of the union of the separate components is apparent. *C,* An exploded view depicts the morphological identity that each of the three component bones—ilium, ischium, and pubis—brings to the triradiate cartilage (E, epiphysis; M, metaphysis; D, diaphysis).

lar, and triradiate cartilage functionally accommodates progressive expansion of the acetabular concavity in response to proximal femoral growth. Thus, the major function of the triradiate-acetabular cartilage is to facilitate a radial increase in absolute size of the acetabulum while maintaining a spherical congruency with the femoral head.

The triradiate cartilage in the newborn is wide relative to the size of the hip bones. As the hip develops, the widths of the arms progressively narrow until they are approximately 5 to 6 mm wide throughout most of childhood and adolescence. Standard anteroposterior radiographs restrict interpretation of the triradiate cartilage to the composite radiolucency of the superior arms and are difficult to obtain because of the obliquity of the acetabulum and the superimposition of the capital femoral ossification center. Direct views of the acetabulum permit a fuller appreciation of its true appearance (Fig. 2).

As the child reaches adolescence, secondary ossification centers analogous to those seen in long bones develop within the arms of the triradiate cartilage (Fig. 3).[23] These epiphyses expand toward the periphery of the acetabulum, contributing to a greater depth and surface area for femoral articulation. Radiographically interpreted as os acetabuli in the adolescent, they represent coalescence of secondary ossification centers, transforming each bipolar growth plate of

the triradiate cartilage into two separate growth plates of mirroring morphology and antipodal growth potential.[22, 24] They fuse at about the age of 18 years.[21] Enlargement of the ischiopubic junction is evident radiographically and should not be misinterpreted as an osteochondrosis or healing stress fracture.

PROXIMAL FEMUR

Several features contribute to the unique structure and intricacy of the proximal femur. These include the emergence of three ossification centers from a composite chondroepiphysis, a ligamentous attachment to the acetabulum that emanates from the center of the proximal articular surface, and the intracapsular course of the limited capital femoral blood vessels. Coupled with the continuum of the articular cartilage with the hyaline growth cartilage, an inelastic capsular girding, and muscular action rotating the femur on an axis separate from the medullary cortex, both the biomechanics and structural dynamics of the proximal femur are complex.

As in the acetabulum, the femoral blastema is apparent during the fourth week of embryonic life in the 15-mm embryo. With the appearance of the chondrocyte phenotype, matrix elaboration is initiated. Primary ossification of the anlage is initiated centrally in the anlage and proceeds both proximally and distally along the shaft of the femur. Although circumferential ossification characterizes the central diaphysis of the femur, primary ossification of the diaphyseal shaft initially remains incomplete medially and posterior at the site of the lesser trochanter, notching the top of the diaphyseal cylinder (Fig. 4).

The proximal femur is a composite structure at birth, with the greater trochanter, the lesser trochanter, and the capital femur a common mass of cartilage (Fig. 5). Within this synchondrous epiphysis, numerous cartilage canals are present that provide a basis for nutrition of the cartilage initially and later establish a conduit for cell lineages that support the differentiation of bone. These vessels penetrate the chondroepiphysis of the proximal femur in the 39-mm embryo and elaborate in complexity and volume with continued development of the chondroepiphysis.[25, 26]

The normal morphology of the proximal femur features a spherical femoral head, variable anteversion, virtually no neck, and a neutral articulotrochanteric distance (i.e., the height of the trochanter is similar to that of the femoral articulating surface). During ensuing developmental periods, this distance becomes positive commensurate with the elongation of the femoral neck.

The hip capsule attaches along the intertrochanteric region superiorly, anteriorly, and posteriorly and just above the lesser trochanter at the inferior margin. Proximally, the capsule attaches at the interface of bone and hyaline cartilage just beyond the fibrocartilaginous labrum on the acetabular side, making the rim and its transverse acetabular ligament intracapsular structures. The greater and lesser trochanters, although differentiating as indivisible regions of the chondroepiphysis, during development assume extracapsular, apophyseal function, similar in many respects to the tibial tuberosity.

Ossification begins in the capital femur 4 to 6 months postnatally, although a range of 2 to 10 months would be

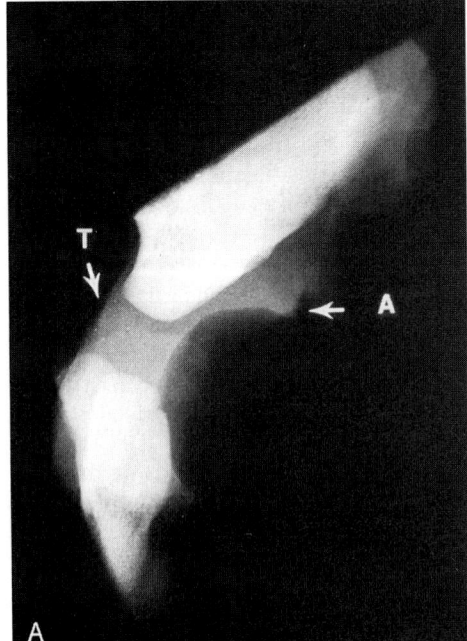

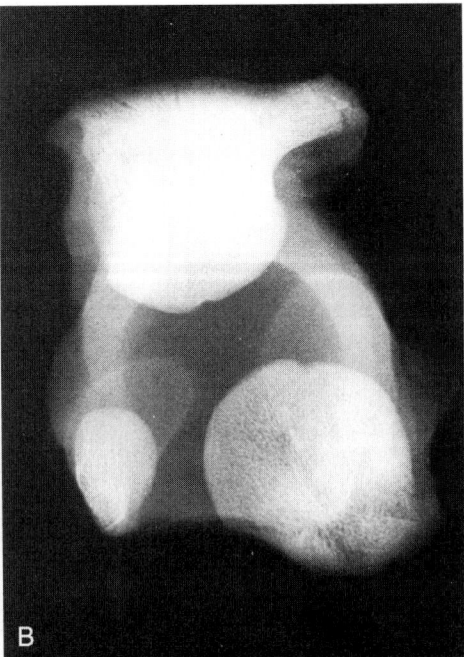

Fig. 2. Direct radiographic views of the acetabulum. This permits a clear assessment of the developmental patterns. *A,* Duplication of a standard anterior view does not allow a full appreciation of the acetabulum from this stillborn neonate. In this radiograph, both the acetabular (A) and triradiate (T) cartilages are apparent. *B,* A radiograph perpendicular to the acetabular fossa provides an appreciation for the cartilaginous component and growth potential of the acetabulum. Note the shadow of the femoral articular circumference defined as well. *C,* As the skeleton matures, the bipolar areas of growth cartilage separating the pelvic bones narrow. This view shows the appearance of the triradiate cartilage at 4 years.

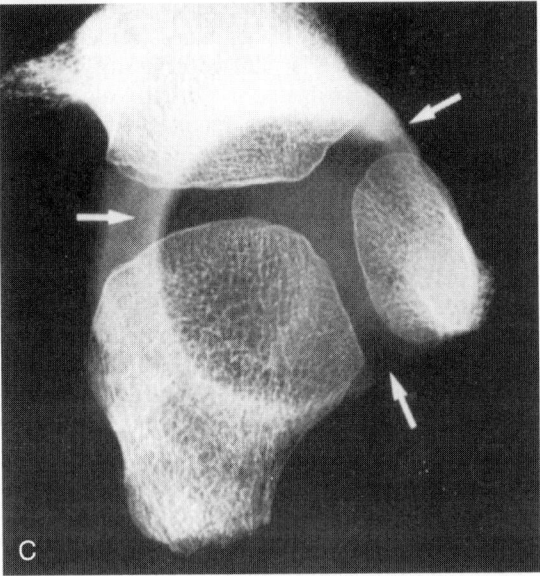

within normal limits. The ossification center expands centrifugally, eventually conforming to the hemispheric shape of the articular contour. Ossification of the secondary center is coordinate with enhanced growth of the medial aspect of the metaphysis. The femoral neck elongates over the ensuing 6 to 12 months. Although a significant amount of hyaline cartilage initially links the greater trochanter and the capital femoral intraepiphyseal centers, elongation of the neck results in increasing separation despite the original continuity. As the neck develops, the superior articular surface of the capital femur attains a more proximal position relative to the greater trochanter, which is still largely composed of cartilage, firmly establishing a positive articulotrochanteric distance.

Increased growth of the medial physis leads to a more specific definition of the capital femoral physis as well. Continued expansion of the secondary ossification center results in its flattening at the juxtaposition with the physis, transforming the original round shape into a hemispherical shape and establishing a bipolar growth zone between the capital femur ossification center and the metaphysis (Fig. 6). Laxity in the hip capsule decreases, and the medial physis, in response to normal hip joint mechanics, begins to angulate and also to develop mammillary processes. Akin to interlocking bone and cartilage pegs, they give the physis an undulated appearance, reaching their maximum height between the ages of 6 and 13 years. Although shear strength of the capital epiphyseal plate is dependent on the perichondrial zone of Ranvier during infancy, after 3 years of age the predominant support for resisting shear shifts to the interlocking morphology.[26–28]

Development and maintenance of secondary centers delimit the physis to a more consistent range of strains and mediate biomechanical stimuli as a summative rather than

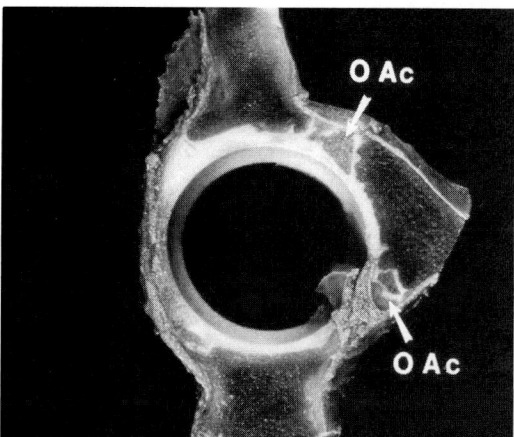

Fig. 3. Adolescent development of the triradiate cartilage. Individual margins of the separate pelvic bones can be clearly seen. The os acetabuli (O Ac) are distinguished by a marrow similar in appearance to epiphyses of long bones.

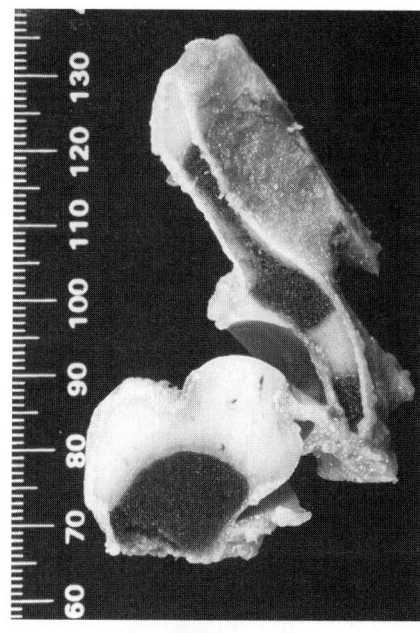

Fig. 5. Proximal aspect of femur. At birth, the entire proximal aspect of the femur is composed of cartilage. It is not possible to separately distinguish regional morphologies such as the greater trochanter from the capital femoral epiphysis.

an acute signal. The idea of compression enhancing bone formation and the dynamics of focal pressure imparted by an ossicle in the middle of volume of cartilage have been explored as a model for site specificity of secondary center formation.[29] Germane to the concept of secondary center development is stress transduction through dissimilar mediums. Cartilage (articular-epiphyseal) to bone (metaphysis) conduction will differ from cartilage (articular) to bone (secondary center) to cartilage (physis) to bone (metaphysis) in not only signal but in stress and strain profiles as well, particularly in shear. Mammillary process development relies on restitution of neutral strain and stress abatement.

Skeletal tissue morphology reflects a sustained effort to retain and exaggerate the reserve zone matrix. Such production heightens the quiescent state of the physeal chondrocyte, suppresses the transition of the metaphyseal morphotype, and extends the regional growth potential. Maximum height may be an extrusion of the biological

potential to react to stress in such a condition and may reflect organismal variation. Animals attaining the distinction of height feature larger and more complex mammillary processes at their physes.

Continued longitudinal and interstitial growth of the femoral neck results in elongation and thinning of the intraepiphyseal area at 3 to 4 years of age, although a posterosuperior region remains as a definite mass of cartilage between the greater trochanter and the femoral head (Fig. 7). During this time, the greater trochanter develops a secondary center of ossification directly above the lateral metaphysis that is initiated from a single center or rapidly

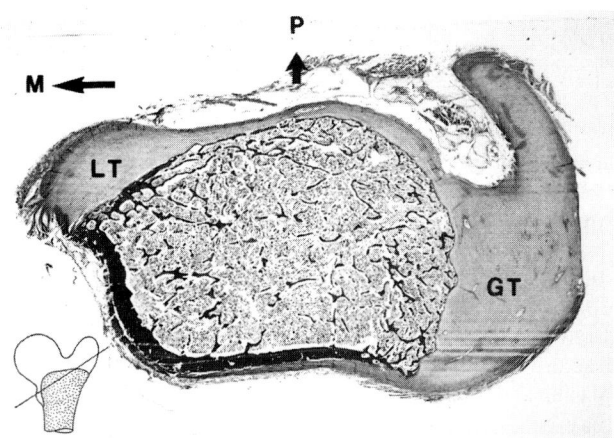

Fig. 4. The hyaline cartilage of the greater and lesser trochanters and the capital epiphysis as a common mass. The lesser trochanter (LT) in this stillborn, full-term infant is continuous with the hyaline cartilage of the greater trochanter (GT). Medial (M) and posterior (P) aspects, as well as plane of section, are indicated.

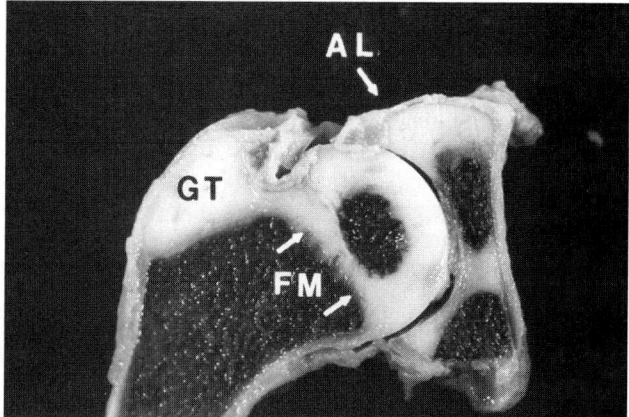

Fig. 6. By 1 year, continued centrifugal expansion of the capital femoral ossification center results in flattening at its interface with the femoral shaft metaphysis (FM). Such development establishes a growth plate that facilitates directional extension perpendicular to the new physis *(white arrows)*. Continuity between the capital femur and the greater trochanter (GT) is maintained on the superior aspect of the femoral neck. The acetabular labrum (AL) plays an important role as a hip stabilizer.

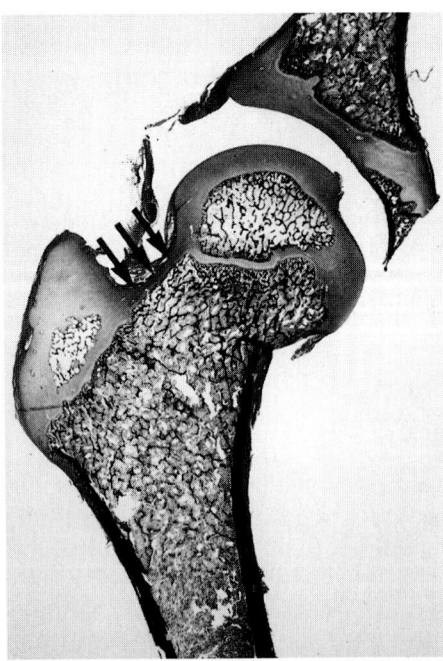

Fig. 7. Thinning of the superior aspect of the femoral neck. Thinning of the superior aspect of the femoral neck (three *bold arrows)* characterizes the period of development between 3 and 4 years. By this time, the capital femoral epiphysis has attained a nearly hemispherical profile, domed to a subchondral articular margin, and flattened at its physeal interface.

coalesces from multiple, small ossific foci. The metaphysis demonstrates enhanced medial trabecular patterning along its superior neck in conjunction with an increasing intertrochanteric distance, reflecting the faster growth rate of the capital physis compared with that of the greater trochanter. As tensile forces accommodate bone differentiation without antecedent hyaline cartilage,[30, 31] distraction osteosynthesis at the femoral neck potentiates bone formation with sustained vascular supply and integrates formative modeling as a mechanistic continuum for bone growth.[32]

Expansion of the greater trochanter and enlargement of the ossification center of the capital epiphysis continue over the period of 5 to 8 years. The greater trochanter often develops an additional ossification center near the proximal end of the trochanter, which rapidly fuses with the main center. An area juxtaposed to the fovea capitis develops a distinct indentation in the ossification center. By the end of this stage of development, the proximal femur has formed the final anatomic contours of anteversion, the functionally separate femoral head and trochanter, and the neck-shaft angle.

The neck angle of the femur at birth averages 138 degrees, increasing to 145 degrees at 1 year. After the infant begins to walk, it gradually thereafter declines until reaching the average adult angle of 120 degrees.[33] Most of the subsequent growth through adolescence will comprise the remodeling of trabecular patterns and the integrated enlargement of the capital femur and the trochanters.

Femoral torsion angle, from which anteversion is determined, is formed by the intersecting planes of the femoral condyles with a line drawn through the femoral neck and femoral head centers. If the plane of the head-neck axis passes anterior to the condylar plane, it is termed *anteversion;* if it passes posteriorly, it is called femoral *retroversion.* Femoral anteversion at birth ranges from +15 degrees to +53 degrees, gradually decreasing until the adult values of +14 degrees are attained.[34–36]

The intraepiphyseal fibrous growth plate that emerged at 3 to 4 years of age maintains a significant fibrocartilaginous component and, as alluded to earlier, continues to form bone by a membranous rather than an endochondral mechanism. A fairly abrupt histological change, sometimes associated with an osseous extension analogous to the osseous ring of the zone of Ranvier, demarcates the lateral portion of the capital femoral physis from the intraepiphyseal physis. The cell columns are obliquely oriented away from the center of the intraepiphyseal region and follow tensile stress patterns. As its major function, the intraepiphyseal region provides a basis for widening of the neck together with elongation and modeling. After femoral neck fracture, damaged cellular function could lead to a narrow, deformed femoral neck.

The period from 13 to 16 years of age is characterized by rapid growth, which may account for an increased susceptibility to slipped capital femoral epiphysis. It is also marked by the physiological closure of the physis. Of the three active growth regions of the proximal femur, the capital femoral physis is the first to close. The process begins centrally with an increasing thickness of the subchondral epiphyseal plate followed by a similar thickening of the trabecular bone of the metaphysis. Because chondrocytes of the growth plate form occasional clones rather than cell columns, a general attenuation of plate dynamics occurs, resulting in a thinning of the growth plate. The dense osseous plates on either side of the physis join together by small bridges that gradually become larger. The fusion progresses centrifugally, eventually incorporating the entire capital femoral epiphysis. As coalition nears completion in the capital femur, a similar process begins in the greater trochanteric physis. After the union of the metaphyseal bone with the separate epiphyses, final modeling of the remaining hyaline matrix of the capital physis establishes a subarticular, subchondral bone interface with only articular cartilage remaining.

VASCULAR SUPPLY

The proximal femur is notably disposed to vascular variation and remains uniquely susceptible to vascular disorders at any and all stages of postnatal development and growth. It is essential to understand the changing patterns of macroscopic and microscopic circulation in the context of proximal femoral development to adequately appreciate the role of the vascular supply in normal physiological development and the consequence of ischemic changes encountered in slipped femoral capital epiphysis, femoral neck fracture, traumatic hip dislocation, developmental hip dysplasia, and Legg-Calvé-Perthes disease. The predisposition may be ascribed primarily to the development of an intracapsular course for the increasingly limited blood vessels that supply the femoral head.

The extracapsular blood supply to the proximal femur is derived principally from the medial and lateral circumflex

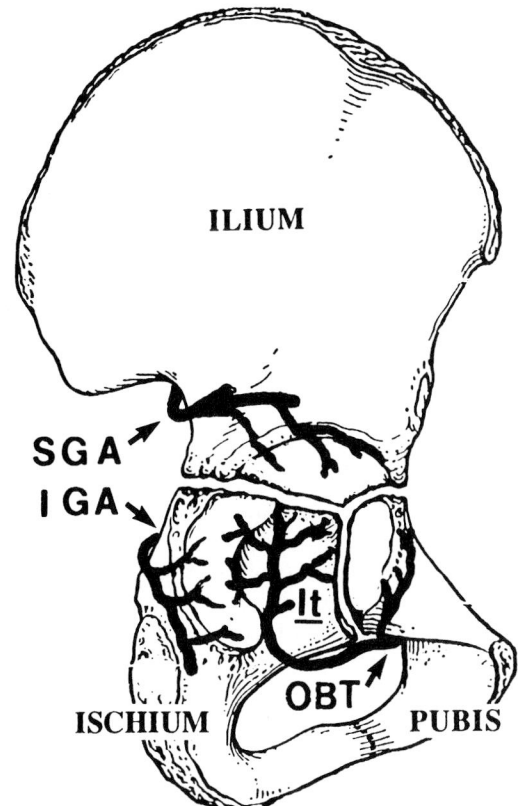

Fig. 8. Arterial supply to the developing acetabulum. Arterial supply to the developing acetabulum is derived from branches of the internal iliac artery. The superior aspect is supported by branches from the superior gluteal artery (SGA), whereas the posterior aspect receives its vascular supply from the inferior gluteal artery (IGA). The floor of the acetabulum, the artery to the ligamentum teres (lt), and the pubic portion of the acetabulum are nourished by branches of the obturator artery (OBT). (Adapted from Ulloa I: Embryonic and fetal development of the vascular system of the proximal end of the femur and acetabulum in man. Z Orthop 1962; 96:306; Grant JCB: An Atlas of Anatomy. Baltimore, Williams & Wilkins, 1972.)

cant periosteal capillary network embraces the inferior aspect of the neck region as well as the diaphyseal portion of the proximal femur. The medial, posterior, and lateral aspects of the ring are a continuation of medial femoral circumflex artery, whereas the lateral circumflex artery forms the anterior aspect of the ring.

The predominant blood supply of the proximal femur, regardless of the stage of postnatal development, is derived from the deep (profunda) femoral artery. The lateral circumflex artery displays little variation, arising from the profunda artery 90% of the time, whereas the medial circumflex artery, although from the profunda in 30% of specimens, more often arises as an independent vessel directly from the main femoral trunk.[28]

During the first year of life, the lateral circumflex branches supply a considerable portion of the anterior chondroepiphysis. After passing laterally and anterior to the iliopsoas, the lateral femoral circumflex artery divides into several terminal branches that ascend as lateral and anterior cervical branches to the femoral head and neck. With the development and elongation of the neck, however, the lateral circumflex artery increasingly supplies the greater trochanter, the anterior femoral neck, and metaphysis and decreasingly contributes to the intracapsular capital femoral circulation (Fig. 9).

The medial femoral circumflex artery passes posteriorly between the iliopsoas and pectineus muscles and then between the medial capsule and the obturator externus muscles. Branches provide vascular support for the medial inferior aspect of the neck between the inferomedial capsular insertion and the lesser trochanter. A small branch courses along the anterior capsular insertion. The major portion of the medial circumflex artery, however, traverses the poste-

arteries. Anastomoses of the vessels are present around the hip joint, particularly over the capsule and along anterior and posterior peritrochanteric regions. With anastomotic connections, compromise of one or more major extracapsular vessels at specific areas has potential to jeopardize functional flow in adjacent regions by a process akin to siphoning. Development and branching patterns of vessels to a great extent reflect biological demand. Vascular beds in the proximal femur encircle, anastomose, and balance separate arterial sources and venous returns that are necessary to support the metabolic demands of the developing femur. Should an element of the supply side be affected, arterial imbalance may initiate arterial flow dynamics that change not only the pattern but also the direction of flow. Marked arterial imbalance has potential for contributing to venous stasis with regional distribution.

In the 2-month-old embryo, both extracapsular circumflex arteries to the proximal femur, the acetabular artery as a branch from the obturator to the acetabular fossa, and the artery to the ligamentum teres are present (Fig. 8).[37] The medial and lateral circumflex arteries anastomose to form a ring around the femoral neck base, from which a signifi-

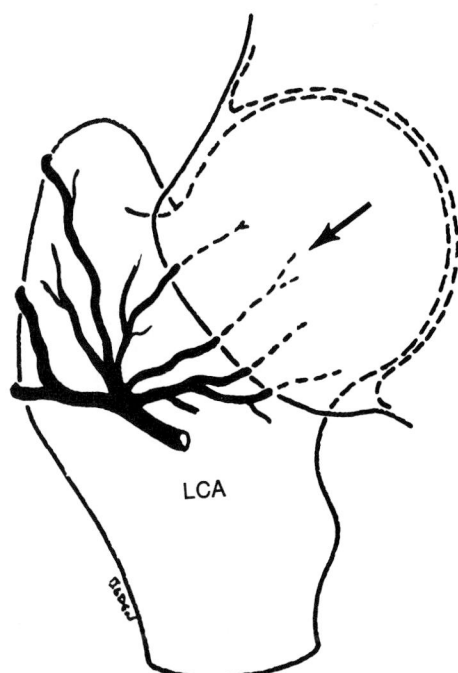

Fig. 9. Lateral circumflex artery. The lateral circumflex artery (LCA) primarily supplies the greater trochanter but does send anterior, intracapsular branches as well to the femoral head.

rior intertrochanteric notch as the intraepiphyseal artery and eventually crosses over to the anterosuperior aspect of the intertrochanteric groove, where it anastomoses with the terminal ramifications of the lateral circumflex artery.

At birth, the two circumflex arteries supply approximately equal portions of the greater trochanter, the capital femoral hyaline cartilage, and physis, with the medial supplying the posterior aspect and the lateral supplying the anterior half. Attachment of the hip capsule remains relatively constant, resulting in a relatively medial displacement of the capital femoral epiphysis and necessitating changing circulation patterns. The lateral circumflex artery increasingly becomes the predominate blood supply to the developing intracapsular metaphysis. As the articular surface and the underlying epiphysis gradually overlap the anterior and the inferior metaphysis, fewer areas remain where the anterior vessels can penetrate. By 3 to 5 years of age, the anterior branches supply only the metaphysis, whereas the posteriorly located medial circumflex branches assume the primary role for vascular support of the capital femoral epiphysis throughout its development.

The medial artery establishes two important posterior circulations. Sometimes referred to as ascending cervical arteries,[28] the posterior inferior artery arises from the medial circumflex artery near the lesser trochanter, penetrates the hip capsule, and courses along the inferior femoral neck. The more important system, the posterosuperior arterial system, penetrates the hip capsule and courses along the superior region of the femoral neck, often composed of two or more arteries. The ascending arteries anastomose to form a subsynovial ring on the femoral neck surface at the articular cartilage margin. Even during the perinatal period, several large vessels entering the chondroepiphysis characterize the superior region (Fig. 10). The posteroinferior artery, which unlike the posterosuperior system is usually a single-vessel system, courses in a much more mobile retinacular reflection, sending off minimal branches to the underlying epiphysis and metaphysis but never directly crosses the growth plate.

ARTICULATION-CAPSULAR AND LIGAMENTOUS CONSTRAINT

The articulation of the proximal femur with the acetabulum is classified as an enarthrosis, or ball-and-socket joint. Such conformation permits extensive mobility through a wide range of functional motion. Although it is conceptually useful to consider the articulation as a spherical mechanical bearing, mammalian joints develop incongruities inherent to both an adaptive loading history and the relative position of the joints.[38, 39] During early development, when substantial portions of both the femur and acetabulum are composed of cartilage, precision of fit between the separate components is less critical to the dynamics of articulation than when a more static conformation is acquired. Were joint surfaces to remain incongruent during large stresses of weight, the articular surfaces would rapidly deteriorate. Fortunately, the compliance of the cartilaginous surfaces of the separate joint components coupled with synovial fluid accommodates the necessary apposition during the load phase of articulation. Because many of the properties of synovial lubrication depend on contact with articular surfaces, incongruencies may bear some functional role in distribution of synovial fluid.[40]

During the early condensation of the limb axis, an investment of mesodermal cells surrounds the bones as periosteum and the joints as capsule. Essentially continuous along the contour of the skeletal axis, the morphology is clearly demarcated at the transition of capsule and periosteum. Whereas the periosteum is strongly adherent to the diaphyseal and metaphyseal aspect of the developing bone, the capsule is inadherent and inelastic, spanning and sustaining the joint as an articulation of two separate entities. Attachment occurs at the separate metaphyses of the femur and the acetabulum, within which is supported a vascular synovium. Although the collagenous capsule is inelastic, its sites of attachment are morphologically dynamic enough to permit growth and continued expansion of the articular surfaces without restricting motion. The hip joint capsule is reinforced by the iliofemoral, pubofemoral, and ischiofemoral ligaments, and yet remains sensitive to stretch and serves as a mechanism for muscular feedback and pain.

The iliofemoral ligament (Bigelow's ligament) resembles an inverted Y. The apex of the ligament originates from the anteroinferior iliac spine and traverses the anterior aspect of the hip joint before dividing as a broad, thickened longitudinal band that attaches along the anterior intertrochanteric line. The iliofemoral ligament limits hyperextension and lateral rotation of the hip joint and is taut in full extension. Full extension of the hip exposes the capsule and ligaments to a twisting and shortening effect that forces the head onto the acetabulum and may increase intracapsular pressure, especially when a hemarthrosis is present.[41] The dynamics of such action may warrant consideration of the biomechanical imposition that an emergence of postnatal hip extension brings to a structure that has developed under the protracted mechanical bias of flex-

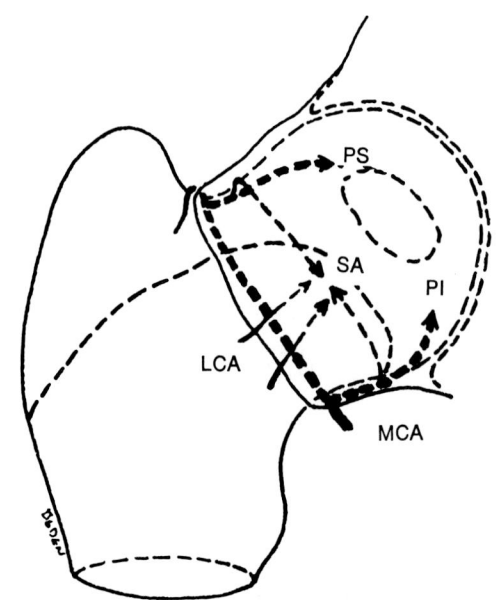

Fig. 10. Several large vessels entering the chondroepiphysis characterize the superior region. A subsynovial intracapsular anastomosis (SA) is derived from posterosuperior (PS) and posteroinferior (PI) branches of the medial circumflex artery (MCA). The lateral circumflex artery (LCA) contributes little anteriorly to this anastomosis.

ion. Little information is available detailing the relative set point of capsular fibroblast matrix elaboration with respect to chondrocyte matrix synthesis. In this regard, taking into account the inelastic nature of ligament with respect to the moldable cartilage matrix, a posterosuperior compressive force may develop as a result of ligamentous tethering. Anatomically, this restrictive force would be most pronounced during a transition from flexion to extension, suggesting that inherent genetic competence may be one factor that determines the capacity for balance between the two tissue phenotypes, especially during developmental periods of shallow acetabular depth.

CONCLUSION

Successful development and maturation of the hip require progressive integration of varying congenital, environmental, and morphological stimuli over an extensive span of time to ensure that the physiology of the adult joint will accurately reflect the paired function of the separate components. Development remains a continuum of proactive and reactive biological events that sustain capacity to render mechanical competence to the hip in static posture or ambulation, withstanding changing loads through adaptive modeling. It is this dynamic component of the developing hip that confers mobility to a spectrum of human and nonhuman morphotypes.

Because growth and development of both the acetabulum and the proximal femur are dependent on cell and tissue mechanisms of endochondral ossification, initially small differences in structures may lead to large-scale divergence over a course of progressive development. Understanding normal morphology of the developing hip brings a certain prognostic value to clinical assessment by extending a basis for recognizing how aberrant immature structures might later compromise adult tissue biomechanical performance.

REFERENCES

1. Streeter GL: Development horizons in human embryos. A review of the histogenesis of cartilage and bone. Contr Embryol Carn Inst 1949; 33:149.
2. Bardeen CR, Lewis WH: The development of the limbs, body-wall and back in man. Am J Anat 1901; 1:1.
3. Shubin N, Tabin C, Carroll S: Fossils, genes, and the evolution of animal limbs. Nature 1997; 388:639.
4. Saunders JW, Gasseling MT: Ectodermal-mesenchymal interactions in the origin of limb symmetry. In Fleischmajer R, Billingham RA (eds): Epithelial-Mesenchymal Interactions. Baltimore, Williams & Wilkins, 1968, p 78.
5. Pinot M: Le role du mesoderme somitique dans la morphogenese precoce des membres de l'embryon de Poulet. J Embryol Exp Morphol 1970; 23:109.
6. Geduspan JS, Solursh M: A growth-promoting influence from the mesonephros during limb outgrowth. Dev Biol 1992; 151:242.
7. Strayer LM Jr: Embryology of the human hip joint. Clin Orthop 1971; 74:221.
8. Brickell PM, Tickle C: Morphogens in chick limb development. Bioessays 1989; 11:145.
9. Brockes JP: Retinoids, homeobox genes, and limb morphogenesis. Neuron 1989; 2:1285.
10. Eichele G: Pattern formation in vertebrate limb. Curr Opin Cell Biol 1990; 2:975.
11. Bryant SV, Gardiner DM: Retinoic acid, local cell-cell interactions, and pattern formation in vertebrate limbs. Dev Biol 1992; 152:1.
12. Fuhr G, Richter E, Zimmerman H, et al: Cell traces: Footprints of individual cells during locomotion and adhesion. Biol Chem 1998; 379:1161.
13. Zimmermann H, Hagedorn R, Richter E, et al: Topography of cell traces studied by atomic force microscopy. Eur Biophys J 1999; 28:516.
14. Parkinson D: Human spinal arachnoid septa, trabeculae, and "rogue strands." Am J Anat 1991; 192:498.

15. Lewis EB: A gene complex controlling segmentation in *Drosophila.* Nature 1978; 276:565.
16. Dolle P, Izpisua-Belmonte JC, Falkenstein H, et al: Coordinate expression of the murine Hox-5 complex homeobox containing genes during limb pattern formation. Nature 1989; 342:767.
17. Duboule D, Dolle P: The structural and functional organization of the murine HOX gene family resembles that of *Drosophila* homeotic genes. EMBO J 1989; 8:1497.
18. Lewin SO, Opitz JM: Fibular A/hypoplasia: Review and documentation of the fibular developmental field. Am J Med Genet 1986; 2:215.
19. Ganey TM, Ogden JA, Carey T, et al: Morphologic and histologic characterization of Fibular Dimelia. J Pediatr Orthop, 2000; 9:24.
20. Gardner E, Gray DM: Prenatal development of the human hip joint. Am J Anat 1950; 87:163.
21. Ponseti IV: Growth and development of the acetabulum in the normal child. J Bone Joint Surg 1978; 60:575.
22. Ogden JA: Skeletal Injury in the Child, 3rd ed. New York, Springer-Verlag, 2000.
23. Ogden JA: Hip development and vascularity: Relationship to chondroosseous trauma in the growing child. In The Hip. St. Louis, MO, CV Mosby, 1981, vol 9.
24. Zander G: Os acetabuli and other bony periarticular calcifications at the hip joint. Acta Radiol (Stockh) 1943; 24:317.
25. Ganey TM, Love SM, Ogden JA: Development of vascularization in the chondroepiphysis of the rabbit. J Orthop Res 1992; 10:496.
26. Ogden JA: Changing patterns of proximal femoral vascularity. J Bone Joint Surg Am 1974; 56:941.
27. Chung SMK, Batterman SC, Brighton CT: Shear strength of the human femoral capital epiphyseal growth plate. J Bone Joint Surg 1976; 58:94.
28. Chung SMK: Embryology, growth, and development. In Steinberg ME (ed): The

Hip and Its Disorders. Philadelphia, WB Saunders, 1991.
29. Carter DR, Wong M: Mechanical stresses and endochondral ossification in the chondroepiphysis. J Orthop Res 1988; 6:148.
30. Ilizarov GA: Basic principles of transosseous compression and distraction osteosynthesis. Ortop Travmatol Protez 1971; 32:7.
31. Ilizarov GA: The tension-stress effect on the genesis and growth of tissues. Part I. The influence of the rate and frequency of distraction. Clin Orthop 1989; 238:249.
32. Ganey TM, Ogden JA, Sasse J, et al: Basement membrane composition of cartilage canals during development and ossification of the epiphysis. Anat Rec 1995; 241:425.
33. Hensinger RN: Standards in Pediatric Orthopedics. New York, Raven Press, 1986.
34. Chung SMK: Hip Disorders in Infants and Children. Philadelphia, Lea & Febiger, 1981.
35. Walker JM: Comparison of normal and abnormal human fetal hip joints: A quantitative study with significance to congenital hip disease. J Pediatr Orthop 1983; 3:173.
36. Watanabe RS: Embryology of the human hip. Clin Orthop 1974; 98:8.
37. Ulloa I: Embryonic and fetal development of the vascular system of the proximal end of the femur and acetabulum in man. Z Orthop 1962; 96:306.
38. Bullough PG, Goodfellow JW, Greenwald AS, et al: Incongruent surfaces in the human hip joint. Nature 1968; 217:1290.
39. Goodfellow JW, Bullough PG: Studies on age changes in the human hip joint. J Bone Joint Surg Br 1968; 50:222.
40. Greenwald AS: Biomechanics of the hip. In Steinberg ME (ed): The Hip and its Disorders. Philadelphia, WB Saunders, 1991, p 357.
41. Ogden JA: Injury to growth mechanisms of the immature skeleton. Skeletal Radiol 1981; 6:237.

DEVELOPMENTAL DYSPLASIA OF THE HIP: DIAGNOSIS AND TREATMENT OF THE NON-AMBULATOR

section 9

chapter 16

John M. Roberts

Summary

- Clinical differentiation of subluxation from dislocation is critical.
- Pathoanatomic obstructions to reduction become worse in the untreated dislocation.
- Reducibility of dislocation determines initial treatment.
- Abduction devices (harness, brace, cast) maintain (not obtain) reduction.
- Appropriate imagery (ultrasonography, radiography, arthrography) helps monitor treatment.
- Closed reduction is usually successful before walking age.
- Possible complications of treatment include redislocation and avascular necrosis of the femoral capital epiphysis.

Developmental dysplasia of the hip (DDH) is an abnormal formation of the hip joint, the result of multiple factors affecting growth. At the time of diagnosis, one of the following types most likely defines the abnormality: dislocation, dislocatable, subluxation, subluxatable, or acetabular dysplasia.

Developmental dislocation means that no contact exists between the articular surfaces of the femoral head and the acetabulum. A dislocatable hip implies that the femoral head rests in a position of total or partial contact with the articular surface of the acetabulum but can be positioned so that all contact is lost. Developmental subluxation means that partial contact is maintained between articular surfaces, but the femoral head is not centered in the acetabulum (the center of rotation of the femoral head does not coincide with the center of rotation of the acetabulum). A subluxatable hip can be positioned so that contact between the articular surfaces is decreased but not eliminated. A hip may be dysplastic without dislocation or subluxation; the acetabulum is shallow and oriented more vertically than normal.

Precise identification of the type of malformation in a specific patient is critical to selecting appropriate treatment. As well, the age and gender of the patient may influence choice of treatment and eventual outcome. Untreated or inadequately treated, one abnormality can lead to another, even during the relatively short period from birth to walking age covered in this chapter.

The incidence of developmental dislocation requiring definitive treatment is probably one to two cases per thousand live births.[1] There is wide variation among ethnic groups. Prevalences of 2% to 20% are reported in Central Europe. Prevalences between 0.2% and 2.0% have been found in Northern Europe and North America. The incidence is lowest among Chinese and black Africans. In some countries, the use of ultrasonography for screening the hips of newborns has produced a much higher apparent incidence of DDH. Recently, Bialik et al[2] reported a sonographic incidence of 55 per thousand compared with a true incidence of 5 per thousand requiring treatment. Ninety percent of the sonographically pathological hips developed normally without treatment.

DDH is six times more frequent in females than males. The left hip alone is involved in 60% of cases, the right hip in 20%, and both hips in 20%. If one child has DDH, the risk to each subsequent sibling is approximately 6%; if one parent has DDH, the risk to each newborn is 12%; if one parent and one child have DDH, the risk to subsequent children increases to 36%. There is a 40% concordance in identical twins. It follows that risk factors include female gender, positive family history, and involvement of the left hip.

Other risk factors are manifestations of fetal packing: first born baby (50% to 60% of patients with DDH); breech presentation (16% have DDH); congenital muscular torticollis[3] (8% to 20% have DDH); congenital subluxation (hyperextension) of knees; and oligohydramnios. Postnatal positioning of a newborn's lax hip joint in adduction may be harmful; a strong message to avoid swaddling comes from the higher prevalence in areas where this custom is practiced (among Native Americans, northern Italy).

PATHOGENESIS

The inheritance pattern of DDH is considered multifactorial. Wynne-Davies[4] suggested that the increased joint laxity could be a dominant pattern and acetabular dysplasia polygenic.

At birth, the capsule of the hip joint is a loose sleeve that may allow the femoral head to ride out of the socket onto the acetabular rim (subluxation) or beyond (dislocation). A deficient superior and posterior rim of the acetabulum contributes to instability. There is disagreement as to whether the rim abnormality represents a growth deficiency[5, 6] (neolimbus) or inversion of a more developed acetabular labrum.[7, 8] The size of an inverted limbus may vary in extent from a marginal structure to an extensive curtain covering a major portion of the articular surface of the acetabulum (Fig. 1). In any case, the dislocated hip lies in a capsular pocket formed by distention of the capsule superiorly and posteriorly.

In most newborns, the dislocated femoral head can be lifted over the acetabular rim to be repositioned in the acetabulum. Once the flexor (iliopsoas), adductor (adductor longus, adductor brevis, pectineus), and medial hamstring muscles (gracilis, semitendinosus, semimembranosus) become contracted, reduction is prevented. The anterior capsule becomes an obstruction as it is held against the articular surface of the acetabulum by the purse-string action of

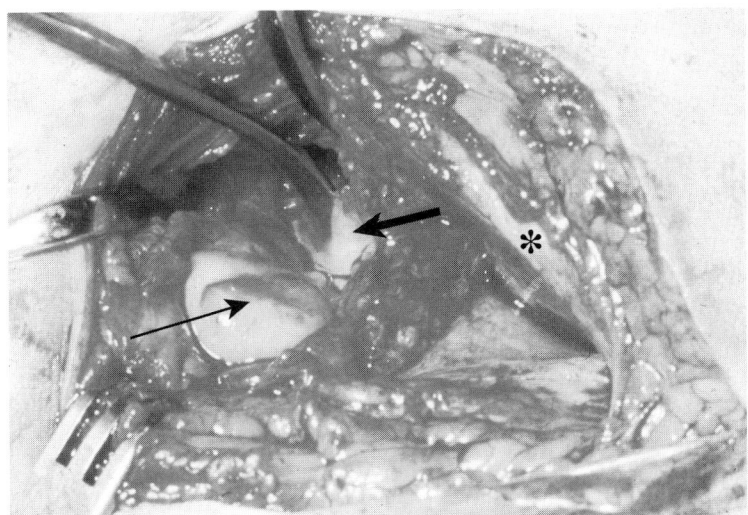

Fig. 1. Pathoanatomy of left DDH at time of anterior-approach open reduction. The joint capsule has been opened and the ligamentum teres excised. The tip of the dural elevator lies underneath the inverted limbus *(large arrow)*. Note the flattening of the medial aspect of the femoral head *(small arrow)*. *Iliac crest.

the iliopsoas in its course to insert in the lesser trochanter (Fig. 2). A constricted isthmus forms between the tight anterior capsule and the inverted limbus. The cartilaginous femoral capital epiphysis is often larger than the isthmic opening to the true acetabulum. As well, intra-articular structures obstruct reduction: the ligamentum teres is hyperplastic, the pulvinar is hypertrophic, and the transverse ligament crossing between the arms of the horseshoe-shaped acetabulum is thick and tight (Table 1).

Structural abnormalities of the acetabulum and upper femur pose problems in maintaining reduction. The femoral head, flattened medially, may skid upward and backward in a shallow, more vertically oriented, acetabulum, particularly if there is deficiency of the rim. With the hip extended and rotated laterally, increased anteversion of the upper femur may contribute to anterior subluxation. A

good understanding of the many-faceted pathoanatomy of DDH is essential to interpretation of clinical features.

CLINICAL FEATURES

The pathognomonic sign of developmental dislocation of the hip remains Ortolani's "segno dello scotto," a palpable jump of the femoral head over the acetabular rim.[9] The flexed and adducted hip is held gently with one hand (the examiner's right hand for the patient's left hip, or vice versa) with the long finger down and hooked over the tip of the trochanter while the examiner's other hand steadies the pelvis (Fig. 3). Gentle elevation of the proximal femur brings the dislocated femoral head over the edge of the acetabulum and into the socket. Abduction of the hip at this point usually maintains the femoral head in the reduced position. The Ortolani sign is a sensation similar to that of driving an automobile over a speedbump in the road. It is especially important that the infant be completely relaxed in order to find this valuable sign.

The provocation Barlow sign[10] is the reverse maneuver in which the femoral head is guided, with a jump, from a position of reduction to a position of dislocation beyond the rim of the acetabulum. Gentle downward pressure on the thigh is applied with the hip in adduction and flexion. The Barlow maneuver may give a feeling of instability or pistoning without the jump of a frank dislocation, thereby identifying the subluxatable hip.

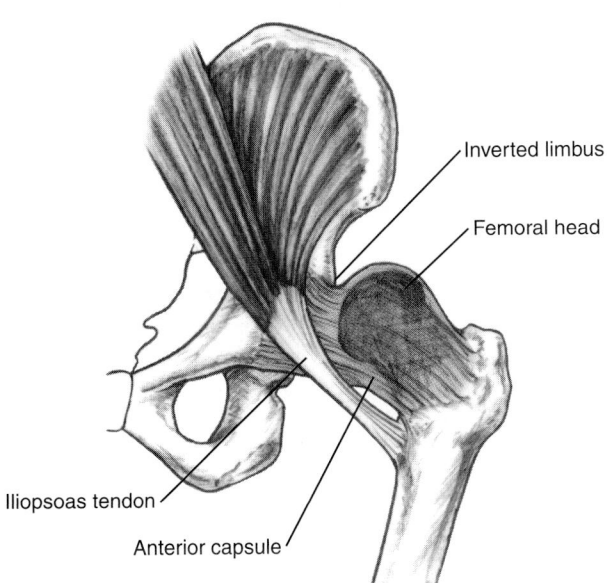

Inverted limbus

Femoral head

Iliopsoas tendon

Anterior capsule

Fig. 2. Drawing. This is a schematic drawing of the relationships of the inverted limbus, anterior capsule, and the iliopsoas tendon to the dislocated femoral head.

TABLE 1. OBSTRUCTIONS TO REDUCTION OF DDH
• Inverted limbus (neolimbus)
• Anterior capsule
• Muscle contracture:
Iliopsoas
Hip adductors
Medial hamstrings
• Hypertrophied ligamentum teres
• Hyperplastic pulvinar
• Transverse acetabular ligament

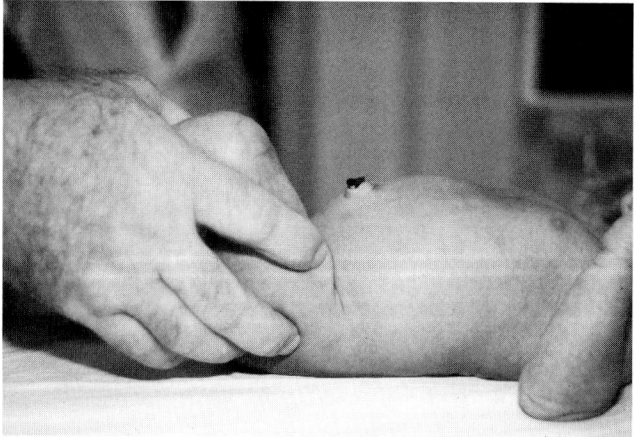

Fig. 3. Position. These are the proper positions of the examiner's hand and the infant's hip when the examiner is eliciting the Ortolani or Barlow sign.

As the child's hip matures during the first 6 months of life, the Ortolani and Barlow signs gradually disappear in the untreated hip. The flexor, adductor, and hamstring muscles become contracted and prevent reduction or displacement of the femoral head relative to the acetabulum. Instead, there is limitation of abduction of the hip joint. If both hips are dislocated and irreducible, there is bilateral limitation of abduction, more difficult to appreciate than in the unilateral dislocation. The Galeazzi sign is positive in the unilateral, but not in the bilateral, dislocation: the knees lie at different levels when the patient is placed supine with hips and knees flexed to 90 degrees. Nelaton's line is an imaginary line from the tip of the trochanter through the ipsilateral anterosuperior iliac spine. A high trochanter is found by medial extrapolation of Nelaton's line: if it passes through the umbilicus or above, the alignment of the trochanter relative to the pelvis is probably normal; if the medial extrapolation passes below the umbilicus, the trochanter is abnormally high. As a sign of DDH, asymmetrical skin creases of the thigh are notoriously unreliable, but gluteal creases at different levels may indicate proximal displacement of the upper femur on the side of the proximal crease. Ruwe et al[11] described a technique for clinical assessment of femoral anteversion. The patient is positioned prone with the hip extended and the knee flexed to

90°; the hip is rotated medially until maximum prominence of the greater trochanter is felt, and anteversion is measured by the angle between the tibial shaft and the true vertical.

INVESTIGATION

Options for imagery include ultrasonography, radiography, dynamic arthrography, computed tomography (CT) scan, and magnetic resonance imaging (MRI) (Table 2). Ultrasonography shows the nonossified femoral head and its relationship to the acetabulum quite well in the infant up to 4 months of age. It has the advantage of being a real-time study and avoids radiation. As well, deep sedation or anesthesia is not required. Beginning at age 4 months, an anteroposterior radiograph is useful for estimating the depth of the acetabulum. As soon as the ossific nucleus for the femoral capital epiphysis appears, the relationship of the femoral head to the acetabulum can be assessed. Dynamic arthrography is an invasive procedure, performed with the patient under general anesthesia; it is very useful in assessment of the quality of closed reduction and, in some cases, subsequent appraisal of postreduction remodeling. CT scanning is used by some to confirm maintenance of reduction in the casted infant younger than 1 year of age. The disadvantages of MRI are expense and the need for anesthesia in the infant, without providing a dynamic study.

ULTRASONOGRAPHY

Graf, an Austrian orthopaedic surgeon, introduced the use of ultrasonography for the diagnosis of developmental dysplasia of the hip in infants.[12] He constructed a classification based on angles measured in the coronal plane. The alpha angle compares the vertical reference line representing the anterior border of the ilium with a line tangent to the roof of the acetabulum. The beta angle compares the index line with a line through the acetabular labrum. Graf maintained that an alpha angle less than 43 degrees indicated dislocation, an angle between 43 and 50 degrees indicated subluxation, an angle between 50 and 60 degrees could be found in immature hips without being pathological and an angle greater than 60 degrees was normal.

Harcke et al[13, 14] in the United States and Terjesen et al[15] in Norway showed that instability of the hip could be demonstrated by dynamic ultrasonography. Harcke showed

		TABLE 2. IMAGERY OF DDH		
Method	**Indications**	**Advantages**		**Disadvantages**
Ultrasonography	Infant < 4 mo	No anesthesia Dynamic study No radiation		Overread Overtreatment
Radiography	Infant > 4 mo	Quantitative assessment: (acetabular index, center-edge angle)		Radiation exposure Cartilage radiolucent Static study
Arthrography	Closed reduction	Shows joint surfaces Dynamic study		Radiation exposure Requires anesthesia Invasive procedure
CT scan	Assess reduced hip in cast	Identifies posterior redislocation		Radiation exposure

encroachment of the femoral capital epiphysis on the posterior rim of the acetabulum when the Barlow maneuver was carried out in a subluxatable hip. Terjesen's bony rim percentage (BRP) compared the distance from the acetabular floor to the lateral bony rim of the acetabular roof with the distance from the acetabular floor to the lateral joint capsule. Terjesen maintained that the BRP represented the percentage of the femoral head covered by the osseous acetabular roof and that all unstable hips had a BRP below the limit of normal (44% in girls and 47% in boys). Terjesen's BRP is not the same as Reimers' index[16] which measures the portion of the femoral head medial to Perkins' line[17] compared with the diameter of the femoral head. Ultrasonography uses as reference the anterior border of the ilium, whereas Perkins' line on the anteroposterior radiograph is a vertical line drawn at the lateral edge of the acetabulum.

Early on, ultrasonography was used in some centers to screen all newborn infants.[2, 15] Other centers developed programs to evaluate hips in high-risk infants, e.g., positive family history, breech presentation, torticollis, plagiocephaly, oligohydramnios, hyperextended knees.[14, 18, 19] A subset of hips with normal clinical examination but abnormal ultrasonography findings was then recognized. At first, these hips were treated actively, but more recently, some workers have chosen to observe clinically stable hips, even with ultrasonographic abnormality, until reevaluation by physical examination and radiography when the patient reaches 4 months of age. Castelein et al[20] showed that only four hips ultimately required treatment in a cohort of 144 neonatal hips, which were clinically stable but had ultrasonographic abnormalities initially. Terjesen et al[21] found 306 infants with ultrasonographic abnormalities who were clinically normal; at 4 to 5 months 291 had developed normal hips without treatment, and 15 infants achieved normalcy after subsequent treatment in an abduction splint. At this time, clinical instability (the Ortolani or Barlow sign) remains the primary indication in the newborn for definitive treatment, even in the case of an abnormal ultrasonographic examination.

Ultrasonography is a convenient method for confirming maintenance of closed reduction in a Pavlik harness.[22, 23] The study can be performed successfully without removing the abduction device. If a hip becomes redislocated and remains held in the abnormal position, posterior rim deficiency of the acetabulum may become worse. To avoid such damage, ultrasonography is performed weekly until the reduction stabilizes.

Ultrasound examination is useful as a no-risk procedure to reassure parents and treating physician that a hip "click" need not be treated. Bond et al[24] showed in a prospective study of 50 infants with hip clicks that the average alpha angle was 62 degrees in the clicking hips compared with 63 degrees in the uninvolved hips. All hips had more than 50% femoral head coverage by the acetabulum. All hips were stable on dynamic ultrasonography.

Currently, primary indications for ultrasonography include confirmation of clinical impression, reassurance of stability in normal at-risk or clicking hips, and monitoring of treatment in the Pavlik harness. As Catterall[18] emphasized in 1994, the cornerstone of diagnosis is the physical examination (Fig. 4).

RADIOGRAPHY

Radiographs become useful when an infant reaches the age of 4 to 6 months. The Y line of Hilgenreiner is drawn through the triradiate cartilages at the most distal point of the ilium in each acetabulum (Fig. 5). The acetabular index describes the direction of the acetabular roof relative to the Y line of Hilgenreiner: a line is drawn through the edge of the acetabulum medial and downward through the distal point of the ilium in the triradiate cartilage. Tonnis[25] found that in girls younger than 2 years of age, acetabular indices greater than 36 degrees indicated mild dysplasia, and indices greater than 41 degrees indicated severe dysplasia. Errors in the determination of the acetabular index can be caused by rotation of the pelvis and flexion/extension variations of the pelvis when the anteroposterior view is taken. Portinaro et al[26] found that if the rotation of the pelvis is confined to +/- 5 degrees, the maximum error induced by rotation is 3 degrees; if flexion/extension of the pelvis is confined to +/- 10 degrees, the maximum error induced is 3 degrees. Broughton et al[27] found inter- and intraobserver errors of +/- 6 degrees for the acetabular index. A decrease in the acetabular index during the first year after reduction indicates a favorable prognosis.

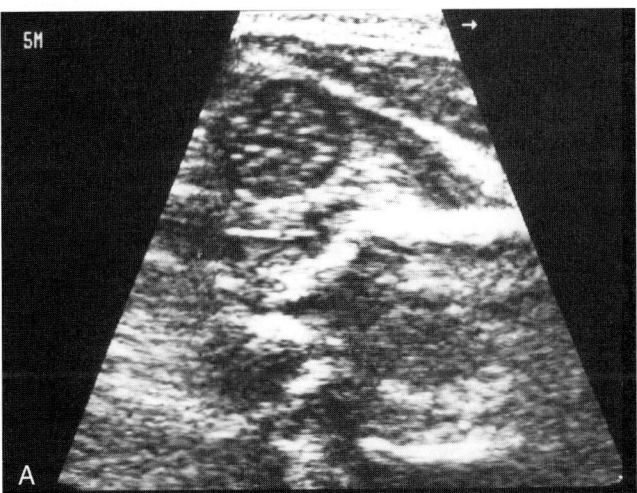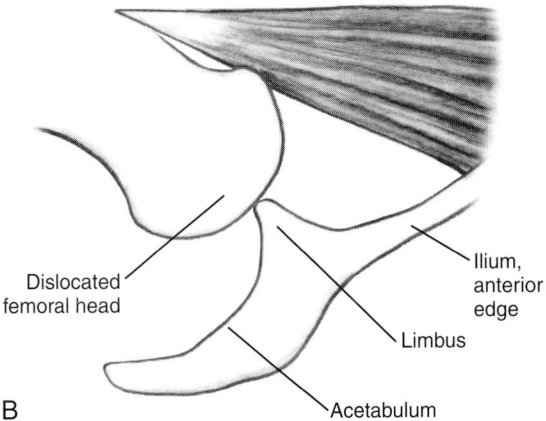

Fig. 4. View. Shown is the dislocation of the femoral head on ultrasonography in coronal plane *(A)*; see *B* for details.

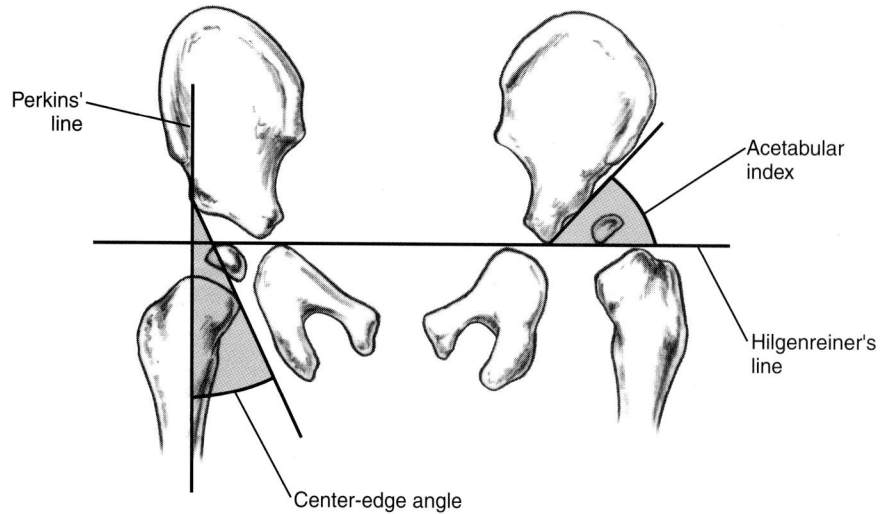

Perkins'
line

Acetabular
index

Hilgenreiner's
line

Center-edge angle

Fig. 5. Drawing. This is a schematic drawing of the anteroposterior radiogram of an infant's pelvis with left DDH showing the acetabular index and the center-edge angle.

The structure of the teardrop (medial wall of the acetabulum) also has prognostic significance. A persistent V shape indicates thickening of the acetabular floor, which implies an incomplete reduction.[28] Albinana et al[29] found that hips with a persistent V-shaped teardrop were usually Severin class IV at the time of skeletal maturity, predictive of a poor prognosis for adult years.

In some cases, the femoral capital epiphysis has started to ossify by the time the first radiograph is made at 4 to 6 months. The relationship of the femoral head to the acetabulum can then be ascertained. Perkins' line is drawn at the edge of the acetabulum perpendicular to the Y line of Hilgenreiner. The center edge angle of Wiberg[30] compares a line drawn through the ossific nucleus of the femoral capital epiphysis and the edge of the acetabulum with Perkins' line. A center edge angle of more than 20 degrees indicates successful reduction. The relationships of the ossific nucleus of the femoral capital epiphysis to Perkins' line and to a horizontal line placed at the edge of the acetabulum define Tonnis'[1] classification of DDH: group I means that the ossific nucleus is medial to Perkins' line; group II means that the ossific nucleus is lateral to Perkins' line but distal to the horizontal line at the edge of the acetabulum; group III means that the ossific nucleus is lateral to Perkins' line and lies at the edge of the acetabulum; and group IV means that the ossific nucleus is superior to the edge of the acetabulum. Group I signifies a normal or reduced hip; group II may be either a subluxated or dislocated hip; groups III and IV are most likely dislocated.

DYNAMIC ARTHROGRAPHY

Severin[8] popularized the use of arthrography for the assessment of DDH. Contrast material is introduced into the hip joint through an anterior, medial, or lateral approach. An image intensifier enables dynamic assessment. The arthrogram is most helpful at the time of reduction. Before manipulation, obstructions can be identified. The shape and position of the limbus can appear as a rounded eminence at the rim or an in-folding of labrum and capsule that lies between the acetabulum and the femoral head. The isthmus

between the limbus and the anteroinferior capsule is narrowed. Hyperplasia of the ligamentum teres, the transverse ligament, and the pulvinar can often be visualized. Indentation of the anteroinferior capsule by the iliopsoas tendon can be seen as a filling defect..

After reduction, the remaining gap between the articular surface of the femoral head and the acetabulum is measured by the transverse diameter of the intervening dye pool. This is an important factor in the quality of reduction. The risk of avascular necrosis climbs to 25% if the gap measures more than 6 mm.[1]

The dynamic arthrogram also provides accurate assessment of stability of reduction, a guide to the optimum position for postreduction immobilization. The "safety zone" of Ramsey et al[31] is defined as the range of motion from 50 degrees of abduction to the point at which the hip redislocates when it is adducted. Similarly, the flexed and abducted hip can be carried into extension, the physician noting the point at which the femoral head redislocated. Additionally, the effect of extending the knee on the reduced hip can be appraised. Tightening the hamstrings by extension of the knee may force the femoral head out of the acetabulum. In such cases, the postreduction cast should hold the knee in flexion and hold the hip reduced in moderate abduction and flexion.

At time of subsequent cast change or removal, dynamic arthrography may be used to estimate stability and the extent of soft-tissue remodeling. In a successful response to reduction, the inverted limbus of the acetabulum remodels to contain the femoral head.[32] As well, attrition of the hyperplastic ligamentum teres, pulvinar, and transverse ligament occurs. The femoral head comes to lie in contact with the medial wall of the acetabulum, without a gap between the articular surfaces.

COMPUTED TOMOGRAPHY SCAN

The use of a CT scan for patients younger than 1 year of age is usually limited to assessing a formal closed reduction and casting. After the patient has recovered from general anesthesia, isometric contraction of the hip flexors and adductors can cause redislocation, even in a well-applied cast. An anteroposterior radiograph, while useful in determining the position of the femoral head relative to the acetabulum in the coronal plane, cannot rule out a recurrent posterior dislocation. CT scan cuts through the affected hip will indicate whether the femoral head is anterior or posterior to the acetabular rim. Three-dimensional reconstruction from a CT scan is used mostly to assess deformity in the older child.

MAGNETIC RESONANCE IMAGING

Kashiwagi et al[33] developed a classification of DDH based on MRI. In type A, the femoral head is displaced posteriorly but still lies in contact with the inner wall of the acetabulum (subluxation). In type B, the center of the femoral head lies at the edge of the acetabulum (severe subluxation). In type C, the femoral head is displaced posterior to the acetabular edge (dislocation). A rounded or inverted configuration of the posterior limbus can be visualized. But the authors conceded that MRI is expensive, requires sedation, and is impractical to perform in all patients with DDH. Similarly, Fisher et al[34] showed that the MRI demonstrated qualitative information not available on plain films but did not recommend routine use in the evaluation of DDH.

DIFFERENTIAL DIAGNOSIS

Differentiation of adventitious clicks from a true Ortolani or Barlow sign may be problematic, particularly for the inexperienced clinician. Sources of clicks include impingement of the iliopsoas tendon on the anterior aspect of the upper femur, impingement of the iliofemoral aponeurosis on the greater trochanter, and impingement of the hamstrings on the femoral condyles. Clicks usually resolve with rapid growth of the patient during the first year. No treatment is required. Stability can be confirmed by dynamic ultrasonography.

The clinical finding of a high trochanter is not pathognomonic of a dislocated hip. It is also found in infantile coxa vara[35] and proximal focal deficiency (PFFD). In coxa vara and PFFD, the femur is truly short in overall length from femoral head to distal condyles. Coxa vara may be misdiagnosed as DDH in the neonatal hip when the femoral head is not yet ossified on radiographs and the trochanter appears proximal to the acetabulum; ultrasonography or arthrography will show the femoral head reduced in the acetabulum. In PFFD, the femoral head may be present and reduced, or it may be absent. Other deficiencies in the same limb may be noted: short fibula, absent toes, instability of the knee (deficient cruciate ligaments), and limitation of eversion/inversion of the foot (tarsal coalition). Moreover, the thigh in PFFD is usually very short.

MANAGEMENT

If physical examination of a newborn's hip(s) (Fig. 6) reveals a positive Ortolani sign, indicating easy reducibility of a dislocated hip, the patient is placed in an abduction device to maintain reduction until the hip stabilizes by soft-tissue remodeling. Currently in North America, the most popular device is the Pavlik harness (Fig. 7).[22, 23, 36] It

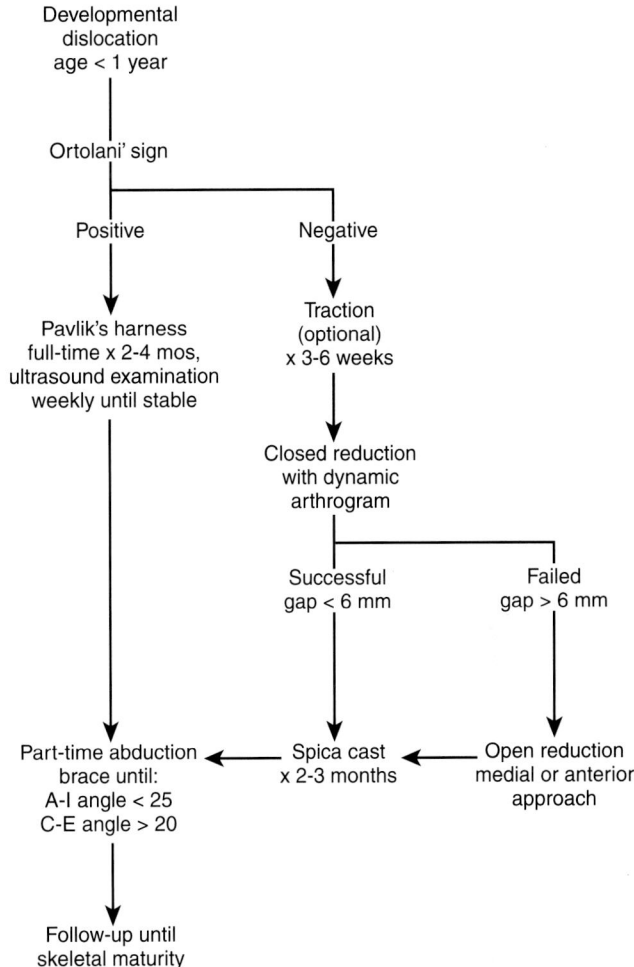

Treatment of Developmental Dislocation Under Walking Age

Fig. 6. Algorithm. This outlines treatment of developmental dislocation of the hip in the patient younger than walking age.

consists of a circumferential band placed at the nipple line to which shoulder straps and lower extremity stirrups are attached. The stirrups are adjusted so that each hip is held in 100 to 110 degrees of flexion and between 25 and 50 degrees of abduction. It is important to gauge flexion of the hip by the anterior surface of the thigh. The posterior surface of the thigh may lead one to think that there is more hip flexion than actually exists. A circumferential strap just distal to the knee, which attaches to the medial longitudinal and lateral longitudinal stirrup straps, is carefully adjusted so that the medial longitudinal strap cannot move laterally over the front of the knee with consequent loss of hip abduction. The circumferential leg strap should not chafe skin in the popliteal fossa as the patient flexes and extends the knee through a limited range. If the hip is flexed too much in the harness, there is danger of femoral neuropathy. If the hip is abducted too much, there is danger of avascular necrosis of the femoral capital epiphysis. If too much adduction is allowed, the hip may redislocate. It is helpful to confirm reduction with ultrasonography, easily done without removing the harness.

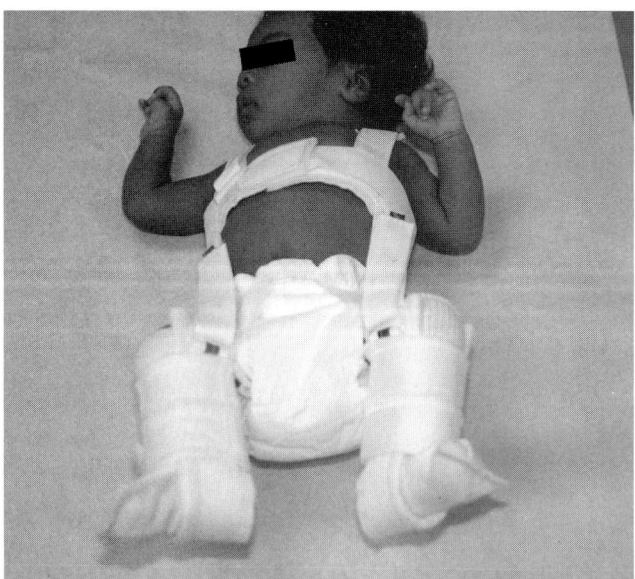

Fig. 7. Infant in a Pavlik harness. The harness has been applied to maintain closed reduction.

The parents are instructed in diapering, bathing, and clothing their baby without removing the harness, worn continuously until the reduction stabilizes after 3 to 4 weeks. In the beginning, the patient returns weekly for physical examination and ultrasonography to make sure that the hip remains reduced. Once the hip feels stable to clinical examination, confirmed by dynamic ultrasonography, the stirrups can be adjusted so that both hips are brought down to a position of 90 degrees of flexion. Harness treatment is continued for not less than 2 months. A longer period in the harness may be indicated for the child with generalized joint laxity whose hip stabilizes slowly. A longer period may also be needed if the initiation of treatment is delayed. The Pavlik harness is appropriate up to the age of 6 months. Thereafter, the child may overpower the harness with active motion of the extremities. Alternative devices include the Frejka pillow and the von Rosen splint, both of which tend to force the hips into more abduction than desired.

After the period of full-time splinting, part-time abduction splinting, either in harness or a removable plastic orthosis, may be continued in order to stimulate deepening of the acetabulum with growth. Beginning at age 4 months, an anteroposterior radiograph of the pelvis is made, taking care to position the patient with pelvis and lower extremities in neutral rotation. The acetabular index is measured. If the ossific nucleus has appeared in the femoral capital epiphysis, the center edge of angle of Wiberg is measured as well. Abduction splinting at night and naptime is continued until the acetabular index decreases to less than 25 degrees and the center edge angle increases to more than 20 degrees. Radiographs are repeated at reasonable intervals in order to follow development of the hip joint.

If examination of the newborn reveals a Barlow-positive dislocatable or subluxatable hip but the femoral head rests in the position of reduction in the acetabulum, the hip can be observed for 2 to 4 weeks to see if it will stabilize spontaneously.[37] If repeated clinical examination, confirmed by dynamic ultrasonography, indicates a stable reduced hip, observation continues until an anteroposterior radiograph is made at 4 months of age. If acetabular dysplasia is present, part-time abduction splinting is advised to stimulate deepening of the acetabulum until the acetabular index is less than 25 degrees and the center-edge angle is greater than 20 degrees on serial radiographs.

An irreducible dislocated hip, in a patient younger than 1 year of age, is treated by gentle manipulative closed reduction with the patient anesthetized. The use of prereduction traction for 3 to 6 weeks is controversial. Many patients used to be treated with traction in an effort to minimize the risk of avascular necrosis and increase the chance of successful reduction. Recent studies[38, 39] have indicated similar results whether traction is used or not. If traction is used, some apply split Russell's traction with the hip extended to stretch out the iliopsoas muscle. Others apply traction in a position of hip flexion with knees extended to stretch out medial hamstrings.

It is helpful to carry out closed reduction with simultaneous dynamic arthrography, using an image intensifier (Fig. 8).[8, 40] Before manipulation, 30% water-soluble radio-opaque material is injected intra-articularly. The femoral head is then positioned in the isthmus between the inverted limbus and the tight anteroinferior capsule. If the remaining gap or pool of dye between the articular surface of the femoral head and the acetabulum exceeds 6 mm, the attempt at closed reduction is aborted, and open reduction is carried out (during the same anesthesia if prior approval for this option has been obtained from the parents). If closed reduction is successful, with a gap less than 6 mm, a spica cast is applied to hold the hip in 100 to 110 degrees of flexion and no more than 50 to 60 degrees of abduction. One should be very careful to mold the cast posterior to the trochanter to help stabilize the reduction. The cast may end at the knees if prior examination of the reduced hip did not show loss of reduction with extension of the knee or rotation of the hip medially or laterally. If extension of the knee or rotation caused loss of reduction, the cast is extended to the supramalleolar level bilaterally.

After the infant has awakened from anesthesia, a CT scan through the casted hip is obtained to confirm maintenance of reduction in the sagittal plane (Fig. 9). The postreduction cast is continued for 8 to 12 weeks. Shoulder straps crossed in the back are attached to the proximal trim line of the cast to keep the infant down in the cast in order to maintain the desired amount of hip flexion. Instructions in cast care are given to the parents. If the cast becomes soaked with urine, skin sores may develop. Gortex liners are helpful.[41] Change of cast requires general anesthesia with attendant risks.

Stability is assessed by clinical examination when the spica cast is changed or finally removed. At that time, a regimen of part-time abduction splinting is begun if the center-edge angle is less than 20 degrees or the acetabular index is greater than 25 degrees. As the child approaches 1 year of age, closed reduction of an untreated or persistently dislocated hip may become more difficult. If gentle closed reduction with adequate centering fails (medial dye pool

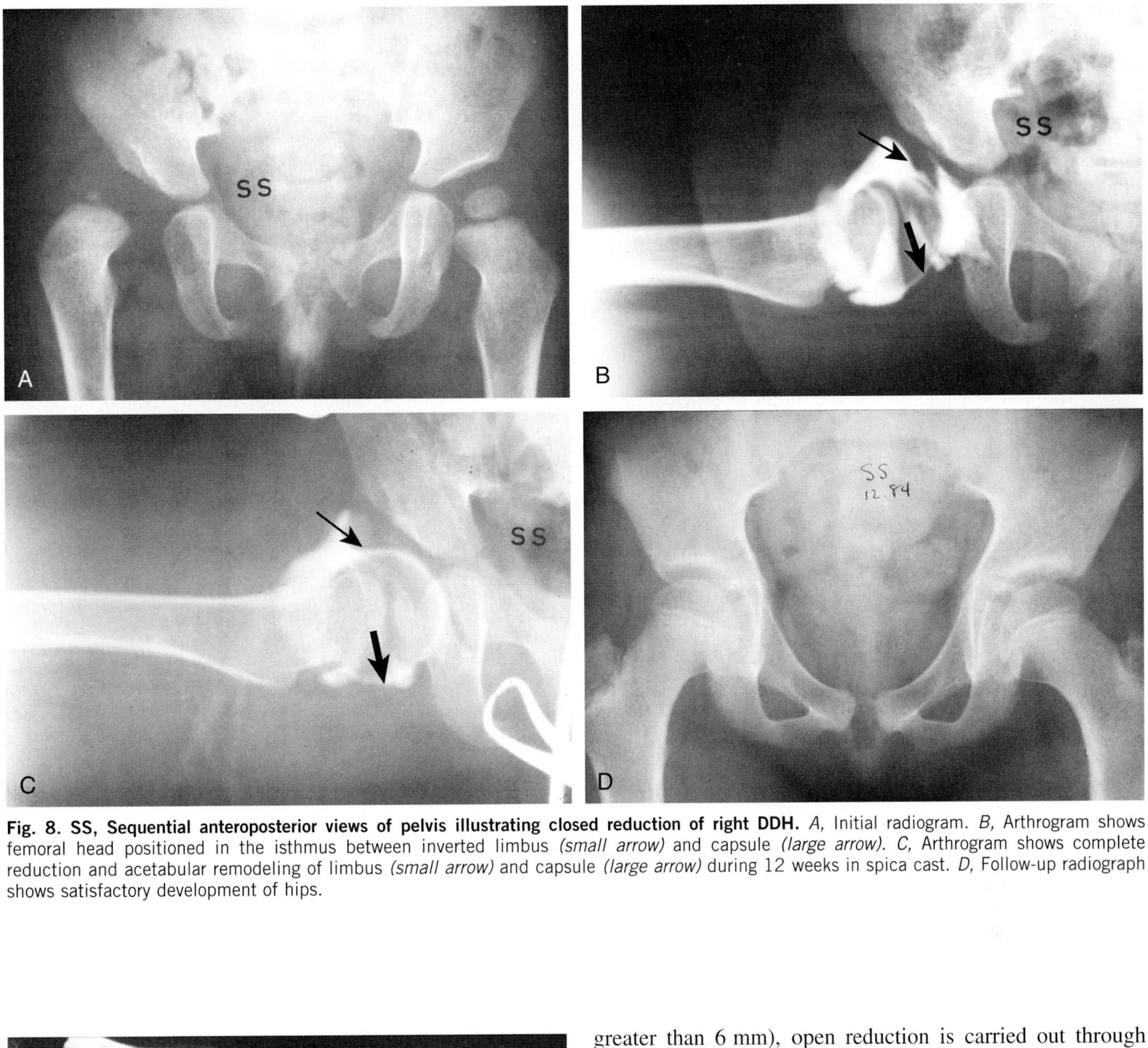

Fig. 8. SS, Sequential anteroposterior views of pelvis illustrating closed reduction of right DDH. *A,* Initial radiogram. *B,* Arthrogram shows femoral head positioned in the isthmus between inverted limbus *(small arrow)* and capsule *(large arrow). C,* Arthrogram shows complete reduction and acetabular remodeling of limbus *(small arrow)* and capsule *(large arrow)* during 12 weeks in spica cast. *D,* Follow-up radiograph shows satisfactory development of hips.

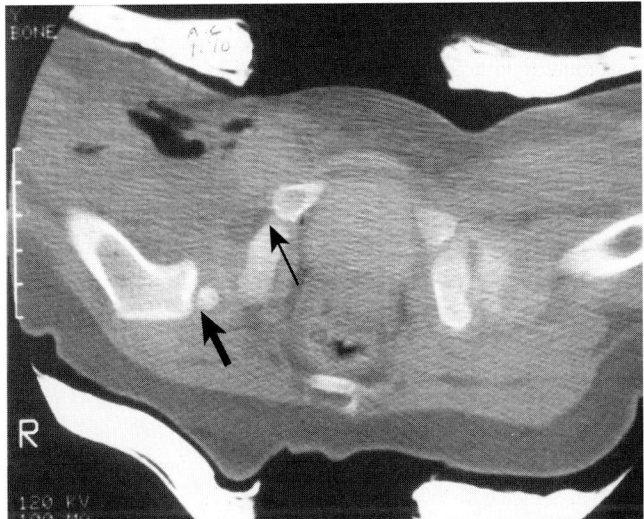

Fig. 9. CT scan. Scan shows redislocation of left hip after closed reduction and casting. *Large arrow,* dislocated (posterior) femoral head; *small arrow,* triradiate cartilage.

greater than 6 mm), open reduction is carried out through either the medial or anterior approach.

The medial approach, variously described,[42–46] may be carried out through tissue planes posterior to the adductor brevis, between the adductor brevis and adductor longus, or anterior to the adductor longus. A short transverse or longitudinal incision is made over the origin of the adductor longus. Through the chosen tissue plane, the insertion of the iliopsoas into the lesser trochanter is identified with blunt finger dissection. Hemostasis is obtained with a cautery, attempting to avoid injury to the circumflex femoral vessels. The entire iliopsoas tendon is lengthened by Z-plasty or released selectively by transecting the psoas portion of the tendon. The anterior capsule is incised with a T, placing the transverse arm parallel to the anterior edge of the acetabulum. Through the capsular incision, the femoral head can be visualized and reduced into the acetabulum. The adductor muscles are released as needed to increase the safety zone of reduction. After wound closure, a bilateral hip spica cast is applied with shoulder straps and extension to supramalleolar levels to maintain a safe position of reduction (usually abduction), external rotation, and flexion. The cast is continued for 8 to 12 weeks. Thereafter, the postoperative regimen following closed reduction is the same as described earlier.

An anterior open reduction is carried out through an incision placed one fingerbreadth distal and parallel to the anterior third of the iliac crest, extending medially to a point anterior to the femoral neurovascular bundle. After retraction of the mobilized distal flap, the interval between the sartorius and tensor fascia lata is found by blunt palpation. The superficial femoral nerve is mobilized and protected. The origin of the tensor fascia lata with the periosteum of the external surface of the anterior third of the ilium is reflected to expose the dislocated hip encased in the capsular sleeve. The iliopsoas tendon, descending medially to the joint capsule, is identified and lengthened at the pelvic brim by transection of the psoas portion or released near the lesser trochanter to enable transfer to the anterior capsule at time of wound closure.

The capsule is opened with a T-shaped incision, placing the horizontal portion parallel to and just below the anterior rim of the acetabulum. The vertical portion of the T extends distally in line with the femoral neck. Reflection of the capsular flaps exposes the femoral head and the hyperplastic ligamentum teres leading down through the isthmus to the transverse ligament at the bottom of the true acetabulum. The anterior approach affords exposure of the limbus superiorly and posteriorly. The ligamentum teres is excised, and the transverse ligament is incised. The hypertrophic pulvinar is partly excised, being careful to obtain hemostasis by using a cautery. An inverted limbus should be carefully everted, with radial cuts anteriorly and posteriorly as required. After reduction of the femoral head, the lateral capsular flap is brought medially to suture to the anterior rim of the acetabulum. The medial transposition of the lateral flap should eradicate the redundant pocket in the superior and posterior capsule. Partial excision of the pocket by removing a V-shaped wedge may be required. The medial capsular flap may be imbricated over the sutured lateral capsule or partly removed if stability of the reduced hip is not threatened. Sometimes it is possible, during capsular closure, to pass an interrupted suture through the lateral capsule and the outside surface of the edge of the everted limbus to maintain the limbus in the corrected position.

The wound is closed in layers, and the patient is placed in a one-and-a-half-hip spica cast with the hip abducted, extended, and medially rotated, usually the position of stability after anterior approach open reduction. A CT scan is obtained through plaster to confirm reduction after the patient is awakened from anesthesia. The cast is continued for 2 to 3 months, after which part-time abduction splinting is used until the acetabular index decreases to less than 25 degrees and the center edge angle increases to more than 20 degrees.

The goal of treatment in the patient's first year of life is to obtain a complete and stable reduction as soon as possible and as gently as possible.[47, 48] When this occurs, the femoral head is captured in the acetabulum, and deepening of the acetabulum is stimulated by contact with the femoral head. If femoral anteversion causes subluxation anteriorly and laterally when the hip is extended for weight bearing,

acetabular dysplasia may persist. In such cases, prolonged night-time bracing or secondary operative procedures may be indicated at an age older than 12 months.

COMPLICATIONS

Maintenance of reduction in harness or cast introduces risks of redislocation, avascular necrosis of the femoral capital epiphysis, or femoral neuropathy (Table 3).[36, 47] Contributing factors include the pathoanatomy of a specific hip and the position required to maintain reduction. Most authors caution that the hip should not be positioned in more than 50 to 60 degrees of abduction in order to avoid growth inhibition or avascular necrosis of the proximal femur. Ramsey et al[31] described a "safety zone" between too little abduction, which would lead to redislocation, and too much abduction, which would lead to avascular necrosis. Similarly, too little flexion would allow redislocation, but too much flexion might cause compression of the femoral nerve with consequent numbness of skin on the anterior thigh and weakness of active knee extension. While the patient is still anesthetized following closed reduction, it is useful to find the limits of the safety zone by using flexion/extension and adduction/abduction positioning to find where the hip redislocates in terms of the limits of abduction (50 to 60 degrees) and flexion (100 to 110 degrees). If the zone is too constricted, it may be widened by flexor or adductor releases.

Treatment of redislocation involves prompt re-reduction and application of spica cast with better molding under the trochanter and careful attention to the position of the hip as the cast is applied. Selective muscle releases (adductor longus, adductor brevis, iliopsoas) are to be considered. If redislocation occurs following a second attempt at closed reduction, open reduction by either a medial or anterior approach is indicated.

A large infolded limbus may not remodel. It continues to be interposed between the articular surface of the femoral head and acetabulum so that the femoral head remains dislocated because no contact exists between articular surfaces. The upper femur will stand out from the acetabulum on follow-up radiographs. Rather than assume subluxation associated with anteversion, one should be careful to rule out interposition of limbus with arthrography.

When dislocation persists in a hip still held in flexion and abduction by a Pavlik harness or spica cast, increased deformation of the posterior rim of the acetabulum occurs from the pressure of the femoral head and the strap-like ligamentum teres running up to it from the bottom of the

TABLE 3. COMPLICATIONS OF TREATMENT OF DDH
• Redislocation
• Persistent subluxation after successful reduction:
Acetabular dysplasia
Femoral anteversion
• Avascular necrosis of upper femur
• Infection after invasive procedures
• Femoral nerve compression
• Skin breakdown under casts

acetabulum. Posterior rim deficiency increases the difficulty of subsequent reduction. Viere et al[49] noted that dislocated hips that did not reduce in Pavlik's harness were more likely to require subsequent open reduction. Jones et al[50] found that 13 out of 19 hips required surgery to obtain stable, located hips after failure of reduction in a Pavlik harness (Pavlik's disease). Furthermore, persistent posterior acetabular deficiency may destabilize a previously reduced hip after innominate osteotomy or derotation osteotomy of the upper femur. The message is clear: an abduction device, whether harness or orthosis, should be limited to maintaining reduction rather than obtaining reduction. It is prudent to apply a Pavlik harness only to infants who have Ortolani-positive hips, indicating easy reducibility.

The relative tightness of the isthmic ring formed by the infolded limbus and the taut anteroinferior capsule may present a significant barrier at the entrance of the acetabulum. Severin[8] has shown that the constriction ring dilates if the femoral head is held against it. But others have shown that if the distance between the articular surface of the femoral head and medial wall of acetabulum is too great (manifestation of a tight ring), avascular necrosis becomes a greater risk. Race and Herring[51] showed that the gap should not exceed 7 mm. Tonnis[1] showed that the risk of avascular necrosis increases from 6% to 25% when the gap exceeds 6 mm.

The diagnosis of avascular necrosis is made on serial radiographs during the months following reduction. The criteria of Salter et al[52] include failure of the ossific nucleus of the femoral head to appear within 1 year after reduction, failure of growth of an existing ossific nucleus within 1 year after reduction, broadening of the femoral neck within 1 year after reduction, increased radiographic bone density followed by fragmentation of the femoral head, and residual deformity of the femoral head and neck when reossification is complete (coxa magna, coxa plana, coxa brevis).

Avascular necrosis is classified by Kalamchi and MacEwen[53] as follows: type I—involvement of the epiphysis alone, with fragmentation and usually good recovery of femoral head shape; type II—growth inhibition of the lateral portion of the subcapital growth plate, which may cause progressive coxa valga; type III—involvement of the proximal epiphysis and the central part of the subcapital growth plate, causing coxa brevis with overriding trochanter contributing to a gluteus medius limp in later years; type IV—extensive involvement of the entire epiphysis and growth plate, causing severe coxa brevis (Fig. 10). Treatment of residual deformities resulting from avascular necrosis is usually carried out when the patient is older than walking age, beyond the scope of this chapter.

Segal et al[54] have questioned whether one should wait until the ossific nucleus appears in the femoral capital epiphysis before attempting closed reduction. They offer evidence that closed reduction of the unossified femoral head increases the risk of avascular necrosis, compared with hips reduced later after the appearance of the ossific nucleus. This suggests that the ossific nucleus protects the overlying cartilage from potentially damaging compression. However, Luhmann et al[55] confirm early reports that age at time of closed reduction is not a factor. Assuming that reduction is gentle and that positioning for maintenance of

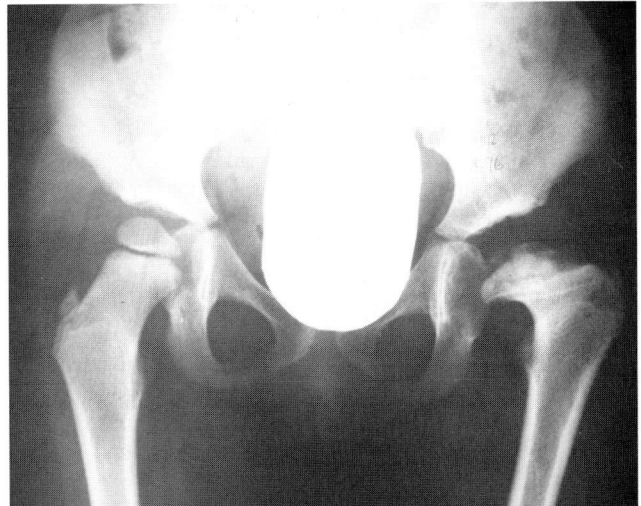

Fig. 10. Type IV avascular necrosis of the left femoral capital epiphysis. This is after repeated closed reduction attempts followed by open reduction and upper femoral osteotomy.

reduction is appropriate, the authors believe that reduction should be carried out when the dislocation is diagnosed.

RESULTS

The literature indicates that 90% to 95% of Ortolani- or Barlow-positive hips respond to treatment in the Pavlik harness before 4 months of age. In 1988, Grill et al[56] reported the results of 3611 hips in 2636 patients treated with a Pavlik harness and examined 1 to 9 years later by a European Paediatric Orthopaedic Society study group. In Tonnis grade II and III hips, the reduction rate was 92%. In 79 Tonnis grade IV hips, the rate of avascular necrosis was 16%. Overall, the avascular necrosis rate was 2.4%.

Fujioka et al[57] reported the results of 150 hips that were monitored for more than 20 years after treatment with a Pavlik harness; 35 hips (22%) showed variable grades of deformity of the femoral head or neck or both. Results were defined by Severin's classification: 106 hips class I, 10 hips class II, 30 hips class III, 8 hips class IV, and 4 hips class V. Clinical results were measured by the Japanese Orthopaedic Association scale; scores were 97.46 ± 5.63 for all hips.

In 1994, Malvitz and Weinstein[5] reported the results of 152 hips in 119 patients managed by closed reduction and monitored for an average duration of 30 years. The average Iowa hip score was 91 points (range 38 to 100 points). Thirty-five hips were rated Severin class I, 35 class II, 28 class III, 53 class IV, and 1 class V. Growth disturbance in the proximal femur was noted in 91 hips (60%). Sixty-five hips (43%) had radiographic evidence of osteoarthritis. Seventeen hips had undergone total hip replacement arthroplasty. The importance of obtaining a concentric reduction early on and avoiding growth disturbance was emphasized.

Complete reduction as the best predictor of success was echoed in papers by Chen et al,[58] Tanaka et al,[32] and Forlin et al.[59] Weintroub et al[60] compared the growth and development of dislocated hips reduced in early infancy with those of a group of normal controls; they showed that a dislocated hip, properly reduced, tends to develop normally at a more rapid rate over a longer period. However, a delay in development may indicate the need for a secondary surgical procedure.

In 1997, Morcuende et al[45] reported the long-term outcome after medial-approach open reduction in 93 hips in 76 children. The average age at time of operation was 14 months, but the range was from 2 to 50 months. The average age at follow-up was 11 years, with the range from 4 to 23 years. Sixty-six hips (71%) had excellent or good results; 24 (26%) had fair results; three (3%) had poor results according to the Severin classification system. However, growth deformities were more prevalent than anticipated: 22 hips (24%) had type II avascular necrosis, 13 hips (14%) had type III, 3 (3%) had type IV, and 2 (2%) had nonclassified lesions. The authors make the point that the unanticipated large number of hips with type II lesions (growth inhibition of the lateral portion of the subcapital physis) can be ascribed to the emergence of this complication over a longer follow-up.

Mankey et al[44] reviewed the results of open reduction by Ludloff's technique performed in 66 hips in 63 children who had operations at an average age of 12 months (2 to 63 months) and who were monitored for 6 years (range 2 to 13 years). In 33% of the hips, pelvic osteotomy was performed subsequently for acetabular dysplasia. As well, avascular necrosis was noted in 10 hips (13%). Even in the best of hands, a medial-approach open reduction fails to avoid growth disturbances either in the femur or acetabulum.

Anterior-approach open reduction is performed infrequently in infants younger than walking age because closed reduction with or without muscle lengthening is often successful. In 1995, Wenger et al[61] reported the results of open reduction with femoral shortening and frequently pelvic osteotomy in children younger than 2 years of age. The five hips treated (patients younger than 1 year of age) were teratological dislocations in three patients with dysmorphic conditions (arthrogryposis, congenital muscular dystrophy, and Pierre-Robin syndrome). The results in all five hips were reported as satisfactory at 5 to 11 years follow-up.

REFERENCES

1. Tonnis D: Congenital Dysplasia and Dislocation of the Hip in Children and Adults. New York, Springer-Verlag, 1984.
2. Bialik V, Bialik GM, Blazer S, et al: Developmental dysplasia of the hip: A new approach to incidence. Pediatrics 1999; 103:93.
3. Walsh JJ, Morrissy RT: Torticollis and hip dislocation. J Paediatr Orthop 1998; 18:219.
4. Wynne-Davies R: Heritable Disorders in Orthopaedic Practice. Oxford, England, Blackwell Scientific Publications, 1973.
5. Malvitz TA, Weinstein SL: Closed reduction for congenital dislocation of the hip: Functional and radiographic results after an average of thirty years. J Bone Joint Surg Am 1994; 76:1777.
6. Weinstein SL, Ponseti IV: Congenital dislocation of the hip: Open reduction through a medial approach. J Bone Joint Surg Am 1979; 61:119.
7. Scaglietti O, Calandriello B: Open reduction of congenital dislocation of the hip. J Bone Joint Surg Br 1962; 44:257.
8. Severin E: Congenital dislocation of the hip: Development of the joint after closed reduction. J Bone Joint Surg Am 1950; 32:507.
9. Ortolani M: Un segno poco noto et la sua importanza per la diagnosi precoce di prelussazione congenita dell'anca. Ferrara, Italy, Fatti dell'accademia medica, 1936.
10. Barlow TG: Early diagnosis and treatment of congenital dislocation of the hip. J Bone Joint Surg Br 1962; 44:292.
11. Ruwe PA, Gage JR, Ozonoff MB, et al: Clinical determination of femoral anteversion: A comparison with established techniques. J Bone Joint Surg Am 1992; 74:820.
12. Graf R: New possibilities for the diagnosis of congenital hip joint dislocation by

ultrasonography. J Paediatr Orthop 1983; 3:354.
13. Grissom LE, Harcke HT: Sonography in congenital deficiency of the femur. J Paediatr Orthop 1994; 14:29.
14. Harcke HT, Kumar SJ: Current concepts review: The role of ultrasound in the diagnosis and management of congenital dislocation and dysplasia of the hip. J Bone Joint Surg Am 1991; 73:622.
15. Terjesen T, Bredland T, Berg V: Ultrasound for hip assessment in the newborn. J Bone Joint Surg Br 1989; 71:767.
16. Reimers J: The stability of the hip in children. Acta Orthop Scand 1980; 184:1.
17. Perkins G: Signs by which to diagnose congenital dislocation of the hip, 1928. Clin Orthop 1992; 274:3.
18. Catterall A: The early diagnosis of congenital dislocation of the hip. J Bone Joint Surg Br 1994; 76:515.
19. Hensinger RN: The changing role of ultrasound in the management of developmental dysplasia of the hip (DDH). J Paediatr Orthop 1995; 15:723.
20. Castelein RM, Sauter AJM, de Vlieger M, et al: Natural history of ultrasound hip abnormalities in clinically normal newborns. J Paediatr Orthop 1992; 12:423.
21. Terjesen T, Holen KJ, Tegnander A: Hip abnormalities detected by ultrasound in clinically normal newborn infants. J Bone Joint Surg Br 1996; 78:636.
22. Hangen DH, Kasser JR, Emans JB, et al: The Pavlik harness and developmental dysplasia of the hip: Has ultrasound changed treatment patterns? J Paediatr Orthop 1995; 15:729.
23. Montgomery GBH, Harcke HT, Bowen JR, et al: The management of dislocated hip with Pavlik harness: Treatment and ultrasound monitoring. J Paediatr Orthop 1997; 17:189.
24. Bond CD, Hennrikus WL, DellaMaggiore

ED: Prospective evaluation of newborn soft-tissue hip "clicks" with ultrasound. J Paediatr Orthop 1997; 17:199.
25. Tonnis D: Normal values of the hip joint for the evaluation of x-rays in children and adults. Clin Orthop 1976; 119:39.
26. Portinaro NMA, Murray DW, Bhullar TPS, et al: Errors in measurement of acetabular index. J Paediatr Orthop 1995; 15:780.
27. Broughton NS, Brougham DI, Cole WG, et al: Reliability of radiologic measurements in the assessment of the child's hip. J Bone Joint Surg Br 1989; 71:6.
28. Smith JT, Matan A, Coleman SS, et al: The predictive value of the development of the acetabular teardrop figure in developmental dysplasia of the hip. J Paediatr Orthop 1997; 17:165.
29. Albinana J, Morcuende JA, Weinstein SL: The teardrop in congenital dislocation of the hip diagnosed late. J Bone Joint Surg Am 1996; 78:1048.
30. Wiberg G: Studies on dysplastic acetabula in congenital dislocation of the hip joint. Acta Chir Scand 1939; 83:58.
31. Ramsey PL, Lasser S, MacEwen G: Congenital dislocation of the hip: Use of the Pavlik harness in the child during the first six months of life. J Bone Joint Surg Am 1976; 58:1000.
32. Tanaka T, Yoshihashi Y, Miura T: Changes in soft tissue interposition after reduction of developmental dislocation of the hip. J Paediatr Orthop 1994; 14:16.
33. Kashiwagi N, Suzuki S, Kasahara Y, et al: Prediction of reduction in developmental dysplasia of the hip by magnetic resonance imaging. J Paediatr Orthop 1996; 16:254.
34. Fisher R, O'Brien TS, Davis KM: Magnetic resonance imaging in congenital dysplasia of the hip. J Paediatr Orthop 1991; 11:617.
35. Weinstein JN, Kuo KN, Millar EA: Con-

genital coxa vara: A retrospective review. J Paediatr Orthop 1984; 4:70.

36. Mubarak S, Garfin S, Vance R, et al: Pitfalls in the use of the Pavlik harness for treatment of congenital dysplasia, subluxation, and dislocation of the hip. J Bone Joint Surg Am 1981; 63:1239.

37. Gardiner HM, Dunn PM: Controlled trial of immediate splinting vs. ultrasonographic surveillance in congenitally dislocatable hips. Lancet 1990; 336:1553.

38. Kahle WK, Anderson MB, Alpert J, et al: The value of preliminary traction in the treatment of congenital dislocation of the hip. J Bone Joint Surg Am 1990; 72: 1043.

39. Quinn RH, Renshaw TS, DeLuca PA: Preliminary traction in the treatment of developmental dislocation of the hip. J Paediatr Orthop 1994; 14:636.

40. Liu JSC, Kuo KN, Lubicky JP: Arthrographic evaluation of developmental dysplasia of the hip: Outcome prediction. Clin Orthop 1996; 326:229.

41. Wolff CR, James P: The prevention of skin excoriation under children's hip spica casts using the Gorotex pantaloon. J Paediatr Orthop 1995; 15:386.

42. Fergusson AB Jr: Primary open reduction of congenital dislocation of the hip using a median adductor approach. J Bone Joint Surg Am 1973; 55:671.

43. Ludloff K: The open reduction of the congenital hip dislocation by an anterior incision. Am J Orthop Surg 1913; 10: 438.

44. Mankey MG, Arntz CT, Staheli LT: Open reduction through a medial approach for congenital dislocation of the hip. J Bone Joint Surg Am 1993; 75: 1334.

45. Morcuende JA, Meyer MD, Dolan LA, et al: Long-term outcome after open reduction through an anteromedial approach for congenital dislocation of the hip. J Bone Joint Surg Am 1997; 79:810.

46. Tumer Y, Ward WT, Grudziak J: Medial open reduction in the treatment of developmental dislocation of the hip. J Paediatr Orthop 1997; 17:176.

47. Gabuzda GM, Renshaw TS: Reduction of congenital dislocation of the hip. J Bone Joint Surg Am 1992; 74:624.

48. Smith WS, Badgely CE, Orwig JB, et al: Correlation of postreduction roentgenograms and thirty-one-year follow-up in congenital dislocation of the hip. J Bone Joint Surg Am 1968; 50:1081.

49. Viere RG, Birch JG, Herring JA, et al: Use of the Pavlik harness in congenital dislocation of the hip. J Bone Joint Surg Am 1990; 72:238.

50. Jones G, Schoenecker PL, Dias LS: Developmental hip dysplasia potentiated by inappropriate use of the Pavlik harness. J Paediatr Orthop 1992; 12:722.

51. Race C, Herring JA: Congenital dislocation of the hip: An evaluation of closed reduction. J Paediatr Orthop 1983; 3:166.

52. Salter RB, Kostuik J, Dallas S: Avascular necrosis of the femoral head as a complication of treatment for congenital dislocation of the hip in young children: A clinical and experimental investigation. Can J Surg 1969; 12:44.

53. Kalamchi A, MacEwen GD: Avascular necrosis following treatment of congenital dislocation of the hip. J Bone Joint Surg Am 1980; 62:876.

54. Segal LS, Boal DK, Borthwick L, et al: Avascular necrosis after treatment of DDH: The protective influence of the os-

sific nucleus. J Paediatr Orthop 1999; 19: 177.

55. Luhmann SJ, Schoenecker PL, Anderson AM, et al: The prognostic importance of the ossific nucleus in the treatment of congenital dysplasia of the hip. J Bone Joint Surg Am 1998; 80:1719.

56. Grill F, Bensahel H, Canadell J, et al: The Pavlik harness in the treatment of congenital dislocating hip: Report on a multi-center study of the European Paediatric Orthopaedic Society. J Paediatr Orthop 1988; 8:1.

57. Fujioka F, Terayama K, Sugimoto N, et al: Long-term results of congenital dislocation of the hip treated with the Pavlik harness. J Paediatr Orthop 1995; 15:747.

58. Chen, I-H, Kuo KN, Lubicky JP: Prognosticating factors in acetabular development following reduction of developmental dysplasia of the hip. J Paediatr Orthop 1994; 14:3.

59. Forlin E, Choi IH, Guille JT, et al: Prognostic factors in congenital dislocation of the hip treated with closed reduction. J Bone Joint Surg Am 1992; 74:1140.

60. Weintroub S, Green I, Terdiman R, et al: Growth and development of congenitally dislocated hips reduced in early infancy. J Bone Joint Surg Am 1979; 61:125.

61. Wenger DR, Lee C-S, Kolman B: Derotational femoral shortening for developmental dislocation of the hip: Special indications and results in the child younger than two years. J Paediatr Orthop 1995; 15:768.

DIAGNOSIS AND TREATMENT IN THE AMBULATORY CHILD WITH DEVELOPMENTAL DYSPLASIA OF THE HIP

George T. Rab

Summary
- Children younger than 6 to 9 years with unilateral dislocations or those younger than 6 with bilateral dislocations should be considered for treatment.
- Subluxation and/or persistent dysplasia on radiographs should be surgically treated.
- Concentric reduction of the hip and satisfactory range of motion are prerequisites to surgical correction of dysplasia.
- Osteotomies do not specifically correct dysplasia; they provide the mechanical stability for remodeling to correct dysplasia.
- Many surgical approaches are possible depending on the site of maximum deformity and the preference of the surgeon. All procedures require careful technique and experienced judgment.
- Salvage techniques for older children with symptoms can be beneficial, but surgery for asymptomatic hips in children older than 10 to 12 years is generally not indicated.

Walking children with developmental dysplasia of the hip (DDH) have a variety of biological and mechanical problems ranging from the untreated dislocation to complex deformities of dysplasia after treatment or avascular necrosis (AVN). There are common features to evaluation and treatment plans, and many operative procedures are applied widely to the diverse manifestations of dysplasia. However, surgeons should recognize the high level of judgment and experience required to attempt treatment of more complicated cases. Treatment of this group of patients by inexperienced orthopaedic surgeons is not recommended.

HISTORICAL REVIEW

- During approximately 1900 to 1940, Adolph Lorenz from Vienna popularized the closed method of hip reduction and casting in extreme positions for stability. There was a high incidence of AVN.
- In 1955 Karl Chiari introduced his salvage iliac osteotomy for subluxation and acetabular dysplasia.
- In 1958 Paul Pemberton of Utah described an acetabuloplasty by rotating the iliac portion of the hip downward, thus reducing subluxation and decreasing the capacity of the oversized acetabulum.
- In 1961 Robert B. Salter introduced innovative surgical correction of dysplasia by reorientation of the acetabulum based on landmark studies of acetabular dysplasia in piglets.
- In 1972 James R. Gage and Robert B. Winter linked a formal, monitored prereduction traction program to a dramatic reduction in AVN. Their study also included casting in Salter's "human position," which may have confused the reasons for improved results.

- Robert Bucholz and John A. Ogden (1978) and Ali Kalamchi and G. Dean MacEwen (1980)[1] clarified the causes of AVN and introduced a useful clinical classification.
- Ignacio Ponseti and colleagues, from Iowa, produced a series of studies on normal acetabular development and remodeling of the acetabulum after reduction. This provided a basis for understanding the natural history of DDH after treatment at various ages.
- In the late 1980s, Sherman Coleman (Utah), Malcolm Menalaus (Australia), and others questioned the value of prereduction traction and suggested that well-documented reduction and casting in flexion ("human position") are the prime factors for reducing AVN.

PATHOANATOMY

As the child with hip dislocation, subluxation, or dysplasia reaches walking age and beyond, opportunities for nonsurgical management diminish greatly. This is due in part to the continuation of soft-tissue contracture, which renders closed treatment impossible. In addition, the lack of concentric reduction impedes acetabular and femoral head development and leads to progressive dysplasia. The problems of developmental dysplasia are a continuum, but most experts recognize distinct entities that are grouped to make description and decision-making easier (Fig. 1).

DISLOCATION

The femoral head is completely dislocated from the acetabulum. This usually occurs at or near the time of birth, although there are documented cases of late dislocation associated with ligament laxity and persistent acetabular deformity. Because concentric, mobile joint surfaces have not been in contact with one another, both the acetabulum and femoral head exhibit deformity. The acetabulum is shallow, with a sloping roof and a blunted, deformed limbus. The anteroposterior diameter may decrease and, in late cases (older than 3 to 4 years), may almost resemble a gothic arch. Varying amounts of anterior wall deficiency are seen. The ligamentum teres is hypertrophic (occasionally ruptured) and adherent to the fovea, and the capsule may drape across the anterior one-half of the acetabulum and become adherent to it, completely hiding the articular cartilage in this region. The femoral head is invariably small with medial flattening, and the ligamentum teres dents the medial head as well. This is often called a "bullet-shaped" femoral head.

SUBLUXATION

The femoral head drifts from its ideal concentric position and rests, noncentered, against the superior acetabular articular surface. It is always displaced laterally but may be

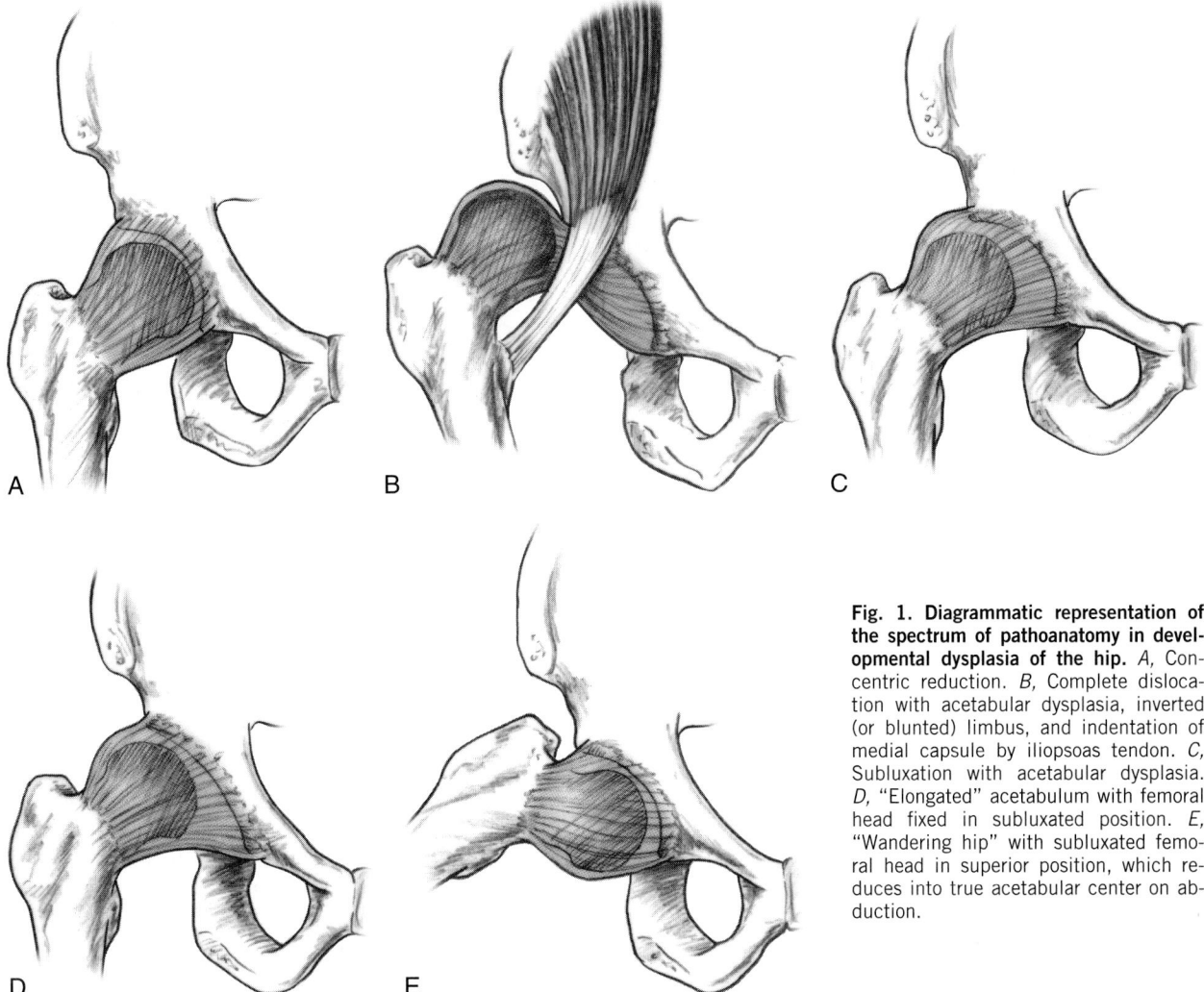

Fig. 1. Diagrammatic representation of the spectrum of pathoanatomy in developmental dysplasia of the hip. *A*, Concentric reduction. *B*, Complete dislocation with acetabular dysplasia, inverted (or blunted) limbus, and indentation of medial capsule by iliopsoas tendon. *C*, Subluxation with acetabular dysplasia. *D*, "Elongated" acetabulum with femoral head fixed in subluxated position. *E*, "Wandering hip" with subluxated femoral head in superior position, which reduces into true acetabular center on abduction.

either anterior or posterior to its optimum position. Capsular laxity and articular dysplasia are the typical causes of subluxation and are usually self-perpetuating. That is, the instability allowed by a loose capsule allows nonconcentric pressure to retard growth and ossification of the acetabulum and leads to increasing dysplasia, which facilitates increasing subluxation. Femoral head deformity may play a role, as may increased femoral anteversion, but most of the dysplasia associated with subluxation is acetabular. Subluxation is most common after treatment of dislocation (either by closed or open means), but it can be seen in older children with no history of early problems ("primary acetabular dysplasia").

DYSPLASIA

Abnormal growth patterns allow persistent anatomical deformities of either the femoral or acetabular components of the hip joint. Normal growth of the cartilage joint anlage and correct patterns of ossification appear to depend on physiological application of force across a mobile, concentric joint. Too little force leads to the atrophic dysplasia seen in the neglected hip with persistent dislocation. Excessive force applied asymmetrically (subluxation) deforms

cartilage and retards ossification, so the deformed anlage remains at high risk during growth. Biological laxity can allow subluxation, and persistent subluxation causes dysplasia. Dysplasia patterns depend on the mechanical stimulus. A hip that subluxates superiorly may eventually develop a blunting of the anterosuperior limbus and acetabular rim, with an elongated appearance on standard radiograph. In abduction, the femoral head remains displaced into the deformed portion of the acetabulum. Alternately, a lax hip may develop generalized acetabular enlargement and elongation, with superior migration with the leg in extension and inferior reduction with the leg abducted (Coleman termed this the "wandering hip").

NATURAL HISTORY (UNTREATED)

Complete dislocations that remain untreated are generally pain free until degenerative changes ensue between the femoral surface and the false acetabulum. This may occur in late middle age, although some patients have a normal life span without disabling pain. Trendelenburg's gait and limb length difference persist for the lifetime. Reconstruction in adults often requires acetabular bone graft augmen-

TABLE 1. CLINICAL FINDINGS SUMMARY		
Hip abduction	Asymmetrical, reduced to 70 degrees or less	May be normal (laxity)
Limb length	+ Galleazzi's sign (short femur when flexed)	Rarely found before 12 months or with subluxation only
Limp	Trendelenburg's, hyperlordosis	Limp is always painless

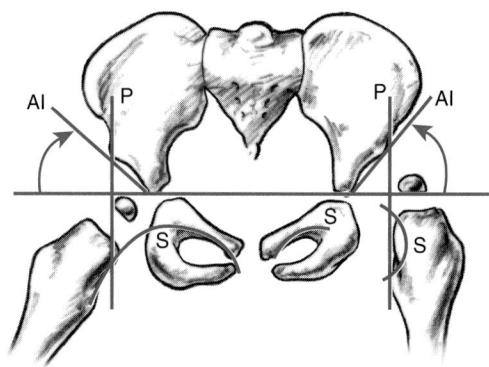

Fig. 2. Determination of radiographic lines and indexes used to assess degree of subluxation and acetabular dysplasia. The description, significance, and range in normal patients are in Table 2.

tation, femoral shortening, and customized small components.

Subluxation (true instability) generally increases during growth, leading to persistent dysplasia, which encourages increasing subluxation. In adolescence, the fibrotic hip capsule generally limits migration of the femoral head, but the degenerative changes from articular incongruence may lead to pain.

Dysplasia may worsen or resolve depending on the stability of the joint. If a concentric, stable reduction is achieved in the first 4 to 6 years of life, dysplasia may remodel with a normal or near-normal hip at maturity. If instability (subluxation) persists, dysplasia generally progresses and the result at maturity is a subluxated, frequently painful hip.

CLINICAL FEATURES

SIGNS AND SYMPTOMS

Children just beginning to walk with a dysplastic or dislocated hip may appear completely normal to parent and physician, but clinical signs develop rapidly with increasing weight and maturation (Table 1). When the hip dislocates, the lack of a stable fulcrum reduces the efficiency of all the gluteal muscles, producing increased lumbar lordosis and a Trendelenburg gait. Bilateral dislocations produce a characteristic waddling gait. Pain is always absent when dislocation is complete but may be present in older children with subluxation (usually older than 10 years) or after multiple unsuccessful surgical attempts at correction. Neglected or multiply operated cases may have thigh atrophy.

PHYSICAL EXAMINATION

The most important physical finding is lack of passive abduction of the hip. It may be subtle in cases of mild subluxation or in young children with dislocations who have significant ligament laxity. Loss of abduction that was once normal is strong evidence of progressive subluxation, even when radiographs are equivocal.

Well-recognized signs of pistoning and reduction that are seen in the newborn are absent in walking-age children, but the Galleazzi sign (asymmetrical height of knees when the knees and hips are flexed) is usually detectable.

Children who have had surgical treatment can have physical abnormalities despite successful surgery. Thigh atrophy is common, and lack of abduction may be seen in older children who have achieved concentric reduction. After pelvic osteotomies, impingement against the anterior acetabulum causes decreased flexion.

RADIOGRAPHIC DETERMINATION OF DYSPLASIA AND SUBLUXATION

Radiographic studies depend on the patient's age and the degree of previous treatment.[2] For diagnostic purposes, complete dislocations are easily appreciated in the walking child because the proximal femoral epiphyseal nucleus is

TABLE 2. RADIOGRAPHIC FINDINGS SUMMARY			
Line/angle	Drawing	Normal	Abnormal
Hilgenreiner's line	Horizontal between triradiate cartilages		
Perkin's line	Vertical (perpendicular to Hilgenreiner's line) through acetabular edge		
Acetabular index	Angle between Hilgenreiner's line and line between triradiate cartilage and acetabular edge	<25 degrees at 12 months of age, decreasing to 20 degrees at 36 months	>30 degrees at age 12 months or failure to decrease (remodel) over 2–3 years
Center-edge angle	Angle between Perkins' line and a line between acetabular edge and center of epiphysis	~22 degrees at 12 months, 30 degrees at 24 months	<20 degrees or grossly asymmetrical
Shenton's line	Curved line along medial femoral neck, and the inferior margin of the superior pubic ramus	Smooth curve	Broken line (may be unreliable because of femoral position)
"Teardrop"	Formed by cortex of acetabular fossa, cotyloid notch, and inner pelvis	Concave, progressive narrowing	Thick, convex, and not remodeling 6–12 months after reduction

visible, even if delayed in appearance. A more important role of plain radiographs is the longitudinal assessment of dysplasia, especially of the acetabulum. Serial acetabular index measurements, center-edge determinations, and qualitative evaluation of the "teardrop" are helpful for decision-making after reduction[3] (Fig. 2). Some surgeons place great emphasis on specific numerical indices of dysplasia, whereas others are content to interpret films qualitatively in the context of physical exam findings.

There is no completely accurate method of assessing three-dimensional (3-D) acetabular or femoral dysplasia using standard radiographs. The surgeon exploring an untreated 3-year-old developmental dislocation will ultimately make decisions based on the surgical anatomy and not the radiograph.

INVESTIGATION

USE OF ROUTINE RADIOGRAPHIC VIEWS

For most patients, a true anteroposterior pelvis radiograph is the appropriate routine view. Rotation can distort acetabular anatomy. Older children may be standing, but if there is leg-length inequality an appropriate lift should be used. Abduction-internal rotation views tend to simulate the congruence achieved by femoral varus osteotomy, but it is questionable whether the rotational aspect is accurate. Abduction views are particularly helpful in defining the "wandering hip" with an enlarged acetabulum, which reduces in abduction. True lateral and false-profile lateral views are useful in older children for planning pelvic osteotomy.

After reduction, plain radiographs may not show anterior or posterior subluxation occurring in the spica cast.

ARTHROGRAPHY

Arthrography is a useful tool when closed reduction is performed. Besides assuring the surgeon that the joint is actually reduced, it defines the depth of reduction, anatomy of the superior limbus, and potential obstacles to reduction such as an enlarged ligamentum teres or hypertrophic foveal contents (Fig. 3). When these features are present, repeat arthrography at 2 to 4 months can indicate whether or not sufficient remodeling has occurred (see later discussion). Routine arthrography is otherwise of little clinical use in decision-making.

COMPUTED TOMOGRAPHY AND 3-D COMPUTED TOMOGRAPHY RECONSTRUCTIONS

Computed tomography (CT), or regular tomography, can be helpful after closed or open reduction when there is suspicion of posterior subluxation, which is poorly visualized in a cast by routine radiograph.

Three-dimensional CT reconstruction can provide remarkable insight into the anatomical issues of dysplasia in older children. It is clearly most useful when planning surgical treatment for a child who has undergone previous surgery, especially previous pelvic osteotomy, where it can give information that cannot be determined by other methods (e.g., direction of subluxation, degree of acetabular erosion). Descriptive classifications of hip subluxation by 3-D CT are not clinically useful currently but may lead to

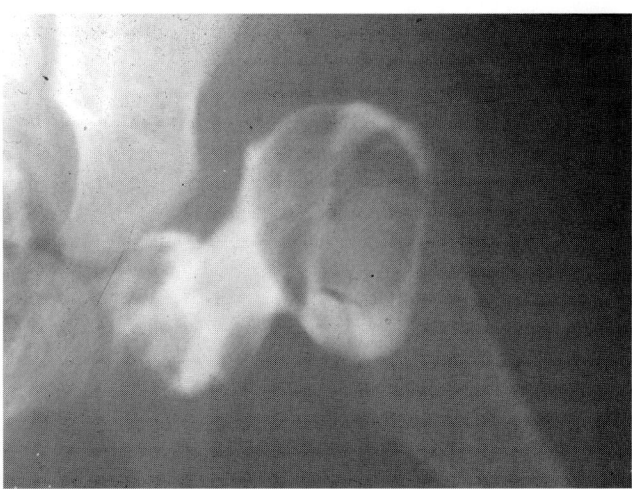

Fig. 3. Arthrogram of a dislocated hip. This view after an attempted closed reduction shows a lack of concentric positioning, subluxation, redundant ligamentum teres in the acetabular fossa, and a deep indentation of the inferior capsule from the iliopsoas tendon.

better understanding of the progressive disease of dysplasia.[4]

MAGNETIC RESONANCE IMAGING

Magnetic resonance imaging (MRI) is very sensitive for diagnosing medial synovial fluid pooling when the hip is subluxated and also allows imaging of the nonossified acetabular roof, which may be present in cartilage even when acetabular index is high on conventional radiograph. Clinicians differ on the significance of these findings for treatment selection. I have found little value of MRI in hip dysplasia.

MANAGEMENT

TREATMENT OPTIONS: DISLOCATIONS

Developmental dislocations should be treated by reduction as soon as they are discovered, with several limitations. Certain diseases may be associated with dislocations because of physiological or neurological abnormalities (e.g., diastrophic dysplasia, arthrogryposis, meningomyelocele, Down syndrome). These pathological (nondevelopmental) dislocations require a different decision-making process than the typical developmental dislocation. To complicate the issue further, children with syndromes may have concurrent developmental dislocations that should be treated; for example, occasionally treatable dislocation occurs in sacral-level meningomyelocele patients.

After 6 to 9 years of age, the chances of successfully correcting the extreme secondary dysplasia associated with dislocation decrease, and the resulting surgical outcome may be predictably worse than the natural history of untreated dislocation. There is no consensus about the upper age for surgical treatment of dislocation. Many textbooks suggest an upper limit of 6 years for bilateral dislocations and 9 years for unilateral, but these are empiric limits often based on anecdotal results and limited follow-up (Fig. 4).

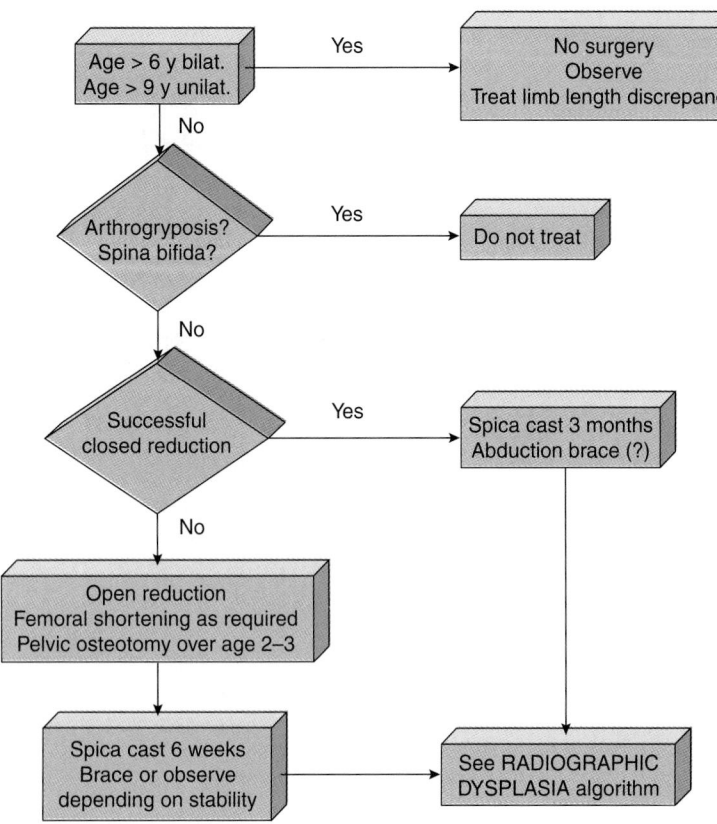

Fig. 4. Dislocation after walking age.

TREATMENT INDICATIONS

Treat the following:

- Children younger than 5 to 9 years with unilateral dislocation.
- Children younger than 5 to 6 years with bilateral dislocations.

  Do not treat the following:

- Children older than 2 to 3 years with arthrogrypotic dislocations, especially if bilateral.
- Children with spina bifida and hip dislocations, except in rare circumstances.
- Children older than 6 to 9 years with painless untreated developmental dislocations.

Closed Reduction and Spica Cast
Pros and Cons

Closed reduction and spica casting can be a useful technique until the child is several years old. Historically, open reduction was the standard approach for children of walking age, but reports of the long-term success of closed technique have firmly established it as a treatment option.[5] Closed reduction may not be possible as children age or the reduction may not be stable, but these issues can be decided rapidly under an anesthetic. Prolonged casting and brace immobilization are essential for a good result, and there may be social or medical limits on the duration of spica casting that sway the surgeon toward the use of open techniques.

Priorities

Successful closed reduction requires a deep anesthetic with relaxation. Once reduced, the hip must be stable in a position that is primarily flexed, with abduction limited to 40 to 45 degrees. Arthrography is helpful to define anatomy of the reduction, although it does not initially need to demonstrate a complete, deep reduction as long as it confirms stability and position opposite the triradiate cartilage. Spica cast immobilization for 3 months or more, followed by abduction bracing, is advisable.

Controversies

The use of prereduction traction is a highly controversial issue.[6] Initially advocated as a method to reduce the incidence of AVN after closed reduction, traction became widely used in the same era as did the use of the "human" or flexed position for postreduction casting. The dramatic decrease in AVN may, in retrospect, be related to the improved casting position, but decades passed before surgeons cautiously began eliminating the traction regimen without observing the feared increase in AVN. Although a body of literature supports reduction without traction, some surgeons continue to use it.

Open Reduction
Pros and Cons

Open reduction is the mainstay of treatment for developmental dysplasia in the walking-age child. Although it can be performed through a number of surgical approaches, anterior open reduction is most popular. It frequently requires extensive experience and judgment and meticulous anatomical dissection. There is no "cookbook" approach to open reduction. The surgeon must be prepared to modify the approach, add femoral or pelvic procedures, and otherwise alter the operation on the spot, depending on findings and stability after reduction. An improperly performed open reduction is worse than no treatment at all, and salvage may be difficult or impossible.

Priorities

The surgeon should be sufficiently experienced or have such experience immediately available to make the complex decisions about correction of concurrent dysplasia as it is encountered in the operating room. The surgical approach and dissection must be planned to define the anatomical features of the dislocation and to deal with those that either impede reduction (such as an adherent anterior capsule) or limit postoperative stability. A deep reduction must be obtained and maintained after open reduction. The hip will not "settle in" if inadequate surgery is done. Compression of the reduced joint must be subjectively assessed and femoral shortening performed if the reduction is too tight. Especially in older children (3 years and older), pelvic osteotomy may be required to maintain stability of the reduction during casting. Compulsive, persistent follow-up radiographs must confirm reduction and its maintenance, especially in the first 4 to 6 weeks, because early subluxation invariably leads to fibrosis and reduction failure.

Controversies

Surgical approach is usually anterior, through the interval defined by a Smith-Petersen incision, although a transverse skin incision is far more cosmetic than the traditional vertical scar. Although the iliac apophysis may be split, this is unnecessary unless pelvic osteotomy is also performed. The rare younger patient who has an obviously reducible hip that is unstable because of a tight iliopsoas may be approached medially (Ludloff's or Ferguson's techniques), but correction of superior deformities (limbus) is difficult through this incision.

Management of the limbus itself is controversial, especially because surgeons cannot agree on the exact pathoanatomy. It has been described as "inverted," and some surgical texts show an instrument hooked beneath it to "evert" it. However, others (including myself) believe it is "bunched up" and compressed and will remodel after reduction. Excision of the limbus is currently condemned because it contains material that will eventually ossify to form the acetabular rim. Several radial incisions may enlarge a constricted limbus that is blocking adequate reduction.

In North America, reconstruction by some form of capsulorrhaphy is common, whereas in Europe many surgeons excise portions of the capsule and rely on healing and fibrosis to generate a neocapsule. There does not appear to be a clear-cut advantage to either approach, with the exception that an excessively tight anterior capsulotomy can cause posterior subluxation in a dysplastic hip.

Open Reduction/Femoral Shortening
Pros and Cons

Femoral shortening osteotomy is not an isolated procedure for DDH. It is used in conjunction with open reduction to reduce the compressive loading after reduction. Its most important advantage is the dramatic reduction in risk of AVN when femoral shortening is used.[7] Shortening is frequently necessary in 12- to 18-month-old patients and more so with increasing age. Other than the additional scar and the need for internal fixation, there are probably few disadvantages to a properly performed femoral shortening. In general, if a surgeon is considering the procedure, the hip is better with it. The introduction of an additional procedure to a complex open reduction introduces more room for error, such as allowing malposition of the femoral fragment.[8]

Priorities

The femur should be shortened sufficiently (usually 1.5 to 2.0 cm) so that, once reduced, there is no compression of the joint. Additional shortening may be appropriate if an innominate osteotomy is to be performed simultaneously. Internal fixation (with a small-fragment plate) is essential for anatomical control of fragment position. Usually two incisions are used (anterior for the reduction and lateral for the femoral shortening), and closure of the lateral wound is best completed before the final reduction is achieved because of the manipulation required to close the wound later. The plate is usually small enough that it becomes incorporated within the femoral shaft, and routine removal is unnecessary.

Controversies

There is little understanding of the role of articular pressure on acetabular remodeling. Femoral shortening may reduce this pressure enough that acetabular growth differs from that which follows closed reduction. The decision to shorten is usually a subjective one, with difference of opinion about whether, and how much, to shorten. There is no scientific evaluation of the advantages of varus-shortening osteotomy over simple longitudinal shortening. There is also no agreement whether or not to change the rotational position of the proximal femur because the role of anteversion in causing or maintaining instability is poorly understood.

Open Reduction/Pelvic Osteotomy (with or Without Femoral Shortening)
Pros and Cons

At open reduction, acetabular dysplasia may be severe enough that pelvic osteotomy is performed concurrently. Sometimes, reorientation of the acetabulum is essential to initial postoperative stability after the reduction. At other times, because of advanced age or relative dysplasia, the surgeon may perform acetabular reconstruction because the pelvis is exposed and surgery is convenient, although not essential, at that time. Usually, femoral shortening is required in a hip undergoing open reduction that has extensive dysplastic changes.

Physiological remodeling of acetabular dysplasia occurs after stable concentric reduction of the hip. Pelvic osteotomy may be necessary to achieve that stability. However, if pelvic osteotomy is performed as a routine in younger patients (younger than 2 years), physiological remodeling may not be given an adequate chance to occur. After 3 years of age, nearly all patients will require correction of the acetabulum, and timing is the main issue.

Whether or not the surgeon is prepared to attempt correction of acetabular pathology at open reduction and femoral shortening depends not only on the disease but also the experience of the surgeon. The addition of each step adds 3-D complexity to an already complex operation and increases the risk of posterior subluxation and other complications.

Priorities

A surgeon planning combined open reduction, femoral shortening, and pelvic osteotomy must be skilled at each procedure alone before attempting them in combination. If the femoral shortening includes any derotation of femoral anteversion, the degree of correction should generally be reduced to compensate for the reduced posterior coverage introduced by acetabular procedures. Children should be at least 18 months old for successful pelvic osteotomy.

Controversies

The choice of pelvic osteotomy depends on the acetabular pathology at surgery; radiographs are generally less helpful than direct observation. Selection between individual procedures may be subjective. A spacious, stretched acetabulum can be improved by Pemberton pericapsular osteotomy, and the femoral shaft fragment removed for shortening can function as the graft. More typically, the acetabulum is small and deficient anteriorly and superiorly, and simple reorientation by Salter osteotomy improves the stability in a weightbearing position. Some acetabula are so deficient and malformed that no pelvic procedure is logical. In these cases, open reduction and prolonged casting may allow development of the acetabulum that can be secondarily reoriented by late pelvic osteotomy. Many surgeons have

preferences for individual procedures and perform them for a wide variety of pathology without specific tailoring to the observed disorder.

TREATMENT OPTIONS: RADIOGRAPHIC DYSPLASIA IN THE YOUNGER CHILD
Indications (Fig. 5)

- Children with radiographic dysplasia after closed or open reduction that fails to remodel over a period of 4 to 6 years.
- Children older than 6 years with radiographic acetabular dysplasia.
- Children older than 10 years with painful dysplasia and subluxation that can be reduced concentrically.
- Some children older than 10 to 12 years with asymptomatic subluxation and dislocation.

Role of Open Reduction in Subtle Subluxation

Some femoral heads are subluxated into the superior elongated portion of the acetabulum and do not descend deeply on abduction. This is particularly frequent in children who have undergone open reduction, because aggressive fibrous tissue can form after early subluxation and block the fovea. All reconstructive osteotomies for subluxation must be preceded by a complete, concentric reduction. In some cases, this is achieved by simply abducting the hip under general anesthesia, but in other cases a formal open reduction may be required as a prerequisite to osteotomy. Children with significant loss of motion generally have fixed subluxation requiring repeat open reduction.

Femoral Varus Osteotomy
Pros and Cons

Femoral varus osteotomy is indicated when the proximal femoral element of dysplasia (excess anteversion and coxa valga) is radiographically greater than the acetabular dysplasia. This is a subjective determination, widely variable between evaluators. The distinction between valgus and anteversion is difficult because most apparent valgus is an artifact of external rotation. On internal rotation, the neck-

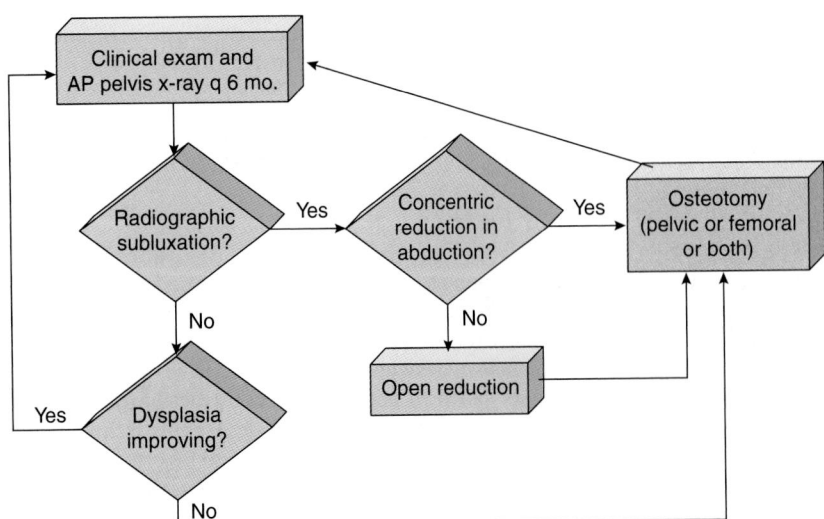

Fig. 5. Radiographic dysplasia after walking age.

shaft angle appears normal. If femoral varus osteotomy improves hip stability, acetabular dysplasia will remodel, especially before 4 years of age.[9]

Significant Trendelenburg's limping occurs after femoral varus osteotomy, especially in older children. This usually improves, but in teenagers it can become permanent. Shortening of the leg is almost inevitable, although in children younger than 8 to 10 years there may be sufficient overgrowth that normal leg length is ultimately restored. With growth, remodeling of varus is inevitable unless the degree of varus is excessive (neck-shaft angle of 110 degrees or less), in which case the undesirable overcorrection may remain.

The type of implant used generally means that a second operation for hardware removal is necessary. Sometimes this can be combined with acetabular surgery if dysplasia persists.

Priorities

Femoral osteotomy must be preceded by a concentric reduction of the hip, and there must be full range of motion of the hip. If motion is limited, adduction of the distal fragment is the expected result, and the child will be worse than if no surgery was performed. Trendelenburg's gait is minimized by limiting age to 6 years. Rigid fixation and careful radiograph control of osteotomy geometry are essential. A spica cast may be used to supplement fixation in younger children. The degree of varus should be limited so that the neck-shaft angle is greater than 110 degrees in children younger than 4 years and 120 degrees in older children. Excessive varus does not remodel completely and can be associated with atraumatic epiphyseal slippage. Results in patients with preexisting AVN are unpredictable.

Controversies

It is not understood why femoral osteotomy increases hip stability to a sufficient degree that dysplasia improves. Certainly, there is some redirection of muscle forces and a different surface contacts the acetabulum, but the extent of these changes may be minor.

The ability of femoral osteotomy to correct excessive anteversion by derotation is controversial and questionable.

In the DDH patient, advocates of derotation imply that the distal femur will remain in an anatomically normal position and the femoral neck will rotate to a more retroverted position. When the same operation is used to correct abnormal arc of hip motion, the expected result is to change the functional leg position during activity. Both outcomes cannot logically be correct.

Pelvic Osteotomy (Salter's, Pemberton's, Triple Innominate)

Reconstructive osteotomies of the acetabulum (Fig. 6) fall into two groups: those that reorient the acetabulum in space (Salter's, triple innominate), and those that alter the acetabular configuration (Pemberton's and variants). They have many features in common, but each has particular applications and limits. All are appropriate for skeletally immature patients. Once the triradiate cartilage has closed, other reorientation procedures (such as Ganz's osteotomy; see later discussion) are used.

Pros and Cons

All of the pelvic osteotomy procedures are designed to improve radiographic and anatomical acetabular dysplasia. This is generally accomplished by reducing subluxation. Pelvic procedures do not suddenly correct or eliminate dysplasia; they provide the increased stability against subluxation that provides an environment in which physiological remodeling reduces dysplasia. They are indicated when acetabular dysplasia and subluxation are present and the child still has sufficient growth remaining to allow remodeling of the dysplasia.

The reorientation osteotomies attempt to bring the acetabular surface more in line with weightbearing forces; this usually means more superior coverage. Anterior acetabular deficiency is common in this age group, and Salter's osteotomy improves anterior coverage as well. The Salter procedure, in particular, has anatomical limits to its redirection and rarely improves center-edge angle by more than 15 degrees. For patients who require more redirection, cutting the pubic and ischial bones allows 3D repositioning as required at the expense of greater surgical complexity and risk. These procedures work best when the acetabulum is

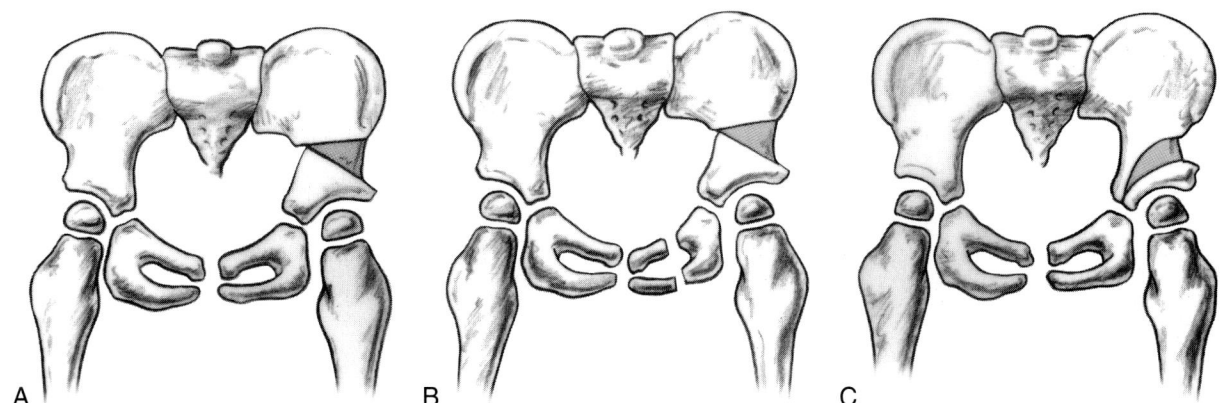

Fig. 6. Reconstructive pelvic osteotomies of the hip for skeletally immature children. *A,* Salter's innominate osteotomy. *B,* Triple innominate osteotomy. *C,* Pemberton's pericapsular osteotomy.

small and shallow but spherical, with marginal deficiency. They require a minor second procedure to remove internal fixation (usually threaded Steinmann's pins).

Pemberton's procedure changes acetabular shape and volume by hinging the superior acetabulum laterally and anteriorly through the triradiate cartilage. Because this cartilage must be open for the flexibility to perform this operation, the absolute upper age for use is 10 to 12 years or younger.[10] Younger ages than this are preferable to ensure cartilage flexibility. The ideal patient for this procedure is a child with a radiographically elongated acetabulum whose hip reduces deeply and inferiorly when abducted (a "wandering hip"). The change in shape when a 3-D concave surface is folded is complex, more akin to a crease than to the idealized reduction in size illustrated in drawings. The effect can be like a gabled roof placed on a sphere. This may give transient stiffness of the hip, but it is the increased stability afforded the hip that quickly encourages reliable remodeling and improvement of the dysplasia.

A limp will be present for 3 to 6 months postoperatively because the abductor muscles must be stripped from the ilium. Some surgeons believe that pelvic osteotomy is conceptually more difficult than femoral osteotomy, but that probably reflects the widespread experience most orthopaedists have with femoral procedures.

Priorities

A concentric reduction (ability of the femoral head to descend into the depths of the true acetabulum) and a good range of abduction are the most important prerequisites for pelvic osteotomy. If these are absent, open reduction and mobilization are necessary before application of pelvic surgery.

The surgeon should ensure that the limited correction of Salter's osteotomy will be sufficient to eliminate subluxation. In mild cases this is self-evident, but preoperative radiographs of the hip flexed 25 degrees and abducted 15 degrees can help determine success. More severe subluxation will require the increased correction afforded by triple innominate osteotomy or addition of other procedures such as femoral varus osteotomy.

Salter's osteotomy (or triple innominate osteotomy) should never be performed bilaterally and simultaneously. This renders the pelvis mechanically unstable. Only after healing and clinical recovery should the second side be corrected in bilateral cases.

An open triradiate cartilage is a necessity for Pemberton's osteotomy. Although open, this structure in late childhood may be relatively rigid, making the hinging necessary for correction difficult to obtain.

Controversies

The upper age limit for these procedures to enhance remodeling is not well defined but probably is 10 to 12 years. Beyond this age, they function to redistribute articular pressures, but they cannot be expected to affect remodeling reliably.

There are many patients in whom either Salter's or Pemberton's osteotomies might be used depending on the surgeon's preference. Both operations can successfully be repeated if required, but at some point a more extensive approach should be considered. Likewise, a subjective preoperative decision must be made about whether correction will be sufficient to correct subluxation, particularly with Salter's osteotomy. Radiographs may help (see prior discussion), but in borderline cases the surgeon must be prepared to mobilize the reoriented distal fragment by cutting the pubis (Sutherland's modification) or ischium and pubis (triple innominate osteotomy).

TREATMENT OPTIONS: SYMPTOMATIC DYSPLASIA IN THE OLDER CHILD
Indications and Age Ranges (Fig. 7)
- Children younger than 10 to 12 years with significant radiographic dysplasia.
- Children older than 10 years with symptomatic dysplasia and/or subluxation.
- Some children older than 10 to 12 years with asymptomatic subluxation and dislocation.

Femoral Osteotomy
For most patients, femoral osteotomy at this age causes

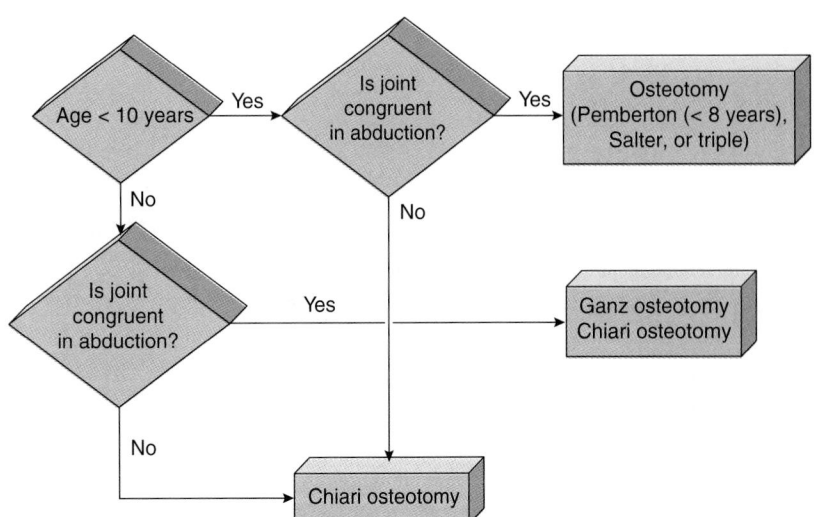

Fig. 7. Symptomatic dysplasia in the older child.

persistent limp and poor resolution of dysplasia (see prior discussion). It is generally not indicated except as an occasional adjunct to acetabular reconstruction. Concurrent distal transfer of the greater trochanter may help minimize limp.

Pelvic Osteotomy (Salter's, Triple Innominate, Ganz's, and Variants)
Pros and Cons
For most children younger than 6 to 8 years, relatively standardized Salter's or Pemberton's osteotomies are sufficient to reconstruct a dysplastic acetabulum safely. In older children, residual dysplasia may be too severe to expect correction with Salter's osteotomy. More aggressive reorientation by triple innominate[11] or Ganz's osteotomies is dependent on the patient's age. All reorientation procedures are more successful when acetabular deficiency is greater than acetabular deformity, so that a congruent hip with good support during weightbearing is achieved.

Priorities
If the child has had previous femoral or acetabular surgery, subluxation may be posterior or anterior in addition to lateral. Unless this is clear, 3-D CT can be very helpful in providing guidance for customizing later reconstructive procedures.

Because these are reconstructive osteotomies, relative congruency of surfaces is required for success. A poorly reduced hip or one with a widened or elongated profile will not improve. Salvage procedures should be used if such a hip causes symptoms.

Controversies
Surgery for older children with DDH is controversial. The potential for poor results and complications is high, so surgery is often based on symptoms (pain) rather than radiographic appearance. Not all children with troublesome dysplasia experience successful reconstruction. Multiple unsuccessful operations can render a hip permanently stiff or painful, and the surgeon must recognize when to stop. At about age 10, there is a transition in goals from creating a more normal hip to improving a painful hip. At that point, salvage procedures discussed later become more appropriate than reconstructive procedures.

Nevertheless, as imaging techniques improve and surgical procedures are refined, there is an understandable enthusiasm in some centers to reconstruct the seriously dysplastic hip that is asymptomatic. Currently, there are insufficient long-term studies to either support or refute this approach.

TREATMENT OPTION FOR SALVAGE OF INCONGRUENT HIPS
Indications and Contraindications
- Indicated in children older than 10 years with painful dysplasia and subluxation (chief indication).
- Indicated in some children older than 10 to 12 years with asymptomatic subluxation and dislocation.
- Generally not indicated in the presence of degenerative changes or flexion less than 90 degrees.

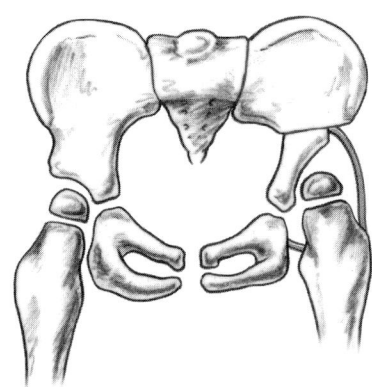

Fig. 8. Chiari's osteotomy is a "salvage," rather than reconstructive, procedure. Its success depends on the ability of the raw cancellous iliac surface to adhere to the capsule, so that the capsule undergoes metaplasia and becomes part of the articular weightbearing surface.

Note that patients with dysplasia but reducible hips are best treated by reconstructive procedures mentioned previously.

Chiari's Osteotomy
Pros and Cons
Chiari's osteotomy (Fig. 8) is a displacement of the intact hip and capsule medially beneath a raw cut through cancellous iliac bone. Ideally, the cut is made just at the superior attachment of capsule to the ilium, so the proximal bone is in direct contact with capsule and quickly fills in the area between. The capsule undergoes metaplasia into fibrocartilage, and the proximal iliac fragment becomes a weight-bearing extension of the insufficient acetabulum, functioning as a shelf to limit further subluxation proximally. The main indication for Chiari's osteotomy is pain, and it can be quite effective at achieving lasting pain relief.

Because it is a salvage procedure, Chiari's osteotomy is done without relocating a subluxated hip. Its purpose is to block further subluxation and resolve pain. Opening the hip joint at the same time is contraindicated because it lessens the inherent stability provided by the capsule and often leads to a bad result. Occasionally, the subluxated femoral head will be so proximal that the osteotomy cannot be done without entering the sacroiliac joint.

Priorities
Patients should have pain to justify subjecting them to Chiari's osteotomy. It is too significant a procedure to perform on the basis of radiographic criteria alone. Restricted abduction leads to a poor result. A patient with a Trendelenburg limp before Chiari's osteotomy will have one postoperatively. Trochanteric transfer may be combined with Chiari's osteotomy, or an alternate lateral approach, including trochanteric osteotomy, can be used (see later discussion).

The position and angle of the cut are critical to success. It must be initiated just at the attachment of the capsule to the ilium, in the "groove" just under the reflected head of the rectus femoris. If it is too low, stiffness and pain will result. The cut should angle upward slightly (10 to 15 degrees) for best femoral coverage (Fig. 9), but excessive

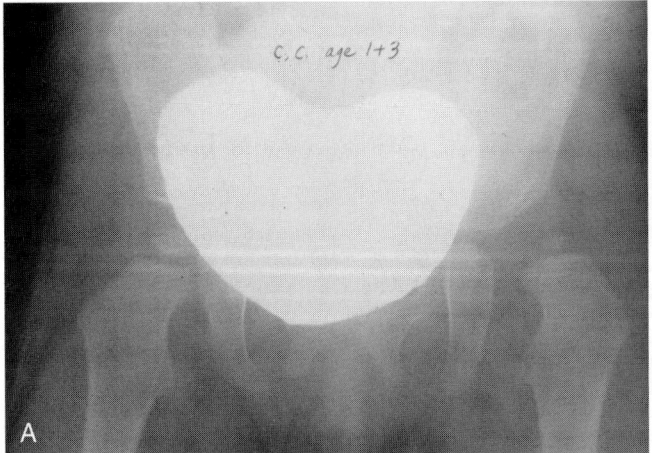

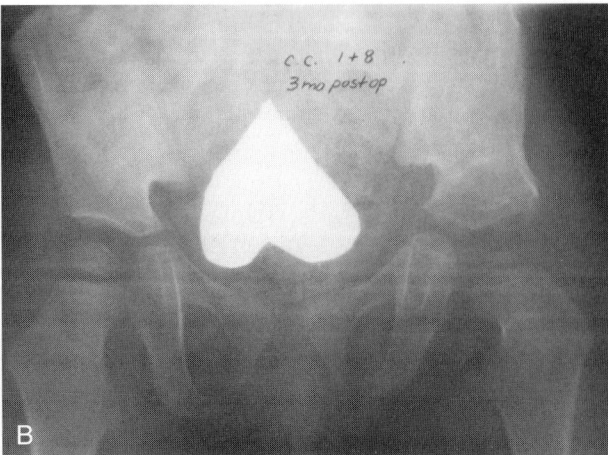

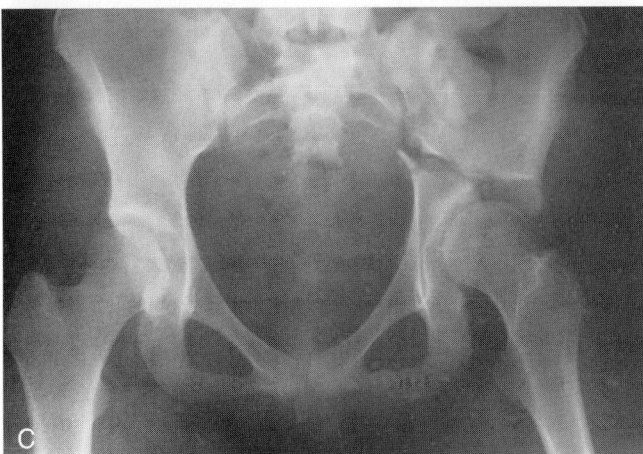

Fig. 9. Radiograph immediately following Chiari's osteotomy. Note upward tilt of osteotomy cut, position just above capsule, and medial displacement of distal fragment.

angle will exacerbate late limp. The straight cut described by Chiari may allow posterior displacement of the distal fragment, so some surgeons make a curved cut. This must be kept cylindrical (the cut planes must be parallel), and not conical, to allow displacement of the fragment.

Open reduction and capsulotomy should not be performed at the same sitting as Chiari's osteotomy. The procedure is contraindicated if significant degenerative changes are present.[12]

Controversies

As originally described, the cut is a simple transverse one. Attempts to modify the shape of the cut to make it more physiological have met with mixed success, sometimes blocking smooth displacement while failing to measurably change the outcome.

An aspect of Chiari's osteotomy that may be overlooked is the medial displacement of the hip joint afforded by the procedure. Because this occurs by hinging at the pubic symphysis, there is slight loss of posterior and superior coverage in the anatomical acetabulum, which is compensated by the cancellous "shelf" that forms postoperatively.

Reconstruction of a severely dysplastic hip by total joint arthroplasty may be simpler after Chiari's osteotomy because there is a larger surface for cementing the acetabular component. This empiric observation has not been confirmed by outcome studies.

Acetabular Shelf Procedures

Much of the discussion of these procedures is covered in the prior section on Chiari's osteotomy. In general, shelf operations (Fig. 10) are more likely to be used when minimal subluxation is accompanied by severe acetabular dysplasia and when the improvement of acetabular coverage is a higher priority than pain relief. Chiari's procedure is better for painful hips with significant subluxation.

Pros and Cons

Acetabular shelf procedures have a long and controversial history in the treatment of DDH. Like the Chiari osteotomy, an acetabular shelf can produce a mechanical block that limits subluxation with relief of pain. Shelf procedures are simpler and less invasive than Chiari's osteotomy.

A major negative to the procedure is the high rate of ultimate resorption of the graft material, which usually signifies clinical failure as well.

Priorities

Because of the high failure rate, acetabular shelf should be used cautiously for treatment of pain and not simple radiographic dysplasia. A theoretical exception to this might be the application of a shelf for a temporary goal (demonstrated subluxation during the active phase of collapse in AVN).

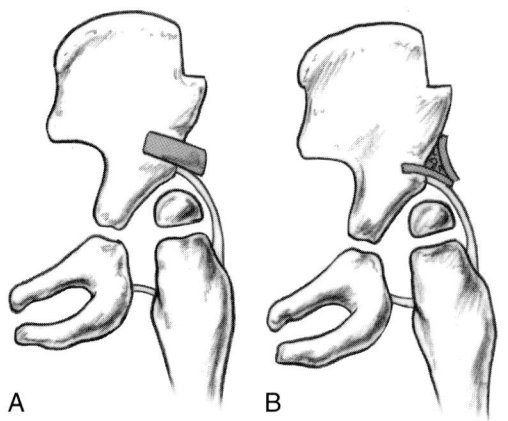

Fig. 10. Variations of the acetabular shelf procedure. *A,* Ghormley shelf uses the anterior superior iliac spine. *B,* Staheli shelf uses the reflected head of the rectus femoris to hold corticocancellous graft against the acetabulum.

Controversies

The shelf material has been varied, including cancellous or corticocancellous strips, allograft, and tricortical iliac crest graft, and long-term studies have not differentiated among them. Conceptually, graft, which is mechanically loaded, has been assumed to remain (or at least resorb more slowly), but that has not been proven scientifically.

TREATMENT OPTIONS FOR THE MULTIPLY OPERATED OR FAILED HIP
Decision-Making

The complex decision to continue operative management of a multiply operated dysplastic hip requires a clear understanding of likely goals and surgical limits. Factors to consider include the following:

- Age: complete success is unlikely in patients older than 10 years.
- Stiffness: do not attempt treatment until motion is recovered.
- Pain: a painful dysplastic hip, if mobile, is potentially treatable.
- Bilaterality: this is a relative contraindication to treatment.

SPECIFIC SURGICAL PROCEDURES

CLOSED REDUCTION: SPICA CAST
Planning and Technique

Satisfactory closed reduction of a hip after walking age is never predictable before the induction of general anesthesia. For that reason, a surgeon who is unprepared to proceed with open reduction, femoral shortening, and even pelvic reorientation osteotomy should not attempt closed reduction (see Chapter 9–16). Use of traction is controversial (see prior discussion).

The procedure itself differs little from its use in younger children. Immobilization in flexion, with no more than 40 degrees of abduction, should be the goal. Because ossification of the femoral head makes its location visible, arthrography is optional. Adductor tenotomy may be considered if

its use allows a more stable reduction in the position noted previously, but it should not encourage the surgeon to place the hip in more abduction than would not otherwise be acceptable. Immobilization for at least 12 weeks, followed by prolonged abduction bracing, is recommended.

Basic Surgical Approach to Anterior Hip and Pelvis

Most operations used for DDH require exposure of the anterior pelvis and hip. These generally rely on the Smith-Petersen approach, but a far more cosmetic skin incision can be made with excellent visualization. A small transverse inguinal incision suffices for open reduction, whereas a more extended, more oblique skin incision laterally over the iliac crest is appropriate for pelvic osteotomies (Fig. 11A).

After the skin is mobilized and the lateral femoral cutaneous nerve isolated, the interval between sartorius and tensor is developed, exposing the rectus (see Fig. 11B). The straight head of rectus femoris may be tagged or cut; there is no agreement on this point. The abductors are swept laterally with a periosteal elevator, and the iliopsoas is swept medially, exposing the capsule with the reflected head of the rectus femoris along its superior margin (see Fig. 11C).

It is unnecessary to strip the iliac crest for simple open reduction. If pelvic osteotomy is performed, the anterior interval should be developed fully before the iliac apophysis is incised and the pelvis stripped subperiosteally (see Fig. 11D). The classic iliac crest exposure uses a longitudinal apophyseal incision along the top of the pelvis. It should be made sharply with a single deep cut using a scalpel. Alternatively, some surgeons incise the periosteum longitudinally just lateral to the outer edge of the apophysis and pull the entire apophysis medially off the top of the pelvis to expose the inner table. Packing with a sponge usually quickly stops bleeding. A right-angle clamp can be carefully worked along the inner and outer pelves posteriorly to expose the sciatic notch subperiosteally.

OPEN REDUCTION (ANTERIOR APPROACH, MEDIAL APPROACH)
Planning, Approach, and Technique

Standard open reduction is performed through an anterior approach (see prior discussion). Exposure of the pelvis is unnecessary. The capsule must be thoroughly exposed, particularly medially and inferiorly (Fig. 12A). The psoas tendon is always contracted, and its tendinous portion should be incised. Although I use a T incision in the capsule (see Fig. 12B), there is no evidence of superiority of any capsulotomy method. The ligamentum teres, if not ruptured, is sharply incised from the femoral head. Its stump can be useful in finding the center of the true acetabulum, which can be surprisingly inferior in position.

Exposing the acetabulum is the most difficult portion of the procedure. Frequently, the anterior capsule lies adherent over the anterior half of the acetabulum and must be carefully eased up with a Kidner ("peanut") dissector (see Fig. 12C). If the joint is full of fibrous material, all of it must be gently excised or the hip will not reduce. In the inferior acetabulum, the large transverse acetabular ligament must be sectioned (I use a Mayo scissors).

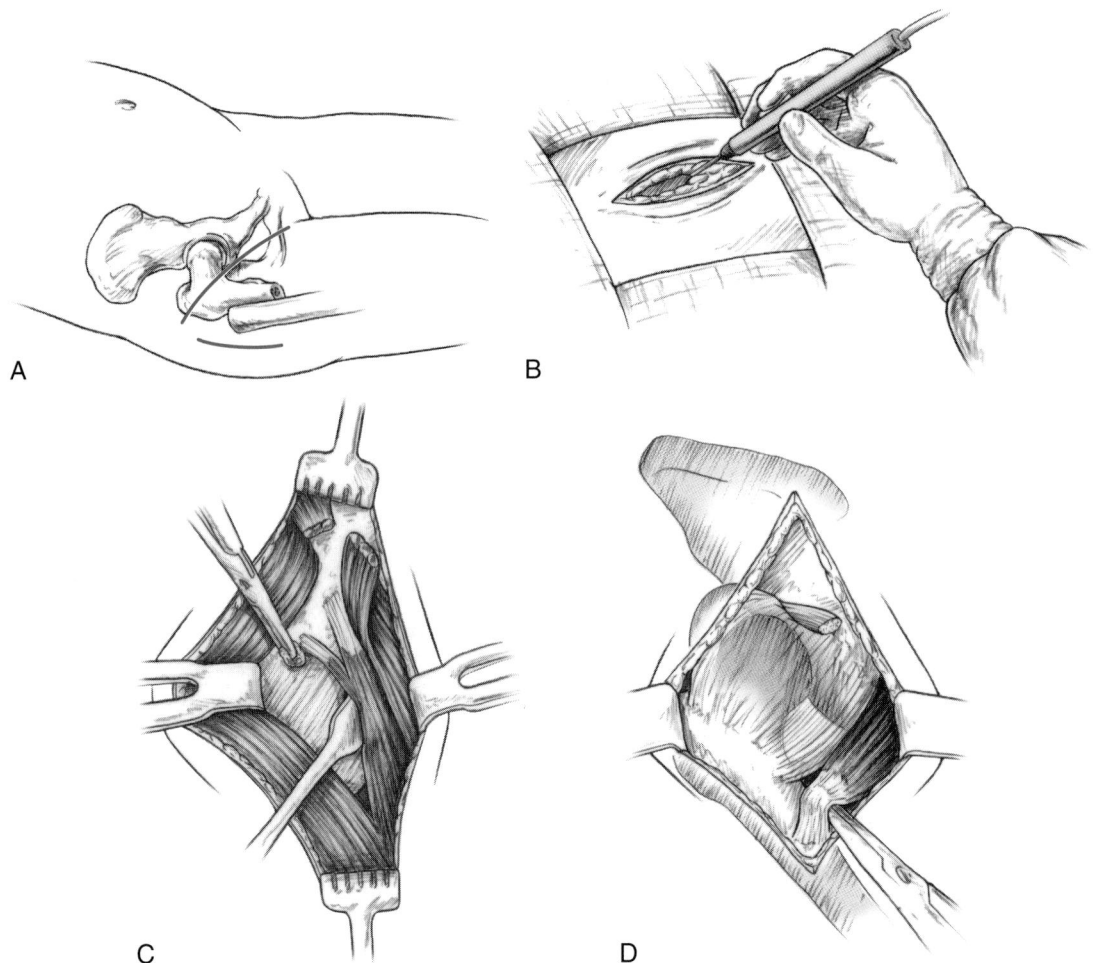

Fig. 11. Basic anterior approach to the hip joint and pelvis used for most procedures described. See text for further discussion.

After a trial reduction, the femur should be shortened (see later discussion) if the tension is too great. If the hip must be held in too much flexion to maintain stability, a Salter osteotomy or other pelvic procedure should be considered. I find reorientation more likely to be useful at open reduction, but occasionally the Pemberton procedure is an option. Neither correction should be too extreme because of the risk of posterior subluxation.

Capsulorrhaphy (see Fig. 12D) is a controversial subject; some surgeons are compulsive about it and some are not. I have attempted both ways and doubt there is much difference in results, with the exception that a very tight anterior capsulorrhaphy can force the femoral head out posteriorly. In older children with severe dysplasia, a smooth pin through the hip for 4 weeks can provide stability.

FEMORAL SHORTENING
Planning, Approach, and Technique
Femoral shortening is easiest through a separate lateral approach. After exposing the bone subperiosteally, place a four-hole plate on the femur just distal to the trochanteric apophysis, and predrill and tap the proximal two holes. Make a transverse osteotomy and excise sufficient femoral shaft (usually 2 cm) so that tension will disappear (check the overlap by gently pulling on the distal fragment while

the femoral head is reduced). Secure the distal segment to the plate with a clamp (Fig. 13), reduce the hip, and check (and adjust) anteversion before securing the remaining holes in the plate. I rarely add varus to the osteotomy unless the child is older than 5 to 6 years; otherwise, the technique is the same. The lateral wound should be completely closed before finishing the final portions of the reduction and anterior wound closure. Postoperative casting for 6 weeks is standard but should be modified by requirements of the open reduction.

FEMORAL VARUS OSTEOTOMY
Planning, Approach, and Technique
Femoral varus osteotomy in young children is best planned by observing stability under fluoroscopy in the operating room. This allows assessment of direction of subluxation as well as degree of anteversion (determined with the hip flexed 90 degrees). Fixation by a pediatric hip screw system is conceptually straightforward since the device courses up the center of the femoral neck, and rigid fixation is of intermediate importance because spica casting is used postoperatively. In the rare older child undergoing isolated femoral osteotomy, more attention should be given to stability and trochanter position postoperatively; radiographic tracings and cutouts are useful for this as well as

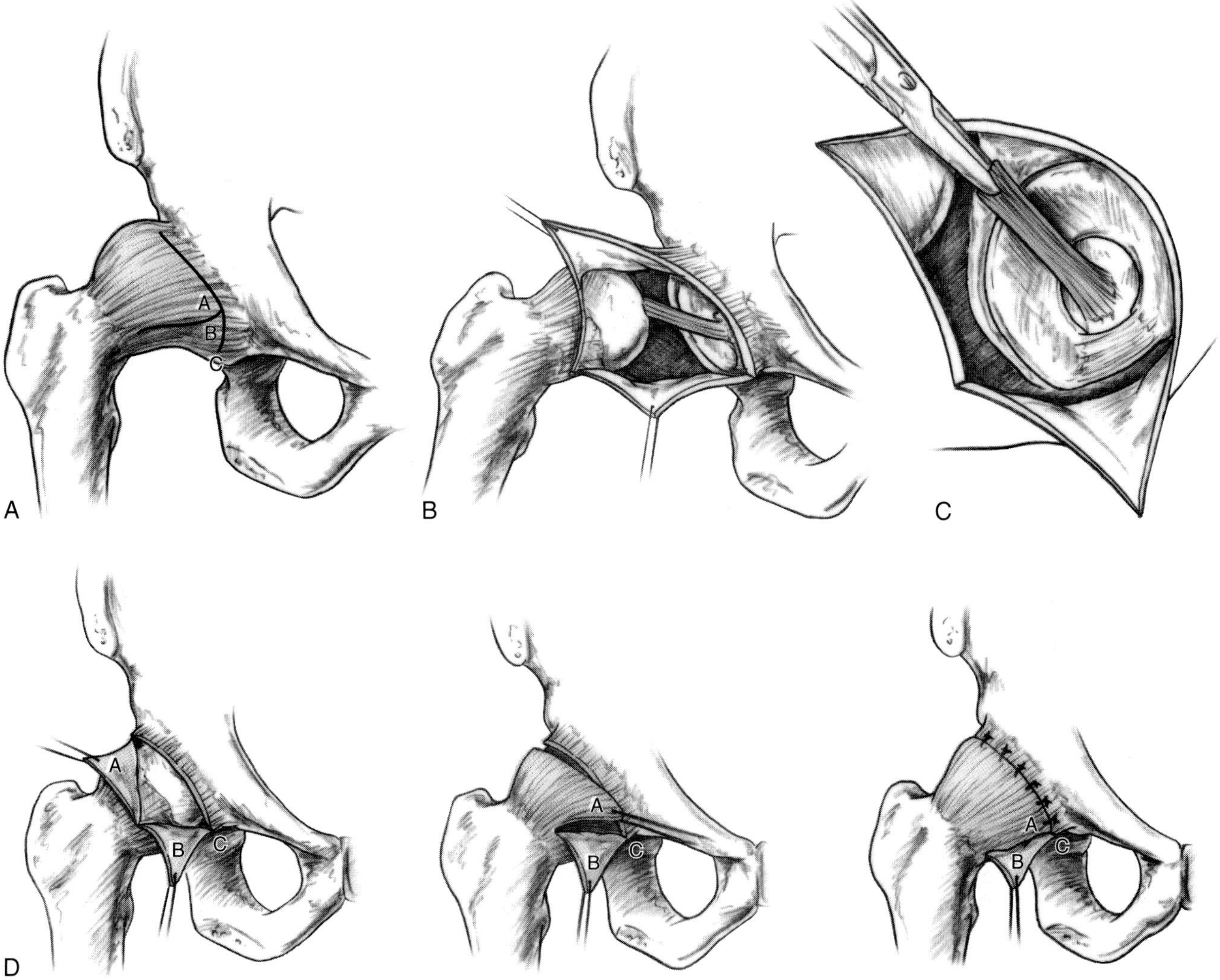

Fig. 12. *A–D*, **Open reduction and capsulorrhaphy of the hip.** See text for further discussion.

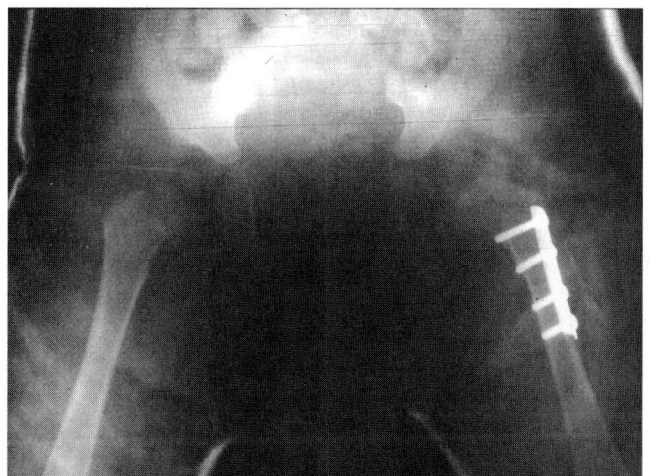

Fig. 13. Femoral shortening osteotomy. This is secured with a four-hole plate; it is an option when performing open reduction in the older child.

for planning the angle of insertion of the many devices that are used for fixation.

Femoral osteotomy for DDH is best performed with the limb free using a straight lateral approach. An anteroposterior C-arm allows excellent visualization of anatomy, with frog lateral obtained by flexing the hip. The vastus lateralis should be reflected from its posterior attachment to avoid denervating it, cauterizing posterior perforating vessels as they are identified. Any standard fixation device of appropriate size may be used, but it is essential to gain rotational stability of the proximal fragment by "interfacing" the surface of the osteotomy cut, particularly when a hip screw device is used (the fragment can spin on the screw). If there is a question of stability, an interfragmentary screw or wire can be placed.

SALTER'S OSTEOTOMY
Planning, Approach, and Technique
The Salter osteotomy is a forward and outward rotational redirection of the distal pelvis (containing the acetabulum),

using local iliac bone graft and threaded Steinmann's pin fixation. It has been carefully described in the literature, and its technique is highly standardized, with wise emphasis on the necessity of a concentric reduction as a prerequisite. Although the reduction does not specifically have to be present on preoperative standing radiographs, it must be obtainable under fluoroscopy in the operating room when the hip is only slightly abducted (15 degrees) and flexed (25 degrees). There must also be good abduction beyond this point. If these criteria are not met, the operation will fail.

Salter's osteotomy is performed through an anterior exposure of the ilium, with subperiosteal exposure of the sciatic notch (right-angle clamps inserted into the notch from medial and lateral should touch). The iliopsoas tendon should be lengthened. The most difficult portion of the procedure is passing the Gigli saw and making the cut in the ilium at the level of anterior superior spine. Saw passage can be facilitated by passing a red rubber catheter or dental tape as a preliminary tracer and using this to pull the saw through. When sawing, an assistant can spread the soft tissues and help to protect them. The saw cut should be a little more proximal (higher) on the lateral ilium, so that a squared surface accepts the bone graft when the osteotomy is displaced.

The distal fragment spins on the contact point of the symphysis, and the distal fragment should be pulled slightly anterior. It must not slide posterior. If the hip capsule is intact, abduction/external rotation/extension positioning will tend to displace the distal fragment appropriately. If the capsule is opened, displacement is difficult, even with a tenaculum. The surgeon must be gentle but persistent and resist the temptation to use a lamina spreader or pull the proximal ilium proximally. The best bone grafts for older children are taken with a saw rather than a bone cutter (as for the Pemberton osteotomy discussed later) and carefully shaped with a rongeur. The graft should have a 30-degree wedge (the maximum correction with Salter's osteotomy). Internal fixation should be achieved with two Steinmann's pins; some surgeons prefer radiograph control, although with experience this is unnecessary. The iliac crest should be closed before cutting off the pins because they must protrude enough to be easily palpable for removal after 6 weeks.

PEMBERTON'S PERICAPSULAR OSTEOTOMY
Planning, Approach, and Technique
Pericapsular osteotomy is performed through an anterior approach to the ilium. Periosteum should be elevated back to the sciatic notch, but it is not necessary to pass behind it as in the Salter osteotomy. It is essential to strip the periosteum distally to the triradiate cartilage; this can be felt clinically as a resistance to further elevation. Care is taken to not damage the cartilage.

A small curved osteotome is used to score the iliac cuts on the internal and external tables of the ilium. These cuts begin at the anterior inferior spine and curve behind the acetabulum but short of the sciatic notch until they reach the triradiate cartilage. This is done under direct vision, with help from the image intensifier. (Tilted to view from a slightly medial oblique direction, the radiograph gives a better profile of the ilium and cut and stays out of the

surgeon's way.) The lateral cut should be a little higher than the medial; after the surgeon gains experience with the technique, cuts can be modified to allow more lateral tilting by limiting the medial cut and enlarging the lateral cut. Once the cortex is scored, a large curved osteotome is advanced around the acetabulum under image control while being guided by the scores in the cortical bone. A large spherical Smith-Petersen gouge (thinned if necessary) is ideal for this. As the cut nears the triradiate cartilage, the osteotome itself can be used to pry the dome fragment down carefully. A small curved osteotome is useful to complete this cut to, but not through, the triradiate cartilage.

A wedge-shaped iliac graft is removed using a saw from the superior portion of the pelvis. One must be careful not to score beyond the tip of the graft, or the ilium can fracture. The graft is shaped using a rongeur to fit the curved osteotomy site, and the site is wedged open to receive the graft. A smooth lamina spreader can be helpful at this point. Some surgeons make a small recess in the site to stabilize the graft, but I have found that this may weaken the ilium and cause late loss of position. Steinmann's pin fixation is not required but may be used if the surgeon is unsure of graft stability. Spica casting is used for 5 to 6 weeks.

TRIPLE INNOMINATE OSTEOTOMY
Planning, Approach, and Technique
Triple innominate osteotomy is a specialized, complex mobilization of the entire acetabulum, allowing 3D reorientation into any position required for coverage. The superior cut and graft fixation are made in the fashion of Salter's osteotomy, but the pubis and ischium are also cut, freeing the acetabulum for extensive redirection. Steel makes the pubic cut through an inguinal incision and the ischial cut through the buttock. Tönnis et al[13] used a posterior gluteal approach for the ischial cut. The ischial cut can also be performed anteromedially through a subinguinal incision, between the adductor magnus and obturator externis. In all cases, it is wise to remove a 1.5- to 2.0-cm wedge from the ischium to facilitate medial displacement of the acetabulum as it is rotated. It is possible to overcorrect the rotation of the fragment, causing instability in a different plane.

CHIARI'S OSTEOTOMY
Planning, Approach, and Technique
Chiari's osteotomy is performed through an anterior approach with the pelvis exposed subperiosteally. Expose the entire inner and outer tables back to the sciatic notch, as for a Salter osteotomy. Image intensifier control is necessary. Identify and peel back the reflected head of the rectus femoris to expose the insertion of the superior capsule on the pelvis. This is the correct site for the osteotomy, and it should be confirmed by radiograph. A pin inserted from this point upward 15 degrees (not to be exceeded) helps when orienting the osteotomy.

Chiari[14] originally used a wide osteotome and made a single transverse cut, but many surgeons have modified the procedure by making a dome-like series of cuts over the acetabulum. This is easiest using two half-inch osteotomes. The dome must be cylindrical rather than conic or the osteotomy will not displace. The use of malleable retractors along the inner table protects the pelvic contents because the inner cortex must be fully cut for the osteotomy to displace. The posterior portion of the osteotomy is most safely made using a Gigli saw through the sciatic notch, as described for a Salter osteotomy. Once completed, the osteotomy should be medially displaced by abducting the hip; 50% displacement is appropriate. It may be held in an abduction spica cast or, more commonly, fixed with one to two cancellous screws to allow early mobilization. Crutches are used for 4 to 6 weeks to allow consolidation of the osteotomy site.

If Trendelenburg's gait is present before Chiari's osteotomy, it will persist or be made worse if the angle of the osteotomy is too high. The trochanter may be advanced at surgery to minimize this effect. Alternatively, the surgical approach can be direct lateral, with osteotomy of the trochanter and reflection of the abductor group proximally on the ilium. This allows direct exposure of the osteotomy site, and the trochanter is advanced during the closure.[15]

ACETABULAR SHELF PROCEDURES
Planning, Approach, and Technique

Shelf procedures are most frequently performed when subluxation is mild and acetabular dysplasia significant. An ideal candidate has an aspherical acetabulum, with superolateral deficiency, which is mildly subluxated but incongruent when abducted (making redirection inappropriate). The same approach is used as for Chiari's osteotomy, except the inner table of the pelvis is not exposed. As with the Chiari procedure, the shelf is placed at the top of the capsule as identified by the reflected head of the rectus femoris and by radiograph. The shelf material may be a variety of iliac crest preparations. The most common shelf procedure currently performed is the Staheli slotted acetabular augmentation, using corticocancellous chips.[16]

Staheli shelf is designed to restore at least 35 degrees of center-edge angle by augmenting the acetabulum. The base of the shelf is a slot, carefully formed at the superior margin using an upwardly directed 4.5-mm drill to make holes about the superior margin, which are connected with a rongeur. The slot extends anteriorly or posteriorly as required for coverage. Layers of corticocancellous strips (cortex down) are placed into the slot, along the capsule, and held there by suturing the reflected head over them. They are augmented by a cancellous bone buttress. Immobilization in a spica cast for 6 weeks is followed by protected weightbearing as the shelf matures.

COMPLICATIONS

INCOMPLETE REDUCTION, PERSISTENT SUBLUXATION

Persistent subluxation suggests that either complete reduction (closed or open) was not obtained at the time of surgery or the surgical treatment selected was insufficient to correct dysplasia. Treatment is by repeat surgery.

Incomplete reduction can follow closed or open treatment. After closed reduction, a "wide" reduction, in which the femoral head can be shown arthrographically to be "docked" beneath the superior limbus, may be temporarily acceptable if a follow-up arthrogram at 6 weeks demonstrates a deep, concentric reduction. This type of reduction

can be thought of as a ball resting on a doughnut, and soft-tissue remodeling is often rapid. If the repeat arthrogram does not show a deep reduction with remodeling of the labrum, open reduction is imperative.

Incomplete reduction after an open reduction is actually a technical failure to achieve or maintain reduction rather than a complication itself. However, recognition that a reduction is initially inadequate, rather than initially adequate with delayed subluxation, requires good radiographs and interpretation.

REDISLOCATION

Resubluxation and redislocation must be treated promptly, particularly after open reduction. Simple reorientation of the femur and casting in the new position may suffice if performed within the first few weeks after the initial reduction, but the surgeon should not avoid prompt repeat open reduction if necessary.

Once the subluxation has been controlled, the surgeon must determine the cause. Ligament laxity may respond to prolonged casting or bracing. Soft-tissue instability and loss of position in the cast are appropriately treated. Deficiencies of the acetabulum may respond to long-term casting and bracing, followed later by acetabular reorientation.

STIFFNESS

Prolonged stiffness after reduction of a dislocated hip generally is a sign of either unrecognized subluxation or early AVN. A stiff hip must be allowed to regain mobility before additional surgical treatment is carried out, usually by eliminating all immobilization and observing the child for 6 to 18 months. The exception to this guideline is the early recognition of subluxation, at which point repeat open reduction may be an option.

FEMORAL GROWTH DISTURBANCE

Disorders of physeal growth are fairly common after treatment of DDH and are particularly troublesome after closed reduction and femoral varus osteotomy. They may occur early, usually associated with AVN. However, late appearance (after 8 to 10 years) is possible, generally taking the form of lateral growth arrest and gradual development and progression of coxa valga. This can lead to late dysplasia in a child whose hip initially appeared to be improving. Treatment is by repeat femoral varus osteotomy. Long-term follow-up is mandatory.

AVN

AVN after treatment of DDH can take many forms, some insignificant and some with major consequences for the limb.[17] In its minimal form, AVN is a transient lucency or irregularity of the proximal femoral ossification center that spontaneously resolves without sequelae. More extensive AVN may cause sufficient femoral head deformity to cause subluxation, which can be exaggerated by the preexisting laxity and dysplasia.[1] The combination of a deformable femoral head (from AVN) and subluxation can be devastating and should be treated.[18] Options include repositioning and casting, abduction bracing, or operative treatment of subluxation such as Salter's osteotomy (Fig. 13). Treatment selection follows the same general rules as for DDH, but subluxation and femoral collapse are transient issues in

AVN, and a more conservative approach may be tried first.

Articular deformity and growth arrest from AVN can cause coxarthrosis, coxa breva, and limb inequality.

LOSS OF FIXATION: FEMORAL

Loss of position after femoral osteotomy is rare unless a pediatric screw device is used, in which case the proximal fragment can spin on the screw, distorting the femur from its desired orientation. Repeat osteotomy may be necessary. To avoid this, careful interference fit between fragments is necessary, or an interfragmentary screw or pin can be used. Spica casting is appropriate whenever the surgeon questions the quality of fixation. Nonunion is rare but may require repeat fixation and bone grafting.

LOSS OF FIXATION OR EARLY GRAFT COLLAPSE: PELVIC

Loss of position is most common after Salter's, Pemberton's, or triple innominate osteotomy. It may be due to improper graft placement, graft collapse, or poor fixation in the case of Salter's or triple innominate osteotomy. Actual nonunion is exceedingly rare. When detected in the first 10 to 14 days, it may require repeat operation, but after that time it is probably wisest to let the osteotomy heal, rehabilitate the patient, and observe for 3 to 6 months. Repeat osteotomy can then be performed if appropriate.

INFECTION

Infection of the hip joint after reduction may be delayed in its clinical appearance because of spica casting and prophy-

TABLE 3. COMPLICATION SUMMARY					
Complication	Cause	Clinical Manifestation	Reducing Risks	Possible Outcomes	Treatment Options
Incomplete reduction, persistent subluxation.	Reduction not obtained at surgery. Insufficient surgery to correct dysplasia.	Early stiffness.	Use arthrogram to check stability of closed reduction. Expose entire acetabulum at open reduction. Careful radiograph assessment.	Progressive subluxation. Progressive dysplasia. Loss of abduction. Trendelenburg's limp.	Manipulation, closed reduction, spica cast (early). Repeat open reduction.
Redislocation.	Insufficient duration of casting. Ligament laxity.	Stiffness. Foreshortening and adduction of limb.	Treat promptly. Assess degree of dysplasia preoperatively.	Persistent complete dislocation. Trendelenburg's gait. Short limb.	Determine the cause. Long-term casting and bracing. Late acetabular reorientation.
Stiffness.	Unrecognized subluxation or early avascular necrosis.	Early stiffness.	Observe for 6–18 months.	See persistent subluxation, avascular necrosis.	Allow to regain mobility before additional surgery. Repeat open reduction.
Femoral growth disturbance.	Presumed vascular or compressive injury to femoral physis.	Coxa valga with late appearance (after 8–10 years).	Unknown. Adequate femoral shortening may reduce compressive risks.	Coxa valga may lead to progressive dysplasia.	Repeat femoral osteotomy. Long-term follow-up is mandatory.
Avascular necrosis.	Some insignificant and some with major consequences. Transient lucency or irregularity of the proximal femoral ossification center.	Stiffness. Femoral head ossification irregularity and deformity. Radiographic subluxation.	Radiographic subluxation should be treated.	Resolution without sequelae. Femoral head deformity with coxarthrosis. Trendelenburg's gait. Limb inequality.	Repositioning and casting, abduction bracing, or operative treatment of subluxation such as Salter's osteotomy. Late: limb equalization, trochanter transfer.
Loss of fixation: femoral.	Proximal fragment can spin on the screw of a hip screw device.	Pain. Progressive loss of bone position by radiograph.	Spica casting is appropriate whenever the surgeon questions the quality of fixation. Interfragmentary screw or wire.	Abnormal range of motion. Persistent or progressive dysplasia.	Prolonged casting if position is satisfactory. Repeat osteotomy may be necessary.
Loss of fixation or early graft collapse: pelvic.	Loss of position is most common after Salter's, Pemberton's, or triple innominate.	Early change of radiograph position. Loss of correction. Persistent radiographic acetabular dysplasia.	Use tricortical graft. Supplement fixation with wire if required. Postoperative spica cast and restricted weight-bearing.	Persistent dysplasia.	Let osteotomy heal, rehabilitate patient, and observe for 3–6 months. Repeat osteotomy.
Infection.	Contamination at surgery. Bacteremia. Erosion of fixation pin through skin.	Stiffness, pain, and loss of joint space. May be delayed in its clinical appearance because of spica casting and prophylactic antibiotics.	Careful surgical technique. Prophylactic antibiotics when indicated. High index of suspicion with early aspiration or exploration.	Osteomyelitis. Persistent drainage. Loss of position.	Surgical débridement, cultures, and appropriate antibiotics.
Sciatic nerve palsy.	Direct surgical injury. Hematoma. Posterior displacement of pelvic osteotomy.	Immediate or gradual loss of sensory and motor function.	Avoid posterior displacement of osteotomies.	Prompt surgical correction.	Exploration and nerve repair. Hematoma drainage. Repositioning of osteotomy.
Narrowing of the pelvis.	Certain pelvic osteotomies may narrow the pelvis.	Interference with childbirth. Bilateral surgery exaggerates the effect.	If possible, correct dysplasia by 6–8 years of age.	Persistent problems for as long as 8 years.	Corrected by remodeling. Cesarean section.

lactic antibiotics. It is detected by stiffness, pain, and loss of joint space and must be treated with surgical débridement, cultures, and appropriate antibiotics. Although osteomyelitis after osteotomy in children is rare, a high index of suspicion and early aspiration or reexploration is appropriate because of the difficulty in controlling chronic pelvic osteomyelitis.

SCIATIC NERVE PALSY

This feared complication can have many causes. Direct surgical injury to the nerve is possible; usually the surgeon will be aware of specific intraoperative incidents that make this likely, and exploration and nerve repair should be considered. Hematoma collection is suspected if bleeding was brisk or if the palsy develops slowly postoperatively; observation or decompression are options, depending on speed and severity of progression. Posterior displacement of Salter's, triple innominate, or Chiari's osteotomies can cause sciatic palsy; treatment is prompt surgical correction.

NARROWING OF THE PELVIS

Certain pelvic osteotomies, particularly the Chiari osteotomy and variants, triple innominate osteotomy, and, to a lesser extent, Salter's osteotomy may narrow the pelvis and interfere with childbirth for as long as 8 years before being corrected by remodeling. Bilateral surgery exaggerates this effect.

RESULTS/FUNCTIONAL GAINS

A meaningful discussion of results and outcomes is difficult in this group of patients because of the extreme diversity of age, biological diversity of disease, and responses to surgery. However, certain generalizations can be made[19]:

- Children with DDH who are never treated have a painless limp.
- Some patients with untreated DDH and many with treated DDH will eventually experience coxarthrosis.
- Successful closed reduction after walking age can result in excellent hip function, but the presence of degenerative changes and growth abnormalities is significant.[20]
- Surgical treatment of dysplasia, if successful, can result in better short- and midterm function than if treatment was not performed.
- Unsuccessful surgical treatment of dysplasia often results in a worse hip than if nothing had been done.
- So-called salvage operations for symptomatic DDH are generally successful in controlling pain for one to two decades.

REFERENCES

1. Kalamchi A, MacEwen GD: Avascular necrosis following treatment of congenital dislocation of the hip. J Bone Joint Surg Am 1980; 62:876.
2. Scoles PV, Boyd A, Jones PK: Roentgenographic parameters of the normal infant hip. J Pediatr Orthop 1987; 7:656.
3. Smith JT, Matan A, Coleman SS, et al: The predictive value of the development of the acetabular teardrop figure in developmental dysplasia of the hip. J Pediatr Orthop 1997; 17:165.
4. Kim HT, Wenger DR: The morphology of residual acetabular deficiency in childhood hip dysplasia: Three-dimensional computed tomographic analysis. J Pediatr Orthop 1997; 17:637.
5. Kerry RM, Simonds GW: Long-term results of late non-operative reduction of developmental dysplasia of the hip. J Bone Joint Surg Br 1998; 80:78.
6. Kahle WK, Anderson MB, Alpert J, et al: The value of preliminary traction in the treatment of congenital dislocation of the hip. J Bone Joint Surg Am 1990; 72:1043.
7. Schoenecker PL, Strecker WB: Congenital dislocation of the hip in children. Comparison of the effects of femoral shortening and of skeletal traction in treatment. J Bone Joint Surg Am 1984; 66:21.

8. Wenger DR, Lee C-S, Kolman B: Derotational femoral shortening osteotomy for developmental dislocation of the hip: Special indications and results in the child younger than 2 years. J Pediatr Orthop 1995; 15: 768.
9. Kasser JR, Bowen JR, MacEwen GD: Varus derotation osteotomy in the treatment of persistent dysplasia in congenital dislocation of the hip. J Bone Joint Surg Am 1985; 67:195.
10. Faciszewski T, Kiefer GN, Coleman SS: Pemberton osteotomy for residual acetabular dysplasia in children who have congenital dislocation of the hip. J Bone Joint Surg Am 1993; 75:143.
11. de Kleuver M, Kooijman MA, Pavlov PW, et al: Triple osteotomy of the pelvis for acetabular dysplasia: Results at 8 to 15 years. J Bone Joint Surg Br 1997; 79:225.
12. Windhager R, Pongracz N, Schönecker W, et al: Chiari osteotomy for congenital dislocation and subluxation of the hip. Results after 20 to 34 years follow-up. J Bone Joint Surg Br 1991; 73:890.
13. Tönnis D, Behrens K, Tscharani F: A modified technique of the triple pelvic osteotomy: Early results. J Pediatr Orthop 1981; 1:241.

14. Chiari K: Medial displacement osteotomy of the pelvis. Clin Orthop 1974; 98:55.
15. Kowamura B, Hosono S, Yokogushi K: Dome osteotomy of the pelvis. In Tachdjian MO (ed): Congenital Dislocation of the Hip. New York, Churchill-Livingstone, 1982, p 609.
16. Staheli L: Technique: Slotted acetabular augmentation. J Pediatr Orthop 1981; 1: 321.
17. Kruczynski J: Avascular necrosis of the proximal femur in developmental dislocation of the hip. Incidence, risk factors, sequelae and MR imaging for diagnosis and prognosis. Acta Orthop Scand Suppl 1996; 268:1.
18. Bar-On E, Huo MH, DeLuca PA: Early innominate osteotomy as a treatment for avascular necrosis complicating developmental hip dysplasia. J Pediatr Orthop 1977; 6:138.
19. Weinstein SL: Natural history and treatment outcomes of childhood hip disorders. Clin Orthop 1997; 344:227.
20. Malvitz TA, Weinstein SL: Closed reduction for congenital dysplasia of the hip. Functional and radiographic results after an average of thirty years. J Bone Joint Surg Am 1994; 76:1777.

section
9
chapter
18

COMPLICATIONS IN THE TREATMENT OF HIP DYSPLASIA

Perry L. Schoenecker

Summary

- The consequence of complications, which cause shortening and/or stiffness, may be far worse than an untreated dislocated hip.
- Complications may result from failure of diagnosis, failure to achieve and maintain reduction, nonphysiological positioning, lack of normal growth and development, and/or technical errors.
- Reduction by any technique must involve physiological positioning, careful surgical approach, and long-term evaluation.
- Persistent use of a Pavlik harness, without satisfactory reduction of a dislocation, may compromise subsequent treatment by closed reduction.
- Redislocation most often results from inadequate soft-tissue management.
- Careful surgical dissection and achievement of anatomic reduction without undue soft-tissue tension or compression of the femoral head within the acetabulum can minimize the risk of avascular necrosis.
- Femoral and/or pelvic osteotomy should be used to enhance stability of an anatomic reduction or correct anatomic deficiencies, not to effect reduction.

The objectives in the treatment of developmental hip dysplasia (DDH) are to do the following:

- Achieve an anatomic reduction.
- Maintain the reduction.
- Establish normal growth and development.

When selecting a treatment option, the associated complications and their potential for harm must be considered. Failure to recognize a dislocation is an obvious complication. Once a dislocation is recognized, treatment is begun. Reduction must be anatomic, concentric, and without excess force or pressure. Failure to do so may potentiate hip dysplasia and further complicate treatment. Even with optimal initial management, normal growth and development of the hip may not occur.

COMPLICATIONS OF REDUCTION TECHNIQUES

REDUCTION BY PAVLIK'S HARNESS

In the first few weeks of life, Pavlik's harness treatment of the Ortolani-positive hip will be successful in 70% of infants.[1, 2] This is substantially different from the 90% and greater success rate sometimes quoted, which includes hips that are subluxable (Barlow positive), not dislocated. An appropriately applied harness holds the hip in approximately 100 degrees of flexion and restricts adduction but does not force abduction. A common error is having the flexion straps too medial, which tends to internally rotate and adduct the leg. By adjusting the flexion-abduction position, a dislocated hip can usually be satisfactorily positioned over the true acetabulum. Excessive flexion may result in femoral nerve palsy secondary to compression of the nerve under the inguinal crease.

Harness usage may be complicated by failure to recognize that the unstable femoral head is not reduced into the true acetabulum. Ultrasound imaging correlated with the clinical exam will accurately show the location of the femoral head relative to the posterior acetabulum.[3–5] The transverse ultrasound image is best for demonstrating whether the femoral head is reduced in the acetabulum or is subluxed over the posterior rim of the acetabulum (Fig. 1). The unreduced hip, continuously splinted in flexion, is slowly driven laterally and posteriorly. Abduction is not restricted, falsely suggesting that the hip is reduced. Prolonged inappropriate use of the Pavlik harness results in a variable degree of flattening of the posterior-lateral acetabulum, which complicates future treatment.[6] If after a 4- to 5-week trial of the Pavlik harness the femoral head has not stabilized within the acetabulum, the Pavlik harness should be discontinued and another method of treatment used to treat the dislocation.[6, 7]

CLOSED REDUCTION AND SPICA CAST APPLICATION

Closed reduction and spica cast application are indicated for infants who present after 6 to 8 months of age and for those in whom Pavlik's harness treatment failed. Closed reduction is not recommended for teratological dislocations or dislocation after open reduction because of the high rate of failure to achieve stable anatomic reduction.

Adequacy of the reduction must be confirmed.[8] Failure to recognize posterior positioning of the femoral head can produce iatrogenic deformity similar to that described with the Pavlik harness. The quality of reduction is confirmed with conventional radiograph and/or arthrogram (Fig. 2). On a true anteroposterior (AP) pelvis film, the distance from the medial wall of the acetabulum to the proximal femoral metaphysis should not vary by more than 2 to 3 mm when the normal and dislocated sides are compared. A difference of greater than 4 mm suggests pathological lateralization with subluxation and/or redislocation. The center of a femoral head, which is anatomically reduced, will always be located below Hilgenreiner's line. Arthrographic evidence of an unstable reduction includes a narrowed isthmus with an inverted or blunted labrum, which obstructs entrance of the femoral head into the acetabulum, and/or excess pooling of contrast medially. Computed tomography (CT) images taken at the level of the acetabulum are optimum for documenting the AP position of the femoral head.

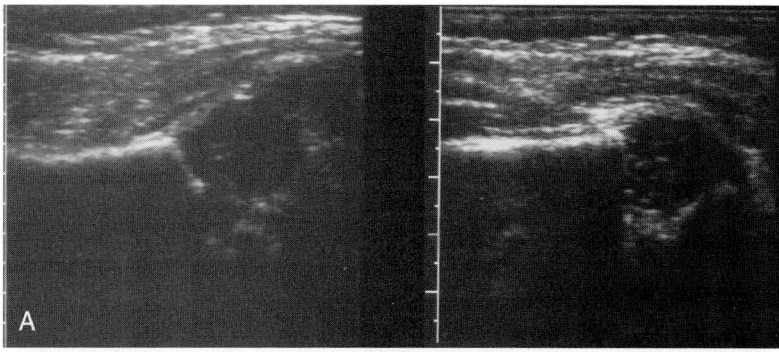

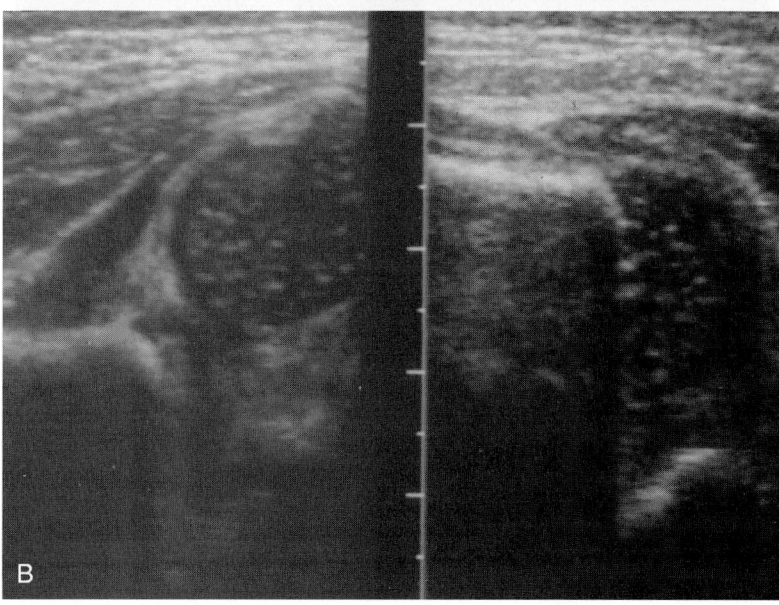

Fig. 1. Ultrasound images of reduced and dysplastic hips. *A,* The left ultrasound image shows a coronal view of a reduced hip; the corresponding transverse image is on the right. In both views, the femoral head sits within the acetabulum directly across from the triradiate cartilage. *B,* This dysplastic hip demonstrates poor coverage on the coronal image. The hip is laterally subluxed. The transverse image shows the head dislocated over the posterior acetabular lip.

Attention to detail is essential in the application of a spica cast. Care must be taken in positioning the extremities during cast application to ensure that the hip is held in an appropriate position. Abduction of at least 45 degrees but not more than 60 degrees and hip flexion of approximately 90 to 110 degrees reproduces the "human" position. This position is a balance between stable reduction and the least risk of femoral head vascular compromise. Flexion,

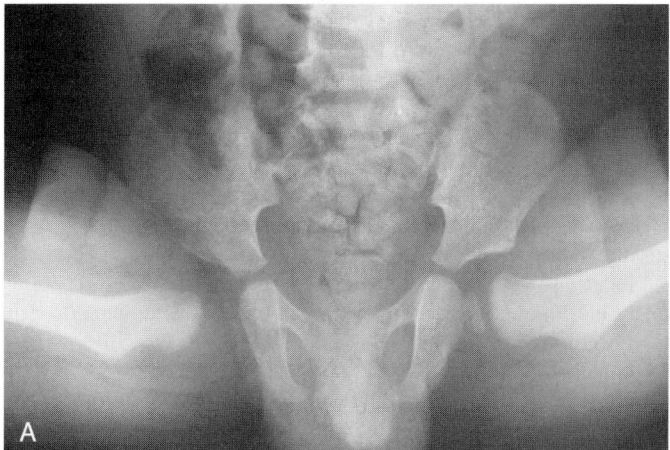

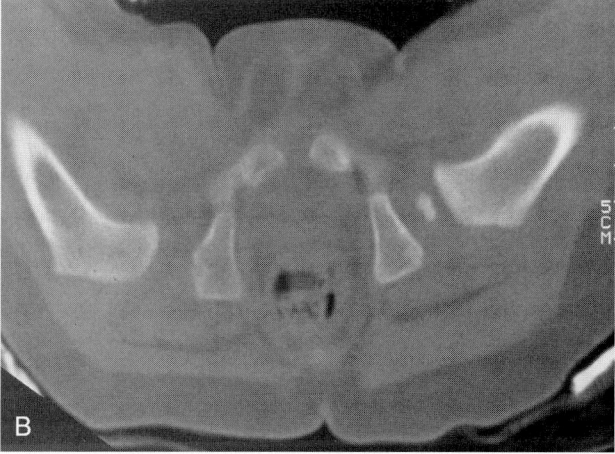

Fig. 2. Documentation of femoral head position after closed reduction. *A,* Anteroposterior pelvis film after closed reduction. The ossification center should be positioned at or below Hilgenreiner's line. The distance from the femoral metaphysis to the acetabulum should not vary more than 2 to 4 mm between the normal and reduced hip. A greater difference suggests lateral subluxation. If the dislocated side appears closer to the acetabulum, it is likely dislocated posteriorly. *B,* A follow-up computed tomography scan through the hip shows the femoral head posterior to the acetabulum. This may be difficult to detect with plain films alone.

without adequate abduction, places the head in a position where posterior dislocation can occur. Knee flexion should be between 60 degrees and 90 degrees, which increases hip stability by decreasing hamstring tension. The spica cast must extend to the rib cage proximally and below the knees distally. The cast should extend posteriorly and medially along the buttock with pressure directed anteriorly, molding the posterior portion of the spica cast on the dislocated side. This maneuver supports the proximal femur and limits the tendency for recurrent posterior dislocation.

Plain films at the time of cast application and 7 to 10 days later must confirm the achievement and maintenance of a successful closed reduction. CT imaging, particularly after initial reduction, is also recommended to confirm the anatomic AP relationship of the femoral head within the acetabulum. Patient factors that may contribute to failed closed reduction include capsular laxity, increased femoral anteversion, and acetabular deficiency. Technical factors include lack of adequate abduction and cast insufficiency. Redislocation that is detected in the first few days after initial closed reduction might be considered for a second closed reduction, particularly if the initial closed reduction was assessed as a relatively stable anatomic reduction.[9] An open reduction will be needed in most other children.[10, 11] Late recognition (>2 weeks) of redislocation while in a spica cast is a technically challenging problem. The dislocated femoral head deforms the posterolateral acetabulum. The anterior soft tissues (capsule, hip flexors) also shorten. Subsequent open reduction must include a release of these anterior structures and may require additional osteotomy to correct secondary deformities. The anterior capsule must not be overtightened, or the femoral head may be forced posteriorly. Less hip flexion (approximately 30 degrees) is used because of the already shortened anterior structures and to avoid posterior subluxation that is more likely with greater flexion.

COMPLICATIONS OF MEDIAL APPROACH OPEN REDUCTION

The medial approach allows access only to those medial structures that may prohibit complete reduction, such as the adductor musculature, psoas tendon, and medial capsule, but does not permit capsulorrhaphy.[12-14] The medial circumflex vessels, which course along the medial capsule, may be injured. Redislocation after a medial approach should be treated with open reduction from an anterior approach.[12, 13]

COMPLICATIONS OF OPEN REDUCTION

Open reduction is necessary for the patient in whom other treatment approaches have failed. It is considered a primary procedure in the older infant and in those with a teratological dislocation. The obstacles to anatomic reduction, which can be successfully addressed by this approach, include hip flexor muscles, capsule, intra-articular soft tissues, and labrum. Inadequate management of these obstacles by appropriate release may result in open reduction failure. Inadequate soft-tissue exposure is a common error. The medial capsule must first be satisfactorily exposed to facilitate an adequate release. Fractional lengthening of the psoas tendon is usually necessary to provide ample exposure of the medial capsule before capsulotomy. The medial capsule

must be completely incised. The hypertrophied pulvinar and excess ligamentum teres can then be removed. The contracted transverse acetabular ligament is transected. These steps are critical in obtaining reduction of the femoral head into the true acetabulum. A competently performed anteromedial capsulotomy helps avoid the error of misidentification of an inverted labrum as the medial wall of the acetabulum; otherwise, the femoral head will remain unreduced or in the false acetabulum (Fig. 3). A major technical error occurs if the labrum is excised in an attempt to fit the femoral head into the acetabulum. Loss of the labrum potentiates instability and acetabular dysplasia.

The redundancy of the superior and lateral capsule must be recognized. The capsule must be dissected free from its attachment to the abductor muscles to the lateral pelvis. Failure to do so makes capsulorrhaphy more difficult. The redundant lateral capsule must be obliterated for successful repair. An abnormal capsular attachment around the femoral head and neck, which acts like a leash or excess bulk around the femoral head, may also block adequate reduction. This abnormal capsular attachment must be carefully but adequately dissected for reduction of the femoral head.

Once anatomic reduction has been achieved, soft-tissue tension must be assessed. The femoral head should not be forced into the acetabulum. Femoral shortening allows effective lengthening of the structures extrinsic to the hip, which may produce undue compression of the femoral head in the acetabulum. This minimizes the potential for both redislocation and avascular necrosis (AVN) and is most often necessary in high dislocations and in children older than 24 months.[15, 16]

The addition of femoral and/or pelvic osteotomy should be considered if the femoral head reduction cannot be maintained with the limb in a reasonably anatomic position.[17-20] These procedures must not be substituted for insufficient open reduction, or failure is ensured. Failure to identify and correct significant femoral and/or acetabular dysplasia at the time of open reduction increases the risk of subluxation and/or redislocation. As with closed reduction, careful positioning and cast application can minimize these risks. Plain films, taken after cast application, are essential. CT imaging may be useful if the hips cannot be visualized adequately on plain films or if posterior subluxation is a risk, such as after open reduction for failed Pavlik's harness or closed treatment.[8] Follow-up films at 7 to 10 days are recommended to ensure no loss of reduction or osteotomy position.

Redislocation is possible even after a satisfactory open reduction.[12-19] Immediate repeat open reduction is appropriate in the first 1 to 2 weeks after open reduction. If redislocation is not recognized for several weeks after open reduction, a different treatment strategy is indicated. Any immobilization should be discontinued. The child should be allowed unlimited use of the involved extremity to encourage resolution of the hip flexion contracture that is typically present. Only after several weeks or months should another open reduction be planned. It is essential to determine the cause of failure. Most failures stem from insufficient anterior and medial release and failure to achieve a concentric reduction into the true acetabulum. A previously unrecognized deformity of the proximal femur

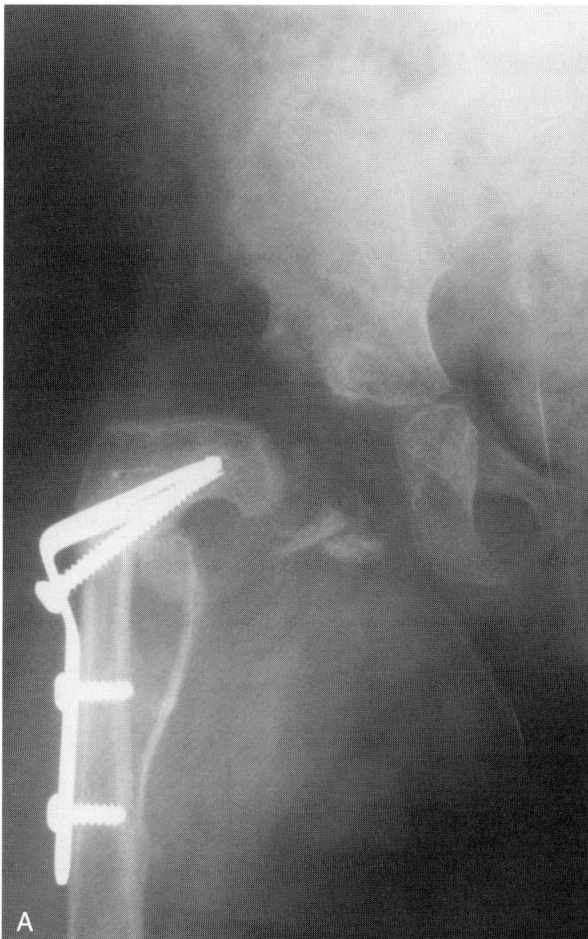

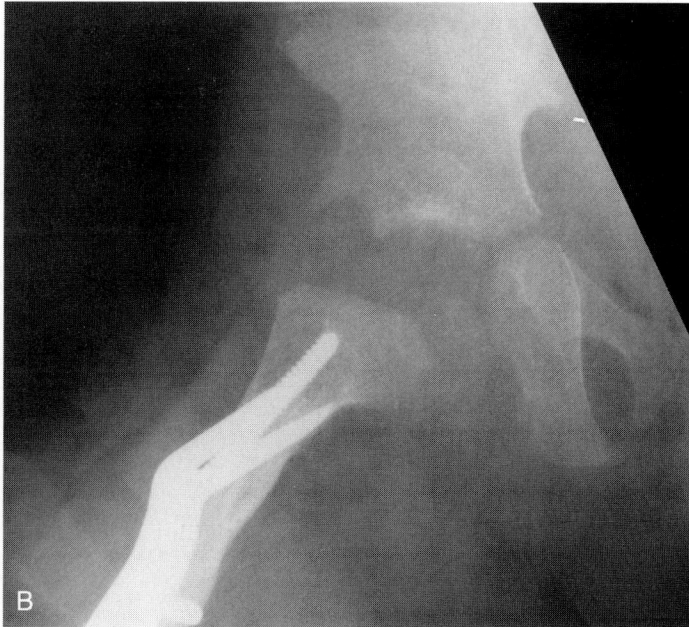

Fig. 3. The femoral head must be reduced in the true acetabulum. *A,* An open reduction of the right hip has been attempted. Femoral and pelvic osteotomies were performed as well. The femoral head was erroneously reduced into the false acetabulum and is too lateral. *B,* Open reduction and femoral osteotomy have been redone. The femoral head is now within the true acetabulum. The revision femoral osteotomy repositioned the femur within the acetabulum. At the initial open reduction, the medial capsule had not been adequately incised, leaving the femoral head unreduced. The previous Pemberton-type pelvic osteotomy hinged on the edge of the true acetabulum rather than the triradiate cartilage. Osteotomy cannot substitute for inadequate reduction.

or acetabulum may contribute to redislocation. Femoral or pelvic osteotomy may enhance stability.

Iatrogenic instability (and subsequent redislocation) can occur secondarily to redirectional osteotomy of the femur (relative overcorrection of femoral anteversion and/or valgus deformity). This posteroinferior subluxation is further potentiated when the femoral osteotomy is combined with a pelvic osteotomy and/or overzealous capsular repair. Excess medial displacement of the distal fragment during a proximal femoral osteotomy effectively shortens the femoral neck. While the proximal fragment readily reduces into the acetabulum, the redundant medial soft tissue levers the femoral head out of the acetabulum (Fig. 4). Restoration of femoral neck length balances the soft-tissue tension and stabilizes the osteotomy and the reduction. Less frequently, a pelvic osteotomy may require revision.[20] Displacement of a bone graft with loss of coverage may require revision.

COMPLICATIONS RELATED TO AVN

PREVALENCE

AVN is the most serious complication resulting from the treatment of hip dysplasia. Involvement of the femoral capital epiphysis alone may cause minimal morbidity. If, however, the growth plate is involved, severe growth disturbance may occur, and the prognosis is guarded. Every

method used to reduce a dislocation has a risk of AVN. A normal hip, held in a nonphysiological position, can also be subject to AVN.[21]

The reported prevalence of AVN in association with closed treatment of DDH varies according to the criteria used and the length of follow-up. Severe AVN, which involves both the epiphysis and metaphysis of the proximal femur, occurs in 2% to 6%.[9, 10, 22–26] A lesser degree of AVN occurs in 25% to 33% of hips, which produces irregular ossification, believed to be an ischemic event involving only the epiphysis with little or no subsequent growth abnormality.[25, 26]

AVN, ranging from 10% to 66%, has been reported after medial open reduction.[12, 13, 27] Controversy exists over the relative importance of preserving the medial circumflex vessels.[13, 27] Experimental work suggests that after release of the tight medial soft tissues, the relatively greater abduction allowed may stretch the vessels and is more likely an explanation for AVN than direct injury to the medial circumflex vessels.[28]

Open anterior or iliofemoral reduction is associated with 0% to 37% rate of AVN.[15, 17, 18, 29] The earliest clinical sign typically is persistent stiffness after cast removal. A stiff hip with evidence of AVN is likely to remain so for weeks to months after open reduction. Other than relative increased femoral head density, there often are minimal ra-

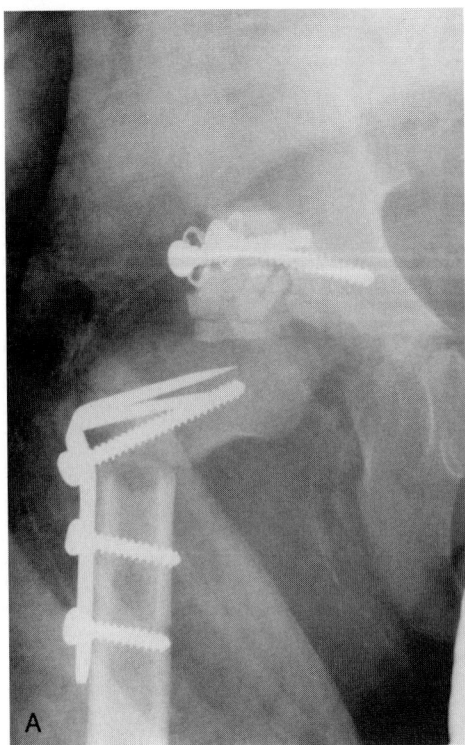
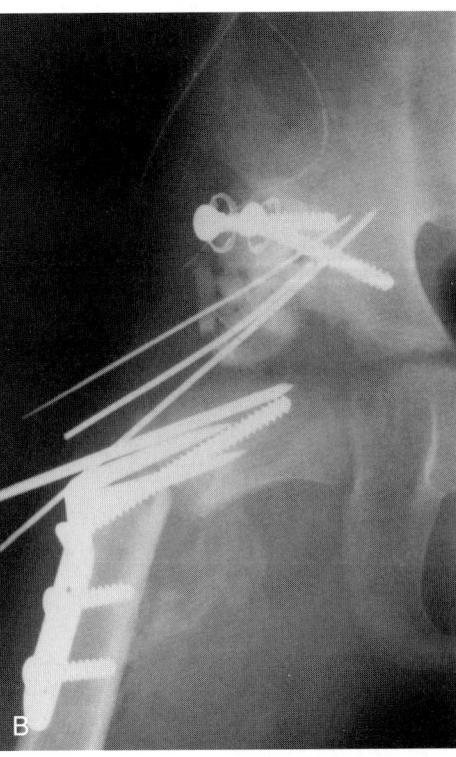

Fig. 4. Medial displacement of the femoral shaft may potentiate instability. *A*, This patient had an open reduction with femoral and pelvic osteotomy. The distal femoral fragment has been shifted too far medially, effectively shortening the femoral neck. When the leg is adducted, as shown here, the femoral head is displaced laterally, and subluxation occurs. The shortened femoral neck can lever against the soft tissues of the remaining capsule and result in subluxation or dislocation. A relatively short neck can result from excess varus or medial displacement or osteotomy too high in the femur. *B*, Revision of the femoral osteotomy to correct the medial displacement corrects the subluxation caused by the medial soft tissues.

diographic changes. Early radiographic signs of AVN do not correlate with final radiographic outcome. Some hips with minimal signs have had disastrous results. Several years of follow-up are necessary to detect changes resulting from AVN.

AVOIDANCE OF AVN

AVN can be minimized by taking steps to obtain a stable, anatomic reduction of the dislocated hip with minimal force, which in turn will maximize postreduction blood flow into the relatively soft cartilaginous femoral head. The severity of the dislocation, ease of reduction, patient age, surgical approach necessary for reduction, and position necessary for stable reduction are important factors. The safest reduction is one that is gentle, avoids extreme position, and is mindful of the vascular structures at risk.

The risk of AVN with Pavlik's harness treatment or any abduction orthosis is related to the extent to which the hip is held in abduction. It should not be held in abduction, only limited in adduction.[30]

After closed reduction, extreme abduction must be avoided and the safe zone of reduction respected. Prereduction traction and adductor tenotomy have been used to protect the femoral head. The extent to which each affords protection is unclear. In 1972, Gage and Winter reported on the effectiveness of prereduction traction as a way to reduce the incidence of AVN; however, the effect of traction alone is not clearly distinguished from that of variable positions used during cast immobilization.[25] Several other reports were unable to demonstrate clearly effectiveness of prereduction traction.[10, 22, 31] In a 1998 review of 20 years' experience, using a treatment protocol, which included 2 to

3 weeks of traction before attempted reduction, Luhmann and Schoenecker et al[24] reported a 3% incidence of AVN. Despite the lack of clear indications that traction alone was responsible for reduction of ischemic insult, prereduction traction is widely used.[32] Studies are even less clear (more controversial) regarding the role of traction in reducing the need for open reduction.

Once reduction has been obtained, the position of cast immobilization becomes an important factor to minimize the risk of AVN. The Lorenz position, which places the hips in extreme abduction, must be avoided.[33]

The unossified femoral head may be at greater risk of AVN, suggesting that open reduction be delayed until ossification is present.[34] However, some hips do not ossify until after 12 months of age. For these hips, the risks of delay in reduction and increasing dysplasia must be weighed against the risk of AVN.

AVN of the proximal femur may result from injury to the medial circumflex vessels during exposure or sectioning of the medial capsule. An extensive release along the posterolateral capsule may injure the posterior vessels entering the epiphysis. Osteotomy of the femur performed too close to the base of the neck also increases risk of AVN (Fig. 5).[35]

AVN of the acetabulum may occur when a pericapsular osteotomy is performed in conjunction with open reduction. The soft-tissue dissection necessary for exposure may compromise blood supply to the periacetabular fragment. A Pemberton-type osteotomy performed too close to the acetabulum may potentiate necrosis of the fragment. In time, the lateral edge of the acetabular fragment may subside, resulting in residual acetabular dysplasia.

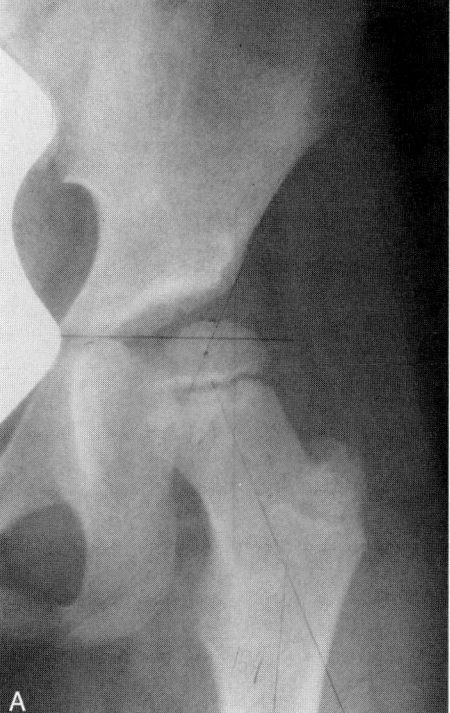 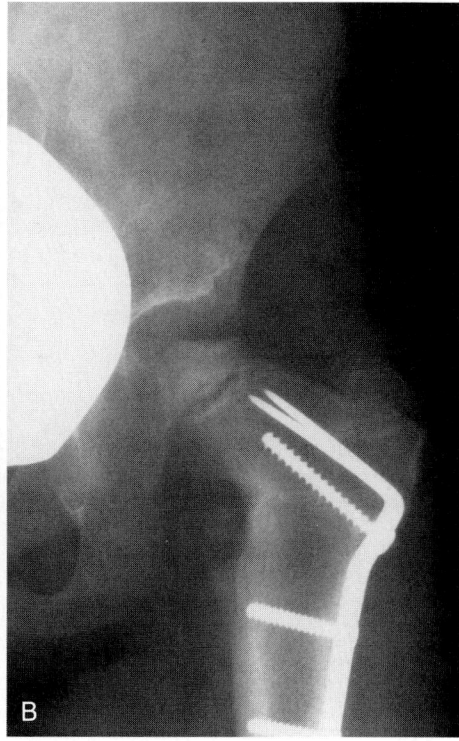

Fig 5. Osteotomy in femoral neck resulting in avascular necrosis (AVN). *A,* This child had residual subluxation. A femoral varus osteotomy was performed. *B,* This film taken 6 months later shows changes of AVN. The osteotomy has been performed above the lesser trochanter through the base of the femoral neck. Osteotomy performed too high on the femur may injure the circumflex vessels directly or indirectly by increased intracapsular pressure from bleeding or traction from displacement.

DETECTION OF AVN

After successful reduction of a dislocated hip, growth and development of the proximal femur and acetabulum should normalize. Infant hips should demonstrate progressive ossification of the femoral head comparable to the normal hip. Delay in this process, greater than 1 year by Salter's criteria, indicates vascular compromise to some degree.[9] Most normal infant hips will demonstrate growth arrest lines after reduction. Because the proximal femoral cartilage model is continuous with that of the greater trochanter, the usual growth arrest line will parallel the femoral neck horizontally as well as obliquely along the lateral neck.[36] Asymmetry along these lines is suggestive of partial growth arrest. The pattern and severity will vary with the nature of the vascular insult.

AVN should be suspected if, after a seemingly uncomplicated open reduction, with or without concomitant osteotomy, pain and stiffness occur. Typically, no clear cause is evident. The femoral head appears well located, although at times it may appear slightly inferior in position within the acetabulum. Healing of any osteotomy is not delayed. The bone of the pelvis and proximal femur may appear osteopenic. The pain may be severe enough to interfere with rehabilitation. If the femoral head does not appear to be avascular (no increased density relative to the surrounding bone, absence of any fragmentation of an ossified femoral head), then the prognosis is favorable for a satisfactory recovery. However, hips with radiographic changes suggestive of AVN have a guarded prognosis.

Four patterns of growth disturbance are described.[37, 38] These reflect the extent of involvement and the potential for recovery and late deformity. Transient ischemia of the entire femoral head may occur. Typically, a transient vascular insult is reversible and causes minimal, if any, necrosis. Full recovery is expected. Total ischemia of the femoral head with growth arrest produces a short femoral neck with a high greater trochanter (Fig. 6). Functional coxa vara develops along with as much as 5 cm of limb length inequality. Ischemia of the lateral portion of the head may cause partial growth arrest, which may result in valgus deformity from more rapid growth of the medial area of the neck compared with the lateral area. Acetabular dysplasia may persist because of the increased compression forces at the lateral edge of the developing acetabulum. The femoral head usually becomes aspherical, and acetabular dysplasia persists. These changes are slow to develop and may take years to become apparent. Ischemia of the medial femoral head with growth arrest will result in shortening of the medial neck (coxa breva) and varus. These hips have the poorest prognosis. Coxa vara, trochanteric overgrowth, and limb length shortening, typically more than 5 cm, may result. These changes are often slow to evolve with growth, taking several years to become apparent.[39] Residual hip dysplasia with degenerative changes may occur in the last three patterns of AVN.

The optimum treatment of AVN is prevention.[40] Should AVN occur, the treatment is directed at correcting the secondary deformities. Coxa vara is treated by proximal femoral valgus osteotomy. Valgus deformity of the proximal femur, often associated with subluxation, is corrected by proximal femoral varus osteotomy. If performed before age 4 or 5 years, this may be sufficient treatment. The older child with acetabular dysplasia may require a pelvic osteotomy as well. Proximal positioning of the greater tro-

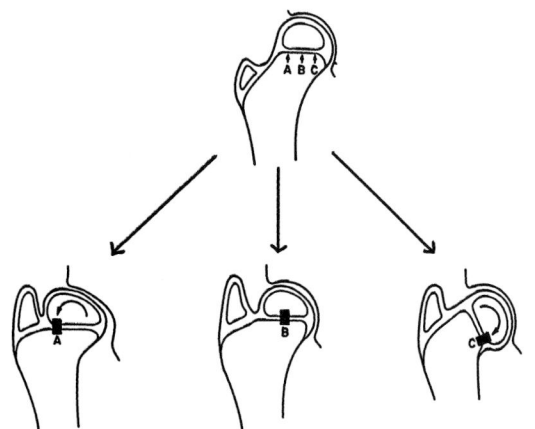

Fig. 6. Growth disturbance. The physis of the femoral head and the physis of the neck are contiguous in the infant and young child (upper view). Interruption of blood supply to the growing proximal femur produces deformity dependent on the zone that is involved. Transient ischemia may be reversible, with little sequelae. Total head ischemia, causing growth arrest, results in a uniformly short femoral neck with a relatively high greater trochanter (lower center view). Limb length inequality is a major concern. Involvement of the lateral physis and apophysis results in a valgus femoral neck (lower left view). Lateral subluxation may be a persistent problem and may potentiate acetabular dysplasia. Involvement of the medial physis results in a varus femoral neck with relative overgrowth of the trochanter (lower right view). Although acetabular dysplasia is often minimal, the mechanical inefficiency of the hip and limb shortening are serious concerns.

chanter contributes to abductor weakness. This may result from AVN or may be secondary to a varus osteotomy. Greater trochanteric apophyseodesis may be considered but is technically difficult to accomplish in young children and not very effective beyond age 8 years. Distal and lateral transfer of the greater trochanter may be effective in the older child. Limb length inequality of less than 3 cm can be managed by appropriately timed distal femoral epiphyseodesis. Beyond 3 to 4 cm, lengthening of the femur may be considered. A stable hip without significant dysplasia is a prerequisite. Lengthening of the femur in the face of noted acetabular dysplasia will potentiate hip instability and potentiate subluxation.

FAILURE TO ESTABLISH NORMAL GROWTH AND DEVELOPMENT

All treated hips should be monitored to skeletal maturity. Problems related to AVN, growth disturbances, and limb length inequality might not be apparent for several years. Late subluxation and acetabular dysplasia do occur (Fig. 7). Reconstructive procedures such as femoral and/or redirectional pelvic osteotomy may correct such deformities before significant degenerative changes occur.

OTHER TECHNICAL ERRORS

NEUROVASCULAR INJURY
Because of their potential for serious long-term consequence, certain technical errors deserve special attention, specifically femoral neurovascular, external iliac, and sciatic nerve injuries. Although these complications are rare, they can be devastating. These structures are at greatest risk during dissection about the pelvis. Most injuries are due to traction or compression on nerves or blood vessels. Exposure of the sciatic notch, medial wall of the pelvis, and superior pubic ramus presents the greatest risk. Injury may also occur during exposure or retraction of the psoas tendon, particularly in a tight hip.

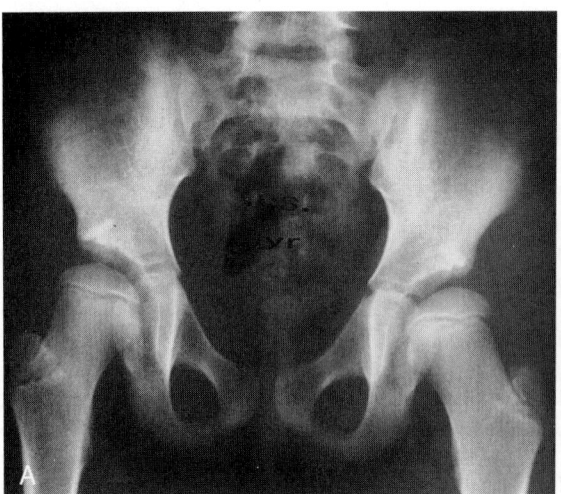
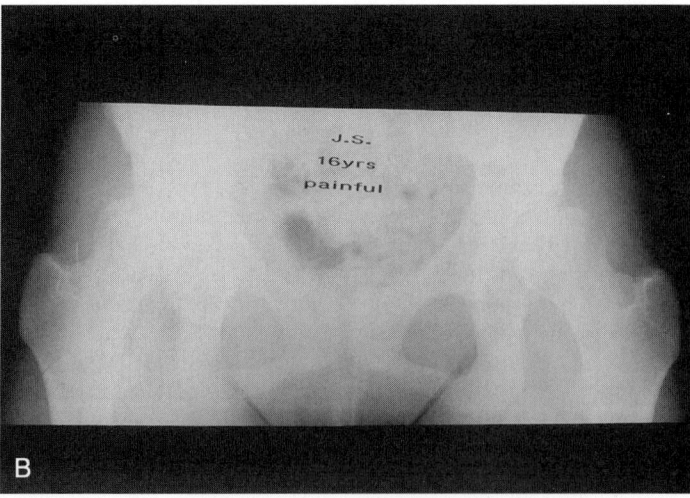

Fig. 7. Dysplasia. Dysplasia that does not resolve in early childhood may result in progressive deterioration and pain in adolescence. *A,* This child had bilateral developmental hip dysplasia, treated with closed reduction as an infant. Mild subluxation was noted at 3 years of age. At age 6, the child remains asymptomatic with mild subluxation and persistent dysplasia. *B,* By age 16 the patient had pain on a daily basis. Subluxation has increased bilaterally, and acetabular coverage is poor. A seemingly mild abnormality, noted in a young child, may progress. All hips requiring active treatment, as in infants and children, should be considered at risk for late dysplasia and monitored at reasonable intervals throughout childhood and adolescence. Pain is not a reliable indicator of a hip at risk. Dysplasia that has not shown resolution by the time of triradiate cartilage closure is not expected to resolve without treatment. Earlier intervention with femoral and/or pelvic redirectional osteotomy should be considered rather than continued observation of an increasing deformity.

Most instances of acute hemorrhage result from avulsion of periosteal vessels, which can be controlled by electrocautery, bone wax, or temporary packing. Injury to an external iliac vessel, although uncommon, must be treated as a surgical emergency. Packing with Gelfoam soaked in epinephrine may provide temporary tamponade until the vessel can be adequately exposed either through a transperitoneal or retroperitoneal approach. Should major vessel injury occur, the hemodynamic status of the child and adequacy of limb perfusion must be assessed to determine the safety and wisdom of completing the planned procedure.

Most serious nerve injuries involve the sciatic nerve. Exposure of the sciatic notch in preparation for osteotomy presents a risk, particularly compression by retractors placed around the notch. Osteotomy cuts into or near the notch must be completed with care. Displacement of the bone fragment may also cause sciatic nerve injury. Evoked potential monitoring should be considered in high-risk patients and procedures. Most of these injuries are neurapraxias and will show gradual improvement and/or full recovery.

The femoral nerve is protected to some extent by the psoas muscle and tendon. Traction injury may occur during exposure of the superior pubic ramus for osteotomy, usually in an older child or adolescent. The femoral nerve may also be compressed during excess hip flexion either in a Pavlik harness or spica cast.

OSTEOTOMY ERRORS

Appropriate selection and execution of these procedures are requisite for success.[17,20] The risk of AVN after femoral or pelvic osteotomy has been discussed. The risk of inadvertent penetration of the acetabulum while performing or fixing a periacetabular osteotomy can be reduced by adequate exposure, use of image intensification, and clear understanding of the anatomy. Overzealous correction by either a pelvic or femoral osteotomy may limit hip range of motion, which must also be avoided.

REFERENCES

1. Moran ME, Kim DJ, Mubarak SJ: Results of early treatment of the unstable newborn hip with the Pavlik harness. Presented at the annual meeting of Pediatric Orthopedic Society of North America, Memphis, TN, 1994.
2. Warner WC, Morrissy RT: Treatment of congenital dislocation of the hip with the Pavlik harness. Presented at the annual meeting of American Academy of Orthopedic Surgery, New Orleans, LA, 1990.
3. Mubarak S, Garfin S, Vance, R, et al: Pitfalls in the use of the Pavlik harness for treatment of congenital dysplasia, subluxation and dislocation of the hip. J Bone Joint Surg Am 1981; 63:1239.
4. Viere RG, Birch JG, Herring JA, et al: Use of the Pavlik harness in congenital dislocation of the hip. An analysis of failures of treatment. J Bone Joint Surg Am 1990; 72:238.
5. Harding MGB, Harcke HT, Bowen JR, et al: Management of dislocated hips with Pavlik harness treatment and ultrasound monitoring. J Pediatr Orthop 1997; 17: 189.
6. Jones GT, Schoenecker PL, Dias LS: Developmental hip dysplasia potentiated by inappropriate use of the Pavlik harness. J Pediatr Orthop 1992; 12:722.
7. Harris IE, Dickens R, Menelaus MB: Use of the Pavlik harness for hip displacements: When to abandon treatment. Clin Orthop Rel Res 1992; 281:29.
8. Smith BG, Kasser JR, Hey LA, et al: Post reduction computed tomography in developmental dislocation of the hip. Part I: Analysis of measurement reliability. Part II: Predictive value for outcome. J Pediatr Orthop 1997; 17:626.
9. Zionts LE, MacEwen GD: Treatment of congenital dislocation of the hip in children between the ages of one and three years. J Bone Joint Surg Am 1986; 68: 829.
10. Quinn RH, Renshaw TS, DeLuca PA: Preliminary traction in the treatment of developmental dislocation of the hip. J Pediatr Orthop 1994; 14:636.
11. Schoenecker PL, Dollard PA, Sheridan JJ, et al: Closed reduction of developmental dislocation of the hip in children older than 18 months. J Pediatr Orthop 1995; 15:763.
12. Mankey MG, Arntz CT, Staheli LT: Open reduction through a medial approach for congenital dislocation of the hip. A critical review of the Ludloff approach in sixty-six hips. J Bone Joint Surg Am 1993; 75: 1334.
13. Castillo R, Sherman FC: Medial adductor open reduction for congenital dislocation of the hip. J Pediatr Orthop 1990; 10:335.
14. Weinstein SL, Ponseti IV: Congenital dislocation of the hip: Open reduction through a medial approach. J Bone Joint Surg Am 1979; 61:119.
15. Schoenecker PL, Strecker WB: Congenital dislocation of the hip in children. Comparison of the effects of femoral shortening and of skeletal traction in treatment. J Bone Joint Surg Am 1984; 66:21.
16. Ryan MG, Johnson LO, Quanbeck DS, et al: One-stage treatment of congenital dislocation of the hip in children three to ten years old: Functional and radiographic results. J Bone Joint Surg Am 1998; 80:336.
17. Salter RB, Dubos JP: The first fifteen years personal experience with innominate osteotomy in treatment of congenital dislocation and subluxation of the hip. Clin Orthop 1974; 98:72.
18. Berkeley ME, Dickson JH: Surgical therapy for congenital dislocation of the hip in patients who are 12–36 months old. J Bone Joint Surg 1984; 66:412.
19. Gibson PH, Benson MKD: Congenital dislocation of the hip: Review at maturity of 147 hips treated by excision of the limbus and derotation osteotomy. J Bone Joint Surg Br 1982; 64:169.
20. McKay DW: Pemberton's innominate osteotomy. Indications, techniques, results, pitfalls and complications. In Tachdjian MO (ed): Tachdjian's Congenital Dislocation of the Hip. New York, Churchill Livingstone, 1982, p 543.
21. Schoenecker PL, Bitz DM, Whiteside LA: The acute effect of position of immobilization on capital femoral epiphyseal blood flow. A quantitative study using the hydrogen washout technique. J Bone Joint Surg Am 1978; 60:899.
22. Kahle WK, Anderson MB, Alpert J, et al: The value of preliminary traction in the treatment of congenital dislocation of the hip. J Bone Joint Surg Am 1990; 72:1043.
23. Camp J, Herring JA, Dworezynski C: Comparison of inpatient and outpatient traction in developmental dislocation of the hip. J Pediatr Orthop 1994; 14:9.
24. Luhmann SJ, Schoenecker PL, Anderson AM, et al: The prognostic importance of the ossific nucleus in the treatment of congenital dysplasia of the hip. J Bone Joint Surg Am 1998; 80:1719.
25. Gage JR, Winter RB: Avascular necrosis of the capital femoral epiphysis as a complication of closed reduction of congenital dislocation of the hip: A critical review of twenty years' experience at Gillette Children's Hospital. J Bone Joint Surg Am 1972; 54:373.
26. Salter RB, Kostuik J, Dallas S: Avascular necrosis of the femoral head as a complication of treatment for congenital dislocation of the hip in young children: A clinical and experimental investigation. Can J Surg 1969; 12:44.
27. Kalamchi A, Schmidt TL, MacEwen GD: Congenital dislocation of the hip: Open reduction by the medial approach. Clin Orthop 1982; 169:127.
28. Fisher EH, Beck PA, Hoffer MM: Necrosis of the capital femoral epiphysis and medial approaches to the hip in piglets. J Orthop Res 1991; 9:203.
29. Thomas IH, Dunin AJ, Cole WG, et al:

Avascular necrosis after open reduction for congenital dislocation of the hip: Analysis of causative factors and natural history. J Pediatr Orthop 1989; 9:525.

30. Suzuki S, Yamamuro T: Avascular necrosis in patients treated with the Pavlik harness for congenital dislocation of the hip. J Bone Joint Surg Am 1990; 72:1048.

31. Brougham DI, Broughton NS, Cole WG, et al: Avascular necrosis following closed reduction of congenital dislocation of the hip: Review of influencing factors and long-term follow-up. J Bone Joint Surg Br 1990; 72:557.

32. Fish DN, Herzenberg JE, Hensinger RN: Current practice in use of prereduction traction for congenital dislocation of the hip. J Pediatr Orthop 1991; 11:149.

33. Ogden JA: Changing patterns of proximal femoral vascularity. J Bone Joint Surg Am 1974; 56:941.

34. Segal LS, Boal DK, Borthwick L, et al: Avascular necrosis following treatment of DDH: The protective influence of the ossific nucleus. Presented at the annual meeting of Pediatric Orthopedic Society of North America, Miami, FL, 1995.

35. Tonnis D: Congenital Dysplasia and Dislocation of the Hip in Children and Adults. New York, Springer-Verlag, 1987, p 268, and 342.

36. O'Brien T, Millis MB, Griffin PP: The early identification and classification of growth disturbance of the proximal end of the femur. J Bone Joint Surg Am 1986; 68:970.

37. Bucholz RW, Ogden JA: Pattern of ischemic necrosis of the proximal femur in nonoperatively treated congenital hip disease. In The Hip: Proceedings of the Sixth Open Scientific Meeting of the Hip Society. St. Louis, MO, CV Mosby, 1978, p 43.

38. Kalamchi A, MacEwen GD: Avascular necrosis following treatment of congenital dislocation of the hip. J Bone Joint Surg Am 1980; 62:876.

39. Malvitz TA, Weinstein SL: Closed reduction for congenital dysplasia of the hip: Functional and radiographic results after an average of thirty years. J Bone Joint Surg Am 1994; 76: 1777.

40. Robinson HJ, Shannon MA: Avascular necrosis in congenital hip dysplasia: The effect of treatment. J Pediatr Orthop 1989; 9:293.

section
9
chapter
19

LEGG-CALVÉ-PERTHES

Daniel R. Cooperman

Summary

- Legg-Calvé-Perthes disease is an acquired disorder of the proximal femoral epiphysis characterized by cartilage hypertrophy and bony necrosis.
- The cause is unknown. The pathology suggests repeated bouts of ischemia in the proximal femoral epiphysis.
- The disease most commonly affects males, who are from 4 to 8 years of age and of small stature, with very delayed bone ages.
- The children present with hip stiffness, thigh atrophy, limp, and sometimes complaints of pain during the early stages and may develop bony deformity of the hip joint late in the disease.
- The prognosis for the hip joint is primarily related to the age of the patient at the onset of disease (with younger patients doing better), the amount of the femoral head involved (with the partially involved hip doing better than the completely involved hip), and the presence or absence of femoral subluxation (subluxation correlating with poor outcomes.)
- Treatment is controversial. Some but not all experts believe that containment treatment is necessary for obtaining good results in high-risk patients.

Legg-Calvé-Perthes disease is an acquired disorder of chondrogenesis and osteogenesis in the proximal femoral epiphysis. The exact cause is unknown, but the disease almost certainly results from epiphyseal ischemia, which leads to cartilage hypertrophy and bone necrosis. Collapse of the epiphysis is often seen, which can result in permanent bony deformity. It is classified as an osteochondrosis, as are other disturbances of osteogenesis and chondrogenesis seen in growing children, including Köhler's disease (tarsal navicular), Panner's disease (capitellum), Freiberg's infarction (second metatarsal head), and Osgood-Schlatter disease (tibial tubercle).

Avascular or ischemic necrosis of the proximal femoral epiphysis is not unique to Legg-Calvé-Perthes disease. It can be found as a complication of sickle cell disease, steroid treatment, femoral neck fracture, hip joint infections, and other processes. Only idiopathic avascular necrosis in children is Legg-Calvé-Perthes disease.

Legg-Calvé-Perthes disease has carried many names since it was discovered in 1909.[1] Some names honor its discoverers: Perthes' disease, Legg-Perthes disease, Legg-Calvé-Perthes disease, Calvé-Waldenström-Legg-Perthes disease. Some are descriptive, such as osteochondritis coxae juvenilis, osteochondritis deformans, coxa plana, pseudocoxalgia, and osteochondral trophopathy of the hip. Most authors now favor the name Legg-Calvé-Perthes disease or Perthes' disease.

EPIDEMIOLOGY

Perthes' disease occurs in 1 of 1500 children. It is four times more common in males than in females. The process most often occurs in children from 4 to 8 years of age, although it also occurs from 2 to 12 years of age. It is bilateral in 10% of cases. It is thought to occur in a *susceptible* child. Such a child is extremely active, is of small stature, and has a profoundly delayed bone age. Bone age frequently lags behind chronological age by 1 to 3 years.[2]

Perthes' disease is more common in Japanese, Eskimo, and Central European populations and less common in blacks, native Australians, American Indians, and Polynesians.[3] There is disagreement about whether there is a significant genetic component within families. Most physicians agree that if there is a genetic component to the disease, it is subtle.[2]

HISTORICAL REVIEW

In 1909, Arthur T. Legg presented the paper "An Obscure Affection of the Hip Joint" at the American Orthopaedic Association. He described a previously unreported hip condition that he differentiated from tuberculosis of the hip joint. Jacque Calvé of France, Georg Perthes of Germany, and Henning Waldenström of Sweden also described this condition between 1909 and 1910.[4] Legg, Calvé, and Perthes were convinced the process was distinct from tuberculosis of the hip joint. Waldenström was not. Waldenström's misimpression about etiologic factors cost him eponymic immortality. In 1921, Dallas Phemister discovered that ischemic necrosis of bone was the predominant pathologic factor.[5] In 1922, Waldenström described the roentgenographic evolution of Perthes' disease (Table 1).[6] In 1953, Stig Jonsater[7] took biopsy samples from 34 patients and described the cartilaginous and bony pathologic factors. During the first half of the 20th century, many world-renowned centers treated these patients with 1 to 4 years of enforced recumbency in hospitals, as outlined by Goff in his classic monograph.[4] The results of recumbency and non-weightbearing ambulatory bracing were widely reported during the 1940s, 1950s, and 1960s.[7a, 7b] These reports are hard to understand, as authors used very different definitions of what a good, fair, and poor outcome was. In 1964, Mose[8] published a reproducible radiographic outcome measure for patients with Perthes' disease using templates etched with multiple concentric circles. The Mose method brought order to the reporting of outcomes in Legg-Calvé-Perthes disease. Many patients develop aspherical femoral heads following non-weightbearing treatment, and many of these had unsatisfactory clinical outcomes in long-term follow-up studies. Physicians sought a concept other than non-weightbearing for treatment. Many chose containment. Harrison and Menon (1966),[9] Harrison, Turner, and Nicholson (1969),[10] and Petrie and Bitenc (1971)[11] reported on patients treated in devices that enforced hip abduction and internal rotation in an effort to contain or place the femoral head in the depths of the acetabulum. Physicians hoped that the soft, flattened femoral head frequently seen in Perthes' disease would be molded by the round acetabulum. Braces and casts were applied that were worn for months, sometimes years. Soeur et al (1952)[12] and later Axer (1965)[13] proposed a femoral osteotomy to contain the head. Axer believed that it had many advantages over recumbency or ambulatory brace treatment, especially the short treatment time. In 6 weeks, the osteotomy could heal and the child would rapidly begin full and unrestricted weightbearing. Salter[14] suggested a pelvic osteotomy to accomplish the same goal. In 1971, Catterall[15] published a comprehensive classification scheme to be used during the early stages of Perthes' disease. This scheme describes the extent and location of femoral head involvement. Catterall correlated his classification scheme with outcomes in both treated and untreated patients. In 1981, Stulberg et al[16] combined the Mose classification with an assessment of acetabular shape. This provides more information about long-term outcome than the Mose system used alone. Salter and Thompson (1984)[17] as well as Herring et al (1992)[18] have proposed systems to augment or replace the Catterall system, which can be very difficult to use.[19] Catterall et al,[20] Ippolito and Ponseti,[21] and Ponseti et al[22] reported on biopsy and necropsy material in Perthes' disease. They all suggested that Perthes' disease is preceded by a systemic disease of cartilage, which may predispose children to avascular necrosis.

Recently, Martinez et al[23] and Meehan et al[24] questioned the efficacy of a popular containment orthosis, the Scottish-Rite abduction orthosis, for treating severely involved patients. They remind us that there is still much to learn about the results of treatment of Perthes' disease because

TABLE 1. WALDENSTRÖM ROENTGENOGRAPHIC STAGING OF PERTHES' DISEASE AND RELATED PATHOLOGY

Stage	Duration	Radiograph Appearance	Pathology
Initial	6 months	Increased head-socket distance	Necrosis of most or all epiphyseal bone and marrow
		Subchondral thinning	Vascular invasion of dead bone
		A dense epiphysis that is homogeneous	Epiphyseal cartilage hypertrophy
		Metaphyseal cysts are rare	Epiphysis is soft when punctured with biopsy trocar
Fragmentation	8 months	Subchondral fracture appears	Dead bone resorbed with live bone replacing it
		Epiphysis is alternately dense and porous	Unossified physeal cartilage streams into metaphysis, making cysts
		Metaphyseal cysts are common	Epiphyseal cartilage hypertrophy
			Epiphysis is alternately soft and hard when punctured with biopsy trocar
Reparative	51 months	Normal bone appears in area of previous resorption	Dead bone resorbed as live bone replaces it
		All sclerotic bone removed as epiphysis becomes homogeneous	
Growth	Until maturity	Hip evolves toward adult shape	Presumed normal
Definite	Adult hip	Final shape of hip	Presumed normal

the natural history of the process is poorly understood. The treatment of Perthes' disease creates more controversy than the treatment of any other childhood hip disease.

PATHOGENESIS

ETIOLOGY

Perthes' disease results from ischemia in the proximal femoral epiphysis. The cause is unknown. It may be arterial, related to trauma, transient synovitis, or congenital anomalies. It may be venous; for decades authors have reported sluggish flow in the venous side. Liu and Ho[25] recently demonstrated profound venous congestion in 32 patients with unilateral Perthes' disease when comparing the involved and uninvolved hips. Arterial flows were nearly equivalent. Hyperviscosity of blood[26] has been suggested as a cause of venous congestion, as has thrombophilia,[27] an increased tendency to clot, or a decreased ability to lyse clots. Either could lead to secondary intraepiphyseal infarction. There are many suggestions concerning the cause of Perthes' disease and no consensus in the medical community.

PATHOLOGY

The pathology in Perthes' disease has been defined by biopsy and a few necropsy specimens (see Table 1).[7, 20–22] In the *initial* stage, there is epiphyseal bone and marrow necrosis, vascular invasion of the necrotic epiphysis, and epiphyseal cartilage hypertrophy. Jonsater states that the epiphysis is physically soft when a biopsy trocar is passed into it. In the *fragmentation* stage, dead bone is being replaced with live bone and unossified physeal cartilage streams into the metaphysis, forming cysts. In the *reparative* stage, all dead bone is removed. The epiphysis becomes homogeneous again. The bone necrosis seen in most specimens appears to be the result of multiple infarctions, not of a single infarction, as necrotic bone is layered with necrotic repair bone.[28] Most authors believe that multiple bouts of infarction are necessary to cause Perthes' disease.

The epiphyseal cartilage is also abnormal, with disordered collagen fibrils, abnormally increased proteoglycan concentrations, and a decrease in structural glycoproteins. It is suggested that Perthes' disease is preceded by a generalized disorder of cartilage metabolism.[20–22] Blood vessels that nourish the epiphysis must flow through cartilage to reach the epiphysis. If this cartilage framework is unstable, occlusion could occur, resulting in ischemia. A pathologic condition is cartilage seen on the affected side in Perthes' disease and also on the *unaffected* side in unilateral disease. On the unaffected side, there is a decrease in articular cartilage thickness and an increase in epiphyseal cartilage height, a narrowing of the physis, and disorder in endochondral ossification when compared with a normal hip. With careful examination of radiographs[29] in unilateral Perthes' disease, the "normal" opposite side is slightly flattened 50% of the time. Because the cartilage of the uninvolved hip is abnormal in Perthes' disease, it is reasonable to assume that the cartilage of the involved hip was abnormal prior to the onset of Perthes' disease. This suggests that Perthes' disease is preceded by a disorder of cartilage.[20–22]

PATHOLOGY AND CLINICAL DISEASE

Salter states that there are two forms of Perthes' disease, based on animal studies and clinical observation. The first type is clinically silent and benign. It results from a single infarction of bone. The infarction is followed by necrosis of epiphyseal bone and marrow. New blood vessels invade the epiphysis after infarction, resorbing dead bone and laying down new bone. If the pace of resorption and the pace of new bone formation are balanced, the dead bone is completely replaced with live bone in a benign fashion. There is no change in femoral head shape. There are no symptoms. If the pace of resorption outstrips the pace of new bone formation, weightbearing causes the necrotic epiphysis to collapse. This leads to crushing of the bone and the new blood vessels in the newly revascularized epiphysis. A painful subchondral fracture and clinical disease results from the second infarction, according to Salter.

CLASSIFICATION SCHEMES DURING ACTIVE DISEASE

Three classification schemes are used during active disease: the Catterall, the Salter-Thompson, and the Herring.

The Catterall system is based on the geographic distribution of epiphyseal abnormalities using anteroposterior and lateral radiographs. In Catterall type I involvement, less than a quarter of the epiphysis is involved. In type II, less than half the epiphysis is involved. In type III, almost all the epiphysis is involved, and in type IV the total proximal femoral epiphysis is affected (Fig. 1). Catterall assigned prognosis based on the extent of involvement and the presence of "risk factors," which have negative prognostic significance. These risk factors include lateral subluxation of the femoral head, calcification lateral to the epiphysis, Gage's sign (a radiolucent V in the lateral portion of the epiphysis), and a horizontal physis.

The Salter-Thompson scheme identifies the extent and location of the subchondral fracture frequently seen in Perthes' disease. If the fracture spans less than 50% of the epiphysis, it is an "A"; more than 50%, it is a "B."

The Herring system hinges on lateral pillar involvement. Herring defines the lateral 15% to 30% of the epiphysis seen on the anteroposterior radiograph as the lateral pillar. He assigns patients to three groups depending on whether the lateral pillar is uninvolved (Herring A), less than 50% involved (Herring B), or more than 50% involved (Herring C).

The Catterall and Herring systems are easy to use late in the fragmentation stage when all necrotic bone has identified itself. Unfortunately, this is too late to make treatment decisions. Consequently, physicians try to predict where collapse will occur using the subtle changes in density that precede fragmentation and collapse. This can be difficult. Van Dome et al[30] found that the Catterall classification appeared to change in 40% of hips presenting before the fragmentation stage and in only 6% that presented during the fragmentation stage. Christenson et al[19] found considerable inter- and intraobserver disagreement when using the Catterall system. The Catterall and Herring systems are difficult to use because Perthes' disease is a continuum, not a disease with three or four distinct, mutually exclusive presentations. There are certainly dozens of recognizable patterns of deformity that vary according to patient age and

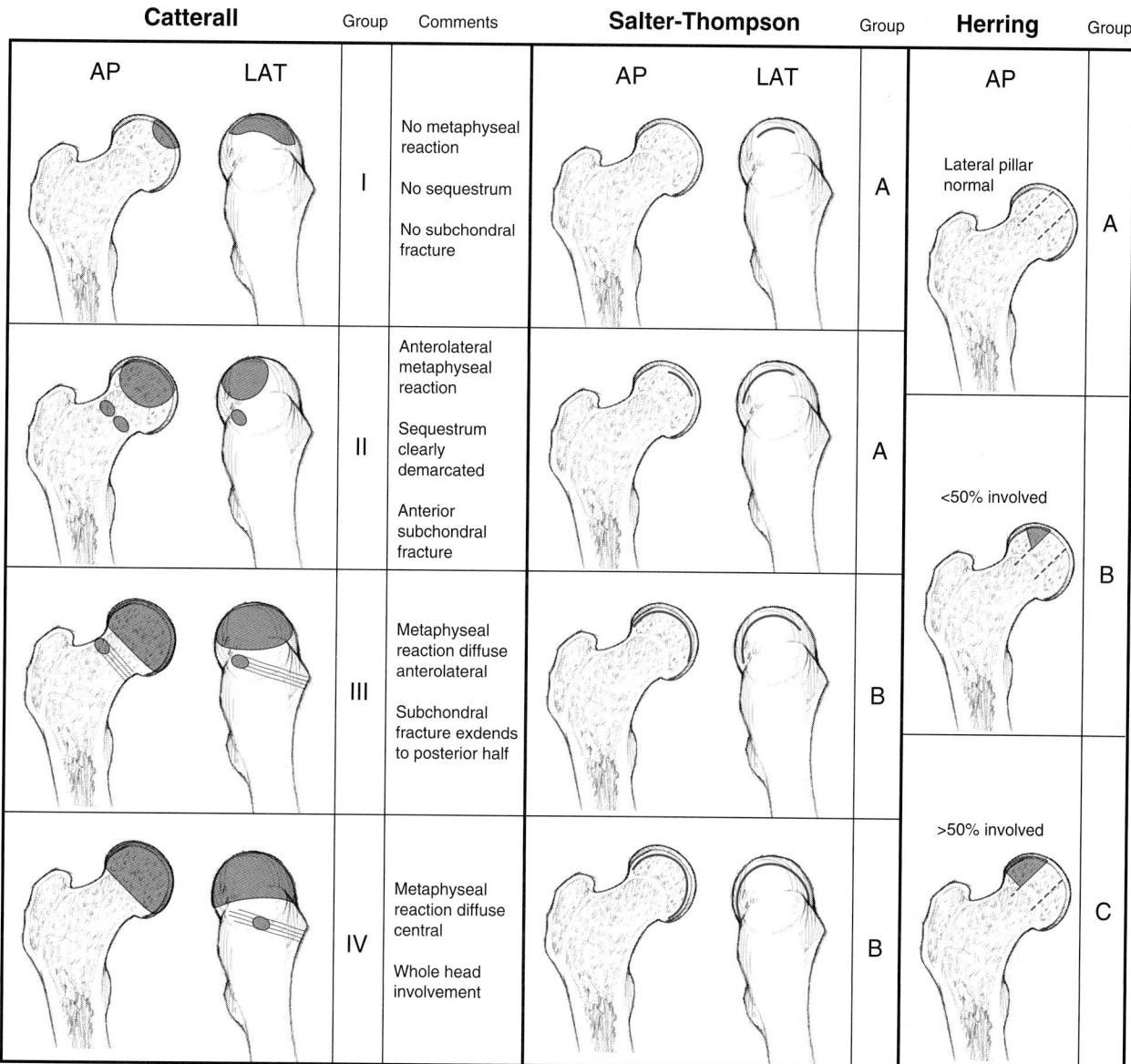

Fig. 1. Classification schemes. These schemes are used during the active phase of Perthes' disease.

the severity of ischemia. These authors have chosen a few points along the continuum to serve as markers. They are useful but not perfect markers.

The Salter-Thompson system relies on identifying the subchondral fracture that attends most cases of Perthes' disease. Unfortunately, an experienced observer like Catterall can find the fracture only 25% to 30% of the time. Salter and Thompson can find it just 66% of the time. When it is present, it is useful, because fragmentation occurs under the fracture and nowhere else. When it is not present, other signs must be used.

RISK FACTORS
Catterall's concept of risk factors is important. Subluxation is an especially important risk factor. Arthrograms[31] have

demonstrated that lateral and proximal subluxation of the femur is essentially a reflection of femoral head deformity and not related to true subluxation. As the head flattens and enlarges, the proximal femur appears to migrate proximally and laterally. For this reason, Axer strongly suggested that the term *pseudosubluxation* be used. I consider a lateral subluxation to be significant if the lateral subluxation ratio is greater than 1.5 to 1.0 (Fig. 2). I consider superior subluxation significant if Shenton's line is broken. Subluxation identifies a femoral head that is deformed. Calcification lateral to the epiphysis has a similar implication. The calcification is still "in the epiphysis." However, the epiphysis is no longer rounded, so the calcification looks lateral to the epiphysis. This sign complements subluxation as a sign of femoral deformity.

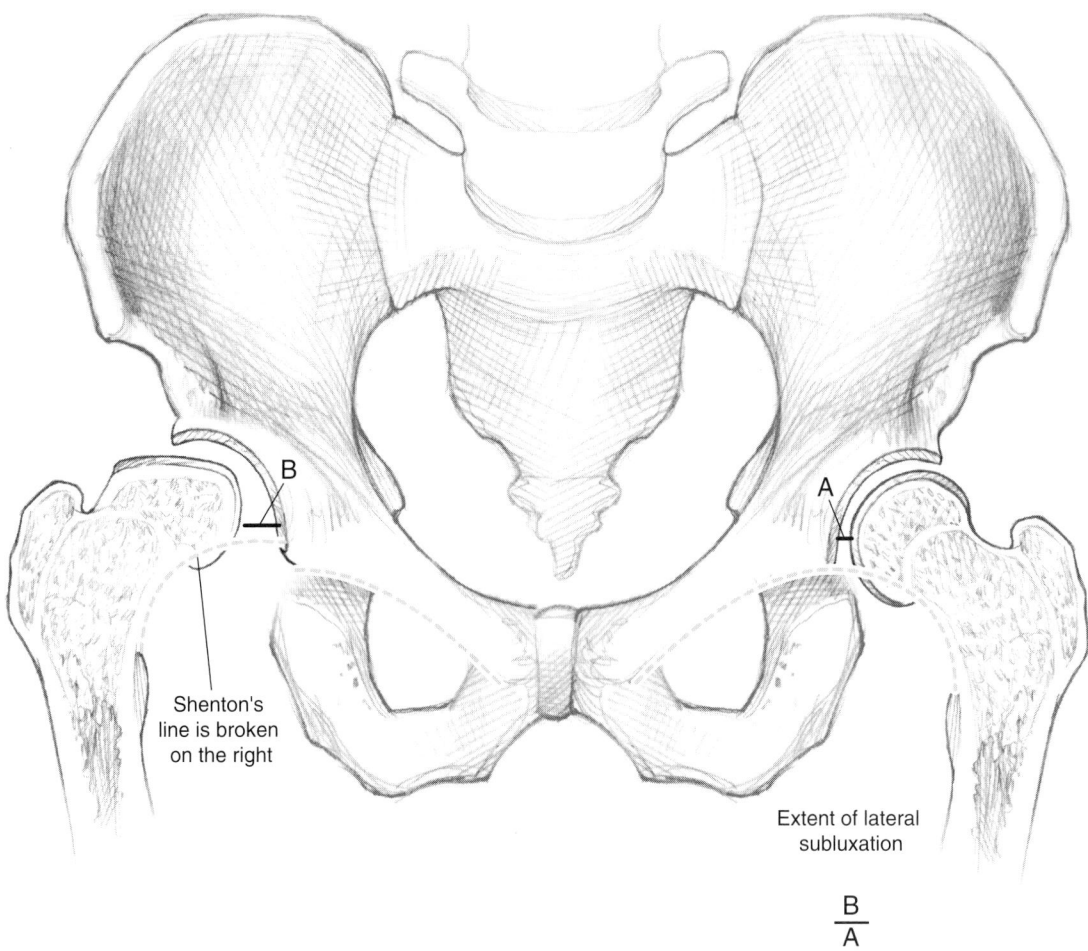

Shenton's
line is broken
on the right

A

Extent of lateral
subluxation

$$\frac{B}{A}$$

Fig. 2. View. The right hip is subluxated laterally and proximally.

CLASSIFICATION SCHEMES AFTER SKELETAL MATURITY

Two classification schemes are used after skeletal maturity: the Mose and the Stulberg.

Mose proposed using circular templates to evaluate the shape of the femoral head at skeletal maturity[8] (Fig. 3). He defined a "good" outcome as a spherical head (less than 1 mm of deviation from circular on the anteroposterior and lateral radiograph). Those that deviate up to 2 mm have a "fair" outcome, and those that deviate by more than 2 mm have a "poor" outcome.

Stulberg et al[16] proposed a five-part rating system to predict long-term performance (Fig. 4). Types I and II have a Mose good femoral head and congruent acetabula. They have normal hip function. Type III and type IV have Mose's fair and Mose's poor femoral heads, with congruent acetabula. These patients develop arthritis in their fifth, sixth, and seventh decades. Type V hips have Mose's poor heads and incongruent acetabula. These patients develop arthritis prior to the fifth decade.

All patients with Mose's good outcomes have normal hip function in the longest follow-up study in the medical literature.[32] Patients with all other outcomes develop arthritis, if monitored long enough.

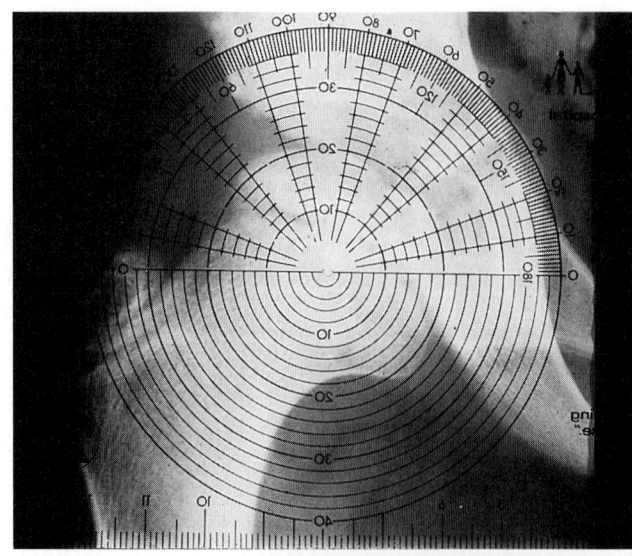

Fig. 3. Mose's template centered on femoral head. The head varies by 2 mm from circular. This is an example of a Mose fair outcome.

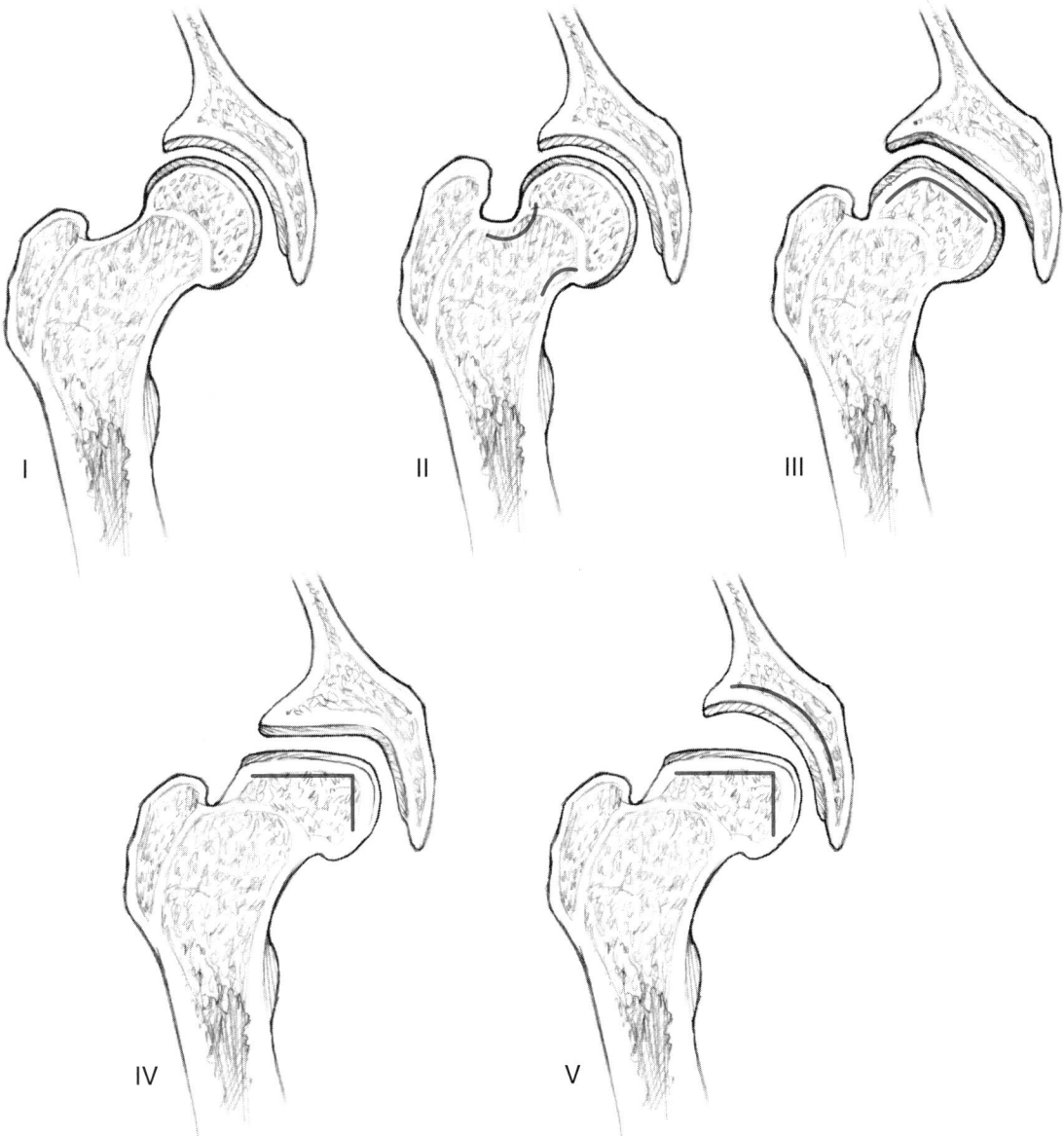

Fig. 4. Views. I, Normal hip. II, Mose's good head with some variation from normal, such as a short femoral neck. III, Mose's fair or poor head. Mushroom-shaped or triangular with congruent acetabulum. IV, Mose's poor head. Square head with congruent acetabulum. V, Mose's poor head, with incongruent acetabulum.

CLINICAL FEATURES

The onset of Perthes' disease is insidious, beginning with intermittent limping. It is frequently painless. Many months may pass before children are brought to medical attention. When complaints of pain exist, many patients report discomfort in the groin and anteromedial thigh, which is the obturator nerve distribution. Occasionally, patients complain of ipsilateral knee pain only and deny any groin or thigh pain. Symptoms are exacerbated by activity and palliated by bedrest. Early in the disease, the physical examination will demonstrate a limp that is a combination of a Trendelenburg limp and an antalgic limp. The affected side demonstrates decreased hip abduction and decreased hip rotation with internal rotation being absent and external rotation being decreased from the normal side. Much of the loss of the range of motion is due to muscle spasm. Range of motion may increase dramatically after a day or two of bedrest. Mild to moderate thigh atrophy is common. Late in the disease, hip adduction and flexion contractures do not palliate dramatically with bedrest, as contractures become more fixed. As patients near adulthood, it is uncommon to demonstrate muscle contracture, although patients with nonspherical femoral heads may have restricted motion.

INVESTIGATION

RADIOGRAPHS

Plain radiographs are usually adequate to diagnose Perthes' disease, even in the early stages. The first signs of Perthes' disease are lateralization of a femoral head that is slightly smaller than the opposite side. The affected side appears smaller because growth has temporarily ceased. It is lateralized secondary to cartilage hypertrophy. Next, increased density is noted. This may be apparent rather than real, due to a relative decrease in density of the normal surrounding bone secondary to disuse. The density of the affected epiphysis does not change because the necrotic epiphysis cannot respond to disuse. There may be a real increase in density, as the newly revascularized epiphysis has new bone laid down upon necrotic bone yet to be resorbed. Other radiographic changes in Perthes' disease are listed in Table 1 and Figure 1.

TECHNETIUM SCANNING

Bone scanning can make the diagnosis of Perthes' disease more quickly than plain radiography.[33] The avascular necrosis of Perthes' disease is evidenced by decreased isotope uptake, which can be noted on both the anteroposterior and the lateral views of the hip. Some authors have proposed staging systems based on bone scan, but these systems are not in wide use.

MAGNETIC RESONANCE IMAGING

Magnetic resonance imaging (MRI) can diagnose Perthes' disease more quickly than plain radiographs. There is disagreement about whether MRI is faster or more sensitive than bone scanning in establishing a diagnosis. Certainly it provides excellent detail concerning the true shape of the femoral head, acetabulum, femoral cartilage, and acetabular cartilage. It is seldom used for making treatment decisions.

ARTHROGRAPHY

The hip arthrogram is a useful and occasionally used tool. Before MRI, it was the definitive way to characterize the true shape of the cartilaginous femoral head. Schiller and Axer[34] used arthrograms to identify the extent of flattening and lateralization of the epiphysis and used this information to make clinical decisions. Today, MRI can provide the same information noninvasively. Arthrograms can be used to provide dynamic views of coverage in patients with badly deformed femoral heads (Figs. 5 to 7).

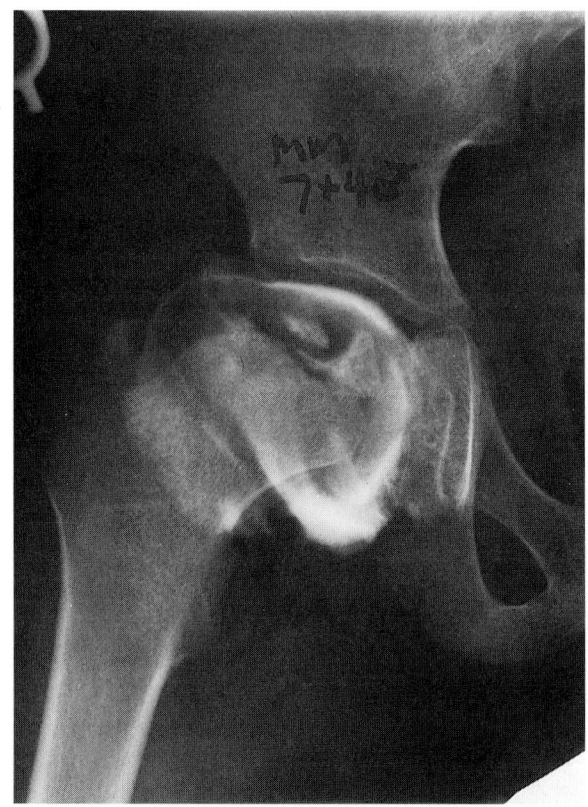

Fig. 6. Patient No. 1. An arthrogram demonstrates flattening of the femoral head.

DIFFERENTIAL DIAGNOSIS

Perthes' disease is a common problem in boys of short stature between 4 and 8 years of age with a unilateral hip problem causing a painless or near painless limp of many months' duration. In addition, if these boys have limited hip abduction and internal rotation combined with modest thigh atrophy and a delayed bone age, Perthes' disease is

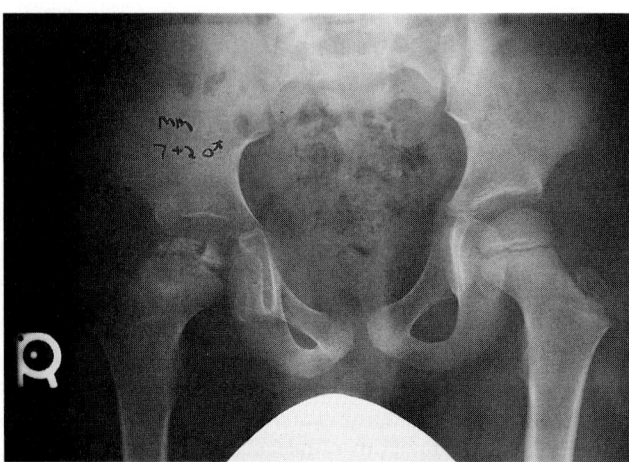

Fig. 5. Patient No. 1. The right hip is significantly subluxated laterally and proximally.

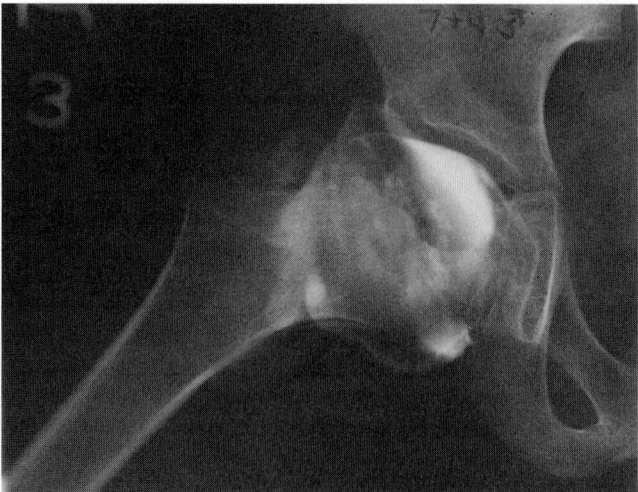

Fig. 7. Patient No. 1. Abduction and internal rotation place the flattened femoral head within the acetabulum "containing" it.

likely. Add this to radiographs demonstrating a fragmented, small, lateralized proximal femoral epiphysis with a small metaphyseal cyst or two, and the diagnosis of Perthes' disease is assured. There are, of course, other processes that affect the hips of children that might mimic some aspects of Perthes' disease, so a rather broad differential diagnostic list should be familiar.

TOXIC SYNOVITIS

Toxic synovitis is a self-limiting acute synovitis often seen in boys less than 4 years of age. It lasts from 3 to 10 days. In general there is acute onset of pain. There is minimal thigh atrophy. Most cases of toxic synovitis clear with bedrest and anti-inflammatory medications in a few to 5 days. If the synovitis lasts longer than 10 days, a bone scan can be used to rule out Perthes' disease.

HIP JOINT INFECTION

Pyogenic arthritis can be confused with toxic synovitis and Perthes' disease. In pyogenic arthritis, the patient is acutely ill with a fever, an increased white blood cell count, and increased erythrocyte sedimentation rate. These are not seen in Perthes' disease. In infection, children tend to hold their hips in flexion, abduction, and external rotation to create the largest possible hip joint volume. In Perthes' disease, hip adduction is more common. An ultrasonogram can be useful in identifying an effusion, which may require aspiration. The diagnosis of infection is suggested when the aspirated fluid has an extremely high white blood cell count or bacteria present on Gram's stain.

JUVENILE RHEUMATOID ARTHRITIS

Occasionally monarticular juvenile rheumatoid arthritis will present as arthritis at one hip. Children with this condition will frequently have a limp and hip pain of insidious onset. They may demonstrate signs of chronicity, such as thigh atrophy. Aspiration can reveal surprisingly high white blood cell counts. Juvenile rheumatoid arthritis can be confused with early Perthes' disease, toxic synovitis, or pyogenic arthritis. A careful history revealing fevers and a rash combined with blood test results such as a positive antinuclear antibody test or changes suggestive of uveitis[35] on a slit lamp examination can confirm the diagnosis of juvenile rheumatoid arthritis.

BILATERALITY

Bilateral Perthes' disease is seen in 10% of patients. It would be very uncommon, however, to see bilateral Perthes' disease presenting with both hips at the same Waldenström stage (see Table 1). When bilateral and symmetrical hip disease resembling Perthes' disease presents, it is most often a bone dysplasia such as multiple epiphyseal dysplasia or spondyloepiphyseal dysplasia. In both settings, there may be a history of family members with short stature and early hip and knee arthritis. Additionally, plain radiographs of the knees and spine should be abnormal in spondyloepiphyseal dysplasia and normal in patients with Perthes' disease. Hypothyroidism is a rare cause of radiographs suggestive of bilateral Perthes' disease. A careful physical examination and appropriate laboratory tests should diagnose cretinism.

JUVENILE OSTEONECROSIS

There are many causes of juvenile osteonecrosis other than Perthes' disease. Hemoglobinopathy such as sickle cell disease and thalassemia are often encountered. Osteonecrosis can also be seen in idiopathic thrombocytopenia purpura and hemophilia. A careful history will usually suggest these hematological disorders, which may also be suspected from routine blood testing. Gaucher's disease is occasionally confused with Perthes' disease, but a careful history and an appropriate physical examination and blood tests should make this diagnosis. Perthes'-like changes can be seen following treatment of developmental hip dysplasia, traumatically dislocated hips, femoral neck fracture, hip joint infection, and certain neoplasms such as leukemia, lymphoma, and eosinophilic granuloma. A history, clinical examination, and laboratory studies such as bone scans, computed tomographic scan, bone marrow aspiration, and routine blood tests can be used to identify these problems.

MANAGEMENT

Some general rules determine prognosis in patients with Perthes' disease: (1) younger patients do better than older ones; (2) partial head involvement is less destructive than whole head involvement; and (3) proximal and lateral subluxation is a bad sign. There is confusion about the natural history of Perthes' disease because these factors are difficult to quantitate. It is not known whether bone age or chronological age is a better measure of "age." The modern classification schemes during the active phase of Perthes' disease do not adequately account for the extent of femoral head involvement because they describe only a few points along the continuum of the disease. Also, these schemes are difficult to apply consistently, and *none* factor in cartilage abnormalities that may play an important role in outcome. Proximal and lateral subluxation are reflections of femoral head flattening, but the best way to measure or grade flattening is not known. The difficulty in defining these terms makes the natural history of Perthes' disease difficult to understand and the effects of treatment especially difficult to understand. Consequently, there is considerable disagreement in the medical community about the efficacy of treatment of Perthes' disease.

I believe that there are patients who would benefit from one of the three basic types of treatment.

SYMPTOMATIC TREATMENT

Most patients with Perthes' disease have synovitis early in the initial stage. Bedrest and occasional administration of anti-inflammatory drugs are used to provide comfort and increase range of motion. Almost all patients benefit from this type of treatment.

CONTAINMENT TREATMENT

"Failure to introduce the head completely into the acetabulum will result in unequal compression on various aspects of the epiphysis and high and low spots with resulting deformation. If the femoral head is *contained* within the acetabular cup, then like jelly poured into a mold, the head should be the same shape as the cup when it is allowed to come out after reconstitution."[10] This notion has been expressed for decades. It served as justification for treating all patients with Perthes' disease prior to 1970. Since then, practitioners have learned that some patients develop round femoral heads without treatment, some need containment, and others have femoral heads that are so severely deformed that containment does not work (see Table 2).

Most containment treatment is preceded by efforts to maximize hip range of motion. Bedrest, traction, physical therapy, anti-inflammatory medications, and occasional soft tissue lengthenings are used.

A variety of braces and surgical procedures have been designed to provide containment. The braces provide either hip abduction and internal rotation (Petrie's[11] casts, Newington's abduction orthosis[36]) or abduction and hip flexion (Scottish Rite orthosis[36]). The brace is worn until the active phase of the disease subsides and healing begins (when fragmentation ends and the reparative phase begins). This point can be identified on a radiograph when the first puff of new bone is seen in the epiphysis where necrotic bone had previously been resorbed. This can be 6 to 24 months from the onset of symptoms. Surgery can contain the head. Currently, many different types and combinations of femoral and pelvic osteotomies are used to contain the hip, especially varus derotation osteotomy and innominate osteotomy. Following surgery, no bracing is necessary. Consequently, the "time in treatment" is much shorter than with bracing. Once the operation has healed, children can have full and unrestricted activities. Rab et al[37] investigated the femoral acetabular relationship using finite element analysis. They determined that the femoral head was 120% of a hemisphere whereas the acetabulum was 75% of the hemisphere. This suggests that "containment" of the entire head is impossible, as the head is "too big" to be contained. This led to some skepticism about containment treatment, especially in patients with whole head involvement.[24,25] In spite of this, containment is the most often invoked concept when treatment is undertaken to improve femoral head shape.

Braces and surgery are equally effective for most patients who need containment. The treatment offered should suit the child and family, as there are considerable differences between surgery and bracing treatments.

SALVAGE SURGERY

When the reparative stage begins, the epiphysis is no longer deformable. Containment will not cause the head to become more round. If the hip is misshapen and symptomatic, surgery can be offered to compensate for its shape (see Complications).

PROBLEM PATIENTS

Patients with whole femoral head involvement who are between 6 and 10 years of age at the onset of disease with significant subluxation and patients who are older than 10 years at the onset of disease represent problematic cases. Treatment can be offered, but expectations must be limited. Results are frequently disappointing. Whether the results of treatment are worse than the outcome with no treatment at all has not been established.

Occasionally, younger patients can have much worse outcomes than their age at presentation or pattern of involvement would suggest. These patients cannot be identified in advance. It may be that they have a disease different in pathogenesis than typical Perthes' disease, or possibly they have much more severe cartilaginous involvement and this cannot be appreciated on the radiograph. When these patients are seen in clinical practice, it causes doubt about all that is known about the typical child with Perthes' disease.

COMPLICATIONS

Complications of brace treatment in patients with Perthes' disease are rare. Occasionally knee stiffness or pain and hip abduction contractures are encountered. After treatment is discontinued, the problems usually resolve rapidly. Varus derotation osteotomy and innominate osteotomy are the most popular surgeries for Perthes' disease patients. These procedures share some general risks, including (1) adverse reaction to anesthesia, (2) infection, (3) damage to nerves

TABLE 2. INDICATIONS FOR CONTAINMENT TREATMENT IN PERTHES' DISEASE		
Patients Who Do Well with No Treatment	**Patients Who Benefit from Treatment**	**Patients Who May Do Poorly with or Without Treatment**
Partial head involvement* without subluxation, age <8 y†	Partial head involvement with subluxation, age <8 y	Whole head involvement with subluxation, age 6–10 y
Whole head involvement‡ with no subluxation, age <6 y	Partial head involvement with or without subluxation, age 8–10 y	Age >10 y
	Whole head involvement with subluxation, age <6 y	
	Whole head involvement without subluxation, age 6–10 y	
	SUBLUXATION	
	1. Significant lateral subluxation—greater than 1.5 to 1.0 lateral subluxation ratio	
	2. Significant superior subluxation—Shenton's line broken	

* Catterall I and II disease.
† All ages are chronological ages at onset of disease.
‡ Catterall III and IV disease.

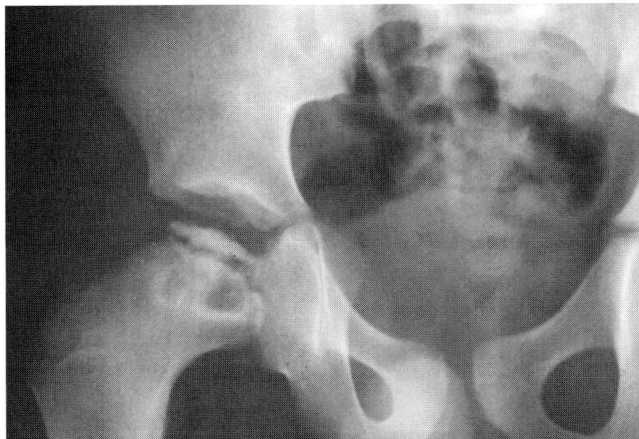

Fig. 8. Patient No. 2. This shows complete collapse of the epiphysis with metaphyseal cysts. There is insignificant lateral subluxation and no proximal subluxation.

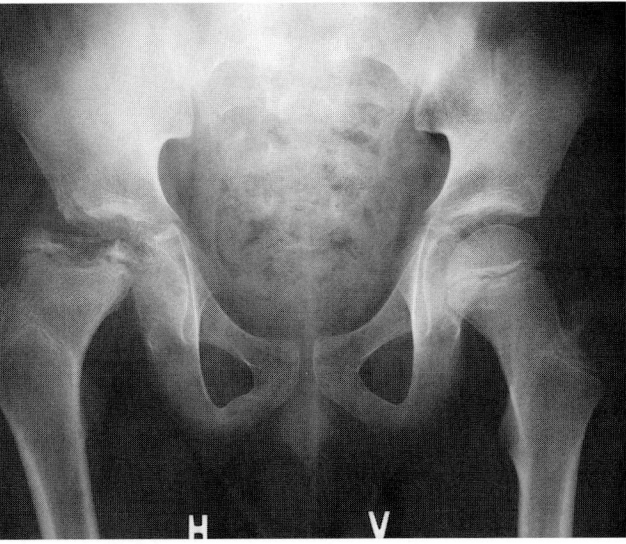

Fig. 10. Patient No. 3. This shows partial head involvement with significant lateral and proximal subluxation. The patient is treated with crutches. (From Cooperman DR, Stulberg SD: Clin Orthop Rel Res 1986; 203:289.)

and blood vessels in the surgical field, and (4) delayed or nonunion at the osteotomy site.

There are complications peculiar to innominate osteotomy. They are lengthening of the ipsilateral leg and loss of alignment at the operative site. The site is fixed with two or three large threaded wires, but fixation is in the cancellous bone of the pelvis and can be tenuous. If the cortical bone on the medial wall of the pelvis above and below the osteotomy is not well aligned, the distal fragment may settle into the proximal fragment and correction may be lost. Also, incomplete release of the iliopsoas at the pelvic brim can increase pressure within the hip joint, causing stiffness and flattening of the femoral head.

Varus derotation osteotomy has certain specific risks associated with it. A Trendelenburg gait is almost always seen immediately following surgery. If normal remodeling of the femoral head and neck do not occur, this Trendelenburg limp can be permanent, unless a second operation is offered. Varus alignment also shortens the ipsilateral leg

about 1.5 cm. If more than 10 or 15 degrees of derotation are added to the osteotomy, external rotation of the foot will evidence itself initially. If the femoral head becomes round and growth proceeds normally, the foot should rotate back to a neutral position. If the femoral head does not remodel sufficiently, permanent external rotation deformity of the lower extremity may result. In both innominate and

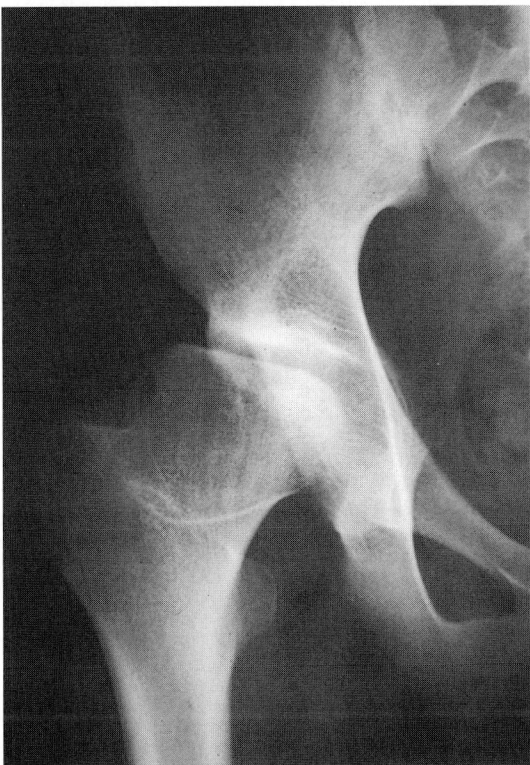

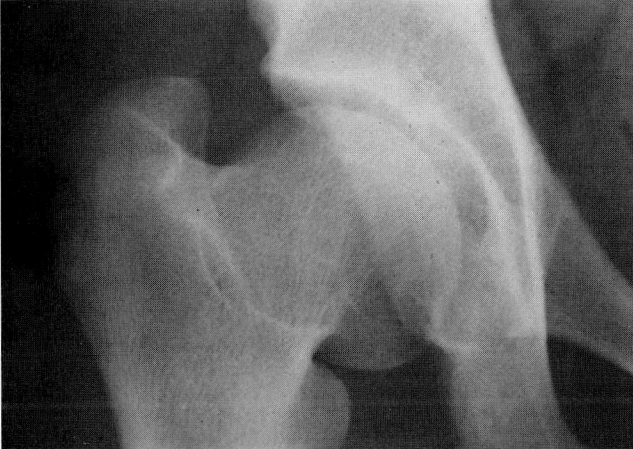

Fig. 9. Patient No. 2. This shows a Mose good head, Stulberg's 2 outcome. The head is round, and the neck has suffered a growth arrest. The trochanter is overriding.

Fig. 11. Patient No. 3. This shows a Mose poor, Stulberg's 4 outcome with a flat femoral head and flat acetabulum. (From Cooperman DR, Stulberg SD: Clin Orthop Rel Res 1986; 203:289.)

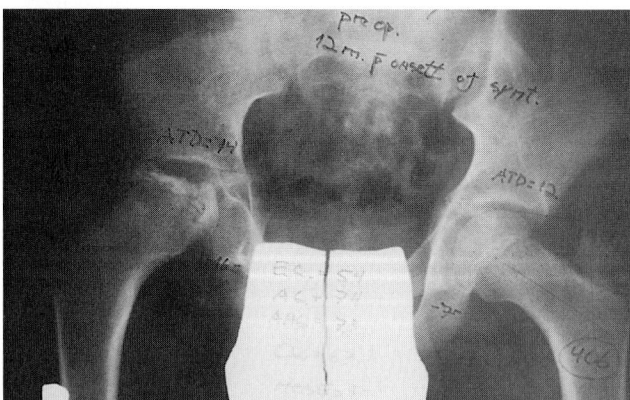

Fig. 12. Patient No. 4. This shows partial head involvement in a 10-year-old male patient in the fragmentation stage. He has significant lateral and proximal subluxation. He is at risk for a poor outcome. (From Cooperman DR, Stulberg SD: Clin Orthop Rel Res 1986; 203: 289.)

femoral osteotomy, a secondary anesthetic procedure is necessary for hardware removal.

Biological complications also occur in Perthes' disease. These occur with or without treatment and as such are more closely related to poor outcomes than to complications of treatment.

Femoral neck growth arrest is occasionally seen in patients with Perthes' disease. This will result in apparent overriding of the greater trochanter and a leg length discrepancy (Figs. 8 and 9). A Trendelenburg limp can result if the tip of the trochanter is proximal to the superior articular surface of the femoral head. This biological problem can be considerably exacerbated if a varus derotation osteotomy has been performed. A trochanteric advancement and a contralateral distal femoral epiphysiodesis may be necessary to correct this problem.

Osteochondritis dissecans complicates Perthes' disease.[38] This process may liberate a bony fragment into the hip joint and cause hip pain. If this occurs, excision of the fragment is recommended.

Occasionally, patients undergo such severe collapse that the hip becomes grossly incongruous. One type of incongruous outcome has been labeled hinged abduction. In this setting, the femoral head is so misshapen that abduction causes most of the medial aspect of the head to be pried away from the medial wall of the socket. Experts vary on the best approach to this problem. Recommendations include valgus osteotomy, Chiari's osteotomy, cheilectomy, and shelf procedure. The range of options suggests that no option is particularly attractive.

RESULTS OF TREATMENT

Results of treatment need to be compared to the natural history of the disease to be meaningful. Salter did this in a 1980 report.[14] He studied a group of 38 patients treated

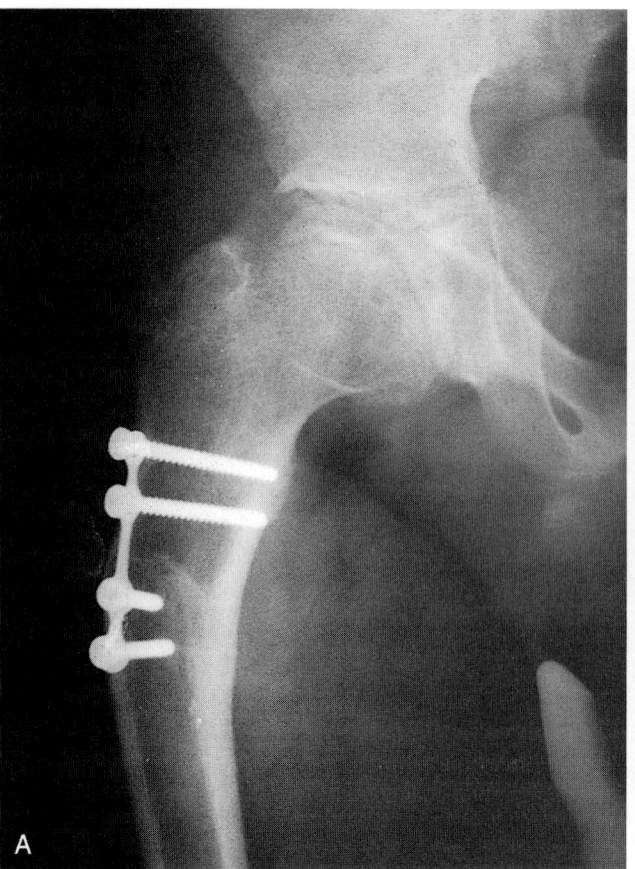

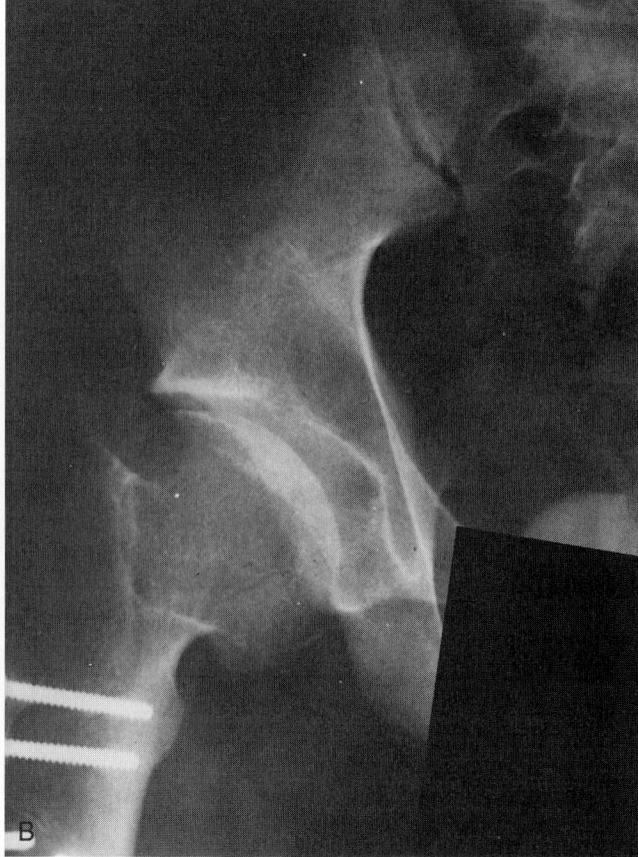

Fig. 13. Patient No. 4. Approaching skeletal maturity *(A)* and at skeletal maturity *(B)* a Mose good, Stulberg's 2 outcome can be seen following varus derotation osteotomy. (From Cooperman DR, Stulberg SD: Clin Orthop Rel Res 1986; 203:289.)

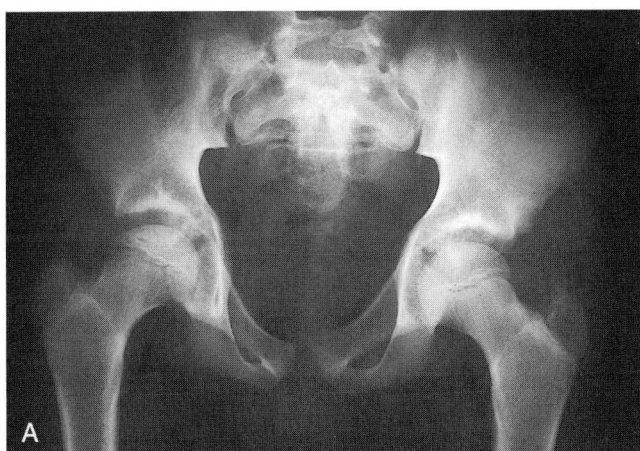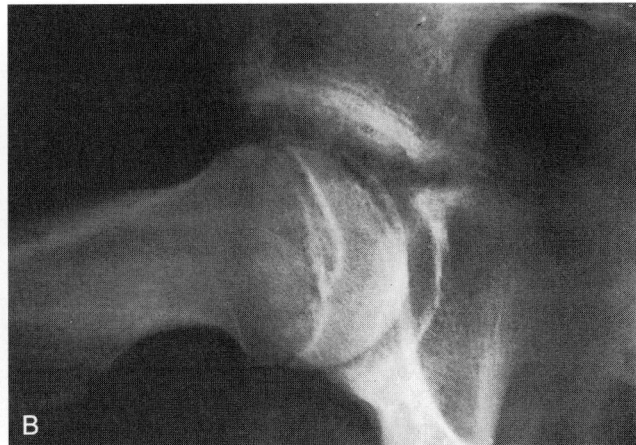

Fig. 14. Patient No. 5. This shows a 13-year-old male early in the fragmentation phase with insignificant proximal *(A)* and lateral *(B)* subluxation. Note his subchondral fracture. (From Stulberg SD, Cooperman DR: J Bone Jt Surg Am 1981; 63:1095.)

with non-weightbearing, noncontainment methods (average age at onset was 7 years). At maturity, this group of patients had 37% Mose's good results, 29% Mose's fair, and 34% Mose's poor. A second group was studied that consisted of 110 patients. All had Salter-Thompson B disease and all were older than 6 years of age, with an average age of 8. All had loss of containment. Salter recommends treatment for all children older than 6 years with Salter-Thompson B disease with a loss of containment. All these patients underwent an innominate osteotomy, and that resulted in 77% Mose's good, 17% Mose's fair, and 6% Mose's poor outcomes.

Cooperman and Stulberg[36] reported a multicenter study in 1986. Seventy-two patients were treated with crutches and a cork lift on the opposite foot. This was essentially a nontreatment group. Fifty-eight patients were treated with a Scottish Rite orthosis (a waist belt attached to two thigh cuffs enforcing hip abduction and allowing free flexion and extension). Forty-eight patients were treated with a Newington abduction orthosis (a long leg brace enforcing abduction and internal rotation) and 70 with femoral osteotomies. Patients under 8 years of age with Catterall's I and II lesions without subluxation did equally well in all four groups. The authors concluded that none needed treatment, as crutches are essentially no treatment. In patients 8 years

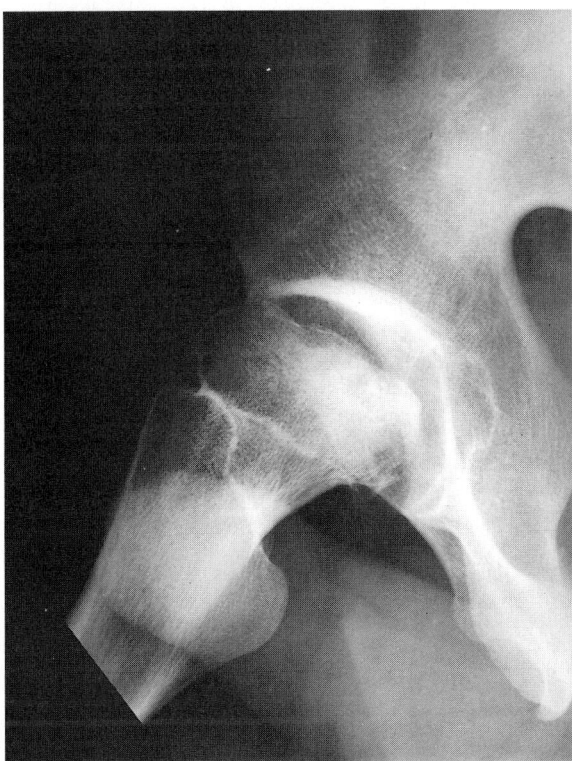

Fig. 15. Patient No. 5. This patient was treated with crutches. He has a Stulberg 5 outcome. (From Stulberg SD, Cooperman DR: J Bone Jt Surg Am 1981; 63:1095.)

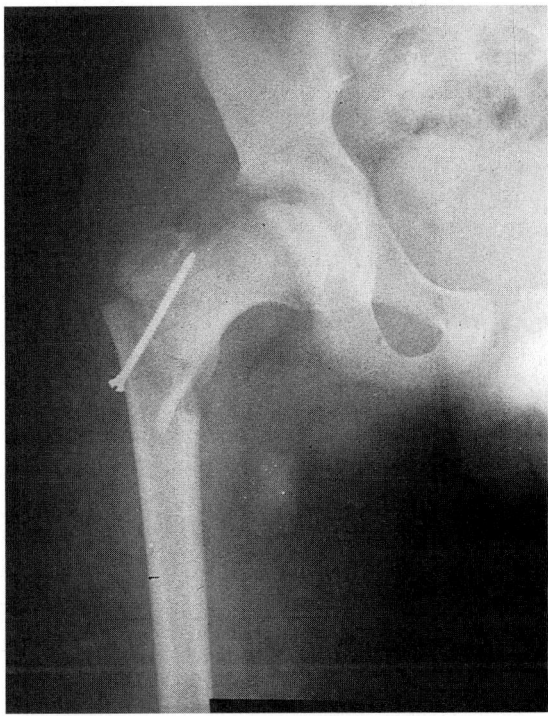

Fig. 16. Patient No. 6. A 12-year-old in the initial stage s/p varus derotation osteotomy. (From Stulberg SD, Cooperman DR: J Bone Jt Surg Am 1981; 63:1095.)

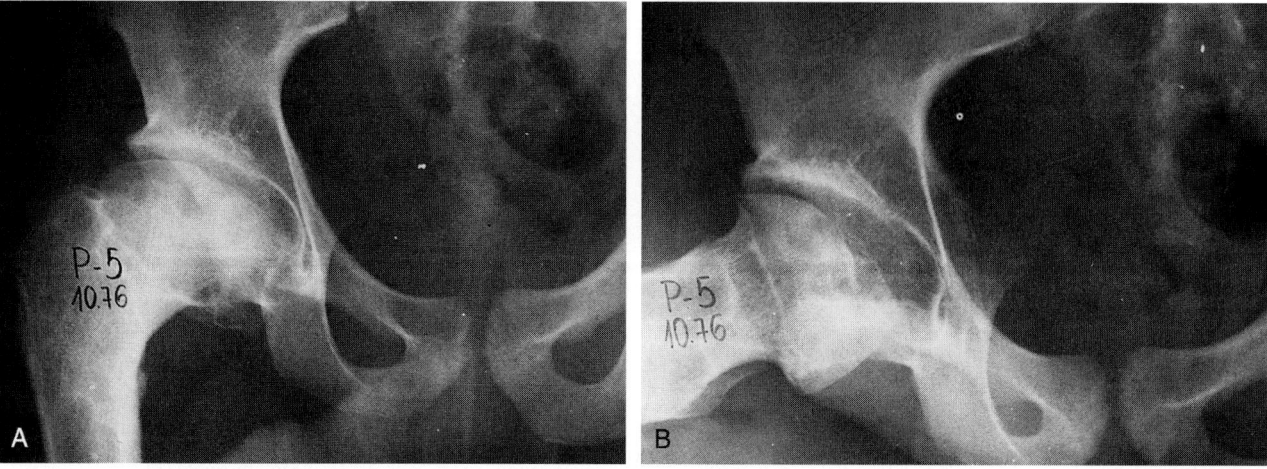

Fig. 17. Patient No. 6. At maturity, the patient has a Stulberg 5 outcome. He has evidenced considerable collapse and no remodeling (*A* and *B*).

of age and younger with Catterall's I and type II involvement with significant subluxation, the containment groups (both braces and varus derotation osteotomy) fared better than the crutch-walking group, and all containment groups fared equally well. In patients 8 to 12 years of age with partial head involvement with or without subluxations, all containment methods were superior to crutch-walking (Figs. 10 to 13). Patients older than 12 years of age with partial head involvement fared poorly with or without treatment (Figs. 14 to 17). Patients younger than 8 years old with total head involvement (Catterall's III or IV) did better with varus derotation osteotomies than with braces or crutches. In the group of patients older than 8 years with whole head involvement, all three containment methods were superior to crutch walking, but numbers were small.

These studies suggest that containment works for certain patients. Significant subluxation is a sign of femoral head flattening and needs treatment. Increasing age is a poor prognostic sign, as the disease begins to resemble adult idiopathic avascular necrosis, where collapse is not followed by reconstitution. Containment plays no role in the treatment of adult idiopathic avascular necrosis. As children age (>10 years) their disease more closely resembles adult idiopathic avascular necrosis, in that the prognosis for remodeling is poor.

Girls do worse than boys. They are more likely to have more severe involvement at any given age compared with boys and they have fewer years to remodel. The prognosis for girls is always guarded.

Functional assessment of children and young adults demonstrates normal or near normal function in most patients after the acute phase of Perthes' disease subsides. Patients do well for decades even with considerable deformity. This fact has occasioned some experts to forego containment treatment. These authorities await more certain information about prognosis and response to treatment than exists today. Other experts treat aggressively with containment treatment based on the literature and personal experience. The treatment of Perthes' disease causes more controversy than the treatment of any other childhood hip disorder.

REFERENCES

1. Harbin M, Zollinger R: Osteochondritis of the growth centers. Surg Gynecol Obstet 1930; LI:145.
2. Herring JA: Legg-Calvé-Perthes Disease. AAOS Monograph Series, 1996.
3. Thompson GH, Salter RB: Legg-Calvé-Perthes disease: Current concepts and controversies. Orthop Clin North Am 1987; 18:617.
4. Goff CW: Legg-Calvé-Perthes Syndrome and Related Osteochondroses of Youth. Springfield, Charles C. Thomas, 1954, p 3.
5. Phemister DB: Operation for epiphysitis of the head of the femur (Perthes' disease): Finding and result. Arch Surg 1921; 2: 221.
6. Waldenström H: The definite form of the coxa plana. Acta Radiol 1922; 1:384.
7. Jonsater S: Coxa plana: A histo-pathologic and arthrographic study. Acta Orthop Scand 1953; Suppl XII.
7a. Ratliff AHC: Perthes' disease. J Bone Joint Surg Br 1967; 49:102.
7b. Snyder CH: A sling for use in Legg-Perthes disease. J Bone Joint Surg 1947; 29: 524.
8. Mose K: Legg-Calvé-Perthes Disease: A Comparison Between Three Methods of Conservative Treatment. Universitets Rorlaget Aarhus, 1964.
9. Harrison MH, Menon MP: Legg-Calvé-Perthes disease: The value of roentgenographic measurement in clinical practice with special reference to the broomstick plaster method. J Bone Joint Surg Am 1966; 48:1301.
10. Harrison MH, Turner MH, Nicholson FJ: Coxa plana: Results of a new form of splinting. J Bone Joint Surg Am 1969; 51: 1057.
11. Petrie JG, Bitenc I: The abduction weight-bearing treatment in Legg-Calvé-Perthes' disease. J Bone Joint Surg Br 1981; 53:54.
12. Soeur R, Berchmans E, Simonart J, et al: Pathologenie et classement des osteochondrites en general. Acta Orthop Belg 1952; 18:51.
13. Axer A: Subtrochanteric osteotomy in the treatment of Perthes' disease: A preliminary report. J Bone Joint Surg Br 1965; 47:489.
14. Salter RB: Legg-Perthes disease: The scientific basis for the methods of treatment and their indications. Clin Orthop 1980; 150:8.
15. Catterall A: The natural history of Perthes' disease. J Bone Joint Surg Br 1971; 53:37.

16. Stulberg SD, Cooperman DR, Wallenstein R: The natural history of Legg-Calvé-Perthes disease. J Bone Joint Surg Am 1981; 63:1095.
17. Salter RB, Thompson GH: Legg-Calvé-Perthes disease: The prognostic significance of the subchondral fracture and a two-group classification of the femoral head involvement. J Bone Joint Surg Am 1984; 66:479.
18. Herring JA, Newstatt JB, Williams JJ, et al: The lateral Pillar classification of Legg-Calvé-Perthes disease. J Pediatr Orthop 1992; 12:143.
19. Christensen F, Soballe K, Ejsted R, et al: The Catterall classification of Perthes' disease: An assessment of reliability. J Bone Joint Surg Br 1986; 68:614.
20. Catterall A, Pringle J, Byers PD, et al: A review of the morphology of Perthes' disease. J Bone Joint Surg Br 1982; 64:269.
21. Ippolito E, Ponseti I: The role of epiphyseal cartilage and physis of the proximal femur in the pathogenesis of LCPD. Mapfre Med 1995; 6:16.
22. Ponseti IV, Maynard JA, Weinstein SL, et al: Legg-Calvé-Perthes disease: Histochemical and ultrastructural observations of the epiphyseal cartilage and physis. J Bone Joint Surg Am 1983; 65:797.
23. Martinez AG, Weinstein S, Dietz FR: The weightbearing abduction brace for the treatment of Legg-Perthes disease. J Bone Joint Surg Am 1992; 74:12.
24. Meehan PL, Angel D, Nelson JM: The Scottish-Rite abduction orthosis for the treatment of Legg-Perthes disease. J Bone Joint Surg Am 1992; 74:2.
25. Liu SL, Ho TC: The role of venous hypertension in the pathogenesis of Legg-Perthes disease: A clinical and experimental study. J Bone Joint Surg Am 1991; 73:194.
26. Kleinman RG, Bleck EE: Increased blood viscosity in patients with Legg-Perthes disease: A preliminary report. J Ped Orthop 1981; 1:131.
27. Glueck CJ, Crawford A, Roy D, et al: Association of antithrombotic factor deficiencies and hypofibrimolysis with Legg-Perthes disease. J Bone Joint Surg Am 1996; 78:3.
28. Inoue A, Freeman MAR, Vernon-Roberts B, et al: The pathogenesis of Perthes' disease. J Bone Joint Surg Br 1976; 58:453.
29. Harrison MH, Blakemore ME: A study of the "normal" hip in children with unilateral Perthes' disease. J Bone Joint Surg Br 1980; 62:31.
30. Van Dom BE, Crider RJ, Noyes JD, Larsen LJ: Determination of the Catterall classification in Legg-Calve-Perthes disease. J Bone Joint Surg Am 1981; 63:906.
31. Gershuni DH, Exer A, Hendel D: Arthrography as an aid to diagnosis, prognosis, and therapy in Legg-Calvé-Perthes disease. Acta Orthop Scand 1980; 51:505.
32. McAndrew MP, Weinstein SL: A long-term follow-up of Legg-Calvé-Perthes disease. J Bone Joint Surg Am 1984; 66:860.
33. Fisher RL, Roderique JW, Brown DC, et al: The relationship of isotopic bone imaging findings to prognosis in Legg-Perthes disease. Clin Orthop Rel Res 1980; 150:23.
34. Schiller MG, Axer A: Hypertrophy of the femoral head in Legg-Calvé-Perthes syndrome. Acta Orthop Scand 1972; 43:45.
35. Nguyen QD: Saving the vision of children with juvenile rheumatoid arthritis associated with uveitis. JAMA 1998; 280:1133.
36. Cooperman DR, Stulberg SD: Ambulatory containment treatment in Perthes' disease. Clin Orthop Rel Res 1986; 203:289.
37. Rab GT, Wyatt M, Sutherland DH, et al: A technique for determining femoral head containment during gait. J Ped Orthop 1985; 5:8.
38. Wood JB, Klassen RA, Peterson HA: Osteochondritis dissecans of the femoral head in children and adolescents: A report of 17 cases. J Ped Orthop 1995; 15:313.

section 9 chapter

20

SLIPPED CAPITAL FEMORAL EPIPHYSIS

Scott A. Hoffinger

Summary
- Slipped capital femoral epiphysis (SCFE) is common and can present as frequently as 1 in 400 males.
- SCFE often presents as vague knee or thigh pain and is often diagnosed weeks after the onset of symptoms.
- SCFEs are classified as stable or unstable, with a higher rate of avascular necrosis (AVN) among unstable cases.
- In situ pinning is recommended for all stable and most unstable cases.

SCFE is a common adolescent disorder that has been implicated as a cause of adult osteoarthritis of the hip.[1, 2] Fortunately, current treatment permits reproducible, good results in the majority of cases.

Although common terminology refers to slippage of the epiphyseal portion of the proximal femur, the epiphysis is actually held within the acetabulum, and the femoral neck that displaces anteriorly and proximally relative to the femoral head. This causes an acquired retroversion of the proximal femur, resulting in the typical clinical presentation of a shortened, externally rotated, lower extremity.

INCIDENCE

The incidence of SCFE has been reported to differ widely in a variety of subgroups. White girls have a risk of 1.64:100,000,[3, 4] and white boys have an incidence of 1:988, when age most at risk is considered.[5] According to Kelsey,[3] the cumulative risk (incidence x number of years at risk) is as high as 1:400 for black males. Loder et al[6] have also shown considerable racial variation. They reported a frequency of 0.1 for Indo-Mediterraneans and a high of 4.5 for the Polynesian population relative to white individuals (1.0). There is a suggestion that patients in northern latitudes may have a seasonal variation in presentation, with symptoms more likely to develop in the summer months.[5, 7] Slipped epiphysis is also believed to have a genetic component, expressed as autosomal-dominant with variable penetrance, and a positive family history can increase the risk of developing a slip to 7%.[8]

Many patients present with bilateral SCFE, and others develop contralateral slipping during the remainder of their growth[5, 6, 9–14]: one-fifth of patients have bilateral SCFE at presentation,[11, 13, 14] and up to 43% may develop a contralateral slip before the end of growth for a total bilateral rate of 34% to 61%.[6, 11] However, 92% of patients who develop late contralateral slippage are asymptomatic, and most of these slips are mild in severity.[13] Stasikelis et al[6, 14, 15] have shown that patients who develop bilateral slips tend to be younger, male, and more skeletally immature. Although the majority of patients who develop contralateral slips do so in the first 18 months after presentation, all patients should be monitored radiographically until physeal closure.[6, 13]

ETIOLOGICAL FACTORS

Excess weight is a significant element in many patients with SCFE and may be the primary etiologic factor in some.[6, 10, 14, 16, 17] In the study of Loder et al,[6, 7] 87% of children had above-average weight, with 63% over the 90th percentile. The average age at presentation was 12 years for girls and 13.5 years for boys, with heavier children presenting younger.

SCFE may be related to endocrine disorders. Hypothyroidism, hypopituitarism, hyperparathyroidism, renal failure, rickets, treatment with growth hormone, radiation therapy, and altered sex hormone ratios due to genetic mosaicism have all been reported.[18–26] However, the significance of these findings in healthy children with normal endocrinological profiles has been questioned. Mann et al[24] found 20% of endocrinologically normal patients with SCFE had at least one abnormal blood hormone level. Wilcox et al[26] reported decreased T_3 in 25% of patients, decreased testosterone in 76% of patients, and decreased growth hormone in 87% of clinically normal patients with SCFE. Other authors have found no abnormalities in growth hormone, testosterone, estradiol, or urinary estrogen levels.[18, 27] Harris[21] and Oka et al[28] showed that estradiol strengthened the physeal plate, and growth hormone and testosterone decreased its strength. Wilcox et al and Harris suggested that it is the ratio of these hormones and not absolute levels that influences physeal strength. Brenkel et al[18] also believed that these hormone levels played a role, possibly through somatomedin. Recommendations for the need for endocrinological testing vary from all patients[29] to patients who have a symptomatic endocrine abnormality.[24] It appears that a thorough history and physical examination can provide valuable information regarding which patients require referral or testing. Patients whose presentation is atypical, particularly patients younger than 10 years, should be screened for endocrinological disease, especially hypothyroidism.

Patients with chronic renal disease often have bilateral involvement, and the risk of progression is high. It is recommended that these patients be closely observed radiographically during a 2-month period of medical management. If they are able to quickly come under good medical control, then they can continue to be observed. However, if their hyperparathyroid status cannot be made stable medically, then bilateral pinning should be considered.[23] Patients who are on thyroid replacement therapy should also be considered for prophylactic bilateral pinning because of the high incidence of bilaterality.[29, 30]

PATHOPHYSIOLOGY

SCFE is a mechanical as well as a biochemical event. Bright et al[16] noted that rat proximal tibiae had a "period of weakness" in prepubescence. They noted that subfailure loads of 50% produced microcracks that made subsequent slipping easier. Male rats also failed with less stress than female rats, just as in humans. Physeal biopsy samples in human SCFE show disruption of the orderly progression of chondrocyte maturation.[31, 32] The cells are not lined up in rows but rather are grouped in clusters. The slipping occurs in the zone of cell hypertrophy but may extend into the zone of provisional calcification.[17, 32] Ultrastructural examination and results of matrix staining have shown changes in the matrix composition[33, 34] as well as increased chondrocyte degeneration and death.[33]

Chung et al[17] noted that the physis may fail on a purely mechanical basis. They studied failure of human pediatric proximal femora and found that the perichondrial ring was important for physeal stability under age 3 years. Over that age the mamillary processes assumed a greater significance and disruption of the perichondrial ring was not needed for failure in older children. Chung and Gelberman et al[17, 35] believed that mechanical factors, coupled with retroversion of the femoral neck, and increased weight could result in failure loads during fast walking or running. No underlying physeal or biochemical abnormality was required.

CLINICAL PRESENTATION

Three distinct modes of patient presentation have been noted: (1) chronic, with symptoms present for more than 3 weeks; these patients are able to walk; (2) acute, with symptoms present for fewer than 3 weeks; these patients may be unable to walk; and (3) acute on chronic, with the patients experiencing an acute exacerbation of their chronic symptoms.

The clinical significance of these presentations was not appreciated until Loder et al[36] stressed the importance of physeal stability. These investigators introduced the term "unstable" for slips in which the patient could not bear weight. Instability had a profound effect on the eventual clinical result, especially in terms of AVN. Fifty-three percent of the unstable hips had a poor result, and only one of the stable slips (4%) had a poor result. The unstable hips had a 47% rate of AVN, and none of the stable hips developed AVN. Similar results were noted by Kallio et al,[37] who defined unstable as either the inability of the patient to bear weight or the demonstration of an effusion by ultrasonography. These studies point out the precarious nature of the blood supply to the femoral epiphysis, which can become disrupted at the time the slip becomes unstable, and explains the poor clinical results that may not be reflected in the duration of symptoms.

PHYSICAL EXAMINATION

Patients with a chronic, stable SCFE often present with a multimonth history of limping, perhaps more appreciated by the parent than the patient. They may complain of knee pain, and it is crucial in all patients 10 to 14 years of age with knee or thigh pain to test for SCFE. Examination will demonstrate the lower extremity lying in external rotation. Flexion of the hip results in obligatory external rotation due to the new relationship between the femoral epiphysis and the femoral neck. Decreased internal rotation is best

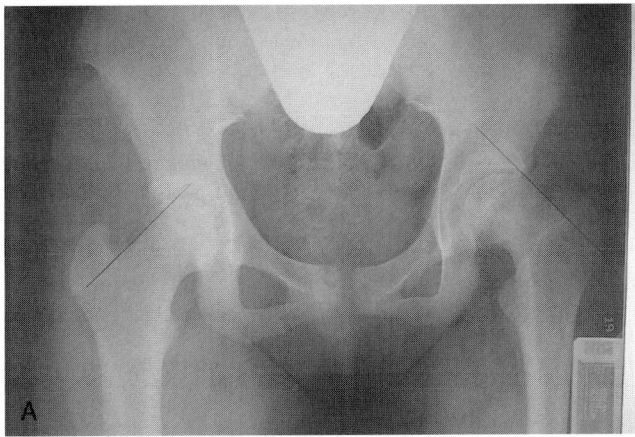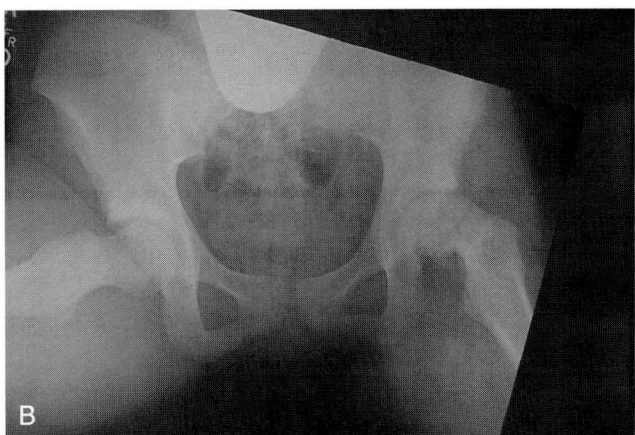

Fig. 1. Anteroposterior and frog lateral pelvis radiographs. *A* and *B* demonstrate slipping of the left capital femoral epiphysis. Klein's line on the superior border of the femoral neck intersects no epiphysis on the left compared with the right normal side.

demonstrated with the patient prone and the knee flexed. Internal rotation to end range will often reproduce the patient's symptoms. Evaluation of gait shows a limp that combines shortened limb "fall-off" with a mild Trendelenburg lurch. This latter finding is caused by the decreased mechanical efficiency of the abductors due to the relative coxa breva secondary to posterior epiphyseal displacement and pain. A pre-slip should be considered in patients with this clinical presentation but no apparent slip on radiograph. No actual slipping has occurred in a pre-slip, but both the gross and microscopic changes can be found in the physis, and slipping is likely to be the next step in the process. These patients may have radiographic widening or irregularity of the physis combined with osteopenia of the proximal femur.

RADIOGRAPHY

Radiographs confirm the diagnosis of SCFE. Additional studies, such as a technetium bone scan, can be used in patients with a suspected pre-slip. Radiographic evaluation consists of anteroposterior and frog lateral views of the pelvis to allow comparison with the uninvolved hip as well as to ensure that a simultaneous contralateral slip is not missed. All post-treatment follow-up films should also include both views of the pelvis because of the risk of bilateral slipped epiphyses. Patients who present with unilateral hip radiographs should have pelvic films before surgery. Radiographic findings include widening of the proximal femoral physis, posterior slipping of the epiphysis, femoral osteopenia, and a metaphyseal "blanch sign" caused by the superimposition of the posterior portion of the epiphysis over the upper femoral metaphysis.[38] Klein's line, along the superior femoral neck,[39] intersects less epiphysis on the involved side and may pass superior to the entire femoral epiphysis (Fig.1). In more chronic slips, rounding of the superior edge of the metaphysis and new bone formation on the inferior side are seen. The extent of slip is measured from routine radiographs. Measurements from ultrasonography and computed tomography (CT) scan have also been described.[37, 40]

Patients with an unstable slipped epiphysis may be too uncomfortable to tolerate moving the hip for ideal films. These patients can be assessed with computed tomography scan[40] if the initial plain film is not acceptable.

The severity of slippage of the femoral epiphysis along with stability must be considered in determining the likely prognosis and choosing appropriate treatment. The most widely used radiographic measure is the lateral head shaft angle described by Southwick[41] (Fig. 2). The angulation between a line drawn along the physis and one along the

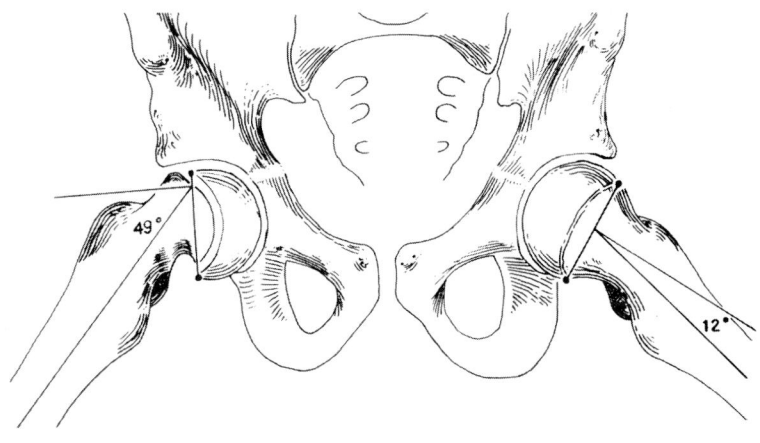

Fig. 2. Measurement of head-shaft angle. If both sides are slipped, 12 degrees is subtracted from the measurement to simulate a nonslipped contralateral side. (From Aronsson D, Carlson W: Slipped capital femoral epiphysis: Prospective study of fixation with single screw. J Bone Joint Surg Am 1992; 74:811.)

femoral shaft—the head shaft angle—is measured on the lateral film. The measurement of the normal side is then subtracted from the slipped side, and the slip angle is determined. Twelve degrees is used as a standard measure when both sides have slipped.[41, 42] Southwick considered slips less than 30 degrees mild, 30 to 70 degrees severe, and slips more than 70 degrees extremely severe. Other investigators[9, 43, 44] have modified Southwick's angles to 30 degrees, 30 to 50 degrees, and over 50 degrees as measurements of mild, moderate, and severe slips. Another classification describes the percentage of the epiphyseal movement relative to the metaphysis, with up to 33% being mild, 34% to 50% being moderate, and more than 51% being severe.[45] Crawford[10] recommends this system and uses 0% to 33% as mild, 34% to 66% as moderate, and more than 67% as severe. Regardless of the system used, it is important to measure the degree of slippage accurately so that the patient can be monitored for any changes in slip angle.

NATURAL HISTORY

A correlation between extent of femoral head deformity and osteoarthritis of the hip has been demonstrated by Stulberg et al,[2] Goodman et al,[1] Jerre,[12] Boyer et al,[9] and others.[43, 44] Unfortunately, this has resulted in some forms of management with high complication rates having worse outcomes than those with untreated disease.[9, 44, 46, 47] Remodeling of the femoral neck can occur,[48–51] and range of motion (ROM) may increase significantly even in the absence of radiographic bony remodeling.[49, 50] These factors, along with an appreciation of the importance of physeal stability, have allowed the development of better treatment algorithms for SCFE patients.

TREATMENT

The goal of treatment in SCFE is to stabilize the epiphysis and prevent further displacement while avoiding complications, most notably AVN and chondrolysis. Acute, unstable slipped epiphyses have a much higher incidence of AVN than stable slips, which is a reflection of the acuity of slip and not the treatment. However, certain types of management can increase the likelihood of these complications.

Spica Cast. Spica casting can be successful in preventing further slippage in the majority of cases and may prove beneficial in preventing sequential, bilateral slips.[45] However, studies have reported up to an 18% prevalence of continued slippage and a 53% prevalence of chondrolysis[45, 47, 52] that may develop in the noninvolved hip.[53] The difficulty of applying a hip spica cast on a markedly overweight teenage patient has also decreased the enthusiasm for this technique.

STABLE SLIPPED EPIPHYSES

Open Bone Graft Epiphyseodesis. This procedure can be safely performed in skilled hands and provides for rapid closure of the physis in as few as 10 weeks postoperatively.[47, 54, 55] The procedure is technically difficult and has associated complications, including thigh numbness, heterotopic ossification, and relatively great blood loss. These complications, along with prolonged operating times, have made this procedure less popular.[56, 57]

Pinning In Situ. This is the procedure of choice for chronic, stable slipped epiphyses of any extent. Reports consistently show that reduction of a chronic slipped epiphysis can increase the risk of AVN[9, 44, 46] and that even the most severe slips can be pinned in situ.[58] Attention must be paid to the technical aspect of the procedure in order to avoid pin penetration, continued slipping, fracture, and other complications (see the upcoming section titled Technique).

ACUTE, UNSTABLE SLIPPED EPIPHYSES

It appears that closed reduction of the acute, unstable slip does not cause AVN.[59, 60] However, many unstable slips have a prodromal period of limp and thigh pain indicating a preexisting chronic slip. The severity of the chronic slip is unknown and must be inferred from a radiographic assessment of the femoral neck. If reduction is attempted, over-reduction of the chronic component can increase the risk of AVN.[9, 61–64] Because the natural history of a mild slip is favorable, there is no need to reduce any slip completely if there are radiographic signs of remodeling. Rhoad et al[59] reported a study of 10 unstable slips that underwent operative reduction after bone scanning. None of the four hips with normal bone scans developed AVN even though three were reduced from grade III to grade I slips. Six other hips had abnormal pretreatment bone scans, and five developed AVN, again implying that the vascular status of the epiphysis had already been determined at the time of presentation. Until a study is reported that shows no difference in the incidence of AVN following reduction of unstable slips compared with those that are pinned in situ, caution should be exercised in attempting to reduce unstable hips beyond the acute component. There is some evidence that if reduction is carried out within the first 24 hours following an acute slip, rates of AVN are less.[63] However, all reductions in Rhoad's study were performed after 24 hours with no apparent ill effect.

Prior reports with multiple pins implicated this method as a cause of unsatisfactory results.[65] Walters and Simon[66] showed that persistent pin penetration was a significant risk factor for the development of chondrolysis. Several other authors subsequently showed that unrecognized pin penetration is common.[67, 68] Multiple pins also reduce the chance of achieving one ideally placed screw[65] and provide no more than 33% increased strength.[69] Adequate visualization with the fluoroscope is essential to avoid persistent pin penetration. Transient pin penetration during the procedure has not been associated with increased complications.[70]

Technique

The operation can be performed either on a fracture table or with the leg draped free on a radiolucent table. The hip must be well visualized by fluoroscopy in all planes before the patient is prepared. Moving the hip, the patient, and the x-ray unit may all be needed to allow appropriate visualization. If the patient is positioned on a fracture table and there is difficulty in obtaining the lateral view, an unscrubbed assistant can manually control the leg, remove it from the leg holder, and move the hip through a ROM and into the frog, or Lauenstein's, lateral position. In the unusual circumstance that adequate visualization of the hip cannot be obtained, the hip can be pinned under computed tomography guidance.[71]

Using fluoroscopy, lines are drawn overlying the femoral neck, which bisect the epiphysis, perpendicular to the upper femoral physis in both anteroposterior and lateral projections (Fig. 3). The intersection of these lines determines the starting point of the guide pin. The entry point for the guide pin in a slipped epiphysis will be on the anterior proximal femur, not lateral as in a hip fracture. The starting point will be further anterior the greater the severity of the slip (Fig. 4).[72–74] A stainless steel cannulated screw of at least 6.5-mm diameter is used.[65, 75] Titanium has the

disadvantage that screw removal is more difficult due to osseointegration.[75, 76] Although Steinmann's pins have been used, complications are fewer with the larger threads of a screw.[77]

The technical goal of pinning is a single screw perpendicular to the physis, with three to five intraepiphyseal threads, the tip in the exact center of the epiphysis, yet not within 2 mm of the articular surface (Fig. 5). The guide pin is initially placed percutaneously and advanced toward the center of the epiphysis, checking both anteroposterior

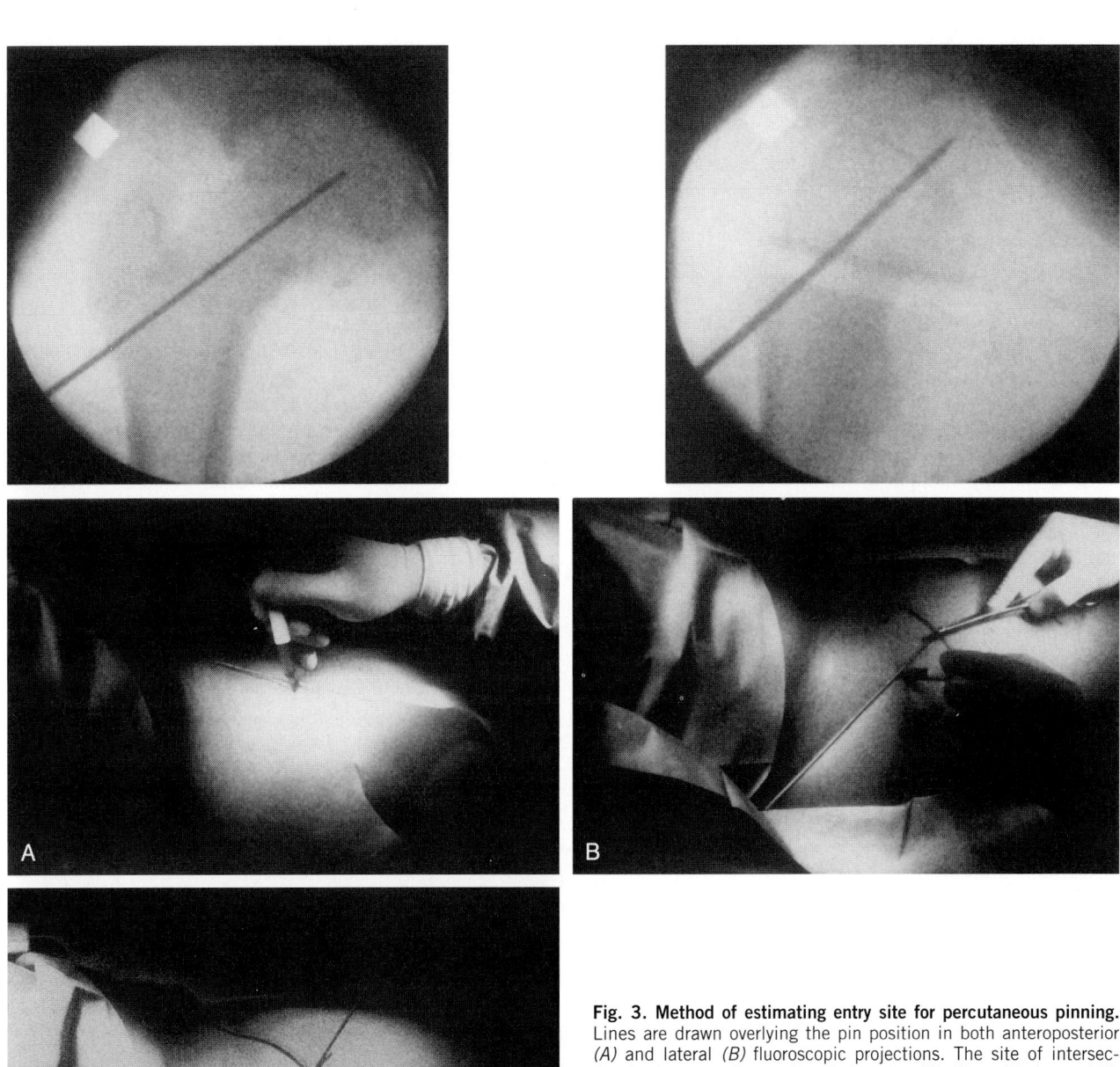

Fig. 3. Method of estimating entry site for percutaneous pinning. Lines are drawn overlying the pin position in both anteroposterior (A) and lateral (B) fluoroscopic projections. The site of intersection is the approximate site of pin entry (C). (From Lindaman LM, Canale ST, Beaty JH, et al: A fluoroscopic technique for determining the incision site for percutaneous fixation of slipped capital femoral epiphysis. J Pediatr Orthop 1991; 11:397.)

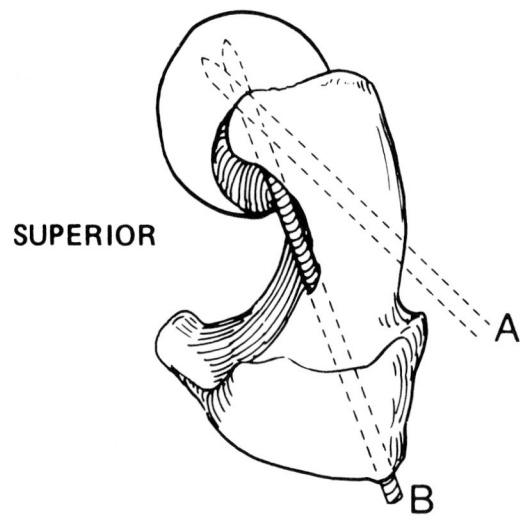

Fig. 4. Views. A greater amount of slipping requires a more anterior entry site for pinning *(A)*. Direct lateral entry such as in *B* increases the risk of poor pin placement by exiting posteriorly near the blood supply and reentering the femoral epiphysis. (From Riley PM, Weiner DS, Gillespie R: Hazards of internal fixation in the treatment of slipped capital femoral epiphysis. J Bone Joint Surg Am 1990; 72: 1500.)

and lateral radiographic projections. This may take several passes to accomplish. In severe slips, osteopenia of the most proximal portion of the femoral neck may lead to decreased holding strength of the screw, and a less perpendicular approach may be needed to allow for stronger bone in the femoral neck. It is important to avoid exiting the femoral neck posteriorly and then reentering the epiphysis. It is also best to avoid the posterior, superior quadrant of the head as its vascularity may be critical.[78] In a mild slip or pre-slip, the entry point may be on the lateral upper femur. In these cases, entry should be above the lesser trochanter and without multiple starting holes to reduce the risk of proximal femur fracture. Other pin complications include femoral neck fracture,[79] upper femoral growth disturbance in young children,[80] and progression despite a

well-placed screw.[81] Complications are more common with poorly placed screws.

Following placement of the screw, several techniques can be used to ensure that the tip is within bone. These include injecting dye through the screw, an arthrogram, or the "approach withdraw phenomenon" described by Moseley.[82] Using the latter technique, the hip is put through a complete range of internal and external rotation under fluoroscopic control. The screw tip will be seen to approach the articular surface as the hip is rotated internally. The screw tip must then be seen to withdraw as the hip is further rotated internally. Multiple views and projections are necessary to prevent inadvertent pin penetration despite routine radiographs that show the pin safely within bone (Fig. 6). If limited ROM does not allow the hip to rotate, then the x-ray unit should be rotated. This should also be done in flexion and extension to verify that in no projection does the screw continue to approach the articular surface without eventually withdrawing.

Aftercare

The studies of Kibiloski et al[69] showed that a slipped epiphysis fixed with a screw does not approach the strength of the intact upper femur. Although some authors allow immediate weightbearing,[83] a period of restricted weightbearing with crutches seems wise. The patient is seen, and radiographs are taken at 1 week and again at 6 weeks following surgery, at which time full weightbearing is resumed. Follow-up visits are scheduled at 12 weeks and every 3 to 6 months thereafter until bilateral physeal closure is seen radiographically. Contact sports must be restricted until the slipped epiphysis shows physeal closure, usually 5 to 13 months after the pinning.[65, 84]

Most authors no longer recommend prophylactic pinning of the contralateral hip, because hardware complication rates of 13% to 26% have been reported.[68, 85] The presence of clinical symptoms, radiographic evidence of slipping, or underlying metabolic disease such as hypothyroidism are indications for contralateral pinning. Because most contralateral slips are mild in severity and are asymptomatic, radiographic follow-up is mandatory.

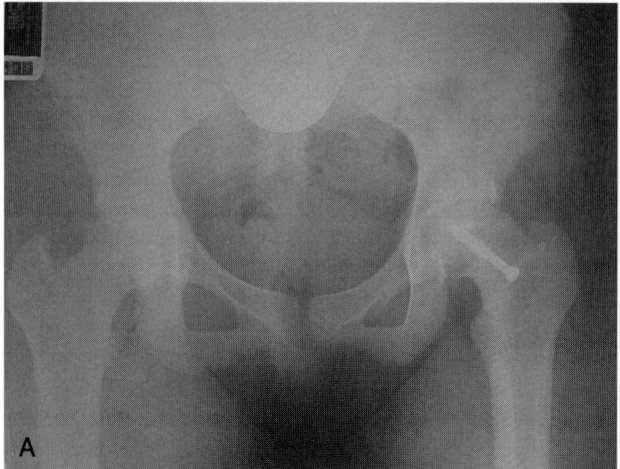
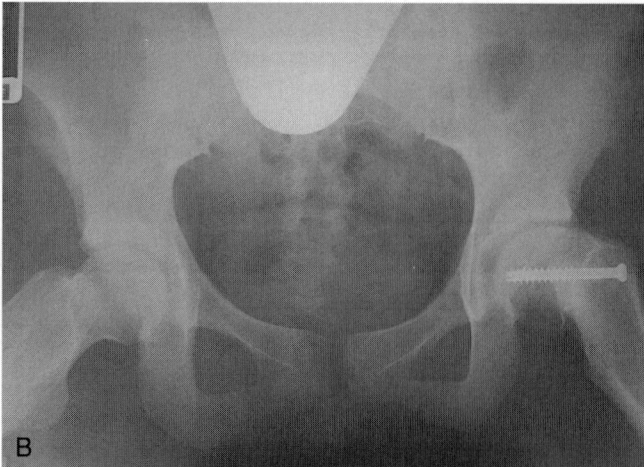

Fig. 5. Views. These are anteroposterior *(A)* and frog lateral *(B)* radiographs of a well-placed pin in SCFE.

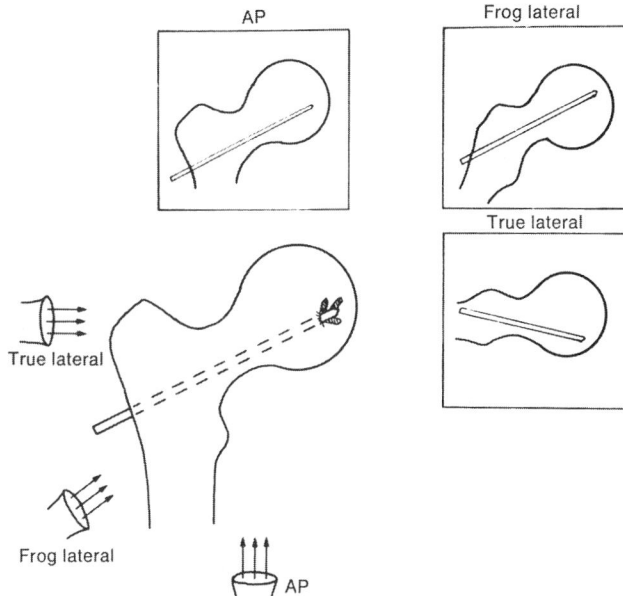

Fig. 6. Pin placement. Pins that protrude from the femoral head can easily appear to be "in" radiographically. To minimize this, a perfectly centered pin is the goal. The "approach withdraw phenomenon" or some other method should be used to ensure there is no persistent pin protrusion. (From Walters R, Simon S: Joint destruction: A sequel of unrecognized pin penetration in patients with slipped capital femoral epiphyses. In The Hip: Proceedings of The Eighth Open Scientific Meeting of The Hip Society. St. Louis, CV Mosby, 1980, p 145.)

With meticulous attention to detail, in situ fixation of stable SCFEs with placement of a single screw can result in reproducibly good results. Aronsson and Carlson,[83] Ward et al,[84] Rhoad et al,[59] and Aronsson and Loder[42] reported a total of 183 stable hips treated with a single screw with no cases of chondrolysis and no AVN. Unstable slips are more challenging to treat as the blood supply may be compromised. This same group of authors treated 27 cases of unstable slipped epiphysis, with seven cases of AVN and no chondrolysis. These results are still better than reports following the use of multiple pins.[65, 86]

Screw removal is more difficult than it looks, with many failures and an average operative time of 1 hour and blood loss of 127 mL.[68, 75, 76] Most surgeons are now leaving these single screws in place unless the patient is symptomatic. If screw removal is to be undertaken, closure of the physis should be clearly documented prior to the attempt.

Complications

Chondrolysis is defined as a decrease in joint space of more than 2 mm[42] or a joint space less than 50% of the normal side.[87] Earlier reviews of chondrolysis were clouded by the use of multiple different treatments, including reduction, traction, spica casting, acute osteotomies, large nails, and multiple pins, in stable and unstable slips.[47, 86, 88, 89] Chondrolysis was reported to be more frequent in blacks and in girls, with a frequency as high as 50% in black girls.[88–90] Although more recent data continue to point to a higher incidence in girls,[91] the reported higher frequency in

African-Americans has been questioned and may reflect differences in surgeon experience in particular locations.[42, 91, 92] Single pin techniques, decreased use of traction, and the absence of attempted reduction or casting will permit more accurate comparisons of outcomes. There are few recent data to suggest that the incidence of chondrolysis is higher in African-American patients.

The pathophysiology of chondrolysis is an autoimmune phenomenon with immune complexes in the synovial fluid. Variable studies have reported higher immunoglobulin M concentrations.[93, 94] Synovial biopsy samples show chronic inflammation.[53, 90, 93, 94] Chondrolysis appears more likely to occur in hips with more severe slips and persistent pin penetration.[66, 89] Chondrolysis can also exist before treatment. If suspected, technetium bone scanning can be confirmatory and may be predictive, showing increased uptake over the joint and decreased uptake in the greater and lesser trochanters.[87]

The treatment of chondrolysis includes decreased weight-bearing, anti-inflammatory medication, and gentle ROM therapy. Should this fail, complete capsulectomy and continuous passive ROM can be tried, but the long-term results in patients with chondrolysis are often poor, and arthrodesis may be necessary.[10, 53, 89, 90]

AVASCULAR NECROSIS

The blood supply to the immature hip arises from the medial femoral circumflex artery that supplies the lateral ascending cervical artery, which then gives off a lateral epiphyseal artery as well as metaphyseal branches. All branches of the lateral ascending artery originate from a vessel that crosses the capsule at the trochanteric fossa and may be at risk during certain procedures.[95] Because the physis forms a barrier to intraosseous blood supply to the epiphysis, the most important part of the vascular supply is along the posterior neck and head, entering at the perichondrial ring to supply the ossification center. It is suspected that this vascular supply is interrupted in cases of unstable SCFE. Intraosseous blood supply is richest in the posterosuperior femoral neck and head; therefore, screws placed in that area can have a deleterious effect on the vascularity of the epiphysis.[78]

AVN has been shown to be largely a result of the slip itself in unstable hips, but reduction of a chronic slip,[12, 96, 97] poor screw placement, and exiting the femoral neck posteriorly and reentering the epiphysis can all contribute to its development. Should AVN develop, collapse is likely, with resulting secondary pin protrusion into the joint. The fixation must be withdrawn at that point to ensure an already difficult situation is not compounded by persistent intra-articular hardware.

Results in patients with AVN are poor, with worsening hip joint deterioration as the length of follow-up increases. Krahn et al[98] showed that all hips had degenerative changes on radiograph at an average follow-up of 31 years; 41% of his patients had undergone reconstructive surgery as adolescents or young adults.

OSTEOTOMY

The results of pinning in situ are consistently better than those of acute osteotomy.[9, 12, 44, 46, 86, 96] Increased ROM is

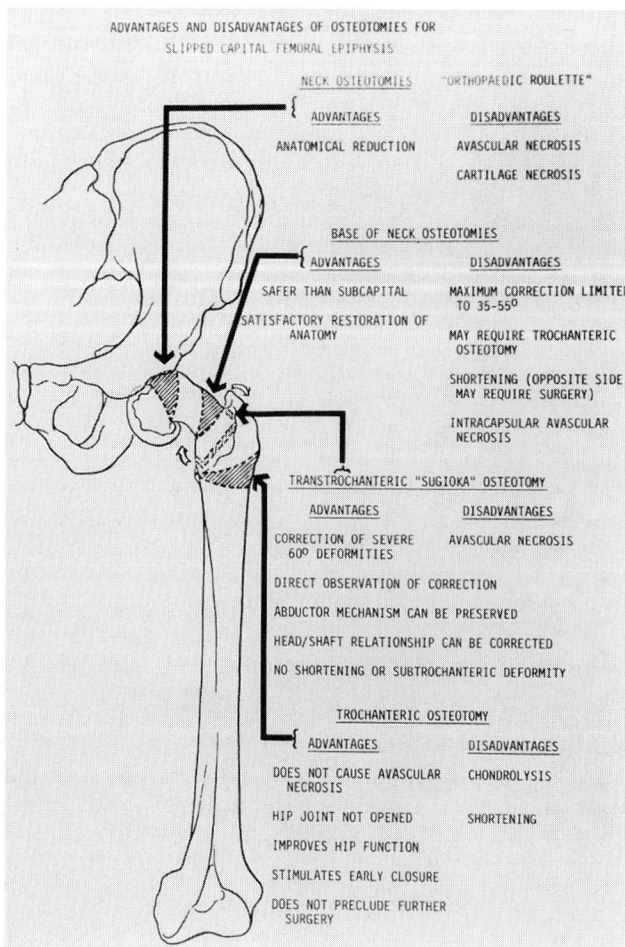

ADVANTAGES AND DISADVANTAGES OF OSTEOTOMIES FOR
SLIPPED CAPITAL FEMORAL EPIPHYSIS

NECK OSTEOTOMIES   "ORTHOPAEDIC ROULETTE"

ADVANTAGES   DISADVANTAGES

ANATOMICAL REDUCTION   AVASCULAR NECROSIS

CARTILAGE NECROSIS

BASE OF NECK OSTEOTOMIES

ADVANTAGES   DISADVANTAGES

SAFER THAN SUBCAPITAL   MAXIMUM CORRECTION LIMITED
TO 35-55°

SATISFACTORY RESTORATION OF
ANATOMY   MAY REQUIRE TROCHANTERIC
OSTEOTOMY

SHORTENING (OPPOSITE SIDE
MAY REQUIRE SURGERY)

INTRACAPSULAR AVASCULAR
NECROSIS

TRANSTROCHANTERIC "SUGIOKA" OSTEOTOMY

ADVANTAGES   DISADVANTAGES

CORRECTION OF SEVERE   AVASCULAR NECROSIS
60° DEFORMITIES

DIRECT OBSERVATION OF CORRECTION

ABDUCTOR MECHANISM CAN BE PRESERVED

HEAD/SHAFT RELATIONSHIP CAN BE CORRECTED

NO SHORTENING OR SUBTROCHANTERIC DEFORMITY

TROCHANTERIC OSTEOTOMY

ADVANTAGES   DISADVANTAGES

DOES NOT CAUSE AVASCULAR   CHONDROLYSIS
NECROSIS

HIP JOINT NOT OPENED   SHORTENING

IMPROVES HIP FUNCTION

STIMULATES EARLY CLOSURE

DOES NOT PRECLUDE FURTHER
SURGERY

Fig. 7. Sites of osteotomy in slipped capital femoral epiphysis. Although proximal sites of osteotomy are more anatomic, the risk of complications is substantially increased when compared with intertrochanteric or subtrochanteric osteotomies. (From Clin Orthop Rel Res 1979; 141:17.)

common following in situ treatment of SCFE. Osteotomy is a reconstructive procedure that should be reserved for those patients who have residual deformity and limitation of motion at least 1 year after pinning of the slipped epiphysis. Most of these patients will have slip angles of at least 50 degrees.[10, 96, 99] The goal of osteotomy is to improve function by improving ROM. As yet there are insufficient data to show a sufficiently low complication rate and significantly increased longevity of the hips to recommend the prophylactic osteotomy to prevent the development of degenerative joint disease.

The most appropriate anatomic site for correction of the slip deformity is at the level of the physis. This procedure can lead to a good outcome.[100, 101] However, most studies report dismal results with high rates of AVN and poor clinical outcomes in up to 59% of patients (Fig. 7).[47, 96, 102]

A compensatory base of femoral neck osteotomy can improve ROM but does not truly restore normal anatomy. This procedure can be done at the intra- or extra-capsular level, with lower rates of AVN reported following the extracapsular osteotomy.[102–104]

The surgical complication rates of osteotomy decrease as one moves further distally. However, the three-dimensional conceptualization of the operative correction needed to improve motion becomes more difficult.[41, 105] Intertrochanteric osteotomy creates less deformity for the total joint surgeon than does the subtrochanteric osteotomy, but if translation of the subtrochanteric femoral shaft is minimized, angulation can be managed in the case of future arthroplasty. Southwick's biplane osteotomy corrects the retroversion and the apparent varus with an anterolaterally-based osteotomy. Although chondrolysis can result, the cartilage tends to reconstitute over time. Chondrolysis may occur less frequently with today's stronger internal fixation rather than postoperative spica casting.[41, 106, 107] Millis[108] has used the Imhauser intertrochanteric flexion osteotomy, which utilizes an anteriorly based wedge to correct the retroversion by creating a more normal, valgus neck shaft angle. This procedure should be easier to conceptualize and has a low complication rate.

SCFE remains a challenging condition to treat. Prompt diagnosis of these patients, identification of contralateral slips, good visualization in the operating room, and meticulous technique can lead to reproducible good outcomes in chronic, stable slips and help reduce the chance of complications in the acute, unstable cases, which are, fortunately, less common.

REFERENCES

1. Goodman DA, Feighan JE, Smith AD, et al: Subclinical slipped capital femoral epiphysis: Relationship to osteoarthrosis of the hip. J Bone Joint Surg Am 1997; 79:1489.
2. Stulberg SD, Cordell LD, Harris WH, et al: Unrecognized childhood hip disease: A major cause of idiopathic osteoarthritis of the hip. In The Hip: Proceedings of the Third Open Scientific Meeting Of The Hip Society. St. Louis, CV Mosby, 1975, p 212.
3. Kelsey J: The incidence and distribution of slipped capital femoral epiphysis in Connecticut. J Chron Dis 1971; 23:567.
4. Kelsey JL, Keggi KJ, Southwick WO: The incidence and distribution of slipped capital femoral epiphysis in Connecticut and Southwestern United States. J Bone Joint Surg Am 1970; 52:1203.
5. Jerre T, Karlsson J, Henrikson B: Incidence of physiolysis of the hip: A population-based study of 175 patients. Acta Orthop Scand 1996; 67:53.
6. Loder R: The demographics of slipped capital femoral epiphysis: An international multicenter study. Clin Orthop 1996; 322:8.
7. Loder R: A worldwide study on the seasonal variation of slipped capital femoral epiphysis. Clin Orthop 1996; 322:28.
8. Montsko P, DeJonge T: Slipped capital femoral epiphysis in 6 of 8 first-degree relatives. Acta Orthop Scand 1995; 66: 511.
9. Boyer DW, Mickelson MR, Ponseti IV: Slipped capital femoral epiphysis: Long-term follow-up. J Bone Joint Surg Am 1981; 63:85.
10. Crawford AH: Current concepts review: Slipped capital femoral epiphysis. J Bone Joint Surg Am 1988; 70:1422.
11. Hagglund G, Hansson LI, Orderberg G, et al: Bilaterality in slipped capital femoral epiphysis. J Bone Joint Surg Br 1988; 70:179.
12. Jerre T: A study in slipped upper femoral epiphysis with special reference to late

functional and roentgenological results and the value of closed reduction. Acta Orthop Scand 1950; 6:1.

13. Jerre R, Billing L, Hansson G, et al: Contralateral hip in patients primarily treated for unilateral slipped capital femoral epiphysis. J Bone Joint Surg Br 1994; 76:563.

14. Loder RT, Aronsson DD, Greenfield ML: The epidemiology of bilateral slipped capital femoral epiphysis. J Bone Joint Surg Am 1993; 75:1141.

15. Stasikelis PJ, Sullivan CM, Phillips WA, et al: Slipped capital femoral epiphysis: Prediction of contralateral involvement. J Bone Joint Surg Am 1996; 78:1149.

16. Bright RW, Burstein AH, Elmore SM: Epiphyseal plate cartilage: A biomechanical and histological analysis of failure modes. J Bone Joint Surg Am 1974; 56: 688.

17. Chung SM, Batterman SC, Brighton CT: Shear strength of the human femoral capital epiphyseal plate. J Bone Joint Surg Am 1976; 58:94.

18. Brenkel IJ, Dias JJ, Davies TG, et al: Hormone status in patients with slipped capital femoral epiphysis. J Bone Joint Surg Br 1989; 71:33.

19. Fidler MW, Brook CG: Slipped upper femoral epiphysis following treatment with human growth hormone. J Bone Joint Surg Am 1974; 56:1719.

20. Forrester-Brown M: Slipping of the upper femoral epiphysis. J Bone Joint Surg 1941; 23:256.

21. Harris WR: The endocrine basis for slipping of the upper femoral epiphysis. J Bone Joint Surg Br 1950; 32:5.

22. Hirano T, Stamelos S, Harris V, et al: Association of primary hypothyroidism and slipped capital femoral epiphysis. J Pediatr 1978; 93:262.

23. Loder RT, Hensinger RN: Slipped capital femoral epiphysis associated with renal failure osteodystrophy. J Pediatr Orthop 1997; 17:205.

24. Mann DC, Weddington J, Richton S: Hormonal studies in patients with slipped capital femoral epiphysis without evidence of endocrinopathy. J Pediatr Orthop 1988; 8:543.

25. Primiano GA, Hughston JC: Slipped capital femoral epiphysis in a true hypogonadal male (Klinefelter's mosaic XY/XXY). J Bone Joint Surg Am 1971; 53: 597.

26. Wilcox PG, Weiner DS, Leighley B: Maturation factors in slipped capital femoral epiphysis. J Pediatr Orthop 1988; 8: 196.

27. Razzano CD, Nelson C, Eversman J: Growth hormone levels in slipped capital femoral epiphysis. J Bone Joint Surg Am 1972; 54:1224.

28. Oka M, Miki T, Hama H, et al: The mechanical strength of the growth plate under the influence of sex hormones. Clin Orthop Rel Res 1979; 145:264.

29. Wells D, King JD, Roe TR, et al: Review of slipped capital femoral epiphysis associated with endocrine disease. J Pediatr Orthop 1993; 13:610.

30. Loder RT, Wittenberg B, Desilva G: Slipped capital femoral epiphysis with endocrine disorders. J Pediatr Orthop 1995; 15:349.

31. Ippolito E, Mickelson MR, Ponseti IV: A histochemical study of slipped capital femoral epiphysis. J Bone Joint Surg Am 1981; 63:1109.

32. Ponseti I, McClintock R: The pathology of slipping of the upper femoral metaphysis. J Bone Joint Surg Am 1956; 38:71.

33. Agamanolis D, Wiener D, and Lloyd J: Slipped capital femoral epiphysis: A pathological study II—an ultrastructural study of 23 cases. J Pediatr Orthop 1985; 5:47.

34. Mickelson MR, Ponseti IV, Cooper RR, et al: The ultrastructure of the growth plate in slipped capital femoral epiphysis. J Bone Joint Surg Am 1977; 59:1076.

35. Gelberman RH, Cohen MS, Shaw BA, et al: The association of femoral retroversion with slipped capital femoral epiphysis. J Bone Joint Surg Am 1986; 68: 1000.

36. Loder R, Richards BS, Shapiro PS, et al: Acute slipped capital femoral epiphysis: The importance of physeal stabilty. J Bone Joint Surg Am 1993; 75:1134.

37. Kallio PE, Mah ET, Foster BK, et al: Slipped capital femoral epiphysis: Incidence and clinical assessment of physeal instability. J Bone Joint Surg Br 1995; 77:752.

38. Steel HH: The metaphyseal blanch sign of slipped capital femoral epiphysis. J Bone Joint Surg Am 1986; 68:920.

39. Klein A, Joplin RJ, Reidy JA, et al: Roentgenographic features of slipped capital femoral epiphysis. AJR Am J Roentgenol 1951; 66:361.

40. Cohen MS, Gelberman RH, Griffin PP, et al: Slipped capital femoral epiphysis: Assessment of epiphyseal displacement and angulation. J Pediatr Orthop 1986; 6:259.

41. Southwick W: Osteotomy through the lesser trochanter for slipped capital femoral epiphysis. J Bone Joint Surg Am 1967; 49:807.

42. Aronsson D, Loder R: Slipped capital femoral epiphysis in black children. J Pediatr Orthop 1992; 12:74.

43. Carney BT, Weinstein SL: The natural history of untreated chronic slipped capital femoral epiphysis. Clin Orthop 1996; 322:43.

44. Carney BT, Weinstein SL, Noble J: Long-term follow-up of slipped capital femoral epiphysis. J Bone Joint Surg Am 1991; 73:667.

45. Betz R, Steel H, Emper WD, et al: Treatment of slipped capital femoral epiphysis with spica cast. J Bone Joint Surg Am 1990; 72:587.

46. Hansson G, Billing L, Hogstedt B, et al: Long-term results after nailing in situ of slipped upper femoral epiphysis: A 30-year follow-up of 59 hips. J Bone Joint Surg Br 1998; 80:70.

47. Howorth MB: Slipping of the upper femoral epiphysis. J Bone Joint Surg Am 1949; 31:734.

48. Jones JR, Paterson DC, Hillier TM, et al: Remodeling after pinning for slipped capital femoral epiphysis. J Bone Joint Surg Br 1990; 72:568.

49. O'Brien ET, Fahey JJ: Remodeling of the femoral neck after in situ pinning for slipped capital femoral epiphysis. J Bone Joint Surg Am 1977; 59:62.

50. Siegel D, Kasser JR, Sponseller P, et al: Slipped capital femoral epiphysis: A quantitative analysis of motion, gait, and femoral remodeling after in situ fixation. J Bone Joint Surg Am 1991; 73:659.

51. Wong-Chung J, Strong M: Physeal remodeling after internal fixation of slipped capital femoral epiphysis. J Pediatr Orthop 1991; 11:2.

52. Hurley J, Betz R, Loder R, et al: Slipped capital femoral epiphysis: Prevalence of late contralateral slip. J Bone Joint Surg Am 1996; 78:226.

53. Lowe HG: Avascular necrosis after slipping of the upper femoral epiphysis. J Bone Joint Surg Br 1961; 43:688.

54. Herndon CH, Heyman CH, Bell DM: Treatment of slipped capital femoral epiphysis by epiphyseodesis and osteoplasty of the femoral neck. J Bone Joint Surg Am 1963; 45:999.

55. Weiner DS, Weiner S, Melby A, et al: A 30-year experience with bone graft epiphyseodesis in the treatment of slipped capital femoral epiphysis. J Pediatr Orthop 1984; 4:145.

56. Irani RN, Rosenzweig AH, Cotler HB, et al: Epiphyseodesis in slipped capital femoral epiphysis: A comparison of various surgical modalities. J Pediatr Orthop 1985; 5:661.

57. Ward WT, Wood K: Open bone graft epiphyseodesis for slipped capital femoral epiphysis. J Pediatr Orthop 1990; 10:14.

58. Herman MJ, Dormans JP, Davidson RS, et al: Screw fixation of grade III slipped capital femoral epiphysis. Clin Orthop Rel Res 1996; 322:77.

59. Rhoad RC, Davidson RS, Heyman S, et al: Pretreatment bone scan in SCFE: A predictor of ischemia and avascular necrosis. J Pediatr Orthop 1999; 19:164.

60. Fahey JJ, O'Brien ET: Acute slipped capital femoral epiphysis. J Bone Joint Surg Am 1965; 47:1105.

61. Casey BH, Hamilton HW, Bobechko WP: Reduction of acutely slipped upper femoral epiphysis. J Bone Joint Surg Br 1972; 54:607.

62. Fairbank TJ: Manipulative reduction in slipped capital femoral epiphysis. J Bone Joint Surg Br 1969; 51:252.

63. Peterson MD, Weiner DS, Green NE, et al: Acute slipped capital femoral epiphysis: The value and safety of urgent manipulative reduction. J Pediatr Orthop 1997; 17:648.

64. Rattey T, Piehl F, Wright JG: Acute slipped capital femoral epiphysis: Review of outcomes and rates of avascular necrosis. J Bone Joint Surg Am 1996; 78:398.

65. Blanco JS, Taylor B, Johnston II CE: Comparison of single-pin vs. multiple pin in treatment of slipped capital femoral epiphysis. J Pediatr Orthop 1992; 12:384.

66. Walters R, Simon SR: Joint destruction: A sequel of unrecognized pin penetration in patients with slipped capital femoral epiphyses. In Riley LH Jr (ed): The Hip: Proceedings Of The Eighth Open Scientific Meeting Of The Hip Society. St. Louis, CV Mosby, 1980, p 145.

67. Bennet GC, Koreska J, Rang M: Pin placement in slipped capital femoral epiphysis. J Pediatr Orthop 1984; 4:574.

68. Greenough CG, Bromage JD, Jackson AM: Pinning of slipped capital femoral epiphysis: A trouble-free procedure? J Pediatr Orthop 1985; 5:657.

69. Kibiloski LJ, Doane RM, Karol LA, et al: Biomechanical analysis of single- vs. double-screw fixation in slipped capital femoral epiphysis at physiological load levels. J Pediatr Orthop 1994; 14:627.

70. Zionts LE, Simonian PT, Harvey Jr JP: Transient penetration of the hip joint during in situ cannulated-screw fixation of slipped capital femoral epiphysis. J Bone Joint Surg Am 1991; 73:1054.

71. Ebraheim N: Percutaneous computed tomography stabilization of moderate to severe slipped capital femoral epiphysis. Orthopedics 1991; 14:859.

72. Crider RJ, Krell T, Mcguire M, et al: Anterolateral approach for moderate to severe slipped capital femoral epiphysis. J Pediatr Orthop 1988; 8:661.

73. Morrissy RT: Slipped capital femoral epiphysis technique of percutaneous in situ fixation. J Pediatr Orthop 1990; 10:347.

74. Nguyen D, Morrissy RT: Slipped capital femoral epiphysis: The rationale for the technique of percutaneous in situ fixation. J Pediatr Orthop 1990; 10:341.

75. Vresilovic EJ, Spindler KP, Robertson WW, et al: Failures of pin removal after in situ pinning of slipped capital femoral epiphysis: A comparison of different pin types. J Pediatr Orthop 1990; 10:764.

76. Lee TK, Haynes RJ, Longo JA, et al: Pin removal in slipped capital femoral epiphysis: Unsuitability of titanium devices. J Pediatr Orthop 1996; 16:49.

77. Laplaza FJ, Burke SW: Epiphyseal growth after pinning of slipped capital femoral epiphysis. J Pediatr Orthop 1995; 15:357.

78. Brodetti A: The blood supply of the femoral neck and head in relation to the damaging effects of nails and screws. J Bone Joint Surg Br 1960; 42:794.

79. Baynham G, Lucie R, Cummings R: Femoral neck fracture secondary to in situ pinning of slipped capital femoral epiphysis: A previously unreported complication. J Pediatr Orthop 1991; 11:187.

80. Segal LS, Davidson RS, Robertson Jr WW, et al: Growth disturbances of the proximal femur after pinning of juvenile slipped capital femoral epiphysis. J Pediatr Orthop 1991; 11:631.

81. Denton JR: Progression of a slipped capital femoral epiphysis after fixation with a single cannulated screw. J Bone Joint Surg Am 1993; 75:425.

82. Moseley C: The approach withdraw phenomenon in the pinning of slipped capital femoral epiphysis. Orthop Trans 1985; 9:497.

83. Aronsson D, Carlson W: Slipped capital femoral epiphysis: Prospective study of fixation with single screw. J Bone Joint Surg Am 1992; 74:810.

84. Ward WT, Stefko J, Wood KB, et al: Fixation with a single screw for slipped capital femoral epiphysis. J Bone Joint Surg 1992; 74:799.

85. Emery RJ, Todd RC, Dunn DM: Prophylactic pinning in slipped upper femoral epiphysis: Prevention of complications. J Bone Joint Surg Br 1990; 72:217.

86. Howorth MB: Treatment and slipping of the capital femoral epiphysis. Clin Orthop 1966; 48:53.

87. El-Khoury GY, Mickelson MR: Chondrolysis following slipped capital femoral epiphysis. Radiology 1997; 123:327.

88. Cruess RL: The pathology of acute necrosis of cartilage in slipping of the capital femoral epiphysis. J Bone Joint Surg Am 1963; 45:1013.

89. Maurer RC, Larsen IJ: Acute necrosis of cartilage in slipped capital femoral epiphysis. J Bone Joint Surg Am 1970; 52:39.

90. Tillema DA, Golding JSR: Chondrolysis following slipped capital femoral epiphysis in Jamaica. J Bone Joint Surg Am 1971; 53:1528.

91. Spero CR, Masciale JP, Tornetta III P, et al: Slipped capital femoral epiphysis in black children: Incidence of chondrolysis. J Pediatr Orthop 1992; 12:444.

92. Kennedy JP, Weiner DS: Results of slipped capital femoral epiphysis in the black population. J Pediatr Orthop 1990; 10:224.

93. Eisenstein A, Rothschild S: Biochemical abnormalities in patients with slipped capital femoral epiphysis and chondrolysis. J Bone Joint Surg Am 1976; 58:459.

94. Morrissy RT, Kalderon AE, Gerdes MH: Synovial immunofluorescence in patients with slipped capital femoral epiphysis. J Pediatr Orthop 1981; 1:55.

95. Chung SM: The arterial supply of the developing proximal end of the human femur. J Bone Joint Surg Am 1976; 58:961.

96. Jerre R, Hansson G, Wallin J, et al: Long-term results after realignment oper-

97. Lowe HG: Necrosis of articular cartilage after slipping of the capital femoral epiphysis: Report of six cases with recovery. J Bone Joint Surg Br 1970; 52:108.

98. Krahn TH, Canale ST, Beatty JH, et al: Long-term follow-up of patients with avascular necrosis after treatment of slipped capital femoral epiphysis. J Pediatr Orthop 1993; 13:154.

99. Crawford AH: The role of osteotomy in the treatment of slipped capital femoral epiphysis. J Pediatr Orthop 1996; 5:102.

100. Fish JB: Cuneiform osteotomy of the femoral neck in the treatment of slipped capital femoral epiphysis: A follow-up note. J Bone Joint Surg Am 1994; 76:46.

101. Nishiyama K, Sakamaki T, Ishii Y: Follow-up study of subcapital wedge osteotomy for severe slipped capital femoral epiphysis. J Pediatr Orthop 1989; 9:412.

102. Gage JR, Sundberg AB, Nolan DR, et al: Complications after cuneiform osteotomy for moderately or severely slipped capital femoral epiphysis. J Bone Joint Surg Am 1978; 60:157.

103. Abraham E, Garst J, Barmada R: Treatment of moderate-to-severe slipped capital femoral epiphysis with extracapsular osteotomy. J Pediatr Orthop 1993; 13:294.

104. Kramer WG, Craig WA, Noel S: Compensating osteotomy at the base of the femoral neck for slipped capital femoral epiphysis. J Bone Joint Surg Am 1976; 58:796.

105. Whiteside LA, Schoenecker PL: Combined valgus derotation osteotomy and cervical osteoplasty for severely slipped capital femoral epiphysis. Clin Orthop Rel Res 1978; 132:88.

106. Frymoyer JW: Chondrolysis of the hip following Southwick osteotomy for severe slipped capital femoral epiphysis. Clin Orthop Rel Res 1974; 99:120.

107. Rao JP, Francis AM, Siwek CW: The treatment of chronic slipped capital femoral epiphysis by biplane osteotomy. J Bone Joint Surg Am 1984; 66:1169.

108. Millis MB, Murphy SB, Poss R: Osteotomies of the hip in the prevention and treatment of osteoarthritis. Instr Course Lect 1996; 45:209.

section 9
21
chapter

CONGENITAL DEFORMITIES OF THE KNEE

James H. Beaty, William C. Warner, Jr, and S. Terry Canale

Summary

- Bipartite patella is usually asymptomatic and is often a coincidental finding on radiographs obtained for other reasons; for symptomatic patients, nonoperative treatment (restriction of competitive activities, nonsteroidal anti-inflammatory drugs, and a short-arc exercise program) is usually sufficient.
- Conservative management is recommended for discoid meniscus because of the likelihood of degenerative changes in the knee joint after meniscectomy. If partial meniscectomy is required, arthroscopic techniques can be used.
- Popliteal cysts are usually unilateral, occur between the ages of 1 and 14 years, are more common in males than in females, and usually resolve spontaneously within 1 to 2 years.
- Congenital dislocation of the knee includes a spectrum of deformities ranging from hyperextension to total displacement, for which treatment is usually nonoperative.
- Most patients with congenital absence of the anterior cruciate ligament are asymptomatic; for symptomatic patients, treatment usually consists of observation or bracing.
- Congenital dislocation of the patella may be unilateral or bilateral and has been reported in association with other abnormalities, such as arthrogryposis and Down's syndrome; recommended treatment is surgery, which should be done as early as feasible.
- Nail-patella syndrome is a rare dysplasia that may require surgical treatment consisting of a combination of proximal and distal patellar realignments, quadricepsplasties for extension contractures, and full posterior and capsular releases for flexion deformities.

CONGENITAL DISLOCATION AND SUBLUXATION OF THE KNEE

Congenital knee dislocation (recurvatum) (CKD) is rare[1]; its reported incidence ranges from 0.017 to 0.7 occurrences per 1000 births. Some authors estimated that congenital hip dislocation (CHD) is 40 to 80 times more common than CKD of the knee.[2–5] CKD is two to three times more frequent in females than in males, the right and left knees are equally affected, and about one-third of patients have bilateral dislocations.

The cause of CKD is unknown, although several theories have been proposed (Table 1).

CKD occurs in association with other skeletal anomalies in 82% to 88% of patients,[2–4, 6] most often CHD, congenital deformities of the feet, and congenital dislocation of the elbow (Table 2).

CLASSIFICATION

Congenital dislocation of the knee includes a spectrum of conditions that usually are classified according to the severity of the deformity (Fig. 1 and Table 3).

Carlson and O'Connor[6] also identified three types of patients with CKDs: those with an isolated dislocation, those with multiple dislocations, and those with known syndromes. Ferris and Jackson[7] described four children with six "congenital snapping knees," in whom anterior subluxation of the tibia on the femur occurred with knee extension and spontaneously reduced with knee flexion. These children had no marked recurvatum deformity, and knee flexion was not restricted by quadriceps fibrosis. All four, however, had other major clinical anomalies and anterior cruciate ligament insufficiency. The most obvious clinical sign was an audible and palpable "clunk" that accompanied both subluxation and reduction. Curtis and Fisher[9] described 10 knees in five children with a similar condition they called "heritable congenital tibiofemoral subluxation."

CLINICAL EXAMINATION

The hyperextension of the knee is distinctive, and the diagnosis can be easily made by visual inspection (Fig. 2). Knee flexion is limited, and the knee can be extended further than its hyperextended position. Lateral radiographs demonstrate either partial displacement (subluxation) or complete dislocation of the tibia on the femur, with the tibial plateau sloped posteriorly (Fig. 3). Anteroposterior views show associated lateral and rotary subluxation and valgus deformity of the knee. The ossification centers of the proximal tibia and distal femur usually are hypoplastic or occasionally absent.

TREATMENT

The treatment of congenital hyperextension and subluxation of the knee depends on the severity of the deformity and the age at which treatment is begun.[4, 6, 10, 11] Most series report excellent or good results with nonoperative treatment

---

TABLE 1. CAUSES OF CONGENITAL KNEE DISLOCATION

- Birth trauma[14]
- Fetal molding[19]
- Hypoplasia and attenuation of anterior cruciate ligament[14]
- Quadriceps contracture[12]
- Intrauterine ischemia similar to compartment syndrome[10]
- Heredity[4, 16]

TABLE 2. ANOMALIES ASSOCIATED WITH CONGENITAL KNEE DISLOCATION

Skeletal
- Congenital hip dislocation (45%)
- Congenital foot deformities (31%)
- Congenital elbow dislocation (10%)

Other
- Cleft palate and cleft lip
- Spina bifida
- Hydrocephalus
- Down's syndrome
- Cryptorchidism
- Angiomata
- Facial paralysis
- Imperforate anus

if treatment is begun early and no other anomalies or syndromes are present. If multiple lower limb deformities are present, the knee dislocation should be treated before any of the other deformities.[6, 12, 13] Ko et al[12] reported successful concomitant treatment of CKD and CHD with the Pavlik harness.

In newborns with mild or moderate hyperextension or subluxation, serial manipulation and casting should begin as soon as possible. The knee is manipulated and casted every 2 weeks in as much flexion as can be easily obtained. Forceful casting in flexion has been cited as a cause of posterior sloping of the tibial plateau. After 90 degrees of flexion is obtained by casting, the knee can be maintained in flexion in a Pavlik harness. Lateral subluxation of the knee is a contraindication to the use of a Pavlik harness because the harness will aggravate the lateral subluxation.

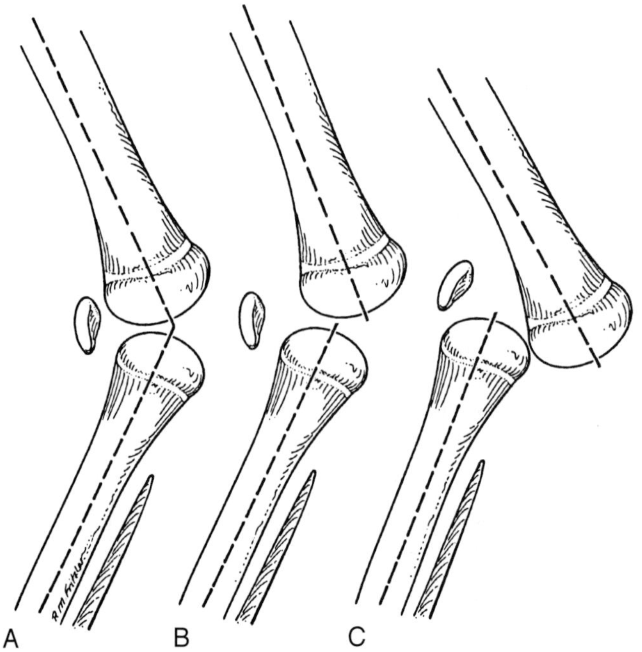

If the subluxation or dislocation cannot be reduced by serial manipulation, surgery usually is necessary.[6] Skin or skeletal traction has been used to reduce the dislocation and obtain 45 degrees of knee flexion before a casting program is begun. Most often, however, open reduction and quadricepsplasty are required. Surgery should be done before the infant begins to try to walk, preferably at about 6 months of age. Several procedures have been described for the treatment of CKD, but all involve lengthening of the quadriceps mechanism and release of the anterior capsule. The V-Y lengthening of the quadriceps tendon described by Curtis and Fisher[9] is most commonly used (Fig. 4). Roy and Crawford[14] described a percutaneous quadriceps lengthening technique in which the fascia overlying the rectus portion of the quadriceps is released through a small stab incision made one to two patellar lengths superior to the patella in the midline. Medial and lateral stab incisions are then made at the superior border of the patella for release of the medial and lateral quadriceps and the retinaculum. In older children, full flexion may not be obtained, and a femoral or tibial osteotomy may be necessary.

CONGENITAL ABSENCE OF THE ANTERIOR CRUCIATE LIGAMENT

Congenital absence of the anterior cruciate ligament (ACL) is rare. Although this condition was initially described in association with CKD, it is not known whether the absence of the ACL is primary or secondary. Several authors reported absence of the ACL as a distinct, solitary entity.[15, 16] It also has been reported in association with other limb disorders.[17–21] Absence of the ACL may or may not cause symptoms. Physical examination usually reveals a positive anterior drawer test and at least a grade 3 Lachman's sign. Radiological evidence of hypoplasia of one or both tibial spines is suggestive of congenital ligament deficiency. The

Fig. 1. Classification of congenital knee dislocation according to severity. *A,* Hyperextension. *B,* Subluxation. *C,* Dislocation. (Redrawn from Curtis BH, Fisher RL: Congenital hyperextension with anterior subluxation of the knee: Surgical treatment and long-term observations. J Bone Joint Surg Am 1964; 51:255.)

TABLE 3. CLASSIFICATION OF CONGENITAL KNEE DISLOCATION

Grade	Description
I	Congenital hyperextension Minimal or no subluxation of tibia on femur 15–20 degrees of hyperextension Can be passively manipulated into 45–90 degrees of flexion
II	Congenital subluxation Epiphysis of tibia displaced forward on anterior aspect of femoral condyles, with some contact between tibial and femoral articular surfaces 25–45 degrees of hyperextension Can be passively flexed only to neutral position
III	Congenital dislocation Upper tibial epiphysis totally displaced in front of femoral condyles, no contact between articular surfaces

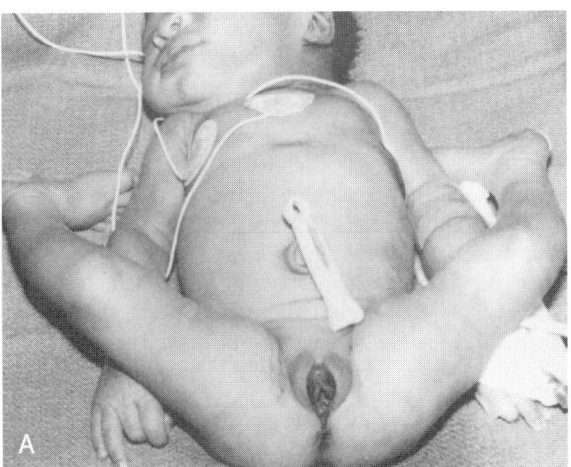
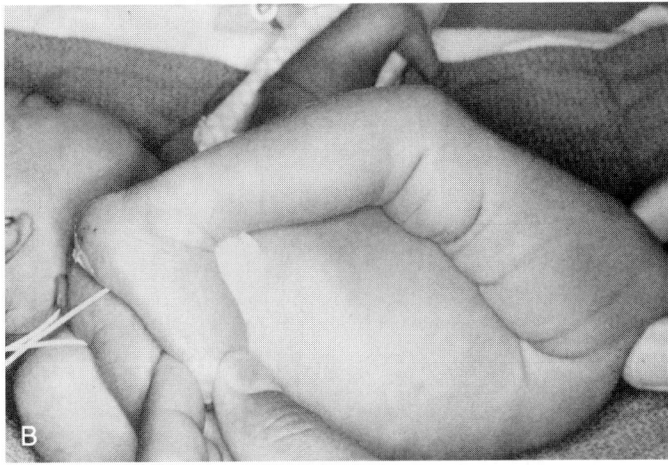

Fig. 2. Congenital knee dislocation. *A,* Newborn with congenital knee dislocation. *B,* Note prominence of femoral condyles posterior to anteriorly dislocated tibia and fibula. (Photographs courtesy of Dr. Jay Cummings, reproduced from Beaty JH: Congenital anomalies of the foot and lower extremity. In Canale ST, Beaty JH [eds]: Operative Pediatric Orthopaedics, 2nd ed. St. Louis, MO, CV Mosby, 1995.)

intercondylar notch is V-shaped or shallow, and the lateral femoral condyle may be hypoplastic.

In patients with tibial or femoral dysplasia, the diagnosis is important because subluxation or dislocation of the knee has been reported after femoral lengthening when the ACL is absent.[18] Before femoral lengthening is done, radiographs should be carefully scrutinized for any evidence of absence of the ACL. Because most patients with congenital absence of the ACL are asymptomatic or have only mild symptoms and because the natural history is unknown, treatment usu-

ally consists of observation or bracing for symptomatic patients.

CONGENITAL DISLOCATION OF THE PATELLA

The congenitally dislocated patella is dislocated laterally and cannot be reduced by closed manipulation. The condition may be unilateral or bilateral, and a familial tendency

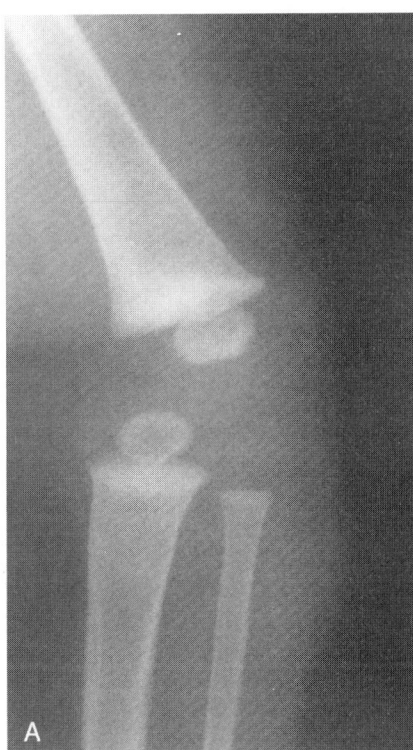
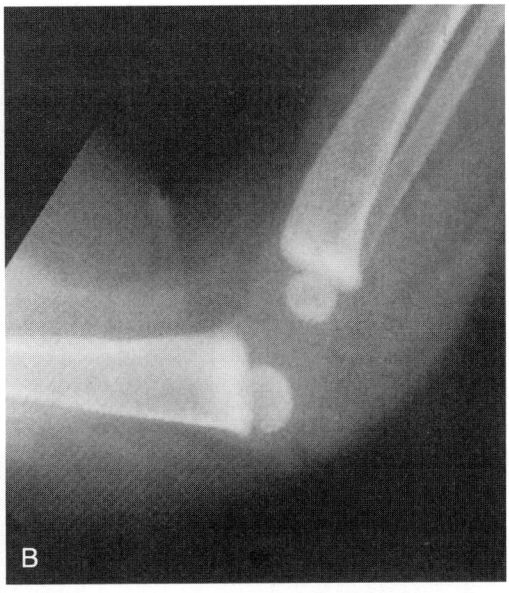

Fig. 3. Congenital knee dislocation. Radiographic appearance. *A,* Medial displacement of tibia and fibula is evident on anteroposterior view. *B,* Lateral view shows anterior dislocation of tibia on femoral condyle. (From Beaty JH: Congenital anomalies of the foot and lower extremity. In Canale ST, Beaty JH [eds]: Operative Pediatric Orthopaedics, 2nd ed. St. Louis, MO, CV Mosby, 1995.)

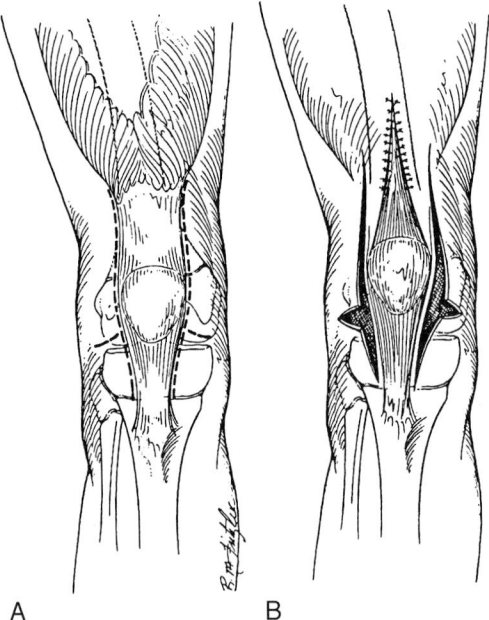

Fig. 4. Curtis and Fisher technique for correction of congenital knee dislocation. *A,* Incisions to release anterior capsule medially and laterally as well as medial and lateral retinaculum of quadriceps mechanism. *B,* Correction after soft-tissue release and lengthening of rectus femoris muscle. (From Beaty JH: Congenital anomalies of the foot and lower extremity. In Canale ST, Beaty JH [eds]: Operative Pediatric Orthopaedics, 2nd ed. St. Louis, MO, CV Mosby, 1995.)

has been reported. The condition also has been reported in association with other abnormalities, including arthrogryposis and Down's syndrome.[22]

The patella is dislocated on the lateral side of the lateral femoral condyle and is hypoplastic and misshapen; the lateral femoral condyle is flattened anteriorly.[23] The vastus lateralis muscle may be absent, and the iliotibial band may be attached to the patella.[24] Varying degrees of genu valgum are present, and the tibia tends to rotate externally and subluxate laterally. With the patella dislocated, the quadriceps flexes the knee and externally rotates the tibia.

Because the patella is small at birth and is not ossified until 2 to 3 years of age, the diagnosis often is overlooked.[25, 26] Congenital patellar dislocation should be suspected in an infant with a fixed flexion deformity of the knee and excessive lateral rotation of the tibia. Usually the knee cannot be actively extended from a flexed position because of the altered pull of the quadriceps muscles. The femoral condyles can be palpated, and the patella can be located above the fibular head. Radiographs usually are not helpful until the age of 3 to 5 years because of the lack of patellar ossification. Before this age, lateral radiographs show a loss of the normal quadriceps soft-tissue shadow. The use of ultrasonography has been suggested for evaluation of the unossified patella.[27]

When the patella remains dislocated, walking often is delayed and difficult because of the loss of active knee extension. Secondary articular and bony changes occur in the patella, lateral femoral condyle, and intercondylar notch (Fig. 5). The valgus stress stretches the medial collateral ligament, and the capsule on the medial and anteromedial aspects of the joint becomes hypertrophic.[28-30]

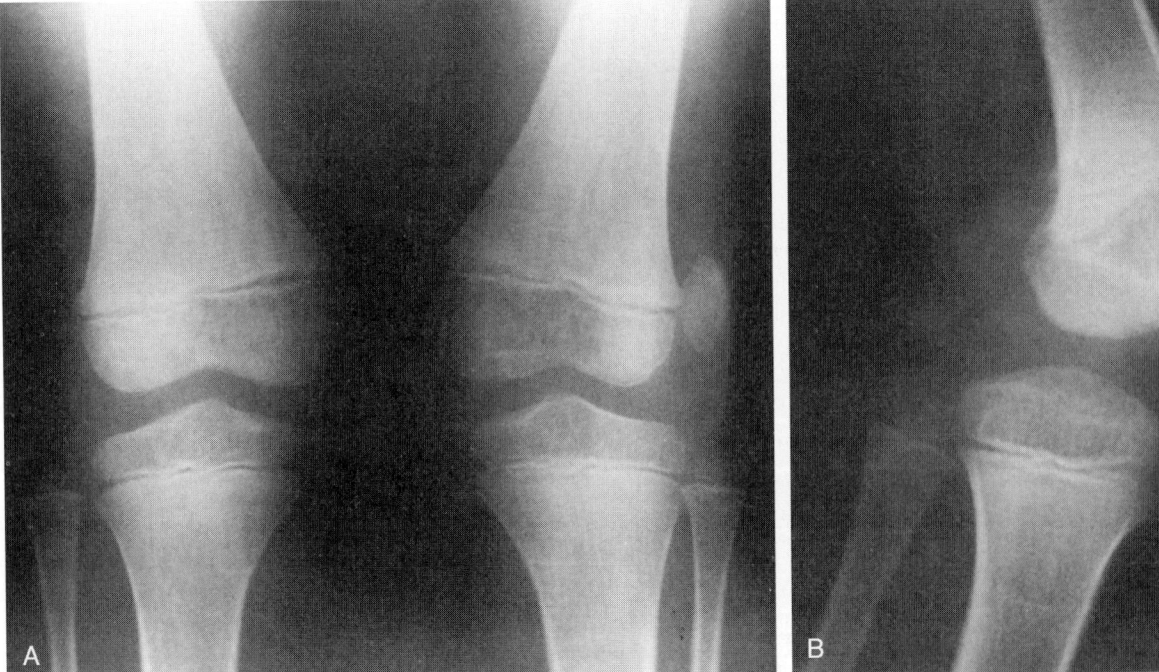

Fig. 5. Untreated congenital dislocation of the left patella in a 5-year-old boy. *A,* Anteroposterior view shows fixed lateral dislocation. *B,* On lateral view, patella appears absent because of superimposed femoral condyles. (From Beaty JH: Congenital anomalies of the foot and lower extremity. In Canale ST, Beaty JH [eds]: Operative Pediatric Orthopaedics, 2nd ed. St. Louis, MO, CV Mosby, 1995.)

Closed reduction is impossible, and the deformity can be corrected only by surgery.[25] Because the severity of the deformity is directly related to the length of time it remains uncorrected, surgery should be performed as soon as the diagnosis is made. Correction usually requires extensive lateral release, medial imbrication, and, if necessary, transfer of the semitendinosus to the patella as a check rein.[31, 32]

Gordon and Schoenecker[33] used a modification of the extensive release procedure described by Stanisavljevic et al[25] for treatment of fixed, painful lateral dislocation in 11 patients (17 knees) (average age, 7 years 9 months). In skeletally immature patients, the entire patellar tendon was transferred medially, and in skeletally mature patients the tibial tubercle was transferred medially. At an average follow-up of 5 years, all patients reported marked increases in activity and relief of pain.

NAIL-PATELLA SYNDROME

Nail-patella syndrome (hereditary onychoosteodysplasia) is a rare dysplasia with four characteristic findings: dysplasia of the fingernails, hypoplasia or absence of the patella, radial head dislocations, and iliac horns.[26, 27, 34–41] Nephropathy accompanied by mild proteinuria also is a common manifestation of this syndrome. Farley et al[36] reported glaucoma in three generations of family members with nail-patella syndrome. Other skeletal deformities such as foot abnormalities, most commonly a clubfoot deformity,[38] shoulder girdle dysplasia,[39] and clavicular horns[41] have been reported. The fingernails are either hypoplastic or absent, but the toenails usually are not involved. Involved fingernails have splitting, spooning, and ridging; there are lesser degrees of changes in the fingernails on the ulnar side of the hand. The thumbnails are always involved. Iliac horns, considered pathognomonic of the disease, are bilateral smooth bony outgrowths from the posterior ilium. They cause no symptoms, have no effect on gait, and need no treatment.

The patella is either hypoplastic or absent and may be abnormally shaped and unstable. Contracture of the quadriceps muscles and atrophy of the vastus medialis are common. Hypoplasia of the femoral condyles and an intercondylar synovial septum also have been reported,[40] as have late degenerative changes of the knee joint. Guidera et al[38] reported the best surgical results with combined proximal and distal patellar realignments, quadricepsplasties for extension contractures, and full posterior and capsular releases for flexion deformities. Femoral osteotomies were required in some patients for residual deformities.

BIPARTITE PATELLA

The patella may arise from two or more centers of ossification. If a separate center of ossification does not fuse with the main body of the patella, it is attached to the patella by fibrocartilaginous tissue, resulting in bipartite patella.[42, 43] Most ossicles are superolateral, but lateral, medial, and inferior lesions have been reported (Table 4).

Bipartite patella is bilateral in about 40% of patients, usually is asymptomatic, and often is a coincidental finding on radiographs obtained for some other reason.[44, 45] Pain in the superolateral pole of the patella usually is caused by an

TABLE 4. CLASSIFICATION OF BIPARTITE PATELLA (SAUPE)

Type	Description
I	Inferior pole (5%)
II	Lateral margin (20%)
III	Superolateral pole (75%)

overuse syndrome, such as chondromalacia, rather than by bipartite patella.[46–48] Occasionally, excessive lateral tension from the vastus lateralis results in hypermobility of the bipartite patella.[49–51] Hypermobility can be determined by the "squatting position test," in which a skyline view of patella is obtained with the patient in a squatting position. Occasionally, a superolateral lesion can be mistaken for an acute patellar fracture. Bone scanning may be helpful in making the diagnosis of a fracture of the superolateral pole of the patella.

Restriction of competitive activity, use of nonsteroidal anti-inflammatory drugs, and a program of short-arc exercises generally allow resolution of symptoms. Repetitive microtrauma may fracture the synchondrosis and produce pain[43, 52]; this usually resolves with 3 weeks of knee immobilization. If symptoms persist after nonoperative treatment, surgery may be indicated (Table 5).

Excision of a bipartite patella rarely is indicated, except for persistent pain in older adolescents and young adults who have not responded to conservative treatment and who wish to continue competitive sports.

DISCOID MENISCUS

A discoid meniscus is disk shaped rather than semilunar, as are normal menisci. The two most widely accepted causes of discoid meniscus are those proposed by Smillie[53] and Kaplan.[54] Smillie suggested that the discoid meniscus resulted from an arrest at varying stages of embryological meniscal development. He divided discoid lateral meniscus into three forms: primitive, intermediate, and infantile. Kaplan, however, found no cartilaginous disk representing the meniscus at any stage of human embryological development nor in any comparative anatomic dissections. He believed that the meniscus formed normally but that, instead of its normal attachments to the posterior tibial plateau, it was attached to the lateral surface of the medial femoral condyle by the meniscofemoral ligament (Wrisberg's ligament). Because of the abnormal attachment, knee extension pulls the lateral meniscus into the intercondylar area. According to Kaplan, constant mediolateral motion

TABLE 5. SURGERY FOR BIPARTITE PATELLA

Excision of the accessory fragment
Lateral retinacular release
Subperiosteal release of vastus lateralis
Open reduction and internal fixation with bone grafting of the fragment

and irritation of the lateral meniscus transforms an initially normal, semilunar meniscus into a thick fibrocartilaginous mass, or discoid meniscus.

A fourth type of discoid meniscus—the ring-shaped meniscus—has been described[55, 56] but appears to be extremely rare.

Discoid menisci often are asymptomatic. Wrisberg's ligament types are most likely to be symptomatic. Symptoms usually occur by 6 to 8 years of age.

SYMPTOMS OF DISCOID MENISCUS

- Snapping or clicking in the knee.
- Sensation of giving way or catching.
- Palpable "clunk" during the last 15 to 20 degrees of extension of the flexed knee.
- Fullness along lateral joint line.
- Joint effusion.
- Thigh atrophy.

Plain radiographs show widening of the lateral joint space compared with the other side. Flattening of the lateral femoral condyle and cupping of the lateral aspect of the tibial plateau also are suggestive of discoid meniscus. Magnetic resonance imaging (MRI) is the diagnostic method of choice (Fig. 6).[57–61]

The characteristic MRI appearance of symptomatic discoid menisci in children is a diffusely thick meniscus with a slab configuration and diffusely increased intrameniscal signal that may or may not extend to the joint surface.

In children, conservative management of discoid meniscus is recommended because of the well-documented occurrence of degenerative knee joint changes after meniscectomy.[62–64] A short period of immobilization is followed by restriction of activities and progressive quadriceps-strengthening exercises. If the knee frequently locks or if function is significantly impaired, surgery is indicated.[64a] The type of surgery depends on the type of lesion identified at surgery (Table 6).[58, 65–67] Good results have been reported after saucerization and partial meniscectomy of asympto-

TABLE 6. CLASSIFICATION OF DISCOID MENISCUS

Type	
Wrisberg's ligament	No attachment to the tibial plateau posteriorly
	Only posterior attachment is through the lateral meniscofemoral ligament, resulting in a hypermobile lateral meniscus
Complete	Intact attachments
	Not hypermobile
Incomplete	Differs from the complete type only in size

Adapted from Watanabe M, Takeda S, Ikeuchi H: Atlas of Arthroscopy, 3rd ed. Berlin, Springer-Verlag, 1979. Used with permission.

matic, stable lesions,[67, 68, 68a] but in hypermobile Wrisberg's-type lesions, partial meniscectomy results in an unstable meniscal rim. In this Wrisberg type, in which the posterior ligamentous attachments are not intact, treatment may include peripheral repair of the discoid meniscus and partial meniscectomy or total meniscectomy.

The controversy continues over total or partial meniscectomy, open or arthroscopic technique, and even type of arthroscopic technique.[68b] Washington et al[69] suggested that total meniscectomy may offer the best prognosis, for a longer period of time, for symptom-free knees in patients 16 years old or younger. In their group of 15 patients (18 knees), 17 years after total meniscectomies, 10 patients had excellent results, three had good results, and five had fair results. In their report of arthroscopic meniscectomy of discoid lateral meniscus in 17 adolescents, Aglietti et al[70] found no correlation between meniscal type, type of meniscectomy (partial or total), and clinical and radiographic results. At an average 10-year follow-up, 12 of 17 patients had excellent results, four had good results, and one had a fair result. Conversely, Smith et al[71] reported fair or poor results in 40% of 43 knees at an average of 6.5 years after total or partial meniscectomy. Because of persistent symp-

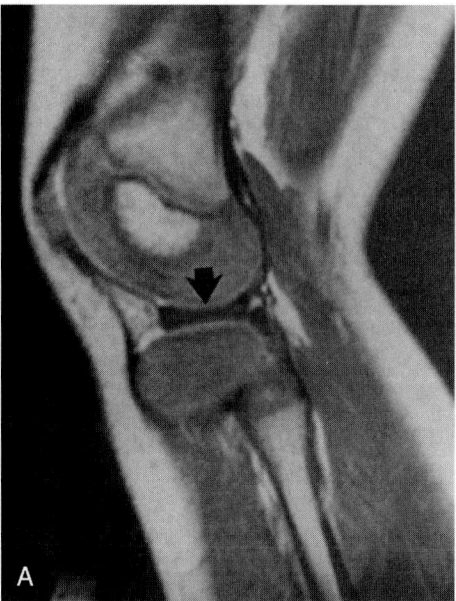
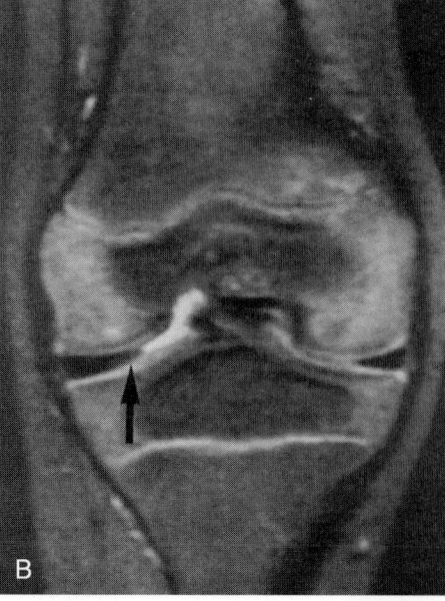

Fig. 6. Magnetic resonance image of discoid meniscus in a 3-year-old boy. *A,* Sagittal proton density image shows abnormally thick lateral meniscus. *B,* Fat-suppressed, coronal proton density image demonstrates extension of discoid meniscus centrally *(arrow)* into weightbearing portion of lateral compartment. (From Witte D: Magnetic resonance imaging in orthopaedics. In Canale ST [ed]: Campbell's Operative Orthopaedics, 9th ed. St. Louis, MO, CV Mosby, 1998.)

toms and evidence of osteoarthrosis in many of their patients, Räber et al[72] recommended that total meniscectomy in children be avoided whenever possible.

Arthroscopic techniques for removal of the discoid meniscus in one piece or two pieces have been described, each with its proponents. Kim et al[73] advocated a one-piece removal because the operating time is short (less than 20 minutes), the procedure is less aggressive than conventional partial meniscectomy techniques (piecemeal removal or morcellation), there is less damage to the cartilage, and there is less formation of foreign bodies. Their technique uses three nonstandard knee portals: lateral patellofemoral axillary portal, far anteromedial portal, and low anterolateral portal. The central portion of the meniscus is removed in one piece, and the meniscal rim is reshaped and smoothed.

Ogata[74] described a technique for two-piece excision of a discoid meniscus in which the torn meniscus is divided into anterior and posterior pieces for removal. According to him, disadvantages of one-piece removal include the difficulty of working in the confined space within the compartment, especially for the posterior incision; the difficulty of determining the width of the rim to be retained; and the large portal required for removal of a large piece of meniscus. Piecemeal arthroscopic excision, although easier, has several disadvantages: it is time consuming; the frequent use of instruments such as a basket forceps increases the risk of damage to the articular surface and the intact pe-

ripheral rim of the meniscus; and there is the possibility of leaving pieces of excised meniscus in the joint. He cited several advantages of the two-piece excision. First, the procedure is easier because the posterior portion can be easily seen after the anterior piece is removed. Second, the extent of intrasubstance disease can be evaluated with a transverse cut to the midportion of the meniscus, allowing accurate determination of the width of the rim to be retained. Third, a large portal is not required for removal of the two pieces.

POPLITEAL CYSTS

Popliteal cysts usually arise between the semimembranosus and gastrocnemius tendons and represent an enlargement of the bursa between these two muscles. Popliteal cysts usually are unilateral, occur between the ages of 2 and 14 years, and are more common in males than in females.[75, 76] In a review of 393 MRI studies of children's knees, De Maeseneer et al[77] found popliteal cysts in 25 (6.3%.) The lesion usually is distal to the popliteal crease and is prominent with the knee hyperextended. MRI[78] and ultrasonography[79] have been reported for evaluation of popliteal cysts. Most popliteal cysts in children are isolated bursal sac formations and are not related to disease in the knee joint; they rarely are symptomatic. Treatment is conservative, and surgery usually is not indicated for popliteal cysts in children.[80, 81] Most cysts resolve spontaneously within 1 to 2 years.

REFERENCES

Dislocation and Subluxation of the Knee

1. Muhammad KS, Koman LA, Mooney JF III, et al: Congenital dislocation of the knee: Overview of management options. J South Orthop Assoc 1999; 8:93.
2. Curtis BH, Fisher RL: Congenital hyperextension with anterior subluxation of the knee: Surgical treatment and long-term observations. J Bone Joint Surg Am 1964; 51:255.
3. Johnson E, Audell R, Oppenheim WL: Congenital dislocation of the knee. J Pediatr Orthop 1987; 7:194.
4. Katz MP, Grogono BJ, Soper KC: The etiology and treatment of congenital dislocation of the knee. J Bone Joint Surg Br 1967; 49:112.
5. Neibauer JJ, King DE: Congenital dislocation of the knee. J Bone Joint Surg Am 1960; 42:207.
6. Drennan JC: Congenital dislocation of the knee and patella. Instr Course Lect 1993; 42:517.
7. Carlson DH, O'Connor J: Congenital dislocation of the knee. Am J Roentgenol 1976; 127:465.
8. Ferris BD, Jackson AM: Congenital snapping knee: Habitual anterior subluxation of the tibia in extension. J Bone Joint Surg Br 1990; 72:453.
9. Curtis BH, Fisher RL: Heritable congenital tibiofemoral subluxation: Clinical features and surgical treatment. J Bone Joint Surg Am 1970; 52:1104.

10. Ferris B, Aichroth P: The treatment of congenital knee dislocation: A review of nineteen knees. Clin Orthop 1987; 216: 136.
11. Haga N, Nakamura S, Sakaguchi R, et al: Congenital dislocation of the knee reduced spontaneously or with minimal treatment. J Pediatr Orthop 1997; 17:59.
12. Ko JY, Shih CH, Wenger DR: Congenital dislocation of the knee. J Pediatr Orthop 1999; 19:242.
13. Oishi T, Sugioka Y, Matsumoto S, et al: Congenital dislocation of the knee: Its pathologic features and treatment. Clin Orthop 1993; 278:187.
14. Roy DR, Crawford AH: Percutaneous quadriceps recession: A technique for management of congenital hyperextension deformity of the knee in the neonate. J Pediatr Orthop 1989; 9:717.

Congenital Absence of the Anterior Cruciate Ligament

15. Barrett GR, Tomasin JD: Bilateral congenital absence of the anterior cruciate ligament. Orthopedics 1988; 11:431.
16. Johansson E, Aparisi T: Congenital absence of the cruciate ligaments: A case report and review of the literature. Clin Orthop 1982; 162:108.
17. Johansson E, Aparisi T: Missing cruciate ligament in congenital short femur. J Bone Joint Surg Am 1983; 65:1109.
18. Kaelin A, Hulin PH, Carlioz H: Congeni-

tal aplasia of the cruciate ligaments: A report of six cases. J Bone Joint Surg Br 1986; 68:827.
19. Thomas NP, Jackson AM, Aichroth PM: Congenital absence of the anterior cruciate ligament: A common component of knee dysplasia. J Bone Joint Surg Br 1985; 67: 572.
20. Tolo VT: Congenital absence of the menisci and cruciate ligaments of the knee: A case report. J Bone Joint Surg Am 1981; 63:1022.
21. Torode IP, Gillespie R: Anteroposterior instability of the knee: A sign of congenital limb deficiency. J Pediatr Orthop 1983; 3: 467.

Dislocation of the Patella

22. McCall RE, Lessenberry HB: Bilateral congenital dislocation of the patella. J Pediatr Orthop 1987; 7:100.
23. Gunn DR: Contracture of the quadriceps muscle: A discussion on the etiology and relationship to recurrent dislocation of the patella. J Bone Joint Surg Br 1964; 46: 492.
24. Jeffreys TE: Recurrent dislocation of the patella due to abnormal attachment of the ilio-tibial tract. J Bone Joint Surg Br 1963; 45:740.
25. Stanisavljevic S, Zemenick G, Miller D: Congenital, irreducible, permanent lateral dislocation of the patella. Clin Orthop 1976; 116:190.
26. Zeier FG, Dissanayke C: Congenital dislo-

cation of the patella. Clin Orthop 1980; 148:140.

27. Walker J, Rang M, Daneman A: Ultrasonography of the unossified patella in young children. J Pediatr Orthop 1991; 11: 100.

28. Green JP, Waugh W: Congenital lateral dislocation of the patella. J Bone Joint Surg Br 1968; 50:285.

29. Jones RDS, Fisher RL, Curtis BH: Congenital dislocation of the patella. Clin Orthop 1976; 119:177.

30. Støren H: Congenital complete dislocation of patella causing serious disability in childhood: The operative treatment. Acta Orthop Scand 1965; 36:301.

31. Langenskiöld AL, Ritsilä V: Congenital dislocation of the patella and its operative treatment. J Pediatr Orthop 1992; 12:315.

32. Gao GX, Lee EH, Bose K: Surgical management of congenital and habitual dislocation of the patella. J Pediatr Orthop 1990; 10:255.

33. Gordon JE, Schoenecker PL: Surgical treatment of congenital dislocation of the patella. J Pediatr Orthop 1999; 19:260.

Nail-Patella Syndrome

34. Beals RK, Eckhardt AL: Hereditary onycho-osteodysplasia (nail-patella) syndrome: A report of nine kindreds. J Bone Joint Surg Am 1969; 51:505.

35. Duncan JG, Souter WA: Hereditary onycho-osteodysplasia. The nail patella syndrome. J Bone Joint Surg Br 1964; 45: 242.

36. Farley FA, Lichter PR, Downs CA, et al: An orthopaedic scoring system for nail-patella syndrome and application to a kindred with variable expressivity and glaucoma. J Pediatr Orthop 1999; 19:624.

37. Garces MA, Muraskas JK, Muraskas EK, et al: Hereditary onycho-osteo-dysplasia (HOOD syndrome): A report of two cases. Skeletal Radiol 1982; 8:55.

38. Guidera KJ, Satterwhite Y, Ogden JA: Nail patella syndrome: A review of 44 orthopaedic patients. J Pediatr Orthop 1991; 11:737.

39. Loomer RL: Shoulder girdle dysplasia associated with nail patella syndrome: A case report and literature review. Clin Orthop 1989; 238:112.

40. Yakish SD, Fu FH: Long-term follow-up of the treatment of a family with nail-patella syndrome. J Pediatr Orthop 1983; 3:360.

41. Yarali HN, Erden GA, Karaarslan F, et al: Clavicular horn: Another bony projection in nail-patella syndrome. Pediatr Radiol 1995; 25:549.

Bipartite Patella

42. Insall J: Current concepts review: Patellar pain. J Bone Joint Surg Am 1982; 64:147.

43. Ogden JA, McCarthy SM, Joke P: The painful bipartite patella. J Pediatr Orthop 1982; 2:263.

44. Carter SR: Traumatic separation of a bipartite patella. Injury 1989; 20:244.

45. DeLee JC, Dickhaut SC: The discoid lateral meniscus syndrome. J Bone Joint Surg Am 1982; 64:1068.

46. Bourne MH, Bianco AJ Jr: Bipartite patella in the adolescent: Results of surgical excision. J Pediatr Orthop 1990; 10:69.

47. Casscells SW: Chondromalacia of the patella. J Pediatr Orthop 1982; 2:560.

48. Halpern AA, Hewitt O: Painful medial bipartite patellae. Clin Orthop 1978; 134: 180.

49. Ishikawa H, Sakurai A, Hirata S, et al: Painful bipartite patella in young athletes: The diagnostic value of skyline views taken in squatting position and the results of surgical excision. Clin Orthop Rel Res 1994; 305:223.

50. Mori Y, Okumo H, Iketani H, et al: Efficacy of lateral retinacular release for painful bipartite patella. Am J Sports Med 1995; 23:13.

51. Ogata K: Painful bipartite patella: A new approach to operative treatment. J Bone Joint Surg Am 1994; 76:573.

52. Green WT Jr: Painful bipartite patella: A report of three cases. Clin Orthop 1975; 110:197.

Discoid Meniscus

53. Smillie IS: The congenital discoid meniscus. J Bone Joint Surg Br 1948; 30:671.

54. Kaplan EB: Discoid lateral meniscus of the knee joint: Nature, mechanism, and operative treatment. J Bone Joint Surg Am 1957; 39:77.

55. Monllau JC, León A, Cugat R, et al: Ring-shaped lateral meniscus. Arthroscopy 1998; 14:502.

56. Noble J: Congenital absence of the anterior cruciate ligament associated with a ring meniscus: Report of a case. J Bone Joint Surg Am 1975; 57:1165.

57. Auge W II, Kaeding CC: Case report: Bilateral discoid medial menisci with extensive intrasubstance cleavage tears: MRI and arthroscopic correlation. Arthroscopy 1994; 10:313.

58. Barnes CL, McCarthy RE, Vander-Schildden JL, et al: Discoid lateral meniscus in a young child: Case report and review of the literature. J Pediatr Orthop 1987; 8:707.

59. Hamada M, Shino K, Kawano K, et al: Usefulness of magnetic resonance imaging for detecting intrasubstance tears and/or degeneration of lateral discoid meniscus. Arthroscopy 1994; 10:645.

60. Silverman JM, Mink JH, Deutsch AL: Discoid menisci of the knee: MR imaging appearance. Radiology 1989; 173:351.

61. Stark JE, Siegel MJ, Weinberger E, et al: Discoid menisci in children: MR features. J Comp Assist Tomogr 1995; 19:608.

62. Manzione M, Pizzutillo PD, Peoples AB, et al: Meniscectomy in children: A long-term follow-up study. Am J Sports Med 1983; 11:111.

63. Medlar RC, Mandiberg JJ, Lyne ED: Meniscectomies in children: Report of long-term results (mean, 8.3 years) of 26 children. Am J Sports Med 1980; 8:87.

64. Zaman M, Leonard MA: Meniscectomy in children: Results in 59 knees. Injury 1981; 12:425.

64a. Fujikawa K, Iseki F, Mikura Y: Partial resection of the discoid meniscus in the child's knee. J Bone Joint Surg Br 1981; 63:391.

65. Aichroth PM, Patel DV, Marx CL: Congenital discoid lateral meniscus in children: A follow-up study and evolution of management. J Bone Joint Surg Br 1991; 73:932.

66. Dickhaut SC, DeLee JC: The discoid lateral-meniscus syndrome. J Bone Joint Surg Am 1982; 64:1068.

67. Fritschy D, Gonseth D: Discoid lateral meniscus. Int Orthop 1991; 15:145.

68. Dimakopoulos P, Patel D: Partial excision of discoid meniscus: Arthroscopic operation of 10 patients. Acta Orthop Scand 1990; 61:40.

68a. Vandermeer RD, Cunningham FK: Arthroscopic treatment of the discoid lateral meniscus: Results of long-term follow-up. Arthroscopy 1989; 5:101.

68b. Watanabe M, Takeda S, Ikeuchi H: Atlas of Arthroscopy, 3rd ed. Berlin, Springer-Verlag, 1979.

69. Washington ER, Root L, Liener UC: Discoid lateral meniscus in children: Long-term follow-up after excision. J Bone Joint Surg Am 1995; 77:1357.

70. Aglietti P, Bertini FA, Buzzi R, et al: Arthroscopic meniscectomy for discoid lateral meniscus in children and adolescents: 10-year follow-up. Am J Knee Surg 1999; 12:83.

71. Smith CF, Van Dyk GE, Jurgutis J, et al: Cautious surgery for discoid menisci. Am J Knee Surg 1999; 12:25.

72. Räber DA, Friederich NF, Hefti F: Discoid lateral meniscus in children: Long-term follow-up after total meniscectomy. J Bone Joint Surg Am 1998; 80:1579.

73. Kim S-J, Yoo J-H, Kim H-K: Arthroscopic one-piece excision technique for the treatment of symptomatic lateral discoid meniscus. Arthroscopy 1996; 12:752.

74. Ogata K: Arthroscopic technique: Two-piece excision of discoid meniscus. Arthroscopy 1997; 13:666.

Popliteal Cysts

75. Baker ND: Evaluation of popliteal cysts. Rheum Dis Clin North Am 1991; 17:803.

76. Baker WM: On the formation of synovial cysts in the leg in connection with disease of the knee joint. St Bart Hosp Rep 1977; 13:245.

77. De Maeseneer M, Debaere C, Desprechins B, et al: Popliteal cysts in children: Prevalence, appearance and associated findings at MR imaging. Pediatr Radiol 1999; 29: 605.

78. Fielding JR, Franklin PD, Kustan J: Popliteal cysts: A reassessment using magnetic resonance imaging. Skeletal Radiol 1991; 20:433.

79. Szer IS, Klein-Gitelmann M, DeNardo BA, et al: Ultrasonography in the study of prevalence and clinical evolution of popliteal cysts in children with knee effusions. J Rheumatol 1992; 19:458.

80. Dinhamn JM: Popliteal cysts in children: The case against surgery. J Bone Joint Surg Br 1975; 57:69.

81. Massari L, Faccini R, Gupi L, et al: Diagnosis and treatment of popliteal cysts. Chir Organi Mov 1990; 75:245.

KNEE DISORDERS IN ADOLESCENCE

Scott A. Hoffinger

Summary

- The knee is the most frequently injured joint in adolescent sports.
- Medial meniscal tears are the most common internal derangement seen.
- Patellofemoral problems are best managed nonoperatively.
- Anterior cruciate ligament (ACL) injuries are becoming more common in both boys and girls, and ligament reconstruction can be performed in selected skeletally immature patients.
- Tibial eminence fractures are difficult fractures that often leave the patient with some degree of laxity.
- Osteochondritis dissecans (OCD), usually involving the lateral side of the medial femoral condyle, has a favorable natural history if the articular surface is intact and the patient is young.

The knee is a frequent source of complaints in the adolescent patient both from overuse injuries as well as acute trauma. However, the knee is also the most common presenting site for osteosarcoma and a frequent source of referred pain in patients with slipped capital femoral epiphysis. Because these latter conditions are more urgent and require aggressive treatment, they must always be kept in mind when evaluating an adolescent patient with knee pain.

INCIDENCE

Pritchett[1] found that 20% of high school football players will sustain at least one injury per season and 13% will have injuries involving the knee. Of those with internal derangement, 59% will have further injury to that same knee, and 87% of those with patellar injuries will suffer reinjury. DeHaven and Lintner[2] studied 4500 young athletes and noted that, among those younger than 13 years, the most common injury was a fracture of the tibia or fibula, followed by internal derangement. For those between ages 13 and 15 years, patellofemoral disorders were most common, followed by internal derangement. Internal derangement was the most common injury suffered only for those older than 16 years. Males also suffered more internal derangement than females, whose most common injury was patellofemoral. This latter may reflect the sports chosen, because football, an exclusively male sport in their study, was the most common sport in which injury occurred.

LIGAMENT INJURIES/PHYSEAL INJURIES

The knee lacks the inherent bony stability of a joint such as the hip and thus requires the ligaments to maintain

stability while allowing a significant degree of mobility (Fig. 1). With open physes, a varus or valgus stress may result in a Salter type I or II fracture of the distal femur or, less commonly, proximal tibia rather than a ligamentous injury. These injuries will usually have more swelling and point tenderness and may be seen as a widening of the physis on radiograph. These fractures require casting. The distal femoral fracture may be particularly unstable and should be monitored for displacement. Both injuries should be followed up long term to ensure there is no physeal arrest.

MEDIAL COLLATERAL LIGAMENT

A valgus or clipping type injury will result in stress on the medial collateral ligament (MCL). If enough stress is applied, the ligament may rupture and secondary restraints are then loaded. These include the posterior capsule and the ACL. Isolated grade I or II MCL injuries can be treated expectantly with a period of protected weightbearing, a free hinged knee brace if quite tender, and return to sport when the range of motion (ROM) is full and there is no pain. Isolated grade III injuries (i.e., without anterior cruciate instability) will require at least 4 weeks of protection in a hinged knee brace and protection when returning to sport.[3]

ANTERIOR CRUCIATE LIGAMENT

ACL injuries are becoming more common or at least more commonly recognized in the pediatric athlete. When they occur in young children, they present a treatment dilemma. Stanitski et al[4] found that, although acute hemarthrosis before age 12 is as likely to represent a meniscal tear as an ACL injury, after that age ACL injury becomes more common. In either age group, as in adults, acute hemarthrosis is an indicator of significant intra-articular injury. The natural history of skeletally immature patients with an ACL-deficient knee is generally poor, especially if they wish to return to sports.[5, 6] McCarroll et al[6] noted that only seven of 16 young patients treated nonoperatively returned to sports, and all experienced recurrent episodes of giving way, effusions, and pain. Conversely, of 24 pediatric athletes who were repaired surgically, all returned to sports and 22 were able to continue participating long term. The most common sport for ACL injury was football for males and basketball for females.

In the young athlete with an ACL injury, a rehabilitation program is begun with weightbearing as tolerated and an ACL brace. If they are unable to return to sports or have symptoms of instability with activities of daily living, then surgical reconstruction is considered. If they are younger than 12 years, one must consider changing sports or taking time off until a physiological type repair can be undertaken. Alternatively, one can perform an "over the top"

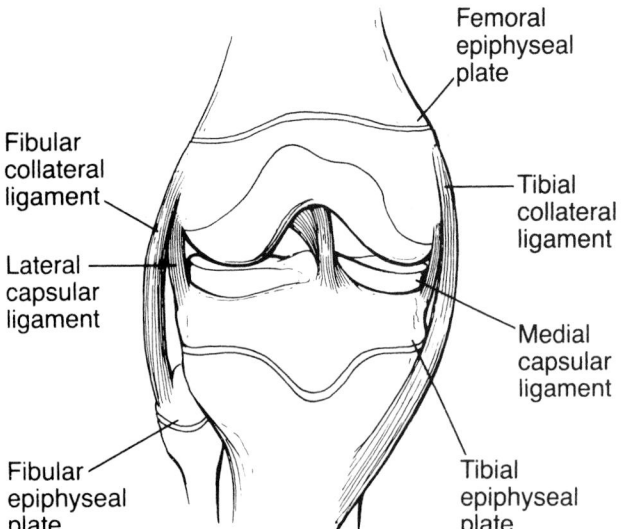

Fig. 1. Ligaments of the knee in relation to the physes. (From Stanitski CL, DeLee J, Drez D: Pediatric and Adolescent Sports Medicine. Philadelphia, WB Saunders, 1994.)

type of repair without violating the physis. Because the distal femur and proximal tibia together represent 70% of the growth of the lower extremity, contributing 1.6 cm per year to longitudinal growth, it may be best if repair in a very young patient is delayed. However, frequent episodes of giving way uncontrolled by bracing will put the menisci at risk, and delay may prove harmful in this regard.

ACL reconstruction can be performed in the teenager over bone age 13 who has persistent symptoms and wishes to return to sports. The risk and consequences of physeal injury are lessened as the patient approaches skeletal maturity. Many immature patients have been operated on with good results.[6, 7] McCarroll et al[6] used an extra-articular repair in athletes younger than 13 with no difference in result compared with an intra-articular repair in those older than 13. Lipscomb and Anderson[7] reported on intra-articular repair in athletes with open physes with only one apparent physeal complication. This patient had limb length inequality, not angular deformity. The authors attributed this to the staples used to fix the repair, not to the semitendinosus graft or the bony tunnels needed. Fortunately, the tunnels in the upper tibia and distal femur required for ACL reconstruction are fairly central; therefore, a physeal arrest of the distal femur may simply result in a fish tail deformity and not appreciably affect limb length or angular growth. Also a tendon graft in an appropriately sized hole may function similar to a fat graft and create a barrier to bony physeal bar formation. If intra-articular repair is to be performed, grafts involving bone plugs appear to be contraindicated.[7] Preoperative discussion with the family should center more on long-term function than the upcoming sports season.

TIBIAL EMINENCE
Children between the ages of 8 and 13 may suffer a fracture of the intercondylar eminence of the tibia at the insertion of the ACL rather than rupture the ACL. These frac-

tures have been classified into three types depending on the degree of displacement (Fig. 2).[8, 9] Types I and II can be treated nonoperatively. The knee is tapped for blood, and lidocaine is instilled to both reduce the pain and allow casting in extension. Extension decreases the tension on the anterior cruciate and allows the fragment to reduce better into the upper tibial epiphysis. Care is taken not to hyperextend the knee, which may result in vascular compromise when swelling recurs. The amount of extension is a subject of controversy. Some suggest complete extension because the lateral femoral condyle helps reduce the fragment in the terminal 5 degrees.[10] However, Meyers and McKeever[9] recommended 20 degrees of flexion to correspond to the point of minimum tension on the ACL. The reduction can be observed radiographically or arthroscopically. The knee is casted for 6 weeks, and a therapy program is started.

Type III fractures should be treated the same way. However, if the piece is still displaced or it appears the anterior horn of the lateral meniscus is under the edge, then repair is indicated. This can be done arthroscopically or open but requires drill holes through the upper tibia and fixation with PDS or other absorbable sutures. Alternatively, one can use either an intraepiphyseal screw or one that crosses the physis but is removed early. Stiffness is quite common, and casting in extension should be used for no more than 4 weeks followed by protected ROM in a hinged brace.

Follow-up studies show residual anterior translation of the tibia (51% with positive anterior drawer), but most patients are asymptomatic and are able to return to sports without bracing.[11] However, loss of some motion is common in type III injuries; 27 of 45 patients in Baxter and Wiley's[11] study lost more than 10 degrees of extension.

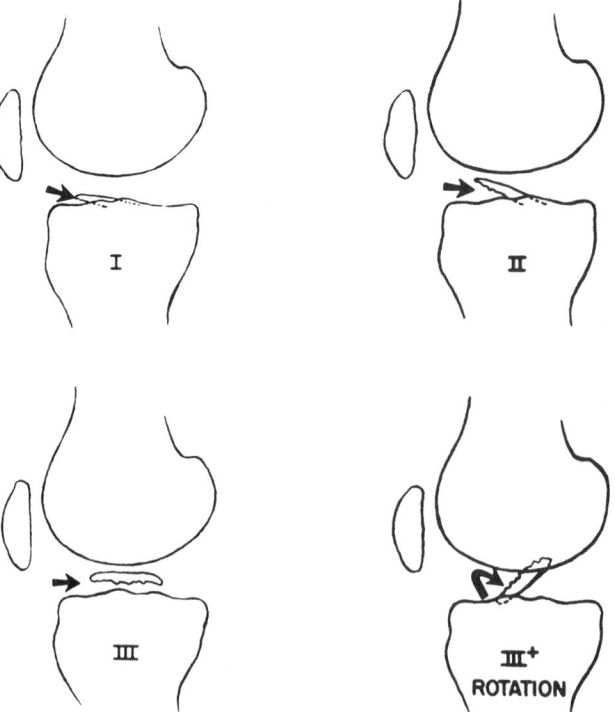

Fig. 2. Classification of tibial eminence fractures. (From Meyers M, McKeever F: J Bone Joint Surg Am 1970; 52:1677.)

OSGOOD-SCHLATTER DISEASE

Osgood-Schlatter disease is the result of repetitive, tensile stress at the insertion of the patellar tendon on the tibial tubercle and attempts at osseous repair.[12] It is much more common in athletes than in non-athletic individuals.[13] This condition should be easily diagnosed based on history and physical exam, with tenderness directly over the tibial tubercle. Radiographs are important only if there is a question about neoplasm, but nighttime pain, worsening symptoms, or swelling and warmth should prompt radiographic evaluation. When growth ceases, the patient will become asymptomatic. Before then, the symptoms will wax and wane. Treatment consists of activity modification, avoidance of inciting activities (running stairs, jumping, deep knee bends), anti-inflammatory medication, ice applications when irritated, and hamstring and quadriceps stretching. During an acute flare, splinting and casting may enhance the athlete's return to sport.

SINDING-LARSEN-JOHANSSON DISEASE

Sinding-Larsen-Johansson disease, or jumper's knee, is a traction tendinitis caused by inflammation at the distal pole of the patella at the origin of the patellar ligament. This condition is similar to Osgood-Schlatter disease, although anatomically there is no apophysis at this site. Sinding-Larsen-Johansson disease occurs in active patients, many of whom play basketball, volleyball, or soccer.[14] Examination shows tenderness exactly at the distal pole of the patella. Concomitant Osgood-Schlatter disease may be present in certain cases. The examiner should also look for knee flexion contracture and hamstring or quadriceps tightness. Radiographs may show fragmentation. Treatment consists of activity modification, stretching of tight tendons if present, icing and anti-inflammatory drugs when symptomatic, and potentially a period of casting if recalcitrant. If these measures do not help, it may be necessary for the patient to refrain from vigorous activities for a prolonged period.

BIPARTITE PATELLA

This condition presents with anterior knee pain and tenderness over the patella itself rather than at the patellofemoral joint. Saupe classified the location of the synchondrosis: type I, at the inferior pole (5%); type II, at the lateral margin (20%); and type III, the most common, at the superior lateral quadrant (75%) (Fig. 3).[15] Symptoms should respond to treatment for any of the anterior knee tension syndromes (Osgood-Schlatter disease, Sinding-Lar-sen-Johansson disease, patellar tendinitis), specifically activity modification, anti-inflammatory medication, ice application, and stretching. If these treatments fail or if the lesion separates, then excision of the fragment or, if large, internal fixation with local bone, can be undertaken.[16, 17]

PATELLAR DISLOCATION

Patellar dislocation usually results from an external rotation maneuver over a planted foot. The patella dislocates laterally in the majority of cases. If the knee swells dramatically, then investigation for osteochondral fracture, most likely occurring with the dislocation, should be undertaken. If no fracture is present, the swelling may indicate a significant retinacular tear.

After reduction, the initial treatment for patellar dislocation consists of a period of immobilization. Splinting or casting for 3 to 4 weeks is more effective than a simple patellar brace.[18] The goal is to prevent recurrence, likely in up to 44%, and as many as 27% may eventually undergo surgical repair. Unsatisfactory results can be observed in more than 50% of patients, leading some to suggest a more surgically aggressive approach.[19] Therapeutic exercises should be started in the cast with quad setting and leg lifts. After immobilization, formal physical therapy with quadriceps exercises will be important.

Some patients may have predisposing anatomic factors, including genu valgum, increased femoral anteversion, external tibial torsion, tight iliotibial band, and pes planus. Patients without predisposing factors have a better result after the initial dislocation. Those with anatomic factors may experience redislocation and require surgical intervention. The type of surgery chosen should be based on the patient's particular anatomic risk factors. One approach for all patients is not wise. Some patients will require lateral release and medial reefing, whereas others may need tibial tubercle transfer or its equivalent.[20]

ANTERIOR KNEE PAIN

Anterior knee pain is an extremely common complaint in adolescents and has many varied causes. One of the more common sources of discomfort is the patellofemoral articulation. Maltracking, again a result of anatomic factors such as rotational malalignment, genu valgum, tight lateral structures, or weak vastus medialis, can result in increased contact pressure, especially on the lateral patellar facet. Stanitski's[21] five-point plan is a good way to approach these patients: (1) factor identification, (2) factor modification,

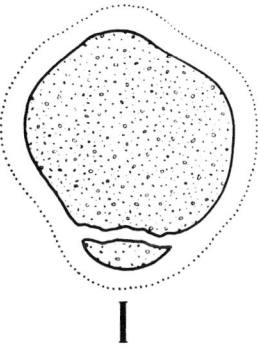 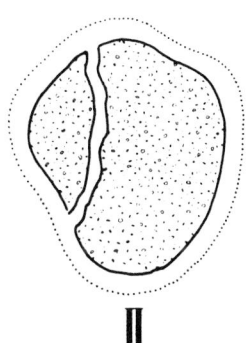 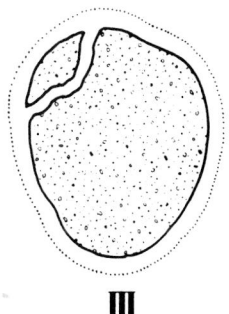

Fig. 3. Types of bipartite patellae. (From Ogden JA: Skeletal Injury in the Child. Philadelphia, Lea & Febiger, 1982.)

I   II   III

(3) pain control, (4) progressive rehabilitation, and (5) maintenance.

On first evaluation the patient should be examined for these anatomic factors. Those that can be corrected, such as flexible flatfoot, tight lateral retinaculum, or weak or imbalanced quadriceps, should be addressed. Radiographs are helpful to rule out other causes of pain, such as tumor or OCD. A sunrise or Merchant's view may not be particularly helpful on the first visit because it is likely not to change the initial management. Avoiding overuse is stressed, and playing while in pain should be discouraged. Isometric quadriceps exercises and limited arc quads to prevent further damage to the patellofemoral articulation should be instituted. Anti-inflammatory medication should also prove useful.

If conservative measures fail and radiographs are normal, care should be taken before proceeding to surgical intervention. If there is still evidence of patellar maltracking despite rigorous attention to exercise, then a soft-tissue balancing procedure might be indicated. Results are not uniformly good, and overzealous lateral release with medial reefing can result in medial patellar dislocation; therefore, one should be judicious in its use.[22]

MENISCAL INJURIES

The importance of the menisci to the long-term function of the knee is now understood, and complete meniscectomies are rarely performed. Like ACL injuries, the increased vigor of adolescent sport has made these injuries more common.[4, 23] Meniscal tears are uncommon before 10 years of age but become much more common after the age of 14. The most common tear is a longitudinal tear of the medial meniscus.[24]

Presenting symptoms and signs are similar to those in the adult, with intermittent swelling, potential giving way, and joint line tenderness, but adolescents can also experience other conditions less common in adults, confusing the diagnosis (patellofemoral pain, OCD). Diagnosis can be made clinically, using magnetic resonance imaging (MRI) or arthroscopically. Clinical diagnosis will reflect the skill and experience of the examiner. Conversely, MRI has a significant false-positive rate possibly because of the common finding of high signal within the healthy medial meniscus. Thus, some investigators strongly recommend against its use in the adolescent population, preferring clinical examination and arthroscopy instead. When identified, treatment is as for adult patients, with repair whenever feasible.

DISCOID MENISCUS

This entity presents as a snapping knee often with an audibly loud, intra-articular clunk. The cause of the discoid meniscus is believed to be abnormal development as a result of hypermobility, not a lack of embryological remodeling.[26] Watanabe et al[27] classified discoid meniscus into three types (Fig. 4): type I, complete with no central hollow; type II, incomplete with the meniscus extending further across the plateau but not completely; and type III, the Wrisberg ligament type with posterior instability.

Presenting symptoms are usually mechanical. The child may have a loud snap or pop, and the examiner may notice momentary subluxation of the tibia as this occurs. Because of the hypermobility, these menisci are subject to tears. When this occurs the symptoms may include locking and pain. Radiographs may show flattening of the lateral condyle. MRI should show the meniscus to be discoid.

Treatment of a symptomatic discoid meniscus is arthroscopic "saucerization" with débridement of the central portion, leaving a rim of 6 to 8 mm.[28] Leaving a broader rim can lead to recurrent tearing. The unstable type III meniscus and any remaining peripheral tears should be repaired. Vandermeer and Cunningham reported that 28% of patients required further surgery for recurrent tears.[29]

OSTEOCHONDRITIS DISSECANS

OCD is a condition of uncertain cause that appears to be the result of cyclic, cumulative stress to the subchondral bone, with resulting fracture, inflammation, and vascular compromise. This leads to softening of the bone and an increased susceptibility of the chondral surface to crack. The bone fragment may break free and become a loose body. The most common location is the lateral surface of the medial femoral condyle, but any surface of the femur or even patella can be involved. It is unclear whether this is the result of repetitive trauma on a previously normal area or trauma to an area with abnormal vascularity or other anatomic architecture.

Presenting symptoms are activity-related pain, mild swelling, possible effusion, and occasionally clicking, catching, and locking. The area over the lesion, if one can

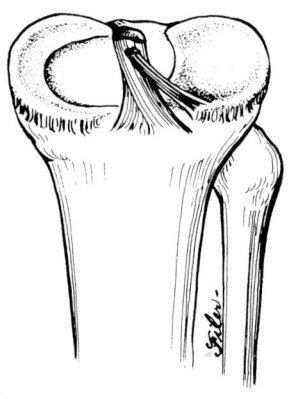
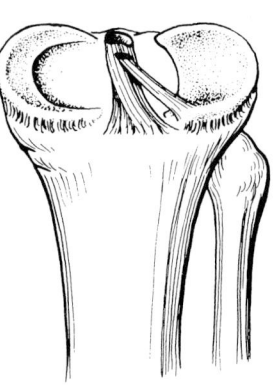
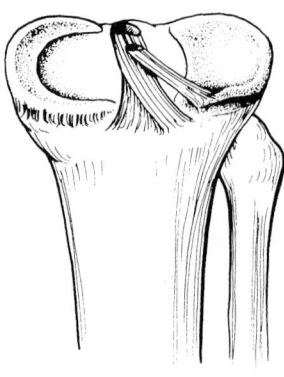

Fig. 4. Classification of discoid menisci. (From Ogden JA: Skeletal Injury in the Child. Philadelphia, Lea & Febiger, 1982.)

I

II

III

find it on examination, will be tender. Radiographs will show a subchondral lucency and possibly a lucent halo around an area of bone. This may not appear on a simple anteroposterior or lateral view, and a notch view will have the highest yield on plain radiographs.

After identification, MRI will show the extent of the lesion, but information regarding the viability of the area and whether the lesion is simply an ossific variant can be obtained from a technetium bone scan. Cahill[30] classified OCD into five stages based on radiographic and bone scan findings. In stage 0, radiographs and bone scan are normal. The diagnosis of OCD can be made only in retrospect, or the case is a normal ossific variant. In stage I, radiographs are abnormal but bone scan is normal. This also may represent a normal variant. In stage II, there is increased uptake on the bone scan. Stage III OCD demonstrates increased bone scan in the lesion and the femoral condyle. Stage IV OCD shows increased uptake in the adjacent tibial plateau as well, indicating a long-standing lesion that has incited a response on the apposing articular surface.

Treatment of OCD depends on the age of the patient, location and viability of the lesion, whether the articular cartilage surface is intact, and whether the osteochondritic piece is free (Fig. 5). For asymptomatic patients with radiographic changes noted incidentally, no treatment is necessary. If the lesion is large, then bone scan is helpful to determine whether the radiographic changes are simply an ossific variant. For intact lesions (i.e., those with an intact cartilage surface), treatment is to minimize local trauma and prevent shear forces on the lesion. Depending on location, this will require activity restriction and may require periods of non-weightbearing to decrease forces and to help enforce decreased activity in this usually very athletic, and motivated, population. More posterior lesions often do not require crutch walking. Casting is best avoided because of the beneficial effects of movement on the nutrition of joint cartilage.[15, 31]

The period of reduced activity and the time required for healing are quite variable and not well reported. Cahill[30] used limited bone scanning at 4-month intervals and indicated that symptom resolution along with scintigraphic activity reduction to a stage II level is needed to declare healing. He reported an average time to healing of 10 months in juvenile OCD. Others believe that drilling of the lesion can speed up healing and allow an earlier return to full activity.[30]

For lesions without an intact cartilage surface, the synovial fluid seems to be an impediment to healing, and surgical intervention is more often needed. In these cases or in

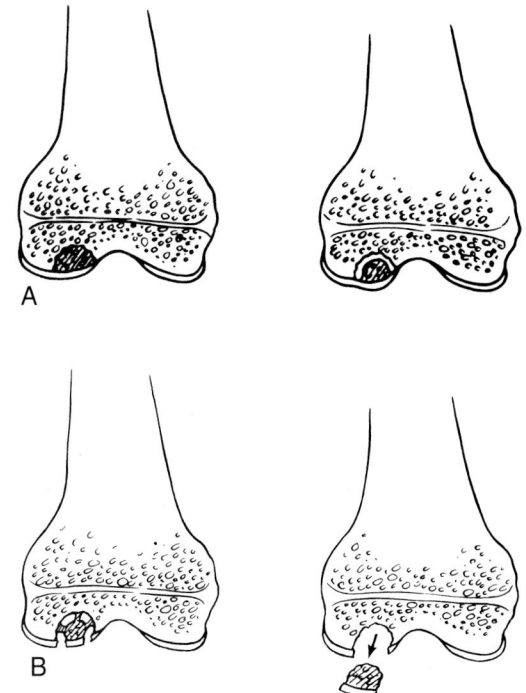

Fig. 5. Osteochondritis dissecans. The condition is shown with and without an intact articular cartilage surface, progressing to loose body formation. (From Stanitski CL, DeLee J, Drez D: Pediatric and Adolescent Sports Medicine. Philadelphia, WB Saunders, 1994.)

recalcitrant cases with an intact cartilage surface, drilling is the next step. If during arthroscopic evaluation the lesion is noted to be loose, then curettage of the base, replacement of the subchondral bone and cartilage surface, and fixation with either absorbable, buried, or retrograde pins is needed. The most severe category is that in which the bone has broken free and formed a loose body. If the lesion is large and/or on the weightbearing surface, then every attempt should be made to refit the piece back into its original location. This is a technically difficult procedure because, as a result of remodeling, the loose body no longer fits perfectly, and some refashioning is required.

For the rare individual in whom these procedures fail, techniques of cartilage cell grafting or cartilage and subchondral bone plugs hold promise. Fortunately, however, the prognosis in younger adolescents is much better than in adults, for whom these latter procedures are more commonly needed.

REFERENCES

1. Pritchett JW: A statistical study of knee injuries due to football in high school athletes. J Bone Joint Surg 1982; 64:240.
2. DeHaven KE, Lintner DM: Athletic injuries: Comparison by age, sport, and gender. Am J Sports Med 1986; 14:218.
3. Micheli L, Foster T: Acute knee injuries in the immature athlete. Instructional Course Lectures 1993; 41:473.
4. Stanitski CL, Harvell JC, Fu F: Observa-

tions on acute knee hemarthrosis in children and adolescents. J Pediatr Orthop 1993; 13:506.
5. Eiskjar S, Larsen ST: Arthroscopy of the knee in children. Acta Orthop Scand 1987; 58:273.
6. McCarroll JR, Rettig AC, Shelbourne KD. Anterior cruciate ligament injuries in the young athlete with open physes. Am J Sports Med 1986; 16:44.

7. Lipscomb AB, Anderson A: Tears of the anterior cruciate ligament in adolescents. J Bone Joint Surg 1986; 68:19.
8. Meyers MH, McKeever FM: Fractures of the intercondylar eminence of the tibia. J Bone Joint Surg 1959; 41:209.
9. Meyers MH, McKeever FM. Fractures of the intercondylar eminence of the tibia. J Bone Joint Surg 1970; 52:1677.
10. Roberts JM: Avulsion fractures of the

proximal tibial epiphysis. In Kennedy JC (ed): The Injured Adolescent Knee. Baltimore, Williams & Wilkins, 1979, p 141.

11. Baxter MP, Wiley JJ: Fractures of the tibial spine in children: An evaluation of knee stability. J Bone Joint Surg Br 1988; 70:228.

12. Stanitski CL: Anterior knee pain syndromes in the adolescent. Instructional Course Lectures 1994; 43:211.

13. Kuju UM, Kvist M, Heinonen O: Osgood-Schlatter's disease in adolescent athletes. Am J Sports Med 1985; 13:236.

14. Medler RC, Lyne D: Sinding-Larsen-Johansson disease: Its etiology and natural history. J Bone Joint Surg 1978; 60:1113.

15. Stanitski CL, DeLee J, Drez D: Pediatric and Adolescent Sports Medicine. Philadelphia, WB Saunders, 1994.

16. Green WT: Painful bipartite patellae: A report of three cases. Clin Orthop 1975; 110:197.

17. Weaver J: Bipartite patellae as a cause of disability in the athlete. Am J Sports Med 1977; 5:137.

18. Maenpaa H, Lehto MU: Patellar dislocation. The long-term results of nonoperative management in 100 patients. Am J Sports Med 1997; 25:213.

19. Cefield RH, Bryan R: Acute dislocation of the patella: Results of conservative treatment. J Trauma. 1977; 17:526.

20. Eilert R: Adolescent anterior knee pain. Instructional Course Lectures 1993; 41: 497.

21. Stanitski CL: Knee overuse disorders in the pediatric and adolescent athlete. Instruct Course Lectures 1993; 41:483.

22. Hughston JC, Deese M: Medial subluxation of the patella as a complication of lateral retinacular release. Am J Sports Med 1988; 16:383.

23. Andrish J: Meniscal injuries in children and adolescents: Diagnosis and management. J Am Acad Orthop Surg 1996; 4: 231.

24. Fu FH, Baratz M: Meniscal injuries. In DeLee JC, Drez D Jr (eds): Orthopaedic Sports Medicine: Principles and Practice. Philadelphia, WB Saunders, 1994, vol 2, p 1146.

25. Stanitski CL: Correlation of arthroscopic and clinical examinations with magnetic resonance imaging: Findings of injured knees in children and adolescents. Am J Sports Med 1998; 26:2.

26. Kaplan EB: Discoid lateral meniscus of the knee joint: Nature, mechanism, and operative treatment. J Bone Joint Surg 1957; 39:77.

27. Watanbe M, Takeda S, Ikeuchi H: Atlas of Arthroscopy. Tokyo, Igaku-Shoin, 1979, p 88.

28. Hayashi LK, Yamaga H, Ida K, et al: Arthroscopic meniscectomy for discoid lateral meniscus in children. J Bone Joint Surg 1988; 70:1495.

29. Vandermeer RD, Cunningham FK: Arthroscopic treatment of the discoid lateral meniscus: Results of long-term follow-up. Arthroscopy 1989; 5:101.

30. Cahill B: Osteochondritis dissecans of the knee: Treatment of juvenile and adult forms. J Am Acad Orthop Surg 1995; 3: 237.

31. Bradley J, Dandy DJ: Osteochondritis dissecans and other lesions of the femoral condyles. J Bone Joint Surg Br 1989; 71: 518.

LEG DEFORMITIES

Arthur Pappas, Errol Mortimer

Summary
- Identification of a lower extremity deformity in a child should initiate a comprehensive assessment for cause and associated disorders.
- Congenital deformities are frequently associated with other anomalies in the ipsilateral or contralateral limb, upper extremities, or viscera.
- Developmental deformities may be benign or associated with a systemic metabolic disorder or bone dysplasia.
- Post-traumatic deformities may progress, remain stable, or improve.
- Management must address joint stability, bone deformity, and limb length inequality. Limb function should take priority over appearance.

Deformities of the lower extremity represent a broad spectrum of clinical entities ranging in severity from trivial, requiring only reassurance, to the most complex problems addressed by the orthopedic surgeon.

The surgeon must be able to discriminate between the benign deformities and those that are progressive and require intervention. In most cases, this can be accomplished with a thorough history and physical examination supplemented by judicious use of plain radiographs. Occasionally, the correct diagnosis and management can be made only with more sophisticated investigations, including specific imaging modalities, biochemical studies, and genetic consultations.

Deformities that develop in the first years of life are frequently physiological and self-limited. These include genu varum and valgum, femoral anteversion, rotational contractures of the hips, and tibial torsion. Pathological diagnoses, such as Blount's disease, rickets, neuromuscular disorders, or osteochondrodysplasias, must be ruled out.

Congenital malformations of the lower extremity are usually not self-limited. All require prolonged observation, and most will require some form of reconstructive or corrective surgery. These deformities include angular and rotational deformities, longitudinal deficiencies, and bony dysplasias.

HISTORICAL REVIEW

Diagnoses have not changed in many years. Rickets is much less common than it was prior to routine supplementation of milk with vitamin D. Congenital malformations have remained rare throughout the decades except for a brief epidemic related to the use in Canada and Europe of thalidomide in pregnant women in the early 1960s.

In contrast, the treatment of developmental deformities and congenital malformations has undergone significant changes in recent decades. The benign natural history of many developmental deformities has been better documented, which allows the orthopedic surgeon to simply observe many of the problems, which were previously treated with prolonged bracing or shoe modification.

An important advance in the management of congenital malformations has been the evolution of the biology and surgical technique of limb lengthening and deformity correction. Several external fixation systems have been developed that allow gradual correction of complex bone and joint deformities, including substantial limb length discrepancy (LLD). The sophistication and performance of prosthetic lower limbs have also progressed significantly in recent years.[1, 2] Materials used are lighter and stronger, allowing children to participate more easily in usual activities. Although excellent functional results can be expected with good surgical technique and advanced prosthetic materials, the availability of reconstructive alternatives has made amputation a less common choice than it was a decade ago.

EPIDEMIOLOGY

Evaluation of lower extremity deformities is one of the most common reasons for pediatric orthopedic referral. The majority of children referred have benign physiological deformities. The incidence of true limb deficiencies is much smaller. The overall incidence is approximately 6.0 per 10,000 live births. Overall, 205 heritable limb deficiencies and 165 skeletal dysplasias have been described.[3]

CLINICAL FEATURES
General

A comprehensive musculoskeletal examination must be performed when any significant deformity is noted. This includes evaluation of the structure and function of all extremities and the spine. The examination should include limb symmetry, proportions of the proximal segment compared with the distal segment, and range-of-motion of all joints. Abnormal cutaneous markings such as café-au-lait spots and spinal dimples or hairy patches should be noted. Facial features, especially the location of the ears, the distance between the eyes, and the formation of the midface and jaw, should be observed because these are commonly abnormal in syndromes and skeletal dysplasias.

Plain radiographs may be helpful in distinguishing physiological from pathological deformities. Full lower-extremity anteroposterior films (bilateral hips to ankles on a 17- or 36-inch film) should be obtained on any child with a significant congenital malformation or a significant varus or valgus deformity. The child should be positioned with the patellae facing forward (not the foot) in order to obtain consistent, reproducible images. In the case of an unossified patella, its center can be identified with a lead bead. This allows accurate determination of the degree of angulation as measured by the femorotibial angle, which can be used for future comparison. The mechanical axis of the limb, defined by the straight line from the center of the femoral head to the center of the ankle, can also be used to monitor angular deformities. It is somewhat more variable in children than in adults. The normal mechanical axis passes near the medial tibial spine at the knee. Its position is easily monitored over time to determine if a deformity is improving or worsening. Long-leg radiographs also allow evaluation of multiple bones and joints in order to rule out a generalized bony dysplasia. If this is suspected, addi-

tional films of the upper extremities and spine should be obtained.

ROTATIONAL DEFORMITIES
General

In-toeing may represent the single most common presenting complaint to the pediatric orthopaedic surgeon. Its treatment is controversial and is frequently dictated more by philosophy than scientific data. Its cause is usually attributed to femoral anteversion, tibial torsion, or metatarsus adductus. Soft-tissue causes include internal rotation contractures of the hips and dynamic overactivity of the tibialis posterior muscle. The physician must understand the causes and natural history and must be able to rule out other pathological gait patterns related to an underlying neurological disease such as cerebral palsy or muscular dystrophy.

Assessment

A complete physical examination must be performed to rule out muscle spasticity or weakness in either the upper or lower extremities. The spine and gluteal cleft should be inspected for congenital scoliosis or evidence of underlying spinal anomalies (lipoma, meningocele, cyst, or diastematomyelia) that may cause a muscle imbalance. The skin should be inspected for lesions suggestive of neurofibromatosis. Neurological examination should inspect strength and reflexes in all major motor groups.

The child's gait is the most important element of the examination. The foot progression angle is frequently used to evaluate the presence and magnitude of in-toeing (Fig. 1) and should be documented at each visit. It is defined as the angle made by the axis of the foot relative to the direction of motion of the child.[4] By convention, positive values represent out-toeing, and negative values represent in-toeing. The foot progression angle changes with the age of the child and ranges from −5 to 20 degrees.

In-toeing is typically attributed to some combination of femoral anteversion, internal tibial torsion, and metatarsus adductus. Overactivity or contracture of the tibialis posterior can also cause the foot to swing inward; this is often confused with tibial torsion. The position of the patellae during ambulation is very helpful. If the patella is directed

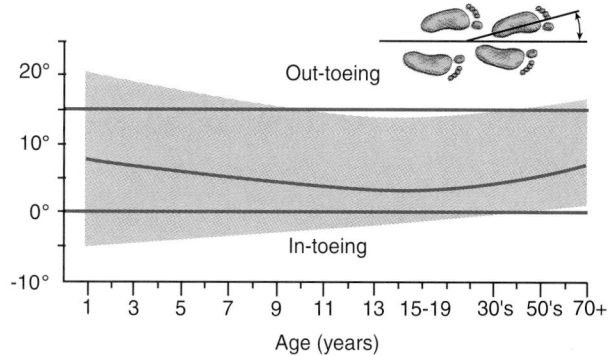

Fig. 1. Foot-progression angle. This describes the angle made by the long axis of the foot relative to the progression of the child. (Staheli L: Rotational problems in children. In Schafer M (ed): Instructional Course Lectures XLIII, Rosemont, IL, AAOS, 1992, p 201.)

medially, this signifies that there is an element of femoral anteversion or internal rotation contracture of the hip. Tibial torsion may or may not be present. If the patella is directed forward, the hip is not usually the cause. Overactivity of the tibialis posterior muscle causes the foot to turn in during the swing phase of gait and when the foot strikes the ground. Overactivity of the abductor hallucis causes a dynamic metatarsus adductus that is usually most apparent during stance phase.

To assess rotation, the hips should be examined with the child prone on the examining table (Fig. 2). Each lower extremity should be rotated internally and externally. In infancy, external rotation of the hips is normally greater than internal rotation. During the toddler years, this pattern gradually reverses and, by about age 4 to 5 years, internal and external rotation should be symmetric. Subsequently, internal rotation is slightly greater than external.

Internal and external tibial torsion may be assessed in two ways. With the child prone and the knees flexed to 90 degrees, the position of the relaxed hindfoot relative to the axis of the femur is determined (Fig. 3). This is the thigh-foot angle, which is normally positioned neutrally at birth and increases to the adult position of 20 degrees of external rotation by about age 8 years. Tibial rotation may also be measured by assessing the transmalleolar axis (Fig. 4), which is the angle between the medial and lateral malleolus relative to the coronal plane of the femoral condyles. This angle is normally greater than 15 degrees of external rotation. Internal tibial torsion is a common cause of intoeing in the toddler years.

The shape of the foot is inspected for overall shape and contour. The lateral border of the foot should be straight; if it is not, it should be passively and actively correctible by stroking the lateral border of the foot. Metatarsus adductus typically arises in infancy as forefoot adduction and usually resolves with stretching exercises or, occasionally, correc-

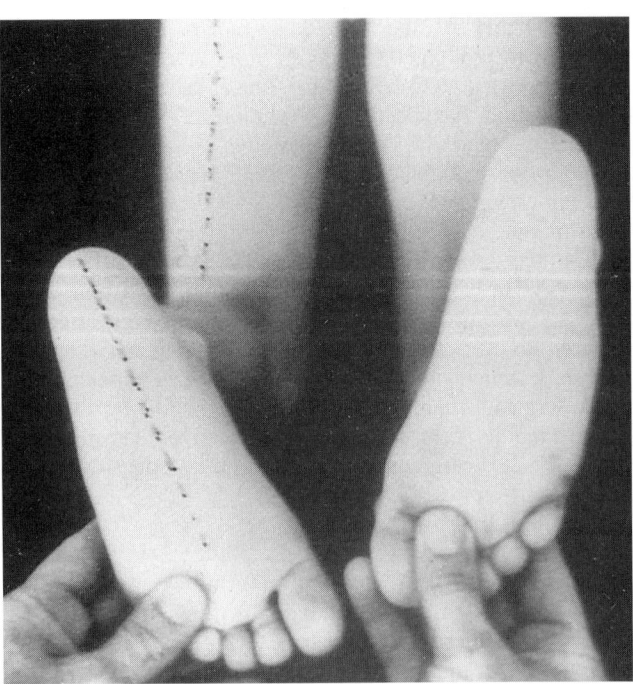

Fig. 3. View. The femur is placed in neutral rotational alignment. The long axis of the foot is shown by the dotted line.

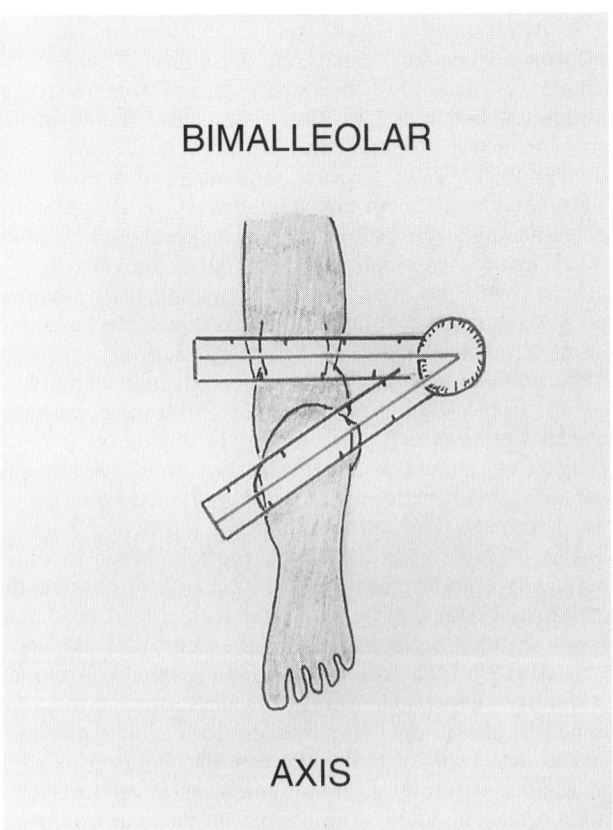

Fig. 4. View. The transmalleolar or bimalleolar axis is obtained by manually establishing the malleolar prominences compared with the neutrally aligned femur. The transmalleolar axis determines the degree of rotation occurring in the ankle joint.

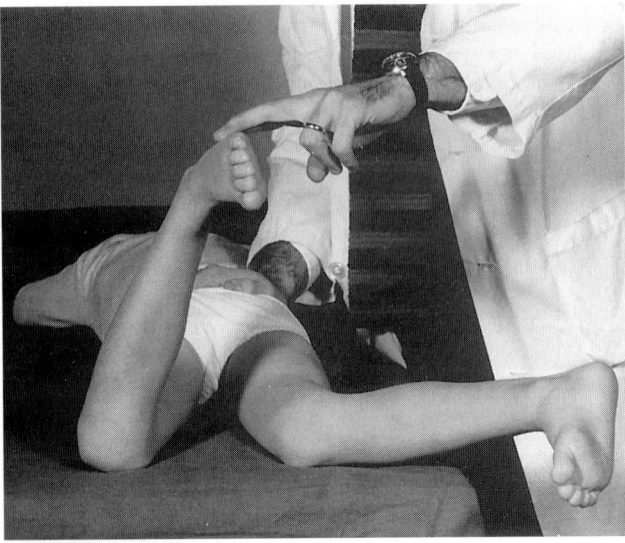

Fig. 2. View. The examiner must place one hand on the patient's pelvis to prevent pelvic rotation, which could alter the measured range of motion. External rotation is demonstrated.

tive casting. When it persists during the toddler years, it is unsightly and may cause falling. It almost always resolves spontaneously by age 3 to 4 years and may be assisted with an ankle foot orthosis.

Femoral Anteversion

Femoral anteversion is a common cause of in-toeing after infancy. It refers to anterior angulation of the femoral neck relative to the coronal plane of the femoral condyles (Fig. 5). In adulthood, the femoral neck is normally anteverted between 10 and 15 degrees. Normal infants may have up to 45 degrees of anteversion, which gradually decreases to the adult value by about age 6 to 8 years. Persistent femoral anteversion, also referred to as femoral antetorsion, causes the leg to rotate internally during ambulation. It will also be measured as greater internal than external rotation of the hip when the child is examined prone. The gait will demonstrate internal rotation of the entire extremity, and the patella will point medially. Internal rotation contractures of the hips may have an identical clinical appearance. They can be distinguished from each other by performing a rotation study using computed tomograph (CT) scan. The orientation of the proximal femur is compared to the distal femoral intercondylar axis to obtain an accurate measurement. This study is performed only to assist with preoperative planning, not for routine evaluation.

Tibial Torsion

Tibial torsion is usually noted before or soon after a child begins to walk. It may be related to intrauterine positioning or may represent a normal physiological stage of development of the lower extremities. It is often bilateral and symmetric. Clinically, the foot appears rotated internally relative to the position of the knee, especially the patella. Tibial torsion is often associated with metarsus adductus or physiological genu vara; the combination of the deformities can be striking. The range of normal tibial torsion is quite variable; up to 20 degrees of internal tibial torsion is normal in infants. The transmalleolar axis normally becomes more externally rotated during childhood, resulting in 15 to 20 degrees of external tibial torsion by adolescence. In a child with isolated internal tibial torsion, the feet will turn in but the patellae will not because the inward rotation occurs below the knees.

Treatment for Femoral Anteversion and Tibial Torsion

Devices such as twister cables, external rotation (e.g., Denis Browne) splints, and shoe wedges have been used extensively to treat these deformities. Nevertheless, the family should be reassured that the natural history of these deformities is spontaneous resolution in more than 90% of cases. Physical therapy to achieve a normal heel-toe gait, correct any contractures, and alter poor sitting and walking habits may assist the corrections that normally accompany physiological maturation. There are convincing data that the deformities will not lead to later morbidity, such as knee pain, or accelerated osteoarthritis of the hip or knee.[4–6]

The use of various orthopedic devices is controversial because there are few objective data to prove their efficacy. Whereas derotation braces may facilitate soft-tissue stretching, their direct effect on bone is not well substantiated. Denis Browne splints may occasionally be useful prior to walking age for severe torsion. Twister cables supplemented by gait training can be helpful for the occasional child whose in-toeing leads to frequent falling. These devices are rarely of any value in treating children with an underlying neurological disease or bony dysplasia.

Older children with residual anatomical deformities can usually overcome their problem by consciously altering the gait later in childhood or adolescence, which leaves very few children who actually require active treatment. Physical therapy to stretch the hip capsule may assist the older child.

Severe debilitating deformities that cannot be corrected with physical therapy can be corrected with femoral or tibial osteotomies during adolescence. In the authors' experience, this is rarely indicated. Surgery for femoral anteversion should be considered for the child with more than 80 degrees of internal hip rotation and less than 15 degrees of external hip rotation. The two most common surgical alternatives include proximal femoral osteotomy with a dynamic screw or blade plate and distal femoral osteotomy with external fixation. The former has the advantage of having fewer associated complications, especially refracture, and the latter has the advantage of being adjustable after the patient is off the operating table. Osteotomies for tibial torsion should always be distal to the tubercle in children to avoid injury to the proximal growth plate.

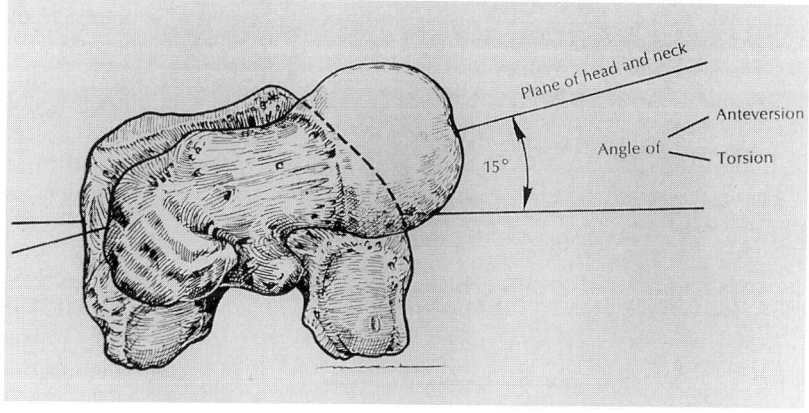

Fig. 5. Femoral version. It is arbitrarily determined as the angle between the long axis of the femoral neck and the coronal plane of the femoral condyles.

Screws, plates, or external fixation may be used. The last has the advantage of being easily adjusted at the bedside if derotation has led to peroneal nerve injury from over-stretching.

ANGULAR DEFORMITIES

Angular deformities may be acquired or congenital. Many acquired angular deformities of early childhood are physiological. When congenital, they usually indicate a true pathological condition. Congenital deformities are grouped into posteromedial, anterolateral, and anteromedial (also see the section on congenital limb deficiencies).

Developmental Deformities

Physiological angular deformities usually present between ages 18 months and 3 years but occasionally may present as early as 9 or 10 months. Physiological genu varum (bowleg) reaches its peak at 6 months and may persist until 2.5 yrs. The extremity usually then overcorrects and by age 3 to 4 years may adopt a valgus (knock-knee) appearance.[7, 8] This usually resolves within the following 2 years but may persist, especially in females and obese patients. Pathological diagnoses may present at any time, and the differential diagnosis of genu varum or valgum must always be considered (Table 1). Children's heights should be measured and plotted on a growth curve. Abnormal short stature associated with a bone dysplasia or metabolic disease may not appear until the child is 1 or 2 years of age.

Genu Varum

A careful history and physical examination will often lead to the correct diagnosis. Hypophosphatemic rickets may be associated with a positive family history. Vitamin D-deficient rickets is uncommon but may be seen in children who are nourished primarily with breast milk into their toddler years. Children with either physiological bowing or Blount's disease may give histories of early walking, heavy weight, and progression of the deformity. Children with physiological bowlegs, rickets, and Blount's disease may look identical on physical examination but can often be distinguished from each other on radiographs.

Physiological bowlegs can appear to be a significant disabling disorder. The combination of bowlegs and the

marked internal tibial torsion that is often present is unsightly and may lead to frequent falling. Historically, most children with significant bowlegs were treated with braces that applied a valgus corrective force. Even relatively severe physiological bowlegs will frequently correct spontaneously without any specific treatment, providing that the growth plates are undisturbed (Fig. 6). The difficulty is in predicting which children's deformities will resolve and which will progress. This is often impossible in the first 2 to 3 years of life and follow-up every 4 to 6 months is necessary until complete resolution.

Blount's disease is caused by dysplastic changes in the posteromedial aspect of the proximal tibial physis and epiphysis. Two forms exist, infantile and adolescent. Although some anatomical and pathological features are similar in the two groups, other features, such as frequent bilaterality and associated tibial torsion in the infantile form, suggest that they are not identical diseases.[9] The precise cause is not known, but heredity, early walking, increased body weight, and early varus alignment of the limb play a role. The deformity is not purely varus; it frequently involves internal rotation and mild apex anterior angulation. A small LLD may be present.

Radiographs of children with physiological genu varum demonstrate bowing in the femur and tibia, relatively symmetric involvement bilaterally, normal widths of the growth plates, and absence of the characteristic medial proximal tibial beak. Both the distal femoral and proximal tibial metaphyses often appear beaked in normal children younger than 18 to 24 months. Levine and Drennan[10] studied the predictive value of measuring the metaphyseal-diaphyseal (M-D) angle of the tibia to differentiate between physiological bowing and Blount's disease. Drennan associated an angle greater than 11 degrees with increased risk of developing Blount's disease. More recently, it has been reported that 16 degrees is more specific.[11] Schoenecker observed that it is the relative degree of femoral to tibial bowing that is most sensitive and specific and has shown that Blount's disease is likely if the ratio of the femoral M-D angle to tibial M-D angle is greater than 1.

Langenskiold[12] documented the progressive radiographic deformity of the medial proximal tibial growth plate (Fig. 7), progressing from isolated beaking to sloping of the entire medial plateau with arrest of the medial growth plate.

The classic radiographic findings of rickets arise from failure of the cartilaginous growth plate to ossify. They include thickening of the physis (the distance between the metaphysis and the epiphysis); cup-shaped, irregular metaphyses; irregular metaphyseal trabecular bone pattern; and diminished density of the cortices (Fig. 8).

Treatment

Treatment depends on the cause of the bowing. Infantile Blount's disease can be treated with a brace that applies a valgus corrective force at the knee. It has been reported to be effective for children with severity up to Langenskiold grade II.[13, 14] If the deformity does not resolve, a proximal tibial osteotomy is indicated before age 4 years, after which permanent growth plate damage is more likely to occur (Fig. 9). Parents should be advised of the significant

TABLE 1. DIFFERENTIAL DIAGNOSIS OF GENU VARUM/ GENU VALGUM	
Genu varum	**Genu valgum**
Blount's disease (infantile, adolescent)	Juvenile rheumatoid arthritis
Rickets (Vitamin D-deficient, resistant)	Fibrous dysplasia
Achondroplasia	X-linked hypophosphatemia
Pseudoachondroplasia	Renal osteodystrophy
Multiple epiphyseal dysplasia	Marfan's syndrome
Metaphyseal chondrodysplasia	Osteogenesis imperfecta
Osteogenesis imperfecta	Congenital short femur

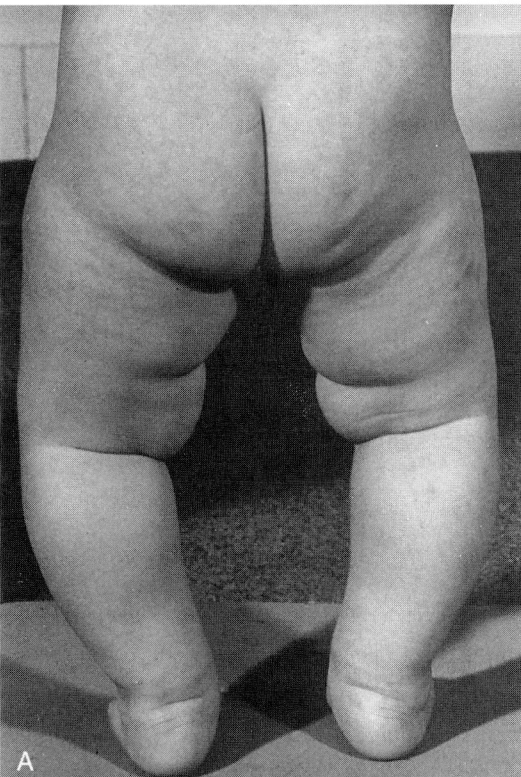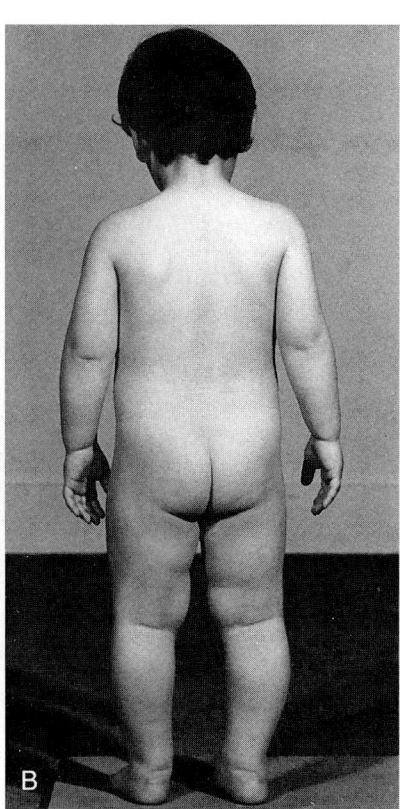

Fig. 6. Views. *A,* Spontaneous correction in the 2-year-old patient. *B,* Improvement of genu varum and internal tibial torsion.

risk of recurrence, especially if the child presents with a more severe deformity. Slight overcorrection into valgus should be achieved at the time of surgery. Common surgical alternatives include pin fixation, plate and screw fixation, external fixation, and hemiepiphysiodesis.[15, 16]

Recurrence is more common if the tibial osteotomy is performed after age 5 years. It may be due to persistence of the underlying disorder or, in severe cases, to physeal bar formation in the medial proximal tibial physis. This should be evaluated with CT or magnetic resonance imaging (MRI) to determine its extent. Resection of the bony bar should be attempted in younger children. If this is impossible or unsuccessful, completion of the physeal arrest, elevation of the medial tibial plateau, and limb length-

ening may be considered as indicated by the individual's age and degree of deformity.

Treatment of rickets is primarily medical by providing the nutritional supplements that are lacking or treating the underlying renal disorder. Mild-to-moderate deformities can be expected to remodel rapidly, but severe deformities may require surgical correction if they do not correct with medical treatment.

Genu Valgum
Genu valgum presents less frequently than genu varum. A small amount of femorotibial valgus angulation (up to 10 degrees) may be physiological as the bowleg deformity of early childhood resolves. Genu valgum may be measured

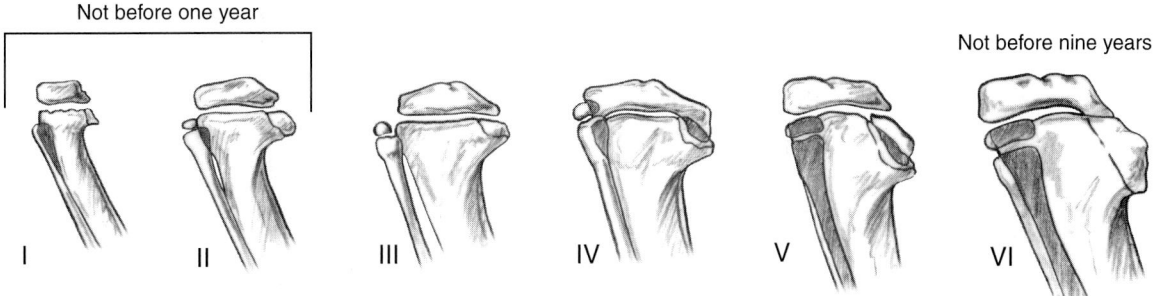

Fig. 7. Chart. Interobserver reliability is unpredictable in groups II–IV, reducing the clinical significance of this classification system. (Redrawn from Langenskiold A, Risk EB: Tibia vara [osteochondrosis deformans tibial]: A survey of seventy-one cases. J Bone Joint Surg Am 1964; 46: 1405.)

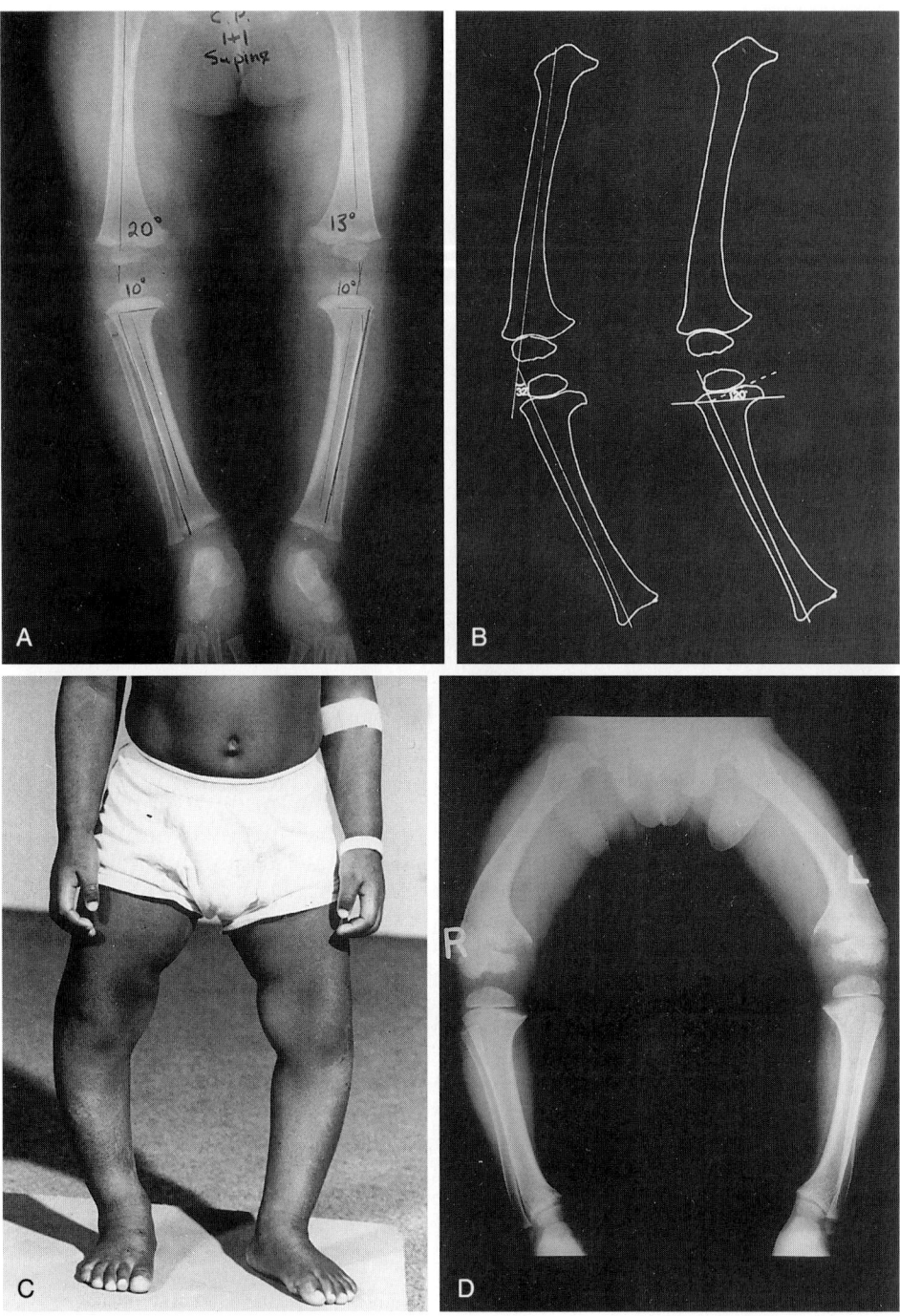

Fig. 8. View. *A,* Physiological bow-leg has a normal metaphyseal-diaphyseal angle. The tibiofemoral angle is unreliable because of knee ligament laxity. *B,* The metaphyseal-diaphyseal angle is established by the intersection of a line through the transverse plane of the proximal tibial metaphysis with a line perpendicular to the long axis of the tibial diaphysis. *C,* Persistence of genu varum in a 2-year-old patient requires radiographic assessment. *D,* The abnormally wide radiolucent physis and the metaphyseal trumpeting are pathognomonic of rickets. (Courtesy of Kenneth Guidera, MD.)

clinically as the femorotibial angle or as the distance between the medial malleoli when the knees are together. The normal distance between the malleoli is up to 9 or 10 cm. These are good approximations of the severity of the deformity, but if more accurate measurements are necessary, radiographs should be obtained. In most cases, physiological genu valgum resolves spontaneously. By the time a child reaches 6 or 7 years the mechanical axis of the lower extremities (defined as a straight line from the center of the hip to the center of the ankle) achieves its adult position.

Pathological causes lead to genu valgum less commonly than to genu varum. Fractures of the proximal tibia are notorious for causing progressive valgus deformity during the following 1 to 2 years. Osteochondromata or enchondromata of the proximal tibia or fibula may cause this deformity. Renal osteodystrophy and some epiphyseal and metaphyseal dysplasias may also cause knock knees. If the deformity is congenital, longitudinal deficiency of the fibula must also be considered. Although there are no natural history studies that precisely correlate residual angular deformity, whether varus of valgus, with development of

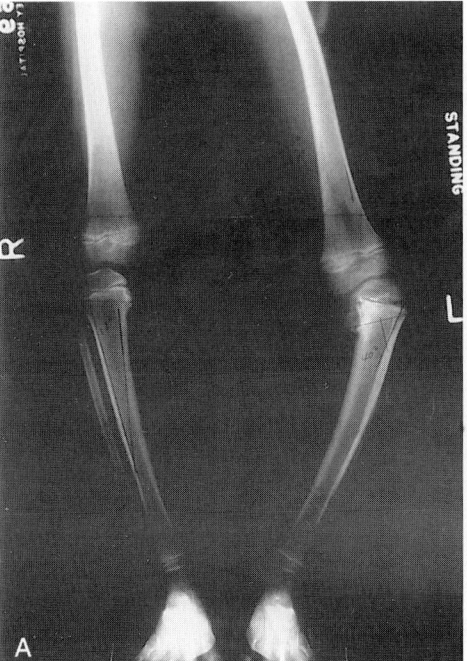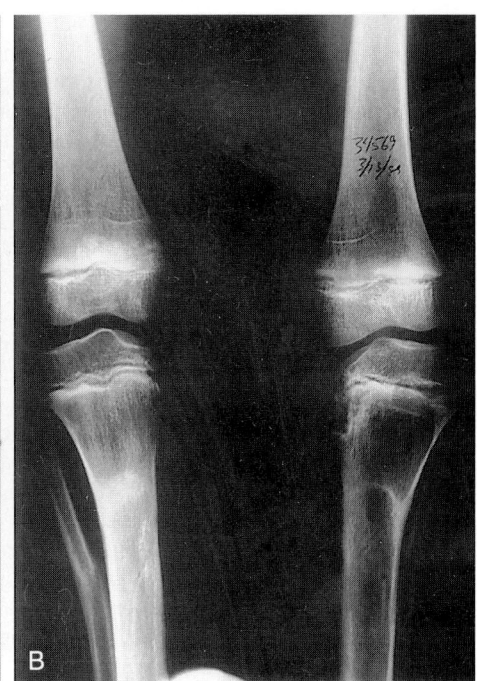

Fig. 9. Views. *A,* A 6-year-old female with bilateral tibia vara demonstrates left lateral tibial subluxation. *B,* Films obtained 3 years later illustrate the effectiveness of the oblique proximal tibial osteotomies. (Courtesy of James C. Drennan, MD.)

early osteoarthritis, most clinicians agree that any deformity in excess of 15 to 20 degrees should be treated. Bracing is indicated for younger children; however, its efficacy has not been proved. Night-time bracing may be better tolerated by the patient than full-time bracing. Hemiepiphysiodesis with staples can be used to correct the deformity.[17, 18] Completion of epiphysiodesis at the time of staple removal eliminates the risk of excessive rebound of the correction.

If an osteotomy is performed, it is usually done at the level of the proximal tibia, but careful analysis of the deformity may indicate the distal femur as the site where the correction should be performed. Hemiepiphysiodesis is a less invasive procedure but must be carefully timed to be successful. It may be used in the tibia, femur, or both.

Post-Traumatic Deformities

Post-traumatic angular deformities of the lower extremities may occur as a result of three mechanisms: asymmetric growth plate stimulation, asymmetric growth plate inhibition, or malunion of the fracture. These occur much more frequently in the lower extremity than in the upper extremity. Any fracture that affects the growth plate must be monitored for at least 2 years or until the physician has confirmed normal growth. Pappas[19] reviewed 101 fractures involving the proximal and distal tibial epiphyses and observed four patterns of growth variation: (1) symmetric stimulation leading to overgrowth (n = 5); (2) asymmetric stimulation leading to angular deformity (n = 10); (3) symmetric deceleration or cessation leading to shortening (n = 35); (4) asymmetric deceleration or cessation leading to angular deformity (n = 52). Changes in growth dynamics were frequently not appreciated until several months after injury. Careful observation shows that changes in growth velocity may be nonlinear. For example, one 7-

year-old patient who sustained a distal tibial fracture demonstrated 50% deceleration of growth the first year, 75% deceleration of growth the second year, and no further distal tibial growth subsequently. Similarly, in general, a period of transient postinjury overgrowth was usually followed by a period of normal growth or even decelerated growth. This underlines the importance of carefully monitoring growth patterns for several years after injury.

Angular deformities occasionally occur as a result of asymmetric overgrowth. Fractures of the proximal tibial metaphysis are best known for causing valgus deformities by this mechanism. First reported by Cozen,[20] these fractures have since received great attention. The injury may appear innocuous but can develop valgus deformities for up to 17 months after injury.[21] It is unclear how this occurs, but it is most likely related to asymmetric stimulation of the medial proximal tibial growth plate. Other proposed mechanisms include tethering of the lateral tibial growth plate by the fibula, soft-tissue interposition, and inadequate initial reduction. The natural history of this deformity is spontaneous improvement over 2 to 3 years. Corrective osteotomy should be deferred at least this long, if possible.[22]

Fractures involving the distal femur and proximal tibia are at high risk of causing angular deformities and LLD[23] due to physeal injury and growth deceleration. This occurs more frequently with Salter III and IV fractures but may also occur in the less severe Salter I or II fractures. Distal femoral growth arrest is especially common after fracture because the normal physis has an undulating shape, and fractures may pass through several zones of the growth plate. In younger children, the periosteum is very thick, and the force necessary to fracture the physis may be sufficient to damage it permanently. Hresko and Kasser[24] reported on 7 children with nonphyseal femoral fractures who had associated occult physeal fractures that were identified only at an average of 1 year 10 months after injury when a significant angular deformity developed.

Scrupulous treatment to achieve an anatomical reduction is necessary for Salter III and IV fractures to minimize the development of physeal bars. This may be achieved either open or closed. After anatomical reduction, fractures are best fixed with appropriately sized wires or screws. Cannulated screws in the metaphysis or the epiphysis are useful when a closed reduction can be achieved. If the fixation must cross the growth plate, smooth wires should be used and removed at the earliest possible time, preferably within 4 to 6 weeks of insertion. Additional cast immobilization may be necessary.

Partial or complete physeal arrest may occur despite the surgeon's best efforts. If a complete physeal arrest occurs, a pure LLD will occur without angulation. The predicted limb length inequality should be calculated on the basis of the individual's bone age and growth-remaining data. The magnitude of the predicted discrepancy dictates whether treatment will include observation, use of a shoe lift, contralateral epiphysiodesis, or limb lengthening. If the growth arrest is incomplete, an angular deformity may develop. This will depend on the skeletal age of the individual and the size of the bony bar. If the bar is small and central, the remainder of the growth plate may overcome the tethering effect of the bar; angular deformity may be avoided. Peripheral bars and larger bars have a greater propensity to cause angular deformities. Treatment is necessary to avoid progression of the deformity.

Evaluation and treatment of post-traumatic physeal bridges have been reviewed extensively.[25, 26] The geography of the bar may be assessed by plain radiography, polytomography, CT scan, or MRI. Multi-axial imaging modalities provide a better understanding of the three-dimensional anatomy. Peripheral bars are more readily accessible, but they cause a high recurrence rate due to iatrogenic injury. Resection of a central bar requires a metaphyseal window adjacent to the growth plate and removal of the bar with a bur. A dental mirror may facilitate visualization. Physeal bars occupying up to 50% of a physis may be removed successfully. The defect created is usually filled with locally harvested fat, but silicone and methylmethacrylate may also be used. If the bar is greater than 50% of the area of the physis, the likelihood of success is much less, and surgical completion of the growth arrest may be necessary if sufficient growth remains to cause a significant deformity. The projected LLD after completion of the growth arrest must then be calculated. Treatment options then include observation for a small projected discrepancy and contralateral epiphysiodesis or ipsilateral limb lengthening for a larger discrepancy. Any child with a growth arrest must be monitored until skeletal maturity.

The acceptable amount of angular malunion depends on the age of the child, the affected bone, the location of the fracture, and the direction of angulation. The younger the child, the greater the capacity to remodel. Malunions adjacent to a joint and in its plane of motion remodel very readily in younger children. Femoral fractures in children younger than 6 years will completely remodel up to 20 degrees of angulation in the coronal plane and 30 degrees

of angulation in the sagittal plane. Remodeling in the tibia is less reliable. Less than 5 degrees of varus or 10 degrees of valgus should be present at the end of growth.

Fractures of the tibia and fibula have particular importance when the fibula remains intact. Two situations may occur. If the fibula is uninjured, it tends to cause varus angulation of the tibia, which must be addressed when the cast is applied. Usually, a modest valgus mold to the cast compensates for the deforming force of the fibula. Frequent follow-up is initially necessary to ensure the fracture does not angulate in the cast. The fibula may also undergo plastic deformation, and this usually leads to a valgus deformity. This is usually adequately treated with a well molded cast.

Angular deformities caused by overgrowth, growth deceleration, or malunion should not immediately be addressed surgically unless the deformity is severe. The potential for remodeling of a malunion to occur must be carefully considered. If there is at least 2 years of growth remaining and the physis is healthy, it may be appropriate to observe the individual until skeletal maturity, allowing the full potential for remodeling to occur. However, correction of a deformity by manipulating the behavior of a physis with a hemiepiphysiodesis requires a period of ongoing growth. Excessive delays in treatment for observation may result in loss of the opportunity to use this method.

Congenital Posteromedial Bow

This idiopathic congenital malformation presents at birth with an obvious tibial and fibular bow, limb shortening, and impressive calcaneovalgus foot deformity (Fig. 10). It is an isolated unilateral deformity with no other associated lesions or syndromes. There is a soft-tissue contracture of the posterior and lateral structures of the lower leg that improves with growth. The lower half of the tibia is most affected, and growth of the distal tibial physis is decreased. Its clinical course is relatively benign, considering the appearance at birth. The angular deformity usually corrects spontaneously, leaving a modest LLD and sometimes a small valgus deformity of the distal tibia. Ankle motion usually remains slightly decreased, often in both dorsiflexion and plantarflexion. Congenital posteromedial bow must be distinguished from an anterolateral bow associated with congenital pseudarthrosis of the tibia. Plain radiographs demonstrate the apex of the deformity to be medial in the anteroposterior view and posterior on the lateral view. The quality of the bone is normal.

Pappas[27] reviewed 33 patients with this problem and documented its severity and natural history. The angular deformity ranged from 25 to 70 degrees. This corrected completely or nearly completely in almost all cases, with 50% of the deformity correcting in the first 2 years of life. The medial bow generally corrects less completely than the posterior component. The common residual deformity is an LLD that usually ranges from 4 to 5 cm but may be as high as 6.9 cm. The percentage of shortening relative to the normal tibia is constant and allows early prediction of ultimate LLD.

Treatment involves application of corrective casts or passive stretching in infancy to correct the foot deformity. This usually resolves completely within the first 6 to 12

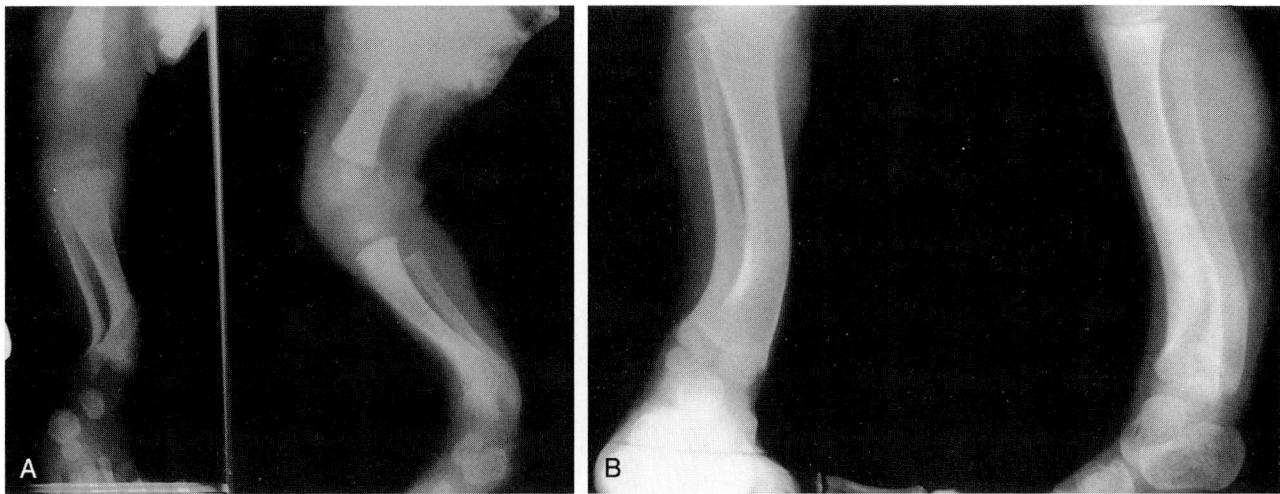

Fig. 10. Spontaneous improvement. This posterior bowing can be accurately measured by using the proximal and distal tibial growth plates. *A,* Newborn radiographs. *B,* Shows greater improvement in the sagittal plane at 2 years of age.

months of life. Tibial osteotomy is not recommended until remodeling is complete, because correcting the deformity surgically does not seem to affect the LLD. If the residual angular deformity is not significant, and the LLD is small, a contralateral epiphysiodesis may be done to equalize the limb lengths. Otherwise, combined angular correction and limb lengthening is preferred.

Congenital Pseudarthrosis of the Tibia and Congenital Anterolateral Bow

Congenital anterolateral bow is almost always the first manifestation of congenital pseudarthrosis of the tibia (CPT) or an equivalent preceding lesion. At birth, radiographs may show a fracture to be present or may show narrowing or sclerosis without a fracture or pseudarthrosis. Approximately 50% of congenital pseudarthroses of the tibia are associated with neurofibromatosis, although at birth there may not be any other manifestations of the disease, such as café-au-lait spots, cutaneous neurofibromata, or hemihypertrophy. Only 1% to 2% of individuals with neurofibromatosis have CPT. Pathological specimens show hamartomatous fibrous tissue around and invading the dysplastic bone to a variable extent proximally and distally. CPT may also occasionally be associated with fibrous dysplasia, and both diagnoses should be considered. In a series of 43 individuals with anterolateral bowing, Tuncay et al[28] identified 5 patients whose anterolateral bowing resolved spontaneously without any treatment or prophylactic bracing. These individuals had no identifiable syndrome or stigmata of neurofibromatosis or fibrous dysplasia. Early callus formation and subperiosteal new bone formation on the posteromedial concavity were good prognostic signs.

Boyd classified six types of congenital pseudarthrosis (Fig. 11, Table 2). Type II is the most common and the type usually associated with neurofibromatosis. Radiographs demonstrate narrowing of the tibia, usually in the distal third, with loss of the medullary canal. Other researchers distinguish only three general groups.[29] The dysplastic type shows narrowing and angulation of the tibia and sometimes of the fibula. The tibia may be fractured at

birth but frequently fractures only after the child begins to ambulate. The cystic type does not show narrowing of the tibia but does show cystlike lucencies in the affected portions of the bone. Angulation may not be present at birth but develops in the first months of life. Fracture usually occurs by age 8 months. The late type presents after age 5 years. The leg is initially normal but subsequently develops an LLD and a fracture with minimal trauma. A pseudarthrosis ensues.

Unlike congenital posteromedial bow, the natural history of congenital anterolateral bow is progression. Individuals born with congenital anterolateral bow without fractures must be braced from infancy to attempt to avoid fracturing, which almost invariably results in pseudarthrosis. An ankle-foot orthosis with an anterior shell is typically used until skeletal maturity. Osteotomy of the tibia to correct malalignment is absolutely contraindicated because it too invariably leads to pseudarthrosis. Children born with a pseudarthrosis should be braced initially until they may be safely subjected to operation.

Healing the pseudarthrosisis is notoriously difficult. Even after successful healing, the refracture rate is high. Numerous surgical procedures have been described for the child with CPT. Simple bracing or casting always fails to heal a

TABLE 2. BOYD'S CLASSIFICATION OF CONGENITAL PSEUDARTHROSIS	
Type	**Characteristics**
I	Anterior bow, congenital abnormalities (clubfoot)
II	Anterior bow with hourglass constriction of tibia. Associated with NFB
III	Cystic changes in tibia
IV	Sclerosis of tibia without narrowing
V	Dysplasia of fibula +/− tibial pseudarthrosis
VI	Intraosseous neurofibroma (?factitious)

NFB = neurofibromatosis.

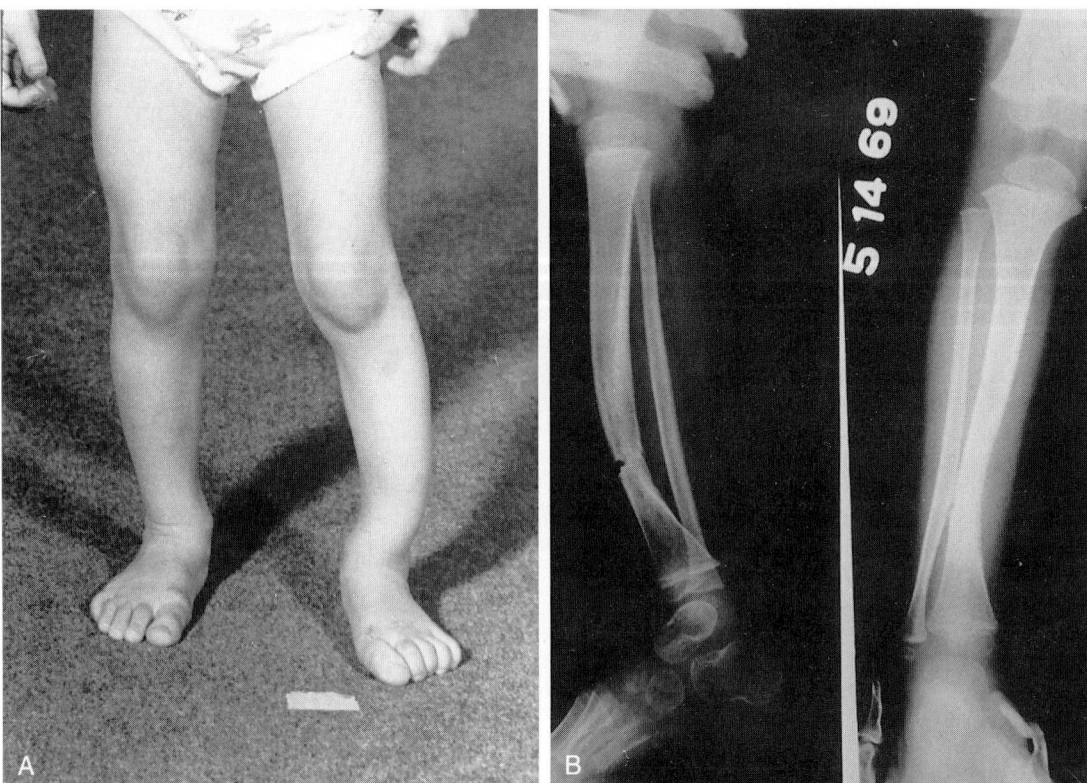

Fig. 11. Views. *A,* A 3-year-old patient with neurofibromatosis presents with anterolateral tibial bowing. *B,* Boyd's type II pseuarthrosis is noted on radiographs. Williams' intramedullary rodding led to a successful long-term outcome.

pseudarthrosis, and bone grafting is necessary. Fracture fixation with plates and screws is rarely successful, even when supplemented with bone graft. Intramedullary fixation has a reported 80% initial healing rate when autogenous cancellous bone is used for grafting, although many will later refracture.[30] Most consider this the gold standard initial procedure for CPT. For those cases that fail to unite, two main techniques have been utilized. Free vascularized fibular grafting has been reported with a greater than 90% incidence of initial healing.[31] Shortcomings of this procedure include difficulties treating the associated limb length discrepancy and the inability to easily repeat the procedure due to limited donor sites.

Several strategies have been used with ring external fixators.[32, 33] The fixator is applied first, and the diseased bone is resected. The diseased hamartomatous soft tissues, including the periosteum, should also be locally resected. The bone ends are approximated and bone-grafted. The tibia may be lengthened at a remote site, usually proximally if necessary. The fixator may be removed after adequate healing, and long-term bracing until skeletal maturity is recommended. Initial healing rates have been reported to be 90% or more, but about 50% can be expected to refracture. The advantages of this technique include the ability to repeat the procedure if necessary after refracture and to simultaneously address limb length discrepancy and angular deformity. Despite newer methods, treating CPT remains among the most difficult challenges in pediatric orthopedics, with high failure rates due to refracture, deformity, and stiffness of the foot and ankle.

Amputation is recommended for those cases in which stable healing cannot be achieved. The result is reliable, and function is nearly always excellent with rehabilitation. The indications for amputation are not clear and are becoming increasingly uncertain as reports of reconstruction become increasingly optimistic. However, despite the availability of highly technical equipment and methods, a role for amputation remains for the multiply operated unhealed tibia or a stiff or painful dysfunctional ankle. Both Syme's amputation and below-knee amputation have been recommended. The former has the advantage of providing an end-bearing stump and preserving maximum limb length. The pseudarthrosis does not usually interfere with function but may make prosthetic fitting slightly more difficult.

Enchondromatosis

Multiple enchondromatosis (Ollier's disease) is considered to be a condition of bone dysplasia, not of bony neoplasia. There is no tendency toward heritability. The lesions are usually predominantly or exclusively unilateral but may involve any bone of the upper or lower extremity. They may be monomelic. The long bones are more commonly involved. Enchondromas usually arise in the metaphyses of bones as stippled radiolucent lesions, which may possess a pattern of longitudinal calcific striations. They rarely arise in the epiphyses. They are believed to arise when dysplastic chondrocytes originating in the growth plate deposit in these areas. They fail to undergo normal enchondral calcification and produce islands of mature hyaline cartilage. In a small number of cases, they may undergo malignant degeneration to chondrosarcoma in adulthood, and close follow-up throughout life is mandatory.

Abnormal growth of the physis leads to angular deformities and LLD. The mechanism of growth inhibition is believed to be due either to the inherent abnormality of the growth plate cartilage or to a tethering effect on the epiphyseal cartilage by an abnormally thick periosteal sleeve. The apex of angular deformities is always on the side where the metaphyseal involvement by the enchondroma is greatest. The deformities are progressive, and the outcome is difficult to predict.

Maffucci's syndrome is Ollier's disease with subcutaneous hemangiomata. The skin lesions are not necessarily anatomically related to the bone lesions. Individuals with Maffucci's syndrome tend to have more severe involvement of the skeleton with enchondromata. They also are at greatly increased risk of developing both musculoskeletal and visceral malignancies and must be monitored very closely.

Treatment involves surgical correction of the angular deformity and the limb length discrepancy. There are no clearly established criteria for timing corrective osteotomies. Most authors agree that deformities should not be allowed to exceed about 20 to 25 degrees. When an enchondroma is resected, careful attention must be paid to the proximity of the physis to avoid iatrogenic injury. Recurrence is common if the child is still growing, and families should be aware that procedures might have to be repeated near the end of growth. Overcorrection is not recommended because of the difficulty in determining the magnitude of overcorrection that will result in appropriate alignment at the end of growth. Problems with bone healing have not been noted, either with osteotomy or lengthening.

Shapiro[34] reported on 21 patients and found 80% of the femora and 42% of the tibiae to develop angular deformities. Epiphysiodesis of the unaffected limb limited LLD, but partial epiphyseal arrest to correct deformity was ineffective. He noted three causes of recurrent angulation: (1) persistence of the lesion at the growth plate; the osteotomy is directed at correcting the angular deformity, not eliminating the lesion; (2) inadequate correction of the deformity; intraoperative and immediate postoperative radiographs must be critically evaluated to ensure that an adequate correction was achieved; (3) loss of correction postoperatively; poor quality of the affected bone may make stable fixation difficult. Osteotomy and fixation should be outside the area of the enchondroma whenever possible.

Osteochondromatosis

Hereditary multiple exostoses (osteochondromatosis) is a heritable dysplasia of bone characterized by multiple sessile or pedunculated osteochondromas that occur primarily in the metaphyses of long bones. Osteochondromatosis is transmitted in an autosomal-dominant pattern. The lesions arise as a result of a defect in the periphery of the affected growth plate, causing enchondral ossification to occur outside the limit of the normal metaphysis. The lesion arises adjacent to the growth plate but migrates toward the diaphysis as the bone grows. The exostosis possesses its own growth cartilage cap and continues to enlarge until skeletal maturity is reached.

Abnormalities of bone growth include angular deformity and longitudinal growth inhibition. These appear to be related to multiple factors. The presence of the osteochondroma leads to abnormal metaphyseal remodeling, which may create an angular deformity. In two-bone limb segments, the exostosis may impinge mechanically on the second bone or apply tension to the adjacent interosseous membrane, creating an angular deformity or subluxation of the adjacent joint. This occurs most frequently in the distal forearm and distal leg. Treatment of this problem primarily involves resection of the deforming osteochondroma. The deformity may remodel if sufficient growth remains. Otherwise, the deformity may be corrected with an osteotomy, with shortening of the unaffected bone or lengthening of the affected bone. If there is an associated LLD, simultaneous lengthening and deformity correction with an external fixator may be appropriate.

Individuals with multiple osteochondromatosis tend to have shorter than average stature. It is unclear whether this is due to multiple physeal involvement or a related genetic predisposition. If the limb growth inhibition results in limbs of equal length, no treatment is necessary. If there is a resulting LLD, an epiphysiodesis or limb lengthening procedure may be indicated. Schmale et al[35] reviewed the findings in 113 individuals in 46 families with multiple osteochondromatosis. They found that 70% had a lesion in the distal femur, 71% had a lesion in the proximal tibia, and 27% had a lesion in the proximal fibula. Only two individuals had a deformity of the ankle, and 10% had an LLD that was greater than 2 cm. Overall, 74% of the individuals had at least one lesion removed; these patients averaged three operative procedures each.

Hemihypertrophy

Various terms have been used to denote hypertrophy: including congenital hemihypertrophy, congenital hypertrophy, pure total hemihypertrophy, unilateral hypertrophy, hemigigantism, partial gigantism, congenital asymmetry, and others. There is no widely accepted definition of the term nor classification of the disease.

No definitive guidelines exist for distinguishing between mild idiopathic hypertrophy and mild atrophy. To confuse the matter further, there is a certain amount of asymmetry in the normal population, and the point at which asymmetry can be considered abnormal has not been satisfactorily established.

Pappas and Nehme[36] surveyed 376 subjects and found that the average asymmetry varied with age. At 1 year, the average lower extremity asymmetry averaged 0.4 cm, and the asymmetry reached a maximum of 1.1 cm at maturity, with 95% of the population falling within these figures. The description of "normal" can overlap that of abnormal asymmetry; i.e., a 1-year-old with a 0.4-cm discrepancy may be at the upper limit of normal or may have hypertrophy. In diagnosing hypertrophy in an otherwise normal individual, factors other than absolute differences, including the progression of the discrepancy, the size of each lower limb relative to the rest of the body and to each other, and the relative percentage of lengthening that the discrepancy represents, must be evaluated. The authors established a convention to define abnormal asymmetry as a 5% or greater difference in size. This percentage was applied to length and circumference measurements. For the femur of average length, this means a 0.7-cm discrepancy at year 1, 1.3 cm at 5 years, 1.8 cm at year 10, and 2.3 cm by year 18. For the average-length tibia, 5% represents 0.6 cm at year 1, 1.0 cm at 5 years, 1.4 cm at year 10, and 1.8 cm at year 18.

Hypertrophy of the lower extremity can exist as hypertrophy in length or in circumference or in both. Many instances of hypertrophy localized to a limb segment have a clear cause, such as inflammation (e.g., juvenile rheumatoid arthritis), prior trauma (shortening or overgrowth), neurological impairment (actually hemiatrophy), or tumors. In addition, several syndromes have a predictable association with hemihypertrophy, including Russell-Silver, Beckwith-Wiedemann, neurofibromatosis, and Klippel-Trenaunay syndrome. However, the most common form of true hemihypertrophy is idiopathic. This is associated with true enlargement of one-half of the body in both length and girth. The paired viscera may also be affected. Approximately 5% of individuals with hemihypertophy have intra-abdominal malignancies, the most common being Wilms' tumor. Because the association is well known, its frequency is often mistaken to be higher, and reassurance of the family is important. Treatment of the limb length inequality is usually best done with an epiphysiodesis.

FIBULAR HEMIMELIA

Fibular hemimelia (hypoplasia or aplasia of the fibula) is the most common longitudinal deficiency of the lower extremity. It may present with an LLD or with anteromedial bowing of the tibia, with a skin dimple at the apex of the deformity (Fig. 12). Either the proximal or distal end may be affected. The occurrence is sporadic, and the incidence is approximately 1 in 10,000.[37]

Abnormalities of the foot and ankle joint are often its most striking features. The foot is frequently positioned in severe valgus and is often missing one or two lateral rays. Abnormalities of the ankle include valgus instability and a ball-and-socket-ankle conformation. The latter is a result of associated tarsal coalition that occurs in up to 50% of affected individuals. Children frequently have some degree of ipsilateral deformity of the femur, including shortening, mild valgus of the distal femur, and anteroposterior knee instability due to a deficient anterior cruciate ligament. In a review of 291 patients with congenital unilateral extremity shortening, 129 had shortening of the fibula.[38] All individuals with a deficiency of the fibula were noted to have some additional lower extremity malformation. The spectrum of malformations included virtually all lower extremity malformations.

Achterman and Kalamchi[39] classified fibular hemimelia into three groups (Fig. 13). Type Ia is a short fibula, with the proximal fibula situated below the tibial physis and the distal physis above the talar dome. Type Ib is deficient by 30% to 50%, and the foreshortened lateral malleolus does not support the talus in the mortise. Type II is total or near total absence of the fibula. There may be a vestigial distal malleolar anlage that is not readily evident on plain radiograph.

Investigations at birth should include radiographs of both

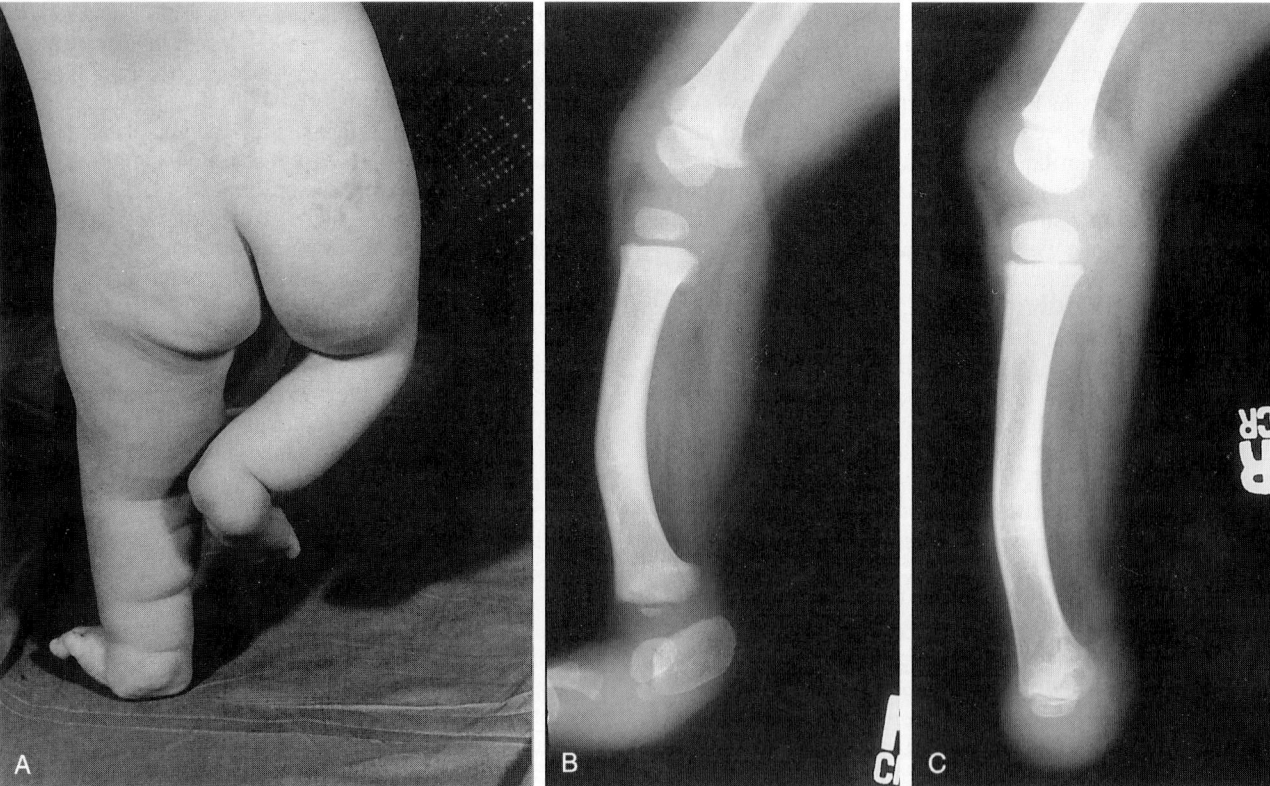

Fig. 12. Views. *A,* Fibular hemimelia may have an associated proximal focal femoral deficiency. Note the marked eversion of the hindfoot. *B,* Lateral radiograph demonstrates severe hindfoot eversion and absence of lateral rays. *C,* Lateral radiograph following Boyd's amputation with spontaneous improvement in anterior fibular bowing. (Courtesy of James C. Drennan, MD.)

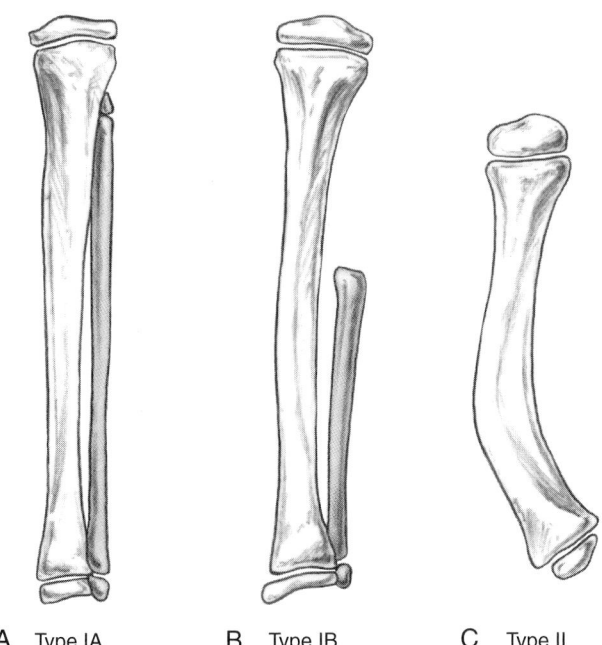

A Type IA   B Type IB   C Type II

Fig. 13. Achterman-Kalamchi classification. This classification of congenital deficiency of the fibula has significant clinical implications. (From Achterman C, Kalamchi J: Congenital absence of the fibula. J Bone Joint Surg Br 1979; 61:133.)

lower extremities, including the feet and the pelvis, to look for associated anomalies. The majority of patients will have anomalies of the femur. This may be a subtle valgus malalignment or a severe proximal focal femoral deficiency (PFFD). Individuals with a significant femoral deficiency should be treated as having a PFFD, with the fibular abnormality being secondary. The femoral intercondylar notch may be shallow with flattening of the proximal tibial spines. Radiographs of the foot frequently show the lateral fourth and fifth rays to be completely absent. Congenital tarsal coalition is not usually evident at birth but will become evident as ossification of the tarsal bones progresses. It may be useful to obtain an MRI of the ankle and leg to determine if there is a fibrocartilaginous lateral malleolus. If one is present, it may be used to stabilize the foot below the tibia. In its absence, correction of the valgus position is more complex.

When planning treatment, consideration of all the elements of the deformity is essential. This includes LLD, valgus knee deformity, anteromedial bowing of the tibia, ankle valgus, ankle instability, and deformity of the foot. Treatment is divided into two main alternatives, amputation and reconstruction. Traditionally, treatment has depended on two major factors, the predicted overall LLD and the ability to stabilize the ankle. The integrity of the foot has also been considered an important element in the decision to salvage the limb.[40] Growth inhibition is constant during development of the limb, so the percent shortening of the limb at maturity can often be predicted at birth. In the past, greater than 35% overall shortening of the limb at maturity has been considered the reasonable limit beyond which limb lengthening is excessively difficult and complications unacceptable.[41] However, modern limb lengthening techniques have made this number controversial.

When amputation is selected for the child with isolated longitudinal deficiency of the fibula, the family can be ensured that function is excellent with essentially unrestricted ability to participate in sports. If the amputation is performed when the child seems nearly ready to walk, the child will typically develop skills at an age that parallels or nearly parallels age-matched cohorts.[4] Gait is essentially normal. Syme's or Boyd's amputation provides an optimal end-bearing stump that is easily fitted with a prosthesis. Stump overgrowth is not a problem. The only significant problem has been instability of the heel pad with Syme's amputation. Many authors favor Boyd's amputation, which retains a thin sliver of the calcaneus attached to its native heel pad.

The advantages of reconstructing the limb are obvious, and the availability of the Ilizarov apparatus has made it technically more feasible. Psychological stresses resulting from the complexity and long duration of limb reconstruction has been an important reason for some to advocate amputation. Although significant transient mental problems have been documented, these have been shown to abate with time,[42, 43] and long-term psychological injury has not been noted. Birch et al[44] found excellent physical function and psychological health in 10 patients who underwent Syme's amputation for fibular deficiency. The authors concluded that this should be the standard against which lengthening should be compared in order to justify its recommendation.

Current techniques of limb reconstruction are based on limb lengthening and deformity correction using external fixation. A review by Catagni and Guerreschi provides an excellent summary of the elements of the deformity that must be considered.[45] The status of the femur, the hip, and the knee joint must be given particular attention as femoral reconstruction may present additional challenges to reconstruction of the lower leg. Associated acetabular dysplasia may have to be treated, particularly if significant femoral lengthening will be necessary, as the hip may be at greater risk of subluxation. Distal femoral valgus deformity nearly always requires correction to avoid malalignment of the limb. It may also contribute to patellofemoral instability. Anteroposterior instability secondary to cruciate deficiency is not usually a clinical problem but may contribute to tibiofemoral subluxation or dislocation during lengthening.

Catagni prefers to use a classification modified from that of Dal Monte and Donzelli.[46] Three grades are identified, I–III, based on severity. For the least severe (grade I), a single tibial lengthening near skeletal maturity is recommended. Simultaneous correction of angular deformity depends on the severity of the deformity. In this grade, the foot does not usually require reconstruction. For the moderately severe (grade II), a limb extension orthosis is used until the first limb lengthening at age 10 to 12 years. The ankle mortise is reconstructed by pulling the calcaneus into varus and transporting the fibula distally. Angular correction of the lower leg is performed but may recur. A second lengthening is anticipated near skeletal maturity to correct the residual limb length discrepancy and angular deformity.

Correction of the most severe (grade III) is complex and requires multiple steps. The function of the ankle is compromised; the ankle should undergo open reduction in infancy. Corrective casting from birth may facilitate this. A limb extension orthosis is used until the next stage. The age at the first lengthening may be the toddler years or when the child is 5 to 6 years. If a severe angular deformity exists, only a modest lengthening should be performed. If there is less angular deformity, the lengthening may be more ambitious. At the next stage, femoral angular deformity correction and femoral lengthening are added to tibial and possibly foot and ankle reconstruction. This requires a frame that extends from the femur to the foot and may be supplied at age 8 to 10 years. Two additional stages may be required to complete the correction. An additional ankle arthrodesis is sometimes indicated if the foot is painful or malpositioned. Paley[47] addressed the problem of ankle valgus by assessing the ankle's position in maximal valgus and performing a corrective supramalleolar varus focal dome osteotomy such that the position of maximal valgus of the ankle places the foot in neutral alignment with the axis of the tibia. Treatment by this technique is extremely challenging and should be attempted only by those most familiar with the disorder and the corrective device they are using. Although good results are often obtained, knee and ankle stiffness frequently affect function in the more severe grades. Results may be expected to be as good or better with reconstruction as with amputation for the less severe grades but probably not as good for the most severe limb deficiencies.

TIBIAL HEMIMELIA

Congenital longitudinal deficiency of the tibia is an extremely rare condition (1/10[6]). The condition is obvious at birth, presenting with marked shortening of the limb, equinovarus foot deformity, and duplication or deletion of rays. Knee and ankle instability are variable but often severe. It is often associated with split hands ("lobster-claw deformity") and cardiac and renal anomalies. Other musculoskeletal abnormalities include PFFD, hip dysplasia, vertebral anomalies, duplicated femoral segments, and anomalies of the radius, ulna, and digits.[48] When associated with split hands, it is usually bilateral and associated with an autosomal-dominant inheritance pattern. It has also been seen as an isolated anomaly in two siblings with a postulated autosomal-recessive inheritance.

Tibial hemimelia was classified by Jones et al[49] and reviewed by Schoenecker et al[48] (Fig. 14). It includes four major groups. In type 1, the tibia is radiographically absent at birth; in type 1a it remains absent during growth, and in type 1b a hyoplastic proximal tibia develops during infancy. In both types the distal femur is markedly hypoplastic. In type 2, the proximal tibia is present but hypoplastic, and the distal femur is nearly normal. Type 3 is least common and demonstrates a short segment of tibial diaphysis with poorly defined proximal and distal articulations. Type 4 is a distal tibiofibular diastasis with a small limb length discrepancy. The clubfoot is the most striking feature in this type.

When evaluating these children, the most important determination to make is the presence of a functioning quadriceps mechanism and proximal tibial anlage. This may be determined by physical examination but often requires additional imaging. Plain radiographs will show a bony anlage in type 2, but arthrography, computed tomography, ultrasonography, or MRI may be necessary to distinguish between type 1a and 1b deformities. If the quadriceps is

Type	Radiological description	Number of limbs
1 A	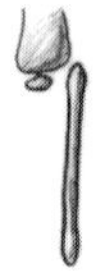 • Tibia not seen • Hypoplastic lower femoral epiphysis	6
1 B	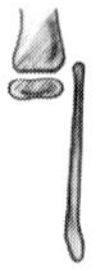 • Tibia not seen • Normal lower femoral epiphysis	12
2	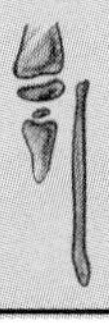 • Distal tibia not seen	5
3	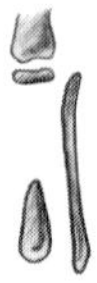 • Proximal tibia not seen	2
4	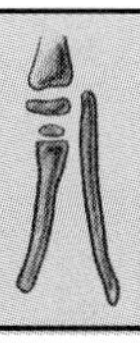 • Diastasis	4

Fig. 14. Jones' classification. This establishes clinical and radiographic features that assist in developing treatment options. (From Jones D, Barnes J, Lloyd-Roberts GC: Congenital aplasia and dysplasias of the tibia with intact fibula. J Bone Joint Surg Br 1978; 60: 31.)

functional, consideration should be given to reconstructing the limb with a fibular transposition or tibiofibular synostosis. Brown[50] advocated centralization of the fibula into the femoral condylar notch. This procedure has had mixed results if the quadriceps is present. If the quadriceps is absent, successful reconstruction of the limb is even less likely.

Achieving ankle stability is another major problem in all but the type 4 deficiencies. Long-term bracing and repeated surgeries are required to maintain an acceptable foot position. Even then, the function is usually poor, leading most authors to recommend ablation of the foot by Syme's or Boyd amputation in the majority of types 1, 2, and 3.

It is commonly accepted that centralization of the fibula in the absence of an adequate extensor mechanism will lead to uniformly poor results due to a high incidence of knee flexion contracture. Loder[51] performed a meta-analysis of all reported cases in the English-language literature of fibular transfer for longitudinal deficiency of the tibia. There were 75 type 1a and 12 type 1b tibiae. Thirty-nine type 1a tibiae ultimately underwent knee disarticulation due to uncontrolled flexion contractures. In contrast, varus-valgus instability was the more significant problem with the type 1b; it was easily managed with the prosthesis used for the simultaneous foot amputation.

An alternative to the Brown fibular centralization procedure is a proximal tibiofibular synostosis. This requires the presence of a functional articulation between the distal femur and proximal tibia. It can therefore be used in some type 1b and in type 2 deformities. The synostosis has the advantage of utilizing the functional original knee joint while providing maximal leg length and function.

Treatment of type 3 deficiencies depends on the development of the proximal and distal joints as well as on the position of the foot. If the position of the foot can be aligned appropriately, it may be retained and a limb extension prosthesis used. Alternatively, a Syme, Boyd, or Chopart amputation may be performed to provide very good function with a below-knee prosthesis.

The ankle in type 4 deformities can usually be stabilized. Open reduction of the diastasis is usually necessary, followed by prolonged bracing. The knee is usually stable or can be rendered stable with a brace or surgery. The substantial limb length discrepancy is the remaining problem, and this can be treated with appropriately staged lengthening procedures. As with all complex lengthenings, complications remain significant. For more severe foot deformities associated with a large LLD, primary below-knee amputation or foot ablation procedures remain viable alternatives.

Reconstruction with an external fixator has also been attempted for types 1, 2, and 3. The approach requires simultaneous or sequential correction of all elements of the deformity. The knee flexion contracture can be corrected, the foot position reduced, and the tibia, if present, straightened and lengthened. This technique is extremely demanding, and there has been very limited experience with it.

CONGENITAL LONGITUDINAL DEFICIENCY OF THE FEMUR

Longitudinal deficiencies of the femur represent a spectrum of anomalies, ranging from simple shortening of an otherwise normal femur to complete absence of the femur, with associated abnormal development of the pelvis and multiple anomalies of the knee, leg, and foot. Many cases are bilateral (15%), and most are associated with ipsilateral fibular deficiencies (60% to 70%).

Proximal focal femoral deficiency is a misnomer because it is not only the proximal femoral region that is affected. The diaphysis and distal femur are also abnormal. At birth, the thigh is short and bulky with an obvious LLD. The quadriceps musculature may be hypoplastic, creating a funnel-shaped thigh. The hip is typically positioned in flexion, abduction, and external rotation. The action of the psoas and hamstrings exaggerates this position, especially if there is a site of pseudarthrosis. Frequently there is a valgus alignment of the distal femur, and the knee ligaments are unstable. The anterior cruciate ligament is usually deficient. Other associated anomalies are present in at least 65% to 70% of cases.

There are two general types of congenital longitudinal deficiency of the femur: with or without an osseous defect. If there is an osseous defect, it is usually referred to as PFFD. If there is no defect, some authors refer to the deformity as a congenital short femur (CSF), a subset of PFFD. The CSF group represents a heterogeneous population with varying amounts of shortening and structural abnormalities. However, they have in common the presence of a relatively normal hip and knee with all osseous structures present. There is usually moderate coxa vara, diaphyseal bowing, and valgus orientation of the distal femoral condyles. The ultimate length of the femur ranges from 60% to 90% of the normal side, with a limb length discrepancy from 5 to 20 cm. The cruciate ligaments are deficient, resulting in knee instability. The treatment goal in this group is achieving equal limb lengths and restoring normal limb alignment.

In true PFFD, not all bony elements of the femur are present. The milder deficiencies are represented by a proximal femoral pseudarthrosis with varying degrees of coxa vara with or without acetabular dysplasia. The ischiopubic structures may be hypoplastic. The distal femur, when present, usually has a valgus orientation with hypoplasia of the lateral condyle. The cruciate ligaments, especially the anterior cruciate, are frequently absent. The more severe deficiencies have no femur, with a severely dysplastic acetabulum that articulates with the tibia. The fibula is often absent, and the foot may have the characteristics of fibular hemimelia. The major challenge is rendering the hip and knee stable and suitable for prosthetic fitting.

Identifying the specific type of PFFD may be difficult or impossible at birth by plain radiograph due to the inability to characterize the unossified portion of the limb. Additional imaging modalities, including MRI or arthrography, may assist in classifying the type of PFFD present.

Numerous classifications exist for PFFD. Pappas' classification is based on the evaluation of 139 femora in 125 patients (Table 3). It contains nine classes whose degree of severity decreases with the class. Class I is complete absence of the femur, and class IX is a hypoplastic or congenital short femur. This classification includes both CSF and PFFD and a comprehensive description of their specific subtypes. Associated malformations and prognosis are detailed in this review.

The Aitken classification is commonly used because of its simplicity and its implications for treatment. It includes four groups, types A to D. There is no classification for the congenital short femur.

In type A, the femur is short with coxa vara. The acetabulum is normal, and there is an adequate femoral head. Early in life, the proximal portion of the femur is cartilagi-

TABLE 3. PAPPAS' CLASSIFICATION	
Class 1	Congenital absence of the femur
Class II	Proximal femoral and pelvic deficiency
Class III	Proximal femoral deficiency with no osseous connection between femoral shaft and head
Class IV	Proximal femoral deficiency with disorganized fibro-osseous disconnection between femoral shaft and head
Class V	Midfemoral deficiency with hypoplastic proximal and distal development
Class VI	Distal femoral deficiency
Class VII	Hypoplastic femur with coxa vara and sclerosed diaphysis
Class VIII	Hypoplastic femur with coxa valga
Class IX	Hypoplastic femur with normal proportions

nous, and the distal portion is bony. The cartilaginous portion ossifies, but a pseudarthrosis often develops in the subtrochanteric region. This undergoes progressive varus deformity but may ossify spontaneously.

In type B, the femoral head is present and is typically situated in a mildly dysplastic acetabulum. Ossification of the femoral head is markedly delayed. There is a pseudarthrosis between the proximal femur and the short femoral diaphysis component. Unlike type A, this type does not heal spontaneously.

In type C, the acetabulum is severely dysplastic. The femoral head is absent or represented by a small cartilaginous tuft. The femoral shaft is severely shortened, and the hip is markedly unstable.

Type D is the most severe form of PFFD. Both the acetabulum and femoral head are absent. The femoral shaft is very short and severely deformed, and there is no tuft in the proximal segment to represent the femoral head. The femur may be represented by only the femoral condyles.

Current management of these deformities is changing. Stabilization of the hip with either fusion or osteotomy and correction of major LLD by rotationplasty, prosthetic fitting, or limb lengthenings are the basic principles of management. When the PFFD is bilateral, children achieve a remarkable degree of coordination and ambulate easily without surgery or prostheses. For these individuals, prosthetic use is often more cosmetic than functional and for achieving social acceptance. Reconstructive surgery has traditionally been discouraged for these patients because of the high risk of diminishing function. Surgery of the foot and ankle may be indicated to facilitate prosthetic fitting.

For less severe deformities (Pappas IV–IX; Aitken A, B), especially if unilateral, reconstruction may be considered. Because the femoral head and acetabulum are present, hip instability, if present, may be corrected with a pelvic osteotomy. Ossification of the proximal femoral osseous defect must be achieved prior to or during the first lengthening procedure. This should be delayed until about age 2 or 3 years, at which time the osseous defect may have ossified spontaneously. Consolidation of the pseudarthrosis may be achieved using either internal or external fixation, depending on whether lengthening is being done. If there is a persistent pseudarthrosis and bone stock is poor, bone grafting may be necessary. Varus deformity should be corrected simultaneously.

The projected LLD at maturity is another important consideration in planning treatment. This can be determined as soon as the cartilaginous portions of the affected limb are ossified sufficiently to accurately measure its length. Growth inhibition is usually constant throughout growth. If the affected femur is 50% short at birth, it can be expected to be 50% short at maturity. Gillespie and Torode[54] (Fig. 15) recommended that limb lengthening be considered for children whose affected femur is at least 60% of the length of the normal femur. However, this recommendation was made in the era of the Wagner technique, and modern methods of limb lengthening are more predictable in achieving larger lengthenings.

If the patient is a good candidate for lengthening, a modest lengthening of 5 cm may be considered at an early age. It is well tolerated, and bone regeneration is reliable. The proximal varus and distal valgus deformities can be

corrected simultaneously. Frequently, the proximal varus deformity may be corrected acutely at the beginning of the procedure, and the distal valgus deformity may be corrected gradually or acutely at the end of the lengthening. Stability of the knee must be considered because deficiency of the anterior cruciate ligament may lead to subluxation or dislocation of the knee. This can be achieved by crossing the knee with the external fixator. Additional staged lengthenings must be anticipated to achieve equal limb lengths. Contralateral epiphysiodesis may also be used to make limb length equality easier to achieve.

For more severe deformities (Pappas I–III, Aitken C, D), attempts to reconstruct the limb anatomically are much more difficult. Absence of a true hip joint, stiffness of the hip and knee, large LLD, and associated deformities may make this goal virtually impossible to achieve. Prosthetic fitting is used, and this may be done in several different manners. The first prosthetic limb is usually fitted when the child is attempting to pull to the standing position. A limb extension prosthesis utilizes the intact foot without surgical modification of the limb. A prosthetic platform is incorporated in the artificial limb for attachment to the foot. This method is useful in childhood, but integration of an adult foot into this type of prosthesis makes it unacceptably bulky. The alternatives are either to perform a Syme or Boyd amputation or to subject the lower leg to a Van Ness rotation or similar procedure and use the ankle as the knee joint. When the femoral segment is very small, fusion of

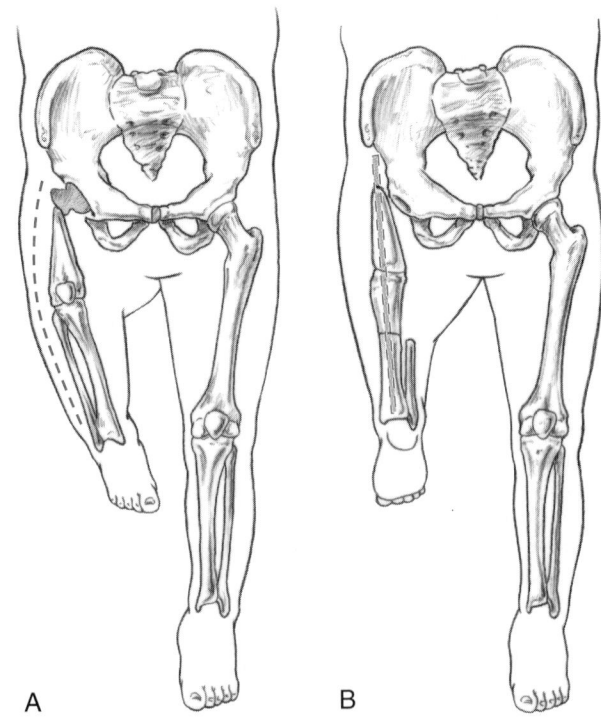

Fig. 15. Van Ness rotationplasty requires fusion of the knee. *A,* The rotational correction can be performed through the knee at the time of knee fusion. (Torode IP, Gillespie R: Rotationplasty of the lower limb for congenital defects of the femur. J Bone Joint Surg Br 1983; 65:570.) Line drawing demonstrates proximal focal femoral deficiency and the recommended incision *(line of dashes). B,* Line drawing demonstrates intramedullary rodding and reversal of foot alignment. (Torode IP, Gillespie R: J Bone Joint Surg Br 1983; 65:572. Fig. 7).

the knee is the most common procedure performed. This provides a more stable limb for prosthetic fitting than if the knee is left intact. Fusion is usually accompanied by ablation of the foot to facilitate prosthetic fitting. Although fusing the knee and amputating the foot provides a stable limb, it necessitates the use of an above-knee prosthesis.

Alternatively, reconstructing the limb with a van Ness rotationplasty[55] depends on the integrity of the foot and ankle. The distal limb is rotated 180 degrees through the tibia, allowing the ankle to function as a knee, with the foot functioning as the "below-knee" stump. In this position, ankle dorsiflexion translates into knee flexion (see Fig. 15). Results of this technique were limited due to spontaneous derotation of the limb.

Gillespie and Torode[56] modified the original technique by fusing the knee and performing most of the rotation there, leaving a relatively small amount of rotation at a mid-diaphyseal tibial site. The resultant proximal limb segment, composed of the femur and tibia, provides better characteristics for prosthetic fitting and weightbearing than leaving both the hip and knee unfused. Krajbich[57] modified this procedure by performing the entire rotation through the knee and transferring all muscle insertions so that their pull is in a straight line across the rotated knee. The advantages of this method of reconstruction include a biological knee powered by the patient's muscles, a stump capable of proprioception, and the psychological benefit of the foot being retained. Most children may be considered candidates for rotationplasty, the major contraindication being a stiff or malformed foot or ankle that is not capable of providing a functional and mobile distal stump.

When the femur is short and the hip is dysplastic, an unstable gait frequently results. Prosthetic fitting is difficult, and ambulation is inefficient. Iliofemoral fusion may be done in order to increase hip stability and improve gait. In this situation, the knee is left mobile to function as the hip moving in a single flexion-extension plane but substantially improving function and cosmesis. A Chiari osteotomy may be done concurrently to provide a bed for the fusion. Although this procedure provides hip stability, it has the disadvantage of diminishing useful hip motion. Some believe that this is better ignored and allow stability to develop 2 degrees to muscle strengthening.

REFERENCES

1. Michael JW: Overview of prosthetic feet. In Greene WB (ed): Instructional Course Lectures XXXIX. Park Ridge, IL, American Academy of Orthopaedic Surgeons, 1990, p 367.
2. Michael JW: Current concepts in above-knee socket design. In Greene WB (ed): Instructional Course Lectures XXXIX. Park Ridge, IL, American Academy of Orthopaedic Surgeons, 1990, p 373.
3. Wilson GN: Heritable limb deficiencies. In Herring JA, Birch JG (eds): The Child With a Limb Deficiency. Rosemont, IL, American Academy of Orthopaedic Surgeons, 1998.
4. Staheli LT: Rotational problems in children. In Schafer M (ed): Instructional Course Lectures XLIII. Rosemont, IL, American Academy of Orthopaedic Surgeons, 1994, p 199.
5. Wedge JH, Munkacsi I, Loback D: Anteversion of the femur and idiopathic osteoarthrosis of the hip. J Bone Joint Surg Am 1989; 71:1040.
6. Hubbard DD, Staheli LI, Chew DE, et al: Medial femoral torsion and osteoarthritis. J Ped Orthop 1988; 8:540.
7. Engel GM, Staheli LT: The natural history of torsion and other factors influencing gait in childhood: A study of the angle of gait, tibial torsion, knee angle, hip rotation, and development of the arch in normal children. Clin Orthop 1974; 99:12.
8. Greene WB: Genu varum and genu valgum in children. In Schafer M (ed): Instructional Course Lectures XLIII. Rosemont, IL, American Academy of Orthopaedic Surgeons, 1994, p 151.
9. Carter JR, Leeson MC, Thompson GH, et al: Late-onset tibia vara: A histopathologic analysis: A comparative evaluation with infantile tibia vara and slipped capital femoral epiphysis. J Pediatr Orthop 1988; 8:187.
10. Levine AM, Drennan JC: Physiologic bowing and tibia vara: The metaphyseal-diaphyseal angle in the measurement of bow-leg deformities. J Bone Joint Surg Am 1982; 64:1158.
11. Feldman MD, Schoenecker PL: Use of the metaphyseal-diaphyseal angle in the evolution of bowed legs. J Bone Joint Surg Am 1993; 75:1602.
12. Langeskiold A, Risk EB: Tibia vara (osteochondrosis deformans tibial): A survey of seventy-one cases. J Bone Joint Surg Am 1964; 46:1405.
13. Richards BS, Katz DE, Sims JB: Effectiveness of brace treatment in early infantile Blount's disease. J Pediatr Orthop 1998; 18:374.
14. Raney EM, Topoleski TA, Yaghoubian R, et al: Orthotic treatment of infantile tibia vara. J Pediatr Orthop 1998; 18:670.
15. Greene WB: Instructional course lectures: Infantile tibia vara. J Bone Joint Surg Am 1993; 75:130.
16. Martin SD, Moran MC, Martin TL, et al: Proximal tibial osteotomy with compression plate fixation for tibia vara. J Pediatr Orthop 1994; 14:619.
17. Bowen JR, Torres RR, Forlin E: Partial epiphysiodesis to address genu varum or genu valgum. J Pediatr Orthop 1992; 12:359.
18. Bowen JR, Leakey JL, Zhang ZZ, et al: Partial epiphysiodesis at the knee to correct angular deformity. Clin Orthop 1985; 198:184.
19. Pappas: Unpublished data.
20. Cozen L: Fracture of the proximal portion of the tibia in children followed by valgus deformity. Surg Gynecol Obstet 1953; 97:183.
21. Zionts LE, MacEwen GD: Spontaneous improvement of post-traumatic tibia valga. J Bone Joint Surg Am 1986; 68:680.
22. Zionts LE, MacEwen GD: Spontaneous improvement of post-traumatic tibia valga. J Bone Joint Surg Am 1986; 68:680.
23. Beaty JH, Kumar A: Current concepts review: Fractures about the knee in children. J Bone Joint Surg Am 1994; 76:1870.
24. Hresko MT, Kasser JR: Physeal arrest about the knee associated with non-physeal fractures in the lower extremity. J Bone Joint Surg Am 1989; 71:698.
25. Birch JG: Surgical technique of physeal bar resection. In Ellert RE (ed): Instructional Course Lectures XLI. Rosemont, IL, American Academy of Orthopaedic Surgeons, 1992.
26. Peterson HA: Review: Partial growth plate arrest and its treatment. J Pediatr Orthop 1984; 4:246.
27. Pappas AM: Congenital posteromedial bowing of the tibia and fibula. J Pediatr Orthop 1984; 4:525.
28. Tuncay IC, Johnston CE II, Birch JG: Spontaneous resolution of congenital anterolateral bowing of the tibia. J Pediatr Orthop 1994; 14:599.
29. Tachdjian MO: In Pediatric Orthopedics. Philadelphia, WB Saunders, 1990 2nd ed, p 658.
30. Anderson DJ, Schoenecker PL, Sheridan JJ, et al: Use of an intramedullary rod for the treatment of congenital pseudarthrosis of the tibia. J Bone Joint Surg Am 1992; 74:161.
31. Weiland AJ, Weiss A-PC, Moore JR, et al: Vascularized fibular grafts in the treatment of congenital pseudarthrosis of the tibia. J Bone Joint Surg Am 1990; 72:654.
32. Fabry G, Lammens J, Melkebeek J, et al: Treatment of congenital pseudarthrosis with the Ilizarov technique. J Ped Orthop 1988; 8:67.
33. Paley D, Catagni M, Argnani F, et al: Treatment of congenital pseudoarthrosis of the tibia using the Ilizarov technique. Clin Orthop 1992; 280:81.

34. Shapiro F: Ollier's disease. An assessment of angular deformity, shortening and pathological fracture in twenty-one patients. J Bone Joint Surg Am 1982; 74:95.

35. Schmale GA, Conrad EU, Raskind WH: The natural history of hereditary multiple exostoses. J Bone Joint Surg Am 1994; 76:986.

36. Pappas AM, Nehme A-M: Hemihypertrophy and hemiatrophy. Clin Orthop 1979; 144:198.

37. Froster UG, Baird PA: Congenital defects of lower limbs and associated malformations: A population-based study. Am J Med Genet 1993; 45:60.

38. Pappas AM, Hanawalt BJ, Anderson M: Congenital defects of the fibula. Orthop Clin North Am 1972; 3:187.

39. Achterman C, Kalamchi A: Congenital absence of the fibula. J Bone Joint Surg Am 1979; 61:133.

40. Oppenheim WL: Fibular deficiency and the indications for Syme's amputation. Prosthet Orthot Int 1991; 15:131.

41. Herring JA: Syme amputation for fibular hemimelia: A second look in the Ilizarov era. In Eilert RE (ed): Instructional Course Lectures. Rosemont, IL, American Academy of Orthopaedic Surgeons, 1992.

42. Ghoneem HF, Wright JG, Cole WG, et al: The Ilizarov method for correction of complex deformities: Psychological and functional outcomes. J Bone Joint Surg Am 1996; 78:1480.

43. Morton AA: Psychological considerations in the planning of staged reconstruction in limb deficiencies. In Herring JA, Birch JG (eds): The Child With a Limb Deficiency. Rosemont, IL, American Academy of Orthopaedic Surgeons, 1998.

44. Birch JG, Walsh SJ, Small JM, et al: Syme amputation for the treatment of fibular deficiency. J Bone Joint Surg Am 1999; 81:1511.

45. Catagni MA, Guerreschi F: Management of fibular hemimelia using the Ilizarov method. In Herring JA, Birch JG (eds): The Child With a Limb Deficiency. Rosemont, IL, American Academy of Orthopaedic Surgeons, 1998.

46. Dal Monte A, Donzelli O: Tibial lengthening according to Ilizarov in congenital hypoplasia of the leg. J Pediatr Orthop 1987; 7:135.

47. Paley D: AAOS meeting, 1999.

48. Schoenecker PL, Capelli AM, Millar EA, et al: Congenital longitudinal deficiency of the tibia. J Bone Joint Surg Am 1989; 71:278.

49. Jones D, Barnes J, Lloyd-Roberts GC: Congenital aplasia and dysplasias of the tibia with intact fibula: Classification and management. J Bone Joint Surg Br 1978; 60:31.

50. Brown FW: Construction of a knee joint in congenital total absence of the tibia (paraxial hemimelia tibia): J Bone Joint Surg Am 1965; 47:695.

51. Loder RT: Fibular transfer for congenital longitudinal deficiency of the tibia (Brown procedure). In Herring JA, Birch JG (eds): The Child With a Limb Deficiency. Rosemont, IL, American Academy of Orthopaedic Surgeons, 1998.

52. Pappas AM: Congenital abnormalities of the femur and related lower extremity malformations: Classification and treatment. J Pediatr Orthop 1983; 3:45.

53. Aitken GT: Proximal femoral focal deficiency: Definition, classification and management. In Aitken GT (ed): Proximal femoral focal deficiency: A congenital anomaly. Washington DC, National Academy of Sciences, 1969.

54. Gillespie R, Torode IP: Classification and management of congenital abnormalities of the femur. J Bone Joint Surg Br 1983; 65:557.

55. van Ness CP: Rotation-plasty for congenital defects of the femur: Making use of the ankle of the shortened limb to control the knee joint of a prosthesis. J Bone Joint Surg Br 1950; 32:12.

56. Torode IP, Gillespie R: Rotationplasty of the lower limb for congenital defects of the femur. J Bone Joint Surg Br 1983; 65:569.

57. Kraybich JI: Rotationplasty in the management of proximal femoral focal deficiency. In Herring JA, Birch JG (eds): The Child with a Limb Deficiency. Rosemont, IL, American Academy of Orthopaedic Surgeons, 1998.

section
9
chapter
24

CLUBFOOT

Alain Diméglio and Frédérique Diméglio

Summary

A Philosophy for Treatment: 10 Recommendations

- The foot must be assessed accurately at birth.
- Treatment is urgent, and each day can make a difference.
- The parents must be available, cooperative, and clearly informed of the treatment plan.
- Orthopaedic treatment should not be stubbornly continued if it fails to produce desirable results; in this case, the need for an operation is clear.
- A complete knowledge of the physiopathology of clubfoot is essential to the proper performance of functional treatment. Rehabilitation must follow the progressive states of correction.
- The physiotherapist has an essential role to play as a contact person for parents, to whom he or she must give accurate and coherent information as well as reassurance.
- Daily manipulations plus use of a passive motion machine can substantially decrease the need for surgery. A passive motion machine makes physiotherapy more effective.
- Training of orthopaedists and therapists treating clubfoot is essential and must be performed on a continuing basis. Videos are useful to improve know-how and avoid gross rehabilitation errors.
- Surgery has a place in the treatment of clubfoot, but it should not be the only modality of treatment. It is, rather, one phase in a strategy aimed at controlling the foot throughout growth. Surgery must be integrated in the framework of treatment, that is, preceded by active and strict manipulation treatment and supplemented by relentless rehabilitation.
- Sequelae of treatment are often disabling, with a stiff, atrophic foot. They often are the consequence of treatment that had not started well, and rarely of the progression of a neurological disease.

The oldest existing written description of clubfoot and its treatment is ascribed to Hippocrates (460–377 BC). In 1575, Ambroise Paré described the deformity. His treatment consisted of manipulations and bandaging. In 1784, Lorenz performed the first Achilles tenotomy. The first detailed description of pathoanatomy of clubfoot was published by Antonio Scarpa in 1803.[54] In 1816, Delpech gave a beautiful description of the three-dimensional deformity.[16] In 1889, Farabeuf analyzed the morphology of the talus.[30] Codvilla, in 1906, published the first posterior and medial release.[10] In 1930, Denis Browne described his special splint, and Kite used plaster casts with encouraging re-

sults.[39–41] In 1971, Turco published the first results of the one-stage posterior and medial release with internal fixation.[64, 66] Since the 1970s, a growing number of surgeons have advocated early soft-tissue release.[6, 12, 17, 18, 44–46, 59–61]

All investigators agree that the so-called idiopathic clubfoot is a diagnosis by exclusion, as is idiopathic scoliosis. It is essential to always search for a cause. The clinical assessment must not be limited to an orthopaedic examination, however. It must be pediatric in a general sense; the examiner must (1) assess the neurological status of the child, (2) check for spinal dysraphism, (3) consider the possibility of an aborted form of neurological disease, such as a congenital myopathy or minimum arthrogryposis, and (4) carefully check the face and the hands of the child. The neonatal ultrasonographic examination is essential today to check the axis of the cord and the condition of the brain and of the heart.

Some diseases may unveil themselves incidentally. A stiff hindfoot should lead the examiner to suspect an invisible neonatal hindfoot coalition. In fact, clubfoot covers a wide spectrum of situations with an infinite number of nuances, from extreme stiffness to complete suppleness. Classification is required but it is inevitably arbitrary. In order to provide a framework for discussion and to assess the results objectively, clubfoot is now codified by order of increasing severity, on a scale ranging from 0 to 20, from extreme mildness to major severity, so that the condition of the foot to be treated can be quickly established.[22]

ETIOLOGY

The pathogenesis and biomechanics of clubfoot are not really well-known. As it grows during intrauterine life, the foot inevitably goes through a phase of physiological equinus before the 12th week. Then it unfolds gradually until it assumes a normal position.

The following four theories attempt to explain the clubfoot condition.

1. *The foetal developmental arrest in the fibula phase.* Bohm postulated that the cause of a clubfoot was an arrest in embryonic development.[5]
2. *The postural theory,* also called extrinsic compression theory, is highly disputable.
3. *The neuromuscular theory,* put forward by Ponseti and Uhthoff, states that a pathological process affects some muscles and is associated with the appearance of fibrotic sheaths.[31, 37, 38, 50]
4. *The malformation theory* holds that the talus is abnormal, especially its neck and head. This deformity becomes a focus of retraction.[36, 56]

The overall incidence rate of talipes equinovarus in the general population is 1.24 per 1000 live births. In their review of the genetic aspect of clubfoot, Cowell and Wein conclude that idiopathic talipes equinovarus is primarily caused by a multifactorial inheritance system, which is modified by intrauterine environmental factors and possibly is affected by a gene acting in a dominant fashion.[11]

PHYSIOPATHOLOGY OF THE FOOT

Scarpa describes the deformity (Fig. 1) as a subluxation of the talocalcaneonavicular complex[54] that leads to a fixed exaggeration of the normal equinovarus position of the foot (Fig. 2). It results from an abnormal relationship between the talus and the os calcis and in a medial displacement of the navicular. Retraction of the muscles, tendons, and ligaments then occurs around this deformity. The posterior tibial muscle and Achilles tendon play a key role in locking the hindfoot in varus and equinus (Fig. 3).

A clubfoot combines inward rotation of the calcaneus and of the foot in equinus and varus, with the forefoot closing up on the heel and the entire foot on the leg. The posterior tibial muscle, regarded as one of the key muscles in clubfoot, displaces the navicular and, along with it, the entire calcaneo-forefoot block, which then comes into varus, adduction, and equinus. The triceps, flexor hallucis longus, and anterior tibialis muscles also take part in this three-dimensional deformity.[25, 55]

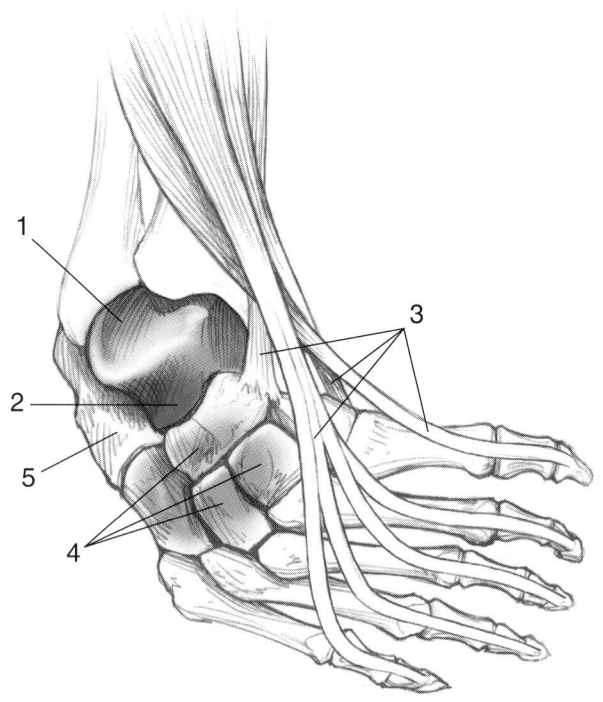

Fig. 2. Diagram. Note the different deformities: 1, equinus in the ankle; 2, talus deformity; 3, Retraction of tibionavicular ligament, anterior tibialis, and long common extensor; 4, Adduction of the forefoot; 5, Inversion of the calcaneus.

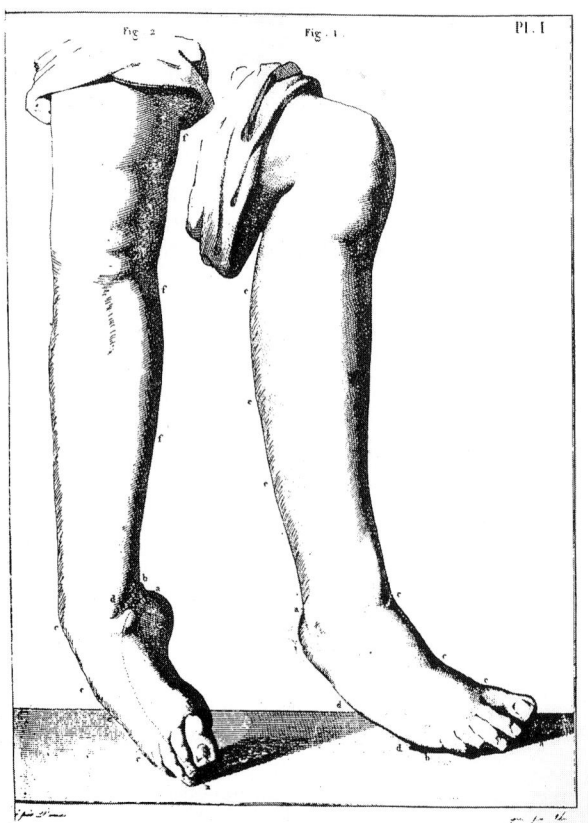

Fig. 1. Diagram. Note the three-dimensional deformity: equinus, varus, and supination. Clubfoot is characterized by a disequilibrium between the lateral column dependent from the calcaneus and the medial column dependent from the talus. For Catterall, the term "varus" is no longer acceptable but is, for the most part, a consequence of forefoot supination and cavus, both of which can be identified. (From Delpech JM: De l'orthomorphie: Considérations sur la difformité appelées pieds bots. Ed Gabon, Montpellier, 1816.)

ANATOMIC FACTS

The following four anatomic facts are associated in this condition:

1. There is a critical relationship between the four bones of the hindfoot—the calcaneus, talus, cuboid, and navicular (Fig. 4). They form the subtalar complex, which should be examined in a broader perspective. The four bones share a continuous joint space. Locking of the hindfoot in equinovarus automatically causes supination of the calcaneo-forefoot block. The foot moves as a whole, as demonstrated by inversion and eversion. Equinus, varus, adduction, and supination in clubfoot are isolated from one another only for intellectual practicality and easier understanding. In fact, they are interrelated and cannot be dissociated.

2. The foot is made of two columns; the talus-dependent column and the calcaneus-dependent column. Restoring proper divergence between the talus and the calcaneus restores the balance between these two columns.[6] As growth in the clubfoot progresses, the lateral column tends to develop much more than the medial column, resulting in the kidney-shaped deformity. Contraction progresses anteroposteriorly, mainly in the tibiotarsal, subtalar, and midtarsal joints, and sometimes in the forefoot.

3. The talus is a peculiar bone, with no tendinous attachments. The calcaneo-forefoot block is an anatomic entity extending from the os calcis to the phalanges. It moves as a block around the talus, by means of the

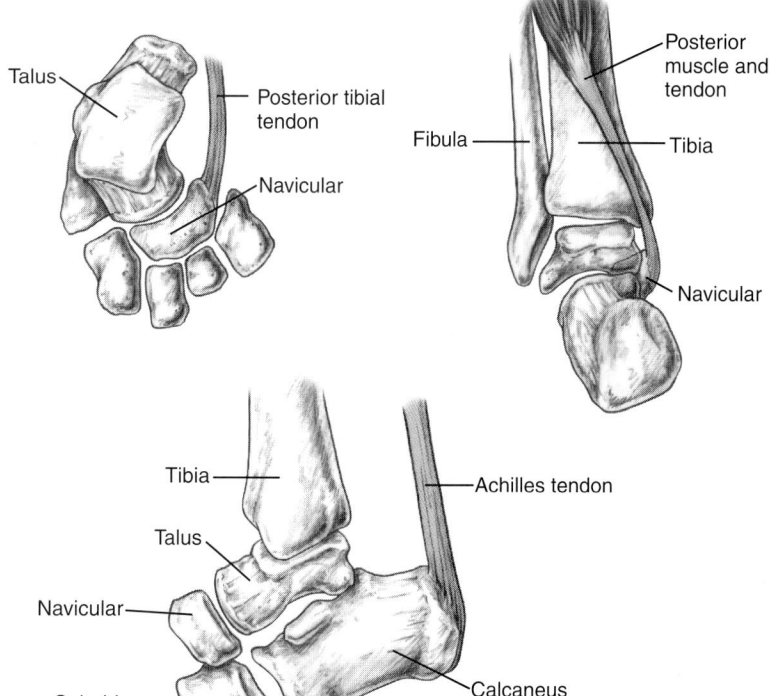

Fig. 3. Diagram. The deformity is increased by the retraction of the Achilles tendon and the posterior tibialis muscle, which act in synchronization.

interosseous talocalcaneal ligament, which acts as a central pivot similar to the cruciate ligaments in the knee.

4. Growth in the foot is characterized by the apposition between hard and soft—between the ossified and non-ossified parts, between fragile structures like the growth cartilage and relatively tough structures like the ossified parts of bones. Each muscle has its own elastic potential. The triceps surae has limited lengthening capacity, and this restriction creates the risk of the tarsal break in the case of major fixed equinus.

CLINICAL ASSESSMENT

Nothing should be done before the foot is clinically assessed.[19] Assessment is an essential stage of management. The deformity of the foot does not herald its reducibility. Palpation is the most important element; nothing can replace touch with an experienced hand. The examiner:

1. Feels the calcaneal contour to determine whether the calcaneus is in place or not.
2. Assesses the lateral aspect of the talus on the anterolateral dorsum of the foot.
3. Tries to reduce the foot in the horizontal (rotation of the calcaneo-forefoot block and adduction), sagittal (equinus), and frontal (varus) planes.
4. Tests muscle tone; reducibility of the foot is essential to success.

Classification of clubfoot distinguishes four categories (Fig. 5), benign, moderate, severe, and very severe.[22] A scale ranging from 0 to 20 has been established, as follows:

- *Grade I:* From 0 to 5; benign, or soft-soft feet are totally reducible feet.

- *Grade II:* From 5 to 10; moderate or soft-stiff feet are reducible, partly resistant feet.
- *Grade III:* From 10 to 15, severe or stiff-soft feet are resistant, partly reducible feet.
- *Grade IV:* From 15 to 20, very severe or stiff-stiff feet are virtually irreducible.

To determine the severity score, the four main parameters are graded for each of 4 possible points (highest total score being 16 points): (1) equinus, (2) hindfoot varus, (3)

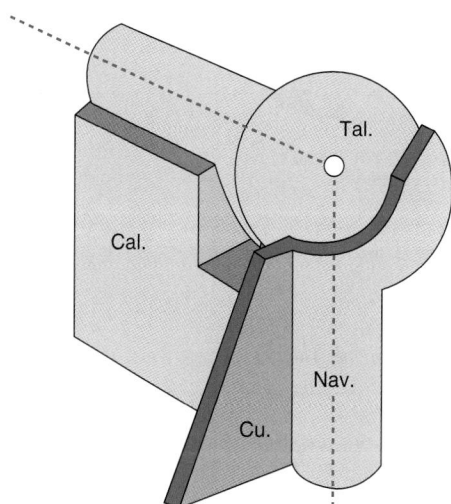

Fig. 4. Diagram. Talus, calcaneus, cuboid, and navicular are involved in the same articulation. The concept of the subtalar joint must include the midtarsal joint. The calcaneocuboid joint is an articulation of stability; the talonavicular joint is an articulation of mobility.[69]

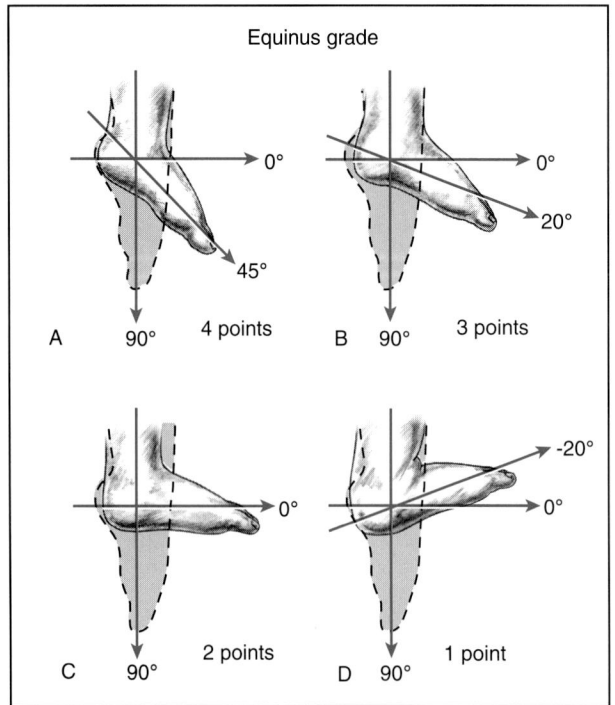

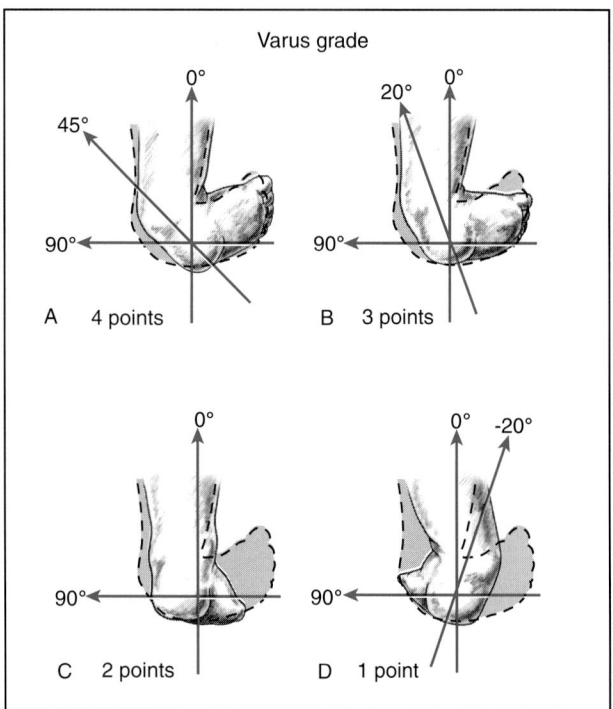

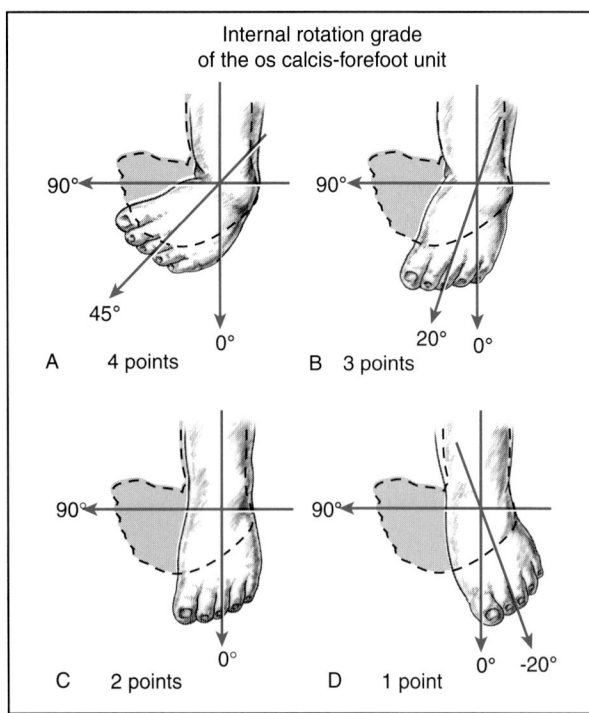

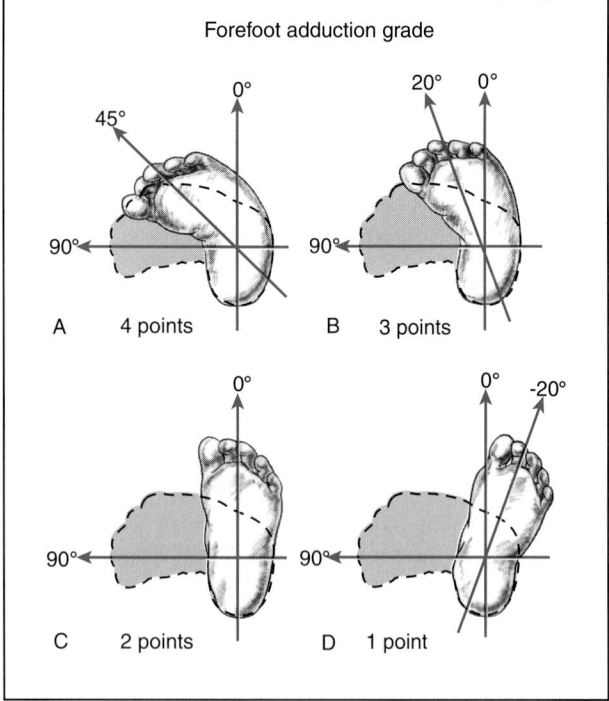

Fig. 5. Diagram and table. Classification of clubfoot.

internal rotation of the calcaneo-forefoot block, and (4) adduction of the forefoot relative to the hindfoot. In addition, four pejorative points may be added to the score if the following unfavorable physical findings are found (highest total score 20 points):

- 1 point for the medial skin crease.
- 1 point for the posterior skin crease.
- 1 point for cavus deformity.

- 1 point for global hypertonia of the baby (or muscles that appear to be fibrous, or suspected severe amyotrophy).

This classification is very useful. It allows monitoring the effectiveness of the orthopaedic treatment each day. The success of manipulations is increased as the foot becomes reducible. This classification allows monitoring the evolution of reducibility throughout treatment.

					TOTAL
Equinus	1	2	3	4	
Varus	1	2	3	4	
Internal rotation	1	2	3	4	
Forefoot add	1	2	3	4	
Posterior crease	1				
Medial crease	1				
Cavus deformity	1				
Muscle quality	1				
				SCORE /20:	

Fig. 5. *(Continued).*

RADIOGRAPHIC ASSESSEMENT

Plain radiographs only show the position in which the foot lies. Stress radiographs identify fixed deformity. Two radiographs are of value. A lateral view with the foot in maximum dorsiflexion should have the fibula superimposed on the tibia. Breeching of the calcaneocuboid or cubometatarsal joints suggests false correction with a rocker-bottom foot. A stress anteroposterior radiograph with the foot in eversion shows the alignment of the calcaneocuboid joint and whether there is a divergence between the talus and calcaneus.

Ultrasonography may be useful to demonstrate a persistent talonavicular dislocation before age 1 year.

PHYSIOTHERAPY AND FUNCTIONAL TREATMENT

GENERAL CONSIDERATIONS

It is our opinion that the physiotherapy of clubfoot is urgent and compulsory and must be performed immediately. In reality, each team has its own principles, and the approaches may be different and sometimes contradictory. However, the functional manipulation plus splinting or successive casting methods have the same fundamental goals: (1) operating on as few clubfeet as possible and (2) when surgery is inevitable, limiting its extent as much as possible.

The value of physiotherapy differs according to the individual school of treatment. Some believe in its utility and perform it consistently, but others regard it as only an auxiliary method that helps differentiate reducible feet from feet that require surgery. Other teams are skeptical about the usefulness of manipulation, thinking that the fibrous retraction is so tough that a surgical knife is needed to release them. Still others believe that the method is difficult to use for geographic or financial reasons.

In fact, manipulating a clubfoot requires a good deal of experience, and a physiotherapist working far from a specialist hospital may not be experienced in the technique. Because of the low incidence rate of clubfoot (1 in 800

births), each practitioner treats only one case every 2 years! Rehabilitation is easier if the family lives close to a university hospital or other major medical center. The daily physiotherapeutic care is demanding and time-consuming. It sometimes lasts more than a year and is expensive. It would be difficult to implement in a health system such as that of the United States. The treatment plan for clubfoot must therefore consider cultural and economic conditions in each country.

Physiotherapy and manipulations are definitely urgent. They could even be started right after birth, as long as the foot has some degree of reducibility. The aim is to quickly reduce the deformity without going so fast as to damage the foot. There is no way to catch up on lost time, and the first days after birth are precious.

PRACTICAL METHOD AND REQUIREMENTS

The practitioner must be guided by the following two fundamental notions:

The Foot Is Fragile During the Neonatal Period

Only 35% of the foot is ossified. The cartilaginous midfoot is the first part to be damaged by improper manipulation. There is a high risk of false correction and rocker-bottom foot deformity. Paradoxically, cartilaginous bones are soft and flexible, whereas the fibrous structures are very tough. The functional method aims at releasing the retracted soft tissue around the posterior tibialis muscle and Achilles tendon and to thus restore the muscle balance of the hindfoot. As long as the tuber of the os calcis is displaced proximally, the deformity is not corrected. The talus is exposed to a great extent by the equinus deviation. It is not visibly crushed, and the talar dome is flattened by varus and equinus. This deformity of the talus can be increased by inappropriate manipulation. The varus deformity persists as long as there is some equinus, and adduction will not subside as long as there is some equinovarus.

Effective manipulation requires a mental vision of the anatomic pattern of clubfoot. The calcaneo-forefoot block and the navicular must be derotated around the talus, and the calcaneus must be lowered posteriorly and raised anteriorly. This may seem like a theoretical exercise, but it is quite complicated in practice.

Correction Must Be Progressive and Gradual

Starting in the horizontal plane, correction proceeds with the adduction of the forefoot and the derotation of the calcaneo-forefoot block, then in the sagittal plane in varus and equinus. The correction is based on the fundamental principle that the calcaneus is involved in the three components of deformity: equinus, varus, and adduction. The posterior tuberosity of the calcaneus is raised and its distal part lowered in adduction and inversion under the talus. The calcaneus is therefore set in equinus, varus, and adduction. The navicular is displaced medially relative to the talar head and may articulate with the medial malleolus. The navicular and calcaneus are normally linked by the spring ligament and move together around the talar head during eversion movements.

The following three changes must be made to correct the deformity:

1. The navicular must be moved from its set medial position on the medial malleolus.
2. The distal part of the calcaneus, which is associated with the head of the talus, must be mobilized.
3. The posterior part of the calcaneus, which is displaced proximally and laterally, must be brought back medially and distally.

Equinus, varus, and adduction all play a part and are combined in a single deformity. Equinus cannot be completely corrected if varus is not, and vice versa.

Any manipulation, however, *must not:*

- Force the foot.
- Try to correct supination by lowering the first metatarsal bone, which causes an aggravation of cavus.[50]
- Twist the midtarsal joint.

There are two methods of French clubfoot manipulation: the functional method developed by Bensahel with Guillaume and the staff of Robert Debré Hospital, and the method developed by Seringe at Saint Vincent-de-Paul Hospital. The Robert Debré method was described by Bensahel and Guillaume in detail in fundamental articles in the *Journal of Pediatric Orthopaedics*.[3, 4] The description of clubfoot correction given here is largely patterned on this method combined with our own experience. The method implemented by Seringe is slightly different. He uses the same principles as the functional method but also proposing the use of rigid corrective splints; this method has been extensively described in many documented articles.[57, 58]

The talus must be firmly held throughout manipulation. The functional manipulation method is sequential and includes:

- Decoaptation of the navicular from the medial malleolus.
- Abduction of calcaneo forefoot block around the talus.
- Correction of equinus.

These manipulations must be performed at least once every day in articular decoaptation in order to avoid excessive pressure and stress of fibrous soft tissue on the cartilage. The maximum amplitude of correction can be obtained, without nociceptive reactions, while the baby is sleeping.[24] This four-step breakdown is very useful and its sequence should be respected. However, as already mentioned, the bones of the hindfoot are interdependent. As in golf or tennis, the trainer breaks down the movements into steps for pedagogical convenience, but the actual movement is a smooth, harmonious sequence that requires experience and many years of work.

Muscle stimulation and a bandage complete the manipulations. The systematic position of a clubfoot, downwards and inwards, hinders proper contraction of the peroneal muscles. In fact, the exaggerated distance from the insertion of these muscles in no case makes eversion easier. Therefore, active rehabilitation is performed right from the first manipulation with the foot in a position that is corrected as far as possible, in order to bring the peroneal muscle insertions closer and to facilitate eversion.

Stimulation is performed with the fingertips or a toothbrush all along the lateral aspect of the foot and the leg. The mother is requested to "tickle" the baby's bandaged foot as often as possible, at the level of the fifth toe. "Global chain" movements are also performed when the baby is awake.

Trying to establish full correction at once is a temptation that must be withstood, because it may eventually produce resistant edema, which stiffens the foot and seems to foster fibrosis. However, even if edema does appear, the foot must still be lightly bandaged and raised. Removing the bandage, even for a day, could cause major regression of clinical gains, especially in newborns.

THE PASSIVE MOTION MACHINE METHOD

The passive motion machine must be used during the first days of life and as often as possible during the first 3 months (Fig. 6). This machine was introduced by Metaizeau in Nancy in 1988, and it has been used only in highly specialized facilities.[23] The prototype could be used only for children at least 4 months old. However, we at the Montpellier school considered that the period between birth and the fourth month was a crucial and precious one. Frédérique Bonnet[23] suggested that components of the machine should be miniaturized to be used on newborns.

The machine in itself is not sufficient to correct clubfoot; it is part of a strategy in which the functional rehabilitation method plays a key role. The machine is used to potentiate the effects of the functional method and as a complement to the manipulation treatment. This method is supported by a regional organization aimed at training physiotherapists who treat clubfeet throughout Languedoc-Roussillon. A video learning method is used, as well as repeated training of physiotherapists specializing in pediatric orthopaedics.

To connect a baby to the passive motion splint, a small sole must be placed under the foot and attached to the machine. The sole will be better attached if it is narrower than the foot. An appropriate bandage must be made with foam and various types of adhesive tape.

RESULTS OF FUNCTIONAL TREATMENT

Bensahel and associates reviewed 338 clubfeet from 1974 to 1978.[3, 4] After a treatment using functional rehabilitation, they obtained good results in 48% of patients, acceptable

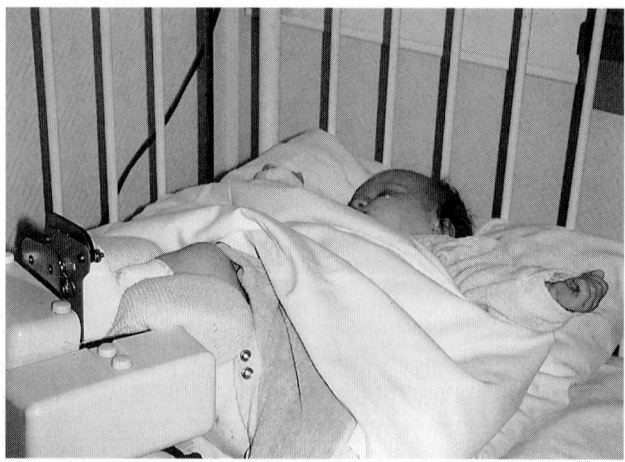

Fig. 6. View. Passive motion machine can be used more than 15 hours a day. Correction is gentle and atraumatic when the baby is sleeping.

results in 29%, and poor results in 23%. Supplementary surgery was therefore required in 52% of cases. Used as a complement to the functional method, surgery gives good results in 86% of patients, fair results in 10%, and poor results in 4%.

In the Seringe series, initial reducibility played a key role.[57, 58] Grade II, moderate (soft-stiff) clubfeet responded to the functional treatment in 67% of cases, grade III, severe (stiff-soft) clubfeet in 57% of cases, and grade IV, very severe (stiff-stiff) clubfeet in 30% of cases. The physiotherapist has a major influence. Only 30% of clubfeet treated by specialist physiotherapists required operation, compared with 58% of those treated by nonspecialist are operated. No cases of softer feet (soft-stiff) that were treated by a specialist physiotherapist required surgery, compared with 40% of those managed by a nonspecialist.

The method we use at Montpellier Hospital (functional treatment plus passive motion machine and plaster) combines the manipulations of the functional method with passive machine and the plaster as early as the first days of life.[23, 24] The first contact with the child's parents is critical. They expect clear explanations. We have to ensure that they understand what the treatment is about, trust us, and therefore cooperate with treatment. The rehabilitation scheme proposed to them must take their potential as givers of treatment into account. The baby must be completely relaxed both for manual functional rehabilitation and for manipulation on the Kinetec machine, with the knee and the hip flexed. Rehabilitation aims at correcting the foot in the various planes of space, and correction must be maintained by a relatively loose bandage.

From 1991 to 1997 at Montpellier Hospital, 200 clubfeet were treated with intensive physiotherapy in combination with a passive motion machine. For all categories, 74% of feet were never operated on. Of the 26% of feet operated on, 14% underwent the so-called conventional procedures, posterior-plantar-medial release; 11% had simple posterior release; and 1% required an extensive operation (i.e., a lateral release of the calcaneocuboid joint)

Of the 41 feet grade IV, very severe (stiff-stiff) feet treated at Montpellier Hospital (Fig. 7), 46% (19) were not operated. For the remaining 54% (22), surgical treatment was distributed as follows:

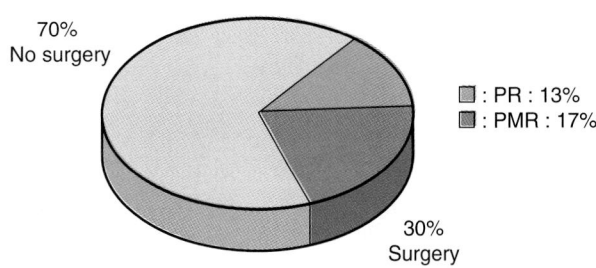

111 severe feet out of 200 feet with intensive physiotherapy

70% No surgery

■ : PR : 13%
■ : PMR : 17%

30% Surgery

Fig. 8. Chart. Grade III: No surgery was performed in 70% of severe clubfeet. Posterior release (PR) was performed in 13%, and posterior medial release (PMR) in 17%.

- Limited posterior release, 12%.
- Conventional posterior-medial release, 32%.
- Extensive surgery, 2%.

Of the 111 feet grade III, severe (stiff-soft) feet (Fig. 8), 70% (78) were not operated on. For the remaining 30% (33), surgical treatment was distributed as follows:

- Limited posterior release, 13%.
- Conventional posterior-medial release, 17%.

Of the 48 feet grade II, moderate (soft-stiff) feet treated at Montpellier Hospital (Fig. 9), treatment with manipulations plus use of the passive motion machine was effective in 100% of cases.

In an experiment, use of this treatment achieved a reduction in the number of surgical cases each year. The rate of surgical procedures decreased from 40% in the first series (1991 to 1992) to 12% in the last series (1997) (Fig. 10) The effectiveness of the machine is obvious (Figs. 11 and 12). Our results show that well-performed, organized, supervised orthopaedic treatment that is coordinated by a unit set up in the department of pediatric orthopaedics and that involves strict compliance with the guidelines of the functional method can noticeably reduce the number of surgical procedures. There are few disadvantages and no occurence of skin disorder, growth cartilage crush, or false reduction. This perfect synchronization between functional treatment and passive motion machine makes surgery less frequent, more elective, and less extensive. The passive motion ma-

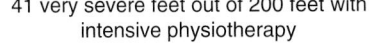

41 very severe feet out of 200 feet with intensive physiotherapy

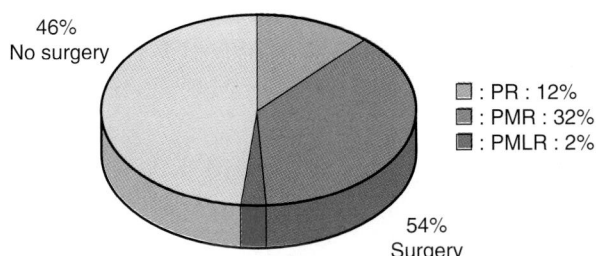

46% No surgery

■ : PR : 12%
■ : PMR : 32%
■ : PMLR : 2%

54% Surgery

Fig. 7. Chart. Grade IV: No surgery was performed in 46% of very severe clubfeet. Posterior release (PR) was performed in 12%, posterior-medial release (PMR) in 32%, and posterior-medial lateral release (PMLR) in 2%.

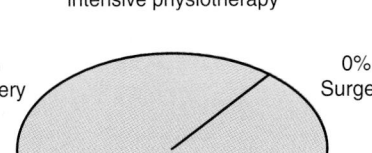

48 moderate feet out of 200 feet with intensive physiotherapy

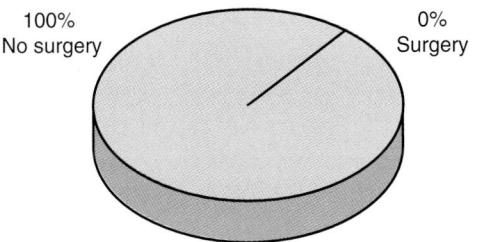

100% No surgery

0% Surgery

Fig. 9. Chart. Grade II: 100% of clubfeet were not operated on.

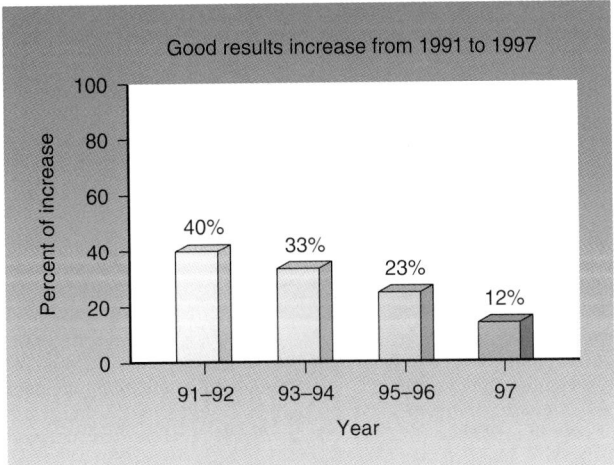

Fig. 10. Chart. The learning curve in treatment is essential. In 1991 to 1992, 40% of club feet were operated on, but in 1997, only 12%.

chine optimizes orthopaedic treatment and makes it more effective.

The economic aspect of such treatment deserves consideration. The treatment method is very demanding because it requires many daytime hospitalizations during the first 3 months of life. However, these expenses are offset by the number of cases in which surgery is avoided. Surgery also involves casts, not to mention the risks of recurrences and complications. One physiotherapist can treat and follow 50 children with clubfeet a year and save 38 children a year from surgery; the therapist's salary for 1 year corresponds to the cost of the surgical treatment for 10 clubfeet.

THE PLASTER CAST METHOD

The plaster cast method was developed by Kite and Ponseti.[39–42, 50] The latter believes that clubfoot is akin to fibrous collagen diseases, such as Dupuytren's disease. In his opinion, surgical release cannot abolish an infiltrating, torpid, and recurrent process.

As early as birth, it is urgent to immobilize and correct the foot in order to put the ligaments to rest and to let the inflammatory storm abate. Ponseti believes that stretching the ligaments and manipulating the foot daily is a fatal mistake, because repetitive manipulations stimulate cell proliferation. In his approach, immobilization in casts has the advantage of relaxing the ligaments by gradually unfolding the foot.

This theory is paradoxical in the view of physiotherapists, whose primary function is to mobilize joints. This philosophy is therefore the opposite of that of Salter, who always considered that a joint had to be kept moving to preserve its cartilage. Therefore, it is difficult to find a way through a complex body of contradictory information.

Kite and Ponseti emphasize the following points:

1. The casts can be made without the use of general anesthesia.
2. The knee must always be included in the cast.
3. The equinus must be preserved.

A set of three plaster casts are made at 2-week intervals. On the 45th day, percutaneous tenotomy of the Achilles tendon is performed. Then manipulations are continued, sometimes with the use of splints. In imperfectly responding cases, Ponseti proposes transplantation of the anterior tibialis muscle onto the lateral aspect of the foot later during growth, at age 2 or 3 years. He states that this treatment solves 80% of problems and regards conventional clubfoot surgery as too aggressive.

The cast, including the knee, progressively derotates the foot and the calcaneo-forefoot block. This may be a useful method when the family cannot make daily commutes for treatment. The cast, also called a "braking cast," primarily helps reduce the horizontal component of the deformity. It cannot correct posterior retraction, however, especially not equinus and varus.

After the series of casts, some surgeons proceed with manipulations and bandages, using splints at nights. Others believe that the casts provide the best correction achievable. They propose early surgery, as early as the fourth month, to release the resistant fibrous structures, particu-

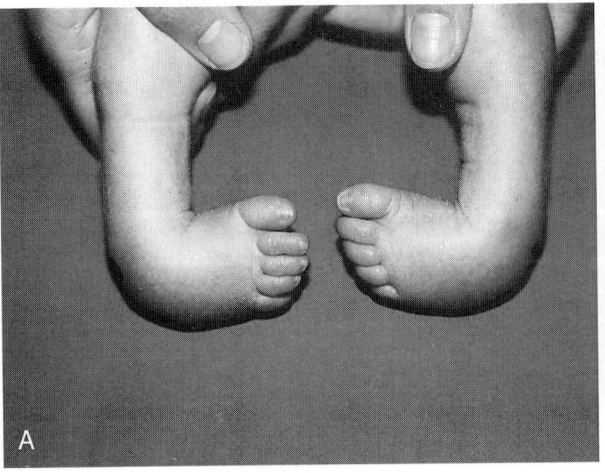
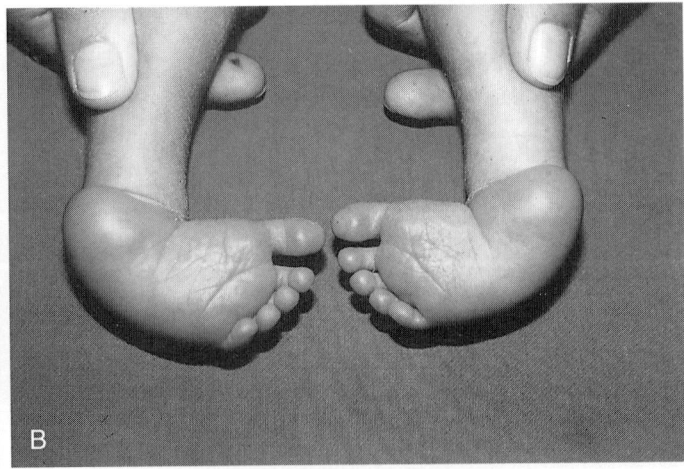

Fig. 11. View. Bilateral stiff-stiff foot was treated with manipulations and passive motion machine.

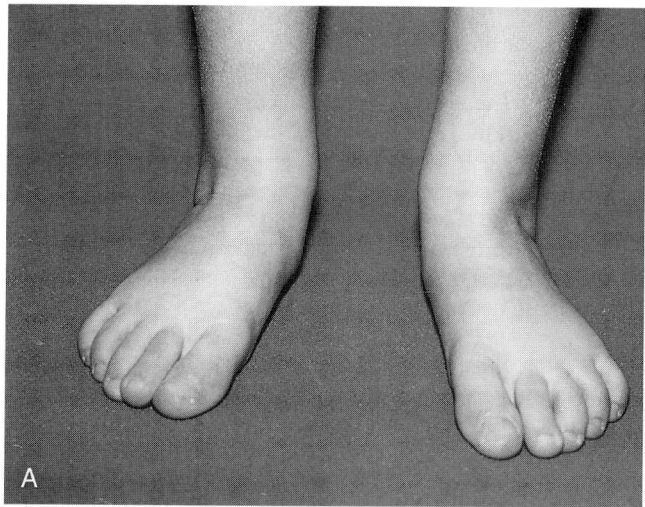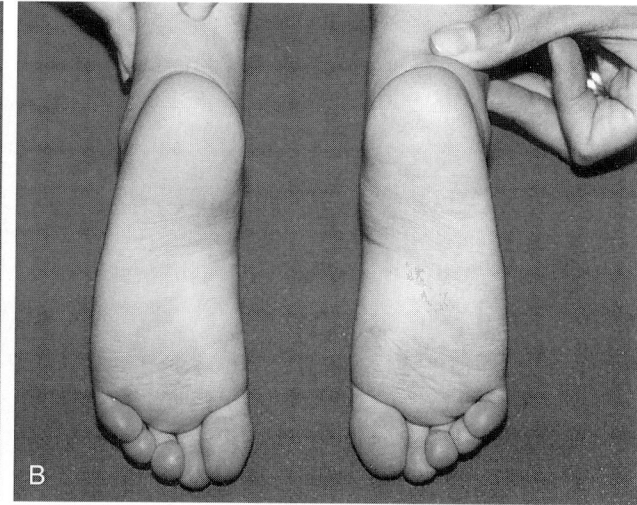

Fig. 12. View. Results of patient in Figure 11 at 5 years of age.

larly the posterior ones. This procedure includes posterior release with lengthening of Achilles tendon, posterior lengthening of all tendons, and sometimes subtalar capsulotomy.[18]

The use of plaster casts is a popular method for treatment of clubfoot in Europe, where a survey revealed that 80% of surgeons preferred them to conventional manipulation.

SURGICAL TREATMENT

INDICATIONS AND TIMING

Surgical treatment is required when the orthopaedic treatment is no longer effective and progress has come to a halt. The first 3 months of life are crucial, as progress is less evident after that. The assessment on the third month is important. It may reveal either one of two situations that will require a decision:

- The functional plus passive motion machine treatment must be continued because it is effective, and surgery can be avoided.
- Or the orthopaedic treatment can be continued to maintain the progress made, with the knowledge that surgery will be required. In this case, the date of the surgical treatment will be chosen by the surgeon.

Some teams prefer operating on the feet when the child is 6 months, others at 9 months or 12 months. Various surveys have shown no significant difference in results when feet were operated on after 6 months. The date of surgery varies according to the surgeon's experience.[14] A high proportion of children with clubfeet undergo surgery between 6 and 9 months of age. Surgery during the neonatal period and before 6 months of age is appealing in principle, but there is a high rate of recurrence, and fibrous reactions are very intensive during the first months of life. It is impossible to maintain the correction achieved. We no longer contemplate this kind of surgery.[52, 53]

GENERAL PRINCIPLES

Surgery follows three basics principles:

1. It is a plastic surgery. The sheaths and tendons must be preserved with the same care as in hand surgery. Any lengthening of the white portion of a muscle inevitably leads to fibrosis. In order to release a retracted muscle, it is better to perform lengthening at the junction of the red and white portions, double intermuscular recession, as in surgery for cerebral palsy. This procedure has been well described by Atar and colleagues.[1]
2. The more the foot has been reduced previously, the easier and more limited surgery becomes. The preoperative manipulations and casts prepare the skin and reduce the deformity.
3. The extent of surgery depends on the severity of the deformity. Surgery must be selective à la carte.[3] There is a place for limited surgery.[6, 19] A total plantar-lateral-medial-posterior release is not required for every clubfoot.[7, 21]

OPERATIVE TECHNIQUES

Surgery proceeds in several steps: posterior release, plantar release, and midtarsal release follow a hierarchic sequence. We prefer starting with posterior release and then, if needed, proceed with plantar and midtarsal release.[19-21, 65-68]

Several types of incision are described: medial L incision or Cincinnati incision and a double posterolateral and medial incision, which we prefer.[12]

In surgery to treat clubfeet, four structures must absolutely be preserved:

- The interosseous ligament.
- The medial collateral ligament.
- The bifurcate ligament.
- The tendon sheaths.

Posterior Release

This consists (Figs. 13 and 14) of a posterolateral incision, opening of the peroneal muscle sheath with a section of

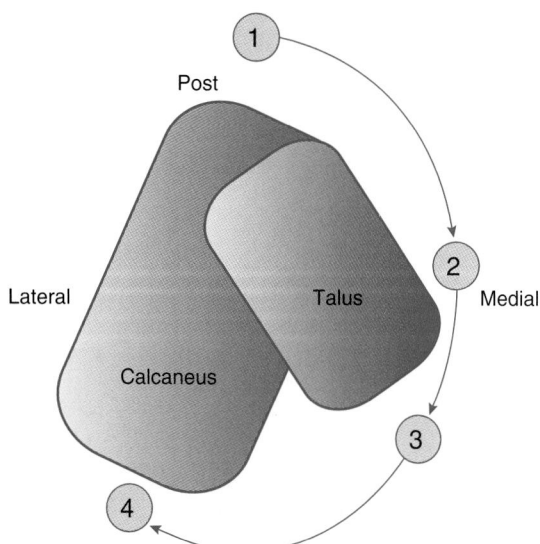

Fig. 13. Diagram. Surgery starts with posterior release. Plantar, medial, and eventually, if necessary, midtarsal releases are performed à la carte. The extent of surgery depends on the severity and the rigidity of the deformity.

the posterolateral knot, tibiotarsal and posterior subtalar capsulotomies, double intermuscular recession of the flexor hallucis longus and, if required by the extent of retraction, double intermuscular recession of the tibialis posterior and the flexor digitorum longus muscles. The posterior-medial edge must be totally released, including resection of the posterior part of the medial collateral ligament. At the end of dissection, the talus fits into the tibiotarsal groove. The upper and medial part of its dome is often deformed, giving a mirror image of the extent of equinus and varus. The posterior tibial neurovascular pedicle must be carefully dissected to release it from its sheath of fibrosis. After careful location of the entrance of the calcaneal canal, the medial and posterior aspects of the calcaneus must be released posterior to the neurovascular pedicle to better correct the varus deviation.

In moderate forms of clubfoot, posterior release may be sufficient. Some feet have a minor degree of equinus. In some cases, posterior release may avoid lengthening of the Achilles tendon. If the posterior release is not sufficient, a profile radiograph with the foot in dorsiflexion shows a persistent lack of divergence between the talus and the calcaneus. In this case, the surgeon should proceed with plantar and medial releases.

Plantar Release

In our opinion, plantar release (Fig. 15) is the fundamental step for severe forms of clubfoot. It should be not timid but accurate and complete, very much like a real Steindler procedure.[63, 67]

After a medial incision is made and the posterior tibial neurovascular pedicle is located at the entrance of the calcaneal canal, the origin of the abductor hallucis on the medial aspect of the calcaneus is dissected. Dissection is then extended to the sole of the foot to release the plantar muscles, which continue the fibrous lamina of the triceps.

Complete release of the abductor hallucis causes a forward displacement by at least 2 cm. After the muscle is detached from the medial aspect of the calcaneus, it must be dissected from the vascular pedicle. The plantar fascia, flexor digitorium brevis, and abductor digiti minimi pedis are completely released from the heel. The plantar release is an "advancement plasty" of the abductor hallucis and plantar muscles. In addition, the long plantar ligament must be divided in the region of the calcaneocuboid joint.

After the plantar release, medial release is very easy. The foot is becoming "soft and reducible."

Medial Release

This step always include the release of the posterior tibialis muscle with its ramifications reaching out to the sole of the foot. This long dissection allows addition of some length, and at the end of the procedure, the distal portion can be reinserted on the navicular. The release of the talonavicular joint includes the revision of Henry's knot and progressive reduction.

If the deformity is severe, dissection should be continued under the plantar aspect of the midtarsal joint. After exposure of the peroneus longus, the calcaneocuboid joint should be opened. The interosseus ligament, the deep portion of the medial deltoid ligament, and the bifurcate ligament must be respected.

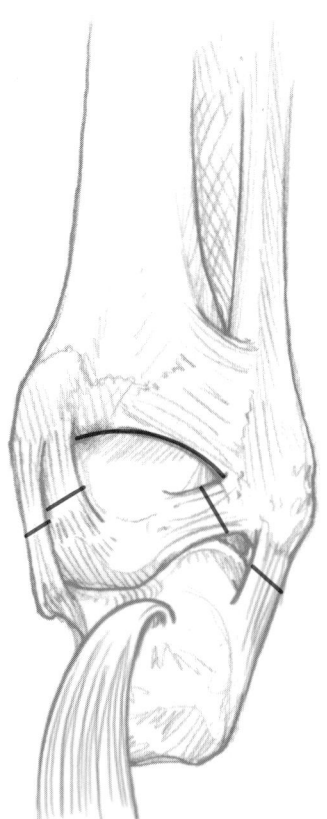

Fig. 14. Diagram. Posterior release. Release of the peroneal muscle sheath and of the calcaneofibulae ligament are essential. Release of the subtalar joint must be limited. The surgeon should avoid cutting the interosseus ligament.

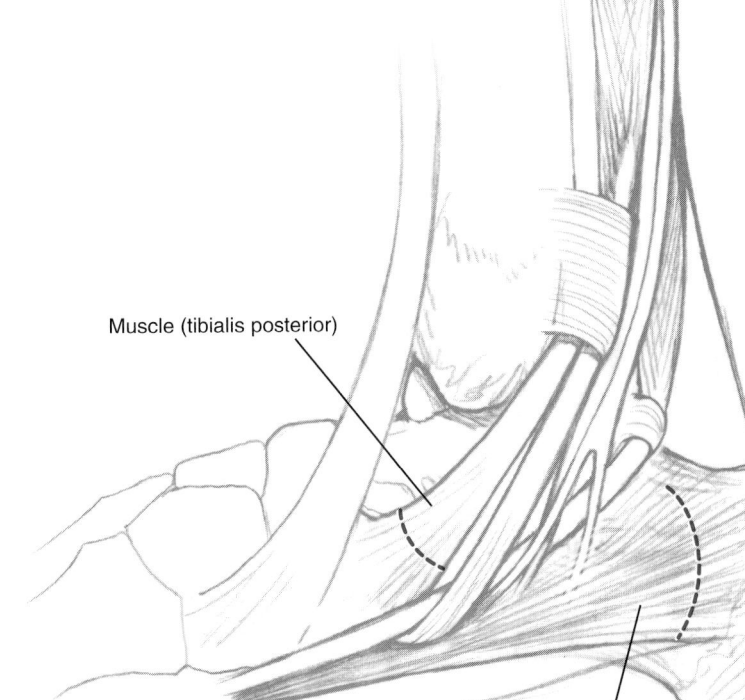

Fig. 15. Diagram. Plantar and medial release. After dissection of the vessels and nerves, plantar release is performed. A substantial advancement of the abductor hallucis muscle and of the plantar muscle must be obtained. With preservation of the sheath and the medial collateral ligament, the distal part of the posterior tibialis is released. Sheaths of the tendons must be preserved. The surgeon should avoid lengthening the muscle in the white portion. Plantar release must be performed before talonavicular release.

Muscle (tibialis posterior)

Plantar muscle and abductor muscle Hallucis

Confirmation of Reduction

The deformity of the foot is reduced at the end of these various steps. It is not necessary to make a counterpart incision on the lateral aspect of the foot, in the calcaneocuboid region, to reduce the lateral column; this additional lateral procedure only has limited indications. Several signs confirm reduction:

- The hindfoot is in light valgus.
- The talus is well balanced in the tibiotarsal groove.
- A straight lateral column.
- A deployed midtarsal joint.

Fixation and Cast Application

It is essential to fix the medial column with a pin inserted posteroanteriorly: the Kirshner wire is placed posteriorly in the long axis of the talar body, which is internally rotated in the ankle mortise. (This technical procedure is recommended by Carroll.[6–8]) The incisions are closed after release of the tourniquet. If the Achilles tendon has been lengthened (its suture should be performed with the foot angled at 90 degrees), the fixation pin should be buried.

A light cast, more similar to a semirigid bandage, must be used to maintain reduction. It must be renewed on the eighth day and kept on for 2 months with the knee included in the cast, and then another month without including the knee. The pin is removed at the end of the third month.

POSTOPERATIVE REHABILITATION

Surgically correcting a foot is one thing, and maintaining correction another. Rehabilitation becomes much easier once retraction is abolished. It is up to the physiotherapist to maintain mobility and prevent recurrence. It is advisable to use the passive motion machine, which makes handling much easier during this period. The foot must be mobilized in all planes, including plantar-flexion. It is essential to stimulate the peroneal muscles to avoid inward rotation during walking. The physiotherapist's work is easier once the baby can stand.

After the child has learned to walk, additional exercises can be added, such as walking on tip toe and walking on the heel, or with the foot attached to small plates of wood resembling miniature skis to stimulate the dorsiflexors and evertor muscles. Everything must be done to restore the best possible mobility, both passive and active. Inward rotation must be countered, and the parents must be instructed not to let the child sleep on the belly, because in that position the feet are locked in plantar-flexion. Splints may be prescribed for the night in order to avoid a recurrence of equinus. Shoes with a strong counter and a straight or antivarus inner edge should be proposed.[24]

ASSESSMENT DURING GROWTH

An objective assessment is required, but it is not easy after only 1 or 2 years. When the navicular starts ossifying around age 5 years, it becomes easier to perform a radiographic evaluation of the foot, which must then be repeated at 10 years. The functional assessment must take into account (1) the deformities of the hindfoot (varus or valgus) (2) the mobility of the subtalar joint, which is often reduced by half, (3) the mobility in plantar and dorsal flexion, and (4) the overall axis of the lower limb.

A radiographic assessment is obviously essential to assessment. The divergence between the talus and calcaneus must be assessed on anteroposterior and profile views, but the general morphology of the bones must also be checked, especially a flattened talus or a subluxation of the navicular, which always is a bad sign.

The functional assessment consists of evaluation of (1) the gait on tiptoes and on the heels, (2) the way the child goes down stairs, stands on one foot, can (or cannot) jump a rope, and walks on an irregular ground, (3) the wear of the shoes, (4) the unrolling of the foot, and (5) calf atrophy. The examiner should look for a recurvatum knee, which may conceal the equinus of the foot; a weakness of the triceps, which always causes problems; and weak toe flexors.

Assessment methods are well described by Lehman and Seringe in Epeldegui's book.[26] This very comprehensive examination made at ages 5 years and 10 years allows correction of some good results that relapse. The relative mobility of the feet is often surprising: Even when dorsiflexion and plantar-flexion are correct, pronation and supination are more frequently limited than expected. Talus foot is always invalidating; only 50% of children can walk on tiptoes after surgery.

COMPLICATIONS
Relapse
Surgery for clubfoot is difficult, and recurrence is always disastrous. This is probably the most extensive type of foot surgery, and it involves devastating actions like lengthening, the opening of tendon sheaths, and capsulotomies. The relapse rate is 20%.[13, 28, 43]

Surgical cuts are always a cause of fibrosis. Surgery for relapsed clubfoot can have only very modest goals and should be used only for salvage. The margin between success and failure after surgery is very narrow. Reduction must be accurate to within millimeters. The best surgery is the one that allows one to perform all actions at the same time (Fig. 16).

The many causes of recurrence can be summed up as follows:

1. The severity of the foot plays a major role. The risk of recurrence is higher in severe stiff-stiff feet than in moderate, reducible feet such as soft-stiff feet.
2. The surgeon's lack of experience is an important factor. This complex surgery requires long practice and highly elaborate tactical and technical skills.
3. Timid surgery inevitably leads to recurrence. On the contrary, massive and extensive surgery can be a cause of stiffness and overcorrection. The golden mean is difficult to find.
4. There is always a risk of leaving a cause undetected, such as tarsal coalition, a neurological disease, or a degenerative disease such as Charcot-Marie-Tooth-Hoffman syndrome or spinal dysraphism.
5. The lack of postoperative monitoring is fatal. Retention of the foot in a splint and manipulation must be continued after surgery. Watchful observation must never cease. It is an error to believe that clubfoot surgery solves all problems once and for all.

When recurrence has been established, all the problems must be identified. Recurrence can be *moderate*, merely

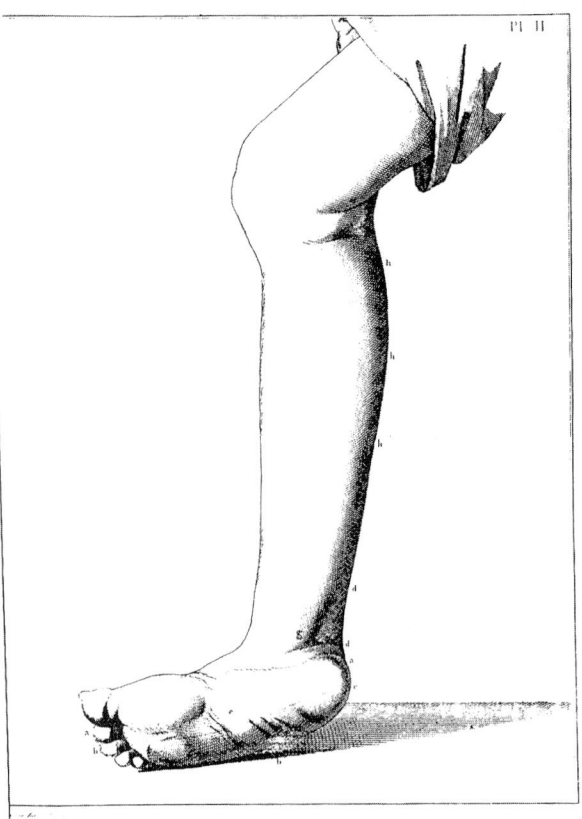

Fig. 16. Relapsed clubfoot: equinus, varus, supination, and cavus are combined. Plantar release is essential. Correction of the disequilibrium between the medial column and the lateral column is necessary. (From Delpech JM: De l'Orthomorphie: Considérations sur la difformité appelées pieds bots. Ed Gabon, Montpellier, 1816.)

consisting in forefoot adduction or a defect in dorsiflexion. Such minor deformities should be accepted, and the temptation of a second procedure should be resisted. It is difficult to put a figure on these cases of moderate recurrence, but they make up about 10% of cases.

Alternatively, recurrence may be *extensive* and may cause walking disorders. Second surgery is then necessary. Its result greatly depends on the previous procedure. If initial surgery was limited, there is hope that the situation can be corrected and an acceptable result achieved. If the first procedure has been extensive and mutilating, however, second surgery is bound to be difficult and unrewarding and to yield inevitably mediocre results.

Preoperative Assessment
It should consist of the following steps:

1. The condition of the muscles must be assessed, and the remaining strength of the triceps and of the flexor muscles beneath the fibrosis must be checked.
2. The condition of the skin, especially in the region of the os calcis, can be a critical factor in healing.
3. The trophic condition of the foot must be assessed. One should check its warmth and sensation and feel for the pulse of the dorsal and posterior tibial arteries.
4. Radiographic assessment is essential to appreciate the condition of bones: flattening of the talus and dorsal

dislocation of the navicular always have a poor prognosis.

5. Checking for plantar retraction is essential. Tarraf and Carroll emphasize this aspect of the problem, believing that plantar contracture retraction is a primary factor in recurrence.[7, 63]

Surgery for relapse of clubfoot is always dangerous. It entails a risk for the skin and the blood vessels. Advice should be sought from a plastic surgeon, and a preoperative arteriographic study should be performed to check the integrity of the blood vessels.[33, 62] The preoperative arteriograph is required for three reasons:

- The first operation may have cut off a vessel or increased its fragility.
- There is vascular abnormality in 20% of clubfeet.[33, 62]
- Second surgery will inevitably be time-consuming, and it may require repeated use of a pneumatic tourniquet.

Technical Precautions

For recurrent clubfoot, two strategies are available: a total second surgery or a limited surgery.

Total Second Surgery. This often requires posterior, medial, plantar, midtarsal, and lateral releases. A few precautions must be taken:

1. A new approach should be chosen and, if possible, the second cut should be performed in a healthy area; for instance, a lateral incision can be performed if the initial surgery was done through a large medial incision.
2. Further lengthening of the Achilles tendon can only increase its weakness.
3. The tendons are often fibrosed, especially if they have been lengthened in the calcaneal canal during initial surgery, or if the tendon sheaths have been open or excised.
4. The posterior tibialis muscle is often fibrotic. It must be definitively detached from the navicular, and it may have to be attached to another muscle, for example, to strengthen the triceps, or transplanted through the interosseous membrane.

Plantar release is always necessary. It must be extensive and is a fundamental step in this second surgery. If the abductor hallucis is too extensively fibrosed, it must be sacrificed.

Midtarsal release must be total, and an extensive approach on the lateral aspect of the foot may have to be chosen to realign the lateral column, using calcaneal or cuboid osteotomy and reaching to the hidden aspect of the talus. The lateral and medial columns absolutely must be pinned. This second surgery is unrewarding and often disappointing. Of course, the effort and the extent of surgery should be tailored to the degree and severity of recurrence. The tourniquet must be removed at the end of the operation to check the condition of blood vessels.

Limited Surgery. Limited surgery is another option for relapse of clubfoot. In some cases, the hindfoot seems to be in a correct condition; that is, there is no varus deviation, although the dorsal or plantar flexion of the foot is limited. There is often a medial deviation with adduction.

In such cases, surgery can involve only the midtarsal joint, based on Evans' philosophy.[28]

Limited surgery generally consists of:

1. Release of the talonavicular dislocation, with a fixation wire.
2. Extensive plantar release.
3. Release of the lateral column with calcaneal or cuboid osteotomy.

Other maneuvers are possible, such as the transplantation of the tibialis anterior to the lateral aspect to try to obtain a plantigrade foot. Ippolito and Ponseti believe that this procedure may correct many jeopardized feet.[35] This limited surgery is possible when there is an active supination during the swing phase, accompanied by increasing adductus and forefoot supination.

Surgery of the forefoot to correct adduction is not sensible, and it entails a risk of additional stiffness in the only area of the foot that is not harmed. In many cases, forefoot adduction must be accepted. Residual deformity of the forefoot in most clubfeet is secondary to residual deformity of the hindfoot. Metatarsal osteotomies are rarely indicated; we do not recommend the procedure of Heyman.

Recommendations

There should be no illusion about surgery of relapsed clubfoot. Although it corrects the morphology of the foot, it causes new areas of stiffness. The aim is to obtain a plantigrade, functional, painless foot. An objective analysis of the results is often disappointing. In most cases, there is a limitation of hindfoot mobility. The foot does not move well during a step. Pronation and supination are virtually nonexistent, and the arc of mobility in the sagittal plane never exceeds 30 degrees. It is difficult to know what will become of these feet in the long term, after 20 or 30 years.

We have no experience with Illizarov's method of second surgery, a gradual procedure that requires time and a lot of experience. This method may be valuable aid after

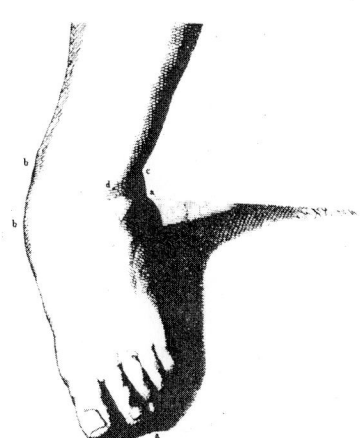

Fig. 17. Overcorrection is the result of extensive surgery. The lateral column is shortened and the medial column is too long. Lengthening of the lateral column is recommended. (From Delpech JM: De l'Orthomorphie: Considérations sur la difformité appelées pieds bots. Ed Gabon, Montpellier, 1816.)

multiple previous operations. Triple-arthrodesis surgery aimed at joint fusion is always possible at the end of growth. However, if recurrence appears around 5 or 6 years of age, it is better to take the risk of surgery for release than to wait until triple arthrodesis can be performed. Bone deformities tend to worsen with time. The result of triple arthrodesis can be highly uncertain in case of talar deformity. Fortunately, the children's functional adaptations are often surprising, and the results of clubfoot surgery, however poor, remain acceptable and compatible with normal life.

Recurrence of clubfoot can be avoided with experience, surgery tailored to each individual case, watchful and rigorous postoperative monitoring, and the preparation for sur-gery with manipulation or casts. The decision to operate again must be given a great deal of thought.

Hypercorrection

Hypercorrection is a difficult deformity to treat. Overcorrection must be avoided through preservation of the deep portion of the deltoid ligament, the interosseus ligament between the talus and the os calcis. The navicular must not be overdisplaced laterally. The valgus of the hindfoot can be corrected by an osteotomy of the os calcis. The shortening of the lateral column must be treated by a lengthening of the os calcis as described by Evans and Mosca.[3] Stabilization of the subtalar joint with a Grice procedure is necessary in severe overcorrection (Fig. 17).

REFERENCES

1. Atar D, Lehman WB, Grant AD, et al: Fractional lengthening of the flexor tendons in clubfoot surgery. Clin Orthop 1991; 267:9.

2. Attenborough CG: Congenital talipes equinovarus. J Bone Joint Surg Br 1966; 48:31.

3. Bensahel H, Guillaume A, Czukonyi Z, et al: Results of physical therapy for idiopathic clubfoot: A long-term follow-up study. J Pediatr Orthop 1990; 10:189.

4. Bensahel H, Guillaume A, Csukonyi Z, et al: The intimacy of clubfoot: The ways of functional treatment. J Pediatr Orthop 1994; 3:155.

5. Bohm M: The embryologic origin of clubfoot. J Bone Joint Surg 1929; 11:229.

6. Carroll NC: The pathoanatomy of congenital clubfoot. Orthop Clinic North Am 1978; 9:225.

7. Carroll NC: Clubfoot. In Morrissy RT (ed): Pediatric Orthopaedics. Philadelphia, JB Lippincott, 1990, 3rd ed.

8. Carroll NC: Controversies in the surgical management of clubfoot. Instr Course Lect 1996; 45:331.

9. Catterall A: A method of assessment of the clubfoot deformity. Clin Orthop Relat Res 1991; 264:48.

10. Codvilla A: Sulla cura del piede equino varo congenito: Nuovo metodo di cura cruenta. Archivo Orthopedica 1906; 23:245.

11. Cowell JR, Wein BK: Genetic aspects of clubfoot. J Bone Joint Surg Am 1980; 62:1381.

12. Crawford AH, Marxen JL, Osterfeld DL: The Cincinnati incision: A comprehensive approach for surgical procedures of the foot and ankle in children. J Bone Joint Surg Am 1982; 64:55.

13. Crawford AH, Gupta AK: Clubfoot controversies: Complications and causes for failure. Instr Course Lect 1996; 45:339.

14. Cummings RJ, Lovell WW: Current concepts review: Operative treatment of congenital idiopathic clubfoot. J Bone Joint Surg Am 1988; 70:1108.

15. Deitz FR, Ponsei IV, Buckwalter JA: Morphometric study of clubfoot. J Pediatr Orthop 1983; 3:311.

16. Delpech JM: De l'Orthomorphie: Considérations sur la difformité appelées pieds bots. Ed Gabon, Montpellier 1816.

17. Depuy J, Drennan JC: Correction of idiopathic clubfoot: A comparison of results of early versus delayed posteromedial release. J Pediatr Orthop 1989; 9:44.

18. De Sanctis N, Nunziata R: Long-term results of a modified radical posterior release in moderate to severe clubfoot. J Pediatr Orthop B 1993; 1:158.

19. Diméglio A: Le pied bot. Montpellier, Sauramps Médical diffusion Vigot, 1985.

20. Diméglio A, Bonnel F, Pous JG: La croissance du pied. In Idiopathic Club Foot. Montpellier, Sauramps Médical, 1986.

21. Diméglio A: Strategic errors in surgery for Clubfoot. In Epeldegui T (ed): Update and Controversies on Clubfoot. Madrid, A Madrid Vicente ediciones, 1993, p 223.

22. Diméglio A, Bensahel H, Souchet Ph, et al: Classification of clubfoot. J Pediatr Orthop B 1995; 4:129.

23. Diméglio A, Bonnet F: Orthopaedic treatment and passive motion machine: Consequences for the surgical treatment of clubfoot. J Pediatr Orthop B 1996; 5:173.

24. Diméglio A, Bonnet F: Rééducation du pied bot varus equin. Encycl Méd Chir (Elsevier, Paris) Kinésithérapie-Médedine physique-Réadaptation, 26-428-B-10, 1997, 12p.

25. Diméglio A, Herrisson Ch, Simon L: Le pied de l'enfant et de l'Adolescent. Paris, Masson, 1998.

26. Epeldegui T: Update and Controversies on Clubfoot. Madrid, A Madrid Vicente ediciones, 1993, p 223.

27. Epeldegui T, Delgado M: Acetabulum pedis. Part I: Talocalcaneonavicular joint socket in clubfoot. J Pediatr Orthop B 1995; 4:11.

28. Evans D: Relapsed clubfoot. J Bone Joint Surg Br 1961; 43:722.

29. Evans D: Calcaneo-valgus deformity. J Bone Joint Surg Br 1975; 57:270.

30. Farabeuf LH: Interventions dans les pieds bots. In Precis de Manuel Opératoire. Paris, Masson, 1889, p 834.

31. Feldbrin Z, Gilai AN, Ezra E, et al: Muscle imbalance in the aetiology of idiopathic club foot: An electromyographic study. J Bone Joint Surg Br 1995; 77:596.

32. Handelsman JE, Baladamante ME: Neuromuscular studies in clubfoot. J Pediatr Orthop 1981; 1:23.

33. Hootnick DR, Levinsohn EM, Crider RJ, et al: Congenital arterial malformations associated with clubfoot. Clin Orthop 1982; 167:160.

34. Husson A: An anatomical and functional study of the tarsus. PhD dissertation, Leiden University, 1961.

35. Ippolito E, Ponseti IV: Congenital clubfoot in the human fetus: A histological study. J Bone Joint Surg Am 1980; 62:8.

36. Irani RN, Sherman MS: The pathological anatomy of clubfoot. J Bone Joint Surg Am 1963; 45:45.

37. Isaacs H, Handelsman JE, Badenhorst M, et al: The muscles in clubfoot: A histological, histochemical, and electron microscopic study. J Bone Joint Surg Br 1977; 59:465.

38. Kawashima T, Uhthoff HK: Development of the foot in prenatal life in relation to idiopathic club foot. J Pediatr Orthop 1990; 10:232.

39. Kite JH: Non-operative treatment of congenital clubfeet. Southern Med 1930; 23:337.

40. Kite JH: Some suggestions on the treatment of clubfoot by casts: AAOS Instructional Course Lecture. J Bone Joint Surg Am 1963; 45:406.

41. Kite JH: The Clubfoot. New York, Grune & Stratton, 1964.

42. Kite JH: Nonoperative treatment of congenital clubfoot. Clin Orthop 1972; 84:29.

43. Lehman WB, Atar D, Grant AD, et al: Treatment of failed clubfoot surgery. J Pediatr Orthop B 1994; 3:168.

44. McKay D: New concept and approach to clubfoot treatment. Section I: Principles and morbid anatomy. J Pediatr Orthop 1982; 2:347.

45. McKay D: New concept and approach to clubfoot treatment. Section II: Evaluation and results. J Pediatr Orthop 1983; 3:10.

46. McKay D: New concept and approach to clubfoot treatment. Section III: Principles and morbid anatomy. J Pediatr Orthop 1983; 3:141.

47. Magone JB, Torch MA, Clark RN, et al: Comparative review of surgical treatment of the idiopathic clubfoot by three different procedures at Columbus Children's Hospital. J Pediatr Orthop 1989; 9:49.

48. Masse P: Le traitement du pied bot par la méthode "Fonctionnelle." In Cahier d'enseignement de la SOFCOT. Paris, Expansion Scientifique, 1977, 3:51.

49. Ponseti IV, El-Khoury GY, Ippolito E, et al: A radiographic study of skeletal deformities in treated clubfeet. Clin Orthop 1981; 160:30.

50. Ponseti IV: Congenital clubfoot. Fundamentals of Treatment. Oxford, Oxford University Press, 1996.

51. Ponseti IV: Current concepts review: Treatment of congenital clubfoot. J Bone Joint Surg Am 1992; 74:448.

52. Pous JG, Carlioz H: Le pied bot varus équin congénital. Cahiers d'enseignement de la SOFCOT 1977, N°3. Collection J. Duparc. Expansion scientifique Française.

53. Pous JG, Carlioz H: Le pied bot varus équin congénital. Cahiers d'enseignement de la SOFCOT 1993, N°43. Collection J. Duparc. Expansion scientifique Française.

54. Scarpa A: A Memoir on Congenital Clubfeet of Children (translated from Italian by J. W. Wishart). Edinburgh, Constable, 1818.

55. Scott WA, Hosking SW, Catterall A: Clubfoot: Observations on the surgical anatomy of dorsiflexion. J Bone Joint Surg Br 1984; 66:71.

56. Shapiro F, Glimcher MJ: Gross and histological abnormalities of the talus in congenital clubfoot. J Bone Joint Surg Am 1979; 61:522.

57. Seringe R, Atia R: Pied bot varus equin congénital idiopathique: Résultats du traitement "fonctionnel" (269 pieds). Rev Chir Orthop 1990; 76:490.

58. Seringe R, Chedeville R: Traitement non Chirurgical. In Le pied bot varus équin congénital. Cahiers d'enseignement de la SOFCOT 1993, N°43. Collection J. Duparc. Expansion scientifique Française.

59. Simons GW: The Clubfoot. New York, Springer-Verlag, 1994.

60. Simons GW: Complete subtalar release in clubfoot. Part I: A preliminary report. J Bone Joint Surg Am 1985; 67:1056.

61. Simons GW: Complete subtalar release in clubfeet. Part II: Comparison with less extensive procedure. J Bone Joint Surg Am 1985; 67:1044.

62. Sodre H, Bruschini S, Mestriner LA, et al: Arterial abnormalities in talipes equinovarus as assessed by arteriography and the Doppler technique. J Pediatr Orthop 1990; 10:101.

63. Tarraf YN, Carroll NC: Analysis of the components of residual deformity in clubfeet presenting for reoperation. J Pediatr Orthop 1992; 12:207.

64. Turco VJ: Clubfoot. New York, Churchill Livingstone, 1981.

65. Turco VJ: Present management of idiopathic clubfoot. J Pediatr Orthop B 1994; 3:149.

66. Turco VJ: Resistant clubfoot: One-stage posteromedial release with internal fixation: A follow-up report of a fifteen-year experience. J Bone Joint Surg Am 1979; 61:805.

67. Weintroub S, Kermosh O: Comparative evaluation of initial surgical procedures in clubfoot. J Pediatr Orthop B 1994; 3:171.

68. Yngve DA, Gross RH, Sullivan JA: Clubfoot release without wide subtalar release. J Pediatr Orthop 1990; 10:473.

69. Husson A: Anatomical and functional study of the tarsus. Ph.D. dissertation, Leiden University, 1961.

VERTICAL TALUS

section 9
chapter 25

Marek Napiontek

Summary
- Vertical talus is a rare disorder, often coexisting with neurological and genetic syndromes.
- The diagnosis must be confirmed radiographically.
- Treatment of vertical talus is difficult. Nonoperative treatment almost always fails.
- The primary treatment option is one-stage open reduction with tendon lengthening and transposition in the first year of life.

DEFINITION

Vertical talus is an anatomic or radiographic description of the position of the talus in the ankle joint in the sagittal plane. Synonyms include congenital vertical talus (CVT), congenital flatfoot, congenital convex pes valgus, rockerbottom foot, and talipes convex pes valgus. The talus is in fixed plantar flexion in the ankle joint, and there is dorsal and lateral dislocation of the midfoot in relation to the talus and calcaneus. It results in the clinical appearance of convex planovalgus foot with shortening of the Achilles tendon and extensors. The disorder may be associated with a variety of conditions. It may be a primary congenital deformity (known as CVT) occurring as an idiopathic form or associated with multiple malformation syndromes; an in utero deformation; or a component of chromosome aneuploidy states. It may also be secondary to neuromuscular abnormalities such as a peripheral or central nervous system disease or may occur after prolonged bedrest, as an iatrogenic deformation after nonoperative treatment of congenital clubfoot, and with a deficient tibialis posterior tendon.

HISTORICAL REVIEW

Theodor Essau in 1856 was the first to describe the pathological anatomy of CVT,[1] whereas Henken in 1914 presented its radiological and clinical picture.[2] Lamy and Weissman in 1939, in the English literature, described the malformation and its treatment.[3]

EPIDEMIOLOGY

The frequency of occurrence of the deformity has not been clearly determined. Pick and Chicote-Campos,[4] on the basis of the data found in the literature, stated that it comprises

0.24% to 0.4% of all foot deformities. Jacobsen and Crawford,[5] in a study at an orthopaedic clinic for major foot disorders, determined that less than 4% are due to CVT. A vertical talus constitutes 10% of foot deformities in those with myelomeningocele. The deformity affects boys more often than girls. In half of the cases, the defect affects only one foot. Hereditary and familial occurrence is rare; it is found mainly in idiopathic CVT.[6]

PATHOGENESIS

ETIOLOGY

The cause is unknown but is explained by some as a neuromuscular imbalance in utero. Drennan and Sharrard[7] thought that CVT in patients with myelomeningocele was due to an imbalance between a weak tibialis posterior muscle and strong dorsiflexors, whereas Specht[8] found deficient intrinsic muscles. Approximately, one-half of cases of CVT are associated with systemic neurological, muscular, or skeletal disorders, such as arthrogryposis, spina bifida, mental retardation, Down syndrome, and trisomies 13 to 15 and 18.

Isolated CVT can be transmitted as an autosomal-dominant trait with variable expression and incomplete penetrance.[9]

PATHOLOGICAL ANATOMY

The hindfoot is locked in equinus, and the talus generally assumes a vertical position relative to the ankle joint. Displacement through the transverse tarsal articulation includes medial column dislocation, with the navicular moving dorsally and laterally relative to the talar head and neck. There is similar displacement of the cuboid relative to the anterior part of the calcaneus when the lateral column of the foot is involved. The forefoot is abducted and may also demonstrate pronation or supination.[10] The navicular becomes triangular in shape, and the plantar half is hypoplastic. Eventually, secondary osseous and articular surface changes occur, especially in the calcaneotalonavicular and calcaneocuboid joints. Shortening of the lateral column of the foot may also affect the outcome of surgical treatment.

Midtarsal displacement is associated with contracture of the posterior, dorsal, and lateral ligaments, tendons, and capsular structures, and the medial soft-tissue structures are frequently overstretched. Shortening of the Achilles tendon and peroneal muscles may be found. Both the shortened peroneal muscles as well as the attenuated tibialis posterior muscle may displace anterior to their malleolus, causing them to act as pedal dorsiflexors.[11] This may be an additional factor decreasing the push-off power in an untreated deformity. Shortening of the extensors of all the toes as well as of the tibialis anterior muscle is observed.

DIAGNOSIS

The defect is diagnosed as soon as the infant is born, especially if the deformity occurs in association with genetic and chromosomal disturbance syndromes. Often the acquired (Lichtblau's[12] group 3) or idiopathic (Hamanishi's[6] group 5) type is overlooked, because in these cases postural calcaneovalgus deformity is erroneously diagnosed. It is essential to take a lateral radiograph in full plantar flexion. The foot is considered a true CVT only if the first metatarsal, lateral cuneiform, or navicular remain dorsally dislocated onto the talar head (Figs. 1 and 2).

CLINICAL FEATURES

CVT is characterized by equinus position of the hindfoot, abduction of the forefoot, and flattening or convexity of the expected medial longitudinal arch. The most prominent part of the sole is the talar head and anterior part of the calcaneus. The convexity on the medial border of the foot is the protruding navicular bone (my intraoperative observation). Diminished calf girth and, in older children, a characteristic position of the toes, with the second toe rising vertically and overriding the third and great toes, are also part of the clinical presentation. CVT can be considered as comprising a group of rotational disturbances, in which the subtalar complex, consisting of the calcaneus, cuboid, and navicular together with the cuneiforms, metatarsals, and phalanges, rotates outward in the horizontal and coronal planes. Additionally, a part of the subtalar complex anterior to the calcaneus (but without it) rotates more in the same planes and dorsally in the sagittal plane. Observations concerning forefoot supination in CVT were made by Król and Marciniak[10] and may have clinical importance, especially in attempted correction of the hindfoot equinus and eversion. The deformity is not correctable by normal means.

INVESTIGATIONS

The navicular does not ossify until 2.5 years of age. In newborns and infants, lateral radiographs using the ossification center of the medial[13] or lateral[14] cuneiform can demonstrate the abnormal relationship of the midfoot to the long axis of the plantar flexed talus. However, on the same view, the ossific nucleus of the talus may have a rounded contour, making measurements difficult. Careful observation of the soft tissue on the plantar surface of the foot will delineate the rocker-bottom deformity.

RADIOGRAPHS

Standard anteroposterior (AP) and lateral radiographs should be obtained, with older children in a standing position and younger children in a simulated weightbearing position. Additionally, plantar flexion lateral views are necessary to confirm the talonavicular dislocation. A lateral radiograph in maximum dorsiflexion confirms the fixed equinus position of the calcaneus and talus relative to the tibia (shortening of the Achilles tendon and aids decision-making about its lengthening). A talar axis–first metatarsal base angle and calcaneal axis–first metatarsal base angle[10] provide information about differentiation between oblique talus and navicular displacement and tendo Achilles shortening. An AP view demonstrates abduction of the forefoot at the midtarsal joint and also in the Lisfranc joint. Interestingly, the AP talocalcaneal angle generally is in an acceptable range[15] (a mean of 34 degrees[16]). In toddlers the talus acquires an hourglass shape as a result of the pressure that the navicular bone exerts on its neck. The anterior part of the calcaneus becomes slim and bent in a beak-like fashion and looks like a Dutch clog.[10] Lateral and AP

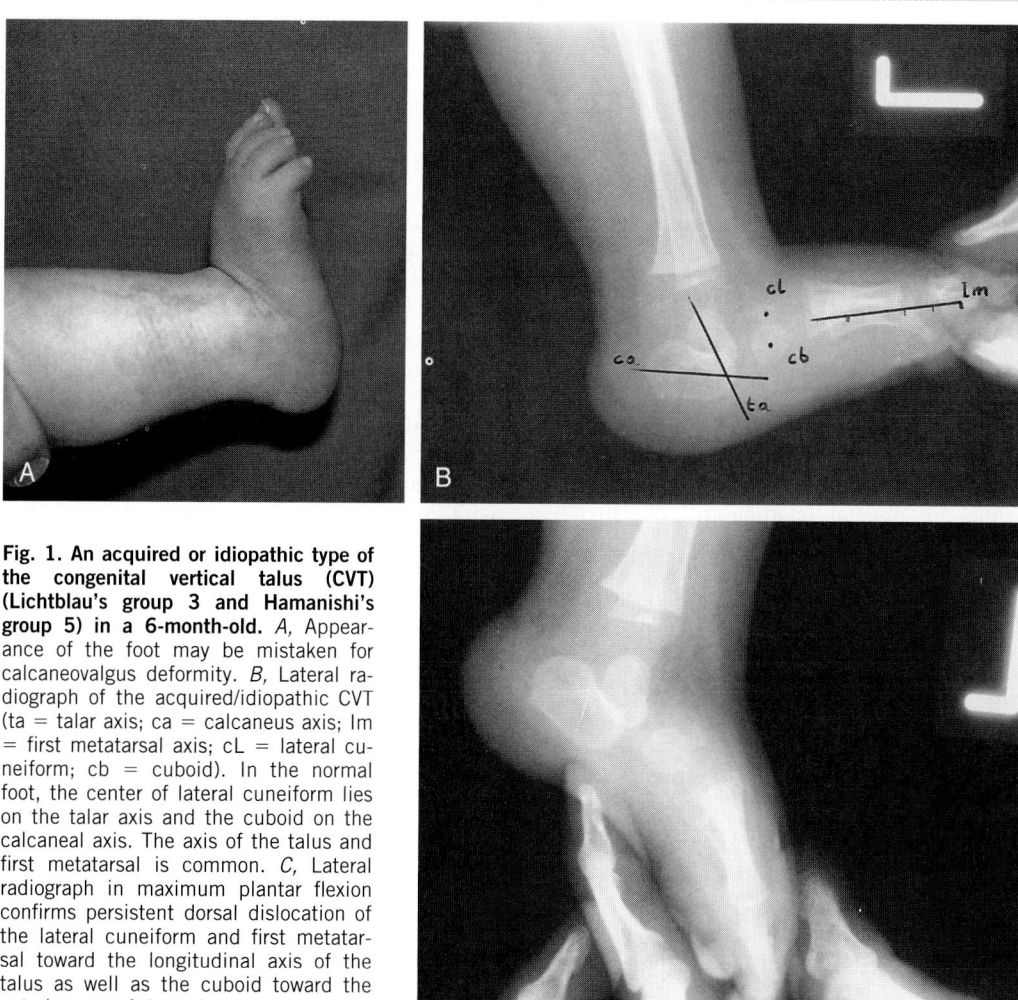

Fig. 1. An acquired or idiopathic type of the congenital vertical talus (CVT) (Lichtblau's group 3 and Hamanishi's group 5) in a 6-month-old. *A,* Appearance of the foot may be mistaken for calcaneovalgus deformity. *B,* Lateral radiograph of the acquired/idiopathic CVT (ta = talar axis; ca = calcaneus axis; lm = first metatarsal axis; cL = lateral cuneiform; cb = cuboid). In the normal foot, the center of lateral cuneiform lies on the talar axis and the cuboid on the calcaneal axis. The axis of the talus and first metatarsal is common. *C,* Lateral radiograph in maximum plantar flexion confirms persistent dorsal dislocation of the lateral cuneiform and first metatarsal toward the longitudinal axis of the talus as well as the cuboid toward the anterior part of the calcaneus.

radiographs reveal dorsal and lateral dislocations, respectively, of the navicular in relation to the talar head and cuboid to the anterior part of the calcaneus.

Napiontek[16] introduced a method of evaluation, but its use for appraising the outcome of the treatment is applicable only in older children. In deformities of neurogenic origin, the characteristic thin and elongated shapes of the talus and calcaneus are apparent.

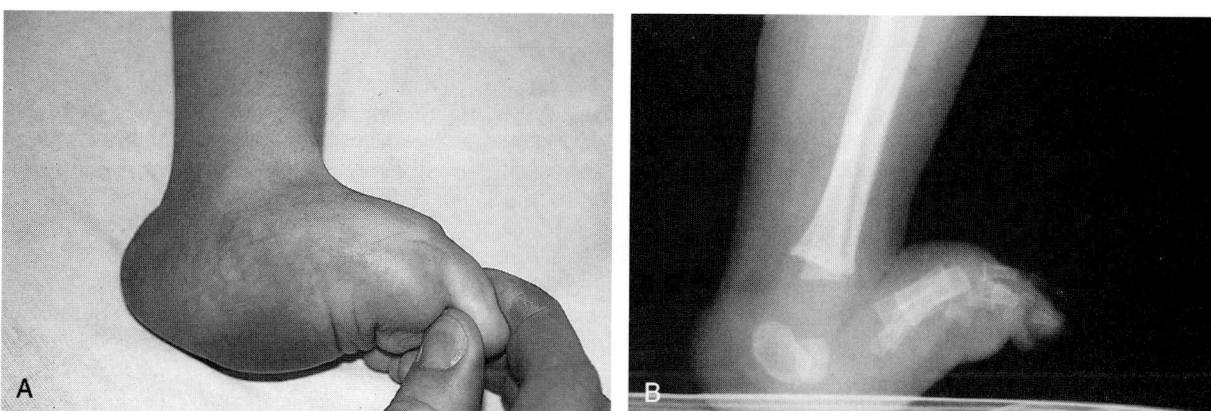

Fig. 2. A teratogenic type of congenital vertical talus (CVT) (Lichtblau's group 1) or CVT associated with neural tube defects and spinal anomalies (Hamanishi's group 1). *A,* Extreme rocker-bottom deformity in an untreated 3 year-old girl. *B,* Lateral radiograph of the same foot immediately after birth.

ULTRASONOGRAPHY

This technique can be a useful supplement to radiological evaluation in infants.[17] Hamel and Becker[18] developed a method of assessing talonavicular malalignment before ossification of the navicular.

CLASSIFICATION OF THE DEFORMITY

Etiological classifications established independently by Lichtblau[12] and Hamanishi[6] are the most useful. The former is simple and practical; the latter is more detailed.

LICHTBLAU'S CLASSIFICATION

Group 1—teratogenic type: genetic cause, often familial history, bilateral, associated defects (developmental dislocation of the hip, mental retardation); recognized at birth as "Persian slipper deformity"; foot rigid and resistant to passive manipulation; tight extensors and heel cord.

Group 2—neurogenic type: muscle imbalance, myelomeningocele or neurofibromatosis, unilateral; seems correctable in the infant; more rigid in the older child.

Group 3—acquired type: from temporary malposition in utero, not familial; no other defects except an opposite equinovarus foot or developmental dislocation of the hip; unilateral; partially correctable and not severely rigid (may be mistaken for calcaneovalgus foot); hindfoot may not be fixed in equinus; extensors permit manipulation of the forefoot into equinus.

HAMANISHI'S CLASSIFICATION

Group 1: CVT associated with neural tube defects and spinal anomalies; varying degrees of paralytic imbalances of the extrinsic and intrinsic muscles, which are believed to initiate the deformities, and an intrauterine postural effect may fix them secondarily.

Group 2: CVT associated with a wide variety of neuromuscular disorders without spinal anomalies (including arthrogryposis multiplex congenita, neurofibromatosis, and cerebral palsy).

Group 3: CVT as a major part of the skeletal abnormalities of known malformation syndromes (including Freeman-Sheldon syndrome).

Group 4: CVT with chromosomal aberrations.

Group 5: idiopathic CVT subdivided into four types based on the patterns of other skeletal abnormalities and inheritance: (A) intrauterine molding or deformation; (B) digitotalar dysmorphism; (C) familial occurrence of CVT or oblique talus; and (D) sporadic and unassociated.

OTHER CLASSIFICATION SYSTEMS

Two other classification systems offer additional insight into the problems. Król and Marciniak[10] divided severe and mild types of CVT into two groups: those with forefoot supination and those with forefoot pronation. Coleman and Jarrett[19] divided the deformity into two groups as well: those with and those without a dislocation in the calcaneocuboid joint. In their opinion, the deformity accompanied by a dislocation in this joint is more difficult to treat.

DIFFERENTIAL DIAGNOSIS

In newborns, the calcaneovalgus foot, especially with forefoot abduction, can be misdiagnosed as CVT. A radiograph may not prove helpful because, in a lateral view, the ossification center of the talus may be nearly spherical and the navicular is invisible. In older children, flexible or paralytic flatfoot (especially with shortening of the Achilles tendon) with the oblique talus on a lateral standing radiograph can imitate CVT. Additionally, vertical talus arising later in childhood secondary to a neuromuscular disorder such as poliomyelitis or cerebral palsy should be considered.

MANAGEMENT

The treatment of CVT should begin immediately after birth with serial manipulation and casting. Stretching casts should not be applied for more than 6 to 12 weeks, and this kind of treatment should be considered preparatory to surgical management. The frequency and duration are similar to those used in congenital talipes equinovarus. The above-knee plaster cast is applied in maximum plantar flexion and supination of the foot. In prevalent opinions, the nonoperative treatment is successful in few cases.

OPERATIVE TREATMENT

The last 20 years have brought one-stage operative procedures[15, 16, 20–26] consisting basically of open reduction of the dislocated joints and lengthening of the Achilles tendon, peroneals, and extensors. Stabilization with Kirschner wire is obligatory. The operation is best performed during the first year of life with the Cincinnati approach,[20] because it ensures the best view of the anatomic structures of the hindfoot and midfoot.

TECHNIQUE USED BY THE AUTHOR

This technique is recommended for children aged 3 months to 2.5 years. With the child placed prone, the Cincinnati approach is used. However, in children older than 18 to 24 months, because of problems with wound closing, the double incision, either posteromedial and lateral or posterolateral and medial, is highly advisable (Fig. 3).

The Lateral Release

The belly of the short toe extensors is released. The sheaths of the peroneal tendons are opened, and the tendons are lengthened by a Z-technique, distal to the lateral malleolus. Whereas the calcaneocuboid joint is completely opened, the talonavicular joint is opened only from its lateral side. The talocalcaneal interosseous ligament and the calcaneofibular ligament are cut, and the joints between the talus and the calcaneus are opened.

The Posterior Release

These steps are followed by lengthening of the Achilles tendon by a Z-technique, which may be troublesome because the belly of the triceps surae may extend considerably, causing shortness of the tendinous part. Posterior capsulotomy of the ankle joint is optional and depends on correction of the hindfoot equinus. During the posterior capsulotomy, both the posterior talofibular ligament and the posterior fibers of the deltoid ligament are divided.

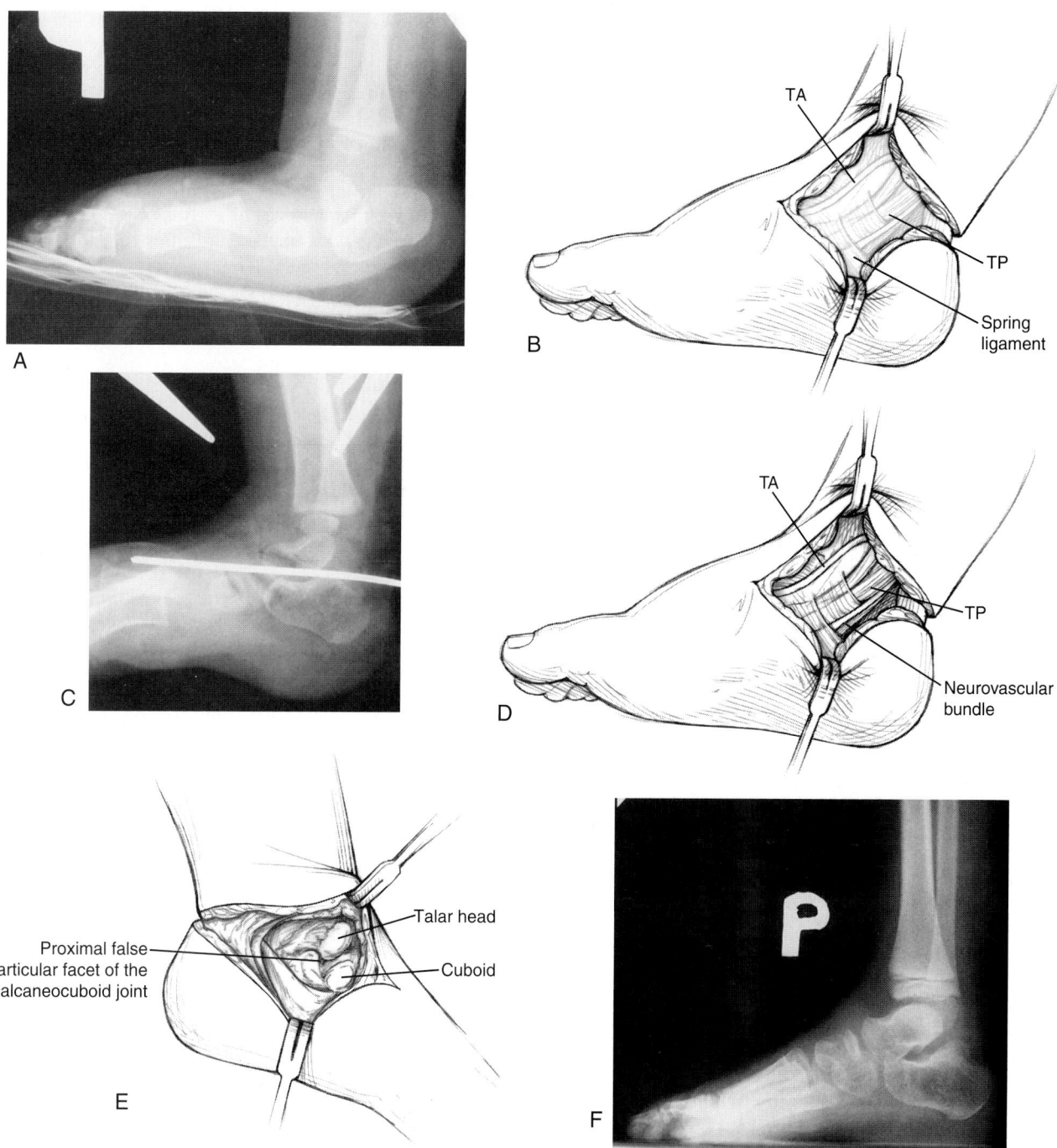

Fig. 3. Proper reduction of the acquired/idiopathic congenital vertical talus with a one-stage surgical procedure. *A*, Lateral radiograph before surgery in 1-year-old girl. *B*, An intraoperative view after medial release (TA = cut tibialis anterior tendon; TP = cut tibialis posterior tendon; *arrow* indicates spring ligament). *C*, Intraoperative radiograph with Kirschner's wire acting as a lever, reducing the talus and navicular. *D*, Medial side of the foot after reduction (TA = tibialis anterior tendon transposed through the hole in spring ligament; TP = shortened tibialis posterior tendon). *E*, Lateral side of the foot after reduction (*arrow* indicates where the proximal false articular face of the calcaneocuboid joint is displaced dorsally). *F*, Result 4 years later.

The Medial Release

On the medial border of the foot, the sheath of the tibialis posterior tendon is opened and the tendon is shortened by a z-technique. The tendons of the flexor digitorum longus and flexor hallucis longus are identified just below the talar head and navicular and are separated from the spring liga-ment. The spring ligament is then incised longitudinally (exactly as the sheath of the posterior tibial muscle tendon runs), adding a transverse incision at the level of the talo-navicular joint, which should be proximal to the most prominent spot (navicular). After revealing the head of the talus, all tendinous and capsular components dorsal to the midtarsal joint should be cut completely. This is followed by releasing the attachment of the anterior tibial muscle tendon and by lengthening of the contracted tendon of the extensor digitorum longus. This maneuver is best done from a separate dorsal incision above the ankle joint to lengthen the tendon by a Z-technique because the tendon is common to all toes. In some incorrigible deformities, the capsule and ligaments between the talus and calcaneus should be cut using the complete subtalar release. This release allows a three-dimensional reduction of the subtalar complex in relation to the talus, equalizing the medial and lateral rays of the foot. This occurs because, during the talonavicular reduction, the calcaneus moves a bit forward in relation to the talus.

Reduction

After such a release, the Kirschner wire is inserted into the real center of the talar head but not into the center of its false articular surface. The wire comes out through the posterior surface of the talus. The wire acts as a lever, enabling one to direct the talus precisely onto the navicular. After the reduction, the wire exits on the dorsum of the foot. The reduction should be monitored radiologically, particularly when the surgeon is not experienced in the procedure. The appearance of the calcaneocuboid joint indirectly testifies to the correct talonavicular reduction because of the plantar displacement of the cuboid. The entire anterior part of the calcaneus is revealed. The displacement is so great that it seems incorrect. Particular attention should be paid to talonavicular reduction in the horizontal plane. The difference in length between the medial and lateral rays of the foot is why obtaining the correct shape of the foot in the horizontal plane (i.e., neutral position of the forefoot) is always associated with medial displacement of the navicular bone in relation to the head of the talus.[16] A correct reduction in this plane may leave the surgeon somewhat dissatisfied because of some persistent abduction of the forefoot. It can be corrected with open wedge osteotomy of the anterior part of the calcaneus but only after the talonavicular joint has been stabilized. Otherwise, an iatrogenic medial dislocation of the navicular may ensue. The calcaneocuboid joint and thus the lateral ray of the foot sometimes require stabilization with Kirschner's wire. Whereas stabilization of the lateral ray of the foot is only occasionally necessary, calcaneotalar stabilization is mandatory.

The last stage consists of transposition of the tibialis anterior tendon through an opening made in the spring ligament at the level of the talar head proximal to its transverse incision. After the transposition and suturing, the tendon forms a loop, which lifts the talar head dorsally. The procedure is completed with shortening of the tibialis posterior tendon and suturing of the lengthened tendons when they are tense. The above-knee plaster cast is applied for 6 weeks. Then, after removing the Kirschner wires (without anesthesia), the below-knee plaster cast is applied for another 8 weeks. Normal shoes are worn immediately after cast removal, with standard support of the longitudinal arch. In paralytic deformity, an ankle-foot orthosis may be worn.

TECHNIQUES COMPLEMENTARY TO OPEN REDUCTION

- Resection of the navicular bone,[27] which is especially useful in arthrogrypotic CVT in small children.
- Extra-articular talocalcaneal arthrodesis according to Grice, which can be used at 2.5 years of age and thereafter.
- Opening wedge of the anterior part of the calcaneus, as used by myself, sometimes as early as 6 months of age.
- Opening wedge with fibular graft inserted into the calcaneocuboid joint.[28]
- Transposition of tendons (e.g., the peroneus brevis onto the tibialis posterior tendon in paralytic deformity).

SALVAGE PROCEDURES

- Resection of the talar head and severing of the tendons.
- Dega's technique: resection of the talar head and closing wedge osteotomy of the anterior part of the calcaneus.[29]
- Triple arthrodesis.

COMPLICATIONS

Nonspecific complications are associated with incompetence and tight plaster cast applied after the procedure. It may result in skin necrosis, avascular necrosis of the bones, or compartment syndrome.

Specific complications are associated with the nature of the deformity. It may result in skin deficiency on the anterolateral aspect of the foot after correction of the deformity or in stretch and occlusion of the dorsalis pedis artery after reduction of the stiff deformity. The latter may result in skin necrosis and avascular necrosis of the talus or navicular. Avascular bone necrosis not only develops as a result of vascular inefficiency, but it is probably also an effect of the pressure in the talonavicular joint after its reduction. It is caused by elongation of the first ray of the foot. Weakening of the push-off power can be a result of overcorrection of the equinus position of the hindfoot (tendo Achilles overlengthening) and a seemingly calcaneal position of the hindfoot, caused by lack of reduction and dorsal dislocation of the forefoot (in the sagittal plane, the forefoot is shifted up in relation to the hindfoot).[16] In some cases, Grice's extra-articular arthrodesis can result in overcorrection, especially when there is primary supination of the forefoot.[16]

RESULTS FROM THE LITERATURE

Almost all authors report advantages of the one-stage procedure consisting of soft-tissue release, open reduction, tendon lengthening, and stabilization with Kirschner wires.[15, 16, 21–25, 30] The number of feet evaluated in one article ranged from 10 to 36. Most authors report good or satisfactory results with this method of treatment. Unfortunately, most studies include vertical tali with heterogeneous causes, including myelomeningocele and cerebral palsy patients. Additionally, only two of the mentioned articles contain radiographic criteria for evaluation of the talonavicular displacement. None, however, presents criteria for evaluation of the cuboid displacement toward the anterior part of the calcaneus. The criteria for clinical and radiographic evaluation are different.

COMMENTS

Open reduction can be used in all types of deformities regardless of cause. Varying the technique according to cause is possible in older children, in whom the muscular balance may be determined. It consists of extending the release and transposing the tendons, which is done in patients with myelomeningocele or cerebral palsy.

In some forms of CVT, such as Lichtblau's group 1 (teratogenic) or Hamanishi's groups 2 (arthrogrypotic), 3 (malformation syndromes), and 4 (chromosomal aberrations), reconstruction of the normal anatomic relations is associated with such tension of the soft tissues that occlusion of the vessels on the dorsum of the foot, caused either by lengthening and narrowing or too intense pressure of the talar head onto the navicular bone, may ensue. These may interfere with blood supply, causing problems with wound healing or avascular necrosis, mainly within the navicular and talar head. For this reason, in these types of deformities, talonavicular reduction or lengthening of the lateral ray of the foot through an opening wedge osteotomy of the anterior part of the calcaneus is not advisable. In small children, it seems safer to consider naviculectomy, which will loosen the foot, equalize the rays, and enable an easy reduction. In children between 4 and 6 years of age, resection of the talar head with closing wedge osteotomy of the anterior part of the calcaneus with tendo Achilles lengthening[29] is a better solution. In patients with total arthrogryposis or myelomeningocele, cutting the contractured tendons will not be a mistake.

In the future, the natural history of the etiologically different types of CVT should be studied because, as some authors[14, 16] confirmed, persistent talonavicular dislocation coexists with a correct shape and good function of the foot. Similar radiographic and clinical criteria for homogeneous type of the deformity should be used.

REFERENCES

1. Osmond-Clarke H: Congenital vertical talus. J Bone Joint Surg Br 1956; 38:334.
2. Henken R: Contribution a l'étude des formes osseuses du piedplat valgus congenital. Paris, Lyons, 1914.
3. Lamy L, Weissman L: Congenital convex pes valgus. J Bone Joint Surg 1931; 21:79.
4. Pick CF, Chicote-Campos F: Der angeborene Plattfuss mit Talus verticalis. Stuttgart, Ferdinand Enke Verlag, 1979.
5. Jacobsen ST, Crawford AH: Congenital vertical talus. J Pediatr Orthop 1983; 3:306.
6. Hamanishi C: Congenital vertical talus: Classification with 69 cases and new measurement system. J Pediatr Orthop 1984; 4:318.
7. Drennan JC, Sharrard WJW: The pathological anatomy of convex pes valgus. J Bone Joint Surg Br 1971; 53:455.
8. Specht EE: Congenital paralytic vertical talus. An anatomical study. J Bone Joint Surg Am 1975; 57:842.
9. Stern HJ, Clark RD, Stroberg AJ, et al: Autosomal dominant transmission of isolated congenital vertical talus. Clin Gen 1989; 36:427.
10. Król J, Marciniak W: Pes planus taloflexus congenitus: Patologia i obraz kliniczny [Congenital flatfoot: Its pathology and clinical picture]. Chir Narz Ruchu Ortop Pol 1966; 31:587.
11. Patterson WR, Fitz DA, Smith WS: The pathologic anatomy of congenital pes valgus. J Bone Joint Surg Am 1968; 50:458.
12. Lichtblau S: Congenital vertical talus. Bull Hosp Joint Diseases 1978; 39:165.
13. Eyre-Brook AL: Congenital vertical talus. J Bone Joint Surg Br 1967; 49:618.
14. Clark MW, D'Ambrosia RD, Ferguson AB: Congenital vertical talus. J Bone Joint Surg Am 1977; 59:816.
15. Daumas L, Filipe G, Carlioz H: Le pied convexe congenital. Technique et resultats de la correction operatoire en un seul temps. Rev Chir Orthop Appareil Moteur 1995; 81:527.
16. Napiontek M: Congenital vertical talus: A retrospective and critical review of 32 feet operated on by peritalar reduction. J Pediatr Orthop B 1995; 4:179.
17. Schlesinger AE, Deeney VFX, Caskey PF: Sonography of the nonossified tarsal navicular cartilage in an infant with congenital vertical talus. Pediatr Radiol 1989; 20:134.
18. Hamel J, Becker W: Sonographische Diagnostik bei Talus verticalis im Sauglings- und Kleinkindesalter. Ultraschall Klin Prax 1995; 9:185.
19. Coleman SS, Jarrett J: Congenital vertical talus: Pathomechanics and treatment. J Bone Joint Surg Am 1966; 48:1026.
20. Crawford AH, Marxen JL, Osterfeld DL: The Cincinnati incision: A comprehensive approach for surgical procedures of the foot and ankle in childhood. J Bone Joint Surg Am 1982; 64:1355.
21. DeRosa P, Ahlfeld S: Congenital vertical talus: The Riley experience. Foot Ankle 1984; 5:118.
22. Dodge LD, Ashley RK, Gilbert RJ: Treatment of the congenital vertical talus: A retrospective review of 36 feet with long-term follow-up. Foot Ankle 1987; 7:326.
23. Raab P, Krauspe R: One-stage procedure for surgical correction of congenital vertical talus. In Epeldegui T (ed): Flatfoot and Forefoot Deformities. Madrid, Vicente Ediciones, 1995, p 253.
24. Seimon LP: Surgical correction of congenital vertical talus under the age of 2 years. J Pediatr Orthop 1987; 7:405.
25. Stricker S, Rosen E: Early one-stage reconstruction of congenital vertical talus. Foot Ankle Int 1997; 18:535.
26. Tachdjian MO: Pediatric Orthopedics. Philadelphia, WB Saunders, 1972, p 1359.
27. Stone KH: Congenital vertical talus: A new operation. Proc R Soc Med 1963; 56:12.
28. Marciniak W: Die operative peritalare Reposition mit verlongerung des lateralen Fussstrahles bei angeborenen Plattfuss [Talus verticalis]. Beitr Orthop Traumatol 1987; 34:426.
29. Dega W: Pes planus taloflexus congenitus: Wrodzona plaskosc stopy [Pes planus taloflexus congenitus: Congenital flattening of the foot]. Chir Narz Ruchu Ortop Pol 1955; 20:281.
30. Oppenheim W, Smith C, Christie W: Congenital vertical talus. Foot Ankle 1985; 5:198.

section
9
chapter
26

TARSAL COALITION

Tomas Epeldegui

Summary

- Tarsal coalition may be of osseous, cartilaginous, or fibrous tissue.
- The incidence of tarsal coalition is approximately 1% of the general population.
- The onset of symptoms is most common in the preadolescent age group.
- The diagnosis of tarsal coalition can be confirmed by radiography, computed tomography, or magnetic resonance imaging.
- Calcaneonavicular and talocalcaneal bars are the most frequent forms of coalition.
- Conservative management is recommended when the onset of clinical symptoms is recent.
- The type of surgical management depends on the size of the bony bridge, the presence or absence of subtalar osteoarthritis, and the degree of hindfoot valgus deformity.

Tarsal coalition is a congenital deformity that results in the connection of two or more bones in the foot that share a common synovial joint lining. Connections can be of osseous (synostosis), cartilaginous (synchondrosis), or fibrous (syndesmosis) tissue. An osseous bridge may also be acquired secondary to articular disorders (tumors, arthritis).[1] Tarsal coalition may be partial or total.

Tarsal coalitions were first described by Buffon in 1750. Such anomalies have also been noted in a pre-Columbian Indian skeleton. Cuveilhier first described the calcaneonavicular coalition in 1829. Sloman made an important radiographic contribution to the diagnosis of calcaneonavicular coalitions when he observed that a 45 degree internal oblique view demonstrates this form of osseous bridge.[2] Zuckerkandl reported the talocalcaneal coalition in 1877.

Robert Jones defined the peroneal spastic flatfoot in 1897. Harris and Beath reported the association of tarsal coalition and peroneal spastic flatfoot in 1947.[3, 4] Currently, radiographic imaging as well as computed tomography (CT), magnetic resonance imaging (MRI), and scintigraphy have increased our understanding of the anatomic changes and clinical findings of this congenital anomaly.

ETIOLOGY

EMBRYONIC FOOT DEVELOPMENT

Knowledge of the development of the skeleton of the foot is essential to understanding the pathogenesis and etiologic factors involved in tarsal coalition.[5] The embryonic period, related to "developmental horizons" reported by Gardner,[6] is a critical period and includes 23 stages. The phases of blastemal condensation, initial chondrification, and preliminary joint formation occur within the embryonic period (7 weeks after ovulation) and the foot resembles that of adults in detail. Blastemal tarsal condensation occurs in stages 17 and 18 and includes three to four digital prolongations. Anomalies in the number of skeletal elements arise very early in intrauterine life, probably 4 to 5 weeks after ovulation. All elements except the sesamoids undergo chondrification by stage 23. Homogenous interzones "and intermediate cell masses" become three-layered, with cavities lined with synovial tissue that appear in the middle of the three layers during the 9th and 11th week of gestation (60 mm). The tarsal bones develop with endochondral ossification. Many tarsal bones ossify postnatally, the last of these being the navicular. Gardner noted several forms of tarsal coalition before the specimen reaches the length of 73 mm. Pfitzner noted that accessory ossicles were commonly found in the area of tarsal coalition[7] and felt that these accessory bones were responsible for bar formation. Kawashima and Uhthoff [8] reported that joint cavities with synovial linings permitting movements appeared around the 11th week and they concurred with Gardner's observation that talocalcaneal bridges could be found during the 9th and 10th week but became less common in older specimens. They attributed this to failure of or delay in differentiation of mesenchymal tissue into more specialized tissue between the posterior portion of the sustentaculum tali and the corresponding part of the talus during the 7½ to 8½ postovulatory week. They differentiated coalitions into complete bars (bony or cartilaginous) that could be located intra-articularly, extra-articularly, or both, and incomplete coalitions. They agreed with Gardner's conclusion that the change in the biomechanical environment after birth may cause the chondral bridge to break down before completion of ossification in some cases.

GENETICS

Tarsal coalitions are generally found as isolated deformities. Tarsal bars have been reported in other congenital disorders. Coincident ipsilateral limb deformities include talipes equinovarus, fibular hemimelia, and proximal focal femoral deficiency. Apert's syndrome, mesomelic dysplasia, otopalatodigital syndrome, and Nevergelt-Perlman syndromes are examples of generalized syndromes. Tarsal coalitions have been described in different generations of the same family. Leonard[7] reviewed the families of 31 Scottish patients with tarsal coalitions and found some type of tarsal coalition in 33% of parents and 47% of siblings. He concluded that the coalition was a multifactorial disorder of autosomal dominance with nearly full penetrance. In his study, all first-degree relatives with tarsal coalitions were asymptomatic.

INCIDENCE AND CLASSIFICATION

The true incidence of tarsal coalitions in the general population is unknown. Radiographic studies performed on young males prior to admittance into the army found an prevalence between 0.4% and 2%.[3, 9] The incidence may actually be higher, since tarsal coalition can occur in asymptomatic feet. Pfitzner reported a 6% incidence in human skeletons emphasizing talocalcaneal and calcaneonavicular coalitions. Kawashima and Uhthoff[8] also noted a higher incidence of prenatal cartilaginous talocalcaneal coalitions than have been reported in clinical studies.

The two most common forms of tarsal coalition involve the calcaneus and talus or the calcaneus and navicula and account for the vast majority of symptomatic feet. Talocalcaneal coalitions are slightly more common. The coexistence of two or more forms of coalition in the same foot is infrequent but has been reported. Approximately 60% of calcaneonavicular and 50% of talocalcaneal coalitions occur bilaterally.[10] The literature suggests a male preponderance of 60% to 80%.[11–13]

PATHOMECHANICS

The skeleton of the human foot contains two osseous columns. The medial column is composed of the talus, the navicular bone, the three cuneiform, and the medial three metatarsi and toes. The lateral column includes the calcaneus, the cuboid bone, and the fourth and fifth metatarsi and toes. The two columns intersect at the level of the talocalcaneonavicular joint. This joint has been described as a distal ankle joint because the movement of the tibiotalar joint complements the movement of the talocalcaneal joint in such a way that plantar flexion is coupled with inversion and dorsiflexion associated with eversion of the foot.[14] This combined movement is the result of the anatomy of the Chopart joint in which the calcaneocuboid and talonavicular axes act jointly to create a divergent angle.

Helicoidal movement occurs around the talar head as a result of the different axes. The entire foot moves around the talar head, which is contained within a ball and socket joint, sometimes described as "acetabulum pedis," formed by the talocalcaneonavicular joint and its ligaments.[15] During ambulation, the subtalar joint permits both a gliding and a rotatory motion. During dorsiflexion, the calcaneus glides distally and externally in the horizontal plane while the joint rotation permits eversion of the hindfoot. This can produce eversion of the foot and can result in a flatfoot and the development of a secondary contracture of the peroneal muscles. When one of the components of the talocalcaneonavicular joint is blocked or loses its elasticity, the movement of the foot around the talar head is interrupted or limited. This restriction of motion is especially pronounced in cases of talocalcaneal coalition and to a lesser degree in calcaneonavicular coalition. Restriction of subtalar motion by the coalition both limits the distal gliding of the calcaneus, forcing the heel bone into valgus, and blocks the navicular from gliding dorsally over the convex talar head.

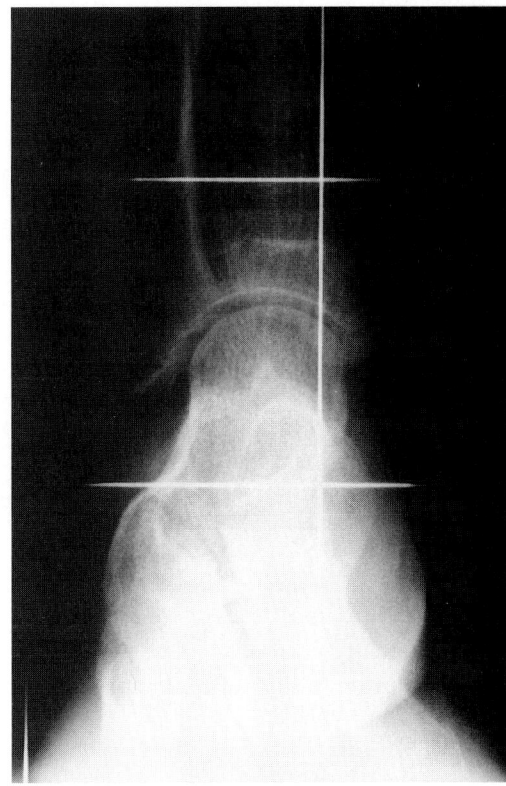

Fig. 1. Anteroposterior radiograph of the ankle joint. This shows a ball and socket ankle joint in a patient with talocalcaneal tarsal coalition. The round shape of the talar dome may compensate for limited subtalar movement.

To compensate for the limited movement of the joint, a complementary movement is required at the nearest joint. This explains the association of tarsal coalition with a ball and socket ankle joint, which is frequently associated with a tarsal coalition (Fig. 1). However, other attempts at compensation can also be observed at the Chopart joint which can develop a spherical profile, converting it into a ball and socket joint to overcome the limitation of movements (Fig. 2).

The nonosseous bars in early childhood may ossify and cause further restriction in joint motion. This may explain why tarsal coalitions have a delayed onset of symptoms. The talonavicular coalition ossifies between 3 and 5 years of age. The calcaneonavicular coalition most commonly ossifies between 8 and 12 years of age and the talocalcaneal bars ossify between 12 and 16 years of age.[16] These ages correspond with the most common times that the different types of coalition become symptomatic.

CLINICAL FEATURES

Tarsal coalition may present radiographically without clinical symptoms. Discomfort or pain is the most frequent complaint, is usually not severe, and develops at ages concordant with the ossification time of the bars. This explains the frequent diagnosis during the preadolescent period, particularly with talocalcaneal coalition.[17] The patients may

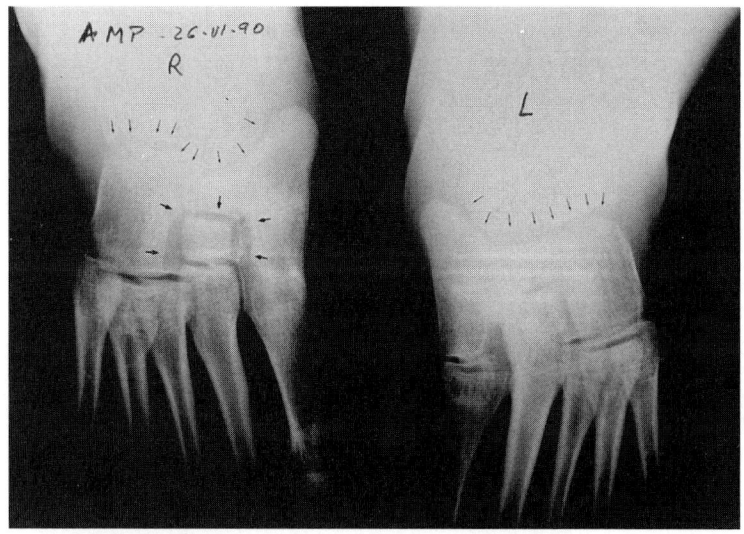

Fig. 2. Anteroposterior radiograph of the foot. This is a Chopart joint adaptation to a tarsal coalition. In the right foot, intercuneiform coalition generates advanced dynamic solicitations, trying to compensate the movement. In the left foot is a talocalcaneal coalition. The round shape of the Chopart joint when compared with the left foot is a consequence of adaptive changes to increase the movements compensating the blocked subtalar joint.

also refer to a previous history of recurrent ankle sprains as their chief clinical complaint.

PHYSICAL EXAMINATION

Restricted subtalar movement is generally observed. Stiffness and pes planovalgus are associated with tarsal pain and are the result of restriction of motion of the talocalcaneonavicular joint described in the pathomechanics. A varus deformity has also been reported.[18] However, spasm or stiffness in the peroneal muscles can develop secondary to the hindfoot eversion and may be aggravated by running. Pain may be secondary to peroneal muscle spasm. In addition, the heel may fail to rotate into hindfoot varus when the patient stands on tip-toes. A medial longitudinal plantar arch may not develop when the first metatarsophalangeal joint is hyperextended in stance position (Jack's test). Calf atrophy is also frequently observed.

Symptoms may differ depending on the anatomic location of the bar. The patient with a calcaneonavicular bar refers pain to the area of the coalition and may retain partial subtalar movement. As symptoms progress, a peroneal spastic flatfoot may develop. In some cases, a bony prominence may be observed on the dorsum of the midfoot close to the talonavicular joint. This protuberance corresponds to the radiographic bony beak observed on the neck of the talus.

One-third of patients with a talocalcaneal bar have complete restriction of subtalar joint movement. This may cause increased peroneal muscle contracture during demanding exercises, and this activity may also increase the pain. Two-thirds of patients present with a bony prominence slightly posterior to the medial malleolus. Tinel's sign can be elicited by tapping the bony eminence. One third of patients have occasional sensory disturbances on the plantar aspect of the foot.[19] This explains why the bony prominence can be considered to cause tarsal tunnel syndrome, particularly in adolescent athletes. A varus deformity of the hindfoot has also been reported with this form of bridge.

RADIOLOGY

Anteroposterior, lateral, internal oblique, and axial radiographic projections of the foot should be obtained. A weightbearing anteroposterior view of the ankle may demonstrate an associated ball and socket joint.

Anteroposterior Projection. This view provides information concerning several coalitions, including talonavicular, intercuneiform, and calcaneocuboid bars. In general it does not aid in the diagnosis of the most common forms of coalitions.

Lateral Projection. Weightbearing lateral radiographs can show the indirect signs of restriction of talocalcaneonavicular joint movement. Talar beaking describes a prominence on the dorsum of the talar neck, which can vary from a slight prominence to a significant bony spur. Talar beaking has been found in 70% of valgus feet with tarsal coalition.[20] The presence of this hypertrophic spur should lead the physician to suspect the existence of a tarsal coalition. Occasionally a spur on the dorsal surface of the navicular bone can be found. Harris and Beath[1] describe an accessory tarsal bone found at the anteromedial process of the os calcis, which they term *calcaneus secondarius*. A very long anteromedial process extending from the calcaneal head can also be an indirect sign of a calcaneonavicular bar ("anteaters sign").[21] Multiple tarsal coalitions may also be observed on this projection (Fig. 3).

Oblique Projection. The 45-degree internal oblique view described by Slomann[2] is the most likely radiographic projection to confirm the presence of a calcaneonavicular coalition (Fig. 4). This view is definitive when a true bony bridge is present, and additional complementary studies are not necessary to determine the surgical treatment. Doubts of the diagnosis may still exist when the union is a synchondrosis.

Calcaneal Axial View (Harris' Projection).[1] This view can demonstrate talocalcaneal coalition of both the medial and posterior facets but is rarely used today because of the technical difficulties in obtaining adequate visualization of

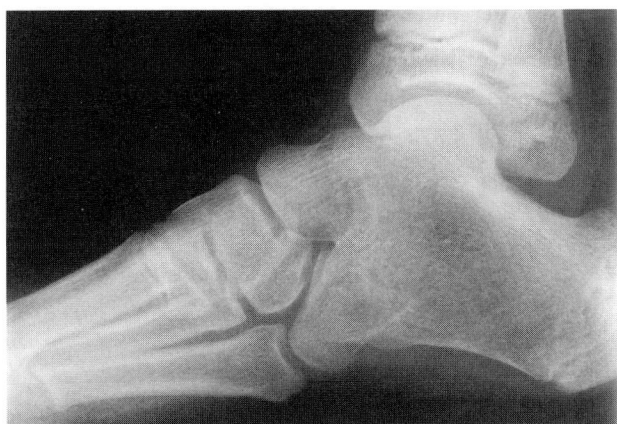

Fig. 3. Radiograph. These are talocalcaneal, talonavicular and calcaneocuboid and intercuneiforms, multiple coalition in the same foot.

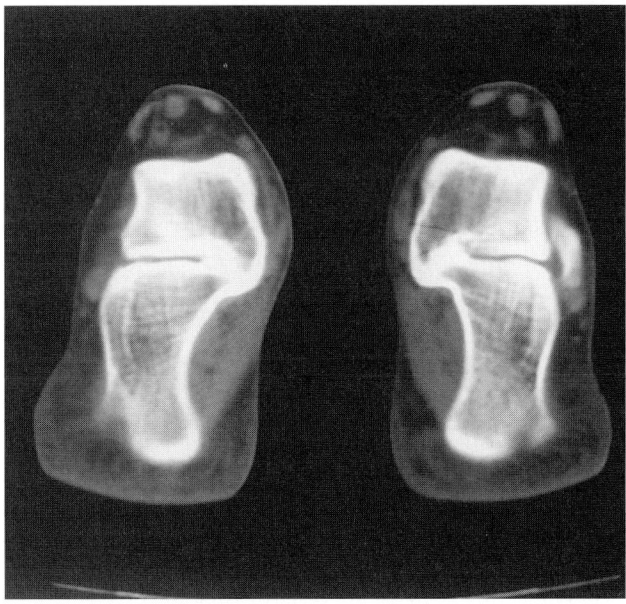

Fig. 5. Coronal cut of CT scan. This is a case of an bilateral talocalcaneal coalition. The bar and valgus of the os calcis may be evaluated.

the subtalar joint. Any radiographic obliquity of the middle facet is considered evidence of a coalition in the area of the sustentaculum tali. Indirect signs that support the presence of a talocalcaneal bar are sclerotic changes at the level of the medial facet or secondary degenerative changes.

COMPUTED TOMOGRAPHY

Computed tomography (CT) complements standard radiographic views in cases in which the suspected diagnosis cannot be confirmed.[22] Sections obtained in the coronal plane are particularly helpful in visualizing talocalcaneal coalitions, particularly involving the medial facet, which is the most common location. The amount of fusion of the individual subtalar joint can also be demonstrated. The CT scan allows visualization of single or multiple bars and facilitates quantifying the joint surface involved in the bony bridge (Fig. 5). The coronal projection allows the degree of valgus of the os calcis to be evaluated with respect to the talus and tibiotalar joint. CT scans confirm the diagnosis of an osseous bar in a talocalcaneal coalition, but doubts may still remain if the bar is cartilaginous.

MAGNETIC RESONANCE IMAGING

Magnetic resonance imaging (MRI) is less commonly indicated but has the advantage of being able to demonstrate the existence of cartilaginous or fibrous union.[23] It is indicated when there is persistence of clinical symptoms accompanying difficulty in confirmation of the diagnosis by radiographs or CT scan. The presence of a cartilaginous or fibrous bar can occur in both talocalcaneal and calcaneonavicular conditions. The MRI scan does not provide any additional information for the diagnosis or treatment when the coalition is osseous.

SCINTIGRAPHY

Bone scans are not specific, but they focus attention to the area of the hindfoot where coalition may be present (Table 1).[24]

DIFFERENTIAL DIAGNOSIS

Painful flexible flatfeet can present with a sensation of stiffness but without the dynamic demonstration of osseous hindfoot block or peroneal contracture with sustained spasticity. Adolescent flatfeet may also become painful after repeated sprains or traumatic arthritis.

The examiner should be aware that tarsal coalition may be part of a variety of syndromes, including fibular and tibial hemimelia, proximal focal femoral deficiency, talipes equinovarus, and Apert's syndrome. It is important that the entire musculoskeletal spectrum of these syndromes be clinically evaluated. A characteristic example can be the association with fibular hemimelia. This syndrome can include a tarsal coalition with an accompanying ball and socket ankle joint, leg length discrepancy, and hypoplasia of the external femoral condyle with insufficiency of the

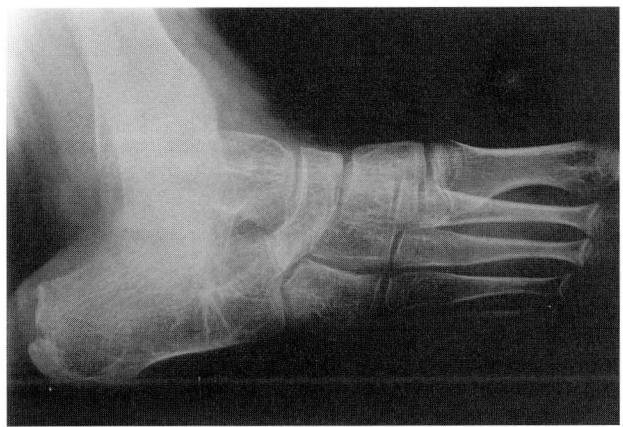

Fig. 4. Radiograph. The calcaneonavicular coalition is well appreciated by a Slomann oblique projection.

	Scintigraphy	Radiology	CT-scan	MRI
TABLE 1. RECOMMENDED PROCEDURES TO CONFIRM THE DIAGNOSIS THROUGH IMAGING TECHNIQUES				
Calcaneonavicular Coalition	Nonspecific	* Oblique projection (Slomann)	Plantar cut	Nonspecific Recommended for fibrous or cartilaginous coalition
Talocalcaneal Coalition	Nonspecific	Calcaneal projection (Harris)	* Coronal cut † Valgus of the calcaneus	Nonspecific Recommended for fibrous or cartilaginous coalition
Multiple Tarsal Coalition	Nonspecific	* Dorsoplantar and lateral projection	Transaxial view	Nonspecific

* Usually confirm the diagnosis.
† Relevant information for surgical decision.

anterior cruciate ligament.[25] Stiff and painful feet may also be found in some rheumatic and inflammatory conditions. Cases secondary to subtalar arthrodesis, infections, or tumors constitute remaining factors to be ruled out in a differential diagnosis of these tarsal unions.[16] When rheumatoid arthritis affects the tarsal joints, it induces peroneal spasm with resultant valgus deformity.

TREATMENT

Treatment is restricted to symptomatic coalitions. Chance radiologic findings do not require orthopaedic intervention.

NONOPERATIVE TREATMENT

Conservative management is generally recommended as the initial form of treatment. The program may vary according to the intensity of the symptoms. In mild or moderate cases, foot supports may be used that combine an insole with plantar support coupled with a supination wedge of the shoe heel. When effective, this approach should allow the patient to carry out normal activity.

Patients who present with a peroneal spastic flatfoot require immobilization in a non-weightbearing plaster cast. General anesthesia may be needed to appropriately apply the plaster immobilization with the hindfoot inverted and the forefoot supinated. The initial non-weightbearing plaster cast should be worn for 3 to 4 weeks and can be followed by a similar cast applied without anesthesia for an additional month. Additional casting has not proven to be advantageous. When the pain is relieved by immobilization, it is necessary to initiate physical therapy to regain the mobility and flexibility of the hindfoot. A power-building program for hindfoot inverters and forefoot supinators is begun after motion has been regained.

OPERATIVE TREATMENT

Surgical management must be considered when conservative care is unsuccessful. The operative options vary according to the location and type of coalition. The algorithm given in Figure 6 may assist in making treatment decisions.

Calcaneonavicular Coalition

The operative treatment of calcaneonavicular coalition includes resection of the osseous bar between the two bones when the bar is detected prior to the onset of secondary degenerative change.[26] This approach was suggested by Badgley in 1927 and later described by Cowell.[27]

Technique. The bar is approached by an Ollier incision, with care taken to protect the sural nerve. The extensor digitorum brevis muscle is identified and detached from its proximal origin on the dorsal surface of the calcaneus. This exposes the tarsal coalition, and a 1 cm rectangular block is resected with an osteotome to completely sever the bony bridge. Care must be taken to avoid iatrogenic damage to neighboring joints. The muscle belly of the short extensor is introduced into the cavity resulting from the resection and acts as an interposed soft tissue barrier to reformation of bone. Its suture is brought out on the non-weightbearing medial aspect of the foot. A non-weightbearing cast is used for 3 weeks and progressive weightbearing is then introduced. Re-education of the movement of the hindfoot and midfoot is mandatory during the final recuperation phase.

Talocalcaneal Coalition

Bar resection is the preferred surgical option for talocalcaneal coalition. Preoperative requirements that must be met include the following:

Joint Area Involved. Determination of the amount of the subtalar joint involved in the coalitions must be made. The area of coalition must be less than 50% of the area of combined middle and posterior facets to consider bar resection. When the coalition's surface is greater than 50%, the possibility of a favorable outcome from bone resection combined with interposed soft tissue is unlikely. The articular surfaces of the hindfoot bones also contain growth cartilage, and it is unlikely that a normal subtalar joint will develop when the resection exceeds 50%. Similar to the calcaneonavicular coalition, the resection must be wide enough to remove the entire bridge.

Subtalar Osteoarthritis. The presence of osteoarthritis can be radiographically demonstrated by joint sclerosis, narrowing, and deformity. The arthritis can set off a chain of irreversible mechanical alterations that will not disappear following bar resection. In this situation, resection is optional but may aide in correction of hindfoot valgus at the time of triple arthrodesis. The presence of a palpable medial hindfoot prominence associated with a tarsal tunnel syndrome also can serve as an indication for resection of the coalition.

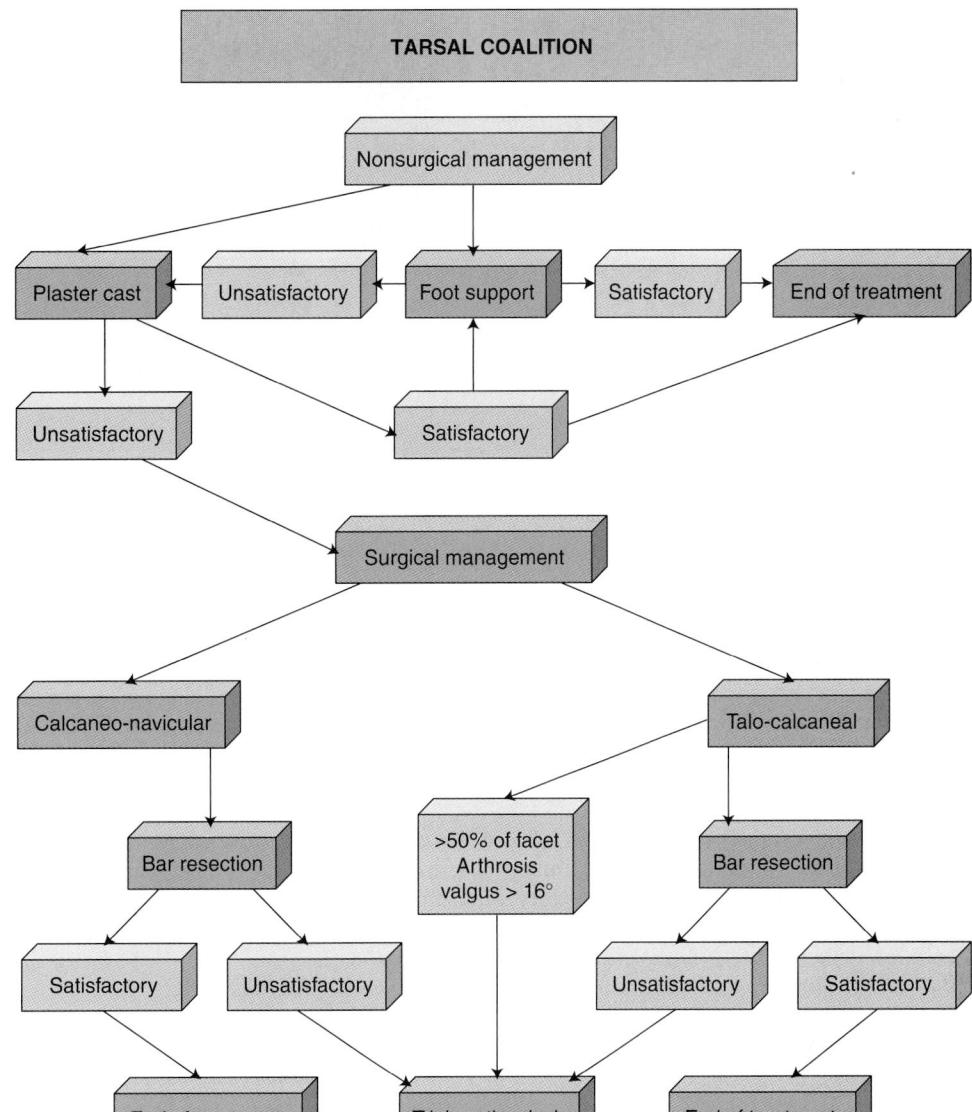

TARSAL COALITION

Nonsurgical management

Plaster cast — Unsatisfactory — Foot support — Satisfactory — End of treatment

Unsatisfactory — Satisfactory

Surgical management

Calcaneo-navicular — Talo-calcaneal

Bar resection — >50% of facet Arthrosis valgus > 16° — Bar resection

Satisfactory — Unsatisfactory — Unsatisfactory — Satisfactory

End of treatment — Triple arthrodesis — End of treatment

Fig. 6. Algorithm for treatment decisions.

Valgus of the Os Calcis. The valgus angle of the os calcis can be measured from the CT coronal cuts and provides important preoperative information. Retrospective studies of surgical outcomes have demonstrated that poor clinical results are associated with a preoperative hindfoot valgus that exceeds 16 to 18 degrees.

The radiographic presence of talar beaking is not considered a contraindication to resection surgery of either calcaneonavicular or talocalcaneal bars. Satisfactory results of surgery have been reported when this adaptive bone change has been present.

In summary, contraindications to resection of the bony bridge include involvement of more than 50% of the surface of the posterior astragalocalcaneal joint; radiographic signs of osteoarthritis of the subtalar joint; and a hindfoot valgus greater than 16 degrees.[9, 19, 20, 28] When these contraindications exist, a more radical surgical treatment should be adopted, such as a triple arthrodesis.

Techniques. The surgical approach of talocalcaneal bar resection is performed through a medial incision based over the sustentaculum tali. The flexor hallucis longus is exposed and retracted plantarward. The tibialis posterior and the flexor digitorum longus and neurovascular bundle are retracted dorsally. The capsules of the posterior and anterior subtalar joints are identified and opened, allowing the definition of the length of the bony bridge, which may obliterate the medial facet. Resection of the bar is performed using osteotomes, drills, or rongeurs. The resection must be complete and circumferentially expose subtalar joint cartilage before the joint can be assessed for restoration of movement. The raw surfaces of the osteotomy are covered with bone wax and the iatrogenic cavity is filled with autogenous fat graft (Figs. 7 through 10).

Postoperative management includes a non-weightbearing plaster immobilization for 3 to 4 weeks. The cast is removed and the patient instructed in initiation of hindfoot

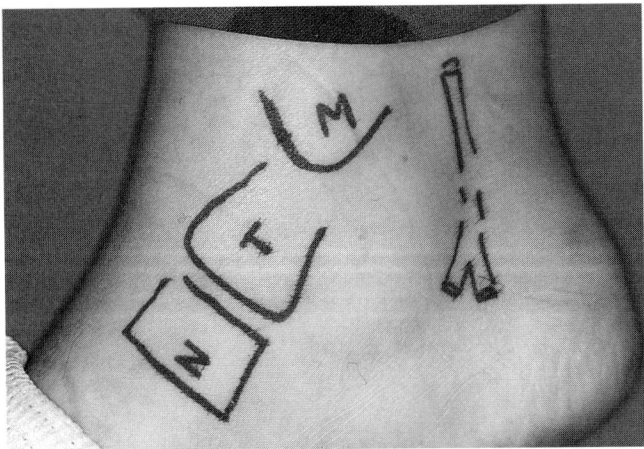

Fig. 7. **Anatomical references for surgical resection of a talocalcaneal coalition.** M: medial malleolus; T: talus; N: navicular; and, on the right, the neurovascular bundle.

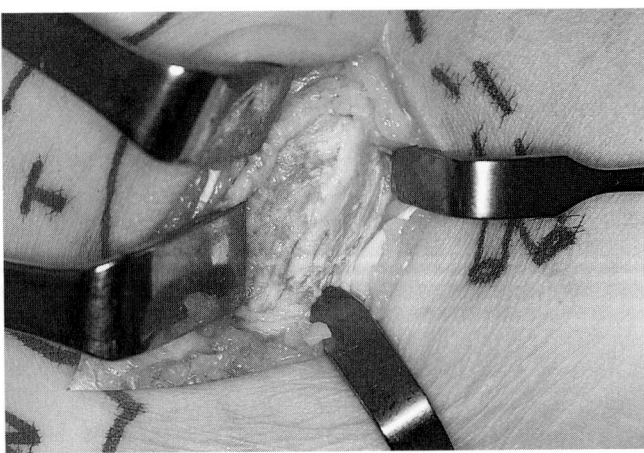

Fig. 9. The bone bar delimited.

and midfoot motion with non-weightbearing being maintained until the 6th week. The start of weightbearing should be gradual, recognizing that pain and stiffness are signs that the non-weightbearing period may need to be prolonged.

Triple Arthrodesis

Triple arthrodesis is the surgery of choice in cases in which conservative management or limited surgical resection are likely to result in unsatisfactory outcomes. It is indicated for talocalcaneal coalitions when there is evidence of degenerative arthritis, involvement of more than 50% of the posterior subtalar joint, or calcaneovalgus of more than 16 degrees.[13, 20] It is also considered the defini-

tive surgery after bar resection has failed for both talocalcaneal and calcaneonavicular coalitions. Currently its use has decreased, since additional diagnostic studies have led to more accurate diagnosis. The fact that younger patients now have diagnostic confirmation of the coalition also contributes to the infrequent use of this surgical approach.

Os Calcis Osteotomy

Carroll[29] has suggested os calcis osteotomy as an alternative to a triple arthrodesis in cases with degenerative osteoarthritis. This alternate method of treatment can lead to clinical improvement.[30] Wilde and Davidson suggest that the procedure should be more frequently performed.

OUTCOME

Most authors report a high rate of good results with both conservative and surgical treatment.

NONOPERATIVE TREATMENT

Reports of nonoperative treatment are less frequent than reports of studies of operative management. Takakura has reported 68% good results with nonoperative treatment in talocalcaneal coalitions. Gonzalez noted that the actual in-

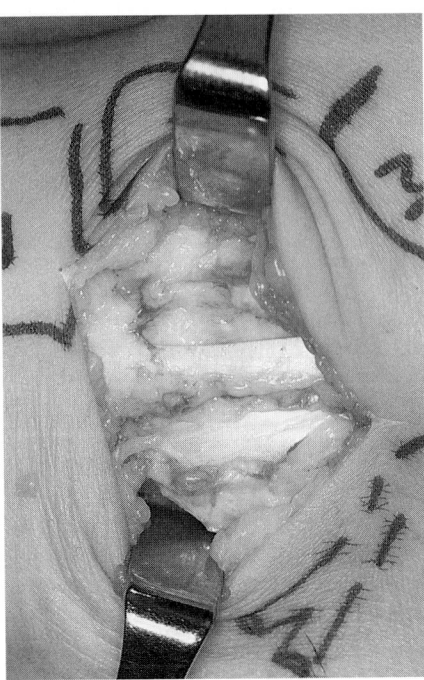

Fig. 8. Identification of flexor tendons.

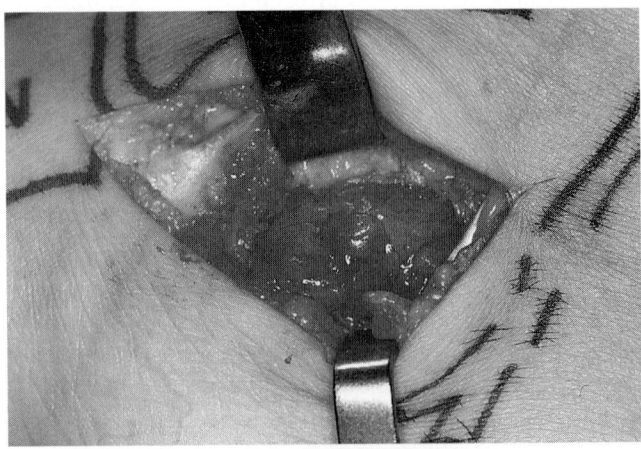

Fig. 10. Cavity filled with fat.

cidence of good results is not known in calcaneonavicular resection. Mosier also reported favorable outcomes with nonoperative treatment in both calcaneonavicular and talocalcaneal coalitions.

OPERATIVE TREATMENT

Most results have very satisfactory outcomes. Jayakumar and Cowell[16] also found good outcomes following bony resection. Resection of the calcaneonavicular coalition has a high degree of successful results, varying from 68 to 96%. The best results were found in patients whose age was between 1 and 15 years.[11, 31, 32] The presence of talar beaking did not change the good results.

The results of resection of talocalcaneal coalition are only slightly less optimistic, varying between 77 and 80%.[9, 12, 33] Wilde et al,[20] however, were more precise in their criteria, and only 50% of their patients had a favorable result. They stressed that extension of the coalition so that more than 50% of the posterior facet was involved, coupled with hindfoot valgus of more than 16 degrees, led to unfavorable outcomes. In this series, only 40% of the patients had preoperative indications for bar resection, whereas the remaining 60% underwent triple arthrodesis.

Davidson[28] analyzed a series of 17 coalitions and divided them into four groups according to the degree of valgus of the os calcis. Four feet responded to nonoperative treatment. Cases in group 3 (18 degree valgus) and seven feet in group IV (25 degree valgus) had poor results with resection of the talocalcaneal bar.

REFERENCES

1. Harris RI, Beath T: Etiology of peroneal spastic flat foot. J Bone Joint Surg Br 1948; 30:624.
2. Slomann HC: On coalitio calcaneo-navicularis. J Orthop Surg 1921; 3:586.
3. Mosier KM, Asher M: Tarsal coalitions and peroneal spastic flat foot. J Bone Joint Surg Am 1984; 66:976.
4. Daumas L, Morin C, Leonard JC: Les synostoses congénitales du tarse. Arch Pediatr 1996; 3:900.
5. O'Rahilly R, Gray DJ, Gardner E: Chondrification in the hands and feet of staged human embryos. Contrib Embryol 1957; 36:183.
6. Gardner E: Prenatal development of the skeleton and joint of the human foot. J Bone Joint Surg Am 1959; 44:847.
7. Leonard MA: The inheritance of tarsal coalition and its relationship to spastic flatfoot. J Bone Joint Surg Br 1974; 56:520.
8. Kawashima T, Uhthoff HK: Prenatal development around sustentaculum tali and its relation to talocalcaneal coalitions. J Pediatr Orthop 1990; 10:238.
9. Scranton PE: Treatment of symptomatic talocalcaneal coalition. J Bone Joint Surg Am 1987; 69:533.
10. Drennan JC: Tarsal coalition. Instruct Course Lect 1996; 45:323.
11. González P, Kumar SJ: Calcaneonavicular coalition treated by resection and interposition of the extensor digitorum brevis muscle. J Bone Joint Surg Am 1990; 72:71.
12. Olney BW, Asher MA: Excision of symptomatic coalition of the middle facet of the

talocalcaneal joint. J Bone Joint Surg Am 1987; 69:539.
13. Stormont DM, Peterson HA: The relative incidence of tarsal coalition. Clin Orthop 1983; 181:28.
14. Elftan H, Manter J: The evolution of the human foot, with especial reference to the joints. J Anat 1935; 70:56.
15. Epeldegui T, Delgado E: Acetabulum pedis. Part I: Talocalcaneonavicular joint socket in normal foot. Pediatr Orthop 1995; 4B:1.
16. Jayakumar S, Cowell HR: Rigid flatfoot. Clin Orthop 1977; 122:77.
17. Badgley CE: Coalition of the calcaneus and the navicular. Arch Surg 1927; 15:75.
18. Comfort TK, Johnson LO: Resection for symptomatic talocalcaneal coalition. J Pediatr Orthop 1998; 18:283.
19. Takakura Y, Sugimoto K, Tanaka Y, et al: Symptomatic talocalcaneal coalition. Clin Orthop 1991; 269:249.
20. Wilde PH, Torode IP, Dickens DR, et al: Resection for symptomatic talocalcaneal coalition. J Bone Joint Surg Br 1994; 76:797.
21. Rouvreau PH, Puliquen JC, Langlais J, et al: Synostoses et coalitions tarsiennes chez l'enfant: Etude de 68 cas chez 47 patients. Rev Clin Orthop 1994; 80:252.
22. Clarke DM: Multiple tarsal coalitions in the same foot. J Pediatr Orthop 1997; 17:777.
23. Wechsler RJ, Schweitzer ME, Deely DM, et al: Tarsal coalition: Depiction and characterization with CT and MR imaging. Radiology 1994; 193:447.

24. Lima RT, Mishkin F: The bone scan in tarsal coalition: a case report. Pediatr Radiol 1996; 26:754.
25. Bettin D, Karbowski A, Schwering L: Congenital ball-and-socket anomaly of the ankle. J Pediatr Orthop 1996; 16:492.
26. Cowell, HR: Talocalcaneal coalition and new causes of peroneal spastic flatfoot. Clin Orthop 1972; 85:16.
27. Cowell HR: Extensor brevis arthroplasty. In Proceedings of the American academy of Orthopaedic surgeons. J Bone Joint Surg Am 1970; 52:820.
28. Davidson R: Clinical outcome of tarsal coalition as it relates to valgus deformity. Presented in POSNA annual meeting, Cleveland, May, 1998.
29. Carroll NC: The pediatric foot. In Dee R, Hunst LC, Grumber M (eds): Kottneiers Principles of Orthopaedic Practice. New York, McGraw-Hill, 1998, p 822.
30. Cain TJ, Hyman S: Peroneal spastic flatfoot: Its treatment by osteotomy of the os calcis. J Bone Surg 1978; 60:527.
31. Chambers RB, Cook TM, Cowell HR: Surgical reconstruction for calcaneonavicular coalition. J Bone Joint Surg Am 1982; 64:829.
32. Swiontkowski MF, Scranton PE, Hansen S: Tarsal coalitions: Long-term results of surgical treatment. J Pediatr Orthop 1983; 3:287.
33. McCormack TJ, Olney B, Asher M: Talocalcaneal coalition resection: a 10-year follow-up. J Pediatr Orthop 1997; 17:13.

FLEXIBLE FLATFOOT, METATARSUS ADDUCTUS, SKEWFOOT

Vincent S. Mosca

Summary
- Flatfoot is ubiquitous at birth and present in approximately 20% of adults.
- Flexible flatfoot rarely causes pain and disability unless associated with a short Achilles tendon.
- The longitudinal arch develops spontaneously during the first decade of life.
- There is no evidence that shoes or orthoses have any effect on the development of the arch.
- Surgery is rarely, if ever, indicated for flexible flatfoot.
- Surgery may be indicated for flexible flatfoot with a short Achilles tendon when nonsurgical treatment has failed to relieve the pain and callosities under the head of the plantar flexed talus. Joint preserving techniques should be employed.
- Metatarsus adductus is a very common neonatal foot shape.
- Prognosis for spontaneous correction of metatarsus adductus deformity is excellent.
- Flexibility is the key prognostic feature in metatarsus adductus.
- Serial casting is employed for partly flexible and rigid deformities of metatarsus adductus.
- Surgery is rarely, if ever, indicated for metatarsus adductus.
- Medial cuneiform and cuboid osteotomies are the procedures recommended for the rare situation of an older child with disability related to residual deformity of metatarsus adductus.
- Skewfoot is a rare and poorly defined foot shape that combines the forefoot deformity of metatarsus adductus with the hindfoot deformity of flatfoot.
- The incidence, cause, and natural history of skewfoot are unknown.
- Nonoperative treatment of skewfoot with serial casting should be employed, using lack of flexibility as the indication (as in metatarsus adductus).
- Disability in the older child with skewfoot is similar to that in children with flexible flatfoot with a short Achilles tendon.
- Surgery is indicated for skewfoot when nonsurgical treatment has failed to relieve the pain and callosities under the head of the plantar flexed talus. Joint preserving techniques should be employed to correct the hindfoot and midfoot deformities. Lengthening of the Achilles tendon is almost routinely required.

FLEXIBLE FLATFOOT

A flatfoot is characterized by excessive lowering of the longitudinal arch. The point at which a low normal arch becomes a flatfoot is unknown, however, because there are no universally accepted clinical or radiographic definitions of the average height, or the normal range of heights, of the longitudinal arch. Despite the lack of a strict definition, all practitioners agree that some arches are lower than others. Controversy about the definition, cause, natural history, and treatment of flatfoot has abounded for many decades.

Harris and Beath[1] found flatfoot in 23% of the 3600 adults they examined, and they subclassified these feet. Flexible flatfoot, which accounted for approximately two thirds of these feet, was "regarded as the normal contour of a strong and stable foot" and "of little consequence as a cause of disability." A flexible flatfoot with a short Achilles tendon, which was found in about 25% of the feet, was a common cause of pain and disability.[2] The remaining 9% were rigid flatfeet and were most often caused by tarsal coalitions. Some of these were painful.

Flexible flatfoot is present at birth, is much more common in children than adults, and tends to run in families. Footprint[3] and radiographic[4] studies have confirmed that the longitudinal arch develops spontaneously during the first decade of life. The average height of the arch increases and the normal range of arch heights narrows with age.

PATHOGENESIS
The height of the longitudinal arch is determined by the shapes of the bones and the laxity of the ligaments of the foot.[5] Muscles are important for balance and function, but not for structure. It is not known when the Achilles tendon contracture develops in those affected individuals.

CLINICAL FEATURES
The primary deformity of a flatfoot is excessive eversion of the subtalar complex. This creates two clinical deformities: valgus alignment of the hindfoot and planus alignment of the midfoot. Valgus positioning of the calcaneus under the talus is one component of eversion of the subtalar complex. Eversion also consists of (1) external rotation of the calcaneus under the talus, creating out-toeing; (2) abduction and dorsiflexion of the navicular on the head of the talus, which, combined with plantar flexion of the talus, produces a midfoot sag or lowering of the longitudinal arch; and (3) dorsiflexion of the calcaneus in relation to the talus but with plantar flexion of the calcaneus in relation to the tibia. The lateral column, or border, of the foot is short in relation to the medial column. Supination of the forefoot on the hindfoot is a second deformity that exists in a flatfoot. It accounts for the simultaneous ground contact of all of the metatarsal heads. There is free mobility of the subtalar complex in a flexible flatfoot. This is manifested by elevation of the longitudinal arch and inversion of the hindfoot

to varus during toe-standing (Fig. 1). The ankle can be dorsiflexed at least 10 degrees above neutral in the benign flexible flatfoot. Proper assessment for contracture of the Achilles tendon is performed with the subtalar joint inverted to neutral and the knee extended.

INVESTIGATION

Radiographs are not necessary to diagnose flexible flatfoot. They are helpful in the diagnosis of rigid flatfoot. Radiographs of the flexible flatfoot with a short Achilles tendon are helpful in the preoperative assessment of deformity and should always be performed in weightbearing.

DIFFERENTIAL DIAGNOSIS

Flexible flatfoot is ubiquitous at birth and is a component of the positional calcaneovalgus foot deformity. It must be differentiated from congenital vertical talus at birth, however. In the latter deformity, the subtalar complex cannot be inverted and the longitudinal arch cannot be created by passive manipulation. Progress flattening and rigidity of the longitudinal arch occurs in 1% of the population between the ages of 8 and 12 years. Tarsal coalition is the usual cause.

MANAGEMENT

The natural history is that there will be a spontaneous increase in the height of the longitudinal arch in most flatfooted children. The prognosis for untreated individuals with flexible flatfeet is excellent for long-term comfort and function. The focus must, therefore, be on education rather than intervention.

Despite these facts, attempts have been made to create an arch in the child's foot by nonoperative and operative means. With the now-known natural history of arch development in children, it is not surprising that uncontrolled studies have reported the efficacy of corrective shoes and arch supports in the creation of the longitudinal arch in children. However, two controlled, prospective, randomized studies found no efficacy of these interventions over natural history alone,[6, 7] and studies from developing countries have found a higher prevalence of flatfeet, some of which were painful and had restricted mobility, in shod compared with unshod children.[8, 9]

Some children with flexible flatfoot have diffuse and poorly localized, activity-related pain in the leg or foot. Shoe inserts have been shown to relieve or diminish these symptoms as well as to increase the useful life of shoes that would otherwise be worn unevenly. These effects have been observed without a documented alteration in the height of the arch.[10, 11]

Some children with flexible flatfoot with a short Achilles tendon have pain with weightbearing or callosities, or both, under the head of the talus. A contracted heel cord prevents normal dorsiflexion of the ankle during gait. The talus remains plantar-flexed and the dorsiflexion stress is shifted to the talonavicular joint. The soft tissues under the head of the talus are subjected to excessive direct axial loading and shear stress. A rigid arch support will only increase the pressure under the head of the talus. An aggressive Achilles tendon stretching program may relieve symptoms by increasing the range of ankle dorsiflexion.

Surgery is rarely, if ever, indicated for flexible flatfoot. Nevertheless, an exhaustive list of operative procedures to correct flatfoot has been proposed during the last century.[12] Most procedures have been abandoned because of failure to achieve or maintain correction of deformity or to relieve symptoms. All long-term follow-up studies of arthrodesis of even small midtarsal joints in children have documented the development of degenerative arthrosis at adjacent, unfused joints.[12]

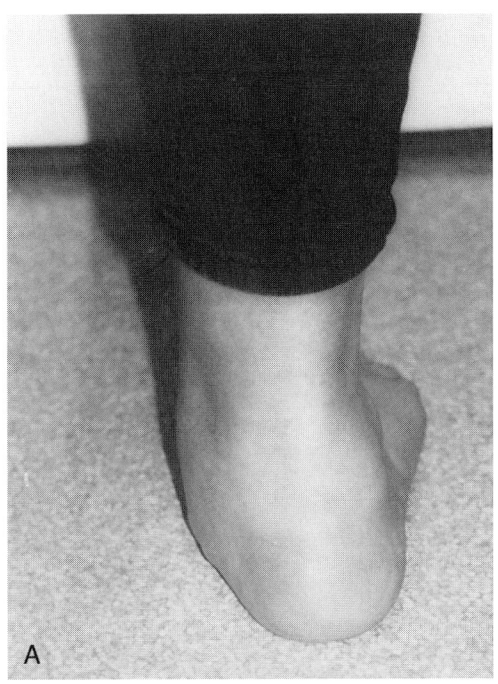 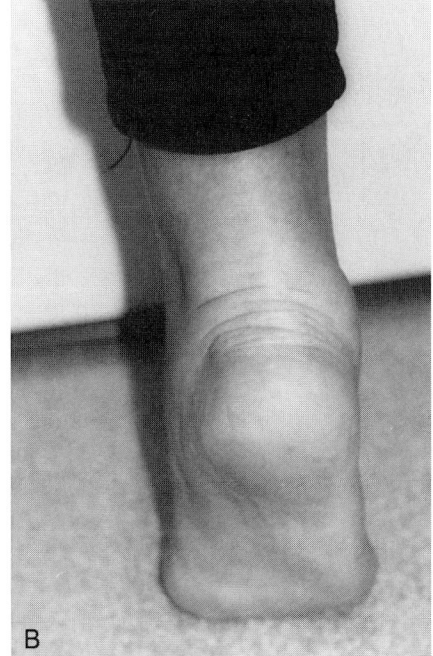

Fig. 1. Flexible flatfoot. *A,* Valgus alignment of the hindfoot with abduction of the midfoot and flattening of the longitudinal arch. *B,* Inversion of the hindfoot to varus with elevation of the longitudinal arch during toe-standing. (From Mosca VS: Flexible flatfoot and skewfoot. In Drennan JC [ed]: The Child's Foot and Ankle, New York, Raven Press, 1992, pp 355–376.)

A   B

Surgery is occasionally indicated for flexible flatfoot with a short Achilles tendon when prolonged attempts at nonoperative management have failed to relieve the pain and callosities under the head of the plantar-flexed talus. The Achilles tendon must be lengthened. In addition, severe foot deformity should be corrected by one of the described osteotomy procedures, the only techniques that have been shown to correct and maintain correction of deformity while avoiding arthrodesis. The posterior calca-neal displacement osteotomy[13] creates a compensatory deformity to improve the valgus alignment of the hindfoot. It often improves the shape of the foot and relieves pain, although it does not directly address and correct the eversion deformity of the subtalar complex. The calcaneal lengthening osteotomy[14, 15] corrects all components of even severe eversion deformity at the site of deformity, restores the function of the subtalar complex, relieves symptoms, and is, therefore, the procedure of choice (Fig. 2). It also

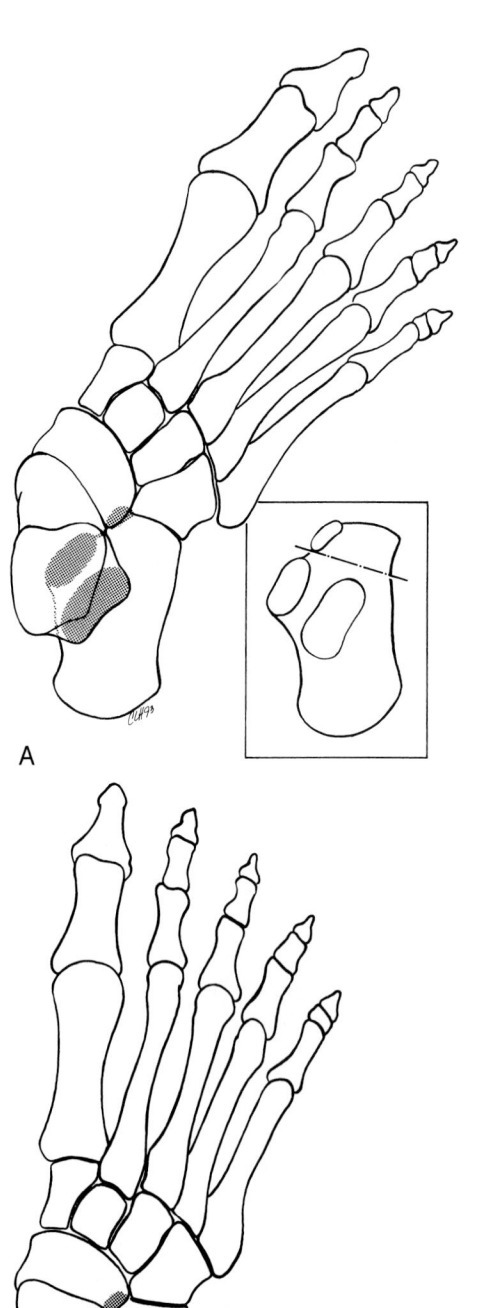

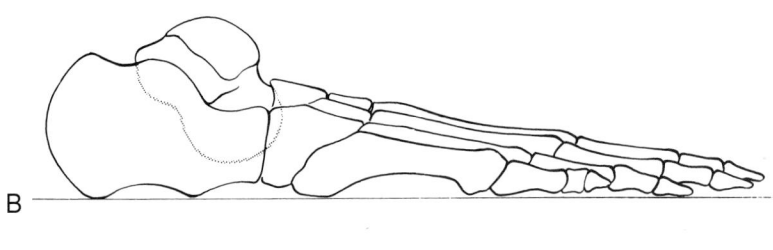

Fig. 2. Calcaneal lengthening osteotomy. *A,* Dorsal view of a flatfoot. Oblique dashed line indicates position of the osteotomy exiting between the anterior and middle facets of the calcaneus. *B,* Lateral view of a flatfoot. Plantar-flexion of the talus and calcaneus creates a sag of the midfoot. *C,* Dorsal view shows correction of all components of the deformity with the trapezoid-shaped graft in place. *D,* Lateral view shows correction of all components of the deformity with the graft in place. (From Mosca VS: Calcaneal lengthening for valgus deformity of the hind-foot: Results in children who had severe, symptomatic flatfoot and skewfoot. J Bone Joint Surg Am 1995; 77:500.)

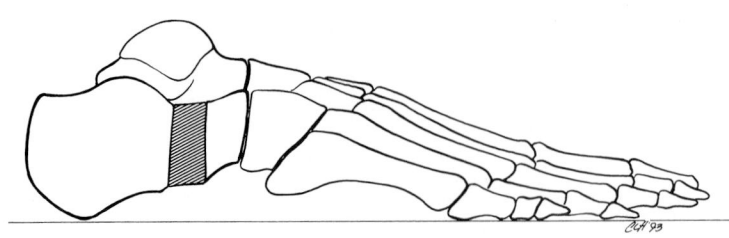

has the best reported long-term results of any procedure that has been used to correct flatfoot.[16] Rigid supination of the forefoot, if present, must be recognized and treated concurrently with a procedure on the medial column of the foot, such as an osteotomy of the medial cuneiform or first metatarsal bone.

METATARSUS ADDUCTUS

Metatarsus adductus and metatarsus varus are terms that have been used to describe the most common congenital foot deformity, which is characterized by medial deviation of the forefoot on the hindfoot. There are actually three different foot deformities that share this feature. Confusion exists concerning their differentiation and nomenclature. Metatarsus adductus is the term used most commonly to describe a benign deformity in which medial deviation of the forefoot on the hindfoot is combined with neutral to slight valgus alignment of the hindfoot. Although metatarsus varus is the term used by some authors to describe the same deformity, it can also be used to refer to a rare foot deformity characterized by medial deviation with supination of the forefoot on the hindfoot. The lateral border of the foot is convex and the base of the fifth metatarsal is prominent in both of these conditions. Both terms have been used to describe a rare foot deformity now commonly referred to as skewfoot, which combines medial deviation of the forefoot on the hindfoot with severe valgus deformity of the hindfoot.

The incidence of metatarsus adductus has been reported at between 0.1% and 12%.[17, 18] The wide range reflects the lack of a strict definition. The long-term disabilities of metatarsus adductus in adulthood have not been reported. The natural history of metatarsus adductus is for spontaneous correction in 86% to 89% of cases.[19, 20] The rate may actually approach 95% when broad inclusion criteria are employed. The flexibility rather than the severity of the deformity correlates with prognosis for spontaneous correction.[21]

PATHOGENESIS
Although many theories have been proposed, the cause of metatarsus adductus remains unknown. In utero positioning and familial transmission may account for some cases. Congenital deformity of the medial cuneiform bone, consisting of a trapezoidal shape with medial tilt of the first metatarsal-cuneiform joint, is a likely cause, particularly for those cases that do not correct spontaneously (Fig. 3).[22]

CLINICAL FEATURES
Medial deviation of the forefoot on the hindfoot is best seen by viewing the plantar aspect of the foot and noting the alignment of the lateral border (Fig. 4A). The severity of the deformity can be determined by using Bleck's heel bisector method; however, the flexibility of the deformity is the more important feature to assess.[23] The foot is flexible if the forefoot can be passively corrected into abduction (Fig. 4B) and is partly flexible if it can be passively corrected to neutral. It is inflexible, or rigid, if it cannot be passively corrected to neutral.

There is frequently a dorsal-plantar skin crease on the medial aspect of the foot. The ankle has full dorsiflexion

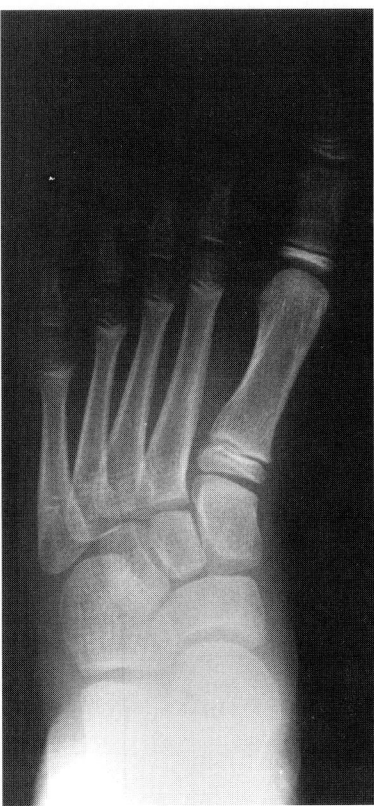

Fig. 3 Metatarsus adductus. Trapezoid-shaped medial cuneiform with medial deviation of medial cuneiform-first metatarsal joint. (From Cappello T, Mosca VS: Metatarsus adductus and skewfoot. Foot Ankle Clin 1998; 3:1.)

and plantar-flexion mobility. The hindfoot is in neutral to slight valgus alignment and there is normal mobility of the subtalar joint.

INVESTIGATION
Radiographs are not necessary for diagnosis. The radiographic classification system proposed by Berg[24] is flawed and prone to error.[25]

DIFFERENTIAL DIAGNOSIS
The differentiation of metatarsus adductus, metatarsus varus, and skewfoot may not be possible in infancy, but there should be no confusion of these conditions with clubfoot. The latter deformity is characterized by medial deviation of the forefoot as well as rigid equinus, cavus, and varus of the ankle, midfoot, and hindfoot.

MANAGEMENT
Flexible metatarsus adductus resolves spontaneously. Serial long leg casting should be employed for those feet in children between 6 and 12 months of age that are partly flexible and rigid.[19, 21] The deformity will usually be corrected in 6 to 8 weeks (three to four casts). A holding device, such as a reverse or straight last shoe, should be used at night for several months thereafter to prevent recurrence of deformity. One can anticipate 90% good results in the treated feet at long-term follow-up and no need for surgery, even with mild to moderate residual deformity.[19]

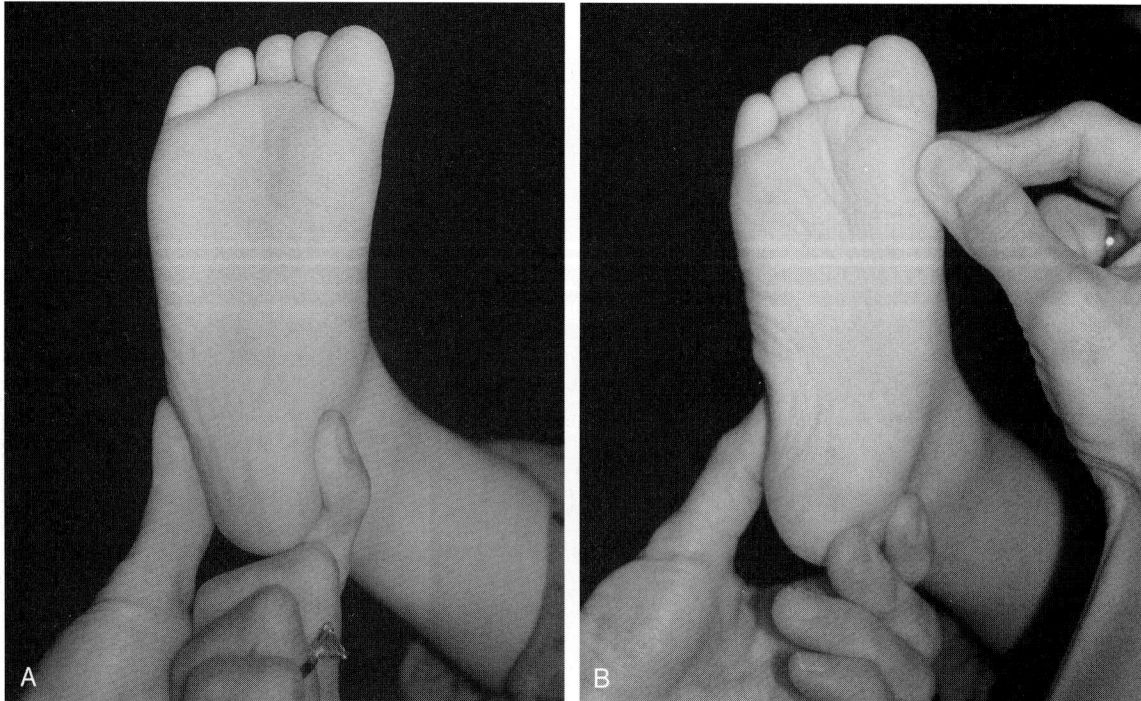

Fig. 4. Metatarsus adductus. *A*, Plantar view shows convex lateral border. *B*, Flexible deformity passively correctable into abduction. (From Cappello T, Mosca VS: Metatarsus adductus and skewfoot. Foot Ankle Clin 1998; 3:1.)

Surgery is rarely, if ever, needed. However, severe deformity in the older, untreated child may cause pain, callus formation, and shoe fitting problems. The techniques of tarsometatarsal capsulotomies and of osteotomies at the base of the metatarsals are associated with high rates of complications.[12] An opening wedge osteotomy of the trapezoid-shaped medial cuneiform treats the deformity at the site of deformity and is associated with few risks or complications. Concurrent osteotomies at the base of the lesser metatarsals or a closing wedge osteotomy of the cuboid bone may be necessary.[26, 27]

SKEWFOOT

Skewfoot is the term used to describe a rare and poorly defined foot shape that combines the forefoot deformity of metatarsus adductus with the hindfoot deformity of flatfoot.[12] It is generally discussed in relation to metatarsus adductus, although disability because of the condition is most often related to the hindfoot deformity. It has had many appellations in the literature, including metatarsus adductus, metatarsus varus, serpentine foot, and Z-foot. The unifying and defining features are the severity of the components of the deformity and the resistance to treatment.[28–30] Very little is known about this deformity, including the strict definition, prevalence, cause, natural history, and effective treatment.

PATHOGENESIS
Idiopathic and iatrogenic skewfoot deformities exist. The cause is unknown.

CLINICAL FEATURES
It is difficult to differentiate skewfoot from metatarsus adductus in infancy. Medial deviation of the forefoot with a midfoot crease is common to both conditions. Assessment of the degree of valgus deformity of the hindfoot in such small feet is neither reliable nor important for early management. The deformity is more apparent in the older child and adolescent. In the older age groups, the deformity often more closely resembles a flatfoot.

INVESTIGATION
The radiographic classification system proposed by Berg[24] is flawed and prone to error.[25] A weightbearing anteroposterior radiograph of the foot in the older child (Fig. 5A) reveals abduction at the talonavicular joint, adduction at Lisfranc's joint, and a trapezoid medial cuneiform with medial deviation of the cuneiform–first metatarsal joint. The weightbearing lateral view (Fig. 5B) reveals plantar flexion of the talus and calcaneus, dorsiflexion at the talonavicular joint, and plantar flexion at Lisfranc's joint. It is these opposite direction deformities in the interval between the hindfoot and forefoot in both planes that characterize skewfoot.[12, 15]

DIFFERENTIAL DIAGNOSIS
The unanswered question is whether skewfoot is metatarsus adductus with excessive hindfoot valgus or a flatfoot with excessive forefoot adductus.

MANAGEMENT
One cannot clearly differentiate skewfoot from metatarsus adductus in infancy and one cannot correct valgus defor-

mity of the hindfoot nonoperatively. It is, therefore, reasonable to manage skewfoot with serial casting of the forefoot deformity based on its flexibility as is recommended for metatarsus adductus. Care must be taken to avoid excessive valgus stress on the already everted subtalar joint during manipulation and casting. Reverse last shoes and Denis Browne bars should likewise be avoided because of their tendency to apply valgus stress on the subtalar joint.[24]

The Achilles tendon is contracted in most of the persistent and symptomatic skewfeet in older children and adolescents. These patients resemble symptomatic patients with flexible flatfoot with a short Achilles tendon. They have pain with weightbearing and callosities under the head of the talus.[12, 15, 31] Additional pain and callosities may be present at the first metatarsal head and the base of the fifth metatarsal. There is no role for rigid arch supports, which will only increase the pressure under the head of the rigidly plantar-flexed talus. An aggressive Achilles tendon stretching program may relieve symptoms by increasing the range of ankle dorsiflexion.

Surgery is occasionally indicated for skewfoot when prolonged attempts at nonoperative management have failed to relieve the pain and callosities under the head of the plantar-flexed talus.[12, 15, 31] Suggestions for operative treatment can be found in the literature,[32] but most are based on theory and not on a review of operative results.[12] The recommendations include tarsometatarsal capsulotomies or osteotomies at the base of the metatarsals for correction of the forefoot deformity combined with subtalar arthrodesis. High rates of complications, including degenerative osteoarthrosis, have been reported at long-term follow-up of these procedures.[12] The largest reported series on the operative management of skewfoot deformity recently documented good correction of all components of the deformity and relief of symptoms at short-term follow-up using alternative techniques that importantly avoid arthrodesis of the hindfoot.[31] A medial cuneiform opening wedge osteotomy for correction of the forefoot adductus was combined with the calcaneal lengthening osteotomy for correction of the hindfoot deformity (see Fig. 5). Achilles tendon lengthening was required. Long-term follow-up is forthcoming, but good results are anticipated because of the favorable intermediate-term results that have been reported for each of the individual procedures.

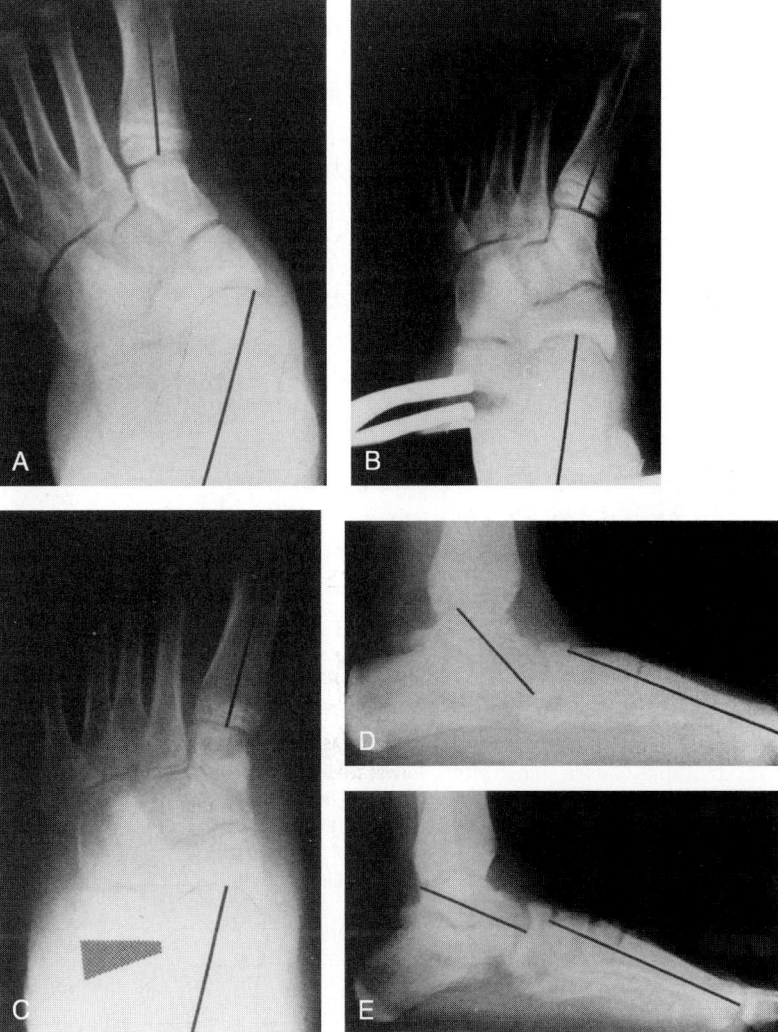

Fig. 5. Painful skewfoot deformity in a 13 year old boy corrected by means of a calcaneal lengthening osteotomy, medial cuneiform opening wedge osteotomy, and Achilles tendon lengthening. *A,* AP view shows abduction at the talonavicular joint, adduction at Lisfranc's joint, and a trapezoid-shaped medial cuneiform with medial deviation of the cuneiform-first metatarsal joint. *B,* Laminar spreader in calcaneal osteotomy shows good correction of the malalignment of the subtalar complex. Medial cuneiform deformity is better visualized on this image. *C,* Hatched area highlights the calcaneal graft. The bone graft wedge in the medial cuneiform has corrected that deformity. *D,* Preoperative lateral view shows plantar flexion of the talus and calcaneus, dorsiflexion at the talonavicular joint, and plantar flexion at Lisfranc's joint. *E,* Postoperative correction of deformities. (From Mosca VS. Flexible flatfoot and skewfoot. In Drennan JC [ed]: The Child's Foot and Ankle. New York, Raven Press, 1992, pp. 355–376.)

REFERENCES

1. Harris RI, Beath T: Army Foot Survey: An Investigation of Foot Ailments in Canadian Soldiers, Vol 1. Ottawa, National Research Council of Canada, 1947.
2. Harris RI, Beath T: Hypermobile flat-foot with short tendo Achilles. J Bone Joint Surg Am 1948; 30:116.
3. Staheli LT, Chew DE, Corbett M: The longitudinal arch: A survey of eight-hundred and eighty-two feet in normal children and adults. J Bone Joint Surg Am 1987; 69:426.
4. Vanderwilde R, Staheli LT, Chew DE, et al: Measurements on radiographs of the foot in normal infants and children. J Bone Joint Surg Am 1988; 70:407.
5. Basmajian JV, Stecko G: The role of muscles in arch support of the foot: An electromyographic study. J Bone Joint Surg Am 1963; 45:1184.
6. Gould N, Moreland M, Alvarez R, et al: Development of the child's arch. Foot Ankle 1989; 9:241.
7. Wenger DR, Mauldin D, Speck G, et al: Corrective shoes and inserts as treatment for flexible flatfoot in infants and children. J Bone Joint Surg Am 1989; 71:800.
8. Sim-Fook L, Hodgson AR: A comparison of foot forms among the non-shoe and shoe-wearing Chinese population. J Bone Joint Surg Am 1958; 40:1058.
9. Rao UB, Joseph B: The influence of footwear on the prevalence of flat foot: A survey of 2300 children. J Bone Joint Surg Br 1992; 74:525.
10. Basta NW, Mital MA, Bonadio O, et al: A comparative study of the role of shoes, arch supports, and navicular cookies in the management of symptomatic mobile flat feet in children. Int Orthop 1977; 1:143.
11. Theologis TN, Gordon C, Benson MKD: Heel seats and shoe wear. J Pediatr Orthop 1994; 14:760.
12. Mosca VS: Flexible flatfoot and skewfoot. In Drennan JC (ed): The Child's Foot and Ankle. New York, Raven Press, 1992, p 355.
13. Koutsogiannis E: Treatment of mobile flat foot by displacement osteotomy of the calcaneus. J Bone Joint Surg Br 1971; 53:96.
14. Evans D: Calcaneo-valgus deformity. J Bone Joint Surg Br 1975; 57:270.
15. Mosca VS: Calcaneal lengthening for valgus deformity of the hindfoot: Results in children who had severe, symptomatic flatfoot and skewfoot. J Bone Joint Surg Am 1995; 77:500.
16. Phillips GE: A review of elongation of os calcis for flat feet. J Bone Joint Surg Br 1983; 65:15.
17. Wynne-Davies R: Family studies and the cause of congenital club foot: Talipes equinovarus, talipes calcaneovalgus and metatarsus varus. J Bone Joint Surg Br 1964; 46:445.
18. Hunziger UA, Largo RH, Duc G: Neonatal metatarsus adductus, joint mobility, axis and rotation of the lower extremity in preterm and term children 0–5 years of age. Eur J Pediatr 1988; 148:19.
19. Ponseti IV, Becker JR: Congenital metatarsus adductus: The results of treatment. J Bone Joint Surg Am 1966; 48:702.
20. Rushforth GF: The natural history of hooked forefoot. J Bone Joint Surg Br 1978; 60:530.
21. Farsetti P, Weinstein SL, Ponseti IV: The long-term functional and radiographic outcomes of untreated and non-operatively treated metatarsus adductus. J Bone Joint Surg Am 1994; 76:257.
22. Morcuende JA, Ponseti EV: Congenital metatarsus adductus in early human fetal development: A histologic study. Clin Orthop 1996; 333:261.
23. Bleck EE: Metatarsus adductus: Classification and relationship to outcomes of treatment. J Pediatr Orthop 1983; 3:2.
24. Berg EE: A reappraisal of metatarsus adductus and skewfoot. J Bone Joint Surg Am 1986; 68:1185.
25. Cook DA, Breed AL, Cook T, et al: Observer variability in the radiographic measurement and classification of metatarsus adductus. J Pediatr Orthop 1992; 12:86.
26. Anderson DJ, Schoenecker PL, Blair VP III, et al: Combined lateral column shortening and medial column lengthening in the treatment of severe forefoot adductus. Orthop Trans 1991; 15:665.
27. Kling TF, Schmidt TL, Conklin MJ: Open wedge osteotomy of the first cuneiform for metatarsus adductus. Orthop Trans 1991; 15:106.
28. Peabody CW, Muro F: Congenital metatarsus varus. J Bone Joint Surg Am 1933; 15:171.
29. McCormick DW, Blount WP: Metatarsus adductovarus: "Skewfoot." JAMA 1949; 141:449.
30. Kite JH: Congenital metatarsus varus: Report of 300 cases. J Bone Joint Surg Am 1950; 32:500.
31. Mosca VS: Skewfoot deformity in children: Correction by calcaneal neck lengthening and medial cuneiform opening wedge osteotomies. J Pediatr Orthop 1993; 13:807.
32. Peterson HA: Skewfoot (forefoot adduction with heel valgus). J Pediatr Orthop 1986; 6:24.

section 9

chapter 28

BUNIONS

Heidi M. Stephens

Summary

- Bunions are a common forefoot disorder with multiple causes, most often associated with constrictive shoewear.
- Nonoperative treatment involves relieving pressure with wide footwear.
- Operative intervention should be considered only for pain symptoms.
- The hallux valgus and intermetatarsal angles measured on weightbearing radiographs are used in surgical decision-making.
- To avoid complications from bunion surgery, both patient and procedure selection must be careful.

DEFINITION

Hallux valgus is a complex deformity of the first ray. Typically, the first metatarsal lies in varus relative to the lesser metatarsals (metatarsus primus varus). The metatarsal head is prominent, often with an enlarged median eminence and bursa formation. The hallux itself lies in valgus and is commonly pronated. Crowding of the second toe is common. Another term for hallux valgus, "bunion," is derived from the Latin word for turnip because of the appearance of the inflamed metatarsal head.

HISTORICAL REVIEW

It is well recognized that hallux valgus is virtually absent in unshod or barefoot societies.[1] Beginning in the early 1900s, in Europe and the United States, procedures were developed to surgically correct painful hallux valgus. As early as 1933, Verbrugge[2] reported that there were 153 different described surgeries for hallux valgus. The number of procedures continues to grow as surgeons seek to improve their surgical outcomes. There are several reasons for the large number of procedures for hallux valgus, including surgeon's preference for and modifications of techniques and variability in the anatomy of the deformity from foot to foot. Every procedure has potential complications, and patient satisfaction following hallux valgus surgery has not always met surgeons' expectations. Although hundreds of separate procedures have been described to surgically treat symptomatic hallux valgus, these procedures generally fall into several discrete categories. These categories of procedures and specific examples of techniques within each category will be discussed. Specific indications and contraindications for various procedures and known complications will be noted.

EPIDEMIOLOGY/ PATHOGENESIS

Contributing factors in the development of hallux valgus include intrinsic (genetic) and extrinsic (environmental) factors. Women far outnumber men presenting with hallux valgus. Adolescent hallux valgus is relatively uncommon and is generally associated with a strong family history. The incidence of hallux valgus increases with age and use of shoewear with high heels and/or a pointed toebox.[1]

CLINICAL FEATURES

The anatomy relevant for hallux valgus is not limited to the first metatarsal phalangeal joint where the most obvious component of the deformity exists. Pathoanatomy as far proximal as the knee and hindfoot may contribute to development and treatment. Genu valgum as well as hindfoot valgus and pronation (pes planovalgus) predispose the development of hallux valgus and may be associated with a higher rate of recurrence postoperatively. At the level of the tarsometatarsal (TMT) joint, the obliquity and mobility of the articulation have important implications in the development of hallux valgus.[3] The distal metatarsal articular angle and the congruence of the metatarsophalangeal (MTP) joint are significant anatomic features that will be discussed later.

The dynamic forces around the first MTP joint include the intrinsic and extrinsic flexor and extensor tendons. The sesamoid complex and the balance between the abductor and adductor hallucis muscles are also integral components of the first MTP joint position and function.[4]

PATIENT EVALUATION

A thorough history is the first element of evaluation of a patient with a painful hallux valgus deformity. Pain is the crucial element in the history. A patient who has a visible deformity but no pain is a poor surgical candidate. "Cosmetic" hallux valgus surgery frequently leads to unsatisfied patients. The location, timing, severity, and duration of the pain symptom need to be documented. Pain may exist over the medial eminence, within the joint, or under the first or second MTP joints. Exacerbating factors should be identified. Shoewear and activity questions need to be asked. There must be alignment of goals and expectations between the surgeon and the patient.[4]

The physical examination should begin with observation of the patient's gait and shoewear on entering the examination room. Overall limb alignment should be evaluated for evidence of excessive valgus at the knee or at the hindfoot level. Pronation and metatarsus adductus should be noted if present. The skin should be inspected for erythema or bursal swelling over the median eminence, which would indicate chronic pressure and inflammation. Calluses under the second MTP joint are often associated with hypermobility of the first ray or an excessively long second metatarsal relative to the first (Morton's foot). Any osteotomy of the first metatarsal undertaken in a patient who has a callus under the second MTP joint preoperatively may lead to further stress transfer and pain beneath the second metatarsal head postoperatively. The second metatarsal joint should be checked for painful instability. It is not uncommon to correct hallux valgus in order to allow reduction of a painful subluxed or dislocated second toe. The first metatarsocuneiform joint should be manipulated to determine whether hypermobility or painful crepitus is present. Either finding may suggest the use of a Lapidus procedure. The range of motion of the MTP joint should be documented in both the deformed and the passively corrected position. The neurovascular status of the foot should be carefully examined. A patient with lack of protective sensation may be a poor surgical candidate because of lack of compliance with non-weightbearing as well as the increased risk of stress transfer in the insensate foot. If pulses are not palpated, noninvasive vascular studies or vascular consultation is recommended before proceeding with surgery. Finally, the mood, affect, and general mental status of the patient may be factors in the treatment decision.[4, 5]

INVESTIGATION

The standard views for evaluation of a patient with hallux valgus are weightbearing anteroposterior and lateral views. There are standard radiographic angular measurements that should be recorded for any hallux valgus (Fig. 1). These include the hallux valgus angle (HVA), the intermetatarsal angle (IMA), and the distal metatarsal articular angle (DMAA). Normal values for these angles are as follows: HVA less than 15 degrees, IMA less than 9 degrees, and DMAA less than 9 degrees. The first metatarsocuneiform joint obliquity should also be noted. Obliquity of less than 8 degrees from the perpendicular of the long axis of the first metatarsal is considered normal.[3,4]

If excessive obliquity or hypermobility of the first metatarsocuneiform joint has been identified, an additional "strapped" weightbearing radiographic view should be obtained. Both an oblique metatarsocuneiform joint and a round metatarsal head predispose to hallux valgus. A metatarsocuneiform articulation that is perpendicular to the long axis of the metatarsal shaft is more stable and is associated

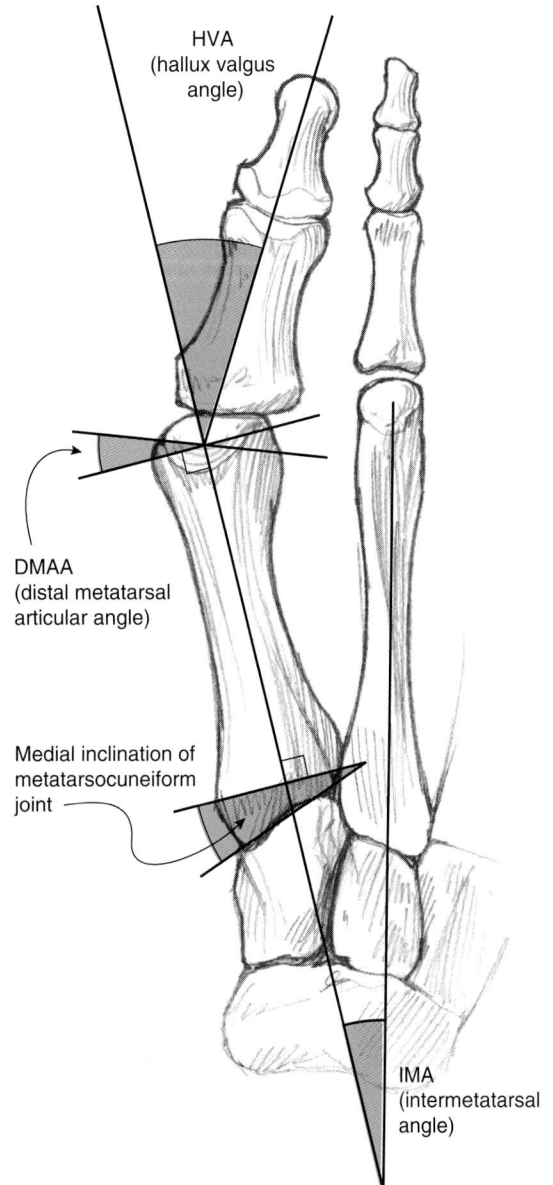

HVA
(hallux valgus
angle)

DMAA
(distal metatarsal
articular angle)

Medial inclination of
metatarsocuneiform
joint

IMA
(intermetatarsal
angle)

Fig. 1. Radiographic measurements for hallux valgus. This is a schematic of the common radiographic measurements used to evaluate a hallux valgus deformity.

with hallux rigidus, not hallux valgus. This is even more true when a facet exists between the first and second metatarsal bases.[5]

General radiographic features to recognize include evidence of arthritis or previous trauma or deformities other than the hallux valgus, such as midfoot collapse. The second metatarsal should be inspected for length relative to the first metatarsal and for evidence of medial cortical hypertrophy. A second metatarsal that is longer than the first will be likely to develop additional stress after a first metatarsal osteotomy, especially a proximal osteotomy in which dorsiflexion may inadvertently occur. Medial cortical hypertrophy preoperatively indicates that the weightbearing of the first metatarsal is already being shifted to the second

metatarsal. Many surgeries may worsen the stress transfer. The size of the medial eminence and arthritic changes in the MTP joint should be noted. The position of the sesamoids and presence of hallux valgus interphalangeus provide useful information on the nature of the deformity. The DMAA and congruence of the joint may suggest a procedure that translates the distal metatarsal instead of rotating the metatarsal into alignment to maximize postoperative joint function.[6]

Congruence of the metatarsal joint is important in considering surgical intervention. If the MTP joint is congruent in the preoperative radiograph, the relationship between the metatarsal and the phalanx should be preserved. Procedures such as a chevron osteotomy and an Akin procedure are best for congruent joints. If the MTP joint is incongruent preoperatively, then a distal soft-tissue or proximal osteotomy will help to restore more anatomical relationships between the metatarsal and the phalanx (congruence).[4, 5] The major determinants for which surgical procedure to perform are the radiographic parameters IMA and HVA, not congruence. Sometimes a congruent MTP joint is seen with a very high IMA and HVA. In this case, a proximal osteotomy and distal soft-tissue procedure would be done, realizing that there will likely be some loss of MTP motion because of the disruption of the MTP joint congruence.

DIFFERENTIAL DIAGNOSIS

Complaints of pain in or around the first MTP joint may be caused by a variety of conditions, including arthritis, hallux rigidus, sesamoid disorders, and gout. Although the deformity associated with hallux valgus often makes the differential diagnosis clear once a physical examination is performed, these other painful conditions may coexist. A painless hallux valgus in a first ray afflicted with gout will not improve symptomatically following corrective surgery for the hallux valgus. A careful history and physical examination are all that is necessary to make a definitive diagnosis of hallux valgus.

MANAGEMENT
Conservative Management

A trial of conservative management is recommended in all patients with symptomatic hallux valgus. The main component of conservative treatment is properly fitting shoewear that accommodates the deformity. Night splints and bunion socks are of limited value in preventing progression of deformity. Patient education plays a major role in nonoperative treatment. Many patients simply wear shoes that do not fit. A useful in-office tool consists of outlining the patient's weightbearing foot and superimposing an outline of the shoe. The shoe should be ¼ to ½ inch or less smaller than the foot. An in-office Brannock device to measure the foot accurately can also be used to educate the patient as to true shoe size. Many patients believe their feet are still the size they were when they were a teenager. Typically, the forefoot spreads, and the shoe size increases with age. Patients should be instructed to wear a flat shoe that fits the width of the foot based on the above technique. Only if conservative treatment fails should surgical management be considered.[1, 4, 5]

Surgical Management
Distal Soft-Tissue Procedures/Ostectomy

At the level of the MTP joint, the simplest and most straightforward procedures include ostectomy of the median eminence (Silver's procedure) and soft-tissue correction (modified McBride's procedure). These procedures are rarely indicated alone and are often combined with other procedures such as metatarsal osteotomies. Silver's procedure is typically indicated for a deformity in which there is an excessively large median eminence and an intermetatarsal angle in the normal range. The ostectomy is performed through a medial approach and consists of resection of the excessive bone just medial to the sagittal sulcus with reefing of the medial capsule.[7] There are several types of medial capsular incision and repair or reefing. Three of the most common types include a vertical capsular incision that ellipses capsular tissue, creation of an L-flap with a distal vertical incision and a dorsal horizontal limb, and a transverse incision ellipsing some dorsal capsular tissue.

The distal soft-tissue procedure most commonly consists of a lateral release combined with medial capsular reefing, with or without median eminence ostectomy (Fig. 2). The lateral release involves release of the conjoint tendon from the lateral sesamoid and the proximal phalanx and release of the lateral capsule. This procedure will improve the hallux valgus angle but will have little lasting impact on the intermetatarsal angle. For this reason, this procedure is rarely indicated alone and is more commonly combined with a proximal bony correction.[8, 9]

The lateral release is performed through a first-web incision. The conjoined tendon is dissected off of the sesamoid and the base of the proximal phalanx laterally and attached dorsally to the periosteum of the distal metatarsal. The lateral capsule is released to allow passive correction of the hallux relative to the metatarsal. Finally, the medial capsule is reefed to hold the correction (Fig. 3).[4, 5]

Postoperatively, the patient is allowed weightbearing as tolerated in a bunion dressing. The bunion dressing is changed weekly for 6 weeks, followed by a range-of-motion program. The most common complications are over- or undercorrection or excessive medial eminence resection.

Distal Osteotomies. There are dozens of described distal first metatarsal osteotomies. In general, these translational procedures are indicated for a deformity with an intermetatarsal of around 13 degrees or less and an HVA less than 30 degrees (unless the metatarsal osteotomy is combined with a proximal phalangeal osteotomy or Akin's procedure). The distal osteotomies most commonly translate the metatarsal head rather than rotate the metatarsal head into a corrected position. This translation maintains the preoperative congruency of the joint. A joint that is incongruent preoperatively will not be improved with a translational osteotomy and may perhaps be better treated with a rotational-type procedure that will change the congruence. Several of the more common distal metatarsal osteotomies include the chevron (or Austin), Mitchell, and closing wedge procedures.[10–12] Most orthopaedists favor the chevron procedure because it minimizes the amount of first metatarsal

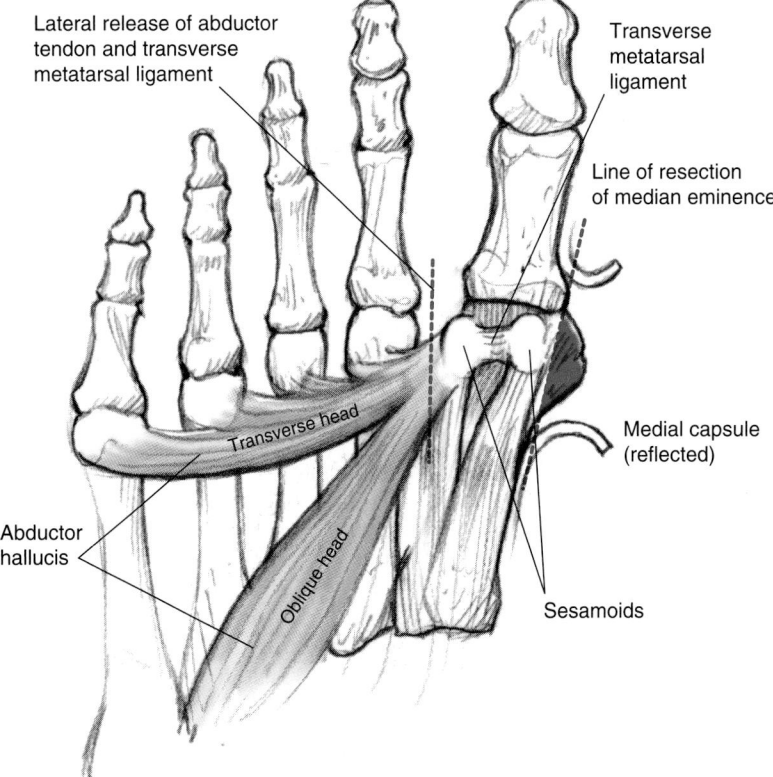

Fig. 2. Lateral release and median eminence resection. The pertinent anatomy of the hallux metatarsal phalangeal joint is illustrated. The modified McBride procedure involves release of the conjoint tendon and lateral capsule and resection of the median eminence.

Lateral release of abductor tendon and transverse metatarsal ligament

Transverse metatarsal ligament

Line of resection of median eminence

Transverse head

Medial capsule (reflected)

Abductor hallucis

Oblique head

Sesamoids

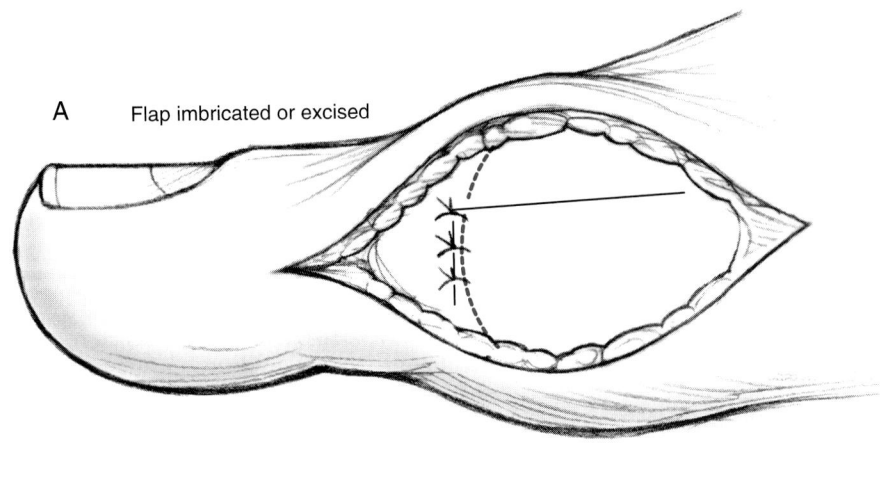

A Flap imbricated or excised

Fig. 3. Capsular incisions and repair.
This is a lateral view of hallux medial
skin incision. Dotted line = MTP joint.

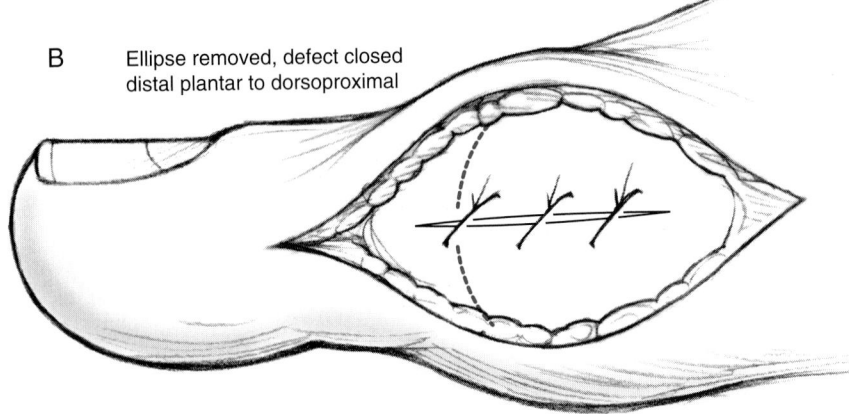

B Ellipse removed, defect closed
distal plantar to dorsoproximal

shortening. The chevron cut is also inherently stable, which decreases the likelihood of dorsiflexion malunion (Fig. 4).

The chevron procedure is performed through a medial incision centered at the first MTP joint. The median eminence is resected just medial to the sagittal sulcus as in the Silver procedure. A V- (or chevron) shaped osteotomy is made in the horizontal plane with the apex distal. The amount of capsular stripping of the distal metatarsal is kept to a minimum to avoid osteonecrosis of the metatarsal head. The metatarsal head is then translated laterally 4 to 6 mm. This osteotomy is typically stable; however, fixation with an absorbable pin or K-wire is useful to ensure maintenance of correction.[13, 14] The prominent step-off bone on the proximal side of the osteotomy is resected in line with the medial border of the foot. The medial capsule is reefed to correct the HVA. Further correction of the HVA by a lateral release is relatively contraindicated because of a high rate of osteonecrosis of the metatarsal head when these procedures are combined.[4, 10, 11] Performing the lateral release through the first MTP joint with a chevron is believed by some to be acceptable as no additional lateral soft-tissue stripping is necessary. Another option to combine with a chevron to improve the toe alignment is an Akin proximal phalangeal osteotomy (discussed later).

In a foot in which there is an abnormally high DMAA, a modification of the chevron osteotomy (Reverdin's method)

may be required. The chevron is angled distally to prevent excessive shortening. A dorsal wedge of 1 to 2 mm is removed medially to allow the articular surface to rotate back into normal alignment. The chevron is translated and rotated through the chevron cut to correct a milder deformity, or it may be used without translation laterally as an adjunct to a proximal osteotomy (double osteotomy). The choice of whether the correction needs the double osteotomy depends on the magnitude of the IMA.[5]

The Mitchell and closing wedge–type distal osteotomies are associated with at least several millimeters of first metatarsal shortening. Excessive first metatarsal shortening, especially in a patient with Morton's foot, will lead to stress transfer to the second metatarsal head. In severe cases, stress fractures of the second metatarsal and severe metatarsalgia may develop.

Postoperative Care. A bunion dressing is applied at surgery, and the patient is weightbearing on the heel for only the first 2 weeks. Sutures are removed, and full weightbearing is allowed in a postoperative shoe after replacement of a bunion dressing at week 2. Bunion dressings are continued until week 4. At week 4, the patient is instructed in MTP range-of-motion exercises, and a full-time Velcro bunion splint can be substituted for the bunion dressing to allow bathing. As long as the hallux position appears stable, the splint is used only at night. Loose shoewear may

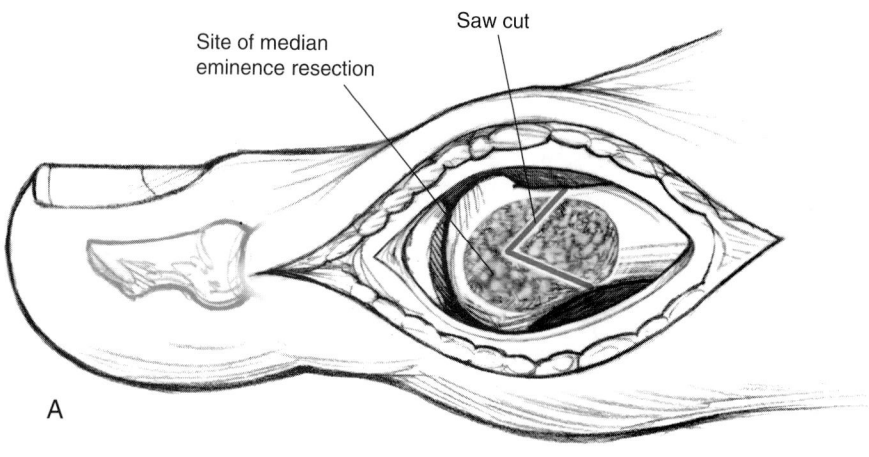

Site of median
eminence resection

Saw cut

A

Fig. 4. Chevron distal osteotomy. *A,* After the median eminence is resected, a transverse V-shaped saw cut is made with the apex approximately 1 cm from the joint surface. *B,* The metatarsal head is translated 4 to 6 mm, and the prominent medial step-off is resected in line with the medial border of the foot.

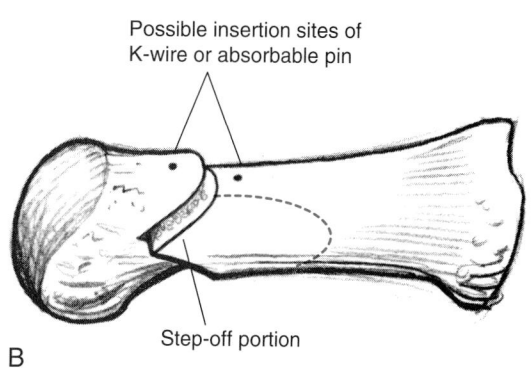

Possible insertion sites of
K-wire or absorbable pin

Step-off portion

B

be resumed once the daytime splinting or dressing is discontinued. The most common complications are avascular necrosis of the metatarsal head, nonunion or malunion of the osteotomy, and shortening of the metatarsal.

Proximal Osteotomies. Proximal osteotomies are necessary when the IMA is 14 to 15 degrees or more, especially when there is a significant HVA. The proximal osteotomies generally correct the high IMA by rotating the divergent first metatarsal shaft into a corrected position. It is quite common to combine a proximal metatarsal osteotomy with a distal soft-tissue procedure in order to correct the HVA.[9, 15–18] The proximal osteotomy rotates the first metatarsal shaft into a position more parallel to the second metatarsal shaft in the horizontal or anteroposterior plane while maintaining the alignment in the vertical or lateral plane. The most common proximal metatarsal osteotomies are the crescentic dome osteotomy and the proximal chevron osteotomy. The most common complications of the proximal osteotomy are shortening and dorsiflexion malunion of the first metatarsal.[19, 20] Either of these complications can lead to second metatarsal stress transfer and possible metatarsalgia and/or second metatarsal stress fracture. Unlike the chevron osteotomy, osteonecrosis is not a concern in the proximal osteotomies. Proximal osteotomies can be used as salvage procedures for the undercorrected hallux valgus (Fig. 5).[21]

If a distal procedure is being combined with the dome osteotomy, it should be completed first. A skin incision is made dorsally, centered over the first metatarsal extending from the palpable metatarsocuneiform joint about 4 cm distally. Subperiosteal exposure of the base of the metatarsal allows marking before creating the osteotomy. The dome cut is marked 1 cm distal to the TMT joint, the predrilled hole for the fixation screw is marked at 2 cm distal to the TMT joint, and a longitudinal alignment line is made down the shaft at the level of the osteotomy to assess the correction achieved intraoperatively.

Fixation of the osteotomy is generally with a small fragment screw in a lag mode. A 4-mm partially threaded screw is easy to use and requires the use of a single drill. The gliding screw hole is made first at the 2-cm mark, aiming proximally. The dorsal screw hole should be countersunk to prevent screwhead prominence. The angle of the drill must be very shallow with respect to the metatarsal shaft. The drill should also angle somewhat laterally to ensure purchase within the proximal metatarsal once the osteotomy is rotated into corrected position. The crescentic dome osteotomy is performed 1 to 1.5 cm distal to the metatarsocuneiform joint using a curved saw blade. The saw should be placed on the metatarsal shaft at an angle that subtends the difference between being perpendicular to the sole of the foot and perpendicular to the shaft of the metatarsal. The convexity of the dome cut is distal, although in initial descriptions it was convexity-proximal. The convexity-distal technique allows better purchase of the fixation device in the proximal metatarsal fragment and also allows freer rotation of the distal metatarsal. Using the longitudinal line as a guide and a Hohmann retractor as a

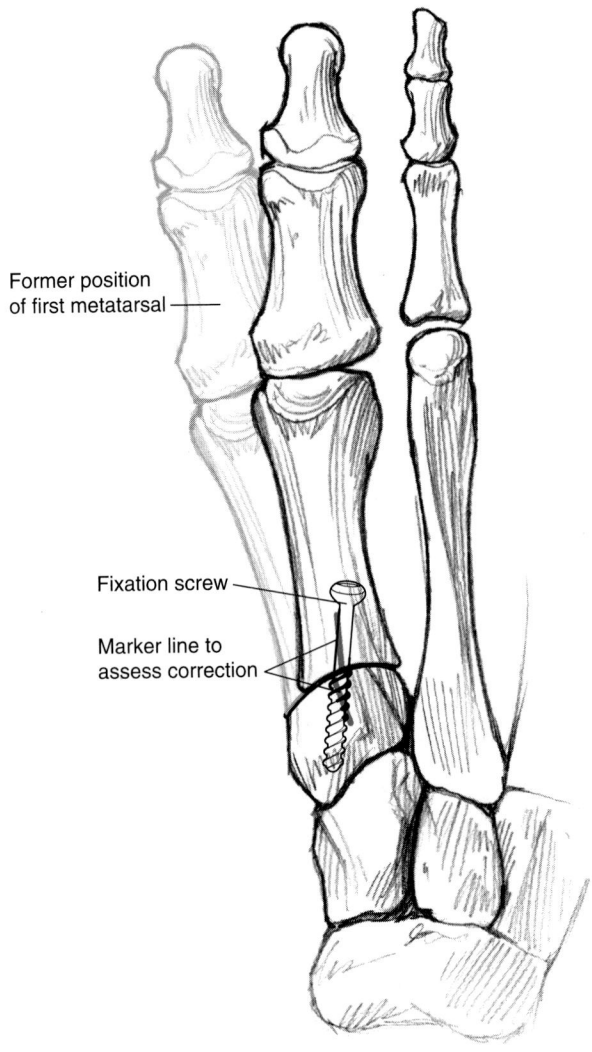

Former position of first metatarsal

Fixation screw

Marker line to assess correction

Fig. 5. Proximal dome osteotomy. This is a schematic of correction achieved with a proximal crescentic osteotomy fixed with a lag screw.

lever in the first intermetatarsal space, the metatarsal is rotated into a corrected position. The drill hole is completed across the osteotomy. The hole is measured and tapped, and the lag screw is inserted. Care must be taken not to allow dorsiflexion of the osteotomy.[9, 19, 20] Actually, translating the distal fragment a few millimeters plantarly may be useful in maintaining weightbearing on the first metatarsal head.

The proximal chevron has become popular as a more rigid and stable proximal osteotomy. A chevron cut is made with the apex distal about 1.5 cm from the TMT joint. The osteotomy is rotated or tilted laterally to correct the IMA. Fixation with a screw from proximal to distal is preferred.[15–17]

Postoperative Care. A bunion dressing is applied at surgery, and the patient is non-weightbearing for the first 2 weeks. Sutures are removed, and heel-only weightbearing is allowed in a postoperative shoe after replacement of a bunion dressing at week 2. Bunion dressings are continued until week 4. At weeks 4 to 6, the patient is instructed in MTP range-of-motion exercises, and a full-time Velcro bunion splint can be substituted for the bunion dressing to

allow bathing. A postoperative radiograph is also checked for assessment of bony healing. As long as the position appears stable, weightbearing is advanced, and splinting may be night splinting only. Loose shoewear may be resumed once the daytime splinting or dressings are discontinued. Complications include nonunion and malunion, shortening, and over- or undercorrection of the deformity.

Arthrodesis Procedures

There are two arthrodesis procedures that can be used in treatment of hallux valgus. The first MTP arthrodesis and the cuneiform first metatarsal arthrodesis (Lapidus' procedure) have very specific indications.

A first MTP arthrodesis was initially described in 1852 by Broca[22] for the treatment of hallux valgus. This fusion is currently used as a primary procedure for patients with arthritis of the joint and neuromuscular abnormality involving the limb. Arthritis may be rheumatoid arthritis, osteoarthritis, or post-traumatic arthritis. MTP arthrodesis remains a reliable salvage for failed bunion surgery.[23] The weightbearing function of the first ray is preserved with an MTP fusion. Relative contraindications for MTP fusion include

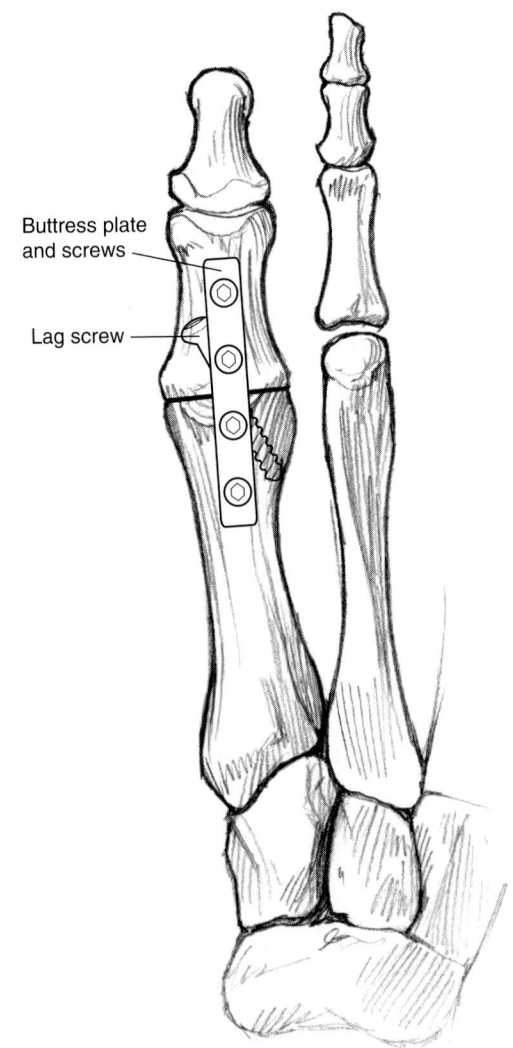

Buttress plate and screws

Lag screw

Fig. 6. MTP arthrodesis. This is the postoperative appearance of hallux first metatarsal phalangeal fusion using a buttress plate and lag screw.

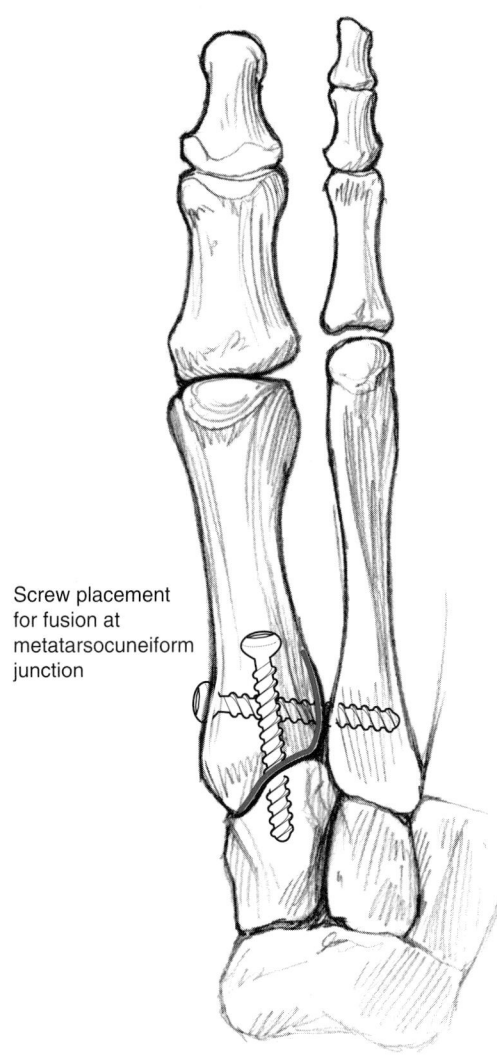

Screw placement for fusion at metatarsocuneiform junction

Fig. 7. Lapidus' procedure. This is an illustration of Lapidus' first tarsometatarsal arthrodesis.

arthritis of the cuneiform first metatarsal or interphalangeal joints and insensitivity of the foot (Fig. 6).

The first MTP fusion is carried out through a dorsal incision centered over the joint. The extensor hallucis longus tendon is retracted laterally, and the capsule is incised in line with the skin incision. The base of the proximal phalanx and the distal articular surface of the metatarsal are resected. The method of resection may be planar cuts or conical cuts using specially designed reamers. The planar cuts typically cause less shortening of the first ray. The position of the arthrodesis should be in about 10 to 15 degrees of physiological valgus and in about 10 degrees of dorsiflexion relative to the floor. The toe should be neutral with respect to pronation or supination. A K-wire is used to hold the position while a lag screw is placed from distal to proximal across the arthrodesis site. A four- or five-hole one-third semitubular dorsal buttress plate adds stability to the fusion and is recommended.[4, 5]

Postoperative care involves heel-only weightbearing until the sutures are removed at 2 weeks. The patient may then bear weight as tolerated in a postoperative shoe or a walking cast for an additional 3 to 4 weeks. A radiograph is

taken at 5 to 6 weeks, and the patient is allowed to wean back into regular shoewear. Complications include nonunion or malunion.

Arthrodesis of the first metatarsocuneiform joint combined with a distal soft-tissue procedure was initially described in 1911 by Albrecht[24] but popularized by Lapidus[25] as effective treatment of hallux valgus with severe metatarsus primus varus. Typically, candidates for the Lapidus procedure are younger patients with an IM angle greater than 15 degrees and an oblique, hypermobile first metatarsocuneiform joint.[3] Hypermobility of the first metatarsocuneiform articulation is the primary current indication for this procedure, although this is not a use that was identified by Lapidus. Contraindications include a nonhypermobile metatarsocuneiform joint and a lesser metatarsus primus varus deformity (Fig. 7).

The distal soft-tissue procedure is performed as previously described. A longitudinal incision is made centered over the metatarsocuneiform joint. The capsule is also incised longitudinally. The curved joint surfaces are taken down to viable cancellous bone. Care is taken to remove more bone from the lateral and plantar aspect of the joint to allow correction. A lag screw is placed dorsally from

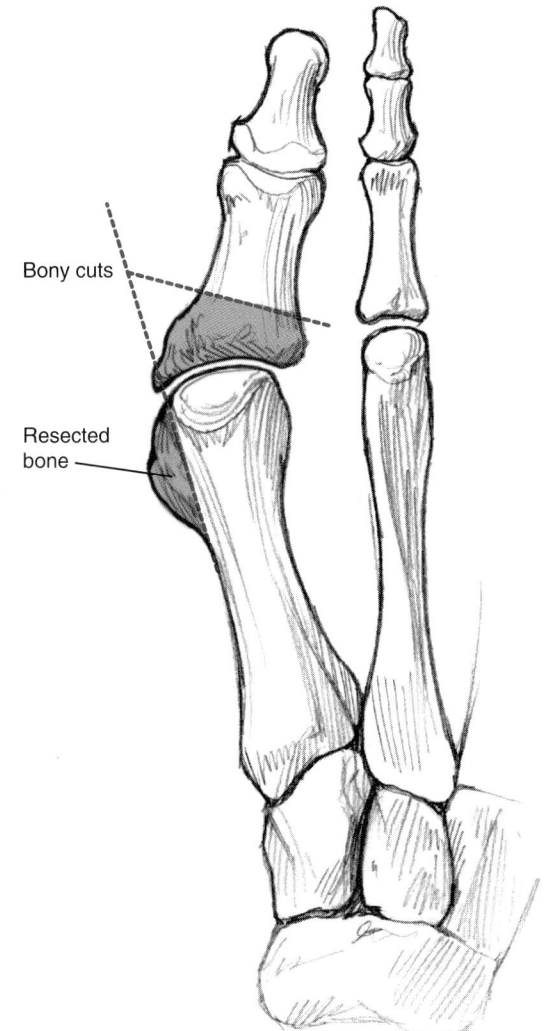

Bony cuts

Resected bone

Fig. 8. Keller's procedure. This is a schematic of bony cuts performed in a Keller resection arthroplasty.

the first metatarsal into the cuneiform. A second lag screw is used to prevent rotation and to hold correction of the IMA. The second screw goes from the medial aspect of the base of the first metatarsal into the base of the second metatarsal or the middle cuneiform.[3] Some choose to remove this second screw after the fusion has healed and prior to allowing weightbearing.

Postoperatively, the patient is generally non-weightbearing for 4 to 6 weeks, and a short leg cast or walker boot is used. Once a solid arthrodesis is noted radiographically, normal shoewear and weightbearing are allowed. Nonunion is the major complication, with rates up to 20%.

Phalangeal Procedures

Osteotomy or ostectomy of the proximal phalanx of the hallux is occasionally indicated in the treatment of hallux valgus.

The Akin procedure was first described in 1925.[26] The original description included excision of the median eminence of the metatarsal along with a medially-based closing wedge osteotomy of the base of the phalanx. The Akin procedure is performed through a medial incision centered over the MTP joint. The osteotomy can be fixed with suture, temporary K-wire, or absorbable pins. The primary indication for the Akin procedure is a hallux valgus interphalangeus deformity. Another indication is a patient with a congruent joint with inadequate correction of the HVA using the chevron osteotomy alone. Nonunion is a possible complication.

The Keller ostectomy was first described in 1887 but popularized by Keller in 1912.[5, 27] The current indications for this procedure are limited because of predictable complications including cock-up deformity of the great toe and stress transfer to the lesser rays.[28] An elderly patient with severe pain and deformity who would not tolerate a more extensive surgery or a longer recovery period is about the only good indication for the Keller procedure in the treatment of hallux valgus. Occasionally, the Keller ostectomy is used to salvage a failed bunion surgery (Fig. 8).[23]

Through a medial incision centered over the MTP joint, the medial eminence and the proximal third of the proximal phalanx are resected. The continuity of the flexor via the plantar plate is maintained if possible by suturing the plantar plate to the residual proximal phalanx. The joint is stabilized with a large K-wire or Steinmann pin. Capsule interposition may be a useful arthroplasty.

Postoperatively, the patient can bear weight as tolerated in a bunion dressing and a postoperative shoe. The pin is pulled at week 3 to 4, and normal shoewear is resumed by about week 6 or when swelling allows.

SUMMARY

Despite a large number of described procedures and variations for the treatment of hallux valgus, new ideas continue to emerge. There is no single procedure; rather, every patient and every deformity must be evaluated independently in order to select the correct treatment.

REFERENCES

1. Coughlin MJ, Thompson FM: The high price of high-fashion footwear. AAOS Instruct Course Lect 1995; 44:371.
2. Verbrugge J: Pathogenie et traitment de l'hallux valgus. Bull Mem Soc Belge d'Othop 1967; 54:103.
3. Sangeorzan BJ, Hansen ST Jr: Modified Lapidus procedure for hallux valgus. Foot Ankle 1989; 9:262.
4. Coughlin MJ: Hallux valgus. J Bone Joint Surg Am 1996; 78:932.
5. Mann R, Coughlin M: Adult hallux valgus. In Mann R, Caughlin M (eds): Surgery of the Foot and Ankle. St. Louis, Mosby, 1993, p 167.
6. Coughlin MJ: Hallux valgus in men: Effect of the distal metatarsal articular angle on hallux valgus correction. Foot Ankle Int 1997; 18:463.
7. Silver D: The operative treatment of hallux valgus. J Bone Joint Surg 1923; 5:409.
8. McBride ED: The McBride bunion hallux valgus operation: Refinements in the successive surgical steps of the operation. J Bone Joint Surg Am 1967; 49:1675.
9. Mann RA, Rudicel S, Graves SC: Repair of hallux valgus with distal soft-tissue procedure and proximal metatarsal osteotomy: A long-term follow-up. J Bone Joint Surg Am 1992; 74:124.
10. Johnson KA, Cofield RH, Morrey BF:

Chevron osteotomy for hallux valgus. Clin Orthop 1979; 142:44.
11. Shereff M: Chevron osteotomy for hallux vagus. Curr Ther Foot Ankle Surg 1993; 46:9.
12. Saunders M: Complications of hallux valgus surgery: Iatrogenic hallux varus soft-tissue reconstruction. Foot Ankle Clin 1998; 3:1.
13. Winemaker MJ, Amendola A: Comparison of bioabsorbable pins and Kirschner wires in the fixation of chevron osteotomies for hallux valgus. Foot Ankle Int 1996; 17: 623.
14. Gill LH, Martin DF, Coumas JM, et al: Fixation with bioabsorbable pins in chevron bunionectomy. J Bone Joint Surg Am 1997; 79:1510.
15. Sammarco GJ, Brainard BJ, Sammarco VJ: Bunion correction using proximal chevron osteotomy. Foot Ankle 1993; 14:8.
16. Easley ME, Kiezbzak GM, Hodges-Davis W, et al: Prospective, randomized comparison of proximal crescentic and proximal chevron osteotomies for correction of hallux valgus deformity. Foot Ankle Int 1996; 17:307.
17. Sammarco GJ, Russo-Alesi FG: Bunion correction using proximal chevron osteotomy: A single incision technique. Foot Ankle Int 1998; 19:430.

18. Markbreiter LA, Thompson FM: Proximal metatarsal osteotomy in hallux valgus correction: A comparison of crescentic and chevron procedures. Foot Ankle Int 1997; 71:6.
19. Conklin M: Complication of hallux valgus surgery: Persistent or recurrent hallux valgus deformity and complications of metatarsal osteotomies. Foot Ankle Clin 1998; 3:19.
20. Richardson EG: Complications after hallux valgus surgery. Instr Course Lect 1999; 48:331.
21. Kitaoka HB, Patzer GL: Salvage treatment of failed hallux valgus operations with proximal first metatarsal osteotomy and distal soft-tissue reconstruction. Foot Ankle Int 1998; 19:127.
22. Broca P: Des difformites de la partie anteriere du pied produite par Factin de la chaussure. Faction Chaussure 1852; 27:60.
23. Kitaoka HB, Patzer GL: Arthrodesis versus resection arthroplasty for failed hallux valgus operations. Clin Orthop 1998; 347: 208.
24. Albrecht GH: The pathology and treatment of hallux valgus [in Russian]. Tusk Vrach 1911; 10:14.
25. Lapidus PW: Operative correction of the metatarsus varus primus in hallux valgus. Surg Gynecol Obstet 1934; 58:183.

26. Akin OF: The treatment of hallux valgus: A new operative procedure and its results. Med Sentinel 1925; 33:678.

27. Keller WL: The surgical treatment of bunions and hallux valgus. N Y Med J 1912; 95:696.

28. Beskin L: Akin's phalangeal osteotomy for bunion repair. Curr Foot Ankle Surg 1993; 54:7.

LIMB LENGTH DISCREPANCY

Ellen M. Raney and Amira A. Helal

section 9 chapter 29

Summary
- The goal of treatment of limb length discrepancy is to improve function and quality of life.
- Treatment should be individualized.
- Use a team approach.
- The treatment team should consider the importance of body image.
- Do not let technology triumph over reason.

The goal of treatment of limb length discrepancy is to achieve functional status in the areas of strength, range of motion, ambulation, and activities of daily living. Cosmesis should be considered to preserve an adequate body image.

TREATMENT GOALS, INDICATIONS, AND CONTRAINDICATIONS

The treatment of patients with limb length discrepancy is highly individualized. However, it is useful to consider broad treatment categories based on the predicted discrepancy at the completion of growth (Table 1). The patient's anticipated adult height should be considered also.

Small discrepancies in leg lengths (<2 cm) can be well tolerated.[1] A shoe lift of less than 1 cm can be placed inside a shoe. Larger lifts can be added to the exterior of the shoe. Such lifts are cosmetically unappealing and frequently are refused by adolescents. An attractive alternative for many patients with a small but significant discrepancy is epiphysiodesis to slow the growth of the longer leg. The main advantage of epiphysiodesis is that it is a relatively

minor surgery with a brief recovery. Disadvantages include a reduction in overall adult height and the necessity to operate on the longer, usually more normal, leg. The same is true for shortening procedures, which are most commonly reserved for cases in which the window of opportunity for an epiphysiodesis has passed.

Lengthening procedures are a viable option for larger discrepancies (>4 cm). Although the results can be quite satisfactory, these procedures should be approached with caution. Lengthening procedures have a notoriously high complication rate. A candidate for lengthening must be able to tolerate the procedure physically and emotionally. The patient, as well as the parents, must be a willing participant in the process. The patient and family must be prepared for a long course of treatment. Lengthening can be performed as a staged procedure if the discrepancy is too large to be corrected in one treatment session.

The multidisciplinary approach with involvement of a pediatrician, psychologist, and social services has been found to be of tremendous help to the orthopaedic surgeon in maintaining the health and well-being of these children during the lengthening process.

Contraindications to lengthening include an unstable joint on either end of the bone segment to be lengthened. This could exacerbate the instability and lead to dislocation. Patients with deformity secondary to metabolic bone disease may be able to undergo lengthening at a slower rate with longer time healing.[2]

The lengthening of extremities in people with severe growth-limiting dysplasias, such as achondroplasia, has not gained wide popularity in this country. European surgeons have been more aggressive in this area. These patients usually undergo at least six separate lengthening procedures (femurs, tibiae, humeri).

Extremely large discrepancies in the lower extremities are in some cases better managed with amputation during infancy. This is especially true in patients with severe deformities in addition to shortening. The severity of the deformity may be more than is appreciated radiographically because of the paucity of ossification in the infant. A prosthesis can be much more functional than a lengthened extremity, which is weak or stiff. Support and counseling should be provided to parents as they face this difficult decision.

TABLE 1. TREATMENT OPTIONS BASED ON ANTICIPATED LEG LENGTH DISCREPANCY AT COMPLETION OF GROWTH	
Leg Length Discrepancy, cm	Treatment
0–2	Observation or shoe lift
2–4	Epiphysiodesis
4–17	Lengthening
>17	Amputation

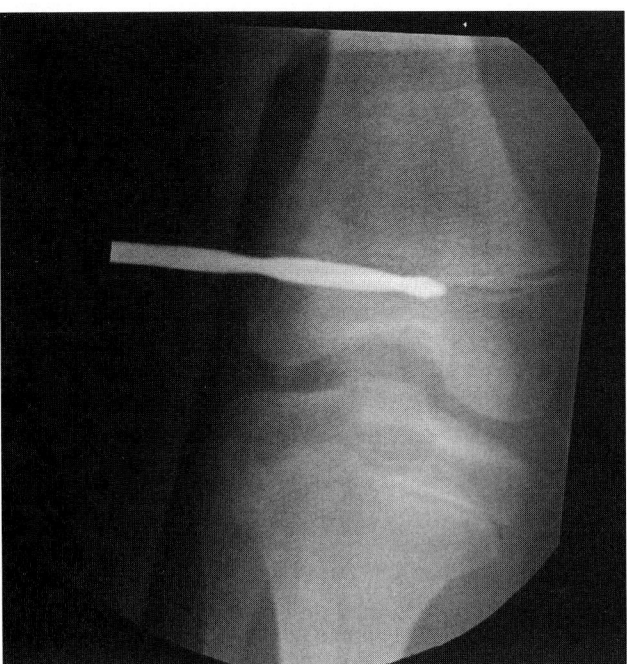

Fig. 1. Epiphysiodesis technique. A radiograph of a distal femur shows a drill bit crossing the distal femoral physis.

PATHOLOGY

Numerous pathological entities can lead to limb length inequality. Categories include congenital, post-traumatic, infectious, and metabolic diseases. These conditions are discussed elsewhere in this text. Each cause has implications for the quality of the soft tissues and bone, as well as the overall physical and emotional health of the patient.

EPIPHYSIODESIS

The most essential element in an epiphysiodesis is timing. The timing is based on at least three serial lower extremity scanograms taken at 6-month intervals. The measurements are then placed on the straight line graph as described by Mosely[3] or the growth-remaining curves of Anderson and Green.[4]

TECHNIQUE

The procedure is technically straightforward. The classic technique of epiphysiodesis was described by Phemister.[5] A cortical window of bone is removed to allow access to the physis. The physis becomes visible as a white line. The physis is then removed with curets under direct vision.

The percutaneous method of epiphysiodesis has recently gained popularity. Minimal soft-tissue disruption is required, leading to less stiffness and smaller scars. This may be performed with a drill or curet (Fig. 1).[6-8] Because this is most commonly performed in the distal femur and proximal tibia, the approaches are straight medial and lateral. The level of the physis is visualized under image intensification. Through a percutaneous incision, a drill is inserted directly across the physis. The drill is then withdrawn and redirected anteriorly and posteriorly in a fan-shaped pattern (Fig. 2). Withdraw the drill bit completely before redirecting it to prevent breakage of the drill bit. Care must be taken to avoid unintentionally exiting the bone in any direction. Entering the joint anteriorly is a hazard. The neurovascular bundle lies posteriorly. In the procedure description by Canale, the purpose is to create a central bridge,[7] whereas that described by Timberlake leaves the central column intact and creates lateral physeal bridging.[8] Unless the projected growth remaining from the proximal tibia is more than 2 cm at the time of epiphysiodesis, the fibula does not usually require epiphysiodesis. The fibula may be approached though the same incision as the proximal tibia. Avoid the peroneal nerve.

POSTOPERATIVE MANAGEMENT

Following the open technique, patients are usually placed in a removable knee immobilizer for 4 to 6 weeks for protection of the weakened area while weightbearing.[1] Minimal postoperative immobilization is required following the percutaneous procedure. Patients can usually resume full activity by 6 weeks.

COMPLICATIONS

The overwhelming cause of poor results from epiphysiodesis is an error in timing. The results of epiphysiodesis with the Phemister technique were reviewed by Blair. A timing error was noted in 41 of 67 patients. In the majority of these patients, the correct time for epiphysiodesis was

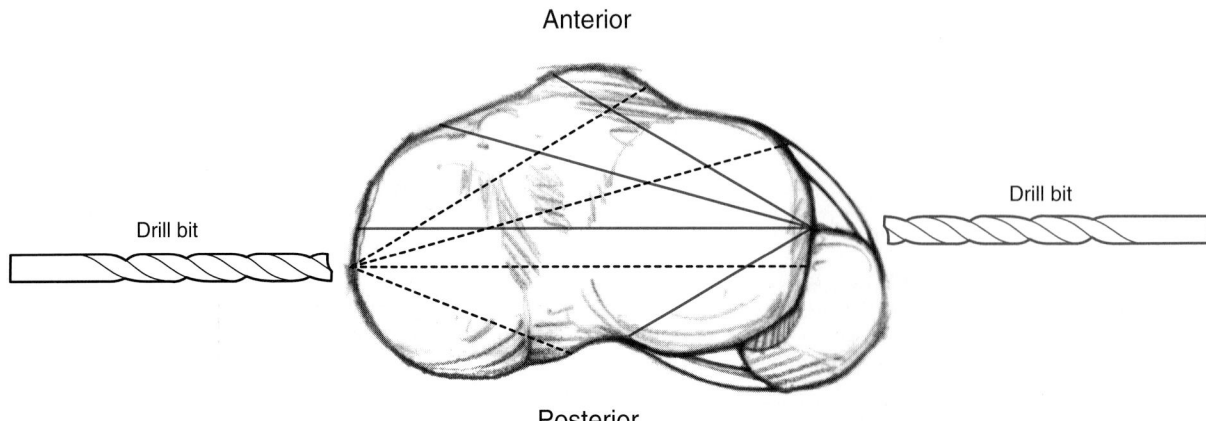

Fig. 2. Drilling pattern. This cross-section representation of proximal tibial physis demonstrates a fan-shaped pattern of drilling.

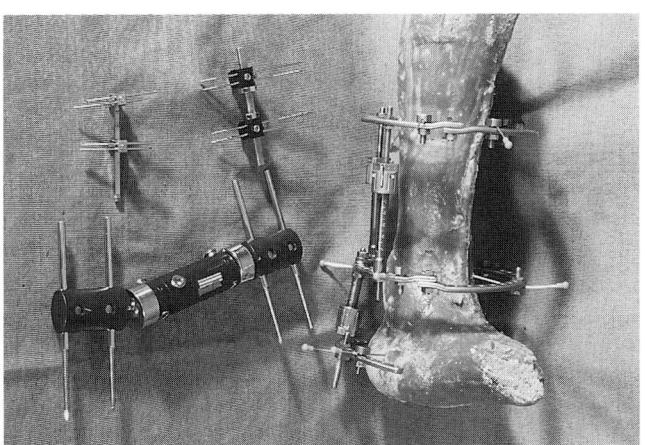

Fig. 3. External fixation devices. These are representative types of external fixation devices, clockwise from upper left: Minihoffman, Orthofix, Ilizarov, EBI.

commonly performed for a length discrepancy between the radius and ulna. Such discrepancies frequently produce symptomatic loss of motion and grip strength. Care must be taken to maintain range of motion, as stiffness is poorly tolerated in the upper extremity.

TECHNIQUE

Stabilization for distraction osteogenesis is generally provided by an external fixation device. Several types of external fixation devices are available (Fig. 3). Preoperative planning is essential. Maximal stability is achieved by having points of fixation in each bone segment near the osteotomy site and as far from the osteotomy site as possible (Fig. 4).

The type of fixation device used is generally determined by surgeon preference. The authors have come to favor a circular frame because of the versatility and ability to address deformities in several planes. Hinges can be placed to

missed as the patients were followed in routine clinical appointments.[9] Incomplete fusion of the physis is an uncommon complication. Incomplete fusion rates of 1 in 56 and 10 in 67 have been reported following open epiphysiodesis.[1, 9] Incomplete fusion was not identified in preliminary reports of percutaneous epiphysiodesis.[7, 8] If left untreated, incomplete fusion could lead to an angular deformity or continued length discrepancy. With early detection, this problem is easily treated by surgical ablation of the remaining open physis prior to the development of a clinically significant deformity. This complication is best avoided by meticulous surgical technique.

LENGTHENING

The concept of lengthening limbs through skeletal traction was introduced by Codivilla in 1904.[10] Wagner[11] used an external fixation device to distract a diaphyseal osteotomy. Fixation was converted to a plate and screws with iliac crest bone grafting after adequate length was obtained.

Current limb-lengthening techniques are based primarily on the research efforts of Gavril Ilizarov. He described *distraction histiogenesis*, which refers to the regeneration of tissue by gradual distraction force. When specifically referring to bone lengthening, the term *distraction osteogenesis* is also used. Distraction osteogenesis is the most common lengthening method currently employed. Ilizarov has shown with animal experimentation that the factors producing optimal bone regeneration are stable fixation, a distraction rate of 1 mm per day divided into at least four intervals, active muscle function, and normal weightbearing.[12] The time to radiographic union is frequently referred to in terms of the healing index. The number of treatment days (or months) required is divided by the number of centimeters lengthened. De Bastiani noted an average healing index of 38 days per centimeter in a series of 100 patients with healing indices ranging from 24 days/cm in the humerus to 41 days/cm in the tibia.[13] Healing indices have been noted to decrease with longer lengthenings.[14]

Limb length discrepancy can also occur in the upper extremities, although upper extremity discrepancy is often well tolerated. Humeral lengthening can be performed for marked shortening. Lengthening of the forearm is most

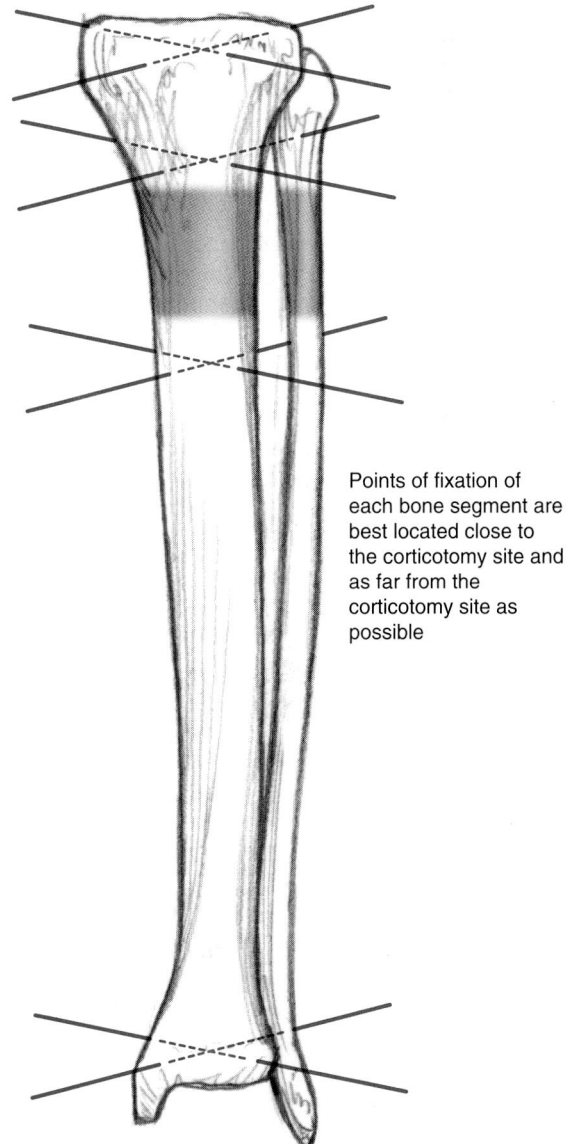

Points of fixation of each bone segment are best located close to the corticotomy site and as far from the corticotomy site as possible

Fig. 4. Points of fixation. This is a diagram of tibial Ilizarov device with points of fixation at either end of each bone segment.

allow angular correction concomitant with lengthening. Ideally, the frame is sized to the patient and assembled preoperatively.

The circular frames employ transfixation wires. Application of tension along the wire yields stability. The wire can be placed at any level along the bone. Thorough knowledge of the cross-sectional anatomy is essential. Neurovascular structures are obviously avoided. Tendons should not be penetrated. Muscles are placed in maximum excursion prior to penetration by flexing or extending the adjacent joint. This manipulation decreases tethering of the muscles. The wires are separated by at least 60-degree angles to enhance stability. Half-pins can be employed where the anatomy does not allow transverse fixation (e.g., proximal femur).

The simplicity of a monolateral frame is preferred by some surgeons. In certain instances, such as metacarpal lengthening, the anatomy may favor a monolateral device. The same principles of planning apply: maintain stability and preserve anatomy. The frame is preassembled or sized preoperatively. A template or the actual frame is used as a guide through which holes are drilled and screws are inserted. This is necessary to ensure that the screws are in proper alignment for attachment to the frame. Most monolateral frames require parallel screw insertion.

For ease of application, external fixation devices are initially applied to the intact bone. The device is then partially removed while a corticotomy is performed. This allows the corticotomy site to be moved freely. With use of the circular frame the hinges are removed. With the monolateral device the bar (or frame) is removed. Following the corticotomy, the frame is reattached, restoring the bone to its natural alignment.

A corticotomy involves cutting the cortex of the bone without entering the medullary canal and therefore damaging the medullary blood supply. Periosteal stripping is kept to a minimum. The healing potential is thus maintained as much as is possible. Cuts are made with an osteotome rather than a power saw to minimize tissue necrosis. An incomplete corticotomy is made and the remaining intact bone is fractured. The irregular surface of the corticotomy also increases the surface area for healing. Corticotomies are performed through the metaphyseal bone when possible. A latency period of 5 to 7 days is recommended prior to commencing distractions to allow organization of the hematoma. The optimal distraction rate is 1 mm per day divided into at least four intervals. Distractions are usually performed by the patient.

POSTOPERATIVE MANAGEMENT

Physical therapy to maintain range of motion and strength is essential (Fig. 5). Ilizarov theorized that active use of the limb was vital to new bone formation.[12] Certainly, a stiff lengthened extremity is not a desired functional outcome. Weightbearing is also beneficial to new bone formation (Fig. 6). Orthoses (static and dynamic) are used liberally on the joints above and below the lengthening site to prevent contractures and allow weightbearing (Fig. 7).

The fixation device is removed when the lengthened site appears stable radiographically. The authors protect the lengthened area with a removable orthosis until the medullary canal has reformed, indicating sufficient remodeling.

Lengthening of the femur over an intramedullary nail with either a circular or a monolateral fixator has also been described. The advantages are a decrease in the total time the patient spends in an external fixator, which facilitates rehabilitation, and reduction of the risk of fracture by the presence of an intramedullary rod. Paley[15] reported good results in 30 of 32 femurs lengthened in such a fashion. Interestingly, the length of time to healing was not reduced, despite intramedullary reaming.

COMPLICATIONS

The introduction of various lengthening procedures revolutionized the approach to the child with limb length discrepancy. The more liberal use of such therapy, however, has been hampered by the potential for numerous complications arising during lengthening or even after removal of the device.

A complication of treatment is best regarded as any untoward occurrence that takes place during lengthening or after the procedure is completed. Although this may lead to

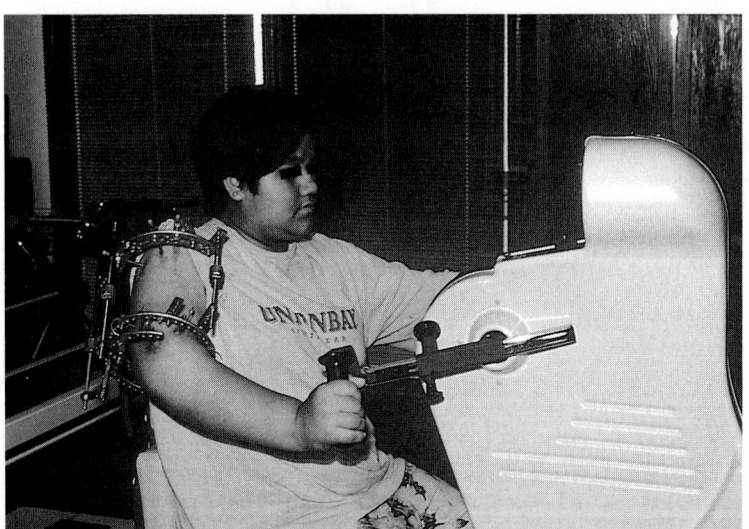

Fig. 5. Active use is encouraged. A patient undergoing humeral lengthening performs upper extremity cycling exercise.

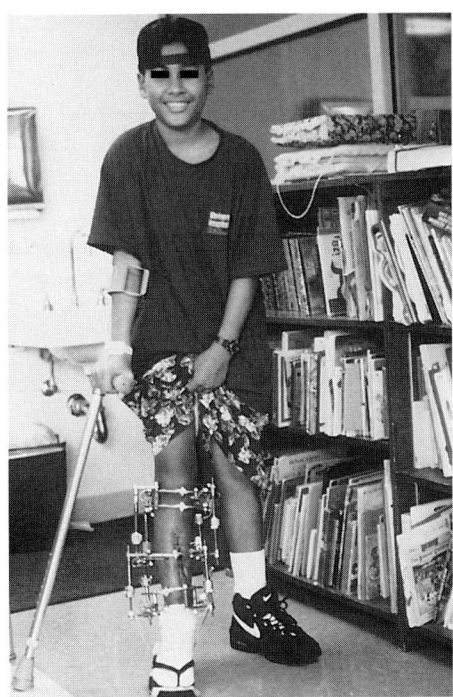

Fig. 6. Weightbearing is encouraged. A patient undergoing femoral lengthening walks with a cane.

higher reported rates of complications, it allows physicians to have a better understanding of problems arising as a result of lengthening. It is hoped that assessing the risk for such occurrences and anticipating problems will ultimately minimize or prevent many of the sequelae.

The reported rates of complication vary from as low as 15% to as high as 250%.[16,17] The wide variations are attributed to the lack of consensus in defining complications, the cause and degree of the discrepancy or deformity being corrected, the lengthening device used, and the surgeon's experience using it. A learning curve clearly exists, as demonstrated by Dahl et al.[18]

Complications arising during the course of lengthening may involve almost any organ system. The most common areas are the following:

- Musculoskeletal.
- Infectious.
- Neurological.
- Vascular.
- General.

Musculoskeletal

Stiffness. Joint stiffness is common and may have a deleterious effect on the outcome. Stiffness should be prevented by aggressive therapy and splinting when necessary. Permanent contractions occur at a rate of 1% to 7%.[19] Soft-tissue releases are required in certain instances.

Joint Instability. Joint subluxation or dislocation can frequently be prevented by maintaining an adequate range of motion. A joint that is subjected to the forces of distraction while not in a neutral position is more likely to sub-

lux. Management includes splinting, decreasing the distraction rates, and possible surgical stabilization.[20]

Nonunion. Poor callus formation can be an indicator of incipient nonunion (Fig. 8). Management consists of encouraging weightbearing and decreasing the lengthening rate if poor callus formation is noted. Additionally, bone healing can be stimulated by alternating several days of compression with several days of distraction across the lengthening site.[21] Recalcitrant nonunion may require bone grafting.

Fracture. Late fractures through the lengthening site are usually seen as small stress fractures, which can be managed nonoperatively. The authors have also noted fractures of the femur while patients are undergoing Ilizarov treatment of the tibia and vice versa. The cause is thought to be a combination of disuse osteopenia and a lever arm created by the fixation device. Stiffness at the knee may also contribute to this problem. These cases were able to be managed with an orthotic thigh cuff added to the frame.[22] Malunion, osteoporosis, and growth arrest have also been among the reported complications (Fig. 9).[23–25]

Infectious

Pin track infection is by far the most commonly seen complication, with greater than 100% occurrence rate in some studies.[18] The variances in the reported incidences are due to the definitions used. Some authors report only those infections requiring intravenous antibiotics.[14] Most infections are superficial or simple bacterial colonization that promptly respond to oral antibiotics and local wound care. Deeper wound infections, cellulitis, or even osteomyelitis occur less commonly but are well recognized and poten-

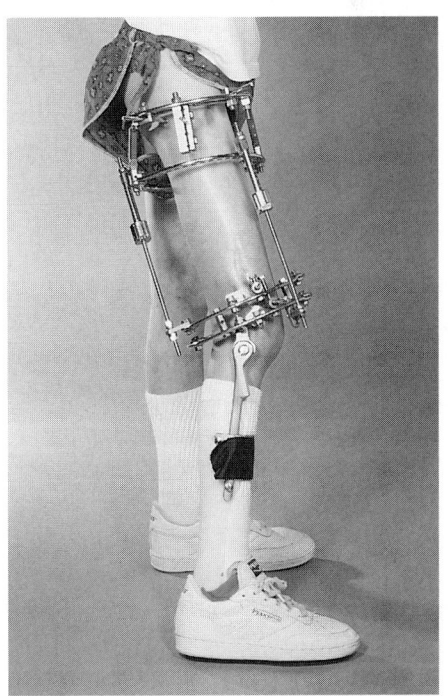

Fig. 7. Orthoses are useful during lengthening. This is a patient undergoing femoral lengthening. Spring-loaded hinges encourage knee extension. Ankle-foot orthosis maintains plantigrade foot position.

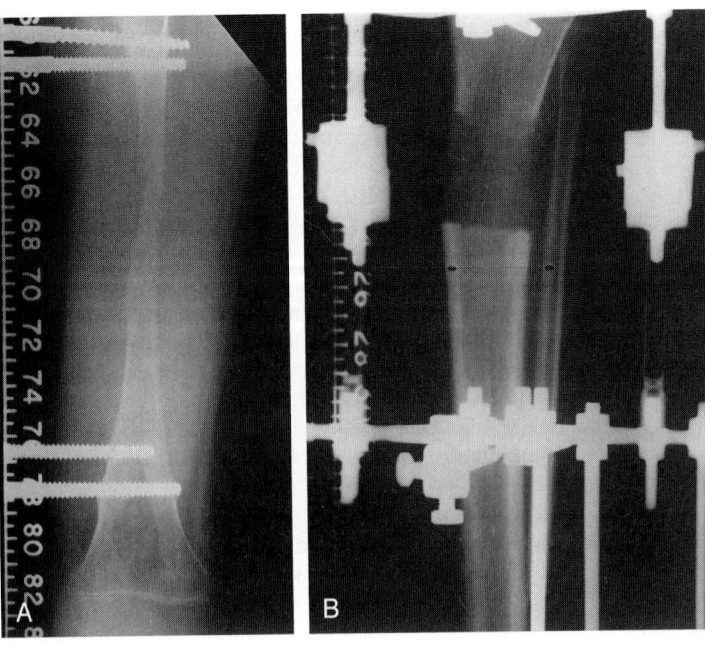

Fig. 8. Callus formation. *A,* Poor formation. Femoral lengthening with callus demonstrates attenuated appearance and "peppermint stick"–shaped ends. *B,* Good formation. Tibial lengthening with healthy, even callus, demonstrating good healing potential.

tially more serious. In such cases, prompt and aggressive parenteral antibiotics become necessary. Surgical débridement may be required.

The incidence of infection is decreased by meticulous daily cleansing of the pin sites. This is best performed by the patient. Protocols vary from simple soap and water to antiseptics or diluted hydrogen peroxide. The skin around the pin sites should not be under tension. The sites often require release with a local anesthetic.

Neurological

Transient neuropathy, whether clinically manifested or detected only by electrophysiological testing, is a very common complication, occurring in as many as 30% of patients.[26, 27] The most common mechanism is believed to be nerve stretching. Neuropraxias noted during distraction can frequently be managed by decreasing the distraction rate. Occasionally, permanent nerve damage can ensue. Neuropraxias noted immediately after frame application may be an indication of nerve injury by pin placement and necessitate evaluation and possible pin removal.

Vascular

Vascular complications are less common but more potentially serious problems. Bleeding can occur intraoperatively owing to either the osteotomy or wire placement. Edema of the extremity being lengthened is almost universal and can be a source of discomfort throughout the lengthening period.[28] Deep venous thrombosis has been reported[19, 25] but not frequently enough to warrant anticoagulant prophylaxis. Compartment syndrome is a rare occurrence but constitutes a surgical emergency requiring immediate fasciotomy and decompression.[18, 28, 29]

General

Hypertension. This is one of the most interesting problems reported in children undergoing lengthening for limb discrepancies.[26, 30–32] The mechanism is believed to be a result of nerve stretching, particularly of the sciatic nerve, which stimulates catecholamine release and subsequent elevation in blood pressure. A renal etiology cannot, however,

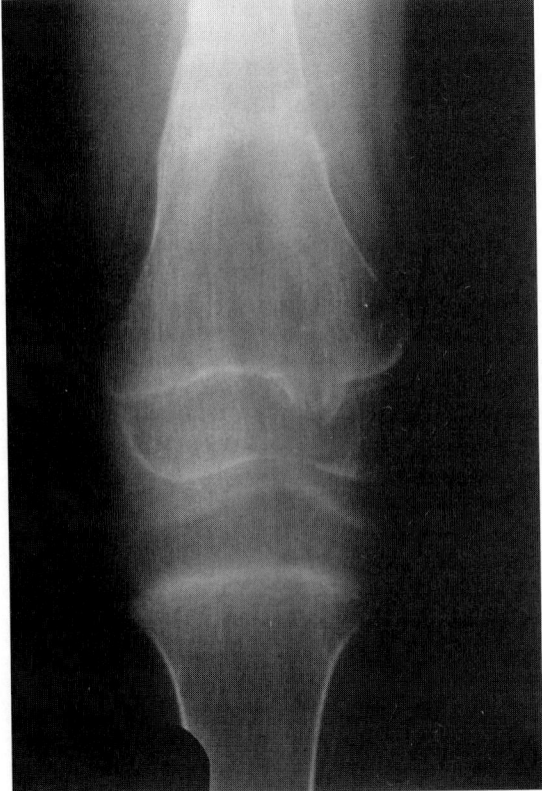

Fig. 9. Growth arrest. A central growth arrest in the patient in Figure 8A was noted 3 months after removal of an external fixator for femoral lengthening. The most distal pins site is visible, notably several centimeters away from the physis.

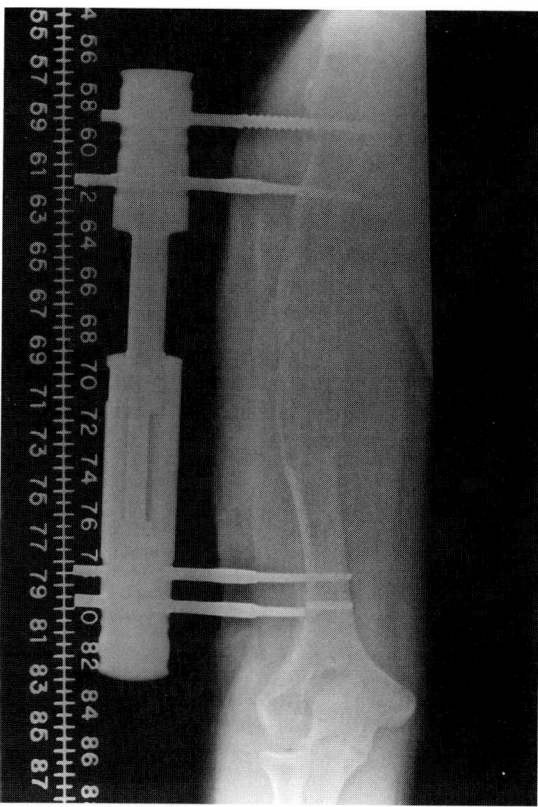

Fig. 10. Hardware failure. This shows a humerus lengthening with broken screw distally.

ized. Some patients have elected to have scar revision surgery. A variety of miscellaneous complications have been recognized, including hardware failure (pin or wire breakage), reflex sympathetic dystrophy, or dermatitis due to antiseptic solutions (Fig. 10).

FEMORAL SHORTENING

Shortening is a viable alternative in patients with a moderate leg length discrepancy. The primary advantage versus a lengthening procedure is that shortening is done as a single operation rather than a process that continues for months. Shortening of the bone necessarily creates loss of muscle tension and therefore weakening. The patients require a knee immobilizer or crutches postoperatively. Most patients are able to walk independently by a few weeks. Cybex testing at 1 year following closed femoral shortening demonstrated strength at least equal to the opposite leg in 8 of 10 patients.[36] Shortening of more than 7 cm is not recommended because of excess weakness. Additional considerations include the necessity to operate on the longer leg, which is usually the more normal leg, and a reduction in overall height.

SHORTENING TECHNIQUE

A subtrochanteric osteotomy is frequently employed. Cast immobilization is not required if adequate internal fixation via a blade plate is obtained, and the patient is sufficiently cooperative for crutch ambulation and limited weightbearing. The proximal femur is exposed via a standard lateral approach. The chisel for a blade plate is inserted. The bone is then sectioned with an oscillating saw, and a section of bone of an appropriate length is removed. The chisel is exchanged for the blade plate, which is impacted into the proximal fragment and then secured to the distal fragment with screws inserted with compression technique.

Alternatively, a closed femoral shortening procedure can be performed. This procedure is technically demanding. Following insertion of an intramedullary guidewire and reaming of the canal, an intramedullary saw is inserted, and a midshaft osteotomy is performed from the inside out. A second parallel cut is then made more proximally.[37] The section is then split vertically with backcutting osteotomes. The fragments are displaced laterally. The rod is then introduced. The main advantage of the closed technique over the subtrochanteric osteotomy is a reduction in the size of the scar. The main disadvantage is difficulty controlling rotation. Rotational problems have been noted in 10% of these patients.[37]

CONCLUSION

Limb deformities and limb length discrepancies in children frequently present a challenge to the pediatric orthopaedic surgeon. Their causes are various and treatment options numerous. For successful outcome, it is imperative that management be tailored to the child's individual needs. The multidisciplinary team approach has, once again, proved to be an important factor in obtaining optimal results.

be ignored, as evidenced by the excellent response to therapy with angiotensin-converting enzyme inhibitors.[33] Often the hypertension in such patients remains asymptomatic, hence the importance of careful blood pressure monitoring, especially in the early period after distractions are initiated.

In some patients, blood pressure elevation can be quite significant and potentially serious, requiring either slowing or even temporary cessation of distractions. The use of antihypertensive agents becomes necessary if continuation of the process is imperative because of factors such as imminent consolidation of the osteotomy site. The authors have noted hypertension more frequently in patients with arthrogryposis.

Psychological Changes. A wide variety of psychosocial problems have been reported.[34] The development of anxiety, depression, disturbed sleep, and even aggressive behavior are easy to understand in a child who is subject to prolonged hospitalization or enduring chronic pain. Suicide attempts have also been reported on occasion.[35] Low self-esteem and lack of family or social support are among the important contributing factors.

In the authors' institution, all potential lengthening candidates are carefully screened prior to surgery with special emphasis on pre-existing emotional imbalance or social maladjustments. Every attempt is made to identify a solid support system in both the family and the community.

Others. Scarring is an anticipated result of lengthening with an external fixation device. Treatment is individual-

REFERENCES

1. Stephens DC, Herrick W, MacEwen GD: Epiphysiodesis for limb length inequality. Clin Orthop 1978; 136:41.

2. Stanitski DF: Treatment of deformity secondary to metabolic bone disease with the Ilizarov technique. Clin Orthop 1994; 301: 38.

3. Mosely CF: A straight line graph for leg length discrepancies. Clin Orthop 1978; 136:33.

4. Anderson M, Green W, Messner M: Growth and predictions of growth in the lower extremities. J Bone Joint Surg Am 1963; 45:1.

5. Phemister DB: Operative arrestment of longitudinal growth of bones in the treatment of deformities. J Bone Joint Surg 1933; 15:1.

6. Ogilvie JW: Epiphysiodesis: Evaluation of a new technique. J Pediatr Orthop 1986; 6:147.

7. Canale ST, Russell TA, Holcomb RL: Percutaneous epiphysiodesis: Experimental study and preliminary clinical results. J Pediatr Orthop 1986; 6:150.

8. Timberlake R, Bowen R, Guille J, et al: Prospective evaluation of fifty-three consecutive percutaneous epiphysiodeses of the distal femur and proximal tibia and fibula. J Pediatr Orthop 1991; 11:350.

9. Blair V, Walker S, Sheridan J, et al: Epiphysiodesis: A problem of timing. J Pediatr Orthop 1982; 2:281.

10. Codivilla A: On the means of lengthening, in the lower limbs, the muscles and tissues which are shortened through deformity. Am J Orthop Surg 1904; 2:353.

11. Wagner H: Operative lengthening of the femur. Clin Orthop 1978; 136:125.

12. Ilizarov G: Clinical application of the tension-stress effect for limb lengthening. Clin Orthop 1990; 250:8.

13. De Bastiani G, Aldegheri R, Renzi-Brivio L, et al: Limb lengthening by callous distraction (callotasis). J Pediatr Orthop 1987; 7:129.

14. Noonan KJ, Leyes M, Forriol F, et al: Distraction osteogenesis of the lower extremity with use of the monolateral external fixation. J Bone Joint Surg Am 1998; 80:793.

15. Paley D, Herzenberg JE, Paremain G, et al: Femoral lengthening over an intramedullary nail. J Bone Joint Surg Am 1997; 79:1464.

16. Sproul JT, Price CT: Recent advances in limb lengthening I: Clinical advances. Orthop Rev 1992, 21:307.

17. Paley D: What orthopaedic surgery can do for your patients. Contemp Pediatr 1992, 9:63.

18. Dahl MT, Gulli B, Berg T: Complications of limb lengthening: A learning curve. Clin Orthop 1994, 301:10.

19. Eldridge JC, Bell DF: Problems with substantial limb lengthening. Orthop Clin North Am 1991, 22:625.

20. Guidera KJ, Hess WF, Highhouse KP, et al: Extremity lengthening: Results and complications with the Orthofix system. J Pediatr Orthop 1991, 11:90.

21. Ilizarov GA: Pseudarthroses and defects of long tubular bones. In Transosseous Osteosynthesis: Theoretical and Clinical Aspects of the Regeneration and Growth of Tissue. Berlin, Springer-Verlag, 1992, p 453.

22. Guidera KG, Raney EM, Ganey T, et al: Ilizarov treatment of congenital pseudarthrosis of the tibia. J Pediatr Orthop 1997; 17:668.

23. Bonnard C, Favard L, Sollogoub I, et al: Limb lengthening in children using the Ilizarov method. Clin Orthop 1993, 293:83.

24. Osterman IK, Merikanto J: Diaphyseal bone lengthening in children using Wagner device: Long-term results. J Pediatr Orthop 1991, 11:449.

25. Vizkelety TL, Marschalko P: Limb lengthening operations. Acta Chir Hung 1993, 33:55.

26. Karger C, Guille JT, Bowen R: Lengthening of congenital lower limb deficiencies. Clin Orthop 1993, 291:236.

27. Galardi G, Comi G, Lozza L, et al: Peripheral nerve damage during limb lengthenings: Neurophysiology in five cases of bilateral tibial lengthenings. J Bone Joint Surg Br 1990, 72:121.

28. Velasquez RJ, Bell DF, Armstrong PF, et al: Complications of use of the Ilizarov technique in the correction of limb deformities in children. J Bone Joint Surg Am 1993, 75:1148.

29. Tjernstrom B, Olerud S, Karlstrom G: Direct leg lengthenings. J Orthop Trauma 1993, 7:543.

30. Taleb YA, Hamden J, Ahmed M: Orthopaedic causes of hypertension in pediatric patients. J Bone Joint Surg Am 1982, 64: 291.

31. Whitehall ZH, Hakala MW: The hypertension of femoral lengthening: A canine experimental model. Surg Forum 1976, 27: 525.

32. Yosipovitch ZH, Palti Y: Alterations in blood pressure during leg lengthening: A clinical and experimental investigation. J Bone Joint Surg Am 1967, 49:1352.

33. Helal A, Guidera KJ, Campos A, et al: Hypertension following orthopaedic surgery in children. J Pediatr Orthop 1993, 13:773.

34. Faber FWM, Keessen W, van Roermard PM: Complications of leg lengthening: 46 procedures in 28 patients. Acta Orthop Scand 1991, 62:327.

35. Hrutkay JM, Eilert RE: Operative lengthening of the lower extremity and associated psychological aspects: The Childrens Hospital experience. J Pediatr Orthop 1990, 10:373.

36. Chapman ME, Duwelius PJ, Bray TJ, et al: Closed intramedullary femoral osteotomy. Clin Orthop 1993, 287:245.

37. Winquist R, Hansen S, Pearson R: Closed intramedullary shortening of the femur. Clin Orthop 1978; 136:54.

NEUROMUSCULAR

WALTER B. GREENE

CEREBRAL PALSY: OVERVIEW AND MANAGEMENT OF SPINAL DEFORMITIES

section 10 chapter 1

Steven E. Koop

Summary
Cerebral palsy is a disorder of the brain that:
- Is nonprogressive (some prefer the term static encephalopathy).
- Develops during gestation, at delivery, or shortly after birth (onset up to 18 months of age).
- Causes permanent impairment of motor function that may secondarily lead to progressive contractures and bony deformities.
- May be associated with learning disabilities, mental retardation, speech impairment, visual deficits, hearing loss, and swallowing disorders.

PATHOGENESIS

Cerebral palsy is secondary to an injury, disease, or developmental abnormality of the brain. Prematurity, with its associated risk of intraventricular hemorrhage, is the most common cause of cerebral palsy. Anomalous brain development, pre- and postnatal cerebral infections (e.g., cytomegalovirus, bacterial meningitis), trauma, and birth hypoxia are additional causes.[1] However, in many cases, the definite cause cannot be identified.

Some causes of cerebral palsy such as Rh incompatibility or maternal rubella infection can be eliminated; however, even with sophisticated maternal health care, the prevalence of cerebral palsy has remained stable at about 2 per 1000 live births during most of this century. The reason for this consistent prevalence is that, although neonatal care had advanced considerably, now infants of very low birth weight (500 to 1000 g) commonly survive, but this group of neonates is at significantly greater risk for cerebral palsy.

CLASSIFICATION

Individuals with cerebral palsy are classified according to the neurological type, anatomic pattern, and functional consequence of the motor abnormality.

Classification by neurological groups include the following:

- Spasticity is characterized by exaggerated response of muscles to stretch reflexes.
- Dyskinesia includes the involuntary movements of athetosis, dystonia, and ataxia. Subgroups of athetosis include the following: ballismus (uncontrolled involuntary movement of proximal joints), chorea (involuntary movement of fingers or distal joints), and tension athetosis (typically extension patterns that can be broken by repetitive motion of the involved joint).[2] Ataxia is characterized by lack of balance and uncoordinated movement. Dystonia is intermittent and severe distorted posturing of the limbs, neck, or trunk.

- Hypotonia: many neonates with cerebral palsy are floppy or hypotonic and then progress to a spastic or athetoid status. However, some children with cerebral palsy have persistent muscle hypotonia.

Anatomic patterns include hemiplegia, diplegia, triplegia, and quadriplegia.

- Hemiplegics have involvement on one side of the body (i.e. ipsilateral upper and lower extremity spasticity).
- Diplegics have much greater involvement of the lower than the upper extremities.
- Triplegics typically have involvement of both lower extremities and a single upper extremity.
- Quadriplegics have extensive involvement of all extremities. Head and trunk control is also affected in this group, and another term for this is total body involvement.

Functional classification is based on the degree to which motor tasks can be performed. This varies from being unable to sit without support to being able to walk considerable distances without external support. Hemiplegics invariably function as community ambulators. Diplegics commonly walk at either a household or community functional level but may require a walker or crutches for balance support. A large proportion of quadriplegic patients are wheelchair dependent.

The prognosis for walking can be predicted by assessing neonatal reflexes and motor milestones. A child with cerebral palsy is unlikely to achieve independent walking function if

- At the age of 12 months, neonatal reflexes such as the asymmetric and symmetric tonic neck reflexes persist and the parachute reaction has not developed.
- At the age of 20 months, head control has not developed.
- At the age of 4 years, independent sitting has not developed.

A child with cerebral palsy will generally be able to walk (with or without support) if

- At the age of 9 months, head control has developed.
- At the age of 24 months, the child is able to sit independently.

DEVELOPMENT OF MUSCULOSKELETAL DEFORMITIES

As they grow, infants and children gradually develop control over extremity and trunk muscles, and they gradually learn how to accomplish "developmental milestones" such as sitting, walking, and running. Increased motor control is the result of neurological maturation, environmental stimulation, and repeated activity trials. A child with cerebral palsy also demonstrates neurological maturation, although the end point of development will vary with the nature and severity of neurological dysfunction.

Muscle contracture and joint deformities are common in children with cerebral palsy who have spasticity. Muscle imbalance between agonists and antagonists develops in these children as a result of various factors, including limb postures, cross-sectional area of muscle, and degree of spasticity. Muscle elasticity and flexibility are reduced, and in time a true contracture of the muscle develops as muscle growth fails to keep pace with bone growth. The range of motion for the affected joint is thereby reduced.

Bone growth is also responsive to asymmetric muscle forces, and normal patterns of growth may be disturbed. The normal resolution of infantile torsions may not occur, and abnormal bony torsions may develop. Joint instability, subluxation, and dislocation may develop, leading to incongruent joint surfaces and degenerative arthritis.

Although often overlooked, muscle weakness is implied in the term "palsy," and even the more "spastic" muscle in children with cerebral palsy is typically weak compared with strength in normal children. Muscle weakness also contributes to the development of musculoskeletal deformities. This is particularly true in the spine, where reduced trunk control, asymmetric tone, and compromised balance mechanisms reduce the ability to control the spinal column, leading to deformities in the frontal plane (scoliosis) and in the sagittal plane (lordosis and kyphosis).[2]

The impact of neurological function during growth and development becomes evident when the prevalence of hip dysplasia and spine deformity are compared between children with normal neurological function and those with cerebral palsy. The incidence of hip dysplasia, including dislocation, is 1 to 2 per 1000 in the general population. In cerebral palsy, the likelihood of hip dislocation is closely linked to the pattern and severity of neurological involvement. It is uncommon in hemiplegia (<5%) and diplegia (5% to 20%) and common in quadriplegia (20% to 50%).[2] Progressing beyond subluxation is uncommon in hemiplegics and diplegics, but the majority of subluxations in quadriplegics eventually progress to dislocation. The prevalence of a significant idiopathic scoliosis (curve magnitude >30 degrees) in the general population is 1 per 1000. The prevalence of scoliosis in cerebral palsy is greater and varies with neurological impairment; curves greater than 30 degrees occur in approximately 15% of children with quadriplegia.[3-5]

DIFFERENTIAL DIAGNOSIS

Cerebral palsy is heterogenous, and many conditions are similar in part. An essential component of cerebral palsy is the presence of a *static* brain anomaly. Therefore, an important component of the diagnostic evaluation is the detection of progressive neurological disorders, some of which are treatable. Severe cerebral palsy is usually apparent, but mild forms may present as a problem of in-toeing or toe walking. A history of delay in developmental milestones coupled with spasticity in the plantar flexors and upper extremity (elbow flexion and forearm pronation while walking) suggests a hemiplegic pattern of cerebral palsy. Idiopathic toe walkers are characterized by normal motor milestones and either no spasticity or abnormal tone limited to the plantar flexors.

Subsequent chapters describe the consequences for the upper and lower extremities. The remainder of this chapter focuses on spinal deformities.

CLINICAL FEATURES OF SCOLIOSIS

The first signs of spinal deformity in cerebral palsy are changes in posture, particularly when seated, and changes in the shape of the trunk. Excessive kyphosis makes a child lean forward and makes it difficult to look at the surrounding environment. Scoliosis results in decompensation to one side and the need for propping on an arm or the side of a chair. This limits the use of that extremity for other functional activities. Decompensation to one side coupled with pelvic obliquity will shift the sitting pressures to one side, concentrating in small areas such as the tissues directly over the ischial tuberosity or greater trochanter. Although protective sensation is preserved in cerebral palsy, motor or verbal limitations may make it impossible for a child to change positions and relieve pressure or to ask for help in the presence of pain.

Distortion of the rib cage associated with scoliosis is known to impair pulmonary function; however, cross-sectional data on pulmonary function are lacking for children with cerebral palsy. The most severe deformities develop in quadriplegia, and these patients may have additional intrinsic lung damage associated with gastric reflux and poor secretion control, causing repetitive aspiration.[6]

Spinal deformities in cerebral palsy are often accompanied by hip problems. A common finding is a windswept deformity in which one hip is adducted, internally rotated, and flexed while the other is abducted and externally rotated. The windswept deformity is often associated with pelvic obliquity and unilateral hip subluxation or dislocation (adducted side); however, the child with scoliosis may also have either no hip dysplasia or bilateral dislocations. In addition, treatment of the hip deformities usually does not affect progression of a scoliotic deformity.

INVESTIGATION

The typical curve pattern in nonambulating cerebral palsy patients is a long, C-shaped thoracolumbar curve that extends into the pelvis. Independent ambulators are more likely to have curve patterns similar to those observed in idiopathic scoliosis.

An anteroposterior and lateral radiograph may be done with the patient standing or sitting. With good standing balance, a standing radiograph should be done. Otherwise, radiographs made in a sitting position are preferred, even though wheelchairs and other seating devices provide support, which reduces the severity of the deformity. It is more difficult to position children with cerebral palsy in a reproducible posture that allows consistent quantification of their spinal deformity. The resultant variation in Cobb's measurements makes it difficult to ascertain whether a curvature is truly increasing or remaining stable in patients with cerebral palsy.

MANAGEMENT

The goals of treating spinal deformities in cerebral palsy are the same regardless of whether nonoperative or operative methods are used: obtain a level pelvis and center the trunk over the pelvis.[7-9] These goals lead to a stable and durable sitting posture, prevent skin breakdown, and free the upper extremities for functional tasks of everyday life.

Nonoperative management consists of external support, either a custom-made thoracolumbar-sacral orthosis or a specially designed wheelchair. Very little, however, is known about the long-term efficacy of orthotic management of spinal deformities in cerebral palsy. Studies to determine the effects of bracing are difficult because of the variation in neurological involvement, age at onset, curve size and patterns, and amount of time these children are able to wear a brace. Studies show that bracing scoliosis in cerebral palsy is not nearly as effective as bracing children with idiopathic curvatures. Alternatively, performing a long fusion in a young child is also problematic. In these children, the purpose of the brace is to try to delay the need for operation.

There is a tendency among parents and physicians to delay operative management of spinal deformities in children with cerebral palsy. Parents do not want their child to experience the pain of surgery, and physicians are aware of the magnitude of the surgical event and the frequent complications. Studies demonstrate that the average cerebral palsy curve magnitude at operation is 60 to 70 degrees, much larger than would be tolerated for idiopathic scoliosis.[10-14] Excessive delay results in larger deformities that are even more difficult to manage.

Indications for surgery include the following:

- Curvature greater than 40 degrees with growth remaining.
- Pain or loss of functional sitting.

PREOPERATIVE INVESTIGATION

The best method to assess flexibility of curvatures in these patients is a supine anteroposterior radiograph while traction is applied. Performing this "stretch" film on a Risser table is best because longitudinal traction and lateral correction forces can be applied.

Complications after spinal surgery in patients with cere-bral palsy are relatively common.[7-14] Pneumonia, bleeding, pseudarthrosis, and infection are particularly problematic (Table 1). Preoperative investigation may minimize these risks. Pulmonary function tests may not be practical; however, for patients with severe curvatures, arterial blood gases may reveal chronic carbon dioxide retention, and a chest radiograph may show evidence of intrinsic lung changes. Some seizure medications affect the clotting mechanism. For example, valproic acid may cause a coagulopathy similar to von Willebrand's disease.[6] In addition to the usual clotting studies, measuring the bleeding time may demonstrate a problem.

Malnutrition secondary to feeding difficulties is a special concern because it increases the rate of infection.[6, 9] Screening studies for protein deficiency include a lymphocyte count, serum albumin, and possibly serum transferrin and prealbumin.

OPERATION

To achieve the goal of a level pelvis and balanced trunk in cerebral palsy patients, several decision-making principles must be applied that are different from those used for idiopathic scoliosis. Fusions must be more extensive than the measured curve intervals, often must extend from the upper thoracic spine to the pelvis, and should be supported by instrumentation that applies corrective and fixation forces to as many vertebrae as possible.[7, 8, 11] These principles are necessary because of trunk weakness and poor balance, pelvic obliquity, and relatively osteopenic bone found in patients with cerebral palsy.

Posterior spinal fusion with segmental instrumentation and bone graft from the second or third thoracic vertebra to the low lumbar area in the ambulatory patient or to the sacrum in the nonambulatory patient is appropriate when flexibility studies demonstrate that curve magnitudes can be reduced to less than 50 degrees and pelvic obliquity can be minimized (Fig. 1). For more severe curves, anterior multi-level diskectomy and fusion increase flexibility and decrease the likelihood of pseudarthrosis. The anterior fusion should be combined with the posterior procedure because multiple studies demonstrated high rates of failure for isolated anterior fusions.[7, 8, 10, 12-14] Whether the anterior fu-

Complication Type	Ferguson and Allen[8]	Lonstein and Akbarnia[11]	Stanitsky et al[13]	Swank et al[14]	Cassidy et al[15]
Blood loss					
Anterior only		1500 mL			906 mL
Posterior only		2230 mL			2040 mL
Anterior and posterior combined			3700 mL		
Pseudarthrosis rate					
Anterior only		72%			
Posterior only	6.5%	40%		None	40%
Anterior and posterior combined		None		None	10%
Wound infection or problems	8.7%	3%	3.9%		5.8%
Pulmonary			19.6%	8%	7%
Urinary tract infections			15.7%		13%
Instrumentation failure	15%			8%	10%
Deaths (related to surgery)	2.1%		3.9%		

TABLE 1. COMPLICATION RATES FOR SPINE FUSION SURGERY IN CEREBRAL PALSY

* The complication rates for spine fusion surgery in cerebral palsy are much higher than those found in surgery for idiopathic scoliosis.

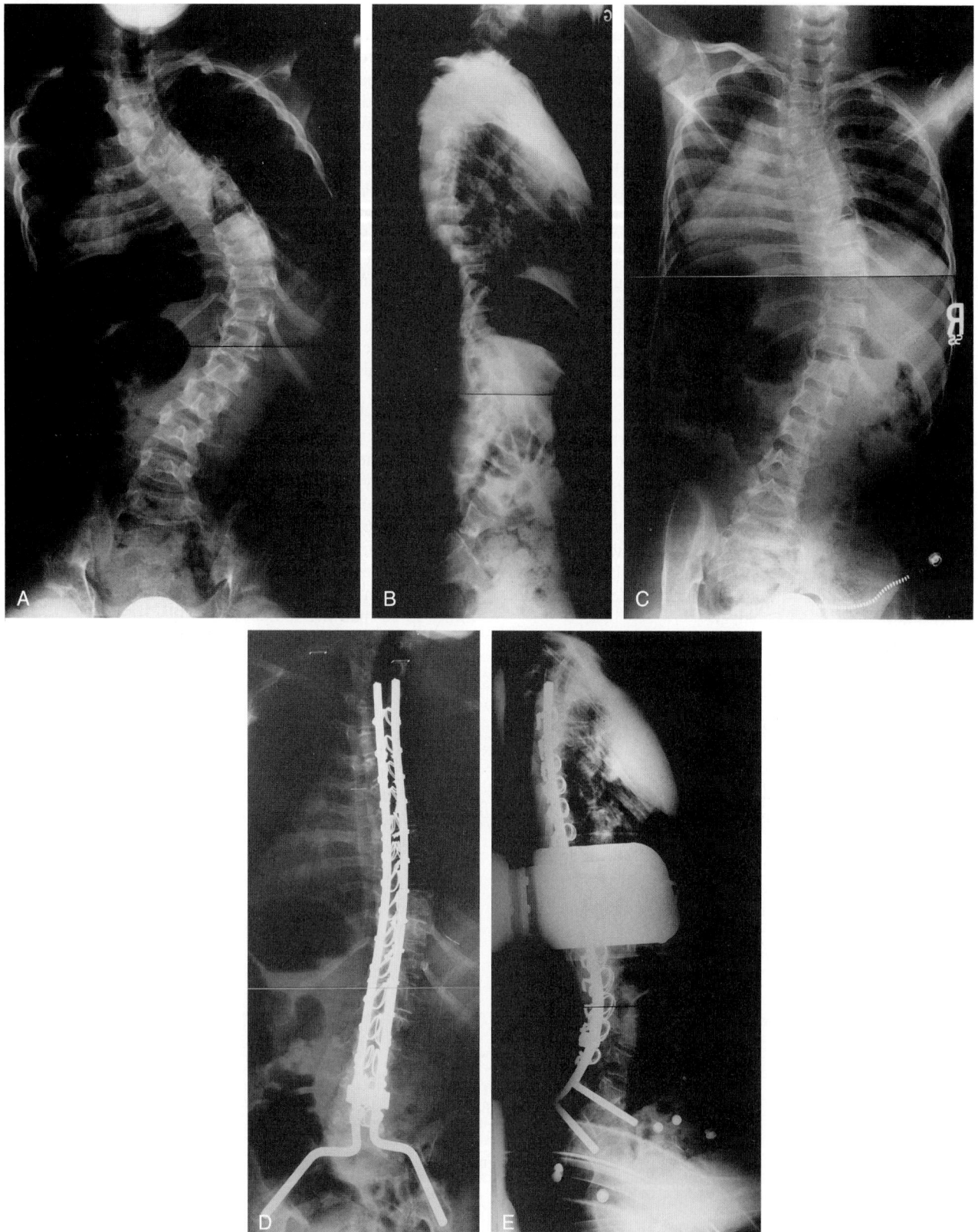

Fig. 1. Surgical intervention for severe scoliosis in cerebral palsy. *A*, Unsupported sitting AP roentgenogram. *B*, Unsupported sitting lateral roentgenogram. *C*, Supine AP traction study demonstrating curve flexibility. *D*, Sitting AP roentgenogram 1 year after surgery. *E*, Sitting lateral roentgenogram 1 year after surgery.

sion should be instrumented is less clear. The combined anterior and posterior fusions may be done in a single operative event.[12]

Anesthesiologists familiar with complex spine surgery are essential. Many children will need intensive postoperative care, including brief mechanical ventilator support and parenteral nutrition.

COMPLICATIONS

Complications after spinal surgery in patients with cerebral palsy are relatively common (see Table 1).[7–14] Blood loss during neuromuscular spine surgery can be large and can lead to coagulopathy. Postoperative respiratory compromise is common, and the risk of pneumonia can be minimized by short-term mechanical ventilation. Wound infections are a particular risk in the presence of malnutrition. Pseudar-

throsis rates can be reduced to a baseline risk of 3% to 5% by making good preoperative decisions and using careful technique and secure segmental instrumentation.

RESULTS

The majority of parents and health care workers who have documented the onset of pain, loss of functional abilities, and respiratory or gastrointestinal compromise with the appearance and progression of spinal deformity believe that surgery improves the function and quality of life for a child with cerebral palsy.[7, 10, 11, 13] The benefits are less certain when the need is less evident.[15] This might include the severely retarded who cannot report symptoms and adults with long-standing intrinsic pulmonary compromise that may not be improved even by reducing the spinal deformity.

REFERENCES

1. Aicardi J, Bax M: Cerebral palsy. In Aicardi J (ed): Diseases of the Nervous System in Childhood. London, Mac Keith Press, 1998, 2nd ed, p 210.
2. Koop SE: Orthopaedic aspects of static encephalopathies. In Miller G, Ramer J (eds): Static Encephalopathies of Infancy and Childhood. New York, Raven Press, 1992, p 95.
3. Madigan RR, Wallace SL: Scoliosis in the institutionalized cerebral palsy population. Spine 1981; 6:583.
4. Thometz JG, Simon SR: Progression of scoliosis after skeletal maturity in institutionalized adults who have cerebral palsy. J Bone Joint Surg Am 1988; 70:1290.
5. Rosenthal RK, Levine DB, McCarver CL: The occurrence of scoliosis in cerebral palsy. Dev Med Child Neurol 1974; 16: 664.
6. Winter S: Preoperative assessment of the

child with neuromuscular scoliosis. Orthop Clin North Am 1994; 25:239.
7. Boachie-Adjei O, Lonstein JE, Winter RB, et al: Management of neuromuscular spinal deformities with Luque segmental instrumentation. J Bone Joint Surg Am 1989; 71:548.
8. Ferguson RL, Allen BL: Considerations in the treatment of cerebral palsy patients with spinal deformities. Orthop Clin North Am 1988; 19:419.
9. Jevsevar DS, Karlin LI: The relationship between preoperative nutritional status and complications after an operation for scoliosis in patients who have cerebral palsy. J Bone Joint Surg Am 1993; 75:880.
10. Bonnett C, Brown JC, Grow T: Thoracolumbar scoliosis in cerebral palsy. J Bone Joint Surg Am 1976; 58:328.
11. Lonstein JE, Akbarnia BA: Operative treatment of spinal deformities in patients

with cerebral palsy or mental retardation. J Bone Joint Surg Am 1083; 65:43.
12. O'Brien T, Akmakjian J, Ogin G, et al: Comparison of one-stage versus two-stage anterior/posterior spinal fusion for neuromuscular scoliosis. J Pediatr Orthop 1992; 12:610.
13. Stanitski CL, Micheli LJ, Hall JE, et al: Surgical correction of spinal deformity in cerebral palsy. Spine 1982; 7:563.
14. Swank SM, Cohen DS, Brown JC: Spine fusion in cerebral palsy with L-rod segmental spinal instrumentation: A comparison of single and two-stage combined approach with Zielke instrumentation. Spine 1989; 14:750.
15. Cassidy C, Craig CL, Perry A, et al: A reassessment of spinal stabilization in severe cerebral palsy. J Pediatr Orthop 1994; 14:731.

section
10
chapter
2

GUIDELINES FOR MANAGING LOWER EXTREMITY PROBLEMS IN CEREBRAL PALSY

Michael D. Aiona

Summary

- Lower extremity dynamic and anatomic deformities are the result of muscle imbalance.
- The goal of treatment is to maximize function and prevent pain.
- Understanding the interrelationship of joints facilitates recognition of primary versus secondary deformities.
- Three-dimensional gait analysis assists in defining deformities and treatment options.
- Correct as many of the dynamic and anatomic deformities in one surgical setting as possible.
- Rapid mobilization will minimize weakness and facilitate early return to function.
- Recurrence of deformity may occur with growth and may require repeat intervention.

Patients with cerebral palsy have varying degrees of motor impairment. The severity and type of motor disorder determine the functional level of the patient and the potential development of specific deformities. Nonambulatory patients are more likely to have severe hip dysplasia, scoliosis, and joint contractures. Treatment goals for these patients are prevention of pain, maintenance of functional sitting, and development of transfer and self-care skills. The ambulatory patient is less likely to have significant hip dysplasia; however, dynamic gait deformities lead to increased energy consumption and joint pain secondary to abnormal mechanical loading. Treatment is directed at correction of the dynamic deformities, joint contractures, and bony deformities that interfere with function.[1]

This chapter reviews the common deformities affecting lower extremity function. Although the specific problems of each joint are described separately, one must recognize that functions of the lower extremity joints are interrelated. Treatment recommendations must address all of the identified abnormalities.

HISTORICAL REVIEW

All too often surgical treatment in the past addressed single-joint deformities with multiple sequential operations. Technological advances in gait analysis have improved the evaluation and treatment of the lower extremities by assisting in the identification of joint deviations and interactions. Knowledge of the interrelationships of muscle abnormalities and mechanical factors has led to multilevel correction at a single operation. This provides obvious psychological benefits for the child and also minimizes the risk of an isolated correction causing a secondary deformity at an adjacent joint.

PATHOGENESIS: CLINICAL FEATURES

Different levels of muscle strength, spasticity, and coordination create an imbalance of forces across joints. With growth, this imbalance of forces contributes to the development of static and dynamic deformities. The static deformities include the following:

1. Varying degrees of hip instability.
2. Rotational deformities of the femur and tibia.
3. Fixed contractures of the hip, knee, ankle, and foot.

Dynamic deformities interfere with gait by altering joint kinematics and kinetics at multiple levels.[2]

INVESTIGATION

The initial evaluation should include a review of the birth history, associated medical problems, and motor development. The physical exam must include the upper extremity because the degree of its impairment affects the ability to use assistive devices. Static lower extremity measurements include range of motion of the hip, knee, and ankle in all planes, presence of contractures, and structural alignment of the foot. Measuring range of motion using two-finger pressure as opposed to forceful, slow stretch provides more useful information because it more closely parallels joint abnormalities during walking. Dynamic measurements should include evaluation of muscle tone and strength. Gait disturbances will reflect the degree of motor control impairment and the presence of a movement disorder. Radiographs of the hips and other joints as needed complete the assessment.

Interpretation of the physical findings requires caution because the patient's spasticity and neurological control may vary. Factors that may heighten the degree of spasticity include anxiety (particularly common at the child's first visit), an intercurrent viral illness, fatigue, and speed of walking.

The necessity of instrumented gait analysis in planning treatment is controversial. At a minimum, one should be knowledgeable concerning normal kinesiology and the abnormal primary and secondary deviations observed in cerebral palsy.

Instrumented gait lab analysis simultaneously documents the three-dimensional motion of all three joints. Concurrent electromyographic (EMG) data can provide information regarding phasic and dysphasic muscle activity. Kinetic data reflect the power generation during gait and assist in distinguishing compensatory versus primary abnormalities. Multiplane gait deviations are difficult to identify by visual assessment alone. Furthermore, muscle activity and kinetic data are not available with mere observation of gait.[2] Differences between the recommended treatment plans based on clinical observation alone and those after computerized three-dimensional gait analysis have been documented.[3]

TREATMENT PRINCIPLES

Tendon lengthenings, releases, and transfers balance the muscle forces across joints. Osteotomies and arthrodeses correct the anatomic deformities. The principles of treatment are the following:

1. Identification and treatment of all correctable abnormalities with single-stage surgery.
2. Immobilizing joints in a functional position (maximuming hip/knee extension with the ankle at right angles).
3. Minimizing postoperative immobilization to maintaining strength.
4. Intensive therapy to regain function after cast removal.
5. Appropriate splinting and bracing.

Age influences the timing of surgery. One must balance the greater potential for remodeling and relearning at a younger age against the real potential for recurrent deformity with growth. Many studies have documented the loss of initial correction with bony and soft-tissue procedures in patients younger than 6 years. The older patient has a diminished chance for recurrence but also has less ability to adapt to a different muscle balance. Generally, patients with greater neurological involvement have a greater rate of recurrence.

MUSCLE STRENGTHENING

Muscles in patients with cerebral palsy can be strengthened through a well-directed physical therapy program. Strengthening a weak quadriceps muscle results in improved gait kinematics with increased knee extension. Transferring muscles to substitute for weak or nonfunctional muscles provides additional functional strength.

MUSCLE LENGTHENING

To reduce the strong deforming force, one can lengthen or release the dominant musculotendinous unit. Lengthening shifts the arc of motion of the joint to a more functional

position with theoretically no ultimate effect on the power-generating capacity of the muscle. Releasing the muscle diminishes its deforming force while maintaining some residual function.

Three techniques are commonly used to lengthen the musculotendinous unit. Lengthening the tendon may be performed as an open or percutaneous procedure. Open techniques allow specific control of the amount of lengthening. Percutaneous methods rely on controlled stretching of the tendon by a less extensive procedure; however, control of the amount of lengthening is not as precise. Neither procedure theoretically affects excursion or strength of the muscle.

A third technique is cutting an aponeurosis. This allows stretching of the underlying muscle and lengthening of the musculotendinous unit while retaining its continuity (Fig. 1). This "fractional lengthening technique" is commonly used for the semimembranosus, biceps femoris, and gastrocnemius muscles.

HIP

Hip stability depends on the bony architecture and balance of forces across the joint. The hip abductors and extensors must balance the forces of the flexors and adductors. In the patient with cerebral palsy, the spastic adductors and hip flexors are typically the dominant deforming forces. As the femur is repeatedly adducted and flexed, the femoral head will displace laterally and superiorly. The lack of a concentric reduction causes secondary dysplasia of the acetabulum and proximal femur. Untreated, patients frequently progress from subluxation to dislocation and pain (Fig. 2). Nonambulatory patients are more likely to have dislocated hips. Prevention is the best treatment because successful salvage of the dislocated hip is difficult.[4]

The migration percentage is a radiographic assessment of hip stability and a quantitative measurement of the amount of femoral head subluxation. Lines are drawn at right angles to the Hilgenreiner line at the medial and lateral edges of the femoral head and the lateral edge of the acetabulum (Fig. 3). The percentage of femoral head uncovered by the acetabulum (A/A+B × 100) is reproducible; however, a significant change must be greater than 10% to account for interrater and positioning variability. Through sequential

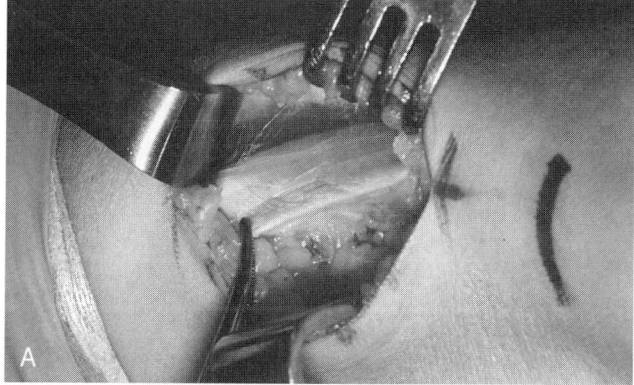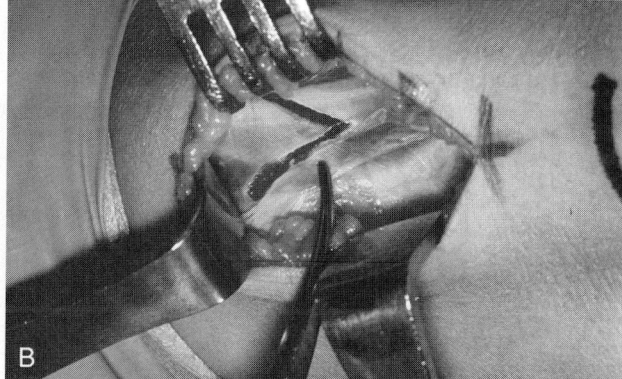

Fig. 1. View. *A,* Exposure of the gastrocnemius, revealing the aponeurosis of the muscle. *B,* Intramuscular aponeurosis lengthening showing the muscle remaining intact.

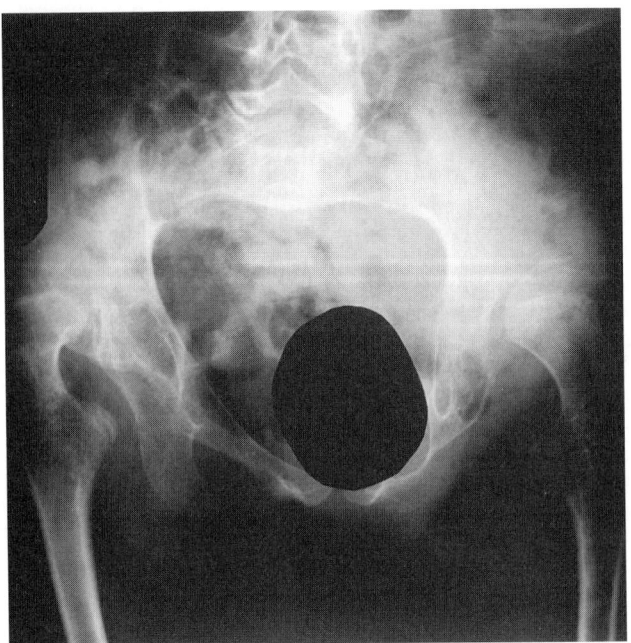

Fig. 2. Long-term follow-up of untreated at-risk hips. They are painful, dislocated, with fixed deformity.

radiographs, instability is identified. Hips with a migration percentage less than 25% are stable; those with a migration percentage greater than 70% will dislocate if left untreated. A progression of 10% in those hips with percentages within these limits is indicative of instability and requires treatment. Clinical findings of limited abduction and a migration percentage greater than 35 to 40 degrees may be an indication for treatment even without documented progression.[5]

The age of the patient and the degree of bony deformity determine the treatment. Most patients younger than 4 years stabilize with a muscle-balancing procedure consisting of an adductor release and psoas tenotomy. The goal of the adductor release is to obtain 40 to 45 degrees of passive abduction in the operating room. This may require release of the adductor longus, gracilis, and brevis or a more limited release in less severe contractures. Children in the 4- to 7-year age range with a migration percentage greater than 40% need a proximal femoral varus shortening osteotomy to correct the associated bony deformity along with the muscle releases. In this age group, reduction of the deforming muscle forces and correction of the proximal femoral deformity induce acetabular remodeling if the center edge angle (CEA) is greater than 5 to 10 degrees. However, once the patient has reached 8 years of age or if the CEA is less than 0 degrees, the potential for remodeling secondary acetabular changes is insufficient.[6] In this situation, a concomitant acetabular procedure is required to achieve stability and prevent future subluxation. An additional radiographic sign is the maturation of the sourcil (eyebrow in French), which should develop a rather uniform density of the subchondral bone in the superior acetabulum, and the lack of this may indicate the need for an acetabular procedure.[8] In complex hips, a three-dimensional computed axial tomography scan may assist in preoperative planning by defining the location of the acetabular deficiency, the amount of femoral anteversion, and the shape of the femoral head.[9]

Postoperatively, patients are immobilized for 4 to 6 weeks in a spica cast with the lower extremities in a functional position of 30 to 40 degrees of abduction, full hip, and knee extension and the ankle at 90 degrees. Pain and antispasm medications postoperatively and after cast removal provide comfort and enhance cooperation during rehabilitation. Physical therapy is directed toward regaining joint motion and muscle strength and improving function. The use of knee immobilizers and abduction pillows at night helps to prevent recurrent contractures (Table 1).

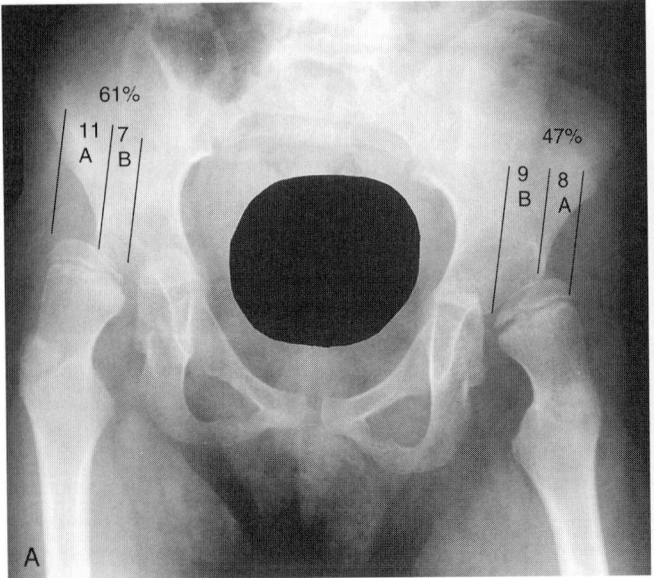
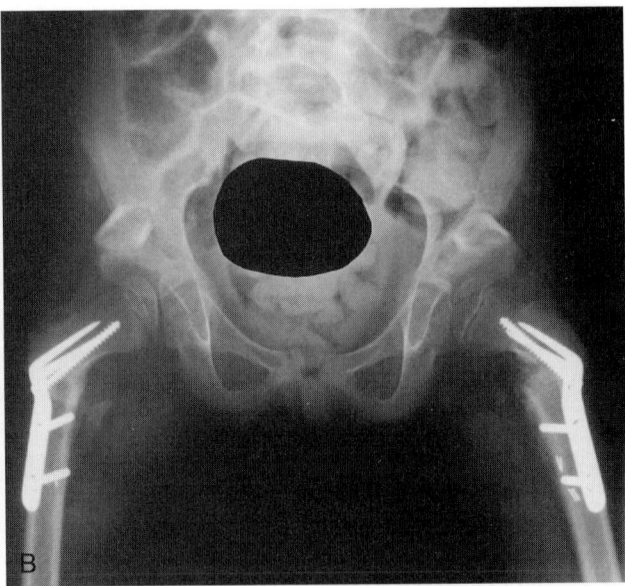

Fig. 3. View. *A,* Preoperative radiograph of unstable hips with migration percentage of 61% and 47%. *B,* Postoperative radiograph after bilateral proximal femoral varus osteotomies and Albee's acetabuloplasty showing improved coverage.

TABLE 1. MANAGEMENT OF THE HIP

| Migration % | Nonoperative Treatment | Age | Surgical Treatment | | Postoperative Management |
			Soft Tissue	Bony	
<25%	Abduction pillow and positioning	All ages	None		
25% <X <70%	If progressive, will eventually dislocate	<4 years	ADIP		Cast LLC with removable abduction bar for 2–4 weeks Nighttime abduction brace
		4 years <X <8 years	ADIP	PFVRSO	Spica cast 6 weeks PT to regain function after cast removal Nighttime abduction brace
		>8 years	ADIP	PFVRSO, acetabular procedure (shelf or periacetabular osteotomy)	As above
>70%	Will result in progressive dislocation		ADIP ± proximal hamstring release	As above	As above
>100% "round femoral head"			As above	As above	As above

General guidelines to follow in the assessment and treatment of the hip. ADIP, adductor and iliopsoas release; PFVRSO, proximal femoral varus shortening osteotomy; PT, physical therapy; LLC, long-leg cast.

A painful dislocated hip in an older patient makes seating and positioning difficult. Significant femoral head deformity mandates selection of a salvage procedure. Arthrodesis will eliminate the pain in the joint, but the loss of motion will make sitting and positioning difficult and will predispose the patient to fractures and pressure sores. A repositioning shortening valgus osteotomy moves the femoral head away from the acetabulum and corrects the adduction deformity. The soft tissues are addressed by incorporating shortening with the osteotomy to functionally lengthen the muscles. Pain relief, however, after this procedure is more variable, and there is a possibility of recurrence. Alternatively, resection arthroplasty removes the deformed femoral head and attempts to maintain motion. The keys to success are resection below the level of the lesser trochanter and postoperative traction to reduce the risk of proximal migration of the limb. Pain often improves slowly, and it may take up to 1 year for the soft tissues to "accommodate" the new position. Heterotopic ossification may adversely affect pain relief and limb motion (Table 2).

The windblown hip syndrome is distinguished by an adduction deformity of one hip and fixed abduction of the contralateral hip. The associated pelvic obliquity makes seating and perineal care difficult. Furthermore, scoliosis

TABLE 2. MANAGEMENT OF DEFORMED DISLOCATED HIP

Migration %	Soft Tissue	Procedure	Postoperative Management	Advantages	Disadvantages
>100%	ADIP, proximal hamstring release	Hip fusion	Spica cast 6 weeks PT to regain function after cast removal	Predictable pain relief	Stiffness with potential positioning difficulty Nonunion Fracture Need for casting
	As above	Proximal femoral resection	Traction for 2–4 weeks PT to regain function in seating and positioning	More mobility of joint	Heterotopic ossification Persistent pain Need for traction postoperatively
	As above	Proximal valgus shortening osteotomy	Spica cast 6 weeks PT to regain function after cast removal	Improved positioning of hip No radical shortening	Persistent mild pain

Treatment must be individualized along with surgeon preference and experience. ADIP, adductor and iliopsoas release; PT, physical therapy.

may aggravate the windblown pelvic deformity. In addition to treating the adducted hip, the abducted side must be addressed with a varus shortening osteotomy or abductor soft-tissue release to prevent rapid recurrence of the deformity. Postoperative management consisting of casting and therapy is similar to other hip interventions.

Dynamic hip deformities are classified by the primary plane of deviation. Spastic adductors cause coronal plane deformity and a scissoring gait, with the limbs adducting and crossing the midline. Limb advancement is compromised. If the patient is ambulatory, only the adductor longus and gracilis muscles are released, and patients are returned to previous function as soon as tolerated. Nighttime abduction bracing is thought to be important in preventing recurrence. Adductor transfers should not be done because the operation is more complicated, requires longer immobilization, and is more likely to cause asymmetric gait.[10]

In the sagittal plane, excessive hip flexion in stance phase is common. Exaggerated lumbar lordosis and compensation by distal joints are necessary to maintain an upright posture. If a hip flexion contracture of greater than 15 to 20 degrees is present, an intramuscular release of the psoas at the pelvic brim gains an average of 7 degrees of stance phase hip extension with an associated increase in step length.[11] Postoperative management is prone lying and early mobilization. If the release is performed at the level of the lesser trochanter, weakness of hip flexion may occur.

The combination of retained femoral anteversion and dynamic imbalance of the rotators causes internal rotation gait deformity. This places the flexion/extension axis of rotation at the knee to be out of plane with the line of progression. Circumduction, crouch position, and diminished stride length may occur. Muscle-balancing procedures for excessive hip internal rotation are unpredictable. Therefore, osteotomy to correct the femoral anteversion is preferred. The goal of surgery is to achieve a static rotational profile that favors external rotation. The location of the corrective osteotomy may be proximal or distal. If hip extension is decreased during the stance phase of gait, then a proximal rotational femoral osteotomy above the lesser trochanter functionally lengthens the iliopsoas and corrects both flexion and rotation deformities. If hip subluxation is present, then simultaneous correction may be achieved with a proximal femoral varus rotational osteotomy. If the sagittal plane deformity is minimal (less than 10 degrees of flexion contracture), then a distal rotational osteotomy can be performed. The distal osteotomy is technically simpler to perform with minimal blood loss, although concerns of the patellofemoral alignment have been raised.

With stable internal fixation, casting is not necessary, and earlier walking is allowed. Walking mechanics are improved in most patients. Improvement in the transverse plane alignment may also decrease sagittal plane deviations and restore the normal ankle-knee mechanical couple.

KNEE

Sagittal plane deformities may be present in stance and swing phase. Crouch gait is defined as the lack of full knee extension during stance phase. The functional impact of persistent knee flexion while walking is increased energy consumption and the potential development of patellofemoral pain. Separating primary from secondary causes of crouch can be challenging. Hamstring spasticity and tightness are primary factors. Weakness of plantar flexion at the ankle (calcaneus gait) or persistent hip flexion can secondarily cause crouch gait. In these situations, the knee must mechanically compensate as the patient balances the ground reaction force across joints to maintain an upright posture. Primary and secondary conditions may be present in various degrees and combinations. Regardless of cause, treatment must include strengthening of the quadriceps muscle complex (the weak muscle).

If the hamstrings are the causative factor, lengthening will balance the forces across the knee. Medial hamstring lengthening is achieved by fractional lengthening of the gracilis and semimembranosus muscles and lengthening or tenotomy of the semitendinosus muscle. A fractional lengthening of the biceps femoris muscle is performed if initial medial hamstring lengthening does not achieve a popliteal angle of less than 20 to 30 degrees. Postoperative management includes casting of the knee in full extension with immediate mobilization and ambulation. The casts are removed once the patient is confidently walking, usually at 2 to 4 weeks. Nighttime use of knee immobilizers maintains extension. Sciatic nerve paresthesia and reflex sympathetic dystrophy may develop, particularly in patients with a preoperative fixed knee flexion contracture. In this situation, therapy may be difficult to perform because patients are reluctant to ambulate and exercise.[12]

The gains from surgery are improved knee extension in stance and swing phase with improved gait parameters such as velocity. Recurrence may occur in younger patients (younger than 8 years), although it is less likely in independent ambulators. Potential secondary effects of isolated hamstring lengthening include stiff knee gait, because spasticity of the quadriceps muscles may become the dominant force across the knee. Resulting hamstring weakness may increase anterior pelvic tilt and hip flexion, because the balance of forces across the hip are altered. Treatment is concomitant iliopsoas release over the pelvic brim if more than 15 degrees of hip flexion contracture is present. The hip kinematic changes, however, may be secondary to weakness of the hip extensors.

Genu recurvatum during midstance may be caused by an equinus posture of the ankle exaggerating the plantar flexion/knee extension couple. Lengthening the hamstrings in this situation exacerbates the knee deformity. Treatment is directed at the equinus deformity as outlined elsewhere. Progression to a fixed hyperextension deformity of the knee is difficult to correct. Early recognition and prevention are the keys to success.

A stiff knee gait during swing results in the lack of normal swing-phase knee flexion and delayed timing of peak knee flexion. The patient has difficulty clearing the stiff, extended limb, decreased walking velocity, and diminished shock absorption with uneven weight transfer during stance. Physical examination typically reveals a tight rectus femoris muscle (positive Ely's test). If the rectus femoris muscle is inappropriately active throughout swing phase, transfer of the rectus femoris muscle medial and posterior to the axis of knee rotation will eliminate its deforming extension force and augment knee flexion. The distal attachment may be to the sartorius, semitendinosus, or gracilis muscle. Cast or brace immobilization for approximately 2 to 3 weeks allows healing. Physical therapy is performed to gain knee flexion while maintaining knee extension during stance phase. Most investigators report variable gains of 7 to 15 degrees of swing-phase knee flexion; however, predicting outcome by physical examination measures and EMG activity varies widely.[13, 14]

ANKLE

Equinus, the most common abnormality of the ankle, causes a diminished weightbearing surface area and increased pressure over the metatarsal heads in stance phase along with functional dropfoot in swing phase. Secondary surrounding joint deformity may develop, including talonavicular subluxation, excessive heel valgus, and genu recurvatum. In a young child, initial treatment is prevention with appropriate bracing and physical therapy. Botulinum toxin injections and serial casting may reduce tone and equinus, although surgery will be necessary in a high percentage of patients.[15]

For a fixed contracture in a child older than 6 to 8 years, surgical lengthening is often the best option. The type of procedure depends on identifying the contribution of each muscle to the deformity. If the equinus corrects beyond neutral (90 degrees) with knee flexion (positive Silverskiold's test), then an isolated gastrocnemius lengthening is performed at its musculotendinous junction (Vulpius/Baker slide). If equinus persists even with knee flexion, then a traditional Z or "slide" lengthening of the Achilles tendon

should be performed[16] (Table 3). Postoperative management starts with a weightbearing cast for 4 to 6 weeks. Braces maintain correction and may improve walking if strength of the dorsiflexors is insufficient.

Satisfactory results correlate with maintenance of strength and the function of two ankle rockers (controlled stance-phase dorsiflexion and push-off power). Because this muscle complex produces 36% of the power generated in gait, inappropriate lengthening (excessive or when not indicated) can cause calcaneus deformity (excessive ankle dorsiflexion in stance) with resultant crouch gait. The undesirable outcome of weakening of the triceps surae complex may occur in up to 30% of patients, requiring brace treatment, which will only partially restore second rocker and will not improve push-off power. One must be aware of midstance knee flexion causing an apparent toe-toe gait pattern unrelated to equinus. Careful examination of the ankle and knee along with a thorough gait evaluation should prevent this error in assessment.

FOOT

Equinovarus, most often seen in hemiplegic patients, is characterized by hindfoot inversion and equinus. The major deforming forces are the triceps surae combined with some pattern of anterior tibialis and/or posterior tibialis spasticity. The functional deficit is abnormal pressure over the lateral border of the foot with callus formation and pain. Treatment must address the imbalance between the inverters and evertors of the foot. An overactive posterior tibialis can be lengthened or transferred. If the peroneals are

TABLE 3. MANAGEMENT OF EQUINUS DEFORMITY			
Procedure	Advantages	Disadvantages	Posttreatment Management
Botulinum toxin injection	Nonoperative Does not permanently weaken muscle Delays the need for surgery	Short-term effect (6 weeks to 6 months) Requires reinjection to maintain results Does not prevent need for surgery	Casting and AFO bracing
Serial casting	Nonoperative Does not permanently weaken muscle	Return visits for casting (up to 4–6×) Correction may be of short duration Could create midfoot break with poor casting technique	AFO once correction obtained
Z-lengthening	Lengthens tendon Amount lengthened is controlled No muscle lengthening	Large potential for overcorrection and development of weakness	Casting at 90 degrees for 6 weeks Fixed AFO worn day and night for 2 months AFO of choice
Percutaneous lengthening	Small incision Less pain/scarring "Sheath" remains intact Muscle tension maintained	Uncontrolled lengthening with potential for complete disruption	As above
Gastrocnemia aponeurosis lengthening if positive Silverskiold test	Differential lengthening Addresses the pathological muscle Maintains power of tendo-Achilles complex	Technically more difficult Unable to adjust amount of lengthening	Casting for 6 weeks AFO of choice

Although listed separately, some treatments may occur in sequence, and the indications for each procedure may exist despite treatment with another listed approach. AFO, ankle-foot orthosis.

TABLE 4. MANAGEMENT OF EQUINOVALGUS FOOT DEFORMITY			
Procedure	Advantages	Disadvantages	Postoperative Management
Medial displacement cal-caneal osteotomy Calcaneal neck lengthening	Simple technically Preserves joint motion Addresses midfoot path	May not address the midfoot pa-thology Technically difficult Soft-tissue reefing medially nec-essary Must rebalance the muscle forces across the joint Unpredictable results	Casting for 6–8 weeks Non-weightbearing casting 4–6 weeks with weightbearing in casts for 4–6 weeks
Subtalar arthrodesis	Predictable correction Muscle balance not necessary to maintain correction	Loss of motion Unable to accommodate abnor-mal loading driven by more proximal joints	Casting 6–8 weeks May bear weight in 2–3 weeks

The treatment of the equinus deformity should follow the treatment options listed in Table 3.

strong (grade 4+), lengthening of the posterior tibialis will allow the evertors to function and reduce the influence of the posterior tibialis tendon. If the anterior tibialis is over-active, then a split anterior tibialis transfer to the cuboid will balance the foot.[17] If the anterior and posterior tibialis muscles are overactive, then a split transfer of the anterior tibialis and lengthening of the posterior tibialis are indi-cated. If the peroneals are weak, then a split posterior tibialis transfer to the peroneus brevis will augment the everting force.[18] Any residual equinus deformity is treated as described previously. Six weeks of casting allows ten-don healing. Eighty to 85% of patients improve; failures involve technical factors (loosening of transfer) and inap-propriate patient selection (fixed deformity and inappropri-ate transfer of a weak muscle).

With an equinovalgus deformity, the triceps surae is overactive and ultimately becomes contracted. The role of the peroneals is less clear. Treatment of the bony deform-ity as opposed to soft-tissue realignment is more predict-able. The foot "breaks" through the midfoot with subluxa-tion of the talonavicular joint and prominence of the talar head medially, causing pain and brace fitting difficulties. With time, the medial column of the foot becomes long relative to the lateral column. Degenerative changes may also develop. Indications for treatment include the follow-ing:

1. To make the foot brace tolerant if adjustments fail to accommodate the deformity.
2. To make the patient brace free.

3. To provide pain relief.
4. To treat progressive deformity.

Treatment is directed at the components of the defor-mity: the equinus, the excessive valgus of the calcaneus, and the midfoot subluxation.

If the valgus deformity of the calcaneus is fixed, a me-dial displacement osteotomy improves the foot contact pat-tern by correction of the hindfoot. If the deformity is flexi-ble, calcaneal neck lengthening corrects the valgus positioning while reducing the navicular on the talus. Con-comitant soft-tissue procedures are performed to balance the muscle forces. The theoretical advantage of these extra-articular procedures is the maintenance of subtalar joint motion.[19] Results are less predictable, because the defor-mity may recur through the joint, requiring further surgery for correction.

Talocalcaneal arthrodesis is the proven method for pre-dictable permanent correction of the deformity. Internal fix-ation to hold the corrected position and autologous bone graft to achieve fusion address the problems with the previ-ous techniques (Grice's procedure). Long-term follow-up of hindfoot fusions reveal excellent functional outcomes de-spite the loss of motion.[20] Once the foot is corrected, the equinus component is addressed as previously defined (Ta-ble 4).

Satisfactory results of 80% to 85% are reported with all of these procedures. Poor results are related to the final position of the foot. Intraoperative radiographs films may assist in determining the bony correction obtained.

REFERENCES

1. Renshaw TS, Green NE, Griffin PP, et al: Cerebral palsy: Orthopedic management. J Bone Joint Surg Am 1995; 77:1590.
2. Gage JR, DeLuca PA, Renshaw TS: Gait analysis: Principles and applications. J Bone Joint Surg Am 1995; 77:1607.
3. DeLuca PA, Davis RB, Ounpuu S, et al: Alterations in surgical decision making in patients with cerebral palsy based on 3-D gait analysis. J Pediatr Orthop 1997; 17: 608.
4. Cooperman DR, Bartucci E, Dietrick E, et al: Hip dislocation in spastic cerebral palsy: Long-term consequences. J Pediatr Orthop 1987; 7:268.
5. Miller F, Dias RC, Dabney KW, et al: Soft tissue release for spastic hip subluxa-tion in cerebral palsy. J Pediatr Orthop 1997; 17:571.
6. Brunner R, Bauman JU: Long-term effects of intertrochanteric varus-derotation osteot-omy on femur and acetabulum in spastic cerebral palsy: An 11-18 year F/U study. J Pediatr Orthop 1997; 17:585.
7. Shea KG, Coleman SS, Carroll K, et al: Pericapsular osteotomy to treat a dysplas-tic hip in cerebral palsy. J Bone Joint Surg Am 1997; 79:1342.
8. Miller F, Girardi H, Lipton G, et al: Re-construction of the dysplastic hip with peri-ileal pelvic and femoral osteotomy followed by immediate mobilization. J Pe-diatr Orthop 1997; 17:592.

9. Lundy DW, Ganey TM, Ogden JA, et al: Pathologic morphology of the dislocated proximal femur in children with cerebral palsy. J Pediatr Orthop 1998; 18:528.

10. Scott A, Chambers C, Cain TE: Adductor transfers in cerebral palsy: Long term results studied by gait analysis. J Pediatr Orthop 1996; 16:741.

11. Sutherland DH, Zilberfarb JL, Kaufman KR, et al: Psoas release at the pelvic brim in ambulatory patients with cerebral palsy: Outcome technique and functional outcome. J Pediatr Orthop 1997; 17:563.

12. DeLuca PA, Ounpuu S, Davis RB, et al: Effect of hamstring and psoas lengthening on pelvic tilt in patients with spastic diplegic cerebral palsy. J Pediatr Orthop 1998; 18:712.

13. Chambers H, Lauer A, Kaufman K, et al: Prediction of outcome after rectus femoris surgery in cerebral palsy: The role of cocontraction of the rectus femoris and vastus lateralis. J Pediatr Orthop 1998; 18:703.

14. Miller F, Cardosa Dias R, Lipton G, et al: Effect of rectus EMG pattern on outcome of rectus femoris transfers. J Pediatr Orthop 1997; 17:603.

15. Corry IS, Cosgrove AP, Duffy CM, et al: Botulinum toxin A compared with stretching casts in the treatment of spastic equinus: A randomized prospective trial. J Pediatr Orthop 1998; 18:304.

16. Yngve D, Chambers C: Vulpius and Z lengthening. J Pediatr Orthop 1996; 16:759.

17. Barnes MJ, Herring JA: Combined split anterior tibial tendon transfer and intramuscular lengthening of the posterior tibial tendon. J Bone Joint Surg Am 1991; 73:734.

18. O'Byrne JM, Kennedy A, Jenkinson A, et al: Split tibialis posterior transfer in the treatment of spastic equinovarus foot. J Pediatr Orthop 1997; 17:481.

19. Mosca V: Calcaneal lengthening for valgus deformity of the hindfoot. J Bone Joint Surg Am 1995; 77:500.

20. Tenuta J, Shelton YA, Miller F: Long-term follow-up of triple arthrodesis in patients with cerebral palsy. J Pediatr Orthop 1993; 13:713.

CEREBRAL PALSY: UPPER EXTREMITY

section 10 chapter 3

William B. Strecker

Summary

- Children with cerebral palsy present different surgical challenges as it relates to upper extremity.
- They normally will attempt to use the hand, but, because of spasticity of certain muscles, they are unable to place the hand in a functional position.
- Surgical intervention to improve hand position and, therefore, aid in function is usually gratifying to child, parents, and physician.

In his seminal 1862 treatise, Little[1] first described the association of perinatal anoxia and subsequent "spastic rigidity of the limbs of newborn children," what is now referred to as static encephalopathy or cerebral palsy. Little's description of the upper extremity in children with this condition is still appropriate today: "The upper extremities were sometimes held down by preponderating actions of pectorals, teres major and teres minor, and latissimus dorsi; the elbows are semiflexed, the wrist partially flexed, pronated and the fingers incapable of perfect voluntary direction" (Fig. 1).

Careful examination is required before determining treatment options. Unlike other evaluations, this needs to be one of observation rather than palpation. How the child performs certain tasks and patterns of movement must be assessed. Evaluation of the patient is usually based on serial examinations. The pattern of spastic responses (i.e., elbow flexion, forearm pronation, wrist flexion) can be helpful.

The use of dynamic electromyography (D/EMG) to identify whether a muscle is spastic and its phasic firing pattern has been described[2, 3]; however, D/EMGs are technically demanding, requiring equipment and trained personnel to perform and evaluate, and their value has yet to be deter-

mined. The use of selective nerve blocks has also been advocated, especially to determine whether antagonist muscles have sufficient strength to function.[4, 5] This has been found more useful in the brain injury or stroke patient than in the child with cerebral palsy. Clinical observation offers the best assessment as to which muscle groups are functioning at specific times. Decisions are based on evaluations by an experienced surgeon and therapist and parental observation. Specific issues that must be addressed include whether the extremity is used for activities; which muscles are spastic and interfere with function; and which muscles are producing deformities and may be useful as an augmentation transfer.

Various criteria have been proposed as guidelines for selection of surgical candidates. Voluntary use of the hand or attempted use is probably the most useful.[6, 7] If a child attempts to use the hand, then operative procedures may facilitate hand function. However, it must be remembered that surgical procedures cannot induce function. Intelligence has been proposed as a guideline, but this has not been established. Sensibility has also been recommended as a surgical candidate selection criterion; however, although most patients have some impairment, it does not seem to affect the clinical results. Age and hand placement have also been reported as factors, but neither of these seem to alter results. Athetosis and dystonia are relative contraindications to surgery, but operative procedures can be predictability performed in a patient with spasticity and concomitant athetoid movements.

Management of these children is conducted on many levels. Physical and occupational therapy is beneficial in maintaining joint mobility and facilitating motor maturation. Orthotics, although useful in the lower extremities, have limited use in the upper extremity. They are cumbersome and insensate and tend to interfere with hand

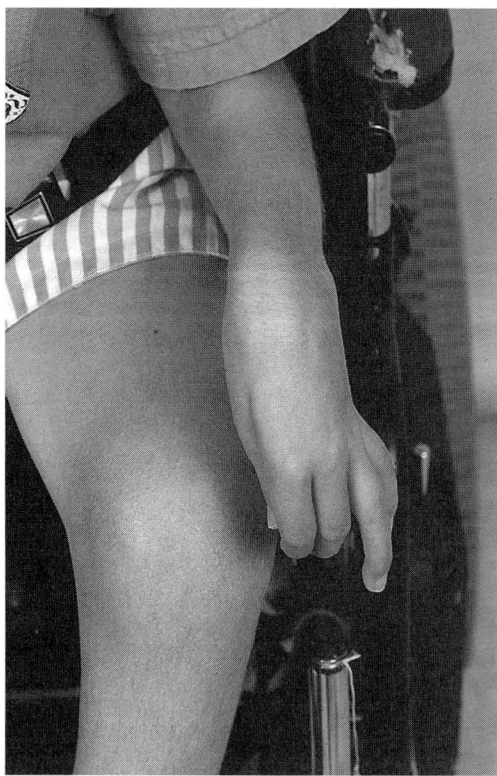

Fig. 1. Typical posture of spastic upper extremity. The elbow is flexed, forearm pronated, wrist flexed, and thumb adducted.

function. Various medications[8] have been used in the management of cerebral palsy, including benzodiazepines, dantrolene sodium, and, more recently, botulinum-A toxin (Botox)[9] and baclofen.[10]

The objective of upper extremity surgery is to release the deforming force and reposition the extremity, placing it in a more functional position. Surgical procedures are, therefore, directed toward weakening the spastic muscle, which may be accomplished by musculotendinous lengthening, neurectomy, or reduction osteotomy; augmentation tendon transfers to enhance weak muscles; release of joint contractures, and arthrodesis as a salvage procedure. None of these procedures correct the spasticity or lack of fine motor coordination but rather reposition the extremity, placing it in a more functional and aesthetic position. Weakening the spastic muscle is the most common procedure and is usually done by lengthening the muscle tendon unit either at its origin, midsubstance, or insertion. Neurectomy effects weakening by paralyzing the muscle. This is most often used in brain injury and stroke patients but can selectively be used in cerebral palsy patients. Augmentation tendon transfers are performed less frequently than lengthening (weakening) procedures. Tendon transfers are less predictable in this patient population, and "re-education" can be more challenging. The ideal tendon for transfer is one that is known to be firing "in-phase" and contributing to the deforming force.

There are two general indications for surgical intervention: to facilitate care or hygiene and to improve hand function. The single most useful determinant to the latter is if the patient attempts to voluntarily use the hand during daily activities, and either its position or spasticity interferes with this. Voluntary initiation of use has proved more useful to predict outcome than intelligence, age, sensation, or extent of spasticity.

OPERATIVE PROCEDURES

The most commonly used muscle releases and tendon transfers are now discussed. Most children with cerebral palsy require augmentation tendon transfers because of underlying muscle weakness.

SHOULDER

The most common deformity is adduction and internal rotation secondary to overactivity of the subscapularis and pectoralis major muscles. As a result, the arm is held toward the side and internally rotated. Although this muscle pattern is commonly seen, it rarely causes a functional or hygiene problem. Surgical release is indicated for severe deformities (i.e., abduction less than 45 degrees and external rotation of less than 10 degrees).

The procedure is performed through a deltopectoral incision. The pectoralis major is lengthened in a Z fashion. The subscapularis is then released from its insertion. If external rotation is still restricted, then the contracted anterior joint capsule is released. Postoperatively, the child is immobilized in a shoulder spica for 6 weeks, and then active range of motion (ROM) is begun.

ELBOW FLEXION

Elbow flexion contractures greater than 90 degrees interfere with the use of crutches, the ability to reach for objects, dressing, and other two-handed activities. Elbow flexion may be viewed as an aesthetic problem when there is exaggerated flexion with running, walking, or activities. The brachioradialis is thought to be the most spastic elbow flexor followed by the biceps and the brachialis, respectively.[3] Various procedures have been advocated comprising three categories: neurectomy of the musculocutaneous nerve,[11] release of spastic elbow flexors,[12] and release of the flexor-pronator mass from its origin.[13]

Neurectomy of the musculocutaneous nerve is useful only after a nerve block has demonstrated improved elbow function. This procedure will not correct a fixed elbow flexion contracture. Lengthening the spastic elbow flexors can decrease an elbow flexion contracture. Although this usually is the preferred method, Z-lengthening of the biceps can reduce elbow flexion so much that bringing the hand to the mouth is difficult. Release of the flexor-pronator origin will provide some decrease in elbow flexion contracture as well as release wrist and finger flexion deformities. It is a technically more difficult procedure and only addresses the elbow contracture secondarily; therefore, it is usually not indicated. Augmentation tendon transfer is usually not needed because gravity will assist movement into extension.

ELBOW FLEXION RELEASE

A transverse or S-shaped incision is made across the antecubital fossa. The lacertus fibrosis is identified and released with care to protect the medial antebrachial cutaneous nerve. The paratenon is stripped from the biceps tendon in mild or dynamic flexion contractures. Z-lengthening is required in severe contractures (i.e., those fixed contractures of greater than 90 degrees). The brachialis muscle is then fractionally lengthened at the musculotendinous junction. In severe cases, the brachioradialis is detached from its origin. Anterior capsulotomy is usually not required.

The arm is immobilized in a long-arm cast at 45 degrees flexion for 4 weeks and then in a splint for a subsequent 2-week period during which ROM therapy is begun. Occasionally, night splinting is used for 6 to 8 weeks as deemed necessary.

FOREARM PRONATION

Pronation deformity of the forearm is caused by spasticity of the pronator teres and quadratus muscle. In a child, this can be a disabling problem in that it places the hand in an ineffectual position and interferes with grasping objects and two-handed activities. Several muscle lengthening-releasing procedures have been advocated, including the flexor-pronator slide, pronator tenotomy, and pronator quadratus release. Tendon transfers have included the flexor carpi ulnaris (FCU) to extensor carpi radialis longus or brachiaradialis. Rerouting the pronator teres through the interosseous membrane, creating a supinating force, is also useful.[14, 15] Children with mild pronation deformity who are able to supinate to neutral usually require only a musculotendinous release of the pronator teres at its insertion. For most children with pronation deformity, the preferred treatment is a pronator reroutement. This procedure not only releases the deformity force but redirects it, creating the desired activity.

PRONATOR TERES REROUTING

A longitudinal midforearm incision is made, and the interval between the brachioradialis and the extensor carpi radialis brevis (ECRB) is developed. Care is taken to protect the radial sensory nerve. The pronator teres insertion is sharply dissected with a 2-cm strip of periosteum. The interosseous membrane is exposed and dissected free from the radius. The mobilized pronator teres is then redirected through the interosseous space in a volar to dorsal direc-

tion. The tendon is then reattached to the radius dorsolaterally at the level of its origin with a suture anchor.

Postoperatively, the arm is immobilized in a long-arm cast with the elbow at 90 degrees, forearm in 60 degrees supination, and wrist at neutral for 4 weeks. A splint is fabricated, and ROM instituted. For the first 2 weeks, the splint is worn full time except while performing ROM. The splint is then worn at night for the next 2 weeks, at which time all splinting is discontinued (Fig. 2).

WRIST AND FINGER FLEXION

Wrist flexion with or without ulnar deviation is commonly seen. Not only is it aesthetically displeasing to these children, but it also interferes with finger flexion and grasping. The FCU is the primary spastic wrist flexor, but the flexor carpi radialis (FCR) and palmaris longus (PL) have also been implicated. The finger flexors can also produce a wrist flexion deformity. With the wrist in a neutral position, if the fingers are clenched and the patient is unable to extend them, then the flexor digitorum sublimis (FDS) and/or flexor digitorum profundus are contributing factors to the wrist flexion deformity; the FDS is usually the greater offender. Ulnar deviation is not only caused by the FCU, but the extensor carpi ulnaris (ECU) may cause ulnar deviation and wrist flexion in a pronated forearm.

Several procedures to lengthen wrist and finger flexors have been described, including flexor pronator slide, fractional or Z-lengthening of tight flexors, or sublimis to profundus (STP) transfers.[16] It is important to recognize that lengthening of finger flexors reduces the flexor tendon excursion, digital flexion, and, therefore, power. Z-lengthening and STP transfers are most useful in the severe contractures. To prevent intrinsic plus deformity, neurectomy of the motor branch of the ulnar nerve is usually required with STP transfers. Fractional lengthening usually adds 2 cm of length and allows the musculotendinous unit to "seek its own" length. This is the preferred procedure when indicated.

If wrist flexion is mild and ulnar deviation significant, then the ECU must be addressed. In these instances, the ECU is detached at its insertion and transferred to the

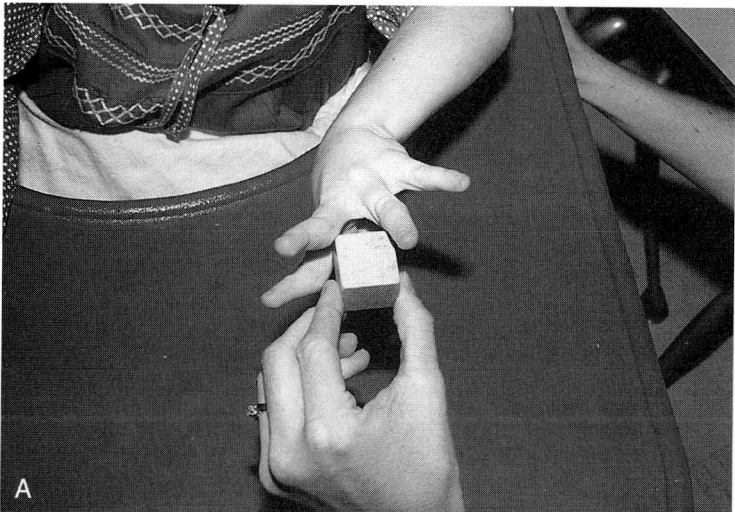
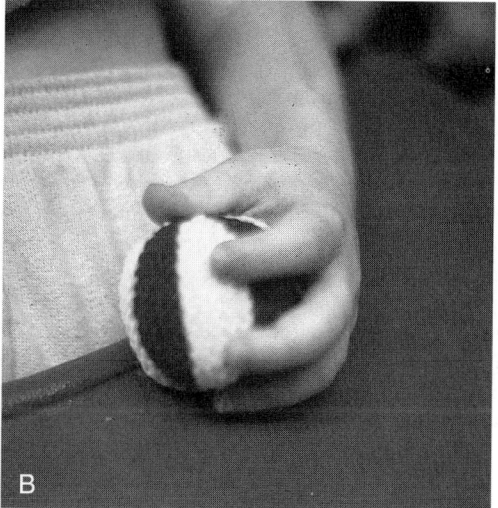

Fig. 2. Reversed pronated grasp. *A,* Preoperative view. *B,* Postoperative pronator reroutement. Note the excellent position for two-hand tasks.

ECRB with concomitant fractional lengthening of the FCU. The FCU is the principle wrist flexor and can be lengthened by musculotendinous fractional lengthening or Z-lengthening or by using it as an augmentation transfer to assist wrist extension. When both the FCR and FCU contribute to the flexion posture, it is important that the continuity of one be maintained. Usually the FCU is transferred and the FCR is fractionally lengthened.

If the wrist extensors are weak and are unable to maintain extension despite release of the flexion deformity, tendon transfer is indicated.[17] Wrist extension facilitates grasping. If the patient is unable to extend the wrist with fingers flexed, then weakness is usually present. Several transfers have been proposed, including brachioradialis, pronator teres, FCR, and FDS. The FCU transfer is the most appealing because it releases a deforming force and provides an excellent donor. This is usually transferred to the ECRB. A wrist extension posture is to be avoided; therefore, it is important that the transfer be tensioned so that the wrist is in a neutral to slight flexion position against gravity. This is in contrast to tensioning the wrist in extension, which is the technique used when transferring the FCU for nonspastic conditions.

FRACTIONAL LENGTHENING OF THE FLEXORS

Through a longitudinal volar incision, the musculotendinous junctions of the wrist and finger flexors are exposed. The tendon of each involved muscle is incised at one or two sites as needed. It is important that this be done proximally enough so that sufficient muscle is present to maintain the muscle-tendon continuity. The wrist and digits are then passively extended, providing adequate length and allowing the musculotendinous unit to "seek its own level."

The wrist is immobilized in 25 degrees of extension, metaphalangeal (MP) joints in neutral, and fingers slightly flexed for 4 weeks. Then a splint is fabricated, and ROM is begun. Immobilization is removed at 6 weeks. and splinting is done at night for the following 2 to 4 weeks.

FLEXOR CARPI ULNARIS TO EXTENSOR CARPI RADIALIS BREVIS

A longitudinal volar incision is made over the FCU. It is detached from the pisiform and mobilized proximally to its neurovascular bundle. A second dorsal incision is made over the ECRB proximal to the extensor retinaculum. The FCU is then routed subcutaneously around the ulnar side of the forearm and weaved through and sutured to the ECRB. Tension is adjusted so that the wrist is maintained in neutral to slight flexion against gravity. Care is taken to avoid abutment of tendon junction and extensor retinaculum.

Postoperatively, a long-arm cast is applied with the forearm in 45 to 60 degrees of supination and the wrist in 10 degrees of dorsiflexion for 4 weeks. A splint is then applied for 2 weeks while ROM is begun and then at night for 2 weeks.

EXTENSOR CARPI ULNARIS TO EXTENSOR CARPI RADIALIS BREVIS

A dorsal midline incision is made. The ECU is detached at its insertion on the base of the fifth metacarpal and mobilized proximally. It is then transferred subcutaneously and sutured to the ECRB as previously described for the FCU transfer. The postoperative protocol is the same as previously described.

ARTHRODESIS

In a child with severe flexion deformity who does not require wrist motion to accomplish finger extension by tenodesis, wrist fusion can be considered. This is particularly true in those children who are having problems dressing because of difficulty in navigating a flexed wrist through a shirt or jacket sleeve. If skeletally mature, a standard wrist arthrodesis can be performed. In those children who are skeletally immature, wrist arthrodesis is performed by epiphyseal fusion.

THUMB-IN-PALM DEFORMITY

The thumb-in-palm deformity is the most noticeable and the most functionally disabling of the upper extremity deformities. The thumb is flexed and adducted into the palm. This position hinders grasping activities. A thumb-in-palm deformity interferes with the remaining digits, so that during digital extension the thumb blocks entry of objects in the palm, and during flexion it precedes the other digits into the palm, interfering with grasp. The spastic intrinsic muscles, including the flexor pollicis brevis, first dorsal interosseous, and particularly the adductor pollicis, are the primary cause of this deformity. The extensor pollicis longus (EPL) usually has satisfactory function in these children, as evidenced by interphalangeal joint extension in the face of metacarpal and phalangeal adduction, but the EPL also acts as a secondary thumb adductor.

The goal of treatment is to get the thumb out of the palm so that it no longer interferes with the function of the fingers and to place it in a position to facilitate grasp. To this end, it is necessary to release the spastic intrinsic muscles and augment this with a tendon transfer. The adductor pollicis longus, flexor pollicis brevis, and first dorsal interosseous are always released; sometimes release of opponens pollicis and abductor pollicis brevis must also be performed. It is preferred that these muscles are released at their origin, maintaining the continuity of the muscle-tendon unit.

Numerous augmentation tendon transfers have been described in conjunction with the release,[18, 19] including brachioradialis, PL, ECRB or ECRL, FCR, FCU, and FDS. One or more of these may be transferred to the abductor pollicis longus and extensor pollicis brevis to position the thumb out of the palm. As previously noted, the EPL has been observed to function during activity causing interphalangeal joint extension, although the first ray is adducted and flexed. It is, therefore, believed that the EPL is an ideal transfer because it both relieves a deforming force and augments an active muscle.[20]

EPL REROUTING

This is always performed with a concomitant intrinsic release. A palmar incision is made along the thenar crease from the base of the index finger to the volar carpal ligament. The adductor pollicis is exposed between the common digital nerve to the index and long fingers and the flexor tendons to the long finger. It is dissected from its origin on the third metacarpal; care is taken not to injure the deep palmar arch and motor branch of the ulnar nerve where it enters the muscle. Complete detachment is necessary. Proximally, the opponens pollicis and abductor pollicis brevis are detached from their origin on the volar carpal ligament.

A second incision is made dorsally along the first metacarpal and proximal phalanx of the thumb. The EPL is transected distally and dissected proximally to release soft-tissue attachments of the extensor hood. It is tagged for future transfer. The first dorsal interosseous is sharply dissected off the ulnar aspect of the thumb metacarpal. Care is taken not to injure the princeps pollicis artery proximally.

A third incision is made dorsally proximal to Lister's tubercle and the EPL tendon is delivered into this wound. The forearm fascia is released proximally. A small curved hemostat is then passed from the second wound through the first dorsal compartment, emerging in the third incision. The EPL is grasped and pulled distally through the first dorsal compartment. It is then passed around the abductor pollicis longus and sutured through a transverse tunnel in the MP capsule under enough tension to hold the thumb extended. If the MP joint can be passively hyperextended

the tunnel is located proximally to the MP joint and a Kirschner wire is placed across the joint for 4 weeks to prevent hyperextension. The tendon is then sutured back to the extensor hood and the distal stump and tensioned to position the interphalangeal joint in neutral.

Postoperatively, the patient is placed in a short-arm thumb spica for 4 weeks. Any Kirschner wire is then removed, a splint fabricated, and ROM begun. At 6 weeks, splinting is discontinued except for night splinting.

SUMMARY

It is important that careful serial examinations be performed before any surgical consideration. Because of the protein manifestation in children with cerebral palsy, there can be no "cookbook" approach. Usually, for any functional improvement to be made, the child must be trying to voluntarily use the extremity. Our experience has been that, with careful selection, appropriately performed surgical intervention has consistently led to improved function. In the child for whom surgery was performed to enable care, all caregivers noted that the child's care and positioning were facilitated with surgery. It must be remembered that our goal is to better position the hand, even though we are unable to change the underlying neurological problem (Fig. 3).

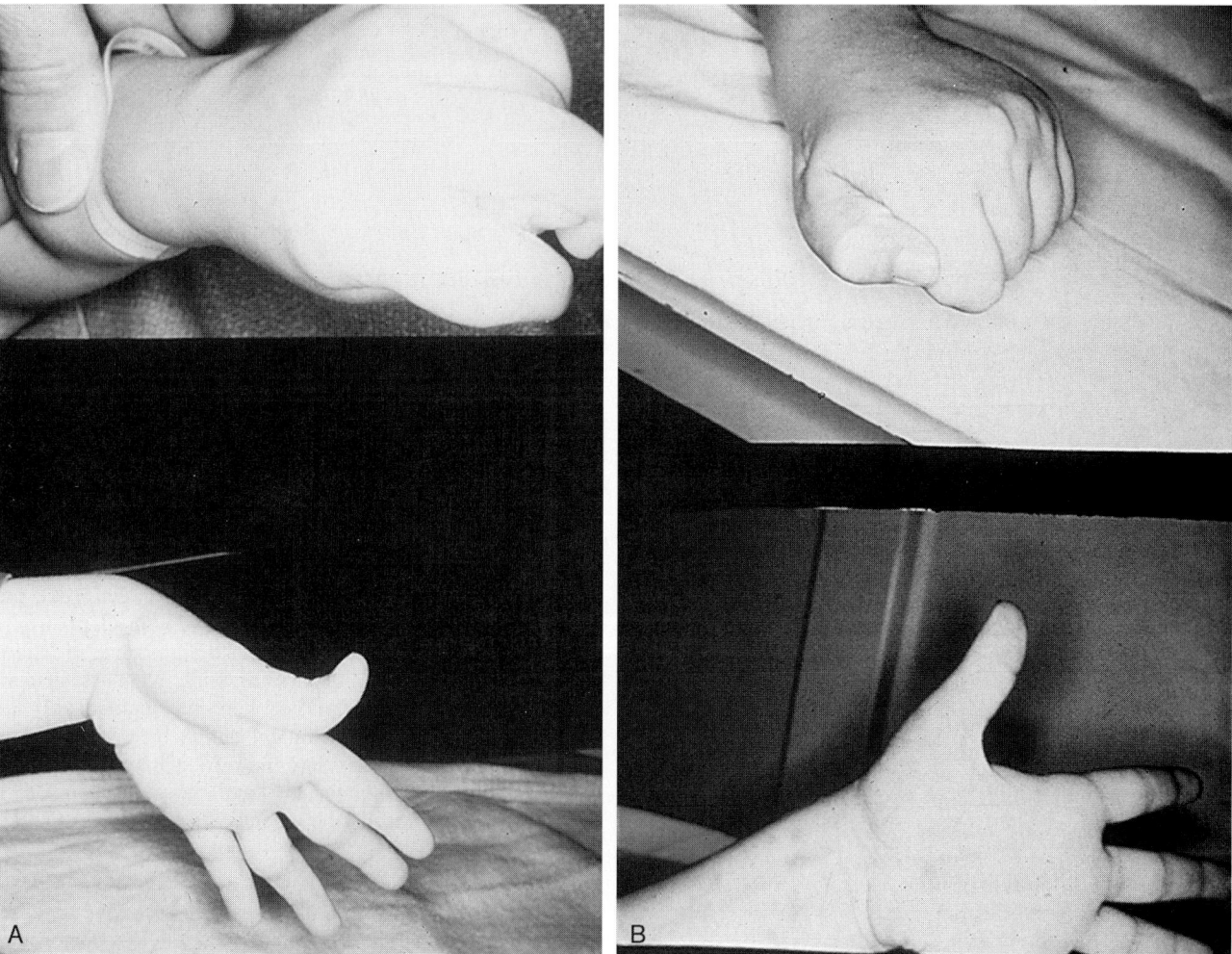

Fig. 3. Hand position. *A*, Preoperative view. Note that in flexion the thumb assumes a position that blocks placement of an object in the hand and in extension is not in a position to grasp. *B*, Postoperative position of thumb in flexion and extension.

REFERENCES

1. Little WJ: On the influence of abnormal parturition, difficult labours, premature birth, asphyxia neonatorum, on the mental and physical condition of the child, especially in relation to deformities. Trans Obstet Soc (London) 1862; 3:293.
2. Hoffer M, Perry J, Melkonian Konian GJ: Dynamic electromyography and decision-making for surgery in the upper extremity of patients with cerebral palsy. J Hand Surg 1979; 4:424.
3. Keenan MAE, Haider TT, Stone LR: Dynamic electromyography to elbow spasticity. J Hand Surg Am 1990; 15:607.
4. Braun RM, Hoffer MM, Mooney V, et al: Phenol nerve blocks in the treatment of acquired spastic hemiplegia in the upper limb. J Bone Joint Surg Am 1973; 55:580.
5. Keenan MAE, Tomar E, Stone L, et al: Percutaneous phenal blocks of the musculocutaneous nerve to control elbow flexor spasticity. J Hand Surg Am 1990; 15:340.
6. Manske PR: Cerebral palsy of the upper extremity. Hand Clin 1990; 6:697.
7. Samilson RL: Principles of assessment of the upper limb in cerebral palsy. Clin Orthop 1966; 47:105.
8. Nogen AG: Medical treatment for spasticity in children with cerebral palsy. Child Brain 1976; 2:304.
9. Koman LA, Mooney JF III, Smith B, et al: Management of cerebral palsy with botulinum-A toxin: Preliminary investigation. J Pediatr Orthop 1993; 13:489.
10. Van Hemert JCJ: A double-blind comparison of baclofen and placebo in patients with spasticity of cerebral palsy origin. In Feldman R, Young RR, Koella WP (eds): Spasticity: Disordered Motor Control. Chicago, Yearbook, 1980, p 41.
11. Hoffer MM: Cerebral palsy. In Green DP (ed): Operative Hand Surgery. New York, Churchill-Livingstone, 1993, 3rd ed, p 215.
12. Mital MA, Sakellarides HT: Surgery of the upper extremity in the retarded individual with spastic cerebral palsy. Orthop Clin North Am 1981; 12:127.
13. Page CM: An operation for the relief of flexion contracture in the forearm. J Bone Joint Surg 1923; 5:233.
14. Sakellarides HT, Mital MA, Lenzi WD: Treatment of pronator contractures of the forearm in cerebral palsy by changing the insertion of the pronator radii teres. J Bone Joint Surg Am 1981; 63:645.
15. Strecker WB, Emanual JP, Dailey L, et al: Comparison of pronator tenotomy and pronator rerouting in children with spastic cerebral palsy. J Hand Surg Am 1988; 13:540.
16. Braun RM, Vise GT: Sublimis to profundus tendon transfers in the hemiplegic upper extremity. J Bone Joint Surg Am 1973; 55:873.
17. Beach WR, Strecker WB, Coe J, et al: The results of the Green transfer in the treatment of patients with spastic cerebral palsy. J Pediatr Orthop 1991; 11:731.
18. House JH, Gwathney FW, Fidler MO: A dynamic approach to the thumb-in-palm deformity in cerebral palsy. J Bone Joint Surg Am 1981; 63:216.
19. Keats S: Surgical treatment of the hand in cerebral palsy: Correction of the thumb-in-palm and other deformities. Report of nineteen cases. J Bone Joint Surg Am 1965; 47:274.
20. Manske PR: Redirection of extensor pollicis longus in the treatment of spastic thumb-in-palm deformity. J Hand Surg Am 1985; 10:53.

section **10** chapter **4**

FRIEDREICH'S ATAXIA AND RETT'S SYNDROME

Hubert Labelle

Summary

- Friedreich's ataxia is a recessively inherited spinocerebellar degenerative disease and is the most frequent hereditary ataxic syndrome.
- The hallmark of the disease is an ataxic gait presenting in a child or adolescent with weak or absent deep tendon reflexes.
- The key orthopedic features are scoliosis and occasionally pes cavovarus. Surgery may be required to treat the scoliotic deformity.
- Rett's syndrome is a progressive encephalopathy of undetermined cause developing only in girls after age 6 to 18 months.
- The hallmark of the disease is a progressive loss of intellectual function and motor skills after a normal period of development.
- The key orthopedic features are scoliosis and occasionally hip subluxation and pes equinus. Surgery may be required to treat the scoliotic deformity.

FRIEDREICH'S ATAXIA

DEFINITION

More than 57 hereditary ataxic syndromes have been reported to date. Friedreich's ataxia is the most common type and is best described as a progressive spinocerebellar degenerative disease characterized by ataxia. To facilitate differentiation from the numerous clinical variants of hereditary ataxias, it is described as an autosomal-recessive ataxia with an age of early onset, progressive, with weak or absent deep tendon reflexes and a predominant spinocerebellar incoordination.[1]

HISTORICAL REVIEW

Few eponyms in neurology are as closely identified with a disease as the one described by Nicolaus Friedreich in a series of five classic articles published between 1863 and 1877.[2] Friedreich was born July 31, 1825, in Germany; he studied biology and medicine under the guidance of Rudolf Virchow at the University of Würzburg, in his hometown. His early clinical descriptions were not immediately accepted as being of a new clinical entity, but eventually the French School of Neurology, led by Charcot, was convinced and proposed the term "maladie de Friedreich" in 1882, the year of Friedreich's death.

EPIDEMIOLOGY

The disease is inherited as an autosomal-recessive trait, and the abnormal gene has been mapped on the centromeric region of chromosome 9 by genetic linkage.[3] Although rare, Friedreich's ataxia has a worldwide geographic distribution. Its prevalence is approximately 1 in 100,000, and the incidence ranges from 1 in 25,000 to 50,000. Males and females are equally affected.

PATHOGENESIS

The cause of Friedreich's ataxia is a gene mutation on chromosome 9. The exact biochemical abnormality produced by the defective gene has not yet been identified. The metabolic disturbance created by the abnormal gene leads to various anatomic lesions, which are responsible for the clinical features of the disease. The anatomic lesions found at autopsy or biopsy in the peripheral and central nervous system of patients with typical Friedreich's ataxia are moderate to marked loss of large myelinated fibers and a minimal loss of small fibers in the peripheral nerves. In the spinal cord, anterior horns and cranial motor nerves appear normal, but there is a significant loss of large myelinated fibers in the posterior columns and in the cerebellum. The cerebral cortex and white matter are normal.

CLINICAL FEATURES

The most frequent initial symptom and presenting complaint is ataxia in a child or adolescent presenting with an abnormal gait pattern and difficulty standing still or running. The key orthopedic features are scoliosis, pes cavus, and muscle weakness. To isolate Friedreich's ataxia from the large number of other ataxic syndromes, Geoffroy et al[4] proposed a classification system, later modified by Harding,[5] which is now universally accepted:

Group I: typical Friedreich's ataxia.
    Ia: complete picture.
    Ib: incomplete picture.
Group IIa: atypical Friedreich's ataxia.
Group IIb: not Friedreich's ataxia.

Typical Friedreich's ataxia (groups Ia and Ib) can be characterized by a number of primary, constant symptoms and signs that are present in 100% of cases and are essential for diagnosis. In addition, some secondary signs are present in more than 90% of cases. Finally, a large number of accessory symptoms and signs may be prevented but cannot be used to establish a diagnosis. Patients in group Ib are identical to those in group Ia except that they do not have the pes cavus deformity. Group IIa patients differ from group I patients mainly because of lack of progression of ataxia and a very mild degree of scoliosis. Group IIb is heterogenous; specifically, dysarthria, posterior column signs, and muscle weakness are lacking.

The primary symptoms and signs needed for diagnosis are onset of symptoms before age 20 years, progressive ataxia, absent knee and ankle jerks, extensor plantar responses, decreased motor nerve conduction velocity in upper limbs with small or absent sensory action potentials, and dysarthria. The secondary symptoms and signs present in most cases but not essential for diagnosis are scoliosis, pyramidal weakness in lower limbs, absent reflexes in upper limbs, distal loss of joint position and vibration sense in lower limbs, and abnormal electrocardiogram (ECG) caused by a progressive hypertrophic cardiomyopathy. Finally, the accessory symptoms and signs present in less than 50% of patients are optic atrophy, nystagmus, distal muscle weakness and wasting, partial deafness, pes cavus, and diabetes.

Scoliosis appears to be a constant finding, although it is not always present at diagnosis. Males and females are equally affected and left-sided curves are as frequent as right-sided curves, as is the case in many neuromuscular conditions. The curve pattern, however, is more closely related to that of idiopathic scoliosis, with a clear predominance of double structural thoracic and lumbar curves followed by single thoracic or lumbar curve (Fig. 1). The classic C-shaped thoracolumbar curve pattern usually associated with neuromuscular diseases is found in only 15% to 20% of cases reported.[6–8]

Curve progression is variable. A significant correlation has been found between progressive curves and early onset of disease or early appearance of curves before puberty.[8] When the disease onset is before age 10 years and scoliosis occurs before age 15 years, most curves progress to greater than 60 degrees and require surgical intervention. When the disease onset is after age 10 years and the scoliosis occurs after age 15 years, curve progression is not as severe; most do not reach 40 degrees by skeletal maturity and, consequently, progression is rare.

Because no correlation has been detected among progressive curves, degree of muscle weakness, level of ambulatory function, and duration of the disease process, it is postulated that the pathogenesis of the scoliotic deformity is related to the disturbance of equilibrium and postural reflexes. This disturbance may also be operative in idiopathic scoliosis.

An increased thoracic kyphosis has been reported in 40% to 60% of scoliotic deformities. However, studies

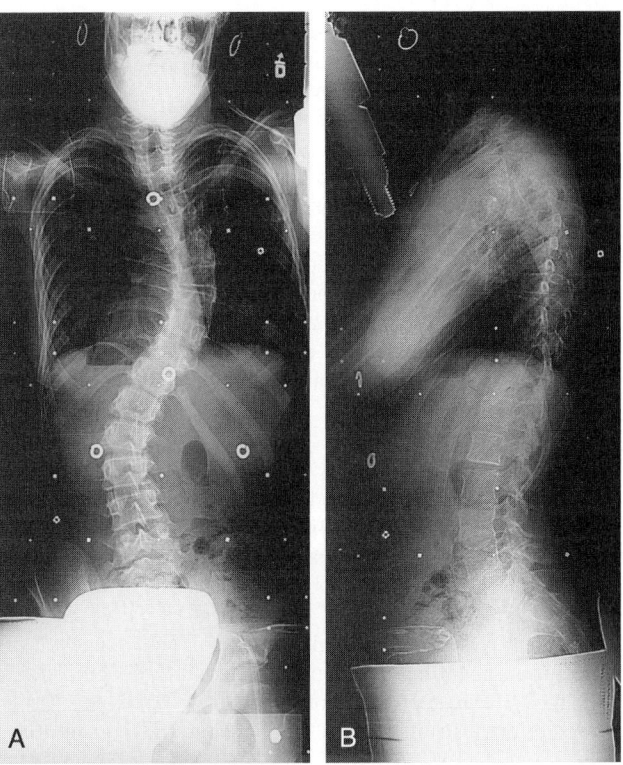

Fig. 1. Friedreich's ataxia. *A,* Anteroposterior radiograph of an adolescent female. This double structural thoracic and lumbar curve pattern is the most frequent. *B,* Lateral radiograph of the same patient. Note the thoracic hypokyphosis and lumbar hypolordosis associated with the scoliotic curves and the high thoracic kyphosis above the scoliotic segment.

using three-dimensional reconstructions of the spine revealed that the scoliotic deformity is frequently hypokyphotic and that kyphotic deformities are located above the scoliotic segment in the upper thoracic area or at the thoracolumbar junction between two curves. Kyphosis tends to appear later in the course of the disease, many years after the appearance of a scoliotic deformity.[1]

Pes cavovarus occurs in less than 50% of affected individuals and is caused by muscle weakness and imbalance.[9] It progresses slowly and may be accompanied by an equinus deformity. In most cases, the deformity is mild and does not significantly impair walking. Progression may be noted after loss of ambulation.

Muscle weakness is symmetric, slowly progressive in the first decades and rapidly progressive when functional ambulation is lost. It initially involves the proximal lower limb muscles; the upper limbs and trunk remain relatively spared.[10] Ataxia is relentlessly progressive, usually leading to loss of ambulation in the second decade. Death from cardiomyopathy occurs in the third or fourth decade.

INVESTIGATION

Nerve conduction studies show decreased sensory and motor conduction velocity in the peripheral nerves. Pulmonary function studies show evidence of restrictive lung disease proportional to the severity of scoliosis. The ECG in adults typically shows a progressive hypertrophic cardiomyopathy pattern. Laboratory tests are usually normal except for evidence of chemical diabetes mellitus in 40% of patients.

MANAGEMENT

Nonoperative treatment of scoliosis has generally been unsuccessful and is not recommended.[6–8] A thoracolumbosacral orthosis (TLSO) may be tried in progressive and moderate curves below 40 degrees to slow the rate of progression. However, it is often poorly tolerated and may interfere with walking because it prevents compensatory truncal movements necessary for balance and movement. Surgery is the only treatment alternative that can clearly alter the progression by providing curve correction and stabilization. An adequate preoperative investigation is important, with careful evaluation for cardiomyopathy. Pulmonary function tests are mandatory. During anesthesia, careful monitoring of the cardiopulmonary function should be instituted.

The indications for surgery are similar to those for adolescent idiopathic scoliosis and include progressive curves with a Cobb angle greater than 40 degrees in the frontal plane. Curves less than 40 degrees should be monitored; those more than 60 degrees should be treated surgically; and those between 40 to 60 degrees can be either monitored or treated surgically. In the latter case, treatment decisions are based primarily on the patient's age at disease onset, age when the scoliosis was first recognized, and evidence of curve progression.[8]

Posterior instrumentation and fusion with a multirod, hook, and screw system is the treatment of choice when surgery is indicated. The instrumentation should not extend down to the sacrum, except for C-shaped thoracolumbar curves with associated pelvic obliquity. In all other curves, the lower level of instrumentation should be selected using the same criteria as idiopathic scoliosis (see Chapter 9–11). Fusion and instrumentation should be extended high in the thoracic area to prevent the development or deterioration of a kyphosis above the scoliotic segment. Anterior surgery with or without instrumentation, usually followed by posterior instrumentation, should be limited to rigid curves greater than 60 degrees associated with poor sitting balance.

Pes cavovarus is usually mild in ambulatory patients and does not require treatment. In selected cases, muscle stretching and ankle-foot orthoses may be useful in delaying progression and in stabilizing the foot and ankle during standing or walking. More rigid and severe deformities can occur in patients who are wheelchair bound and have lost significant muscle strength of the lower limbs. In these cases, surgery will improve cosmesis but will not restore function. For the occasional ambulatory patient with a more severe deformity, the surgical treatment recommended is the same as outlined for Charcot-Marie-Tooth disease (see Chapter 10–7).

RETT'S SYNDROME

DEFINITION

Rett's syndrome is a progressive encephalopathy of undetermined cause that is observed only in girls after a period of normal development through the first 6 to 18 months of life. The abnormal neurological development starts with hypotonia, followed by ataxia, and finally spasticity. It is characterized by a progressive loss of intellectual function and fine and gross motor skills.

HISTORICAL REVIEW

In 1966, Andreas Rett of Vienna was the first to recognize this syndrome as a specific entity and to report on studies of 22 girls in the German literature.[11] Rett provided an extensive English language account of Rett's syndrome in 1977, but the syndrome became widely recognized only in 1983, when Hagberg et al[12] reported a series of 35 patients from several countries. Hagberg et al confirmed the truly international character of this entity and recognized Rett's pioneering work.

EPIDEMIOLOGY

The occurrence of Rett's syndrome in females only has led to the hypothesis that it is an X-linked dominant disorder that is lethal in males.[13] As in Friedreich's ataxia, this syndrome is rare but has a worldwide geographic distribution. The incidence is estimated between 1 in 10,000 to 15,000 live female births.

PATHOGENESIS

The genetic basis and the biochemical abnormality produced by the defective gene have not yet been identified. Postmortem studies reveal diffuse atrophy, reduced brain weight, and nonspecific cerebral hemispherical changes.

CLINICAL FEATURES

The most frequent initial symptom is the sudden deterioration of intellectual function and fine and gross motor skills appearing in girls between age 1 and 2 years after a period of apparently normal development. This includes symptoms of autism, dementia, seizure disorder, loss of verbal skills, as well as truncal and gait ataxia, loss of purposeful hand function, and the appearance of stereotypic hand movements. The key orthopedic features include scoliosis, coxa valga, foot abnormalities, and lower extremity contractures.[14,15]

There are nine necessary criteria for Rett syndome[13]:

1. Normal prenatal and perinatal period.
2. Normal psychomotor development through the first 6 months of life.
3. Normal head circumference at birth.
4. Deceleration of head growth after 5 months of age.
5. Loss of acquired hand skills between 6 and 30 months of age.
6. Psychomotor retardation.
7. Stereotypic hand movements.
8. Gait and truncal ataxia between ages 1 and 4 years.
9. Tentative diagnosis until 2 to 5 years of age.

Each individual affected with this disorder passes through four clinical stages. Stage 1 (early-onset stagnation) occurs between 6 to 18 months and is characterized by an arrest of developmental progress with no other specific clinical finding. This is followed by stage II (rapid destruction) occurring between 1 to 4 years of age in which a rapid developmental deterioration occurs over weeks to months. Acquired verbal and hand functions are lost, associated with personality changes such as dementia with autistic features and appearance of stereotypic hand movements, ataxic gait, irregular breathing, and seizures. Stage III (pseudostationary) evolves from the preschool through the early school years. It is marked by a period of apparent stabilization with regression of autistic features but persistence of mental retardation as well as gait and truncal ataxia. Ultimately, between ages 5 to 15 years, stage IV (late motor deterioration) will be dominated by loss of ambulatory function and the appearance of spasticity, muscle wasting, and orthopaedic manifestations of the disorder. Life expectancy is probably decreased, but many individuals have survived into their third or fourth decade.

The most common orthopaedic abnormality is *scoliosis*, which is present in more than 80% of patients at stage IV (Fig. 2).[16-19] Information is lacking on the natural history of scoliosis in Rett's syndrome. In general, however, long, sweeping C-shaped thoracolumbar curves will develop, sometimes with pelvic obliquity. The age at presentation varies between 4 to 18 years (average, 8 years). Scoliosis is of neurogenic origin and develops earlier than idiopathic scoliosis. Curve progression is usually more rapid, and early hypotonia, muscle weakness, and an early appearance of stage IV have been shown to correlate with an increased risk of progression. However, not all patients have curves progressing beyond 40 degrees and, therefore, will not require treatment. Sagittal plane deformities are frequent with hypokyphosis and hypolordosis in the scoliotic segments and kyphosis in the high thoracic area.

The natural history of other orthopaedic manifestations is also poorly known.[14, 15] *Coxa valga* is frequent and may progress to hip subluxation or dislocation in a small number of individuals. Various *foot deformities*, such as equinus, equinovarus, or equinovalgus have been reported in 10% to 20% of patients. *Fractures* of the upper and lower extremities after minimal trauma may occur in association with osteopenia when ambulatory function has been lost.

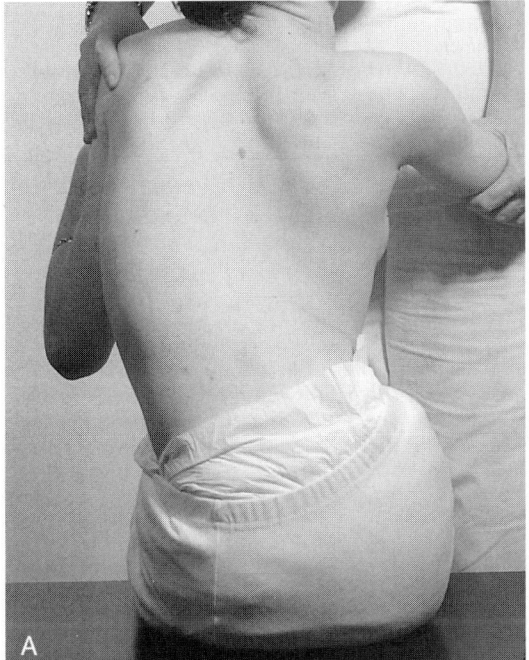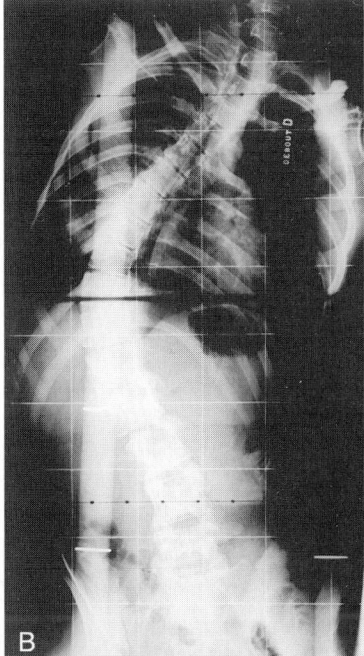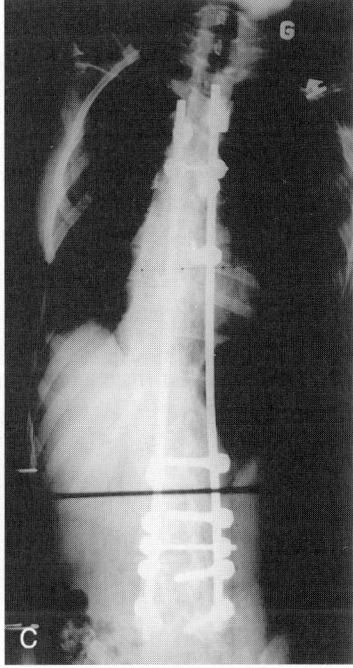

Fig. 2. Rett's syndrome. *A*, The trunk deformity of a young adolescent female. *B*, Anteroposterior radiograph of the same patient illustrating the typical C-shaped thoracolumbar curve pattern. *C*, Postoperative radiograph of the same patient after posterior instrumentation and fusion with a multirod, hook, and screw system.

INVESTIGATION

In the absence of a specific biological marker, the diagnosis of Rett's syndrome is based on the clinical characteristics of the disease. Epileptiform activity detected by electroencephalogram (EEG) is almost always present at diagnosis, and the EEG in relationship to breathing activity may be abnormal. Computed tomography and magnetic resonance imaging reveal cortical atrophy. Other laboratory and imaging study results are usually normal.

MANAGEMENT

Rett's syndrome is relatively new as a distinct entity. Currently, there is no cure for the disease, and firm conclusions regarding the efficacy of orthopedic treatment cannot be made with certainty.[17] Bracing of flexible scoliotic curves between 20 and 40 degrees with a TLSO may be useful in slowing curve progression and should be tried if it does not impair ambulatory or respiratory functions. Surgical correction to stabilize progressive curves greater than 40 degrees is recommended and may improve the quality of life as in other encephalopathies such as cerebral palsy. Autologous bone grafting with posterior instrumentation and a multirod, hook, and screw system is the treatment of choice, with extension of fusion to the pelvis for patients with pelvic obliquity. Anterior surgical release with posterior instrumentation and fusion should be limited to rigid curves greater than 60 degrees. As in other progressive neurological disorders, careful evaluation of pulmonary function and seizure control is mandatory in the pre- and postoperative periods. Treatment of hip subluxation and dislocation should follow the same principles as for cerebral palsy (see Chapter 10–2). Finally, Achilles tendon lengthening may be required in selected cases.

REFERENCES

1. Labelle H, Duhaime M, Allard P: Spinal deformities in Friedreich's ataxia. In Weinstein SL (ed): The Pediatric Spine: Principles and Practice. New York, Raven Press, 1994, p 999.
2. Friedreich N: Ueber degenerative atrophie der spinalen hinterstrange. Virchows Arch Pathol Anat 1863; 26:391.
3. Chamberlain S, Shaw J, Rowland A, et al: Mapping of mutation causing Friedreich's ataxia to human chromosome 9. Nature 1988; 334:248.
4. Geoffroy G, Barbeau A, Breton G, et al: Clinical description and roentgenologic evaluation of patients with Friedreich's ataxia. Can J Neurol Sci 1976; 3:279.
5. Harding AE: Friedreich's ataxia: A clinical and genetic study of 90 families with an analysis of early diagnostic criteria and intrafamilial clustering of clinical features. Brain 1981; 104:589.
6. Cady RB, Bobechko WP: Incidence, natural history, and treatment of scoliosis in Friedreich's ataxia. J Pediatr Orthop 1984; 4:673.

7. Daher YH, Lonstein JE, Winter RB, et al: Spinal deformities in patients with Friedreich's ataxia: A review of 19 patients. J Pediatr Orthop 1985; 5:553.
8. Labelle H, Tohmé S, Duhaime M, et al: The natural history of scoliosis in Friedreich's ataxia. J Bone Joint Surg Am 1986; 68:564.
9. Thomson GH: Neuromuscular disorders. In Morrissey RT, Weinstein SL (eds): Lovell and Winter's Pediatric Orthopaedics. Philadelphia, Lippincott-Raven, 1996, p 558.
10. Beauchamp M, Labelle H, Duhaime M, et al: Natural history of muscle weakness in Friedreich's ataxia and its relation to loss of ambulation. Clin Orthop Rel Res 1995; 311:270.
11. Rett A: Über ein eigenartiges Hirnatrophisches Syndrome bei Hyperammonaemie in Kindersalter. Wien Med Wochenschr 1966; 116:723.
12. Hagberg B, Aicardi J, Dias K, et al: A progressive syndrome of autism, dementia, ataxia, and loss of purposeful hand use in girls: Rett's syndrome: Report of 35 cases. Ann Neurol 1983; 14:471.
13. Trevathan E, Naidu S: The clinical recognition and differential diagnosis of Rett syndrome. J Child Neurol 1988; 3(suppl): S6.
14. Guidera K, Borrelli J, Raney E, et al: Orthopaedic manifestations of Rett syndrome. J Pediatr Orthop 1991; 11:204.
15. Loder R, Lee C, Richards B: Orthopaedic aspects of Rett syndrome: A multicenter review. J Pediatr Orthop 1989; 9:557.
16. Bassett G, Tolo V: The incidence and natural history of scoliosis in the Rett syndrome. Dev Med Child Neurol 1990; 32: 963.
17. Basset G: Rett syndrome. In Weinstein SL (ed): The Pediatric Spine: Principles and Practice. New York, Raven Press, 1994, p 1089.
18. Holm V, King H: Scoliosis in the Rett syndrome. Brain Dev 1990; 12:151.
19. Lindström J, Strokland E, Hagberg B: Scoliosis in Rett syndrome. Spine 1994; 14:1632.

ANTERIOR HORN CELL DISEASES

John R. Fisk and David Hatfield

Summary

- Poliomyelitis has four distinct stages.
- Poliomyelitis has had and continues to have an enormous social and economic impact.
- Eradication strategies for poliomyelitis are in place and appear to be working.
- Awareness and treatment options for post-polio syndrome remain a challenge.
- Establishing a diagnosis of spinal muscle atrophy is primarily prognostic.
- Therapy for spinal muscle atrophy is usually symptomatic, although spinal curvatures should be addressed aggressively.
- The diagnosis of spinal muscle atrophy may be confused with muscular dystrophies.
- Respiratory failure secondary to pulmonary infection is the most common cause of death in patients with spinal muscle atrophy.

Anterior horn cells are large motor neurons located in the ventral portion of the spinal cord. These cells with their axons constitute one part of the motor unit (Fig. 1). The other portion is the muscle fiber. The health and function of a muscle fiber is dependent on the normal health and function of its anterior horn cell. When the connection of the motor neuron via its axon and motor end plates to the muscle fibers is lost, whether by trauma or disease, the muscle fibers will die. Poliomyelitis, a viral illness affecting the anterior horn cell, and spinal muscular atrophy, a hereditary degenerative disease of the anterior horn cell, are discussed in this chapter.

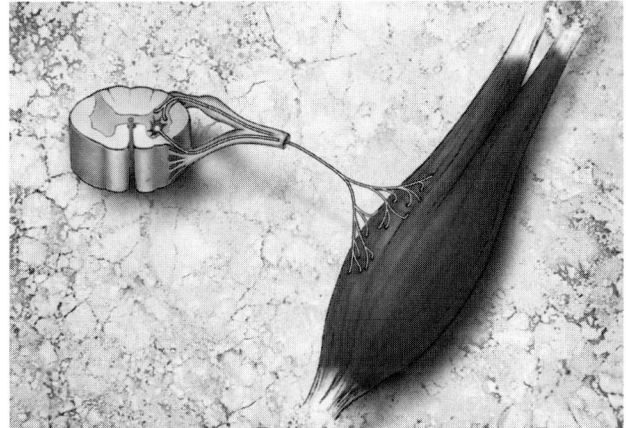

Fig. 1. Anterior horn cell. The motor unit consists of the anterior horn, its axon, and associated muscle fibers.

POLIOMYELITIS

The polioviruses are small, RNA-containing enteroviruses of which there are three subtypes. Type I accounts for 85% of cases of the paralytic illness.[1] After oral-oral or fecal-oral spread, viruses multiply in the pharynx and intestine during a 1- to 3-week incubation period. Blood-borne dissemination then occurs. The virus continues to be excreted in the saliva for 2 or 3 days and in the feces for a further 2 or 3 weeks. During this time, the infection is very contagious, and household infection rates can reach 100%. Most infections, however, are asymptomatic or self-limiting "flu-like" illnesses, with less than 5% of infected individuals experiencing motor weakness.[2] Similar illnesses known collectively as acute flaccid paralysis have been associated with other enteroviruses, particularly Coxsackie A and B and echoviruses.[3]

The poliovirus invades the motor neurons selectively via receptors that allow this virus to enter an axon and then migrate to the anterior horn cell. In patients experiencing paralysis, more than 95% of the motor neurons are affected, but not all of the infected cells die.

Adaptations to necrosis of the anterior horn cell are so effective that up to 50% of the original number of motor neurons can be lost without the muscle losing clinically normal strength. These adaptations include terminal axon sprouting to support orphaned muscle fibers and muscle fiber hypertrophy. A single motor neuron that initially stimulated 1000 muscle cells might eventually innervate 5000 to 10,000 cells, creating a giant motor unit. These adaptations are neither static nor permanent. After recovery from the acute illness, there is an ongoing process of remodeling of the motor units that consists of both denervation and reinnervation. It is this process of remodeling and constant repair that allows the motor units to achieve a steady state of muscle strength. When this steady state is disrupted, new muscle weakness occurs.[4]

Worldwide incidence and distribution of poliomyelitis have changed radically since the introduction of effective vaccinations (Fig. 2). Although many orthopaedic surgeons do not have experience with poliomyelitis, the increasing opportunities for international outreach and the emergence of the post-poliomyelitis syndrome demand an understanding of this important disease.

HISTORICAL PERSPECTIVE

Acute paralytic poliomyelitis has likely been a part of human history since biblical times and may even date to 18th-dynasty Egypt (1580–1350 BC).[5] The first epidemic in North America was in 1894. During the epidemic of 1916, fear of this illness changed how families would allow their children to play with others during the summer months. There was an early understanding of how it was

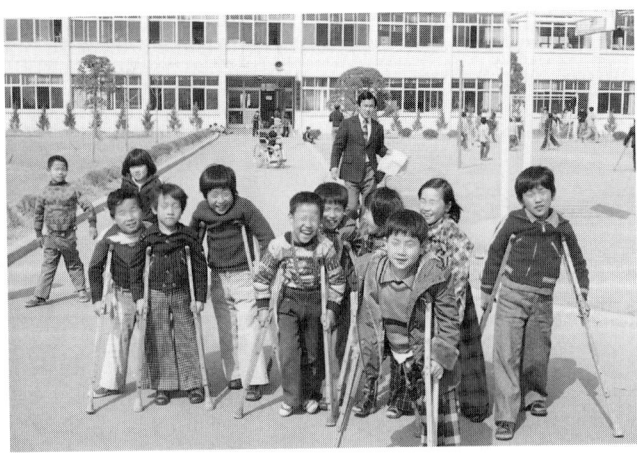

Fig. 2. Asian children post-polio. Western countries and many Asian countries no longer have acute infections.

spread, but not how to prevent it. Franklin Delano Roosevelt contracted this illness on August 11, 1921. The story of how he dealt with the disease is famous (Fig. 3). Through his efforts and those of Basil O'Connor, a friend and administrator of Warm Springs, Georgia and, later, the Foundation for Infantile Paralysis, money was raised and research supported. John Enders was awarded the Nobel Prize for developing techniques of growing the virus on monkey kidney cell cultures, a process that allowed Jonas Salk to develop the first effective vaccination. On April 24, 1954, the field trials of the Salk vaccine were begun: 1.8 million children participated in what was the largest clinical trial in history.

The Salk vaccine is a killed virus injection. Sabin followed in 1961 with an inactivated virus oral vaccine. The results were dramatic. There were 55,000 reported cases of poliomyelitis in the United States in 1954 and only 200 3 years later (Fig. 4).

The last case of infection caused by a wild virus in the Western Hemisphere was in 1991.

CLINICAL COURSE

Poliomyelitis can be divided into four distinct stages: acute illness, period of recovery, stable disability, and post-poliomyelitis syndrome. Traditionally, orthopaedic surgeons were involved in the care and treatment of children in the stable phase. Recently the role has expanded to include the needs of the population suffering from the fourth stage, post-poliomyelitis syndrome.

Poliomyelitis has been called the Great Educator. The generation of orthopaedists who were the mentors of those now actively in practice did little else in their pediatric clinics than correct deformities and restore function to children affected by the epidemic of past times. Today's physicians, if trained in the West, may feel overwhelmed when confronted by the perplexing issues presented by paralytic poliomyelitis residua. *Campbell's Operative Orthopaedics*[6] has almost 100 pages related to the surgery of poliomyelitis. The procedures are for the most part not difficult. The decision-making process on what to do and when to do it is the greater challenge.

Each affected child is different because of different combinations of paralysis. For example, one can see a child with a totally flail leg (Fig. 5) who is able to walk brace-free or a child with upper limbs so weak that the child cannot support the body weight and who somehow manage to use crutches to walk. Manual muscle testing should be thorough and reproducible to identify muscles that are deficient and muscles that are strong enough to transfer. Muscles that are transferred lose one grade. With the exception of those transferred only for stability, all must be grade 4 or better, on a scale of 1 to 5, to be able to function adequately after transfer.

Before beginning treatment of any individual, the surgeon must have a plan based on priorities and the child's environment. The needs of someone who culturally spends most of his or her time squatting or sitting on the floor are quite distinct from those of one who must climb onto a school bus and sit on furniture throughout the day. When first seeing a child who has had poliomyelitis, it is all too easy to focus on a single deformity. The orthopaedist must focus on functional goals rather than a single deformity. A systematic approach to establishing treatment priorities is needed.[7] The priorities for management are, by and large,

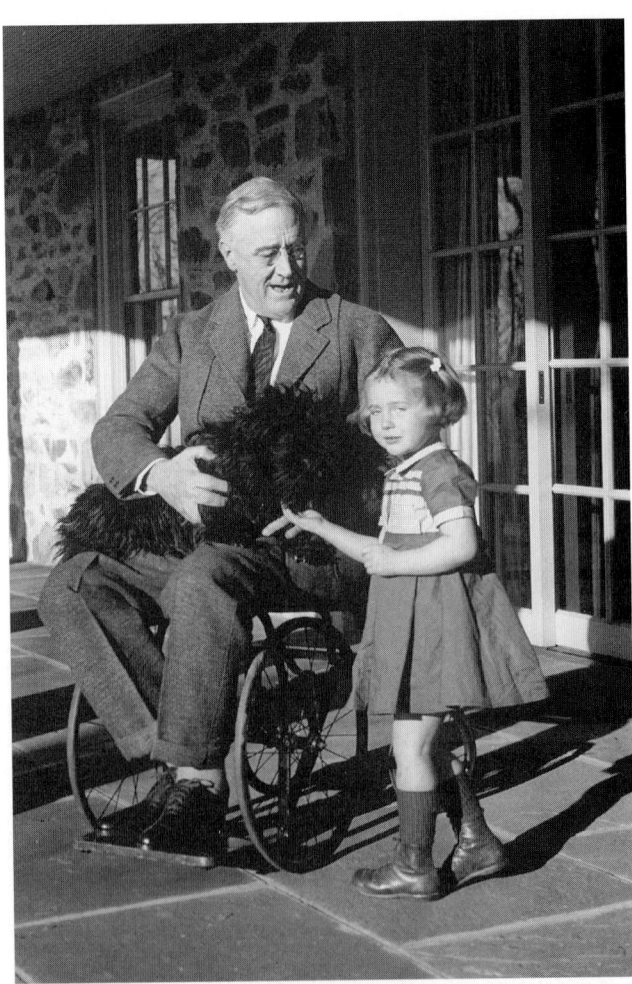

Fig. 3. Franklin Delano Roosevelt. This is one of the only two photographs showing his disability after poliomyelitis. (From the Franklin D. Roosevelt Library.)

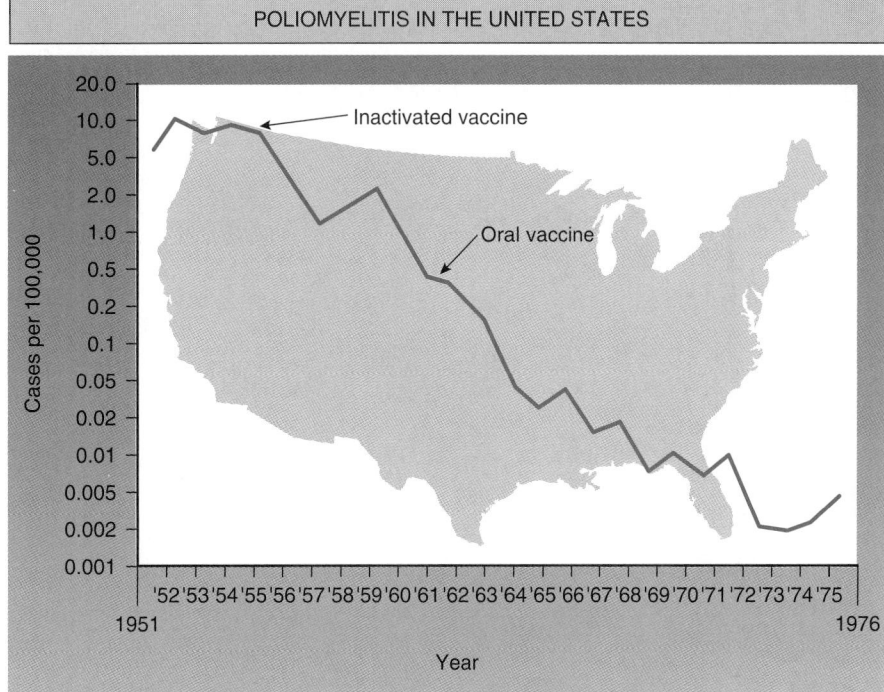

POLIOMYELITIS IN THE UNITED STATES

Inactivated vaccine

Oral vaccine

Cases per 100,000

'52 '53 '54 '55 '56 '57 '58 '59 '60 '61 '62 '63 '64 '65 '66 '67 '68 '69 '70 '71 '72 '73 '74 '75

1951

1976

Year

Fig. 4. Poliomyelitis in the United States. The decline in cases since 1954 documents the effectiveness of the vaccinations.

sequential: (1) get the child walking; (2) correct factors that will create deformity with growth; (3) consider factors that will obviate or reduce a lifetime dependency on external bracing; (4) correct upper extremity problems; (5) treat scoliosis.

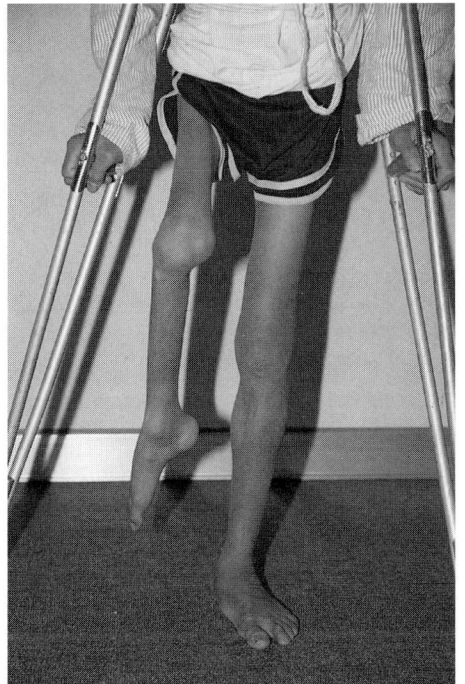

Fig. 5. Flail leg. The level of associated disability varies greatly depending on the social structure of the patient's environment.

In the developing world, treatment priorities based on functional goals appropriate to an individual's environment using locally available technologies will help the greatest numbers of those in need.[8]

TREATMENT RECOMMENDATIONS
Acute Illness
During the acute stage of infection, the emphasis is support and comfort of the patient. Working during the epidemics before development of the vaccination, Sister Elizabeth Kenny, an Australian nurse, advocated an intensive program to provide comfort that emphasized hot packs and positioning for the acute muscle pains. Few of the modern ventilator technologies are more effective than was the iron lung (Fig. 6). Patients with paralysis of respiratory muscles and, in the case of bulbar involvement, the diaphragm require long-term ventilator support.

Period of Recovery
During the recovery stage, positioning and maintaining range of motion are critical.[9] Those muscle fibers left orphaned and without innervation die and become fibrotic. Significant contractures will develop unless there are aggressive efforts to prevent them.

Period of Stable Disability
Get the Child Walking. During the stable stage, or the stage of chronicity, deformities and disabilities can be addressed. Keeping in mind the treatment priorities outlined earlier, it is important to get the child walking and not overemphasize striving for walking perfection. Huckstep concluded, as a result of his personal experience with 5000 patients, that death before maturity in developing countries is usually the result of failing to treat the child who is only

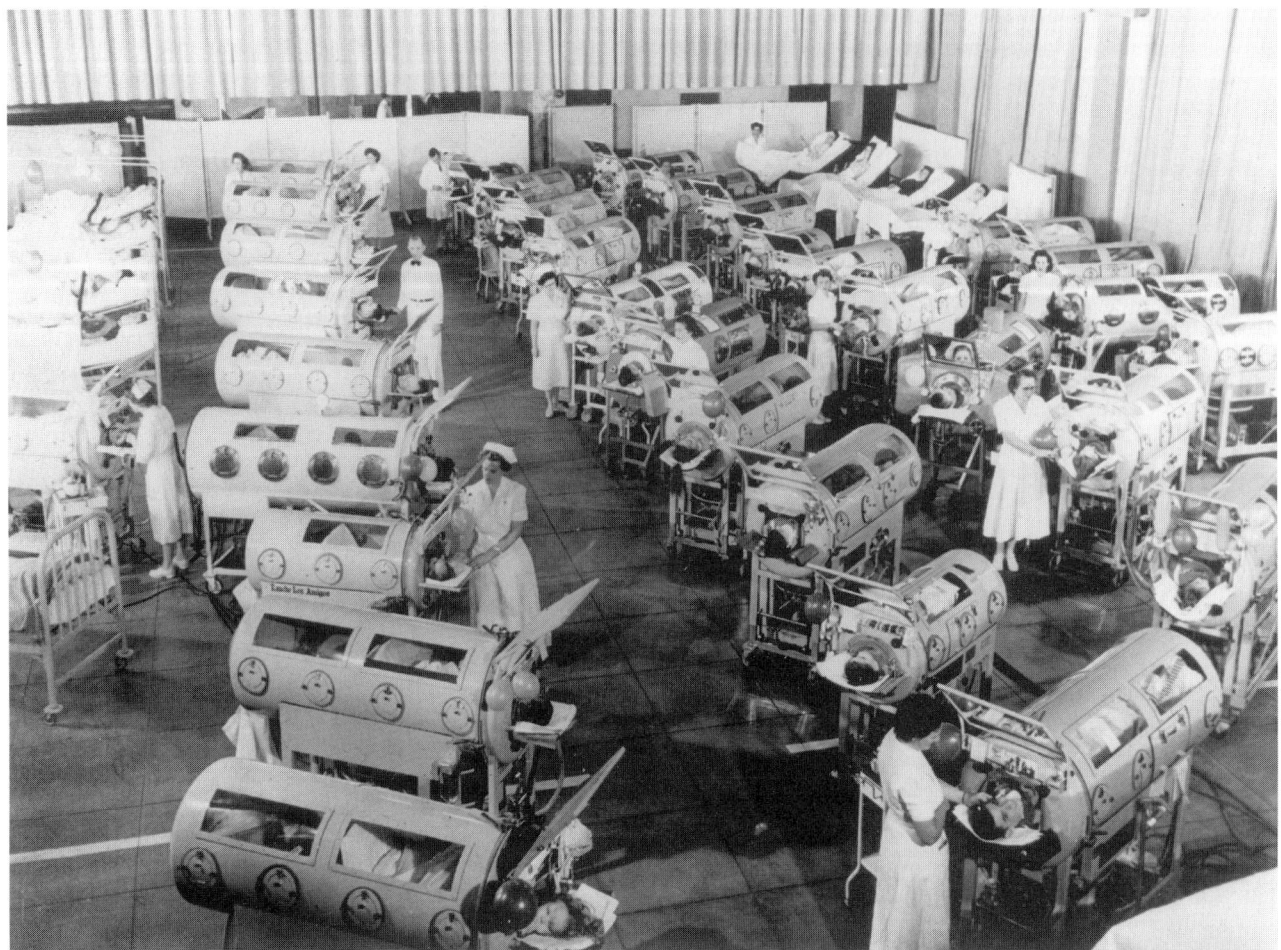

Fig. 6. Iron lung. It is effective for treating respiratory paralysis. A commonly used device in the prevaccination era. (Courtesy of March of Dimes.)

able to crawl. Most children with poliomyelitis, however, when able to be upright and walking with supports, or following surgery, are accepted by the community, educated by parents and relatives, and employable when they reach maturity. The child can be up on his or her feet with the minimal contracture correction necessary and the simplest braces. Simple subcutaneous tenotomies and bracing will often restore function much more efficiently than complicated surgical reconstructive procedures. The contracture releases required early are most often the hip flexors and abductors, the fascia lata distally, and the heel cord. The extent and duration of the deformities will dictate the techniques chosen.

Prevent Deformities. As a child begins to walk, he or she should be assessed to focus on those problems that, as the child grows, commonly result in deformity. At the foot, for example, equinus deformity and dropfoot develop from paralyzed dorsiflexors, foot valgus results from unbalanced peroneals, and equinovarus can be secondary to an unbalanced tibialis posterior or calcaneus due to absent gastrosoleus function. Cavus deformities are secondary to intrinsic muscle weakness.

At the knee, hyperextension occurs as a result of weak hamstrings and/or the floor reaction force of a fixed equinus contracture. A dangling leg is minimally func-

tional, but a child may do quite well with crutches. When the leg is supported orthotically, ambulation may be possible without crutches, freeing the upper extremities for more useful functions, as well as stimulating better growth of the flail leg.

Leg length discrepancy, another common deformity of growth and development, varies in its acceptability in different cultures. In the West, 2.5 cm is considered a reasonable upper limit; however, a far greater leg length difference is usually tolerated elsewhere (Fig. 7). It is not surprising to find children with 6 to 8 cm differences who are largely unconcerned and assume the associated limp to be inevitable.

A great deal has been written about hip instability. There are many tendon transfers and bony procedures designed to restore lost stability; however, a hip that is stiff from many surgical procedures may be less functional than one that is unstable yet very flexible, especially in cultures accustomed to floor sitting.

Decrease Bracing. Once the child is walking with confidence, and anticipated deformities cared for, one needs to ask, "Can the child be made brace-free or can bracing be decreased?" (Fig. 8). The most important antigravity muscles are the quadriceps, the hip extensors, and the gastrosoleus group. A child with absent quadriceps function can

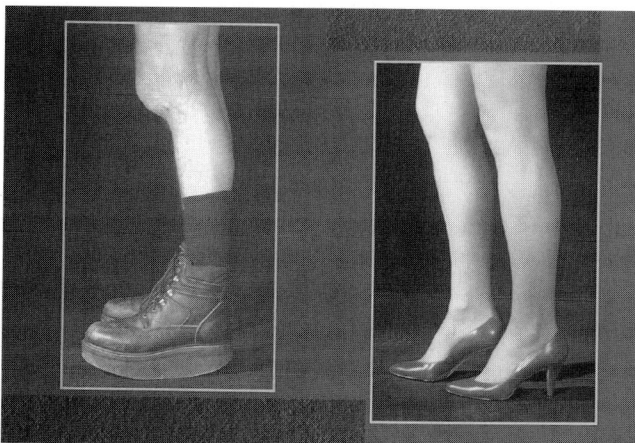

Fig. 7. Leg length inequality. The functional and cosmetic effect of a leg length inequality varies greatly as to the age, sex, and society of the individual.

walk brace-free provided he or she has hip extensors, ankle plantar flexors, or a combination of both. These muscles will allow him or her to maintain the knee in extension during midstance. The ligaments and joint capsule can provide passive stability and passive extension during midstance but over time may become stretched, allowing hyperextension. If the knee cannot be prevented from buckling, surgical procedures may restore the lost stability. They generally address plantar movements around the ankle or extension osteotomy at the knee. Hamstring transfers, for extension, frequently cause limited flexion at the knee, making squatting difficult. There are many choices to

help relieve the paralytic post-poliomyelitis patient from having to use a long-leg orthosis.[6]

Upper Extremity. Stabilizing a flail shoulder frequently provides a significant improvement in the function of the elbow and hand. Transfers about the elbow may improve the ability to position the hand in space. Transfers about the hand may restore opposition or pinch and greatly improve its function. In addition, the clinician should not ignore the importance of the child's use of the upper extremities to support the body weight with crutches, or of shifting trunk weight by leaning on the arm of a wheelchair.

Scoliosis. Spinal deformity is common in all neuromuscular diseases occurring in skeletally immature children (Fig. 9). The deformities in poliomyelitis tend to remain flexible longer than in other neuromuscular diseases. Standard indicators for treatment of scoliosis with proven progression should be followed. Orthotic management alone is rarely successful; however, it may stall progression of a curve until more growth has been attained. Supporting a collapsing trunk with a corset does not prevent curve progression, although many patients claim an improved sense of support while using a corset.

Surgery is indicated to stop progression and provide trunk support when the curves warrant. Curves greater than 55 degrees generally progress. It has long been taught that stabilizing the lumbar spine may decrease the patient's ability to walk. Recent reports challenge this concept. A stabilized pelvis may be better able to propel a flail lower extremity.

In summary, the decisions in the surgical treatment of poliomyelitis are more difficult than the procedures them-

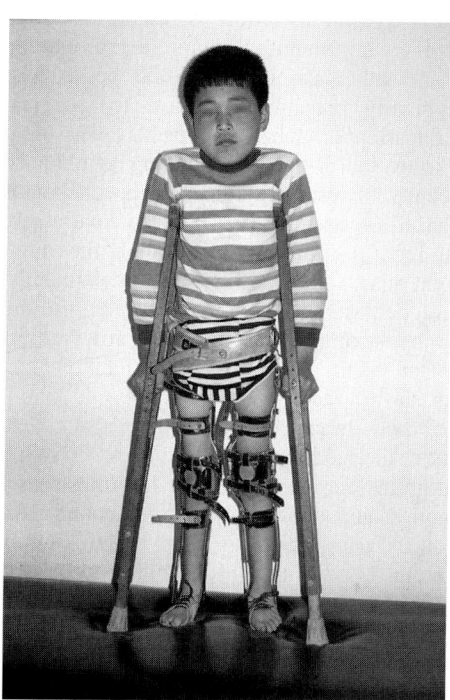

Fig. 8. KAFO. Knee-ankle-foot orthoses were once common in the recovery stage after paralysis. They rarely remained necessary after tendon transfers.

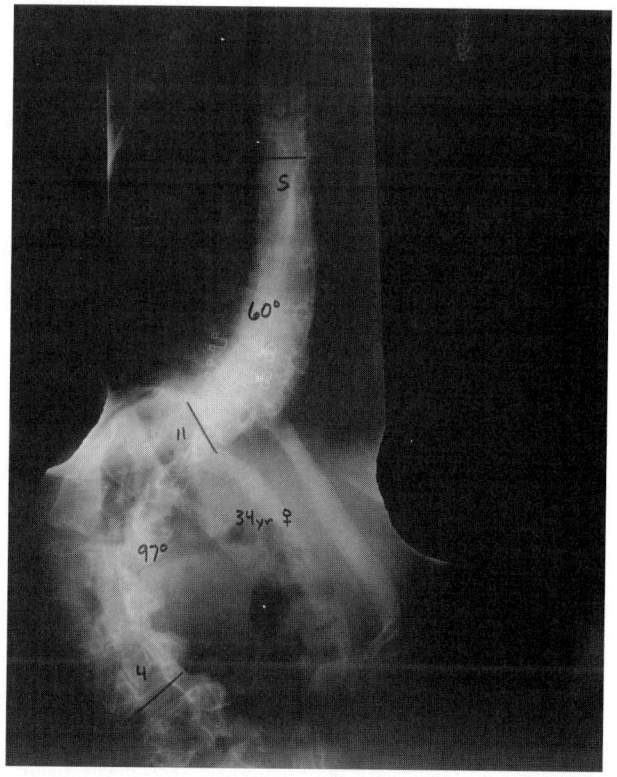

Fig. 9. Scoliosis. This shows a typical paralytic curve pattern with oblique pelvis.

selves. Although there are well-established patterns of disease, each patient is different.[10] Proceeding cautiously is best when there is doubt about what effect a procedure will have in a given patient.

POST-POLIOMYELITIS SYNDROME

The existence of a fourth stage of poliomyelitis was initially disputed, but it is now clear that poliomyelitis has a fourth stage. It is neither a new disease nor a recrudescence of the acute infection, but another aspect of a paralytic disease caused by the neural damage resulting from the original viral illness. It deserves the distinct title post-poliomyelitis syndrome because it marks a substantial functional change in its victims many years after they thought they had recovered from their original illness.

Post-poliomyelitis syndrome produces a cluster of symptoms in individuals who developed poliomyelitis, on average, 33 years earlier. Symptoms may include fatigue, muscle and joint pain, reduced exercise tolerance, impairment of activities of daily living, limb atrophy, cramps, and fatigue. They exclude musculoskeletal symptoms due to back injuries, radiculopathy, compression neuropathies, and other medical, neurological, orthopaedic, or psychiatric illness.[10] The stability experienced in stage 3 ends, and this onset of new symptoms begins for 20% to 40% of individuals who had paralytic poliomyelitis (Fig. 10).

Post-poliomyelitis syndrome is not a new disorder. It was described in the French medical literature in 1875.[11] Jean Martin Charcot, the 19th century neuropathologist, hypothesized that after an initial disease of the spinal cord, individuals might experience new weakness caused by overuse of the involved muscles. His observations are surprisingly relevant to the current understanding of post-poliomyelitis syndrome. The normal degeneration and regeneration process of axon sprouts results in loss of innervation when surviving giant motor neurons can no longer metabolically support this process. In the non-poliomyelitis individual, significant attrition of motor neurons does not occur until a person reaches the age of 60 years or more. In the

patient with poliomyelitis, however, the stressed anterior horn cell is vulnerable to earlier degenerative changes. Post-poliomyelitis individuals are functioning with such a diminished motor neuron pool that any loss of motor-neuron units results in a loss of function.

It is estimated that 40% of poliomyelitis survivors will experience new symptoms an average of 30 to 40 years after their acute illness. Forty percent of the estimated 640,000 survivors in the United States and 20 million worldwide will be at risk. For these individuals, the essence of good medical care is to relieve symptoms, improve muscle function, and improve the individual's sense of well-being. This management strategy is frequently referred to as "bracing and pacing."[12]

There is a distinct post-poliomyelitis personality. Children who often spent months away from their families in rehabilitation institutions frequently developed a strong inwardly directed power to overcome their adversity. The "use it or lose it" coaching of their therapists, at a time when there was a naturally occurring motor unit recovery, reinforced the development of the classic type-A personality. Years later, age-matched studies comparing post-poliomyelitis persons with non-poliomyelitis persons have shown a much higher achievement level in those recovering from paralysis. These people struggled to rid themselves of their braces and when they had, considered themselves recovered. Many feel they are normal in spite of clinically evident weakness. Thus, as this group of overachievers are confronted with a progressive loss of function beyond that which we all experience with advancing age, it is little wonder that one of the primary symptoms is depression. There is also a major reluctance to admit the need for additional interventions.

There are a number of principles for aiding the post-poliomyelitis syndrome patient. First is accurate diagnosis. Amyotrophic lateral sclerosis, for example, can present with similar symptoms. More common disorders, such as rotator cuff tears, meniscal tears, nerve entrapment syndromes, and other disorders, should be excluded. These people typically present with great fear of an uncertain future. Education on what to expect is very helpful. They need to know that what is happening to them is neither a recrudescence of the infection nor psychosomatic. Treatment is based on early identification of overused muscles.[12] Adequate rest, pacing oneself through the day, judicious aerobic exercise, correction of biomechanically unsound joints, and occasionally bracing are required. Joints, once stabilized by stronger muscles, may now require external support. But, with individuals who feel that they at one time had surmounted the impossible and had rid themselves of their braces, moving them back into external support is easier said than done.

Nonfatiguing aerobic programs for improved cardiovascular function and control are recommended. If such exercise produces pain that lasts more than 20 minutes, then the individual is causing muscle injury and should proceed at a slower rate (J. Perry, personal communication). Exercise can help to maintain strength and, in some underutilized muscles, improve strength.

It was formerly taught that degenerative joint disease and pain were unusual in poliomyelitis. It was felt that in spite of joint instability, weakness decreased stresses on

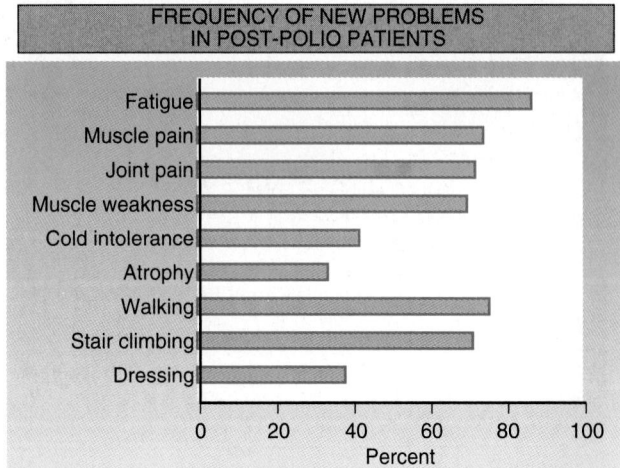

Fig. 10. Frequency of new problems in post-polio patients. These are the presenting complaints of a post-polio population. (Copyright 1998 by Scientific American, Inc. All rights reserved.)

joints. Joint pain does occur following poliomyelitis, but the numbers requiring total joint arthroplasties are never the less small. Over a 16-year period, only 11 of more than 2000 patients receiving total knee arthroplasty at one institution had a history of poliomyelitis.[13]

SPINAL MUSCULAR ATROPHY

Spinal muscular atrophy involves the spontaneous degeneration of anterior horn cells leading to weakness or paralysis. It is the second most common cause of childhood muscular disturbance following Duchenne's muscular dystrophy.

Originally, two types were recognized. Werdnig-Hoffmann disease was the name applied to the infantile form, which results in early death (Table 1). Similar symptoms with a later onset were known as Kugelberg-Welander disease. In an effort to standardize the nomenclature, the syndrome has been divided into SMA I through III.[14]

SMA I is characterized by onset before the age of 6 months with death before 2 years from respiratory failure. This corresponds with Werdnig-Hoffman in the older nomenclature.[15] SMA II, also known as the chronic infantile form, has an onset of symptoms at 6 to 18 months of age. These children characteristically have normal motor milestones initially but never gain the ability to walk. After an early progression in weakness, they may remain static for long periods. Patients with types I and II disease will present as floppy infants.[16] SMA III (corresponding to Kugelberg-Welander disease) has an onset after 18 months of age with symptoms possibly not appearing until later in the first decade. It then will show a long, slow progression.

Although spinal muscle atrophy is usually regarded as a recessively inherited disorder, there appear to be forms that are inherited as autosomal dominant. There is disagreement about whether SMA I or SMA II presents with the greatest frequency. Although SMA I may be more frequent, it is also associated with early death, and so SMA II is seen more frequently in reported series. Despite the grouping of patients into SMA I through III, there is a spectrum of disease rather than distinct disease entities.

The survival motor neuron (SMN) and neuronal apoptosis inhibitor protein (NAIP) genes have been associated with spinal muscular atrophy.[17, 18] The disease has been associated with a variable number of deletions in a small portion of chromosome 5 (5q11.2-q13.3 locus).[19] Muscle weakness and disease progression in spinal muscular atrophy probably results from the inappropriate persistence of normally occurring programmed cell death of motor neurons.

PRESENTATION

The initial presentation is with hypotonia and significant muscle weakness. There may be a fine tremor of the fingers and fasciculations of the tongue. Proximal muscles are affected more than distal ones. Lower extremity involvement is more common than upper extremity. Sensation and intellectual function are not affected. Initially the diagnosis may be confused with muscular dystrophy. The two diseases can be differentiated by electromyographic and nerve conduction studies. Electromyograph shows neuropathic changes. Nerve conduction velocities are normal. Muscle biopsy demonstrates changes consistent with denervation.

TREATMENT

The treatment of all forms of spinal muscle atrophy is supportive rather than curative. The severely affected child with spinal muscle atrophy may have little need for orthopaedic surgery. Patients with SMA II and III are best treated using a team approach of physicians, orthotists, and physical therapists to achieve functional goals.

Scoliosis and hip instability are the most troubling orthopaedic problems. Most children with infantile spinal muscular atrophy are unable to walk. Coxa valga due to the lack of weightbearing and muscle imbalance may lead to subluxation or dislocation of the hip. Treatment consisting of hip osteotomy may help preserve a comfortable stable platform on which to sit. A flexible hip that is dislocated is better than a stiff hip from multiple surgical procedures. Patients with the juvenile form are able to walk for many years. Bracing may help prolong this function.

The spinal deformity may have a profound effect on pulmonary function. In a skeletally immature child, once the curve is recognizable, it will continue to progress. The severity of the curve usually corresponds to the severity of weakness and atrophy. Bracing may help to slow curve progression, but spinal stabilization is ultimately required in almost all adolescent patients. Curve progression can rarely be controlled and chest wall deformity secondary to the orthosis may result.[20] Goals for surgery include improved sitting ability and maintenance of respiratory function. It is important to achieve a balanced trunk that is centered over a level pelvis. This outcome may require fusion to the pelvis. Surgical indications and techniques parallel those appropriate for other neuromuscular conditions.

CONCLUSION

The anterior horn cell and its axon is only half of the neuromotor unit. It is intuitive to think that loss of neuronal function will cause weakness. Very significant functional disabilities result from diseases affecting these cells in the spinal cord, whether it is from infection or degeneration. The secondary effect of unbalanced muscle strength in the skeletally immature child is deformity of the spine and of the long bones. Preventing and treating these deformities helps minimize functional loss. This is where the orthopaedic surgeon frequently gets involved. However, all of these patients have multiple needs; consequently, the importance of the role of the orthopaedist as a member of a larger team must be emphasized.

TABLE 1. HISTORY OF SPINAL MUSCULAR ATROPHY	
1891	Werdnig first described an infantile condition with generalized weakness.
1893	Hoffman contributed further descriptions.
1956	Kugelberg and Welander described a juvenile form with a less progressive nature.
1990	Survival motor neuron (SMN) and neuronal apoptosis inhibitor protein (NAIP) genes were located.

REFERENCES

1. Sabin AB: Poliomyelitis. In Horsfass FC, Tamm I (eds): Viral and Rickettsial Infections in Man, 5th ed. Philadelphia, JB Lippincott, 1980, p 1348.
2. Jobelt B, Lipton HL: Enterovirus infections. In Vinken PJ, Bruyn GW, Klowers HL, et al (eds): Handbook of Clinical Neurology, vol 56: Viral Diseases. Amsterdam, Elsevier Science Publishers BV, 1989, p 314.
3. Gear JH: Nonpolio causes of polio-like paralytic syndromes. Rev Infect Dis 1984; 6:S379.
4. Halsted LS: Post-polio syndrome. Sci Am 1998; 278:42.
5. Trojan DA, Cashman NR: Current trends in Post-Poliomyelitis Syndrome. New York, Milestone Medical Communications; 1996, p 5.
6. Canale ST (ed): Campbell's Operative Orthopaedics, 9th ed. St. Louis, Mosby-Year Book, 1998, p 3972.
7. Watts HG, Gillies H: A Practical Guide to the Orthopaedic Management of Children with Residua of Paralytic Poliomyelitis. New York, Orthopaedics Overseas Publication, Botit Publishing, 1992.
8. Huckstep RL: Appropriate surgery and appliances for patients with deformities and paralysis in developing countries. AAOS Instr Course Lect 1992; 41:461.
9. World Health Organization: Guidelines for the Prevention of Deformities in Polio. WHO Publication 91.1, Geneva, 1995.
10. Halstead LS, Wiechers DO (eds): Research and Clinical Aspects of the Late Effects of Poliomyelitis. White Plains, NY. March of Dimes, 1987.
11. Hull HF: Paralytic polio: seasoned strategies, disappearing disease. Lancet 1994; 343:1131.
12. Perry J, Fontaine JD, Mulroy S: Findings in post-poliomyelitis syndromes. J Bone Joint Surg Am 1995; 77:1148.
13. Patterson BM, Insall JN: Surgical management of nonarthritis of arthroplasty. J Arthroplasty 1992; 7:419.
14. The International SMA Consortium Meeting Report. Neuromuscular Disorders 1992; 2:423.
15. Zerres K, Rudnik-Schoneborn S, Forrest E, et al: A collaborative study on the natural history of childhood and juvenile onset proximal spinal muscular atrophy (type II and III SMA): 569 patients. J Neurol Sci 1997; 146:67.
16. Carter GT, Abresch RL, Fowler W, et al: Profiles of neuromuscular diseases: Spinal muscular atrophy. Am J Phys Med Rehabil 1995; 74:S150.
17. Brzustowicz LM, Lehner T, Castillo LH: Genetic mapping of chronic childhood-onset spinal muscular atrophy to chromosome 5q11.2-13.3. Nature 1990; 344:540.
18. Sommerville MJ, Hunter AB, Aubry HL, et al: Clinical application of the molecular diagnosis of spinal muscular atrophy: Deletions of neuronal apoptosis inhibitor protein and survival motor neuron genes. Am J Med Genet 1997; 69:159.
19. Campbell L, Potter A, Ionatius J, et al: Genomic variation and gene conversion in spinal muscular atrophy: Implications for disease process and clinical phenotype. Am J Hum Genet 1997; 61:40.
20. Robinson D, Galasko CSB, Delaney C, et al: Scoliosis and lung function in spinal muscular atrophy. Eur Spine J 1995; 4: 268.

section 10 chapter 6

MYELOMENINGOCELE

John V. Banta

Summary
- The incidence of spina bifida in the United States is estimated to be 0.5 to 1 per 1000 live births. This disorder affects the brain and spinal cord and musculoskeletal and genitourinary systems.
- The prenatal diagnosis can be made by means of ultrasonographic examination. Prenatal, maternal ingestion of folate provides a 70% protective effect against neural tube defects.
- Treatment objectives include early closure of the spinal defect to prevent sepsis, ventriculoperitoneal shunting to control hydrocephalus, and orthopaedic procedures to correct or prevent deformity and enhance mobility.
- The major socioeconomic impact on adult survivors consists of restricted mobility, social isolation, contractures, spinal deformity, pressure sores, and genitourinary complications often resulting in repeated costly hospitalization.[1, 2]
- The long-term goals of treatment are the correction of congenital deformities, prevention of contractures and spinal deformity, promotion of mobility, providing urinary and bowel continence, and encouraging social interaction and independent living.

Spinal dysraphism and *neural tube defects* are generic terms referring to failure of closure of the midline spinal elements and the resultant brain and spinal cord abnormalities. Myelomeningocele is the most common type of neural tube defect. Children with myelomeningocele have failure of closure of the posterior laminar arches and at birth have dorsal herniation of a cerebral spinal fluid sac containing an incompletely formed spinal cord referred to as a neural placode. The lesion is incompletely covered with skin and is subject to rupture during or after birth (Fig. 1).

Depending on the location and extent of the lesion, children with myelomeningocele have variable dysfunction of the spinal cord with associated loss of motor and sensory function. Most frequently, there is paralysis affecting all nerve roots distal to the lesion. Myelomeningocele also disrupts normal circulation of the cerebral spinal fluid with resulting hydrocephalus and, if untreated, marked expansion of the skull. Type II Chiari's malformation of the hindbrain, with inferior displacement of the cerebral tonsils and the inferior lobes of the cerebellum, frequently occurs in myelomeningocele. Owing to the hydrocephalus, the central canal of the spinal cord, which normally closes during fetal development, often remains open. Syringomyelia is present in approximately 20% of cases.

Other types of spinal dysraphism are less common. Me-

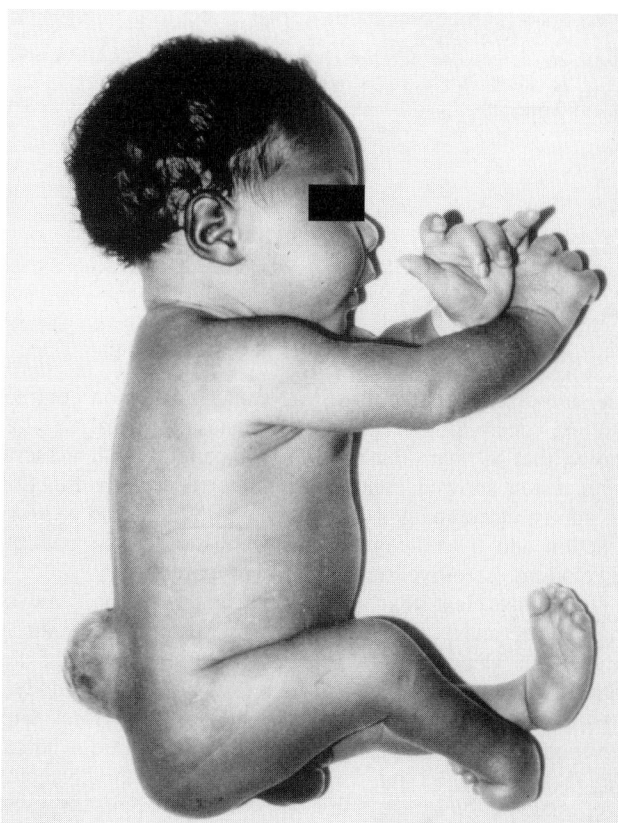

Fig. 1. Newborn child with a mid-lumbar level myelomeningocele prior to closure. Position of the lower extremities would suggest intact hip flexors, intact hamstring function in the right knee, and possible intact or spastic activity of the left quadriceps muscle. Bilateral talipes equinovarus deformities are present.

rica and detailed anatomic descriptions were completed by Dutch anatomists in the 17th century. Surgical treatment was largely unsuccessful until 1956, when the first successful shunt for the control of hydrocephalus was developed by Spitz and Holter. In 1959, a team of physicians and surgeons in Sheffield, England developed an interdisciplinary team approach to treat the affected newborn infant. Early testing of amniotic fluid α-fetoprotein for prenatal detection was refined in 1977. Subsequent testing of maternal serum levels of α-fetoprotein was also helpful in prenatal screening; however, the false-negative rate of this test approached 20%. Ultrasonographic techniques were perfected in the early 1980s to visualize the spinal defect during pregnancy.

In 1986, two further ultrasonographic signs of intracranial anomalies were detected: the lemon sign, describing a concave contour of the frontal bones, and the banana sign, describing the anterior curving of the cerebellar hemispheres plus the obliteration of the cisterna magna.[5] In 1991, the protective effect of preconceptual maternal ingestion of folate was established in two randomized double-blinded trials. A daily 0.4-mg dose of folate provides a 70% protective effect in the prevention of neural tube defects.[6]

PATHOGENESIS

The cause of neural tube defects is multifactorial. Proven causes include maternal ingestion of sodium valproate, exposure to hyperthermia, maternal diabetes, and the chromosome abnormalities trisomy 18 and triplody.[3] A genetic factor is implicated, since the risk of recurrence to a couple with one affected child is 1 in 30 and increases to 1 in 10 with two affected children.[7] The actual role of folate is not clear. Current investigations center on the methionine synthase enzyme and the mutation 677 C to T in the 5,10 methylene tetrahydrofolate reductase gene on chromosome lp363.[8]

The pathogenesis of myelomeningocele, as first hypothesized by von Recklinghausen in 1886, is probably disruption of the closure of the neural grove folds between postovulatory days 20 and 24. The anterior neuropore (corresponding to the junction between the brain and the spinal cord) closes at about day 24 (failure of which results in anencephaly) and the caudal neuropore (corresponding to the level of the second sacral vertebra) closes at approximately day 26. Secondary neurulation occurs distal to the posterior neuropore in the tail bud, whose mesenchyme develops somite pairs 30 to 34, which form the coccyx and remaining sacral vertebrae.[9] Abnormal secondary neurulation in the caudal region is the cause of sacral agenesis, more commonly referred to as the *caudal regression syndrome*. In rare cases, myelomeningocele is associated with some degree of caudal regression as evidenced by abnormal formation or segmentation of the sacrum and lower lumbar vertebrae.

In summary, defects in the closure of the neural tube may result in a wide spectrum of deformity ranging from total anencephaly (which is incompatible with life) to cervical, thoracic, lumbar, or sacral level defects. The resultant neurological loss largely determines the functional outcome of the child and the resultant neurological functional level determines the indicated orthopaedic treatments. The differ-

ningoceles are herniations of the meninges containing cerebral spinal fluid but no neural elements. These patients usually have no neurological symptoms at birth but are at increased risk for tethered cord syndrome. Occult forms of dysraphism include elongated conus with a tight filum terminale and dermal sinus tracts. Lipomyelomeningocele is characterized by lumbosacral lipomas having variable extension of the lipoma into the conus medullaris and accompanying nerve roots. Children with lipomyelomeningocele typically have normal skin coverage and a soft, eccentric swelling in the lower back from the lipomatous tissue and spina bifida. The dorsal skin also may have a faint hemangioma or possibly a dimple or small area of hypertrichosis. Lipomyelomeningocele is not associated with hydrocephalus but may present with variable levels of motor and sensory loss depending on the extent of the lesion.[3]

Diastematomyelia is a rare form of dysraphism characterized by a midline bony or cartilaginous septa or spur that divides the spinal cord. The current theory of the pathogenesis of this anomaly refers to it as the *split cord syndrome*.[4] The skin over this defect often contains an area of hypertrichosis, and radiographs demonstrate widening of the pedicles at the level of the lesion.

HISTORICAL REVIEW

Skeletal remains with neural arch defects have been recognized in Bronze Age specimens in Europe and North Af-

ential diagnosis of neural tube defects includes the obvious open defect myelomeningocele as well as the less obvious closed or covert lesions, including lipomeningocele and diastematomyelia. The child with myelomeningocele frequently has hydrocephalus and Chiari's II malformation. Lipomyelomeningocele, diastematomyelia, and other occult types of spinal dysraphism are not associated with hydrocephalus or hindbrain anomalies.

PHYSICAL EXAMINATION

The neurological examination is critical in establishing treatment goals. In addition to flaccid motor paralysis, many patients exhibit spasticity due either to upper motor neuron lesions above the spinal defect (static encephalopathy, cord syrinx) or to reflex activity in segments of the spinal cord below the level of the lesion.[10]

The initial physical examination should note the presence of any congenital scoliosis, pelvic obliquity, dislocation or contracture of the hips, and contractures of the knee, ankle, and foot. The neurological examination should assess the voluntary manual muscle strength grades 0 to 5 with the functional motor level defined as the lowest nerve root demonstrating antigravity function (Table 1).

Establishing the functional motor level is essential to planning the mobility expectations for the child as well as anticipating the long-term mobility goals. Functional ambulation can be defined as[11]:

Community: walk inside and outside, may need orthoses or crutches and wheelchair for long trips.
Household: only walk indoors, independent transfers, wheel-chair for some indoor and all outside activities.
Nonfunctional: walk as a therapy exercise only, wheelchair for all mobility.
Nonambulatory: wheelchair-bound but may self-transfer.

Walking ability is dependent on many factors, including the patient's neurological level and age, independent sitting balance, scoliosis, and energy cost. Of these factors, the neurological level is the most important determinant of long-term ambulatory function[12] (Table 2).

In a more recent Scandinavian study, 50% of the nonwalkers had neurological abnormalities such as syringomyelia or Chiari's malformation. Decreased walking ability

TABLE 2. AMBULATION POTENTIAL BY MOTOR LEVEL	
Motor Level	**Percent Ambulation (n = 163)**
Thoracic–L1–L2	0
L3	54
L4	67
L5	80
Sacral	100

was associated with scoliosis, age, and hip flexion contracture in decreasing relevance.[13] Long-term analysis has shown that as many as one-third of patients with a sacral level lesion showed continued decline in walking function as adults, accompanied by decline in motor and sensory function and by skin breakdown, with half of the patients developing osteomyelitis of the lower extremity.[14]

It is now clear that, with increasing age, the "law of mass" becomes a critical factor. Specifically, muscle strength is dependent on the cross-sectional area of the muscle, whereas the body mass is measured by the body's cross-sectional diameter plus the height. Therefore, with advancing age, strength increases by the square whereas the mass increases by the cube.[15] Thus, with advancing age, many adolescents convert to a wheelchair for more rapid, less energy-consuming mobility. Based on these factors, the orthotic algorithm given in Table 3 can be used to determine the expected bracing requirements depending on the child's functional motor level.

TREATMENT GUIDELINES

FOOT

The most common deformities are equinus, calcaneus, planovalgus, and paralytic vertical talus. Treatment objectives are to provide a plantigrade mobile foot that will allow for regular shoe wear and provide a stable platform for self-transfers and walking. Early careful, well-padded casting may allow for delay in surgical correction until 9 to 12 months of age when the foot attains adequate size. Surgery should be planned such that when postoperative casting is concluded, the child can be immediately placed into the proper orthoses to allow upright stance and appropriate night splints to prevent recurrent deformity. Because of the high prevalence of motor imbalance and spasticity, a radical release with tendon resection rather than lengthening provides a better outcome. Complete posterior, midfoot, and forefoot release is required to realign the varus, adductus, and supination deformity and talectomy should be reserved as a second-stage revision of hindfoot equinus and varus.[16] Even at the sacral level, orthotic support is required to prevent insidious recurrent deformity, skin ulceration, and potential osteomyelitis.[17] Tendon transfer is appropriate when it is absolutely clear that there is no spastic component to the muscle. Anterior tibial transfer to correct calcaneal deformity illustrates this problem, in which the surgical procedure fails to achieve the desired goal due to unrecognized spasticity.[18] Arthrodesis of tarsal bones in the anesthetic foot is rarely indicated, as the risk of neuro-

TABLE 1. FUNCTIONAL CLASSIFICATION OF MOTOR PARALYSIS		
Level	**Function**	**Probable Muscle**
Thoracic	None	None
L-1	Hip flexion weak	Iliopsoas
L-2	Hip flexion strong	Iliopsoas plus sartorius
L-3	Knee extension	Quadriceps
L-4	Knee flexion	Medial hamstrings
L-5	Foot dorsiflexion/eversion	Anterior tibialis plus peronei
Sacral	Foot plantar flexion	Gastrocsoleus plus posterior tibialis

Data from Samuelsson L, Skoog M: Ambulation in patients with myelomeningocele: A multivariate statistical analysis. J Pediatr Orthop 1988; 8:569.

TABLE 3. ORTHOTIC GUIDELINES

Level	Muscle	Age 2–5 Years	Age 5–10 Years	Age 10+ Years
Thoracic	Flail	Parapodium or HKAFO	Parawalker with/without wheelchair or HKAFO	Wheelchair
L1–2	Hip flexors	Parapodium or RGO or HKAFO	RGO with/without HKAFO	Wheelchair
L3–4	Quadriceps, medial hamstrings	RGO	KAFO	Possibly wheelchair
L5	Hip abductors, medial/lateral hamstrings	AFO	AFO	Possibly floor reaction AFO
S1	Hip extensors	AFO	AFO	AFO
S2–4	All of above	AFO	AFO	AFO

AFO, ankle and foot orthosis; HKAFO, hip, knee, and ankle orthosis (pelvic band for upper lumbar patients, more extensive support for thoracic patients); KAFO, knee, ankle, and foot orthosis; Parapodium, standing frame articulated at hip and knee to allow standing or sitting; Parawalker, swivel-based platforms mounted below parapodium to allow forward motion by swinging of upper trunk and arms; RGO, reciprocating gait orthosis with cable connection between mobile hip joints to assist reciprocal gait with crutch assist.

pathic arthropathy of the ankle joint following subtalar and triple arthrodesis frequently is observed with increasing age of the patient (Fig. 2). Preoperative radiographs should include standing views of the ankle to exclude valgus deformity of the ankle. Surgical management of foot deformity is summarized in Table 4.

KNEE

Flexion contracture is the most common knee deformity with the greatest prevalence in the patient with a thoracic level lesion. Late progressive contracture is common in the older child who discontinues walking. Contracture greater than 20 degrees commonly results in breakage of the orthosis and prepatellar skin breakdown. Surgical release should achieve some recurvatum, as recurrent contracture is common in skeletally immature patients. Surgical treatment usually requires lengthening or tenotomy of the hamstring tendons and release of the posterior capsule of the knee.[19]

Children with spastic or synergistic motor function may develop an extension contracture of the knee. This is best treated by V-Y lengthening of the quadriceps tendon in those with quadriceps function or by early tenotomy in children who lack voluntary function of the quadriceps. Any surgery about the lower extremity that requires casting has the attendant risk of skin breakdown at the heel and prepatellar regions

Patients with mid-lumbar level weakness develop a characteristic gait pattern. Abductor weakness results in an abductor lurch, increased valgus thrust at the knee, and excessive trunk rotation to advance the body over the weightbearing limb. The absent or weak plantar flexors result in increased ankle dorsiflexion during midstance, a resultant knee flexion moment, and apparent knee valgus. The end result is stress on the medial ligaments and articular cartilage, anteromedial rotatory instability, and crouched gait (Fig. 3A).[20]

Gait analysis studies suggest that the use of an ankle-foot orthosis is excessive for ankle dorsiflexion and crouch gait. Orthotic support also increases motion in the transverse plane at the knee joint, which may be deleterious in

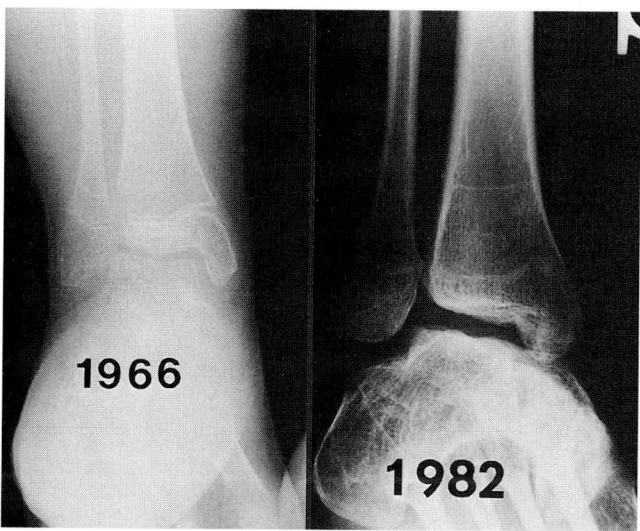

Fig. 2. Mortise views of the ankle. A child had undergone a subtalar arthrodesis at the age of 7 years on the left in 1966; the resultant dissolution of the talar dome within 16 years on the right.

TABLE 4. SURGICAL MANAGEMENT OF FOOT DEFORMITY

Deformity	Treatment
Equinovarus	Initial treatment: Radical release of hindfoot, midfoot, and forefoot. Late or recurrent deformity: calcaneal cuboid enucleation, or fusion, talectomy
Calcaneus	Anterior tibial transfer to os calcis, or extensor tendon
Paralytic convex pes valgus	Open reduction with tendo-Achilles and extensor tendon lengthening, transfer peroneus brevis or longus to posterior tibialis
Ankle valgus	Tendo-Achilles tenodesis to fibula, selective medial physeal staple or screw fixation of distal tibia in patients younger than 8 years, supramalleolar osteotomy after physeal closure[1, 22]

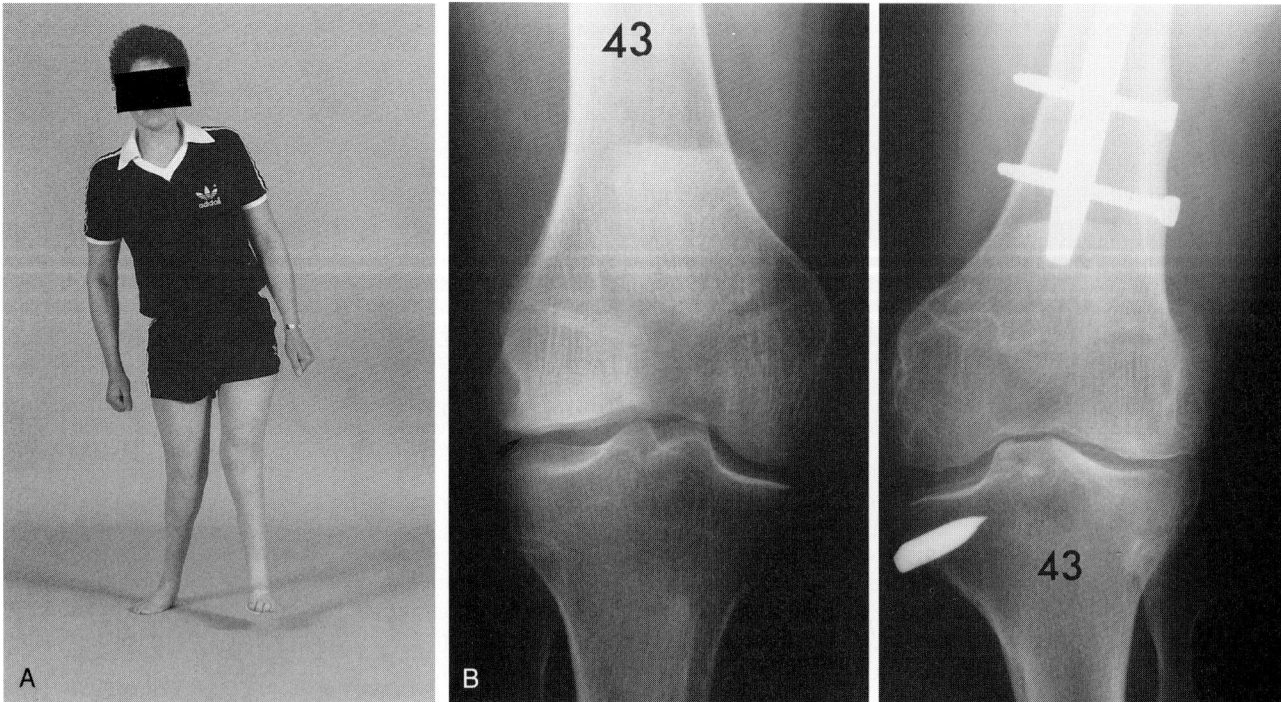

Fig. 3. Views. *A*, A 43-year-old male with a fifth lumbar motor level demonstrating the characteristic gluteal weakness, trunk shift, and flexion valgus deformity of the right knee in stance phase. *B*, Radiographs of the knees of the same patient demonstrating early degenerative changes at the knee joint. He had previously sustained a mid-diaphyseal left femoral fracture.

the older patient.[21] Therefore, in those patients with increased knee laxity, conversion to knee-ankle-foot orthosis with a free knee joint may prevent later arthritic changes (Fig. 3B).

HIP

The early controversy concerning aggressive surgical intervention for paralytic dysplastic and dislocated hips was clarified by a study of 116 children by Menelaus who concluded that extensive surgery was best reserved for those patients with antigravity quadriceps function in both lower limbs. Children presenting with higher levels of paralysis were best treated by release of tendon and soft-tissue contractures to allow for mobile hips for sitting as well as standing. Combined surgical procedures under one anesthetic were recommended not only to reduce hospital costs but also to aid in minimizing the risk of immobilization osteoporosis, fractures, and skin breakdown and to minimize the deleterious effects on growth and development caused by numerous hospitalizations.[22] The presence of the femoral head within the acetabulum did not affect the ability to ambulate,[23] and neither hip dislocation nor hip flexion contracture was related to muscle imbalance in a large multicenter study of 1061 children.[24] Numerous studies substantiate the fact that the functional neurological level is the most important determinant of walking ability.[25] Most femoral osteotomies are reserved for correction of flexion or angular deformities. Because of the gluteal weakness, the pelvic bone mass is not as well developed as in children of comparable age with normal motor control. As a consequence, major pelvic reconstruction procedures such as a Chiari pelvic osteotomy do not provide long-term

hip stability.[26] It has been proposed that reduction of a unilateral hip dislocation in a child with myelomeningocele will prevent subsequent pelvic obliquity and the development of scoliosis; however, as in cerebral palsy, the pelvic obliquity relates to the scoliosis and not to the presence or absence of hip dislocation.[27] Therefore, major reconstructive surgery of the hip is best reserved for the child with unilateral involvement and near-normal motor power. General surgical guidelines for hip surgery should include not only the patient's age, motor level, and cognitive abilities but also a realistic assessment of the child's long-term potential for ambulation (Table 5).

In the older child with lordoscoliosis and severe fixed hip flexion contracture, appropriate sitting balance can be restored by means of a subtrochanteric posterior wedge resection osteotomy to allow extension of the femur below the fixed contracture. Caution must be exercised, however, to calculate the effective range of motion of the hip joint preoperatively, since extension is gained at the expense of the same degree of passive flexion of the hip joint. Occasionally, a femoral head resection with soft tissue interposition and postoperative traction is indicated for the child with an ankylosed hip that prevents proper sitting balance; however, heterotopic bone formation is a possible complication of this procedure. In summary, the major goal of hip surgery is to achieve a painless mobile hip and not a reduced hip that is both stiff and painful.

SPINE

Scoliosis. Scoliosis in children with myelomeningocele may be congenital or developmental in origin. The major predictive factors for developmental scoliosis are the neuro-

TABLE 5. GUIDELINES FOR HIP SURGERY		
Motor Level	Functional Expectation	Procedure
Thoracic	Mobile hips, self-transfers	Soft tissue releases, rare intertrochanteric extension osteotomy
L1–2	Upright stance early years, self-transfers	Soft tissue releases, rare varus osteotomy
L3–4	Walking first decade, continued ambulation markedly decreased in adolescence	? Transfer iliopsoas or external oblique to greater trochanter, adductor to ischium, femoral osteotomy
L5	Good functional expectations	Muscle transfer plus femoral and occipital pelvic osteotomy
Sacral	Best prognosis	Any of the above but caveat: Preserve mobility and prevent stiffness

logical level and the level of the last intact laminar arch.[28] The tethered cord syndrome has been implicated as a causative factor for scoliosis, but, to date, there have been no long-term clinical studies to substantiate this hypothesis. The prevalence of scoliosis relates directly to the motor level, ranging from 20% in sacral levels to 94% in thoracic levels. The average rate of progression of deformity is 5 degrees per year in the preadolescent patient.[29]

Brace treatment for paralytic scoliosis is difficult. Any anesthetic truncal skin will not tolerate isolated corrective forces; therefore, a total contact spinal orthosis is preferred. Bracing may slow the progression of deformity but will not be effective for curves greater than 45 degrees.[30] The orthosis may temporarily assist in sitting balance, thus freeing the upper extremities, but close monitoring of structural curves approaching 50 degrees should be done every 6 to 10 months, recording the structural deformity on supine bending radiographs. Once the curve exceeds 50 degrees on forced bending, surgery is indicated.

The results of posterior arthrodesis alone have been historically poor owing to the deficient laminar arches, poor skin coverage, and high rate of perioperative complications. Circumferential, anterior, and posterior arthrodesis with posterior segmental spinal instrumentation has been most effective in obtaining curve correction, a solid arthrodesis, and elimination of pelvic obliquity (Fig. 4).[31, 32] The introduction of better fixation devices allows anterior fusion of only some thoracolumbar and lumbar curves. Recently, posterior arthrodesis alone, augmented by pedicle screw fixation, was reported,[33] but long-term follow-up studies are not yet available.

Scoliosis surgery for myelomeningocele has the highest associated perioperative complication rates reported in the treatment of neuromuscular scoliosis. Therefore, detailed preoperative planning is essential to assess shunt patency by computed tomography scan and the spinal cord by magnetic resonance imaging for unrecognized severe Chiari's deformities, syrinx formation, lipomas, or split cord malformations (Fig. 5). Preoperative urodynamic studies as well as nutritional assessment is critical. In addition to paralysis and uncontrolled hydrocephalus, adherence of the neural

placode at the site of repair of the lesion may be implicated in the development of smaller curves. Small, nonstructural curves in association with headaches, back pain, spasticity, altered urinary or motor function, progressive foot deformity, or rapid increase in spinal curvature may be due to tethering, and neurosurgical consultation should be obtained prior to performing spinal arthrodesis.[34] For those patients presenting with larger structural curves and severe spasticity of the lower extremities, rhizotomy or distal cordectomy may be indicated at the time of the posterior fusion.

The patient is in the best physiological condition at the time of the first surgical procedure; therefore, whenever possible, anterior and posterior arthrodeses should be performed in one stage. Earlier reports indicated that extending the fusion to the pelvis resulted in patients' losing the ability to ambulate. In retrospect, many patients in these reports were children in the early second decade treated by a posterior arthrodesis and Harrington instrumentation followed by recumbency and casting. Current surgical techniques provide rigid stability of the spine, and by the age of 10 years, children with midlumbar to thoracic level paralysis are self-selecting a wheelchair for enhanced, more energy-efficient mobility.

With modern implants, spinal fusion can be limited to the lower lumbar spine for those curves not extending to the pelvis. There is a 5% reported incidence of spondylolisthesis in children with myelomeningocele, however,[35] and the long-term effects of the lever arm of a fusion on the few remaining motion segments in the insensate lumbar spine are not known.

Kyphosis. The prevalence of kyphosis is between 10% and 15% of all patients. The deformity is most often a severe and rigid lumbar deformity with wedging of the apical vertebra but may also be a long, sweeping flexible kyphosis that corrects on hyperextension of the spine. The latter deformity can be managed with a total contact orthosis during the early years of growth followed by anterior-release, interbody fusion, and posterior arthrodesis at a later age. The former deformity presents a formidable surgical challenge because the overlying skin is often severely compromised. In these cases, the kyphotic deformity is amenable to a direct posterior approach with transection of the distal dural sac and rudimentary placode followed by resection/decancellation of selective apical vertebral bodies to correct the deformity. A limited fusion at the level of the resection/decancellation is performed in younger children. With increasing age, the fusion must be extended to include the entire spine, as deformity above the level of resection with further growth is inevitable. It is important to note the fact that the central canal of the spinal cord remains open in these patients and often serves as an additional route for decompression of spinal fluid. The cord should not be tied off at the time of transection, as fatalities have been reported. Rather the dural sac should be oversewn with watertight closure distal to the level of the resected end of the spinal cord.

For the older child of 4 years of age, resection of the upper limb of the kyphotic deformity, which includes the lordotic segment immediately cephalad to apical vertebra, is indicated.[36] Fixation by means of a double right-angle contoured Luque rod inserted into the first sacral foramina

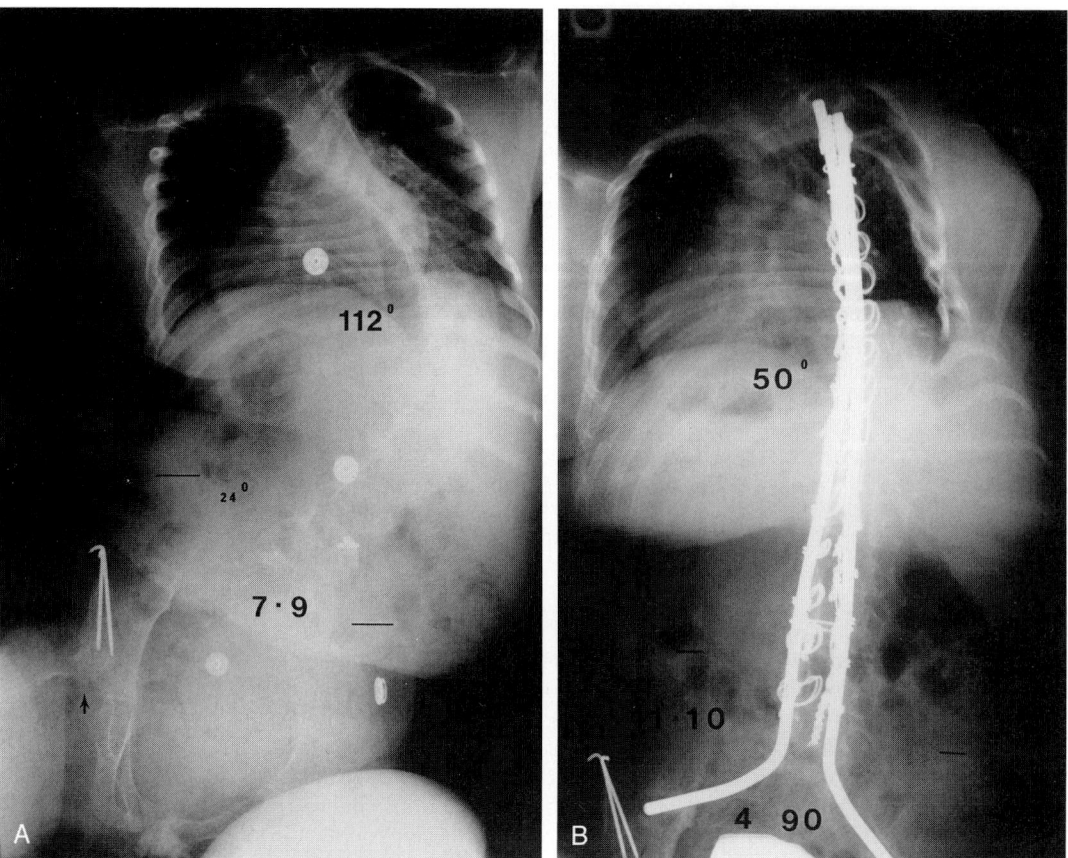

Fig. 4. Views. *A,* Anteroposterior radiograph of a 7-year, 9-month-old child with a 112-degree-long sweeping thoracolumbar scoliosis. Note the unsuccessful attempted surgical reconstruction for the right hip, which remains dislocated. *B,* Anteroposterior radiograph of the same child following a two-stage anterior T4-L5 fusion followed by a second-stage posterior arthrodesis from T3 to the pelvis, utilizing the Luque-Galveston technique of segmental spinal fixation.

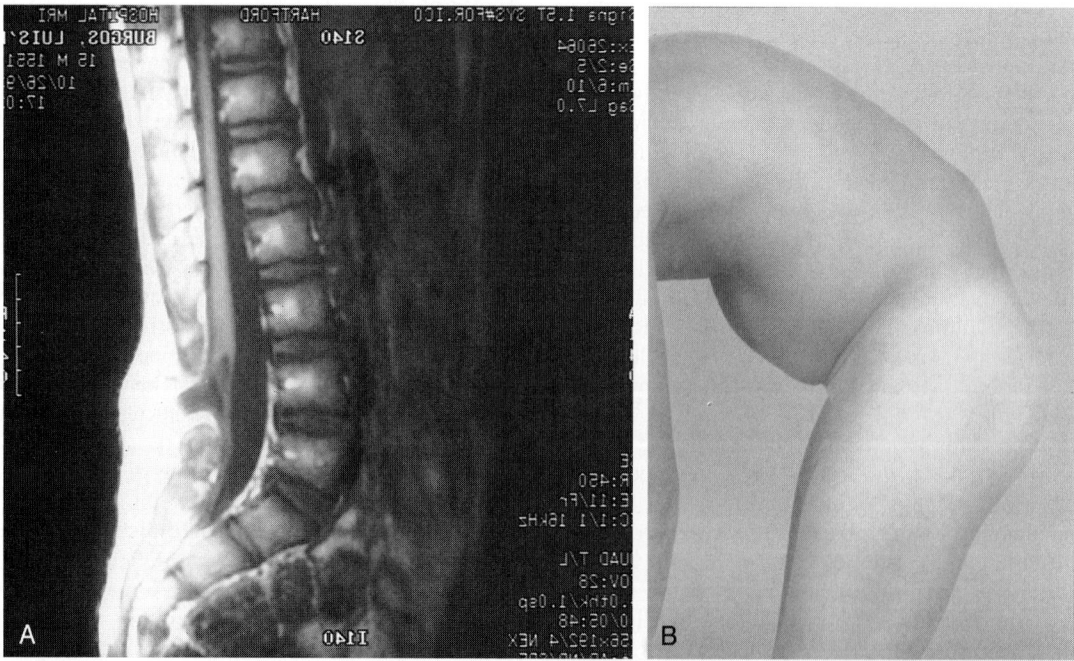

Fig. 5. Views. *A,* Magnetic resonance image of the lumbar spine demonstrating a low-lying conus medullaris with posterior adherence to a lipoma. *B,* Clinical photograph of the same child demonstrating the mid-lumbar skin-covered swelling of the lipoma.

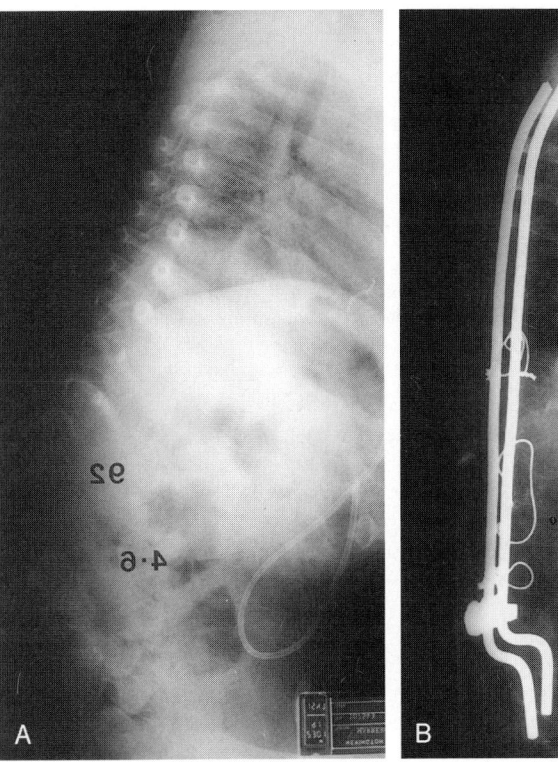

Fig. 6. Radiographs. *A,* Lateral radiograph of a 4-year, 6-month-old male with a 92-degree midlumbar kyphosis. *B,* Lateral radiograph of the same child 2 years later demonstrating the correction obtained following resection of the upper limb of the kyphotic segment. Fixation with two Luque rods contoured to fit through the first sacral foramina was used to restore normal sagittal alignment. Merseline tapes had been used to secure the upper thoracic laminar arches to the rods with spinal fusion only at the level of the kyphosis to allow for further longitudinal spinal growth.

provides optimal fixation of the lower spinal segment and pelvis and can be attached with sublaminar wires beneath the intact cephalad lamina (Fig. 6).[37] In contrast to acquired kyphotic deformity caused by trauma or sepsis, the aorta in children with congenital kyphosis spans the kyphotic defect, but the kidneys are often within the concavity of the deformity; thus meticulous dissection and hemostasis are required.[38]

COMPLICATIONS

Latex allergy is a serious, potentially lethal complication for patients with myelomeningocele. Even the most purified latex products have a residual 2% latex protein allergen. A 27 Da NRL protein has been identified in sensitized patients. The prevalence of latex allergy has been estimated to range from 34% to 64%.[39] In addition, these children also demonstrate a cross-sensitivity to ethylene oxide–exposed products as well. It is postulated that children develop sensitization to these agents as a result of repeated surgical procedures as well as repeated catheterizations. In addition to obtaining a complete history from the patient and family, there is an increased risk of latex allergy in any child with a history of atopy. Therefore, the best prophylaxis against latex reaction is to provide a totally latex-free environment in both the operating room and the outpatient clinic areas.[40]

Skin ulcers on the back are directly related to anesthetic skin, and kyphotic spinal deformity on the pelvis to scoliosis and pelvic obliquity, and on the lower extremities to weightbearing pressures. The major causes of pressure sore formation in the ambulatory child are due to foot deformity, restricted foot and ankle motion, and arthrodesis of the foot.[41]

Fractures are common in the child with high-level paralysis because of muscle weakness and subsequent decreased bone mineralization. Joint contractures and prolonged immobilization following surgery are additional predisposing factors. Most fractures in myelomeningocele children are diaphyseal or metaphyseal fractures of the femur and tibia. The most common clinical presentation of a fracture in an insensate limb is painless swelling, overlying warmth, and a low-grade fever. Beside obvious diaphyseal and metaphyseal fractures, there can be subtle physeal fractures not readily identifiable on initial radiographs that may become apparent 7 to 14 days later as periosteal new bone formation or juxtaepiphyseal bone resorption, which may mimic sepsis or neoplasia. Most diaphyseal and metaphyseal fractures respond to immobilization with soft bulky splints, frequent change of position to prevent pressure sore formation, and rapid return to external orthoses that provide support and allow weightbearing yet permit skin inspection.

Physeal fractures also occur in these children as a result of repetitive stress. The pathophysiology of these injuries is somewhat similar to that of Charcot's arthropathy. A typical presentation is an indolent onset of swelling in the region of the involved physis. Physeal fractures may require a longer period of cast immobilization.[42]

The evolution of multidisciplinary clinics to offer competent, integrated advice has provided the best medical management for these individuals. Current financial constraints in the delivery of health care resulting in the disbanding of such integrated clinics have resulted in increased morbidity, with a noted increase in the rate of amputation and nephrectomy in older patients.[43]

REFERENCES

1. Beaty JH, Canale ST: Orthopaedic aspects of myelomeningocele, in Current Concepts Review, J Bone Joint Surg Am 1990; 72: 626.

2. Kinsman SL, Doehring MC: The cost of preventable conditions in adults with spina bifida. Eur J Pediatr Surg 1996; 6(Suppl 1):17.

3. Shurtleff DB, Lemire RJ: Epidemiology, etiologic factors, and prenatal diagnosis of open spinal dysraphism. Neurosurg Clin North Am 1995; (6):183.

4. Pang D: Split cord malformation. In Disorders of the Pediatric Spine. New York, Raven Press, 1995, p 203.

5. Babcock C J: Ultrasound evaluation of the prenatal and neonatal spina bifida. Neurosurg Clin North Am 1995; 6:203.

6. Wald NJ: Folic acid and neural tube defects: The current evidence and implications for prevention. Ciba Foundation Symposium 181, Neural Tube Defects. West Sussex, England, John Wiley & Sons, 1994, p 192.

7. Seller MJ: Risks in spina bifida, annotation. Dev Med Child Neurol 1994; 36: 1021.

8. Minns RA: Folic acid and neural tube defects. Spinal Cord 1996; 34:460.

9. O'Rahilly R, Muller F: Neurulation in the normal human embryo. Ciba Foundaton Symposium 181, Neural Tube Defects. West Sussex, England, John Wiley & Sons, 1994, p 70.

10. Gothkelch N: Aspects of the surgical management of myelomeningocele: A review article. Dev Med Child Neurol 1986; 28: 525.

11. Hoffer MM, Feiwell E, Perry R, et al: Functional ambulation in patients with myelomeningocele. J Bone Joint Surg Am 1973; 55:137.

12. Asher M, Olsen J: Factors affecting the ambulatory status of patients with spina bifida cystica. J Bone Joint Surg Am 1983; 65:350.

13. Samuelsson L, Skoog M: Ambulaton in patients with myelomeningocele: A multivariate statistical analysis. J Pediatr Orthop 1988; 8:569.

14. Brinker MR, Rosenfeld SR, Feiwell E, et al: Myelomeningocele at the sacral level. J Bone Joint Surg Am 1994; 76:1293.

15. Banta JV: The Orthopaedic History of Spinal Dysraphism II, The Modern Surgical Treatment, Review article, Journal of Developmental Medicine and Child Neurology, 1996; 38,954.

16. Neto JC, Dias LS, Gabrieli AP: Congenital talipes equinovarus in spina bifida: Treatment and results. J Pediatr Orthop 1996; 16:782.

17. Harris MB, Banta JV: Cost of skin care in the myelomeningocele populaton. J Pediatr Orthop 1990; 10:355.

18. Bliss DG, Menelaus MB: The results of transfer of the tibialis anterior to the heel in patients who have a myelomeningocele. J Bone Joint Surg Am 1986; 68:1258.

19. Marshall PD, Broughton NS, Menelaus MB, et al: Surgical release of knee flexion contractures in myelomeningocele. J Bone Joint Surg Br 1996; 78:912.

20. Williams JJ, Graham GP, Dunne KB, et al: Late knee problems in myelomeningocele. J Pediatr Orthop 1993; 13:701.

21. Thomson JD, Ouunpu S, Davis RB, et al: The effects of ankle foot orthoses in the ankle and knee in persons with myelomeningocele. J Pediatr Orthop 1999; 19:27.

22. Menelaus MB: The hip in myelomeningocele: Management directed toward a minimum number of operations and a minimum period of immobilization. J Bone Joint Surg Br 1976; 58:448.

23. Feiwell E, Downey DS, Blatt T: The effect of hip reduction on function in patients with myelomeningocele. J Bone Joint Surg Am 1978; 60:169.

24. Broughton NS, Menelaus MB: The natural history of hip deformity in myelomen-fjingocele. J Bone Joint Surg Br 1993, 75: 760.

25. Fraser RK, Hoffman EB, Sparks LJ, Buccimazza SS: The unstable hip and mid lumbar myelomeningocele. J Bone Joint Surg Br 1992; 74:143.

26. Mannor DA, Weinstein SL, Dietz FR: Long term follow-up of Chiari pelvic osteotomy in myelomeningocele. J Pediatr Orthop 1996; 16:769.

27. Keggi JM, Banta JV, Walton C: The myelodysplastic hip and scoliosis. Dev Med Child Neurol 1992; 34:240.

28. Piggott H: The natural history of scoliosis in myelomeningocele. J Bone Joint Surg Br 1980; 62:54.

29. Muller EB, Nordwall A: Prevalence of scoliosis in children with myelomeningocele in Western Sweden. Spine 1992; 17: 1097.

30. Muller EB, Nordwall A: Brace treatment of scoliosis in children with myelomeningocele. Spine 1994; 19:151.

31. Osebold WR, Mayfield JK, Winter RB, et al: Surgical treatment of paralytic scoliosis associated with myelomeningocele. J Bone Joint Surg Am 1982; 64:841.

32. McMaster MJ: Anterior and posterior instrumentation and fusion of thoracolumbar scoliosis due to myelomeningocele. J Bone Joint Surg Br 1987; 69:20.

33. Rodgers WB, Frim DM, Emans JB: Surgery of the spine in myelodysplasia: An overview. Clin Orthop Rel Res 1997; 338: 19.

34. Banta JV, Drummond D, Ferguson RL: Teatment of neuromuscular scoliosis. In Zuckerman JD (ed): Instructional Course Lecture, vol 48. American Academy of Orthopaedic Surgeons, Rosemont, IL, 1999, p 557.

35. Stanitsky CL, Stanitsky DF, LaMont RL: Spondylolisthesis in myelomeningocele. J Pediatr Orthop 1994; 14:586.

36. Lintner S, Lindseth RE: Kyphotic deformity in patients who have a myelomeningocle. J Bone Joint Surg Am 1994; 76: 1301.

37. Jwarner WC, Fackler CD: Comparison of two instrumentation techniques in treatment of lumbar kyphosis in myelodysplasia. J Pediatr Orthop 1993; 13:704.

38. Fromm B, Carstens C, Niethard FU, et al: Aortography in children with myelomeningocele and lumbar kyphosis. J Bone Joint Surg Br 1992; 74:691.

39. Niggemann T, Moers A, Seidel U, et al: Risk factors for latex allergy in patients with spina bifida. J Clin Exp Allergy 1996; 26:934.

40. Birmingham PK, Dsida RM, Grayhack JJ, et al: Do latex precautions in children with myelodysplasia reduce intraoperative allergic reactions? J Pediatr Orthop 1996; 16: 799.

41. Maynard MJ, Weiner LS, Burke SW: Neuropathic foot ulceration in patients with myelodysplasia. J Pediatr Orthop 1992; 12:786.

42. Banta JV: Fractures in the myelomeningocele child. In Letts RM (ed): Management of Pediatric Fractures. New York, Churchill Livingstone; 1944, p 1063.

43. Kaufman BA, Terbrock A, Winters N, et al: Disbanding a multidisciplinary clinic: Effects on the health care of myelomeningocele patients. Pediatr Neurosurg 1994; 21:36.

HEREDITARY SENSORY MOTOR NEUROPATHIES

Brian G. Smith

Summary
- These neuropathies are characterized by demyelination of peripheral nerves and distal motor weakness.
- The inheritance pattern is variable, although often autosomal dominant.
- The clinical manifestations are variable, even within families.
- Electrophysiological studies typically demonstrate delay in nerve conduction.
- Typical deformities include cavovarus feet and claw toes.
- Appropriate treatment can maximize walking function and minimize foot deformity.

DEFINITION

The heredity sensory motor neuropathies (HSMNs) comprise a group of inherited disorders characterized by progressive motor and sensory neuropathies producing distal extremity weakness and deformity. Formerly known as Charcot-Marie-Tooth disease (CMT) and peroneal muscular atrophy, these conditions demonstrate delays in nerve conduction studies (NCSs) and are identified by genetic defects involving duplications, primarily on chromosomes 1 and 17.

HISTORICAL REVIEW

1886: Jean Martin Charcot and Pierre Marie in Paris and Howard Henry Tooth in England separately described CMT.

1959: Dwyer described calcaneal osteotomy for hindfoot varus.

1968: Dyck and Lambert provided first comprehensive classification scheme for CMT.

1975: Classification of seven types by Dyck, adopted by most neurologists and geneticists.[1]

1990s: Explosion of information on molecular genetics and identification of genetic defects in the HSMNs.

PATHOGENESIS

The HSMN disorders affect approximately 125,000 people in the United States, with an incidence of about 1 in 2500.[2] Although originally thought to be primarily of autosomal-dominant inheritance, advancements in genetic research in the past decade now document transmission via the recessive and sex-linked modes of inheritance as well.

The primary defect of the HSMN disorders is demyelination of peripheral nerves. The duplication on chromosome 17 in CMT 1A includes the gene for peripheral myelin protein 22 (PMP-22). PMP-22 comprises about 2% to 5% of the total myelin protein and is found in the compact myelin of Schwann's cells.[3] Analysis of genetic mutations and histological findings in other HSMNs suggests that PMP-22 has a role in myelin composition of axons and Schwann cells.[3, 4] Although the precise role of PMP-22 is not known, it may be involved in the adhesion of axons and Schwann cells.[3, 4]

The myelin protein zero (MPZ) gene on chromosome 1 encodes the protein PO, a glycoprotein that composes 50% of peripheral myelin protein. Point mutations in the MPZ gene have been identified in CMT 1B.[3]

Connexin 32 (Cx32) is a gap junction protein. Gap junctions are intercellular aqueous channels permitting the cytoplasmic passage of ions between adjacent cells. The precise function of Cx32 in peripheral nerves remains elusive,[5] but analysis of mutations in patients with CMT X reveals abnormalities in the X chromosome at q13.1, the location of the Cx32 gene.

GENETIC FEATURES

Although originally thought to be much higher, fully 76% of cases of HSMN are autosomal dominant.[6] New mutations often account for a significant portion of the remainder of CMT cases discovered each year.

CLASSIFICATION

The original classification schemes were based on electrophysiological differences and the amount of delay on NCSs.[7] Within the last decade, genetic analysis has guided classification, and a new system based on the genetic defect has been developed (Table 1).[1, 5]

CMT 1A is the most common HSMN, comprising 50% to 60% of cases.[2] It is also known as hypertrophic, demyelinating, and axonal-type CMT. Patients with CMT 1A demonstrate moderate to severe slowing on motor and NCSs. NCS slowing in CMT patients is evident 2 years before the clinical manifestations of the disease and remains stable 5 years after the onset of symptoms.[3] The severity of slowing on NCSs does not correlate with the clinical severity of the disease. However, the reduction of compound muscle action potentials does correlate with clinical involvement.[3] Likewise, the degree of NCS delay in CMT 1A patients can vary widely, even between family members. Even greater than the variability of conduction delay is that of the clinical manifestations in CMT 1A patients, even in those with similar conduction disorders.[8]

Peripheral nerve biopsies in CMT 1A patients show demyelination, remyelination, and hypertrophic changes characterized by "onion bulb" formation of circumferentially aligned Schwann's cells around axonal internodes.[3, 6] In

TABLE 1. HEREDITARY SENSORY MOTOR NEUROPATHIES						
CMT Subtypes	**Genetic Locus/ Disorder**	**Gene Product**	**Age at Onset**	**Initial Symptoms**	**Nerve Conduction Velocity**	**Pathological Features**
CMT 1A	17p11.2-12 duplication	PMP-22	First, second decades of life	Distal leg weakness	Moderately to severely slowed	"Onion bulbs"; decreased number of myelinated fibers
CMT 1B	1q22.23 point mutation	PO	First decade of life	Distal leg weakness	Moderately to severely slowed	"Onion bulbs"; decreased number of myelinated fibers
CMT 1C	Unknown	Unknown	First decade of life	Distal leg weakness	Moderately to severely slowed	"Onion bulbs"; decreased number of myelinated fibers
Dejerine-Sottas disease	17p11.2-12 duplication/ mutation	PMP-22	Early childhood	Severe muscle weakness	Severely slowed	More severe than CMT 1
CMT X	X q13.1 point mutation	Cx32	First, second decades of life	Distal leg weakness	Slowed	Decreased number of myelinated fibers
CMT 2	1 p unknown	Unknown	Second, third, or later decade	Distal leg weakness	Normal to slightly slowed	Axonal degeneration; decreased number of large myelinated fibers

CMT, Charcot-Marie-Tooth disease.

slender CMT 1A patients, the hypertrophied peripheral nerves may be palpable (ulna, peroneal) or even visible (greater auricular nerve).[8]

CMT 1B is also autosomal dominant but is much less common than CMT 1A and has been documented in only a handful of families worldwide.[5] CMT 1C is also autosomal dominant and very rare. Its genetic defect has not been determined, mapping neither to chromosome 17 nor chromosome 1.[2, 3]

Accounting for about 10% to 20% of HSMNs, X-linked CMT (CMT X) may occur in X-linked dominant (CMT X1) or X-linked recessive (CMT X2) forms. Conduction delay in these patients is intermediate.[7] The absence of male-to-male transmission and the tendency for males to be more affected than females typify these disorders.[6] Clinical symptoms appear in the first two decades. Fifty percent of female carriers are asymptomatic.[6]

CMT 2 is inherited as an autosomal-dominant condition. At the time this chapter was written, the affected gene was unidentified, although some studies suggested a linkage to the short arm of chromosome 1.[6] NCSs distinguish between CMT 1 and CMT 2 patients; the latter group has nerve conduction velocities (NCVs) only mildly to moderately decreased, often 80% to 90% of normal but never less than 60% of normal. The clinical manifestations of the neuronal degeneration of CMT 2 patients are similar to the electrophysiological findings with a later age of presentation, often not until the fourth decade, with less severe symptoms.

Originally classified as HSMN type III in 1975, Dejerine-Sottas disease was described as a more severe HSMN with an autosomal-recessive inheritance pattern. Molecular genetics studies now cast doubt that Dejerine-Sottas disease is a single entity, because the genetic findings in "diagnosed" patients are so heterogeneous.[6] Dejerine-Sottas disease patients have thin or absent myelin sheaths, typically present in the first decade, are more severely involved with a more progressive course, and have profoundly decreased NCVs.[7]

CLINICAL FEATURES

Charcot and Marie described the primary clinical features of HSMNs more than 100 years ago. These include a progressive lower extremity weakness and muscular atrophy that produces muscle imbalance, foot and ankle deformities, and gait impairment.[8, 9] The typical patient with CMT 1A presents in late childhood or adolescence with complaints of tripping and falling, frequent ankle sprains, alteration of gait to accommodate a footdrop, foot pain or difficulty wearing shoes, or generalized clumsiness.[8] Specific early complaints related to foot problems may include weakness, painful corns and calluses, difficulty finding comfortable shoes, heel pain, ankle instability, and claw toe deformities.[9]

Patients with severe lower extremity[3] involvement originally were described as having inverted champagne bottle legs by Charcot and Marie (also known as stork leg appearance). Only about 20% of CMT patients are severely disabled to the point of being nonambulatory.[6]

Upper extremity involvement occurs later and often after lower extremity signs are well established. A slow progression of weakness involving the intrinsic muscles impairs fine motor control, may cause frequent cramps, and eventually causes claw hand deformities. Approximately two-thirds of patients with CMT experience hand symptoms, which begin in the second or third decade or later.[10]

Common clinical findings include diminished or absent deep tendon reflexes; lower extremity weakness; foot deformities, including claw or hammer toe deformities; and hand weakness. Sensory examination findings include preservation of pain and temperature sensation with impairment of light touch, proprioception, and vibration.[2] Balance problems and tremors are also common.[2]

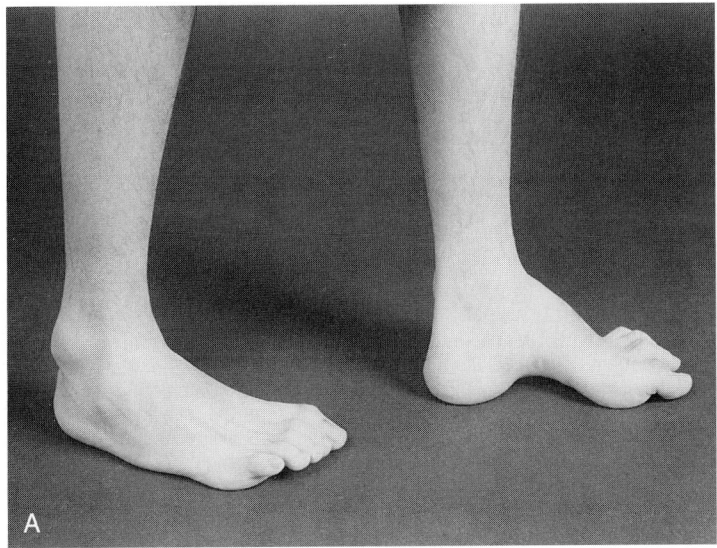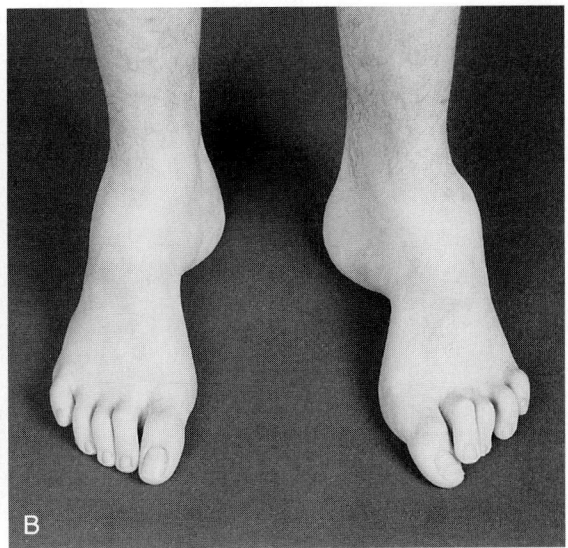

Fig. 1. Charcot-Marie-Tooth disease. A 13-year-old boy with severe cavovarus foot deformities. Clinical appearance from the medial side *(A)* and frontal view *(B)* demonstrating cavus and forefoot deformities.

Associated conditions in CMT patients include hip dysplasia and scoliosis. Walker et al[11] documented hip dysplasia in 6% of 100 patients with CMT. Dysplasia was more frequent in girls and more common in patients with CMT 1.

Scoliosis occurs more frequently than previously identified in CMT patients. In a review of 100 patients, Walker et al reported an incidence of 37%.[12] Kyphosis occurred with or without scoliosis in nearly 20% of patients. Spinal deformity was found more commonly in girls and in patients with CMT 1. Four of the 37 patients in the study required treatment.[12]

The hallmark of CMT is a progressive cavus foot with elevation of the medial longitudinal arch. Pes cavus is often associated with claw toe deformity and hindfoot varus (Fig. 1). Associated problems include lateral ankle instability, painful corns and calluses, difficulty with shoe wear, and impairment of balance and gait.[9] A flexible deformity that is initially flexible often becomes fixed and rigid and more symptomatic as the weakness progresses (Fig. 2).

The pathogenesis of the cavus foot has been a source of interest and controversy for many years. One theory proposes that weakness of intrinsic muscles of the foot causes hyperextension of the metatarsophalangeal joints, claw toe deformities, and a windlass effect with plantar flexion of the metatarsals and progressive contracture of the plantar fascia.[9] Another theory is based on cavus resulting from a relatively strong peroneus longus muscle causing plantar flexion of the first metatarsal in the presence of a weakened anterior tibialis muscle. The cavus and hindfoot varus is exacerbated by the overpull of the posterior tibialis over the relatively weak peroneus brevis.[10]

INVESTIGATION

CMT is diagnosed on the basis of a history and physical exam consistent with signs and symptoms of a peripheral neuropathy. Family history is often positive. Electromyographic studies and particularly NCVs are highly reliable for the confirmation of diffuse and uniform slowing, a defining characteristic of HSMNs.[8] Blood tests for genetic diagnosis of CMT 1A and CMT X are available.

The characteristic radiographic findings of pes cavus, forefoot adduction, hindfoot varus, and plantar flexion of the first metatarsal are demonstrated on standing radiographs of the foot (see Fig. 2).

DIFFERENTIAL DIAGNOSIS

Like CMT patients, those with distal spinal muscular atrophy (SMA) demonstrate distal weakness and atrophy with preservation of sensation. Foot deformities and contractures are common, and this disorder may also be inherited in a autosomal-dominant or autosomal-recessive manner.[7] Electrophysiological studies demonstrate distal motor degeneration in the presence of normal NCVs.[7] CMT also may be confused with distal SMA and Refsum's disease.[3, 7]

The differential diagnosis of a cavus foot deformity is varied and includes congenital, developmental, and neuromuscular causes. Bilateral cavus feet might occur secondary to spinal cord tumors, spinal dysraphia, diastematomyelia, polio, and Friedreich's ataxia. Unilateral cavus foot deformities should prompt consideration of a tethered spinal cord, polio, crush injury to the foot, and residuals of deep posterior compartment syndrome.[9] Idiopathic pes cavus should be a diagnosis of last resort.[13]

MANAGEMENT

Evaluation of gait and assessment of the flexibility of the hindfoot are essential in evaluating these foot deformities in CMT. Coleman described a test in which a 1-inch block is placed along the lateral border of the forefoot to demonstrate both flexibility of the hindfoot and the contribution of forefoot plantar flexion to the hindfoot varus[14] (Fig. 3).

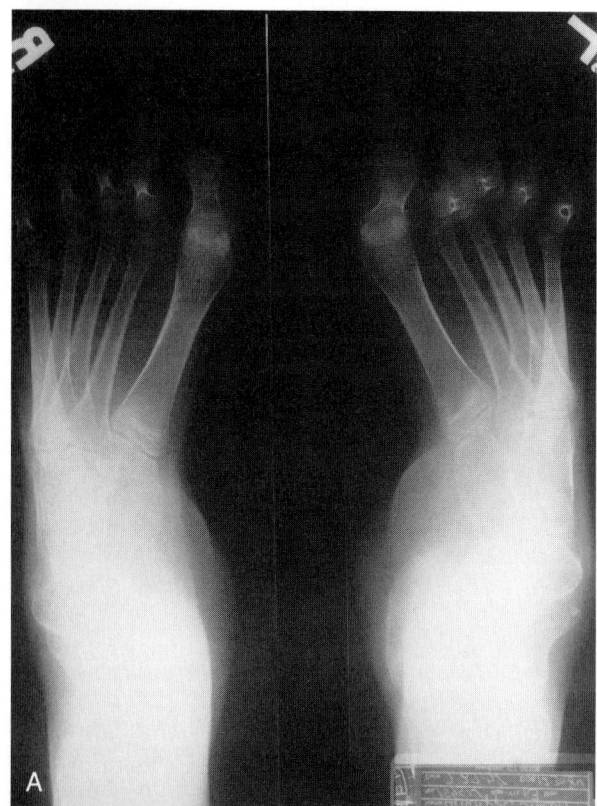

Fig. 2. **Charcot-Marie-Tooth disease.** Standing preoperative radiographs of patient in Figure 1. *A,* Anteroposterior view of both feet. *B,* True lateral film of ankle. *C,* True lateral film of forefoot depicting the severe forefoot adduction. Note also on lateral film the decrease in Hibbs' calcaneal–first metatarsal angle (normal, 140 degrees) (angle H) and increase in Meary's first metatarsal-calcaneus angle (normal, 0 to 10 degrees) (angle M).

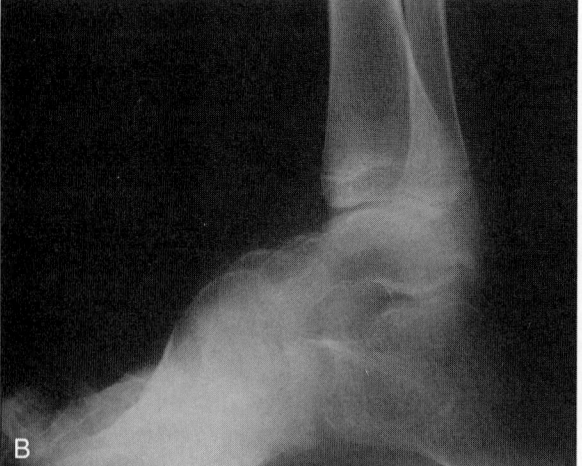

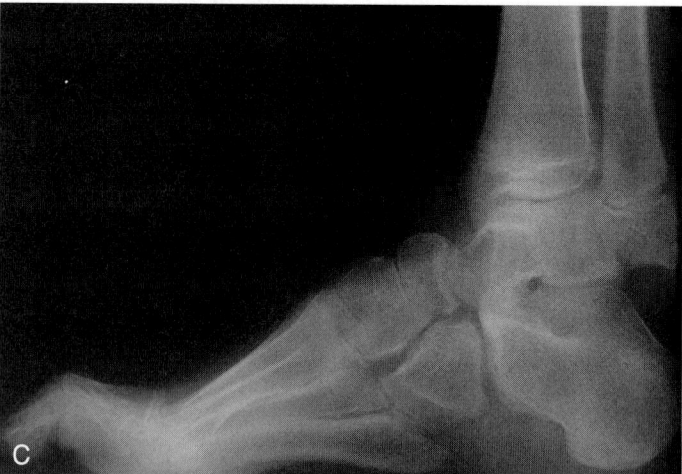

Flexible foot deformities can be managed by bracing or shoe modifications. Nonoperative options for the flexible cavovarus foot include a stretching program of the plantar fascia, extra-depth shoes to accommodate claw toes, an orthotic with a lateral heel wedge to minimize hindfoot varus, and, for patients with footdrop, an ankle-foot orthosis.[9] Because of the progressive nature of CMT, nonoperative treatment may not have long-term therapeutic benefit.

Operative treatment of pes cavus has evolved considerably in the last 75 years. The most common soft-tissue procedure is plantar fasciotomy with subsequent serial casting to correct cavus deformity. Restoring muscle balance by tendon transfer may improve function and minimize recurrent deformity. Muscle-balancing procedures include transfer of the posterior tibialis muscle through the interosseous membrane to the dorsum of the foot (usually middle cuneiform) to assist with dorsiflexion in the presence of a weak anterior tibialis muscle. Transfer of the peroneus longus muscle to the brevis muscle may restore lateral eversion strength. The modified Jones procedure includes transfer of the extensor hallucis longus to the first metatarsal to retain its dorsiflexion power while minimizing metarsophalangeal hyperextension and plantar flexion of the first ray. Arthrodesis of the interphalangeal joint of the great toe is done at the same time to prevent flexion deformity (Fig. 4). Heel cord lengthening may be appropriate, providing that standing lateral radiographs do not demonstrate calcaneal cavus (excessive calcaneal declination).[9]

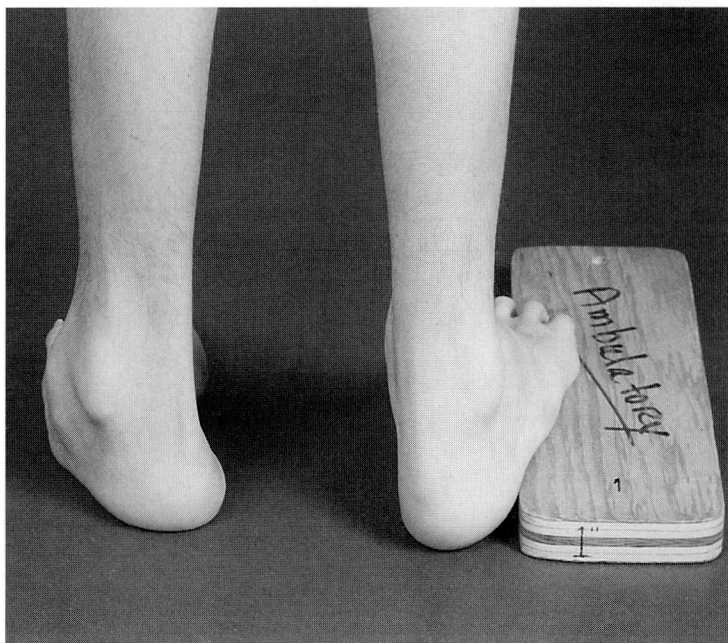

Fig. 3. Charcot-Marie-Tooth disease. Same patient as in Fig. 1. Significant hindfoot varus is evident in stance on left with correction of varus on right foot by a modified Coleman block test.

Bony procedures are necessary to correct fixed deformity. To correct a claw toe deformity, a Girdlestone-Taylor transfer of the flexor digitorum longus to the toe extensors with arthroplasty of the metaphalangeal and proximal interphalangeal points may be indicated. Radiographic assessment of Hibbs' angle and apex location has been suggested as a means to determine the site of corrective osteotomies in rigid cavus feet. Pes cavus located in the forefoot or midfoot may be addressed by dorsiflexion osteotomy through the proximal metatarsals in the skeletally mature foot or by closing dorsal wedge osteotomy in the midfoot tarsal area[9] (see Fig. 4).

Calcaneal osteotomies for pes cavovarus include the classic lateral closing wedge osteotomy, which Dwyer described in 1959. Other alternatives include a calcaneal slide osteotomy shifting the proximal portion laterally.[9] For calcaneal cavus, a crescentic sliding posterior displacement osteotomy may be the best option.[14]

The salvage procedure for correction of a severe deformity in mature feet is the triple arthrodesis. The Ryerson technique is most commonly used, in which appropriate wedges are removed from the talonavicular, subtalar, and calcaneal-cuboid joints laterally so as to correct forefoot adduction and hindfoot varus. The Lambrinudi triple arthrodesis may be performed in patients with fixed midfoot or forefoot equinus.[10] Internal fixation is used to maintain position and promote arthodesis. Given that CMT patients have decreased proprioception and impaired balance, appropriate tendon transfers to balance the foot or continued bracing is necessary to optimize outcome.[15] Scoliosis and hip dysplasia may be asymptomatic. Regular physical exams and screening radiographs should detect the problem.

Upper extremity involvement in patients with CMT is milder than lower extremity involvement. The primary problems affecting hand function include lack of opposition, weak pinch, and clawing of fingers. Simple occupational therapy measures such as splinting or grip modifications may minimize dysfunction for most patients. Tendon transfers may be appropriate in the relatively few patients who are severely involved.[16] However, these patients should understand that the muscle weakness is progressive.

COMPLICATIONS

The progression of distal atrophy and weakness also tends to compromise or complicate outcome of surgery about the foot in patients with CMT. Inadequate plantar release and overlengthening of the Achilles tendon are pitfalls to be avoided.[14] Osteotomies about the midfoot for fixed cavus deformities may be at risk for delayed union or nonunion, loss of fixation or position, and injury to the blood supply to the forefoot.[14] Dwyer's closing lateral wedge osteotomy may shorten the heel and cause excessive pressure at the base of the fifth metatarsal.[14]

Triple arthrodesis has a higher complication rate in CMT patients. Wukich and Bowen reported a 15% pseudarthrosis rate in their series of 22 patients (34 feet) undergoing triple arthrodesis, mostly at the talonavicular joint.[17] Furthermore, 60% of the patients in this study developed either over- or undercorrection, contributing to persistent deformity, asymmetric weightbearing, and an increased likelihood of callosities, pain, and poor outcome.[17] Drennan and Wetmore[15] obtained follow-up averaging nearly 21 years in 16 CMT patients undergoing 30 triple arthrodeses. They found that the results significantly declined with time. The long-term results of triple arthrodesis patients were "poor" in their study, primarily secondary to increased osteoarthritis at the ankle joint.[15] Similarly, Wukich and Bowen[17] reported that 68% of patients with triple arthrodeses had fair or poor outcomes at an average of 12 years postoperatively. The progressive nature of the peripheral neuropathy with in-

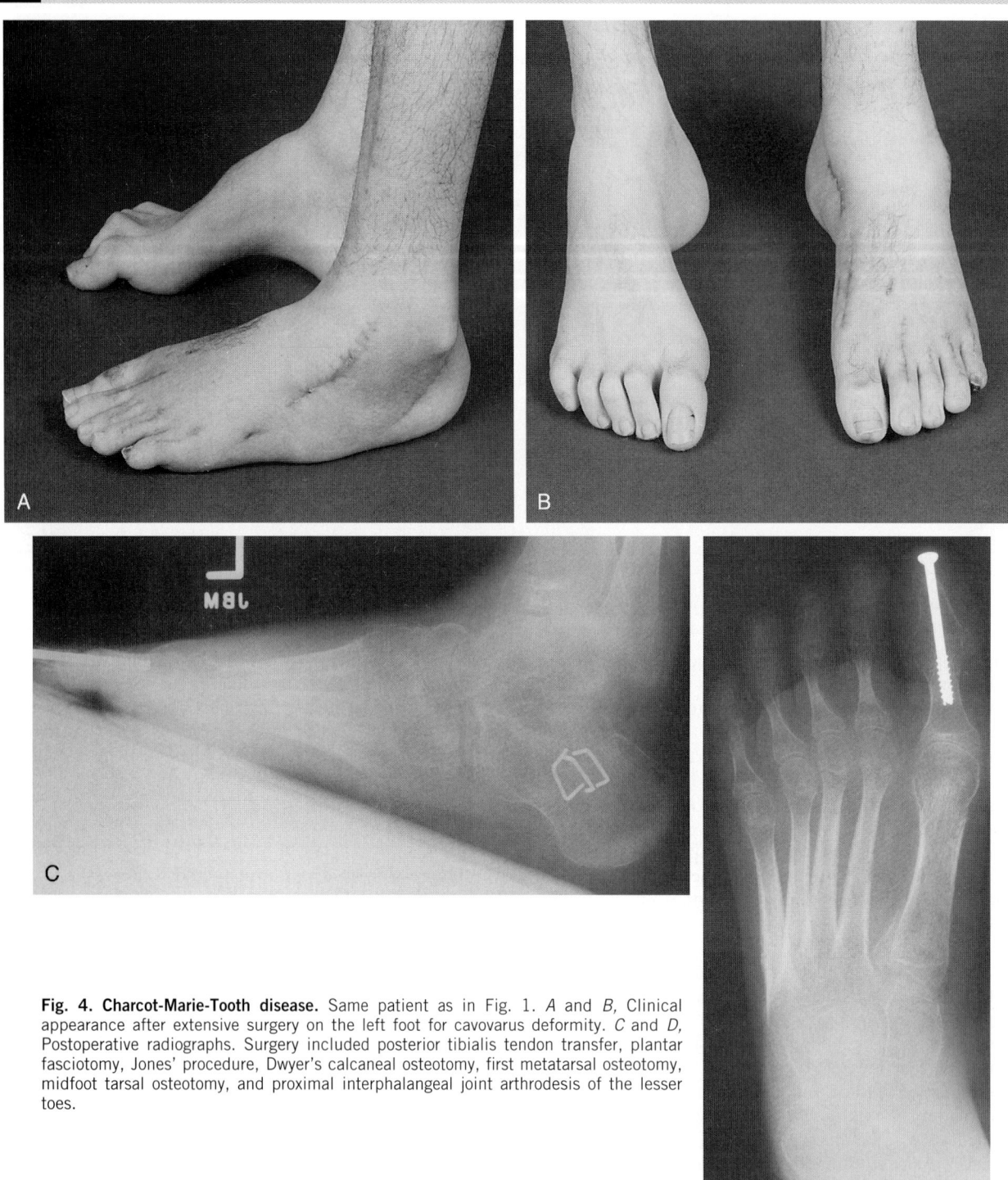

Fig. 4. Charcot-Marie-Tooth disease. Same patient as in Fig. 1. *A* and *B*, Clinical appearance after extensive surgery on the left foot for cavovarus deformity. *C* and *D*, Postoperative radiographs. Surgery included posterior tibialis tendon transfer, plantar fasciotomy, Jones' procedure, Dwyer's calcaneal osteotomy, first metatarsal osteotomy, midfoot tarsal osteotomy, and proximal interphalangeal joint arthrodesis of the lesser toes.

creasing weakness and impaired sensation in the presence of a fixed hindfoot served to increase loading at the ankle joint and cause early degeneration.[15] These authors and others suggested that early soft release coupled with tendon transfers and nonarticular osteotomies for correction of deformity may help prevent further deformity and the need for triple arthrodesis in CMT patients.[18]

Complications of surgical procedures in CMT patients

also are related to the peripheral neuropathy inherent in the disorder. For example, Kumar et al[19] experienced a high incidence of neurological problems in a series of CMT patients undergoing hip osteotomies for dysplasia. Likewise, intraoperative spinal cord monitoring in CMT patients undergoing spinal fusion surgery may be unreliable because of the peripheral neuropathy, requiring use of the intraoperative wake-up test to ensure safety.[10]

REFERENCES

1. Birouk N, Gouider R, Guern L, et al: Charcot-Marie-Tooth disease type 1A with 17p11.2 duplication. Brain 1997; 120:813.
2. Ionasescu V: Charcot-Marie-Tooth neuropathies: From clinical description to molecular genetics. Muscle Nerve 1995; 18:267.
3. Murakami T, Garcia C, Reiter L, et al: Charcot-Marie-Tooth disease and related neuropathies. Medicine 1996; 75:233.
4. Thomas P, King R, Small J, et al: The pathology of Charcot-Marie-Tooth disease and related disorders. Neuropathol Appl Neurobiol 1996; 22:269.
5. Harding A: From the syndrome of Charcot-Marie and Tooth to disorders of peripheral myelin proteins. Brain 1995; 118: 809.
6. Ouvrier R: Correlation between the histopathologic, genotypic and phenotypic features of hereditary peripheral neuropathies in childhood. J Child Neurol 1996; 11: 133.
7. England J, Garcia C: Electrophysiologic studies in different genotypes of Charcot-Marie-Tooth disease. Curr Opin Neurol 1996; 9:338.
8. Njegovan M, Leonard E, Joseph F: Rehabilitation medicine approach to Charcot-Marie-Tooth disease. Clin Podiatr Med Surg 1997; 14:99.
9. Holmes J, Hansen S: Foot and ankle manifestations of Charcot-Marie-Tooth disease. Foot Ankle 1993; 14:476.
10. Thompson G: Hereditary motor sensory neuropathies. In Morrissy R, Weinstein S (eds): Lovell and Winter's Pediatric Orthopaedics. Philadelphia, Lippincott-Raven, 1996, vol I, p 561.
11. Walker J, Nelson K, Heavilon J, et al: Hip abnormalities in children with Charcot-Marie-Tooth disease. J Pediatr Orthop 1994; 14:54.
12. Walker J, Nelson K, Stevens D, et al: Spinal deformity in Charcot-Marie-Tooth disease. Spine 1994; 19:1044.
13. Samilson R, Dillow W: Cavus, cavovarus and calcanocavus. Clin Orthop Rel Res 1983; 177:125.
14. Thometz J, Garcia J: Cavus deformity. In Drennan J (ed): The Child's Foot and Ankle. New York, Raven Press, 1992, p 343.
15. Wetmore R, Drennan J: Long term results of triple arthrodesis of Charcot-Marie-Tooth disease. J Bone Joint Surg Am 1989; 71: 417.
16. Wood V, Huene D, Nguyen J: Treatment of the upper limb in Charcot-Marie-Tooth disease. J Bone Joint Surg Br 1995; 20: 511.
17. Wukich D, Bowen J: A long-term study of triple arthrodesis for correction of pes cavovarus in Charcot-Marie-Tooth disease. J Pediatr Orthop 1989; 9:433.
18. Roper B, Tibrewal S: Soft tissue surgery in Charcot-Marie-Tooth disease. J Bone Joint Surg Br 1989; 71:17.
19. Kumar S, Marks H, Bowen J, et al: Hip dysplasia associated with Charcot-Marie-Tooth disease in the older child and adolescent. J Pediatr Orthop 1985; 5:511.

section 10 chapter 8

MUSCULAR DYSTROPHY

Michael D. Sussman

Summary

- Duchenne's muscular dystrophy (DMD) is an uncommon X-linked condition involving progressive loss of functional muscle and replacement with fibrofatty tissue.
- The genetic basis of DMD and Becker's muscular dystrophy (BMD), a related but milder condition, is an abnormality of dystrophin, a protein that stabilizes the myofiber membrane.
- Affected boys will walk late (after age 18 months), lose their ability to walk by age 11 to 12 years, after which they become progressively more disabled as a result of their muscle weakness. They usually die by age 20 as a result of respiratory muscle insufficiency.
- One issue facing the orthopaedic surgeon is the development of lower extremity contractures toward the end of the walking phase, which can be treated with contracture release in a select group of patients.
- The major orthopaedic issue is the development of scoliosis, which is seen in 90% of patients beginning at age 11 to 13 years and will progress to severe disabling deformity if not treated by spinal instrumentation and fusion.
- Spinal instrumentation and fusion of those patients in whom scoliosis develops should be undertaken as soon as the curve is identified, because the natural history in DMD is continued progression, which is relatively unaltered by any nonoperative intervention.

DMD is a genetically inherited disease of muscle with characteristic clinical, histological, and biochemical findings. It is caused by an abnormality in the gene for dystrophin, a cell membrane–associated protein, resulting in a total absence of dystrophin in muscle as well as in other tissues where dystrophin is also produced. In a very similar but related condition, known as BMD, there is also an alteration in the gene for dystrophin. However, in this case, a smaller dystrophin molecule in a smaller than normal amount is produced. These two conditions are referred to as "dystrophinopathies."[1]

HISTORICAL REVIEW

Although there were a few reports in the early 19th century of isolated patients with what probably was DMD, the seminal publication was by Guillaume Benjamin Amand Duchenne, who described his first case in 1861 and published 13 cases in 1868, including clinical photographs and muscle biopsies. Duchenne accumulated further cases, described the clinical course, and made particular note of the enlarged but weak muscles that he recognized were due to an excessive amount of fibrofatty tissue.[2] Subsequent studies over the next 130 years refined this original description and clarified the X-linked nature of the condition. However, they added little to our understanding of this condition until Kunkel, Hoffman, and their colleagues identified dystrophin as the underlying cause in 1988.[1]

EPIDEMIOLOGY

DMD is relatively rare; its incidence varies between two and three per 10,000 male live births. Of these cases, 70% to 80% can be traced to preceding generations, and the remainder are new mutations. It is thought that many of these new mutations arise in the sperm cell line on the paternal side of the mother of affected boys.[3]

PATHOGENESIS

Muscle functions in affected patients seem to be normal very early in life; however, with the passage of time and with growth, there is progressive deterioration of muscle both functionally and histologically. The progressive nature of this condition characterizes it as a dystrophy, whereas conditions involving structural abnormalities of muscle that are relatively static are known as myopathies.

HISTOLOGICAL APPEARANCE

Although DMD and BMD progress at different rates, the histological changes are virtually indistinguishable using standard histological stains. The characteristic changes include necrosis of muscle fibers as evidenced by marked variation in fiber diameter, the appearance of nuclei centrally rather than peripherally, and clusters of lymphocytes. There is also infiltration with fibrofatty tissues, which becomes more marked with time so that in the teenage years there may be a predominance of fibrofatty tissue with just a few remaining muscle fibers (Fig. 1).

MOLECULAR BASIS OF DMD AND BMD

The cause of DMD and BMD is an abnormality in the gene for the cell membrane–associated protein dystrophin.[1, 4] Dystrophin is a very large protein that contains 3685 amino acids (compared with approximately 1000 amino acids in each collagen chain). In DMD two-thirds of the patients demonstrate large deletions from the gene, and one-third demonstrate other genetic abnormalities not easily detected by the usual clinical techniques, including point mutations, small deletions, or partial duplications. How-

ever, whether there is a large deletion that is clinically detectable or a small deletion or mutation, the common factor in DMD is that the deletion begins within a triplet nucleotide sequence, which codes for a specific amino acid, so that the reading frame of the messenger RNA (mRNA) is disrupted. When the gene is respliced, either a nonsense protein is produced that is rapidly degraded or the transcription of the mRNA is interrupted so that a truncated protein is produced. In either situation, no normal dystrophin is synthesized. In BMD, there are also deletions from the dystrophin gene, but these deletions occur between triplets, usually within a noncoding (intron) sequence, which do not disrupt the reading frame so that a smaller than normal dystrophin in smaller quantity is produced that is able to be incorporated into the cell membrane[4] (Fig. 2).

Dystrophin and several other associated proteins, known as the dystrophin-associated proteins (DAPs), stabilize the muscle fiber membrane and presumably link the actin cytoskeleton to the extracellular matrix via merosin.

The absence of dystrophin leads to increased fragility and instability of the myofiber membrane and results in increased serum levels of creatine kinase (CK) resulting from leakage of CK along with other intracellular components.[5, 6] An elevated level of CK is not a cause of the disease but is a marker for muscle cell membrane instability and a strong indicator of DMD or BMD. This myofiber membrane fragility leads to chronic degeneration of the muscle, and, although there is regeneration of muscle fibers, ultimately the regenerative process is exhausted and muscle mass is lost and replaced with fibrofatty tissue. Leakage of cellular contents stimulates a mast cell–mediated inflammatory response, which leads to the marked intramuscular fibrosis, severely impairing muscle function. Another factor in the muscle dysfunction resulting from the absence of normal dystrophin is a disruption of intracellular pathways that supply the energy, which supports muscle function.[1] When dystrophin is absent, there is an associated reduction of the levels of the DAPs by 90%. Isolated abnormalities of the DAPs, which include dystroglycans, syntrophins, and sarcoglycans such as adhalin, are found in up to 20% of patients with limb-girdle dystrophies,[7] dem-

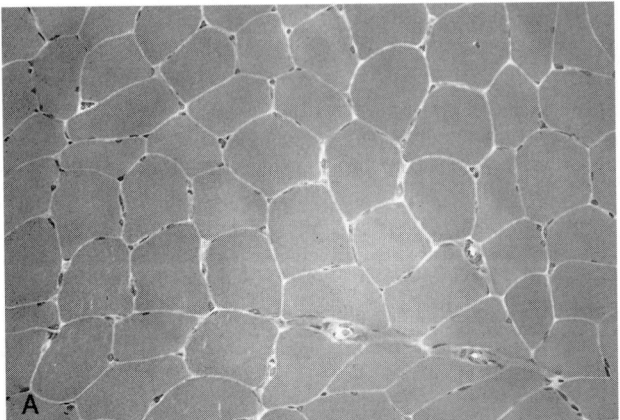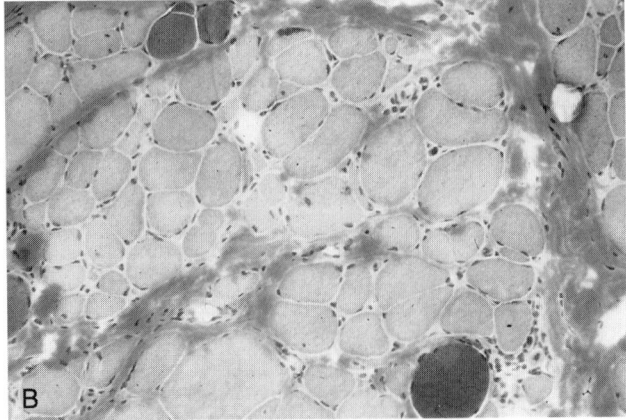

Fig. 1. Muscle cross-sections with trichrome stain. *A,* Normal muscle. Note the regularity of the muscle fiber diameter, peripheral nuclei, and minimal fibrous tissue. *B,* Duchenne's muscular dystrophy. Note the marked variation in fiber diameter, presence of central nuclei, and marked fibrosis between muscle fascicles. In more advanced disease, the muscle fibers are almost totally replaced with fibrofatty tissue. (From Staheli LT: Pediatric Orthopedic Secrets. Philadelphia, Hanley & Belfus, 1998, p 367.)

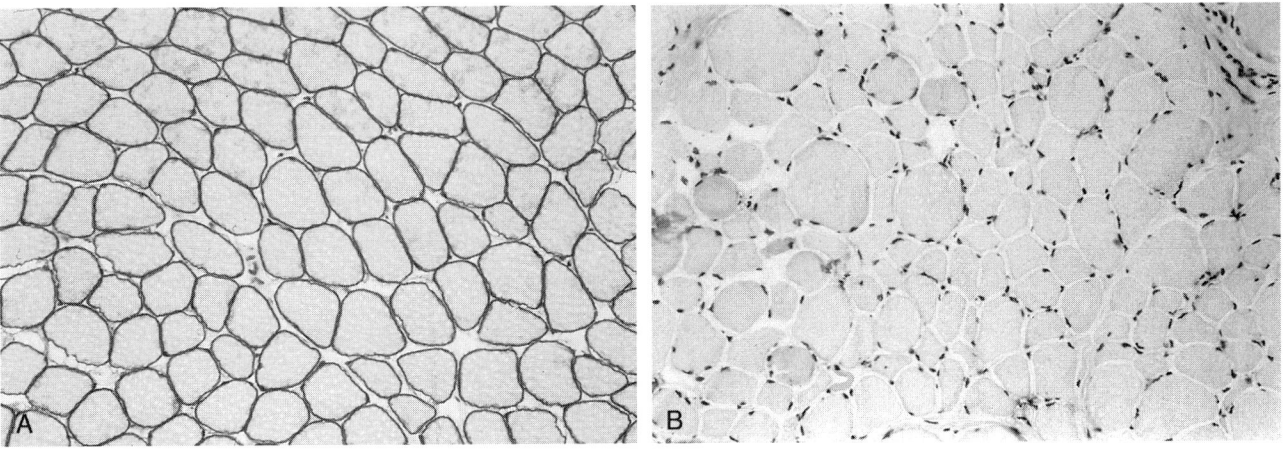

Fig. 2. Muscle stained with antibody to dystrophin. *A,* Normal view. Note the regular intense staining of the myofiber membrane throughout section. *B,* Duchenne's muscular dystrophy showing complete absence of staining of myofiber membrane with antibody to dystrophin.

onstrating the importance of these DAPs in muscle function.[8] Therefore, the associated deficiency in these DAPs further compromises muscle function.

GENETICS

The dystrophin gene is located on the X chromosome at the locus Xp21. Therefore, DMD and BMD are inherited as X-linked recessive traits.[3] A female carrier will pass the condition to half of her male children and the carrier state to half of her female children. Affected males rarely reproduce.

CLINICAL FEATURES

AGE 0 TO 4 YEARS

Affected newborns appear normal. During the first few months of life, infants with DMD do not demonstrate any major clinical abnormalities. However, with growth, weakness becomes noticeable. Walking is significantly delayed and usually begins after the age of 18 months. When an affected infant is held suspended in the prone position at 6 months, he will be able to extend the legs fully. By 18 months, however, one will note a significant droop of the legs.

By age 1 to 2 years, one may begin to note the presence of characteristic calf enlargement. This "pseudohypertrophy" is enlargement of the muscle resulting from infiltration with fibrofatty tissue (Fig. 3). Boys with DMD walk with a wide-based gait, increased lumbar lordosis, and a Trendelenburg-type shift of the trunk toward the stance-phase limb. This gait pattern becomes evident by age 4 or 5 years and becomes more pronounced over the next few years. Patients with DMD almost never are able to run normally or climb stairs reciprocally without a handrail.

They always have trouble rising from the floor and use the so-called Gowers maneuver to achieve this (Fig. 4). This maneuver is demonstrated by all boys with DMD, and although it is characteristic of this disease, it is not diagnostic, because children with proximal muscle weakness from other causes will also rise from the floor using the Gowers maneuver. Observation of a child rising from the floor is an excellent screening test for weakness of the

pelvic girdle and quadriceps muscles. Shoulder girdle weakness can be demonstrated by the Meryon sign. The examiner places his or her hands in the axillae of the child and lifts him upward. Because of the muscle weakness, the child will slip through the examiner's hands. This sign is usually not positive until after age 5 years.

Patients may have cognitive deficits, particularly in the areas of expressive language. Many of these children have learning disabilities and will require special education, although some boys will be relatively normal cognitively.

AGE 4 TO 8 YEARS

During this time, affected boys fatigue easily and begin to show increasing lumbar lordosis and increasing side-to-side truncal shift during gait (Trendelenburg's gait) (Fig. 5).

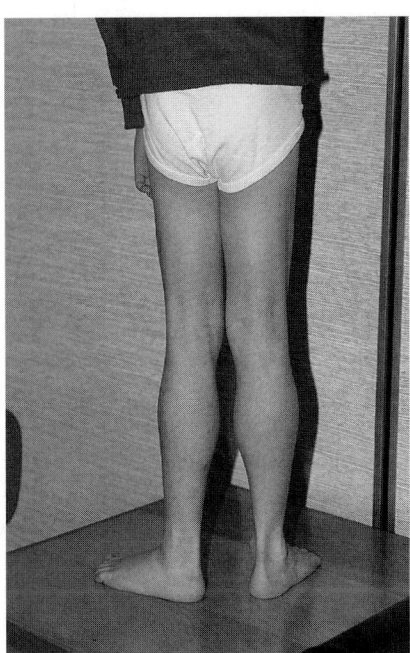

Fig. 3. Duchenne's muscular dystrophy. A 6-year-old boy with Duchenne's muscular dystrophy demonstrates marked calf hypertrophy.

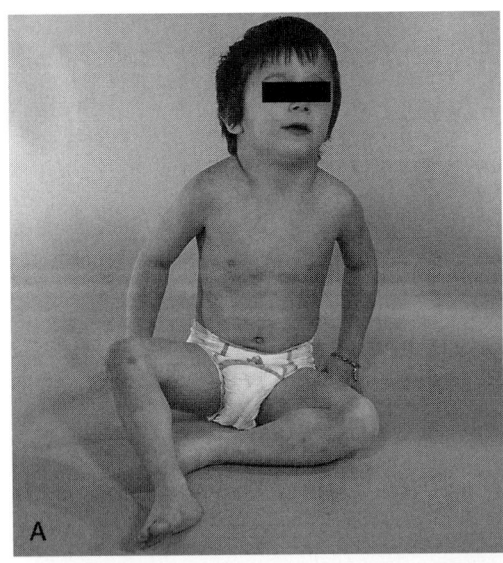

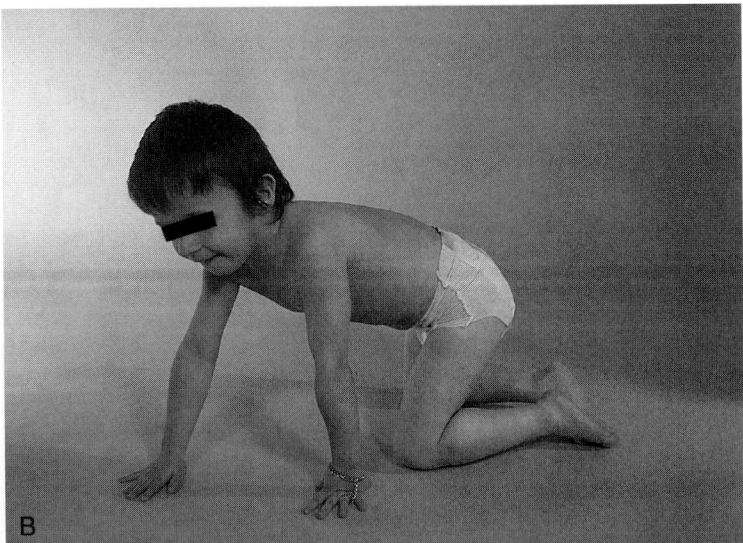

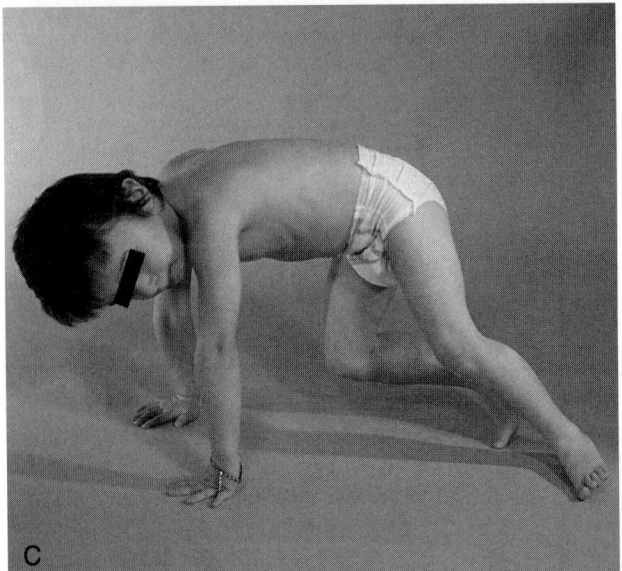

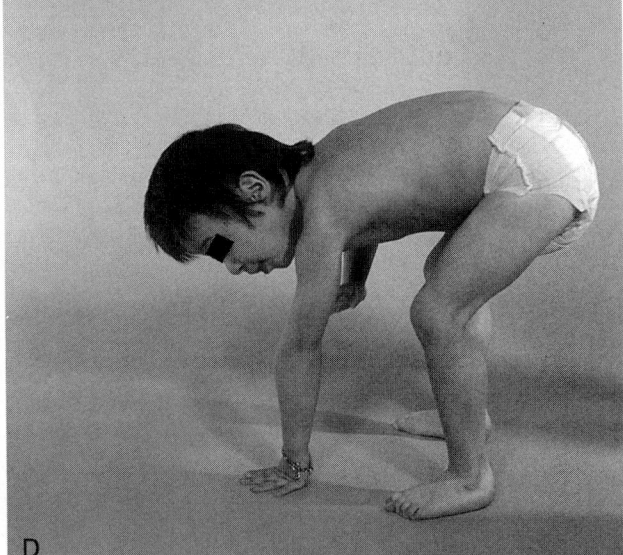

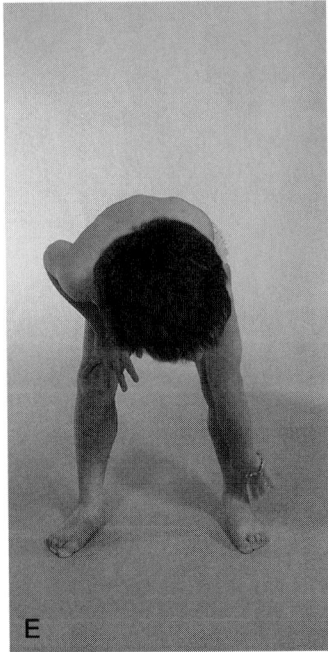

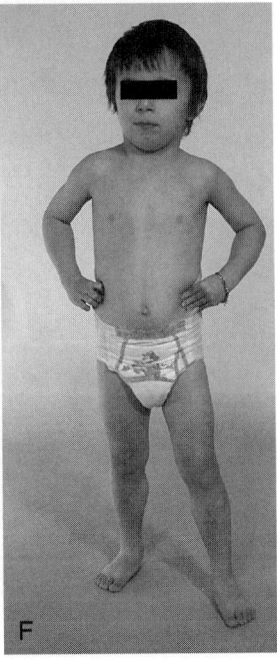

Fig. 4. Gowers' maneuver. A 5-year-old boy with Duchenne's muscular dystrophy demonstrates Gowers' maneuver. *A*, The patient is sitting on the floor. *B*, The first action the patient takes to rise from the floor is to roll over and assume the prone position. *C*, The patient next extends the knees to rise into the so-called "bear position." *D*, The patient begins to extend the hips to achieve upright position. *E*, The patient uses a hand on his thigh to help maintain knee extension and bring the trunk upright over the extended knees. *F*, The patient finally achieves an upright position.

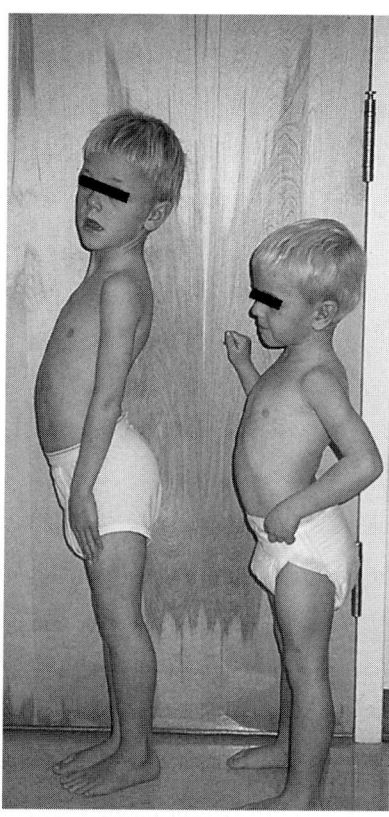

Fig. 5. Duchenne's muscular dystrophy. Brothers, 4 and 6 years old, with Duchenne's muscular dystrophy show wide-based stance and increased lumbar lordosis.

spinal lordosis, which seems to stabilize the spine and prevent scoliosis.[11]

Untreated scoliosis increases inexorably and is associated with pelvic obliquity and truncal decompensation,[12] resulting in significant pain and sitting instability, which leads to loss of the ability to perform any activities of daily life because of the patient's need to use the upper extremities to support himself while sitting. As these curves progress, they extend into the pelvis, causing significant degrees of pelvic obliquity (Fig. 6). As the curvature is increasing, the muscle weakness is also progressing, so that pulmonary function diminishes by 4% per year with an additional 4% for each 10 degrees of thoracic scoliosis.[13] By the age of 15, patients generally have a vital capacity less than 35% of predicted.[14]

At the same time, patients may gain significant amounts of weight, further increasing the difficulty in caring for them. Some affected boys have associated gastrointestinal problems (because of the lack of dystrophin in the smooth muscle of the gut), including decreased gastric emptying and constipation.[15] As it becomes more difficult for them to eat, most patients will lose weight and ultimately become thin.

The least involved muscles are the distal muscles of the forearm and hand and the bulbar innervated muscles of the face. It has been noted that the extraocular muscles seem to be totally unaffected.

The pulmonary dysfunction continues to worsen. However, because of their reduced activity, patients have little in the way of pulmonary symptoms until they reach the

They also experience early heel rise and an equinus position of the foot during the stance phase of gait. With progressive quadriceps weakness, usually after age 6, they also lose the knee flexion at weight acceptance and maintain full knee extension throughout the entire stance phase.[9]

Contractures will begin to be seen in this stage in the hip flexors, iliotibial band, knee flexors, and Achilles tendon in the lower extremity and at the elbow flexors in the upper extremity.

AGE 8 TO 12 YEARS

As the disease progresses, the gait abnormality becomes more marked, the contractures continue to worsen, and the quadriceps become progressively weaker, so that extensor lag develops at the knee and knee flexion contracture appears. The combination of the development of 10 to 15 degrees of knee flexion contracture along with significant weakness of the quadriceps leads to a loss of the ability to stand and walk.

AGE 12 YEARS AND OLDER

By this age, most patients are unable to stand independently and are full-time wheelchair users. Scoliosis develops between age 11 and 13 in about 90% of DMD boys. This is usually a thoracolumbar scoliosis associated with a generalized kyphosis, with the major convexity to the side of the dominant hand.[17] Those DMD patients in whom scoliosis does not develop demonstrate an associated total

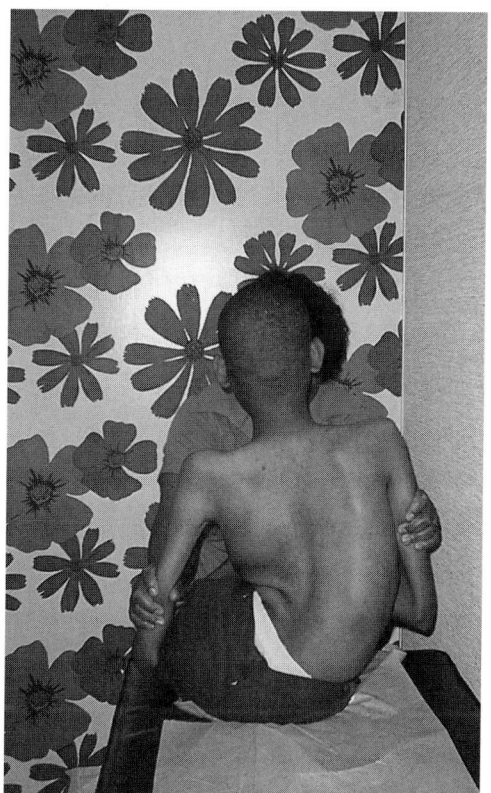

Fig. 6. Severe untreated scoliosis in an 18 year old.

point of decompensation, which occurs when their vital capacities are less than 20% of predicted.

Patients die between the ages of 16 and 21 years either from a pulmonary infection that they are unable to clear or from progressive pulmonary failure.[16] Severe cardiomyopathy occurs in a small subset of patients and may be a major factor in their death. One study demonstrated cardiomyopathy in female carriers.[17]

DIAGNOSIS

When there is a positive family history, there will be a high index of suspicion, appropriate diagnostic tests can be undertaken quickly, and the diagnosis is usually made early. In contrast, in a child with no family history, the diagnosis will have to be suspected by the physician before appropriate diagnostic tests can be undertaken; consequently, diagnosis may be delayed. Therefore, it is imperative to be acquainted with the clinical signs so that appropriate diagnostic studies can be instituted when a patient does present. A study in England reported a series of patients who initially were referred to the orthopaedist at a mean age of 3 years; none were accurately diagnosed by the consultant orthopaedist at the initial presentation, and the average delay in diagnosis after initial referral to an orthopaedist was 2 years.[18]

Clinical signs are as follows:

Motor delay: most boys will walk at the age of 18 months or later.

Clumsiness: patients will never have a smooth gait and will walk with a wide-based gait with increased lumbar lordosis. Boys will be unable to run and not be able to keep up with their peers.

Inability to climb stairs: patients with DMD are never able to climb steps in a normal reciprocal fashion without the aid of a handrail.

Appearance: patients will generally have increased lumbar lordosis, pes planus, and in most, but not all, patients the pseudohypertrophy of the calf can be appreciated.

Gowers' maneuver: patients will demonstrate the utilization of the Gowers maneuver to rise from the floor.

Deep tendon reflexes will be present until the muscle weakness progresses to a degree at which the muscle is no longer able to respond. This is later in the course of the disease.

LABORATORY INVESTIGATIONS

Normal serum levels of CK in most laboratories range between 120 and 250. Patients with DMD and BMD will have levels ranging from 7000 to 15,000 or greater, so that the elevation is unequivocal. Mildly elevated CK may occur occasionally in normal children, so that if the elevation is mild the tests should be repeated. If a consistent mild elevation of CK is documented, the patient should be investigated for other types of muscle disease such as limbgirdle dystrophy, facioscapulohumeral muscular dystrophy, Emery-Dreifuss dystrophy, or other muscle diseases.

If the CK is greater than 5000 and the history is consistent with a slowly progressive onset of disease, the patient is likely to be affected with DMD or BMD. To be absolutely certain, blood should then be sent for DNA analysis of the dystrophin gene. In about two-thirds of patients, there is a large deletion in the dystrophin gene that is easily identified. However, in the remaining one-third, there is only a small deletion or point mutation that is not detectable with routine DNA studies, so that additional investigations may need to be pursued.

If the patient has a high CK and negative DNA studies for dystrophin, the next diagnostic step that can be done is a muscle biopsy. However, if there is a family history of DMD/BMD or if the clinical findings are characteristic and the CK is higher than 5000, a presumptive diagnosis of DMD or BMD can be made and biopsy is not essential unless the parents feel strongly that an absolute diagnosis is critical. In performing the muscle biopsy, one should take care that an adequate specimen containing sufficient viable muscle is removed. Because the biopsy requires general anesthesia in children of this age, precautions should be taken, because patients with DMD as well as other muscle diseases are prone to *malignant hyperthermia,* a problem that can be avoided by recognizing the risk and avoiding inciting agents such as succinylcholine. An updated supply of sodium dantrolene for intravenous use should always be available when operating on these patients, because this agent is effective in treating malignant hyperthermia if it occurs.[19] The muscle specimen should not be placed in fixative but should be taken directly to a laboratory familiar with histological analysis of muscle disease, where it will be frozen for histochemical analysis and adenosine triphosphatase staining as well as immunohistochemical staining for dystrophin. Tissue can also be sent for Western blot to assess the quantity of dystrophin in the muscle tissue and to distinguish between DMD (no dystrophin) and BMD (reduced quantity of abnormal dystrophin). Standard histology should also be done.

Once the diagnosis is made, appropriate genetic counseling should be provided to parents as well as to other possible heterozygotes in the family. If the patient's DNA studies are positive for deletions in the dystrophin gene, then identification of female carriers in the family by the DNA testing can be done, and genetic counseling is much more precise.

In the absence of a positive DNA test, linkage studies can be done to demonstrate whether possible heterozygotes carry the X chromosome with the abnormal dystrophin gene or a normal X chromosome. If a known heterozygote is pregnant and this person has an identifiable deletion in the dystrophin gene, then prenatal DNA testing by amniocentesis or chorionic villus sampling can be done for prenatal diagnosis. If the mother is one of the 30% without an obvious deletion, then linkage studies may be done.

DIFFERENTIAL DIAGNOSIS

BMD

BMD is allelic with DMD (i.e., the genetic defect resides on the same dystrophin gene), but in the case of BMD, a smaller dystrophin is produced in lesser quantities. This has a similar but less profound effect as the complete absence of dystrophin, so that the diseases progress at a slower rate. Immunohistochemical staining of the muscle for dystrophin will show spotty staining of the cell membrane, as opposed to no staining in DMD, and Western blot analysis will show a reduced quantity of a smaller dystrophin molecule.

Although differentiating between Becker and Duchenne dystrophy by laboratory studies may be helpful for prognostication, patients are treated on the basis of their clinical findings.

The important clinical differentiating finding is that BMD patients generally present after age 8, whereas DMD patients generally present with their initial problems between the ages of 2 and 4. There is a higher incidence of cardiomyopathy in Becker dystrophy, so that making this precise diagnosis may be important.

DERMATOMYOSITIS

Dermatomyositis may cause profound progressive generalized muscle weakness. Historically, these patients have normal early motor development and then develop relatively acute onset of weakness associated with skin changes, the most characteristic of which is a malar flush. Patients with dermatomyositis have an elevated erythrocyte sedimentation rate and increased levels of serum CK. In fact, this is the only entity other than DMD in which there is massive elevation of serum CK. The diagnosis can be confirmed by skin and muscle biopsy, which show the characteristic inflammatory changes of dermatomyositis. Many patients will have spontaneous regression of their disease. In the 20% to 30% with persistent and severe involvement, treatment with corticosteroids may be appropriate.

SPINAL MUSCULAR ATROPHY

Patients with type III spinal muscular atrophy will have onset of weakness during childhood with predominantly proximal musculature involvement, and it may initially be confused with DMD. Examination, however, will reveal absent deep tendon reflexes and presence of fasciculations, which are a manifestation of the spontaneous firing of the degrading anterior horn cells and can be seen most easily in the tongue and outstretched fingers. By having the patients hold their arm and fingers extended and placing a piece of paper on the outstretched hands, hand fasciculations will be accentuated and more easily appreciated. Blood studies in spinal muscular atrophy (SMA) show normal CK and normal DNA for abnormalities of dystrophin. However, there is a DNA test for spinal muscular atrophy that is positive in 95% of patients with types I, II, and IIIA spinal muscular atrophy and in 50% to 66% of patients with type IIIB spinal muscular atrophy. Electromyography studies can also distinguish SMA from DMD and BMD.

EMERY-DREIFUSS DYSTROPHY

Many patients with Emery-Dreifuss dystrophy probably continue to be classified as having DMD. Although these patients present a similar clinical picture to DMD and BMD, they have only mild elevation of CK. They do not show the marked pseudohypertrophy and do have some other unique characteristics such as a tendency to develop contractures early, particularly equinus, elbow flexion, and neck extension contractures. Emery-Dreifuss dystrophy patients may have conduction defects on electrocardiogram, and these conduction problems may have fatal consequences. Patients with Emery-Dreifuss dystrophy will be negative for DNA evidence of dystrophin abnormality but will show evidence of abnormality in the gene emerin. Unfortunately, however, this test is not yet clinically available.[20]

LIMB-GIRDLE DYSTROPHY

Limb-girdle muscular dystrophy, rather than being a single disease, represents a group of progressive muscular dystrophies. They are characterized by progressive loss of muscle strength without pseudohypertrophy and mild to significant elevation of serum CK. About 20% of the cases can be classified by histochemical analysis of muscle biopsy specimens on the basis of abnormalities of the sarcoglycans such as adhalin or other components of the dystrophin-sarcoglycan complex.[7] In addition, one subtype, limb-girdle type 2A, is due in most cases to a mutation of the proteolytic enzyme calpain-3, which makes it the only muscular dystrophy resulting from an abnormality in an enzyme rather than a structural protein.[3]

MANAGEMENT

Patients with DMD and other associated muscle diseases are best managed in a multidisciplinary clinic setting. Included among the team are the orthopaedic surgeon, pediatric neurologist, developmental pediatrician, physical therapist, occupational therapist, social worker, orthotist, equipment specialist, and a Muscular Dystrophy Association of America representative (the MDAA funds most MD clinics). In addition, consultants should be available to handle associated pulmonary problems and monitor pulmonary function, and a cardiologist should be standing by for assessment of cardiomyopathy, particularly if any surgery is contemplated.

MEDICAL AND PHARMACOLOGICAL TREATMENT

Although a variety of pharmacological agents have been assessed over the years, the only medication that has been objectively demonstrated to influence the natural course of the disease is prednisone. Prednisone at a dosage of 0.75 mg/kg/day (not every other day) has been shown to reduce the loss of muscle strength in 5- to 15-year-old DMD patients and to increase muscle mass. The effects were seen within 10 days, plateaued at 3 months, and were sustained for the 18 months of the study.[21] The persistence of this improvement for longer than 18 months has not yet been published, but long-term data have showed maintenance of benefits with prolongation of walking and a decrease in the need for scoliosis surgery. The most significant side effect that led to discontinuation of treatment was weight gain (S. Pandya and R. T. Moxley III, personal communication, 2000). The disadvantages of prednisone are its side effects, such as weight gain, hypertension, personality changes, and development of acne. Although strength is improved, it is not clear that function is similarly enhanced, because the additional weight gain may counterbalance the influence on muscle strength. In addition, the influence on bone density and development of osteoporosis have not been investigated. Because of these significant questions regarding side effects, the administration of prednisone is not universally recommended. Deflazacort, a corticosteroid similar to prednisone, is thought to be as effective but has fewer side effects. It is currently unavailable in the United States but is undergoing a trial in Canada.

GENETIC TREATMENT

Because DMD is a genetic disease wherein the gene product is absent rather than abnormal, there is the possibility of introducing the normal gene into affected patients. In an experimental study, the dystrophin gene was introduced into the fertilized ova of dystrophin-deficient mice. The gene was linked with a CK promoter, so that dystrophin would be expressed in muscle tissue as well as other tissues where CK is expressed. All animals derived from these zygotes produced greater than normal amounts of dystrophin in muscle and remained clinically and histologically normal.[22] Furthermore, in these genetically treated mice, the levels of all the dystrophin-associated proteins were restored to normal from the very low levels seen in the absence of dystrophin.[8] A smaller than normal "mini-dystrophin" gene has been introduced with some success to both mice and dogs by an adenovirus vector.[23, 24]

It is, however, a huge technological jump to introduce the gene into a mature animal as opposed to a zygote. There are associated problems of reaction to the viral vector and possible immunological reaction to a dystrophin, which may be recognized as a foreign protein in DMD patients who have never synthesized dystrophin. However, when the technological hurdle of introducing genes into a mature mammalian species is overcome, muscular dystrophy will then become a curable disease. It is, however, likely that changes in the muscle that have accumulated up until the time gene transfer is accomplished will not be reversed, and muscle fibrosis will persist. In this situation, early diagnosis will be critical, so that newborn testing of CK might be instituted as a screening procedure in infants or prenatal diagnosis might be done in fetuses at risk.

Stimulation of the synthesis of utrophin, a protein similar to dystrophin, seems to replace the function of the missing dystrophin and correct the clinical disease in MDX mice.[25] Therefore, there is interest in pharmacologically stimulating the utrophin gene in DMD patients. Because this is upregulation of a protein already present, this would avoid much of the complexity and potential risk of introducing a dystrophin gene. However, whether utrophin can truly substitute for dystrophin is not completely clear at this point.

There has also been interest in replacing the dystrophin gene by injection of normal fetal myoblasts. This is done by multiple injections directly into muscle and is accompanied by administration of cyclosporine to suppress rejection. Interestingly, cyclosporine alone has been shown to alleviate symptoms in DMD. However, this regimen has not been successful in humans as it was in mice and is not recommended.[5, 26]

Another potential approach is utilization of bone marrow transplantation, wherein in addition to hematopoietic stem cells, mesenchymal stem cells, which have the capability to differentiate into muscle, are introduced after marrow ablation by cytotoxic drugs and radiation.[27] Although this approach may be possible, risk as well as cost is high, and this regimen has not yet been used in humans for DMD or BMD.

An innovative new approach to treatment may be the administration of the antibiotic gentamicin, which has a side effect of suppressing premature stop codons that are responsible for the disease in about 15% of DMD patients. This has been successful in the MDX mouse, which pos-sesses this stop codon mutation, but has not yet been reported in patients.[28]

MANAGEMENT

STAGE 1: AGE 0 TO 4 YEARS (DIAGNOSTIC PHASE)

During this stage, patients will be recognized as having delayed motor skills by their parents and present to their primary health care providers, who in turn may refer them to the orthopaedic surgeon for diagnosis. When there is a positive family history, a diagnosis will be ascertained quickly. However, when there is a negative family history, diagnosis will take longer. Once the diagnosis is determined, this devastating information must be presented to the family with sensitivity and clarity. The presenter should be knowledgeable about the natural history so that accurate information can be provided to the family. There should be a note of optimism introduced based on the tremendous advances occurring in the treatment of genetic disease. Ongoing counseling and family support by clinic members should be instituted.

STAGE 2: AGE 4 TO 8 YEARS (QUIESCENT PHASE)

During this phase, a patient's motor skills will begin to deviate from their peers. They will have trouble keeping up in recreational activities and should be provided with alternative recreational outlets that are more individual rather than team based. An example of an activity that tends to be very positive for these patients is swimming. Patients may have problems in school and should be tested for learning disabilities. Many of these patients have problems in the area of expressive language, and adaptations may need to be made in their learning program to deal with this.

If they begin to develop contracture of the Achilles tendon, as manifested by less than 5 to 10 degrees of passive dorsiflexion with the knee extended, then ankle-foot orthoses (AFOs) should be fitted for use during sleep. These should be molded at 90 degrees rather than in a dorsiflexed position so that they will be easier to tolerate. AFOs should not be used for ambulation, because the limitation of ankle motion that they impose will adversely affect balance and the overall ability to ambulate. Isolated Achilles tenotomy or lengthening should be avoided if possible because, once the ground reaction force of the equinus contracture tendon is lost, boys will be unable to stand without a knee-AFO (KAFO).

STAGE 3: AGE 8 TO 12 YEARS (LOSS OF AMBULATION)

As the disease progresses, patients acquire a more wide-based gait with a greater degree of abductor lurch (shifting the trunk over the stance-phase extremity). They have difficulty walking up and down steps and finally lose this ability. They also have increasing difficulty getting up from the floor or from a low chair and should be provided with a higher chair to make it easier to get from a sitting to a standing position. Walking will cease when knee flexion contracture develops and the quadriceps are unable to prevent the flexed knee from collapsing during the single-limb stance. This can be dealt with by prescription of KAFOs with a locking knee of a design that the patient can operate independently. Use of KAFOs will allow continued ambulation, although this will primarily be household or exercise ambulation. Both a manual and a power wheelchair should be provided at this time so that boys will continue to have independent mobility.

Stretching, as directed by the physical therapist, has been advocated to prevent or minimize contracture. However, there are no objective studies to demonstrate that stretching exercises will reverse or even slow the relentless progression of contracture in these patients.

Multiple tendon lengthenings have been advocated when contractures become clinically significant.[29] Knee flexion contracture greater than 20 degrees is frequently the reason why patients are no longer able to be placed into their KAFOs. Siegel et al[30] recommended release of the rectus femoris from the anterior inferior iliac spine, a section of the iliotibial band, release and lengthening of the hamstrings (tenotomy of semitendinosus and gracilis and fractional lengthening of semimembranosus and biceps femoris), and Achilles tendon lengthening or tenotomy when contracture begins to develop.[30] After these multilevel releases, patients will require a KAFO to stand and continue household ambulation.[31]

It has been recommended that when the Achilles tendon is lengthened or tenotomized, transfer of the tibialis posterior to the middorsum of the foot prevents subsequent development of progressive equinovarus, which occurs in spite of the Achilles tenotomy. An alternative approach that I have used (which has not been verified on long-term follow-up but seems promising on short-term follow-up) is tenotomy of the tibialis posterior, flexor digitorum longus, and flexor hallucis longus along with Achilles tenotomy.

Only selected patients benefit by contracture release surgery. There must be sufficient motivation on the part of the patient as well as sufficient trunk strength in the face of developing contracture to make multiple releases worthwhile. There are strong advocates, particularly in Europe, of prophylactic lengthening at age 6 or 7 years of the gracilis, alone or in combination with other hamstring tendons, to prolong ambulation.[32–34]

STAGE 4: AGE 12 TO 16 YEARS (FULL-TIME SITTING/DEVELOPMENT OF SPINAL DEFORMITY)

The onset of spinal deformity usually occurs between the ages of 11 and 13 years and can be ascertained by sitting anteroposterior spine radiographs that should be taken at regular intervals beginning at about age 10 years. There is almost universal agreement among orthopaedists who deal with DMD patients that the best approach to treatment of scoliosis in these patients is early posterior instrumentation and fusion of the spine.[35] A variety of seating systems and spinal orthoses have been used to try to control curvatures in DMD patients, but they have been universally and uniformly unsuccessful.[36] In contrast to other neuromuscular diseases, in which it may be advantageous to delay the progression of deformity by bracing, there is a significant disadvantage to delaying surgery in patients with DMD for the following reasons:

Sufficient spinal growth has occurred by age 11 years to allow a posterior fusion.

The muscle in these patients becomes quite fibrotic and stiff as they age, so that the dissection becomes more difficult, with increased blood loss in older patients, and correction is more difficult, resulting in more severe residual curvature.

The greatest risk of surgery is postoperative pulmonary insufficiency with pneumonia. Pulmonary function decreases significantly between the ages of 11 and 16, so that the older the patient in surgery, the higher is the risk for serious postoperative pulmonary complication.[14]

Therefore, once one ascertains a consistent curvature, patients should be offered surgery, because delaying surgery will significantly increase the risk to the patient and compromise the goal of establishing a stable trunk balanced over a level pelvis.[37]

It is generally agreed that fusion should extend to the upper thoracic spine, and thoracic kyphosis should be maintained to maintain the center of mass of the head forward. By achieving this, patients can usually maintain head control using the stronger neck extensors. If the thoracic spine is placed in relative lordosis, the head is thrown backward, and the neck flexors are too weak to maintain independent head control. There is no consensus on the degree of distal extension of the fusion. Some investigators, including myself, believe that when patients are stabilized before the development of significant deformity, and with pelvic obliquity less than 10 degrees, then fusion to L5 is sufficient and late progression does not occur through the L5-S1 joint.[38, 39] Other investigators, however, disagree and recommend that all patients be stabilized to the pelvis and fused to the sacrum.[40]

Before operation, a patient should have thorough cardiac and pulmonary evaluation, anesthetic agents that are known to be associated with malignant hyperthermia should be avoided, and intravenous sodium dantrolene should be available. Hypotensive anesthesia will reduce blood loss and should be used.[41] If the forced vital capacity (FVC) is greater than 50%, patients are at relatively low risk for pulmonary problems. However, if FVC is less than 35%, risk of postoperative pulmonary complications is significant.[14, 37] Patients should be treated with a segmental type of instrumentation system so that they can be mobilized rapidly after the surgery and should be sitting on the first or second postoperative day so that they can maintain head control. It is generally advisable for patients to spend at least the first 24 hours postoperatively in an intensive care unit so that ventilatory issues can be addressed if necessary (Fig. 7).

Providing spinal stabilization significantly improves the quality of life for these patients during their teenage years.[42] Boys with DMD in whom scoliosis develops and who do not have spinal stabilization have a tremendous amount of difficulty sitting, require the use of their arms for trunk stability, and therefore lose activities of daily living (ADL) skills. In addition, those patients undergoing spinal stabilization will have better maintenance of pulmonary function and a longer life span.[43] However, the major rationale for performing spinal fusion is the significant improvement in quality of life in those patients having a stable, balanced spine.[42]

Other issues during this time relate to the further loss of independence as a result of the progressive muscle weakness and contracture. Aids for feeding will be necessary,

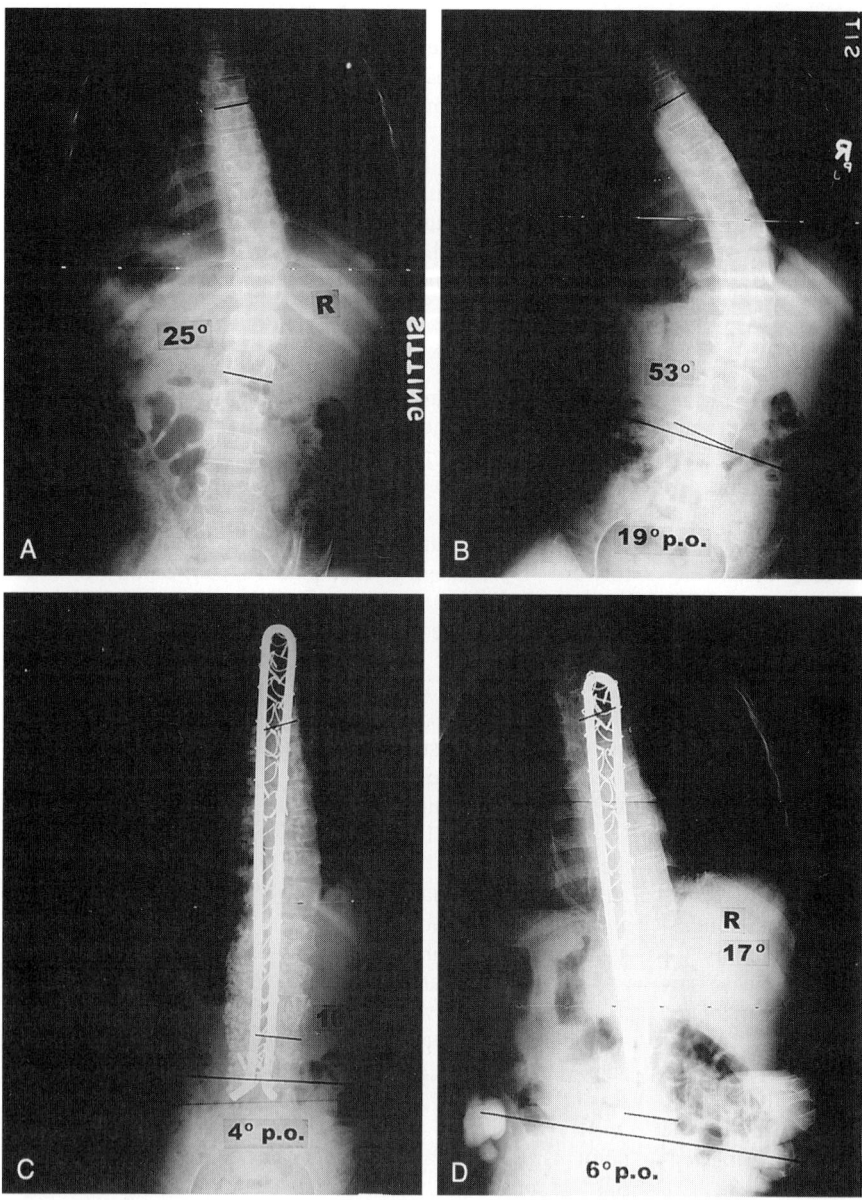

Fig. 7. Duchenne's muscular dystrophy. These are serial spinal radiographs of a patient with Duchenne's muscular dystrophy. *A,* At age 11 years 6 months, patient demonstrates 25-degree scoliosis from T6 to L2 with a level pelvis. *B,* At age 12 years 1 month, patient shows doubling of scoliotic deformity in a 7-month period of time. Patient at this point also has increased pelvic obliquity to 19 degrees. *C,* Sitting spinal radiographs at age 12 years 2 months, 1 month after Luque's fusion using unit rod with sacral bars removed from T3 to L5. Scoliosis is reduced to 16 degrees and pelvic obliquity to 6 degrees. *D,* The same patient at age 15 years 4 months, 3 years 2 months postoperatively showing maintenance of curve correction at 17 degrees and minimal increase of pelvic obliquity to 6 degrees. The patient continues to sit comfortably full time; however, earlier surgery would have allowed more complete correction of pelvic obliquity.

such as an elevated lap tray or an elevated table from which the patient can eat. To maintain independent mobility, patients will require a power wheelchair with a control system that the patient can operate, appropriate seat cushions to distribute pressure, and inserts to provide lateral support to the trunk. Families may need to be supplied with a lift for the home setting, because patients are unable to assist with transfers. In addition, patients will need almost total assistance with basic ADLs, such as dressing, feeding, and toileting, as time progress.

STAGE 5: AGE 16 YEARS AND OLDER

In the older teenager, the major issues are those relating to the progressive loss of self-care skills and pulmonary function as well as planning for end of life. The natural history of this disease is that pulmonary function will continue to decrease, and few patients will survive past their 20th birthday without ventilatory support. The usual terminal event is an overwhelming respiratory infection that cannot be cleared because of the patient's poor pulmonary func-

tion. Alternatively, some patients will experience progressive loss of pulmonary function with hypoxia and hypercarbia and succumb much more slowly. Technology exists to significantly prolong the life of these patients by providing ventilatory support.[16] Initially, night Bi-PAN systems may provide appropriate support for several years. Ultimately, patients will require full-time ventilatory support, and the only way to provide this in a reasonable fashion is via tracheostomy, usually when their FVC approaches 10%. Small, portable ventilators are available that attach to wheelchairs. Patients treated in this fashion may survive well into the third or fourth decade of life but may ultimately succumb to cardiomyopathy or ventilatory complications. Discussions, therefore, should be undertaken with families by the midteenage years, at the very latest, regarding their wishes if an acute pulmonary infection occurs (i.e., advanced directive). Once a patient is aggressively treated with intubation, they often survive this otherwise terminal episode but, as a result, may require permanent assisted ventilation. Therefore, families should be prepared to make the choice of how they would like to proceed when such a crisis occurs.

CONCLUSION

Caring for patients with DMD is demanding but extremely satisfying. Although currently there is no cure for the disease, there is a significant amount one can contribute toward the child's function and happiness. In addition, a knowledgeable and skilled clinical team provides a tremendous amount of support to the families who care for these severely handicapped young men with this devastating degenerative disease.

REFERENCES

1. Hoffman E, Fishbeck K, Brown R, et al: Characterization of dystrophin in muscle-biopsy specimens from patients with Duchenne's or Becker's muscular dystrophy. N Engl J Med 1988; 318:1363.
2. Jay V: On a historical note: Duchenne of Boulogne. Pediatr Dev Pathol 1998; 3:254.
3. Online Mendelian Inheritance in Man (MIM no. 310200). Baltimore, MD, Johns Hopkins University. Retrieved October 7, 1999 at http://www.ncbi.nlm.nih.gov/omim/.
4. Monaco AP: Detection of deletions spanning the Duchenne muscular dystrophy locus using a tightly linked DNA segment. Nature 1985; 316:842.
5. Pagel C, Morgan J: Myoblast transfer and gene therapy in muscular dystrophies. Microsc Res Tech 1995; 30:469.
6. Vilquin J, Brussee V, Asselin I, et al: Evidence of MDX mouse skeletal muscle fragility in vivo by eccentric running exercise. Muscle Nerve 1998; 21:567.
7. Duggan D, Gorospe J, Fanin M, et al: Mutations in the sarcoglycan genes in patients with myopathy. N Engl J Med 1997; 336:618.
8. Matsumura K, Lee C, Caskey C, et al: Restoration of dystrophin-associated proteins in skeletal muscle of MDX mice transgenic for dystrophin gene. FEBS Lett 1993; 320:276.
9. Khodadadeh S, McClelland M, Patrick J, et al: Knee moments in Duchenne muscular dystrophy. Lancet 1986; 2:544.
10. Johnson E, Yarnell S: Hand dominance and scoliosis in Duchenne muscular dystrophy. Arch Phys Med Rehabil 1976; 57:462.
11. Gibson D, Wilkins K: The management of spinal deformities in Duchenne muscular dystrophy: A new concept of spinal bracing. Clin Orthop 1975; 108:41.
12. Smith A, Koreska J, Moseley C: Progression of scoliosis in Duchenne muscular dystrophy. J Bone Joint Surg Am 1989; 71:1066.
13. Kurz L, Mubarak S, Schultz P, et al: Correlation of scoliosis and pulmonary function in Duchenne muscular dystrophy. J Pediatr Orthop 1983; 3:347.
14. Miller F, Moseley C, Koreska J: Pulmonary function and scoliosis in Duchenne dystrophy. J Pediatr Orthop 1988; 8:133.
15. Barohn R, Levine E, Olson J, et al: Gastric hypomotility in Duchenne's muscular dystrophy. N Engl J Med 1988; 319:15.
16. Vianello A, Bevilacqua M, Salvador V, et al: Long-term nasal intermittent positive pressure ventilation in advanced Duchenne's muscular dystrophy. Chest 1994; 105:445.

17. Politano L, Nigro V: Development of cardiomyopathy in female carriers of Duchenne and Becker muscular dystrophies. JAMA 1996; 275:1335.
18. Read L, Galasko C: Delay in diagnosing Duchenne muscular dystrophy in orthopaedic clinics. J Bone Joint Surg Br 1986; 68:481.
19. Forst R, Kronchen-Kaufmann A, Forst J: Duchenne muscular dystrophy: Contracture preventative operations of the lower extremities with special reference to anesthesiologic aspects. Klin Padiatr 1991; 203:24.
20. Tsuchiya Y, Arahata K: Emery-Dreifuss syndrome. Curr Opin Neurol 1997; 10:421.
21. Griggs R, Moxley R III, Mendell J, et al: Duchenne dystrophy: Randomized, controlled trial of prednisone (18 months) and azathioprine (12 months). Neurology 1993; 43:520.
22. Cox G, Cole N, Matsumura K, et al: Overexpression of dystrophon in transgenic MDX mice eliminates dystrophic symptoms without toxicity. Nature 1993; 364:725.
23. Karpati G, Gilbert R, Petrof B, et al: Gene therapy research for Duchenne and Becker muscular dystrophies. Curr Opin Neurol 1997; 10:430.
24. Wells D, Wells KE, Asante EA, et al: Expression of human full-length and mini-dystrophin in transgenic MDX mice: Implications for gene therapy of Duchenne muscular dystrophy. Hum Mol Genet 1995; 4:1245.
25. Tinsley J, Deconinck N, Fisher R, et al: Expression of full-length utrophin prevents muscular dystrophy in MDX mice. Nat Med 1998; 4:1441.
26. Morgan J: Cell and gene therapy in Duchenne muscular dystrophy. Hum Gene Ther 1994; 5:165.
27. Gussoni E, Soneoka Y, Strickland C: Dystrophin expression in the MDX mouse restored by stem cell transplantation. Nature 1999; 401:390.
28. Barton-Davis E, Cordier L, Shoturma D, et al: Aminoglycoside antibiotics restore dystrophin function to skeletal muscles of MDX mice. J Clin Invest 1999; 104:375.
29. Smith S, Green N, Cole R, et al: Prolongation of ambulation in children with Duchenne muscular dystrophy by subcutaneous lower limb tenotomy. J Pediatr Orthop 1993; 13:336.
30. Siegel I, Miller J, Ray R: Subcutaneous lower limb tenotomy in the treatment of pseudohypertrophic muscular dystrophy. J Bone Joint Surg Am 1968; 50:1437.

31. Vignos P, Wagner M, Karlinchak B: Evaluation of a program for long-term treatment of Duchenne muscular dystrophy. Experience at the University Hospitals of Cleveland. J Bone Joint Surg Am 1996; 78:1844.
32. Forst R, Forst J: Importance of lower limb surgery in Duchenne muscular dystrophy. Arch Orthop Trauma Surg 1995; 114:106.
33. Goertzen M, Baltzer A, Voit T: Clinical results of early orthopaedic management in Duchenne muscular dystrophy. Neuropediatrics 1995; 26:257.
34. Rideau Y, Duport G, Delaubier A, et al: Early treatment to preserve quality of locomotion for children with Duchenne muscular dystrophy. Semin Neurol 1995; 15:9.
35. Sussman M: Advantage of early spinal stabilization and fusion in patients with Duchenne muscular dystrophy. J Pediatr Orthop 1984; 4:532.
36. Seeger B, Sutherland A, Clark M: Orthotic management of scoliosis in Duchenne muscular dystrophy. Arch Phys Med Rehabil 1984; 65:83.
37. Miller F, Moseley C, Koreska J: Spinal fusion in Duchenne muscular dystrophy. Dev Med Child Neurol 1992; 34:775.
38. Mubarak S, Morin W, Leach J: Spinal fusion in Duchenne muscular dystrophy: Fixation and fusion to the sacropelvis? J Pediatr Orthop 1993; 13:752.
39. Rice J, Jeffers B, Devitt A, et al: Management of the collapsing spine for patients with Duchenne muscular dystrophy. Ir J Med Sci 1998; 167:242.
40. Alman B, Kim H: Pelvic obliquity after fusion of the spine in Duchenne muscular dystrophy. J Bone Joint Surg Br 1999; 81:821.
41. Fox H, Thomas C, Thompson A: Spinal instrumentation for Duchenne's muscular dystrophy: Experience of hypotensive anesthesia to minimize blood loss. J Pediatr Orthop 1997; 17:750.
42. Bridwell K, Baldus C, Iffrig T, et al: Process measures and patient/parent evaluation of surgical management of spinal deformities in patients with progressive flaccid neuromuscular scoliosis (Duchenne's muscular dystrophy and spinal muscular atrophy). Spine 1999; 24:1300.
43. Galasko C, Delaney C, Morris P: Spinal stabilization in Duchenne muscular dystrophy. J Bone Joint Surg Br 1992; 74:210.

NEUROFIBROMATOSIS TYPE 1

Walter B. Greene

Summary

- Neurofibromatosis 1 is a common genetic disease with multiple clinical manifestations.
- The appearance and severity of the clinical problems are typically progressive.
- Scoliosis is the most common orthopaedic problem.
- Dystrophic scoliosis in these patients can be difficult to treat.
- Anterolateral bowing of the tibia, pseudarthrosis of the tibia, and overgrowth of an extremity are other orthopaedic problems.

DEFINITION

Neurofibromatosis type 1 (NF1), also called peripheral neurofibromatosis or von Recklinghausen's disease, is a common genetic disorder that causes tumors to grow along various types of nerves and, in addition, affects the development of nonnervous tissues such as bone and skin.[1] By contrast, neurofibromatosis type 2 (NF2) is a different and relatively uncommon genetic disorder characterized by acoustic neuromas and other sites of cranial and spinal nerve schwannomas.

HISTORICAL REVIEW

Although many authors published descriptions of NF1 throughout the 18th century, it was Friedrich von Recklinghausen's classic 1882 study that characterized the disorder and the neural origin of the tumors. Public attention to NF1 was stimulated by theater productions about Joseph Merrick, the "elephant man," who was misdiagnosed in 1909 as having von Recklinghausen's disease. It is now known that Merrick had Proteus' syndrome.

The past two decades are significant for identification of the NF1 gene and for multicenter, collaborative studies. Even though many questions remain, these two factors have significantly expanded our knowledge of NF1.

EPIDEMIOLOGY

NF1 is an autosomal-dominant disorder that affects about 1 in 4000 people.[2] New mutations account for about half of the cases and are mostly of paternal origin. Penetrance is complete; however, the severity of the disorder varies greatly, even within the same family. Clinical manifestations of NF1 typically progress with age.

PATHOGENESIS

The NF1 gene is located on the long arm of chromosome 17 at band q11.2 and is quite large, spanning 350 Kb of genomic DNA. A large number of NF1-specific germline mutations have been reported; however, no clear pattern has emerged that correlates the different mutations with the different clinical phenotypes.

Neurofibromin, the NF1 protein product, has been identified in all parts of the brain (especially pyramidal and Purkinje cells) and in neurons, oligodendrocytes, dorsal root ganglia, and Schwann's cells of peripheral nerves.[2] Neurofibromin has also been localized to keratinocytes and melanocytes in developing human skin.

The functions of the NF1 gene and neurofibromin have not been elucidated, but data are accumulating that NF1 acts as a tumor suppressor gene and, as such, plays an important role in the control of cell growth and differentiation. The central portion of the NF1 gene shows homology to guanosine triphosphatase (GTPase) activating proteins, and the resultant part of neurofibromin is involved in the regulation of *ras* proteins that are critical for the control of cell proliferation.

CLINICAL FEATURES

The criteria for diagnosing NF1 were established by a 1987 National Institutes of Health consensus conference and reaffirmed in a 1997 study (Table 1).[3] The two hallmarks of NF1 are neurofibromas and the café au lait spots (CLSs) (Fig. 1).

The clinical manifestations of NF1 and their prevalence are listed in Table 2. Variability in prevalence depends on the mean age of the population (some NF1 lesions increase with age), whether the study was population based or derived from specialty clinics, and the criteria used to define the clinical feature. Clinical problems may be severe, but some NF1 patients are minimally affected.

Neurofibromas are benign tumors composed of fibroblasts, axons, Schwann-like cells, perineural cells, mast cells, and extracellular matrix. These lesions may occur at any site where cranial, spinal, or peripheral nerves are present. The prevalence of neurofibromas is age dependent, and virtually all NF1 patients older than 40 years demonstrate discrete neurofibromas.[4] Growth of neurofibromas is unpredictable and includes periods of rapid growth and periods of quiescence or even indefinite stability.

Cutaneous or dermal neurofibromas are slightly raised lesions that have a soft, somewhat gelatinous consistency on palpation. These lesions move with the skin, typically appear in the preadolescent years, may number in the hundreds, and frequently cause cosmetic problems but do not transform into malignant tumors. Subcutaneous or nodular

TABLE 1. DIAGNOSIS CRITERIA FOR NEUROFIBROMATOSIS TYPE 1 (NF1)

Presence of Two or More of the Following:

Six or more café au lait spots
    5 mm or larger before puberty
    ≥15 mm or larger after puberty
Freckling in the axilla or groin
Optic glioma (tumor of the optic pathway)
Two or more Lisch nodules (benign iris hamartomas)
Two or more neurofibromas of any type or one or more plexiform neurofibroma
A distinctive bony lesion
    Dysplasia of the sphenoid bone
    Dysplasia or thinning of long bone cortex
A first-degree relative with NF1

toms such as decreased endurance, a dropped-foot gait, and abductor lurch.

Malignant peripheral nerve sheath tumors (MPNSTs), formerly called "neurofibrosarcomas" or "malignant schwannomas," result from malignant degeneration of a plexiform neurofibroma. These tumors are aggressive and invasive. Localized pain, an enlarging mass, or progressive neurological symptoms are suggestive of an MPNST in an NF1 patient. However, progressive neurological symptoms may also occur with "benign" growth of a plexiform neurofibroma.

Optic gliomas are the most common central nervous system (CNS) tumor in NF1 patients.[4, 6] Any part of the optic tract may be involved. Only about one-third are symptomatic; problems typically begin during the first decade. An enlarging optic glioma may cause dimness of vision, visual field defects, headache, vomiting, anorexia, and

neurofibromas are beneath the skin, are uncommon before puberty, are commonly a source of pruritus and pain, and may cause paresthesia.

Plexiform neurofibromas are congenital lesions characterized by diffuse hypertrophy of the involved nerves but with preservation of the nerves' fascicular organization. The prevalence of plexiform neurofibroma is 20% to 30% in clinical reports but increases to 40% when imaging studies are routinely obtained.[4–7] These lesions may involve the dermis or may arise in the deeper structures. Palpation of dermal lesions provokes an image of a "bag of worms." Plexiform neurofibromas may cause disfigurement and hyperpigmentation of the overlying skin. These lesions may also cause diffuse hypertrophy of the soft tissue and bone, with a result ranging from an isolated macrodactyly or small leg length discrepancy to gigantism of the entire extremity. Craniofacial plexiform neurofibromas may cause severe facial disfigurement.

Plexiform neurofibromas may remain static or may grow at any age. These lesions are particularly prone to expand during puberty. Enlargement of a plexiform neurofibroma may cause neurological dysfunction, with resultant muscle and sensory abnormalities manifested by signs and symp-

TABLE 2. CLINICAL MANIFESTATIONS OF NEUROFIBROMATOSIS TYPE 1 AND THEIR APPROXIMATE FREQUENCY	
Manifestation	**Frequency (%)**
Nervous System	
Cutaneous neurofibroma	75–90
Plexiform neurofibroma	20–40
Malignant peripheral nerve sheath tumors	1–4
Optic glioma	15
Symptomatic	5
Central nervous system associated	
Learning disabilities	30–65
Hyperintense T_2 signal	60–70
Precocious puberty	1–3
Seizures	6
Sphenoid wing dysplasia	11
Spinal cord associated	
Dumbbell-shaped neurofibroma	
Dural ectasia	
Pseudomeningoceles	
Cutaneous	
Café au lait macules (≥6)	80–99
Inguinal or axillary freckling	80
Xanthogranulomas	2
Hemangiomas	6
Craniofacial	
Lisch nodules	60–100
Facial asymmetry	8
Congenital glaucoma	0.5
Cardiovascular	
Congenital heart defect	2
Hypertension	Common
Skeletal	
Scoliosis	25
Congenital bowed tibia	2–4
Macrodactyly	
Leg length discrepancy	
Short stature	
Subjective Effects	
Cosmetic problems	40
Psychological/social problems	40

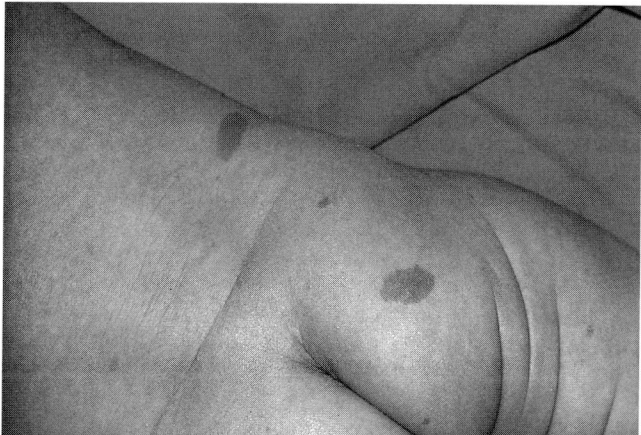

Fig. 1. Typical café au lait spots. This 3-month-old child was subsequently diagnosed with neurofibromatosis type 1.

Compiled from Gutmann et al,[3] Friedman and Birch,[4] Huson,[5] Riccardi,[6] Samuelsson and Axelsson,[7] Goldberg et al,[8] and North et al.[9]

nystagmus.[8] Precocious puberty in NF1 patients is associated with optic gliomas.[4]

Learning disabilities are common in children with NF1.[9] The mean IQ of NF1 patients ranges from 89 to 94. Mental retardation (IQ less than 70) is approximately twice as frequent as in the general population. A particular profile of cognitive deficits has not been associated with NF1, but individual patients may have a specific learning disability or attention-deficit/hyperactivity disorder.

Intracranial hyperintense T_2 signals are common in children with NF1.[9] The cause of these magnetic resonance imaging (MRI) signals is unclear, but abnormal myelin is a possibility. These hyperintense T_2 signals tend to disappear during the second and third decades of life. In the absence of neurological deficits, these MRI findings do not correlate with macrocephaly or other clinical manifestations of NF1.

Neurofibromas and other spinal cord manifestations of NF1 contribute to the abnormal pressure phenomenon affecting vertebral growth and stability. A "dumbbell" plexiform neurofibroma may cause widening of the neural foramen, scalloping of the posterior vertebral body, and instability of the spine.

Café au lait spots are hyperpigmented, tan-colored macules that may be present at birth and occur in virtually all children with NF1 before the age of 6 years (see Fig. 1).[3, 9] CLSs are characterized by giant melanosomes on electron microscopy. Their size and number increase with age; therefore, to be diagnostic, CLS must be *larger than 15 mm* after puberty (see Table 1).

Axillary and inguinal freckling is a good diagnostic marker for NF1. These 2- to 4-mm hyperpigmented spots may be congenital but typically appear and increase later in life. Freckling is also common in the neck and in the submammary region in women.

Juvenile-onset xanthogranuloma in NF1 may be associated with juvenile chronic myeloid leukemia, but the risk is low and does not warrant routine bone marrow aspirates.[3]

Lisch's nodules (benign hamartomas of the iris) are uncommon during early childhood but are found in virtually all adults with NF1. Slit-lamp examination is often required to detect these nodules, but their presence is helpful in confirming the diagnosis of NF1.

In children with NF1, hypertension is usually secondary to renal artery stenosis or, uncommonly, pheochromocytoma. Essential hypertension is more common in adults. Blood pressure monitoring should be routine in NF1 patients.

Scoliosis is the most common orthopaedic manifestation of NF1.[10, 11] Dystrophic and nondystrophic patterns of curvature are observed. The features of dystrophic NF1 scoliosis include a short curve with marked angulation and rotation, spindling (penciling) of the ribs and transverse processes, vertebral scalloping, foramina enlargement, defective pedicles, and, on occasion, subluxation of the vertebrae (Fig. 2).[10–15] Dystrophic scoliosis is resistant to bracing and is frequently associated with a neurofibroma. Nondystrophic scoliosis in NF1 has radiographic features similar to those of idiopathic scoliosis; however, when this type of curvature appears at a relatively young age, there is a tendency for a worse prognosis and for development of dystrophic features.[10]

Anterolateral bowing of the tibia is a congenital deformity that is often associated with NF1 (Fig. 3). The defor-

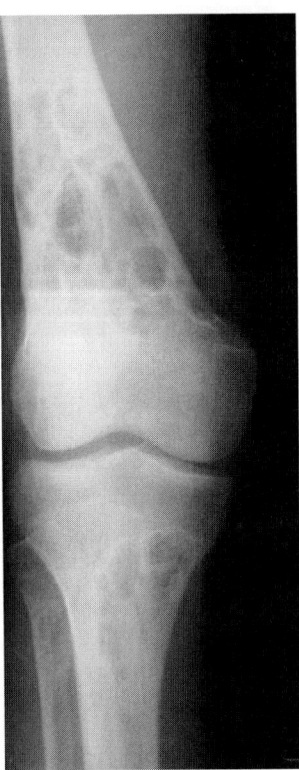

Fig. 2. Extensive cystic lesions in the distal femur and proximal tibia. Similar findings were found in the opposite extremity of this 17-year-old boy with neurofibromatosis type 1. No masses were palpated. Despite ominous appearance, the patient experienced only mild aching in the knee with extended walking.

mity often progresses to pseudarthrosis of the tibia, a condition that is difficult to treat. Patients with NF1 may also experience pseudarthrosis of other bones, including the fibula, radius, ulna, and clavicle. Fortunately, this is uncommon.

Short stature is common. NF1 patients achieve a mean height of approximately the 5th to 10th percentile.[5] Musculoskeletal problems such as leg length discrepancy and scoliosis account for only part of the short stature.

Skeletal lesions of the long bones range from scalloping of the cortex to cystic lesions that may appear quite ominous despite their asymptomatic nature (see Fig. 2). The cause of these lesions is uncertain, but MRI studies suggest that the lesion is mostly fibrous tissue.

Physicians should be aware and supportive of the cosmetic and psychological problems that may occur in NF1 patients. Counseling should be arranged when appropriate.

The occurrence of malignant neoplasms is significantly higher in NF1 patients than in the general population (probably two to three times). Many questions remain unresolved, but the tumor suppressor function of the NF1 gene and the "two-hit" phenomenon undoubtedly play a role in the development of these neoplasms.[2] Malignant peripheral neural sheath tumors, pheochromocytoma, juvenile chronic myeloid leukemia, Wilms' tumor, and rhabdomyosarcoma are more common during childhood.[8] In adults, typical NF1 tumors may develop, but other types of malignancies are also more prevalent.[16]

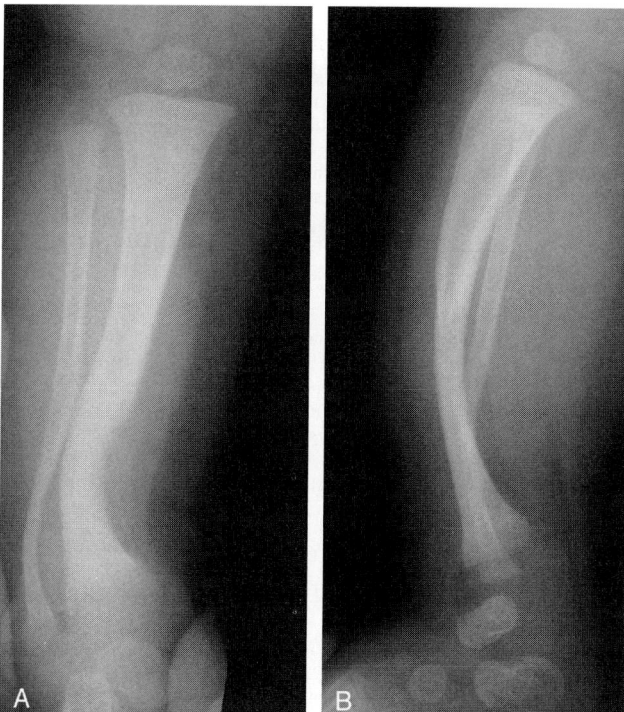

Fig. 3. Anterolateral bowing of the tibia. The patient is a 3-month-old girl with multiple café au lait spots. Anteroposterior *(A)* radiograph and *(B)* lateral radiograph of the tibia.

DIFFERENTIAL DIAGNOSIS

Anterolateral bowing and congenital pseudarthrosis of the tibia have a high association with NF1, and infants with this deformity should be evaluated thoroughly for NF1. Because the clinical features of NF1 are not always manifested during early childhood, these patients should be periodically reexamined for the possibility of NF1. NF1 also should be considered in children with macrodactyly, limb overgrowth, and dystrophic scoliosis.

Disorders that may be confused with NF1 include familial CLSs, Proteus' syndrome, McCune-Albright syndrome, Watson's syndrome, Bannayan-Riley-Ruvalcaba syndrome, and multiple lentigines syndrome. Orthopaedic surgeons are likely to encounter two disorders in this list. Proteus' syndrome is characterized by macrocephaly, facial asymmetry, varicosities, hemangiomas, lipomas, lymphangiomas, leg length discrepancy, macrodactyly, and distinctive gyriform lesions on the plantar aspect of the foot. McCune-Albright syndrome is characterized by hyperpigmented skin macules, multiple areas of fibrous dysplasia, precocious puberty, and other endocrine disorders.

MANAGEMENT

Anterolateral bowing of the tibia should be managed with long-term, prophylactic bracing when the child begins to bear weight. This minimizes the considerable risk of progression to a "congenital" pseudarthrosis, a very difficult problem to treat. Management of pseudarthrosis of the tibia, leg length discrepancy, and other related problems is discussed in other chapters.

Nondystrophic scoliosis in NF1 is managed by the same principles used in idiopathic scoliosis. Dystrophic scoliosis is different.[10–15] Brace therapy is ineffective, and early stabilization should be done (Fig. 4). Risk factors for more rapid and severe progression include early age at onset, abnormal kyphosis, severe vertebral rotation, vertebral scalloping, and major penciling of the ribs.[12] Preoperative evaluation should include an MRI or computed tomography myelogram to define the presence of problems such as neurofibromas, vertebral scalloping, and dural ectasia as well as radiographs of the cervical spine to exclude instability that would compromise induction of anesthesia.[13, 17]

The risk of pseudarthrosis after spine fusion is significantly increased in NF1 patients.[14, 15] The presence of either increased kyphosis, severe curvatures, or marked dystrophic bony changes requires an anterior and posterior fusion to reduce the rate of pseudarthrosis. Rigid, segmental fixation of the posterior fusion is preferred in all patients; however, dystrophic changes in the lamina or pedicles may make stabilization difficult.

COMPLICATIONS

Because the rate of pseudarthrosis after spinal fusion is so high, postoperative bracing should be considered even if an anterior and posterior spinal fusion was done. Neurological deficits may be secondary to a variety of causes, including vertebral instability, growth of a plexiform neurofibroma, or a spinal deformity such as an angulated kyphosis. Anterior decompression is required in the latter case.

Manifestations of NF1 are unpredictable. These patients should be routinely evaluated by a physician who is knowledgeable about the numerous, potential problems these patients may experience.

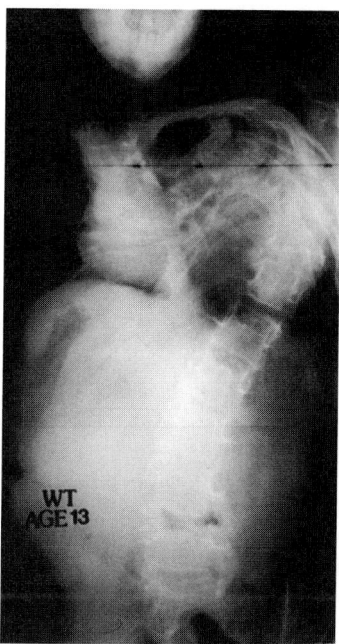

Fig. 4. Dystrophic scoliosis. The patient is a 13-year-old boy with neurofibromatosis type 1. Curvature measured 20 degrees at age 10 years and increased to 153 degrees at this time. (Photograph courtesy of Robert W. Gaines, MD.)

REFERENCES

1. National Neurofibromatosis Foundation: Diagnosing and Managing NF1 and NF2. Http://www.nf.org.
2. Shen MH, Harper PS, Upadhyayam M: Molecular genetics of neurofibromatosis type 1 (NF1). J Med Genet 1996; 33:2.
3. Gutmann DH, Alysworth A, Carey JC, et al: The diagnostic evaluation and multidisciplinary management of neurofibromatosis 1 and neurofibromatosis 2. JAMA 1997; 278:51.
4. Friedman JM, Birch PH: Type 1 neurofibromatosis: A descriptive analysis of the disorder in 1,728 patients. Am J Med Genet 1997; 70:138.
5. Huson SM: Neurofibromatosis 1: A clinical and genetic overview. In Huson SM, Hughes RAC (eds): The Neurofibromatoses: A Pathogenetic and Clinical Overview. London, Chapman and Hall Medical, 1994, p 160.
6. Riccardi VM: Neurofibromatosis: Phenotype, Natural History and Pathogenesis, 2nd ed. Baltimore, MD, Johns Hopkins University Press, 1992.
7. Samuelsson B, Axelsson R: Neurofibromatosis: A clinical and genetic study of 96 cases in Gothenburg, Sweden. Acta Derm Venereol Suppl (Stockh) 1981; 95:67.
8. Goldberg Y, Dibbern K, Klein J, et al: Neurofibromatosis type 1—An update and review for the primary pediatrician. Clin Pediatr 1996; 35:545.
9. North KN, Riccardi V, Samango-Sprouse C, et al: Cognitive function and academic performance in neurofibromatosis: 1. Consensus statement from the NF1 cognitive disorders task force. Neurology 1997; 48: 1121.
10. Crawford AH: Pitfalls of spinal deformities associated with neurofibromatosis in children. Clin Orthop 1989; 245:29.
11. Crawford AH, Bagamery N: Osseous manifestations of neurofibromatosis in childhood. J Pediatr Orthop 1986; 6:72.
12. Funasaki H, Winter RB, Lonstein JB, et al: Pathophysiology of spinal deformities in neurofibromatosis. J Bone Joint Surg Am 1994; 76:692.
13. Kim HW, Weinstein SL: Spine update: The management of scoliosis in neurofibromatosis. Spine 1997; 22:2770.
14. Sirois JL, Drennan JC: Dystrophic spinal deformity in neurofibromatosis. J Pediatr Orthop 1990; 10:522.
15. Winter RB, Moe JH, Bradford DS, et al: Spine deformity in neurofibromatosis: A review of one hundred and two patients. J Bone Joint Surg Am 1979; 61:677.
16. Zöller M, Rembeck B, Akesson HO, et al: Life expectancy, mortality and prognostic factors in neurofibromatosis type 1. A twelve-year follow-up of an epidemiological study in Gröteborg, Sweden. Acta Derm Venereol 1995; 75:136.
17. Yong-Hing K, Kalamchi A, MacEwen GD: Cervical spine abnormalities in neurofibromatosis. J Bone Joint Surg Am 1979; 61:695.

ARTHROGRYPOSIS

R. M. Bernstein and William L. Oppenheim

Summary

- Arthrogryposis is a general term referring to a group of unrelated diseases that have multiple congenital joint contractures as a common feature.
- Arthrogryposis multiplex congenita (amyoplasia) represents the most common form.
- Establishing an accurate diagnosis facilitates the formulation of a rational treatment plan for a particular patient.
- Recurrence of deformity after operative intervention that is done prior to skeletal maturity is common and expected.
- Despite severe physical involvement, children with amyoplasia are usually extremely motivated and are known for developing unique methods of manipulating their environments.

The term "arthrogryposis" comes from the Greek words *arthro,* meaning joint, and *gryp,* meaning curved. It is a descriptive term applied to patients with multiple, nonprogressive, congenital joint contractures. Because multiple joint contractures represent a general phenotypic appearance common to a large number of heterogeneous syndromes, it is necessary to differentiate these syndromes to anticipate the natural history, to formulate a rational treatment plan, and to provide genetic counseling for individual families. To date, more than 150 entities have been subsumed under the term arthrogryposis.[1]

Unfortunately, confusion has arisen because the term is also used in the literature to denote a particular entity also referred to as "classical" arthrogryposis—arthrogryposis multiplex congenita, or amyoplasia. This syndrome is represented by symmetric limb involvement, normal intelligence, and absence of genetic transmission (Fig. 1). To avoid this problem in this chapter, the term arthrogryposis is used to describe the phenotypic appearance of multiple joint contractures, and the "classical" disease is called amyoplasia (Table 1).

EPIDEMIOLOGY

Arthrogryposis of some form occurs once in about 3000 live births; amyoplasia occurs once in every 10,000 live births.[3] Whereas amyoplasia is sporadic, other types of arthrogryposis, such as distal arthrogryposis (types I and II), appear to be autosomal-dominant.

TABLE 1. EVOLUTION OF AMYOPLASIA AS A SYNDROME		
Otto	1841	First clinical description of arthrogryposis.
Stern	1923	Coined the term "arthrogryposis multiplex congenita."
Hall	1982	Described distal arthrogryposis.
Hall	1983	Delineated amyoplasia as a specific disorder[2]

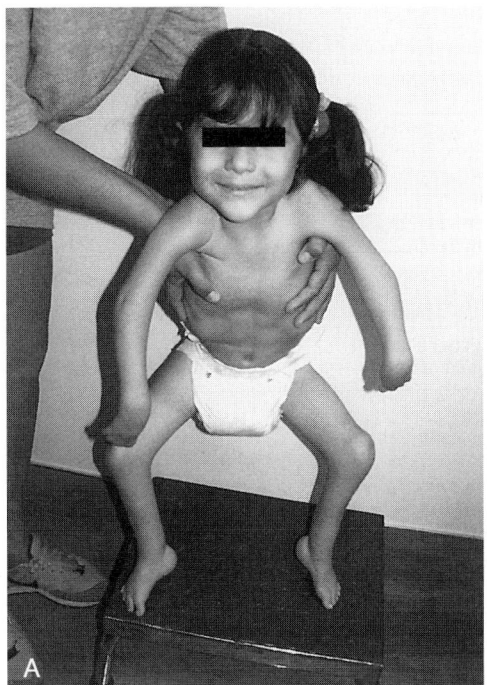
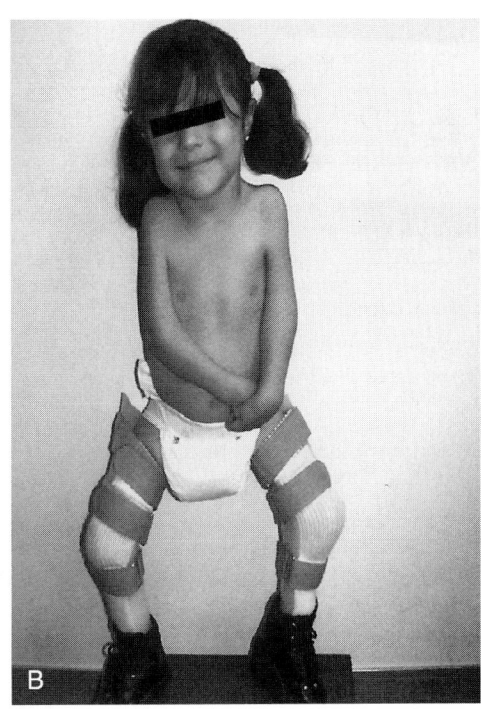

Fig. 1. Amyoplasia. This 5-year-old girl exhibits many of the characteristic features of amyoplasia. *A,* Note the dimpling of the skin over the extensor surface of the elbow and a lack of flexion creases in the cubital fossae, the internal rotation of the shoulders, and the palmar flexion and ulnar deviation of the hands and wrists. *B,* Despite the fixed flexion deformities of the lower extremities and feet, the patient has been fitted with bilateral knee-ankle-foot orthoses and shoe wedges to allow standing and walking.

PATHOGENESIS

Given the large number of syndromes associated with arthrogryposis, it is clear that its cause is multifactorial. The development of congenital joint contractures may be the result of a decrease in fetal movement (fetal akinesia), resulting in periarticular fibrosis and limited motion. Potential causes of fetal akinesia include neural tube defects, anterior horn cell dysfunction, lack of peripheral nerve myelination, and muscle abnormalities such as congenital muscular dystrophy and congenital myopathies. Other causes of fetal akinesia include connective tissue disorders, uterine crowding, intrauterine vascular compromise, and maternal problems such as multiple sclerosis, diabetes, myasthenia gravis, and drug ingestion.

This theory of fetal akinesia is supported by animal models in which fetal movement is arrested by the use of a paralyzing agent such as curare. The resultant offspring are born with the phenotypic appearance of arthrogryposis.

In amyoplasia, the muscles are usually hypoplastic and replaced with fibrous tissue, resulting in a decrease in the number of muscle fibers (Fig. 2). The interpretation of muscle biopsies have varied, suggesting both a myopathic and neuropathic etiology. A decrease in the number of anterior horn cells (dysgenesis), without a concurrent increase in microglial cells, supports the theory of a central nervous system defect in many cases.

CLINICAL FEATURES OF AMYOPLASIA

Although amyoplasia generally presents with symmetric involvement of all four limbs (84%), it has been described with only the lower limbs involved (11%) and, less commonly, with only upper limb involvement (5%).[4] Typical upper extremity involvement includes internal rotation and adduction of the shoulders, extended elbows, flexed and ulnarly deviated wrists, internally flexed fingers, and adducted thumbs. The shoulders are internally rotated and adducted with weak function of the deltoid. The elbows are extended, and the biceps and brachialis are unable to flex the elbow. The wrists are flexed and ulnarly deviated, the fingers are partially but rigidly flexed, and the thumbs are usually adducted. Common deformities at the hip include accompanying flexion and adduction contractures, with hip dislocation in one-third of patients. The knees may be flexed or (less commonly) extended. Congenital subluxation or dislocation of the knee may occur. The feet commonly exhibit a rigid equinovarus deformity, although congenital vertical talus may also be seen.

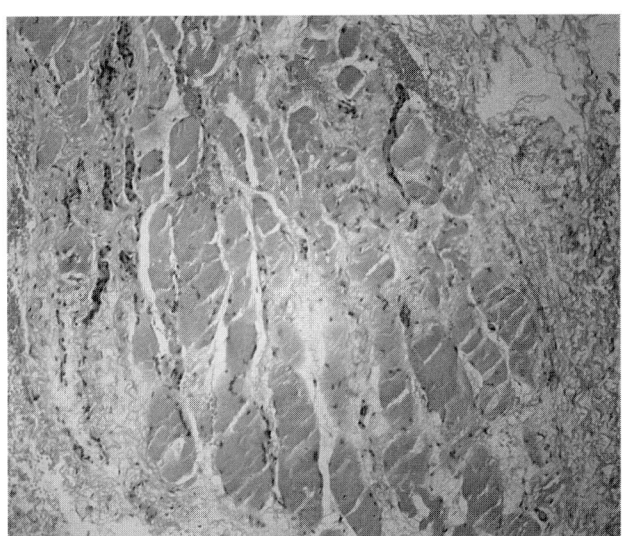

Fig. 2. Section of muscle. From a child with arthrogryposis, showing normal and atrophic skeletal muscle with area of gross fibrosis.

TABLE 2. DIAGNOSTIC TESTS		
Test	Result in Amyoplasia	Differential Diagnosis
Creatine phosphoki- nase	Normal	Congenital muscular dystrophy.
Muscle biopsy	Variable	May help differentiate a neuropathic from a myopathic disease.
Nerve conduction studies	Normal	
EMG	Normal 50%	May distinguish between a neurogenic and my- opathic abnormality in amyoplasia.
CT scan of the head	Normal	Useful to evaluate chil- dren with central ner- vous system (CNS) in- volvement.
Chromosomal studies	Normal	Useful in children with multisystem defects or CNS involvement.

Along with the limited range of motion is a firm, inelastic end point of motion. (The trunk is largely spared, although scoliosis may develop later in one-third of cases.) Because of diminished muscle mass, the limbs take on a fusiform appearance. Normal skin creases over the joints are absent, and webbing across the elbows or knees may be present. Skin dimpling is frequently seen over the extensor surfaces of subcutaneous joints. Sensation is intact, but deep tendon reflexes are often diminished or absent.

A large midline facial hemangioma (nevus flammeus) and mild micrognathia may be present. Hypoplasia of the labial folds in female patients, inguinal hernia and cryptorchidism in male patients, abdominal wall defects, gastroschisis, and bowel atresia have been reported in association with amyoplasia.

Given the number of congenital syndromes that include features of arthrogryposis, the clinician must always search for additional congenital abnormalities and visually inspect the spine and neck for evidence of dysraphism. Motor and sensory examinations should be carefully documented, and the range of motion of all joints should be recorded.

Further Diagnostic Testing
Radiographs of the spine and hips should be obtained to rule out dysraphism or dislocation. Radiographs of other suspicious areas should be obtained as needed.

The necessity of obtaining additional laboratory studies in patients with obvious amyoplasia is controversial. However, if the diagnosis of amyoplasia is in question, a geneticist knowledgeable in the arthrogryposes should be consulted. Table 2 lists tests that may be useful.

DIFFERENTIAL DIAGNOSIS
The following list includes the more common diseases to be considered in the differential diagnosis of arthrogryposis:

Distal arthrogryposis type I.
  Overlapping fingers/ulnar deviation.

Distal arthrogryposis type IIa–e:
  a. Cleft palate, short stature.
  b. Ptosis; ophthalmoplegia; hard, woody muscles.
  c. Cleft lip, cleft palate.
  d. Scoliosis.
  e. Trismus.
Multiple pterygium syndrome.
Whistling face syndrome (Freeman-Sheldon syndrome).
Sacral agenesis.
Contractural arachnodactyly.
Skeletal dysplasia.
  Diastrophic dysplasia.
  Metatropic dysplasia.
Myopathy.
  Central core.
  Nemaline.
Fetal alcohol syndrome.
Myelomeningocele.
Myotonic dystrophy.
Spinal muscular atrophy.
Congenital muscular dystrophy.
Larsen's syndrome.
Möbius' syndrome.
Turner's syndrome.
Nail-patella syndrome.

MANAGEMENT

GENERAL MANAGEMENT
A general algorithm for contractures is shown in Figure 3. The management of joint contractures in amyoplasia involves the orthopaedist, physical and occupational therapists, and a developmental specialist. All joint abnormalities need to be considered together, as it is a common error to focus on the lower extremities and overlook the upper limb distortions and limitations that, in the final analysis, often constitute the greater disability for the patient. Con-

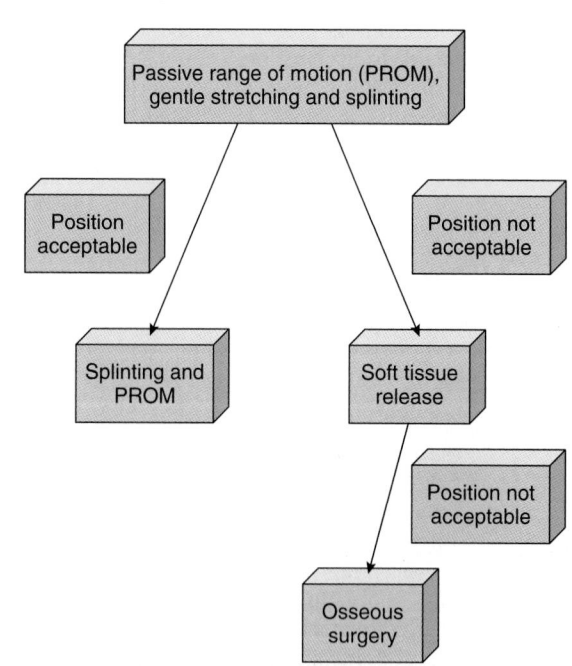

Fig. 3. Algorithm. For management of joint contractures.

tractures in a child with amyoplasia noted at birth should be treated initially with gentle stretching and range of motion. Long-term splinting with lightweight orthoses may delay the recurrence of deformities.

REGIONAL MANAGEMENT
Hip
Hip flexion contractures occur in many amyoplasia patients. Gentle stretching should be initiated as early as possible. In the most significant contractures, the patient is unable to compensate with lordosis of the lumbar spine, making walking difficult. Contractures exceeding 45 degrees require surgical release, but patients with lesser contractures may benefit as well.

The prevalence of hip dislocation is from 15% to 30%. Because the dislocation is usually teratological (a congenital dislocation that is not reducible by gentle manipulation at birth), the results of closed reduction have been uniformly poor, resulting in stiff hips with unacceptably high rates of redislocation. In the past, treatment of hip dislocation was controversial.

Treatment options included acceptance of the dislocation, closed reduction, open reduction from an anterior approach, and open reduction from a medial approach.

Open reduction may be no panacea. There is always concern of converting a dislocated supple hip into a reduced, but stiff hip. With unilateral hip dislocation, there is general agreement that an open reduction should be performed between 3 months and 1 year of age. This may prevent difficulties associated with pelvic obliquity and leg length discrepancy. Whether the open reduction is performed by a medial or anterior approach depends on surgeon preference. Most surgeons utilize the anterior approach, but Staheli et al[5] reported good results with the medial approach. In children older than 2 years of age, femoral shortening and pelvic osteotomy may facilitate an open reduction.

If both hips are dislocated, open reduction is more controversial. Bilateral hip dislocations with symmetrical deformities have not been shown to prevent walking in children with amyoplasia. Even when the hip is successfully reduced, children do not walk normally. Thus, some authors recommend acceptance of bilateral dislocations. Conversely, Szoke and coworkers,[6] recommending open reduction of both hips through a medial approach, reported good results.

Results from open reduction of the hip vary widely. The best results were reported by Szoke et al, utilizing the medial approach. Others have supported the use of the anterior approach with femoral shortening, but the patient populations have not been homogenous. It is clear that results vary with the severity of the disease. Complications of open reduction include redislocation, stiffness, and osteonecrosis.[6,7]

Knee
In patients with amyoplasia, 60% to 85% have involvement of the knee with either a flexion deformity or, less commonly, a hyperextension contracture. In one study,[8] all children with extension contractures were community walkers, whereas only 50% with flexion contractures achieved this level of function. Extension deformities can be treated with casting to improve flexion. However, once flexion is

achieved, maintaining extension and preventing progression to a flexion contracture may be difficult. Occasionally, a V-Y quadriceps plasty is necessary to obtain knee flexion.

Knee flexion deformities are more difficult to treat. Options include manual stretching, casting, soft-tissue release, gradual extension in a circular frame, and extension osteotomy. In the study by Murray and Fixsen,[8] only 7 of 26 knee flexion deformities responded to therapy and splinting. Fractures from overzealous manipulation have been reported; thus, it is important for therapy and casting to be performed judiciously. Care also must be taken to prevent posterior subluxation as the knee is extended. This may be accomplished by using antisubluxation cast hinges to pull the proximal tibia forward as the knee is extended.

Posterior release has been successful in younger patients. It generally includes release of the medial and lateral hamstrings, a posterior capsulotomy, and release of the posterior cruciate ligament. This operation can be performed through medial and lateral longitudinal incisions or by utilizing a posterior Z-plasty incision. Because the neurovascular bundle cannot be lengthened, repeated cast wedging is implemented postoperatively to slowly bring the knee into full extension.

The use of a circular frame fixator to correct knee flexion deformities has been reported with some success. Brunner and coworkers[9] reported significant improvement with the use of the Ilizarov frame over time. Complications included frequent pin site infections and recurrence of the deformity over time.

Distal femoral supracondylar shortening and extension osteotomy can improve the position of the leg but does not change the position of the joint. The advantage is that when the bone is shortened, tension on the neurovascular structures and skin is reduced. In addition, varus, valgus, or rotational deformities may also be addressed. The osteotomy also produces a "dog-leg" deformity that may be unacceptable to the parents, and recurrence of the deformity in skeletally immature patients is the rule, with knee flexion recurring at about 1 degree per month.[10] This procedure should be reserved for patients approaching skeletal maturity or when lesser methods have failed.

Foot
Foot deformities in amyoplasia include clubfeet and congenital vertical tali (congenital convex pes valgus). The deformities are usually severe and rigid. Serial manipulation and casting may partially improve the clubfoot but are not effective in congenital vertical talus.

Surgical correction of the clubfoot should be performed prior to walking. The surgical options include posterior medial and lateral releases, talectomy, circular frame correction and, in the older child, triple arthrodesis. Niki et al[11] reported their results with surgical release and casting. The mean age at surgery was 7 months. Recurrence was noted in 73% of feet, and further surgery was required in 48% of the patients.

Numerous authors have suggested primary or secondary talectomy. Removing the talus effectively lengthens the soft tissues, allowing the foot to be brought out of equinus. There is wide acceptance in the literature that it is a useful technique in relapsed clubfeet, although some authors have suggested its use as the primary procedure.[12, 13] The disadvantages of talectomy are tibiocalcaneal incongruity and

TABLE 3. RESULTS OF CLUBFOOT SURGERY	
	Satisfactory (Plantigrade, Braceable Foot)
Talectomy[12, 13, 16]	50%–82%
PMR[11, 13]	31%–95%
Circular frame[9]	63% "improved"

TABLE 5. REPORTED COMPLICATIONS OF FOOT SURGERY IN ARTHROGRYPOSIS[16, 18]
Wound slough.
Avascular necrosis of the talus.
Recurrence.
Malignant hyperthermia.

the loss of stability of the medial column of the foot. Thus, recurrent equinus and progression of mid- and forefoot adductus are common. One way to potentially avoid the midfoot deformity is to combine the talectomy with a stabilizing fusion of the calcaneocuboid joint.

Circular frame correction of the resistant clubfoot is currently gaining acceptance. After a limited soft-tissue release, frame components are applied separately to the tibia, hindfoot, and midfoot and then connected by interposed distracters. Some surgeons prefer the use of hinges, but these need to be placed perfectly. In our experience, with a limited soft-tissue release and no hinges, the foot gives way at the level of the releases, localizing the correction to these areas. It is important to include a wire through the distal tibial epiphysis that is connected to the tibial frame. This prevents the distal tibial epiphysis from being separated by the distraction.

Feet with persistent deformity at or near the end of growth may be managed by a triple or pantalar arthrodesis. The method must be tailored to the particular deformity, and wedges of bone usually must be removed to place the foot in the plantigrade position.

Results in the treatment of clubfoot in amyoplasia are not comparable to the results for idiopathic clubfeet, but surgery does produce a plantigrade foot that allows bracing and ambulation (Tables 3 and 4).

The publications regarding congenital vertical talus involve diverse populations that include some patients with "arthrogryposis" and diverse methods of the postoperative evaluation.[14–19] Thus, the best method of treating congenital vertical talus in children with arthrogryposis multiplex congenita has not been determined (Table 5).

Upper Extremity

The problems involving the upper extremity in children with amyoplasia are complex. Contractures are treated initially with gentle manipulation. In children with severe diffuse weakness, the use of orthotics and training by an occupational therapist may be the best approach, especially if the child is older and has already adapted to the limb positions. For example, many children learn to feed themselves without elbow flexor function by utilizing the edge of the table as a balanced arm feeder, or the odd positioning of the hands may allow grasping between them. Preexisting function must never be sacrificed in order to obtain a more "normal"-appearing upper extremity.

Surgery can be performed to increase the elbow range of motion, to change the position of the humerus, and to position the wrist. Because the shoulder is often medially rotated, a simple external rotation osteotomy may improve the position of the hand in space.

Improvement in elbow function may be obtained by a V-Y triceps tendon lengthening and posterior elbow release and by transferring muscles to allow for elbow flexion when passive range of motion is present. Candidate muscles for transfer to enhance elbow flexion include the triceps, the pectoralis major, and the Steindler flexorplasty.[20] A triceps transfer usually results in an elbow flexion contracture and may cause difficulty in reaching the perineum or using crutches. The Steindler flexorplasty is a relatively simple procedure. However, the flexor-pronator mass is often nonfunctional in these patients. Even when successful, the range of motion and strength gained are marginal, but balancing this is the fact that small gains are usually utilized to maximum advantage by these bright and innovative patients. The pectoralis transfer is promising, but the biceps is frequently of poor quality, requiring either a fascia lata graft or flexor carpi ulnaris graft to connect the transferred muscle to the forearm.[21]

The wrist in arthrogryposis presents two issues: the wrist extensors are often absent, and the wrist is frequently positioned in marked flexion. It is important to address contraction at both the wrist and fingers at the same time. Stabilizing the wrist (usually in 5 to 20 degrees of palmar flexion) may greatly aid in both the function and appearance of the upper extremity. Lengthening tight finger and wrist flexors, release of the volar wrist capsule, and, when feasible, transfer of a wrist flexor to augment wrist extension is preferred (Tables 6 and 7).

TABLE 4. COMPLICATIONS OF CLUBFOOT SURGERY			
	Posteromedial Release[11]	Talectomy[12]	Circular Frame[9]
Recurrence	73%	21%	41%
Infection[17]			"Common"

TABLE 6. RESULTS OF UPPER EXTREMITY TREATMENT			
	Preoperative E/F*	Postoperative E/F*	Mean ROM Improvement
Posterior elbow release[22]	10°/30°	49°/88°	39°
Triceps transfer[22]	0°/60°	37°/120°	13°

* Elbow extension/flexion.

TABLE 7. POTENTIAL COMPLICATIONS OF UPPER EXTREMITY SURGERY[20]
Loss of bimanual opposition.
Recurrence of deformity.
Ineffective transfers.
Nerve palsy.

TABLE 8. COMPLICATIONS OF SPINE SURGERY	
Pseudarthrosis	17%–43%
Curve progression	17%–57%
Infection	0%–14%

Spine

Scoliosis develops in up to 35% of patients with amyoplasia but is usually not present at birth. Vertebral anomalies are generally not present; therefore, periodic evaluation of the spine is necessary for all patients. Most publications involve patients with arthrogryposis from a variety of causes. Early curve onset, a paralytic curve pattern, and pelvic obliquity are poor prognostic signs for curve progression. A brace may be helpful in delaying surgery. In one series, progression occurred at an average of 6.5 degrees per year.[23] If the curve is greater than about 50 degrees, spinal fusion should be considered. Left untreated, a progressive scoliosis may result in debilitating spinal deformity. A combined anteroposterior approach may be necessary if the curve is large and extremely rigid. Postoperative loss of correction is similar to that in idiopathic patients. Surgery is less successful in obtaining correction in arthrogryposis than in idiopathic scoliosis, with correction averaging about 35% in one series[24] (Table 8).

REFERENCES

1. Hall JG: Genetic aspects of arthrogryposis. Clin Orthop 1985; 194:44.
2. Hall JG, Reed SD, Driscoll EP: Amyoplasia: A common, sporadic condition with congenital contractures. Am J Med Gen 1983; 15:571.
3. Hall JG: Arthrogryposis multiplex congenita: Etiology, genetics, classification, diagnostic approach, and general aspects. J Pediatr Orthop B 1997; 6:159.
4. Sells JM, Jaffe KM, Hall JG: Amyoplasia, the most common type of arthrogryposis: The potential for good outcome. Pediatrics 1996; 97:225.
5. Staheli LT, Chew DE, Elliott JS, et al: Management of hip dislocations in children with arthrogryposis. J Pediatr Orthop 1987; 7:681.
6. Szoke G, Staheli LT, Jaffe K, et al: Medial-approach open reduction of hip dislocation in amyoplasia-type arthrogryposis. J Pediatr Orthop 1996; 16:127.
7. Gruel CR, Birch JG, Roach JW, et al: Teratologic dislocation of the hip. J Pediatr Orthop 1986; 6:693.
8. Murray C, Fixsen JA: Management of knee deformity in classical arthrogryposis multiplex congenita (amyoplasia congenita). J Pediatr Orthop B 1997; 6:186.
9. Brunner R, Hefti F, Tgetgel JD: Arthrogrypotic joint contracture at the knee and the foot: Correction with a circular frame. J Pediatr Orthop B 1997; 6:192.
10. DelBello DA, Watts HG: Distal femoral extension osteotomy for knee flexion contracture in patients with arthrogryposis. J Pediatr Orthop 1996; 16:122.
11. Niki H, Staheli LT, Mosca VS: Management of clubfoot deformity in amyoplasia. J Pediatr Orthop 1997; 17:803.
12. Green ADL, Fixsen JA, Lloyd-Roberts GC: Talectomy for arthrogryposis multiplex congenita. J Bone Joint Surg Br 1984; 66:697.
13. Segal LS, Mann DC, Feiwell E, et al: Equinovarus deformity in arthrogryposis and myelomeningocele: Evaluation of primary talectomy. Foot Ankle 1989; 10:12.
14. Drennan JC: Congenital vertical talus. J Bone Joint Surg Am 1995; 77:1916.
15. Clark MW, D'Ambrosia RD, Ferguson ABJ: Congenital vertical talus. J Bone Joint Surg Am 1977; 59:816.
16. Guidera KJ, Drennan JC: Foot and ankle deformities in arthrogryposis multiplex congenita. Clin Orthop 1985; 195:93.
17. Dias LS, Stern LS: Talectomy in the treatment of resistant talipes equinovarus deformity in myelomeningocele and arthrogryposis. J Pediatr Orthop 1987; 7:39.
18. Adelaar RS, Williams RM, Gould JS: Congenital convex pes valgus: Results of an early comprehensive release and a review of congenital vertical talus at Richmond Crippled Children's Hospital and the University of Alabama at Birmingham. Foot Ankle 1980; 1:62.
19. Seimon LP: Surgical correction of congenital vertical talus under the age of 2 years. J Pediatr Orthop 1987; 7:405.
20. Doyle JR, James PM, Larsen LJ, et al: Restoration of elbow flexion in arthrogryposis multiplex congenita. J Hand Surg 1980; 5:149.
21. Dungl P: Reconstruction of Elbow Flexion with M. Pectoralis in Arthrogryposis Multiplex Congenita Type I. Madrid, European Pediatric Orthopedic Society, 1998.
22. Axt MW, Niethard FU, Doderlein L, et al: Principles of treatment of the upper extremity in arthrogryposis multiplex congenita type I. J Pediatr Orthop B 1997; 6:179.
23. Herron LD, Weston GW, Dawson EG: Scoliosis in arthrogryposis multiplex congenita. J Bone Joint Surg Am 1978; 60:293.
24. Daher YH, Lonstein JE, Winter RB, et al: Spinal deformities in patients with arthrogryposis. Spine 1985; 10:609.

ACQUIRED CEREBROSPASTIC DISORDER: STROKE, BRAIN INJURY

John D. Hsu

Summary

- In traumatic brain injury, orthopaedic involvement includes treatment of skeletal trauma and assistance in the management of spasticity and joint contractures.
- Upper extremity tightness and contractures can be improved by nonoperative measures (ranging, stretching, and splinting) or by surgical release of appropriate structures.
- In the lower extremity, resection of heterotopic bone is an important procedure.
- Release or lengthening of structures in the lower extremity can correct dynamic deformities.

The functional needs of patients with an acquired cerebrospastic disorder continue to be a challenge to orthopaedic surgeons involved in their rehabilitative care.[1–3]

In most instances, these events are generally unplanned, and traumatic brain injury or stroke often disables a normally functioning individual. Fortunately, some of these changes are transient and temporary. Unfortunately, permanent residual cerebral defects may cause significant motor, sensory, cognitive, and functional disability. Mobility, self-care, and the ability to communicate may be affected and impaired.

TRAUMATIC BRAIN INJURY

In traumatic brain injury (TBI), children have a better prognosis than adults, and young adults have a lower mortality rate and are better qualified for survival than older adults. Fortunately, the majority of patients who survive a head injury can make substantial neurological recovery.[4, 5] A large proportion of TBI patients can be expected to become ambulatory and capable of self-care activities (Fig. 1).

STROKE

Timing is important because it is generally recognized that no further spontaneous neurological recovery may be expected 6 months after a stroke. Motor control and muscle tone are important contributors to balance reactions and, when present, enhance the patient's potential for ambulation.[6]

NONSURGICAL TREATMENT

Spasticity, a velocity-dependent increase in stretch reflex activity, accompanies many upper motor neuron disease processes, including stroke and TBI. Therefore, strategies

that are useful adjuncts for the treatment of muscle overactivity can be used initially to treat this patient population.

Pharmacological agents are available to treat spasticity. These medications are an adjunct to physical therapy, serial casting, or muscle-lengthening procedures, and training of antagonist muscle groups and reduce muscle overactivity by reducing excitability of motor pathways at the level of the central nervous system (CNS), the neuromuscular junction, and the muscle (H. Levenson, personal communication, 2000).

Local blocks affecting the muscle (the neuromuscular block) or close to the nerve innervating the muscle (perineural block) can be achieved with local anesthetic agents and neurolytic alcohols (phenol and ethanol). Botox or botulinum toxin, which causes a presynaptic block of acetylcholine release, can be used to decrease spasticity in a muscle group for a duration of 3 to 6 months with longer relief of symptoms and less pain from the procedure in comparison to neurolytic alcohols. Baclofen (Lioresal) is now available in oral and intrathecal formulation for pump implant to reduce CNS-mediated spasticity. New drugs such as tizanidine have emerged as contenders for treatment of spasticity of spinal and cerebral origin.

Fortunately, there have been many recent developments with the schemas and medications just mentioned. All of these measures have assisted the patient with spasticity of various causes to return to partial or near self-care, to work, and to independent living.[7]

TBI: ASSESSMENT

GLASGOW COMA SCALE

The Glasgow Coma Scale (Table 1) is recognized as a predictor of global outcome. The scoring is based on the degree of coma present. Testing is done with three major categories: (1) eye opening, (2) motor response, and (3) best verbal response. For instance, if eye opening is spontaneous, with the patient responding to and obeying verbal commands, oriented, and able to converse, then the score is high and the prognosis for recovery is good. In contrast, when the eye opening response occurs as a result of painful stimuli, testing shows flexion withdrawal patterns, and the patient makes incomprehensible sounds, then the score is low. For the individual person, the higher the score, the more likely it is that the patient will make a greater functional recovery.[8]

RANCHO LOS AMIGOS SCALE OF COGNITIVE FUNCTION

A disability rating scale has been developed at Rancho Los Amigos Hospital based on the level of cognitive functioning and behavior (Table 2). This scale defines eight levels of cognitive functioning, ranging from level 1 (no re-

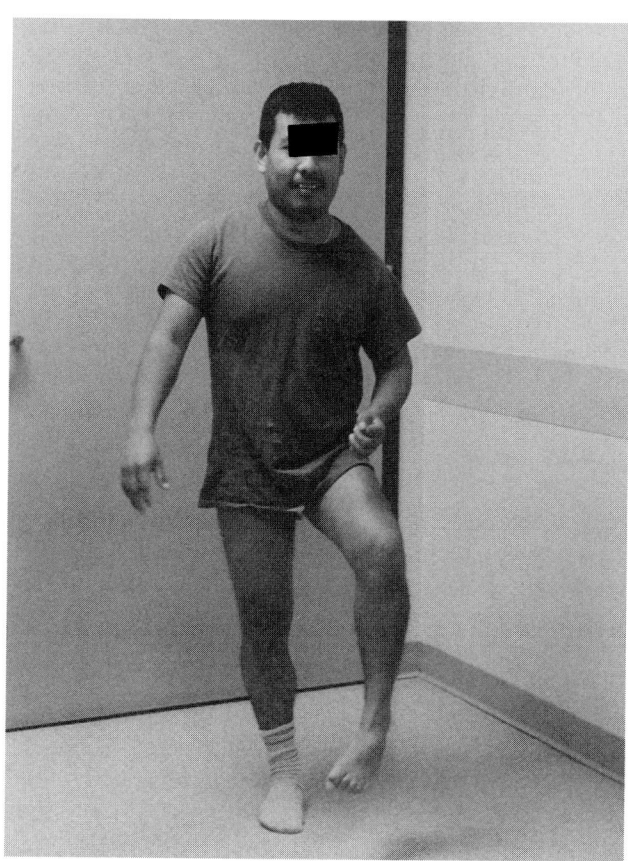

Fig. 1. Traumatic brain injury. Note posturing. Left shoulder and elbow are flexed as are left wrist and fingers. In the lower extremity, the left leg is lifted up so as to clear the ground. The foot is in equinovarus.

TABLE 1. GLASGOW COMA SCALE*

Variable	Score
Eye Opening	
Spontaneously	4
To speech	3
To pain	2
None	1
Best Verbal Response	
Oriented to person, place, and time	5
Confused but able to converse	4
Inappropriate words	3
Incomprehensible sounds	2
None	1
Best Motor Response	
Obey commands	5
Purposefully tries to remove a painful stimulus	4
Flexion to pain	3
Extension to pain	2
None	1

* Measures depth or quality of the coma.
From Jones C: Glasgow Coma Scale. Am J Nurs 1979; 79:1551.

ORTHOPAEDIC CONSIDERATIONS

The orthopaedic surgeon who sees the patient is required to assess a person who may be unable to communicate, may be in a decerebrate state, and may have fractures and joint injuries in addition to the brain insult. The goal is to minimize further damage to the bony and joint structures as well as to the surrounding tissues.[11, 12] As the person recovers and the sequelae from the traumatic event stabilize, the orthopaedic surgeon becomes involved in trying to maintain or restore function. Thus, orthopaedic involvement can by categorized as follows:

1. Treatment of fractures and/or joint injuries of the spine and extremities.
2. Assistance in the management of spasticity and joint contractures.

TABLE 2. RANCHO LOS AMIGOS: LEVEL OF COGNITIVE FUNCTIONING

Level	Description
I	No response
II	Generalized response
III	Localized response
IV	Confused, agitated
V	Confused, inappropriate
VI	Confused, appropriate
VII	Automatic, appropriate
VIII	Purposeful, appropriate

From Hagen C, Malkmus D, Durham P: Levels of cognitive functioning. In Rehabilitation of the Head Injured Adult. Comprehensive Physical Management. Downey, CA, Professional Staff Association of Rancho Los Amigos Hospital, 1979.

sponse) to level 8 ("purposeful and appropriate"). A lower scale gives a poorer prognosis, and a score at level 5 ("confused and appropriate, nonagitated"), with the patient being alert, able to respond to simple commands fairly consistently, and having gross attention to the environment but highly distractible, indicates that the patient may be able to take sufficient direction so that the rehabilitation program can be initiated.[9]

At level 6, the patient is confused but has goal-directed behavior dependent on external input for direction. This person may show a vague recognition of some staff members and has increased awareness of basic needs. With further progression to level 7 ("automatic, appropriate"), the patient appears to be oriented within the surroundings and can go through a daily routine automatically with minimal to no confusion. Recall is shallow, and judgment remains impaired. At level 8, the person is alert, oriented, and able to recall and integrate past and recent events, being aware of the surroundings and culture. The level is deemed purposeful and appropriate. This person can show carryover for new learning. Within the physical capabilities, return to independent living, driving, and work may be possible.

To plan treatment as a member of the rehabilitation team, it is important that the orthopaedic surgeon know the patient's prognosis and progress as well as the underlying scientific basis of the problems and issues encountered.[10]

ACUTE PHASE

ACUTE FRACTURES AND JOINT DISLOCATIONS OF THE SPINE AND EXTREMITIES

In an acute setting, the role of the orthopaedic surgeon is limited. Although it is important to identify these injuries in a patient, priorities for life-saving measures—maintenance of airway, resuscitation, and control of bleeding—take precedence. The goal is to minimize further damage to the bony and joint structures as well as to the surrounding tissues.

If possible, internal fixation is desirable to facilitate rehabilitation and to minimize the high rate of complications associated with traction and partial immobilization. It should be remembered that approximately 10% to 15% of fractures and joint dislocations may be missed during the acute phase.[13]

RECOVERY/STABLE PHASE

Permanent upper and lower extremity joint deformities should be corrected. The goal is to improve existing and remaining function and, when there is no fixed deformity, to provide care directed at the control of spasticity. Release of an overactive muscle to improve extremity and joint alignment can aid function and benefit the patient's outlook significantly.

SHOULDER

SHOULDER SUBLUXATION

Acutely, flaccidity of the shoulder musculature may cause subluxation at the shoulder with resultant pain. A sling or other type of shoulder support can be helpful.[14] With the cooperation of the patient, musculature could also be strengthened by an exercise program, providing there is sufficient motion in the shoulder. Shoulder arthrodesis is seldom needed and, when performed, can significantly limit the residual function.

SHOULDER TIGHTNESS

Increase in muscle tone leads to the development of a shoulder joint contracture. Specifically, when the tightness is in the pectoralis major muscle, stretching and ranging followed by further stretching can be attempted to improve the function. If the shoulder tightness persists, subscapularis tendon release is indicated.[15]

ELBOW

ELBOW FLEXION CONTRACTURE

Mild elbow flexion contracture can be improved by ranging, stretching, and splinting. Persistent, unremitting forces in elbow flexion lead to a "frozen" elbow joint. If severe, moisture will collect in the flexor crease region and cause a malodorous infection. Permanent elbow flexion contracture can be alleviated by surgical release at the elbow using biceps tenotomy or by musculocutaneous neurectomy. A musculocutaneous nerve block may temporarily improve, and perhaps prevent, severe elbow flexion contraction secondary to spasticity.

ULNAR NERVE NEURITIS AT THE CUBITAL TUNNEL

Persons suffering from stroke or hemiplegia are prone to sit for prolonged periods of time and use a wheelchair. When this occurs, the medial aspect of the elbow can rest on the armrests for several hours during the day. The ulnar nerve may become irritated by this constant pressure. Ulnar nerve conduction studies confirm the clinical findings. Nonoperative treatment is performed by repositioning the elbow, padding the armrests, use of an elbow support (Heelbo), and encouraging motion and activity. When the problem persists and the ulnar nerve neuritis causes hand weakness and muscle wasting, it is appropriate to transfer the ulnar nerve anteriorly.[16]

WRIST AND HAND

WRIST-HAND-FINGER FLEXION CONTRACTURES

The person with selective motion in the wrist and hand needs an aggressive therapy program that includes stretching and splinting. Residual deformities need to be dealt with surgically.

In the mild case, the following surgical procedures are recommended:

1. Fractional lengthening of the wrist flexors and deep finger flexors.
2. Fractional lengthening or release of the superficial finger flexors.
3. Transfer of the flexor carpi ulnaris to the dorsum of the hand.

For severe cases, when the residual position of the hand becomes a clenched fist as a result of fixed finger contractures and persistent spasticity of both the superficial and deep finger flexors, the sublimus-to-profundus transfer operation is indicated. Release or lengthening of the flexor carpi radialis and flexor carpi ulnaris may also be required.

SEVERE THUMB CONTRACTURES

Severe thumb contractures may occur in conjunction with severe wrist and finger contractures. Thus, release by fractional lengthening or Z-plasty may be indicated and combined with other surgical procedures.

LOWER EXTREMITY

Orthopaedic procedures for the lower extremity include the following:

1. Operations that assist a person to transfer, stand, and walk better.
2. Procedures that assist a more dependent person in other activities such as sitting, assisted transfers, toileting, and maintaining personal hygiene.

Tendon transfers are used to remove deforming spastic forces so that the dynamic pull causing deformity can be removed and used for more purposeful and more stable functions such as standing and walking. This can be accomplished by whole- or partial-muscle transfers. Frequently, these procedures can be made after an initial trial of casting and tone-reducing medication. Temporary relief can be obtained with systemic drugs such as baclofen, local infiltrations such as nerve blocks using lidocaine, or at motor points using botulinum toxin. Temporary relief lasting a few hours to several months can be obtained. Sometimes the improved position can be maintained by cast immobilization. These recent developments in therapeutics have taken preference over the use of open phenol blocks, which require meticulous surgical dissection and identification so that sensory nerves are not included in the phenol injection and harmed.

Several operations that may assist in maintaining or improving extremity and joint function are discussed next.

RESECTION OF HETEROTOPIC BONE

The most common site for heterotopic bone formation is around the hip joint. The diagnosis can be confirmed and the course after the development of heterotopic ossification can be monitored by laboratory and radiographic studies (Fig. 2).[11, 18] With maturity of the ossification process, heterotopic bone that interferes with joint motion and function can be safely excised. It is important to know the exact location of the heterotopic bone that is to be excised. Vital structures such as major blood vessels may be adjacent or encased in the mass. Computed tomography scans serve as a useful guide to the surgeon, and three-dimensional reconstruction pictures give the exact location of how the extraosseous calcified mass may relate to the joint and to other structures. Although the chance of recurrence may be high, general improvement of motion can be obtained and sufficient range of motion maintained so that key tasks and important functional recovery may be restored.

Heterotopic ossification can also occur at the knee joint. Excision is warranted when it interferes with sitting and standing.

CORRECTION OF DYNAMIC DEFORMITIES
Hip Procedures

Spasticity in the hip flexors and adductors causes deformities that interfere with standing and walking. The surgical procedure of choice to relieve hip flexor spasticity is psoas release or lengthening. When scissoring also occurs, usu-

ally spasticity of the adductor muscles has increased. Adductor tenotomy followed by obturator neurectomy should be considered. When both deformities occur, the surgical releases can include both procedures.[19]

KNEE

HAMSTRING-LENGTHENING PROCEDURES

Open surgical procedures behind the knee to lengthen the semimembranosus, semitendinosus, and biceps femoris may alleviate a dynamic knee flexion deformity. This procedure also improves walking and allows a person to stand straighter. Postoperatively, the surgical correction needs to be maintained by casting the knee in the extended position. When the casts are removed, the use of knee splints may be necessary to maintain the corrected position, especially at night.[20]

SELECTIVE QUADRICEPS RELEASE

Inadequate knee flexion during the swing phase may result in a stiff-legged gait. Rectus femoris transfer or quadriceps release or lengthening is the surgical procedure of choice.

ANKLE AND FOOT DEFORMITIES

EQUINUS DEFORMITY

The surgical procedure of choice is a tendo-Achilles lengthening for the recalcitrant case in which cast correction cannot yield satisfactory results. The goal is to achieve a plantigrade foot, which generally can be accomplished by a percutaneous procedure, which reduces the risk of morbidity. It is important for an ambulatory person to resume walking as soon as possible. Thus, postoperative ambulation in the cast becomes desirable. Correction of severe, fixed, or recurrent equinus contractures may require Z-type lengthening of the Achilles tendon as well as posterior ankle capsulotomy.[22]

SEVERE VALGUS OR PRONATION OF THE FOOT

The peroneal longus tendon, when spastic and unopposed, causes a severe valgus or pronation deformity of the foot, especially during stance phase. Transfer to the heel or to the dorsum of the foot may alleviate this problem.

PERSISTENT EQUINOVARUS OF THE FOOT AND ANKLE

Posterior tibial tendon procedures include conventional tendon transfer, split posterior tibialis tendon transfer, and fractional lengthening. The action of the posterior tibial muscle should be assessed with a varus or equinovarus deformity of the foot and ankle. When the posterior tibial works in phase, it can be weakened by a split posterior tibialis tendon transfer.[27] However, the posterior tibial muscle is generally not the only muscle causing the deformity and generally acts in conjuction with the anterior tibialis and long toe extensors. Thus, when a foot is correctable by other means, the surgical procedure of choice to correct residual posterior tibial spasticity is release of the posterior tibial tendon at the level of the distal third of the leg by fractional lengthening.

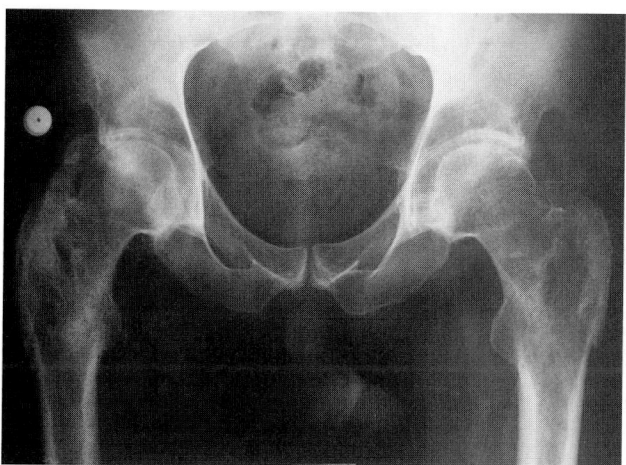

Fig. 2. Radiograph of pelvis showing heterotopic ossification in hip.

PERSISTENT VARUS OF THE FOOT AND ANKLE

Other operations to correct varus deformity of the foot that have been used successfully weaken the anterior tibial muscle and distribute its forces. The split anterior tibial tendon transfer has been successful,[24, 25] especially when walking (dynamic) electromyographic studies show it to be working in phase. A similar correction may be possible with transfer of the entire muscle to the middle of the forefoot, and the latter procedure has been used more often with improved anchoring and fastening techniques.[26]

PALLIATIVE CARE OF THE LOWER EXTREMITY

CONTRACTURE RELEASES

Contracture releases as palliative procedures may be used to facilitate care. Improved hygiene and ability to maintain self-care activities can facilitate overall management.

For the severely disabled, totally dependent patient with a very poor residual cognitive level, one of the basic needs is to promote good perineal hygiene to prevent or minimize the possibility of acquiring ischial and sacral pressure sores. There is a need to minimize moisture collection in the groin and buttock regions. A regularly scheduled turning program and assistive sitting device are important. Contracted hip adductors and hip flexors may impede these activities and make sitting activities difficult. Surgical release of hip contracture to improve positioning can serve a very useful function. Neurectomy, when combined with hip adductor releases, improves the chance to maintain the corrected position.

PROXIMAL HAMSTRING RELEASES

Hip extension contractures prohibit sitting and warrant consideration of proximal hamstring releases. This should be followed by range-of-motion exercises and restoration of sitting activities.

DISTAL HAMSTRING RELEASES

Contraction of the hamstrings with a persistent hip flexion contracture makes transfers difficult and comfortable sitting impossible, despite the acceptability of the "90-90" position for a patient who cannot achieve the standing position. Thirty degrees of range can be safely gained by lengthening of the hamstrings and posterior capsule release. Further extension can cause knee subluxation or peroneal nerve stretching; the latter could give unbearable paresthesias to the patient whose cognitive senses have diminished.

ANKLE AND FOOT RELEASES

The lateral malleolus can rub against the side bars of wheelchair leg rests. Skin breakdown may occur when the foot is in equinovarus. Ulcerations against bony prominences, especially the prominent talar head, are most likely to be seen in more severe instances. Surgical correction of this deformity includes releasing the anterior and posterior tibial tendon and lengthening the Achilles tendon. After cast immobilization, the foot and ankle need to be positioned in a neutral position and supported by ankle-foot orthoses.[27] Tendon transfers at this phase are not indicated.

TOE FLEXOR RELEASES

Toe flexors can become tight when associated with repositioning of the ankle in dorsiflexion. Distal releases are indicated and can be accomplished by distal tenotomy of the toe flexors.

ACKNOWLEDGMENT

I thank Janet Hirsch for typing this chapter.

REFERENCES

1. Garland DE, Waters RL: Orthopedic evaluation in hemiplegic stroke. Orthop Clin North Am 1978; 9:291.
2. McCollough NC III: The role of the orthopedic surgeon in the treatment of stroke. Orthop Clin North Am 1978; 9:305.
3. Savinelli R, Timm M, Montgomery J, et al: Therapy evaluation and management of patients with hemiplegia. Orthop Clin Rel Res 1978; 131:15.
4. Sandel ME, Labi MLC: Outcome prediction: Clinical and research perspectives. STAR Phys Med Rehabil 1990; 4:409.
5. Stylianos S: Late sequelae of major trauma in children. Pediatr Clin North Am 1998; 45:853.
6. Keenan MA, Perry J, Jordan C: Factors affecting balance and ambulation after stroke. Orthop Clin Rel Res 1984; 182:165.
7. Reiter F, Danni M, Lagalla G, et al: Low-dose botulinum toxin with ankle taping for the treatment of spastic equinovarus foot after stroke. Arch Phys Med Rehabil 1998; 79:532.
8. Jones C: Glasgow Coma Scale. Am J Nurs 1979; 79:1551.
9. Hagen C, Malkmus D, Durham P: Levels of cognitive functioning. In Rehabilitation of the Head Injured Adult: Comprehensive Physical Management. Downey, CA, Professional Staff Association of Rancho Los Amigos Hospitals, 1979.
10. Perry J: Scientific basis of rehabilitation. Instruct Course Lectures, Am Acad Orthop Surg 1985; 34:385.
11. Kishwaha VP, Garland DE: Extremity fractures in the patient with a traumatic brain injury. J.A.A.O.S., 1998; 6;298.
12. Davis JW, Phreaner DL, Hoyt DB, et al: The etiology of missed cervical spine injuries. J Trauma 1993; 34:342.
13. Garland DE, Bailey S: Undetected injuries in head-injured adults. Orthop Clin 1981; 155:162.
14. Krempen JF, Silver RA, Hadley J, et al: The use of the Varney brace for subluxating shoulders in stroke and upper motor neuron injuries. Orthop Clin Rel Res 1977; 122:204.
15. Braum RM, West F, Nooney V, et al: Surgical treatment of the painful shoulder contracture in the stroke patient. J Bone Joint Surg Am 1971; 53:1307.
16. Davis FA, Hsu JD: Use of ulnar nerve transposition in the adult brain injured patient. Orthop Trans 1996; 19:850.
17. Bidner SM, Rubins IM, Desjardins JV, et al: Evidence for a humoral mechanism for enchanted osteogenesis after head injury. J Bone Joint Surg Am 1990; 72:1144.
18. Hsu JD, Sakimura I, Stauffer ES: Heterotopic ossification around the hip joint in spinal cord injured patients. Orthop Clin 1975; 112:165.
19. Pinzur MS: Surgical correction of lower extremity problems in patients with brain injury. J Head Trauma Rehabil 1996; 11:69.
20. Keenan MAE, Kozin SH, Berlet AC: Manual of Orthopaedic Surgery for Spasticity. New York, Raven Presss, 1993.
21. Waters RL, Perry J, Garland DE: Surgical correction of gait abnormalities following stroke. Orthop Clin Rel Res 1978; 131:54.

22. Hsu JD, Hoffer MM: Posterior tibial tendon transfer anteriorly through the interosseous membrane. Orthop Clin Rel Res 1978; 131:202.
23. Green NE, Griffin PP, Shiavi R: Split posterior tibial-tendon transfer in spastic cerebral palsy. J Bone Joint Surg 1983; 65: 748.
24. Hoffer MM, Reiswig JA, Garrett AM, et al: The split anterior tibial tendon transfer in the treatment of spastic varus hindfoot of childhood. Orthop Clin North Am 1974; 5:31.
25. Edwards P, Hsu JD: SPLATT combined with tendo Achilles lengthening for spastic equinovarus in adults: Results and predictors of surgical outcome. Foot Ankle 1993; 14:335.
26. Garceau GJ, Manning KR: The anterior tibial tendon transfer. J Bone Joint Surg 1947; 29:1044.
27. Hsu JD, Jackson R: Treatment of symptomatic foot and ankle deformities in the nonambulatory neuromuscular patient. Foot Ankle 1985; 5:238.

section 10 chapter 12

PEDIATRIC SPINAL CORD INJURY: LONG-TERM MANAGEMENT

John P. Lubicky

Summary

- This condition has a major socioeconomic/public health impact because of its life-altering effects in many areas and the need for ongoing health management.
- The effects of growth influence a number of the consequences of spinal cord injury (SCI).
- Management goals must emphasize the need for independence and mobility and awareness that constant vigilance to avoid or recognize and then treat the complications of SCI is a lifelong chore.
- The importance of education and socialization as well as efforts for eventual transition to adult life must be stressed.
- Pediatric SCI patients are best managed by a multidisciplinary team.

INTRODUCTION

DEFINITION

SCI is a condition in which damage to the spinal cord causes its function to be either completely or incompletely lost. A complete SCI is one in which all sensory and motor function is lost below the level of the lesion. In an incomplete SCI, some normal cord function is preserved below the level of the lesion. SCI can be caused by trauma (e.g., spinal fractures or dislocations, penetrating wounds), by tumors of the spine or spinal cord, as a result of medical and surgical interventions (e.g., scoliosis surgery, repair of coarctation of the aorta), or by other disease processes (e.g., transverse myelitis, Guillain-Barré syndrome). Malfunction of the spinal cord sets up a cascade of physiological processes that can then cause abnormalities in multiple organ systems.

HISTORICAL REVIEW

Modern treatment of SCI, at least for adults, began in England during World War II, when a spinal care unit was initiated at Mandeville with Sir Ludwig Guttman as its director. This center became the Stoke Mandeville Hospital Spinal Unit. Subsequent contributions by Bedbrook in England and Munro and Bors in the United States further focused on the proper treatment of SCI. The work of Rusk and Young and others eventually led to the establishment of the first model SCI system in the United States, a data base created under the auspices of the National Institute for Disability and Rehabilitation Research for adult patients.[1, 2]

Noting the unique factors that affect children with SCI, Steel in the late 1970s persuaded the Shriners Hospitals for Children to develop comprehensive care for children with SCIs. Subsequently, three regional SCI centers within the Shriners system were developed and began a close cooperation with the Model System. Currently, the largest data base on spinal cord injury patients is maintained through the cooperation of Model Spinal Cord Injury Care System (MSCICS) and the Shriners Hospitals for Children Spinal Cord Injury Centers data base (NSSCID). More than a decade of experience with pediatric spinal cord injury led to a symposium and eventual publication of a monograph covering virtually all aspects of the care of pediatric SCI in 1996.[3]

EPIDEMIOLOGY

Approximately 7600 to 10,000 new SCI cases occur per year in the United States, of which 3% to 5% occur in persons younger than 15 years. Trauma causes 85% to 90% of the cases. Of all injuries, about two-thirds are complete lesions and one-third are incomplete. Tetraplegia occurs in 40% and paraplegia in 60%. Males predominate in the traumatic group, although there is not much of a gender difference in very young children with SCIs. Unfortunately, over the recent past, violence resulting in penetrating injuries such as gunshot wounds is now responsible for a larger percentage of SCIs.[4]

PATHOGENESIS

SCI results from either anatomic and/or physiological disruption of the spinal cord. The initial injury sets off a cascade of events that results in an autodestructive biochemical process known as the secondary injury, which causes further damage to the cord. Various pharmacological measures, especially high-dose corticosteroids given close to the time of injury, have been shown to limit further damage and perhaps enhance recovery. In general, if neurological improvement after a complete SCI does not occur within the first hours after the incident, the prognosis for recovery is very poor. Overall life expectancy is shortened and is affected by the level of injury.[5]

CLINICAL FEATURES

Clinical manifestation of SCI after the acute phase treatment depends on the level of the lesion. A detailed physical examination is needed to determine motor and sensory function as well as to identify other consequences of SCI such as spasticity, the presence of musculoskeletal abnormalities (e.g., spinal deformity, contractures, hip dislocation), pressure ulcers, bowel and bladder function, and so on. Remaining muscle function and strength can be used to determine subsequent function.

INVESTIGATIONS

From an orthopaedic perspective, various imaging studies are the most helpful in evaluating musculoskeletal problems associated with SCI. Plain radiographs are useful in evaluating spinal deformity, the status of hip reduction/dysplasia, and established heterotopic ossification. Changes in neurological function/level may be evaluated by spinal magnetic resonance imaging (MRI) to rule out the development of a syringomyelia or continued pressure on the spinal cord from bony fragments, disk herniation, or spinal canal malalignment. Bone scans may be helpful in identifying early cases of heterotopic ossification not yet visible on plain radiographs. Urological management uses renal and bladder ultrasonography, contrast-enhanced radiographs, and nuclear scans as well as urodynamics and urinalysis/urine cultures to evaluate genitourinary tract function and disease.

DIFFERENTIAL DIAGNOSIS

The diagnosis of SCI and its type after a traumatic incident is generally straightforward. In young children, the presence of SCI without radiographic abnormality (SCIWORA) after a traumatic incident is a peculiarity that occurs because of the elasticity and flexible nature of the spinal column in this age group. This phenomenon exists because the extreme elasticity of the ligaments and disk bonds between the vertebrae allows the spinal column itself to elongate more than the spinal cord, causing injury to the substance of the spinal cord. This entity, SCIWORA, was described before the common usage of MRI, which has now shown, in many of these cases, that actually, ligaments or disks have been disrupted. Identification of this was not possible before this imaging technique. In the future, SCIWORA will be used less frequently because of enhanced imaging techniques that identify heretofore unidentifiable injury to various components of the spinal column. Identifying the exact cause of nontraumatic SCI (e.g., Guillain-Barré syndrome and transverse myelitis) is important for prognostication and risk of recovery/recurrence. A very small number of cases may be of hysterical cause.

COST OF MANAGEMENT OF SCI

Overall, the costs of managing a patient with SCI, not only through the acute phase of the injury but for a lifetime, are quite high. Data for this can be gathered from the MSCICS and NSSCID data bases. As can be expected, the care for a tetraplegic patient is higher than that for a paraplegic patient. It has been found that utilization of nursing home care accounted for only 0.6% of children with SCI compared with 5.8% of adults. Charges for acute care of a high tetraplegic patient average about $150,000, with subsequent acute rehabilitation costing about $136,000. For a Frankel D paraplegic (patients with useful sensory and motor function), charges for acute care averaged $46,000, with an additional $44,000 spent for acute rehabilitation. Rehospitalization for complications resulting from SCI is common, but there does not appear to be any statistical difference in the likelihood of rehospitalization when comparing tetraplegic and paraplegic patients at varying time intervals from the date of injury.

Over the course of a lifetime, those with SCI incurred two broad categories of costs: direct costs: and indirect costs Direct costs include various levels of medical care, home modifications, equipment supplies, attendant care, and vocational rehabilitation services, among others. Total direct costs depend on the age at injury and the level of injury. For example, cost over a lifetime for a 10-year-old with a high tetraplegic SCI can range from $1.4 to $2.2 million. In contrast, a Frankel D paraplegic patient's direct costs range from $254,000 to $415,000. Indirect costs are potential costs and include lost wages and fringe benefits and productivity. The prediction of indirect costs for children is difficult because the prediction is usually based on current income, which children do not generally have at the time of their injury. Again, using the example of a 10-year-old with a high tetraplegic SCI, estimated indirect costs over a lifetime can range from $654,000 to $2,000,000, whereas a Frankel D paraplegic patient's indirect costs can range from $445,000 to $1,400,000. (In all of these discussions, the amounts are in 1994 dollars.) It is clear that management of all aspects of injury over a lifetime is quite expensive. To decrease the cost, careful monitoring of health status and prevention of and prompt treatment of complications of SCI are needed. Additionally, an emphasis should be placed on the need for SCI patients to continue their education and become gainfully employed.[6, 7]

COMPLICATIONS

Many potential complications can arise in patients with SCI. It is beyond the scope of this chapter to comment on all of them. However, a few important complications are now discussed briefly.

Pressure Ulcers

Pressure ulcers, formerly known as pressure sores and decubitus ulcers, occur frequently. These can range from temporarily reddened areas of skin to very deep sores that are associated with osteomyelitis of the underlying bone (Fig. 1). Several classifications have been developed to better describe and rank them according to severity. From the Model Systems experience, 32% of patients experience pressure ulcers during the acute care and rehabilitation phases of their treatment; however, the majority are not severe. Pressure ulcers during this phase occur in the following areas in order of frequency: sacrum, heels, and ischium. At an average time of 2 years after injury, about 9% of patients experience pressure ulcers. The occurrence at this stage in order of frequency is ischium, sacrum, and greater trochanter. Pressure ulcers can interfere significantly with rehabilitation and the achievement of mobility and independence in activities of daily living.[8-10] Therefore,

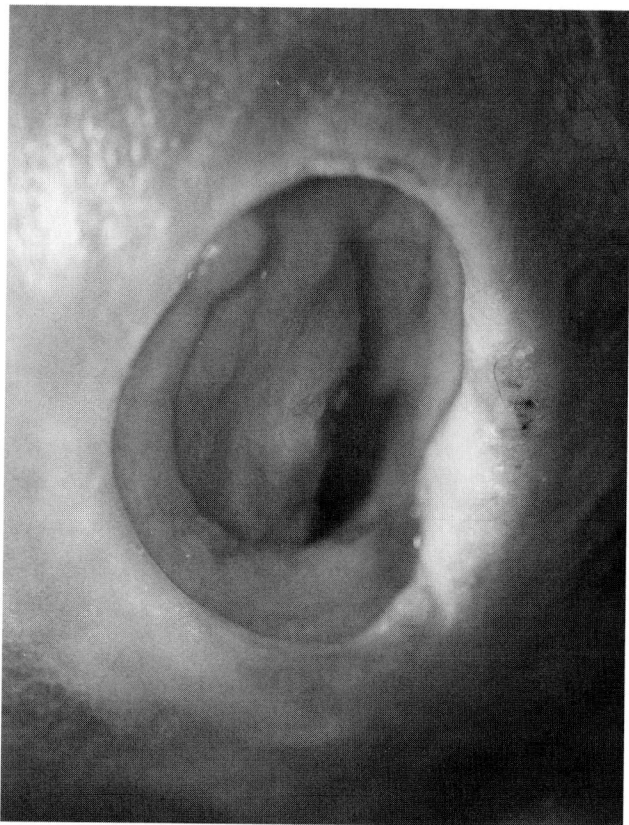

Fig. 1. Severe infected ischial pressure ulcer. This ulcer has eroded down to the bone and is associated with osteomyelitis of the ischium.

prevention is very important, and to that end, education of the patient and caregivers is of utmost importance. Measures to prevent pressure ulcers include the development of skin tolerance, skin inspection, equipment (e.g., cushions), positioning techniques, hygiene, and nutrition. The more mild and moderate types of pressure ulcers may be managed by nonoperative measures.[11, 12] However, when the ulcers become deep and result in cavities beneath the skin that are associated with soft-tissue or bony infection, surgical treatment consisting of débridement and closure is necessary. Various surgical techniques can be used in this regard. More severe ulcers require extensive surgery and also require that patients be recumbent for prolonged periods of time until the entire site heals completely.[13, 14]

Spasticity

Spasticity is a neurological condition in which there is increased involuntary muscle tone resulting from altered control of the stretch reflex, causing excessive flexor and/or extensor muscle activity. The pathological process that causes this is a loss of the inhibiting effects on the stretch reflex from the pyramidal system, which in the normal situation modulates the stretch reflex. Spasticity occurs in about 75% of adults and in 50% of children with SCI, and this problem appears to be more common in those with incomplete lesions. Spasticity occurs on average 6 weeks after cervical SCI and 10 weeks after thoracic SCI. The severity of spasticity, precluding any other intercurrent factors, plateaus approximately 2 years after injury. Spasticity

can be severe and can cause pain, sleep disturbances, pressure ulcers, and hip dislocation. Spasticity may cause muscle imbalance with subsequent abnormal positioning of the lower extremities. This may, for example, contribute to the development of hip dislocation. Contributing factors to periodic worsening of spasticity include urinary tract infections and bladder stones, pressure ulcers, paronychias, and soft-tissue trauma. Some degree of spasticity, however, can be useful in the performance of some functions, (e.g., standing transfers).[15]

Management of spasticity involves eliminating inciting causes and daily stretching of affected muscles. Further treatment can include the oral administration of baclofen, diazepam, and clonidine. However, spasticity may worsen in patients otherwise well controlled by these oral medications if some of the just-mentioned inciting causes are present. For those who have spasticity that is not adequately controlled by oral medication, intrathecal baclofen, dorsal root rhizotomy, muscle injections of botulinum toxin or phenol, or surgical releases may become necessary.[16-18]

Latex Allergy

Latex allergy was recognized as the cause of a number of otherwise unexplained incidents of intraoperative anaphylactic reactions, some of which were fatal, in children who had multiple congenital anomalies, especially urological and myelodysplastic anomalites.[19-21] The allergy seems to be caused by early and repeated exposure to natural rubber protein, which occurs in latex urinary catheters and other medical devices. The diagnosis of latex allergy is made by a history of an immediate-type hypersensitivity reaction as well as by various laboratory tests (radioallergosorbent test, radioimmunosassay). These tests have varying sensitivity and specificity because of the substances being tested. Therefore, the most significant confirmatory evidence is that of a known allergic reaction of a specific patient to a natural rubber product. At least 16% to 18% of patients with SCI have latex allergy. The main treatment for latex allergy is to avoid contact with any latex substances. Beyond that, medical treatment includes the acute administration of epinephrine for an acute allergic reaction and other measures (e.g., prophylactic medications such as diphenhydramine, methylprednisolone, and ranitidine) for situations that place a patient at risk.[22-25]

ORTHOPAEDIC COMPLICATIONS

After the acute phase of the injury, which may include high-energy fractures of long bones in addition to spinal trauma, a number of abnormalities of the musculoskeletal system can occur. Minimal trauma may cause pathological fractures as a result of osteopenia that exists in nonambulatory patients, who may also have some other issues, such as poor nutrition, that can contribute to the bone resorption. Generally, these fractures heal rapidly, and many can be treated with minimal immobilization.[26, 27] As mentioned in the Spasticity section, joint contactures can occur as a result of muscle imbalance but also may be fostered by positioning. Early institution of range of motion and stretching, as well as appropriate splinting, helps to maintain functional range of motion and avoid contractures that interfere with function.[28] Muscle imbalance and contractures can lead to hip dislocation[29] (Fig. 2).

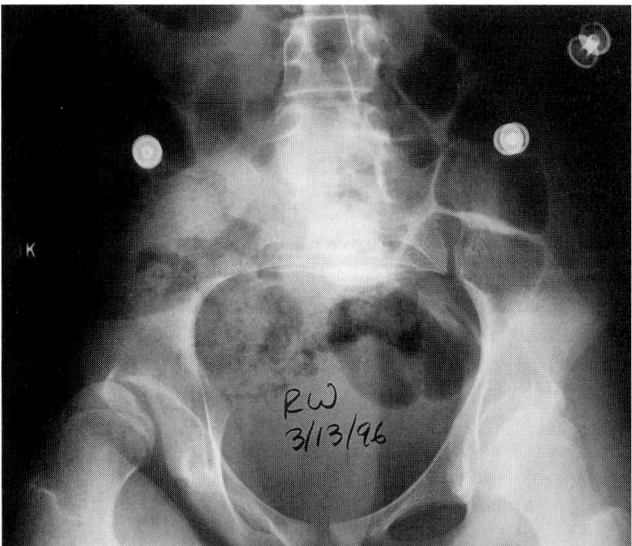

Fig. 2. Hip dislocation. This is an anteroposterior radiograph of the pelvis of an adolescent girl with a recent dislocation of the right hip associated with increased spasticity and decreased range of motion of the hip. Subsequent right hip reconstruction, including soft-tissue releases, proximal femoral osteotomy, and acetabuloplasty, restored near-normal passive range of motion of the hip and decreased spasticity.

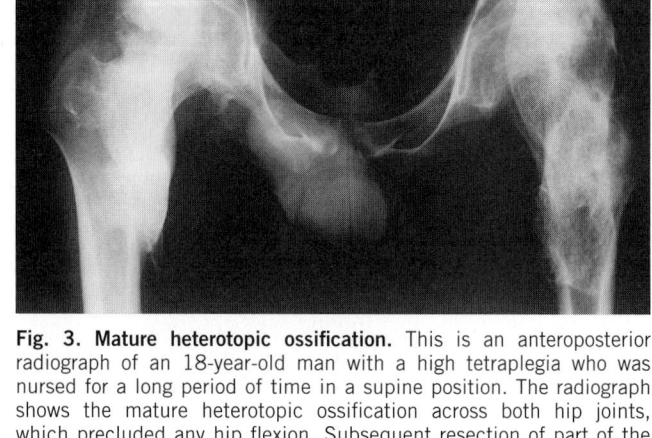

Fig. 3. Mature heterotopic ossification. This is an anteroposterior radiograph of an 18-year-old man with a high tetraplegia who was nursed for a long period of time in a supine position. The radiograph shows the mature heterotopic ossification across both hip joints, which precluded any hip flexion. Subsequent resection of part of the heterotopic bone bilaterally resulted in the ability to flex the hips beyond 90 degrees and allowed the patient to assume a normal sitting position.

Heterotopic ossification occurs in 20% to 30% of adults at an average of 6 months after SCI; however, only 3% to 10% of children with SCI experience it at an average time of 14 months after injury. Its occurrence may produce pain and swelling and may eventually lead to decrease in range of motion, with actual ankylosis of the affected joint. Medical management includes medications such as indomethacin and etidronate disodium and radiation therapy. For established mature bony heterotopic ossification, surgical excision is indicated to restore joint motion. It appears now that simply waiting 1.5 years from the time of injury is sufficient to prevent recurrence after surgical intervention regardless of what is seen on a bone scan[30] (Fig. 3).

Spinal deformity is a particular problem in children with SCI. This can result from the malunion of a spinal fracture, from complications from the surgical treatment of a spinal fracture or dislocations, or, most commonly, from paralysis. The particular type of spinal deformity, its development, and its severity are intimately linked with skeletal maturity at the time of injury. Although the incidence of a spinal deformity developing in a skeletally immature child is high, not every child will acquire a paralytic deformity. Factors that are important in the development of progressive deformity include a complete injury associated with no useful function in the lower extremities. Bracing young, immature children with flexible curves may help with positioning to achieve comfortable and appropriate posture; however, braces cannot affect the natural history of paralytic curves. For children older than 10 years who have scoliotic curves greater than 50 degrees, spinal fusion and instrumentation are indicated to provide permanent leveling of the pelvis and correction and stabilization of the spinal deformity[31, 32] (Fig. 4).

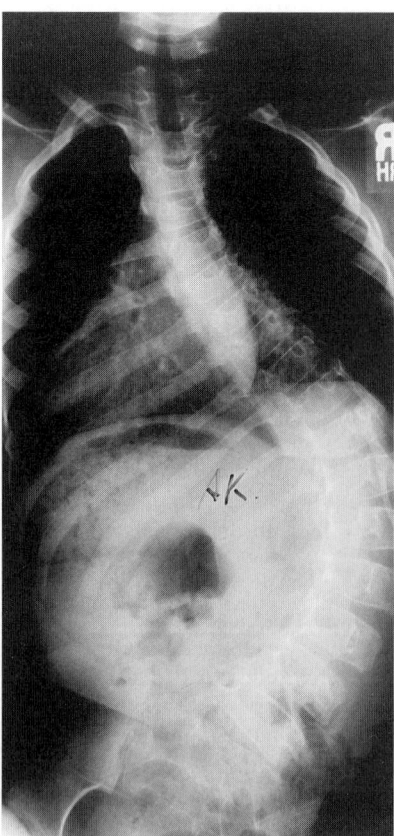

Fig. 4. Progressive scoliosis. This is an anteroposterior sitting radiograph of a 10-year-old girl with upper thoracic paraplegia. She experienced progressive scoliosis with significant pelvic obliquity that interfered with sitting.

Rehabilitation

The overall goal of rehabilitation of an SCI patient is to maximize his or her functional abilities. To do this properly, a focus on the whole person, including the socioeconomic situation and degree of impairment, is necessary. This is best accomplished using a team approach, with professionals along with family/caregivers and the patient. It is important to remember that the goals of handicapped people may be different than those of the professionals caring for them. The following functions are ranked according to importance by handicapped people: communication, activities of daily living, mobility, and walking.[33–35] Physical rehabilitation should start immediately after SCI, with maintenance of range of motion, strengthening of functioning muscles, and development of self-care skills using a different level of neurological function. These interventions need to be developmentally based in pediatric patients to correspond with the patients' developmental stage. Upright posture should be offered to all patients who can tolerate this, especially the very young, with the understanding that those with significantly impaired motor function will eventually and most commonly use the wheelchair as their main method of mobility. The standing position

and walking, if possible, will be aided by appropriate bracing and, occasionally, surgery, which may include procedures such as tendon transfers, releases, osteotomies, and implantation of electrodes for stimulation.[35–37]

Although management of medical problems and physical rehabilitation are extremely important, equal focus must be placed on development and maintenance of life skills. Independent living and education are extremely important. It appears that life satisfaction in adult patients who were injured as children depends on educational level, employment status, and long-term health management. These factors do not seem to be affected by the level of injury. Independence, education, and employment, as well as other aspects of socialization, make a smooth transition to adulthood more likely than if these factors are overlooked. However, extraneous factors may interfere with achieving independent living and employment opportunities.[38, 39]

RESULTS

The management of SCI patients can be both challenging and rewarding for the patient and caregivers. Cooperative efforts by all involved ensure the best chance for a successful outcome.

REFERENCES

1. Thomas JP: The model spinal cord injury concept: Development and implementation. In Stover SL, DeLisa JA, Whiteneck GG (eds): Spinal Cord Injury: Outcomes From the Model Systems. Gaithersburg, MD, Aspen Publishers, 1995, p 1.
2. Bedbrook GM: Spinal injuries with tetraplegia and paraplegia. J Bone Joint Surg Br 1979; 61:267.
3. Betz RR, Mulcahey MJ (eds): The Child With a Spinal Cord Injury. Rosemont, IL, American Academy of Orthopaedic Surgeons, 1996.
4. Vogel LC, DeVivo MJ: Etiology and demographics. In Betz RR, Mulcahey MJ (eds): The Child With a Spinal Cord Injury. Rosemont, IL, American Academy of Orthopaedic Surgeons, 1996, p 3.
5. Bracken MB, Shephard MJ, Holford TR, et al: Administration of methylprednisolone for 24 or 48 hours or tirilazad mesylate for 48 hours in the treatment of acute spinal cord Injury. JAMA 1997; 277:1597.
6. DeVivo MJ, Whiteneck GG, Charles ED Jr: The economic impact of spinal cord injury. In Stover SL, DeLisa JA, Whiteneck GG (eds): Spinal Cord Injury: Clinical Outcomes from the Model Systems. Gaithersburg, MD, Aspen Publishers, 1995, p 234.
7. DeVivo MJ, Kartus PL, Rutt RD, et al: The influence of age at the time of spinal cord injury on rehabilitation outcome. Arch Neurol 1990; 47:687.
8. Yarkony GM: Pressure ulcers: A review. Arch Phys Med Rehabil 1994; 75:908.
9. Yarkony GM, Kirm PM, Carlson C, et al: Classification of pressure ulcers. Arch Dermatol 1990; 126:1218.
10. Shea JD: Pressure sores: Classification and management. Clin Orthop 1975; 112:89.
11. Seymour RJ, Lacefield WE: Wheelchair

cushion effect on pressure and skin temperature. Arch Phys Med Rehabil 1985; 66:103.
12. Vogel LC: Medical management of pressure ulcers. In Betz RR, Mulcahey MJ (eds): The Child With a Spinal Cord Injury. Rosemont, IL, American Academy of Orthopaedic Surgeons, 1996, p 293.
13. Lewis VL Jr, Bailey MH, Pulawski G, et al: The diagnosis of osteomyelitis in patients with pressure sores. Plast Reconstr Surg 1988; 81:229.
14. Apple DF, Murray HH: Surgical management of pressure ulcers. In Betz RR, Mulcahey MJ, (eds): The Child With a Spinal Cord Injury. Rosemont, IL, American Academy of Orthopaedic Surgeons, 1996, p 305.
15. Vogel LC: Spasticity: Diagnostic workup and medical management. In Betz RR, Mulcahey MJ (eds): The Child With a Spinal Cord Injury. Rosemont, IL, American Academy of Orthopaedic Surgeons, 1996, p 261.
16. Penn RD, Kroin JS: Long-term intrathecal baclofen infusion for treatment of spasticity. J Neurosurg 1987; 66:181.
17. Snow BJ, Tsui JK, Bhatt MH, et al: Treatment of spasticity with botulinum toxin: A double blind study. Ann Neurol 1990; 28: 512.
18. Apple DF, Murray HH: Spasticity: Surgical management. In Betz RR, Mulcahey MJ (eds): The Child With a Spinal Cord Injury. Rosemont, IL, American Academy of Orthopaedic Surgeons, 1996, p 269.
19. D'Astous J, Drouin MA, Rhine E: Intraoperative anaphylaxis secondary to latex in children who have spina bifida. Report of 2 cases. J Bone Joint Surg Am 1992; 74: 1084.
20. Emans JB: Allergy to latex in patients

who have myelodysplasia: Relevance for the orthopaedic surgeon. J Bone Joint Surg Am 1992; 74:1103.
21. Anaphylactic reactions during general anesthesia among pediatric patients: United States Jan 1990–Jan 1991. MMWR Morb Mortal Wkly Rep 1991; 40:437.
22. Levy DA: Report of the International Latex Conference: Sensitivity to latex in medical devices. Allergy 1993; 48 (suppl): S1.
23. Vogel LC, Shrader T, Lubicky JP: Latex allergy in children and adolescents with spinal cord injury. J Pediatr Orthop 1995; 15:517.
24. Levy DA, Choipin D, Pecquet C, et al: Allergy to latex. Allergy 1992; 47:579.
25. American Academy of Allergy and Immunology: Task force on allergic reactions to latex. Committee report. J Allergy Clin Immunol 1993; 92:16.
26. Betz RR, Triolo RJ, Hermida VM, et al: The effect of functional neuromuscular stimulation on bone mineral content in lower limbs of spinal cord injured children. Presented at the annual meeting of the American Spinal Injury Association Seattle, WA, April 1991.
27. Lee JJ, Lyne ED: Pathological fractures in severely handicapped children and young adults. J Pediatr Orthop 1990; 10:497.
28. Tynan, M: Joint contractures in children with spinal cord injury. In Betz RR, Mulcahey MJ (eds): The Child With a Spinal Cord Injury. Rosemont, IL, American Academy of Orthopaedic Surgeons, 1996, p 339.
29. Rink P, Miller F: Hip instability in spinal cord injury patients. J Pediatr Orthop 1990; 10:5.
30. Betz RR: Heterotopic ossification. In Betz RR, Mulcahey, MJ (eds): The Child With

a Spinal Cord Injury. Rosemont, IL, American Academy of Orthopaedic Surgeons, 1996, p 345.

31. Lubicky JP, Betz RR: Spinal deformity in children and adolescents with spinal cord injury. In Betz RR, Mulcahey MJ (eds): The Child With a Spinal Cord Injury. Rosemont, IL, American Academy of Orthopaedic Surgeons, 1996, p 363.

32. Godfried DH, Vogel LC, Lubicky JP: Spinal deformity in pediatric spinal cord injury patients. Presented at the annual meeting of the Pediatric Orthopaedic Society, Banff, Alberta, Canada, May 1997.

33. Nelson MR, Tilbor AG, Frieden L, et al: Introduction to pediatric rehabilitation. In Betz RR, Mulcahey MJ (eds): The Child With a Spinal Cord Injury. Rosemont, IL, American Academy of Orthopaedic Surgeons, 1996, p 461.

34. Hoffer MM, Feiwell E, Perry J, et al: Functional ambulation in patients with myelomeningocele. J Bone Joint Surg Am 1973; 55:137.

35. Hall DM, Johnson SL, Middleton J: Rehabilitation of head injured children. Arch Dis Child 1990; 65:553.

36. Vogel LC, Lubicky JP: Ambulation in children and adolescents with spinal cord injuries. J Pediatr Orthop 1995; 15:510.

37. Kelly MA, Stokes KS: Standing and ambulation for the child with paraplegia or tetraplegia. In Betz RR, Mulcahey MJ (eds): The Child With a Spinal Cord Injury. Rosemont, IL, American Academy of Orthopaedic Surgeons, 1996, p 519.

38. Anderson CJ, Johnson KA, Klaas SJ, et al: Pediatric spinal cord injury: Transition to adulthood. J Voc Rehab 1998; 10:103.

39. Vogel LC, Klaas SJ, Lubicky JP, et al: Long-term outcomes and life satisfaction of adults who had pediatric spinal cord injury. Arch Phys Med Rehabil 1998; 79: 1416.

FOOT AND ANKLE

CHARLES L. SALTZMAN

LIGAMENT INJURIES OF THE FOOT AND ANKLE

David A. Porter

Summary
- These injuries are common, occur in younger persons, and cause short- and long-term disabilities.
- Nonoperative treatment is effective for most lateral ankle sprains, stable syndesmosis sprains, stable medial ankle sprains, and stable midfoot sprains.
- Operative treatment is required for unstable syndesmosis sprains, unstable medial sprains, and unstable midfoot sprains.
- The natural history is influenced by the type of injury (stable versus unstable), the location of the injury (lateral ankle versus medial ankle, syndesmosis, and midfoot), and associated injuries (occult fractures).
- Occult injuries are common and often misdiagnosed.
- Treatment options are becoming well established.

ANKLE SPRAIN

DEFINITION

The isolated lateral ankle sprain involves a ligament injury to the anterior talofibular ligament (ATFL), the calcaneofibular ligament (CFL), and rarely the posterior talofibular ligament (PTFL) (Fig. 1A). The medial ankle sprain involves a ligament injury to the superficial and deep deltoid ligaments. The syndesmosis sprain involves a ligament injury to the interosseous membrane, the anterior and posterior inferior tibiofibular ligament (AITFL and PITFL), and the superficial and deep deltoid ligaments, and often a high fibula fracture (Maissoneuve fracture) (Fig. 2, Fig. 3). The stable syndesmosis sprain without a fibula fracture is often termed a "high ankle sprain." This injury also often involves injury to the anterior deltoid ligament (see Fig. 2A). A midfoot sprain involves a ligament injury to the tarsometatarsal (TMT) ligaments (Lisfranc joints) and is often termed a "Lisfranc" dislocation or sprain (Fig. 4D and E, Fig. 5).

HISTORICAL REVIEW

1815: Jacque Lisfranc[1] (surgeon in Napoleon's army) describes injury to midfoot and amputation at TMT joint.

1840: Maisonneuve[2] describes classic fibula fracture with syndesmosis rupture.

1949: First published report on lateral ankle reconstruction.[3]

1960s: Peroneal tendon used for reconstruction of ATFL.[4, 5]

1988: Jackson et al[6] describe mechanism of isolated deltoid ligament injury.

1990s: Increased interest in nonoperative treatment for acute "unstable" lateral sprains; recognition for need to immobilize in dorsiflexion for proper ligament healing.

EPIDEMIOLOGY

An average of 27,000 ankle sprains occur each day in the United States, most commonly related to athletics.

Ten percent of ankle sprains are medial sprains and 10% involve a significant syndesmosis injury.

Midfoot sprains compose 0.2% of all fractures and 7% to 8% of all complex foot and ankle problems. As many as 20% are missed or misdiagnosed. Most sprains are related to motor vehicle accidents and athletics. There is an average of one injury per 55,000 persons per year.

PATHOGENESIS

The mechanism of injury helps identify and explain the injury and, therefore, must be obtained in the history. These injuries result from rotational and angular movements of the foot and ankle that exceed the tensile strength of the ligament.

Lateral Ankle Sprain

The mechanism involves a plantar flexion and simultaneous inversion to the ankle. Typically, this occurs just as the patient begins to load the ball of the foot. Often this injury occurs with landing associated with a jump or a fall. The mortise alignment with the ankle in neutral (90-degree angle between leg and plantar surface of foot) is very stable (a box [the talus] inside a box [the fibula and tibia]). However, as the ankle goes into plantar flexion, the talus advances anteriorly and is "unlocked" from the tibia/fibula mortise. Because the anterior talus is wider than the posterior talus, as the ankle is plantar flexed, a "looseness" between the talus and the mortise is created. It is important to understand that the ATFL is tight in plantar flexion, whereas the CFL is the most taut in neutral. This difference likely explains why the ATFL is the most commonly injured ligament among lateral ankle sprains. Statistically, the ATFL is the weakest of the ankle ligaments.

Medial Ankle Sprains

Medial ankle sprains can occur from several mechanisms: abduction, external rotation, or a combination of these two. A pure abduction force will cause a deep deltoid injury, whereas a primary external rotation force will create an anterior deltoid injury (see Fig. 2A). A combination of the two forces can disrupt both ligaments and result in more severe injuries involving the lateral side of the ankle (e.g., fibula or the syndesmosis) (see Fig. 2A–C).

Syndesmosis Sprain

A syndesmosis sprain requires a significant amount of force and always involves external rotation. Typically, this injury involves both abduction and external rotation with dorsiflexion (see Fig. 2A–C).

Midfoot Sprain

A midfoot sprain typically involves one of three mechanisms of injury. In a motor vehicle accident, axial loading

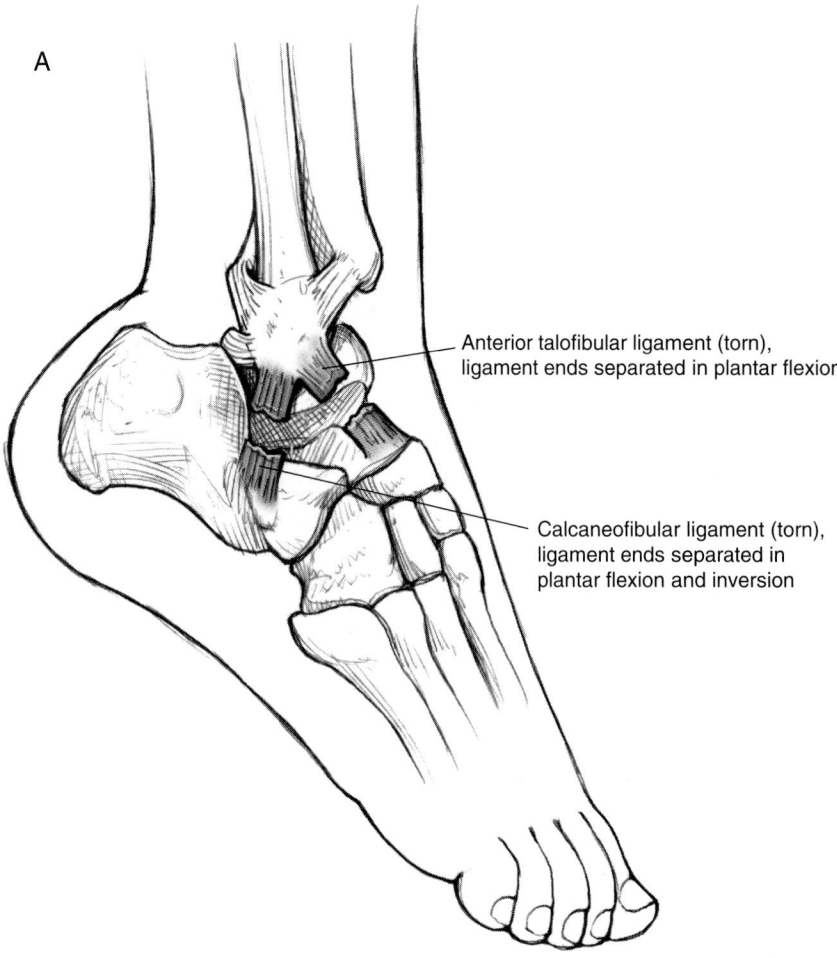

A

Anterior talofibular ligament (torn),
ligament ends separated in plantar flexion

Calcaneofibular ligament (torn),
ligament ends separated in
plantar flexion and inversion

Fig. 1. Lateral ankle sprain. *A*, Grade III lateral ankle sprain anatomic injury. Note the lack of opposition of the anterior talofibular ligament (ATFL) and the calcaneofibular ligament (CFL) with the foot/ankle in plantar flexion and inversion. *B*, Grade III lateral ankle sprain. Note the complete opposition of the ATFL and the CFL with the foot/ankle in dorsiflexion and neutral eversion.

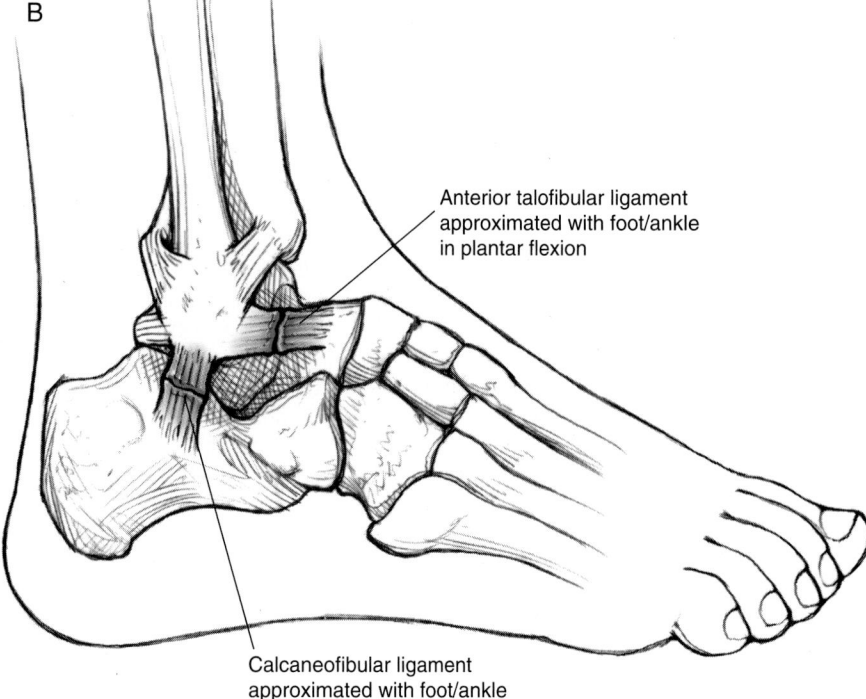

B

Anterior talofibular ligament
approximated with foot/ankle
in plantar flexion

Calcaneofibular ligament
approximated with foot/ankle
in eversion

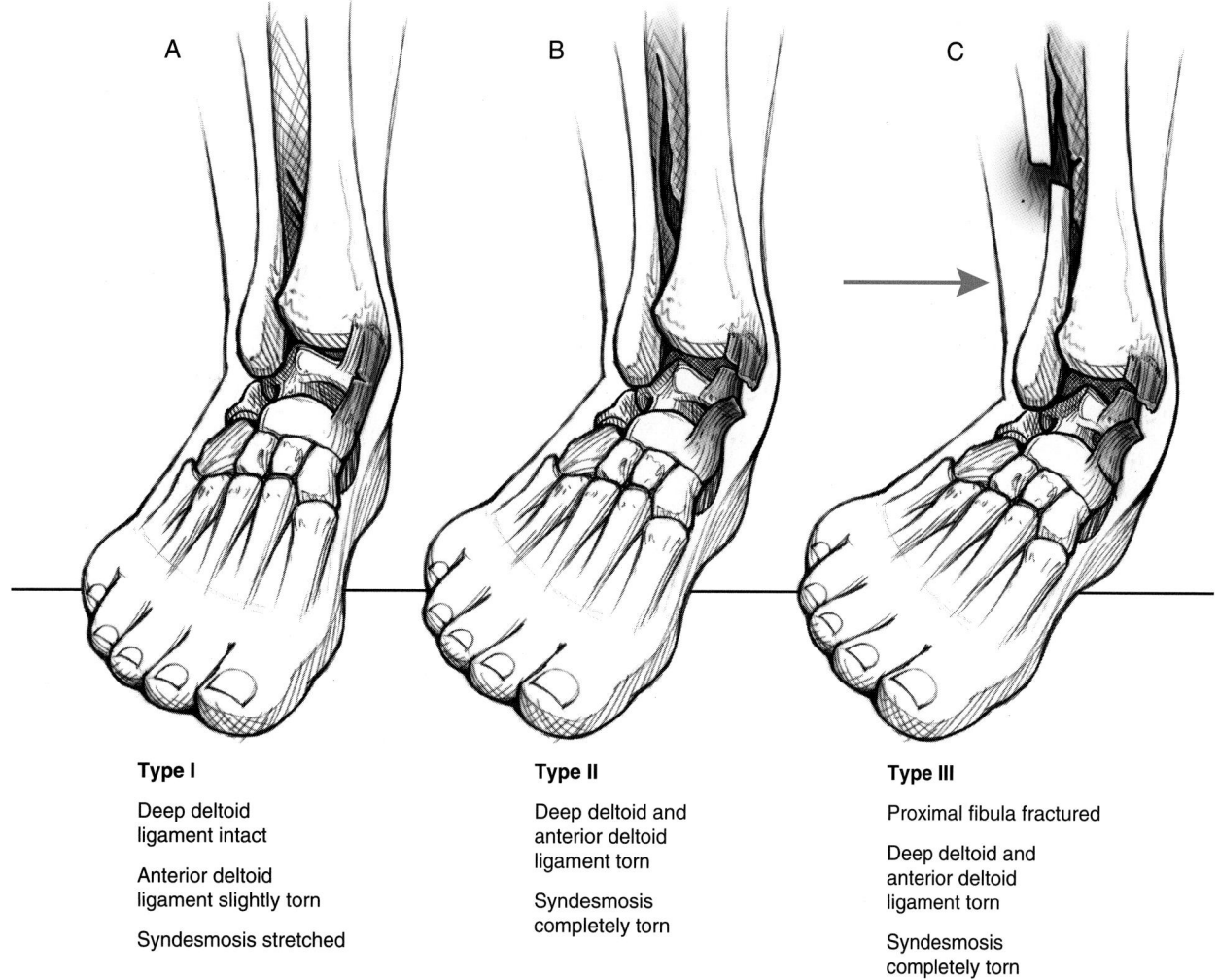

Type I

Deep deltoid
ligament intact

Anterior deltoid
ligament slightly torn

Syndesmosis stretched

Type II

Deep deltoid and
anterior deltoid
ligament torn

Syndesmosis
completely torn

Type III

Proximal fibula fractured

Deep deltoid and
anterior deltoid
ligament torn

Syndesmosis
completely torn

Fig. 2. Syndesmosis sprain. *A*, Stable syndesmosis sprain without fracture. Note stretching and injury to the anterior deltoid and anterior interior tibiofibular ligaments with external rotation and eversion. *B*, Occult syndesmosis disruption and deltoid ligament disruption. *C*, Syndesmosis disruption with fibula fracture (Maisonneuve's injury).

of the plantar flexed foot on the brake occurs by the floorboard collapsing, driving the foot into forced dorsiflexion. This high-energy mechanism is often associated with multiple trauma and fractures to the foot and lower extremity. The other two common mechanisms involve less energy and often only a ligamentous disruption, which can be a difficult diagnostic dilemma. One low-energy mechanism involves a fall or step off an uneven surface (e.g., falling down a step on a plantar-flexed foot or even stepping off a curb and missing the step) (see Fig. 4B–D). The other low-energy mechanism occurs in sports, most commonly football. An athlete gets caught in a pile-up, and another player lands on the back of the injured athlete's heel with the foot in an equinus position (see Fig. 4A, C, D). The mechanism in each of these situations involves a dorsal dislocation of the foot at the TMT ligament and often abduction of the forefoot at the TMT joint (see Fig. 4C, D). The plantar ligaments are much stronger than the dorsal ligaments, thus explaining why plantar dislocations are rare.

CLINICAL FEATURES

The clinical presentation of a ligament injury to the foot and ankle can be very similar to that of a bony injury. It

takes a careful and thorough examination to determine the exact anatomic injury. Unfortunately, the tendency can be to categorize all of these injuries as "ankle sprains." However, the prognosis and management of these injuries can greatly vary; therefore, complete and prompt recovery is entirely dependent on making the correct diagnosis and initiating the proper treatment plan.

Lateral Ankle Sprain

This injury is characterized by a twisting injury to the involved ankle. The patient often recalls a "pop" with immediate pain and swelling. Depending on the degree of injury, the patient may or may not be able to bear weight on the extremity (Table 1). The swelling in the first hour can often reveal the degree of injury. A grade I injury will have little or no ecchymosis and minimal swelling, whereas a grade II injury has a characteristic swelling the size of a golf ball located at the ATFL (just anterior to the distal tip of the fibula). Likewise, a grade III injury has diffuse immediate swelling both laterally and medially and clinically appears as a fracture. Typically, the orthopedist sees the patient 1 to 3 days after the injury. However, it is important to question the patient about the extent of the

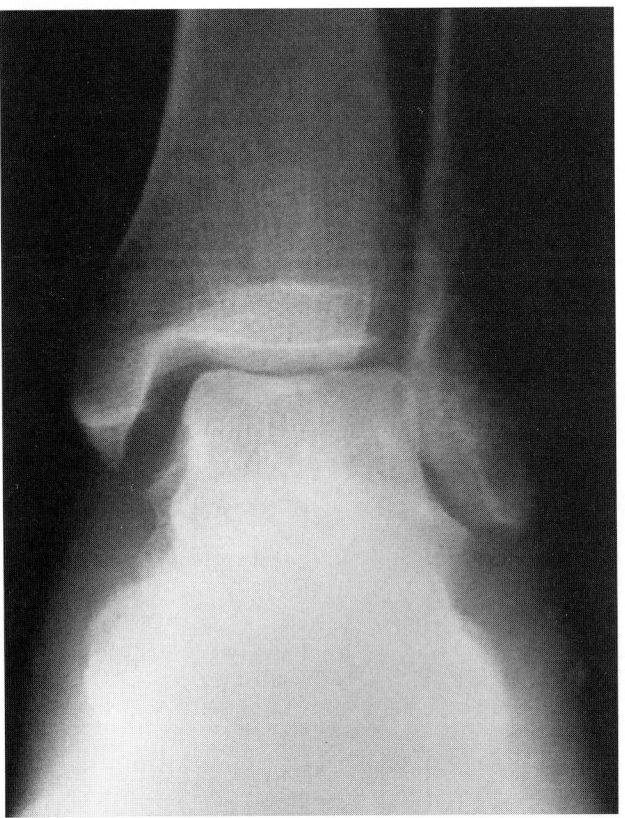

Fig. 3. Unstable syndesmosis. An anteroposterior radiograph demonstrates this type of injury. Note the wide medial clearspace and wide tibia-fibia interval.

swelling in the first hour to assist in establishing the degree of the sprain. At 1 to 3 days, a grade I sprain will have mild to moderate swelling with no medial swelling, whereas a grade II sprain will likely have both medial and lateral swelling, often with frank pitting edema. Grade III sprains after 1 to 3 days have 1+ to 2+ pitting edema. Table 1 describes the anterior drawer and talar tilt test findings, which are the hallmarks of classifying lateral ankle sprains.

After an examination of the patient's swelling, it is important to properly perform the stability exam. The anterior drawer test is performed with the patient relaxed and the ankle in plantar flexion, because the ATFL is tight in plantar flexion (Fig. 6). Particular attention is paid to the amount of excursion of the talus on the tibia, the quality of the end point, and the presence or absence of a suction sign as well as the patient's response to the test. A positive suction sign (see Fig. 6) denotes a complete rupture of the ATFL. Next, the talar tilt test is performed with the ankle in neutral dorsiflexion. It is important to stabilize the entire

hindfoot (calcaneus, talus, and navicular) as one unit, so that the motion detected is in the ankle and not the transverse tarsal joint (talonavicular and calcaneocuboid) or subtalar joint. Attention is paid to the amount of motion and the quality of the end point. Both tests need to be compared with the opposite, uninjured ankle to determine whether there is pathological laxity. Tenderness will exist directly over the ATFL (just anterior to the distal tip of the fibula) with all grades of the lateral ankle sprain. Grade II and grade III sprains will demonstrate tenderness over the CFL (just below the tip of the fibula and medial to the peroneal tendons). Tenderness in the CFL is harder to isolate than at the ATFL and difficult to differentiate from peroneal tendon pain. It should be noted that all grade II and grade III sprains will have some degree of medial pain and swelling, particularly if seen 1 to 3 days after injury. The medial symptoms are due to impaction of the medial neck of the talus on the anterior distal border of the medial malleolus (Fig. 7). This impaction injury can sometimes lead to bony contusions in the acute setting and spur development in the chronic setting. This medial pain should not be confused with a medial ankle sprain. It should also be noted that all grade II and grade III sprains will have pain at the distal tibiofibular ligament and anterolateral ankle capsule and should not be confused with a syndesmosis sprain. The external rotation test and the squeeze test will be negative.

Medial Ankle Sprain

A twisting injury is also characteristic of this ankle injury. However, if asked, the patient often describes the mechanism of injury as motion in which "the foot went out and the ankle went in." The patient is less likely to describe a "pop" but notes severe medial pain and medial swelling. Medial sprains are more painful, and weightbearing is more difficult than a comparable grade of a lateral sprain. Even a grade I sprain can cause the patient to be unable to bear weight. Tenderness is the most important aspect of the physical examination. Remarkable tenderness will be found over the deltoid ligament and the distal tip of the medial malleolus. Abduction stress can elicit increased excursion compared to the opposite side, but this fact is difficult to rely on because the patient has significant pain with this maneuver if the ligament is injured. External rotation stress testing is a very important maneuver with medial ankle sprains. The proximal leg is stabilized, and the foot and ankle are externally rotated within the ankle mortise. This maneuver stresses the anterior deltoid ligament and the syndesmosis ligament concurrently. Pain medial or anteromedial reflects a medial sprain, whereas pain in this location plus pain throughout the lower leg (interosseous membrane) reflects a syndesmosis sprain and possibly a

Grade	Anterior Drawer	Talar Tilt	ATFL	CFL
	TABLE 1. LATERAL ANKLE SPRAINS			
I	Negative	Negative	Stretched	No injury
II	Increased, poor end point, positive suction sign	Negative	Torn	Stretched
III	Increased, poor end point, positive suction sign	Increased, poor end point	Torn	Torn

ATFL, anterior talofibular ligament; CFL, calcaneofibular ligament.

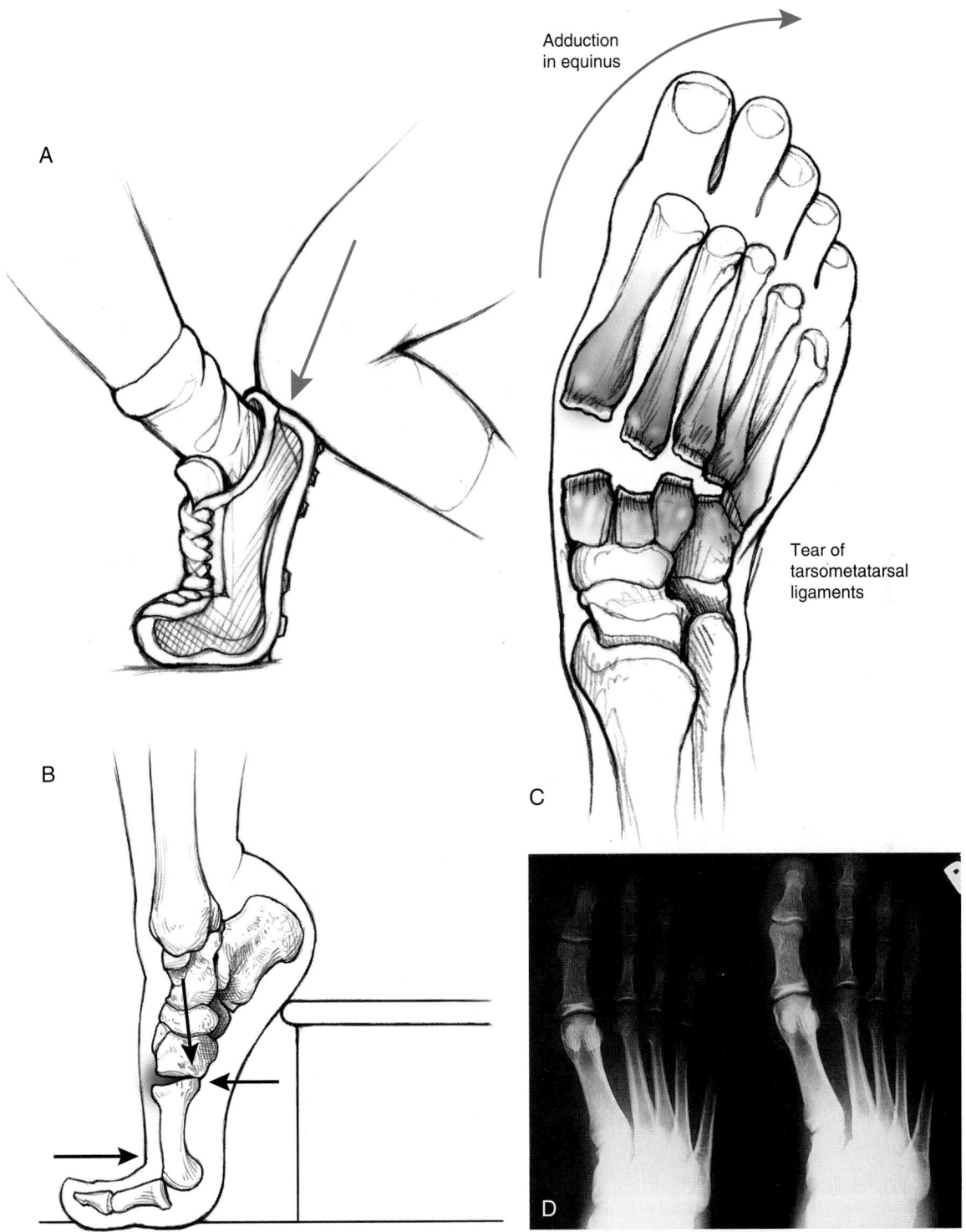

Adduction
in equinus

Tear of
tarsometatarsal
ligaments

Fig. 4. Lisfranc's dislocation. *A*, Mechanism of midfoot injury in football (Lisfranc's dislocation). *B*, Axial loading forces resulting in midfoot injury (Lisfranc's dislocation). *C*, Lisfranc's dislocation. *D*, Standing bilateral comparison anteroposterior radiographs of the feet demonstrate Lisfranc dislocation on the right and stable midfoot on left.

Maisonneuve fracture. A lateral sprain will not have pain with abduction or external rotation stressing.

Syndesmosis Sprain

This injury results from an abduction, external rotation, and dorsiflexion mechanism to the ankle and lower leg. The pain is severe and noted both medially and laterally up the anterolateral leg. The patient is unable to bear weight with this injury and recognizes the injury as being severe, perhaps the "worst sprain I have ever had." Significant pain with the external rotation test, pain at least halfway up the anterolateral leg, and palpable tenderness over the deltoid are hallmarks of the syndesmosis sprain. Pain will also be noted in the ankle while squeezing the fibula and tibia

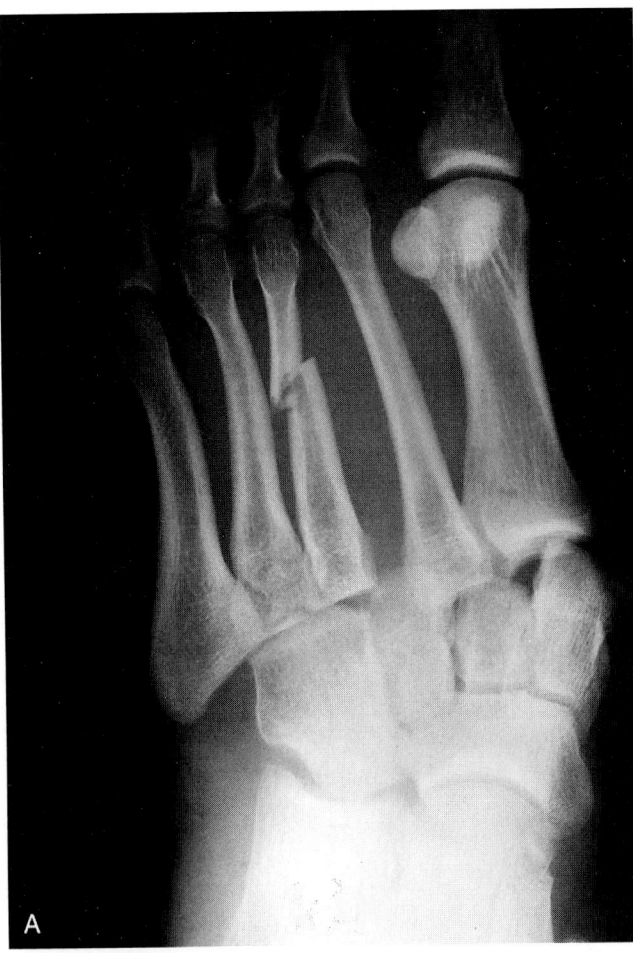
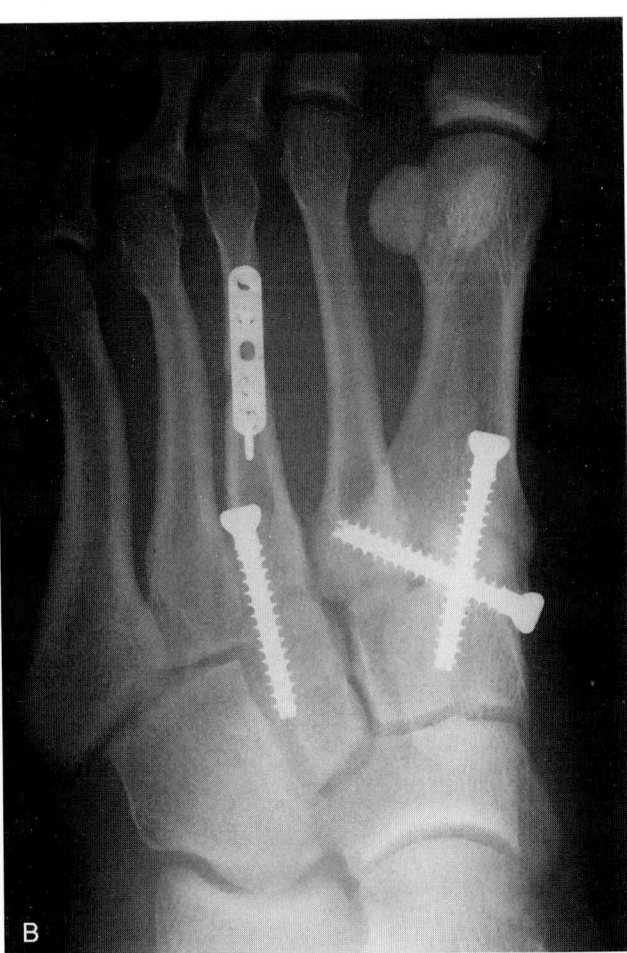

Fig. 5. Lisfranc's fracture dislocation. *A*, Anteroposterior radiograph demonstrates Lisfranc's fracture dislocation. Note the malalignment and the tarsometatarsal joints and third metatarsal fracture. *B*, Anteroposterior radiograph demonstrates Lisfranc's fracture dislocation in *A* after open reduction and internal fixation.

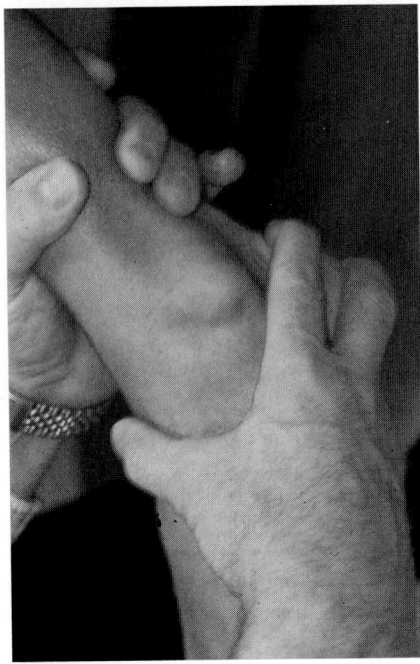

Fig. 6. Anterior drawer test. This demonstrates a positive suction sign in a patient with a torn anterior talofibular ligament during anterior drawer test.

proximally (squeeze test). Pain over the ATFL and CFL is mild except when the entire leg is extremely swollen. In this setting, the external rotation test is the most important test. The examiner must not miss this injury because of its poor long-term prognosis if not diagnosed and treated properly.

Midfoot Sprain

The patient reports severe pain at the dorsal midfoot and an inability to bear weight on the injured extremity. In the first hour, the swelling may be mild, but over time the foot demonstrates rather tense swelling. Blistering can develop after 12 to 24 hours. Crepitation will be present if there is an associated fracture. Pain with palpation is severe over the TMT joint, especially at the base of the second metatarsal and at the second, medial cuneiform ligament (Lisfranc's ligament). If the swelling is mild and the diagnosis is in question, abduction stress of the forefoot will elicit characteristic pain. Local anesthetic may be required to examine for instability in the midfoot with stressing.

INVESTIGATION

Weightbearing radiographs of the foot (midfoot sprain) or ankle (lateral ankle sprain, medial ankle sprain, syndesmo-

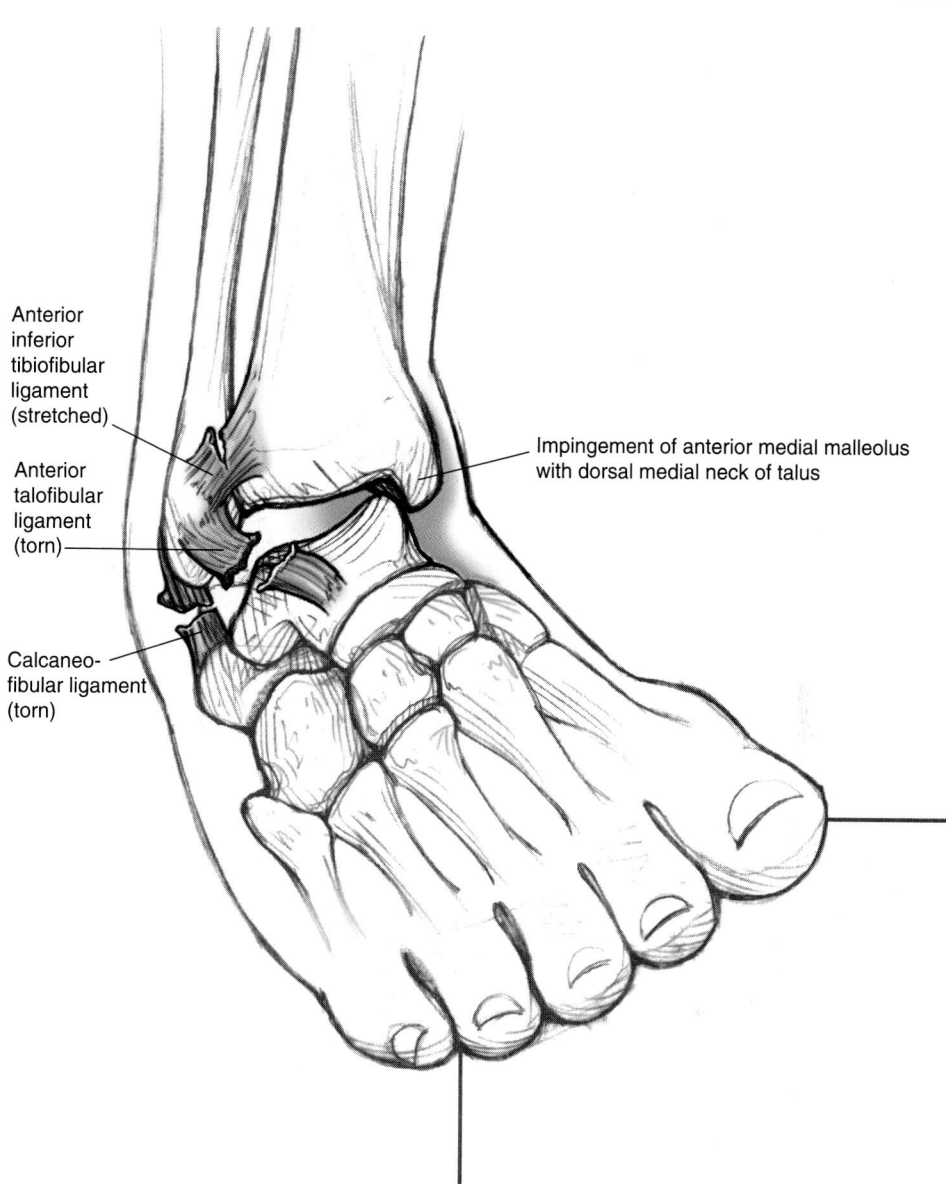

Anterior inferior tibiofibular ligament (stretched)

Anterior talofibular ligament (torn)

Calcaneofibular ligament (torn)

Impingement of anterior medial malleolus with dorsal medial neck of talus

Fig. 7. Lateral ankle instability with anteromedial impingement. This shows anteromedial spurring results. Note concomitant injury to anteroinferior tibiofibular ligament.

sis) are the primary imaging tools. Weightbearing gives physiological stress to the ligaments and helps in determining subtle ligament disruption. Comparison radiographs can be helpful if the injury films are questionable, but they are not routinely used. Special attention to the foot radiographs should be given for a "fleck" sign (a small fleck of bone at the base of the second metatarsal indicating disruption of the Lisfranc ligament). A radiograph of the entire tibia and fibula should be obtained if a Maissoneuve fracture (syndesmosis injury with a proximal fibula fracture) is suspected.

Stress Radiographs

Stress radiographs can be particularly helpful in assessing stable versus unstable medial and syndesmosis sprains. Stress radiographs can prove helpful in determining chronic lateral ankle instability, although they are not routinely used to determine treatment (see Management section). Weightbearing anteroposterior radiographs of the foot are used as stress radiographs for midfoot sprains. Comparison films are used routinely in all settings in which stress radiographs are deemed necessary.

Magnetic Resonance Imaging

Magnetic resonance imaging (MRI) can be a useful adjunct in isolated cases. Routine use of MRI is not necessary in the injuries presented. MRI can be very helpful in cases involving a severely sprained ankle with an unknown mechanism of injury and a high index of suspicion for an unstable medial or syndesmosis sprain with negative stress radiographs. An unstable syndesmosis sprain will have injury, edema, and separation of the interosseous membrane well above the ankle along with disruption of the deltoid ligament (deep and anterior). An unstable medial ankle sprain will demonstrate complete disruption of the deep and anterior deltoid without disruption or significant edema in the interosseous membrane. Intra-articular gadolinium is seldom used in the foot and ankle. MRI can also be beneficial to discover bone contusions and subtle osteochondral lesions of the talus or tibia in patients with acute or chronic ankle trauma.

Computed Tomography

In the acute setting, computed tomography (CT) is not indicated unless there is an associated fracture (e.g., anterior process fracture of calcaneus [see Fig. 10], lateral process fracture of talus [see Chapter 3–20], or osteochondral fracture of talus—see Chapter 4–6) or suspected fracture with an abnormal radiograph. The CT scan is very useful for delineating small avulsion or compression fractures, classifying osteochondral fractures or osteochondral lesions (OCLs) identified on plain radiographs, and further identifying loose bodies or spurring in the chronic setting. The CT scan is used in the chronic setting when a bone scan has suggested an occult fracture or stress fracture and when the uptake is located in the subtalar joint. A CT arthrogram is used primarily to assess cartilage integrity of the ankle. CT is not routinely used in midfoot sprains because they cannot be done with weightbearing. Use of the CT scan for concomitant fracture of the midfoot with a Lisfranc dislocation is helpful to delineate the fracture pattern and detect occult fractures.

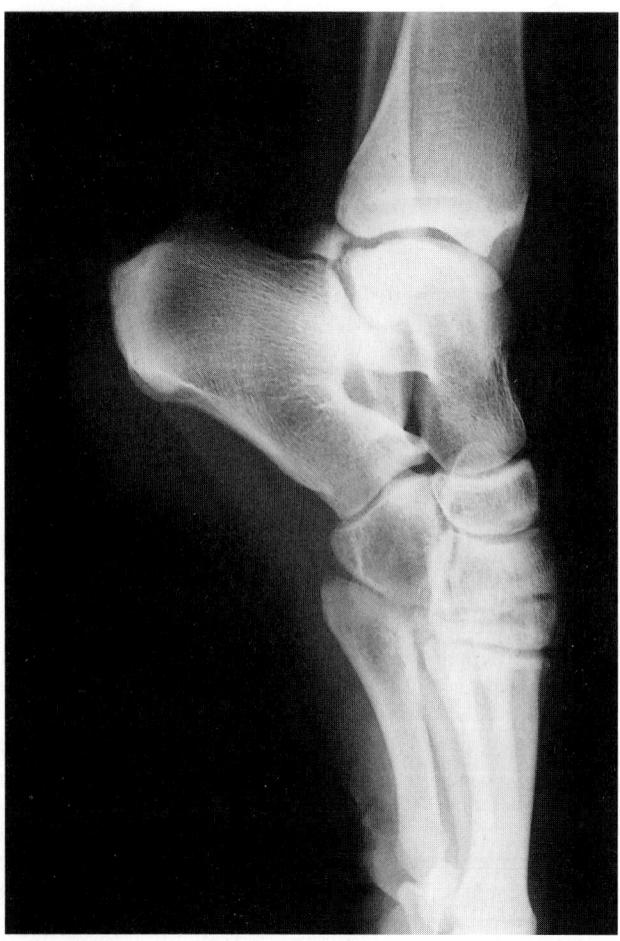

Fig. 8. Posterior process fracture of talus (os trigonum). Lateral radiograph of the ankle in maximal plantar flexion demonstrates posterior ankle impingement with os trigonum.

Bone Scan

Nuclear medicine bone scans are very useful in the patient with chronic ankle pain whose primary complaint is pain rather than instability. A negative bone scan rules out any significant bony cause for the pain. If the bone scan demonstrates asymmetric increased uptake in the painful ankle, further imaging is usually required to delineate the bony source of the uptake and pain. When the increased uptake is localized to the subtalar joint, the bone scan is followed by a CT scan, whereas when the uptake is in the ankle and the radiographs demonstrate no fractures, loose bodies, or OCLs, the bone scan is followed by an MRI. The MRI in this setting is especially useful in determining bone contusions and subtle OCLs.

DIFFERENTIAL DIAGNOSIS

The most common diagnosis for a ligament injury to the foot and ankle is an "ankle sprain." Therefore, this discussion will cover all aspects of the differential diagnosis in relation to grade I to grade III ankle sprains.

Grade I Ankle Sprain (No Ecchymosis and Minimal Swelling)

Grade I lateral ankle sprain.
Bifurcate ligament sprain.
TMT sprain (fourth, fifth, lateral Lisfranc).
Grade I Lisfranc's sprain.
Apophyseal nonunion fifth metatarsal.
Metatarsal stress fracture (fourth or fifth).
Navicular stress fracture.
Tarsal coalition.
Os trigonum (posterior impingement).
Anterior ankle impingement (medial or lateral).

Diagnostic Keys. The specific location of pain, as determined by anatomic palpation, is the key to the diagnosis. The involved structure will be tender, and all other structures should be minimally tender or nontender. The ability to perform a discrete anatomic exam of each of these structures is of paramount importance.

The grade I lateral ankle sprain is tender at the ATFL, the bifurcate ligament sprain is tender over the anterior process of the calcaneus, and the "lateral Lisfranc" is tender at the fourth and fifth TMT joint and with stressing these joints. The Lisfranc sprain is tender at the base of the first and second TMT joints.

Apophyseal nonunion is tender at the base of the fifth metatarsal, and radiographs demonstrate a nonunited fifth metatarsal apophysis (Fig. 9). The fourth or fifth metatarsal stress fracture is tender at the metaphyseal-diaphyseal junction of the involved bone with a fracture noted on radiographs (see Chapter 4–4).

The navicular stress fracture, almost exclusively seen in athletes, is signaled by pain at the "N spot" (tenderness just lateral to the anterior tibial tendon over the dorsal navicular bone) and usually requires a bone scan and CT for detection and classification of the fracture (see Chapter 4–4).

Tarsal coalition presents with decreased subtalar motion, especially with talocalcaneal coalition. Patients will have tenderness over the calcaneal navicular interval laterally (calcaneonavicular) or sustentacular tali medially (talocalca-

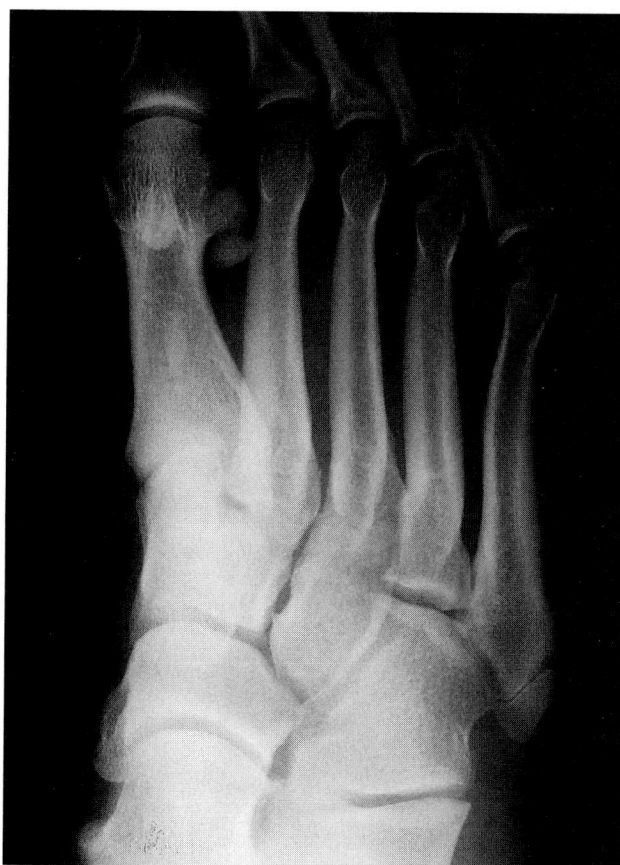

Fig. 9. Fifth metatarsal apophyseal fracture nonunion. This nonunion is demonstrated on an oblique radiograph of the foot.

neal). Radiographs demonstrate the calcaneonavicular bar on the oblique view and on an axial view of the calcaneus for the talocalcaneal coalition (see Chapter 9–26). A CT scan is used for delineation of the coalition.

Posterior ankle impingement presents with tenderness directly over the posterior process of the talus. The os trigonum can be seen on the lateral radiograph (see Fig. 8).

Anterior ankle impingements are usually characterized by chronic ankle pain. Anteromedial impingement involves a palpable medial talar neck spur, pain with forced dorsiflexion, medial gutter spurring on the AP ankle radiograph, and talar neck spurring on either the lateral ankle film or an oblique view of the foot. The anterolateral impingement is a soft-tissue impingement from chronic lateral instability or inadequate rehabilitation after a lateral ankle sprain (grade I to III).[7, 8] Tenderness is localized to the anteroinferior tibiofibular ligament (AITFL) and is increased by dorsiflexion with concomitant palpation on the ligament. Radiographs are normal.

Grade II Ankle Sprain (Ecchymosis, Moderate Swelling [Medial or Lateral], Pain with Weightbearing)

Grade II lateral ankle sprain.
Anterior process fracture calcaneus.
Lateral process fracture of talus.
Osteochondral fracture of talus/tibia.

Peroneal tendon dislocation/subluxation.
Medial tendon tear (posterior tibial/flexor hallucis).
Unstable Lisfranc sprain.
Medial ankle sprain (stable or unstable).
Stable syndesmosis sprain.
Fifth metatarsal avulsion fracture.
Fibula fracture.
Achilles tendon rupture.

Diagnostic Keys. The grade II lateral sprain causes a golf ball–size swelling over the ATFL in 1 to 2 hours, has a positive suction sign on anterior drawer (see Fig. 6), and causes moderate medial pain at the anterior border of the medial malleolus. The grade II lateral sprain presents with pain at the medial neck of the talus with a negative squeeze test and a negative external rotation test, while having normal radiographs.

The anterior process fracture has ecchymosis principally on the lateral ankle and dorsolateral foot with pain isolated to the anterior process (inferior and distal to the sinus tarsi). The fracture can be seen on the lateral ankle radiograph (Fig. 10) or the oblique radiograph of the foot. A CT scan of both feet is typically needed to delineate the extent of the articular involvement.

The symptoms of a lateral process fracture are similar to those of a grade II lateral sprain. The fracture is common among snowboarders. Bony tenderness is difficult to localize because the process is not subcutaneous, but one should note that tenderness is most intense just distal to the tip of the fibula. The fracture can be seen well on the oblique view of the ankle, just distal to the tip of the fibula (see Chapter 3–20). A CT scan is needed to determine optimal treatment and the extent of subtalar joint involvement.

Osteochondral lesions of the talus (see Chapter 4–6) have been previously called osteochondritis dissecans, osteochondral fractures of the talus, and talar dome lesions. However, these injuries are now called osteochondral lesions of the talus to encompass all lesions on the dome of the talus. Most patients with this injury have a history of traumatic ankle injuries. The patient complains of recurring injury secondary to "giving way." Other patients can

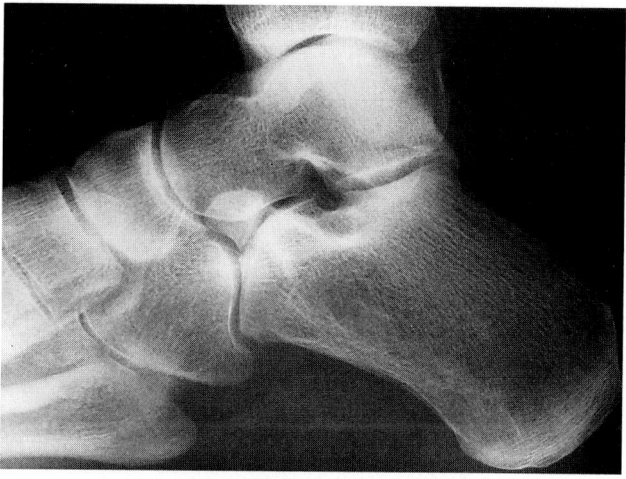

Fig. 10. Anterior process fracture of the calcaneus. This type of fracture is demonstrated on a lateral radiograph of the foot.

present with OCLs secondary to metabolic reasons (e.g., steroid use, coagulopathy, deep-sea diving). Osteochondral lesions of the talus are often associated with ankle instability. The bony tenderness is difficult to palpate because of its intra-articular location. Medial lesions are posterior and can sometimes be appreciated by plantar flexing the ankle and palpating the medial dome. The lateral lesions are anterior and more easily palpated with the ankle plantar flexed. Although radiographs reveal the lesion on the dome of the respective side of the talus, the posteromedial lesion can be better visualized with the ankle in slight plantar flexion. If the lesion can be seen on plain radiographs, then a CT scan is preferable for bony delineation of the lesion and to determine whether the lesion is attached or unattached.

Peroneal tendon dislocation or subluxation involves the peroneus longus anteriorly slipping over the posterolateral lip of the fibula (see Chapter 11–3). This injury, although common among skiers, can be see in any sport. Tenderness is present along the posterior border of the fibula rather than the anterior fibula, as in a lateral ankle sprain. The instability of the tendon can be demonstrated clinically by passively placing the foot and ankle in plantar flexion and eversion (to relax the tension on the tendon) and then gently pulling the peroneus longus out from behind the fibula. Radiographs of this injury are commonly negative.

Tendon tears of the flexor hallucis longus (see Chapter 11–3) or posterior tibial tendon are rare in the acute setting. These tendons should be visualized on an MRI if done for a medial ankle sprain. Posterior tibial tendon insufficiency is covered elsewhere (see Chapter 11–7).

An unstable midfoot sprain must be suspected in any patient with a large swollen foot after trauma. The swelling can be from an ankle sprain, but exquisite tenderness at the base of the first and second metatarsal on the dorsum of the foot is a Lisfranc dislocation until proven stable. Standing, bilateral comparison AP radiographs will be diagnostic (see Figs. 4 and 5). MRI and CT can be obtained but are often not necessary to make the diagnosis.

A medial ankle sprain, even if stable, is a severe injury. The patient often has difficulty bearing weight without assistance and has significant swelling throughout the ankle but most severe medially. Tenderness is localized and very exquisite over the deltoid ligament, both the anterior and deep deltoid. There will be pain with the external rotation test but not with the squeeze test. If the deltoid is completely ruptured (grade III, unstable), there will be increased excursion with the external rotation test and with abduction stress. This injury may be documented with stress radiographs of the involved and uninvolved ankles.

Stable Syndesmosis Sprain. The history is helpful if it can distinguish among external rotation, abduction, and dorsiflexion mechanisms of injury. This injury must be suspected in the significant sprain and in patients who report difficulty with ambulating and who have severe pain with both the external rotation stress and the squeeze test. Comparison stress radiographs can differentiate between stable and unstable sprains. An MRI can document the syndesmosis injury but cannot always differentiate the stable from the unstable sprain.

The fifth metatarsal avulsion fracture can be confused with a grade II sprain because there is lateral pain and

ecchymosis, and if seen 2 to 3 days after injury, the swelling can be diffuse (primarily over the lateral foot). Tenderness at the base of the fifth metatarsal and the oblique radiograph of the foot confirm the diagnosis. However, if ankle radiographs only are obtained, the fracture cannot always be easily seen.

Fibula Fracture. Weber's A or B fractures can present very similar to a grade II sprain. Tenderness is bony at the lateral malleolus, not at the ligaments. Although the lateral ligaments may have some tenderness, it is not the maximal point. Radiographs of the ankle confirm the diagnosis and determine the degree of displacement and thus the treatment (see Chapter 3-19).

Achilles Tendon Rupture. An ankle sprain is the most common initial diagnosis in patients with a neglected rupture.[9] The history is of hearing a "pop," having been kicked, or having been hit in the back of the leg during eccentric loading of the foot and ankle. No plantar flexion with the gastrocnemius squeeze test (Thompson's test[10]) confirms the diagnosis. Often there is a palpable defect in the midsubstance of the tendon if the patient is examined within 2 to 3 days of the injury (see Chapter 11–3).

Grade III Ankle Sprain (Diffuse Ecchymosis, Severe Pitting Edema Up the Leg, Severe Pain with Weightbearing)

This sprain can have concomitant injuries; they present identically for each of these diagnoses, and careful palpation and careful review of appropriate radiographs are essential to avoid incomplete or incorrect diagnosis.

Grade III lateral ankle sprain.
Anterior process fracture of calcaneus.
Lateral process fracture of talus.
Osteochondral fracture of talus/tibia.
Peroneal tendon dislocation/subluxation.
Medial tendon tear (posterior tibial/flexor hallucis).
Unstable Lisfranc sprain.
Medial ankle sprain (stable or unstable).
Unstable syndesmosis sprain (± Maissoneuve fracture).
Fibula fracture ± deltoid disruption.
Ankle fracture (bimalleolar, trimalleolar, pilon).
Achilles rupture.
Calcaneus fracture.
Talar neck fracture.

Diagnostic Keys. The grade III lateral ankle sprain has immediate diffuse swelling and ecchymosis because of the complete rupture of the ATFL and the CFL. This injury should be considered an ankle dislocation. The exam is similar to that for a grade II sprain with an increase in the excursion of the talar tilt test. There is a higher rate of associated injuries.

The anterior process fracture, lateral process fracture, osteochondral fracture, and peroneal tendon dislocation present similarly to that noted for grade II ankle sprain. These injuries typically present as occult associated injuries in conjunction with a grade III lateral sprain, syndesmosis sprain, or an ankle fracture.

A medial tendon rupture is an associated injury in conjunction with a severe medial ankle sprain, a syndesmosis sprain, an ankle fracture, or a calcaneus fracture.

An unstable Lisfranc sprain was noted previously (see

Grade II Ankle Sprain). It is common to have associated fractures (multiple trauma or metatarsal fractures) and blistering of the foot (see Fig. 5).

The unstable syndesmosis sprain is a severe ankle injury that must not be missed. It should be suspected and ruled out with any severe ankle sprain. The examination is the same as noted previously, but with more tenderness, inability to bear full weight, and swelling at least halfway up the leg. The radiographs can reveal widening of the medial clear space or widening of the tibula-fibula interval (unstable syndesmosis; see Fig. 3). The Maissoneuve injury also has a fracture of the proximal fibula. The treating physician must be aware that the non-weightbearing (NWB), unstressed radiograph of the ankle can be normal. A stress radiograph will demonstrate the occult unstable sprain.

A fibula fracture in this setting also often has a disruption of the deltoid ligament. The exam will be remarkable for tenderness both medially (over the deltoid ligament) and laterally (over the distal fibula). The radiograph must be examined closely to assess the medial clear space. Widening of the medial clear space indicates complete disruption of the deltoid ligament.

An ankle fracture in this setting can be very severe and involves at least two malleoli (bimalleolar and trimalleolar) or the tibial plafond (pilon) (see Chapters 3–18 and 3–19). Bony tenderness, severe swelling (often blistering), and an inability to bear weight are the hallmarks of these fractures. The classification of the fracture is determined radiographically.

A calcaneus fracture and talar neck fracture must be considered in the differential diagnosis of the grade III sprain (see Chapter 3–20). The calcaneus fracture will have exquisite tenderness over the calcaneal tuberosity both medially and laterally. The talar neck fracture presents with tenderness just anterior to the ankle joint along the course of the talar neck. The lateral ankle or foot radiograph is best for identifying these fractures. Bohler's angle is decreased (less than 20 degrees) with a calcaneus fracture. The calcaneus fracture is also seen with an axial view of the heel. The talar neck fracture can be subtle if it is not displaced. The fracture line typically is at the junction of the body and the neck.

MANAGEMENT
Lateral Ankle Sprain: Acute
The management of lateral ankle sprains follows the same principles and goals regardless of the degree of the sprain. A functional rehabilitation program with bracing and limited intermittent immobilization is used. The patient is started immediately on Achilles tendon stretching and aggressive peroneal tendon strengthening. After patients can ambulate well without assistance, they begin proprioception retraining exercises. Within 1 to 2 days of injury, patients are started on a biking program to assist in muscle rehabilitation and strengthening, maintenance of aerobic fitness, and early proprioception retraining. As they become more comfortable, patients are progressed to StairMaster (Kirkland, WA) exercises and then to functional progression exercises and back to work or sport.

The degree of immobilization and bracing depends on the grade of the injury (see Table 1). More specifically, the method of immobilization depends on whether the sprain is

TABLE 2. LISFRANC'S (MIDFOOT) FRACTURE DISLOCATION RESULTS/ COMPLICATIONS		
Complication	%	
Compartment syndrome	<10	
Vascular injury	<5	
Screw breakage	<10	Wire breakage, rate higher
Amputation	<10	
Skin loss/injury	0–20	
Nerve injury	0–10	With surgery and with casting
Chronic pain	50–75	
Stiffness	50–100	
Good–excellent	40–60	Better with anatomic alignment
Fair–poor	40–60	Increased poor results with joint injury, poor alignment
Arthrosis	30–100	Increased rate with less anatomic reduction

stable (grade I) or unstable (grade II or III). The grade I stable sprain is braced either with a lace-up brace or a stirrup brace depending on the activity level of the patient. The stirrup brace provides more protection and stability but less range of motion and less comfort in a shoe. The unstable sprain (grades II and III) is much more prone to long-term laxity, because the ligament has been completely ruptured. Positioning of the foot and ankle allows the ligament to heal at an anatomic length (see Fig. 1B).[11] Any plantar flexion or inversion results in healing of the ligament with laxity (see Fig. 1A). Therefore, the worst treatment for the unstable sprain is crutches and NWB with an elastic wrap. I use a removable walking boot for all patients with unstable lateral ankle sprains. Inside the boot is placed a Cryo/Cuff (AirCast, Summit, NJ) to control edema, allow immediate weightbearing without crutches, and yet maintain neutral dorsiflexion of the ankle. The boot is worn day and night until the ankle is stable (1 to 2 weeks for grade II and 2 to 3 weeks for grade III). The patient is allowed to wean out of the boot (first in the daytime) while full weightbearing with a brace (typically a stirrup brace) but continues wearing the boot at night for an additional 2 weeks. The boot is removed three to four times a day to perform the rehabilitation exercises noted previously. The boot is worn initially for stationary biking and stair-stepping exercises. Later when weaning out of the boot, the patient wears a brace while exercising. Casting the foot in neutral dorsiflexion can also be used but does not allow concomitant range of motion and Achilles tendon strengthening.

Operative treatment of the acute sprain is reserved for the following conditions: (1) an acute sprain in a person with chronic disabling instability that requires surgical reconstruction in spite of the recent injury; (2) an acute grade II or III sprain with an associated injury that required operative intervention (e.g., osteochondral fracture of the talus, lateral process fracture of talus, or peroneal tendon dislocation). Some authors advocated repair of the lateral ligaments in the young competitive athlete with greater than 15 degrees of talar tilt on a stress radiograph and greater than 10 mm of anterior translation on anterior drawer.[12] I have not used this criterion to perform primary repair of the lateral ankle ligaments.

Lateral Ankle Sprain: Chronic

Management of chronic lateral ankle instability is more complex, and surgical reconstruction has a more involved role. Initially, it is important to determine whether the patient's complaint is pain or instability. The chronic unstable ankle is often not painful. If pain is the primary complaint, the treating physician must consider an occult fracture (see prior discussion of differential diagnosis for ankle sprains, especially anterior ankle impingement, OCL talus, painful os trigonum, and navicular stress fracture). It is also important to determine whether the patient's complaint of instability is mechanical (giving away because of laxity) or functional (giving away as a result of weakness, neurological factors, or Achilles tightness).[13-16] Harrington[17] noted that reconstruction of the lateral ligaments in patients with mild to moderate varus arthritis can improve pain.

Medial Ankle Sprain

Although medial ankle sprains are much less common than lateral sprains, the severity and temporary impairment are much greater. Isolated medial ankle sprains are almost exclusively stable. Unstable medial sprains are almost exclusively associated with a syndesmosis disruption or a fibula fracture. Therefore, only management of the stable medial sprain is presented. The same treatment plan is used for this sprain as for grade II and grade III lateral sprains with one exception: use of posterior tibial tendon strengthening rather than peroneal strengthening.

Syndesmosis Sprain

The stable syndesmosis sprain is treated with immobilization (cast versus removable boot). I prefer boot immobilization to allow for concomitant range of motion and posterior tibial tendon strengthening. Early use of a short articulating ankle-foot orthosis may allow earlier return to sport and work. Unstable syndesmosis injuries (grade II or III) require anatomic reduction. I favor surgical stabilization for grade II and grade III injuries. Some specialists favor cast immobilization with the foot in internal rotation for grade II injuries. Anatomic reduction must be obtained and maintained for 8 to 12 weeks to allow for healing of the interosseous membrane and deltoid ligament.

Midfoot Sprain

Early reports suggested adequate results despite residual radiographic deformity. Today, anatomic alignment must be the goal, and satisfactory results are possible in most cases.[18] Nonoperative treatment is appropriate only for stable acute injuries with no radiographic malalignment (see Fig. 4D). Nonoperative treatment includes immobilization for 3 to 6 weeks with either a cast or walking boot. Surgical intervention is indicated if malalignment is noted on the AP or lateral foot radiographs (see Fig. 5). If a high index of suspicion exists with normal radiographs, then fluoroscopic evaluation under anesthesia and stability assessment are recommended.

Procedures for Chronic Lateral Ankle Instability

Procedures are indicated for chronic lateral ankle instability during sport activity or with activities of daily living.

Associated anterior ankle impingement, OCL talus, painful os trigonum, loose bodies, and peroneal tendon tears/instability can be concomitant.

Arthroscopy of the ankle before reconstruction for associated pathology is often required.

Brostrom/Gould reconstruction is used in competitive athletes and in young patients (younger than 25 to 30 years) with strong native tissue (ATFL and CFL), no previous reconstructive procedures, and without generalized ligamentous laxity.

Brostrom/Evans or Chrisman-Snook reconstruction is used for older adults (older than 30 years) with poor local tissue, heavy laborers, possibly large athletes (heavier than 250 to 300 pounds, e.g., football linemen), and patients with generalized ligamentous laxity and revision surgery.

Patients with varus heel alignment may require a lateral closing wedge osteotomy at reconstruction.[19] The osteotomy is added if the heel cannot be passively placed in neutral or slight eversion.

Postoperative rehabilitation: immobilized in walking cast or removable boot for 4 weeks and peroneal strengthening. The athlete then progresses from bike riding to Stair-Master (Kirkland, WA) to running and then to functional progression. The athlete can return to sports after completing functional progression. Return to work for the sit-down job can be 1 to 2 weeks; return to sports and heavy manual labor will be 2 to 4 months.

Brostrom's Reconstruction with Gould's Modification

Consider ankle arthroscopy before reconstruction to address impingement, OCL, and so on.

Incorporate anterolateral portal into lateral incision along Langerhans' line for cosmesis (for younger patients with intact peroneal tendons).

Reattach ligaments into bony trough with drill holes to give firm reconstruction with less risk of later stretching out.[16]

Suture CFL with hindfoot in eversion and ankle in slight plantar flexion, suture ATFL with same hindfoot eversion but with ankle in dorsiflexion.

Always use Gould modification[20] (inferior extensor retinaculum to lateral fibula; Fig. 11).

Brostrom/Evans Reconstruction

Consider ankle arthroscopy before reconstruction to address impingement, OCL, and so on.

Longitudinal incision: warn patient of potential poor cosmesis.

One-half of the peroneus brevis tendon is routed through a fibular tunnel and then lateral to the fibula and is tied back on itself at the tunnel origin; incise lateral periosteum so tendon lies "flat" on fibula without prominence.

Begin drill hole at confluence of ATFL, CFL origin on fibula, proceed proximal and posterior, protect peroneals while drilling.

Suture tenodesis with hindfoot in neutral, not eversion, and ankle in neutral dorsiflexion; possible to give eversion contracture with this procedure and require later release.

Procedures for Syndesmosis Disruption

These are indicated for unstable (complete disruption) syndesmosis injury.

Associated deltoid disruption and high fibula fracture (Maissoneuve fracture) are common.

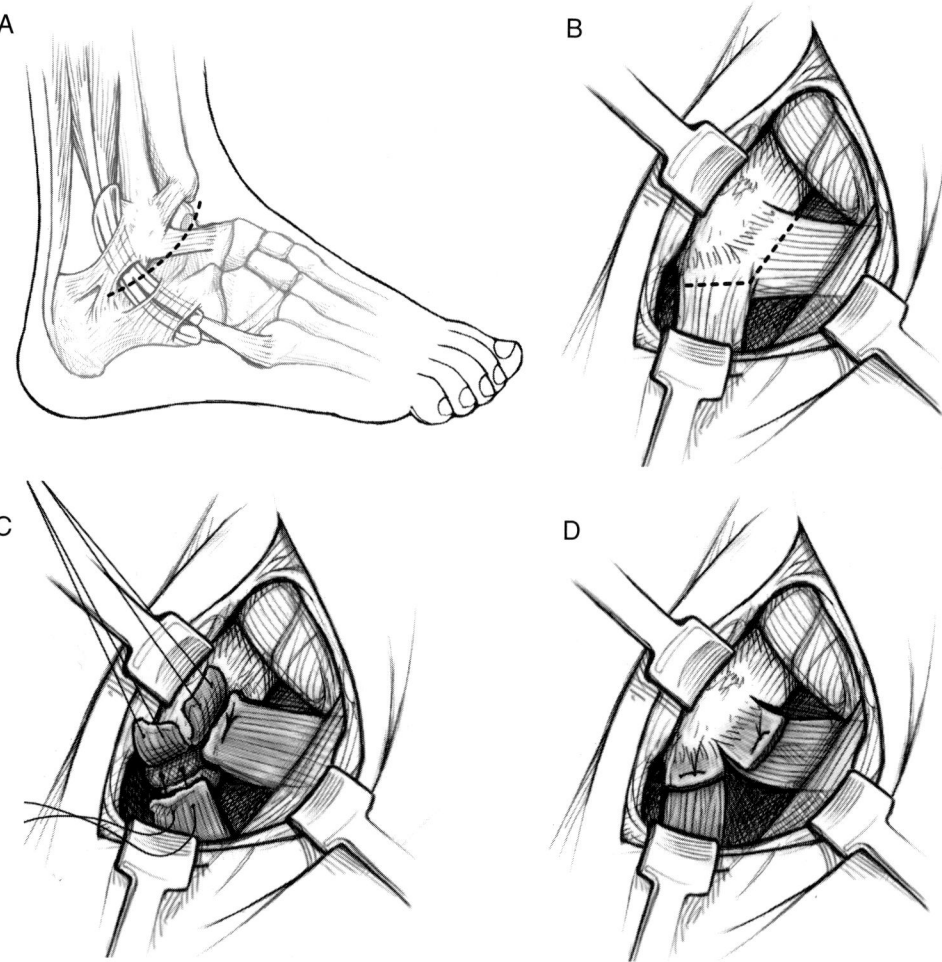

A

B

C

D

Fig. 11. Brostrom-Gould procedure. *A,* Anterolateral incision. *B,* Arthrotomy leaving a 3.0-mm cuff at the fibula. The proximal stump of the ligament is elevated. *C,* The distal stump of the ligament is sutured into the fibula. *D,* The proximal origin is imbricated into the dorsal stump. Inferior extensor retinaculum is then sutured into the lateral fibular periosteum.

Open reduction of syndesmosis and distal tibial-fibular articulation may be necessary to ensure anatomic reduction of the fibula in tibial incisura.

Open repair of deltoid may be necessary to obtain anatomic medial alignment: one to two screws (3.5 to 4.5 mm) placed across syndesmosis just above the ankle joint through three to four cortices.

Open reduction and internal fixation (ORIF) of fibula fracture is necessary if it is near the ankle joint.

Postoperative rehabilitation: cast versus fracture boot for 6 to 10 weeks, NWB for 2 to 4 weeks, screws removed at 12 to 16 weeks. Return to work for the sit-down job can be 1 to 2 weeks; return to sports and heavy manual labor is 4 to 5 months.

Author's preference: two 4.5-mm cannulated screws through three cortices with four-hole one-third tubular plate removed at 12 weeks; commonly repair deltoid ligament, immobilized in a fracture boot for 8 weeks, 2 weeks NWB; stirrup brace for 3 months after boot.

ORIF Syndesmosis with or Without Fibula Fracture
Arthroscopy before ORIF is typically not needed.

I prefer open repair of all medial ligaments to ensure abduction and external rotation stability and repair of deep deltoid (abduction stability) and anterior deltoid (external rotation stability).

Medial Ankle Repair (Deltoid Ligament Repair)
Isolated repair is rarely indicated. This is used with syndesmosis ORIF or with distal fibula fracture ORIF.

Anteromedial incision is necessary to allow visualization of ankle joint and repair anterior deltoid.

If midsubstance rupture has occurred, then intrasubstance repair is performed with absorbable size 0 suture.

If there is soft-tissue avulsion off the medial malleolus, then repair to bone should be performed with small trough and drill holes.

Rehabilitation is the same as with ORIF syndesmosis.

Procedures for Midfoot Ligament Disruption (Lisfranc's Dislocation)
This is indicated for unstable TMT ligament injury (>2 mm displacement or unstable on exam under anesthesia).

Associated fractures of the metatarsals can occur.

Anatomic reduction of each TMT joint must be obtained and maintained; this is best achieved with open reduction (see Fig. 5).

Make a dorsal S incision at the base of the first or second interspace; make a second incision as necessary.

Screw fixation is most rigid (3.5 to 4.5 mm); a solid screw is the standard, but a cannulated screw is commonly used.

Postoperative rehabilitation: removable boot allows early

range of motion to counteract potential stiffness, NWB for 6 weeks, protected weightbearing for 3 to 4 weeks. Screw removal is controversial (12 to 16 weeks versus not removing). Return to work for the sit-down job can be 1 to 2 weeks; return to sports and heavy manual labor is 4 to 5 months.

Author's preference: 4.5-mm cannulated screws removed at 12 weeks (acute ORIF) to 16 weeks (ORIF 2 to 6 weeks after injury).

RESULTS AND COMPLICATIONS
Lateral Ankle Sprain

The results with nonoperative treatment of acute lateral ankle sprains is very good. Lateral ankle laxity can be demonstrated in 40% to 60%,[21, 22] but symptomatic instability is typically 10%.[21] Peroneal tendon weakness can be present in 20%,[22] but the rate of peroneal tendon tears is not reported. Degenerative arthritis should be less than 20%.[21, 23] A semirigid ankle stabilizer has been shown to reduce the risk of lateral ankle injuries in basketball.[24]

Anatomic repairs to reconstruct the lateral ligaments give good to excellent results in 80% to 90% of patients; recurrent instability is present in 5% to 13%, primarily those with generalized ligamentous laxity.[25, 26] Patients with uncorrected hindfoot varus also have a higher failure rate. Between 85% and 95% of patients return to sports after reconstruction, and most return to work.[25, 26] Complications are minimal; neuromas develop in approximately 5% of patients.[25, 26]

Results after the Brostrom-Evans reconstruction are less favorable.[27, 28] Subjectively, there is a 60% to 80% good to excellent result; 5% to 45% of patients complain of some instability. Objectively, early ankle arthrosis can be seen in up to 90% of patients at 10 years follow-up and 50% will have changes in the subtalar joint.

Medial Sprain

The results depend on obtaining and maintaining anatomic alignment to the medial ankle and associated injuries at the time of the ligament sprain. Most individuals have slight valgus hindfoot alignment. Therefore, any residual medial instability is disabling. Average time to return to sports with an initially stable high ankle sprain (anterior deltoid, deep deltoid, and distal syndesmosis) is 6 weeks. Longterm instability is uncommon, but chronic pain is common even if there is no persistent instability. The high incidence of associated injuries may be related to the high rate of chronic pain. Outcome data are not available for this injury. Return to sport was 12 weeks in the one reported case.[6]

Syndesmosis Sprain

Outcome data are strikingly limited in this injury. The return to sport and heavy labor is 6 to 12 weeks if anatomic reduction is maintained.[29–32] Pain and stiffness are noted in 25% to 40% of patients with anatomic reduction[31, 33] and in 100% of those with inadequate reduction. Arthrosis has not been documented in long-term studies, but I believe that inadequate reduction will lead to near 100% degenerative arthritis. Anatomic reduction will lessen but not alleviate these changes.

Midfoot Sprain

The results for midfoot sprain (see Table 2) depend on the final anatomic alignment (including the maintenance of the longitudinal arch),[34] the alignment at the TMT joint (see Investigation), and the degree of injury present at the TMT joint surface.[34–38] That is, better results occur if anatomic alignment is obtained and maintained. Better outcomes are associated with maintenance of the longitudinal arch. These findings are true whether the original displacement is severe or subtle. Arntz et al[35] also noted better outcomes after closed injuries than open midfoot sprains. Orthosis management is common even with good to excellent outcomes. Chronic pain and radiographic arthrosis are common even after anatomic reduction. However, the outcomes appear to be improving with the advent of ORIF, attention to anatomic reduction, and early motion. Controversy still exists regarding the need to remove screws and the timing of removal. Anatomic reduction obtained within 4 weeks of the injury gives much better outcomes. Delayed surgery after 8 weeks gives poor outcomes.

SUBTALAR SPRAIN

HISTORICAL REVIEW

1962: First reported case of subtalar instability with stress tomograms.

1960s: Chrisman and Snook surgically treat patients with subtalar instability; subtalar tilt shown on plain radiographs.

1970s: Mechanism of injury, either inversion or internal rotation.

1980s: Ligamentous cutting studies demonstrate instability.

1990s: Stress Broden's view advocated for documentation; triligamentous versus modified Brostrom method for surgical reconstruction.

Subtalar sprain is an isolated diagnosis that has recently drawn interest. Because the diagnosis and management are still unproven, I have added this special section. It is thought that isolated subtalar sprains represent less than 1% of all ankle sprains. The mechanism of injury is indistinguishable from that of a lateral ankle sprain. However, isolated disruption of the subtalar ligaments requires neutral or slight dorsiflexion of the ankle with inversion. Subtalar dislocation typically involves a severe internal rotation force, and this mechanism may also play a role in isolated subtalar sprains.[39] The diagnosis cannot clinically be distinguished from lateral ankle instability in the acute or chronic setting. The calcaneofibular, lateral talocalcaneal, and cervical ligaments are the primary lateral subtalar stabilizers. The interosseous ligament and inferior extensor retinaculum play a role in stabilization also. The interosseous ligament lies in the triplane axis of rotation of this joint and is not necessarily injured if the instability is rotational. The inferior extensor retinaculum is sutured to the fibular periosteum in the Gould modification of the Brostrom procedure to provide added subtalar stability; thus, it may have some role in stability. Diagnostically, stress tomograms and stress Broden's view have been advocated to confirm the diagnosis. To date, a consensus has not been reached on the optimal means to confirm the diagnosis. Management of the acute subtalar sprain is the same as for the acute lateral ankle sprain. Management of the isolated chronic instability is not well established. Non-operative treatment is similar to that for lateral ankle instability (e.g., peroneal tendon strengthening, bracing, and proprioception retraining). Tendon transfer procedures have been used as in lateral ankle reconstruction (Chrisman-Snook), and Clanton and Schon[40] proposed the triligamentous reconstruction. I prefer the modified Brostrom for this condition. However, isolated chronic subtalar instability is rare. Results of treatment have been good regarding stability. Complications include wound healing problems and stiffness, especially limitation of inversion. I expect more consensus will develop regarding the diagnosis and management of this injury. Also, it may be that many patients who are thought to have sinus tarsi syndrome have subtle subtalar instability.

REFERENCES

1. Lisfranc J: Nouvelle Method Operatoire pour l'Amputation Partielle du Pied dans son Articulation Tarso-Metatarsienne: Methode Precedes des Nombreuses Modifications qu'a Subies Celle de Chopart. Paris, Gabon, 1815.
2. Maisonneuve JG: Recherches sur la fracture du perone. Arch Gen Med 1840; 7:165.
3. Leonard MH: Injuries of the lateral ligaments of the ankle. A clinical and experimental study. J Bone Joint Surg Am 1949; 31:373.
4. Evans DL: Recurrent instability of the ankle—A method of surgical treatment. J R Soc Med 1953; 46:343.
5. Watson-Jones R: Recurrent forward dislocation of the ankle joint. J Bone Joint Surg Br 1952; 34:519.
6. Jackson R, Wills RE, Jackson R: Rupture of the deltoid ligaments without involvement of the lateral ligaments. Am J Sports Med 1988; 16:541.
7. Ferkel RD, Karzel RP, Del Pizzo W, et al: Arthroscopic treatment of anterolateral impingement of the ankle. Am J Sports Med 1991; 19:440.
8. McCarroll JR, Schrader JW, Shelbourne KD, et al: Meniscoid lesions of the ankle in soccer players. Am J Sports Med 1987; 15:255.
9. Porter DA, Mannarino FP, Snead D, et al: Primary repair without augmentation for early neglected Achilles tendon ruptures in the recreational athlete. Foot Ankle Int 1997; 18:557.
10. Thompson TC, Doherty GH: Spontaneous rupture of tendon of Achilles: A new clinical diagnostic test. J Trauma 1962; 2:126.
11. Smith R, Reischl S: Treatment of ankle sprains in young athletes. Am J Sports Med 1986; 14:465.
12. Clanton TO, Porter DA: Primary care of foot and ankle injuries in athletes. Clin Sports Med 1997; 16:435.
13. Brand RL, Black HM, Cox JS: The natural history of inadequately treated ankle sprain. Am J Sports Med 1977; 5:248.
14. Freeman MAR, Dean MRE, Hanham IWF: The etiology and prevention of functional instability of the foot. J Bone Joint Surg Br 1965; 47:678.
15. Renstrom P: Persistently painful sprained ankle. J Am Acad Orthop Surg 1994; 2:270.
16. Renstrom P, Kannus P: Management of ankle sprains. Oper Tech Sport Med 1994; 2:58.
17. Harrington KD: Degenerative arthritis of the ankle secondary to long-standing lateral ligament instability. J Bone Joint Surg Am 1979; 61:354.
18. Meyerson M: Tarsometatarsal joint injury. Subtle signs hold the key. Phys Sports Med 1993; 21:97.
19. Dwyer FC: Osteotomy of the calcaneum for pes cavus. J Bone Joint Surg Br 1959; 41:80.
20. Gould N, Seligson D, Gassman J: Early and late repair of the lateral ligament of the ankle. Foot Ankle 1980; 1:84.
21. Lofvenberg R, Karrholm J, Lund B: The outcome of nonoperated patients with chronic lateral instability of the ankle: A 20-year follow up study. Foot Ankle 1994; 15:165.
22. Bosien WR, Staples OS, Russell SW: Residual disability following acute ankle sprains. J Bone Joint Surg Am 1955; 37:1237.
23. Boszotta H, Sauer G: Die chronische fibulare brandinsuffizienz am oberen sprungelenk spatergegrisse nach modifizierter Watson-Jones plastik. Unfallchirurg 1989; 92:11.
24. Sitler M, Ryan J, Wheeler B, et al: The efficacy of a semi-rigid ankle stabilizer to reduce acute ankle injuries in basketball. A randomized clinical study at West Point. Am J Sports Med 1994; 22:454.
25. Karlsson J, Bergsten T, Lansinger O, et al: Reconstruction of the lateral ligaments of the ankle for chronic lateral instability. J Bone Joint Surg Am 1988; 70:581.
26. Karlsson J, Bergsten T, Lansinger O, et al: Surgical treatment of chronic lateral instability of the ankle joint. A new procedure. Am J Sports Med 1989; 17:268.
27. Rosenbaum D, Becker H-P, Sterk J, et al: Functional evaluation of the 10-year outcome after modified Evans repair for chronic ankle instability. Foot Ankle 1997; 18:765.
28. Karlsson J, Bergsten T, Lansinger O, et al: Lateral instability of the ankle treated by the Evans procedure: A long term clinical and radiological follow up. J Bone Joint Surg Br 1988; 70:476.
29. Hopkinson WJ, St. Pierre P, Ryan JB, et al: Syndesmosis sprains of the ankle. Foot Ankle 1990; 10:325.
30. Boytim MJ, Fischer DA, Neumann L: Syndesmotic sprains of the ankle. Foot Ankle 1991; 19:294.
31. Taylor DC, Englehardt DL, Bassett FH: Syndesmosis sprains of the ankle: The influence of heterotopic ossification. Am J Sports Med 1992; 20:146.
32. Fritschy D: An unusual ankle injury in top skiers. Am J Sports Med 1989; 17:282.
33. Edwards GS, DeLee JC: Ankle diastasis without fracture. Foot Ankle 1984; 4:305.
34. Faciszewski T, Burks R, Manaster BJ: Subtle injuries of the Lisfranc joint. J Bone Joint Surg Am 1990; 72:1519.
35. Arntz C, Veith R, Hansen S: Fractures and fracture-dislocations of the tarsometatarsal joint. J Bone Joint Surg Am 1988; 70:173.
36. Wilpuolla E: Tarsometatarsal fracture dislocations. Acta Orthop Scand 1973; 44:335.
37. Wilson DW: Injuries of the tarso-metatarsal joints. J Bone Joint Surgery Br 1972; 54:677.
38. Brunet JA, Wiley JJ: The late results of tarsometatarsal joint injuries. J Bone Joint Surg Br 1987; 69:437.
39. Dias LS: The lateral ankle sprain: An experimental study. J Trauma 1979; 19:266.
40. Clanton TO, Schon LC: Athletic injuries to the soft tissues of the foot and ankle. In Mann RA, Coughlin MJ (eds): Surgery of the Foot and Ankle, 6th ed. St. Louis, MO, CV Mosby, 1993, p 1128.

ANKLE ARTHRITIS DIAGNOSIS AND MANAGEMENT

Nicholas A. Abidi and Sheldon S. Lin

Summary
- The most common cause of ankle arthritis is traumatic injury.
- Realignment osteotomies are considered with mild arthritis and deformity.
- Ankle arthrodesis relieves pain in approximately 90% of patients.
- The long-term effect of ankle fusion on pain and function remains unclear.
- Initial results with uncemented total ankle replacements are promising.

Ankle arthritis can develop from many pathways: post-traumatic, septic, rheumatological, or osteoarthritic. The absence of a low friction articular cartilage surface results in inflammation with joint synovitis, osteophyte formation, limitation of motion and, most significantly, pain.

Nonoperative techniques are used initially to reduce pain and improve patient function. This starts with oral medications, shoe inserts, or external modifications and progresses to bracing.

Several operative techniques have been devised to eliminate pain associated with arthritis. These include joint space débridement of osteophytes, distal tibial osteotomies, distraction arthroplasty, total ankle replacement, and ankle arthrodesis. Total joint arthroplasty has not yet enjoyed the widespread success in the ankle joint that it has in other major joints in the body.[1–3]

Arthrodesis of the ankle joint remains a reliable procedure for the relief of painful conditions, including osteoarthritis, post-traumatic arthritis, rheumatoid arthritis, and complications of septic arthritis. A variety of ankle arthrodesis techniques have been described over the years.[4–16] This chapter discusses the pathophysiology, causes, and management of ankle arthritis.

HISTORICAL PERSPECTIVE

Ankle procedures for problems related to arthritis are widely performed in the United States. Although arthritis is distinctly less common in the ankle than in the hip and knee, it is an equally disabling condition. Stauffer[17] reported that only 6% of all cases of disabling degenerative joint disease of a major lower extremity involve the ankle. Trauma was the underlying etiological factor in virtually all of their cases of ankle joint degeneration. In their series of more than 300 cases of disabling ankle degeneration, only two patients were unable to attribute their disability to a history of a past fracture or recurrent ankle ligament injury. Stauffer noted a bimodal age distribution, with post-traumatic degenerative joint disease following ankle fracture reaching a peak in the 4th decade and following recurrent ankle sprains peaking in the 6th decade.

Increased understanding of the relationship of suboptimal anatomic restoration to the development of post-traumatic arthritis has led to improved operative reduction and therefore better patient outcome after ankle fracture. Ramsey and Hamilton, in 1976,[17a] demonstrated that a 1 mm lateral subluxation of the talus resulted in a 40% reduction of surface contact of the weightbearing surface of the tibiotalar joint. Phillips et al, in 1985,[18] noted the correlation of poor outcome with an abnormal talocrural angle. Weber and Simpson[19] popularized the concept of ankle joint reconstruction in patients after a malunited ankle to reduce the risk of post-traumatic arthritis. In 1990, Marti et al[20] validated this concept by demonstrating almost no progression of arthritis of the ankle joint, after successful correction of a malunion.

CLINICAL FEATURES

EVALUATION OF THE PATIENT WITH ANKLE PAIN
History
The physician should ascertain which patient activities induce ankle pain as well as what their expected level of functioning will be in the future. Care should be taken to determine whether a patient has global or isolated ankle pain with activity. Anterior ankle pain with stair climbing or descent can be a sign that the patient simply has ankle impingement. The presence of pain that awakens the patient from sleep or is present at rest should be ascertained. Symptoms present at these times typically signify advanced degenerative arthritis, or other disease processes (e.g., neuropathy).

Physical Examination
Comparisons should be made between the affected and unaffected ankles. Evaluation begins with inspection of lower extremity alignment and determination of limb length discrepancy. Malalignments of the spine, hip, or knee can affect the ankle and lead to ankle pain due to abnormal positioning of the foot relative to the limb or discrepancies of heel strike between limbs. These malalignments must be ascertained during the preoperative planning with consideration given to addressing proximal deformities with osteotomy, arthroplasty, or arthrodesis prior to distal deformities. This concept is critical in patients with rheumatoid arthritis. Alternatively, a flexion contracture in an ipsilateral knee will increase the anterior impingement force across a painful ankle with limited dorsiflexion.[21] Replacing the knee may allow the foot to reach a more plantigrade position and relieve stresses experienced at the ankle joint and obviate ankle surgery.

Typically, the foot lies with 20 to 30 degrees of external rotation relative to the tibia.[22] This position should be maintained postoperatively. The unaffected extremity can serve as a standard for comparison of external rotation in the patient.

An examination includes assessment for a joint effusion, range of motion, and ligament stability in addition to skin integrity, temperature, and neurovascular status. Accurate ankle range of motion should be determined with the subtalar joint held in neutral position. Several functional analyses documented a mean of 70 degrees of total sagittal plane motion. Subjects required 56 degrees of sagittal plane motion for stair descent and 27 degrees for walking on level surfaces.[23–26]

Assess the tendons that surround the ankle. Injuries to these structures can be mistaken for internal ankle disorders. Injections of local anesthetic into symptomatic joints, tendons, or nerves can help pinpoint areas of involvement. Injection of local corticosteroids can result in tendon damage and should not be performed.

Preoperative assessment of the foot also includes careful inspection of the subtalar joint. Inversion and eversion motion of the subtalar joint of each limb should be compared. Crepitus of the subtalar joint should be investigated preoperatively as an additional source of hindfoot pain. Failure to recognize subtalar arthritis can lead to persistent postoperative pain after ankle arthrodesis. Advanced radiographic studies or selective joint injections can help ascertain the clinical significance of subtalar pain versus ankle pain.

INVESTIGATIVE SECTION

RADIOLOGICAL EVALUATION
Preoperative Evaluation
Standard evaluation of ankle pathology includes radiographic determination of deformity and degeneration of joint surfaces. Joint space obliterations are best assessed with weightbearing radiographs. Three views are the most useful for determining joint space narrowing and osteophyte formation: standing lateral (Fig. 1A), anteroposterior, and mortise views (Fig. 1B).

True tibiotalar and tibiopedal motion can be assessed pre- and postoperatively by using stress dorsiflexion and plantar flexion lateral radiographs.[27, 28]

Computed tomography (CT) scanning alone or in combination with arthrography can be used to assess joint space defects and degenerative changes and determine the location of painful osteophytes.

Bone scans can be used to verify clinical findings and to evaluate contiguous joint pathology (subtalar, talonavicular, and calcaneocuboid joints) preoperatively. Although very sensitive, bone scans are regarded as being nonspecific tests. They do not differentiate between the various causes of inflammation. These secondary imaging modalities provide useful information when preexisting hardware is present in the region in question.

Postoperative Radiographic Evaluation
An obvious concern addressed by postoperative imaging includes the presence of union of the arthrodesis site. This can frequently be determined by plain radiography. With questionable radiographs in a patient who has persistent pain postoperatively, CT scanning and tomography should be used to evaluate the fusion mass.

EVALUATION TOOLS AND HISTORICAL RESULTS
Scoring systems of the foot and ankle provide standardized methods of evaluating and comparing patient function pre- and postoperatively. Two prominent and widely used methods for evaluating patients functioning with ankle pathology have been described. The earlier classic study of

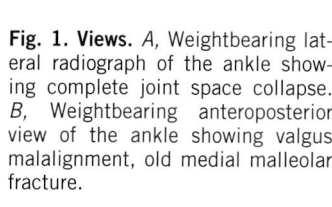

Fig. 1. Views. *A*, Weightbearing lateral radiograph of the ankle showing complete joint space collapse. *B*, Weightbearing anteroposterior view of the ankle showing valgus malalignment, old medial malleolar fracture.

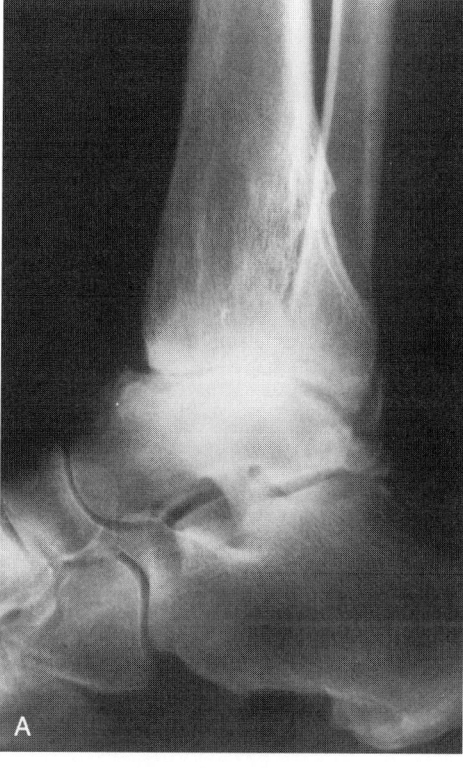

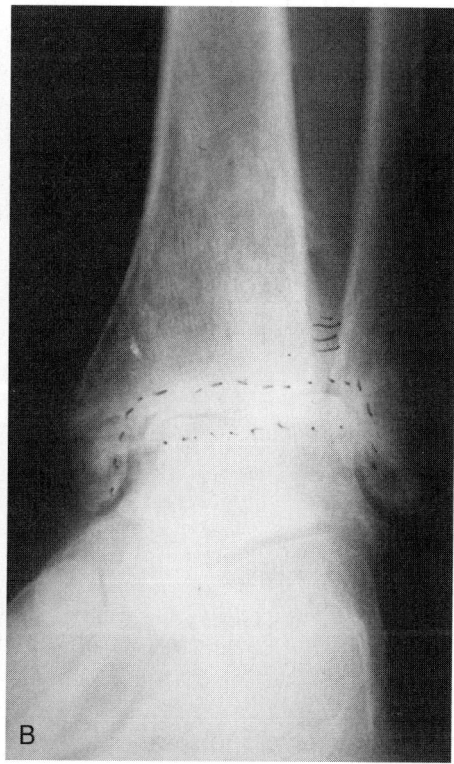

patient function and gait analysis after ankle arthrodesis was published by Mazur et al.[27] Mazur devised a widely accepted scoring system for evaluation of patient function before and after ankle fusion (Table 1). Patients in Mazur's study had an average preoperative score of 40.3 ± 11.2 points and an average postoperative score of 80.0 ± 8.9 points (p <0.01). The maximum possible postoperative score was 90 points (secondary to the loss of ankle motion in the sagittal plane after arthrodesis).

A more recent scoring system incorporates subjective and objective factors into numerical scales to describe function, alignment, and pain (Table 2).[29] After a review of the literature and the consensus of a committee of the American Orthopaedic Foot and Ankle Society, a 100-point scoring system was devised for evaluation of the ankle and hindfoot. Alignment of the foot can affect the patient's knee function and therefore the gait.[30] It should be noted that functional evaluation systems do not evaluate all aspects of a procedure, such as the rates of pseudarthrosis.

The most recent scoring system introduced for assessing patients with osteoarthritis of the ankle is the Ankle Osteoarthritis Scale (Table 3).[31] This instrument has been proven as a valid and reliable measurement tool for assessing the degree of pain and disability experienced by patients with osteoarthritis of the ankle. It is based on a visual analogue scale as measured along a series of 100 mm long bars. The responses are filled out by patients. Each category's score is tabulated, all of the responses are added together for each subsection of pain or disability, and the overall percentage is calculated from the maximum possible outcome for each category. The Ankle Osteoarthritis Scale was validated against the (1) Western Ontario McMaster University Osteoarthritis Index, a disease-specific scale for osteoarthritis and (2) the SF-36 (Medical Outcome Study 36 Question Short Form), an internationally accepted general health survey. This newer measurement tool has not been widely utilized as yet for a large clinical series but shows great promise.

TABLE 1. CLINICAL OUTCOME AFTER ANKLE ARTHRODESIS: GRADING SYSTEM (WEARING SHOES)

Pain

None, or patient ignores it	50
Slight when going up or down stairs or walking long distances (no restriction of activities of daily living)	45
Moderate when going up or down stairs or walking long distances; none during level gait; occasional non-narcotic medication needed	40
During level gait, with more pain on stairs; none at rest; daily medication used	25
At rest or at night in addition to during walking; narcotic medication required	10
Continuous, regardless of activity	0
Disabled because of pain	0

Total _____

Function

Limp, antalgic
None	6
Slight	4
Moderate	2
Marked	0

Total _____

Distance
Unlimited	6
4–6 blocks	4
1–3 blocks	2
Indoors only	1
Bed-chair	0
Unable to walk	0

Total _____

Support
None	6
Cane, long walks only	5
Cane, full time	3
2 canes or crutches	1
Walker required or unable to walk	0

Total _____

Hills (up)
Climbs normally	3
Climbs with foot externally rotated	2
Climbs on toes or by side-stepping	1
Unable to climb hills	0

Total _____

Hills (down)
Descends normally	3
Descends with foot externally rotated	2
Descends on toes or by side-stepping	1
Unable to descend	0

Total _____

Stairs (up)
Climbs normally	3
Needs banister	2
Steps up with normal foot only	1
Unable to climb stairs	0

Total _____

Stairs (down)
Descends normally	3
Needs banister	2
Steps down with normal foot only	1
Unable to descend stairs	0

Total _____

Ability to rise on toes (stability)
Able to rise on toes × 10 repetitions	5
Able to rise on toes × 5 repetitions	3
Able to rise on toes × 1 repetition	1
Unable to rise on toes	0

Total _____

Running
Able to run as much as desired	5
Able to run but limited	3
Unable to run	0

Total _____

Range of motion

Dorsiflexion beyond neutral
40 degrees	5
30 degrees	4
20 degrees	3
10 degrees	2
5 degrees	1
0 degrees	0

Total _____

Plantar flexion
40 degrees	5
30 degrees	4
20 degrees	3
10 degrees	2
5 degrees	1
0 degrees	0

Total _____

From Mazur et al: Ankle arthrodesis. J Bone Joint Surg Am 1979, 61:964.

TABLE 2. AOFAS CLINICAL ANKLE-HINDFOOT RATING SCALE (100 POINTS TOTAL)

PAIN (40 points)

None	40
Mild, occasional	30
Moderate, daily	20
Severe, almost always present	0

FUNCTION (50 points)

Activity limitations, support requirement

No limitations, no support	10
No limitation of daily activities, limitation of recreational activities, no support	7
Limited daily and recreational activities, cane	4
Severe limitations of daily and recreational activities, walker, crutches, wheelchair, brace	0

MAXIMUM WALKING DISTANCE, BLOCKS

Greater than 6	5
4–6	4
1–3	2
Less than 1	0

WALKING SURFACES

No difficulty on any surface	5
Some difficulty on uneven terrain, stairs, inclines, ladders	3
Severe difficulty on uneven terrain, stairs, inclines, ladders	0

GAIT ABNORMALITY

None, slight	8
Obvious	4
Marked	0

SAGITTAL MOTION (flexion plus extension)

Normal or mild restriction (30 degrees or more)	8
Moderate restriction (15–29 degrees)	4
Severe restriction (less than 15 degrees)	0

HINDFOOT MOTION (inversion plus eversion)

Normal or mild restriction (75–100% normal)	6
Moderate restriction (25–74% normal)	3
Marked restriction (less than 25% normal)	0

ANKLE-HINDFOOT STABILITY (anteroposterior, varus-valgus)

Stable	8
Definitely unstable	0

ALIGNMENT (10 points)

Good, plantigrade foot, ankle-hindfoot well aligned	10
Fair, plantigrade foot, some degree of ankle-hindfoot malalignment observed, no symptoms	5
Poor, nonplantigrade foot, severe malalignment, symptoms	0

Reprinted with permission from Kitaoka HB, et al: Clinical rating systems for the ankle-hindfoot, midfoot, hallux, and lesser toes. Foot Ankle 1994, 15(7): 349.

DIFFERENTIAL DIAGNOSIS

Intra-articular pathologic lesions must be distinguished from surrounding **joint tendinitis and bursitis**. This can be achieved with diagnostic testing such as magnetic resonance imaging or with injection of local anesthetic.

Primary osteoarthritis of the ankle is rare.[32] It is predominant in Japanese society, perhaps because of the style of sitting.[33] It is a diagnosis of exclusion. It has been addressed successfully with low tibial osteotomy.[34]

Post-traumatic osteoarthritis is the most common form of ankle arthritis. Post-traumatic disease can be present after intra-articular fractures or improper joint biomechanics after extra-articular fractures. Frequently, deformity is present in the joint. The extent of bone loss after trauma and joint space collapse can be assessed with weightbearing radiographs and CT scans.

Avascular necrosis must be considered in cases in which sclerosis of the talar dome is present. Patients may have a history of talar neck fracture, steroid or alcohol usage, or nonspecific injuries. Avascular necrosis of the talus can result in progressive segmental collapse and an increasing amount of particulate matter into the joint. Often these loose bodies cause periodic episodes of inflammation and locking of the ankle. An arthrodesis requires extensive débridement of sclerotic, dead bone to expose adequately perfused bone. Insufficient débridement of sclerotic bone results in high rates of nonunion and delayed unions after arthrodesis attempts.[35, 36]

Systemic inflammatory diseases such as **rheumatoid arthritis** should be excluded prior to considering operative intervention. Ankle arthritis can be effectively treated with a medical regimen prior to considering surgical intervention, particularly during a flare of the disease. The majority of patients with rheumatoid arthritis test positive for rheumatoid factor. In addition, the diagnosis of rheumatoid arthritis requires the presence of certain other symptoms: morning stiffness, multiple joint swelling, rheumatoid nodules, and joint erosion on radiographs.[37] As many as 16% of patients with rheumatoid disease have presented with forefoot pain as their initial manifestation of the condition.[38]

Patients with absence of rheumatoid factor in the serum, but manifestations of inflammatory arthritis are classified as having **seronegative arthropathy**. The four major disorders include **ankylosing spondylitis**, **psoriatic arthritis**, **Reiter's syndrome**, and **inflammatory bowel arthritides**. These patients can have inflammation or enthesopathies at the insertion of tendons, joint capsules, fascia, and ligaments. Patients fitting this description have (1) negative rheumatoid factor, (2) oligoarthritis involving large joints of the lower extremity, (3) radiographic evidence of sacroiliitis and/or spondylitis, (4) familial aggregation, (5) HLA-B27 presence in certain patients, especially those with ankylosing spondylitis and Reiter's syndrome, (6) enthesopathies, and (7) extra-articular clinical characteristics.[39] Extra-articular manifestations of seronegative spondyloarthropathy include psoriasiform nail or skin lesions, ocular inflammation, genital tract ulceration or infection, gastrointestinal ulceration or infection, erythema nodosum, thrombophlebitis, and aortitis or aortic valve insufficiency.

Metabolic and infectious causes of arthritis must be considered as well. This can include **gonococcal disease, Lyme disease,** and **gouty uricemia**.

Infectious causes can have cryptic origins with insidious or acute onset. Patients should be questioned about possible exposure to disease sources for sexually transmitted diseases and insect bites. Clinical laboratory tests or joint aspirates for crystals, cell count, or culture should be performed in cases requiring diagnostic confirmation.

Screening bloodwork in patients with inflammatory pattern, metabolic, or infectious type arthritis suggested by bilateral or diffuse complaints include screening radiographs; serologies including but not limited to complete blood count (CBC), erythrocyte sedimentation rate (ESR), C reactive protein (CRP), serum uric acid level, rheumatoid factor, anti-nuclear antibody, HLA-B27, and Lyme titers. Laboratory testing must be correlated with clinical findings to devise an appropriate treatment plan. Clinicians should

TABLE 3. ANKLE OSTEOARTHRITIS PAIN SCALE*

A. Name: _____ **Age:** _____ **Gender:** _____ **Weight:** _____ **Occupation:** _____

Pain

The line next to each item represents the amount of pain you typically had in each situation. On the far left is "No pain" and on the far right is "The worst pain imaginable". Place a mark on the line to indicate how bad your *ankle* pain was in each of the following situations during the *past week.* If you were not involved in one or more of these situations, mark that item NA.

B. How Severe Was Your *Ankle* Pain:

			NA
1. At its worst?	No pain _____	Worst pain imaginable	____
2. Before you get up in the morning?	No pain _____	Worst pain imaginable	NA ____
3. When you walked barefoot?	No pain _____	Worst pain imaginable	NA ____
4. When you stood barefoot?	No pain _____	Worst pain imaginable	NA ____
5. When you walked wearing shoes?	No pain _____	Worst pain imaginable	NA ____
6. When you stood wearing shoes?	No pain _____	Worst pain imaginable	NA ____
7. When you walked wearing shoe inserts or braces?	No pain _____	Worst pain imaginable	NA ____
8. When you stood wearing shoe inserts or braces?	No pain _____	Worst pain imaginable	NA ____
9. At the end of the day?	No pain _____	Worst pain imaginable	NA ____

_____/_____ = _____%

B. Name: _____ **Date:** ____/____/____

Disability

The line next to each item represents the amount of difficulty you had performing an activity. On the far left is "No Difficulty" and on the far right is "So difficult unable". Place a mark on the line to indicate how much difficulty you had performing each activity because of your *ankle* during the past week. If you did not perform an activity during the past week, place a "X" in the column under the heading NA.

C. How Much Difficulty Did You Have:

			NA
1. Walking around the house?	No difficulty _____	So difficult unable	NA ____
2. Walking outside on uneven ground?	No difficulty _____	So difficult unable	NA ____
3. Walking four or more blocks?	No difficulty _____	So difficult unable	NA ____
4. Climbing stairs?	No difficulty _____	So difficult unable	NA ____
5. Descending stairs?	No difficulty _____	So difficult unable	NA ____
6. Standing on tip toes?	No difficulty _____	So difficult unable	NA ____
7. Getting out of a chair?	No difficulty _____	So difficult unable	NA ____
8. Climbing up or down curbs?	No difficulty _____	So difficult unable	NA ____
9. Walking fast or running?	No difficulty _____	So difficult unable	NA ____

_____/_____ = _____%

* The scale consists of 18 items. Patients respond by placing a mark along a 100 mm horizontal line to depict their level of pain or disability for the described condition. Each subscale, pain (A) or disability (B), consists of nine items. The sums of the responses for the nine-item subscales are tallied to generate each subscale's total score and the overall score. In cases of "not applicable," the responses are dropped so that normalized total scores are calculated. (From Domsic RT, Saltzman CL: Ankle osteoarthritis scale. Foot Ankle 1998; 19:466.)

also consider that a disease process may not be immediately identified in laboratory testing and that patients may need to be retested periodically.

PATHOGENESIS

Arthritis of the ankle is routinely seen in the practice of Orthopaedic Surgery. Unlike in other major lower extremity joints, primary osteoarthritis is a rare phenomenon in the ankle.[34] Joint failure (loss of articular cartilage) is attributed to several causes: stress overload of articular surfaces (commonly seen in post-traumatic arthritis), the presence of an inflammatory process (e.g., rheumatoid arthritis), or the presence of an underlying infection.

Post-traumatic arthritis of the tibiotalar joint typically occurs after an ankle, tibial plafond, or talus fracture (or some combination thereof). Osteochondral injuries (49% in one series) after an ankle fracture are typically underestimated.[40] The presence of a pilon fracture implies a significant degree of energy involvement and cartilage or soft tissue injury. Talus fractures are noted to result in a significant incidence of post-traumatic arthritis of the ankle (33%) and/or subtalar joints (66%). Avascular necrosis of the talus commonly occurs after a fracture and leads to additional segmental collapse and tibiotalar arthritis.[41]

Abnormal ankle biomechanics is a critical factor in the development of ankle arthritis. In an experimental setting,[42] the investigators reported a significant reduction of joint contact area (42%) with a 1 mm lateral talar shift. Zindrick et al[43] documented a 49% increase in mean articular pressure with a 2 mm lateral talar shift. Macko et al[44] reported significant experimental alteration in joint reaction forces with a loss of the posterior malleolar fragment. It is evident that anatomic restoration of fibular rotation and length (as well as stabilization of the syndesmosis)[20] is critical to minimize the incidence of post-traumatic arthritis. Less common causes of ankle arthritis include the inflammatory condition of rheumatoid arthritis, seronegative arthritides, and crystalline arthropathies (gout, pseudogout). An infectious process such as a septic ankle may lead to cartilage loss and joint deterioration.

Characterization of normal and pathological joint physiology is necessary to understand the treatment of ankle arthritis. The development of post-traumatic arthritis or primary arthritis is often indistinguishable and may be analyzed in similar light.

The hip and the knee joint are common sites for primary osteoarthritis (incidence which increases with age). In contrast, this phenomenon is rare in the ankle joint. Studies made of articular cartilage lesion of a random series of necropsies reveal a low incidence of primary ankle osteoarthritis. Meachin[45] analyzed 45 left ankle joints from a random series of adult necropsies. Although foci of fibrillation were common in the ankle joint, only 1 of 20 ankles from subjects older than 70 years of age and none of subjects younger than this demonstrated any regions of full-thickness cartilage defect with osteoarthritis. Muehleman et al[46] evaluated 50 cadavers (mean age, 76 years; range, 36 to 94) and noted that only 18% of the ankles were grade III/IV osteoarthritis, compared with 66% of the knee joints. Huch et al[47] noted similar results with only 5 of 78 (6%) ankle joints (average age, 47 years) and 9 of 36 (25%) knees demonstrating full-thickness defects. It is evident that the majority of articular cartilage of the normal ankle joint is highly resistant to clinically demonstrable osteoarthritis.

Several hypotheses have been advanced to explain the rarity of primary ankle osteoarthritis. First, in the normal-level walking, the resultant forces transmitted by the hip, knee, and ankle joint are approximately equal.[48] Therefore, the rarity of ankle osteoarthritis cannot be attributed to smaller resultant forces.

One hypothesis is that the cartilage in the hip and knee joint becomes weaker with age, whereas that in the talus retains its mechanical properties. Kempson[49] demonstrated that the tensile fracture stress of the femoral head cartilage of the hip decreased significantly with age in comparison with the talar cartilage of the ankle, which shows little change. The tensile stiffness decreases more in the femoral

head cartilage than in the talar cartilage with increased age. It is suggested that the progressive fatigue failure causes the reduction in articular cartilage properties with age in the hip and knee, but not in the ankle. These results offer a possible explanation for the observation that primary osteoarthritis rarely occurs in the ankle except secondary to traumatic conditions.

Another significant difference noted between the knee and ankle chondrocytes was also reported in matrix metalloproteinase (MMP) production. Only MMP-8 has been identified to be capable of cleavage at the second site of aggrecan and is thought to be essential. Chubinskaya et al[50] analyzed the presence and distribution of MMP-3 and MMP-8 from two different joints from normal human donors. MMP-8 was detected in the untreated cartilage from the normal knee joint but not in the untreated cartilage from the normal ankle joint. The fact that ankle cartilage, which has a low incidence of osteoarthritis, does not express MMP-8, whereas knee cartilage, which has a high incidence of osteoarthritis, does constitutively express MMP-8 suggests that MMP-8 might be one of the key enzymes in the pathogenesis of osteoarthritis.

MANAGEMENT TECHNIQUES

NONOPERATIVE TREATMENT

Conservative therapy for arthritis of the ankle typically starts with shoe inserts or modification. A shoe with a cushioned heel and a rocker-bottomed sole has been shown to be of benefit in the early phase of treatment of these patients.[51] Later treatment can include the use of a molded ankle foot orthosis or a double upright type brace attached to the patient's shoe.[52]

Medications are frequently used to augment mechanical modes of treatment. Nonsteroidal anti-inflammatory drugs can help to relieve pain and inflammation. Patients should be screened for contraindications to nonsteroidal anti-inflammatory drugs and have serum and urine chemistries performed if chronic use is contemplated. Intra-articular injections of steroid and anesthetic combinations can be used to decrease intra-articular inflammation. The authors prefer to space these injections 3 months apart and to limit the total number of injections to three.

Final conservative treatment can consist of placing the patient into a walking cast for 6 weeks. This has been suggested as a trial to determine patient acceptance and possibility of pain relief from a fusion operation.[51] Patients with rheumatoid arthritis have been noted to occasionally undergo spontaneous fusion when casted.

SURGICAL TREATMENT
Palliative Ankle Débridement

Ankle joint débridement is commonly performed arthroscopically for early arthritis. This technique permits direct visualization of intra-articular and intracapsular structures, thus allowing accurate diagnostic evaluation and the opportunity for immediate therapeutic intervention.

Removal of impinging osteophytes by arthrotomy or arthroscopy has provided effective relief of pain.[56] Originally coined as "athletes ankle",[53] this entity has also been termed "footballer ankle."[54] It is commonly seen in athletes, and several large series have documented a high prevalence of impinging spurs in football players (up to 45%),[54] and in dancers (up to 59.3%).[55] The proposed mechanism consists of extreme ankle dorsiflexion with resultant anterior joint impingement and posterior joint distraction. It is theorized that repetitive anterior ankle impingement causes anterior subperiosteal hemorrhages and subsequent sclerotic bone growth.

Indications. Specific indications for ankle débridement include impinging osteophytes, synovitis, adhesions, loose bodies, ossicles, and chondral defects.[1, 56–64] Ankle débridement may also be useful in patients with previous ankle fractures (with adequate reduction) who note persistent pain and/or synovitis. Analysis of several clinical series has documented the role and outcome of arthroscopic ankle débridement for treatment of early arthritis and impingement syndrome.[55–57, 65–69]

Results. Few studies exist that document patient outcome after ankle arthroscopy for diffuse ankle degenerative joint disease. Ogilvie-Harris and Sekyi-Otu[68] reported on the results of ankle arthroscopy performed on 23 patients with ankle osteoarthritis. Statistically significant improvement was documented in 17 of 27 ankles with relation to pain, swelling, stiffness, limp, and activity level. However, similar findings were not noted in patients with feelings of instability. The authors concluded that arthroscopic débridement offers some clinical relief in patients with osteoarthritis alone, without ankle instability.

Loong et al[66] reported their experience with a series of 84 patients who had undergone arthroscopy for chronic ankle pain after failing conservative treatment. This series included multiple diagnoses, including transchondral fractures, synovitis, loose bodies, ligament instability, anterior impingement syndrome, osteochondral defect, and osteoarthritis. Patients with osteoarthritis of the ankle achieved only good to fair results. In contrast, patients with a majority of other diagnoses experienced excellent results.

In a study by Feder and Schonholtz[65] of a series of 30 arthroscopic cases with at least 24 months of follow-up, 9 patients had a preoperative diagnosis of post-traumatic osteoarthritis with or without a loose body. Only six were rated both functionally and subjectively, with two good, three fair, and one poor result. The authors concluded that patients with a chondral or osteochondral defect experienced significantly better outcome after arthroscopic intervention.

The findings of Loong et al,[66] Ogilvie-Harris and Sekeyi-Out,[68] and Feder and Schonholz[65] are similar and confirm the concept that arthroscopic débridement of an arthritic ankle is useful but may result in limited improvement. Poor results are noted in patients with significant ankle instability with diffuse arthritis.

Precise recreation of ankle joint anatomical relationships after rotational ankle fractures has a major influence on patient outcome. One series[70] reported 85% good-to-excellent results after reconstruction of an ankle malunion. Factors associated with favorable patient outcome include position of the talus in the mortise, stability of the syndesmosis, correct length of the fibula, and condition of the joint surface at the time of reconstruction. It is evident that "all components of the malunion need to be corrected, the goal being full restoration of normal anatomy."[20] Ankle reconstruction should be considered as an alternative to arthrodesis for patients with a malunited ankle fracture and minimal osteoarthritis (Fig. 2A to C).[19, 20, 70, 71]

Clinical results support the concept that late reconstruction of the malunited ankle provides pain relief and improved patient function.[19, 20, 71–73] Weber and Simpson[19] reported good and excellent results at average follow-up of 11.2 years in 17 of 23 patients who underwent an ankle reconstruction (fibular lengthening). Only one of the six patients experienced poor results necessitating an ankle fusion. Marti et al[20] analyzed 31 malunited ankle fractures treated with reconstructive osteotomies and achieved subjectively 71% and objectively 77% good-to-excellent results. Offierski et al[71] examined 11 patients who had undergone reconstruction of malunited ankle fractures. Ten were rated fair to good and one was rated as having poor outcome. Similar results were noted by other series.[74] Twenty of 26 patients reported satisfactory results and the ability to resume their preinjury level of activity at an average of 6 years' follow-up.

Ankle Arthrodesis

Arthrodesis for painful arthritic ankle is the gold standard by which all other treatment options are measured. When achieved, this is a highly successful operation that reliably returns the patient to high level of activity by alleviating pain and deformity.[8, 28]

Patient outcome after ankle arthrodesis has been analyzed using objective questions with an ankle rating system.[27] Mazur et al[27] evaluated 12 patients who underwent unilateral ankle arthrodesis for post-traumatic injury. The authors found that all patients functioned well under the conditions of normal daily living while wearing shoes. The patients were pain-free, able to return to work, and able to participate in leisure sports activities, long-distance walking, and hill or stair climbing. Younger patients were even able to jog.

The position of an ankle arthrodesis is critical for an ideal clinical outcome.[8, 22, 30] Mann[8, 22] stated that the goal of an ankle arthrodesis is to create a plantigrade foot that resembles the uninvolved extremity. Recommended position for an ankle fusion consists of slight external rotation (5 to 10 degrees) and slight valgus (5 to 8 degrees) alignment of the heel.[8, 22, 30] Comparison to the contralateral limb is useful in determining actual position.

Another recommendation is positioning the center of the talar dome posterior to the midline of the tibia. This concept, theoretically, reduces the moment arm at the arthrodesis site and improves gait. No study has documented any clinical advantages with posterior positioning of the foot relative to the tibia.

One major complaint after ankle arthrodesis is the significant loss of mobility. Biomechanical studies[21] of patients with multiple lower extremity involvement (e.g., ipsilateral painful stiff knee or hip) have documented significant gait alteration with shorter steps during ambulation and increased demand on the ankle joint.

The loss of ankle joint mobility is usually compensated with an increased hindfoot or midfoot motion.[10] Despite this phenomenon, patients with an ankle arthrodesis report limited ability to walk barefoot or on uneven ground.[27] Gait analysis and cadaveric studies[74] documented significantly increased stress on the contiguous joints after an

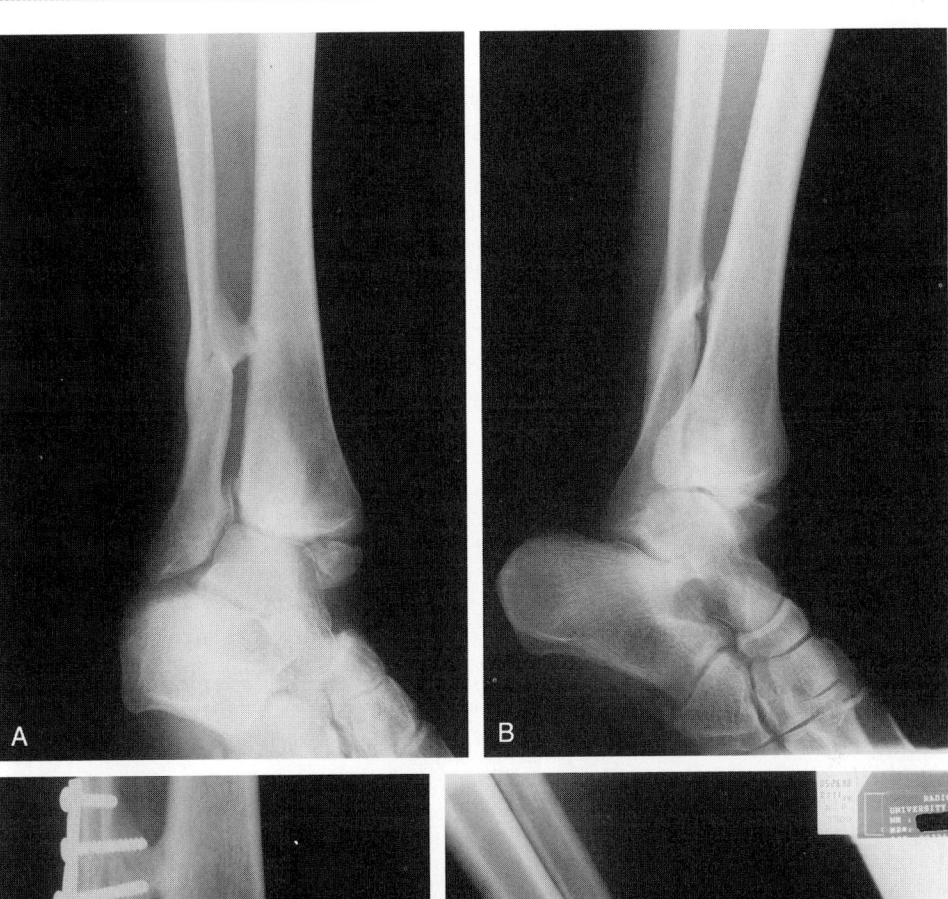

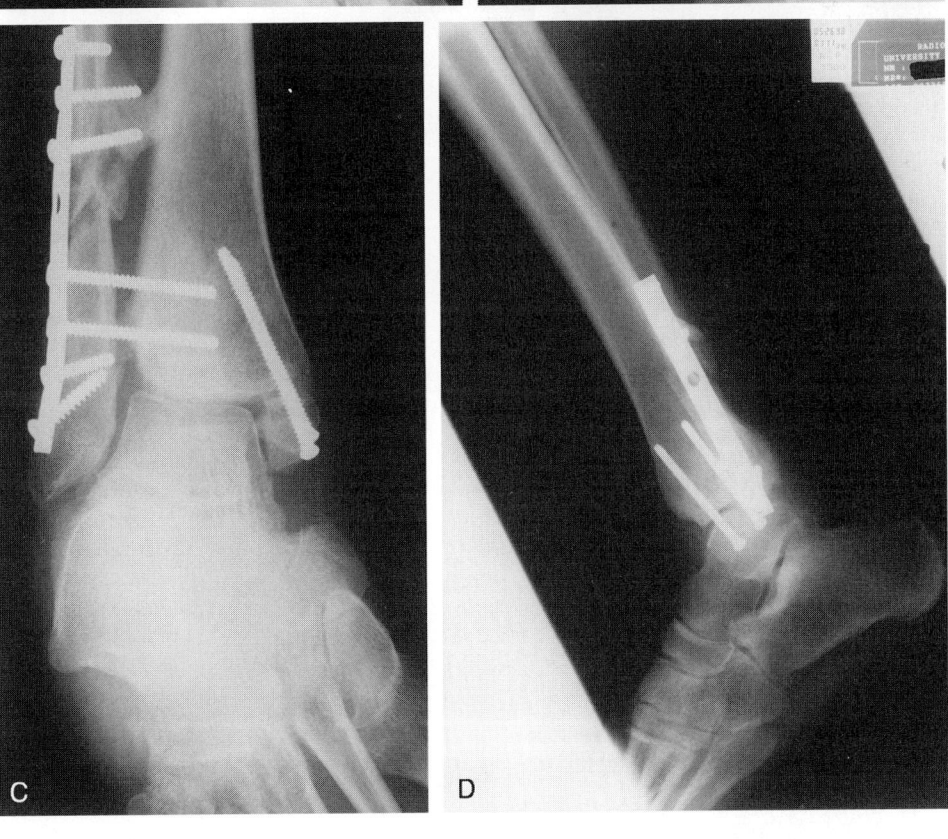

Fig. 2. 33-year-old incarcerated male who sustained closed trimalleolar ankle fracture, untreated for 9 months. *A*, Mortise radiograph revealing a malunited ankle fracture. *B*, Lateral radiograph of the malunited ankle. *C*, AP radiograph demonstrating a united ankle with good joint alignment in a clinically asymptomatic patient. *D*, Lateral postoperative radiograph confirming alignment of the fibula and reduction of the medial malleolar fragment.

arthrodesis. The long-term effects of increased stress on contiguous joints after ankle arthrodesis have not been ascertained but, intuitively, this may result in increased wear and arthritis.

Although ankle arthrodesis has been performed for more than 100 years, no single technique has demonstrated universal acceptance. Because of the significant complication rate and number of nonunions,[35] many variations of a given technique for achieving ankle arthrodesis have been described. These techniques differ in the surgical approach, method of débridement, application of interpositional or onlay graft, and method of fixation. To effectively understand the general concepts, four commonly used techniques (compressive external fixator, arthroscopic débridement, mini-open method, author's preferred method) are discussed in the treatment of ankle arthritis.

External Fixation. Patients with ankle pain due to arthritis that is resistant to conservative management are suitable surgical candidates. Early techniques of arthrodesis carried high rates of nonunion until the application of an external fixator by Charnley.[5] Current indications for the use of an external fixator include the presence of a pre-existing infection (e.g., septic arthritis, infected total ankle replacement or hardware).[12] It has also been suggested for fixation for patients with extreme osteoporosis after disuse.

The optimal configuration of external fixation has been argued in the past. The Calandruccio external fixator uses a triangular configuration to provide stability and compression across the tibiotalar joint (Fig. 3A to C).[7] It does not rely on the Achilles tendon to serve as a tension band configuration. Its fixation pins are placed through the neck of the talus, the tibia, and the calcaneus. This triangular arrangement provides optimal resistance to torsional forces.

Sagittal plane motion occurs more frequently with inadvertent weightbearing. An alternative method of external fixation involves the use of a unilateral device that provides optimal resistance to dorsiflexion and plantar flexion at the tibiotalar joint.[16] The fixation pins with the unilateral

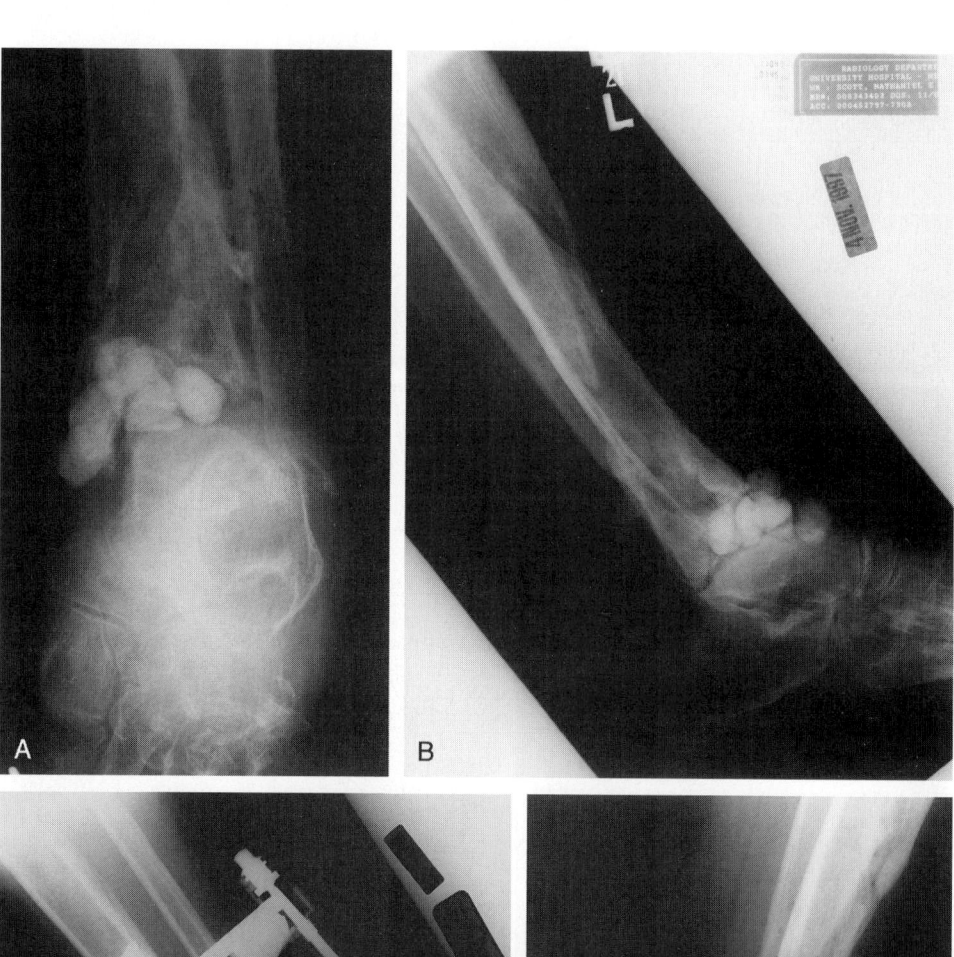

Fig. 3. 30-year-old incarcerated male who sustained a pilon fracture that went on to become infected with MRSA osteomyelitis of the distal tibia. *A*, AP significant bone loss in the distal tibia. *B*, Lateral significant bone loss in the distal tibia with antibiotic beads. *C*, After placement of external fixator for ankle arthrodesis. *D*, Successful arthrodesis achieved after 4 months.

device are also of a larger diameter than the Calandruccio external fixator pins. The unilateral ankle external fixator pins are placed into the medial aspect of the tibia, calcaneus, and the neck of the talus.

External fixation permits patients to bear weight for the first 8 weeks after the operation without any adverse effects on the rate of union. After removal of the external fixator, they are placed into a walking cast for 4 weeks. This technique avoids postoperative osteopenia and results in an arthrodesis rate of 92%.[7]

Ratliff conducted a retrospective study of 59 ankles that had undergone compression arthrodesis with a Charnley external fixator, with 1- to 9-year follow-up. He noted 61% excellent, 18% good, 19% fair, and 2% poor outcomes in this patient population. Six patients had a limp, and two had persistent pain due to unrecognized subtalar arthritis. A significant rate of complications related to pin tract infection developed in this patient population from the use of an external fixator.

Arthroscopically-Assisted Arthrodesis. Myerson et al[11] proposed another technique for ankle arthrodesis that utilized an arthroscopically-assisted method of joint débridement. This technique may only be utilized on ankles with minimal deformity, but substantial arthritic pain.

The arthroscopic procedure is performed through two or, occasionally, three portals. One portal is medial to the tibialis anterior tendon and the other is lateral to the extensor digitorum longus tendons or peroneus tertius tendon. A third portal can be placed to remove debris that is generated during denuding of the articular surfaces. The joint space is distracted with a noninvasive distractor or a unilateral external fixator. A 4.5-mm bur and curets are used to denude the articular surfaces. Compression of the joint surfaces can be carried out with internal or external fixation; preferably, two cannulated screws are used across the tibia, fibula, and talus. The first is introduced from the lateral aspect of the tibia and placed into

the neck of the talus. This is an area of high density within the talus and therefore can provide excellent fixation. The second screw is placed from the medial malleolus into the lateral aspect of the talus. Patients are maintained on non-weightbearing status for 5 weeks postoperatively. They are allowed to bear weight at that point until the joint is fused.

Myerson et al[11] compared arthroscopically-assisted arthrodesis to the standard, open technique. Patients who underwent the arthroscopic technique achieved union at 8.7 weeks on average. Patients who underwent arthrodesis by a conventional open technique using similar fixation methods fused, on average, by 14.5 weeks. Fusion rates were similar for both techniques.

Recently, Paremain et al[75] advocated the "mini-open" technique, which utilizes enlarged arthroscopic portals for exposure and removal of cartilage. The "mini-open" method decreased the amount of soft tissue stripping necessary in standard open techniques and permitted radiographic fusion by a mean of 6 weeks. The authors switched to this technique because they felt that it was less technically demanding than the arthroscopic technique.

Case Report. A case of a 65-year-old patient with post-traumatic arthritis demonstrates adequate screw fixation (Figs. 4 and 5). The patient went on to a successful arthrodesis 10 weeks after surgery and currently ambulates with a single axis cushion heel shoe with a rocker bottom without a limp.

In patients with compromised soft tissue in the anterior or lateral aspects of the ankle or with nonunions, alternative techniques must sometimes be relied on. Gruen and Mears[76] have described the successful use of an angled blade plate inserted through a posterior approach for tibiotalar, tibiotalocalcaneal, or tibiocalcaneal arthrodesis. The use of a retrograde intramedullary nail has also been described successfully in patients with soft tissue compromise, failed arthrodesis, and diabetic neuropathy.[77, 78]

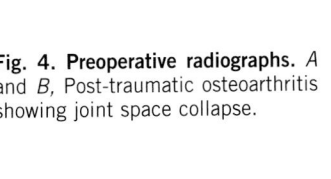

Fig. 4. Preoperative radiographs. *A* and *B*, Post-traumatic osteoarthritis showing joint space collapse.

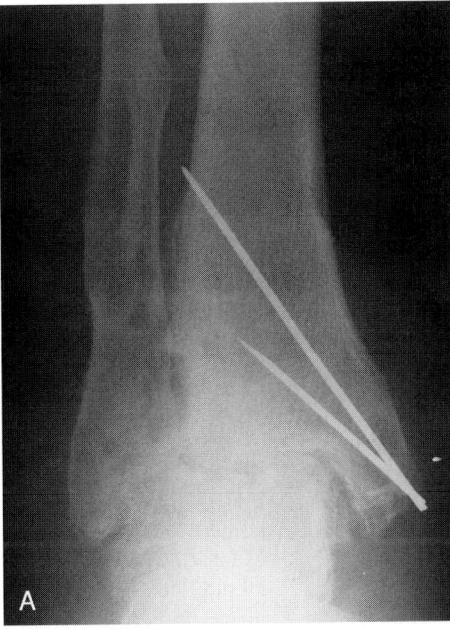

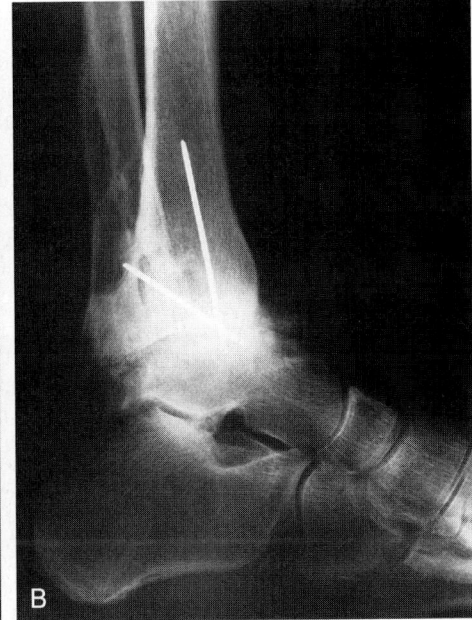

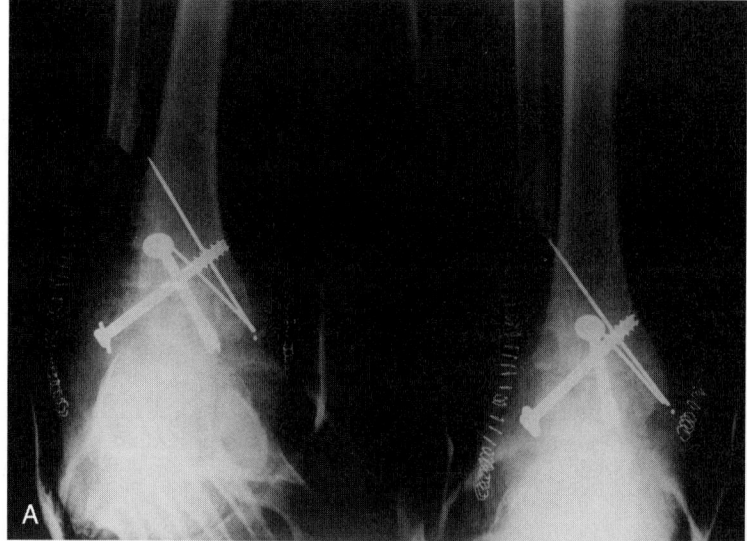

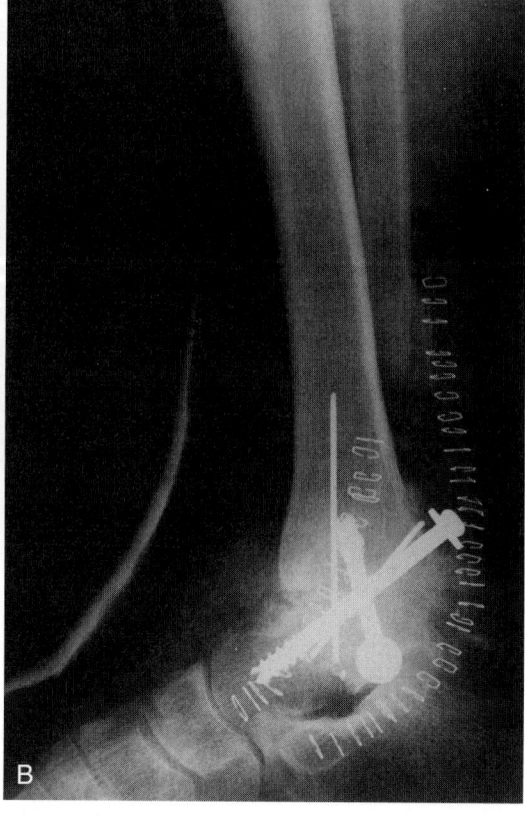

Fig. 5. Immediate postoperative radiographs. These show screw placement that maximizes compression and minimizes rotation at the arthrodesis site. A third screw is added from the neck of the talus laterally through the medial malleolus when possible.

COMPLICATIONS OF ANKLE ARTHODESIS

The most commonly encountered complication with ankle arthrodesis is nonunion. In a study by Frey et al at USC,[35] 78 ankle arthrodeses were reviewed with an average of 4 years of follow-up in an effort to determine which factors predisposed patients to developing nonunions. They determined that complications occurred in 44 patients (56%) consisting of 32 (41%) nonunions, 7 (9%) infections, 2 (3%) nerve injuries, 2 (3%) malunions, and 2 (3%) wound problems. Risk factors associated with nonunion in this series include severity of fracture, evidence of avascular necrosis of the talus, infection, major medical problems, and history of open injuries. Factors not associated with nonunion include age, past history of subtalar or triple arthrodesis, and technique. The diagnosis of combined plafond and talus fracture gave the worst prognosis, followed by Hawkins II or III talar fractures. Other studies have noted similar risk factors associated with nonunion. Holt et al[6] noted three conditions (avascular talus, pyarthrosis, and spasticity) that placed the patient at risk for nonunion. The rate of successful fusion for patients who had one of these three risk factors was 38%; of the 19 patients who did not have one of these risk factors, only 1 had a delayed union, for a successful fusion rate of 93%. Large-fragment screw fixation led to higher rates of union. This may be due to less soft tissue stripping associated with this technique compared with plating or better compression provided by the screw technique.

Nonunion after ankle arthrodesis has also been associated with smoking. In a case-control study,[79] the relative risk of nonunion after ankle arthrodesis was determined for smokers versus nonsmokers. In patients without any other risk factors, the risk of nonunion for smokers was 16 times the risk of nonunion in nonsmokers. The effects of nicotine on peripheral circulation and of hydrogen cyanide and carbon monoxide on the oxygen-carrying capacity of hemoglobin have all been cited as possible causes of cigarettes' influence on arthrodesis. The period of cessation of smoking prior to surgery necessary to clear some of its toxic effects is unclear. One study has suggested that 1 week prior to surgery might provide enough time to clear the radicals and thrombotic components from the blood stream.[80]

There are few articles that discuss the treatment of pseudarthrosis or nonunion of the ankle joint. Kirkpatrick et al[81] reported successful arthrodesis in 9 of 11 patients who sustained a pseudoarthrosis after failed ankle fusion. Seven of the 11 were treated using a transfibular approach that allowed excision of the fibrous tissue and sclerotic bone, decortication of the medial malleolus, and fixation of the tibia to the talus with cancellous screws and onlay/inlay fibula graft. Kitaoka[82] reported a union rate of 78% for treatment of nonunion following an attempted ankle arthrodesis after failure of total ankle replacement.

INFECTIONS

The infection rate after an attempted ankle arthrodesis has ranged from 0% to 28%.[8, 27, 83–87] The recommendations of Mann and coworkers to minimize an infection include a meticulous technique, removal of all devitalized tissue, adequate homeostasis, and use of intravenous antibiotics.[8, 88] The prevention of hematoma formation and minimizing the incidence of skin sloughs by using a full-thickness flap, adequate length of incision (to reduce tension), and a snug dressing are critical for an ideal outcome.

ARTHRITIS IN CONTIGUOUS JOINTS

In addition to the common complications (nonunion, infection), other unique problems of ankle arthrodesis include the development of stress fractures and the progression of arthritis into the surrounding joints.

A stress fracture occurs secondary to mechanical fatigue of the bone when it is subjected to "repetitive loading." Two clinical series have documented this rare complication in patients months after a solid arthrodesis.[89, 90] Lidor et al[89] reported on a series of 12 patients who had a stress fracture of the tibia and one patient who had a fracture of the fibula after ankle or foot arthrodesis. All but one of the fusion sites had fused prior to the occurrence of the stress fracture. The stress fracture that occurred in patients after arthrodesis was seen in the middle to distal aspect of the fibula.

Factors related to ankle arthrodesis that may contribute to stress fracture include increased bending forces transmitted to a distal tibia associated with decreased mechanical strength of bone,[91] loss of normal shock absorption mechanism, disuse osteopenia, decreased bone strength of the distal tibia compared with the talus, and magnified forces secondary to gait pattern changes of foot malposition.[92] In general, a stress fracture is treated nonoperatively with a reduction of the amount of repetitive stress to the bone. Most stress fractures healed uneventfully.

Gait analysis and cadaveric studies have shown that an ankle fusion does increase stress to the contiguous joints. Unfortunately, few clinical series exist that determine whether this increased stress has any clinical significance long term. Morrey and Weideman[93] reported 30 patients (at an average of 7.3 years after surgery) having virtually no subtalar motion and motion of 13 degrees at the Chopart joint after ankle arthrodesis. Similar findings of decreased subtalar joint motion were also noted in 23 of 31 patients of Ratliff's series.[13] The reason for the loss of motion after an ankle fusion was not ascertained.

With regard to the Chopart joint, Morrey and Weideman did not note the development of significant arthritis. Even for those patients with radiographic evidence of arthritis, the clinical symptoms (of pain and function) did not correlate with radiographic findings. Intuitively, an ankle fusion may increase the stress and motion of contiguous joints; however, its clinical significance appears to be minimal.

Alternative Treatment Methodologies

Joint Distraction. Distraction of the arthritic ankle joint has been advocated as a technique to improve joint alignment, minimize joint space narrowing, and delay or prevent an arthrodesis procedure.[94] Distraction of the joint is theorized to alter articular hydrostatic pressure and allow regeneration of articular cartilage. Concomitant correction of the joint malalignment allows improved physiological joint contact forces.

Valburg et al[95] documented that ankle distraction resulted in intermittently fluctuating joint hydrostatic pressures. Similar fluctuations in vitro resulted in increased proteoglycan synthesis in osteoarthritic cartilage.[96]

In a retrospective study of 11 patients, distraction across the ankle joint for 3 months with an Ilizarov device provided moderate pain relief and improved range of motion at 20 months' follow-up.[95] The presence of an equinus contracture preoperatively correlated with poor patient outcome. Insufficient patient outcome studies exist to support routine use of the Ilizarov distraction technique.

Distal Tibial Osteotomies. Ankle injuries or primary osteoarthritis resulting in varus deformity of the ankle joint can lead to excessive articular cartilage wear of the medial ankle joint surfaces. Primary osteoarthritis is much more predominant in Japan and may be related to style of sitting.[34] It is postulated to arise from hypoplasia of the medial malleolus and medial tibia. Alternatively, post-traumatic arthritis can result in varus deformity of the ankle joint as well. In younger patients with painless passive range of motion and relatively well preserved lateral ankle joint articular cartilage, an attempt should be made to avoid arthrodesis.

Takakura et al[34] performed a study of 18 patients with primary osteoarthritis. The tibiotalar joint space was narrowed medially, with tenderness and pain localized to this area during weightbearing. The lateral tibiotalar joint was well preserved during weightbearing. Arthroscopy confirmed the presence of articular cartilage in 13 patients. Radiographic grading was stage 2 to 3 in the majority of patients.

The surgical technique for supramalleolar osteotomy was performed to achieve 4 to 5 degrees of valgus alignment. Anteromedial opening osteotomies were performed on all 18 subjects at an average of 5 cm from the tip of the medial malleolus. The fibula was cut at the same level. Patients noted substantial relief of pain and improved ambulation with little change in joint mobility. Overall results were excellent in six patients, good in nine, fair in three, and poor in none. Although studies have demonstrated good outcome for patients with primary osteoarthritis, no data exist to support its use for patients with varus deformity arising from post-traumatic arthritis.

Total Ankle Arthroplasty. Total ankle arthroplasty (TAA) has been proposed as an alternative to arthrodesis in the management of painful arthritis of the tibiotalar joint. Historically, the tibiotalar arthrodesis carries a significant number of complications.[93, 97–99] A review of a large series of arthrodeses revealed relatively high rates of nonunion (20%), and unsatisfactory end results (28%).[5, 100] Sacrificing the ankle motion also places great stress on the contiguous joints (knee, midtarsal).[27]

Prior to its routine application, the clinical outcome and longevity of TAA must be judged against the current gold standard, tibiotalar arthrodesis. First, if success is judged by "pain relief," TAA must achieve comparable results with total pain relief in at least 59% to 75% of patients at 15-year follow-up.[27, 101, 102] Ratliff[13] reported good or subjective results in 46 of 52 ankle arthrodeses at long-term follow-up. TAA must demonstrate a satisfactory durability, particularly in young patients with post-traumatic arthritis.

The initial series of cemented ankle arthroplasty with short-term results were generally encouraging.[103–108] Unfortunately, medium- and long-term patient follow-up revealed considerable complications, including implant failure, component loosening and subsidence, and impingement.[2, 104, 106–113]

The Mayo total ankle replacement, a cemented constrained design, was initially noted to have 72% good or excellent results after 2 years' follow-up in 102 patients.[108] Survivorship analysis of Mayo total ankle replacement was estimated at 5-, 10-, and 15-year rates of 79%, 65%, and 61%, respectively.[3] A recent series[2] confirmed this estimate with approximately one third (36%; 57) of 160 total ankle arthroplasties having failed after a mean follow-up period of 9 years.

Additional series studying total ankle replacement other than the Mayo design confirm poor long-term survivorship. Bolton-Maggs et al[113] reported satisfactory results in only 13 of 41 total ankle arthroplasties performed with the Imperial College/London Hospital (ICLH) implant after a mean of 5.5 years. Takakura et al[117] reported the results of 25 arthroplasties at 8 years' (mean) follow-up. Six patients experienced good outcome, whereas 9 noted fair and 10 noted poor outcome.

The complications associated with a cemented, constrained ankle arthroplasty include component loosening, talar component subsidence into the cancellous talar body, and the need for improved tibial component fixation. Because of high rates of complication and reoperation, constrained ankle arthroplasty (i.e., Mayo) is not recommended for osteoarthritis of the ankle.[2]

Recent advances with cementless, porous, in-growth designs have been described (Fig. 6).[114–117] In an independent, retrospective study, Lin et al[118] evaluated patient outcome after implantation of an uncemented, semiconstrained New Jersey LCS Ankle, Buechel-Pappas TAA (Endotech, South Orange, NJ) (Fig. 7A&B). This prosthesis required minimal bone resection and consisted of titanium alloy tibial and talar components with an ultra-high molecular-weight polyethylene (UMPWE) liner between the two components. The undersurface had a sintered bead porous coating. At an average follow-up of 54 months, according to the criteria of Mazur,[27] the results were excellent in 13 TAAs (43.3%), good in 6 TAAs (20%), fair in 6 TAAs (20%), and poor in 5 TAAs (16.6%). The mean dorsiflexion was 4.8 degrees, and the mean plantar flexion was 16.2 degrees. This paper showed two failures, necessitating a revision of one prosthesis and fusion of another ankle with iliac crest bone graft interposed between the tibia and talus.

In another series by Pyevich et al,[115] a retrospective clinical outcome study was conducted on 100 of the first patients who had received a semiconstrained, uncemented Agility TAA (DePuy, Inc., Warsaw, IN). This uncemented device consists of a titanium tibial component with an UMPWE liner and a chrome cobalt talar component. The implantation procedure for the Agility requires creation of a distal tibiofibular synostosis for a stable base of support. Eighty-five ankles were available for intermediate follow-up at an average of 4.8 years after implantation. Forty-seven TAAs (55%) caused no pain according to the patients; 24 (28%) caused mild pain; 14 (16%) caused moderate pain; and none caused severe pain. Seventy-eight of the 82 surveyed patients (95%) would have the operation again. The average American Orthopaedic Foot and Ankle Society (AOFAS) clinical ankle-hindfoot score[29] for the patients in the study was 85 points. Postoperative complications included plantar flexion contractures, tibiofibular synostosis nonunions, and tibial and talar component migration. Of the total 100 first Agility implantations, there have been 5 revision arthroplasties, with one of these requiring arthrodesis for persistent pain. The stability of the tibial component of the Agility prosthesis correlated with the achievement of a solid tibiofibular synostosis.

Kofoed[116] performed a retrospective review on 20 uncemented Scandanavian Total Ankle Replacements (S.T.A.R., Waldemar Link GmbH&Co, Hamburg, Germany) that were implanted over 4 years. Primary arthritis was diagnosed in four ankles, post-traumatic arthrosis in 14 ankles, and hemochromatosis in two ankles. The uncemented replacement utilizes a stainless steel (L 316) talar cap and distal tibial

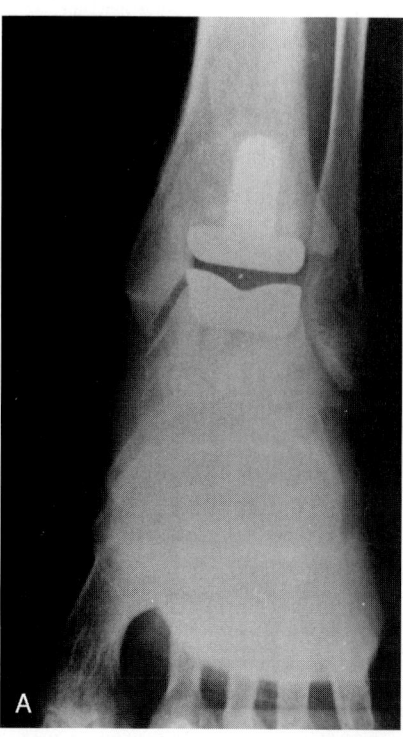
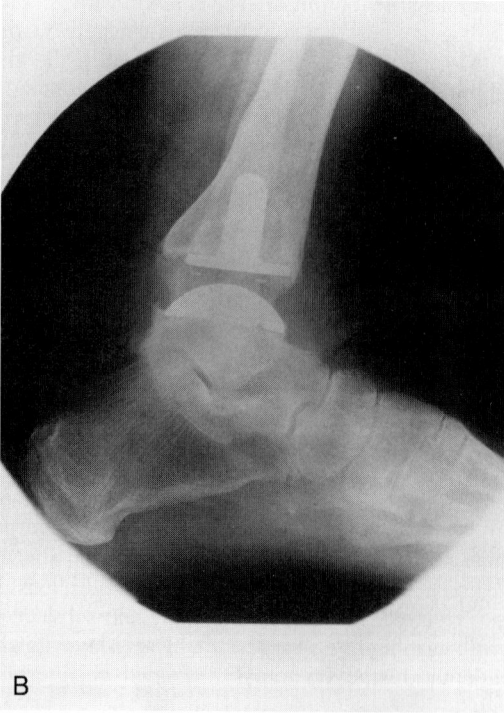

Fig. 6. AP and lateral radiographs. These show cementless total ankle arthroplasty (Buechel-Pappas) showing appropriate alignment.

A   B

base, with a 1.5 mm thick polyethylene floating meniscal spacer. The nonarticular surfaces are porous, coated with hydroxyapatite. At an average 4.1 years' follow-up, the ankle pain and function scores had changed from 27.5 preoperatively to 91.8 at follow-up. There were 17 excellent, 1 good, and 2 unacceptable results. There were no cases of tibial loosening. In one patient, there was tibial and talar subsidence in the third postoperative month, which did not progress further with longer follow-up. One patient required revision for subsidence 1 year after implantation. Newer trials are currently underway.

The early results of these uncemented TAAs are promising, but because of unknown long-term survivorship, current indications should be limited to older patients with low demands, bilateral ankle arthritis, or diffuse hindfoot arthritis requiring simultaneous hindfoot arthrodesis.

CONCLUSION

After conservative measures of treating ankle arthritis such as brace and shoewear modifications have failed, operative intervention should be considered. Initial operative treatment for focal arthritic complaints might consist of ankle cheilectomy or arthroscopic joint débridement of impinging osteophytes. Ankle arthrodesis is an effective means of treating patients with global, disabling ankle arthritis. Arthroscopic arthrodesis or the "mini-open" techniques can be used for patients with minimal deformity. Open arthrodesis can be used for patients with significant ankle deformity and malalignment preoperatively. Blade plate and retrograde nail fixation can be used for revision arthrodesis. Careful examination of all of the lower extremity joints, alignment, and gait should be carried out preoperatively. This will help determine what the overall effect of ankle arthrodesis will be on a patient. Prior to arthrodesis, the relationship of the hindfoot to the forefoot should be evaluated. A plantigrade foot position can be obtained by placing the heel in 5 to 7 degrees of valgus, externally rotating the ankle by 5 to 10 degrees and displacing the talus posteriorly. Appropriate positioning of the foot during arthrodesis can help avoid altering the patient's gait significantly and also preserve hip and knee function.

REFERENCES

1. McGuire MR, Kyle RF, Gustillo RB, et al: Comparative analysis of ankle arthroplasty versus ankle arthrodesis. Clin Orthop 1988; 226:174.
2. Kitaoka HB, Patzer GL: Clinical results of the Mayo total ankle arthroplasty. J Bone Joint Surg Am 1996; 78:1658.
3. Kitaoka HB, Patzer GL, Ilstrup DM, et al: Survivorship analysis of the Mayo total ankle arthroplasty. J Bone Joint Surg Am 1994; 76:974.
4. Barr JS, Record EE: Arthrodesis of the ankle joint. N Engl J Med 1953; 248:53.
5. Charnley J: Compression arthrodesis of the ankle and shoulder. J Bone Joint Surg Br 1951; 33:180.
6. Holt ES, Hansen ST, Mayo KA, et al: Ankle arthrodesis using internal screw fixation. Clin Orthop 1991; 268:21.
7. Malarkey RF, Binski JC: Ankle arthrodesis with the Calandruccio frame and bimalleolar onlay grafting. Clin Orthop 1991; 268:44.
8. Mann RA, VanManen JW, Wapner KL, et al: Ankle fusion. Clin Orthop 1991; 268:49.
9. Mears DC, Gordon RG, Kann SE, et al: Ankle arthrodesis with an anterior tension plate. Clin. Orthop 1991; 268:70.
10. Morgan CD, Henke JA, Bailey RW, et al: Long-term results of tibiotalar arthrodesis. J Bone Joint Surg Am 1985; 67: 546.
11. Myerson MS, Quill G: Ankle arthrodesis: A comparison of an arthroscopic and an open method of treatment. Clin Orthop 1991; 268:84.
12. Newman A: Ankle fusion with the Hoffman external fixation device. Foot Ankle 1980; 1:102.
13. Ratliff AH: Compression arthrodesis of the ankle. J Bone Joint Surg Br 1959; 41:524.
14. Scranton PE: Use of internal compression in arthrodesis of the ankle. J Bone Joint Surg Am 1985; 67:550.
15. Wang GJ, Shen WJ, McLaughlin RE, et al: Transfibular compression arthrodesis of the ankle joint. Clin Orthop 1993, 289:223.
16. Thordarson DB, Markolf KL, Cracchiolo A: External fixation in arthrodesis of the ankle. J Bone Joint Surg Am 1994; 76: 1541.
17. Stauffer RN: Intra-articular ankle problems. In Evarts CM (ed): Surgery of the Musculoskeletal System, vol. 4. New York, Churchill-Livingstone, 1990, p 3868.
17a. Ramsey PL, Hamilton W: Changes in tibiotalar area of contact caused by lateral talar shift. J Bone Joint Surg Am 1976; 58:356.
18. Phillips WA, Schwartz HS, Keller CS, et al: A prospective, randomized study of the management of severe ankle fractures. J Bone Joint Surg Am 1985; 67:67.
19. Weber BG, Simpson LA: Corrective lengthening osteotomy of the fibula. Clin Orthop 1985; 199:81.
20. Marti RK, Raaymaker ELFB, Nolte PA: Malunited ankle fractures. J Bone Joint Surg Br 1990; 72:709.
21. Hintermann B, Nigg BM: Influence of arthrodesis on kinematics of the axially loaded ankle complex during dorsiflexion plantarflexion. Foot Ankle 1995; 16:1995.
22. Mann RA: Biomechanical approach to the treatment of foot problems. Foot Ankle 1982; 2:205.
23. Murray MP, Drought AB, Kary RC: Walking patterns of normal man. J Bone Joint Surg Am 1964; 46:335.
24. Sammarco GJ, Burstein AH, Frankel VH: Biomechanics of the ankle: A kinematic study. Orthop Clin 1973; 4:75.
25. Stauffer RN, Chao EYS, Brewster J: Force and motion analysis of the normal, diseased and prosthetic ankle joint. Clin Orthop 1977; 127:189.
26. Wright DG, Desai SM, Henderson WH: Action of the subtalar and ankle joint complex during the stance phase of walking. J Bone Joint Surg Am 1964; 46:361.
27. Mazur JM, Schwartz E, Simon SR: Ankle arthrodesis. J Bone Joint Surg Am 1979; 61:964.
28. Mann RA, Rongstad KM: Arthrodesis of the ankle: a critical analysis. Foot Ankle 1998; 19:3.
29. Kitaoka HB, Alexander IJ, Adelaar RS, et al: Clinical rating systems for the ankle-hindfoot, midfoot, hallux and Lesser. Foot Ankle 1994; 15:349.
30. Buck P, Morrey BF, Chao EYS: The optimum position of arthrodesis of the ankle. J Bone Joint Surg Am 1987; 69:1052.
31. Domsic RT, Saltzman CL: Ankle osteoarthritis scale. Foot Ankle 1998; 19:466.
32. Katcherian DA: Treatment of ankle arthrosis. Clin Orthop 1998; 349:48.
33. Demetriades L, Strauss E, Gallina J: Osteoarthritis of the ankle. Clin Orthop 1998; 349:28.
34. Takakura Y, Tanaka Y, Kumal T, et al: Low tibial osteotomy for osteoarthritis of the ankle. J Bone Joint Surg Br 1995; 77:50.
35. Frey C, Halikus NM, Vu-Rose T, et al: A review of ankle arthrodesis: Predisposing factors to non-union. Foot Ankle 1994; 15:581.
36. Manoli A, Beals TC, Hansen ST: Technical factors in hindfoot arthrodesis. Instr Course Lect 1997; 46:347.
37. Geppert MJ, Mizel MS: Management of heel pain in inflammatory arthritides. Clin Orthop 1998; 349:93.
38. Thomas WH: Rheumatoid arthritis of the ankle and foot. AAOS Instr Course Lect 1979; 28:325.
39. Schumacher HR: *Primer on the Rheumatic Diseases*. Atlanta, Arthritis Foundation, 1988, p 355.
40. Lantz BA, McAndrews M: Effect of concomitant chondral injuries accompanying operatively reduced malleolar fractures. J Orthop Trauma 1991; 5:125.

41. Thordarson DB, Triffon MJ, Terk MR: Magnetic resonance imaging to detect avascular necrosis after open reduction and internal fixation of talar neck fractures. Foot Ankle 1996; 17:742.

42. Ramsey PL, Hamilton WC: Changes in tibiotalar area of contact caused by lateral talar shift. J Bone Joint Surg Am 1976; 58:356.

43. Zindrick MR, Hopkins GE, Knight GW, et al: The effect of lateral talar shift upon the biomechanics of the ankle joint. Orthop Trans 1985; 9:332.

44. Macko VW, Mathews LS, Zwirkoski P, et al: The joint-contact area of the ankle: The contribution of the posterior malleolus. J Bone Joint Surg Am 1991; 73:347.

45. Meachim G: G cartilage fibrillation at the ankle joint in Liverpool necropsies. J Anat 1975; 119:601.

46. Muehleman C, Bareither D, Huch K: Incidence of human osteoarthritis in the joints of lower extremity. FASEB J 1995; 9:A967.

47. Huch K, Kuettner KE, Dieppe P: Osteoarthritis in ankle and knee joint. Semin Arthritis Rheum 1997; 26:667.

48. Unsworth A: Tribology of human and artificial joints. Proc Inst Mech Eng 1991; 205:163.

49. Kempson GE: Age-related change in the tensile properties of human articular cartilage: A comparative study between the femoral head of the hip joint and talus of the ankle joint. Biochim Biophys Acta 1991; 1075:223.

50. Chubinskskaya S, Huch K, Mikecz K, et al: Chondrocyte matrix metalloproteinase 8: Up-regulation of neutrophil collagenase by IL-1 beta in human cartilage from knee and ankle joint. Lab Invest 1996; 74:232.

51. Scranton PE: Overview of ankle arthrodesis. Clin Orthop 1991; 268:96.

52. Schon LC, Ouzounian TJ: The ankle. In Jahss MH (ed): Disorders of the Foot and Ankle, vol 2. Philadelphia, W.B. Saunders, 1991, p 1417.

53. Morris LH: Athletes ankle. J Bone Joint Surg 1943; 25:220.

54. McMurray TP: Footballers ankle. J Bone Joint Surg Br 1950; 32:68.

55. Stoller SM, Hellmat F, Kleiger B: A comparative study of the frequency of anterior ankle impingement exostosis of the ankle in dancers and nondancers. Joint Ankle 1984; 4:201.

56. Scranton PE, McDermott JE: Tibiotalar spurs: A comparison of open versus arthroscopic debridement. Foot Ankle 1992; 13:125.

57. Hawkins RB: Arthroscopic treatment of sports-related anterior osteophytes in the ankle. Foot Ankle 1988; 9:87.

58. Ferkel RD, Fischer SP: Progress in ankle arthroscopy. Clin Orthop 1989; 240:210.

59. Amendola A, Petrik J, Webster-Bogart S: Ankle arthroscopy: Outcome in 79 consecutive patients. Arthroscopy 1996; 12:563.

60. Dijk CNV, Scholte D: Arthroscopy of the ankle. Arthroscopy 1997; 13:90.

61. Martin DF, Baker CL, Curl WW, et al: Operative ankle arthroscopy: Long term follow-up. Am J Sports Med 1989; 17:16.

62. McGinty JB: Arthroscopic removal of loose bodies. Orthop Clin North Am 1982; 13:313.

63. Stetson WB, Ferkel RD: Ankle arthroscopy: I. Techniques and complications. J Am Acad Orthop Surg 1996; 4:17.

64. Stetson WB, Ferkel RD: Ankle arthroscopy: II. Indications and results. J Am Acad Orthop Surg 1996; 4:24.

65. Feder KS, Schonholtz GJ: Ankle arthroscopy: Review and long term results. Foot Ankle 1992; 13:382.

66. Loong TW, Mitra AK, Tan SK: Role of arthroscopy in ankle disorders: Early experience. Ann Acad Med Singapore 1994; 23:348.

67. Meislin RJ, Rose DJ, Parisien S, et al: Arthroscopic treatment of synovial impingement of the ankle. Am J Sports Med 1993; 21:186.

68. Ogilvie-Harris DJ, Sekyi-Otu A: Arthroscopic debridement for osteoarthritic ankle. Arthroscopy 1995; 11:433.

69. Ogilvie-Harris DJ, Mahomed N, Demaziere A: Anterior impingement of the ankle treated by arthroscopic removal of bony spurs. J Bone Joint Surg Br 1993; 75:437.

70. Rosen H: Reconstructive procedures about the ankle joint. In Jahss MH (ed): Disorders of the Foot and Ankle, vol. 3. Philadelphia: W.B. Saunders, 1991, p 2593.

71. Offierski CM, Graham JD, Hall JH, et al: Late revision of fibular malunion in ankle fractures. Clin Orthop 1982; 171:145.

72. Weber BG: Lengthening osteotomy of the fibula to correct a widened mortice of the ankle after fracture. Int Orthop 1981; 4:289.

73. Yablon IG, Leach RE: Reconstruction of malunited ankle fractures. J Bone Joint Surg Br 1989; 71:521.

74. Gellman H, Leninan M, Halikis N, et al: Selective tarsal arthrodesis: An in vitro analysis of the effect on foot motion. Foot Ankle 1987; 8:127.

75. Paremain GP, Miller SD, Myerson MS: Ankle arthrodesis: Results after the miniarthrotomy technique. Foot Ankle 1996; 17:247.

76. Gruen GS, Mears DC: Arthrodesis of the ankle and subtalar joints. Clin Orthop 1991; 268:15.

77. Kile TA, Donnelly RE, Gehrke JC, et al: Tibiotalocalcaneal arthrodesis with an intramedullary device. Foot Ankle 1994; 15:669.

78. Pinzur MS, Kelikian A: Charcot ankle fusion with a retrograde locked intramedullary nail. Foot Ankle 1997; 18:699.

79. Cobb TK, Gabrielsen TA, Campbell DC, et al: Cigarette smoking and nonunion after ankle arthrodesis. Foot Ankle 1994; 15:64.

80. Lind J, Kramhoft M, Bodtker S: The influence of smoking on complications after primary amputations of the lower extremity. Clin Orthop 1991; 267:211.

81. Kirkpatrick JS, Goldner JL, Goldner RD: Revision arthrodesis for tibiotalar pseudoarthrosis with fibular onlay-inlay graft and internal screw fixation. Clin Orthop 1991; 268:29.

82. Kitaoka HB: Salvage of nonunion following ankle arthrodesis for failed total ankle arthroplasty. Clin Orthop 1991; 268:37.

83. Parisien JS, Vangsness T: Operative arthroscopy of the ankle. Clin Orthop 1985; 199:46.

84. Hagen RJ: Ankle arthrodesis: Problems and pitfalls. Clin Orthop 1986; 202:152.

85. Moeckel BH, Patterson BM, Inglis AE, et al: Ankle arthrodesis: A comparison of internal and external fixation. Clin Orthop 1991; 268:78.

86. Dent CM, Patil M, Fairclough JA: Arthroscopic ankle arthrodesis. J Bone Joint Surg Br 1993; 75:830.

87. Helm R: The results of ankle arthrodesis. J Bone Joint Surg Br 1990; 72:141.

88. Mann RA, Chou LB: Tibiocalcaneal arthrodesis. Foot Ankle 1995; 16:401.

89. Lidor C, Ferris LC, Hall R, et al: Stress fracture of the tibia after arthrodesis of ankle or hindfoot. J Bone Joint Surg Am 1997; 79:558.

90. Mitchell JR, Johnson JE, Collier BD, et al: Stress fracture of the tibia following extensive hindfoot and ankle arthrodesis: a report of three cases. Foot Ankle 1995; 15:445.

91. Huid I, Rasmussen O, Jensen NC, et al: Trabecular bone strength profile at the ankle joint. Clin Orthop 1985; 199:306.

92. Carmines DV, Nunley JA, McElhaney JH: Effect of ankle taping on the motion and loading pattern of the foot for walking subject. J Orthop Res 1988; 6:223.

93. Morrey BF, Weideman GP: Complication and long term results of ankle arthrodesis following trauma. J Bone Joint Surg Am 1980; 62:777.

94. Roermund PMV, Valburg AAV, Duivemann E, et al: Function of stiff joints may be restored by ilizarov joint distraction. Clin Orthop 1998; 348:220.

95. Valburg AAV, Roermund PMV, Lammens J, et al: Can ilizarov joint distraction delay the need for an arthrodesis of the ankle. J Bone Joint Surg Br 1995; 77:720.

96. Lafeber FP, Veldhuijzen JP, VanRoy JL, et al: Intermittent hydrostatic compressive force stimulates exclusively the proteoglycan synthesis of osteoarthritc human cartilage. Br J Rheumatology 1992; 31:437.

97. Davis RJ, Millis MB: Ankle arthrodesis in the management of traumatic ankle arthrosis: A long term retrospective series. J Trauma 1990; 20:674.

98. Lance EM, Paval A, Fries I, et al: Arthrodesis of the ankle. Clin Orthop 1979; 142:146.

99. Leicht P, Kofoed H: Subtalar arthrosis following ankle arthrodesis. Foot Ankle 1992; 2:89.

100. Johnson EW, Boseker EH: Arthrodesis of the ankle. Arch Surg 1968; 97:766.

101. Said E, Hunka L, Siller TN: Where fusions stand today. J Bone Joint Surg Br 1978; 60:211.

102. Vahvanen V: Arthrodesis of the talocrural or pantalar joints in rheumatoid arthritis. Acta Orthop Scand 1969; 40:642.

103. Evanski PM, Waugh TR: Management of arthritis of the ankle: An alternative to arthrodesis. Clin Orthop 1977; 122:110.

104. Groth HE: Total ankle replacement with the Oregon Ankle–evaluation of 44 patients followed for 2–7 years. Orthop Trans 1983; 7:488.

105. Kofoed H: Cylindrical cemented ankle arthroplasty: A prospective series with long term follow-up. Foot Ankle 1995; 16:474.

106. Lachiewicz PF, Inglis AE, Ranawat CS: Total ankle replacement in rheumatoid arthritis. J Bone Joint Surg Am 1984; 66:340.

107. St. Newton E: Total ankle arthroplasty. J Bone Joint Surg Am 1982; 64:104.

108. Stauffer RN, Segal NM: Total ankle arthroplasty: Four years experience. Clin Orthop 1981; 160:217.

109. Stauffer RN: Total ankle replacement. Arch Surg 1977; 112:1105.

110. Samuelson KM, Freeman MA, Tuke MA: Development and evolution of ICLH ankle replacement. Foot Ankle 1982; 3:32.

111. Herberts P, Goldie IF, Korner L, et al: Endoprosthetic arthroplasty of ankle joint: A clinical and radiological follow-up. Acta Ortho Scand 1982; 53:683.

112. Dini AA, Bassett FH: Evaluation of the early results of Smith total ankle replacement. Clin Orthop 1980; 146:228.

113. Bolton-Maggs BG, Sudlow RA, Freeman MAR: Total ankle arthroplasty: A long-term review of the London Hospital experience. J Bone Joint Surg Br 1985; 67:785.

114. Buechel FF, Pappas MJ, Iorio LJ: New Jersey low contact stress total ankle replacement: Biomechanical rationale and review of 23 cementless cases. Foot Ankle 1988; 8:279.

115. Pyevich MT, Saltzman CL, Callaghan JJ, et al: Total ankle arthroplasty: A unique design. J Bone Joint Surg Am 1998; 80:1410.

116. Kofoed H: Biological fixation of ankle arthroplasty. Foot 1995; 5:27.

117. Takakura Y, Tanaka Y, Sugimoto K, et al: Ankle arthroplasty: A comparative study of cemented metal and uncemented ceramic prosthesis. Clin Orthop 1990; 252:209.

118. Lin SS, Drazala MR, Eng K: Independent Evaluation of Buechel-Pappas Second Generation Cementless Total Ankle Arthroplasty. American Orthopaedic Foot and Ankle Society, Winter Meeting, New Orleans, LA, 1998.

RECOMMENDED READING

Aaron AD: Ankle fusion: A retrospective review. Orthopedics 1990; 13:1249.

Abdo R, Wasilewski S: Ankle arthrodesis: A long term study. Foot Ankle 1992; 13:307.

Ala-Kokko L, Baldwin CT, Moskowitz RW: Single base mutation in type II procollagen gene (COL2A1) as a cause of primary osteoarthritis associated with a mild chondrodysplasia. Proc Natl Acad Sci U S A 1990; 87:6565.

Braly WG, Baker JK, Tullos HS: Arthrodesis of the ankle with lateral plating. Foot Ankle 1994; 15:649.

Cooper PS, Posteraro A, Nowak MD: Ankle arthrodesis: Compression generation and torsional stability of the cross and parallel screw techniques. American Orthopaedic Foot and Ankle Society 27th Annual Meeting, San Francisco, 1997.

Ferkel RD, Guhl JF, Buecker V, et al: Complication in ankle arthroscopy: Analysis of first 518 cases. Orthop Trans 1993; 16:726.

Flock TJ, Ishikawa S, Hecht PJ, et al: Heel anatomy for retrograde tibiocalcaneal roddings: A roentgenographic and anatomic analysis. Foot Ankle 1997; 18:233.

Fosang AJ, Last K, Neame PJ, et al: Neutrophil collagenase (MMP-8) cleaves at the aggrecanase site E373-A374 in the interglobular domain of cartilage aggrecan. Biochem J 1994; 304:347.

Friedman RL, Glisson RR, Nunley JA: A biomechanical comparative analysis of two techniques for tibiotalar arthrodesis. Foot Ankle 1994; 15:301.

Guhl JF: Traumatic and degenerative arthritis. In Guhl JF (ed): Ankle Arthroscopy: Pathological and Surgical Technique. Thorofare, NJ, SLACK, 1988:122.

Harper MC: Malunited ankle fracture realignment. In Johnson KA (ed): The Foot and Ankle. New York: Raven Press, 1994, p 451.

Holderbaum D, Malamud CJ, Moskowitz RW: Human cartilage from late stage familial osteoarthritis transcribes type II collagen mRNA encoding a cysteine in position 519. Biochem Biophys Res Commun 1993; 192:1169.

Hulth A: Does osteoarthrosis depend on growth of the mineralized layer of cartilage? Clin Orthop 1993, 287:19.

Jimenez SA, Dharmavaram RM: Genetic aspects of osteoarthritis. Ann Rheum Dis 1994; 53:789.

Kleiger B: Anterior tibiotalar impingement syndrome in dancers. Foot Ankle 1992; 3:69.

Kuettner KE: Biochemistry of articular cartilage in health and disease. Clin Biochem 1992; 25:155.

Lohmander LS, Hoerrner LA, Dahlberg L, et al: Stromelysin, tissue inhibitor of metalloproteinases and proteoglycan fragments in human knee joint fluid after injury. J Rheumatol 1993; 20:1362.

Lohmander LS, Neamy PJ, Sandy JD: The structures of aggrecan fragments in human synovial fluid. Arthritis Rheum 1993; 36:1214.

Lohmander LS, Saxne T, Heinegard DK: Release of cartilage oligomeric matrix protein (COMP) into joint fluid after knee injury and in osteoarthritis. Ann Rheum Dis 1994; 53:8.

Moore TJ, Prince R, Pochatko D, et al: Retrograde intramedullary nail for ankle arthrodesis. Foot Ankle 1995; 16:433.

Pelletier JP, Faure MP, DiBattista JA, et al: Coordinate synthesis of stromelysin, interleukin-1 and oncogene proteins in experimental osteoarthritis: An immunohistochemical study. Am J Pathol 1993; 142:95.

Rolfe B, Nordt W, Sallis JG, et al: Assessing fibular length using bimalleolar angular measurements. Foot Ankle 1989; 10:104.

Salter RB, Simmonds DF, Malcolm BW, et al: The biological effects of continuous passive motion on the healing of full thickness defects in articular cartilage: An experimental investigation in the rabbit. J Bone Joint Surg Am 1980; 62:1232.

Salter RB, Field P: The effects of continuous compression on living articular cartilage: An experimental investigation. J Bone Joint Surg Am 1960; 42:31.

Sandy JD, Flannery CR, Neame PJ, et al: The structure of aggrecan fragment in human synovial fluid; evidence for the involvement in osteoarthritis of novel proteinase which cleave the Glu 373-ala 374 bond of interglobular domains. J Clin Invest 1992; 89:1512.

Sarkisian JS, Cody GW: Closed treatment of ankle fractures: New criterion for evaluation. A review of 250 cases. J Trauma 1976; 16:323.

Schneider D: Arthroscopic ankle fusion. Arthroscopic Video J, 1983.

Thordarson DB: Ankle fusion with internal fixation. Tech Orthop 1993; 8:44.

TENDINOPATHIES OF THE FOOT AND ANKLE

Scott T. McMullen and Timothy C. Fitzgibbons

Summary
- Tendinopathies of the foot and ankle affect a wide range of patient profiles, ranging from young athletic individuals to older patients with more sedentary lifestyles.
- The most likely cause, mechanical overload of the soft-tissue regions, has a significant role in the development of these painful syndromes. Single traumatic events contribute along with more long-standing repetitive forces.
- Treatment options focus on limitation of the involved mechanical overload as well as potential correction of structural/anatomic abnormalities.

DEFINITION

Tendinopathies of the foot and ankle are painful conditions related to soft-tissue inflammation of peritendinous structures, focal tendon degeneration and dysfunction, and acute tendon injuries, including dislocation, fissuring, partial tears, and complete ruptures. The primary areas of clinical concern focused on in this chapter are the Achilles tendon and the peroneal tendon complex. Also discussed are disorders involving the anterior tibial tendon and flexor hallucis longus (FHL) tendon. The posterior tibial tendon may have significant involvement; however, this is covered in more detail in Chapter 11–7.

EPIDEMIOLOGY

Tendinopathies of the foot and ankle occur in a wide patient population base, ranging from young athletic individuals to older, more sedentary patients who experience peritendinous inflammation and frank tendon degeneration. Historically, Achilles tendon ruptures are the third most frequent major tendon disruption.[1] In the past, the peroneal tendon complex has had little focus. Over time it has been investigated further and is now a more widely accepted

cause of lateral ankle pain. Pathology involving the FHL tendon may occur in patients involved in rigorous dance activities.

PATHOGENESIS

Tendinopathies of the foot and ankle are believed to occur as a result of functional and mechanical overload. Inflammatory changes may develop within the tissues and frank degeneration may also occur; however, the likely cause is multifactorial. Rupture of the tendon substance may also occur with traumatic events, including both rupture of normal tendon substance as a result of severe mechanical overload and ruptured degenerative tendon substance with less forceful loading. Table 1 lists the involved tissues, and the descriptive terminology varies depending on the tissues involved.[2]

Very little scientific information directly correlates a specific activity, its duration, and the development of tendinopathy. Lysholm and Wiklander[3] described a direct relationship occurring in runners. Intrinsic factors such as structural malalignment, systemic inflammatory conditions, muscle imbalance, and extrinsic factors of mechanical overload may play a role.

PERONEAL TENDON PROBLEMS

DEFINITION

Disorders involving the peroneal tendon complex may lead to lateral ankle pain, swelling, and limited function. Diagnostic potentials are listed in Table 2. When dealing with lateral ankle pain, one should have a high index of suspicion regarding the peroneal tendon complex as a potential source of the symptoms.

PATHOGENESIS
Anatomy
The peroneus longus (p. longus) and peroneus brevis (p. brevis) muscles compose the lateral compartment of the leg

TABLE 1. TENDON PATHOLOGY	
Terminology	**Tissue Involvement**
Tenosynovitis, peritendinitis, peritenonitis	Tendon sheath: peritenon, mesotenon, and epitenon
Tendinitis	Tendon/endotenon
Tendinosis	Tendon/endotenon, tendon insertion

Adapted from Almekinders LC: Tendinitis and other chronic tendinopathies. J Am Acad Orthop Surg 1998; 6:57.

TABLE 2. DEVELOPMENT OF TENDON PATHOLOGY
Intrinsic factors
Structural malalignment
Motor/muscle abnormality
Tendon degeneration
Systemic inflammatory condition
Extrinsic factors
Mechanical overload
Single event
Repetitive event
Duration
Frequency

and originate proximally, with innervation being the superficial peroneal nerve. The tendinous structures begin in the middle aspect of the leg and course distally with the p. brevis anterior to the p. longus (Fig. 1). A common synovial sheath begins several centimeters proximal to the tip of the lateral malleolus. The tendons then travel through a fibro-osseous tunnel composed of the superior peroneal retinaculum, the posterior talofibular ligament, the calcaneal fibular ligament, the posteroinferior tibial-fibular ligament, and the retromalleolar sulcus of the distal fibula. The retromalleolar sulcus may have depths ranging from negligible to approximately 3 mm.[4] The superior peroneal retinaculum originates from the periosteum of the posterior-lateral aspect of the distal fibula, closely associated with a small rim of tissue resembling fibrocartilage. The quality of retinacular tissue ranges from a very thin covering to a tough fibrous band.[5] Davis et al[6] described five distinctly different insertional variations of the superior peroneal retinaculum. Distal to the superior peroneal retinaculum, the tendons travel in separate synovial sheaths. The inferior peroneal retinaculum originates approximately 2 to 3 cm distal to the tip of the fibula and may be continuous with the inferior extensor retinaculum of the foot. The p. brevis inserts onto the tuberosity of the base of the fifth metatarsal. The p. longus emerges from its sheath to enter the cuboid tunnel created by the cuboid groove and long plantar ligament and enters a second synovial sheath before it terminates on the plantar lateral aspect of the base of the first metatarsal and medial cuneiform.

Anatomic variations may contribute to pathological entities. Distal extension of the p. brevis muscle belly beyond the common synovial sheath may contribute to a stenosis and tenosynovial inflammation. The peroneus quartus muscle may be present in up to 22% of patients. Its origin is a variant in the lateral compartment; the peroneal tubercle is the typical insertion.[7] The round or oval accessory bone located within the p. longus tendon is known as the os peroneum. It may be present in up to 20% of individuals, with a slightly higher frequency in males than females.[8] The os peroneum may be single, bipartite, or multipartite.

Biomechanics

The peroneal tendons exert a plantar flexion and eversion force. However, the component of total plantar flexion force is minimal compared with the gastroc-soleus complex. Their main function as everters of the hindfoot is more significant in terms of overall work provided. This function helps to balance those forces of the posteromedial flexor tendon complex.[9] The p. longus is also an important plantar flexor of the first ray and is a key component in creation of deformities with neuromuscular imbalance. The vascular supply of the peroneal tendons arises from two posterolateral vincula, one for the p. longus and one for the p. brevis, originating from the posterior peroneal artery. No zone of hypovascularity has been found.[10]

CLINICAL FEATURES

Pathology of the peroneal tendons may range from tenosynovial inflammation to frank tendon fissuring, degeneration, and rupture. This may be related to repetitive activities under normal anatomic situations; however, variations may

predispose to the development of disorders as listed in Table 3.

Patients with peroneal tendon disorders describe pain on the posterior lateral ankle with radiation into the lateral hindfoot/midfoot and distal leg areas. Swelling and pronounced tenosynovial inflammation may be present. Palpation may also reveal localized warmth. Palpation should begin several centimeters proximal to the tip of the distal fibula and proceed along the course of the peroneal tendon complex, noting areas of maximal tenderness. Palpation should continue distally to both the insertion of the p. brevis as well as through the cuboid groove and on to the plantar surface of the midfoot. Pain may be aggravated by passive/active inversion and plantar flexion or eversion and dorsiflexion. Decreased eversion strength may also be present in severe cases or if rupture has occurred; however, this is a less reliable finding.

With ongoing tenosynovial inflammation, tendon degeneration, fissuring, and rupture may occur. Acute traumatic ruptures of relatively normal tendon substance have been reported but are extremely uncommon.[11] The most common degeneration involves the p. brevis, which is trapped under the p. longus in the retromalleolar sulcus. This process may be further exacerbated by instability of the superior peroneal retinaculum. Fissuring of the p. longus tendon is less common and, when present, typically occurs more distally in the region of the peroneal tubercle or cuboid groove. Patients with peroneal tendinopathies may complain of a sense of giving way of the lateral ankle area consistent with functional instability with or without mechanical ankle instability. They may also experience a sense of catching in the posterolateral ankle and hindfoot area.

Examination of the Ankle

Structures should be evaluated in both standing and nonstanding positions. In addition to inspection and palpation, motion, strength, and mechanical instability should be evaluated. The use of a small amount of lidocaine (Xylocaine, 1%) may be very helpful. A decrease in pain with intra-sheath injection further confirms the diagnosis of pain localized to the peroneal tendon complex.

INVESTIGATION

Plain radiographs should be obtained as the initial screening tool. Anteroposterior (AP), lateral, and mortise radiographs of the ankle, standing if possible, may reveal osseous abnormalities (fracture, lesion, arthrosis) and soft-tissue swelling. Standing AP and oblique radiographs of the foot may be helpful because both peroneal tendons terminate within the midfoot. A calcaneal view is helpful when dealing with a history of hindfoot trauma. One should look for

TABLE 3. PREDISPOSING FACTORS
Anterolateral ankle instability
Varus hindfoot
Valgus hindfoot with subfibular impingement
Calcaneus fracture with subfibular impingement
Anomalous distal peroneus brevis muscle belly
Peroneus quartus muscle

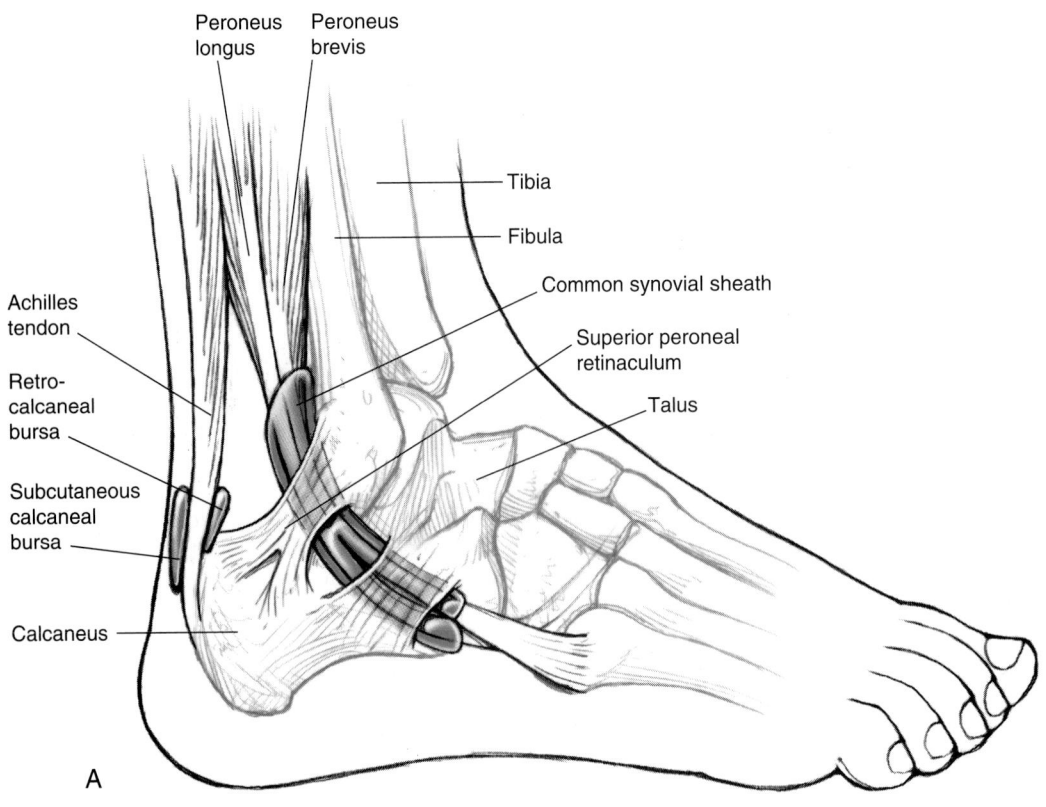

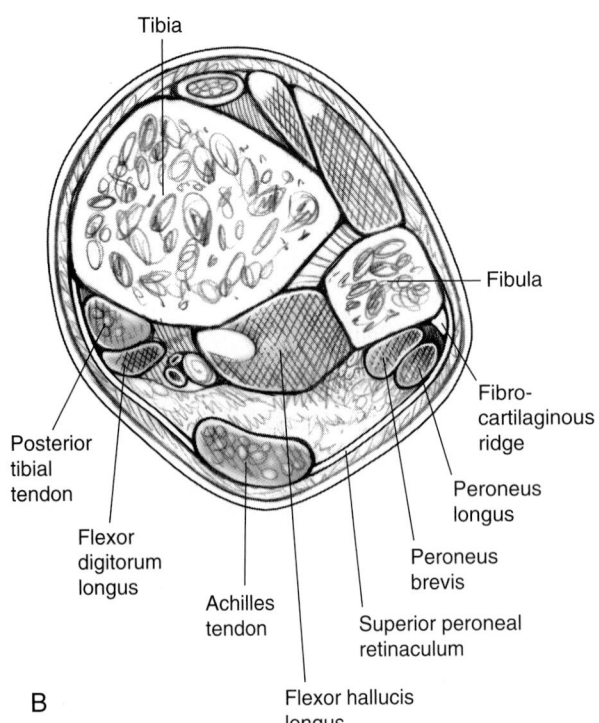

Fig. 1. Tendon anatomy. *A,* Lateral ankle. *B,* Cross-sectional anatomy.

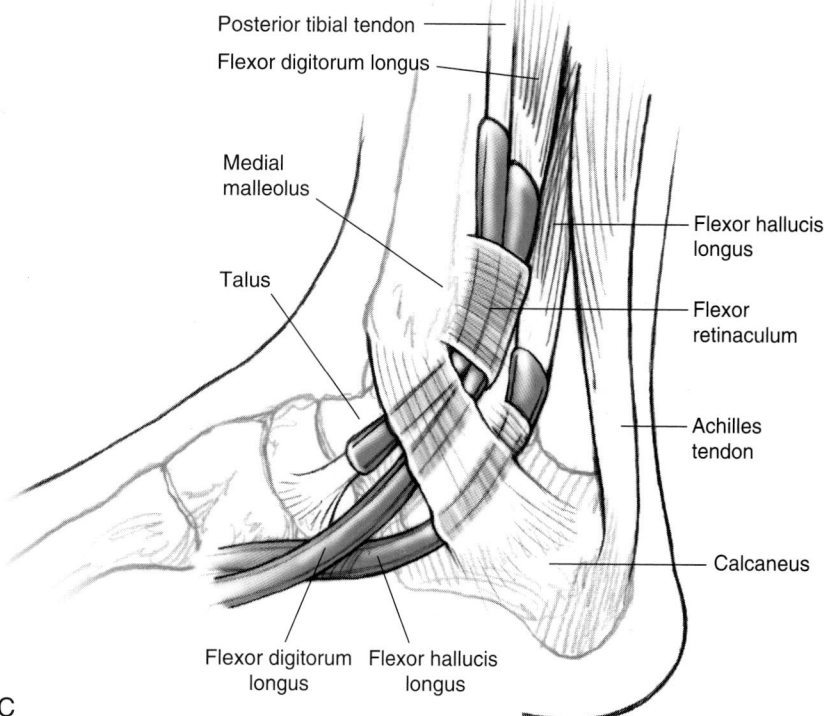

Fig. 1. *C*, Medial ankle.

C

an os peroneum in the region of the cuboid groove. Proximal migration or separation of a multipartite os indicates disruption of the p. longus tendon. New bone formation about the os may indicate recent trauma.[8] A small rim avulsion fracture from the posterolateral distal fibular surface can be seen with osseous disruption of the superior peroneal retinaculum, which is discussed later.

With a detailed physical examination, plain radiographs, and a high index of suspicion, disorders of the peroneal complex can be diagnosed. In diagnostic dilemmas, more sophisticated studies can be helpful. Options include peroneal tenography, ultrasonography, computed tomography (CT), and magnetic resonance imaging (MRI). Peroneal tenography allows for the visualization of structures within the peroneal tendon sheath; however, it is invasive, and with the advent of noninvasive MRI, its role is becoming more limited. Ultrasonography may reveal changes of tendon thickening and rupture. However, this may be highly variable depending on the skill of the ultrasonographer, and its overall role remains limited at this time. CT scanning shows excellent osseous detail, and soft-tissue windows may assist in the diagnosis of tenosynovial inflammation and complete tendon rupturing. However, partial tendon injuries may be elusive with this imaging modality.

MRI offers excellent soft-tissue visualization of both extratendinous and intratendinous material, although false-negative scans still occur. Variations of the magnetic field may be used to augment visualization. Khoury et al[12] nicely correlated MRI and surgical findings. Their most common MRI finding was a linear or round area of increased signal intensity in the tendon substance on the axial T_1- and T_2-weighted images. Longitudinal areas of intratendinous hyperintensity were seen on sagittal images.

Contrast between low and high signal intensities is well shown on T_1-weighted images. The T_2-weighted images depict abnormal fluid associated with pathological processes. In Khoury's study, increased signal intensity of peroneal tendon disorder was observed both on T_1- and T_2-weighted images. It was brighter on T_1-weighted images, and T_2-weighted images readily depicted the increased signal intensity in all patients.

DIFFERENTIAL DIAGNOSES

The differential diagnoses of peroneal tendon problems are listed in Table 4. The patient history should include information regarding the exact location, frequency, intensity,

TABLE 4. DIFFERENTIAL DIAGNOSES OF PERONEAL TENDON PATHOLOGY

Peroneal tendinopathy
  Tenosynovitis
  Tendon degeneration
  Tendon rupture
Peroneal tendon instability
True ankle joint pathology
  Synovitis and impingement
  Osteochondritis dissecans
Fracture
  Distal fibula
  Lateral talar process
  Anterior process of calcaneus
  Base of fifth metatarsal
  Calcaneal fracture with lateral wall displacement
Anterior lateral ankle instability
Tumor

and duration of the painful symptoms; distant or recent trauma; findings of swelling; and any successful or unsuccessful treatment attempt. The examination should focus on the distal leg, ankle, and foot area, looking for point tenderness, swelling and warmth, instability (peroneal tendon, ankle joint), and structural deformity.

MANAGEMENT

The mainstay of treatment of peroneal tendon disorders is nonoperative. Limitation of mechanical stresses plays a significant role. The use of anti-inflammatory medication may aid in the control of pain and swelling. For mild cases with a neutral or slightly varus hindfoot, a heel lateral wedge is used. Symptoms associated with subfibular impingement and a valgus hindfoot may benefit from medial support and posting. For moderate cases, protection is obtained with a laced ankle stabilizing orthosis. For more severe cases, a removable walking boot or true walking cast is used. During active treatment, weightbearing activities should be limited as pain dictates. Each option should be tried for a minimum of 3 to 4 weeks before considering it a success or failure.

With tenosynovial inflammation, the very limited use of a small amount, 0.25 to 0.5 mL, of a soluble corticosteroid agent may be considered. However, care should be taken to avoid intratendinous injection, and repeated injections should not be performed.

Ongoing symptoms may require surgical intervention.

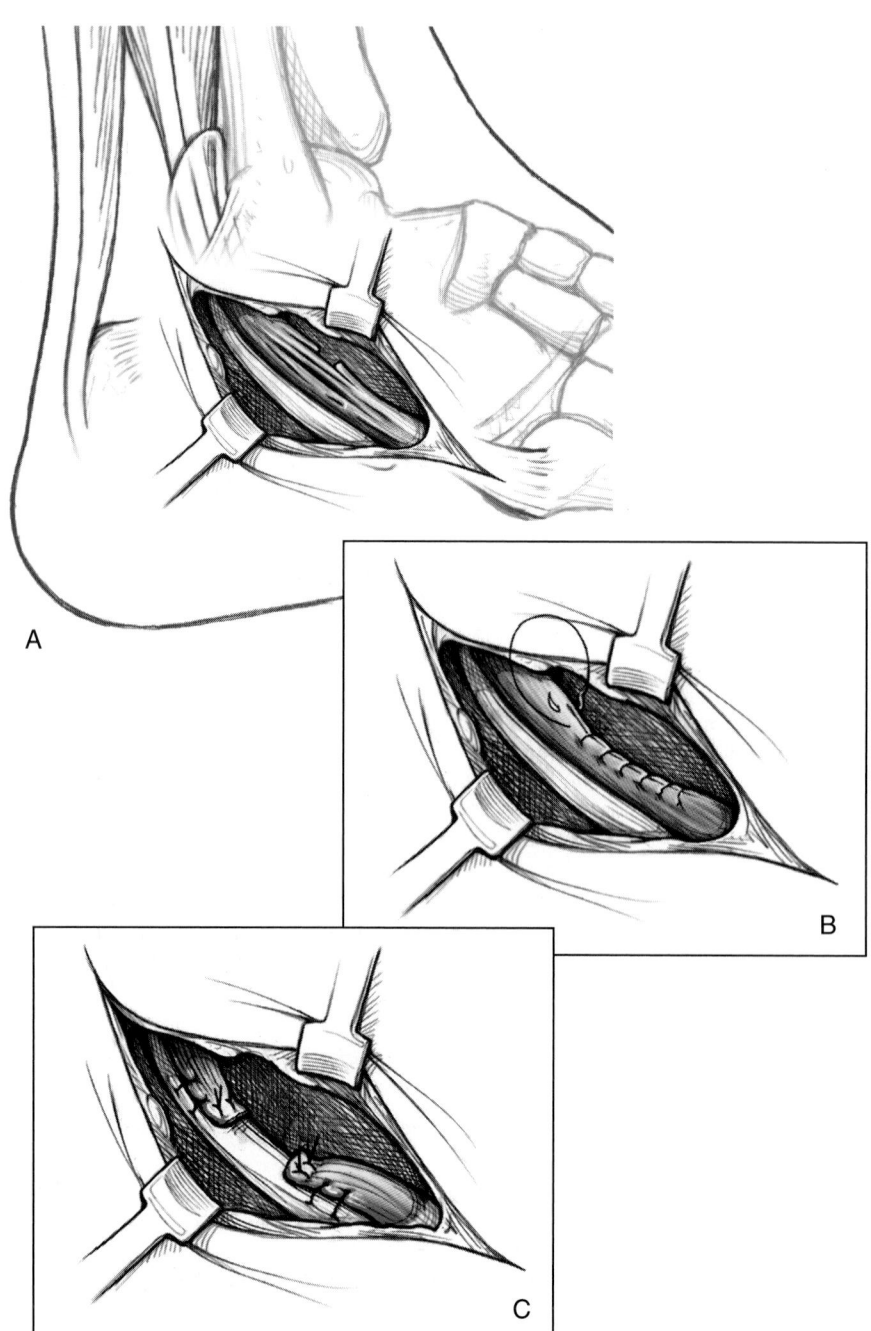

Fig. 2. Peroneal tendon disorders. *A*, Degeneration and fissuring of peroneus brevis. *B*, Tubularization of peroneus brevis after débridement. *C*, Tenodesis of peroneus brevis to peroneus longus after resection.

The surgical plan should include options for correcting all disorders encountered. The incision is planned to cover the area of tendon disorder and may begin several centimeters proximal to the tip of the lateral malleolus and extend as far distal as the cuboid groove and even onto the plantar aspect of the midfoot. Limited subcutaneous flaps are developed; care is taken to protect the sural nerve and its branches in the posterior flap. The integrity of the superior peroneal retinaculum should be directly inspected. The ankle is put through a range of motion to investigate for gross or subtle incompetency. The tenosynovial sheaths are opened, including the retinacular structures if needed. Tenosynovial inflammation is excised, and the tendon should be inspected thoroughly on all aspects for signs of degeneration and fissuring. Areas of abnormal tendon appearance should be débrided sharply. Grading is based on the amount of cross-sectional area involved: grade I, less than 50%; grade II, greater than 50%.[13] After débridement of grade I lesions, the tendon is tubularized in running fashion with a small absorbable suture. Grade II lesions require complete tendon débridement and tenodesis proximally and distally with an 0-0 nonabsorbable or slowly absorbing suture. Care is taken to create a smooth margin in a location proximal or distal to the fibular groove and superior peroneal retinaculum to prevent impingement (Fig. 2).

A symptomatic os peroneum may be excised as indicated with repair of the residual p. longus tendon or with complete débridement of the tendon and tenodesis to the p. brevis. With chronic peroneal tendon degeneration and complete disruption, additional options include tenodesis to the lateral calcaneus or reconstruction with a tendon graft such as the plantaris or FHL.

The retinacular structures should be carefully repaired and reconstructed as needed. Wound closure is performed in a layered fashion, and postoperative immobilization is performed using a non-weightbearing short-leg splint for approximately 10 to 14 days. After this, activities and immobilization depend on the extent of surgical intervention. With tenosynovectomy, a laced splint or immobilization in a removable walking boot for approximately 2 to 4 weeks is used. With tendon reconstruction or superior peroneal retinacular reconstruction, immobilization in a removable walking boot is continued for a minimum of 4 weeks, with initiation of early gentle passive range of motion exercises to avoid scar formation.

COMPLICATIONS/PITFALLS

With loss of peroneal function, imbalance may arise with overpull of the posterior medial flexor tendon complex, creating structural deformity. Surgical complications include infection, soft-tissue healing problems, traumatic injury to the sural nerve and its branches, iatrogenic tendon injury, and inadequate reconstruction of the superior peroneal retinaculum. Complications are minimized with strict attention to surgical detail, particularly to reconstruction of the superior peroneal retinaculum.

RESULTS

With a high index of suspicion of peroneal tendon disorder, successful results can be achieved. Basset and Speer[14] monitored eight athletes for an average of 7.9 years after débridement of p. longus tendon injuries; ankles became

asymptomatic and patients returned to full activity. Krause and Brodsky[13] reported on 20 patients who underwent surgical reconstruction. Their patients reported that, on average, 79% of their preoperative pain was relieved by surgery. The average American Orthopaedic Foot and Ankle Society ankle hindfoot score overall was 85; similar results were noted when comparing tenodesis versus tendon repair. A slightly higher functional level was seen in nonworkers' compensation patients versus workers' compensation patients.

PERONEAL TENDON INSTABILITY

DEFINITION

Instability of the peroneal tendon complex occurs when the peroneal tendons are no longer securely restrained in their retromalleolus sulcus and fibro-osseous tunnel. Instability of the peroneal tendon complex as a result of dysfunction or injury of the superior peroneal retinaculum can be an illusive diagnosis and a cause of ongoing lateral ankle pain. Peroneal tendon instability may occur as a result of a single forceful traumatic event; however, contributing factors such as anterolateral ankle instability or congenital variations such as a shallow retrofibular sulcus may lead to instability on a more chronic basis.[15]

PATHOGENESIS
Anatomy

The superior peroneal retinaculum anatomy (see Fig. 1) was previously described. Acute injury occurs when there is maximum tension on the peroneal complex. A sudden dorsiflexion stress with reflex contraction may be the most common cause; however, plantar flexion with eversion or inversion stresses may also play a role.[15] Skiers may be prone to this injury as the tip of the ski digs into the snow, creating an unexpected dorsiflexion moment across the ankle.[5, 15] A more chronic condition may arise when anterolateral ligament instability leads to fissuring of the p. brevis by the longus tendon, causing the brevis to splay over the posterolateral fibular ridge under a lax superior peroneal retinaculum.[16] Surgical cases reveal the superior peroneal retinaculum elevated from the lateral surface of the fibula, usually with the periosteum included as the superior peroneal retinacular fibers blend with the periosteum and not the fibrocartilagenous rim.[5] In none of the cases reported was the retinacular tissue actually torn. Initially, three grades were described, with grade I injuries being unstable only under tension and grade II and grade III injuries being very unstable.[5] A fourth type includes avulsion of the superior peroneal retinaculum from the posterior insertion on the calcaneus with anterior displacement of the tendons[5, 17] (Fig. 3).

CLINICAL FEATURES

Acute disruption of the superior peroneal retinaculum creates lateral ankle pain and swelling. The patient may experience a sense of popping over the distal fibula. Within the first several hours, swelling may be localized to the posterolateral ankle region, but with time the entire lateral ankle becomes swollen, potentially obscuring the diagnosis.[5] Palpation elicits tenderness at the superior peroneal retinaculum. Dorsiflexion and active eversion may create

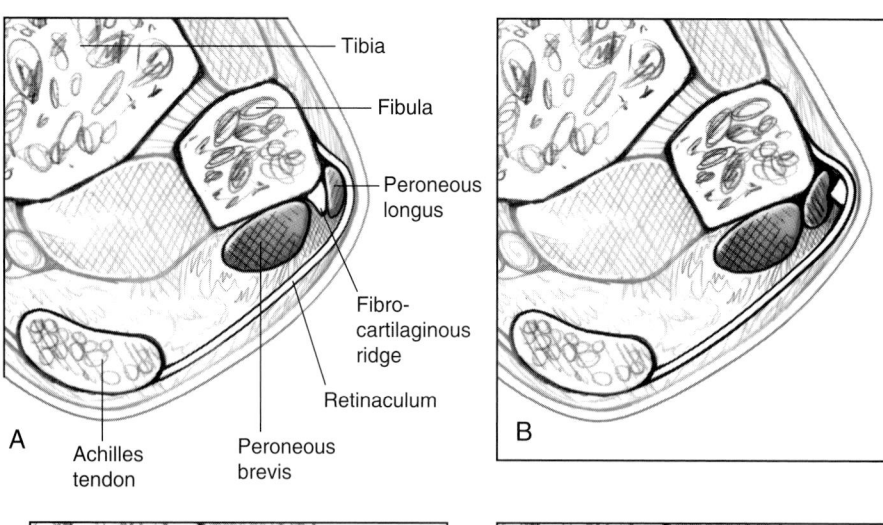

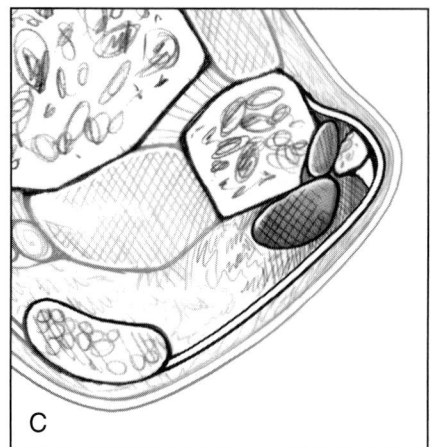

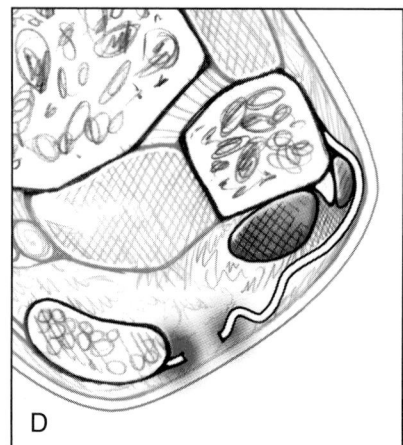

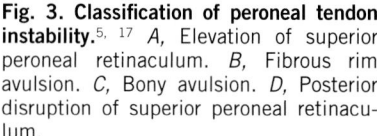

Fig. 3. Classification of peroneal tendon instability.[5, 17] *A*, Elevation of superior peroneal retinaculum. *B*, Fibrous rim avulsion. *C*, Bony avulsion. *D*, Posterior disruption of superior peroneal retinaculum.

discomfort. Subluxation may also be noted. In the acute situation, this is difficult to demonstrate because of local swelling and apprehension.[18]

Posterolateral ankle pain occurs with chronic tendon subluxation and may create posterolateral ankle pain and an associated sense of catching or snapping in this region. Anterolateral ankle pain may occur if there is associated ankle instability and impingement. With frequent turning of the ankle, patients may actually sense the tendon complex traveling over the posterolateral fibular ridge. Provocative testing includes active dorsiflexion/eversion. Plantar flexion/inversion may also reproduce symptoms of peroneal instability.

INVESTIGATION

Standing AP, lateral, and mortise radiographs may reveal a small rim avulsion fracture corresponding to a grade III injury. It may be best visualized on the mortise view.[19, 20] This finding may occur in 15% to 50% of cases. CT or MRI may be obtained when the specific diagnosis is in question; however, clinical findings are the mainstay of diagnosing this injury.

DIFFERENTIAL DIAGNOSES

The differential diagnoses of peroneal tendon complex instability correspond to those of true peroneal tendinopathy and were previously described (see Table 4).

MANAGEMENT

Nonoperative treatment includes immobilization in a well-molded plaster short-leg walking cast. However, surgical repair of the superior peroneal retinaculum remains the mainstay of treatment. The retinaculum may be reattached to the posterolateral surface of the fibula through drill holes or with a suture anchor. A small bony avulsion fragment may also be included in the repair, if present. Surgery is done in either a lateral or prone position; a curvilinear incision is centered over the superior peroneal retinaculum. Care is taken to protect the sural nerve and its branches. The retinaculum is reattached to the prepared surface of the distal fibula using an 0-0 nonabsorbable suture through drill holes or with suture anchor. The central aspect of the retinaculum should be repaired if open, and the skin is approximated in a layered fashion. The extremity is splinted in a short-leg stirrup splint with a footplate in a position of slight plantar flexion and eversion. Patients are non-weightbearing for 2 weeks and then move into either a short-leg walking cast or a removable walking boot for an additional 2 to 4 weeks. Activities are then increased initially in an ankle support. The support may be discontinued as symptoms allow.

In cases of chronic tendon instability, a period of immobilization may help to improve symptoms related to tenosynovial inflammation but will not allow for correction of the instability, and early recurrence of symptoms is expected. More than 20 surgical procedures have been described for treatment of chronic tendon instability.[15] The repairs are grouped into categories depending on tissues used: either bone or soft tissue. The goal of treatment is to correct a disorder without sacrificing normal anatomic structures if possible.

Reconstruction of the superior peroneal retinaculum may be possible as previously described for acute injury. This has the advantage of using the native soft-tissue structures without sacrificing uninvolved areas. If possible, this should be used. If retinacular tissues are significantly attenuated, direct repair and attachment are not possible. Additional soft-tissue augmentation may be needed. In 1932 Elis Jones[21] described a method using a thin strip of Achilles tendon, which is left attached distally and is brought through a drill hole in the distal fibula, reconstructing the retinacular structures. An alternative soft-tissue reconstruction includes rerouting under the calcaneal fibular ligament. Both of these augmentations involve the use of normal anatomic structures, and both have been shown to be clinically successful[13, 15] but do run the risk of causing difficulties with the donor tissue.

Bony procedures involve deepening the retrofibular sulcus or creation of a bone block. Groove-deepening procedures are performed when the retrofibular sulcus is believed to be contributing to the instability. A medially based cortical hinge flap may be elevated and fashioned with either an osteotome or saw with dimensions approximately 3 cm in length by 1 cm in width. Through this window, cancellous bone is removed. The cortical window is then hinged inward.[22] Deepening procedures removing the posterior cortex of the fibula may create sharp edges, leading to additional tendon disorder. Bone block procedures use sections of the distal fibula to impede dislocation of the peroneal tendon complex.[23] This sacrifices distal fibular anatomy and has potential for failure of union and internal fixation and does not directly correct the underlying soft-tissue disorder.

After surgical reconstruction, soft tissues are closed in a layered fashion. Postoperatively, patients are immobilized in a short-leg stirrup plaster splint with a footplate for approximately 2 weeks. Patients are then maintained in a short-leg fiberglass non-weightbearing cast until approximately 4 to 6 weeks postoperatively. Ambulation is then advanced in a removable walking boot and then a stabilizing ankle sleeve.

COMPLICATIONS

Peroneal tendon instability without accurate diagnosis and treatment will lead to ongoing tendon injury. Over time, this may lead to tendon fissuring and frank tendon rupture. Surgical complications include local wound healing problems, infection, and injury to the sural nerve and its branches. Insufficient reconstruction of the retinacular tissue may lead to ongoing instability. Bone block procedures may be complicated by nonunion and failure of internal fixation and tendon impingement. A groove-deepening procedure creating rough edges may lead to direct tendon wearing. Rerouting procedures into the calcaneal fibular ligament may lead to lateral ankle instability if the ligamentous structure is not reconstructed properly. Use of a split Achilles tendon transfer may be complicated by local symptoms within the Achilles tendon area and its insertion. When placing drill holes in the distal fibula, care must be taken to leave adequate bone bridge to prevent cortical fracture and incompetency of the reconstruction. With attention to detail, the complication rate is expected to be low.

RESULTS

Overall external results may be obtained with reconstruction of the restraining structures of the peroneal tendon complex. Although the redislocation rate is low, it has been reported. In the 73 patients whom Eckert and Davis[5] operated on and monitored for longer than 6 months, three experienced redislocation and underwent subsequent reconstruction with additional soft-tissue procedures. With a combination of soft-tissue reconstruction and a groove-deepening procedure, no dislocations have been reported.

ACHILLES TENDON PATHOLOGY

DEFINITION

The Achilles tendon is the most famous of all human tendons because of its description in ancient Greek mythology and the disability associated with its rupture. In modern days, with the increasing participation in recreational sports, the incidence of Achilles tendon disorders has increased. Although acute rupture can be a significant disabling and even career-ending injury, with the more modern surgical techniques and early mobilization, return to normal function has become more common. Perhaps the most difficult Achilles tendon problem facing today's orthopaedist is the treatment of the degenerative processes, especially distal Achilles tendon insertional pain.

PATHOGENESIS
Anatomy

The Achilles tendon is formed by the convergence of the gastrocnemius and soleus muscles. It is the strongest, largest, and thickest tendon in the human body. As the tendon traverses toward its attachment in the posterior calcaneus, the Achilles fibers spiral laterally approximately 90 degrees. The Achilles tendon does not have a true synovial sheath but rather a peritenon, which covers the tendon, allowing approximately 1.5 cm of tendon glide (see Fig. 1). A cross-section of the leg demonstrates the location of the Achilles tendon directly posteriorly. It also demonstrates the proximity of the Achilles tendon medially to the posterior tibial artery, vein, and posterior tibial nerve as well as to the flexor hallucis muscle and tendon, which is of clinical significance in surgical treatment, especially of chronic ruptures.[24–26]

A cross-section of the Achilles tendon itself reveals that the peritenon is divided into a parietal and visceral level, and mesotenon connects the outer parietal layer to the inner visceral layer and also is the site for vascular infiltration.

The insertion of the Achilles tendon is of clinical significance because of its importance in surgical procedures dealing with degenerative processes of the Achilles tendon. As noted, the tendon itself spirals laterally 90 degrees, becomes rounded and narrow above the calcaneus, but then broadens and inserts in a perpendicular fashion into the posterior calcaneus approximately 2 to 5 cm distal to the tip of the superior calcaneal tuberosity. In the end, the fibers associated with the gastrocnemius insert primarily laterally, whereas the soleus contribution inserts primarily medially. The posterior superior calcaneal tuberosity varies in its size and can contribute to pressure of the tendon against the posterior counter of the shoe. The bursae of the posterior heel include the retrocalcaneal bursa, which overlies the posterior superior tuberosity. It has been described as being horseshoe shaped and is consistently found between the anterior margin of the tendon and the posterior superior calcaneal process. A second bursa, which is a pretendon or adventitial bursa, lies between the Achilles tendon and the skin. This is the bursa that becomes inflamed in the so-called pump bump syndrome. A Haglund deformity is an excessively prominent posterosuperior calcaneal tuberosity and can contribute to the pump bump syndrome. Haglund's deformity and pump bump syndrome are used interchangeably.

The blood supply to the Achilles tendon comes from multiple sources.[27] The tendon itself receives its blood supply from muscular branches. Distal supply tends to be from the osseous and periosteal vessels near the insertion site. The blood supply to the tendon at its distal third is sparse and thus the cause of this being the most common site for tendon degeneration and rupture. The tendon also receives nourishment from the peritenon, which has blood supply as described previously.

Histology
The Achilles tendon has a histological appearance similar to that of other tendons in the body. The tendon consists of fascicles separated by thin films of endotenon. The tendon itself is composed of mature fibroblasts called tenocytes. These tenocytes are embedded in an extracellular matrix consisting of collagen, elastin, mucopolysaccharides, and glycoproteins. With age, there is a decrease in the diameter, density, and cellularity of the collagen fibrils.

Biomechanics
The biomechanics of the Achilles tendon are relatively straightforward in that the tendon is a musculotendinous complex that crosses the knee, ankle, and subtalar joints. Although its primary function is plantar flexion of the ankle, this complex also contributes to flexion of the knee and supination of the subtalar joint. The Achilles tendon complex also has a function in stabilization of the hindfoot in normal gait.[28]

Much has been written about the biomechanical properties of tendons and their response to immobilization and stress. Enwemeka and others[28, 29] showed that there is a benefit to early mobilization in terms of tendon healing and tendon regeneration. This is important in balancing the period of time the tendon is immobilized after surgical repair to when active tendon function is allowed. It appears clear that controlled tendon function is justified and helpful in the postoperative treatment of Achilles tendon ruptures.

INVESTIGATION
There is no substitute for a thorough history and physical examination of the patient. Whether the problem is an acute rupture or a progressive degeneration, patients' verbal description of symptoms is the most helpful piece of information in establishing a diagnosis. Physical examination also is extremely important, especially in localizing the problem and determining the effect of active and passive motion on the symptoms.

The role of the plain AP and lateral radiographs is limited in pure tendon injuries but can be of help in calcified and Achilles tendon attachment problems. The evaluation of the prominence of the posterosuperior calcaneal process is also important and aided by the plain radiograph. Historically, before the advent of CT and MRI, the xeroradiogram was believed to be helpful in assessing a tendon injury because of its emphasis on soft-tissue clarity. This, however, has become obsolete with newer imaging techniques.

The CT was initially helpful in allowing some assessment of soft tissues. The MRI and its superior ability to assess soft-tissue defects and degenerating processes has replaced the CT as a first-line imaging modality.

Tenography of the Achilles tendon has been used in diagnosis and treatment of Achilles tendon ruptures. Dye injection allows documentation of tendon apposition. Other than this, there is probably no other use for tenography.

The current role of ultrasonography remains uncertain. There is no question that it can be helpful in assessing not only tendon partial and complete rupture but also degenerative processes. However, with the increased anatomic definition achievable with MRI, the information from the MRI is probably more helpful.[30, 31] Although an argument can be made on cost effectiveness, most orthopaedists now tend to depend on the MRI as the primary imaging device for evaluation of Achilles tendon injuries.

Because of the extremely low water content of all tendons, they appear black on all MRI images regardless of whether a T_1- or T_2-weighted spin echo is used. Developments in MRI pulse sequence technology have optimized the contrast between dark tendon signals and abnormal increase in water content, which helps characterize most pathological processes.

Imaging the Achilles tendon is most commonly accomplished in a sagittal and axial plane. The axial plane allows the best assessment of the tendon morphology, including tendon thickness and absence of tendon signal. The sagittal plane is believed to give the best depiction of the full extent of the abnormality. At present, MRI appears to be the imaging technology of choice for Achilles tendinopathies, although most diagnoses can be made on the basis of a good history and a careful clinical examination.

DIFFERENTIAL DIAGNOSIS
The differential diagnosis and treatment of various Achilles tendon problems are summarized in Table 5. The tendinitis classification described by Puddu et al[32] and Almekinders[2] has been used.

Tendon inflammation and degeneration problems are those tendon problems that involve the Achilles tendon itself and not its attachment to the calcaneus. Achilles tendinitis is an inflammation of the peritenon. This is usually a more acute condition that occurs commonly in the running athlete. Patients typically present with localized swelling, warmth, and tenderness in the Achilles tendon itself.

TABLE 5. DIFFERENTIAL DIAGNOSIS AND TREATMENT: TENDINOPATHIES AND RUPTURES OF THE ACHILLES TENDON

Problem	Definition	Signs and Symptoms	Nonsurgical Treatment	Surgical Treatment
Tendon inflammation and degeneration	Pure tendinitis (inflammation of the peritenon)	Local tenderness, swelling and warmth with occasional crepitation	Rest, NSAIDs, physical therapy, 0.5-inch lift in shoe, walking boot with 0.5-inch lift	Saline distention injection Decompression peritenon Multiple small incisions
	Tendinosis (degeneration, thickening, microtearing, calcification)	Thickening and palpable nodules; pain with active plantar flexion; positive MRI	Same as above except longer	Excision of diseased portion of tendon; severe cases: FHL transfer or augmentation
	Combination of both			
Insertional pain	Haglund deformity (plump bump syndrome)	Swollen inflamed superficial bursa; prominent posterior/superior calcaneal tuberosity	NSAIDs, local treatment, 0.5-inch lift in shoe, pad or modify shoe counter	Aggressive posterosuperior calcaneal bone resection
	Retrocalcaneal bursitis	Pain squeezing anterior to tendon; seen usually in combination with attachment pain	Rest, NSAIDs, PT, 0.5-inch lift in shoe	Bone resection plus decompression of bursa
	Degenerative Achilles attachment pain	Pain at attachment; large inflamed soft-tissue mass	Rest, NSAIDs, PT, walking boot with 0.5-inch lift as long as 6 months	Aggressive bone resection plus tendon débridement through various surgical approaches; excise distal tendon and tendon transfer in severe cases
Tendon rupture	Preruptue (tendinitis)	Tendinitis symptoms	Rest, PT, NSAIDs, 0.5-inch lift	Occasionally tendinitis surgical options
	Complete or partial rupture	Inability to flex against gravity, positive Thompson test, positive defect	Long-leg cast in equinus 1 month, short-leg cast progressing to neutral and with progressive weightbearing for 2 months, walking boot with 0.5-inch lift 1 month, 0.5-inch lift in shoe 6 months	Primary repair, modified Kessler technique
	Chronic neglected rupture	± defect, ± Thompson test, difficulty with plantar flexion against gravity, hyperdorsiflexion	Walking boot with 0.5-inch lift for 6 months	Tendon advancement, tendon turn-down, tendon excision with FHL or FDL transfer

NSAID, nonsteroidal anti-inflammatory drugs; MRI, magnetic resonance imaging; FHL, flexor hallucis longus; PT, physical therapy; FDL, flexor digitorum longus.

True Achilles tendinitis tends to occur in the younger patient with less chance for degenerative changes. This occurs commonly after some type of increase in activity, such as increasing mileage in a long-distance runner.

Tendinosis is the disorder of the Achilles tendon in which there is some degeneration in the substance of the tendon itself. This tends to occur in older individuals and is commonly less activity-related. Patients complain of chronic pain and eventual thickening and occasional nodular formation in the tendon itself. This is believed to be due to degeneration in the substance of the tendon with occasional secondary calcification. Commonly, patients present with a combination of both tendinitis and tendinosis. This is believed to be an acute inflammation superimposed on a chronic degenerative process.

It is important to differentiate the tendinitis problems from the more chronic tendinosis problems. Length of recovery time is usually linked to the duration of symptoms. Acute cases tend to subside faster than chronic cases. Tendon rupture is also a differential diagnosis that must be ruled out in tendinitis cases.

Tendon attachment or insertional Achilles tendon problems with posterior heel symptoms tend to be among the most difficult problems facing orthopaedic surgeons. Many of these patients present with significant disabling symptoms and have had long periods of failed conservative treatment. Haglund deformity occurs simply as a result of a prominence at the posterosuperior calcaneal tuberosity with pressure on the posterior counter of the shoe. This problem is probably only seen in its pure sense in the young adolescent patient. Later in life, it is commonly associated with degenerative disorders of the Achilles tendon and retrocalcaneal bursitis. Retrocalcaneal bursitis is an inflammation of the bursa anterior to the Achilles tendon. Although this can present as a separate entity, it is commonly associated with a generalized degenerative posterior Achilles tendon insertional problem.

Patients with insertional pain not only have pain with pressure of the shoe against the thickened swollen Achilles tendon attachment but also have discomfort with function of the tendon depending on the amount of tendon degeneration present. In the younger patient with the more acute problem, passive dorsiflexion of the foot tends to increase the symptoms. Focal pressure on the tendon attachment causes symptoms. These patients do not always present with large, swollen deformities. More commonly, there is some swelling of the distal Achilles tendon and secondary calcification. These patients present with a thickened posterior hindfoot with difficulty with shoe wear. Pain with arising from bed or a sitting position is common with this condition.

Rupture of the Achilles tendon can be divided into three different types. The first type is the prerupture state. These patients present with symptoms of Achilles tendinitis, and, as described previously, are usually young athletes who have increased their level of activity (e.g., increasing mileage in their running habits). Symptoms of localized pain, tenderness, and pain in the Achilles tendon may be a prodrome to eventual rupture. Patients with acute rupture classically describe an event occurring during sporting activity. The symptoms can occur with a sudden planting of the foot and change of direction. The rupture commonly occurs with the activity of sudden plantar flexion. In any event, patients usually describe very acute pain with localization to the Achilles tendon. Commonly, they feel "like I've been shot" or kicked in the leg.

Physical examination reveals an inability to plantar flex against gravity. When the patients are placed prone on the table with their feet extending over the end of the table, a palpable defect is noted. The Thompson test involves squeezing the posterior calf and observing obligatory ankle plantar flexion. It is performed initially on the uninjured side and then compared with the injured side. A positive Thompson test occurs when squeezing the gastrocsoleus muscles fails to produce any plantarflexion of the foot.

Delayed or neglected ruptures occur in those patients in whom the initial diagnosis of a partial or complete rupture is missed and in patients with chronic degenerative changes and tendinosis of the tendon in which the rupture is gradual rupture. In this chapter, we consider a delayed rupture to be any rupture that is recognized 6 weeks or longer since the acute injury. These patients have more subtle symptoms. Some are able to walk quite well without a limp. However, when truly tested for the ability to stand on their toes against gravity, they have difficulty. The Thompson test may or may not be positive. Commonly, the patients have a notable hyperdorsiflexion ability on the affected side compared with the nonaffected side. This is, of course, due to the increased length of the tendon. A palpable defect may or may not be present.

The differential diagnosis in Achilles tendon rupture problems involves ruptured versus nonruptured conditions. Patients with acute Achilles tendinitis sometimes can be difficult to differentiate from those patients with a true rupture. Also, patients with an acute rupture of their plantaris tendon have symptoms similar to an Achilles tendon rupture. Physical examination reveals the tendon is intact and the pain, although initially in the medial aspect of the hindfoot, commonly then becomes more proximal in the area where the retracted plantaris tendon is present. The so-called musculotendinous injury can be similar to an Achilles tendon rupture. These patients have a similar clinical episode, yet their tendon appears to be intact clinically and their symptoms tend to be in the more proximal portion of

the calf. There is believed to be an actual musculotendinous injury or defect, and this is treated nonsurgically.

MANAGEMENT

Patients with tendinopathies and tendon insertional problems are initially given a thorough history and physical examination and undergo initial standing AP and lateral plain radiographs. Initial treatment includes thorough education about the problem and its chronicity, rest and avoidance of strenuous activities, nonsteroidal anti-inflammatory medication, and physical therapy. Physical therapy includes initial modality treatment followed by gradual stretching and strengthening exercises. Shoe modifications include the use of a 2-inch lift in an existing shoe. In patients with Haglund deformity, a pedorthist can split the posterior counter of the shoe and pad this for decompression of the inflamed superficial bursa. In more acute or severe cases, patients can be placed in a short-leg removable walking boot with a prebuilt 2-inch lift. This allows daily range of motion and prevents ankle stiffness, yet facilitates rest of the inflamed tendon. Although a short-leg cast can be considered, ankle stiffness can occur, and we have found the short-leg brace to be more acceptable. Weightbearing can be gradually allowed. In chronic tendinosis cases, patients can use these walking devices on a daily basis for as long as 6 months and lead relatively normal lives while the slow progress of healing occurs. Although commonly performed, injection in and around the tendon does promote degeneration, and this increases the chance of rupture. We recommend against injection for tendinitis and insertional tendon problems.

Initial treatment as described previously can be used for at least 6 weeks for tendinitis and at least 6 months for tendinosis and insertional problems. In failures of conservative treatment, further evaluation and treatment are warranted. At this point, an MRI of the tendon can be obtained. The purpose of the MRI is to look for signal changes within the tendon or its insertion site consistent with rupture or degeneration and to help with preoperative planning (Fig. 4).

Surgical treatment for Achilles tendinitis and Achilles tendon insertional problems has been well described and debated in the literature.[15, 33–42] The extent of the contributions to the literature demonstrates the complexity of the problem and the frustrations by orthopaedic surgeons in surgical treatment. In surgical treatment for pure tendinitis, the common surgical denominator seems to be decompression of the tendon. This can be accomplished by longitudinal release of the peritenon or with multiple, even percutaneous, transverse incisions in the peritenon. The goal in patients with pure tendinitis is decompression followed by rest and immobilization. In those patients with tendon degeneration, surgical options become more plentiful. Surgical exposure includes posteromedial incisions, posterolateral incisions, a combination of posteromedial and posterolateral incisions, central tendon splitting incisions, and posterior hockey stick incisions.

In patients with pure Haglund's deformity, aggressive resection of the posterosuperior calcaneal tuberosity is all that is necessary and can usually be performed through a posteromedial or posterolateral incision, or both. In most cases, however, this syndrome does not occur without

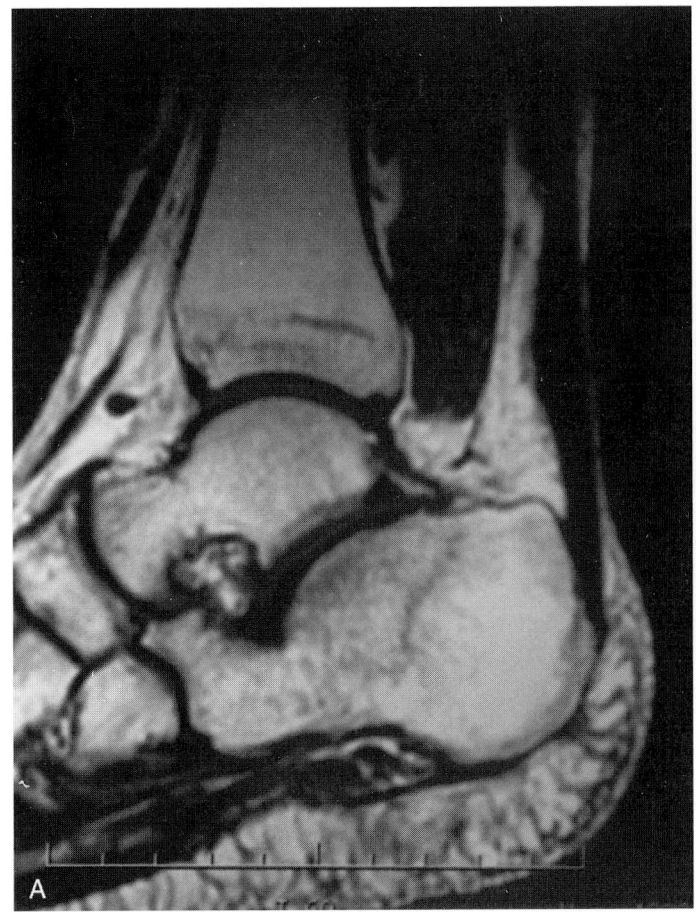

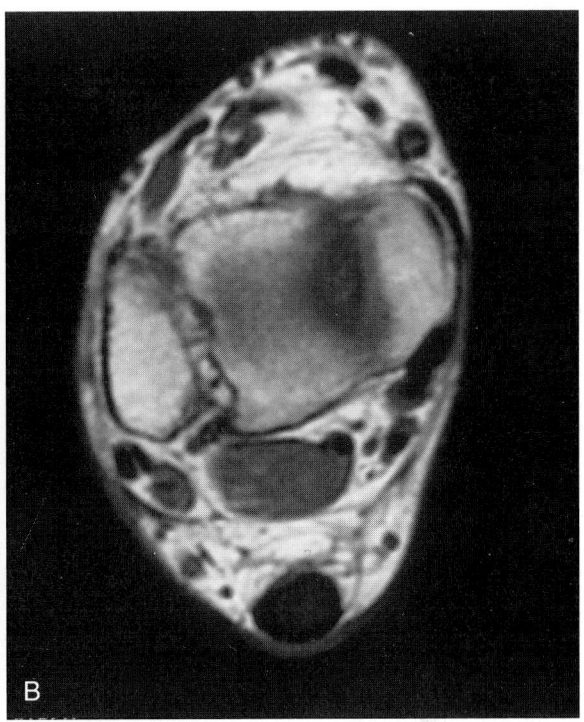

Fig. 4. Chronic degenerative tendinosis. *A*, Sagittal view of thickened enlarged tendon. *B*, Magnetic resonance image, coronal view, of patient with chronic degenerative Achilles tendinosis.

Achilles tendon involvement; therefore, some form of tendon débridement is usually necessary. Common to all surgical approaches appears to be aggressive bone resection followed by tendon débridement with or without excision.

The importance of aggressive bone resection in any Achilles tendon insertional problem has been well described by Jones and James.[37] Less aggressive bone resections, even in minor cases of pump bump syndrome in adolescents, prove to be unsuccessful. Keck and Kelly[43] described calcaneal osteotomy as another alternative in patients with large posterior/superior tuberosity. Tendon débridement can be performed through a variety of techniques depending on the severity of the disease process. Clain and Baxter[44] recommended a central tendon splitting incision with or without partial detachment of the tendon. Sammarco and Taylor[33] also recommended this procedure. Medial, lateral, and direct posterior incisions also have been demonstrated to accomplish the desired effect. A portion of the tendon that is degenerated should be longitudinally divided and excised. If necessary, tendon detachment should be performed. If more than one-third of the tendon is detached, at a minimum the tendon should be reattached, usually using suture anchors. Again, we recommend aggressive bone resection in combination with aggressive tendon débridement, or a satisfactory result will not occur.

The real controversy occurs in those patients with severe degenerative-type Achilles tendon insertional problems. In our experience, many of these patients, even with aggressive bone resection and tendon débridement, simply do not do well. Débriding and repairing an already degenerative tendon raises the question as to whether this is adequate treatment. The patients' continued pain postoperatively may be related to the persistent existence of the degenerated tendon. For that reason, more aggressive treatment, which includes complete detachment of the Achilles tendon, excision of the degenerated distal portion of the tendon, and aggressive bone resection, has been performed. This is followed by transfer of the flexor hallucis tendon, as described by Wapner et al[45] for chronic ruptures. Early reports suggest that this procedure may provide more reliable improvement to the problem of diffuse degenerative insertional Achilles tendinosis.

Postoperative treatment includes immobilization for the period of time considered necessary for the particular procedure performed. Most patients are placed in a short-leg compressive dressing with plaster splints initially. At 7 to 10 days, this is converted to a short-leg fiberglass nonweightbearing cast. In patients with FHL tendon transfers, this is kept on for at least 1 month followed by a series of cast changes, bringing the foot to neutral to allow ambulation. The patient eventually progresses to a removable walking boot with a prebuilt 2-inch lift. At 3 to 4 months, this is then converted to a shoe with a 2-inch lift for at least 6 months. For those patients with less aggressive tendon débridements, immobilization in a splint for 7 to 10 days followed by a removable walking boot is probably adequate.

Management of the patient with Achilles tendon ruptures can be more straightforward. A thorough history and physical examination is most important, but in our practice many patients undergo MRI evaluation (Fig. 5). In patients with a pre- or partial rupture, nonsurgical treatment can be used with immobilization in either a removable walking boot, as noted previously, or perhaps a short-term short-leg fiberglass cast. Patients with complete or partial ruptures are given the option of surgical versus nonsurgical treatment.[46] In our practice, nonsurgical treatment includes 4 weeks in a long-leg cast with the foot in equinus nonweightbearing, 4 weeks in a short-leg cast with the foot in less equinus with no or partial weightbearing, and finally 4 weeks in a short-leg walking cast. This is followed by a period of time in a removable walking boot with a 2-inch lift and eventually a shoe with a 2-inch lift. Patients are given information on re-rupture risk and potential strength deficits and are at least given the option of nonsurgical treatment.

Most patients with any level of recreational or work-related activities undergo surgical exploration and repair.[47, 48] Surgical morbidity in most patients is minor, although wound healing can be a problem. With meticulous handling of the soft tissues, primary wound healing usually occurs. Surgical exploration is performed through a posteromedial or a posterolateral incision. Primary repair using a modified Kessler technique with a nonabsorbable suture is performed. The "fanned" plantaris tendon to promote a serosal layer over the suture repair is used when possible.

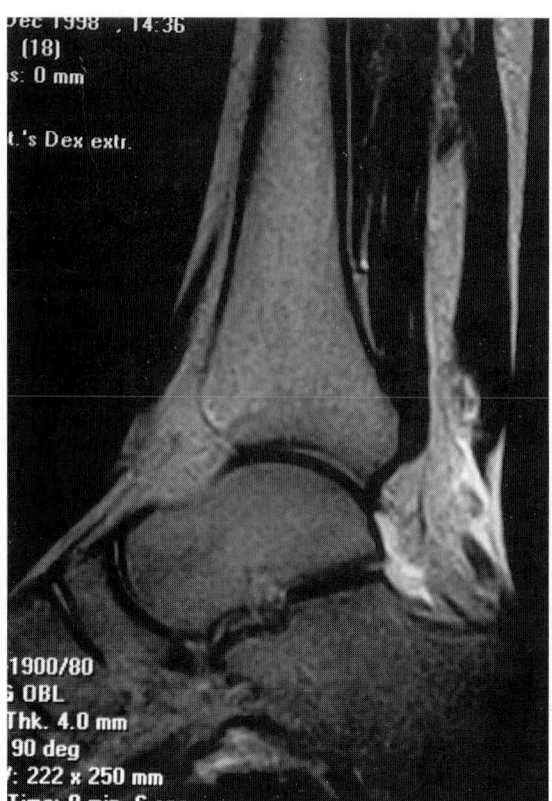

Fig. 5. Complete rupture of Achilles tendon. The sagittal view of a magnetic resonance image is shown.

Patients are immobilized with the foot in moderate equinus in a short-leg fiberglass cast for 1 month followed by progressive cast change, bringing the foot to neutral position and progressive weightbearing. Weightbearing is started as soon as possible depending on the quality of the repair. Studies, as noted previously, showed that early weightbearing can promote tendon strength and healing. A removable walking boot with a 2-inch lift can be used as early as 4 to 6 weeks depending on repair. A shoe with a 2-inch lift is used for 3 to 6 months after this.

In chronic or neglected ruptures, primary repair is used when possible but not at the expense of long periods of maximum equinus of the foot. V-Y advancement of the musculotendinous complex or turn-down procedures have been used.[49] Recently, however, we used Wapner et al's[45] technique with transfer of the FHL tendon. Flexor digitorum longus (FDL) tendon transfers and augmentations have also been described and can be used successfully.[35, 50] Postoperative immobilization of these patients, unfortunately, must be longer. Occasionally, a short period of time in a long-leg fiberglass cast with the foot in equinus can be used but is usually avoided. All patients eventually are graduated from a cast to a removable walking boot with a 2-inch lift.

COMPLICATIONS

For problems of tendinitis and insertional tendinopathies, the surgical options, although available, are not clearly predictable and dependable. For that reason, conservative care should always be the recommended initial treatment. Patients should be instructed on the length of time that these problems take to respond and be encouraged to be patient. Complications of surgery can include wound healing problems as well as rupture or rerupture of the tendon, sympathetic and disuse dystrophy, and joint stiffness. In patients with Achilles tendon ruptures, conservative treatment has been shown to be effective and should be given as an option to patients. Patients who intend to return to strenuous activities probably are best treated with surgical apposition of the tendon and early mobilization when possible to promote joint stiffness.

RESULTS

The results of surgical treatment for all of the conditions involving the Achilles tendon have been acceptable but not overwhelming. Kvist and Kvist[39] reported good or excellent results in 96% of 182 patients for operative treatment of chronic tendinitis. The results in surgery of Haglund's deformity have been variable. Nesse and Finsen[40] noted pain persisting in 12 of 35 heels. Sammarco and Taylor[33] reported more acceptable results in Haglund's deformity in the nonathlete. The results in patients with degenerative chronic insertional problems of the Achilles tendon have not been reliable, and thus resection of the distal portion of the tendon with augmentation of the FHL or FDL tendon has gained popularity. However, good prospective studies comparing options are lacking.

The results of both nonoperative and operative treatment of Achilles tendon ruptures have been well reported and are nearly equivalent. The risk of rerupture and the post-treatment strength of the Achilles tendon are slightly decreased in those patients treated nonsurgically. Primary repair is recommended for patients desiring return to more strenuous activities.

SUMMARY

Problems of the Achilles tendon, especially the more difficult chronic tendinopathies and tendon attachment problems, can be a challenge to the orthopaedic surgeon. Knowledge of the anatomy and various surgical and nonsurgical options are important. Most patients with chronic nonrupture problems can and should be treated nonsurgically, but in refractory cases aggressive surgical treatment may be required. Tendon augmentation with the FHL can be considered. Achilles tendon ruptures in the athletic population are generally treated with an acute repair and more rapid mobilization. However, nonsurgical treatment remains a viable option. Early protected mobilization of the healing tendon appears associated with an earlier and more reliable return of function.

FHL TENDON PATHOLOGY

DEFINITION

The FHL tendon courses through a synovial sheath and fibro-osseous tunnel in the posterior medial ankle and hindfoot area. It may be subjected to intense mechanical forces and can be a source of posterior ankle pain. Tenosynovitis of the FHL tendon may occur along with thickening and triggering of the tendon complex.

EPIDEMIOLOGY

Symptoms may develop in the FHL tendon area after a twisting injury to the ankle, isolated calcaneal fracture involving the sustentaculum tali, and repetitive plantar flexion/dorsiflexion activity. Ballet dancing appears to be one activity that may add increased risk for problems in this region, and the FHL tendon has been termed the Achilles tendon of the dancer's foot.[51]

PATHOGENESIS
Anatomy

The tendon travels distally through its fibro-osseous tunnel under the flexor retinaculum along the medial surface of the calcaneus in close proximity to the neurovascular bundle and underneath the sustentaculum tali (see Fig. 1B and C). Distally in the plantar medial midfoot, the sheaths of the FHL and FDL cross and interdigitate at the master knot of Henry. The tendon inserts at the plantar base of the distal phalanx of the great toe (see Fig. 1C).

Repetitive plantar flexion and dorsiflexion activities may create tenosynovial inflammation surrounding the FHL. A low-lying FHL muscle belly may also be pulled into the tendon sheath, creating impingement and increased pressure and thereby further exacerbating tenosynovial inflammation. Partial tearing or thickening within the tendon substance may contribute to nodule formation and triggering of the hallux, known as *hallux saltans*.[52, 53] In extreme cases of tenosynovial inflammation, the FHL may become locked within the sheath.

Biomechanics

The course of the FHL tendon is plantar/medial to the ankle and hindfoot axis of rotation, and thus it exerts a plantar flexion and inversion moment. Its distal function is plantar flexion of the metatarsophalangeal (MTP) and interphalangeal joints of the hallux.

CLINICAL FEATURES

Pathology involving the FHL tendon will create pain in the posterior ankle and posterior medial hindfoot. One may sense a catching or triggering phenomenon, which may be related to tearing or thickening of the tendon within its sheath.[52] Physical examination will reveal tenderness along the course of the FHL tendon, beginning slightly proximal to the ankle level and potentially proceeding distally through the area of the flexor retinaculum. Placing the ankle through a range of motion may also reproduce triggering. With the ankle held stationary, active motion of the hallux in direct palpation over the FHL tendon may further exacerbate symptoms. Pseudohallux rigidus occurs as the tendon becomes locked within its sheath and is demonstrated by showing limited dorsiflexion of the hallux MTP joint when the ankle and knee are held in a position of maximum extension.[51, 53] Posteromedial ankle pain reproduced with rapid, forceful passive plantar flexion raises suspicion of FHL tendinopathy.

INVESTIGATION

Radiological studies may reveal associated osseous abnormalities; however, the diagnosis of FHL tendon disorder is primarily clinical. Plain radiographs obtained should be standing AP, lateral, and mortise views of the ankle. The lateral view may reveal prominent posterior talar process or an os trigonum. A symptomatic os trigonum may occur as an isolated entity, but it may also contribute to FHL tenosynovitis. With a history of hindfoot fracture, a calcaneal view may reveal structural changes within the calcaneus contributing to symptoms. MRI scanning may assist when the diagnosis is less certain. However, it must be remembered that some fluid in the tendon sheath is a normal finding.

DIFFERENTIAL DIAGNOSES

The differential diagnosis of tenosynovitis of the FHL tendon is listed in Table 6 and includes those entities creating posterior ankle region and posterior medial hindfoot region pain.

MANAGEMENT

The mainstay of treatment involves rest and the use of anti-inflammatory agents. Involvement in dance activities should be modified to avoid at risk maneuvers. With ongoing symptoms, a period of immobilization in a removable walking boot or cast may be beneficial. Persistent significant symptoms may warrant surgical intervention. Surgery is directed at release of the constricting FHL tendon sheath. A curvilinear incision is made in the posteromedial ankle over the FDL tendon. Strict care must be taken to avoid injury to the neurovascular bundle. The most direct route is through the FDL tendon sheath anterior to the neurovascular bundle. This also lessens the risk of injury to the medial calcaneal nerve branches. The tendon sheath should be opened from its proximal extent to at least the sustentaculum. Localized tenosynovial inflammation may be excised in sharp fashion. An associated symptomatic os trigonum should be excised. Closure is performed in a

TABLE 6. DIFFERENTIAL DIAGNOSES OF POSTERIOR MEDIAL ANKLE/HINDFOOT PAIN
Flexor hallucis longus tenosynovitis
Fracture of posterior process of talus
Symptomatic os trigonum
Posterior tibial tendon tenosynovitis
Achilles tendon pathology/retrocalcaneal pain
Subtalar joint pathology
Arthrosis
Coalition
Tumor

layered fashion, and again strict care must be taken to avoid injury to the neurovascular structures. Patients are mobilized non-weightbearing for approximately 10 to 14 days in a short-leg splint or walking boot followed by gradual progression of range of motion and weightbearing activities.

ANTERIOR TIBIAL TENDON

Pathology involving the anterior tibial tendon may lead to pain in the region of the anteromedial ankle area as well as pain extending down to the midfoot area.

PATHOGENESIS

Tenosynovial inflammation of the anterior tibial tendon typically is brought on by repetitive dorsiflexion and plantar flexion activities and is associated with irritation from overlying footwear. Rupture of the anterior tibial tendon is rare; however, it can occur when there is a forceful contraction against a forcibly plantar-flexed foot.

Anatomy

The tibialis anterior originates in the proximal leg from the pretibial surface, and innervation is from the deep peroneal nerve. The tendon courses underneath the retinacular structures and is noted to be quite prominent in the anterior ankle region. Its insertion is on the dorsal and medial aspects of the medial cuneiform and the base of the first metatarsal.

Biomechanics

The anterior tibial tendon is a forceful dorsiflexor of the ankle and invertor of the foot.

CLINICAL FEATURES

Pain is localized over the course of the anterior tibial tendon. Active dorsiflexion against resistance may elicit discomfort. Symptoms will be exacerbated with direct palpation over the tendon as well. Care should be taken to examine for associated ankle joint swelling and true ankle joint tenderness consistent with interarticular disorder. With rupture of the anterior tibial tendon, a palpable defect will be evident and retraction of the proximal segment into the distal leg may be felt as a palpable thickening. Dorsiflexion weakness will also be noted. Etiological investigation involving the anterior tibial tendon is limited. Plain radiographs, including standing AP, lateral, and oblique views of the ankle and foot, may reveal additional disorder. MRI may be of benefit when a rupture is considered and the level of the retraction of the proximal fragment is unknown.

DIFFERENTIAL DIAGNOSES

Differential diagnoses include true joint disorder of the ankle or midfoot, and with isolated weakness one should consider more proximal neurological compression syndromes.

MANAGEMENT

Rest and anti-inflammatory drug use is recommended. If external factors are involved, shoe or boot modifications should be instituted. Use of supportive ankle sleeves may exacerbate symptoms because of direct pressure over the anterior tibial tendon region. With more pronounced symptoms, immobilization in a removable walking boot may assist in abatement of symptoms. For chronic cases a leaf-spring ankle-foot orthosis can be used.

Surgical reconstruction may be performed with direct reattachment if there has been little retraction of the tendon substance. A split turn-down procedure of the proximal segment has been described for midsubstance rupture.

REFERENCES

1. Weiner AD, Lipscomb PR: Rupture of muscles and tendons. Minn Med 1956; 39: 731.
2. Almekinders LC: Tendinitis and other chronic tendinopathies. J Am Acad Orthop Surg 1998; 6:57.
3. Lysholm J, Wiklander J: Injury in runners. Am J Sports Med 1987; 15:168.
4. Edwards ME: Relation of peroneal tendons to fibula, calcaneus and cuboideum. Am J Anat 1928; 42:213.
5. Eckert WR, Davis EA Jr: Acute rupture of the peroneal retinaculum. J Bone Joint Surg Am 1976; 58:670.
6. Davis WH, Sobel M, Deland J, et al: The superior peroneal retinaculum: An anatomic study. Foot Ankle 1994; 15:271.
7. Sobel M, Levy M, Bhone W: Congenital variations of the peroneus quartus muscle: An anatomic study. Foot Ankle 1990; 11: 81.
8. Sobel M, Pavlov H, Geppert M, et al: Painful os peroneum syndrome: A spectrum of conditions responsible for lateral foot pain. Foot Ankle 1994; 13:112.
9. Clark HD, Kitaoka HB, Ehman RL: Peroneal tendon injuries. Foot Ankle 1998; 19: 280.
10. Sobel M, Geppert M, Hannafin J, et al: Microvascular anatomy of peroneal tendons. Foot Ankle 1992; 13:469.
11. Kilkelly FX, McHale KA: Acute rupture of the peroneus longus tendon in a runner: A case report and review of the literature. Foot Ankle Int 1994; 15:567.
12. Khoury N, El-Khoury GY, Saltzman CA, et al: Peroneus longus and peroneus brevis tears: MRI imaging evaluation. Radiology 1996; 200:833.
13. Krause JO, Brodsky JW: Peroneus brevis tendon tears: Pathophysiology, surgical re-
construction, and clinical results. Foot Ankle Int 1998; 19:271.
14. Basset FH, Speer KP: Longitudinal rupture of the peroneal tendon. Am J Sports Med 1993; 21:354.
15. Clanton TO, Schon LC: Athletic injuries to the soft tissues of the foot and ankle. In Mann R, Coughlin M (eds): Surgery of the Foot and Ankle. St. Louis, MO, CV Mosby, 1993, 6th ed, vol 27, p 1095.
16. Sobel M, Geppert M, Warren W: Chronic ankle instability as a cause of peroneal tendon injury. Clin Orthop Rel Res 1993; 296:187.
17. Oden RR: Tendon injuries about the ankle resulting from skiing. Clin Orthop 1987; 216:63.
18. Mason RB, Henderson EJP: Traumatic peroneal tendon instability. Am J Sports Med 1996; 24:652.

19. Murr S: Dislocation of the peroneal tendons with marginal fracture of the lateral malleolus. J Bone Joint Surg Br 1961; 43: 563.

20. Moritz JR: Ski injuries. Am J Surg 1959; 98:493.

21. Jones E: Operative treatment of chronic dislocation of the peroneal tendons. J Bone Joint Surg 1931; 14:574.

22. Zoellner G, Clancy W Jr: Recurrent dislocation of the peroneal tendon. J Bone Joint Surgery Am 1979; 61:292.

23. Kelly RE: An operation for chronic dislocation of the peroneal tendons. Br J Surg 1920; 7:502.

24. Saltzman CL, Teursch DS: Achilles tendon injuries. J Am Acad Orthop Surg 1998; 6:316.

25. Perry JR: Contemporary approaches to the Achilles tendon. In Myerson MS (ed): Foot and Ankle Clinics. Philadelphia, WB Saunders, 1997.

26. Perry JR: Achilles tendon anatomy. In Myerson MS (ed): Foot and Ankle Clinics. Philadelphia, WB Saunders, 1997, p 363.

27. Carr AJ, Norris SH: The blood supply of the calcaneal tendon. J Bone Joint Surg Br 1989; 71:100.

28. Curwin SL: Biomechanics of the tendon and the effects of immobilization. In Myerson MS (ed): Foot and Ankle Clinics. Philadelphia, WB Saunders, 1997, p 371.

29. Enwemeka CS, Spielholz NI, Nelson AJ: The effect of early functional activities on experimentally tenotomized tendons in rats. Am J Phys Med Rehabil 1998; 67: 264.

30. Deutsch AL, Lund PJ, Mink GH: MR imaging and diagnostic ultrasound in the evaluation of Achilles tendon disorders. In Myerson MS (ed): Foot and Ankle Clinics. Philadelphia, WB Saunders, 1997, p 391.

31. Neuhold A, Stiskal M, Kainberger F, et al: Degenerative Achilles tendon disease: Assessment by magnetic resonance and ultrasonography. Eur J Radiol 1992; 14:213.

32. Puddu G, Ippolito E, Postacchini F: A classification of Achilles tendon disease. Am J Sports Med 1976; 4:145.

33. Sammarco GJ, Taylor AL: Operative management of Haglund's deformity in the nonathlete: A retrospective study. Foot Ankle 1998; 19:724.

34. Plattner P, Mann R: Disorders of tendons. In Mann RA (ed): Surgery of the Foot and Ankle. St. Louis, MO, CV Mosby, 1993, 6th ed, vol 19, p 805.

35. Mann RA, Chou L: Effective intervention for Achilles tendinitis and tendinosis. J Musculoskel Med 1988; 15:57.

36. Myerson MS, McGarvey W: Disorders of the insertion of the Achilles tendon and Achilles tendinitis. J Bone Joint Surg Am 1998; 12:1814.

37. Jones DC, James SL: Partial calcaneal osteotomy for retrocalcaneal bursitis. Am J Sports Med 1984; 12:72.

38. Jones DC: Tendon disorders of the foot and ankle. J Am Acad Orthop Surg 1993; 1:87.

39. Kvist H, Kvist E: The operative treatment of chronic calcaneal peritenonitis. J Bone Joint Surg Br 1980; 62:353.

40. Nesse E, Finsen V: Poor results after resection of Haglund's heel. Analysis of 35 heels in 23 patients after three years. Acta Orthop Scand 1994; 65:107.

41. Saltzman CL, Thermann H: Achilles tendon problems. In Pfeffer GB, Frey CC (eds): Current Practice in Foot and Ankle Surgery. New York, McGraw-Hill, 1993, p 194.

42. Schepsis AA, Leach RE: Surgical management of Achilles tendinitis. Am J Sports Med 1987; 15:308.

43. Keck SW, Kelly PJ: Bursitis of the posterior aspect of the heel: Evaluation of surgical treatment of 18 patients. J Bone Joint Surg Am 1995; 47:267.

44. Clain MR, Baxter DE: Achilles tendinitis. Foot Ankle 1992; 13:482.

45. Wapner KL, Hecht PJ, Mills RH Jr: Reconstruction of neglected Achilles tendon injury. Orthop Clin North Am 1995; 26:249.

46. Cetti R, Christensen SE, Ejsted R, et al: Operative versus nonoperative treatment of Achilles tendon rupture: A prospective randomized study and review of the literature. Am J Sports Med 1993; 21:791.

47. Mandelbaum BR, Myerson MS, Forster R: Achilles tendon ruptures: A new method of repair, early range of motion, and functional rehabilitation. Am J Sports Med 1995; 23:392.

48. Wapner KL: Acute repair of the Achilles tendon. In Johnson KA (ed): Master Techniques in Orthopaedic Surgery: The Foot and Ankle. New York, Raven Press, 1994, p 299.

49. Calhoun JH: Delayed repair of the Achilles tendon. In Johnson KA (ed): Master Techniques in Orthopaedic Surgery: The Foot and Ankle. New York, Raven Press, 1994, p 311.

50. Mann RA, Holmes GB Jr, Seale KS, et al: Chronic rupture of the Achilles tendon: A new technique of repair. J Bone Joint Surg Am 1991; 73:214.

51. Hamilton WG: Stenosing tenosynovitis of the flexor hallucis longus tendon and posterior impingement upon the os trigonum in ballet dancers. Foot Ankle 1982; 3:74.

52. Samarco TJ, Miller EH: Partial rupture of the flexor hallucis longus tendon in classic ballet dancers: Two case reports. J Bone Joint Surg Am 1979; 61:149.

53. Hamilton W: Foot and ankle injuries in dancers. In Mann RA, Coughlin M (eds): Surgery of the Foot and Ankle. St. Louis, MO, CV Mosby, 1993, 6th ed, vol 29, p 1241.

THE RHEUMATOID FOOT AND ANKLE

Judith F. Baumhauer

Summary

- Approximately 5 million people suffer from rheumatoid arthritis.[1]
- Patients with rheumatoid arthritis have[2]
    Six times the probability of severe limitation of activity
    Four times as many days of restricted activity.
    Ten times the work disability rate of the general population.
    Three times the cost of medical care.
    Twice the rate of hospitalization.
    Four times the number of ambulatory visits to a physician than does an age- and gender-matched population without the disease.
- Rheumatoid arthritis begins in the feet in 17% of patients.
- Eighty-nine percent to 94% of patients with rheumatoid arthritis have foot or ankle symptoms during the course of their disease process.[3, 4]
- The diagnosis of rheumatoid arthritis is based on clinical, laboratory, and radiographic criteria and may be insidious in onset, contributing to the difficulty in diagnosis.
- Symptomatic rheumatoid joint involvement of the foot most commonly affects, in order, the forefoot, talonavicular, subtalar, calcaneal cuboid, and ankle joints.
- Goals of treatment include relief of pain, prevention and/or correction of deformity, and improvement and/or preservation of function.
- Initial treatment begins with drug therapy and nonoperative modalities (physical therapy, orthoses, shoe modifications, brace wear, and walking aids). Treatment may then progress to surgical procedures as necessary.
- Morbidity impact studies demonstrate that, with more effective medical and surgical management and better rehabilitative strategies for people with rheumatoid arthritis, significant benefits are seen in the patients, their families, and society.[5]

DEFINITION

Rheumatoid arthritis is a systemic inflammatory disease process of unknown cause, mediated in part by the interaction of antigens, antibodies, complement, and immune complexes. Its major distinctive feature is a chronic symmetric, erosive synovitis of peripheral joints leading to progressive joint destruction, deformity, and disability. Extraosseous manifestations of rheumatoid arthritis, although less common, include rheumatoid nodules, pericarditis, lymphadenopathy, arteritis, scleritis, neuropathy, splenomegaly, bursitis, and tendinopathy.

HISTORICAL REVIEW

In the 1800s, Garrod coined the term *rheumatoid arthritis,* differentiating it from other rheumatic diseases.[6]

A number of epidemiological studies have proven that the foot and ankle tend to be preferentially affected during the course of the disease process. Because of the weight-bearing function of these joints, this leads to greater pain, dysfunction, and disability than upper extremity involvement.

The current era of surgical management was ushered in by Hoffman, who in 1911 first advocated resection of the metatarsal heads through a plantar incision for claw toes. Since then, a wide variety of techniques have been described for correction of fixed contractures of the forefoot secondary to rheumatoid arthritis.[7] These techniques include a variation on bone resection such as partial proximal phalangectomies, Keller's resection arthroplasty, and plantar condylectomies.[8] Surgical approaches have ranged from dorsal to plantar incisions with or without soft-tissue advancement flaps for plantar metatarsal head coverage.

The next evolution included artificial implants in the foot. Because of their excellent results in the hand, silicone implants were used in the foot; the early published reports were presented in the 1980s.[9] With the development of silicone synovitis, loss of toe alignment, and weightbearing function,[10] arthrodesis procedures for the first metatarsophalangeal (MTP) joint became more commonly performed.

Rheumatoid involvement of the hindfoot joints results in pain, heel valgus, forefoot varus, and midfoot collapse potentially leading to symptomatic ankle malalignment, limited motion, and pain. The surgical approach to the hindfoot historically consisted of stabilization through arthrodesis, traditionally involving the talonavicular, calcaneal cuboid, and subtalar joints (triple arthrodesis).[11] Recognizing the potential for increased stress at adjacent joints after fusion, the pendulum has swung to limited single or double arthrodesis of affected symptomatic joints.[12]

Although thought to be less commonly symptomatic, ankle involvement surgically consisted of an ankle arthrodesis. Total ankle arthroplasty has, in the past, been plagued with loosening, wear, and bone loss. Newer designs have been fabricated, and long-term studies are being performed and reviewed with cautious optimism in the low-demand rheumatoid arthritic patient population.[13]

EPIDEMIOLOGY

Rheumatoid arthritis afflicts approximately 1% of the adult population worldwide. The disease presents in the foot in 17% of patients and involves the foot in 89% of patients at some time during the course of the disease process.[3] The forefoot is thought to be the most commonly affected, followed by the talonavicular, subtalar, calcaneal cuboid, and ankle joints. A 1994 prevalence study found a higher number of ankle problems related to lack of motion rather than pain.[4] The disease prevalence increases with age, and it affects women twice as much as men. The more common age presentation is between the fourth and sixth decades. In the United States, age, lack of formal education, and lower socioeconomic class correlate with both the incidence and poor prognosis of rheumatoid arthritis. The patient with rheumatoid arthritis faces increasing functional disability. One study reported that, at 17 years of disease duration, 80% of patients were moderately disabled.[14] Patients with rheumatoid arthritis are at increased risk for work disability within 10 years after the onset of disease (50% able to work) and a drastic reduction in earnings (up to 60% in those with moderate rheumatoid arthritis compared with normal individuals). In the United States, patients with rheumatoid arthritis have three times the cost of medical care, twice the hospitalization, and four times the number of ambulatory visits to a physician as does an age- and gender-matched population.[15]

Significant advances have been made in the understanding of the inflammatory process leading to joint destruction and rheumatoid arthritis. The initiating event remains elusive but most likely involves endothelial cell expression of adhesion molecules in response to specific cytokines. This triggers monocyte and lymphocyte migration into the synovial tissue. As well, additional chemotactic factors are released, inducing neutrophil accumulation into this space. Inflammatory and regulatory cytokines such as interleukin-1, tumor necrosis factor-α and growth factors are produced by activated synovial macrophages, resulting in chondrocyte and synovial fibroblastic release of proteinases, leukotrienes, prostaglandins, and reactive oxidases. These factors cause cartilage degradation and bone resorption. This self-perpetuating process induces synovial tissue angiogenesis and massive synovial hyperplasia or pannus formation.[16]

Gender and immune susceptibility appear to be major determinants in the development of rheumatoid arthritis. Hormonal influences are reflected by the increased female-male ratio of 2:1. Additional evidence includes the clinical remission of rheumatoid arthritis in pregnancy with a relapse after delivery as well as a decrease of incidence of rheumatoid arthritis in patients using oral contraceptives or postmenopausal hormones.[17]

Rheumatoid arthritis is strongly associated with the class II major histocompatibility complex, HLA-DR4. Specific subtypes of HLA-DR4 predict a more severe clinical course. Sequences of amino acids found on the β chain hypervariable region have been linked with rheumatoid arthritis and are collectively referred to as the rheumatoid arthritis susceptibility sequence or shared epitope.[18]

PATHOANATOMY

The classic structural changes associated with rheumatoid arthritis of the forefoot include dorsally dislocated metatarsal phalangeal joints of the lesser toes, plantar callosities under prominent metatarsal heads, and hallux valgus deformity of the great toe. These alignment abnormalities are due to the cellular inflammatory process previously de-scribed, resulting in synovitis and capsular and ligamentous laxity of the MTP joints. Through continued weightbearing, dorsiflexion stress leads to subluxation of the destabilized lesser MTP joints. The intrinsic muscles then lie dorsal to the flexion/extension axis, resulting in a loss of both MTP joint flexion and interphalangeal (IP) joint extension. Continued mechanical and intrinsic muscle dorsiflexion force leads to dislocation of the second, third, fourth, and fifth metatarsal phalangeal joints, with the proximal phalanx lying to rest on the dorsal neck of each respective metatarsal. Subsequently, the plantar fat pad, which is anchored to the proximal phalanx base, is pulled distally. The metatarsal heads herniate through the weakened plantar capsule, placing the metatarsal heads in a subcutaneous position without any fat pad protection during weightbearing, leading to increased focal plantar pressures and callus formation.

Synovitis, capsular, and ligamentous laxity of the hindfoot leads to flattening of the longitudinal arch in 50% of patients with a typical progressive valgus deformity.[19] Posterior tibial tendinopathy has been suggested in the literature as a primary cause of the valgus deformity. However, electromyographic studies demonstrated that the tibialis posterior musculature produces prolonged activity during the gait cycle in an attempt to stabilize longitudinal arch. Gait analysis has revealed an increased valgus of the hindfoot during weightbearing, leading to decreased plantar flexion and increased dorsiflexion of the ankle joint, delayed heel rise, shortened stride length, and decreased walking velocity.[20]

CLINICAL FEATURES

Patients with rheumatoid arthritis and forefoot arthropathy typically present with pain from callosities because of prominent plantar metatarsal heads, a hallux valgus deformity with a prominent medial eminence, and dorsally subluxated or dislocated MTP joints of the lesser toes accompanied by dorsal proximal interphalangeal (PIP) joint irritation from shoe wear. The complaints typically are pain under the metatarsal heads and difficulty in finding adequate toe box height for footwear. Patients with hindfoot rheumatoid arthropathy complain of pain in the "ankle region." When specifically examined, this typically is in the region of the sinus tarsi and subtalar joint. The patient may or may not have noticed a progressive deviation of the heel into valgus associated with an increased pronation deformity through the midfoot and forefoot. With excessive valgus deformity of the hindfoot, fibular pain resulting from stress fractures may be the primary complaint. A breakdown of the medial heel counter is evident on inspection of the shoe.

Ankle involvement may be secondary to the severe hindfoot valgus or may be a primary complaint. Decreased motion, not pain, is the most common problem.[4] The decrease in ankle motion secondary to arthritic involvement tends to lead to decreased functional capabilities during ambulation and stair climbing.

Physical examination includes inspection, looking for rheumatoid nodules and cysts, plantar and dorsal callosities, and splinter nail hemorrhages suggestive of rheumatoid vasculitis. A sensory examination of the cutaneous nerves and palpation of the dorsalis pedis and tibial artery supply to the foot are performed. Peripheral neuropathy can occur secondary to arteritis of the vasovasorum of the cutaneous nerves. A complete motor examination will delineate any tendon dysfunction. A global weakness in the lower extremities may be suggestive of spinal cord compression secondary to cervical spine instability. Tendon ruptures in the foot are rare but may occur and must be ruled out.

Focal palpation of the hindfoot, midfoot, and forefoot delineates painful joints. The midfoot joints typically have radiographic changes; however, they are not symptomatic and rarely require surgical intervention. Particular joints to be palpated include the MTP joints, the area of the sinus tarsi and subtalar joint, and the talonavicular, calcaneal cuboid, ankle, and IP joints. These joints are then placed through a range of motion to determine the flexible versus fixed nature of the deformities. In addition to range-of-motion examination of the foot and ankle, the hip and knee similarly should be examined. Excessive genu valgum can lead to compensatory hindfoot valgus and forefoot varus. An examination should be repeated during weightbearing to assess the degree of lower extremity malalignment. Examination of the patient during walking is quite helpful to identify the typical shuffled gait, shortened stride length, and decreased walking velocity. Table 1 summarizes the complete physical examination components and abnormalities found in examination of the rheumatoid foot and ankle.

INVESTIGATION

Early in the disease process the diagnosis is suggested by clinical findings of unilateral arthritis, progressing to characteristically symmetric arthritis of the small peripheral joints associated with morning stiffness lasting at least 1 hour. Laboratory tests typically performed include rheumatoid factor (positive in 85% of patients with rheumatoid arthritis) and an erythrocyte sedimentation rate (commonly elevated). The fluorescent antinuclear antibody test is positive in only 45% of patients with rheumatoid arthritis. Complement levels are increased in the acute phase of rheumatoid arthritis and decreased in patients with rheumatoid arthritis and vasculitis. C-reactive protein is increased in greater than 90% of patients with rheumatoid arthritis. C-reactive protein is elevated in many acute disease processes and, therefore, is not a specific diagnostic test for rheumatoid arthritis. The standard radiographs recommended for evaluation of the rheumatoid foot and ankle include weightbearing anteroposterior, lateral, and oblique views of the foot, anteroposterior ankle, and tibial calcaneus (Morrey) (Figs. 1 to 3). Features detected on these plain films include soft-tissue swelling and proliferation, juxta-articular and diffuse osteoporosis, marginal bony erosions, joint space narrowing, subluxation and malalignment, ankylosis, reactive sclerosis around healing erosions, and osteophytes in severely damaged joints.

Up to 81% of patients with erosions on hand and feet films also show damage in the cervical spine.[21] These defects should be carefully sought on foot radiographs. Such findings, correlated with clinical findings of neck pain or symptoms and signs of neurological abnormalities, suggest the need for lateral cervical spine radiographs in flexion and extension, looking for cervical instability.

Additional studies providing diagnostic information include magnetic resonance imaging (MRI) when diffuse

synovitis is apparent clinically and specific delineation of a joint involvement is unclear (Fig. 4A and B). A computed tomography (CT) scan can aid in evaluating joint involvement, and selective joint injections of lidocaine with or without cortisone may allow localization of painful joints when the specific joint is difficult to identify by palpation alone.

DIFFERENTIAL DIAGNOSIS

Because rheumatoid arthritis may present as a soft-tissue mass around the joint or as an invasive destructive lesion within a joint, differential diagnosis includes tumors, infection, and other inflammatory arthropathies, including autoimmune diseases and gout. After a thorough history and physical examination and appropriate radiographic tests, laboratory evaluations, including a complete blood count with white blood cell count differentiation, erythrocyte sedimentation rate, and C-reactive protein, should be obtained. Primary diagnosis will be based on a needle aspiration or core biopsy of the soft-tissue mass. In rheumatoid arthritis

TABLE 1. CLINICAL FEATURES TO BE INCLUDED IN THE PHYSICAL EXAMINATION OF THE FOOT AND ANKLE IN THE RHEUMATOID PATIENT

Inspection	Range of Motion
General	Hip joint
Rheumatoid nodule cysts	Knee joint
Callosities	Ankle joint
Nail splinter hemorrhages	Subtalar joint
Forefoot	Transverse tarsal joints
Dorsal lateral subluxated/dislocated MTP 2–5	MTP joints (1–5)
Hallux valgus	IP joints (1–5)
Metatarsus primus varus	**Palpation (tenderness)**
Distal migration of the plantar fat pad	MTP joints (1–5)
Plantar callosities under metatarsal heads	Sinus tarsi
PIP joint irritation	Talonavicular
Medial eminence irritation of the great toe	Calcaneal cuboid
IP joint hyperextension (chisel toe)	Ankle joints
IP joint pronation (helix tortus)	IP joints
Hindfoot	Distal fibula for stress fracture
Valgus alignment	**Standing Inspection**
Diffuse swelling	Growth plate alignment
Cutaneous Nerve Exam	Leg rotation
Peripheral neuropathy secondary to arteritis of the vaso vasorum	Knee deformity
	Leg length discrepancy
	Pelvic obliquity
Peripheral Pulses	**Gait Inspection**
Dorsalis pedis and posterior tibial arteries	Shuffled gait
	Shortened stride length
Motor Function Examination	Decreased walking velocity
Tendon strength	Hindfoot valgus
Spinal cord compression of C1-2 instability	Loss of arch with pronation deformity

MTP, metatarsophalangeal; PIP, proximal interphalangeal; IP, interphalangeal.

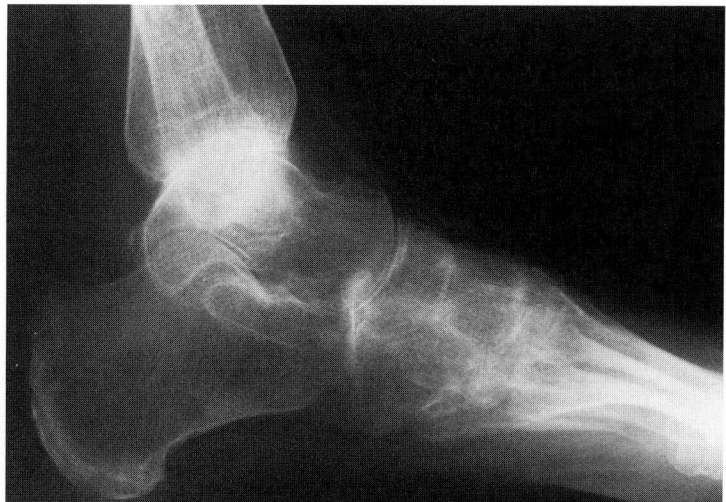

Fig. 1. Joint space narrowing. Standing lateral radiograph of the foot demonstrates joint space narrowing of the subtalar, calcaneocuboid, and midfoot joints.

the histology reveals synovial tissue angiogenesis and hyperplasia. Special staining techniques can be performed to search for rheumatoid factor in the specimen undergoing biopsy. Cultures obtained at biopsy will yield no growth. Gout has classic findings of needle-shaped urate crystals located within polymorphonuclear neutrophils. They show negative birefringence with polarized microscopy not present in rheumatoid arthritis.

MANAGEMENT

GENERAL

The initial treatment of the symptomatic patient with rheumatoid arthritis in the forefoot, hindfoot, or ankle consists of optimizing medical management of the disease. The traditional pyramidal approach to pharmacological agents

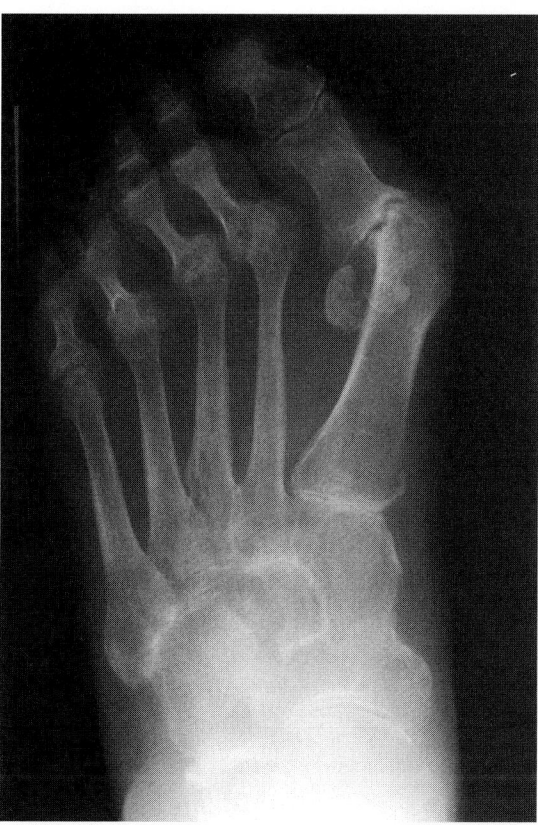

Fig. 2. Erosive changes. Standing anteroposterior radiograph of the foot demonstrates erosive changes of metatarsophalangeal joints 1 to 5 with lateral subluxation.

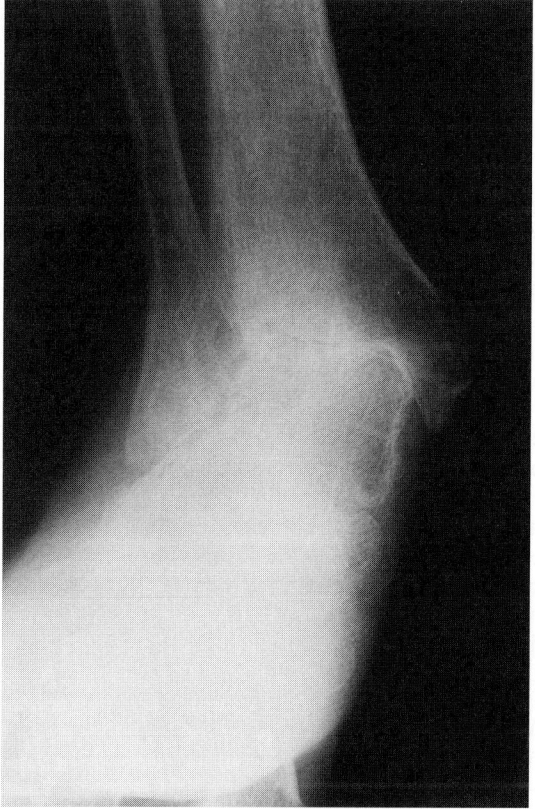

Fig. 3. Distal fibular erosion and impingement. Standing anteroposterior radiograph of the ankle demonstrates distal fibular erosion and impingement secondary to severe hindfoot valgus with less severe ankle valgus. Note the large cyst involving the medial malleolus.

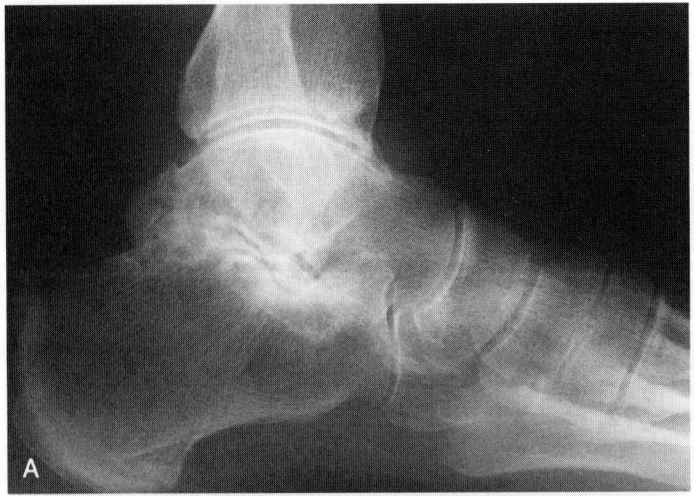

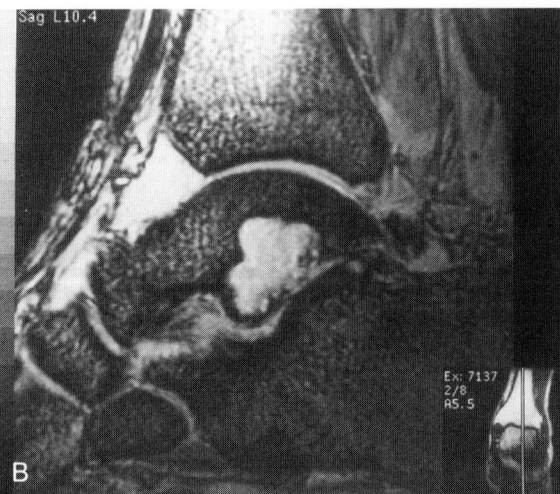

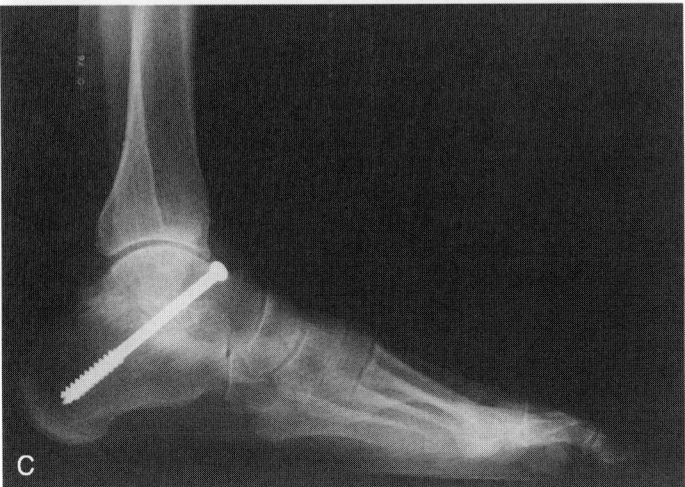

Fig. 4. Erosions of subtalar joint. *A*, Standing lateral radiograph of the foot demonstrating erosions of the subtalar joint, with a large cyst of the talar body. Note the small osteophyte at anterior aspect of the distal tibial with preservation of the remainder of the ankle joint. *B*, Sagittal magnetic resonance image of the ankle and hindfoot demonstrating large cystic lesions of the talar body extending into the subtalar joint. Fluid is present in the ankle joint. *C*, Standing lateral radiograph of the foot demonstrating single 7.3-mm cannulated screw fixation of the subtalar joint.

begins with nonsteroidal anti-inflammatory drugs and progresses to disease-modifying medications (corticosteroids, hydroxychloroquine [Plaquenil], gold, D-penicillamine) and finally cytotoxic agents (azathioprine, cyclophosphamide, and methotrexate).[22] Different agents are undergoing trials as new data become available in the pathophysiology of this disease process.

Nonoperative Treatment

Local corticosteroid injections for the treatment of synovitis may decrease pain and swelling. The duration of relief is variable and based on the degree of deformity and severity of joint disease.

Range-of-motion exercises continue to be prescribed to maintain mobility of the MTP, hindfoot, and ankle joints in the rheumatoid patient. No studies are available reporting on the success of this treatment in regard to prolonged function or pain relief. Moist heat may be helpful for chronic pain. With concurrent problems of neuropathy or vasculitis, modalities such as contrast baths using extremes in temperature should be avoided.

Orthotic management has three principal modes of action: corrective, supportive, and accommodative. Corrective effects are primarily achieved in the growing child. Supportive effects are used in the flexible foot to reestablish foot alignment and weightbearing. Accommodative effects are implemented with fixed deformities and directed toward relief of painful pressure areas through cushioning and redistribution of plantar forces. In rheumatoid arthritis with isolated synovitis and flexible forefoot deformities, supportive effects can be used. A metatarsal pad proximal to the metatarsal head can eliminate weight from the area and decrease the mechanical forces, allowing the synovitis within the joint to subside. As the disease process progresses from a flexible to a fixed stage, accommodative orthoses are necessary. Total contact inserts made of flexible material such as cork, foam, and soft plastics are designed to absorb shock and permit the physiological motions of the foot during walking. Viscoelastic polymers can be placed underneath the prominent metatarsal heads, providing additional cushioning. Shoe modifications can include an extended steel shank built into the sole of the shoe to decrease forces across the MTP joints. A rocker sole may be added to an extended steel shank modification to allow forward propulsion during walking. A high toe box can accommodate PIP joint contractures. Stretching of the shoe in regions of bony prominences such as the hallux and PIP joints may decrease irritation of the skin over these areas. In the rare case of symptomatic midfoot arthritis in the rheumatoid patient, similar orthotic and shoe modifications can be used to decrease the forces across the midfoot.

Symptomatic arthritis of the hindfoot, including the subtalar, talonavicular, and/or calcaneocuboid joints, may be improved with cushioned rubber or crepe soles to provide shock absorption during heel strike. With a supple hindfoot deformity, a University of California Biomechanics Laboratory insert may limit the motion across the irritated joints and provide for a better functional position of the foot during ambulation. A fiberglass–reinforced medial heel counter and/or a medial heel wedge built onto the sole of the shoe or orthotic may decrease fibular impingement symptoms from excessive hindfoot valgus.

Walking aids, including crutches, canes, and walkers, will decrease the stress on the foot and ankle. Patients with rheumatoid arthritis usually have upper extremity afflictions as well. Therefore, prolonged use of these ambulatory aids may be difficult.

Two types of braces traditionally have been used to aid in the control of pain and improve foot alignment of the hindfoot and ankle in patients with rheumatoid arthritis. A custom-molded ankle foot orthosis with an anterior clamshell component can allow for a portion of the weightbearing to be carried at the level of the calf and decrease the amount of force seen across the ankle and hindfoot joints. The problem with these polypropylene devices is the potential irritation of the soft tissues over bony prominences against the rigid plastic mold. An alternative is a double upright brace built onto a shoe with either a leather calf corset or polypropylene front and back component to the calf. This similarly will reduce weight applied through the ankle and hindfoot joints and avoid skin irritation. The ankle articulation can be fixed or hinged based on the degree of deformity and ankle symptoms. These braces can be used in patients with fixed or flexible deformities. With additional shoe modifications, the fixed deformities can be supported and accommodated to provide a stable foot to floor contact in the nonsurgical candidate.

OPERATIVE TREATMENT

In patients with severe pain or significant deformity, an inability to wear shoes, or resistance to conservative treatment, surgical intervention is indicated. The goals of surgical treatment are the same as for nonoperative management and include pain relief, correction or accommodation of the deformity, and preservation or restoration of function.

Preoperative planning is essential in this patient population with a systemic disease process. Cervical spine instability should be sought and treated before surgery of the foot or ankle. Physical therapy consultation may be necessary preoperatively because of upper extremity involvement and the need for ambulatory aids to modify weightbearing postoperatively. It is recommended that nonsteroidal anti-inflammatory drugs and aspirin be stopped 1 week before surgery to avoid excessive bleeding or hematoma formation. Although methotrexate had been thought to delay wound healing, current literature has found no delay in wound healing times. Therefore, it can be continued during the course of surgical treatment. Stress doses of perioperative corticosteroids for patients taking steroids is a controversial subject and is based on daily dose, disease severity, and surgical procedure. Rheumatology and anesthesiology

consultation on the subject before surgery is helpful to address this issue. The contralateral limb should have adequate pain control, with appropriate brace and footwear to support the operative limb during healing.

The goals of surgical forefoot reconstruction are to reestablish alignment of the MTP joints and weightbearing function of the great toe, restore adequate padding under the metatarsal head area, and correct fixed deformities of the lesser toes. The surgical options can be divided into operations for the hallux and those of the lesser MTP joints.

Surgery for hallux in patients with rheumatoid arthritis includes resection arthroplasty, Silastic or total toe replacement, and arthrodesis of the MTP joint. Resection arthroplasty has traditionally included either metatarsal head excision (Mayo's resection) or, more commonly, proximal phalanx base resection (Keller's). Through gait analysis and long-term follow-up studies, resection arthroplasty results have been unsatisfactory because of recurrence, poor weightbearing function of the great toe, transfer metatarsalgia, forefoot instability, and the development of a cock-up toe deformity of the hallux (Tables 2 and 3).

Replacement arthroplasty of the first MTP joint has continued to evolve over the past 30 years. The advantages of the procedure include preservation of motion and excellent relief of pain.[34] The disadvantages include material failure of the implant leading to silicone-induced synovitis and osteolysis.[35] There is a loss of strength and weightbearing function of the great toe as a result of shortening and subluxation.

The results of joint replacement arthroplasty are quite variable because of the many factors involved, including type of implant, patient population, age and functional abilities of the patient, duration of follow-up, and presence of associated deformities of the foot. Because of the high biomechanical demands placed on the first MTP joint and the complex articulations of the joints of the foot, routine use of joint replacement arthroplasty cannot be recommended until good and excellent results have been achieved consistently over time.

Because of long-term failures of resection arthroplasty and the variable results with replacement arthroplasty, the current trend in treatment is arthrodesis of the first MTP joint. A variety of arthrodesis techniques have been described and include multiple Steinmann pin fixation, crosslag screw stabilization, and dorsal compression plating (Fig. 5A and B). Fusion rates range from 90% to 100% despite the type of fixation used (see Table 3). As a result of improved weightbearing function of the first MTP joint, the complication of transfer metatarsalgia is minimal. Complications are due to technical errors of malposition (hallux varus or valgus), IP joint arthritis, and nonunion (see Table 2).

Surgical goals in the reconstruction for the lesser toes include realignment of the MTP and interphalangeal joints, relocation of the plantar fat pad, and improved ability to wear shoes. The mainstay of treatment has been resection arthroplasty of the MTP joint through metatarsal head resection alone or in combination with proximal phalanx excision. Excellent results have been obtained through either a dorsal longitudinal or a plantar transverse incision. Although a transverse plantar incision has the advantage of

TABLE 2. COMPLICATIONS OF FOREFOOT SURGERY IN THE RHEUMATOID PATIENT: CAUSES AND POTENTIAL SOLUTIONS

Complication	Cause	Potential Solution
Valgus or varus malalignment first MTP joint (up to 50%)	Excisional arthroplasty with destabilization Spontaneous arthrodesis after excisional arthroplasty	Revision arthrodesis first MTP joint
Recurrent metatarsalgia	Inadequate metatarsal head resection Residual plantar spike of metatarsal Poor arc of resection of metatarsals Excisional arthroplasty of first MTP joint with lateral transfer of weight Exacerbation of systemic rheumatoid disease (cyst or inflammatory mass)	Dorsal-distal to plantar proximal lesser metatarsal head excision Entire lesser metatarsal head excision Arthrodesis first MTP joint to improve weight-bearing Continued medical management of rheumatoid disease
First IP joint pain/deformity	First MTP arthrodesis with preoperative IP joint pain First MTP joint arthrodesis in less than 15 degrees of valgus First MTP joint arthrodesis in less than 20 degrees of dorsiflexion	Preoperative assessment of IP joint of hallux Arthrodesis of first MTP joint in adequate valgus and dorsiflexion (recommended 15 degrees valgus; 25 to 30 degrees dorsiflexion in relationship to shaft)
First MTP nonunion (5%–10%)	Inadequate immobilization Inadequate surgical fixation	Often asymptomatic If symptomatic: Revision with improved surgical fixation (plates/screws; crossed screws; Steinman pins) and postoperative immobilization

Surgery includes resection arthroplasty (Keller), first metatarsophalangeal (MTP) arthrodesis, and metatarsal head with or without proximal phalanx base resections of the lesser toes. IP, interphalangeal.

TABLE 3. RESULTS OF FOREFOOT SURGERY IN THE RHEUMATOID PATIENT

Study	Number of Feet	Follow-Up Duration	Conclusion

Beaucham et al (1984)[26]	34 (first MTP arthrodesis)	28 months (8–56 months)	Pain relief/improvement
			  33/34 arthrodesis
			  39/30 excisional arthroplasty

	30 (excisional arthroplasty first MTP)	48 months (6–47 months)	Balance improvement
			  13/34 arthrodesis
			  4/30 excisional arthroplasty
			Walking distance all improved
			Shoe fitting (of patients requiring custom shoes)
			  6/21 normal shoes after arthrodesis.
			  7/16 normal shoes after excisional arthroplasty

Mann and Thompson (1984)[27]	18 (first MTP arthrodesis)	4.1 years (2–7.25 years)	14/18 excellent (no pain, normal shoes) 2/18 good (no pain, open toed shoes) 2/18 fair (some pain) 0/18 poor (no improvement)

Raunio et al (1987)[28]	30 (arthrodesis)	31 ± 8 months	Functional evaluation†
			  28/30 excellent, good, or fair
			Anatomical evaluation†‡
			  25/30 excellent, good, or fair
			  23/30 better/much better
			  4/30 unchanged
			  3/30 worse

	35 (excisional arthroplasty)	44 ± 30 months	Functional evaluation†
			  28/35 excellent, good, or fair
			Anatomical evaluation†‡
			  27/35 excellent, good, or fair
			  28/35 better/much better
			  4/35 unchanged
			  3/35 worse

* Surgery includes resection arthroplasty (Keller), first MTP arthrodesis with or without lesser toe resection arthroplasty.
† Causes of dissatisfaction (not significantly different between groups): persistent pain in first MTP joint, persistent bunion, deformity recurrent, great toe hyperextension, poor first MTP motion, swelling, or other discomfort.
‡ Specific criteria not provided.
MTP, metatarsophalangeal.

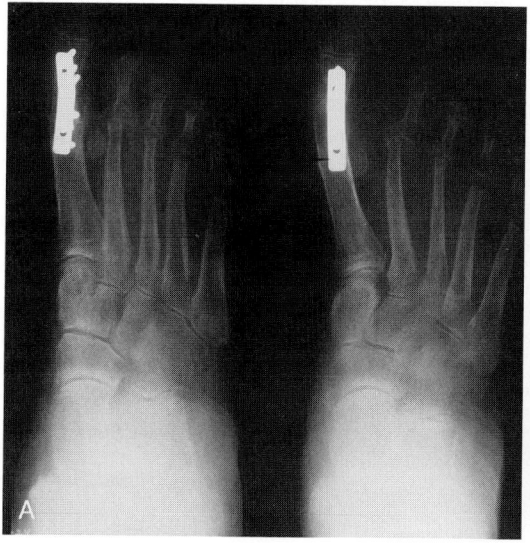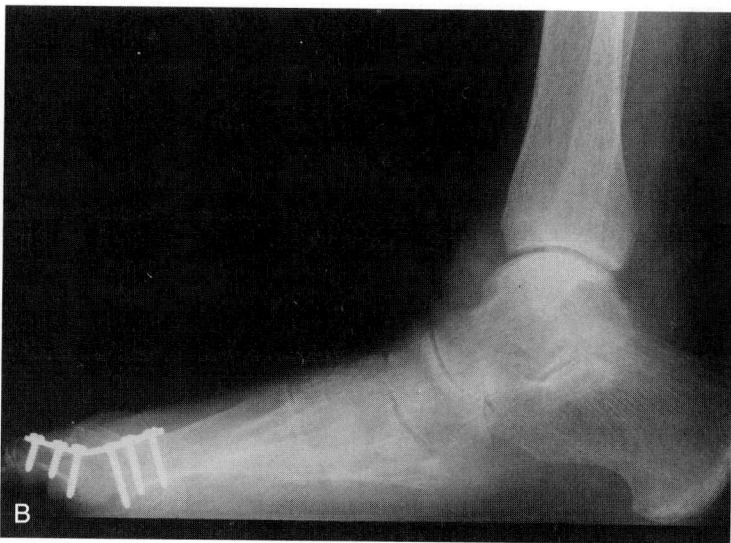

Fig. 5. Reconstructed forefoot. *A* and *B,* Standing anteroposterior, lateral, and oblique radiographs after forefoot reconstruction with first metatarsophalangeal arthrodesis and metatarsal head resection of toes 2 to 5.

ease of approach, the authors reporting on the largest series of plantar incisions for the foot do not advocate routine use of plantar incisions for procedures that are normally performed adequately through a dorsal approach.[36]

There are several key technical points leading to the improved results during metatarsal head excision for lesser toe deformity. Adequate resection of the entire metatarsal head with beveled cuts angled dorsal distal to plantar proximal decreases the incidence of residual plantar prominences. A gentle decreasing arc in the length of the second through fifth metatarsal is performed to mimic the physiological MTP joint break. The metatarsal of the great toe should be no more than 2 mm longer than the second toe. Closed osteoclasis can be performed of the PIP joints when fixed deformities are present. Smooth 0.062-mm Kirschner's wires are placed from the toe tip across the MTP joint to maintain alignment and stabilization of the lesser toes. These longitudinal pins may remain for 6 weeks postoperatively.

Hindfoot arthropathy associated with rheumatoid arthritis has been observed in 72% of females and 58% of males. In other studies examining disease duration and hindfoot involvement, 8% were found to be symptomatic when diagnosed with rheumatoid arthritis within 5 years and 25% of patients with a disease of greater than 5 years. It appears that hindfoot arthropathy secondary to rheumatoid arthritis occurs with increasing prevalence as the disease process progresses. CT scan results examining the hindfoot found subtalar involvement in 29% of patients with rheumatoid arthritis, talonavicular involvement in 39%, and calcaneocuboid joint arthropathy in 25%.[23] As a result of the coupled motion of the hindfoot complex, isolated joint disease is uncommon. With adult rheumatoid arthritis, a valgus deformity occurs through the hindfoot with a compensatory forefoot varus and abduction. These deformities can begin as flexible deformities and progress to a fixed nature. Surgical intervention has consisted of single or triple arthrodeses stabilizing the affected joint(s) with internal fixa-

tion to obtain a plantigrade foot. Bone graft may or may not be used. Fixation with 6.5 mm or larger partially threaded cancellous screws is currently recommended, although staple fixation has been used successfully in the past to achieve a stable union (see also Fig. 4C). The postoperative protocol includes a non-weightbearing short-leg cast for 6 weeks, progressing to a short-leg weightbearing cast or brace for an additional 6 weeks or until radiographic union is identified (Table 4).

Technical factors affecting outcome include the ability to restore the hindfoot to 5 to 10 degrees of valgus, stable fixation, preparation of bleeding bone surfaces to avoid a nonunion, and recognized adjacent joint disease, primarily the ankle joint, to avoid continued pain (Table 5).

COMPLICATIONS
Forefoot Surgery

There is a discrepancy in the literature regarding the recommended surgical treatment for the forefoot in a patient with rheumatoid arthritis. This major discrepancy is in treatment of the first MTP joint with an arthrodesis versus a resection arthroplasty (see Tables 2 and 3). Although resection arthroplasty, excision of the base of the proximal phalanx of the great toe, initially gave good results, long-term follow-up has demonstrated recurrent malalignment of the great toe and transfer metatarsalgia as the primary complications of this procedure. Vahvanen et al[24] found 50% of patients who underwent excisional arthroplasty of the great toe experienced valgus or varus malalignment. The first MTP joint also may spontaneously ankylose in these patients. The salvage of this situation would consist of a surgical arthrodesis in an acceptable first MTP joint position. The current recommended position for arthrodesis of the first MTP joint is approximately 15 degrees of valgus to decrease interphalangeal joint irritation and 25 to 30 degrees of dorsiflexion in relationship to the metatarsal shaft with neutral rotation. With malalignment of the great toe either through excisional arthroplasty or iatrogenic

TABLE 4. RESULTS OF TRIPLE ARTHRODESIS IN THE RHEUMATOID PATIENT

Study	No. of Feet	Follow-Up	Conclusions	Criteria
Adam and Ranawat (1976)[30]	44 hindfoot procedures 16 arthrodesis	Overall: 4 years (range, 4 months–12.5 years)	14/16 good 1/16 fair 1 1/16 poor	Retrospective study Pain relief Alignment Radiographic union
Vahvanen (1964)[11]	290	3.7 years (range, less than 1 to more than 7 years)	Good results, 85.5% Fair results, 8.6% Poor results, 5.9%	Retrospective review Functional assessment Swelling, pain, ROM Alignment
Wigren (1987)[31]	25	4.5 years (range, 6 months–11 years)	25 total pain relief (100%)	Retrospective review Pain relief
Cracchiolo et al (1990)[32]	27	44.1 months (range, 24–80 months)	92% satisfactory results	Retrospective review (Dowel technique) Patient satisfaction with operation Additional criteria Examined Pain Ability to walk Physical examination Radiographs
Figgie et al (1993)[33]	49	7–13 years (mean, 5 years)	90% satisfaction 94% decreased pain 85% increased activity 80% improvement of ambulatory status 83% complete relief of pain	Retrospective review Subjective pain scale Record activity level (non-ambulator, household, community, unlimited ambulator) PE-LE alignment, ROM Radiographs reviewed

ROM, range of motion; PE, physical examination; LE, lower extremity.

means, metatarsalgia of the lesser toes can occur. Surgical correction of the malalignment through revision arthrodesis is recommended. Additional causes of recurrent metatarsalgia include inadequate resection of the lesser metatarsal heads, leaving a residual plantar spike of bone, poor arc of resection of the lesser metatarsals, or the development of plantar cyst or soft-tissue inflammatory mass. If the lesser metatarsal heads are prominent with the residual spike of bone or have a poor arc of resection, revision surgery can be performed.

IP joint arthritis can develop after arthrodesis of the first MTP joint. A first MTP arthrodesis position in less than 15 degrees of valgus or less than 20 degrees of dorsiflexion may lead to increased stress across the IP joint during walking.[25] Salvage may consist of a revision of the arthrodesis position or fusion of the IP joint or both. Nonun-

TABLE 5. COMPLICATIONS OF TRIPLE ARTHRODESIS IN THE RHEUMATOID PATIENT: CAUSES AND POTENTIAL SOLUTIONS

Complication	Cause	Potential Solution
Nerve injury (sural nerve) Delayed wound healing (5%–15%)	Lateral approach Poor soft-tissue technique Extensive dissection Medications (prednisone)	Careful approach Careful handling of soft tissues
Progression of ankle joint symptoms (11%–20.7%)	Excessive valgus positioning with arthrodesis	Plantigrade foot positioning
	Unrecognized preexisting ankle disease	Preoperative assessment of ankle symptoms, disease
	Excessive dissection violating the ankle joint ligament and capsular structures	Soft-tissue exposure confined to subtalar talonavicular and calcaneocuboid joints
Superficial wound infection (10%)	Medications (prednisone) Poor soft-tissue technique	Meticulous soft-tissue handling Antibiotic coverage with local wound care
Nonunion (9.3% T-N, 6.5% C-C)	Inadequate surgical stabilization Inadequate postoperative immobilization	Improved surgical stabilization Postoperative casting/bracing
Avascular necrosis	Excessive dissection Concurrent vasculitis	Careful soft-tissue dissection Preoperative recognition

T-N, talonavicular; C-C, calcaneocuboid.

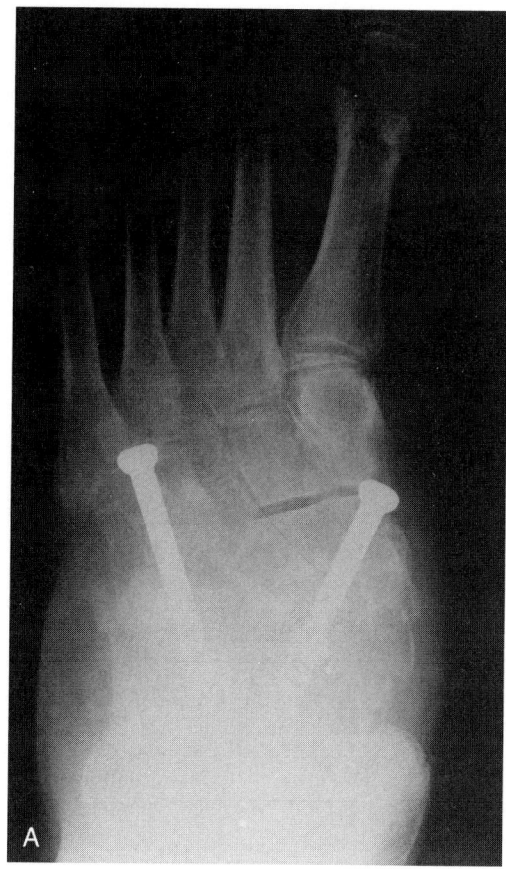

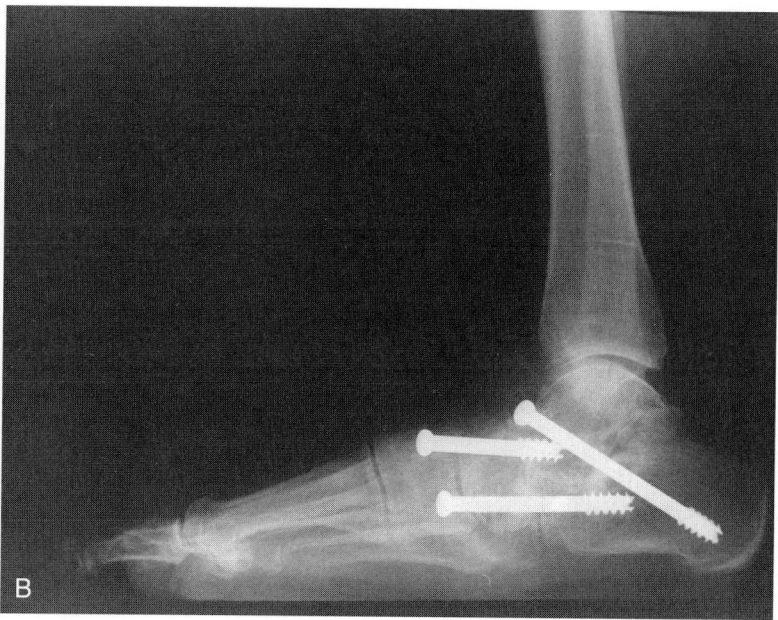

Fig. 6. Results after triple arthrodesis. *A* and *B*, Standing anteroposterior and lateral radiograph of the foot after a triple arthrodesis using three 7.3-mm cannulated screws for fixation.

ion of the first MTP joint may occur in 5% to 10% of attempted fusions. The cause of this may be secondary to inadequate immobilization or surgical fixation, and often this is asymptomatic. If symptomatic, revisions with improved surgical stabilization to include a plate and/or screw construct, cross screws, or Steinmann's pins with improved postoperative immobilization may be performed.

Wound or pin tract infection has occurred in a rare number of cases of forefoot surgery. Local wound care with or without antibiotics has provided an adequate solution to this problem.

The overall results of forefoot surgery in the rheumatoid patient population are based primarily on pain relief, function, and shoe fitting. Critical assessment of the available publications is difficult secondary to a combination of factors, among them inclusion of populations other than those with rheumatoid arthritis, collapse over surgical procedure, arthrodesis or excisional arthroplasty of the first MTP joint, and incomplete description of the criteria used to obtain the results. Some generalities can be inferred from the literature on forefoot surgery for the first MTP joint regardless of the technique used. First, patients are provided pain relief through surgical intervention of the forefoot. Second, with the incorporation of a first MTP joint arthrodesis, weightbearing function of the foot is improved, as has been demonstrated by pedobarograph analysis. This results in improved patient balance and decreased incidence of transfer metatarsalgia. The long-term follow-up studies of excisional arthroplasty of the first MTP joint (Keller's) suggest it results in increased great toe malalignment, transfer

metatarsalgia with pain, and more difficulty with shoe wear issues.

HINDFOOT SURGERY

The literature has reported several complications with a triple arthrodesis (see Table 5). Results of isolated talonavicular arthrodesis and triple arthrodesis are presented in Tables 4 and 6, respectively. Nonunion has been reported to occur in up to 15% of patients and may involve the talonavicular, calcaneocuboid, and/or subtalar joint. Nonunion of the talonavicular joint is most common, occurring in 3% to 5% of cases. The suggested causes of nonunion include inadequate exposure and an isolated lateral incision without the use of a medial incision. The lack of internal fixation without the use of screws or staples is another cause. Some believe that a bone graft supplement is necessary to prevent nonunion in cases of severe valgus deformity. Malunion or malalignment with residual valgus deformity has been reported to occur in 8% to 14% of patients undergoing a triple arthrodesis. This results in persistent lateral impingement of the calcaneus by the fibula, the potential for tibial neuritis, and the development of ankle pain. The potential cause of malalignment, again, may be the use of an isolated lateral incision for excision of all three hindfoot joints. Kitaoka[37] commented that with an isolated lateral approach more lateral bone than medial bone may be removed, leading to residual valgus malalignment. Additional causes include inadequate internal fixation with screws or staples, insufficient correction of the forefoot varus after subtalar stabilization, and an unrecognized naviculocunei-

TABLE 6. RESULTS OF TALONAVICULAR ARTHRODESIS IN THE RHEUMATOID PATIENT			
Study	No. of Feet	Follow-up	Criteria
Elbaor et al (1976)[29]	26 (RA) 5 (OA)	5 years (range, 1–13 years)	Pain (mild or absent), 30/35 Improved ambulation, 31/35
Ruff and Turner (1984)[12]	10	38.5 months (range, 9–92 months)	7 good, 3 fair (based on radiographic fusion, clinical malalignment, patient symptoms)

RA, rheumatoid arthritis; OA, osteoarthritis.

form and/or tarsometatarsal joint subluxation contributing to the valgus deformity. Care must be taken to produce a plantigrade foot position after stabilization of the subtalar joint through correction of the transverse tarsal joints. With distal fixed involvement of the naviculomedial cuneiform and/or tarsometatarsal joints, extension of the arthrodesis to include these joints may be prudent. The sural nerve can be injured through the lateral approach to the sinus tarsi, and care must be taken to protect this nerve and its branches. Delayed wound healing has been reported to occur in 5% to 15% of triple arthrodeses cases. Poor soft-tissue technique, extensive dissection of the soft tissues, and preoperative medications such as prednisone may contribute to delayed healing. Eleven to 21% of patients reported in the literature have had progression of the ankle joint symptoms after a triple arthrodesis. Contributing causes include excessive valgus positioning of the hindfoot during arthrodesis, unrecognized preexisting ankle disease, and excessive dissection violating the ankle joint ligaments and capsular structures, resulting in potential ankle malalignment or injury. Figgie et al[33] reported an increased incidence of ankle pain in patients with valgus malalignment of 10 degrees or more (62%), whereas the incidence of ankle symptoms in patients with hindfoot arthrodeses positioned in less than 10 degrees of valgus were 2.5%. This reemphasizes the goal of plantigrade foot positioning without excessive valgus. Additionally, progression of ankle joint symptoms can be avoided by recognizing preoperative disease and informing the patient of the potential complications through informed consent. When the patient experiences pain preoperatively, one should consider a pantalar arthrodesis. Soft-tissue exposure should be confined to the subtalar, talonavicular, and calcaneocuboid joints, avoiding violation of the ankle joint. Superficial wound infections were found in 10% of rheumatoid patients undergoing a triple arthrodesis. Potential causes are similar to those for delayed wound healing and include preoperative medications such as prednisone and poor soft-tissue handling techniques. Perioperative antibiotic coverage is recommended. The treatment of superficial wound infections includes additional antibiotic coverage with local wound care. A rare complication reported by Kitaoka[37] is avascular necrosis of the talus. A potential cause of avascular necrosis is excessive dissection in the region of the talus and potentially concurrent vasculitis.

REFERENCES

1. Burra G, Katchis S: Rheumatoid arthritis of the forefoot. Rheum Dis Clin North Am 1998; 24:173.
2. Markenson JA: Worldwide trends in the socioeconomic impact and long term prognosis of rheumatoid arthritis. Semin Arthritis Rheum 1991; 21:4.
3. Vainio K: The rheumatoid foot: A clinic study with pathologic and rheumatologic comments. Ann Chir Gynaecol 1956; 45:1.
4. Michelson J: Foot and ankle problems in rheumatoid arthritis. Foot Ankle Int 1994; 15:608.
5. McDuffie FC: Morbidity impact of rheumatoid arthritis on society. Am J Med 1985; 78:1.
6. Garrod AE: A treatise on rheumatism and rheumatoid arthritis. Griffin London 1890. In Haynie RL, Yakel J (eds): Perioperative management of rheumatoid patient. J Foot Ankle Surg 1996; 35:94.
7. Hoffman P: An operation for severe grades of contracted or clawed toes. Am J Orthop Surg 1911; 9:441.
8. Richardson EG: Rheumatoid foot. In Crenshaw AH (ed): Campbell's Operative Orthopaedics. St. Louis, MO, CV Mosby, 1992, vol 4, p 2763.
9. Cracchiolo A III, Swanson A, Swanson GD: The arthritic great toe metatarsophalangeal joint: A review of flexible silicone implant arthroplasty from two medical centers. Clin Orthop 1981; 157:64.
10. Sheriff MJ, Janss MH: Complications of Silastic implant arthroplasty in the hallux. Foot Ankle 1980; 1:95.
11. Vahvanen VA: Rheumatoid arthritis in the pantalar joints: A follow-up study of triple arthrodesis on 292 adult feet. Acta Orthop Scand 1964; 107:3.
12. Ruff ME, Turner RH: Selective hindfoot arthrodesis in rheumatoid arthritis. Orthopaedics 1984; 7:49.
13. Pyerich MT, Saltzman CL, Callaghan JJ, et al: Total ankle arthroplasty: A unique design. Two to twelve year follow-up. J Bone Joint Surg Am 1998; 80:1410.
14. Wolfe F: Fifty years of antirheumatic therapy: The prognosis of rheumatoid arthritis. J Rheumatol 1990; 17:24.
15. Felts W, Yelin E: The economic impact of the rheumatoid diseases in the United States. J Rheumatol 1989; 16:867.
16. Firestein GS: The immunopathogenesis of rheumatoid arthritis. Curr Opin Rheumatol 1991; 3:398.
17. Van Zeben D, Hazes JM, Vandenbrouche JP, et al: Diminished incidence of severe rheumatoid arthritis associated with oral contraceptive use. Arthritis Rheum 1990; 33:1462.
18. Arnett FC: Histocompatibility typing in the rheumatic diseases. Diagnostic and prognostic implications. Rheum Dis Clin North Am 1991; 20(2):371.
19. Spiegel TM, Spiegel JS: Rheumatoid arthritis in the foot and ankle: Diagnosis, pathology and treatment: The relationship between foot and ankle deformity and disease duration in 50 patients. Foot Ankle 1982; 2:318.
20. Keenan M, Peabody TD, Gronley JK, et al: Valgus deformity of the feet and characteristics of gait in patients who have rheumatoid arthritis. J Bone Joint Surg Am 1991; 73:237.
21. Winfield J, Yang A, Williams P, et al: Prospective study of the radiological changes in hands, feet and cervical spine in adult rheumatoid diseases. Ann Rheum Dis 1983; 42:613.
22. Smyth CJ, Hanson RW: Rheumatologic view of the rheumatoid foot. Clin Orthop Rel Res 1997; 340:7.

23. Seltzer SE, Weissman BN, Adams DF, et al: Computed tomography of the hindfoot with rheumatoid arthritis. Arthritis Rheum 1985; 28:1234.

24. Vahvanen V, Piirainen H, Kettunen P: Resection arthroplasty of the metatarsophalangeal joints in rheumatoid arthritis. Scand J Rheumatol 1980; 9:257.

25. Fitzgerald JAW: A review of long term results of arthrodesis of the first metatarsophalangeal joint. J Bone Joint Surg Br 1969; 51:488.

26. Beaucham CG, Kirby T, Rudge SR, et al: Fusion of the first metatarsophalangeal joint in forefoot arthroplasty. Clin Orthop Rel Res 1984; 190:249.

27. Mann RA, Thompson FM: Arthrodesis of the first metatarsophalangeal joint for hallux valgus in rheumatoid arthritis. J Bone Joint Surg Am 1984; 66(5):687.

28. Raunio P, Lehtimäki M, Eerola M, et al: Resection arthroplasty versus arthrodesis of the first metatarsophalangeal joint for hallux valgus in rheumatoid arthritis. Rheumatology 1987; 11:173.

29. Elbaor JE, Thomas WH, Weinfeld MS, et al: Talonavicular arthrodesis for rheumatoid arthritis of the hindfoot. Orthop Clin North Am 1976; 7:821.

30. Adam W, Ranawat C: Arthrodesis of the hindfoot in rheumatoid arthritis. Orthop Clin North Am 1976; 7:827.

31. Wigren A: Operative treatment with special regard to the hindfoot. Rheumatology 1987; 11:100.

32. Cracchiolo A, Pearson S, Kitaoka H, et al: Hindfoot arthrodesis in adults utilizing a dowel graft technique. Clin Orthop Rel Res 1990; 257:193.

33. Figgie MP, O'Mally MJ, Ranawat C, et al: Triple arthrodesis in rheumatoid arthritis. CORR 1993; 292:250.

34. Cracchiolo A III, Swanson A, Swanson GD: The arthritic great toe metatarsophalangeal joint: A review of flexible silicone implants arthroplasty from two medical centers. Clin Orthop 1981; 157:64.

35. Shereff MJ, Jahss MH: Complications of Silastic implant arthroplasty in the hallux. Foot Ankle 1980; 1:95.

36. Richardson EG, Brotzman SB, Graves SC: The plantar incision for procedures involving the forefoot. J Bone Joint Surg Am 1993; 75:726.

37. Kitaoka HB: Rheumatoid hindfoot. Orthop Clin North Am 1989; 20:593.

THE DIABETIC FOOT

section 11 chapter 5

Naomi Laird, Mark Slovenkai, and Charles L. Saltzman

Summary

- Diabetic foot complications can have an enormous social and economic impact on a patient's life.
- Tight glycemic control and proper patient foot education are the keys to prevention.
- Often, the complications progress insidiously and are well established before diagnosis.
- Peripheral neuropathy plays a leading role in the development of foot complications.
- Differentiating between Charcot's arthropathy and osteomyelitis is essential for determining appropriate care.
- In the United States approximately 50% of all nontraumatic amputations are related to end-stage complications of diabetes.

Diabetes mellitus affects approximately 15.7 million people in the United States, or 5.9% of the population,[1] of which less than 10% are type 1 and more than 90% are type 2.[2] It is estimated that 5.4 million of these patients are undiagnosed and remain asymptomatic for many years until diabetic complications surface. Death rates among middle-aged adults with diabetes are twice as high as those of nondiabetic patients of the same age.

Complications from diabetes tend to progress insidiously and are often well established at the time of diagnosis. Common long-term complications related to diabetes mellitus include retinopathy, nephropathy, neuropathy, heart disease, hypertension, stroke, peripheral vascular disease, neurogenic bladder, sexual dysfunction, infection, and diabetic foot disorders. The 1999 U.S. health care cost for treatment

of diabetes was estimated by the American Diabetes Association as $44 billion related to medical costs and another $54 billion related to disability, time lost from work, and premature mortality.

Foot problems account for approximately 20% to 25% of all hospital admissions for diabetic patients.[3] Approximately 50% of all nontraumatic amputations are related to end-stage complications of diabetes, many of which could have been prevented with early recognition, intervention, and patient education. The hardship incurred by the diabetic patient can have a tremendous economic impact, produce huge stresses on family and social relations, and sometimes predicate a complete change in lifestyle.

PATHOGENESIS

NEUROPATHY

Most diabetic foot problems are related to neuropathy. Of the three anatomically defined types of peripheral neuropathy (autonomic, sensory, and motor), *sensory neuropathy* is the leading factor in diabetic foot complications. The loss of protective sensation combined with mechanical insult undetected by the patient results in skin breakdown. The patient does not feel pain, the condition is often not perceived as worrisome, and appropriate medical care is frequently delayed. Education of the patient as well as the physician is paramount to the prevention of devastating complications.

The exact mechanism for complications caused by diabetes mellitus continues to be somewhat elusive and may be multifactorial. Diabetes affects the eyes (including the retina and cataracts), nerves, kidney, and aorta. These tissues are permeable to glucose; as glucose concentrations in the blood increase, so do the concentrations of intracellular glucose and byproducts of glucose metabolism.[4, 5] In the polyol pathway, glucose is catalyzed by the enzyme aldose reductase into sorbitol. Sorbitol is believed to be a tissue toxin and has been linked to retinopathy, nephropathy, neuropathy, aortic disease, and cataracts.[5] An accumulation of sorbitol inhibits neural synthesis of *myo*-inositol and suppresses phosphoinositide metabolism, which ultimately leads to a decrease in Na+, K+, and -ATPase activity.[4–6]

A second theory suggests the mechanism of diabetic neuropathy is related to glycosylation of proteins. Numerous proteins are affected by glycosylation, including fibrin, collagen, and lipoproteins, and the glycoprotein recognition system of hepatic endothelial cells. The effects of glycosylation on the low-density lipoprotein cause the lipoproteins to be not recognized by the normal receptors, leading to an increased half-life of low-density lipoproteins. Glycosylated collagen is less soluble and resists degradation by collagenase, trapping low-density lipoprotein at rates two to three times greater than normal collagen, which may be related to basement membrane thickening, tight waxy skin, and limitation of joint motion. Advanced glycosylation end products are formed.

During periods of hyperglycemia, the formation of sorbitol and advanced glycosylated end products is associated with the loss of myelinated and unmyelinated fibers, wallerian degeneration, and blunted nerve fiber reproduction.[4] A study by Partanen and colleagues[6] indicated that axonal degeneration may be a major factor in the cause of neuropathy due to decrease of the amplitudes of the sensory and motor responses, indicating axonal destruction. This decrease was more pronounced than the slowing of nerve conduction velocities, which is an indicator of demyelination. Reichard et al[7] found similar results. Both groups found that patients with poor glycemic control had greater incidences of neuropathy. Their results suggest that early insulin therapy for type 2 diabetes mellitus may have some neuroprotective effects. Furthermore, the Diabetes Control and Complications Trial has shown that complications caused by diabetes mellitus can be significantly reduced with tight glycemic control.[8]

Motor neuropathy typically results in intrinsic muscle atrophy, weakness, loss of function, motor imbalance, and contracture, leading to foot deformity. Claw toe deformity is most common. This common deformity leads to pressure under the metatarsal head due to weak intrinsic tendons, contracted and unbalanced extrinsic tendons, hyperextension of the proximal phalanx, and dislocation of the metatarsophalangeal (MTP) joints. The deformity leads to increased plantar pressures under the metatarsal heads and on the dorsum of the toes, both of which conditions can result in ulceration. Less commonly, mononeuropathy of the peroneal nerve can produce footdrop, which, if left untreated, can result in a fixed equinus deformity. Typical symptoms of extrinsic motor neuropathy include foot slapping, toe dragging/catching when walking, and poor coordination of legs and hands.

Autonomic neuropathy is seen as a late complication but may subclinically preface many of the other, more obvious, changes. Difficulty with testing peripheral sympathetic function makes determining the local level of involvement challenging. Clearly though, the effects of global diabetic autonomic neuropathy are great, with a 5-year mortality rate three times higher than that of patients without autonomic dysfunction. In the extremities, the clear clinical effects of autonomic neuropathy involve decreased thermal regulation and loss of normal sweating of the skin of the foot, resulting in thick, dry, scaly skin and nail deformities. The thick dry skin becomes less pliable, cracks easily, and provides entry for bacterial pathogens.

The pathophysiology of microangiopathy is complex, and the role of sympathetic dysfunction is just becoming recognized. Recent-onset diabetes is characterized by an increased tissue blood flow that is partially normalized by improved glycemic control. However, as the duration of diabetes increases, microvascular blood flow decreases, and autoregulation is lost. This pattern can be observed in diverse microvascular beds, including the eye, kidney, and skin, supporting diabetic disturbance of a basic microvascular control mechanism. There is convincing evidence that increased peripheral flow in diabetes is due to precapillary vasodilation, causing capillary hyperperfusion and, ultimately, capillary hypertension. Capillary hypertension is evident within 1 year of the diagnosis of type 1 diabetes and improves with intensified glycemic control. Capillary hypertension stimulates microvascular endothelial cells to produce more extracellular matrix proteins, leading to a thickening of the capillary basement membrane. Capillary sclerosis results, with limited microvascular blood flow, dysfunctional autoregulation, and clinical microangiopathic disease. In the foot, this results in nutritive difficulties and likely affects skin healing, fracture development, and healing and response to infection.

Charcot's neuroarthropathy may be related to motor and autonomic neuropathy. Muscle weakness leading to muscle imbalance, combined with decreased sweating, increased arteriovenous shunting, edema, and increased bone blood flow, may contribute to Charcot's neuroarthropathy.[9]

ARTERIOSCLEROTIC DISEASE

Arteriosclerotic disease is more common in diabetic patients, occurs at an earlier age, is more diffuse, accelerates faster, and is more extensive than in nondiabetic patients. Pathologically, the arterial intima and media typically show changes. In the diabetic patient, plaques develop circumferentially along the length of the vessel, and calcification occurs within the tunica media. This produces a "lead pipe" appearance on a radiograph.[3] These calcified vessels become stiff and noncompliant, making Doppler's pressure measurements inaccurate. The coexistence of diabetes mellitus, lipoprotein elevations, hypertension, and tobacco addiction increase the incidence rate and progression of atherosclerotic disease.[10] Atherosclerosis develops at major bifurcations or areas of posterior fixation or sharp angulation. A commonly affected area for diabetic patients is the popliteal trifurcation and the distal runoff of these vessels.

Lower extremity ischemia occurs more frequently in diabetic patients. Ischemia is classified as functional or critical. Functional ischemia is experienced as claudicatory pain with exercise, related to an imbalance between blood flow demand and supply. Critical ischemia has been strictly defined as recurrent resting pain, persisting for more than 2 weeks, that either requires analgesics or is related to ulceration or gangrene of the foot or toes.[10] Although these concepts are convenient for delineating the general condition of the limb, clinically these two types frequently overlap. In the diabetic patient with peripheral neuropathy and loss of sensory cues, rest pain may not be a prevalent clinical symptom. Patients with significant ischemia should undergo routine noninvasive vascular studies and possible magnetic resonance angiography or arteriography to assess the severity of disease and necessity of vascular reconstruction.

BIOMECHANICS

A variety of structural changes in the foot is associated with diabetic foot complications. These changes can accelerate callus formation, ulceration, infection, and amputation. These changes can be static or dynamic. The dynamic changes are the hardest to sort out in the clinical setting and require heightened awareness and thoughtful evaluation by the clinician.

Glycosylation of tendons and ligaments has a detrimental effect on joint range of motion. Decreased range of motion at any joint can change the biomechanics of gait and transfer load in abnormal ways. In particular, limited motion at the talocrural joint due to tightness of the gastrocnemius/ soleus complex decreases dorsiflexion and typically leads to increased forefoot plantar pressures.

A study by Oppenheim and colleagues[11] found that diabetic patients with moderate-to-severe neuropathy were significantly less stable than normal subjects. Poor stability can potentially increase the risk of injury due to loss of balance and falling. If this is combined with a static structural change (such as partial forefoot amputation or midfoot Charcot's neuroarthropathic deformity) (Fig. 1), the patient is at increased risk of further injury. The clinician must evaluate the diabetic patient's gait pattern and standing to determine if some measure of orthotic treatment will be helpful in preventing devastating complications.

CLINICAL FEATURES AND MANAGEMENT

PERIPHERAL NEUROPATHY

Diabetic peripheral neuropathy is one of the most common complications of diabetes. Paradoxically, the initial development of peripheral neuropathy may be painful. Signs and symptoms may involve a constellation of sensations including numbness, paresthesias, dysesthesias, burning (especially at night), sharp shooting pains, and tingling. Typically the symptoms are bilateral and in a stocking-and-glove pattern.

The insensate foot plays the leading role in the development of complications ending with amputation. The lack of protective sensation can permit a small, seemingly benign injury to go undetected and without medical attention. Poorly fitting shoes and repetitive pressure from underlying bony prominences can cause ulceration.

Peripheral neuropathy causes dry skin, callus development, ulcerations, fissures, claw toe deformities, and hair growth loss. Test for sensitivity or hypersensitivity with light touch, pin prick, pinwheel, and vibration. Vibratory perception may be evaluated using the tuning fork (128 cps) or a variable-frequency vibrometer. Ankle and knee reflexes should be evaluated. Ankle reflex is normally the first to become absent.

Use of the Semmes-Weinstein monofilaments may be the simplest and most reliable quantitative test. The monofilaments vary by thickness, stiffness, and area at the tip. They are graded by the amount of pressure necessary to cause the filament to buckle, which is expressed on a logarithmic scale. A fairly predictable force can be applied to the skin with a given monofilament size by placing the monofilament perpendicular to the surface of the foot and applying pressure until the filament buckles (Fig. 2). The patient is asked to respond when the monofilament is felt. Areas

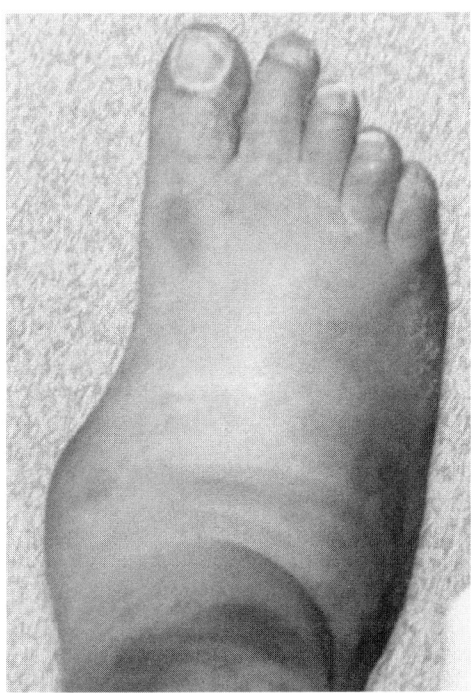

Fig. 1. Charcot's midfoot arthropathy. Note the deformity on the medial aspect of the foot.

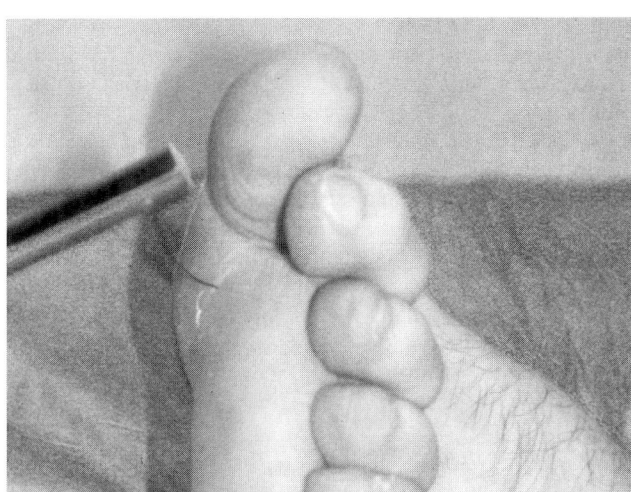

Fig. 2. Semmes-Weinstein 5.07 monofilament. This demonstrates enough pressure applied to buckle the monofilament.

tested include the plantar aspect of the great toe, the base of the fifth toe, the plantar aspects of the metatarsal heads, the medial and lateral midfoot, the plantar aspect of the heel, and the medial and lateral edges of the foot. Calloused areas are avoided. Protective sensation has been lost and the patient is at risk for ulceration if the patient cannot detect the 5.07 monofilament.[12, 13] The Semmes-Weinstein monofilaments are not perfectly predictive of impending problems, and patients who feel the 5.07 monofilament may still be at risk of ulceration and Charcot's arthropathy.

Treatment for painful peripheral neuropathy is currently aimed at symptomatic relief. Many of the pharmacological agents used are marginally successful in alleviating the painful symptoms of peripheral neuropathy. Topical capsaicin cream is sometimes helpful with burning pain and hyperesthesia. Cold soaks and massage are occasionally helpful. Current systemic therapies include tricyclic antidepressants, anticonvulsants, antiarrhythmics, local analgesics, and narcotics. Problematic adverse effects such as dry mouth, orthostatic hypotension, and arrhythmogenic potential can result from use of these agents.[14]

Tricyclic antidepressants include imipramine, desipramine, amitriptyline, and nortriptyline. These drugs act to block pain transmission pathways centrally and block norepinephrine and serotonin re-uptake.[14] Amitriptyline and imipramine primarily block serotonin pathways, whereas desipramine and nortriptyline primarily block norepinephrine re-uptake. Amitriptyline has been shown to be 60% to 75% effective in symptom relief of painful peripheral neuropathy.[15] Gabapentin is gaining popularity because of fewer adverse side effects.

Morello and colleagues[15] found that both amitriptyline and gabapentin decreased peripheral neuropathic pain with similar efficacy and rates of adverse effects. Amitriptyline is usually titrated slowly from 25 mg/day to 75 mg/day. Gabapentin is titrated slowly from 300 mg/day to as high as 3600 mg/day or the maximally tolerated dose.[14] Kumar and associates[16] conducted a study using transcutaneous electrotherapy and amitriptyline combination therapy. They found significant relief of painful symptoms with the combination of the two, indicating that electrotherapy may play a role in relieving painful peripheral neuropathy. Other drugs presently being studied, which may bring about relief, include aldose reductase inhibitors, neural growth factors, antioxidants, and alpha-lipoic acid. A 7-month multicenter, randomized, controlled trial with alpha-lipoic acid showed no significant change in symptoms.[17]

Tight glycemic control, as shown by the Diabetes Control and Complications Trial, may prevent peripheral neuropathy. Narcotics should be avoided if possible because of their addictive potential. Amitriptyline and nortriptyline are the first line of drug therapy because of their low cost. Gabapentin is a good alternative for patients for whom amitriptyline has failed or for whom it is contraindicated because of unstable angina, congestive heart failure, premature ventricular contractions, sustained arrhythmia, or conduction system disease.[14]

DIABETIC FOOT ULCERS

The most common reason diabetic patients seek medical attention is foot ulcers. It is estimated that 15% of people with diabetes develop one or more foot ulceration in the course of their disease. Diabetes is the leading cause of nontraumatic amputation of the lower extremities, and as many as 24% of diabetic patients with foot ulcers require an amputation. Unfortunately, the rates of amputation of the lower extremity in diabetic patients continue to rise rather than fall despite many advances made in the treatment of diabetes.

Recognizing and determining the mechanisms leading to diabetic foot ulcers is crucial to the selection of appropriate treatment and prevention of further ulceration. The most common location of diabetic foot ulcers is the plantar surface of the forefoot. Plantar ulcers are caused by abnormal or prolonged pressures applied to an insensate neuropathic foot. Common foot deformities (e.g., claw toes and Charcot's midfoot) contribute to the development of high focal pressure and ulcer formation. Ulcers formed on the sides and dorsal aspects of the foot are usually due to shoe pressure. Posterior heel ulcers most frequently occur during hospitalizations and are related to increased heel pressure while lying in bed. The tissue surrounding the posterior, medial, and lateral aspects of the heel is immobile and not designed for weightbearing. Because of this natural deficiency of soft-tissue coverage, a heel ulcer can lead to osteomyelitis rather quickly. Heel ulcers often do not respond well to traditional treatment for diabetic foot ulcers, commonly requiring surgical intervention with débridement, bony resection, and amputation.[3]

Phases. A brief review of wound healing is important for understanding the process of normal healing and recognizing when a wound is not progressing as expected. Further treatment is based, in part, on where in the healing process the wound has stalled. There are four phases in the wound-healing process.[18, 19]

Phase one involves the initial injury and rapid hemostasis. Wound edges retract and contract, compressing small vessels. Platelets aggregate and release cytokines and growth factors, causing the clotting cascade to be activated. Vasodilatory substances are released, initiating the migration of neutrophils.

The inflammatory phase begins when the complement system is activated, releasing chemotactic factors and other mediators. Granulocytes migrate to the wound, followed by lymphocytes, which control bacterial growth. Macrophages, the main inflammatory cells, invade the wound and phagocytose wound debris. The macrophages also stimulate fibroblast reproduction, neovascularization, and release of more chemotactic factors.

The proliferative phase begins with an increase of fibroblastic and endothelial cell migration to the wound. Epithelialization involves the production of extracellular matrix by epithelial cells. These cells form at the wound edges and progress across the wound, forming more normal layers of the epidermis. New vessel formation occurs, giving an erythematous appearance at the wound edges. Initially, collagen is laid down in an unorganized pattern.

The remodeling or *final phase* begins with the migration of keratinocytes. This phase reorganizes the collagen and improves the tensile strength. Over time, scarring contracts, and there is a return to more normal skin integrity.

Chronic wounds do not follow the organized process of normal wound healing. Diabetic foot ulcers seem to stall in either the inflammatory or proliferative phase. Why some of these ulcers remain relatively unchanged for weeks, months, or years and others go on to deep infection remains a mystery. Because of the unpredictability of foot ulcers, no ulcer should go untreated or be allowed to remain stagnant. Failure to progress is a signal for the practitioner to ask, "Where in the healing process is the ulcer stalled and why? Is the pressure being relieved? Is infection present? Is the patient being compliant? Is surgical intervention necessary?"

Classifications. Diabetic foot ulcers are a primary precursor to infection and amputation. Grading or classifying the ulcer may aid in determining appropriate treatment and best outcome for the patient. The Wagner classification is the most widely accepted and used system in clinical practice for the grading of diabetic foot ulcers. This classification was developed by Wagner and Meggitt in the 1970s and provides common language for communication among clinicians. The Wagner classification system has six grades, the first four pertaining to the depth of the ulcer and presence of infection: grade 0, no open lesion; grade 1, superficial; grade 2, deep; and grade 3, deep with infection. Vascular status is rated in the last two grades: grade 4 is partial gangrene, and grade 5 is global foot gangrene.[3, 20]

Brodsky[3] proposed a modification of the Wagner classification based on depth and ischemia. According to this scheme, grade 0 is a foot "at risk," a foot that has had a history of ulceration or disease that could lead to ulceration; grade 1, superficial ulceration and not infected; grade 2, deep ulceration exposing tendon or joint, with or without infection; and grade 3, extensive ulceration with exposed bone and/or deep infection or abscess. Ischemia is classified separately. These grades are combined with an ischemia classification: grade A, not ischemic; grade B, ischemia without gangrene; grade C, partial forefoot gangrene; and grade D, complete foot gangrene.

A third classification, the University of Texas Diabetic Wound Classification System, grades and stages ulcers as follows: grade 0, a pre- or postulcerative site that is healed; grade 1, superficial through the epidermis, or epidermis and dermis, but not penetrating to bone, tendon, or joint; grade 2, penetrated to tendon or capsule; and grade 3, penetrated to bone or into the joint. Each grade is further staged: stage A, clean not infected; stage B, nonischemic infected; stage C, ischemic noninfected; and stage D, infected ischemic wound.[21] All the grading systems are beneficial for helping understand where a wound lies in the spectrum of disease, helping identify appropriate therapy, and predicting outcome.

Evaluation. Treatment of diabetic foot ulcers involves an initial careful physical examination. All wounds must be inspected, palpated, and probed to determine the depth and extent of the wound: its odor, location, appearance, and temperature. Probe the ulcer, looking for tracks leading to tendon, abscess, bone, or into the joint. The authors of this chapter ask a series of simple questions: Does the wound have a foul odor? What color is the drainage (if any) from the ulcer? Is there granulation tissue in the base of the ulcer? How much callus is surrounding the ulceration, and can this be inhibiting collagen matrix formation? Are there areas of eschar or necrosis? What has been the treatment to date?

The clinician can evaluate the vascular system by looking for hair growth on the toes, checking capillary refill and palpating for the presence of dorsalis pedis pulse and posterior tibial pulse. The presence of a pulse does not mean focal ischemia does not exist. The absence of this pulse may mean that further vascular evaluation is required.

Determining the presence of infection is vital. Perhaps the best indicator of infection is a recent loss of normal glycemic control. All ulcers are superficially colonized; thus, swabbing every ulcer is not useful and can be misleading. Infected ulcers usually drain; tend to be deeper than grade 1; have surrounding erythema, cellulitis, and varied amounts of edema; and the patient may have generalized foot and leg swelling or lymphadenitis. Probing to bone in this setting is strongly predictive of osteomyelitis. Initial radiograph may be negative for osteomyelitis. Limb- or life-threatening infections should be treated with broad-spectrum intravenous antibiotics and hospitalization. Local infections not involving bone can be treated initially with outpatient oral therapy and reevaluated in 48 to 72 hours.

Treatment. The first line of treatment for any ulcer is relief of pressure. Relief of all mechanical stress is imperative to successful healing. Treatment depends on the grade and location of the ulcer, presence of infection, compliance of the patient, success of previous treatments, and the skill of the clinician. Options for pressure relief (off-loading) include bedrest, healing sandals, custom full-contact inserts, bivalved ankle-foot orthoses, total contact casting (TCC), and cast boots of various types. Bedrest can aid in the healing process of ulcerations; however, this is not a benign treatment. The negative effects of bedrest include deconditioning and risks of thrombosis/embolism and pneumonia. Complete bedrest is not generally recommended. Patients with foot ulcers should not be treated in their own shoes, which cannot accommodate dressings and are often heavily contaminated with bacteria.

Crutches, a walker, and especially a wheelchair may assist with off-loading. Total non-weightbearing is usually quite difficult for the patient with peripheral neuropathy. The patient often has trouble with maintaining balance on the other, often insensate, foot. Moreover, the patient frequently cannot detect when the injured foot is on the floor.

Frequent follow-up is important for patients with diabetic foot ulcers in order to assess treatment efficacy and evaluate for unrecognized infection. The ulcer can be traced on nonexposed radiograph and documented in the patient's chart. Maximum length and width dimensions can also be recorded for quick reference. With this method, clinicians can recognize ulcers not responding to treatment.

Ulcer treatment begins with débridement. Sharp débridement to "saucerize" the hyperkeratotic rind surrounding the ulcer should be performed. Removal of this tissue allows the clinician to establish the true size of the ulcer and relieve shear stresses to allow development of new peripheral granular tissue. Débridement alone is not sufficient treatment; it must be combined with off-loading. Solutions such as Dakin's (hypochlorite) solution, acetic acid soaks, hydrogen peroxide, and povidone-iodine solutions should be avoided; these solutions can be toxic to tissues.

Selecting a dressing should be aimed at establishing the optimal wound healing environment, providing a barrier to infection, and protecting against further damage. Cost must also be considered; the clinician must address this because patients may be reluctant to admit that they cannot afford the selected therapy. Treatment options include moist saline gauze, silver sulfadiazine cream, petrolatum gauze, and hydrocolloids to prevent drying out. Newer treatments available and under investigation are cultured human dermis, granulocyte colony stimulating factor, growth factor, platelet derivative (becaplermin), ketanserin, hyperbaric oxygen therapy, and electrical stimulation. Studies have compared newer forms of dressing—such as the calcium alginate glycyl-histidyl-lysine-Cu2$^+$ complex topical gel, collagen-alginate dressing, polyurethane foam, and polyurethane gel dressing—with the traditional saline gauze dressing. The majority of these studies found no significant difference in healing between the groups.[22] Dermal replacements, consisting of allogeneic fibroblasts grown on a resorbable matrix, may soon be available in the United States; they have been approved in Australia, England, Canada, Denmark, Finland, Norway, the Netherlands, and New Zealand.[23, 24] Dermal replacements may be an alternative for the patients for whom skin grafting is needed.

TCC remains the "gold standard" treatment for diabetic neuropathic foot ulcers. Studies have shown that plantar ulcers heal quicker with TCC.[25–27] Shaw and associates[25] found three mechanisms that allow TCC to off-load the plantar aspect of the forefoot: (1) transfer of approximately 30% of the load from the leg to the cast wall, (2) increased load sharing by the heel, and (3) creation of a cavity by the foam covering the forefoot, which removes the load from the metatarsal heads. This study indicates that TCC is excellent treatment for forefoot ulcers but may not be ideal for heel ulcers. Other studies, however, do indicate that TCC may be effective in healing heel ulcers, with prolonged casting.[26] A cast is contraindicated in the presence of infection, severe arterial insufficiency, or poor patient compliance. Ulcers on the sides and dorsa of feet are usually from shoe pressure and do not respond as well to circumferential casting. Heel ulcers may respond to an ankle-foot orthosis designed to relieve heel pressure.

Care must be taken when applying and removing a total contact cast; this usually requires a skilled clinician (Fig. 3). Do not overpad; as the padding compresses in the cast, the foot can shear within the cast and develop new ulcerations. A closed toe cast is most desirable. The closed environment may aid in healing and limit toe motion. Claw toe deformities increase pressure on the metatarsal heads. Placing the toes in slight plantar flexion decreases hyperextension of the MTP joints and plantar pressure on the metatarsal heads. Selective padding of the malleoli, the anterior aspect of the tibia, the dorsum of the toes, and any prominent bony areas such as from Charcot's deformity is recommended. Initially, the cast is changed weekly and then, depending on drainage, at 2- to 3-week intervals.

Complication can occur from TCC. Movement inside the cast may cause new superficial blisters or ulceration. Care must be taken to examine the insensate foot at each cast change. TCC can usually continue when superficial complications arise. When problems arise, reevaluate the padding procedure, and ensure that the foot is fully dorsiflexed during application of each cast. If a new ulcer appears, the patient is usually placed into a cast boot with a soft, full-contact liner.

Patients with tight Achilles tendons are at risk for ulcerations of the forefoot. A study by Armstrong and associates[28] indicated percutaneous lengthening of the Achilles tendon reduces plantar pressures on the forefoot. This technique may be combined with TCC and can be performed with a local anesthetic in the office.

After successful healing, the clinician should apply new prevention strategies. Custom inserts, extra-depth shoes, custom shoes, ankle-foot orthosis, or surgical intervention to repair claw toe or Charcot's deformity may be advisable. The initial phase after removal from a cast is the time when an ulcer is most likely to recur. This period requires

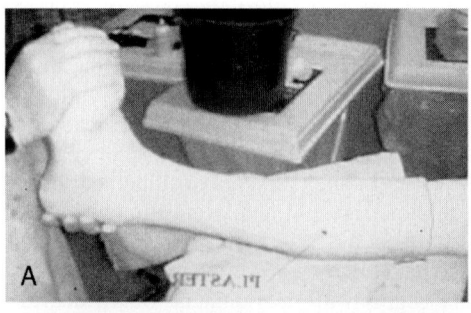
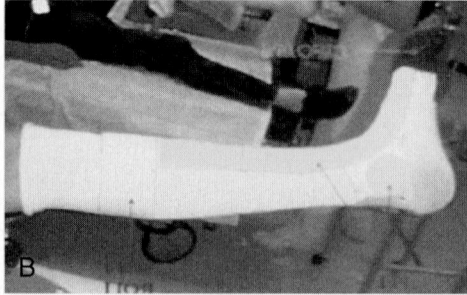
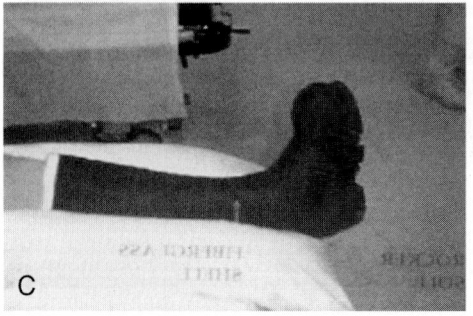
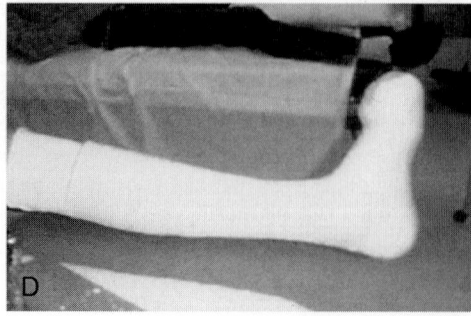

Fig. 3. Total contact cast. *A,* Application of lamb's wool between toes, cast sock, felt padding, and Sifoam. *B* and *C,* Plaster application using 4-inch orthoflex, 30-inch plaster splint, and fast-setting plaster rolls covered in a carapace of fiberglass with a walking base application.

vigilant attention to shear stress control and activity limitation.

Failure of the diabetic foot ulcer to heal or recurrent ulcers may be an indication for surgical intervention. The forefoot is the most common area of involvement. Claw toe deformity often causes ulcers on the dorsum of the proximal interphalangeal joint, at the plantar aspect of the metatarsal head, or the tip of the toe. As long as osteomyelitis does not exist, these deformities often respond to correction. For toe-tip ulcers, a simple flexor tenotomy may be helpful. In less flexible cases, preferably after ulcer closure, hemiresection procedures generally work. Metatarsophalangeal plantar ulcers may respond to a simple plantar condylectomy, a procedure usually performed after ulcer healing. Ulcerations of the hallux occur often at the plantar-medial aspect and are caused by hallux valgus and hallucal pronation. Pressure may be relieved by partial resection of the condyle, standard metatarsal osteotomy and realignment, hemiresection of the base of the hallux (Keller's procedure), or phalangeal base osteotomy. In these patients, osteotomies are not routinely performed because of concerns regarding healing. Ulcerations under the first metatarsophalangeal joint can lead quickly to osteomyelitis of the sesamoid bones and of the first metatarsal head. Ulcerations in this area may require resection of the medial sesamoid or, in highly selected cases, dorsiflexion osteotomy of the first metatarsal. All forefoot procedures can be combined with an Achilles tendon lengthening or a gastrocnemius fascial slide.

Charcot's deformities increase the risk of foot ulceration from the development of focally increased pressure. Large bony prominences that appear at the plantar-medial or lateral aspects of the foot sometimes cause large ulcerations (Fig. 4). Surgical options include realignment arthrodesis or removal of the bony protuberances (exostectomy).

Lateral foot ulcerations are most often caused by hindfoot varus deformity and are found over the base of the fifth metatarsal. Resection of the bony prominence may lead to further problems such as loss of function of the peroneus brevis or increased pressure on the new bony prominence. If flexible, the hindfoot deformity may be corrected by a custom AFO. Other patients may require correction of the hindfoot deformity with calcaneal osteotomy, or if midtarsal deformity coexists, a triple arthrodesis.

CHARCOT'S JOINTS

Charcot's neuroarthropathy is a destructive condition that can progress rapidly, resulting in severe debilitating deformity, leading to ulceration, infection, and amputation of the foot and ankle. Jean-Martin Charcot first described this condition in 1868 when he found the neuropathic component associated with syphilis. In 1936, Jordon found the association of Charcot's joint with diabetes mellitus.[3, 29-31] The most common theories regarding the pathophysiology of Charcot's joint suggest that there are vascular and traumatic components. The belief is that autonomic neuropathy leads to increased blood flow to the area, resulting in increased bone resorption and subsequent osteopenia. Combined with abnormal stresses on the foot from motor neuropathy and undetected injury from sensory neuropathy, all these conditions are thought to lead to development of Charcot's foot in diabetes. Typically, a patient with Charcot's joint has been diagnosed with diabetes for 10 years, is older, and is overweight,[29, 30] although Charcot's joint can be the first sign of diabetes mellitus.[3] Charcot's joint develops in approximately 1% to 2.5% of diabetic patients; approximately 30% of those patients develop Charcot's joints bilaterally.[3, 30]

Presenting signs of Charcot's joint are relatively painless swelling and erythema of the foot and ankle. Deformity, if present, may be a fracture, subluxation, dislocation, or fracture/dislocation of sudden or insidious onset.

Staging of Charcot's Joints. Staging was first described by Eichenholtz in 1966. His system was based on radiographic appearance as the joint progressed from the initial occurrence through the healing process. Stage I is an acute inflammatory process. The patient presents with a painless, edematous, and erythematous foot. Radiographs show fragmentation or dislocation (Fig. 5A). All too often, this stage goes unrecognized by the clinician or is thought to be an infection. Stage II is coalescence, during which the reparative process begins. Edema, erythema, and warmth decrease, and radiographs show coalescence and resorption of bony fragments and new bone formation (see Fig. 5B). Stage III is the consolidation stage of healing. Mature bone is noted on radiograph (see Fig. 5C) and, clinically, inflammation resolves. The patient is usually left with a fixed deformity.

Management. The goal is to ultimately achieve a plantigrade, clinically stable foot that can fit into a shoe or brace. Healing can be a long and tiresome process, frustrating for the patient and physician. Reasonable goals and expectations need to be set early, and the patient must ensure compliance during the healing process in order to optimize results and decrease complications. Nonoperative treatment should be attempted before any surgical procedures are considered.

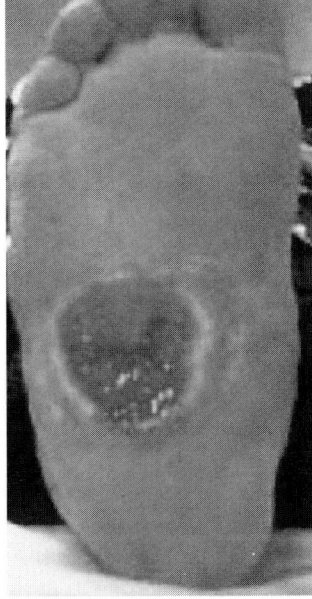

Fig. 4. Charcot's mid-foot arthropathy. This has a plantar ulcer.

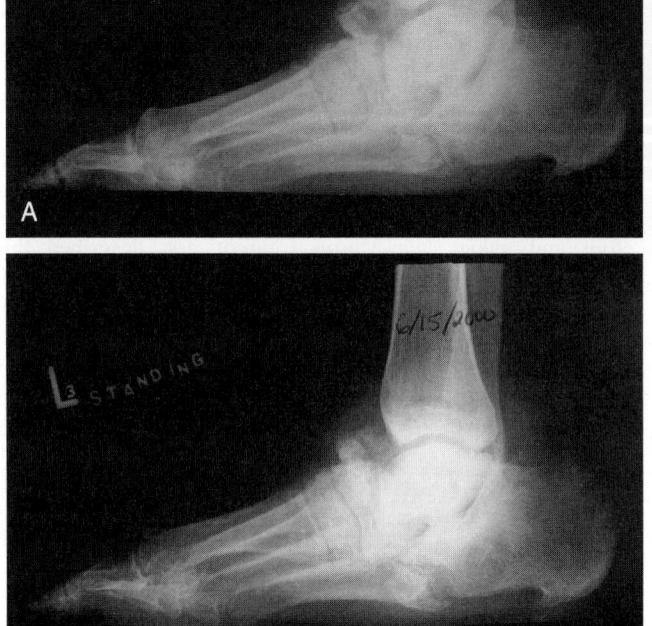

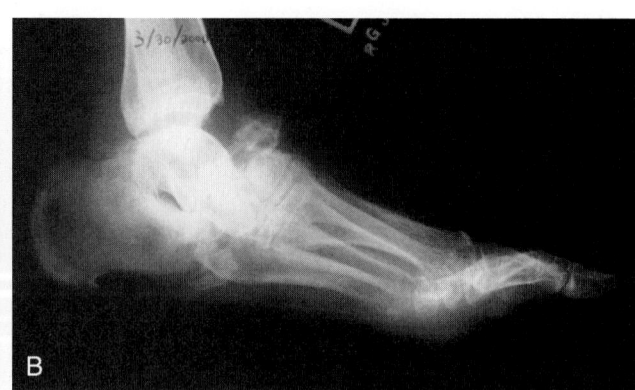

Fig. 5. Views. *A,* Radiograph of Charcot's arthropathy, stage I, dissolution, showing osseous fragmentation and dislocation. *B,* Radiograph of same patient in stage II, coalescence of Charcot's arthropathy, showing osseous coalescence and resorption of bony fragments. *C,* Stage III resolution, showing bony consolidation and remodeling, leaving a fixed deformity.

The initial treatment involves non-weightbearing TCC, rest, and elevation. There is rapid edema reduction, and the first cast change should be done within the first week. Individual leg volume decreases will determine the cast change interval. A general guideline is to change the cast at 1 week, 3 weeks, 6 weeks, 9 weeks, and 12 weeks.

Periodic radiographic evaluation can aid in determining the progress from Eichenholtz stage I to stage II. Clinical evaluation will reveal decreased edema, erythema, and warmth, with minimal daily variations in swelling. Commercially available volumeters or skin thermistors can help this assessment. The examiner can palpate increased stability of the foot by manual stress testing. Cast boots and prefabricated braces are available and may be an alternative for a patient for whom casting is contraindicated. The disadvantage of the brace is the lack of a custom fit and potential slippage. Some deformities do not fit into any of the "off-the-shelf" braces.

When a Charcot joint has advanced into stage II and volume fluctuations are minimal, the foot can be placed in a removable, bivalved, full-contact AFO or Charcot's Restraint Orthotic Walker (CROW) (Fig. 6). The CROW is a custom orthosis that is removable. It has a rocker bottom to aid in ambulation and can have a wedge or out-flare added to achieve proper ground reaction forces. This custom-molded device can accommodate severe deformity.

Some authors recommend the use of the patellar tendon–bearing brace (PTB),[32] whereas others discourage use of this brace for Charcot's joints.[3] Saltzman et al[33] found that the PTB decreased mean peak forces to the hindfoot by 32%; with extra padding, the forces were decreased by 37%. The forces in the midfoot area were not decreased more than in a shoe alone. This study indicated that the PTB may be useful for hindfoot Charcot's joints but not for midfoot or forefoot Charcot's joints. The problem with the PTB, though, is poor patient acceptance and the risk of ulceration over the patellar tendon, a potentially devastating complication in this patient population.

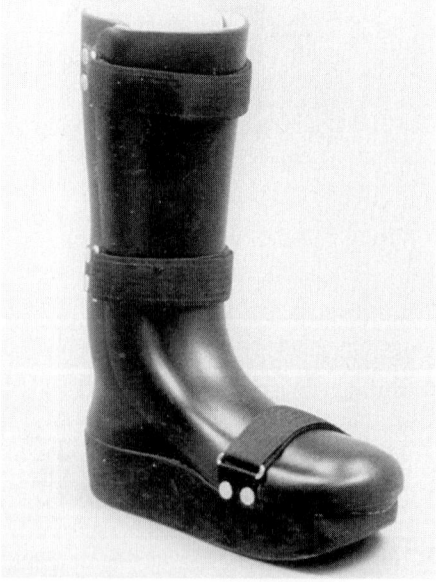

Fig. 6. Charcot's restraint orthotic walker. This is a bivalved full contact ankle-foot orthosis.

Eichenholtz stage III is reached when a Charcot joint is clinically stable and has achieved bony consolidation on radiograph evaluation. This usually occurs some time between 6 and 18 months after initial presentation. Treatment at this stage varies by the severity and location of the deformity. The patient is fitted with a custom dual-density accommodative insole and appropriate footwear, such as an extra-depth shoe, a custom-made shoe, or a properly fitting jogging or walking shoe. Most patients can fit into a properly fitted off-the-shelf shoe with custom accommodative inserts. Referral to an orthotist or pedorthist who is experienced with Charcot's joints is advantageous. Patients with severe hindfoot deformity may require a permanent CROW or a posterior-shell AFO with molded insole.

Complications. Complications associated with Charcot's joints include chronic ulcerations, infection, osteomyelitis, and severe uncontrollable deformity. The ulcerations should be treated initially as discussed earlier in this chapter. Once healed, surgical intervention may be necessary. Infection usually results from a nonhealing ulcer and must be treated with appropriate antibiotics and surgical intervention such as débridement or amputation. On healing, correction of the deformity may be necessary with a realignment arthrodesis or excision of the bony prominence.

INVESTIGATION

INITIAL SCREENING AND PHYSICAL EXAMINATION

Evaluation of the diabetic patient should begin as the patient enters the examination room. Observe the patient's gait, whether the pelvis is level, foot placement, and slapping of the foot (footdrop) with ambulation. Then examine the shoes for wear pattern and for nails or other objects that may cause harm to the foot.

Documentation of the evaluation (Fig. 7) is important for comparison at follow-up visits and for monitoring progression of diabetic foot complications. Observe the skin for trauma, erythema, dryness, calluses, and edema. Check especially between web spaces. Dry skin can crack, providing an avenue for bacteria. Erythema may indicate cellulitis or irritation from a shoe or from where a brace is rubbing. Calluses can have an infection or ulceration beneath them. Edema could be an indication of cellulitis, arterial or venous insufficiency, or development of Charcot's joint. Palpate the skin temperature with the back of your hand. A red, hot, and swollen extremity may indicate infection or Charcot's joint. Elevation of the extremity may cause the erythema to resolve; this simple technique can help differentiate cellulitis from infection and erythema from Charcot's joint. Erythema from cellulitis does not resolve with elevation. Furthermore, a break in skin integrity in the region of redness strongly suggests infection.

An ulcer's outline should be traced onto acetate and placed in the patient's chart, or a photograph should be taken and placed in the chart. Measure and document the length, width, and depth of the ulcer. Make note of any underlying structures seen or probed. Look for an ulcer track by probing the ulcer with a blunt instrument or cotton-tipped applicator. Probing to bone should heighten suspicion for osteomyelitis. Document any drainage and its color and odor. Palpate for lymphadenopathy. Evaluate the nails for discoloration, thickened mycosis, in-curving, or paronychial infections. Is hair growth of a normal pattern, or has it decreased? Palpate the pulses, including the dorsalis pedis and posterior tibial pulses, and check for capillary refill. An absence of or delayed capillary refill is indicative of venous insufficiency, and absent pulses indicate peripheral arterial disease.[29]

Sensory examination should be documented. The Semmes-Weinstein monofilament 5.07 may be used for evaluation of protective sensation (see the earlier section on Peripheral Neuropathy). Diagram the areas of decreased sensation in the patient's chart.

Examine active and passive range of motion at the ankle and hallux as well as mobility or instability of the midfoot. In particular, determine the amount of allowable dorsiflexion of the ankle, a potential major factor in the development of mid- and forefoot problems. Assess resisted range of motion of dorsiflexion, inversion, eversion, and motion of the extensor hallux longus and flexor hallux longus. Evaluate for deformities such as claw toe, hammer toe, hallux valgus and hallux rigidus, hindfoot varus, and collapse of the longitudinal arch, often seen with Charcot's joints.

FOCUSED VASCULAR EXAMINATION

Vascular evaluation is often necessary to determine the healing potential of the diabetic patient. Patients with non-healing ulcers or nonpalpable pulses require further vascular evaluation. Arterial Doppler's ultrasound pressure measurements are most commonly used. Doppler ultrasound is a good screening device but often should not be used as the sole determinant of healing potential in diabetic patients. Vascular assessment often requires a combination of objective data and clinical vascular expertise.

A screening evaluation using the ankle-to-brachial index is widely employed. This involves dividing the ankle pressure on each side by the higher of the two brachial artery pressures. The severity of occlusive disease is indicated by the values determined. Normal values should be equal to or greater than 1, and values less than 0.9 are considered abnormal.[10] Rest pain usually occurs with values between 0.3 and 0.5. Patients with calcified vessel walls may have a falsely elevated index. False values should be suspected if elevated to 1.3 or greater and/or does not match the patient's clinical picture. Patients with normal values should have palpable ankle pulses.

Segmental pressures taken at different levels of the leg can aid in determining the level of the occlusive disease. Measurements taken from the thigh, upper calf, and immediately above the ankle are taken, and a gradient is determined. Gradients greater than 20 mm Hg between sites indicate occlusive disease.

A leg with a calf pressure of 65 to 70 mm Hg can usually heal a below-knee amputation; pressures below 50 mm Hg decrease the healing potential to approximately 40%. An ankle pressure greater than 40 mm Hg is a good indicator of healing at this level. Ankle pressures less than 30 to 40 mm Hg are a poor indicator of potential for healing of partial foot amputations. Transcutaneous oxygen measured with laser Doppler below 40 mm Hg and abso-

DIABETIC FOOT EVALUATION

Patient's Name _____ DOB __/__/__ Clinical Chart# _____

Diabetes Mellitus: Type 1/Type 2 # of Years with DM _____

Treatment: Insulin Oral Diet

Tobacco Use: Yes / No Pack years _____ ETOH use: Amount _____

Co-morbidity: Peripheral Neuropathy_____, Nephropathy _____, Retinopathy _____, CAD _____,
Peripheral vascular disease _____.

History of: Numbness _____, Paresthesia/Dysesthesia _____, Absence of pain with injury _____

Exam:

1. Gait:

2. Skin: Dry/scaly   Keratosis (callus) location:

   Temperature - warm/cool   Dependent rubor

   Ulceration: size - L _____ x W _____ x D _____

   Drainage: Purulent/Clear/Serous   Odor: Left/Right

   Erythema: Location_____   Decrease with elevation?   Yes/No

   Lymphadenopathy: Location _____

3. Nails _____ Hair growth _____ Toe web space _____

4. Pulses: Dorsalis pedis–R____ L ____, Posterior tibialis–R____ L ____ Cap Refill–R____ L____

7. Sensory Exam: Semmes- Weinstein (5.07)   L/R
   A = absent   P = present   D = decreased

8. Range of motion   Right/Left

   Ankle

   Hallux

9. Resisted range of motion: Right/Left

10. Deformities:

Fig. 7. Sample clinical intake form. This is for diabetic foot evaluation.

lute toe systolic pressure below 45 mm Hg are considered abnormal, and toe or skin pressures less than 30 mm Hg suggest poor healing potential.[10, 21]

Segmental plethysmography recorders measure changes in volume of the limb by evaluating the waveform of arterial inflow. As occlusive disease progresses, the normal triphasic wave pattern flattens and loses the characteristic notch. Segmental plethysmography can reveal monophasic flow patterns in the patient with stiff arteries due to calcification.

The Duplex scan can evaluate blood flow of peripheral arteries in the lower extremity. A pulsed Doppler is combined with real-time B-mode ultrasonographic imaging. This technique enables the evaluation of velocity patterns at a particular point along the vessel. The Duplex scan assigns color to indicate the mean velocity at the chosen point. Red and blue indicate flow toward and away from the transducer, representing real-time flow patterns. The Duplex scan is useful from the aorta to the tibial branches and may also help with imaging the venous system.

IMAGING
Radiographs

Radiographs are the first imaging choice in the arsenal of diagnostic studies when evaluating the diabetic foot. Radiographs have limited use when evaluating for acute osteomyelitis but are helpful later in the disease. Infection may be identified by periosteal reaction, lytic cavities, or radiodense sequestra. Osteolysis may be seen on plain film in the distal forefoot to mid-metatarsal level, usually as "penciling" of the distal metatarsal or a vanishing phalanx.[3] This suggests an underlying neuropathic disorder and is thought to reflect sympathetic nerve–induced hyperemia and bone resorption. Charcot's joints may be seen on radiographs as fracture/dislocations or fragmentation of bone. Early on, Charcot's changes may not be easily identified or may present simply as localized osteopenia.

Nuclear Medicine Imaging

Technetium 99m bone scans are highly sensitive and remain positive 2 to 4 weeks after the onset of infection. Whereas a negative scan can strongly exclude the diagnosis of osteomyelitis, a positive result is not specific for infection and can reveal uptake from fractures or Charcot's joints. Gallium 67 citrate becomes positive early in the infection process, approximately 24 to 48 hours after the onset of infection, and returns to normal approximately 6 weeks after treatment. Gallium 67 citrate has a low sensitivity for small-bone infection, relatively poor resolution, and requires a large amount of purulent material and active white cell phagocytosis to image properly. Gallium scans also become positive with cellulitis, arthritis, and fractures, so the usefulness in this testing is low.

Indium 111-labeled white blood cell scans are believed to be a specific, valuable tool in the evaluation of osteomyelitis. In this test, the patient's white cells are tagged with indium 111, which then localizes to areas of bone infection seen with osteomyelitis. A method used to improve sensitivity is to combine the indium scan with a technetium bone scan. This simultaneous dual-window imaging approach is particularly helpful in differentiating a Charcot joint from infection. When comparing the two scan results, if the area positive on indium overlies the same positive area on the technetium scan, then osteomyelitis is a likely diagnosis. Should the positive area of the indium localize in the soft tissue or more superficially to the area of uptake on the technetium scan, then cellulitis or abscess may be the diagnosis. If the delayed-phase technetium scan is hot and the indium scan is not, then the patient likely has a Charcot fracture or dislocation. Not infrequently, bone biopsy is required to make a definitive diagnosis.

Magnetic Resonance Imaging

Magnetic resonance imaging has become a standard option in the evaluation of infection in the diabetic foot. The magnetic resonance image is more sensitive than the bone scan and detects osteomyelitis sooner, but certain limitations exist. Any condition causing an increase in intramedullary edema causes a change in bone marrow signal, making it difficult to differentiate between osteomyelitis and bone edema from Charcot's joint, acute injury, tumor, or healing fracture.[3, 34] The image can differentiate cellulitis

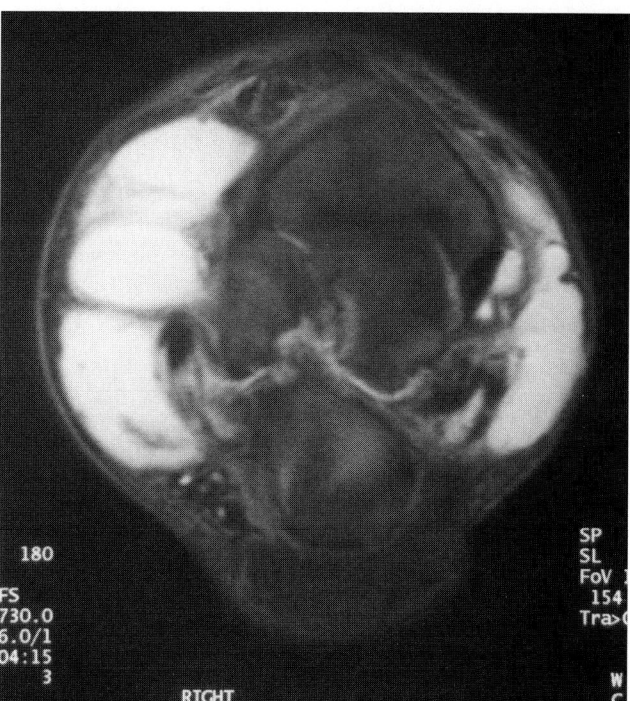

Fig. 8. Magnetic resonance image. A right foot and ankle define multiple abscesses on the medial and lateral aspects of the hindfoot.

from osteomyelitis and is particularly helpful in delineating abscesses (Fig. 8).

Computed Tomography

Computed tomography was once the best means of identifying osteomyelitis, providing multiplanar and three-dimensional images of body structures by computer enhancement and magnification of subtle chemical and density differences. Although tomography is helpful in evaluating cortical bone and sequestra, soft-tissue tumors, subtle or complex fractures, and intra-articular abnormalities, it has difficulty in determining the transition zone between infection and normal tissue. Computed tomography has largely been supplanted by magnetic resonance imaging and currently has a limited role in diabetic foot evaluation.

COMPLICATIONS

INFECTION

The primary cause of hospitalization for complications of diabetes is related to lesions of the foot. In the United States alone, more than 50,000 lower extremity amputations are performed annually at a cost of over $1 billion.[35] Diabetic foot infections are typically polymicrobial and include gram-positive cocci, gram-negative bacilli, and anaerobes.[36, 37] The most common organisms are *Staphylococcus aureus*, *Streptococcus*, group A and B streptococci, gram-negative *Pseudomonas*, *Acinetobacter*, *Enterobacter*, *Escherichia*, *Klebsiella*, and anaerobic *Bacteroides*, *Peptostreptococcus*, *Clostridium*, and *Prevotella*.[37–40] These organisms may work synergistically and cause great and rapid destruction in compromised hosts.

Factors that influence healing of diabetic foot infections include bacterial load, vascular impairment, immunocompromised state from neutrophil depletion or dysfunction, and nutritional status. The usual signs of infection are often absent in the diabetic foot. Fever, chills, and elevated leukocyte count are not common and, if present, may indicate a systemic illness. Elevation of normal glycemic control is probably the best systemic indicator of infection. Laboratory assessment can include a complete blood cell count with differential, erythrocyte sedimentation rate, acute metabolic profile, and C-reactive protein. However, these studies are less helpful in identifying or following a diabetic foot infection than in nondiabetic infections. Radiographic evaluation is often initially normal.

The clinical diagnosis of infection should be based initially on a history of recent loss of glycemic control and the physical findings of erythema, cellulitis, increased drainage and, occasionally, tenderness. Probing a sinus tract to the bone is a strong indicator for underlying osteomyelitis.[41] Another indicator of underlying osteomyelitis in a diabetic foot is the development of a "sausage toe" deformity associated with ulceration.[42]

Antibiotic therapy should be broad spectrum and directed toward the most likely combination of gram-positive cocci, gram-negative rods, and anaerobes. Rarely is the infection caused by a single microbial organism. Traditionally, broad spectrum antimicrobial therapy (Table 1) included two to three drugs such as an aminoglycoside, a β-lactamase–resistant penicillin, and metronidazole. Aminoglycoside antimicrobials should be used with caution because of neph-

rotoxicity. Diabetic patients often already have impaired renal function. Aztreonam may be substituted for the aminoglycoside.

Third-generation cephalosporins have increased coverage for gram-negative organisms; there is less coverage for gram-positive organisms. Ceftazidime provides coverage against *Pseudomonas aeruginosa*. Imipenem, a carbapenem, is active against *Pseudomonas* as well as gram-positive staphylococci and enterococci. Combination drugs are often required in diabetic foot infections because of their broad spectrum coverage. Examples of the combination drugs are piperacillin/tazobactam, ampicillin/sulbactam, and ticarcillin/clavulanic acid.[3, 43, 44]

Diamantopoulos and associates[45] found that the combination of intravenous ciprofloxacin 300 mg/12 hours and intravenous clindamycin 600 mg/8 hours was found to have positive results as an empirical and definitive treatment of severe diabetic foot infections. Clindamycin has activity against aerobic and anaerobic cocci; it is not active against gram-negative rods.

An aggressive organism often found with diabetic foot infections is enterococcus. Almost all strains of enterococci display some level of antibiotic resistance, often to multiple antibiotics. Vancomycin may be an alternative to penicillin; however, there is an ever-increasing emergence of vancomycin-resistant enterococcus. A penicillin β-lactamase inhibitor (ampicillin-sulbactam) in combination with gentamicin has been shown to be active in vitro against β-lactamase,

TABLE 1. BROAD SPECTRUM ANTIBIOTIC THERAPY FOR DIABETIC FOOT INFECTIONS

Antibiotic	Coverage	Adult Dose Range
Fluoroquinolones		
Ciprofloxacin	Empiric therapy	250–750 mg po bid 200–400 mg IV q 12 hours
Levofloxacin	Empiric therapy	500 mg po/IV q day
Antiparasitic		
Metronidazole	Anaerobes	500 mg IV/po q 6 hours
Aminoglycoside		
Gentamicin	Broad spectrum	1 mg/kg IV/IM monitor peaks and troughs
First-Generation Cephalosporin		
Cefazolin	Gram-positive	0.5–1.5 g IV/IM q 6–8 hours
Third-Generation Cephalosporin		
Ceftriaxone	Gram-negative	1–2 g IV/IM q 24 hours
Cefotaxime	Gram-negative	1–2 g IV/IM q 6–8 hours
Ceftazidime	Gram-negative & *Pseudomonas*	1–2 g IV q 8–12 hours
Carbapenem		
Imipenem	*Pseudomonas*, gram-positive Staphylococcus enterococci	250–1000 mg IV q 6–8 hours
Combination Agents		
Amoxicillin & clavulanate	Broad spectrum	500–875 mg po bid
Ampicillin & sulbactam	Broad spectrum	1.5–3 g IM/IV q 6 hours
Ticarcillin & clavulanate	Broad spectrum	3.1 g IV q 4–6 hours
Piperacillin & tazobactam	Broad spectrum	3.375 g IV q 4–6 hours
Other Antimicrobial Agents		
Vancomycin	Broad spectrum	1 g IV q 12 hours
Clindamycin	Aerobic & anaerobic cocci Not gram-negative rods	150–400 mg po q.i.d. or 600–900 mg IV q 8 hours
Aztreonam	Substitute for gentamicin	0.5–2 g IV/IM q 6–12 hours

TABLE 2. DIFFERENTIAL DIAGNOSIS CHART

Condition	Radiologic and Vascular Studies	Laboratory Tests	Nonsurgical Treatment	Surgical Treatment
I. Infection	Doppler to determine vascularity	CBC/differential, CRP, sedimentation rate, metabolic profile, blood glucose	Appropriate condition below	
a. Cellulitis	Radiograph, MRI, CT, bone scan may or may not help. Does elevation resolve erythema?	As above	Broad spectrum antibiotic	
b. Abscess	As above	As above, plus culture and sensitivity	Broad spectrum IV/PO intraoperative antibiotics, adjust pending cultures	I&D, possible excision or partial amputation
c. Osteomyelitis	As above	As above, plus intraoperative culture and sensitivity	Broad spectrum IV/PO antibiotics, adjust pending C&S × 6 weeks of treatment	Excision of infected bone, possible toe/ray amputation, transmetatarsal amputation, below-knee amputation
II. Charcot joint	Radiograph, MRI, consider bone mineral density testing	Blood glucose, CBC/differential, CRP, sedimentation rate, metabolic profile	Total contact cast, CROW, may need custom inserts	Eventual fusion or bony-prominence resection
III. Dysvascular	Doppler, vascular consult			Revascularization

MRI: magnetic resonance imaging; CT: computed tomography; CBC: complete blood cell count; CRP: C-reactive protein; IV: intravenous; PO: oral; C&S: culture + sensitivity; CROW: Charcot's restraint orthotic walker.

producing penicillin-resistant strains.[46] Vancomycin-resistant enterococcus may require surgical intervention.

Pexiganan may be a next alternative for antibiotic therapy in diabetic foot infection. In clinical trials, pexiganan displayed broad spectrum in vitro antimicrobial activity against organisms isolated from infected diabetic foot ulcers in 835 outpatients. These trials found pexiganan to have broad spectrum antimicrobial activity against gram-positive aerobes, gram-negative aerobes including *Pseudomonas*, *Enterobacter*, *Klebsiella*, *Escherichia*, and *Flavobacterium* species as well as anaerobic organisms isolated from the ulcers.[40] Pexiganan did not display cross-resistance with other antibiotics commonly used for diabetic foot ulcers.

Granulocyte colony-stimulating factor (GCSF) has been investigated for its ability to enhance healing in diabetic foot infection.[47] GCSF, an endogenous hemopoietic growth factor, increases the release of neutrophils from the bone marrow, improving neutrophil function. The recombinant form of GCSF is presently used to treat neutropenia induced by chemotherapy and has been studied for efficacy with diabetic foot infections. The results indicate that patients who received GCSF therapy along with antibiotic therapy had quicker eradication of pathogens, earlier resolution of cellulitis, shorter hospitalizations, and less intravenous antibiotic therapy than the placebo counterparts.

OVERVIEW

Diabetic foot infection treatment is based on clinical signs and symptoms of increasing blood glucose levels, erythema, cellulitis, tenderness, fever, and chills. Laboratory studies, such as complete blood cell count with differential, C-reactive protein, erythrocyte sedimentation rate, and metabolic profile, may or may not be helpful. The suspicion of osteomyelitis by either probing to bone or "sausage toe" deformity should be investigated further. Plain films are often normal; bone scans are nonspecific. False-negative results for technetium 99m bone scans occur with poor vascular supply to the extremity.[37] Magnetic resonance imaging is more sensitive than bone scan, can identify osteomyelitis and abscess, and is helpful with surgical planning but tends to overrepresent the distribution of intramedullary infection. Simultaneous dual window nuclear imaging with technetium 99 and indium 111-labeled white blood cells can help differentiate osteomyelitis from Charcot's arthropathy.

Cultures and biopsy may be helpful. A superficial swab culture of the wound is not indicative of the deep-seated infection, whereas cultures obtained from the base of the ulcer after débridement are usually more representative. Biopsy performed intraoperatively through a separate incision is the most reliable technique.

Treatment of diabetic foot infections begins with broad spectrum antimicrobial therapy, often with intravenous antibiotics. These needs to be combined with good wound care, consisting of drainage of all abscesses, regular dressing changes, débridement, rest, and pressure relief. In the presence of osteomyelitis or abscess, surgical intervention is often required.

FOREIGN BODIES IN THE DIABETIC FOOT

The combination of neuropathy, poor vision, and decreased flexibility can lead to foreign body trauma to the diabetic foot. Patient education is essential in preventing unnecessary injury and infection. Proper shoe wear is also invaluable in protecting the diabetic patient's feet.

FRACTURES

Diabetic patients are at increased risk of complications from ankle fractures because of peripheral neuropathy, vascular insufficiency, hyperglycemia, and other comorbid conditions. A simple fracture normally treated by casting for 6 weeks can progress to a Charcot joint. The decision to treat a fracture surgically versus nonsurgically in this group of patients can be difficult. A study of ankle fractures compared diabetic patients with nondiabetic patients with similar fractures treated by surgical intervention; the study found that diabetic patients were at increased risk of infection.[48] The patients at greatest risk were those who had poor compliance with diabetic treatment and chronic hyperglycemia. Another study[49] found that diabetic patients with ankle fractures had a 2.76 times greater risk of complications than the control group when treated with surgical intervention. Care must be taken when treating a diabetic patient with an ankle fracture. The diabetic patient often needs a longer time in a cast for consolidation to occur and, generally, should be protected for twice as long. In this setting, it is critical that the clinician educate the patient and family repetitively regarding weightbearing status and monitor the patient's leg closely for subtle signs of infection or delayed healing.

MANAGEMENT

GENERAL GUIDELINES FOR FOOT EVALUATION

The American Diabetes Association annually issues clinical practice recommendations. These guidelines provide essential aspects of diabetic foot care, with the intent to identify the foot "at risk," initiate preventive care and treatment, and reduce the need for amputation.[51]

According to these guidelines, a comprehensive screening examination should be performed at least annually, with examination of the patient's legs and feet, including between all the toes. The vascular, neurological, and musculoskeletal systems must be evaluated. The high-risk foot, once determined, should be evaluated at each visit. The patient at risk for developing foot ulcers is the patient who has lost protective sensation or who has peripheral vascular disease. Factors that increase risk further are deformities of the foot and ankle, including Charcot's joint, hammer toes, claw toes, and nail/skin abnormalities such as dry, scaly skin. The musculoskeletal examination should include gait evaluation and range of motion at the ankle and the hallux. Soft-tissue examination for skin breakdown should also be performed.

The vascular examination includes palpation of pulses in the lower extremities and skin inspection for changes indicating ischemia. Should a patient have claudication symptoms or nonhealing wounds, a vascular consultation should be requested.

A neurological examination should include methods to determine loss of protective sensation. This may be performed in many ways. The American Diabetes Association recommends using the 5.07 (10-g) Semmes-Weinstein monofilament. The insensate patient must be involved in an ongoing program of education. The patient must be placed in appropriate footwear.

Patient education is extremely important in the prevention of foot complications. Low-risk patients must be educated concerning foot hygiene, proper footwear, prevention of foot trauma, the need to stop smoking, and appropriate action to take when problems arise. High-risk patients and family members should be taught daily foot care and understand the implication the loss of protective sensation has, regarding the foot and resulting injury.

The clinician must recognize and provide prompt and appropriate care when an ulcer has developed. It is important to determine the mechanism causing the ulcer; accurately describe the ulcer by measuring its depth, width, and length; identify underlying structures that are exposed and/or involved; assess for purulent exudate, necrosis, sinus tracts, and odor; assess for surrounding signs of edema, cellulitis, abscess, and fluctuation; exclude systemic infection; perform a vascular evaluation; and probe for bone.

Radiological evaluation is performed as appropriate. Deep specimens may be obtained by curettage of the base of the wound for culture and sensitivity. A bone biopsy sample may be needed.

All abscesses must be incised and drained. Débridement must extend to noninfected tissue and must be repeated until a healthy soft-tissue bed is obtained. Appropriate wound aftercare is important, but the use of topical agents for treating diabetic foot ulcers is controversial. Prolonged soaking of the foot in water is not recommended.

Pressure relief is extremely important. Crutch ambulation, TCC, diabetic bracewear, orthotics, and special healing shoes are all important means of alleviating pressure and mechanical stress to the area of the ulcer. Once healing has occurred, evaluation for the best means of prevention must occur. Referral to clinicians who specialize in bracing and shoe wear, such as an orthotist or pedorthist, is appropriate. A study by Pinzur and colleagues,[52] with the American Orthopaedic Foot and Ankle Society Shoe Survey of Diabetic Patients, found that only 25% of the diabetic foot patients surveyed received prophylactic intervention for foot orthoses and/or protective shoes.

In cases of inadequate circulation, vascular reconstruction may be appropriate. Vasodilator drugs have not been shown to be helpful with diabetic foot ulcers, and vasoconstrictor drugs should not be used.

Tight blood glucose control is the main goal in the overall care of the diabetic patient. Increasing or widely fluctuating blood glucose control is an indicator of infection. Prolonged hyperglycemia may decrease the patient's ability to fight infection.

Recognition of a Charcot joint is extremely important. An acutely swollen foot with no bony abnormalities on radiograph and no break in skin integrity may indicate early Charcot changes.

PATIENT EDUCATION

Patient education guidelines listed below are recommendations from the Diabetes Committee of the American Orthopaedic Foot and Ankle Society[12]:

1. Do not walk barefoot.
2. Do not use corn or callus removers.
3. Bathe the foot daily with mild soap.
4. Use a soft brush to clean around the nails.

5. Dry the feet with special attention to the web spaces. Use lamb's wool between the toes if the web space skin remains moist or becomes macerated.
6. Use oil, lotion, or lanolin cream to avoid dryness.
7. Use socks that absorb perspiration and breathe (cotton or natural fibers).

The American Orthopaedic Foot and Ankle Society Classification

Risk category O. Normal-appearing foot with normal sensation with or without minor deformity. Basic foot education, yearly examinations, and normal footwear and laced shoes are recommended.

Risk Category 1. Normal-appearing foot, insensate, and no deformities. Daily foot self-examination, at-risk patient education, and pressure-dissipating noncustom inserts that should be replaced every 6 months are recommended. Appropriate shoes include Oxford soft-leather laced shoes of adequate size to accommodate pressure-dissipating accommodative insoles or foot orthoses. Follow-up should be every 6 months.

Risk Category 2. Insensate foot with deformity, without a history of or presence of ulcer. Daily foot self-examination, at-risk patient education, custom-fabricated pressure-dissipating accommodative foot orthoses, inlay depth, soft-leather adjustable lacing shoes, clinical evaluation for any new-onset skin or nail pathological condition, and follow-up monitoring by physician or nurse every 4 months are recommended.

Risk Category 3. Insensate foot with deformity and history of ulcer. Daily foot self-examination, scheduled clinical examinations at designated intervals (varying with magnitude of deformity), at-risk patient education, custom-fabricated pressure-dissipating accommodative foot orthoses, inlay depth, soft-leather adjustable lacing shoes, follow-up monitoring by physician or nurse every 2 months, immediate clinical evaluation with any new onset of skin or nail pathological conditions, and possible referral to an orthopaedic foot and ankle surgeon are recommended.

Skin and Nail Care

Due to autonomic neuropathy, the skin becomes excessively dry and cracks more easily. The patient should apply lotion to the dry areas once to twice daily while avoiding the area between the toes. A thin layer of petroleum jelly applied after a shower or bath can trap in the hydration absorbed by the skin.

Regular nail care should be performed either by the patient or a professional. A straight nail clipper can be used to trim the nail transversely. This is done to avoid skin overgrowth at the borders. Rounding the nail can lead to ingrown toenails. If the nail becomes thick or the patient has poor eyesight, a professional should be used.

Shoes and Custom Orthoses

Appropriate footwear is an important aspect of the care of the diabetic patient. Properly fitted shoes can decrease shear, which causes skin breakdown, and relieve pressure from mild deformities. For example, pressure can be relieved from the dorsum of the toes with an extra-depth shoe when the patient has developed a claw toe deformity. With the inclusion of an accommodative insert, plantar pressures may be relieved. Properly fitting shoe wear can protect the feet from extraneous injury.

Currently, Medicare provides reimbursement for one pair of extra-depth shoes and three pairs of inserts, or one pair of custom-molded shoes plus two additional pairs of inserts, each year for patients with high-risk feet.[51] Properly fitted shoes should not have to be broken in; a diabetic patient can develop skin breakdown in a short time. The shoes should match the foot and allow room for inserts. The patient should, however, remove the new shoes periodically to inspect the foot for areas of irritation and slowly progress to longer time in the shoes.

Orthotic intervention may include custom-molded inserts designed to off-weight high-pressure areas and accommodative shoe wear. Rigid orthoses made of hard plastic, acrylic, graphite, and Rohadur are contraindicated for the insensate foot of the diabetic patient. These do not absorb shock or decrease pressure areas, and this is required for the diabetic patient. Custom shoes are occasionally necessary. Diabetic patients should have at least two pairs of properly fitted shoes and inserts so they can alternate shoes daily or even during the day.

THE TEAM

Diabetes mellitus is a multisystem disease often requiring many specialists. The difficult task is coordinating the team, especially when not all its members are within the same clinic. All too often, certain aspects of diabetic care are overlooked. Education of patients and physicians is continuing in an effort to improve the care of the diabetic patient and ultimately decrease the complication rate.

REFERENCES

1. National Diabetes Information Clearing House: Diabetes statistics in the United States. NIH Publication 99–3892, 1999.
2. Eldelman SV, Henry RR: Diabetes statistics. In Eldelman SV, Henry RR (eds): Diagnosis and Management of Type 2 Diabetes, 3rd ed. Caddo, OK, Professional Communications, 1999, p 11.
3. Brodsky JW: The diabetic foot. In Coughlin MJ, Mann RA (eds): Surgery of the Foot and Ankle, 7th ed. St. Louis, Mosby, 1999, p 895.
4. Clark CM, Lee DA: Drug therapy: Prevention and treatment of the complications of diabetes mellitus. N Engl J Med 332:1210, 1995.
5. Foster DW: Diabetes mellitus. In Isselbacher KJ, Braunwald E, Wilson JD, et al (eds): Harrison's Principles of Internal Medicine, 13th ed. New York, McGraw-Hill, 1994, p 1994.
6. Partanen J, Niskanen L, Lehtinen J, et al: Natural history of peripheral neuropathy in patients with non–insulin dependent diabetes mellitus. N Engl J Med 89:94, 1995.
7. Reichard P, Nilsson BY, Rosenqvist U: The effect of long-term intensified insulin treatment on the development of microvascular complications of diabetes mellitus. N Engl J Med 304:309, 1993.
8. The Diabetes Control and Complication Trial Research Group: The effects of intensive diabetes therapy on the development and progression of neuropathy. Ann Intern Med 122:561, 1995.
9. Cavanagh PR, Ulbrecht JS: Biomechanics of the diabetic foot: A quantitative approach to the assessment of neuropathy, deformity and plantar pressure. In Jahss MH (ed): Disorders of the Foot and Ankle, 2nd ed. Philadelphia, WB Saunders, 1991, p 1864.

10. Queral LA: Evaluation and treatment of vascular insufficiency. In Jahss MH (ed): Disorders of the Foot and Ankle, 2nd ed. Philadelphia, WB Saunders, 1991, p 399.

11. Oppenheim U, Kohen-Raz R, Alex D, et al: Postural characteristics of diabetic neuropathy. Diabetes Care 22:328, 1999.

12. Pinzur MS, Slovenkai MP, Trepman E: Guidelines for diabetic foot care. Foot Ankle Int 20:695, 1999.

13. Caputo GM, Cavanagh PR, Ulbrecht JS, et al: Current concepts: Assessment and management of foot disease in patients with diabetes. N Engl J Med 331:854, 1994.

14. Low PA, Dotson RM: Symptomatic treatment of painful neuropathy. JAMA 280:1863, 1998.

15. Morello CM, Leckband SG, Stoner CP, et al: Randomized double-blind study comparing the efficacy of gabapentin with amitriptyline on diabetic peripheral neuropathy pain. Arch Intern Med 159:1931, 1999.

16. Kumar D, Alvaro MS, Julka IS, et al: Diabetic peripheral neuropathy. Diabetes Care 21:1322, 1998.

17. Ziegler D, Hanefeld M, Ruhnau KJ, et al: Treatment of symptomatic diabetic polyneuropathy with the antioxidant alpha-lipoic acid. Diabetes Care 22:1296, 1999.

18. American Diabetes Association: Consensus development conference on diabetic foot wound care. Diabetes Care 22:1354, 1999.

19. Trott AT: Surface injury and wound healing. In Trott AT (ed): Wounds and Lacerations, 2nd ed. St. Louis, Mosby–Year Book, 1997, p 20.

20. Levine SE, Myerson MS: Management of ulceration and infection in the diabetic foot. In Myerson MS (ed): Foot and Ankle Disorders, vol I. Philadelphia, WB Saunders, 2000, p 411.

21. Armstrong DG, Lavery LA, Harkless LB: Validation of a diabetic wound classification system. Diabetes Care 21:855, 1998.

22. Mason J, O'Keeffe C, McIntosh A, et al: A systematic review of foot ulcer in patients with type 2 diabetes mellitus: Prevention. Diabetic Med 16:801, 1999.

23. Phillips TJ: Tissue-engineered skin. Arch Dermatol 135:977, 1999.

24. Bello YM, Phillips TJ: Recent advances in wound healing. JAMA 283:716, 2000.

25. Shaw JE, Hsi W-L, Ulbrecht JS, et al: The mechanism of plantar unloading in total contact casts: Implications for design and clinical use. Foot Ankle Int 18:809, 1997.

26. Wertsch JJ, Frank LW, Zhu H, et al: Plantar pressures with total contact casting. J Rehabil Res Dev 32:205, 1995

27. Laing PW, Cogley DI, Klenerman L: Neuropathic foot ulceration treated by total contact casts. J Bone Joint Surg Br 74:133, 1991.

28. Armstrong DG, Stacpoole-Shea S, Nguyen H, et al: Lengthening of the Achilles tendon in diabetic patients who are at high risk for ulceration of the foot. J Bone Joint Surg Am 81:535, 1999.

29. Pinzur MS: Benchmark analysis of diabetic patients with neuropathic (Charcot) foot deformity. Foot Ankle Int 20:564, 1999.

30. Myerson MS: Diabetic neuroarthropathy. In Myerson MS (ed): Foot and Ankle Disorders, vol I. Philadelphia, WB Saunders, 2000, p 439.

31. Armstrong DG, Lavery LA: Elevated peak plantar pressures in patients who have Charcot arthropathy. J Bone Joint Surg Am 80:365, 1998.

32. Guse ST, Alvine FG: Treatment of diabetic foot ulcers and Charcot neuropathy using the patellar tendon–bearing brace. Foot Ankle Int 18:675, 1997.

33. Saltzman CL, Johnson KA, Goldstein RH, et al: The patellar tendon–bearing brace as treatment for neurotrophic arthropathy: A dynamic force monitoring study. Foot Ankle 13:14, 1992.

34. Fears RL, Gleis GE, Seligson D: Diagnosis and treatment of complications. In Browner BD, Levine AM, Jupiter JB, et al (eds): Skeletal Trauma, 2nd ed. Philadelphia: WB Saunders, 1998, p 543.

35. Pittet D, Wyssa B, Herter-Clavel C, et al: Outcome of diabetic foot infections treated conservatively. Arch Intern Med 159:851, 1999.

36. Lypsky BA, Pecoraro RE, Larson SA, et al: Out-patient management of uncomplicated lower-extremity infections in diabetic patients. Arch Intern Med 150:790, 1990.

37. Eckman MH, Greenfield S, Mackey WC, et al: Foot infections in diabetic patients: Decision and cost-effectiveness analyses. JAMA 273:712, 1995.

38. Tentolouris N, Jude EB, Smirnof I, et al: Methacillin-resistant *Staphylococcus aureus*: An increasing problem in a diabetic foot clinic. Diabetic Med 16:767, 1999.

39. Hill SL, Holtzman GI, Buse R: The effects of peripheral vascular disease with osteomyelitis in the diabetic foot. Am J Surg 177:282, 1999.

40. Ge Y, MacDonald D, Henry MM, et al: In vitro susceptibility to pexiganan of bacteria isolated from infected diabetic foot ulcers. Diagn Microbiol Infect Dis 35:45, 1999.

41. Grayson ML, Gibbons GW, Balogh K, et al: Probing to bone in infected pedal ulcers: A clinical sign of underlying osteomyelitis in diabetic patients. JAMA 273:721, 1995.

42. Rajbhandari SM, Sutton M, Davies C, et al: "Sausage toe": A reliable sign of underlying osteomyelitis. Diabetic Med 17:74, 2000.

43. Zeillemaker AM, Veldkamp KE, van Kraaij MG, et al: Piperacillin/tazobactam therapy for diabetic foot infection. Foot Ankle Int 19:169, 1998.

44. Lipsky BA, Baker PD, Landon GC, et al: Antibiotic therapy for diabetic foot infections: Comparison of two parenteral-to-oral regimens. Clin Infect Dis 24:643, 1997.

45. Diamantopoulos EJ, Haritos D, Yfandi G, et al: Management and outcome of severe diabetic foot infections. Exp Clin Endocrinol Diabetes 106:346, 1998.

46. DeBakey ME, McCollum CH: Acquired diseases of the aorta. In Rakel RE (ed): Conn's Current Therapy. Philadelphia, WB Saunders, 1998, p 248.

47. Gough A, Clapperton M, Rolando N, et al: Randomized placebo-controlled trial of granulocyte colony-stimulating factor in diabetic foot infection. Lancet 350:855, 1997.

48. Flynn JM, Rodriguez-del Rio F, Piza PA: Closed ankle fractures in the diabetic patient. Foot Ankle Int 21:311, 2000.

49. Blotter RH, Connelly E, Wasan A, et al: Acute complications in the operative treatment of isolated ankle fractures in patients with diabetes mellitus. Foot Ankle Int 20:687, 1999.

50. Zoorob RJ, Hagen MD: Guidelines on the care of diabetic nephropathy, retinopathy and foot disease. Am Fam Physicians 56:2021, 1997.

51. American Diabetes Association: Position statement: Preventive foot care in people with diabetes mellitus. Diabetes Care 21:2178, 1998.

52. Pinzur MS, Shields NN, Goelitz B, et al: American orthopaedic foot and ankle society shoe survey of diabetic patients. Foot Ankle Int 20:703, 1999.

NERVE PROBLEMS OF THE FOOT AND ANKLE

Lew C. Schon, Ilan Cohen, and Mark E. Easley

Summary

- Nerve problems of the foot and ankle are frequently underdiagnosed and inadequately treated.
- Certain cases will become chronic and may at times be part of a broader chronic regional pain syndrome (type 2).
- Diagnosis is made on clinical bases but is supported by electrodiagnostic studies and, occasionally, imaging studies.
- Nonoperative treatment of chronic cases involves eliminating the offending activity and using bracing, desensitization, and chemical agents such as tricyclic antidepressant (TCA) medications, antiepileptic drugs (AEDs), and serotonin uptake inhibitors.
- For chronically compressed nerves, a surgical nerve release may be warranted.
- Several surgical options exist for injured nerves that do not respond to release or for nerves that have been stretched, crushed, and/or partially or completely transected. These options include revision release, a vein-wrap procedure, transection, and containment or peripheral nerve stimulation (PNS).

Nerve problems of the foot and ankle are often overlooked and misdiagnosed. It is not uncommon for a nerve problem to coexist with another more readily apparent orthopaedic musculoskeletal condition that may distract the examiner's attention from the less obvious nerve injury. Many of these nerve insults are self-limiting and resolve with time. Several nerve conditions are more persistent and may require nerve-directed treatment. This chapter presents terminology that aids in understanding of the symptoms, describes primary and end-stage nerve syndromes, and reviews nonoperative and surgical treatment modalities.

BACKGROUND

TERMINOLOGY

The specific terms used to describe the various conditions are relevant for prognosis and treatment. They are as follows:

Neuralgia denotes any nerve pain of certain or uncertain origin. Neuralgia can be nociceptive, i.e., produced by a repetitive painful stimulus of the peripheral nerve. *Ectopic neuralgia* results from abnormal electrical discharges originating along the course of the nerve due to nerve compromise. These abnormal discharges occur without provocation, unlike the physically triggered nerve impulses in nociceptive neuralgia.

Neuritis describes nerve disorder secondary only to an inflammatory process.

Nerve entrapment indicates a nerve that is compressed or restricted.

A *neuroma* is a disorganized fibroneural tissue mass that forms at the site of a nerve transection or laceration. A *neuroma-in-continuity* is a neuroma that occurs within an intact nerve in response to internally damaged fascicles, resulting in a distal portion of the nerve that no longer functions properly.

Neurapraxia refers to a nerve that has been stretched or compressed without organic damage to the nerve or its surrounding connective tissue. Neurapraxia will eventually heal, although in some cases it may take as long as 6 months for complete recovery. *Axonotmesis* is a more serious nerve injury with internal axonal damage. *Neurotmesis* is the most severe injury, in which both the neural elements and the supportive connective tissue around it have been damaged. Of these three types of injuries, neurotmesis has the worst prognosis.

Neuropathy refers to nerve dysfunction secondary to a systemic disease affecting the peripheral nervous system.

The term *complex regional pain syndrome* (CRPS), introduced by the International Association for the Study of Pain, has replaced the terms reflex sympathetic dystrophy, Sudeck's atrophy, and causalgia.[1] CRPS is divided into two types. Type 1 is defined as neuropathic pain with manifestations of sympathetic influence not associated with a specific nerve injury. Type 2 is similar to type 1 but is associated with a specific nerve injury.

Central pain syndrome is pain caused by a lesion or dysfunction in the central nervous system.

There are various terms used to describe the character of neuropathic pain. They are as follows:

Allodynia is pain evoked by a stimulus that usually does not produce a painful response.

Analgesia is the absence of pain in response to a stimulus that would normally produce a painful response.

Anesthesia dolorosa is pain in a site that is numb, the pain typically occurring after a nerve transection.

Dysesthesia is a spontaneous or evoked unpleasant and abnormal neuralgic sensation.

Deafferentation pain is pain in the area innervated by or surrounded by a surgically or traumatically transected nerve.

Hyperalgesia is an increased response to a normally painful stimulus.

Hyperesthesia is increased sensitivity due to stimulation.

Hypoesthesia is decreased sensitivity to any stimulation.

Hyperpathia is an extremely painful response to a stimulus.

Paresthesia is an abnormal sensation that is either spontaneous or evoked. If a paresthesia is painful, it is called a *dysesthesia*.

EPIDEMIOLOGY

Neuromas may occur at any age, from late adolescence and beyond. According to Kenzora,[2] traumatic neuromas of the foot and ankle are found in patients 16 to 60 years old (mean age, 36 years). The reported male:female ratio in his series was 1:2.5, but more epidemiological data need to be gathered before any conclusion can be drawn from these numbers. The natural history of patients with chronic neuralgia remains a mystery because there are no long-term studies regarding various causes and their final outcomes. It is interesting to note that symptomatic neuromas are typically not seen in the very old or very young.

PATHOGENESIS

NERVE DAMAGE AND NEUROMA FORMATION

A nerve may be damaged traumatically by one or more mechanisms.[3] Its direct continuity may be disrupted by a partial laceration or a complete transection, or the inner neural elements may be injured without the presence of an overt anatomic lesion, as with external compression either acute (as in a crush injury) or chronic (as in an entrapment neuropathy). In the latter condition, the nerve is typically trapped underneath or within tight bands of fibrotic or scar tissue, but it may also be compressed by a space-occupying lesion such as a ganglion cyst or a soft-tissue tumor. Bony prominences may also contribute to neural compression.

Another type of injury originates from within the nerve, as when the nerve is stretched beyond its physiological properties of elasticity, resulting in varying degrees of axonal damage. A mild acute ankle sprain or a mild twisting injury of the foot may result in severe chronic neuralgia. In addition to such an acute event, chronic or recurrent stretch also plays a role in triggering a chronic neuralgia. Tarsal tunnel syndrome, for example, is a chronic neuralgic condition of the posterior tibial nerve (TN) and its branches that is often seen in feet with a valgus deformity of the hindfoot, because the nerve that courses along the medial aspect of the ankle tends to be stretched.

Axonal injury initiates a reparative response. If the neuron remains intact, the distal part of the damaged axon is gradually absorbed in a process called wallerian degeneration.[4] The proximal part of the axon that maintains a potential for regeneration eventually sprouts and, if it encounters an empty endoneural tube in its proximity, it will grow within it at a rate of 1 to 2 mm per day in an attempt to restore the inner architecture of the nerve.[5] The resulting functional outcome depends on the percentage of the axons that manage to find their way distally and to regenerate in a normal, physiological fashion. If, however, displacement has occurred between the nerve endings, the sprouting axons may be unable to reach the distal endoneural tubes. They will then continue to elongate and proliferate at the site of injury, forming a neuroma,[6] a mass of disorganized tissue containing axons and connective tissue. Neuromas contain different types of cells, including Schwann's cells, macrophages, fibroblasts, and myofibroblasts that have contractile properties and are thought to contribute to neuroma pain by causing the collagen matrix to contract around unmyelinated nerve fibers.[7] The risk of neuroma formation may be reduced by early exploration and end-to-end repair of a lacerated or transected nerve. Painful neuromas are those that contain sensory fibers; injuries of pure motor nerves are not associated with pain.[8] However, the mechanism of pain is not fully understood.

Neuromas are classified into three types: neuromas-in-continuity, neuromas in completely severed nerves, and amputation-stump neuromas.[9]

Neuromas-in-continuity can be subdivided into spindle neuromas (in which the perineurium is intact) and lateral neuromas (with partial disruption of the perineurium and neuromas after nerve repairs). The spindle neuroma forms in response to chronic irritation or compression. Examples in the foot include Morton's interdigital neuroma and neuroma of the lateral branch of the deep peroneal nerve over the dorsal prominence of the navicular. Despite its name, it is not a true neuroma because the thickening involves only the epineurium and not the nerve fibers. This enlargement is caused by proliferation of the fibrous connective tissue. There is, however, experimental evidence that crushed nerves may produce a true neuroma-in-continuity with regenerating axons that grow out of their neurotubular sheaths but remain confined within the epineurium.[10]

Lateral neuromas and transection (type 2) neuromas result from partial nerve lacerations, as seen in penetrating or iatrogenic trauma.[11] Surgical procedures not uncommonly associated with iatrogenic nerve injury with subsequent formation of neuromas include ankle arthroscopies, internal fixation of ankle fractures, excisional biopsy of ganglia, metatarsal osteotomies, sesamoid excision, and removal of hardware.[12] The anatomic variations of the superficial sensory nerves around the ankle and the dorsum of the foot, as well as careless dissection habits, contribute to the magnitude of this problem.

Amputation stump neuromas, those from completely severed nerves, may occur in intact limbs when a nerve is transected as well as in amputated limbs. They may cause substantial functional impairment not only because they are subjected to friction and pressure from external sources such as a brace or prosthesis (nociceptive neuralgia) but also because they are sometimes associated with spontaneous pain (ectopic neuralgia).[13] A unique example is the phenomenon of phantom limb pain, in which the pain or paresthesia is perceived in a distribution area that is distal to the amputation site. These neuromas may at times require revision transection and sometimes burial or transposition of the nerve.[14]

For both partial and complete nerve transections, the best method of avoiding neuromas is to be careful with surgical exposure. Also, when evaluating an extremity that has been injured, identification of a nerve injury allows the decision process for considering repair to begin. Finally, if there is nerve injury, repair of the nerve using meticulous microsurgical techniques is warranted.

Severe chronic nerve irritation is not always associated with a visible neuroma. In cases of crush or chronic and acute stretching injuries, the nerve at the time of exploration often has a normal macroscopic appearance. Such is also the case with many nerves released for a diagnosis of "entrapment neuropathy," a diagnosis not always substantiated even in cases of revision surgery. A typical patient is the one treated by repeated releases of the tarsal tunnel, with each intervention being followed by increased deterioration of the condition and worsening of symptoms. Included in this category are all cases of chronic neuralgia classified as idiopathic, ones with no identifiable triggering event or injury. It may be that dysfunction of the nerve in these intriguing cases is the result of subtle microanatomic or physiological changes, but the answers are not yet known, and such patients pose a challenge to foot and ankle surgeons and pain management specialists as well, because they are difficult to treat and the prognosis is often guarded.

CHRONIC PAIN

Pain is not only an isolated perception of a noxious stimulus acting on the periphery and carried to the somatosensory cortex in the brain (nociceptive pain). Other forms of pain have been recognized, including central, psychological, and behavioral pain.[15] Moreover, the seemingly simple nociceptive response is really very complex because the signal of pain is subjected to central modulation at different levels along its path so that what is perceived might be very different from what was originally recorded by the peripheral pain receptor.[16]

Noxious stimuli are detected by receptors located at the ending of myelinated A-delta and unmyelinated C-afferent pain fibers. The signals are then carried to the nociceptive neuron in the dorsal horn, ascend along the spinal cord, cross the midbrain, and finally reach the somatosensory cortex.[17] These signals may be subjected to peripheral inhibition through stimulation of large myelinated A-beta touch and pressure fibers. These fibers also terminate at the dorsal horn where they exert their inhibitory effect and block the signals of pain from being transmitted to the central nervous system. This concept is known as the gate mechanism of pain, and it is used by treatment modalities for chronic pain management such as desensitization, transcutaneous electrical nerve stimulation (TENS), and implanted PNS.[18]

PRIMARY NERVE PROBLEMS

THE TN AND ITS BRANCHES
Anatomy
The TN is one of the two main branches of the sciatic nerve. It courses along the deep posterior compartment in the leg and along the posteromedial aspect of the ankle where it is confined within a fibro-osseous tunnel called the tarsal tunnel. The roof of the tunnel is formed by the flexor retinaculum, which stretches from the posterior aspect of the medial malleolus to the posterior processes of the talus and calcaneus and attaches to the sheaths of the posterior tibial, flexor digitorum longus, and flexor hallucis longus tendons. The TN in the tarsal canal is accompanied by the tibial artery and one or two veins that lie in a very intimate relationship with the nerve and are sometimes found to be intertwined around the nerve. The nerve divides into the medial plantar nerve (MPN), the lateral plantar nerve (LPN), and the medial calcaneal nerve (MCN) branches. Cadaveric dissections have demonstrated that the bifurcation into the two main branches (MPN and LPN) occurs within the tarsal canal in 69% to 96% of cases and proximal to the canal in the remainder (Fig. 1). In 60% of the cases, the MCN has more than one branch. These branches may arise from the TN, MPN, or LPN, originating proximal to the canal in 70% of the cases and within the canal or distal to it in 30%.

The LPN gives off the first branch (FBLPN) that courses obliquely anterior to medial calcaneal tuberosity and travels between the deep fascia of the abductor hallucis (ABH) and the quadratus plantae muscles. It then courses laterally and divides into three branches that innervate the medial calcaneal periosteum/quadratus plantae, the flexor digitorum brevis, and the abductor digiti quinti. The MPN lies anterior to the LPN, and both MCN and FBLPN lie medial in relation to these two branches. MPN and LPN divide further distally into plantar branches that innervate the intrinsic muscles of the foot and provide plantar sensation.

TN Entrapment (Tarsal Tunnel Syndrome)
Overview. Tarsal tunnel syndrome is defined as compression or compromise of the TN or its branches underneath the flexor retinaculum. Some cases are idiopathic, but an identifiable cause may be found in more than 80% of patients; approximately one-third of cases is related to trauma or post-traumatic arthritis.[19–21] Pathological findings compressing the nerve in the canal include scar tissue, ganglions, other soft-tissue tumors, varicosities, inflammatory synovitis, aberrant muscle bellies, exostoses or fracture fragments, and bony prominences related to talocalcaneal coalitions.[20, 21] Tarsal tunnel syndrome has also been associated with valgus malalignment of the hindfoot, either

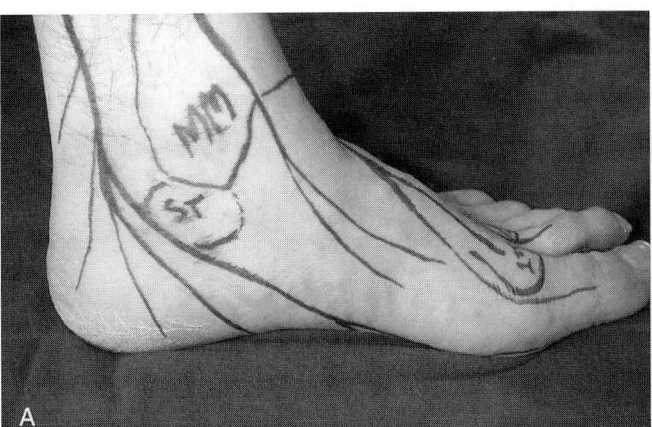
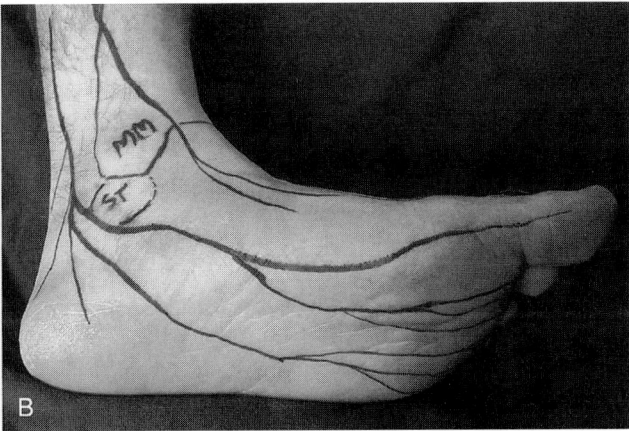

Fig. 1. The tibial nerve. It courses medially behind the tibia just posterior to the tibial artery. It branches into the medial plantar nerve, the lateral plantar nerve, and the medial calcaneal nerve(s) in the region of the medial malleolus calcaneal axis. *A,* Lateral view. *B,* Plantar view.

fixed or dynamic, that stretches the nerve.[3] Compartment syndromes after calcaneal fractures are another etiological factor.[22, 23]

The symptoms are described as medial or posteromedial foot and ankle pain, exacerbated by activity and relieved by rest, radiating into the plantar aspect of the foot distally or to the medial calf proximally. The pain is characterized as burning, tingling, electric, shooting, or numbing. The clinician should check the alignment of the foot, noting any varus or valgus that may affect the TN. Ankle and subtalar range of motion is assessed to rule out arthritis or tarsal coalition. Active range-of-motion and strength testing should be performed to determine whether there is more proximal nerve compression or tendon dysfunction (e.g., posterior tibialis tendinitis) that may mimic tarsal tunnel syndrome. Intrinsic muscle wasting and clawtoe deformities, which are late signs of TN dysfunction, are typically not found at presentation. The medial aspect of the ankle and the sole of the foot are palpated and percussed along the course of the nerve and its branches. Sensory testing is done with the monofilament test, side-to-side light-touch comparison, or two-point discrimination. There is often decreased sensation of the plantar aspect of the foot. Radiculopathy must be ruled out by means of inspection of the spine and appropriate clinical tests. Finally, if objective findings are equivocal, the evaluation should be completed by dynamic testing. The patient is asked to perform the type of activity that usually reproduces the symptoms, and the patient is then reexamined in the same fashion.

Radiographs and computed tomography are used to assess the alignment and bone and joint disorder (e.g., coalition) (Fig. 2), and magnetic resonance imaging (MRI) is used to detect soft-tissue disorders, including space-occupying lesions and tendinitis. Electrodiagnostic findings consistent with tarsal tunnel syndrome may include prolonged distal latency or decreased amplitudes on nerve conduction studies. Axonal denervation may be seen on electromyography as a more advanced finding. There is, however, controversy among clinicians and researchers regarding the accuracy of these studies in confirming the diagnosis of tarsal tunnel syndrome. Electrodiagnostic studies are nevertheless

a useful modality for ruling out both radiculopathy and peripheral neuropathy.[19, 24]

Treatment. TN entrapment can be managed nonoperatively or surgically.

Nonoperative. Nonsteroidal anti-inflammatory medications and steroid injections may be used in cases associated with inflammation. Different pharmacological agents, including vitamin B_6, TCAs (e.g., amitriptyline), and AEDs (e.g., gabapentin), may be tried to alleviate the symptoms. Venous congestion may be treated with compression stockings. Pitting edema should be evaluated by an internist and reduced by treating the underlying systemic disorder.

When the syndrome is caused by flexible overpronation of the foot, the alignment should be restored using a medial longitudinal arch support or an ankle stirrup brace.[25] Ganglions may be reduced in size by a single attempt at aspirating the cyst, but great care must be taken not to injure the nerve or blood vessels. As a rule, symptomatic space-occupying lesions do not resolve with nonoperative treatment, and they may need to be removed surgically.[19]

Surgical. Release should include the superficial fascia, the flexor retinaculum, and the deep fascia of the ABH distally to release the MPN, LPN, and FBLPN. The tarsal canal should be explored for space-occupying lesions, but neurolysis should not routinely be performed because it tends to increase postoperative scarring around the nerve. The authors of this chapter generally do not recommend manipulating the artery and the veins that accompany the TN (Fig. 3). In addition, the perineural fat should be left intact to minimize the possibility of postoperative scarring. The wound should de closed with 4-0 Vicryl sutures for the subcutaneous tissues and 4-0 nylon sutures for the skin.

If the nerve is heavily encased in scar tissue, it should be released by careful and meticulous dissection using magnifying loupes. We advocate protecting the nerve from adhesion re-formation in these cases by adding a barrier technique. Our preference is to perform a vein-wrap procedure, using either a saphenous vein autograft or an umbilical vein allograft, placing the vein partially or entirely around the nerve, depending on the location and degree of scarring. If the nerve, at the time of exploration, is severely

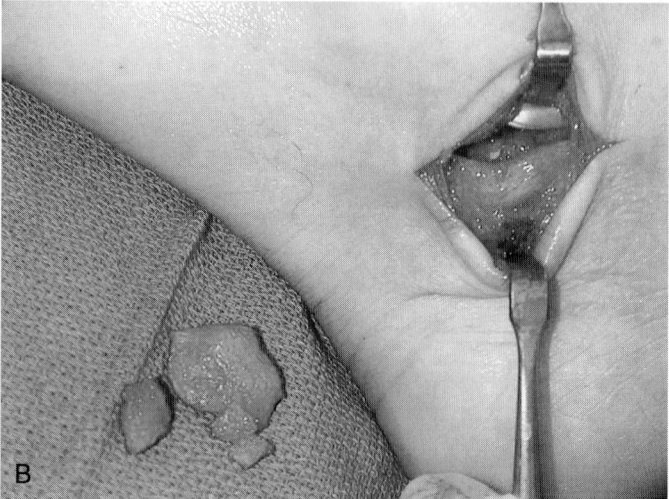

Fig. 2. A tarsal coalition. It is identified as a cause for medial ankle nerve symptoms. *A*, Preoperative radiograph. *B*, Intraoperative photograph.

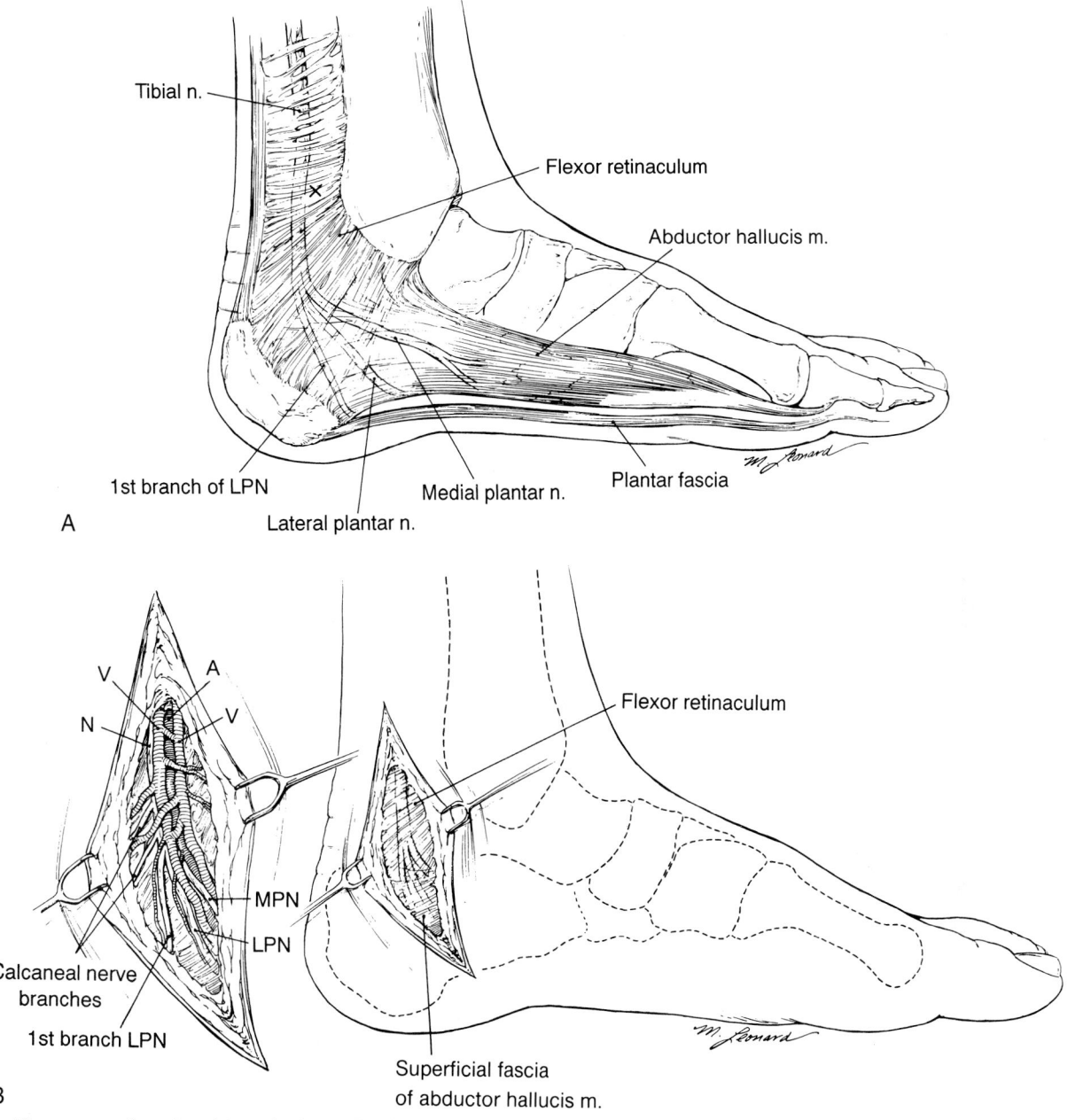

Fig. 3. The exposure for a tarsal tunnel release. The intimate relationship between the nerve and the artery and the vein(s) is demonstrated. (From Schon LC: Tarsal tunnel release. In Myerson M [ed]: Current Therapy in Foot and Ankle Surgery. St. Louis, Mosby-Year Book, 1993, p 174.)

damaged or if a neuroma is present, other surgical procedures may be warranted (see below).

Results. Surgical release of the tarsal tunnel has reported success rates that vary from 44% to 90%, but most series are relatively small, and follow-up periods are short. Pfeiffer and Cracchiolo[26] reported results in 32 feet with 8 years of follow-up; there was only a 44% success rate. Sammarco and colleagues[27] found a 57% satisfaction rate in seven cases. Bailie and Kelikian[28] reviewed 34 feet with tarsal tunnel release; the overall rate of substantial improvement was 73%. These results are similar to the 78% success rate reported by Mann.[20] The best results are achieved when a space-occupying lesion is identified and removed. The failed cases have either persistent pain or recurrence of the symptoms some time after decompression. Failure may result from one of the following:

Incorrect diagnosis. Other causes of posteromedial ankle pain may include tendinitis of the tibialis posterior tendon, posterior ankle impingement and symptomatic os trigonum, ankle arthritis, and lumbar radiculopathy.

Inadequate surgical release. The decompression may be insufficient either proximally or distally, or a space-occupying lesion may be overlooked. Percussion paresthesias distal to the surgical scar may imply an incomplete distal decompression.

Substantial internal damage to the nerve. In this situation, additional decompression attempts to relieve pain would be futile. Distal zones of numbness with ectopic neuralgia (spontaneous "shooters"), deafferentation phenomenon (increased sensitivity of the nerves adjacent to the zone of the damaged nerve), and anesthesia dolorosa (a zone of numbness that is painful to touch) are all indicative of internal nerve damage.

Scar formation around the nerve (adhesive neuralgia). The typical presentation is recurrent pain after some initial period of relief. A history of wound compromise or infection after decompression may also suggest excessive perineural scarring. Decreased range of motion and symptoms reproduced with active and passive ankle motion support this diagnosis, as does a thickened, tender, immobile scar associated with focal percussion paresthesias.

A revision tarsal tunnel release may be attempted with a chance of a good outcome, provided that there is no major internal nerve damage. The best results are obtained in patients who had previous incomplete proximal or distal decompression of the flexor retinaculum.[3, 29] Adhesive neuralgia at revision may require (or "possibly require") a barrier procedure because, otherwise, the expected outcome is uniformly poor. Internally damaged nerves may be best treated by PNS (see the later section on Peripheral Nerve Stimulation).

MPN Entrapment (Jogger's Foot)

The MPN gets compressed between the deep fascia of the ABH muscle and the medial tuberosity of the navicular in its path from underneath the flexor retinaculum toward the master Henry knot. MPN entrapment is associated with repetitive stress in hyperpronated feet with a valgus hindfoot and is typically seen in runners and military recruits.[30–33] The patient complains of medial arch pain radiating to the three medial toes. Symptoms are activity-related (usually running) and are sometimes related to the use of a new insert for the correction of pes planus.[33] During examination, symptoms may be reproduced by palpation along the MPN and may be aggravated by heel rise that causes the ABH muscle to tighten. Occasionally, dynamic testing (by having the patient run on a treadmill before the examination) induces latent symptoms. The patient is examined in the weightbearing position to assess for contributing deformity. Areas of external compression on the nerve may be identified by having the patient stand on the orthosis. A foot deformity and a medial navicular prominence may be seen on radiographs. Electrodiagnostic studies are not always helpful in a distal nerve entrapment because the studies consist of static testing performed on a dynamic disorder.[34] Nonoperative management is often successful with shoe modification to compensate for overpronation, an orthosis that provides arch support without pressure and activity modification. Operative treatment is indicated for resistant cases and includes release of the ABH fascia and the calcaneonavicular ligament at Henry's knot.[33] A favorable outcome may be expected as suggested by anecdotal reports, but large series are not available.

LPN Entrapment

The LPN has been shown by electrodiagnostic studies to be the most compromised nerve in tarsal tunnel syndrome.[35] This vulnerability has been attributed to its oblique anatomic course in a separate tunnel.[36] Isolated LPN entrapment is possible, and it is managed in the same way as tarsal tunnel syndrome.

Entrapment of the FBLPN (Baxter's Nerve)

This isolated entity is responsible for the symptoms in up to 20% of patients with chronic insertional plantar fasciitis.[34, 37] Compression of the nerve occurs between the deep fascia of the ABH and the quadratus plantae muscle and occasionally at the long plantar ligament or flexor digitorum brevis levels. Contributing factors include hyperpronation, ABH hypertrophy, accessory muscles, and aberrant bursae.[37, 38] The patient complains of chronic heel pain aggravated by activity, sometimes even without direct heel pressure. The pain radiates to the medial ankle or to the lateral aspect of the foot and typically does not respond to the management protocol for plantar fasciitis. Examination may reveal heel valgus or foot pronation and, compared with insertional plantar fasciitis, the point of maximal tenderness is usually located more proximally on the medial aspect of the heel.[3, 33, 35] Eversion of the foot may reproduce the symptoms, and weakness of the abductor digiti quinti can be present. Electrodiagnostic studies are helpful in detecting nerve compromise, as was demonstrated by Schon and colleagues.[34] Nonoperative treatment is the same as that for tarsal tunnel syndrome, and local injections can reduce nerve irritation caused by surrounding inflammation.[33] Surgical intervention, indicated for patients who do not respond to nonoperative measures, involves decompression of the nerve by release of the superficial and deep fascia of the ABH and decompression of the adjacent plantar fascia. A small portion of the fascia is excised to avoid recurrence (Fig. 4). The procedure provides satisfactory relief to 85% of patients.[37]

MCN Branches Entrapment

Several authors[35, 39] have claimed that involvement of these branches contributes to chronic heel pain, but the issue is controversial. Others attribute the symptoms to the FBLPN. However, post-traumatic neuromas of the calcaneal branches can pose a problem and, on occasion, need to be excised.

DEEP PERONEAL NERVE
Anatomy

The nerve branches from the common peroneal nerve and courses between the extensor hallucis longus and the extensor digitorum longus muscles up to approximately 1 cm above the ankle, where it divides into a motor branch supplying the extensor digitorum brevis muscle and a sensory branch that innervates the dorsum of the first web space (Fig. 5).

Entrapment (Anterior Tarsal Tunnel Syndrome)

Pathogenesis and Etiology. The most common site of entrapment is between the inferior edge of the extensor retinaculum and the bony structures underneath, the talus and navicular. Compression may also occur at the superior retinacular edge, where the nerve is crossed by the extensor hallucis longus tendon, or at the point where the extensor hallucis brevis tendon crosses the nerve.[40]

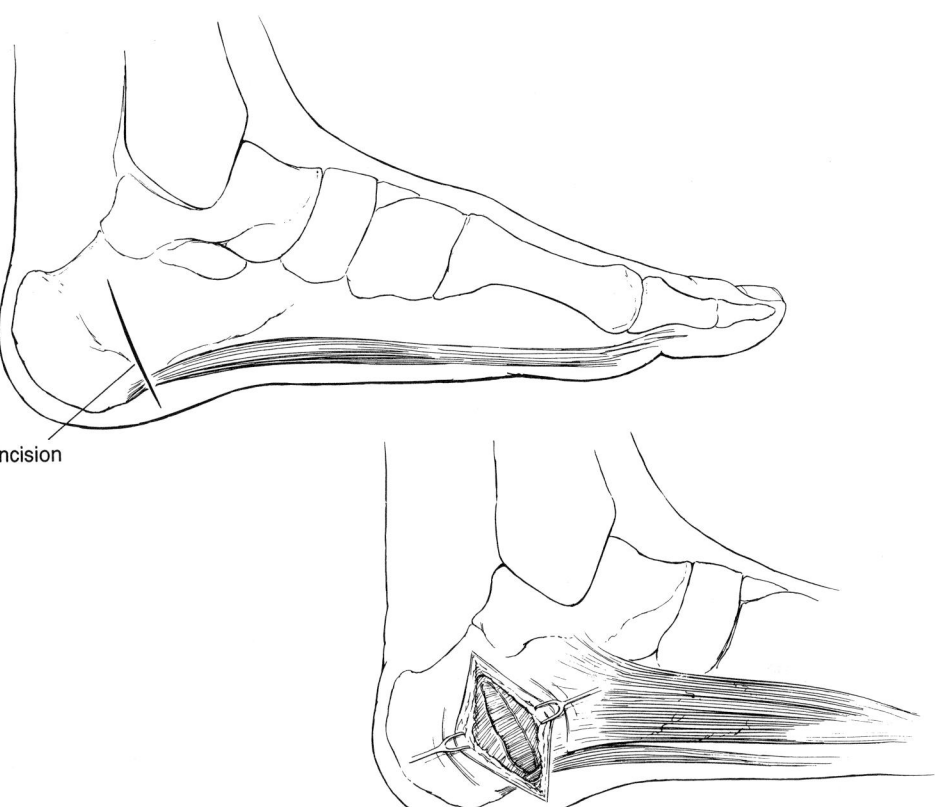

Fig. 4. Release of the first branch of the lateral plantar nerve. *A,* Incision over the lateral plantar nerve. *B,* Release of the deep fascia of the abductor muscle, followed by resection of a small portion of the plantar fascia. (From Schon LC: Tarsal tunnel release. In Myerson M [ed]: Current Therapy in Foot and Ankle Surgery. St. Louis, Mosby-Year Book, 1993, p 179.)

Incision

Causative factors include trauma, arthritis, dorsal osteophytes, excessive and prolonged ankle plantarflexion, tight shoewear, ganglions, and soft-tissue tumors.[32, 40]

Diagnosis (History, Physical Examination, Diagnostic Studies). The patient complains of dorsal foot pain radiating into the first web space. The pain may be related to tight shoewear or to other forms of local pressure on the

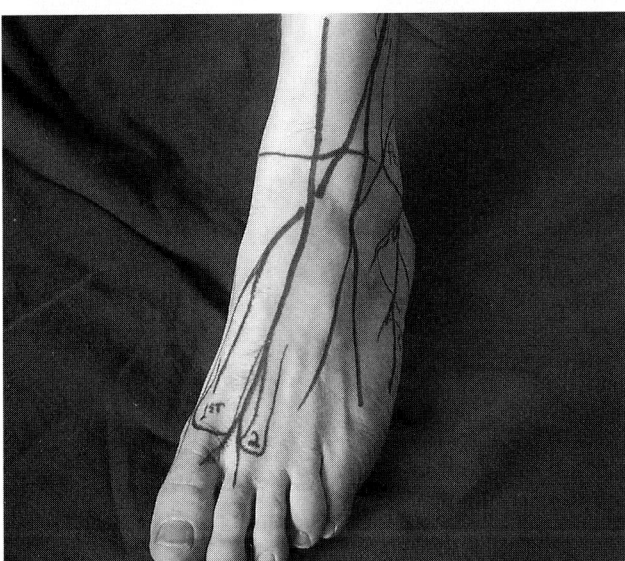

Fig. 5. The deep peroneal nerve. It courses within the anterior compartment and then anterior to the ankle. After providing a motor branch to the extensor digitorum brevis, it provides sensation to the first web space dorsally.

anterior aspect of the ankle. There may be a history of trauma or recurrent ankle sprains. Symptoms aggravated by activity are suggestive of exertional compartment syndrome.

On physical examination, the area of maximal tenderness, identified by palpation, is usually located at the inferior extensor retinaculum. Osteophytes and ganglions can be felt along the course of the nerve. The pain can sometimes be reproduced in full-ankle dorsiflexion or plantarflexion. The neurological examination may reveal diminished sensation in the first web space or weakness and atrophy of the extensor digitorum brevis muscle.[41] The ankle joint should be tested for stability. Because instability may stretch the nerve and lead to symptoms, dynamic testing may be needed if symptoms occur only during physical activity.

Radiographs may identify compressing osteophytes or exostoses. Electrodiagnostic studies can help rule out peripheral neuropathies or proximal involvement (double-crush injuries) and may differentiate between proximal and distal compression within the canal.[41] However, a study with normal results does not contraindicate surgery. Local diagnostic nerve blocks confirm the diagnosis. Anterior compartment syndrome is assessed by compartment pressure measurements after a treadmill stress test.

Management. Nonoperative measures include activity modification, accommodative shoewear, ankle bracing for instability, pharmacological agents, and steroid injections. Surgery is considered when all nonoperative therapies have been unsuccessful. Surgical intervention consists of releasing the extensor retinaculum carefully to preserve its proximal portion to avoid bowstringing, resection of osteophytes, ankle ligament reconstruction for associated instability, and fasciotomy in the presence of an anterior compartment syndrome. At times, it may be necessary to release the extensor hallucis brevis tendon.[33]

Results. Dellon[41] reported an 80% satisfactory outcome rate in 20 patients with surgical decompression. Poor results are usually associated with internal nerve damage (crush/neuroma) and with systemic neuropathies.

SUPERFICIAL PERONEAL NERVE
Anatomy
The superficial peroneal nerve (SPN) courses in the lateral compartment of the leg and then travels through a tunnel of deep fascia situated approximately 8 to 12 cm proximal to the lateral malleolus. It then divides into the medial cutaneous branch that supplies sensation to the dorsomedial aspect of the foot and ankle and the intermediate cutaneous branch that innervates the dorsolateral skin of the foot and ankle (Fig. 6).[42, 43]

Entrapment
Etiology and Pathogenesis. This uncommon syndrome may be idiopathic or associated with ankle instability, direct trauma, ganglions and other soft-tissue tumors, exertional anterior compartment syndrome, muscle herniation, ankle edema, and fibular fractures.

Two types of injury should be considered. First, compression of the nerve beneath the fascia at the fibrous tunnel level may be exacerbated by static muscle herniation or by dynamic herniation that can be seen with exertional anterior compartment syndrome or after a fasciotomy. Second, with traction of the intermediate cutaneous branch with ankle instability and recurrent ankle sprains, the branch is trapped at the site of exit from under the deep fascia.

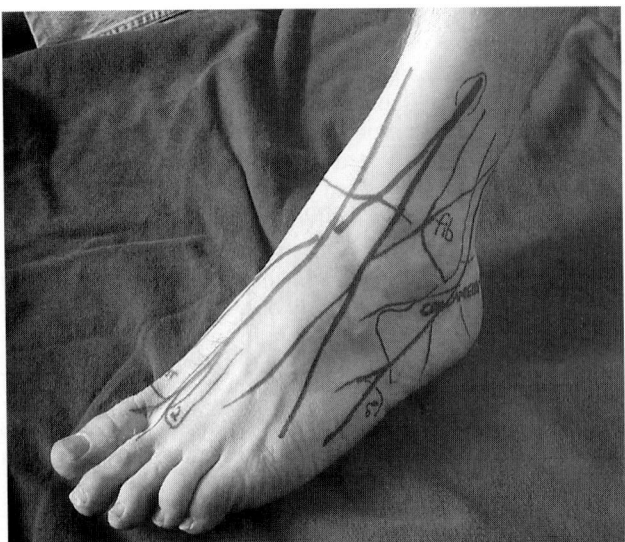

Fig. 6. Superficial peroneal nerve. After providing motor nerves to the peroneal muscles, the SPN runs either in the lateral or anterior compartment and pierces the fascia as one or two terminal sensory branches. The most medial, called the dorsal medial cutaneous nerve, innervates the medial skin of the dorsum of the foot. The intermediate dorsal cutaneous nerve provides sensation for the second through the fourth toes and dorsum of the foot.

Diagnosis (History, Physical Examination, Diagnostic Studies). The patient complains of pain along the anterolateral aspect of the ankle and foot associated with paresthesias or numbness. Any previous sprain or trauma should be recorded, and a previous fasciotomy should be noted as well.

Palpation along the course of the SPN reveals the point of maximal tenderness and can identify a muscle herniation, a fascial defect, or a bony prominence. Percussion produces paresthesias in the nerve's distribution.[32, 43] Three provocative diagnostic tests were described by Styf.[44] Palpation of the nerve is performed during active ankle dorsiflexion/eversion and then during plantarflexion/inversion. The ankle is finally tested in plantarflexion/inversion without nerve palpation. Stability of the joint must also be assessed.

Radiographs may diagnose fracture fragments or bony prominences. Electrodiagnostic studies can detect SPN compromise and rule out peripheral neuropathy. Local diagnostic blocks are helpful in confirming the diagnosis. Compartment pressures should be measured if exertional compartment syndrome is suspected.[43]

Management. Nonoperative measures include ankle bracing, peroneal muscle strengthening, lateral shoe wedges, pharmacological agents, TCAs, AEDs, and local steroid injections.

Surgery consists of nerve release at the fibrous tunnel, resection of exostoses, extensive compartment fasciotomy when indicated, and ankle ligament reconstruction in the presence of instability.[35, 43]

Results. A success rate of 75% can be expected after adequate decompression.[43]

SAPHENOUS NERVE
Anatomy
The nerve courses with the superficial femoral artery after branching from the femoral nerve. It penetrates the subsartorial fascia approximately 10 cm proximal to the medial femoral condyle and divides into the infrapatellar and sartorial branches. The infrapatellar branch courses anteriorly, superficial to the insertion of the pes anserinus, to innervate the skin over the proximal tibia just distal to the knee joint. This branch is often injured with the anterior surgical approach to the knee joint during total knee replacement. The sartorial branch descends along the medial tibial border accompanied by the greater saphenous vein, and it divides again approximately 15 cm proximal to the medial malleolus into two branches innervating the skin of the medial ankle and the medial foot (Fig. 7).

Entrapment
Etiology and Pathogenesis. The most common point of entrapment is at the level of the subsartorial fascia above the knee, and the pain may radiate distally along the distribution area. Direct trauma or any surgery may damage the nerve internally or entrap it in scar tissue.

Diagnosis (History, Physical Examination, Diagnostic Studies). The patient complains of medial foot and ankle pain, but the point of maximal tenderness is located over the subsartorial canal. MRI or ultrasonography may diagnose soft-tissue masses. A diagnostic block is recommended. Somatosensory evoked potentials may also aid in diagnosis.[45]

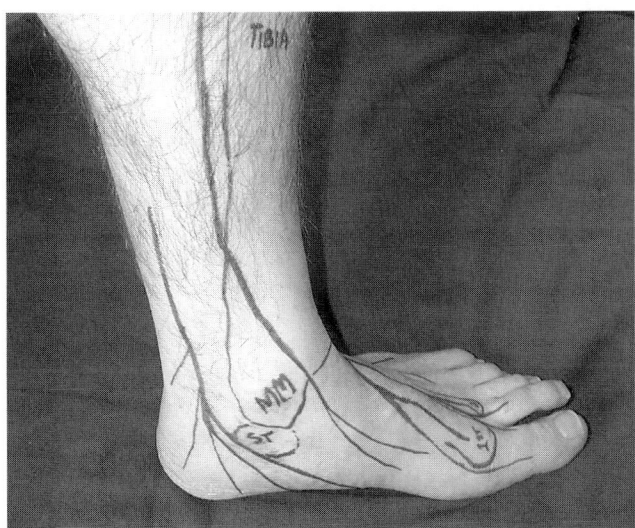

Fig. 7. The saphenous nerve. It runs along the posteromedial border of the tibia. Proximally, the nerve travels with the femoral artery and then pierces Hunter's fascia. The infrapatellar branch courses around the sartorius muscle to innervate the medial aspect of the knee. Distally, it runs along the medial tibia and then courses anteriorly over the talocrural articulation.

Management and Results. Local steroid injections provide satisfactory pain relief in 38% to 80% of the patients.[46, 47] The remainder may require surgical release through the anterior aspect of Hunter's canal with division of the subsartorial fascia.[45, 48]

SURAL NERVE
Anatomy

The medial sural nerve originating from the TN and the lateral sural nerve branching from the peroneal nerve combine in the distal leg to form the sural nerve coursing along the lateral aspect of the ankle. It then divides just proximal to the ankle into a lateral branch and a posterior branch. The lateral branch supplies the skin of the lateral ankle and anastomoses occasionally with the SPN. The posterior branch innervates the skin of the outer heel and the lateral foot up to the proximal part of the fifth metatarsus (Fig. 8).[49]

Entrapment

Etiology. Common causes of sural nerve compromise include ankle sprains, fractures of the fifth metatarsal base or calcaneus, ganglions, Achilles' or peroneal tendinitis, edema, and iatrogenic surgical trauma.[50]

Diagnosis (History, Physical Examination, Diagnostic Studies). Pain is localized to the lateral foot and ankle and is associated with dysesthesias and paresthesias. Previous surgery and symptoms of ankle instability should be noted. Palpation may reveal tenderness and a positive Tinel's sign along the nerve. The ankle and hindfoot should be stressed in inversion to identify a dynamic entrapment. Plain radiographs rule out bony abnormalities. MRI may be needed to evaluate soft-tissue masses. Electrodiagnostic studies yield only occasionally positive results. A local anesthetic block may aid in diagnosis but, if pain relief is not achieved, the block must be repeated more proximally, and the anastomosing fibers of the SPN should be numbed as well.

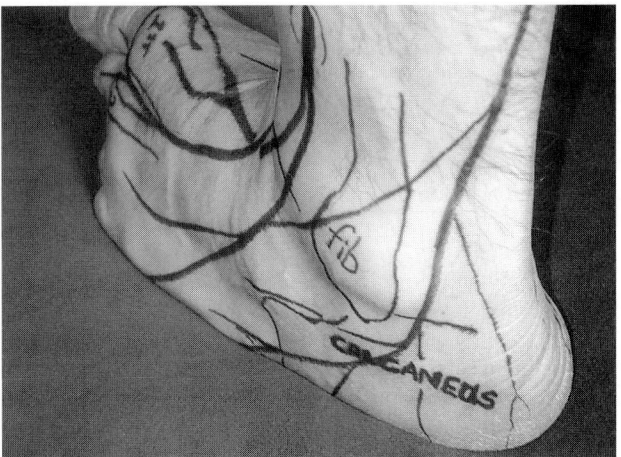

Fig. 8. The sural nerve. It is near the midline of the posterior leg, just superficial to the fascia. In the lower quarter of the leg, it begins to lie within the sulcus between the peroneal tendon sheath and the Achilles tendon. It becomes the lateral dorsal cutaneous nerve in the foot, innervating the lateral border of the foot.

Management. Nonoperative treatment includes nonsteroidal anti-inflammatory medications, vitamin B_6, TCAs, and AEDs. In the presence of ankle instability, ankle bracing, shoe wedges, and physical therapy may prove effective. Surgery consists of nerve release from scar tissue or constrictive structures.

Results. No large series are available. Surgical decompression typically results in pain relief when a specific site of nerve compression has been identified.[51] Lateral stabilization of an unstable ankle may relieve sural neuralgia even without decompressing the nerve.[52]

INTERDIGITAL NEURALGIA (MORTON'S NEUROMA)
Anatomy

The interdigital nerve is stretched over the anterior edges of the transverse metatarsal ligament and the coalesced portion of the plantar fascia (Fig. 9).

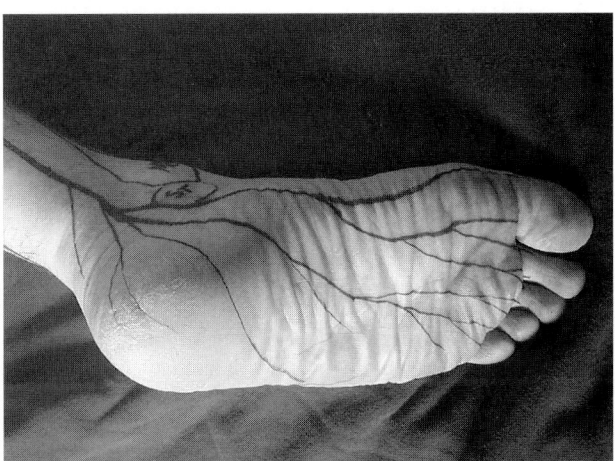

Fig. 9. The interdigital nerves. They are distal branches of the medial plantar nerve and the lateral plantar nerve.

Entrapment

Pathogenesis and Etiology. High-heeled shoes may exacerbate the entrapment because hyperextension of the metatarsophalangeal (MTP) joints increases the nerve tethering by the transverse metatarsal ligament.[3] Histological findings include nerve fiber degeneration, perineural fibrosis, and deposition of amorphous eosinophilic material.[53] The third and the second web spaces are the most commonly affected sites.

Contributing factors include direct plantar trauma, thickening of the ligament, ganglion and soft-tissue tumors in the web space, hammertoe or clawtoe deformities with MTP joint instability, a hypermobile first ray with transfer metatarsalgia, bursae or inflammation within the web space, and MTP joint synovitis.[3, 54, 55]

Diagnosis (History, Physical Examination, Diagnostic Studies). The differential diagnosis is proximal nerve compromise, metatarsal stress fracture, and MTP joint disorders, including synovitis, instability, and degenerative or inflammatory arthritis.[56]

Patients usually experience burning plantar foot pain between the metatarsal heads. The pain is activity-related and radiates into the toes. It is aggravated by weightbearing in tight toebox, high-heeled shoes. The symptoms may be reproduced by palpating the plantar interspace distal to the metatarsal heads. A positive Mulder's sign is highly suggestive of interdigital neuralgia.[57] To elicit this sign, the clinician palpates the interspace with one hand and transversely compresses the metatarsal heads with the other hand. A click should be appreciated, and symptoms should be reproduced. This click has to be differentiated from other clicks that may occur from subluxation of tendons or intrinsic musculature. Any lesser toe deformities are noted, and the MTP joints are assessed for mobility and stability. Decreased sensation may be found in the adjacent aspect of the affected toes.

Radiographs define malalignment and degenerative changes in the toes and MTP joints. Ultrasonography and MRI may assist in diagnosis by showing enlarged nerves, but interpretation of the findings is still controversial.[58-60] Diagnosis is best confirmed with a local block proximal to the web space along the common digital nerve.

Management. Nonoperative therapies include using wide-toebox, low-heeled shoes, soft soles or inserts, and metatarsal pads. The latter may occasionally exacerbate the symptoms. Steroid injections may provide long-term relief, but they should be used cautiously because of side effects, including fat-pad atrophy and MTP joint capsule attenuation. Only 20% to 60% of patients experience long-term relief with nonoperative measures alone.

The surgical approach may be either dorsal[61] or plantar.[62] Most surgeons favor the dorsal approach for primary cases, reserving the plantar approach for revision surgery because it is associated with skin and fat-pad complications. The transverse metatarsal ligament is transected, and the interdigital nerve is excised 3 cm proximal to the ligament.[63] The patient has to be informed that, as a result of the surgery, excision of the nerve will inevitably result in numbness of the toes. Although this is usually well tolerated by the patient, it may occasionally be annoying. In rare cases, the patient may develop anesthesia dolorosa or deafferentation pain. Because of the ablative nature of the surgery for this type of compression neuropathy, some clinicians have recommended transecting the ligament without excising the nerve.[64, 65] This interesting approach limits the potential symptomatic neuroma formation with chronic neuralgia. The efficacy of this release has not been well tested.

Results. Reported success rates for primary common digital nerve resection are from 60% to 96%.[61, 66-68] The best results are obtained in isolated third-web-space neuralgia. Transection of the ligament alone yields 80% to 85% satisfactory results.[65, 69, 70] Revision surgery is associated with a less predictable outcome. Patient dissatisfaction from either no improvement or from worsening of the symptoms ranges from 24% to 40%.[3, 61, 68, 71]

CHRONIC NERVE PROBLEMS

Patients with chronic nerve pain (neuralgia) usually have a multiple neurological symptoms and findings. The complaints may be unusual, intense, or severe, but the clinical examination may be less or more dramatic or appear nonanatomic or inconsistent with standard musculoskeletal disorder. It is often only on closer scrutiny that a logical profile evolves. The profile can be additionally blurred because nerve problems are often found in patients with chronic trauma or chronic surgical failure. Thus, patience and an open mind are required when evaluating for treatable lesions.

DIAGNOSIS
History

A thorough history must be obtained. A history of trauma or previous surgery is usually but not always present.[72] The trauma may have been "open" (penetrating or degloving injury, previous surgery) or "closed" (crush, sprain, or twisting injury). A fracture may also have occurred. How each event impacted the patient's pain is important. New features with different events should be noted.

The patient with a chronic nerve problem typically complains of marked pain along the distribution of a peripheral nerve. The pain is often described as tingling or burning and it radiates proximally or distally. The pain may worsen with pressure from the shoe/brace or the floor, and pressure from a mattress and/or bedsheets at night may cause severe discomfort (nociceptive neuralgia). Sometimes, to be able to sleep, a patient has to wear socks or have a protective cradle or boot around the foot. Episodes of severe, spontaneous, and short-term "ectopic" pain unrelated to touch or pressure ("shooters") may also be present and may vary in frequency and intensity (ectopic neuralgia). Note whether the pain and its radiation pattern are consistent with the neuroanatomy, i.e., whether the symptoms may be attributed to a specific nerve territory or whether they are diffuse. The latter is suggestive of sympathetically mediated pain and may be associated with other sympathetic symptoms such as perceptions of inappropriate temperature changes in the extremity (e.g., "the leg feels ice cold"), changes in color of the skin, recurrent episodes of swelling not necessarily related to gravity or activity, and abnormal skin moisture. The presence of a primary nerve lesion categorizes the chronic neuralgia with or without sympathetically mediated pain as a CRPS type 2.[73] In the absence of such a nerve lesion, the clinical presentation is defined as a CRPS type 1.

The possibilities of more than one nerve being involved or in more than one location for a single nerve must be kept in mind. Pain along the distribution of two separate nerves that share a common origin without a clear history of trauma to both suggests a neural insult in a more proximal location and, thus, represents a CRPS type 2. A single nerve may also be injured at two levels, thereby resulting in a double crush. A herniated disc in the lumbar spine may, for instance, exacerbate the pain associated with a distal peripheral nerve lesion. Evaluation of the spinal cord or the brain might therefore be warranted in the presence of bilaterality, gait imbalance, radiculopathy, and symptoms of motor involvement such as muscle weakness, spasticity, tremor, or involuntary muscle activity.

Physical Examination

Inspection of the feet, performed with the patient in both weightbearing and non-weightbearing postures, may reveal foot deformities and malalignment, joint contractures or instability, osseous prominences, and soft-tissue lesions. The patient's gait is observed because it may aggravate and accentuate dynamic deformities or reveal patterns of antalgic avoidance. The presence of previous surgical scars is noted as well as their exact locations with respect to the anatomic path of the nerves of the foot (posterior tibial, saphenous, deep and superficial peroneal, and sural nerves and their branches).

All nerves are systematically palpated and percussed. Areas of tenderness along the course of a nerve, with local pressure reproducing the patient's pain or a positive Tinel's sign in a nonregenerating nerve, are indicative of chronic nerve compromise. Sensation should be carefully assessed, and areas of abnormal perception (zones of hyperesthesia, dysesthesia, allodynia, decreased sensation, total numbness, and anesthesia dolorosa) should be mapped. The Semmes-Weinstein monofilament test is more sensitive than the routine manual evaluation and may detect subtle sensory abnormalities in light-touch and deep-pressure thresholds in the early phases of neural deterioration.[74]

Assess the motor function of all muscle groups. It may be found to be pathological in combined motor and sensory neuropathies, in lumbar radiculopathy, and with involvement of the TN, which is the only nerve in the foot that has a motor component. Weakness of the posterior tibial tendon due to partial or complete tear is associated with a pes planovalgus deformity and may aggravate a tarsal tunnel syndrome by exerting traction on the TN or by causing its branches to become compressed against the shoe or the floor. Signs of sympathetic involvement (including diffuse swelling, changes in skin color/temperature, increased sweating or dry skin, atrophic changes in the skin or toenails, continuous pain and allodynia, or hyperalgesia) should be recorded. However, a positive response to a sympathetic block is a prerequisite to diagnosing sympathetic involvement.[75] The spine should be examined to rule out radiculopathy or a double crush. Finally, evaluate the vascular status of the involved extremity, especially if surgery is an option.

Imaging Studies

Radiographs and sometimes a computed tomography scan may be needed to rule out a bone disorder as a potential cause of nerve compromise. Nerves may be compressed or irritated by bony prominences, exostoses, coalitions, nonunions, and malunions. Decreased bone radiodensity is not helpful in assessment because it is a nonspecific finding that may be associated with disuse atrophy and sympathetic dysfunction. Increased uptake in the delayed phase of a three-phase technetium bone scan represents increased bone metabolism and can be found in CRPS, but the relevance of this scan as a diagnostic study is controversial.[76] MRI may diagnose soft-tissue lesions that compress the nerves, and it may occasionally diagnose a nerve tumor or a large neuroma.[77] It is useful in failed cases of TN release for evaluating the contents of the tarsal tunnel and ruling out other disorders.[78] An MRI of the spine may be indicated with associated back symptoms or radiculopathy.

Nerve Blocks

A series of local peripheral nerve blocks is probably the most informative investigative study in the evaluation of nerve pain. It helps localize the involved nerve and the pathways of pain signal transmission. It can also help predict the immediate outcome of a nerve transection and allows the patient to experience some of the numb feeling after surgical denervation.[79] Unfortunately, it does not mimic the result of a surgical transection nor does it reveal the potential adverse sequelae of the deafferentation phenomenon.

If pain is suspected to originate from a mechanical problem such as an arthritic joint or a chronically inflamed tendon, it must be ruled out first by injecting the appropriate mechanical structure. The nerve block is performed proximal to the area of tenderness; if done properly, it should result in numbness in the whole distribution area. Complete pain relief should then follow. If this is not the case, the block may be repeated more proximally and include adjacent nerves in order to rule out aberrant pathways and interneural anastomoses, which are common especially along the distribution path of the sural nerve.[80] If pain relief is still not achieved, the peripheral nerve might not be the main contributor to pain, and other potential sources should be evaluated. A sympathetic block is used to detect sympathetically mediated pain, and an epidural block may be helpful in diagnosing radicular pain.

Electrodiagnostic Studies

Nerve conduction studies in conjunction with electromyography may provide useful information about the location and the degree of severity of nerve compromise. It is good to distinguish between external nerve compression and intraneural disorder and assesses the degree of intraneural damage. If internal damage is found to be substantial, nerve release or vein wrap procedures may not be good options, and better results may be anticipated with nerve transection and burial or PNS. Electrodiagnostic studies may also identify peripheral neuropathy, spinal radiculopathy, or a double crush.[81]

Differential Diagnosis

Space-occupying lesions, such as ganglia or inclusion cysts that externally compress the nerve, and bony outgrowths such as exostoses must be ruled out. Pain from a neuroma should be differentiated from that originating from underlying arthritis, and radicular pain must be differentiated from a peripheral neuralgia. The clinician should inquire about backache and previous back problems when obtaining the patient history. Include an examination of the back, a modified Lassegue or straight-leg-raising test, and a thorough and systematic neurological examination of both lower extremities. In case of doubt, additional studies such as electromyography or an MRI of the spine may be required. Symptoms of CRPS should be noted because they differ in both treatment and prognosis. Nerve pain may be from any type of chronic neuropathy secondary to a systemic disease. Finally, attention must be given to determining concomitant structural or musculoskeletal problems, which are often overlooked in patients with chronic nerve pain.

MANAGEMENT
Nonoperative Treatment

Shoe Modification and Orthoses. A shoe should be large enough to avoid excessive pressure on the foot but not so large that it shifts around the foot. Soft and pliable shoes or open sandals are usually recommended. Local pressure may sometimes be relieved by stretching, cushioning doughnut-shaped pads, or custom protective orthoses.

Immobilization. Immobilization may provide short-term relief of nerve pain, but it is often only partially effective in the long run. There are many modes of immobilization that patients with severe neuralgia cannot tolerate, which can complicate any foot and ankle surgery that requires strict immobilization as part of the postoperative regimen.

Pharmacological Agents. Medications exert their pain-modulating effects through peripheral and central pain pathways.[72, 73]

Oral sympatholytics include phenoxybenzamine (Dibenzyline), prazosin (Minipress), terazosin (Hytrin), and clonidine (Catapres). Their mode of action is unknown. They are either β-blockers or α-adrenergic in their sympathetic activity and are indicated for patients exhibiting a sympathetic component or symptoms of vasomotor instability. Side effects include hypotension, sedation, and sexual dysfunction. Clonidine is an α_2-adrenergic agonist that can be administered locally through patches containing 0.1 to 0.3 mg/day. It carries the potential risk of skin irritation.

Nonsteroidal anti-inflammatory medications have a limited place in nerve pain control, unless there is a related inflammatory component that contributes to it.

Steroids may be taken orally, parenterally, or by local injection. Their mode of action is discussed in the section on local blocks. When used systemically (especially for a long time), steroids may cause peptic ulcers, erosive gastritis, osteoporosis, diabetes, Cushing's syndrome, avascular necrosis, cataracts, and life-threatening immunosuppression. Abrupt discontinuation in a patient chronically taking steroids may result in acute addisonian crisis (adrenal insufficiency).

Vitamin B_6 has been used to improve nerve function and decrease symptoms, although there is no evidence of its effectiveness. The daily dose is 100 to 150 mg. It is safe but, when given in excess, may induce a peripheral neuropathy.

TCAs include amitriptyline (Elavil), nortriptyline (Pamelor), and desipramine (Norpramin). They act at lower doses than medications required for depression management by enhancing serotonin effects on the central nervous system, thereby diminishing central pain perception. Side effects include hypotension, sedation, urinary retention, constipation, dry mouth, blurred vision, weight gain, and nightmares.

Serotonin reuptake inhibitors include trazodone (Desyrel), fluoxetine (Prozac), paroxetine (Paxil), and sertraline (Zoloft). The effect is similar to that of TCAs because they all increase the level of serotonin in the brain's synapses. Side effects include insomnia, sedation, agitation, and sexual dysfunction.

Opioid analgesics decrease pain by inhibiting the release of presynaptic neurotransmitters and by modifying their postsynaptic effect. The major concerns are tolerance and potential addiction. Long-acting narcotics such as methadone and oxycodone (OxyContin) are recommended for managing chronic pain.

Calcium channel blockers include nifedipine (Procardia), verapamil (Calan), and diltiazem (Cardizem). They reduce nerve hypersensitivity by inhibiting calcium-ion exchange across the axonal membrane. Associated vasomotor instability may benefit from their effect on smooth muscle. Side effects include hypotension, edema, and constipation.

Antiarrhythmics include lidocaine given by repeated infusions and its oral derivatives mexiletine and flecainide. The presence of a second- or third-degree atrial ventricular block is a contraindication. Side effects include gastrointestinal upset and dizziness.

AEDs include carbamazepine (Tegretol), phenytoin (Dilantin), clonazepam (Klonopin), and gabapentin (Neurontin). They suppress ectopic neuronal activity. Potential side effects include dysphoria, drowsiness, confusion, and gastrointestinal upset.

Topical agents, aside from the clonidine patches, include capsaicin cream (a substance P inhibitor), ketamine cream, and local anesthetics such as lidocaine ointment and patches.

Physical Therapy. Desensitization has been shown to be effective in chronic neuralgia.[82] This form of perception reeducation is performed by rubbing, percussing, and massaging the hypersensitive areas until a gradually increasing tolerance to touch and pressure is achieved. The mechanism of action is unknown, but it is believed to block the transmission along pain fibers by stimulation of inhibitory pathways within the nerve (i.e., the gate mechanism of pain). A second indication for physiotherapy in the presence of chronic nerve problems is the early stages of CRPS type 2. In such a patient, physiotherapy (including heat, hydrotherapy, ultrasonography, and desensitization) combats the symptoms and potential sequelae of the sympathetically mediated component of the disease. The physiotherapy is administered in conjunction with mild analgesics and nonsteroidal anti-inflammatory medications. Another important task of the physiotherapist is to maintain joint mobility, strength, and overall conditioning during the time the patient with a chronic nerve problem is incapacitated.

TENS. TENS is best used as an adjunct with other nonoperative measures; its success rate is 33% when used as a single modality but increases to 44% when combined with other modalities.[83] It is believed to achieve pain control by activating inhibitory mechanisms through stimulation of large myelinated nerve fibers (the gate mechanism). It usually provides only partial, temporary relief.

We have found that patients who respond to a TENS unit will also be good candidates for PNS. The TENS unit gives patients an opportunity to get acquainted with the tingling sensations associated with electrical stimulation, and it may help discern some of the few individuals who respond to stimulation by paradoxical exacerbation of their symptoms. Thus, patients who have increased pain with a TENS unit are probably not good candidates for PNS. Failure to gain adequate pain relief with TENS, however, should not preclude a patient from having a PNS device implanted because they may still do well with the more focused method of PNS. However, this is a controversial issue; other investigators have had different experiences.[84]

Nerve Blocks. A lidocaine injection is a powerful diagnostic tool, but it has minimal therapeutic value in itself unless used in conjunction with a corticosteroid.[85] Local injection of steroids is widely used, and it can offer long-term pain relief in post-traumatic neuromas as well as in interdigital neuromas. The mode of action of steroids is uncertain. Theories include softening of the surrounding scar, a local anti-inflammatory effect, and decreased ectopic neural activity via reduction of the action potential of nerve fibers through stabilization of axonal membranes. Repeated injections may be needed to achieve the maximal therapeutic effect.[86] Caution must be exercised when subcutaneous injections are used because they may cause local tissue atrophy.

Sympathetic blocks may be helpful for patients with CRPS because they uncouple the combined sympathetic and sensory responses to noxious stimuli that result in additive inappropriate responses, thus breaking the pain cycle. The sympathetic block should be initiated early in the disease process and may be repeated every other day if a patient has some response. During the time the block is effective, the patient should perform activities or physical therapy, maintain some limb function, and avoid secondary problems such as contracture, osteopenia, and atrophy.

Pain Management Centers. The patient with chronic neuralgia may benefit from a multidisciplinary approach that deals not only with the pain itself but also with the associated psychological and psychosocial aspects of the problem, such as generalized stress, depression, addiction to narcotic medications, issues of low self-esteem, unemployment, lack of family support, and so on. The pain clinic uses a team approach of specialists skilled in a multimodality management of chronic pain. The orthopaedist is a member of that team and should reevaluate the patient periodically to rule out treatable musculoskeletal or nerve lesions.[87]

Surgical Treatment

Prevention of neuroma formation can be achieved by using meticulous dissection to avoid inadvertent injuries to peripheral nerves in the course of surgery. Whenever a nerve has been injured, whether by trauma or iatrogenically, attempt to repair the nerve by suturing the epineurium. Distal, small sensory nerve branches in the foot usually do not require repair. In such cases, the risks associated with surgical exploration and the likelihood of finding and success-fully repairing the nerve must be taken into consideration. Results in large nerves may be improved with fascicular repair using microsurgical techniques, but this procedure may not be applicable to the relatively small nerves in the foot and ankle. If the distal part is damaged or scarred, the damaged section can be bypassed using a nerve graft. Once a neuroma is present, management becomes problematic, with less predictable results and lower success rates. Nonoperative treatment should always be tried first; even if it does not result in full resolution, partial relief is often enough to abort the need for a surgical intervention. Surgery should be considered only for patients who do not respond to nonoperative measures. A neuroma can be approached surgically in two different ways: (1) by resecting the neuroma with an additional procedure (burial into muscle or bone) to decrease the chances of disorganized axonal regeneration or (2) by inhibiting the pain signals transmitted along the nerve with PNS.

When planning surgery, all associated musculoskeletal factors that may contribute to nerve compromise should be considered and need to be corrected either primarily or concurrently during nerve surgery. Severe cases that do not respond to any of the above-mentioned modalities may be considered for spinal cord stimulation or for spinally administered opioids via an implanted pump. Despite all efforts, some of these complex patients with recalcitrant pain may require amputations. The results of amputation in such cases are highly variable and controversial.

Once chronic pain is established, there are many nerve procedures that may be used in the attempt to control the pain: neurolysis, revision neurolysis, revision neurolysis with a barrier procedure, neuroma or nerve transection, and PNS.

Nerve Release (Neurolysis). In this procedure, the nerve is released either primarily or as a revision. Depending on the previous history and surgeries, the nerve may appear normal, scarred, partially transected, or distorted. The release may be simple, or it may be an incredibly meticulous and prolonged procedure. Therefore, results vary from case to case.

Indications. The procedure may be successful if external compression or impingement is present and if the nerve itself is inherently intact. Potential causes of external compression include bony fragments or prominences, soft-tissue cysts and tumors, rheumatic synovitis, muscle impingement, engorged varicose veins, scar tissue, and incomplete release during previous surgery.

Results. The outcome of surgical treatment for chronic neural pain and revision neurolysis after a primary failure is less favorable than that of primary neurolysis for an acute nerve entrapment. The patients who tend to do better after revision surgery are those with incomplete primary release. In one study, 24 patients with chronic postsurgical tibial neuralgia were reviewed.[29] Evaluation was performed with a pain score using a visual analogue scale ranging from 0 (= no pain) to 10 (= pain so intense that amputation is requested) and a functional score ranging from 0 (= full function) to 10 (= necessity of a wheelchair). The average pain score improved from 9 to 6, and the average functional score improved from 8 to 6. Of the 24 patients, 12 returned to work in lighter-duty occupations compared with their work before nerve compromise; 12 patients remained unemployed.

Nerve Transection. This procedure may be performed after previous transection or as a last-resort attempt at controlling the pain. The concept is that by interrupting the conduits that carry the pain signal, the pain level will be improved. Unfortunately, in some cases, the newly traumatized nerve end will eventually resume the role of the pain generator, and the benefits of this procedure are lost. In other cases, the pain signal is not regenerated from the distal end of the nerve, but it originates in a chronic condition from the proximal, spinal nerve body, and the benefits of this procedure are either short-lived or never realized.

Indications. Most transections in the foot are performed in combination with containment (e.g., burial into muscle or bone) to improve pain resolution and minimize recurrence of a symptomatic neuroma. The most popular site for a simple transection without containment remains the web space for the treatment of a symptomatic interdigital neuroma.[88] Other terminal sensory branches in the lower extremity, such as the infrapatellar branch of the saphenous nerve, may be approached in this manner.

Technique. It is recommended that the nerve be approached proximally to the site of the previous transection and, after it is identified, traced distally until the neuroma is located. The neuroma is then mobilized, gently pulled, and sharply transected proximally, allowing the nerve to retract into the surrounding soft tissues.

Results. Primary transection in the foot is associated with a success rate of 65% to 83%. Revision surgery has a less favorable outcome, with satisfactory pain relief ranging from 50% to 81%.[12, 61, 68, 71, 89, 90]

Transection with Containment. The concept behind this procedure is that the nerve ending that had been generating the pain signal is placed into a more protective or healthier bed. The new environment may anatomically or physiologically minimize the development of a recurrent symptomatic neuroma.

Indications. The procedure is indicated for a failed nerve release or revision release, for a chronic traumatic/iatrogenic transection or a failed surgical transection, and for an injured nerve in a mechanically vulnerable location.

Technique. Many techniques of containment have been described in the literature, but none seem to offer an optimal and predictable outcome. The techniques include burial into muscle, fat, bone, or vessels; nerve repair or grafting; proximal implantation into a different nerve (centrocentral anastomosis); proximal implantation into the same nerve; epineural closure (suture, biocompatible glue); proximal nerve ligation (suture, radioactive materials); nerve stump capping; physical tip ablation (freezing, cautery, electrocoagulation, CO_2 laser beam photocoagulation); chemical tip ablation (alcohol, phenol, formaldehyde); nerve crushing, and so on.[88] We prefer to contain the nerve within muscle because the muscle provides a soft, protective barrier. After the nerve is dissected proximally, the distal end is secured with an epineurial suture. With a curved or right-angle hemostat, a pathway is created deep within the belly of an adjacent muscle. The hemostat is then used to grasp the end of the suture and is then withdrawn from the muscle. The end of the protruding nerve is then transected and allowed to retract within the muscle (Fig. 10). A second choice is transection and burial into bone. The challenge with this procedure is to create a passageway in bone that

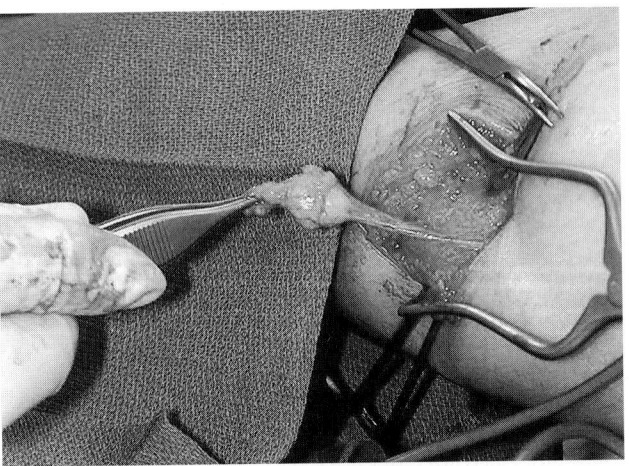

Fig. 10. The neuroma. It is identified, and the hemostat is passed to lead the nerve into the muscle belly.

is easy for through-and-through threading of the nerve. One method is to plan a drill hole from one cortex to another, i.e., in a straight rather than curved line.

Results. In one study,[72] 61 procedures were performed in 53 patients, with an average follow-up of 30 months. On a scale ranging from 0 (= no pain) to 10 (= pain so intense that amputation is requested), the average pain score improved from 8.5 to 4.8. On a scale ranging from 0 (= full function) to 10 (= necessity of a wheelchair), the average dysfunction score improved from 7.6 to 4.7. The work status improved in 45% of the patients. The best results were obtained in patients treated for neuroma or nociceptive neuralgia (pain produced by mechanical stressing). In chronic cases associated with crush or stretch and idiopathic cases (especially with ectopic neuralgia—sudden, severe, spontaneous, unprovoked pain), the outcome was less favorable. A 82% success rate was reported by Dellon and MacKinnon[91] using a similar technique in 78 patients monitored for 31 months. They recommended using deeper rather than superficial muscles. They also advised using muscles that had limited excursions that would be less likely to cause additional nerve traction with movement.

Neurolysis with Barrier Procedure. The primary or revision neurolysis may be followed by a procedure that in theory would protect the nerve from rescarring in a traumatized or unhealthy soft-tissue bed. Thus, the barrier procedure should protect the nerve from the ingrowth of scar tissue.

Indications. Adhesive neuralgia is a condition in which the nerve is entrapped in scar tissue. The typical scenario of a patient with adhesive neuralgia is that of a nerve release, which produced temporary relief, followed by recurring (or worsening) symptoms within 2 to 24 months. The operative scar is hypertrophic, immobile, and tender. Ankle motion (in tibial neuralgia) or adjacent joint motion reproduces the pain and dysesthesias.

Different types of barriers have been used (including fat, silicone, and so on) with variable success rates. Our preferred method is the vein wrap, using an autologous saphenous vein graft. Alternatively, a glutaraldehyde-preserved umbilical vein may be used, but this graft is bulky and less well suited to use with smaller-diameter nerves, such as those in the foot.

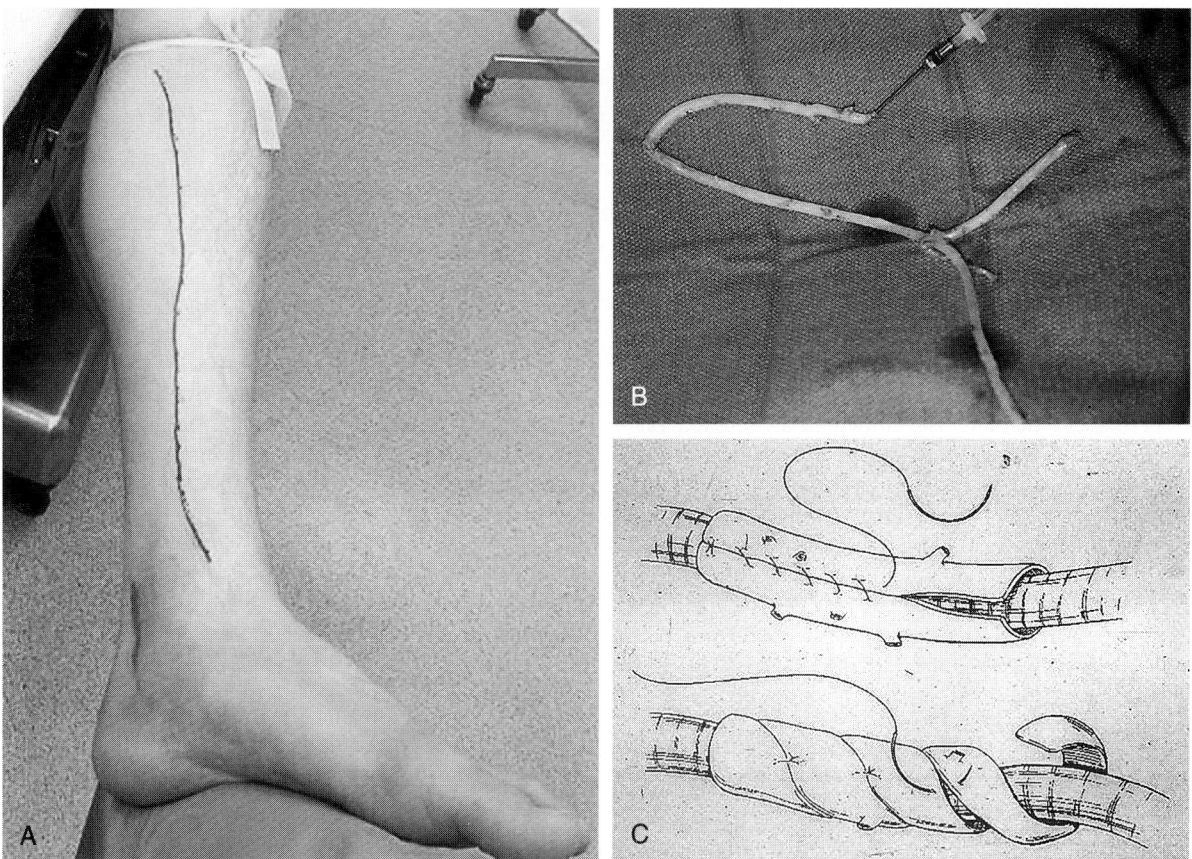

Fig. 11. The vein wrap procedure. *A,* The saphenous vein is marked preoperatively. *B,* The vein is harvested, and its small branches are clamped during distention of the vein with lidocaine. *C,* The vein is split and wrapped in a barber-pole fashion around the nerve. (From Schon LC, Easley ME: Chronic pain. In Myerson MS [ed]: Foot and Ankle Disorders. Philadelphia, WB Saunders, 2000, p 851.)

Technique. Preoperatively, the saphenous vein is palpated using a tourniquet, and the course of the vein is drawn on the skin with a permanent marker (Fig. 11A). Intraoperatively, the affected nerve is then explored and meticulously released from the entrapping scar. After completing the nerve release, the saphenous vein is harvested from the medial leg, and all the small feeder vein branches are clamped (see Fig. 11B). The vein is removed and distended with lidocaine for 15 to 20 minutes to block the sodium pump and keep the vein from contracting. The vein is split longitudinally, wrapped loosely around the nerve in a "barber-pole" fashion with the endothelial side facing the nerve, and secured in place by sutures (see Fig. 11C). If the nerve is narrow, the vein can simply be applied longitudinally around it. If most of the scar tissue is superficial to the nerve, the vein may be sewn in an open fashion over the nerve, isolating it from the more superficial scar tissues. This minimizes the surgical trauma to the nerve and preserves the more normal tissue bed so that it may continue to provide nutrition to the nerve.

Results. Easley and Schon[92] monitored 25 patients undergoing this procedure for 24 months (average); 68% were satisfied with the procedure. The average pain score (scale, 0 to 10) improved from 8.7 to 4.6, and the dysfunction score (scale, 0 to 10) improved from 7.3 to 4.4. Of the 18 previously nonworking patients, 10 were able to work after surgery. Similar results were reported by Gould et al[93] for 64 patients monitored for 31 months. There was a 63%

patient satisfaction rate, and the average pain score improved from 8.7 to 6.1. However, 25% of patients noted an increase in symptoms.

PNS. PNS is believed to act through activation of the gate mechanism of pain (see the earlier discussion on chronic pain). The electrical current (or associated magnetic field) stimulates large myelinated A-beta fibers that exert an inhibitory effect on nociceptive signals carried from the periphery. This inhibition takes place at the level of the spinal cord, in the dorsal horns where the ascending tracts carrying pain signals to the brain are located. The clinical potential of peripheral stimulation was demonstrated by Wall and Sweet[94] in 1967, and it was in the same year that Shealy and colleagues[95] reported their preliminary results with spinal cord stimulation. PNS was first used to treat chronic neuralgia in the upper extremity. Recently, technique and device modifications have led to improved attempts in the lower extremities.

Indications. Any patient with chronic peripheral neuralgia for whom nonoperative and surgical attempts to control the pain have failed is a potential candidate for PNS. Previous surgical interventions may include any type of nerve release, repair, transection, rerouting, grafting, or implantation of a spinal cord stimulator. PNS may be used either as an isolated procedure or as an adjunct to other types of surgical intervention such as nerve release, neuroma resection, transfer of a transected nerve, and even a vein wrap in the most severe cases. Using a dual-lead transmitter, stimulation may be applied simultaneously to more than one nerve. It may also be used bilaterally.

Contraindications. Contraindications include infection or ulceration at the site of implantation and the presence of a pacemaker (due to possible electronic cross-talk between the two devices). Other electronic devices, such as a spinal cord stimulator or other PNS device, represent a relative contraindication because the complication of cross-talk can be avoided with proper preoperative planning in most cases. The presence of a peripheral neuropathy or of symptoms and signs of sympathetically mediated pain (CRPS type 2) do not preclude the use of the stimulator.[72]

Technique. Before surgery, the patient is examined, and painful zones on the extremity are mapped and marked with a permanent marker. The drawings are copied on a rubber foot and ankle model to facilitate intraoperative discussion with the patient. Surgery is performed under general anesthesia. The chosen site for implantation of the lead is always above the ankle level and preferably proximal to the area of actual nerve damage. Dissection is carried down to the fascia. A longitudinal rectangular fascial graft is then harvested and sewn to the lead. The nerve is explored and released. The wound edges are injected with a long-acting local anesthetic while the tissues are irrigated to avoid inadequately anesthetizing the nerve. The lead is applied to the nerve and connected to a temporary external signal generator. The patient can be temporarily reversed from

anesthesia for a wake-up test in which the lead is adjusted on the nerve to achieve maximal coverage/pain relief (Fig. 12A). These adjustments are guided by verbal input from the patient. After the optimal position for the lead is found, it is sewn in place to the epineurium (see Fig. 12B), and the patient is reanesthetized. A permanent signal generator is implanted in a subcutaneous pocket in the thigh (see Fig. 12C). It is connected to the lead by a wire that is passed through a subcutaneous tunnel created between the two points. The wire is secured in place by an anchoring suture, and the wound is copiously irrigated and closed in the regular fashion.[72] This procedure also can be performed in two stages: first, implantation of leads to external battery and second, implantation of permanent battery after a week of ambulation.

Complications. PNS is an electronic device with mechanical parts. It has to function as a watertight unit in a liquid environment. Moreover, the device is designed so that it may be operated and programmed transcutaneously with a remote control unit. This complexity carries a substantial potential for malfunction. Fortunately, however, technical problems have been overcome, including electrode migration, wire breakage, generator site pain, crosstalk between bilateral devices, and infection. Infection is a serious complication that requires removal (at least temporary) of the device and reinsertion after resolution. One drawback of PNS is that if a patient's symptoms do not

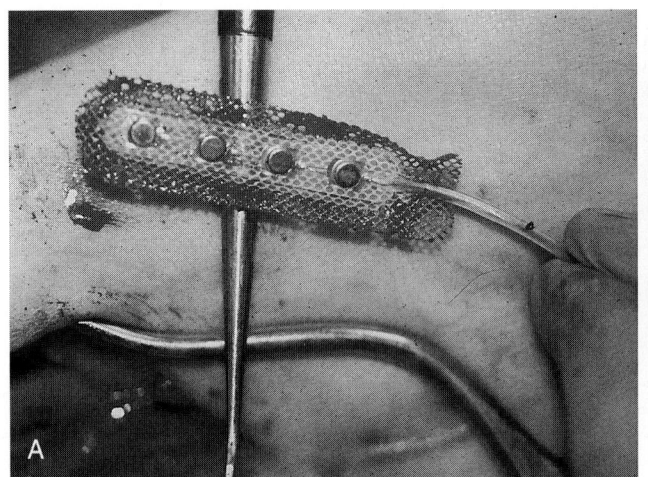

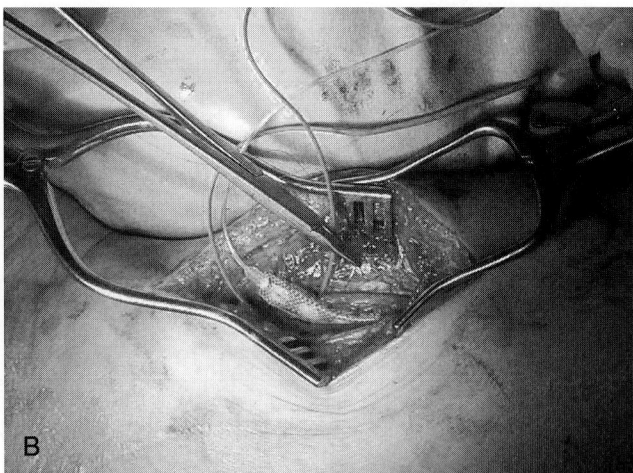

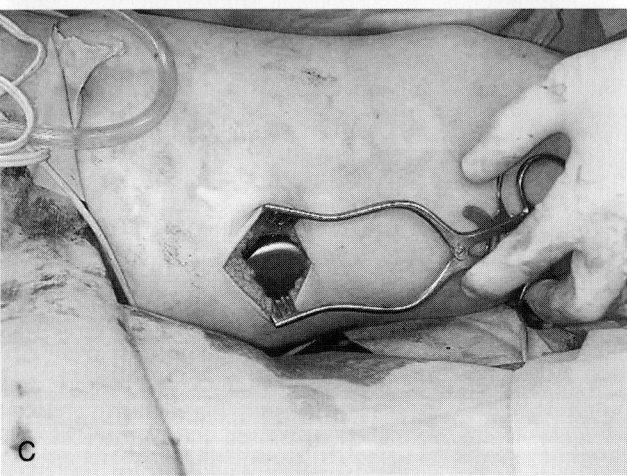

Fig. 12. View. The tibial nerve has been released, the wound edges have been anesthetized, and the patient is reversed from anesthesia. During the wake-up test, the lead *(A)* is meticulously positioned so that there is optimum pain relief. Then the lead is sutured to the epineurium *(B)*. The pulse generator is then inserted into the thigh *(C)*.

improve, and continued long-term stimulation is necessary, the pulse generator (whose average life is 3 years) may need to be changed periodically. Each battery change involves minor revision surgery (usually under local anesthesia) in the thigh but still carries a potential risk for complications. "Heavy users" that need currents of greater amplitude (more than 3 amps) to obtain pain relief may wear out the battery in the pulse generator earlier, sometimes within 1 year.

Results. Overall, our patients managed with PNS have experienced an average of 40% improvement in pain level, and overall improvement in ambulation, sleep, and medication needs has been noted. In such severe cases, a 10% improvement can be very substantial to the patient.

SUMMARY

Nerve problems of the leg, ankle, and foot may resolve spontaneously or with nonoperative treatment. Medications such as TCAs and AEDs are helpful in managing patients with neuralgia. For patients who do not respond to tincture of time and nonoperative modalities, surgery is considered. The initial surgery is typically a neurolysis, which usually

improves the patient's condition if there is a nerve entrapment. For patients with more devastating trauma (especially those involving a crush, transection, or severe stretching mechanism) or multiple failed previous surgeries, more complex surgeries may be warranted. If a nerve release was incomplete, extending the release may be beneficial. If the nerve was transected and the end of the nerve remained mechanically vulnerable (i.e., nociceptive neuralgia), a revision of the nerve transection with burial more proximally (out of the zone of mechanical vulnerability) is considered. For patients with adhesive neuralgia, in which initial nerve release provided temporary relief, or for patients in whom postoperative infection or wound problems increased the scarring, a revision release and vein wrapping are warranted. For patients with ectopic neuralgia, especially when there is anesthesia dolorosa, deafferentation phenomenon, and CRPS type 2, PNS is an option. A spinal cord stimulator may also be used as an end-stage salvage attempt when all other peripheral nerve surgeries have failed. In many of these chronic cases, the involvement of a pain center can be very helpful in providing a multimodality approach to symptomatic relief.

REFERENCES

1. Merskey H, Bogduk N: Relatively generalized syndromes. In Classification of Chronic Pain: Descriptions of Chronic Pain Syndromes and Definitions of Pain Terms, 2nd ed. Seattle, International Association of the Study of Pain, Task Force on Taxonomy, IASP Press, 1994, p 39.
2. Kenzora JE: Sensory nerve neuromas leading to failed foot surgery. Foot Ankle 1986; 7:110.
3. Mann RA, Baxter DE: Diseases of the nerves. In Mann RA, Coughlin MJ (eds): Surgery of the Foot and Ankle, 6th ed. St. Louis, Mosby-Year Book, 1993, p 543.
4. Lehman RA, Hayes GJ: Degeneration and regeneration in peripheral nerve. Brain 1967; 90:285.
5. Corner EM: The structure, forms and conditions of the ends of divided nerves: With a note on regeneration neuromata. Br J Surg 1918; 6:273.
6. Santi MD, Botte MJ: Nerve injury and repair in the foot and ankle. Foot Ankle Int 1996; 17:425.
7. Battista AF, Lusskin R: The anatomy and physiology of the peripheral nerve. Foot Ankle 1986; 7:65.
8. Devor M, Wall PD: Type of sensory nerve fibre sprouting to form a neuroma. Nature 1976; 262:705.
9. Sunderland S: Nerves and Nerve Injuries, 2nd ed. New York, Churchill Livingstone, 1978.
10. Herndon JH, Hess AV: Neuromas. In Gelberman RH (ed): Operative Nerve Repair and Reconstruction. Philadelphia, JB Lippincott, 1991, p 1525.
11. McGrath MH, Polayes IM: Posttraumatic median neuroma: A cause of carpal tunnel syndrome. Ann Plast Surg 1979; 3:227.
12. Kenzora JE: Symptomatic incisional neuromas on the dorsum of the foot. Foot Ankle 1984; 5:2.

13. Herndon JH: Neuromas. In Green DP, Hotchkiss RN (eds): Operative Hand Surgery, 3rd ed. New York, Churchill Livingstone, 1993, p 1387.
14. Wilson RL: Management of pain following peripheral nerve injuries. Orthop Clin North Am 1981; 12:343.
15. Cousins MJ, Bridenbaugh PO: Neural blockade. Clinical Anesthesia and Management of Pain, 2nd ed. Philadelphia, JB Lippincott, 1988.
16. Bonica JJ: Neurophysiologic and pathologic aspects of acute and chronic pain. Arch Surg 1977; 112:750.
17. Wall PD, Melzack R: Textbook of Pain, 3rd ed. New York, Churchill Livingstone, 1994.
18. Melzack R, Wall PD: Pain mechanisms: A new theory. Science 1965; 150:971.
19. Cimino WR: Tarsal tunnel syndrome: Review of the literature. Foot Ankle 1990; 11:47.
20. Mann RA: Tarsal tunnel syndrome. Orthop Clin North Am 1974; 5:109.
21. Takakura Y, Kitada C, Sugimoto K, et al: Tarsal tunnel syndrome: Causes and results of operative treatment. J Bone Joint Surg Br 1991; 73:125.
22. Myerson M, Quill GE Jr: Late complications of fractures of the calcaneus. J Bone Joint Surg Am 1993; 75:331.
23. Saxby T, Myerson M, Schon L: Compartment syndrome of the foot following calcaneus fracture. Foot 1992; 2:157.
24. Cotton FJ: Old os calcis fractures. Ann Surg 1921; 74:294.
25. Francis H, March L, Terenty T, et al: Benign joint hypermobility with neuropathy: Documentation and mechanism of tarsal tunnel syndrome. J Rheumatol 1987; 14:577.
26. Pfeiffer WH, Cracchiolo A III: Clinical results after tarsal tunnel decompression. J Bone Joint Surg Am 1994; 76:1222.

27. Sammarco GJ, Chalk DE, Feibel JH: Tarsal tunnel syndrome and additional nerve lesions in the same limb. Foot Ankle 1993; 14:71.
28. Bailie DS, Kelikian AS: Tarsal tunnel syndrome: Diagnosis, surgical technique, and functional outcome. Foot Ankle Int 1998; 19:65.
29. Skalley TC, Schon LC, Hinton RY, et al: Clinical results following revision tibial nerve release. Foot Ankle Int 1994; 15:360.
30. Murphy PC, Baxter DE: Nerve entrapment of the foot and ankle in runners. Clin Sports Med 1985; 4:753.
31. Stein M, Shlamkovitch N, Finestone A, et al: Marcher's digitalgia paresthetica among recruits. Foot Ankle 1989; 9:312.
32. Schon LC, Baxter DE: Neuropathies of the foot and ankle in athletes. Clin Sports Med 1990; 9:489.
33. Schon LC: Nerve entrapment, neuropathy, and nerve dysfunction in athletes. Orthop Clin North Am 1994; 25:47.
34. Schon LC, Glennon TP, Baxter DE: Heel pain syndrome: Electrodiagnostic support for nerve entrapment. Foot Ankle 1993; 14:129.
35. Beskin JL: Nerve entrapment syndromes of the foot and ankle. J Am Acad Orthop Surg 1997; 5:261.
36. Kaplan PE, Kernahan WT: Tarsal tunnel syndrome: An electrodiagnostic and surgical correlation. J Bone Joint Surg Am 1981; 63:96.
37. Baxter DE, Pfeffer GB: Treatment of chronic heel pain by surgical release of the first branch of the lateral plantar nerve. Clin Orthop 1992; 279:229.
38. Rondhuis JJ, Huson A: The first branch of the lateral plantar nerve and heel pain. Acta Morphol Nederl Scand 1986; 24:269.
39. Tanz SS: Heel pain. Clin Orthop 1963; 28:169.

40. Gessini L, Jandolo B, Pietrangeli A: The anterior tarsal syndrome: Report of four cases. J Bone Joint Surg Am 1984; 66: 786.

41. Dellon AL: Deep peroneal nerve entrapment on the dorsum of the foot. Foot Ankle 1990; 11:73.

42. Sarrafian SK: Anatomy of the Foot and Ankle: Descriptive, Topographic, Functional. Philadelphia, JB Lippincott, 1983.

43. Styf J: Entrapment of the superficial peroneal nerve: Diagnosis and results of decompression. J Bone Joint Surg Br 1989; 71:131.

44. Styf J: Diagnosis of exercise-induced pain in the anterior aspect of the lower leg. Am J Sports Med 1988; 16:165.

45. Tranier S, Durey A, Chevallier B, et al: Value of somatosensory evoked potentials in saphenous entrapment neuropathy. J Neurol Neurosurg Psychiatry 1992; 55: 461.

46. Mozes M, Ouaknine G, Nathan H: Saphenous nerve entrapment simulating vascular disorder. Surgery 1975; 77:299.

47. Romanoff ME, Cory PC Jr, Kalenak A, et al: Saphenous nerve entrapment at the adductor canal. Am J Sports Med 1989; 17: 478.

48. Kopell HP, Thompson WAL: Peripheral Entrapment Neuropathies, 2nd ed. Huntington, NY, Robert E Kreiger Publications Inc, 1976.

49. Lawrence SJ, Botte MJ: The sural nerve in the foot and ankle: An anatomic study with clinical and surgical implications. Foot Ankle Int 1994; 15:490.

50. Starosta D, Sacchetti AD, Sharkey P: Calcaneal fracture with compartment syndrome of the foot. Ann Emerg Med 1988; 17:856.

51. Pringle RM, Protheroe K, Mukherjee SK: Entrapment neuropathy of the sural nerve. J Bone Joint Surg Br 1974; 56:465.

52. Schon LC, Baxter DE: Heel pain syndrome and entrapment neuropathies about the foot and ankle. In Gould JS (ed): Operative Foot Surgery. Philadelphia, WB Saunders, 1994, p 192.

53. Graham CE, Graham DM: Morton's neuroma: A microscopic evaluation. Foot Ankle 1984; 5:150.

54. Awerbuch MS, Shephard E, Vernon-Roberts B: Morton's metatarsalgia due to intermetatarsophalangeal bursitis as an early manifestation of rheumatoid arthritis. Clin Orthop 1982; 167:214.

55. Chandler JT, Davis WH, Anderson RB: Instability of the second metatarsophalangeal joint presenting as second webspace interdigital neuroma. Presented at the 26th Annual Meeting of the American Orthopaedic Foot and Ankle Society, Atlanta, February 25, 1996.

56. Borges LF, Hallett M, Selkoe DJ, et al: The anterior tarsal tunnel syndrome: Report of two cases. J Neurosurg 1981; 54: 89.

57. Mulder JD. The causative mechanism in Morton's metatarsalgia. J Bone Joint Surg Br 1951; 33:94.

58. Redd RA, Peters VJ, Emery SF, et al: Morton neuroma: Sonographic evaluation. Radiology 1989; 171:415.

59. Resch S, Stenstrom A, Jonsson A, et al: The diagnostic efficacy of magnetic resonance imaging and ultrasonography in Morton's neuroma: A radiological-surgical correlation. Foot Ankle Int 1994; 15:88.

60. Terk MR, Kwong PK, Suthar M, et al: Morton neuroma: Evaluation with MR imaging performed with contrast enhancement and fat suppression. Radiology 1993; 189:239.

61. Mann RA, Reynolds JC: Interdigital neuroma: A critical clinical analysis. Foot Ankle 1983; 3:238.

62. Richardson EG, Brotzman SB, Graves SC: The plantar incision for procedures involving the forefoot: An evaluation of one hundred and fifty incisions in one hundred and fifteen patients. J Bone Joint Surg Am 1993; 75:726.

63. Amis JA, Siverhus SW, Liwnicz BH: An anatomic basis for recurrence after Morton's neuroma excision. Foot Ankle 1992; 13:153.

64. Dellon AL: Treatment of recurrent metatarsalgia by neuroma resection and muscle implantation: Case report and proposed algorithm of management for Morton's neuroma. Microsurgery 1989; 10:256.

65. Diebold PF, Delagoutte JP: [True neurolysis in the treatment of Morton's neuroma]. Acta Orthop Belg 1989; 55:467.

66. Friscia DA, Strom DE, Parr JW, et al: Surgical treatment for primary interdigital neuroma. Orthopedics 1991; 14:669.

67. Rasmussen MR, Kitaoka HB, Patzer GL: Nonoperative treatment of plantar interdigital neuroma with a single corticosteroid injection. Clin Orthop 1996; 326:188.

68. Johnson JE, Johnson KA, Unni KK: Persistent pain after excision of an interdigital neuroma: Results of reoperation. J Bone Joint Surg Am 1988; 70:651.

69. Dellon AL: Treatment of Morton's neuroma as a nerve compression: The role for neurolysis. J Am Podiatr Med Assoc 1992; 82:399.

70. Gauthier G: Thomas Morton's disease—a nerve entrapment syndrome: A new surgical technique. Clin Orthop 1979; 142:90.

71. Beskin JL, Baxter DE: Recurrent pain following interdigital neurectomy: A plantar approach. Foot Ankle 1988; 9:34.

72. Schon LC, Easley ME: Chronic pain. In Myerson MS (ed): Foot and Ankle Disorders. Philadelphia, WB Saunders, 2000, p 851.

73. Pedowitz WJ, Berberian WS: The multiply operated foot and regional pain syndromes. Foot Ankle Clin 1998; 3:129.

74. Weinstein S: Fifty years of somatosensory research: From the Semmes-Weinstein monofilaments to the Weinstein Enhanced Sensory test. J Hand Ther 1993; 6:11.

75. Campbell JN: Complex regional pain syndrome and the sympathetic nervous system. In Campbell JN (ed): Pain 1996—An Updated Review. Seattle, International Association of the Study of Pain, IASP Press, 1996, p 89.

76. Kozin F, Soin JS, Ryan LM, et al: Bone scintigraphy in the reflex sympathetic dystrophy syndrome. Radiology 1981; 138: 437.

77. Erickson SJ, Quinn SF, Kneeland JB, et al: MR imaging of the tarsal tunnel and related spaces: Normal and abnormal findings with anatomic correlation. AJR Am J Roentgenol 1990; 155:323.

78. Zeiss J, Fenton P, Ebraheim N, et al: Magnetic resonance imaging for ineffec-

tual tarsal tunnel surgical treatment. Clin Orthop 1991; 264:264.

79. Abadir AR: Diagnostic nerve blocks. In Omer GE Jr, Spinner M, Van Beek AL (eds): Management of Peripheral Nerve Problems, 2nd ed. Philadelphia, WB Saunders, 1998, p 65.

80. Ortiguela ME, Wood MB, Cahill DR: Anatomy of the sural nerve complex. J Hand Surg Am 1987; 12:1119.

81. Wilbourn AJ, Shields RW Jr: Generalized polyneuropathies and other nonsurgical peripheral nervous system disorders. In Omer GE Jr, Spinner M, Van Beek AL (eds): Management of Peripheral Nerve Problems, 2nd ed. Philadelphia, WB Saunders, 1998, p 648.

82. Grant GH: Methods of treatment of neuromata of the hand. J Bone Joint Surg Am 1951; 33:841.

83. Long DM: Electrical stimulation for the control of pain. Arch Surg 1977; 112:884.

84. Masear VR, Bonatz E: Painful neuromas of the lower extremity and postneurectomy pain. In Omer GE Jr, Spinner M, Van Beek AL (eds): Management of Peripheral Nerve Problems, 2nd ed. Philadelphia, WB Saunders, 1998, p 151.

85. Devor M, Govrin-Lippmann R, Raber P: Corticosteroids suppress ectopic neural discharge originating in experimental neuromas. Pain 1985; 22:127.

86. Smith JR, Gomez NH: Local injection therapy of neuromata of the hand with triamcinolone acetonide: A preliminary study of twenty-two patients. J Bone Joint Surg Am 1970; 52:71.

87. Schultz D: Indications for utilization of a pain clinic. In Omer GE Jr, Spinner M, Van Beek AL (eds): Management of Peripheral Nerve Problems, 2nd ed. Philadelphia, WB Saunders, 1998, p 120.

88. Botte MJ, Tran HN, Copp SN, et al: Traumatic neuromas of the foot and ankle. Foot Ankle Clin 1998; 3:71.

89. Tupper JW, Booth DM: Treatment of painful neuromas of sensory nerves in the hand: A comparison of traditional and newer methods. J Hand Surg Am 1976; 1: 144.

90. Lam PWC, Anderson CD, Easley ME, et al: Preliminary results of peripheral nerve stimulation for intractable lower extremity nerve pain. Presented at the International FES Society 6th Vienna International Workshop on Functional Electrostimulation: Basics, Technology, Application. Vienna, Austria, September 18, 1999.

91. Dellon AL, MacKinnon SE: Susceptibility of the superficial sensory branch of the radial nerve to form painful neuromas. J Hand Surg Br 1984; 9:42.

92. Easley ME, Schon LC: Peripheral nerve vein wrapping for intractable lower extremity pain. Foot Ankle Int 2000; 21:492.

93. Gould JS, Hart TS, O'Brien TS, et al: Outcome analysis of vein wrapping for intractable painful nerves in continuity. Presented at the 12th Annual Summer Meeting of the American Foot and Ankle Society, Hilton Head, SC, June 28, 1996.

94. Wall PD, Sweet WH: Temporary abolition of pain in man. Science 1967; 155:108.

95. Shealy CN, Mortimer JT, Reswick JB: Electrical inhibition of pain by stimulation of the dorsal columns: Preliminary clinical report. Anesth Analg 1967; 46:489.

ACQUIRED ADULT FLATFOOT DEFORMITY

Jonathan T. Deland and Il Hoon Sung

Summary

- Acquired adult flatfoot produces debilitating, progressive deformity.
- Conservative treatment can be successful, especially in the short term; however, progressive deformity may still occur.
- Surgical treatment has best results in earlier stages.
- Hindfoot arthrodesis used in later stages is helpful but often leaves patients with significant limitations.

Acquired adult flatfoot is a progressive deformity. Although the term can include flatfoot deformity acquired from other causes,[1–4] such as arthrosis, trauma, or neuropathic feet, for this chapter it specifically refers to the deformity associated with failure of the posterior tibial tendon and supporting ligaments. Failure of the tendon is usually gradual, with considerable degeneration of the tendon found at surgery (Fig. 1). The flatfoot deformity is common at the level of the talonavicular joint and hindfoot but also occurs at the naviculocuneiform[5] and metatarsotarsal joints.[6] Most often, the ligaments do not undergo acute rupture but gradually elongate, especially at the spring ligament complex[7,8] (the plantar and superomedial calcaneonavicular ligaments).[9]

Adult acquired flatfoot represents a progressive collapse of the medial longitudinal arch.[10–13] Pain first occurs medially because of failure of the tendon. In later stages, once the tendon has failed, the medial pain can resolve, but lateral pain develops from progressive deformity. Acquired adult flatfoot is in general a disease of middle to older age, with a peak incidence at 55 years of age. Although occur-

ring in both sexes, it is more prevalent in women. At first thought to be a rare problem,[14,15] with recognition of how to diagnose the disease, it has become increasingly recognized as not uncommon.[16] Its true incidence is unknown.

Although authors have described a progressive flatfoot deformity, its association with failure of the posterior tibial tendon has only become widely recognized within the past 20 years.[7,17–19] Mann[1] and Johnson[19] described the failure of the tendon and the associated flatfoot deformity. Failure of the tendon was treated with a FDL tendon transfer.[10,11,18] Despite providing some pain relief, this did not correct the deformity, which can still progress. Fusions were used for symptomatic nonflexible deformity[20–24]; they provided correction, although the patients had limitations of stiffness.[25] The medial slide (MS), described by Lord[26] and Koutsagannis[27] and popularized by Myerson,[13] has been performed in addition to the tendon transfer to treat the flatfoot deformity and the tendon failure. Lengthening of the lateral column by placing a bone graft near the calcaneocuboid (CC) joint was originally described by Evans[28] in adolescents with flatfoot deformity; this procedure provides considerable correction of deformity[29–31] at the expense of pressure in the CC joint.[32] Direct repair or reconstruction of the ligaments to support the arch[33–36] has not been successful as an isolated treatment, and its utility, even with an osteotomy, can be questioned. Adult progressive flatfoot deformity remains a challenging entity to treat. It presents with different amounts of deformity and at different locations. Progress is still being made in being able to achieve better correction and better function of the foot.

PATHOGENESIS

The cause of failure of the tendon and ligaments of the arch is most likely multifactorial. Some patients relate the beginning of the medial pain to a traumatic incident, but this is not the majority of patients. Obesity has been noted more frequently in these patients than in the general population.[37] In our experience, obesity is common and present in the majority of patients. Similarly, a preexisting flatfoot is common and may place increased stress on the tendon and medial soft tissues. Increased stress promotes failure of the tendon and arch. Once deformity progresses, further progression is likely. A zone of hypovascularity in the posterior tibial tendon has been noted at the level of the medial malleolus.[38] Ruptures do occur at this location as well as distal to it. The tendon also takes a significant turn at this level.[19] There does not appear to be any one causative factor that unites all patients with adult acquired flatfoot deformity. Some biological propensity to degeneration of collagen may be another factor,[39] which has not yet been elucidated. Adult progressive flatfoot is a combination of biological factors and physical stress that results in degeneration of the soft tissues and progressive deformity.

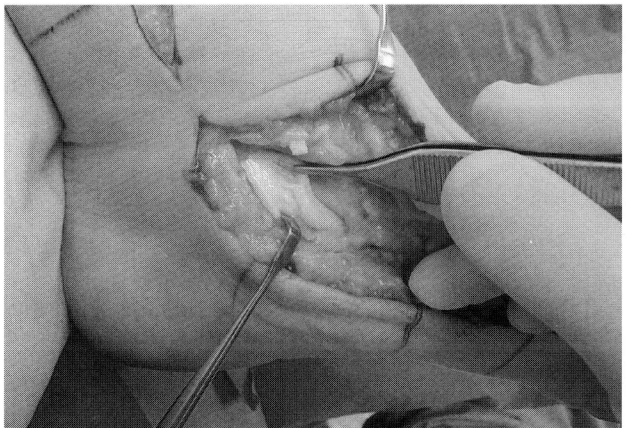

Fig. 1. Pathologic features. This is a posterior tibial tendon. Note the enlargement and fissuring of the tendon and the irregularity and longitudinal splitting of the tendon.

CLINICAL FEATURES

The most common symptom early in the course of the disease is pain over the posterior tibial tendon just distal and inferior to the medial malleolus. Once failure of the tendon has occurred, the pain can dissipate. Patients may then go through a period without significant pain, believing their problem has resolved, except perhaps noting a weakness in the arch. They may or may not notice collapse of the arch as it is occurring. In later stages when the deformity has progressed sufficiently, lateral impingement at the subtalar joint and fibula can occur from what has been described as the peritalar subluxation of the foot. The foot subluxates about the talus in a lateral and dorsal direction. Symptoms therefore depend on the stage of disease. The most widely accepted clinical staging system has been presented by Myerson.[40] Our preferred staging is similar (Table 1). In stage I, patients have minimal or no detectable deformity, with medial pain and swelling about the tendon. This stage is most often not just a tenosynovitis about the tendon; failure within the tendon has occurred. In stage II, patients have definite deformity with valgus angulation of the heel but a flexible hindfoot. In stage III, contracture and rigidity in the hindfoot have occurred with limited inversion of the triple joint complex, constituting a fixed deformity. Finally, in stage IV, deformity has occurred in the foot and also at the level of the ankle, with valgus tilting of the talus from failure of the deltoid ligament.

With the patient sitting on the examining table, the tendon can be palpated just distal to the medial malleolus. The tendon is tender early in the disease, commonly between the medial malleolus and navicular. Triple joint motion (inversion and eversion) should be measured and compared with that of the opposite foot by passively inverting the entire foot about the talus, starting with the foot and ankle in neutral position. The testing of strength in the posterior tibial tendon and muscle is done by a combined inversion plantarflexion motion of the foot against the examiner's hand, which is placed on the medial forefoot. This strength should be manually felt by the examiner, with the foot beginning from an everted position and going

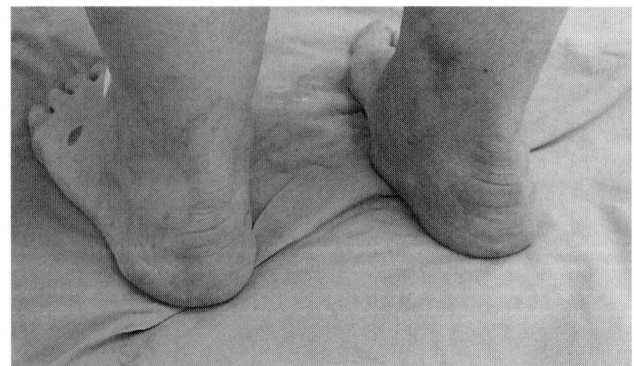

Fig. 2. Clinical photograph. This shows collapse of the longitudinal arch.

toward neutral and plantarflexion. By doing this, contribution from the anterior tibialis muscle is excluded.[40,41] Having the patient practice the motion on the opposite foot first is helpful. The alignment of the foot is then observed with the patient standing. The examiner can look at the height of the arch and determine if there is any collapse of the midfoot with abduction of the forefoot (Figs. 2 and 3). On the posterior view, the valgus of the heel (Fig. 4) can be compared with that of the opposite foot. This is an important assessment; hindfoot valgus cannot be easily measured by x-ray film. A single stance heel-rise test should then be performed. This needs to be demonstrated to the patient. The patient leans against the wall; then, lifting one foot off the ground, the patient attempts to go up on the toes of the involved foot. Difficulty in going up on the toes or poor inversion of the heel will be noted in a foot with significant failure of the tendon. Comparison should be made with the normal foot. A positive single stance heel-rise test is not pathognomonic for failure of the posterior tibial tendon; pain or deformity in the foot from other causes can give a positive test result. Tenderness along the posterior tibial tendon and weakness on inversion muscle testing can make the diagnosis of the adult acquired flatfoot from posterior tibial tendon insufficiency in its earlier stages. At a later stage, weakness of inversion and deformity are noted.

TABLE 1. CLINICAL STAGING		
Stage	**Characteristics**	**Surgical Treatment**
I	Tendon failure with inversion weakness; no or minimal deformity	Reconstruction of tendon ± MS osteotomy
II	Flexible deformity with increased heel valgus ± abduction of the mid- and forefoot	Reconstruction of tendon. MS osteotomy ± Evans osteotomy or subtalar arthrodesis
III	Fixed deformity (lack of passive inversion)	Talonavicular, talonavicular + calcaneocuboid, or triple arthrodesis
IV	Valgus tilt of talus within ankle mortise	Brace, triple arthrodesis risks increased deformity at the ankle. No good treatment.

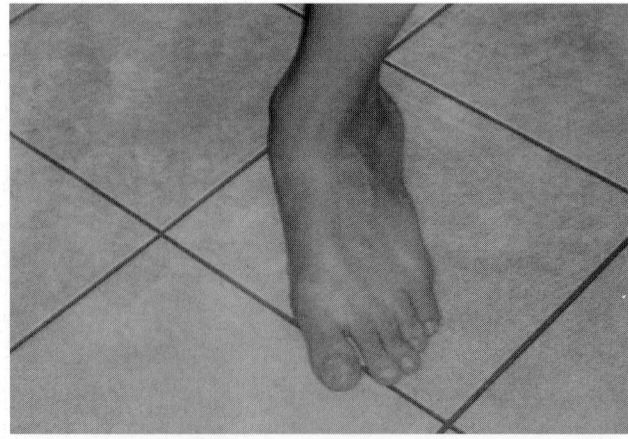

Fig. 3. Clinical photograph. This shows abduction deformity of the foot.

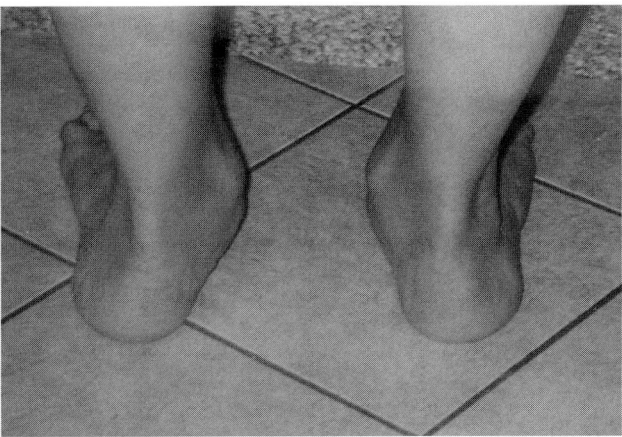

Fig. 4. Clinical photograph. This shows valgus deformity of the heel.

INVESTIGATION

In patients with posterior tibial tendon insufficiency, routine radiographs of the foot should be taken. These include a standing anteroposterior (AP), standing lateral, and supine oblique view of the foot. A standing AP view of the ankle should also be taken for patients with deformity to determine if there is any valgus tilting of the talus within the ankle mortise (Fig. 5). Deformity anywhere along the arch can be noted, and the talonavicular, naviculocuneiform, and/or metatarsotarsal joints should be examined on the lateral view for collapse. The standing lateral x-ray film should be examined for a sag at each one of these locations (Fig. 6). On the AP view, lateral subluxation of the foot can be seen by exposure of the medial talar head and displacement of the navicular laterally on the talar head (Fig. 7). This AP uncoverage angle can be measured by a technique described by Sangeorzan.[30] The collapse of the arch on the lateral view can be measured by the distance from the inferior medial cuneiform to the base of the fifth metatarsal and compared with that of the opposite foot.[42] The sag of the arch can also be measured by the talar first metatarsal angle on the lateral view. With a supine oblique

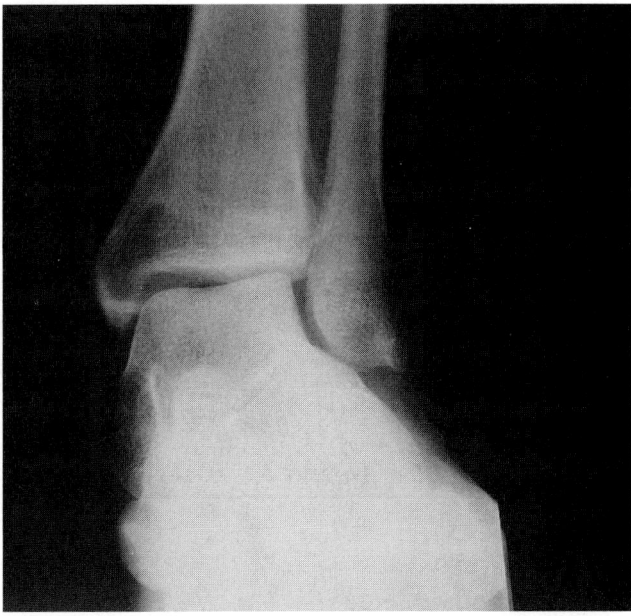

Fig. 5. Weightbearing AP radiograph. Ankle joint shows talar tilt.

view, presence of midfoot lesions such as arthroses should be sought.

A magnetic resonance image (MRI) study is a useful tool for assessing abnormal conditions of the tendons and other soft tissues of the foot (Fig. 8).[43-45] It is, however, not mandatory for diagnosis of failure of the posterior tibial tendon. Moderately high-resolution MRI can be helpful if the diagnosis is in question. For example, in a patient with persistent tenosynovitis, the tendon may be intact or minimally degenerated. The MRI can be used to confirm the lack of degeneration or tear in the tendon. High-resolution MRI is also helpful in identifying tears in the spring ligament complex (Fig. 9), which can occur without significant disorder in the posterior tibial tendon. Such scans should be performed with 1.5 TESLA units and not in an open MRI. Scanning should be done on one foot at a time to give high-quality images.

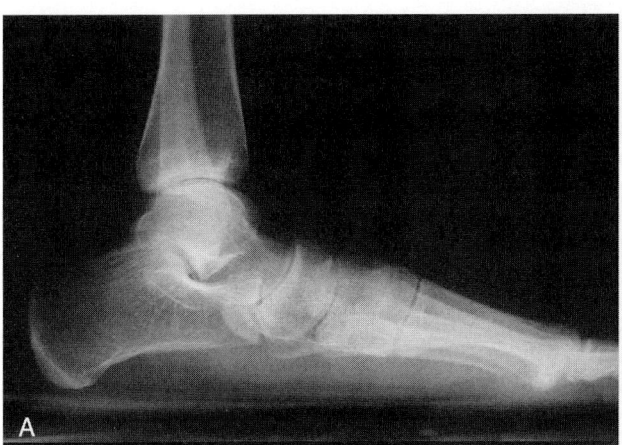
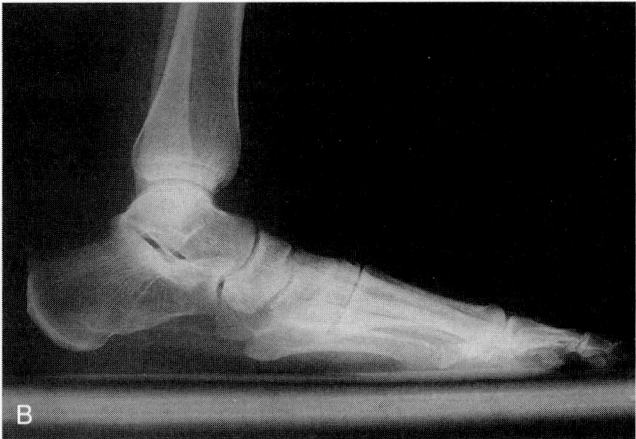

Fig. 6. Weightbearing lateral radiographs of the foot. These are sites of the deformity: at the talonavicular joint *(A)* and at the naviculocuneiform and metatarsotarsal joints *(B)*.

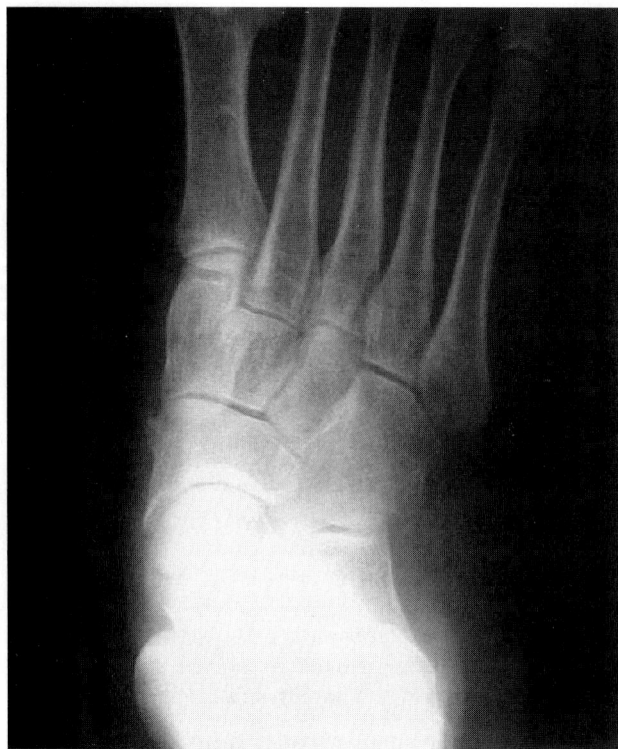

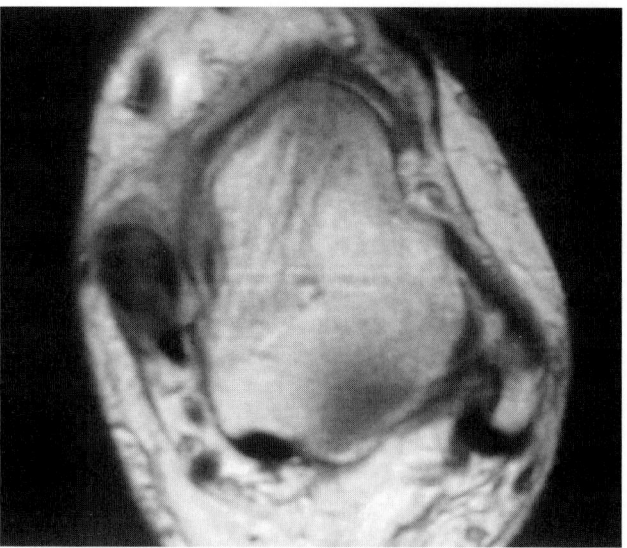

Fig. 8. MRI of abnormal posterior tibial tendon. Axial image shows low signal intensity in the tendon.

Fig. 7. Weightbearing AP radiograph of the foot. This shows subluxation of the talonavicular joint.

DIFFERENTIAL DIAGNOSIS

An adult acquired flatfoot can have causes other than failure of the posterior tibial tendon and associated ligaments. An acquired flatfoot can be from arthritis in the midfoot, which is not necessarily associated with failure of the posterior tibial tendon. Progressive collapse of the arch also occurs in patients with neuropathy, commonly diabetic patients. Therefore, patients with a history of diabetes or other possible causes of neurological involvement such as alcoholism should be examined for neuropathy. Medial ankle pain can be from degenerative changes and spurs at the medial ankle. It is possible to have degenerative changes at the ankle joint and adult acquired flatfoot simultaneously, although usually one of them is responsible for the symptoms. Location of the tenderness and, if necessary, differential lidocaine injections can be helpful in determining which (or both) is responsible for the symptoms.

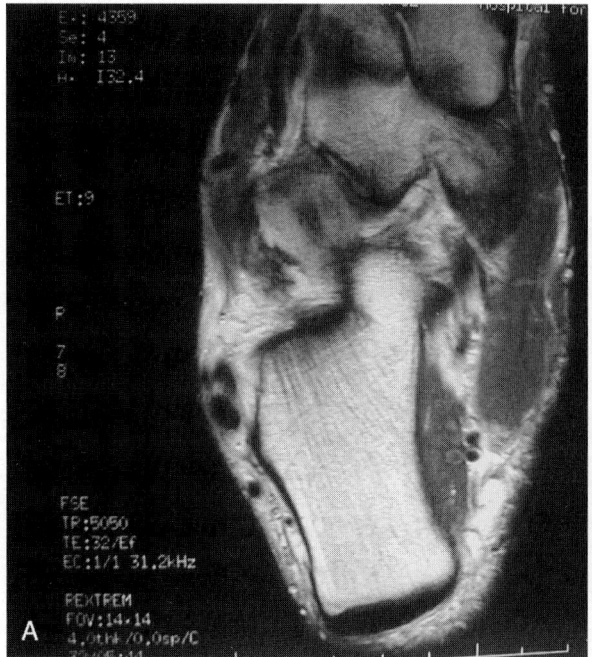

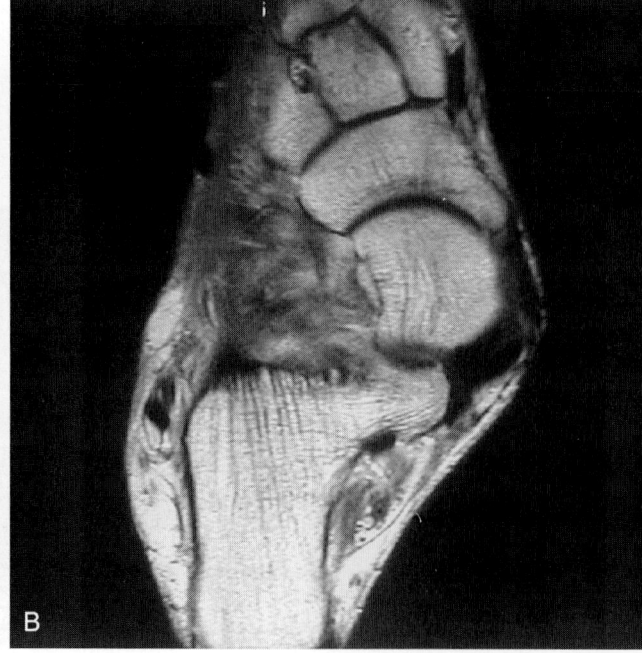

Fig. 9. MRI of abnormal spring ligament. This shows inferior portion (A) and superomedial portion (B). Note the disruption of the continuity of the fibers and low signal intensity.

MANAGEMENT

NONOPERATIVE

Patients can be managed conservatively.[46] However, the use of orthotics, braces, or casts has not been shown to prevent progression of deformity once it starts. These devices can be useful in lessening symptoms, but patients should not be told that progressive deformity will be halted. Patients without significant deformity and minimal weakness on manual muscle testing or patients with medical contraindications for surgery are particularly appropriate for conservative treatment.[46, 47] The use of a walking cast for 4 to 6 weeks can dissipate symptoms. Orthotics with medial longitudinal arch support and a medial heel wedge may or may not lessen symptoms. Often, an ankle level brace is helpful. For patients with more deformity, an ankle-foot orthosis will give added support if the patient can tolerate its use. This brace can be made with a posterior trim or ankle hinge to allow some ankle motion. Less supportive but easier to tolerate are canvas or leather lace-up ankle supports.

OPERATIVE DECISION-MAKING

If the correct procedure is chosen, surgical management is effective in relieving medial pain and mitigating progression of the deformity in stage I or II disease. The type of surgical management is contingent on the stage and type of deformity (Fig. 10). In stage I, a flexor digitorum tendon transfer is performed. This can be performed with a calcaneal osteotomy in order to assist the tendon transfer and should correct any increased heel valgus. In cases with no detectable deformity or in unusual cases, such as a cavus foot where varus alignment of the heel occurs, the osteotomy is omitted, or less displacement of the calcaneus is performed. The osteotomy and transfer are also used in stage II where minimal forefoot abduction is present (Fig. 11). For stage II patients with considerable abduction at the level of the talonavicular joint, various procedures have been used. A lateral column-lengthening Evans procedure can be added to the MS osteotomy for more correction of deformity (Fig. 12).[48] Alternatively, a lateral column-lengthening can be done by fusion of a CC joint with bone graft at the joint to provide the lengthening (Fig. 13). Some surgeons prefer this treatment to the Evans as it avoids the possibility of arthritis at the CC joint. The authors' preference is to not fuse the CC joint, as degenerative changes after a combined MS and modified Evans procedure have not been a common problem, and patients without a fusion in their hindfoot usually have fewer remaining symptoms and/or better function. In a comparative study, patients with fusion of the CC joint had more remaining symptoms than those with a combined MS and modified Evans osteotomy.[49] Other authors perform a subtalar fusion, particularly in less active or older patients. In stage III disease, the contracture is such that significant inversion motion is not possible. Therefore, a tendon transfer cannot restore active inversion. In these patients, a fusion becomes necessary if the symptoms cause considerable limitation on ambulation. Fusion of the subtalar joint can be done if significant forefoot varus (elevation of the

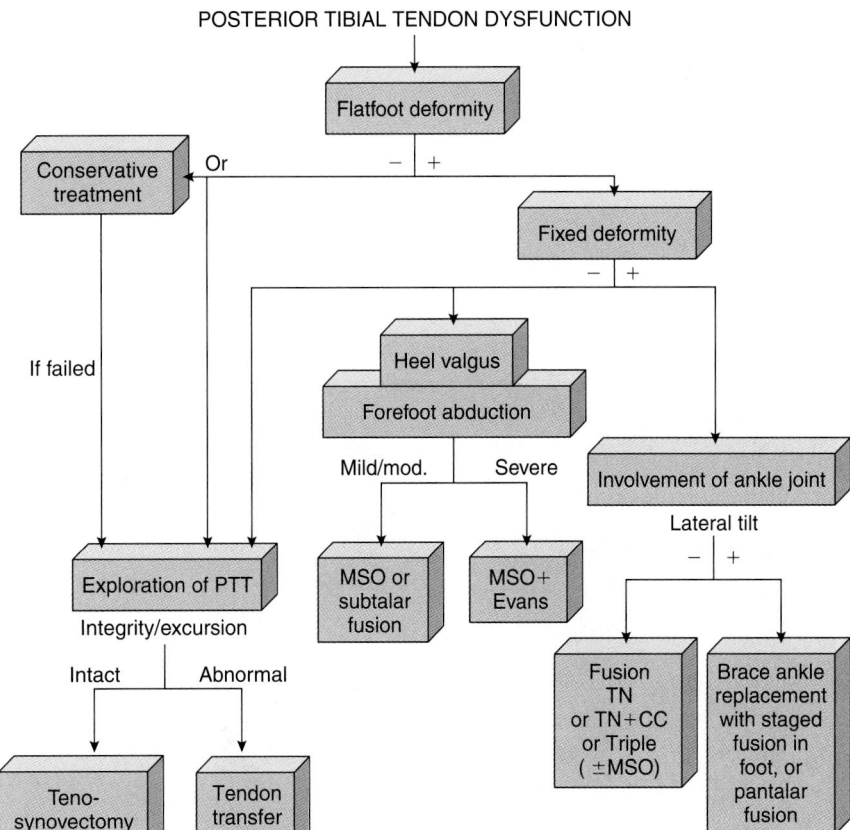

Fig. 10. Algorithm. Chart shows diagnosis and treatment of PTTD.

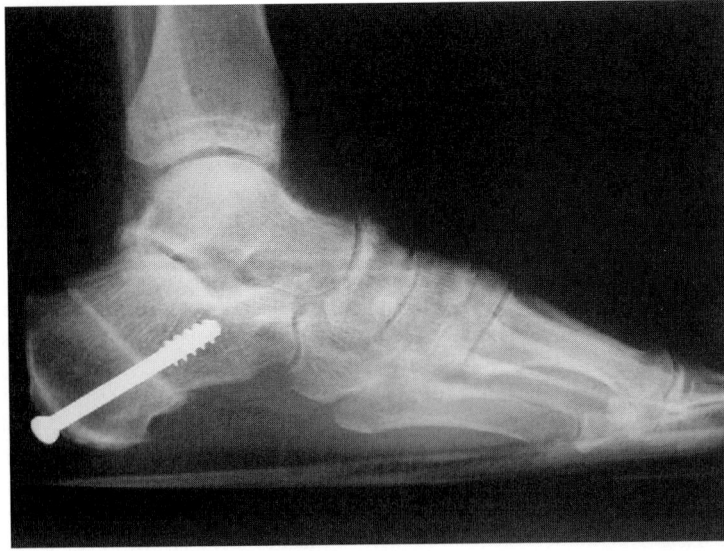

Fig. 11. Postoperative weightbearing lateral radiograph of the foot. The medial slide calcaneal osteotomy.

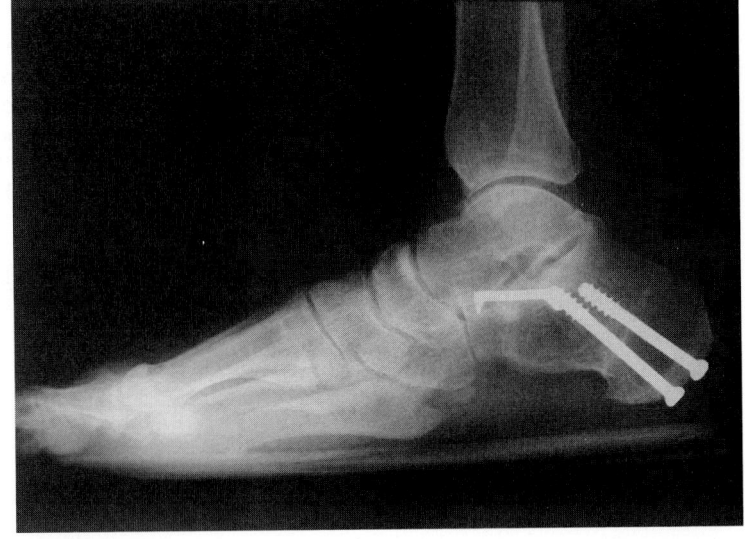

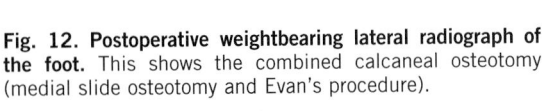

Fig. 12. Postoperative weightbearing lateral radiograph of the foot. This shows the combined calcaneal osteotomy (medial slide osteotomy and Evan's procedure).

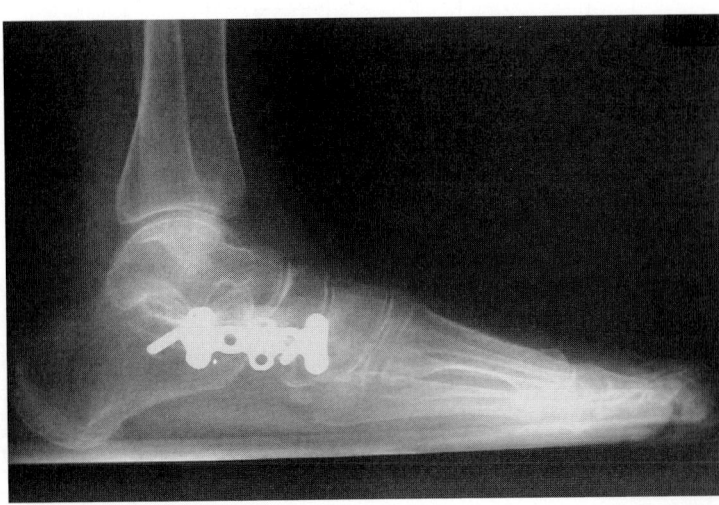

Fig. 13. Postoperative weightbearing lateral radiograph of the foot. This shows the calcaneocuboid distraction arthrodesis.

first metatarsal more than 10 degrees) is not present. If more deformity is present, correction will need to be done through the talonavicular joint, where considerable correction can be gained but more loss of motion occurs. This can be done in the form of a single, double (talonavicular and CC), or triple arthrodesis. Choice of fusion should provide correction of deformity, resulting in a plantigrade foot without excessive valgus or varus of forefoot or hindfoot. An MS osteotomy can be added to gain further correction of the heel in a triple or subtalar arthrodesis if further correction is needed.

STANDARD SURGICAL TECHNIQUE

An FDL tendon transfer (Fig. 14) is performed through a medial incision along the posterior tibial tendon, beginning 6 cm above the level of the ankle and continuing to the level of the proximal first metatarsal on the medial side of the foot. The tendon is inspected. Most commonly, there is degenerative change in the tendon so that 50% or more of the tendon is involved, often with longitudinal split side of the tendon and/or gross enlargement. In this circumstance, a tendon transfer is performed. The tendon is tenodesed proximally to the FDL, and the posterior tibial tendon is excised distal to the tenodesis. The FDL is identified at the level of the inferior talar head, and exposure of the tendon is continued distally. There is usually an interconnection between the flexor hallucis longus and FDL that can be left intact.[50,51] Alternatively, the two tendons can be tenodesed together. The FDL is detached distally. It can be either left in its own sheath or passed through the posterior tibial

tendon sheath. It is then brought through a drill hole in the navicular from plantar to dorsal and tied back on to the stump of the posterior tibial tendon. In the majority of cases, there is some deformity in the foot present, and therefore an MS calcaneal osteotomy is added or, in the case of considerably more deformity, an Evans along with an MS osteotomy.

The MS osteotomy is performed through a lateral oblique incision just behind the level of the sural nerve. Blunt dissection is used to avoid injury to the nerve branches. The lateral calcaneal wall is exposed, and an oblique osteotomy is made anterior to both the superior tuberosity of the calcaneus and the inferior calcaneal tuberosity approximately midway through the body of the posterior calcaneus. The osteotomy is mobilized with a laminar spreader and elevator so that it can be displaced approximately 1 cm medially. After displacement, it is pinned and inspected. For fixation, a partially threaded large cancellous cannulated screw is placed from the posterior medial heel across the osteotomy site, being careful to aim the screw somewhat laterally and thereby stay within the calcaneus (Fig. 15). If necessary, the Evans procedure is performed through a separate longitudinal incision just above the level of the peroneal tendons at the anterior calcaneus. The CC joint is identified, and the lateral wall of the anterior calcaneus is exposed, and retractors are placed. An osteotomy is made with a saw perpendicular to the plantar aspect of the foot, about 1.5 cm proximal to the CC joint (Fig. 16, top arrow). A blunt laminar spreader is used to distract the osteotomy for correction of the flatfoot. When the laminar

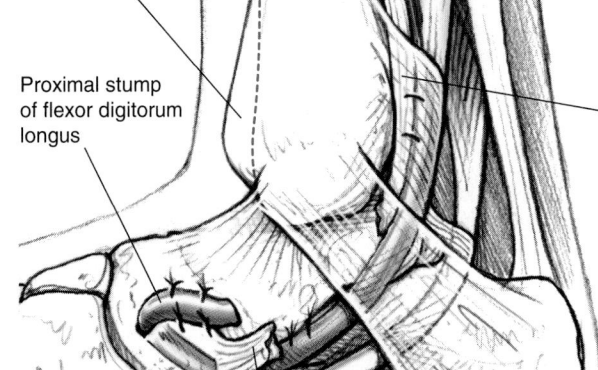

Fig. 14. Diagram. This shows the flexor digitorum longus transfer through a drill hole in the navicular.

Reshape anterior margin of tibia

Proximal stump of flexor digitorum longus

Flexor digitorum longus

Posterior tibialis tendon

Detached end of posterior tibialis tendon

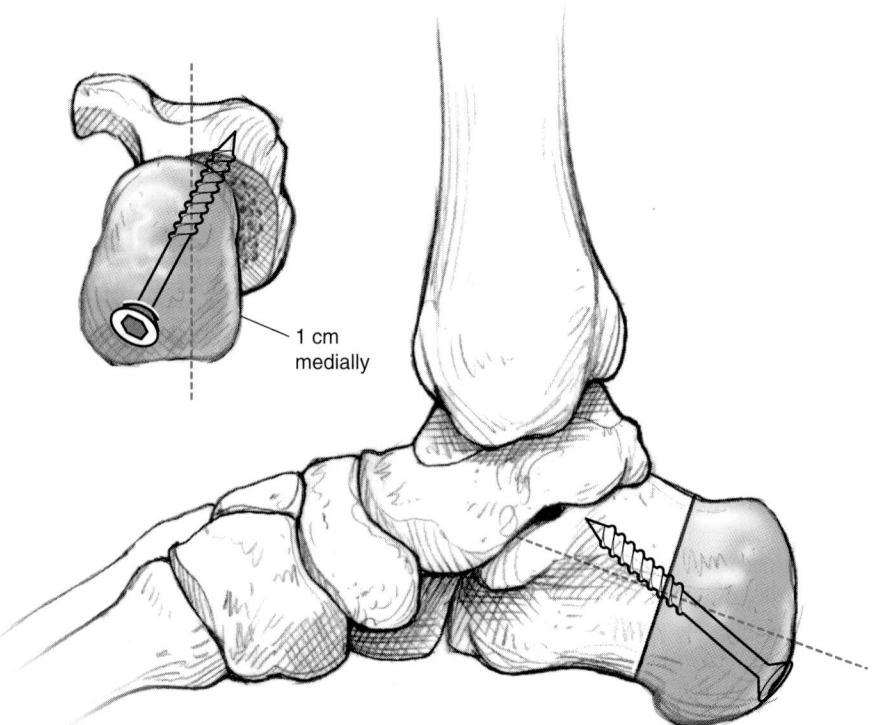

**1 cm
medially**

Fig. 15. Diagram. This shows the medial slide calcaneal osteotomy. The amount of the medialization is adjustable, depending on the severity of the heel.

Fig. 16. Diagram. This shows the combined calcaneal osteotomy; the medial slide osteotomy and Evan's procedure.

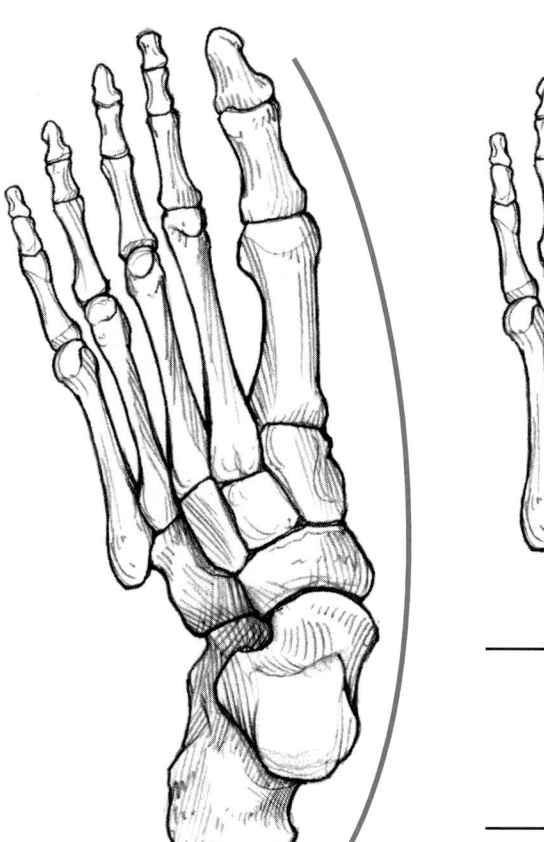

spreader is placed, the first ray is held down even with the level of the fifth metatarsal so that elevation of the first ray is minimized and the cuboid is elevated. The amount of correction is inspected clinically and on radiograph so that overcorrection and undercorrection are avoided. An AP fluoroscan or plain radiograph with simulated weightbearing is helpful. A tricortical bone graft is placed at the osteotomy site to maintain the correction once the spreader is removed. The bone graft is usually 7 to 10 mm. Fixation is used, commonly a screw or staple. Radiographs are made to confirm proper alignment of the foot and placement of the fixation.

The CC distraction arthrodesis (Fig. 17A) is performed through an incision similar to the Evans but continued more distally over the body of the cuboid. The joint surfaces are resected with a saw or osteotome perpendicular to the plantar aspect of the foot. Distraction is performed for correction, judged by the alignment of the foot and centering the talus in the talonavicular joint on the AP fluoroscan. A laminar spreader and iliac bone graft are used. Healing of the fusion can be difficult. Therefore, particular attention is given to a good fit for the graft and good fixation that is now commonly performed with a cervical H-plate and screws. Because of difficulty in healing and remaining symptoms, our preference is the combined Evans/MS osteotomies.

Fusion of the talonavicular and CC joints is performed through anteromedial and sinus tarsi longitudinal incisions. Curets and osteotomes are used to resect these joint surfaces just into the subchondral bone but preserving the contour of the joints. Fixation of the talonavicular joint is accomplished with compression screws or staples and fixation of the CC joint with one or two staples. The subtalar fusion is fixed with a compression screw that can be placed either from the neck of the talus down or from the distal posterior heel up into the talus. With a triple arthrodesis (Fig. 18) one subtalar screw is sufficient, but with a subtalar fusion often two screws are used to prevent rotation. Most important in all these fusions is placing the foot in the normal plantigrade position, avoiding over- or undercorrection when the fixation is inserted. The proper alignment is the normal physiological standing position, 5 degrees of heel valgus with the first metatarsal head neither dorsiflexed nor plantarflexed in comparison with the fifth metatarsal head. Undercorrection with residual excessive heel valgus will encourage persistent lateral impingement. Overcorrection results in excessive lateral weightbearing and greater stiffness in the foot and is to be carefully avoided. For aftercare, the fusions are kept non-weightbearing for 6 to 8 weeks and gradually progressed to full weightbearing, with the hard cast being used for a total of 12 weeks. The cast is discontinued when radiographs con-

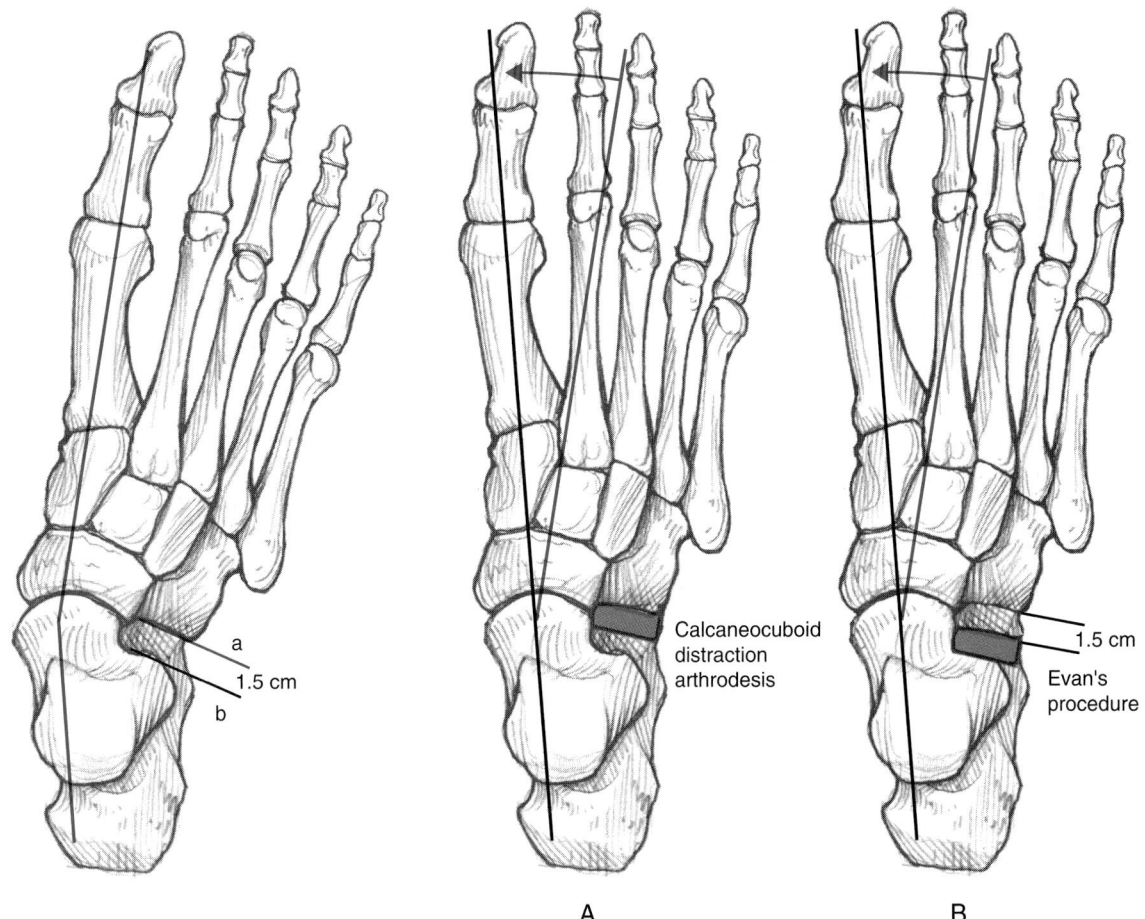

A   B

Fig. 17. Diagram. The lateral column-lengthening procedures use tricortical iliac bone graft; the calcaneocuboid distraction arthrodesis *(A)* and Evan's procedure *(B)*.

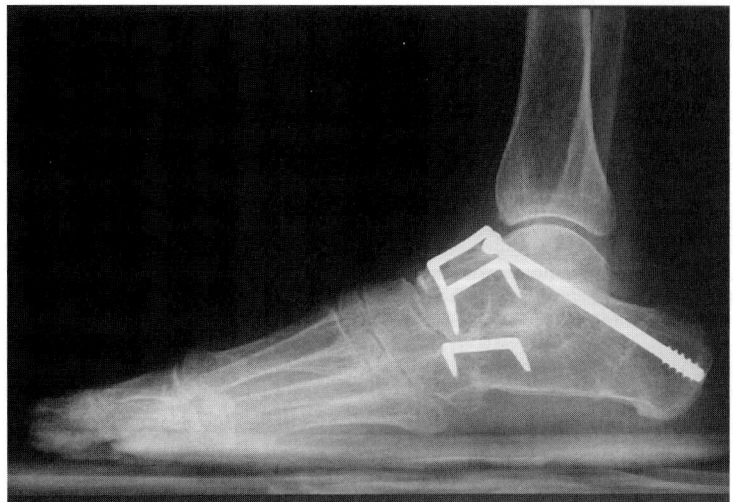

Fig. 18. Postoperative weightbearing lateral radiograph of the foot. This shows the triple arthrodesis. Note the medial slide osteotomy that was necessary in this case to avoid excessive heel valgus.

firm solid union. Aftercare of the tendon transfer and osteotomy consists of non-weightbearing, with the foot held in some plantarflexion and inversion until 6 weeks, when weightbearing is started with a removable or hard cast. By 10 weeks, the patient is begun on range-of-motion exercises with more vigorous strengthening exercises being done after 4 to 5 months after surgery.

RESULTS

The results of an isolated tendon transfer in feet with deformity showed resolution of the medial pain but lack of correction of the deformity.[10-12] Over time, the deformity is likely to progress and the procedure to fail. Initial reviews of the FDL transfer with MS osteotomy showed correction of the deformity on both AP and lateral views, although not necessarily full correction. In our experience, the osteotomy can correct mild-to-moderate heel valgus but not significant abduction at the midfoot. Because the foot retains full motion, remaining symptoms are minimal as long as adequate correction of bony alignment is achieved. Active inversion of the foot is improved, but full inversion strength is not restored. Greater strength is achieved in those feet with better bony correction and physical therapy. Using the American Orthopaedic Foot and Ankle Society hindfoot outcome score, these patients were graded at follow-up in the range of 85 on a 100-point scale, indicating good ambulatory function with minimal pain. For most, physical therapy resistive exercises to increase inversion and plantarflexion strength is helpful once the tendon transfer is well healed at 4 to 5 months.

In the initial report of the modified Evans procedure with the MS, Pomeroy and Manoli[48] showed considerable correction of the deformity and the maintenance of good function. No subsequent degenerative arthritis of the CC joint or need to fuse the CC joint was reported, but the follow-up was short. The AOFAS score was similar to the result of the MS calcaneal osteotomy. The CC distraction arthrodesis was reviewed as an alternative to the triple arthrodesis[52] and showed more remaining motion in the foot than a triple arthrodesis. Authors have noted difficulty

in healing, and nonunions have been reported. Good correction is achieved, but no AOFAS outcome hindfoot scale has been published for comparison. In the authors' experience, some of these patients can have significant discomfort remaining. Subtalar fusions have shown good resolution of pain, but in our experience patients with either one of these hindfoot fusions do not compare favorably with calcaneal osteotomy patients. Results of patients treated with a triple arthrodesis have suggested that this is a salvage procedure, after which significant discomfort remains when walking on uneven ground or with increased activities.

Because these procedures are done for different amounts of deformity, comparison of the results is problematic. It would be expected that the results of a tendon transfer with a calcaneal osteotomy (as long as adequate correction is achieved) would be superior to that of a fusion in the hindfoot. A recent study compares results of the combined osteotomies (Evans and an MS), CC distraction arthrodesis, and triple arthrodesis. The AOFAS hindfoot scores were significantly lower in those patients with arthrodesis (the CC distraction arthrodesis or triple arthrodesis). Questions directly measuring function, such as any limitation of walking distance or the ability to get enough exercises, showed a consistently higher score in osteotomy patients compared with fusion patients. This suggests that the surgical treatment of the adult acquired flatfoot deformity is best performed before fusions are required. If near-normal motion remains in the triple joint complex, and there is a choice between a fusion and nonfusion procedure, the nonfusion procedure is preferred as long as good bony correction is obtained and proper alignment of the foot is achieved.

Direct repair or reconstruction of the spring ligament without an osteotomy for correction to bony alignment has yet to be consistently successful. If lateral tilting of the talus within the ankle mortise is present, the patient is at risk for increasing deformity and ankle arthritis. A triple arthrodesis performed in the setting of weak deltoid or lateral tilt of the talus risks increased deformity and arthritis, compromising the benefits of surgery. Lateral tilting of the talus has been noted in patients after triple or subtalar arthrodesis that was not present prior to those procedures. When the symptoms of deformity and arthritis in the ankle necessitate treatment there, the use of a pantalar arthrodesis offers quite a restricted ability to ambulate. The limitations are such that an ankle replacement may be preferable to a pantalar arthrodesis. The results of triple or pantalar arthrodesis underscore the importance of early and adequate treatment of the adult acquired flatfoot.

REFERENCES

1. Mann RA: Acquired flatfoot in adults. Clin Orthop 1983; 181:46.
2. Myerson MS: Acquired flatfoot in the adult. Adv Orthop Surg 1989; 2:155.
3. Goldner JL, Keats PK, Bassett FH III, et al: Progressive talipes equinovalgus due to trauma or degeneration of the posterior tibial tendon and medial plantar ligaments. Orthop Clin North Am 1974; 5:39.
4. Pedowitz WJ, Kovatis P: Flatfoot in the adult. J Am Acad Orthop Surg 1995; 3: 293.
5. Mann RA: Rupture of the tibialis posterior tendon. Instr Course Lect 1984; 33:302.
6. Henceroth WD II, Deyerle WM: The acquired unilateral flatfoot in the adult: Some causative factors. Foot Ankle 1982; 2:304.
7. Kaye RA, Jahss MH: Tibialis posterior: A review of anatomy and biomechanics in relation to support of the medial longitudinal arch. Foot Ankle 1991; 11:244.
8. Sung I, Deland JT, Potter HG: Posterior tibial tendon insufficiency: Which ligaments are involved? Presented at the annual Summer meeting of the American Orthopaedic Foot and Ankle Society, Puerto Rico, 1999.
9. Davis WH, Sobel M, DiCarlo EF, et al: Gross, histological and microvascular anatomy and biomechanical testing of the spring ligament complex. Foot Ankle Int 1996; 17:95.
10. Mann RA, Thompson FM: Rupture of the posterior tibial tendon causing flatfoot: Surgical treatment. J Bone Joint Surg Am 1985; 67:556.
11. Funk DA, Cass JR, Johnson KA: Acquired adult flatfoot secondary to posterior tibial tendon pathology. J Bone Joint Surg Am 1986; 68:95.
12. Johnson KA, Strom DE: Tibialis posterior tendon dysfunction. Clin Orthop 1989; 239:196.
13. Myerson MS, Corrigan J, Thompson F, et al: Tendon transfer combined with calcaneal osteotomy for posterior tibial tendon insufficiency: A radiological investigation. Foot Ankle Int 1995; 16:712.
14. Key JA: Partial rupture of the tendon of the posterior tibial muscle. J Bone Joint Surg Am 1953; 35:1006.
15. Kettelkamp BB, Alexander HH: Spontaneous rupture of the posterior tibial tendon, J Bone Joint Surg Am 1969; 51:759.
16. Gould N, Schneider W, Takamara A: Epidemiological survey of foot problems in the continental United States: 1978–1979. Foot Ankle 1980; 1:8.
17. Mann RA, Specht LH: Posterior tibial tendon ruptures: Analysis of eight cases. Foot Ankle 1982; 2:350.
18. Jahss MH: Spontaneous rupture of the tibialis posterior tendon: Clinical findings, tenographic studies and a new technique of repair. Foot Ankle 1982; 3:158.

19. Johnson KA: Tibialis posterior tendon rupture. Clin Orthop 1983; 177:140.
20. Clain MR, Baxter DE: Simultaneous calcaneocuboid and talonavicular fusion: Long-term follow-up study. J Bone Joint Surg Br 1994; 76:133.
21. Harper MC, Tisdel CL: Talonavicular arthrodesis for the painful adult acquired flatfoot. Foot Ankle Int 1996; 17:658.
22. Kitaoka HB, Ptzer GL: Subtalar arthrodesis for posterior tibial tendon dysfunction and pes planus. Clin Orthop 1997; 345: 187.
23. Vogler HW: Triple arthrodesis as a salvage for end-stage flatfoot. Clin Podiatr Med Surg 1989; 6:591.
24. Sammarco GJ: Technique of triple arthrodesis in treatment of symptomatic pes planus. Orthopedics 1988; 11:1607.
25. Astion DJ, Deland JT, Otis JC: Motion of the hindfoot after simulated arthrodesis. J Bone Joint Surg Am 1997; 79:241.
26. Lord JP: Correction of extreme flatfoot: Value of osteotomy of os calcis and inward displacement of posterior fragment (Gleich operation). JAMA 1923; 81:1502.
27. Koutsogiannis E: Treatment of mobile flatfoot by displacement osteotomy of the calcaneus. J Bone Joint Surg Br 1971; 53:96.
28. Evans D: Calcaeo-valgus deformity. J Bone Joint Surg Br 1975; 57:270.
29. Phillips GE: A review of elongation of os calcis for flat feet. J Bone Joint Surg Br 1983; 65:15.
30. Sangeorzan BJ, Mosca V, Hansen ST Jr: Effect of calcaneal lengthening on relationships among the hindfoot and forefoot. Foot Ankle 1993; 14:136.
31. Anderson AF, Fowler SB: Anterior calcaneal osteotomy for symptomatic juvenile pes planus. Foot Ankle 1984; 4:274
32. Cooper PS, Nowak MD, Shaer J: Calcaneocuboid joint pressure with lateral column lengthening (Evans) procedure. Foot Ankle Int 1997; 18:199.
33. Deland JT, Arnoczky S, Thompson FM: Adult acquired flatfoot deformity at the talonavicular joint: Reconstruction of the spring ligament in an in vitro model. Foot Ankle 1992; 13:327.
34. Cracchiolo A III: Evaluation of spring ligament pathology in patients with posterior tibial tendon rupture, tendon transfer, and ligament repair. Foot Ankle Clin 1997; 2: 297.
35. Thordarson DB, Schmotzer H, Chon J: Reconstruction with tenodesis in an adult flatfoot model. J Bone Joint Surg Am 1995; 77:1557.
36. Gazdag AR, Cracchiolo III: Rupture of the posterior tibial tendon: Evaluation of injury of the spring ligament and clinical assessment of tendon transfer and ligament repair. J Bone Joint Surg Am 1997; 79: 675.
37. Holmes GB, Olney BW: Triple arthrodesis

with lateral column lengthening for treatment of severe planovalgus deformity. Foot Ankle Int 1995; 16:395.
38. Frey C, Shereff M, Greenidge N: Vascularity of the posterior tibial tendon. J Bone Joint Surg Am 1990; 72:884.
39. Hamlin CR, Kohn RR, Luschin JH: Apparent accelerated aging of human collagen in diabetes mellitus. Diabetes 1975; 24:902.
40. Myerson MS: Adult acquired flatfoot deformity: Treatment of dysfunction to the posterior tibial tendon. J Am Acad Orthop Surg 1996; 78:780.
41. Mann RA: Flatfoot in adults. In Mann RA, Coughlin MJ (eds): Surgery of the Foot and Ankle, St. Louis, Mosby–Year Book, 1993, 6th ed, vol 1.
42. Beals TC, Pomeroy GC, Manoli A II: Posterior tendon insufficiency: Diagnosis and treatment. J Am Acad Orthop Surg 1999; 7:112.
43. Alexander IJ, Johnson KA, Berquist TH: Magnetic resonance imaging in the diagnosis of disruption of the posterior tibial tendon. Foot Ankle 1987; 8:144.
44. Conti S, Michelson J, Jahss M: Clinical significance of magnetic resonance imaging in preoperative planning for reconstruction of posterior tibial tendon ruptures. Foot Ankle 1992; 13:20.
45. Rosenberg ZS, Cheung Y, Jahss MH, et al: Rupture of posterior tibial tendon imaging with surgical correlation. Radiology 1988; 169:229.
46. Chao W, Wapner KL, Lee TH, et al: Nonoperative management of posterior tibial tendon dysfunction. Foot Ankle Int 1996; 12:736.
47. Sferra JJ, Rosenberg GA: Nonoperative treatment of posterior tibial tendon pathology. Foot Ankle Clin 1997; 2:261.
48. Pomeroy GP, Manoli A II: A new operative approach for flatfoot secondary to tibialis posterior tendon insufficiency: A preliminary report. Foot Ankle Int 1997; 18: 206.
49. Deland JT, Page A, Sung I: Functional results of different procedures used in posterior tibial insufficiency. Presented at the annual summer meeting of the AOFAS, Puerto Rico, 1999.
50. Wapner KL, Hecht PJ, Shea JR, et al: Anatomy of second muscular layer of the foot: Consideration selection in transfer for Achilles and posterior tibial tendon reconstruction. Foot Ankle Int 1994; 15:420.
51. Sarrafian SK: Anatomy of the Foot and Ankle. Philadelphia, JB Lippincott, 1983, p 157.
52. Sands A, Grujic L, Sangeorzan B, et al: Lateral column lengthening through the calcaneo-cuboid joint: An alternative to triple arthrodesis for correction of flatfoot. Presented at the 25th Annual Meeting of the AOFAS, Orlando, FL, 1995.

MIDFOOT ARTHRITIS

Steven A. Herbst, Douglas Beaman, Lisa DeGnore, and Charles L. Saltzman

Summary

- Midfoot arthritis is a debilitating condition. Among its causes are post-traumatic degenerative joint disease, primary osteoarthritis, inflammatory arthropathy, and neuroarthropathy.
- Patient diagnosis, pertinent medical history, and expectation affect outcome of both operative and nonoperative management.
- Nonoperative management consists of orthotics to accommodate deformity and control instability. Decrease in midfoot stresses can be achieved with carbon fiber/steel shank inserts, rocker-bottoms, and bars.
- If nonoperative management fails, operative management can be pursued, usually consisting of fusion of the involved joints. Correction of deformity is desirable.

The human foot is a highly complex structure, commonly divided into three regions: hindfoot, midfoot, and forefoot. The midfoot consists of the bones and joints spanning from the Lisfranc (or tarsometatarsal) joints through the intercuneiform joints. This set of complex articulations is responsible for the transfer of force from heel to toe during locomotion. The midfoot may develop arthritis primarily or secondary to chronic instability, traumatic injury, or inflammatory disease. The exact incidence of primary midfoot arthritis in the general population is unknown; however, it may be more common than previously recognized. As the population ages, the incidence is very likely to rise. Midfoot instability tends to develop insidiously as a result of a subtle, often generalized ligamentous laxity. The repetitive abnormal mechanics may lead to degenerative changes in the joint cartilage, ultimately resulting in severe arthropathy. Traumatic injury to the midfoot often occurs in active young to middle-aged males and is usually due to sports injury, a fall from a height, a crush injury, or a motor vehicle accident.[1] Less commonly, osteoporotic older patients can injure the midfoot from slipping off a stair or curb onto a plantar flexed foot. Arthritis resulting from acute trauma to these joints can follow and sometimes accounts for pain and substantial loss of productivity in the work force. The natural history after severe traumatic injury to the midfoot is unclear but frequently results in significant disability and pain despite treatment. The variables affecting outcome seem to be severity of injury, quality of reduction, and presence or absence of significant crush component.[2]

Treatment of midfoot arthritis begins with conservative measures, including shoe modifications, activity restriction, arthritis medication, and weight loss. Despite these measures, dysfunction frequently persists, and surgical intervention is often considered. The usual surgical treatment is arthrodesis of the involved joints.

HISTORICAL REVIEW

Very little has been written historically on the treatment of midfoot arthritis. The standard of care for years has been orthotic treatment. The earliest publications on surgical treatment dealt mainly with post-traumatic arthritis. In 1972 Wippula noted that patients tend to function well despite the development of arthrosis; therefore, primary arthrodesis was not indicated. More recent literature suggests that surgical management (arthodesis, correction of deformity/instability) can improve patient function and satisfaction in symptomatic patients.[2-7]

ANATOMY/PATHOGENESIS

The midfoot is composed of multiple articulations and ligamentous connections between adjacent tarsal bones and metatarsal bases. Three distinct articular compartments are present: medial, containing the first metatarsocuneiform joint; central, containing the second and third metatarsocuneiform joints and intercuneiform joints; and lateral compartment, containing the cubometatarsal joints. This forms the basis of a columnar division of the foot into medial, central, and lateral. A complex and variable ligamentous configuration consisting of dorsal, plantar, and interosseous ligaments provide a stout soft-tissue envelope. The three cuneiforms and cuboid form a transverse arch with the apex at the third metatarsocuneiform articulation.[8]

Midfoot motion has been quantitated in the sagittal plane and in rotation, with approximately 10 degrees occurring in both planes at the cubometatarsal joints and considerably less (0.6 to 3.5 degrees) at the cuneiform-metatarsal joints. Motion occurs at the naviculocuneiform (2.1 to 7.3 degrees) articulation but decreases from medial to lateral.[9] The planes of motion and forces exerted on the foot are responsible for the typical deformity of pronation, dorsiflexion, and abduction seen with midfoot arthrosis.

The first metatarsocuneiform joint is stabilized in weightbearing primarily by its plantar ligament. A clinical study has shown that, in the asymptomatic foot, first metatarsocuneiform motion averages 4.4 degrees in the sagittal plane, and thumb hyperflexibility correlated with increased motion.[10] Multiple variables, including angle of the first and second intermetatarsals, patient sex and age, elbow and knee hyperextension, and distal cuneiform shape did not correlate with first metatarsocuneiform motion. The morphology of this joint is variable, and descriptions have been based on the medial inclination, lateral radiographic slope, and type of articular facet with the second metatarsal.

The second metatarsal base is recessed between the medial and lateral cuneiforms by approximately 8 mm and 4 mm, respectively. The strong, oblique interosseous Lisfranc ligament connects the second metatarsal base with the medial cuneiform. This ligament is approximately 8 to 10 mm in length and 5 to 6 mm thick and is the largest in the tarsometatarsal complex. This is the strongest plantar ligament and connects the medial cuneiform to the second and third metatarsal bases.[8] The bony, ligamentous structure of the second tarsometatarsal joint provides the primary stabilization of the midfoot. In the cadaver foot, dorsolateral displacement of this joint results in considerable loss of contact area; a 3-mm displacement causes a 38.6% decrease in articular contact.[11] It remains to be shown whether this abnormal contact correlates with arthrosis or pain.

A cadaver investigation of the tarsometatarsal joints found that as loads increased on the leg contact forces increased in the medial three joints, whereas loads up to twice body weight did not increase contact forces in the lateral two joints. This may help to explain the small incidence of symptomatic arthritis in the cubometatarsal articulation.

Several reports attempted to correlate joint reduction accuracy with clinical results, finding that poor results occurred with greater inaccuracy.[2, 12, 13] Only one report found good results with nonanatomic reduction.[14] Moreover, despite good surgical technique and acceptable reduction, many have reported post-traumatic arthritis and pain in treated patients with up to a 50% prevalence of chronic symptoms. Injuries and dysfunction of the Lisfranc joint can have a significant human and economic impact.

CLINICAL FEATURES

HISTORY OF ILLNESS

In evaluating midfoot problems, a good clinical history is key. Details of injury and activity, occupation, expectations, and symptoms should, of course, be included. However, it is important to remember that systemic medical problems often affect the foot as well as the outcome of treatment. A thorough history of illness, surgery, medications, allergies, social factors, and family should be obtained and a review of systems performed.

SIGNS AND SYMPTOMS

Pain is the most common presenting complaint. Most will complain of increased problems, including pain and swelling with prolonged activity, with stair climbing, and while on uneven ground. Deformity may cause difficulty with shoe wear and calluses as a result of pressure against bony prominences. Women may be unable to wear high-heeled shoes. If there has been an associated neurological injury from a traumatic event, patients may complain of burning, dysesthetic pain that worsens at night.

PHYSICAL EXAMINATION

The physical examination includes evaluating both feet for comparison. Gait should be evaluated with the patient barefoot, looking for stride length as well as mechanics. A standing examination of both feet is important to determine the degree and location of deformity. The most common deformity after trauma is abduction and flattening of the foot through the Lisfranc joints. The sitting examination of both feet includes determination of the deformity flexibility, motion measurements, neurovascular and skin assessment, and careful palpation of each midfoot joint. Skin is examined for color, texture, swelling, scars, deformity, nail and hair growth, and venous changes. Range of motion is compared with that of the normal foot; pronation and supination may be diminished, and the motion may elicit pain. The midfoot can be stressed with a pronation-abduction maneuver. Palpation of all areas of the foot, ankle, and lower leg is important in accurate diagnosis. It is necessary to carefully distinguish and palpate each joint in the complex as well as each metatarsal. In particular, alignment of

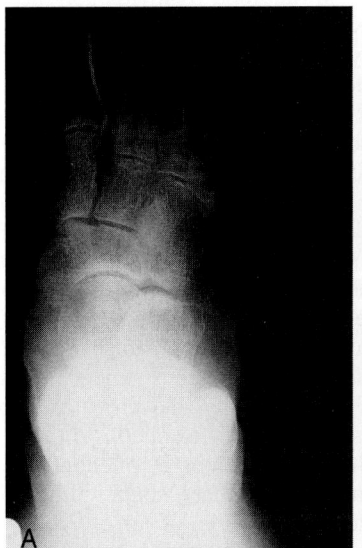 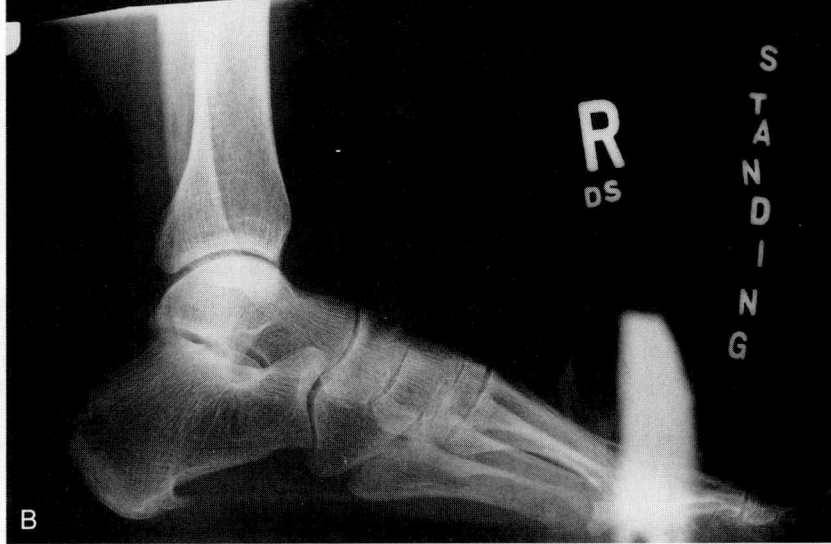

Fig. 1. Symptomatic midfoot arthritis. These are preoperative anteroposterior and lateral radiographs of a 55-year-old woman with symptomatic midfoot arthritis. She presented with persistent pain after incurring a subtle Lisfranc injury, which was treated late with excision of bony avulsion fracture. Note that radiographs are relatively unremarkable.

the metatarsal heads should be determined while the patient is seated. Sensation in all nerve distributions, pulses, and capillary refill should be examined.

INVESTIGATION

The radiographic evaluation of the arthritic midfoot includes standing anteroposterior, lateral, and oblique radiographs (Fig. 1). Weightbearing views may be considered stress views and may uncover subtle instability. It is useful to image both feet to determine the degree of deformity, which can be assessed by measurement of the anteroposterior talus–first metatarsal, talus–second metatarsal, and lateral talus–first metatarsal angles. In cases with deformity, there is often loss of talar head coverage by the navicular bone.

Occasionally, it is difficult to determine the extent of arthritis with the use of plain radiographs and physical examination. Although controversial, in these cases a bone scan or computed tomography scan can be useful on a preoperative basis (Fig. 2). Computed tomography may be particularly helpful with delineating the extent of disease. These imaging modalities should be carefully interpreted and used in conjunction with the physical examination, which is useful to repeat on separate occasions. Some authors discussed the use of selective injections of local anesthetic under fluoroscopic control (G. El-Khoury and C. L. Saltzman, personal communication, 1998); however, this can be difficult to perform accurately and painful to the patient and may be misleading because of the lack of predictable synovial compartmentalization of the midfoot joints.

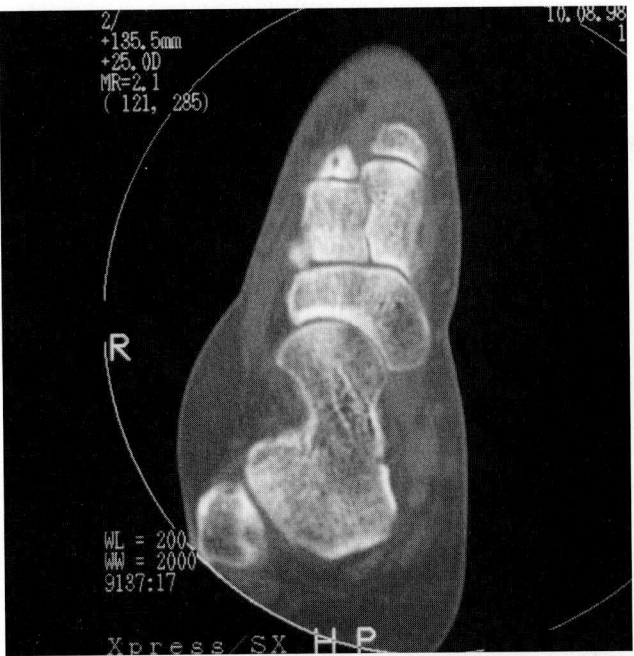

Fig. 2. Degenerative joint disease (DJD). This is a preoperative computed tomography scan (reconstruction in the plane of the sole of the foot) of the same patient as in Figure 1 shows intercuneiform DJD as well as metatarsocuneiform DJD at the first and second metatarsocuneiform joints.

Magnetic resonance imaging may prove helpful as cartilage sequences improve. Cartilage integrity and presence of synovial thickening and/or effusion may aid in the diagnosis of painful feet with poor localization. Magnetic resonance imaging may also show soft-tissue (i.e., tendon) inflammation, which may complicate the diagnosis.

Selective aspiration (cell count, Gram stain, crystal analysis) and selective blood chemistries/serologies to rule out infection, crystal arthropathy, and inflammatory disease are indicated as based on history and physical exam.

DIFFERENTIAL DIAGNOSIS FOR MIDFOOT ARTHRITIS

OSTEOARTHRITIS

Arthritis of the tarsometatarsal complex occurs as primary degenerative arthritis as well as after trauma. In one series, patients with primary arthritis tended to be older (60 years versus 40 years) and have a larger extent of disease and greater deformity compared with those with post-traumatic arthritis.[3] Primary arthritis may, however, affect only one joint and be without deformity. Dorsal osteophytes are typically present with severe involvement, but they can also be present in isolated joint involvement and cause nerve impingement symptoms as a result of peroneal nerve branch compression. Despite advances in the treatment of injuries to the tarsometatarsal joints, post-traumatic arthritis continues to be prevalent. This is observed even after presumably subtle injuries, possibly secondary to articular cartilage damage. Factors associated with the development of post-traumatic arthritis include persistent malalignment, especially with collapse of the medial longitudinal arch, and demonstrable articular injury.[13]

INFLAMMATORY ARTHRITIS

Rheumatoid arthritis is the most common inflammatory arthritic disorder affecting the foot. The midfoot typically does not present with the significant involvement that is seen in the forefoot and hindfoot. Synovitis may be present in up to two-thirds of patients with chronic rheumatoid disease.[15] Joint ankylosis may occur but is usually not of functional significance. Involvement of the medial column, particularly the first metatarsocuneiform joint, may lead to instability and subsequently contribute to a flatfoot deformity and/or the development of a hallux valgus deformity.

The seronegative spondyloarthopathies are a group of inflammatory disorders similar to rheumatoid arthritis and include ankylosing spondylitis, psoriatic arthritis, and Reiter's syndrome. They are characterized by a nonspecific inflammatory process involving synovial joints, tendon sheaths, joint capsules, tendon and ligament bony attachments (entheses), and fibrocartilaginous structures. The process is typically of low intensity and chronic, associated with fibrosis and ossification, differentiating it from rheumatoid arthritis. Although the foot is often affected, the midfoot is rarely involved in these conditions. Enthesopathy is common; a frequent site of involvement is the plantar fascia origin, with resultant heel pain. Whereas the rheumatoid foot demonstrates generalized osteopenia, loss of joint space, and bony destruction, the seronegative disorders do not typically have severe osteopenia but do have periarticular calcifications, periostitis, bony erosions, joint ankylosis, subchondral sclerosis, and calcification at entheses.

Ankylosing spondylitis primarily involves the axial skeleton. Calcaneal entheses are most commonly affected in the foot. Approximately 90% of white people with this disorder are HLA-B27–positive. Reiter's syndrome, also commonly HLA-B27–positive, and psoriatic arthritis are similar both clinically and radiographically. Both may present with a more acute course than ankylosing spondylitis. Reiter's syndrome commonly affects the foot but in an asymmetric pattern, whereas psoriasis tends to be symmetric and also affects the hands. Reiter's syndrome can affect the hindfoot and midfoot, with the development of bony ankylosis. The classic Reiter's triad of urethritis, conjunctivitis, and arthritis is infrequently seen; most patients exhibit only certain components of the triad. The arthritic process in psoriasis usually follows the cutaneous manifestations, but is present before skin involvement in 10% to 20% of patients. The juvenile with seronegative spondyloarthropathy often presents with lower extremity involvement. Midfoot involvement was observed clinically in 15 of 40 patients, with an average age of 11.2 years in one study.[17] Spontaneous fusion of joints in the midfoot may occur, and bracing or orthoses may be helpful to maintain a plantigrade foot during the active stage of the disease.

CRYSTAL-INDUCED ARTHRITIS

Gout and pseudogout are crystalline deposition disorders that may present with foot involvement. Although the initial presentation is typically not in the midfoot, in late stages, they often can cause a diffuse destructive/lytic process through the midfoot. Crystal-induced arthritis should be kept in the differential diagnosis for patients presenting with a permeative destructive arthritic process of the midfoot, no history of trauma, infection or neuropathy, and normal ligamentous laxity.

Gout involves the intra-articular presence of monosodium urate crystals, which are needle shaped and negatively birefringent under a polarizing microscope. It results from a disorder of purine metabolism but also may occur in certain diseases and with medications that elevate the serum uric acid. Gout is more frequent in men than women and typically presents with an acute arthritis or periarticular inflammatory reaction of the first metatarsophalangeal joint. This joint is involved in 50% to 75% of initial attacks, and 90% of patients will have involvement of this joint at some point. An acute attack is manifested by severe pain, swelling, erythema, and warmth about the involved joint, typically lasting for several days before subsiding. Attacks frequently occur during the postoperative period. Diagnosis can often be made on a clinical basis, and crystal analysis of joint fluid can confirm the diagnosis. Serum uric acid level may be normal. Radiographs are typically normal with an initial attack but may later demonstrate periarticular erosions or lesions on both sides of the joint. Joint destruction may occur in chronic cases. With improved awareness of the disease, in developed nations, chronic tophaceous gout is now rare.

Pseudogout results from calcium pyrophosphate dihydrate crystal deposition in joints or periarticular tissue, causing an inflammatory reaction. Crystals are of variable shape and have weak positive birefringence under the polarizing microscope. Radiographs may demonstrate fine intra-articular calcifications, but joint destruction is uncommon. The metatarsophalangeal joints are most commonly affected in the foot, and treatment is symptomatic with medical management of acute synovitis. If severe joint involvement occurs, the process may be similar to degenerative arthritis or neuroarthropathy with bony fragmentation.

NEUROARTHROPATHY

Neuroarthropathy, defined as a progressive degenerative and destructive arthropathy occurring secondary to loss of joint sensory innervation, causes significant disability in the foot. Disorders associated with neuropathic arthropathy include diabetes, syphilis, syringomyelia, pernicious anemia, leprosy, spina bifida, congenital insensitivity to pain, Charcot-Marie-Tooth disease, and idiopathic and other causes of peripheral neuropathy. Diabetes is currently the most common cause in this country, and neuroarthropathy occurs in approximately 0.15% to 2.5% of diabetics. The midfoot is the most common location of involvement, representing 60% to 70% of cases in the foot and ankle.[18] The typical patient experiences a relatively painless swelling of the midfoot, without skin lesions, that progresses to a rocker-bottom deformity with extrusion of the cuboid plantarward and dorsolateral subluxation of the metatarsocuneiform joints.

MANAGEMENT

NONOPERATIVE

Nonoperative treatment modalities (Table 1) for midfoot osteoarthritis include shoe modifications, orthotic management, use of nonsteroidal anti-inflammatory drugs, activity modification, and weight reduction. The central shoe modification is application of a rocker-bottom sole with or without stiffening provided by an extended steel shank or full-length carbon fiber insert. An ankle-foot orthosis with a full-length footplate will provide additional support for more severe involvement. A custom or off-the-shelf orthotic device may be useful to provide cushioning, support of the longitudinal arch, and metatarsal head relief, but patients with deformity may not tolerate arch support because of a plantar bony prominence. Shoe wear modifications, padding, and skip-lacing techniques can help decrease pressure from dorsal osteophytes. The goal of nonoperative treatment is to decrease motion and forces across the midfoot and pressure relief over bony prominences.

Treatment of inflammatory or crystal-induced arthritis involves greater focus on the systemic cause of the midfoot disorder. Rheumatoid patients are treated with nonsteroidal agents, disease-modifying drugs, and a host of immune suppressors, depending on the individual patient's response to medication. Patients with gout are treated with nonsteroidal agents or colchicine, purine metabolism and/or excretion-modifying drugs and rest, elevation, and ice for symptomatic relief.

The orthotic/shoeing approaches are essentially the same as for osteoarthritis, except that particular vigilance is required in patients with severe rheumatoid disease. These patients often have wrist and hand or hip involvement,

TABLE 1. SUGGESTED TREATMENT STRATEGY OF BOTH OPERATIVE AND NONOPERATIVE MANAGEMENT

Treatment Type	Indications	Specific Treatment	Expected Outcome
Nonoperative	Initial therapy Poor surgical candidate	NSAIDS Treatment of systemic conditions Temporary immobilization Shoewear modifications Orthotics	Painless, shoeable/braceable foot without ulceration
Operative (no deformity)	Failed nonoperative treatment	Fusion of involved joints Osteophyte removal	Same
Operative (deformity)	Failed nonoperative treatment	Fusion of involved joints ± osteotomy and/or structural bonegrafting	Same
Operative (instability ± deformity)	Failed	Fusion of involved joints Structural grafting if deformity present	Same

NSAIDs, nonsteroidal anti-inflammatory drugs.

which makes donning and doffing their shoes difficult. Shoes can be modified with an extended tongue and Velcro closures to help keep these patients able to apply their footwear independently. Concomitant forefoot problems should be considered when writing a prescription for a rheumatoid patient with midfoot problems. An extra-deep shoe is usually mandatory, and soft seamless material should be considered for patients with fragile skin.

The neuroarthropathic midfoot typically collapses into a rocker-bottom deformity with a plantar prominence. A plantar medial deformity with forefoot abduction results with medial and central column involvement. If there is lateral column involvement, a complete rocker-bottom deformity will result, with dorsal subluxation of the entire forefoot.

Initially these feet are treated with non-weightbearing casts, typically total contact casts that are changed frequently to avoid skin ulceration from volume reduction that naturally follows cast immobilization. For the average patient, this involves changing the cast at 3 days after presentation, then after 1 week, 3 weeks, and 6 weeks, and so on. When the volume stabilizes, a mold is taken for a full-contact, bivalved ankle-foot orthosis. This is used until the midfoot achieves stability (4 to 18 months after presentation). The vast majority of midfoot neuroarthropathic feet become stable and can be managed with long-term bracing (custom ankle-foot orthosis) or, for patients with minimal deformity, with a custom multilaminar orthotic device in extra-depth, split, or custom shoe wear. Ultimately, treatment is based on achieving pressure relief of bony prominences, minimizing shear forces, and providing stability. Patient education in this process is critical. The primary goal is avoidance of skin breakdown and ulceration. In the face of ulceration, meticulous nonoperative management with close patient follow-up is generally successful.

OPERATIVE

Operative treatment is indicated when nonoperative modalities are exhausted and the patient is unable to perform daily activities. Similar basic strategies are used for all the different causes of midfoot arthritis with a few salient ex-

ceptions. Rheumatoid patients, especially those who are steroid dependent, are at increased risk of wound difficulties. In these patients in particular, every attempt should first be made to try all nonoperative modalities. If those attempts fail, and surgery is performed, the soft tissues must be handled meticulously, incisions spaced widely, and dissections limited. Another patient population that deserves special concern includes those with unstable midfoot neuroarthropathy. If surgery is planned, these patients need to understand that the risks include an increased potential for deep infection and that the goal of surgery is to make them braceable and avoid recurrent skin breakdown.

Osteophyte resection is performed when symptoms are secondary to nerve impingement or skin irritation from the prominence. Arthrodesis of the involved joints is otherwise indicated. Generally agreed-on surgical principles regarding midfoot arthrodesis have evolved. These include realignment and fusion of deformity/instability, and in patients without deformity an in situ fusion is performed. All joints with symptomatic arthritis or part of the deformity should be included. Longitudinal incisions are used, with protection of the cutaneous nerves. Rigid internal fixation with meticulous joint preparation is necessary. Bone graft can be used to fill spaces and maintain alignment.

The operative approaches to the midfoot are based on joint involvement. Single-joint arthritis can be approached directly dorsal to the joint and dorsomedial to the first tarsometatarsal joint. Recommendations vary regarding the approach to multiple joints. An accepted method is to approach the first tarsometatarsal joint dorsomedially, the second and third tarsometatarsal joints through an incision centered between the second and third metatarsals, and the fourth and fifth tarsometatarsal joints between the fourth and fifth metatarsals. The cubometatarsal joints are sometimes not fused but rather treated with hemiresection of joint surfaces to preserve motion (Fig. 3).

An in situ arthrodesis is performed in feet without deformity. All articular cartilage is removed from the involved joints, and the subchondral bone is feathered with a small osteotome or drilled with a small-caliber bit. Internal fixation is achieved with the use of interfragmentary screws to

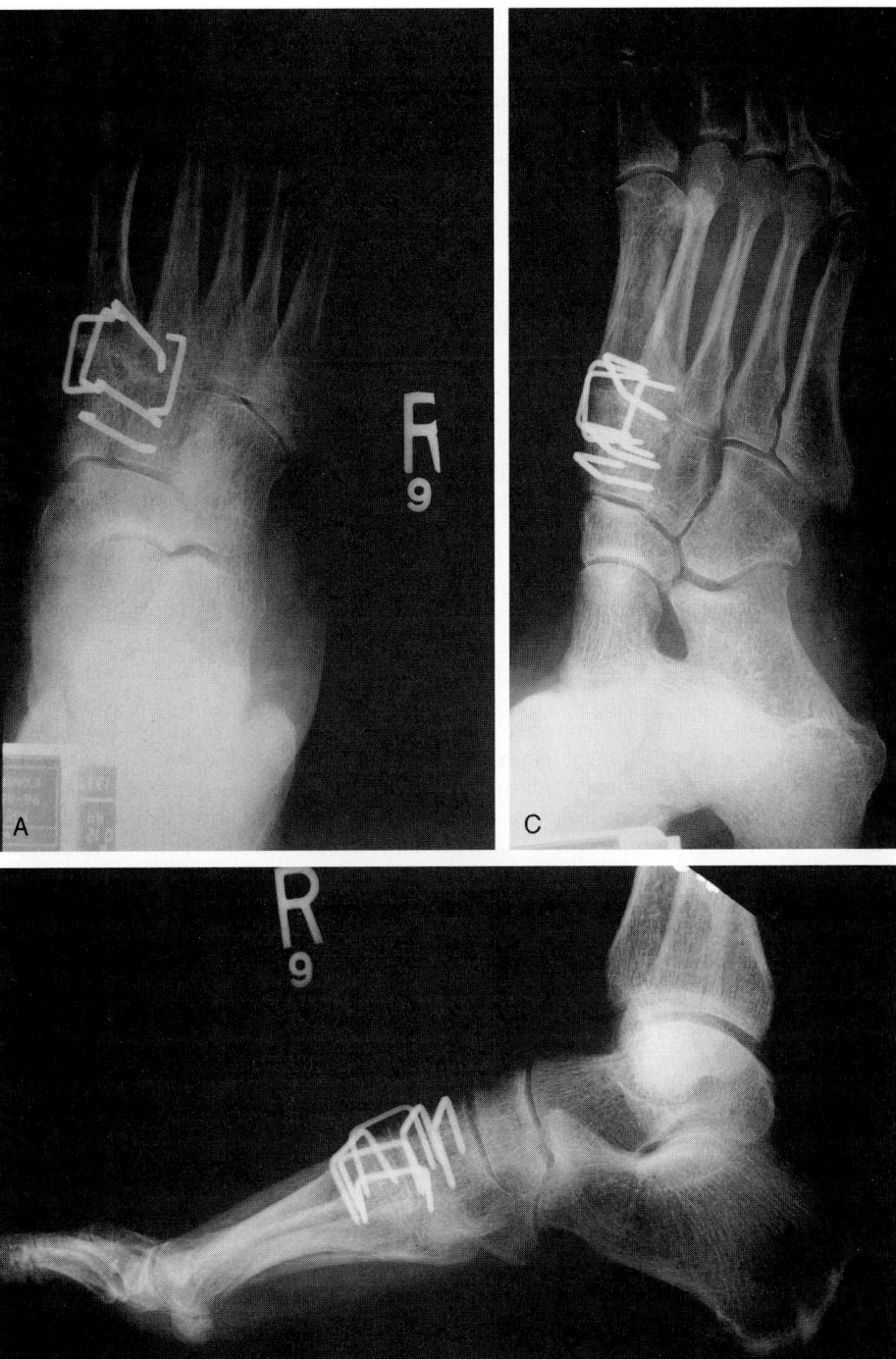

Fig. 3. Four-month postoperative radiographs (anteroposterior, lateral, oblique) after successful fusion. The patient in Figure 1 had relief of 50% of pain but had persistent deep peroneal nerve dysesthesia secondary to the initial injury.

provide compression where possible. Interfragmentary compression may cause malalignment in certain circumstances such as between cuneiforms or with an isolated naviculocuneiform joint. In these circumstances, the advantages of interfragmentary compression (reliable fusion, decreased need for bone graft) must be weighed against the disadvantage of changing the mechanics of the foot.

Fixation with 3.5- to 4.5-mm screws usually works well in the midfoot, although small staples, large-diameter smooth pins and even plantar or medial plates can be used.

Screw patterns vary, but generally fixation proceeds from proximal to distal and from medial to lateral if the naviculocuneiform or intercuneiform joints are involved. It is beneficial to retain the cuboid-lateral cuneiform articulation to allow some residual lateral midfoot motion. The intercuneiform joints are also generally retained unless involved in the arthritic process or deformity.

In patients undergoing naviculomedial cuneiform arthrodesis, the navicular-middle cuneiform joint may need to be released or included to obtain satisfactory compression.

It is critical to maintain the metatarsal heads at a symmetric level. However, in isolated first metatarsocuneiform arthrodesis when there is shortening of the medial column, it may be necessary to plantar flex the first metatarsal compression to increase its weightbearing role.

Deformity correction often requires bony resection medially and occasionally lengthening of the lateral soft tissues, particularly the peroneus brevis tendon. The use of a small external fixator on the lateral column can be helpful to assist with the correction. It has been recommended to correct any deformity, particularly if there is more than 2 mm or 15 degrees of displacement. Bone graft may be necessary to fill any bony defects or gaps. Fixation, as with an in situ arthrodesis, can be accomplished with interfragmentary screw fixation. The use of medial column plating is helpful to maintain alignment in severe deformity.[6]

A subset of patients with midfoot arthritis presents with extensive pathology involving a considerable portion of the medial column, from the talonavicular joint to the medial cuneiform or first metatarsal. Often this results from significant trauma, particularly involving the tarsonavicular and surrounding joints. Occasionally, there is collapse of only the lateral portion of the navicular bone. A variable degree of involvement may be present within the central and lateral columns.

Treatment in these cases is complex because of the extent of disease. Surgical treatment alternatives include inlay or interpositional iliac crest bone grafting. The inlay technique involves the creation of a medial or dorsal rectangular slot from the talus to the involved cuneiforms or metatarsal bases. This can be formed with a bur, and a tricortical graft is inlaid with distraction of the foot. The involved joints are not prepared separately but are spanned by the graft. Fixation may be achieved with screws through the graft into the midfoot and hindfoot or with the use of the mini fragment or small fragment implant sets. In patients with osteopenic bone, supplementary external fixation may be useful in the early phases of graft incorporation. Simultaneous arthrodesis of the calcaneocuboid joint in these cases will lend stability to the fusion mass.

The interpositional technique includes resection of the affected bone segment and replacement with tricortical iliac crest graft. The use of two grafts to fill the segment, with the superior side of the crest positioned dorsally, has been advocated. Fixation can be achieved with screws or with a plate spanning the defect and gaining screw purchase both proximal and distal to the graft. Postoperative care with either technique requires immobilization and non-weight-bearing for a minimum of 2 to 3 months. Often graft incorporation requires up to 6 months, and premature weightbearing may lead to loss of fixation and nonunion.

The neuroarthropathic midfoot typically collapses into a rocker-bottom deformity with a plantar prominence. A plantar-medial deformity with forefoot abduction results with medial and central column involvement. If there is lateral column involvement, a complete rocker-bottom deformity will result, with dorsal subluxation of the entire forefoot.[18] By current standards, the surgical indications in the neuroarthropathic midfoot include recurrent ulceration despite exhaustive nonoperative care and unbraceable deformity. The goal of treatment is to obtain an ambulatory, ulcer-free, and shoeable plantigrade foot, thus avoiding the need for amputation. A stable deformity with a plantar bony prominence associated with recurrent or chronic ulceration is managed with an exostectomy of the offending bone.[19] Arthrodesis is indicated in patients with severe or unstable deformity.[17, 20, 21]

In this population, arthrodesis must be considered with caution because of the potential for severe complications, and only compliant patients with adequate vascular supply without infection should be considered. Contraindications include ongoing infection, gangrene, and (arguably) active neuroarthropathy with bony resorption or fragmentation. As always, surgical reconstruction includes preoperative planning, careful attention to surgical technique, meticulous soft-tissue handling, and strict postoperative management. Longitudinal incisions are used to expose the deformity, which is realigned by taking down the involved joints, and with osteotomies if fixed deformity is present. Internal fixation must be rigid and may be achieved with plates and interfragmentary screw fixation. Percutaneous Achilles tendon lengthening is frequently necessary.

COMPLICATIONS

The complications of midfoot arthrodeses are (1) wound breakdown, (2) nerve injury, (3) nonunion, (4) continued pain, and (5) new areas of high pressure and pain. Wound breakdown is associated with skin fragility, long-term prednisone use, nutritional or vascular problems, and aggressive intraoperative retraction. Nerve injury is often partially the result of the original injury, perineural scarring and fibrosis after midfoot arthrodesis, and the associated immobilization. The terminal branches of both the superficial and deep peroneal branches are "at risk." Longitudinal incisions away from these generally palpable structures, careful intraoperative retraction, and avoidance during skin closure decrease the likelihood of nerve entrapment. All patients should be informed preoperatively that these surgeries carry the intrinsic risk of nerve dysfunction postoperatively, including the possibility of hypoesthesia, dysesthesia, or paresthesia.

In addition to wound or nerve problems, nonunion is always a risk, despite optimal surgical treatment. Patient factors and surgeon-controlled factors may influence the likelihood of obtaining a satisfactory early fusion. Patient factors include inherent vascularity and innervation, smoking history, and compliance with postoperative weightbearing restrictions. Surgical factors include identification of the correct joints to fuse, removal of sufficient cartilage and subchondral bone to obtain fusion, realignment into corrected position, use of autologous graft or similarly inductive and conductive graft when necessary, adequate stabilization of joints, and substantial postoperative immobilization. Some arthrodeses procedures proceed well, the patient's foot heals within a few months, and the patient then presents with a new pain in the same foot. Usually this is due to a fusion of the midfoot in such a way that increases focal weightbearing and pressure under the foot. This may occur under the first ray, with excessive force on the metatarsosesamoid joint, under an isolated central metatarsal from an isolated plantar flexed metatarsal, or on the lateral side of the forefoot from fusion of the lateral midfoot in supination. To avoid these difficulties, the surgeon must strive to fuse the midfoot with the plane of the metatarsal heads oriented perpendicular to the long axis of the tibia.

RESULTS

The outcome of orthotic treatment of midfoot arthritis depends largely on the appropriateness of the prescription and the expertise of the orthotist in fitting the prescription. The importance of good, two-way open communication between the orthotist and the physician cannot be overemphasized. In general, the physician has the best concept of the bony and articular anatomy, the source of pain, and the mechanical environment to reduce or eliminate provocative motions. The orthotist will try to fill the prescription to meet the needs of the patient and the physician, but needs to be apprised of the physician's anatomic and mechanical concerns. After fitting, patients should be seen by both the physician and the orthotist on multiple occasions until the orthotic fits well and the shoe is modified appropriately. Common problems include (1) too steep a rocker-bottom or roller sole, (2) setting the rocker-bottom or roller too far forward on the sole, (3) not enough stiffening to the shoe, (4) too hard of a material at the interface of the orthotic and the skin, and (5) insufficient medial support within the in-depth shoe. If an inshoe orthotic fits well but does not relieve pain, then an ankle-foot orthosis may be required.

Three studies provided data on the outcome of midfoot arthrodesis for primary and post-traumatic degenerative arthritis. In one report, 40 patients monitored for an average of 6 years had a 93% satisfaction rate. The union rate was 98%, or 176 of the 179 joints involved achieved union.[3] Correction of deformity, as measured by both the change in the anteroposterior and lateral talus-first metatarsal angle, was approximately 8 degrees in both planes. In the other report, 32 patients with post-traumatic arthritis had considerable improvement in their American Orthopaedic Foot and Ankle Society score, with only one asymptomatic nonunion. The extent or location of the arthrodesis, patient age, need for revision surgery, and work-related status of the original injury were shown to have no significant effect on outcome.[5] The most frequent complications in both series included, neuroma formation, metatarsalgia related to malunion, and wound slough. Malunion occurred in seven

of the combined total of 72 patients and involved plantar flexion of the second metatarsal in all as well as the third or first metatarsal in four. Of these seven patients, two underwent operative treatment with a dorsal closing-wedge osteotomy and five were managed successfully with a metatarsal pad or cushioned insole.

In a separate study of the use of medial column plating, the outcome of nine patients with severe deformity has been reported. All obtained fusion and reliable correction of deformity with good or excellent results in seven, fair results in one, and one Charcot foot, which was noted to be difficult to grade.[6]

In a series of 21 Charcot feet undergoing arthrodesis in the midfoot and hindfoot, limb salvage was obtained in eighteen. Seventy percent of ulcers healed at an average of 6 weeks, with no midfoot ulcer recurrence. Fusion in successful cases was achieved in approximately 5 months. Two patients experienced nonunion, with hardware failure, and two underwent a below-knee amputation for postoperative osteomyelitis. Other complications included wound dehiscence, recurrent deformity, forefoot ulceration, and death. Overall, surgery-related complications occurred in 38% of cases (8/21). Of the salvaged feet, 87% were able to wear extra-depth, wide-toe box, and off-the-shelf shoes with inserts.[20]

Exostectomy has been reported to be successful as well.[19] In a series of 12 patients, 11 healed with no subsequent breakdown; one required repeat exostectomy and eventual Syme's amputation.

In another report, Schon et al[18] developed a new classification system based on location and severity of the deformity for Charcot feet and then described their novel treatment approach for these problems. In their series, four of 131 patients were acutely operated on secondary to impending skin compromise with a 50% complication rate. The remaining 127 were managed conservatively, 86 successfully. Forty-one eventually required intervention for recurrent ulceration. The majority underwent biplanar arthrodesis and correction of deformity. Twelve of 37 had wound complications; seven of 37 required additional surgery. All but one foot was managed with regular or orthopaedic footwear; eight feet required bracing. Ninety percent of patients were satisfied without reservation. They reported no amputations.[18]

REFERENCES

1. Hardcastle PH, Reschauer R, Kutscha-Lissberg E, et al: Injuries to the tarsometatarsal joint: Incidence, classification and treatment. J Bone Joint Surg Br 1982; 64:349.
2. Myerson MS, Fisher RT, Burgess AR, et al: Fracture dislocations of the tarsometatarsal joints: End results correlated with pathology and treatment. Foot Ankle 1986; 6:225.
3. Mann RA, Prieskorn D, Sobel M: Midtarsal and tarsometatarsal arthrodesis for primary degenerative osteoarthritis or osteoarthritis after trauma. J Bone Joint Surg Am 1996; 78:1376.
4. Sangeorzan BJ, Veith RG, Hansen ST: Salvage of Lisfranc's tarsometatarsal joint by arthrodesis. Foot Ankle 1990; 10:193.

5. Komenda GA, Myerson MS, Biddinger KR: Results of arthrodesis of the tarsometatarsal joints after traumatic injury. J Bone Joint Surg Am 1996; 78:1665.
6. Horton GA, Olney BW: Deformity correction and arthrodesis of the midfoot with a medial plate. Foot Ankle 1993; 14:493.
7. Johnson JE, Johnson KA: Dowel arthrodesis for degenerative arthritis of the tarsometatarsal (Lisfranc) joints. Foot Ankle 1986; 6:243.
8. dePalma LD, Santucci A, Sabetta SP, et al: Anatomy of the Lisfranc joint complex. Foot Ankle 1997; 18:356.
9. Ouzounian TJ, Sheref MJ: In vitro determination of midfoot motion. Foot Ankle 1989; 10:140.
10. Fritz GR, Prieskorn D: First metatarsocu-

neiform motion: A radiographic and statistical analysis. Foot Ankle 1995; 16:117.
11. Ebraheim NA, Yang H, Lu J, et al: Computer evaluation of second tarsometatarsal joint dislocation. Foot Ankle 1996; 17:685.
12. Wilson DW: Injuries of the tarso-metatarsal joints: Etiology, classification and results of treatment. J Bone Joint Surg Br 1972; 54:677.
13. Arntz CT, Veith RG, Hansen ST: Fractures and fracture-dislocations of the tarsometatarsal joint. J Bone Joint Surg Am 1988; 79:173.
14. Brunet JA, Wiley JJ: The late results of tarsometatarsal joint injuries. J Bone Joint Surg Br 1987; 69:437.
15. Vidigal E, Jacoby R, Dixon A, et al: The

foot in chronic rheumatoid disease. Ann Rheum Dis 1975; 34:292.

16. Guerra J, Resnick D: Arthritides affecting the foot: Radiographic-pathologic correlation. Foot Ankle 1982; 2:325.

17. Levi S, Ansell BM, Klenerman L: Tarsometatarsal involvement in juvenile spondyloarthropathy. Foot Ankle 1990; 11:90.

18. Schon LC, Easley ME, Weinfeld SB: Charcot neuroarthropathy of the foot and ankle. Clin Orthop Rel Res 1998; 349:116.

19. Brodsky JW, Rouse AM: Exostectomy for symptomatic bony prominences in diabetic Charcot feet. Clin Orthop Rel Res 1993; 296:21.

20. Early JS, Hansen ST: Surgical reconstruction of the diabetic foot: A salvage approach for midfoot collapse. Foot Ankle 1996; 17:325.

21. Bono JV, Roger DJ, Jacobs RL: Surgical arthrodesis of the neuropathic foot. Clin Orthop Rel Res 1993; 296:14.

22. Myerson MS, Henderson MR, Saxby T, et al: Management of midfoot diabetic neuroarthropathy. Foot Ankle 1994; 15:233.

section 11 chapter 9

DISORDERS OF THE FIRST RAY

Brian G. Donley and E. Greer Richardson

Summary
- Problems of the first ray are common.
- The major causal factors related to hallux valgus are faulty footwear and familial predisposition.
- Nonoperative treatment for deformity is rarely efficacious.
- First metatarsophalangeal deformity without arthritis is generally treated with a confirmation of soft-tissue and bony realignment procedures.
- First metatarsophalangeal arthritis can be treated with partial resection arthrodesis.

An estimated 43 million Americans have foot problems, costing approximately $5.3 billion annually. Of women between 20 and 60 years of age, more than 75% have some type of foot deformity. The National Center for Health Statistics, in their 1990 National Health Survey, reported that 51 of every 1000 persons reported "trouble with bunions."

HALLUX VALGUS

The most frequent great toe problem is hallux valgus, a lateral deviation of the hallux. However, frequently there are multiple components to the deformity: varus deformity of the first metatarsus, bunion formation, hypertrophy of the medial eminence, arthritis of the first metatarsophalangeal (MTP) joint, hammertoe, corns, calluses, and metatarsalgia (Fig. 1). If the valgus deformity of the great toe is severe, it can crowd the second toe and cause overlapping or underlapping of the second toe and possibly subluxation or dislocation of the second MTP joint.[1, 2]

ETIOLOGY

No single cause of hallux valgus can be isolated. Evidence supports that hallux valgus is familial, especially when it occurs during adolescence. A major factor in the development of hallux valgus in many patients is footwear. Anatomic and structural abnormalities that have been implicated in the development of hallux valgus include pronated flatfeet, abnormal insertion of the posterior tibial tendon, increased obliquity of the first metatarsomedial-cuneiform joint, an abnormally long first ray, incongruous articular surfaces of the first MTP joint, and excessive valgus tilt of the articular surface of the first metatarsal head or the proximal phalangeal articular surface or both. Once the hallux valgus angle (HVA) increases to 30 degrees or more, pronation of the great toe may result, which signals a likely progression of deformity (Fig. 2).

EVALUATION

History

A careful history is the first step in the evaluation of hallux valgus. The patient's occupation and recreational activities, as well as choice of shoe wear, can be important factors in determining whether surgical treatment is indicated. A patient whose occupation requires long periods of standing or walking or who is a competitive athlete may not be able to return to presurgical levels of activity. If the patient's choice of shoe wear is ill-suited to the size and shape of the foot, surgical correction of the hallux valgus deformity will still leave the patient unable to wear the shoes he or she desires, or the deformity will likely return.

Physical Examination

The entire foot should be thoroughly examined while the patient is standing, sitting, and lying supine. Particular attention should be given to the remainder of the forefoot. Corns, calluses, warts, interdigital neuromas, bunionettes, hammertoes, and clawtoes should be identified. Although pain and deformity may be relieved after correction of the hallux valgus, the result can be compromised if symptoms in the lesser toes or metatarsals are not identified preoperatively. Ranges of motion of the ankle, subtalar, transverse tarsal, and MTP joints should be evaluated. The approximate amount of correction that can be obtained with surgery, with maintenance of satisfactory range of motion, can be determined by attempting to correct the hallux vaglus deformity (reducing the first MTP joint as congruously as possible) and then moving the great toe in dorsiflexion and plantarflexion. Crepitation may be felt if the MTP joint is

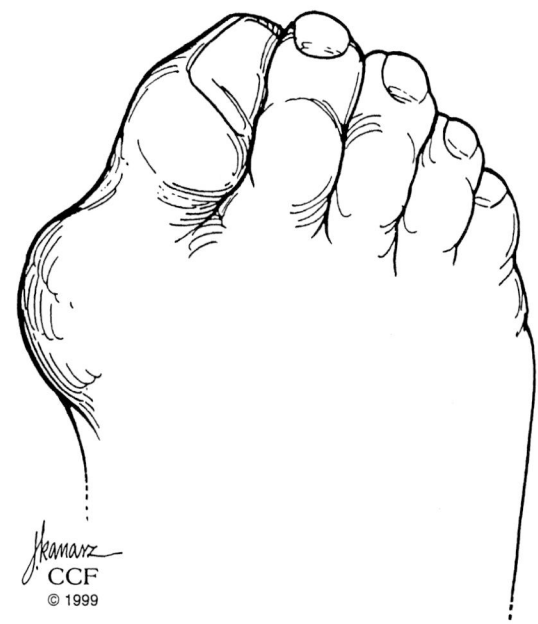

Fig. 1. Hallux valgus and deformities often associated with it. ©1999 CCF from Joe Kanasz.

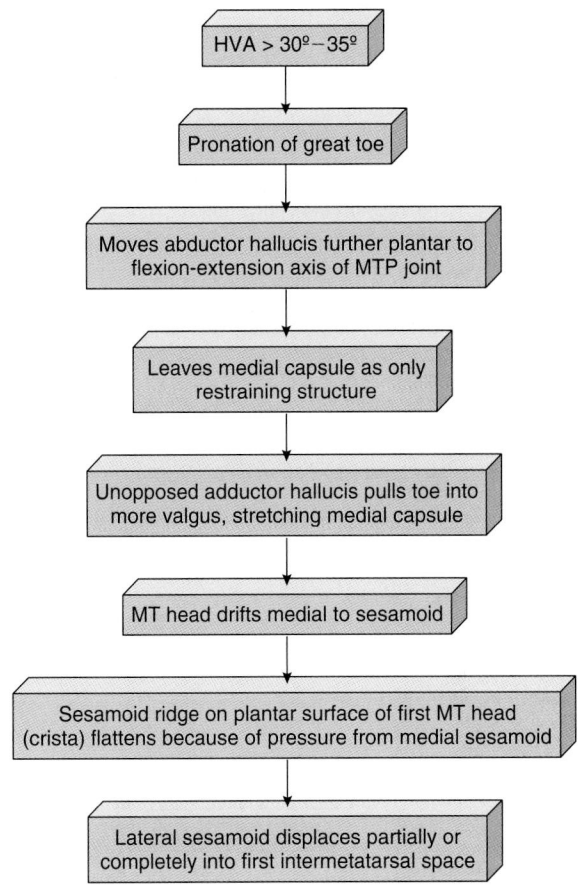

Fig. 2. Progression of hallux valgus deformity.

arthritic. The neurovascular status of the foot also should be carefully evaluated.

Radiographic Examination

Standard radiographs for evaluation of hallux valgus should include standing (weightbearing) dorsoplantar and lateral views, non-weightbearing oblique view, and sesamoid view. Several radiographic angles are used to help determine the severity of the deformity (Table 1). The HVA and the intermetatarsal angle (IMA) are most frequently cited as guidelines for treatment decisions, but interobserver measurements of the HVA can vary significantly.[3]

Surgical decisions should be based on clinical observation and serial radiographs rather than on subtle differences in radiographic measurements.[1–4]

Other radiographic findings include the relative lengths of the first and second metatarsals, congruency of the first MTP joint, position of the sesamoids, shape of the first

Angle	Measured On	Location	Importance	Normal
	TABLE 1. RADIOGRAPHIC ANGLES USED FOR EVALUATION OF HALLUX VALGUS DEFORMITY			
Hallux valgus	Standing dorsoplantar view	Between long axes of first proximal phalanx and first metatarsal, bisecting their diaphysis	Identifies degree of deformity at the MTP joint	Less than 15 degrees
First-second intermetatarsal	Standing dorsoplantar view	Between long axes of first and second metatarsal, bisecting shafts of first and second metatarsals	Not influenced by overresection of medial eminence; not accurate for postoperative evaluation of distal osteotomies	Less than 9 degrees
Distal metatarsal articular	Standing dorsoplantar view	Angle of line bisecting metatarsal shaft with line through base of distal articular cartilage cap	Offset of angle is predisposing factor in development of hallux valgus	10–15 degrees
Hallux interphalangeus	Standing dorsoplantar view	Between long axes of first proximal phalanx and first distal phalanx, bisecting their diaphysis	Identifies degree of deformity at the IP joint	Less than 8 degrees
Phalangeal articular	Standing dorsoplantar view	Articular angle of base of proximal phalanx in relation to longitudinal axis	Offset of angle is predisposing factor in development of hallux valgus	7–10 degrees

MTP, metatarsophalangeal; IP, interphalangeal.

TABLE 2. RADIOGRAPHIC FINDINGS IN HALLUX VALGUS

Variable	Findings
Sesamoid position	Amount of displacement of the tibial sesamoid relative to a reference line that bisects the long axis of the first MT shaft: Grade 0, no displacement Grade 1, less than 50% overlap Grade 2, more than 50% overlap Grade 3, complete displacement beyond line
Congruent joint	No lateral deviation of proximal phalanx on MT head
Incongruent joint	Lateral deviation of proximal phalanx on MT head, ranging from minimal to severe subluxation
Shape of MT head	Flat, predisposed to hallux rigidus and DJD Round, predisposed to hallux valgus and intrinsic instability Dome shaped, predisposed to intrinsic stability

MT, metatarsal; DJD, degenerative joint disease.

metatarsal head (Table 2), and arthritic changes (joint space narrowing, osteophyte formation, and subchondral cyst).

TREATMENT

Initially, most patients can be treated nonsurgically with appropriate shoe modifications, exercises, and activity adjustments. Surgical treatment of hallux valgus for cosmetic reasons alone is seldom indicated. Severe, painful deformity that prevents reasonable function is an indication for surgical treatment.

More than 150 surgical procedures have been described for correction of hallux valgus, and determining the appropriate procedure or combination of procedures is perhaps the most difficult aspect of treatment. Although all of the components of the hallux vaglus deformity should be considered in the choice of a surgical procedure, the hallux valgus deformity can be divided into four types to help determine appropriate treatment: congruent joint, incongruent joint, hypermobility of the metatarsocuneiform joint, or arthrosis of the first MTP joint. A number of treatment algorithms have been developed to assist in treatment decision-making[1, 3, 5] (Fig. 3).

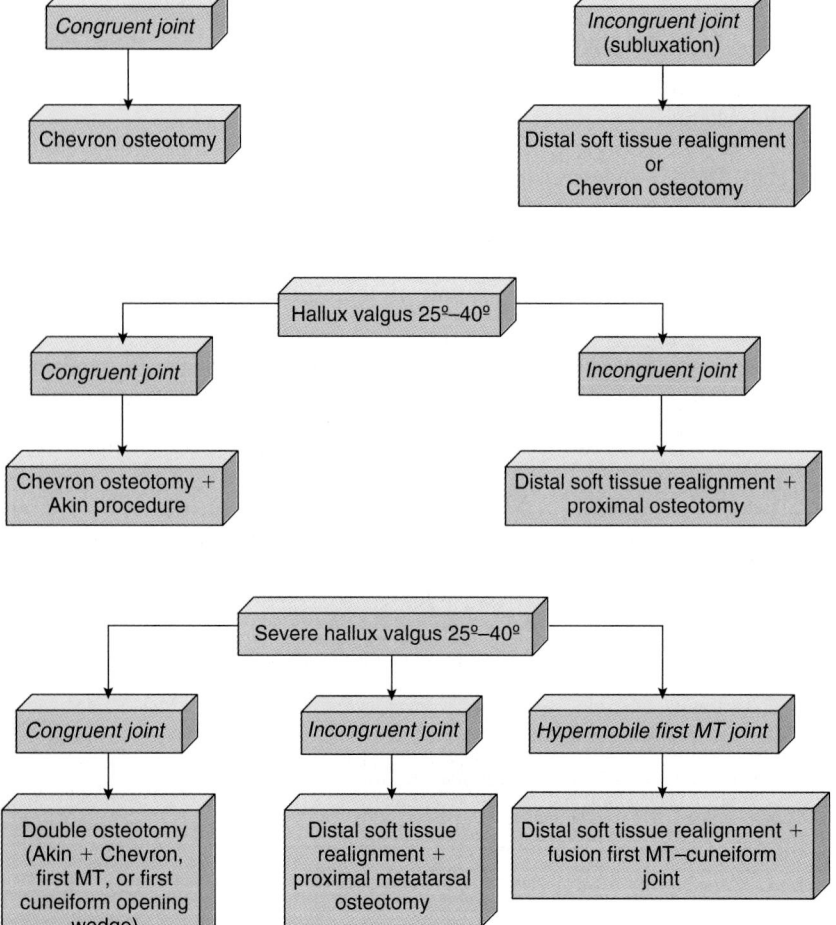

Fig. 3. Treatment algorithm for hallux valgus. (Modified from Mann RA: Instr Course Lect 1990; 39:3.)

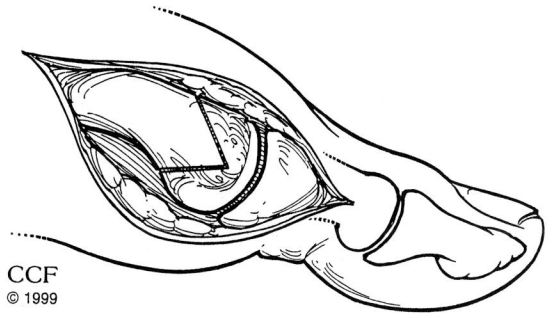

Fig. 4. Chevron osteotomy. The angle of the osteotomy cuts is 60 to 90 degrees, providing a large stable surface area. ©1999 CCF from Joe Kanasz.

Distal Soft-Tissue Procedure, With or Without Proximal Crescentric or Chevron Osteotomy or Metatarsal-Cuneiform Joint Fusion

A distal soft-tissue procedure to release the contracted structures on the lateral side of the MTP joint, combined with removal of the medial eminence exostosis, is most appropriate for a patient younger than 50 years with an HVA of 15 to 25 degrees, an IMA of less than 13 degrees, and no degenerative changes at the MTP joint. The adductor hallucis tendon, the lateral joint capsule, and the transverse metatarsal ligament are released through a dorsal web space dissection. A medial midline approach allows removal of the exostosis and plication of the medial capsule. Recurrence of the deformity is the most common complication when a fixed IMA angle is not corrected by the soft-tissue procedure. Iatrogenic hallux varus and cock-up deformity also may occur.

If the IMA is more than 13 degrees, a proximal crescentric or proximal chevron osteotomy is recommended, because a distal procedure is less likely to obtain satisfactory corrections. The osteotomy is made approximately 1 cm distal to the metatarsocuneiform joint to obtain adequate correction.[6–8] In a patient with a hypermobile metatarsocuneiform joint, arthrodesis of the metatarsocuneiform joint should be added to the soft-tissue procedure instead of a proximal metatarsal osteotomy.

Distal Chevron Osteotomy

Currently, the most widely used distal metatarsal osteotomy is the chevron osteotomy[9–14] (Fig. 4), which includes (1) medial eminence removal, (2) a V-shaped intracapsular osteotomy through the first metatarsal head, (3) lateral displacement of the capital fragment, (4) removal of the resulting projection of the first metatarsal, and (5) medial capsulorrhaphy. Fixation of the osteotomy with one or two Kirschner's wires, a cortical screw, or a biodegradable pin adds stability to the osteotomy. With some modifications, such as more proximal placement of the apex of the osteotomy in the metatarsal head, the chevron osteotomy can be used for more severe deformities (up to 35 degrees of hallux valgus and up to 15 degrees of first to second intermetatarsal diversion). Johnson, who popularized the chevron osteotomy, also modified it by changing the length and position of the limbs of the osteotomy in the metatarsal head and using a 2.7-mm screw for fixation, which

extended the indications for the osteotomy to severe deformities with intermetatarsal angles of up to 15 or 16 degrees.

Proximal Phalangeal Osteotomy

The Akin proximal phalangeal osteotomy[15] (Fig. 5) is used to treat valgus deformity in the hallux (hallux valgus interphalangeus). It is made at the base of the proximal phalanx, 3 to 4 mm distal to the articular surfaces. The osteotomy must be distal enough to avoid violating the MTP joint. Usually a medially based wedge of 3 to 5 mm is removed, and the osteotomy is stabilized with sutures, Kirschner's wires, or biodegradable pins. This osteotomy should not be used alone for treatment of an incongruent joint, because the deformity is almost certain to recur or progress.[16]

Resection Arthroplasty

Resection (Keller's) arthroplasty is performed for low-demand patients with severe deformity and/or arthritis. It is done through a medial midline incision, through which a proximally based flap is created, the medial eminence is removed, and the proximal third of the proximal phalanx is excised. If possible, the short flexor tendons should be reattached to the proximal phalanx through a drill hole. The medial capsule is plicated, and longitudinal pins are used to stabilize the MTP joint.

Arthrodesis

Arthrodesis of the first MTP joint is most commonly indicated for patients with degenerative or rheumatoid arthritis or neuromuscular disease, recurrent hallux valgus, or post-traumatic hallux valgus.[17] The joint surfaces can be cut flat, or a ball-and-socket configuration can be created with or without specialized reamers. The ideal position for fusion is approximately 15 degrees of valgus and 10 to 15 degrees of dorsiflexion in relation to the plantar aspect of the foot.

Fusion of the metatarsocuneiform joint is indicated for severe metatarsus primus varus, moderate hallux valgus deformity associated with hypermobility of the first ray, generalized ligamentous laxity, and hypermobility in an adolescent and symptomatic degenerative arthritis of the metatarsocuneiform joint. Myerson et al[18] reported good results in 77% of 67 patients with metatarsocuneiform arthrodesis, despite frequent complications of nonunion (9.5%), need for screw removal (30%), and development of dorsal bunions (7%).

COMPLICATIONS OF HALLUX VALGUS SURGERY

Despite the numerous reports of complications of hallux valgus surgery, most patients obtain satisfactory results and are pleased with them. The most common complications, regardless of procedure, are incomplete correction and recurrence of the hallux valgus deformity. Both of these are often technique related, and their likelihood can be decreased by careful attention to surgical technique and preoperative surgical decision-making.

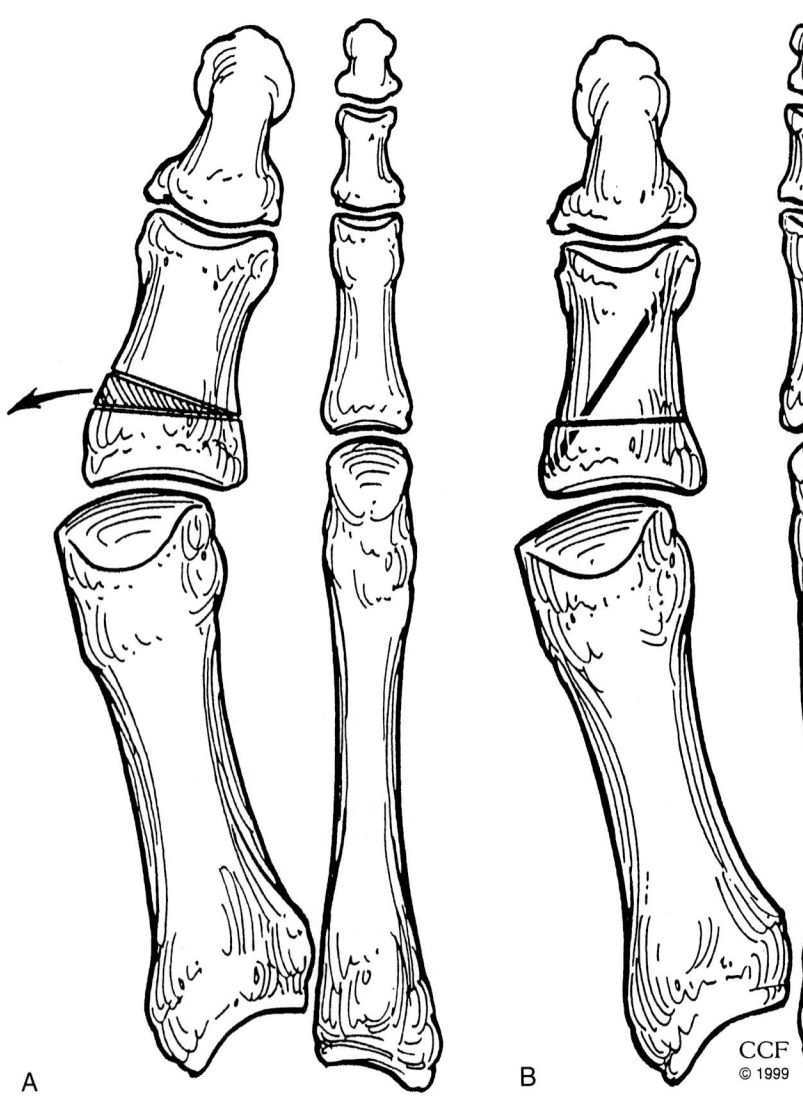

A

B

Fig. 5. Akin osteotomy. Phalangeal closing wedge osteotomy (*A*) and final position of hallux (*B*). ©1999 CCF from Joe Kanasz.

CCF
© 1999

JUVENILE OR ADOLESCENT HALLUX VALGUS

A symptomatic hallux vaglus deformity is uncommon in children and adolescents. Although the deformity may have developed at an early age, the patient often does not seek treatment until adulthood. In juvenile or adolescent hallux valgus, the HVA and IMA usually are not as severe as in adults, and the medial eminence rarely is enlarged. Adolescent hallux valgus deformity is more common in girls, and approximately 75% of patients have a family history of hallux valgus. In determining treatment, the presence of open physes as well as the possibility of joint hypermobility must be considered in these patients.

TREATMENT

Initially, nonsurgical treatment can relieve most symptoms, but progression of the deformity and pain often make surgery necessary. The indications for surgical correction of a hallux valgus deformity in an adolescent are not firmly established, nor is the timing of the procedure during adolescence agreed on. Debate continues regarding whether the procedure should be postponed until the physes of the phalanx and metatarsal are closed, whether radiographic confirmation of progression should be documented before recommending surgery, and whether pain should be a primary indication for operative treatment as in adults. Several well-documented series recommend operative correction only for adolescents with painful, progressive deformity after the physes are closed. In contrast, other well-documented, retrospective studies indicate that surgery before 15 years of age, with or without open physes, yields the best long-term results, especially if preservation of normal MTP motion is considered an essential element of acceptable results.

As in adult patients, the surgical procedure must correct all components of the deformity. Coughlin[19] devised algorithms for determining the treatment of young patients with mild hallux valgus deformities (HVA of 25 degrees or less) (Fig. 6), moderate deformities (HVA of 25 to 40 degrees)

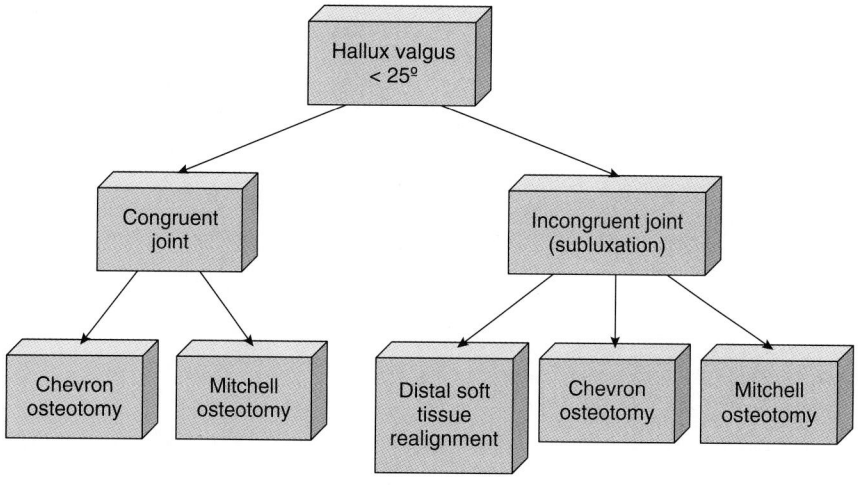

Fig. 6. Treatment algorithm for mild juvenile hallux valgus deformity. (From Coughlin MJ: Juvenile bunion. In Mann RA, Coughlin MJ [eds]: Surgery of the Foot and Ankle. St. Louis, MO, Mosby–Year Book, 1993, 6th ed, p 297.)

(Fig. 7), and severe deformities (HVA of more than 40 degrees) (Fig. 8). Depending on its size, the medial eminence may or may not require excision. An IMA of 10 degrees or more requires a metatarsal osteotomy. If the IMA is corrected to 6 degrees or less and the HVA to 15 degrees or less, the likelihood of unattractive, symptomatic recurrence is rare.[20] The most difficult combination of deformities to correct includes hypermobile flatfoot, metatarsus primus varus, and hallux valgus; recurrence is common. Often proximal metatarsal osteotomy, distal metatarsal osteotomy, or both are required. Patients and parents should be fully advised that no operative procedure can always avoid recurrence of the deformity in this population.

Mitchell Osteotomy

The Mitchell extra-articular osteotomy (Fig. 9) obtains correction by lateral displacement and angulation of a distal metaphyseal osteotomy.[21] Because it is slightly more proximal than a chevron osteotomy, it allows more correction. The most common complication after this osteotomy is metatarsalgia (25% to 40%), often caused by displacement,

dorsal angulation, or shortening of the metatarsal. Plantar angulation at the osteotomy site and rigid internal fixation will help avoid this complication.

Double and Triple Osteotomies

More recently, because many patients with juvenile or adolescent hallux valgus have congruent MTP joints, double and triple osteotomies have been recommended for correction of the deformity.[22]

Peterson and Newman[22] recommended an opening wedge proximally and a closing wedge distally to correct the abnormal distal metatarsal articular angle (DMAA) and IMA (Fig. 10). They reported excellent correction in 13 of 15 feet in patients ranging in age from 12 to 21 years treated with a double osteotomy.

For severe deformities in adolescents, Coughlin[23] recommended a triple osteotomy (Fig. 11), which includes a medial cuneiform opening wedge osteotomy, a distal metatarsal osteotomy to correct the abnormal distal metatarsal articular angle, and an Akin osteotomy. Coughlin reserved this procedure for patients with markedly splayed forefeet and widened first to fifth metatarsal angle of more than 30

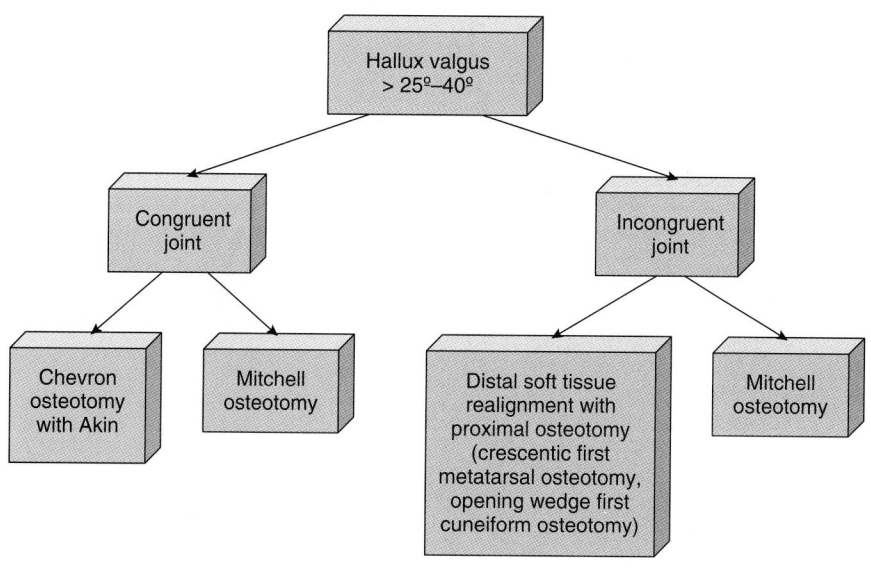

Fig. 7. Treatment algorithm for moderate juvenile hallux valgus deformity. (From Coughlin MJ: Juvenile bunion. In Mann RA, Coughlin MJ [eds]: Surgery of the Foot and Ankle. St. Louis, MO, Mosby–Year Book, 1993, p 297.)

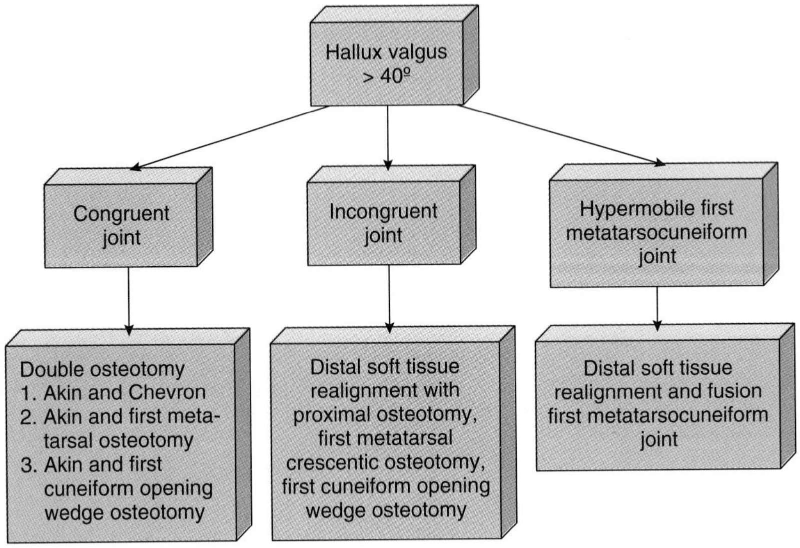

Hallux valgus
> 40º

Congruent
joint

Incongruent
joint

Hypermobile first
metatarsocuneiform
joint

Double osteotomy
1. Akin and Chevron
2. Akin and first meta-
   tarsal osteotomy
3. Akin and first
   cuneiform opening
   wedge osteotomy

Distal soft tissue
realignment with
proximal osteotomy,
first metatarsal
crescentic osteotomy,
first cuneiform opening
wedge osteotomy

Distal soft tissue
realignment and fusion
first metatarsocuneiform
joint

Fig. 8. Treatment algorithm for severe juvenile hallux valgus. (From Coughlin MJ: Juvenile bunion. In Mann RA, Coughlin MJ [eds]: Surgery of the Foot and Ankle. St. Louis, MO, Mosby-Year Book, 1993, p 297.)

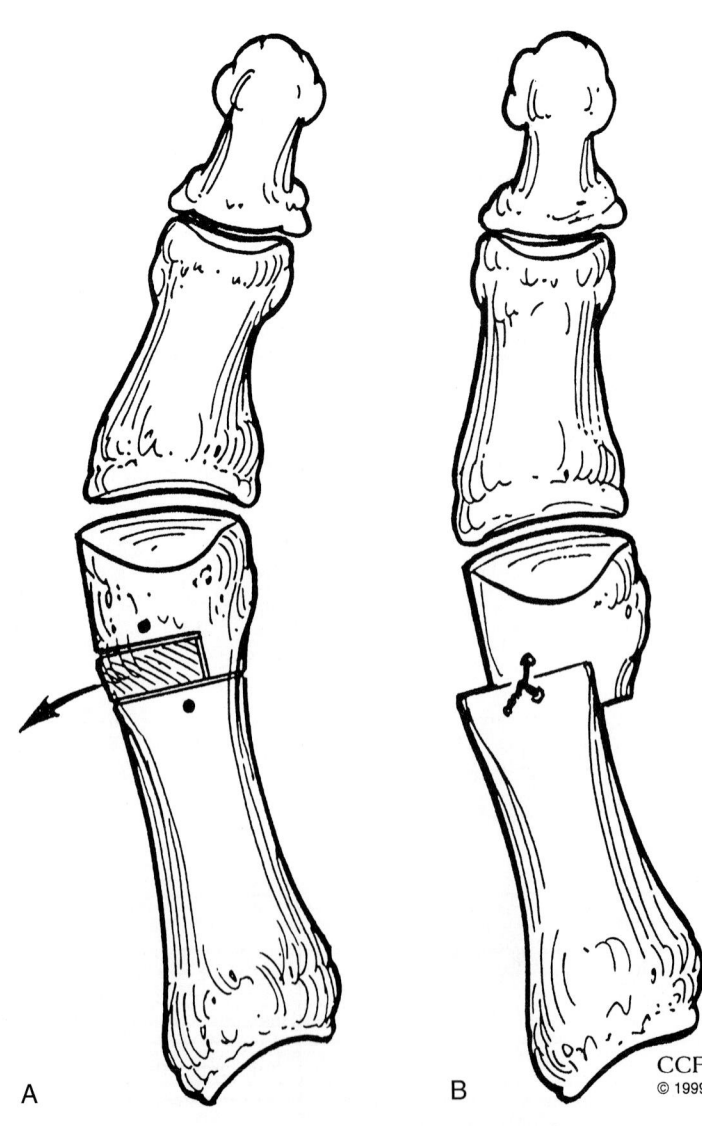

Fig 9. Mitchell osteotomy. *A,* Excision of bone from between osteotomies. *B,* Displacement of capital fragment and tying of sutures. ©1999 CCF from Joe Kanasz.

A   B

CCF
© 1999

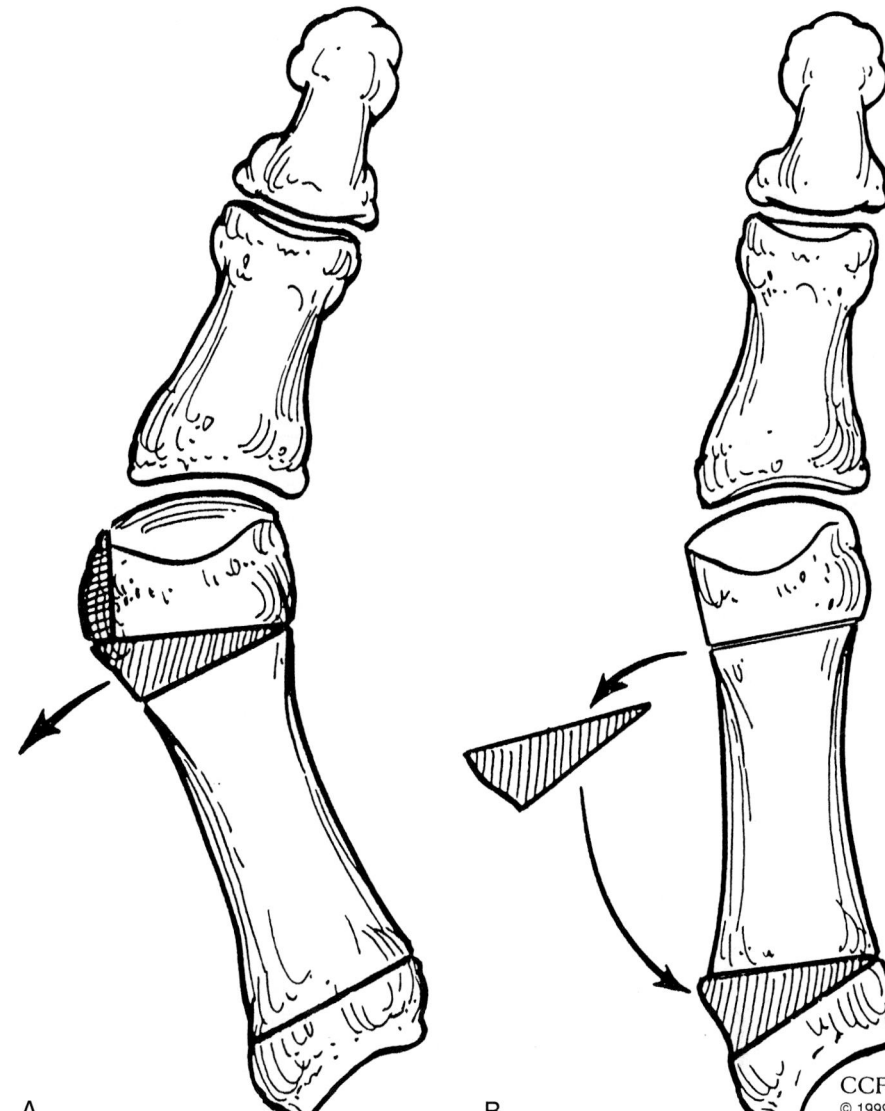

Fig. 10. Double first metatarsal osteotomies. ©1999 CCF from Joe Kanasz.

A

B

degrees, excessive first-to-second IMA of more than 15 degrees, HVA of more than 35 degrees, and a distal metatarsal articular angle of more than 15 degrees.

With either double or triple osteotomies, extreme care must be taken to avoid excessive soft-tissue dissection, which can lead to devascularization of a portion of the metatarsal. Care also must be taken not to disturb metatarsal or phalangeal physes. Multiple osteotomies may create instability with displacement and eventual malalignment or malunion.

RECURRENT HALLUX VALGUS

ETIOLOGY

Recurrent hallux valgus is the most common complication after hallux valgus surgery. It is most often caused by the choice of an inappropriate procedure, a failure to obtain adequate correction, or continued use to shoe wear that is too tight. Inadequate or inappropriate postoperative management may result in failure even when the surgery was

properly chosen and performed. Certain preoperative conditions, such as arthritis, diabetes, and concomitant foot deformities, may predispose a patient to recurrence of the hallux valgus deformity, and these should be considered in the choice of procedure.

TREATMENT

The magnitude and rigidity of the recurrent deformity are guides to treatment. As a rule, a deformity that occurred after a soft-tissue procedure should not be treated with another soft-tissue procedure unless the deformity is completely flexible (the hallux can be easily reduced into varus and the first metatarsal freely translates laterally by manual pressure). First web space dissection, lateral release, and repeat medial capsular imbrication with manual lateral displacement of the first metatarsal are recommended only in patients with mild, flexible deformity.

When the DMAA is increased in recurrent hallux valgus, reducing the hallux will place the phalanx incongruously on the metatarsal head. The phalanx will rest in varus on

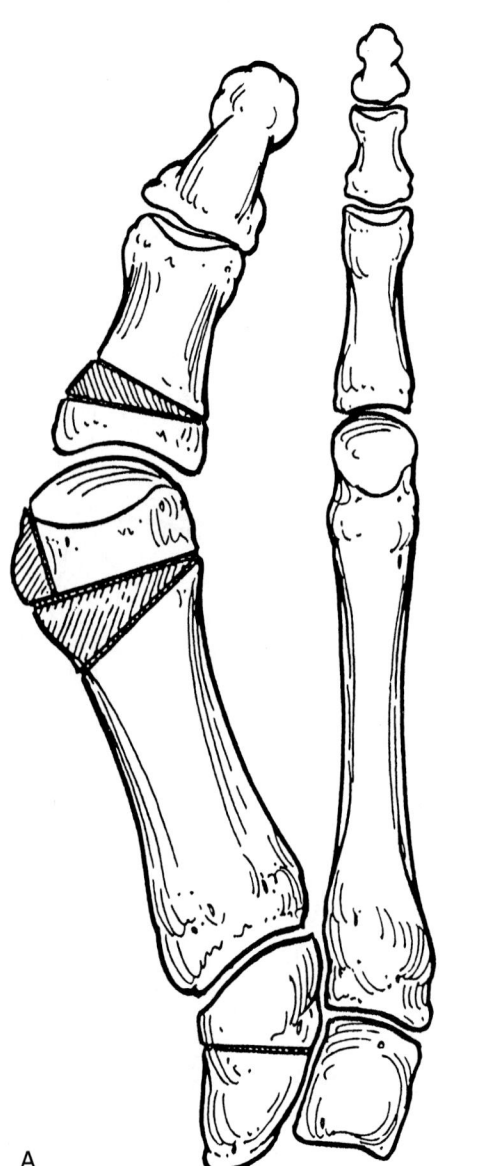

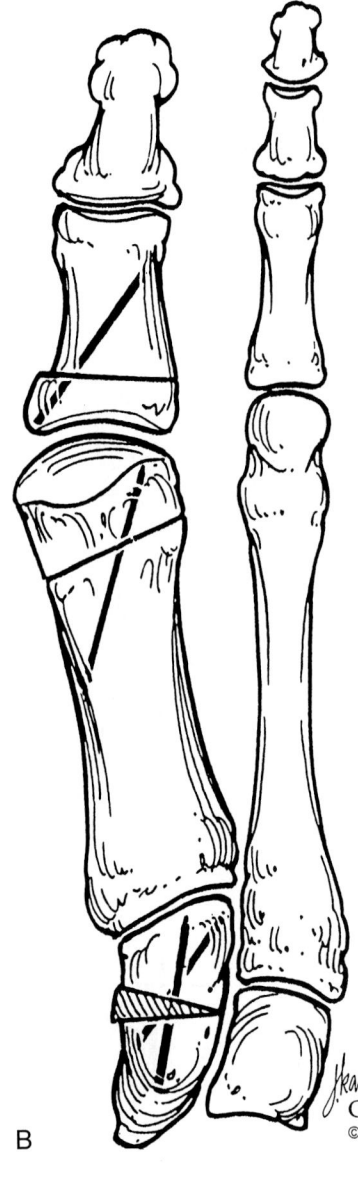

Fig. 11. Triple osteotomies. *A,* A closing wedge osteotomy of the distal end of the metatarsal with exostectomy of the medial eminence and opening wedge osteotomy of the first cuneiform and closing wedge osteotomy of proximal phalanx. *B,* Final corrective position of hallux. ©1999 CCF from Joe Kanasz.

the first metatarsal head and will leave the lateral aspect of the first metatarsal head uncovered. This deformity can be corrected with medial capsulorrhaphy, distal metatarsal closing wedge osteotomy, and first web space dissection with lateral soft-tissue release.

Recurrent deformities after osteotomies generally require repeat osteotomies for correction. For malunion of a chevron osteotomy, Richardson and Donley[2] recommended a "broomstick" osteotomy to allow correction of all planes of deformity and to preserve as much length as possible. Recurrent deformity after basilar metatarsal osteotomy should be treated with a second basilar metatarsal osteotomy, medial capsular imbrication of the first metatarsophalangeal joint, and first web space dissection with release of the contracted lateral structures. A combination of chevron and Akin osteotomies can be used for greater correction of valgus deformity.[16] For severe recurrent deformity, arthrodesis of the first MTP joint is often the most appropriate operation. Resection (Keller's) arthroplasty can be used for correction of recurrent deformity in elderly patients who

have limited physical demands on their feet and have some degree of osteoarthritis at the first MTP joint.

HALLUX VARUS

Hallux varus deformity is defined radiographically by a negative metatarsophalangeal angle in the axial plane and clinically by abduction (medial deviation) of the hallux on the first metatarsal. However, often sagittal and coronal plane deformities exist along with the axial plane deformity. Usually the MTP joint is extended, the interphalangeal (IP) joint is flexed in the sagittal plane, and the phalanx is supinated in the coronal plane (Fig. 12).

ETIOLOGY

Although numerous causes exist,[24–26] acquired hallux varus most commonly occurs after surgical correction for hallux valgus. The incidence of hallux varus after hallux valgus surgery has ranged from 2% to nearly 13%.[25, 27, 28] Hallux varus occurs because of soft-tissue or bony imbalance that

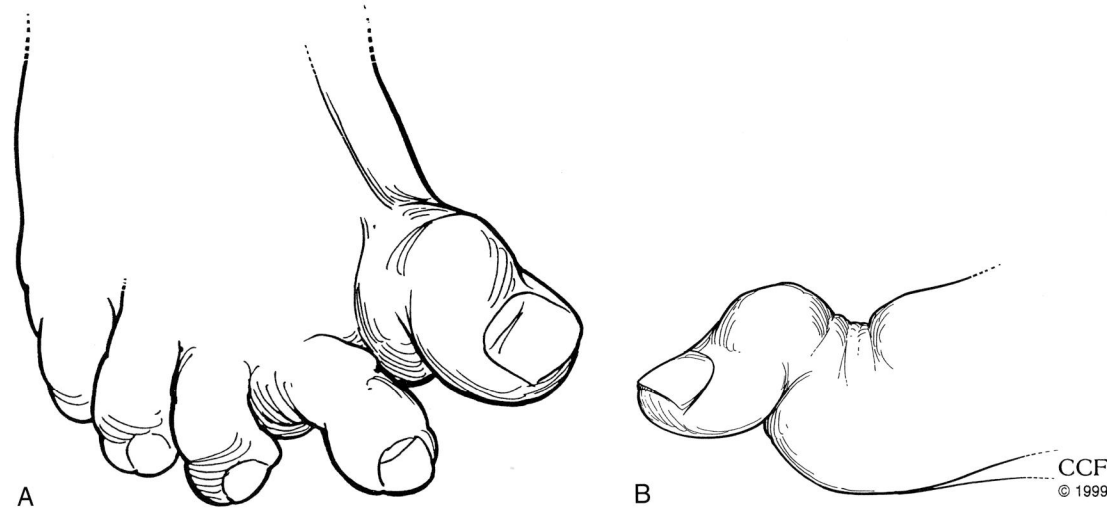

Fig. 12. Hallux varus deformity. *A*, Extension of metatarsophalangeal joint. *B*, Flexion of interphalangeal joint in sagittal plane. ©1999 CCF from Joe Kanasz.

allows the normal musculotendinous forces of the MTP joint to exert a varus deforming force. Although hallux varus may occur after any hallux valgus surgery including proximal and distal metatarsal osteotomies, it has been associated with the McBride procedure in which the fibular sesamoid is removed (Table 3).

Hallux varus may also be related to overly aggressive attempts to correct hallux valgus deformity. Excessive release of the lateral MTP joint structures, excessive tightening of the medial MTP joint capsule, excessive resection of the medial eminence, and overcorrection of the IMA are the most common causes of hallux varus. Although a single cause is unlikely to lead to hallux varus, a combination of these factors leads to a bony and soft-tissue imbalance,

which allows the normal musculotendinous forces of the MTP joint to exert a progressive varus-deforming force.

Hallux varus also may be caused by a number of conditions, including osteoarthritis, trauma, rheumatoid arthritis, psoriatic arthritis, poliomyelitis, Charcot-Marie-Tooth disease, congenital absence of the fibular sesamoid, and avascular necrosis of the metatarsal head.

PHYSICAL EXAMINATION

Common complaints in patients with hallux varus are unsightly deformity, pain, difficulty with shoe wear, weakness with push-off, instability of the MTP joint, metatarsalgia, and numbness of the toes. On physical examination, a noticeable gap usually is present between the first and second toes. In some patients, in addition to the varus posture of the toe, the MTP joint is extended and the IP joint is flexed ("snake in the grass" deformity). Medially, the extensor hallucis longus tendon may be shaped like a bowstring and taut. Plantar palpation of the MTP joint may reveal a medially displaced tibial sesamoid. With fixed deformities in which the toe is supinated in the coronal plane, a dorsal keratosis often is present at the IP joint.[7] The longer a patient has had the deformity, the more likely that range of motion of the MTP and IP joints will be restricted and the deformity will be painful.

RADIOGRAPHIC EXAMINATION

On radiographs, the MTP angle often is negative, and the IMA angle is small or negative. Medial subluxation of the tibial sesamoid, absence of the fibular sesamoid, degenerative changes of the MTP joint, and the amount of medial metatarsal head removed with medial eminence resection also can be evaluated on radiographs.

TREATMENT

The best treatment for acquired hallux varus, of course, is prevention. Initially, patients with hallux varus should be treated conservatively with splinting, taping, or footwear modifications. Anti-inflammatory medications, if not contraindicated, may decrease pain. Flexible hallux varus usu-

		Hallux Varus (%)
Study	**Procedure**	
Hansen (1974)	McBride	13
Thordarson and Leventen (1996)	Crescentic osteotomy plus modified McBride	10
Easley et al (1996)[10]	Distal soft-tissue procedure plus proximal crescentic osteotomy	10
	Distal soft-tissue procedure plus proximal chevron osteotomy	12
Mann and Coughlin (1993)[1]	Distal soft-tissue procedure plus fibular sesamoidectomy	8
Mann et al (1992)[7]	Distal soft-tissue procedure plus proximal metatarsal osteotomy	12
Pochatko et al (1994)	Lateral release plus chevron osteotomy	5
Peterson et al (1994)	Distal first metatarsal osteotomy plus adductor tendon release	2

TABLE 3. OCCURRENCE OF HALLUX VARUS AFTER SURGERY FOR HALLUX VALGUS

ally is symptomatic only when it is severe (more than 25 degrees), because the hallux impinges against the shoe. Fixed hallux varus is symptomatic when moderate or severe (more than 10 degrees), especially when it is associated with sagittal plane deformities of MTP extension and IP flexion. The radiographic deformity may not correlate with the clinical deformity, and many patients are able to tolerate even relatively severe deformities with footwear and activity modifications.[29]

Early recognition of the deformity is important. If hallux varus is recognized early after a soft-tissue procedure for hallux valgus correction, weekly dressings and tapings of the hallux in a valgus position of 15 degrees may correct the deformity; however, treatment must begin within the first 4 to 6 weeks and continue for 3 months.[2] If the deformity is not recognized or treated for 2 months or longer after surgery, surgical correction usually is required.

To determine the appropriate procedure for correction of acquired hallux varus, both the IP and MTP joints must be evaluated in both the axial and sagittal planes, and deformities should be classified as either supple (passively correctable) or fixed (Table 4). Because degenerative joint disease of the MTP joint precludes all surgical management except for resection arthroplasty or arthrodesis, the foot must be evaluated clinically and radiographically for evidence of degenerative arthritis.[30]

Procedures to correct hallux varus include soft-tissue release and realignment, tendon transfers, metatarsal and proximal phalangeal osteotomies, resection and implant arthroplasties, and arthrodesis.

If a mild supple deformity is recognized early, soft-tissue release may be all that is necessary. However, soft-tissue release alone rarely is successful, and usually a bony procedure or tendon transfer is necessary.[31, 32] Regardless of

TABLE 5. SOFT-TISSUE RELEASE AND REALIGNMENT PROCEDURES FOR HALLUX VARUS

Study	Procedure
McBride (1935)	Lengthening of abductor tendon, reinforcement of lateral structures of MTP joint
Hawkins (1971)[27]	Medial V capsulotomy, mobilization of tibial sesamoid, transfer of abductor tendon deep to FHB through drill hole in proximal phalanx
Poehling and DeTorre (1982)	Transfer of EHL, IP joint fusion (modified Jones procedure)
Johnson and Spiegl (1984)	Transfer of EHL to plantar lateral aspect of proximal phalanx combined with IP joint fusion
Jahss (1991)	Transfer of free tendon graft using plantaris, peroneus tertius, or long toe extensor (if EHL is severely damaged)
Mann and Coughlin (1993)[1]	Transfer portion of EHL to proximal phalanx without IP fusion
Tourne et al (1995)	Release of abductor tendon insertion and reconstruction of "lateral ligament" of MTP joint with 1.5-mm elastic polyethylene terephthalate suture
Myerson & Komenda (1996)[32]	Transfer of EHB to metatarsal shaft
Richardson and Donley (1998)[2]	Medial capsulotomy in coronal plane, placement of sesamoids in proper position, skin closure only, Kirschner-wire stabilization of hallux in 10–15° valgus

what other surgical procedures are performed for correction of hallux varus, soft-tissue release is an essential first step to correct the balance of the tight medial deforming forces and the loose lateral capsular and musculotendinous structures. A number of techniques have been described for soft-tissue release and realignment (Table 5), with and without tendon transfer or tibial sesamoidectomy.

For hallux varus caused by overcorrection of the IMA by metatarsal osteotomy (metatarsal malunion), surgical options include (1) a second metatarsal osteotomy through the apex of the metatarsal deformity, with the addition of a tendon transfer if the varus deformity is not completely corrected; (2) a takedown of the osteotomy site and realignment of the metatarsal, along with medial capsule release and realignment; and (3) a reverse Akin procedure to correct the hallux varus through a lateral closing wedge or concentric osteotomy. When degenerative changes of the MTP joint are present or deformities of the MTP joint are fixed, a resection arthroplasty or arthrodesis is indicated.

HALLUX RIGIDUS

Hallux rigidus in adults is caused by progressive degenerative arthritis of the first MTP joint characterized by painful motion, especially dorsiflexion. A mechanical or biological insult to the articular surface is the usual initiating mechanism, resulting in bone formation about the dorsal, medial, and lateral metatarsal head and occasionally on the dorsal aspect of the proximal phalanx. Hallux rigidus in adolescents is characterized by osteochondritis dissecans–like changes in the articular cartilage.

TABLE 4. GENERAL GUIDELINES FOR OPERATIVE TREATMENT OF HALLUX VARUS

	Deformity	
Deformity	**Degenerative Changes or Fixed Deformity MTP Joint**	**Supple Deformity MTP Joint**
Fixed Deformity IP Joint	MTP joint fusion or resection arthroplasty*	EHL transfer, IP joint fusion
Supple Deformity IP Joint	MTP joint fusion or resection arthroplasty*	Mild or short duration: correction dressing and splinting program or soft-tissue realignment procedure. Moderate or severe with longer duration: split EHL transfer without IP fusion, EHL transfer with IP joint fusion.

MTP, metatarsophalangeal; IP, interphalangeal; EHL, extensor hallucis longus.
* A soft-tissue realignment procedure usually is necessary before these corrective procedures.

PHYSICAL AND RADIOGRAPHIC EXAMINATION

Pain with activity and footwear is the most common complaint. Physical examination findings include a painful dorsal prominence over the metatarsal head (usually lateral), increased bulk around the MTP joint, and limited dorsiflexion. Arthritic changes, such as squaring-off of the MTP joint, sclerosis, osteophyte formation, and cyst formation, are visible on radiographs. Patients complain of dorsal pain with extremes of both dorsiflexion and plantar flexion of the MTP joint.

TREATMENT

Nonoperative treatment can include the use of a wide toe-box shoe to accommodate the enlarged joint, a rigid sole with a rocker or roller-bottom, a full-length carbon fiber insert to limit first MTP motion, and nonsteroidal anti-inflammatory medications. Intra-articular steroid injection may provide temporary relief of pain, but this should be used carefully, because repeated injections can accelerate the degenerative process. Surgery is indicated if symptoms become disabling.

Surgical options include cheilectomy,[33–36] osteotomy,[37] arthrodesis,[38] and resection arthroplasty. Cheilectomy (Fig. 13) is indicated for patients with mild to moderate arthrosis; approximately 70% of patients have satisfactory results at 5-year follow-up. Generally, all the osteophytes around the metatarsal head are removed to allow approximately 70 degrees of dorsiflexion at surgery. If this amount of dorsiflexion cannot be obtained after cheilectomy, dorsiflexion osteotomy of the proximal phalanx can be added. Mann and Clanton[35] recommended removal of 20% to 30% of the dorsal metatarsal head. For severe arthritis, MTP joint arthrodesis can reliably relieve pain but at the expense of motion.[38] Resection arthroplasty may be appropriate for patients with low functional demands, but instability after this procedure can result in transfer metatarsalgia.

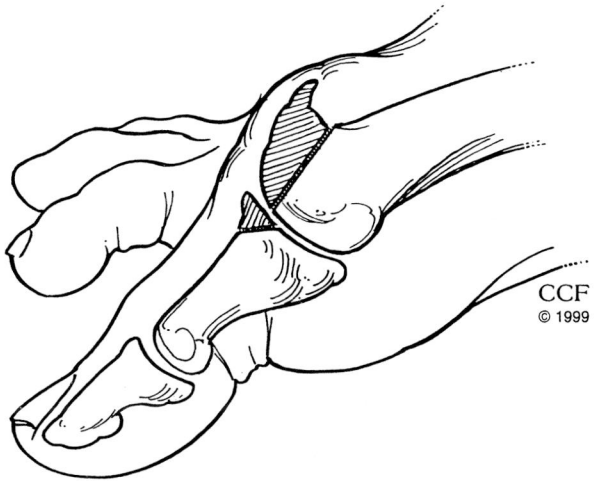

Fig. 13. Line of resection of dorsal cheilectomy and removal of osteophyte from dorsal proximal phalanx. ©1999 CCF from Joe Kanasz.

SESAMOID PROBLEMS

Although these small bones may seem inconsequential, when they are injured they can cause disabling pain. The sesamoids can be injured by acute trauma, such as forced dorsiflexion or a fall from a height, and activities such as racket sports, football, soccer, basketball, volleyball, running, and sprinting can result in overuse injury from repetitive stress. Arthritic inflammation, chondromalacia, flexor hallucis brevis tendinitis, osteochondritis dissecans, and fracture must be considered when there is persistent pain in the first MTP joint.[39, 40]

ANATOMY

The two sesamoids are embedded in the tendons of the short flexor of the great toe and are held together by the intersesamoid ligament and the plantar plate, which inserts on the base of the proximal phalanx of the hallux. The medial (tibial) sesamoid, which usually is larger than the lateral (fibular sesamoid) rests in the medial facet (sulcus) of the first metatarsal head and is more impacted by weightbearing than the lateral sesamoid, which rests in the lateral facet. The hallucal sesamoids function to absorb weightbearing pressure, reduce friction, and protect tendons when they are vulnerable. They are important to the dynamic function of the great toe and act as a fulcrum to increase the mechanical force of the flexor hallucis brevis and longus tendons.

PHYSICAL EXAMINATION

Sesamoid disorders are characterized by localized pain beneath the first metatarsal head during weightbearing. Physical examination demonstrates tenderness to palpation and restriction of motion because of pain. Swelling, diminished strength in plantar flexion, and gradual loss of active and passive dorsiflexion, as well as reactive synovitis of the first MTP joint, may be present. Sesamoid-related pain must be differentiated from tenosynovitis of the flexor hallucis longus tendon.

RADIOGRAPHIC EXAMINATION

Anteroposterior and medial and lateral oblique radiographic views are more helpful than the standard lateral view of the foot. An axial sesamoid view should be obtained if a pathological condition of the sesamoid is suspected. Radiographs can help identify acute fractures, whose sharp, irregular borders differ from the smooth cortical edge of bipartite sesamoids. Bipartite medial sesamoid is much more frequent than bipartite lateral sesamoid.[41] If radiographs are normal, a bone scan may be helpful to identify stress fracture; a marked difference in uptake between the sesamoids of one foot compared with the other is significant.[42] Magnetic resonance imaging can be helpful if osteomyelitis is suspected.[43]

TREATMENT

Whether the problem is sesamoiditis (acute or chronic inflammation), osteochondrosis, stress fracture, or acute fracture, the initial treatment is conservative. Sesamoiditis may respond to nonsteroidal anti-inflammatory medication or intra-articular steroid injection. For an acute or stress fracture, limiting the range of motion of the MTP joint with taping and using a metatarsal pad and a stiff-soled shoe is often sufficient, although it may take many months for discomfort to subside.

Surgical treatment for painful sesamoid disorders that do not respond to conservative treatment involves partial or complete resection of one or both sesamoids. Excision of both sesamoids should be avoided unless absolutely necessary, because hallux valgus or cock-up deformity of the toe may result. (Occasionally, a young adult man may require resection of both sesamoids because of unrelenting symptoms of inflammatory arthritis.) The medial sesamoid is excised through an inferomedial incision; care is taken to protect the sensory branch of the medial plantar nerve. The lateral sesamoid usually is excised through a plantar incision just lateral to the lateral sesamoid, although a dorsolateral first interspace incision can be used.

Because total sesamoidectomy produces a mechanical defect in the flexor hallucis brevis muscle tendon unit by reducing this muscle's flexion moment arm at the MTP

joint,[44] some authors recommended consideration of partial excision. Two-thirds of either sesamoid can be removed without disturbing the ligamentous attachments, and this seems to relieve pain just as well as total sesamoidectomy.[2]

If an intractable plantar keratosis develops beneath the medial sesamoid, sesamoid shaving is an alternative to sesamoid excision if there is normal mobility of the first metatarsal. Mann and Wapner[45] suggested that shaving is superior to excision because postoperative morbidity is less. They described removing the plantar half of the sesamoid and smoothing the sharp edges with a rongeur.

Autologous bone grafting for nonunion of the sesamoid also may be an alternative to sesamoid excision in selected patients (usually high-performance athletes).[46]

ACKNOWLEDGMENT

We gratefully acknowledge the assistance from Kay Daugherty, editor, and Joe Kanasz, artist, in the preparation of this chapter.

REFERENCES

1. Mann RA, Coughlin MJ: Adult hallux valgus. In Mann RA Coughlin MJ (eds): Surgery of the Foot and Ankle. St. Louis, MO, Mosby Year-Book, 1993, 6th ed, p 167.

2. Richardson EG, Donley BG: Disorders of the hallux. In Canale ST (ed): Campbell's Operative Orthopaedics. St. Louis, MO, Mosby-Year Book, 1998, 9th eds p 1621.

3. Mann RA: Decision making in bunion surgery. AAOS Instr Course Lect 1990; 40:3.

4. Schneider W, Knahr K: Metatarsophalangeal and intermetatarsal angle: Different values and interpretation of postoperative results dependent on the technique of measurement. Foot Ankle Int 1998; 19: 532.

5. Mann RA: Disorders of the first metatarsophalangeal joint. J in Assoc Orthop Surg 1995; 3:34.

6. Dreeben S, Mann RA: Advanced hallux valgus deformity: Long-term results utilizing the distal soft tissue procedure and proximal metatarsal osteotomy. Foot Ankle Int 1996; 17:142.

7. Mann RA, Rudicel S, Graves SC: Repair of hallux valgus with a distal soft-tissue procedure and proximal metatarsal osteotomy. J Bone Joint Surg Am 1992; 74:124.

8. Thordarson DB, Leventen EO: Hallux valgus correction with proximal metatarsal osteotomy: Two-year follow-up. Foot Ankle 1992; 12:321.

9. Donnelly RE, Saltzman CL, Kile T, et al: Modified chevron osteotomy for hallux valgus. Foot Ankle 1994; 15:642.

10. Easley ME, Kiebzak GM, Davis WH, et al: Prospective, randomized comparison of proximal crescentic and proximal chevron osteotomies for correction of hallux varus deformity. Foot Ankle 1996; 17:1.

11. Johnson JE, Clanton TO, Baxter DE, et al: Comparison of chevron osteotomy and modified McBride bunionectomy for correction of mild to moderate hallux valgus deformity. Foot Ankle 1991; 12:61.

12. Mann RA, Donatto KC: The chevron osteotomy: A clinical and radiographic analysis. Foot Ankle Int 1997; 18:255.

13. Markbreiter LA, Thompson FM: Proximal metatarsal osteotomy in hallux valgus correction: A comparison of crescentic and chevron procedures. Foot Ankle Int 1997; 18:71.

14. Sammarco GJ, Brainard BJ, Sammarco VJ: Bunion correction using proximal chevron osteotomy. Foot Ankle 1993; 14:8.

15. Beskin JL: Akin's phalangeal osteotomy for bunion repair. In Myerson M (ed): Current Therapy in Foot and Ankle Surgery. St. Louis, MO, Mosby-Year Book, 1993, p 54.

16. Mitchell LA, Baxter DE: A chevron-Akin double osteotomy for correction of hallux valgus. Foot Ankle 1991; 12:7.

17. Coughlin MJ: Arthrodesis of the first metatarsophalangeal joint. Orthop Rev 1990; 19: 177.

18. Myerson M, Allon S, McGarvey W: Metatarsocuneiform arthrodesis for management of hallux valgus and metatarsus primus varus. Foot Ankle 1992; 13:107.

19. Coughlin MJ: Evaluation and treatment of juvenile hallux valgus. Contemp Orthop 1990; 21:169.

20. Scranton PE, Zuckerman JD: Bunion surgery in adolescents: Results of surgical treatment. J Pediatr Orthop 1984; 4:39.

21. Canale PB, Aronsson DD, Lamont RL, et al: The Mitchell procedure for the treatment of adolescent hallux valgus. J Bone Joint Surg Am 1993; 75:1610.

22. Peterson HA, Newman SR: Adolescent bunion deformity treated with double osteotomy and longitudinal pin fixation of the first ray. J Pediatr Orthop 1993; 13: 80.

23. Coughlin MJ: Hallux valgus. Instr Course Lect 1997; 46:357.

24. Davies MS, Parker BC: Idiopathic hallux varus. Foot Ankle 1995; 16:210.

25. Donley BG: Acquired hallux varus. Foot Ankle Int 1997; 18:586.

26. Granberry WM, Hickey CH: Idiopathic adult hallux varus. Foot Ankle 1994; 15: 197.

27. Hawkins FB: Acquired hallux varus: Cause, prevention and correction. Clin Orthop 1971; 76:169.

28. Johnson KA, Saltzman CL, Frisca DA: Hallux varus. In Gould JS (ed): Operative Foot Surgery. Philadelphia, WB Saunders, 1994, p 28.

29. Trnka JH, Zehl R, Hunderford M, et al: Acquired hallux varus and clinical tolerability. Foot Ankle Int 1997; 18:593.

30. Skalley TC, Myerson MS: The operative treatment of acquired hallux varus. Clin Orthop 1994; 306:183.

31. Clark WD: Abductor hallucis tendon transfer for hallux varus. J Foot Surg 1984; 23:146.

32. Myerson MS, Komenda GA: Results of hallux varus correction using an extensor hallucis brevis tenodesis. Foot Ankle 1996; 17:21.

33. Geldwert JJ, Rock GD, McGrath MP, et al: Cheilectomy: Still a useful technique for grade I and grade II hallux limitus/rigidus. J Foot Surg 1992; 31:154.

34. Hattrup SJ, Johnson KA: Subjective results of hallux rigidus following treatment with cheilectomy. Clin Orthop 1988; 226: 182.

35. Mann RA, Clanton TO: Hallux rigidus: Treatment by cheilectomy. J Bone Joint Surg Am 1988; 70:400.

36. Pfeffer GB: Cheilectomy. In Thompson RC (ed): The Foot and Ankle: Master Techniques in Orthopaedic Surgery. New York, Raven Press, 1994, p 119.

37. Citron N, Neil M: Dorsal wedge osteotomy of the proximal phalanx for hallux rigidus: Long-term results. J Bone Joint Surg Br 1987; 69:835.

38. O'Doherty DP, Lowrie IG, Magnussen PA, et al: Management of the painful first

metatarsophalangeal joint in the older patient. J Bone Joint Surg Br 1990; 72:839.

39. Coughlin MJ: Sesamoid pain: Causes and surgical treatment. Instr Course Lect 1990; 39:23.

40. Taylor JA, Sartoris DJ, Huang GS, et al: Painful conditions affecting the first metatarsal sesamoid bones. Radiographics 1993; 13:817.

41. Frankel JP, Harrington J: Symptomatic bi-partite sesamoids. J Foot Surg 1990; 29: 318.

42. Chism R, Peyser A, Milgrom C: Bone scintigraphy in the assessment of the hallucal sesamoids. Foot Ankle Int 1995; 16: 291.

43. Rahn KA, Jacobson FS: Pseudomonas osteomyelitis of the metatarsal sesamoid bones. Am J Orthop 1997; 26:365.

44. Aper RL, Saltzman CL, Brown TD: The effect of hallux sesamoid excision on the flexor hallucis longus moment arm. Clin Orthop 1996; 325:209.

45. Mann RA, Wapner KL: Tibial sesamoid shaving for treatment of intractable plantar keratosis. Foot Ankle 1992; 13:196.

46. Anderson RB, McBryde AM Jr: Autogenous bone grafting of hallux sesamoid nonunions. Foot Ankle Int 1997; 18:293.

section 11
chapter 10

PROBLEMS OF THE LESSER TOES

Sylvia Resch

Summary

- Minor toe operations have traditionally been left to the less experienced surgeon and given low priority on the operation room lists, but this has changed with the development of foot surgery as a subspecialty.
- The function of the lesser toes is balance and propulsion. Together with the metatarsals they are a part of the body's shock absorption system.
- Toe deformity is a great problem for a large number of patients and is caused by normal shoe wearing; systemic diseases such as rheumatoid arthritis, diabetes, and neurological disorders; infection; and trauma.
- Treatment should be aimed at restoring toe function and making normal shoe wearing possible.
- There is a high incidence rate of medicolegal claims concerning toes.[1]

Whereas the first ray of the foot, including the hallux, has been the subject of intense interest for many decades, the lesser toes and their metatarsals have been thought to be less important, with rather little function. Indeed, when the foot is studied in its non-weightbearing state, one might well conclude that lesser toe function is quite limited and thus not as important. The function of the lesser toes becomes obvious on standing and in propulsion. Their purpose is to stabilize the foot firmly on the ground with the help of the muscles acting on the toes, thus achieving balance, and to maintain this balance on push-off. It has been shown that this function is compromised in patients with diabetes,[2, 3] thus aggravating the amount of weight the ball of the foot must endure during walking.

As muscle balance is such an intrinsic part of the function of the lesser toes, it can be easily understood that the shod foot gives rise to deformity through inhibition of normal muscle action. The deformities then lead to problems wearing normal shoes, which can be of great importance to the patient.

HISTORICAL REVIEW

The Pobble Operation, so called after Edward Lear's poem about the pobble who had no toes,[4] has been used in the past to eliminate problems with the toes by simply amputating them. These operations were often considered minor and left to inexperienced surgeons. Recent biomechanical studies show that the toes are essential for good balance and propulsion.[5] With the advent of foot surgery as a subspecialty, more interest has been shown in the toes. Instead of simple and more destructive phalangectomies, foot surgeons now recommend ligament and tendon transfers. A great deal of interest has been focused on the problems of the lesser toes, most often the second toe.[6, 7]

EPIDEMIOLOGY

Problems of the lesser toes most often concern deformity. The amount of deformity is correlated to gender (female), age, and the use of shoes.[8] It is estimated that 50% of women older than 60 years will have some deformity of the toes.[9] Deformity of the lesser toes is very common in patients with rheumatoid arthritis, and indeed can be the first sign of the disease. In arteriosclerosis, the lesser toes are often the first to become ischemic. The majority of foot ulcers are found on the toes, usually because of trauma associated with an ill-fitting shoe.[10] Some conditions are hereditary and can be found in childhood, such as curly toes.

PATHOGENESIS

DEFORMITY

The function of the lesser toes depends on the delicate balance in the supportive structures, which allow stability and propulsion in final push-off. As in the fingers, the plantar and dorsal tendons and the extrinsic and intrinsic muscles surround the joints of the toe to place it in position for push-off. When the muscles are perfectly balanced, the toes maintain their natural positions. Acquired deformities are common among shod people. When the foot is confined in a shoe, the function of the toes is partially inhibited. This eventually leads to relative atrophy of primarily the intrinsic foot muscles—the lumbricals, the interossei, and the short flexors and extensors—with deformity as a result. Undoubtedly, there is a certain hereditary structure in the musculature of the foot, which could explain why there is a familial predisposition to deformity. It is worth noting that while shoes as such, regardless of style, lead to a tendency to structural changes in the toes, narrow shoes with too little room naturally exacerbate pain and discomfort, even if they are not to blame for the deformity. It has also been shown that female gender increases the tendency to deformity and is an independent factor, along with amount of time shoes have been worn.[8]

TRAUMA

Even in the parts of the world, now increasingly less common, where shoes are not worn, people cannot avoid foot and toe problems. Instead of acquired deformities, trauma and infection lead to pathology.[11] In shoe-wearing societies, trauma also plays a role in problems of the lesser toes. Turf toe is a well-known phenomenon, consisting of a distal contusion of a lesser toe, acquired through longitudinal trauma in the shoe. Aside from direct fractures of the toes, trauma also plays a role in the pathogenesis of lesser toe problems in the case of deformity after compartment syndrome. Prolonged increased compartment pressure of the calf muscles or the muscles of the foot lead to cavus foot and clawing of the lesser toes.

SYSTEMIC DISORDERS

The lesser toes can be affected by systemic disorders. Rheumatoid arthritis frequently debuts in the feet and may lead to swelling of the toes as well as instability of the metatarsophalangeal (MTP) joints leading to claw and hammer toes. Other forms of arthritis, such as gout and pyrophosphate deposits, are also found in the lesser toes.

Diabetes is a very serious contributor to pathological conditions in the lesser toes. Diabetic neuropathy affects the sensory nerves, the sympathetic nerves, and the muscular fibers. Thus diabetic neuropathy often leads to muscular atrophy, which results in cavus foot and clawing of the toes. Poor sympathetic innervation affects the ability of the foot to sweat and changes the effect of friction on the skin. Sensory neuropathy allows trauma from the shoes and floor to go unnoticed by the patient, often leading to ulcers on the toes. The combination of a numb foot with deformity in standard shoes is often implicated in diabetic foot ulcers. Approximately 2% to 8% of diabetic patients with neuropathy will develop osteopathy (osteoarthropathy, Charcot's foot). This can affect all parts of the foot, including the toes, but is an unusual cause of deformity.

CONGENITAL OR PEDIATRIC DEFORMITIES

Congenital disorders such as clubfoot can lead to problems of the lesser toes. Curly toes, a benign flexion of the toes, is congenital, as are constriction bands and digiti quinti varus.

NONSPECIFIC ARTHRITIS

A condition receiving more attention recently is instability of the second toe, also called crossover toe. This is thought to be the result of a nonspecific arthritis of the second MTP joint.

IATROGENIC CONDITIONS

Multiple operations are common in attempts to correct structural deformities of the toes. Any adjustment in one toe will affect the function of all the other toes. This can be the result of pressure (interdigital clavus), changes in the distribution of weightbearing because of changes in length, and changes in the position of toes adjacent to the one operated on. With each additional operation to the foot, the results become more and more unpredictable.

CLINICAL FEATURES

For practical purposes, the pathology of the lesser toes can be divided into deformities of the toes themselves, as well as metatarsalgia due to structural changes in the foot; Morton's toe, which includes both interdigital neuroma and nonspecific arthritis of the MTP joint; skin conditions, including corns and keratoses; and nail problems.

DEFORMITY

Lesser-toe deformities are caused by various combinations of flexion and extension contractures of the proximal interphalangeal (PIP) and distal interphalangeal (DIP) joints (Fig. 1). The common terminology is explained in the figure. All of these deformities are initially stable in the MTP joint. For various reasons, such as arthritis, an instability may develop in the MTP joint, which in severe cases can cause subluxation of the joint. Differentiating between a common hammer toe deformity and one with additional subluxation of the MTP joint is important, since treatment is not the same.

A special case of MTP joint subluxation is crossover toe. This condition is generally found in the second toe. Because of a nonspecific arthritis of the MTP joint, the lateral supporting structures of the joint become lax and allow the toe to cross over the big toe. This is a very difficult situation to remedy. Various procedures have been described (see Management).[12–14]

The deformed toes' inability to exert pressure on push-off, thus transferring the weight to the metatarsal heads, leads in many cases to very painful metatarsalgia. Among painful foot conditions, this one rated highest in Visual Analog Scale score for pain.[15] Atrophy of the plantar fat pad, found in old age and rheumatoid arthritis, also leads to abnormal pressure on the metatarsal heads, leading to plantar keratosis and severe pain on weightbearing.

MORTON'S NEUROMA

Interdigital nerve entrapment in the foot is most commonly found in the interdigital space between the second and third and the third and fourth metatarsal heads.[16] The patient presents with a burning, shooting pain at this location, often with radiation to the corresponding lesser toes. The pain can be severe and is always exacerbated by simultaneous weightbearing and shoe wearing. The patient must stand still and often removes the shoe and massages the foot in some way. Typically the pain localization is diffuse in the beginning, becoming more well localized as the condition progresses. If the pain is more pronounced in

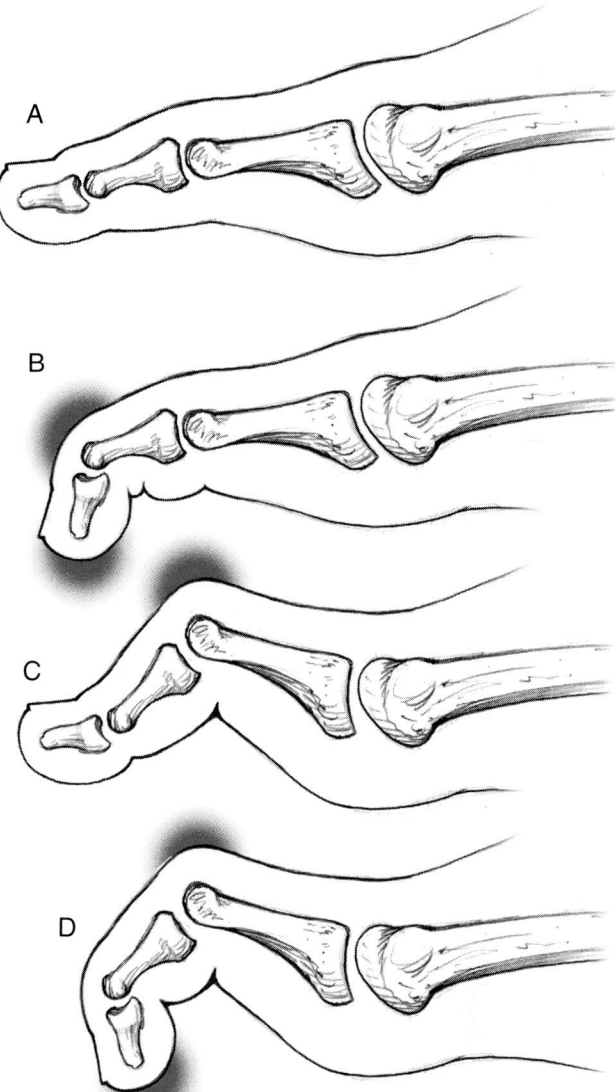

Fig. 1. Common deformities of the lesser toes. Areas that tend to develop corns are indicated. *A,* normal toe; *B,* mallet toe; *C,* hammer toe; *D,* claw toe.

barefoot walking, this speaks against Morton's neuroma, indicating metatarsalgia. Neuromas in two adjacent interdigital spaces are not uncommon. The pathogenesis is thought to be a combination of the bursa between the metatarsal heads and the tight intermetatarsal ligament (Fig. 2). The exact location of the bursa has been discussed, and locations both dorsal to and plantar to the neuroma have been described. The neuroma is histologically a traumatic neuroma, not a tumor.[17] Although ultrasonography, magnetic resonance imaging, and injection of local anesthetic have been used to diagnose the condition, most cases can be diagnosed by clinical history and the typical, often radiating pain described by the patient when the interdigital space is compressed in a dorsoplantar and mediolateral fashion simultaneously. Feeling a click during this maneuver (Mulder's click) strengthens the diagnosis.[18] Corticosteroids can be used successfully at an early stage, but treatment is generally operative (see Management).

SKIN PROBLEMS

The skin of the foot must withstand a great deal of pressure, especially shear forces, often confined in a moist environment. This leads to numerous skin problems. Barefoot walkers have problems with infections and trauma.

Hard corns (Fig. 3) are hyperkeratotic lesions over bony prominences, commonly over the dorsal aspect of the PIP joints, especially in conjunction with toe deformity. These can be extremely painful and can develop a bursa, which can become inflamed or infected. Only reduction of pressure can reduce the corn. This can be achieved by reducing external pressure, as by shoe modification, or internal pressure, by excision of the underlying bony prominence. Simple excision of the corn is only a temporary procedure (see Management).

Interdigital clavus, or soft corn, is the development of pressure changes in the skin between the toes when the condyles of adjacent toes lie too close together, especially when confined in a shoe. The moisture between the toes

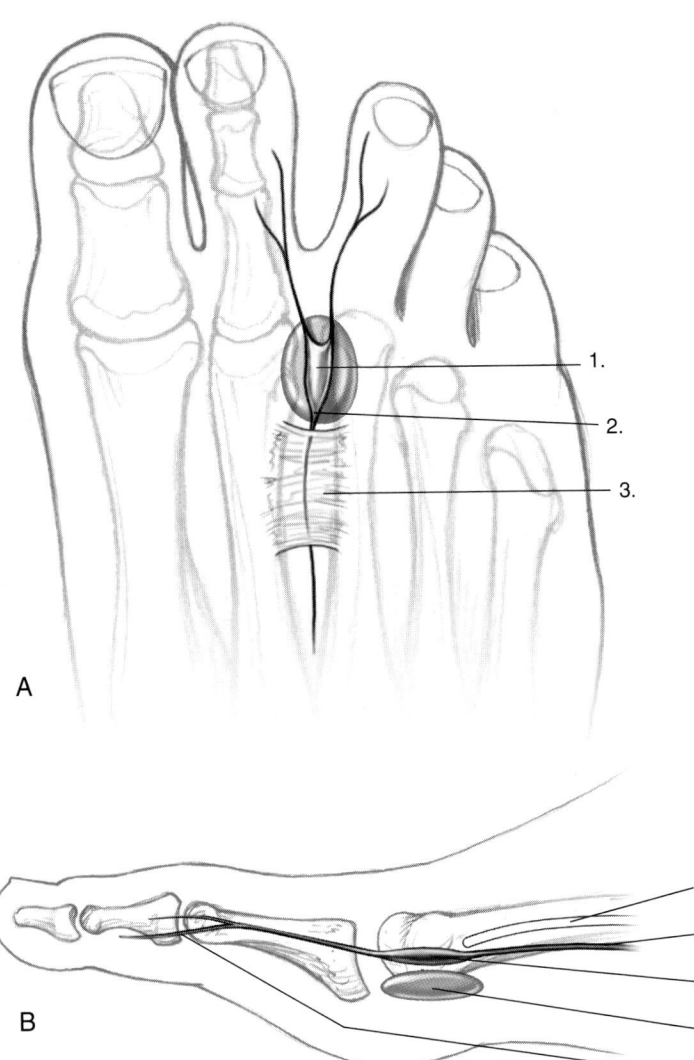

A

B

Fig. 2. Pathogenesis of Morton's neuroma. The relationship between the intermetatarsal ligament, the intermetatarsal bursa, and the nerve bifurcation shows how a traumatic neuroma might result if the bursa is enlarged. *A*, Intermetatarsal bursa (1), Morton's neuroma (2), intermetatarsal ligament (3). *B*, Intermetatarsal ligament (1), intermetatarsal portion of the nerve (2), neuroma (3), intermetatarsal bursa (4), digital nerve branch (5).

softens the hyperkeratotic layer. In some patients, a sinus can develop to the web space, which can result in major plantar abscesses in diabetic patients. Treatment principles are the same as for hard corns.

Intractable plantar keratosis leading to metatarsalgia is a major problem for many patients. This is due to insufficiency of the supporting structures of the forefoot, which leads to increased pressure under the metatarsal heads on weightbearing. Common deformities such as hallux valgus contribute by reducing the amount of weightbearing under the first ray. A hyperkeratotic lesion forms. It can develop to the extent that it produces the effect of a foreign body. Conservative treatment to reduce the amount of hyperkeratotic tissue will help, but definitive treatment must include redistribution of weight under the forefoot and is not always easily solved.

FOOT ULCERS IN SYSTEMIC DISEASE

Although the biomechanical mechanisms are the same as in the development of corns and hyperkeratosis, the addition of ischemia in *arteriosclerotic* and *diabetic* patients radi-

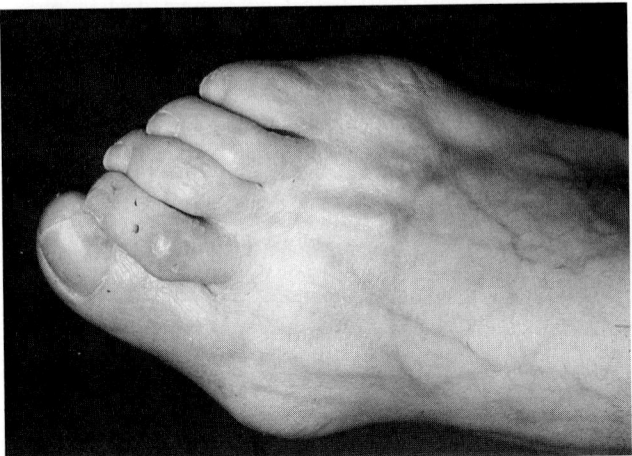

Fig. 3. Hard corn. A typical hard corn located over the dorsal PIP joint in hammer toe.

cally affects the approach to the problem of foot ulcers. In addition, patients with diabetes of a duration of more than 10 years have neuropathy in practically all cases, which also affects diagnosis, prognosis, and treatment. In diabetic patients, foot ulcers are often asymptomatic until they are well developed, since the patient has poor sensibility. It is vital that **all** diabetic patients have their feet checked regularly and that they be taught to do this themselves **every day**. Ischemic nondiabetic patients often have severe pain, leading to faster discovery of the lesions. A special form of hyperkeratotic plantar lesion in diabetic neuropathy, known as mal perforans ulcer, deserves special mention (Fig. 4). These lesions develop in areas under pressure in neuropathic feet. Since the neuropathy is sensory, the patient does not feel anything. The sympathetic aspects of the neuropathy lead to decreased sweating, which increases the shear pressure. A sinus develops between the skin and the bony prominence and fills with fluid. Eventually, the sinus breaks through, often presenting with a 1- to 2-mm hole in the middle of a hyperkeratotic lesion. In fact, the ulcer is often 20 to 30 mm in diameter under the skin. Treatment must keep this in mind (see Management).

Interdigital corns also take on quite other proportions in diabetic patients. The development of infection in the corns is not uncommon and can have disastrous consequences. As mentioned earlier, web space infections can result. These are often the first stages of abscess formation that can affect the whole foot. Although such infections can be treated operatively and medically, almost half lead to some form of amputation.[19]

In the clinical assessment of the patient with systemic disease, the distal circulation must always be kept in mind before plans are made for surgery.

NAILS

Ingrown toenail, or unguis incarnatus (onychocryptosis), is often found in youngsters, sometimes in diabetic patients. It is an inflammatory process in the nail fold, usually of the large toe, but sometimes found in the other toes. Often, but not always, both nail folds are affected. The shape of the nail bed, environmental conditions such as humidity, pressure from the shoe, and to some extent improper trimming of the nail cause the condition. When the inflamma-

tion becomes infected, it is very painful, inhibiting the youngster from sports and so on. In the beginning, conservative management with warm soaks, introduction of a mesh of some kind under the inflamed corner, open shoes, and modification of activity can give good results. If the condition is persistent, or infection ensues, operative management may be necessary.

Fungal infections (onychomycosis) are quite common and rarely symptomatic. The patient finds the nails unsightly and may have problems with snagging of hosiery. Clinical diagnosis is often easy, but at times a culture sample taken at the most proximal part of the infected nail may lead to diagnosis, although these can be negative even in the presence of fungus. Treatment has been difficult, leading to recurrence in a large proportion of cases, even when such a drastic measure as avulsion of the entire nail has been undertaken. Recently, the systemic antimycotic agent terbinafine was introduced. Treatment for 3 months is required and has been successful in 70% of cases. It is expensive, however, and carries potential of side effects.

Subungual exostosis, although not a nail condition, usually presents as a nail problem. The exostosis may develop post-traumatically or be an osteochondroma of the distal phalanx. This condition is most common in the big toe and presents as a painful nail, which can be deformed. Radiographs are diagnostic and operation with exision of the exostosis is recommended.

Malignant melanoma can develop under the nails and should not be forgotten as a differential diagnosis to hematoma under the nails, turf toe, and other discolorations.

INVESTIGATIONS

CLINICAL EVALUATION

An adequate clinical evaluation is still the mainstay of investigation. The foot must be examined both in the relaxed state and on weightbearing. It is important to find the precise location of pain and tenderness, or to describe it as diffuse if such is the case. Pain radiation should be noted. The general appearance of the foot and visible deformities are described. Any lesions or pressure marks attributable to shoes should be noted. As in all examinations of the extremities, peripheral circulation should be assessed by pal-

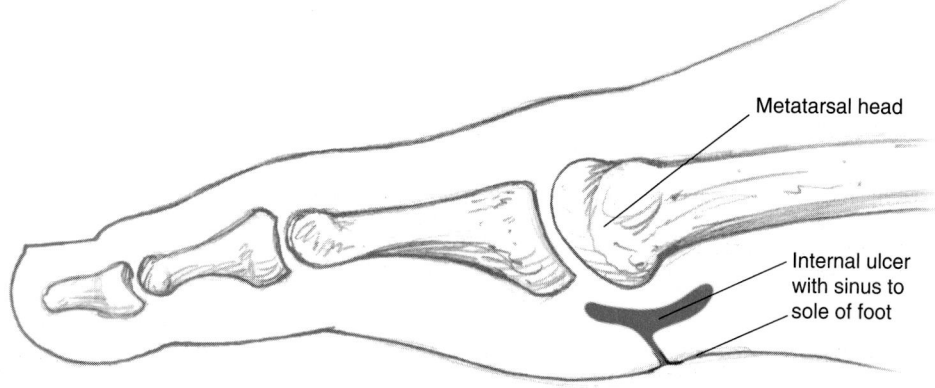

Fig. 4. Mal perforans ulcer. Mal perforans ulcer is produced by shear forces under the metatarsal head. A small sinus is the first manifestation of a larger subcutaneous ulcer.

Metatarsal head

Internal ulcer with sinus to sole of foot

pation of the distal arteries (posterior tibial artery, anterior tibial artery, and dorsal pedal artery), temperature evaluation, and capillary refilling. This is obviously of special importance in patients with suspected arteriosclerosis or diabetes. Adequate peripheral circulation is vital when surgery is being considered.

A neurological evaluation should be done. The use of the 5.07 size Semmes-Weinstein monofilament (0.54 mm) has been shown to be a good screen for diabetic neuropathy. In addition, the absence of hair on the toes and muscular atrophy may disclose neuropathy.

Since rheumatoid arthritis often manifests in the small joints of the feet, signs of swelling and inflammation in the joints should be looked for.

It is important to have the patient walk barefoot over the floor. It is then possible to evaluate whether the lesser toes are used in propulsion and balance.

An inspection of the patient's shoes may give a clue as to the cause of certain deformities and of ulcers in diabetic patients.

IMAGING

Plain radiographs are usually essential. They give valuable hints as to the underlying cause for deformity, such as post-traumatic changes, subungual exostosis, and arthritic changes with cysts. They are also necessary when planning surgery for deformities that show dorsal subluxation in the MTP joints, which affect the type of surgery recommended. In diabetic and other neuropathic feet, plain radiographs are essential. More than one foreign body has been found to explain symptoms. Indeed, it is not unusual for such a finding to be the first indicator of diabetes. Plain radiographs should be used liberally.

Angiography is used when assessing an ischemic foot prior to possible reconstructive vascular surgery.

Magnetic resonance imaging has been shown to be useful in the evaluation of the lesser toes. Its main use is in soft-tissue diagnosis, such as in Morton's neuroma (Fig. 5).[20] When the clinical diagnosis of Morton's neuroma is unclear, or when it is difficult to establish which web space

houses the neuroma, magnetic resonance imaging can be of use. Infections in diabetic patients can also benefit from such an evaluation to rule out deep abscesses.

Isotope scanning can be used at times. It can show a stress fracture in a metatarsal bone as a differential diagnosis to Morton's neuroma.

Computed tomography, although seldom used for conditions of the lesser toes, has its place in the evaluation of the forefoot. Declination of the metatarsal heads can be identified and form a differential diagnosis to Morton's neuroma.

Ultrasonography has been used to aid in the diagnosis of Morton's neuroma [20] and in locating foreign bodies.

FOOT PRESSURE MEASUREMENT

Modern, office-based computerized systems of recording pressure under the foot are now available. Although these systems leave much to be desired for scientific purposes, they offer a way of making the activity under the foot visible to the patient and the doctor. It has been shown, for example, that patients with neuropathic diabetes use their small toes very little during gait. One often sees areas of relatively increased pressure under the metatarsal heads. Although absolute values for destructive pressures vary from system to system, sequential foot prints in a single patient can give some idea of the pathology and effectiveness of treatment. These systems are not necessary in day-to-day practice.

DISTAL BLOOD PRESSURE

Distal pressure measurement by Doppler ultrasonography is an essential part of every investigation if there is the slightest suspicion of circulatory disturbance. We know that a distal pressure of the ankle of less than 70 mm Hg is often not compatible with healing below the ankle. The measurements should be done both at the ankle and at the big toe. False high pressure can be found in extremely stiff arteries. Raising the foot and palpating the level above the heart at which one feels no pulse can give an indication of the actual blood pressure.

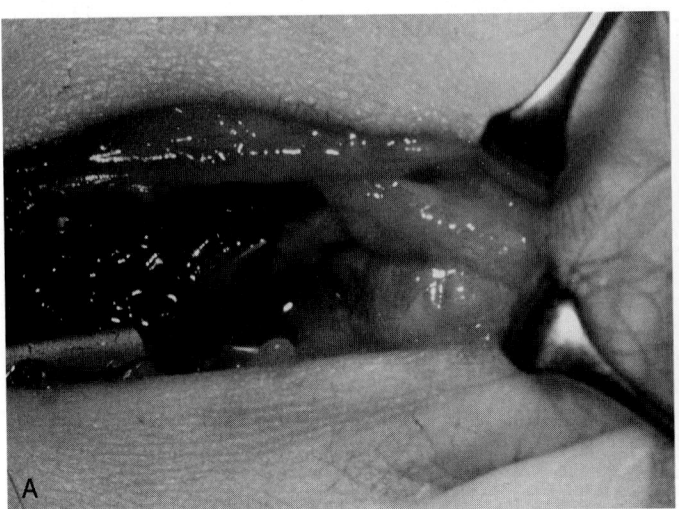 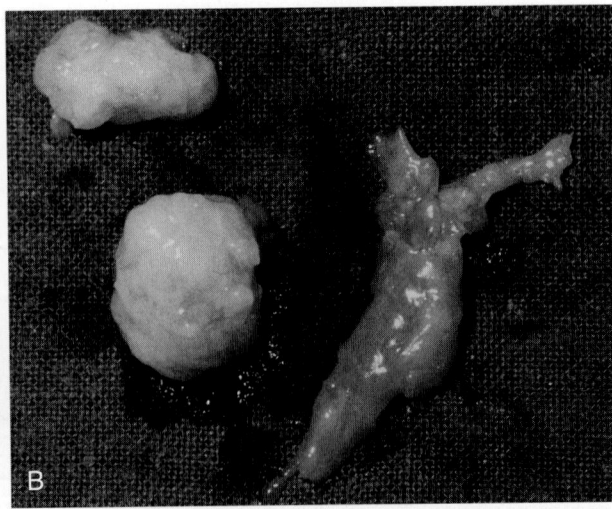

Fig. 5. Morton's neuroma. *A,* At surgery, the toes are pointing to the right. *B,* After removal, the neuroma is to the right, the bursa to the left, and fat tissue above.

LABORATORY WORK

Most ordinary deformities of the lesser toes do not require extensive laboratory work. When there is suspicion of a systemic disorder, laboratory tests pertaining to that disorder may be relevant. Rheumatoid arthritis and diabetes are the systemic disorders most commonly found in foot conditions. Bacterial culture may be necessary in treating infections, and fungal cultures may be required to motivate a patient to undergo 3 months of expensive antimycotic therapy.

TEST WITH LOCAL ANESTHETIC

An excellent test for Morton's neuroma is the test with local anesthetic, and it is especially useful when it is difficult to decide which web space is affected. One to 2 mL of local anesthetic agent is injected in the suspected web space between the metatarsal heads. The patient is asked to walk around for about 20 minutes. If the affected space has been injected, the pain will cease.

MANAGEMENT

As in many deformities and diseases of the foot, both a nonoperative and an operative approach can be used. Which is most appropriate for the particular patient depends on many factors: the severity of the disorder, the risk of complications, the age of the patient, the patient's sensitivity to esthetic aspects, and financial issues. It is important to remember that recovery after surgery to the foot is often prolonged, with weeks and even months of swelling and shoe problems being the rule rather than the exception.

NONOPERATIVE

Shoe adjustments are the obvious approach to problems of deformity that are mild, or in elderly patients in whom the risks associated with surgery are increased. It is usually wearing the shoe that causes pain and discomfort in patients with toe deformities such as hammer and claw toes. An extra-depth toe box or custom shoes can do a great deal to alleviate symptoms. The use of pads and straps may provide some comfort. In metatarsalgia, a rocker-bottom sole and special inserts can help alleviate symptoms. When the pain is due to Morton's neuroma, inserts tend to increase pain and discomfort, since the pressure of the metatarsal pad is right under the neuroma.

Routine foot care with paring of callus and proper trimming of nails is highly recommended for patients with diabetes and arteriosclerosis. In addition to increasing comfort for these patients, who often are poor candidates for surgery, regular attention to the feet leads to the discovery of lesions in time for curative measures.

If the foot conditions are caused by systemic disease, it is obviously necessary to regulate the underlying disease. No matter how good the foot care is and how adequate the surgery, a diabetic patient without proper metabolic control will not be definitely healed. Patients with rheumatoid arthritis need to be treated medically. Underlying causes for infections such as edema must be treated.

Most fractures and dislocations of the toes can be treated nonoperatively. Frank dislocations and severely angulated shaft fractures are reduced under local anesthesia. A fractured toe is then taped to the neighboring toe to give it some stability and decrease pain. Intra-articular fractures are generally left to heal without operative reduction, and a fibrous ankylosis will often result. Occasionally, it may be necessary to do a phalangectomy as for hammer toe or a fusion if symptoms persist. It is important to point out to the patient that the toe will be swollen and painful for quite some time, often 3 weeks or longer.

OPERATIVE TREATMENT

A bloodless field should be used whenever possible. For resection of the interdigital nerve in Morton's neuroma, a bloodless field is mandatory. Many foot operations bleed postoperatively. It is more comfortable for the patient to change the dressing after 3 days. I find that a fairly large number of wounds require up to 3 weeks to heal, and prefer to leave the sutures in for that long. Weightbearing should be allowed whenever possible. A special shoe with a firm sole that can be adjusted over the dressings can make it possible for the patient to walk. Putting some weight on the foot will compress the venous sinuses in the arch of the foot and help reduce postoperative edema. When not walking, patients should sit with the foot elevated.

Small Toe Deformity. Hammer toe, mallet toe, claw toe, and curly toe are examples. The choice of operative treatment depends on the contracture and amount of passive correction possible (Table 1).[4]

Flexible Deformity. If the deformity is mild and correctable, a *soft-tissue procedure* can be used. This applies also to curly toe deformity, a mallet toe deformity in children. A flexor tenotomy can be performed through a mid-lateral incision at the level of the middle phalanx. A sharp blade is introduced and turned in a plantar direction, dividing the flexor tendon. Flexor to extensor transfer has also been used but is more complex and does not improve results in curly toes.[21] Through a midlateral incision, the flexor tendon is divided as far distally as possible. It is then brought up dorsally to the extensor tendon and sutured in place.[4] It is also possible to divide the flexor tendon longitudinally,

TABLE 1. TREATMENT OF SMALL TOE DEFORMITY*

Deformity	Procedure
PIP joint mobile, MTP joint normal	Flexor tenotomy (curly toe) or flexor-to-extensor transfer
PIP joint fixed, MTP joint mobile	Fusion or excision of PIP joint
PIP joint fixed, MTP joint fixed, subluxed	Fusion or excision of PIP joint, extensor tenotomy, dorsal capsulotomy, collateral ligament release at MTP joint
PIP joint fixed, severe MTP joint dislocated, fixed†	Excision of base of proximal phalanx and/or part of metatarsal head, PIP joint fusion or excision
Failed PIP excision arthroplasty	PIP joint fusion

* Author's preferred treatment options depending on the severity of the deformity.
† Very difficult to treat; author recommends consulting a specialist on foot surgery.
MTP, metatarsophalangeal; PIP, proximal interphalangeal.

bringing half up on each side of the toe, then suturing it in place into the extensor hood.

Fixed Deformity. Since the deformity is usually fixed in adults, the most common procedures involve bony correction. The procedure, which is either an excision arthroplasty or an arthrodesis, is done at the contracted joint. A transverse skin incision is made over the affected joint. If the callus is large, it may be removed with an elliptical incision. I find that an extension of the incision proximally on the side of the toe makes for a better, more atraumatic approach. The extensor tendon is divided and the cartilage surfaces are exposed. For an *arthrodesis*, the cartilage is removed with a nibbler or a power bur and the toe is fixed with a Kirschner wire applied in a retrograde fashion. Some authors advocate two wires to control rotation.[4] A small degree of flexion in the PIP joint is preferable. If there is a tendency toward subluxation of the MTP joint, a

dorsal capsule release and extensor tenotomy with fixation through the MTP joint may be considered.[22] The wire is left in place 3 to 4 weeks. The approach is the same for an excision arthroplasty. The distal end of the proximal phalanx is excised at the juncture of the neck and head. The surgeon should be sure that the entire head and condyles are removed, but not remove any shaft, and should check by reduction that the deformity is corrected. Enough should be excised to allow the toe to be straight, but not so much that the toe becomes wobbly. This procedure allows for a stable fibrous pseudarthrosis and works well for the majority of patients. Arthrodeses can be done at both the PIP and the DIP joints if necessary in claw toes. If there is significant subluxation of the MTP joint, correction by the above-described methods will be difficult. Procedures such as those described for crossover toe deformity can be considered (Fig. 6).

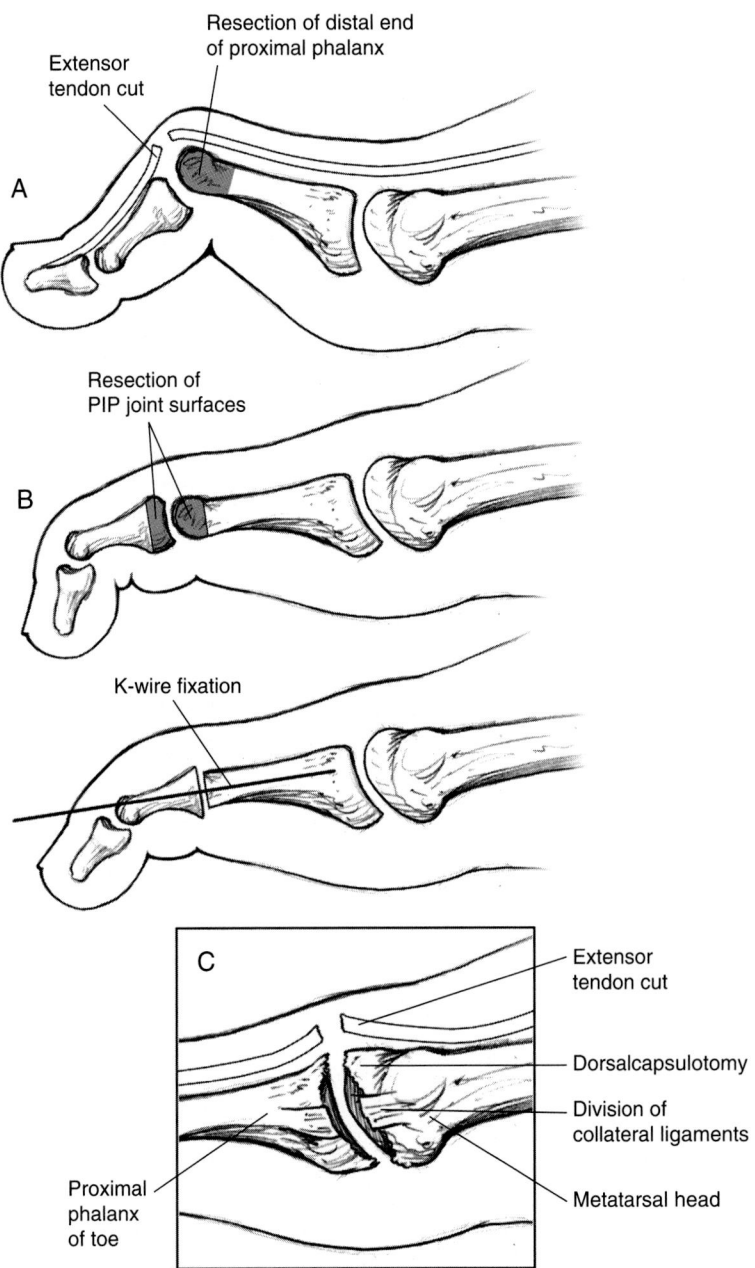

Fig. 6. Surgical procedures for fixed deformity of the lesser toes. *A*, Proximal interphalangeal (PIP) joint arthroplasty with excision of the distal end of the proximal phalanx and extensor tenotomy. *B*, PIP joint fusion with Kirschner wire fixation in slight flexion. *C*, Additional release at the metatarsophalangeal joint: dorsal capsule, extensor tendon, collateral ligaments.

Crossover Deformity of the Second Toe. Crossover toe deformity seems to affect mainly the second toe. The main pathology is subluxation or complete dorsal displacement of the toe at the MTP joint, often combined with hammer toe deformity. A soft-tissue correction at the MTP joint has been suggested, such as extensor digiti longus lengthening, resection of extensor digiti brevis, dorsal capsulotomy, collateral ligament release, and decompression by partial resection of the metatarsal head or of the base of the proximal phalanx. The procedure is difficult and the results are still ambiguous.[7, 14, 23]

Interdigital Clavus, Soft Corns. The condyles causing the corns are removed. A radiograph of the foot in the shoe can demonstrate the offenders if necessary, although a clinical examination is usually enough. A small incision is made over the condyle and a bur or small chisel is used to remove the condyle. I find that a suture in the collateral ligament is necessary if this ligament has been divided. Otherwise, the toe may deviate after surgery.

Morton's Neuroma. Morton's neuroma is generally best treated surgically. Usually resection of the affected nerve is required. There have been recommendations to perform only a release of the intermetatarsal ligament, but there are no studies to show which method gives best results. In cases in which the nerve is macroscopically not affected, such an approach might be possible. In my experience, the diagnosis of Morton's neuroma is often delayed,[17] sometimes by several years, and there are obvious macroscopic changes in the nerve. The resulting paresthesia does not seem to bother most patients, possibly because many already have traumatic paresthesia. Since the dissection is done very close to the vascular structures, it is not advisable to explore and resect the nerve in the adjacent web spaces as well. Because of the chronic inflammation, the structures are not always easy to separate, and the blood vessels may be inadvertently damaged, compromising the blood supply to the middle toe. Either a dorsal or a plantar incision may be used. The plantar incision is more uncomfortable for the patient initially but heals well. This approach discloses the neuroma well, although the plantar fat pad may be difficult to retract. The dorsal approach causes fewer initial wound problems and with training is just as easy. I prefer it, partly because the tension in the intermetatarsal ligament is easier to judge. I use the plantar approach in cases of reoperation for amputation neuromas that are located more proximally and harder to locate from a dorsal approach.

A 4-cm-long incision is placed dorsally in the appropriate web space beginning at the interdigital fold (Fig. 7). After subcutaneous dissection, a metatarsal spreader is used to give access. Pressure on the plantar side of the web space will usually push the intermetatarsal bursa into the space. Typically, it is about the size of a pea. The intermetatarsal ligament is then located and sharply divided. The interdigital nerve is seen. It courses distally over the bursa, where it is often split into numerous parts and divided into the two dorsal nerve branches, which course into the respective toes. It can sometimes be easier to

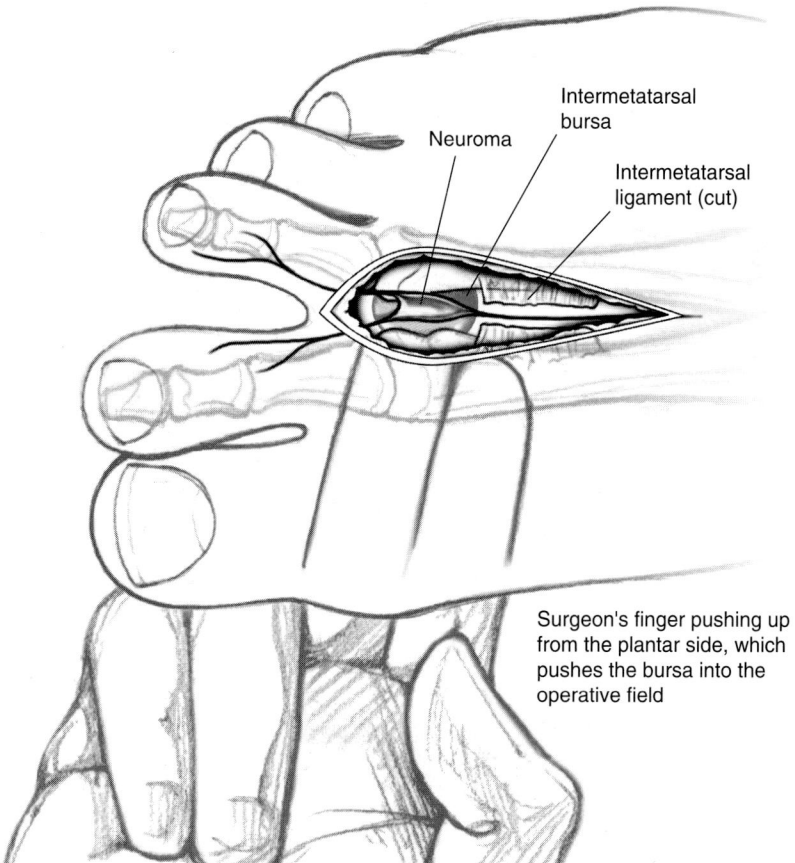

Fig. 7. Schematic view of dorsal approach to excision of Morton's neuroma. The author usually pushes up under the web space with a finger, which pushes the bursa with the neuroma overlying it into view.

Neuroma / Intermetatarsal bursa / Intermetatarsal ligament (cut) / Surgeon's finger pushing up from the plantar side, which pushes the bursa into the operative field

begin the dissection distally and follow it proximally. The distal branches are then cut and the nerve and bursa are dissected free. The proximal nerve is cut well proximally. One must be sure that it retracts. At times, scar tissue can tether the nerve plantarly under the metatarsal and lead to a traumatic amputation neuroma. Bleeding can be a problem. I often release the tourniquet to find major bleeders. Only skin is sutured. A microscopic evaluation to confirm the removal of neuroma is valuable. Full weightbearing is allowed immediately. Usually pain relief is immediate and striking.

Ingrown Toenail. A number of surgical possibilities exist, from amputation of the distal phalanx,[24] to total removal of the nail matrix,[25] to partial surgical removal of the nail matrix. Removal of only the skin fold has also been done. Most recently, phenolization of the nail plate has been shown to have good effect.[26] The toe is anesthetized with local anesthetic without epinephrine. It is exsanguinated. A bloodless field is necessary to identify the nail matrix. In surgical removal, a small 5-mm incision is made at the proximal corner of the nail on the affected side (Fig. 8). A special straight scissors aids in cutting the nail from distal to proximal through the matrix under the cuticle. With a straight forceps, the surgeon removes the nail edge and matrix by gently rolling it like opening a sardine can. This prevents the matrix from tearing off. The fold wherein the matrix lies is then removed. A moist dressing is applied. After 2 days, the patient may change the dressing himself or herself by putting the foot in lukewarm foot bath, bandages and all. The bandages are easily removed after a few minutes. The foot is dried and a new dressing is applied. This can be done daily, and most will heal quickly, with a scab forming within a week. No sutures are needed. Phenolization seems to give equivalent results and lead to quicker healing. Anesthesia and exsanguination are as already described. No incision is made. The nail is cut and the cut is continued under the cuticle, which has been gently lifted to avoid damage. A fine chisel can be used here. Instead of removing the matrix and nail fold, the surgeon applies 80% liquefied phenol on an orange stick for 2 minutes to the nail bed, swabs it dry, and reapplies it for an additional minute. No evidence shows that flushing is necessary. Moist dressings are used, and the patient is seen again within a week.[27]

There is some discussion whether it is advisable to operate on ingrown toenails when there is an ongoing infection. Although it is naturally more appealing to operate in an inactive phase, I find that this is often impossible to achieve. The infections persist as long as the nail is ingrown and an "uninfected window of opportunity" is impossible to find. The operative procedure can be carried out while the patient is being treated with antibiotics. If the infection is severe, it may be advisable to see the patient after a few days. I have not used phenol in infected cases.

Severe Nail Deformity. In some cases, the deformity of the nail is so severe that it causes the patient great trouble with shoes. Both in fungal infections that have resisted treatment and in other deformities, the entire nail bed, including a portion of the distal phalanx, may be removed. The plantar tissue is then advanced around the tip of the toe and sutured to the former cuticle.

COMPLICATIONS

The complications associated with surgery of the lesser toes are those found in all surgical procedures: risk of infection and delayed healing. In the toes, special attention should be paid to the circulatory status. Since these deformities become more prevalent in the elderly, there is also an increased risk that the circulation will not be adequate for healing. It is estimated that healing requires four times the circulatory capacity of the maintenance of intact skin.

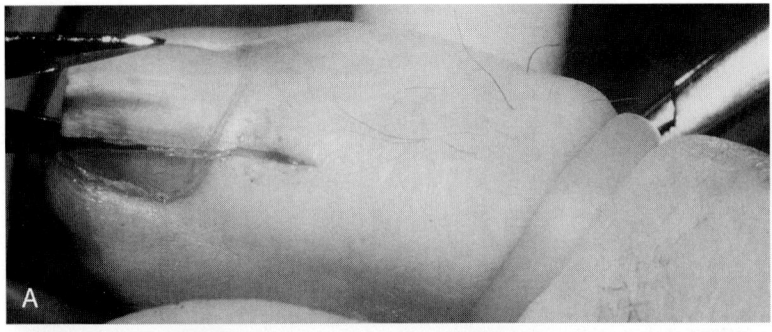
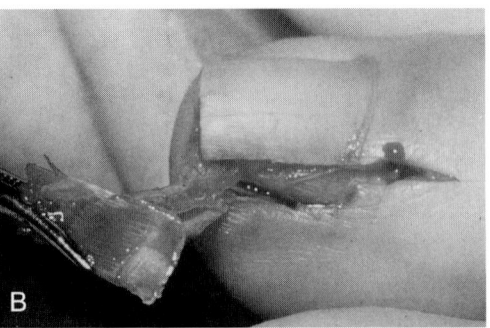
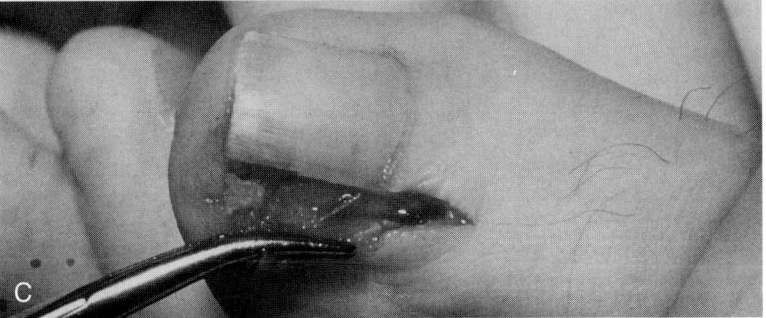

Fig. 8. Partial nail matrix removal in ingrown toenail. *A,* An incision is placed at the lateral edge of the nail bed and the nail is split with flat, sharp scissors through the nail matrix. *B,* The nail with matrix is removed with a gentle rotating motion to remove it completely. *C,* Under the incision is the pocket in which the nail matrix has been, which must be removed. Note the tourniquet for a bloodless field.

In very old patients, it is often advisable to chose nonoperative treatment. In diabetic patients, there is also an increased risk of infection, especially if there is an ulcer to be treated. Complications to infection can be disastrous, with spreading of the infection and incipient ischemia, sometimes even resulting in amputation. It is wise to be in full control and to make sure that the patient can be relied upon to report untoward events before proceeding with surgery. As in all foot surgery, bony healing takes time, especially if it is measured in radiographic changes. There is the possibility of failure to unite in fusions. On the other hand, fibrous fusions are usually sufficient to take care of the patient's symptoms. Recurrence of the deformity, while not a complication as such, is not unusual. The fine balance of structures required for the lesser toes to practice their function is not easily restored, and the forces acting on them are great. When the balance between the toes is disturbed, weight is transferred from one toe to another. This can lead to transfer metatarsalgia, a very painful condition with pressure and calluses under one or several of the metatarsal heads. This is a fairly common complication to surgery of the great toe, reported in up to 20% of patients with proximal first metatarsal osteotomies.[28] The incidence rate associated with other procedures has not been reported but has been seen clinically.

RESULTS

Few prospective randomized studies of surgery of the lesser toes, indeed of foot surgery in general, exist. To my knowledge, only one double-blind randomized study of toe surgery has been published.[21] By using the same incision for both surgeries of curly toes and having follow-up done by a different surgeon, it could be shown that simple flexor tenotomy had the same effect as a flexor-to-extensor tendon transfer procedure. There are numerous retrospective reports and operative descriptions. In general, success rates are reported to be 80% to 90% in primary procedures. It is commonly accepted that the success rate of reoperations decreases. Every effort should be made to make the first operation the last one.

REFERENCES

1. Glyn Thomas T: Medical litigation and the foot. Foot 1991; 1:3.
2. Mueller MJ, Minor SD, Sahrmann SA, et al: Differences in the gait characteristics of patients with diabetes and peripheral neuropathy compared with age-matched controls. Phys Ther 1994; 74:299.
3. Cavanagh PR, Derr JA, Ulbrecht JS, et al: Problems with gait and posture in neuropathic patients with insulin-dependent diabetes mellitus. Diabet Med 1992; 9:469.
4. Grace D: The lesser rays. In Helal B, Rowley D, Cracchiolo A III, et al (eds): Surgery of Disorders of the Foot. London, Martin Dunitz, 1996, p 335.
5. Hughes J, Clark P, Klenerman L: The importance of the toes in walking. J Bone Joint Surg Br 1990; 72:245.
6. Bhatia D, Myerson M, Curtis M, et al: Anatomical restraints to dislocation of the second metatarsophalangeal joint and assessment of a repair technique. J Bone Joint Surg Am 1994; 76:1371.
7. Coughlin M: Subluxation and dislocation of the second metatarsophalangeal joint. Orthop Clin North Am 1989; 20:535.
8. Shine IB: Incidence of hallux valgus in a partially shoe-wearing community. Br Med J 1965; 1:1648.
9. Hardy RH, Clapham CR: Observations on hallux valgus. Based on a controlled series. J Bone Joint Surg Br 1951; 33:376.
10. Larsson J, Apelqvist J: Toward less amputations in diabetic patients: Incidence, causes, cost, treatment and prevention. Review Acta Orthop Scand 1995; 66:181.
11. Jeliffe DB, Humphreys J: Lesions of the feet in African soldiers. J Trop Med Hyg 1952.
12. Coughlin M: Crossover second toe deformity. Foot Ankle 1987; 8:29.
13. Johnson J, Price T: Cross over second toe deformity: Etiology and treatent. J Foot Surg 1989; 28:417.
14. Myerson M: Arthroplasty of the second toe. Semin Arthrop 1992; 3:31.
15. Turan I, Lindgren U: Moire topography in the care of foot deformities. J Foot Surg 1985; 5:339.
16. Gauthier G: Thomas Morton's disease: A nerve entrapment syndrome. Clin Orthop 1979; 142:90.
17. Resch S, Stenström A, Jónsson À, et al: The diagnostic efficacy of magnetic resonance imaging and ultrasonography in Morton's neuroma: A radiological-surgical correlation. Foot Ankle 1994; 15:88.
18. Mulder JD: The causative mechanism in Morton's metatarsalgia. J Bone Joint Surg Br 1951; 33:94.
19. Eneroth M, Apelqvist J, Stenström A: Clinical characteristics and outcome in 233 diabetic patients with deep foot infections. Foot Ankle Int 1997; 18:716.
20. Erickson SJ: Interdigital (Morton) neuroma: High-resolution MR imaging with a solenoid coil. Radiology 1991; 181:833.
21. Hamer A, Stanley D, Smith T: Surgery for curly toe deformity: A double-blind, randomized, prospective trial. J Bone Joint Surg Br 1993; 75:662.
22. Richardson EG: Lesser toe abnormalities. In Canale T (ed): Campbell's Operative Orthopaedics. St Louis: Mosby–Year Book, 1998, 9th ed, vol II, p 2729.
23. Richardson G: Realignment of the overlapping second toe. In Johnson KA (ed): Master Techniques in Orthopedic Surgery: The Foot and Ankle. New York, Raven Press, 1994, p 135.
24. Dixon GJ: Treatment of ingrown toenail. Foot Ankle 1983; 3:254.
25. Zadig F: Obliteration of the nailbed of the great toe without shortening of the terminal phalanx. JAMA 1950; 92:229.
26. Beaton D, Kriss S, Blacklay P, et al: Ingrowing toenails: A patient evaluation of phenolization versus wedge excision. Chiropodist 1990; 55:62.
27. Rendall G: The nails. In Helal B, Rowley D, Cracchiolo A III, et al (eds): Surgery of Disorders of the Foot. London, Martin Dunitz, 1996.
28. Resch S, Stenström A, Reynisson K, Jonsson K: Results after chevron osteotomy and proximal osteotomy for hallux valgus: A prospective randomized study. Foot 1993; 3:99.

ORTHOTIC MANAGEMENT OF FOOT AND ANKLE PROBLEMS

Donald G. Shurr and Chris Fellner

Summary
- Diabetic foot ulcers are one of the most common reasons for admission to an acute care hospital bed.
- Incomplete understanding of the problems will lead to inadequate foot and ankle treatment.
- Trauma produced by poor shoe fit can lead to major limb amputation.
- Centers for Disease Control estimates that 85% of foot and leg amputations may be prevented by proper foot care and properly fitted shoes.
- Successful outcomes occur when the orthopaedic physician and orthotist share a common understanding of the biomechanical problems and all people involved, including the patient, share an understanding of the solutions and prescription.

The orthotic management of the foot and ankle demands a complementary relationship between the orthopaedic physician and the orthotist. This relationship involves a mutual understanding of the roles and treatment options that each may recommend so that treatment is understood and accepted by the patient. Patient compliance is often influenced by the way the orthopaedist and orthotist approach the clinical problems, acting in concert. Also critical are any changes in necessary shoeing or dress, necessitated by the wearing of special shoes or clothes to allow prescribed treatment devices to be worn in an effort to alter any pathological or painful foot and ankle problems.

The purpose of this chapter is to describe the processes by which the physician and orthotist deal with myriad foot and ankle problems. It includes examination of the relevant biomechanical studies that form the basis of the modern practice of orthotics. It also includes a brief review of materials available and their relevant properties. Completed devices, including advantages and disadvantages of custom-molded foot and ankle orthoses, are then discussed. Finally, a study of the essence of prescription writing includes discussion of the elements of a meaningful and descriptive orthotic prescription, one that can be interpreted by the clinical orthotist and will provide the patient with the properly designed foot or ankle orthosis.

BIOMECHANICS: THE BASIS FOR CLINICAL ORTHOTIC MANAGEMENT

Orthoses for the foot and ankle provide assistance in several ways:

1. Correction of deformity, if flexible, and accommodation if fixed, which may include distal deformities from other joints

2. Control of motion, generally to allow motion and to provide a stop
3. Augmentation of muscle weakness, either flaccid or spastic
4. Augmentation of ligamentous weakness, from grade 1 through rupture
5. Transfer of weightbearing proximally or better distribution of pressure
6. Proprioception, which may affect control of the knee.

Most orthoses for the foot and ankle use one or more of the just-stated purposes. It is not unusual to provide orthotic solutions for patients that take away other more normal motions or motors in order to complete the treatment. This is "robbing Peter to pay Paul" and is very common, even with the most modern orthotic treatment.

In most instances, it is advantageous to correct a flexible deformity, returning the joint or joints to a more normal anatomic position. Theoretically, this then allows the orthosis to hold the affected joint in its more normal alignment. Biomechanically, this reduces the abnormal or deforming forces on the joints and should reduce the associated pain occurring with the flexible deformity. Sometimes the correction of flexible deformities is more art than science, particularly when the deformity has taken place over a long period of time and the changes have occurred very gradually. In such cases, it is not unusual to fabricate an intermediate orthosis, followed by the more corrected one, because the return to near normal may be more successful when done in steps or stages over time.

Normally, the anatomic structures act in concert to allow desired motion and to stop unwanted or painful motion near the limits of each joint. This process includes the bones, ligaments, tendons, and structural designs, such as the shape of the dome of the talus. When any of these structures break down, an orthosis might be indicated to help restore these normal restraints. An example of such an orthosis is a custom-molded, solid-ankle ankle-foot orthosis (AFO), used to prohibit ankle dorsiflexion in the patient with osteochondritis dissecans of the dome of the talus. If properly aligned and fabricated, the limitation of dorsiflexion on the ankle joint precludes the talar dome from being loaded in the area of the defect, while allowing weightbearing and ambulation on the injured ankle.

Orthoses may be used in cases of weakness caused by flaccid or spastic conditions. Worldwide, poliomyelitis is the principal cause when flaccid paralyses are raised, but in North America diabetic neuropathy is currently far more common. Spastic conditions often seen include stroke, head injury, and spinal cord injury. The presence or absence of sensory involvement further confounds these cases, because skin breakdown can preclude a design or strategy that would have succeeded had it not been for the loss of sensation.

Ligamentous laxity of the midfoot or ankle can be challenging to control with orthotic management. Key to treatment of such problems is the degree of the strain, the patient's weight and activity level, and any cosmetic needs included in the patient's vocation or avocation. Tradeoffs to produce cosmesis can result in an inadequate biomechanical solution, allowing further deterioration of the affected ligaments.

Problems involving painful weightbearing of the foot represent a large percentage of patients seen on any busy foot service. The biomechanical evaluation of these patients needs to identify any abnormal anatomy, either present or absent, and to rule out any treatable disease processes before orthotic prescription. These common problems include metatarsalgia, heel pain, and any abnormal pressures taken on the first or fifth metatarsal heads. Treatment of these problems may involve the use of soft, rigid, or semirigid insoles, shoe modifications, or, in severe cases involving diabetes, the concept of proximally transferring patient weight onto the leg or thigh.

CLINICAL FEATURES AND BIOMECHANICS

Although it is necessary to know the diagnosis before initiating orthotic treatment, it is also critical to understand fully the nature and extent of the functional impairment. This understanding will provide a basis for the development of an orthotic "blueprint" or treatment plan. This blueprint forms the beginning of the discussion between physician and orthotist to ensure that both know what goals are to be achieved. It also provides a point from which further discussion or information gathering might occur. Any questions or problems need to be addressed before the impression taking, because it is after this point that the biomechanics, alignment, and component choices have already been made. New information after this point in time will necessitate refabrication of the device or process, adding cost to the orthosis and wasting time toward the delivery of the device to the patient.

Support in the literature exists for much of what is commonly seen in foot clinics. Rogers and Cavanagh[1] found that pressures under the head of the second metatarsal were higher when a Morton's foot structure (MFS) was present. This is thought to be due to the foreshortened first metatarsal and the lack of incremental loading of the first. They concluded that MFS predisposes these feet to problems associated with excessive localized foot pressure. Basford and Smith[2] described 25 of 96 patients in their study who would not wear insoles given to them for purpose of study. The patients reported that the insoles made the shoe fit too tightly. These individuals could not benefit from the insoles because they would not wear them in their shoes. This study reinforces that shoeing in many cases is as important as any insole, because without the "right" shoe the insole will not be given a chance.

Perry et al[3] documented that the risk of amputation resulting from diabetes is 15 times greater than in the general population. The type of shoes and inserts worn may influence this outcome. They concluded that leather-soled shoes produce plantar pressures equal to barefoot

pressures while walking on wooden floors. Crepe-soled shoes reduce plantar surface pressures by 31%.

Nyska et al[4] studied the plantar foot pressures between high-heel and low-heel shoes. They found that high-heel shoes decreased the forces on the heel, lateral forefoot, and midfoot and increased the pressures on the medial forefoot and hallux. The magnitude of the increase was 40% from low heel to high heel. The authors suggested that the high medial load may further contribute to the deformity called hallux valgus.

Clark et al[5] evaluated 36 different shoes with varied midsole hardness, heel flare, and heel height for the effects on hindfoot motion during running. Results showed that shoes with softer midsoles allowed more pronation and hindfoot motion than either medium or dense midsoled shoes. Shoes without outflares allowed more motion than shoes with soles of either 15 or 30 degrees of outflare. Heel height had no effect on frontal plane motion, as expected.

Frey et al[6] studied 356 women to evaluate trends in shoe wear and the effects on development of foot deformities and pain. The majority of the women tested wore shoes that were too small and too tight, and had increased in shoe size since the age of 20 years. Few of the participants had had their feet measured before new shoe purchase in the preceding 5 years.

Many foot problems are due to increased plantar pressure and shear forces. Shear forces have always been recognized but are difficult to measure. Shoe modifications and orthoses have been documented to reduce plantar pressure. Wong et al.[7] measured pressure and shear forces on 22 barefoot individuals wearing cotton socks or silicone-insole socks. Silicone socks were superior to cotton socks in reducing horizontal shear and their friction coefficients. Further study may show whether individuals with pathological feet and skin conditions benefit to the same extent as those with healthy feet and skin.

In 1998, Foto and Birke[8] evaluated multidensity orthotic materials used in the footwear of patients with diabetes. Results demonstrated that all materials tested experienced losses in performance throughout the testing period; the greatest loss occurred in the first 10,000 cycles. Of all the materials tested, poron plus Plastazote #2 and Spenco plus Microcel Puff Lite showed the lowest dynamic compression set over the 100,000 cycles of testing. Material development continues today and, it is hoped, will lead to an improved spectrum of orthotic material choices.

Ulcers of the plantar surface of the heel are common and particularly troublesome and difficult to treat. Studies using total contact casting reveal that pressures on the plantar surface of the foot are more easily reduced on the metatarsal heads than on the heel. However, Armstrong and Stacpoole-Shea[9] studied the healing of heel ulcers using a variety of modalities. Of note was that all other devices reduced the pressure better than a depth shoe. Although not great, the total contact cast reduced heel pressures better than off-the-shelf boots, but only 33% less than a baseline sneaker. Total contact cast is thought to allow shear reduction, decreased plantar pressure over time, and a protected wound environment.

Ashry et al[10] used an in-shoe sensor array to measure peak pressures on the plantar surface of 11 diabetic feet

TABLE 1. ORTHOTIC MATERIALS

Materials	Specific Properties	Indications	Advantages and Disadvantages
Thermoplastics Polypropylene	Requires positive model Requires high temperature	Lower limb orthoses Used for strength	Heat malleable; shrinkage Rigidity; fractures with repeat cycles; stress rises with cyclic loading after 10,000 cycles
Polyethylene Thermasetting resins	For vacuum forming Uses base materials to produce strength	Used as veneer Strong, lightweight material: prosthetics	Flexible: cracks with use High strength-weight ratio; difficult to heat relieve once cured
Closed-cell foams (Plastazote)	Heat moldable	FO or lining AFOs	Soft and easily moldable; will bottom out in relatively short time
Open-cell foams Cork (thermo)	Shock absorption Heat moldable	FO or lining AFOs Often used in combination with leather	Long lasting; may be ground or layers added; difficult to clean; may crack after long usage (dries out)

FO = foot orthosis; AFO = ankle-foot orthosis.

using five different combinations of shoes and insole modifications and materials. These strategies included depth shoes with Plastazote insoles, with and without metatarsal pads and with and without a medial longitudinal arch pad. All strategies except that of no insole reduced the plantar pressures, but no other strategy showed superior pressure reduction compared with the others.

BASIC MATERIAL CHOICES AVAILABLE IN ORTHOTICS

Once the evaluation is complete and the prescription has been written and discussed, the design of the orthosis must be considered. Items that may impact on design include the patient's weight and activity level, the vocation or avocation and any cosmetic concerns (including shoes), and the elements that might impact adversely on the proposed design. Integral to the design is the material of choice, which often can act as an adjunct to the chosen design. Materials can impact weight, strength, flexibility, necessary thickness, and various degrees of cushioning, off-loading, or load transfer.

Historically, the choices of materials were few. Initially,

natural products were used, such as tree bark and wood. Later, as metals came along, iron, brass, tin, and leather were the materials of choice. The 1940s saw the introduction of aluminum and resins used for veneers. In 1968, Dr. Gordon Yates ushered in a new era when he introduced the United States to polypropylene. Today many plastics abound, with new types introduced everyday. Plastics allow custom molding and endless change possibilities as the patient grows or as conditions change (Table 1).

MANAGEMENT

The orthotic management of ankle and foot problems often includes the use of custom-molded above-the-ankle orthotics or AFOs (Table 2). These should be used only when other more conservative devices have failed or when it is obvious that the clinical problem requires a longer or larger lever arm to provide the necessary corrective forces. It is also imperative that all parties agree with the plan so that the patient has prior knowledge that a different shoe may be necessary.

Classically, AFOs were made from metals, either iron or later aluminum or steel. Because these devices demanded a

TABLE 2. ANKLE-FOOT ORTHOSES

Orthosis	Indications	Advantages	Disadvantages	Material of Choice
Solid ankle	DF, evertor, and plantar-flexor weakness	Stability, worn in shoe	Eliminates ankle-foot motion	Polypropylene
Leaf spring	DF and evertor weakness	Cosmetic, worn in shoe	Little frontal plane control	Polypropylene
Clamshell	Used to transfer load from foot-ankle to leg	Stability	May require larger shoe; not volume-change friendly	Polypropylene with polyethylene tongue or front
CROW	End-stage foot disease	Allows ambulation; volume friendly; requires no shoe; restricts foot motion	Cosmesis; requires custom inserts remade	Copolymer
Posterior opening articulated/adjustable	PTTD; pronation of midfoot, talonavicular subluxation/dislocation	Worn in shoe; stability	Takes time to adjust to new midfoot weightbearing areas	Polypropylene
Solid ankle articulated	OCD of talar dome; OA of ankle joint	Allows some volitional PF; offers ML control	Joints wear out with larger patients	Polypropylene or laminates (carbon)

DF = dorsiflexion; CROW = Charcot restraint orthotic walker; PTTD = posterior tibial tendon dysfunction; OCD = osteochondritis dissecans; OA = osteoarthritis; PF = plantar flexion; ML = medial-lateral.

stirrup for attachment to the shoe, they were quite heavy and condemned the wearer to one corrected shoe, unless multiple AFOs were made or split stirrups were used. These split stirrups were not designed for heavy users and frequently failed. This is not meant to demean the modern use of metal AFOs, because they do represent a clear option today when heavy-duty use is anticipated.

The advantages of metal AFOs include adjustability, strength, flexibility in leg volume changes in patients who have persistent volume swings, and the ability to fit a chronically swollen foot into an off-the-shelf shoe. The disadvantages include weight, cosmesis, restriction to a single shoe, and the lack of a total contact fit (Fig 1).

The concept of a trial or temporary orthosis should include consideration of an all-metal device. Clearly, the widest choices of joints and other components still rest with metal. When the medical condition may be changing, for better or worse, the metal joints, in particular the bi-channel ankle joint, offer the most options. Cosmesis remains the main deterrent to the use of metal AFOs.

Since 1968, polypropylene has become the mainstay material of choice for custom-molded AFOs. Early experiences with polypropylene proved its usefulness for a large variety of orthotic applications, both adult and pediatric. By using polypropylene, total-contact orthoses were avail-

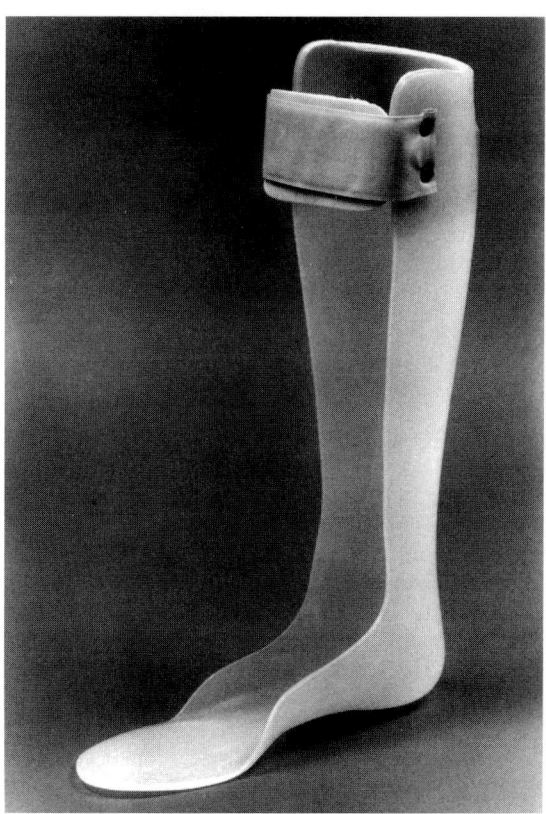

Fig. 2. Solid-ankle ankle-foot orthosis made of polypropylene.

able, and these orthoses were, therefore, virtually adjustable for the lifetime of the device. Via selective heating, changes could be made over the life of the device as changes in the anatomy of the patient occurred. In addition, the AFO could be placed in many shoes, making it invisible to most eyes.

Early reports by Engen, Sarno, and Stills demonstrated the various designs and clinical uses for polypropylene. The first reports by Engen demonstrated the utility of the design and material. The trim lines, or the length that the edges of the plastics were trimmed, dictated the stiffness of the ankle motion as well as the control of frontal plane motion. Cutting the trim line posterior to the malleoli allowed truer ankle motion in early swing phase, introducing the concept of a toe pick-up orthosis or a leaf spring. Biomechanically, the plantar flexors deform the plastic into plantar flexion at late stance phase, allowing the plastic to rebound in early swing phase, thus clearing the toe. These designs are currently used for neurological absence of ankle dorsiflexors to slow or stop forward rotation of the tibia in midstance and to assist with painful late stance–phase dorsiflexion as in arthritis of the ankle or osteochondritis of the talus and in other nonspecific situations in which the goal is to slow the anterior rotation of the tibia on the talus. Solid-ankle designs, with the trim lines cut in front of the malleoli, also are of benefit to the patient with posterior tibial tendon dysfunction (PTTD). This long trim line on the medial side of the orthosis prevents the midfoot from rolling into pronation in stance phase and stops the gradual deformity and pain. Assuming the Achilles tendon

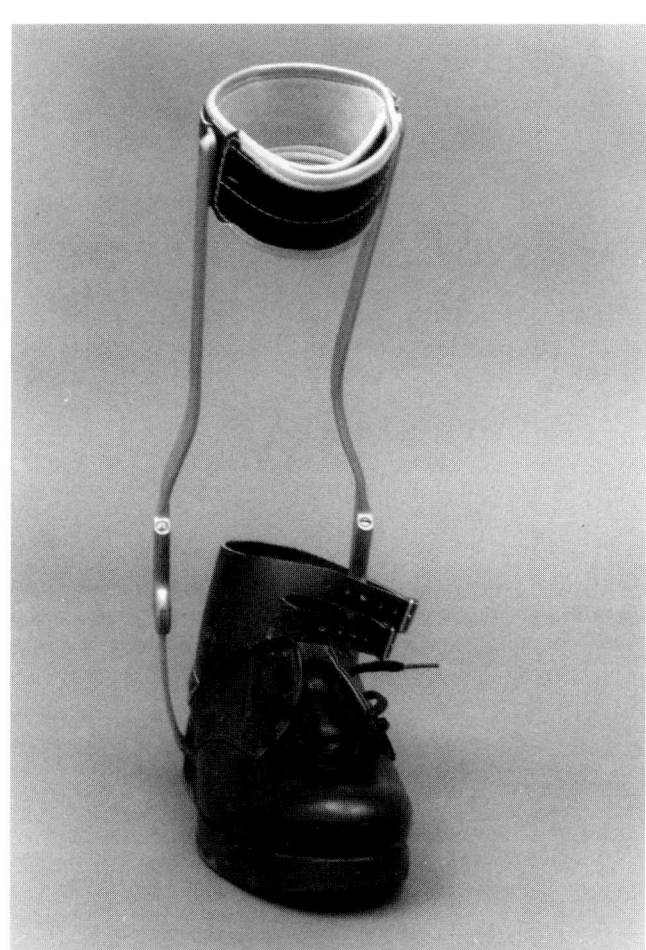

Fig. 1. Metal ankle-foot orthosis.

is not tight and the ankle can be moved passively into dorsiflexion, a near plantigrade position of the device allows nearly normal gait (Fig. 2). For patients with moderate to severe PTTD, a posterior-opening, articulated, custom-molded AFO is indicated (Fig. 3). This AFO allows sagittal plane motion while restraining or supporting the motion of the midfoot in the frontal plane. This AFO may be needed as an intermediary device, because full hindfoot neutral position can be quite painful for the patient with severe PTTD. It also requires a well-constructed, broad-heeled tie oxford shoe to assist in midfoot pronation control.

If needed, another design option is the clamshell front, which may be added for patients who have Achilles tendon tightness or spasticity or who are quite large, making positioning maintenance difficult. The clamshell design also allows the orthotist to apply some of the patient's weight to the leg, thus off-loading the bottom of the foot (Fig. 4).

Motion of the ankle or subtalar joints can also be reduced with the use of a leather-lined custom-molded, plastic AFO. This AFO boot has been shown in our studies to reduce motion in both the sagittal and frontal planes. Because of the leather lacer, it is adjustable and comfortable for patients with unstable volume. This device provides the stability of a plastic AFO and the adjustability of the leather lacer. Patients must have good enough hand strength to be able to lace and tighten the strings or have someone available who can perform that function (Fig. 5).

The Charcot restraint orthotic walker (CROW) is a solid-

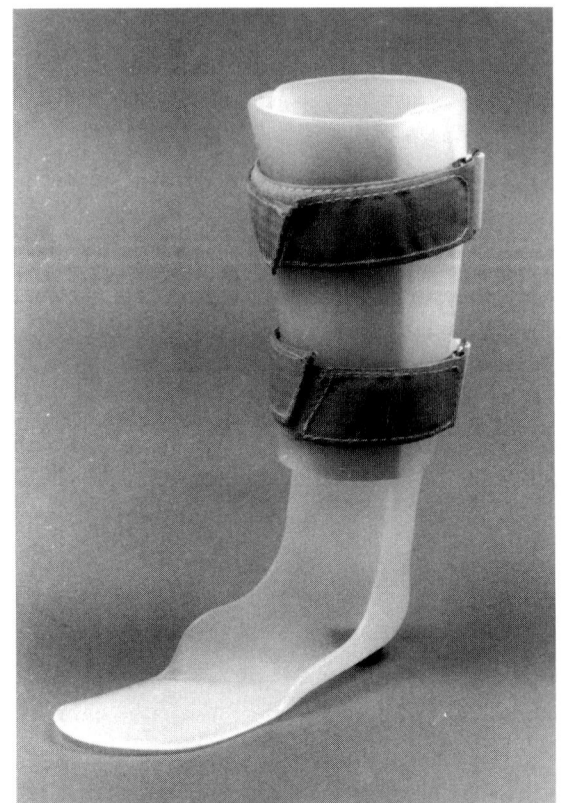

Fig. 4. Custom-molded clamshell ankle-foot orthosis.

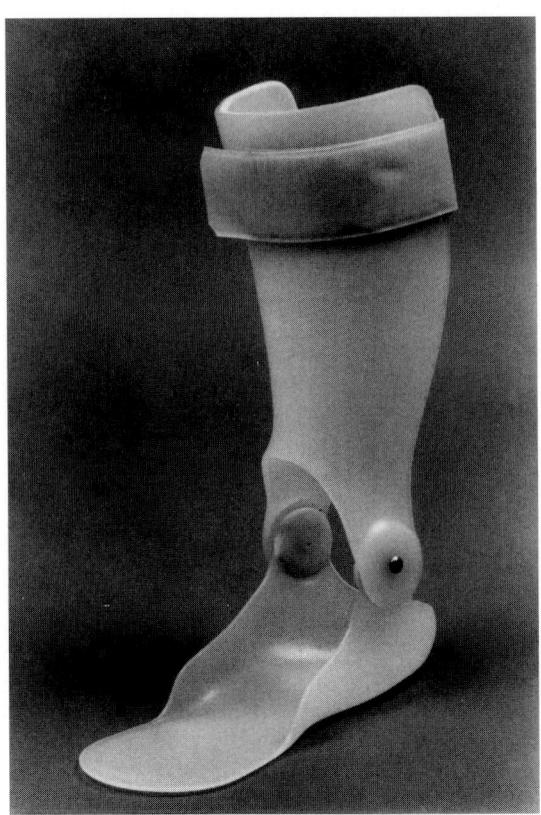

Fig. 3. Posterior-opening, articulated, custom-molded ankle-foot orthosis.

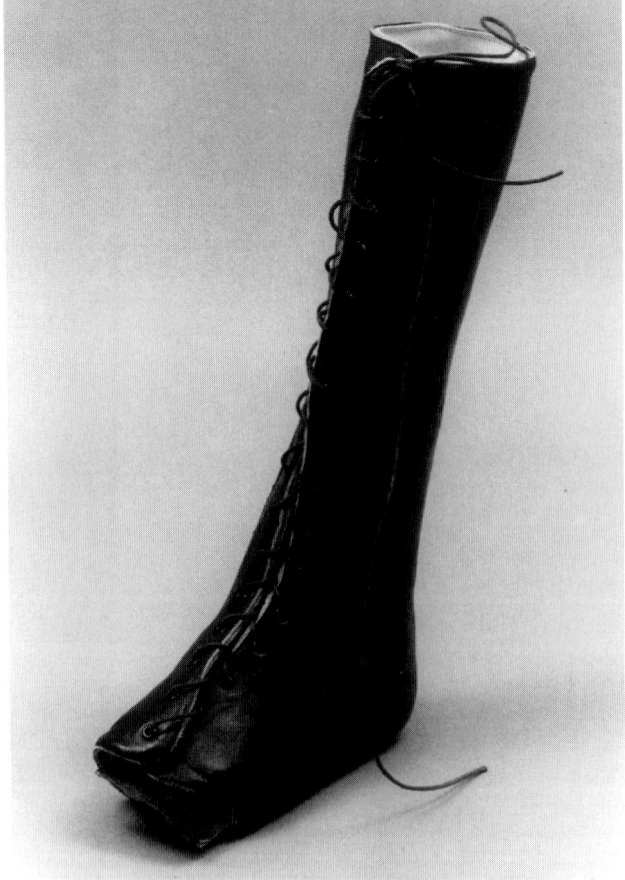

Fig. 5. Custom-molded, leather-lined, plastic ankle-foot orthosis.

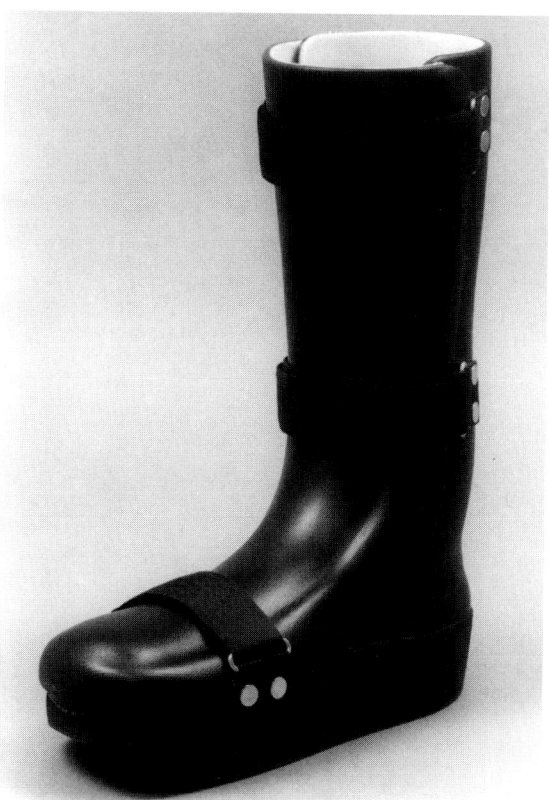

Fig. 6. Charcot restraint orthotic walker.

ankle, custom-molded AFO with a pretibial shell used originally for diabetics with end-stage feet. The CROW does, however, have a limited use for nondiabetics in cases of chronic plantar ulcers, unstable columns, and painful ankle and subtalar problems recalcitrant to other forms of orthotic treatment (Fig. 6).

Many off-the-shelf walkers, boots, and braces are available. We have found them helpful as short-term solutions. However, the lack of total contact fitting limits their utility. The use of a soft, comfortable plantar liner can improve comfort and fit.

CONCLUSIONS

The foot presents many varied challenges for both the orthopaedic surgeon and the clinical orthotist. Accurate and complete treatment of all involved diseases will afford the patient the most certain opportunity for functional restoration. An open dialogue among the physician, orthotist, and patient offers the best chance for compliance. A well-written and complete orthotic blueprint allows all players to proceed and progress toward mutually accepted goals. Follow-up ensures continual evaluation of progress toward these goals.

REFERENCES

1. Rogers MM, Cavanagh PR: Pressure distribution in Morton's foot structure. *Med Sci Sports Exerc* 1989; 21:23–28.
2. Basford JR, Smith MA: Shoe insoles in the work place. *Orthopedics* 1989; 12: 285–289.
3. Perry JE: The use of running shoes to reduce plantar pressures in patients who have diabetes. *J Bone Joint Surg Am* 1995; 77a:1819–1828.
4. Nyska M: Plantar foot pressures during treadmill walking with high-heel and low-heel shoes. *Foot Ankle Int* 1996; 17:662–666.
5. Clark TE: The effects of shoe design parameters on rearfoot control in running. *Med Sci Sports Exerc* 1983; 376–381.
6. Frey C, Thompson F, Smith J, et al: *American Orthopaedic Foot and Ankle Society women's shoe survey.* Foot Ankle 1993; 14:78–81.
7. Wong PY: Effects of silicone-insole socks on pressure distribution and shear force of the foot. Chang Kend I Hsueh Tsa Chih 1998; 21:20–27.
8. Foto JG. Birke JA: Evaluation of multi-density orthotic materials used in footwear for patients with diabetes. Foot Ankle Int No. 12, December, 1998; 19:836–841.
9. Armstrong DG, Stacpoole-Shea S: Total contact casts and removable cast walkers: Mitigation of plantar heel pressure. J Am Podiatr Med Assoc 1999; 89:50–53.
10. Ashry HR, et al: Effectiveness of diabetic insoles to reduce foot pressures. J Foot Ankle Surg 1997; 36:268–271.

HAND AND PERIPHERAL NERVE SOFT-TISSUE AND BONE INJURIES

PETER J. STERN

NAIL BED AND FINGERTIP INJURIES

Robert L. Bass

Summary

- Nail bed and fingertip injuries are so common that their true incidence defies accurate analysis.
- Associated distal phalanx fractures are common and need appropriate treatment, either by débridement or more rarely stabilization.
- Associated flexor and/or extensor tendon injuries can occur and need appropriate management along with treatment of the nail bed and fingertip injury.
- Accurate evaluation of injured structures is essential to formulation of an appropriate treatment algorithm.
- The avoidance of nail deformity, stiffness, and a sensitive fingertip is the goal of therapy.
- The simplest procedure that lends itself to these ends is most appropriate.

HISTORICAL REVIEW

Historically, nail bed injuries were treated by débridement and dressing changes, and thus healing by secondary intention. This frequently caused deformed nail plates and sensitive, scarred fingertips, as noted by Flatt in 1955.[1] As early as 1929, recommendations for repair of the injury by grafting from the toes or other digits was considered. In 1957, Schiller recommended the replacement of the nail plate for support of associated phalanx fractures, and to allow for optimal regrowth of the nail.[2] In 1967, Kleinert et al[3] classified nail bed injuries and developed a management algorithm. In 1984, Zook et al[4] published their experience with primary repair of nail bed injuries. Based on this report and experience, primary repair is considered the standard of care at this time.

Fingertip injuries can be treated in a variety of ways depending on multiple variables, including extent of soft tissue loss, associated bony injury or loss, digit involved, age of patient, timing of evaluation and treatment, and treatment preferences of the surgeon involved. Coverage techniques include open treatment,[5] skin grafting, local flaps, cross-finger flaps, thenar flaps, pedicled flaps, and even free flaps. Open treatment works well when no bone is exposed and the soft tissue defect is less than 1 cm in diameter. Multiple follow-up studies show the efficacy of this treatment.[5–7] Patton[8] reported split-thickness skin grafting for fingertip injuries in 1969. Follow-up studies of full thickness skin grafting include those by O'Malley,[9] Lie et al,[10] Mack,[11] and Schenck and Cheema.[12] The volar V-Y flap was first described by Tranquilli-Leali in 1935,[13] and popularized in 1970 by Atasoy et al.[14] The lateral digital flap was introduced by Kutler[15] in 1944, and revised by Fisher[16] in 1967. The thenar flap was first described by Gatewood in 1926.[17] Subsequent modifications of this technique have been described by Flatt,[18] Barton,[19] and Smith

and Albin.[20] Cross finger flaps were initially reported on by Gurdin and Pangman[21] in 1950, followed by Cronin[22] and Tempest.[23] Subsequently, many authors have described modifications, including innervation of these flaps and the use of "reversed" cross-finger flaps.[24] First dorsal metacarpal artery pedicle flaps were described Foucher and Braun[25] for coverage of thumb tip injures. Sherif[26] has further delineated the anatomy and use of this flap. The neurovascular island flap first described by Littler[27] requires the transfer of an island of soft tissue from the ulnar aspect of the ring or middle finger across the palm to resurface the thumb. Reversed digital artery flaps (homodigital island flap) have been described and used by Sapp and Allen.[28] This technique uses an island of skin on the side of the proximal phalanx of the injured digit, supplied in a retrograde fashion to cover fingertip injuries. Homodigital island flaps and their utility were recently evaluated by Lanzetta and Mastropasoua.[29] Very distal neurovascular island flaps have been described and reported on by Tsai and Yeun[30] for coverage of volar oblique fingertip amputations. In 1993, Kamai et al[31] described a thenar free flap for fingertip reconstruction, based on the superficial palmar branch of the radial artery and the palmar cutaneous branch of the median nerve.

As one can see, the variety and number of techniques for fingertip coverage is long. The preceding list is not all-inclusive but does exemplify the wide selection of techniques available. The most common techniques include open treatment, skin grafting, and local and regional flaps and are the basis for the remainder of this chapter.

PATHOGENESIS

Fingertip injuries may be one of the most common and underestimated injuries, from both work- and leisure-related activities. Hand and upper extremity minor trauma account for a very high percentage of ambulatory emergency room visits. Of these injuries, nail bed and fingertip injuries constitute a very high percentage. Many of these injuries, unfortunately, are not treated by individuals with expertise in musculoskeletal trauma. This aspect emphasizes the need for appropriate evaluation and treatment selection.

CLINICAL FEATURES

Nail bed injuries can be characterized by anatomic location, either involving the sterile or germinal matrix. They also have been classified, by Kleinert et al,[3] into six categories: simple lacerations, crushing lacerations, avulsive lacerations, lacerations with associated fractures, lacerations with loss of skin and pulp, and fingertip amputations. Zook et al[4] did an extremely complete study of almost 300 nail bed injuries categorized by location and mechanism of injury, all treated in a similar fashion. They categorized the injuries anatomically, as distal, middle, or proximal nail bed, and dorsal or palmar nail fold. The categories used in this study included simple lacerations, crush injuries, and avulsion injuries. Also noted was the fact that nail bed injuries occurred in association with fingertip injuries more frequently than isolated nail bed injuries in a ratio of 6 to 1.

Either in association with nail bed injuries or alone, fingertip injuries are frequently described by angles and levels of amputations. The angles of injury or partial amputation are described as volar oblique, dorsal oblique, or transverse. The important aspect of differentiating level of injury is to identify whether or not bone is exposed.

INVESTIGATION

In addition to a thorough clinical examination, standard radiographic analysis is indicated in the evaluation of all fingertip injuries. It is also important to inquire whether amputated pieces of digits have been recovered. Skin can be deflated and applied as a full-thickness graft and nail matrix can likewise be reattached. Patient related factors, including occupation, handedness, avocation, pre-existing hand problems, and the presence of systemic disease, all play a role in the formulation of the most appropriate algorithm for injury management.

TREATMENT GOALS

The goal of treatment of injury to the fingertip is a painless, aesthetically acceptable fingertip with durable and sensate skin. The goal of treatment of nail bed injuries is a normal-appearing, stable, nail plate. Tables 1 and 2 outline the most common injury types for nail bed and fingertip injuries with their associated treatment indications, advantages, disadvantages, and contraindications.

PROCEDURES AND POSTOPERATIVE CARE

NAIL BED INJURIES

Nail bed injuries can be adequately treated by primary suture repair using 6-0 or 7-0 plain or chromic gut to repair the nail matrix component and 5-0 nylon to repair the laceration of associated pulp skin. This technique is the same for simple lacerations and stellate types (Fig. 1). If a small portion of nail bed is still attached to a piece of sharply amputated nail plate, the combined amputated part can be reapproximated without unnecessary damage to the small piece of nail bed.

Nail bed injuries associated with nail bed loss can be treated by thin split-thickness nail bed graft (0.018 to 0.028 cm). This can be obtained freehand using a No. 15 scalpel blade (Fig. 2). The graft is thin enough to be translucent. It is rotated into the site of the defect and sewn in place with 6-0 or 7-0 absorbable suture. If there is not enough uninjured nail bed from the digit that has the defect, a similar procedure can be used to harvest split-thickness nail bed graft from the great toe after a traumatic nail plate removal. This, however, creates donor site morbidity in a previously uninjured area.

Postoperatively, antibiotic ointment and xeroform gauze are placed over the area of repair or grafting and tucked beneath the eponychial fold to prevent adherence of the fold. If the nail plate is minimally injured, it may be replaced to help splint the soft tissues, but this is optional.

		TABLE 1. NAIL BED INJURIES		
Type	**Treatment Options**	**Advantages**	**Disadvantages**	**Contraindications**
Simple laceration	Primary nail bed approximation with 6-0, 7-0 chromic sutures with loupe magnification	Simple technique Good results, reliability	None	None
Crush/stellate injury	Primary nail bed approximation with 6-0, 7-0 chromic sutures with loupe magnification	Native nail bed tissue provides best chance for normal nail growth	Small fragments difficult to approximate Injured tissue somewhat fragile	Substance loss of nail bed matrix
Avulsion	Split-thickness graft:	Technically relatively simple:	Negligible	If defect is greater than one half of total nail bed area
	From adjacent uninjured nail bed	Allows repair with native tissue; low donor site morbidity	Donor site morbidity, harvesting from previously uninjured donor site	If donor site deformity not desired or warranted
	From other donor site, e.g., great toe	Same as above except increased donor site morbidity, harvesting from previously uninjured donor site		
	Vascularized nail bed graft	Technically difficult; significant alteration of donor site/increased morbidity	Increased morbidity	No microsurgical skill or equipment available

TABLE 2. FINGERTIP INJURIES

Type	Treatment Options	Advantages	Disadvantages	Contraindications
Soft tissue without bone exposed <1 cm²	Healing by second intention	Simple, effective wound contracture Brings in normal sensate skin Complete healing in 3–5 weeks	Few	None
>1 cm²	FTSG from hypothenar eminence	Less contraction than STSG; more durable than STSG Low donor site morbidity	Requires removal of normal tissue from donor site Loss of graft Behaves as "biologic dressing"	Defect wider than 2 cm Exposed tendon Exposed bone Multiple digits
Soft tissue with bone exposed	Shortening, primary closure	Simple, provides good function, minimizes number and complexity of procedures	Further loss of digit If nail bed not fully ablated, problematic nail bed remnants Possibility of tendon dynamic problems, "quadriga," "lumbrical plus digit"	>5 mm sterile matrix
Local flaps (type dependent on obliquity of tissue loss)	V-Y [Atasoy] (transverse or dorsal oblique)	Local tissue of same structure functions as that tissue lost Simple	Distal edge of flap can normally be advanced ~1 cm If distal edge sewn under tension, can lead to hook nail deformity	Amputations in which more soft tissue lost proximally (volar oblique)
	Kutler (transverse)	Local tissue of similar structure, function	Flaps are small Difficult to advance Suture lines meet directly over tip, palmar aspect of pulp	Amputation in which more soft tissue lost proximally (volar oblique)
Regional flaps	Cross-finger flaps	Preserve length and obtain coverage in amputations with volar oblique angle Allow replacement of substantial pulp loss	Unappealing donor site in females and dark-skinned persons	Arthritis, rheumatoid arthritis, diabetes; vasospastic disorders
	Thenar flaps	Preserve length and obtain coverage in amputations with volar oblique angle Allow replacement of substantial pulp loss	Unappealing donor site in females and dark-skinned persons	Relative contraindication: age >40 years

FTSG, full-thickness skin graft; STSG, split-thickness skin graft.

A bulky soft dressing is applied and the fingertip is splinted. The dressing is changed after 5 days. The initially placed xeroform gauze should be left in place. Local wound care can then be carried out by gentle daily cleansing with saline or dilute peroxide solution. After about 1 week, the nail bed becomes nontender and only a light dressing need be applied.

FINGERTIP INJURIES

In injuries less than 1 cm² with soft-tissue loss and no bone exposed, débridement and healing by secondary intention provides excellent results. All devitalized edges are sharply and carefully removed and a contoured piece of xeroform gauze is applied followed by a soft dressing. After 5 days, the original dressing is removed and daily wet to dry dressing changes are begun with reapplication of xeroform gauze and a light dressing. Wound granulation and contracture can take 3 to 5 weeks. An interesting but similar technique using a Hyphean finger cap to injuries of even larger dimensions has been proved to be effective.[2]

Larger defects, without exposed bone, can be covered by full-thickness grafting techniques. One of the most commonly used areas is the hypothenar eminence region. An ellipse of skin approximately 2 × 6 cm can be taken from the hypothenar region, with the dorsal margin of the limit being at the junction of the palmar and dorsal skin (Fig. 3). After the skin ellipse is incised at its distal margin, one can harvest it and nearly completely defat it by using a skin hook for traction and sharply elevating the skin graft at the dermal subcutaneous fat level. Care should be taken not to

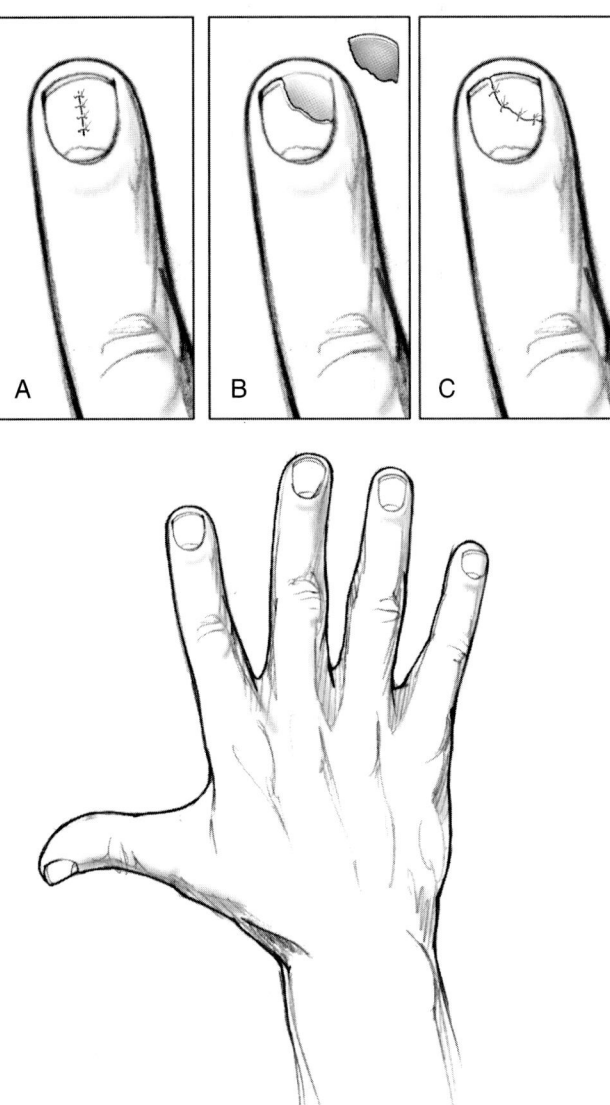

Fig. 1. Nail bed lacerations and repairs. *A,* Simple laceration repaired with interrupted absorbable sutures. *B,* Nail bed laceration with portion of nail bed adherent to nail. *C,* Composite nail bed/nail plate piece sutured back in place.

flexion crease in the midline of the digit. One carefully mobilizes the flap under loupe magnification, with digital tourniquet control, by incising the skin and dermis with a scalpel. Then the fibrous septa that anchor the pulp to the underlying distal phalanx can be carefully divided with a scalpel or sharp iris scissors. Then to mobilize the deepest aspect of the flap, from the distal aspect of the wound, a No. 15 scalpel blade is used to fully release the flap from the periosteum by sweeping along the volar aspect of the distal phalanx. After the flap is fully mobilized distally, the distal margin can be sewn to the nail bed with 5-0 nylon suture or a long-acting absorbable suture such as a polydioxanone suture. The digital tourniquet can be released to check adequacy of flap perfusion. If the flap has inadequate inflow, it should be released distally, the digit shortened slightly, and the flap then replaced in a position of less tension. After adequate inflow to the flap is confirmed, the remaining incisions can be closed loosely with 5-0 or 6-0 nylon (Fig. 5).

Regional flaps, including cross-finger flaps and thenar flaps, can be used with oblique soft-tissue injuries when there is more volar than dorsal soft-tissue loss such that local flap coverage would be insufficient (Fig. 6). The standard cross-finger flap is outlined as a rectangle over the middle phalanx of the donor digit. This rectangle can then be contoured to better fit the defect after it is elevated. The longitudinal axis of the "hinge" of the flap is the mid-

perforate the graft. This is best accomplished by rolling the graft over the index finger, keeping it under maximal tension with the skin hook, and using sharp scalpel blades. After the skin graft is harvested, it is contoured to fit the defect and sewn in place with multiple 5-0 nylon sutures. Several of the sutures should be left long for tying down a bolster of gauze over the graft for even compression (Fig. 4). This dressing should be left in place for 10 to 14 days. At that time, sutures can be removed and a light dressing applied.

For fingertip injuries with more tissue loss dorsally than volarly, the V-Y flap (Tranquilli-Leali flap), popularized by Atasoy, is an excellent alternative.[14] The critical factor that must be assessed is whether there is enough tissue for distal advancement. The distal edge of the flap can be advanced only about 1 cm. The flap is patterned with the distal margin of the flap or base of the triangle as the wound margin. The apex of the flap is at the distal digital

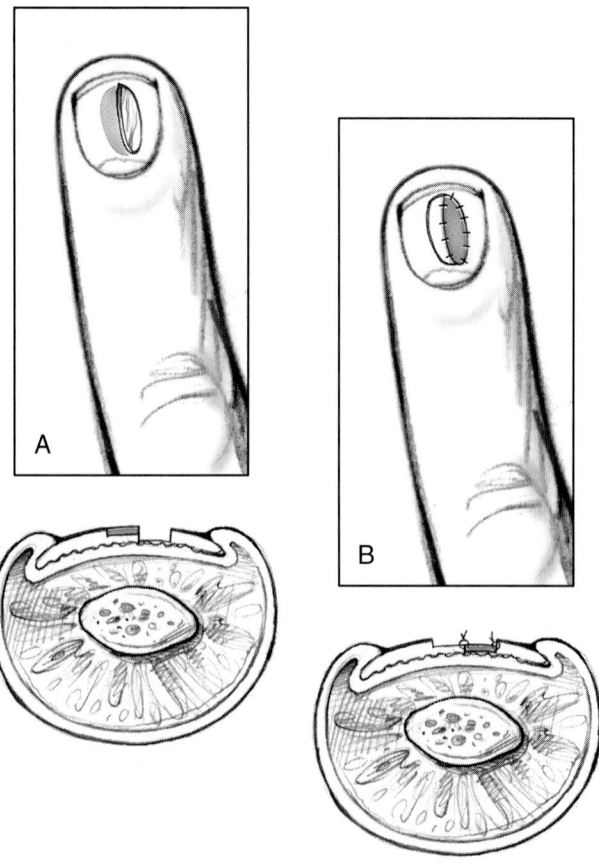

Fig. 2. Nail bed laceration with substance loss of nail matrix. *A,* Injury with loss of sterile matrix portion (coronal and axial views). *B,* Depiction of donor site adjacent split-thickness nail bed graft (shaded area) and repair with graft sutured in place.

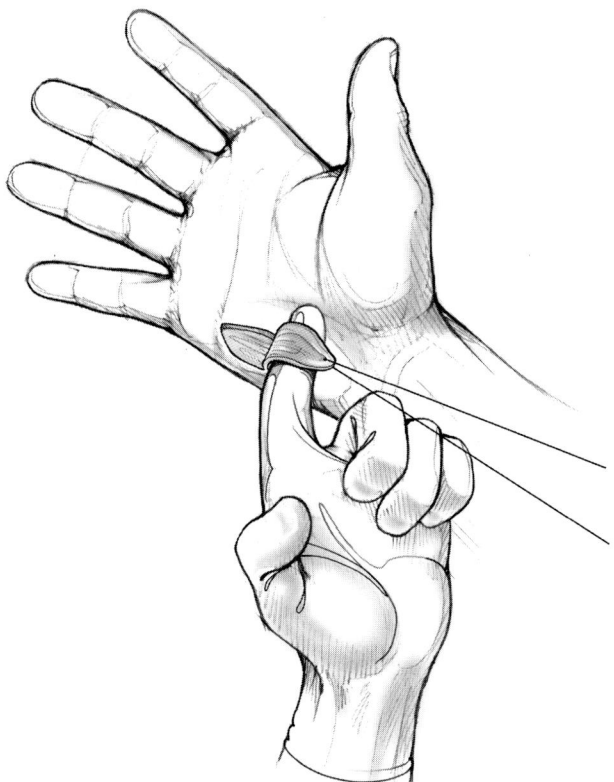

Fig. 3. Technique for harvesting full-thickness skin graft from ulnar border of hand.

lateral line adjacent to the injured digit. The skin is incised on three sides of the rectangle, leaving the hinge intact. The incision is carried down to the level of the peritoneum, which must be protected. The flap is elevated towards the

"hinge" side. To obtain full length of the flap, Cleland's ligaments deep to the hinge side of the flap need to be carefully released, with care taken not to injure the underlying digital artery. Then an appropriately sized full-thickness skin graft is harvested from the groin or upper inner arm by the same technique shown in Figure 3. The skin graft is then sewn in place over the donor defect with several sutures left long to allow for a bolster to be tied in place. The elevated flap can then be sewn in place over the defect of the injured digit. Light dressings are applied. The flap is divided under local anesthesia at 12 to 14 days, and the divided margin can be left open to close secondarily or closed primarily. Subsequently, digital range of motion exercises are instituted to minimize digital stiffness.

Thenar flaps are another option for digital tip loss. They are best used in younger patients or children, when the defect of the finger is angled volarly with exposure of the tuft of the distal phalanx but the entirety of the palmar pulp is not lost. The standard thenar flap is achieved by flexing the injured digit into the palm, and the dimensions of the flap are patterned to fit the soft tissue defect of the digit. A proximally based flap is then raised at the level of the palmar fascia/subcutaneous fat junction. At this juncture, a full-thickness skin graft the size of the donor defect is sewn into place prior to insetting the flap. Finally, the elevated flap is sewn in place, covering the defect in the digit. A light dressing is applied, and the hand is splinted. The flap is then divided after 12 to 14 days under local anesthesia. Subsequently, digital range of motion exercises are instituted.

COMPLICATIONS

Complications from surgery on nail bed injuries are poorly documented. The development of an infection can ad-

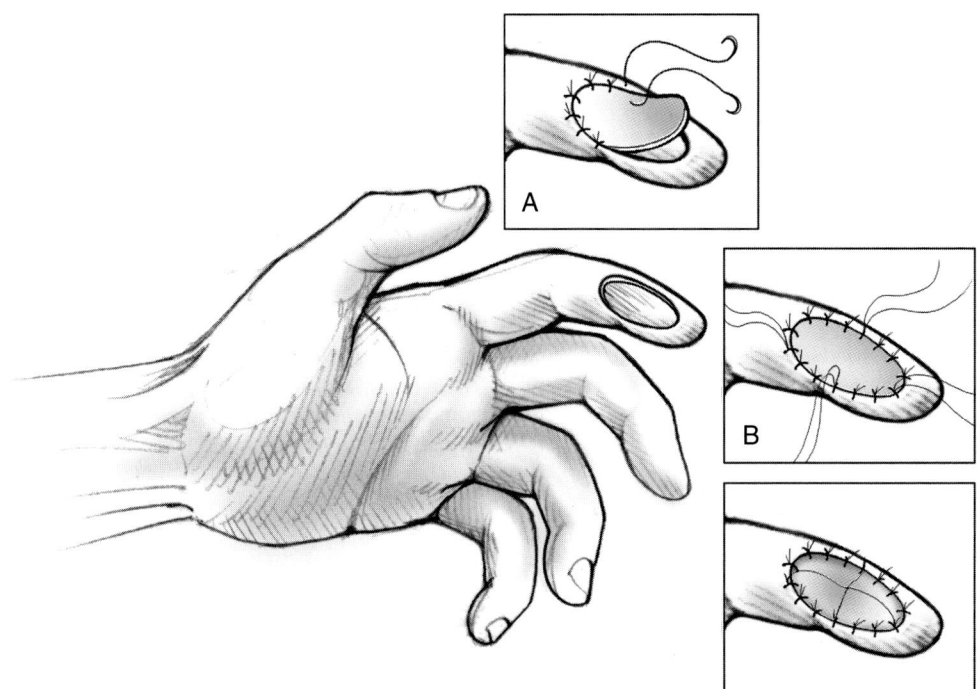

Fig. 4. Full-thickness skin grafting for fingertip injury. *A*, Full-thickness skin graft (harvested as in Fig. 3) being sutured into place. *B*, Graft fully sutured in place with several sutures left long to hold cotton bolster securely in place.

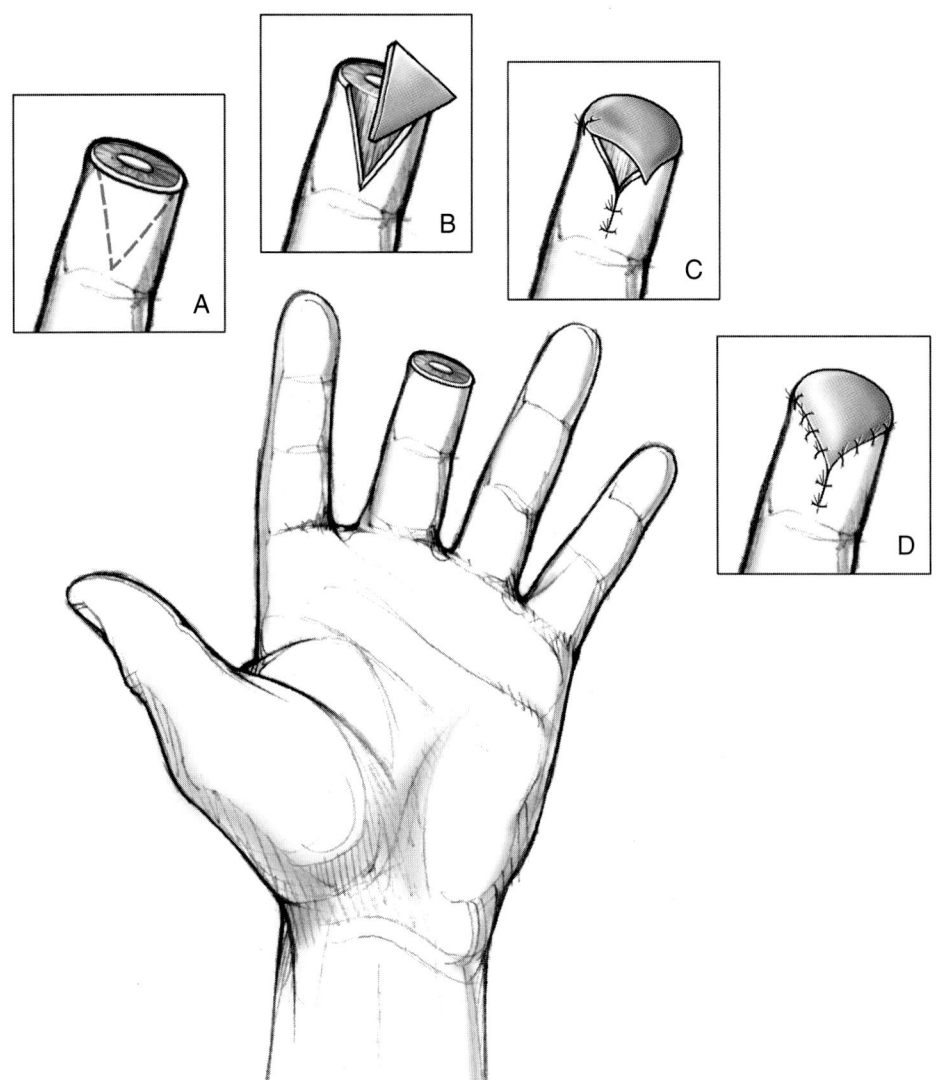

Fig. 5. V-Y flap. *A,* Outline of triangular flap. *B,* Flap incised and fully mobilized. *C,* Initial inset of flap. *D,* Flap fully inset with multiple sutures.

versely affect the outcome.[4] As in any infection, débridement and antibiotics with secondary coverage are necessary. Complications in fingertip reconstruction include infection and digital joint stiffness. Digital joint stiffness is particularly noted in the use of thenar flaps. However, Grab et al[32] reported satisfactory results in patients ranging from 2 to 76 years of age. When performing a thenar flap, one must take care to appropriately flex the metacarpophalangeal joint to prevent undesirable proximal interphalangeal joint stiffness. A splint should be used to maintain this metacarpophalangeal flexion until division of the flap is performed. Digital joint stiffness is not as much of a problem in cross-finger flaps. This is considered one of the reasons to perform a cross-finger flap instead of a thenar flap.

OUTCOMES AND RESULTS

Zook et al[4] monitored 184 nail bed repairs for 6 months or longer. Evaluation took into account shape surface charac-

teristics, splitting, and the appearance of the eponychial fold. All split nails, nails with less than two-thirds adherence, and very rough nails were considered major deformities. Other deformities were considered minor. The sum of minor and major variations for each fingertip was used to determine a grade of excellent, very good, good, fair, or poor for each result. An excellent result was a repaired nail identical to the opposite nail. Very good nails exhibited one minor variation. A nail with a good result had two minor variations, whereas one with a fair result had three minor variations or one major variation. A nail with a poor result exhibited more than three minor or one major variation. Fifty-five percent excellent, 24% very good, 11% good, 2% fair, and 8% poor results were found. Kleinert et al[3] reviewed nail bed injuries and their secondary deformities in a classic article in 1967. This paper reviews the complications, including split nails, poorly adherent nails, bone spurs causing cracked nails, ingrown nails, wide nails, protruding nails, and malaligned nails. This review also details methods of correction of these deformities.

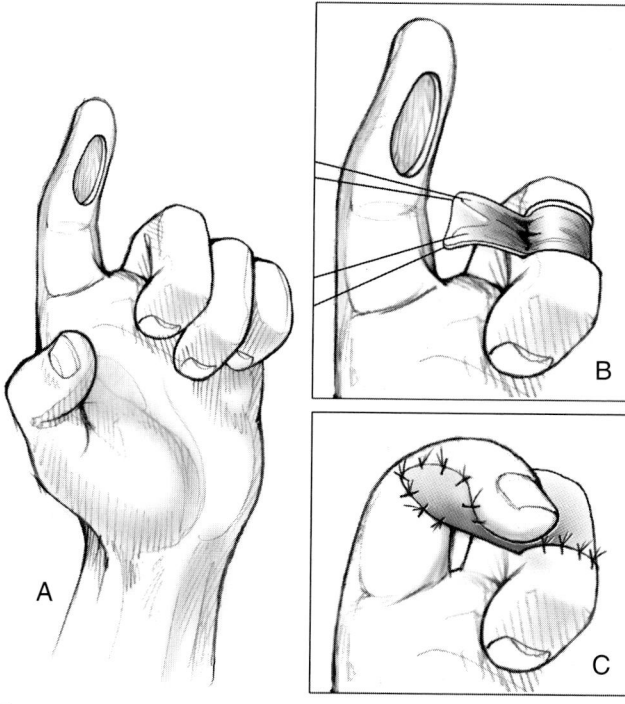

Both reports recommend the best way to avoid these complications by primary and accurate repair of injured nail beds.

Long-term follow-up of fingertip injuries are not well documented in the literature. Digital hypersensitivity and cold intolerance are common for the first 12 months. However, accurate determination as to the extent and the duration of these symptoms has not been determined in clinical follow-up studies. One noted problem in volar V-Y flaps that are sewn to the remaining nail matrix under too much tension is a hook nail deformity. The nail bed is drawn distally and poor bony support causes the hook deformity. Attempts at correction include further shortening of the nail matrix and provision of soft tissue coverage to augment the pulp of the digit. Alternatively soft tissue in the form of a cross-finger flap with a bone graft can be attempted to add bony support as well as soft tissue coverage. These procedures usually improve the hook deformity, but complete correction is uncommon. Most patients who undergo standard cross-finger flaps have a return of protective sensibility (8 mm two-point discrimination), but the sensibility is always less than normal. Only half of patients older than 40 years have return of protective sensibility.[33]

Fig. 6. Cross-finger flap. *A*, Injury. *B*, Elevation of flap. *C*, Flap inset.

REFERENCES

1. Flatt AE: Minor hand injuries with bone joint surgery. J Bone Joint Surg Br 1955; 37:117.
2. Schiller C: Nail replacement in fingertip injures. Plast Reconstr Surg 1957; 19:521.
3. Kleinert HK, Patcha SM: The deformed nail, a frequent result of failure to repair nailbed injuries. J Trauma 1967; 7:177.
4. Zook EG, Guy RJ, et al: A study of nail-bed injuries: causes, treatment, prognosis. J Hand Surg Am 1984; 9:247.
5. Louis DS, Palmer AK, Burney RE: Open treatment of digital tip injuries. JAMA 1980; 244:697.
6. Lee LP, Lam PY: A simple and efficient treatment for fingertip injuries. J Hand Surg Br 1995; 20:63.
7. Sturman M: Late results of fingertip injuries. J Bone Joint Surg 1963; 45:289.
8. Patton HS: Split skin graft from hypothenar area for fingertip avulsions. Plast Reconstr Surg 1969; 43:426.
9. O'Malley TS: Full thickness skin grafts in finger amputations. WIS Med J 1934; 33:337.
10. Lie MK: Free full thickness skin graft from the palm to cover defects of the fingers. J Bone Joint Surg Am 1970; 52:559.
11. Mack GR: Free palmar skin grafts for resurfacing digital defects. J Hand Surg Am 1981; 6:565.
12. Schenck RR, Cheema TA: Hypothenar skin grafts for fingertip reconstruction. J Hand Surg Am 1984; 9:750.
13. Tranquilli-Leali: Ricostruzione dell'apice falangi ungueali mediante autoplastica volare peduncolata per scorrimento. Infortin Traum Lav 1935; 1:186.
14. Atasoy E: Reconstruction of the amputated fingertip with a triangular volar flap. J Bone Joint Surg Am 1970; 52:911.
15. Kutler W: A method for repair of finger amputation. Ohio State Med J 1944; 40:126.
16. Fisher RH: The Kutler method of repair of fingertip amputations. J Bone Joint Surg Am 1967; 49:317.
17. Gatewood R: A plastic repair of fingertip defects without hospitalization. JAMA 1926; 187:1479.
18. Flatt AE: The thenar flap. J Bone Joint Surg Br 1957; 39:80.
19. Barton NJ: A modified thenar flap. Hand 1975; 7:150.
20. Smith RJ, Albine R: Thenar "H-flap" for fingertip injuries. J Trauma 1976; 16:778.
21. Gurdin M, Pangman WJ: The repair of surface defects of fingers by transdigital flaps. Plast Reconstr Surg 1950; 5:368.
22. Cronin JD: The cross-finger flap: A new method of repair. Am Surg 1951; 17:419.
23. Tempest MN: Cross-finger flaps in the treatment of injuries to the fingertip. Plast Reconstr Surg 1952; 9:205.
24. Atasoy E: Reversed cross-finger flaps. J Hand Surg 1980; 5:572.
25. Foucher G, Braun JB: A new island flap transfer from the dorsum of the index to the thumb. Plast Reconstr Surg 1979; 63:344.
26. Sherif MM: First dorsal metacarpal artery flap in hand reconstruction: II. Clinical application. J Hand Surg Am 1994; 19:32.
27. Littler JW: Neurovascular pedicle method of digital transposition for reconstruction of the thumb. Plast Reconstr Surg 1953; 12:303.
28. Sapp JW, Allen RJ: A reversed digit artery island flap for the treatment of fingertip injuries. J Hand Surg Am 1993; 18:528.
29. Lanzetta M, Mastropasoua B: Versatility of the homodigital triangular island flap in fingertip reconstruction. J Hand Surg Br 1995; 20:824.
30. Tsai TM, Yeun JC: A neurovascular flap for volar-oblique fingertip amputations: Analysis of long-term results. J Hand Surg Br 1996; 21:94.
31. Kamai K, Ide Y: A new thenar free flap. Plast Reconstr Surg 1993; 92:1380.
32. Grab JB, Beasley RW: Fingertip reconstruction. Hand Clin 1985; 1:667.
33. Kleinert HE, McAllister CG, et al: A critical evaluation of cross finger flaps. J Trauma 1974; 14:756.

FLEXOR TENDON INJURIES

Fraser J. Leversedge and John G. Seiler III

Summary

- Primary tenorrhaphy of flexor tendon lacerations, regardless of injury zone, is the preferred method of treatment.
- Zone II repairs require a precise knowledge of anatomy, meticulous technique, and strict adherence to postoperative rehabilitation protocols.
- To optimize results, especially following zone II repairs, a supervised program employing passive range of motion with an extension block splint is necessary.
- Complications, including tendon adhesions, digital contractures, and repair disruption, may cause a suboptimal result.

"It is not difficult to suture tendons and prepare the ground for sound union; the real problem is to obtain a freely sliding tendon capable of restoring good function."

R. Guy Pulvertaft, 1948[1]

"The process of tendon repair and the technic of tendon suture and tendon graft are two of the major problems of present day surgery."

Mason and Shearon, 1932[2]

Successful treatment of flexor tendon injuries remains one of the most difficult problems in hand surgery. Although these injuries have historically been associated with significant hand impairment, new treatment methods have greatly improved patient outcomes. Still, it is often difficult to solve the paradox of necessary tendon repair and free soft-tissue gliding. Current investigations continue to explore strategies that allow differential soft-tissue incorporation in the clinical setting. The purpose of this chapter is to review the anatomy of the flexor tendon apparatus, the physiology of tendon repair, techniques currently used to suture flexor tendons, and modern aftercare regimens.

HISTORICAL REVIEW

Nearly 100 years ago, Erich Lexer emphasized meticulous surgical technique in repairing flexor tendons.[3] Bunnell stressed the importance of strict atraumatic technique in the handling of tendons and surrounding tissues, aseptic protocol, a bloodless field, and careful assistance. He later added that the use of sharp instruments, good lighting, and a comfortable working position for the surgeon would enhance surgical outcomes. He also coined the term "no man's land" to describe the region of the finger where the results of primary tendon repair were poor.[4, 5] The disappointing functional results led Bunnell and many of his contemporaries to recommend delayed tendon grafting as the treatment for zone II tendon injuries.

Based on observations of canine tendon healing, in 1932, Mason and Shearon described a two-stage tendon repair process. An "exudative phase" of approximately 21 days is characterized by a gelatinous exudative interconnection of the repair site and an adhesive continuity between the sheath and peritendinous tissues. Subsequently a "formative phase" occurs, during which time the tendon cells proliferate into the callus with a proportional increase in the tensile strength of the repair site related to the loads applied across the tendon.[2] Lindsay, in 1959, investigated flexor tendon healing in chickens and concluded that the peritendinous tissues participated extensively in the repair process—by cellular differentiation, proliferation, and migration into the repair site. In 1962, Potenza described an extrinsic mechanism of repair showing adhesion formation and obliteration of the tendon's gliding surface following intrasynovial tendon repair and complete post-repair immobilization in a canine model. Only minimal repair response was observed at the tendon ends; rather dense fibrous adhesions occurred at points of disruptions in the peritendinous tissues. These adhesions were viewed as a vital source of vascular ingrowth for the healing tendons.[6]

Basic scientific studies have attempted to further evaluate the roles of intrinsic and extrinsic repair mechanisms, both for primary flexor tendon repair and for associated methods of delayed flexor tendon grafting, crucial pulley reconstruction, and repair of the surrounding tissues such as the tendon sheath.[7–18] The advancing fields of molecular and cellular biology have permitted further study of the tendon repair response and the interaction with surrounding tissues. Prevention of motion-limiting adhesions continues to be investigated with the potential for the use of biologic and synthetic barriers to adhesion formation.[19–21]

ANATOMY

The flexor digitorum superficialis (FDS) arises from multiple points on the volar surface of the humerus, ulna, and radius. By the middle third of the forearm, the superficialis muscle belly has divided into four bundles, which in turn further divide into a superficial and a deep layer, the superficial layer sending its tendons to the long and ring fingers and the deeper layer extending tendons to the index and small fingers. In the forearm, the distinct FDS muscle bundles allow independent flexion of the digits. The oval-shaped superficialis tendon lies palmar to the flexor digitorum profundus (FDP) tendon along its course until entering the digital sheath. The FDP has a common muscular origin, which often results in recruitment of multiple digits during active flexion. At the level of the A1 pulley, the superficialis tendon flattens out and splits to allow the deeper profundus tendon to pass distally to its insertion at the distal phalanx. In the digit, the bifurcating limbs of the superficialis tendon rotate away from the midline and wrap around the profundus tendon with half of the fibers crossing on the palmar surface of the phalanx (known as the chiasma tendinum of Camper)[22] to insert dorsal to the profundus tendon on the palmar surface of the proximal half of the middle phalanx. The remaining fibers continue distally to insert as respectively named radial and ulnar slips onto the base of the middle phalanx.

In an effort to accurately describe tendon injuries, Kleinert and Verdan classified tendon injuries by anatomic zones (Fig. 1).[23] The tendons begin in the distal third of the forearm and course distally through five anatomic zones. Zone V begins at the muscle-tendon junction and extends to the proximal wrist crease and the entrance to the carpal canal. Nine flexor tendons and the median nerve enter the carpal canal and zone IV deep to the transverse carpal ligament. The region, from the distal edge of the transverse carpal ligament to the start of the digital fibro-osseous sheath (zone III) is described as the lumbrical zone. Zone II begins at the level of the metacarpal neck, concurrent with the origin of the flexor sheath, and extends to the insertion of the FDS tendon within the digit. Distal to the FDS insertion is zone I.

The flexor pollicis longus (FPL) takes its broad origin from the volar surface of the middle and distal third of the radius and from the radial third of the interosseous membrane. The FPL enters its digital sheath proximal to the entrance to the carpal canal and continues distally to insert at the base of the distal phalanx of the thumb after passing between the two sesamoids at the volar plate of the metacarpophalangeal (MCP) joint.

PULLEYS OF THE DIGIT

Within the hand, flexor tendon fascicles are covered by a thin visceral and parietal adventitia, or paratenon, which contains synovial-like fluid. At the base of each digit, the tendons enter a synovial-lined fibro-osseous tunnel, which

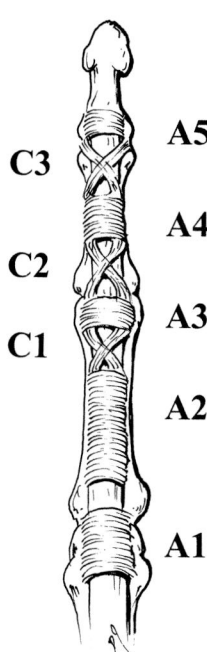

Fig. 2. Pulleys of the digit. These are annular (A1–A5) and cruciform pulleys (C1–C3), which provide a biomechanical advantage by maximizing the efficiency of joint rotation and force transmission.

provides both a biomechanical advantage and a source of tendon nutrition.[24]

Condensations of the synovial sheaths form at strategic points along the digit and work in conjunction with the palmar aponeurosis pulley and the transverse carpal ligament to maximize efficiency of joint rotation and force transmission. Five annular pulleys and three cruciform pulleys have been described.[22] Biomechanical studies have concluded that the A2 and A4 annular pulleys are the most important.[24-26] The A1, A3, and A5 pulleys originate from the palmar plates of the MCP, proximal interphalangeal (PIP), and distal interphalangeal (DIP) joints, respectively. The A2 and A4 pulleys are continuous with the periosteum of the proximal aspect of the proximal phalanx and of the middle third of the middle phalanx, respectively. The cruciform pulleys are relatively thin and accordion onto adjacent annular pulleys during finger flexion. The cruciform pulleys are located between A2 and A3 (C1), between A3 and A4 (C2), and between A4 and A5 (C3) (Fig. 2).[24]

PULLEYS OF THE THUMB

Three pulleys, the A1, A2, and oblique pulleys, comprise the pulley system of the thumb. The A1 pulley is located at the level of the MCP joint, attaching to the volar plate and the base of the proximal phalanx. The oblique pulley is oriented in a distal and radial direction at the level of the diaphysis of the proximal phalanx. The distal A2 pulley overlies the interphalangeal joint, taking its origin from the volar plate.

The flexor sheath and pulley apparatus maintain an optimal moment arm between the flexor tendon and the joint center of rotation. Any tendon bowstringing produced by pulley insufficiency will increase the effective moment arm.

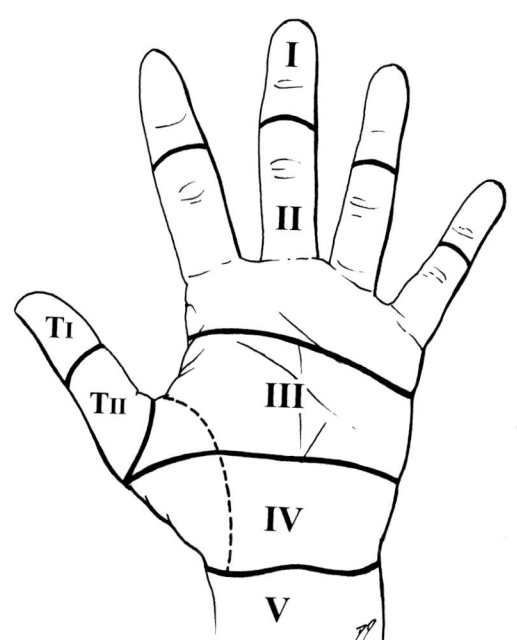

Fig. 1 Classification of flexor tendon injuries by anatomic zones.

VASCULAR SUPPLY

The flexor tendon has three primary sources of vascular supply.[25–29] The paratenon contains longitudinally aligned vessels within its substance.[30] The mesotendon, or sheath equivalent, represents a dual source of nutrition through its vascular contributions and a mechanism of synovial diffusion. Finally, the osseous insertions of each tendon provide a third source of vascular supply.

BIOLOGY

CURRENT CONCEPTS OF FLEXOR TENDON REPAIR

The process of tendon repair evolves through three phases: inflammatory, reparative, and remodeling.[2, 6, 31, 32] Following tendon suture, an inflammatory response involves the formation of a fibrin clot and migration of macrophages and other inflammatory cells to the repair site. Associated release of growth factors and chemotactic factors such as fibronectin occurs.[17, 33, 34] In the 2 cm area surrounding the repair, cells within the epitenon proliferate and migrate to the repair site.[14, 35] At approximately 10 days following repair, the gliding surface has been restored.[16, 36] The strength of the repair site during this stage is related to the strength of the tendon suture method.[16]

A reparative phase, lasting approximately 28 days, follows the initial inflammatory period. This phase has been characterized primarily by the intense production of collagen by epitenon cells, which forms a dynamic scaffolding across the repair site.

A later remodeling phase is characterized by collagen remodeling and decreased rates of cell division. Increased tensile strength reported at the repair site is consistent with the structural remodeling of collagen fibrils and revascularization of the repair site.[2, 6, 7, 14, 16, 32, 37]

Restoration of flexor tendon gliding surface and tensile strength following repair is also dependent on postoperative rehabilitation methods. Early tendon mobilization has been demonstrated to limit peritendinous adhesion formation and to improve the repair site healing response, tendon excursion, and tensile strength.[36, 38–44] Particularly, tendon excursion and tensile strength were observed to improve with increased frequency and duration of postoperative mobilization exercises. A dose-response curve for postoperative mobilization has been confirmed in prospective clinical trials.[45]

During early phases of tendon healing, repair site strength is primarily dependent on the strength of suture method. To permit earlier active tendon mobilization, various new suture methods have been developed to provide increased strength. Initial repair site strength is directly related to the intrinsic properties of the type of suture used, the number of suture strands traversing the repair site, and the number of grasping loops incorporated into the repair.[41, 46–48] The addition of an epitendinous finishing suture has been shown to be of benefit, both providing added tensile strength and smoothing the repair site.[49]

Rehabilitation protocols that employ early active tendon mobilization are designed to be used with newer multistrand, multigrasp suture methods and compliant patients. These programs increase early linear tendon excursion and apply increased loads to tendon repair sites. Although still under investigation (TE Trumble and JG Seiler, unpublished data), it is hoped that by increasing early tendon excursion, the formation of peritendinous adhesions will diminish and later function will improve. Further early load application to the repair site may enhance the tendon repair process. If excessive loads are applied to the repair site, then tendon repair gap formation or repair site rupture may occur.

CLINICAL FEATURES

HISTORY

Injury to the flexor tendons results from multiple causes. Structures associated by proximity may also be injured, and therefore a thorough, well-documented history and physical examination are imperative. Information such as occupation, hand dominance, tetanus status, and other pertinent medical history may assist in both preoperative planning and postoperative rehabilitation. Time from injury should be established. In cases of open injury, time to presentation may preclude immediate operative repair, owing to the need for initial wound irrigation and débridement. The mechanism of injury is important to predicting the nature of surgical treatment. A laceration caused by the gripping of a knife blade may place the tendon transection more distal to the skin defect with the digits held in extension at the time of surgery.

CLINICAL EXAMINATION

Evaluation of gross wound contamination and involvement of bony, neurovascular, and soft tissues is important for operative decision making. The wound location is considered for incorporation into a more formal digital exposure. Neurovascular evaluation should be conducted before infiltration of the affected region with local anesthetic.

Assessment of tendon continuity is done by both direct visualization (at the point of laceration, if applicable) and by clinical evaluation based on a knowledge of tendon anatomy. FDP assessment is performed with the dorsum of the affected digit placed flat on a firm surface with the MCP and PIP joints blocked in extension. Ability to actively flex the DIP joint in this position indicates that the FDP tendon is intact. Although the FDP is the only flexor of the DIP joint, it also acts as a secondary flexor to the PIP joint. Therefore, to assess the function of the FDS, the FDP must be restrained. This is done by blocking the profundi to the nonaffected digits in full extension while the patient attempts to flex the PIP joint of the free digit. Examination should also be done for painful flexion, which often indicates a partial tendon injury.

CLASSIFICATION

TENDON LACERATION

Transection or laceration injuries to flexor tendons are defined by their zone of injury and as complete or incomplete transections. These anatomic divisions allow the surgeon to plan for repair.

TENDON AVULSION

Isolated avulsion of the insertion of the FDS tendon from the proximal phalanx is extremely rare. Avulsion of the

TABLE 1. CLASSIFICATION OF FLEXOR TENDON AVULSION INJURIES

Type	Injury	Prognosis
I	FDP retraction proximal to A1 pulley	Poor
II	FDP retraction to PIP joint	Moderate
III	FDP retraction to A4 pulley	Good
IIIA	Type III injury with subsequent dissociation and retraction of tendon from bony fragment	Poor

FDP, flexor digitorum profundus; PIP, proximal interphalangeal.

FDP tendon at its insertion on the distal phalanx is more common, particularly in sporting activities. This avulsion injury most commonly occurs in young males participating in sports. The mechanism is of a sudden forced extension of a flexed digit, such as occurs while attempting to grasp the shirt or collar of a fleeing opponent (hence the term "rugger jersey finger"). These eccentric contractions result in applied loads that are sufficient to rupture the flexor insertion. The ring finger is the most commonly involved digit.

A classification system for FDP bony avulsion injuries is important, as it emphasizes the variation in both prognosis and treatment choices based on the level of tendon retraction, the remaining sources of nutrition to the avulsed tendon, and the nature of the potential bony avulsion fragment. Leddy and Packer[50] have described a useful scheme of three main types of bony FDP avulsion injuries (types I, II, and III), which is supplemented by a fourth, rare type IIIA injury described by Robins and Dobyns in 1975 (Table 1).[51, 52] For all types of avulsion injuries, preoperative radiographs facilitate accurate injury assessment.

Type I

Type I injuries involve an avulsion of the FDP insertion and subsequent retraction of the tendon and its bony attachment beneath the A1 pulley and into the palm. In doing so, the tendon is stripped of its regional source of vascular supply and is removed from the intrasynovial environment. Owing to the significant compromise of tendon nutrition and of the resulting contracture from prolonged retraction of the tendon into the palm following this type of injury, operative repair within 7 to 10 days is recommended.

Type II

Type II injuries are characterized by an avulsion of the profundus insertion with retraction to the level of the PIP joint. Prognosis is improved relative to the type I injuries because of the more distal retention of the vinculae and their associated vascular supply. The continuity of the synovial sheath remains intact, thus providing a source of synovial fluid diffusion. Early anatomic repair is preferred.

Type III and Type IIIA

In type III injuries, a large bony avulsion occurs from the distal phalanx and is trapped from retracting proximally by the A4 pulley. In contrast to types I and II injuries, the vinculae and synovial sheath remain in continuity. Conver-

sion of this injury to an unusual type IIIA lesion occurs when avulsion of the profundus tendon from the fracture fragment itself allows the tendon to retract proximally, comparable to that of a type I or type II injury.[51, 52]

PROCEDURE

PREOPERATIVE PLANNING

Surgical repair of flexor tendons is done in an operating room setting. Preoperatively, we routinely administer an intravenous dose of a first-generation cephalosporin (and an aminoglycoside if the wound is grossly contaminated). Tetanus toxoid and/or tetanus immunoglobulin are administered when indicated. Tendon repairs are done using optical magnification (2.5–3.5× loupe magnification).

GENERAL PRINCIPLES
Incision

In general, a midaxial or a Bruner-type incision is preferred for adequate exposure of the affected area; however, original lacerations should be incorporated into the exposure when feasible (Fig. 3). Meticulous hemostasis is imperative during dissection.

Tendon Retrieval

The divided tendon ends are localized and brought into the laceration site using windows created in the membranous portion of the flexor tendon sheath.[53, 54] Often, hemorrhage within the sheath identifies the retracted tendon. If the tendon has retracted proximally, a transverse incision is made in the palm to identify the proximal tendon. A pediatric feeding tube, passed retrograde from the initial wound, may be sutured to the proximal tendon end, allowing delivery of the tendon into the digit with retraction of the feeding tube. The distal tendon end is located by direct exposure and flexion of the distal digit.

Throughout the procedure, tendon handling is minimized. Disruption of the epitenon promotes adhesion formation. Following delivery of the transected tendon ends

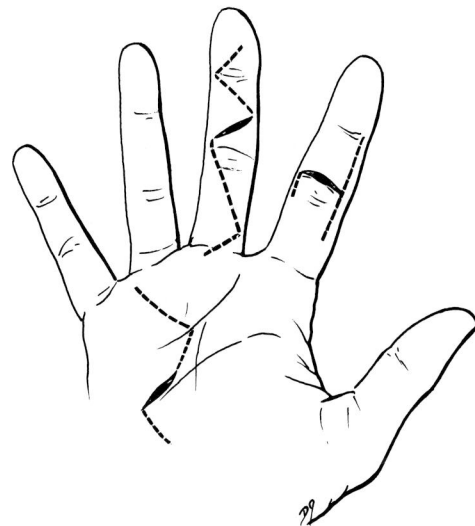

Fig. 3. Surgical incision. This shows incorporation of lacerations or skin wounds into surgical incisions. Volar zig-zag (Bruner's) or midaxial incisions are both acceptable.

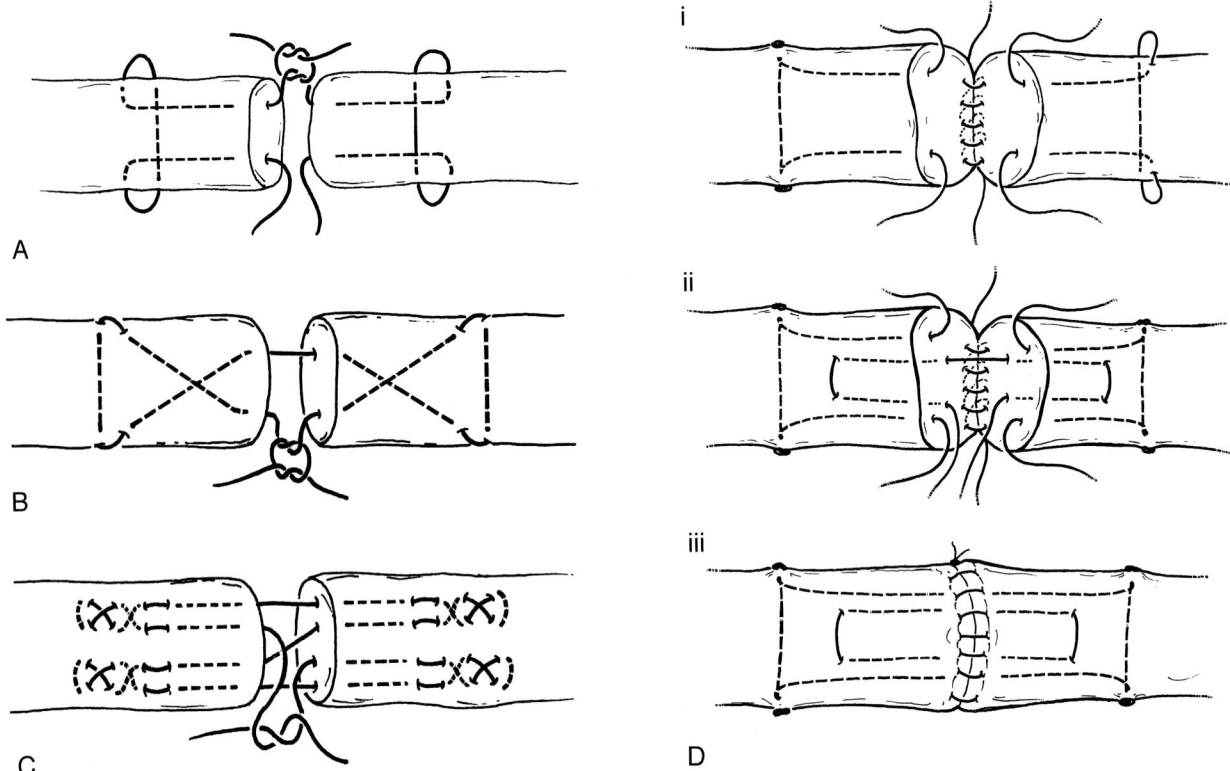

Fig. 4. Suture methods. *A*, Modified Kessler's (two sutures) technique. *B*, Kleinert's modification of Bunnell's technique. *C*, Savage's (modified four-strand) technique. *D*, Strickland's four-strand technique: basic two-strand core suture (i) is supplemented by a central horizontal-mattress suture (ii) and is finished with a peripheral epitendinous running-lock stitch (iii).

into the laceration site, Keith's needles or 20-gauge hypodermic needles are placed transversely through the tendon approximately 2 cm proximal and distal to the transected ends and into the surrounding soft tissue. With both ends of the flexor tendons anatomically configured and in a stable position, flexor tendon repair can be completed.

Suture Technique

Currently we use a multistrand, multigrasp repair that is of sufficient strength to allow early active tendon mobilization (Fig. 4). We have found it helpful to repair the dorsal tendon using the epitendinous suture prior to placing the core suture.[55] This technical modification allows accurate tendon coaptation and eliminates the need to rotate the tendon to place the back wall epitenon sutures. The core sutures are placed next. Finally, the repair is finished with a running, unlocked 6-0 nylon epitendinous suture that smoothes the tendon ends and encloses the core suture knots within the site of repair. Preservation of the crucial pulleys is imperative to minimize tendon bowstringing and to minimize loss of grip strength. Reconstruction or repair of the A2 and A4 pulleys should be done to provide improved biomechanical function and to prevent significant tendon bowstringing.

SPECIAL CONSIDERATIONS IN REPAIR

ZONE I

Zone I injuries, distal to the FDS insertion, involve the FDP tendon only. Lacerations are repaired by direct end-to-end suture or, if insufficient distal tendon stump is avail-

able, by tendon advancement and reinsertion into the distal phalanx. In general, minimal retraction of the lacerated tendon occurs due to the stabilizing effect of the vinculae. The functionally important A4 pulley should be preserved and if the pulley is rendered incompetent by injury, then reconstruction should be done. Direct end-to-end repair is done using a standard combined core and epitendinous suture method. If less than 1 cm of distal stump remains or if the residual tendon stump is incapable of stable suture repair, then tendon advancement of up to 1 cm may be done.[56] The distal tendon is débrided and a periosteal flap is raised distal to the palmar plate at the base of the distal phalanx. Our preference for tendon reinsertion is by a modified Bunnell pull-out wire and button technique (Fig. 5). An oblique drill hole is made from the raised periosteal flap and directed dorsally. A 3-0 Prolene suture (double-armed, straight needles) is placed in a single, crisscross or nonlocking fashion into the proximal tendon stump. The free suture ends are then passed through the bony tunnel and tied over a well-padded, dorsally placed button. The tendon should not be advanced too far within the distal phalanx because a DIP joint flexion contracture could result. Postoperatively, a standard protocol of controlled active or early passive motion is used. The pull-out suture is removed at 6 weeks.

ZONE II

Repair of zone II injuries often requires more extensile exposure of the digit. Full-thickness skin and subcutaneous tissue flaps should be raised to limit the risk of skin necrosis. The A2 and A4 pulleys should be preserved.

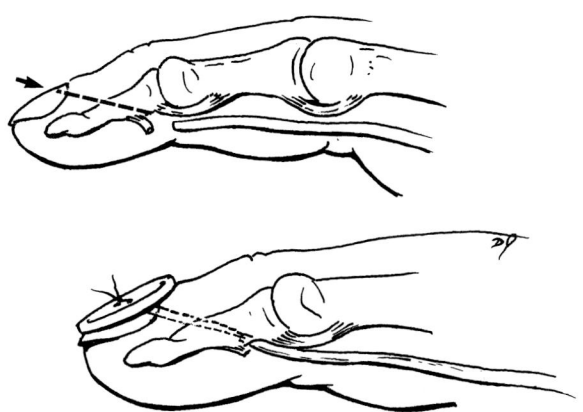

Fig. 5. Pull-through suture technique for zone I injuries. A single, nonlocking permanent suture (3-0 Prolene) is placed in the end of the distal tendon stump. The suture is passed through an oblique drill hole in the distal phalanx, and the distal tendon is advanced into a prepared cancellous trough within the base of the distal phalanx. The suture is tied over a well-padded button dorsally.

The proximal tendon may not be visible in the wound and one or a combination of techniques may be used for tendon recovery. "Milking" the tendon from each end with the wrist and MCP joints flexed may allow delivery of the proximal tendon into the wound. A fine tendon grasper can be used to retrieve tendons that are retained locally within the digital sheath. Tendons that have retracted into the palm have lost the stabilizing effect of their vincular attachments and may require a separate incision in the palm to locate the retracted tendon. A no. 5 pediatric feeding tube can be passed antegrade and temporarily sutured to the retracted tendons; it is then drawn distally and a repair is done using a core suture method with 4-0 braided nonabsorbable suture, supplemented by a running epitendinous suture of 6-0 nylon.

If transection of both FDS and FDP tendons occurs, we prefer to repair the FDS first, and then the FDP. It is imperative to re-establish the correct orientation of the superficialis and profundus tendons prior to repair. Lacerations of the FDS tendon proximal to its decussation are repaired using a core suture technique with 4-0 Dacron suture. The repair is finished with a running 6-0 nylon epitendinous suture. Those injuries distal to its split are repaired using horizontal mattress sutures of 4-0 braided Dacron suture.

ZONE III

Flexor tendon injuries in zone III may involve multiple complete and/or incomplete lacerations and may be associated with neurovascular compromise. Transected tendons are repaired and rehabilitated using the same principles as followed for zone I and II injuries with core and epitendinous suture methods.

ZONE IV

Injuries to the flexor tendons within the carpal canal, or zone IV, are less common due to the sheltered location of the tendons and median nerve. Each tendon should be identified and separately examined. Primary repair is indicated for all tendons. A core suture method using 4-0

braided Dacron suture is recommended. The epitendinous suture is not critical at this level, and the transverse carpal ligament is not repaired.

ZONE V

Injuries within zone V usually involve the laceration of multiple tendons and may be associated with neurovascular injury, particularly to median and ulnar nerves and radial and ulnar vessels. Early primary repair is recommended. Postoperatively, a standard early passive motion rehabilitation protocol is used unless repair of neural or vascular structures indicates an alternative method of rehabilitation.

FLEXOR POLLICIS LONGUS

In zone I injuries of the thumb, treatment principles are similar to those used with the digits. Up to 1 cm of tendon advancement may be done, with reinsertion into an osseous tunnel drilled into the distal phalanx. In unusual cases, additional tendon length may be gained by Z-lengthening of the FPL proximal to the wrist or by "fractional lengthening" at the musculotendinous junction. These methods will increase tendon length by 2 to 3 cm but will weaken the strength of FPL flexion.[57]

The A2 pulley is located in zone I and is preferentially preserved. The oblique and A1 pulleys are the biomechanically more important, however, as an intact oblique or first annular pulley can maintain functional tendon excursion.[58]

An appreciation for the comparative anatomy of thumb and digits is important in considering zone II injuries.[22] There are only one tendon (FPL) and two pulleys (oblique and A1) to consider. Only one pulley is required to prevent significant bowstringing. Often, significant retraction of the transected FPL is prevented by intact vinculae. If the vinculae are disrupted, the lacerated tendon will retract into the carpal canal or proximal to the wrist.

FLEXOR DIGITORUM PROFUNDUS AVULSION INJURIES
Type I

Adequate exposure of the tendon sheath and neurovascular bundles is done from the A2 pulley distal to the FDP insertion by a Bruner-type incision when necessary. If the profundus tendon has retracted proximally, a transverse incision is made in the distal palmar crease to expose the FDP tendon. A small pediatric feeding tube is passed retrograde and is anchored to the tube by suture and is passed distally. The tendon may be reattached to its insertion site by creation of a bony trough in the distal phalanx and suture fixation over a padded dorsal button (see description of zone I surgical repair). The pull-out suture is removed 6 weeks postoperatively, and standard rehabilitation for flexor tendon repair is followed.

Type II

Treatment of type II injuries is similar to that of type I injuries. The retracted tendon and bone fragment (if present) are identified and a transverse incision is made in the sheath distal to the A2 pulley and the tendon is passed to its insertion at the distal phalanx within the fibro-osseous sheath, as described earlier. A delay in treatment may result in a myostatic contracture or adhesion formation at

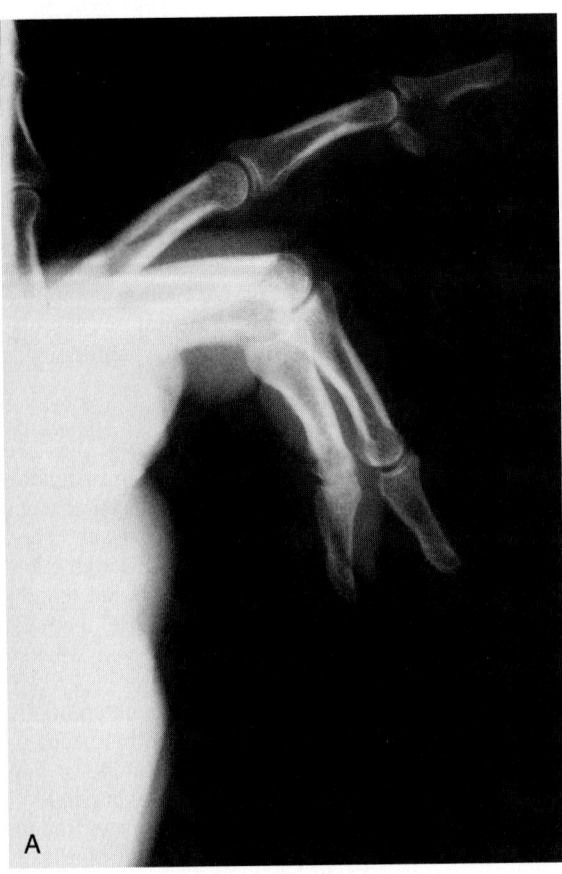
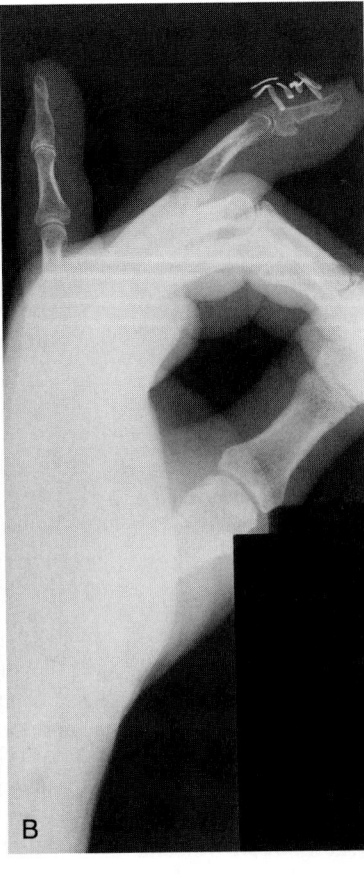

Fig. 6. Flexor digitorum profundus (FDP) avulsion injuries. These are lateral radiographs of a type III FDP avulsion injury. *A,* Injury radiograph. *B,* Postoperative radiograph demonstrating articular surface reduction and repair using a pull-through suture method.

the PIP joint, requiring intraoperative assessment and surgical proximal interphalangeal joint release.

Type III and Type IIIA

Open reduction and internal fixation of the bony fragment is preferred for type III or IIIA injuries, followed by subsequent retrieval and reinsertion of the avulsed tendon as recommended for type I or II injuries (based on the level of tendon retraction). Postoperative management is unchanged for type III injuries (Fig. 6).

PARTIAL TENDON LACERATIONS

Establishing consistent and accurate percentage estimates of incomplete lacerations of the flexor tendon is difficult. The study by Cooney et al and other studies suggest that an increased risk of triggering, entrapment, or rupture is associated with lacerations involving greater than 60% of the cross-sectional area of the tendon and recommend surgical intervention for those lacerations exceeding this value.[59] We recommend flap excision for partial flexor tendon lacerations involving 50% or less of the tendon's cross-sectional area. If the laceration is greater than 50%, then a traditional core suture method is used.

POSTOPERATIVE MANAGEMENT

Postoperative management of flexor tendon injuries is initiated with preoperative counseling as to individual expectations, realistic goals, and the need for commitment to rehabilitation. Historically, poor functional results have been

associated with postoperative immobilization (which encourages peritendinous adhesion formation), more severe injuries, and patient noncompliance. Contemporary investigations suggest that early motion facilitates intrinsic tendon repair, minimizing adhesion formation.[35, 37, 38, 41, 60–62] Individualized therapy and modified splinting may be indicated for contracture, associated neurological injury, or predicted patient noncompliance (i.e., in children).

Zone IV and V repairs are treated with early passive mobilization and extension block splinting for a total of 6 weeks. The wrist is positioned at 30 degrees of palmar flexion, the MCP joints at 45 degrees of flexion, and the interphalangeal joints in extension.

For zone I, II, and III injuries, we prefer two frequently used rehabilitation programs: a controlled active extension and passive flexion protocol described by Kleinert et al, and a controlled passive flexion motion technique described by Duran and Houser; and an early active motion protocol.

ACTIVE EXTENSION, PASSIVE FLEXION (KLEINERT)

Kleinert et al[63, 64] described a protocol of active extension and passive flexion using a dorsal extension blocking splint with the wrist positioned at 45 degrees of palmar flexion, the MCPs at 30 degrees of flexion, and the interphalangeal joints at 10 degrees of flexion (Fig. 7). A rubber band is attached to the involved finger nail and to a volar wrist band, allowing a patient to actively extend the digit with recoil of the rubber band causing passive flexion. If the rubber band traction is too tight or full passive extension is

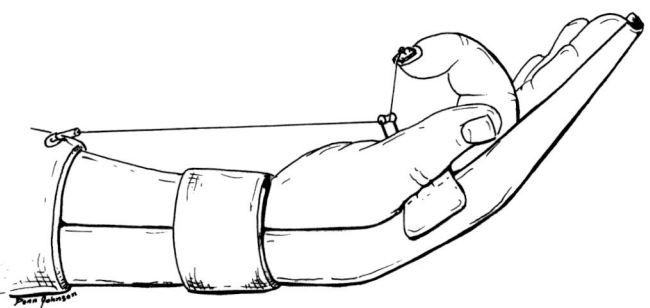

Fig. 7. Postoperative management. Illustration of the Kleinert splint, modified with a roller-bar or palmar pulley, used for a protocol of active extension and passive flexion.

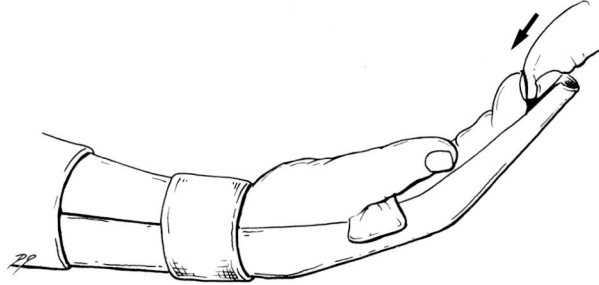

Fig. 8. Postoperative management. Illustration of a dorsal blocking splint used in the Duran and Houser protocol of passive flexion and passive extension.

not achieved, a PIP joint contracture may develop. The dorsal blocking splint is removed at approximately 4 weeks, replaced by a wrist band to anchor the rubber band, which is used to provide passive flexion for a further 3 to 4 weeks. Progressive active digital flexion is started at 7 to 8 weeks postoperatively, with a return to normal hand activities by 10 to 12 weeks.

CONTROLLED PASSIVE MOTION (DURAN AND HOUSER)

The controlled passive motion protocol, described by Duran and Houser in 1975,[65, 66] uses a dorsal extension blocking splint and a careful regimen of passive flexion and active extension exercises starting immediately following surgery for 4 weeks. These passive mobilization exercises were designed to create 3 to 5 mm of tendon excursion for the purpose of limiting peritendinous adhesion formation. The wrist, MCP, and interphalangeal joints are held by Velcro straps in 20 degrees of palmar flexion, 50 degrees of flexion, and extension positions, respectively. Exercises are done twice daily. In the 5th week, active flexion and extension of the wrist and digits is initiated. The dorsal splint is replaced between exercise sessions. Splinting is discontinued at 6 weeks. By 8 to 12 weeks, progressive strengthening exercises and normal hand activities are pursued (Fig. 8).

OUTCOMES

CLINICAL ASSESSMENT

Multiple assessment systems have been proposed to evaluate the functional outcomes of flexor tendon repair. In 1976, the American Society for Surgery of the Hand developed and recommended a method calculating the sum of the angular flexion of the MCP, PIP, and DIP joints and subtracting any extension deficit for each joint.[67] This was done for both active and passive flexion and was done with the hand in a clenched fist position. Total active motion and total passive motion could then be determined and compared to designated "normal" values or used to determine the percentage of active motion regained by surgical treatment. A "normal" total active motion was considered to be 260 degrees; or a summation of 85 degrees (MCP), 110 degrees (PIP), and 65 degrees (DIP).

Another classification system is that of Strickland and Glogovac.[68] They proposed a modified assessment method from that of the American Society for Surgery of the Hand

based on reasoning that motion of the MCP joint was not directly dependent on extrinsic flexor action. Their formula is as follows:

$$\frac{\text{Total active motion (PIP + DIP)} - \text{extension lag}}{175 \text{ degrees}} \times 100$$

$$= \% \text{ of normal active PIP + DIP motion}$$

RESULTS

Variations in reporting criteria and in repair methods and rehabilitation programs provide little consistency for comparing outcomes of flexor tendon repair. In general, however, results of zone II flexor tendon repair continue to be complicated by unsatisfactory rates of decreased digital motion requiring secondary tenolysis, functional deficit, and tendon rupture. Strickland, in 1985, reported on 71 consecutive cases in 58 patients undergoing primary flexor tendon repair followed by an early postoperative mobilization protocol. Overall, 25% excellent, 31% good, 27% fair, 13% poor, and 4% rupture rates were recorded.[69] These results are comparable to those presented by Duran and Houser[66] in 1975 and by Lister[62] in 1977. More recently, Silverskiold reported on 46 consecutive patients (55 injured digits) who underwent primary flexor tendon repair using a modified Kessler core suture and epitendinous cross-stitch method followed by early mobilization. All patients, except for 2 reported tendon ruptures, demonstrated greater than 70% return of active motion at 6 months postoperatively.[41]

COMPLICATIONS

Nonoperative management of partial flexor tendon lacerations may be associated with delayed rupture, triggering, or entrapment of the involved tendon. Despite careful adherence to proposed indications for repair of partial injuries, rupture may occur following excessive force placed across the tendon. Triggering and entrapment result from the mobile tendon flap becoming ensnared in a tear of the surrounding synovial sheath.

Complications associated with direct primary or delayed primary tendon repair include perioperative infection, tendon rupture, limitation of digital motion, peritendinous adhesion formation, flexion contracture, and tendon bowstringing.

Tendon rupture may result from many factors, including problems with the surgical method and poor postoperative compliance with therapy. Tendon ruptures occur most commonly at approximately 10 days postoperatively but may occur as late as 6 to 8 weeks following repair. Poor surgical technique and noncompliance with postsurgical management may also be responsible for poor digital function. Flexion contracture, extension lag, and loss of digital flexion have all been described. Tendon bowstringing results from traumatic crucial pulley loss (particularly A2 or A4).

REFERENCES

1. Pulvertaft RG: Repair of tendon injuries in the hand. Ann R Coll Surg 1948; 3:3.
2. Mason ML, Shearon CG: The process of tendon repair. An experimental study of tendon suture and tendon graft. Arch Surg 1932; 25:615.
3. Kleinert HE, Spokevicius S, Papas NH: History of flexor tendon repair. J Hand Surg Am 1995; 20:S46.
4. Bunnell S: Reconstructive surgery of the hand. Surg Gynecol Obstet 1924; 39:259.
5. Bunnell S: Repair of nerves and tendons of the hand. J Bone Joint Surg 1928; 10:1.
6. Potenza AD: Tendon healing within the flexor digital sheath in the dog: An experimental study. J Bone Joint Surg Am 1962; 44:49.
7. Urbaniak JR, Bright DS, Gill LH, et al: Vascularization and the gliding mechanism of free flexor tendon grafts inserted by the silicone rod method. J Bone Joint Surg Am 1974; 56:473.
8. Eiken O, Lundborg G, Rank F: The role of the digital synovial sheath in tendon grafting. Scand J Plast Reconstr Surg 1975; 9:182.
9. Matthews P: The fate of isolated segments of flexor tendons within the digital sheath: A study in synovial nutrition. Br J Plast Surg 1976; 29:216.
10. Eiken O, Hagberg L, Rank F: The healing process of transplanted digital tendon sheath synovium. Scand J Plast Reconstr Surg 1978; 12:225.
11. Lundborg G, Rank F: Experimental intrinsic healing of flexor tendons based upon synovial fluid nutrition. J Hand Surg Am 1978; 3:21.
12. Lundborg G, Holm S, Myrhage R: The role of the synovial fluid and tendon sheath for flexor tendon nutrition. Scand J Plast Reconstr Surg 1980; 14:99.
13. Gelberman RH, Vande Berg JS, Lundborg GN, et al: Flexor tendon healing and restoration of the gliding surface: An ultrastructural study in dogs. J Bone Joint Surg Am 1983; 65:70.
14. Manske PR, Gelberman RH, Vande Berg J, et al: Flexor tendon repair: Morphological evidence of intrinsic healing in vitro. J Bone Joint Surg Am 1984; 66:385.
15. Lundborg G, Rank F, Heinau B: Intrinsic tendon healing. Scand J Plast Reconstr Surg 1985; 19:113.
16. Gelberman RH, Khabie V, Cahill CJ: The revascularization of healing flexor tendons in the digital sheath. J Bone Joint Surg Am 1991; 73:868.
17. Duffy FJ, Seiler JG, Heigrueter CA, et al: Intrinsic mitogenic potential of canine flexor tendons. J Hand Surg Br 1992; 17:275.
18. Nishida J, Seiler JG, Amadio PC, et al: Flexor tendon-pulley interaction after annular pulley reconstruction: A biomechanical study in a dog model in vivo. J Hand Surg Am 1998; 23:279.
19. Hagberg L: Exogenous hyaluronate as an adjunct in the prevention of adhesions after flexor tendon surgery: A controlled clinical trial. J Hand Surg Am 1992; 17:132.
20. Wiig M, Abrahamsson SO, Lundborg G: Tendon repair: cellular activities in rabbit deep flexor tendons and surrounding synovial sheaths and the effects of Hyaluronan: An experimental study in vivo and in vitro. J Hand Surg Am 1997; 22:818.
21. Hanff G, Hagberg L: Prevention of restrictive adhesions with expanded Polytetrafluoroethylene diffusible membrane following flexor tendon repair: An experimental study in rabbits. J Hand Surg Am 1998; 23:658.
22. Kaplan EB: Functional and Surgical Anatomy of the Hand, 2nd ed. Philadelphia, J.B. Lippincott, 1965.
23. Kleinert HE, Verdan C: Report of the Committee on tendon injuries. J Hand Surg Am 1983; 8:794.
24. Doyle JR, Blythe WF: The finger flexor tendon sheath and pulleys: Anatomy and reconstruction. In American Academy of Orthopaedic Surgeons: Symposium on Tendon Surgery in the Hand. St. Louis, C.V. Mosby, 1975.
25. Cleveland M: Restoration of the digital portion of a flexor tendon and sheath in the hand. J Bone Joint Surg 1933; 15:762.
26. Lin GT, Amadio PC, An K-N, et al: Functional anatomy of the human digital flexor pulley system. J Hand Surg Am 1989; 14:949.
27. Berkenbusch H: Flexor tendon nutrition. Hand Clin 1985; 1:13.
28. Arai H: Flexor tendon nutrition. Hand Clin 1985; 1:13.
29. Mayer L: The physiologic method of tendon transplantation. Surg Gynecol Obstet 1916; 22:182.
30. Edwards DAW: The blood supply and the lymphatic drainage of tendons. J Anatomy 1946; 80:147.
31. Strickland JW: Flexor tendon injuries: I. Foundations of treatment. J Am Acad Orthop Surg 1995; 3:44.
32. Flynn JE, Graham JH: Healing following tendon suture and tendon transplants. Surg Gynecol Obstet 1962; 10:467.
33. Amiel D, Gelberman RH, Harwood F, et al: Fibronectin in healing flexor tendons subjected to immobilization or early controlled passive motion. Matrix 1991; 11:184.
34. Gelberman RH, Stenberg D, Amiel D, et al: Fibroblast chemotaxis after tendon repair. J Hand Surg Am 1991; 16:686.
35. Gelberman RH, Amiel D, Gonsalves M, et al: The influence of protected passive mobilization on the healing of flexor tendons: A biochemical and microangiographic study. Hand 1981; 13:120.
36. Gelberman RH, Manske PR, Akeson WH, et al: Flexor tendon repair. J Orthop Res 1986; 4:119.
37. Gelberman RH, Woo S L-Y, Lothringer K, et al: Effects of early intermittent passive mobilization on healing canine flexor tendons. J Hand Surg Am 1982; 7:170.
38. Gelberman RH, Menon J, Gonsalves M, et al: The effects of mobilization on the vascularization of healing flexor tendons in dogs. Clin Orthop 1980; 153:283.
39. Aoki M, Kubota H, Pruitt DL, et al: Biomechanical and histologic characteristics of canine flexor tendon repair using early postoperative mobilization. J Hand Surg Am 1997; 22:107.
40. Takai S, Woo S L-Y, Horibe S, et al: The effects of frequency and duration of controlled passive mobilization on tendon healing. J Orthop Res 1991; 9:705.
41. Silverskiold KL, May EJ: Flexor tendon repair in zone II with a new suture technique and an early mobilization program combining passive and active flexion. J Hand Surg Am 1994; 19:53.
42. Kubota H, Manske PR, Aoki M, et al: Effect of motion and tension on injured flexor tendons in chickens. J Hand Surg Am 1996; 21:456.
43. Tanaka H, Manske PR, Pruitt DL: Effect of cyclic tension on lacerated flexor tendons in vitro. J Hand Surg Am 1995; 20:467.
44. Pruitt DL, Tanaka H, Aoki M, et al: Cyclic stress testing after in vivo healing of canine flexor tendon lacerations. J Hand Surg Am 1996; 21:974.
45. Gelberman RH, Nunley JA, Osterman AL, et al: Influences of the protected passive mobilization interval on flexor tendon healing. Clin Orthop Rel Res 1991; 264:189.
46. Winters SC, Gelberman RH, Woo S L-Y, et al: The effects of multiple-strand suture methods on the strength and excursion of repaired intrasynovial flexor tendons: A biomechanical study in dogs. J Hand Surg Am 1998; 23:97.
47. Thurman RT, Trumble TE, Hanel DP, et al: Two-, four-, and six-strand zone II flexor tendon repairs: An in situ biomechanical comparison using a cadaver model. J Hand Surg Am 1998; 23:261.
48. Savage R, Risitano G: Flexor tendon repair using a "six strand" method of repair and early active mobilization. J Hand Surg Br 1989; 14:396.
49. Lin GT, An KN, Amadio PC, et al: Studies of running suture for flexor tendon repair in dogs. J Hand Surg Am 1988; 13:553.
50. Leddy JP, Packer JW: Avulsion of the profundus tendon insertion in athletes. J Hand Surg 1977; 2:6.
51. Robins PR, Dobyns JH: Avulsion of the insertion of the flexor digitorum profundus tendon associated with fracture of the dis-

tal phalanx. A brief review. In: American Academy of Orthopaedic Surgeons Symposium on Tendon Surgery in the Hand. St. Louis, C.V. Mosby, 1975.

52. Smith JH: Avulsion of the profundus tendon with simultaneous intraarticular fracture of the distal phalanx: Case report. J Hand Surg 1981; 6:600.

53. Lister GD: Incision and closure of the flexor tendon sheath during tendon repair. Hand 1983; 15:123.

54. Lister GD: Indications and techniques for repair of the flexor tendon sheath. Hand Clin 1985; 1:85.

55. Sanders WE: Advantages of "epitenon first" suture placement technique in flexor tendon repair. Clin Orthop 1992; 280:198.

56. Malerich MM, Baird RA, McMaster W, et al: Permissible limits of flexor digitorum profundus tendon advancement: An anatomical study. J Hand Surg Am 1987; 12:30.

57. Urbaniak JR: Repair of the flexor pollicis longus. Hand Clin 1985; 1:69.

58. Zissimos AG, Szabo RM, Yinger KE, et al: Biomechanics of the thumb flexor pulley system. J Hand Surg Am 1994; 19: 475.

59. Cooney WP, Weidman K, Malo D, et al: Management of acute flexor tendon injury in the hand. Am Acad Orthop Surg Instruct Course Lect 1985; 34:373.

60. Gelberman RH, Woo S L-Y, Amiel D, et al: Influences of flexor sheath continuity and early motion on tendon healing in dogs. J Hand Surg Am 1990; 15:69.

61. Chow JA, Thomas LJ, Dovelle S, et al: Controlled motion rehabilitation after flexor tendon repair and grafting. A multicentre study. J Bone Joint Surg Br 1988; 70:591.

62. Lister GD, Kleinert HE, Kutz JG, et al: Primary flexor tendon repair followed by immediate controlled mobilization. J Hand Surg Am 1977; 2:441.

63. Kleinert HE, Kutz JE, Atasoy E, et al: Primary repair of flexor tendons. Orthop Clin North Am 1973; 4:865.

64. Kleinert HE, Kutz JE, Cohen MJ: Primary repair of zone 2 flexor tendon lacerations. In American Academy of Orthopaedic Surgeons Symposium on Tendon Surgery in the Hand. St. Louis, C.V. Mosby, 1975, p 91.

65. Cannon NM, Strickland JW: Therapy following flexor tendon surgery. Hand Clin 1985; 1:147.

66. Duran RJ, Houser RG: Controlled passive motion following flexor tendon repair in zones 2 and 3. In American Academy of Orthopaedic Surgeons Symposium on Tendon Surgery in the Hand. St. Louis, C.V. Mosby, 1975, p 105.

67. American Society for Surgery of the Hand: Clinical Assessment Committee Report. Presented March 10, 1976.

68. Strickland JW, Glogovac SV: Digital function following flexor tendon repair in zone II: A comparison of immobilization and controlled passive motion techniques. J Hand Surg Am 1980, 5:537.

69. Strickland JW: Results of flexor tendon surgery in zone II. Hand Clin 1985; 1:167.

---

section **12** chapter **3**

EXTENSOR TENDON INJURIES

Mary Lynn Newport

Summary

- Approximately 66% of extensor tendon lacerations are associated with other injuries (fracture, skin loss, or joint capsule damage), thereby increasing the complexity of treatment for most extensor injuries.
- Distal injuries (zones I to IV) fare poorly compared with injuries in proximal zones (zones V to VII).
- The average loss of flexion is greater than the average loss of extension, producing significant hand dysfunction.
- Careful attention to preoperative diagnosis, intraoperative repair technique, and postoperative rehabilitation protocol is important to achieving a good functional outcome.

The extensor mechanism of the hand constitutes a complex and delicate interplay between the intrinsic and extrinsic systems to allow smooth, coordinated motion of the digits. Despite this complexity, the significance of traumatic extensor tendon injuries is often minimized or the injuries are missed. In reality, these injuries can and do cause significant hand dysfunction. The same care and attention given to flexor tendon injuries should also be devoted to extensor injuries.

Until recently, there was a general dictum that extensor injuries did universally well, and if there was a problem, it could be easily rectified by tenolysis. That in fact is not the case when the literature and clinical results are viewed critically.[1-4]

It is easy to understand how these injuries can prove difficult: over the digit, the extensor mechanism covers bone on three sides and has very limited excursion because of the interconnection between intrinsic and extrinsic muscles. In addition, there is little subcutaneous tissue to promote gliding. All of these factors produce adhesions and, hence, finger dysfunction that includes loss of extension *and* loss of flexion.[4] Although chronic deformity has been evaluated, relatively little research has been aimed at acute injuries of the extensor mechanism until the recent, significant increase in interest in these injuries.

HISTORICAL REVIEW

The first modern discussion of the results of extensor tendon laceration was by Miller in 1942.[2] Between then and 1990, only 11 reports concerning this injury or the results of different rehabilitation protocols were published in the English literature.[4] Static treatment postoperatively with a cast generally produced suboptimal results, whereas later reports of dynamic splinting techniques showed better results. In 1990, Newport et al,[4] using a grading system based on Miller's work (Table 1), discussed the results of static splinting in a large group of patients, showing that injuries in the distal zones fared poorly (40% good/excellent results) compared with injuries in the more proximal zones (65% good/excellent results), that intrasynovial injuries (zone VII) had results equivalent with those of injuries in zones VI and VIII (67% good/excellent results compared with 66% and 63%, respectively), and that there was a significant loss of *flexion* as well as extension as a result of

TABLE 1. MILLER'S CLASSIFICATION (MODIFIED) FOR EVALUATION OF RESULTS AFTER EXTENSOR TENDON REPAIR

Result	Total Extension Lag, Degrees	Total Loss Flexion, Degrees
Excellent	0	0
Good	≤10	≤20
Fair	11–45	11–45
Poor	≥45	≥45

this injury.[4] In fact, loss of flexion—both in average number of degrees and in number of digits affected—was greater than the loss of extension. A number of reports since then have looked at different active and dynamic rehabilitation protocols,[5–7] the biomechanics of injury and repair,[8, 9] and new suture techniques.[10]

PATHOGENESIS

Most extensor tendon injuries occur secondary to direct trauma. Approximately one-third are simple injuries with straightforward skin and tendon lacerations. Two-thirds, however, are associated with concomitant injuries, including significant soft-tissue damage, fracture, or flexor tendon injury.[4]

The extensor mechanism is divided into nine zones for the fingers and five for the thumb (Fig. 1). The odd-numbered zones occur over joints (except for zone IX over the mid-forearm) and the even-numbered zones over bone. Knowledge of the zone of injury can help direct acute care and rehabilitation choices as well as provide understanding of potential outcome and complications.

Blunt trauma can also cause extensor mechanism injury. Most disruptions of the extensor tendon at the distal interphalangeal (DIP) joint ("mallet finger") are secondary to forced hyperflexion or hyperextension of the joint. Closed trauma can also injure the extensor mechanism at the proximal interphalangeal (PIP) joint, resulting in loss of PIP extension and possible boutonnière deformity. The usual mechanism of injury is either direct blow to the dorsum of the PIP joint, which ruptures the central slip, or forced hyperflexion of the PIP joint.

The sagittal bands in zone V can be injured by direct trauma or by acute flexion of the metacarpophalangeal (MCP) joint. Rupture of the sagittal band (usually on the radial side of the joint) may result in extensor tendon subluxation ulnarly into the intermetacarpal valley. This limits the mechanical advantage of the tendon to extend the joint. The patient is not able to attain extension from a flexed position but may be able to maintain extension after the MCP has been passively extended as the tendon slides back to the dorsum of the MCP joint.

CLINICAL FEATURES

Injury in zones I through IV will prevent the patient from fully extending the interphalangeal (IP) joints of the digit. Examination should include adequate visualization of the tendon proximal and distal to the zone of injury. Most

extensor tendon lacerations occur with the finger in a flexed position: the injured area is pulled proximally when the hand is extended during examination. Any patient who cannot fully extend the joints distal to the site of injury, has pain on extension, or cannot painlessly resist a gentle flexion force by the examiner should be considered to have an extensor tendon laceration until proved otherwise. The wound should be extended as necessary to gain adequate visualization.

Injury to zones V through IX will prevent the patient from independently extending the MCP joint of the digit. The examiner should be observant for two potential sources of confusion for these proximal injuries: (1) Care should be taken to ensure that MCP extension does not occur via an intact, adjacent juncture tendinum for injuries in zone VI proximal to the junctura. This can be done reliably only through direct visualization. (2) IP extension through the intrinsic muscles should not be mistaken for an intact proximal extensor tendon. This can be evaluated by asking the patient to extend the MCP joints while keeping the IP joints flexed. Differential diagnoses to consider are radial nerve injury, in which a patient cannot actively extend the fingers but has a normal tenodesis effect in the fingers during passive wrist flexion and extension; locked trigger finger, in which the patient cannot actively or pas-

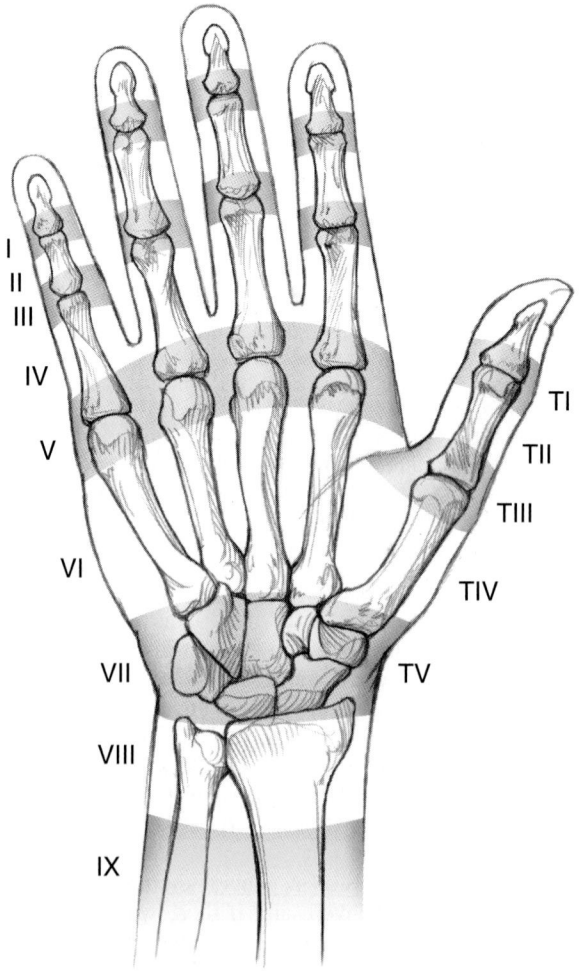

Fig. 1. View. This shows extensor tendon zones.

sively move the finger; and sagittal band rupture, in which the patient cannot actively attain MCP extension but can maintain it if the finger is passively extended.

TREATMENT

NONOPERATIVE

Closed mallet and boutonnière injuries can and should be treated acutely in a nonoperative fashion under most circumstances. Doyle[11] divides mallet fingers into four categories (Table 2). Treatment for the different categories is generally similar: splinting of only the DIP joint in 0 degrees of extension. The PIP joint is always left free so it does not become stiff. Care should be taken not to hyperextend the DIP joint when splinting because this may disrupt the blood supply to the dorsal skin, resulting in skin breakdown, the most common treatment complication of mallet finger.[12] Dorsal splints are good to use for this injury because they allow near normal function of the hand, leave the finger pad free for touch, and are well accepted by patients. Other options include using an aluminum and foam splint volarly or a commercially available slip-on Stack splint (Link America, Inc., Hanover, NJ). Open reduction and internal fixation (ORIF) of mallet fractures can be problematic and, some argue, unnecessary.[13] The fracture fragments are often extremely small and may already be compromised by comminution. In general, if the joint subluxation can be corrected, transarticular fixation without a direct dorsal approach may be all that is necessary and avoids the complications of ORIF. If the joint cannot be reduced, open reduction of the joint and indirect approximation of the extensor mechanism through a tendon pullout suture volarly and pinning of the joint will achieve a congruous, stable joint.

Closed central slip injuries of the extensor mechanism overlying the PIP joint are also treated nonoperatively. If seen initially, the diagnosis can be made if there is a high degree of suspicion for this injury. Patients with this injury will have a fusiform PIP joint swelling, just as in ligament sprains. The mechanism of injury is often similar. However, the patient with extensor tendon rupture will be tender dorsally over the joint and will have pain with resisted finger extension or may not be able to extend fully. Treatment includes splinting of the PIP joint alone (usually dorsally), which encourages free motion of the DIP joint to allow gliding of the lateral bands. Flexion of the DIP joint pulls the entire extensor mechanism distally, better approximating the torn tendon overlying the PIP joint. If this injury is not treated early, the injury to the central slip allows the PIP joint to fall into flexion. This attenuates the triangular ligament holding the lateral bands in a dorsal position. They then slip volarly, increasing the flexion moment on the PIP joint, resulting in a flexion posture of the joint. The volarly subluxed lateral bands produce an increased extension force on the DIP joint. The resultant DIP hyperextension combined with PIP flexion is the typical boutonnière deformity.

Sagittal band ruptures often occur as the result of minimal trauma. There is little pain and almost no swelling. The patient notes a finger stuck in flexion at the MCP joint. These patients are usually able to maintain extension if the finger is positioned there passively, but they are unable to actively attain extension because the extensor tendon has slipped into the intermetacarpal valley and does not have a sufficient moment arm to extend the finger. Conservative treatment can be successful if the injury is very recent—within a day or two—and involves immobilizing the MCP joint in full extension, leaving the IP joints free for motion. This is maintained for 4 to 6 weeks. If the injury is not recent, surgical reconstruction should be considered. Often, the injury is old enough that the sagittal band on the contralateral side has shortened and needs to be released to centralize the extensor tendon over the MCP joint. The injured side is primarily repaired with fine, absorbable suture. The hand is immobilized as described earlier.

TABLE 2. TREATMENT OF EXTENSOR INJURIES (CLOSED AND OPEN) ZONES I–VII		
Injury	**Definition**	**Treatment**
Zone I—mallet		
Subclass I	Soft tissue, avulsion off distal phalanx	Splint DIP, dorsal or volar
II	Laceration	Irrigation, débridement, direct repair with tenodermodesis, transarticular Kirschner's wire
III	Deep avulsion	Irrigate and débride, skin coverage, Kirschner's wire
IV	Significant fracture	
	a. Transepiphyseal	Splint
	b. <1/2 articular surface No subluxation	Splint, possible Kirschner's wire
	c. >1/2 with subluxation	Kirschner's wire, consider indirect reduction
Zone III—boutonnière Laceration	Central slip rupture	Gain full passive extension, then splint for 6 weeks, DIP free
Zone I–II		Irrigate and debride joint as necessary, tenodermodesis, Kirschner's wire
		Splint for 6 weeks, AROM of PIP
III–IV		Irrigate and debride joint as necessary, modified Kessler's or Bunnell's, no Kirschner's wire
		Dynamic splinting or active motion as possible
V–VII		Modified Bunnell's repair
		Dynamic splint or active motion

OPERATIVE

Extensor tendon lacerations should be treated with primary repair when possible. Concomitant injury (fracture, open joint capsule) should be treated appropriately. Injuries over joints should be carefully evaluated to be certain the joint capsule has not been violated. If direct inspection does not reveal the open joint but there is high suspicion, methylene blue, radiographic dye, or sterile saline can be injected into the joint (away from the laceration) to see if any fluid leaks from the disrupted capsule. All fractures need to be fully evaluated with radiographs. A patient with an open joint or open fracture should be taken on an emergency basis to the operating room for débridement, ORIF as necessary, and tendon repair. For extensor tendon injuries not associated with open joints or open fractures, the tendon repair can be done on a delayed primary basis after the wound has been cleaned, the skin loosely approximated, and the hand or finger splinted appropriately.

Extensor tendon repair in zones I and II can be technically challenging. The tendon is very thin, has no excursion, and holds sutures poorly. The tenodermodesis method of McFarlane and Hampole[14] is probably the easiest and

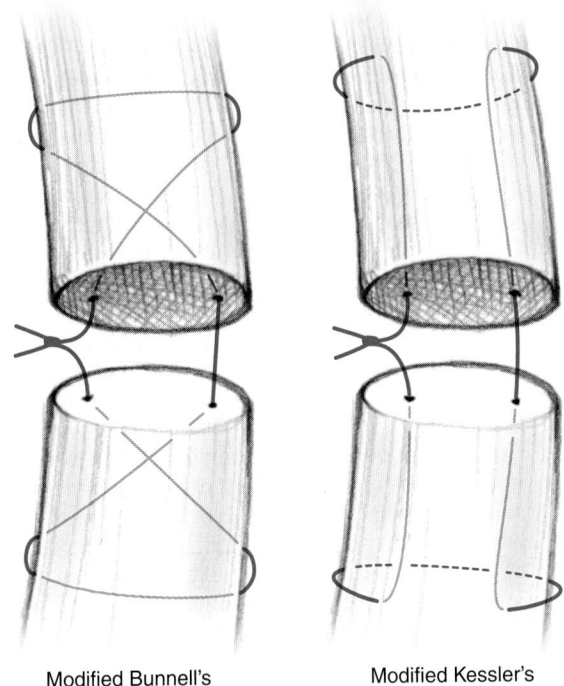

Modified Bunnell's   Modified Kessler's

Fig. 2. Operative repair techniques for extensor tendon injuries. *A,* Modified Bunnell's technique; *B,* Modified Kessler's technique; *C,* Grasping technique.

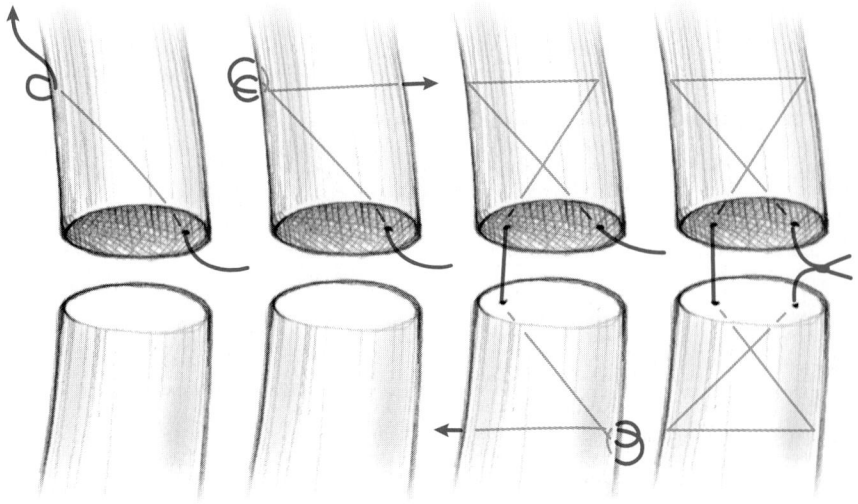

Grasping technique

most reliable repair technique. In this method, the tendon and skin are approximated together in a mattress or figure-of-eight fashion using nonabsorbable suture material. The repair and postoperative care are made easier by transfixing the DIP joint with a percutaneous Kirschner's wire. This allows wound care without placing stress on the tendon repair. The sutures remain in place for 2 to 3 weeks; the Kirschner wire, protected by a volar or dorsal splint, remains in place for 6 weeks. PIP motion is encouraged during the entire postoperative period.

Injuries in zones III and IV are treated with primary repair. The wound is extended as necessary to obtain adequate visualization of the tendon ends. Biomechanically, the modified Kessler or Bunnell techniques (see Fig. 1) are similar in strength and shortening.[9] Both appear strong enough to allow early motion. All principles of tendon repair—adequate exposure, gentle handling of tendon fragments, use of a strong core suture of nonabsorbable material—are followed.

Injuries in zones V through IX can also be treated on a delayed primary basis if there is no open joint or fracture. The suture technique of choice is the modified Bunnell or the grasping modification of the Bunnell technique (Fig. 2).[8, 10] This new repair technique is 25% stronger than the modified Bunnell repair and is strong enough to allow early active (protected) motion.

POSTOPERATIVE REHABILITATION

Static splinting has been a mainstay of extensor tendon rehabilitation and, in certain circumstances, is the treatment of choice. The potential difficulties are obvious, however. With thin tendon closely approximated to bone and skin, both of which are often injured along with the tendon, adhesion formation can occur. The wide area of tendon to bone over the phalanges makes injuries in the distal zones particularly troublesome. Studies using static splinting have uniformly produced results inferior to those using more active protocols.[5, 6] As a consequence, static splinting is not recommended unless other factors preclude the need for gliding—factors such as patient compliance or severe bone or skin injury not adequately stabilized by the original procedure. It is also for these reasons that stable internal fixation, which will allow early tendon gliding, is recommended whenever feasible.

Studies of dynamic splinting showed that the extensor tendons could withstand the forces associated with gliding, as have biomechanical studies.[5, 6, 8, 9] Results have improved in injuries in the more proximal zones and in zones III and IV.[15] Dynamic splinting can be cumbersome, however, and difficult for some patients to manage (Fig. 3).

Active postoperative rehabilitation protocols are easier to manage for compliant patients, produce excellent results, and allow better overall hand function between exercise periods. The tendon repair techniques recommended in this chapter are theoretically strong enough to withstand the forces of early active motion, and clinical results seem to indicate that repair rupture and tendon elongation occur with less frequency compared with static or dynamic splinting. Evans' early short arc active motions protocol[16] keeps the patient in a splint in extension between exercise periods. For injuries in zones III and IV, just the affected finger is splinted in 0 degrees extension at the IP joints. Several times per day, the patient switches to an exercise splint with 30 to 40 degrees of flexion built in and actively flexes and extends within the confines of the splint. Total active motion for the PIP and DIP joints increased from 111 degrees for statically immobilized fingers to 132 degrees for fingers treated with short arc active motion. The rates of good and excellent results improved from 42% for static immobilization (compared with 40% for Newport's series[4]) to 65% for mobilized injuries. For more proximal injuries, Evans uses a program that combines dynamic splinting (rubber bands passively return the fingers to an extended position while allowing the patient to actively flex them) and short arc active motion. This improved the results from 189 degrees of total active motion (MCP + PIP + DIP − extension lag) for statically splinted injuries to 248 degrees with the combined tendon gliding program.

Static splinting continues to be widely used, but the results of tendon gliding programs, passive or active, have clearly shown improved results and must be considered for all patients. The effort and cost are greater than for simple static splinting, but the improvements in time lost from work, residual hand dysfunction, and need for reconstructive surgery seem to make this procedure very much worthwhile.

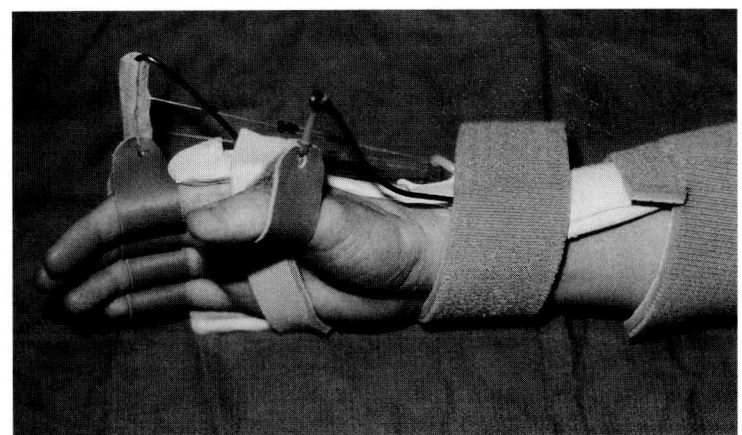

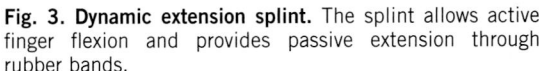

Fig. 3. Dynamic extension splint. The splint allows active finger flexion and provides passive extension through rubber bands.

REFERENCES

1. Kelly AP Jr: Primary tendon repairs: A study of 789 consecutive tendon severances. J Bone Joint Surg Am 1959; 41:581.

2. Miller H: Repair of severed tendons of the hand and wrist. Surg Gynecol Obstet 1942; 75:693.

3. Littler JW: The finger extensor mechanism. Surg Clin North Am 1967; 47:415.

4. Newport ML, Blair WF, Steyers CM Jr: Long-term results of extensor tendon repair. J Hand Surg Am 1990; 15:961.

5. Evans RB, Burkhalter WE: A study of the dynamic anatomy of extensor tendons and implications for treatment. J Hand Surg Am 1986; 11:774.

6. Browne EZ Jr, Ribik CA: Early dynamic splinting for extensor tendon injuries. J Hand Surg Am 1989; 14:72.

7. Hung LK, Chan A, Chang J, et al: Early controlled active mobilization with dynamic splintage for treatment of extensor tendon injuries. J Hand Surg Am 1990; 15:251.

8. Newport ML, Williams CD: Biomechanical characteristics of extensor tendon suture techniques. J Hand Surg Am 1992; 17:272.

9. Newport ML, Pollack GR, Williams CD: Biomechanical characteristics of suture techniques in extensor zone IV. J Hand Surg Am 1995; 20:650.

10. Newport ML, Waters SN: A new suture technique for extensor tendon repair. J Hand Surg Am. Accepted for publication.

11. Doyle JR: Extensor tendons: Acute injuries. In Green DP, Hotchkiss RN, Pederson WC (eds): Operative Hand Surgery. New York, Churchill Livingstone, 1999, 4th ed, p 1950.

12. Stern PJ, Kastrup JJ: Complications and prognosis of treatment of mallet finger. J Hand Surg Am 1998; 23:329.

13. Wehbe MA, Schneider LH: Mallet fractures. J Bone Joint Surg Am 1984; 66:658.

14. McFarlane RM, Hampole MK: Treatment of extensor tendon injuries of the hand. Can J Surg 1973; 16:366.

15. Saldana MJ, Choban S, Westerbeck P, et al: Results of acute zone III extensor tendon injuries treated with dynamic extension splinting. J Hand Surg Am 1991; 16:1145.

16. Evans RB: Immediate active short arc motion following extensor tendon repair. Hand Clin 1995; 11:483.

section **12** chapter **4**

TENDINITIS OF THE HAND AND WRIST

Stephen H. Lacey

Summary

- Inflammatory conditions of tendons in the hand and wrist are among the most common disorders in an orthopaedic surgeon's practice.
- The goals of treatment are to relieve pain and preserve function in the most practical and efficient manner.
- Surgeons should look for other disorders, such as diabetes, Dupuytren's contracture, and anatomic variations.
- When treating these apparently routine disorders, surgeons must avoid complacency. Relatively minor problems can turn into major ones if complications occur.
- Primary management is usually nonoperative but should not be so prolonged that it results in unnecessary inconvenience and secondary changes of disuse and contracture.

PATHOGENESIS

Modern usage of the term "tendinitis" provides a convenient, although technically inaccurate, means of describing all inflammatory conditions involving tendons and their sheaths that are brought on by overuse or trauma. More accurately, inflammation of the paratenon (Fig. 1) should be defined as "paratenonitis," and involvement of the inner substance of the tendon should be defined as "tendinitis." The paratenon becomes inflamed when tendons rub against resistant structures such as bone or thickened ligaments. Tenovaginitis, tenosynovitis, and peritendinitis are terms synonymous with inflammation of the paratenon. When only the inside of the tendon is involved, "tendinitis" describes an inflammatory cellular response to the disruption of intratendinous fibers. Here, the midsubstance of the tendon undergoes microfailure as a result of excessive force (mechanical overload) or age-related collagen degeneration. Tendinitis results when the secondary inflammatory response occurs in the paratenon.[4]

Tendinitis is a common cause of pain in the hand and wrist. It has become pervasive in our society, affecting athletes, manual laborers, keyboard operators, homemakers, assembly line workers, and even computer game enthusiasts.[1, 2] Orthopaedic surgeons may be called on to evaluate patients at any time during the course of the disorder. It is important to take an accurate history and to document objective findings. Atypical symptoms should alert the surgeon to look for other disorders or etiologies, such as occult tumors.[3] These data are critical when and if legal or work-related issues arise later.

ANATOMY

All extrinsic tendons providing hand and wrist movement cross the wrist. Traveling within narrow tunnels to reach their insertion sites, they are vulnerable to compression, shear, and excessive wear (Fig. 2). Crowding can be secondary to bony prominences, fracture fragments, or extra tendons within these tunnels. Extrinsic tendons of the thumb are vulnerable to attrition, because tendons originating in the forearm must cross over axially aligned structures or change direction around bony pulleys to reach the

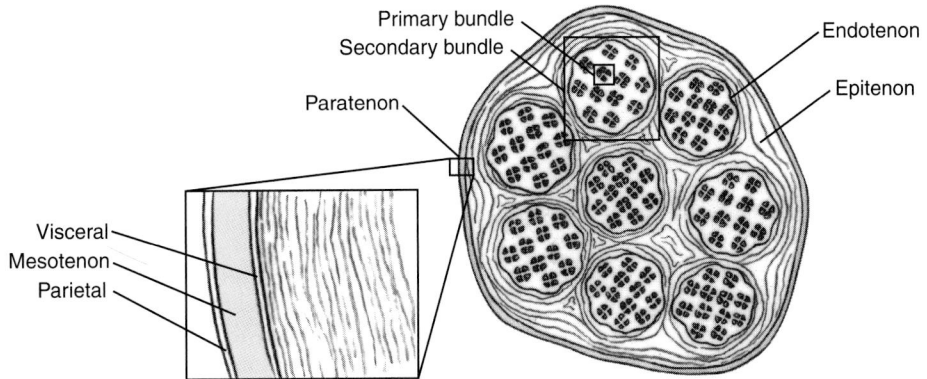

Fig. 1. Transverse section of a tendon.

thumb. Thus, the abductor pollicis longus (APL) and extensor pollicis brevis (EPB) cross over the radial wrist extensors before reaching the thumb. Likewise, the extensor pollicis longus (EPL) must turn acutely around Lister's tubercle (Fig. 3). Similar areas exist at the scaphoid tuberosity, where spurs can cause chronic tenosynovitis of the flexor pollicis longus and rupture, as in Mannerfelt's syndrome (Fig. 4).[5] Tenosynovitis of the flexor tendons within the carpal canal can be induced by the vice-like narrowing of a thickened transverse carpal ligament on one side and enlarged arthritic carpal joints on the other. Also, the hook of the hamate is a source of tendinitis or tendon rupture when its normally smooth concave radial surface is altered by fracture.[6]

TREATMENT

The majority of cases of tendinitis respond to nonoperative management (Table 1). The initial focus should be on reducing or eliminating activities leading to worsening of the condition. Alteration or modification of mechanical factors includes the use of splints, rest, or ergonomic changes to reduce overload. Nonsteroidal anti-inflammatory drugs (NSAIDs) may control pain but do not appear to correct the problem as long as abnormal mechanical factors exist. Steroid injections are helpful but can be complicated by

subcutaneous atrophy, loss of skin pigmentation, and tendon rupture. Although release of constricting tunnels is the foundation of surgical treatment, it is not without risk. Complications are summarized in Table 2.

STENOSING FLEXOR TENOSYNOVITIS (TRIGGER FINGER)

One of the most common forms of tendinitis is trigger finger. There are idiopathic changes in the first annular pulley that lead to restriction of the gliding motion of the flexor tendons. Sampson et al[7] have shown increased numbers of chondrocytes in the inner, or friction, layer of the A1 pulley. Type III collagen is also present in the involved pulleys. These ultrastructural changes may be due to a metaplastic response by soft tissue to repetitive loading.

Clearly, there is an association with diabetes. Chammas and colleagues[8] noted that 20% of diabetic patients had trigger digits and that some patients had involvement of multiple digits. Blyth and Ross[9] reported that, of 100 patients operated on for trigger finger, 18 were diabetics.

Injection of corticosteroid into the tendon sheath is a reliable treatment for trigger finger. Marks and Gunther[10] showed that 84% of trigger fingers and 92% of trigger thumbs were free of symptoms after a single injection of triamcinolone (average follow-up 3.5 years). Diabetic patients respond less favorably to corticosteroid injections. Griggs et al[11] reported that only 50% of diabetic patients treated with injection had resolution of triggering. They

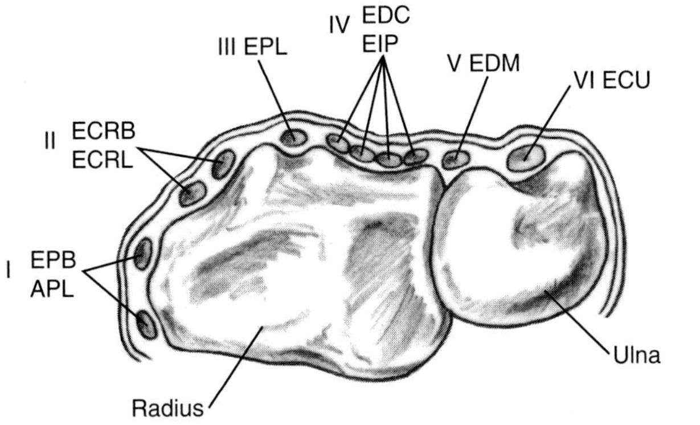

Fig. 2. The six dorsal compartments of the wrist. (EPB, extensor pollicis brevis; APL, abductor pollicis longus; ECRB, extensor carpi radialis brevis; ECRL, extensor carpi radialis longus; EPL, extensor pollicis longus; EDC, extensor digitorum communis; EIP, extensor indicis proprius; EDM, extensor digiti minimi; ECU, extensor carpi ulnaris.)

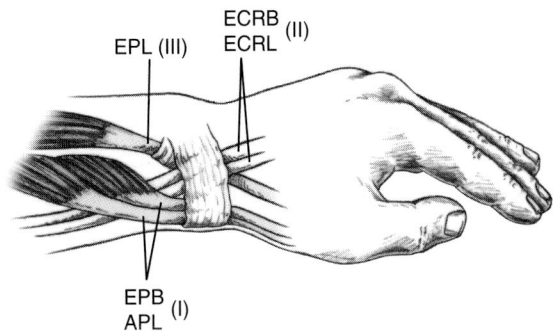

Fig. 3. Intersection syndrome. This shows location of the intersection syndrome at the crossover point of the extensor pollicis brevis (EPB) and abductor pollicis longus (APL) with the extensor carpi radialis brevis (ECRB) and extensor carpi radialis longus (ECRL). (EPL, extensor pollicis longus.)

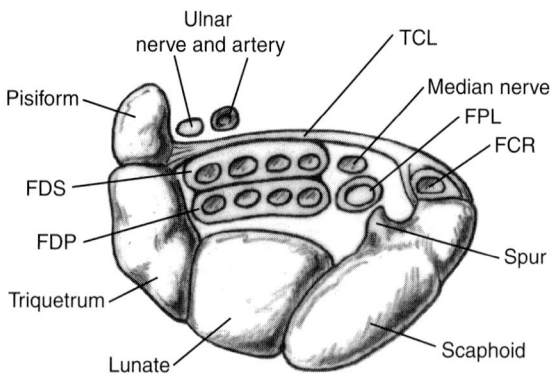

Fig. 4. Contents of the carpal canal at the level of the proximal carpal row. A spur (osteophyte) protrudes from the scaphoid, fraying the flexor pollicis longus (FPL) (Mannerfelt's syndrome). The median nerve is just above the FPL. (TCL, transverse carpal ligament; Lu, lunate; Sc, scaphoid; Tr, triquetrum; P, pisiform; FCR, flexor carpi radialis.)

also found that insulin-dependent diabetic patients had a higher incidence of multiple digit involvement and required surgical release more often than non–insulin-dependent diabetic patients.

When nonoperative measures fail to relieve triggering, A1 pulley release is appropriate. Currently, the most popular technique consists of an open approach, direct visualization of the A1 pulley, and release with a sharp instrument such as a scalpel, scissors, or small meniscotome. It is important to release enough of the A1 pulley but to avoid extending the release too far distally to include the A2 pulley.

The surgeon should be able to locate the A1 pulley accurately for each digit by using external landmarks. There are two popular techniques for localizing the A1 pulleys. The mathematical laws of nature popularized by Fibonacci dictate that the combined lengths of the middle

and distal phalanges (P2 + P3) are about equal to the entire length of the proximal phalanx (P1) (Fig. 5). As the A1 pulley resides at the base of P1, the combined length can be found by measuring a distance proximally from the proximal interphalangeal flexion crease equal to P2 + P3. Another method relies on the flexion creases of the palm (Fig. 6). The index finger A1 pulley is at the level of the midpalmar crease; the middle finger is between the distal and middle creases; and the ring and little fingers are at the level of the distal palmar crease. For the thumb, the A1 pulley is at the flexion crease of the metatarsophalangeal (MP) joint.[12] Surgeons prefer various incisions, including small transverse, oblique, and longitudinal incisions. To avoid contractures, longitudinal incisions should not cross flexion creases.

Percutaneous release of the A1 pulley has become popular. This can be done safely in a clean treatment room in the office, provided that the surgeon has practiced on cadaveric hands. Many surgeons are reluctant to release the A1 pulley of the thumb or the index this way because of the proximity of the digital nerves. Pope and Wolfe[13] showed in a cadaveric study that the digital nerves to the index and thumb are within 2 or 3 mm of the entry site of the cutting needle. The digital nerves of the ulnar three digits are aligned more along the longitudinal axis, thus allowing a safer approach with the percutaneous technique (see Fig. 6).

The diabetic trigger finger deserves special attention. Early surgical intervention is appropriate in diabetic patients because they are prone to joint contractures if the trigger finger is allowed to persist. Furthermore, release of the A1 pulley may not solve triggering in the diabetic patient. After A1 pulley release, the surgeon should ask the patient to actively flex the involved finger. If triggering persists, the surgeon should be prepared to do a reduction tenoplasty.[14] This can be accomplished by resection of one arm of the flexor digitorum sublimis tendon or removal of the central third of the profundus tendon.

TABLE 1. EXTENSOR TENOSYNOVITIS				
Diagnosis/Location	Chief Complaint	Findings	Tendon(s)	Treatment
De Quervain's tendinitis, first compartment	Pain with use of thumb, soreness radial styloid	Positive Finkelstein's test, tender radial styloid	APL, EPB	Splinting, NSAIDs, injection, release first compartment
ECU tendinitis, sixth compartment	Pain near ulnar styloid	Tender, thick ulnar styloid region	ECU	Splinting, NSAIDs, injection, release sixth compartment
EPL tendinitis, third compartment	Pain dorsal wrist, snapping of thumb	Tenderness, swelling at Lister's tubercle	EPL	Splinting, NSAIDs, release third compartment, no injection, relocate EPL outside compartment
EDC tendinitis, fourth compartment	Pain over dorsal central wrist	Swelling, crepitus, tenderness of fourth compartment	EDC, EIP	Splinting, NSAIDs, injection, release fourth compartment, tenosynovectomy
EDM tendinitis, fifth compartment	Pain on wrist flexion, use of fifth finger	Tenderness radial to ulnar head	EDM	Splinting, NSAIDs, release fifth compartment
Intersection syndrome	Pain, swelling, snapping forearm	Crepitus, pain at intersection zone	APL, EPB, ECRL, ECRB	Splinting, NSAIDs, injection, release second compartment and remove extra APL

APL, abductor pollicis longus; ECRB, extensor carpi radialis brevis; ECRL, extensor carpi radialis longus; ECU, extensor carpi ulnaris; EDC, extensor digitorum communis; EDM, extensor digiti minimi; EIP, extensor indicis proprius; EPB, extensor pollicis brevis; EPL, extensor pollicis longus; NSAIDs, nonsteroidal anti-inflammatory drugs.

TABLE 2. SURGICAL COMPLICATIONS			
Condition	Failure to Correct Pathology	Nerve Injury	Tendon Problems
Trigger digit	Incomplete release of A1 pulley	Digital nerve(s)	A2 pulley release and bowstringing
Trigger thumb	Incomplete release of A1 pulley	Radial digital nerve	Release of oblique pulley, bowstringing
De Quervain's tendinitis	Incomplete release, separate tunnel EPB	Superficial radial nerve and branches	Tendon instability and subluxation
ECU tendinitis	Incomplete release	Dorsal branch of ulnar nerve	Potential instability of ECU, volar subluxation
Extensor pollicis longus tendinitis	Failure to remove bone spurs at Lister's tubercle	Superficial radial nerve and branches	Tendon rupture
Intersection syndrome	Failure to release APL fascia or remove accessory tendons	Superficial radial nerve and branches	Recurrent bursitis of APL
FCR tendinitis	Incomplete release, failure to débride trapezial groove	Palmar cutaneous branch of median nerve	FCR tendon rupture

APL, abductor pollicis longus; ECU, extensor carpi ulnaris; EPB, extensor pollicis brevis; FCR, flexor carpi radialis.

De QUERVAIN'S TENDINITIS

Traditional anatomic drawings show a single compartment on the radial side of the distal radius enclosing two tendons: the EPB and the APL (see Fig. 2). This arrangement occurs in about 20% of dissected specimens. More commonly, there are additional tendons within the compartment, or there are septa within the compartment creating a small isolated tunnel for the EPB. Other disorders in the vicinity of the first dorsal compartment can be confused with De Quervain's tendinitis. Scaphoid fractures typically are tender on palpation of the snuffbox, and basilar arthritis of the thumb causes pain distal to the first dorsal compartment.

Finkelstein's test is helpful but should be done carefully because it can elicit a great deal of pain and may be painful even for normal patients (Fig. 7).[15] It is performed by having the patient hyperflex the thumb and trap it in the palm with the other fingers. Then the examiner deviates the wrist ulnarward. If significant constriction exists in the compartment, the patient will have pain in the region of the radial styloid. This maneuver should elicit pain well before reaching complete ulnar deviation. The examiner should repeat the test on the opposite wrist for comparison. Typical findings also include a nodule at the distal edge of

the first dorsal compartment. Radiographs are important for excluding other conditions that produce pain in this area, such as scaphoid fracture, radioscaphoid arthritis, and basilar arthritis of the thumb.

Injections of corticosteroid with or without splinting and physiotherapy usually give dramatic relief. If palpation reveals tenderness directly over the dorsal portion of the first compartment, there is probably a separate tunnel for the EPB, and the injection should be given only in this region. Accurate injection of corticosteroid correlates well with relief of symptoms.[16] Louis[17] reported a variation of Finkelstein's test that is useful for patients who present with persisting symptoms after surgical release. The examiner holds the thumb metacarpal in abduction while acutely flexing only the MP joint. This will cause pain when the separate tunnel for the EPB tunnel is still intact.

Obviously, surgical treatment should release the area of stenosis. The thickened extensor retinaculum is released completely, preserving some palmar sheath as a shelf to block subluxation of the tendons. It is common to find multiple slips of the APL. It is important also to identify the most dorsal tendon within the released compartment(s). The surgeon can be assured that there has been adequate decompression of the compartment(s) when traction on the

Fig. 5. Application of the Fibonacci series to locating the A1 pulley. The Fibonacci sequence as it applies to nature is that the sum of the preceding two units equals the next unit. This makes the length of P1 essentially equal to the combined length of P2 and P3. The reference point is the proximal interphalangeal crease. Not all of the pulleys are labeled.

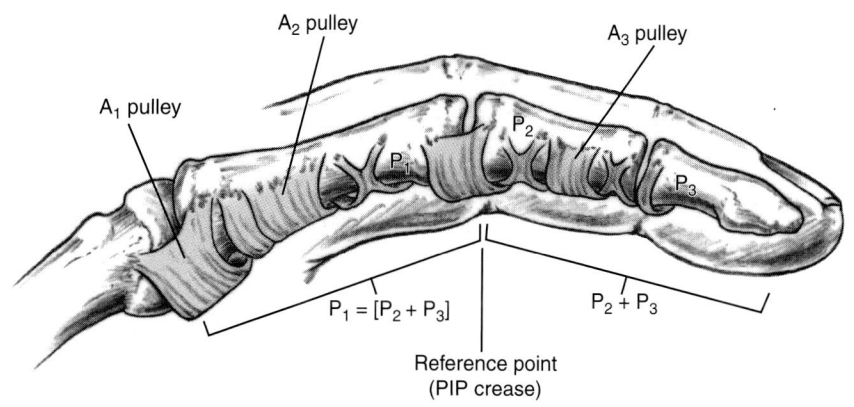

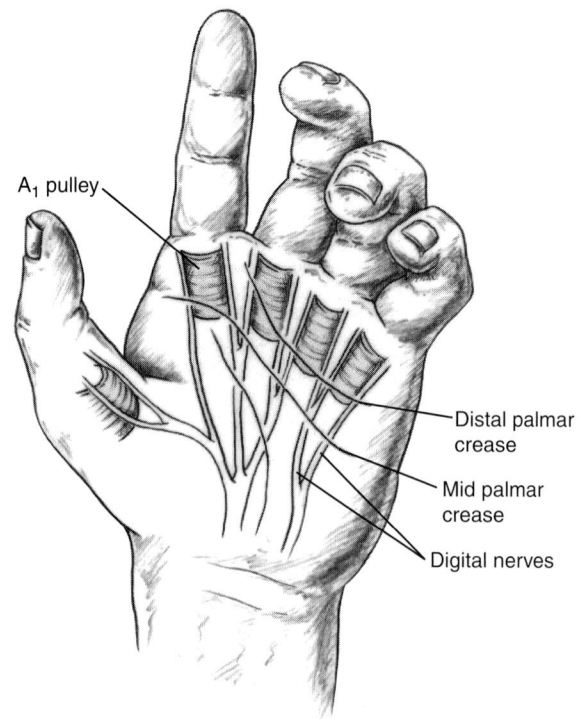

Fig. 6. Alternate means of locating the pulleys. Note the proximity of the digital nerves.

most dorsal tendon in the first compartment extends the MP joint of the thumb (Fig. 8).

Whether the incision is longitudinal, transverse, or angled, the surgeon must look for and carefully protect the superficial radial nerve and its branches. This requires attention to detail, meticulous technique, and gentle handling of the tissues. Radial sensory neuritis or neuroma can be a disastrous complication of this procedure and can lead to reflex sympathetic dystrophy.

Special consideration should be given to those cases affecting working women. Arons[18] cautioned about a surgical approach in these patients. He reported that among 16 women referred postoperatively, there were 23 associated diagnoses, ranging from lateral epicondylitis to carpal tunnel syndrome and 14 complications. There were significant problems in returning these women to work. Even in a group of 11 women referred preoperatively, there were 8 associated diagnoses. Only 3 of the 11 women in the second group underwent surgery.

INTERSECTION SYNDROME

This disorder is a bursitis of the APL at a point proximal to the wrist where the APL and EPB cross the radial wrist extensors about 4 cm proximal to the wrist (see Fig. 3).[19] It occurs in anyone who repetitively manipulates the wrist while gripping or handling objects. Canoeists, kayak enthusiasts ("rower's wrist"), and laborers develop this disorder. The distinguishing feature of this disorder is crepitus that is often audible with combined motions of the wrist and thumb. Although NSAIDs, splinting, or injections of corticosteroids help in most of these cases, some require release

of the second dorsal compartment and the fascia of the APL or removal of an accessory slip of the APL.

EXTENSOR CARPI ULNARIS TENDINITIS

This disorder is less common than other tendinopathies about the wrist but must be differentiated from triangular fibrocartilage tears, instability of the extensor carpi ulnaris (ECU), and the rare condition of tenosynovitis of the extensor digiti minimi (EDM). If the usual conservative measures do not relieve symptoms, surgical release of the sixth compartment is usually curative. Although some authors have cautioned that release of the retinaculum of the 6th compartment without repair can lead to destabilization of the distal radioulnar joint,[20] studies by Kip and Peimer[21] showed that it is not necessary to repair the retinaculum and that simple release is all that is necessary.

EPL TENDINITIS

This disorder results from wear at Lister's tubercle where the EPL turns acutely toward the thumb.[22] Sharp edges of bone from Colles' fractures are a common cause of tendinitis or rupture of this tendon. Overuse and repetitive thumb movements, especially combined with wrist motion, can also cause this condition.[23] Cortisone injections may lead to rupture of an already compromised tendon and should be avoided. If splinting is not effective, the surgeon should shave Lister's tubercle down to a smooth surface, close the retinaculum over the bone, and relocate the EPL outside the third compartment.

EDM TENDINITIS

This unusual condition usually follows trauma to the wrist area. Patients with EDM tendinitis complain of pain over the fifth compartment on combined gripping or extension movements of the hand.[24] The differential diagnoses include triangular fibrocartilage tear and ECU tendinitis. Musicians who use the fifth finger repetitively are prone to developing this condition. A helpful test is to have the patient flex the fifth finger and the wrist simultaneously

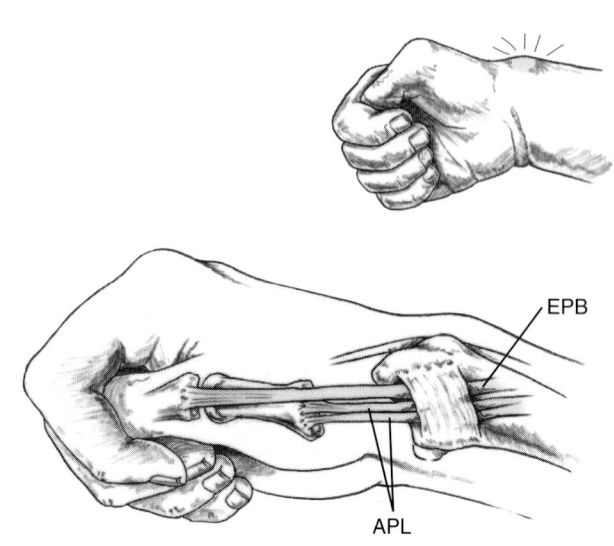

Fig. 7. Finkelstein's test.

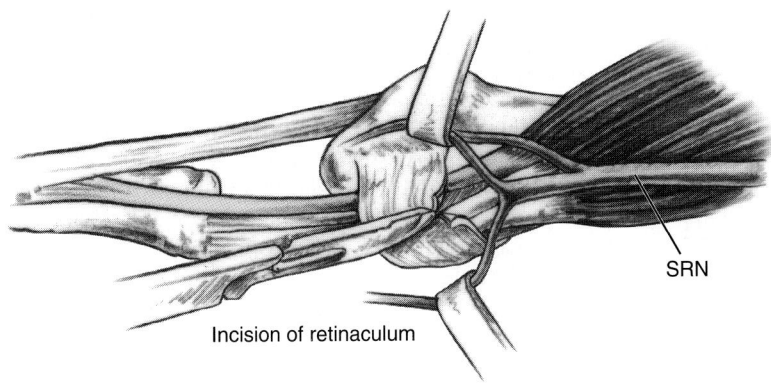

Incision of retinaculum

SRN

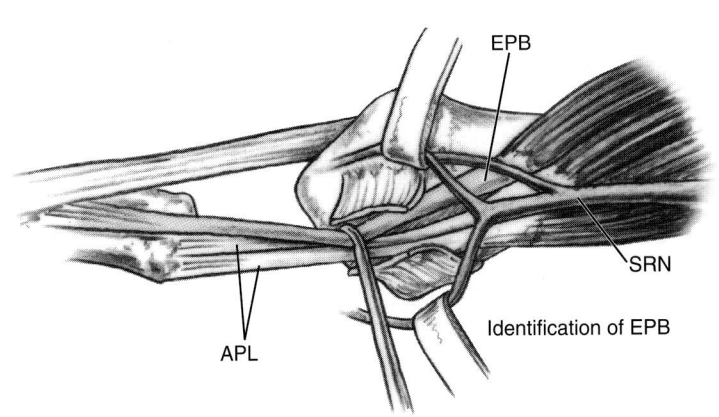

EPB

SRN

APL

Identification of EPB

Fig. 8. De Quervain's tendinitis. *Top,* Release of the first compartment, preserving some of the volar retinaculum and protecting the superficial radial nerve. *Bottom,* Identification of the separate tunnel for the extensor pollicis brevis (EPB) and placing traction on the tendon to make sure it extends the thumb metatarsal joint. (APL, abductor pollicis longus; SRN, superficial radial nerve.)

and then extend the fifth finger against resistance. If the patient experiences pain over the fifth compartment, tendinitis of the EDM probably exists. Conservative treatment is usually effective. When surgery is necessary, the surgeon should look for anomalous tendons or encroachment of the EDM muscle belly within the compartment. The discovery of two tendons within the fifth compartment at surgery is not unusual and is not a pathological finding.

EXTENSOR DIGITORUM COMMUNIS TENDINITIS

Several factors can lead to tendinitis within the fourth dorsal compartment. Most cases of extensor digitorum communis (EDC) tendinitis are associated with rheumatoid arthritis. In nonrheumatoid patients, crowding within the compartment can come from carpal bossing at the carpometacarpal junction, osteophytes, residua of fractures, and anomalous or enlarged muscles. The muscle belly of the extensor indicis proprius is normally within the fourth dorsal compartment but becomes pathological when overuse results in hypertrophy and crowding.

Tenosynovitis can be caused by the presence of an extensor digitorum manus muscle.[25] These unusual muscles arise from the dorsal wrist or the metacarpals and travel within the fourth compartment, usually inserting into the extensor hood of the index or middle fingers. Enlargement can cause crowding within the fourth compartment, or teno-

synovitis can result from impingement against the retinaculum. Although decompression of the muscle by retinacular release is usually all that is necessary, particularly large muscles or ones that have undergone degeneration may require excision.

Treatment of tendinitis of the EDC presents a challenge. Prolonged extension block splinting may help the patient to limit the use of the wrist and metacarpophalangeal joints and thus the EDC. If surgical treatment becomes necessary, decompression of the fourth compartment may be combined with tenosynovectomy. Preservation of at least part of the extensor retinaculum prevents extensor tendon bowstringing. Interposition of the extensor retinaculum between the extensor tendons and underlying structures provides a barrier to further irritation of the tendons.

FLEXOR CARPI RADIALIS TENDINITIS

Flexor carpi radialis (FCR) tendinitis occurs within the tight fibrous tunnel formed by the scaphoid tuberosity, the trapezium, and the transverse carpal ligament.[26] Patients typically have localized tenderness directly over the FCR tendon just proximal to the scaphoid tuberosity. Pain can be elicited by acute passive extension of the wrist or active flexion and radial deviation against resistance. Radiographs may demonstrate scaphotrapezial trapezoid arthritis, calcification near the scaphoid tuberosity, or irregularities of the trapezial groove. Carpal tunnel views and computed tomography scans can provide more detailed images of osteophytes or abnormalities of the trapezial ridge. Nonoperative treatment includes splints, modification of activities, and NSAIDs. If there is evidence of impingement caused by osteophytes or bony irregularities, corticosteroid injections may hasten tendon rupture. Surgery should focus on release of the FCR tunnel, lysis of adhesions, and removal of spurs within the trapezial groove. As is true of other operations in this area, the palmar cutaneous nerve is vulnerable to injury as well as volar branches of the superficial radial nerve.[27]

FLEXOR CARPI ULNARIS TENDINITIS

This may be indistinguishable from pisotriquetral arthritis, another cause of pain on the ulnar side of the wrist. These two disorders are common in racquet sports. Both may present with crepitus on wrist motion. Occasionally, radiographs will demonstrate calcific densities in the flexor carpi ulnaris tendon. Moving the pisiform under compression against the triquetrum may elicit pain in pisotriquetral ar-

thritis. Although nonoperative measures are usually successful, excision of the pisiform will likely provide relief for either condition if these measures fail.[28]

LINBURG'S SYNDROME

Patients with pain in the distal anterior forearm near the wrist may have Linburg's syndrome.[29] This disorder may be overlooked or confused with FCR tendinitis. It is due to connections between the profundus tendon of the index finger and the flexor pollicis longus. Patients cannot independently flex the interphalangeal joint of the thumb without flexing the distal interphalangeal joint of the index. As the examiner blocks flexion of the distal interphalangeal joint of the index, the patient, on attempting to flex the thumb interphalangeal joint, will feel pain at the wrist and be unable to flex the thumb. Although temporarily helpful, corticosteroid injection in the region of the flexor pollicis longus tendon sheath at the wrist is not curative. Exploration and lysis of connections between the tendons are appropriate treatments.

REFERENCES

1. Casanova J, Casanova J: Nintendinitis (letter). J Hand Surg Am 1991; 16:181.
2. Kiefhaber R, Stern PJ: Upper extremity tendinitis and overuse syndromes in the athlete. Clin Sports Med 1992; 11:39.
3. Fromm B, Martini A, Schmidt E: Osteoid osteoma of the radial styloid mimicking stenosing tenosynovitis: A case report. J Hand Surg Br 1992; 17:236.
4. Clancy WF: Tendon trauma and overuse injuries. In Leadbetter WB, Buckwalter JA, Gordon SL (eds): Sports-Induced Inflammation: Clinical and Basic Science Concepts. Park Ridge, IL, American Academy of Orthopaedic Surgeons, 1990, p 609.
5. Mannerfelt L, Norman O: Attrition ruptures of flexor tendons in rheumatoid arthritis caused by bony spurs in the carpal tunnel: A clinical and radiological study. J Bone Joint Surg Br 1969; 51:270.
6. Milek MA, Boulas HJ: Flexor tendon ruptures secondary to hamate hook fractures. J Hand Surg Am 1990; 15:740.
7. Sampson SP, Badalamente MA, Hurst LC, et al: Pathobiology of the human A1 pulley in trigger finger. J Hand Surg Am 1991; 16:714.
8. Chammas M, Bousquet P, Renard E, et al: Dupuytren's disease, carpal tunnel syndrome, trigger finger, and diabetes mellitus. J Hand Surg Am 1995; 20:109.
9. Blyth MJ, Ross DJ: Diabetes and trigger finger. J Hand Surg Br 1996; 21:244.
10. Marks MR, Gunther SF: Efficacy of cortisone injections in treatment of trigger fin-

gers and thumbs. J Hand Surg Am 1989; 14:722.
11. Griggs SM, Weiss AP, Lane LB, et al: Treatment of trigger finger in patients with diabetes mellitus. J Hand Surg Am 1995; 20:787.
12. Bugbee WD, Botte MJ: Surface anatomy of the hand: The relationships between palmar skin creases and osseous anatomy. Clin Orthop 1993; 296:122.
13. Pope DF, Wolfe SW: Safety and efficacy of percutaneous trigger finger release. J Hand Surg Am 1995; 20:280.
14. Seradge H, Kleinert HE: Reduction flexor tenoplasty: Treatment of stenosing flexor tenosynovitis distal to the first pulley. J Hand Surg 1981; 6:543.
15. Finkelstein H: Stenosing tendovaginitis at the radial styloid process. J Bone Joint Surg 1930; 12:509.
16. Zingas C, Failla JM, Van Holsbeeck M: Injection accuracy and clinical relief of de Quervain's tendinitis. J Hand Surg Am 1998; 23:89.
17. Louis DS: Incomplete release of the first dorsal compartment: A diagnostic test. J Hand Surg Am 1987; 12:87.
18. Arons MS: De Quervain's release in working women: A report of failures, complications, and associated diagnoses. J Hand Surg Am 1987; 12:540.
19. Grundberg AB, Reagan DS: Pathologic anatomy of the forearm: Intersection syndrome. J Hand Surg Am 1985; 10:299.
20. Spinner M, Kaplan EB: Extensor carpi ulnaris: Its relationship to the stability of the

distal radio-ulnar joint. Clin Orthop 1970; 68:124.
21. Kip PC, Peimer CA: Release of the sixth dorsal compartment. J Hand Surg Am 1994; 19:599.
22. McMahon MS, Posner MA: Triggering of the thumb due to stenosing tenosynovitis of the extensor pollicis longus: A case report. J Hand Surg Am 1994; 19:623.
23. Bonatz E, Kramer TD, Masear VR: Rupture of the extensor pollicis longus tendon. Am J Orthop 1996; 25:118.
24. O'Rourke PJ, O'Sullivan T, Stephens M: Extensor tendon sheath stenosis resulting in triggering of the little finger. J Hand Surg Br 1994; 19:662.
25. Patel MR, Desai SS, Bassini-Lipson L, et al: Painful extensor digitorum brevis manus muscle. J Hand Surg Am 1989; 14:674.
26. Bishop AT, Gabel G, Carmichael SW: Flexor carpi radialis tendinitis I: Operative anatomy. J Bone Joint Surg Am 1994; 76:1009.
27. Gabel G, Bishop AT, Wood MB: Flexor carpi radialis tendinitis II: Results of operative treatment. J Bone Joint Surg Am 1994; 76:1015.
28. Palmieri TJ: Pisiform area pain treatment by pisiform excision. J Hand Surg Am 1982; 7:477.
29. Linburg RM, Comstock BE: Anomalous tendon slips from the flexor pollicis longus to the flexor digitorum profundus. J Hand Surg 1979; 4:79.

WRIST INSTABILITY

Subir Jossan and Scott W. Wolfe

Summary
- This chapter presents a review of anatomy and carpal kinematics.
- This chapter outlines a general classification system.
- It specifies aids in diagnosis and radiographic findings.
- It presents treatment alternatives for common injury patterns.

Carpal instability is defined by abnormal carpal bone kinematics or kinetics that occurs during physiological load. Carpal instability is generally secondary to traumatic disruption of the bony or ligamentous stabilizers of the carpus. Chronic pain, weakness, and degenerative arthritis may be the end result of untreated instability patterns.

ANATOMY

The carpus consists of eight bones arranged in two rows. The proximal row consists of the scaphoid, lunate, triquetral, and pisiform. The pisiform is a sesamoid bone and is not considered a functional part of the proximal row. The distal row consists of the trapezium, trapezoid, capitate, and hamate.

Normal carpal function depends on a well-balanced intrinsic and extrinsic ligament system. The intrinsic ligaments originate and insert on the carpus, whereas the extrinsic (or capsular) ligaments course between the radius and the carpus.[1] The proximal row interosseous ligaments are C-shaped and bind neighboring carpal bones via their dorsal, palmar, and proximal edges. The ligaments are thick dorsally and palmarly but have a thin membranous central portion.[2] The dorsal capsular ligaments include the dorsal radiocarpal and dorsal intercarpal ligaments (Fig. 1A). The palmar capsular ligaments include the radioscaphocapitate, radiolunate (long and short), radioscapholunate, ulnolunate, and ulnotriquetral. The radioscaphocapitate and triquetrocapitate ligaments form a V across the midcarpal joint, referred to as the deltoid ligament. The long and short radiolunate ligaments, described by Berger et al,[3] are critical stabilizers of the lunate and proximal carpal row (Fig. 1B). The radioscapholunate ligament (ligament of Testut) was once thought to be a prime stabilizer of the carpus, but is now more widely recognized as a vascular conduit to the scapholunate interosseous ligament.

The tendons responsible for wrist movement are located far from the center of motion of the wrist (the head of the capitate) to maximize their moment arm and their mechanical effect on wrist motion. Conversely, the digital flexor and extensor tendons are located centrally, diminishing their effect on wrist motion. Normal wrist flexion and extension includes a 150-degree arc of motion. Approximately half of this motion occurs at the radiocarpal joint and half at the midcarpal joint.[4]

KINEMATICS

Navarro proposed that the carpus behaved as three longitudinal columns, defining the scaphoid as the lateral column, the lunate and distal row as the central column, and the triquetrum as the medial column. The scaphoid functioned as the critical stabilizing link of the carpus and was responsible for coordinating the complex kinematics of the individual carpal bones. Weber expanded on this concept by emphasizing the load-transmitting function of the central column and ability of the relatively "unloaded" triquetrohamate joint to coordinate the motions of the carpus. The unique "helicoidal" surface of this joint created a force couple that simultaneously extended the triquetrum and lunate during ulnar deviation, while forcing the hamate and capitate to translate dorsally. Similarly, in radial deviation, the triquetrum slid proximally and rose dorsally on the helicoidal face of the hamate and into conjoint palmar flexion.

In their 1972 article, Linscheid et al[5] called our attention to the important "intercalated segment" of the carpus in reference to the scaphoid, lunate, and triquetrum. The authors contended that kinematics of the carpus is perhaps better described in terms of carpal rows than carpal columns, a theory attributed to Destot in 1925. The proximal carpal row was demonstrated to have no tendon insertions and motion of the row to be dependent entirely on mechanical and ligamentous constraints. Thus, the proximal row can be thought of as "intercalated" between a relatively fixed distal carpal row and the forearm (Fig. 2). In the uninjured state, motions of the three proximal carpal row bones are always in the same direction, albeit at different magnitudes, regardless of the direction of hand motion. Disruption of the interosseous ligaments between the bones of the proximal carpal row predictably causes carpal instability. Lichtman et al[6] further described the "oval ring" of the carpus to emphasize the critical additional "mobile links" between the proximal and distal carpal rows at the scaphotrapezial and triquetrohamate joints and the fact that injury anywhere along the ring would disrupt normal carpal kinematics.

Although the exact mechanism may be debated, the position of the proximal carpal row changes from that of flexion in radial deviation to extension in ulnar deviation. This normal motion of the intact proximal row must be understood before considering abnormal motion within the row when ligament or bony injury occurs.

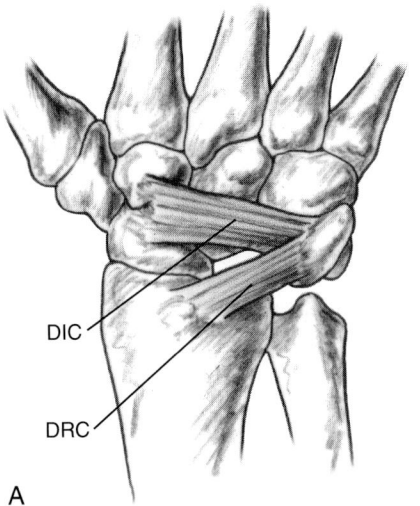

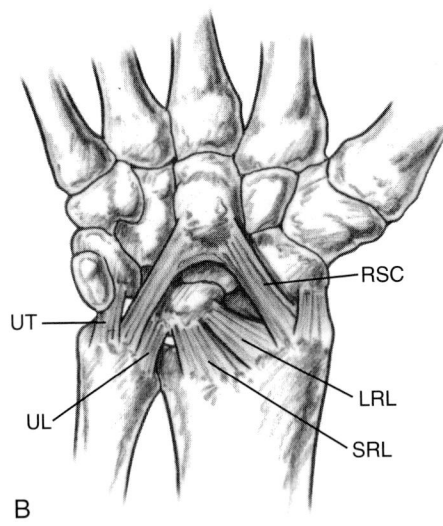

Fig. 1. Extrinsic ligaments of the wrist. *A,* Dorsal capsular ligaments, including the dorsal intercarpal ligament and the dorsal radiocarpal ligament. *B,* The palmar extrinsic ligaments. Note the stout long and short radiolunate ligaments.

MECHANISM OF INJURY

Mayfield[7] described four progressive stages of perilunate instability using a cadaveric model. Hyperextension injury to the carpal ligaments was reproducibly demonstrated by loading a wrist to failure in a position of dorsiflexion, ulnar deviation, and intercarpal supination. The carpus failed first at the scapholunate interosseous ligament and, with increasing loads, in a clockwise fashion about the lunate until complete lunate dislocation had occurred. He also noted that ulnar-sided loading with the carpus in a hyperpronated position caused isolated triquetrolunate injury.

CLASSIFICATION

Classification of carpal instabilities is controversial, and a comprehensive classification scheme has not been universally adopted. Dobyns et al[8] described two general patterns of instability based primarily on the integrity of the interosseous ligaments of the intercalated segment or proximal carpal row. Dissociative carpal instability (CID) refers to a ligamentous or bony disruption within the proximal row that allows the bones within the row to dissociate from one another. Nondissociative carpal instability (CIND) refers to similar patterns of instability that occur without a break in the continuity of the proximal carpal row. CID is the most common group of carpal instabilities within which scapholunate interosseous ligament ruptures predominate (Fig. 3).

Isolated scapholunate ligament injury uncouples the proximal carpal row and initiates a condition known as "rotatory subluxation of the scaphoid."[9] Watson et al[9] recognized a spectrum of injury to this ligament, ranging from abnormal kinematics of the scaphoid with heavy activities to the full-blown collapse pattern of dorsal intercalated segment instability (DISI). An injury to the scapholunate ligament is necessary but not sufficient to result in a DISI pattern. Additional ligament injury or gradual attenuation must occur to the secondary extrinsic stabilizers of the lunate before DISI will be manifested.[10] DISI is defined by abnormal extension of the lunate, and when secondary to scapholunate disruption, the scaphoid assumes a flexed posture, whereas the remainder of the proximal carpal row extends (Fig. 4).

Injury to the triquetrolunate ligament can result in CID. Isolated injury to this ligament causes painful kinematic aberrations between the triquetral and the lunate but is insufficient to cause volar intercalated segment instability (VISI). Additional injury or attenuation to the dorsal radiotriquetral or ulnar arm of the deltoid ligament is necessary to permit VISI.[11] VISI is characterized by abnormal flexion of the lunate and an increased capitolunate angle (see Fig. 4). Generally, the scapholunate angle remains normal or decreased in this pattern.

CIND patterns can be caused by many entities, including ligamentous laxity, capitolunate instability (CLIP)[11a], and malunited distal radius fractures. As previously stated, the abnormality is within the extrinsic ligaments that connect the distal radius and ulna to the carpus and not within the intercarpal ligaments that connect bones within each carpal row. CIND conditions may result in dorsal or volar flexion of the entire proximal row; therefore, both VISI and DISI

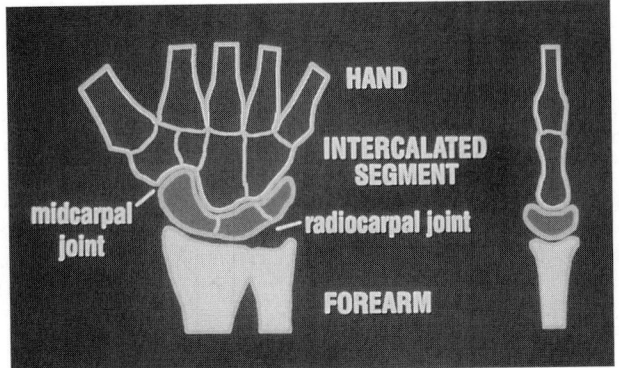

Fig. 2. Proximal carpal row. The proximal carpal row is "intercalated" between the relatively fixed distal carpal row bones and the two bones of the forearm. It has no tendon attachments and is thus entirely dependent on mechanical contact and ligamentous restraints to guide its motion.

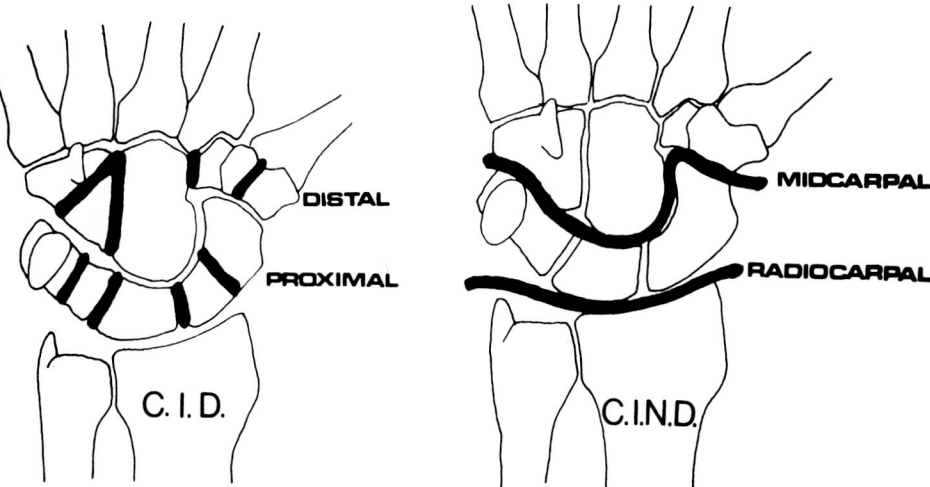

Fig. 3. Dissociative and nondissociative instability patterns. Dissociative carpal instability occurs when there has been a bony or soft-tissue disruption within the proximal carpal row. A nondissociative instability may present with identical abnormal postures of the carpal bones (volar intercalated segment instability or dorsal intercalated segment instability), but there is no ligamentous disruption within either carpal row. (From Cooney WP, Wright TW, Dobyns JH: Carpal instability nondissociative. In The Wrist. St. Louis, MO, CV Mosby, 1998, p 551.)

patterns are possible with nondissociative injuries. These instability patterns, also referred to in the literature as "midcarpal" instability patterns, are frequently manifested by a painful and dramatic transition of the proximal carpal row from a flexed position to an extended position (or vice versa) with radioulnar deviation. CLIP is a rare form of CIND caused by congenital ligament laxity of the capitolunate complex, which allows displacement of the capitate from the lunate with forceful activities. Adaptive carpal instability is defined as a posture assumed by the carpus in response to a dorsal or volar malunion of the distal radius and is a nondissociative instability variant.

Radiocarpal instability is a rare form of carpal instability wherein the entire carpus is shifted in reference to the forearm. It has been described in dorsal, volar, ulnar, and radial variants. The entity may result from fracture dislocations, inflammatory arthritis, scaphoid or lunate dislocation, or dorsal carpal dislocation. Radiocarpal instability requires a near-complete disruption of the extrinsic ligament support of the carpus, and ulnar translocation is the most common type.[12] Taleisnik[13] emphasized the importance of distinguishing between two variants of ulnar translocation based on the integrity of the scapholunate interosseous ligament. In type I ulnar translation, the entire carpus is shifted in an ulnar direction, as is often seen in rheumatoid arthritis. In the second variant, the carpus is translocated through a disrupted scapholunate ligament, leaving the scaphoid in its normal position.[13]

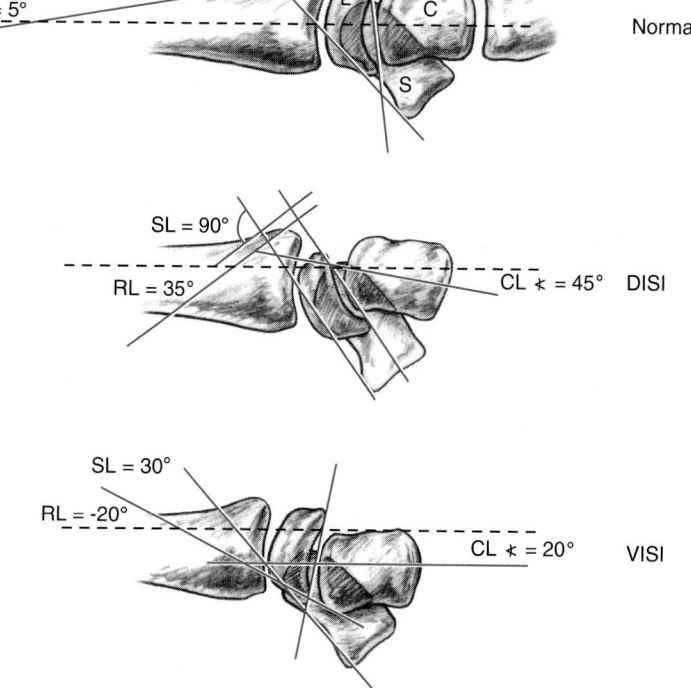

Fig. 4. Normal and abnormal carpal postures. In the uninjured wrist, the capitate and longitudinal axis of the radius are colinear. In dorsal intercalated segment instability, the lunate extends (more than 15 degrees), and the capitate translates dorsally. The scaphoid flexes and the scapholunate angle is increased (more than 70 degrees). In volar intercalated segment instability patterns, the lunate is characteristically flexed (more than 15 degrees volar), and the scapholunate angle is generally decreased (25 to 30 degrees).

Complex carpal instabilities refer to combination instability patterns such as those seen with perilunate and lunate dislocations, axial disruptions of the carpus, and scaphocapitate syndrome. In these situations, carpal posture and kinematics are variable, and treatment must be individualized.

Finally, the distinction between static and dynamic instability patterns should be made. Dynamic instabilities are those that are manifested only during forceful activities, thus requiring stress or dynamic imaging studies for detection. Static deformities are present and detectable with standard radiographic views.

DIAGNOSIS

HISTORY AND PHYSICAL EXAMINATION

The initial history should document the mechanism of injury and associated complaints, including pain, weakness, giving way, and presence of a click or pop with motion. Physical examination may reveal point tenderness, pain at the extremes of motion, and abnormal carpal motion with provocative maneuvers. Many specific examination techniques have been described to assist in the detection of interosseous ligament injury, including the scaphoid shift test and the shear, shuck, and compression tests for lunotriquetral instability. A complete description of each of these techniques is beyond the scope of this chapter.

Watson et al[9] described the scaphoid shift test as an essential component of the examination for rotatory subluxation of the scaphoid. The test is performed with the examiner's ipsilateral thumb on the scaphoid tubercle. During radial deviation in an uninjured wrist, the scaphoid tubercle will flex against the examiner's thumb. With scaphoid instability, the proximal pole of the scaphoid will be moved dorsally out of the elliptical scaphoid fossa of the radius during radial deviation and will reduce with a dramatic "clunk" on relief of thumb pressure. Kleinman described the shear test for lunotriquetral instability. With the forearm in neutral, the examiner's contralateral thumb is placed on the dorsal lunate and the ipsilateral thumb is placed on the volar pisotriquetral complex. If dorsovolar shear force causes palpable laxity that reproduces the patients' symptoms, the test is considered positive.

IMAGING STUDIES

Standard radiographs include a posteroanterior (PA) and lateral view of the involved wrist and comparison radiographs of the opposite wrist. Oblique radiographs are generally not helpful for soft-tissue injuries. Stress views include radial and ulnar deviation PA views as well as lateral views in full flexion and full extension. An AP film taken during forceful grip helps to profile the scapholunate joint and will occasionally widen the scapholunate interval after injury.

In suspected scapholunate injuries, a scapholunate interval on the PA film of 3 mm or greater is considered abnormal, especially if asymmetric. The so-called "cortical ring sign" refers to the superimposition of the scaphoid tubercle on the scaphoid waist in the PA view, and it occurs with abnormal flexion of the scaphoid. A lateral film in full wrist flexion that demonstrates minimal or no lunate flexion and a marked increase in the scapholunate angle (more than 90 degrees) is virtually diagnostic of a scapholunate ligament disruption (Fig. 5). DISI is defined

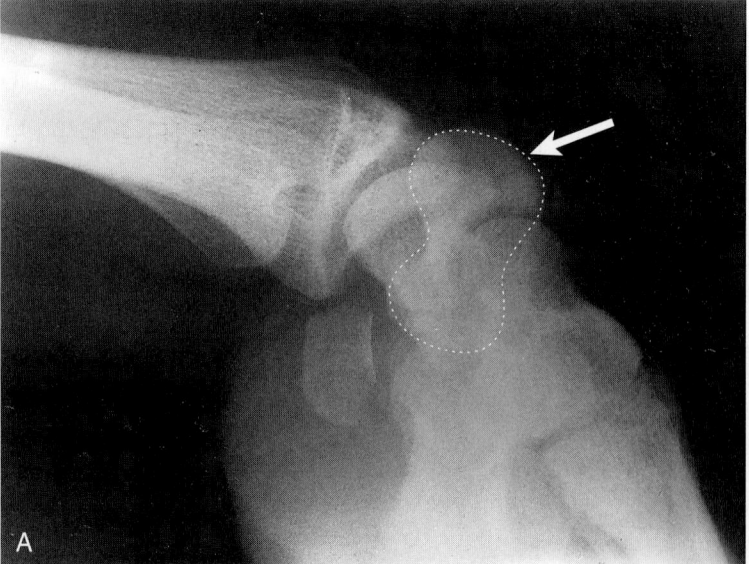
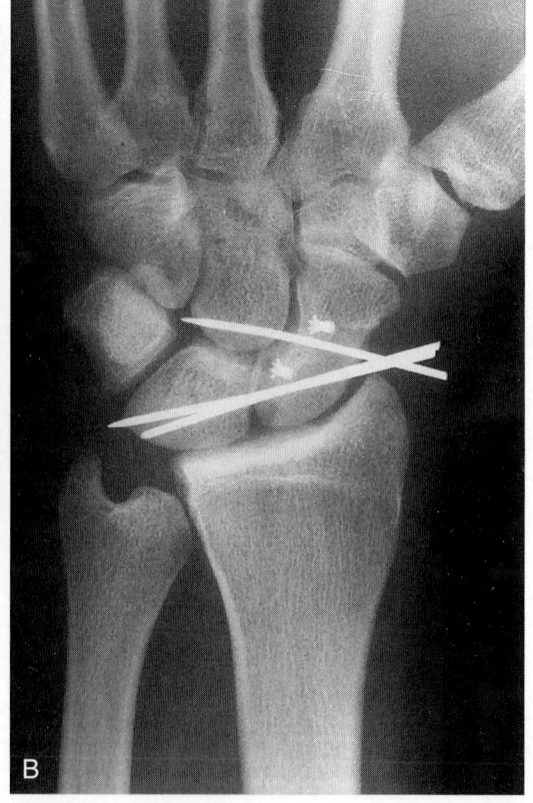

Fig. 5. Scapholunate injuries. *A,* This patient presented 1 year after a fall with a painful click in the wrist. Posteroanterior (PA) and lateral radiographs were entirely normal. A full-flexion lateral radiograph demonstrates lack of lunate flexion and a dorsally subluxated scaphoid *(arrow).* This is diagnostic of scapholunate ligament incompetence. *B,* PA view after scapholunate ligament repair and dorsal capsulodesis.

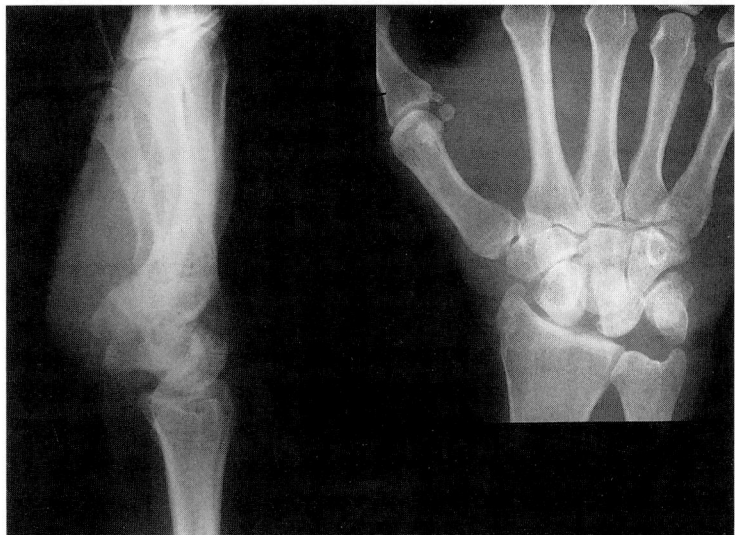

Fig. 6. Type II ulnar translocation. Note the widened scapholunate interval and the near loss of contact between the lunate and the lunate fossa of the distal radius.

by a radiolunate angle of greater than 15 degrees of extension on a true lateral radiograph. The scapholunate angle (measured as the angle between the longitudinal axes of both bones on a true lateral radiograph) is defined as abnormal if it is greater than 70 degrees (normal = 30 to 60 degrees).

Specific radiographic abnormalities seen in volar intercalated segment instability include a flexed scaphoid on the PA view and a triangular-shaped lunate, secondary to its narrow dorsal pole. The cortical ring sign may be positive. In dissociative injuries, the triquetrum is extended on the lateral film, whereas the remainder of the proximal carpal row is flexed. A positive Mayersbach sign is seen, in which the distance between the ulnar head and the triquetrum is decreased. A step-off between the triquetrum and lunate may be present but is not considered diagnostic of triquetrolunate injury. On the lateral radiograph, the scapholunate interosseous angle is usually less than 30 degrees.[14]

Ulnar translocation of the carpus also has specific radiographic findings, as noted by McMurtry et al.[15] The distance from the center of the head of the capitate to the longitudinal axis of the ulna, divided by the length of the third metacarpal, yields a ratio predictive of ulnar translation. On the PA film, the lunate may have little apparent contact with the lunate fossa of the radius. In type II ulnar translation, the scapholunate interval is abnormally widened (Fig. 6).

Ancillary tests may be helpful in the diagnosis of carpal instability. Dynamic instability requires dynamic cine- or fluoroscopic examination of the wrist, if stress static views are nondiagnostic. Bone scans may aid in determining whether an occult fracture is present. Arthrography, once believed to be diagnostic of intercarpal ligament disruption, lacks specificity and is not a highly accurate aid to physical diagnosis. Computed tomography scanning may be useful for delineation of occult fractures, and magnetic resonance imaging may be helpful in detecting interosseous ligament disruption.

Arthroscopy has been criticized by some to be overly sensitive but, when correlated with precise physical findings, probably gives the highest diagnostic yield. Concurrent intraoperative fluoroscopic examination of the scaphoid shift test allows visualization of normal and abnormal carpal kinematics. Arthroscopy has the advantage of determining partial tears of ligaments, visualizing mild degenerative changes in the carpal bones, as well as providing the opportunity for treatment at diagnosis. Arthroscopy carries a greater potential for complication, including nerve and tendon injury.

MANAGEMENT

SCAPHOLUNATE DISSOCIATION

Although infrequently diagnosed in the acute stage, acute scapholunate dissociations should be treated aggressively to avoid long-term complications of instability and degenerative change. Some authors recommend closed manipulation and percutaneous pinning, with or without arthroscopy, for injuries less than 3 weeks old. The capitate and entire distal row may be translated in a volar direction by dorsally applied thumb pressure to realign the lunate into neutral posture. The scapholunate gap can also be manually compressed. The scapholunate and capitolunate joints may then be pinned with multiple Kirschner's wires in a percutaneous fashion (Fig. 7). Because it is difficult to precisely align the scaphoid and lunate percutaneously, most authors recommend open repair of complete scapholunate interosseous ruptures combined with dorsal capsulodesis.[16]

Chronic scapholunate dissociation requires a more individualized approach, depending on the chronicity of the injury, the mobility of the carpal bones, and the presence or absence of degenerative change. For those patients without degenerative changes on radiographs and with minimal scapholunate widening, a dorsal capsulodesis with ligament repair is appropriate[16] (Fig. 8). Several authors prefer intercarpal arthrodesis (scaphotrapezial-trapezoid or scaphocapitate) for chronic scapholunate injuries, particularly if the scaphoid or lunate is not reducible or if the scapholunate ligament remnant is of poor quality. Although the kinematic changes and load transfer after different intercarpal

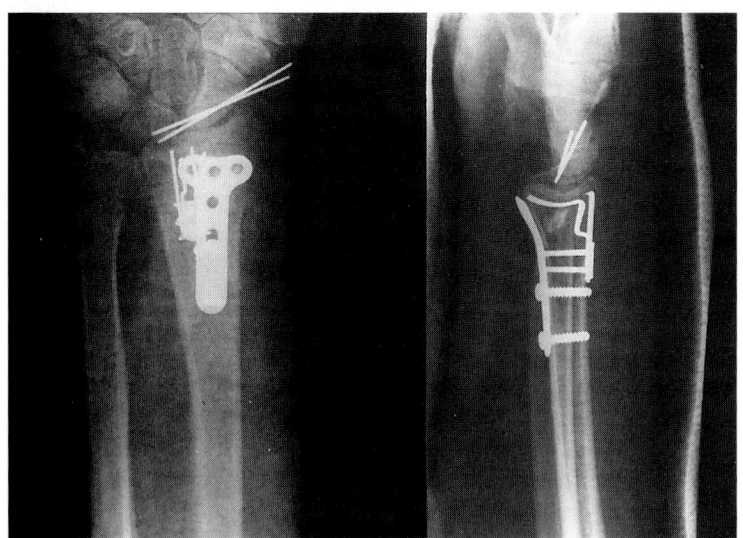

Fig. 7. Pinning of scapholunate joint. Postoperative radiograph demonstrates reduction and pinning of scapholunate joint and simultaneous internal fixation of the distal radius fracture.

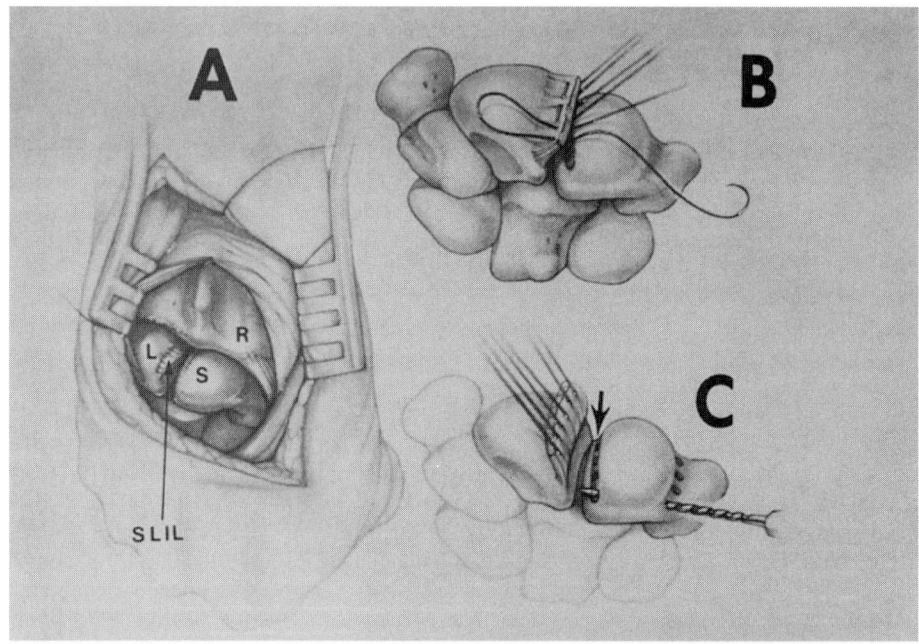

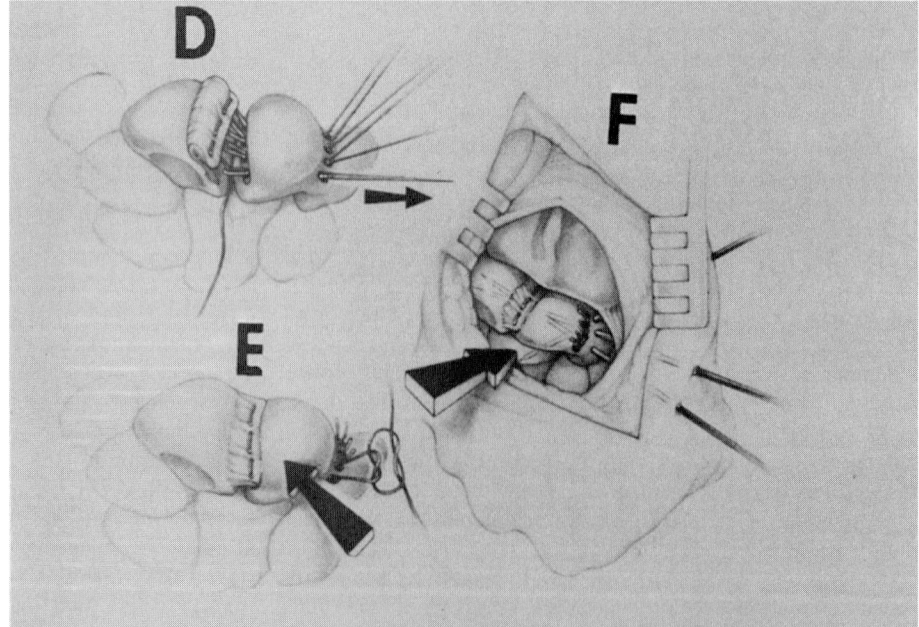

Fig. 8. Technique for open repair of acute scapholunate interosseous ligament injuries. The procedure is augmented with a dorsal capsulodesis. (Reproduced with permission from Lavernia CJ, Cohen MS, Taleisnik J: Treatment of scapholunate dissociation by ligamentous repair and capsulodesis. J Hand Surg Am 1992; 17:355.)

fusions have been extensively studied and are controversial, it is reasonable to assume that any fusion that crosses the midcarpal joint will predictably reduce global wrist motion by approximately 50% and should be considered a salvage procedure.

If arthritic changes are present, radiocarpal or midcarpal arthrodesis may be required. Studies showed that proximal row carpectomy compares favorably with intercarpal arthrodesis in both motion and grip strength at medium-term follow-up.[17] With pancarpal degenerative change, complete wrist arthrodesis is a reliable salvage procedure to restore hand function and reduce or eliminate pain.

TRIQUETROLUNATE DISSOCIATION

Acute triquetrolunate injuries are less common than scapholunate injuries. Acute injuries without volar intercalated segment instability may be treated in the majority of cases in a well-molded short-arm cast for 4 weeks. Chronic isolated triquetrolunate injuries without VISI may be treated with triquetrolunate arthrodesis. Symptomatic dissociative VISI requires operative repair in most cases. Although it is difficult to restore precise triquetrolunate alignment and kinematics, an attempt at repair of the triquetrolunate ligament in the acute situation with dorsal as well as volar capsulodesis is reasonable. The goal of the procedure is to prevent excessive volar flexion of the proximal row. If arthritic change or chronic fixed deformity is present, triquetral-hamate-capitate-lunate (four corner) arthrodesis is preferred. Isolated triquetrolunate arthrodesis cannot correct a VISI deformity and is specifically contraindicated in this situation.

Treatment for nondissociative (CIND) patterns is even more controversial.[18] These patients usually present with a volar flexed instability pattern. Many patients in this category have generalized ligamentous laxity and usually have normal arthroscopic and arthrographic findings. Treatment should include a short course of splinting or casting for acute painful episodes followed by a full course of physical therapy for strengthening. For those patients in whom a prolonged course of conservative therapy fails, consideration of an anterior and posterior capsular imbrication and pinning may be given. Midcarpal arthrodesis is reserved for select patients with chronic disabling wrist pain.[19] Unlike dissociative instability, the condition has not been demonstrated to progress to degenerative change.

Malunited distal radius fractures may result in nondissociative instability patterns, most commonly manifested as a DISI pattern. Corrective osteotomy of the malunited radius is the treatment of choice. The treatment of the underlying radius malunion is warranted. If chronic, the dorsiflexion instability pattern may not fully correct after radial realignment, but symptomatic improvement is generally predictable.

REFERENCES

1. Mayfield JK, Johnson RP, Kilcoyne RF: The ligaments of the human wrist and their functional significance. Anat Rec 1976; 186:417.
2. Ruby LK: Wrist biomechanics. In Eilert RE (ed): Instructional Course Lectures. Park Ridge, IL, American Academy of Orthopaedic Surgeons, vol 41, p 25.
3. Berger H, Landsmeer JMF: The palmar radiocarpal ligaments: A study of adult and fetal human wrist joints. J Hand Surg Am 1990; 15:847.
4. Ruby LK, Cooney WP III, An KN, et al: Relative motion of selected carpal bones: A kinematic analysis of the normal wrist. J Hand Surg Am 1988; 13:1.
5. Linscheid RL, Dobyns JH, Beabout JW, et al: Traumatic instability of the wrist. J Bone Joint Surg Am 1972; 54:1262.
6. Lichtman DM, Schneider JR, Swafford AR, et al: Ulnar midcarpal instability: Clinical and laboratory analysis. J Hand Surg Am 1981; 6:515.
7. Mayfield JK: Patterns of injury to carpal ligaments: A spectrum. Clin Orthop 1984; 187:36.
8. Dobyns JH, Linscheid RL, Macksoud W, et al: Carpal instability, nondissociative. In Proceedings of the American Academy of Orthopaedic Surgeons. Park Ridge, IL, American Academy of Orthopaedic Surgeons, 1987, p 108.
9. Watson H, Ottoni L, Pitts EC, et al: Rotary subluxation of the scaphoid: A spectrum of instability. J Hand Surg Br 1993; 18:62.
10. Meade TD, Schneider LH, Cherry K: Radiographic analysis of selective ligament sectioning at the carpal scaphoid: A cadaver study. J Hand Surg Am 1990; 15: 855.
11. Horii E, Garcia-Elias M, An KN, et al: A kinematic study of luno-triquetral dissociations. J Hand Surg Am 1991; 16:355.
11a. Louis DS, Hankin FM, Greene TL, et al: Central carpal instability–capitate lunate instability. Orthopaedics 1984; 7:1693.
12. Viegas SF, Patterson RM, Ward K: Extrinsic wrist ligaments in the pathomechanics of ulnar translation instability. J Hand Surg Am 1995; 20:312.
13. Taleisnik J: Current concepts review. Carpal instability. J Bone Joint Surg Am 1988; 70:1262.
14. Taleisnik J: Carpal instability. J Bone Joint Surg Am 1988; 70:1262.
15. McMurtry RY, Youm Y, Platt AE, et al: Kinematics of the wrist: Part II. Clinical applications. J Bone Joint Surg Am 1978; 60:955.
16. Lavernia CJ, Cohen MS, Taleisnik J: Treatment of scapholunate dissociation by ligamentous repair and capsulodesis. J Hand Surg Am 1992; 17:354.
17. Wyrick JD, Stern PJ, Kiefhaber TR: Motion-preserving procedures in the treatment of scapholunate advanced collapse wrist: Proximal row carpectomy versus four-corner arthrodesis. J Hand Surg 1995; 6:965.
18. Wright TW, Dobyns JH, Linscheid RL, et al: Carpal instability non-dissociative. J Hand Surg Br 1994; 19:763.
19. Lichtman DM, Bruckner JD, Culp RW, et al: Palmar midcarpal instability: Results of surgical reconstruction. J Hand Surg Am 1993; 18:307.

NONUNION OF THE SCAPHOID

Randall W. Culp

Summary

- Scaphoid fractures are common and constitute 60% to 70% of all carpal fractures. Nonunion rates vary from 5% to 50%.
- Risk factors for nonunion include fracture displacement, carpal instability, comminution, and proximal pole location.
- Symptomatic scaphoid nonunions have a high probability of progressive degenerative changes.
- Scaphoid nonunions are classified based on displacement, carpal instability, and degenerative changes.
- Stable internal fixation and bone grafting comprise the recommended treatment for most nonarthritic scaphoid nonunions.

Among all wrist injuries, the incidence of fractures of the scaphoid is second only to that of the distal radius.[1] Scaphoid fractures constitute 60% to 70% of all carpal bone fractures. A scaphoid fracture becomes a nonunion when it fails to unite within 6 months of injury. Reported rates of nonunion vary from 5% to 50%. It has been estimated that there are 17,250 to 34,500 nonunions per year despite proper treatment. Because most nonunions occur in young men in their second or third decade, prolonged treatment[2] may also create significant economic hardship.

The criterion for successful treatment is a functional outcome superior to the natural history of scaphoid nonunion. Symptomatic nonunions have a high probability of progressive degenerative changes and persistent symptoms.[3, 4] The procedure of choice for most nonunions consists of open reduction, bone grafting, and fixation, which can achieve both union and a functional outcome.[5]

RISK FACTORS

Union requires prompt diagnosis, bone apposition, adequate blood supply, and fracture immobilization. Fracture displacement of only 1 mm markedly increases the risk of nonunion for those fractures treated nonoperatively (Fig. 1). Among scaphoid fractures treated with immobilization, the nonunion rate is only 5% if nondisplaced but ranges from 46% to 92% if displaced.

Carpal instability is now recognized as a risk factor for nonunion. The presence of a dorsiflexed intercalated segment instability on initial radiographs is a harbinger of potential nonunion (Fig. 2A and B).

Fracture type and location also affect the risk of nonunion. Comminuted fractures have been associated with increased risk of nonunion. Proximal pole fractures have the highest risk of nonunion and are the slowest to unite. Of the three fracture patterns described by Rüsse (transverse, horizontal oblique, and vertical oblique), the vertical oblique pattern, in which the fracture line is almost parallel to the long axis of the radius, has the highest risk of nonunion.

Studies of the vascular supply to the scaphoid demonstrated that the proximal 80% of the bone, including the entire proximal pole, is supplied by a distal and dorsal branch of the radial artery.[6] Thus, avascular necrosis, particularly of the proximal pole, may play a role in nonunion because of inadequate blood supply.

Finally, late diagnosis and inadequate immobilization can cause nonunion. Early diagnosis requires a high index of suspicion and adequate radiographs. Patients with snuffbox tenderness and negative initial radiographs require at the least repeat films in 2 weeks when some resorption of the fracture site may facilitate diagnosis. There is continued debate as to the relationship of the type of immobilization to risk factors for nonunion. Some studies indicated that scaphoid fractures should initially be treated in a long-arm cast. Others suggested that short-arm casting is sufficient.

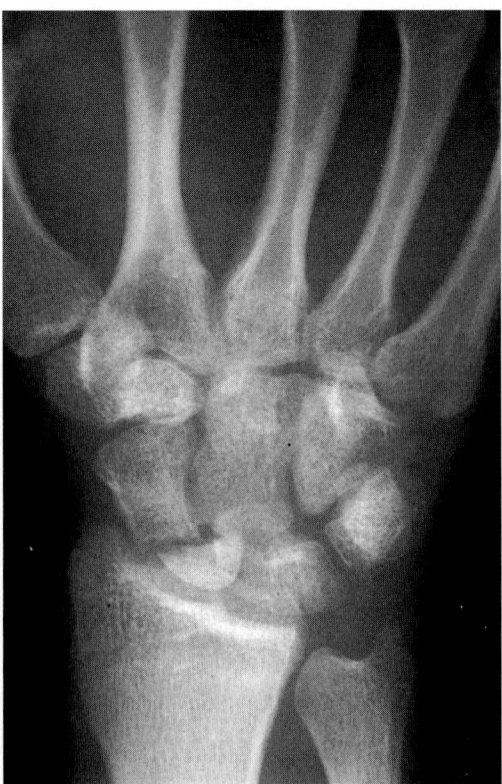

Fig. 1. Displaced proximal pole scaphoid fracture. This is a posteroanterior radiograph.

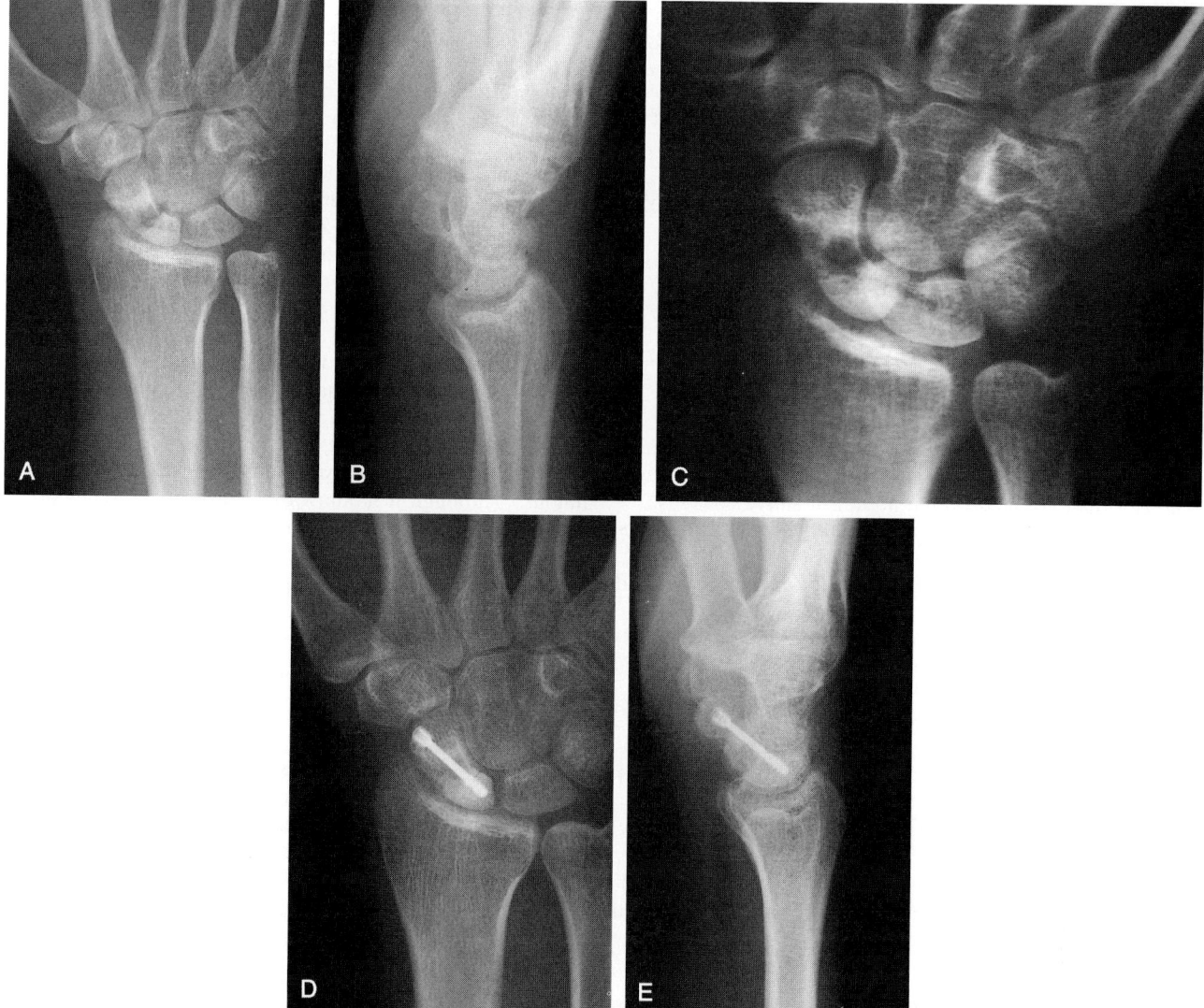

Fig. 2. Carpal instability. Posteroanterior (PA) radiograph *A*, demonstrating scaphoid nonunion. *B*, Lateral radiograph. Dorsiflexed intercalated segment instability (DISI) instability pattern. Note extended posture of lunate on the lateral view. *C*, Tomograph demonstrating scaphoid nonunion. Note cystic changes. *D*, PA radiograph demonstrating healed fracture with Herbert screw and wedge bone joint. *E*, Lateral radiograph demonstrating healed fracture. Note correction of DISI.

There is also debate regarding whether the thumb should be included in the immobilization and regarding its relationship to nonunion. The most important issue referable to immobilization is that it should be continued until union is radiographically confirmed.

NATURAL HISTORY

The earlier literature suggested that certain patients with scaphoid nonunions functioned quite satisfactorily. However, most recent studies indicated that untreated scaphoid nonunion eventually leads to posttraumatic osteoarthritis.

In patients with symptomatic nonunion, Mack et al[3] showed that progressive radiographic changes and increasing osteoarthritis occur with time. Between 5 and 10 years, cystic sclerotic changes are confined to the scaphoid. Radiocarpal arthritis developed in the second decade. After more

than 20 years, generalized osteoarthritis of the wrist was found. Ruby et al[4] found similar findings radiographically, but these radiographic changes did not necessarily correlate with symptoms.

Not all scaphoid nonunions are symptomatic. Asymptomatic nonunions are often discovered incidentally in radiographs taken for other purposes. Controversy continues to surround the appropriate management of the patient with an asymptomatic nonunion of the scaphoid.

Scaphoid nonunions can be divided into five distinct types based on the presence or absence of displacement, carpal instability, and degenerative changes (Table 1). Treatment is based on classification type.

Type I: simple nonunion. Simple nonunion is stable, is nondisplaced, and has no degenerative changes.

Type II: unstable nonunion (see Figs. 1 and 2A–C). Unsta-

TABLE 1. TYPES OF SCAPHOID NONUNION		
Type	Name	Characteristics
I	Simple	No displacement No degenerative change
II	Unstable	Displacement >1 mm or scapholunate angle >70 degrees
III	Early arthritic	Radioscaphoid arthritis
IV	Scaphoid nonunion advanced collapse (SNAC wrist)	Radioscaphoid arthritis and midcarpal arthritis
V	SNAC wrist plus	Pain carpal arthritis

ble nonunion is characterized by significant displacement (greater than 1 mm) or instability (scapholunate angle greater than 70 degrees) but no degenerative changes.

Type III: nonunion with early degenerative changes. Radioscaphoid arthritis is present with joint space narrowing, subchondral sclerosis, and beaking of the radial styloid process.

Type IV: scaphoid nonunion advanced collapsed (SNAC) wrist. Arthritis of radioscaphoid and midcarpal joint is present.

Type V: scaphoid nonunion advanced collapse plus (SNAC plus). Advanced degenerative changes are present to include the radiolunate joint.

DIAGNOSTIC IMAGING

Plain radiographs remain the cornerstone of initial and follow-up imaging. Posteroanterior lateral, ulnarly deviated (scaphoid view), and oblique radiographs are obtained. These views are assessed for nonunion, displacement, instability, and arthritic changes. For the assessment of scaphoid healing, plain radiographs may be inadequate. Care must be taken not to mistake overlap of the fragments for healing.

If doubt exists as to healing, tomographs or computed tomography (CT) scans are recommended. Tomography is taken in five planes with 2-mm cuts. A CT scan with 1.0- to 1.5-mm cuts in the longitudinal axis of the scaphoid serves the same purpose. Both techniques permit accurate assessment of healing, displacement, and degenerative changes.

If a bone graft of a nonunion is planned but avascular necrosis is suspected, a magnetic resonance imaging (MRI) scan is obtained (Fig. 3A and B). Avascular necrosis of the scaphoid, particularly the proximal pole, is an important predictor of success of surgery to correct scaphoid nonunions.[7] Although it is known that plain radiographs do not accurately demonstrate true avascular necrosis, a decrease in marrow intensity in T_1-weighted images on MRI has been shown to have a high specificity for avascular necrosis.[8]

NONOPERATIVE TREATMENT

NO INTERVENTION

According to some reports, established nonunions, particularly if stable and without carpal collapse, may not require any treatment because they can remain with minimal symptoms. Elderly patients who have low-demand upper extremity requirements in this radiographic category may not require treatment.

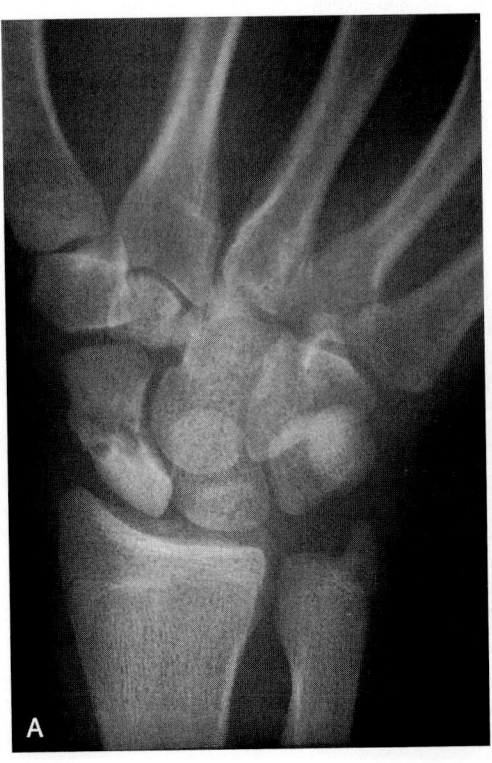

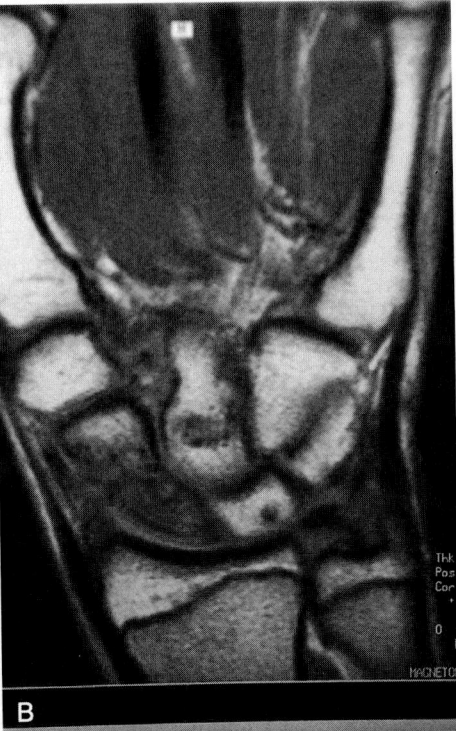

Fig. 3. *A*, Scaphoid nonunion and increased density of the proximal pole. Posteroanterior radiograph. *B*, Magnetic resonance imaging scan shows decreased signal in the proximal pole, which is consistent with avascular necrosis.

CASTING

Cast immobilization has been shown to promote union of the stable, nondisplaced nonunions. Casting can also be used in combination with other forms of treatment, including electrical stimulation. Prolonged immobilization (greater than 6 months), unfortunately, has a significant impact not only on the patient's wrist motion but also on the quality of life and productivity.

ELECTRICAL STIMULATION

Electrical stimulation has been used as an alternative to surgical care or as an adjunct, but its usefulness remains controversial.[1] Some studies showed it to be more efficacious than other nonoperative modalities.[9] Although the current supportive evidence is inconclusive, pulsed electromagnetic fields have been recommended for the treatment of nondisplaced nonunions without carpal instability of less than 5 year's duration. This treatment, combined with plaster immobilization, has yielded an 80% healing rate initially, although more recent studies have seemed to demonstrate a lower success rate. It is known that this treatment is not as effective as bone grafting techniques and does not correct scaphoid collapse.

OPERATIVE TREATMENT

INDICATIONS

Evidence indicates that post-traumatic osteoarthritis increases in patients with scaphoid nonunion. It is believed that few nonunions remain stable, nondisplaced, and free of arthritis after 10 years.[3, 4] Accordingly, even asymptomatic patients with stable, undisplaced nonunions should be advised of the possibility of late degenerative changes. For these reasons, fragments that are grossly displaced or unstable because of ligamentous or osseous disruption should be treated with open reduction and internal fixation.[1, 10] Surgery is also recommended for most young, healthy patients even if they are free of symptoms, because of the evidence linking scaphoid nonunion with osteoarthritis.

A variety of surgical procedures have been described for the treatment of scaphoid nonunion, including standard bone grafting, vascularized bone grafting, internal fixation, and salvage procedures. No single procedure is appropriate for all nonunions, but treatment is dictated by the presence of displacement, instability, and arthritic changes.

SURGICAL APPROACH

Studies of the arterial anatomy of the scaphoid have provided relevant information on the various operative approaches to best preserve the intraosseous blood supply.[6] Eighty percent of the intraosseous vascularity and the entire proximal pole are supplied through branches of the radial artery entering through the dorsal ridges. Twenty percent of the bone receives its blood supply from volar radial arterial branches at the distal tuberosity. The volar surgical approach has been found to best preserve the important dorsal ridge vessels.[11]

Another important consideration is the location of the nonunion. Middle-third waist nonunions should be approached through the volar approach to protect the blood supply. However, small proximal poles are best approached through a dorsal incision.[11a] This allows the proximal pole

fragment to be stabilized with pins or screws. Because the blood supply has usually been completely divided in this type of a fracture, the dorsal approach is not likely to add additional compromise to the osseous blood supply.

Type I: Scaphoid Nonunion

In situ volar inlay bone grafting, as described by Rüsse, either from the iliac crest or the distal radius, is the procedure of choice for this type of nonunion. Although originally described without supplemental pin fixation,[1, 7, 10, 12–14] today most authors recommend supplemental fixation for both stable and unstable nonunion.[1, 5] This prevents micromotion at the nonunion site and adds little surgical morbidity. It should be noted that some authors espoused a dorsal inlay approach and bone grafting.

Type II: Scaphoid Nonunion

Because this nonunion demonstrates an instability pattern, a wedge or interposition bone graft is required in addition to internal fixation, as described by Fernandez.[15]

The scaphoid often assumes a "humpback" deformity (angulation in the sagittal plane with the apex pointing dorsally), which may be due to initial displacement or chronic resorption of the fracture site. Interposition of bone graft in the volar wedge-shaped defect is necessary to restore length and correct carpal instability. Stable internal fixation of both fragments and the interposed bone graft is mandatory.

A variety of internal fixation devices have been described including K-wires, ASIF screws, Herbert's screws, mini-Herbert's screws, cannulated ASIF and Herbert-Whipple screws, and the Accutrac screw. Internal fixation can decrease the duration of immobilization required to achieve union, thus allowing early range of motion. It should be noted that 82% to 100% success rates have been described with these devices (Table 2).[5, 14–17]

Each device has its advantages and disadvantages. K-wires are easy to insert and can be used with avascular changes but do not provide compression of the nonunion. ASIF screws provide excellent compression but have constraints because of the size of the osseous fragments and the possibility of intra-articular head placement. The Herbert screws, initially designed for scaphoid fractures, have a narrow diameter and subchondral containment intra-articularly but can be technically difficult to insert (see Fig. 2A–E).

Proximal pole unstable nonunions are particularly challenging. A small proximal pole fracture is more likely to be avascular and take longer to heal. If the fragment is especially small, it can be excised if the dorsal scapholunate ligament is intact. K-wires or mini-Herbert's screws are often used. It is this nonunion for which the use of vascularized distal radius pedicle bone grafting is becoming increasingly popular.[18, 19]

Type III: Scaphoid Nonunion

Surgical options for type III nonunions include radial styloidectomy alone, radial styloidectomy with interpositional bone grafting, or a salvage procedure such as a proximal row carpectomy.[20] Although radial styloidectomy alone may provide only temporary relief of pain because it does not prevent radial migration of the distal carpal row, it

TABLE 2. RATES OF UNION ACHIEVED WITH VARIOUS BONE-GRAFTING PROCEDURES				
Study	Procedure	No. Patients	Union Rate (%)	Mean Time to Union (weeks)
Warren-Smith and Barton[14]	Rüsse graft	28	61	18.0
Green[7]		45	75	22.0
Stark et al[13]		43	81	N/A
Cooney et al[1]		66	88	N/A
Hooning van Duyvenbode et al[12]		N/A	93	N/A
Fernadez[15]	Fernandez graft K-wire fixation	6	100	10.2 (cast 8 weeks)
Stark et al[5]		151	97	17.0
Warren-Smith and Barton[14]	Herbert screw	22	82	12.0
Herbert and Fisher[16]		77	86	28.0 (cast 4 weeks)
Sukul et al[17]	A-O screw	42	91	27.9
Zaidemberg et al[19]	Vascularized graft	11	100	6.2

N/A, not applicable.

certainly carries low morbidity. It can be performed through an open incision or arthroscopically.

Most patients at this stage are candidates for interpositional bone grafting and radial styloidectomy. The theory is that if bone union can be obtained, further degenerative changes may be prevented.

Proximal row carpectomy is a well-recognized procedure for scaphoid nonunion with favorable results as long as 20 years after surgery. It is appropriate for established nonunions not suitable for bone grafting.

Type IV: Scaphoid Nonunion

Surgical options for type IV nonunion are scaphoid excision with midcarpal arthrodesis (SLAC wrist procedure) or wrist arthrodesis. Proximal row carpectomy is generally not indicated when arthritic changes are noted at the head of the capitate.

Type V: Scaphoid Nonunion

Wrist arthrodesis is the surgical treatment of choice for type V symptomatic nonunions of the scaphoid.

REFERENCES

1. Cooney WP III, Dobyns JH, Linscheid RL: Nonunion of the scaphoid: Analysis of the results from bone grafting. J Hand Surg 1980; 5:343.

2. Osterman AL, Mikulics M: Scaphoid nonunion. Hand Clin 1988; 14:437.

3. Mack GR, Bosse MJ, Gelberman RH, et al: The natural history of scaphoid nonunion. J Bone Joint Surg Am 1984; 66:504.

4. Ruby LK, Stinson K, Belsky MR: The natural history of scaphoid nonunion: A review of fifty-five cases. J Bone Joint Surg Am 1985; 67:428.

5. Stark HH, Rickard TA, Zemel NO, et al: Treatment of ununited fractures of the scaphoid by iliac bone grafts and Kirschner-wire fixation. J Bone Joint Surg Am 1988; 70: 982.

6. Gelberman RH, Menon J: The vascularity of the scaphoid bone. J Hand Surg 1980; 5:508.

7. Green DP: The effect of avascular necrosis on Rüsse bone grafting for scaphoid nonunion. J Hand Surg Am 1985; 13:216.

8. Trumble TE: Avascular necrosis after scaphoid fracture: A correlation of magnetic resonance imaging and histology. J Hand Surg [Am] 1990; 15:557.

9. Bora FW Jr, Osterman AL, Woodbury DF, et al: Treatment of nonunion of the scaphoid by direct current. Orthop Clin North Am 1984; 15:107.

10. Rüsse O: Fracture of the carpal navicular: Diagnosis, non-operative treatment, and operative treatment. J Bone Joint Surg Am 1960; 42:759.

11. Botte MJ, Mortensen WW, Gelberman RH, et al: Internal vascularity of the scaphoid in cadavers after insertion of the Herbert screw. J Hand Surg Am 1988; 13: 216.

11a. DeMaagd RL, Engber WD: Retrograde Herbert screw fixation for treatment of proximal pole scaphoid nonunions. J Hand Surg Am 1989; 149:996.

12. Hooning van Duyvenbode JF, Keijser LC, Hauet EJ, et al: Pseudarthrosis of the scaphoid treated by the Matti-Rüsse operations: A long-term review of 77 cases. J Bone Joint Surg Br 1991; 73:603.

13. Stark A, Brostom LA, Svartengren G: Scaphoid nonunion treated with the Matti-Rüsse technique: Long-term results. Clin Orthop 1987; 214:175.

14. Warren-Smith CD, Barton NJ: Nonunion of the scaphoid: Rüsse graft vs Herbert screw. J Hand Surg [Br] 1988; 13:83.

15. Fernandez DL: A technique for anterior wedge-shaped grafts for scaphoid nonunions with carpal instability. J Hand Surg Am 1984; 9:733.

16. Herbert TJ, Fisher WE: Management of the fractured scaphoid using a new bone screw. J Bone Joint Surg Br 1984; 66:114.

17. Sukul DM, Johannes EJ, Marti RK: Corticocancellous grafting and an AO/ASIF lag screw for nonunion of the scaphoid: A retrospective analysis. J Bone Joint Surg Br 1990; 72:835.

18. Sheetz KK, Bishop AT, Berger RA: The arterial blood supply of the distal radius and ulna and its potential use in vascularized pedicled bone grafts. J Hand Surg Am 1995; 20:902.

19. Zaidemberg C, Siebert JW, Angrigiani C: A new vascularized bone graft for scaphoid nonunion. J Hand Surg Am 1991; 16: 474.

20. Culp RW, McGuigan FX, Turner MA, et al: Proximal row carpectomy: A multicenter study. J Hand Surg Am 1993; 18:19.

METACARPAL AND PHALANGEAL NONUNIONS

William B. Geissler

Summary

- The rate of metacarpal and phalangeal nonunions in the hand is very low, ranging from 1 to 10 per 1000 fractures.
- The occurrence of nonunion correlates with initial fracture displacement and reduction, fracture configuration, and the extent of soft-tissue damage.
- Joint stiffness, contracture, and tendon adhesions are frequent complications of metacarpal and phalangeal nonunions.
- Treatment principles include stable internal fixation to allow early pain-free range of motion, simultaneous release of joint and tendon adhesions, and immediate intensive rehabilitation.

INTRODUCTION

Fortunately, nonunions of the metacarpals and phalanges of the hand are rare.[1] The ability to achieve and maintain fracture reduction depends on several factors, including fracture configuration, amount of displacement, and associated soft-tissue damage. Inability to maintain a stable adequate reduction may lead to fracture (cast) disease characterized by pain, brawny edema, and deformity with muscle imbalance. If left untreated, the injury may progress to a nonunion. Because nonunions have a painful range of motion with bony deformity, they are frequently complicated by joint contractures, stiffness, and tendon adhesions. Dysfunction may not be limited to the involved digit because of the quadriga effect of the flexor digitorum profundus tendon if it is involved.

Several factors may play a role in the pathogenesis of a nonunion: an inherently poor blood supply secondary to traumatic soft-tissue injury or operative devascularization, persistent fracture displacement or distraction resulting from soft-tissue interposition, and continued motion at the fracture site despite immobilization or internal fixation.[2] Severe bone loss, fracture comminution, and infection may lead to nonunion.

Patients with nonunion of the metacarpal or phalanx present with the clinical signs of advanced fracture disease. The area over the fracture site may be tender to palpation. Motion is frequently painful, which leads to joint contractures as the patient seeks to avoid terminal flexion and extension. Bony deformity leads to muscle imbalance with contractures and tendon adhesions. The digits and hand stay persistently swollen, further limiting motion. Nonunions are clinically unstable to manual stress testing, which may be demonstrated on plain radiographs. Radiographic signs of nonunion include persistent or enlarging radiolucent fracture lines, mushrooming of the fracture ends, sclerosis of the fracture margins, sealing of the intra-medullary canal, submarginal cyst formation, and generalized osteopenia.

GOALS, INDICATIONS, AND CONTRAINDICATIONS

The treatment of nonunions emphasizes the basics of fracture management, including stable internal fixation to allow early range of motion for intensive rehabilitation.[3] Functional recovery cannot be achieved without restoration of a stable osseous framework; therefore, rigid implants are necessary. Kirschner's wires alone are usually inadequate. The need for stability must also be balanced with preservation of blood supply and respect for the soft tissues. Dissection and implants must be as unobtrusive as possible to minimize their effect on the closely adhered tendons. Joint and tendon contractures are addressed simultaneously with bone reconstruction.

Indications for surgery include a painful nonunion of the metacarpal joint or phalanx, as demonstrated by radiographs, causing limitation of function. Contraindications to immediate internal fixation include uncontrolled infection. Control of the infection is necessary before implant fixation and bone grafting.

A relative contraindication involves the patient with severe neurological involvement with no hand function and no pain.

A nonunion is defined as a fracture failing to unite in the anticipated time frame or when there is no radiographic progression of healing. Management of nonunions of the metacarpal and phalanx depends on its classification (Table 1).

PROCEDURE

Metacarpal nonunions are approached using a dorsal incision. The incision is placed to the side of the metacarpal to avoid incorporation of the mobile extensor tendons with the fracture and skin, following the concept of "one wound, one scar." Although rotational deformity is unacceptable, metacarpal shortening up to 4 mm is well tolerated.[4] In a patient with secondary intrinsic scarring, it may be feasible to leave the metacarpal slightly short to manage the soft-tissue contracture more easily (Figs. 1 and 2). Oblique and spiral fractures longer than twice the diameter of the bone may be stabilized by two or more miniscrews (2.0 or 2.7 mm).[5] However, screws alone are usually insufficient in nonunions because of bone loss. Hypertrophic nonunions are usually stabilized with 2.0-mm reconstruction plates with their lower profile to limit adhesions. The bending strength of a plate is proportional to the cube of its thickness. In nonunions in which extensive bone loss exists, thicker 2.7-mm minidynamic compression plates

TABLE 1. TREATMENT OPTIONS

Type	Indications	Treatment	Outcome
Hypertrophic	Fracture: unstable, displaced; needs stability to unite Intact vascularity	Stable internal fixation Bone graft optional	Metacarpal: minimal loss of motion
Oligotrophic	Delayed union Usually seen in slightly displaced intra-articular fractures	Compressive fixation Salvage: arthrodesis arthroplasty	Decreased range of motion, usually extension
Atrophic	Fracture ends avascular Absence of bony reaction Usually extensive bone loss	Excision avascular bone ends Bone carpentry Stable internal fixation	Decreased range of motion: flexion/extension
Infected	Bacterial enzymatic degradation Loss of vascularity	Excise infected tissue Internal fixation/bone grafting Eliminate dead space once infection controlled	Decreased range of motion, depending on associated soft-tissue involvement

may be necessary. Plates must be of sufficient length for screws to purchase three or four cortices on either side of the fracture. They are applied dorsally on the tension side of the bone where dorsal angulation tends to occur.[6] When a fracture is near the diaphyseal-metaphyseal junction, T, L, or minicondylar plates may be used to allow placement of more screws in the metaphysis than a straight plate.[7]

Minicondylar plates are more versatile because they have a lower profile and may be placed laterally as well.[8] In infected nonunions, necrotic bone and soft tissue are extensively débrided. External fixation or transverse Kirschner's wires, pinning the distal fragment to the adjacent metacarpal, temporarily stabilizes the fracture. The fracture is then bone grafted and stabilized, eliminating dead space once

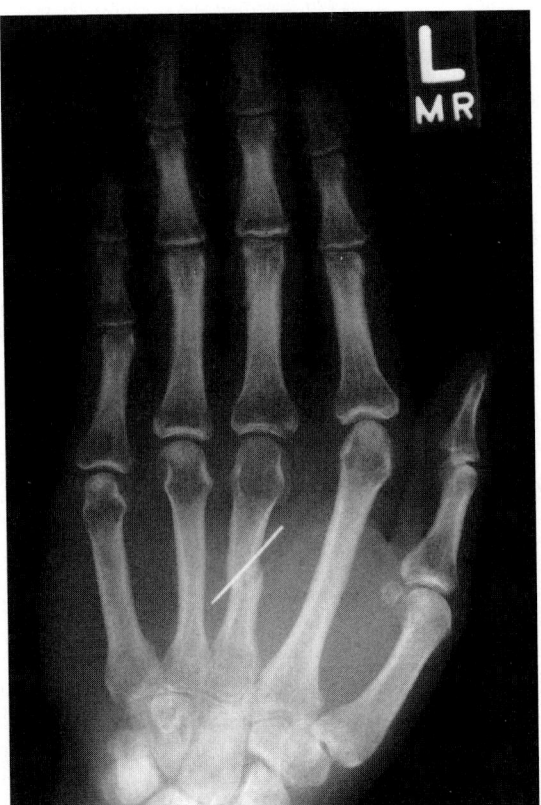

Fig. 1. Hypertrophic nonunion of the long metacarpal. This is an anteroposterior radiograph. The patient experienced a crush injury, resulting in a compartment syndrome of the hand, which was decompressed, and the fracture was pinned at an outside hospital. Close inspection shows that the Kirschner wires do not actually cross the fracture site. The patient had hypertrophic nonunion resulting from instability. The fracture can heal if adequately stabilized.

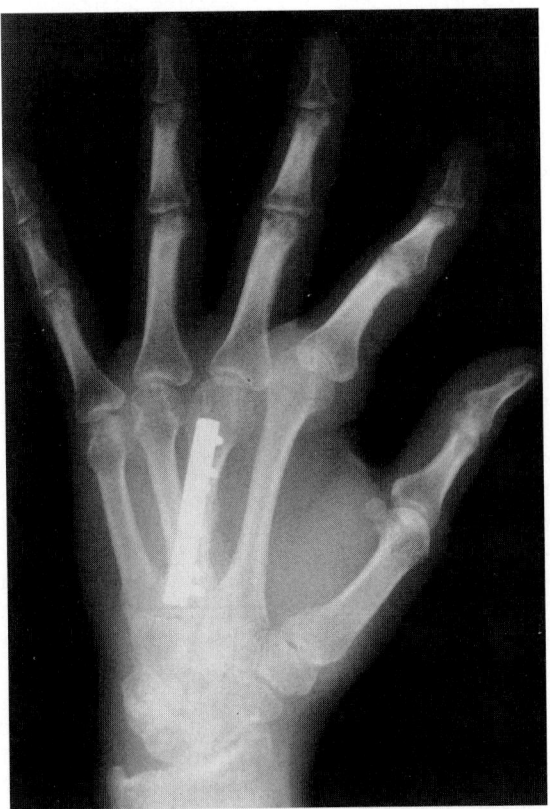

Fig. 2. Stabilization of fracture with 2.0-mm plate. The patient had intrinsic contractures resulting from the crush injury and involvement of the deep motor branch of the ulnar nerve. The metacarpal was stabilized slightly short to address more easily the associated intrinsic contractures, which were released at the same setting.

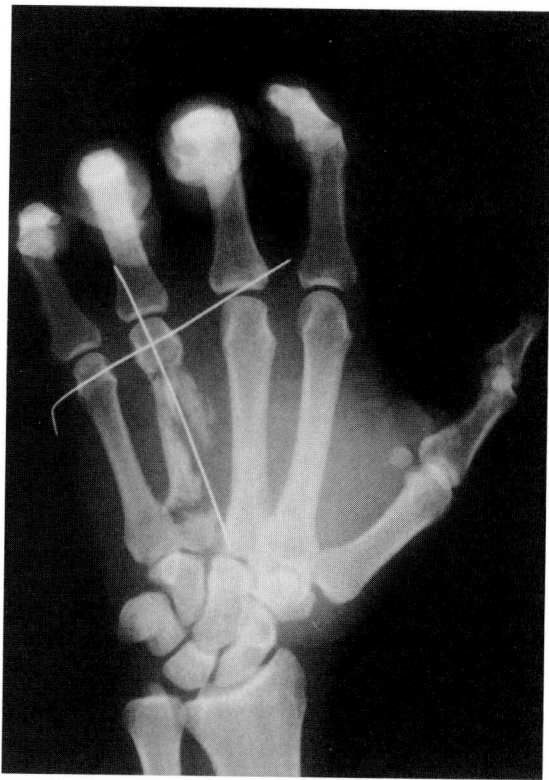

Fig. 3. Atrophic nonunion secondary to crush injury with extensive bone loss. This anteroposterior radiograph was taken approximately 3 months after patient was stabilized at another hospital.

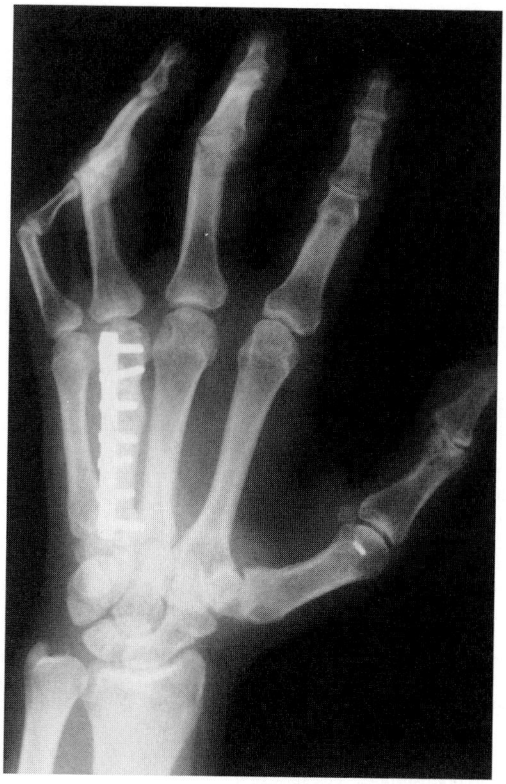

Fig. 4. Reconstruction of ring metacarpal. The ring metacarpal was reconstructed with a bicortical iliac crest bone graft and stabilized with a 2.0-mm plate. A thumb adduction contracture was simultaneously released.

the infection is under control. The distal radius or olecranon processes are ideal locations for bone graft when a small amount of graft is needed. Cancellous bone may be compressed in a syringe to enhance its structural stability. The iliac crest is used if larger amounts of bone graft are required, particularly when the majority of the metacarpal needs to be reconstructed (Figs. 3 and 4).[9]

The midaxial incision is preferred in nonunions of the phalanges, particularly in the zone 2 flexor tendon area. Incisions and implants should be placed as unobtrusively as possible to minimize scarring of the mobile gliding tendons. The lateral band may be excised when the extrinsic extensor tendon is intact during application of the implant. The 2.0- or 1.5-mm minicondylar plate is ideal for phalangeal nonunions, particularly those involving the metaphyseal-diaphyseal junction because of its low profile and lateral application.

Joint contractures and adhesions are simultaneously released. The insertion of the extrinsic common extensor tendon into the dorsal base of the middle phalanx should be left intact to prevent a boutonnière deformity. The transverse and oblique fibers of the dorsal hood may be excised, preserving 4 to 6 mm of the central slip proximal to the interphalangeal joint. This "uncouples" the intrinsic and extrinsic extensor systems to enhance potential for recovery of lost motion. Sometimes only the check rein ligament is all that needs to be released in proximal interphalangeal flexion contractures.

TABLE 2. COMPLICATIONS		
Complication	**Cause**	**Treatment**
Plate fatigue fracture	Thin plate	Replace with thicker plate (dynamic compression plate)
	Plate hole over fracture	Bone graft, bone stimulator
Loss of fixation	Short plate	Replace with longer plate, not necessarily thicker
	Osteopenia	May need different configuration (straight to T plate)
		Bone graft, bone stimulator
		Supplement with external fixation
		Use larger screws
Joint contracture	Prolonged immobilization	Tenolysis with metal removal
	Unstable fixation	Emphasize proximal interphalangeal extension
	Residuals of injury	Immediate range of motion

Amputation is reserved for dysfunctional digits. Every effort is made to preserve the thumb. Implants are removed at the discretion of the patient and surgeon and allow a second opportunity for joint tenolysis.

COMPLICATIONS

Complications relate to continued nonunion despite operative intervention.[10] As in other fractures, it is a race between how long it takes the bone to heal and how long the implant holds the fracture (Table 2).

OUTCOME

The single most effective treatment for nonunions is prevention. Traumatic or operative devascularization, fracture displacement, soft-tissue interposition, bone loss, and infection are factors that the surgeon must consider when managing these injuries. Early intervention when these factors are present will result in improved results compared with delayed reconstruction. The management of nonunions, in comparison to that of acute fractures, has the disadvantage of overcoming soft-tissue complications associated with the delay in fracture healing.

REFERENCES

1. Stern PJ, Wiser MJ, Reilly DG: Complications of plate fixation in the hand skeleton. Clin Orthop 1987; 214:59.
2. Heim U: The treatment of nonunion in the bones of the hand. In Chapchal G (ed): Pseudoarthroses and Their Treatment. Stuttgart, George Thiem, 1979, p 168.
3. Jupiter JB, Koniuch MP, Smith RS: The management of delayed union and nonunion of the metacarpals and phalanges. J Hand Surg Am 1985; 10:457.
4. Freeland AE, Jabaley ME, Hughes JL: Stable Fixation of the Hand and Wrist. New York, Springer-Verlag, 1986.

5. Ford DJ, El-Hadidi S, Lunn PG, et al: Fractures of the metacarpals: Treatment by AO screws and plate fixation. J Hand Surg Br 1987; 12:34.
6. Dabezies EJ, Schulte JP: Fixation of metacarpal and phalangeal fractures with minimal plates and screws. J Hand Surg Am 1986; 11:283.
7. Segmuller G: Surgical Stabilization of the Skeleton of the Hand. Baltimore, Williams & Wilkins, 1977.
8. Buchler U, Fischer T: Use of a minicondylar plate for metacarpal and phalangeal

periarticular injuries. Clin Orthop 1987; 214:53.
9. Leung PC: Use of an intramedullary bone peg in digital replantations, revascularizations and toe transfers. J Hand Surg 1981; 6:281.
10. Butler B, Neviaser RJ, Adams JP: Complications of treatment of injuries to the hand. In Epps CP (ed): Complications in Orthopaedic Surgery. Philadelphia, JB Lippincott, 1994, p 359.

section 12 chapter 8

GENERAL ASPECTS OF MICROVASCULAR TISSUE REPLANTATION

Peter J. Evans and David S. Ruch

Summary
- Hand injuries account for up to 30% of all work-related injuries, and digital amputations occur three to four times more frequently at work.
- Traumatic amputation of limbs and digits results in significant socioeconomic losses.
- Care in the assessment of the socioeconomic, psychological, and physical aspects of an amputation injury must be individualized to obtain a satisfactory outcome.
- When replantation is undertaken, an integrated team of surgeons, operating room staff, nurses, and therapists is required.
- Now that the rate vascular patency exceeds 80% in replantations, the intraoperative and postoperative management of associated soft-tissue injury has become the limiting factor in successful outcomes for replanted structures.

Completely severed parts (limbs, hands, and fingers) are being reattached with increasing reliability and in more centers than ever before. Replantation is no longer an investigational procedure, and patency and viability of a replanted part in more than 80% of cases are a result of the advances in microsurgical instrumentation, materials, and techniques. Later advances in postoperative management, including reduction in hospital stays and progressive therapy, have decreased the initial economic impact of replantation surgery and improved the functional outcomes.

Several technical and socioeconomic challenges remain in replantation surgery. Optimal function of injured muscles, nerves, tendons, ligaments, and joints after replantation is now the most difficult surgical problem. A growing understanding of the outcomes of replantation surgery, based on the severity of injury, patient co-morbidities, and socioeconomic factors, will aid physicians and patients in the decision to choose replantation.

HISTORICAL REVIEW

Although replantation was successfully performed in a laboratory setting at the turn of the twentieth century, clinical replantation did not occur until more than 50 years later.[1-3] The term *microsurgery* arose from the work by Jacobson and Suarez,[4] who in 1960 presented their paper on the experimental anastomosis of 1- to 2-mm vessels to the

American College of Surgeons. Subsequently, Chen and colleagues[5] published the first report of an arm replantation, and Malt and McKhann[6] followed with a report on two cases of arm replantation, the first of which was performed in 1962. Smaller, digital vessels were first clinically repaired in 1963 by Kleinert and associates[7]; but the first successful replantation of a thumb was performed 5 years later by Komatsu and Tamai.[8] Microvascular reconstruction for amputated parts was initiated in 1969 by Cobbett,[9] who described the first successful toe-to-hand transfer. This effort was furthered by Manktelow, with his work on "Functioning Free Muscle Transfer," presented in 1982 to the American Society for Surgery of the Hand.

Over the past 40 years, advances in the technical aspects of replantation, including microvascular repair (microinstruments, microsuture, operating microscope), bone-shortening techniques (permitting tension-free anastomoses and wound closure), postoperative monitoring, and prevention of thrombosis, have led to the maximization of the survival of the replanted part.

PATHOGENESIS

Most amputations occur in the workplace, and the type and frequency vary according to region, time of year, and status of the economy. In rural areas, farming injuries are more common, but in industrial regions, conveyer belt and punch press injuries predominate. Although conflicting data exist, rapid upswings in the economy can often be temporally related to an increase in industrial injuries, a trend thought mainly to be due to rapid implementation of a less experienced work force. In adults, digital injuries occur three to four times more frequently at work. In children, unfortunately, digital avulsion amputations are twice as common as clean-cut amputations.[10]

CLINICAL FEATURES

Terminology must be clarified in regard to amputation injuries. In *complete amputation*, the part retains no connection to the patient; reattachment of that part is referred to as *replantation*. *Incomplete amputation* describes a part that has no arterial supply but retains some soft-tissue connection (skin, nerve, and tendon); reattachment of that part is referred to as *revascularization*. Revascularized parts are potentially more viable because an adequate venous drainage may exist, but the procedure may be more difficult to perform because (1) a two-teamed approach cannot be implemented and (2) at times, bone cannot be readily shortened to allow repair of débrided structures.

Ring avulsion injuries can be classified according to Urbaniak and colleagues[11] (Table 1). It is of utmost importance to realize that the clinical appearance of the amputated part and remaining stump in the emergency room may not predict the potential for a successful replantation. A detailed examination of the remaining stump is impossible. Active bleeding, hematoma, and tattered or avulsed skin flaps can often lead to an overestimation of the severity of the injury, whereas "cleaner-looking" injuries often hide longitudinal injuries to tendons, nerves, or arteries. Therefore, the patient and family should be advised that the outcome is uncertain until after surgery.

TABLE 1. MODIFIED URBANIAK CLASSIFICATION OF RING AVULSION INJURIES

Class I	Adequate circulation. Standard bone and soft-tissue treatment sufficient.
Class II	IIA: Inadequate arterial circulation, but bones, tendons, nerves, veins are intact. IIB: Inadequate venous circulation, but bones, tendons, nerves, arteries are intact.
Class III	Complete degloving or complete amputation.

Modified from Urbaniak JR, Roth JR, Nonley JA, et al: The results of replantation after amputation of a single finger. J Bone Joint Surg Am 1985; 67:611.

INVESTIGATIONS

The patient should undergo triage as for any trauma. If the amputated part is associated with other bodily injuries, the appropriate trauma work-up and precautions should be implemented. If the amputation is the sole injury, orthogonal roentgenograms of the amputated part and remaining stump, blood typing and cross-matching, and other age-appropriate investigations are done.

GOALS, INDICATIONS, AND CONTRAINDICATIONS

The goal of treatment of a patient with an amputated part is the return of that patient to as close to preinjury status as possible with the least amount of psychological, physical, and socioeconomic morbidity as possible. The goal of replantation is the same, with the addition that the function after replantation must be better than that of a prosthesis or an amputation, and that any difference must be worth the incurred morbidity.

Implicit in these goals is the requirement of a dedicated replantation team that can accurately assess and treat such injuries. Surgeons should be trained in the hand and upper extremity, should be comfortable with fracture management, tendon and nerve repair, and soft-tissue coverage, and should be able to perform microvascular anastomoses with a greater than 90% patency rate in 1-mm vessels. As noted, an experienced support staff in the operating room, intensive care unit, and ward is essential to good outcomes.

Even in the most experienced centers, the decision to replant an amputated part is often difficult. Table 2 lists several factors that have been identified to help define the indications for and contraindications to replantation.[1] Although absolute indications and contraindications are not always present for each factor, the most clearly identified descriptors are given.

PROCEDURE

MANAGEMENT AND TRANSPORTATION OF PATIENT AND AMPUTATED PART

Treatment at the scene of the injury and the first medical contact should follow standard trauma protocols, with any life-threatening injuries treated first. The patient must be hemodynamically stable, and stump bleeding must be controlled. The stump is cleaned of gross contamination and

TABLE 2. GENERAL GUIDELINES FOR MICROVASCULAR REPLANTATION

Factor	Indication	Contraindication
Age	• Any part in children. • No upper limit.	• Insufficient strength or coordination anticipated for rehabilitation.
Severity of injury	• Clean, sharp guillotine. • Minimal local crush. • Avulsion with minimal vascular injury (class II).	• Extensive crush or avulsion (class III). • Segmental injuries. • Extensive contamination with soil bacteria (farm).
Level of amputation	• Humerus, elbow, proximal forearm. • Thumb, any level. • Single or multiple digits distal to flexor digitorum superficialis.	• Humerus close to shoulder. • Just above, through, or just below the elbow. • Single digit proximal to flexor digitorum superficialis insertion, especially index or small finger, or through proximal interphalangeal joint.
Interval between amputation and revascularization	• <6 hours warm ischemia, <12 hours cold ischemia, proximal to palm	• >8 hours warm ischemia, >30 hours cold ischemia, digits.
Multiple or bilateral amputations	• Replant at least two digits in the ring and long finger positions. • Bilateral replants fare better than prostheses; if impossible, use available digits to replant one side.	
Segmental injuries to injured part Patient's general condition	• Few. • Young, healthy.	• Vascular failure rate high. • Associated injuries requiring prolonged life-saving operations. • Preexisting vascular disease, such as diabetes, rheumatoid arthritis, lupus, or other collagen vascular diseases. • Excessive anesthetic risk. • Psychiatric illness responsible for amputation, with poor chance of control.
Patient's rehabilitation potential	• Intelligent, well-motivated.	• Mentally challenged or unable to participate in therapy.
Economic factors Other	• Unclear.	• Unclear. • Preexisting deformity or disability severe enough to preclude satisfactory function.

wrapped in a sterile compression bandage. Bleeding usually stops with complete amputations as vessels contract, but partial vessel lacerations may have persistent bleeding. Blind applications of clamps should be avoided because neurovascular damage may result. Temporary use of regulated pneumatic tourniquets or blood pressure cuffs can be helpful, but elastic or cloth tourniquets can risk potential ischemia and neurovascular damage.

The completely amputated part should be cleaned of any gross contamination with sterile saline and then cooled. Cooling is performed by either of two methods (Fig. 1). The part (1) is wrapped in gauze soaked in sterile saline or lactated Ringer's solution and then placed in a plastic bag, which is sealed, or (2) is fully immersed in a bag containing sterile saline or lactated Ringer's solution. With either method, the bag is placed in iced water in an insulated container, with care taken to avoid direct contact of the part with the ice to prevent freezing of the part. Dry ice should never be used. Preparation of a major amputated part (including muscle) requires even more attention to cooling, and initial complete immersion of the bagged part in iced water for 20 to 60 minutes to achieve rapid cooling is advised. The amputated part or parts should be labeled and kept with the patient at all times.

The incompletely amputated part requires special treatment. The injured limb should be wrapped in gauze soaked in sterile saline, and a padded splint applied to provide comfort and avoid kinking of the vascular pedicle. Ice packs are placed on the devascularized portion.

After the patient and injured limb are stabilized, the patient is transported to a center that can evaluate and treat such injuries, with a goal of less than 2 to 3 hours of ischemia time.

PREOPERATIVE PLANNING AND PREPARATION

Once the patient with an amputation arrives at a replantation center, optimal management involves two teams, one for the patient and one for the amputated part. The patient's history, physical examination, and roentgenograms are reviewed, and the patient is stabilized, given prophylactic broad-spectrum antibiotics and tetanus prophylaxis if required, and consulted in regard to the treatment options and outcomes. Simultaneously, examination and preparation of the amputated part are performed. If feasible, the amputated part is taken to the operating room immediately, cleaned, and evaluated.

SURGICAL MANAGEMENT
Anesthesia

Upper arm and lower extremity amputations require general anesthesia, but regional anesthesia can be used for most other amputations. The advantage of regional anesthesia, used as either the primary anesthetic or an adjunct to

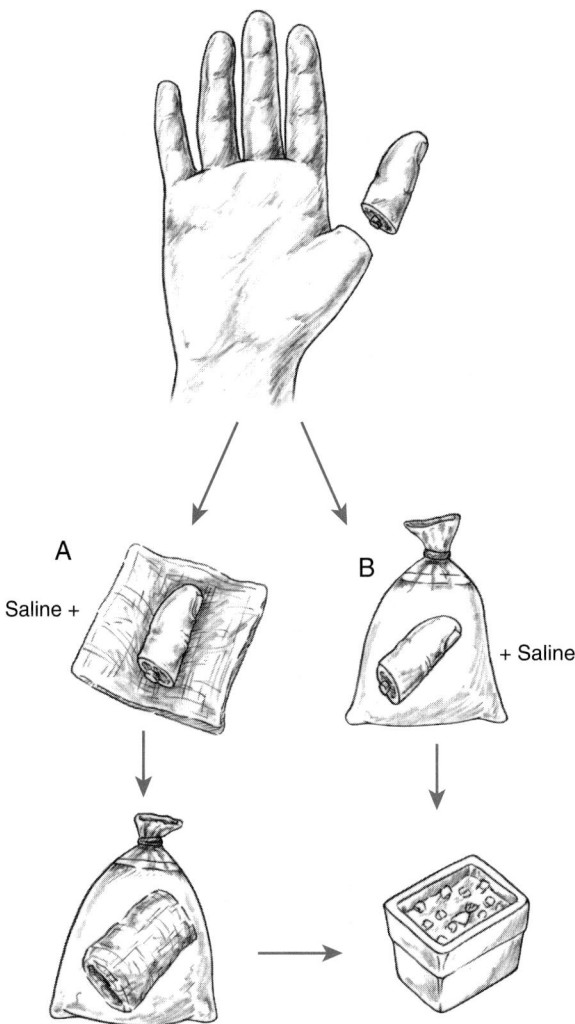

Fig. 1. Cooling technique for transportation of amputated parts. Digits should be cleaned of any gross contamination and then prepared by one of two techniques. The part is wrapped in sterile gauze soaked in physiological solution, then placed in a plastic bag, which is sealed *(A)* or is fully immersed in a bag containing sterile physiological solution *(B)*. The bag is placed in iced water in an insulated container, direct contact of the part with the ice being avoided to prevent freezing of the part.

general anesthesia, is the sympathetic blockade, which enhances peripheral blood flow and reduces vasospasm.

Microsurgical Instrumentation

Numerous microsurgical instruments are commercially available, and the selection is made in part at the surgeon's discretion.[12] Instruments should be simple, corrosion-resistant, and fabricated with nonglare material, and should approximate accurately (Fig. 2). Scissors and needle holders should have nonlocking spring mechanisms and should be long enough to rest comfortably in the thumb–index finger web space. Sufficient length will minimize intrinsic muscle fatigue, decrease hand tremors, and help reduce technical errors.

Forceps. Smoothly functioning forceps capable of holding without tearing are essential. Their tips should vary from 0.2 mm to 0.6 mm. A variety of specialized forceps

are available for vessel dilation, stretching, and tissue manipulation.

Scissors. Adventitial scissors are straight, and dissecting scissors have a gentle curve. Tips may be pointed or slightly blunted; the latter are preferable for the less experienced surgeon because they decrease inadvertent injury of the patient (vessel damage) and surgical colleagues. Handles may be straight, rounded, or flared. Many of the newer microscissors are counterbalanced for better "feel" and maneuverability.

Needle Holders. Most microsurgeons prefer specialized needle holders, with finely forged tips and smooth action, to jewelers' forceps. Needle holders come with straight or curved jaws. A gently curved jaw facilitates handling, allowing one to rotate the needle through the vessel wall by rolling the handle between the thumb and forefinger. Locking needle holders should be avoided.

Clamps. Single and double clamps in several sizes are available for vessel approximation or hemostasis. Vessel clamps are designed to hold the vessel, to prevent bleeding, and to allow rotatory approximation. Disposable single and double clamps of varying size and pressure are now available and are suitable for 0.4-mm to 2.0-mm vessels. The

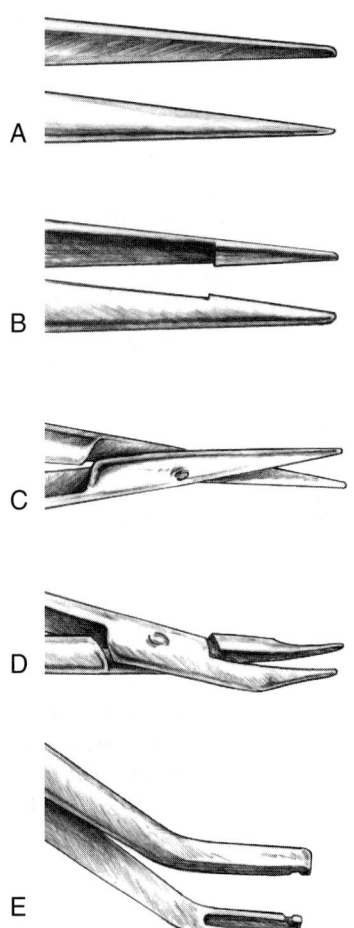

Fig. 2. Basic microsurgical instruments. These are suture *(A)* handling/tying and tissue-manipulating forceps. Specialized *(B)* vessel-dilating forceps. Straight *(C)* or curved *(D)* adventitial or dissecting scissors. Straight or curved *(E) (inset)* nonlocking needle holder for suturing.

TABLE 3. OPERATIVE SEQUENCE FOR LIMB REPLANTATION

1. Tagging of vessels, nerves, and tendons.
2. Débridement.
3. Bone shortening and fixation.
4. Repair of extensor tendons.
5. Anastomosis of arteries.
6. Repair of nerves.
7. Anastomosis of veins, preferably two for every artery.
8. Repair of flexor tendons.
9. Skin closure or coverage.

perfect clamp has enough tension to hold the vessel without damage and jaws 1.5 to 2.0 times wider than the diameter of the vessel. A clamp with excessive pressure would damage the intima and media, later possibly producing thrombosis. *One should avoid using double bar clamps to overcome tension during vessel approximation.*

Suture Material and Needles. As a basic rule, the surgeon should choose the smallest needle capable of passing through the vessel wall without bending and the smallest suture strong enough to approximate the vessel. Standard blunt-tipped, noncutting needle sizes range in diameter from 50 to 135 μm and in cord length from 2 to 5 mm. Suture material in sizes 8-0 to 11-0 (35 to 14 μm) is available on most needles.

Magnification. The choice of magnification relates to vessel size. Large vessels in the proximal forearm or arm may be repaired reliably by many surgeons using loupe magnification (2.5× to 6.0×). Because magnification requires concomitant increases in light to be effective, it is often simpler to use an operating microscope than higher-power loupes and headlamp. Gross dissection may be facilitated by the use of loupe magnification of 3.5× to 4.5×; the vessel repair is then accomplished with the operating microscope at 6.0× to 30.0×. Inspection of the vessel under high power is essential to prevent inadvertent anastomosis of a damaged vessel.

Sequence of Replantation and Techniques

The sequence varies slightly with the level and mechanism of amputation but can be generally summarized (Table 3). For replantation of multiple digits, most surgeons find it most time-efficient to repair like structures on each digit prior to repairing the next structure on any single digit.

Preparation of the Amputated Part

Dissection is performed on an ice-filled pan, the pan wrapped with plastic and a sterile sheet, with the use of loupe magnification, microscopic magnification, or both. Careful débridement is performed, and the nerves, arteries, veins, and tendons are identified and tagged. Longitudinal, slightly dorsally placed midlateral incisions on each side of a digit provide quick and safe access to the neurovascular bundle and allow veins to be located within the subdermal layer (Fig. 3). In more proximal amputations, standard extensile incisions can be made. Bone shortening is performed (if the amputated part has the longer bone segment) to allow for tension-free anastomoses. For fingers, two in-

tramedullary K-wires are placed in a retrograde fashion through the fracture site in final preparation for replantation.

If the amputation mechanism was crush or avulsion, the arterial system should be perfused with heparinized Ringer's or saline solution through a small silicone catheter. If there is no return flow or there is distal extravasation of perfusate, successful revascularization is unlikely.

Preparation of the Remaining Limb

In general, rigid skeletal fixation is performed prior to vascular repair in cases involving skeletal trauma. In critical injuries, arterial and venous shunting may be used to prevent excessive warm ischemia. Wounds are explored under loupe magnification, with use of a tourniquet to provide a bloodless field. Extensile incisions are made that incorporate traumatic wounds. If clinically indicated, fasciotomy is performed. Dead and necrotic tissue is excised, and wound margins are trimmed. Transected and injured structures, if not easily recognizable, are identified proximally and distally in normal tissue, mobilized, and tagged with vascular tapes, loops, or sutures as described for the part. Sutures are placed, but they are not tied if lacerated flexor tendons are adjacent to or would interfere with vascular anastomoses. If performed after vascular repair, tendon approximation is possible without additional dissection, and damage to the vessel repair is minimized. Performing tendon repair before vessel anastomosis may make exposure of the anastomotic site more difficult because of finger, hand, or wrist position or the presence of the tendon itself.

The periadventitial plane is identified proximal and distal to the transection site to allow rapid and safe dissection. Vessels are dissected from surrounding tissues, and atraumatic vascular clamps are placed on either side of the repair site. Manipulation of the media or intima is mini-

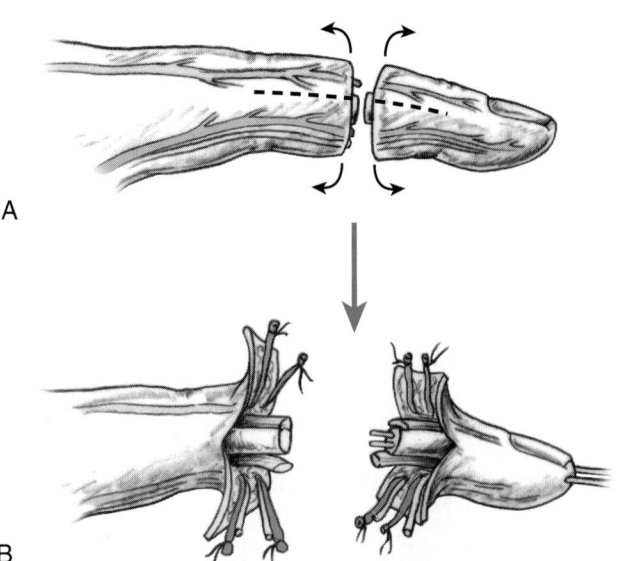

Fig. 3. Exposure and preparation of the amputated part and stump. *A,* The volar neurovascular bundle and dorsal veins are exposed through slightly dorsal midaxial incisions. *B,* All structures are then tagged, and retrograde K-wires are placed in the bone of the amputated part.

mized. The periadventitial tissue is removed so that the vessel wall and lumen can be visualized easily and debris does not interfere with the passing or tying of sutures. Both portions of the vessel are inspected to determine whether the intima and media are suitable for anastomosis. Hemorrhage within the media, intimal disruption, multiple stellate tears, and telescoping of the intima are ominous findings that require additional resection back to "normal" vessel. Intimal damage itself is an important but not definitive factor in long-term patency. However, intimal damage is the most easily recognizable external sign of local trauma, may indicate significant additional damage, and is associated with a higher rate of thrombosis. Therefore, it is good practice to resect the vessel until relatively normal intima is visualized.

Bone Shortening and Fixation

Although some surgeons prefer to not shorten the skeleton for replantations and choose to perform vein grafts, most recommend bone shortening to maximize cortical contact and stability and avoid extra anastomoses and potentially decreased patency rates. To allow tension-free vessel and nerve repair, shortening of 0.5 to 1.0 cm in the hand and digits and up to 2 to 4 cm proximal to the wrist is recommended. The thumb poses a unique dilemma, and shortening of the amputated part, not the stump, is recommended to provide good bone stock in case the replant fails.

Several methods of fixation have been utilized, each of which has inherent advantages and disadvantages. Simple, quick, reliable fixation is usually the best, because vascular and soft-tissue problems, not bone problems, are responsible for poor outcomes. The site of the amputation may tend to favor one method of fixation over another.

For most diaphyseal- or metadiaphyseal-level amputations in the hand, double axial K-wire fixation is recommended (Fig. 4). K-wires are usually placed in the amputated part as mentioned, and both are then driven across the fracture, one usually across the joint proximally for early added stability until the soft tissues stabilize. The

following advantages of this mode of fixation have been described[1]:

- It is simple and quick.
- Less bone exposure is required.
- Less skeletal mass is required for fixation.
- Rotational deformity of the replanted digit can be easily corrected.
- Reshortening after fixation is facilitated if required for nerve, vessel or skin approximation.

For metaphyseal-level amputations, either double axial K-wire fixation or a 90-90 intraosseous wiring technique with 24-gauge wire is recommended. Wire techniques require greater exposure but allow for earlier motion and stability at this level. Amputations through the joint frequently damage the articular surface irreparably, and arthrodesis or, rarely, immediate silicone joint replacement may be indicated. More proximal upper extremity and lower extremity amputations should undergo standard osteosynthesis techniques.

Extensor Tendon Repair

The extensor tendons should be repaired with one or two horizontal mattress 4-0 nonabsorbable braided sutures. In cases in which the extensor tendons are absent or extensively damaged, acute reconstruction is not advisable, and arthrodesis of interphalangeal joints or secondary tendon grafting is recommended.

Arterial Anastomosis
End-to-End Vascular Repair

A primary end-to-end repair can be performed if excessive tension at the anastomotic site can be avoided.[12] In sharp, nonsegmental injuries or when minimal artery has been resected, a tension-free anastomosis after resection of damaged vessel ends is usually accomplished by moderate proximal and distal mobilization of the artery.[12]

The use of colored background material during anastomosis improves visualization and handling of suture, de-

Fig. 4. Digital bone fixation. *A,* Diaphyseal fractures are most easily stabilized by K-wires, one of which crosses the joint above, and one crosses below for added stability. *B,* Metaphyseal fractures are best stabilized with intraosseous wires. *C,* Thumb metacarpophalangeal joint fixation with an intraosseous screw is conveniently performed. *D,* Most arthrodeses, however, can be readily stabilized by a crossed K-wire technique.

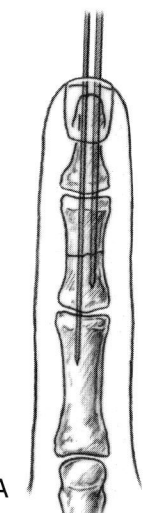
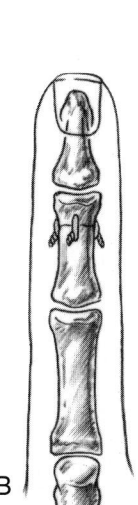
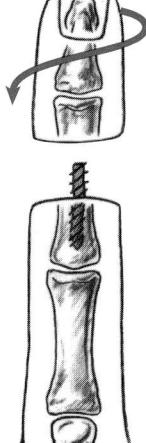
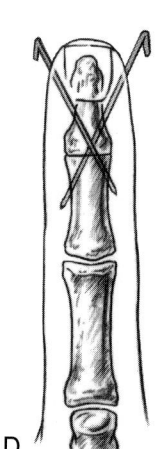

A   B   C   D

creases glare, and increases contrast. Vessel-approximating clamps can be used to hold the vessel in position, not to overcome excessive tension. Access to the anastomotic site is facilitated by bar clamps oriented with the open end away from the primary surgeon for initial suture placement. Under the operating microscope, tension is adjusted, the vessel is exposed, lumens are irrigated with heparinized saline, and debris or loose adventitial tissue is removed. A final inspection of the intima is made, and if the vessel is suitable, the anastomosis is begun.

After ensuring that the vessel is not twisted and that tension is not excessive, the surgeon places stay sutures at 120 degrees. Sutures to approximate the front wall are placed by halving the distance with each suture, with the use of a triangulation technique (Fig. 5). The bar vessel-approximating clamp is rotated 180 degrees (open end toward the primary surgeon), and the back wall is similarly approximated. Forearm-level injuries are repaired with nonabsorbable 7-0, 8-0, or 9-0 sutures, and distal vessels are repaired with 9-0, 10-0, or 11-0 sutures.

When the anastomosis is complete, it is inspected and the clamp is removed. Additional sutures may be necessary, but early leaks often stop spontaneously or can be stopped by placement of fat over the anastomosis. Technical errors in performing anastomoses can also cause turbulence and thrombosis. Patency may be confirmed by direct observation or by patency testing. Systemic intraoperative heparin may be given as one or two 2000- to 5000-unit boluses immediately before the tourniquet is released.

Vascular Grafts for Arterial Repair

Vein grafting should be used without hesitation to overcome excessive tension when a damaged vessel cannot be mobilized to achieve end-to-end reapproximation after appropriate débridement.[12] Although two anastomoses are necessary, patency rates are not significantly lower, in spite of the use of vein grafts in more severe injuries. As in the lower extremity, reverse interposition vein grafts are frequently used in the arm. Other graft types exist, including nonreversed in situ valvulotomized vein segments and synthetic or allograft material; they are used mostly for revascularization procedures rather than replantation.

Reversed Interposition Autologous Vein Grafting. For radial artery, ulnar artery, or proximal superficial arch injuries, the cephalic vein from the forearm, the distal saphenous or lesser saphenous vein, or a dorsal vein from the foot can be used with equal efficacy. For digital vessels, veins from the volar forearm are excellent donor sources.

At the time of surgery, the ends of the severed artery are dissected and mobilized, and vascular clips are placed to allow later rapid identification. Typically, the vein graft is reversed and placed in position. The more difficult anastomosis is performed first, because the greater freedom allowed by the mobility of the vein graft makes repair easier and prevents technical errors.

Nerve Repair

Following revascularization, the nerves are repaired under the microscope with standard microneurosurgical technique using 8-0 to 10-0 nylon sutures. Digital nerves require only two or three epineural sutures, but more proximal injuries utilize a group fascicular technique with careful matching of the topography of proximal and distal stumps.

In most cases, primary repair following débridement of the cut ends of the nerve is possible after bone shortening. However, if undue tension exists, nerve grafting is indicated. In the upper extremity, the medial antebrachial cutaneous nerve serves as good donor interposition graft, because it can be obtained from the same sterile field.

Venous Anastomosis

The timing of vein repair varies among surgeons. Some prefer to repair veins after extensor tendons as a convenience and to decrease blood loss after arterial repair, especially for multiple digit replantation or if large veins can be repaired. Ideally, two veins should be repaired for every artery anastomosed (at least three per digit) to minimize venous congestion and swelling.[13]

For finger replantations distal to the distal interphalangeal joint, veins may not be repairable, and alternative methods of venous drainage may be utilized.[1] These methods include (1) repair of volar veins, (2) creation of an arteriovenous (AV) fistula by anastomosis of one distal artery to a distal vein, (3) removal of the nail plate followed by scraping of the nail matrix with a cotton applicator and subsequent application of a heparin-soaked pledget every 1 or 2 hours, (4) application of medical-grade leeches, and (5) periodic digital massage of the replanted fingertip.

Flexor Tendon Repair

A two-strand suture method is simple and reliable and allows sutures to be placed in each cut end at the time of initial preparation. Nonabsorbable 3-0 braided sutures should used. The repair should be delayed, however, until after vessel and nerve repair are performed, especially in digits, to avoid finger flexion, which can hinder access during microsurgical repair.

If primary flexor tendon repair is not feasible because of anticipated excess tendon loss after débridement or avul-

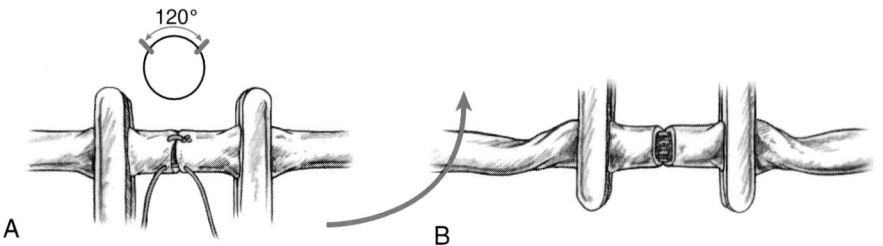

Fig. 5. Vessel repair using a bar clamp and background material. *A*, Placement of initial sutures at 120 degrees and subsequent placement of sutures in the "front wall." *B*, The clamp is then flipped 180 degrees, and the "back wall" is repaired. Fewer sutures are required for smaller vessels than depicted.

A   B

sion, a two-stage silicone rod insertion procedure should be performed. The second stage, consisting of rod removal and free-tendon grafting, can be safely performed 3 months after replantation.

Skin Closure or Coverage

All necrotic skin is débrided. Prior to closure, hemostasis must be achieved to prevent hematoma and subsequent compromise to the underlying vascular repair and the potential for infection. Skin edges should be approximated, without tension, by simple nylon sutures. Midlateral incisions on digits are frequently only partially closed, just enough to prevent vessel or nerve desiccation; they can be left open if required. In cases of skin loss, a local flap or split-thickness skin grafting may be required. Drains should be used proximal to the metacarpophalangeal joints to monitor bleeding and prevent hematoma.

Dressing and Splint

Wound closures are covered with petrolatum-impregnated gauze, fluffed 4×4 gauze (also between fingers in upper extremities), a thick layer of bulky Jones cotton, a plaster splint, and an elastic (Ace) wrap. For replantations involving the hand, the long-arm dressing should keep the hand propped up vertically with either a prefabricated or a plaster-made support. There should be a loop or the plaster should be "petalled" around the hand to protect replanted digits from inadvertent injury (Fig. 6). The hand may be lowered if the arterial flow is reduced, and raised if the venous return is sluggish. All layers of dressing must be carefully placed in a noncircumferential manner to prevent constriction.

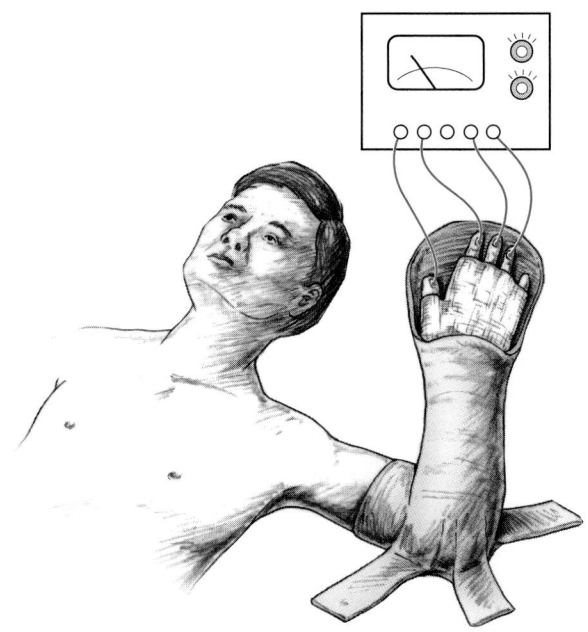

Fig. 6. Postreplantation splinting and monitoring. Hand and digit replantations should be placed in a well-padded splint that allows stable upright placement of the hand and protection from inadvertent injury. Distal temperatures are monitored as an indicator of vascular patency.

POSTOPERATIVE MANAGEMENT
Medication, Diet, and Room Temperature

Patients are advised to eliminate smoking as well as the use of smokeless tobacco and caffeine. The patient is placed in a warm, quiet environment for 1 to 3 days. Dextran 40 infusion is continued at 20 mL/hour for 2 to 4 days, and salicylates (125 mg/day) are administered. If sedation is necessary, chlorpromazine (25 mg PO tid) is used; this agent can act as a vasodilator and prevent vasospasm secondary to anxiety. Narcotic analgesia may be used as necessary. Prophylactic broad-spectrum antibiotics are given for 72 hours.

Systemic heparinization is rarely required, but in cases of crush or avulsion injury, it may be required and should be given to prolong the partial thromboplastin time to 1.5 times normal. Care must be taken to monitor the wound and dressing to avoid excess bleeding.

Replant Monitoring

The circulation in the hand is assessed by its color, pulp turgor, capillary refill, and warmth every hour for 6 hours and then every other hour for 24 hours. A simple, reliable method of monitoring is with a digital thermometer and small surface probes on each finger (see Fig. 6). If the absolute temperature drops below 30°C, or if there is a greater than 2°C to 3°C difference between a replanted digit and an adjacent finger, vascular compromise is present and should be corrected. Other monitoring techniques, such as transcutaneous oxygen measurements, laser Doppler flowmetry, hydrogen washout, and fluorescein perfusion, are expensive and complex and require more technical supervision.

Therapy

Occupational and physical therapy should be instituted early. The postoperative dressing and splint should not be disturbed until the patient's first visit to therapy. With uncomplicated replantations distal to the proximal interphalangeal joint, passive and active flexion can begin at 7 to 10 days. More complex or tenable vascular reconstruction, less stable bony constructs, or unstable soft tissues may require a slower start. Active extension is withheld as in isolated extensor tendon injuries. Therapy, which is required 2 or 3 times per week, includes static and dynamic bracing, edema control, and desensitization of painful neuromas.

COMPLICATIONS AND RESULTS

COMPLICATIONS
Early Complications

Most technical pitfalls can be avoided with careful attention to details (Table 4). Circulatory compromise is the paramount concern, and immediate measures must be taken if it occurs. The highest risk for critical thrombosis is in the first 3 days, but some risk remains for up to 2 weeks, especially in smokers.[14] The dressing should be cut back to ensure that blood-soaked bandages have not become circumferentially constrictive, and the limb reassessed. A decision to return the patient to the operating room should be made within the first 4 to 6 hours of vascular compromise,

TABLE 4. METHODS OF AVOIDING PITFALLS IN REPLANTATION SURGERY	
Pitfall	**Method of Avoidance**
Ischemia	Excise damaged arterial segment.
	Ensure adequate outflow and distal run-off (venous).
	Avoid excess redundancy and tension of artery.
	Avoid tight wound closure.
Venous congestion	Repair two veins for every artery.
	Avoid tight wound closure.
	Avoid excess redundancy, tension, and torsion of vein.
Hematoma	Ensure meticulous hemostasis of vascular branches.
	Drain when possible.
Stiffness	Early therapy.

because success of reoperation diminishes with time. All anastomoses pertinent to the affected part should be reinspected before and after intervention. Failed anastomoses should be cut back and redone, sometimes requiring a search for alternative vessels in the case of veins, or grafting if larger segments are damaged. On the basis of the initial injury and operation and the success of intraoperative findings at the time of reoperation, reamputation is indicated if flow cannot be reliably restored.

Compartment syndrome of the proximal or distal limb, including the hand or foot, can occur and should be managed aggressively with fasciotomies to prevent ischemia, anastomotic failure, and further tissue necrosis. Skin necrosis can occur as a result of secondary necrosis of compromised tissue. Additional débridement, closure, or a local flap or skin graft, or a combination of these measures, may

be required. Infection is uncommon and can be managed with antibiotics, débridement, and drainage as needed.

Late Complications

Nonunion and malunion are infrequent but may require reoperation, bone grafting, and internal fixation. Stiffness is the most common complication; freeing of adherent flexor and extensor tendons or joint releases, including the capsule, collateral ligaments, and volar plate, may be required. For more damaged, painful joints, arthrodesis or interpositional arthroplasty may be indicated. Delayed return of nerve function or neuroma may require reexploration and neurolysis or interpositional grafting. The timing of late reconstruction varies according to the patient's tissue response and motivation, therapy goals, and the surgeon's judgment.

RESULTS

Success of replantation must be measured in terms of vascular survival, sensorimotor return, motion, and, most important, functional use of the replanted part.

Survival of replanted limbs and digits varies with patient and injury factors as outlined previously. Major limb replantation survival rates vary from 40% to 80%. Digits can be expected to survive 86% of the time,[15] thumbs 82%,[16] and pediatric replants 77% (lower due to lower threshold for replantation).[17] Sensation should recover as in isolated nerve injuries of similar mechanism and level. Two-point discrimination recovers on average to 8 to 9 mm for cleanly amputated thumbs and fingers and 11 to 12 mm for avulsion and ragged injuries. Cold intolerance improves after 2 years or longer and may be linked to nerve injury and recovery.

In general, the best results of replantation are achieved in young, motivated patients with sharp, distal amputations (excluding injuries between the metacarpophalangeal and proximal interphalangeal joints).

REFERENCES

1. Goldner RD, Urbaniak JR: Replantation. In Green DP, Hotchkiss RN, Pederson WC (eds): Green's Operative Hand Surgery. Philadelphia, Churchill Livingstone, 1999, vol 3, p 1139.
2. Jobe MT: Microsurgery. In Canale ST (ed): Campbell's Operative Orthopaedics. St. Louis, Mosby, 1998, vol 4, p 3173.
3. Pederson WC, Sanders WE: Principles of microvascular surgery. In Green DP, Hotchkiss RN, Pederson WC (eds): Green's Operative Hand Surgery, 4th ed. Philadelphia, Churchill Livingstone, 1999, vol 2, p 1094.
4. Jacobson JH, Suarez EI: Microsurgery in anastomosis of small vessels. Surg Forum 1960; 11:243.
5. Chen CT, Chien YC, Pao YS: Salvage of the forearm following complete traumatic amputation. Chin Med J 1963; 82:632.
6. Malt RA, McKhann C: Replantation of severed arms. JAMA 1964; 189:716.

7. Kleinert HE, Kasdan ML, Romero JL: Small blood-vessel anastomosis for salvage of severely injured upper extremity. J Bone Joint Surg Am 1963; 45:788.
8. Komatsu S, Tamai S: Successful replantation of a completely cut-off thumb: Case report. Plast Reconstr Surg 1968; 42:374.
9. Cobbett JR: Free digital transfer: Report of a case of transfer of a great toe to replace an amputated thumb. J Bone Joint Surg 1969; 51:677.
10. Kleinert HE, Kleinert JM, McCabe SJ, et al: Replantation. Clin Symp 1992; 43:1.
11. Urbaniak JR, Evans JP, Bright DS: Microvascular management of ring avulsion injuries. J Hand Surg Am 1981; 6:25.
12. Evans PJ, Ruch DS, Patterson Smith B, et al: Management of vascular disorders in the upper extremity. In Chapman MW (ed): Operative Orthopaedics. Philadelphia, Lippincott Williams & Wilkins, 2000.

13. Matsuda M, Chikamatsu E, Shimizu Y: Correlation between number of anastomosed vessels and survival rate in finger replantation. J Reconstr Microsurg 1993; 9:1.
14. Betancourt FM, Mah ET, McCabe SJ: Timing of critical thrombosis after replantation surgery of the digits. J Reconstr Microsurg 1998; 14:313.
15. Urbaniak JR, Roth JH, Nunley JA, et al: The results of replantation after amputation of a single finger. J Bone Joint Surg Am 1985; 67:611–619.
16. Bowen CVA, Beveridge J, Milliken RG, et al: Rotating shaft avulsion amputations of the thumb. J Hand Surg Am 1991; 16: 117.
17. Taras JS, Nunley JA, Urbaniak JR, et al: Replantation in children. Microsurgery 1991; 12:216.

section 12 chapter 9
REGIONAL FLAPS
Robert J. Goitz and Matthew M. Tomaino

Summary
- Knowledge of coverage options for the hand and upper extremity may facilitate optimal treatment of soft-tissue defects.
- The dorsal skin over the index finger at the level of the proximal phalanx is vascularized by the first dorsal metacarpal artery and can be harvested as an axial pattern island flap for coverage of thumb defects.
- A fasciocutaneous flap can be fashioned from the volar or dorsal forearm based on septocutaneous perforators from the radial artery or posterior interosseous artery to provide coverage of elbow or hand defects.
- A fillet flap can be fashioned from a nonsalvageable digit to provide coverage of soft-tissue defects of the remaining digits or hand.

INTRODUCTION

The subcutaneous position of many vital structures in the upper extremity makes them vulnerable to injury, which may expose tendon, nerve, bone, or joint. Optimal treatment of hand and wrist injuries often necessitates early motion to minimize stiffness and scar adherence. However, healing of injured tissues and the introduction of early motion therapy is predicated on a well-vascularized and healed soft-tissue envelope. At times free tissue transfer may be required, but knowledge of the multiple regional flaps available in the upper extremity may allow early coverage, therapy, and functional return without microvascular reconstruction.[1]

GENERAL PRINCIPLES

Consideration of treatment options requires a thorough understanding of the soft-tissue defect. First, the viability of the wound bed must be evaluated. Exposed but viable fat, fascia, and paratenon may be optimally treated with a simple skin graft or may even heal by secondary intention. If the exposed bed is unable to support a skin graft or heal with dressing changes, then coverage with local soft tissue should be considered. The surrounding skin and subcutaneous tissue, if they are not traumatized and are of adequate size, may provide optimal coverage through the use of rotation or transposition flaps. The defect created by the donor site should not create any further functional deficits, however. For example, the first web space must remain mobile to allow for the extensive motion of the thumb metacarpal. Skin grafts in this area may scar and contract, resulting in restricted thumb mobility. If the wound bed is unable to support a skin graft, heal by secondary intention, or be adequately covered with local tissue, a regional flap may be an appropriate choice.

FIRST DORSAL METACARPAL ARTERY FLAP

ANATOMY

Dorsal skin extending along the second metacarpal to the level of the proximal interphalangeal (PIP) joint is supplied by the first dorsal metacarpal artery (FDMA). This artery is a branch of the radial artery exiting just distal to the extensor pollicis longus but just before entering the first dorsal interosseous (DIO) muscle. The FDMA travels superficial to the DIO fascia and has been shown to be quite reliable.[1, 2]

INDICATIONS

The FDMA flap is a neurovascular island flap incorporating the entire dorsal skin of the index proximal phalanx with the vascular pedicle based just distal to the carpometacarpal joint. It is most often used to resurface defects on the thumb,[3] especially tip amputations (Fig. 1A). It may also be rotated as far ulnarly as the dorsal distal ring metacarpal.[4] A dorsal sensory branch may be included to provide sensibility.

As an extension of the FDMA flap, dorsal skin over the index metacarpal as well as the proximal phalanx may be elevated and transposed to cover first web space defects[5] (Fig. 2) or distal ulnar hand defects.

PREOPERATIVE PLANNING

The size, position, and extent of the defect will dictate whether the FDMA flap will adequately cover the area. Consideration of the pedicle length and pivot point at the base of the carpometacarpal joint is critical to preoperative planning. If there is any soft-tissue trauma at the base of the first and second metacarpals, the FDMA can be assessed by Doppler ultrasonography to ascertain its presence.

TECHNICAL DETAILS

The size of the flap should incorporate at least a 10% increase over the size of the defect to account for shrinkage of the fasciocutaneous flap. All of the dorsal skin of the index proximal phalanx may be elevated, from the metacarpophalangeal joint to the PIP joint.

Dissection occurs distal to proximal, superficial to the paratenon at the level of the proximal phalanx and deep to the fascia of the DIO muscle at the level of the second metacarpal (see Fig. 1B to D). The FDMA does not need

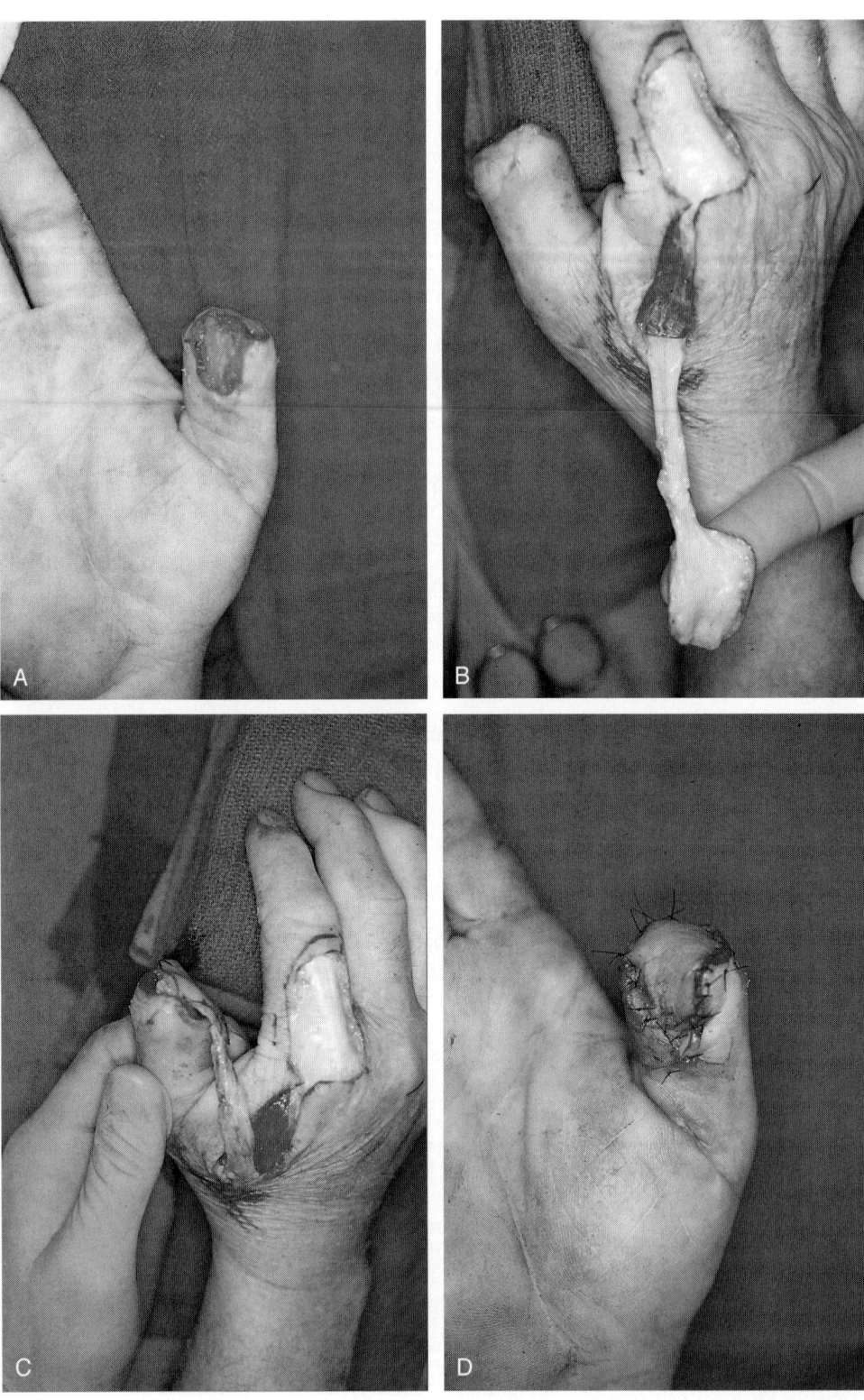

Fig. 1. First dorsal metacarpal artery flap. *A,* This 52-year-old man sustained an amputation of the right thumb through the interphalangeal joint. After débridement, closure could not be performed without additional shortening of the proximal phalanx. *B,* A first dorsal metacarpal artery (FDMA) flap was elevated. The skin from the proximal phalanx was harvested, including the fascia from the first dorsal interosseous muscle. The pedicle can be seen running into the skin flap. *C,* Paratenon has been preserved over the extensor apparatus to the index finger to allow full-thickness skin grafting. The skin flap based on the FDMA is easily passed beneath the subcutaneous tunnel from its pivot point at the base of the thumb and index metacarpals to the thumb tip. *D,* The FDMA skin flap has been inset, preserving the entire length of the thumb proximal phalanx. This enabled the patient to have a useful thumb for pinch.

to be visualized because dissection is deep to the fascia and the artery is located between the fascia and subcutaneous fat. The donor defect is covered with a full-thickness skin graft.

An axial pattern flap is extended proximally to the base of the first and second metacarpals, incorporating the entire dorsal skin over the second metacarpal and proximal phalanx. Usually transposition flaps are considered random pattern flaps, which require adherence to a 1:1 ratio of length to base.[6] However, because this flap has a known axial blood supply (the FDMA), it can sustain a greater ratio.

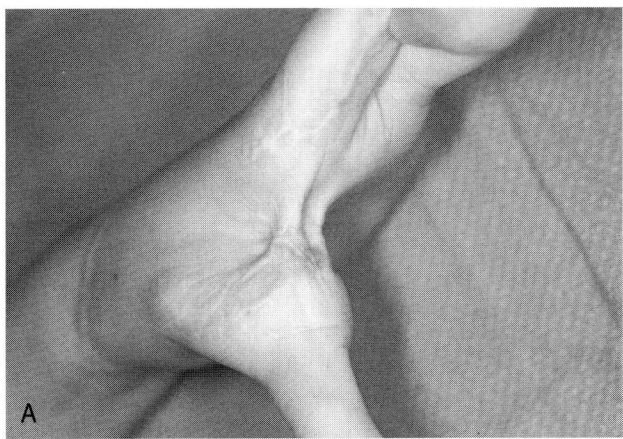
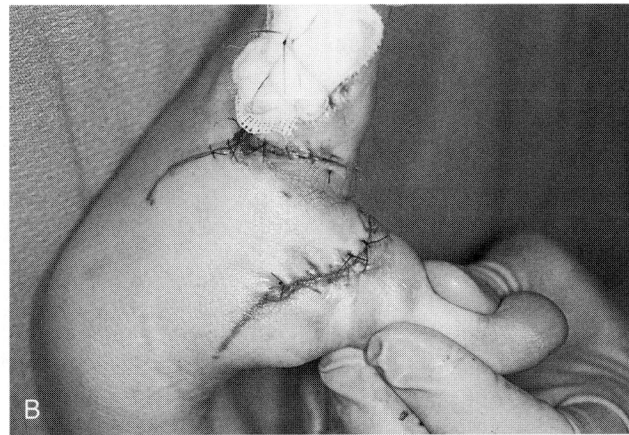

Fig. 2. Dorsal index finger transposition flap to the first web space. *A,* This 11-year-old boy had a toe-to-thumb transfer and skin grafting in the first web space 7 years ago. He complained of pain and limitation of thumb abduction secondary to first web space contracture. Dorsal skin, subcutaneous tissue, and first dorsal interosseous muscle fascia are harvested as a proximally based flap from the base of the index and middle metacarpal. *B,* Transposition to the first web space provides improved contour and motion of the thumb.

RADIAL FOREARM FLAP

ANATOMY
The entire volar forearm skin and subcutaneous tissue are supplied by the radial artery through intermuscular septal perforators that travel between the brachioradialis and the flexor carpi radialis.[7, 8] Venous drainage occurs through vena comitantes and multiple subcutaneous veins. This flap may be harvested as a fascial[9] or fasciocutaneous flap.[10]

INDICATIONS
The radial forearm flap may be used to cover elbow defects through anterograde flow or hand/wrist defects through retrograde flow via the superficial and deep arches

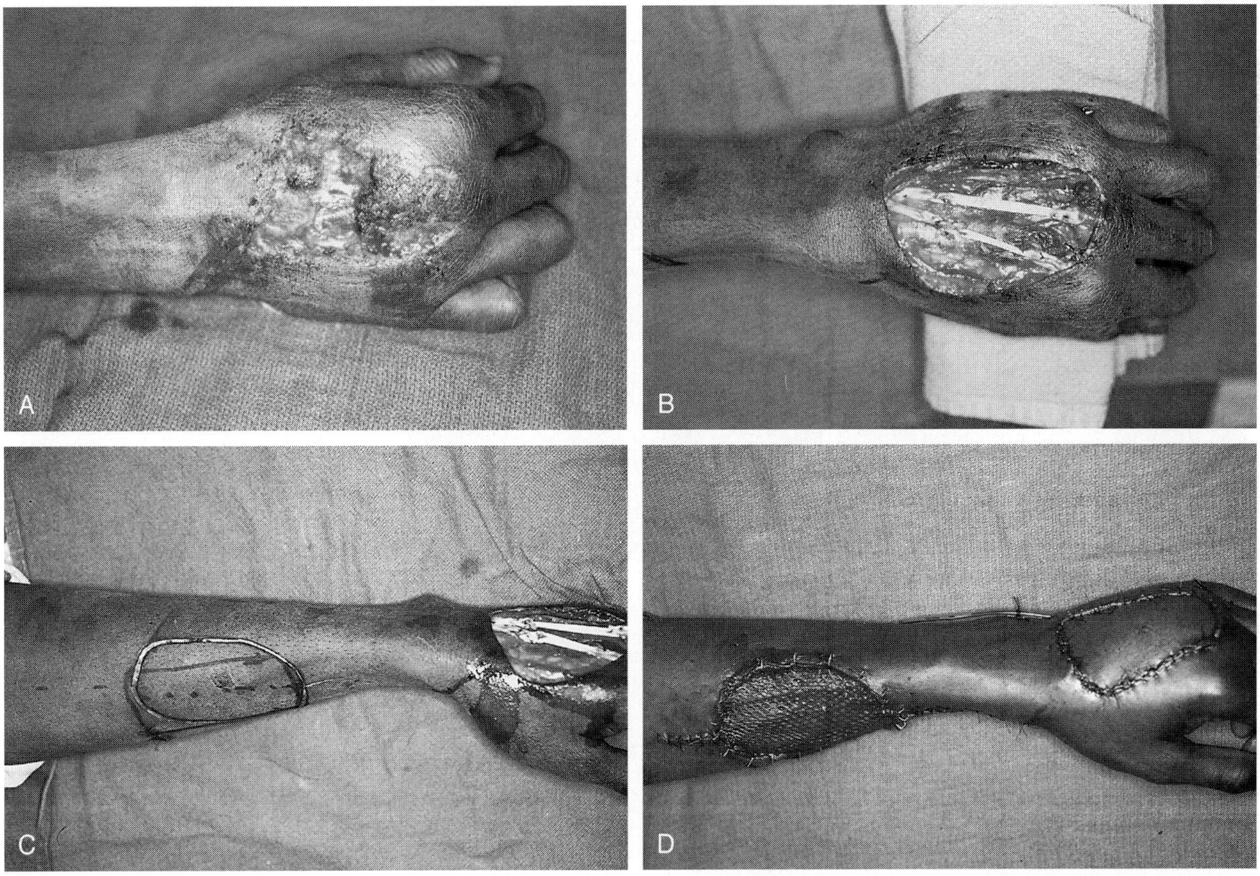

Fig. 3. Radial forearm flap. *A,* This 28-year-old man was involved in a motor vehicle accident and sustained composite tissue loss to the dorsum of the hand with loss of the index and long finger extensor tendons. *B,* After débridement, extensor tendons are exposed. *C,* The flap is designed, and its axis is centered over the radial artery. *D,* The flap is inset into the dorsum of the hand, and the donor defect is covered with a split-thickness skin graft.

of the hand (Fig. 3). Donor defects of between 4 and 6 cm in width may be closed primarily.

PREOPERATIVE PLANNING

It is critical to assess the vascular supply to radial fingers by performing an Allen test before raising the flap because some patients have an incomplete superficial arch with the primary arterial supply from the radial artery to the thumb and index finger.

TECHNICAL DETAILS

The flap is centralized over the course of the radial artery and designed as an ellipse to maximize potential closure and contour of the defect site. The size of the flap is determined by the addition of 10% to the size of the recipient defect to account for shrinkage of the fasciocutaneous flap. A suture or gauze sponge may be used to assess the rotational potential of the flap and the length of the pedicle required to reach the defect from the pivot point adequately. The flap is harvested by making an incision through the skin, subcutaneous tissue, and fascia on the outline of the flap. Dissection is performed in the subfascial plane to the level of the intermuscular septum bounded by the brachioradialis and the flexor carpi radialis. The radial artery is then temporarily occluded proximally to assess digital viability before permanent ligation of the

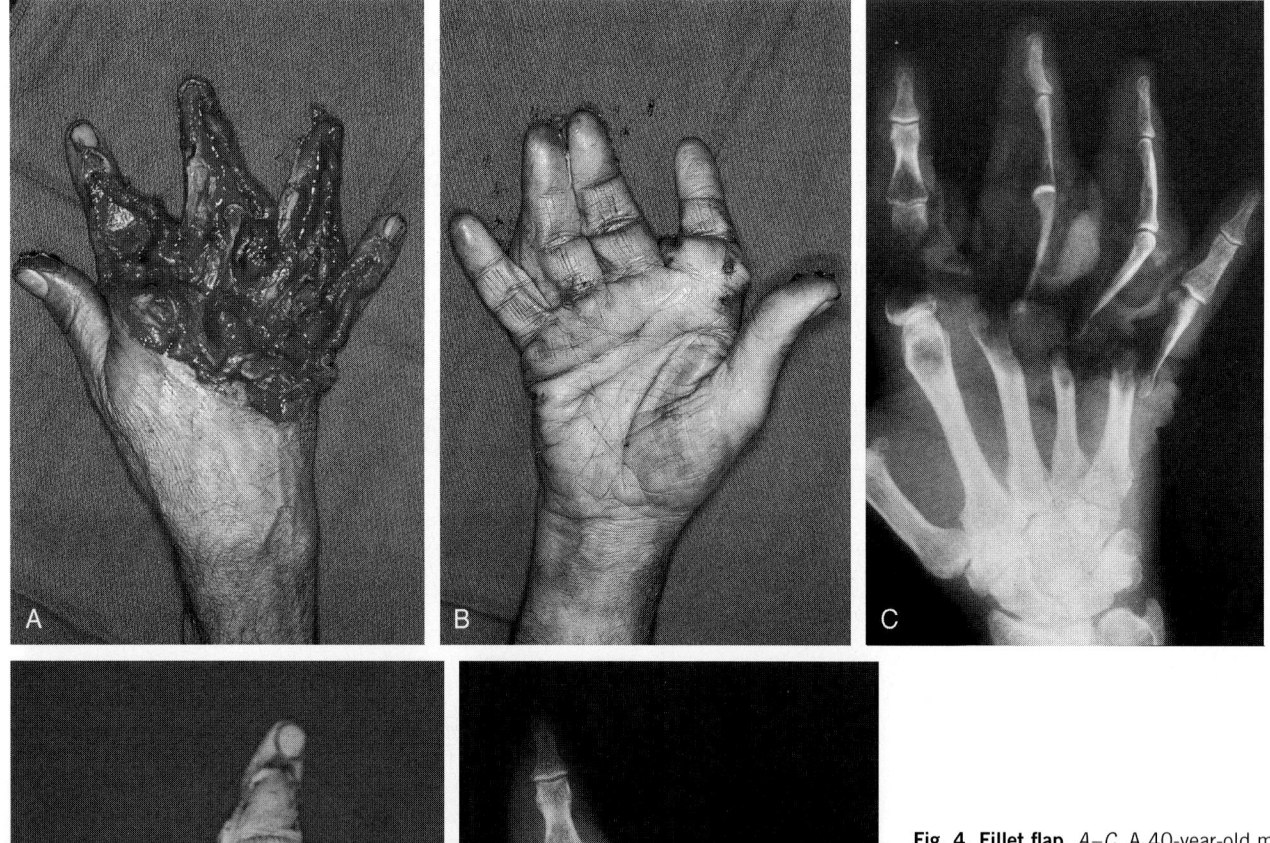

Fig. 4. Fillet flap. *A–C,* A 40-year-old man sustained a grinder injury to the dorsum of the right hand, resulting in loss of the dorsal skin, extensor tendons, and a majority of phalangeal bones. *D–E,* Reconstruction of the index finger and volar hand skin from the nonsalvageable middle, ring, and small fingers. In addition, flexor tendons were used as tendon graft to reconstruct the extensor mechanism, and bone from the middle phalanx of the ring and small fingers was used to restore bony stability to the index proximal phalanx.

radial artery. Release of the intermuscular septum is then performed just dorsal to the radial artery.

The flap is then rotated into position and inset. A skin graft is often required to cover the donor site. The more proximal forearm skin has more redundancy and greater potential for primary closure of the donor site; therefore, the radial forearm flap should be harvested as proximal as possible. In addition, the paratenon must not be violated over the distal volar tendons to facilitate skin grafting of the donor defect.

FILLET FLAP

ANATOMY

The fillet flap refers to the use of sensate viable skin from an unsalvageable digit to provide coverage to a remaining traumatized digit or hand.[11] Generally, digital skin with an intact proximal blood supply from the base can be used for salvage purposes. Digital skin is vascularized through a series of communicating branches from the proper digital vessels. This arcade of vessels allows a digit to remain viable on one vessel. The metacarpal arteries also contribute to the vascularity of a digit through their dorsal supply.

INDICATIONS

When severe hand trauma results in a nonreconstructable digit, it should be used to provide donor parts for reconstruction of the remaining salvageable digits and hand. This includes the use of skin for soft-tissue coverage and the use of tendons, nerves, and bone for graft (Fig. 4).

PREOPERATIVE PLANNING

To assess the size of skin available, the length of the digit from the web space to the nail fold is measured. The width of the flap is equal to the circumference of the digit. The pulp is often not included because of its bulk, but it may be of benefit if a cavity exists.

TECHNICAL DETAILS

All nonviable tissue is débrided from the traumatized digit. A longitudinal incision is made along the digit adjacent to the recipient defect. The skin and subcutaneous tissue, along with the remaining neurovascular structures, are removed from the underlying bone and tendons. The flap is rotated over the defect site and sutured into position. If greater length is required to reach a defect, the base of the skin flap can be incised, creating a neurovascular island flap.[12,13] The remaining amputated parts may be used for graft.

POSTOPERATIVE MANAGEMENT

Initially, limited immobilization is often beneficial after the use of regional flaps to maximize soft-tissue healing. Edema control such as elevation or bulky dressings is used to minimize swelling and tension on the skin repair. Early motion can minimize scar adherence and stiffness and is often instituted 1 week postoperatively. However, skin grafts may require 2 to 3 weeks of immobilization for optimal healing.

COMPLICATIONS

One disadvantage of the use of local and regional flaps for coverage is their potential involvement in the zone of injury. This may result in unexpected marginal flap necrosis. The regional flaps outlined previously are considered highly reliable. However, complications are often associated with incomplete take of the skin graft over the donor site, especially over exposed tendons.[14–16] Maintenance of the paratenon is critical for optimal healing of skin graft over tendons.

REFERENCES

1. Goitz RJ, Westkaemper JG, Tomaino MM, et al: Soft-tissue defects of the digits: Coverage considerations. Hand Clin 1997; 13:189.

2. Sherif MM: First dorsal metacarpal artery flap in hand reconstruction: Anatomical study. J Hand Surg Am 1994; 19:26.

3. Foucher G, Brown J-B: A new island flap transfer from the dorsum of the index to the thumb. Plast Reconstr Surg 1979; 63: 344.

4. Sherif MM: First dorsal metacarpal artery flap in hand reconstruction: II. Clinical application. J Hand Surg Am 1994; 19:32.

5. Earley MJ, Milner RH: Dorsal metacarpal flaps. Br J Plast Surg 1987; 40:333.

6. Spinner M: Fashioned transpositional flap for soft tissue adduction contracture of the thumb. Plast Reconstr Surg 1969; 44: 345.

7. Lister G: The theory of the transposition flap and its practical application in the hand. Clin Plast Surg 1981; 8:115.

8. Foucher G, Van Genechten F, Merle F, et al: A compound radial artery forearm flap in hand surgery: An original modification of the Chinese forearm flap. Br J Plastic Surg 1984; 37:139.

9. Cavanagh S, Pho RWH: The reverse radial forearm flap in the severely injured hand: An anatomical and clinical study. J Hand Surg Br 1992; 17:501.

10. Soutar DS, Tanner NSB: The radial forearm flap in the management of soft-tissue injuries of the hand. Br J Plast Surg 1984; 37:18.

11. Angrigiani C, Grilli D, Dominikow D, et al: Posterior interosseous reverse forearm flap: Experience with 80 consecutive cases. Plast Reconstr Surg 1993; 92:285.

12. Bunnell S: Injuries of the hand. In Bunnell S (ed): Surgery of the Hand, 4th ed. Philadelphia, JB Lippincott, 1964, p 612.

13. Alpert BS, Buncke H: Mutilating multidigital injuries: Use of a free microvascular flap from a non-replantable part. J Hand Surg 1978; 3:196.

14. Idler RS, Mih AD: Soft-tissue coverage of the hand with a free digital fillet flap. Microsurgery 1990; 11:215.

15. Bardsley AF, Soutar DS, Elliot D, et al: Reducing morbidity in the radial forearm flap donor site. Plast Reconstr Surg 1990; 86:287.

16. Liang MD, Swartz WM, Jones FF: Local full-thickness skin-graft coverage for the radial forearm flap donor site. Plast Reconstr Surg 1994; 93:621.

DISTANT FLAPS: PEDICLE AND FREE

Neil J. Wells and Douglas P. Hanel

Summary
- In the last 25 years, flaps have become the main-stay of treatment of difficult wounds and an important part of orthopaedic surgery.
- The objective of using a flap is wound coverage to provide healing of a useful limb.
- The indications are extensive soft-tissue loss with exposed vital structures (nerve, tendons, bone, or joint), unstable scars, coverage of poorly vascularized beds, or restoration of specialized function (sensation or motor unit).
- The goal is to provide vascularized tissue to promote healing and decrease the chance of infection.
- Careful planning, including patient selection, wound preparation, and flap choice are crucial in flap survival.
- Wound coverage with a flap within 1 week after injury improves outcome.

A flap is tissue used to cover a defect. A flap has its own blood supply and is not reliant on its recipient bed for survival. They are classified according to tissue type (skin, muscle, bone, or composite); blood supply, random or axial (based on arterial pedicle); and method of transfer (advancement, rotation, transposition, tubed, or free). Distant pedicle flaps, although of historical interest, have now been largely replaced by free flaps, which require microsurgical anastomosis. The frequency of the use of free flaps has increased dramatically in recent years because the familiarity and success with these flaps has increased.

Since the first reported successful free flap in 1973, vast literature on flap anatomy and clinical results has appeared.[1,2] Early microsurgical reconstruction of complex open extremity trauma significantly decreased the infection and nonunion rate.[3] In the multisystem injured patient with soft-tissue problems, it is essential for a collaborative approach on early fracture stabilization and wound coverage by an orthopaedic surgeon and a specially trained microsurgeon. This emphasizes the need for even the general orthopaedic surgeon not trained in microsurgery to have an understanding of the prerequisites, timing, and available options for soft-tissue reconstruction.

HISTORICAL REVIEW

Combined fracture and flap reconstruction developed during World Wars I and II, where the importance of adequate débridement, immobilization, and delayed closure was recognized. Osteomyelitis during this era was as high as 80%, and in 1965 Brown advocated early coverage.[4] In 1972, McGregor and Jackson described the pedicled groin flap

and defined the difference between random and axial flaps. During the 1970s, the operating microscope was developed. Daniel and Taylor in 1972 described the first free tissue transfers with microsurgery.[5] Since then, there has been a rapid growth of various flap options, with most muscle being described. Godina (1986) showed that early microvascular flap coverage of complex extremity trauma decreased the infection rate from 20% to 1.5%. May and Mathes in 1982 described their experience in the treatment of osteomyelitis with free flaps.[6,7]

CLINICAL SITUATIONS

The application of distant flaps in orthopaedics is seen generally in three clinical situations. The first and most common is in trauma, in which there is extensive soft-tissue injury and/or exposure of bone or other vital structures. This situation is most common in distal tibial fractures (Gustilo IIIB; see discussion of tibial fractures in Chapter 3–18 for more details). In these cases, there are generally long bone injuries (tibia/fibula, radius/ulna) with exposed structures that are not amenable to direct closure or skin grafting. In these situations, it is important that the extent of muscle, tendon, and neurovascular damage is well documented, since these are important in determining the treatment options and prognosis.

The second situation is in cases of chronic osteomyelitis in the lower extremity, in which the patient has a draining sinus with surrounding unhealthy tissue (indurated, scarred, immobile skin) and exposed bone. In these cases, radical débridement of the sinus, the unhealthy local tissue, and the infected bone often leaves a wound that requires the addition of healthy tissue from a distance for closure.

The third situation is in cases of tumor resection, in which functional elements, such as bone, functioning muscle, or soft-tissue bulk, have been sacrificed and need to be reconstructed to provide a more functional limb.

INVESTIGATIONS

As for all surgical patients, full examination of the individual and more specifically the recipient and donor sites is mandatory when free tissue transfer is being considered. Particular attention should be given to the bony skeleton, soft-tissue deficit, vascular tree, and any other structural injuries (nerves, joints, and tendons). It is important to establish whether limb salvage using a free tissue transfer is indicated and, if so, what flap is best suited for the defect. In making a decision, one must be familiar with the functional outcome of amputation, since an insensate nonfunctioning hand or foot is not worth salvaging when the rehabilitation process and potential outcome are considered.

The wound itself needs to be inspected for size dimensions, thoroughness of débridement, and the relation of the defect to the vascular pedicle. The vascular tree can be assessed by Doppler flow clinically or by angiography—several authors routinely do preoperative angiography, whereas others rely only on the location of injury and results of clinical examination. In either case, it is essential for careful intraoperative examination of the potential vessels being considered for anastomosis, and a back-up option should be available.

The bony skeleton needs to be assessed with radiographs before and after fracture fixation. Computed tomography, magnetic resonance imaging, and technetium-labeled erythrocyte or indium III–labeled leukocyte bone scans are utilized as needed based on the clinical situation. The donor site must be examined to ensure that no scars or abnormalities exist that might impair the use of this flap in free tissue transfer.

TREATMENT GOALS, INDICATIONS, AND CONTRAINDICATIONS FOR DISTANT AND FREE FLAPS

When the surgeon is faced with a wound of any kind, he or she must consider all options for closure (primary, secondary, skin graft, local flap, or distant flap) and should proceed with a flap only when the other, simpler options are not suitable. The goal in all cases is healing without infection or unstable scar.

The indications for using a flap include the following:

1. Coverage of skin and soft-tissue loss with exposed vital structures (such as nerves, tendons, bone, and joints).
2. Coverage of unstable scar in cases of burns, radiation, ischemia, and scar contracture.
3. Coverage when a skin graft may hamper later reconstructive procedures, such as tendon reconstruction.
4. Treatment of osteomyelitis with skin breakdown and draining sinuses.
5. Restoration of specialized tissue necessary for function (such as sensation in the hand or foot, tendons, or bone).
6. Restoration of contour and form (esthetics).

The advantages of a free flap as opposed to a pedicle flap include the following:

1. Less restriction in choice of donor site, and therefore improved cosmesis at both donor and recipient sites.
2. Ability to mobilize adjacent joints, therefore less stiffness.
3. Free flaps can be carried out in a single procedure, unlike distant pedicle flaps, which are multistaged.
4. Possible better vascularity in the transferred tissue.

With all the recent advances in microsurgery and an increasing familiarity and comfort with the techniques, the contraindications to free flaps are few and most are best described as reservations. In patients with systemic illnesses such as peripheral vascular disease and diabetes, the risk of failure is thought to increase (although many recent articles have shown that this is no longer a significant contraindication).[8,9] Poor local recipient vessels preclude their use and necessitate a vein graft, which increases failure rates. A hand or foot supplied by a single vessel risks the viability of the extremity, if there is a problem with the anastomosis.

Absolute contraindications to the use of a free flap include the following:

1. Inability of the institution to support the operative and postoperative management of a microsurgical program.
2. Poor functional potential.
3. Other reliable and simpler means are unavailable.
4. Patient is unwilling to cooperate with postoperative care.
5. Other medical or surgical problems preclude a lengthy operation.

The disadvantages of free flaps include the following:

1. A longer, more difficult operation.
2. Donor site problems.
3. Special equipment and specialized training.
4. A 10% to 25% re-exploration rate with 5% to 10% failure rate.

Selection of the donor flap depends on the size of the defect, the qualities needed in the flap, the vascular pedicle anatomy, cosmesis, and the surgeon's familiarity with the flap. Table 1 lists most of the flaps commonly used and describes the vascularity, advantages, disadvantages, and indications for each. Although many are listed as only pedicle flaps, most have been used as free flaps; however, these are infrequent and not part of the standard repertoire.

PROCEDURE

PREPARATION

Careful preoperative planning is essential. Preoperatively, the patient needs to be well hydrated and medically stabilized. The tissues required and the possible flap options need to be identified.

On the day of surgery, the operating room and the patient need to be kept warm to decrease vasoconstriction. Positioning of the patient requires attention to padding vital structures while allowing access to both surgical sites. An operating microscope or surgical loupes greater than 4× magnification and microsurgical instruments with microvascular clamps are required for the anastomosis.

TECHNICAL DETAILS

The operation has three components: preparation of the wound and the recipient vessels (recipient site), harvesting of the free flap (donor site), and the microvascular anastomoses.

Recipient Site Preparation

There are two key principles for management of the recipient site. First, all nonviable tissue must be débrided and the wound irrigated with pulsed saline to decrease the contamination. Second, careful dissection of the recipient vessels must be carried out with the aid of magnification. The site for anastomosis should be out of the local zone of injury, which will help make this dissection easier and will

TABLE 1. COMMON DISTANT FLAPS

Location	Flap	Classification	Vascular Pedicle	Qualities	Uses	Disadvantages
Trunk	**Latissimus dorsi**	Muscle	Thoracodorsal artery	Large pedicle, good length Large, thin muscle Easily contours Serratus can be added Functioning muscle Skin paddle 30–40 cm TRAM skin can be used	F: tibial defects, forearm, amputation stumps P: shoulder, elbow flexion, spine, anterior chest	Scar visible Repositioning intraoperatively Requires STSG if muscle alone
	Rectus abdominis	Muscle	Superior epigastric artery Inferior epigastric artery	Skin available Easily accessible Large pedicle	P: mediastinum P: groin, pelvis F: leg	Scar noticeable Abdominal weakness
	Serratus anterior	Muscle	Thoracodorsal artery	Multiple slips Small Bone-rib Latissimus dorsi combined	F: foot P/F: mandible	Scar long and noticeable Challenging to elevate because of multiple slips Bulky skin flap
	Groin	Cutaneous	Superficial circumflex iliac artery Deep circumflex iliac artery	Hidden donor scar Bone-iliac crest	P/F: hand-thumb/dorsum F: tibial defects	Dependant position if pedicled Bulky
	Parascapular	Cutaneous	Descending branch of circumflex scapular artery	Combine with scapular for large area Large pedicle Bone-lateral border of scapula	F: arm, leg	May require STSG at donor site Visible scar Repositioning in operating room often necessary
	Scapular	Cutaneous	Transverse branch of circumflex scapular artery			
Head and neck	**Temporoparietal**	Fasciocutaneous	Superficial temporal artery	Thin, pliable Good pedicle Hidden scar	F: dorsum hand, dorsum foot	Requires STSG at recipient site
Arm	**Lateral arm**	Fasciocutaneous	Posterior radial collateral artery	Thin skin Reliable long pedicle Large vessels innervated	F: foot, hand	Visible scar Sensory nerves posterior cutaneous of arm and forearm often damaged

	Type	Artery	Features	Uses	Disadvantages
Radial forearm	Fasciocutaneous	Radial artery	Sensate via lateral antebrachial nerve; Bone: radius; Tendon: palmaris longus	P: hand; F: foot, ankle	Visible scar; May require STSG for donor site; Radius fracture with bone harvest; ? Ischemia to hand; Same as radial forearm
Ulnar artery	Fasiocutaneous	Ulnar artery	Thin, pliable; Sensate via cutaneous nerve	P: hand; F: foot	
Leg					
Gastrocnemius	Muscle	Medial or lateral sural artery	Pedicle; Simple elevation	P: knee and proximal tibia	Short length; Needs STSG to flap or defect
Gracilis	Muscle	Branch of medial circumflex femoral artery	Thin muscle; Can innervate; Inconspicuous donor site	F: multiple uses; P: groin	Small pedicle
Soleus	Muscle	Branch of posterior tibial artery	Can be split and slid over tibia; Can be based distally	P: mid-tibial, small defects	Often damaged during initial trauma; Unreliable if based distally
Dorsalis pedis	Cutaneous	Dorsalis pedis artery	Bone: metatarsal; Extensor tendon available; Can be sensate; Thin, pliable	P: foot, ankle; F: hand, face	Donor site morbidity. STSG to cover donor site. Incorporates with difficulty, especially if bone is harvested.
Peroneal	Fasciocutaneous	Peroneal artery	Composite with fibula	P: leg reconstruction; F: forearm, jaw	Need wide pedicle for transposition flaps
Plantar	Fasciocutaneous	Medial plantar artery		P: foot	Donor scar on plantar aspect of foot; Short arc of rotation
Posterior tibial	Fasciocutaneous	Post-tibial artery	Can innervate with sural nerve; Thin, pliable skin	P: mid-leg	Donor defect; Small arc
Thigh (medial and lateral)	Fasciocutaneous	Perforating branches of superficial femoral artery; Perforator of profunda femoris	Sensate medial and lateral cutaneous nerve; Take fascia and fat alone	F: foot, hand	Visible scar

F, free flap; P, pedicle flap; STSG, split-thickness skin graft; TRAM, transverse rectus abdominis muscle.

decrease the complications at the microvascular anastomosis. Preparation of the recipient site should be done prior to harvesting of the donor site, to accurately establish the size of the defect, the required vascular pedicle length, and whether vein grafts are necessary. Often this is done simultaneously with two surgical teams.

Harvesting of the Donor Site

The keys to harvesting the donor flap are making sure this is the most appropriate flap and the raising of the flap in an atraumatic fashion. When marking out the dimensions of the flap, it is important to include the thickness of the flap and any convexity of the recipient site in these measurements, as they increase the size of the flap required to fill the defect.

During flap elevation, hemostasis is required to allow good visualization of the pedicle. The flap should be raised until its only vascular supply is the pedicle. At this time, the flap should be left in situ and the microsurgeon should have the microscope and the recipient vessels ready for immediate anastomosis. The flap donor vessels are transected and the flap is transferred to the recipient site while covered with a cool moist sponge.

Microvascular Anastomosis

The anastomosis needs to be done atraumatically and with careful observation to ensure that no twisting, kinking, or redundancy of the vessels occurs. Once the anastomosis is completed and patency verified, the flap is sutured into place, and a well-padded dressing and splint are applied to protect the anastomosis from pressure, tension, and kinking. Prior to the patient's leaving the operating room, the flap is checked to make sure the blood flow was not altered while the dressing was applied.

POSTOPERATIVE MANAGEMENT

The first 5 postoperative days are a critical phase in flap survival and therefore have led to numerous rituals of management specific to the idiosyncrasies of each microsurgeon. Generally, the patient is kept on a caffeine- and nicotine-free diet while on bedrest in a warm room. The flap is monitored hourly (for at least the first 24 hours) to assess for vascular compromise. Since most vascular problems arise in the venous system and are initially difficult to diagnose, numerous clinical and mechanical methods have been developed to diagnose impending flap failure. A combination of clinical examination (flap color, capillary refill, and temperature [if skin is present]) combined with direct monitoring of the vascular flow by techniques such as ultrasonic or laser Doppler monitoring, digital plethysmography, photoplethysmography, transcutaneous oxygen tension monitoring, or radioisotope clearance assays.

Pharmacotherapy with low-dose aspirin for at least 1 month is used to prevent thrombus formation and spasm at the anastomosis. Some practitioners use low molecular weight dextran both for intravascular volume expansion and for its antiplatelet and anticoagulation effects. Heparin is reserved for salvage situations because of the complications associated with anticoagulation (flap hematoma formation and donor site bleeding).

COMPLICATIONS AND RESULTS

COMPLICATIONS

Although vascular compromise is the major complication of concern to the microsurgeon, complications can occur at the donor and recipient sites.

Anastomosis

Vascular compromise occurs in 10% to 20% of cases with a greater than 50% salvage with early intervention.[10]

The initial treatment of a vascularly compromised flap includes the following:

1. Ensuring adequate circulation (normotensive, euvolemic).
2. Examining the dressing to loosen or remove constrictive areas.
3. Repositioning the patient if the pedicle is being compressed.
4. Examining the recipient site for signs of hematoma and, if found, releasing the flap to allow evacuation.

If this fails or if there is any doubt, then **immediately return to the operating room,** and do the following:

1. Remove all sutures and elevate the flap.
2. Remove the hematoma with normal saline.
3. Examine the pedicle for kinking or compression and for level of occlusion.
4. Examine the anastomosis by opening it and checking flow. Do not hesitate to redo the anastomosis if no other inflow or outflow source of obstruction can be found. **Do not rely on pharmacotherapy or other modalities to salvage a failing flap; exploration is a must.**

Donor Site

Complications at the donor site include the following:

Unsightly scar. There is an increased likelihood of scar if the donor flap was large, with the resulting increased tension on the wound closure. This can be avoided by not exceeding the known limitations of the flap or by choosing a different flap.

Seroma/hematoma. This complication is more common in sites of large muscle flaps with large potential space. It is best avoided by good hemostasis and adequate drainage.

Infection. There is a low risk of infection. The likelihood can be decreased with good technique and no crosscontamination with the recipient site.

Contour irregularity. Nearly all flaps leave some irregularity. This is best managed by preparing the patient in advance.

Recipient Site

Complications at the recipient site include the following:

Partial flap failure. Failure is not uncommon in pedicle flaps at the distal end. This is best avoided by choosing the flap appropriately and not exceeding its vascular territory. If failure occurs, allow the area to become well defined and then tangentially excise the tissue and skingraft it, if possible.

Nonunion. Nonunion is often associated with infection.

This is increased if the flap is done later than 7 days after injury (increase from 5% to 30% in open tibial fractures). Treatment should include removal of infected bone, good fixation, antibiotics, and bone grafting as necessary.

Infection. Risk of infection is increased by 10% (up to 60%) if flap coverage is done later than 1 week after injury. This is best avoided by radical débridement at the initial procedure and by early flap coverage. Once infection occurs, radical débridement of all contaminated tissue is required.

SPECIFIC FLAPS
Gracilis Muscle Flap

The gracilis muscle can be used as a muscle or musculocutaneous flap via pedicle or free transfer (Fig. 1).[11] Its narrow contour, easy accessibility in the supine position, and minimal donor morbidity have made it a common choice for distal tibial and ankle fractures.

Anatomy. The gracilis muscle arises from the inferior ramus of the pubis and inserts on the medial aspect of the tibia. It is innervated by a branch of the anterior division of the obturator nerve, which enters the muscle near its dominant vascular pedicle, the medial femoral circumflex artery, and its vena comitans, between 8 and 12 cm from the muscle origin. The vascular pedicle can be 4 to 6 cm long and 1 to 2 mm in diameter.

Dissection. The leg is abducted and externally rotated and a line is drawn between the palpable origin of the adductor longus and the tibial tuberosity. The gracilis lies just posterior to this. The surgeon incises down to the gracilis muscle and incises the fascia overlying it and lifts it off posteriorly. Next, the surgeon dissects anteriorly to separate the gracilis muscle from the adductor longus. The secondary pedicle (approximately two thirds of the muscle length from the origin) is identified and ligated. The distal part of the muscle is bluntly dissected and transected. Next, the surgeon elevates the muscle from distal to proximal off the deep adductor magnus muscle. At the level of the main pedicle, the surgeon carefully separates the adductor longus and adductor magnus muscles and follows the pedicle to its origin. The origin of the muscle is divided, then the neurovascular pedicle, and the muscle is transferred to the recipient site.

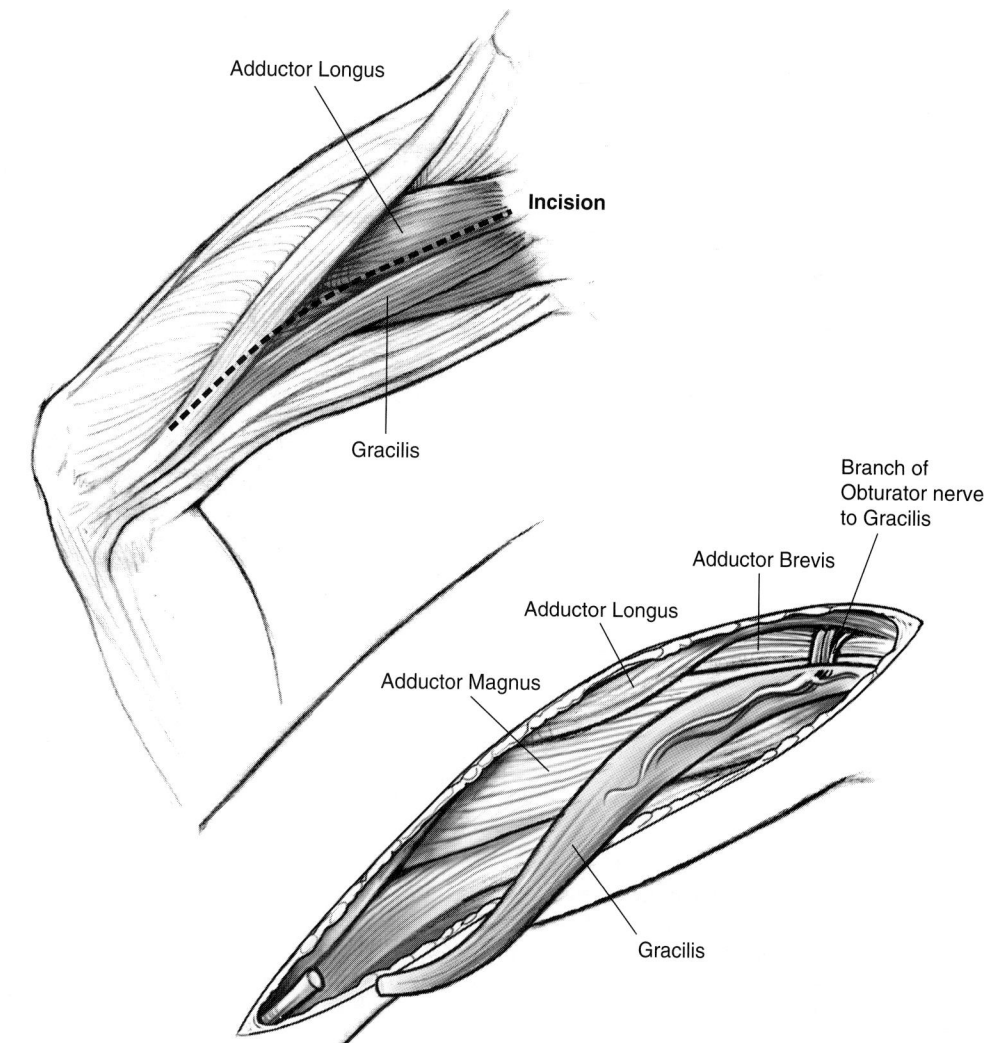

Fig. 1. The gracilis muscle flap.

Latissimus Dorsi Muscle Flap

The latissimus dorsi muscle has been used extensively for soft-tissue reconstruction because of its large size, thin pliable shape, and long reliable large pedicle. It can be used as either a muscle or musculocutaneous flap (Fig. 2).

Anatomy. The latissimus dorsi muscle arises from the iliac crest and thoracolumbar fascia and extends up the back in a triangular shape to insert along the bicipital groove of the humerus. The dominant pedicle for the latissimus dorsi is the thoracodorsal artery, which is a terminal branch of the subscapular artery.[12] The thoracodorsal vascular bundle enters the deep surface of the muscle 8 to 12 cm from its insertion in the humerus.

Dissection. The patient is placed in a lateral decubitus position with sandbags to protect the brachial plexus. The anterior border of the muscle from axilla to iliac crest is identified and a skin incision is made just posterior to this. The muscle is separated superficially from the skin and then the anterior margin is dissected off the chest wall and serratus anterior muscle. The inferior aspect is transected at the required length and elevation is continued posteriorly to

elevate the muscle off the posterior chest wall. The muscle is then detached at its medial origin and lifted superiorly.

The vascular pedicle to serratus anterior is identified and this can be followed to identify the thoracodorsal pedicle, which is palpable in the muscle. The vessels to the serratus anterior are divided (unless the serratus is to be included in the flap). Dissection is carried proximally along the pedicle to the circumflex scapular branch origin. The pedicle can be transected proximal or distal to this branch, depending on requirements for pedicle length, diameter, and the need for an interposition T-shaped graft. The incision is closed primarily over a suction drain.

Scapular and Parascapular Flaps

Scapular and parascapular flaps can be used individually or combined using both the transverse (scapular) and descending (parascapular) branches of the circumflex scapular artery (Fig. 3).[13, 14] The skin and subcutaneous layer varies in thickness depending on the size of the individual and is more difficult to dissect in obese patients.

Anatomy. The scapular and parascapular flaps overlie

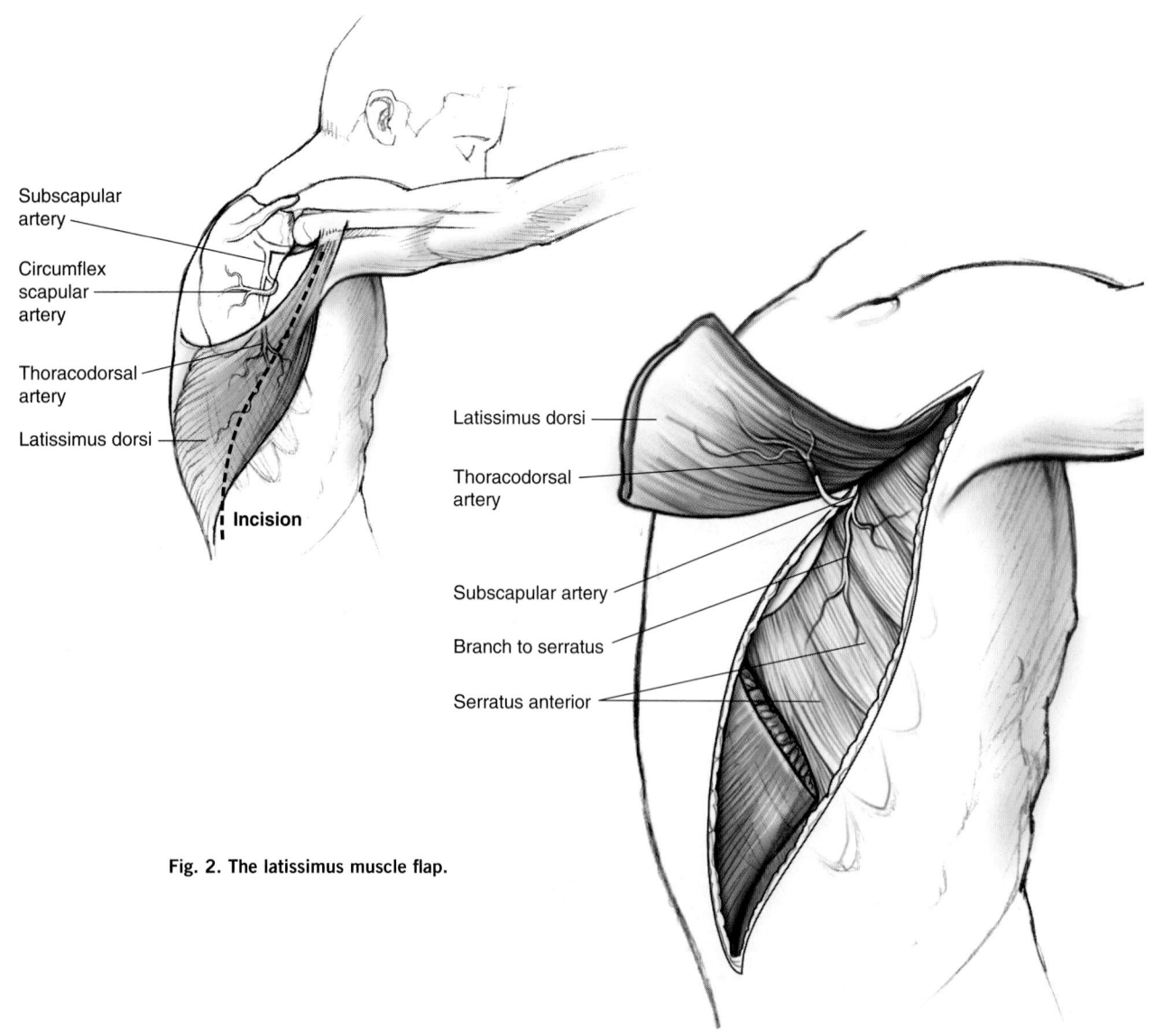

Subscapular artery

Circumflex scapular artery

Thoracodorsal artery

Latissimus dorsi

Incision

Latissimus dorsi

Thoracodorsal artery

Subscapular artery

Branch to serratus

Serratus anterior

Fig. 2. The latissimus muscle flap.

the scapula and receive their blood supply from the circumflex scapular artery, which leaves the thoracodorsal artery and runs between the teres major and teres minor muscles in the triangular space to emerge in the subcutaneous tissue.

Dissection. The patient is placed in a lateral decubitus position with the arm draped free. The triangular space is palpated and Doppler ultrasonography is used to identify the transverse and descending branches. The flap can then be centered over either or both branches. Alternatively, the flap can be designed over the mid-portion of the scapula and extended to 2 cm from the vertebral spinous processes to 2 cm posterior to the posterior axillary line and from 2 cm inferior to the scapular spine to 2 cm superior to the tip of the scapula.

The inferior and medial borders of the flap are incised down to the fascia and the flap is elevated laterally. The inferior border is elevated off the teres major until the superior edge of teres major, and then the pedicle is identified as it enters the triangular space. The rest of the skin flap is incised and elevated, so that the pedicle is remaining. The pedicle is then followed into the triangular space, where numerous branches arise along the medial side of the pedicle to supply the lateral border of the scapula.

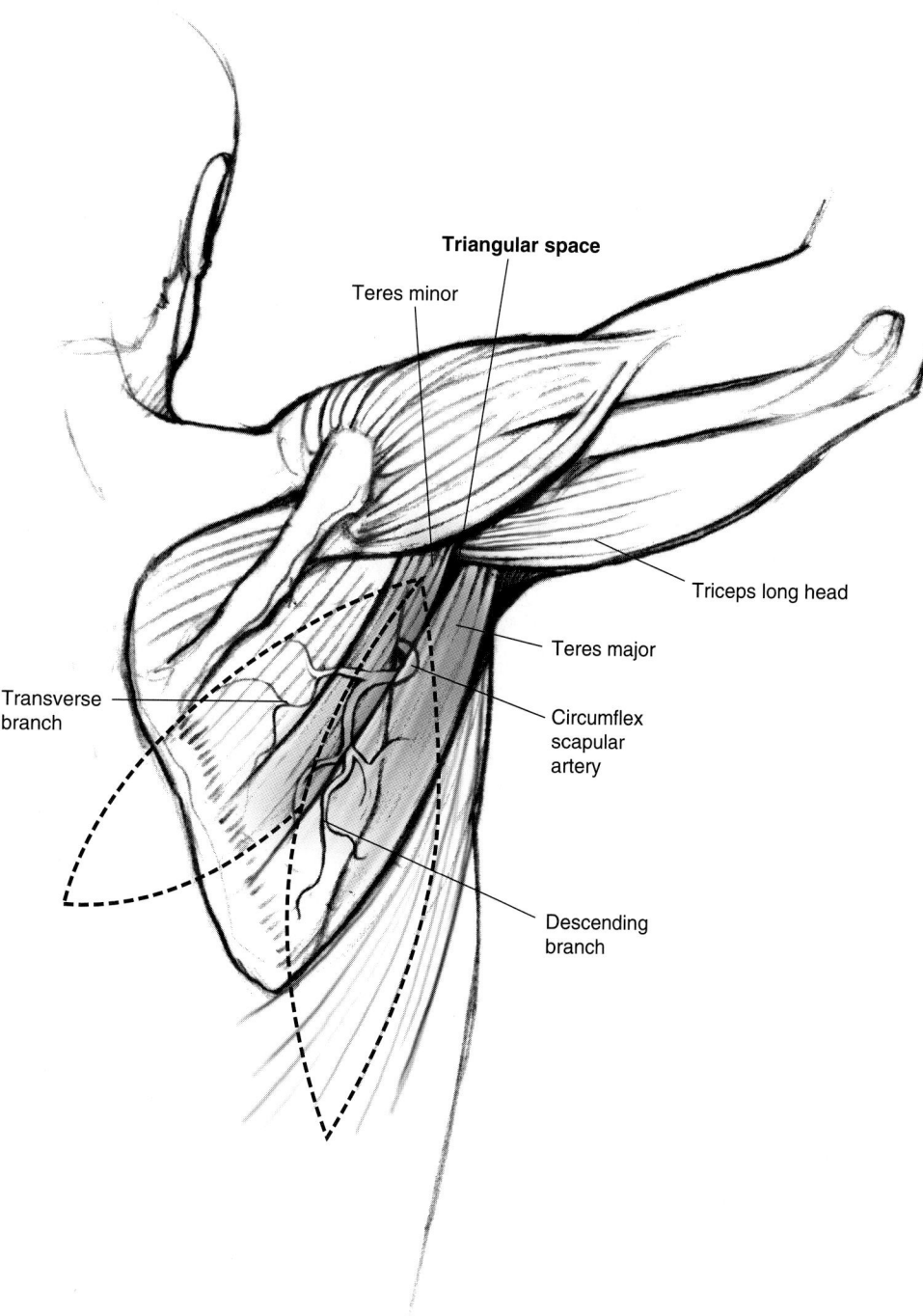

Fig. 3. The scapular and parascapular flaps.

These will need to be divided to allow access to the main pedicle. The pedicle is then transected as required.

Lateral Arm Flap

The lateral arm flap is useful for the coverage of complex wounds of the hand because of its thin, pliable nature and its ability to be innervated (Fig. 4).[15] It also may be harvested from the ipsilateral arm.

Anatomy. The flap overlies the lateral intermuscular septum and can extend down to the lateral epicondyle. The blood supply is via the posterior radial collateral artery (PRCA), a branch of the profunda brachii artery at the level of the insertion of the deltoid muscle. The PRCA runs with the posterior cutaneous nerves of the arm and forearm in the intermuscular septum posterior to the brachioradialis. It sends numerous cutaneous branches along its course, which supply the flap.

Dissection. The flap is centered over a line drawn between the deltoid insertion and the lateral epicondyle. The posterior aspect of the flap is incised through the fascia overlying the triceps. The fascia is then dissected off the triceps and left contiguous with the lateral intermuscular septum. The posterior radial collateral artery is identified within the septum and followed proximally to the profunda brachii along the deltoid insertion. The posterior cutaneous nerve of the arm is identified entering the flap, and the radial nerve is identified and protected as it runs anteriorly to the brachioradialis. Next, the anterior aspect of the flap is elevated in a similar fashion, between the brachialis and its fascia, in a posterior direction to the intermuscular septum. The PRCA is divided distally and the flap is elevated off the bone until the proximal end with adequate pedicle length is obtained. The wound is closed primarily if possible.

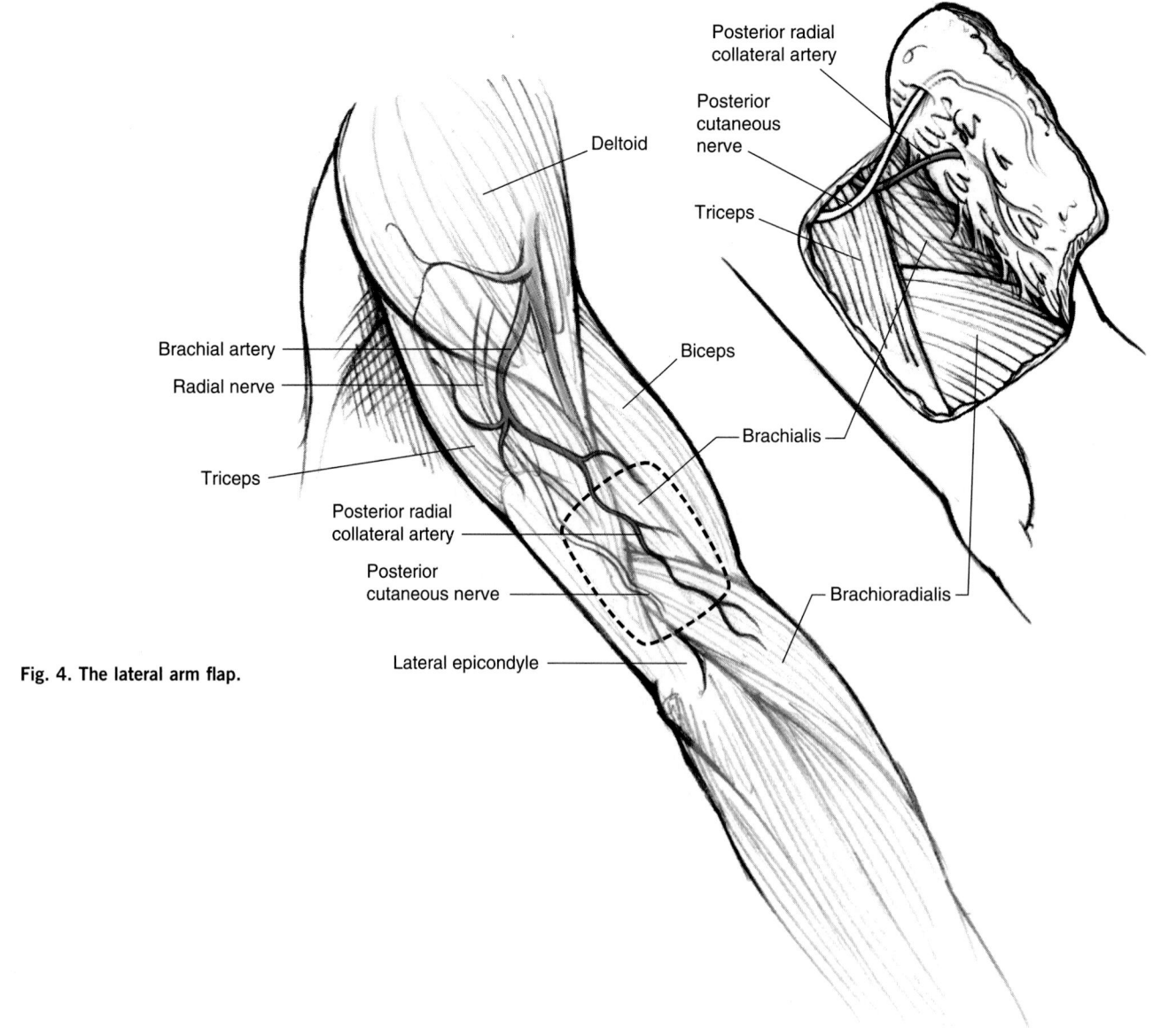

Fig. 4. The lateral arm flap.

OUTCOME

Assessing the results and outcomes of all the different flap options, techniques, and clinical uses is impossible because the results are inherently linked to the underlying coverage problem. Despite this, most institutions are now reporting a success rate of greater than 90%. Studies that have examined donor site morbidity showed that despite problems, patients were pleased with the procedure.

There is now extensive research on outcomes for cases in which a free flap was done for open tibial fractures.[3, 16] Several authors have shown that early soft-tissue reconstruction decreases the cost and duration of hospitalization and results in better joint motion and better psychological status.[17, 18]

It must be remembered, however, that the rehabilitation of a mangled extremity can take up to 2 years and that this is significantly longer than for some amputations. The ability to reconstruct the limb must be balanced by the patient's needs and commitment to rehabilitation. If the patient is unable or unwilling to dedicate this amount of time, then amputation may be the best option. The surgeon should remember that just because reconstruction can be done, does not always imply that it should be done.[19, 20]

REFERENCES

1. Khouri RK, Cooley BC, Kunselman AR, et al: A prospective study of microvascular free-flap surgery and outcome. Plast Reconstr Surg 1998; 102:711.
2. Shaw WW: Microvascular free flap: The first decade. Clin Plast Surg 1983; 10:3.
3. Godina M: Early microsurgical reconstruction of complex trauma of the extremities. Plast Reconstr Surg 1986; 78:285.
4. Brown RF: The management of traumatic tissue loss in the lower limb; especially when complicated by skeletal injuries. Br J Plast Surg 1965; 18:26.
5. Daniel RK, Taylor GI: Distant transfer of an island flap by microvascular anastamoses. Plast Reconstr Surg 1973; 52:111.
6. May JW, Gallico GG, Lukash FN: Microvascular transfer of free tissue for closure of bone wounds of the distal lower extremity. N Engl J Med 1982; 306:253.
7. Mathes SJ: The muscle flap for management of osteomyelitis. N Engl J Med 1982; 306:294.
8. Cooley BC, Hanel DP, Anderson RB, et al: The influence of diabetes upon free tissue transfer: Flap survival and microvascular healing. Ann Plast Surg 1992; 29:58.
9. Cooley BC, Hanel DP, Ma L, et al: The influence of diabetes upon free-flap transfer: The effect of ischemia on flap viability. Ann Plast Surg 1992; 29:65.
10. Hidalgo DA, Jones CS: The role of emergent exploration in free tissue transfer: A review of 150 consecutive cases. Plast Reconstr Surg 1990; 86:492.
11. Giordano PA, Abbes M, Pequignot JP: Gracilis blood supply: Anatomical and clinical re-evaluation. Br J Plast Surg 1990; 43:266.
12. Bartlett SP, May JW, Yaremchuk MJ: The latissimus muscle flap: A fresh cadaver study of the primary neurovascular pedicle. Plast Reconstr Surg 1981; 67:631.
13. Gilbert A, Teot L: The free scapular flap. Plast Reconstr Surg 1982; 69:601.
14. Nassif TM, Vidal L, Bovet JL, et al: The parascapular flap: A new cutaneous microsurgical free flap. Plast Reconstr Surg 1982; 69:591.
15. Yousif NJ, Warren R, Matloub HS, et al: The lateral arm fascial free flap: Its anatomy and use in reconstruction. Plast Reconstr Surg 1990; 86:1138.
16. Gustilo RB, Mendoza RM: Results of treatment of 1400 open fractures. In Gustilo RB (ed): Management of Open Fractures and Their Complications. Philadelphia, WB Saunders, 1982, pp 202–208.
17. Irons GB, Fisher J, Schmitt EH: Vascularized muscular and musculocutaneous flaps for management of osteomyelitis. Orthop Clin North Am 1984; 15:473.
18. Khouri RK: Free flap surgery: The second decade. Clin Plast Surg 1992; 19:757.
19. Bondurant FJ, Cotler HB, Buckle R, et al: The medical and economic impact of severely injured lower extremities. J Trauma 1988; 28:1270.
20. Caudle RJ, Stern PJ: Severe open fractures of the tibia. J Bone Joint Surg 1987; 69:801.

section **12** chapter **11**

RHEUMATOID ARTHRITIC HAND

Andrew L. Terrono

Summary
- Goals of surgery in the rheumatoid arthritic hand are pain relief, improved function, slowing of disease progression, and improved appearance.
- Nearly all the procedures performed for this disorder fall into the following categories: tenosynovectomy, synovectomy, tendon surgery, arthoplasty, and arthodesis.
- The patient's medical, social, and economic conditions are key considerations, and a team approach to treatment is needed.

1. Morning stiffness in and around joints lasting at least 1 hour before maximal improvement.
2. Soft-tissue swelling of three or more joint areas.
3. Swelling (arthritis) of the proximal interphalangeal (PIP), metacarpophalangeal (MP), or wrist joints.
4. Symmetric arthritis.
5. Subcutaneous nodules.
6. Positive test for RA.
7. Radiographic erosions or periarticular osteopenia in hand or wrist joints.

Rheumatoid arthritis (RA) is a systemic condition that affects 1% of the population. The criteria for diagnosis were revised in 1988 and include

Criteria 1 through 4 must be present for at least 6 weeks: four or more criteria must be present. Another definite cause of arthritis must not be present to diagnose RA alone.[1]

Deformities, joint destruction, and pathological anatomy are the result of the diseased and hypertrophied synovial tissue altering its surroundings. Rheumatoid synovium destroys articular cartilage, invades subchondral bone, and stretches the soft tissues that support the involved joint. It also surrounds and invades the flexor and extensor tendons. This results in disruption of the normal architecture of the hand and wrist and loss of the normal delicate balance of flexor and extensor forces across adjacent joints of the hand-wrist unit.

RA involvement in the hand can be divided into tendon involvement (flexor and extensor tendons) and joint involvement (wrist joint, MP joints, and thumb and finger joints). Nearly all of the surgical procedures performed on the rheumatoid hand and wrist fall into one of following groups: tenosynovectomy, synovectomy, tendon surgery, and salvage surgery (arthroplasty and arthrodesis). The goals of surgery are pain relief (most important), improved function, slow disease progression, and improved appearance.[2, 3]

GENERAL APPROACH

Patients are allowed to express all of their problems, including pain and functional deficits. They are asked specifically what they cannot do and what they would like to do. Physical examination of the entire upper extremity is performed. Active and passive range of motion of the digits, wrist, forearm, elbow, and shoulder is recorded. Areas of tenosynovitis, synovitis, tenderness, and instability are sought. Signs and symptoms of carpal tunnel syndrome are sought. Neutral posteroanterior, lateral, and oblique radiographs, including those of the wrist and hand, to evaluate the radiocarpal and distal radioulnar joints, MP joints, and interphalangeal (IP) joints, are obtained. However, radiographs do not always correlate well with the clinical picture. The radiographs may show severe destruction, but symptoms may be minimal.

The surgeon must take the patient's medical, social, and economic condition into consideration. A team approach is needed, including the patient, hand surgeon, rheumatologist, and hand therapist. Cervical spine and temporomandibular joint involvement may not be obvious but can influence the anesthetic management and should be evaluated preoperatively. Nonsteroidal anti-inflammatory drugs can alter platelet function and are stopped before surgery.

In general, pain and nerve compression are alleviated first. Preventive surgery such as tenosynovectomy takes precedence over joint reconstruction; however, joints must be mobile for tendon reconstruction to succeed. Unless the MP joints can be extended passively, any transfer will become adherent. The more reliable procedures should be done first (such as wrist or thumb MP fusion). Deformity does not always equal loss of function, and that must be evaluated. Proximal joints are usually corrected first. For example, wrist alignment is corrected at the same time or before MP joint surgery, and MP subluxation is corrected at or before extension deformities of the PIP joint. The results of a combined procedure may fall short. Combined procedures such as multiple MP arthroplasties performed with tendon reconstruction will, in general, not do as well as an isolated MP arthroplasty with intact tendons.

TENOSYNOVITIS

Tenosynovitis is common and may occur months before joint disease. The three common sites of involvement are the extensor retinaculum (Fig. 1), the flexor retinaculum (Fig. 2), and digital flexor sheaths. Rheumatoid tenosynovitis can cause pain, decreased tendon excursion, and tendon rupture. Tenosynovectomy can prevent secondary problems if done early. Fifty percent to 70% of patients with tenosynovitis have been found to have infiltration of the tendon by tenosynovium at the time of prophylactic tenosynovectomy.[4]

Tenosynovitis in the carpal tunnel can cause median nerve compression. The swelling can cause limited active motion; however, secondary joint stiffness can occur, limiting passive motion. Medical management, rest, splinting, and steroid local injection may also result in remission. However, if there is no improvement after 4 to 6 months of appropriate medical management, tenosynovectomy is indicted. Symptoms and signs of carpal tunnel syndrome, loss of active motion, and tendon rupture are also indications for surgery. The goal of flexor tenosynovectomy is to make active and passive finger flexion equal.

To perform a dorsal tenosynovectomy a straight incision is made just to the ulnar side of the midline. The posterior interosseous nerve on the floor of the fourth compartment is resected. The extensor retinaculum is open in the fourth or sixth compartment. The septum between the compartments is incised from the inside to open the involved compartments. The extensor pollicis longus (EPL) is protected as it crosses obliquely across the wrist. Hypertrophied synovium is removed from each extensor tendon sheath in a systematic manner. If an area of tendon appears so attenuated or frayed that tendon rupture appears imminent, the tendon at risk can be sutured to an adjacent extensor tendon above and below the area of damage, or the frayed and attenuated areas can be imbricated. Next, the wrist joint is evaluated. If wrist and or distal radioulnar joint (DRUJ) synovitis is present, the joint is opened, and a synovectomy and bone spike removal are performed. (See Synovectomy section.)

If possible, half of the retinaculum should be retained over the extensor tendons. The other half is passed deep to the extensor tendons and sutured in place to provide a smooth gliding surface beneath the tendons. The extensor

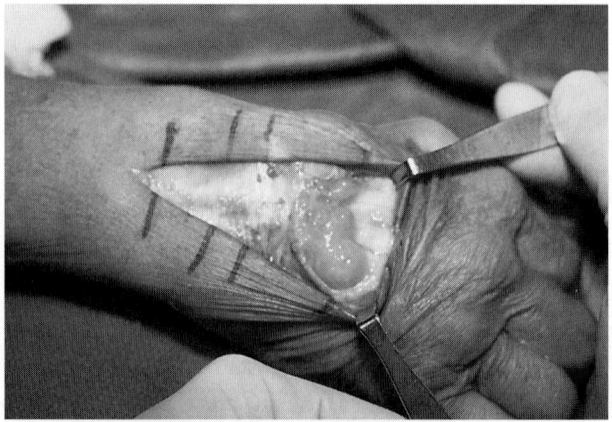

Fig. 1. Dorsal tenosynovitis extending distal to the extensor retinaculum.

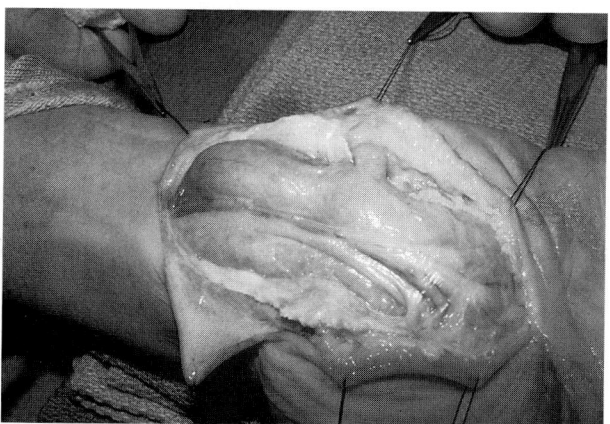

Fig. 2. Volar tenosynovitis. Exposure is achieved using an extended carpal tunnel approach. Skin retraction sutures are used to gently retract the skin.

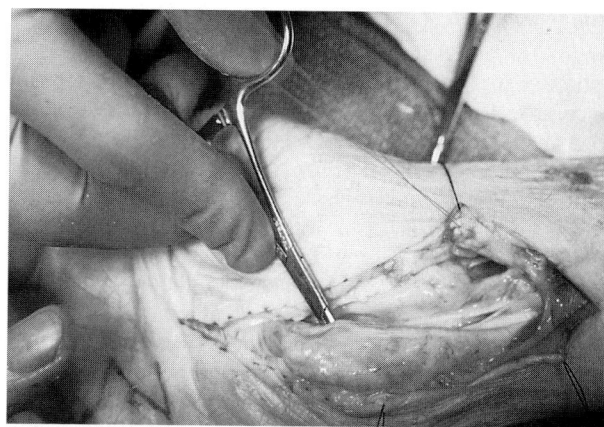

Fig. 3. Flexor tenosynovectomy. During flexor tenosynovectomy, unsuspected flexor digitorum profundus ruptures were found. However, good flexor function was present preoperatively; therefore, the tendons were not separated.

carpi ulnaris (ECU) tendon may be stabilized or relocated in a dorsal position by a narrow segment of the retinaculum. If there is a passively correctable radial deviation wrist deformity, the ECU may be transferred to the extensor carpi radialis longus (ECRL).[5] Preoperatively, to evaluate whether the relocated ECU will function, place the forearm in supination and evaluate wrist extension. If the ECU functions as an extensor in this position, it will function appropriately in the relocated position. If not, an ECRL transfer is indicated.

Complications after dorsal tenosynovectomy are infrequent but include skin necrosis, delayed skin healing, tendon adhesions and, rarely, tendon rupture.[6] The most serious complication after dorsal tenosynovectomy is skin necrosis or loss. Hematoma is the most frequent cause for delayed skin healing. A drain should be used routinely to prevent a hematoma. The skin is closed without tension. Occasionally, postoperative adhesions may result either in an extensor lag of the MP joints or in loss of active finger flexion. If a significant extensor lag develops, a dynamic dorsal extension splint is used. Loss of motion after dorsal tenosynovectomy occurs more often in those patients whose tendons are found to be in poor condition at surgery and in those with multiple joint involvement. Tenolysis after dorsal tenosynovectomy rarely is necessary. However, if significant impairment of function persists after 6 months of therapy, tenolysis should be considered.

To perform a wrist flexor tenosynovectomy an extended carpal tunnel incision, which is extended 4 to 5 cm proximal to the wrist crease, is used. Careful median nerve decompression is performed. Tenosynovectomy is performed for the flexor pollicis longus (FPL) and each flexor digitorum sublimis (FDS) and the flexor digitorum profundus (FDP), usually as a group. Occasionally, unsuspected ruptures of the deep flexor tendons may be discovered (Fig. 3). Therefore, it is critical that the function of the flexor tendons is known before surgery. If the FDP tendons are functioning by pulling through scar tissue, complete removal of all diseased tissue is not performed. After tenosynovectomy, the floor of the carpal canal is inspected for protruding bone spurs. Traction is applied to each flexor

tendon to check finger motion. Smooth motion of the fingers and thumb should be present. If smooth motion of the tendons is not present, the involved tendon must be explored as far distally as necessary to remove the nodules. After removal of the nodule, the defect in the tendon is repaired with interrupted fine sutures.

Rheumatoid "trigger finger" involvement can vary from localized to diffuse tenosynovitis with or without nodules (Fig. 4). The diseased tenosynovium surrounding the tendon is excised. However, the annular pulleys are preserved, narrowed if necessary, to prevent bowstringing of the flexor tendons. Traction is applied to the flexor tendons to confirm smooth gliding and equal active and passive motion. Gentle manipulation of stiff joints can be performed to restore passive joint motion. If after a complete tenosynovectomy there is still catching, excision of one slip of the FDS tendon can be resected to decompress the fibroosseous canal to allow free excursion of the tendons.[7] The entire superficial flexor tendon may be excised if it is severely diseased and prevents complete "pull-through" of the profundus tendon. Postoperatively, finger motion is started early, usually the day after surgery.

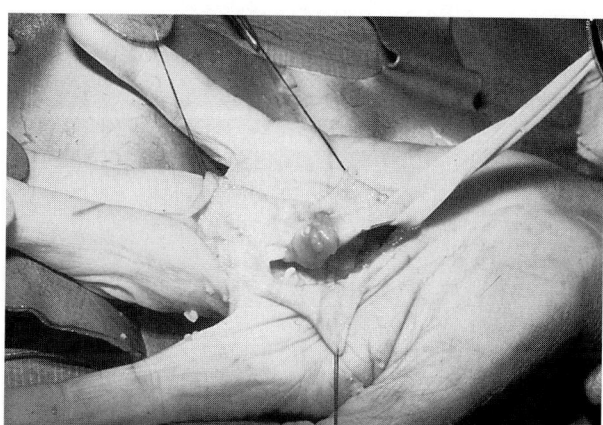

Fig. 4. Flexor tenosynovitis. This nodule in the palm caused by flexor tenosynovitis will impede flexor tendon function.

TENDON RUPTURES

Tendon ruptures are common complications of RA. The ruptures can be secondary to attrition on a bone prominence, direct tendon invasion of tenosynovium, or ischemia from increased pressure in an enclosed space (dorsal wrist, carpal tunnel, or flexor sheath)[8–11] Attrition ruptures of the extensor tendons occur most frequently at either the distal end of the ulna or at Lister's tubercle. Attrition ruptures of the flexor tendons occur most commonly on the volar aspect of the wrist, where they contact the scaphoid. Any bone can be involved.[8, 9] The most common ruptures are the extensor digiti quinti (EDQ) and EPL and FPL. The factors leading to a single tendon rupture, unless corrected, are often responsible for subsequent ruptures. Multiple extensor tendon ruptures (especially those that occur in rapid sequence) are usually the result of attrition against a bone spike on the ulnar, as described by Vaughan-Jackson[12] (Fig. 5). Similar findings can be seen with rupture of the FPL on the volar scaphoid (Mannerfelt lesion)[9] and subsequent flexor digitorum rupture of the index and middle finger (Fig. 6).

Although the correct diagnosis of tendon rupture usually is not difficult, it requires both an observant patient and an informed physician. Tendon ruptures usually are painless and commonly follow trivial hand use or activity. RA patients who become accustomed to frequent variations and limitations of hand function are apt to delay medical attention unless the functional loss after a tendon rupture is obvious to them or is quite significant. Sudden loss of finger extension or flexion, alteration of digital posture, and lack of active motion can also be seen. Evaluation for tenosynovitis and bone prominence is performed. Each tendon's function is evaluated against resistance. Isolated ruptures of the EDQ, EPL, or FPL may cause only limited functional loss and, therefore, may go unrecognized or be overshadowed by more significant deformities.[13]

Other conditions that mimic extensor tendon rupture should be excluded before surgery to restore extensor power to the fingers is performed. The most common of these is MP joint dislocation. The lack of passive MP joint extension and the difficulty seeing the extensor tendons on the dorsal aspect of the hand make the differential diagnosis between the MP joint dislocation and extensor tendon rupture difficult. The second condition to be excluded is displacement of the extensor tendons into the valleys between the metacarpal heads. When this occurs, extensor force is lost because the tendons now lie volar to the axis of motion of the MP joints. The patient cannot actively extend the MP joints from a flexed position. If passive MP extension is possible, the patient is able to maintain MP joint extension. This is not always the case, and occasionally it is necessary to explore the tendons at the level of the wrist at the time of MP arthroplasty to verify their continuity. The treatment for subluxation of the extensor tendons is relocation over the MP joints with or without MP joint arthroplasty. Of those conditions simulating multiple extensor tendon rupture, the least common but most difficult condition to diagnose is paralysis of the extensor muscles secondary to posterior interosseous nerve compression as the result of elbow synovitis. Patients with posterior interosseous nerve compression, in addition to the absence of active finger extension, usually demonstrate some radial deviation of the wrist because of paralysis of the extensor carpi ulnaris muscle. If passive MP extension and wrist flexion are present, the best diagnostic test is the tenodesis test, noting the presence or absence of MP joint extension as the wrist is flexed. Patients with multiple extensor tendon ruptures usually have dorsal tenosynovitis

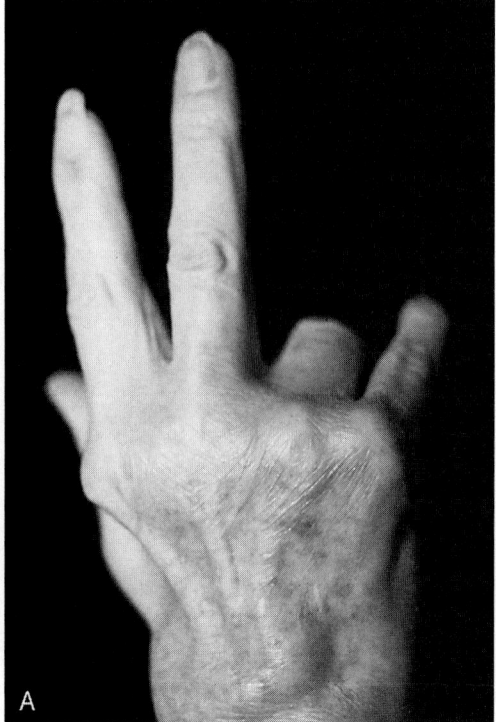

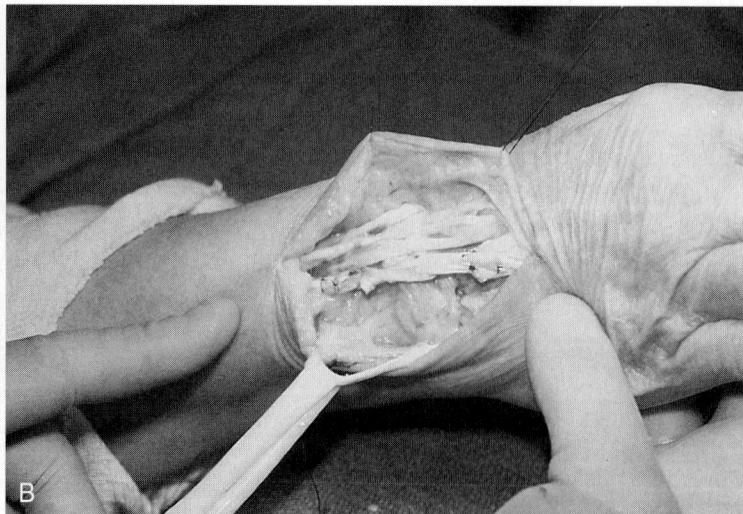

Fig. 5. Triple extensor rupture. *A*, Preoperative view of triple extensor rupture, including the extensor digiti quinti and extensor digitorum communis to the small and ring finger. *B*, This was treated with an intercalated graft using the palmaris longus.

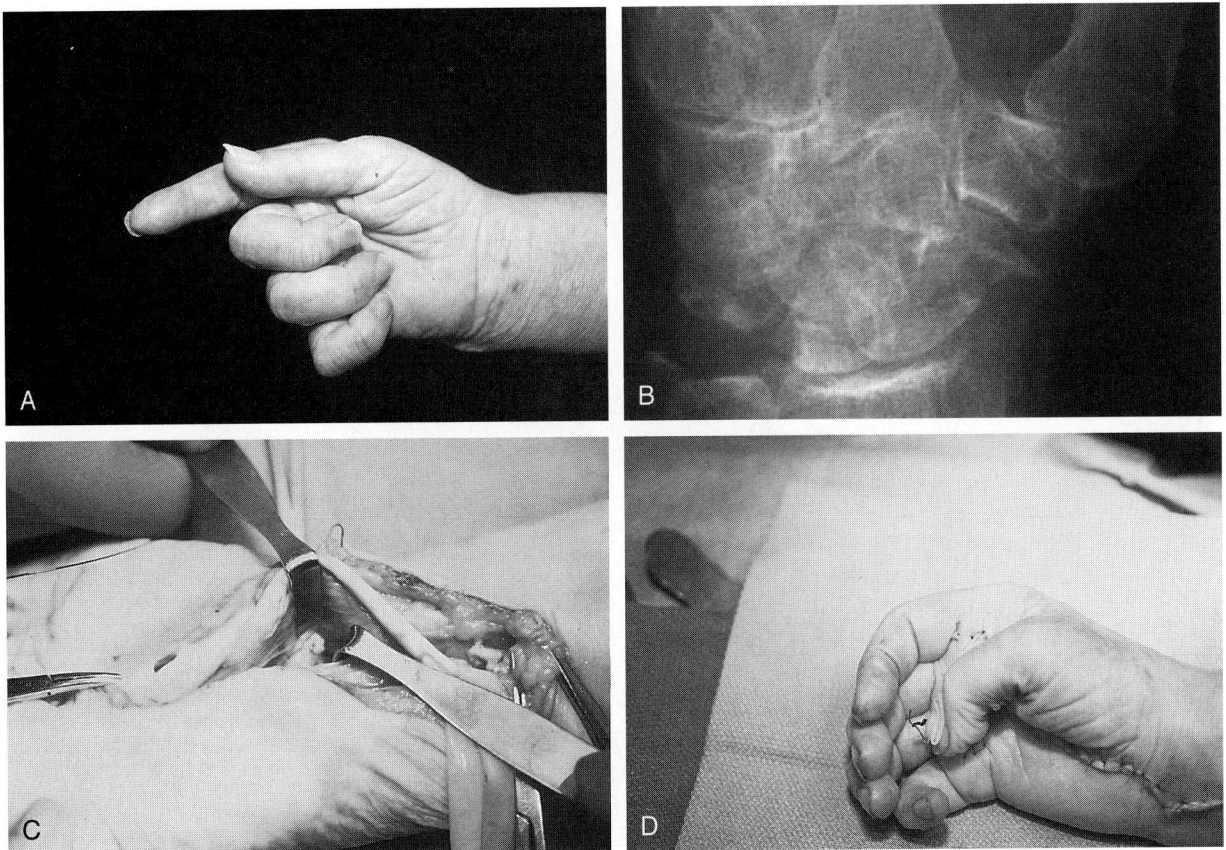

Fig. 6. Inability to flex the thumb interphalangeal (IP) joint and index finger proximal IP and distal IP joints. *A,* Attempt at making a fist, and the thumb IP joint and index finger do not flex. *B,* The scaphoid spur (Mannerfelt lesion) is seen on the oblique view. *C,* A scaphoid spur is seen in the base of the extended carpal tunnel incision. *D,* An intercalated graft for the flexor pollicis longus tendon is performed, and the flexor digitorum profundus index is attached to the middle finger FDP.

or a prominent distal ulna, which predisposes to extensor tendon rupture, whereas patients with posterior interosseous nerve compression may not.[13]

The differential diagnosis of flexor rupture includes a fixed hyperextension deformity or stiffness of the interphalangeal joint or a tendon nodule or tenosynovitis, limiting active flexion. A rare compression neuropathy such as an anterior interosseous nerve compression can also simulate tendon rupture. The differential is evaluated as with extensor ruptures. Passive motion of the finger must be present to conclude that tendons are ruptured. After a flexor tendon rupture is recognized, the site of rupture must be determined. Flexor tendon ruptures can occur at the wrist, in the palm, and within the finger. Palpation for fullness (or lack thereof) within the finger can be useful in this regard. Ultimately, surgical exploration is necessary to determine the exact site.

The treatment options for RA patients with tendon ruptures are removal of the cause of the rupture, with restoration of tendon function through direct repair (rare), intercalated graft (see Figs. 5 and 6) (if muscle not contracted), attaching to adjacent tendon (Fig. 7), tendon transfer, or fusion of the involved joints (Tables 1 and 2). Tendon surgery is different in RA and non-RA patients, and these differences must be considered when planning tendon surgery to reconstruct rheumatoid tendon ruptures. Among the

differences are that the joints may be stiff or unstable, the tendon bed is often not optimal and compromises tendon excursion, the tendons to be transferred may have been weakened by ischemia or by tenosynovial invasion, and the tenodesis effect, which enhances tendon function, may be lost as a result of compromised adjacent joint motion.[4]

In the case of extensor tendon ruptures, direct repair is rarely possible. (see Table 1). In such cases suture of the distal tendon stump to an adjacent tendon (see Fig. 7) or a bridge graft (see Figs. 5 and 6) is performed. Donors for tendon transfer include extensor indicis proprius, wrist extensors or flexors (limited excursion) if the wrist is fused, EPL (if thumb MP is fused), and the FDS.[2] The graft should be put in "tight" because the muscle will gradually stretch postoperatively. The tension must be sufficient so that when the wrist is flexed moderately, the fingers are maintained in complete extension, and when the wrist is extended moderately, the MP joints flex only 20 to 30 degrees. Intercalated or "bridge" grafts can be useful, particularly to maintain independent motion (EDQ) or in multiple ruptures. Bora et al[14] reported excellent results using the palmaris longus to bridge the extensor tendon defect after multiple tendon ruptures.

With respect to flexor tendon ruptures, it is not always possible to achieve active Finger flexion. The best results are from attrition ruptures in the palm or wrist and the

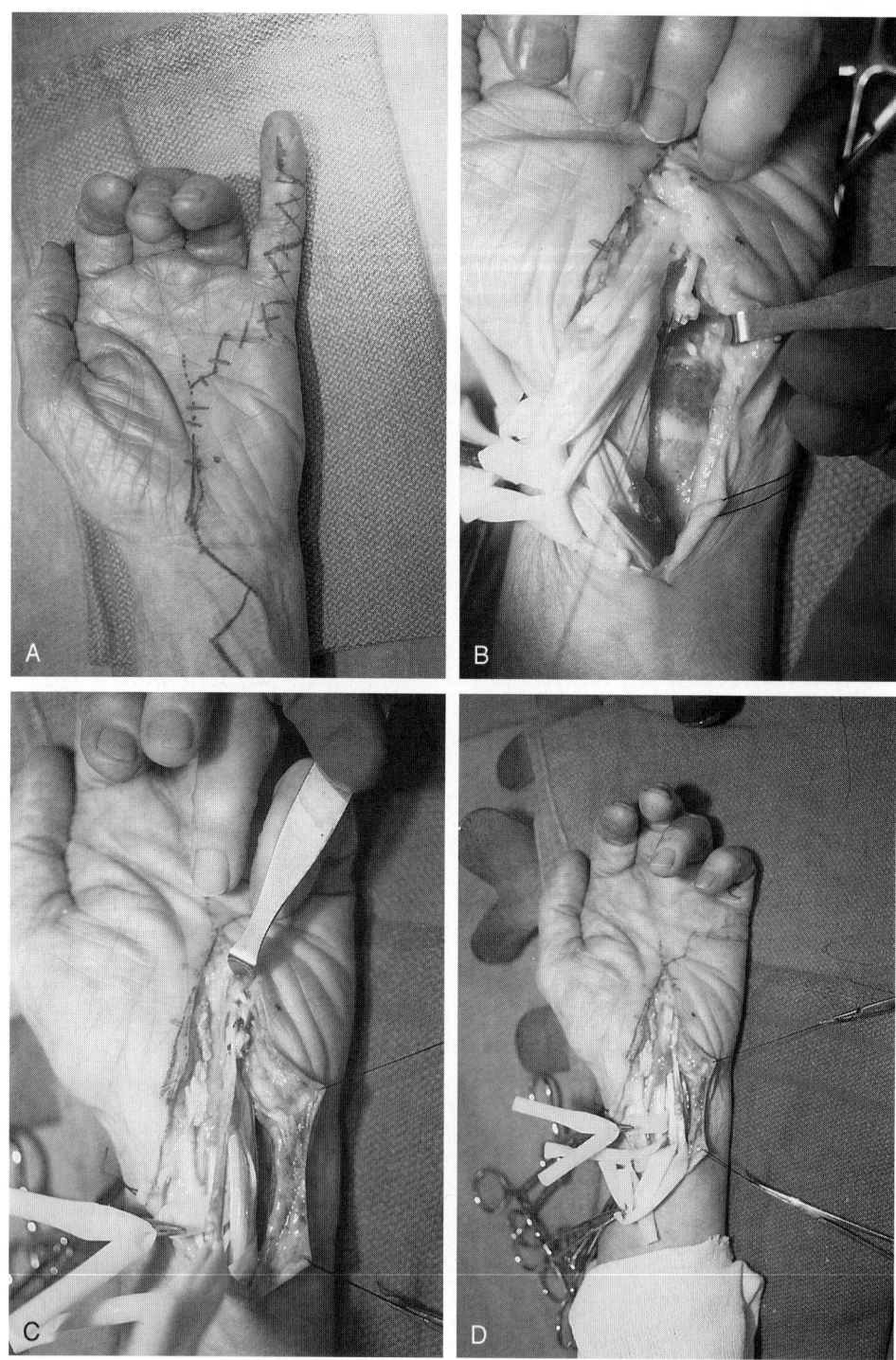

Fig. 7. Inability to flex the small finger. *A,* The small finger has lost the normal semiflexed posture, indicating a flexor tendon rupture. The appropriate incision that may be needed is drawn out. *B,* Spur on the ulnar caused the attrition ruptures of the flexor digitorum profundas (FDP) and flexor digitorum sublimus of the small finger. Note distal stump of FDP attached to the suture. *C,* The FDP of the small finger is woven into the FDP of the ring finger. *D,* Resting posture of the hand is restored.

worst result is secondary to tenosynovium in the finger.[8] The treatment should match the degree of functional loss (see Table 2). A volar wrist synovectomy can be done when a flexor tenosynovectomy is indicated to prevent destruction of the deep volar ligaments and secondary rotation of the scaphoid.[15]

JOINTS

Synovial hypertrophy within the joint stretches the supporting structures, including the collateral ligaments and cap-

sule and, in the digit, the volar plate and extensor mechanism. Subchondral erosion causes cartilage and bone loss and collapse (Fig. 8). The position of the joint is related to the balance of forces across the joint. The treatment of joints involved in RA depends on the symptoms of pain, loss of function, and appearance. The options for treatment include synovectomy, tendon function restoration, arthroplasty, and arthrodesis.

In the wrist, the middle of the scaphoid at the radioscaphocapitate ligament, the ulnar styloid, the ulnar head,

TABLE 1. OPTIONS FOR EXTENSOR TENDON RUPTURES

Rupture Type	Option
Ruptures, all	Dorsal tenosynovectomy Remove bone spikes Retinacular relocation to cover bone Ulnar head resection as necessary
Single rupture	Primary repair Adjacent suture Intercalated graft EIP transfer
Double rupture usually EDC (ring and small), EDQ	See above plus EIP transfer
Triple rupture	See above plus FDS (mid) through IOM or around side Wrist extensor, especially if wrist fusion EPL if MP fusion
Quadruple rupture	See above plus Another FDS

EDC, extensor digitorum communis; EDQ, extensor digiti quanti; EIP, extensor indicis proprius; FDS, flexor digitorum sublimis; IOM, interosseous membrane; MP, metacarpophalangeal; EPL, extensor pollicis longus.

and triangular fibrocartilage (TFCC) frequently are the earliest to be involved by rheumatoid synovitis.[15] This will eventually lead to a shortened, radially rotated, volar subluxed carpus, with a supinated hand, prominent distal ulna, and subluxed ECU. This results in imbalance of the extensor tendons, radial shift of the metacarpals, and ulnar deviation of the fingers.[16] This wrist deformity will influence ulnar deviation of the MP joints.[17]

In the MP joints synovial proliferation occurs in the recess between the metacarpal head and collateral ligament attachment, resulting in dysfunction of the collateral ligaments. Ultimately, the MP joints will have volar subluxation or dislocation and ulnar deviation. Wrist deformity,[17] flexor and extensor tendon forces, intrinsic muscle imbalance, and the forces of gravity and pinch all influence MP joint position.[18]

PIP joint synovitis stretches the extensor mechanism, which may result in a boutonnière deformity that is difficult to reconstruct. Alternatively, the synovium may stretch out the volar plate and a swan-neck deformity can result.

SYNOVECTOMY

Synovectomy is indicated for pain with persistent localized synovitis despite relatively good medical control, including steroid injections over a 6- to 9-month period, whose radiographs show minimal changes.[6] There are no studies that demonstrate conclusively that synovectomy will change the natural course of rheumatoid disease. The contraindications include a fixed deformity, minimal motion with no pain, or severe radiograph changes.

For the wrist, I agree with the traditional recommendations but would perform a synovectomy for patients with more advanced radiographs, especially in younger patients with bilateral involvement and if they are undergoing other

wrist surgery (see Fig. 8). Long-term follow-up reviews of wrist synovectomy found consistent and dramatic relief of pain and varying loss of wrist motion.[19, 20] Arthroscopic synovectomy has been performed, but its benefit is not clear. When a distal radioulnar joint synovectomy is performed, the TFCC is preserved if possible. The TFCC remnants can be tightly closed to the dorsal ulnar corner of the radius to help correct the carpal supination. The wrist is splinted in neutral and the forearm fully supinated for approximately 3 weeks. A longer period of splinting may be necessary if there is excessive wrist ligament laxity.

MP joint synovectomy is often combined with soft-tissue reconstruction, including extensor relocation, ligament reconstruction, and intrinsic release or transfer. Crossed intrinsic transfer is another method to restore finger alignment and prevent recurrent ulnar drift.[21] Synovectomy with soft-tissue reconstruction is indicated for persistent MP synovitis in patients with early volar subluxation and ulnar drift. Such a procedure may slow the progression of the disease in a young patient. Another indication is the inability to extend the MP joint actively because of complete dislocation of the extensor tendons but maintenance of active extension if the MP joints are extended passively.

MP joint synovectomy for a single joint may be performed through a longitudinal incision and on multiple joints usually through a transverse incision. Usually, the joint is exposed with an incision through the ulnar sagittal band. Intrinsic release is performed, if necessary. In the small finger, the abductor digiti quinti is a strong ulnar-deforming muscle that must be released, but the flexor digiti quinti is not.[22] Synovectomy is performed. The radial

TABLE 2. OPTIONS FOR FLEXOR TENDON RUPTURES

Rupture Type	Option
Ruptures, all	Determine location Tenosynovectomy CTR if in wrist Remove bone spikes Cover bone Match treatment with loss
Rupture at wrist, palm	Primary repair Adjacent suture Intercalated graft FDS transfer (middle)
Single FDS or FDP rupture in digit	See above Do not reconstruct FDS with intact FDP Usually do not reconstruct FDP with intact FDS If FDP is ruptured, stabilize DIP as needed
FDP and FDS rupture in digit	See above Rarely staged reconstruct (need good joints) If joints involved, consider fusion If index or middle, especially if MP involved, consider fusion
Multiple ruptures	See above plus Try to establish FDP function

CTR, carpal tunnel release; FDS, flexor digitorum sublimis; FDP, flexor digitorum protundus; MP, metacarpophalangeal.

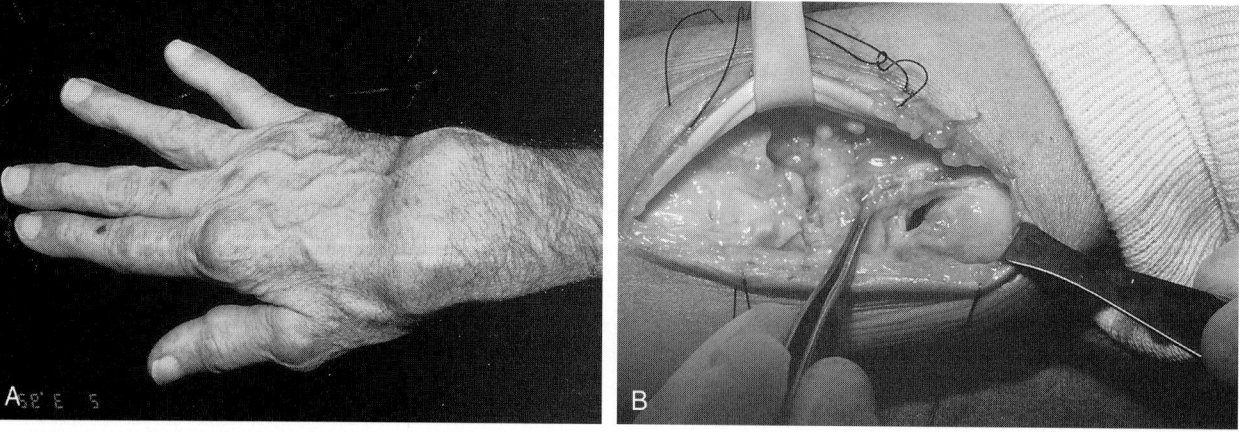

Fig. 8. Wrist and distal radioulnar joint (DRUJ) pain and synovitis. *A,* Obvious dorsal wrist synovitis. *B,* Synovectomy of the wrist and DRUJ is performed after failed nonoperative treatment.

collateral ligament can be imbricated. The extensor mechanism is repositioned by imbricating the radial side. If the mechanism still subluxates ulnarly, it can be secured[23] by attaching a slip of extensor tendon around the collateral or through the capsule or by attaching the extensor tendon to the proximal phalanx through the drill holes. Active motion is begun 1 to 2 days postoperatively, and a program of dynamic and static splinting similar to that after MP joint arthroplasty is used for 4 to 8 weeks. The fingers are protected during the exercises and are splinted in extension between exercise periods. Long-term splinting and carefully supervised therapy are important in preventing the postoperative recurrence of deformity.[2]

Synovectomy of the PIP joint is performed earlier than that of other joints and has relatively little morbidity.[24] One reason is that the results of PIP joint arthroplasty are less reliable than those of MP joint arthroplasty, and PIP joint fusion can be disabling. Also, the PIP joint is more stable than the MP joint, and recurrent deformity after synovectomy is less common than after MP joint synovectomy.

SALVAGE
Wrist

Historically, fusion has been the reconstructive procedure of choice for the rheumatoid wrist.[2, 25] Intramedullary fixation with a pin or rod has developed to be the most useful technique[26, 27] (Fig. 9). Wrist fusion is indicated in patients who are likely to place high demand on the wrist after

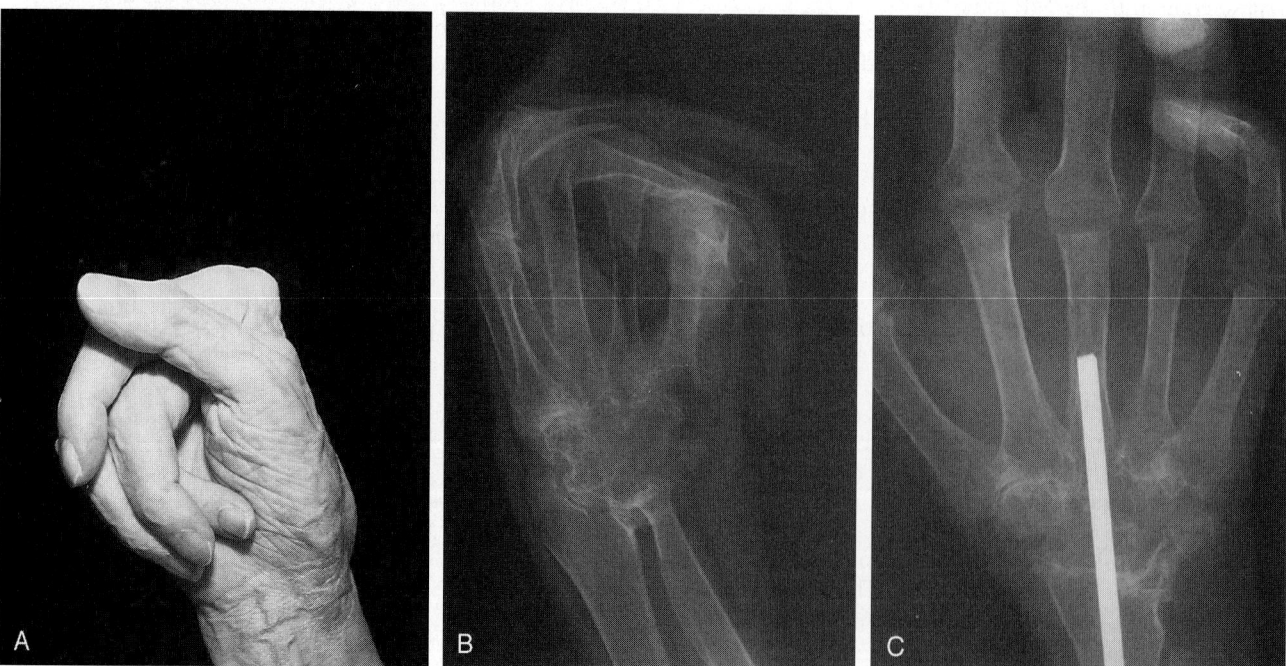

Fig. 9. Severe metacarpophalangeal (MP) and wrist joint involvement. *A,* Severe MP joint involvement with flexion of the MP joints and significant functional disability. *B,* Radiograph shows marked wrist involvement and MP flexion. *C,* As a first step, a wrist fusion using an intramedullary rod in the middle metacarpal and distal ulna excision was performed. After the wrist fused, MP arthroplasties were performed and significantly improved function.

surgery (i.e., use ambulatory aids) or have significant wrist deformity or instability, poor wrist extensor tendon function, or poor bone stock.

After appropriate preparation of the articular surface, fixation is performed. Fixation with one or two Steinmann's pins' fixation in the radius and between the metacarpals is usually preferred. Two smaller pins allow the wrist to be placed in slight extension. One or two small staples or an obliquely placed Kirschner wire may be used to provide additional fixation of the radiocarpal joint if necessary. Use of a plate is not routine because of bone quality and skin problems. If there is severe loss of carpal bone stock, the Steinmann pin is introduced into the third metacarpal to provide stability. If the MP joints are dislocated and MP joint arthroplasties are indicated, the rod can be drilled through the distal end of the metacarpal and countersunk proximally, and an MP joint arthroplasty can be performed subsequently (see Fig. 9). This method requires that the wrist be fused in a neutral position, which is an excellent wrist position for most rheumatoid patients. The position of the wrist can be varied only 5 to 10 degrees by adjusting the direction of the pin as it is driven into the radius. The position of the wrist cannot be altered after the rod has been inserted. The single rod, albeit large in diameter, may not provide secure control of rotation of the carpus to the distal radius.[2]

Partial wrist fusion has applications in rheumatoid wrist disease.[28] Limited wrist fusion is useful in those rheumatoid patients whose disease has destroyed the radiocarpal joints but has left the midcarpal joints relatively unaffected or the reverse. Limited fusion of the involved joints combined with a synovectomy of the less involved joints may relieve pain, yet preserve 25% to 50% of wrist motion.

When a proximal row fusion is performed, usually the radius, scaphoid, and lunate bones are fused (Fig. 10). If the articular surface of the scaphoid is preserved, the fusion may be limited to the radiolunate articulation alone.[28] Autologous bone graft (distal ulna, metacarpal heads, or distal radius) is packed between the individual bones to be fused.

Complications of wrist fusion include pseudarthrosis, deep wound infection, superficial skin necrosis, median nerve or superficial radial nerve compression, fracture of the healed fusion, and pin migration.

In the mid-1970s, Swanson et al[29] developed the silicone rubber wrist arthroplasty for reconstruction of the rheumatoid wrist. However, fracture, silicone synovitis, unpredictable results, and difficulty of revision have made this an uncommon procedure.[30–32] Total wrist arthroplasties have been used with inconsistent results.[33, 34] Candidates for wrist arthroplasty include patients who will have low demand on the wrist after surgery and those with wrist extensors in good condition, minimal wrist deformity, or good bone stock. Bilateral wrist arthroplasties are not encouraged. Those patients who do undergo wrist arthroplasty and require crutches as an ambulatory aid should use only forearm or platform crutches. Patients with arthroplasties should use wrist splints for any activity that will place stress on the wrist.

DRUJ

Involvement of the DRUJ is a common cause of disability in the rheumatoid wrist. Distal ulna excision alone may be indicated in the patient whose symptoms are limited to the DRUJ and whose radiocarpal joint is stable and functional, even when the radiocarpal joint shows significant destruction on radiographs.[35] For this reason, distal ulna

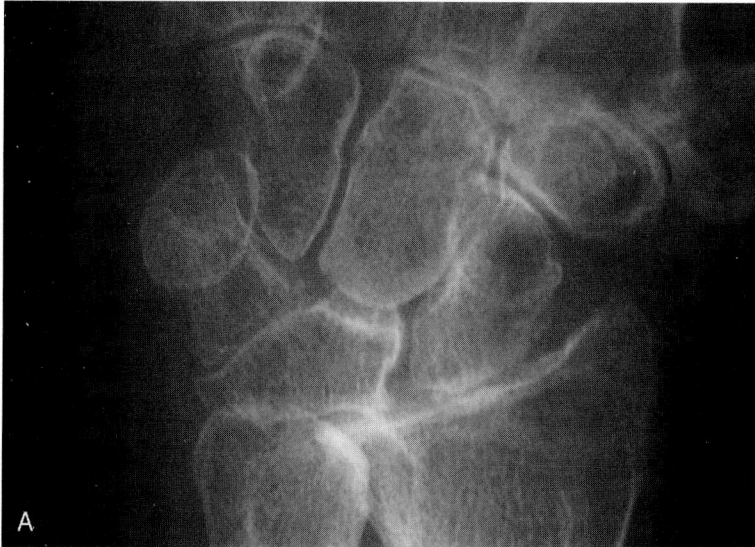

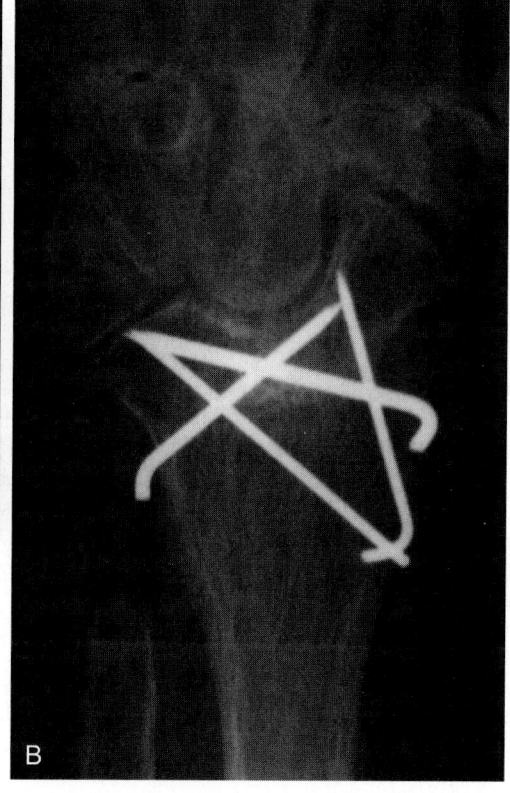

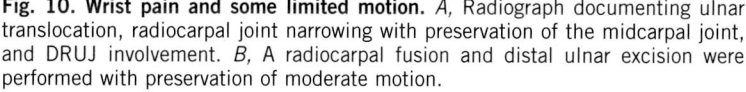

Fig. 10. **Wrist pain and some limited motion.** *A,* Radiograph documenting ulnar translocation, radiocarpal joint narrowing with preservation of the midcarpal joint, and DRUJ involvement. *B,* A radiocarpal fusion and distal ulnar excision were performed with preservation of moderate motion.

TABLE 3. OPTIONS FOR TREATMENT OF INVOLVED THUMB JOINTS		
IP Joint	**MP Joint**	**CMC Joint**
Synovectomy Fusion Flexor tenodesis (½ FPL) Restore FPL function Joint release	Synovectomy Restore EPL function EPL rerouting Volar capsulodesis/sesamoidesis Ligament repair/reconstruction Fusion Arthroplasty	LRTI: partial trapezial resection LRTI: total trapezial resection (if good wrist bone stock) Fusion (lupus)

IP, interphalangeal; MP, metacarpophalangeal; CMC, carpometacarpal; LRTI, ligament reconstruction and tendon interposition; FPL, flexor pollicis longus; EPL, extensor pollicis longus.

excision and reconstruction of the triangular fibrocartilage and the distal radioulnar joint (see DRUJ synovectomy) are performed frequently in the wrist affected by RA. It is important to use soft-tissue reconstruction to correct supination of the carpus and subluxation of the distal ulna.[36]

There has been renewed interest in fusion of the distal ulna to the sigmoid notch of the radius with resection of a segment of ulna to allow rotation of forearm (the Sauve-Kapandji procedure).[37] The Sauve-Kapandji procedure may be better for younger patients with painful DRUJ dysfunction because it provides stable fixation of the ulnar head, preserves ulnocarpal support, restores forearm rotation, may prevent ulnar translocation, and results in a better appearance than does distal ulna resection.[37] I have found that the Sauve-Kapandji procedure does not prevent or correct ulnar translocation in the rheumatoid patient. Radiocarpal fusion is preferred for patients with established or impending ulnar translocation (see Fig. 10).

The most frequent complication after distal ulna excision is painful forearm rotation. This often will respond to prolonged splinting and a supervised gentle motion exercise program. If the symptoms do not remit after several months and there is instability of the distal ulna, soft-tissue stabilization can be considered.

MP Joint

Patients with advanced MP joint disease, especially those with a fixed flexion deformity, are candidates for MP arthroplasties. The principles of MP joint arthroplasty are as follows. Wrist deformity must be corrected before MP surgery. Soft-tissue release must be adequate (intrinsics only if necessary). Excision of the volar plate can be very helpful in cases of severe MP joint flexion and allows access to the flexor tendons for a limited tenosynovectomy. Bone resection must be at least the size of the implant but not excessive (see Fig. 9). Appropriate implant size is such that it is not wider than the joint and allows adequate space without buckling. The radial collateral ligament should be repaired with slight overcorrection of deformity. The capsule should be preserved and closed. Postoperative splinting is important. Dynamic and static splints may be used. Postoperatively, the effective arc of motion is increased and moved toward extension. However, motion gradually decreases with time. Ulnar deviation improves but increases (usually to between 10 degrees and 30 degrees) with time. Pain relief and patient satisfaction are good. The complications of MP joint arthroplasty include infection,

implant subluxation, implant breakage, limited motion, and recurrent deformity.[2]

THUMB DEFORMITIES

The thumb in RA can assume a number of different positions. Each joint may or may not be passively correctable and is subsequently divided into early, moderate, and advanced deformities. In the early deformity both MP and IP joints are passively correctable. In a moderate deformity one joint is fixed, and in advanced deformity both joints are fixed. In the typical thumb deformity, the adjacent joints assume opposite positions. If this is not the case, one should look for tendon ruptures. Although the deformities are of interest and understanding their progression is helpful, the treatment programs may be considered at each joint rather than by the type of deformity (Table 3). The most common deformity is the boutonnière or type 1 deformity with MP joint flexion and IP joint hyperextension (Fig. 11). This deformity is caused by loss or weakness of MP joint extension as the result of extensor pollicis brevis (EPB) stretching and EPL rupture or subluxation. The second most common deformity, swan-neck or type III deformity, is characterized by metacarpal adduction and the MP joint hyperextension and distal joint flexion (Fig. 12). The first web space may become contracted. The primary cause is usually subluxation of the carpometacarpal (CMC) joint. The third most common deformity is the gamekeeper's, or type IV, deformity. It is characterized by lateral deviation

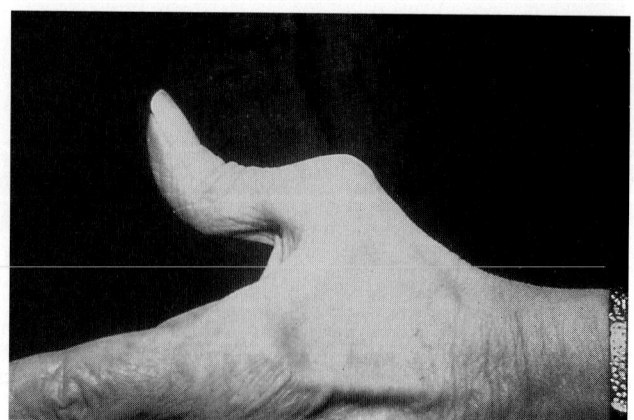

Fig. 11. Most common thumb deformity with metacarpophalangeal joint flexion and interphalangeal joint extension.

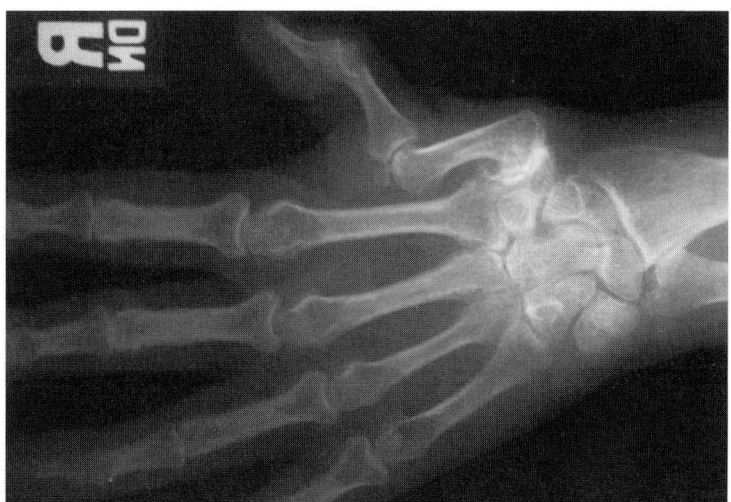

Fig. 12. View. This is a radiograph of the type II thumb deformity initiated at the carpometacarpal (CMC) joint with interphalangeal joint flexion, metacarpophalangeal (MP) joint extension, metacarpal flexion, and a narrowed first web space. This was treated with a ligament reconstruction and tendon interposition, CMC arthroplasty, and MP fusion.

with abduction at the MP joint associated with metacarpal adduction. This deformity is similar in appearance to type III deformity but differs in that the origin is at the MP level, where the ulnar collateral ligament is stretched by synovitis. The metacarpal adduction is secondary to the MP deformity, and the CMC joint is not subluxed. Arthritis mutilans can involve the thumb such that the IP and MP joints are quite unstable and deviate either laterally or into hyperextension.[38]

A suggested treatment plan is given in Table 4. In the early type I deformity, increasing the extensor power at the MP joint is the goal. The EPL can be rerouted to increase the extension force at the MP joint. This is combined with a synovectomy. The EPL is transected distal to the MP joint and sutured through the dorsal capsule or to the base of the proximal phalanx. Good results are maintained for approximately 5 years and then deformity tends to recur. For moderate and advanced type I deformities MP joint

fusion in approximately 10 degrees flexion is the procedure of choice. In the advanced cases with a severely involved hand, an arthroplasty of the MP is indicated. However, motion gradually decreases and instability of the ulnar collateral ligament occurs.[38]

For a swan-neck (type III) deformity, a CMC arthroplasty with trapezial resection and ligament reconstruction and tendon interposition is used.[39] A formal adductor release rarely is necessary. The MP joint is usually treated with a fusion. However, a restraint for hyperextension (capsulodesis or sesamoidesis) can be performed if there is significant flexion.

FINGER DEFORMITIES

Two finger deformities commonly occur in RA. These are the so-called swan-neck (Fig. 13) and boutonnière (Fig. 14) deformities. Other deformities can occur, including lateral deformities secondary to instability of the PIP joint or bone

Joint	Early	Moderate	Advanced
		TABLE 4. SUGGESTED TREATMENT PLAN FOR THUMB DEFORMITY	
		Type I Boutonnière	
IP	—	—	Fusion
MP	Synovectomy	Fusion	Arthroplasty
	EPL rerouting	Occasionally arthroplasty	
		Type III Swan-Neck	
MP	—	Fusion	Fusion
		Volar capsulodesis/sesamoidesis	
CMC	Trapezial resection and LRTI	Trapezial resection and LRTI	Trapezial resection and LRTI
		Type IV Gamekeeper's	
MP	Synovectomy	Fusion	Fusion
	Reconstruction collateral ligament	Occasionally synovectomy and ligament reconstruction	
		Adductor fascia release prn	Adductor fascia release prn
		Arthritis Mutilans	
IP	Fusion & bone graft		
MP	Fusion & bone graft		

IP, interphalangeal; MP, metacarpophalangeal; CMC, carpometacarpal; LRTI, ligament reconstruction and tendon interposition; prn, as necessary.

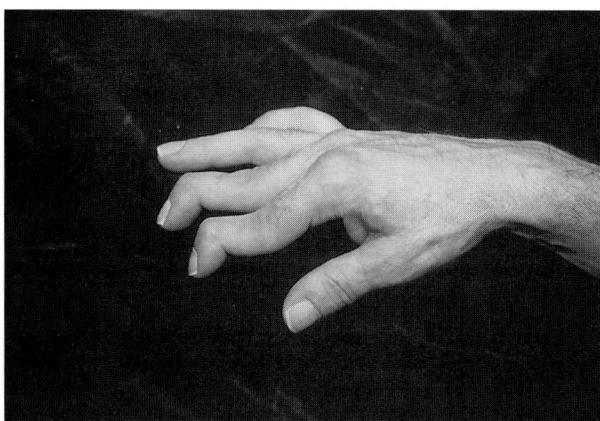

Fig. 13. Swan-neck deformity of the finger with proximal interphalangeal (IP) joint hyperextension and distal IP and metacarpophalangeal flexion.

Type	Characteristics
1	Full range of motion
	No functional limitations
2	Intrinsic tightness
	Limited PIP motion only with an extended MP joint with ulnar deviation corrected
3	Stiff PIP in all positions of MP joint
4	Severe arthritic changes

TABLE 5. CLASSIFICATION SYSTEM OF THE FINGER SWAN-NECK DEFORMITY

PIP, proximal interphalangeal; MP, metacarpophalangeal.

loss as seen in arthritis mutilans. Adjacent fingers may have opposite deformities. Many factors determine the cause of these deformities as well as the extent of functional loss that they produce.[11] The swan-neck deformity is characterized by PIP joint hyperextension with distal IP (DIP) and MP joint flexion, whereas the boutonnière deformity is the reverse.

Although all swan-neck deformities have a superficial resemblance to each other, they vary considerably. The initiating event can be at the MP, PIP, or DIP joint. The adjacent joint assumes the opposite deformity. The most severely involved joint is usually the cause. Each joint must be assessed for active and passive motion, stability, and joint destruction. Intrinsic tightness is evaluated. The significant functional loss associated with this deformity is related directly to the loss of motion at the PIP joint. Classifying these deformities serves as the basis for treatment[40] (Table 5). Each joint must be evaluated for needing treatment, and proximal deformities must be corrected. PIP extension deformities are reconstructed after or at the same time as MP joint arthroplasty, because any residual extension at the PIP joint has a beneficial effect on achieving MP joint flexion after MP joint arthroplasty.

If the DIP joint involvement is the cause of the swan-neck deformity, DIP fusion is usually the most effective treatment. Management of the PIP joint (Table 6) for stages 1 to 3 includes restoring PIP flexion (intrinsic release as needed, PIP joint manipulation, skin release, and lateral band mobilization) and restricting hyperextension (silver ring splint, dermadesis, and FDS tenodesis). If active PIP flexion is limited preoperatively, function of the flexor tendons must be demonstrated by active motion or traction on the tendons. When there is radiographic evidence of advanced intra-articular changes, a salvage procedure is needed (fusion or arthroplasty). Fusion is recommended in the index finger, where stability is particularly important. If the MP joints require arthroplasty, fusion at the PIP joint is recommended. In the swan-neck deformity, PIP arthroplasty works well as long as flexion is restored. Poor lateral ligament support and/or associated flexor tendon ruptures also are indications for fusion.

The boutonnière deformity has three components: flexion of the PIP joint, hyperextension of the DIP joint, and hyperextension of the MP joint. It usually begins with PIP synovitis, which stretches the extensor mechanism. As a result, the central slip is unable to maintain full extension of the joint. The lateral bands displace volarly and become fixed in this position. Shortening of the oblique retinacular ligament results in hyperextension and limited active flexion of the DIP joint. As the flexion deformity of the PIP joint increases, the patient compensates with hyperextension of the MP joint. Functional loss as a result of the boutonnière deformity may remain minimal until the late stages. For this reason, the treatment of early boutonnière deformity should be simple and involve minimal risk. Salvage surgery (fusion or arthroplasty) should be performed only for the severe fixed deformities. The operative approach to the rheumatoid boutonnière deformity depends on the degree of severity. Boutonnière deformities can be classified as mild, moderate, or severe on the basis of the degree of flexion of the PIP joint, the presence of passive correctability of this joint, and the status of the PIP joint surfaces[41] (Table 7). PIP flexion deformities are reconstructed before or at the same time as MP joint arthroplasty, because any residual flexion deformity at the PIP joint has an adverse effect on achieving MP joint flexion after MP joint arthroplasty.

Treatment has three parts: regaining passive PIP extension, maintaining active extension, and regaining DIP flex-

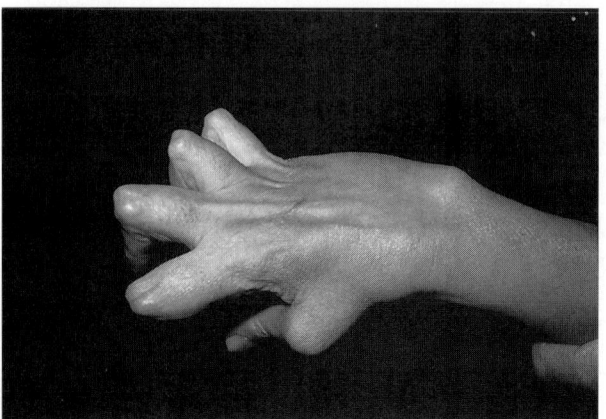

Fig. 14. Severe boutonnière deformity of all fingers. This is best treated with proximal interphalangeal joint fusion.

TABLE 6. OPTIONS FOR TREATMENT OF SWAN-NECK DEFORMITY IN FINGERS

Type	MP Joint	PIP Joint	DIP Joint
1		Splint Dermadesis FDS sling Littler ORL reconstruction	Exercise Fusion
2	Intrinsic stretching Intrinsic release	See above	Fusion
3	See above plus MP joint reconstruction as needed	See above plus PIP joint manipulation Skin release Lateral band mobilization Check flexor tendons	Fusion
4	See above	See above plus Arthroplasty Fusion	Fusion

MP, metacarpophalangeal; PIP, proximal interphalangeal; FDS, flexor digitorum sublimis; ORL, oblique retinacular ligament.

TABLE 7. OPTIONS FOR TREATMENT OF BOUTONNIÈRE FINGER DEFORMITY

Stage	PIP Joint	DIP Joint
Stage I mild (PIP lag <20 degrees) (DIP flexion limited with full PIP extension)	Dynamic splinting Injection vs synovectomy	Extensor tenotomy
Stage II, moderate PIP lag <30 to 40 degrees MP slight hyperextension	Correct any wrist flexion first Extensor reconstruction	Extensor tenotomy
Stage III, severe PIP fixed flexion contracture >30 degrees	Fusion (standard) Arthroplasty	Extensor tenotomy

PIP, proximal interphalangeal; DIP, distal interphalangeal; MP, metacarpophalangeal.

ion. Early in the condition the lack of DIP flexion may be the major complaint. Any operative treatment of this mild boutonnière deformity should not jeopardize existing function. Dynamic extension splinting for the PIP joint is used to restore the balance of the finger. If the disability persists, an oblique extensor tenotomy over the middle phalanx is performed. This method does not risk loss of PIP joint flexion and increases the extensor force on the PIP joint. For a more severe deformity the extensor force must be increased. The central slip is shortened (3–6 mm), the lateral bands are brought dorsally, and an extensor tendon tenotomy is done simultaneously. Unless this is done, there is a risk of restoring PIP extension but markedly limiting DIP flexion. Extensor mechanism reconstruction is recommended for patients with moderate progressive deformity if several criteria are met: good dorsal skin, relatively smooth joint surfaces, intact and functioning flexor tendons, and, of course, passive correctability of the PIP joint. Flexion deformity at the wrist should be corrected before attempting to restore PIP joint extension. Adjustment of the tension of the central slip is very important. It should be possible to flex the PIP joint passively 70 or 80 degrees after the central slip has been reattached. A Kirschner wire is placed across the PIP joint to maintain full extension for 3 to 4 weeks. The joint is protected with a reverse knuckle-bender splint during the day and a padded aluminum splint at night for several weeks. In severe deformities with poor joint surfaces, the recommended salvage treatment is fusion. PIP arthroplasty is not encouraged, and the results are not as good as in swan-neck deformity.

REFERENCES

1. Harris ED Jr: Etiology and pathogenesis of rheumatoid arthritis. In Kelly WN, Harris ED Jr, Ruddy S, et al (eds): Textbook of Rheumatology, 4th ed. Philadelphia, WB Saunders, 1993, p 833.
2. Feldon P, Terrono AL, Nalebuff EA, et al: Rheumatoid arthritis and other conennective tissue diseases. In Green DPHRN, Pederson WC (eds): Green's Operative Hand Surgery, 4th ed. New York, Churchill Livingstone, 1999, p 1651.
3. Nalebuff EA: Rheumatoid hand surgery—update. J Hand Surg 1983; 8:678.
4. Smith RJ: Tendon transfers for rheumatoid arthritis. In Smith RJ (ed): Tendon Transfers of the Hand and Forearm. Boston, Little, Brown, 1987, p 215.
5. Clayton ML, Ferlic DC: Tendon transfer for radial rotation of the wrist in rheumatoid arthritis. Clin Orthop 1974; 100:176.
6. Millender LH, Nalebuff EA: Preventative surgery—tenosynovectomy and synovectomy. Orthop Clin North Am 1975; 6:765.
7. Ferlic DC, Clayton ML: Flexor tenosynovectomy in the rheumatoid finger. J Hand Surg 1978; 3:364.
8. Ertel AN, Millender LH, Nalebuff EA, et

al: Flexor tendon ruptures in patients with rheumatoid arthritis. J Hand Surg [Am] 1988; 13:860.

9. Mannerfelt LG, Norman O: Attrition ruptures of flexor tendons in rheumatoid arthritis caused by bony spurs in the carpal tunnel. A clinical and radiological study. J Bone Joint Surg Br 1969; 51:270.

10. Moore JR, Weiland AJ, Valdata L: Tendon ruptures in the rheumatoid hand: Analysis of treatment and functional results in 60 patients. J Hand Surg [Am] 1987; 12:9.

11. Tubiana R, Valentin P: The physiology of the extension of the fingers. Surg Clin North Am 1964; 44:907.

12. Vaughan-Jackson OJ: Rupture of extensor tendons by attrition at the inferior radioulnar joint. Report of two cases. J Bone Joint Surg Br 1948; 30:528.

13. Nalebuff EA: The recognition and treatment of tendon ruptures in the rheumatoid hand. In AAOS Symposium on Tendon Surgery in the Hand. St. Louis, MO, CV Mosby, 1975, p 255.

14. Bora FW, Osterman AL, Thomas VJ, et al: The treatment of ruptures of multiple extensor tendons at the wrist level by a free tendon graft in the rheumatoid patient. J Hand Surg [Am] 1987; 12:1038.

15. Taleisnik J: Rheumatoid synovitis of the volar compartment of the wrist joint: Its radiological signs and its contribution to wrist and hand deformity. J Hand Surg 1979; 4:526.

16. Taleisnik J: Rheumatoid arthritis of the wrist. Hand Clin 1989; 5:257.

17. Shapiro JS: The etiology of ulnar drift. A new factor. J Bone Joint Surg Am 1968; 50:634.

18. Wilson RL, Carlblom ER: The rheumatoid metacarpophalangeal joint. Hand Clin 1989; 5:223.

19. Thirupathi RG, Ferlic DC, Clayton ML: Dorsal wrist synovectomy in rheumatoid arthritis—a long term study. J Hand Surg 1983; 8:848.

20. Allieu Y, Lussiez B, Ascencio G: The long-term results of synovectomy of the rheumatoid wrist: A report of 60 cases. Fr J Orthop Surg 1989; 3:188.

21. Oster LH, Blair WF, Steyers CM, et al: Crossed intrinsic transfer. J Hand Surg Am 1989; 14:963.

22. Flatt AE: The Care of the Arthritic Hand, 5th ed. St. Louis, MO, Quality Medical Publishing, 1995.

23. Zancolli EA: Pathomechanics and correction of the arthritic ulnar drift before and after cartilage destruction. In The Structural and Dynamic Bases of Hand Surgery, 2nd ed. Philadelphia, JB Lippincott, 1979, p 325.

24. Lipscomb PR: Synovectomy of the distal two joints of the thumb and fingers in rheumatoid arthritis. J Bone Joint Surg Am 1967; 49:1135.

25. Dupont M, Vainio K: Arthrodesis of the wrist in rheumatoid arthritis. A study of 150 cases. Ann Chir Gynecol Fenn 1968; 57:513.

26. Mannerfelt LG, Malmsten M: Arthrodesis of the wrist in rheumatoid arthrtis. A technique without external fixation. Scand J Plast Reconstr Surg 1971; 5:124.

27. Clayton ML: Surgical treatment at the wrist in rheumatoid arthritis. A review of thirty-seven patients. J Bone Joint Surg Am 1965; 47:741.

28. Chamay A, Della S: Radiolunate arthrodesis in rheumatoid wrist: 21 cases. Ann Hand Surg 1991; 10:197.

29. Swanson AB, deGroot-Swanson G, Maupin BK: Flexible implant arthroplasty of the radiocarpal joint. Surgical technique and long-term study. Clin Orthop 1984; 187:94.

30. Stanley JK, Tolat AR: Long-term results of Swanson Silastic arthroplasty in rheumatoid wrist. J Hand Surg Br 1993; 18:381.

31. Haloua JP, Collin JP, Schernberg F, et al: Arthroplasty of the rheumatoid wrist with Swanson implant. Long-term results and complications. Ann Chir Main 1989; 8:124.

32. Smith RJ, Atkinson RE, Jupiter JB: Silicone synovitis of the wrist. J Hand Surg Am 1985; 10:47.

33. Meuli HC, Fernandez DL: Uncemented total wrist arthroplasty. J Hand Surg Am 1995; 20:115.

34. Rettig ME, Beckenbaugh RD: Revision total wrist arthroplasty. J Hand Surg Am 1993; 18:798.

35. Gainor BJ, Schaberg J: The rheumatoid wrist after resection of the distal ulna. J Hand Surg Am 1985; 10:837.

36. Moller M: Forty-eight cases of caput ulnae syndrome treated by synovectomy and resection of the distal ulna. Acta Orthop Scand 1973; 44:278.

37. Taleisnik J: The Sauve-Kapandji procedure. Clin Orthop 1992; 275:110.

38. Terrono A, Millender L: Surgical treatment of the boutonnière rheumatoid thumb deformity. Hand Clin 1989; 5:239.

39. Burton RI, Pellegrini VD Jr: Surgical management of basal joint arthritis of the thumb. Part II: Ligament reconstruction with tendon interposition arthroplasty. J Hand Surg Am 1986; 11:324.

40. Nalebuff EA: The rheumatoid swan-neck deformity. Hand Clin 1989; 5:203.

41. Nalebuff EA, Millender LH: Surgical treatment of the boutonnière deformity in rheumatoid arthritis. Orthop Clin North Am 1975; 6:753.

section 12 chapter 12

OSTEOARTHRITIS OF THE HAND

David R. Steinberg

Summary

- Osteoarthritis is a leading cause of chronic impairment of the hand, affecting one-fourth of the population.
- The majority of cases are due to primary (idiopathic) osteoarthritis.
- The key objectives of treatment are restoration of function and amelioration of pain.
- Most cases of distal interphalangeal (DIP) joint involvement, and some cases of thumb carpometacarpal (CMC) joint involvement, respond well to conservative treatment.
- Surgical options are limited for DIP joint and proximal interphalangeal (PIP) joint osteoarthritis; a variety of techniques are available to treat thumb CMC joint arthritis.

The hand is a unique instrument that must perform fine manipulation as well as power grip and pinch. Independent digital motion and strength may be severely affected by osteoarthritis, leading to pain, deformity, and a decreased ability to perform activities of daily living. Although it is often difficult to restore the hand to its premorbid state, the judicious use of conservative and surgical treatments, along with appropriate rehabilitation protocols, can often improve function to a significant extent.

Osteoarthritis is one of the most common conditions affecting the hand. Lawrence reported a prevalence of 15% to 28% in a population older than 45 years of age.[1] It occurs in peri- and postmenopausal women 10 times more frequently than in men. Osteoarthritis usually develops in the 5th and 6th decades, with an increasing incidence in the aging population.

Surgical intervention is most commonly performed for the symptomatic thumb CMC joint, or basal joint. Gervis[2] first described trapeziectomy in 1949. Froimson[3] recommended tendon interposition after trapezial resection to prevent thumb metacarpal shortening. Silicone hemiarthroplasty and total joint arthroplasty were first described in the 1970s.[4, 5] Eaton and Littler,[6] Thompson,[7] and Burton and Pellegrini[8] emphasized the importance of ligament reconstruction to improve joint stability.

PATHOGENESIS

Osteoarthritis is a progressive deterioration of cartilage within the joint (refer to Chapter 6-2 for a complete discussion). In the hand, this most often occurs as primary degenerative osteoarthritis with polyarticular involvement. Secondary osteoarthritis affects isolated joints that have sustained cartilage damage from trauma or sepsis. Erosive osteoarthritis is a more aggressive form of the disease that has a predilection for the PIP joints. Ligamentous laxity is believed to play a key role in the development of basal joint arthritis. Attenuation or disruption of the anterior oblique ligament leads to dorsoradial subluxation, which causes abnormal cartilage loss and eburnation initially in the palmar joint surfaces.[9] Subsequently, the entire joint surface becomes involved, and marginal osteophytes develop.

CLINICAL PRESENTATION

Primary osteoarthritis involves the DIP joint most often, followed by the thumb basal joint (85% and 65%, respectively).[9] Patients with thumb CMC joint involvement complain of pain at the base of the thumb and thenar eminence. Swelling, crepitus, dorsoradial subluxation, and occasional ganglion formation occur as the disease progresses. CMC joint tenderness and a positive axial grind test result are pathognomonic for basal joint arthritis. Chronic CMC joint subluxation may lead to secondary metacarpal adduction contracture and metacarpophalangeal (MCP) joint hyperextension. Carpal tunnel syndrome, de Quervain's tenosynovitis, and scaphotrapeziotrapezoid arthritis must be considered in the differential diagnosis. Radiographs reveal joint space narrowing and subchondral sclerosis (Fig. 1), which may progress to severe joint deformity and subluxation.

The patient with interphalangeal arthritis presents with gradual swelling and stiffness, with varying degrees of pain. Progression of the disease may lead to flexion deformities and radial or ulnar deviation with collateral ligament attenuation (Fig. 2). Inflamed synovium and marginal osteophytes present as Bouchard's nodes in the PIP joint and Heberden's nodes in the DIP joint. These should not be confused with mucous cysts, which are ganglia that develop at the DIP joint or thumb interphalangeal joint in conjunction with an osteophyte. These are usually located lateral to the terminal tendon and may produce a longitudinal groove of the nail.

Erosive osteoarthritis usually occurs in middle-aged women and has a higher predilection for the interphalangeal joints. The DIP joint is involved in 75% of cases and the PIP joint in 50%.[10] Patients complain of severe pain,

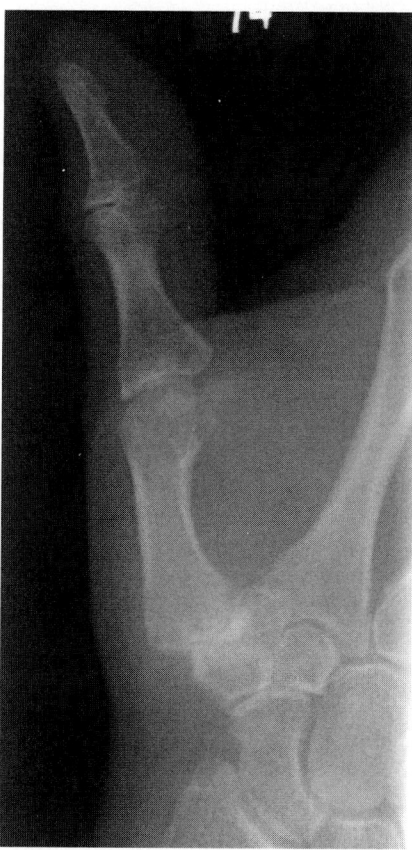

Fig. 1. Pantrapezial osteoarthritis. Moderate degenerative changes include loss of carpometacarpal joint space, subchondral sclerosis, lateral subluxation of the metacarpal, and similar involvement of the scaphotrapezial, scaphotrapezoidal, and trapeziotrapezoidal joint spaces.

swelling, stiffness, and deformity. Progressive destruction of the interphalangeal joints is seen on the radiograph (Fig. 2B).

INVESTIGATION

Standard posteroanterior and lateral radiographs of the hand should be included in the evaluation of osteoarthritis. The CMC joint stress view will demonstrate excessive laxity. Robert's hyperpronation or Bett's view provides the clearest unobstructed look at the basal joint. Carpal tunnel syndrome may coexist and can be evaluated by electrodiagnostic testing. If an inflammatory arthritis is in the differential diagnosis, especially in the case of erosive osteoarthritis, appropriate blood studies may prove useful. The small joints of the hand usually do not lend themselves to aspiration for crystal analysis.

TREATMENT GOALS, INDICATIONS, AND CONTRAINDICATIONS

The treatment of osteoarthritis of the hand usually begins with nonsurgical management. This includes anti-inflammatory medication, splint immobilization, and hand therapy. Oral nonsteroidal anti-inflammatory medications effectively reduce inflammation in various stages of arthritis. Intra-

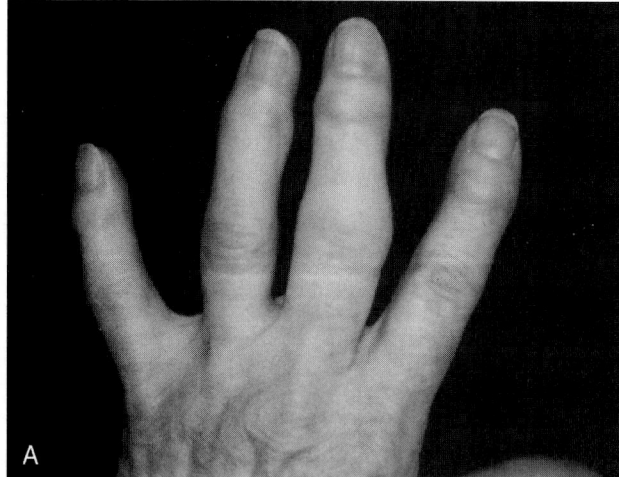

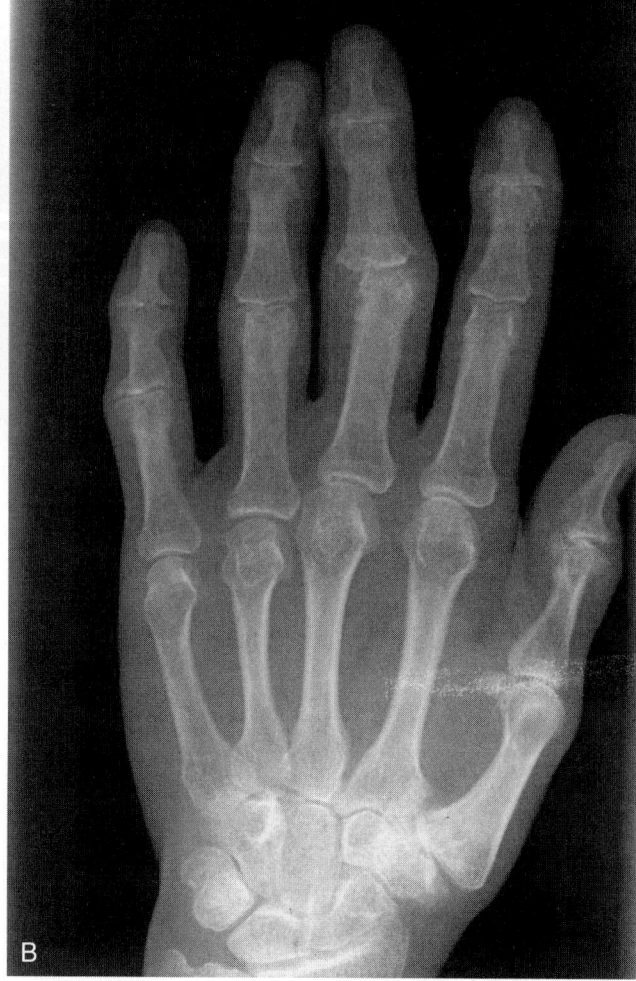

Fig. 2. Erosive osteoarthritis. *A,* Clinical presentation, with Heberden's and Bouchard's nodes. *B,* Radiographic appearance, with involvement of distal interphalangeal, proximal interphalangeal (PIP), thumb interphalangeal, and carpometacarpal joints and more advanced destruction of the long finger PIP joint.

articular corticosteroid injections may be helpful in recalcitrant cases of basal joint and, occasionally, PIP joint arthritis. The clinician should avoid excessive administration of intra-articular steroids, which may accelerate cartilage degeneration. Patients will respond more favorably when pharmacological treatment is combined with temporary or intermittent immobilization. The interphalangeal joint of the thumb and DIP joints of the fingers can be treated with small aluminum or orthoplastic splints. A forearm-based opponens (thumb spica) splint effectively protects the thumb basal joint but may interfere with normal use of the hand. Some patients prefer a hand-based splint, although this allows some motion at the CMC joint. The hand therapist can monitor exercises and administer treatments such as hot paraffin, which will maintain joint mobility. Thenar strengthening may compensate for laxity of the basal joint. The therapist also provides adaptive aids to assist patients in performing certain basic activities, such as buttoning clothing, opening jars, and manipulating zippers. This conservative treatment program is designed to minimize pain, decrease inflammation, and restore function. Recently developed pharmacological agents, including glucosamine/chondroitin sulfate, and intra-articular hyaluronic acid sub-

stitutes, have not been adequately tested in the treatment of hand arthritis.

Pain that is unresponsive to conservative therapy is the most common indication for surgery. Weakness and deformity that interfere with hand function may also be corrected with surgical reconstruction. Severely debilitated individuals or patients with relatively normal or compensated hand function may not be appropriate surgical candidates. Significant degenerative changes as seen on the radiograph are not an absolute indication for surgery, as the level of symptoms may not correlate with the radiographic findings.

PROCEDURES

BASAL JOINT

Many surgical techniques have been described for basal joint arthritis,[11-13] including ligament reconstruction, trapezial resection (partial or complete), metacarpal osteotomy, hemiarthroplasty, interpositional arthroplasty, and total joint arthroplasty. A radiographic staging system may assist the surgeon in choosing the appropriate procedure (Table 1). Stage I disease, with minimal cartilage destruction, may be amenable to ligament reconstruction. Stage II arthritis may

TABLE 1. STAGING OF BASAL JOINT ARTHRITIS	
Stage	Description
I	Pain, laxity, positive carpometacarpal joint grind test
	Mild subluxation on radiograph
II	Crepitus, subluxation
	Trapeziometacarpal joint degenerative changes
III	Pantrapezial arthritis
IV	Metacarpophalangeal joint arthritis in addition to trapeziometacarpal joint involvement

From Burton RI. Basal joint arthrosis of the thumb. Orthop Clin North Am 1973; 4(2):331.

be treated with hemitrapeziectomy, and total trapeziectomy is indicated for stage III disease. These procedures can be performed alone or in combination with interposition or other arthroplasty techniques. One procedure currently favored by many hand surgeons is the ligament reconstruction tendon interposition arthroplasty.[8] Burton has described modifications to his original technique (Figs. 3 and 4).[14]

The specific surgical techniques for these various procedures are beyond the scope of this chapter. Principles common to many of these approaches include the following:

- Dorsoradial incision.
- Isolation of branches of the radial sensory nerve and the radial artery as it passes deep to the first dorsal compartment.
- Arthrotomy between the abductor pollicis longus and extensor pollicis brevis tendons.
- Trapeziectomy with preservation of the flexor carpi radialis tendon.
- Ligament reconstructions employing either free palmaris longus grafts or split or whole flexor carpi radialis tendons (distally based), or distally-based abductor pollicis longus tendons.
- Use of excess tendon graft after ligament reconstruction as soft-tissue interposition.
- Stabilization of the thumb metacarpal bone to the index metacarpal bone with K-wires.
- Postoperative care consisting of 4 to 6 weeks of immobilization, followed by supervised hand therapy.
- Removal of K-wires at 4 weeks.

The hypermobile MCP joint must also be addressed during CMC reconstruction. Just as there are multiple techniques for the CMC joint, different approaches have been described for the MCP joint. Joints with less than 20 degrees of hyperextension can be treated with K-wire fixation in slight flexion. Moderate hyperextension (up to 30 degrees) can be corrected with volar plate advancement or MCP joint arthrodesis. Arthritic MCP joints are fused in approximately 10 degrees of flexion.

There are certain cases in which CMC arthrodesis is preferred over arthroplasty. Young laborers who require significant strength and patients with generalized joint laxity (e.g., those with Ehlers-Danlos syndrome) are ideal candidates for CMC fusion (Fig. 5). Patients must be warned of the associated loss of mobility; most troublesome is the inability to completely flatten the hand because of the fixed palmar abduction of the thumb metacarpal joint. CMC arthrodesis is contraindicated in patients who require arthrodesis of the MCP joint.

PIP JOINT

Satisfactory surgical treatment of the arthritic PIP joint remains problematic. Motion, which is important for grip, can be preserved only with arthroplasty. This is most commonly performed with silicone implants (Fig. 6). Resection arthroplasty, metalloplastic implants, and autogenous joint transfer have also been described.[15] This procedure is indicated in the ulnar two or three digits with adequate bone stock, soft-tissue coverage, and functional flexor tendons and can be performed with either a dorsal or a palmar approach. The dorsal approach allows correction of extensor mechanism imbalance in swan-neck and boutonnière deformities. The palmar approach allows preservation of the central slip, which leads to earlier active motion.[16] Resection arthroplasty alone may be indicated in the very young patient or in cases of active septic arthritis. PIP arthroplasty should not be performed in a digit that also has an MCP arthroplasty as this leads to significant instability.

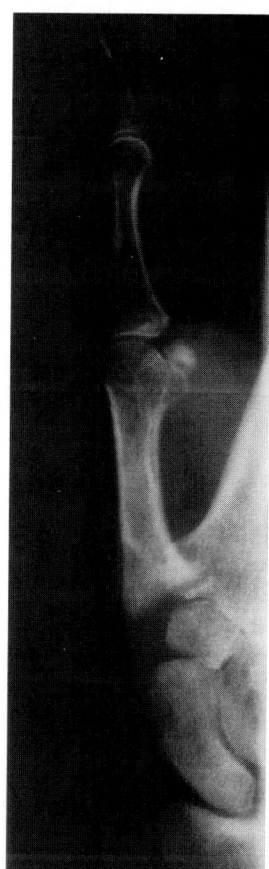

Fig. 3. Ligament reconstruction tendon interposition, radiographic appearance. Joint space is maintained, and the thumb metacarpal joint sits over the scaphoid without lateral subluxation.

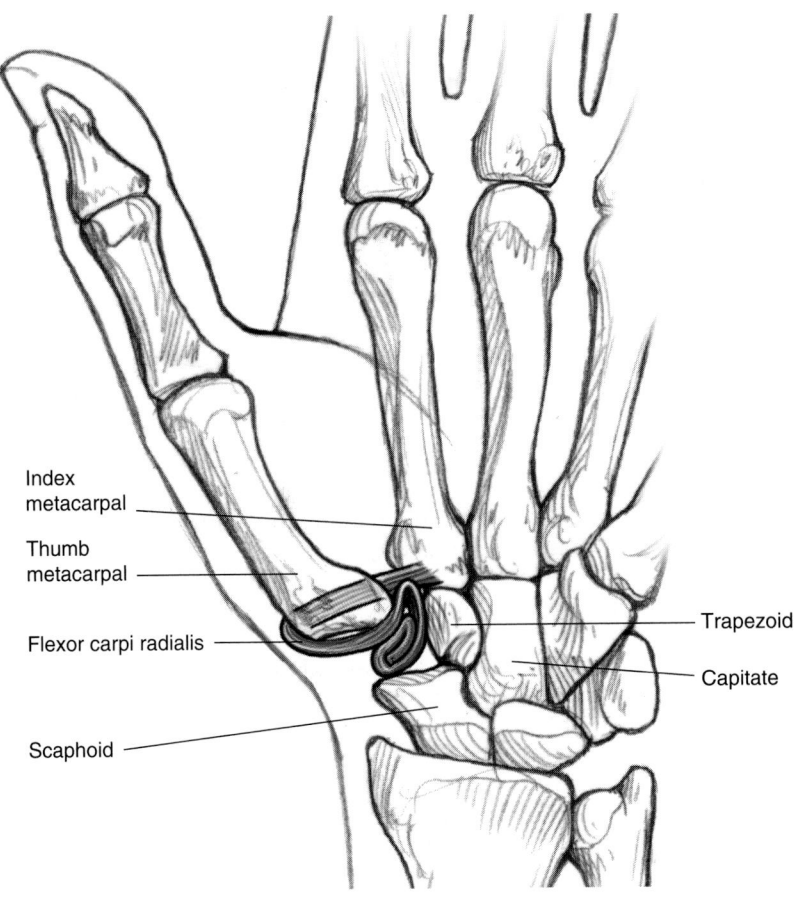

Index
metacarpal

Thumb
metacarpal

Flexor carpi radialis

Scaphoid

Trapezoid

Capitate

Fig. 4. Ligament reconstruction tendon interposition, schematic. The flexor carpi radialis tendon pulled taut through the hole in the thumb metacarpal bone and sutured back onto itself, with the excess rolled to fill the trapezial space.

Arthrodesis is the procedure of choice in the index finger, where a stable PIP joint is required to withstand high lateral forces during key pinch. Failed PIP arthroplasties, poor bone stock, ligamentous instability, and soft-tissue contractures are other indications for arthrodesis. Recommendations for fusion position of the index finger range from 10 degrees to 40 degrees and from 25 degrees to 55 degrees for the ulnar digits. Fusion can be accomplished with tension band, K-wires, interosseous wiring, intramedullary screws, plates, and external fixators (see Chapter 12-15).

DIP JOINT

The most effective treatment of mucous cysts is excision combined with débridement of marginal osteophytes. If the cyst has caused significant attenuation of the overlying dorsal skin, the surgeon may need to design a local rotational flap to ensure adequate soft-tissue coverage of the joint. There is a significant recurrence rate with isolated excision of the cyst and with aspiration. Because of the superficial location of the DIP joint, aspiration may increase the risk of septic arthritis. Stable joints with unremitting pain or unstable DIP joints may require arthrodesis, which can be performed with two K-wires or an intramedullary screw (Fig. 7). The optimal position for fusion ranges from 0 degrees to 15 degrees of flexion.

COMPLICATIONS AND RESULTS

COMPLICATIONS

Injury to neurovascular structures can occur during basal joint surgery. Although the radial sensory nerve and radial artery are at greatest risk, branches of the lateral antebrachial cutaneous nerve, palmar cutaneous nerve, and occasionally median nerve can also be injured. Poor technique can compromise the results of CMC reconstruction. Both joint surfaces of the trapezium must be inspected; radiographs will not always reveal degenerative changes in the scaphotrapezial joint. MCP joint laxity should be evaluated preoperatively and treated appropriately.

Silicone arthroplasty of the CMC joint was associated with bone resorption, implant settling, and subluxation in 25% of cases in one study.[17] Bone resorption has also been reported in 20% to 35% of silastic PIP implants at 2 to 4 years after surgery; the clinical significance of these radiographic changes is unclear.[18] Total joint arthroplasty has been associated with 10% to 44% incidence of loosening.[11, 19] Trapezial resection and tendon interposition procedures have been associated with reduced pinch strength and significant settling of the metacarpal joint.[3] Some loss of the trapezial space also has been described after the ligament reconstruction tendon interposition arthroplasty, although patient satisfaction remained high.[20]

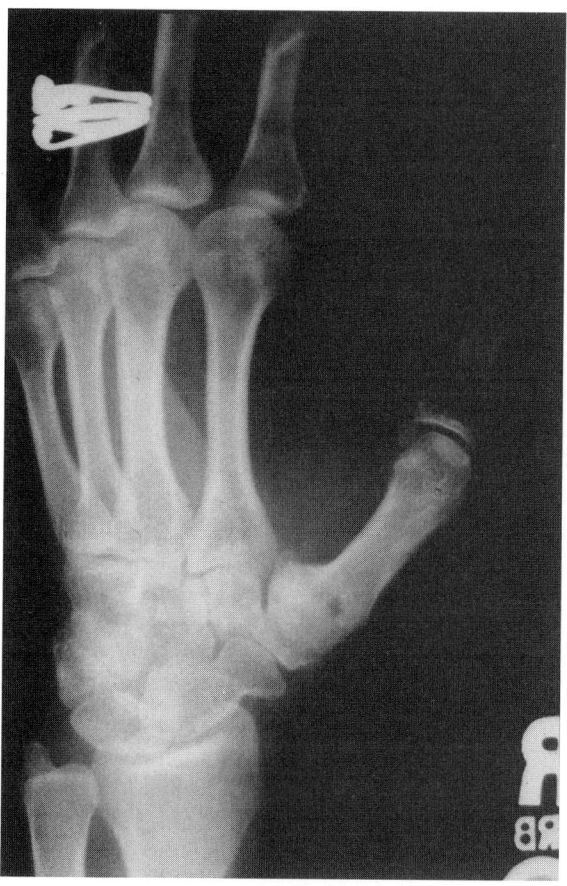

Fig. 5. Thumb carpometacarpal joint fusion. The K-wires used to maintain arthrodesis have been removed.

Complications of arthrodesis include nonunion, painful hardware, and the potential need for prolonged immobilization. Problems specifically associated with basal joint arthrodesis include inability to flatten the hand, increased risk of arthrosis or arthritis in metaphalangeal and scaphotrapezial joints, and MCP joint hypermobility.

RESULTS

The surgeon should examine the patient more than once before proceeding with surgical reconstruction, making sure that the patient's symptoms, and not only the radiographs, justify operative intervention. Clear lines of communication will ensure that both the patient's and the surgeon's expectations are met.

CMC Joint

Trapezial resection, soft-tissue interposition arthroplasty, and silicone implant arthroplasty have been associated with metacarpal settling and weak pinch.[17, 21] Silicone synovitis and fragmentation have also been reported in the thumb.

Thumb basal joint arthrodesis has resulted in 75% to 100% patient satisfaction at 4 to 6.5 years' follow-up. Clinical range of motion is not significantly affected, and grip and pinch strength are similar to that of the contralateral hand.[22]

Patients undergoing ligament reconstruction in association with CMC resection arthroplasty have demonstrated good to excellent function, with significant pain relief and improved strength.[7, 8, 20] Progressive improvement may occur as late as 1 year after surgery. Numerous reports of variations of this procedure, with follow-up ranging from

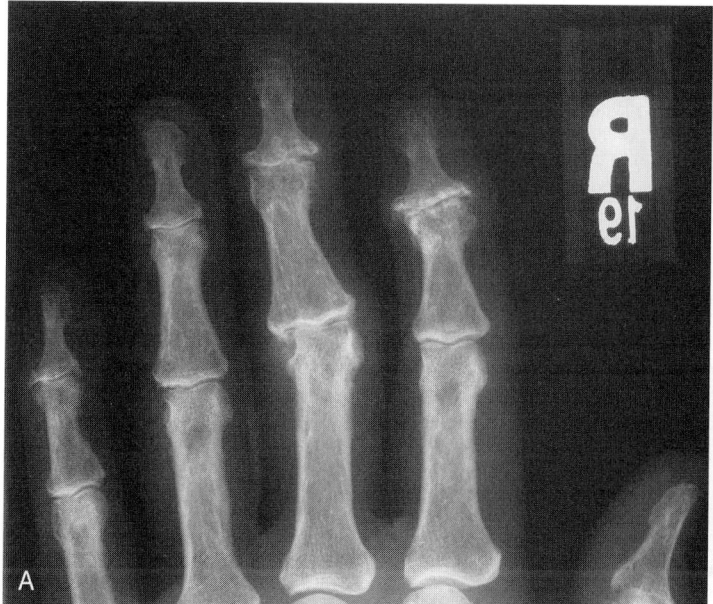

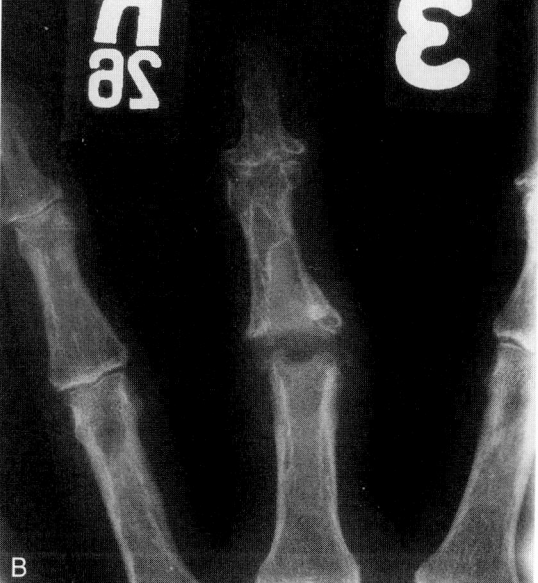

Fig. 6. A stiff, painful long finger proximal interphalangeal (PIP) joint. *A,* Preoperative appearance. *B,* Postoperative appearance of the PIP joint silicone arthroplasty.

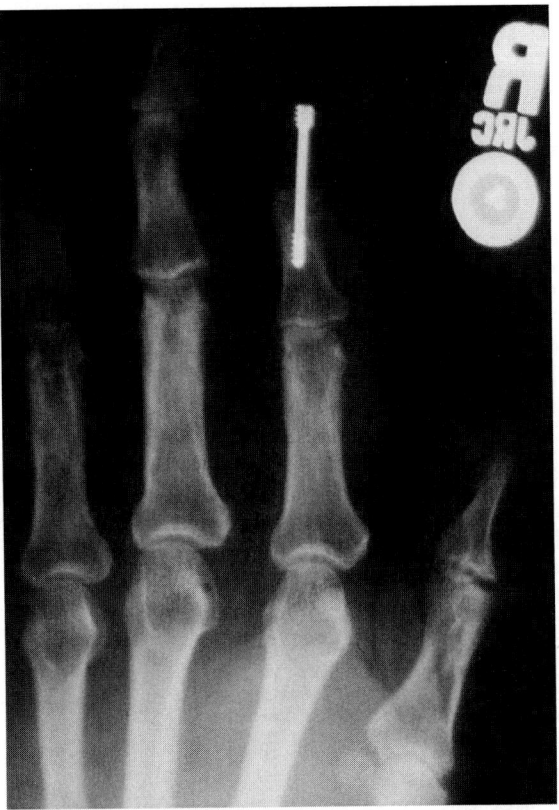

Fig. 7. Distal interphalangeal joint fusion. This is for post-traumatic osteoarthritis with an intramedullary screw.

1.5 to 8 years, have described 85% to 92% symptom resolution with 19% to 30% increase in grip and pinch strength.[11]

PIP Joint

Silicone implants for PIP joint osteoarthritis have demonstrated largely favorable results. In 26 implants monitored for approximately 4 years, mean total arc of motion was 56 degrees with a negligible extension deficit.[18] Lin et al,[16] using a palmar approach, reported a 50% decrease in extension deficit, with a mean total arc of 46 degrees; 97% of patients experienced significant pain relief.

Arthrodesis is well tolerated in the index and long fingers. Jones and Stern[23] reported a low rate of pseudoarthrosis with the tension band technique.

DIP Joint

The current recommended treatment of mucous cysts is very successful. When only the cyst is aspirated or excised, there is a 25% to 50% recurrence rate. The addition of surgical débridement of the joint and osteophyte excision results in near elimination of this problem.[24]

REFERENCES

1. Lawrence JS: Generalized osteoarthrosis in a population sample. Am J Epidemiol 1969; 90:381.
2. Gervis WH: Excision of the trapezium for osteoarthritis of the trapeziometacarpal joint. J Bone Joint Surg Br 1949; 31:537.
3. Froimson A: Tendon arthroplasty of the trapeziometacarpal joint. Clin Orthop Rel Res 1970; 70:191.
4. Swanson AB: Disabling arthritis at the base of the thumb. J Bone Joint Surg Am 1972; 54:456.
5. de la Caffiniere J: Trapeziometacarpal arthroplasty by total prosthesis. Hand 1979; 11:41.
6. Eaton RG, Littler JW: Ligament reconstruction for the painful thumb carpometacarpal joint. J Bone Joint Surg Am 1973; 55:1655.
7. Thompson JS: Surgical treatment of trapeziometacarpal arthrosis. Adv Orthop Surg 1986; 10:105.
8. Burton RI, Pellegrini VD Jr: Surgical management of basal joint arthritis of the thumb II: Ligament reconstruction with tendon interposition arthroplasty. J Hand Surg Am 1986; 11:324.
9. Pellegrini VD Jr: Osteoarthritis at the base of the thumb. Orthop Clin North Am 1992; 23:83.
10. Marmor L, Peter JB: Osteoarthritis of the hand. Clin Orthop Rel Res 1969; 64:164.
11. Calandruccio JH, Jobe MT: Arthroplasty of the thumb carpometacarpal joint. Semin Arthroplasty 1997; 8:135.
12. Lane LB: Atlas of the Hand Clinics: Carpometacarpal Joint. Philadelphia, WB Saunders, 1997, vol 2.
13. Burton RI: Basal joint arthrosis of the thumb. Orthop Clin North Am 1973; 4:331.
14. Burton RI: Ligament reconstruction tendon interposition arthroplasty. In Lane LB (ed): Atlas of the Hand Clinics: Carpometacarpal Joint. Philadelphia, WB Saunders, 1997, p 77.
15. Steinberg DR, Gupta R: Proximal interphalangeal joint arthroplasty. Semin Arthroplasty 1997; 8:120.
16. Lin HK, Wyrick JD, Stern PJ: Proximal interphalangeal joint silicone replacement arthroplasty: Clinical results using an anterior approach. J Hand Surg Am 1995; 20:123.
17. Pellegrini VD Jr, Burton RI: Surgical management of basal joint arthritis of the thumb I: Long-term results of silicone implant arthroplasty. J Hand Surg Am 1986; 11:309.
18. Pellegrini VD, Burton RI: Osteoarthritis of the proximal interphalangeal joint of the hand: Arthroplasty or fusion? J Hand Surg Am 1990; 15:194.
19. van Cappelle HGJ, Elzenga P, van Horn JR: Long-term results and loosening analysis of de la Caffiniere replacements of the trapeziometacarpal joint. J Hand Surg Am 1999; 24:476.
20. Lins R, Gelberman R, McKeown L, et al: Basal joint arthritis: Trapeziectomy with ligament reconstruction and tendon interposition arthroplasty. J Hand Surg Am 1996; 21:202.
21. Amadio P, Millender L, Smith R: Silicone spacer or tendon spacer for trapezium resection arthroplasty: Comparison of results. J Hand Surg 1982; 7:237.
22. Schwendeman L, Stern P: Trapeziometacarpal joint fusion. In Lane LB (ed): Atlas of the Hand Clinics: Carpometacarpal Joint. Philadelphia, WB Saunders, 1997, p 169.
23. Jones BF, Stern PJ: Interphalangeal joint arthrodesis. Hand Clin North Am 1994; 10:267.
24. Eaton RG, Dobranski AI, Littler JW: Marginal osteophyte excision in treatment of mucous cysts. J Bone Joint Surg Am 1973; 55:570.

POST-TRAUMATIC THUMB RECONSTRUCTION

Guy Foucher

Summary

- A patient with thumb amputation has an estimated 40% impairment of the hand.
- Reconstructive goals include a thumb that is not painful, is stable, has good sensibility, has sufficient length for pinch, and has acceptable cosmetic appearance.
- Among the many techniques available and the many factors influencing decision making, level of amputation and patient age are of special relevance.
- Microsurgery has provided new techniques through compound tissue transfer from the foot, but classic techniques such as distraction, lengthening, pollicization, and web deepening are useful alternatives.

Post-traumatic thumb amputation is a major hand mutilation, frequently associated with radial finger amputations. Acutely, replantation has been a major advance, but it is not always possible. When the part is not available, the trauma is beyond repair, or the replantation has failed, reconstruction remains a major challenge for the hand surgeon. It should be performed without a lengthy delay to decrease disability and facilitate integration in daily activity.

HISTORICAL REVIEW

Littler[1] extensively reviewed the history of thumb reconstruction, a field in which he himself has been a major contributor. Nicoladoni[2] introduced two techniques, namely osteoplastic reconstruction (even if he did not complete the procedure, stopping before bone grafting) and toe transfer through the pedicle method. Both of them provided poor sensibility. Guermonprez[3] was among the first to pollicize a finger, a technique refined later by the island principle, thanks to Gosset and Sels[4] and Littler.[5] A mobile and sensitive thumb was obtained, at the price of sacrificing a finger. Matev[6] originated the technique of progressive distraction lengthening, maintaining good sensibility and improving length.

A major step was Buncke's[7] introduction of microvascular techniques, allowing free toe-to-hand transfer. First- and second-toe transfers were followed by refined techniques allowing improved thumb appearance and minimizing donor site morbidity.[8, 9]

CLINICAL FEATURES

Careful history and examination are of paramount importance. Sex, hand dominance, associated diseases, occupation and leisure activities, and date and type of trauma need to be recorded.

We use a psychologist, present at consultation, to help us assess motivation, compliance, functional and cosmetic desires, and psychological status.

The level of amputation, quality of the skin (on the stump and in the web), sensibility and presence of pain at the stump level, and function of the remaining joints (mainly the thumb carpometacarpal) and thenar muscles all must be assessed. In case of associated finger mutilation, any stump is carefully examined because it may be considered for pollicization.

INVESTIGATIONS

A plain radiograph film of the hand is usually adequate except in heavy trauma, when a precise knowledge of hand vascularization is helpful; in such cases, an arteriogram is usually mandatory.

GOALS, INDICATIONS, AND CONTRAINDICATIONS

GOALS

Basic qualities of a reconstructed thumb remain a matter of controversy, but we developed a 200-point scoring system to allow comparison of different types of reconstruction[10] (Table 1).

INDICATIONS AND CONTRAINDICATIONS

Indications and contraindications are outlined in Table 2.

RELEVANT FACTORS IN DECISION MAKING

A long delay between mutilation and reconstruction frequently leads to adaptation and could preclude any attempt at reconstruction.

Age is a major limit for any technique using nerve repair at the recipient site. Avulsion injury may be a contraindication because recipient nerve injury is often extensive. Associated diseases (vascular or neurological) and smoking habits are relative contraindications for some microvascular techniques. Occupational and leisure activities (e.g., sports, music), motivations, compliance, functional and cosmetic desires, and psychological status need to be assessed.

Level of amputation is a major limitation of some techniques (Fig. 1). In the absence of the thumb carpometacarpal joint, only pollicization of a normal finger will provide a good pinch. In contrast, amputation at the metacarpophalangeal joint (MPJ) level is rarely an indication for pollicization because other techniques can be used without the sacrifice of a normal finger.

TABLE 1. SCORING SYSTEM TO COMPARE RECONSTRUCTION TYPES			
Stability of bone (vascularized) and skin	20	Nail	
Painless (including cold)	20	Appearance	10
Mobility (Kapandji score)	15	Size	3
Web	10	Shape	2
Sensibility	20	Dystrophy	3
Fine pinch	10	Dorsal scar	2
Length (relative)	20	Opinion of the patient	15
Strength pinch	20	Donor site morbidity	
Grasp	10	Functional	15
		Cosmetic	5
			200

When the fingers are stiff, the length of the thumb has to be carefully measured to allow distal pinch.

Finally, possible reconstruction must be precisely explained to the patient. Advantages and drawbacks, function, and appearance must all be discussed.

PROCEDURES

PREOPERATIVE PLANNING

All procedures need careful planning and classic instruments of hand surgery, including tourniquet, bipolar coagulation, loupes, and sometimes an operative microscope. If provision of skin for the first web is insufficient, a flap is mandatory before or at the same stage as the thumb reconstruction. For microsurgical transfer, preoperative warming of the patient with core temperature monitoring is necessary.

TECHNICAL DETAILS
Web Deepening

Web deepening is a simple and classic technique. It consists in some type of Z-plasty and could be combined with second proximal ray amputation in case of useless index stump.

Osteoplastic Thumb Reconstruction

Osteoplastic technique encompasses three steps that can be combined: a distant skin flap, a bone graft, and an heterodigital island skin flap (to provide sensibility). Composite free or island tissue transfer, associating the skin flap and a

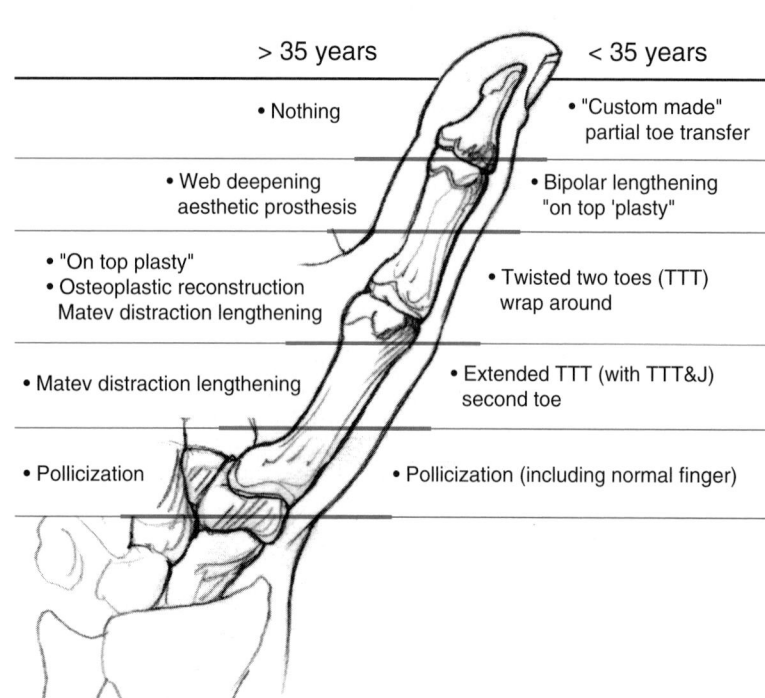

Fig. 1. Indications for thumb reconstruction. Indications are based on patient age and level of amputation.

> 35 years   < 35 years

- Nothing
- "Custom made" partial toe transfer
- Web deepening aesthetic prosthesis
- Bipolar lengthening "on top 'plasty"
- "On top plasty"
- Osteoplastic reconstruction Matev distraction lengthening
- Twisted two toes (TTT) wrap around
- Matev distraction lengthening
- Extended TTT (with TTT&J) second toe
- Pollicization
- Pollicization (including normal finger)

TABLE 2. INDICATIONS AND CONTRADICTIONS

Methods	Indications	Contraindications	Advantages	Drawbacks
No treatment	Exclusion Poor status	Young, well motivated Manual worker Musician	Simplicity	Major disability
Cosmetic prosthesis	Surgery impossible or refused	Manual worker Musician	Appearance	No sensibility No stability (except if fixed on osteointegrated devices)
Web deepening	Distal amputation		Simplicity No hospitalization	Limited relative lengthening
Osteoplastic reconstruction	Age >40 years Avulsion	No island flap available	No hospitalization	Multiple stages Poor appearance Unstable skin Bone resorption No added mobility
Progressive lengthening	Good stump At least two-thirds of metacarpal Adolescent or young adult	Painful stump Insufficient length	Good sensibility No bone resorption No hospitalization	Multiple stages Long time off No added mobility Adduction contracture pin track infection Limited lengthening (40–100%)
Pollicization of normal finger	No first CMCJ No thenar muscles	Major mutilation	Good mobility Good circulation One stage Good mobility Preserved sensibility	Decreased hand strength Inconstant cortical integration Decreased breadth of hand
Pollicization of a mutilated finger	Stump of sufficient length available Good vessel and nerve	Many fingers involved Painful stump Insufficient skin cover or padding	Preserved sensibility Good circulation If index, improve web depth and appearance One stage	Decreased hand strength No added mobility Inconstant cortical integration
Great toe	No other toe available (frostbite, congenital)	No microvascular skill or equipment	Strength and mobility Appearance ±	Donor site
Second toe	Several rays involved Amputation through first metacarpus	No microvascular skill or equipment	Donor site	Appearance (slender)
Wrap-around	Amputation near MPJ	No microvascular skill or equipment Growing child	Relative simplicity Great toe not sacrificed Appearance Long and stiff thumb	Iliac bone graft Bone resorption No mobility No growth potential Donor site healing problem
Twisted two toes	Isolated amputation near MPJ or through distal metacarpus	No microvascular skill or equipment	Growth potential Mobility No great toe sacrifice Stable donor site cover Appearance	Technically demanding
Bipolar lengthening	Remaining proximal one-third of proximal	No microvascular skill or equipiment	No iliac bone graft "short" thumb Good web grasp	Limited growth potential Appearance ±
Custom-made partial toe	Isolated thumb amputation Special demand (musician)	No microvascular skill or equipment	Appearance Presence of nail	Technically demanding

CMCJ, carpometacarpal joint; MPJ, metacarpophalangeal joint.

vascularized bone graft, could save one step, provide good sensibility, and avoid bone resorption. A compound forearm flap, based on the radial artery[11] or the anterior interosseous artery,[12] have been described.

Progressive Lengthening

The technique includes an osteotomy (or a corticotomy) with insertion of an external fixator, allowing progressive lengthening. After a week to allow skin healing, a 1- to

2-mm lengthening is provided each day, controlling pain, distal skin blanching, and pin tolerance. If one wants to avoid secondary bone grafting, the fixator must be left in place until there is solid union and cortical bone is visible from the regenerate. Otherwise, after obtaining the desired length, a bone graft is inserted. When indicated, a web deepening could be combined with second ray amputation, the metacarpal being used for bone graft. It is classically performed at the metacarpal level, but we found it useful to do it at the phalangeal level as well, thereby avoiding the pitfall of intrinsic traction and web deepening. A 100% lengthening is possible in children and at the phalangeal level but is rarely obtained at the metacarpal level in adults.

Pollicization
Intact Donor Finger
The finger selected has been a matter of debate. The use of the index finger allows one to pedicle the finger on arteries (radial and ulnar with sacrifice of the radial artery of the middle finger), collateral palmar and dorsal nerves as well as dorsal veins, and tendons. Hartmann's nervous ring around the artery is less frequent than in the other spaces.

Shortening is obtained through sacrifice of the metacarpal, the head being used as the trapezium. Good positioning in abduction and pronation is mandatory, and mobility is provided through repair of abductor pollicis longus and intrinsic muscles. Shortening of extensor and flexor tendons is optional.

Mutilated Finger
The technique is similar. We favor avoiding any dorsal scar and perform all dissections from a palmar incision; if necessary, a short dorsal transverse incision permits a microsurgical vein repair.[13] It is also of paramount importance to dissect the neurovascular bundles as far proximally as necessary to avoid closing the first web. The same technique is used with microsurgical steps in free hand-to-hand stump transfer, a procedure rarely indicated.

Toe Transfer
Microvascular surgery is based on a knowledge of the anatomy of the donor site. A circular scar at the base of the toe is to be avoided through harvesting a dorsal and palmar triangular flap from the foot. Thorough defatting around the vessels and at the base of the toe is the key to

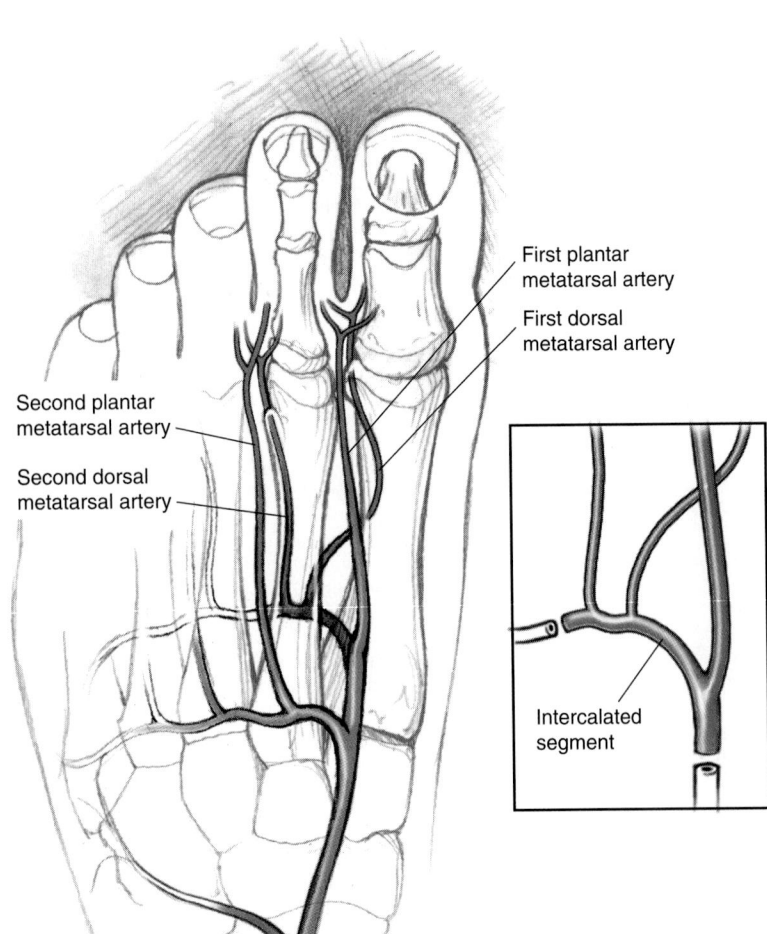

First plantar metatarsal artery

First dorsal metatarsal artery

Second plantar metatarsal artery

Second dorsal metatarsal artery

Intercalated segment

Fig. 2. Arterial anatomy of the first and second space. First dorsal metatarsal artery, first plantar metatarsal artery, second dorsal metatarsal artery, and second plantar metatarsal artery. *Inset,* T-graft interposed in the radial artery.

cosmetic success. The use of at least two arteries of the first and/or second intermetatarsal space avoids postoperative vascular crisis.[14] These arteries are branches of the plantar arcade, which is dissected in continuity with the dorsalis pedis artery (Fig. 2A). An end-to-side anastomosis could be performed. We favor interposition of the dorsalis pedis and plantar arch in the recipient radial artery by two end-to-end sutures, re-establishing a "physiological" flow for the toe and the hand (Fig. 2B). These sutures are usually performed through a transverse incision at the snuff box to avoid a dorsal conspicuous scar. A subcutaneous tunneling allows plenty of space to accommodate donor vessels.

Second Toe Transfer

Four arteries could be used to feed the toe, but the frequently overlooked second plantar metatarsal artery is the more constant in our experience (see Fig 2). If the metatarsophalangeal joint needs to be included to provide sufficient length, the joint has to be tilted palmarly (more than 40 degrees) to avoid a distal Z-deformity and to provide some flexion (Fig. 3). Intrinsic repair and longitudinal K-wire could decrease the tendency of a flexion deformity in this three-phalanx chain.

Partial Toe

For distal-third amputation of the first metacarpus, two techniques are available: the modified "wrap-around"[8, 15] and the "twisted two toes" (TTT).[16] The modified wrap-around consists of harvesting a compound flap from the homolateral great toe. The lateral skin envelope, including the nail and a piece of vascularized bone, is isolated on the vessels of the first space. The longititudinal bone cut (LBC) (Fig. 4)[17] has the advantages of preserving vascularization of the bone and fixation of the skin (through the septa), decreasing the visual projection of the too-large great toenail (the so-called illusion technique[18]), and avoiding first toe shortening.

The TTT is a combination of two flaps lifted on two separated vessels (Fig. 5). From the second toe, a vascularized interphalangeal joint is harvested with flexor and extensor mechanisms based on the second plantar metatarsal artery. From the great toe, the skin envelope and an LBC are isolated on vessels of the first space. Twisting is unnecessary, and a simple "shifting" of the joint in the great toe skin flap is performed using a Kirschner wire for stabilization. This provides a mobile "two-phalanx" thumb. In cases of distal thumb metacarpal amputation, the metatarsophalangeal joint is included and tilted palmarly.

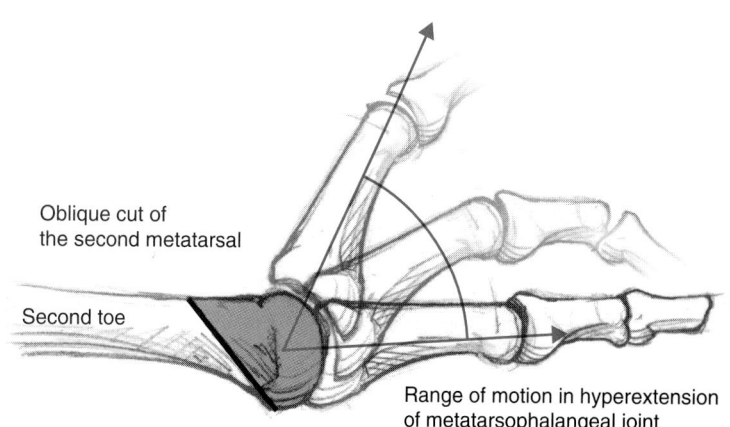

Oblique cut of
the second metatarsal

Second toe

Range of motion in hyperextension
of metatarsophalangeal joint

Fig. 3. Second toe transfer. Tilting of the second metatarsophalangeal joint in second toe transfer provides useful range of flexion and avoids a "ZR" deformity.

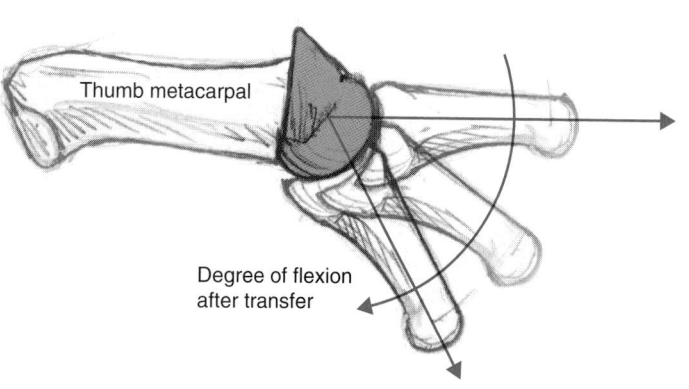

Thumb metacarpal

Degree of flexion
after transfer

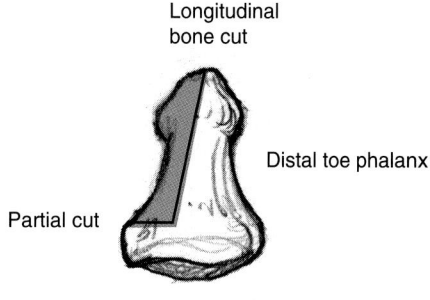

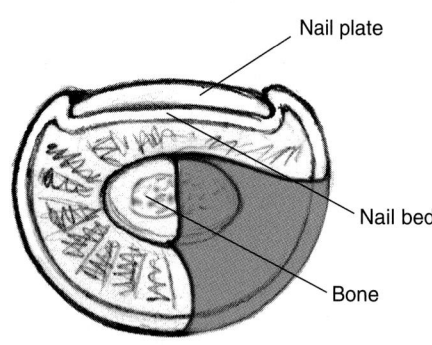

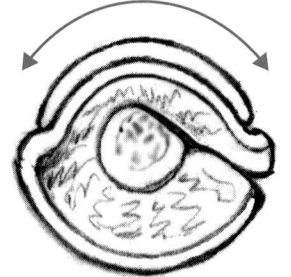

Fig. 4. Technique of longitudinal bone cut on the distal great toe phalanx. The curvature of the nail around the narrow piece of bone decreases the visual projection of the too-large great toe nail, the "illusion technique."

At the donor site level, the second metatarsus is proximally amputated and the filleted second toe provides a stable cover of the great toe with a small nail.

Distal Thumb Amputation

For distal amputation of the thumb, reconstruction could be performed, in selected cases, by tailoring from the great toe the missing thumb tissues: pulp, nail bed or nail complex, and/or bone[9] (Fig. 6).

In a transverse amputation through the proximal third of the proximal phalanx, an alternative to previously described techniques is the "bipolar lengthening,"[19] consisting of a compound transfer from the great toe, taking a skin envelope of the great toe en bloc with the nail complex and an LBC. This provides only a 1.5- to 2-cm lengthening. A web deepening allows a "relative" lengthening of an additional 2 cm (Fig. 6A).

In transverse amputation around the interphalangeal (IP) joint, a similar flap is transferred but without web deepening (Fig. 6B). In oblique dorsal amputation, bone and nail

complex are necessary (Fig. 6C).[20] In oblique palmar amputation, the flap is composed of the pulp, an LBC, and the distal aspect of the nail bed (to provide some support to the nail plate and avoid "parrot beak" deformity) (Fig. 6D). The donor site is covered by a combination of a cross-toe flap (taken from the plantar aspect of the second toe) to cover the dorsum of the great toe and a skin graft harvested from the non-hairbearing area of the instep.

POSTOPERATIVE MANAGEMENT

Each technique and each patient need a specific management but, generally, it is our policy to perform all nonmicrosurgical procedures on an outpatient basis. Elevation of the hand is maintained for 4 to 5 days, depending on the blood flow in the reconstructed thumb. Immobilization is usually maintained for 3 to 4 weeks, and we avoid changing the light cast and the dressing when not necessary. Bone union is usually obtained in 4 to 6 weeks, allowing in-office removal of the Kirschner wire.

The rehabilitation program focuses on re-establishment of passive range of motion through dynamic splinting as well as active motion. Integration of the new thumb could necessitate a formal program of sensory reeducation. After microsurgical operations, we prefer to hospitalize the patient for 5 days to monitor the perfusion of the transfer carefully. We rely mainly on a "Chinese lamp," an ordinary lamp that delivers constant light and heat. Color and, if necessary, capillary refilling are used. Intravenous perfusion is maintained with Dextran, and low-dose aspirin is absorbed orally. The patient is allowed to go home with a light cast on the hand and a special shoe preventing any weightbearing on the forefoot. The K-wire is removed at 4 to 5 weeks, and splinting and active motion begin. In all these cases at 4 to 5 months, when sensibility is recovering, a formal program of sensory re-education is performed.

COMPLICATIONS

Apart from classic complications of orthopaedic surgery each procedure has its own complications.

Osteoplastic thumb reconstruction is frequently plagued by bone resorption except when the bone is maintained vascularized. In our 13 patients with compound forearm flap, none presented such complication but one broke his bone at 2 months and healed with a hypertrophic callus in 5 weeks. Three patients complained about the appearance of their thumb (hairy skin and bulk). Cortical integration of the heterodigital island flap was complete in only 5 patients.

In pollicization of a mutilated finger, in a series of 27 cases[13] we observed three complications: one partial dorsal skin necrosis, one reflex sympathetic dystrophy, and two web "retractions." In fact, preservation of a good first web depends mainly on provision of supple skin and sufficient vascular dissection. We have not seen trophic changes, which occur mainly when a circular scar retracts at the base of the transferred stump; a broken line by sufficient indentations avoids such a complication. Cortical integration can be a problem when reconstruction is performed late.

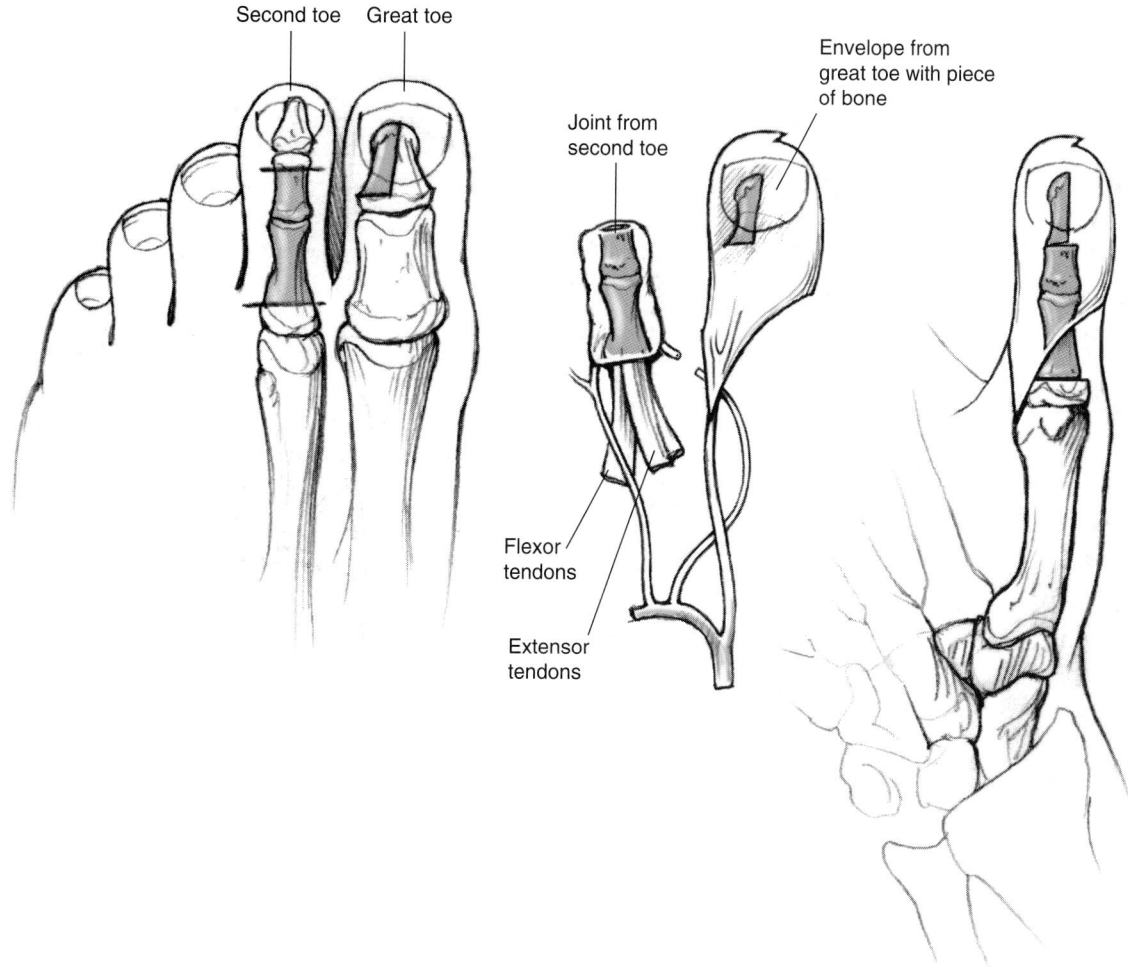

Second toe   Great toe

Joint from
second toe

Envelope from
great toe with piece
of bone

Flexor
tendons

Extensor
tendons

Fig. 5. Twisted two toes technique. The composite joint is taken on the second toe on the plantar artery of the second space. The skin envelope is harvested from the great toe, en bloc with the nail and a piece of bone, based on one or two vessels of the first space.

In our series of 20 progressive distraction lengthenings, we have observed[21] a number of minor complications (25%): pin track infections, pain, distal thumb blanching, loss of length when removing the frame, and slow bone healing. One major complication is progressive narrowing of the first web by angulation of the metacarpus under traction of the powerful adductor. This was observed once but could be avoided through a rigid framework combined with a longitudinal K-wire maintained until the callus is strong enough. The same method avoids progressive flexion of the MPJ in the case of preserved proximal phalanx. Among late complications, insufficient distal soft-tissue coverage was encountered in one case but a vascularized nail transfer allowed to move extra skin on the palmar aspect.

In toe transfer the immediate postoperative course could be complicated by vascular crisis leading to early reoperation (7%). In a personal series of 217 toe transfers, the failure rate was 6%, close to the 4.5% observed by Gu et al[22] in their 300 cases of whole toe transfer. The difference could be explained by the frequent use in our series of partial transfer in which the complexity of the distal dissection explains a higher failure rate (8.5%). However, in the last 7 years, we have not experienced any reoperation or failure, mainly owing to the use of a multiple set of arteries to feed the toe.

In our series, the donor site great toe was not a concern. Occasional pain after strenuous trekking was observed in 3% of cases. Cold intolerance was frequently mentioned (72% of hands and 35% of feet). Proximal second ray amputation gave a good cosmetic result at the donor level, and a dorsal hypertrophic scar was present in only 9%. Barca et al[23] performed a gait analysis in 54 patients after a thumb reconstruction with the great or second toe. Forty involved a wrap-around technique (in 27 the whole distal great toe phalanx was amputated), four involved great toe transfer, and 10 involved second toe transfer. Of those patients treated by a wrap-around, 38.5% presented with hallux rigidus. When the distal phalanx was sacrificed, this problem was less frequent, but there was a clear reduction of the push-off phase of hallux. The group of patients treated by second toe transfer presented some third and fourth metatarsal bone overload with plantar hyperkeratosis at the third metatarsal (20%), fourth metatarsal (10%), or fifth metatarsal (20%) bone. A claw deformity of the third and fourth toes was observed in 20% of these patients. The

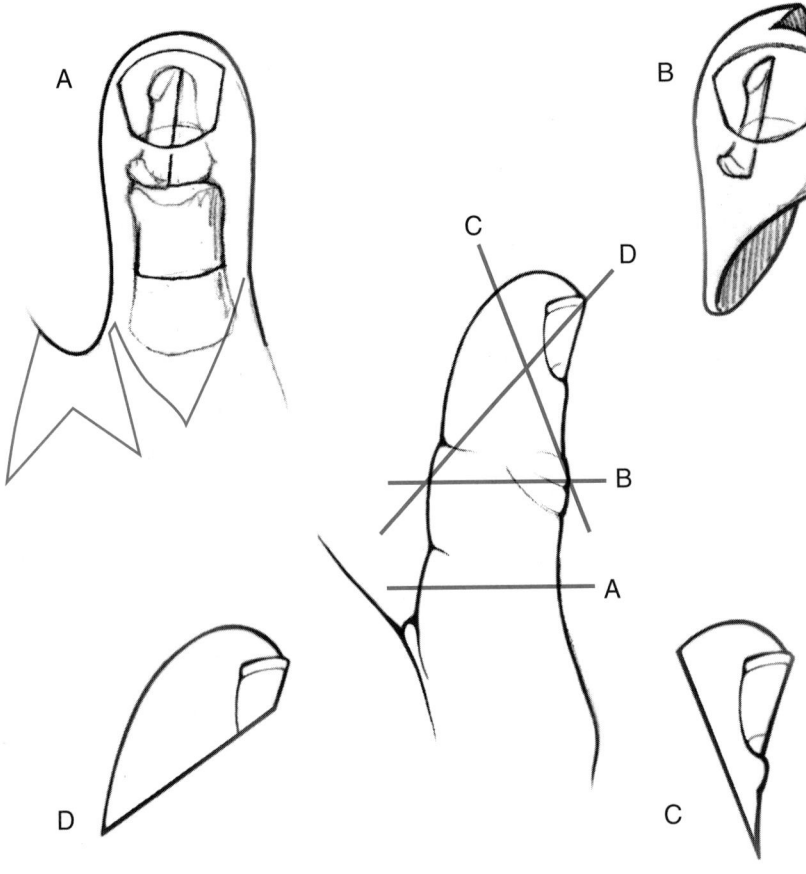

Fig. 6. Partial "custom-made" transfer from the great toe. *A,* Bipolar lengthening with distal lengthening by the partial toe and proximal deepening of the first web. *B,* Technique of reconstruction for transverse amputation around the interphalangeal joint. *C,* Reconstruction in dorsal amputation by compound transfer of nail complex and bone. *D,* Reconstruction of the pulp and distal nail bed by a compound transfer of pulp, bone, and nail bed flap.

four patients who underwent microsurgical reconstruction of the thumb by great toe transfer exhibited an overload of central and lateral metatarsal bones.

In our experience, the second toe has a tendency, at least in adults, to adopt a flexed position, which, in some cases, impedes pulp-to-pulp pinch, necessitating an IP arthrodesis. The classic wrap-around had a tendency to undergo bone resorption, causing a nail horn deformity and unstable palmar skin. With inclusion of a vascularized bone, such complications disappeared. In his series of 30 cases, Lee et al[24] observed one case of total failure, six cases of partial skin necrosis, one bone graft loss, one malunion, and 15 bone graft resorptions.

SHORT-TERM RESULTS AND OUTCOMES

Generally, thumb reconstruction is a rewarding surgery for both patient and surgeon if the indication and surgery are carefully planned and performed.

Concerning pollicization of a mutilated finger, in a review of 27 cases with a mean follow-up of 10 years, the 2-point discrimination (2PD) was less than 10 mm in 89% of patients. Cortical integration was complete in 39%. Opposition to radial fingers was present in 92.5%, but only 41% reached the fifth ray. Daily activity was good in 37%, fair in 41%, and poor in 22%. Cosmesis was acceptable when there was a nail (five cases) or when a great toe nail was microsurgically transferred (three cases).

We also reviewed 17 cases of second toe-to-thumb transfer in adult patients (mean age, 35 years; mean follow-up, 5.7 years). Average 2PD was 11 mm, and average mobility was only 25 degrees with an extensor lag of 31 degrees.

Our experience with wrap-around flaps is not as favorable as Urabaniak's. He obtained good protective sensibility, but "most of his patients had a 2PD of more than 15 mm", with a strength 30% to 50% of normal.[25]

Seven cases of TTT were seen at a mean follow-up of 4.6 years; average mobility was 30 degrees and 2PD, 9 mm.

Among the 47 partial toe transfers, 38 were controlled after a mean interval of 7 years.[26] In a population averaging 34 years of age, mean 2PD was 7 mm, and opposition allowed the thumb to reach the palmar aspect of the fifth finger middle phalanx. Ninety-five percent of patients returned to work, and none remained unemployed. A cosmetic score was developed based on 10 points, taking in account size, shape, nail dystrophy, and dorsal scar (see Table 1). The "trompe l'œil" technique gave a mean score of 7.5 points.

In conclusion, except in acute situations, when replantation remains the best option, thumb reconstruction has to be tailored to each patient, taking into account a number of factors. Microsurgery provides new opportunities, but more classic techniques continue to enjoy good indications. A good reconstruction is not just a good functional thumb from a surgical standpoint; a good balance has to be found with the cosmetic aspect so that patients avoid hiding the thumb in their pocket.

REFERENCES

1. Littler JW: On making a thumb: One hundred years of surgical effort. J Hand Surg 1976; 1:35.
2. Nicoladoni C: Daumenplastik und organischer Ersatz der Fingerspitze. Anticheiropastik und Daktyloplastik). Arch Klin Chir 1900; 61:606.
3. Guermonprez F: Notes sur quelques Résections et Restaurations du Pouce. Paris, Asselin, 1887.
4. Gosset J, Sels M: Technique, indications et résultats de la pollicisation du quatrième doigt. Ann Chir 1964; 48:1005.
5. Littler JW: The neurovascular pedicle method of digital transposition for reconstruction of the thumb. Plast Reconstr Surg 1953; 12:303.
6. Matev IB: Thumb reconstruction in children through metacarpal lengthening. Plast Reconstr Surg 1979; 64:665.
7. Buncke HJ, McLean DH, George PJ, et al: Thumb replacement: Great toe transplantation by microvascular anastomosis. Br J Plast Surg 1973; 26:194.
8. Morrison WA, O'Brien BMcC, MacLeod AM: Thumb reconstruction with a free neurovascular wrap-around flap from the big toe. J Hand Surg 1980; 5:575.
9. Foucher G, Merle M, Maneaud M, et al: Microsurgical free partial toe transfer in hand reconstruction: A report of 12 cases. Plast Reconstr Surg 1980; 65:616.
10. Foucher G, Smith D: Indications in secondary reconstruction of the thumb. In Foucher G (ed): Reconstructive Surgery in Hand Mutilation. London, Martin Dunitz, 1997, p 67.
11. Foucher G, Van Genechten F, Merle M, et al: Single stage thumb reconstruction by a composite forearm island flap. J Hand Surg [Br] 1984; 9:245.
12. Hu W, Martin D, Foucher G, et al: Utilisation du lambeau inter-osseux antérieur en îlot à contrario en chirurgie de la main. A propos de 15 cas. Ann Chir Plast Esthet 1994; 39:288.
13. Foucher G, Rostane S, Chammas M, et al: Pollicization of mutilated fingers. J Bone Joint Surg Am 1996; 78:1889.
14. Foucher G, Moss ALH: Microvascular second toe to finger transfer: A statistical analysis of 55 transfers. Br J Plast Surg 1991; 44:87.
15. Foucher G: Indication du transfert osseux vascularisé en chirurgie de la main. Rev Chir Orthop 1982; 68:38.
16. Foucher G, Van De Kar T: Twisted two toes technique in thumb reconstruction. In Lamb D (ed): Reconstruction of the Thumb. Chapman, 1989, p 275.
17. Foucher G, Binhammer P: Free vascularized toe transfer. In Foucher G (ed): Reconstruction Surgery in Hand Mutilation. London, Martin Dunitz, 1997, p 57.
18. Foucher G, Sammut D: Aesthetic improvement of the nail by illusion technique in partial toe transfer for thumb reconstruction. Ann Plast Surg 1992; 28:195.
19. Foucher G, Chabaud M: The "bipolar lengthening" technique. A modified partial toe transfer for thumb reconstruction. Plast Reconstr Surg 1998; 102:1981.
20. Foucher G, Braun FM, Smith DT: Custom-made free vascularized compound toe transfer for traumatic dorsal loss of the thumb. Plast Reconstr Surg 1991; 87:310.
21. Foucher G, Hultgren T, Merle M, et al: L'allongement digital selon Matev. A propos de 20 cas. Ann Chir Main 1988; 7: 210.
22. Gu YD, Zhang GM, Cheng DS, et al: Free toe transfer for thumb and finger reconstruction in 300 cases. Plast Reconstr Surg 1993; 91:693.
23. Barca F, Santi A, Tartoni PL, et al: Gait analysis of the donor foot in microsurgical reconstruction of the thumb. Foot Ankle Int 1995; 16:201.
24. Lee KS, Chae IJ, Hahn SB: Thumb reconstruction with a free neurovascular wrap-around flap from the big toe: Long-term follow-up of thirty cases. Microsurgery 1995; 16:692.
25. Urbaniak JR: Wrap-around procedure for thumb reconstruction. Hand Clin 1985; 1: 259.
26. Foucher G, Binhammer P: Plea to save the great toe in total thumb reconstruction. Microsurgery 1995; 16:373.

section 12 chapter 14

GAMEKEEPER'S THUMB

Dean G. Sotereanos and Sokratis E. Varitimidis

Summary
- Gamekeeper's thumb is a serious injury to the thumb that may compromise hand function.
- The key objectives are to restore stability and eliminate pain.
- Incomplete tears require conservative treatment.
- Results improve with early surgery.

Injuries to the ulnar collateral ligament (UCL) of the metacarpophalangeal (MP) joint of the thumb are common and in most cases respond well to conservative treatment. Despite adequate treatment, however, chronic post-traumatic instability of the joint is frequent and often disabling. Although Campbell[1] originally introduced it to describe the chronic instability of the UCL in Scottish gamekeepers, the term "gamekeeper's thumb" is applied today in both acute and chronic injuries of the UCL of the thumb MP joint.

PATHOGENESIS

The stability of the MP joint of the thumb is provided by its capsule, its ligaments, and the extensor pollicis brevis tendon. The capsule is a complex fibrous structure that is reinforced by the volar plate inferiorly, by the collateral ligaments ulnarly and radially, and by the extensor pollicis brevis tendon dorsally. The collateral ligaments consist of the proper and the accessory ligament. The proper collateral ligament originates dorsally on the metacarpal head and inserts more volarly on the phalangeal tubercle. During MP flexion the proper ligament is taut and the accessory ligament is relatively lax. The accessory collateral ligament originates just volar to the proper ligament and inserts on the volar plate and sesamoid. The accessory ligament is taut during extension of the joint, and the proper ligament is relatively lax.[2] The collateral ligaments not only provide stability during flexion and extension but also provide dor-

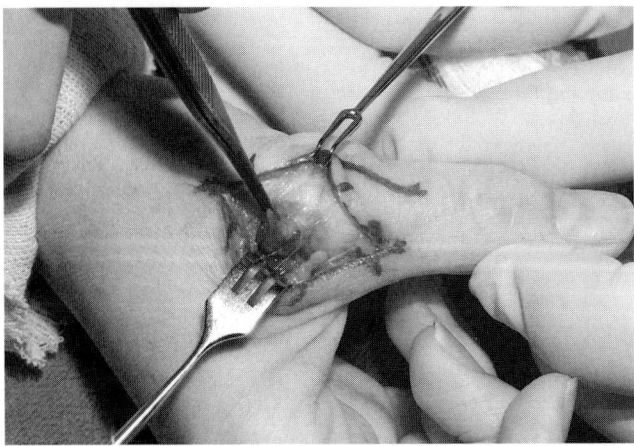

Fig. 1. Stener's lesion. Intraoperative finding. The adductor aponeurosis is interposed between the two stumps of the torn ulnar collateral ligament. Healing is impossible with conservative treatment.

sopalmar stability and prevent palmar subluxation of the proximal phalanx.

Lesions of the ulnar collateral ligament are classified as complete and incomplete ruptures. Differentiation is very important because treatment is significantly different in each category. Complete ruptures of the UCL usually require surgical intervention, whereas incomplete ruptures are treated conservatively with a thumb spica cast.

In complete rupture, the UCL ruptures from the base of the proximal phalanx and becomes trapped beneath the adductor aponeurosis. Because of the displacement, it is impossible for healing to occur. Stener[2] was the first to describe the lesion. He reported on 39 patients with complete rupture of the UCL (Fig. 1) and found that the adductor aponeurosis was interposed in 25.

When the UCL ruptures, in the majority of cases, the tear occurs at the distal part of the ligament, close to its insertion at the base of the proximal phalanx. Bowers and Hurst[3] reported that, in 118 patients with UCL rupture, the tear was found distally in 98 and elsewhere in the substance of the ligament in the remaining 20.

CLINICAL FEATURES

On clinical examination, patients present with pain, swelling, and tenderness of the MP joint and marked weakness in pinch. Pain is more prominent on the ulnar side of the joint, over the injured ligament, and extends from the metacarpal head to the base of the proximal phalanx. A prominent mass near the joint may be the stump of the displaced UCL. Abnormal rotation of the thumb may also be observed. This is because when the UCL is torn, the proximal phalanx can rotate about the axis of the intact radial collateral ligament.

When making the diagnosis, it is important to differentiate between incomplete and complete ruptures of the UCL and also to exclude or confirm any avulsion fracture of the proximal phalanx because treatment and surgical technique are different in each case.

The absence of an end point when stressing the joint is very useful in diagnosis because it suggests a complete tear

of the UCL. The presence of an end point suggests an incomplete rupture of the ligament.

When the joint is stable in flexion and unstable in extension, the proper collateral ligament maintains its continuity, but the accessory collateral ligament and volar plate have ruptured. When the joint is stable in extension and unstable in flexion, the proper collateral is torn but the accessory collateral and volar plate retain their strength and continuity. When there is pronounced instability in both flexion and extension, the entire ulnar complex of ligaments is disrupted (Fig. 2). Stability is defined as an opening of not more than 10 degrees beyond that of the unaffected side. Instability is defined as more than 30 degrees of abduction arc on the stress radiograph compared with the contralateral side.

INVESTIGATION

Plain radiographs must always be taken before stressing the joint to prevent displacement of a previously undisplaced fracture of the base of the proximal phalanx. This can occur when the proximal phalanx is radially deviated. A nondisplaced or minimally displaced (less than 2 mm) avulsion fracture indicates avulsion of the UCL without a Stener lesion. In such a case, application of a thumb spica cast is all that is required. If stress is applied to the joint, a Stener lesion may occur, requiring surgical intervention. After plain radiograph evaluation, the MP joint can be examined under stress. This should be done in both extension and flexion, and no conclusion should be made before the contralateral uninjured thumb is also examined for comparison. The examination can be performed more accurately and with less pain if a local anesthetic is used.

An arthrogram of the MP joint has also been recommended to diagnose and differentiate a UCL tear.[3] The examination depends on the extravasation of contrast into the adductor muscle or along the sheaths of the extensor pollicis brevis and extensor pollicis longus tendons, indicating a capsular rupture. In the presence of a complete ligamentous rupture, the ruptured ligament can be outlined and thus its position defined.

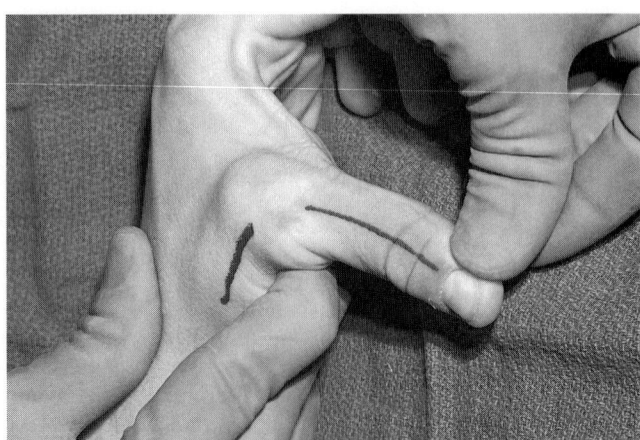

Fig. 2. Clinical examination of a torn ulnar collateral ligament. Abduction of the thumb is beyond normal. The examination is done after injection of a local anesthetic (lidocaine [Xylocaine]) for pain relief.

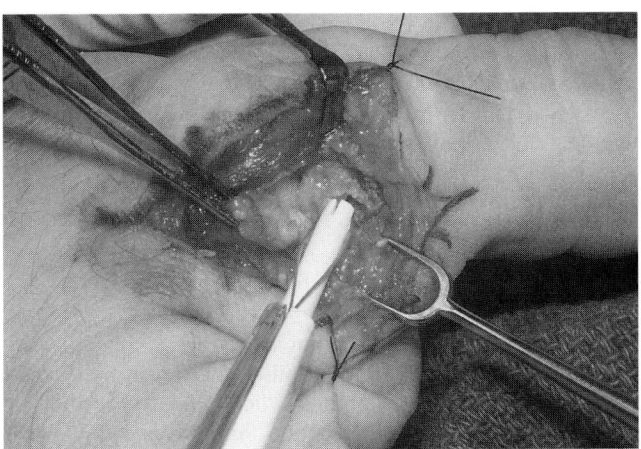

Fig. 3. Placement of a mini bone anchor. After drilling is completed in the proximal part of the proximal phalanx of the thumb, the mini anchor is placed with the assistance of an instrument designed specially for this purpose.

Ultrasonography has also given reliable results.[4] Magnetic resonance imaging is very sensitive in the diagnosis of a UCL tear,[5] but its high cost makes its use limited unless other methods are equivocal.

TREATMENT

Acute incomplete ruptures of the UCL are treated nonoperatively with a thumb spica cast for 4 to 6 weeks. Because there is no Stener's lesion, complete healing of the ligament and normal function can be expected.

Acute complete ruptures of the UCL require surgical treatment with repair of the torn ligament. Conservative treatment in the presence of a complete tear has poor results, and a delay of 4 to 6 weeks may preclude reattachment of the ligament because of fibrosis and granulation tissue that has formed at the site of injury.

REPAIR OF ACUTE COMPLETE RUPTURES OF THE UCL

A curvilinear, 4-cm long incision is made centered over the MP joint on the ulnar side. The sensory branches of the radial nerve are identified and protected. The adductor aponeurosis is transected at its insertion into the extensor pollicis longus. The UCL is then identified. Frequently, the UCL is ruptured at its insertion at the base of the proximal phalanx. If there is a midsubstance tear, repair of the ligament could be done with end-to-end sutures. If there is no ligament distally, the volar ulnar base of the proximal phalanx is roughened with a curet or a bur to ensure an adequate attachment site, necessary for ligament fixation. Then, using a drill bit, one suture anchor is placed in the base of the proximal phalanx[6] and tied into the proximal stump of the UCL (Fig. 3). Excellent ligament-to-bone contact should result. The adductor aponeurosis is then approximated. Any tear of the dorsal capsule should be carefully repaired to prevent volar subluxation. A suture should also be placed between the distal volar portion of the ligament and the volar plate to enhance stability of the

joint. Finally, to secure stability in the postoperative period, a Kirschner wire is passed through the joint while it is held in 20 degrees flexion. The hand is placed in a thumb spica splint, and after sutures are removed a thumb spica cast is applied. No more than 4 weeks of immobilization is necessary. Both the Kirschner wire and the cast are removed at that time. Active motion is started gradually, and unrestricted use of the hand is started at 4 months.

If anchors are not available, the pull-out button technique can be used. Two 3-0 nylon sutures are passed through the stump of the ligament at its corners. The insertion site of the ligament at the proximal phalanx is then roughened. The sutures are placed in Keith's needles and, with the help of a Kirschner wire, are passed across the bone on the radial side and over the skin. Finally, they are tied over a padded button.

RECONSTRUCTION OF CHRONIC COMPLETE RUPTURES OF THE UCL

In chronic complete lesions of the UCL (more than 4 weeks old), there is fibrosis and scarring at the site of the lesion, and many times the ligament is difficult to identify. Various surgical techniques have been described for the treatment of chronic ligament insufficiency: tendon transfer, tendon advancement, free tendon grafts, and finally MP fusion if attempts for reconstruction fail. Sakellarides and DeWeese[7] recommended reconstruction using the extensor

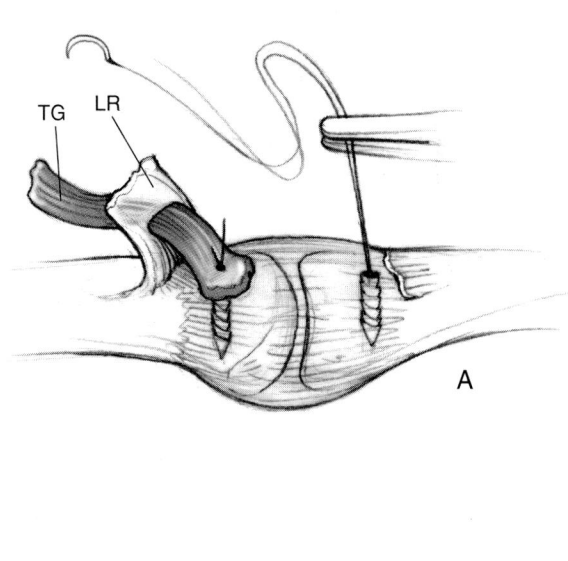

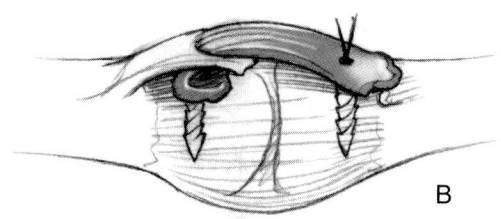

Fig. 4. Reconstruction of the ulnar collateral ligament. Reconstruction is performed using a tendon graft from palmaris longus. The graft is sutured to the ligament remnant proximally and is attached to the proximal phalanx with the use of a bone anchor (TG, tendon graft, LR, ligament remnant).

pollicis brevis tendon. Smith[8] reported excellent results using a tendon graft from the palmaris longus tendon. Neviaser et al[9] achieved good results by advancing the insertion of the adductor pollicis on the proximal phalanx, 1 cm distally.

A Technique Using a Free Tendon Graft

The same exposure used for acute injuries is also used in this technique. The bone surface is roughened at both insertion sites (metacarpal and proximal phalanx), and two anchors are inserted. Any residual ligament is preserved. A small portion of the palmaris longus tendon is then harvested for tendon graft. The bone anchor suture is passed through the end of the tendon graft at the insertion sites. If residual ligament is available, the graft is woven through an incision in the ligament (Fig. 4), and the suture is passed through both the ligament and the tendon graft. The tendon graft is then pulled to the bone and tied. The graft is also sutured to the periosteum and the capsule to augment the repair. The adductor aponeurosis is imbricated to augment the reconstruction further. Before closure of the skin, stability is tested by stressing the MP joint radially. Postoperative treatment and rehabilitation are the same as in the reconstruction of acute ruptures.

COMPLICATIONS AND RESULTS

Complications of reconstruction of the UCL include prolonged stiffness, persistent instability, and bone tunnel fracture. Fusion of the MP joint is the salvage procedure of choice if soft-tissue reconstruction fails or degenerative arthritis develops.

REFERENCES

1. Campbell CS: Gamekeeper's thumb. J Bone Joint Surg Br 1955; 37:148.
2. Stener B: Displacement of the ruptured ulnar collateral ligament of the metacarpophalangeal joint of the thumb. J Bone Joint Surg Br 1962; 44:869.
3. Bowers WH, Hurst LC: Gamekeeper's thumb: Evaluation by arthrography and stress roentgenography. J Bone Joint Surg Am 1977; 59:519.
4. Hergan K, Mittler C, Wolfgang O: Ulnar collateral ligament: Differentiation of displaced and nondisplaced tears with US and MRI imaging. Radiology 1955; 194:65.
5. Spaeth HJ, Abrams RA, Bock GW, et al: Gamekeeper's thumb: Differentiation of nondisplaced and displaced tears with MR imaging. Radiology 1993; 188:553.
6. Weiland AJ, Berner SH, Hotchkiss RN, et al: Repair of acute ulnar collateral ligament injuries of the thumb metacarpophalangeal joint with an intraosseous suture anchor. J Hand Surg Am 1977; 22:585.
7. Sakellarides HT, DeWeese JW: Instability of the metacarpophalangeal joint of the thumb. Reconstruction of the collateral ligaments using the extensor pollicis brevis tendon. J Bone Joint Surg Am 1976; 58:106.
8. Smith RJ: Post traumatic instability of the metacarpophalangeal joint of the thumb. J Bone Joint Surg Am 1977; 59:14.
9. Neviaser RJ, Wilson JN, Lievano A: Rupture of the ulnar collateral ligament of the thumb (gamekeeper's thumb): Correction by dynamic repair. J Bone Joint Surg Am 1971; 53:1357.

section 12 chapter 15

ARTHRODESIS

Edward Diao

Summary

- Arthrodesis is an important technique for managing a variety of hand conditions.
- Osteoarthritis, rheumatoid arthritis, trauma, congenital conditions, and neuromuscular problems are conditions that are amenable to arthrodesis.
- Preoperative assessment of all surrounding joints is important.
- Bone contouring and fixation can be achieved by a variety of means.

The upper extremity is notable for the many small joints that must work together to provide stability, dexterity, and maximal function. It is common for conditions affecting the joint architecture—the cartilage, subchondral bone, and ligamentous supports—to compromise upper extremity function significantly. Broadly speaking, these conditions can be treated, if conservative therapy fails, with arthroplasty or arthrodesis. In the upper extremity, arthrodesis, particularly of the small joints, constitutes a very important tool in the surgeon's armamentarium. This is in contrast to the larger joints, such as the hip, knee, shoulder, and elbow, in which arthrodesis is less commonly performed than arthroplasty.

Arthrodesis is indicated when there is pain, deformity, or instability in post-traumatic arthritis, systemic arthritis, and congenital deformities. Arthrodesis may also be appropriate for neuropathy or myopathy that does not involve primary joint disease. In addition, peripheral nerve palsies or central nervous system defects can impair muscle balance and function in the upper extremity. In these patients with neuromuscular problems, arthrodesis can be performed to control joints that may be mechanically sound but that lack sufficient muscular control to function adequately. Reducing the number of movable joints may also allow the surgeon to use muscle-tendon units as donors for tendon transfers to restore movement to the remaining joints.

When considering arthrodesis, the primary alternative is arthroplasty. In certain joints, arthrodesis is a more reliable procedure than arthroplasty. In part, this is due to the problems of fixation of a "total joint arthroplasty," particu-

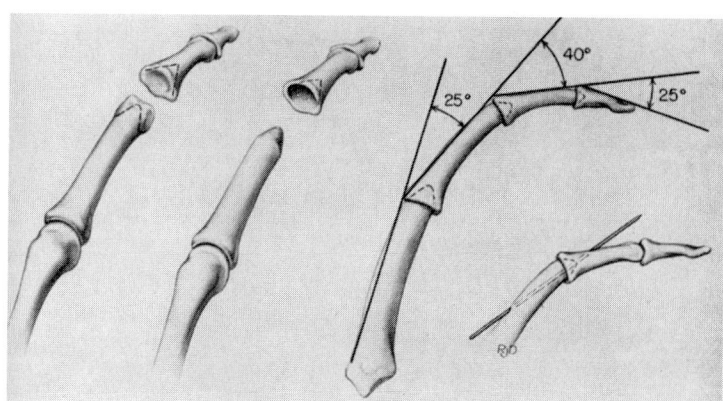

Fig. 1. Cup-and-cone bone preparation. (From Carroll RE, Hill NA: Small joint arthrodesis in hand reconstruction. J Bone Joint Surg Am 1969; 51:1219.)

larly in smaller joints. In other joints, the issue is whether fusion will improve function enough to warrant sacrificing movement. Another consideration is the longevity of the operation that is being contemplated. Arthrodesis is generally a once-in-a-lifetime operation that does not require revision. The decision to perform arthrodesis of one of the joints of the hand or wrist must be based in part on carefully evaluating the neighboring or surrounding joints. For example, interphalangeal joint arthrodesis may be considered only after fully evaluating the metacarpophalangeal and proximal or distal interphalangeal joints. If the carpometacarpal joint is being considered for arthrodesis, the metacarpophalangeal and interphalangeal joints must be evaluated. The status of the neighboring joints has much to do with the immediate success of the arthrodesis and ultimately with the longevity of the reconstruction.

This chapter provides a review of the myriad conventional techniques that have been associated with acceptable results clinically and biomechanically as well as newer techniques that may become more important in the future. Also, arthrodesis of specific joints in the hand and wrist is discussed.

HISTORICAL REVIEW

Historically, solid arthrodesis of the small joints of the hand has been accomplished by a variety of means.[1–6]

Difficulties with standard treatments motivated Carroll and Hill[2] to describe a technique in which the surgeon, rather than simply squaring off the bone ends, removes cartilage and shapes it into a gently rounded "spike" at the base of the distal articular surface. Multiple awl, or drill, holes, were placed at the osteocartilaginous junction of the proximal articular surface, and then these holes were connected with small osteotomes and curets to create a cone-shaped effect. The "cup-and-cone" technique for small joint arthrodesis used Kirschner's wires (K-wires) at the arthrodesis site to hold it in an oblique fashion (Fig. 1). Between 1952 and 1967, Carroll and Hill reported on 635 metacarpophalangeal and interphalangeal joint arthrodeses. There was an overall pseudarthrosis rate of 5%. Elimination of cases of spastic paralysis resulted in an overall pseudarthrosis rate of 2%. Four revisions were required for rotational errors.

In addition to the classic flat-cut bone preparation method, in 1968 Omer[7] described the chevron cut for small joint arthrodesis, which was used for reconstructions of the forearm and hand after acute traumatic peripheral nerve injuries.

The three basic methods of making bone cuts for small joint arthodesis in the hand, therefore, are (1) opposing flat cuts, (3) cup-and-cone cuts, and (3) chevron cuts. Methods of fixation of small joint arthrodesis include wire loop,[8] K-wires[2,9] (Fig. 2), external fixation[10] (Fig. 3), bone plugs and

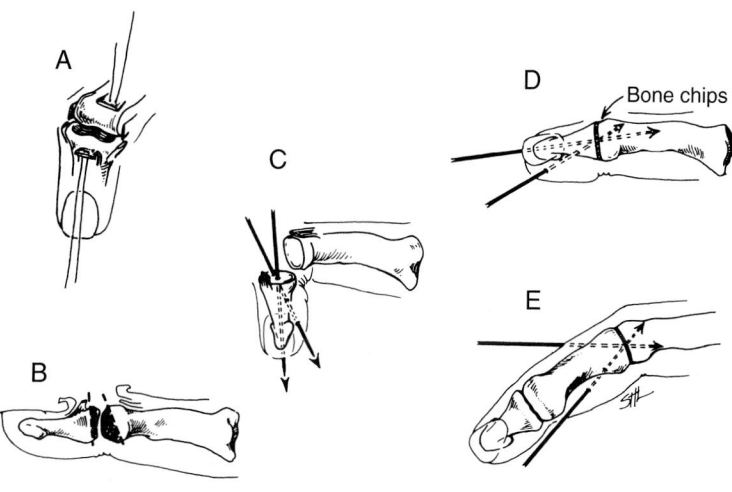

Fig. 2. Crossed K-wires. (From Burton RI, Margles SW, Lunseth PA: Small-joint arthrodesis in the hand. J Hand Surg Am 1986; 11:679.)

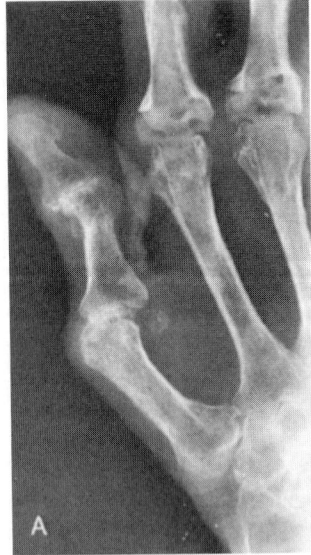
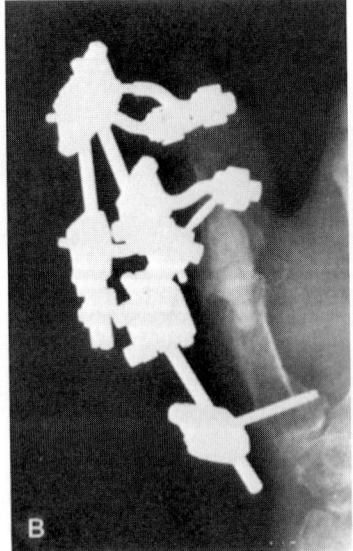
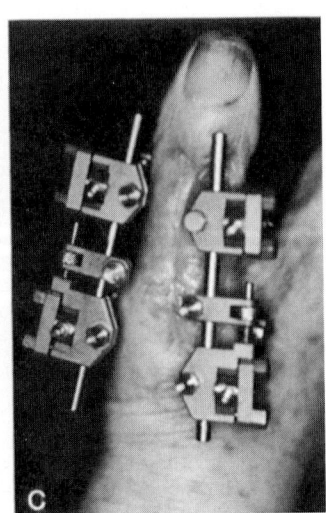

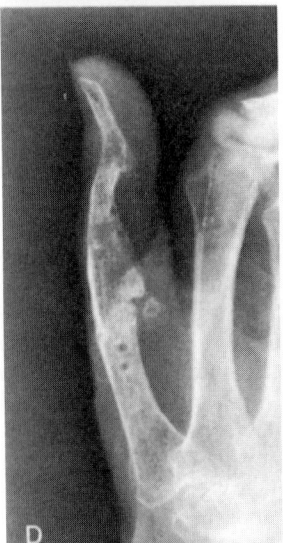

Fig. 3. External fixator technique. (From Bishop AT: Small joint arthrodesis. Hand Clin 1993; 9:685.)

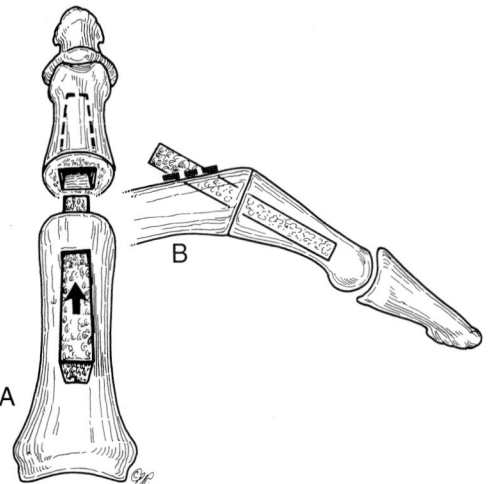

Fig. 4. Moberg's bone plug technique. (From Green DP: Green's Operative Hand Surgery. Philadelphia, Churchill Livingstone, 1999, 4th ed, p 104.)

pins[11] (Fig. 4), nuts and bolts,[12] pins and rubber bands,[13] K-wire/screw[14] (Fig. 5), wire loops/pin[15] (Fig. 6), tension band wire[16] (Fig. 7), Herbert's screw[17] (Fig. 8), and intramedullary polypropylene peg.[18]

INDICATIONS FOR ARTHRODESIS IN THE SMALL JOINTS OF THE HAND

The indications for arthrodesis in the small joints of the hand are consistent with those for arthrodesis in other joints of the body: pain, instability, deformity, and loss of function. Loss of muscle function to control a joint is also a primary reason for arthroplasty. Although arthrodesis is useful as an index procedure, it is also a salvage procedure for those patients who have undergone prior attempts at arthroplasty. The small joints of the hand that are amenable to arthrodesis include the interphalangeal (IP) joints of the fingers (i.e., the proximal IP [PIP] joint and the distal IP [DIP] joints), the metacarpophalangeal (MCP) joints, and

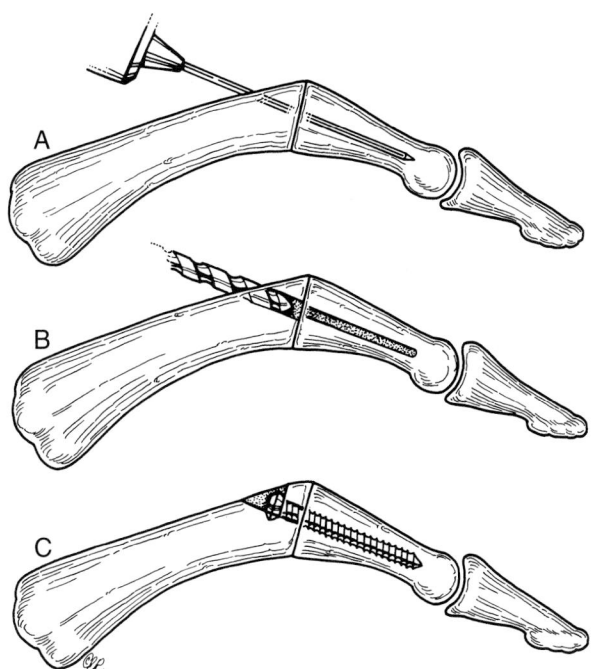

Fig. 5. Lag screw technique. (From Green DP: Green's Operative Hand Surgery. Philadelphia, Churchill Livingstone, 1999, 4th ed, p 100.)

In the DIP joints, a position between 0 degrees of flexion (i.e., full extension) or a small amount of flexion is ideal, although some authors advocated as much as 20 degrees of flexion. Generally, full extension, or near full extension, is the ideal position. In terms of the fingers themselves, the goal is a gentle cascade with more extension on the radial side (i.e., index finger) and more flexion on the ulnar side (i.e., little finger). These rules apply to PIP and metaphalangeal (MP) arthrodesis positions (Fig. 9). Index finger MP arthrodesis should be performed in a position so the thumb can oppose the tip of the index finger to pinch. This is generally approximately 25 degrees. From this position, an increasing amount of flexion (i.e., 5 degrees) at each successive joint may be appropriate, with resulting 40 degrees of MP flexion at the little finger MP joint. In terms

in the thumb the carpometacarpophalangeal (CMC) joint. As mentioned, the alternative procedures in the small joints of the hand that primarily flex and extend include silicone implant arthroplasty or autologous interposition soft-tissue graft arthroplasty. Special considerations for small joint arthrodesis apply to the CMC joint, because the function of this joint involves more than flexion/extension, which is the usual motion of the other small joints of the hand that are candidates for arthrodesis. In the thumb, there are a wider variety of alternatives to arthrodesis.

More specific indications include post-traumatic arthritis, osteoarthritis, systemic arthropathies, and acquired deformity secondary to soft-tissue problems (Table 1).

As stated, the evaluation of a patient's joint as an appropriate candidate for arthrodesis includes careful analysis of the entire extremity and, in particular, the status of the adjacent joints, those proximal and distal to the joint. The natural result of arthrodesis along a finger will be to increase stress in the remaining proximal or distal joint. Therefore, the likelihood of degenerative arthritis developing in the remaining joints is somewhat higher and needs to be taken into consideration when planning the arthrodesis.

OPERATIVE TECHNIQUE

The goals of arthrodesis in the small joints of the fingers are the same regardless of the surgical technique used to achieve them.

POSITION

Gentle flexion of the MCP joints is desirable because the fingers should still be able to grip objects of varying size.

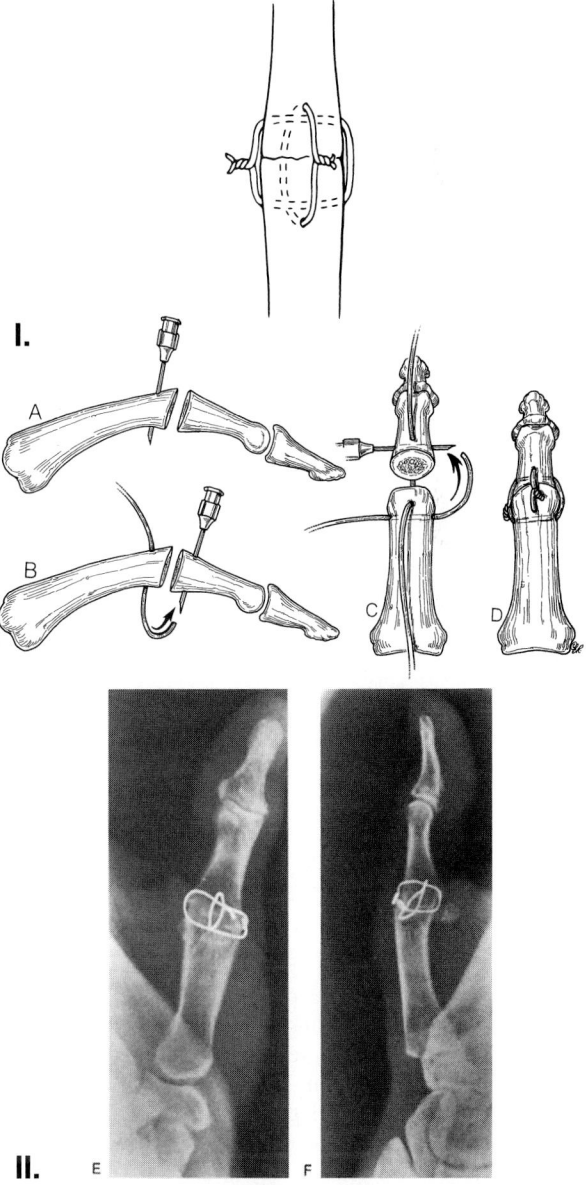

Fig. 6. Interosseous wiring technique. (From Hand Clin 1994; 10: 273; From Green DP: Green's Operative Hand Surgery. Philadelphia, Churchill Livingstone, 1999, 4th ed, p 99.)

A

B

C

D

E

F

I

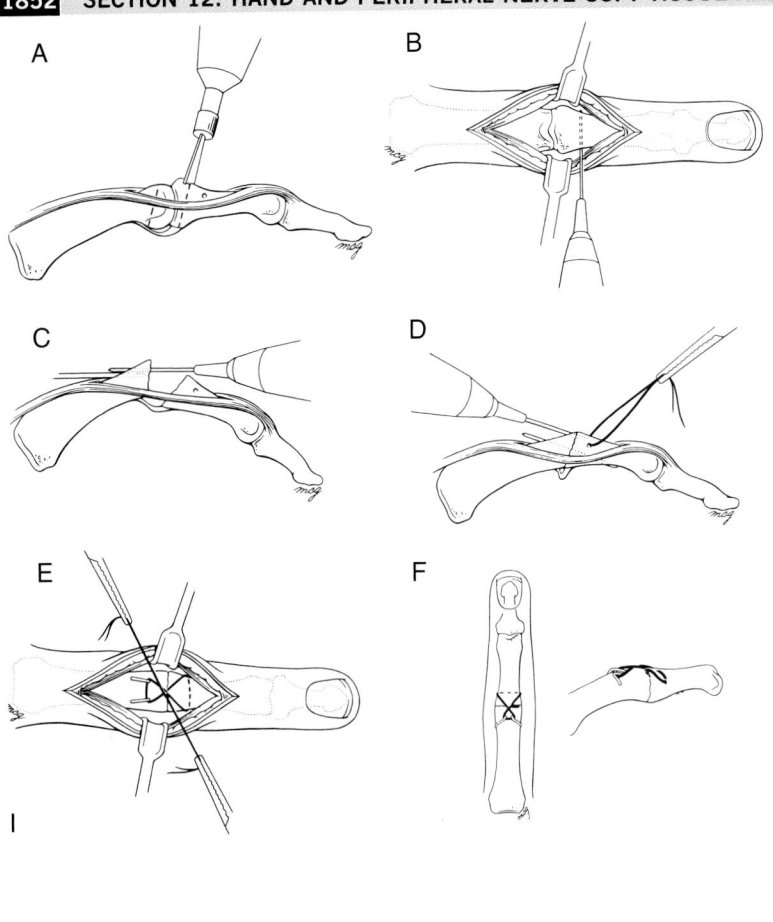

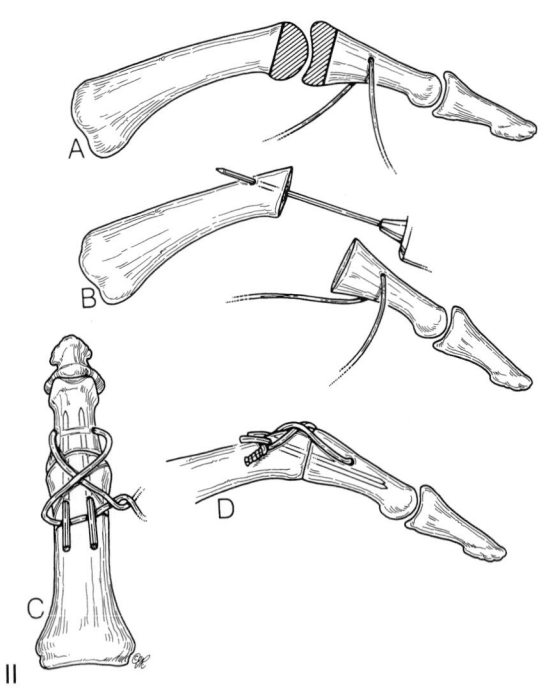

Fig. 7. Tension band wiring technique. (From Stern PJ, Gates NT, Jones TB: Tension band arthrodesis of small joints in the hand. J Hand Surg Am 1993; 18:196; Green DP: Green's Operative Hand Surgery. Philadelphia, Churchill Livingstone, 1999, 4th ed, p 100.)

II

of the PIP joint, the range recommended is from between 20 degrees on the index finger to 55 degrees for the little finger. On average, 40 degrees is recommended, with perhaps a little more flexion (i.e., 50 degrees at the little finger). I believe that 40 degrees is roughly an appropriate angle. It should be emphasized that the optimal position for each joint to be arthrodesed may depend on the particulars of the patient's hand and also the occupational activities that this hand will be required to perform. For example, a patient who handles small manual tools may require greater flexion of joints in the ring and little finger. Alternatively,

a patient who uses the hand in the open position to maintain the palm and fingers flat on a surface may require more extension.

With the index, middle finger, and thumb, one of the goals should be effective pulp-to-pulp pinch with the thumb. Therefore, mild supination of the index and middle finger or pronation of thumb may be helpful. Some of the techniques shorten the fingers slightly, which is acceptable, because if a finger is to be rendered immobile, it is advantageous to have it shortened a little. However, shortening should be avoided in the thumb, in which normal

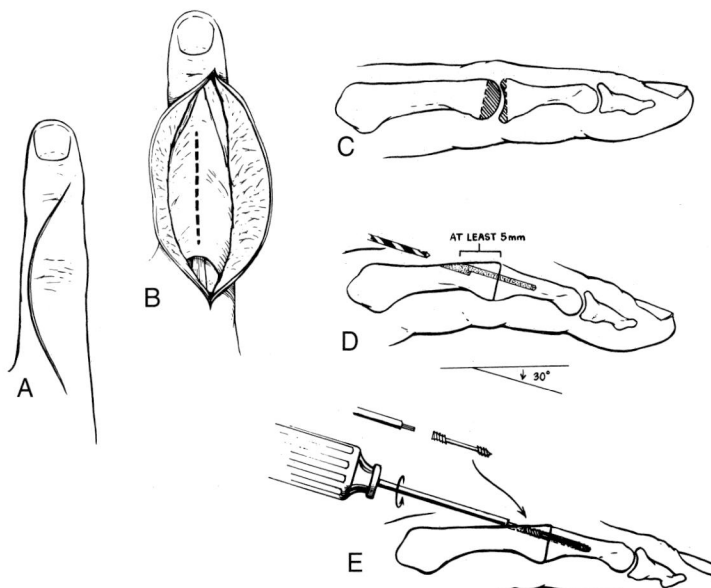

Fig. 8. Herbert's screw technique. (From Ayres JR, Goldstrohn GL, Miller GJ, et al: Proximal interphalangeal joint arthrodesis with the Herbert screw. J Hand Surg Am 1988; 13:601.)

length is desirable. In terms of the MCP joint of the thumb, 5 to 15 degrees of flexion is generally appropriate (Fig. 10).

PREPARATION

Preparation of the arthrodesis site involves exposure of the joint, reflection of the soft tissues, resection of the surrounding soft-tissue envelope and joint capsule, and preparation of the joint surfaces. With the fingers, one of the most expeditious ways to expose the IP or MP joints is through a dorsal approach. In the DIP joint, this can be a proximally based U-shaped flap, with the transverse limb halfway between the lunula, the distal hyponychial fold, and the extension creases at the DIP joint, with the longitudinal limbs roughly along the midaxial line. This affords good exposure of the margins of the joint as well as the

TABLE 1. INDICATIONS FOR ARTHRODESIS	
Type	**Indications**
Post-traumatic arthritis	Sequelae of interarticular fractures
	Sequelae of interarticular dislocations
	Sequelae of interarticular fracture/dislocations
	Sequelae of joint dislocations or fracture/dislocation followed by tendon imbalance (boutonnière or swan-neck deformities)
	Fixed contracture after joint dislocations or fracture/dislocations
	Contractures after burns
	Muscular disorder causing muscle imbalance, compartment syndromes, or post-ischemic contractures
	Contractures after open trauma (i.e., lacerations with skin and soft-tissue adhesions, including tendons, collateral ligaments, or volar plate joint capsule)
Osteoarthritis and systemic arthropathies	Rheumatoid arthritis
	Systemic lupus erythematosus
	Psoriatic arthritis
	Scleroderma
	CREST syndrome
Acquired deformity secondary to soft-tissue problems	Postburn contractures
	Dupuytren's contracture with severe deformities
	Peripheral nerve palsies leading to instability or muscle imbalance
	Central nervous system disorders leading to instability or muscle imbalance
	Salvages of digits with tendon dysfunction (i.e., flexor digitorum profundus disruptions in which a "superficialis" finger is indicated with DIP joint arthrodesis)
	Mallet finger deformity refractory to splint treatment or soft-tissue reconstruction
	Collateral ligament injury, especially thumb MCP joint

CREST syndrome, *c*alcinosis cutis, *R*aynaud's phenomenon, *e*sophageal dysfunction, *s*clerodactyly, and *t*elangiectasia; DIP, distal interphalangeal; MCP, metacarpophalangeal.

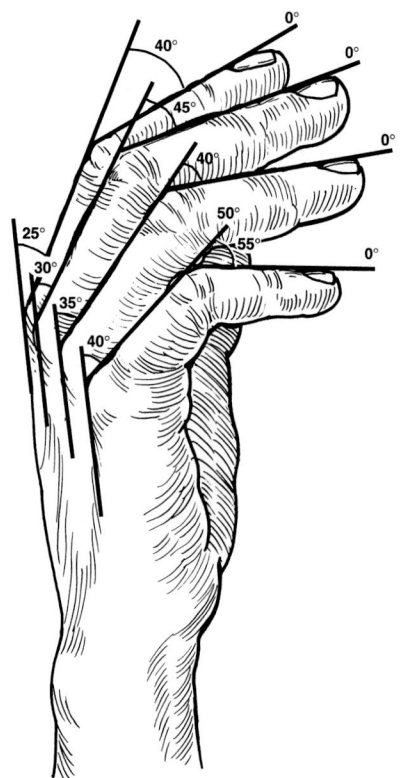

Fig. 9. Preferred positions for arthrodesis of the finger joints. (From Green DP: Green's Operative Hand Surgery. Philadelphia, Churchill Livingstone, 1999, 4th ed, p 96.)

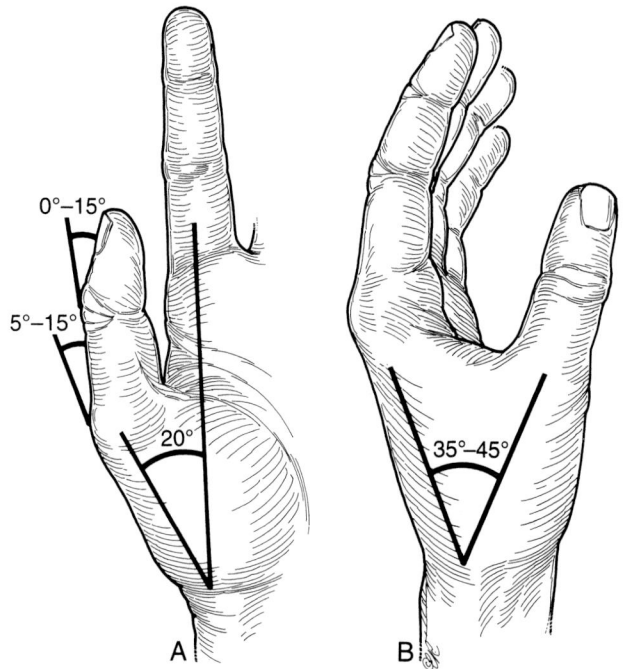

Fig. 10. Preferred position for thumb joint arthrodesis. (From Green DP: Green's Operative Hand Surgery. Philadelphia, Churchill Livingstone, 1999, 4th ed, p 97.)

dorsum of the joint. It is a useful incision for surgery on the DIP joint for conditions such as mallet deformities and mucous cysts. Alternatively, a chevron, or Y-shaped, incision can be used with the proximal longitudinal midline limb joined over the DIP joint by two oblique limbs to expose the joint. An H-type incision can also be used at the DIP joint and may be particularly appropriate for the thumb (Fig. 11). For the PIP joint, the simplest incision is a straight incision or a gentle S-shaped incision over the dorsum of the PIP joint. Exposure, then, is through an extensor tendon longitudinal splitting approach, repaired afterward with a nonabsorbable suture. For exposure of the PIP joint, takedown of the central slip insertion on the base of the middle phalanx is required, but its repair is unnecessary because the middle phalanx will be fused to the proximal phalanx. Reconstruction of the lateral bands is, however, critical to prevent postoperative boutonnière deformity.

The MCP joint is easily exposed through a dorsal approach as well. The skin incision can be longitudinal, S-shaped, or transverse, depending on whether the surgeon is operating on one or multiple joints, as in a patient with rheumatoid arthritis. Exposure of the MCP joint is preferably accomplished not through a central extensor tendon splitting incision, as in the PIP joint, but to one side of the central extensor digitorum communis (EDC) tendon. Therefore, longitudinal division of the sagittal band and extensor hood mechanism is required to gain wide exposure to the MCP joint. After such exposure, reconstruction of the sagittal band and hood mechanism must be performed to pre-

vent subluxation of the EDC, which would result in an extension lag defect in the MCP joint.

METHODS OF FIXATION
Laboratory Studies

Several laboratory studies examined the biomechanical efficacies of various methods of arthrodesis fixation. Wyrsch et al[19] compared tension band and Herbert's screw fixation in DIP joint arthrodesis. The Herbert screw demonstrated significantly greater anteroposterior bending strength and torsional rigidity than did tension bands. This occurred despite fracture or thread penetration at the tip of the distal phalanx in many of the specimens during screw placement. Vanik et al[20] used a cadaver bending test to evaluate fixation of a transverse diaphyseal metacarpal osteotomy using K-wires, interosseous wires, dorsal five-hole plate fixation, and lateral five-hole plate fixation. Interosseous wires per-

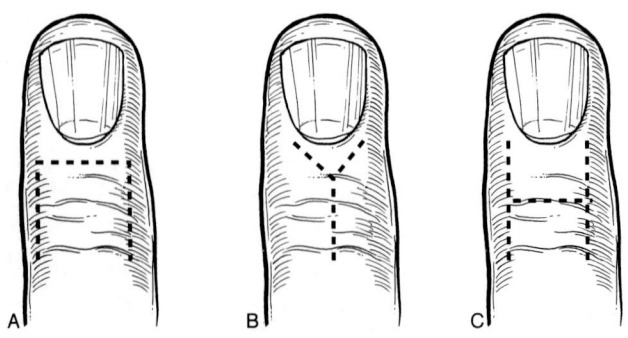

Fig. 11. Surgical approaches to the distal interphalangeal joint. (From Green DP: Green's Operative Hand Surgery. Philadelphia, Churchill Livingstone, 1999, 4th ed, p 104.)

formed the best followed by K-wires. Kovach et al[21] performed a biomechanical study to compare crossed K-wires, tension bands, and a single interosseous loop supplemented by K-wire fixation for PIP joint arthrodesis. Tension bands were found to be the strongest.

Clinical Studies

Stern et al[22] reported on 290 small joint arthrodeses of MCP and PIP joints using tension bands with 0.028- or 0.035-inch K-wires and 25- or 26-gauge stainless steel wires through threaded holes. They reported a 3% nonunion rate, and 9% of the fusions required hardware removal. Four patients had a painless pseudarthrosis at the operation site. The authors concluded that tension bands provided reliable, stable fixation with some compression, and in compliant patients they were able to dispense with external splinting.

Leibovic and Strickland[23] reviewed the Indiana hand experience with small joint arthrodesis. In this series, K-wires were associated with the highest nonunion rate, tension bands had an intermediate nonunion rate, and Herbert's screws had the lowest nonunion rate. They found a 50% failure rate in the plates compared with a 21% failure rate of K-wires, a 5% failure rate of tension bands, and a 0.5% failure rate of Herbert's screws. Traditionally, the most common type of fixation for arthrodesis has been crossed K-wires. In a review by Burton et al,[24] 171 consecutive arthrodeses of small joints of the hand were performed on 134 patients using the technique described by Littler.[25] Excellent alignment of bone surfaces with flat-bone cuts, accurate placement of crossed K-wires, and use of supplemental cancellous bone graft were the hallmarks of this technique. These authors achieved union in 170 of 171 arthrodeses for a nonunion rate of 0.6%. There were no infections and only four delayed unions. Uhl and Schneider[26] reviewed 76 consecutive cases of tension band arthrodesis with a fusion rate of 99%. IJsselstein et al[27] retrospectively reviewed 203 arthrodeses to compare tension bands and various conventional K-wire techniques, including single K-wire, crossed K-wires, and crossed K-wires with interosseous wires. There was an 18% incidence of pin site infection and a 15% reoperation rate in the K-wire groups. There was a 2% rate of infection in the tension band group and a 5% reoperation rate. In their hands, tension bands offered the best results. McGlynn et al[28] used K-wires for fixation of bones prepared by a high-speed bur and achieved bone union in 10 weeks or less in 86% of digits. This modification of the Carroll and Hill technique using a power bur proved effective in these authors' hands. When combined with three K-wires, they found that external mobilization may be unnecessary. Evolving from Kirschner's and interosseous wires, various types of screws, plates, external fixators, and bone plugs have been used to effect arthrodesis. Faithfull and Herbert[29] reviewed use of the Herbert bone screw and achieved a 100% union rate in the small joints of the finger and thumb in 25 patients. Using lag screws, Wright and McMurtry[30] reported a 96% fusion rate in 110 joints in 83 patients. There was a 100% fusion rate at the PIP joint and 96% at the MP joint. Of their four failures, two had infections. In a more recent study by Katzman et al[31] of 51 Herbert's screw arthrodeses in IP joints in patients with

degenerative or post-traumatic arthritis as well as rheumatoid arthritis or mallet finger deformities, solid osseous union occurred in all patients, with an average interval to fusion of 8 weeks. Nine of 33 rheumatoid joints required supplemental K-wires to prevent rotation. There were six complications, mostly in rheumatoid patients.

The first large tension band arthrodesis series in the finger joints was reported by Allende and Engelem.[32] They had a total of 26 digits, with only five complications, two infections, two cases of malunion or delayed union, and only one case of carpometacarpal joint arthrodesis. Büchler and Aiken[33] described plate fixation in 18 patients with severe industrial injuries with segmental bone loss. Plates are useful in more severe cases of post-traumatic joint destruction. Watson and Lovallo[34] described an arthrodesis technique for severe Dupuytren's contraction in which the proximal phalanx was shortened and then arthrodesed at the resultant PIP joint. External fixation techniques were described in two series. Braun and Rhoades[35] described dynamic compression using K-wires and methylmethacrylate to provide dynamic compression for small joint arthrodesis in 31 joints. They had no angular malunions or nonunions and considered this a viable alternative technique. Bishop[36] described the use of commercially available external fixators for arthrodesis.

Teoh et al[37] described an alternative method of A-O screw fixation using an oblique lag screw with a 96% union rate in 23 joints. More recently, biodegradable pins have been introduced in hand surgery. Jensen and Jensen[38] compared biodegradable pins with K-wires. They found no difference in time to union or complication rates. They indicated that biodegradable pins offered certain advantages, because no additional procedures were needed in the 11 patients with them compared with the 12 patients in the K-wire group. Perhaps of more historical interest is the bone peg as a method of bone grafting in those patients with severe bone loss. The original technique described in 1960 by Moberg and Henrikson[39] used bone grafts cut in straight square sections. Baruch and Kahanovich[40] described an angulated bone peg taken from the ulna or iliac crest for patients with bone loss and instability after trauma to the finger and failed arthroplasty.

Stern and Fulton[41] performed a study that specifically examined complications of small joint arthrodesis. They studied 181 arthrodeses of DIP and thumb IP joints. They compared various techniques, including crossed K-pins (111 joints), interfragmentary wires and longitudinal K-pins (43 joints), and Herbert's screws (27 joints). The nonunion rate was similar in each technique. There were 21 nonunions, of which 13 were pain free and six required subsequent arthrodeses (with one amputation and one patient who refused further surgery). Twenty percent of the fused joints had major complications: nonunion, malunion, deep infection, and osteomyelitis. Sixteen percent of patients experienced minor complications such as superficial wound infections, dorsal skin necrosis, cold intolerance, PIP stiffness, paresthesias, and prominent hardware. This study presents a more pessimistic view of the potential complications of small joint arthrodesis. Nonetheless, overall, arthrodesis in small joints of the hand is a very useful and predictable treatment and certainly the best treatment for some of the conditions that require reconstructive surgery.

ARTHRODESIS WITH OPEN PHYSIS

Kowalski and Manske[42] described an open physis technique for arthrodesis in the skeletally immature patient that avoids interference with the growth plate (Fig. 12). This technique was successful in 43 of 47 patients. At the proximal bone involved in the arthrodesis, a sharp blade is used to make progressive cuts perpendicular to the long axis of the shaft and in line with the anticipated plane of arthrodesis; thin layers of articular cartilage are sequentially removed until the bony center of ossification is reached. The surgeon is cautioned not to proceed beyond the ossific nucleus and into the physeal plate itself. Subchondral bone is carefully removed to expose the underlying cancellous bone. On the opposite articular surface a similar procedure is done, and then crossed K-wires are used to fuse the opposing articular surfaces.

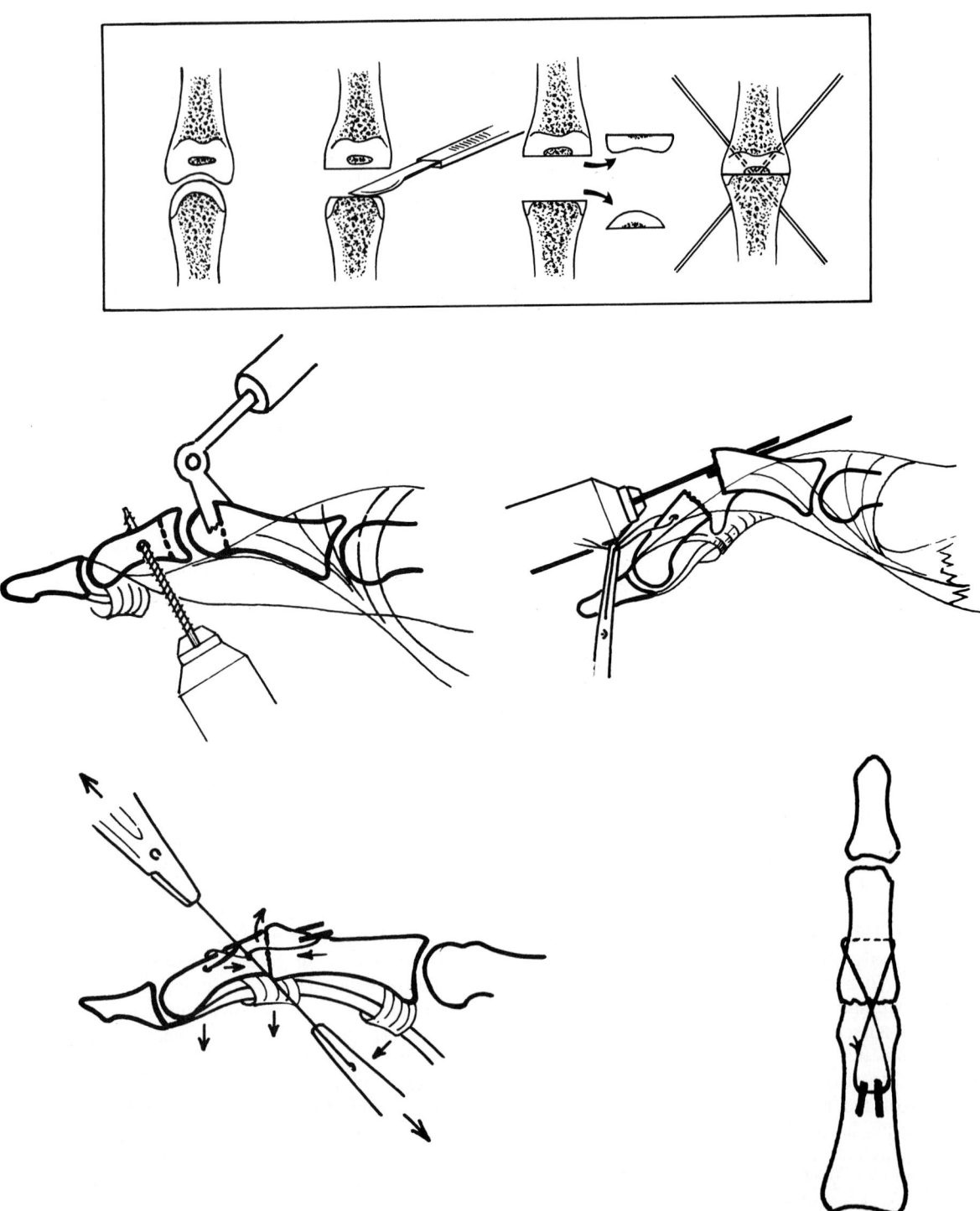

Fig. 12. Arthrodesis with open physis technique. (From Kowalski MF, Manske PR: Arthrodesis of digital joints in children. J Hand Surg Am 1988; 13:875.)

Author's Preferred Technique: DIP Arthrodesis

Either of the most common incisions—the dorsal H type or the inverted-U type—works well. After the skin incision, care is taken to protect the skin flaps and keep the soft-tissue plane deep (i.e., at the level of the epitenon of the terminal tendon, which will decrease the risk of dorsal skin necrosis). The extensor tendon can be divided at the level of the joint and elevated with the capsule to expose the joint. Surgical removal of marginal osteophytes with curets and rongeurs is performed. Sectioning of the collateral ligaments may facilitate exposure of the joint surfaces. Bone can be resected either by curets, oscillating saw, or osteotomes. In the DIP joint, I prefer the flat-bone cut technique to that of the cup-and-cone.

The Herbert screw (Fig. 13) provides excellent bone fixation when bone stock is adequate and the cross-sectional dimensions of the bone are large enough to accommodate the screw. Alternatively, a mini-Herbert's screw can be used for smaller fingers. Preparation with a standard retrograde technique with hand drilling is performed for the core hole, tapping for the screw threads and then placing the appropriately sized screw in a retrograde fashion.

It is critical to place the Herbert screw precisely. It is difficult to revise a screw that has been placed in the wrong position. Intraoperative fluoroscopy is essential for accurate placement of implants. An appropriate depth screw is selected and then placed to provide compression at the arthrodesis site. Splinting is advocated for the first 4 weeks.

Selecting alternative techniques of fixation is determined by the quality and quantity of bone available at the DIP. The surgeon may need to select K-wire instead of screw fixation. I believe that interosseous wires, although they provide good compression, require more significant surgical exposure than do Herbert's screw or K-wire fixation (Fig. 14) and thus have more limited applications.

Author's Preferred Technique: PIP Arthrodesis

The PIP has somewhat different considerations than the DIP. It has larger bones and bone surfaces; therefore, ac-

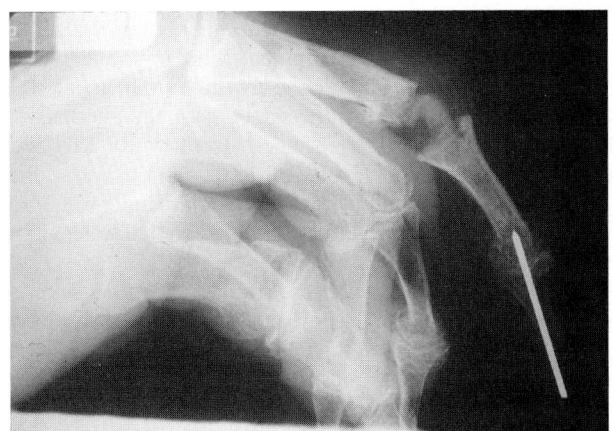

Fig. 14. K-wire fixation. This is one of the arthrodesis techniques for salvage and segmental defects in the DIP joint. Radiographic lateral view of DIP arthrodesis with single longitudinal K-wire fixation. Note the PIP silicone implant arthroplasty in the same digit.

ceptance of screw fixation is not an issue. However, to have good bone purchase at both the head of the screw proximally and the screw threads distally, relatively larger screws must be used in an oblique or intramedullary fashion. Therefore, the bone resection and bone removal that may be required can be significant. Moreover, to use an A-O lag screw, there may be significant cortical bone that

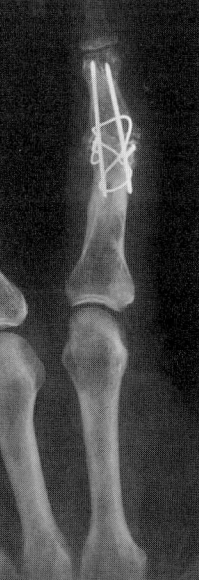

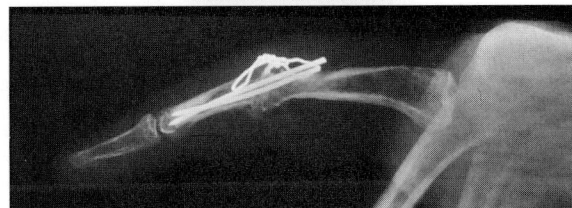

Fig. 15. Arthrodeses with the tension band technique. These are anteroposterior (A) and lateral (B) radiographs. This is a PIP joint fusion of the ring finger.

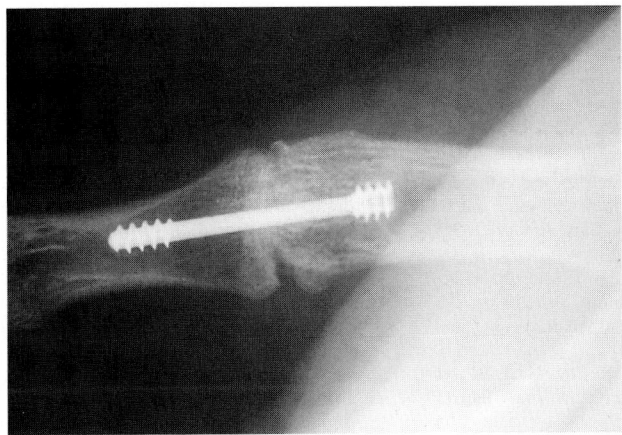

Fig. 13. Herbert's screw fixation for metacarpophalangeal thumb joint arthrodesis.

is removed to allow adequate "seating" of the head of the screw in an anterograde placement with proximal phalangeal bone removal. Therefore, K-wires supplemented by tension bands provide an excellent surgical alternative.[22] There usually is good bone stock to allow for this technique, and minimal bone removal is required. Several clinical studies also support its use as a treatment method, preferentially for PIP arthrodesis (Fig. 15). The technique is illustrated in Figure 7.

The PIP joint is exposed by a longitudinal incision. An extensor tendon splitting approach is followed by removal of the central slip and retraction of the lateral bands along either side. The joint capsule is exposed, and collateral ligament excision is performed as needed to allow exposure of the joint surfaces. Bone can be fashioned either through flat cuts or Carroll and Hill's[2] cup-and-cone tech-

nique. Two longitudinal K-wires, either 0.035 or 0.045 inch, are passed anterograde from the distal metaphyseal portion of the proximal phalanx down the intramedullary space of the middle phalanx to engage the palmar cortex at the midportion of the middle phalanx. Joint angles are determined using the guidelines mentioned previously. A transverse bone tunnel is made with a K-wire in the junction of the proximal one-third to the proximal one-half of the middle phalanx. A 25-gauge wire is passed through the bone tunnel and looped in a figure-of-eight fashion over the longitudinal pins and tightened. The extensor mechanism is repaired with 5-0 nonabsorbable suture, and the skin is closed. Temporary splinting is provided, and, depending on the patient, early mobilization is possible with good bone stock and adequate surgical technique in the compliant patient.

REFERENCES

1. Badger FG: Arthrodesis of the carpo-metacarpal joint of the thumb. J Bone Joint Surg Br 1964; 46:162.
2. Carroll RE, Hill NA: Small joint arthrodesis in hand reconstruction. J Bone Joint Surg Am 1969; 51:1219.
3. Eaton RG, Littler JW: A study of the basal joint of the thumb. J Bone Joint Surg Am 1969; 51:661.
4. Gervis H: Excision of the trapezium for osteoarthritis of the trapezio-metacarpal joint. J Bone Joint Surg Br 1949; 31:537.
5. Leach RE, Bolton PE: Arthritis of the carpo-metacarpal joint of the thumb. J Bone Joint Surg Am 1968; 50:1171.
6. Muller GM: Arthrodesis of the trapeziometacarpal joint for osteoarthritis. J Bone Joint Surg Br 1949; 31:540.
7. Omer GE Jr: Evaluation and reconstruction of the forearm and hand after acute traumatic peripheral nerve injuries. J Bone Joint Surg Am 1968; 50:1454.
8. Robertson DC: The function of the interphalangeal joints. Can J Surg 1964; 7:433.
9. Granowitz S, Vainio K: Proximal interphalangeal joint arthrodesis in rheumatoid arthritis. A follow-up study of 122 operations. Acta Orthop Scand 1966; 37:301.
10. Tupper JW: A compression arthrodesis device for small joints of the hands. Hand 1972; 4:62.
11. Potenza AD: Brief note. A technique for arthrodesis of finger joints. J Bone Joint Surg Am 1973; 55:1534.
12. Ikuta Y, Tsuge K: Micro-bolts and microscrews for fixation of small bones in the hand. Hand 1974; 6:261.
13. Wexler MR, Rousso M, Weinberg H: Arthrodesis of finger joints by dynamic external compression using dorsoventral Kirschner wires and rubber bands. Plast Reconstr Surg 1977; 60:882.
14. Engel J, Tsur H, Farin I: A comparison between K-wire and compression screw fixation after arthodesis of the distal interphalangeal joint. Plast Reconstr Surg 1977; 60:611.
15. Lister G: Intraosseous wiring of the digital skeleton. J Hand Surg Am 1978; 3:427.
16. Segmüller G: Surgical Stabilization of the Skeleton of the Hand. Baltimore, Williams & Wilkins, 1977, p 45.
17. Ayres JR, Goldstrohm GL, Miller GJ, et al: Proximal interphalangeal joint arthrodesis with the Herbert screw. J Hand Surg Am 1988; 13:600.
18. Sanderson PL, Morris MA, Fahmy NR: A long-term review of the Harrison-Nicolle peg in digital arthrodesis. J Hand Surg Br 1991; 16:283.
19. Wyrsch B, Dawson J, Aufranc S, et al: Distal interphalangeal joint arthrodesis comparing tension-band wire and Herbert screw: A biomechanical and dimensional analysis. J Hand Surg Am 1996; 21:438.
20. Vanik RK, Weber RC, Matloub HS, et al: The comparative strengths of internal fixation techniques. J Hand Surg Am 1984; 9:216.
21. Kovach JC, Werner FW, Palmer AK, et al: Biomechanical analysis of internal fixation techniques for proximal interphalangeal joint arthrodesis. J Hand Surg Am 1986; 11:562.
22. Stern PJ, Gates NT, Jones TB: Tension band arthrodesis of small joints in the hand. J Hand Surg Am 1993; 18:194.
23. Leibovic SJ, Strickland JW: Arthrodesis of the proximal interphalangeal joint of the finger: Comparison of the use of the Herbert screw with other fixation methods. J Hand Surg Am 1994; 19:181.
24. Burton RI, Margles SW, Lunseth PA: Small-joint arthrodesis in the hand. J Hand Surg Am 1986; 11:678.
25. Littler JW: Tendon transfers and arthrodesis in combined median and ulnar nerve paralysis. J Bone Joint Surg Am 1949; 31:225.
26. Uhl RL, Schneider LH: Tension band arthrodesis of finger joints: A retrospective review of 76 consecutive cases. J Hand Surg Am 1992; 17:518.
27. IJsselstein C, Hovius SE, ten Have BL, et al: Is the pectoralis myocutaneous flap in intraoral and oropharyngeal reconstruction outdated? Am J Surg 1996; 172:259.
28. McGlynn JT, Smith RA, Bogumill GP: Arthrodesis of small joint of the hand: A rapid and effective technique. J Hand Surg Am 1988; 13:595.
29. Faithfull DK, Herbert TJ: Small joint fusions of the hand using the Herbert bone screw. J Hand Surg Br 1984;9:167.
30. Wright CS, McMurtry RY: AO arthrodesis in the hand. J Hand Surg Am 1983; 8:932.
31. Katzman SS, Gibeault JD, Dickson K, et al: Use of a Herbert screw for interphalangeal joint arthrodesis. Clin Orthop Rel Res 1993; 296:127.
32. Allende BT, Engelem JC: Tension-band arthrodesis in the finger joints. J Hand Surg Am 1980; 5:269.
33. Büchler U, Aiken MA: Arthrodesis of the proximal interphalangeal joint by solid bone grafting and plate fixation in extensive injuries to the dorsal aspect of the finger. J Hand Surg Am 1988; 13:589.
34. Watson HK, Lovallo JL: Salvage of severe recurrent Dupuytren's contracture of the ring and small fingers. J Hand Surg Am 1987; 12:287.
35. Braun RM, Rhoades CE: Dynamic compression for small bone arthrodesis. J Hand Surg Am 1985; 10:340.
36. Bishop AT: Small joint arthrodesis. Hand Clin 1993; 9:683.
37. Teoh LC, Yeo SJ, Singh I: Interphalangeal joint arthrodesis with oblique placement of an AO lag screw. J Hand Surg Br 1994; 19:208.
38. Jensen CH, Jensen CM: Biodegradable pins versus Kirschner wires in hand surgery. J Hand Surg Br 1996; 21:507.
39. Moberg E, Henrikson B: Technique for digital arthrodesis: A study of 150 cases. Acta Chir Scand 1959–1960; 118:331.
40. Baruch A, Kahanovich S: Angulated bone peg. Plast Reconstr Surg 1980; 66:471.
41. Stern PJ, Fulton DB: Distal interphalangeal joint arthrodesis: An analysis of complications. J Hand Surg Am 1992; 17:1139.
42. Kowalski MF, Manske PR: Arthrodesis of digital joints in children. J Hand Surg Am 1988; 13:874.

TENDON TRANSFERS IN THE UPPER EXTREMITY

Jack Choueka and Daniel P. Mass

Summary
- Tendon transfers are performed to substitute for the function of muscles paralyzed or weakened by nerve damage or injury, to replace severed or avulsed tendons, or to correct the balance of the hand.
- The goal is to restore or improve function of the hand without adversely affecting the function provided by the transferred musculotendinous unit.
- Each case must be individualized. The operative plan can usually be determined from a detailed history and physical examination but may require electrodiagnostic studies.
- Considerations in tendon transfers include muscle availability, muscle force, direction of pull, and integrity and mobility of the proposed tendon transfer.
- Postoperatively, tendon transfers should be protected until the patient begins an extensive rehabilitation program, which includes range of motion and strengthening.

Tendon transfers in the upper extremity can restore function to a hand paralyzed by nerve damage or disease. Tendon transfers are most commonly performed for paralysis or weakening of muscle secondary to nerve injury or damage. They are less commonly performed for nerve damage secondary to compressive neuropathies. Another indication is rheumatoid arthritis, in which procedures are undertaken not only to correct an unbalanced hand secondary to progressive deformity but also to replace tendons ruptured by the disease process. In cerebral palsy and strokes, tendon transfers are performed to restore balance to the hand, and in direct trauma (avulsions or lacerations), to restore a tendon's competence.

This chapter concentrates on tendon transfers performed for nerve paralysis in the upper extremity, allowing a more focused discussion on the principles involved in tendon transfers, which are easily extrapolated to other clinical scenarios. Table 1 lists the common abbreviations used in the remainder of the chapter.

Selection of the proper tendon transfer requires a complete understanding of the patient's needs and the disease process. For example, a heavy laborer and a watchmaker have very different requirements and are commonly treated with different transfers for a similar deficit.

Tendon transfers are contraindicated in the patient with poor bony stability, a soft-tissue sleeve that is scarred so as to prevent tendon gliding, or a fixed joint contracture. They should only rarely be performed during the initial trauma procedure. In addition, tendon transfers should be performed with caution in patients who are unwilling or would be unable to participate in the postoperative proto-

col. Most important, the patient and physician must have realistic expectations and must not overestimate the potential of the tendon transfer.

HISTORICAL REVIEW

Tendon transfers were sparsely reported prior to the late 19th century. In 1881, Nicoladoni performed the first tendon transfer in the foot.[1] Although the transfer eventually failed, Nicoladoni prominence as the chairman of surgery at the University of Innsbruck and the overwhelming need for tendon transfers resulting from the recent outbreak of poliomyelitis in Europe set the stage for further development of the technique.[2] In 1893, Drobnik reported on 16 tendon transfers, and soon after, in 1897, Rochet performed the first tendon transfer for cerebral palsy.[2]

In 1914, Leo Mayer published a series on the physiological principles of tendon transfers,[3] which still hold true today; they are as follows:

- Restore the normal relationship between tendon and sheath.
- Course through tissue adapted to gliding of a tendon.
- Imitate normal insertion to bone or cartilage of the original tendon.
- Establish normal tension.
- Have an effective line of traction.

The outbreak of World War I altered the focus of tendon transfers from treatment of poliomyelitis and cerebral palsy in the lower extremity to traumatic reconstruction in the upper extremity. From immediately after World War I to the present, numerous tendon transfers have been described for the various nerve palsies.

CLINICAL FEATURES

LOW MEDIAN NERVE PALSY

Sensory Loss. Volar surface of thumb, index finger, long finger, and half of ring finger.

Motors Lost. First and second lumbricals, opponens pollicis, abductor pollicis brevis, flexor pollicis brevis (superficial half).

Functional Loss. Sensory loss often more disabling than motor loss. One third of patients with low median nerve palsy do not require opposition transfer because the ulnar innervation to the FPB can allow adequate opposition.

Associated Abnormalities. When nerve injury is secondary to laceration, flexor tendons are often involved, and this can affect possible transfer options. If neglected, thenar paralysis can lead to an *adduction* contracture.

General Principles. Opposition transfers should be aimed at positioning the thumb in preparation for grasp because ulnar-innervated intrinsics can flex the thumb. An

TABLE 1. COMMON ABBREVIATIONS USED IN CHAPTER	
Abbreviation	Definition
ADQ	Abductor digiti quinti
APB	Abductor pollicis brevis
APL	Abductor pollicis longus
BR	Brachioradial
DIP	Distal interphalangeal
ECRB	Extensor carpi radialis brevis
ECRL	Extensor carpi radialis longus
ECU	Extensor carpi ulnaris
EDC	Extensor digitorum communis
EDQ	Extensor digiti quinti
EIP	Extensor indicis proprius
EPB	Extensor pollicis brevis
EPL	Extensor pollicis longus
FCR	Flexor carpi radialis
FCU	Flexor carpi ulnaris
FDP	Flexor digitorum profundus
FDS	Flexor digitorum sublimis
FPL	Flexor pollicis longus
IP	Interphalangeal
MP	Metaphalangeal
MCP	Metacarpophalangeal
PIP	Proximal interphalangeal
PL	Peroneus longus
PQ	Pronator quadratus

overzealous transfer can therefore lead to an MP flexion deformity.

Authors' Preferred Transfer. EIP to APB (Burkhalter et al)[4] (Fig. 1).

Other Described Transfers
- FDS of ring finger to APB, with FCU as pulley (Littler).[5]
- ADQ to APB (Huber).[6]
- PL to radial side of MP joint of thumb (Camitz).[7]

HIGH MEDIAN NERVE PALSY

Sensory Loss. Same as for low median nerve palsy, plus radial palm of hand.

Motors Lost. In addition to those lost with low median nerve palsy, FPL, FDS, FDP to the index and long finger, pronator quadratus, and FCR are also lost.

Functional Loss. Thumb opposition and IP flexion, DIP flexion of the index and long fingers. Independent PIP flexion to all fingers.

Associated Abnormalities. Loss of forearm pronation can become disabling.

Authors' Preferred Transfers
- EIP to APB for opposition.
- Side-to-side transfer of FDP of ring and little fingers to FDP of index and middle finger.
- BR to FPL for thumb flexion.

Other Described Transfers. Burkhalter[8]:

- EIP to APB for opposition.
- ECRL to FDP of index and middle finger.
- BR to FPL for thumb flexion.

RADIAL NERVE PALSY

Loss of Sensation. Dorsum of thumb, index finger, long finger, and half of ring finger.

Motors Lost. APL, EPB, ECRB, EPL, EDC, EIP, EDQ, ECU. The ECRL and supinator are affected in high radial nerve palsies.

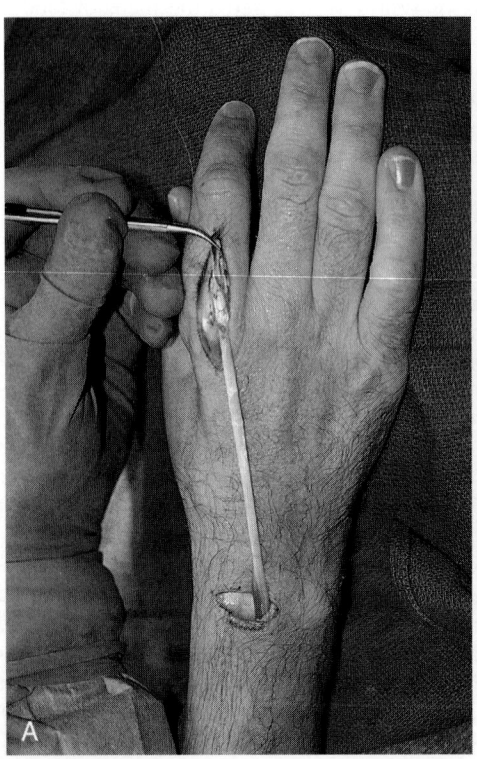
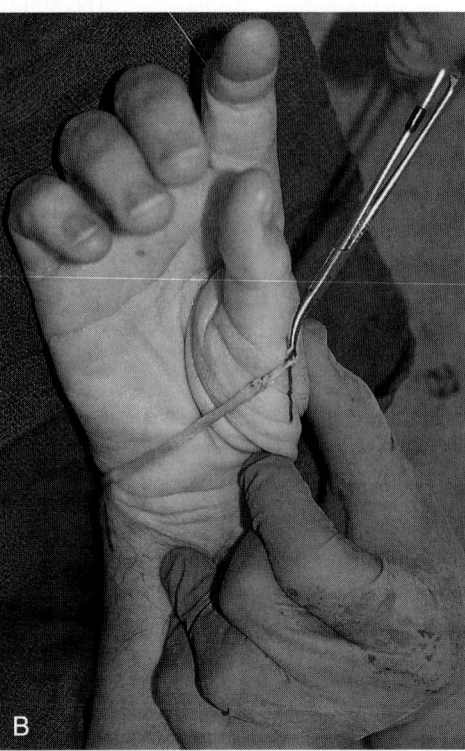

Fig. 1. View. *A,* The EIP is harvested as distally as possible and is brought out proximal to the extensor retinaculum. It is then brought around the ulnar side of the wrist, with care taken to protect the superficial branches of the ulnar nerve, and (*B*) attached to the insertion of the APB.

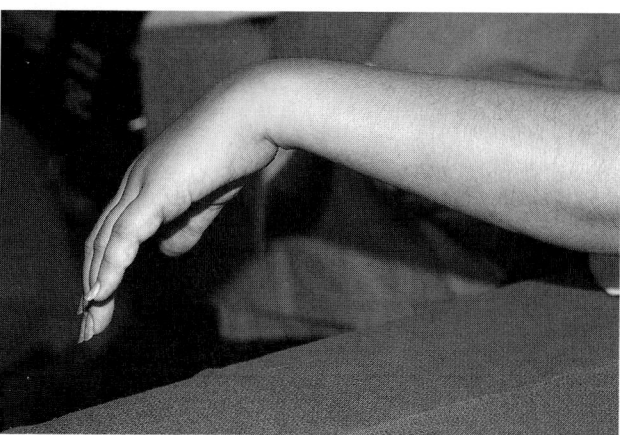

Fig. 2. View. This is radial nerve palsy: inability to extend the wrist or digits at the MP joint.

Functional Loss. Finger and wrist extension. Thumb extension and abduction (Fig. 2).

General Principles. Most profound dysfunction is secondary to the inability to extend the wrist. Transfer should be performed early to act as internal splint, avoiding the need for external devices while nerve is healing.

Associated Abnormalities. Often found in conjunction with humeral shaft fractures at the junction of the middle and distal thirds (Holstein-Lewis fracture).

Authors' Preferred Transfers. Modified from Brand[9] (Fig. 3):

- PT to ECRB for wrist extension ± yoke of ECRL transferred to the fourth metacarpal.
- PL to EPL through the first dorsal compartment, for thumb extension.
- FCR to EDC, through the interosseous membrane, for finger extension.

For low radial nerve palsies, we perform the same transfers without a transfer for wrist extension.

Other Described Transfers. Boyes[10]:

- PT to ECRB and ECRB for wrist extension.
- FCR to APL for thumb abduction.

- FDS (ring) to EPL and EIP for thumb and index extension.
- FDS (middle) to EDC for finger extension.

ULNAR NERVE PALSY

Sensory Loss. Little finger and ulnar half of ring finger.

Functional Loss. Digital abduction and adduction. Weakness of pinch and grasp. Impairment of precision hand function. Asynchronous pattern of finger flexion.

Associated Abnormalities

Froment's Sign.[11] Hyperextension of the thumb IP joint on powerful pinch (Fig. 4).

Jeanne's Sign.[12] Hyperextension of the thumb MCP joint on powerful pinch.

Clawing Deformity. Hyperextension at the MP joint caused by unrestricted extension by the extrinsic extensors. With attempted extension of the PIP or DIP joints, the MP hyperextension increases, tightening the FDS and FDP. With high ulnar nerve palsy, the two flexors are paralyzed, decreasing the clawing deformity.

Authors' Preferred Transfers

- ECRL with palmaris tendon for lengthening to the extensor hood versus volar MP capsulorraphies, depending on the need for strength.
- FDS to first dorsal interosseous to restore index abduction.
- Ring FDS to adductor pollicis to restore thumb adduction.

INVESTIGATION

In addition to a thorough history and physical examination, electrodiagnostic tests can be helpful in determining the most appropriate tendon transfers. Such tests can aid in establishing both the return capacity of a paralyzed muscle and the relative strength of a tendon proposed for transfer.

GOALS

The goal of any tendon transfer is (1) to restore missing or weakened function or (2) to restore balance to the hand without adversely affecting the function of the transferred tendon.

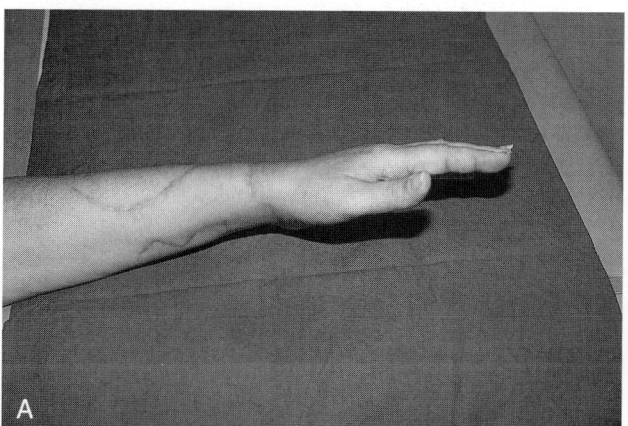
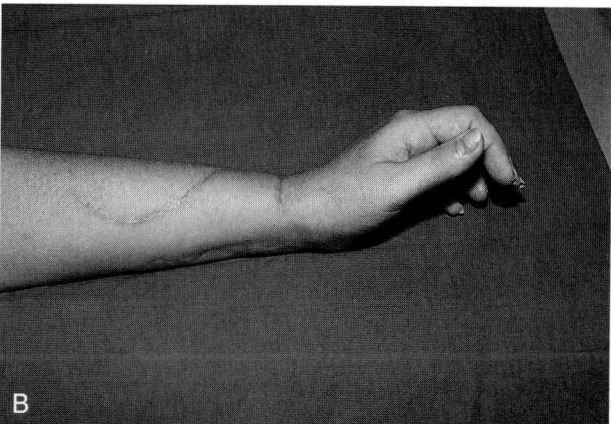

Fig. 3. View. *A,* Active finger extension with wrist neutral. *B,* Active wrist extension allows incomplete finger extension. After transfers, there is active, completely functional wrist, finger, and thumb extension.

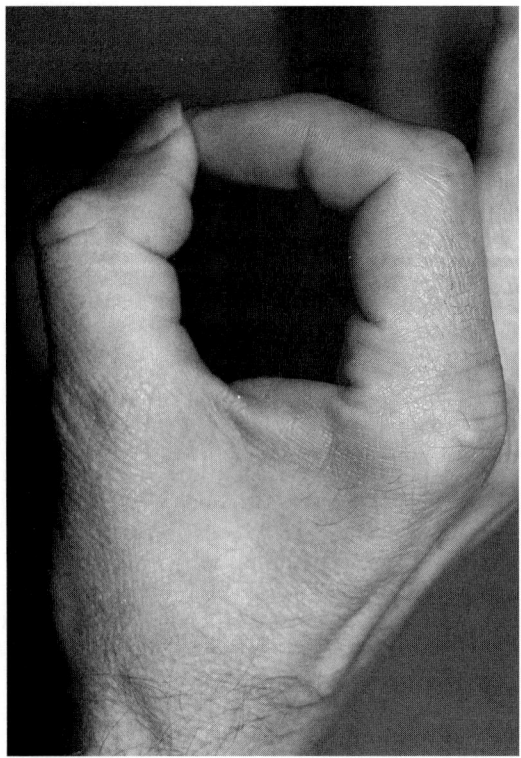

Fig. 4. View. This is Froment's sign, as described in text. Note atrophy of the first dorsal interosseous.

DISADVANTAGES

The main disadvantage of a tendon transfer is the loss of the original function of the transferred muscle. Regardless of the tendons remaining to perform the original function, there is always a measurable loss of strength associated with the sacrifice of a tendon. Another main disadvantage is common inability to transfer the tendon effectively because of trauma, ongoing disease, or lack of available tendons. In these cases, alternatives to the tendon transfers must be considered either in lieu of or in addition to the proposed transfer. These alternatives include neurroraphy, arthrodesis, and tenodesis.

TREATMENT OPTIONS

Neurorrhaphy. Only for peripheral nerve injuries. This procedure can be performed in conjunction with the tendon transfers, which then will act as an internal splint while the muscles are recovering nerve function.[13] This procedure may also restore lost sensation. The best results are seen with sharp lacerations in children younger than 12 years in whom neurorrhaphy is performed within 6 months of injury. Recovery of function after nerve repair is much slower (up to 24 months) than after tendon transfers.

Arthrodesis. Performed either when no transfer is available for a particular function or to provide more potential tendons for transfer. Fusing the wrist allows the use of both wrist extensors for other transfers.

Group Tendon Transfer. Although tenodesis does not allow independent function of the tendon, it is helpful

when there is a shortage of tendons to transfer. Often, groups of tendons are tenodesed in order to accept one transfer. For instance, during tendon transfers for radial nerve palsy, the EDC tendons are tenodesed to each other, and one tendon is transferred into the group, providing joined finger extension.

Intercalary Graft. Used for tendon avulsions when direct repair is unobtainable. Benefits include a more direct anatomic line of pull.

External Splints. Helpful during the wait for tendon transfers, to maintain functional position of the hand and prevent contractures. In radial nerve palsy, a wrist splint in extension along with dynamic finger extension with rubber bands is used (Fig. 5). For ulnar nerve palsy, a lumbrical block splint to prevent MP hypertension is used to prevent the intrinsic minus positioning of the fingers.

SELECTING TRANSFERS

PREREQUISITES FOR TENDON TRANSFERS
Prior to the undertaking of a tendon transfer, certain conditions must be met, as follows:

- Bony stability.
- Full passive joint mobility.
- Acceptable distal sensation.
- Healthy tissue through which tissue can be transferred.
- Normal or near-normal motor strength in donor muscle.
- Acceptable excursion of the transferred muscle.

PLANNING FOR TENDON TRANSFERS
Pragmatically speaking, the surgeon must determine what is lost, what is needed, and, finally, what is available for transfer. If more functions are needed than could be provided by the available tendons, one of the alternatives listed previously should be employed. Next, the procedures must be staged. Staging is usually done by dividing the transfers and performing them in the following order: (1)

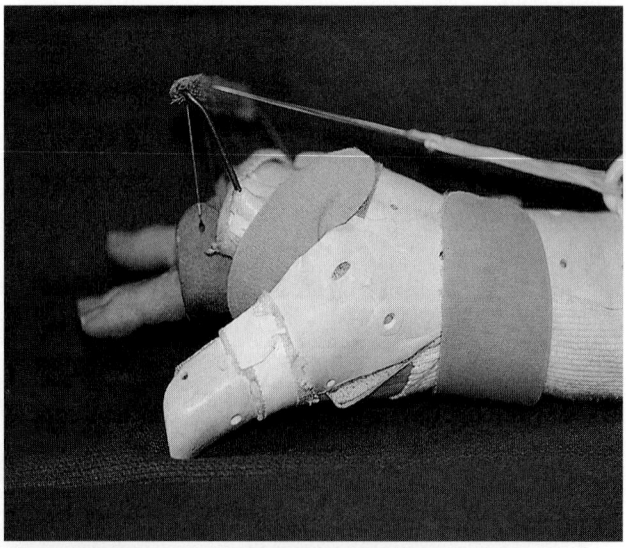

Fig. 5. View. This splint, which maintains the wrist in slight extension with dynamic extension of the fingers, was used both preoperatively and postoperatively for a complete radial nerve palsy.

those on the extensor side of the arm, (2) those on the flexor side, and (3) those that involve both sides. Each case must be individualized, but this division serves as a good general rule.

Multiple transfers have been described for every lost function. It is beyond the scope of this chapter to discuss or even list all of them. Instead, by analyzing the transfers needed for a specific deficit in the following example, we hope to illustrate all the key points involved in both planning and performing tendon transfers.

Example: Radial Nerve Palsy

The first table lists the possible tendons available for transfer in a radial nerve palsy:

What Is Needed	What Would Work	What Is Available
Wrist extension	FPL	FCR
Finger extension	FCR	FCU
Thumb extension	FCU	FDS
Thumb abduction	FDS (I, M, R, S)	PL
	FDP (I, M, R, S)	PT
	PL	
	PT	

The second table shows the matching up (indicated by arrows) of what is needed and the tendon available to perform the authors' preferred method of treatment:

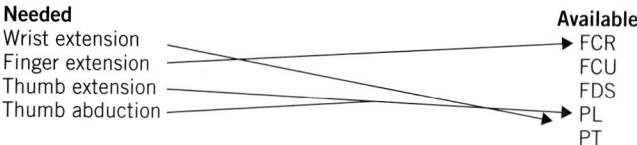

Needed
Wrist extension
Finger extension
Thumb extension
Thumb abduction

Available
FCR
FCU
FDS
PL
PT

PRINCIPLES

The biomechanical principles used to determine any transfer are the same. The transfers recommended in the preceding example for radial nerve palsy are used to review the principles.

Availability. Tendons that cannot be spared from the original function are not used in the transfers. In the example, the FPL and the FDP were excluded because their sacrifice would prevent flexion of the IP joint of the thumb and the DIP joints of the remaining fingers. These tendons alone allow the finger to grasp. Use of the FDS, although weakening grip and causing loss of independence of finger flexion, does not prevent functional finger flexion. In order to retain wrist flexion, only one of the wrist flexors could be transferred. In this example, the FCU was spared because it is the only ulnar deviator of the wrist. Although some prefer the FCU over the FCR, we believe, as Brand[14] does, that the FCU is an essential muscle that should not be sacrificed because it is the sole ulnar deviator of the wrist after loss of the ECU from the radical palsy and is essential in ulnar stabilization of the wrist.

Appropriate Strength. The force a muscle can exert is directly proportional to the cross-sectional area of all its muscle fibers. It is imperative to match as closely as possible donor and recipient muscles in terms of reasonably similar strength. The strength of a muscle is affected by a variety of factors, including stretch or amplitude, direction

of pull, and integrity. In addition, the function of the transfer dictates the necessary strength required. In general, tendons transferred for grasp must be strong, whereas tendons transferred for positioning, such as thumb and finger extensors, need not be as strong so as not to overpower the antagonist muscles.[2]

Appropriate Amplitude. The effectiveness of a muscle's contraction is dictated by its resting length.[15] This principle is well illustrated by its location on the Blix curve.[16] At both extremes of tension, the muscle's ability to contract diminishes. To maximize the effective contraction, donor tendons with appropriate excursions are selected. Finger extension requires 5 cm of excursion, 3 cm at the wrist joint and 2 cm at the fingers. In the example, transfer of the FCU with 4.2 cm of excursion would not be adequate. The FCR, with 5.2 cm of excursion, is a more appropriate transfer and was therefore selected.

The effective amplitude can also be affected by tensioning at the site of attachment. Overtightening or undertightening of the transfer will move the tension to either side of the Blix curve, decreasing effective contraction. As a rule, we provide the transfer with enough tension to maintain the joint it crosses at 60 degrees.

Direction of Pull. The most effective tendon transfer is one with a straight line of pull. When transferring the FDS or FCR for finger extension, one could go either around the forearm muscles or through the interosseous membrane. One could pass the tendon through the interosseous membrane, which is a much straighter direction for the transfer.[17]

Synergy. *Synergistic muscles* are defined as muscles that act in concert to produce a desired motion. Unlike muscles in the lower extremity, muscles in the upper extremity that move joints in opposite directions are often synergistic. For example, passive flexion of the wrist causes finger extension. It is this synergy that allows the FCR to be transferred to the EDC for finger extension.

Integrity. A transferred tendon should have one function. It is unacceptable to split a tendon and transfer the two halves to two other tendons with different functions. It is acceptable, however, to transfer one tendon to two recipients as long as the recipients have the same function. For instance, in this case, the FCR is transferred to all the finger extensors.

Inserting one tendon into two recipients with either different excursions or different functions would cause one of the recipient tendons to be tethered by the other, either decreasing the effective amplitude or changing the direction of pull. For example, transfer of the PT into the both the ECRL and the ECRB would cause the wrist to go into radial deviation on attempted extension. This would occur because in neutral extension, the ECRB would become slack, leaving only the ECRL with an effective insertion. This arrangement, described as a yoke insertion, should be avoided.[14]

Staging. In general, transfers for extension and flexion should not be performed simultaneously. As a rule we like to perform transfer for extension first, followed by transfers for flexion in a second procedure. Transfers that provide both flexion and extension, such as intrinsic transfers, should be performed as a third operation. In the case of radial nerve palsy, it is safe to perform the transfers in one procedure because they are all for extension.

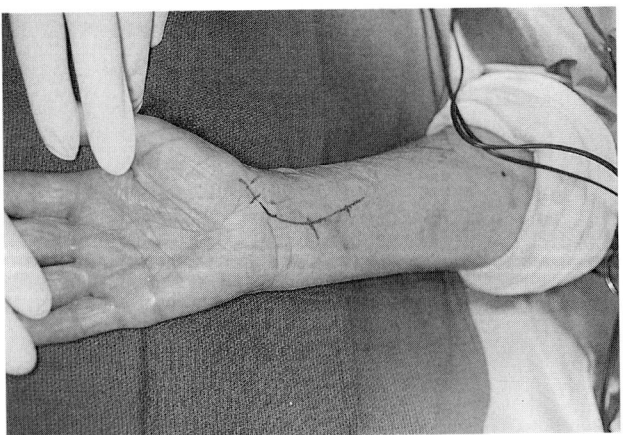

Fig. 6. View. This is a volar harvesting incision for tendon transfers in radial nerve palsy.

Tissue Balance. It is essential that tendons lie beneath healthy tissue that permits gliding. Scar tissue in the area of a tendon transfer risks adhesions, thus decreasing the gliding ability and leading to failure of the transfer.

TECHNIQUE

The procedure can be performed with the use of either regional or general anesthesia. Tourniquet control should always be used. A curved incision is made volarly, beginning at the proximal wrist crease (Fig. 6). The PL and the FCR are harvested at their insertions as distally as possible. The tendon ends are wrapped in moist sponges to prevent desiccation. A dorsal incision is made beginning at Lister's tubercle and extending proximally to expose the insertion of the PT (Fig. 7). The PT is reflected from its insertion into the radius with 1 to 2 cm of periosteum in order to give it extra length.

The EPL tendon is identified distally in the wound and is removed from the third dorsal compartment. It is then transected at the musculotendinous junction. The PL is then passed subcutaneously beneath branches of the superficial radial nerve, in order not to constrict them, and is brought into the proximity of the transected EPL.

The interosseous membrane is then exposed just proxi-

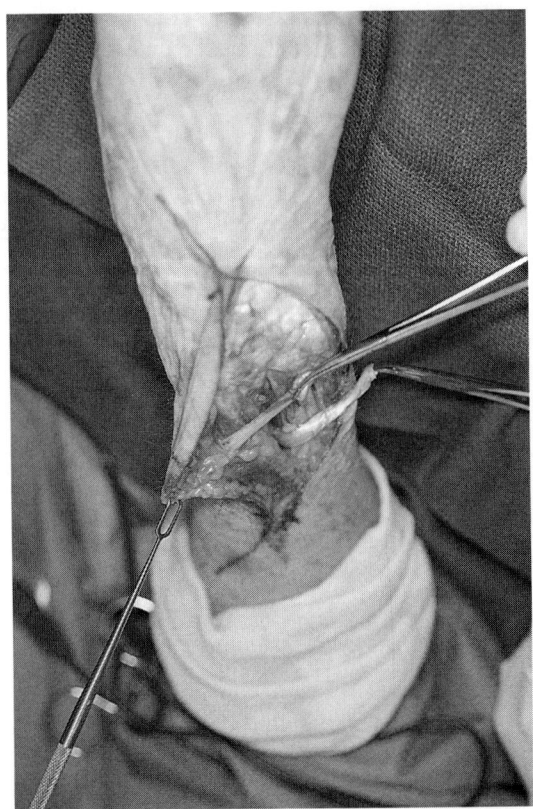

Fig. 8. View. The FCR is brought through the interosseous membrane for transfer to the EDC (proximal tendon held by hemostat). The palmaris longus is transferred to the EPL.

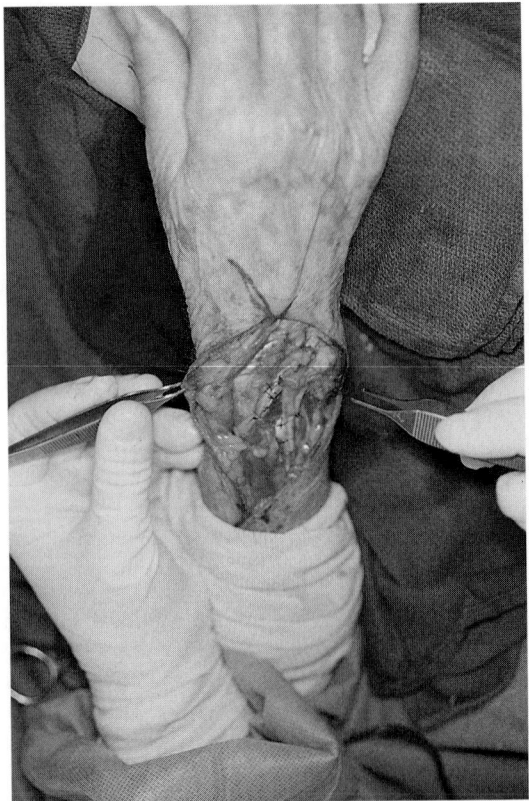

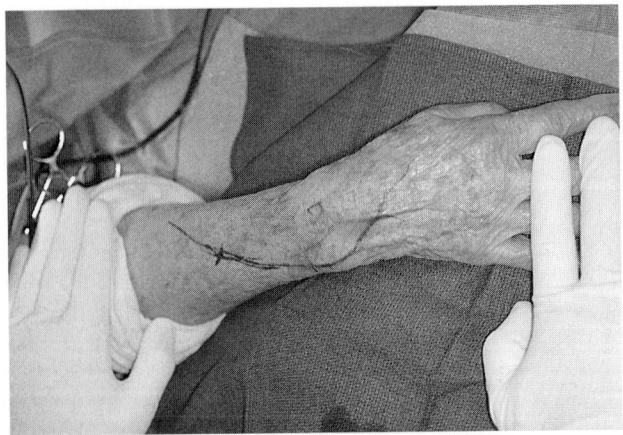

Fig. 7. View. This is a dorsal incision for tendon transfers.

Fig. 9. View. Pulvertaft weaves are used to secure the transfers.

mal to the PQ. The anterior interosseous nerve and artery are protected, and an opening is made in the membrane large enough to prevent constriction of the tendon (Fig. 8). The FCR is passed through the window to the dorsal compartment of the forearm.

With all tendons ready for transfer, the volar wound is closed so as not to affect proper tensioning of the transfers. The transfers are then performed with the use of Pulvertaft[18] weaves and are held in place with 4-0 nylon suture (Fig. 9). The FCR is transferred to the EDC, the PL to the EPL, and the PQ to the ECRB. Before final placement of the sutures, proper tensioning is achieved. Determining the proper tensioning often requires trial and error. One should not hesitate to revise the tension if needed. In general, the transfer should be tight enough to allow a tenodesis effect of finger flexion upon wrist extension while still allowing full finger flexion with the wrist in 30 degrees of extension.

The dorsal wound is closed, and the arm is placed in a splint that maintains the wrist in 45 degrees of extension and the MCPs and the thumb in full extension.

POSTOPERATIVE MANAGEMENT

A long-arm splint is applied with the elbow at 90 degrees, the wrist in 20 degrees of extension, the MPs at full extension, and the PIPs and DIPs free to move.

At 1 week, therapy is started with the wrist in a cock-up splint and the fingers and thumb in dynamic extension. All exercises are performed with the arm in the splint for 6 weeks. Then a strengthening program is started. In general, retraining of muscle function is not necessary, because patients use visual cues to retrain themselves.

COMPLICATIONS

The most common complication of tendon transfers is related to improper tensioning of the transfer. Transfers that are made too loose are difficult to overcome with therapy, whereas those that are made too tight can lead to joint contractures. Adhesions occur when transfers cross through scar tissue.

REFERENCES

1. Erlacher PJ: The development of tendon surgery in Germany: A review of the history and an evaluation of the treatment. Instr Course Lect 1956; 13:110.
2. Smith RJ: Tendon Transfer of the Hand and Forearm. Boston, Little, Brown, 1987.
3. Mayer L: The physiological method of tendon transplantation. Surg Gynecol Obstet 1916; 22:182.
4. Burkhalter WE, Christensen RC, Brown PW: Extensor indicis proprius opponensplasty. J Bone Joint Surg Am 1973; 55:725.
5. Littler JW: Tendon transfers and arthrodeses in combined median and ulnar nerve paralysis. J Bone Joint Surg Am 1949; 31:225.
6. Huber E: Hilfsoperation bei medianuslahmung. Dtsch Chir 1921; 162:271.
7. Camitz H: Uber die behandlung der oppositionslahmung. Acta Chir Scand 1966; 65:77.
8. Burkhalter WE: Early tendon transfers in upper extremity peripheral nerve injury. Clin Orthop 1974; 104:68.
9. Brand PW: Tendon transfers in the forearm. In Flynn JE (ed). Hand Surgery. Baltimore, Williams & Wilkins, 1975, 2nd ed.
10. Boyes JH: Bunnell's Surgery of the Hand. Philadelphia, JB Lippincott, 1970, 5th ed.
11. Froment J: La paralysie de l'adducteur du pouce et le signe de le prehension. Rev Neurol 1914; 28:1236.
12. Jeanne M: La deformation du pouce dans la paralysie cubitale. Bull Mem Soc Chir 1915; 41:793.
13. Burkhalter WE: Restoration of power grip in ulnar nerve paralysis. Orthop Clin North Am 1974; 5:289.
14. Brand PW: Clinical Mechanics of the Hand. St. Louis, CV Mosby, 1985.
15. Omer GE: Determination of physiological length of a reconstructed muscle tendon unit through muscle stimulation. J Bone Joint Surg Am 1965; 47:304.
16. Blix M: Die Lange und die Spannung des Muskels. Skand Arch Physiol 1891; 3:295.
17. Boyes JH: Tendon transfers for radial palsy. Bull Hosp Jt Dis 1960; 21:97.
18. Pulvertaft RG: Suture materials and tendon junctures. Am J Surg 1965; 109:346.

BENIGN BONE AND SOFT-TISSUE TUMORS OF THE HAND AND WRIST

Michael Bothwell and Kevin D. Plancher

Summary

- The dorsal wrist ganglion is the most common dorsal wrist mass, and diagnosis can be made by needle aspiration.
- Neurilemoma is the most common tumor of the peripheral nerve. Nerve dysfunction is rare, and surgical removal with magnification is usually curative.
- Localized nodular tenosynovitis whose treatment is marginal surgical excision has a high recurrence rate.
- Enchondroma accounts for 90% of bone tumor of the hand. Recurrence after treatment with curettage and bone graft is uncommon.
- Giant cell tumor of the distal radius that has expanded beyond its cortical confines requires wide resection and reconstruction.

In this chapter, we discuss frequently encountered soft-tissue and bone tumors of the hand, wrist, and upper extremity. Understanding their incidence, cause, signs and symptoms, differential diagnosis, radiological findings, and pathological appearances will permit effective treatment. Table 1 lists these types of tumors.

SOFT-TISSUE TUMORS

GANGLIA

Ganglia are benign cystic lesions that contain a mucinous, viscous fluid with glucosamine, albumin, globulin, and hyaluronic acid.[1] They are the most common benign soft-tissue tumor of the upper extremity[1, 2] and usually occur in the second through fourth decades of life. Four etiological theories exist.

Cystic formation secondary to mucoid degeneration of connective tissue.

Synovial herniation from a joint.

Cysts that arise from the wrist capsule, which attaches to the scapholunate interosseous ligament and, when stressed, acts as a synovial fluid pump.[2]

Trauma.

DORSAL GANGLIA

Sixty percent to 70% of wrist ganglia are found on the dorsal-ranial surface of the wrist[3] (Fig. 1). They may be small or large and almost always are found over the scapholunate interval. Patients commonly complain of the size of this mass, which may swell and be painful. On physical examination, a firm mass that transilluminates is noted.

Differential diagnoses include extensor digitorum brevis manus, extensor tenosynovitis, and carpal metacarpal boss.

Three forms of treatment include closed rupture, aspiration, and operative intervention.[3] Closed rupture by direct pressure is painful and has a 33% recurrence rate. Richman et al[4] reported that aspiration with multiple needle punctures when combined with 3 weeks of splint immobilization has a 60% failure rate. Without immobilization, the cure rate has been reported to be as low as 13%. Injection of a corticosteroid into the area after aspiration has not been shown to alter recurrence rates.

Surgical treatment of dorsal carpal ganglion should be performed with general or regional anesthesia. Surgical treatment should focus on removing the ganglion cyst and all material between the radial triquetral ligament and dorsal intercarpal ligament. The ganglion is excised with all of its attachments to the joint capsule and scapholunate ligament.[1] Wrist stiffness, injury to the dorsal sensory branch of the radial nerve, and recurrence are the most common complications after surgical excision.[3] The recurrence rates after surgery are reported as high as 10%.[3]

VOLAR WRIST GANGLIA

The second most common site for ganglia is the volar wrist (Fig. 2). These cysts arise from the radiocarpal capsule in the scaphotrapezial joint. The ganglion frequently wraps around the radial artery.

Aspiration is avoided because of possible injury to the radial artery. Before surgical excision, radial artery patency should be confirmed with Allen's test. Complications of this type of excision include injury to the radial artery, lateral antebrachial cutaneous, palmar cutaneous, and superficial radial nerves. Postoperative management is identical to that of dorsal ganglia. Recurrence rates are often higher for volar ganglia because of timid dissection.

FLEXOR TENDON SHEATH GANGLION

Flexor tendon sheath ganglia[5] (Fig. 3) arise at the A-1 pulley of the flexor tendon sheath. Pain may occur when gripping an object. The mass varies in size from 4 to 10

TABLE 1. TUMORS OF THE SOFT-TISSUE AND BONE	
Soft-Tissue Tumors	**Bone Tumors**
Ganglia	Enchondroma
Dorsal	Osteochondroma
Volar	Juxtacortical chondroma
Flexor tendon sheath	Osteoid osteoma
Lipoma	Unicameral bone cyst
Neurilemoma	Aneurysmal bone cyst
Localized nodular tenosynovitis	Giant cell tumor
Aneurysm	
Glomus tumors	
Lipofibromatous hamartoma	

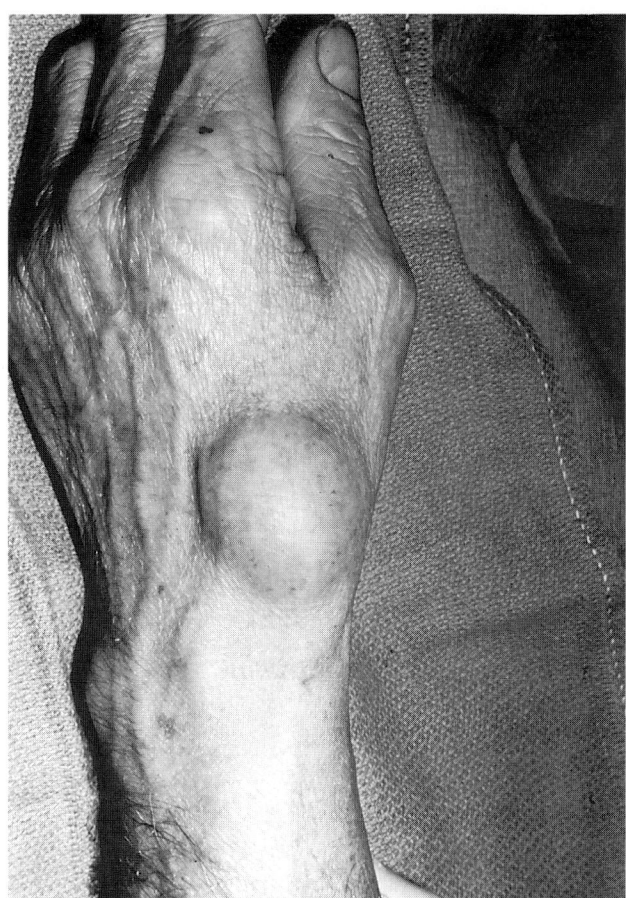

Fig. 1. Dorsal wrist ganglion. Note the dorsal-radial location. Needle aspiration confirms the diagnosis and may be therapeutic. (Courtesy of Peter J. Stern, M.D.)

mm in diameter and is firm. Aspiration is usually effective treatment; surgery is rarely necessary.

LIPOMA

Lipomas (Fig. 4) occur in the third to eighth decade of life and are often noted as a cosmetic concern.[6] Rare in the hand, they occur more frequently in the proximal upper extremity as an asymptomatic mass. When they do occur in the hand, they are usually large, located in the deep palm, where they may cause median nerve compression with a secondary nerve palsy or limit digital flexion.[6]

Radiographic plain films are often useful, revealing the characteristic density of fat, allowing easier diagnosis and evaluation of the extent of the lesion. Magnetic resonance imaging (MRI) and computed tomography (CT) are helpful if the lesion is deep. Electromyography is performed if nerve symptoms are present. Treatment consists of marginal excision of the mass.

NEURILEMOMA (SCHWANNOMA)

Neurilemoma (Fig. 5) is the most common solitary peripheral nerve tumor and arises from the nerve sheath (Schwann's cells).[7] Multiple lesions have been associated with von Recklinghausen's disease. According to Stout,[8] 18% of his patients with a neurilemoma had clinical symptoms of von Recklinghausen's disease. Patients complain of

a painless mass located close to a peripheral nerve; pain is produced when pressure is applied to the mass. These tumors are usually 2 to 3 cm in their longest diameter.

On gross examination, the lesion is spherical and encapsulated. Nerve fascicles run on either side of the tumor and are attenuated by it. Treatment consists of marginal excision, which, using an operating room microscope to identify the perineural tissue, will clarify the tumor-nerve relationship.

NEUROFIBROMA

Neurofibromas arise from the nerve sheath and are intimately associated with nerve fascicles. There are two types of neurofibromas: solitary neurofibroma and neurofibroma of von Recklinghausen's disease. Geschickter[9] noted that only 10% of patients with solitary neurofibromas have neurofibromatosis. Solitary neurofibromas occur in young adults and are typically small and painless lesions. In individuals with von Recklinghausen's disease, there can be associated macrodactyly and malignant degeneration (10% neurofibrosarcoma).[3] No capsule is present in these lesions, thus distinguishing them from neurilemomas. The indications for operative intervention[7] include (1) increasing size or pain, (2) decreasing function, and (3) a subcutaneous lesion with bleeding or ulceration.

Surgical excision with an operating microscope is the

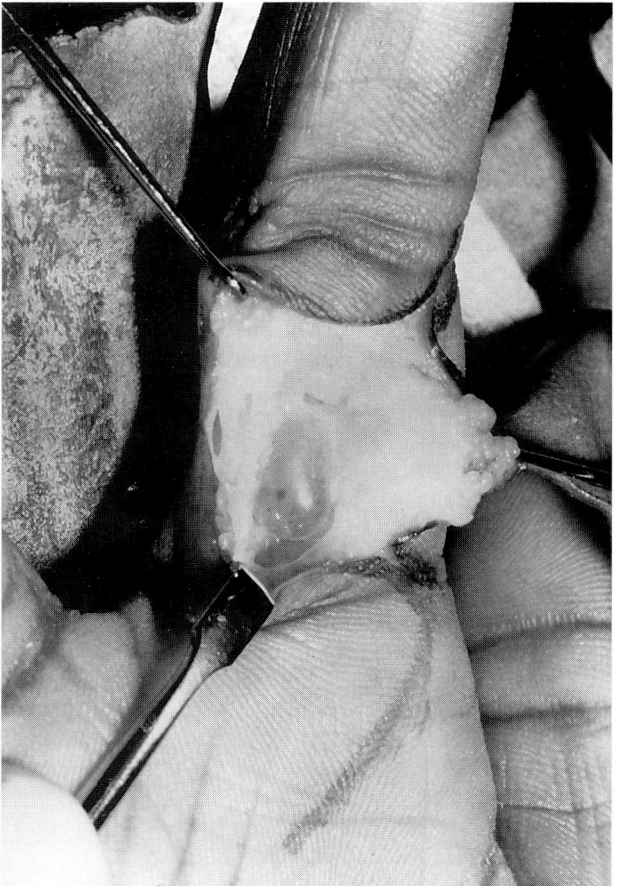

Fig. 2. Volar wrist ganglion. The mass is intimately associated with the radial artery (not seen) and usually arises from the scaphotrapezial-trapezoid or radiocarpal joint. (Courtesy of Peter J. Stern, M.D.)

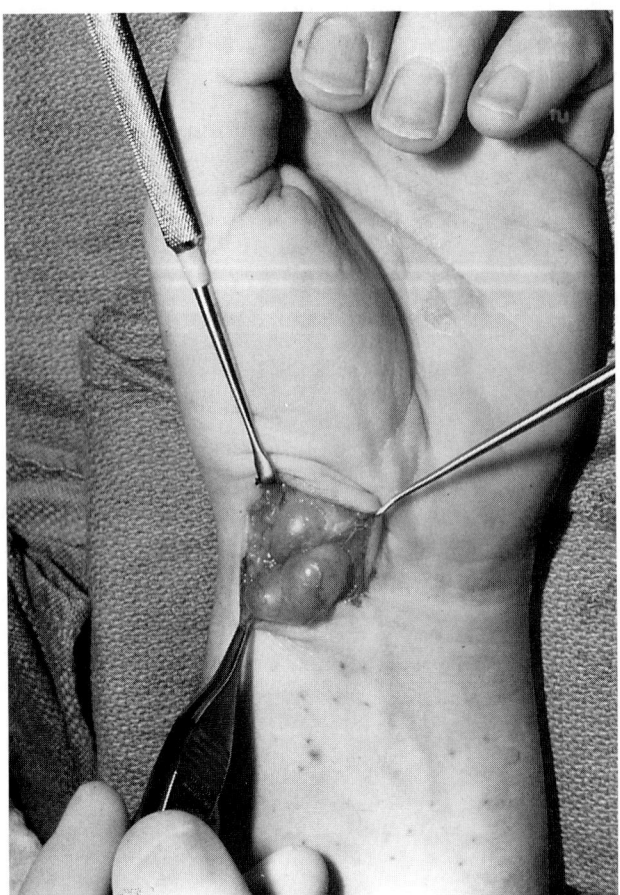

Fig. 3. Flexor tendon sheath ganglion. Operative treatment (depicted here) is rarely necessary and is indicated only if aspiration fails. (Courtesy of Peter J. Stern, M.D.)

treatment of choice. It is extremely difficult, if not impossible, to remove the tumor without creating some neurological deficit because of the intimate association of the tumor and the nerve fascicles. When major nerves are involved, tumor is left behind to preserve function, whereas smaller nerves may be excised to eliminate the lesion. If a major nerve must be excised, then primary repair or nerve grafting is suggested.

LOCALIZED NODULAR TENOSYNOVITIS

Localized nodular tenosynovitis (LNS) (Fig. 6) is also known as giant cell tumor of the tendon sheath, fibrous xanthoma of the synovium, and benign synovium.[10] The localized form is found predominately in the hand and upper extremity, whereas its diffuse form usually presents as a monoarticular synovitis of the lower extremity. LNS and diffuse pigmented villonodular synovitis are histologically similar and believed to be variants of the same process.[10] The cause of LNS is unknown, and recurrence varies from 5% to 50%.[11]

LNS is often noted on the volar aspects of the fingers, adjacent to the distal interphalangeal joint. Its peak incidence is in the fifth decade of life.[12] The lesion is firm, nontender, and lobulated. The duration of symptoms before presentation for treatment may range from several weeks to 30 years, with an average of 2 years.[11]

Plain radiographic examination reveals a lesion with a soft-tissue mass in 50% of the cases.[12] When the lesion is in contact with the cortex, it may cause a pressure indentation erosion. Size can range from 0.5 to 5.0 cm.[11]

Optimal treatment for LNS is not yet known because its symptoms are so benign and rarely cause any functional limitations. When the digit has a decreased range of motion or if the mass is cosmetically displeasing, excision is the treatment of choice. Recurrence is common despite a meticulous excision. Malignant degeneration has not been reported.

GLOMUS TUMORS

The glomus tumor is a benign growth that arises from one of the subcutaneous glomera, which control blood flow.[13] The triad of larcinating pain, pinpoint tenderness, and cold intolerance has been well documented.[3] The tumor can be found anywhere in the body but is most commonly seen in the distal phalanx of the digits. When subungual, there is bluish discoloration beneath the nail, nail ridging, and erosion of the distal phalanx on radiograph. Glomus tumors are rare but, when noted in a subungual location, will cause severe pain with direct pressure or cold. Love's test,[14] which consists of applying pressure over the painful area with the head of a straight pin, is useful to localize the tumor. MRI is useful when patients complain of obscure pain with no other findings.

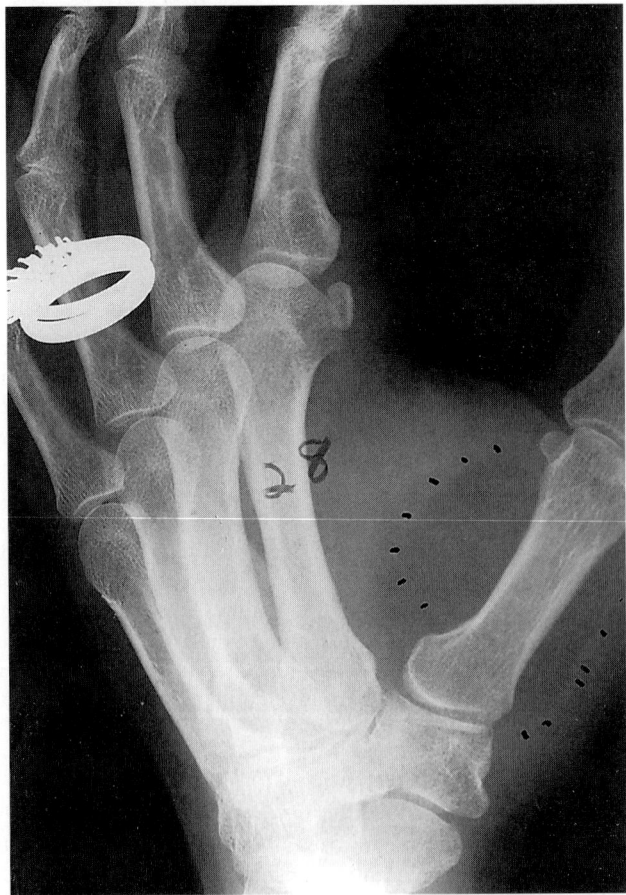

Fig. 4. Radiograph of thenar eminence lipoma. Note the oval fat density between the thumb and index metacarpal. (Courtesy of Peter J. Stern, M.D.)

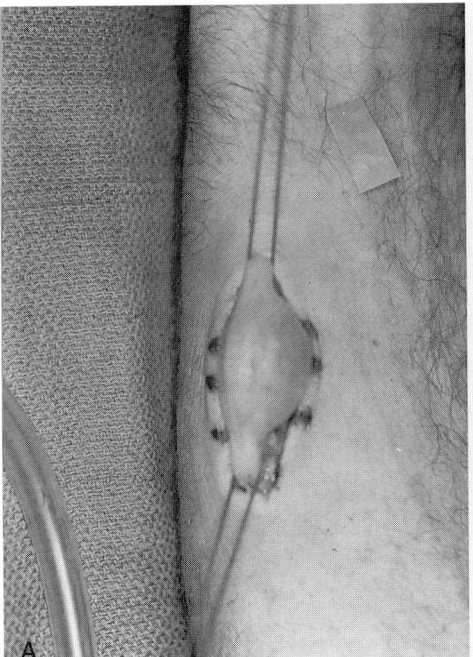 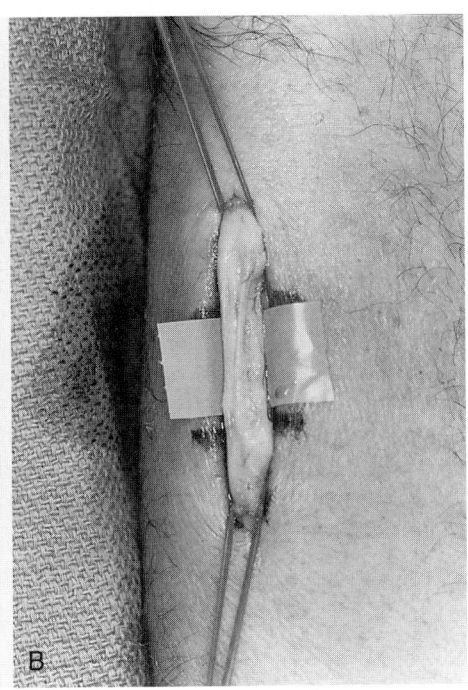

Fig. 5. View. *A,* Neurilemoma of median nerve. The tumor is encapsulated and can be removed with care by marginal excision using magnification. *B,* Following excision. (Courtesy of Peter J. Stern, M.D.)

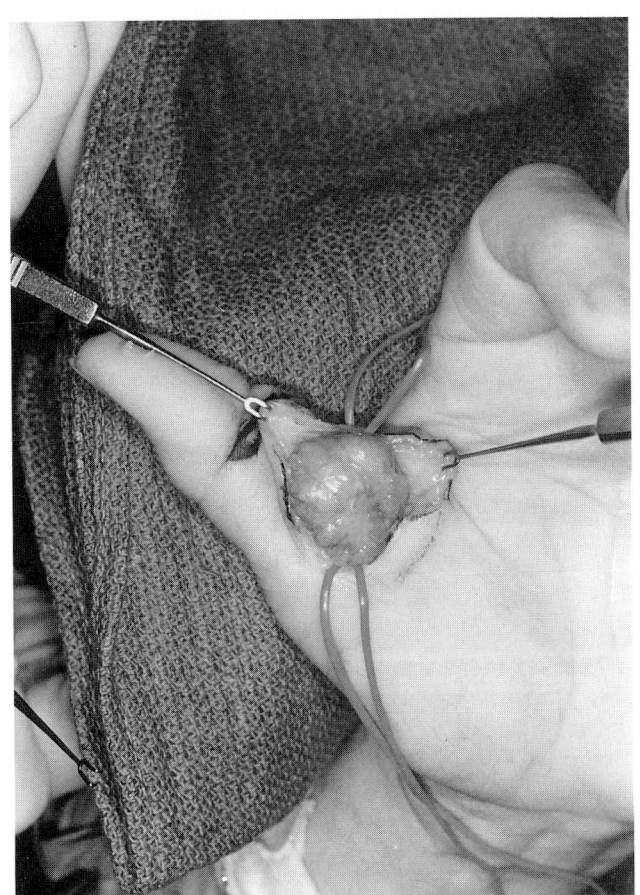

Fig. 6. Localized nodular tenosynovitis at the level of thumb metacarpophalangeal joint. It is lobulated and tan in appearance. The digital nerves are usually adherent to the surface of the tumor and must be identified before excision. (Courtesy of Peter J. Stern, M.D.)

Treatment consists of a marginal surgical excision.[13, 15] Recurrence as high as 24% has been reported. When the lesion is subungual, we remove the nail and mark the lesion with India ink on a separate occasion in the office under local anesthesia. The patient returns to the operating room a day later, and the exact area of concern is labeled and probed without anesthesia. The digit is then anesthetized, and curettage with nail bed repair is performed. With this treatment regimen, our patients have avoided recurrence.

ANEURYSM

Aneurysms are classified as traumatic or nontraumatic. Traumatic aneurysms can be further grouped into true and false aneurysms.

True aneurysms occur after blunt trauma.[16] When in the hand, they occur most commonly in the distal portion of Guyon's canal. Digital artery aneurysms are rare.[17] Damage occurs to the arterial wall media, allowing vascular dilation. The histological finding of an intact arterial wall consisting of muscle and elastin fibers confirms the diagnosis.

False aneurysms occur from a penetrating arterial injury or from a complete rupture of the vessel wall when continuity is maintained by the surrounding soft tissue.[18] Hemorrhage from the vessel results in a contiguous hematoma that forms a fibrous shell adjacent to the vessel.[19]

Some patients with aneurysms complain of the presence of a mass, which may be painful. Others sometimes complain of digital ischemia from emboli, distal nerve symptoms as a result of compression, or digital vasospasm.[20] A complete physical examination should be performed to search for the source of emboli.

Treatment consists of resection.[21] Vascular reconstruction is indicated if there is ischemia distal to the resection.

LIPOFIBROMATOUS HAMARTOMA

Lipofibromatous hamartoma is a rare tumor that causes thickening of the median nerve at the level of the carpal tunnel. It usually appears in childhood as swelling proximal and at the level of the flexor retinaculum. It sometimes will present as carpal tunnel syndrome. It has been associated with macrodactyly and commonly affects the median nerve, although ulnar involvement has been reported.[22] On exploration, there is fusiform enlargement of the nerve. If a biopsy is performed, the lesion reveals excessive fat and fibrous tissue separating normal axons.

Treatment includes nerve decompression. Additional management varies and includes external or internal neurolysis with or without debulking and resection of the tumor.[3] Results vary and are usually better in children. In young children, it has been noted that nerve resection without reconstruction can produce results in which there is no significant motor or sensory deficit.[23]

BONE TUMORS

ENCHONDROMA

Enchondroma (Fig. 7A and B) is the most predominate osseous tumor of the hand and is seen most frequently in the metacarpals and phalanges. It rarely affects the carpal bones and accounts for approximately one-fourth of all benign tumors.[24] Enchondromas can occur at any age, but are most frequently seen in young adults.

Most patients complain of pain or swelling in a finger, and on radiograph a pathological fracture may be noted. Plain radiographs are diagnostic and reveal a centrally located lesion with marked bone expansion. Cortical thinning and calcifications may also be present.

Histologically, this cartilage lesion is lobular and may penetrate the surrounding marrow spaces.[24] The cells are surrounded by a well-defined area of proteoglycan matrix.

Treatment consists of operative intervention but for diagnostic and therapeutic purposes. When a pathological fracture has occurred, there is a debate as to whether to treat the tumor and fracture simultaneously or wait until the fracture heals and perform surgery later. Treatment with curettage and bone grafting is preferred. Malignant degeneration to chondrosarcoma is extremely rare.

OSTEOCHONDROMA

Osteochondroma is the most common benign tumor of bone. It originates in the metaphysis of long bones and may have multiple foci. The tumor typically appears in the second decade of life and predominantly affects males, 1.7 to 1.[25] In the upper extremity, it is commonly located in the proximal humerus as well as the distal radius and ulna. Plain films reveal a peripheral bone projection or growth. There is always a communication of the cortical and cancellous bone, which may contain focal areas of calcification at the site of the osteochondroma. There is often a flaring of the metaphysis of the bone.

Histologically, the surface of the lesion reveals a thin, smooth, translucent, bluish cartilaginous cap.[25] The lesion may be pedunculated or sessile. When pedunculated, the lesion projects away from its nearest joint.

A solitary osteochondroma that is asymptomatic may be monitored clinically. The indications for surgical intervention include functional limitations, cosmesis, and pain. Surgical treatment in children should be limited to osteochondromas, which cause angulatory deformity or limit joint motion. Care should be taken not to injure the

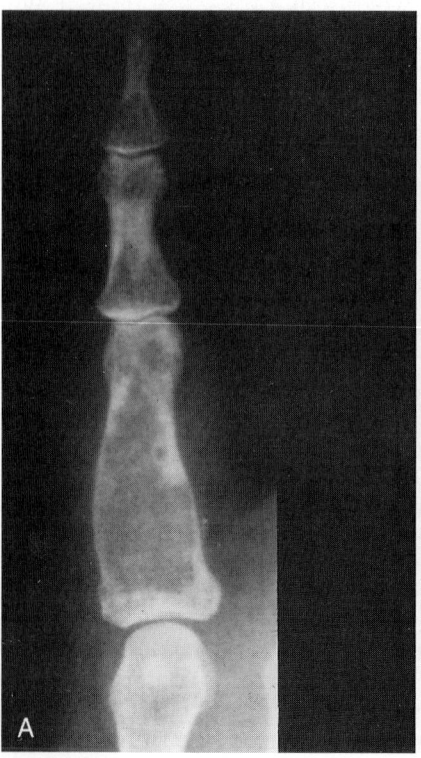
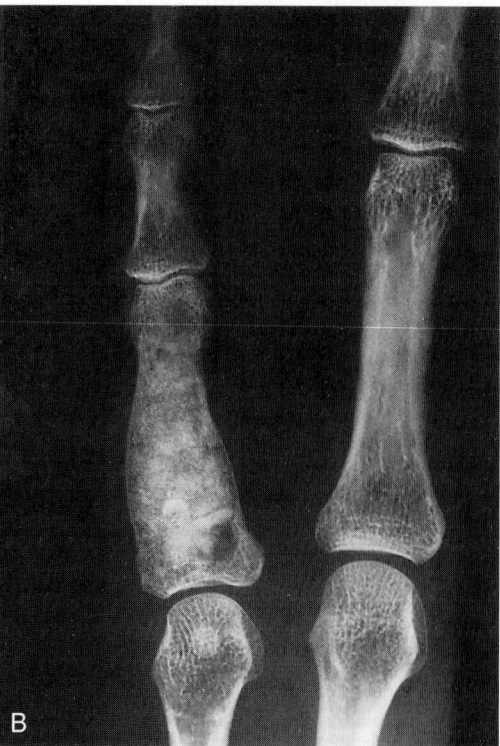

Fig. 7. Radiograph of an enchondroma of the proximal phalanx. *A,* Before surgical intervention. Note the cortical expansion and thinning, the suggestion of calcification, and the lobulated nature of the endosteal surface. *B,* Following treatment with curettage and packing with autogenous bone graft. (Courtesy of Peter J. Stern, M.D.)

physis. Malignant degeneration in solitary osteochondromas is rare.

Multiple osteochondromas cause significant forearm deformities, including ulnar angulation of the distal radius articular surface, ulnar translation of the carpus, and dislocation of the radial head.[26, 27] Aggressive intervention is recommended when any deformity is present. Malignant degeneration in multiple osteochondromas occurs in 10% to 20% of patients.[24]

JUXTACORTICAL (PERIOSTEAL) CHONDROMA

Periosteal chondroma (Fig. 8) is an uncommon benign cartilaginous lesion that forms from the periosteum and erodes into the cortex of the bone. This lesion occurs most frequently in the proximal humerus as well as tubular bones of the hand.[28, 29]

Often a palpable lesion is appreciated on physical examination. Plain radiographs reveal a soft-tissue mass adjacent to the periosteum with a cup- or saucer-shaped cortical indentation with surrounding sclerosis. The lesion may occur in the metaphysis or diaphysis. Calcification of the matrix may often be seen. Radiographically, this lesion may be confused with an osteosarcoma. Gross pathology reveals a well-circumscribed lesion, partly embedded in cortical bone and covered with periosteum. Histologically, the lesion has a blue-white color with a prominent hyaline cartilage component.

Local excision rather than amputation is the treatment of choice for this tumor, which often recurs. When clinical findings confuse the radiological findings, excisional biopsy is indicated before planning a definitive procedure.[28]

OSTEOID OSTEOMA

Osteoid osteoma is a benign solitary osteoblastic lesion containing a central radiolucent nidus, less than 1 cm in diameter that is surrounded by reactive bone. This lesion's peak incidence is in the second decade with a male-female ratio of 3:1. Classically, patients complain of nighttime pain in the involved area.[25] Nonsteroidal anti-inflammatory medication may bring significant pain relief because of the inhibition of prostaglandin synthesis by these tumors. The most common locations in the hand are the proximal phalanges and carpus.[30]

Plain radiographs reveal a small, round lucency surrounded by sclerosis or a cortical reaction. Lesions not demonstrated on plain films require a bone or CT scan. The average duration of symptoms to the onset of treatment is 14 months.[31, 32]

On gross examination, the nidus is red with a granular texture and is very distinctive from the surrounding sclerotic bone.

Treatment by *complete* excision of the nidus eliminates the risk of recurrence and alleviates symptoms.

UNICAMERAL BONE CYST (SIMPLE CYST)

Unicameral bone cysts are benign fluid-filled (serous or serosanguineous) metaphyseal cysts that occur most frequently in the proximal humerus. Its peak incidence is in the first two decades of life, with a male-female ratio of 3:1.[25] The cyst is asymptomatic; pain occurs only when there is an associated pathological fracture. Differential diagnoses are aneurysmal bone cyst and giant cell tumor.

The majority of these lesions present as an incidental finding on routine radiography. Patients may complain of pain, swelling, or stiffness near a joint. Radiographs reveal a large, centrally located metaphyseal lucency that has expanded the cortex. According to Neer et al,[33] these cysts can be classified as either active (located within 5 cm of the growth plate) or inactive (0.5 cm of normal bone between cyst and growth plate).[33]

Grossly, the cystic cavity contains a straw-colored fluid. Partial or complete septation of the cyst may also be seen.

The most common treatment is aspiration and injection of methylprednisone into the lesion with fluoroscopic guidance. Radiographs are taken every 6 weeks to monitor the cyst. After injection, healing may occur after 8 to 12 weeks. The risk of recurrence is about 30% regardless of treatment.[3]

ANEURYSMAL BONE CYST

Aneurysmal bone cyst is a benign, solitary expansile lesion of bone that occurs in the metaphysis of long and flat bones. Its peak incidence is in the second decade of life with a male-female ratio of 1:1.3.[25] Pain and swelling are the most common symptoms.

Plain films reveal a ballooned cystic expansion with a thinned cortex of the affected bone and no significant matrix mineralization.[25] Radiographically, the tumor may appear aggressive and may resemble a giant cell tumor or sarcoma. Subperiosteal bone formation may also be seen. The lesional tissue is hemorrhagic, consisting of unclotted blood. The periphery of the lesion is surrounded by a new layer of periosteal bone.

Treatment consists of excision, curettage, and bone grafting. If the lesion involves an expendable bone, than marginal excision is preferred. Radiation therapy is not indi-

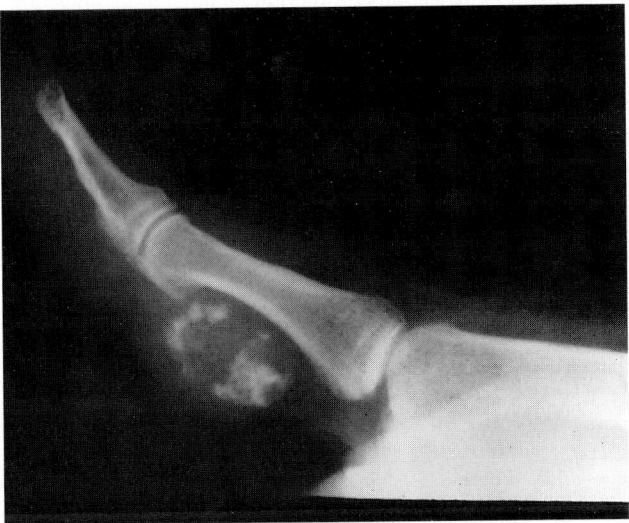

Fig. 8. Radiograph of a periosteal chondroma. Note the calcific mass anterior to the proximal phalanx of thumb and the indentation of the anterior phalangeal cortex. (Courtesy of Peter J. Stern, M.D.)

cated for the treatment of aneurysmal bone cysts of the hand.

GIANT CELL TUMOR OF HAND BONES AND DISTAL RADIUS

Giant cell tumor is an uncommon aggressive neoplasm of the bone (Fig. 9). Its peak incidence is in the third decade of life, with a slight female predominance. Common complaints include pain, swelling, limited range of motion, and weakness of the affected extremity. Pathological fractures are sometimes noted. The distal part of the radius is the third most common site for this tumor, with a 10% occurrence rate.[34]

Plain radiographs reveal an eccentric lytic epiphyseal-metaphyseal lesion. There is neither sclerosis nor a periosteal reaction, and the tumor may thin or erode the cortex. The lesion often shows destruction of cortical and cancellous bone. This lesion may be mistaken for a malignant tumor. Evaluation of giant cell tumor should include a bone scan to rule out multicentricity, a CT scan to determine the cortical or articular violation, a chest CT to rule out metastasis, and an MRI to establish the presence of a secondary soft-tissue component.[3]

There is still some discrepancy regarding how the histological grade of giant cell tumor correlates with its aggressiveness. Regardless of its histological grade, all giant cell tumors of the hand and wrist should be considered aggressive and treated as such.

Local resection or amputation is the treatment of choice for giant cell tumors of the hand.[35] Amputation is a definitive cure and almost eliminates the chance of recurrence. Treatment by curettage and bone grafting is associated with a recurrence rate of up to 90% and is not recommended. Reconstructive surgery with either allograft or autograft after resection may be an option. Cryosurgery for treatment of giant cell tumors has been reported in the literature with some success.[36]

When treating giant cell tumors of the distal radius, the method of curettage and bone grafting has been associated with a high recurrence, particularly if the tumor violates the cortex, ranging from 35% to 80%.[37] Curettage and

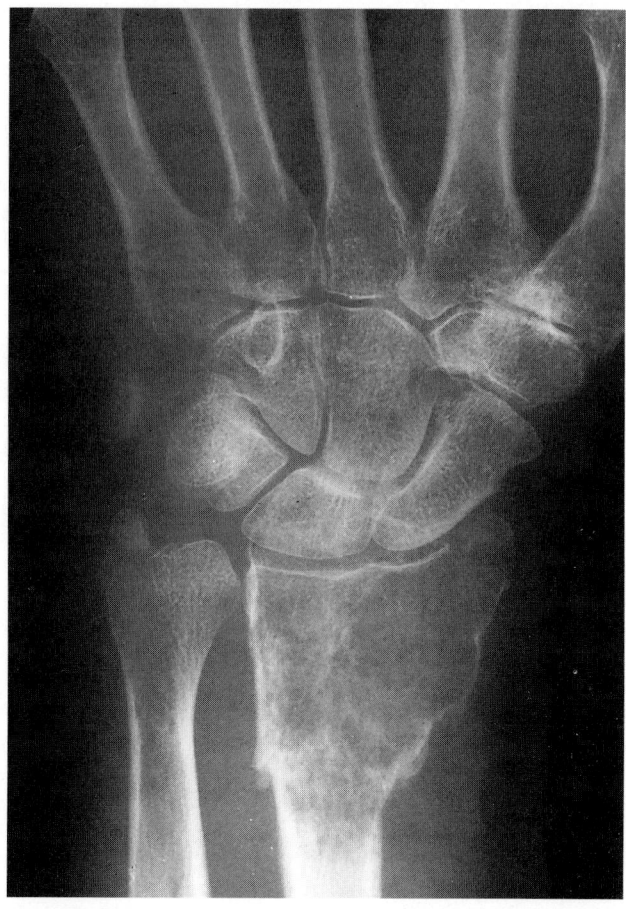

Fig. 9. Radiograph of a giant cell tumor of the distal radius. Note the lucent lesion located in the epiphysis and adjacent metaphyseal, the cortical expansion, the absence of matrix formation, and the sharp transition from tumor to adjacent normal bone. (Courtesy of Peter J. Stern, M.D.)

packing with polymethylmethacrylate are indicated when the cortex remains intact. However, the most frequently used method is en bloc resection, intercalated bone graft, and wrist arthrodesis.[37]

REFERENCES

1. Hooper G: Cystic swellings. In Bogumill GP, Gleegler EJ (eds): *Tumors of the Hand and Upper Limb.* Edinburgh, Churchill-Livingstone, 1993, p 172.

2. Angelides AC, Wallace PF: Ganglions of the hand and wrist. In Green DP (ed): *Operative Hand Surgery,* New York, Churchill-Livingstone, 1993, 3rd ed, p 2157.

3. Dell P, Stern P: Benign and malignant neoplasms of the upper extremity. In Peimer CA (ed): *Surgery of the Hand and Upper Extremity.* New York, McGraw-Hill, 1996, p 2231.

4. Richman JA, Gelberman RH, Engber WD, et al: Ganglions of the wrist and digit: Results of treatment by aspiration and cyst wall puncture. J Hand Surg Am 1987; 12: 1041.

5. Matthews P: Ganglia in the flexor tendon sheaths of the hand. J Bone Joint Surg Br 1973; 55:612.

6. Leffert RD: Lipomas of the upper extremity. J Bone Joint Surg Am 1972; 54:1262.

7. Rosenberg AE, Dick HM, Botte M: Benign and malignant tumors of peripheral nerve. In Gelberman RH (ed): *Operative Nerve Repair and Reconstruction.* Philadelphia, JB Lippincott, 1991, p 1587.

8. Stout AP: The peripheral manifestations of the specific nerve sheath tumor (neurilemoma). Am J Cancer 1935; 24:751.

9. Geschickter CF: Tumors of the peripheral nerves. Am J Cancer 1935; 25:377.

10. Spjut HJ, Dorfman HD, Fechner RE, et al: Tumors of the Bone and Cartilage. Washington, DC, Armed Forces Institute of Pathology, 1971, p 400.

11. Moore JR, Weiland AJ, Curtis RM: Localized nodular tenosynovitis: Experience with 115 cases. J Hand Surg Am 1984; 9: 412.

12. Glowacki K, Weiss AP: Giant cell tumors of the tendon sheath. Hand Clin 1995; 11: 245.

13. Van Geertruyden J, Lorea P, Goldschmidt D, et al: Glomus tumors of the hand. A study of 51 cases. J Hand Surg Br 1996; 21:257.

14. Love JG: Glomus tumors: diagnosis and treatment. Mayo Clin Proc 1994; 19:113.

15. Carroll RE, Berman AT: Glomus tumors of the hand. J Bone Joint Surg Am 1972; 54:691.

16. Kleinert HE, Burget GC, Morgan JA, et al: Aneurysms of the hand. Arch Surg 1973; 106:554.

17. Layman CD, Ogden LL, Lister GD: True aneurysm of digital artery. J Hand Surg 1982; 7:617.

18. Louis DS, Simon MA: Traumatic false aneurysms of the upper extremity. J Bone Joint Surg Am 1974; 56:176.

19. Hentz V, Jackson I, Fogarty D: Case report: False aneurysm of the hand secondary to digital amputation. J Hand Surg 1978; 3:199.

20. Kalisman M, Laborde K, Wolff TW: Ulnar nerve compression secondary to ulnar artery false aneurysm at the Guyon's canal. J Hand Surg 1982; 7:137.

21. McClinton M: Tumors and aneurysms of the upper extremity. Hand Clin 1993; 9: 151.

22. Paletta FX, Senay LC Jr: Lipofibromatous hamartoma of median and ulnar nerve: Surgical treatment. Plast Reconstr Surg 1981; 17:915.

23. Warhold LG, Urban MA, Bora FW Jr, et al: Lipofibromatous hamartomas of the median nerve. J Hand Surg Am 1993; 18: 1032.

24. Gitelis S, McDonald D: Common benign tumors and usual treatment. In Simon M, Springfield D (eds): *Surgery for Bone and Soft-Tissue Tumors.* Philadelphia, Lippincott-Raven, 1998, p 191.

25. Wold L, McLeod R, Sim F, et al: Atlas of Orthopedic Pathology. Philadelphia, WB Saunders, 1990.

26. Burgess RC, Cates H: Deformities of the forearm in patients who have multiple cartilaginous exostosis. J Bone Joint Surg Am 1993; 75:13.

27. Wood VE, Sauser D, Mudge D: The treatment of hereditary multiple exostosis of the upper extremity. J Hand Surg Am 1985; 10:505.

28. Boriani S, Bacchini P, Bertoni F, et al: Periosteal chondroma. J Bone Joint Surg Am 1983; 65:205.

29. Bauer TW, Dorfman HD, Latham JT Jr: Periosteal chondroma. Am J Surg Pathol 1982; 6:631.

30. Bednar M, McCormack R, Glasser D, et al: Osteoid osteoma of the upper extremity. J Hand Surg Am 1993; 18:1019.

31. Doyle LK, Ruby LK, Nalebuff EG, et al: Osteoid osteoma of the hand. J Hand Surg Am 1985; 10:408.

32. Ambrosia JM, Wood LE, Amadio PC: Osteoid osteoma of the hand and wrist. J Hand Surg Am 1987; 12:794.

33. Neer CS, Francis KC, Marcove RC, et al: Treatment of unicameral bone cyst. J Bone Joint Surg Am 1966; 48:731.

34. Seradge H: Distal ulnar translocation in the treatment of giant-cell tumors of the distal end of the radius. J Bone Joint Surg Am 1982; 64:67.

35. Averill R, Smith R, Campbell C: Giant-cell tumors of the bones of the hand. J Hand Surg 1980; 5:39.

36. Marcove R, Lyden J, Hiwas A: Giant cell tumor treated by cryosurgery. A report of 25 cases. J Bone Joint Surg Am 1973; 55: 1633.

37. Vander Griend R, Funderburk C: The treatment of giant-cell tumors of the distal part of the radius. J Bone Joint Surg Am 1993; 75:899.

section
12
chapter
18

KIENBÖCK'S DISEASE

Michell Gerwin

Summary

- The natural history of Kienböck's disease is not well defined.
- The origins of the disease remain controversial.
- Clinical findings tend to be nonspecific; thus, imaging modalities are used to confirm the diagnosis and classify the disease.
- Treatment varies with the stage of disease and (in selected cases) ulnar variance.
- The treatment options are varied.

DEFINITION

Kienböck's disease is osteonecrosis of the carpal lunate. For the purpose of this chapter, terms that have been historically applied to this condition, such as aseptic necrosis, avascular necrosis, and lunatomalacia, are replaced with the term osteonecrosis.

HISTORICAL REVIEW

- Avascular necrosis of the lunate was first described in 1843 by Peste,[1] who noted its collapse in certain cadaver dissections.
- In 1910, a Viennese radiologist, Robert Kienböck,[2] described the radiographic changes and clinical symptomatology associated with osteonecrosis of the lunate; it is with his name that this disease is now associated. He postulated that primary avascularity of the lunate led to its collapse.
- In the 1920s, others cited fracture, with resultant traumatic disruption of the intraosseous or extraosseous blood supply, as an etiologic event.[3]
- In 1928, Hulten[3] noted its association with "ulnar negative" variance and, on this basis, attempted radial shortening to treat Kienböck's disease.[4]
- In the 1950s, other treatments focused on ways of achieving joint unloading, such as ulnar lengthening and capitate shortening. A variety of other techniques were also explored; they were intercarpal arthrodeses, fascial arthroplasties, proximal row carpectomy, and wrist arthrodesis.[5-8]

EPIDEMIOLOGY

Kienböck's disease displays a predilection for the young adult population, people aged 20 to 40 years, but it can also occur in pediatric and elderly patients.

PATHOGENESIS

The cause of osteonecrosis of the carpal bones remains controversial. To date, the pathophysiology of Kienböck's disease is speculative. The essential common pathway in Kienböck's disease is the loss of blood supply to the lunate.

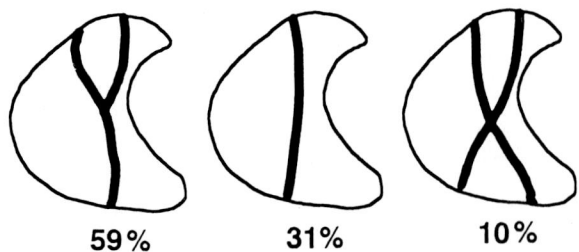

59%   **31%**   **10%**

Fig. 1. The three patterns of intraosseous vascular anastomosis in the lunate bone. Most common is the Y formation, in which two dorsal or volar vessels anastomose with a single opposing vessel. (From Williams CS, Gelberman RH: Vascularity of the lunate. Hand Clin 1993; 9:395; modified from Gelberman RH, Bauman TD, Menon J, et al: The vascularity of the lunate bone and Kienböck's disease. J Hand Surg Am 1980; 5:276.)

PATHOANATOMY

The *lunate* is a semicircular bone that articulates with the radius proximally and the capitate distally. The proximal and distal surfaces are completely covered by articular cartilage. The dorsal and volar radiolunate ligaments attach to the dorsal and palmar surfaces of the lunate, respectively, and provide its vascularity. Injection studies of the extraosseous vascularity of the lunate have demonstrated a consistent volar blood supply and a frequent but inconsistent dorsal blood supply. Palmarly, the radial, ulnar, and palmar branches of the anterior interosseous artery combine to form three transverse arches that supply the lunate. Dorsally, the radial, ulnar, and dorsal branches of the anterior interosseous artery also combine to form three arches. The dorsal blood supply of the lunate, when present, is derived from the proximal two transverse arches over the radiocarpal and intercarpal joints.[9]

Studies of the intraosseous vascularity have demonstrated both palmar and dorsal blood supplies in 74% to 100% of bones.[9–11] A combination of these studies demonstrates a single vascular supply in 7% of lunates.[12] Of the lunates with a dual blood supply, one-third have a single volar vessel and a single dorsal vessel forming an anastomosis, and two-thirds have a three-vessel anastomosis (Fig. 1).[9]

From the knowledge of the vascular anatomy of the lunate, a cause of necrosis can be postulated. It is unlikely that disruption of the extraosseous blood supply would lead to necrosis, because several volar and dorsal arches contribute to vascularity. In lunates with a single nutrient vessel, interruption may lead to necrosis of the entire bone. Similarly, in single-vessel lunates, a coronal fracture could lead to avascularity of the opposite pole (volar or dorsal). Clinically, however, dorsal or volar avascularity is rare, and more commonly, the proximal radial aspect of the lunate or the whole lunate becomes avascular. This observation makes interosseous fracture as a cause of avascularity less likely. Disruption of the nutrient vessel in the lunate with a single nutrient vessel is the most likely cause of Kienböck's disease.

PATHOMECHANICS

The association of ulnar negative variance with lunate osteonecrosis has been brought into question.[4] Although biomechanical studies have correlated increased radiolunate contact stresses with ulnar negative variance,[13] current theory suggests that ulnar negative variance is a predisposing factor and not a primary cause of Kienböck's disease. The theory is based on the numbers of patients with ulnar neutral wrists who have Kienböck's disease and several patients with ulnar negative variance who do not have the disease.

Other investigators have distinguished three types of geometric shapes of the carpal lunate, of which one type is most frequently associated with ulnar negative variance and a fragile trabecular framework. There probably exists a clinical entity "lunate at risk," in which repetitive microtrauma occurs in a lunate that has limited vascularity and the anatomy and physiology of which allow for high loading (ulnar negative variance). Patients often give a history of a single traumatic episode (i.e., extension, axial load) to the wrist, but rarely is there demonstrable force or fracture substantiating the episode as causal. Remarkably, the incidence of osteonecrosis in perilunate dislocations is relatively low.

CLINICAL FEATURES

Kienböck's disease is suspected in the young adult with pain and stiffness over the mid-dorsum of the wrist. Some patients give a history of a recent hyperextension injury, but more describe insidious onset of dull pain centered over the radiolunate joint. The pain is usually exacerbated with activity and partially relieved with rest and immobilization.

Physical examination may demonstrate a radiocarpal effusion, with boggy synovitis over the dorsum of the radiocarpal joint. Flexion and extension are usually limited, and grip strength may be decreased to half of that in the unaffected hand.[14]

INVESTIGATION

Standard posteroanterior radiographs should be obtained in *neutral* forearm positioning to evaluate the lunate and the ulnar variance of the wrist. Increased bone density of the lunate is the earliest sign of avascularity on plain radiographs. Bone scintigraphy may be used to confirm the diagnosis if the plain radiographs are negative. There have been case reports of Kienböck's disease in patients in whom results of initial bone scans were negative but results of magnetic resonance imaging (MRI) were positive.[15] We have not found any recent cases of avascularity of the lunate in which the initial bone scan was negative and a MRI was positive, and so we currently prefer bone scanning as a first-line screening tool because it is more costeffective. MRI is more specific than bone scanning and can be used to confirm the diagnosis or determine the extent of avascularity if this knowledge would influence treatment (Fig. 2).[16]

DIFFERENTIAL DIAGNOSIS
The radiographic differential diagnosis for a radiodense lunate includes transient vascular compromise after fracture-dislocation or dislocation of the carpus. This radiographic appearance resolves 6 to 8 weeks after trauma. Primary

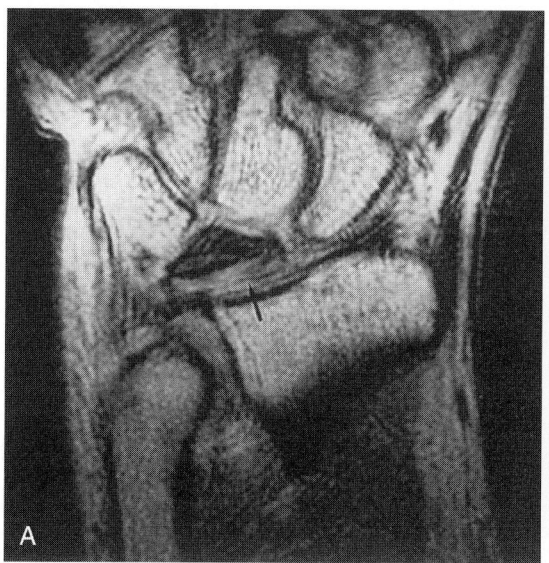
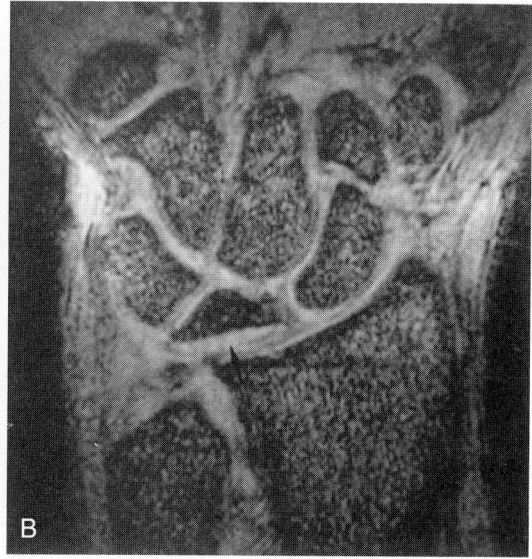

Fig. 2. View. The lunate with osteonecrosis has low signal intensity on both T_1-weighted and T_2-weighted magnetic resonance images. With revascularization, high signal intensity may be seen on T_2-weighted images. (From Gilula LA, Yin Y: Imaging of the Wrist and Hand. Philadelphia, WB Saunders, 1996, p 465.)

osteoarthritis (OA) of the radiocarpal or midcarpal joint can cause sclerosis, cysts, and collapse of the lunate. This disease can be difficult to distinguish from advanced Kienböck's disease; however, a wrist with osteoarthritis does not have proximal migration of the capitate and usually becomes symptomatic in late adulthood. Characteristically, osteoarthritis causes peripheral sclerosis at the articular surfaces as opposed to the diffuse changes seen in Kienböck's disease.

A simple cyst, osteoma, or intraosseous ganglion could mimic Kienböck's disease on plain radiographs but can be distinguished by their well-circumscribed architecture on MRI or trispiral tomography.

GOALS, INDICATIONS, AND CONTRAINDICATIONS

The primary goal of treatment for Kienböck's disease has been to halt progression of collapse of the lunate, later intercarpal collapse, and resultant wrist arthritis. The intervention chosen therefore depends on the stage of the disease.

The classification of Kienböck's disease is based on the radiographic appearance and guides treatment (Fig. 3; Table 1). The classification was first described by Stahl in 1947 and later modified by Lichtman and associates.[17] The prognosis is better for stage I and stage II disease, emphasizing the importance of early diagnosis and treatment.

MANAGEMENT

The management of Kienböck's disease is summarized in Table 2.

NONOPERATIVE CARE

Immobilization has been advocated in *all* stages of Kienböck's disease but has not been shown to halt the progres-

sion of the disease or the bone collapse. Nonoperative treatment of Kienböck's disease has had poor results, with greater than 50% of patients who receive such treatment having daily symptoms.[18] Initial treatment of stage I Kienböck's disease may include immobilization and anti-inflammatory medication. If immobilization does not succeed in alleviating symptoms, surgical intervention should be considered.

OPERATIVE PROCEDURES

The choice of a treatment is based on the stage of the disease, and often, for a given stage, there are several treatment options. Two major radiographic features influence the selection of a surgical treatment. The presence of arthritis commits the surgeon to a salvage procedure, and the presence of *ulnar positive* variance prohibits "joint lev-

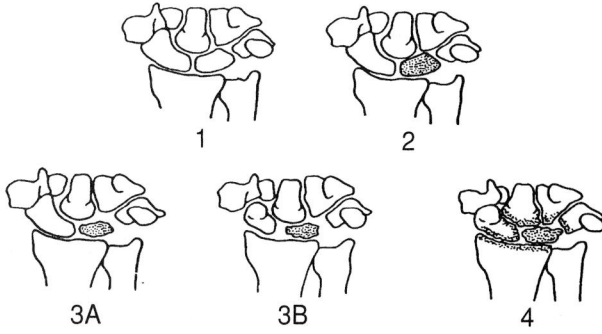

Fig. 3. Radiographic classification of Kienböck's disease. This classification is Lichtman's method: stage I: normal lunate; stage II: sclerosis of the lunate; stage IIIA: sclerosis with fragmentation or collapse of the lunate; stage IIIB: stage IIIA with fixed rotation of the scaphoid; stage IV: degenerative changes in the adjacent intercarpal joints. (From Weiland AJ: Avascular necrosis of the carpus. In Hand Surgery Update. Rosemont, IL, American Academy of Orthopaedic Surgeons, 1996, p 385.)

	TABLE 1. CLASSIFICATION OF KIENBÖCK'S DISEASE	
Stage	**Symptoms**	**Physical Findings**
I	Pain, swelling worse w/activity	Dorsal tenderness, mild loss of grip strength
II	Pain, swelling worse w/activity	Boggy synovitis, mild loss of ROM and grip strength
IIIA	As above w/mild to moderate stiffness	Effusion, moderate loss of ROM and grip strength
IIIB	Stiffness predominates	Moderate to severe loss of ROM and grip strength
IV	Marked pain, swelling, stiffness	Marked loss of ROM and grip strength, crepitus

ROM, range of motion.

eling" procedures such as radial shortening and ulnar lengthening.

Preoperative Planning and Technical Details
Revascularization
The principle behind vascular bundle implantation is that a significant amount of microcirculation exists between the artery and the vein. With implantation of a pedicle into bone, capillary beds proliferate and anastomose with the existing circulation to increase the delivery of osteogenic elements to the bone and accelerate the process of creeping substitution. Revascularization can be used in stage I through stage IIIA Kienböck's disease regardless of ulnar variance. Revascularization is *contraindicated* for stage IIIB or IV disease, because carpal collapse and arthritis cannot be corrected. Pedicled pronator quadratus with radial bone has been described as having success at 7-year follow-up.[19] We prefer transplantation of a vascular pedicle into the lunate, as described by Hori and colleagues.[20]

Vascular Pedicle Transplantation
Before surgery, Doppler examination of the pulses of the second and third dorsal metacarpal arteries is performed. The vessel with the stronger Doppler signal is selected as the donor pedicle. With the use of microscope or loupe magnification, the previously selected vascular bundle (i.e., the artery and its venae comitantes) is dissected as a pedicle, ligated distally with an absorbable suture, and cut at the level of the dorsal digital web space. Avoid "skeletonizing" the artery. The pedicle is then kept moist with 10% lidocaine solution (Xylocaine) while the recipient bed is prepared.

The dorsal capsule is incised over the radiolunate joint, and the dorsal lunate is exposed. A drill hole is made in the nonarticular portion of the lunate from dorsal to volar, through which an 18-gauge needle is passed. Through a small transverse volar wrist counterincision, a 21-gauge needle is next inserted from volar to dorsal *into* the 18-gauge needle now visible through the volar cortex of the lunate, and the 18-gauge needle is withdrawn. The tagging suture on the end of the vascular bundle is then passed through the 21-gauge needle from dorsal to volar to implant the bundle in the lunate, and the needle is withdrawn. The tagging suture is then sutured to the volar capsule to hold the bundle in position within the lunate *without* tension on the pedicle (Fig. 4).

For stage IIIA disease, the necrotic bone should be carefully removed with a burr or curette prior to implantation of the vascular bundle. Iliac crest or distal radius bone chips are then placed in the cavity, and the vascularized pedicle is transplanted through this.

Joint Leveling
Results of joint leveling procedures, which include radial shortening, ulnar lengthening, and capitate shortening, have been encouraging. Joint leveling is indicated in patients with stage I through stage IIIA Kienböck's disease. *Ulnar negative variance is a prerequisite* for radial shortening and ulnar lengthening. Shortening the radius by 2 mm is enough to unload the lunate by 70%. This amount of shortening decreases the radiolunate force while increasing ulnolunate forces by 50% and not affecting the radioscaphoid forces.[13, 21] It is *not* necessary to produce ulnar positive variance. Care must be taken not to overshorten the radius, because distal radioulnar joint incongruity may develop.[22] Radial displacement of the distal fragment along with shortening may help decrease the load across the distal radioulnar joint.[23] If the patient already has ulnar positive variance, a lateral closing or a medial opening wedge osteotomy of the radius measuring 4 to 8 degrees decreases pressure load in the lunate fossa. In contrast, the reverse osteotomy increases radiolunate load.[24]

	TABLE 2. TREATMENT OPTIONS FOR KIENBÖCK'S DISEASE	
Treatment	**Indications**	**Method**
Nonoperative	Stage I disease	Nonsteroidal anti-inflammatory drugs and immobilization
Revascularization	Stage I–IIIA disease	Artery and vein anastomosis
Radial shortening	Stage I–IIIA disease and ulnar negative variance	Osteotomy
Ulnar lengthening	Stage I–IIIA disease and ulnar negative variance	Osteotomy
Radial wedge osteotomy	Stage I–IIIA disease and ulnar negative variance	Osteotomy (closing/opening)
Capitate shortening	Stage I–IIIA disease and ulnar negative variance	Decompression
Intercarpal arthrodesis	Stage IIIB disease	Dorsal approach

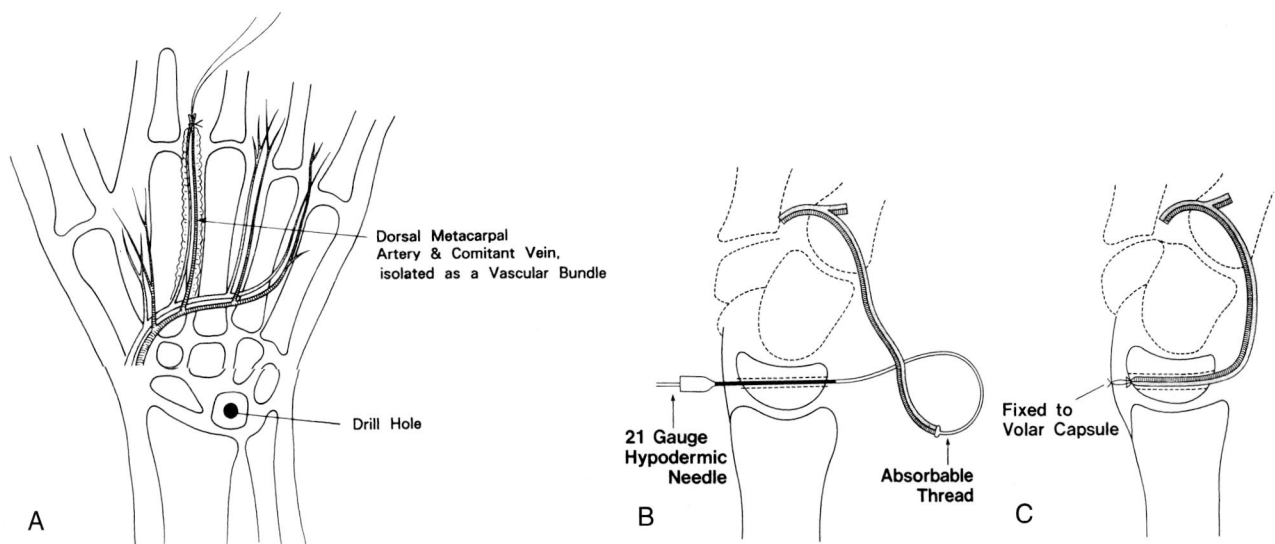

Fig. 4. Vascular pedicle transplantation. *A,* The second dorsal metacarpal artery and vein are isolated as a neurovascular pedicle. A drill hole is made in the lunate from dorsal to volar. *B,* The vascular pedicle is passed through the lunate from dorsal to volar with the assistance of a tagging suture and a 21-gauge needle. *C,* The vascular bundle transplantation is completed. The tagging suture is secured to the volar capsule to prevent withdrawal of the bundle from the lunate. (From Tamai S, Yajima H, Ono H: Revascularization procedures in the treatment of Kienböck's disease. Hand Clin 1993; 9:457.)

An ulnar-lengthening osteotomy accomplishes the *same* goals as radial shortening. Ulnar lengthening produces an intercalary defect that usually requires bone grafting. Drawbacks of ulnar lengthening include bone graft donor site morbidity and a higher risk of nonunion at the osteotomy site.

Capitate shortening has been shown to provide the greatest reduction of compressive forces across the lunate, although it *increases* scaphotrapezial and triquetrohamate forces.[25] The procedure can be performed in an ulnar positive wrist; however, in this situation, capitate shortening involves wrist capsulotomy and therefore more loss of motion than other joint leveling procedures.

Radial Shortening or Radial Wedge Osteotomy

The radius is exposed through a distal Henry approach between the flexor carpi radialis and radial artery. The volar radiocarpal ligaments are *not* disturbed. A six-hole, 3.5-mm dynamic compression (DC) plate is contoured to the volar aspect of the radius as distally as possible to allow the osteotomy to be performed in the radial metaphysis. Placement of the plate too far distally, however, will result in its prominence over the volar lip of the radius. The plate is fixed to the radius with a clamp, and the osteotomy site is marked on the radius at the midpoint of the plate (i.e., between the third and fourth holes); then two of the distal screws are inserted. These two screws are removed, and the plate is temporarily removed. The osteotomy is performed with an oscillating saw to remove a 2-mm segment of bone. Care must be taken to not remove too much radius (Fig. 5).

After the osteotomy, the plate is reattached to the distal radial fragment through the previously made screw holes. If possible, the radial fragment should be displaced *slightly* radially to reduce the forces on the distal radioulnar joint. The remaining screw holes are fastened proximally with use of the dynamic compression aspect of the plate through two of the proximal holes. The radial bone previously removed can be morselized and used as bone graft. Postoperatively, the wrist is immobilized in a removable protective splint until there is radiographic evidence of union.

Ulnar Lengthening

The ulna is approached[26, 27] between the extensor and flexor carpi ulnaris muscles, with care taken to identify and protect the dorsal sensory branch of the ulnar nerve. A six-hole DC plate is contoured to the volar aspect of the distal ulna. Two screw holes are drilled and filled distally with 3.5-mm cortical screws. The osteotomy site is marked just between the third and fourth screw holes and then is cross-hatched to allow for proper rotational positioning after osteotomy. The two previously placed screws and the plate are temporarily removed. The osteotomy is then created with an oscillating saw. Distraction of the osteotomy with a laminar spreader allows for placement of a 3-mm tricortical iliac crest graft. The plate is replaced along the volar surface of the ulna, and the previously drilled screw holes are filled, followed by insertion of the remaining screws. Postoperatively, the arm is put in a short-arm cast full time for 6 to 9 weeks. Armistead and coworkers[26] recommend removal of the plate 1 year after union, to allow the grafted area to become stronger. We rarely remove forearm plates unless a patient complaints of discomfort in the area over the hardware.

Capitate Shortening

The capitate is approached through a straight dorsal longitudinal midline incision. Osteotomy of the capitate is begun with a thin osteotome at the distal margin of the dorsal articular surface of the scaphoid but is not carried to the volar cortex yet. The second cut is made 2 to 3 mm *distal* to the first. Both osteotomies are then continued simultaneously, with the proximal osteotomy completed first. The volar capsule is kept intact as the osteotomized wafer of capitate is removed. The capitate head is then held com-

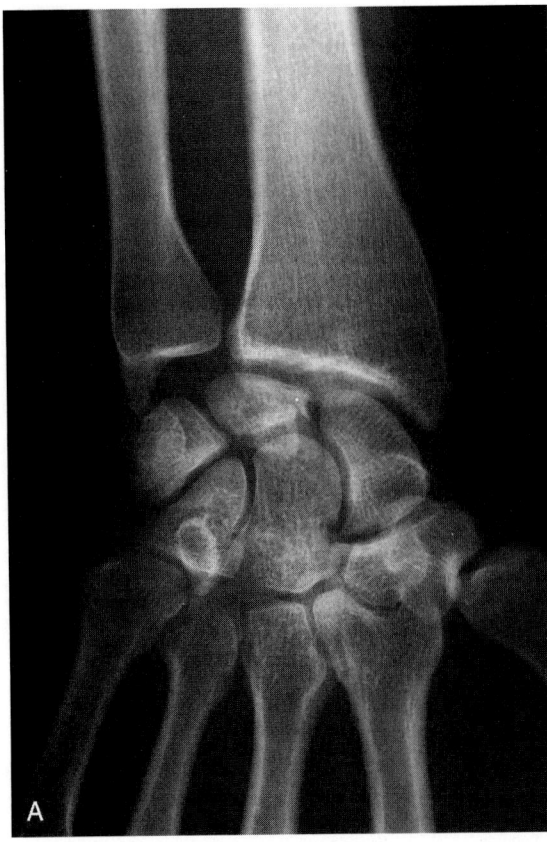
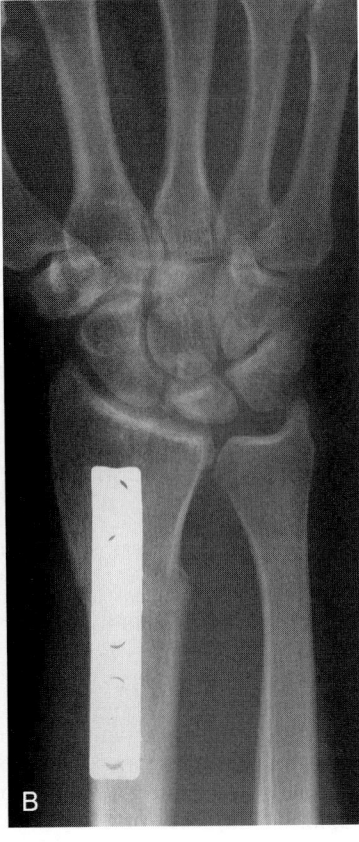

Fig. 5. Radial shortening for Kienböck's disease with a six-hole dynamic compression plate. *A*, Preoperative radiograph of wrist demonstrating ulnar negative variance. *B*, Postoperative radiograph of radial shortening osteotomy.

pressed to the distal pole of the capitate with an elevator while crossed 0.062-inch K-wires are passed retrograde across the osteotomy site. Capitohamate fusion can be performed simultaneously to increase the fusion mass (Fig. 6).

Postoperatively the wrist is immobilized in a short-arm cast for 8 weeks. If radiographs demonstrate early healing of the osteotomy site, the arm is put in a removable wrist splint; if not, another short-arm cast is applied. When complete union is seen radiographically, the pins are removed. Range-of-motion exercises can be begun while the arm is

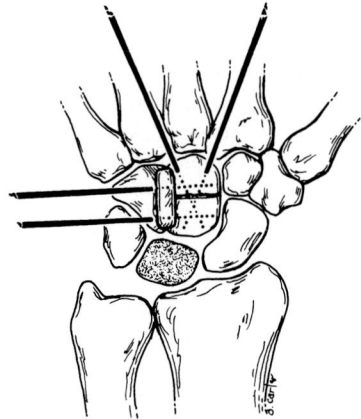

Fig. 6. View. Adjacent surfaces of the hamate and capitate are decorticated and fixed with K-wires along with the osteotomy of the capitate. (From Almquist EA: Capitate shortening in the treatment of Kienböck's disease. Hand Clin 1993; 9:509.)

still in the splint, but the splint should be worn until revascularization of the lunate is seen radiographically.

Resection Arthroplasty with Silicone Implant or Coiled Palmaris Tendon
See the section "Complications and Results" below.

Limited Intercarpal Arthrodesis
Scaphotrapeziotrapezoid (STT) and scaphocapitate (SC) fusions are good options for treatment of stage IIIB Kienböck's disease, especially in the presence of neutral or positive ulnar variance. Both techniques can address the rotatory subluxation of the scaphoid to improve the pattern of carpal collapse in addition to unloading the lunate. SC fusion is technically easier than STT fusion and is usually our first choice. STT and SC arthrodeses have been shown to decrease lunate load an average of 70% compared with capitohamate arthrodesis and to be roughly equal to joint leveling procedures.[21, 25] Fusion of the scaphoid in a neutral or extended position is important to reduce the load on the lunate but may increase load on the radioscaphoid joint.[28]

Experimental wrist kinematics studies have shown loss of motion after either fusion technique to be 15% of flexion and extension and 25% of radioulnar deviation.[29] In vivo values would be expected to be different as a result of postoperative intra-articular fibrosis and, then, later ligament stretching. Experimental studies have shown the ideal radioscaphoid angle for maximal wrist motion to be 41 to 60 degrees after STT fusion and 30 to 57 degrees after SC fusion.[30]

STT Arthrodesis. A transverse incision is made over the STT joint, with care taken to protect branches of the superficial radial nerve and radial artery. The radioscaphoid joint should be inspected for the presence of arthritis, which would preclude STT arthrodesis. Radial styloidectomy is next carried out with 5 mm of the styloid tip removed (this does not affect wrist motion but may lessen first extensor compartment symptoms). The STT joints are decorticated with rongeur, saw, or bur. The trapeziotrapezoid joint is decorticated proximally, with care taken not to disrupt the carpometacarpal joint distally. The lunate is next inspected, and if it is in multiple fragments, it is excised.

A second transverse incision is made 2 cm proximal to the radial styloid, a cortical window is elevated from the radius, and cancellous bone graft is harvested. Two smooth K-wires (0.045- or 0.062-inch) are preset in the trapezoid, and the scaphotrapezial joint is positioned as described by Watson and associates.[31] A periosteal elevator is placed in the scaphotrapezial joint to create a 5-mm space, and the wrist is positioned in 25 degrees of dorsiflexion and 20 degrees of radial deviation. The spacer (periosteal elevator) prevents loss of carpal height due to the decortication. The surgeon then dorsally displaces the scaphoid as far as possible and drives the two K-wires retrograde across the scaphotrapezial joint. This maneuver reduces the scaphoid to about 50 to 60 degrees of volar flexion relative to the long axis of the radius. The previously harvested cancellous graft is then placed across the fusion site (Fig. 7).

SC Fusion. A dorsal midline incision is made over the SC region. Cortical bone is removed from the dorsal two-thirds of the adjacent surfaces of the scaphoid and capitate. Retaining the palmar third of the cortical bone maintains carpal height. The decorticated area is filled with autogenous bone graft, and multiple K-wires are drilled across the fusion site. Care is taken to reduce the scaphoid to the

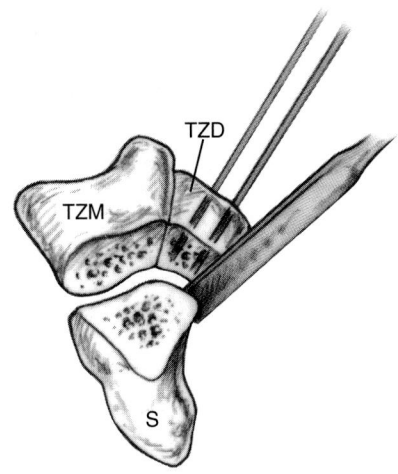

Fig. 7. View. Adjacent surfaces of the scaphoid (S), trapezium (TZM), and trapezoid (TZD) are decorticated to cancellous bone. A 5-mm spacer is placed between the scaphoid and trapezoid, and two K-wires are preset in the trapezoid. The wrist is then positioned in 25 degrees of radial deviation as the distal pole of the scaphoid is displaced dorsally as far as possible. The K-wires are then driven retrograde across the scaphotrapezoid joint. (Redrawn from Watson HK, Pitts EC: Scapholunate dissociation: Treatment by scaphotrapezio-trapezoid arthrodesis. Tech Orthop 1992; 7:30.).

capitate, and intraoperative radiographs should confirm acceptable alignment of scaphoid, capitate, radius, and lunate. If radial deviation past neutral is not possible intraoperatively, then the scaphoid has probably been excessively extended and needs repositioning.

Postoperative Care. After STT or SC fusion, the arm is immobilized in a long-arm thumb spica cast with the index and long fingers in the intrinsic-plus position. After 4 weeks, a short-arm thumb spica cast is applied. Six weeks after surgery, radiographs should demonstrate healing. Once arthrodesis is achieved, the pins are removed, and range of motion is begun.

Wrist Denervation
See the section "Complications and Results" below.

Salvage Procedures: Wrist Arthrodesis and Proximal Row Carpectomy
Treatment of stage IV Kienböck's disease requires a salvage procedure to preserve function and eliminate pain. The best options are proximal row carpectomy and wrist arthrodesis. Proximal row carpectomy is indicated when the articular cartilage of the lunate fossa of the radius and the head of the capitate are in good condition. Although retaining motion, proximal row carpectomy does not provide as strong a grip strength as an arthrodesis. There is no guarantee for any single procedure, and even with proximal row carpectomy, some patients may eventually need wrist arthrodesis.

Some surgeons have advocated that if there is articular loss on the head of the capitate or in the lunate fossa, distraction resection arthroplasty should be performed. In this procedure, the head of the capitate is excised, and the wrist is kept distracted with K-wires. In one series of 11 patients who underwent distraction resection arthroplasty for degenerative arthritis, 25% eventually required wrist arthrodesis.[32]

COMPLICATIONS AND RESULTS

REVASCULARIZATION
Tamai and colleagues[33] reported 51 cases of Kienböck's disease treated with vascular pedicle implantation and followed for an average of 6 years. Five of six wrists with stage I or II disease had good results, and one a fair result. Results in stage III and IV disease were more mixed, even though some patients had bone grafting or limited fusions at the time of revascularization. Seventy-two percent of wrists with stage III disease (not divided into stages IIIA and IIIB) still had a good result. On the average, all the patients in the series had reported improvement in range of motion and grip strength.

JOINT LEVELING
Results of joint leveling procedures, which include radial shortening, ulnar lengthening, and capitate shortening, have been encouraging.

Radial Shortening. Four-year follow-up of radial shortening has demonstrated average increases of 30% in flexion and extension and 50% in grip strength; 87% of patients had good or excellent results.[34–36] Three types of complications are possible after distal radius shortening[18]:

- Nonunion may occur in 4% of cases.
- Excessive shortening can lead to secondary ulnar impaction.
- Ulnar impingement at the distal radial ulnar joint can similarly result from excessive radial shortening.

Radial Wedge Osteotomy. Results of radial wedge osteotomies at 2 years demonstrate a 60% rate of good or excellent results. Even though these results are inferior to the 87% figure for radial shortening,[18] radial wedge osteotomy is a good extra-articular treatment for ulnar-positive wrists and does not limit motion.

Ulnar Lengthening. Results of one series of 60 patients treated with ulnar lengthening demonstrated 90% to be satisfied at 7 years, with pain relief in 86%.[37] Fourteen percent had a delayed union or nonunion, and 8% had symptoms of ulnocarpal impingement or impaction. Donor site morbidity from iliac crest bone grafting, though usually transient, is a frequent occurrence. Plate removal was necessary in 55% of patients, and 5% of patients needed reoperation for nonunion. Despite technically adequate ulnar lengthening, 11% of patients needed further procedures on their wrists, including limited intercarpal fusions and other salvage procedures. In no patients had disease progressed a radiographic stage at follow-up.

Resection Arthroplasty. Long-term results of silicone lunate implantation have demonstrated the incidence of silicone synovitis to approach 50%, with 80% of patients having poor results as a result of either silicone synovitis or dislocation of the prosthesis.[38] Silicone synovitis can destroy joints that otherwise could have been salvaged with a different procedure. The patient with Kienböck's disease tends to be a young, active male who is ill suited for silicone arthroplasty. At this time, we do *not* see a place for silicone lunate arthroplasty in the treatment of Kienböck's disease. Lunate resection and fascial replacement have been almost uniformly unsuccessful because of late carpal collapse and should always be performed in conjunction with a limited intercarpal fusion.[7, 39]

Limited Intercarpal Arthrodesis. Long-term follow-up of close to 5 years for 35 patients undergoing STT arthrodesis has shown 80% to have little or no rest pain and 71% to have no pain with activity.[31] After STT fusion, 30% of wrists may require late lunate excision because of pain, if the lunate was not excised at the time of limited arthrodesis. Nonunion should be treated with a second bone grafting at 3 to 4 months.

Wrist Denervation. Buck-Gramcko[40] reported on wrist denervation alone as treatment of Kienböck's disease. At 6.5 years, 65% of patients had either no pain or pain only with heavy activities. Results were unrelated to the stage of disease at time of surgery, suggesting that the procedure had a true denervation effect. Progression of the lunate changes was seen radiographically in 50% of patients, but only 5 patients showed progressive arthritic changes. Denervation alone is probably not sufficient treatment for Kienböck's disease, but resection of the terminal articular portion of the posterior interosseous nerve should be performed at the time of other procedures if possible.

Wrist Arthrodesis and Proximal Row Carpectomy. Although arthrodesis eliminates motion, it virtually ensures pain relief and good grip strength. The likelihood that subsequent procedures will be required after arthrodesis is low. After wrist fusion, grip strength improves but usually does not return to normal. Pseudarthrosis rates are less than 5%.

After proximal row carpectomy, most patients gain approximately 30 degrees of flexion and extension and achieve at least 50% to as much as 80% of the grip strength in the contralateral hand.[8]

REFERENCES

1. Peste JL: Discussion. Bull Soc Anat 1843; 18:169.
2. Kienböck R (trans. Peltier LF): Concerning traumatic malacia of the lunate and its consequences: Degeneration and compression fractures. Clin Orthop 1980; 149:4.
3. Hulten O: Uber Anatomische der Handgelenknochen. Acta Radiol 1928; 9:155.
4. Kristensen SS, Thomassen E, Christensen F: Ulnar variance in Kienböck's disease. J Hand Surg Br 1986; 11:258.
5. Persson M: Pathogenese und Behandlung der Kienböckschen Lunatum-malazie. Acta Chir Scand 1945; 92.
6. Almquist EE: Capitate shortening in the treatment of Kienböck's disease. Hand Clin 1993; 9:505.
7. Eaton RG: Excision and fascial interposition arthroplasty in the treatment of Kienböck's disease. Hand Clin 1993; 9:513.
8. Imbriglia JE, Broudy AS, Hagberg WC, et al: Proximal row carpectomy: Clinical evaluation. J Hand Surg Am 1990; 15:426.
9. Gelberman RH, Bauman TD, Menon J, et al: The vascularity of the lunate bone and Kienböck's disease. J Hand Surg Am 1980; 5:272.
10. Lee MLH: The intraosseous arterial pattern of the carpal lunate bone and its relation to avascular necrosis. Acta Orthop Scand 1963; 33:43.
11. Panagis JS, Gelberman RH, Taleisnik J, et al: The arterial anatomy of the human carpus. Part II: The intraosseous vascularity. J Hand Surg Am 1983; 8:375.
12. Williams CS, Gelberman RH: Vascularity of the lunate. Hand Clin 1993; 9:391.
13. Palmer A, Werner F: Biomechanics of the distal radioulnar joint. Clinic Orthop 1984; 187:26.
14. Beckenbaugh RD, Shives TC, Dobyns JH, et al: Kienböck's disease: The natural history of Kienböck's disease and consideration of the lunate fractures. Clin Orthop 1980; 149:98.
15. Amadio PC, Hanssen AD, Berquist TH: The genesis of Kienböck's disease: Evaluation of a case by magnetic resonance imaging. J Hand Surg Am 1987; 12:1044.
16. Gerwin M, Potter H, Hotchkiss RN, et al: The use of MRI in the wrist. Presented at the AAOS Annual Meeting.
17. Lichtman DM, Mack GR, MacDonald RI, et al: Kienböck's disease: The role of silicone replacement arthroplasty. J Bone Joint Surg Am 1977; 59:899.
18. Mikkelsen SS, Gelineck J: Poor function after nonoperative treatment of Kienböck's disease. Acta Orthop Scand 1987; 58:241.
19. Braun R: The pronator pedicle bone grafting in the forearm and proximal row. Presented at the 38th annual meeting of the American Society for Surgery of the Hand, March, 1983.
20. Hori Y, Tomai S, Okuda H, et al: Blood vessel transplantation to bone. J Hand Surg Am 1979; 4:23.
21. Trumble T, Glisson RR, Seaber AV, et al: A biomechanical comparison of the methods for treating Kienböck's disease. J Hand Surg Am 1986; 11:88.
22. Nakamura R, Horii E, Imaeda T: Excessive radial shortening in Kienböck's disease. J Hand Surg Br 1990; 15:46.
23. Werner FW, Murphy DJ, Palmer AK: Pressures in the distal radioulnar joint: Effect of surgical procedures used for Kienböck's disease. J Orthop Res 1989; 7:445.
24. Werner FW, Palmer AK, Utter RG: Distal radial osteotomy for the treatment of

Kienböck's disease: A biomechanical study. Orthop Trans 1988; 12:486.

25. Horii E, Garcia-Elias M, Bishop AT, et al: Effect on force transmission across the carpus in procedures used to treat Kienböck's disease. J Hand Surg Am 1990; 15: 393.

26. Armistead RB, Linscheid RL, Dobyns JH, et al: Ulnar lengthening in the treatment of Kienböck's disease. J Bone Joint Surg Am 1982; 64:170.

27. Sundberg SB, Linscheid RL: Kienböck's disease: Results of treatment with ulnar lengthening. Clin Orthop 1984; 187:43.

28. Short WH, Werner FW, Fortino MD, et al: Distribution of pressures and forces on the wrist after simulated intercarpal fusion and Kienböck's disease. J Hand Surg Am 1992; 17:443.

29. Garcia-Elias M, Cooney WP, Linscheid RL, et al: Wrist kinematics after limited intercarpal arthrodesis. J Hand Surg Am 1989; 14:791.

30. Minamikawa Y, Peimer CA, Yamaguchi T, et al: Ideal scaphoid angle for intercarpal arthrodesis. J Hand Surg Am 1989; 17:370.

31. Watson HK, Fink JA, Monacelli DM: Use of the scaphotrapezio-trapezoid fusion in the treatment of Kienböck's disease. Hand Clin 1993; 9:493.

32. Fitzgerald JP, Peimer CA, Smith RJ: distraction resection arthroplasty of the wrist. J Hand Surg Am 1989; 14:774.

33. Tamai S, Yajima H, Ono H: Revascularization procedures in the treatment of Kienböck's disease. Hand Clin 1993; 9: 455.

34. Almquist EE, Burns JF Jr: Radial shortening for the treatment of Kienböck's disease: A 5 to 10 year follow-up. J Hand Surg Am 1982; 8:348.

35. Nakamura R, Horii E, Imaeda T: Excessive radial shortening in Kienböck's disease. J Hand Surg Br 1990; 15:46.

36. Weiss APC, Weiland AJ, Moore R, et al: Radial shortening for Kienböck's disease. J Bone Joint Surg Am 1991; 73:384.

37. Quenzer DE, Linscheid RL: Ulnar lengthening procedures. Hand Clin 1993; 9:467.

38. Alexander AH, Turner MA, Alexander CE, et al: Lunate silicone replacement arthroplasty in Kienböck's disease: A long-term follow-up study. J Hand Surg Am 1990; 15:401.

39. Kato H, Usui M, Minami A: Long-term results of Kienböck's disease treated by excisional arthroplasty with a silicone implant or coiled palmaris longus tendon. J Hand Surg Am 1986; 11:645.

40. Buck-Gramcko D: Denervation of the wrist joint. J Hand Surg Am 1977; 2:54.

section **12** chapter **19**

DUPUYTREN'S CONTRACTURE

Thomas J. Graham and Thomas R. Hunt

Summary
- Dupuytren's disease is thought to be inherited via an autosomal-dominant trait with variable penetrance and influenced by environmental factors.
- Investigation into the biological events critical to the genesis of nodules and the progression of cords has become possible as the fields of molecular biology and genetics have evolved. Growth and maturation factors may hold the key to prevention and treatment.
- Surgery is the mainstay of treatment. Its conceptual simplicity belies the technically challenging nature of the procedure.
- Critical to success is a comprehensive understanding of the normal and altered anatomy and management of critical "resources."

DEFINITION

There are few more characteristic expressions of pathology in the hand than that of Dupuytren's contracture. Its diagnosis is rarely in doubt. Over the past two centuries, little progress has been made toward identifying a nonoperative treatment. Surgery is still the mainstay of treatment for advanced disease.

On a macroscopic level, for the purposes of nomenclature, the quiescent fibrous tissue of the palmar aponeurosis and digital ligamentofascial components are considered as "bands." In the pathological state, when nodules and contractures occur, these entities are termed "cords".[1] Firm nodularity or coalesced cords of tissue in the palm or digit or spanning the web spaces is the hallmark of clinical presentation of Dupuytren's disease (Fig. 1).

Dupuytren's diathesis is a constellation of characteristics that define a subgroup of patients with more severe and aggressive disease, often at several anatomic sites. This subgroup of patients experiences earlier onset (often before age 40) and rapidly progressive contracture in the hands, occasionally involving the radial digits. Garrod's nodes[2] or knuckle pads over the dorsum of the proximal interphalangeal (PIP) joints (Fig. 2) also are more common. Involvement of the plantar fascia of the foot (Ledderhose's contracture) and Buck's fascia of the penis (Peyronie's disease) may also be seen. The prevalence of these ectopic lesions in a series of patients operated for palm and digit contractures was less than 3%.[3]

EPIDEMIOLOGY

Certain factors have demonstrated a high concordance rate with the appearance of Dupuytren's disease. The disease is generally considered to be of genetic origin, inherited by autosomal-dominant transmission with variable penetrance.[4] Despite the inheritance pattern, a positive family history of the disease is appreciated in less than 10% of patients. Those with this association often belong to that special subgroup with Dupuytren's diathesis, referred to earlier. Surprisingly, there are reports of identical twins in which only one twin developed Dupuytren's contracture.[5] This evidence suggests that inheritance is not based on a single mendelian dominant trait but instead on a predisposing allele that confers genetic susceptibility. This and other evidence argue for the importance of environmental influences on the development of Dupuytren's disease.

The true prevalence of Dupuytren's contracture is unknown. Prevalence varies among populations. Mikkelsen[6] examined 16,000 residents of a Norwegian town as part of a mass screening program and found prevalence rates of

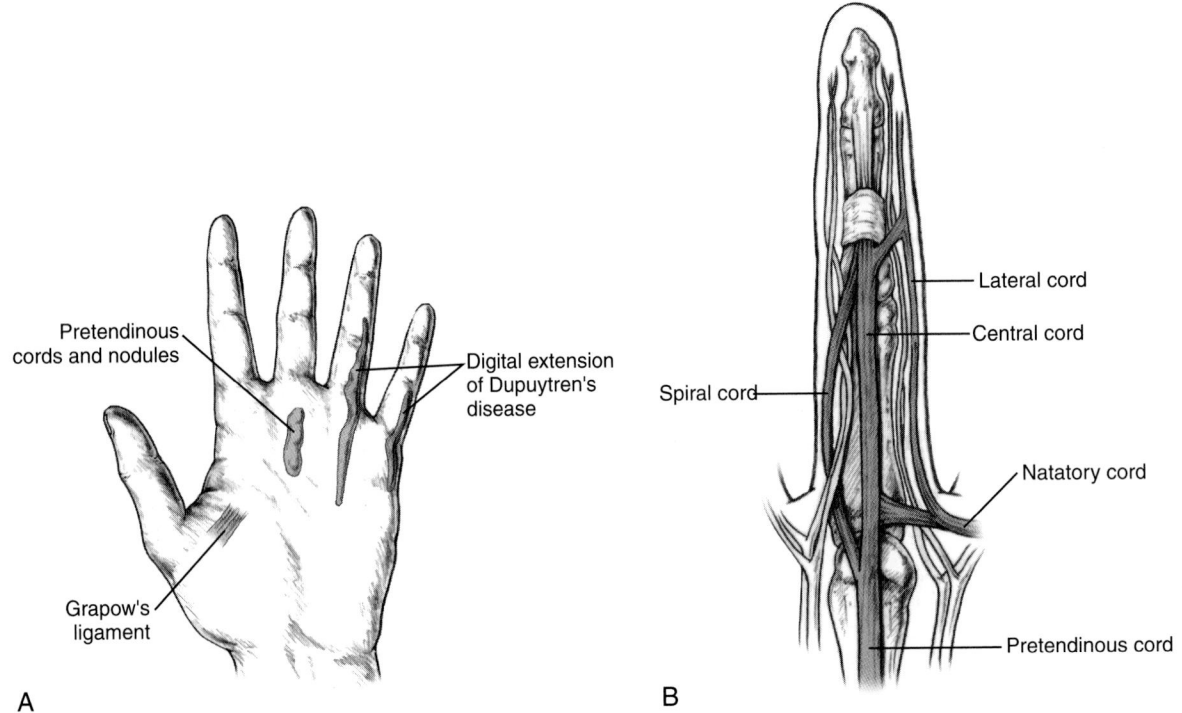

Fig. 1. Dupuytren's contracture. *A,* Depiction of typical sites of involvement of Dupuytren's contracture in the palm and digit. *B,* Summary of the different digital cords. (*B,* Redrawn from McFarlane et al [eds]: Dupuytren's Disease: Biology and Treatment. New York, Churchill Livingstone, 1995, p 555.)

Dupuytren's disease of 9.4% for men and 2.8% for women. Yost et al[7] examined more than 5000 inpatients in New York City and found an overall prevalence of 4.8%. Most investigators found a higher prevalence of the disease in Caucasians, especially in individuals of Northern European ancestry. The prevalence may be as high as 20% in men 60 years of age and older of Northern European origin.[8, 9]

A male predominance is inferred in most studies, although the male-female ratio is variable in published reports, ranging from 2:1 to 10:1. Onset usually occurs in the fifth decade for men and sixth decade for women. In one study of Dupuytren's disease in diabetics, the male-female ratio was equal.[10]

Advancing age is correlated with the development of Dupuytren's contracture. The disease is rare in patients younger than 40 years, and onset is most commonly seen between the ages of 40 and 65 years. However, several reports, replete with supporting histological confirmation, detailed the appearance of the disease in children and teenagers.[11]

There has been exhaustive work on determining what additional epidemiological factors may be associated with the development of Dupuytren's contracture. Three medical problems have received the most significant focus: alcoholism or liver disease, seizure disorders, and diabetes mellitus. Additional pathological associations under investigation include cigarette smoking,[12] HIV infection,[13, 14] local trauma and work injuries[8] (as originally postulated by Dupuytren), and hyperlipidemia.[15]

ALCOHOLISM AND SMOKING

The reported prevalence of alcoholism among patients with Dupuytren's contracture varies from 9% to 78% (averaging approximately 40%), whereas a 20% to 25% prevalence of alcoholism prevails in the general population.[16] Essentially every study focused on the relationship between alcohol and Dupuytren's contracture has shown a greater incidence of excess alcohol consumption in those with the disease. Also, the contractures found in patients consuming significant quantities of alcohol are often severe.[17, 18]

It is debated whether alcohol or its direct effect on the liver is responsible for the increased prevalence of Dupuytren's disease in this population. In a British study, alcoholics and patients with liver disease unrelated to alcohol consumption demonstrated an equally high rate of Dupuytren's contracture. In both groups, the rate was significantly

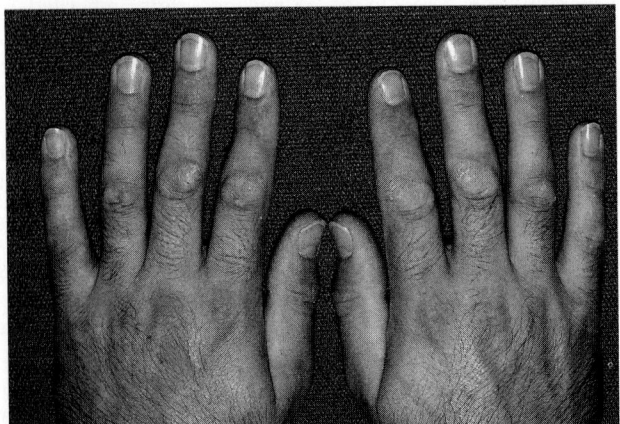

Fig. 2. Garrod's nodes. These nodular thickenings, or knuckle pads, over the dorsum of proximal interphalangeal joints are common.

higher than was noted in controls.[19] It seems likely that regardless of the cause of the hepatic insult, a fundamental change in the ability of the liver to handle its metabolic role enables the basic biological substrates and cellular events of Dupuytren's contracture to be initiated.

Blood flow to the distal extremities is diminished by smoking, and the resulting hypovascular environment may trigger the cascade of events leading to digital contracture. One study evaluated the effects of cigarette smoking and alcohol consumption on 222 patients treated surgically for Dupuytren's contracture and compared them with age- and gender-matched controls. Current cigarette smoking was strongly associated with Dupuytren's contracture requiring surgical correction.[12]

SEIZURE DISORDER

Both seizure disorders and the drugs used to treat them have been associated with the onset of Dupuytren's contracture.[16, 20] Although this population may experience an increased incidence of the disease, the data are conflicting. It appears that the pharmacological agents used to treat seizures are probably not the culprits.[21] Similar to alcoholics, patients with seizure disorders tend to demonstrate more severe contractures.

DIABETES MELLITUS

Dupuytren's disease is quite common in diabetics, with an incidence ranging from 30% to 40%.[22] Some consider Dupuytren's disease to be an early warning sign of diabetes.[23] Its prevalence increases with the duration of the diabetes mellitus but is equal in patients with type 1 and type 2 diabetes and has not been clearly linked to control of blood glucose levels.[10, 24] Some investigators believe microvasculopathy and peripheral neuropathy, complications that may be related more to duration than control of the disease, contribute to the high prevalence of Dupuytren's disease in the diabetic population.

Manifestations of Dupuytren's disease in diabetic patients are usually, but not always, mild. Findings typically include nodularity and thickness in the palm and digits without pronounced cords or joint contractures.[23] Nodules involve the index and long fingers more frequently than is seen in Dupuytren's patients without diabetes.[22]

PATHOGENESIS

The pathogenesis of Dupuytren's contracture is becoming better understood. Investigation into the biological events critical to the genesis of nodules and the progression of cords has become possible as the fields of molecular biology and genetics have matured. We now suspect that digital contracture occurs as the end product of native fibroblast and myofibroblast proliferation, enhanced synthesis of extracellular matrix (collagen and glycosaminoglycans), and myofibroblast contraction controlled by polypeptide growth factors in a genetically susceptible individual, possibly those with chromosomal instability.[25] Indeed, it is these growth factors that may hold the key to the medical treatment and perhaps prevention of this disease.

Growth factors are known to regulate cell growth and differentiation as well as extracellular matrix produc-

tion throughout the body. Platelet-derived growth factor (PDGF), transforming growth factor-beta (TGF-β), beta fibroblast growth factor (βFGF), and others have been implicated in Dupuytren's disease.

Alioto and coauthors[26] outlined a possible model to explain the contribution of growth factors known to be integral in the pathogenesis of Dupuytren's contracture. Microhemorrhages caused by ischemia, trauma, liver disease, or other events stimulate the release of platelets and inflammatory cells. PDGF and TGF-β, released by platelets, stimulate fibroblast proliferation and their differentiation into myofibroblasts as well as extracellular matrix deposition. Inflammatory cells, extracellular matrix, and endothelial cells release cytokines and proteolytic enzymes, which, in turn, result in the release of βFGF, causing further fibroblast proliferation. Genetically induced changes found in Dupuytren's fibroblasts, such as increased receptors and increased receptor sensitivity for these three growth factors, are responsible for excessive cell proliferation and collagen production without normal regulatory controls. This hypovascular environment may then cause more microhemorrhages and progression of the disease state.

This sequence of fibroblast proliferation, collagen synthesis, and contraction of Dupuytren's myofibroblasts may be governed by PDGF or TGF-β autocrine and paracrine feedback loops[27, 28] or by local tissue ischemia. Hueston and Murrell[29, 30] and others believe local tissue ischemia causes release of oxygen-free radicals. These highly reactive free radicals damage the surrounding microvasculature and stimulate fibroblast proliferation, leading to further ischemia and thus a positive feedback loop. The implication of tissue ischemia in the development of Dupuytren's disease may account for a number of epidemiological associations. Cigarette smoking can cause tissue ischemia as can narrowed microvessels in older, male Caucasian and diabetic patients. Advancing age, diabetes, alcohol intake, cigarette smoking, HIV infection, and trauma may result in production of free radicals.[29, 30]

CLINICAL FEATURES

The pathological tissue is superficial and clearly associated with the skin and dermis. There is no excursion with tendon motion, as would be anticipated with nodularity of the flexor system associated with stenosing tenosynovitis. It is also distinct because of its appearance, texture, usual locations, and the fact that it is generally painless except perhaps in its earliest stages. Patients may manifest the initial nodules or cords in various locations other than along the palmar aspect of the ulnar rays, and "pitting" may or may not be observed. There is wide variation in the effect that the cords have on the position and function of the affected digits.

In many patients, the disease is confined to the palm, whereas extension distal to the metacarpophalangeal (MCP) joint crease occurs in others. A minority of patients present with isolated digital involvement. Grapow's ligament (Fig. 3), a transversely oriented cord spanning the volar aspect of the first web space, may limit the span between the index digit and thumb. The degree of flexion contracture at each affected joint can range widely in severity. Rate of disease progression is also unpredictable.

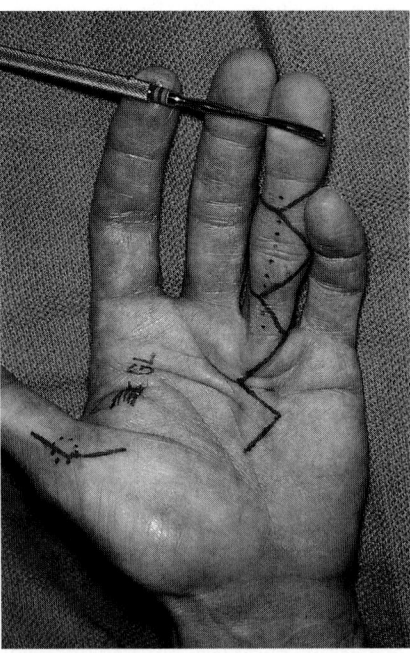

Fig. 3. Multifocal Dupuytren's disease. In addition to significant involvement of the midpalm and ring digit, a Grapow ligament spanned the first web space.

No classification system is used for characterizing Dupuytren's disease. Instead, the clinical distinction between isolated palmar fascia involvement, digital cord presence, or a combination is more meaningful. Accurate assessment of disease severity and expected operative results are based on a thorough description of the pathoanatomy and the magnitude of static flexion contractures.

INVESTIGATION

A thorough history must include questions about the presence of cords on the plantar aspect of the feet and the penis, previous trauma, especially penetrating injury, previous attempts at treatment (injection/aspiration), and family history. There is very little indication for sophisticated imaging or laboratory study. The elements in the history or physical examination that may influence the surgeon to extend the examination to include other modalities would be the recollection of penetrating trauma, significant pain, or atypical location or presentation.

If significant joint flexion contractures are present and release is contemplated, a plain radiographic series is indicated to rule out primary articular disease. If advanced atrophy or symptoms and postures associated with neuropathies exist, electrophysiological studies may be ordered.

MANAGEMENT

The management of Dupuytren's contracture is "binary"; either it is watched with benign neglect or it is surgically excised. To date, there is no effective medical or pharmacological treatment. A number of nonsurgical treatment strategies have been used, ranging from radiotherapy[31] to intralesional injection of steroids, collagenase,[32, 33] or inter-

feron.[34] Steroid injection directly into Dupuytren's nodules has been proposed to control disease progression at an early stage. However, these claims have never been supported scientifically in peer-reviewed publications. As yet, all these medical treatments are of little clinical value.

SURGICAL STRATEGY

The concepts of the surgical treatment for Dupuytren's contracture is straightforward: excise the diseased tissue and release any secondary contractures. This conceptual simplicity belies the technically challenging nature of the surgery. Reduced to its most basic form, the surgical intervention for Dupuytren's contracture is an extended dissection of the neurovascular bundles with excision of all pathological tissue while managing the important "resources" needed for the reconstructive phase, namely the skin.

The surgeon must follow a surgical checklist. The mistake that characterizes the inexperienced surgeon's approach to Dupuytren's release is departure from the systematic, logical progression that he or she exercises for almost all other operations.

First, a familiarity with the predictable locations and patterns of the pathological tissue and its effect on the neurovascular bundles is critical (Fig. 4). Without this understanding, neurovascular structures are at risk and important pathological tissue may be left in situ, resulting in early recurrence of the contracture. Failure to recognize and treat involvement of the septa of Legueu and Juvara[35] or the lateral digital sheet fibers may cause a suboptimal result. Additionally, one must remember the reason why most patients accept the risks of surgery: for the benefit of a straight finger. Although some investigators believe that incremental gains in extension can be achieved with rigorous postoperative rehabilitation (dynamic extension splinting), most often maximum extension is gained during surgery, not during the postoperative therapy phase. The authors advocate thorough release of all tissues volar to the axis of rotation of the affected joints to deliver the maximum benefit from surgery. A PIP joint capsulotomy may be required in cases of severe (more than 60 degrees) joint contracture.

The first step in planning surgical release of Dupuytren's contracture involves skin management and proper placement of incisions. Salient variables that influence the design of the incision include the rays involved, distal extension of the cord, and magnitude of the joint contracture at the MCP and PIP joints. Of these, the extent of the contracture is singular in its challenge for the planning and execution of successful Dupuytren's release.

The approach to each individual ray is rather uniform, with the exceptions of excision of the transverse natatory cord, Grapow's ligament in the first web space, or the extreme ulnar-sided involvement in the small digit. There are some slightly differing strategies when dealing with Dupuytren's disease of the small finger or combined disease in multiple rays. For example, incision planning should take into account the principles of maximum access with minimal dissection and risk to important structures. Surgeons comfortable with the midaxial exposure of the finger may elect to design the digital aspect of the incision in this way provided that most of the disease is unilateral

Fig. 4. Predictable patterns of the pathological tissue. *A,* Drawing of a spiral cord emphasizing displacement of the nerve vascular bundle into a more central and volar location. (Redrawn from McFarlane et al [eds]: Dupuytren's Disease: Biology and Treatment. Churchill, 1990, p 558.) *B,* Intraoperative view showing this relationship (the probe is under the radial digital nerve to the small digit).

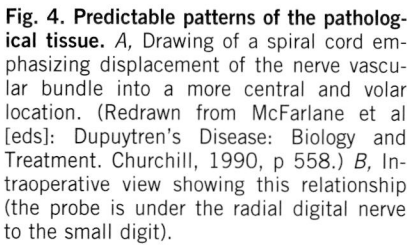

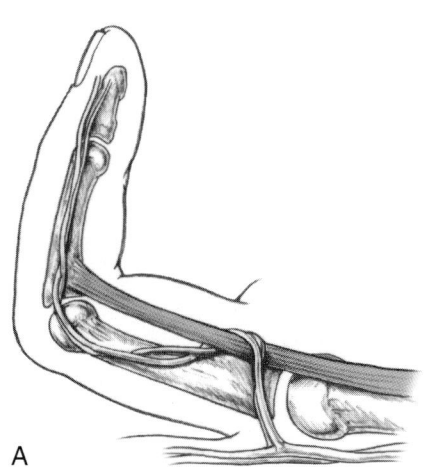

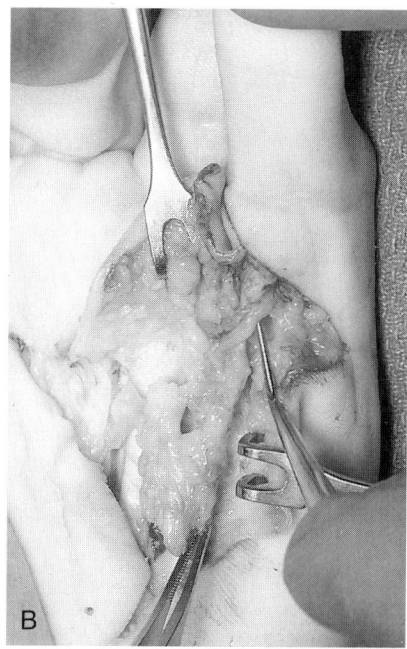

A

B

and there is less than 30 degrees of flexion contracture at the PIP joint.

The "standard" Brunner incision may be inadequate for more extensive contractures. In the more severe cases, consideration must be given to the concepts of lengthening the skin column and mobilizing adjacent skin. The skin column can be lengthened by using V-Y advancement in the transverse dimension (Fig. 5). This is the authors' incision of choice for digits manifesting PIP flexion contractures in the range of 30 to 60 degrees. This is an extremely effective way to gain adequate exposure and cover the fully extended digit. It is limited by the "circumferential area" of digital skin needed to invest the finger's contents.

Options for treatment of contractures exceeding 60 degrees include leaving incisions open, full-thickness skin grafting, complex rotation flaps, and combinations of these techniques. Although the concept of leaving palmar wounds open to heal by secondary intention does not appeal to all surgeons and to very few patients, it is safe and effective.[36, 37] In our experience and that found in the literature, a limited McCash "open palm" technique results in predictable healing with durable, sensate, noncontracted skin. It is highly irregular for a healthy (i.e., nondiabetic) patient to experience any infectious complications during the course of wound healing, and the interval to closure is surprisingly comfortable. There is little substantive change in the rehabilitation regimen when this open palm technique is used. Aside from cleaning and covering the wound, the regular postoperative therapy regimen can proceed without amendment. The open technique should be reserved for the palm in which generous fat over the fibroosseous theca and neurovascular structures prevents their desiccation. All attempts should be made to provide coverage of the digit; however, extremely tight closure of digital skin is not advocated.

Skin grafting has long been advocated by surgeons as a means of providing immediate coverage of palmar defects

and as a deterrent to contracture recurrence. We do not typically advocate skin grafting for isolated palmar skin defects. Because of the potential for donor site morbidity, inferior skin matching, reduced sensibility, hyperpigmentation, and contracture are relatively undesirable possibilities. With other alternatives such as flap rearrangement and the

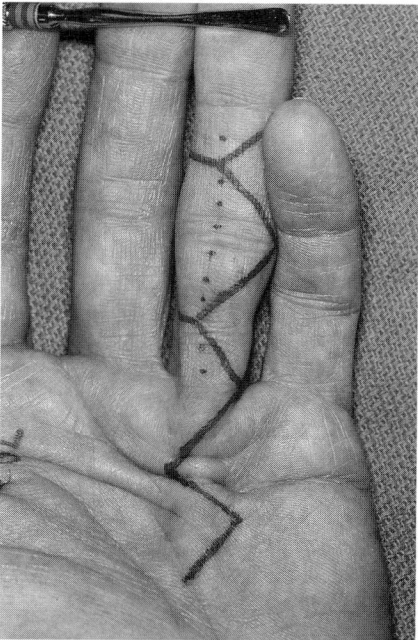

Fig. 5. V-Y advancement technique to lengthen the skin column for moderate flexion deformity. *A,* Palmar view of the V-Y incision. The important parts of the flap design include not crossing the midline with the apex of the lateral-based flap so that it can be advanced into the Y extension and provide the necessary length after digital release. *B,* A view from the medial aspect of the same digit showing the pathological cord and mild to moderate joint contracture.

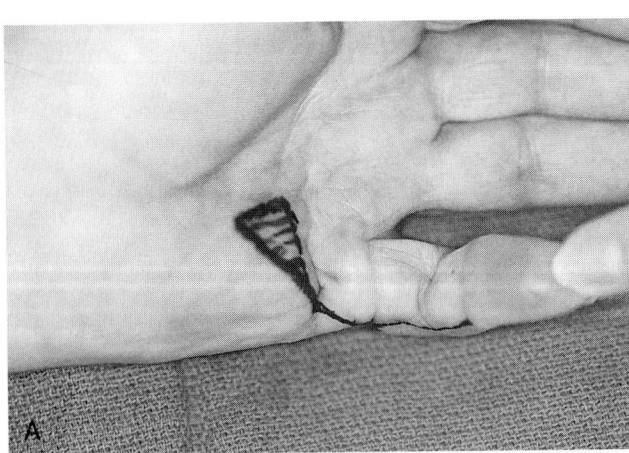
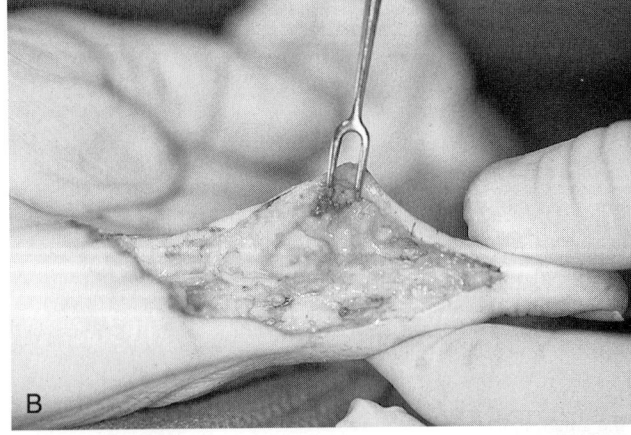
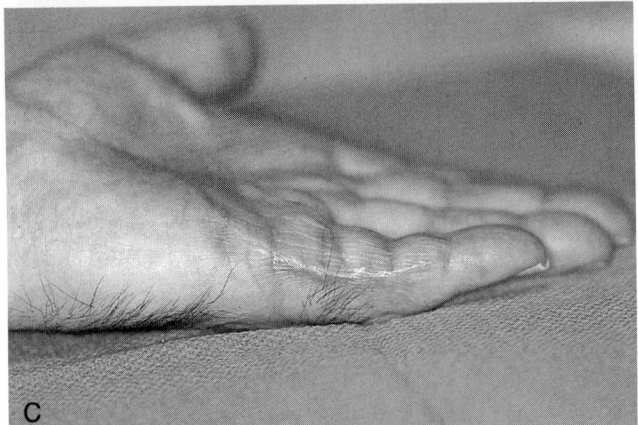
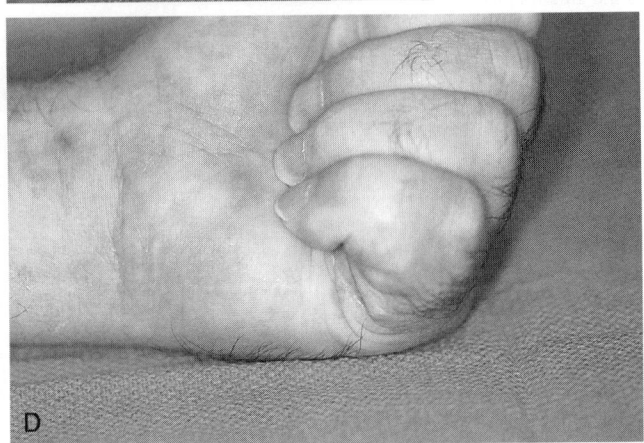

Fig. 6. Clinical series of release of a 60% proximal interphalangeal joint contracture using the J flap. *A,* Drawing of the J incision on the palmar and medial border of the fifth digit. Note the Burow's triangle. *B,* Excellent exposure can be obtained with the midaxial extension of the J incision. *C* and *D,* Appearance of the wound and motion ability one day postoperatively.

open palm technique, skin grafting has an unfavorable risk-benefit profile.

When confronted with extreme contractures about the PIP joint (more than 60 degrees), creative flap fashioning and full-thickness skin grafting is a logical alternative. Our experience has been that rehabilitation in the form of active motion does not need to be significantly altered, although respect for the biology of graft incorporation and vascularization is prudent.

Two special incisions should be described, because they suggest alternatives for specific manifestations of Dupuytren's disease that are not infrequent in their presentation. In both cases, judicious skin management is underscored. The first alternative should be entertained when there is concentration of Dupuytren's disease on the ulnar aspect of the small ray. The second special incision assists in the management of the hand in which multiple digits are involved.

An isolated digital cord of the medial aspect of the fifth digit or more advanced palmar and digital disease concentrated on the ulnar border can be completely excised and the digit covered using the flap. This local advancement flap uses an ulnar midaxial incision over the small finger and a Burow's triangle at the level of the proximal palmar crease (Fig. 6). Used primarily, but not exclusively, for

contractures in which the PIP joint is moderately involved (30 to 60 degrees of contracture), this flap is easy to raise and rotate. It allows the surgeon to operate directly over the cord through its entire length, and almost never requires skin grafting for closure.

When managing Dupuytren's contracture in more than two adjacent rays, the challenges are access to all pathological tissue and maintenance of skin bridge width. The "sickle" incision, as recommended by Raymond Curtis, allows each digit to be handled "on its own merits," while palmar disease can be excised and all wound management alternatives remain available[38] (Fig. 7). We have used this approach on several occasions with success and without skin compromise in the interdigital spaces.

Strategies for making the "peninsulas" of skin between each ray as wide as possible include combining midaxial incisions and traditional Brunner-type approaches or "paralleling" the skin flaps of adjacent digits.

COMPLICATIONS

It is difficult to define the frequency of complications resulting from partial fasciectomy for Dupuytren's contracture, because minor skin slough, transient nerve embarrassment, and incomplete excision are not always reported.

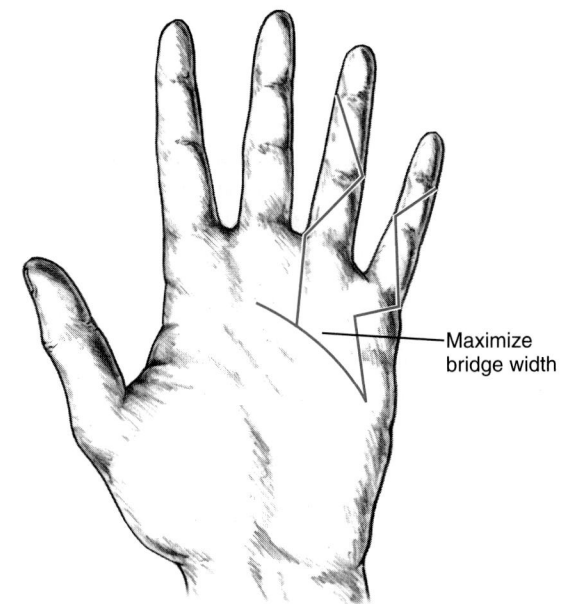

Fig. 7. The universal, or "sickle," incision for Dupuytren's contracture of multiple rays. From this palmar incision, extension to release digital contracture can be performed.

Maximize bridge width

NERVE COMPLICATIONS

Aside from digital loss resulting from ischemia, the most dreaded complication is nerve injury. Because of the intimate relationship of the neurovascular bundle with the pathological tissue, nerve protection is the central focus of Dupuytren's surgery. Inadvertent neurotomy is a recognized complication of this procedure and should be clearly communicated with the patient preoperatively.

Transient postoperative dysfunction of a nerve in continuity is not infrequent. Perineural dissection and direct retraction of the bundle are almost always required during surgery. Additionally, the longitudinal "stretch" placed on the nerve after the digit has been liberated into extension from a flexed posture can cause hypoesthesia.

SKIN COMPLICATIONS

The most common complications are skin-related. Small marginal necrosis occurs but has little lasting affect. Extensive tissue loss can usually result from poor incision planning, excessive or incorrect flap handling, and postoperative hematoma.

Incision planning strategies have already been covered. Simply, the surgeon must understand and respect the random pattern of skin perfusion and avoid jeopardizing vascularity. The correct plane of dissection must also be maintained; the level of the "subdermis" is our target. The transition between diseased tissue and native skin elements is sometimes blurred, placing skin perfusion at risk. In general, biasing toward preservation of a few cell layers under the dermis allows the skin to be nourished by plexus vessels and avoids necrosis.

Significant skin compromise resulting from hematoma is largely preventable. The avoidance of hematoma starts before surgery. Patients are cautioned to discontinue warfarin (Coumadin), aspirin, and nonsteroidal anti-inflammatory

drugs preoperatively. Intraoperatively, we advocate tourniquet deflation and meticulous hemostasis using bipolar cautery and direct pressure before wound closure. We routinely use a drain (removed the day after surgery) together with a compressive dressing. If bleeding and hematoma are concerns, a wound check on the first postoperative day (although a departure from our usual protocol after clean, elective surgery) will minimize this complication.

INCOMPLETE RESOLUTION OF CONTRACTURE AND MOTION

Aside from the unexpected surgical complications described previously, there is one disappointment that the patient and the doctor may share: the inability to obtain full extension of the involved digits. Whether incomplete correction of the contracture should be considered a complication or simply a suboptimal result is open to debate. This result usually takes one of three forms and stems from two different factors: inadequate surgical excision and biological recurrence. We have already stated our bias for achieving complete digital extension in the operating room. In our experience, contracted digits (especially advanced contracture of the PIP joint) do not appreciably improve in the postoperative period if left with a residual flexion contracture. In some cases, there is a "cam" effect that is experienced as the PIP joint nears and slightly exceeds neutral extension. This troublesome finding of a "snapping" of the PIP into hyperextension when the dissected digit is placed in relative extension at the PIP implicates contracture of the more volar fibers of the proper collateral ligament. A judicious collateral ligament release is warranted.

Rapid proliferation of Dupuytren's fascia resulting in suboptimal digital extension may occur after a timid surgical excision or failure to recognize pathological tissue. Often labeled "recurrent Dupuytren's disease," we believe that this is a distinct entity that manifests much earlier than the true biological recurrence discussed later. Not infrequently, the patient notices that there is continued "firmness" in the area of release, just as there was preoperatively. The characteristics of the inflammatory phase of wound healing notwithstanding, there is an accelerated coalescence of Dupuytren's fascia over a course of months. It also appears that this level of disease exceeds the primary status. The very existence of this entity is speculative, and its etiology is likewise conjectural. Perhaps there is an attenuation of the local or humoral factors that mediate the evolution of Dupuytren's contracture.

It is agreed that Dupuytren's contracture can recur. Different from typical postoperative scarring, this is a metachronous lesion.[39] The time course for this type of recurrence, in which complete excision and interval improvement was realized, is on the order of years to decades. Although it usually involves the same rays on which the original operation was performed, this manifestation of the disease may just be following the typical epidemiological pattern. Treatment criteria should be consistent whether for the initial or recurrent contracture.

A patient may also experience loss of digital flexion postoperatively. It is not uncommon for patients with thick, stiff hands and significant small finger PIP contractures to have difficulty regaining full flexion at the small finger distal interphalangeal (DIP) joint, especially if the DIP joint was secondarily hyperextended before surgery. Intensive therapy is the best avenue to follow in treating this problem.

DUPUYTREN'S FLARE

Dupuytren's flare consists of excessive stiffness, uncharacteristic pain, and vasomotor instability involving the operated and sometimes the unoperated digits and has a higher incidence in women.

Some popular, yet unscientific, methods thought to prevent flare include steroid bathing of the wound at the end of the dissection and "automatic" A1 pulley release to diminish the contribution of stenosing tenosynovitis to pain and stiffness.

Once recognized in evolution, Dupuytren's flare should be treated like the early stages of other sympathetically mediated processes. A consistent active and active-assisted motion program should be instituted immediately. This program should be vigorous, emphasizing motion within limits of discomfort. Anti-inflammatory medications and a brief course of oral steroids are extremely helpful in combination with hand therapy. Stellate ganglion blocks are reserved for progressive or severe flare reactions.

The longevity of the flare is variable and is positively influenced by the just-mentioned modalities. Treatment is designed to shorten the "active" phase of the flare and consequently lessen edema, intrinsic fibrosis, and residual stiffness. If recognized and treated early, the flare usually subsides in 4 to 6 weeks. Joint mobility is regained but may require prolonged and intensive therapy.

REFERENCES

1. Luck JV: Dupuytren's contracture: A new concept of the pathogenesis correlated with surgical management. J Bone Joint Surg Am 1959; 41:635.
2. Garrod A: Concerning pads upon the finger joints and their clinical relationships. Br Med 1904; 2:8.
3. Dohlem R: On permanent retraction of the fingers, according to Dupuytren. Rev Rheum 1996; 63:435.
4. Ling RSM: The genetic factors in Dupuytren's disease. J Bone Joint Surg Br 1963; 45:709.
5. Lyall HA: Dupuytren's disease in identical twins. J Hand Surg Br 1993; 18:368.
6. Mikkelsen OA: The prevalence of Dupuytren's disease in Norway. Acta Chir Scand 1972; 138:695.
7. Yost J, Winters T, Fett HC: Dupuytren's contracture: A statistical study. Am J Surg 1955; 90:568.
8. McFarlane RM: Dupuytren's disease: Relation to work and injury. J Hand Surg Am 1991; 16:775.
9. McFarlane RM, Botz FS, Cheung H: Epidemiology of surgical patients. In McFarlane RM, McGrouther DA, Flint MH (eds): Dupuytren's Disease: Biology and Treatment. New York, Churchill Livingstone, 1990, p 201.
10. Arkkila PE, Kantola IM, Viikari JS: Dupuytren's disease: Association with chronic diabetic complications. J Rheum 1997; 24:153.
11. Urban M, Feldberg L, Janssen A, Elliot D: Dupuytren's disease in children. J Hand Surg Br 1996; 21:112.
12. Burge P, Hoy G, Regan P, et al: Smoking, alcohol and the risk of Dupuytren's contracture. J Bone Joint Surg Br 1997; 79:206.
13. Bower M, Nelson M, Gazzard BG: Dupuytren's contracture in patients infected with HIV. BMJ 1990; 300:164.
14. French PD, Kitchen VS, Harris JRW: Prevalence of Dupuytren's contracture in patients infected with HIV. BMJ 1990; 301:967.
15. Sanderson PL, Morris MA, Stanley JK, et al: Lipids and Dupuytren's disease. J Bone Joint Surg Br 1992; 74:923.
16. Hurst LC, Badalamente N: Associated diseases. In McFarlane RM, McGrouther DA, Flint MH (eds): Dupuytren's Disease: Biology and Treatment. New York, Churchill Livingstone, 1990, p 253.
17. Bradlow A, Mowat AG: Dupuytren's contracture and alcohol. Ann Rheum Dis 1986; 45:304.
18. Chum-Kuang S, Patek AJ: Dupuytren's contracture: Its association with alcohol and cirrhosis. Arch Intern Med 1970; 126:278.
19. Noble J, Arafa M, Royle SG, et al: The association between alcohol, hepatic pathology and Dupuytren's disease. J Hand Surg Br 1992; 17:71.
20. Critchley EMR, Vakil SD, Hayward HW, et al: Dupuytren's disease in epilepsy: Result of prolonged administration of anticonvulsants. J Neurol Neurosurg Psychiatry 1976; 39:498.
21. Arafa M, Noble J, Royle SG, et al: Dupuytren's and epilepsy revisited. J Hand Surg Am 1992; 17:221.
22. Chammas M, Bousquet P, Renard E, et al: Dupuytren's disease, carpal tunnel syndrome, trigger finger, and diabetes mellitus. J Hand Surg Am 1995; 20:109.
23. Noble J, Heathcote JG, Cohen H: Diabetes mellitus in the aetiology of Dupuytren's disease. J Bone Joint Surg Br 1984; 66:322.
24. Arkkila PET, Kantola IM, Viikari JS, et al: Dupuytren's disease in type 1 diabetic patients: A five-year prospective study. Clin Exp Rheum 1996; 14:59.
25. Bonnici AV, Birjandi F, Spencer JD, et al: Chromosomal abnormalities in Dupuytren's contracture and carpal tunnel syndrome. J Hand Surg Br 1992; 17:349.
26. Alioto RJ, Rosier RN, Burton RI, et al: Comparative effects of growth factors on fibroblasts of Dupuytren's tissue and normal palmar fascia. J Hand Surg Am 1994; 19:442.
27. Terek RM, Jiranek WA, Goldberg MJ, et al: The expression of platelet-derived growth-factor gene in Dupuytren's contracture. J Bone Joint Surg Am 1995; 77:1.
28. Kloen P, Jennings CL, Gebhardt MC, et al: Transforming growth factor-beta: Possible roles in Dupuytren's contracture. J Hand Surg Am 1995; 20:101.
29. Hueston JT, Murrell GAC: Cell-controlling factors in Dupuytren's contracture. Ann Hand Surg 1990; 9:135.
30. Murrell GAC: Basic science of Dupuytren's disease. Ann Hand Surg 1992; 11:355.
31. Keilholz L, Seegenschmiedt MH, Sauer R: Radiotherapy for prevention of disease progression in early stage Dupuytren's contracture. Int J Radiat Oncol Biol Phys 1996; 36:891.
32. Starkweather KD, Lattuga S, Hurst LC, et al: Collagenase in the treatment of Dupuytren's disease. J Hand Surg Am 1996; 21:490.
33. Hurst LC, Badalamente MA: Nonoperative treatment of Dupuytren's disease. Hand Clin 1999; 15:97.
34. Pittet B, Ruddia-Brandt L, Desmouliere A: Effect of γ-interferon on the clinical and biological evolution of hypertrophic scars and Dupuytren's disease: An open pilot study. Plast Reconstr Surg 1994; 93:1224.
35. Legueu F, Juvara E: Des Aponevrosis de la Paume de la main. Bull Soc Anat Paris Serie 1892; 6:383.
36. Foucher G, Cornil C, Lenoble E, et al: A modified open palm technique for Dupuytren's disease: Short and long term results in 54 patients. Int Orthop 1995; 19:285.
37. Shaw DL, Wise DI, Holms W: Dupuytren's disease treated by palmar fasciectomy and an open palm technique. J Hand Surg Br 1996; 21:484.
38. Carlson CS: Curtis universal incision for Dupuytren's contracture. In Kasdan ML, Amadio PC, Bowers WH (eds): Technical Tips for Hand Surgery. Philadelphia, Hanley and Belfus, 1994, p 91.
39. Zemel NP: Dupuytren's contracture in women. Hand Clin 1991; 7:707.

RADIAL CLUBHAND

Scott H. Kozin

Summary

- The most probable cause of radial clubhand is a defect or abnormal regulation by the apical ectodermal ridge. The majority of causes are sporadic, but the defect may also be caused by teratogens such as thalidomide or radiation.
- The aim of management is to correct functional deficits caused by short or absent radius, short ulna, abnormal muscle anatomy, radial deviation of the wrist, and associated digital abnormalities. Both nonoperative and operative strategies are used.
- Modern surgical methods recognize the importance of the epiphyseal plate and attempt to stretch or release the tight radial structures to allow centralization without excessive force. In addition, lengthening procedures can be used.
- The main preoperative emphasis is to loosen tight radial structures, often with an aggressive stretching and splinting program before surgical intervention.

In 1733, radial clubhand was first described in an autopsy of a newborn infant.[1] Subsequent autopsy observations reported detailed accounts of the anomalous anatomy of the radial clubhand and associated malformations of other body systems. The cause of radial clubhand was discussed in the 19th century as either a congenital defect with disappearance of the primary radial ray anlage or an acquired lesion secondary to syphilis.[2] In 1895, Kummel proposed the cause as abnormal pressure on the embryo along the radial bud between the third and seventh weeks of gestation.[2] At that time, surgeons proposed surgical treatment using an osteotomy of the ulna to correct the deformity or even splitting the distal ulna into a Y configuration and fixing the carpus within the forks.[2, 3] Sayre[3] also suggested preliminary stretching of the soft tissues followed by secondary implantation of the carpus onto the distal ulna. In the 1920s reconstruction of the radius by a bone graft (ulna or tibial) to support the carpus was reported, and in 1945 surgeons performed nonvascularized transplantation of the proximal fibula with its intact growth plate.[4, 5]

In the 1950s, Heikel[2] and Riordan[6] provided valuable insight into radial clubhand, contributing to the classification, associated abnormalities, treatment methods, results, and functional outcome. Heikel[2] removed the radius in newborn rabbits and demonstrated shortening and progressive curvature of the ulna with radial deviation of the wrist during growth. This model provided evidence that the deformity and inhibited growth of the ulna represented a secondary phenomenon related to the absent radius and excessive axial pressure to the growth plate of the ulna. Riordan[6] centralized the carpus and used a fibular graft as a radial substitute, but follow-up evaluation showed lack of fibular growth.

This abridged history of radial clubhand details the problems that still confront the physician treating the child with an absent radius. In this chapter I discuss pathogenesis, clinical features, functional deficits, treatment goals, surgical techniques, results, and complications of radial clubhand as well as innovative techniques that may alter current treatment algorithms.

PATHOGENESIS

Embryogenesis of the upper extremity begins 4 weeks after fertilization as the limb bud forms on the lateral wall of the embryo from the 8th to 10th somites. Limb development occurs in a proximal to distal sequence during embryogenesis.[7] By the eighth week of gestation, embryogenesis is complete and all limb structures are present. Differential growth of the existing structures continues throughout the subsequent fetal stage and birth.

The apical ectodermal ridge (AER) is a thickened layer of ectoderm that caps the developing limb bud. The AER directs differentiation of the underlying mesenchymal tissue and limb formation. Removal of a portion of the AER in chick embryos has produced anomalies similar to radial clubhand.[7] Therefore, a defect or abnormal regulation by the AER is the most probable cause of radial clubhand; the extent of deformity is related to the degree and extent of the AER absence.

The reported incidence of radial clubhand varies between 1:55,000 and 1:100,000 live births.[8] The majority of cases are sporadic without any definable cause. However, exposure to teratogens such as thalidomide and radiation can yield radial deficiencies.[8, 9] Radial clubhand is bilateral in 50% and slightly more common in males than females (3:2).[2, 8, 9] The incidence of radial deficiency within the same family is small, ranging from approximately 5% to 10% of reported cases, and is more common in radial aplasia associated with cardiac abnormalities.[2, 9]

CLINICAL FEATURES

The clinical presentation of radial clubhand varies with the degree of radial deficiency and the presence of associated anomalies. According to the international classification of congenital limb malformations, radial deficiencies are categorized as a longitudinal failure of formation and may be partial or complete.[10] The extent of radial aplasia is divided into four types based on radiograph findings (Table 1).[11]

	TABLE 1. CLASSIFICATION OF RADIAL CLUBHAND	
Type*	Radiograph Findings	Clinical Features
I: short radius	Distal radial epiphysis delayed in appearance Normal proximal radial epiphysis Mild shortening of radius without bowing	Minor radial deviation of hand Thumb hypoplasia is prominent clinical feature requiring treatment
II: hypoplastic	Distal and proximal epiphysis present Abnormal growth in both epiphyses Ulna thickened, shortened, and bowed	Miniature radius Moderate radial deviation of hand
III: partial absence	Partial absence (distal, middle, proximal) of radius Distal one- to two-thirds absence most common Ulna thickened, shortened, and bowed	Severe radial deviation of hand
IV: total absence	No radius present Ulna thickened, shortened, and bowed	Most common type Severe radial deviation of hand

* Because ossification of the radius is delayed in radial clubhand, the differentiation between total and partial absence (types III and IV) cannot be established until approximately 3 years of age.[2] Centralization is required for types II, III, and IV.

BONE AND JOINT ABNORMALITIES

The clinical features of the most common types of radial clubhand (III and IV) are dramatic with abnormalities of the entire limb (Fig. 1). The scapula is often reduced in size, and the clavicle is shorter with an increased curvature.[6] The humerus may or may not be shorter than expected; deficiencies of the capitellum and trochlea are common. Elbow motion is usually diminished more in flexion than extension. The forearm is always decreased in length, because the ulna is approximately 60% of the normal length at birth, and this discrepancy persists throughout the growth period.[2, 9, 10] The ulna is thickened and frequently bowed toward the absent radius with an apex posterior direction, as depicted on the lateral radiograph (Fig. 2).[2,10] Forearm rotation is absent in partial or complete aplasia of the radius.

The wrist is positioned in radial deviation and will eventually develop a perpendicular relationship with the forearm (see Fig. 2).[9, 12, 13] This position further shortens the limb and places the extrinsic flexors and extensors at a mechanical disadvantage, because the tendons must traverse this angle to move the fingers.[10, 13] The articulation between the carpus and ulna does not form a normal joint;

it is usually fibrous but can be lined by hyaline cartilage.[2] The carpal bones are delayed in ossification; the scaphoid and trapezium are often absent or hypoplastic.[2, 9] The status of the radial carpal bones is also related to the degree of thumb hypoplasia (see Chapter 12–22).

The fingers are often stiff, with limited motion at the metacarpophalangeal and interphalangeal joints. The preaxial index and long fingers are often more affected than the ring and small digits.[9]

MUSCLE AND TENDON ABNORMALITIES

Radial clubhand is associated with numerous muscular abnormalities throughout the upper extremity.[2, 6] Shoulder girdle muscles can be hypoplastic or partially absent or can have an abnormal insertion. In the arm, the biceps may be absent or fused to the brachialis muscle.

The forearm demonstrates the most severe abnormalities, primarily in muscles that originate or attach to the radius.

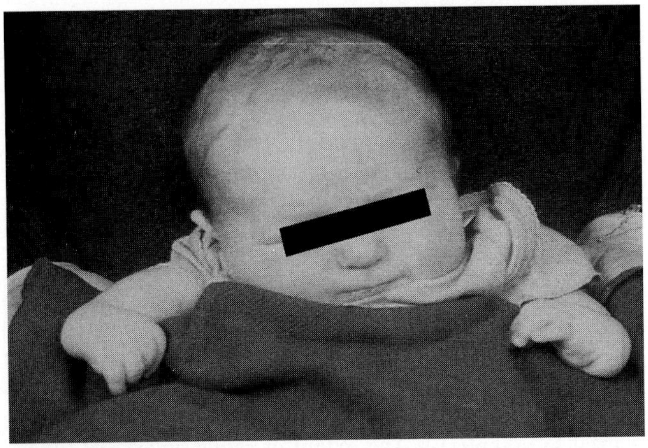

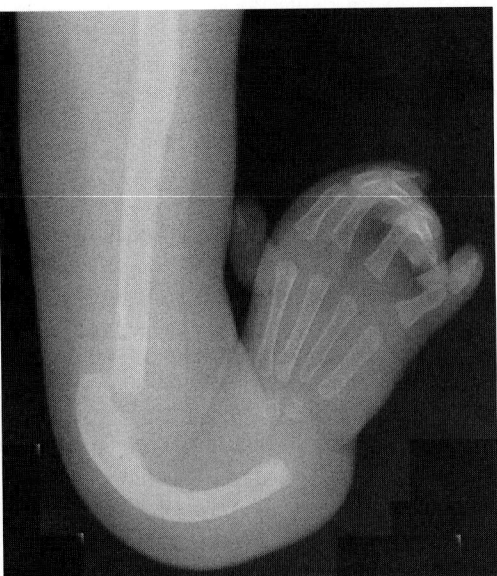

Fig. 1. Clubhand deformity. This is a 3-month-old child with bilateral radial clubhand deformities, perpendicular relationship between forearm and carpus, and absent thumbs.

Fig. 2. Radial clubhand. This is the radiograph appearance of the most common type of radial clubhand (type IV). Ulna is shortened and bowed and thumb is hypoplastic.

The radial wrist extensors are frequently absent or fused. The extrinsic flexors and extensors of the fingers are usually anomalous with abnormal origins and insertions.[2] The flexor and extensor carpi ulnaris, as well as the interossei, lumbricales, and hypothenar muscles, are often normal. The abnormalities of the thumb muscles (extrinsic and intrinsic) are related to the degree of thumb hypoplasia.

NERVE AND ARTERY ABNORMALITIES

The ulnar nerve is normal, but the radial nerve usually terminates at the elbow. An enlarged median nerve substitutes for its absence and supplies a large dorsal branch for sensation to the radial aspect of the hand. This branch is positioned in the fold between the wrist and forearm. An appreciation of this subcutaneous location is critical during surgical incision along the radial aspect of the wrist.[9, 13]

The brachial and ulnar arteries are normal. The radial artery is often absent, and the interosseous arteries remain patent.

ASSOCIATED ABNORMALITIES

Radial deficiency is associated with numerous syndromes. The most common are Holt-Oram (cardiac septal defects), TAR (thrombocytopenia–absent radius), Fanconi's anemia (aplastic anemia), and VACTERL (vertebral, anal abnormalities atresia, cardiac abnormalities, tracheoesophageal fistula, esophageal atresia, renal defects, radial deficiency, and lower limb abnormalities).[2, 10, 11] Additional abnormalities include cleft palate, clubfoot, kyphosis, scoliosis, torticollis, rib deformities, hydrocephalus, and absent ipsilateral lung.[2, 6, 10]

HISTORY AND PHYSICAL EXAMINATION

The history has numerous components, including prenatal, birth, developmental, and hereditary aspects. Potential prenatal factors for radial clubhand are exposure to thalidomide or radiation. A family history of congenital anomalies is important, because radial deficiencies can be hereditary in 5% to 10% of cases. An inquiry into associated systemic anomalies is mandatory, because cardiac (Holt-Oram syndrome), hematological (TAR syndrome, Fanconi's anemia), and renal problems (VACTERL syndrome) can be undiagnosed. These ailments can be life threatening and require accurate identification.

The active and passive motion of the shoulder, elbow, wrist, and digital range of motion is assessed. The ability to flex the elbow for hand-to-mouth function is examined, because this will influence the treatment algorithm. The position of the wrist with respect to the ulna and the ability to correct the radial deviation passively is measured. The thumb is examined for hypoplasia and graded accordingly (see Chapter 12–22).[14]

INVESTIGATIONS

Laboratory analysis includes baseline blood work to assess any acute problems with the kidneys or blood marrow (anemia, thrombocytopenia). In TAR syndrome, the platelet deficiency is present at birth and often resolves by 1 year of age. In contrast, Fanconi's aplastic anemia is not present at birth, develops at 6 to 7 years of age, and is terminal

without bone marrow transplantation. This condition is chromosome-recessive and can be diagnosed before onset by genetic testing, chromosomal fragility, and DNA hypersensitivity. Early diagnosis offers the possibility of producing a sibling with compatible human leukocyte antigens for marrow transplantation.

Plain radiographs to evaluate the degree of radial aplasia and to assess associated abnormalities of the elbow, wrist, and hand are performed. The radial clubhand is classified into four types based on the radiograph appearance (see Table 1 and Fig. 2). However, ossification of the extremity in radial clubhand is delayed, and final determination of complete aplasia of the radius or carpus must be deferred until later.

GOALS, INDICATIONS, AND CONTRAINDICATIONS

The objectives of treatment in radial clubhand are to correct the functional deficit incurred by a short or absent radius, short ulna, abnormal muscular anatomy, and radial deviation of the wrist. Type I radial clubhand has minor radial deviation of the wrist and creates less of a functional problem than types II, III, and IV. In the latter, the wrist assumes severe radial deviation, which further shortens an already undersized forearm, places the extrinsic flexor and extensor tendons at an unfavorable angle, and creates tremendous functional deficits.[2, 10, 13] The digital abnormalities also require consideration, because stiff fingers and a deficient thumb will inhibit grasp, release, and pinch. A hypoplastic or absent thumb requires reconstruction or pollicization, because thumb function directly correlates with use of the radial clubhand (see Chapter 12–22).[2, 14] The functional impairment is far greater in bilateral than unilateral cases.[9]

The basic goals[2, 6, 9, 15] of treatment are to (1) correct the radial deviation of the wrist, (2) balance the wrist on the forearm, (3) maintain wrist and finger motion, (4) promote growth of the forearm, and (5) improve the function of the extremity.

The correction of the radial deviation deformity begins shortly after birth with passive stretching of the taut radial structures. A stiff elbow is also stretched during this time. Splint fabrication is difficult in the newborn and, therefore, is delayed until the forearm is long enough to accommodate a splint. Surgical centralization of the wrist on the ulna remains the standard treatment to correct the radial deviation and is performed at about 1 year of age.

Balancing of the wrist is performed during or after centralization and can be accomplished by tendon and/or bony procedures.[6, 8, 9] Tendon transfers attempt to correct the muscular imbalance and involve advancing the extensor carpi ulnaris or flexor carpi ulnaris to increase its moment arm for ulnar deviation. Other options include transfer of the index and long flexor digitorum superficialis to the dorsum of the wrist or transfer of the flexor and extensor carpi radialis to the ulnar side, or proximal advancement of the hypothenar muscles to the ulna.[10, 13, 16] Bone balance is even more difficult to achieve and requires osseous support to the radial side of the carpus. Initial attempts at nonvascularized transfer of a bone graft were unsuccessful, because continued ulnar growth resulted in loss of support.[6, 15] Recent procedures that involve microsurgical transfer of a vascularized bone graft along with its growth plate (fibula, second toe) are innovative and encouraging.[15, 17]

The maintenance of wrist and finger motion is critical, because stiffness of the wrist reduces the functional capacity of the whole limb.[2] Early attempts to sustain a neutral wrist position involved aggressive notching of the carpus or sharpening of the ulna.[3] These techniques resulted in a straight limb with ankylosis of the wrist and poor outcome.[2] Improved balancing techniques with tendon and/or bone are better methods to retain the wrist on the forearm.[10, 16, 18] Finger motion is difficult to improve despite adequate centralization, because underlying musculotendinous and joint pathology persists.[2] The promotion of growth is an important objective when treating an already shortened forearm segment. Early centralization techniques forcefully placed the wrist on the end of the ulna and either surgically destroyed the epiphyseal plate or placed undo pressure on the growth plate, resulting in early closure with a negative effect on function. It is important to recognize the importance of the epiphyseal plate and attempt to stretch or release the tight radial structures to allow centralization without excessive force. The introduction of distraction histiogenesis (soft tissue and/or bone) and microsurgical epiphyseal transfers has added an additional treatment modality for radial clubhand.[15, 17, 19] Soft-tissue lengthening can be used to stretch the tissues before centralization or bone lengthening can be performed after centralization to decrease the limb length discrepancy.[8, 20]

Although enhanced function is the ultimate goal, cosmesis is improved, which provides an additional psychosocial benefit.[2, 9, 11]

Centralization is indicated in radial clubhand types II, III, and IV with severe radial wrist deviation and insufficient support of the carpus. Thumb hypoplasia is usually addressed at a second stage after wrist centralization. The contraindications for surgical intervention are (1) children with a limited life expectancy, (2) mild deformity with adequate support for the hand (type I), (3) elbow extension contractures, which prevent the hand from reaching the mouth, (4) severe hand defects, and (5) adults who have adjusted to their deformity.[10, 11, 13]

PROCEDURES

PREOPERATIVE PLANNING

Tight radial structures require an aggressive stretching and splinting program before surgical intervention. Failure to elongate the taut radial side will limit the ability to achieve wrist centralization. Preliminary soft-tissue lengthening with an external fixator is an option in recalcitrant cases, in older children with a fixed deformity, and in revision sur-

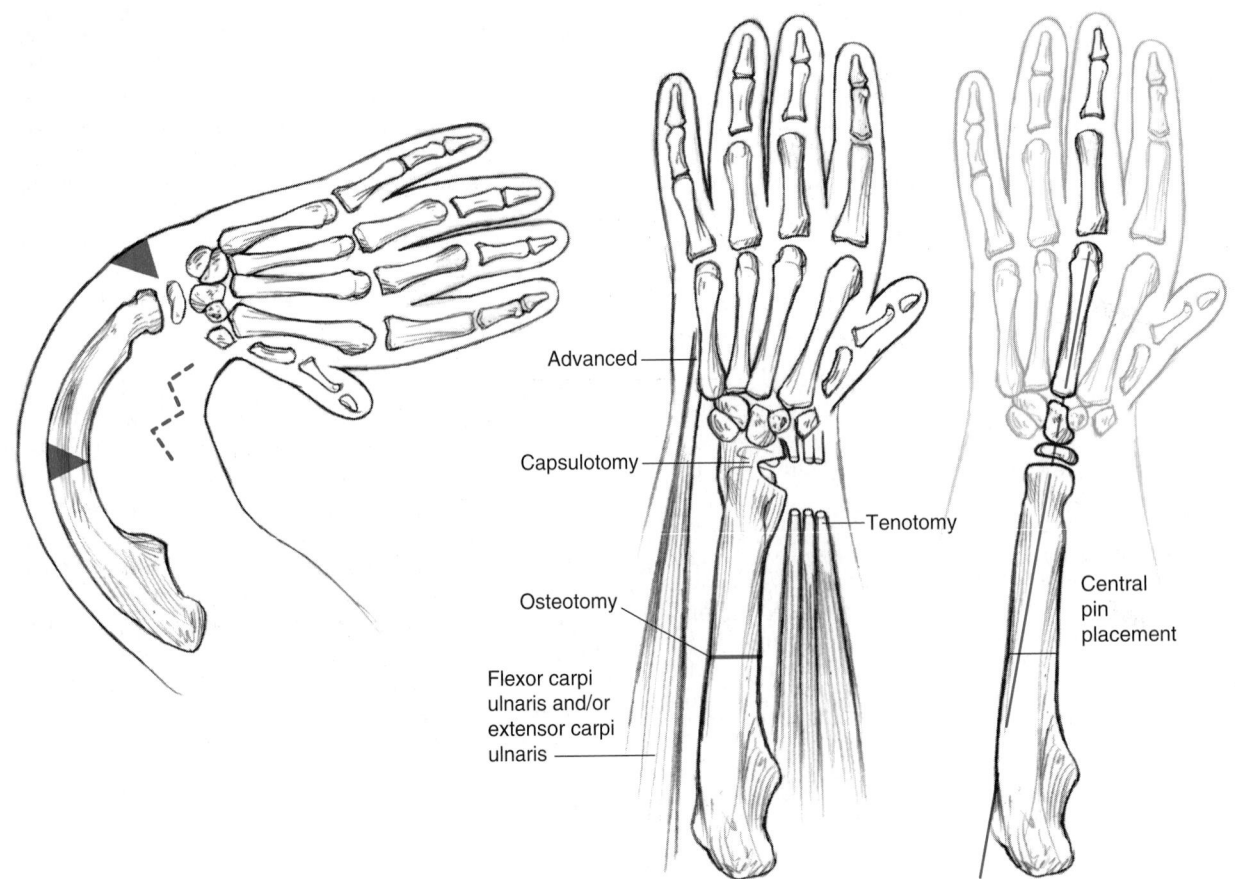

Fig. 3. Centralization. This shows the principles of centralization with release of tight contracted radial structures, centralization of carpus, and tendon transfer to restore balance. Ulnar osteotomy is warranted if bowing is greater than 30 degrees. (From Bayne LG, Klug MS: Long-term review of the surgical treatment of radial deficiencies. J Hand Surg Am 1987; 12:169.)

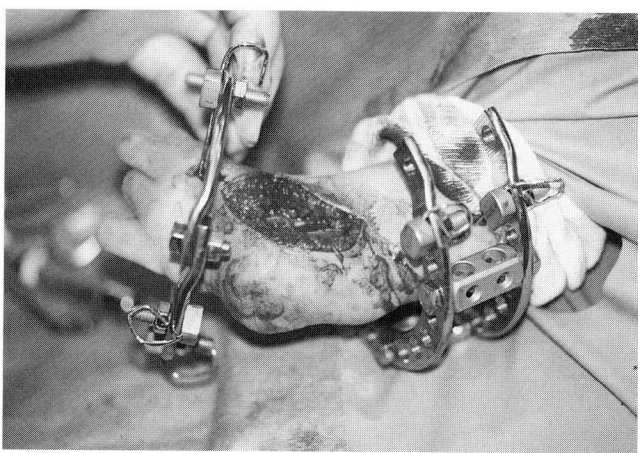

Fig. 4. View. The multiplanar thin-pin external fixator is applied during centralization for soft-tissue and bone lengthening.

gery for recurrent deformity. Radiographs in the anteroposterior and lateral projections, including the elbow and hand, are obtained. The degree of ulnar bow is calculated from the lateral radiograph as an angle formulated between the proximal and distal ulna.[2, 10, 20] Angulation greater than 30 degrees usually requires corrective ulnar osteotomy at time of centralization.

TECHNICAL DETAILS

Centralization of the wrist on to the distal ulna is the standard procedure for radial clubhand types II, III, and IV (Fig. 3). The surgery is performed about 1 year of age. The wrist can be exposed through one or preferably two incisions. The first is a zigzag radial incision. This allows for Z-plasty skin lengthening after centralization. The enlarged median nerve and its anomalous dorsal branch must be identified in the skinfold at the wrist. Aberrant preaxial musculotendinous units and anomalous contracted fibrous bands are identified and released to allow adequate passive correction of the carpus to a neutral position. A second choice of incision is performed beginning at the midline of the wrist dorsally, extending ulnarly in a transverse and elliptical fashion to the volar midline (Fig. 4). This approach allows for excision of redundant skin and subcutaneous tissue. The flexor carpi ulnaris and ulnar neurovascular structures are identified and protected. The carpus is exposed by a transverse incision in the dorsal capsule. The carpus is then reduced onto the distal ulna for centralization. Failure to achieve reduction requires repeat examination of the radial structures for any persistent contracted or fibrotic tissue. In severe cases, adequate reduction cannot be obtained, and alternative measures are necessary. Surgical options include carpectomy, limited shaving of the distal ulna epiphysis while avoiding injury to the growth plate, and corrective closed wedge osteotomy of the ulna, which reduces soft-tissue tension.[11, 13] Another option is application of an external fixator, postoperative distraction, and delayed formal centralization.[8, 20]

Soft-tissue balancing is attempted by dorsal capsular reefing, distal advancement or reefing of the extensor carpi ulnaris insertion, and transfer of the flexor carpi ulnaris to the dorsum. These balancing methods redirect the palmar and radial deviating forces to resist recurrence. The wrist is held reduced by a Kirschner wire placed through the carpus and third metacarpal and into the ulnar shaft. If the ulnar angulation is greater than 30 degrees, a diaphyseal closing wedge osteotomy is performed at the apex of the deformity and is secured with the same Kirschner wire.

POSTOPERATIVE MANAGEMENT

The Kirschner wire is removed 8 to 10 weeks after surgery and active range of motion encouraged. A splint is made and removed for exercises, with gradual weaning from the splint over the next 4 to 6 weeks. A nighttime splint regimen is encouraged until skeletal maturity.

RESULTS AND COMPLICATIONS

RESULTS AND OUTCOME

The results of radial clubhand surgery are difficult to quantify with regard to function. Most children undergo surgery during infancy, which precludes a comparison of function before and after operative intervention. In addition, associated anomalies of the hand (e.g., thumb hypoplasia) often influence use of the extremity.[14] Therefore, the functional results of treatment rely primarily on subjective opinions rather than objective measures.[2] Radiographic or clinical measurements of the deformity can be objectively determined and are based on the ability to achieve and maintain the wrist in a corrected position.

Lamb[9] monitored 31 centralizations for an average of 5 years and measured a preoperative radial deviation of 78 degrees and a follow-up angle of 22 degrees. Bora et al[12] reported on 14 extremities at an average of 14.6 years after centralization and showed a gradual increase in the hand-forearm angle to an average of 25 degrees. Manske et al[13] reported on 21 radial clubhands and measured the hand-forearm angle at 58 degrees preoperatively and 26 degrees at an average 34-month postoperative period. Watson et al[18] monitored 12 centralizations for 10 years and reported a recurrence to an average of 30 degrees. Bayne and Klug[11] observed 53 patients for an average of 8.6 years and reported 81% good or satisfactory results defined as a hand-forearm angle less than 30 degrees. Our long-term results using standard centralization principles have been somewhat disappointing. Eighteen patients monitored for an average of 7 years showed initial significant improvement from a preoperative total angulation (ulnar bow plus hand-forearm angle) of 83 degrees to an immediate postoperative angle of 25 degrees. At follow-up, the total angulation had increased to 59 degrees with a 34-degree loss of correction.[19]

There have been numerous modifications and advances in the technique of centralization. Improved methods to balance the wrist by additional tendon transfers or overcorrecting the wrist into ulnar deviation have been developed.[10, 16] Better attempts at stretching the soft tissue by distraction techniques and bone-lengthening procedures to increase length are also used today (see Fig. 4).[8, 19] In addition, the microsurgical transfer of a viable growth plate (fibula, second toe) to the radial side of the forearm provides a support of the radial carpus that continues growth with time.[15, 17] The technological advances in limb lengthening and microsurgery do add innovative methods to obtain the objectives of treatment. However, the results of these techniques are too limited in number and length of follow-up to draw definitive conclusions.[15, 17, 20]

COMPLICATIONS

Complications from centralization can occur at surgery, during the postoperative period, or during the follow-up period (Table 2).[2, 9–11] Fortunately, these complications are uncommon and continue to decrease as our understanding of the pathoanatomy, degree of soft-tissue contracture, and respect for the epiphyseal plate increases. Recurrence of the deformity is the most common problem after centralization and has numerous causes, including the inability to obtain correction at surgery, inadequate radial soft-tissue release, failure to balance the radial force, and poor splint use.[8, 10, 11, 16, 19] The natural tendency for the shortened

TABLE 2. POTENTIAL COMPLICATIONS AFTER CENTRALIZATION
Necrosis of wound margins
Median nerve injury (iatrogenic or traction)
Vascular compromise (overzealous reduction or pin penetration)
Injury to the growth plate (surgical injury or pressure induced)
Pin tract infection (Kirschner wire or external fixation)
Pin breakage (Kirschner wire or external fixation)
Ulna nonunion (after osteotomy or lengthening)
Ulna fracture (osteotomy site or regenerative bone)
Wrist stiffness (ankylosis or arthrodesis)
Finger stiffness
Recurrence of deformity

radial clubhand to radial deviate for hand-to-mouth use and to position the more functional ulnar border of the hand toward objects to be manipulated can also lead to an increase in deformity.[9]

REFERENCES

1. Petit JL: Histoire de L'Acadamie Royale des Sciences. Paris, Imprimerie Royale, 1733, p 1.
2. Heikel HVA: Aplasia and hypoplasia of the radius. Studies on 64 cases and on epiphyseal transplantation in rabbits with the imitated defect. Acta Orthop Scand Suppl 1959; 39:1–155.
3. Sayre RH: A contribution to the study of clubhand. Trans Am Orthop Assoc 1893; 6:208.
4. Albee FH: Formation of radius congenitally absent: Condition seven years after implantation of a bone graft. Ann Surg 1928; 87:105.
5. Starr DE: Congenital absence of the radius. J Bone Joint Surg 1945; 27:572.
6. Riordan CD: Congenital absence of the radius: 15-year follow-up. J Bone Joint Surg Am 1955; 37:1129.
7. Saunders JW Jr: The proximo-distal sequence of origin of the parts of the chick wing and the role of the ectoderm. J Exp Zool 1948; 108:363.
8. Lourie GM, Lins RE: Radial longitudinal deficiency: A review and update. Hand Clin 1998; 14:85.
9. Lamb DW: Radial clubhand: A continuing study of 68 patients with 117 clubhands. J Bone Joint Surg Am 1977; 59:1.
10. Bora FW Jr, Nicholson JT, Cheema HM: Radial meromelia: The deformity and its treatment. J Bone Joint Surg Am 1970; 52:966.
11. Bayne LG, Klug MS: Long-term review of the surgical treatment of radial deficiencies. J Hand Surg 1987; 12:169.
12. Bora FW Jr, Osterman AL, Kaneda RR, et al: Radial clubhand deformity: Long-term follow-up. J Bone Joint Surg Am 1981; 63:741.
13. Manske PR, McCarroll HR Jr, Swanson K: Centralization of the radial club hand: An ulnar surgical approach. J Hand Surg 1981; 6:423.
14. Kozin SH, Weiss AA, Weber JB, et al: Index finger pollicization for congenital
aplasia or hypoplasia of the thumb. J Hand Surg Am 1992; 17:880.
15. Vilkki SK: Distraction and microvascular epiphysis transfer for radial clubhand. J Hand Surg Br 1998; 23:445.
16. Buck-Gramcko D: Radialization as new treatment for radial clubhand. J Hand Surg Am 1985; 10:964.
17. Tsai TM, Ludvig L, Tonkin M: Vascularized fibular epiphyseal transfer: A clinical study. Clin Orthop 1984; 210:228.
18. Watson HK, Beebe RD, Cruz NI: A centralization procedure for radial clubhand. J Hand Surg Am 1984; 9:541.
19. Damore E, Kozin SH, Thoder JJ, et al: The recurrence of deformity after surgical centralization for radial clubhand. J Hand Surg Am 2000; 25:745.
20. Catagni MA, Szabo RM, Cattaneo R: Preliminary experience with Ilizarov method in late reconstruction of radial hemimelia. J Hand Surg Am 1993; 18:316.

section 12 chapter 21

SYNDACTYLY

John D. Lubahn

Summary
- Syndactyly occurs most frequently between the middle and ring fingers.
- Early release (before 1 year of age) is recommended for index-thumb and ring-small syndactyly to avoid angulatory deformity.
- Surgical release can be improved with a well-designed dorsal commissural flap and liberal use of full-thickness skin grafts.
- "Web creep" (web space contracture) is the most common long-term complication.

Syndactyly, webbed finger, is frequently listed as the most common congenital hand difference, occurring in 1 in 2000 live births.[1, 2] It occurs twice as often in males as females and is 10 times more common in whites than blacks. Syndactyly is most often seen between the long and ring fingers (57%), followed by the ring and small fingers (27%), the index and long fingers (14%), and finally the thumb and index (3%).[3]

HISTORY

Descriptions of syndactyly may be found in writings of Ambroise Paré, Celsius, and Fabricius.[4] Treatment of syndactyly was described as early as 1808. Early (surgical) techniques involved the use of rubber tubes, glass setons, lead beads, and ligatures to separate the fingers and create an epithelial-lined web space.[5] After operative intervention, patients were often left with large, open wounds, which were allowed to heal by secondary intention or longitudinal incisions, which were directly sutured. Poor results were seen. Results became more acceptable with the use of zigzag incisions, skin grafts, and dorsal flaps. In 1810, Zeller[6] first described the use of a dorsal flap for the creation of a web space. A large variety of techniques followed through 1988. These are presented in chronological order with clear drawings in Upton's chapter in McCarthy's *Plastic Surgery*.[5]

PATHOGENESIS

Phylogenetically, syndactyly probably represents persistence of a genetic trait that allowed certain animals to adapt to arboreal or aquatic life.[4] In a human embryo, the developing limb bud begins to appear at 25 days; the hand, between 33 and 36 days. The individual rays can be seen as condensations within this limb bud between 41 and 43 days. The three axes of limb growth are controlled by various growth factors. Proximal to distal development is under the control of the apical ectodermal ridge (AER). The AER elaborates fibroblast growth hormone (2 and 4),

which has been shown to induce finger development.[7] Located more proximal on the developing limb, the zone of polarizing activity, under the control of the sonic hedgehog gene, controls the polarity of radial and ulnar development of the hand. *Wnt-7a* genes control the dorsal-to-palmar orientation of the hand, and *Hox* genes control the development of the AER.[8] These genes direct tissue to become digits. The longitudinal development of the hand and fingers occurs under the direction of apical ectodermal ridge maintenance factor (AERMF).[9] At a genetically predetermined time, the production of this substance ceases. If AERMF continues to be produced, disruption of the interdigital spaces by lysosomal enzymes (apoptosis) does not occur, and either a persistent fetal web remains or some degree of syndactyly develops. This may be partial or complete.

CLASSIFICATION

Syndactyly has been subclassified by geneticists[10] (Table 1). Surgeons, however, tend to use descriptive terms that also may be applied to syndactyly for the purpose of classification. These terms include simple or complex and complete or incomplete. *Simple* implies a connection between two digits by skin alone. An *incomplete,* simple syndactyly includes web fingers, with the web extending a variable distance distally along the length of the finger

TABLE 1. CLASSIFICATION BY GENETICISTS	
Type	**Description**
I	Zygodactyly: the most common form of syndactyly, occurring between the long and ring fingers.
II	Synpolydactyly: syndactyly between the long and ring fingers, including the duplication of ring finger.
III	Ring-small finger syndactyly: usually occurs bilaterally; the distal phalanges may be fused. A rudimentary middle phalanx may occur in the small finger.
IV	Haas-type syndactyly: rare, described by Haas in the *American Journal of Surgery* (1940). Complete syndactyly of all digits occurs, occasionally a sixth metacarpal and/or phalanx may be included, with a cup-shaped hand.
V	Even more rare, this includes the long and ring fingers and the second and third toes. The fourth and fifth metacarpals and metatarsals may be fused.

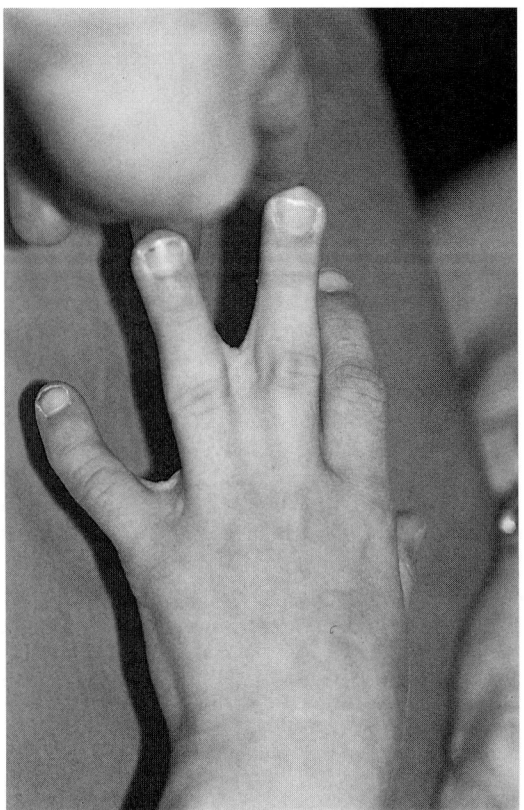

Fig. 1. Simple syndactyly. The skin joins the middle and ring fingers.

(Fig. 1). If the web extends the entire length of the finger, this is termed a complete, simple syndactyly. Complex syndactyly describes a hand in which nerve, tendon, artery, bone, and/or distally the nail are also shared.

CLINICAL FEATURES

Syndactyly may also be seen in association with other more complex syndromes, such as Apert's and Poland's syndromes and conditions such as acrosyndactyly and symphalangia. Apert's syndrome results in premature closure of the cranial sutures and complete, complex syndactyly of the feet and hands.[11] This syndrome is autosomal dominant and affects all races. Although not specifically associated with mental retardation, most children require some special help in school.

Poland's syndrome is defined as the absence of the sternal attachment of the pectoralis major muscles and hypoplasia of the arm, forearm, and hand, and short fingers with either complete or incomplete syndactyly (symbrachydactyly). No known inheritance pattern or other associated anomalies are associated with this condition.

Acrosyndactyly (fenestrated syndactyly) is syndactyly associated with congenital constriction ring syndrome. This is an intrauterine event that occurs after finger separation has begun, resulting in distal ischemia of the fingers and secondary syndactyly at the site of the constriction ring. Epithelial-lined commissures or sinuses are found proximally between the fingers, from the dorsal to palmar surfaces.

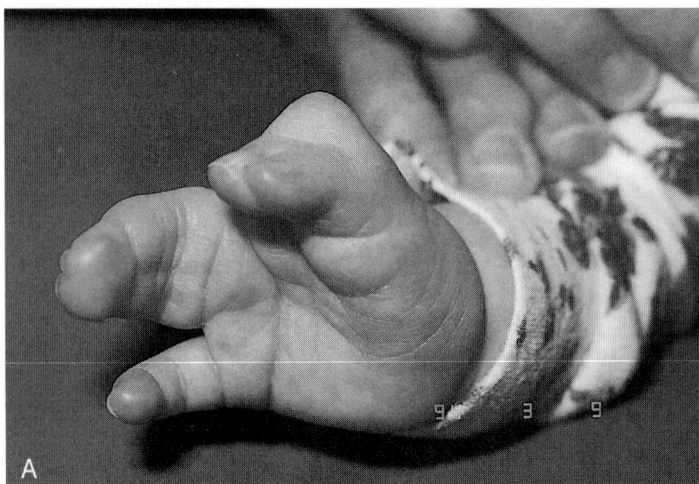

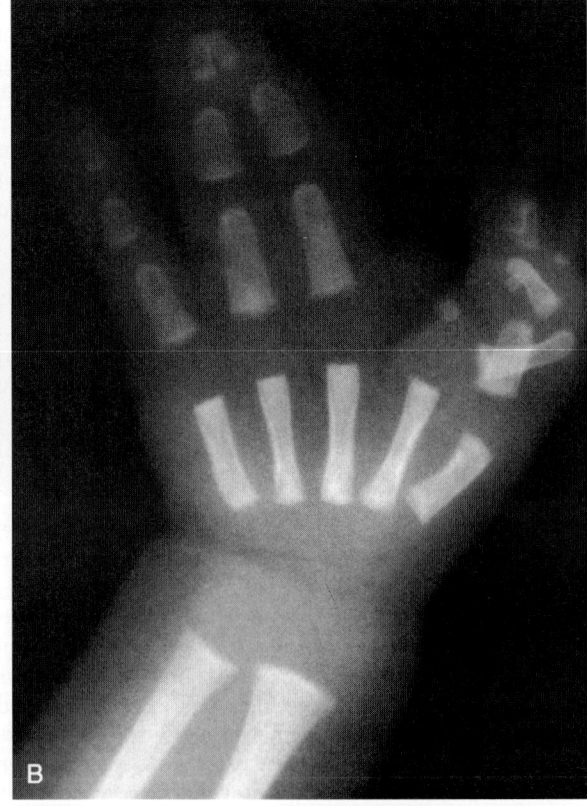

Fig. 2. Complete syndactyly. *A,* Dorsal and palmar views of the hand in complete syndactyly between the long and ring fingers and index and thumb with associated duplication of the thumb. *B,* Anteroposterior radiograph showing the joined distal phalanges of the long and ring fingers as well as the index finger with associated duplication of the thumb. Note the severe flexion deformity of the proximal interphalangeal joint of the index finger.

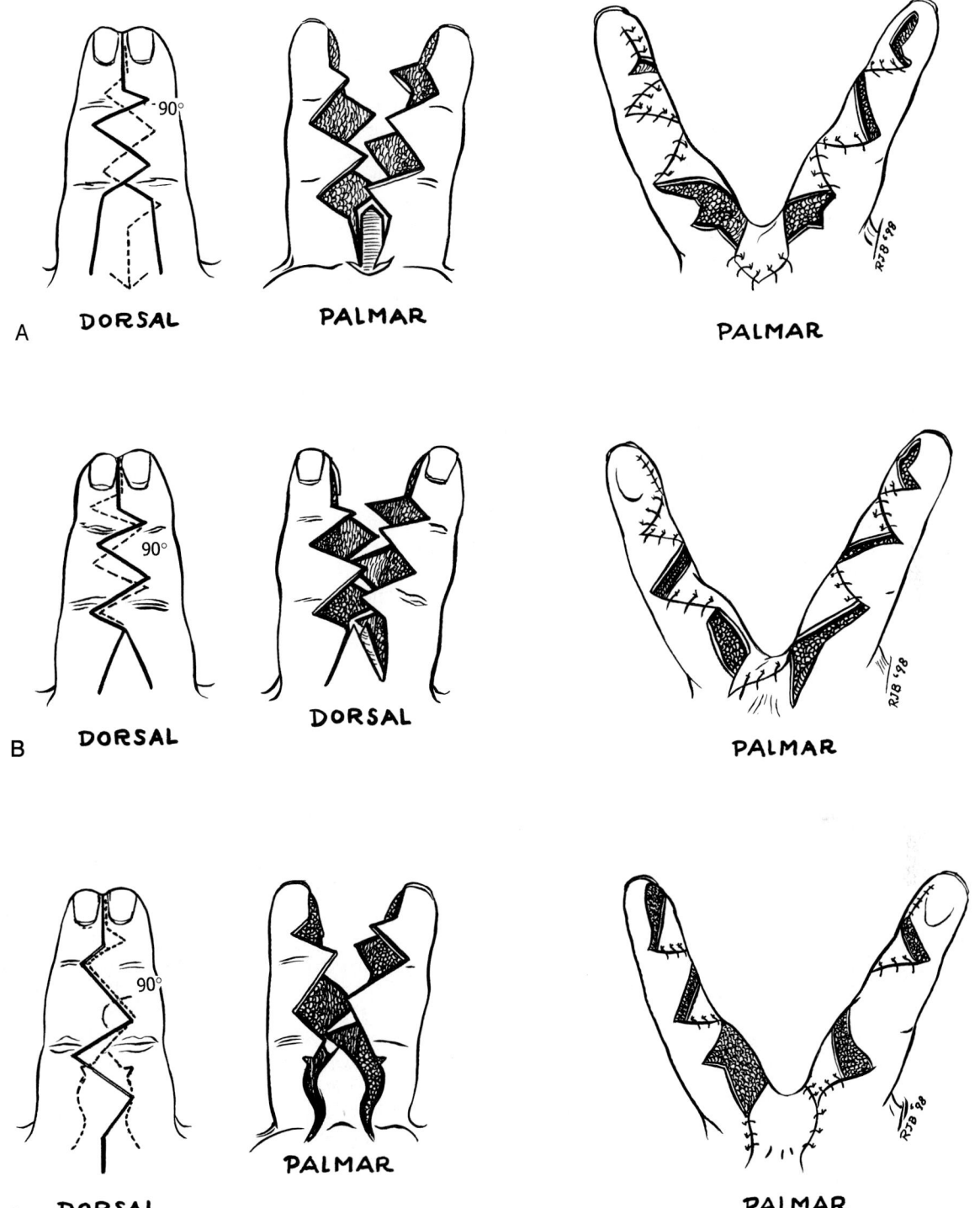

A DORSAL   PALMAR   PALMAR

B DORSAL   DORSAL   PALMAR

C DORSAL   PALMAR   PALMAR

Fig. 3. Zigzag incision. *A,* My preferred incision for syndactyly release using a polyhedron-shaped dorsal flap for creation of the new web space and dorsal palmar flaps, mere images of one another to cover the adjacent fingers. *B,* Same basic incision pattern with triangle-shaped dorsal flap. *C,* "Planaria"-shaped flap.

These represent the degree of web space development present before the constriction band and secondary deformity.

INDICATIONS FOR SURGICAL INTERVENTION

Timing of surgery depends on the health of the patient and the fingers that are involved. Early surgical release is indicated in syndactyly between the thumb and index finger. If untreated, the index will grow toward the thumb and later reconstruction will be difficult, if not impossible (Fig. 2). Likewise, syndactyly between the ring and small fingers may result in fairly early deformity if untreated. If no medical contraindication exists, thumb-index and ring-small finger syndactyly should be released during the first year of life. The index-long and long-ring fingers, however, may grow together more symmetrically, and surgical release can be postponed without worry until age 3 or 4 years.

SURGICAL TECHNIQUE

The patient is placed in the supine position, the hand and arm are prepared and draped, as is the groin, which is used as the donor site for skin graft. Under ideal circumstances, such as simple, incomplete syndactyly, sufficient skin is present to allow direct closure. Such cases are rare, and the current standard is to use skin graft to prevent scar formations.[12]

When two fingers have syndactyly, they are covered by 22% less skin than two individual fingers. This fact is often helpful in explaining to patients and families the necessity of skin graft. Furthermore, interdigital tip-to-tip length is reduced in syndactyly, and the goal of release should be to restore normal length with elastic dorsal skin.[13] Magnification should be used.

Dorsal skin flaps are marked with acute zigzig incisions, with the apex centered over the midline of the joints (Fig. 3A–C). Numerous incisions have been described, but those that tend to be the most consistent include a dorsal flap, which then tapers into the shape of a V or polyhedron. The palmar interdigital incision should be the mirror image of that on the dorsum, placing zigzag corners at the proximal and distal interphalangeal flexor creases of the opposite fingers. As the flaps are raised on the dorsal and palmar surface of the finger, care should be taken to preserve the dorsal veins. In complex syndactyly, with shared nails distally, the technique performed should ensure paronychial symmetry. To accomplish this, local rotation flaps[14] or composite skin from non-weightbearing areas of the foot[15] may be considered. On the palmar surface, the neurovascular structures should be identified and separated. The nerve may be split proximally, if necessary, to the level of the proposed web space. The common digital artery usually branches more distally, particularly in patients with a more complex syndactyly. Either one branch of the artery or the depth of the new web space must be sacrificed. When multiple digits are involved, only one side of a digit should be released at a time.

Deflating the tourniquet before applying the skin graft should be standard procedure. Adequate hemostasis is important, as is a healthy vascular bed to support a skin graft. The skin graft should be harvested from the inguinal region lateral to the femoral pulse to prevent pubic hair growth on the finger. The grafts are sutured in place with 5-0 or 6-0 plain or chromic suture. If the flaps are designed with apices centered over the midline of the joints, the wounds will close except for the proximal-most extent of the wound on each finger adjacent to the web space flap.

The dressing is extremely important. Strips of bismuth-impregnated, nonadherent gauze are cut in strips and applied to the wound over the skin graft in such a fashion that each strip overlaps the other by 5% or 10% of their width, so removal does not result in the graft being pulled loose with each dressing change. Wet cotton is then applied over this layer and secured in place with a heavier suture, or "tie-over." The remainder of the dressing is covered with longitudinal 4 × 4-inch gauze to avoid compression, Kling, Webril, and finally a long arm splint held loosely in place with a Kling wrap and the elbow flexed 90 degrees.

COMPLICATIONS AND RESULTS

The most common complication in the early postoperative period is partial or, in some cases, complete loss of the skin graft. This may occur as a result of infection or hematoma beneath the graft. With time, some degree of web space contracture may once again occur, with secondary scar and possible finger deformity. This phenomenon is referred to as "web creep." Its overall incidence ranges from 7.5% to 60%.[16] Creep is prevented with the liberal use of skin grafts, zigzag incisions, and a well-designed dorsal flap. Hypertrophic scars may develop along the incisions, particularly when all or part of a split-thickness skin graft fails. However, 6 to 12 months after surgery, the scar should have reached a level of maturity at which little change will occur. In more complicated cases, syndactyly deformity may be related to how the skeleton or nail bed has been separated and how each heals and remodels postoperatively. Z-plasty, osteotomy, and nail bed reconstruction are all possible means of reconstruction. Proximal interphalangeal flexion contracture may develop, particularly in complex synpolydactyly. If this occurs, proximal interphalangeal joint (PIPJ) fusion or chondrodesis may be considered; however, many patients will function well with a PIPJ flexion contracture.

REFERENCES

1. Kelikian H: Congenital Deformities of the Hand and Forearm. Philadelphia, WB Saunders, 1974, p 408.

2. Flatt AE: The Care of Congenital Hand Anomalies. St. Louis, MO, CV Mosby, 1977.

3. Lister G: The Hand Diagnosis and Indications, 3rd ed. Edinburgh, Scotland, Churchill Livingstone, 1993, p 484.

4. Tentamy S, McKusick V: The Genetics of Hand Malformation. New York, Alan R. Liss, 1985, p 301.

5. Upton J: Congenital anomalies of the hand and forearm. In McCarthy J (ed): Plastic Surgery, vol. 8. The Hand, part 2. Philadelphia, WB Saunders, 1990, p 5281.

6. Zeller S: Abhandlung über die ersten erscheinungen venerischer lokalkrankheits. Wien, J.G. Binz, 1810.

7. Mahmood R, Bresnick J, Hornbruch A, et al: A role for FGF-8 in the initiation and maintenance of vertebrate limb bud outgrowth. Curr Biol 1995; 5:797.

8. Birch JG: Genetic aspects of limb deficiency. In Herring JA (ed): The Child With a Limb Deficiency. Rosemont, IL, American Academy of Orthopaedic Surgeons, 1998.

9. Scott MP: Hox genes, arms and the man. Nature Genet 1997; 15:117.

10. Matton M, DeBie S, Andrew A: Familial dermatoglyphic analysis in syndactyly type I. J Hand Surg 1981; 6:537.

11. Blank CE: Apert's syndrome (a type of acrocephalosyndactyly)—Observations on a British series of thirty-nine cases. Ann Hum Genet 1960; 24:151.

12. Ekerot L: Syndactyly correction without skin grafting. J Hand Surg Br 1998; 20:330.

13. Eaton CJ, Lister GD: Syndactyly. Hand Clin 1990; 6:555.

14. Buck-Gramcho D: Congenital malformations. In Nigst H, Buck-Gramcho D, Millesi H, et al (eds): Hand Surgery: Vol 1. General Aspects, Elective Surgery. New York, Thieme, 1988, p 1.

15. Ezaki M: Radial polydactyly. Hand Clin 1990; 6:577.

16. Oates SD, Gosain AK: Syndactyly repair performed simultaneously with circumcision: Use of foreskin as a skin graft donor site. J Pediatr Surg 1997; 32:1482.

section
12
chapter
22

THUMB (INCLUDING FLEXED, DUPLICATED, AND HYPOPLASTIC)

Marybeth Ezaki

Summary

- Congenital anomalies of the thumb are common and may be hereditary or nonhereditary.
- Congenital hypoplasia of the thumb is part of the spectrum of radial dysplasia and should trigger a search for associated anomalies.
- Certain segmentation abnormalities of the thumb may occur in association with serious hematological disorders.
- There is no role for corticosteroid injection in the treatment of the pediatric trigger thumb.
- Surgical reconstruction of a child's congenital thumb abnormality requires judgment, an understanding of the developmental anatomy, and the ability to address all components of the deformity at the time of surgical treatment.

Abnormalities of the infant's thumb are relatively common. The majority of the conditions can be grouped into three major categories: flexed, malsegmented, and hypoplastic (Table 1). Some of these conditions occur as isolated conditions; some are associated with other malformations or developmental conditions. The normal development of the human thumb is influenced by many factors and input from genetic loci spread throughout the human genome. For treatment and prognosis purposes, it is important to be aware of and to recognize these relationships.

THE FLEXED THUMB

The four major diagnostic categories that present with a flexed thumb are trigger thumb, spastic thumb, clasped thumb, and arthrogrypotic, or windblown thumb. Careful clinical examination of the hand and the child will lead to the correct diagnosis.

TRIGGER THUMB
Etiology

The infantile form of trigger thumb is usually not present at birth but develops during the first several years of life. The exact cause is unknown but is thought to be related to the complex anatomy at the palmar aspect of the metacarpophalangeal (MCP) joint. The flexor pollicis longus tendon enters the proximal annular pulley at the confluence of intrinsic musculature, sesamoid bones, and tendon sheath. A normal infant maintains a posture of digital flexion, which may predispose the tendon to thicken at this location. Trauma may also play a role.

Clinical Features

Passive extension of the trigger thumb may elicit a click, which may be uncomfortable for the child. More commonly, passive extension of the trigger thumb is limited, and a firm nodule (Notta's node) is palpable at the palmar aspect of the MCP joint. Passive motion of the thumb while palpating the nodule establishes its location within the flexor pollicis longus tendon (Fig. 1).

TABLE 1. THE ABNORMAL THUMB		
Flexed	**Malsegmented**	**Hypoplastic**
Trigger thumb	Nonhereditary forms Wassel's types I–VI	Blauth's types 1–5
Spastic thumb		Miscellaneous
Clasped thumb	Heritable forms Wassel's type VII	
Arthrogrypotic thumb	Triphalangeal Polysyndactyly	

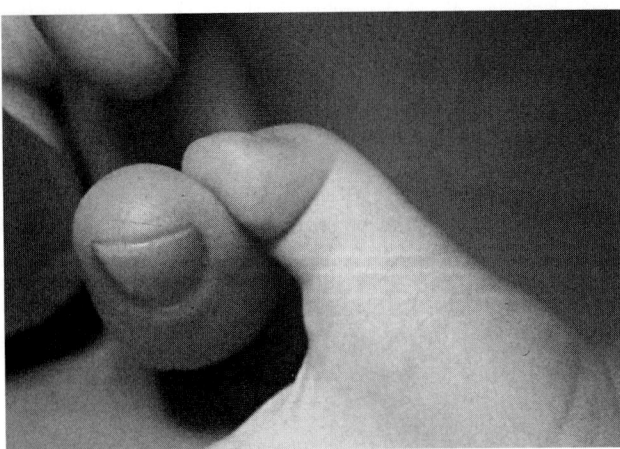

Fig. 1. **Trigger thumb.** This is the clinical appearance.

Associated Conditions

No significant conditions are associated with the diagnosis of a trigger thumb.

Treatment Goals and Indications

Prolonged splinting, ultrasound treatments, and other non-operative treatments have been described, but these do not correct the condition. The results of surgical release are equally good at the age of several years as in infancy. A normal thumb can be expected if the triggering is corrected. There is no place for corticosteroid injection in the pediatric trigger thumb.

Treatment

Treatment of choice is surgical release of the proximal annular pulley sufficient to allow free excursion of the tendon in the sheath.[1] There should be no manipulation of the nodule. The nodule will remodel and decrease in size when the irritating constriction is relieved. Parents will understand the analogy to a callus on the palm caused by an irritating activity. The treatment is to eliminate the source of the irritation and not to excise the callus.

SPASTIC THUMB
Etiology

Spasticity is a manifestation of upper motor neuron dysfunction as a result of cortical malformation, antenatal or perinatal vascular event, injury or infection, or neoplasm.

Clinical Features

The spastic thumb is recognized by increased tone in the intrinsic musculature, which maintains the metacarpal in an adducted position. The spastic thumb is morphologically normal. The MCP joint can be flexed if the extrinsic extensors are weak or can be hyperextended if there is capsular laxity and strong extrinsic extensors (Fig. 2).

Associated Conditions

Developmental delay and sensory impairment, also as a result of the underlying neurological condition, are common in affected children. The sensory impairment has a profound negative effect on the child's attempt to use the hand.[2]

Treatment Goals and Indications

Treatment goals depend on the volitional ability of the child to use the thumb. Release of the spastic muscles can position the thumb outside of the palm to increase function in the child who attempts to use the hand. Surgical repositioning of the thumb can facilitate use as an assist hand or improve hygiene and custodial care in the child who has poor volitional control.

Treatment

A variety of treatment options exist for the spastic hand. Splinting and stretching the thumb are helpful but must be done cautiously so that the MCP joint is not hyperextended. Surgical release of the origins of the spastic muscles, including the short abductor, flexor brevis, opponens pollicis, and both heads of the adductor pollicis, allows the musculature to be recessed and the thumb better positioned for function. Augmentation of extrinsic abduction and extension by tenodesis or by tendon transfer may be needed at a second procedure.[3]

CLASPED THUMB
Etiology

A clasped thumb is due to an inherent malformation of the musculotendinous units that balance the position and function of the thumb. Agenesis or hypoplasia of extensor and abductor muscles and tendons, coupled with inadequate soft-tissue elements and contractures, results in the clinical spectrum of the clasped thumb.[4]

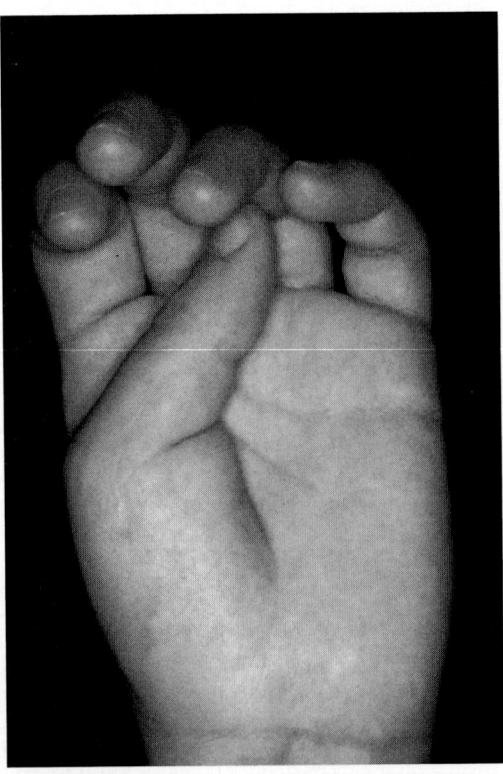

Fig. 2. **Spastic thumb.** This is a child with a spastic thumb in palm posture that limits extension of the entire ray.

Clinical Features

A spectrum of these uncommon thumb conditions come under the category of clasped thumb. The usual finding is a lack of extension of the MCP joint because of congenital absence of the extensor pollicis brevis tendon. Flexion posture of the MCP joint may be due to contracture of the intrinsic musculature. Lack of palmar skin in the more severe cases also limits thumb function (Fig. 3). As the combined extrinsic and intrinsic deficiency becomes more severe and the other fingers become involved, the deformity is referred to as a windblown hand and crosses over into the category of the arthrogypotic thumb.[5]

Associated Conditions

The simpler forms of clasped thumb may occur as isolated conditions with no family history. The more severe deficiencies, which include involvement of the fingers, are related to the diagnostic group of the distal arthrogryposes, which are variably inherited.

Treatment Goals and Indications

The mildest forms of the clasped thumb will respond to passive stretching and then to splinting. If the thumb cannot be passively abducted and extended sufficiently to allow hand function, release of the contracture and exploration and augmentation of the extensor mechanism are indicated.

Treatment

Release of the contracted intrinsic musculature to allow passive positioning of the thumb is accomplished by recession of the origin of the muscles in the palm. Inadequacy of skin may be addressed by web release and flap coverage. Exploration of the dorsum of the thumb may reveal subluxation, hypoplasia, or aplasia of the extensor tendons. A tendon that is present but that lacks excursion indicates that the muscle is inadequate, and a tendon transfer should be performed. Active extension of other fingers may be compromised by the underlying diagnosis. The extensor indicis proprius may be inadequate or absent, and alternative donor tendons should be considered. Extensor digiti quinti is usually reliable as a tendon donor in this situation.

ARTHROGRYPOTIC THUMB
Etiology

In the arthrogrypotic thumb, the musculoskeletal deficiencies are extrinsic and intrinsic. The various forms of arthrogryposis include the "distal" forms and the classic arthrogryposis multiplex congenita. Specific arthrogrypotic conditions have characteristic thumb and hand findings, such as the windblown hand in Freeman-Sheldon, or whistling face, syndrome.

Clinical Features

The thumb MCP joint is flexed, and the skin and soft tissues are tight and nonpliable, with very limited passive motion of the thumb in either direction. The musculotendinous units are fibrotic and the joints contracted and woody. The thumb-index web is usually inadequate, and there is insufficient skin on the palmar aspect of the thumb MCP and interphalangeal (IP) joints. The fingers are variably involved with contractures and fibrotic motor units. Sensation is intact (Fig. 4).

Associated Conditions

The exact cause of arthrogryposis multiplex congenita is unknown. A neural form proposes that lack of innervation of muscles at a crucial time of development leads to abnormal joint cleavage and deformity because of muscle imbalance. A number of the specific types of distal and named-syndrome arthrogryposis are known to be due to genetic defects. Multiple joint and musculotendinous units throughout the limb may be involved.[6]

Treatment Goals and Indications

Most children with arthrogryposis are remarkably adaptable, and not all can benefit sufficiently from surgical care. A careful assessment of the potential function of the thumb is needed before any decision is made to address it surgically. Release of contracture, soft-tissue resurfacing, and change in position of the thumb may be possible, but unforeseen consequences may result if the function of both upper limbs is not considered in its entirety. Arthrodeses should be avoided when possible because of the severe overall limitations in motion.

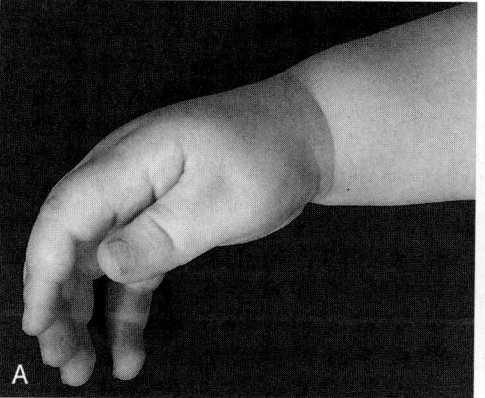 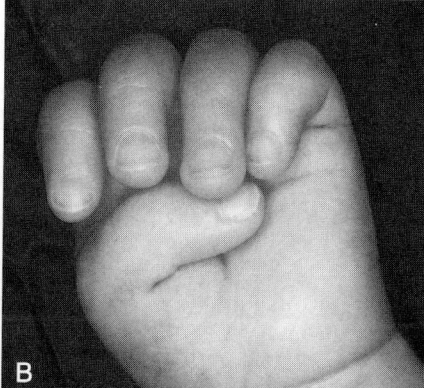 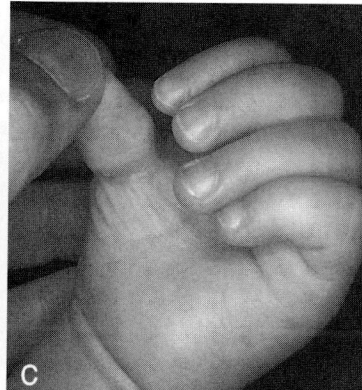

Fig. 3. Clasped thumb. *A*, Absence of the extensor pollicis brevis and some limitation of extension position. *B* and *C*, A clasped thumb with intrinsic and extrinsic deficiencies and inadequate skin coverage.

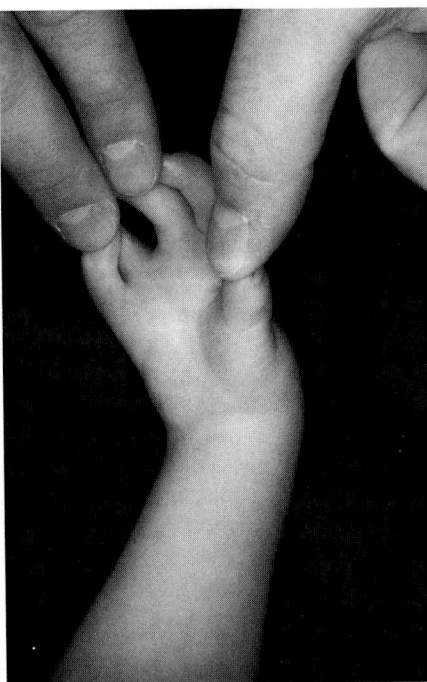

Fig. 4. Arthrogrypotic thumb. The arthrogrypotic thumb shows rigid intrinsic and extrinsic tightness as well as wrist and finger contractures.

Treatment

If the decision is made to approach the arthrogrypotic thumb surgically, all of the deformities should be addressed at that operation. Release of the tight intrinsic musculature, coverage of the web space, stabilization of the MCP joint, and tendon augmentation of extension, if possible, should all be accomplished at one setting.

MALSEGMENTED THUMB

A number of synonyms for these congenital segmentation anomalies exist, including bifid thumb, split thumb, duplicated thumb, radial or preaxial polydactyly, and triphalangeal thumb.

This category of diagnosis is quite broad, and the approach used by geneticists is helpful because it distinguishes those conditions that are associated with other more serious anomalies from those that occur as isolated conditions. The classification also allows prediction of recurrence on a genetic basis.

There are essentially two sorts of radial polydactyly: those that result from a localized error in segmentation near the completion of morphogenesis and those that were genetically preprogrammed to result in a morphologically abnormal thumb. (The first type can be likened to a "ruffle," the latter to a "sprout.")

NONHEREDITARY RADIAL POLYDACTYLY
Etiology

The most common type, the geneticists' group I, occurs sporadically and unilaterally and is the result of excessive segmentation of the radial side of the hand plate. At the completion of formation of the hand plate, the ectoderm normally segments into five digital cusps. The inducing factors elicited by the segmenting ectoderm complete the morphological model of the digit. The differentiation of the mesoderm, progressing from proximal to distal, meets two sets of inducing factors; two smaller, but more or less complete, digital tips result. The level of the juncture of the normal and the abnormal thumb parts determines the Wassel type that results.[7]

Clinical Features

Wassel described six subtypes of this form of malsegmented thumb. This form occurs sporadically and unilaterally, is not heritable, and is not associated with other conditions. This type of thumb has normal proximal parts and split or bifid distal parts. The Wassel type is determined radiographically by counting the number of abnormal bones in the thumb; higher numbers are given to more proximal bifurcation. The exact appearance of the thumb is determined by the level of bifurcation, the degree of symmetry of the parts, the deforming pull of the attached musculotendinous structures, and the inclination of the joint surfaces. The adductor attaches to the ulnar thumb and the abductors to the radial thumbs. The split long flexor and extensor tendons insert eccentrically onto the smaller adjacent thumb tips and may cause a pincer-like appearance (Fig. 5). The ulnar thumb is usually better formed and more functional, although active motion may be significantly limited. The size of the thumb to be reconstructed should be compared with that of the opposite thumb, and the size discrepancy should be pointed out to the parents preoperatively.

Associated Conditions

There are no genetic anomalies, family history, or likelihood of recurrence of the condition in siblings or offspring associated with the Wassel type I through VI thumbs.

Treatment Goals and Indications

The goal of surgical reconstruction is to make the best possible thumb from the available parts. The resulting thumb will not be a normal thumb, and this must be pointed out to the parents. The goals are normal alignment, stability of the joints, sensate and minimally scarred soft-tissue coverage, and some active motion. The thumb will usually be stiff at the interphalangeal joint. A stable, well-aligned, and sensate thumb will appear more normal and function better even if it is slightly smaller than normal. Surgical treatment is recommended for these thumbs provided the child is healthy and there are no associated life-threatening illnesses. All component tissues should be addressed at the time of reconstruction. Soft-tissue flaps should be planned so that the skin innervated by the normal digital nerves is preserved. The thumb ray is aligned by osteotomy when necessary. Collateral ligament reconstruction using a ligamentoperiosteal flap stabilizes the joint.[8] Long flexor and extensor tendons are realigned and reinserted if necessary. Intrinsic muscles are repositioned to exert the appropriate pull on the reconstructed thumb.

By the time a child is 9 months to 1 year of age, the

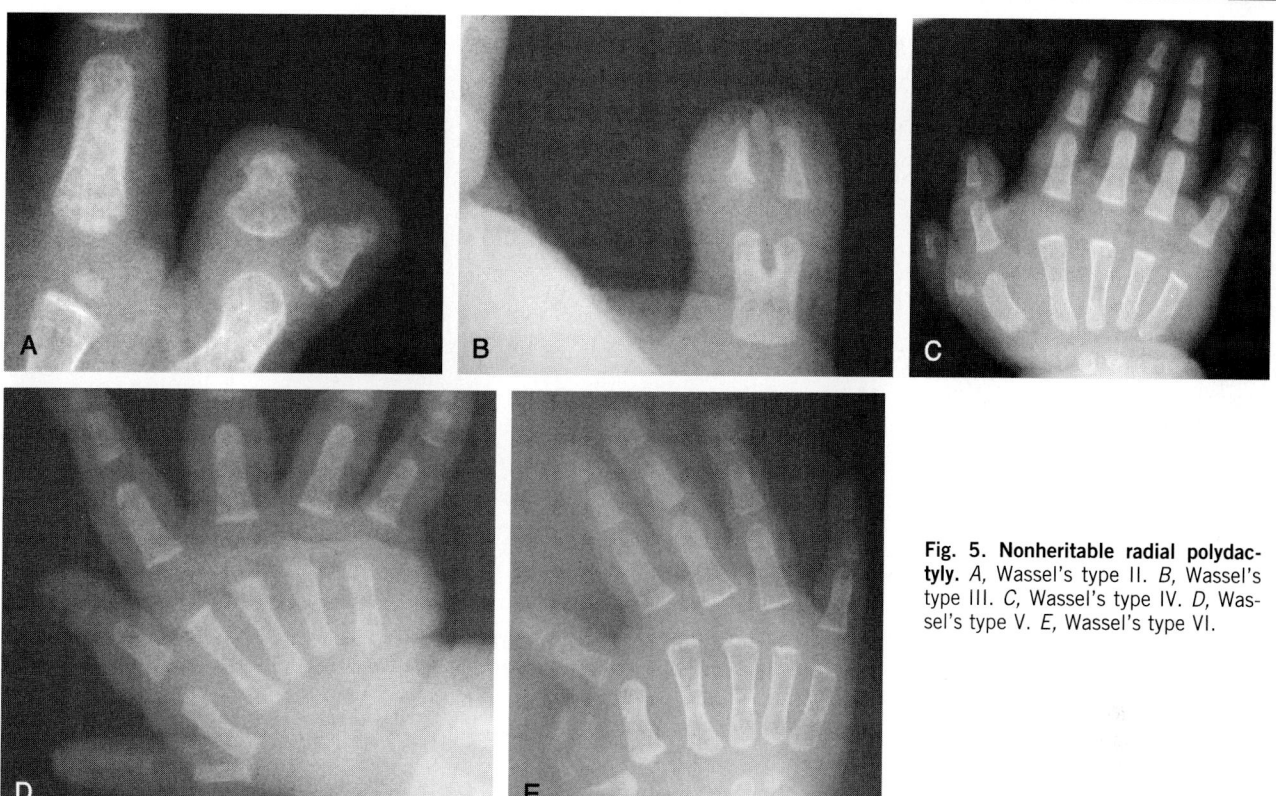

Fig. 5. Nonheritable radial polydactyly. *A*, Wassel's type II. *B*, Wassel's type III. *C*, Wassel's type IV. *D*, Wassel's type V. *E*, Wassel's type VI.

size of the thumb should be large enough to work comfortably to accomplish the reconstruction. The postoperative course includes 4 to 6 weeks of immobilization in a long-arm cast and then use of the hand as tolerated. Long-term problems are related to instability of joints, soft-tissue imbalance, and failure to address the individual components of the deformity at the original procedure.

HERITABLE RADIAL POLYDACTYLY
Etiology
The other broad type of radial polydactyly or duplicated thumb is genetically encoded and thereby likely to be familial, recurrent in siblings or offspring, or associated with other abnormalities. The geneticist classification for these include the opposable triphalangeal thumbs (Wassel's group VII), the nonopposable triphalangeal thumbs, and the thumb polydactyly associated with polysyndactyly. Radial polydactyly that occurs bilaterally is likely to include a triphalangeal component. Wassel noted that these thumbs were different from the others in that they were often bilateral, familial, and associated with other congenital diagnoses. Wassel lumped these into his type VII category. This type is the most common in the Asian population.

Clinical Features
This is a diverse group. The condition is often bilateral. The most common clinical feature is the presence of a triphalangeal component in the abnormal thumb or thumbs. The malsegmentation may be an extra phalanx in a single thumb or a complex polydactyly (Fig. 6).[9]

Associated Conditions
Possible associated conditions include Blackfan-Diamond anemia (with triphalangeal single thumbs), craniofacial abnormalities (with polysyndactyly), and cardiac abnormalities (with opposable and nonopposable triphalangeal thumbs).

Treatment Goals and Indications
These are the same as discussed under Nonhereditary Radial Polydactyly. The triphalangeal component may be an additional phalanx or an additional ossification site within an abnormally shaped phalanx. If the growth plate is in close proximity to the abnormal partial phalanx, correction of alignment may be best postponed until sufficient growth of the digit has occurred. Other procedures include epiphysiodesis to stop longitudinal growth of a segment when adult size has been reached, joint resection or arthrodesis to decrease the number of segments, and resection of abnormal ossicles. The treatment of each thumb must be individualized.[10]

HYPOPLASTIC THUMB

Thumb hypoplasia is a part of the spectrum of radial dysplasia. Abnormal formation of the radial side of the upper limb ranges from slight underdevelopment of the thenar musculature to complete absence of the radius and radial side of the hand. Radial dysplasia is known to be associated with a wide variety of inherited and nonhereditary malformations and syndromes. The timing of development

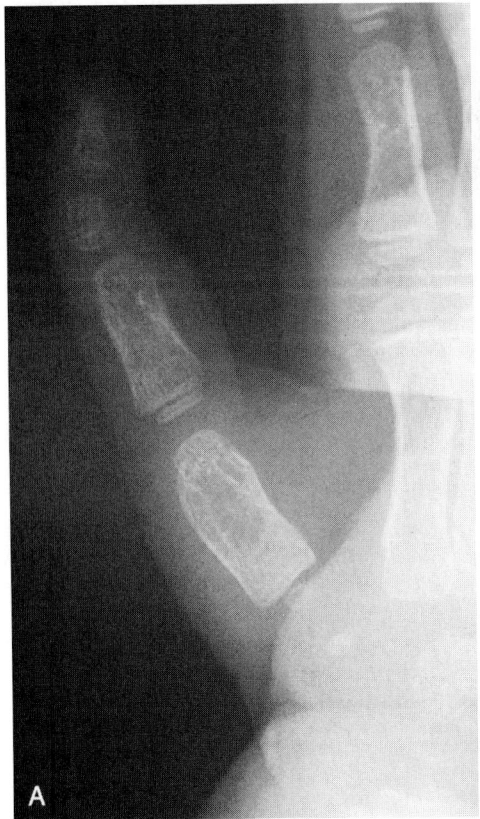

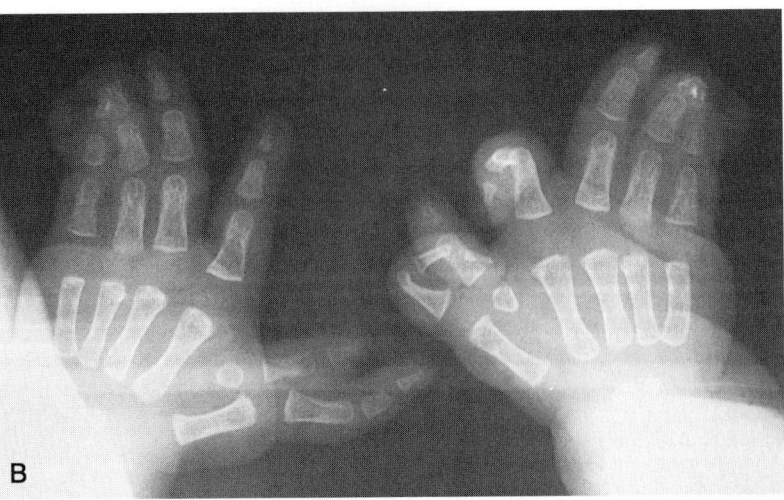

Fig. 6. Heritable radial polydactyly with triphalangism. *A,* Three phalanges in a single thumb. *B,* Triphalangeal radial polydactyly.

of the radius with other organ systems ties these malformations into known clinical associations.

CLINICAL FEATURES

Blauth classified the spectrum of thumb hypoplasia into five main forms; higher numbers indicated additional deficiency to the prior form.[11]

Type I: small to absent thenar muscles, normal bony structure.

Type II: diminished thumb-index web space and incompetent ulnar collateral ligament of the MCP joint; hypoplasia of skeletal elements.

Type III: diminished size of the thumb metacarpal and extrinsic tendon deficiencies; IIIa with a stable carpometacarpal (CMC) joint; IIIb with an unstable CMC joint.

Type IV: the floating thumb.

Type V: the absent thumb.

Abnormalities of the radial side of the carpus usually occur with thumb hypoplasia, but abnormality of the radius itself is not always associated with thumb hypoplasia (Fig. 7).

ASSOCIATED CONDITIONS

Many conditions are associated with radial hypoplasia and, consequently, with thumb hypoplasia. The main systems to be reviewed before surgical care for the thumb are cardiac, hematopoietic, renal, and skeletal. A number of these conditions are known to be caused by genetic errors. These include Holt-Oram syndrome with cardiac malformations, thrombocytopenia–absent radius syndrome, and Fanconi's pancytopenia. A number of chromosomal defects cause radial dysplasia. Radial dysplasia is a component of VAC-TERRL association, involving concurrently developing organ systems; *v*ertebral, *a*nal, *c*ardiac, *t*racheo*e*sophageal, *r*enal, *r*adial, and *l*ower limb abnormalities are associated and may be seen with a single umbilical artery and spinal cord dysraphism.

TREATMENT GOALS AND INDICATIONS

Consideration for the child as a whole involves planning reconstruction of the thumb. The implications of associated diagnoses and the condition of the limb must be addressed first. Restoring a stable, mobile thumb ray for side pinch, tip prehension, and large object stabilization is the goal of treatment. The indications for surgical reconstruction are deficiencies in the function of the thumb in a child who attempts to use the hand and whose associated medical conditions have been addressed and do not pose undue risks for elective hand reconstructive surgery.

TREATMENT

The surgical treatment should address each of the deficient components of the hypoplastic thumb. Opposition transfer to restore palmar abduction, collateral ligament reconstruction, and web space deepening will address type I and type II thumbs. Adding tendon transfers to augment extrinsic

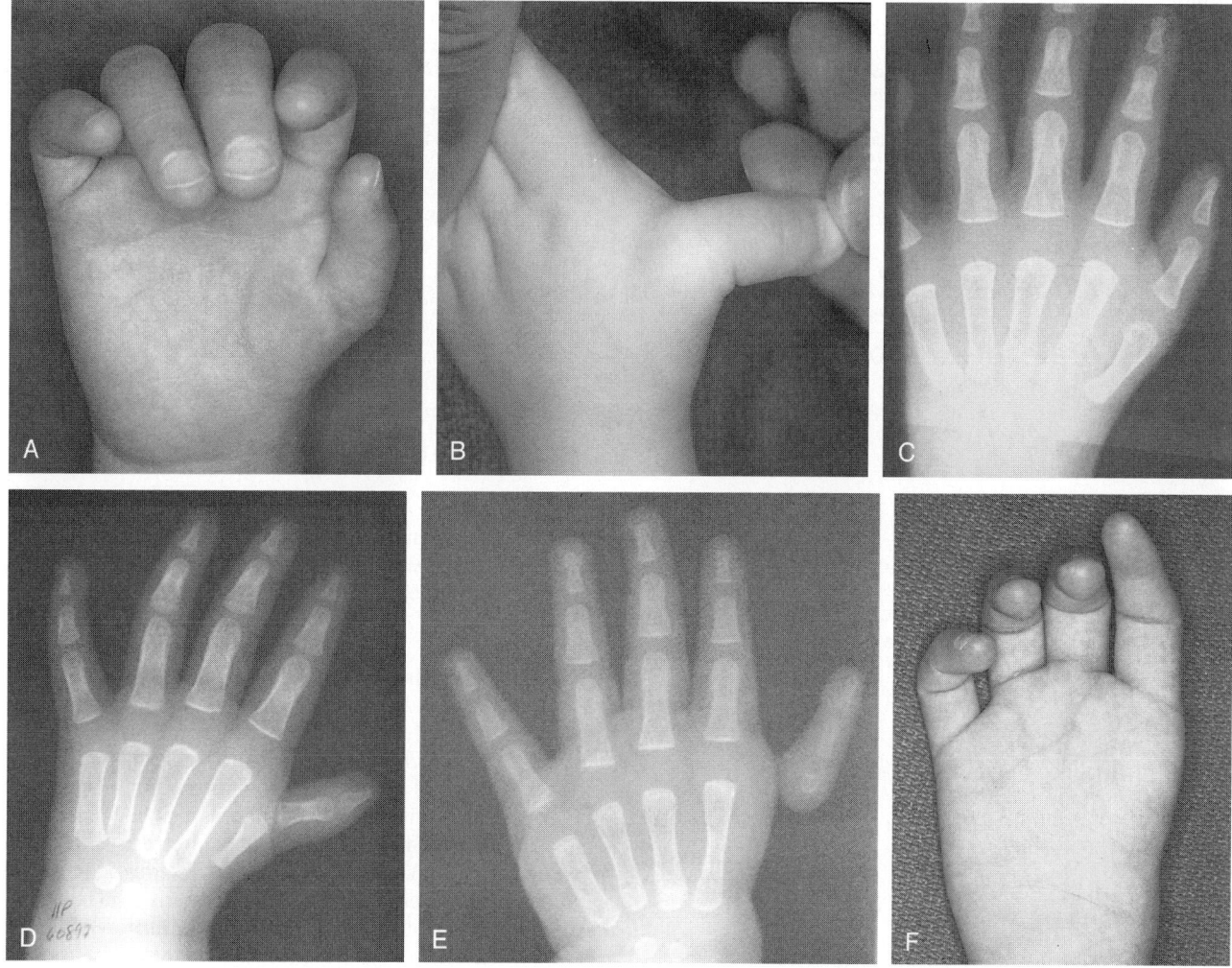

Fig. 7. Thumb hypoplasia. *A* and *B*, Type II hypoplastic thumb with absent thenar musculature and incompetent ulnar collateral ligament. *C*, Type IIIa hypoplastic thumb with additional extrinsic deficiencies and a stable carpometacarpal joint. *D*, Type IIIb hypoplastic thumb with unstable carpometacarpal joint. *E*, Type IV hypoplastic thumb, or "floating thumb." *F*, Type V hypoplastic thumb or absent thumb.

extension will be needed for type IIIa thumbs. Attempted reconstruction of a type IIIb thumb would sacrifice too much of the remaining function of the other fingers, so that the best treatment for function is pollicization of the index finger.[12] Pollicization clearly is the procedure of choice for the floating or absent thumb.[13]

MISCELLANEOUS SMALL THUMBS

Numerous uncommon types of small thumbs are associated with specific syndromes. The "hitchhiker's" thumb in dia-

strophic dwarfism, the small-angled thumb in Rubinstein-Taybi syndrome,[14] and the angled thumb in Apert's syndrome are examples of these "blueprint" abnormalities. Each of these thumbs has its own deficiencies, and treatment must be individualized according to the thumb and the associated condition.

REFERENCES

1. Ger E, Kupcha P, Ger D: The management of trigger thumb in children. J Hand Surg Am 1991; 16(5):944.
2. Van Heest A: Sensibility deficiencies in the hands of children with spastic hemiplegia. J Hand Surg Am 1993; 18:278.
3. House JH, Gwathmey FW, Fidler MO: A

dynamic approach to the thumb-in palm deformity in cerebral palsy. J Bone Joint Surg Am 1981; 63(2):216.
4. Broadbent TR, Woolfe WR. Flexion-adduction deformity of the thumb: Congenital clasped thumb. Plast Reconstr Surg 1964; 34:612.

5. McCarroll HR Jr, Manske PR: The windblown hand: Correction of the complex clasped thumb deformity. Hand Clin 1992; 8(1):147.
6. Kay S: Arthrogryposis. In Green D (ed): Operative Hand Surgery, 4th ed. New York, Churchill Livingstone, 1999, p 473.

7. Wassel HD: The results of surgery for polydactyly of the thumb. A review. Clin Orthop 1969; 64:175.

8. Manske PR: Treatment of duplicated thumb using a ligamentous/periosteal flap. J Hand Surg Am 1989; 14(4):728.

9. Wood VE: Polydactyly and the triphalangeal thumb. J Hand Surg Am 1978; 3(5): 436.

10. Wood VE: Treatment of the triphalangeal thumb. Clin Orthop 1976; 120:188.

11. Blauth W: Der hypoplastiche Daumen. Arch Orthop Unfallchir 1967; 62 (3):225.

12. Manske PR, McCarroll HR Jr, James M: Type III-A hypoplastic thumb. J Hand Surg Am 1995; 20(2):246.

13. Kleinman WB: Management of thumb hypoplasia. Hand Clin 1990; 6(4):617.

14. Wood VE, Rubinstein JH: Surgical treatment of the thumb in the Rubinstein-Taybi syndrome. J Hand Surg Br 1987; 12(2): 166.

PERIPHERAL NERVE INJURIES

section 12 chapter 23

Peter J. L. Jebson

Summary

- Peripheral nerve injury is relatively common and has major socioeconomic consequences.
- A thorough, detailed, and accurate physical examination is essential in evaluation of a suspected peripheral nerve injury.
- Electromyography (EMG) studies provide useful information in the evaluation of late (more than 1 month after injury) peripheral nerve injury but are of very limited value in the early evaluation of a peripheral nerve injury.
- In general, primary peripheral nerve repair yields better functional results than a secondary repair, but an "ideal" secondary repair yields better functional results than a "compromised" primary repair.
- Patient age and mechanism of nerve injury are the most important determinants of the functional result after a nerve repair.
- Precise, tension-free operative repair of a divided nerve provides the best functional result.

It has been estimated that 5% of all patients admitted to a level I trauma center have a peripheral nerve injury.[1, 2] Such injuries are, unfortunately, a common cause of prolonged and often permanent disability and thus have a significant socioeconomic impact. Peripheral nerve injuries occur after penetrating or blunt trauma. The associated bone and soft-tissue injury often influences patient management and outcome. The treatment of a peripheral nerve injury is challenging. The surgeon must have detailed knowledge of the surgical anatomy of peripheral nerves and familiarity with the various techniques of nerve repair and reconstruction.

HISTORICAL REVIEW

Repair of the severed peripheral nerve has gained acceptance only in the last two centuries. Although Galen (130–201 A.D.) did not believe nerve regeneration was feasible, he noted successful cases of nerve repair performed by others. In the 1300s, Guy deChauliac observed such excellent return of function after a repair that "afterward one could not believe that they had been cut."[3] However, the debate regarding nerve regeneration and the source of axons within the distal nerve stump continued until the classic work by Waller[4] and Ramon y Cajal.[5] Waller observed the dissolution of myelin in the entire nerve distal to the site of transection (wallerian degeneration) and the viability of neural tissue that remained connected to the cell body. Using a new silver staining technique, Ramon y Cajal determined axonal regeneration in detail.

The greatest clinical knowledge regarding peripheral nerve injuries has resulted from military conflicts. During the American Civil War, Mitchell was the first to organize and summarize his clinical observations in *Injuries of Nerves*. During World War I, Tinel described the classic finding of regenerating axons that bears his name. Sir Herbert Seddon of Great Britain and Barnes Woodhall of the United States independently studied injuries of the peripheral nervous system during World War II. They performed and analyzed various repair and grafting techniques and established the principle of secondary repair. Seddon[6] developed a functional classification of nerve injuries consisting of three types: neurapraxia, axonotmesis, and neurotmesis. Sir Sidney Sunderland[7] expanded the classification to five types or degrees (Table 1). He also provided detailed analysis of the internal fascicular architecture of peripheral nerves (internal topography). This has been expanded on by others and collectively has led to the concept of matching specific fascicles during repair.[8–10]

With the advent of modern microsurgery, surgeons focused on the mechanical and technical aspects of improving the quality of nerve repair. Researchers developed methods such as histochemical staining, enzyme activity, and electrical stimulation to guide fascicular matching during repair.[11–13] Current emphasis is on the biochemical, humoral, and molecular aspects of neural regeneration as we attempt to gain insight into the critical interactions between regenerating axons and their target cells in hopes of altering or influencing this complex process through pharmacological or genetic intervention. Surgeons have also focused on identifying prognostic factors for recovery after neurorrhaphy, postoperative rehabilitation, and standardized measures of outcome and functional recovery[14–19] (Table 2).

TABLE 1. CLASSIFICATION SYSTEMS FOR NERVE INJURY		
Seddon Classification	**Sunderland Classification**	**Pathology**
Neurapraxia	First degree	Myelin injury or ischemia
Axonotmesis	Second degree	Axons disrupted Endoneurial tubes intact Perineurium intact Epineurium intact
	Third degree	Axons disrupted Endoneurial tubes disrupted Perineurium intact Epineurium intact
	Fourth degree	Axons disrupted Endoneurial tubes disrupted Perineurium disrupted Epineurium intact
Neurotmesis	Fifth degree	Axons disrupted Endoneurial tubes disrupted Perineurium disrupted Epineurium disrupted

TABLE 2. MODIFIED HIGHET METHOD OF ASSESSING THE END RESULT AFTER NERVE REPAIR OR GRAFTING	
Grade	**Description**
Motor Recovery	
M0	No contraction
M1	Return of perceptible contraction in the proximal muscles
M2	Return of perceptible contraction in both proximal and distal muscles
M3	Return of function in both proximal and distal muscles of such a degree that all important muscles are sufficiently powerful to act against gravity
M4	Return of function as a stage 3; in addition, all synergistic and independent movements are possible
M5	Complete recovery
Sensory Recovery	
S0	Absence of sensibility in the autonomous area
S1	Recovery of deep cutaneous pain sensibility within the autonomous area of the nerve
S2	Return of some degree of superficial cutaneous pain and tactile sensibility within the autonomous area of the nerve
S3	Return of superficial cutaneous pain and tactile sensibility throughout the autonomous area, with disappearance of any previous overresponse
S3+	Return of sensibility as in stage 3; in addition, there is some recovery of two-point discrimination within the autonomous area (7–15 mm)
S4	Complete recovery (two-point discrimination, 2–6 mm)

PATHOGENESIS

Injury to a peripheral nerve may occur after any type of trauma. The most common mechanisms involve a laceration, fracture, dislocation, crush injury, or amputation. A combination of injury mechanisms commonly occurs. Unfortunately, peripheral nerve injuries after a gunshot wound are increasing in incidence, particularly in the urban setting.[20] Unlike other injury mechanisms, gunshot wounds cause nerve damage via shock waves, cavitation effects, and direct impact. The resultant nerve injury ranges from a neurapraxia to neurotmesis.[21] Overall, traumatic nerve injuries occur more frequently in men than women at a ratio of 2:1. The nerve most commonly injured in the upper extremity is the radial nerve followed by the ulnar and median nerves.[20]

CLINICAL FEATURES

The clinical features after a peripheral nerve injury vary depending on the mechanism of injury, presence of associated injuries, location and extent of injury (i.e., partial or complete), and the specific nerve involved. Patients may have diminished or absent sensibility within a particular anatomic distribution. They may present with weakness or absent motor function in a particular muscle or motor group. Characteristic limb posturing may also be observed (Fig. 1).

INVESTIGATION

The evaluation of the patient with a suspected peripheral nerve injury begins with a detailed clinical interview and meticulous physical examination. The surgeon should determine the patient's age, hand dominance, and time and mechanism of injury. Associated medical conditions that may influence patient management and outcome should also be identified. A thorough, detailed, and accurate physical examination is mandatory. The extremity should be inspected for signs of crush or contamination. After a gunshot wound, the location of entrance and exit wounds should be identified. The location of an open wound may

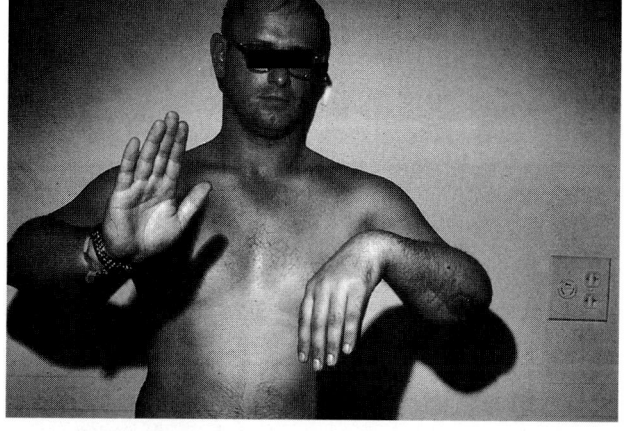

Fig. 1. Peripheral nerve injury. Note the absence of active wrist extension in a patient with disruption of the radial nerve in association with a humeral shaft fracture.

guide a more focused examination of a specific nerve, although the neurovascular status of the entire limb should be carefully assessed.

The assessment of sensibility requires an alert cooperative patient. Sensory testing usually involves the determination of static two-point discrimination (2PD) or the ability to feel a painful stimulus. Alternatively, a 256-Hz tuning fork may be used and is often better tolerated by the patient. The O'Rain wrinkle test may be particularly useful in children, in whom assessment of sensibility can be challenging.[22, 23] When a denervated finger is placed in water, skin wrinkling does not occur.

Motor testing can be performed on a specific muscle or motor group. Thorough knowledge of peripheral nerve anatomy and motor innervation patterns is essential. Muscles should be tested manually for partial or complete loss of function and their power rated. Accurate motor testing is dependent on the absence of associated muscle and tendon injury, presence of joint mobility, and patient cooperation. The results of sensory and motor testing should be compared with the uninjured contralateral extremity if possible.

Radiographs may be necessary if an associated dislocation, fracture, or retained foreign body is suspected. EMG and nerve conduction studies have limited applicability acutely after a nerve injury. For optimal interpretation, these studies should be performed 3 to 4 weeks after injury if clinical circumstances permit.[24] An appropriately performed electrodiagnostic evaluation is invaluable in late-presenting cases or in those with challenging diagnostic problems. Advances in technology have provided high-resolution images of peripheral nerves using magnetic resonance imaging and ultrasonography.[25, 26] However, neither test is routinely used, and their role in the evaluation of peripheral nerve injuries has not been clearly defined.

GOALS, INDICATIONS, AND CONTRAINDICATIONS

The goal of peripheral nerve surgery is to restore the proximal and distal fascicular connections accurately to guide subsequent axonal regeneration and the return of motor function and sensibility to the limb. This may be accomplished via several methods. Primary end-to-end repair, defined as a repair performed within 1 week of the injury, is the preferred treatment choice when conditions permit. However, several criteria must be met: (1) there must be minimal wound contamination, (2) the injured nerve must be located in a well-perfused, viable soft-tissue bed, (3) ideally, the injury should be a sharp transection with no significant crush or avulsion component, (4) there must be an absence of associated injuries that preclude adequate soft-tissue coverage, skeletal stability, or the restoration of circulation at the time of nerve repair, (5) the patient must be metabolically and emotionally stable to undergo the procedure and postoperative rehabilitation, (6) surgical magnification must be available and the operating room team must be familiar with microsurgery. If these conditions are not present, then it is better to delay repair and allow for a better determination of the extent of nerve injury. A secondary nerve repair, defined as any repair performed more than 1 week after injury, performed under favorable conditions is better than a primary repair under

unfavorable terms. If a tension-free repair is difficult or not feasible, the subsequent nerve gap may be overcome by mobilization of the nerve, flexion of adjacent joints, transposition of the nerve, shortening of the extremity, use of a nerve conduit, or nerve grafting.

Mobilization of the nerve can be done for short distances. However, there are limitations for each peripheral nerve. Elongation by 8% to 10% is the safe limit when performing an acute or delayed repair.[27] Overzealous mobilization impedes recovery because of the resultant ischemia and scarring.

Joint flexion may facilitate repair, but the subsequent mobilization will result in tension, altered neural blood flow, and fibrosis. The nerve may be rerouted and transposed to create a more direct anatomic course and facilitate an end-to-end repair in well-vascularized soft tissue. The ulnar nerve at the elbow, the recurrent motor branch of the ulnar nerve at the wrist, and the median nerve at the elbow are best suited for transposition.

Other than replantation, bone shortening is not commonly performed to overcome a nerve gap. Humeral shortening may be indicated when a comminuted fracture and multiple nerves have been injured or if a segmental defect in the ulnar nerve is present in children and adolescents.[27]

Nerve conduits composed of a variety of materials have been used to guide axonal regeneration and overcome a short nerve gap. Successful use of an autologous venous nerve conduit for distal sensory nerve defects has been confirmed in several clinical series.[28] Biological and nonbiological conduits have also been used with limited success.[29] The clinical use of a nerve conduit is currently considered experimental as researchers determine the size of the maximal gap that can be successfully bridged and the outcome of this technique compared with autologous nerve grafting.

Nerve grafting to overcome a gap is the most conventional approach and is indicated when a tension-free repair is not feasible or cannot be facilitated with any of the aforementioned methods. In general, grafting is indicated if two 8-0 sutures do not maintain a tension-free repair with the adjacent joints in neutral position and for a major peripheral nerve defect of 3 cm or more. Several techniques of nerve grafting have been described. The current preferred method is group fascicular (also termed interfascicular) grafting using autologous donor nerve. The sural nerve is the standard donor for grafting of the median, ulnar, and radial nerves. The medial and lateral antebrachial cutaneous nerves, terminal branch of the posterior interosseous nerve, and dorsal cutaneous branch of the ulnar nerve are useful for grafting small defects in the digital nerves.

PROCEDURE

PREOPERATIVE PLANNING
Peripheral nerve surgery should be performed in an operating room environment with a team well versed in microsurgery. Most patients may be scheduled electively within an appropriate time frame after injury. This avoids surgeon fatigue and permits a more controlled setting for microsurgery. Those patients with associated injuries such as open fractures or vascular disruption and secondary limb ische-

mia require more urgent care. General anesthesia is preferred, although a regional anesthesia combined with intravenous sedation may also be used.

For optimal visualization, an operating microscope is preferred. Alternatively, loupe magnification (2.5 to 4.5×) may be used for larger nerves. Appropriate microinstruments are essential, and a bloodless field with limb exsanguination, pneumatic tourniquet control, and the use of bipolar electrocautery should be used.

The entire upper limb should be prepared and draped. The lower extremity should also be incorporated into the operating field if harvesting of the sural nerve is anticipated for nerve grafting. If shortening of bone is being considered to overcome a nerve gap and facilitate a tension-free nerve repair, a saw and instrumentation for skeletal fixation should be available.

TECHNICAL DETAILS

Lacerations or open wounds are incorporated into the skin incision, which is extended proximally and distally in standard fashion. Initial dissection of the injured nerve and surrounding tissues is performed using loupe magnification. It is usually easier to begin the dissection proximal and distal to the zone of injury to facilitate identification of normal anatomy and tissue planes. The injured nerve ends are identified as the surrounding soft tissues are carefully retracted. The operating microscope is brought into the field and the nerve examined. The damaged nerve ends are cut back sharply with a no. 11 scalpel blade or ophthalmic knife until the fascicles appear normal. The nerve is cut perpendicular to the long axis. This is usually performed against a sterile disposable wooden tongue depressor. Microforceps are used to manipulate the nerve gently via the epineurium. The fascicular arrangement and epineurial vessels are carefully identified and used to guide accurate rotational alignment of both nerve ends.

Several techniques have been developed to improve fascicular matching, particularly the identification and separation of specific motor and sensory fascicles. Selective fascicular stimulation with a standard electrical nerve stimulator may be performed in a sedated but awake patient.[12] For best results, the technique must be performed within 3 days of the injury. Nerve stimulation is limited to the positive identification of proximal sensory and distal motor fascicles. Alternatively, individual motor and sensory fibers may be identified in a distal nerve stump for up to 9 days after transection and indefinitely in the proximal stump via histochemical identification of the enzymes acetylcholinesterase and carbonic anhydrase.[11, 13]

The amount of tension anticipated at the repair can be ascertained by reapproximating the nerve ends with microforceps. The neurorrhaphy is performed using nonabsorbable suture. The size of the suture is dependent on the caliber of the nerve. The finest caliber of suture that maintains adequate coaptation and prevents retraction or gapping at the repair site is used. This most commonly involves 8-0, 9-0, or 10-0 suture.

Sutureless methods of nerve repair have also been described. The majority of clinical experience has been with fibrin glue. Successful fibrin glue neurorrhaphy is dependent on the elimination of tension at the repair. The glue is applied as a thin layer three to four times longer than the diameter of the nerve. A small piece of a surgical glove or Esmarch bandage may be wrapped around the repair site to ensure even distribution of the glue and separation from the surrounding tissues.

After repair, the wound is closed over a passive rubber or silicone drain if indicated. A suction drain should not be used because of potential damage to the repair. The patient is kept anesthetized until the extremity has been appropriately immobilized.

The specific technique of nerve repair varies with nerve type, anatomic location of the injury, and surgeon preference. A combination of techniques is often used.

PRIMARY END-TO-END REPAIR
Epineurial Repair

Sutures are placed in the epineurium alone and not the nerve fascicle substance. Several sutures are placed; the number depends on the size of the nerve. For small nerves such as the digital nerve, three to four sutures are sufficient. For larger nerves, eight to 10 sutures may be necessary. Sutures are placed in an orderly fashion; the first suture is placed at the back of the nerve. A second suture is placed 180 degrees from the first suture. Subsequent sutures are placed equidistant between the first two sutures to create equal spacing of the suture within the four quadrants of the repair. The suture is passed through the epineurium proximally and distally and gently tied (Fig. 2). Multiple passes should be avoided. Suture tails are left long to facilitate manipulation and rotation of the nerve. The repair is inspected to verify closure of the epineurium and no fascicular tissue herniation between the sutures.

Group Fascicular Repair

Group fascicular repair requires more delicate instruments and higher magnification than epineurial suture. It is also more technically demanding. Fascicular groups should be identified and matched after careful analysis of the cross-sectional appearance of the nerve ends. Gentle lateral traction is applied on the fascicular groups of each nerve end

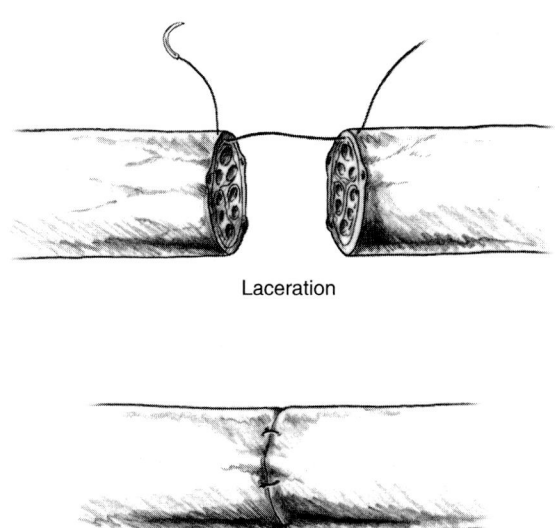

Laceration

Epineurial suture

Fig. 2. Epineurial nerve repair.

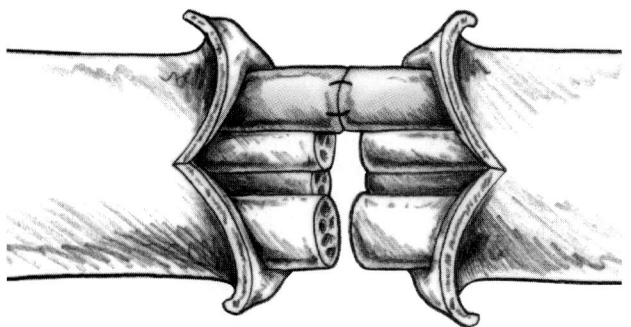

Group fascicular suture

Fig. 3. Group fascicular repair.

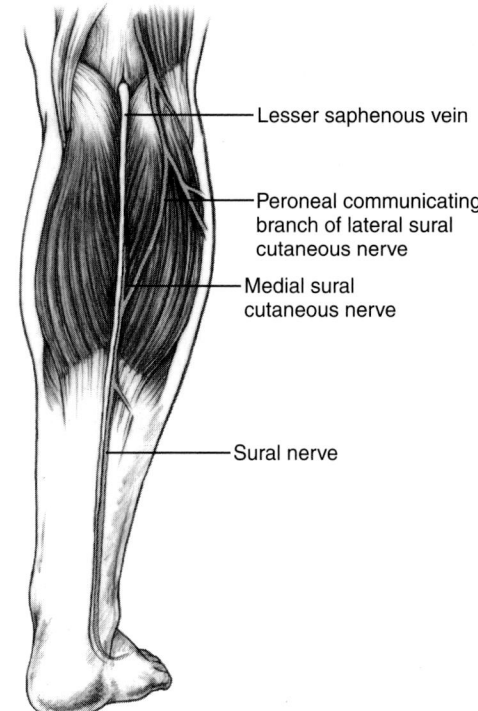

Fig. 5. Nerve grafting. The sural nerve is a common source of graft.

with a microforceps, and the internal epineurium is dissected with a delicate curved microscissor. Each group is isolated for a distance for about 3 to 4 mm. The fascicular groups are sharply trimmed followed by suturing of the interfascicular epineurium with a fine-caliber suture such as 10-0. Alternatively, sutures may be placed at the perineurium of the fascicle if insufficient epineurium is available (Fig. 3).

Individual Fascicular Repair

Individual fascicular repair is rarely performed. The internal epineurium separating individual fascicles is dissected carefully to avoid damaging any interfascicular connections. Usually two 10-0 sutures on a 70- or 50-μm needle placed 180 degrees apart are sufficient for each fascicle (Fig. 4).

FREE NERVE GRAFTING

Wide exposure of the injured nerve is performed. The proximal and distal nerve stumps are identified. The neuroma is sharply resected. Using the operating microscope, microdissection is performed to excise external epineurium and expose fascicular groups. Fascicular groups in both nerve ends are identified. The wound is packed with a saline-soaked sponge, the tourniquet deflated, and hemostasis obtained. The appropriate nerve graft is harvested (Figs. 5 and 6). The size of the defect is determined with the wrist in a neutral position and the elbow extended. An

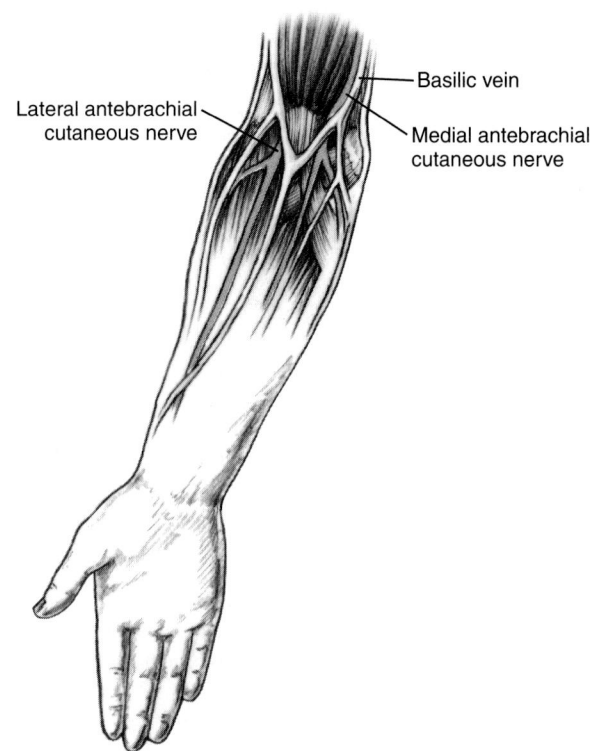

Fig. 6. Nerve grafting. The medial and lateral antebrachial cutaneous nerves are additional sources of graft.

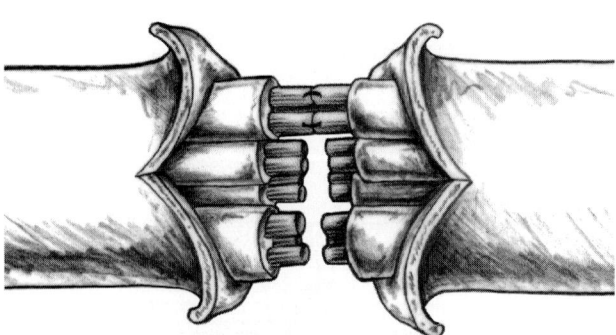

Individual fascicular suture

Fig. 4. Individual fascicular repair.

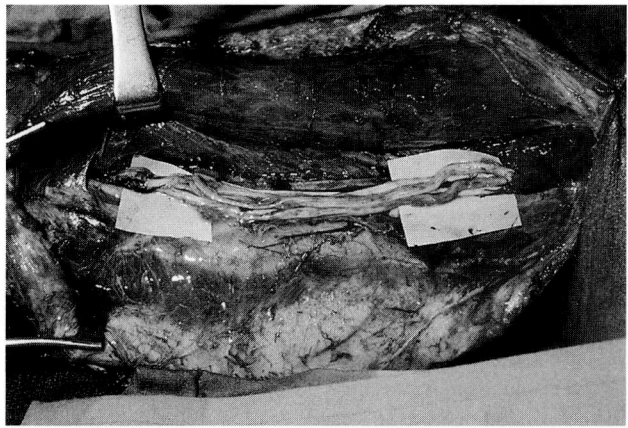

Fig. 7. Sural nerve grafting of a high radial nerve injury with segmental loss after a high-energy gunshot wound.

appropriate length of graft is then gently positioned in the defect with correct rotational alignment (Fig. 7). For small defects, it is easier to match fascicular groups in the nerve ends. With longer gaps, the ends of the graft must be correctly matched within the same quadrant of the nerve ends. The grafts are sutured to the internal epineurium using the minimum number of 10-0 sutures required to obtain a tension-free repair (Fig. 8).

POSTOPERATIVE MANAGEMENT

Nerve repairs are protected in a cast or splint for 3 weeks to permit the development of sufficient strength to tolerate gentle traction.[30] Adjacent joints are often included to avoid inadvertent disruption of the repair. The position of the extremity is best determined intraoperatively by the location of the injury, quality of the repair, and presence of associated injuries.

For nerve grafting proximal to the wrist, the extremity is immobilized with the wrist in neutral and the elbow in 20 degrees of flexion. Immobilization may be discontinued 10

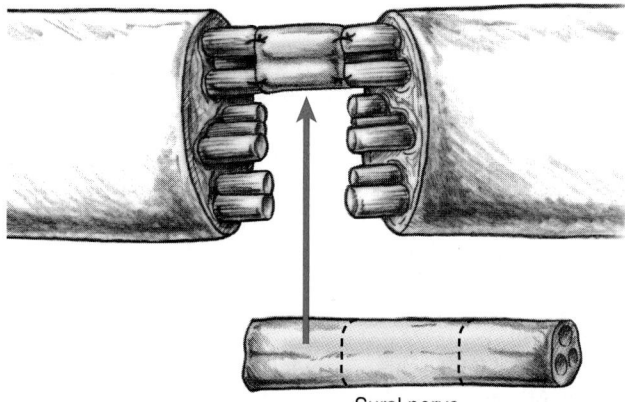

Sural nerve

Fig. 8. Grafting of a nerve defect using interfascicular repair technique.

days postoperatively and gentle mobilization begun with progression to full motion at 3 weeks.

When immobilization is discontinued, a removable custom-fabricated splint or orthosis may be used for an additional 1 to 2 weeks to avoid extreme joint positioning and secondary nerve injury. Rehabilitation involves joint mobilization, avoidance of stiffness, reduction of edema, prevention of contractures, and improved functional use. Strengthening is begun 8 to 12 weeks postoperatively. Sensory reeducation begins when moving touch and 30-cps tuning fork vibration are perceived within the proximal aspect of the denervated area.[16] A desensitization program may be used if painful dysesthesias occur. The assistance of a competent therapist experienced in the rehabilitation of patients with peripheral nerve injuries is essential. The assessment of nerve regeneration during the follow-up period involves verification of an advancing Tinel-Hoffmann sign at the classic rate of 1 inch/month or 1 mm/day and the assessment of specific motor and sensory recovery.

COMPLICATIONS

Hematoma formation, either intraneural or within the wound, is a serious complication that is prevented with appropriate hemostasis and wound drainage. A wound hematoma requires evacuation. Rupture of the neurorrhaphy may occur as a consequence of poor suture technique, inadequate or inappropriate protection of the repair, or premature mobilization with subsequent tension at the repair site. When suspected or recognized in the early postoperative period, exploration with rerepair or grafting is indicated.

The most disheartening of complications is the failure of end-organ regeneration with absent motor function and sensibility, resulting in joint contractures, positional imbalance, and altered limb function. This should be suspected if motor function and sensibility have not returned in an appropriate period of time. Treatment is individualized and may involve resection with nerve grafting, tendon transfers, or a combination of reconstructive procedures.

The formation of a neuroma with radiating pain, paresthesias, and ultimately a chronic pain syndrome can be particularly debilitating. Excision of the neuroma with subsequent grafting or translocation or implantation of the nerve end may be necessary. A painful neuroma may also occur after the harvesting of a nerve graft. An often-underappreciated consequence of harvesting the sural nerve or cutaneous nerves of the forearm is the subsequent sensory deficit. Preoperative block of the nerve with a local anesthetic has been recommended to demonstrate to the patient the anticipated deficit.

SHORT-TERM RESULTS AND OUTCOMES

The results of primary nerve repair are superior to secondary or delayed repair. However, comparing the results of nerve repair or grafting is difficult because of the different repair techniques, heterogeneous patient population, multiple prognostic factors, and dissimilar assessment measures (Table 3).

Patient age and the mechanism of injury are believed to be the prime determinants of functional outcome after nerve repair.[17] The younger the patient, the better is the prognosis. Sharp lacerations have a better prognosis than crush or avulsion injuries.

The four most important factors affecting the outcome of nerve grafting in the upper extremity are patient age, gap size, time delay from injury to grafting, and level of injury (proximal versus distal).[14] In general, age greater than 20 years, a graft larger than 5 cm, a delay longer than 6 months before grafting, and proximal level of injury are associated with less satisfactory outcomes after nerve grafting.

PRIMARY REPAIR
Digital Nerve

Patient age at the time of repair is the main determinant of sensory recovery.[31] Using microsurgical techniques, approximately 75% of patients younger than 20 years of age will achieve a 2PD of less than 6 mm (S4) (see Table 2), whereas only 25% to 50% of adults will have the same recovery level. The results of epineurial and fascicular repair are equivalent.[32, 33] The majority of patients will achieve functional sensory recovery (S3 or better). Some patients will experience persistent hyperesthesias for up to 2 years.

Median Nerve

Age is again the most important determinant of outcome. Children have the best return of motor function and sensibility. Overall, sensibility appears to recover more successfully than motor function. The return of functionally significant intrinsic motor activity occurs in about 50% of patients. Most series report fair (M3, S3) to good (M4, S3+) results in adults.

Ulnar Nerve

The results of ulnar nerve repair distal to the elbow are better than those performed proximally. The prognosis for functional intrinsic muscle return for above-elbow injuries in adults is extremely poor. Approximately 50% of patients will have motor recovery of M4 and sensibility of S3+. An excellent outcome, defined as M5 motor recovery and S4 sensory recovery, occurs in 10% to 15% of patients. There is no difference in the outcome for group fascicular versus epineurial repair.

Radial Nerve

Determining the outcome of radial nerve repairs from the available literature is extremely difficult. In general, below-elbow injuries have a better outcome than above-elbow injuries. Approximately 50% to 70% of below-elbow injuries will achieve a motor recovery level of M3 or better compared with 17% to 50% of above-elbow injuries.

NERVE GRAFTING
Digital Nerve

Patient age at the time of grafting is the most important predictor of outcome. In Frykman and Gramyk's[14] review of six series consisting of 151 cases, 88% of patients achieved useful (S3 or better) sensory recovery, whereas 69% achieved some 2PD. All patients younger than 20 years achieved some 2PD. Up to age 40, all patients achieved useful sensory recovery. Graft length was important; 80% of those patients with a graft smaller than 5 cm achieved at least grade S3 sensibility. Grafting more than 6 months after injury did not appear to affect the results significantly.

Mackinnon and Dellon[29] used polyglycolic tubes as an artificial conduit in 15 patients with a gap between 0.5 and 3 cm. A sensibility of grade S3 or better returned in 86% of patients, whereas 33% achieved grade S4.

Median Nerve

Several studies demonstrated a correlation between sensory and motor recovery after grafting of a median nerve injury.[34, 35] In Frykman and Gramyk's review, 81% achieved grade M3 motor recovery, whereas 79% achieved sensory recovery of S3. Patients younger than 20 years had the best results; 88% achieved useful motor return and 98% achieved useful sensibility. Among patients older than 40 years, 64% achieved useful motor recovery, whereas 58% had useful sensory recovery. Gap length had an effect on motor and sensory recovery. Of those grafts smaller than 5 cm, 95% of patients had useful (M3 or greater) motor recovery, whereas 78% had useful sensory recovery (S3 and greater). For those patients whose gap was greater than 10 cm, only 66% achieved useful motor recovery, whereas 85% had useful sensory recovery. A time delay of greater than 6 months and a proximal level of injury also adversely affected motor and sensory recovery.[14]

Ulnar Nerve

Frykman and Gramyk found that 63% of patients obtained M3 or better motor recovery, whereas 75% achieved a sensory grade of S3 or better. Delaying grafting by more than 6 months after injury and the level of injury affected the results. A gap of more than 10 cm was associated with poor return of sensibility and motor recovery.[14] In the series by Kalomiri et al,[34] 94% of patients achieved useful motor recovery. Similarly, Daoutis et al[36] reported 85% useful motor recovery and 88% useful sensory recovery.

Radial Nerve

In Frykman and Gramyk's review of three series with a total of 60 patients, 78% obtained useful motor recovery, whereas 16% obtained none at all. All of these patients were either older than 40 years, had a gap greater than 10 cm, or sustained a proximal arm injury. All patients younger than 20 years with a graft smaller than 5 cm obtained M3 motor recovery or better. Eighty-one percent of patients whose grafting was performed within 6 months of injury had useful motor recovery. Sensory recovery to the S3 level or better was achieved in all patients younger than 20 years. All patients with a gap length of 5 cm or less had S3+ return compared with 56% of those whose gap was greater than 10 cm. A delay of 6 months did not significantly affect sensory recovery. However, sensory recovery for those injuries above the elbow was poor; only 30% obtained useful sensibility.[14]

Kalomiri et al[34] reported 97% useful motor recovery; 60% achieved a grade M5 in their series of 35 patients. All of the five patients in the series by Daoutis et al[36] achieved grade M3 or better. More recently, Nunley et al[37] reported that 72% of their 20 patients achieved useful motor recovery, with 44% obtaining an M4 or better grade. A better outcome was noted in those patients with injuries of the posterior interosseous nerve compared with high radial nerve injuries.

REFERENCES

1. Noble J, Munro CA, Prasad VSSV, et al: Analysis of upper and lower extremity peripheral nerve injuries in a population of patients with multiple injuries. J Trauma 1998; 45:116.
2. Selecki BR, Ring IT, Simpson DA, et al: Trauma to the central and peripheral nervous systems: Part II. A statistical profile of surgical treatment in New South Wales. Aust N Z J Surg 1977; 52:111.
3. deChauliac G: On Wounds and Fractures (translated by Brennan WA). Unpublished manuscript, Chicago, 1923.
4. Waller AV: Experiments on the glossopharyngeal and hypoglossal nerves of the frog and observations produced thereby in the structure of their primitive fibres. Philos Trans R Soc Lond B Biol Sci 1850; 140:423.
5. Ramon y Cajal S: Degeneration and Regeneration of the Nervous System (translated by May RM). New York, Hafner, 1968.
6. Seddon HG: Three types of nerve injuries. Brain 1943; 66:237.
7. Sunderland S: A classification of peripheral nerve injuries producing loss of function. Brain 1951; 74:491.
8. Jabaley ME, Wallace WH, Heckler FR: Internal topography of major nerves of the forearm and hand: A current view. J Hand Surg 1980; 5:1.
9. Chow JA, Van Beek AL, Bilos ZJ, et al: Anatomical basis for repair of ulnar and median nerves in the distal part of the forearm by group fascicular suture and nerve grafting. J Bone Joint Surg Am 1986; 68:273.
10. Shizhen Z, Xiangluo T, Muzhil L: The microsurgical anatomy of peripheral nerves. In Shizhen Z, Yongjian M, Wencyun Y (eds): Microsurgical Anatomy. Lancaster, England, MTP Press, 1985, p 299.
11. Riley DA, Lang DH: Carbonic anhydrase activity of human peripheral nerves: A possible histochemical aid to nerve repair. J Hand Surg Am 1984; 9:112.
12. Hakstian RW: Funicular orientation by direct stimulation: An aid to peripheral

nerve repair. J Bone Joint Surg Am 1968; 50:1178.
13. Gruber H: Identification of motor and sensory funiculi in cut nerves and their selective reunion. Br J Plast Surg 1976; 29:70.
14. Frykman GK, Gramyk K: Results of nerve grafting. In Gelberman RH (ed): Operative Nerve Repair and Reconstruction. Philadelphia, JB Lippincott, 1991, p 553.
15. Vanderhooft E: Functional outcomes of nerve grafts for the upper and lower extremities. Hand Clinics 2000; 16:93.
16. Dellon AL, Curtis RM, Edgerton MT: Reeducation of sensation in the hand after nerve injury and repair. Plast Reconstr Surg 1974; 53:297.
17. Allan CH: Functional results of primary nerve repair. Hand Clin 2000; 16:67.
18. Steinberg DR, Koman LA: Factors affecting the results of peripheral nerve repair. In Gelberman RH (ed): Operative Nerve Repair and Reconstruction. Philadelphia, JB Lippincott, 1991, vol 1, p 349.
19. Levinthol R, Brown WJ, Rand RW: Comparison of fascicular, interfascicular, and epineurial suture techniques in the repair of simple nerve lacerations. J Neurosurg 1977; 47:744.
20. McAllister RM, Gilbert SE, Calder JS, et al: The epidemiology and management of upper limb peripheral nerve injuries in modern practice. J Hand Surg Br 1996; 21:4.
21. Omer GE Jr: Nerve injuries associated with gunshot wounds of the extremities. In Gelberman RH (ed): Operative Nerve Repair and Reconstruction. Philadelphia, JB Lippincott, 1991.
22. O'Rain S: New and simple test of nerve function in the hand. BMJ 1973; 3:615.
23. Phelps PE, Walker E: Comparison of the finger wrinkling test results to established sensory tests in peripheral nerve injury. Am J Occup Ther 1977; 31:565.
24. Carter GT, Robinson LR, Chang VH, et al: Electrodiagnostic evaluation of traumatic nerve injuries. Hand Clin 2000; 16:1:1.
25. Jarvik JG, Kliot M, Maravilla KR: MR

nerve imaging of the wrist and hand. Hand Clin 2000; 16:13.
26. Filler AG, Kliot M, Howe FA, et al: Application of magnetic resonance neurography in the evaluation of patients with peripheral nerve pathology. J Neurosurg 1996; 85:299.
27. Trumble TE, McCallister WV: Repair of peripheral nerve defects in the upper extremity. Hand Clin 2000; 16:37.
28. Strauch B: Use of nerve conduits in peripheral nerve repair. Hand Clin 2000; 16:123.
29. Mackinnon SE, Dellon AL: Clinical nerve reconstruction with a bioabsorbable polyglycolic acid tube. Plast Reconstr Surg 1990; 85:419.
30. Miller EM: An experimental study to determine the strength of the suture line. Arch Surg 1921; 2:167.
31. Wang WZ, Crain GM, Baylis W, et al: Outcome of digital nerve injuries in adults. J Hand Surg Am 1996; 21:138.
32. Tupper JW, Crick JC, Matteck CR: Fascicular nerve repairs: A comparative study of epineurial and fascicular (perineurial) techniques. Orthop Clin North Am 1988; 19:57.
33. Young L, Wray RC, Weeks PM: A randomized prospective comparison of fascicular and epineurial digital nerve repairs. Plast Reconstr Surg 1981; 68:89.
34. Kalomiri DE, Panayotis N, Soucacos PN, et al: Nerve grafting in peripheral nerve microsurgery of the upper extremity. Microsurgery 1994; 15:506.
35. Walton R, Finseth F: Nerve grafting in the repair of complicated peripheral nerve trauma. J Trauma 1977; 17:793.
36. Daoutis NK, Gerosthathopoulos NE, Efstathopoulus DG, et al: Microsurgical reconstruction of large nerve defects using autologous nerve grafts. Microsurgery 1994; 15:502.
37. Nunley JA, Saies AD, Sandow MJ, et al: Results of interfascicular nerve grafting for radial nerve lesions. Microsurgery 1996; 17:431.

BRACHIAL PLEXUS INJURIES

Peter M. Waters

Summary

- Brachial plexus injuries in the adult are most often secondary to motorcycle or motor vehicle accidents (>80% in most series).[1, 2] Severe injuries can result in profound disability. Forty-four percent of patients in one study lost more than 2 years of work, and only 8% of those patients returned to work within 2 months of injury.[3] Severe plexus injuries are often associated with polytrauma, including neck, head, chest, limb, and vascular injuries. These injuries may be life-threatening[1] and can mask the acute diagnosis of a brachial plexus injury.
- Brachial plexus birth palsies occur in 0.1% to 0.4% of live births. Birth palsies occur most commonly in association with multiparous mothers, high birth weight infants, difficult extractions, and infants in fetal distress at the time of delivery. Most commonly, the upper trunk is involved. If recovery of all muscle groups occurs in the first 6 weeks of life, the outcome is normal. However, if recovery is delayed beyond 2 months of life, some permanent loss will occur, most notably with shoulder abduction and external rotation.[4]
- The goal of treatment is to minimize permanent disability and restore or improve upper limb function.
- The major management decision is whether to microsurgically reconstruct the brachial plexus in patients who do not recover motor function in the first 3 to 6 months after injury. The major factor in outcome is the severity of the original neural injury (avulsion or rupture; degree of injury by Sunderland classification[5]). Other outcome factors are severity of associated injuries, success of surgical interventions, and patient motivation and compliance factors. As would be expected, infants have better rates of recovery than adults, for both spontaneous recovery and postoperative recovery.

HISTORICAL REVIEW

The original written description of an adult traumatic plexus injury may be in the Iliad's 8th song, by Homer. Flaubert published the first anatomic description of a traction injury to the brachial plexus in 1827. Weir Mitchell, in 1872, described the occurrence of causalgia during Civil War traumatic injuries. At the turn of the 20th century, many surgeons described repairs, grafts, and transfers for traumatic plexus injuries: Kennedy (1903), Lange (1912), Fairbank (1913), and Taylor (1920), among others. Scag-

lietti (1942) and Seddon (1975) described post–World War II repairs and were discouraged by the results.

With higher rates of patient survival achieved by improvements in emergency transport systems as well as intensive care of the patient with multiple injuries and by the use of helmets in motorcyclists, surgeons became increasingly disappointed with the natural history of severe traumatic brachial plexus injuries.[1, 2] This situation led Millesi,[2] Narakas,[1, 6] and others to pursue microsurgical reconstruction of the plexus using the advancing medical and surgical technology to improve results. Although the outcomes never reached restoration of normal limb function, they were more positive than amputation or use of a prosthesis. Doi and colleagues[7] described the use of microvascular free muscle transfers to improve upper limb function in severe avulsion injuries.

As early as 1768, Smellie identified the cause of brachial plexus birth palsy as being obstetrical rather than congenital. Duchenne (1861) confirmed the source of the neurological injury to be the plexus. Erb (1875) defined the lesion in the upper trunk. Klumpke (1885) identified the rare lower trunk lesion (C-8–T-1). Clark (1905), Stevens (1934), and others defined the mechanical nature of the traction injuries to the plexus during the birthing process. Narakas and Gilbert and Tassin[8] and others presented their results with microsurgical reconstruction of the infantile brachial plexopathy. Hoffer and associates[9] and Goddard and Fixsen[10] presented results of tendon transfers and osteotomies about the shoulder for secondary reconstruction in the child with chronic plexopathy.

PATHOGENESIS

The majority of injuries to the brachial plexus are secondary to a traction mechanism. High-speed motorcycle and motor vehicle accidents are the most common cause in adults. Falls from a height, especially at the workplace, are also a cause. Traction injuries span the spectrum from upper root and trunk injuries to complete avulsion of all roots. In war zones and certain urban centers, stab and gunshot wounds to the plexus are prevalent.[11] These more commonly affect the upper and middle brachial plexus because the clavicle protects the lower plexus. Although irradiation, thoracic outlet compression, and iatrogenic injury to the brachial plexus also occur, they are not considered here. Associated injuries to the cervical spine, subclavian/axillary vessels, chest, abdomen, head, and limb frequently occur in adult patients.[1, 2] At times, these injuries are life-threatening.

In children, the cause of brachial plexus injury is predominantly related to a traction injury during birth, usually with a vertex presentation and delivery. In this classic shoulder dystocia, the lateral flexion of the neck is used to free the arm from the pubic arch. The injury is most often a postganglionic upper trunk lesion.[4, 6, 8, 12] Injuries also occur with breech delivery and more commonly result in an avulsion of the upper nerve roots.[4] Finally, the causes of brachial injury in adults also apply to children.

CLINICAL FEATURES

Because a high percentage of adults with severe brachial plexus injuries have major associated vascular, skeletal, visceral, and neurological injuries, the clinical presentation and care of those problems dominate patient management in the acute postinjury period. However, it is critical that a thorough neurological examination be conducted as soon as the patient is stable and conscious.

In infants, the injury to the plexus is most often isolated. Associated clavicular and humeral fractures can occur. These may confuse the clinical picture briefly during attempts to sort out a pseudoparalysis from fracture pain and a true palsy. Rarely, there is an associated hemiparesis from central nervous system involvement.

It is imperative to understand the anatomy of the brachial plexus in order to appreciate the physical findings in (Fig. 1). All muscles of the upper extremity except the trapezius are innervated by the brachial plexus. The nerves originate from the fifth through eight cervical and first thoracic nerve roots. Variations occur with contributions from the fourth cervical root (pre–fixed plexus) or less commonly from the second thoracic nerve root (post–fixed plexus). The nerve roots combine to form the trunks, divisions, cords, and eventually the peripheral nerves that supply the individual muscles. Specifically, the C5 and C6 nerve roots form the upper trunk; the C7 nerve root forms the middle trunk; and the C8 and T1 nerve roots form the lower trunk. Each trunk bifurcates into anterior and posterior divisions. The posterior divisions of all three trunks form the posterior cord. The anterior divisions of the upper and middle trunks form the lateral cord. The anterior division of the lower trunk continues as the medial cord.

The major nerves that supply the upper extremity musculature are terminal branches of the cords. The ulnar nerve arises from the medial cord, the radial and axillary nerves from the posterior cord, and the musculocutaneous nerve from the lateral cord. The median nerve arises from contributions from the medial and lateral cords. Motor and sensory losses in each nerve distribution must be thoroughly documented with every patient to define the level and extent of injury as well as to monitor recovery. Patterns of injury can be generally grouped as follows[1, 13, 14]:

- C5-6/upper trunk injury: Results in motor loss or weakness of the deltoid, rotator cuff, subscapularis, biceps, extensor carpi radialis longus, and brachioradialis muscles (Erb's palsy).
- C5-C6-C7: Involves the muscles noted in the previous group as well as the triceps, extensor carpi radialis brevis, and digital extensors.
- Entire brachial plexus: Represents a flail and anesthetic limb associated with a Horner's syndrome.
- C8-T1: A rare injury that represents loss of wrist flexion, finger flexion, and intrinsic hand function (Klumpke's palsy).

The distinction between a preganglionic and postganglionic lesion is important in determining prognosis. Horner's syndrome (injury to the sympathetic chain C8-T1), elevated hemidiaphragm (phrenic nerve), winged scapula (long thoracic nerve), and motor loss of the rhomboids (dorsal scapular), rotator cuff (suprascapular nerve), and latissimus

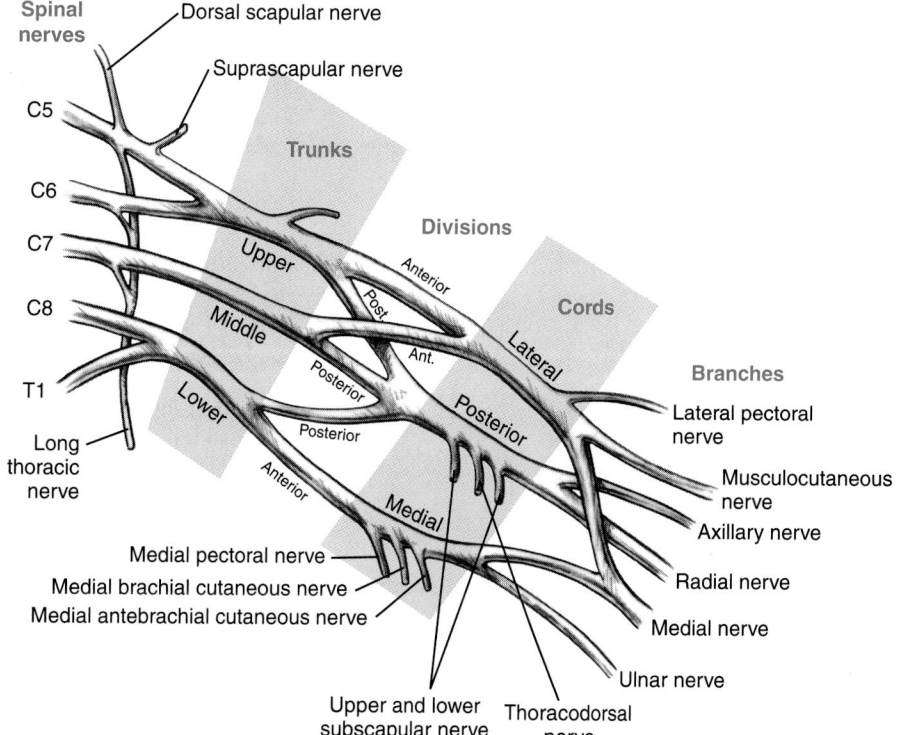

Fig. 1. Normal anatomy of the brachial plexus. (Copyright 1997 American Academy of Orthopaedic Surgeons. Redrawn from J Am Acad Orthop Surg 1997; 5:205.)

dorsi (thoracodorsal nerve) all raise concerns about a pre-ganglionic injury and a poor prognosis.

INVESTIGATION

Serial physical examinations testing motor and sensory function of the affected limb are the most reliable test at present for assessing injury and recovery. In adults, this evaluation involves voluntary muscle and sensory testing. In infants, it requires observation of spontaneous activity and of muscle activity with primitive reflexes (i.e., elbow flexion with Moro reflex), and provocative testing. Plain radiographs may reveal associated fractures (humerus, scapula, clavicle, transverse processes of the cervical spine, ribs) and intrathoracic injuries. The fact that there is significant injury in the anatomic region of the brachial plexus increases the chances of an associated neural injury to the plexus. Computed tomography/myelograms or magnetic resonance imaging (MRI) may aid in diagnosis. The presence of large diverticula or frank meningoceles is diagnostic of avulsion injuries on CT or myelography. The presence of small diverticula, however, was accurate for avulsion injury in only 60% of patients in one series.[21] MRI has a true-positive rate of accuracy similar to that of CT/myelograms and also can visualize associated peripheral nerve injuries.

Electrodiagnostic studies with electromyography and nerve conduction velocity measurements are also used to assess the type and severity of neural injury. If these studies are used, it is best to perform them more than 3 weeks after injury. It is most helpful to assess the paraspinal muscles first in the electromyography study. This assessment distinguishes preganglionic from postganglionic lesions. Denervation potentials in the paraspinal muscles imply a preganglionic lesion, because the posterior branch of the spinal nerve arises adjacent to the cord. If the study must be discontinued because of patient pain, this important information about the level of injury has already been obtained. In terms of nerve conduction velocities, the median and radial nerves are used to assess C6-C7 roots, and the ulnar nerve is used to assess the C8 and T1 roots. Unfortunately, the presence of activity in particular muscles does not mean that the patient will achieve an acceptable level of recovery. Results of these studies must be correlated with physical findings.

The ultimate investigation of brachial plexus injury is surgical exploration. At times, surgery is the most definitive way to assess the type, level, and severity of injury. Often, sensory evoked potentials or motor action potentials are assessed intraoperatively to define peripheral and central nervous system continuity.

GOALS, INDICATIONS, AND CONTRAINDICATIONS

GOALS

The goal of any surgery is to restore or improve upper limb function. Microsurgical reconstruction of the plexus involves the use of neural grafts[1, 6, 8, 11, 12, 14] and transfers[15-17] to provide re-innervation to muscles that otherwise would not recover sufficiently. Although microsurgical reconstruction does not normalize the situation, it may im-prove motor strength and sensory feedback and may lessen dystrophic pain in patients with severe brachial plexopathy. It may also increase the options and success of secondary procedures such as tendon transfers.

Tendon transfers, osteotomies, and joint fusions are meant to correct deformity, stabilize joints, and reset muscle balance in order to improve function. Microvascular muscle transfers are meant to provide muscle strength in desperate situations in which standard neural or musculoskeletal surgical options are limited.

INDICATIONS

Microsurgical exploration and reconstruction are indicated for severe plexus injuries in which spontaneous recovery would result in a painful, hypoesthetic, weak, or dysfunctional limb.[18] Adults who have experienced high-velocity (>60 km/hr) accidents and have flail, anesthetic limbs are candidates for surgical exploration and reconstruction in the first 1 to 3 months after injury.[2] It is presumed these patients have an avulsion injury, especially if Horner's syndrome is present. Infants and adults who do not recover upper trunk function, as indicated by the absence of biceps function in the first 6 months after injury, are candidates for nerve grafting for presumed extraforaminal ruptures (Fig. 2).

Michelow and associates[19] recommended the use of a scoring system for deciding whether to perform nerve reconstruction of infantile palsy. Scoring is based on the return of (1) elbow flexion, (2) elbow extension, (3) extension of the wrist, (4) extension of the fingers, and (5) extension of the thumb. A score of 0 (no function), 1 (partial function), or 2 (normal function) is given for all five parameters. A score of 3.5 or less beyond 3 months of life is an indication for microsurgery. An adult with a rare, lower trunk (C8-T1) lesion is not a candidate for nerve reconstruction because the results of microsurgery in that setting are poor. In an infant, some hand function may return after microsurgery.

Tendon transfers[4, 9, 20] and osteotomies[4, 10, 20] are indicated for patients with chronic plexopathy and limited function. For a donor muscle to function effectively as a transfer, it must be at least grade 4+ out of 5 in strength. Most often, tendon transfer for brachial plexopathy involves the transfer of the latissimus dorsi, teres major, or both to the rotator cuff to improve external rotation and abduction of the shoulder in children. Humeral derotation osteotomies are also used in children with shoulder internal rotation contractures, external rotation weakness, and a deformed glenohumeral joint.[20]

Fusions of the shoulder and wrist are meant to stabilize unstable joints that cannot be dynamically or statically rebalanced by tendon transfers or tenodesis procedures. Transfers of many muscles (pectoralis major, latissimus dorsi, triceps, flexor-pronator origin) have been used to restore elbow flexion. Doi and colleagues[7] advocate the use of double free muscle transfers for prehension following complete paralysis of the plexus. This procedure is used in severe injuries for which tendon transfers are not feasible.

PROCEDURES

Table 1 summarizes the treatments used for brachial plexus injuries.

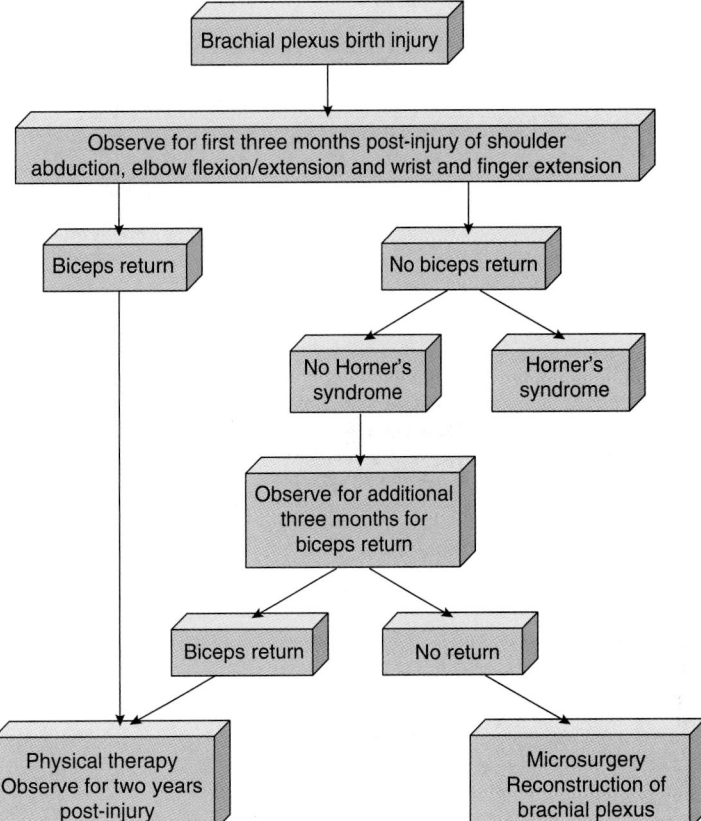

Fig. 2. Algorithm for treatment of patients with incomplete recovery of neural function. (Copyright 1997 American Academy of Orthopaedic Surgeons. Reprinted from Waters P: Obstetrical brachial plexus injuries: Evaluation and management. Journal of the American Academy of Orthopaedic Surgeons 1997; 5:205.)

	Indications	Specific Treatment	Outcome
TABLE 1. TREATMENT OPTIONS FOR BRACHIAL PLEXUS INJURIES			
Nonoperative treatment	Recovery of biceps function by 3 months. Conduction on NCV and no fibrillations on EMG. No meningoceles on myelographic CT.	Maintain passive range of motion of all joints; upper extremity strengthening program; utilization of transcutaneous electrical nerve stimulation or other modalities in adults to lessen neuropathic pain.	Depends on severity of original neurologic injury. Patients with Sunderland[5] class I and II injuries have functional recovery between 2 and 18 months after injury; those with class III injuries may have a weak arm, with pain and cold sensitivity; those with class IV and V injuries have poor spontaneous recovery, frequent RSD.[13]
Microsurgery Nerve grafting Neurotization	1. Root avulsion injury with a flail, insensate arm, Horner's syndrome at 1–3 months after injury.	1. Nerve transfers (neurotizations) of cervical plexus, spinal accessory and/or intercostal nerves with priority to shoulder abduction/external rotation, elbow flexion, and protective sensation of the thumb and index finger.	1. 40% to 75% useful elbow flexion in adults with intercostal transfers. Up to 90% useful elbow flexion in infants. Best results with three nerves, no interposing grafts, and direct repair to the motor branch to the biceps. Comparable results of 40% to 67% useful elbow flexion with spinal accessory transfer.

Table continued on following page

TABLE 1. TREATMENT OPTIONS FOR BRACHIAL PLEXUS INJURIES *Continued*

	Indications	Specific Treatment	Outcome
	2. No return of biceps or upper trunk function by 3–6 months after injury.	2. Nerve grafting from the C-5–C-6 nerve roots to the suprascapular, axillary, radial, and musculocutaneous nerves or respective cords.	2. With nerve grafting 62% to 84% of adults obtain useful elbow flexion with 20% to 76% obtaining some shoulder stability. Results in infants are similar. Best results with short grafts (<5 cm ideal, >10 cm poor) and short time from injury to repair (1–6 months).
Latissimus/teres major tendon transfer to rotator cuff (see Fig. 4)	Shoulder internal rotation contracture and external rotation weakness in a child with chronic plexopathy. Normal glenohumeral joint. Donor muscle with >grade 4+/5 strength.	Release of the pectoralis major tendon via anterior incision; transfer of latissimus dorsi and teres major to rotator cuff insertion at greater tuberosity.	Significant improvement in passive and active range of motion of shoulder, in particular shoulder abduction and external rotation. Significant improvement in Mallet class scores for shoulder abduction, external rotation, and hand to mouth and hand to neck function.
Humeral derotation osteotomy	Shoulder internal rotation contracture and external rotation weakness in a child with chronic plexopathy. Abnormal glenohumeral joint with subluxation, humeral head, and glenoid deformity.	Deltopectoral approach and transverse osteotomy above the level of deltoid muscle insertion. Internal fixation.	Significant improvement in passive and active range of motion of shoulder, in particular shoulder abduction and external rotation. Significant improvement in Mallet class scores for shoulder abduction, external rotation, and hand to mouth and hand to neck function.
Shoulder fusion	Patients with flail shoulders and active elbow flexion. Requires active trapezius and parascapular muscles (serratus anterior).	Various techniques of internal fixation have been successfully used from limited screw fixation to extensive plate fixation. Postoperative SPICA cast immobilization is indicated in the presence of limited fixation, osteopenic bone, and/or an uncooperative patient. Fusion should allow the hand to reach the mouth. Exact position of abduction (0–30 degrees), internal rotation (10–15 degrees), and forward flexion (20–30 degrees) depends on the patient's scapulothoracic motion.	Improves shoulder motion, stability, and function reliably in the appropriate patient.
Elbow flexion tendon transfers Latissimus dorsi Pectoralis major Steindler flexoplasty (pronator-flexor origin transfer) Triceps	>110 degrees passive elbow range of motion, absence of active elbow flexion, and >4+/5 strength in the donor muscle.	Each transfer involves mobilization of the muscle without impairment of neurovascular integrity of the donor. Insertion is into the biceps tendon for pectoralis, latissimus, and triceps. Postoperative protection in a position of elbow flexion is necessary until antigravity strength develops.	Reliable improved active elbow strength and function in 50% to 80% of adults with chronic plexopathy.
Free gracilis muscle transfer	Patients with severe injuries, poor recovery longer than 1 year after injury, and with no available local donor muscles for transfer.	As an elbow flexion transfer, the free gracilis is attached proximally to the coracoid process or clavicle and distally to the biceps tendon. The arterial anastomosis is from the brachial to the gracilis pedicle and neural repair is from the intercostals to the obturator branch to the gracilis. As a double transfer for prehension in complete plexopathy, one free muscle is transferred for elbow flexion and finger extension with innervation by the spinal accessory; the other muscle is used to restore finger flexion with reinnervation by the fifth and sixth intercostals. A shoulder arthrodesis is also performed along with transfer of the third and fourth intercostals to the triceps and the supraclavicular nerve to the median nerve.	Results are preliminary but reveal improved function over those of nonsurgical treatment of these severely affected patients.

MICROSURGERY
Preoperative Planning

In both infants and adults, nerve grafting and nerve transfers have become standard treatment for acute brachial plexus injuries that fail to recover sufficiently in the first 6 months after injury. By means of serial physical examinations, myelographic CT scanning or MRI, and adjunctive electromyography and nerve conduction velocity measurements, the surgeon should be able to identify the majority of patients in whom microsurgery of the plexus is indicated.

At the time of surgery, it is important to be familiar and comfortable with all the possible anatomic variations and potential treatment plans. Because each injury pattern is different, the options of grafting from available healthy nerve roots (Figs. 3 and 4), the use of possible donor grafts (sural, lateral antebrachial cutaneous, ulnar, and so on), and the transfer of donor nerves (intercostal, spinal accessory, cervical plexus, contralateral C7) must all be considered. It is useful for somatosensory evoked potential or nerve action potential evaluation to be available intraoperatively to enable assessment of the integrity of connections between the central and peripheral nervous system and the conductivity of nerve to muscle. At some centers, histological analysis is used to assess the adequacy of proximal and distal neuroma resection.

Technical Details

Initial dissection should be proximal to the neuroma. It is often helpful to identify the phrenic nerve on the anterior surface of the anterior scalene muscle and follow it proximal to find the C5 nerve root. This enables the surgeon to isolate all the nerve roots and trunks. Because restoration of elbow flexion and stabilization of the shoulder are the surgical priorities, transection of the upper trunk or C5 and C6 nerve roots is necessary to determine the viability of the proximal neural stumps. It is at this point that examination of the fascicles under the microscope, histological analysis, or measurements of nerve potentials is helpful.[21]

Exposure distal to the neuroma can often be achieved without a clavicular osteotomy. It is important to identify the suprascapular nerve (as it heads to the suprascapular notch), the lateral cord and musculocutaneous nerve, and the posterior division of the upper trunk and posterior cord. These are the most common distal recipient sites for the sural nerve grafts for restoration of upper trunk function. Also, in infants, grafts may also be placed to the hand, because recovery of some intrinsic hand function can occur in infants. The shorter the nerve grafts, the better the results. The grafts should be attached with 10% to 15% redundancy to optimize healing.

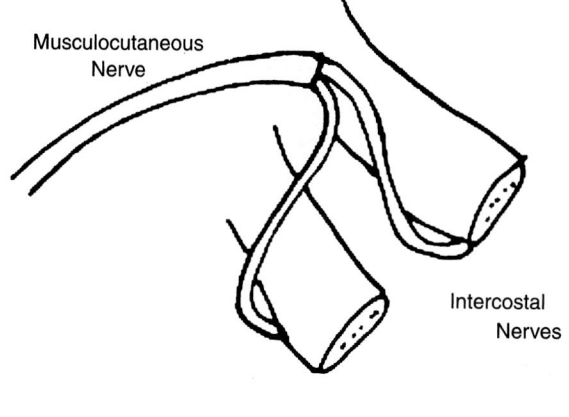

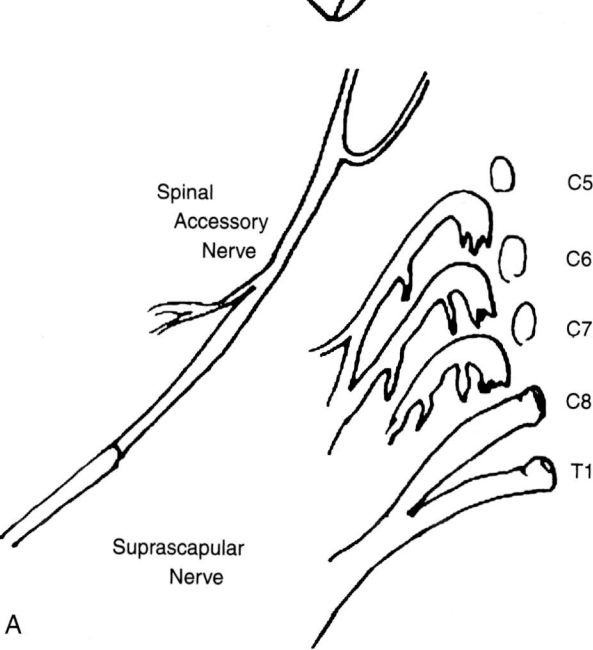

Fig. 3. Illustration of the injury patterns and surgical reconstructions for the more common brachial plexus injuries. *A,* An avulsion injury in which intercostal and spinal accessory nerve transfers are used for reconstruction. *B,* An upper trunk lesion with use of sural nerve grafts for reconstruction of the suprascapular, lateral cord/musculocutaneous nerve, and posterior division of the upper trunk for the axillary and radial nerves. (*A* From Peimer CA: Surgery of the Hand and Upper Extremity. New York, McGraw-Hill, 1996, vol II, p 1452; *B* from Lamb DW [ed]: The Paralyzed Hand. Edinburgh, Churchill Livingstone, 1987, p 116.)

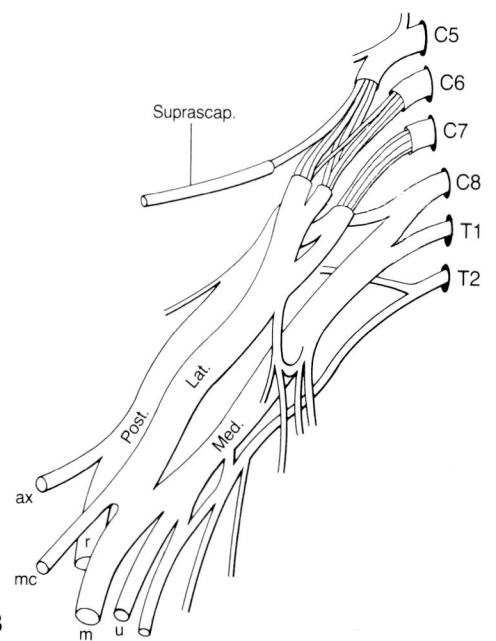

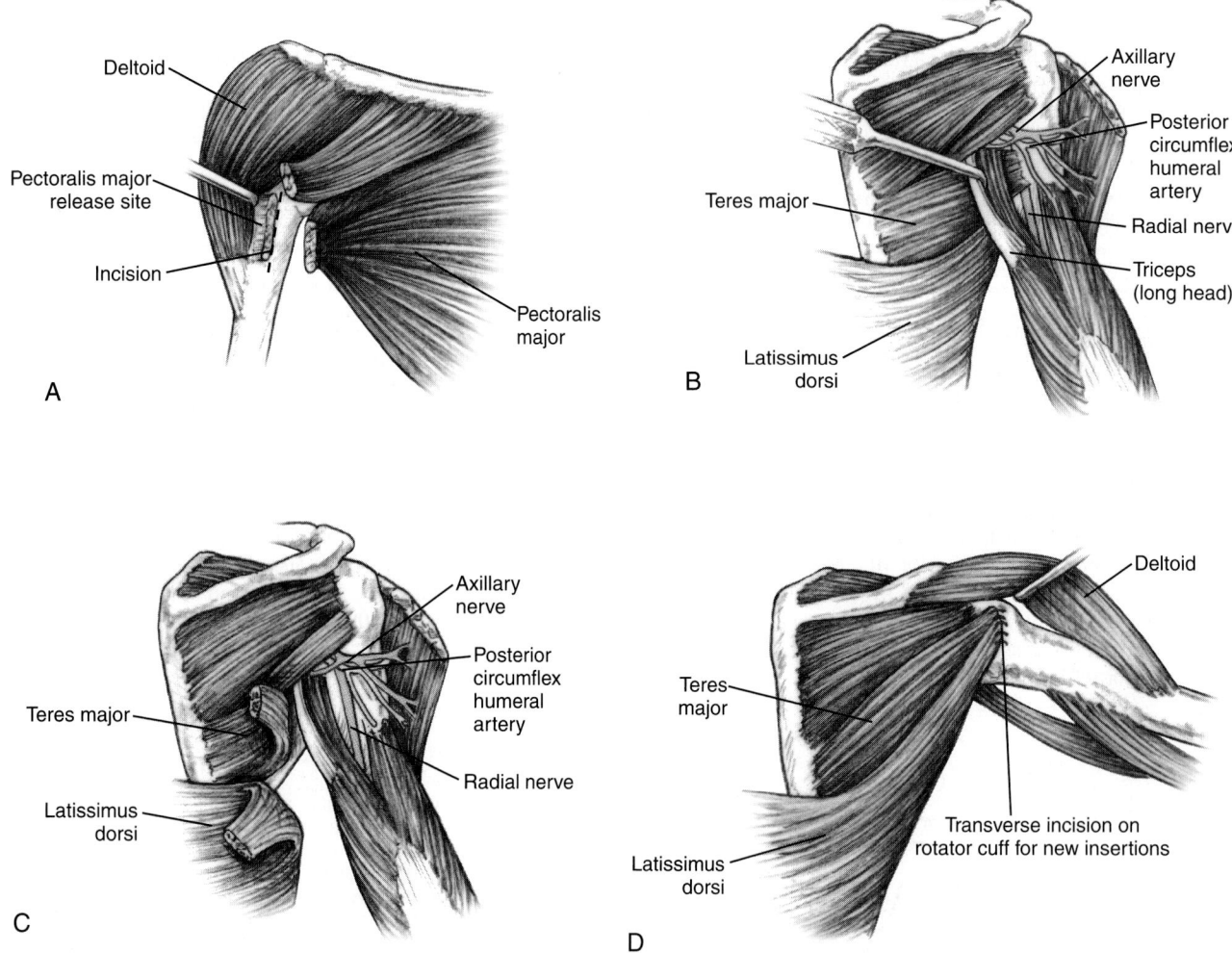

Fig. 4. Illustration. The technique for *(A)* anterior musculotendinous lengthening of the pectoralis major and *(B)* transfer of the latissimus dorsi and teres major tendons to the rotator cuff. The radial and axillary nerves need to be protected with operative exposure and transfer. *C*, Intraoperative photograph of the insertion of the latissimus dorsi tendon tranfer to the rotator cuff tendon. (Redrawn from Hoffer M, Wickenden R, Roper B: Brachial plexus birth palsies. J Bone Joint Surg Am 1979; 60:691.)

POSTOPERATIVE MANAGEMENT

The neural repair is protected for 4 weeks postoperatively. In adults, protection involves a sling and swathe. In children, a Velpeau-type stockinette bandage or a Minerva protection can be used. If there is redundancy of the grafts to prevent tension at the repair sites, postoperative disruption of the repair is less likely. Following the period of neural protection, it is important to regain full passive motion of all joints. Ultimately, neurological recovery takes 6 to 18 months. During that time, it is imperative to prevent the development of joint contractures. Whether the use of peripheral electrical stimulation of the muscles is beneficial in enhancing long-term recovery is unclear.

COMPLICATIONS

Aside from the usual concerns about anesthesia, infection, and bleeding, the most significant complications are worsening of the neurological condition and failure of the procedure to improve the situation. Only microneurolysis has been shown to potentially worsen the situation in cases undergoing late operation. The patient who is aware that microsurgery will not normalize the condition is less likely to be disappointed with less than perfect recovery. As mentioned, the severity of the original neural injury determines the ultimate outcome of neural reconstruction.

RESULTS

Between 50% and 80% of patients undergoing neural reconstruction for elbow flexion and shoulder stabilization had useful outcomes in published studies. Patients with extraforaminal, postganglionic ruptures of the upper trunk do best. Patients with avulsion injuries requiring nerve transfers recover the least.

Tendon transfers,[4, 10, 20] osteotomies,[10, 20] and arthrodesis procedures[13] improve function in infants and adults with chronic plexopathy. Free muscle transfer has had positive short-term results in severe situations.[7]

REFERENCES

1. Narakas AO: Brachial plexus injuries. In McCarthy J (ed): Plastic Surgery. Philadelphia, WB Saunders, 1990, vol 7, p 4776.
2. Millesi H: Brachial plexus injuries, nerve grafting. Clin Orthop 1988; (237):36.
3. Brewerton D, Daniel J: Factors influencing return to work. Br Med J 1971; 4:277.
4. Waters P: Obstetrical brachial plexus injuries: Evaluation and management. J Am Acad Orthop Surg 1997; 5:205.
5. Sunderland S: A classification of peripheral nerve injuries producing loss of function. Brain 1951; 74:491.
6. Narakas AO: Obstetrical brachial plexus injuries. In Lamb DW (ed): The Paralyzed Hand. Edinburgh, Churchill Livingstone, 1987, p 116.
7. Doi K, Sakai K, Kuwata N, et al: Double-muscle technique for reconstruction of prehension after complete avulsion of the brachial plexus. J Hand Surg [Am] 1995; 20:408.
8. Gilbert A, Tassin J: Reparation chirurgicale du plexus brachial dans la paralysis obstetricale. Chirurgie 1984; 110:70.
9. Hoffer M, Wickenden R, Roper B: Brachial plexus birth palsies: Results of transfers to the rotator cuff. J Bone Joint Surg Am 1978; 60:691.
10. Goddard N, Fixsen J: Rotation osteotomy of the humerus for birth injuries of the brachial plexus. J Bone Joint Surg Br 1978; 66:257.
11. Kline D, Judice D: Operative management of selected brachial plexus lesions. J Neurosurg 1983; 58:631.
12. Boome R, Kaye J: Obstetric traction injuries of the brachial plexus: Natural history, indications for surgical repair and results. J Bone Joint Surg Br 1988; 70:571.
13. Krakauer J, Wood M: Adult injuries and salvage. In Peimer C (ed): Surgery of the Hand and Upper Extremity. New York, McGraw-Hill, 1996, p 1411.
14. Alnot J: Traumatic brachial plexus palsy in the adult: Retro- and infra-clavicular lesions. Clin Orthop 1988; 237:9.
15. Narakas AO, Hentz V: Neurotization in brachial plexus injuries, indications and results. Clin Orthop 1988; 237:43.
16. Krakhauer J, Wood M: Intercostal nerve transfer for brachial plexopathy. J Hand Surg Am 1994; 19:829.
17. Kawai H, Kawabata H, Masada K, et al: Nerve repairs for traumatic brachial plexus palsy with root avulsion. Clin Orthop 1988; 237:75.
18. Wynn Parry C: Pain in avulsion of the brachial plexus. Neurosurgery 1984; 15:960.
19. Michelow B, Clarke H, Curtis C, et al: The natural history of obstetrical brachial plexus palsy. Plast Reconstr Surg 1994; 93:675.
20. Waters P, Smith G, Jaramillo D: Glenohumeral deformity secondary to brachial plexus birth palsy. J Bone Joint Surg Am 1998; 50:668.
21. Kawai H, Tsuyuguchi Y, Masada K, et al: Identification of the lesion brachial plexus injuries with root avulsion: A comprehensive assessment by means of preoperative findings, myelography, surgical exploration and intraoperative electrodiagnosis. Neuro-Orthop 1989; 7:15.

section 12 chapter 25

COMPLEX REGIONAL PAIN SYNDROME IN THE UPPER EXTREMITY

Harris Gellman and Evan Collins

Summary

- Although it has been recommended that the terms *reflex sympathetic dystropic* and *causalgia* be replaced by the terms *complex regional pain syndrome type I* and *type II,* the overall analysis of outcomes in patients with chronic pain syndromes has not yet been improved.
- Patients have a similar pattern of clinical symptoms, but type I follows an innocuous injury, and type II follows a known nerve injury.
- Pain may be sympathetically or nonsympathetically mediated.
- For patients with sympathetically mediated pain, the treatment approach should be directed toward inhibiting the abnormality in the α-adrenergic system.
- Patients with sympathetically independent pain, however, where sympathetic blockade is not effective, are much more difficult to treat. Trials of anti-inflammatory medications, such as corticosteroids, nonsteroidal anti-inflammatories, and electroacupuncture, may prove beneficial.
- Overall, there is one fundamental principle: Early recognition and aggressive treatment using an approach incorporating medication, pain management specialists, and occupational or physical therapy is paramount to a successful outcome.

In 1864, Mitchell, a Civil War surgeon, found a number of patients who suffered from chronic, persistent, burning pain after traumatic amputation; he also noted an association with neuroma formation. Mitchell termed this problem *causalgia.*[1] In 1946, Evans treated pain patients successfully with anesthetic blocks and introduced the term *reflex sympathetic dystrophy* (RSD).[1] Newer terminology has been proposed to replace these two terms. The new terminology reflects the belief that the older terms have lost usefulness as clinical designations because they have been used so indiscriminately that it is no longer clear what they mean.[1] The new nomenclature reflects an attempt to classify patients by clinical signs and symptoms rather than by pathophysiology. The term *complex regional pain syndrome* (CRPS) has been introduced in an attempt to accomplish this task. CRPS has been divided into two types: type I to replace the term *reflex sympathetic dystrophy* and type II to replace the term *causalgia.*[1] Both types I and II have the same clinical constellation of symptoms, the same progression of disease stages, and many of the same treatment algorithms. The key distinction between type I and type II is that the latter occurs after a known nerve injury. Type II patients may also respond better to surgical treatment than type I patients. Although a response to sympathetic inhibition may be a characteristic of a particular type of pain syndrome, it is not necessary for diagnosis. Patients whose pain **is** primarily mediated by the sympathetic nervous system are considered to have *sympathetically mediated pain* (SMP), and patients whose pain **is not** primarily mediated by the sympathetic system are considered to have *sympathetically independent pain* (SIP). At different times in the disease process there may be a predominance of SMP or SIP.[2]

Although criteria for these disorders do not include motor disorders, tremor, weakness, and dystonia are frequently seen.[1, 3]

REFLEX SYMPATHETIC DYSTROPHY OF THE UPPER EXTREMITY (CRPS TYPE I)

CRPS type I does not clearly differentiate those pain syndromes that are sympathetically mediated and that respond well to sympathetic interruption from those that do not have sympathetic involvement and, therefore, are much more difficult to treat. Because most of the literature available deals with RSD, the terms *RSD* and *CRPS* will be used interchangeably in this chapter. RSD secondary to nerve injury is synonymous with CRPS type II.

DEFINITIONS

Regardless of the nomenclature used, the diagnosis is always one of exclusion. "CRPS Type I is probably a spectrum of entities that present with similar clinical manifestations, and are often lumped together for the sake of clinical unity."[4] CRPS type I is defined as a disease that develops after an initial innocuous event, the subsequent pain and dysfunction being out of proportion to the initial event, not linked to any specifically documented pathologic process.

The diagnostic criteria are as follows: (1) it follows an initially innocuous event; (2) spontaneous pain, allodynia, and/or hyperesthesia exist beyond the territory of a single peripheral nerve and are disproportionate to the inciting event; (3) there is, or has been, evidence of edema and skin blood flow changes or abnormalities in the pseudomotor activity in that region since the inciting event; and (4) exclusion of the existence of any conditions that could otherwise account for the amount of pain and dysfunction that is present. The diagnostic criteria are the same for type I (RSD) and type II (causalgia) CRPS.

The original term *sympathetically mediated pain* (SMP) was described as "a pain state maintained by the sympathetic nervous system."[5] A newer definition is "any pain state that is maintained by sympathetic efferent innervation, by circulating catecholamines, or by neurochemical action."[2] Therefore, patients who have a positive response to either pharmacologic blockade or to local anesthetic infiltration of the sympathetic nervous system can be considered to have SMP. Those patients who do not respond to either pharmacological or anesthetic blockade are said to have SIP.

CLINICAL PRESENTATION

RSD has been defined as a sympathetically mediated pain syndrome, an active, progressive disease process characterized by pain, edema, and autonomic dysfunction.[6] The pain is often exacerbated by emotional factors. Swelling is the most constant physical finding, which, if not treated early, is often followed by the rapid onset of stiffness. Clinicians experienced treating RSD agree that early diagnosis and treatment are of paramount importance.

Secondary signs, variably present, include osseous demineralization, sudomotor changes, movement disorder, temperature changes, trophic changes, vasomotor changes, discoloration, palmar fibrosis, and hyperhidrosis.[7]

The clinical presentation of RSD varies and is usually divided into three stages of progression based on onset and duration of symptoms.

Stage I is a traumatic phase occurring shortly after the initial noxious event, lasting up to 3 months. Patients usually describe a constant burning pain out of proportion to the initial event. Allodynia and extreme sensitivity to touch are the dominant clinical picture. Pain severity increases during stage I, usually not following a specific dermatomal nerve pattern. Pain may be localized or regional, often spreading from its original site. "Edema initially involving the periarticular portion of the extremity usually begins in the distal region and progresses to a more proximal involvement of that extremity."[1] "Edema and swelling in this region are the most commonly seen clinical manifestation of this problem."[7] Discoloration of the extremity, notably erythema, reflecting alteration in blood flow (autonomic nervous system dysfunction) is also present. Hyperhidrosis (sweating) is commonly seen, and the posture of the affected limb is described as dystonic or protective.

Progression to stage II ("dystrophic phase") occurs within 3 to 9 months of symptoms from the initial event. The predominance of pain as well as marked stiffness of the extremity characterizes this phase. This increase in stiffness reflects the change or alteration of edema from soft to hard. Other changes reflect persistent alterations in blood flow, resulting in increasing warmth followed by cyanosis. Skin changes become evident with loss of skin creases, loss of hair, and a decrease in moisture of the hand. Radiographs often demonstrate spotty periarticular osteopenia.

Stage III "atrophic phase," occurring 9 to 18 months following injury, is characterized by a decrease in complaints of pain with a concomitant increase in overall stiffness and lack of useful function of the involved limb. In general, the extremity is pale, dry, and cool, and the skin has developed a glossy appearance with trophic changes present.[8] Fibrous ankylosis of joints occurs as the edema continues to harden. Autonomic dysfunction becomes fixed, with a constant cool, pale, and dry appearance to the extremity. Trophic changes spread to the deeper tissues. Subcutaneous tissue disappears, with narrowing of the fingers. Radiographs show severe osteopenia. Joint tissues are contracted, thickened, and fibrotic. Muscles are atrophied.

RSD in children shows a similar spectrum of clinical signs and symptoms. Wilder[9] monitored 70 pediatric patients with RSD. Girls predominated, with the lower extremity affected most often. Prognosis for recovery or improvement, however, is better in children than in adults. Additionally, children can develop limb length discrepancy secondary to altered blood flow and trophic changes.[10]

Although staging provides a necessary order to this complex problem, there is no literature to document that all patients develop all of these stages or that these stages progress in a sequential fashion. Recognition of the predominant stage of disease can help direct treatment and may help to predict outcome.

PATHOPHYSIOLOGY

Despite the lack of an accurate animal model and the difficulty of testing etiological theories of RSD, it appears that several factors combine to produce the disease. The exact mechanism whereby the pain response becomes abnormal is not known. Normally, in response to injury there is an activation of the sympathetic nervous system. Sympathetic outflow, initiated by the pain of injury, causes vasoconstriction in the limb, leading to decreased blood loss and swelling. After injury, sympathetic tone decreases, and blood flow of the limb increases, allowing entry of constituents of repair as well as the removal of waste products from the site of injury. If sympathetic tone persists inappropriately, an abnormal feedback mechanism and atypical sympathetic reflex result. This causes tissue edema, resulting in capillary collapse and ischemia, which in turn causes local pain in the injured limb. This pain signal reexcites the sympathetic nerves, and thus a positive feedback circuit becomes established. Currently, there are many theories attempting to explain the abnormal pain response. Livingston described "a vicious cycle of pain, sympathetic disregulation, and cellular damage in the pathogenesis of RSD."[11] He theorized that the activation of nociceptors leads to excitation of an internuclear pool of neurons in the spinal cord that induces an increased activity of the efferent sympathetic system. The subsequent response of vasoconstriction and ischemia stimulates the pain mechanism. Recently, this theory has been revised, suggesting that an unregulated sensitivity of α-adrenoreceptors for catecholamines is responsible. Still other hypotheses seem to suggest that an exaggeration of the peripheral neural inflammatory response to tissue injury is the primary cause of RSD.

Treatment goals are aimed at interruption of this positive feedback loop.[12] For this reason, surgical as well as chemical sympathectomy has been recommended.[12] Sympathetic stimulation has been shown to prolong and enhance abnormal ectopic pain afferents in various experimental situations. Experimentally produced neuromas demonstrate ectopic discharge responsive to sympathetic stimulation[13] and hypersensitivity to chemical, mechanical, and thermal stimuli.[14, 15]

Evidence indicates a possible genetic predisposition in RSD patients resistant to treatment, multiple sclerosis, and narcolepsy as genetically associated neuroimmune disorders.[19] A study reviewing 109 patients suffering from RSD found there was a 3:1 ratio of females to males and an increased risk of disease in those individuals who had family members suffering from this problem.

DIAGNOSIS

The clinical characteristics of CRPS types I and II include complaints of pain and disuse as well as the physical findings of edema, swelling, discoloration, and maintenance of the limb in a dystrophic posture. One or more of the following signs may be found: vasomotor or sudomotor disturbances, edema of the limb, movement disorder, sensitivity to cold, autonomic dysfunction, and trophic changes. Often there is muscle weakness or atrophy. Relief of pain and modification of signs after regional sympathetic blockade are virtually diagnostic of a sympathetically mediated pain disorder. Only one or two of the symptoms and signs accompany many subtle cases of mild RSD, or the entire symptom complex may be vague and confusing, making differential diagnosis difficult.

Aside from these clinical symptoms, the diagnosis of RSD has been supported by other, more objective, data. The most reliable aid to the diagnosis of RSD, in addition to the physical examination, has been the three-phase bone scan.[20] Prior to this bone scan, the finding of periarticular or diffuse mottled demineralization on plain radiographs was used as an aid in the diagnosis of RSD. Because calcium content must be altered 30% to 50% before becoming evident on conventional bone radiographs, the three-phase bone scan will be positive earlier than conventional radiographs. For a scan to be considered diagnostic of RSD, the delayed-phase scan must show diffusely increased activity in the involved joints.[20] In particular, the third phase must demonstrate an increase in uptake to be considered positive (Fig. 1). Mackinnon and Holder[20] found the delayed bone-uptake phase of the three-phase bone scan to have a 96% sensitivity and 98% specificity in detecting RSD. Using stricter criteria for the definition of RSD, Werner and Davidoff[23] found a sensitivity of 50% and a specificity of 92% for the bone-uptake phase. The sensitivity and specificity of the scan was found to be higher when done within 6 months of onset and in patients older than 50 years.

Thermography has also been used in confirming the diagnosis of more subtle cases of CRPS.[26, 27] Thermography is an indirect way of measuring blood flow in an extremity. Increased blood flow to the extremity results in increased temperature. In patients studied using thermography, increased temperature, reflecting increased blood flow, would be considered a positive study. A positive response to a sympathetic block would result in increased temperature and blood flow to the extremity.

Another indirect method used in the evaluation of pain patients is the quantitative pseudomotor reflex test, or resting sweat output test.[28] This test attempts to quantify irregularities in the autonomic nervous system by evaluating the amount of resting sweat. An abnormal resting sweat test reflects an increase in sympathetic autonomic activity, primarily in the noradrenergic system.

PATIENTS AT RISK

RSD has been reported to occur after a multitude of injuries. The prevalence of RSD following distal radius fracture has been reported to occur in up to 20% of patients.[30–33] Patients who developed clinical RSD had the following in common: fractures that required manipulation, fractures associated with ulnar styloid injuries, and fractures that were primarily casted. Elevated intracast pressure seemed to be a common risk factor in most patients studied. The incidence of RSD following spinal cord injury, traumatic brain injury, or stroke has been reported to be approximately 10%. Gellman et al[34] studied 60 consecutive

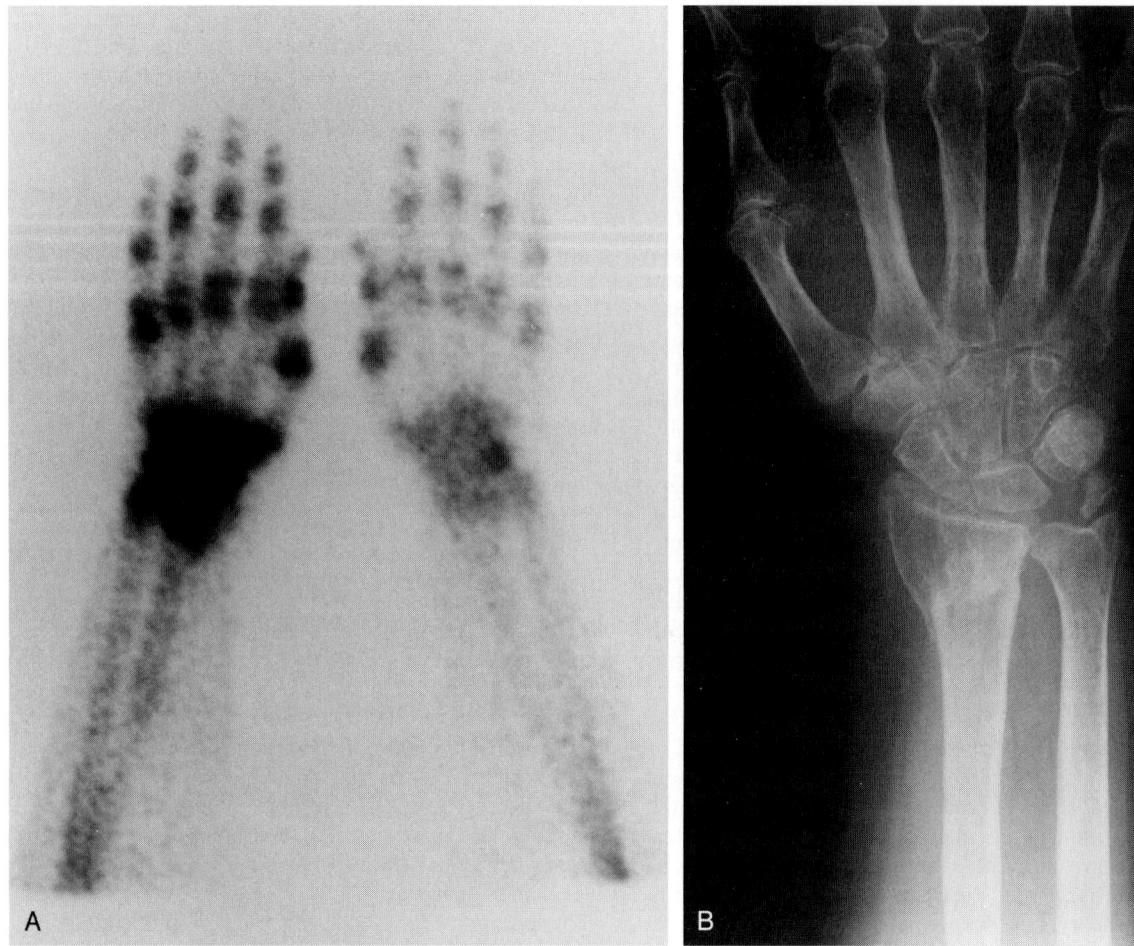

Fig. 1. Views. *A,* Third-phase bone scan. *B,* Radiograph view.

patients with spinal cord injuries; 7 developed diffuse hand pain, swelling, and stiffness; 4 had bilateral involvement; 6 had bone-scan abnormalities.

Considering the large number of potential patients who developed pain syndromes secondary to their primary illness, diagnostic studies that may point out individuals at risk are of benefit. Weiss[36] prospectively studied the prognostic value of the three-phase bone scan as a useful tool in predicting which patients may go on to develop RSD after stroke. Of 22 patients who had three-phase bone scans after stroke, 16 scans were consistent with RSD, with 5 extremities being symptomatic at the time of bone-scan. Of the 11 asymptomatic patients with positive scans, seven (64%) subsequently developed symptoms of RSD. No patient with a negative scan developed RSD. Bone scan, therefore, may be of predictive value in patients after strokes and hemiplegia.

CRPS TYPE II

The association of nerve injuries, especially partial or multiple, with CRPS has been well recognized. Richards[37] analyzed 461 cases of causalgia from World War II experience and found that 83% were in patients with median or tibial

nerve injury. Fifty-three percent had injury to more than one nerve. In 88% of nerve injuries complicated by RSD, the injury was proximal to the elbow or knee.

Nerve compression syndromes such as carpal tunnel syndrome, cubital tunnel syndrome, and herniated cervical disk can be complicated by RSD, with the nerve compression serving as the persistent painful stimulus.

The nerves most commonly involved in injury and the subsequent development of CRPS type II (causalgia) are the median nerve, tibial nerve, superficial radial nerve, ulnar nerve at the wrist, and the saphenous nerve at the knee joint.

TREATMENT

Paramount to the treatment of patients (Fig. 2) suffering from CRPS is early recognition and an aggressive multidisciplinary treatment approach. Early recognition allows prompt initiation of treatment. A high index of suspicion is the key. Delay in treatment not only results in prolonged rehabilitation but also may allow the pain and physical alterations to become established and refractory to treatment. Poplowski and colleagues,[42] in a review of 126 patients with post-traumatic dystrophy, found that the most important factor in predicting improvement with treatment

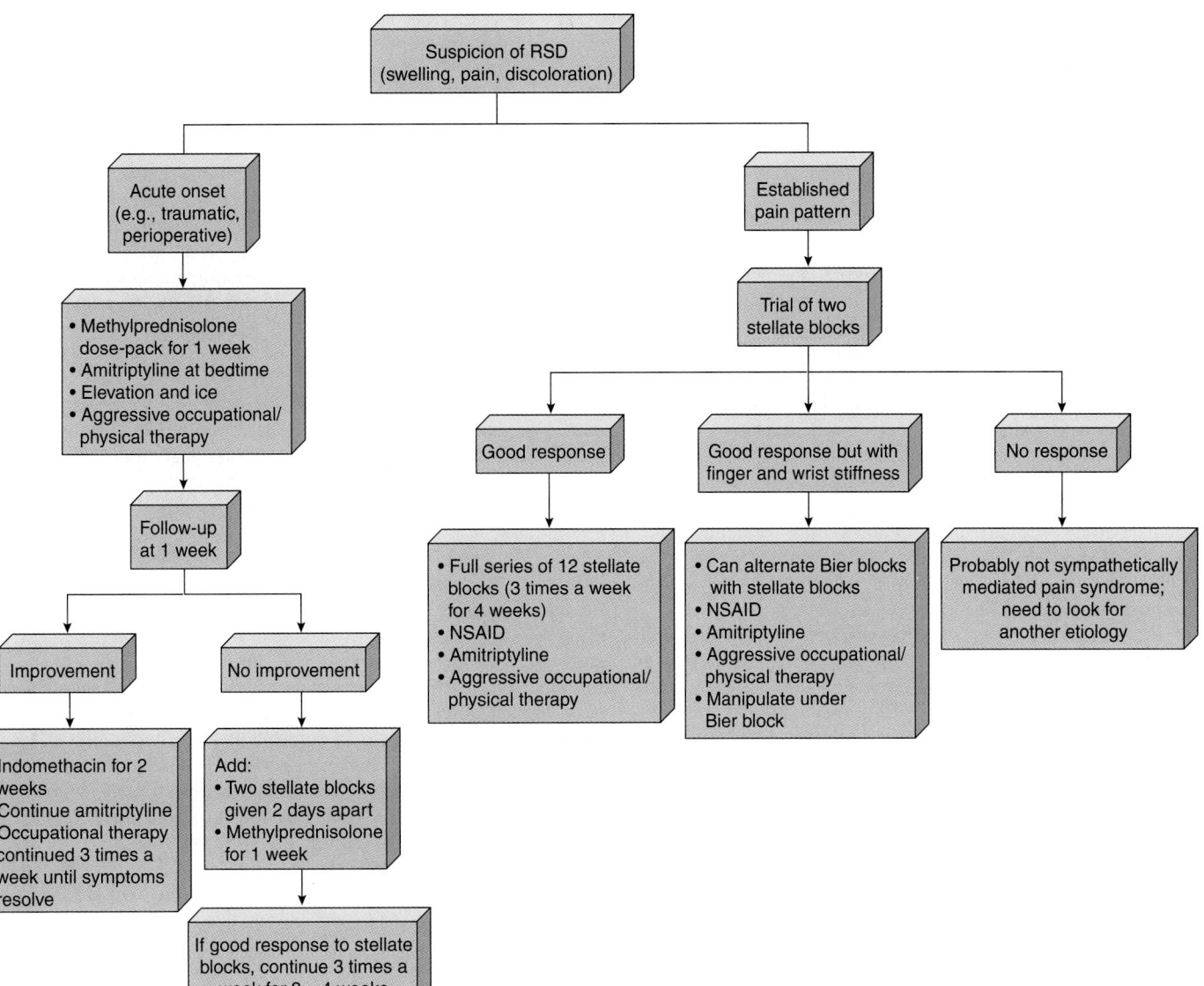

Fig. 2. RSD treatment algorithm. This illustrates decisions for treatment of RSD. (Copyright 1997 American Academy of Orthopaedic Surgeons. Redrawn from J Am Acad Orthop Surg 1997; 5:315.)

was a short interval (less than 6 months) between the onset of RSD and the initiation of treatment.

Occupational and Physical Therapy

The primary role of occupational and physical therapy in the early stages of pain syndromes is to help decrease pain and prevent the development of stiffness. Patients should be treated initially with immobilization and splinting as well as elevation to assist with any edema that is present. Antiedema measures, which include elevation and massage if tolerated, should be incorporated in the treatment algorithm. Passive motion should not be attempted in the early phases of the disease because this would only provoke pain and increase inflammation. Contrast baths have been used effectively in desensitizing these patients and improving blood flow to the extremity.[43] The technique is to place the patient's extremity in warm water for approximately 1 minute and then alternate this with emergence into cold water for approximately 10 minutes or as long as the patient can

tolerate it. This maneuver is repeated as often as the patient can tolerate. For those patients evaluated with stage II or stage III of the disease (with joint stiffness already present), dynamic splinting to improve range of motion may be included in the treatment algorithm. Finally, Watson[44] recommends a stress-loading program of traction and compression exercises. In the 41 patients treated with stress-loading evaluated 3 years later, 88% had relief of pain, 95% had improved range of motion, all had improved grip strength, and 84% returned to the same occupation.

Drug Therapy

Several drugs have shown promise in treatment of patients suffering from CPRS. For those patients who have primarily sympathetically mediated pain, α-adrenergic blockers seem to be most effective. Of the many actions of the sympathetic nervous system, the α-adrenergic action is the most important in its effect as vasoconstrictor in the skin and subcutaneous tissues. Fowler and Moser[45] evaluated the use of phenoxybenzamine to inhibit the adrenergic effects seen in patients suffering from RSD. It was found to be the most effective blocking agent, having the fewest undesirable side effects, and best at eliminating patients' complaints of pain. Ghostine[46] treated patients with CRPS type II (causalgia) with oral phenoxybenzamine and noted pain relief to be significant. The usual recommended starting dose is 10 mg twice a day. The dosage may be increased by 10 mg/day every 2 days until pain is relieved or postural hypotension occurs. The initial dosage should be maintained for at least 5 days before an increase. Treatment usually lasts 6 weeks. In follow-up ranging from 6 months to 6 years, all patients obtained complete relief. Patients treated with phenoxybenzamine must be monitored closely for postural hypotension.[7]

Tabria and coworkers[47] evaluated the role of oral guanethidine in single-dose form for 8 weeks in patients with RSD. The drug functions as a postganglionic adrenergic inhibitor, thus modulating the effect of the sympathetic nervous system on its target organs. They found that guanethedine was effective in alleviating sympathetically mediated pain in their patients. However, side effects included mental depression, loss of appetite, impotence, and orthostatic hypotension.

Propranolol, a β-blocker, may also be used in the treatment of CRPS. It has been shown to be successful in treating patients' pain with fewer side effects, specifically less orthostatic hypotension.[48] This medication is contraindicated in patients with cardiac arrhythmias or asthma.[48]

Clonidine (Catapres) used as a transdermal patch to diminish hyperesthesia in the affected limb has been studied by Davis.[49] Clonidine patches, however, have been shown to be effective only in those patients who have had a positive response to sympathetic blockade.

Calcium channel blockers are a distinct category of medications that are useful in the treatment of CRPS.[50] Nifedipine is the most commonly studied of these medications. Calcium channel blockers have an advantage in that they do not affect the venous capacitance system, thereby decreasing the risk of orthostatic hypotension. Prough[52] reported the use of oral nifedipine in the treatment of 13 patients with RSD. Starting dose was 10 mg three times a day, and it was increased weekly to a maximum of 30 mg three times a day. When a constant level of pain relief was obtained for 3 weeks, the dose was tapered over several days. Of the 13 patients monitored, 7 had complete relief, 2 had partial relief, 3 stopped treatment because of side effects (headache), and 1 was unimproved.

Corticosteroid use in RSD remains controversial. Prednisone has been the most popularly administered steroid, typically given in pulse fashion. Christensen et al[53] also found a good response to high-dose steroids in decreasing edema and in managing pain. The dosage required to achieve this response however, averaged 100 mg per day for several weeks. The risks of complications at such high doses have led some researchers to evaluate different dosing patterns for treatment. Kozin[54] and others[35, 53] have reported good response to systemic corticosteroids using high doses initially (60 to 80 mg a day in divided doses) but then quickly tapering off to achieve the necessary effects. Other authors have had a less impressive response to corticosteroids, however. Wilder et al[9] found no improvement with corticosteroid use. They found pulsed treatment with methylprednisolone (Medrol Dosepak) to be very useful in treating patients diagnosed early (disease of less than 6 months duration) but of limited effectiveness in patients with established disease.

Mood-modifying drugs, such as chlorpromazine (Thorazine), chlordiazepoxide (Librium), trifluoperazine (Stelazine), diazepam (Valium), and Elavil, have been reported to help reduce the pain and complaints in patients with RSD.[55] It should be noted, however, that mood-altering drugs alone are not effective in the treatment of pain syndromes, but they may be used as an adjunct to the primary treatment.

SYMPATHETIC INTERRUPTION

In those patients with primary sympathetically mediated pain, sympathetic interruption can be accomplished through local anesthetics, regional blocks, or surgical ablation. If symptoms are not relieved promptly by oral medications combined with aggressive physical and occupational therapy, treatment should proceed to a trial of stellate ganglion blocks. The response to sympathetic blocks can also be used to define whether or not the RSD is sympathetically mediated. Studies have shown that following stellate ganglion blocks used to confirm the diagnosis, the relief of pain often lasts well beyond the duration of the block.[7] Initially, one or two blocks can be tried to assess effectiveness. If pain relief is good, even temporarily, blocks should be repeated until the pain is controlled, for a maximum of 12 blocks.[7] A second or third series of blocks may be necessary. Patients who do not have relief of pain with stellate ganglion blocks probably have a sympathetically independent RSD; thus, continuing with stellate ganglion blocks would not be beneficial.

In the upper extremity, the stellate ganglion, which lies between the C7 and T1 cervical bodies, is bathed with either 1% lidocaine or 0.25% bupivacaine (Marcaine) to anesthetize the region. A positive response is indicated by a decrease in pain, an increase in blood flow in the extremity, an increase in temperature in the extremity, and Horner's syndrome.[56]

Hanington-Kiff[59] demonstrated the effectiveness of the Bier block technique using guanethidine to act as an inhibitor of the sympathetic system. Ten mg of guanethidine and 25 mL of normal saline are administered using a Bier block double-tourniquet technique. The tourniquet is released after 20 minutes, and relief from both pain and improved blood flow in that region is confirmation that the patient has a sympathetically mediated pain that is responding to the block. However, Jadad et al,[60] in a randomized double-blind study assessing the effectiveness of intravenous regional blocks with guanethidine, did not find a significant difference between the effects of the placebo and guanethidine in any of the outcomes measured, including pain intensity and relief.

SURGICAL SYMPATHECTOMY

Patients with good, but only temporary, pain relief after sympathetic blockade may be considered for surgical sympathectomy. For patients with a primarily sympathetically mediated pain syndrome, surgical sympathectomy has been described as effective, with up to 91% of patients achieving either excellent or good results following an open transthoracic or retroperitoneal surgical sympathetectomy. Olcott,[63] using an open transthoracic or retroperitoneal approach, achieved 74% excellent, 17% good, and 9% poor results in 35 RSD patients at 14 months. Surgical sympathetectomy done endoscopically requires a much shorter hospital stay, however. Robertson[64] treated eight patients with sympathetically mediated pain syndrome with video-assisted thoracic ganglionectomy. A pneumothorax was produced for the procedure and treated with a chest tube. The average hospital stay was 15.4 hours. He reported no intraoperative complications, and surgery time was only 30 minutes. Six of the patients had complete relief or partial relief of their symptoms during an average follow-period of 5 months.

AMPUTATION

Dielissen[65] studied the effectiveness of amputation in relieving the symptoms of RSD in 28 patients who had 34 amputations in 31 limbs. Only two patients were relieved of pain. RSD recurred in the stump in 28 limbs, making most patients unable to wear a prosthesis. Recurrence was most common when amputation was done through a level that was not free of symptoms. Despite the poor results in controlling pain, 24 patients were satisfied with the results of their surgery. Many had felt their situation hopeless before surgery; amputation had improved social function, cured persistent infection, and eliminated painful physical contact with the limb despite the persistence of pain. The authors do not recommend amputation for pain relief because its effectiveness cannot be predicted.

REFERENCES

1. Stanton-Hicks M, Hassenbusch JW: Reflex sympathetic dystrophy: Changing concepts and taxonomy. Pain 1995; 63:127.
2. Wong JY, Wilson PR: Classification of compiled regional pain syndrome. Hand Clinics 1997; 13:319.
3. Schwartzman RJ, Kerrigan J: The movement disorder of reflex sympathetic dystrophy. Neurology 1990; 40:57.
4. Addick JD: Call for clarity: Pain; 1996—an update review. Refresher course in pain management held in conjunction with the 8th World Congress on Pain. IASP Press, 1996, pp 97–99.
5. Roberts JF: Hypothesis on physiologic basis for causalgia and related pain. Pain 1986; 24:297.
6. Amadio PC, Mackinnon SE, Merritt WH, et al: Reflex sympathetic dystrophy syndrome: Consensus report of an ad hoc committee of the American Association of Hand Surgery on the definition of reflex sympathetic dystrophy syndrome. Plast Reconstr Surg 1991; 7:371.
7. Gellman H, Nichols D: Reflex sympathetic dystrophy in the upper extremity. J Am Acad Orthop Surg 1997; 5:313.
8. Wilson PR: Posttraumtic upper extremity reflex sympathetic dystrophy. Hand Clin 1997; 13:367.
9. Wilder RT, Berde CB, Wolohan M, et al: Reflex sympathetic dystrophy in children. J Bone Joint Surg Am 1992; 74:910.
10. Rush PJ, Wilmot D, Saunders N, et al: Severe reflex neurovascular dystrophy in childhood. Arthrit Rheum 1985; 28:952.
11. Livingston W: Pain Mechanisms: A Psychologic Interpretation of Causalgia and Its Related States in London. McMillian, 1944.
12. Bonica J: The Management of Pain with Special Emphasis on the Use of Analgesic Block in Diagnosis, Prognosis, and Therapy. Philadelphia, Lea and Febiger, 1953, p 913.
13. Devor M, Janig W: Activation of myelinated afferents ending in a neuroma by stimulation of the sympathetic supply in a rat. Neurosci Lett 1981; 24:43.
14. Nystrom B, Hoobarth KE: Microelectrode recordings from transected nerves in amputees with phantom limb pain. Neurosci Lett 1981; 27:211.
15. Hu S, Zhu J: Sympathetic facilitation of sustained discharges of polymodal nociceptors. Pain 1989; 38:85.
16. Sato J, Perl ER: Adrenergic excitation of cutaneous pain receptors induced by peripheral nerve injury. Science 1991; 251:1608.
17. Kajander KC, Wakisaka S, Bennett GU: Spontaneous discharge originates in the dorsal root ganglion at the outset of a painful peripheral neuropathy in the rat. Neurosci Lett 1992; 138:225.
18. Woolf CJ: Peripheral nerve injury triggers central sprouting of myelinated afferent. Nature 1992; 355:75.
19. Mailis A, Wade J: Profile of caucasian women with possible genetic predisposition to reflex sympathetic dystrophy: A pilot study. Clin J Pain 1994; 10:210.
20. Mackinnon S, Holder L: The use of three-phase radionuclide bone scanning in the diagnosis of reflex sympathetic dystrophy. J Hand Surg Am 1984; 9:556.
21. Kozin F, Genant HK, Bekerman C, et al: The reflex sympathetic dystrophy syndrome II: roentgenographic and scintigraphic evidence of bilaterality and of periarticular accentuation. Am J Med 1976; 60:332.
22. Kozin F, Soin JS, Ryan LM, et al: Bone scintigraphy in reflex sympathetic dystrophy syndrome. Radiology 1981; 132:437.
23. Werner R, Davidoff G, Jackson D, et al: Factors affecting the sensitivity and specificity of the three-phase technetium bone scan in the diagnosis of reflex sympathetic dystrophy syndrome in the upper extremity. J Hand Surg Am 1989; 14:520.
24. Pollock FE, Koman LA, Smith B, et al: Patterns of microvascular response–associated reflex sympathetic dystrophy. J Hand Surg Am 1993; 18:847.
25. O'Donoghue JP, Powe JE, Mattar AG, et al: Three-phase bone scintigraphy asymmetric patterns in the upper extremities of asymptomatic normals and reflex sympathetic dystrophy patients. Clin Nucl Med 1993; 18:829.
26. Hendler N, Uematsu S, Long D: Thermographic validation of physical complaints in "psychogenic pain" patients. Psychosomatics 1982; 23:283.
27. Low PA, Neumann C, Dyck PJ, et al: Contact thermography in diagnosis of reflex sympathetic dystrophy: A new look at pathogenesis. Thermology 1985; 1:106.
28. Low PA, Amadio PC, Wilson PR, et al: Laboratory findings in reflex quantitative sympathetic dystrophy: A preliminary report. Clin J Pain 1994; 10:235.
29. Sylvest J, Jensen EM, Siggard-Andersen J, et al: Reflex dystrophy: Resting blood flow and muscle temperature as diagnostic criteria. Scand J Rehabil Med 1977; 9:25.
30. Atkins RM, Duckworth T, Kanis JA: Algodystrophy following colles fracture. J Hand Surg Br 1989; 14:161.
31. Field J, Warwick D, Bannister GC: Features of algodystrophy ten years after colles fracture. J Hand Surg Br 1992; 17:318.
32. Field J, Protheroe DL, Atkins RM: Algodystrophy after Colles fractures is associated with secondary tightness of casts. J Bone Joint Surg Br 1994; 76:901.
33. Bickerstaff DR, Kanis JA: Algodystrophy: An under-recognized complication of minor trauma. Br J Rheum 1994; 33:240.
34. Gellman H, Eckert RR, Botte MJ, et al: Reflex sympathetic dystrophy in cervical spinal cord injury patients. Clin Orthop 1988; 233:126.
35. Braus DF, Krauss JK, Strobel J: The shoulder-hand syndrome after stroke: A prospective clinical trial. Ann Neurol 1994; 36:728.
36. Weiss L, Alfano A, Bardfield P, et al: Prognostic value of triple-phase bone scanning for reflex sympathetic dystrophy in hemiplegia. Arch Phys Med Rehab 1993; 74:716.
37. Richards RL: Causalgia: A centennial review. Arch Neurol 1967; 16:339.
38. Stein AH: The relation of median nerve compression to Sudeck's syndrome. Surg Gynecol Obstet 1962; 11:713.
39. Grundberg A, Reagan DS: Compression syndromes in reflex sympathetic dystrophy. J Hand Surg Am 1991; 16:731.
40. Poehling GG, Pollock FE, Koman LA: Reflex sympathetic dystrophy of the knee after sensory nerve injury. Arthroscopy 1988; 4:31.
41. Bennett GJ, Ochoa JL: Thermographic observations on rats with experimental neuropathic pain. Pain 1991; 45:61.
42. Poplowski ZJ, Wiley AM, Murray JF:

Post-traumatic dystrophy of the extremities: A clinical review and trial of treatment. J Bone Joint Surg Am 1983; 65: 642.

43. Bengston K: Physical modalities for complex regional pain syndrome. Hand Clin 1997; 13:443.

44. Watson HK, Carlson L: Treatment of reflex sympathetic dystrophy of the hand with an active "stress loading" program. J Hand Surg Am 1987; 12:779.

45. Fowler FD, Moser M: Use of hexamethonium and dibenzyline in diagnosis and treatment of causalgia. JAMA 1956; 161: 1051.

46. Ghostine SY, Comair YG, Turner DM, et al: Phenoxybenzamine in the treatment of causalgia. J Neurosurg 1984; 60:1263.

47. Tabria T, Shibasaki H, Kuroiwa Y: Reflex sympathetic dystrophy (causalgia) treatment with guanethidine. Arch Neurol 1983; 40:430.

48. Arlet J, Mazieres B: Medical treatment of reflex sympathetic dystrophy. Hand Clin 1997; 13:477.

49. Davis KD, Treede RD, Raja SN, et al: The topical application of clonidine relieves hyperalgesia in patients with sympathetically maintained pain. Pain 1991; 47: 309.

50. Mikkelsen E, Andersson KE, Pedersen OL: The effect of nifedipine on isolated human peripheral vessels. Acta Pharmacol Toxicol 1978; 43:291.

51. Rodeheffer RJ, Rommer JA, Wigley F, et al: Controlled double-blind trial of nifedipine in the treatment of Raynaud's phenomenon. N Engl J Med 1983; 308:80.

52. Prough DS, McLeskey CH, Poehling GG, et al: Efficacy of oral nifedipine in the treatment of reflex sympathetic dystrophy. Anesthesiology 1985; 62:7.

53. Christensen K, Jensen EM, Noer I: The reflex sympathetic dystrophy syndrome response to treatment with systemic corticosteroids. Acta Chir Scand 1982; 148:653.

54. Kozin F, Ryan LM, Carrera GF, et al: The reflex sympathetic dystrophy syndrome III: Scintigraph studies further evidence for the efficacy of systemic corticosteroids, and proposed diagnostic criteria. Am J Med 1981; 1:23.

55. Kleinert HE, Cole NM, Wayne L, et al: Post-traumatic sympathetic dystrophy. Orthop Clin North Am 1973; 4:917.

56. Brown DL: Somatic or sympathetic block for reflex sympathetic dystrophy: Which is indicated? Hand Clin 1997; 13:485.

57. Hobelmann CF, Dellon AL: Use of prolonged sympathetic blockade as an adjunct to surgery in the patient with sympathetic maintained pain. Microsurgery 1989; 10: 151.

58. Linson MA, Leffert R, Todd D: The treatment of upper extremity reflex sympathetic dystrophy with prolonged continuous stellate ganglion blockade. J Hand Surg 1983; 8:153.

59. Hannington-Kiff JG: Pharmacological target blocks in hand surgery and rehabilitation. J Hand Surg Br 1984; 9:29.

60. Jadad AR, Carrol D, Glynn CJ, et al: Intravenous regional sympathetic blockade for pain relief in reflex sympathetic dystrophy: A systematic review and a randomized, double-blind crossover study. J Pain Symptom Manage 1995; 10:13.

61. Hord AH, Rooks MD, Stephens BO, et al: Intravenous regional bretylium and lidocaine for treatment of reflex sympathetic dystrophy: A Randomized double-blind study. Anaesth Analg 1992; 74:818.

62. Ramamurthy S, Hoffman J, Walsh N, et al: Role of tourniquet-induced analgesia in IV regional sympatholysis. Anesthesiology 1986; 65:207.

63. Olcott C, Eltherington LG, Wilcosky BR, et al: Reflex sympathetic dystrophy. The surgeon's role in management. J Vasc Surg 1991; 14:488.

64. Robertson DP, Simpson RK, Rose JE, et al: Video-assisted endoscopic thoracic ganglionectomy J Neurosurg 1993; 79: 238.

65. Dielissen PW, Claassen ATPM, Veldman PHJM, et al: Amputation for reflex sympathetic dystrophy. J Bone Joint Surg Br 1995; 77:270.

NERVE PHYSIOLOGY AND REPAIRS*

Thomas E. Trumble and Wren V. McCallister

Summary

- Nerve conduction is dependent on the flow of ions, which is regulated by voltage-gated channels in the endoneurium.
- Transmission at the neuromuscular junction involves transduction of the action potential from an electrical impulse to a chemical message and back to an electrical impulse. It is proportional to both the intensity and frequency of the stimulus.
- Axonal transport, occurring both anterograde and retrograde, is energy-dependent and is required for communication between the nerve and its target.
- Resorption of motor end plates occurs after denervation and can be inhibited by a calcium-activated neutral protease, calpain.
- The size of the distal fascicle is the most significant factor determining the target of the regenerating growth cone.
- Motor axon sprouts are selective for distal motor nerves, and this may be explained by the presence of a carbohydrate L2/HNK-1, which is preferentially expressed by previously motor axon-associated Schwann's cells in reinnervated peripheral nerves.

Despite the tremendous evolution in the repair and reconstruction of the musculoskeletal system during the last decade, the reconstruction of nerve injuries persists as one of the final frontiers in the repair of the musculoskeletal system. Even with the many technical advances to improve the quality of the surgical techniques with intraoperative magnification, the materials for suturing or bonding nerve ends, and devices for monitoring during surgery, there has been little improvement in the overall results of functional recovery after nerve repair and reconstruction. Efforts to increase our understanding of complex nerve structure and physiology, especially with regard to nerve injury and repair, offer the best hope for future improvements in nerve repair and reconstruction.

FUNDAMENTAL SCIENCE

NEURAL ANATOMY

The three basic elements of peripheral nerves include the epineurium (both external and internal), perineurium, and endoneurium (Fig. 1). The external epineurium consists of the collagenous connective tissues that surround the entire nerve. The internal epineurium is an extension of the external epineurium, which surrounds the nerve fascicles, providing "packing" material to cushion the nerve fascicles. Where nerves cross joints and are, therefore, exposed to greater compressive forces, an increase in the quantity of

internal epineurium is noted. The perineurium forms the lining of the individual fascicles and, as an extension of the blood-brain barrier, is composed of closely packed cells that are united by tight junctions to control intercellular diffusion.[1] In addition, the cells of the perineurium help to block infection and to maintain a positive intrafascicular pressure. The endoneurium surrounds the individual axons and forms the structural component of the Schwann tube. The nutrient vessels of the nerves run longitudinally along the course of the nerve, which facilitates the nerve excursion necessary during joint motion. The perineural vessels enter the endoneurium at oblique angles, which places them at risk for compression. The fascicles are groups of axons within a perineural sleeve whose numbers may vary greatly along the length of any one nerve. Interconnections between fascicles, abundant in the proximal portions of the nerve, form a fascicular plexus. There are very few of these interconnections in the portions of the nerve distal to the knee and ankle, which provides for more consistent neuroanatomy, thereby enhancing the surgeon's ability to align the fascicles properly. There is evidence that adjacent fascicles innervate sites in the extremity that are closely related geographically as opposed to the diverse sites suggested by the long-accepted "internal chaos" theory.[2] Thus, efforts to align the nerves accurately, and thereby preserve their anatomic topography, should result in more accurate reinnervation and a better functional outcome.

NERVE PHYSIOLOGY
Physiology of Peripheral Nerve Conduction

Impulse conduction in peripheral nerves depends on the Na^+/K^+ ATPase, which maintains a resting electrical potential of approximately -70 mV inside the cell. In response to a stimulus at the cell body, an action potential is generated that propagates down the peripheral nerve. At the leading edge of the advancing action potential, depolarizing current begins to open voltage-gated Na^+ channels, and as a result of the increased Na^+ conductance the membrane potential becomes more positive. After a certain threshold membrane potential is achieved, another "all-or-nothing" action potential is generated, and propagation continues. Whereas the rising phase of the action potential depends solely on the voltage-gated Na^+ channels, the falling phase results from the combination of closure of the voltage-gated Na^+ channels and the opening of K^+ channels that restore the resting membrane potential. Once closed, the Na^+ channels briefly remain refractory to stimulation by diffusing positive charge, and this is the mechanism that maintains unidirectional propagation of the action potential.

Physiology of Neuromuscular Transmission

The motor unit is composed of the neuron, its axons, and all the muscle fibers that it innervates, which can vary

---

* Author retains original rights for Figure 1.

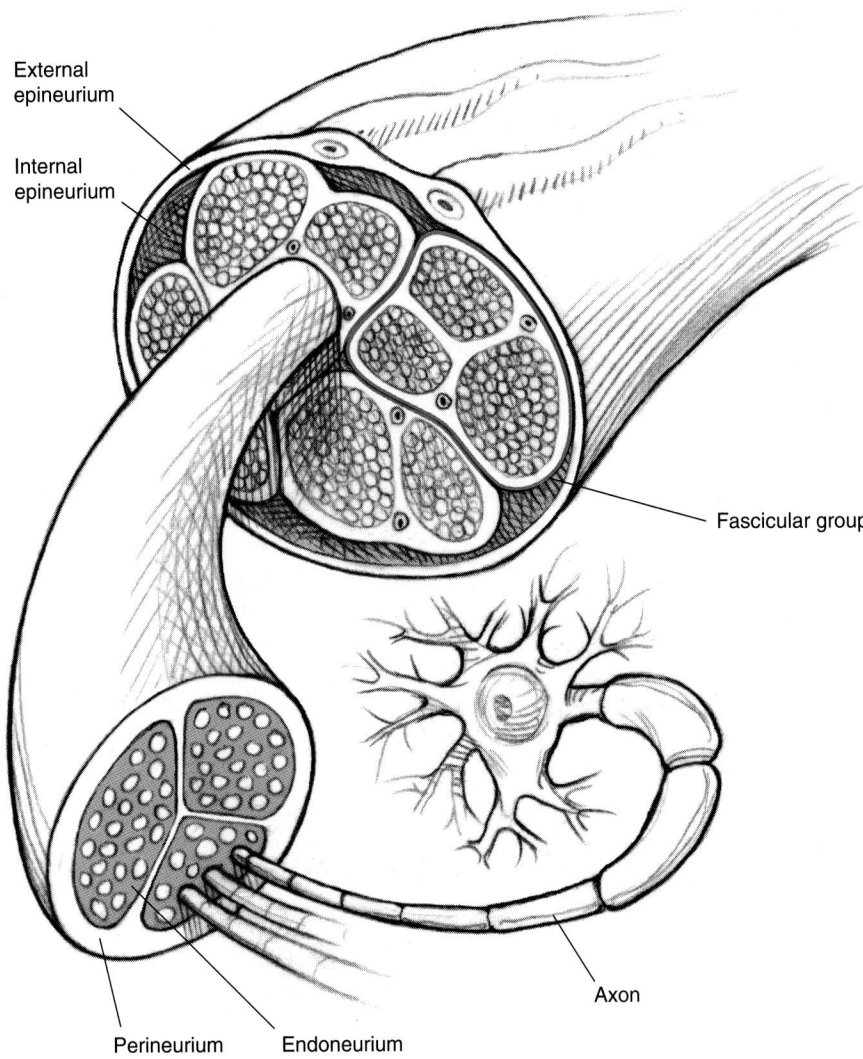

External
epineurium

Internal
epineurium

Fascicular group

Fig. 1. Microscopic organization of peripheral nerve.

Axon

Perineurium   Endoneurium

from 10 to 1000. The critical link between the axons of a motor unit and its innervated muscle fibers is the neuromuscular junction, whose task is to transduce impulses across the physical discontinuity of a synapse. The propagated action potential, on reaching the presynaptic terminal at the neuromuscular junction, stimulates the opening of voltage-gated Ca^{2+} channels, which leads, as a result of Ca^{2+} influx, to exocytosis of vesicles filled with acetylcholine (ACh). The ACh is released into the synaptic cleft at presynaptic regions termed "active zones," which are in apposition to regions of increased receptor density on the postsynaptic membrane. Once released, the ACh binds receptors on the postsynaptic membrane, themselves ion channels that permit the passage of Na^+, resulting in a miniature end-plate potential (MEPP) whose magnitude is proportional to the concentration of ACh. If the stimulus is sufficient, the MEPPs will summate to generate a depolarizing current, the end-plate potential (EPP), which opens voltage-gated Na^+ channels in the membrane region immediately adjacent to the muscle end plate. Thus, having transduced the action potential from an electrical impulse to a chemical message and back to an electrical impulse, the job of the neuromuscular junction is finished, and the

continued conduction of the action potential within the muscle fiber leads to muscle contraction (Fig. 2).

Axonal Transport

Axonal transport occurs in both the anterograde and retrograde directions. Anterograde transport is further categorized as "fast" or "slow." Fast anterograde transport is a mechanism that moves membrane-enclosed vesicles, containing molecules synthesized in the cell body, which are vital to the maintenance of a normal axon, away from the cell body and down the microtubule "railroad track" at a speed of 400 mm/day. The energy for this transport is provided by an ATPase, kinesin, which links traveling organelles with the microtubule for transport. Slow anterograde transport is a transport mechanism that carries cytoskeletal elements at a rate of 0.5 mm/day with the speed of transport related to the size of the axon. Fast retrograde transport is the mechanism that returns scavenged components to the cell body using another ATPase, dynein, which also links the transported materials to the microtubule "railroad." The maintenance of a viable axon is believed to be dependent on "neuron-target communication" mediated by neurotropic factors synthesized by the periph-

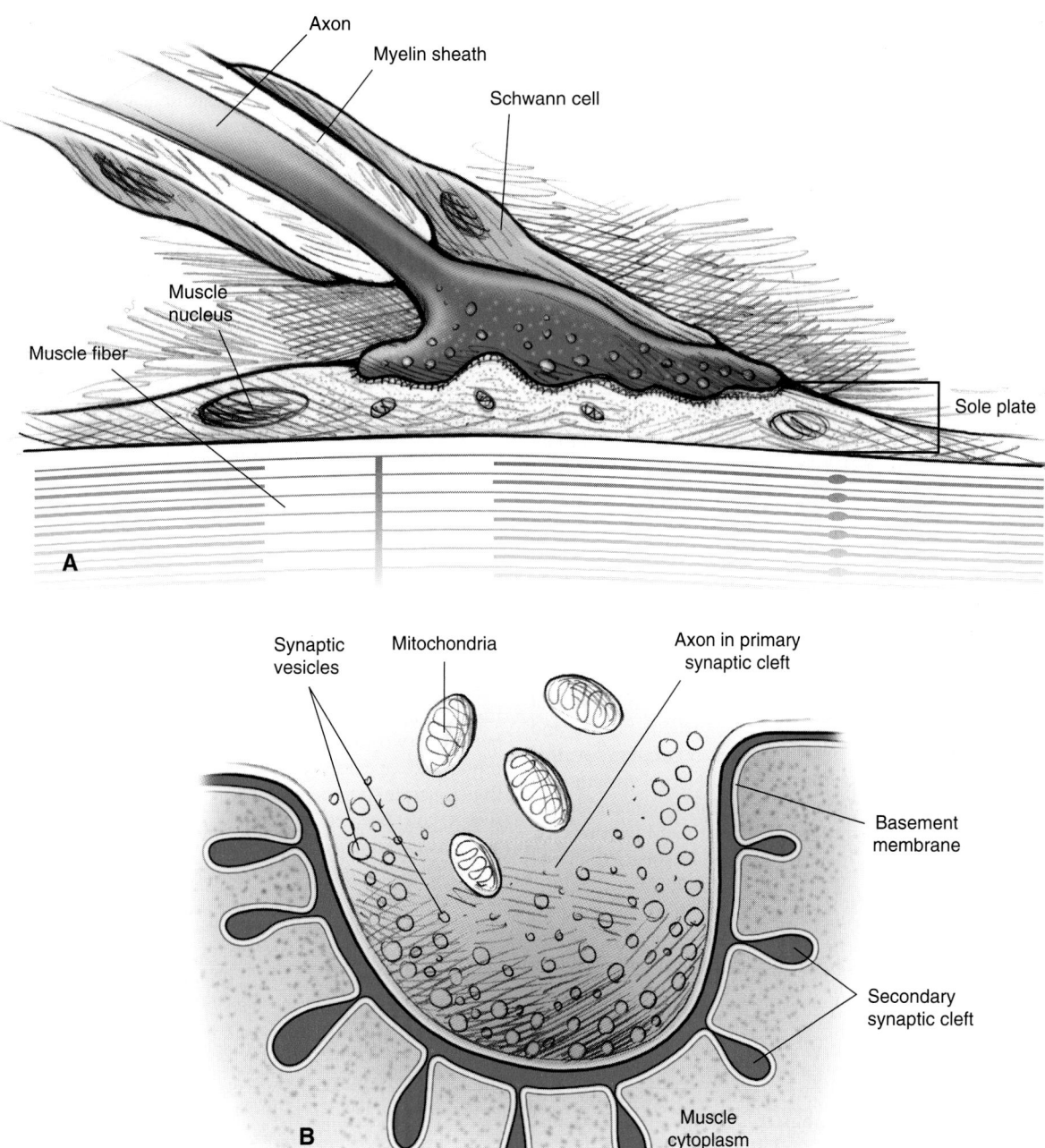

Fig. 2. Features of the neuromuscular junction. *A,* By light microscopy. The nerve terminal axon loses its myelin sheath but is still covered by a Schwann cell. The distal axon lies in an indentation in the muscle membrane. The membrane of the muscle fiber is raised in a mound, the sole plate. This area is rich in cellular organelles although devoid of microfibers. *B,* By electron microscopy. The primary synaptic cleft is further divided by a series of indentations of the muscle fiber membrane, called secondary synaptic clefts. The basement membrane of the muscle is continuous throughout the primary and secondary synaptic clefts. There are numerous synaptic vesicles in the terminal axon. (From Galbraith JA, Myers RR: Impulse conduction. *In* Gelberman RH, ed: Operative Nerve Repair and Reconstruction, 1991, p 30.)

eral target. Fast retrograde transport is the means by which this communication is performed as the neurotropic factors, collected at the distal nerve terminal, are transported to the cell body.

Sensory Receptors

Sensation in the upper extremity relies on three key organelles: (1) Meissner's corpuscles; (2) Merkel's cells; and (3) pacinian corpuscles. Meissner's corpuscles, located in the dermal papillae and especially abundant in the fingertips, are maximally sensitive to vibrations at 30 cps. In addition, they are rapid-adapting sensory receptors and thus well suited for moving two-point discrimination. Merkel's cells, located at the epidermal-dermal junction, are slow-adapting sensory receptors with a small discrete field that is well suited to static two-point testing. These organelles can respond to constant touch or pressure. Widely distributed over the body, the pacinian corpuscles are rapid-adapting sensory receptors that lie in the subcutaneous tissue. They respond best to a stimulus of 250 cps and have a large receptive field, sometimes up to 2 to 3 cm.

NERVE DEGENERATION AND REGENERATION
Wallerian Degeneration
Immediately after nerve injury, a process of wallerian degeneration begins in the distal nerve segment. The process involves macrophage phagocytosis of the Schwann cell tube contents, which prevents obstruction and provides a favorable environment for the regenerating axons.[3] At the first intact node of Ranvier's node proximal to the lesion, the regenerating nerve end sends out sprouts or axonal buds that comprise the regenerating nerve growth cone. Aided by filopodia located at its most distal tip, the growth cone constantly samples the local environment and responds by directing axonal regeneration toward favorable stimuli while withdrawing from stimuli that are unfavorable. One study using a special inbred strain of mouse with delayed axonal degeneration demonstrated that the onset of degeneration is likely dictated by the composition of the axon and not the Schwann cell.[4]

In response to axotomy-induced wallerian degeneration, the metabolism of the neuron increases severalfold to meet the needs of regeneration. A variety of growth factors and cytokines have been implicated in the regulation of this response, termed the cell body reaction. Nerve growth factor has received great research interest and has been shown to inhibit wallerian degeneration, increase neuronal activity, and enhance the rate of regeneration of sensory axons but not that of motor axons.[5] Ciliary neurotropic factor,[6] along with other cytokines and growth factors, has been identified as being involved in nerve regeneration (e.g., brain-derived neurotropic factor, neuroleukin, fibroblastic growth factor, and epidermal growth factor).

Motor End-Plate Degeneration
In response to denervation, a calcium-activated neutral protease, calpain, disrupts the cytoskeletal elements of the motor end plates. Leupeptin inhibits the action of this protease and has been demonstrated in laboratory animals to enhance nerve regeneration by preventing the degradation of the receptors in skeletal muscle.[7] Clinical trials with an oral form of the drug leupeptin are currently being conducted.

Specificity of Nerve Regeneration
Neurotropism is the directed axonal growth up a gradient of diffusible substances produced by the target, the distal end of the nerve. Nerve growth factor, although affecting sensory nerve regeneration, does not directly guide axon regeneration.[8] Still, the axonal buds do preferentially regenerate toward nerve tissue. However, there is no sensory-to-sensory or motor-to-motor specificity; instead, the size of the distal fascicle appears to be the most significant factor determining the target of the regenerating growth cone.[9] In the process of regenerating, motor axons send out multiple axonal buds from any one axon. Research using one fluorescent label that enters the nerve endings innervating skin and another label that enters axonal sprouts innervating muscle has demonstrated that motor axons prune, or eliminate, the axonal sprouts that were mistakenly directed toward sensory nerves.[10] The preference of motor axons for distal motor nerves may be explained by the presence of the carbohydrate L2/HNK-1, which is preferentially expressed by previously motor axon–associated Schwann's cells in reinnervated peripheral nerves.[9]

CLINICAL RELEVANCE AND APPLICATIONS

DIAGNOSTIC STUDIES OF NERVE FUNCTION BASED ON NERVE PHYSIOLOGY
Clinical Tests of Nerve Function
Clinical testing of peripheral nerves is divided into tests of sensation and tests of motor function. Clinical tests of sensation include threshold testing, density testing, and empiric testing. Threshold tests, which determine the level of stimulus required for a response, are the most sensitive tests for nerve compression syndromes in which the number of functioning sensory receptors is normal but their level of activation is depressed. Threshold testing can be accomplished using Semmes-Weinstein monofilaments, fine filaments that exert a discrete amount of pressure on the fingertips for testing, or vibration testing that ranges from low (30 cps) to high (256 cps) frequency. Density tests depend on the fact that there must be a certain number of functioning sensory end organs to be able to discriminate between two stimuli. This ability to interpret the sensory input and accurately distinguish a stimulus consisting of two discrete points requires substantial cortical reinnervation when assayed by both the moving two-point and the static two-point tests. As a result, these tests are best used for evaluating patients who have nearly complete sensory recovery from a nerve injury.

Subjective muscle grading and quantitative strength testing are two clinical tests of motor function. The following subjective staged levels of motor recovery, also devised by the British Medical Research Council, have gained wide clinical acceptance: M0, no muscle activity; M1, contraction without movement; M2, movement of extremity but not against gravity; M3, movement against gravity but not added resistance; M4, movement against both gravity and added resistance but less than normal strength; and M5, normal strength. The surgeon may use quantitative strength testing that relies on measurable data to help accurately compare different techniques of nerve repair. Strength is measured as the isolated force of contracting muscles that have been reinnervated and expressed as a percentage of the normal contralateral side.[11]

Laboratory Tests of Nerve Function
Electrodiagnostic testing includes the use of nerve conduction studies, electromyography (EMG), and somatosensory evoked potentials (SSEPs). Advances in our understanding of nerve physiology have led to the development of more sensitive nerve conduction tests and electromyograms, which have improved the utility of electrodiagnostic testing to the clinician. Measurable delays in nerve conduction velocity (NCV) are produced by injuries that, although not disrupting to axons, can cause focal demyelination with slowing or conduction block. Significant external compression producing partial demyelination is indicated by either

a decrease in nerve conduction across a localized region (e.g., the carpal tunnel) or, conversely, an increase in the delay or latency. On the basis of current understanding of nerve physiology, NCV tests are the most sensitive laboratory test for detecting nerve compression syndromes with demyelination, whereas EMG is most helpful after nerve injury when denervation (i.e., axon loss) occurs. The NCV is usually measured by stimulating a nerve proximally and recording the responses distally over a fixed distance using leads on the digits for sensory fiber conduction and electrodes in or over muscles for motor conduction. In peripheral neuropathies, the nerve conduction is decreased diffusely both proximally and distally in multiple nerves. In contrast, there is only focal slowing with compressive neuropathies. When both compressive and peripheral neuropathies are present, there is focal slowing of one nerve superimposed on a diffuse slowing of multiple nerves. Because latencies (the time between stimulation and recording) include not only nerve conduction time but also neuromuscular junction transmission and muscle fiber conduction, the latencies are reported by convention in milliseconds instead of the velocity (distance in meters/latency or delay in seconds).

Electrodiagnostic Studies for Nerve Injury

About 3 weeks after an injury that does disrupt the nerve axons, either completely or partially, detectable electromyographic changes are produced in the denervated target skeletal muscle. Patients displaying detectable EMG changes will often experience fibrillations, spontaneous insertional activity associated with the implantation of needles into the muscle, and the muscles will demonstrate an inability to voluntarily recruit fibers. With successful reinnervation, the target skeletal muscle develops polyphasic potentials and demonstrates partial voluntary recruitment. Severe nerve compression syndromes can produce axonal disruption resulting in EMG changes.

Somatosensory Evoked Potentials

Again taking advantage of our understanding of nerve physiology, the use of SSEPs involves the application of a stimulus, typically applied to a peripheral nerve, which is conducted along a sensory pathway and results in the production of electrical signals by the contralateral sensory cortex. Measured by electrodes placed on the scalp, a disruption anywhere along the sensory pathway will result in the failure to detect these signals regardless of whether the injury is preganglionic or postganglionic. Aiding in the diagnostic investigation is the fact that preganglionic injuries will demonstrate normal conduction velocities, because the pathway from the neuron to the sensory organelles in the skin remains intact. The SSEP is helpful in differentiating between proximal lesions (e.g., thoracic outlet syndrome and cervical root compression) and distal lesions (e.g., ulnar nerve compression at the elbow). A patient with abnormal SSEPs after stimulation of the small and ring finger but normal NVCs of the ulnar nerve across the elbow most likely has thoracic outlet syndrome with compression of the lower trunk of the brachial plexus and not cubital tunnel syndrome. The surgeon must clearly indicate the specific nerves and muscles to be tested when ordering EMG and NCV studies. One cannot rely on the person performing the study to know all the important clinical

questions needed to diagnose and treat the patient accurately.

NERVE PHYSIOLOGY AND THE TREATMENT OF NERVE INJURIES
Primary Nerve Repairs

The three main categories of primary nerve repair include epineural, group fascicular, and fascicular repairs. Epineural repair, a technique that works well when there is no confusion regarding the proper alignment of the fascicle, involves simply suturing the external epineurium of the nerve. Such a repair is ideal for sharp lacerations with no loss of nerve substance and for partial nerve lacerations when the proper alignment of the nerve is already established[12] (Fig. 3). Group fascicular repairs work best when

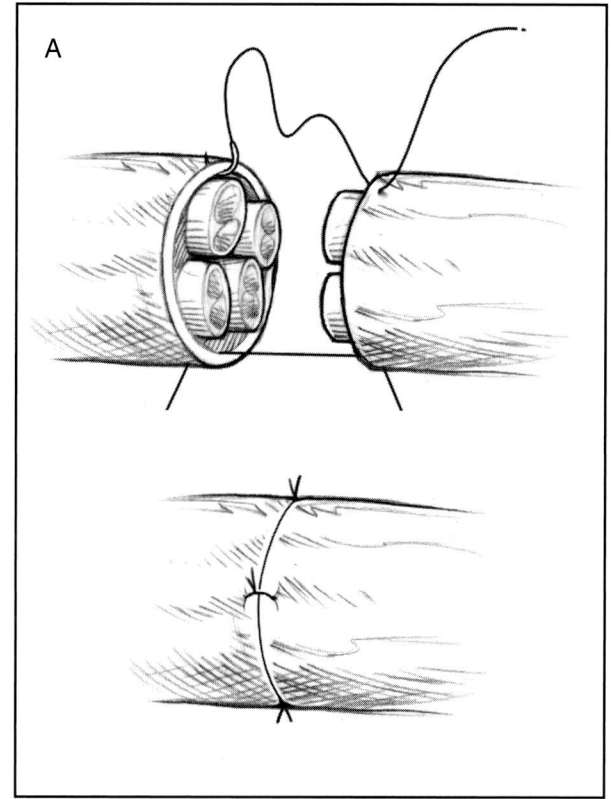

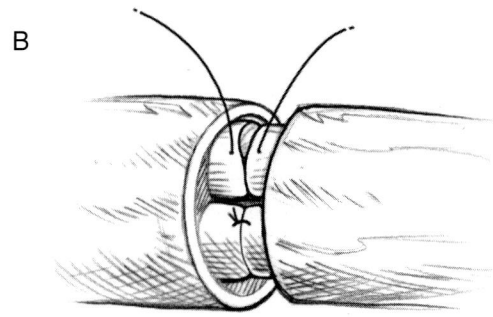

Fig. 3. Epineural repair. *A*, Epineural repairs work well for sharp nerve injuries and partial nerve injuries. *B*, Group fascicular repair provides the best means of matching the fascicles when a segment of the nerve has to be resected because of a crushing component of the injury. (From Garrett WE Jr: Neuromuscular junction. *In* Gelberman RH, ed: Operative Nerve Repair and Reconstruction, 1991, p 74. Copyright Elizabeth Roselius, 1991.)

there has been a crushing component to the nerve injury or a delayed repair requiring the trimming of a portion of the nerve ends.[13] By suturing the fascicular groups, the alignment of the nerve is optimized without the use of excessive numbers of sutures, which can add to the foreign body response and scarring at the site of nerve repair. Fascicular repair is not widely used because of the increased amount of suture material required in the repair site and the difficulty in confirming the actual alignment of the individual fascicles.

Microsutures, using 8-0 nylon for major peripheral nerves and 10-0 nylon for digital nerves, are the most practical means of repairing nerves after most isolated nerve injuries. When multiple cable grafts are required, as in the treatment of brachial plexus injuries, fibrin glue techniques offer the advantage of rapid nerve coaptation.

Secondary Nerve Repairs

Secondary nerve repair involves a means of overcoming gap defects in peripheral nerves and includes techniques such as bone shortening, nerve transposition, joint positioning, nerve elongation, and nerve grafts.

Use of bone shortening is generally limited to cases in which a single bone is present in the upper extremity, most often the humerus.[14] Shortening the humerus is usually used in the treatment of a radial nerve injury with segmental loss that is combined with a delayed union or nonunion of the humerus. The ulnar nerve is the ideal nerve for nerve transposition, especially when combined with elbow flexion for injuries to the ulnar nerve at the level of the elbow. Nerves with extensive branches near the involved joint (e.g., the radial nerve at the elbow) do not gain significant length with transposition.

Joint positioning is one of the most successful means of obtaining increased length for nerve repair; the likelihood of success of joint positioning increases the closer the nerve injury is to the joint.

Nerve elongation offers the potential for an increase of up to 10% in available length along the segment in question (i.e., stretching the nerves). The physiological responses to nerve injury limit the efficacy of nerve elongation in two respects. First, nerves can lose up to 8% of their length within 3 weeks after an injury. Thus, in delayed nerve repairs with no substance loss, nerve elongation will allow for end-to-end repair; however, delayed nerve repairs with segmental loss of the nerve will require other techniques, including nerve grafting. The second limitation when considering how much elongation a nerve can tolerate is not the suture strength but the nerve blood flow.[15] Nerve blood flow is inversely proportional to the tension applied to the nerve. Severe nerve ischemia occurs at only 12% to 15% elongation of the nerve as the blood flow decreases to approximately 30% of baseline. Further indication of the importance of preserving blood flow to the injured nerve is the fact that injured nerves demonstrate a threefold increase in blood flow as part of the reparative process.

Nerve grafting, whether using autografts or allografts, is an important tool in the surgeon's armamentarium.[16] The sural nerve has become the gold standard for use in nerve autografts because of its favorable ratio of axons to epineurium and because the loss of the nerve only produces a small area of sensory deficit on the lateral side of the foot,

which is generally well tolerated. The lateral or medial antebrachial cutaneous nerves may be used for grafting small digital nerves. However, disturbing paresthesias in the forearm can be produced by the loss of these nerves. Thus, we recommend against the use of these nerves as donor nerves.

The limitations in the use of autograft donor nerves, coupled with the fact that the grafting of large nerve defects requires an excessive amount of graft material, has led to extensive research on the use of allograft nerves. Studies confirmed that nerve grafts can survive if the nerve allograft has been properly preserved to maintain cell viability and if the patient is immunosuppressed.[17] Furthermore, immunosuppression does not appear to be required on a permanent basis once the nerve graft has become incorporated by the ingrowth of Schwann cells from the host nerve ends. Despite the promising potential of nerve allografts, the clinical results with autografts still appear to be slightly superior. Thus, although nerve allografts have been a part of clinical investigations, they have not been widely used in the routine clinical setting.

Given that the sural nerve graft is approximately the same size as the fascicular groups of most mixed motor and sensory nerves in the extremities, group fascicular repairs are the favored technique for suturing nerve grafts.[18] The functional results of nerve grafts, both sensory and motor, decreases with increasing delays in grafting and increasing graft length.[11,19] Delays of less than 3 weeks from the time of injury and the use of grafts that are 5.0 cm or less in length provide the optimum results. Using materials that are permanent and biodegradable, several investigators evaluated the use of artificial conduits with or without the impregnation of growth factors, and none of these constructs has proven to be as good as conventional nerve autografts.[19]

Peripheral Nerve Repair Outcomes

The overall status of the extremity has a major impact on the eventual recovery of neural function after the repair of peripheral nerves; the functional recovery is jeopardized by significant injuries to the skin, muscle, tendons, and bony structures. The impact of such injuries derives not only from the direct threat to reinnervation of the injured soft tissues but also from the healing process, which results in the formation of scar tissue. By itself, scar tissue will adversely affect the healing of injured nerves. A critical factor in planning nerve repair is the decrease in functional recovery with increasing times to repair (Fig. 4). As soon as the surgeon has evidence that the nerve has a lesion that disrupts the continuity of the nerve, he or she should complete the nerve repair. Longer delays to surgery are more likely to require a nerve graft that results in two sites of nerve coaptation for the axonal sprouts to traverse, causing decreased specificity of nerve regeneration.

Millesi et al,[18] using interfascicular grafting, reported a 96% to 100% return of sensation throughout an anesthetic area in lesions of the median and ulnar nerves and a 32% to 39% return of two-point discrimination. Earlier series in which epineural suturing was generally used, often without grafting, documented a 46% to 82% return of sensation in previously anesthetic areas and a 4% to 25% return of two-point discrimination. Treating transected median and ulnar nerves with interfascicular grafting, Haase et al reported

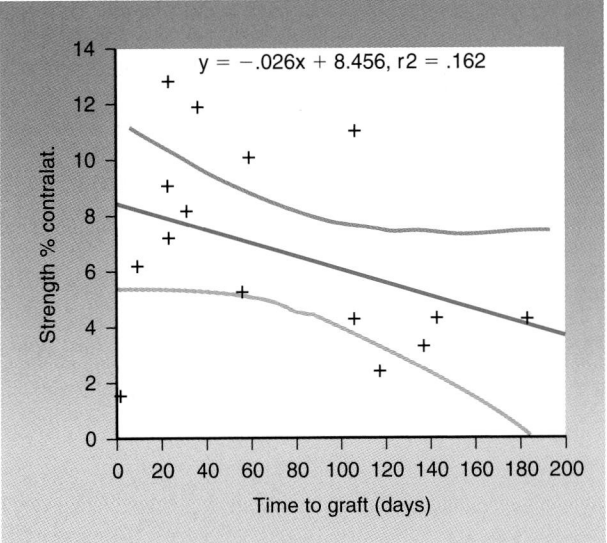

$$y = -.026x + 8.456, r2 = .162$$

Fig. 4. Recovery of muscle strength. In a group of patients requiring nerve grafts for injuries of the radial, median, or ulnar nerves, the recovery of muscle strength decreased with increasing delays to surgery. (From Brushart TM: Mechanical and humoral control of specificity and nerve repair. In Gelberman RH, ed: Operative Nerve Repair and Reconstruction, 1991, p 74. Copyright Elizabeth Roselius, 1991.)

more promising results in more than 60 patients, with 50% to 60% of these patients having return of two-point discrimination and 70% to 97% having return of pain and tactile sensation throughout an anesthetic area. They remarked that their better results could be attributed, at least in part, to their having a relatively younger patient population than those reported in other series.

According to Sunderland,[20] two criteria must be present before fascicular repair or interfascicular grafting can be considered: (1) the fascicular bundle must be large enough for suturing and (2) the fascicle should be sharply localized and sufficiently well defined so that it can be identified and mobilized for repair. Kline[21] noted that these criteria are met in the upper extremity by the radial nerve in the spiral groove and the ulnar nerve at the wrist and the forearm. Although he also indicated that the median nerve often does not meet these criteria, interfascicular grafting in the median nerve has been reported. To assess the possible superiority of one technique over another, careful operative descriptions and postoperative evaluations obtained according to a standardized protocol are mandatory.

Physiology and Repair of Neuromas

Neuromas,[21] whether terminal or in continuity, result from failure of the regenerating nerve growth cone to reach peripheral targets.[22] A neuroma located in an area with little soft-tissue coverage can be so painful as to render the patient's hand or foot useless. A neuroma will be produced, by definition, with every nerve laceration or avulsion that is not repaired. The only way to prevent or minimize neuroma formation is to repair the peripheral nerve. Although there is usually a small neuroma in continuity at the site of any nerve repair, the successful nerve repair results in only a small number of axons being trapped at the repair site in scar tissue and, therefore, unable to reach their target receptors.

The treatment of neuromas generally involves one of the following: excising the neuroma, burying the neuroma, capping the neuroma, or ligating the nerves proximally, ending in painful neuromas. When both nerve ends can be identified and when the repair can be buried under ample soft tissue to provide sufficient mechanical padding, neuroma excision and nerve repair can be very successful. In the absence of convincing evidence to the contrary (several studies have tried to determine whether it is better to bury neuromas in bone or soft tissues), most surgeons prefer to bury the neuroma in a bed with muscle tissue to provide the best padding for the neuroma. Overall, the success rate for burying neuromas is 75%, regardless of the technique. Because revision surgery to rebury the nerve also has a 75% success rate, most patients have relief of pain after one or two attempts at burying a painful neuroma.

Neuromas in continuity generally involve either motor axons in continuity or sensory axons in continuity with disrupted motor fibers. The intact motor fibers may be separated from the disrupted sensory fibers by dissection of the nerve proximal and distal to the nerve repair site. As an aid to help confirm that the intact motor fibers are protected, electrical stimulation may be used when the disrupted sensory fibers in the neuroma are resected and grafted. Less symptomatic are neuromas formed by sensory axons in continuity with disrupted motor fibers, which, in the upper extremity, may be treated with tendon transfers without the need to explore the neuroma. When the motor function is critical compared with the sensory function (e.g., the peroneal nerve), the neuroma can be explored by dissecting the nerve proximal and distal to the site of injury to identify the functioning sensory nerves. The neuroma with the motor nerves can then be resected and repaired with or without a graft.

REFERENCES

1. Lundborg G: Structure and function of the intraneural microvessels as related to trauma, edema formation, and nerve function. J Bone Joint Surg Am 1975; 57:938.
2. Brushart TM: Central course of digital axons within the median nerve of *Macaca mulatta*. J Comp Neurol 1991; 311:197.
3. Bixby JL, Harris WA: Molecular mechanisms of axon growth and guidance. Annu Rev Cell Biol 1991; 7:117.
4. Glass JD, Brushart TM, George EB, et al: Prolonged survival of transected nerve fibres in C57BL/Ola mice is an intrinsic characteristic of the axon. J Neurocytol 1993; 22:311.
5. Ninkina NN, Buchman VL, Akopian AN, et al: Nerve growth factor-regulated properties of sensory neurones in Oct-2 null mutant mice. Brain Res Mol Brain Res 1995; 33:233.
6. Oyesiku NM, Wigston DJ: Ciliary neurotrophic factor stimulates neurite outgrowth from spinal cord neurons. J Comp Neurol 1996; 364:68.
7. Badalamente MA, Hurst LC, Stracher A: Neuromuscular recovery after peripheral nerve repair: Effects of an orally-administered peptide in a primate model. J Reconstr Microsurg 1995; 11:429.
8. Lundborg G, Dahlin L, Danielsen N, et al: Trophism, tropism, and specificity in nerve regeneration. J Reconstr Microsurg 1994; 10:345.

9. Martini R, Schachner M, Brushart TM: The L2/HNK-1 carbohydrate is preferentially expressed by previously motor axon-associated Schwann cells in reinnervated peripheral nerves. J Neurosci 1994; 14: 7180.

10. Brushart TM: Motor axons preferentially reinnervate motor pathways. J Neurosci 1993; 13:2730.

11. Trumble TE, Kahn U, Vanderhooft E, et al: A technique to quantitate motor recovery following nerve grafting. J Hand Surg Am 1995; 20:367.

12. Hurst L, Dowd A, Sampson S, et al: Partial lacerations of median and ulnar nerves. J Hand Surg Am 1991; 16A:207.

13. Cabaud HE, Rodkey WG, McCarroll HR Jr: Peripheral nerve injuries: Studies in higher nonhuman primates. J Hand Surg 1980; 5:201.

14. Trumble TE: In Gelberman RH (ed): Operative Nerve Repair and Reconstruction. Philadelphia, JB Lippincott, 1991, vol 1, p 507.

15. Clark WL, Trumble TE, Swiontkowski MF, et al: Nerve tension and blood flow in a rat model of immediate and delayed repairs. J Hand Surg Am 1992; 17:677.

16. Duel AB: History and development of the surgical treatment of facial palsy. Surg Gynecol Obstet 1933; 56:382.

17. Easterling KJ, Trumble TE: The treatment of peripheral nerve injuries using irradiated allografts and temporary host immunosuppression (in a rat model). J Reconstr Microsurg 1990; 6:301.

18. Millesi H, Meissl G, Berger A: The interfascicular nerve grafting of the median and ulnar nerves. J Bone Joint Surg Am 1972; 54:727.

19. Lundborg G: Neurotropism, frozen muscle grafts and other conduits. J Hand Surg Br 1991; 16:473.

20. Sunderland S: Nerve and Nerve Injuries. Edinburgh, Churchill-Livingstone, 1978.

21. Kline D: Evaluation of the Neuroma-in-Continuity: Management of Peripheral Nerve Problems. Philadelphia, WB Saunders, 1980, p 451.

22. Bora FW, Pleasure DE, Didizian NA: A study of nerve regeneration and neuroma formation after nerve suture by various techniques. J Hand Surg 1976; 1:138.

section
12
chapter
27

MEDIAN NERVE COMPRESSION

Joseph M. Failla

Summary

- The natural history is influenced by the site and severity of compression and is usually progressive sensory or motor loss with decreased hand function.
- Nonoperative treatment is appropriate in mild cases and even in severe cases in the elderly if minimally symptomatic.
- The diagnosis is made by physical examination and electrical testing, with special attention to rule out multiple sites of compression.
- Treatment includes conservative measures and surgery.
- Treatment varies according to the site and severity of compression.

DEFINITION

There are three types of median nerve compression (MNC). Carpal tunnel syndrome (CTS) is intermittent pain, paresthesias, and numbness in the median nerve distribution, with later thenar atrophy and weakness, and permanent loss of median sensation in the hand resulting from compression of the median nerve beneath the transverse carpal ligament (TCL). Pronator syndrome (PS) is pain in the proximal third of the forearm anteriorly, with intermittent median paresthesias and no motor symptoms or permanent loss of sensation, resulting from median nerve compression by various muscle or fascial structures in the proximal forearm. Anterior interosseous nerve syndrome (AINS) is palsy of the flexor pollicis longus, flexor digitorum profundus of the index, and pronator quadratus and is of spontaneous or post-traumatic onset.

EPIDEMIOLOGY

MNC affects both males and females from the 3rd decade until old age. Most patients are not heavy or repetitive laborers, but symptoms can be aggravated by work. There are many associated medical conditions, such as rheumatoid arthritis, diabetes, thyroid dysfunction, and the need for renal dialysis. Incidence in workers using repetitive finger and wrist force is controversial.

PATHOGENESIS

CTS occurs acutely after wrist fracture or dislocation as a result of compression by hematoma or direct nerve contusion or stretch. It can accompany metabolic derangements such as amyloidosis, diabetes mellitus, gout, myxedema, multiple myeloma, acromegaly, and pregnancy. CTS patients have an increased incidence of tendinitis and disk disease.[1] Viral neuritis may cause AINS.[2] Tumors and anomalous muscles may be a localized cause of MNC in the differential diagnosis. Repetitive hand use as an etiological factor is controversial and is beyond the scope of this chapter.

CTS is caused by increased carpal canal pressure, which causes the median nerve to be compressed between the transverse carpal ligament and anteriorly and the flexor tendons and bony floor of the carpal canal posteriorly. Chronically, the nerve develops venous congestion, leaking of fluid interstitially, intrafascicular fibrosis, decreased axoplasmic flow, demyelination with sensory and motor fiber dysfunction, and axon degeneration.[3] Over time there is also external fibrosis of the nerve to surrounding structures within the tunnel, which limits nerve excursion with wrist and upper extremity extreme joint motion and may contribute to neuritis.[4] Experimental studies showed increased carpal canal pressure in all wrist positions in CTS patients compared with controls. These elevated pressures fell to normal levels after carpal tunnel release (CTR).[5] Immediate improvement after CTR suggests a vascular mechanism of nerve insult.

PS is caused by compression of the median nerve by the ligament of Struthers and supracondylar process of the humerus, the lacertus fibrosus, the heads of the pronator muscle or fibrous bands within them, or the tendinous origin of the flexor digitorum superficialis after fracture, soft-tissue trauma, or heavy use of the forearm muscles. Alternatively, it may occur spontaneously. AINS is due to a neuritis, as an element of brachial plexitis, after local fracture or soft-tissue trauma of the forearm. The clinical situations in which the PS and AINS occur are well understood and not speculative.

CLINICAL FEATURES

CTS causes paresthesias and pain in the median distribution of the hand, which are worse at night and referred as far proximally as the shoulder. Symptoms can be aggravated by use of the hand and wrist. Some patients note weakness of grip or pinch. Physical examination shows signs of median nerve irritability with paresthesias to median innervated fingers. Tinel's sign is digital percussion over the median nerve in the region of the wrist flexion crease. Phalen's sign is gravity flexion of the wrist. The carpal tunnel compression test is firm, continuous pressure with both thumb tips over the median nerve in the carpal canal. Sensory testing includes two-point discrimination, vibration, and pressure testing with monofilaments at the digital pulp.[6] Inspection may show thenar wasting, and muscle testing may reveal some loss of abduction strength and loss of thumb opposition (Fig. 1).

PS includes swelling and pain in the proximal forearm over the pronator muscle. Median paresthesias can be present, mostly in the thumb and index finger. Physical examination includes Tinel's sign testing over the median nerve in the region of the pronator muscle bellies, which is

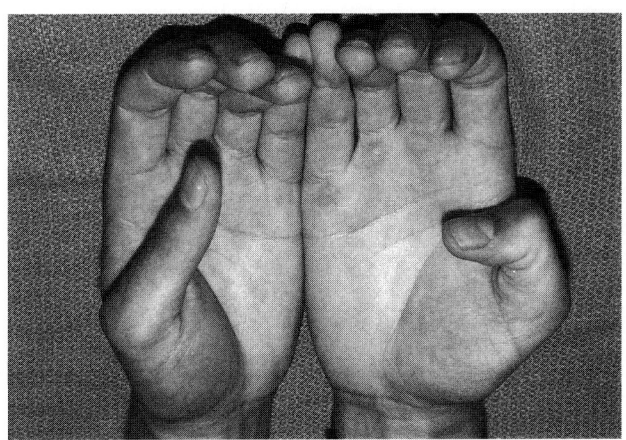

Fig. 2. Incomplete anterior interosseous nerve syndrome palsy. There is associated loss of the right flexor pollicis longus function. Electromyography confirmed involvement of the flexor pollicis longus, flexor digitorum profundus of the index, and pronator quadratus.

often positive. The Phalen sign test can be positive in a minority of patients. Tenderness to palpation of the pronator muscle can reproduce the tenderness felt by the patient, and pain to palpation of the thenar mass is common. Firmness of the pronator muscle is usually present. Median paresthesias elicited with resisted elbow flexion and/or passive pronation implies MNC by the lacertus fibrosus; with resisted pronation, implicates the pronator muscle; and with resisted middle finger flexion, implicates the flexor digitorum superficialis fibrous arch.

AINS includes a history of pain in the shoulder, arm, elbow or forearm, followed by paralysis of either the flexor pollicis longus, flexor digitorum profundus of the index finger, or both. Physical examination shows either partial or complete weakness of the AINS supplied muscles, as tested by resisted distal joint flexion of the thumb and index (Fig. 2). Weakness of the pronator quadratus is also present and, although difficult to test, may be perceptible by testing forearm pronation with the elbow passively flexed to relax the pronator teres. Table 1 provides a summary of these findings.

INVESTIGATION

Knowledge of the general medical condition is important to rule out metabolic causes of CTS, but no specific laboratory test is needed. Radiographs films may show arthrosis or rheumatoid arthritis of the neck, wrist, or fingers or chronic wrist injury (scaphoid nonunion); residual pain in the wrist or digits after CTR could be due to these underlying problems. Electromyography and nerve conduction velocity testing are sensitive and specific for CTS, show severity of nerve involvement, and correlate well with symptoms. However, some consider CTS a clinical diagnosis and base the diagnosis on physical examination, because there are false-negative cases without electrical abnormalities but with severe symptoms in early CTS. Needle testing can be positive for the motor changes in both PS and AINS, but sensory conduction velocity is usually unchanged. In addition, one must rule out other conditions that may simulate CTS (Table 2).

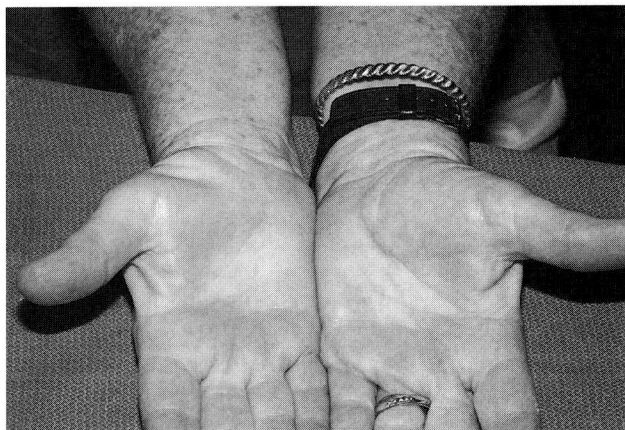

Fig. 1. Carpal tunnel syndrome. These are physical examination findings. Thenar atrophy of right hand secondary to carpal tunnel syndrome is evident.

Examination	CTS	PS	AINS
CT Tinel's sign	+	+ (less than 50%)	−
CT compression test	+	−	−
Phalen's sign	+	+ (approximately 50%)	−
Pronator Tinel's sign	+ (rare)	+	−
Thenar tenderness	+ (rare)	+	−
Palmar wrist tenderness	+	−	−
Weak thenars	+ (late)	−	+ ? MG
Thenar wasting	+ (late)	+ (rare)	−
Weak ulnar intrinsics	−	−	+ ? MG
Weak FPL, FDPII, PQ	−	−	+
Prolonged two-point testing	+ (late)	−	−
Provocative findings (PT, FDS)	−	+	−

TABLE 1. EXAMINATION AND FINDINGS IN MNC

MNC, median nerve compression; MG, Martin-Gruber connection; CT, carpal tunnel; FPL, flexor pollicis longus; FDS, flexor digitorum superficialis; PQ, pronator quadratus; +, present; −, absent.

MANAGEMENT

CARPAL TUNNEL SYNDROME

Conservative treatment for mild CTS is splinting, oral anti-inflammatory drugs, work station modification to avoid awkward positions, and steroid injection, which will relieve symptoms long term in approximately 20% of patients.[7]

TABLE 2. DIFFERENTIAL DIAGNOSIS OF MNC

Condition	Key Findings
Cervical radiculopathy	Neck pain and stiffness
	Bilateral upper extremity symptoms
	No relief after carpal tunnel injection
	Normal sensory latency
	Signs of root irritation on exam
Thoracic outlet syndrome	Sensory and vascular changes in hand
	Symptoms related to shoulder position
	Cervical rib or clavicle malunion
	Ring and little finger involved
Overuse strain phenomenon	Nonanatomic distribution of pain
	No signs of peripheral nerve irritation
Raynaud's phenomenon	Temperature and color changes in hand
	Pain associated with vascular changes
Angina	Pain into left upper extremity
	Associated chest symptoms
Double crush syndrome	CTS coupled with signs of MNC proximally
Median nerve tumor	Local findings at atypical sites

MNC, median nerve compression; CTS, carpal tunnel syndrome.

Corticosteroid injection is the treatment for severe CTS of pregnancy, which does not respond to splinting. This is performed by the patient's obstetrician. An injection that gives temporary relief has diagnostic value and can help differentiate between symptoms caused by CTS and those caused by another site of compression.

With sterile technique the patient is injected with a mixture of 2 mL 1% plain lidocaine and 1 mL steroid solution (e.g., betamethasone, 6 mg/mL) at the wrist flexion crease in a line between the third and fourth metacarpals and ulnar and parallel to the palmaris longus tendon and median nerve. Needle motion with gentle finger flexion confirms accurate placement.

Preoperative Planning

The decision for surgery is individualized, based on the patient's medical condition, age, severity of symptoms, severity of compression, social situation, work needs, expectations, and functional goals. A young patient for whom heavy work or hobbies aggravate symptoms is warned that approximately half of patients will return to the same activity symptom free postoperatively, and that surgery is being done primarily to prevent progression of nerve damage. Cases involving the elderly with pain, paresthesias, and numbness subjectively and thenar wasting and loss of sensibility on physical exam are very special. These patients need to be warned that irreversible fibrosis and axonal loss preclude full recovery and that the pain and paresthesias will be relieved more than the numbness. Diabetics, despite their peripheral neuropathy, can expect substantial relief of sensory symptoms if well localized to the carpal tunnel on physical and electrical testing.

Surgical Approach

Two surgical options exist: standard open and endoscopic CTR. The method chosen depends on the surgeon's experience and expertise; specific training is necessary for the endoscopic method.

The open method is performed under local or regional anesthetic with intravenous sedation and a tourniquet. A linear incision is made over the carpal canal, in a line between the third and fourth metacarpals, from the wrist flexion crease to a level just proximal to the base of the thumb flexion crease (Fig. 3), ulnar to the palmaris longus tendon and its palmar fascial insertion, the median nerve, and the thenar cutaneous nerve, and radial to the ulnar neurovascular bundle. The skin, subcutaneous tissue, palmar fascia, palmaris brevis, and transverse carpal ligament are all sharply incised with a scalpel in the same line. Care is taken, aided by magnification, to look for anomalous motor branching through the TCL, crossing from ulnar to radial, and to avoid damage to the superficial palmar arch and digital nerve branches. The distal forearm fascia and remainder of the TCL proximal to the wrist flexion crease are released under direct vision in the same line. This approach leaves a radial flap of TCL covering the median nerve and prevents bowstringing and scarring to the palmar fascia or subcutaneous tissue.

The standard open method of CTR is the most time tested and the least controversial method. Advantages include a complete view of the median nerve and its potential anomalies, the digital nerves, and the superficial palmar arch. Although patients with ipsilateral ulnar entrapment in

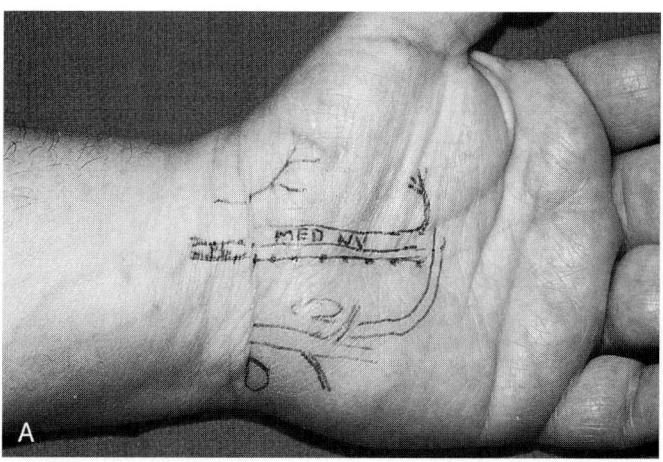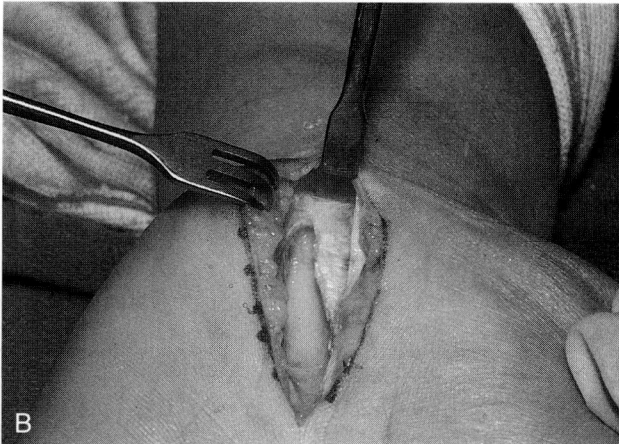

Fig. 3. Surgical technique of open and endoscopic carpal tunnel release (CTR). *A,* Landmarks of open CTR showing an incision (dotted line) between the third and fourth metacarpals, ulnar to the palmaris longus and median nerve (med nv). The thenar cutaneous nerve (top), thenar motor branch (off nerve radially), ulnar artery (bottom), and superficial arch (distal to incision) are marked. *B,* Longitudinal view of the median nerve beneath the radial edge of the cut transverse carpal ligament (TCL), and the proximal TCL before release in direct view proximal to the wrist flexion crease.

Guyon's canal will not require a formal release ulnarly because TCL section also relieves ulnar nerve compression, the need for entering Guyon's canal is facilitated by the standard approach. This approach is also extensile, and if flexor tenosynovectomy or dissection of anomalous muscles or nerve tumors is required, it can easily be accomplished simultaneously. The only potential disadvantage is transient, minimally symptomatic palmar scar sensitivity in most patients. Advocates of endoscopic methods have used this as an impetus for developing their technique.

Endoscopic Release

Endoscopic release can be done with either one proximal incision[8] or with one distal incision and one proximal incision.[9] The advantages include the absence of a palmar scar and possibly a more rapid return to work. Disadvantages include the possibility for incomplete release of the flexor retinaculum, injury to the median or its branches, ulnar nerve injury, superficial arch laceration, and flexor tendon transection.

Complications
Residual Symptoms

The most common complication in both the open and closed methods is residual paresthesias and numbness, present in approximately one-third of patients. This can be due to incomplete release of the TCL or changes in the chronically compressed nerve that preclude full recovery. Postoperative factors are persistent flexor tenosynovitis and scarring of the median nerve under the TCL. Additional factors in the persistence of symptoms is history of heavy laboring jobs, ongoing worker compensation cases, and inability to return to work after surgery.

Some cases of persistent sensory symptoms require reoperation. Reoperation for CTS is done for persistent symptoms that are as severe as or worse than those preoperatively. Results of reoperation, assuming the ligament has previously been completely divided, are unreliable. Neurolysis, tenolysis, tenosynovectomy, epineurotomy, internal neurolysis, or local flap coverage of the median nerve did not routinely relieve symptoms. In one study, only 38 of 131 reoperations (29%) were completely successful.[10]

Palmar Incisional Tenderness

Most patients will have some scar tenderness with hand use after open CTR. This is an expected outcome after any palmar incision and perhaps should not be considered a complication.

Nerve and Vessel Injury

Injury of the palmar cutaneous branch is reported but is also associated with a transverse incision that was obviously carried too radially. This should be avoidable with the standard open linear incision ulnar to the palmar longus. The recurrent motor branch is normally radial to the incision, and with careful distal dissection and vigilance in detecting its variants, damage should be avoidable.

Decreased Grip Strength

Grip strength decreases after open CTR and, in one study, returned to normal approximately 3 months later.[11] The spread of the carpal bones could account for some change in grip strength and wrist pain after CTR, especially in patients with preexisting wrist or thumb carpometacarpal arthrosis, but may also be the mechanism of increasing the space of the carpal canal after CTR.

Reflex Sympathetic Dystrophy

Reflex sympathetic dystrophy is extremely rare after CTR. It occurred in 2 of 107 cases of endoscopic CTR in one study[12] and with a similar low incidence with the open method.[13]

Bowstringing of the Median Nerve

With excessive wrist flexion after open CTR, it is possible for the median nerve to move anteriorly and become scarred to the palmar tissues at the incision. This can be prevented by a postoperative palmar splint in slight wrist extension while the wound heals.

Trigger Finger

Occasionally, very soon postoperatively, the patient experiences a symptomatic trigger finger. This often involves the middle and ring fingers. This may be due to either flexor tenosynovial swelling or anterior translation of the flexor tendons after TCL release. It is treated by steroid injection or surgery if unrelieved.

Infection

Infection in a clean case such as CTR should be less than 1%. The infection rate is higher if associated with a flexor tenosynovectomy or placement of a drain and is higher in diabetic patients.

Results

Modern studies of CTR are outcome studies that compare open and endoscopic methods. Success rates for relief of pain and paresthesias are high with both methods: 98% and 99%, respectively, in one study[26] and 96% and 97%, respectively, in another.[27] Agee et al[8] reported that 85% of patients undergoing the open method and 86% of those undergoing the endoscopic method had relief of tingling at final follow-up. Most young patients with CTS will immediately experience great relief of pain and paresthesias, and most with prior night symptoms report undisturbed sleep soon postoperatively. Sensation of small objects and light touch is also enhanced very quickly. Older patients, however, with long-standing CTS will have relief of pain and paresthesias, but numbness and inability to feel small objects such as coins and buttons will likely remain.

Regarding scar tenderness, two studies showed a higher incidence in the open method[8, 14] but whether this persisted long after the final follow-up period or eventually equalized is not known. Scar sensitivity is an expected result after any palmar incision, and patients should be warned about it preoperatively. The scar usually becomes most tender at approximately 6 to 8 weeks, which corresponds with the time when more vigorous hand use is begun. The tenderness is easily treated with reassurance, and local measures such as a conforming gel pad and gentle scar massage are needed until symptoms abate.

Regarding motor recovery, 65% of the open group and 80% of the endoscopic group had no weakness at final follow-up.[8] One study showed no significant difference in motor recovery between the two groups.[14] A study of open release found improvement in thenar strength and wasting in most patients, but this took more than 2 years to occur in some patients.[15]

Regarding return to work, endoscopic patients returned on average 14 days earlier,[14] 21 days earlier,[8] or at the same time as open-release method patients.[16] One study addressed this question retrospectively and showed that 11 of 28 patients who engaged in heavy labor preoperatively had a poor result and did not return to their original work. What was not addressed is whether or not their symptoms prevented work preoperatively.[17]

PRONATOR SYNDROME AND ANTERIOR INTEROSSEOUS NERVE SYNDROME

Conservative treatment of PS is generally ineffective because of the mechanical isolated nature of the compression. Theoretically, a steroid and lidocaine injection could lessen symptoms or could be diagnostic if it provided some relief; this approach, however, has not systematically been tried. External landmarks are difficult to define for injection about the median nerve in the proximal forearm, and great care must be taken to not inject the nerve or the radial and ulnar arteries. Surgical release of the median nerve resulted in relief of sensory symptoms in 47 of 51 (92%) in one study; poor results were related to the complication of nerve scarring and injury.[18] Another study showed full relief in 28 of 36 (77%) and partial relief in an additional five.[19]

For AINS the first line of treatment is simple observation because it has been shown that many cases will resolve spontaneously. The rationale for spontaneous resolution is that this disease is actually a viral neuritis. Exploration is done if recovery does not occur after a limited period of observation, such as 2 to 3 months.[20] Most patients recover quickly after neurolysis. Complications are minimal with careful nerve dissection.

Operative Approach for Pronator and Anterior Interosseous Syndromes

The incision is begun medial to the biceps tendon, over the median nerve and brachial artery. The incision then curves distally into the antecubital crease and then continues either linearly or in a zigzag fashion in the midline of the anterior forearm, until the junction of the middle and distal thirds. Release begins with finding the median nerve and brachial artery first proximally, deep to the fascia of the arm, near the ligament of Struthers if present. The nerve and artery are traced distally, beneath the lacertus fibrosus, which is completely released. This will reveal the bifurcation of the artery into radial and ulnar arteries, which are both labeled with vessel loops and protected, and the entry of the median nerve between the ulnar and humeral heads of the pronator teres. Fibrous bands connecting the heads or abnormally large muscular vessels can be released at this time. The proximal motor nerve to the pronator teres should be protected as it enters the humeral head. The ulnar head of the pronator teres can be released distally near the radius and the humeral head retracted proximally to reveal the median nerve diving dorsal to the flexor superficialis fibrous arch, which is carefully released. The humeral head may not need to be released if the median nerve can be visualized and protected dorsal to it by retracting the muscle proximally and distally as needed. A common interosseous artery and occasionally a median artery will branch off the radial artery at this level and should be protected. The anterior interosseous nerve will branch off the radial side of the median nerve at the same level and continue distally and radially toward the flexor pollicis longus on the fascia anterior to the flexor profundus muscle bellies.

The PS release is complete after dividing the flexor digitorum superficialis arch. The AINS release begins as the pronator release, because the nerve can branch proximally and run with the median nerve beneath the lacertus and pronator teres and continues more distally. Lesions found at release include compression by the lacertus fibrosus, fibrous bands of either head of the pronator teres, and fibrous bands or anomalous vessels at the flexor digitorum superficialis fibrous arch.

REFERENCES

1. Murray-Leslie F, Wright V: Carpal tunnel syndrome, humeral epicondylitis and the cervical spine: A study of clinical and dimensional relations. BMJ 1976; 5:1439.
2. Parsonage MJ, Turner JWA: Neuralgic amyotrophy: The shoulder girdle syndrome. Lancet 1948; 1:973.
3. Dahlin LB, Rydevik B: Pathophysiology of nerve compression. In Gelberman, RH (ed): Operative Nerve Repair and Reconstruction. Philadelphia, JB Lippincott, 1991, p 847.
4. Wright TW, Glowczewskie F, Wheeler D, et al: Excursion and strain of the median nerve. J Bone Joint Surg Am 1997; 78: 1897.
5. Gelberman RH, Hergenroeder PT, Hargens AR, et al: The carpal tunnel syndrome. A study of carpal canal pressures. J Bone Joint Surg Am 1981; 63:380.
6. Gelberman RH, Szabo RM, Williamson RV, et al: Sensibility testing in peripheral-nerve compression syndromes. J Bone Joint Surg Am 1983; 65:632.
7. Gelberman RH, Aronson D, Weisman MH: Carpal-tunnel syndrome. Results of a prospective trial of steroid injection and splinting. J Bone Joint Surg Am 1980; 62: 1181.

8. Agee J, McCarroll H, Tortosa RD, et al: Endoscopic release of the carpal tunnel: A randomized prospective multicenter study. J Hand Surg [Am] 1992; 17:987.
9. Chow J: Endoscopic release of the carpal ligament: A new technique for carpal tunnel syndrome. Arthroscopy 1989; 5:19.
10. Cobb TK, Amadio PC, Leatherwood DF, et al: Outcome of reoperation for carpal tunnel syndrome. J Hand Surg [Am] 1996; 21:347.
11. Gellman H, Kan D, Gee V, et al: Analysis of pinch and grip strength after carpal tunnel release. J Hand Surg Am 1989; 14: 863.
12. Shinya K, Lanzetta M, Conolly B: Risk and complications in endoscopic carpal tunnel release. J Hand Surg Br 1995; 20: 222.
13. Conolly WB: Pitfalls in carpal tunnel decompression. Aust N Z J Surg 1978; 48: 421.
14. Brown RA, Gelberman RH, Seiler JG, et al: Carpal tunnel release. A prospective randomized assessment of open and endoscopic methods. J Bone Joint Surg Am 1993; 75:1265.

15. Gelberman RH, Pfeffer GB, Gailbraith RT, et al: Results of treatment of severe carpal-tunnel syndrome without internal neurolysis of the median nerve. J Bone Joint Surg Am 1987; 64:896.
16. Bande S, De Smet L, Fabry G: The results of carpal tunnel release: Open versus endoscopic technique. J Hand Surg [Br] 1994; 19:14.
17. Al-Quattan MM, Bowen V, Manktelow RT: Factors associated with poor outcome following primary carpal tunnel release in non-diabetic patients. J Hand Surg [Br] 1994; 19:622.
18. Johnson RK, Spinner M, Shrewsberry MM: Median nerve entrapment syndrome in the proximal forearm. J Hand Surg 1979; 4:48.
19. Hartz CB, Linscheid RL, Gramse RR, et al: The pronator teres syndrome: Compressive neuropathy of the median nerve. J Bone Joint Surg Am 1981; 63:885.
20. Spinner M: The anterior interosseous-nerve syndrome. With special attention to its variations. J Bone Joint Surg Am 1970; 52:84.

section
12
chapter
28

RADIAL NERVE COMPRESSION SYNDROMES

Divya Singh and Thomas Breen

Summary

- While less frequent than compressive neuropathy of the medial or ulnar nerves, compressive neuropathy of the radial nerve does occur.
- Radial tunnel (between the two blocks of the supinator muscle) syndrome, the most common radial nerve compression neuropathy, is often confused with "tennis elbow."
- Radial nerve compressive neuropathy is usually relieved by nonoperative treatment (activity modification, splinting, and nonsteroidal anti-inflammatory drugs).
- Operative treatment is reserved for radial nerve entrapment symptoms not responsive to nonoperative treatment that have been troublesome for more than 3 months.
- Wartenberg's syndrome—mononeuritis of the superficial nervous branch of the radial nerve—can usually be relieved by nonoperative treatment.

ANATOMY

Although involved less than the median and ulnar nerves, the radial nerve can also be affected by compressive neuropa-

thies. Knowledge of radial nerve anatomy is central to understanding the pathophysiology and the treatment of radial compression (Fig. 1). The radial nerve arises from the posterior cord of the brachial plexus, involving roots C5-8 (sometimes T1). Along with the profunda brachii artery, the radial nerve winds posteriorly and laterally along the spiral groove of the humerus, passing beneath the fibrous arch at the origin of the lateral head of the triceps. The nerve passes posterior to anterior approximately 10–12 cm proximal to the elbow, at the lateral intermuscular septum. The nerve follows the lateral border of the brachialis and emerges between the brachialis and brachioradialis, anterior and proximal to the lateral epicondyle. In the arm it supplies the triceps, part of the brachialis (along with the musculocutaneous nerve), the anconeus, the extensor carpi radialis longus (ECRL), and the brachioradialis. About 3 cm proximal or distal to the elbow, it divides into the posterior interosseous nerve (PIN), the superficial radial (sensory) nerve, and the branch to the extensor carpi radialis brevis (ECRB).[1]

The PIN dives between the two heads of the supinator, entering the radial tunnel. The tunnel is formed by the brachialis and biceps tendon medially, the origin of the brachioradialis laterally, and the lateral humeral epicondyle

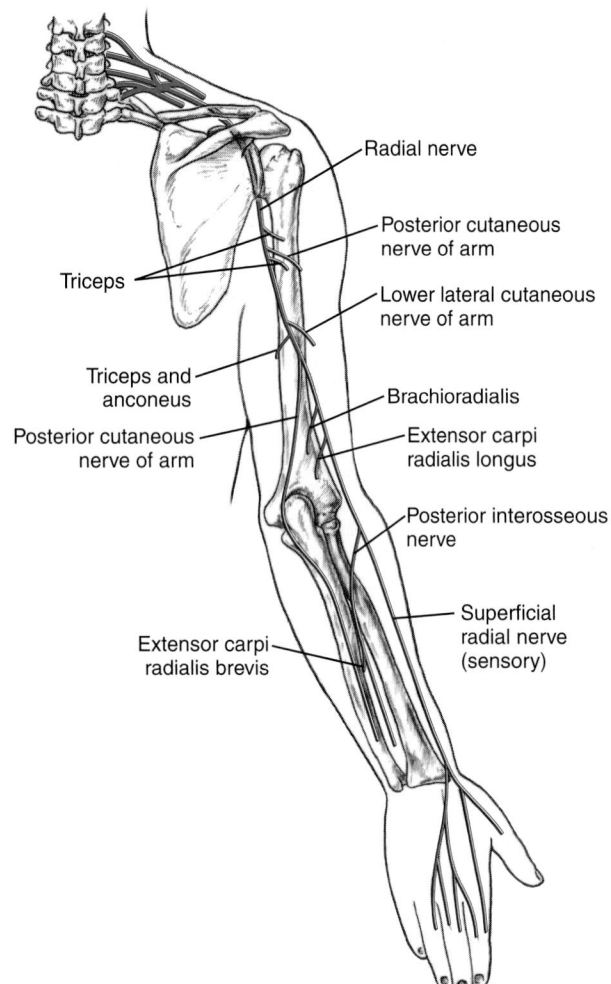

Fig. 1. The course of the radial nerve.

posteriorly. The floor is formed by the radiocapitellar joint capsule.[1] The various sites of compression within the radial tunnel are discussed below. Once the nerve leaves the radial tunnel, it winds along the proximal third of the radius for approximately 4 cm. The nerve is in contact with the periosteum at a bare area at the level of the bicipital tuberosity during supination. After leaving the supinator, the PIN goes on to innervate the wrist, finger, and thumb extensors. Distally, it travels within the fourth dorsal extensor compartment, providing sensory innervation of the wrist capsule and intercarpal ligaments.

The superficial radial nerve proceeds deep to the brachioradialis, running along the radial forearm and parallel to the radial artery in the middle third of the forearm. This nerve exits the fascia and becomes more superficial between the ECRL and brachioradialis tendons. The exit site varies and may be proximal in the mid forearm or distal, a few centimeters proximal to the radial styloid. After the radial sensory nerve crosses the dorsal retinaculum, it divides into five digital dorsal branches, with variable distributions that may include sensation to the thumb dorsum and first web space, the thenar eminence, and the dorsum

of the long, index, and ring to the posterior interphalangeal.

PROXIMAL SITES OF COMPRESSION

"Honeymoon palsy" and "Saturday night palsy" are secondary to acute radial nerve entrapment from external pressure in the axilla. (Proximal compression may also be caused by improper use of crutches).[2] There is weakness of the triceps and brachioradialis and sensory loss (secondary to the posterior cutaneous nerves). Wrist drop results from paralysis of the ECRB, ECRL, and extensor carpi ulnaris (ECU). There is also digital extensor paralysis.[1]

The radial nerve may be compressed at the lateral intermuscular septum, at the junction of the middle and distal thirds of the arm. This site of compression is more common than is recognized and may be associated with displaced humeral fractures or with humeral open reduction and internal fixation (especially if an anterolateral approach is used). Simple neurapraxial injuries to the radial nerve have a good prognosis, usually recovering spontaneously with a month or two. Patients presenting with a humerus fracture and a radial nerve palsy are almost always a neurapraxial injury, whereas radial nerve dysfunction presenting after a fracture reduction may be the result of nerve entrapment within the fracture.

High radial nerve palsies tend to resolve spontaneously. Observation for at least 3 months is indicated. If no recovery is seen on electromyography with persistent symptoms, exploration of the nerve is warranted. In paralysis persisting for more than 18 months, tendon transfers are the most predictable and preferred treatment.[3]

RADIAL TUNNEL SYNDROME/PIN SYNDROME

Although the sites of compression overlap between these two syndromes, the syndromes present distinct clinical pictures. PIN syndrome results primarily in motor loss (partial or complete paralysis of wrist and finger extension); radial tunnel syndrome (RTS) is characterized by pain along the lateral forearm (Fig. 2). Sensation in the hand and forearm is usually intact in both syndromes.

The common sites of compression are (from radial head to supinator muscle)[1, 4]

- Fibrous tissue anterior to the radial head at the entrance of the tunnel.
- Radial recurrent vessels (Henry's leash).
- Leading fibrous edge of the ECRB.
- Proximal edge of the supinator (Frohse's arcade).
- Intramuscular band or the distal edge of the supinator.

RADIAL TUNNEL SYNDROME

This is the most common radial neuropathy.[4] RTS affects middle-aged men and women equally, with an insidious onset.[1] Signs and symptoms include tenderness over the radial tunnel, with pain on palpation at the antebrachial fossa along the site of radial nerve and mobile wad. There may be pain at the lateral epicondyle, which has led to RTS being dubbed "resistant tennis elbow." Patients also

**THE RADIAL TUNNEL
SITES OF POSSIBLE COMPRESSION**

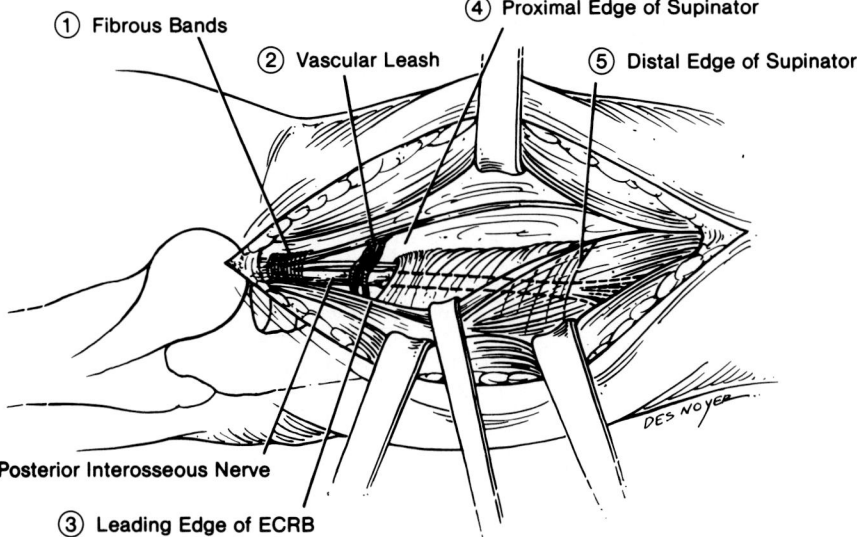

Fig. 2. Anatomy of the radial tunnel. (From Gelberman RH: Operative Nerve Repair and Reconstruction. Philadelphia, JB Lippincott, 1991.)

have pain over the extensor muscle mass when extending the middle finger against resistance (with the wrist in neutral and the elbow in 45 to 90 degrees of flexion) and pain with resisted forearm supination (with the elbow in extension). A positive middle finger test results from tightening the ECRB fascia.[1]

The physical examination is the most useful diagnostic tool. Electromyogram results are nearly always abnormal in PINS and nearly always normal in RTS. Measurement results obtained during resisted supination may be abnormal in RTS.[3] The major differential diagnosis of RTS is lateral epicondylitis. Distinguish between the two based on the point of maximal tenderness: the lateral epicondyle in lateral epicondylitis; the mobile wad and supinator in radial tunnel syndrome.[1]

PIN SYNDROME

Patients with PIN syndrome present with more weakness than paralysis. There may be an inability to extend the metacarpophalangeal joint of the fingers and thumb. Wrist extension is generally preserved, but the wrist deviates radially secondary to paralysis of the ECU and preservation of the ECRL/ECRB.

Causes include repetitive stress (especially pronation/supination) or compression from ganglion or bursae. The proximal edge of the supinator is the most likely cause of compression in PIN syndrome. Men are affected twice as often as women. The onset of weakness is rapid: overnight to weeks, with gradual paralysis of different extensors. It is important to distinguish PIN syndrome from digital or thumb extensor tendon rupture. In PIN syndrome, the extensor tendons are intact and the fingers extend passively at the metacarpophalangeal joint with passive wrist flexion.[5]

Treatment

Nonsurgical. Initial management involves activity modification, splinting with the fingers in extension,[2] and anti-

inflammatory medication. Avoid activities with excessive supination and pronation.

Surgical. Surgery is reserved for symptoms lasting longer than 3 months and not responsive to conservative management. The surgical approach is based on the site of compression (Fig. 3).

Anterolateral Approach. This is the more generalized approach to RTS, allowing exploration of the radial nerve. Begin the incision 5 cm proximal to the elbow crease, along the ulnar border of the mobile wad (brachioradialis and brachialis proximally; ECRB and pronator teres distally), and ligate Henry's leash. Keep the forearm in supination, and free the PIN throughout its course through the supinator. This is the generally preferred approach because of its extensile nature.[1,4]

Posterior Approach. Begin the incision 2 cm distal to the lateral epicondyle and extend it distally for 7 cm. Expose the supinator and, more proximally, the radial nerve. This exposure is limited and useful when the compression has been localized to Frohse's arcade.[4] Splint postoperatively. Begin early range of motion, using a splint for 1 to 2 weeks. Recovery may take 3 to 4 months.

SUPERFICIAL RADIAL NERVE ENTRAPMENT

In 1932 Robert Wartenberg described a mononeuritis of the superficial sensory branch of the radial nerve, an entity he called *cheiralgia paresthetica,* now also known as Wartenberg's syndrome.[6] Possible sites of compression are based on where the nerve becomes more superficial: it emerges between the brachioradialis and the ECRL, and this can vary from midforearm to just proximal to the radial styloid.[3] The distal sites of pain are usually from external sources of compression, such as a watchband. Symptoms include pain, paresthesia, or hyperesthesias over the dorsoradial skin of the hand. Ulnar deviation and frequent pronation/supination

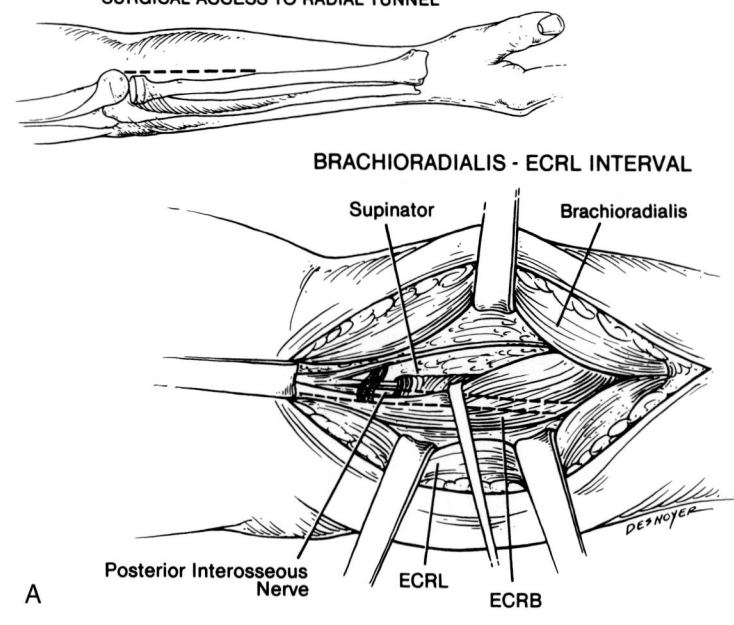

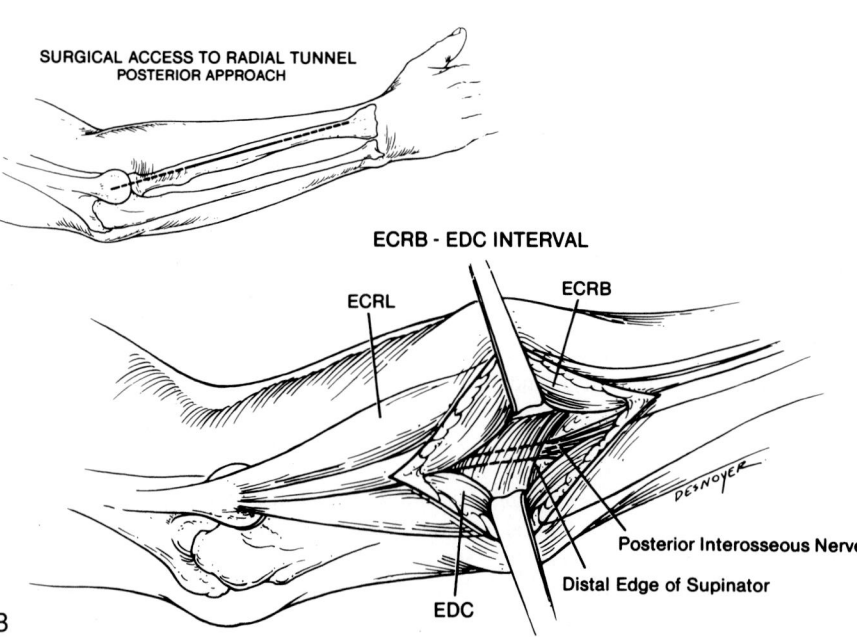

Fig. 3. Surgical approaches for radial tunnel release. (From Gelberman RH: Operative Nerve Repair and Reconstruction. Philadelphia, JB Lippincott, 1991.)

activities aggravate the symptoms. Clinical signs include positive Tinel's and Finkelstein's tests. The differential diagnosis includes intersection syndrome, de Quervain's tenosynovitis, and lateral antebrachial cutaneous nerve irritation (there is often an overlap in sensory distribution between the two nerves). Note that Finkelstein's test may be positive in intersection, de Quervain's, and Wartenberg's syndrome.

Initial treatment consists of removing the offending source of compression, splinting, and desensitization. A cortisone injection may be helpful. In refractory cases, surgical intervention may be necessary. If the compression is more proximal, the nerve can be released between the ECRL and brachioradialis. If the symptoms are more distal, neurolysis, protective isolation (e.g., a vein graft), or ablation can be used.[3]

TERMINAL BRANCH OF THE PIN

The terminal branch of the PIN is in the fourth extensor compartment. Patients present with aching on the dorsum of the wrist, over the fourth dorsal compartment, aggravated by repeated wrist dorsiflexion. Compression may be from a neuroma after nerve graft harvest.

Treatment involves NSAIDs, splinting, and activity modification.[3]

REFERENCES

1. Barnum M, Mastey RD, Weiss APC, et al: Radial tunnel syndrome. Hand Clin 1996; 12:679.
2. Kleinert JM, Mehta S: Radial nerve entrapment. Orthop Clin North Am 1996; 27:305.
3. Osterman AL, Babhulkar S: Unusual compressive neuropathies of the upper limb. Ortho Clin North Am 1996; 27:389.
4. Eversmann WW Jr: Entrapment and compression neuropathies In Green DP (ed): Operative Hand Surgery, 3rd ed. New York, Churchill Livingstone, 1993, p 1454.
5. Gelberman RH: Operative Nerve Repair and Reconstruction. Philadelphia, JB Lippincott, 1991.
6. Ehrlich W, Dellon AL, Mackinnon SE: Cheiralgia paresthetica (entrapment of the radial sensory nerve). J Hand Surg Am 1986; 11:196.

section 12 chapter 29

ULNAR NERVE COMPRESSION

Brian D. Adams

Summary

- Ulnar neuropathy at the elbow is the second most common peripheral nerve entrapment after carpal tunnel syndrome.
- Although it is generally considered a compression neuropathy, the term cubital tunnel syndrome is frequently used to convey its complex pathophysiology.
- Early diagnosis is made by history and physical examination because electrophysiological changes occur late.
- Operative treatment is indicated for neurological deficits or persistent symptoms.
- If atrophy is present, surgery will often not produce complete recovery.
- Selection of one of several effective operative procedures is based on the cause of the neuropathy and surgeon preference.

DEFINITION

Ulnar neuropathy at the elbow is generally considered a compression or entrapment neuropathy; however, a variety of anatomic and physiological factors may contribute to its development. Thus, the term cubital tunnel syndrome is frequently used when a specific cause is not identified. The term tardy ulnar nerve palsy was originally coined to describe a delayed ulnar neuropathy from a post-traumatic valgus deformity of the elbow. Recurrent subluxation or dislocation of the nerve over the medial epicondyle is a known cause of neuritis. However, it is a common and frequently asymptomatic finding.

HISTORICAL REVIEW

In 1878, Panas first documented ulnar nerve compression at the elbow, which he treated by deepening the epicondylar groove. The first anterior nerve transposition is credited to Lausanne in 1897, and 1 year later Curtis[1] was the first to document a subcutaneous transposition, which he performed for a post-traumatic palsy. In 1916, Hunt introduced the term tardy ulnar nerve palsy to convey the de-

layed presentation of a neuropathy after a valgus malunion of the distal humerus. Osborne described the fascia, which often bears his name, that extends between the origins of the two heads of the flexor carpi ulnaris (FCU). Feindel and Stratford[2] further emphasized the ulnar nerve's predisposition to compression as a result of the anatomy near the elbow. They coined the term cubital tunnel syndrome. The various operative treatments currently used have their origins in the first half of the 19th century. Osborne[3] proposed in situ decompression, King and Morgan[4] first described medial epicondylectomy, Adson introduced intramuscular transposition, and Learmonth[5] was the first to advocate submuscular transposition.

EPIDEMIOLOGY

Ulnar neuropathy at the elbow is the second most common peripheral nerve entrapment after carpal tunnel syndrome. Although the majority of cases are idiopathic according to our current understanding of the condition, there may be a specific mechanical cause. Recurrent subluxation or dislocation of the ulnar nerve over the medial epicondyle has been found in up to 16% of the general population and is generally asymptomatic.[6] However, a dislocating nerve is predisposed to friction neuritis, especially in the throwing athlete. Work-related activities involving repetitive elbow flexion and extension may aggravate cubital tunnel syndrome, but no scientific data exist to support work as a true cause or risk factor. Because of its superficial position, the nerve is predisposed to direct compression during a surgical procedure if the arm is improperly positioned or inadequately padded. A valgus malunion of the distal humerus was once a relatively common cause for ulnar neuropathy. A severe flexion contracture of the elbow may also produce a delayed neuropathy. In the current era of high-energy trauma and internal fixation, post-traumatic conditions can involve the nerve through incarceration in callous, heterotopic bone, or scar. Burn patients are also at risk for these problems. Synovitis or osteophytes from arthritis can encroach on the nerve at the epicondylar groove. Similarly, ganglia and other space-occupying lesions can cause compression. Although polyneuropathy often affects the ulnar nerve, the potential for coexisting entrapment at the elbow should also be considered.

ANATOMY AND PATHOGENESIS

The ulnar nerve is a branch of the medial cord of the brachial plexus with its primary contributions from the C7, C8, and T1 nerve roots. Along its course near the elbow, several potential sites for entrapment exist (Fig. 1). The nerve enters this region by passing through the medial intermuscular septum from the anterior to the posterior compartment of the arm to lie on the anterior surface of the medial head of the triceps muscle. The septum is a rare cause of entrapment; however, it marks the proximal extent of the arcade of Struthers, which is frequently implicated in ulnar nerve compression. The prevalence, dimensions, and composition of the arcade are debated, but it is typically described as a 2-cm wide fascial band located approximately 8 cm proximal to the medial epicondyle and composed of fibers derived primarily from the medial intermuscular septum and the enveloping fascia of the triceps.[7] After exiting the arcade, the nerve continues anterior to the medial head of the triceps, which is occasionally prominent or hypertrophic, and with elbow flexion it can compress the nerve against the distal aspect of the septum and the supracondylar ridge of the humerus. The nerve then passes through the epicondylar groove. This fibro-osseous groove is bounded anteriorly by the medial epicondyle, laterally by the olecranon and elbow joint capsule, and medially by a fibroaponeurotic band. On exiting the groove, the nerve passes between the humeral and ulnar heads of the FCU muscle. In the first few centimeters of its course through the muscle, the nerve proceeds deep to a stout fibrous band that connects the superficial surfaces of the two muscle heads. This band is often referred to as Osborne's ligament.[3] The passageway for the nerve beneath this ligament has been named the true cubital tunnel, and it is a frequently implicated site of compression. After the nerve proceeds through the FCU muscle for approximately 2 to 5 cm, it dives under the deep flexor-pronator muscle fascia to lie between the flexor digitorum superficialis and the flexor digitorum profundus muscles in the proximal forearm. This deep fascia is occasionally thickened and presents the most distal site for potential ulnar nerve compression near the elbow.[8]

Any one or a combination of these sites may produce entrapment; however, the pathogenesis of entrapment neuropathy at sites of normal anatomic narrowing is poorly understood. Nerve compression, nerve traction, and conditions intrinsic to the nerve are probably all involved in the process. Fibrosis and thickening of tissues surrounding the nerve or hypertrophy of adjacent muscles, such as the medial head of the triceps or the FCU, are frequently cited as causes of compression. Although hypertrophy of muscle is a natural phenomenon, the stimulation for fibrosis in the absence of notable trauma is unknown. Perhaps fibrosis, especially at the epicondylar groove, is induced by repetitive microtrauma from resting the arm at this site or from an exuberant response to the stresses produced by natural elbow motion. Repetitive throwing accentuates normal stretching of the nerve, especially during the cocking and acceleration phases. Any mechanical tethering of the nerve along its course will accentuate this neural tension. Although nerve subluxation or dislocation is the most common cause for friction neuritis, medial traction spurs and irregularities along the medial joint line can also irritate the nerve.

CLINICAL FEATURES

HISTORY

The history often lacks an inciting event; however, there may have been a traumatic episode or recent change in activity that predisposes to a neuropathy, including a change in occupation or workstation where the patient is chronically leaning on the elbow or holding the elbow flexed. Because the ulnar nerve is relatively exposed at the epicondylar groove, especially if it subluxates over the medial epicondyle, direct trauma as in contact sports can result in nerve contusion. Although this injury usually resolves, it may be the initiating factor of a chronic neuropathy. The nerve may have been damaged during an operative procedure in which the arm was resting on the elbow as a result of improper positioning or inadequate padding.[9]

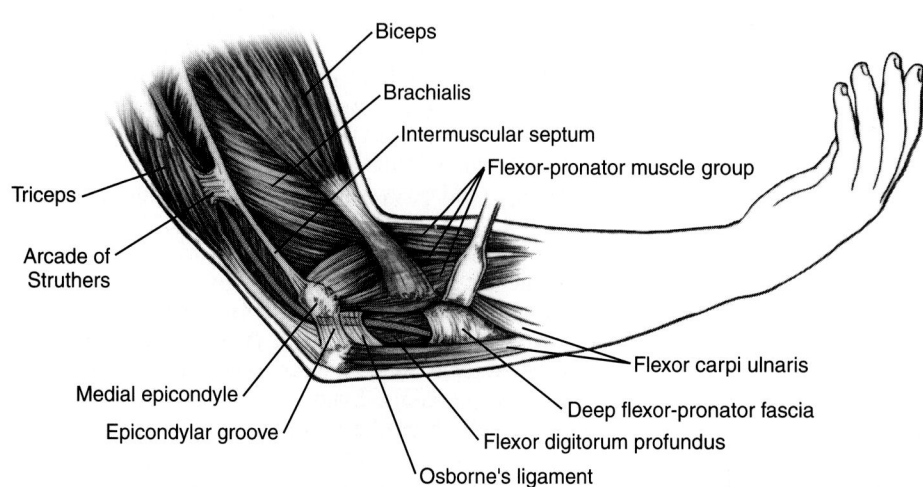

Triceps

Biceps

Brachialis

Intermuscular septum

Flexor-pronator muscle group

Arcade of Struthers

Medial epicondyle

Epicondylar groove

Osborne's ligament

Flexor digitorum profundus

Deep flexor-pronator fascia

Flexor carpi ulnaris

Fig. 1. Course of the ulnar nerve at the elbow and potential sites of compression.

Presenting symptoms vary from mild numbness or paresthesias in the ring and small fingers to severe medial elbow pain. A complaint of cold on the ulnar side of the hand is common. Muscle weakness generally develops after the onset of numbness. Although some individuals report hand fatigue, clumsiness, or difficulty performing certain tasks early on, advanced weakness is typically a late complaint and affects intrinsic function long before any deterioration is noted in the flexor digitorum profundus. Nocturnal paresthesias that routinely awaken the patient are less common with cubital tunnel syndrome than carpal tunnel syndrome. Medial elbow pain is common but is frequently difficult to localize and often associated with radiation into the forearm.

PHYSICAL EXAMINATION

The physical examination should begin at the neck and proceed distally, looking for evidence of cervical disease, brachial plexopathy, and thoracic outlet syndrome. The elbow is inspected for signs of swelling, decreased motion, and an increased carrying angle. Tenderness may be present along the course of the nerve, especially at the epicondylar groove and the proximal portion of the FCU. Observe and palpate for evidence of nerve subluxation or dislocation over the medial epicondyle or a snapping medial head of the triceps muscle. A Tinel sign is sought; however, approximately 25% of asymptomatic people will have a positive test.[10] The elbow flexion test is performed with the elbow maximally flexed and the forearm in supination and wrist in comfortable extension. This test is also falsely positive in up to 24% of the normal population.[10] Applying gentle compression to the nerve at the epicondylar groove with the index and long fingers during the elbow flexion test increases the sensitivity of the examination but may further increase the false-positive rate.

Abnormal two-point discrimination testing indicates a more established neuropathy. Vibratory perception and light touch with Semmes-Weinstein monofilaments are more sensitive tests during the early stage of neuropathy. Atrophy or significant weaknesses of pinch or grip are usually late findings. Intrinsic atrophy is a normal aging process; thus, comparison with the opposite side and the thenar eminence is important. Clawing of the small and ring fingers and increased flexion of the interphalangeal joint of the thumb during pinch (Froment's sign) are indications of chronic neuropathy. Similarly, weakness of the extrinsic small and ring finger flexors occurs very late.

The staging system described by McGowan is the most recognized: grade 1 is a minimal neuropathy without clinically detectable motor weakness, grade 2 is an intermediate neuropathy with noticeable atrophy and measurable weakness, and grade 3 indicates severe neuropathy with intrinsic muscle paresis and claw deformity.[11] Although this classification is well established, it is based only on motor findings, which occur late in the disease, and thus is not helpful in guiding treatment at an early stage.

INVESTIGATION

IMAGING

In most patients, radiographs will be unremarkable and are especially indicated for those with a history of trauma or arthritis and for patients with deformity or abnormal motion. A view profiling the epicondylar groove is particularly useful for identifying osteophytes that encroach on the nerve. Radiographs are also inspected for deformity, callus, and heterotopic bone, which may entrap or displace the nerve. In the throwing athlete, radiographs may demonstrate calcifications inferior to the medial epicondyle in the region of the medial collateral. The role of magnetic resonance imaging is not yet defined.

ELECTRODIAGNOSTIC STUDIES

Electrodiagnosis is helpful in establishing the diagnosis, localizing the level of the compression, and differentiating other or coexisting causes of neuropathy, such as cervical disease or polyneuropathy.[12] However, these studies are not essential when the diagnosis is clinically obvious and the results can be misleading. In patients with classic symptoms but without clinically measurable sensibility or motor deficits, the false-negative rate is upward of 50%. Slowing of motor conduction is considered present when the velocity across the flexed elbow is below 50 m/s or the across-elbow segment is 10 m/s slower than the adjacent forearm segment. A reduction in amplitude of compound muscle action potentials, especially in the abductor digiti minimi, often accompanies slowed motor conduction. Sensory conduction velocity and amplitude are typically measured antidromically (opposite the physiological direction). A reduction in amplitude of the sensory nerve action potential is a sensitive indicator of early ulnar neuropathy.

DIFFERENTIAL DIAGNOSIS

Local problems that can simulate symptoms of ulnar neuropathy include medial epicondylitis and elbow arthritis. Acute or chronic medial collateral ligament injury of the elbow may produce local pain and contribute to neuritis. Because the paresthesias associated with a neuropathy often do not localize to an anatomic distribution, other peripheral nerve entrapments, especially carpal tunnel syndrome, should be considered. Cervical radiculopathy and other spinal lesions, brachial plexopathy, and thoracic outlet syndrome can present with similar symptoms; however, local elbow findings will be absent.

MANAGEMENT

TREATMENT OPTIONS

Patients who present initially with mild to moderate symptoms that have developed recently are candidates for nonoperative treatment. Under these circumstances, the nerve has often been "irritated" by a single episode, such as a direct blow to the nerve, or an increase in time spent with the elbow flexed or resting on the elbow. Nonoperative treatment options include splinting to avoid acute and repetitive elbow flexion, padding to avoid direct pressure on the nerve, and education to avoid irritating postures and positions of the elbow. A simple splinting technique for night use is to wrap a towel around the elbow. Reversing an elbow pad so that it covers the antecubital fossa will also restrict flexion. For daytime use, a custom splint can be fabricated to maintain the elbow in 30 to 40 degrees of flexion.

For the chronic neuropathy associated with muscle weakness, nonoperative treatment is generally not effective. A variety of surgical procedures have been described, each demonstrating good success as a primary surgical procedure. Although surgeon preference is often the deciding factor in selecting a procedure, the operative morbidity of a more extensive procedure should be weighed against its potential advantages. The procedures can be generally divided into two groups: decompression and decompression with transposition. Simple decompression and medial epicondylectomy are procedures that allow the nerve to remain near its normal course. When the nerve is transposed anteriorly, it can be placed subcutaneous, intramuscular, or submuscular. Regardless of the operation chosen, two goals must be met to achieve success. First, all sites of compression must be eliminated (and no new sites created). Second, the nerve's course must allow it to be almost tension free during elbow motion.

OPERATIVE TECHNIQUE

GENERAL PRINCIPLES

Surgery is performed under tourniquet with the use of general or regional anesthesia. Although adequate visualization of the nerve is essential, judicious and careful use of right-angle retractors will allow these procedures to be done with shorter incisions than described originally. The incision is made midway between the medial epicondyle and the olecranon (Fig. 2). At this location, the risk of injury to the medial antebrachial cutaneous nerve is reduced. However, care must be exercised during the subcutaneous dissection to protect its posterior branches, which may cross the elbow anywhere from 6 cm proximal to 6 cm distal to the epicondyle[13] (Fig. 3). Except for simple decompression in which the dissection is typically limited, the nerve is first identified proximally by incising the fascia a few centimeters proximal to the epicondyle and immediately posterior to the medial intermuscular septum. The nerve is gently mobilized with its collateral vessels and tagged with a small Penrose drain. To complete the proxi-

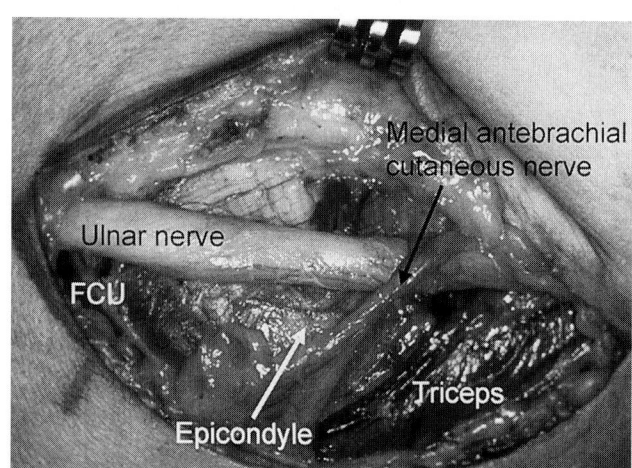

Fig. 3. Prominent medial antebrachial cutaneous nerve coursing through the area of ulnar nerve dissection. (FCU = flexor carpi ulnaris.)

mal release, the arcade of Struthers is incised. The intermuscular septum, especially the distal thicker portion, is excised to prevent its edge from compressing the nerve after transposition. The release continues distally by incising the fibroaponeurotic band at the epicondylar groove and Osborne's ligament at the proximal aspect of the FCU (Fig. 4). The superficial fascia over the FCU is divided several centimeters further and the two muscle heads split bluntly to expose the deep flexor-pronator fascia (Fig. 5). After this fascia is incised, the nerve is mobilized from proximal to distal. Small branches exiting from its deep surface may be encountered at the level of the epicondyle, followed by larger branches that obviously penetrate each head of the FCU. The motor branches are preserved and, if necessary, mobilized proximally by careful interfascicular dissection to allow transposition without tethering. A final inspection should ensure complete freedom of the nerve over the entire length of dissection.

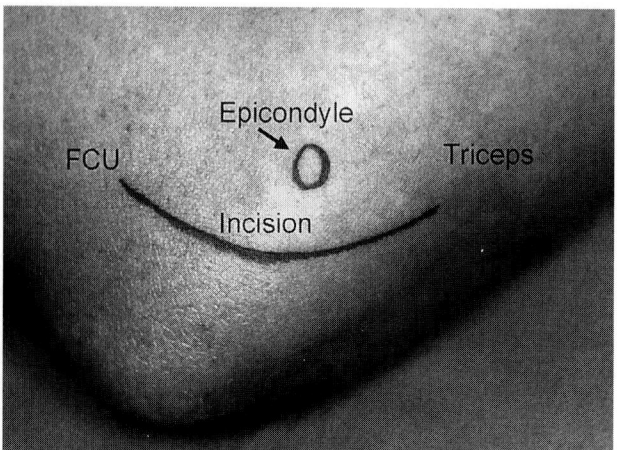

Fig. 2. Operative technique. The incision site is placed well posterior to the medial epicondyle to reduce the risk of injury to cutaneous nerves. (FCU = flexor carpi ulnaris.)

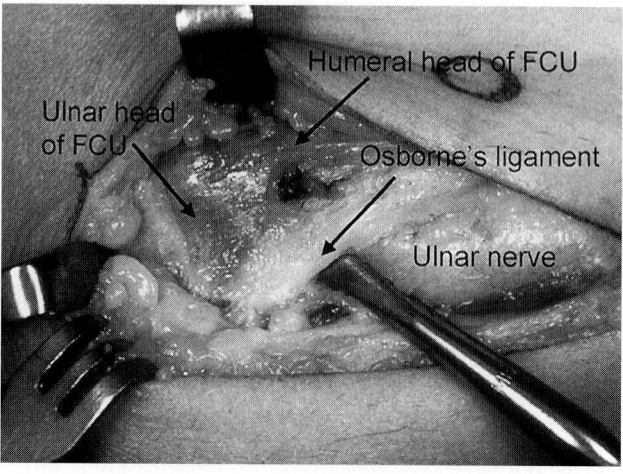

Fig. 4. Osborne ligament. The ligament courses from the medial epicondyle to the olecranon and connects the two heads of the flexor carpi ulnaris (FCU).

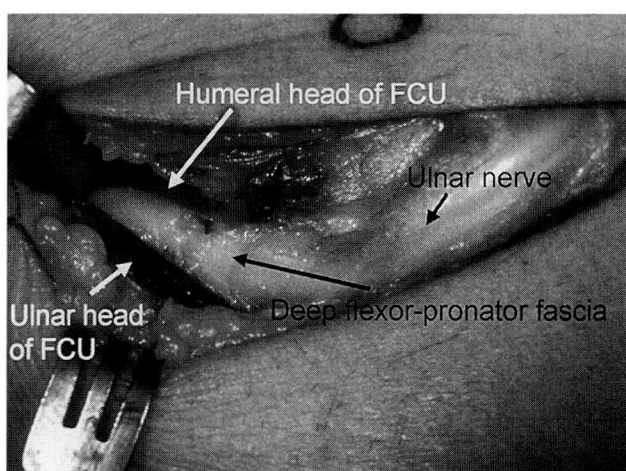

Fig. 5. Exposure of the deep flexor-pronator fascia between the two heads of the flexor carpi ulnaris (FCU). The fascia overlies the ulnar nerve at this site.

SIMPLE DECOMPRESSION

As originally described by Osborne in 1957, the ulnar nerve is decompressed by releasing the fibrous band that bridges the proximal extent of the two heads of the FCU without transposing the nerve.[3] This procedure, sometimes referred to as in situ decompression, is relatively simple and only minimally disturbs the nerve and its vascularity. The risk of anterior nerve subluxation can be reduced by limiting the release distal to a line drawn from the medial epicondyle to the tip of the olecranon. However, some surgeons perform a complete nerve release; if there is a tendency toward subluxation with elbow flexion, then an anterior transposition is performed. Postoperative immobilization is unnecessary, and early return to activities is possible.

MEDIAL EPICONDYLECTOMY

In 1950, King and Morgan[4] described removal of the medial epicondyle to relieve ulnar neuritis. Although all of their patients had post-traumatic conditions, surgeons have since expanded the indications to include idiopathic neuropathy. Theoretically, this procedure requires less dissection for nerve transposition and allows the nerve to seek its own course and thereby reduces nerve tension and irritation caused by a prominent epicondyle.[14] Disadvantages include bone tenderness, flexor-pronator muscle weakness, ectopic bone formation, elbow joint instability, and vulnerability to nerve trauma from loss of the protective epicondyle.

In this technique, structures overlying the nerve are released, but the nerve is not mobilized from its bed. The length of release varies but should extend at least 5 cm proximal and distal to the epicondyle. The medial epicondyle is exposed subperiosteally by detaching the flexor-pronator origin anteriorly and the periosteum posteriorly. The medial epicondyle is removed with a thin osteotome, taking care not to enter the joint or divide the collateral ligament. After the bone surface is smoothed, the tissues are reapproximated over the raw bone to provide a smooth surface for the nerve. Early active motion is encouraged.

SUBCUTANEOUS TRANSPOSITION

Transposing the nerve anteriorly has the potential advantages of removing the nerve from a poor bed and reducing tension in the nerve with elbow flexion. Although mobilizing the nerve impairs blood flow to the nerve, the affect is transient and perhaps minimized if accompanying vessels are brought with the nerve.[15] Subcutaneous transposition is the most common technique used for cubital tunnel syndrome because it is simple and reliable and has few complications.

In this technique, the nerve must be mobilized from the arcade of Struthers to the deep flexor-pronator fascia so that it can assume a gentle curve and not become kinked proximally or distally with transposition.[16] In particular, the medial intermuscular septum must be adequately resected and the nerve released well into the FCU, including interfascicular dissection of its posterior branches. The nerve is transposed 2 to 3 cm anterior to the epicondyle (Fig. 6A–C). The nerve can be stabilized in this position by suturing the deep subcutaneous tissues to the muscle fascia just anterior to the epicondyle or by creating a fasciodermal sling posterior to the nerve. The sling is formed by raising a 1.5 × 1.5-cm flap from the fascia over the flexor-pronator muscle.[17] It can be based either medially or laterally. A medially based flap creates a more compliant sling, whereas a laterally based flap places the smooth, superficial surface of the fascia next to the nerve. Whatever stabilization technique is used, it must not create a new site of compression. A subcuticular closure is performed. Elbow motion is begun early, but full extension is avoided for 3 weeks.

SUBMUSCULAR TRANSPOSITION

Although used routinely by some surgeons, submuscular transposition, which requires greater dissection and is associated with longer postoperative rehabilitation, is perhaps best reserved for young, vigorous people such as athletes and for very thin individuals in whom the nerve is at risk for repeated trauma in a subcutaneous position. This procedure is also the recommended technique for revision surgery.

The technique has changed little since first described by Learmonth in 1942.[5] The nerve is released along its entire course as in a subcutaneous transposition, including resection of the medial intermuscular septum (Fig. 7). In revision surgery, the nerve is identified in both the proximal extent and distal extent of the wound before tracing it centrally into the scarred area. The median nerve is identified. With the median and ulnar nerves protected, a large hemostat is placed under the muscle group just distal to the epicondyle. The flexor-pronator group is released proximally by incising it 1 to 2 cm distal to the epicondyle. Alternatively, the release can be accomplished by elevating its fascial origin subperiosteally from the epicondyle with later suture reattachment through drill holes. The nerve is transposed anteriorly near the median nerve. The flexor-pronator group is then repaired using the appropriate technique. The elbow is immobilized in 90 degrees of flexion. To reduce the risk of nerve adhesions and an elbow flexion contracture, elbow motion should begin within 2 weeks; however, resistive activities should be avoided for 2 months.

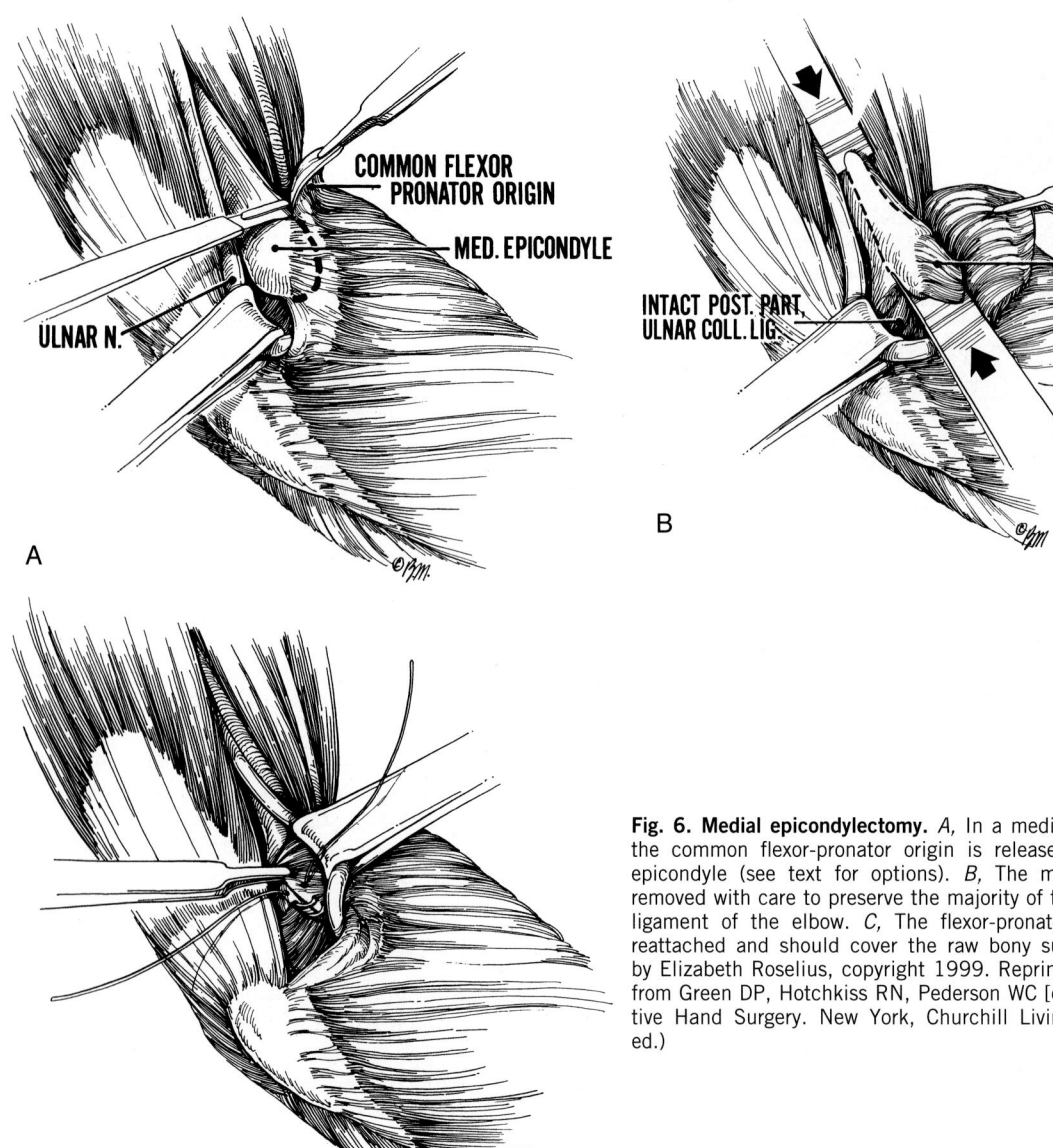

Fig. 6. Medial epicondylectomy. *A,* In a medial epicondylectomy, the common flexor-pronator origin is released from the medial epicondyle (see text for options). *B,* The medial epicondyle is removed with care to preserve the majority of the medial collateral ligament of the elbow. *C,* The flexor-pronator muscle origin is reattached and should cover the raw bony surface. (Illustrations by Elizabeth Roselius, copyright 1999. Reprinted with permission from Green DP, Hotchkiss RN, Pederson WC [eds]: Green's Operative Hand Surgery. New York, Churchill Livingstone, 1999, 4th ed.)

INTRAMUSCULAR TRANSPOSITION

Some surgeons prefer this technique because it avoids placing the nerve in the more vulnerable subcutaneous position and is less extensive than a submuscular transposition. However, intramuscular transposition has generally fallen from favor because of the risk of scarring between the nerve and muscle.[18] Because subcutaneous and submuscular transpositions accomplish nearly the same goals and with less complications, the indication for intramuscular transposition is limited to surgeon preference.

COMPLICATIONS

Complications are minimal when the simplest effective procedure is chosen and performed correctly. Failed surgery is most often attributed to incomplete decompression, especially proximally and distally, and to perineural scarring that produces recurrent compression or traction neuritis.[19, 20] Thus, complete decompression, absence of kinking or surgi-

cally created sites of compression, and free mobility of the nerve must be ensured at the completion of the operation. Early elbow motion promotes nerve gliding and more rapid rehabilitation. Hematoma formation is not uncommon; deflating the tourniquet before closure and cauterizing bleeders is recommended. If oozing remains, a small suction drain should be used for a short period postoperatively. Injury to the medial antebrachial cutaneous nerve may result in hypoesthesia. The medial collateral ligament of the elbow is easily injured in a submuscular transposition. Thus, the ligament must be identified near its origin before the muscle is elevated distally. Posterior subluxation of the nerve over the epicondyle after anterior subcutaneous transposition can be prevented by performing a complete release, placing the nerve sufficiently anterior, avoiding new sources of tethering, and creating an appropriate sling. Proceeding intraoperatively to an anterior transposition is probably the best option when there is a tendency for anterior nerve subluxation after an in situ decompression.

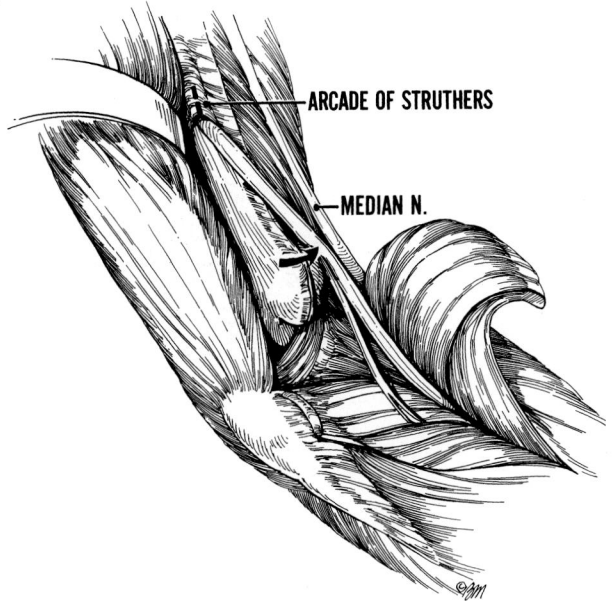

ARCADE OF STRUTHERS

MEDIAN N.

Fig. 7. Submuscular transposition. The flexor-pronator origin has been detached and the ulnar nerve has been transposed medial to the median nerve. (Illustrations by Elizabeth Roselius, copyright 1999. Reprinted with permission from Green DP, Hotchkiss RN, Pederson WC [eds]: Green's Operative Hand Surgery. New York, Churchill Livingstone, 1999, 4th ed.)

RESULTS

In general, operative results depend on the severity of the neuropathy. Improvement can be expected in nearly 100% of patients presenting with mild neuropathy using any of the accepted procedures.[21, 22] In one prospective, randomized comparison of in situ release, subcutaneous transposition, and submuscular transposition for the treatment of cubital tunnel syndrome, there was no statistically significant advantage of any one procedure. However, the results were slightly better in patients undergoing transposition.[21] Most authors conclude that in situ decompression is appropriate only for patients with mild symptoms and a nonsubluxating nerve. Patients with objective weakness and decreased sensibility achieve intermediate results with surgery, whereas those presenting with atrophy have the worst prognosis. Pain and dysesthesias are most reliably improved followed by sensibility. Duration of symptoms affects the outcome only if the neuropathy is severe. Some symptomatic improvement can be expected in a chronic neuropathy associated with atrophy, but the patient should understand that the objectives of surgery are more palliative than curative. Improvement in atrophy occurs in only 17% to 43% of patients.[21] Although revision surgery provides some benefit, the results are unpredictable; residual symptoms are present in 75% of patients. Submuscular transposition is the only revision procedure that has a success rate in excess of 50%.[19, 20]

REFERENCES

1. Curtis BF: Traumatic ulnar neuritis: Transplantation of the nerve. J Nerv Ment Dis 1898; 25:480.
2. Feindel W, Stratford J: The role of the cubital tunnel in tardy ulnar nerve palsy. Can J Surg 1958; 1:287.
3. Osborne GV: The surgical treatment of tardy ulnar neuritis. J Bone Joint Surg Br 1957; 39:782.
4. King T, Morgan FP: The treatment of traumatic ulnar neuritis. Mobilization of the ulnar nerve at the elbow by removal of the medial epicondyle and adjacent bone. Aust N Z J Surg 1950; 20:33.
5. Learmonth JR: A technique for transplanting the ulnar nerve. Surg Gynecol Obstet 1942; 75:792.
6. Childress HM: Recurrent ulnar-nerve dislocation at the elbow. Clin Orthop 1975; 108:168.
7. Al-Qattan, Murray KA: The arcade of Struthers: An anatomical study. J Hand Surg Br 1991; 16:311.
8. Amadio PC, Beckenbaugh RD: Entrapment of the ulnar nerve by the deep flexor-pronator aponeurosis. J Hand Surg Am 1986; 11:83.

9. Rayan GM, Jensen C, Duke J: Elbow flexion test in the normal population. J Hand Surg Am 1992; 17:86.
10. Cooper DE: Nerve injury associated with patient positioning in the operating room. In Gelberman RH (ed): Operative Nerve Repair and Reconstruction. Philadelphia, JB Lippincott, 1991, 1st ed, p 1231.
11. McGowan AJ: The results of transposition of the ulnar nerve for traumatic ulnar neuritis. J Bone Joint Surg Br 1950; 32:293.
12. Hilburn JW: General principles and use of electrodiagnostic studies in carpal and cubital tunnel syndromes. Hand Clin 1996; 12:205.
13. Dellon AL, Mackinnon SE: Injury to the medial antebrachial cutaneous nerve during cubital tunnel surgery. J Hand Surg Br 1985; 10:33.
14. Kuschner SH: Cubital tunnel syndrome. Treatment by medial epicondylectomy. Hand Clin 1996; 12:411.
15. Ogata K, Manske PR, Lesker PA: The effects of surgical dissection on regional blood flow to the ulnar nerve in the cubital tunnel. Clin Orthop 1985; 193:195.

16. Rettig AC, Ebben JR: Anterior subcutaneous transfer of the ulnar nerve in the athlete. Am J Sports Med 1993; 21:836.
17. Eaton RG, Crowe JF, Parkes JC III: Anterior transposition of the ulnar nerve using a non-compressing fasciodermal sling. J Bone Joint Surg Am 1980; 62:820.
18. Kleinman WB, Bishop AT: Anterior intramuscular transposition of the ulnar nerve. J Hand Surg Am 1996; 14:972.
19. Adelaar RS, Foster WC, McDowell C: The treatment of the cubital tunnel syndrome. J Hand Surg Am 1984; 9:90.
20. Broudy AS, Leffert RD, Smith RJ: Technical problems with ulnar nerve transposition at the elbow: Findings and results of reoperation. J Hand Surg 1978; 3:85.
21. Gabel GT, Amadio PC: Reoperation for failed decompression of the ulnar nerve in the region of the elbow. J Bone Joint Surg Am 1990; 72:213.
22. Dellon AL: Review of treatment results for ulnar nerve entrapment at the elbow. J Hand Surg Am 1989; 14:688.

INDEX

ISBN 0-323-01318-X